Taber's®

CYCLOPEDIC MEDICAL DICTIONARY

Edited by

CLAYTON L. THOMAS, M.D., M.P.H.

Consultant in Human Reproduction
Department of Population Sciences
Harvard School of Public Health

Vice President Medical Affairs
Tambrands Inc.

EDITION 15 ILLUSTRATED

Taber's®
CYCLOPEDIC MEDICAL DICTIONARY

F. A. DAVIS COMPANY PHILADELPHIA

Second printing, June 1985
Third printing, March 1986
Fourth printing, November 1986
Fifth printing, November 1987

PRINTED IN THE UNITED STATES OF AMERICA

The editor and publisher have done everything reasonably possible to make this work accurate, up-to-date, and in accord with accepted standards at the time of publication. This work is intended as a general reference, and any guidelines provided should be modified as circumstances demand in the provision of care to each individual person.

Library of Congress Cataloging in Publication Data

Taber, Clarence Wilbur, 1870–1968
Taber's Cyclopedic medical dictionary.

1. Medicine—Dictionaries. I. Thomas, Clayton L., 1921–
. II. Title. III. Title: Cyclopedic medical dictionary.
[DNLM: 1. Dictionaries, Medical. W 13 T113d]
R121.T144 1985 610′.3′21 62-8364
ISBN 0-8036-8309-X
ISBN 0-8036-8308-1 (indexed)

DISTRIBUTORS

United States of America
F. A. DAVIS COMPANY
1915 Arch Street
Philadelphia, Pennsylvania 19103

Atlanta, Georgia
J. A. MAJORS COMPANY
3770-A Zip Industrial Boulevard
P.O. Box 82686
Atlanta, Georgia 30354

Boston, Massachusetts
LOGIN BROTHERS NEW ENGLAND
2 Keith Way
Hingham, Massachusetts 02043

Chicago, Illinois
LOGIN BROTHERS BOOK COMPANY, INC.
1450 West Randolph Street
Chicago, Illinois 60607

Cleveland, Ohio
LOGIN BROTHERS OHIO
1550 Enterprise Parkway
Twinsburg, Ohio 44087

Dallas, Texas
J. A. MAJORS COMPANY
P.O. Box 819074
1851 Diplomat
Dallas, Texas 75381-9074

Houston, Texas
J. A. MAJORS COMPANY
1806 Southgate
Houston, Texas 77030

Los Angeles, California
J. A. MAJORS COMPANY—CALIFORNIA
1220 West Walnut Street
Compton, California 90220

New York, New York
LOGIN BROTHERS NEW JERSEY
P.O. Box 2700A
4 Sperry Road
Fairfield, New Jersey 07006

Philadelphia, Pennsylvania
RITTENHOUSE BOOK DISTRIBUTORS, INC.
511 Feheley Drive
King of Prussia, Pennsylvania 19406

St. Louis, Missouri
MATTHEWS BOOK COMPANY
11559 Rock Island Court
Maryland Heights, Missouri 63043

Canada
McAINSH AND CO., LTD.
2760 Old Leslie Street
Willowdale, Ontario M2K 2X5

Europe
EBS (EUROPEAN BOOKSERVICE)
Flevolaan 36-38, P.O. Box 124, 1380 AC Weesp,
The Netherlands

Australia, New Zealand, Fiji, Papula & New Guinea
HARPER & ROW PTY. LTD.
Corner Frederick Street and Reserve Road
P.O. Box 226
Artarmon NSW 2064
Australia

Mexico, Central America & South America
LIBRERIA INTERNACIONAL, S.A.
Av. Sonora 206
Mexico 11, DF

India
CURRENT TECHNICAL LITERATURE CO. PVT. LTD.
India House, Opp, G.P.O.
Post Box 1374
Bombay 400 001

CONTENTS

INTRODUCTION TO EDITION 15

The original editor of this Dictionary was Mr. Clarence Wilbur Taber. His interest in lexicography began almost a century ago. He would have been 115 years of age had he lived until 1985. As I continue to maintain the goals of excellence and productivity that marked his efforts, I'm certain he would be pleased with this edition, the fifth I have edited.

Thus this edition is dedicated to fulfilling the needs of those in nursing and all others in allied health professions. In keeping with its title, it is comprehensive, and accurate and up-to-date.

In the past, and I hope in the future, my efforts have been aided by those persons who have taken the time to provide constructive criticism. Because perfection is always an elusive goal, readers are requested to write their comments and suggestions to the editor, c/o F. A. Davis Company.

The F. A. Davis Company under the leadership provided by Mr. Robert H. Craven and his son, Robert, has continued application of the expertise required to publish and produce this edition. The company has been extremely well served by Ms. Linda Weinerman and Ms. Linda Hewlings whose excellent work has made possible the translation of my work output into the finished product. My sincere thanks and appreciation are hereby expressed to them.

As expressed in previous editions, my wife, Peggy, provides the support and inspiration that make my efforts in all areas possible. This was particularly evident when she and I were the victims of a terrorist takeover of a plane we were on in Europe in the summer of 1983.

Clayton Lay Thomas, M.D., M.P.H.

SOURCES CONSULTED

A great number of people in a variety of disciplines are directly or indirectly responsible for this edition. The F. A. Davis staff and I have continued to follow the model provided by Mr. Taber in making each edition an improvement over the previous one. This necessitates an unrelenting level of effort and diligence in order to stay abreast of developments in medicine and biology. Thus all available sources of scientific information—books, journals, lectures, film, consulting with nursing and medical experts, television, and use of computers to search medical literature—have been utilized to accomplish this task.

This effort is greatly simplified by using the facilities available in medical and general libraries. I am indebted to the staff of a great number of libraries including the Countway Library at Harvard Medical School and the National Library of Medicine in Bethesda, Maryland.

A number of consultants in various of the allied health sciences and in nursing particularly have taken the time to provide their suggestions for improving this Dictionary. Those persons are assured of my appreciation of their excellent consultative efforts.

Clayton Lay Thomas, M.D., M.P.H.

CONSULTANTS

Charles Christiansen, O.T.R., Ed.D., F.A.O.T.A.
Dean Currier, Ph.D.
Alice M. Donahue, R.N., M.S.N.
Janet D. Donohue, R.N., Ed.D.
Judith A. Erlen, R.N., Ph.D.
Joellen W. Hawkins, R.N., Ph.D., A.S.N.N.
Nancy A. Keller, R.N., M.N.
Thomas Kraker, R.T.R., M.Ed.
Gayle Lyons, R.N., M.S.N.
Carol L. Nichols, R.N., C.N.N., M.S.N.
Linda Rimer, R.N.
James A. Scharff, R.N.C.E.N.
Patricia Schlegel, R.N., B.S., M.A.
Carolyn J. Scott, R.N.
Donna Ayers Snelson, R.N., M.S.N.
Kathy Sullivan, R.N., M.N.
Morris E. Weaver, Ph.D.

(Material supplied by the consultants has been reviewed and edited by Clayton L. Thomas, M.D., Editor, with whom final responsibility rests for the accuracy of content.)

FEATURES AND THEIR USE

Taber's Cyclopedic Medical Dictionary is more than just a medical dictionary. In addition to listing important medical terms, it covers concepts that are vital to the practitioner and student of Nursing and Allied Health. All who work in fields related to health care will find *Taber's* a comprehensive resource tool.

Vocabulary: The vocabulary is updated to meet the ongoing needs of those in the Nursing and Allied Health professions. The Editor and F. A. Davis staff have researched and included new entries reflecting the many changes in the health care professions, approaches to patient care, and aspects of law and ethics.

Pronunciation: More than 95 percent of the main entries are spelled phonetically. Pronunciations are given as simply as possible with most long and short vowels marked diacritically and secondary accents indicated. *Diacritics* are marks over or under vowels. Only two diacritics are used in *Taber's:* the macron ¯ showing the long sound of vowels, as the a in rāte, e in rēbirth, i in īsle, o in ōver, and u in ūnite; and the breve ˘ showing the short sound of vowels, as the a in ăpple, e in ĕver, i in ĭt, o in nŏt, and u in cŭt. *Accents* are marks used to indicate stress upon certain syllables. A single accent ′ is called a primary accent. A double accent ″ is called a secondary accent; it indicates less stress upon a syllable than that given by a primary accent. This difference in stress can be seen in the word an″es-the′si-a.

Spelling: Many words formerly hyphenated are now listed as one word (corticosteroid, gastrointestinal); diphthongs are eliminated where possible; and American rather than British forms are used.

Biographies: For eponymic terms a brief biography is included in brackets immediately following the pronunciation.

Etymology: The etymology for 90 percent of the main entries is presented in brackets following the entry. The major sources of medical terminology are Latin and Greek.

Definitions: The definitions are written in encyclopedic style, offering a comprehensive understanding of the word or concept described. They stand out in a paragraph apart from supplemental material, making it easier to pinpoint the core information. Compound terms are listed under the adjective in most cases.

Masculine and feminine: The singular and masculine form of any noun or pronoun may be read and implied as the plural, feminine, or neuter, as the circumstances may make appropriate.

Alphabetical order: Main entries are alphabetized letter by letter, regardless of spaces that may occur between the words. A comma marks the end of an entry for alphabetical purposes, e.g., **ear, words pert. to** precedes **earache** as well as **ear**

dust. For alphabetical purposes in eponymic terms, the **'s** is ignored, e.g., **Albini's nodules** precedes **albinism.**

Subentries: Subentries are listed under the noun they modify (such as labor, premature or technician, emergency medical), indented from the main entry, and printed in italic typeface.

Abbreviations: Standard abbreviations for entries are included with the definition and also are listed alphabetically throughout the text. Additional abbreviations used for charting and prescription writing are listed in the Appendix. Nonmedical abbreviations used for convenience are listed on page xxx.

Synonyms: Synonyms are listed at the end of the definition. Most synonymous terms have their own complete definition to ease the facility of use. Related terms are indicated by a SEE or RS (related subject) reference. If many related terms are applicable they appear as a separate entry entitled Words pert. to.

Supplemental information: Supplemental information is often included with the definition, and is set apart by a paragraph indent. A heading will often appear with this information. This edition includes a Fact Finding Index listing the entries with the following headings: nursing implications, diagnosis, etiology, first aid, poisoning, prognosis, signs and symptoms, and treatment. Other headings not included in the Fact Finding Index are: caution, contraindications, differential diagnosis, examination, function, incompatibility, indications, pathology, physiology, and therapy.

Illustrations: This edition has 203 illustrations, all of which utilize color to highlight and differentiate portions of the drawings. A list of illustrations appears on page xxv.

Appendix: Detailed information on measurement systems, conversion rules, and scientific notation are contained in the Appendix. Long tables that would interfere with finding words in the text are grouped in the Appendix. Nutrients Present in Food are now placed in one table in the Appendix rather than being spread through the vocabulary. New and revised tables in this edition include: Percentage Solution Tables (apothecaries and metric), Recommended Daily Allowances for Vitamins, Estimated Safe and Adequate Daily Dietary Intakes of Vitamins and Minerals, Mean Heights and Weights and Recommended Energy Intake, Toxic Emergencies, and Nursing Diagnoses. In addition to the directories of Poison Control Centers and Radiological Assistance Centers, this edition lists Burn Centers.

The Interpreter: Questions and statements most often used during examination, in taking a patient's history, and in diagnosis are given in five languages: English, Spanish, Italian, French, and German. The Interpreter is arranged in categories that deal with specific aspects of examination, history, and diagnosis for convenience, and a separate table of contents for The Interpreter helps to quickly locate each section.

FACT FINDING INDEX

Many entries contain supplemental information under a special heading. The following index has been compiled to aid the reader in quickly locating information on: Nursing Implications, Diagnosis, Etiology, First Aid, Poisoning, Prognosis, Signs/Symptoms, and Treatment.

DIAGNOSIS

ETIOLOGY

Etiology

aphonia
aplastic anemia
aptyalia, aptyalism
arevareva
arm, Saturday-night
arteriosclerosis
arthritis
arthritis, rheumatoid
ascites
asphyxia
asteatosis cutis
asthenia, neurocirculatory
asthma
astigmatism
atherosclerosis
atrial fibrillation
atrophy
autism, infantile
backache
battered child syndrome
beriberi
blepharitis
Brodie's abscess
bronchiectasis
bronchitis
bronchopneumonia
bubonic plague
bunion
calculus
cancer
caput succedaneum
carbuncle, carbunculus
cardiospasm
cataplexy, cataplexia
cataracts
cat scratch disease
chill
cholecystitis
cholera
chromidrosis,
chromhidrosis
cirrhosis
coccidioidomycosis
cold, common
colon, irritable
comedo
compensation, failure of
convulsion
cord bladder
corn
craniotabes
cretinism
crib death
croup, membranous
cryptococcosis
cyanosis
dactylitis
deafness
deciduoma, malignant
deformity, gunstock
dengue
dermatitis
dermatitis herpetiformis
dermatitis medicamentosa
dermatitis venenata
dermatitis verrucosa
descensus uteri
diabetes insipidus
diabetes mellitus
diarrhea
diphtheria
Donovania granulomatosis
Down's syndrome
dysentery
dysgenesis, gonadal
dysmenorrhea, primary
dyspnea
ecchymosis
eclampsia
ectopic pregnancy
ectropion
eczema
edema
Ehlers-Danlos syndrome
elephantiasis
emaciation
encephalitis
endometritis
enuresis
epididymitis
epilepsy
epistaxis
erysipelas
erysipeloid
erythema
fever
folliculitis decalvans
freckle
furunculus
gangrene
gastrectasia, gastrectasis
gastritis
gingivitis
glaucoma
glossoplegia
goiter
goiter, exophthalmic
gonorrhea
gout
granuloma inguinale
granulosis rubra nasi
gumboil
Hamman-Rich syndrome
hay fever
headache
heart block
heart failure
hematuria
hemiplegia
hemoglobinuria
hemolytic disease of the
newborn
hemophilia
hemorrhage, cerebral
hemorrhage, uterine
hemorrhagic
nephrosonephritis
hernia
herpangina
heterophoria
hiccough, hiccup
hoarseness
hobnail liver
hyperactivity
hyperemesis gravidarum
hypergenitalism
hyperhidrosis
hyperinsulinism
hyperpnea
hyperptyalism
hypertension
hypertrichosis
hypoglycemia
hysteria
icterus, nonobstructive
impetigo contagiosa
inanition
incompetent palatal
syndrome
incoordination
infection
inflammation
influenza
kala-azar
keratoderma
blennorrhagica
keratosis, seborrheic
kraurosis
labyrinthitis
lactose intolerance
lagophthalmos,
lagophthalmus
laryngitis
laryngitis, acute catarrhal
Leeuwenhoek's disease
Legionnaires disease
leprosy
leptomeningitis
leukemia, chronic
lymphatic
leukemia, chronic
myelocytic
leukorrhea
Lhermitte's sign
lichen planus
Little's disease
liver, abscess of
liver, cirrhosis of
lymphadenitis
lymphadenitis, tuberculous
lymphangitis
lymphogranuloma
venereum
macrocephalia
maduromycosis
malaria

FIRST AID

POISONING

PROGNOSIS

comedo
croup, spasmodic
cryptococcosis
diabetes insipidus
diabetes mellitus
diphtheria
eczema
Ehlers-Danlos syndrome
erysipelas
folliculitis decalvans
gas, vesicant
Gilles de la Tourette's syndrome
gonorrhea
heart, fatty degeneration of
heart, fatty infiltration of
heat exhaustion
hemophilia
hydrocephalus
hypertrophy, pseudomuscular
influenza
intussusception
laryngostenosis, occlusion
leprosy
leukemia, acute lymphatic
leukemia, acute myeloblastic
lichen planus
liver, abscess of
liver, acute yellow atrophy of
liver, amyloid
liver, cancer of
liver, cirrhosis of
lung, edema of
lung abscess
lung collapse
marasmus
measles
meningitis, acute
Minamata disease
mumps
myasthenia gravis
myotonia congenita
nephrosis, lipoid
neuralgia, sphenopalatine
papilledema
Parkinson's disease
peptic ulcer
pericarditis
peritonitis, acute diffuse
peritonitis, chronic
phenol poisoning
phenylketonuria
placenta previa
pneumonia, chronic interstitial
poisoning, potato
poliomyelitis, acute anterior
polyarteritis (nodosa)
prurigo
pyelonephritis
pyloric obstruction and dilatation
Raynaud's disease
Reiter's syndrome
respiratory distress syndrome
Reye's syndrome
rickets
rubella
scabies
sciatica
scleroderma
scurvy
spasm of esophagus
splenitis
steatoma
stomach cancer
stomatitis, aphthous
stomatitis parasitica
stomatitis, ulcerative
strabismus, paralytic
stroke
sycosis
Sydenham's chorea
Tay-Sachs disease
tetany
tonsillitis, acute
trichinosis
typhoid fever
typhus
varicella
verruca
yellow fever

SIGNS/SYMPTOMS

abortion
abruptio placentae
abscess, brain
acapnia
acetonemia
acne vulgaris
acromegaly
actinomycosis
Addison's disease
aeroembolism
alcoholism, acute
alcoholism, chronic
alkalosis, metabolic
alkalosis, respiratory
allergy
amebiasis
amyloid kidney
anaphylactic shock
anaphylaxis
anemia
anemia, pernicious
anesthesia
aneurysm, aortic
aneurysm, arteriovenous
angina pectoris
anilism
anthrax
antimony poisoning
aortitis
apoplexy
appendicitis, acute
appendicitis, chronic
ariboflavinosis
arsenic poisoning
asphyxia
asthenopia
ataxia, locomotor
atrophy, acute yellow
atropine sulfate poisoning
autonomic hyperreflexia
babesiosis
balantidiasis
bismuth poisoning
bites or stings
blackwater fever
blepharitis
boric acid poisoning
botulism
botulism, infant
brain tumor
brass poisoning
Brodie's abscess
bromide poisoning
bronchi, foreign bodies in
bronchiectasis
bronchopneumonia
bruise of head, chest, and abdomen
Buerger's disease
burn, alkali
caffeinism
caisson disease
calculus, renal
calculus, salivary
calculus, urinary
calculus, vesical
cancer
carbon dioxide poisoning
carbon monoxide poisoning
carbon tetrachloride poisoning
carbuncle, carbunculus
carcinoid syndrome
cardiospasm
chancre
chancroid
chilblain
chill
Chinese restaurant syndrome
chloasma
choking
cholecystitis
cholelithiasis
cholera
chorditis nodosa
chromidrosis,

Signs/Symptoms

chromhidrosis
chromium poisoning
cinchophen poisoning
clavicle, dislocation of
clavicle, fracture of
cluster headache
cocaine hydrochloride
poisoning
codeine poisoning
cold, common
colitis, ulcerative
collapse
coma, diabetic
coma, uremic
comedo
compression, cerebral
concussion of brain
contusion
convulsant poisons
copper sulfate poisoning
cord bladder
corn
corrosive poisoning
cramp
cretinism
croton oil poisoning
croup, membranous
croup, spasmodic
cryptococcosis
cyanide poisoning
cyclic vomiting
cyclitis
cystitis
dacryocystitis
death
deer fly fever
delirium tremens
dengue
dermatitis, exfoliative
dermatitis herpetiformis
dermatitis medicamentosa
dermatitis seborrheica
dermatitis venenata
dermatomyositis
descensus uteri
diabetes insipidus
diabetes mellitus
diarrhea, infantile
digitalis poisoning
diphtheria
Diphyllobothrium
latum
diverticulitis, acute
diverticulitis, chronic
drowning
drug addiction
dysentery
dyspnea
ear, foreign bodies in
eclampsia
ectopic pregnancy
eczema
electric shock
emetism
empyema
endocervicitis
endometritis
epididymitis
epiglottitis
epilepsy
ergot poisoning
erosion of cervix uteri
erysipelas
ethmoiditis
faint
fasciolopsiasis
fever
fibroma, uterine
fish poisoning
flames, inhalation of
folliculitis decalvans
food allergies
foot and mouth disease
formaldehyde poisoning
fracture
freezing
frostbite
fumes, nitric acid
furunculus
gallstone
gangrene, dry
gangrene, moist
gas, lewisite
gas, lung irritant
gas, nose irritant
gas, vesicant
gasoline poisoning
gastrectasia, gastrectasis
gastritis, acute
gastritis, chronic
glanders
glossitis, acute
glottis, edema of
goiter, exophthalmic
gonorrhea
gout
granulosis rubra nasi
gumboil
gumma
hay fever
heart, dilation of
heart, fatty degeneration of
heart, fatty infiltration of
heart, fibroid
heart failure
heat exhaustion
hematemesis
hematuria
hemlock poisoning
hemophilia
hemoptysis
hemorrhage
hemorrhage, cerebral
hepatic coma
heroin toxicity
herpangina
herpes genitalis
hip, dislocation of
hip, dislocation of,
backward
hip, dislocation of, forward
histoplasmosis
Hodgkin's disease
human bite
hydropericardium
hyperemesis gravidarum
hyperinsulinism
hyperopia
hyperthyroidism
hypertrophy,
pseudomuscular
hypoglycemia
hypothyroidism
hysteria
icterus, hemolytic
icterus, nonobstructive
ileus
impetigo contagiosa
infection
inflammation
influenza
injury
ink poisoning
insulin shock
internal injury
intestinal obstruction
iodine poisoning
iritis
iron poisoning
jejunum, inflammation of
keratitis interstitial
keratosis pilaris
keratosis, seborrheic
kidney
knee, game
labyrinthitis
laryngitis
laryngitis, acute
catarrhal
laryngitis, atrophic
laryngitis, chronic
laryngitis, syphilitic
laryngitis, tuberculous
laryngostenosis, occlusion
Lassa fever
leprosy
leptomeningitis
leukemia, acute lymphatic
leukemia, chronic
lymphatic
leukemia, chronic
myelocytic
leukorrhea
lichen planus
Little's disease
liver, abscess of

liver, acute yellow atrophy of
liver, amyloid
liver, cancer of
liver, cirrhosis of
lung, edema of
lung abscess
lung collapse
lung collapse, hypostatic
lung collapse, passive
lymphadenia ossea
lymphadenitis
lymphadenitis, tuberculous
lymphangitis
lymphogranuloma venereum
malaria
manganese poisoning
marasmus
Marfan's syndrome
mastitis
mastoiditis
McArdle's disease
measles
meningitis, acute
meningitis, tuberculous
menopause
mercurialism
mercuric chloride poisoning
mercurous chloride poisoning
mercury poisoning
metal fume fever
migraine
miliaria
Minamata disease
molluscum contagiosum
mononucleosis, infectious
mountain fever
mumps
myasthenia gravis
mycosis fungoides
myelitis
myocarditis
myocarditis, acute secondary
myocarditis, chronic
myopathy, facial
myotonia congenita
myxedema
narcotic poisoning
Necator americanus
nephrosis, lipoid
neuralgia, sphenopalatine
neuralgia, trigeminal
neuritis
neuritis, intraocular
neuritis, multiple
neuritis, retrobulbar
nicotine poisoning, acute
nitrous oxide
odontoma, follicular
ophthalmia, sympathetic
opiate poisoning
orchitis
orchitis, syphilitic
orchitis, tuberculous
organic brain syndromes
ornithosis
Oroya fever
orthopnea
osteitis deformans
osteomalacia
osteomyelitis
osteoporosis
oxalic acid poisoning
pachymeningitis, hemorrhagic
pancreatitis, acute
pancreatitis, acute hemorrhagic
pancreatitis, chronic
panniculitis
paralysis, Bell's
parathion poisoning
paratyphoid fever
paresis
Parkinson's disease
paroxysmal cold hemoglobinuria
pediculosis capitis
pediculosis corporis
pediculosis pubis
peliosis
pellagra
pelvic inflammatory disease
peptic ulcer
perforation of stomach or intestine
pericarditis
pericarditis, fibrinous
periostitis
peritonitis, acute diffuse
peritonitis, chronic
pernio
Perthes' disease
pertussis
pharyngitis, acute
pharyngitis, chronic
phenol poisoning
phenylketonuria
phlebitis
phlegmasia alba dolens
phosphaturia
phosphorus
phosphorus poisoning
phrenocardia
pityriasis rosea
placenta previa
plague
pleurisy, diaphragmatic
pneumonia
pneumonia, chronic interstitial
pneumonia, desquamative interstitial
pneumopericardium
pneumothorax
pneumothorax, spontaneous
poison ivy dermatitis
pokeroot poisoning
poliomyelitis, acute anterior
polycythemia vera
polymer fume fever
potassium
potassium chromate poisoning
Pott's disease
pregnancy
progeria
prostatism
pseudoangina
pseudocirrhosis
psittacosis
psoriasis
purpura, idiopathic thrombocytopenic
pyelonephritis
pyemia
pyloric obstruction and dilatation
rabies
ranula
Raynaud's disease
respiratory distress syndrome
retinitis
Reye's syndrome
rheumatic fever
rhinitis, atrophic
rhinitis, chronic hypertrophic
rhinoscleroma
riboflavin
rickets
ringworm
rubella
scabies
scalenus syndrome
scarlet fever
sciatica
scombroid poisoning
scurvy
scurvy, infantile
seasickness
sepsis, puerperal
serum rash
serum sickness
shock
sick sinus syndrome
silver nitrate poisoning
snow blindness
spider, black widow

spider bites or poisoning
spina bifida
splenitis
sprain
sprain of back
sprain of foot
stomach cancer
stomatitis
stomatitis, aphthous
stomatitis, catarrhal
stomatitis, mercurial
stomatitis parasitica
stomatitis, ulcerative
stricture of urethra
stroke
sty(e)
subclavian steal syndrome
suffocation
sulfuric acid poisoning
sycosis
symblepharon
synovitis
syphilis
syphilitic macules
syringomyelia
tabes dorsalis
tapeworm
Tay-Sachs disease
tenosynovitis crepitans
tetany
thromboangiitis obliterans
thrombosis
thrombosis, coronary
thyrotoxicosis
tincture of iodine poisoning
tinea
tin poisoning
tongue-tie
tonsillitis, acute
toxemia
transient ischemic attack
trichiasis
trichinosis
Trichomonas vaginalis
tricuspid atresia
tugging, tracheal
tularemia
turpentine poisoning
typhoid fever
typhus
unconsciousness
undernutrition
uremia
urticaria
uterus, rupture of, in pregnancy
vaginismus
vaginitis
varicella
varicocele
varicose veins
Vincent's angina
wen
wound, bullet
wound, cellulitis of
yaws
yellow fever

TREATMENT

abruptio placentae
abscess, brain
acetaminophen poisoning
acne vulgaris
acrodermatitis enteropathica
acromegaly
Actinomyces israelii
actinomycosis
Adams-Stokes syndrome
Addison's disease
adult respiratory distress syndrome
afibrinogenemia
afterpains
alcoholism, acute
alcoholism, chronic
alkali poisoning
alkalosis, metabolic
alkalosis, respiratory
allergy
alopecia
amebiasis
amenorrhea
ammonia toxicity
anaphylactic shock
anaphylaxis
ancylostomiasis
anemia
anemia, pernicious
aneurysm, aortic
angel's trumpet
angina pectoris
anhidrosis
anthrax
appendicitis, chronic
arevareva
ariboflavinosis
arsenic poisoning
arteriosclerosis
arthritis, gonorrheal
arthritis, rheumatoid
Ascaris lumbricoides
aspirin poisoning
asteatosis cutis
asthenia, neurocirculatory
asthma
ataxia, locomotor
athlete's foot
autonomic hyperreflexia
babesiosis
backache
balantidiasis
Barlow's disease
bartonellosis
bedbug
bedsore
bee sting
Bell's palsy
beriberi
black eye
blister
blister, blood
boil
boric acid poisoning
botulism
botulism, infant
brass poisoning
bronchi, foreign bodies in
bronchiectasis
bronchitis, acute
bronchitis, chronic
bronchopneumonia
Buerger's disease
buphthalmia, buphthalmos
burn
burn, brush
bursitis
caisson disease
calculus, renal
calculus, salivary
calculus, urinary
calculus, vesical
callosity, callositas
cancer
cancrum oris
capillariasis
carbon dioxide poisoning
carbon monoxide poisoning
carbuncle, carbunculus
carcinoid syndrome
cardiospasm
carpal tunnel syndrome
cataracts
cat bite fever
cat scratch disease
celiac disease
chancroid
chiggers
chilblain
cholecystitis
cholelithiasis
cholera
chorditis nodosa
chorea, Sydenham's
choriocarcinoma
chromidrosis, chromhidrosis
chromium poisoning
chronic granulomatous disease
cirrhosis
clavicle, dislocation of
clavicle, fracture of
cluster headache
cocaine hydrochloride

myelocytic
leukorrhea
lichen planus
listeriosis, listerosis
liver, acute yellow atrophy of
liver, amyloid
liver, cancer of
liver, cirrhosis of
liver, inflammation of
lung, edema of
lung abscess
lung collapse
lung collapse, hypostatic
lupus erythematosus, cutaneous
lupus erythematosus, systemic
Lyme disease, Lyme arthritis
lymphadenitis
lymphadenitis, tuberculous
lymphogranuloma venereum
Lysol poisoning
Mace
macroglobulinemia, Waldenström's
malaria
maple syrup urine disease
marasmus
Marburg virus disease
massive collapse of the lung
mastoiditis
Mediterranean fever, familial
Ménière's disease
meningitis, acute
menopause
methyl alcohol poisoning
migraine
miliaria
milium
mitral valve prolapse
mole
molluscum contagiosum
mononucleosis, infectious
morning sickness
morphine poisoning
mucocutaneous lymph node syndrome
mumps
myasthenia gravis
mycetoma
mycosis fungoides
myotonia congenita
myxedema
narcolepsy
narcotism
nasal obstruction
Necator americanus
nephropathy, hypercalcemic
nephropathy, hypokalemic
nephropathy, membranous
nephrosis, lipoid
neuralgia, trigeminal
neuritis, intraocular
neuritis, multiple
neurosis
nevus pigmentosus
nicotine poisoning, acute
nitric acid poisoning
nitrous oxide
nocardiosis
nose, foreign body in
obesity
olecranon, fracture of
ophthalmia, sympathetic
orchitis
organic brain syndromes
ornithosis
Oroya fever
osteitis deformans
osteomalacia
osteomyelitis
otalgia
otosclerosis
oxalic acid poisoning
Paget's disease
Paget's disease, extramammary
paragonimiasis
paraquat
paresis
Parkinson's disease
paronychia
paroxysmal cold hemoglobinuria
pars planitis
patella, fracture of
pediculosis capitis
pediculosis corporis
pellagra
pelvic inflammatory disease
pemphigus
peptic ulcer
perforation of stomach or intestine
pericarditis
perineum, tears of the
peritonitis
peritonitis, acute diffuse
peritonitis, chronic
Peyronie's disease
pharyngitis, acute
pharyngitis, chronic
phencyclidine hydrochloride
phenothiazine
phenylketonuria
pheochromocytoma
phimosis
phlegmasia alba dolens
phycomycosis
pinta
pityriasis rosea
placenta previa
plague
pneumocystis pneumonia
pneumonia, desquamative interstitial
pneumonia, primary atypical
poisoning, arsenic
poisoning, lead
poisoning, potato
poison ivy dermatitis
pokeroot poisoning
polyarteritis (nodosa)
polycystic ovary syndrome
polycythemia vera
polymer fume fever
potbelly
Pott's disease
premenstrual (tension) syndrome
prurigo
pruritus
pseudogout
psoriasis
pterygium, stationary
ptosis, abdominal
puerperal sepsis
pyelonephritis
pyemia
pyloric obstruction and dilatation
pyloric stenosis
quadriplegia
rabies
ranula
Raynaud's disease
Raynaud's phenomenon
Recklinghausen's disease
Reiter's syndrome
relapsing fever
renal failure, acute
respiratory distress syndrome
respiratory failure, acute
retinitis
retinitis pigmentosa
Reye's syndrome
rheumatic fever
rhinitis, acute
rhinitis, atrophic
rhinitis, chronic hypertrophic
rhinoscleroma
rickets
rickets renal
ringworm
rosacea
rubella

LIST OF ILLUSTRATIONS

Illustrations are listed according to the main entry or subentry they accompany. Information in parentheses indicates the aspect shown or additional material illustrated. In most cases, each drawing falls on the same page as the entry it illustrates; however, when there is no space on that page for the illustration, it will appear on the preceding or following page.

LIST OF TABLES

ABBREVIATIONS USED IN TEXT*

ABBR.	abbreviation	gm.	gram
ABNORM.	abnormalities	Gr.	Greek
ADM.	administration	gr.	grain
ADVAN.	advantages	i.e.	that is
Amerind.	American Indian	INCOMPAT.	incompatibility
ANAT.	anatomy	IND.	indications
app.	approximately	I.U.	International Unit
approx.	approximately	Jap.	Japanese
AS.	Anglo-Saxon	kcal.	kilocalorie, Calorie
at. no.	atomic number	kg.	kilogram
at. wt.	atomic weight	L.	Latin
C.	centigrade, Celsius	LL.	Late Latin
C, or Cal.	large Calorie (kilocalorie)	MD.	Middle Dutch
cal.	small calorie	ME.	Middle English
cc.	cubic centimeter	mg.	milligram
CHEM.	chemical	ml.	milliliter
Chem. symb.	Chemical symbol	NA.	Nomina Anatomica
CLASSIF.	classification	NF.	National Formulary
CNS.	central nervous system	OB.	obstetrics
COMP.	composition	O. Fr.	Old French
CONTRA.	contraindication	PATH.	pathology
D.	Dutch	pert.	pertaining
DEVELOP.	development	PHYS.	physical, physiology
DIAG.	diagnosis	pl.	plural
DIFF. DIAG.	differential diagnosis	POSTOP.	postoperative
DISADV.	disadvantages	PROG.	prognosis
dl.	deciliter	q.v.	which see
e.g.	for example	rel.	relating, related
EQUIP.	equipment	RS.	related subjects
esp.	especially	s.	singular
ETIOL.	etiology	Sp.	Spanish
Ex.	example	sp. gr.	specific gravity
EXAM.	examination	SYM.	symptoms
F.	Fahrenheit	SYMB.	symbol
F.A.	first aid	SYN.	synonym
Fr.	French	THERAP.	therapy, therapeutic
FUNCT.	function	USP.	United States Pharmacopeia
Ger.	German		

*Medical and charting abbreviations appear in the Appendix.

A

α. Alpha, q.v., first letter of the Greek alphabet.
Å. *angstrom unit.*
A_2. *aortic second sound.*
a. *accommodation; ampere; anode; anterior; aqua; area; artery.*
a-, an- [Gr., not]. Prefix meaning without, away from, not.
A.A., a.a. *achievement age; Alcoholics Anonymous; amino acid.*
$\overline{\text{aa}}$. [Gr. *ana,* of each]. Prescription sign meaning *the stated amount of each of the substances is to be used in compounding the prescription.*
A.A.A. *American Academy of Allergists; American Association of Anatomists.*
A.A.A.S. *American Association for the Advancement of Science.*
A.A.C.C.N. *American Association of Critical Care Nurses.*
A.A.F.P. *American Academy of Family Practice.*
A.A.G.P. *American Academy of General Practice,* former name of the American Academy of Family Practice.
A.A.I.N. *American Association of Industrial Nurses.*
A.A.M.A. *American Association of Medical Assistants.*
A.A.M.R.L. *American Association of Medical Record Librarians.*
A.A.N.A. *American Association of Nurse Anesthetists.*
A.A.P. *American Academy of Pediatrics.*
A.A.P.A. *American Association of Physicians' Assistants.*
Aaron's sign (ăr'ŏns). [Charles D. Aaron, U.S. physician, 1866–1951] Distress in region of heart or stomach upon pressure over McBurney's point, q.v., in appendicitis.
A.A.R.T. *American Association for Respiratory Therapy.*
ab- [L. *ab,* from]. Prefix meaning from, away from, negative, absent.
Abadie's sign (ă-bă-dēz'). 1. [Charles A. Abadie, Fr. ophthalmologist, 1842–1932] In exophthalmic goiter, spasm of the levator palpebrae superioris. 2. [Jean Abadie, Fr. neurologist, 1873–1946] In tabes dorsalis, insensibility to pressure over the Achilles tendon.
abaissement (ă-bās'mŏn) [Fr., a lowering]. 1. Depression. 2. Synonym for lenticular displacement (couching). 3. Falling.
abalienation (ăb-āl"yĕn-ā'shŭn) [L. *abalienare,* to separate from]. Mental derangement.
A-band. Dark-staining segment of a myofibril muscle fiber. SYN: *anisotropic disk; transverse disk.*
abaptiston (ă"băp-tĭs'tŏn) [Gr. *abaptistos,* not dipped]. Trephine that cannot slip and injure the brain.
abarognosis (ăb"ăr-ŏg-nō'sĭs) [Gr. *a-,* not, + *baros,* weight, + *gnosis,* knowledge]. Loss of ability to sense weight. SEE: *baragnosis.*
abarthrosis (ăb-ăr-thrō'sĭs) [L. *ab,* from, + Gr. *arthron,* joint, + *osis,* condition]. A movable joint or point upon which bones move freely upon each other. SYN: *diarthrosis.*
abarticular [" + *articulus,* joint]. At a distance from a joint.
abarticulation. 1. Dislocation of a joint. 2. Diarthrosis. SYN: *abarthrosis.*
abasia (ă-bā'zē-ă) [Gr. *a-,* not, + *basis,* step]. Motor incoordination in walking. Inability to walk due to impairment of coordination.
a.-astasia. Lack of motor coordination with inability to stand or walk. SYN: *astasia-abasia.*
a. atactica. Uncertain movements in walking.
a., choreic. Abasia associated with chorea of the legs.
a., paralytic. Abasia in which the leg muscles are paralyzed.
a., paroxysmal trepidant. Abasia caused by trembling and sudden stiffening of legs on standing, making walking impossible.
a., spastic. A., paroxysmal trepidant, q.v.
a., trembling; a. trepidans. A., paroxysmal trepidant, q.v.
abasic (ă-bā'sĭk). Pert. to abasia. SYN: *abatic.*
abate (ă-bāt') [L. *ab,* from, + *battere,* to beat]. 1. To lessen or decrease. 2. To cease or cause to cease.
abatement (ă-bāt'mĕnt). Decrease in severity of pain or symptoms.
abatic (ă-băt'ĭk). Pert. to abasia. SYN: *abasic.*
abaxial, abaxile (ăb-ăk'sē-ăl, -sĭl) [L. *ab,* from, + *axis,* axis]. 1. Not in line of axis of the body or a part. 2. At opposite end of the axis of a part.
Abbe's operation (ăb'bāz) [Robert Abbe, U.S. surgeon, 1851–1928] Lateral anastomosis of the intestine.
Abbe-Zeiss apparatus, counting cell hemocytometer. [Ernest Abbe, Ger. physicist, 1840–1905; Carl Zeiss, Ger. optician, 1816–1888] A device for counting blood cells in a specific quantity of blood.
Abbott's method. [Edville G. Abbott, U.S. orthopedic surgeon, 1870–1938] Treatment of scoliosis by a series of plaster jackets.
Abbott-Miller tube. [W. Osler Abbott, U.S. physician, 1902–1943; T. Grier Miller, U.S. physician, b. 1866] A double-channel intestinal tube used to relieve intestinal distention. Commonly called Miller-Abbott tube, q.v.
abdomen (ăb-dō'mĕn, ăb'dō-mĕn) [L., belly]. [NA] That portion of the trunk located be-

tween the chest and the pelvis; the upper portion of the abdominopelvic cavity. Contains the stomach with lower part of esophagus, small and large intestines, liver, gallbladder, spleen, pancreas, and bladder. A serous membrane, the peritoneum, lines this cavity. SEE: *abdominal quadrants* for illus.

a., acute. Medical jargon used to denote any acute abdominal condition demanding prompt surgery.

a., boat-shaped. A., scaphoid, q.v.

a., carinate. A., scaphoid, q.v.

a., navicular. A., scaphoid, q.v.

a. obstipum. Congenital shortness of the rectus abdominis muscle.

a., pendulous. Condition in which the excessively relaxed anterior wall of the abdomen hangs down over the pubis.

a., scaphoid. Condition in which the anterior wall is hollowed, presenting a sunken appearance as in emaciation and some cerebral diseases. SYN: *a., boat-shaped; a., carinate; a., navicular.*

a., surgical. A., acute, q.v.

abdominal (ăb-dŏm′ĭ-năl). Pert. to the abdomen.

abdominal cavity. The cavity within the abdomen. It is lined with a serous membrane, the peritoneum, and contains the following organs: stomach with lower portion of esophagus, small and large intestines (except sigmoid colon and rectum), liver, gallbladder, spleen, pancreas, kidney, and ureter. It is continuous with the pelvic cavity, the two comprising the abdominopelvic cavity. SEE: *abdominal quadrants* for illus.

abdominal crisis. Severe pain in the abdominal area. Usually refers to the pain that occurs during sickle cell anemia crisis or that resulting from syphilis.

abdominal decompression. Technique used in obstetrics to facilitate childbirth. The abdominal area is surrounded by an airtight chamber in which pressure may be intermittently decreased below atmospheric pressure. During labor pains, the pressure is decreased and the uterus is permitted to work more efficiently because the abdominal muscles are elevated away from the uterus.

abdominal examination. INSPECTION: Visual examination of the abdomen is most satisfactorily performed while patient is supine with thighs slightly flexed. In the healthy individual, the abdomen is of an oval form, marked by elevations and depressions corresponding to abdominal muscles, umbilicus, and in some degree by form of adjacent viscera. Is larger relative to size of chest in children than in adults; more rotund and broader inferiorly in females than in males.

Alterations in shape resulting from disease are enlargement (which may be general and symmetrical as in ascites, or partial and irregular from tumors, hypertrophy of such organs as the liver and spleen, or distention of portions of intestines by gas, as the colon in typhoid fever) and retraction (as in extreme emaciation and in several forms of cerebral disease, esp. noticeable in tubercular meningitis of children).

The respiratory movements of abdominal walls bear a certain relation to movements of the thorax and are often increased when the latter are arrested and vice versa; thus abdominal movements are increased in pleurisy, pneumonia, pericarditis, etc., but decreased or wholly suspended when disease causes abdominal pain or in peritonitis.

The superficial abdominal veins are also at times visibly enlarged, indicating an obstruction to the flow of blood, either in the portal system as in cirrhosis or in the inferior vena cava.

AUSCULTATION: Listening to sounds produced in the abdomen. Useful in diagnosing normal sounds produced by peristaltic action of intestines, aneurysm of abdominal aorta, fetal heart sounds, and vascular sounds from placenta. Intestinal sounds may be absent in paralytic ileus, q.v.

PERCUSSION: Patient should be placed in same position as for palpation, and percussion should be for the most part mediate. In exploring abdomen by means of percussion, finger should first be placed immediately below the xiphoid cartilage, pressed firmly down, and carried along the median line toward the pubes, striking it all the way, now forcibly, now gently. The different tones of stomach, colon, and small intestines will be distinctly heard. Percussion should then be made laterally, alternately to one side, then the other, until whole surface is percussed. Abdominal aneurysm gives dullness or flatness over it unless a distended intestine lies above it.

PALPATION: May be performed with tips of fingers, whole hand, or both hands; pressure may be slight or forcible, continuous or intermittent. To obtain greatest amount of information, place patient in supine position with head slightly raised and thighs flexed. The head is supported in order to relax the abdominal wall. It is sometimes necessary to place patient in standing position or leaning forward.

Palpation is of assistance in detecting size, consistency, and position of viscera, existence of tumors and swellings, and whether the tumors change position with respiration or are movable. Also ascertain whether tenderness exists in any portion of the abdominal cavity, if pain is increased or relieved by firm pressure, and if pain is accentuated by sudden release of firm pressure (i.e., rebound tenderness).

Impulse, if one exists, is systolic and expansive, although when situated high there also may be a slight diastolic movement. A thrill is rarely perceptible. Surface of tumor is usually rounded and smooth but may be nodular. Effusion of blood into surrounding tissues may produce lobulations.

abdominal gestation. Abdominal pregnancy. Extrauterine pregnancy in belly cavity.

abdominalgia (ăb-dŏm-ĭn-ăl'jē-ă) [L. *abdomen,* belly, + Gr. *algos,* pain]. Pain in the abdomen.

abdominal inguinal ring. The internal opening of the inguinal canal, bounded inferiorly by the inguinal ligament, medially by the inferior epigastric vessels, and above and laterally by the lower free border of the transversus abdominis muscle. SEE: *canal, inguinal; ring, abdominal; ring, inguinal.*

abdominal quadrants. Four parts or divisions of the abdomen determined by drawing imaginary vertical and horizontal lines through the umbilicus. The quadrants and their contents are:

Right upper quadrant (RUQ): right lobe of liver, gallbladder, part of transverse colon, part of pylorus, hepatic flexure, right kidney, and duodenum; *Right lower q. (RLQ):* cecum, ascending colon, small intestine, appendix, bladder if distended, right ureter, right spermatic duct in male, right ovary and right tube, and uterus if enlarged in female; *Left upper q. (LUQ):* left lobe of liver, stomach, transverse colon, splenic flexure, pancreas, left kidney, and spleen; *Left lower q. (LLQ):* small intestine, left ureter, sigmoid flexure, descending colon, bladder if distended, left spermatic duct in male, left ovary and left tube, and uterus if enlarged in female. SEE: illus.

abdominal reflexes. Contraction of the muscles of the abdominal wall upon stimulation of the overlying skin. Absence of these reflexes indicates damage to the pyramidal tract.

abdominal regions. The abdomen and its external surface are divided into nine regions by four imaginary planes: two horizontal, one at the level of the ninth costal cartilage (or the lowest point of the costal arch), and the other at the level of the highest point of the iliac crest; two vertical, through the centers of the inguinal ligaments (or through the nipples or through the centers of the clavicles) or curved and coinciding with the lateral borders of the two abdominal rectus muscles. SEE: *abdominal quadrants* for illus.

abdominal rings. The apertures in the abdominal wall. *External:* an interval in aponeurosis of external oblique muscle, just above and to outer side of crest of the pubic bone. *Triangular:* about an inch from base to apex and half an inch transversely; provides passage for spermatic cord in the male and round ligament in the female. *Internal* or *deep:* situated in the transversalis fascia, midway between the anterior superior spine of ilium and symphysis pubis, half an inch above Poupart's ligament; oval form, larger in the male. Surrounds spermatic cord in the male and round ligament in the female.

abdominal section. Abdominal incision for any operation on abdominal organs. SYN: *laparotomy,* q.v.

abdomino- (ăb-dŏm'ĭ-nō). Combining form rel. to the abdomen.

abdominocardiac reflex (ăb-dŏm"ĭ-nō-kăr'dē-ăk). A change in heart rate, usually a slowing, resulting from mechanical stimulation of abdominal viscera.

abdominocentesis (ăb-dŏm"ĭ-nō-sĕn-tē'sĭs) [L. *abdomen,* belly, + Gr. *kentesis,* puncture]. Puncture of the abdomen with an instrument for withdrawal of fluid from the abdominal cavity. SYN: *paracentesis, abdominal.*

abdominocystic [" + Gr. *kystis,* bladder]. Pert. to the abdomen and bladder.

abdominogenital (ăb-dŏm"ĭ-nō-jĕn'ĭ-tăl). Pert. to the abdomen and genital organs.

abdominohysterectomy [" + Gr. *hystera,* uterus, + *ektome,* excision]. Removal of uterus through abdominal incision.

abdominohysterotomy (ăb-dŏm"ĭ-nō-hĭs-tĕr-ŏt'ō-mē) [" + " + *tome,* incision]. Incision of the uterus through a surgical opening in the abdomen.

abdominoscopy (ăb-dŏm"ĭ-nŏs'kō-pē) [" + Gr. *skopein,* to examine]. Examination of the abdominal cavity and its contents by use of an endoscope. SEE: *peritoneoscopy.*

abdominoscrotal [" + *scrotum,* bag]. Pert. to the abdomen and scrotum.

abdominoscrotal muscle. Cremaster muscle.

abdominothoracic (ăb-dŏm"ĭ-nō-thō-ră'sĭk) [" + Gr. *thorax,* breastplate]. Pert. to the abdomen and thorax.

abdominothoracic arch. The costal arch; the anterior and lateral boundary between the line dividing the thorax and the abdomen.

abdominouterotomy (ăb-dŏm"ĭ-nō-ū-tĕr-ŏt'ō-mē) [" + *uterus,* womb, + Gr. *tome,* incision]. Abdominohysterotomy.

abdominovaginal (ăb-dŏm"ĭ-nō-văj'ĭ-năl) [" + *vagina,* sheath]. Pert. to the abdomen and vagina.

abdominovesical (ăb-dŏm"ĭ-nō-vĕs'ĭ-kăl) [" + *vesica,* bladder]. Pert. to the abdomen and urinary bladder.

abdominovesical pouch. Peritoneal fold that includes urachal folds.

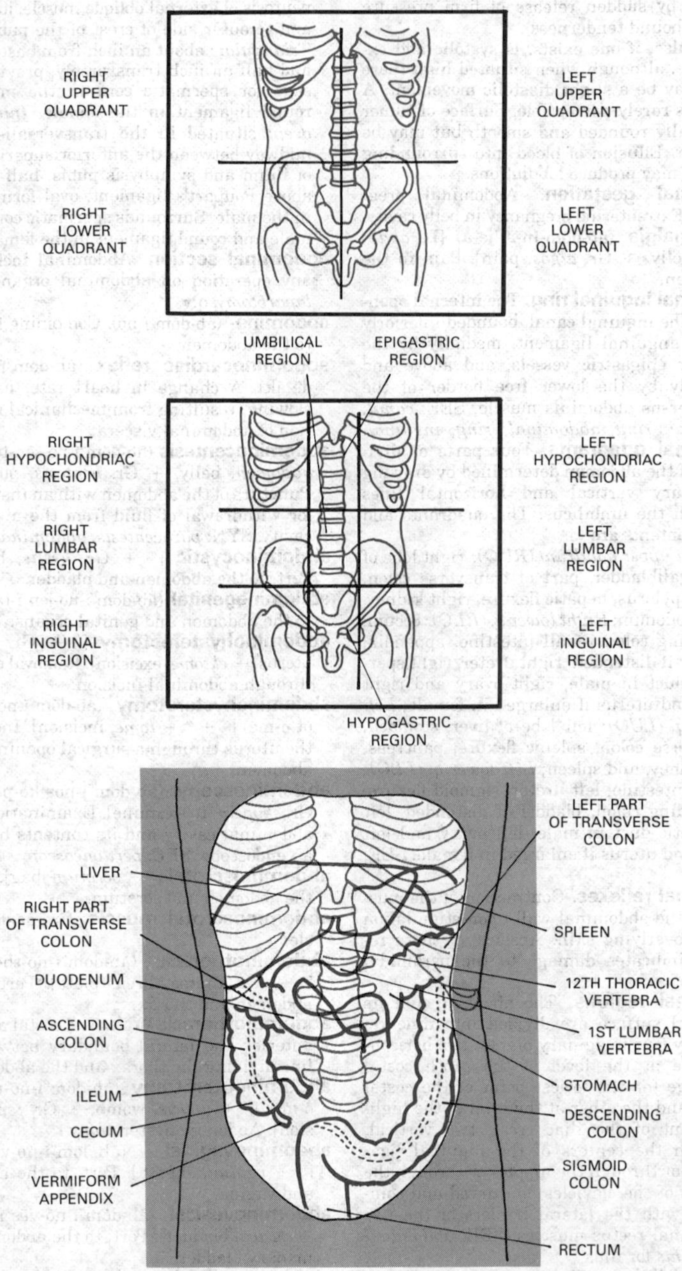

ABDOMINAL QUADRANTS, REGIONS, AND ORGANS

abducens (ăb-dū'sĕnz) [L., drawing away]. Pert. to drawing away from the median line of the body.

a. labiorum. Muscle that elevates angle of mouth. SYN: *caninus muscle; levator anguli oris muscle.* SEE: *Muscles* in *Appendix.*

abducens muscle. Rectus lateralis muscle of eye, which moves the eyeball outward. SEE: *Muscles* in *Appendix.*

abducens nerve. Sixth cranial nerve; it innervates rectus lateralis muscle of eye. SEE: *cranial nerves.*

abducent (ăb-dū'sĕnt) [L. *abducens,* drawing away]. 1. Abducting, leading away from. 2. Abducens.

abducent nerve. Abducens nerve, q.v.

abduct (ăb-dŭkt') [L. *abductus,* led away]. To draw away from the median plane of the body or one of its parts.

abduction (ăb-dŭk'shŭn). 1. The lateral movement of the limbs away from median plane of body, or the lateral bending of the head or trunk. SEE: illus. 2. The movement of the digits away from the axial line of a limb. 3. Outward rotation of the eyes.

abductor (ăb-dŭk'tor). A muscle that upon contraction draws a part away from median plane of body or axial line of an extremity. Opposite of adductor. SEE: *Muscles* in *Appendix.*

Abel's bacillus. [Rudolf Abel, Ger. bacteriologist, 1868–1942] Klebsiella ozaenae; found in ozena, q.v.

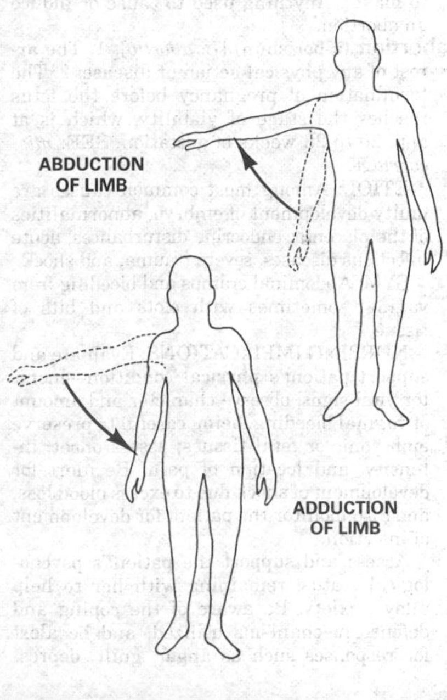

abenteric (ăb-ĕn-tĕr'ĭk) [L. *ab,* from, + Gr. *enteron,* intestine]. Rel. to or involving organs located outside the intestines.

abepithymia (ăb-ĕp-ĭ-thī'mē-ă) [" + Gr. *epithymia,* desire]. Paralysis of the celiac (solar) plexus.

Abernethy, John (ăb'ĕr-nē"thē). British surgeon, 1764–1831.

A.'s fascia. A layer of areolar tissue separating the external iliac artery from the iliac fascia over the psoas muscle.

A.'s sarcoma. A circumscribed, usually malignant, fatty tumor occurring principally on the trunk.

aberrant (ăb-ĕr'ănt) [L. *ab,* from, + *errare,* to wander]. Deviating from normal. SYN: *abnormal.*

aberrant pyramidal tract. Several groups of fibers from the midbrain to the cranial nerve motor nuclei, separating from the main fibers of the cortex.

aberratio (ăb-ĕr-ā'shē-ō) [L.]. Aberration.

a. lactis. Secretion of milk from a site other than the breast.

a. testis. Location of a testis in a position away from the path of normal descent.

aberration (ăb-ĕr-ā'shŭn) [L. *ab,* from, + *errare,* to wander]. 1. Deviation from normal. 2. Imperfect refraction of light rays.

a., chromatic. Unequal refraction of different wavelengths of light through a lens, producing a colored image.

a., chromosomal. Abnormalities in chromosomes with regard to number (aneuploidy, polyploidy) or chromosomal material (translocation, deletion, duplication).

a., diopteric. A., spherical, q.v.

a., distantial. Blurring of a distant object.

a., lateral. Deviation of a ray from the focus measured on a line perpendicular to the axis.

a., longitudinal. Deviation of a ray from the focus measured along the axis.

a., mental. Any deviation from normal mental functions.

a., spherical. Aberration or distortion of an image due to rays entering the peripheral portion of a spherical mirror or lens being refracted differently from those closer to the center. Thus the peripheral rays are focused on the optical axis at a different point from the central rays.

aberrometer (ăb"ĕr-ŏm'ĕ-tĕr) [L. *ab,* from, + *errare,* to wander, + Gr. *metron,* measure]. An instrument for measuring errors in delicate observations or instruments.

abetalipoproteinemia (ā-bā"tă-lĭp"ō-prō"tē-ĭn-ē'mē-ă) [Gr. *a-,* not, + β + *lipos,* fat, + *protos,* first, + *haima,* blood]. A rare inherited disease characterized by absence of plasma β-lipoproteins. There are failure of normal lipid absorption, marked neuromuscular abnormalities, decreased cholesterol, malnutrition, steatorrhea, mental retardation, and retinal degeneration. About 80% of the red blood cells are acanthocytes. Disease usually begins prior to age one and death may occur at an early age. There is no specific treatment. SYN: *acanthocytosis*.

abevacuation (ăb-ē-văk″ū-ā′shŭn) [L. *ab*, from, + *evacuare*, to empty]. 1. Abnormal evacuation, either excessive or deficient. 2. Metastases.

abeyance (ă-bā′ăns) [O. Fr.]. A temporary suspension of activity, sensation, or pain.

abient (ăb′ē-ĕnt). Tending to move away from a stimulus. Opposite of adient.

abiogenesis (ăb-ē-ō-jĕn′ĕ-sĭs) [Gr. *a*-, not, + *bios*, life, + *genesis*, production]. Spontaneous generation of life; theoretical production of living from nonliving matter.

abiogenetic, abiogenous (ăb-ē-ŏ-jĕ-nĕt′ĭk, ăb-ē-ŏj′ĭ-nŭs). Pert. to spontaneous generation.

abiologic, abiological (ā-bī-ō-lŏj′ĭk, -ăl). Not related to biology or the science of life.

abiosis (ăb-ē-ŏ′sĭs) [Gr. *a*-, not, + *bios*, life, + *osis*, condition]. Absence of life.

abiotic (ăb-ē-ŏt′ĭk). Incompatible with life; not viable.

abiotrophy (ăb-ē-ŏt′rō-fē) [″ + ″ + *trophe*, nourishment]. Premature loss of vitality or degeneration of tissues and cells with consequent loss of endurance and resistance.

abirritant (ăb-ĭr′ĭ-tănt) [L. *ab*, from, + *irritare*, to irritate]. Relieving irritation; soothing.

abirritation (ăb″ĭr-rĭ-tā′shŭn). 1. Asthenia, or atony. 2. Decreased response to stimuli.

ablactation (ăb-lăk-tā′shŭn) [L. *ab*, from, + *lactatio*, suckling]. Cessation of milk secretion; weaning.

ablastemic (ă-blăs-tēm′ĭk) [Gr. *a*-, not, + *blastos*, germ, seed]. Not germinal.

ablate (ăb-lāt′) [L. *ablatus*, taken away]. To remove, esp. by excision.

ablatio (ăb-lā′shē-ō) [L., carrying away]. Ablation, removal, detachment.

a. placentae. Premature detachment of a normally situated placenta; abruptio placentae, q.v. SEE: *placenta*.

a. retinae. Detachment of retina. SEE: *retina*.

ablation (ăb-lā′shŭn) [L. *ab*, from, + *latus*, carried]. Removal of a part, as by incision.

ablepharia (ăb-lĕ-fā′rē-ă) [Gr. *a*-, not, + *blepharon*, eyelid]. Congenital absence of or reduction in size of the eyelids.

ablepharon (ă-blĕf′ă-rŏn). Ablepharia.

ablepharous (ă-blĕf′ă-rŭs). Without eyelids.

ablephary (ă-blĕf′ă-rē). Ablepharia.

ablepsia (ă-blĕp′sē-ă) [Gr. *a*-, not, + *blepein*, to see]. Lack of or loss of sight. Blindness.

abluent (ăb′lū-ĕnt) [L. *ab*, from, + *luens*, washing]. An agent possessing cleansing qualities, as a detergent.

ablution (ăb-lū′shŭn). A cleansing or washing.

ablutomania (ă-blū″tō-mā′nē-ă) [L. *ablutio*, a washing, + Gr. *mania*, frenzy]. Compulsion to wash or clean.

abnerval [L. *ab*, from, + *nervus*, nerve]. Away from a nerve, esp. with reference to the passage of an electric current through a muscle away from point where nerve enters the muscle. Opposite of adnerval.

abnormal (ăb-nor′măl) [″ + *norma*, rule]. Deviating from normal. SYN: *aberrant*.

abnormality (ăb″nor-măl′ĭ-tē). Deviation from normal. SYN: *aberration*.

abnormity (ăb-nor′mĭ-tē). 1. Deformity; abnormality. 2. A monstrosity.

abocclusion (ăb″ŏ-kloo′zhŭn). Dentition in which the teeth of the mandible and the maxilla are not in contact.

aborad (ăb-ō′răd) [″ + *oris*, mouth]. Away from the mouth.

aboral (ăb-ō′răl). Opposite to, or away from, the mouth.

abort (ă-bort′) [L. *abortare*, to miscarry]. 1. To expel an embryo or fetus prior to viability. 2. To arrest progress of disease. 3. To arrest growth or development. 4. To discontinue an effort or project before its completion.

abortient (ă-bor′shĕnt) [L. *abortio*, abortion]. 1. Producing abortion. 2. Abortifacient.

abortifacient (ă-bor-tĭ-fā′shĕnt) [″ + *facere*, to make]. Anything used to cause or induce an abortion.

abortion (ă-bor′shŭn) [L. *abortio*]. 1. The arrest of any physical action or disease. 2. The termination of pregnancy before the fetus reaches the stage of viability, which is at app. 20 to 28 weeks of gestation. SEE: *miscarriage*.

ETIOL: Among most common causes are faulty development of embryo, abnormalities of the placenta, endocrine disturbances, acute infectious diseases, severe trauma, and shock.

SYM: Abdominal cramps and bleeding from vagina, sometimes with clots and bits of tissue.

NURSING IMPLICATIONS: Evaluate and support patient's physical condition—monitor vital signs; observe character and amount of vaginal bleeding, being careful to preserve embryonic or fetal tissues; assess onset, intensity, and location of pain. Be alert for development of shock due to excess blood loss, and also monitor the patient for development of infection.

Assess and support the patient's psychological status, remaining with her to help allay anxiety. Be aware of the coping and defense mechanisms utilized, and be alert for responses such as anger, guilt, depression, sadness, happiness, and grief. Provide appropriate support for the patient.

If the patient is to have surgical completion of the abortion, explain the procedure to her.

a., accidental. Abortion that occurs spontaneously.

a., ampullar. Tubal abortion occurring from the ampulla of the oviduct.

a., artificial. Abortion induced or performed purposely, as by a surgeon.

a., cervical. Abortion in which the ovum is retained in the cervical canal.

a., complete. Abortion in which the complete products of conception have been expelled.

a., criminal. Illegal abortion.

a., habitual. Three or more consecutive, spontaneous abortions.

a., imminent. Impending abortion characterized by bleeding and colicky pains that increase. Cervix is usually effaced and patulous.

a., incomplete. Abortion in which part of the products of conception has been retained in the uterus.

a., induced. Abortion brought on intentionally. Abortions may be induced by use of drugs, by use of suction or scraping of lining of uterus for removal of the products of conception, or by injection of sterile hypertonic solutions into the amniotic cavity. SEE: *curettage.*

a., inevitable. Abortion that cannot be halted.

a., infected. Abortion accompanied by infection of retained material with resultant febrile reaction.

a., missed. Abortion in which the fetus has died prior to the twentieth completed week of gestation but the products of conception are retained in the uterus for eight weeks or longer.

a., septic. Abortion in which there is an infection of the products of conception and the endometrial lining of uterus.

a., spontaneous. Abortion occurring without apparent cause.

a., therapeutic. Abortion performed when the mental or physical health of the mother is endangered by continuation of the pregnancy.

a., threatened. The appearance of signs and symptoms of possible loss of fetus. Vaginal bleeding with or without intermittent pain is usually the first sign. If fetus is still alive and attachment to uterus has not been interrupted, pregnancy may continue. Absolute bedrest and sedation recommended, with avoidance of coitus, douches, stress, and cathartics.

a., tubal. 1. A spontaneous abortion in which the fetus has been expelled through the distal end of a uterine tube. 2. The escape of the products of conception into the peritoneal cavity by way of the uterine tube.

abortionist (ă-bor'shŭn-ĭst). One who performs an abortion.

abortive (ă-bor'tĭv) [L. *abortivus*]. 1. Preventing the completion of. 2. Abortifacient; that which prevents the normal continuation of pregnancy. 3. Rudimentary.

abortus (ă-bor'tŭs) [L.]. An aborted fetus.

aboulia (ă-boo'lē-ă) [Gr. *a-*, not, + *boule,* will]. Abulia, q.v.

abrachia (ă-brā'kē-ă) [" + *brachion,* arm]. Congenital absence of arms.

abrachiocephalia (ă-brā"kē-ō-sĕ-fā'lē-ă) [" + " + *kephale,* head]. Congenital absence of arms and head.

abradant (ă-brăd'ĕnt). An abrasive.

abrade (ă-brād') [L. *ab,* from, + *radere,* to scrape]. 1. To chafe. 2. To roughen or remove by friction.

abrasion (ă-brā'zhŭn) [" + *radere,* to scrape]. 1. A scraping away of a portion of skin or of a mucous membrane as a result of injury or by mechanical means, as in dermabrasion for cosmetic purposes. SEE: *avulsion; bruise.* 2. The wearing away of the substance of a tooth. Normally occurs from mastication; may be accomplished by mechanical or chemical means.

abrasive. 1. Producing abrasion. 2. That which abrades.

abreaction (ăb"rē-ăk'shŭn) [" + *re,* again, + *actus,* acting]. In psychoanalysis, release of or discharge of emotional tension by consciously recalling or acting out a painful experience that had been either forgotten or repressed. Abreaction may allow this painful or consciously intolerable experience to become bearable because of the insight gained during the process. The method used to bring about abreaction is termed catharsis, q.v.

abrosia (ă-brō'zē-ă) [Gr.]. 1. Fasting; abstaining from food. 2. A wasting away.

abruptio (ă-brŭp'shē-ō) [L. *abruptus*]. A tearing away from.

a. placentae. Premature detachment of normally situated placenta; ablatio placentae. SEE: *placenta.*

ETIOL: Unknown. May be associated with toxemia, hypofibrinogenemia, and disseminated intravascular coagulation.

PATH: Extravasation of blood between placenta and uterine wall, occasionally between muscle fibers of the uterus.

SYM: Hemorrhage, concealed or evident, or a combination of both. Pain, constant at point of separation of placenta due to blood extruding between muscle fibers. Uterine contraction constant; occasionally tetanic in nature. Increased fetal movements and changes in heart rate until fetal asphyxia and death. Albumin in urine. Anemia.

TREATMENT: In mild cases, rest in bed. In severe cases, shock must first be combated. A soft and partially dilated cervix is an indication for immediate artificial rupture of membranes followed by natural or artificial induction of labor. If the fetus is alive, and if the mother's cervix is firm and not dilated, a cesarean section is the treatment of choice. If the uterus fails to contract after cesarean section, an immediate hysterectomy usually is necessary.

NURSING IMPLICATIONS: Monitor the patient's vital signs, including the fetal heart tones, as ordered. Keep a perineal pad count, including character and amount of blood lost. Administer ordered medications to keep the patient comfortable, and provide calm reassurance that the mother and the baby are being cared for. Prepare the patient for amniotomy and delivery.

abscess (ăb'sĕs) [L. *abscessus*, a going away]. A localized collection of pus in any part of the body. The result of disintegration or displacement of tissue. SEE: illus.; *inflammation; pus; suppuration*.

a., acute. Abscess with local symptoms of inflammation, with fluctuation, and pointing, i.e., about to rupture; also pressure and constitutional symptoms. Inflammation becomes intensified with increased heat, redness, swelling, and edema. Pain becomes throbbing and greater, with impaired loss of function of the part. An elevation appears with fluctuation and softening as it reaches the surface, becoming necrotic and yellow, giving way with evacuation of pus. Pressure symptoms, according to size and depth. In floor of mouth or neck, swelling may cause dyspnea and dysphagia. Constitutional symptoms vary from slight to high fever (fever may be absent in a well walled-off abscess) with chills and sweats if associated with pyemia and septicemia. Any or all general symptoms may be absent in deep-seated abscesses except eventual loss of weight and strength.

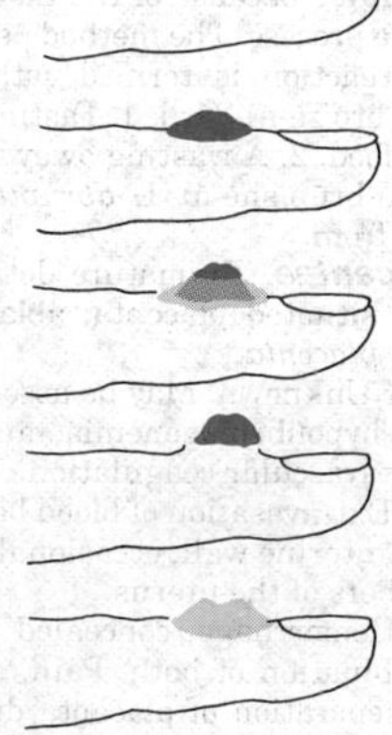

PROGRESSION OF ABSCESS

The abscess may be terminated by pointing, evacuation, and discharge of pus, or it may become inspissated, encapsulated, and at times absorbed. SYN: *a., warm*.

a., alveolar. Abscess about root of a tooth in alveolar cavity. Usually the result of necrosis and infection of dental pulp following dental caries.

a., amebic. 1. Abscess occurring in the liver, developing as a complication of amebic dysentery. Caused by Entamoeba histolytica. 2. Abscess in the brain caused by Entamoeba histolytica.

a., anorectal. Abscess in the tissue near the rectum. SYN: *a., ischiorectal; a., perirectal*.

a., apical. Abscess at the apex of lung or at extremity of root of a tooth.

a., appendiceal, appendicular. Pus formation around an inflamed vermiform appendix.

a., arthrifluent. A wandering abscess, q.v., having origin in a diseased joint.

a., atheromatous. Softening in the wall of a blood vessel as the result of atherosclerosis.

a., axillary. Abscess or multiple abscesses in axilla.

a., bartholin. Abscess of Bartholin's gland.

a., bicameral. Abscess with two pockets.

a., bile duct. Abscess of the bile duct. SYN: *a., cholangitic*.

a., bilharziasis. Abscess in an intestinal wall caused by Schistosoma.

a., blind. Abscess with no external opening, such as a dental granuloma.

a., bone. A., Brodie's, q.v.

a., brain. Intracranial abscess; one involving the brain or its membranes. It is seldom primary but usually occurs secondary to infections of middle ear, nasal sinuses, face, or skull, or from contamination from penetrating wounds or skull fractures. It may also have a metastatic origin arising from septic foci in the lungs (bronchiectasis, empyema, lung abscess), in bone (osteomyelitis), or in the heart (endocarditis). Infection of nervous tissue by the invading organism results in necrosis and liquefaction of the tissue, with edema of surrounding tissues.

Brain abscesses may be acute, subacute, or chronic. Their clinical manifestations depend on part of brain involved, size, virulence of infecting organisms, and other factors. SYN: *a., cerebral; a., intracranial.*

SYM: Severe and persistent headache usually localized over infected area; fever, vomiting, vertigo, malaise, sometimes irritability and other mental symptoms.

TREATMENT: Chemotherapy; surgical intervention may be required.

a., breast. A., mammary, q.v.

a., Brodie's. Suppuration of articular end of a bone, esp. the tibia. SYN: *a., bone.*

a., bursal. Abscess in a bursa.

a., canalicular. Abscess of breast discharging into the milk ducts.

a., caseous. Abscess in which the pus has a cheesy appearance.

a., cerebral. A., brain, q.v. SYN: *a., intracranial.*

a., cheesy. Caseous abscess.

a., cholangitic. Abscess of the bile duct.

a., chronic. Abscess with pus but without signs of inflammation; usually of slow development. Formed by liquefaction of tuberculous tissue. May occur anywhere in or on the body but more frequently in the spine, hips, genitourinary tract, and lymph glands. Symptoms may be very mild. Pain when present is caused by pressure upon surrounding parts. Tenderness often absent. Chronic septic intoxication with afternoon fever may occur. Amyloid disease may develop if the abscess persists for a prolonged period. SYN: *a., cold.*

a., circumscribed. Abscess limited or confined by surrounding tissue.

a., circumtonsillar. Abscess around the tonsil. SYN: *a., peritonsillar; quinsy.*

a., cold. A., chronic, q.v.

a., collar-button. Two pus-containing cavities, one larger than the other, connected by a narrow channel. SYN: *a., shirt-stud.*

a., deep. Abscess arising from below the deep fascia.

a., dental. Abscess beside a tooth, usually near the root.

a., dentoalveolar. Abscess in the alveolar process surrounding the root of a tooth.

a., diffuse. A collection of pus not circumscribed by a well-defined capsule.

a., dry. Abscess that disappears without pointing or breaking.

a., embolic. Abscess due to a septic embolus.

a., emphysematous. Abscess containing air or gas. SYN: *a., tympanitic.*

a., endamebic; a., entamebic. A., amebic, q.v.

a., epidural. A., extradural, q.v.

a., epiploic. Abscess in the omentum.

a., extradural. Abscess on the dura mater.

a., fecal. Abscess containing feces. SYN: *a., stercoral.*

a., filarial. Abscess caused by filaria, q.v.

a., follicular. Abscess forming in a follicle.

a., frontal. Abscess in the frontal lobe of the brain.

a., fungal. Abscess caused by a fungus.

a., gangrenous. Abscess attended with gangrene of surrounding parts.

a., gas. A tympanitic abscess; one containing gas due to presence of gas-forming organisms such as Clostridium perfringens.

a., gingival. Abscess of the gum.

a., glandular. Abscess around a lymph node.

a., gravitation. Abscess in which the pus migrates, sinking to a lower part of the body.

a., helminthic. Abscess due to the presence of a parasitic worm.

a., hematic. Abscess due to an extravasated blood clot.

a., hemorrhagic. Abscess containing blood.

a., hepatic. Abscess of the liver, esp. an amebic abscess.

a., hot. A., acute, q.v

a., hypostatic. A., wandering, q.v.

a., idiopathic. Abscess due to an unknown cause.

a., iliac. Abscess in the iliac region.

a., intracranial. A., brain, q.v. SYN: *a., cerebral.*

a., intradural. Abscess within the layers of the dura mater.

a., intramammary. A., mammary, q.v. SYN: *a., breast.*

a., intramastoid. A mastoid process abscess of the temporal bone.

a., ischiorectal. Abscess in the ischiorectal fossa.

a., kidney. Abscess or multiple abscesses of renal cortex. SYN: *a., renal.*

a., lacrimal. Suppuration of a lacrimal gland.

a., lacunar. Abscess in the urethral lacunae.

a., lateral; a., lateral alveolar. Abscess in periodontal tissue.

a., lumbar. Abscess in the lumbar region.

a., lung. Abscess occurring in the lung.

a., lymphatic. Abscess of a lymph node.

a., mammary. Abscess in the female breast, esp. one involving the glandular tissue. Usually seen during lactation or at time of weaning. SYN: *a., breast; a., intramammary.*

a., marginal. Abscess near the orifice of the anus.

a., mastoid. Suppuration of the mastoid

portion of the temporal bone.

a., mediastinal. Suppuration in the mediastinum.

a., metastatic. Secondary abscess at a distance from focus of infection.

a., migrating. Abscess at a distance from focus of disease with pus along fascial sheaths of muscles. SYN: *a., wandering.*

a., miliary. Small embolic abscess discharging numerous small collections of pus.

a., milk. Mammary abscess during lactation.

a., mother. Primary abscess giving rise to other abscesses.

a., multiple. Group of abscesses accompanying pyemia.

a., nocardial. Abscess caused by Nocardia.

a., orbital. Suppuration in the orbit.

a., ossifluent. Abscess dependent on degeneration of bone tissue.

a., palatal. Abscess in an upper lateral incisor, erupting toward the palate.

a., palmar. Purulent effusion into the tissues of the palm of the hand.

a., pancreatic. Abscess of pancreatic tissue, usually as a complication of acute pancreatitis or abdominal surgery.

a., parafrenal. Abscess on the side of the frenulum of the penis. Usually involves Tyson's gland.

a., parametric; a., parametritic. Abscess between the folds of the broad ligaments of the uterus.

a., paranephric; a., paranephritic. Abscess in the tissues around the kidney.

a., parapancreatic. Abscess in the tissues adjacent to the pancreas.

a., parietal. Periodontal abscess arising in the periodontal tissue other than the orifice through which the vascular supply enters the dental pulp.

a., parotid. Abscess of parotid gland.

a., pelvic. Abscess of the pelvic peritoneum, esp. Douglas' pouch.

a., pelvirectal. Deep rectal abscess.

a., periapical. Periodontal abscess at the root apex of a tooth.

a., pericemental. Alveolar abscess not involving the apex of a tooth.

a., pericoronal. Abscess around the crown of an unerupted molar tooth.

a., peridental. Abscess of periodontal tissue.

a., perinephric. Abscess in tissue about the kidney. SYN: *a., perirenal.*

a., periodontal. Abscess arising in the periodontal tissue (structures of support for teeth).

a., peripleuritic. Abscess in the tissue surrounding the parietal pleura.

a., periproctic. Abscess in the areolar tissue about the anus. SYN: *a., perirectal.*

a., perirectal. A., periproctic, q.v.

a., perirenal. A., perinephric, q.v.

a., peritoneal. Abscess within the peritoneal cavity usually following peritonitis.

a., peritonsillar. Abscess of the tissue around the tonsil capsule. SYN: *a., circumtonsillar; quinsy.*

a., periureteral. Abscess of area around the ureter.

a., periurethral. Abscess in tissue surrounding the urethra.

a., perivesical. Abscess in tissue around the urinary bladder.

a., phlegmonous. An acute abscess in the connective tissue.

a., pneumococcic. Abscess due to infection with pneumococci.

a., postcecal. Abscess situated behind the cecum. SYN: *a., retrocecal.*

a., postmammary. A., retromammary, q.v.

a., prelacrimal. Abscess of the lacrimal bone producing a swelling at inner canthus of eye.

a., premammary. Subcutaneous or subareolar abscess of the mammary gland.

a., primary. Abscess originating at point of infection.

a., prostatic. Abscess within the prostate gland.

a., protozoal. Abscess caused by a protozoon.

a., psoas. Abscess with pus descending in sheath of psoas muscle due to vertebral disease, usually tuberculous in origin.

a., pulmonary. Abscess of the lungs. Nontuberculous suppuration of lung tissue with one or more localized areas of necrosis resulting in pulmonary cavitation.

a., pulp. 1. A cavity discharging pus formed in the pulp of a tooth. 2. An abscess of the tissues of the pulp of a finger.

a., pyemic. A metastatic abscess, usually multiple, due to pyogenic organisms.

a., rectal. Abscess in the rectum.

a., renal. Abscess or multiple abscesses of the renal cortex. SYN: *a., kidney.*

a., residual. Abscess occurring from old inflammatory products at the site of an earlier abscess.

a., retrocecal. A., postcecal, q.v.

a., retromammary. Abscess between the mammary gland and the chest wall.

a., retroperitoneal. Abscess located between the peritoneum and the posterior abdominal wall.

a., retropharyngeal. Abscess of the lymph nodes in the walls of the pharynx. It sometimes simulates diphtheritic pharyngitis.

a., retrovesical. Abscess behind the

bladder.

a., root. Abscess of the root of a tooth. SYN: *a., apical.*

a., sacrococcygeal. Abscess over the sacrum and coccyx.

a., satellite. Secondary abscess arising from and located near the primary abscess.

a., scrofulous. Abscess due to tuberculous degeneration of bone or lymph nodes.

a., secondary. A., embolic, q.v.

a., septicemic. Abscess resulting from septicemia.

a.'s, shirt-stud. Two pus-containing cavities, one larger than the other, connected by a narrow channel. SYN: *a., collar-button.*

a., spermatic. Abscess of the seminiferous tubules.

a., spinal. Abscess due to necrosis of a vertebra.

a., splenic. Abscess of the spleen.

a., stercoral; a., stercoralaceous. Abscess containing feces. SYN: *a., fecal.*

a., sterile. Abscess from which attempts to culture microorganisms are in vain.

a., stitch. Abscess formed about a stitch or suture.

a., streptococcal. Abscess caused by streptococci.

a., subaponeurotic. Abscess beneath an aponeurosis or fascia.

a., subarachnoid. Abscess of the midlayer of the covering of the brain and spinal cord.

a., subareolar. Abscess underneath the areola of the mammary gland, sometimes draining through the nipple.

a., subdiaphragmatic. Abscess beneath the diaphragm. SYN: *a., subphrenic.*

a., subdural. Abscess beneath the dura of brain or spinal cord.

a., subepidermal. Abscess beneath the epidermis.

a., subfascial. Abscess beneath a fascia.

a., subgaleal. Abscess beneath the galea aponeurotica, i.e., the epicranial aponeurosis.

a., submammary. Abscess beneath the mammary gland.

a., subpectoral. Abscess beneath the pectoral muscles.

a., subperiosteal. Bone abscess below the periosteum.

a., subperitoneal. Abscess between the parietal peritoneum and the abdominal wall.

a., subphrenic. A., subdiaphragmatic, q.v.

a., subscapular. Abscess between the serratus anterior and the posterior thoracic wall.

a., subungual. Abscess beneath the distal portion of a fingernail. May follow injuries with pins, needles, or splinters.

a., sudoriparous. Abscess of a sweat gland.

a., superficial. Abscess occurring above the deep fascia.

a., suprahepatic. Abscess in the suspensory ligament between the liver and the diaphragm.

a., sympathetic. Abscess arising some distance from the primary cause.

a., syphilitic. Abscess occurring in the tertiary stage of syphilis.

a., thecal. Abscess in a tendon sheath.

a., thymus. Abscess of the thymus.

a., tonsillar. Acute suppurative tonsillitis.

a., tooth. A., alveolar, q.v.

a., traumatic. Abscess caused by injury.

a., tropical. Amebic abscess of the liver.

a., tuberculous. A., chronic, q.v.

a., tubo-ovarian. Abscess involving both the fallopian tube and the ovary.

a., tympanitic. Abscess that contains air or gas.

a., tympanocervical. Abscess arising in the tympanum and extending to the neck.

a., tympanomastoid. A combined abscess of the tympanum and mastoid.

a., urethral. Abscess of the urethra.

a., urinary. Abscess caused by escape of urine into the tissues.

a., urinous. Abscess that contains pus and urine.

a., verminous. Abscess that is caused by or contains insect larvae or other animal parasites.

a., wandering. Abscess at a distance from focus of disease with pus along fascial sheaths of muscles. SYN: *a., migrating.*

a., warm. A., acute, q.v.

a., worm. Abscess caused by or containing worms.

abscissa (ăb-sĭs'ă) [L. *abscindere,* to cut off]. In a graph of a two-dimensional coordinate system wherein horizontal and perpendicular lines are crossed in order to provide a frame of reference, the abscissa is the horizontal line or x-axis. The ordinate, q.v., is the vertical line or y-axis. SEE: illus.

abscission (ăb-sĭ'zhŭn) [L. *abscindere,* to cut off]. Removal by excision.

absconsio (ăb-skŏn'sē-ō) [L.]. A cavity or fossa.

abscopal (ăb-skō'păl). Concerning the effect of radiation on tissues of the same person or organism at some distance from the actual radiation site or target.

absence (ăb'sĕnz). Brief temporary loss of consciousness, as may occur in petit mal epilepsy, q.v. SYN: *absentia epileptica.*

absence seizure. Seizure in which there is a sudden lapse of consciousness for several seconds. There is usually a blank facial expression that may be accompanied by certain

ABSCISSA

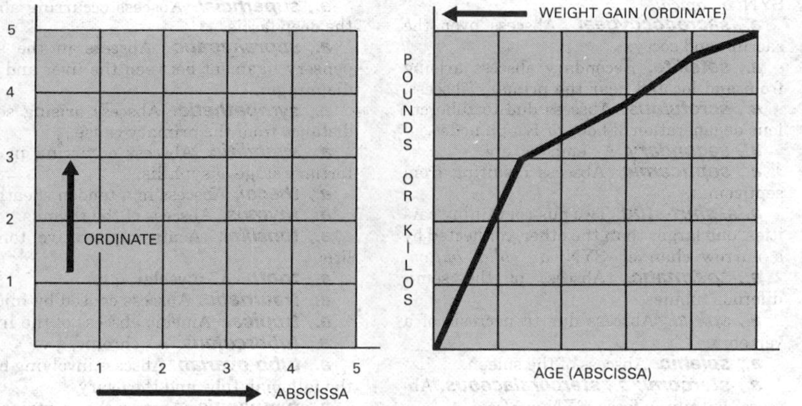

movements such as repeated eye-blinking or lip-smacking. There is no convulsion or fall. This type of attack is characteristic of petit mal epilepsy.

absentia epileptica (ăb-sĕn′shē-ă) [L., absence]. Momentary loss of consciousness. There is no convulsion but there may be transient stereotyped muscle movement. SEE: *absence seizure; epilepsy.*

abs. feb. L. *absente febre,* in the absence of fever.

Absidia (ăb-sĭd′ē-ă). Genus of pathogenic fungi of the order Phycomycetes and the family Mucoraceae. SEE: *phycomycosis.*

absinthe, absinth (ăb′sĭnth) [L. *absinthium,* wormwood]. A liquor, containing oil of wormwood, anise, and other herbs. It is highly toxic, esp. to the nervous system.

absinthism (ăb′sĭn-thĭzm). Deterioration of the nerve centers following excessive use of absinthe.

absolute alcohol. Ethyl alcohol with not more than 1% of water.

absolute scale. Temperature scale in which zero is at the point of absolute zero, q.v. SYN: *Kelvin scale.*

absolute temperature. Temperature measured on the absolute scale, q.v.

absolute zero. The lowest possible temperature, −273.15° C or −459.67° F; equal to zero on the absolute scale.

absorb (ăb-sorb′) [L. *absorbere,* to suck in]. To take in, suck up, or imbibe. SEE: *absorption; adsorption.*

absorbance (ăb-sor′băns). The ability of a material or tissue to absorb the dose of radiation used in x-ray.

absorbefacient (ăb-sor″bĕ-fā′shĕnt) [″ + *facere,* to make]. Causing or that which causes absorption.

absorbent (ăb-sor′bĕnt). 1. A substance that absorbs. 2. Having the power to absorb.

absorptiometer (ăb-sorp″shē-ŏm′ĕ-tĕr) [L. *absorptio,* absorption, + Gr. *metron,* measure]. 1. Instrument for measuring thickness of a layer of liquid, drawn by capillary attraction, between glass plates. 2. Instrument for measuring the absorption of gas by a liquid.

absorption (ăb-sorp′shŭn) [L. *absorptio*]. 1. The taking up of liquids by solids, or of gases by solids or liquids. 2. The taking up of light or of its rays by black or colored rays. 3. The taking up by the body of radiant heat, causing a rise in body temperature. 4. The reduction in intensity of an x-ray beam as it passes through a substance. 5. The passage of a substance through some surface of the body into body fluids and tissues, as the passage of ether through the respiratory epithelium of lungs into the blood during anesthesia, or passage of oil of wintergreen through the skin, the result of several processes: diffusion, q.v., filtration, q.v., osmosis, q.v.

RS: adsorption; chondrolysis; imbibition; osmosis; resorption.

a., colon. Water (important in the conservation of body fluids) and products of bacterial action are normally absorbed esp. in the ascending colon. Some nutrients and drugs are absorbed by the lower bowel. In the human, cellulose is not digested or absorbed but passes from the body as residue. SEE: *fiber.*

a., cutaneous. Absorption through the skin.

a., disjunctive. Separation of a slough by absorption of a layer of adjacent healthy tissue.

a., external. Absorption of material by the skin and mucous membrane.

a., mouth. Some substances, but no food nutrients, can be absorbed from the mouth; some drugs, esp. alkaloids, can be absorbed through the oral mucosa.

a., parenteral. Absorption from a site other than the gastrointestinal tract.

a., pathologic. Absorption into the blood or lymph of substances normally excreted or of a product of disease processes, e.g., pus.

a., percutaneous. A., cutaneous, q.v.

a., protein. In the digestive process, proteins are hydrolyzed to their constituent amino acids in the walls of the intestines. They are transported via the portal vein to the liver and then into the general circulation and to the tissues. Each tissue synthesizes its own form of protein from the amino acids received from the blood.

a., small intestine. The most important absorption of products of digestion occurs in the small intestines, esp. the ileum. Products of digestion absorbed from the gastrointestinal tract pass into either blood or lymph. The mesenteric veins unite to form the portal vein and carry such blood to the liver; the mesenteric lymphatics are called lacteals because during absorption of a fatty meal the lymph they contain looks milky and is called chyle. The lacteals empty into the cisterna chyli and are joined by lymphatics from other parts of the body; the mixed lymph travels, via the thoracic duct, to the subclavian vein, where it empties into the bloodstream.

a., stomach. Absorption of water, alcohol, and some salts through the gastric mucosa.

absorption lines. In spectroscopy, q.v., dark lines of solar spectrum. SYN: *Fraunhofer's lines,* q.v.

absorption spectrum. Spectrum of absorption lines produced when light passes through and is partially absorbed by a substance.

absorptive (ăb-sorp'tĭv). Absorbent.

abstinence (ăb'stĭ-nĕns) [L. *abstinere,* to abstain]. Going without something voluntarily, esp. refraining from indulgence in food, alcoholic beverages, or sexual intercourse.

abstinence syndrome. Partial collapse resulting from withdrawal of alcohol, stimulants, and some opiates. SYN: *withdrawal syndrome.*

abstract (ăb'străkt, ăb-străkt') [L. *abstrahere,* to draw away]. 1. A preparation containing the soluble principles of a drug concentrated and mixed with lactose. 2. A summary or abridgment of an article, book, address, etc.

abstraction (ăb-străk'shŭn). 1. Removal or separation of a constituent from a mixture or compound. 2. Absorption of the mind; inattention or absent-mindedness.

abterminal (ăb-tĕr'mĭ-năl) [L. *ab,* from, + *terminus,* end]. Away from an end and toward the center, said of electric currents in muscles.

abulia (ă-bū'lē-ă) [Gr. *a-,* not, + *boule,* will]. 1. Absence of or inability to exercise will power or initiative. 2. Syndrome of slow reaction, lack of spontaneity, and brief spoken responses. May be part of the clinical picture that accompanies infarction of a cerebellar vessel. SEE: *hypobulia.*

abuse (ă-būs') [L. *abusus,* using up]. Misuse; excessive or improper use.

a., child. Emotional, physical, or sexual injury to a child. May be due to positive action or omission on the part of those responsible for the care of the child.

a., drug. Misuse of drugs, esp. narcotics or psychoactive drugs.

a., spouse. Emotional, physical, or sexual mistreatment of one's spouse.

abuse of the aged. Mental or physical maltreatment or neglect of elderly persons.

abutment (ă-bŭt'mĕnt) [Fr. *abouter,* to place end to end]. The tooth to which a partial denture is anchored.

A.C. *adrenal cortex; air conduction; alternating current; anodal closure; atriocarotid; auriculocarotid; axiocervical.*

Ac. Chem. symb. for actinium.

a.c. L. *ante cibum,* before meals.

acacia (ă-kā'shē-ă). NF. Gum arabic. A dried, gummy exudation from the tree Acacia senegal. Used as a suspending agent or vehicle in pharmaceutical or other industrial products.

acalculia (ă-kăl-kū'lē-ă) [Gr. *a-,* not, + L. *calculare,* to reckon]. Inability to solve mathematical problems.

acampsia (ă-kămp'sē-ă) [" + *kamptein,* to bend]. Inflexibility of a limb; rigidity, ankylosis.

acantha [Gr. *akantha,* thorn]. 1. The spine. 2. A vertebral spinous process.

acanthamebiasis (ă-kăn"thă-mē-bī'ă-sĭs). A very rare disease caused by free-living amebae that ordinarily are found in water, soil, and decaying vegetation. Two genera, Naegleria and Acanthamoeba, have been implicated in causing meningoencephalitis.

Species of Acanthamoeba (A. polyphaga, A. castellani) have been associated with lesions of the eye, skin, and vagina.

acanthesthesia (ă-kăn"thĕs-thē'zē-ă) [" + *aisthesis,* sensation]. A sensation as of a pinprick; a form of paresthesia, q.v.

Acanthia lectularia (ă-kăn'thē-ă lĕk-tū-lā'rē-ă). The bedbug. SYN: *Cimex lectularius.*

acanthiomeatal line. An imaginary line through the acanthion and external meatus.

acanthion [Gr. *akanthion,* little thorn]. Tip of anterior nasal spine.

acantho- [Gr. *akantha,* thorn]. Combining form

meaning thorn, spine.

Acanthocephala (ă-kăn″thō-sĕf′ă-lă) [″ + *kephale,* head]. A class of wormlike entozoa related to the Platyhelminthes, including a few species parasitic in man.

acanthocephaliasis (ă-kăn″thō-sĕf-ă-lī′ă-sĭs). Infestation with Acanthocephala.

Acanthocheilonema perstans (ă-kăn″thō-kī″lō-nē′mă pĕr′stăns). Dipetalonema perstans. A species of filaria that infects wild or domestic animals and occasionally man. In man, the adult worm migrates to the subcutaneous tissue and produces a nodule. The adult worm may, rarely, be seen beneath the conjunctiva.

acanthocyte (ă-kăn′thō-sīt″) [Gr. *akantha,* thorn, + *kytos,* cell]. An abnormal erythrocyte that in wet preparations has protoplasmic projections so that the cell appears to be covered with thorns. SEE: *abetalipoproteinemia.*

acanthocytosis (ă-kăn″thō-sī-tō′sĭs) [″ + ″ + *osis,* condition]. A rare inherited disease characterized by absence of plasma β-lipoproteins. There are failure of normal lipid absorption, marked neuromuscular abnormalities, decreased cholesterol, malnutrition, steatorrhea, mental retardation, and retinal degeneration. About 80% of the red blood cells are acanthocytes. Disease usually begins prior to age one and death may occur at an early age. There is no specific treatment. SYN: *abetalipoproteinemia.*

acanthoid (ă-kăn′thoyd) [″ + *eidos,* form]. Thorny; spiny; of a spinous nature.

acanthokeratodermia (ă-kăn″thō-kĕr″ă-tō-dĕr′mē-ă) [″ + *keras,* horn, + *derma,* skin]. Hypertrophy of the horny portion of the skin of the palms of hands and soles of feet, and thickening of the nails.

acantholysis (ă-kăn-thŏl′ĭ-sĭs) [″ + *lysis,* dissolution]. Any disease of the skin accompanied by degeneration of the cohesive elements of the cells of the outer or horny layer of the skin.

a. bullosa. Obsolete term for epidermolysis bullosa, q.v.

acanthoma (ăk″ăn-thō′mă) [″ + *oma,* tumor]. Benign tumor of the skin. Previously used to denote cancer of skin.

a. adenoides cysticum. A cystic tumor, often familial, occurring on chest, face, and in axillary regions. Tumors contain tissues resembling sweat glands and hair follicles. SYN: *epithelioma adenoides cysticum.*

acanthopelvis, acanthopelyx (ă-kăn″thō-pĕl′vĭs, -pĕl′ĭks) [″ + *pelyx,* pelvis]. A prominent and sharp pubic spine on a rachitic pelvis.

acanthosis (ăk″ăn-thō′sĭs) [″ + *osis,* condition]. Increased thickness of prickle cell layer of skin.

a. nigricans. Rare chronic inflammatory disease of skin in adults sometimes associated with cancer of some internal organ. Characterized by symmetrically distributed hard and soft papillary growths accompanied by hyperpigmentation and hyperkeratosis. SYN: *keratosis nigricans.*

acanthotic (ăk″ăn-thŏt′ĭk). Pert. to acanthosis.

acapnia (ă-kăp′nē-ă) [Gr. *akapnos,* smokeless]. The presence of less than normal amount of carbon dioxide in blood and tissues, e.g., after voluntary overbreathing. SEE: *hyperventilation.*

SYM: Depressed respiration, giddiness, paresthesia, cramps, involuntary contraction of fingers, occasionally convulsions.

acapnial (ă-căp′nē-ăl). Showing or pert. to acapnia.

acarbia (ă-kăr′bē-ă). Diminution of bicarbonate in the blood

acardia (ă-kăr′dē-ă) [Gr. *a-,* not, + *kardia,* heart]. Congenital absence of the heart.

acardiac (ă-kăr′dē-ăk). Having no heart.

acardiacus (ă-kăr-dī′ă-kŭs). A parasitic twin without a heart, therefore utilizing the circulation of its twin. SYN: *acardius.*

acardiotrophia (ă-kăr″dē-ō-trō′fē-a) [″ + ″ + *trophe,* nutrition]. Atrophy of the heart.

acardius. Acardiacus, q.v.

acariasis (ăk″ă-rī′ă-sĭs) [L. *acarus,* mite, + Gr. *-iasis,* condition]. Any disease caused by a mite or acarid. SYN: *acarinosis; acaridiasis.*

a., demodectic. Infection of hair follicles with Demodex folliculorum.

a., psoroptic. Misnomer for psoroptic sarcoptidosis, which affects animals but is rarely seen in man.

a., sarcoptic. Infestation with a burrowing mite, Sarcoptes scabiei, that deposits its eggs in the burrows. SEE: *scabies.*

acaricide (ă-kăr′ĭ-sīd) [″ + *caedere,* to kill]. 1. An agent that destroys acarids. 2. Destroying a member of the order Acarina.

acarid, acaridan (ăk′ă-rĭd, ă-kăr′ĭ-dăn) [L. *acarus,* mite]. A tick or mite; member of the order Acarina.

acaridiasis (ă-kăr″ĭ-dī′ă-sĭs) [″ + Gr. *-iasis,* condition]. Disease caused by a mite. SYN: *acariasis; acarinosis.*

Acarina (ăk″ă-rī′nă). An order of the class Arachnida that includes a large number of species of minute animals known as mites or ticks. Most are ectoparasites, infestation causing local dermatitis with pruritus and sometimes systemic reactions. They also are vectors of a number of diseases. SEE: *Ixodidae; Sarcoptidae; scabies; tick.*

acarinosis (ă-kăr″ĭ-nō′sĭs) [L. *acarus,* mite, + Gr. *osis,* condition]. Disease caused by a mite. SYN: *acariasis; acaridiasis.*

acarodermatitis (ăk″ă-rō-dĕr″mă-tī′tĭs) [″ +

Gr. *derma,* skin, + *itis,* inflammation]. Inflammation of skin caused by a mite.

acaroid (ăk'ă-royd) [" + Gr. *eidos,* resemblance]. Resembling a mite.

acarology (ăk"ă-rŏl'ō-jē) [" + Gr. *logos,* study]. Study of mites and ticks.

acarophobia (ăk"ăr-ō-fō'bē-ă) [" + Gr. *phobos,* fear]. Abnormal fear of mites or worms.

Acarus (ăk'ăr-ŭs) [L., mite]. A genus of mites.

A. folliculorum. Demodex folliculorum, q.v.

A. scabiei. Sarcoptes scabiei. SEE: *Sarcoptidae.*

acarus [L.]. Any mite or tick.

acaryote (ă-kăr'ē-ōt) [Gr. *a-,* not, + *karyon,* nucleus]. Without a nucleus.

acatalasemia (ă"kăt-ă-lă-sē'mē-ă). Acatalasia, q.v.

acatalasia (ă"kăt-ă-lā'zē-ă). A rare inherited disease in which there is an absence of the enzyme catalase. The disease is usually seen in Orientals but may be found in Germans, Swiss, and Israelis. The gingival and oral tissues are particularly susceptible to bacterial invasion with subsequent gangrenous changes and alveolar bone destruction. SYN: *acatalasemia.*

acataleptic (ă-kăt"ă-lĕp'tĭk). 1. Deficient mentally. 2. Uncertain or doubtful.

acatamathesia (ă-kăt"ă-mă-thē'zē-ă) [Gr. *a-,* not, + *katamathesis,* understanding]. 1. Loss of ability to understand spoken words. 2. Inability to comprehend as a result of a brain lesion.

acataphasia (ă-kăt"ă-fā'zē-ă) [" + *kataphasis,* affirmation]. Inability to coherently express thoughts verbally. This condition is due to a cerebral lesion.

acatastasia (ă-kăt-ăs-tā'zē-ă) [Gr. *akatastasis,* disorder]. Irregularity; deviation from normal.

acathexis (ă"kă-thĕks'ĭs) [Gr. *a-,* not, + *kathexis,* retention]. In psychoanalysis, lack of emotion toward a thing or idea that is unconsciously important to the individual.

acathisia (ă"kă-thĭz'ē-ă) [" + *kathisis,* sitting]. Inability to sit down because the thought of doing so causes severe anxiety. Patient has a feeling of restlessness and an urgent need of movement and complains of a feeling of muscular quivering. This symptom may appear as a complication of therapy with antipsychotic tranquilizers such as phenothiazines or reserpine. Also spelled akathisia or akatizia.

acaudal, acaudate (ā-kaw'dăl, -dāt) [" + L. *cauda,* tail]. Having no tail.

ACC. *anodal closure contraction.*

acc. *accommodation.*

acceleration (ăk-sĕl"ĕr-ā'shŭn) [L. *accelerans,* hastening]. 1. Increase in the rapidity of motion or function, as pulse or respiration. 2. Numerical expression of the rate of change in velocity for a given unit of time.

a., angular. Rate of change in velocity per unit of time during circular change in direction.

a., central. A., centripetal, q.v.

a., centripetal. Rate of change in velocity per unit of time while on a circular or curved course.

a., linear. Rate of change in velocity per unit of time while on a straight course.

a., negative. Decrease in the rate of change in velocity per unit of time.

a., positive. Increase in the rate of change in velocity per unit of time.

accelerator (ăk-sĕl'ĕr-ā"tor). Anything that increases action or function. 1. In chemistry, a catalyst. 2. A device that speeds up charged particles to high energy levels to produce X radiation and neutrons.

a., serum prothrombin conversion. ABBR: SPCA. A substance important in blood coagulation; coagulation factor VII. SEE: *coagulation factors.*

accelerator nerves. Sympathetic nerves that contain fibers whose impulses increase rate and force of heartbeat. Postganglionic fibers arise principally in cervical and thoracic ganglia.

accelerator reflexes. Statokinetic reflexes, q.v.

accentuation (ăk-sĕn"chū-ā'shŭn) [L. *accentus,* accent]. Emphasis.

acceptor (ăk-sĕp'tor) [L. *accipere,* to accept]. A compound that unites with a substance freed by another compound, called a donor, q.v.

a., hydrogen. A substance that combines with hydrogen and is reduced when a substrate is oxidized by an enzyme.

a., oxygen. A substance that combines with oxygen and is oxidized when a substrate is reduced by an enzyme.

accessorius (ăk"sĕs-ō'rē-ŭs) [L., supplementary]. Accessory, supplementary, as certain muscles, glands, nerves.

accessory (ăk-sĕs'ō-rē). Auxiliary; assisting. Term applied to a lesser structure that resembles in structure and function a similar organ, as the accessory pancreatic duct (of Santorini) or accessory suprarenal glands. An organ or structure that assists other organs in performing their functions, as accessory reproductive organs.

accessory nerve. Motor nerve made up of a cranial and a spinal part that supplies the trapezius and sternomastoid muscles and pharynx. Accessory portion joins the vagus, to which it supplies its motor and some of its cardioinhibitory fibers. SYN: *eleventh cranial nerve; spinal accessory nerve.*

accessory sign. A nonpathognomonic sign.

accident (ăk′sĭ-dĕnt) [L. *accidens,* happening]. 1. An unexpected event. 2. An unforeseen occurrence of an unfortunate nature; a mishap. 3. An unexpected complicating event in the course of a disease, or following surgery.

a., cerebrovascular. ABBR: CVA. A sudden, unexpected interference in brain function resulting from a vascular disturbance such as cerebral hemorrhage, occlusion of a vessel by a thrombus or embolus, vasospasm, or vasodilation. SYN: *apoplexy; stroke* (def. 4).

a., radiation. Undesired contact or excessive exposure to ionizing radiation.

a., serum. An allergic reaction following the therapeutic introduction of a foreign serum into a hypersensitive individual. SEE: *anaphylaxis.*

accidental (ăk″sĭ-dĕn′tăl). Occurring suddenly, unexpectedly, inadvertently, under unforeseen circumstances.

accident-prone. Said of persons having an unusually high rate of accidents.

accipiter (ăk-sĭp′ĭ-tĕr) [L., a hawk]. A nose bandage with clawlike ends that spread over the face.

ACCl. *anodal closure clonus.*

acclimation, acclimatization (ăk-lĭ-mā′shŭn, ă-klī″mă-tĭ-zā′shŭn) [Fr. *acclimater,* acclimate]. The act of becoming accustomed to a different environment.

acclimatize (ăk-klī′mă-tīz). To become accustomed to a different environment.

accommodation (ă-kŏm″ō-dā′shŭn) [L. *accommodare,* to suit]. ABBR: a.; acc. 1. Adjustment or adaptation. 2. In ophthalmology, the term is applied to a phenomenon noted in receptors in which continued stimulation fails to elicit a sensation or response. 3. The adjustment of the eye for various distances whereby it is able to focus the image of an object on the retina by changing the curvature of the lens. In accommodation for near vision, the ciliary muscle contracts, causing increased rounding of the lens; the pupil contracts and the optic axes converge. These three actions comprise the accommodation reflex. The ability of the eye to accommodate decreases with age. SEE: illus.; *adaptation.*

a., absolute. Accommodation of one eye independent of the other.

a., amplitude of. The difference between refracting power of the eye when accommodating for near and far vision. It is measured in diopters (D) and normally diminishes progressively from childhood to old age. It is approximately 16 D at age 12, 6.5 D at age 30, and 1 D at age 50. SEE: *diopter.*

a., binocular. Accommodation of both eyes jointly.

a., excessive. Greater-than-needed accommodation of the eye.

VISUAL ACCOMMODATION

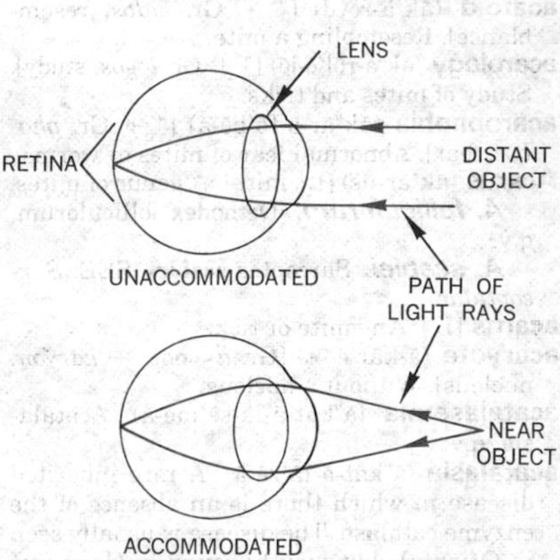

a., histologic. Change in cell form and function due to change in surrounding conditions.

a., mechanism. Method by which curvature of eye lens is changed in order to focus close objects on the retina.

a., negative. Relaxation of ciliary muscle to adjust for distant vision.

a., positive. Contraction of ciliary muscle to adjust for near vision.

a., range of. Distance of vision from its closest to most remote points.

a., relative. The extent to which accommodation is possible for any specific state of convergence of eyes.

a., spasm of. A spasm of the ciliary muscle usually resulting from excessive strain from overuse. Common in myopia.

a., subnormal. Insufficient accommodation.

a., synaptic. Condition in which nerve cells at synapses become less excitable to presynaptic impulses.

accommodation reflex. Contraction of ciliary muscle resulting in rounding of lens, contraction of pupil, and convergence of eyes in accommodation for near vision. SYN: *reflex, near.*

accommodative iridoplegia (ă-kŏm′ō-dā″tĭv ĭr″ĭ-dō-plē′jē-ă). Noncontraction of pupils during accommodation.

accouchement (ă-koosh-mŏn′) [Fr.]. The act of delivery in childbirth; parturition.

a. forcé. Forced delivery, esp. by version, forceps, or other means. Formerly denoted forcible hand delivery.

accoucheur, accoucheuse (ă-koo-shŭr, ă-koo-shĕz′) [Fr.]. An obstetrician or midwife.

accrementition (ăk″rĕ-mĕn-tĭsh′ŭn) [L. *accrescere,* to increase]. Growth of tissues by addition of similar tissue.

accretio (ă-krē′shē-ō) [L.]. Adhesion of parts normally separate from each other.

a. cordis. Condition in which fibrous bands extend from external pericardium to surrounding structures, resulting in angulation and torsion of heart.

accretion (ă-krē′shŭn) [L. *accrescere,* accrue]. 1. Increase by external addition; accumulation. 2. The growing together of parts naturally separate. 3. Accumulation of foreign matter in a cavity.

acculturation. The process in which a member of one culture assumes the values, attitudes, and behavior of a second culture in order to become an accepted member of that culture.

ACD. *absolute cardiac dullness.*

AC/DC. Slang for a bisexual individual.

ACD sol. Citric acid, trisodium citrate, dextrose solution. Anticoagulant used when collecting blood for transfusions.

ACE. *adrenal cortical extract.*

Ace bandage. Trade name for an elastic bandage woven of cotton.

acedia (ă-sē′dē-ă) [Gr. *a-,* not, + *kedos,* care]. Mental state of indifference, insensibility, lack of emotion. SYN: *apathy.*

acenesthesia (ă-sĕn″ĕs-thē′zē-ă) [″ + *koinos,* common, + *aisthesis,* sensation]. Absence of a feeling of well-being, present in such disorders as hypochondriasis and neurasthenia.

acentric (ă-sĕn′trĭk) [″ + L. *centrum,* center]. Not central; peripheral.

A.C.E.P. *American College of Emergency Physicians.*

acephalia, acephalism (ă-sĕ-fā′lē-ă, ă-sĕf′ă-lĭzm) [″ + *kephale,* head]. A developmental disorder in which the head is absent.

acephalo- (ă-sĕf′ă-lō-) [Gr. *a-,* not, + *kephale,* head]. Combining form meaning without a head.

acephalobrachia (ă-sĕf″ă-lō-brā′kē-ă) [″ + ″ + *brachion,* arm]. A developmental anomaly in which head and arms are absent.

acephalocardia (ă-sĕf″ă-lō-kăr′dē-ă) [″ + ″ + *kardia,* heart]. Congenital absence of the head and heart.

acephalochiria (ă-sĕf″ă-lō-kī′rē-ă) [″ + ″ + *cheir,* hand]. Congenital absence of the head and hands.

acephalocyst (ă-sĕf′ă-lō-sĭst) [″ + ″ + *kystis,* bag]. A sterile hydatid cyst.

acephalogastria (ă-sĕf″ă-lō-găs′trē-ă) [″ + ″ + *gaster,* stomach]. Congenital absence of the head, chest, and upper abdomen.

acephalopodia (ă-sĕf″ă-lō-pō′dē-ă) [″ + ″ + *pous,* foot]. Congenital absence of the head and feet.

acephalorhachia (ă-sĕf″ă-lō-rā′kē-ă) [″ + ″ + *rhachis,* spine]. Congenital absence of the head and vertebral column.

acephalostomia (ă-sĕf″ă-lō-stō′mē-ă) [″ + ″ + *stoma,* mouth]. Congenital absence of the head; however, an opening resembling a mouth is present on the superior portion of the body.

acephalothoracia (ă-sĕf″ă-lō-thō-rā′sē-ă) [″ + ″ + *thorax,* chest]. Congenital absence of the head and chest.

acephalus (ă-sĕf′ă-lŭs). A fetus lacking a head.

acerate (ăs′ĕr-āt) [L. *acer*]. Sharp, pointed.

acerbity (ă-sĕrb′ĭ-tē) [L. *acerbus,* sharp]. Astringency combined with acidity.

acervuline (ă-sĕr′vū-lĭn) [L. *acervulus,* a little heap]. Aggregated, occurring in clusters.

acervuloma (ă-sĕr″vū-lō′mă) [″ + *oma,* tumor]. Intracranial tumor containing psammoma bodies.

acervulus (ă-sĕr′vū-lŭs) [L.]. Sandy, gritty, sabulous.

a. cerebri. Gritty matter filling the follicle of the pineal gland. SYN: *brain sand.*

acescence (ă-sĕs′ĕns) [L. *acescere,* to become sour]. 1. Slight acidity. 2. Process of souring.

acescent (ă-sĕs′ĕnt). Slightly acid.

acesodyne (ă-sĕs′ō-dīn) [Gr. *akesis,* cure, + *odyne,* pain]. An agent for relieving pain. SYN: *anodyne.*

acestoma (ă-sĕs-tō′mă) [″ + *oma,* tumor]. The fresh granulations that later form a cicatrix.

aceta (ă-sē′tă). Pl. of acetum.

acetabular (ăs″ĕ-tăb′ū-lăr). Pert. to the acetabulum.

acetabulectomy (ăs″ĕ-tăb″ū-lĕk′tō-mē) [L. *acetabulum,* a little saucer for vinegar, + Gr. *ektome,* excision]. Surgical removal of the acetabulum.

acetabuloplasty (ăs″ĕ-tăb′ū-lō-plăs″tē) [″ + Gr. *plassein,* to form]. Surgical repair and reconstruction of the acetabulum.

acetabulum (ăs″ĕ-tăb′ū-lŭm) [L., a little saucer for vinegar]. 1. The rounded (cotyloid) cavity on the external surface of the innominate bone (os coxae or os innominatum) that receives head of femur. 2. The ventral sucker of the fluke.

acetal (ăs′ĕ-tăl). Chemical combination of an aldehyde with an alcohol.

acetaldehyde (ăs″ĕt-ăl′dĕ-hīd″). CH_3CHO, intermediate in yeast fermentation and metabolism of alcohol. SYN: *acetic aldehyde.*

acetamide (ăs″ĕt-ăm′ĭd). Acetic acid amide, CH_3CONH_2, used in industry for synthesis of chemicals, and as a solvent.

acetaminophen (ă-sĕt″ă-mĭn′ō-fĕn). USP. A synthetic drug with antipyretic and analgesic actions similar to aspirin, used in patients with sensitivity to aspirin. It does not have the anti-inflammatory or antirheumatic actions of aspirin. Trade names for acetaminophen include Tylenol and Datril.

CAUTION: Acute overdose may cause fatal hepatic necrosis.

acetaminophen poisoning. Acute overdose of acetaminophen can cause fatal hepatic necrosis.

TREATMENT: Vigorous procedure to prevent continued absorption of the drug by inducing vomiting or use of gastric lavage. This is followed by oral administration of activated charcoal. Hemodialysis if initiated in the first 12 hours is indicated. N-acetylcysteine is also indicated in treating this condition.

acetanilid (ăs″ĕ-tăn′ĭ-lĭd). A white powder or crystalline substance obtained by interaction of glacial acetic acid and aniline.

ACTION AND USES: Analgesic, antipyretic, and anti-inflammatory. Acute or chronic poisoning may develop due to prolonged administration or drug idiosyncrasy. Because of its toxicity, it is rarely used.

acetanilid poisoning. Symptoms are cyanosis due to formation of methemoglobin, cold sweat, irregular pulse, dyspnea, and unconsciousness. Sudden cardiac failure may occur.

F.A.: In acute poisoning, analeptics such as caffeine, external heat, inhalation of oxygen, gastric lavage or emetics, artificial respiration, blood transfusion. If cyanosis is severe, give methylene blue 1 to 2 mg. per kg. body weight I.V. In chronic poisoning, stop use of drug; iron preparations for secondary anemia. SEE: *Poisons and Poisoning* in *Appendix*.

acetarsol, acetarsone (ăs″ĕ-tăr′sŏl, -sōn). An arsenic compound, acetylaminohydroxyphenylarsonic acid. Contains 27% arsenic. Used in amebiasis and Trichomonas vaginalis infections.

acetate (ăs′ĕ-tāt). A salt of acetic acid.

acetazolamide (ăs″ĕt-ă-zŏl′ă-mīd). USP. A drug that inhibits the enzyme carbonic anhydrase. At one time it was used as a diuretic but more effective drugs are now available. It has been used in treating epilepsy and to reduce intraocular pressure in managing glaucoma. Trade name is Diamox.

acetic (ă-sē′tĭk) [L. *acetum*, vinegar]. Pert. to vinegar; sour.

acetic acid. CH_3COOH. NF. An aqueous solution containing not less than 36% or more than 37% by weight of CH_3COOH. Used as a reagent, a caustic; sometimes taken internally.

Vinegar contains 4 to 6% of this acid. SYN: *acid, ethanoic.*

a.a., glacial. USP. A solution containing not less than 99.5% by weight of acetic acid.

acetic aldehyde. Acetaldehyde, q.v.

acetify (ă-sĕt′ĭ-fī) [″ + *fieri*, to become]. To produce acetic fermentation or vinegar.

acetimeter (ă-sĕ-tĭm′ĕ-tĕr) [″ + Gr. *metron*, measure]. An apparatus that determines the amount of acetic acid in fluid.

acetoacetic acid (ăs″ĕ-tō-ă-sē′tĭk). A ketone body formed when fats are incompletely oxidized, as in diabetes. May appear in the urine in starvation or inadequately treated diabetes mellitus. SYN: *diacetic acid.*

Acetobacter (ă-sē″tō-băk′tĕr) [L. *acetum*, vinegar, + Gr. *bakterion*, little rod]. A genus of nonpathogenic bacteria of the family Pseudomonadaceae.

A. aceti. Species of Acetobacter that transforms wine or cider into vinegar. This produces a stringy substance in the liquid called mother of vinegar.

acetolase (ă-sĕt′ō-lās). An enzyme that catalyzes conversion of alcohol into acetic acid.

acetohexamide (ăs″ĕ-tō-hĕks′ă-mīd). USP. An orally administered hypoglycemic agent.

CAUTION: This drug should be used only in patients with diabetes of the insulin-independent type who cannot be treated with diet alone and who are unwilling or unable to take insulin if weight reduction and dietary control fail.

acetoin (ă-sĕt′ō-ĭn). The substance formed when glucose is fermented by Enterobacter aerogenes. After being oxidized to diacetyl, it provides the characteristic odor of butter.

acetone (ăs′ĕ-tōn). $(CH_3)_2CO$. USP. Dimethyl ketone, a colorless, volatile, inflammable liquid, miscible with water, useful as a solvent, and having a characteristic sweet, fruity, ethereal odor. Found in the blood and urine in diabetes, other metabolic disorders, and after lengthy fasting, produced when the fats are not properly oxidized, due to inability to oxidize glucose in the blood. SEE: *acetoacetic acid; acidosis; ketone; ketonuria; ketosis; test, acetone.*

a. in urine, test for. 1. Wet specially treated paper or stick with urine. If acetone is present, the paper will turn a certain color. These test papers or sticks are commercially available. 2. Take 5 ml. of urine; add a few crystals of ammonium sulfate and dissolve; add a small crystal of sodium nitroprusside, and shake a little. Cover with a layer (about 2 ml.) of strong ammonia. The presence of acetone is indicated by the formation of a purple ring between the layers of liquid. 3. A commercially available tablet is also used for this test.

acetone bodies. Certain substances related to acetone. An example is acetoacetic acid, q.v. SYN: *ketone bodies*, q.v.

acetonemia (ăs″ĕ-tō-nē′mē-ă) [*acetone* + Gr. *haima*, blood]. Large amounts of acetone in blood.

SYM: Abnormal excitement, gradual depression, acidosis.

acetonitrile (ăs″ĕ-tō-nī′trĭl). CH_3CN. Methyl cyanide, a substance found in an increased amount in the urine of persons who smoke three or more cigarettes a day.

acetonuria (ăs″ĕ-tō-nū′rē-ă) [*acetone* + Gr. *ouron*, urine]. The presence of acetone and diacetic bodies in the urine, as in the ketosis of diabetes, starvation, etc., due to incomplete oxidation of fats. Preferred term is *ketonuria*. SEE: *acetone; acidosis; test, acetone*.

acetophenazine maleate (ăs″ĕ-tō-fĕn′ă-zēn măl′ē-āt). USP. An antipsychotic drug of the phenothiazine group. The trade name is Tindal.

acetophenetidin (ăs″ĕ-tō-fĕ-nĕt′ĭ-dĭn). An odorless, white, crystalline substance derived from coal tar. An antipyretic and analgesic. Combined with aspirin and caffeine in some common headache tablets. Excessive use can be toxic and may cause hemolysis of red blood cells. Prolonged use causes serious damage to the kidneys. SYN: *phenacetin*. SEE: *Poisons and Poisoning* in *Appendix*.

acetosoluble (ăs″ĕ-tō-sŏl′ū-bl). Soluble in acetic acid.

acetous (ăs′ĕ-tŭs) [L. *acetum*, vinegar]. 1. Pert. to vinegar. 2. Sour in taste.

acetum (ă-sē′tŭm) [L.]. (pl. *aceta*) 1. Vinegar. 2. A drug dissolved in a weak vinegar solution.

acetyl (ăs′ĕ-tĭl, ă-sēt′ĭl) [″ + Gr. *hyle*, matter]. CH_3CO, the univalent radical.

a. CoA. Acetylcoenzyme A, q.v.

acetylation (ă-sĕt″ĭ-lā′shŭn). The introduction of one or more acetyl groups into an organic compound.

acetylbetamethylcholine (ăs″ĕ-tĭl-bā″tă-mĕth″ĭl-kō′lĭn). A derivative of acetylcholine that is a strong stimulus to the parasympathetic nervous system.

ACTION: Lowers blood pressure, causes vasodilation, stimulates peristalsis, and increases sweating. Used in tachycardia.

acetylcholine (ăs″ĕ-tĭl-kō′lēn). ABBR: ACh. An ester of choline occurring in various organs and tissues of the body. It is thought to play an important role in the transmission of nerve impulses at synapses and myoneural junctions. It is quickly destroyed by an enzyme, cholinesterase. Either excessive or deficient action of acetylcholine at the motor endplates may result in neuromuscular block. SEE: *cholinergic fibers*.

a. chloride. A salt of acetylcholine injected intramuscularly or subcutaneously as a parasympathetic stimulant. It lowers blood pressure by dilating peripheral vessels, and it relaxes smooth muscle spasms. Trade name is Miochol.

acetylcholinesterase (ăs″ĕ-tĭl-kō″lĭn-ĕs′tĕr-ās). ABBR: AChE. Enzyme that stops the action of acetylcholine. It is present in various body tissues including muscles, nerve cells, and red blood cells.

acetylcoenzyme A. A condensation product of coenzyme A, q.v., and acetic acid.

acetylcysteine (ăs″ĕ-tĭl-sĭs′tē-ĭn). USP. Chemical substance that, when it is nebulized and inhaled, liquefies mucus and pus. It is also used experimentally in the treatment of poisoning due to acetaminophen. Trade name is Mucomyst. SEE: *acetaminophen poisoning*.

acetyldigitoxin (ăs″ĕ-tĭl-dĭj″ĭ-tŏk′sĭn). A derivative of digitalis for oral use only. Trade name is Acylanid.

acetylene (ă-sĕt′ĭ-lēn). C_2H_2. A colorless explosive gas with a garlic-like odor.

acetylsalicylic acid (ă-sē″tĭl-săl″ĭ-sĭl′ĭk). ABBR: ASA. Previously used name for aspirin, USP, q.v.

acetylsalicylic acid poisoning. SEE: *aspirin poisoning*.

acetyltransferase (ăs″ĕ-tĭl-trăns′fĕr-ās). Enzyme that is effective in the transfer of an acetyl group from one compound to another.

AcG. *accelerator globulin*, coagulation factor V. SEE: *coagulation factors*.

ACH. *adrenal cortical hormone*.

ACh. *acetylcholine*.

achalasia (ăk″ă-lā′zē-ă) [Gr. *a-*, not, + *chalasis*, relaxation]. Failure to relax; said of muscles, such as sphincters, the normal function of which is a persistent contraction with periods of relaxation.

a. of the cardia. Failure of relaxation of the cardiac sphincter, resulting in difficulty in passage of foods to the stomach. In advanced cases, dysphagia is marked and dilatation of the esophagus may occur. SYN: *cardiospasm*.

a., pelvirectal. Congenital absence of ganglion cells in distal large bowel, resulting in failure of colon to relax.

a., sphincteral. Failure of intestinal sphincters to relax.

AChE. *acetylcholinesterase*.

ache (āk) [AS. *acan*]. 1. A continued pain as distinguished from a sudden or spasmodic pain. May be dull or severe. 2. To suffer continued pain.

acheilia (ă-kī′lē-ă) [Gr. *a-*, not, + *cheilos*, lip]. Congenital absence of one or both lips.

acheiria (ă-kī′rē-ă) [″ + *cheir*, hand]. 1. Congenital absence of one or both hands. 2. Loss of sensation in, with accompanying sense of loss of, one or both hands. May result from temporary or permanent injury or malfunction of sensory mechanism, or may occur in hysteria. 3. Inability to determine to which side of the body a stimulus has been applied. SYN: *achiria*.

acheiropodia (ă-kī″rō-pō′dē-ă) [″ + ″ + *pous*,

foot]. Congenital absence of hands and feet.

achievement age. The age of a person with regard to level of acquired learning, determined by a proficiency test and expressed in terms of the chronological age of the average person showing the same level of attainment. SEE: *age.*

Achilles jerk (ă-kĭl'ēz). [Achilles, hero of the *Iliad,* whose vulnerable spot was his heel because it was from this part that he was suspended when immersed in the river Styx] Achilles tendon reflex, q.v.

Achilles tendon. The tendon of the gastrocnemius and soleus muscles of the leg. SYN: *tendo calcaneus.*

Achilles tendon reflex. Plantar flexion extension of foot resulting from contraction of calf muscles following a sharp blow to the Achilles tendon. The variations and their significance correspond closely to those of the knee jerk. It is exaggerated in upper motor neuron disease and diminished or absent in lower motor neuron disease. The character of the response is influenced by the metabolic rate. Thus attempts have been made to use this reflex as an index of thyroid function. The value of such use is questionable.

achillobursitis (ă-kĭl"ō-bŭr-sī'tĭs) [*Achilles* + L. *bursa,* a pouch, + Gr. *itis,* inflammation]. Inflammation of the bursa lying over the Achilles tendon. SYN: *Albert's disease.*

achillodynia (ă-kĭl"ō-dĭn'ē-ă) [" + Gr. *odyne,* pain]. Pain caused by inflammation between the Achilles tendon and bursa.

achillorrhaphy (ă-kĭl-or'ă-fē) [" + Gr. *rhaphe,* sewing]. Suture of Achilles tendon.

achillotenotomy (ă-kĭl"ō-tĕn-ŏt'ō-mē) [" + Gr. *tenon,* tendon, + *tome,* incision]. Achillotomy, q.v.

achillotomy (ă-kĭl-ŏt'ō-mē) [" + *tome,* incision]. Division of the Achilles tendon. SYN: *achillotenotomy.*

achiria (ă-kī'rē-ă) [Gr. *a-,* not, + *cheir,* hand]. Acheiria, q.v.

achlorhydria (ă"klor-hī'drē-ă) [" + *chloros,* green, + *hydor,* water]. Absence of free hydrochloric acid in the stomach.

ETIOL: May be due to gastric carcinoma, gastric ulcer, pernicious anemia, adrenal insufficiency, chronic gastritis. SEE: *achylia.*

a., histamine-proved. Absence of free acid in gastric secretion even after subcutaneous injection of histamine hydrochloride.

achloride (ă-klō'rīd). A salt other than a chloride; nonchloride.

achloropsia (ă-klō-rŏp'sē-ă) [" + *chloros,* green, + *opsis,* vision]. Color blindness in which green cannot be distinguished. SEE: *deuteranopsia.*

acholia (ă-kō'lē-ă) [" + *chole,* bile]. An absence or decrease of bile or a condition that prevents bile from entering the duodenum.

a., pigmentary. Bile deficiency indicated by clay-colored feces in the absence of jaundice.

acholic (ă-kō'lĭk). Pert. to acholia.

acholuria (ă-kō-lū'rē-ă) [" + *chole,* bile, + *ouron,* urine]. Absence of bile pigments in urine in some forms of jaundice.

achondrogenesis (ă-kŏn"drō-jĕn'ĕ-sĭs) [Gr. *a-,* not, + *chondros,* cartilage, + *genesis,* origin]. Failure of growth of bone, esp. the bones of the extremities.

achondroplasia (ă-kŏn"drō-plā'sē-ă) [" + " + *plasis,* a molding]. Defect in the formation of cartilage at the epiphyses of long bones, producing a form of dwarfism; sometimes seen in rickets. SYN: *chondrodystrophy.*

achroma (ă-krō'mă) [" + *chroma,* color]. An absence of color or normal pigmentation as in leukoderma, albinism, vitiligo. Hereditary, circumscribed skin areas deficient in pigmentation.

achromasia (ăk"rō-mā'zē-ă) [Gr. *achromatos,* without color]. 1. Absence of normal pigmentation of the skin as in albinism, vitiligo, leukoderma. 2. Pallor. 3. The lack of the ability to be stained, said of cells or tissues.

achromate (ă-krō'māt) [Gr. *a-,* not, + *chroma,* color]. A person who is color blind.

achromatic (ăk"rō-măt'ĭk) [Gr. *achromatos,* without color]. 1. Lacking in color. 2. Not dispersing light into its constituent components. 3. Not containing or composed of chromatin. 4. Difficult to stain, with reference to cells and tissues.

achromatic lens. One that transmits light without separating the spectral colors.

achromatin (ă-krō'mă-tĭn). The weakly staining substance of a cell nucleus.

achromatism (ă-krō'mă-tĭzm") [Gr. *a-,* not, + *chroma,* color, + *-ismos,* condition]. Colorlessness.

achromatocyte (ăk"rō-măt'ō-sīt) [Gr. *achromatos,* without color, + *kytos,* cell]. A decolorized red blood cell. SYN: *achromocyte; ghost corpuscle.*

achromatolysis (ă-krō"mă-tŏl'ĭ-sĭs) [" + *lysis,* loosening]. Dissolution of cell achromatin.

achromatophil (ă"krō-măt'ō-fĭl) [" + *philos,* love]. A cell or tissue not stainable in the usual manner.

achromatopsia (ă-krō"mă-tŏp'sē-ă) [" + *opsis,* vision]. Complete color blindness.

achromatosis (ă-krō"mă-tō'sĭs) [" + *osis,* condition]. Condition of being without natural pigmentation. SEE: *achroma.*

achromatous (ă-krō'mă-tŭs). Without color.

achromaturia (ă-krō"mă-tū'rē-ă) [" + *ouron,* urine]. Colorless or nearly colorless urine.

achromia (ă-krō'mē-ă) [Gr. *a-,* not, + *chroma,* color]. 1. Absence of color; pallor. 2. Achromatosis, q.v. 3. Condition in which erythrocytes have large central pale areas; hypochromia.

a., congenital. Albinism, q.v.

achromic (ă-krō′mĭk). Lacking color.

achromophil (ă-krō′mō-fĭl) [″ + ″ + *philos,* love]. Achromatophil, q.v.

achromocyte (ă-krō′mō-sīt) [″ + ″ + *kytos,* cell]. In a blood smear, large, pale, crescent-shaped cells produced from fragile red cells as the bloodfilm preparation is being made. SYN: *crescent bodies; selenoid cells.*

achromotrichia (ă-krō″mō-trĭk′ē-ă) [″ + ″+ *trichia,* condition of the hair]. Lack of color or graying of the hair. SYN: *canities.*

a., nutritional. Grayness of hair due to dietary deficiency.

Achromycin (ăk″rō-mī′sĭn). Trade name for tetracycline, an antibiotic effective in treatment of many bacterial infections.

achroodextrin (ăk″rō-ō-dĕks′trĭn) [Gr. *achroos,* colorless, + *dextrin*]. One of the varieties of dextrin resulting from hydrolysis of starch.

achylia (ă-kī′lē-ă) [Gr. *a-,* not, + *chylos,* chyle]. Absence of chyle or other digestive ferments.

a. gastrica. Complete absence or marked diminution in amount of gastric juice. SEE: *achlorhydria.*

a. pancreatica. Absence or deficiency of pancreatic secretion. Usually a manifestation of chronic pancreatitis.

achylosis (ă″kī-lō′sĭs). Achylia, q.v.

achylous (ă-kī′lŭs) [Gr. *achylos,* without chyle]. 1. Lacking in any kind of digestive secretion. 2. Without chyle.

achymia, achymosis (ă-kī′mē-ă, ăk-ĭ-mō′sĭs) [Gr. *a-,* not, + *chymos,* juice]. Deficiency or absence of chyme.

acicular (ă-sĭk′ū-lăr) [L. *aciculus,* little needle]. Needle-shaped.

acid [L. *acidum,* acid]. 1. Any substance that liberates hydrogen ions (protons) in solution; a hydrogen ion donor. An acid reacts with a metal to form a salt, neutralizes bases, and turns litmus paper red. SEE: *alkali; base; indicator; pH.* 2. A sour substance. 3. The "street" or slang term for LSD, q.v.

a., acetic. CH_3COOH. Substance that gives sour taste to vinegar. Also used as a reagent, and as a caustic; sometimes taken internally. SYN: *a., ethanoic.*

a., acetic, dilute. Solution containing 6% pure acetic acid by weight.

a., acetic, glacial. USP. Solution containing not less than 99.5% of acetic acid by weight.

a., acetoacetic. CH_3COCH_2COOH. A ketone body formed when fats are incompletely oxidized. Appears in urine in abnormal amounts in starvation or inadequately treated diabetes. SYN: *a., acetylacetic; diacetic acid.*

a., acetylacetic. A., acetoacetic.

a., acetylsalicylic. ABBR: ASA. The previously used name for aspirin, USP, q.v.

a., adenylic. A nucleotide formed by condensation of adenosine and phosphoric acid. It is one of the hydrolytic products of nucleic acids and is present in muscle, blood corpuscles, yeast, and other nuclear material. SYN: *adenosine monophosphate.*

a., alginic. An organic acid obtained from species of algae. It is used as a pharmaceutic aid.

a., amino. An organic acid containing one or more NH_2 (amino) groups and a COOH (carboxyl) group. They are the basic building blocks for all of the body's protein elements, and are the end-products of protein digestion or hydrolysis. Certain of these acids are essential in the human body for growth and repair of tissues. Oral preparations of essential amino acids may be used as dietary supplements. SEE: *amino acid.*

a., aminoacetic. NH_2CH_2COOH. A nonessential amino acid, q.v. SYN: *glycine.*

a., aminobenzoic. A., para-aminobenzoic, q.v.

a., aminocaproic. USP. A hemostatic drug. It is a specific antidote for an overdose of a fibrinolytic agent. Trade name is Amicar.

a., aminoglutaric. A. glutamic, q.v.

a., aminosalicylic. A., para-aminosalicylic, q.v.

a., aminosuccinic. A., aspartic, q.v.

a., arsonic. An organic acid that contains the $AsO(OH)_2$ group.

a., arylarsonic. Arsonic acid combined with an aryl radical.

a., ascorbic. USP. $C_6H_8O_6$. A vitamin that occurs naturally in fresh fruits, esp. citrus fruits, and in fresh vegetables. Essential in maintenance of collagen formation, osteoid tissue of bones, and formation and maintenance of dentin. This essential vitamin is used as a dietary supplement and in the prevention and treatment of scurvy. Scurvy develops after approx. 3 months of deficiency of ascorbic acid in the diet. The usefulness of large daily doses (1 to 5 gm. a day) of this vitamin in preventing or treating the common cold in otherwise healthy persons has not been established although it may decrease the severity of symptoms. Continuous treatment with large doses may cause kidney stones to form. SYN: *vitamin C; vitamin, antiscorbutic.*

a., aspartic. $COOHCHNH_2CH_2COOH$. A nonessential amino acid, q.v.; one of the products of pancreatic digestion. SYN: *a., aminosuccinic.*

a., barbituric. $C_4H_4O_3H_2$. A crystalline compound from which phenobarbital and other barbiturates are derived. SYN: *malonylurea.*

a., benzoic. USP. $C_7H_6O_2$. A white crystalline material having a slight odor. Used in keratolytic ointments, and as a food preservative. Saccharin is a derivative of this acid.

a., bile. Any one of the complex acids that occur as salts in bile, e.g., cholic, glycocholic, and taurocholic acids. They give bile its foamy character, are important in the digestion of fats in the intestine, and are reabsorbed from the intestine to be used again by the liver.

a., boric. H_3BO_3. A white crystalline substance that forms in water a very weak acid solution poisonous to plants and animals. Soluble in water, alcohol, or glycerin.

CAUTION: Because of its toxicity, the use of boric acid should be quite limited. It is particularly dangerous because it can be accidentally swallowed by children or used in food because of its physical resemblance to sugar. SEE: *boric acid.*

a., butyric. C_3H_7COOH. An acid having a rancid odor; found in rancid butter, in cheese, perspiration, and cod liver oil.

a., carbolic. Phenol, q.v.

a., carbonic. H_2CO_3. An acid formed from carbon dioxide being dissolved in water.

a., carboxylic. Any acid containing the group COOH. The simplest examples are formic and acetic.

a., chaulmoogric. A cyclic unsaturated fatty acid in chaulmoogra oil, formerly used in treatment of leprosy (Hansen's disease).

a., cholic. An acid formed in the liver by hydrolysis of other bile acids. Important in digestion.

a., chromic. CrO_3. An escharotic sometimes used to remove warts.

a., citric. $C_6H_8O_7$. An acid prepared synthetically or from lemon or lime juice in form of colorless crystals or white crystalline powder. Soluble in water, ether, or alcohol. Used as a preventive of scurvy. Hydrous form is used as a flavoring agent or vehicle.

a., deoxyribonucleic. ABBR: DNA. Deoxyribonucleic acid, q.v.

a., desoxyribonucleic. Former spelling of deoxyribonucleic acid, q.v.

a., diacetic. A., acetoacetic, q.v.

a., 2-3-dihydroxypropanoic. A., glyceric, q.v.

a., ethanedioic. A., oxalic, q.v.

a., ethanoic. A., acetic, q.v.

a., ethylenediaminetetra-acetic. A chelating agent that, in the form of its calcium or sodium salts, is useful in removing certain substances such as lead and digitalis from the body. ABBR: EDTA. SEE: *chelation.*

a., fatty. A carboxylic acid that can be combined with glycerol to form fats; the simplest members of the series are formic and acetic; most typical are stearic and palmitic. A saturated fatty acid has single bonds in its carbon chain, with the general formula $C_nH_{2n}O_2$. An unsaturated fatty acid has one or more double or triple bonds in its carbon chain. In human nutrition, it is felt that by decreasing the intake of saturated fatty acids, cholesterol content of the blood will be decreased.

a., folic. USP. $C_{19}H_{19}N_7O_6$. A member of the vitamin B complex. Found naturally in green plant tissue, liver, and yeast. When produced synthetically, it is identical with pteroylglutamic acid.

CAUTION: Folic acid should not be used in the treatment of pernicious anemia because it does not protect patients against the development of changes in the central nervous system that accompany this type of anemia.

a., formic. HCOOH. The first member of the monobasic fatty acid series. It is a much stronger acid than the others in the series. It occurs naturally in certain animal secretions and in muscle, but it may also be prepared synthetically. It is one of the irritants present in the sting of insects such as bees and ants. SYN: *a., methanoic.*

a., formiminoglutamic. $C_6N_2O_4H_{10}$. An intermediate product in the metabolism of histidine. Its increase in the urine after administration of histidine in patients with folic acid deficiency is the basis for the FIGLU excretion test.

a., gallic. $C_6H_2(OH)_3COOH$. A colorless crystalline acid. It occurs naturally as an excrescence on the twigs of trees, esp. oak trees, as a reaction to the deposition of gall wasp eggs. It is used as a skin astringent and in the manufacture of writing inks and dyes. SYN: *a., 3,4,5-trihydroxybenzoic.*

a., glucuronic. $CHO(CHOH)_4COOH$. An oxidation product of glucose that is present in the urine. Toxic products (such as salicylic acid, menthol, and phenol) that have entered the body through the intestinal system are detoxified in the liver by conjugation with glucuronic acid. SYN: *a., glycuronic.*

a., glutamic. $COOH(CH_2)_2CH(NH_2)$-COOH. A nonessential amino acid formed during protein metabolism. SYN: *a., aminoglutaric.*

a., glyceric. $CH_2OHCHOHCOOH$. An intermediate product of oxidation of fats. SYN: *a., 2,3-dihydroxypropanoic.*

a., glycocholic. $C_{24}H_{39}O_4NHCH_2$-COOH. A bile acid yielding glycine and cholic acid on hydrolysis.

a., glycuronic. A., glucuronic, q.v.

a., hexadecanoic. A., palmitic, q.v.

a., homogentisic. An intermediate product of tyrosine catabolism; found in the urine in alkaptonuria. SYN: *alkapton.*

a., hydriodic. HI. In solution, it is used in various forms of chemical analyses. SYN:

hydrogen iodide.

a., hydrochloric. HCl. An inorganic acid. Normally present in the gastric juice. It destroys fermenting bacteria that might cause intestinal tract disturbances. Five to 10 ml. of a 10% solution of hydrochloric acid in 125 to 250 ml. of water is used in treating hypoacidity or achlorhydria.

CAUTION: When so used, it must be diluted accurately and sipped through a drinking straw. This will prevent the acid from damaging the teeth. SYN: *muriatic acid.*

a., hydrocyanic. HCN. A colorless, extremely poisonous, highly volatile liquid. Occurs naturally in plants. It is obtained synthetically by several methods. Has many industrial uses: electroplating, fumigation, and production of dyes, pigments, synthetic fibers, and plastic. Exposure of man to 200 to 500 parts of acid per 1,000,000 parts of air for 30 minutes is fatal. It acts by preventing cellular respiration. SYN: *hydrogen cyanide; prussic acid.* SEE: *cyanide* in *Poisons and Poisoning* in *Appendix.*

a., hydrosuccinic. A., malic, q.v.

a., hydroxy. An acid containing one or more hydroxyl (OH) groups in addition to the carboxyl (COOH) group.

a., hydroxytoluic. A., mandelic, q.v.

a., imino. An acid formed as a result of oxidation of amino acids in the body.

a., inorganic. An acid containing no carbon atoms. SYN: *mineral acid.*

a., lactic. USP. A mixture of lactic acid, $C_3H_6O_3$, and lactic acid lactate, $C_6H_{10}O_5$, equivalent to a total of not less than 85% and not more than 90%, by weight, of $C_3H_6O_3$. Occurs in sour milk from fermentation of lactose and is formed in muscles during the metabolic changes that occur during strenuous exercise. Lactic acid milk (buttermilk or acidophilus milk) is administered to help prevent growth of putrefactive bacteria in the large intestine. SYN: *2-hydroxypropionic acid.*

a., linoleic. $C_{18}H_{32}O_2$. An unsaturated fatty acid, a dietary essential. First isolated from linseed oil but also found in corn oil. SYN: *a., linolic.*

a., linolenic. $C_{18}H_{30}O_2$. An unsaturated fatty acid, a dietary essential.

a., linolic. A., linoleic, q.v.

a., lysergic. $C_{16}H_{16}N_2O_2$. A crystalline substance, derived from ergot. Its derivative, lysergic acid diethylamide, LSD, is a potent hallucinogen. SEE: *LSD.*

a., malic. $C_4H_6O_5$. Substance found in certain sour fruits such as apples and apricots. Active in aerobic metabolism of carbohydrate. SYN: *a., hydrosuccinic.*

a., malonic. $C_3H_4O_4$. A dibasic acid formed by oxidation of malic acid. Occurs in beets. Active in the tricarboxylic acid cycle in carbohydrate metabolism. Its inhibition of succinic dehydrogenase is the classic example of competitive inhibition.

a., mandelic. $C_8H_8O_3$. A colorless hydroxy acid, q.v. Its salt is used in urinary tract infections. SYN: *a., hydroxytoluic.*

a., methanoic. A., formic, q.v.

a., mineral. A., inorganic, q.v.

a., muriatic. A., hydrochloric, q.v.

a., nicotinic. $C_6H_5NO_2$. A member of the vitamin B complex. Occurs naturally in liver, yeast, milk, cheese, and cereals. Used for prevention and treatment of pellagra. SYN: *niacin.*

a., nitric. HNO_3. A strong corrosive acid prepared from sulfuric acid and a nitrate. It is used in manufacture of explosives and dyes and as a coagulant in testing urine for albumin (Heller's test).

a., nucleic. Any one of a group of high–molecular weight substances found in the cells of all living things. They have a complex chemical structure formed of sugars (pentoses), phosphoric acid, and nitrogen bases (purines and pyrimidines). Most important are ribonucleic acid, q.v., and deoxyribonucleic acid, q.v.

a., 9-octadecenoic. A., oleic, q.v.

a., oleic. $C_{18}H_{34}O_2$. An unsaturated fatty acid found in most organic fats and oils. SYN: *a., 9-octadecenoic.*

a., organic. An acid containing the carboxyl radical COOH.

a., oxalic. $H_2C_2O_4$. The simplest dibasic organic acid. Its potassium or calcium salt occurs naturally in rhubarb, wood sorrel, and many other plants. It is the strongest organic acid and is poisonous. When properly diluted, it is effective in removing ink or rust stains from cloth. It is used also as a reagent. SYN: *a., ethanedioic.*

a., palmitic. $C_{15}H_{31}COOH$. A saturated fatty acid occurring as esters in most natural fats and oils. SYN: *a., hexadecanoic.*

a., pantothenic. $C_9H_{17}NO_5$. One of the B-complex vitamins.

a., para-aminobenzoic. ABBR: PABA. $NH_2C_6H_4COOH$. A member of the vitamin B complex. It is used as a dietary supplement, an antirickettsial drug, a reagent, and a sunscreening agent. It should not be used in persons known to be sensitive to sulfonamides. Inhibits bacteriostatic action of sulfonamides, hence all but topical use is contraindicated during sulfonamide therapy. SYN: *aminobenzoic acid.*

a., para-aminosalicylic. ABBR: PAS. $C_7H_7NO_3$. A white or nearly white and practically odorless powder that darkens when exposed to air or light. An antituberculosis drug, the effectiveness of which is greatly enhanced when used in combination with streptomycin and isoniazid; it is believed to delay development of bacterial resistance. SYN: *aminosalicylic acid*.

a., pectic. An acid derived from pectin.

a., pentanoic. A., valeric, q.v.

a., perchloric. $HClO_4$. A colorless unstable liquid compound; the highest oxygen acid of chlorine.

a., phenic. Phenol, q.v.

a., phenylglycolic. A., mandelic, q.v.

a., phosphoric. An acid formed by oxidation of phosphorus, used as an alkaloidal reagent. The phosphoric acids are: orthophosphoric acid, H_3PO_4; pyrophosphoric acid, $H_4P_2O_7$; metaphosphoric acid, HPO_3; and hypophosphoric acid, $H_4P_2O_6$. The salts of these acids are phosphates.

a., phosphorous. An oxygen acid of phosphorus. The phosphorous acids are: orthophosphorous acid, $H_2(HPO_3)$; pyrophosphorous acid, $H_4P_2O_5$; metaphosphorous acid, HPO_2; and hypophosphorous acid, $H(H_2PO_2)$. The salts of these acids are phosphites.

a., phosphotungstic. $24WO_3 \cdot 2H_3PO_4 \cdot 48H_2O$. The H_2O content may vary. A trigonal crystalline organic acid, the water content of which may vary. Used in the form of its sodium salt in testing for alkaloids.

a., picric. $C_6H_2(NO_2)_3OH$. A yellow crystalline substance that precipitates proteins. Used as a dye and a reagent. SYN: *trinitrophenol*.

a., prussic. A., hydrocyanic, q.v.

a., pteroylglutamic. A., folic, q.v.

a., pyruvic. $CH_3CO \cdot COOH$. An intermediate product of glycolysis in muscle tissues.

a., ribonucleic. ABBR: RNA. A substance found in cytoplasm and chromosomes. It assists in selection and synthesis of proteins from the amino acid sequences.

a., salicylic. USP. $C_7H_6O_3$. A substance that occurs as white needle-shaped crystals or as white crystalline powder. It is used as a local antiseptic or keratolytic agent.

a., saturated fatty. Fatty acid in which the carbon atoms are linked to other carbon atoms by single bonds. SEE: *a., unsaturated fatty; fatty acid*.

a., silicic. An acid containing silica, as H_2SiO_3, H_2SiO_4, or H_2SiO_6. When silicic acid is precipitated, silica gel is obtained.

a., stearic. NF. $C_{18}H_{36}O_2$. A monobasic fatty acid occurring naturally in plants and animals. Used in manufacture of soap and pharmaceutical products such as glycerin suppositories.

a., succinic. $COOH(CH_2)_2COOH$. An intermediate in carbohydrate metabolism.

a., sulfonic. An organic compound of the general formula SO_2OH derived from sulfuric acid by replacement of a hydrogen atom.

a., sulfosalicylic. A crystalline acid soluble in water or alcohol. Used as a reagent for precipitating proteins, as in testing for albumin in urine.

a., sulfuric. H_2SO_4. A colorless, corrosive, heavy liquid prepared from sulfur; used in the production of a great number of industrial products. It is rarely used in medicine. SYN: *vitriol, oil of*.

a., sulfurous. H_2SO_3. An inorganic acid. It is a powerful chemical reducing agent and is used commercially esp. for its bleaching properties.

a., tannic. A glucoside prepared from oak galls and sumac that yields gallic acid and glucose on hydrolysis. SYN: *tannin*, q.v.

a., tartaric. $C_4H_6O_6$. Substance obtained from byproducts of wine fermentation. Widely used in industry in manufacture of carbonated drinks, flavored gelatins, dyes, and metals. Also used as a reagent.

a., taurocholic. A bile acid that yields cholic acid and taurine on hydrolysis.

a., trichloroacetic. $C_2HCl_3O_2$. A caustic crystalline substance.

a., 3,4,5-trihydroxybenzoic. A., gallic, q.v.

a., unsaturated fatty. Organic acid in which some of the carbon atoms are linked to other carbon atoms by double bonds, thus containing less than the maximum possible number of hydrogen atoms. For example, compare unsaturated oleic and linoleic acids with the saturated stearic acid. SEE: *a., saturated fatty; fatty acid*.

a., uric. $C_5H_4N_4O_3$. An important organic constituent of normal urine. Usually occurs in form of salts (urates).

a., valeric. $C_5H_{10}O_2$. An oily liquid of the fatty acid series, existing in four isomeric forms and having a distinctly disagreeable odor. SYN: *a., pentanoic*.

acidaminuria (ăs″ĭd-ăm″ĭ-nū′rē-ă) [L. *acidum*, acid, + *amine* + Gr. *ouron*, urine]. Excess of amino acids in urine.

acid-base balance. The mechanisms by which the acidity and alkalinity of body fluids are kept in a state of equilibrium so that the hydrogen ion concentration, q.v., of arterial blood is maintained at approx. pH 7.35 to 7.45. This is accomplished by action of buffer systems of the blood and the regulatory (homeostatic) functions of the respiratory and urinary systems. Disturbances in acid-base balance result in acidosis, q.v., or alkalosis, q.v. SEE: *pH*.

acidemia (ăs-ĭ-dē′mē-ă) [″ + Gr. *haima*, blood]. Excessive acidity of the blood, due to an uncompensated reduction in circulating alkaline substances or uncompensated increase in circulating acid substances. The hydrogen ion concentration, q.v., of the blood increases, as reflected by a lowering of serum pH values. SEE: *acid-base balance; acidity; acidosis.*

acid fallout. Acid rain, q.v.

acid-fast. Not decolorized easily by acids after staining. Pert. to bacteria that after staining are decolorized by a mixture of acid and alcohol. The acid-fast bacteria retain the red dyes, but the surrounding tissues are decolorized. In clinical medicine, an example of this type of organism is Mycobacterium tuberculosis.

acidifiable (ă-sĭd'ĭ-fī"ă-bl) [" + *fieri,* to be made, + *habilis,* able]. Capable of being transformed to produce an acid reaction.

acidification (ă-sĭd"ĭ-fĭ-kā'shŭn) [" + *factus,* made]. Becoming sour; conversion into an acid.

acidifier (ă-sĭd'ĭ-fī"ĕr) [" + *fieri,* to be made]. Substance that increases the acidity of that to which it is added or exposed.

acidimeter (ăs"ĭ-dĭm'ĕ-tĕr) [" + Gr. *metron,* measure]. Instrument for testing the amount of free acid in a solution.

acidimetry (ăs"ĭ-dĭm'ĕ-trē). Determination of an acid's strength, or of the acidity of a fluid.

acidism, acidismus (ăs'ĭ-dĭzm, ăs"ĭ-dĭz'mŭs) [L. *acidum,* acid, + Gr. *-ismos,* condition]. Poisoning caused by acids introduced from outside the body.

acidity (ă-sĭd'ĭ-tē). 1. The quality of possessing hydrogen ions (protons). SEE: *acid; hydrogen ion; pH.* 2. Sourness.

a. of stomach. Sourness due to fermentation of food in the stomach or over-secretion of acid.

acidocyte (ăs'ĭ-dō-sīt") [" + Gr. *kytos,* cell]. Eosinophil; eosinophilic leukocyte, q.v.

acidocytopenia (ăs"ĭ-dō-sī"tō-pē'nē-ă) [" + " + *penia,* poverty]. Abnormal reduction of number of eosinophils in the blood.

acidocytosis (ăs"ĭ-dō-sī-tō'sĭs) [" + " + *osis,* condition]. Abnormal increase in number of eosinophilic leukocytes in the blood.

acidophil(e) (ă-sĭd'ō-fĭl, -fīl) [" + Gr. *philos,* love]. 1. Capable of being stained by acid stains such as eosin. Said of cells or parts of cells prepared for microscopic study. SYN: *acidophilic; acidophilous.* 2. An acid-staining cell of the anterior pituitary. 3. A bacterial organism that grows well in an acid medium.

acidophilic (ă-sĭd"ō-fĭl'ĭk). 1. Having affinity for acid or pert. to certain tissues and cell granules. 2. Pert. to a cell capable of being stained by acid stains, an eosinophil. SYN: *acidophilous.*

acidophilus milk (ăs"ĭ-dŏf'ĭ-lŭs). Milk fermented by Lactobacillus acidophilus cultures. SEE: *milk.*

acidoresistant (ăs"ĭ-dō-rē-zĭs'tănt). Acid-resisting; said about bacteria.

acidosic (ăs"ĭ-dō'sĭk). Characterized by acidosis.

acidosis (ăs"ĭ-dō'sĭs) [L. *acidum,* acid, + Gr. *osis,* condition]. Excessive acidity of body fluids, due to an accumulation of acids (as in diabetic acidosis or renal disease) or an excessive loss of bicarbonate (as in renal disease). The hydrogen ion concentration, q.v., is increased and thus the pH is decreased. SEE: *acid-base balance; acidemia; buffer; pH.*

a., carbon dioxide. Acidosis resulting from CO_2 retention, as in drowning or decreased respiration.

a., compensated. Acidosis in which the pH of body fluids has been returned to normal. Compensatory mechanisms maintain the normal ratio of bicarbonate to carbonic acid (approx. 20:1) in blood plasma even though the bicarbonate level is decreased.

a., diabetic. Acidosis occurring in advanced stages of uncontrolled diabetes mellitus due to accumulation of ketone bodies, q.v. SEE: *diabetic coma.*

a., hypercapnic. A., respiratory, q.v.

a., hyperchloremic. Acidosis in which there is an abnormally high level of chloride in the blood serum.

a., metabolic. Acidosis resulting from increase in acids other than carbonic acid. Possible causes are excessive ingestion of acids or acid salts, ketosis, severe dehydration, diarrhea, vomiting, renal disease, impaired liver function.

NURSING IMPLICATIONS: Assess patient for symptoms of metabolic acidosis, including nausea and vomiting, diarrhea, headache, changes in level of consciousness, increased rate and depth of respirations, tremors, and convulsions. Measure and record the patient's intake and output, and maintain seizure precautions.

a., renal. Acidosis due to impaired kidney function. The acidosis is induced by excessive loss of bicarbonate or inability to excrete phosphoric and sulfuric acids.

a., respiratory. Acidosis secondary to pulmonary insufficiency resulting in retention of carbon dioxide.

NURSING IMPLICATIONS: Be aware of the symptoms of respiratory acidosis, including weakness, shallow respirations, changes in level of consciousness, and tachycardia. Maintain a patent airway, and assist the patient in coughing and deep breathing exercises in order to increase ventilatory capacity.

acidotic (ăs"ĭ-dŏt'ĭk). Pert. to acidosis.

acid poisoning. Ingestion of a toxic acid. SEE: *acids* in *Poisons and Poisoning* in *Appendix.*

F.A.: Dilute with large volumes of water. Give orally milk, egg white, magnesium oxide, milk of magnesia, lime water, or aluminum hydroxide gel. Avoid carbonates as neutralizers because in the presence of strong acids they will react to produce carbon dioxide gas. This may cause distention and rupture of the stomach. Give demulcents and morphine for pain. CAUTION: The use of emetics and stomach tubes is dangerous.

acid-proof. Acid-fast, q.v.

acid rain. Rain that in passing through the atmosphere is contaminated with acid substances, esp. sulfur dioxide and nitrogen oxide pollutants. SYN: *acid fallout.*

acid salt. A salt formed when only a part of the hydrogen of an acid is replaced by a metal.

acidulate [L. *acidulus,* slightly acid]. To make somewhat sour or acid.

acidulous (ă-sĭd'ū-lŭs). Slightly sour or acid.

acidum (ăs'ĭ-dŭm) [L.]. Acid.

aciduria (ăs-ĭd-ū'rē-ă) [L. *acidum,* acid, + Gr. *ouron,* urine]. The condition of excessive acid in the urine.

aciduric (ăs"ĭ-dū'rĭk) [" + *durare,* to endure]. Capable of growing in an acid medium, but preferring a slightly alkaline medium, as certain bacteria.

acidyl (ăs'ĭ-dĭl). The acid portion of an organic acid that remains when the hydroxyl (OH) group is removed.

acies (ā'sē-ēz) [L., edge]. Margin or border.

acinar (ăs'ĭ-năr) [L. *acinus,* grape]. Rel. to or affecting an acinus, q.v.

acinesia (ăs"ĭ-nē'sē-ă) [Gr. *a-,* not, + *kinesis,* movement]. Akinesia, q.v.

acinesic, acinetic (ăs-ĭ-nē'sĭk, -nĕt'ĭk). Akinetic, q.v.

Acinetobacter (ăs"ĭ-nĕt"ō-băk'tĕr) [Gr. *akinetos,* immovable, + *bakterion,* rod]. A genus of microorganisms widely distributed in nature that are usually nonpathogenic. Acinetobacter luoffi was previously known as Mimapolymorpha and Achromobacter lwoffi. Acinetobacter anitratum was previously known as Herellea vaginicula and Achromobacter anitratum.

acini (ăs'ĭ-nī). Pl. of acinus.

aciniform (ă-sĭn'ĭ-form) [L. *acinus,* grape, + *forma,* shape]. Resembling grapes. SYN: *acinous.*

acinitis (ăs"ĭ-nī'tĭs) [" + Gr. *itis,* inflammation]. Inflammation of glandular acini.

acinose (ăs'ĭ-nōs) [L. *acinosus,* grapelike]. Composed of acini.

acinous (ăs'ĭ-nŭs). Pert. to glands resembling a bunch of grapes, such as acini and alveolar glands. SYN: *aciniform.*

acinus (ăs'ĭ-nŭs) [L., grape]. (pl. *acini*) [NA] Smallest division of a gland; a group of secretory cells surrounding a cavity.

ackee (ă'kē). Akee, q.v.

acladiosis (ăk-lăd"ē-ō'sĭs). An ulcerative skin disease believed to be due to fungi of the genus Acladium.

aclasis, aclasia (ăk'lă-sĭs, ă-klā'zē-ă) [Gr. *a-,* not, + *klasis,* a breaking away]. Abnormal tissue arising from and continuous with a normal structure, as in chondrodysplasia.

a., diaphyseal. Imperfect formation of cancellous bone in cartilage between diaphysis and epiphysis.

aclastic (ă-klăs'tĭk) [" + *klan,* to break]. Not refracting light rays.

acleistocardia (ă-klīs"tō-kăr'dē-ă) [Gr. *akleistos,* not closed, + *kardia,* heart]. Patent foramen ovale of the heart.

acme (ăk'mē) [Gr. *akme,* point]. 1. The highest point, peak. 2. The time of greatest intensity of a symptom or disease process.

acne (ăk'nē) [Gr. *akme,* point]. 1. An inflammatory disease of the sebaceous glands and hair follicles of the skin characterized by comedones, papules, pustules. Cysts and nodules may develop and scarring is common. Usually associated with seborrhea. 2. Acne vulgaris, q.v.

a. artificialis. Acne caused by external disturbance or irritation.

a. atrophica. Acne with residual pitting and scarring.

a., bromide. Characteristic acne caused by bromide.

a. cachecticorum. A type of acne seen in debilitated patients.

a. ciliaris. Acne that affects the edges of the eyelids.

a. conglobata. Acne vulgaris with abscesses, cysts, and sinuses that leave scars.

a., cystic. Acne with cysts containing keratin and sebum.

a. decalvans. Quinquad's disease; a purulent folliculitis of the scalp resulting in irregular bald patches. SYN: *folliculitis decalvans.*

a. frontalis. A. varioliformis, q.v.

a. fulminans. A rare type of acne in teenaged boys. Characterized by inflamed, tender, ulcerative, and crusting lesions of the upper trunk and face. It has a sudden onset and is accompanied by fever, leukocytosis, and an elevated sedimentation rate. About half of the cases have inflammation of several joints.

a., halogen. Acne due to exposure to halogens such as bromine, chlorine, or iodine.

a. indurata. Acne vulgaris with chronic discolored indurated surfaces.

a., keloid. Infection about the hair follicles at back of neck causing scars and thickening of skin.

a. keratosa. Acne vulgaris in which suppurating nodules crust over to form horny plugs. These occur at the corners of the mouth.

a. neonatorum. Acne in the newborn.

a. papulosa. Acne characterized by formation of papules with very little inflammation.

a., petroleum. Acne that may occur in those who work with petroleum and oils.

a. pustulosa. Acne with pustule formation and subsequent deep scars.

a. rosacea. Rosacea, q.v.

a., steroid. Acne caused by systemic or topical use of corticosteroid drugs.

a., summer. Acne that appears only in hot, humid climatic conditions or that is made much worse in such weather. Even though the exact cause is unknown, it is not caused by increased exposure to the sun's rays.

a., tropical. Severe acne caused by or aggravated by living in a hot, humid climate. Skin of the thorax, back, and legs is most commonly affected.

a. urticaria. An acneiform eruption of itching wheals.

a. varioliformis. Vesiculopustular folliculitis that occurs most commonly on temples and frontal margins of the scalp but may be seen on chest, back, or nose.

a. vulgaris. Common acne.

ETIOL: Unknown. Predisposing causes include hereditary or familial tendencies and disturbances in androgen-estrogen balance affecting activity of sebaceous glands. Acne begins at puberty. At that time the increased secretion of androgen in both males and females causes an increase in the size and activity of the pilosebaceous glands. Specific inciting factors may include food allergies, endocrine disorders, therapy with adrenal cortical steroid hormones, and psychogenic factors. Vitamin deficiencies, ingestion of halogens, and contact with chemicals such as tar and chlorinated hydrocarbons may be specific causative factors. The fact that bacteria are important once the disease is present is indicated by the successful results following antibiotic therapy. The lesions may become worse in females during the premenstruum.

SYM: There may be either papules about comedones with black centers, or pustules, or hypertrophied nodules caused by overgrowth of connective tissue. In the indurative type, the lesions are deep-seated and cause scarring. Face, neck, and shoulders are common sites.

PROG: Obstinate and recurrent.

TREATMENT: Local; systemic when indicated. Topical cleansing and peeling (keratolytic) agents; and the use of tetracycline, but this drug should not be used from the fourth fetal month and not prior to age 12 in order to prevent tooth discoloration. The drug 13-cisretinoic acid is being used experimentally. Careful extraction of comedones and incision and drainage of cysts and pustules. Avoidance of conditions known to cause exacerbations.

NURSING IMPLICATIONS: Instruct the patient concerning prevention of obstruction of sebaceous glands by washing skin thoroughly at least three times daily with soap and water; using a soft skin brush to remove oil from the back; avoiding traumatizing pimples; and in applying topical creams. Exposure to moderate sunlight and taking prescribed antibiotics will help to decrease the inflammation. Also encourage the patient to decrease carbohydrate and fat consumption, and to avoid foods that may aggravate the acne. Provide emotional support and understanding, particularly if the patient is an adolescent.

acnegenic (ăk″nē-jĕn′ĭk) [Gr. *akme*, point, + *gennan*, to produce]. Causing or producing acne.

acneiform (ăk-nē′ĭ-form) [″ + L. *forma*, shape]. Resembling acne. Also spelled acneform.

acnemia (ăk-nē′mē-ă) [Gr. *a-*, not, + *kneme*, lower leg.]. Wasting of the calves of the legs.

acnitis (ăk-nī′tĭs) [Gr. *akme*, point, + *itis*, inflammation]. A papular eruption that becomes pustular, leaving slight scars.

acomia (ă-kō′mē-ă) [Gr. *a-*, not, + *kome*, hair]. Baldness. SYN: *alopecia*.

aconite (ăk′ō-nīt) [Gr. *akoniton*]. The dried tuberous root of Aconitum, esp. A. napellus (monkshood) and A. lycoctonum (wolfsbane); a poisonous and very powerful alkaloid. Its action, which is due to the presence of two very potent alkaloids, was well known to the ancients. Aconite is believed to have been used as an arrow poison early in Chinese history and perhaps also by the inhabitants of ancient Gaul. Aconite is no longer used but is of historical interest.

aconitine (ă-kŏn′ĭ-tĭn). The active ingredient in aconite.

aconuresis (ă-kŏn″ū-rē′sĭs) [Gr. *akon*, involuntary, + *ouresis*, urination]. Involuntary voiding of urine. SYN: *enuresis*.

acorea (ă-kō-rē′ă) [Gr. *a-*, not, + *kore*, pupil]. Absence of the pupil of the eye.

acoria (ă-kō′rē-ă) [″ + *koros*, satiety]. 1. Lacking in satisfaction after eating but not from hunger. 2. Gluttony. RS: bulimia; hyperorexia; polyphagia.

acormus (ă-kor′mŭs) [″ + *kormos*, trunk]. 1. Lack of a trunk. 2. A fetal abnormality consisting of a head and extremities without a trunk.

acousia (ă-koo′zē-ă) [Gr. *akousis*, hearing]. The hearing faculty.

acousma (ă-kooz′mă) [Gr. *akousma*, a thing heard]. Nonverbal auditory hallucination.

acousmatagnosia (ă-koos″măt-ăg-nō′sē-ă)

[" + *agnosia*, ignorance]. Inability to understand what is said due to mental or neurological disorder.

acousmatamnesia (ă-koos"măt-ăm-nē'zē-ă) [" + *amnesia*, forgetfulness]. Loss of memory for sounds.

acoustic (ă-koos'tĭk) [Gr. *akoustikos*]. Pert. to sound or to the sense of hearing.

acoustic center. The hearing center in the brain located in the temporal lobe of the cerebrum.

acoustic meatus. The external or internal auditory canal.

acoustic nerve. A nerve consisting of two separate parts: vestibular and cochlear nerves, with superficial origin at junction of pons and medulla. SYN: *auditory nerve; eighth cranial nerve; vestibulocochlear nerve.*

FUNCT: Special senses of hearing and equilibrium. Vestibular and cochlear nerves consist of special somatic afferent fibers. Cells of origin of vestibular nerve are bipolar and lie in the vestibular ganglion, peripheral branches terminating in receptors of semicircular ducts, saccule, and utricle. Cells of origin of cochlear nerve are bipolar and lie in the spiral ganglion, peripheral branches terminating in spiral organ of Corti. The two nerves become joined, enter the internal acoustic meatus with the facial nerve, and then separate.

acousticophobia (ă-koos"tĭ-kō-fō'bē-ă) [Gr. *akoustos*, heard, + *phobos*, fear]. Abnormal fear of loud sounds.

acoustics (ă-koos'tĭks). The science of sound, its production, transmission, and effects.

A.C.P. *American College of Physicians; American College of Pathologists.*

acquired (ă-kwīrd') [L. *acquirere*, to get]. Not hereditary or innate.

acquired immune deficiency syndrome. ABBR: AIDS. The occurrence of immune deficiency in previously healthy individuals. Some of the patients contract a rare form of cancer, Kaposi's sarcoma; some become infected with opportunistic organisms, esp. Pneumocystis carinii. More than 50% of persons who develop AIDS will die from the disease. There is no specific therapy. The etiology of the disease is unknown, but it is thought to be due to an infectious agent, perhaps a virus. Certain groups are esp. at risk of developing this syndrome. Included are highly active homosexual and bisexual men; users of drugs of abuse such as heroin intravenously; Haitians, esp. those who have entered the U.S.A. in the last few years; and patients with hemophilia who have received blood products or blood for clotting factor replacement. Many persons in these populations do not have AIDS, but anyone who develops generalized lymphadenopathy, unexplained weight loss, and thrush should be suspected of having the syndrome. Homosexuals should be warned concerning the effect that having multiple sexual partners has on their risk of developing AIDS. Persons at risk of developing this syndrome should not donate blood. SEE: *Kaposi's sarcoma.*

acquisitus (ă-kwĭs'ĭ-tŭs) [L.]. Acquired.

acral (ăk'răl) [Gr. *akron*, extremity]. Pert. to extremities.

acrania (ă-krā'nē-ă) [Gr. *a-*, not, + *kranion*, skull]. Partial or complete congenital absence of the cranium.

acrasia (ă-krā'zē-ă) [Gr. *akrasia*, bad mixture]. Lack of self-control; intemperance.

acratia (ă-krā'shē-ă) [Gr. *akrateia*, want of power]. Loss of strength or loss of control.

acraturesis (ă-krăt"ū-rē'sĭs) [Gr. *akrates*, powerless, + *ouresis*, urination]. Inability to urinate, or difficulty in urination, as a result of bladder atony or weakness.

Acremonium (ăk"rĕ-mō'nē-ŭm). A genus of fungi, some of which are pathogenic.

acribometer (ăk"rĭ-bŏm'ĕ-tĕr) [Gr. *acribes*, exact, + *metron*, measure]. Instrument that measures minute objects.

acrid (ăk'rĭd) [L. *acer*, sharp]. Burning, bitter, irritating.

acridine (ăk'rĭ-dĭn). A coal-tar hydrocarbon from which certain dyes are prepared.

acriflavine (ăk-rĭ-flā'vĭn). A dye; a derivative of acridine, which is obtained from coal tar. Has been used as a germicide and in urinary tract infections.

acrimony (ăk'rĭ-mō"nē) [L. *acrimonia*, pungency]. Quality of being pungent, acrid, irritating.

acrinia (ă-krĭn'ē-ă) [Gr. *a-*, not, + *krinein*, to separate]. Decreased or absent secretion.

acrisorcin (ăk-rĭ-sor'sĭn). USP. Chemical used in treating tinea versicolor. Trade name is Akrinol.

acritical (ă-krĭt'ĭ-kăl) [" + *kritikos*, critical]. Not marked by a crisis.

acritochromacy (ă-krĭt"ō-krō'mă-sē) [Gr. *akritos*, not distinguishing, + *chroma*, color]. Colorblindness.

acro- (ăk'rō) [Gr. *akron*, extremity]. A combining form meaning extremity, top, extreme point.

acroagnosis (ăk"rō-ăg-nō'sĭs) [" + *gnosis*, knowledge]. Absence of feeling of one's limb.

acroanesthesia (ăk"rō-ăn-ĕs-thē'zē-ă) [" + *an-*, not, + *aisthesis*, sensation]. Lack of sensation in one or more of the extremities.

acroarthritis (ăk-rō-ăr-thrī'tĭs) [" + *arthron*, joint, + *itis*, inflammation]. Arthritis of the hands or feet.

acroasphyxia (ăk"rō-ăs-fĭk'sē-ă) [" + *asphyxia*, pulse stoppage]. Cold, pale condition of hands and feet; symptom of Raynaud's disease.

acroataxia (ăk″rō-ă-tăk′sē-ă) [Gr. *akron,* extremity, + *ataktos,* out of order]. Muscular incoordination involving, or limited to, the fingers and toes.

acrobiology (ăk″rō-bī-ŏl′ō-jē) [″ + *bios,* life, + *logos,* study]. Study of the distribution of airborne organisms and their effects.

acroblast (ăk′rō-blăst) [″ + *blastos,* germ]. A part of the Golgi apparatus in the spermatid from which the acrosome arises.

acrobrachycephaly (ăk″rō-brăk″ĭ-sĕf′ă-lē) [″ + *brachys,* short, + *kephale,* head]. State of having an abnormally short head in the anterior-posterior diameter. Due to fusion of the coronal suture.

acrobystitis (ăk″rō-bĭs-tī′tĭs) [Gr. *akrobystia,* prepuce, + *itis,* inflammation]. Inflammation of the prepuce. SYN: *acroposthitis; posthitis.*

acrocentric (ăk″rō-sĕn′trĭk) [Gr. *akron,* extremity, + L. *centrum,* center]. Pert. to a chromosome in which the centromere is located near one end. At metaphase it has the appearance of a wishbone.

acrocephalia (ăk″rō-sĕf-ā′lē-ă) [″ + *kephale,* head.] Acrocephaly, q.v. SYN: *oxycephalia.*

acrocephalic (ăk″rō-sĕ-făl′ĭk). Pert. to acrocephaly, q.v.

acrocephalosyndactylia, acrocephalosyndactyly (ăk″rō-sĕf″ă-lō-sĭn-dăk-tĭl′ē-ă, -sĭn-dăk′tĭl-ē) [″ + ″ + *syn,* together, + *daktylos,* a finger]. A congenital condition marked by a peaked head and webbed fingers and toes. SYN: *Apert's syndrome.*

acrocephaly (ăk″rō-sĕf′ă-lē) [Gr. *akron,* extremity, + *kephale,* head]. State of having a malformed cranial vault with a high or peaked appearance and a vertical index above 77. SYN: *acrocephalia; oxycephalia.*

ETIOL: Premature closure of the coronal, sagittal, and lambdoidal sutures.

acrochordon (ăk″rō-kor′dŏn) [″ + *chorde,* cord]. A small outgrowth of epidermal and dermal tissue.

acrocinesia, acrocinesis (ăk″rō-sĭn-ē′sē-ă, -sĭs) [″ + *kinesis,* movement]. Excessive movement of the extremities. SYN: *acrokinesia.*

acrocinetic (ăk″rō-sĭn-ĕt′ĭk). Showing excessive motion of the extremities.

acrocontracture (ăk″rō-kŏn-trăkt′ūr) [″ + L. *contrahere,* to draw together]. Contracture of the hands or feet.

acrocyanosis (ăk″rō-sī-ă-nō′sĭs) [″ + *kyanosis,* dark-blue color]. Cyanosis of the extremities. Acrocyanosis of the hands and feet may be normal in the infant within the first hour after birth.

ETIOL: Due to vasomotor disturbances. Seen in catatonia or hysteria.

acrodermatitis (ăk″rō-dĕr-mă-tī′tĭs) [″ + *derma,* skin, + *itis,* inflammation]. Dermatitis of the extremities.

a. chronica atrophicans. Dermatitis of hands and feet that progresses slowly upward on the affected limbs.

a. continua. An obstinate eczematous eruption confined to the extremities.

a. enteropathica. Rare childhood disease with onset between 3 weeks and 18 months. May be fatal if untreated. The genetically determined cause is malabsorption of zinc. Onset is insidious with failure to thrive, diarrhea, loss of hair, and development of vesiculobullous lesions, particularly around body orifices.

TREATMENT: Zinc sulfate given orally will abolish all clinical manifestations of the disease within a few days.

a. hiemalis. A dermatitis occurring in winter, affecting the extremities and tending to disappear spontaneously.

a. perstans. A. continua q.v.

acrodermatosis (ăk″rō-dĕr″mă-tō′sĭs) [Gr. *akron,* extremity, + *derma,* skin, + *osis,* condition]. Any skin disease that affects the hands and feet.

acrodolichomelia (ăk″rō-dŏl″ĭ-kō-mē′lē-ă) [″ + *dolichos,* long, + *melos,* limb]. Condition in which the hands and feet are abnormally long.

acrodynia (ăk″rō-dĭn′ē-ă) [″ + *odyne,* pain]. An infantile disease characterized by lesions of the skin on the hands and feet, swelling of the extremities, digestive disturbances, and itching of hands and feet, which, along with the cheeks and tip of nose, are intensely pink. It is frequently followed by arthritis involving multiple joints and muscle weakness.

ETIOL: Allergic reaction to mercury. SYN: *erythredema; pink disease.*

acroesthesia (ăk″rō-ĕs-thē′zē-ă) [″ + *aisthesis,* sensation]. 1. Abnormal sensitivity of the extremities. 2. Pain in the extremities.

acrogeria (ăk″rō-jĕr′ē-ă) [″ + *geron,* old man]. A condition wherein the skin of the hands and feet shows signs of premature aging.

acrognosis (ăk″rŏg-nō′sĭs) [″ + *gnosis,* knowledge]. Sensory perception of limbs.

acrohyperhidrosis (ăk″rō-hī″pĕr-hī-drō′sĭs) [″ + *hyper,* above, + *hidrosis,* sweating]. Excessive perspiration of hands and feet.

acrohypothermy (ăk″rō-hī″pō-thĕr′mē) [″ + *hypo,* under, + *therme,* heat]. Abnormal coldness of extremities.

acrokeratosis verruciformis (ăk″rō-kĕr″ă-tō′sĭs vĕ-roo′sĭ-for″mĭs) [″ + *keras,* horn, + *osis,* condition; L. *verruca,* wart, + *forma,* form]. Hereditary disease of the skin characterized by warty growths on the extremities, principally on the backs of the hands and on the feet.

acrokinesia (ăk″rō-kĭn-ē′sē-ă) [″ + *kinesis,*

movement]. Excessive motion of the extremities. SYN: *acrocinesia.*

acrolein (ăk-rō'lē-ĭn) [L. *acer,* acrid, + *oleum,* oil]. A volatile liquid produced by dry distillation of glycerin. Irritating to the eyes, it is used in chemical warfare. SYN: *acrylaldehyde.*

acromacria (ăk"rō-măk'rē-ă) [Gr. *akron,* extremity, + *makros,* long]. Abnormal length of fingers. SYN: *arachnodactyly.* SEE: *Marfan's syndrome.*

acromastitis (ăk"rō-măs-tī'tĭs) [" + *mastos,* breast, + *itis,* inflammation]. Inflammation of the nipple. SYN: *thelitis.*

acromegaly (ăk"rō-mĕg'ă-lē) [" + *megas,* big]. A chronic disease of middle-aged persons characterized by elongation and enlargement of bones of the extremities and certain head bones, esp. frontal bone and jaws, accompanied by enlargement of nose and lips and thickening of soft tissues of the face. SYN: *Marie's disease.*

ETIOL: Hyperfunction of the eosinophilic cells of the anterior lobe of the pituitary resulting in excess production of growth hormone. SEE: *somatostatin.*

SYM: Onset of the disease is so gradual that neither the patients nor their associates notice it. Early complaints include muscular pains, headache, sweating. Facial features are enlarged, and mandible and malar bones become prominent with protrusion of orbital ridge. Teeth become widely separated; hands and feet gradually enlarge. About a fourth of the patients will develop diabetes. As the disease progresses, muscular weakness is a serious feature and visual impairment may progress to the point of blindness.

TREATMENT: X-ray therapy or surgery of pituitary gland.

acromelalgia (ăk"rō-mĕl-ăl'jē-ă) [Gr. *akron,* extremity, + *melos,* limb, + *algos,* pain]. Bilateral vasodilation of the vessels of the hands and feet. The skin is reddened, warm, and painful. Cause is unknown. Treatment is symptomatic.

acromelic (ăk"rō-mĕl'ĭk) [" + *melos,* limb]. Pert. to the end of the extremities.

acrometagenesis (ăk"rō-mĕt"ă-jĕn'ĕ-sĭs) [" + *meta,* beyond, + *genesis,* origin]. Abnormal growth of extremities.

acromial (ăk-rō'mē-ăl) [" + *omos,* shoulder]. Rel. to the acromion.

acromial angle. The angle at the edge of the spine of the scapula where it ascends to become the acromion.

acromial process. The acromion, q.v.

acromial reflex. Flexion of forearm with internal rotation of hand resulting from quick blow upon acromion. Elicited in hyperkinetic states.

acromicria (ăk"rō-mĭk'rē-ă) [" + *mikros,* small]. Congenital shortness or smallness of the extremities.

acromioclavicular joint (ă-krō"mē-ō-klă-vĭk'ū-lăr) [" + *omos,* shoulder, + L. *clavicula,* small key]. An arthrodial joint between the acromion and the acromial end of the clavicle.

acromiocoracoid (ă-krō"mē-ō-kor'ă-koyd) [" + " + *korax,* crow, + *eidos,* resemblance]. Pert. to the acromion and coracoid process.

acromiohumeral (ăk-rō"mē-ō-hū'mĕr-ăl) [" + " + L. *humerus,* shoulder]. Pertaining to the acromion and humerus.

acromion (ă-krō'mē-ŏn) [Gr. *akron,* extremity, + *omos,* shoulder]. [NA] The lateral triangular projection of the spine of the scapula that forms the point of the shoulder and articulates with the clavicle. SYN: *acromial process.* SEE: *acromioclavicular joint.*

acromioscapular (ă-krō"mē-ō-skăp'ū-lăr) [" + " + L. *scapula,* shoulder blade]. Pert. to the acromion and scapula.

acromiothoracic (ă-krō"mē-ō-thō-răs'ĭk) [" + " + *thorax,* breastplate]. Pert. to the acromion and thorax.

acromphalus (ăk-rŏm'făl-ŭs) [" + *omphalos,* umbilicus]. 1. Center of navel. 2. Projection of umbilicus, as in beginning of umbilical hernia.

acromyotonia, acromyotonus (ăk"rō-mī-ō-tō'nē-ă, -ŏt'ō-nŭs) [" + *mys,* muscle, + *tonos,* tension]. Myotonia of extremities causing spasmodic deformity.

acronarcotic (ăk"rō-năr-kŏt'ĭk) [L. *acer,* sharp, + Gr. *narkotikos,* benumbing]. Having the property of a narcotic and yet irritant in local effects.

acroneurosis (ăk"rō-nū-rō'sĭs) [Gr. *akron,* extremity, + *neuron,* nerve, + *osis,* condition]. Nervous disorder in the extremities.

acronym (ăk'rō-nĭm) [" + *onym,* name]. Word formed by combining the first letter or letters of a name or a phrase.

Ex.: MASH for *M*obile *A*rmy *S*urgical *H*ospital.

acronyx (ăk'rō-nĭks") [L. *acer,* sharp, + Gr. *onyx,* claw]. An ingrown nail.

acro-osteolysis (ăk"rō-ŏs"tē-ŏl'ĭ-sĭs) [Gr. *akron,* extremity, + *osteon,* bone, + *lysis,* dissolution]. 1. A familial disease in which there is dissolution of the tips of the extremities of young children. There is no history of trauma and spontaneous amputation does not occur. Etiology unknown. 2. An occupational disease seen in workers who come in contact with vinyl chloride polymerization processes. Characterized by Raynaud's phenomenon, scleroderma-like skin changes, and x-ray evidence of bone destruction of the distal phalanges of the hands. Recovery follows after removal from exposure. SEE: *Raynaud's disease.*

acropachy (ăk'rō-păk"ē) [" + *pachys,* thick].

Clubbing of fingers or toes.

acropachyderma (ăk″rō-păk″ē-dĕr′mă) [″ + ″ + *derma,* skin]. Clubbing of the fingers, deformed long bones and thickening of the skin of the scalp, face, and extremities.

acroparalysis (ăk″rō-pă-răl′ĭ-sĭs) [″ + *paralyein,* to disable]. Paralysis of one or more extremities.

acroparesthesia (ăk″rō-păr-ĕs-thē′zē-ă) [″ + *para,* abnormal, + *aisthesis,* sensation]. Sensation of prickling, tingling, or numbness in the extremities.

acropathology (ăk″rō-pă-thŏl′ō-jē) [″ + *pathos,* suffering, + *logos,* study]. Pathology of disease of the extremities.

acropathy (ă-krŏp′ă-thē) [″ + *pathos,* suffering]. Any disease of the extremities.

acrophobia (ăk-rō-fō′bē-ă) [″ + *phobos,* fear]. Morbid fear of high places.

acroposthitis (ăk″rō-pŏs-thī′tĭs) [Gr. *akroposthis,* prepuce, + *itis,* inflammation]. Inflammation of the prepuce of the penis. SYN: *acrobystitis; posthitis.*

acroscleroderma (ăk″rō-sklĕr-ō-dĕr′mă) [Gr. *akron,* extremity, + *scleros,* hard, + *derma,* skin]. Hard, thickened skin condition of toes and fingers. SYN: *sclerodactylia.*

acrosclerosis (ăk″rō-sklĕr-ō′sĭs) [″ + ″ + *osis,* condition]. A scleroderma of the upper extremities, sometimes extending to neck and face. Usually follows Raynaud's disease, q.v.

acrose (ăk′rōs). A sugar prepared synthetically by formaldehyde or glucose condensation.

acrosome (ăk′rō-sōm) [″ + *soma,* body]. The anterior end of the head of the spermatozoon.

acrosphacelus (ăk″rō-sfăs′ĕ-lŭs) [″ + *sphakelos,* gangrene]. Gangrene of digits. May be symptom of Raynaud's disease.

acroteric (ăk″rō-tĕr′ĭk) [Gr. *akroterion,* summit]. Pert. to the outermost parts of the extremities, as the tips of the fingers.

acrotic (ă-krŏt′ĭk). 1. [Gr. *a-,* not, + *krotos,* striking]. Pert. to extreme weakness or absence of the pulse. 2. [Gr. *akrotes,* extreme]. Pert. to the surface of the skin.

acrotism (ăk′rō-tĭzm) [Gr. *a-,* not, + *krotos,* striking, + *-ismos,* condition]. Imperceptibility of the pulse.

acrotrophoneurosis (ăk″rō-trŏf″ō-nū-rō′sĭs) [Gr. *akron,* extremity, + *trophe,* nourishment, + *neuron,* nerve, + *osis,* condition]. Trophoneurosis of extremities with trophic, neuritic, and vascular changes. Usually caused by prolonged immersion in water.

acryl(o)-. Combining form indicating acrylic.

acrylaldehyde (ăk″rĭl-ăl′dĕ-hīd). A volatile liquid produced by dry distillation of glycerin. Irritating to the eyes, it is used in chemical warfare. SYN: *acrolein.*

acrylamide (ă-krĭl′ă-mīd). The amide of acrylic acid, $CH_2CHCONH_2$.

acrylate (ăk′rĭ-lāt). A salt or ester of acrylic acid.

acrylic acid (ă-krĭl′ĭk). A colorless corrosive liquid, $H_2C{=}CHCOOH$. Used in making acrylic polymers, q.v., and resins, q.v.

acrylic resin. General term for various polymers of acrylic acid and their esters. Some of these compounds are used medically as components of contact lenses and dental materials.

acrylonitrile (ăk″rĭ-lō-nī′trĭl). A toxic compound, CH_2CHCN, used in making plastics. SYN: *vinyl cyanide.*

A.C.S., ACS. *American Cancer Society; American Chemical Society; American College of Surgeons; anodal closing sound.*

A.C.S.M. *American College of Sports Medicine.*

act (ăkt). To accomplish a function; the accomplishment of a function.

a., compulsive. The repetitive, ritualistic performance of an act. This may be done despite the individual's attempts to resist the act.

a., impulsive. Sudden action caused by an abnormal impulse or desire.

ACTH. *adrenocorticotropic hormone,* a pituitary hormone that stimulates the cortex of the adrenal glands. SEE: *cortisone.*

actin (ăk′tĭn). One of the two proteins in muscle fiber, the other being myosin.

acting out. Expressing oneself through actions rather than speech.

a.o., neurotic. 1. A form of transference, q.v., in which tension is relieved by responding to a situation as if it were the same situation that originally gave rise to the tension; a displacement of behavioral response from one situation to another. 2. In psychoanalysis, a form of displacement, q.v., in which the patient relives memories rather than expressing them verbally.

actinic (ăk-tĭn′ĭk) [Gr. *aktis,* ray]. 1. Pert. to radiant energy such as x-rays, ultraviolet light, sunlight, particularly the photochemical effects. 2. Pert. to the capability of radiant energy to produce chemical changes.

actinic burns. Burns caused by ultraviolet or sun rays. Treatment as in dry heat burns. SEE: *burn.*

actinic dermatitis. Inflammation and erythema of the skin caused by exposure to radiation.

actinism (ăk′tĭn-ĭzm). That property of radiant energy that produces chemical changes, as in photography or heliotherapy.

actinium (ăk-tĭn′ē-ŭm) [Gr. *aktis,* ray]. A radioactive element. At. no. 89; at. wt. 227. SYMB: Ac.

actino- (ăk′tĭ-nō) [Gr. *aktis,* ray]. Combining form indicating a similarity to a ray or referring to radiation such as x-ray or electromagnetic radiation, e.g., light rays.

Actinobacillus (ăk″tĭ-nō-bă-sĭl′lŭs). Small gram-negative rods that affect mostly domestic animals, but Actinobacillus actinomycetumcomitans has been implicated in endocarditis in man.

actinochemistry (ăk″tĭ-nō-kĕm′ĭs-trē) [″ + *chemeia,* chemistry]. Branch of chemistry concerned with the effects of light rays. SYN: *photochemistry.*

actinodermatitis (ăk″tĭn-ō-dĕr-mă-tī′tĭs) [″ + *derma,* skin, + *itis,* inflammation]. Dermatitis caused by exposure to radiation.

actinogen (ăk-tĭn′ō-jĕn) [″ + *genesis,* production]. Any radioactive element.

actinogenesis (ăk″tĭn-ō-jĕn′ĕ-sĭs). The source or production of radiation.

actinogenic (ăk″tĭn-ō-jĕn′ĭk) [″ + *gennan,* to produce]. 1. Producing radiation. 2. Caused by radiation. SYN: *radiogenic.*

Actinomyces (ăk″tĭn-ō-mī′sēz) [″ + *mykes,* fungus]. A genus of bacteria of the family Actinomycetaceae that contain gram-positive staining filaments. These bacteria cause various diseases in man and animals.

A. antibioticus. A species of Actinomyces from which the antibiotic actinomycin is obtained.

A. bovis. A species of Actinomyces that causes actinomycosis (lumpy jaw) in cattle.

A. israelii. A species of Actinomyces that causes actinomycosis in humans. One clinical form is called lumpy jaw due to the characteristic appearance of the swollen jaw produced by the infection.

TREATMENT: Prolonged therapy with very large doses of penicillin G is required.

Actinomycetales (ăk″tĭ-nō-mī″sĕ-tā′lēz). An order of bacteria that includes the families Mycobacteriaceae, Actinomycetaceae, Actinoplanaceae, Dermatophilaceae, Micromonosporaceae, Nocardiaceae, and Streptomycetaceae.

actinomycete (ăk″tĭ-nō-mī′sēt). Any bacterium of the order Actinomycetales.

actinomycetic (ăk″tĭ-nō-mī-sĕt′ĭk). Pert. to Actinomyces.

actinomycetin (ăk″tĭn-ō-mī-sĕt′ĭn). A lytic substance obtained from Actinomyces; it destroys some gram-positive and gram-negative organisms.

actinomycin A (ăk″tĭn-ō-mī′sĭn). An antibacterial substance obtained from Actinomyces antibioticus, heat-stable and highly toxic, effective against gram-positive organisms. It is orange-colored, and is soluble in alcohol and ether.

actinomycin B. Similar to actinomycin A but not soluble in alcohol. Not used clinically because of its toxicity.

actinomycoma (ăk″tĭ-nō-mī-kō′ma) [Gr. *aktis,* ray, + *mykes,* fungus, + *oma,* tumor]. A tumor produced by actinomycosis, q.v.

actinomycosis (ăk″tĭn-ō-mī-kō′sĭs) [″ + ″ + *osis,* condition]. A noncontagious bacterial disease in animals (lumpy jaw) and man. Infection may be of the cervicofacial, thoracic, or abdominal regions, or may be generalized.

ETIOL: Actinomyces bovis in cattle; Actinomycosis israelii in man. This organism is normally present in the mouth. SEE: *nocardiosis.*

SYM: Formation of slow-growing granulomas, which later break down, discharging viscid pus containing minute yellowish (sulfur) granules.

TREATMENT: Prolonged administration of penicillin is usually effective. Tetracyclines are the second choice. Surgical incision and drainage of accessible lesions is helpful when combined with chemotherapy.

actinomycotic (ăk″tĭn-ō-mī-kŏt′ĭk). Pert. to actinomycosis.

actinon (ăk′tĭn-ŏn) [Gr. *aktis,* ray]. A radioactive isotope of actinium. SYN: *radon*^{219}.

actinoneuritis (ăk″tĭn-ō-nū-rī′tĭs) [″ + *neuron,* nerve, + *itis,* inflammation]. Inflammation of a nerve or nerves resulting from exposure to radium or x-rays.

actinophytosis (ăk″tĭ-nō-fī-tō′sĭs) [″ + *phyton,* plant, + *osis,* condition]. Infection due to Actinomyces.

actinopraxis (ăk″tĭn-ō-prăk′sĭs) [″ + *praxis,* action]. Employment of light or radioactive rays in diagnosis and treatment.

actinotherapy (ăk″tĭn-ō-thĕr′ă-pē) [″ + *therapeia,* healing]. Treatment of disease by rays of light, esp. actinic or photochemically active rays, or by x-rays or radium.

actinotoxemia (ăk″tĭn-ō-tŏk-sē′mē-ă) [″ + *toxikon,* poison, + *haima,* blood]. A toxic reaction produced by an excessive dose of radiation. SEE: *radiation syndrome.*

action (ăk′shŭn) [L. *actio*]. Performance of a function, or process; in pathology, a morbid process.

a., antagonistic. The ability of a drug or a muscle to oppose or resist the action or effect of another drug or muscle. Opposite of synergistic action.

a., astringent. Action in which the tissue cells are contracted or shrunk.

a., bacteriocidal. Action that kills bacteria.

a., bacteriostatic. Action that stops or prevents growth of bacteria without killing them.

a., ball-valve. Intermittent obstruction of a passageway or opening so that the flow of fluid or air is prevented from moving in the normal direction and at the usual rate.

a., calorigenic. Heat produced by the metabolism of food.

a., cumulative. Sudden increased action

of a drug after several doses have been given.

a., drug. SEE: *drug action.*

a., reflex. Involuntary movement produced by sensory nerve stimulation.

a., sparing. The effect of a nonessential nutrient in the diet such that it decreases the requirement for an essential dietary substance.

Ex.: Protein is especially important for tissue growth and development in children. If protein intake is sufficient but caloric intake is inadequate, a protein deficiency will develop. In this situation, the addition of sufficient carbohydrates to the diet is said to spare the protein.

a., specific. The particular action of a drug on another substance or upon an organism or part of that organism.

a., specific dynamic. Stimulation of metabolic rate by ingestion of certain foods, esp. proteins.

a., synergistic. The ability of a drug or muscle to aid or enhance the action or effect of another drug or muscle. Opposite of antagonistic action.

a., thermogenic. The action of a food, drug, or physical agent to cause a rise in output of body heat.

a., trigger. The initiation of activity, physiological or pathological, that may have no relation to the action that started it.

action current. Used in physical therapy. SEE: *action potential.*

action of arrest. The action of decreasing or slowing the function of an organ or cell or a chemical reaction.

action potential. The change in electrical potential of nerve or muscle fiber when stimulated.

activate (ăk′tĭ-vāt). 1. To make active. 2. To make radioactive.

activator (ăk′tĭ-vā″tor) 1. A substance in the body that converts an inactive substance into an active agent, as the action of hydrogen ions on pepsinogen converting it to pepsin. 2. Any substance that specifically induces an activity, such as an inductor or organizer in embryonic development, or a trophic hormone.

active motion. Active range of motion, q.v.

active principle. The chemical substance in a pharmaceutical preparation that is responsible for the effects of the medicine. SEE: *drug action.*

active range of motion. ABBR: AROM. The range of movement at a particular joint that a patient is able to accomplish without assistance. SYN: *active motion.*

active transport. The movement by a cell membrane of molecules against a concentration, electrical, or pressure gradient is accomplished by the process of active transport. An example is the very low concentration of potassium ions in extracellular fluid. Other ions actively transported are sodium, calcium, hydrogen, iron, chloride, iodide, and urate. Several sugars and the amino acids are actively transported.

activities of daily living. ABBR: ADL. The self-care, communication, and mobility skills required for independence in everyday living. SYN: *independent living skills; daily living skills.*

activity (ăk-tĭv′ĭ-tē). The production of energy or motion; the state of being active. One describes a variety of conditions by the use of this word: enzyme activity describes the rate of influence of the enzyme on a particular system; extravehicular activity indicates the actions of space travelers while outside the space vehicle; radiation activity indicates the energy produced by a source of radiation.

a., optical. The rotation of the plane of polarized light when the light passes through a chemical solution.

activity analysis. A process used by occupational therapists to assess the psychosocial, psychodynamic, physical, or developmental characteristics of an activity in determining its utility as a therapeutic modality.

actomyosin (ăk″tō-mī′ō-sĭn). The combination of actin and myosin in a muscle. Upon muscle stimulation, these substances shorten without changing their volume and thus cause contraction of the muscle.

actual (ăk′chū-ăl) [L. *actus*, doing]. Real, existent.

actual cautery. Cautery acting by virtue of its heat and not chemically.

acufilopressure (ăk″ū-fĭ′lō-prĕsh″ŭr) [L. *acus*, needle, + *filum*, thread, + *pressura*, pressure]. Acupressure, q.v., increased by a ligature.

acuity (ă-kū′ĭ-tē) [L. *acuere*, to sharpen]. Clearness, sharpness.

a., visual. Acuteness or sharpness of vision.

acuminate (ă-kū′mĭn-āt) [L. *acuminatus*, sharpened]. Conical or pointed.

acupressure (ăk′ū-prĕsh″ŭr) [L. *acus*, needle, + *pressura*, pressure]. Compression of blood vessels by means of needles in surrounding tissues.

acupressure forceps. Spring-handled forceps for compressing blood vessels.

acupressure needles. Elastic needles for compressing blood vessels.

acupuncture (ăk″ū-pŭngk′chŭr) [″ + *punctura*, puncture]. Technique for treating certain painful conditions and for producing regional anesthesia by passing long thin needles through the skin to specific points. The free ends of the needles are twirled or in some cases used to conduct a weak electric current. Anesthesia sufficient to permit abdominal, thoracic, and head and neck surgery has been produced by the use of acupuncture alone. The patient is fully conscious during the surgery. Explanation of how acupuncture produces these effects is being investigated. Acupuncture as a method of medical investigation (but not for anesthesia) has been known in the Far East for centuries but received little attention in Western cultures until the early 1970s.

acus (ā'kŭs) [L., needle]. A surgical needle.

acusection (ăk"ū-sĕk'shŭn) [" + *secare,* to cut]. Section by an electrosurgical needle.

acusticus (ă-kū'stĭ-kŭs) [Gr. *akoustikos,* hearing]. The acoustic nerve, q.v.

acute (ă-kūt') [L. *acutus,* sharp]. 1. Sharp, severe. 2. Having rapid onset, severe symptoms, and a short course; not chronic.

acutenaculum (ăk"ū-tĕn-ăk'ū-lŭm) [L. *acus,* needle, + *tenaculum,* holder]. A needle holder.

acute necrotizing ulcerative gingivitis. ABBR: ANUG. Trench mouth, q.v.

acute urethral syndrome. Syndrome experienced by women, characterized by acute dysuria, urinary frequency, and lack of significant bacteriuria, i.e., less than 10^{-5} organisms per ml. of urine. Pyuria may or may not be present. The etiology of the syndrome is unknown but it is important to attempt to determine whether or not a specific bacterial infection of the bladder or vagina is present and to treat appropriately.

acutorsion (ăk"ū-tor'shŭn) [" + *torsio,* twisting]. Twisting of an artery with a needle to control hemorrhage.

acyanoblepsia (ă-sī"ă-nō-blĕp'sē-ă) [Gr. *a-,* not, + *kyanos,* blue, + *blepsis,* vision]. Inability to discern blue colors. SYN: *acyanopsia.*

acyanopsia (ă-sī"ă-nŏp'sē-ă). Acyanoblepsia, q.v.

acyanotic (ă-sī"ă-nŏt'ĭk) [" + *kyanos,* blue]. Pert. to the absence of cyanosis.

acyclic (ă-sī'klĭk) 1. Without a cycle. 2. Aliphatic, q.v.

acyclovir (ă-sī'klō-vĭr). An antiviral drug approved for use in herpes simplex infections of the genitals; and herpes infections of the skin of immunocompromised patients. Trade name is Zovirax.

acyesis (ă"sī-ē'sĭs) [" + *kyesis,* pregnancy]. 1. Sterility of the female. 2. Nonpregnancy.

acyl (ăs'ĭl). In organic chemistry, the radical left when the hydroxyl group (OH) is removed from an organic acid.

acylation (ăs"ĭ-lā'shŭn). Incorporation of an acid radical into a chemical.

acystia (ă-sĭs'tē-ă) [" + *kystis,* bladder]. Congenital absence of bladder.

acystinervia, acysteneuria (ă-sĭs"tĭ-nĕr'vē-ă, -nū'rē-ă) [" + " + *neuron,* nerve]. Defective nerve supply to or paralysis of the bladder.

AD. *anodal duration; average deviation; diphenylchlorarsine.*

ad [L. *ad,* to]. In prescription writing, ad indicates that a substance should be added to the formulation up to a specified volume.

ad- [L. *ad,* to]. Prefix indicating adherence, increase, toward, as adduct.

-ad [L. *ad,* to]. Suffix meaning toward, in direction of, as cephalad.

a.d. L. *auris dextra,* right ear.

A.D.A. *American Dental Association; American Diabetes Association; American Dietetic Association.*

A.D.A.A. *American Dental Assistants Association.*

adactylia, adactylism, adactyly (ă"dăk-tĭl'ē-ă, ā-dăk'tĭ-lĭzm, -lē) [" + *daktylos,* finger]. A congenital anomaly consisting of absence of digits of hand or foot.

adamantine (ăd"ă-măn'tĭn) [Gr. *adamantinos*]. Very hard, said of enamel of teeth.

adamantinoma (ăd"ă-măn"tĭ-nō'mă) [" + *oma,* tumor]. A tumor of the jaw, esp. the lower one, arising from the enamel organ. May be partly cystic, partly solid, and may reach a large size; of low-grade malignancy. SYN: *ameloblastoma.*

adamantoblast (ăd'ă-măn'tō-blăst) [Gr. *adamas,* hard surface, + *blastos,* germ]. An enamel cell from which tooth enamel is formed.

adamantoblastoma (ăd"ă-măn"tō-blăs-tō'mă) [" + " + *oma,* tumor]. Overgrowth of an adamantoblast.

adamantoma (ăd"ă-măn-tō'mă) [Gr. *adamas,* hard surface, + *oma,* tumor]. Adamantinoma, q.v.

Adam's apple. The laryngeal prominence formed by the two laminae of the thyroid cartilage. SYN: *pomum Adami; prominentia laryngea* [NA].

Adams-Stokes syndrome. [Robert Adams, Irish physician, 1791–1875; William Stokes, Irish physician, 1804–1878] Altered state of consciousness due to decreased flow of blood to the brain. Caused by any transient interference with cardiac output such as incomplete or complete heart block. The patient may be lightheaded or become completely unconscious and have convulsions.

TREATMENT: Place patient in recumbent position with legs elevated. The long-term treatment consists of implanting a demand-type cardiac pacemaker.

adaptation (ăd"ăp-tā'shŭn) [L. *adaptare,* to adjust]. 1. Adjustment of an organism to a change in environment. 2. Adjustment of the eye to various intensities of light, accomplished by changing size of pupil and accompanied by chemical changes occurring in the rods. 3. In psychology, a change in quality, intensity, or distinctness of a sensation that occurs after continuous stimulation of constant intensity. 4. In dentistry, the proper fitting of dentures or bands to the teeth, or closeness of a filling to walls of a cavity.

a., chromatic. A change in hue or saturation or both resulting from pre-exposure to light of other wavelengths.

a., dark. The adjustment of the eyes for vision in dim light. SYN: *scotopia.*

a., light. Adjustment of the eyes for vision in bright light. SYN: *photopia.*

adapted device. Any tool, implement, or equipment item that has been modified or fabricated to allow persons with limited function to perform daily living tasks or life skills independently.

adapter (ă-dăp'tĕr). 1. A device for joining one part of an apparatus to another part. 2. Device to facilitate connecting electrical supply cords to different receptacles. 3. Device for adapting one type of electrical supply source to the specific requirements of an instrument.

Ex.: An adapter is used to change a 120-volt alternating current to a 12-volt direct current.

adaxial (ăd-ăk'sē-ăl) [L. *ad,* toward, + *axis,* axis]. Toward the main axis. Opposed to abaxial.

ADC. *anodal duration contraction; axiodistocervical.*

add. Prescription abbreviation meaning *let there be added.*

adde (ăd'ē) [L.]. Add, used as a direction in writing prescriptions.

addict (ăd'ĭkt) [L. *addictus,* given over]. One physically or psychologically, or both, dependent on a substance, esp. alcohol or drugs, with use of increasing amounts.

addiction (ă-dĭk'shŭn). Physical or psychological, or both, dependence on a substance, esp. alcohol or drugs, with use of increasing amounts.

Addis count method (ăd'ĭs). [Thomas Addis, U.S. physician, 1881–1949] Method for counting the sediment (casts and cells) in a 12-hour sample of urine.

Addison's disease. [Thomas Addison, Brit. physician, 1793–1860] Disease resulting from deficiency in the secretion of adrenocortical hormones. SYN: *adrenal cortical hypofunction; chronic hypoadrenocorticism.*

ETIOL: Progressive destruction of the adrenal cortex, which is often invaded by chronic infectious diseases as tuberculosis, histoplasmosis, cryptococcosis, and other fungus diseases. Commonly, idiopathic atrophy of the adrenal is the cause.

SYM AND SIGNS: Increased pigmentation of skin and mucous membranes, irregular milk-white patches (vitiligo) on skin, black freckles over head and neck, weakness, fatigability, hypotension, nausea, vomiting, anorexia, weight loss, and occasional hypoglycemia.

PROG: If untreated, the disease will continue a chronic course with progressive but usually relatively slow deterioration; in some patients the deterioration may be rapid. Patients treated properly have an excellent prognosis.

NURSING IMPLICATIONS: Carefully assess the patient for symptoms of an adrenal crisis, such as nausea and vomiting, cyanosis, elevated temperature a sudden drop in blood pressure, weak pulse, and diminished heart sounds. During a crisis, take vital signs every hour. Take blood pressure while the patient is lying down and while standing. During an adrenal crisis, encourage the patient to rest, assist the patient with activities of daily living, limit conversations to conserve the patient's energy, and maintain a careful record of intake and output.

Teach the patient disease management, including protection from infection, increasing salt intake when perspiring, small frequent feedings to decrease the chances of developing hypoglycemia, and correct use of steroid replacement therapy. Patients should wear a Medic Alert pendant or bracelet, q.v., or carry a card stating that they have Addison's disease and indicating the type of steroid therapy they receive. Because stress may precipitate crises, discuss coping and stress management with the patient.

TREATMENT: Adrenocortical hormone therapy is dramatic in its effect and must be given promptly in adrenal crisis in order to prevent death. SEE: *adrenal; epinephrine.*

addisonism (ăd'ĭ-sŭn-ĭzm"). Symptom complex resembling Addison's disease but not caused by disease of the suprarenal glands. There is abnormal skin pigmentation with debility. May be seen in pulmonary tuberculosis.

Addison's planes. Imaginary planes that divide the abdomen into nine regions to aid in the location of internal structures. SEE: *abdominal regions.*

addition (ă-dĭ'shŭn). In chemistry, a reaction in which two substances unite without loss of atoms or valence.

additive (ăd'ĭ-tĭv). In pharmacology, the effect that one drug or substance contributes to the action of another drug or substance. SEE: *synergism.*

a., food. Substance added to food to increase its flavor, storage characteristics, color, aroma, or other qualities.

adducent (ă-dū'sĕnt) [L. *adducere,* to bring

toward]. Causing adduction.

adduct (ă-dŭkt') [L. *adductus,* brought toward]. To draw toward the main axis of body or a limb.

adduction (ă-dŭk'shŭn). 1. Movement of a limb or eye toward median plane of body, or, in case of digits, toward axial line of a limb. SEE: *abduction* for illus.

a., convergent-stimulus. Convergence of eyes upon fixation of gaze on an object at the near point of vision

adductor (ă-dŭk'tor) [L., a bringer toward]. A muscle that draws toward the medial line of the body or to a common center.

adductor reflex. Contraction of adductors of the thigh upon applying pressure to, or tapping, medial surface of thigh or knee.

adelomorphous (ă-dĕl'ō-mor'fŭs) [Gr. *adelos,* not seen, + *morphe,* shape]. Having undefined form. Applied to the central cells of the gastric glands.

adelphotaxis, adelphotaxy (ă-dĕl'fō-tăk"sĭs, -sē) [Gr. *adelphos,* brother, + *taxis,* arrangement]. Grouping of cells in mutual relationships.

adenalgia (ăd"ĕn-ăl'jē-ă) [Gr. *aden,* gland, + *algos,* pain]. Pain in a gland. SYN: *adenodynia.*

adenase (ăd'ĕ-nāz) [" + *-ase,* enzyme]. Enzyme secreted by the pancreas, spleen, and liver that converts adenine, q.v., into hypoxanthine, q.v. SEE: *enzyme.*

adenasthenia (ăd"ĕn-ăs-thē'nē-ă) [" + *astheneia,* weakness]. Deficient glandular functional activity.

adendric, adendritic (ă-dĕn'drĭk, ă"dĕn-drĭt'ĭk) [Gr. *a-,* not, + *dendrites,* rel. to a tree]. Without dendrites, as certain cells in spinal ganglia.

adenectomy (ăd"ĕn-ĕk'tō-mē) [Gr. *aden,* gland, + *ektome,* excision]. Excision of a gland.

adenectopia (ăd"ĕ-nĕk-tō'pē-ă) [" + " + *topos,* place]. Malposition of a gland; a gland in a position other than its normal position.

adenemphraxis (ăd"ĕ-nĕm-frăk'sĭs) [" + *emphraxis,* stoppage]. Obstruction to discharge from a gland.

adenia (ă-dē'nē-ă). Chronic inflammation of a lymph gland with resulting enlargement.

adeniform (ă-dĕn'ĭ-form) [" + L. *forma,* shape]. Like a gland in form.

adenine (ăd'ĕ-nĭn). $C_5H_5N_5$. 6-aminopurine, a solid substance of the uric acid group; one of the two purine bases of ribonucleic acid and deoxyribonucleic acid.

adenitis (ăd"ĕ-nī'tĭs) [" + *itis,* inflammation]. Inflammation of lymph nodes or a gland.

adenization (ăd"ĕ-nĭ-zā'shŭn). Abnormal change into a glandlike structure.

adeno- [Gr. *aden,* gland]. Prefix denoting a gland.

adenoacanthoma (ăd"ĕ-nō-ăk"ăn-thō'mă) [" + *akantha,* thorn, + *oma,* tumor]. Adenocarcinoma in which some cells have undergone squamous metaplasia.

adenoameloblastoma (ăd"ĕ-nō-ă-mĕl"ō-blăs-tō'mă) [" + O. Fr. *amel,* enamel, + Gr. *blastos,* germ, + *oma,* tumor]. Benign tumor of the maxilla.

adenoblast (ăd'ĕ-nō-blăst") [" + *blastos,* germ]. 1. Embryonic cells that produce glandular tissue. 2. Any tissue that produces secretory or glandular activity.

adenocarcinoma (ăd"ĕ-nō-kăr"sĭn-ō'mă) [" + *karkinos,* crab, + *oma,* tumor]. A malignant adenoma arising from a glandular organ.

a., acinar. Adenocarcinoma in which the cells are in the shape of alveoli. SYN: *a., alveolar.*

a., alveolar. A., acinar, q.v.

adenocele (ăd'ĕ-nō-sēl") [" + *kele,* tumor]. A cystic tumor arising from a gland. A tumor of glandular structure.

adenocellulitis (ăd"ĕ-nō-sĕl"ū-lī'tĭs) [" + L. *cella,* small chamber, + Gr. *itis,* inflammation]. Inflammation of a gland and adjacent cellular tissue.

adenochondroma (ăd"ĕ-nō-kŏn-drō'mă) [" + *chondros,* cartilage, + *oma,* tumor]. Adenoma with added characteristics of chondroma.

adenocyst (ăd'ĕ-nō-sĭst") [" + *kystis,* sac]. A cystic tumor arising from a gland.

adenocystoma (ăd"ĕ-nō-sĭs-tō'mă) [" + *kystis,* sac, + *oma,* tumor]. Cystic adenoma.

adenocyte (ăd'ĕ-nō-sīt") [Gr. *aden,* gland, + *kytos,* cell]. A mature secretory cell in a gland.

adenodynia (ăd"ĕ-nō-dĭn'ē-ă) [" + *odyne,* pain]. Pain in a gland. SYN: *adenalgia.*

adenoepithelioma (ăd"ĕ-nō-ĕp"ĭ-thēl-ē-ō'mă) [" + *epi,* on, + *thele,* nipple, + *oma,* tumor]. Tumor consisting of glandular and epithelial elements.

adenofibroma (ăd"ĕ-nō-fī-brō'mă) [" + L. *fibra,* fiber, + Gr. *oma,* tumor]. Tumor of fibrous and glandular tissue (connective tissue) frequently found in the uterus or breast.

adenofibrosis (ăd"ĕ-nō-fī-brō'sĭs) [" + " + Gr. *osis,* condition]. Degeneration of tumor that contains fibrous connective tissue.

adenogenous (ăd"ĕ-nŏj'ĕ-nŭs) [" + *gennan,* to produce]. Originating in glandular tissue.

adenohypophysis (ăd"ĕ-nō-hī-pŏf'ĭ-sĭs) [" + *hypo,* under, + *phyein,* to grow]. The anterior lobe of the pituitary gland, q.v.

adenoid (ăd'ĕ-noyd) [Gr. *adenoeides,* glandular]. Lymphoid; having the appearance of a gland.

adenoidectomy (ăd"ĕ-noyd-ĕk'tō-mē) [" + *ektome,* excision]. Excision of adenoids. SEE: *tonsillectomy.*

NURSING IMPLICATIONS: Carefully monitor the patient's vital signs and observe for symptoms of shock. Inspect the mouth for bleeding, large clot formation, or oozing, and observe the patient for frequent swallowing, which indicates bleeding. Position the patient either prone with head to the side or in a lateral recumbent position to promote drainage. When the operative wound has healed sufficiently, encourage oral intake of cool fluids and soft foods. The patient should be instructed not to gargle until the surgical site has healed.

adenoid hypertrophy. Enlargement of the pharyngeal tonsil occurring commonly in children. May result from infection of Waldeyer's ring or may be congenital.

adenoiditis (ăd″ĕ-noyd-ī′tĭs) [″ + *itis,* inflammation]. Inflammation of adenoid tissue.

adenoids (ăd′ĕ-noyds). Lymphatic tissue forming a prominence on the wall of the pharyngeal recess of the nasopharynx. SEE: *pharyngeal tonsil.*

adenoid tissue. The pharyngeal tonsil, q.v.; adenoids, q.v.

adenolipoma (ăd″ĕ-nō-lĭp-ō′mă) [″ + *lipos,* fat, + *oma,* tumor]. A benign tumor having glandular characteristics but composed of fat.

adenology (ăd″ĕ-nŏl′ō-jē) [″ + *logos,* study]. Study of glands.

adenolymphitis (ăd″ĕ-nō-lĭm-fī′tĭs) [Gr. *aden,* gland, + L. *lympha,* lymph, + Gr. *itis,* inflammation]. Inflammation of a lymph gland. SYN: *lymphadenitis,* q.v.

adenolymphocele (ăd″ĕ-nō-lĭm′fō-sēl) [″ + ″ + Gr. *kele,* tumor]. Cystic dilatation of a lymph node from obstruction.

adenolymphoma (ăd″ĕ-nō-lĭm-fō′mă) [″ + ″ + Gr. *oma,* tumor]. A lymph gland adenoma.

adenoma (ăd″ĕ-nō′mă) [″ + *oma,* tumor]. (pl. *adenomata*) A neoplasm of glandular epithelium.

a., acidophil(ic). A tumor of the pituitary gland whose cells stain with acid dyes. Cause of acromegaly and gigantism. SYN: *a., eosinophil.*

a., basophil(ic). A tumor of the pituitary gland whose cells stain with basic dyes. Cause of Cushing's syndrome.

a., chromophobe. A tumor of the pituitary gland composed of cells that do not stain readily. May cause pituitary deficiency or diabetes insipidus.

a., eosinophil(ic). A., acidophil, q.v.

a., fibroid. Fibroadenoma, q.v.

a., follicular. Adenoma of the thyroid.

a., Hürthle cell. Tumor of the thyroid that contains mostly eosinophil-staining cells. These cells, called Hürthle cells, are usually benign.

a., islet. Nonmalignant neoplasm of the pancreas sometimes containing beta cells. May be cause of hypoglycemia. SYN: *insuloma; a., langerhansian.*

a., langerhansian. A., islet, q.v.

a., malignant. Adenocarcinoma, q.v.

a., papillary. Adenoma in which the alveoli of the adenoma are filled with fluid.

a., pituitary. Adenoma of the pituitary gland.

a., sebaceous. Enlarged sebaceous glands, esp. of the face.

a. sebaceum. Benign tumorlike growths on face developing from epithelium of sebaceous glands that undergo fatty but never colloid metamorphosis. Sometimes associated with mental deficiency.

a., tubular. An adenoma in the form of a tubular gland.

a., villous. Large polyp of the mucosal surface of the large intestine.

adenomalacia (ăd″ĕ-nō-mă-lā′shē-ă) [Gr. *aden,* gland, + *malakia,* softening]. Glandular softening.

adenomatome (ăd″ĕ-nō′mă-tōm) [″ + *oma,* tumor, + *tome,* incision]. Instrument for removing adenoids.

adenomatosis (ăd″ĕ-nō-mă-tō′sĭs) [″ + *oma,* tumor, + *osis,* condition]. The condition of multiple glandular tissue overgrowths.

adenomatous (ăd″ĕ-nō′mă-tŭs). Pert. to adenomas.

adenomere (ăd′ĕ-nō-mēr″) [″ + *meros,* part]. The functional part of a gland.

adenomyoma (ăd″ĕ-nō-mī-ō′mă) [″ + *mys,* muscle, + *oma,* tumor]. A tumor containing glandular and smooth muscular tissue.

adenomyometritis (ăd″ĕ-nō-mī″ō-mĕ-trī′tĭs) [″ + ″ + *metra,* womb, + *itis,* inflammation]. A hyperplastic condition of the uterus that is the result of pelvic inflammation; it grossly resembles an adenomyoma.

adenomyosarcoma (ăd″ĕ-nō-mī″ō-săr-kō′mă) [″ + ″ + *sarx,* flesh, + *oma,* tumor]. Adenosarcoma that includes muscle tissue.

adenomyosis (ăd″ĕ-nō-mī-ō′sĭs) [″ + *mys,* muscle, + *osis,* condition]. Benign invasive growth of the endometrium into the muscular layer of the uterus.

adenoncus (ăd″ĕ-nŏn′kŭs) [″ + *onkos,* tumor]. A tumor or enlargement of a gland.

adenopathy (ăd-ĕ-nŏp′ă-thē) [″ + *pathos,* suffering]. Swelling and morbid change in lymph nodes; glandular disease.

adenopharyngitis (ăd″ĕ-nō-făr″ĭn-jī′tĭs) [″ + *pharynx,* throat, + *itis,* inflammation]. Inflammation of tonsils and pharyngeal mucous membrane.

adenophthalmia (ăd″ĕ-nŏf-thăl′mē-ă) [″ + *ophthalmos,* eye]. Inflammation of the meibomian gland, q.v.

adenosarcoma (ăd″ĕ-nō-săr-kō′mă) [″ + *sarx,* flesh, + *oma,* tumor]. A tumor with adenoma and sarcoma characteristics.

adenosclerosis (ăd″ĕ-nō-sklĕ-rō′sĭs) [″+

sklerosis, hardening]. Glandular hardening.

adenose (ăd'ĕ-nōs). Glandlike.

adenosine (ă-dĕn'ō-sēn). A nucleotide containing adenine and ribose.

a. 3',5'-cyclic monophosphate. ABBR: cyclic AMP. A cyclic form of adenosine. Its synthesis from adenosine triphosphate (ATP) is stimulated by an enzyme, adenylate cyclase (also called cyclic AMP synthetase). Adenosine 3',5'-cyclic monophosphate is important in a wide variety of metabolic responses to cell stimuli.

a. diphosphate, a. 5'-diphosphate. ABBR: ADP. A compound of adenosine containing two phosphoric acid groups. This enzyme is produced during muscle contraction. It is reformed when the muscle relaxes.

a. monophosphate, a. 5'-monophosphate. ABBR: AMP; 5'-AMP. Substance formed by condensation of adenosine and phosphoric acid. It is one of the hydrolytic products of nucleic acids and is present in muscle, red blood cells, yeast, and other nuclear material. SYN *adenylic acid.*

a. triphosphate. ABBR: ATP. A compound of adenosine containing three phosphoric acid groups. An enzyme found in all cells, but particularly in muscle cells. When this substance is split by enzyme action, energy is produced. The energy of the muscle is stored in this compound.

adenosinetriphosphatase (ă-dĕn"ō-sĭn-trī-fŏs'fă-tās). ABBR: ATPase. Enzyme that splits adenosine triphosphate to yield phosphate and energy.

adenosis (ăd"ĕ-nō'sĭs) [Gr. *aden,* gland, + *osis,* condition]. Any disease of a gland, esp. of a lymphatic gland.

adenotome (ăd'ĕ-nō-tōm) [" + *tome,* incision]. Device for excising a gland, esp. the adenoid glands.

adenotonsillectomy (ăd"ĕ-nō-tŏn"sĭl-lĕk'tō-mē) [" + L. *tonsilla,* almond, + Gr. *ektome,* excision]. Surgical removal of the tonsils and adenoids.

adenous (ăd'ĕ-nŭs). Like a gland.

adenovirus (ăd"ĕ-nō-vī'rŭs). One of a group of closely related viruses that can cause infections of the upper respiratory tract. A large number have been isolated.

adenyl (ăd'ĕ-nĭl). The radical $C_5H_4N_5$— present in adenine.

a. cyclase. Enzyme present on most cell surfaces. It catalyzes the production of cyclic AMP (adenosine 3',5'-cyclic monophosphate) from ATP (adenosine triphosphate).

adenylate cyclase (ă-dĕn'ĭ-lāt sī'klās). An enzyme important in the synthesis of adenosine 3',5'-cyclic monophosphate (cyclic AMP) from adenosine triphosphate. SYN: *cyclic AMP synthetase.*

adenylic acid. Adenosine monophosphate, q.v.

adeps (ăd'ĕps) [L.]. Lard; omental hog fat. Used in preparation of ointments.

a. benzoinatus. Benzoinated lard.

a. lanae. Wool fat. Purified anhydrous lanolin from sheep wool. Used as an ointment base.

a. lanae hydrosus. Hydrous wool fat; lanolin.

adermia (ă-dĕr'mē-ă) [Gr. *a-,* not, + *derma,* skin]. Congenital or acquired defect of or lack of skin.

adermogenesis (ă-dĕr"mō-jĕn'ĕ-sĭs) [" + " + *genesis,* production]. Imperfect development of skin.

ADH. *antidiuretic hormone* (vasopressin).

A.D.H.A. *American Dental Hygienists' Association.*

adherence, bacterial (ăd-hēr'ĕns). The property of bacteria that allows them to adhere to specific receptors that are present on some cells but not on others. If bacteria normally present in the intestinal tract did not have this ability, they would be washed out of the intestines.

adherent (ăd-hē'rĕnt) [L. *adhaerere,* to stick to]. Attached to, as of two surfaces.

adhesio (ăd-hē'zē-ō) [L. *adhaesio,* stuck to]. Adhesion.

adhesion (ăd-hē'zhŭn) [L. *adhaesio,* stuck to]. 1. A holding together or uniting of two surfaces or parts, as in wound healing. 2. A fibrous band holding parts together that are normally separated. 3. An attraction to another substance; thus, molecules or blood platelets adhere to each other or to dissimilar materials.

a., abdominal. Adhesion in the abdominal cavity, usually involving the intestines. Caused by inflammation or trauma. If causing great pain or intestinal obstruction, adhesions are treated surgically.

a., pericardial. Adhesion of the pericardial sac. If extensive enough, adhesions may lead to restriction of the normal movement of the heart. SEE: *pericarditis.*

adhesiotomy (ăd-hē"zē-ŏt'ō-mē) [L. *adhaesio,* stuck to, + Gr. *tome,* incision]. Surgical division of adhesions.

adhesive (ăd-hē'sĭv) [L. *adhaesio,* stuck to]. 1. Causing adhesion. 2. Sticky; adhering. 3. That which causes two bodies to adhere.

adhesive inflammation. A serous membrane inflammation making adhesions possible by exudating fibrinous matter.

adhesive tape. USP. A fabric, film, or paper one side of which is coated with an adhesive substance so that it remains in place after application to the skin. SEE: *plaster, adhesive.*

adiadochokinesia, adiadochokinesis (ă-dī"ă-dō"kō-kĭ-nē'sē-ă, -nē'sĭs) [Gr. *a-,* not, + *diadochas,* successive, + *kinesis,* movement]. 1.

Inability to make rapid alternating movements. 2. In neurology, rapid antagonistic movements that cannot be carried out smoothly. Seen in cerebellar disease. RS: asynergia; dysmetria; gait.

adiaphoresis (ă-dī″ă-fō-rē′sĭs) [″ + *diaphorein*, to perspire]. Deficiency or absence of sweat.

adiapneustia (ă″dī-ăp-nū′stē-ă) [″ + *diapnein*, to breathe through]. Failure to sweat; lack of sweat. SYN: *anhidrosis*.

adiastole (ă″dī-ăs′tō-lē) [″ + *diastole*, dilatation]. Imperceptibility of diastole, q.v.

adiathermancy (ă-dī″ă-thĕr′măn-sē) [″ + *dia*, through, + *therme*, heat]. State of being impervious to heat.

adient (ăd′ē-ĕnt) [L. *adeo*, to go toward]. Tending to move toward a stimulus. Opposite of abient.

Adie's syndrome (ā′dēz). [W. J. Adie, Brit. neurologist, 1886–1935] A syndrome characterized by a tonic pupil that responds slowly or not at all to light, accompanied by slow constriction and relaxation in the change from near to distant vision, and impaired accommodation. The affected pupil is frequently larger than the normal pupil. Loss of certain deep tendon reflexes may also be present but there are no other signs of CNS disease. SEE: *pupil, tonic*.

adipectomy (ăd″ĭ-pĕk′tō-mē) [L. *adeps*, fat, + Gr. *ektome*, excision]. Excision of fat or adipose tissue, usually a large quantity.

adipic (ă-dĭp′ĭk). Rel. to adipose tissue, q.v.

adipo-, adip- [L. *adeps*, fat]. Combining forms pert. to fat. See also words beginning with lipo-, lip-.

adipocele (ăd′ĭ-pō-sēl″) [L. *adeps*, fat, + Gr. *kele*, tumor]. A hernia that contains fat or fatty tissue. SYN: *lipocele*.

adipocellular (ăd″ĭ-pō-sĕl′ū-lăr). Containing fat and cellular tissue.

adipocere (ăd′ĭ-pō-sēr″) [″ + *cera*, wax]. A brown, waxlike substance composed of fatty acids and calcium soaps. It is formed in animal tissues that have been buried in a moist place. SYN: *grave wax*.

adipofibroma [″ + *fibra*, fiber, + Gr. *oma*, tumor]. A fibroma and adipoma.

adipogenous, adipogenic (ăd″ĭ-pŏj′ĕn-ŭs, -pō-jĕn′ĭk) [″ + Gr. *gennan*, to produce]. Inducing the formation of fat.

adipoid (ăd′ĭ-poyd) [L. *adeps*, fat, + Gr. *eidos*, resemblance]. Fatlike; lipoid.

adipokinesis (ăd″ĭ-pō-kī-nē′sĭs) [″ + Gr. *kinesis*, motion]. 1. Metabolism of fat with production of free fatty acids. 2. Mobilization and metabolism of body fat.

adipokinetic action. The action of substances to promote formation of free fatty acids from body fat stores.

adipolysis (ăd″ĭ-pŏl′ĭ-sĭs) [″ + Gr. *lysis*, setting free]. The hydrolysis or digestion of fat.

adipometer (ăd″ĭ-pŏm′ĕ-tĕr) [″ + Gr. *metron*, measure]. Instrument for measuring thickness of the skin. Useful in determining thickness of subcutaneous fat layer, therefore used to judge degree of obesity.

adiponecrosis (ăd″ĭ-pō-nĕ-krō′sĭs) [″ + Gr. *nekrosis*, deadness]. Necrosis affecting fatty tissue.

adipose [L. *adiposus*, fatty] Fatty; pert. to fat.

adipose capsule. Perirenal fat.

adipose tissue. Connective or areolar tissue containing masses of fat cells.

adiposis (ăd″ĭ-pō′sĭs) [″ + Gr. *osis*, condition]. Abnormal accumulation of fat in the body. SYN: *corpulence; liposis; obesity*.

a. cerebralis. Obesity due to intracranial disease, esp. of the pituitary.

a. dolorosa. Scattered areas of painful cutaneous nodules or fat accumulations in menopausal women. SYN: *Dercum's disease*.

a. hepatica. Fatty degeneration or infiltration of the liver.

adipositis (ăd″ĭ-pō-sī′tĭs) [L. *adiposus*, fatty, + Gr. *itis*, inflammation]. Infiltration of an inflammatory nature in and beneath subcutaneous adipose tissue.

adiposity (ăd″ĭ-pŏs′ĭ-tē). Excessive fat in the body. SYN: *adiposis; corpulence; obesity*.

adiposogenital dystrophy (ăd″ĭ-pō″sō-jĕn′ĭ-tăl dĭs′trō-fē) [″ + *genitalis*, genital, + Gr. *dys*, bad, disordered, + *trophe*, nourishment]. Combination of adiposity, impaired development of genital organs, and altered secondary sex characteristics. SYN: *Fröhlich's syndrome*.

ETIOL: A disturbance or tumor of the hypothalamus and pituitary gland.

adiposuria (ăd″ĭ-pō-sū′rē-ă) [″ + Gr. *ouron*, urine]. Fat in the urine. SYN: *lipuria*.

adipsia, adipsy (ă-dĭp′sē-ă, -sē) [Gr. *a-*, not, + *dipsa*, thirst]. Absence of thirst.

aditus [L.]. An approach; an entrance.

a. ad antrum. The recess of the tympanic cavity that leads from the epitympanic recess to the tympanic antrum.

a. ad aquaeductum cerebri. The entrance to the sylvian aqueduct, situated at lower posterior angle of third ventricle of brain.

a. ad infundibulum. A small canal leading from the third ventricle into the infundibulum.

a. glottidis inferior. Inferior entrance to the glottis.

a. glottidis superior. Superior entrance to the glottis.

a. laryngis. [NA] Upper aperture of larynx.

adjunct (ăd′jŭnkt). An addition to the principal procedure or course of therapy.

adjuster. Device for holding together the ends of the wire forming a suture.

adjustment [L. *adjuxtare,* to bring together]. 1. Adaptation to a different environment. 2. A change made to improve function or condition.

Ex.: Changing the position of the lenses of a microscope in order to bring the object into focus.

adjuvant (ăd'jū-vănt) [L. *adjuvans,* aiding]. 1. That which assists, esp. a drug added to a prescription to hasten or increase the action of a principal ingredient. 2. In immunology, a variety of substances, including inorganic gels such as alum, aluminum hydroxide, and aluminum phosphate, that increase the antigenic response.

a., Freund's complete. [Jules T. Freund, Hungarian-born U.S. bacteriologist, 1890–1961] A water-in-oil emulsion in which an antigen solution is emulsified in mineral oil with killed mycobacteria to enhance antigenicity. The intense inflammatory response produced by this emulsion makes it unsuitable for use in man.

a., Freund's incomplete. A water-in-oil emulsion in which an antigen solution without mycobacteria is emulsified in mineral oil. On injection, this mixture induces a strong persistent antibody formation.

adjuvant therapy. In cancer therapy, the use of another form of treatment in addition to the primary surgical therapy.

ADL. *activities of daily living,* q.v.

Adler, Alfred. Austrian psychiatrist (1870–1937) who founded the school of individual psychology. SEE: *psychology, individual.*

ad lib. [L. *ad libitum*]. Prescription abbreviation meaning *at pleasure* or *as much as is wanted.*

ad nauseum (ăd naw'sē-ŭm) [L.]. Of such degree or extent as to produce nausea.

adnerval (ăd-nĕr'văl) [L. *ad,* to, + *nervus,* nerve]. Near or toward a nerve.

adneural (ăd-nū'răl) [" + Gr. *neuron,* nerve]. Adnerval.

adnexa (ăd-nĕk'să) [L.]. Accessory parts of a structure.

a. oculi Lacrimal glands.

a. uteri. Ovaries and oviducts.

adnexal (ăd-nĕk'săl). Adjacent or appending.

adnexitis (ăd"nĕk-sī'tĭs) [L. *adnexa,* appendages, + Gr. *itis,* inflammation]. Inflammation of the adnexa uteri.

adnexopexy (ăd-nĕks'ō-pĕk"sē) [" + Gr. *pexis,* fixation]. Fixing the fallopian tube and ovary to the abdominal wall.

adolescence (ăd"ō-lĕs'ĕns) [L. *adolescens*]. The period from the beginning of puberty until maturity. The onset of puberty and maturity is a gradual process and variable among individuals. Thus it is not practical to set exact age or chronological limits in defining the adolescent period.

adolescent (ăd"ō-lĕs'ĕnt). 1. Pert. to adolescence. 2. Young man or woman not fully grown.

adoral (ăd-ō'răl) [L. *ad,* to, + *os,* mouth]. Toward or near the mouth.

ADP. *adenosine diphosphate.*

adrenal (ăd-rē'năl) [L. *ad,* to, + *ren,* kidney]. Originally used to indicate nearness to the kidney. Now used in reference to the adrenal gland or its secretions.

adrenal crisis. Acute adrenocortical insufficiency. CAUTION: Death due to circulatory collapse will result unless the condition is treated promptly and vigorously by instituting corticosteroid therapy. The cause may be a hemorrhage into the adrenal cortex as a result of infection or it may occur at birth, resulting from trauma. In the adult, headache, lassitude, confusion, restlessness, vomiting, and shock progressing to death occur if the cortex is destroyed. Relative adrenal insufficiency can occur in patients for two to three months after discontinuation of adrenocortical hormone therapy. Sudden stress, such as surgery or trauma, can produce a subacute form of adrenal crisis in these patients. SEE: *Addison's disease; Waterhouse-Friderichsen syndrome.*

adrenalectomy (ăd-rē"năl-ĕk'tō-mē) [L. *ad,* to, + *ren,* kidney, + Gr. *ektome,* excision]. Excision of an adrenal gland.

adrenal gland. A triangular-shaped body covering the superior surface of each kidney. It is a gland of internal secretion. SYN: *suprarenal gland.* SEE: illus.

EMBRYOLOGY: The adrenal gland is essentially a double organ composed of an outer cortex and an inner medulla. The cortex arises in the embryo from a region of the mesoderm that also gives rise to the gonads, or sex organs. The medulla arises from ectoderm, which also gives rise to the sympathetic nervous system.

ANAT: The entire gland is enclosed in a tough connective tissue capsule from which trabeculae extend into the cortex. The cortex consists of cells arranged into three zones: the outer zona glomerulosa, the middle zona fasciculata, and the inner zona reticularis. The cells are arranged in a cordlike fashion. The medulla consists of chromaffin cells arranged in groups or anastomosing cords. The two adrenal glands are situated retroperitoneally, each embedded in perirenal fat above its respective kidney. In the adult, the average weight is 5 gm., and the range is 4 to 14 gm. The gland usually is heavier in males than in females.

PHYS: The adrenal medulla synthesizes and stores three catecholamines: dopamine,

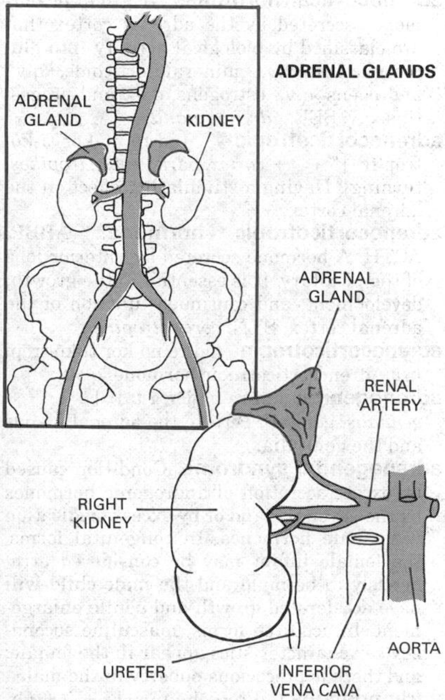

norepinephrine, and epinephrine. Dopamine's chief effects are dilation of systemic arteries, increased cardiac output, and increased flow of blood to the kidneys. The primary action of norepinephrine is to constrict the arterioles and venules with resulting increased resistance to blood flow, elevated blood pressure, and slowing of the heart. Epinephrine constricts vessels in the skin and splanchnic area, dilates vessels in skeletal muscle, increases heart activity, dilates the bronchi by relaxing bronchial musculature, increases level of glucose in the blood by stimulating the production of glucose from glycogen in the liver, increases the amount of fatty acid in the blood, and diminishes activity of the gastrointestinal system. The three catecholamines are also produced in other parts of the body.

The adrenal medulla is under the control of the sympathetic nervous system and functions in conjunction with it. It is intimately related to adjustments of the body in response to emotional states. Anticipatory states tend to bring about the release of norepinephrine. More intense emotional reactions, esp. those in response to extreme stress, tend to increase the secretion of both norepinephrine and epinephrine; epinephrine is important in mobilizing the physiological changes that occur in the "fight or flight" response to emergency situations.

The cortex secretes a group of hormones that vary in quantity and quality. They are all synthesized from cholesterol and contain the basic steroid nucleus perhydrocyclopentanophenanthrene. These compounds are grouped according to their chemical structure and biological activity as follows: glucocorticoids (cortisol, corticosterone), which act principally on carbohydrate metabolism; mineralocorticoids (aldosterone, dehydroepiandrosterone), which affect metabolism of the electrolytes sodium and potassium; androgens (17-ketosteroids), estrogens (estradiol), and progestins (progesterone), all three of which are important in the physiology of reproduction. There is considerable overlap in the biological activity of many of these compounds. SEE: *steroid.*

Almost all body systems are influenced by the action of adrenocortical hormones. Cortisol and cortisone are important in carbohydrate, water, muscle, bone, central nervous system, gastrointestinal, cardiovascular, and hematological metabolism. They are also important anti-inflammatory agents. The principal long-term effect of cortisone and cortisol is catabolic.

The 17-ketosteroids act principally as androgenic and anabolic agents. Aldosterone's principal action is to control sodium and potassium levels in the blood.

PATH: In the medulla, increased secretion of catecholamines occurs when a pheochromocytoma develops. In this condition, the patient develops hypertension, excessive sweating, paroxysmal attacks of blanching or flushing of the skin, tachycardia, headache, anorexia, weight loss, personality changes, signs of increased metabolism, constipation, and postural hypotension. Diagnosis may be confirmed by determining the level of catecholamines or their metabolic end-products in the urine. SEE: *pheochromocytoma.*

In the cortex, when excess secretion of cortical hormones occurs, one of a variety of syndromes may result, depending upon which hormones or group of hormones are increased. If cortisol is increased, the signs of Cushing's syndrome result: obesity with striae and redistribution of fat to produce a "buffalo hump" and "moon face," muscle wasting, osteoporosis, decreased glucose tolerance, atherosclerosis, and systolic hypertension. If the androgens are increased, male sex characteristics are accentuated in the female with voice change, hirsutism, clitoral enlargement, and pronounced muscular development. Baldness and acne will develop in either sex with this condition. It is termed adrenogenital syndrome, q.v.

When aldosterone is elevated, hypertension, low serum potassium, elevated serum sodium, increased urine volume, and, rarely, edema will be present. This is called primary aldosteronism. SEE: *aldosteronism, primary.*

Adrenocortical deficiency may be acute or chronic. The chronic form is called Addison's disease and is characterized by anemia, sluggishness, weakness, weight loss, hypotension, sometimes hypoglycemia, nausea, vomiting, diarrhea, abnormal skin pigmentation, and mental changes. The acute form is called adrenal crisis, q.v. Adrenal crisis due to hemorrhage into the adrenal gland caused by meningococcal infection is called the Waterhouse-Friderichsen syndrome.

Adrenalin (ă-drĕn′ă-lĭn). Trade name for epinephrine, q.v.

adrenaline (ă-drĕn′ă-lēn). British designation for epinephrine, q.v.

adrenalinemia (ă-drĕn″ă-lĭn-ē′mē-ă) [L. *ad,* to, + *ren,* kidney, + Gr. *haima,* blood]. Epinephrine in the blood.

adrenalinuria (ă-drĕn″ă-lĭn-ū′rē-ă) [″ + ″ + Gr. *ouron,* urine]. Epinephrine in the urine.

adrenalism (ă-drĕn′ăl-ĭzm). Illness caused by abnormal function of adrenal glands.

adrenalitis (ă-drē″năl-ī′tĭs) [″ + *ren,* kidney, + Gr. *itis,* inflammation]. Inflammation of the adrenal glands. SYN: *adrenitis.*

adrenalopathy (ă-drē″năl-ŏp′ă-thē) [″ + ″ + Gr. *pathos,* disease]. Disease of the adrenal gland.

adrenarche (ăd″rĕn-ăr′kē) [″ + ″ + Gr. *arkhe,* beginning]. Changes that occur at puberty resulting from effects of increased secretion of adrenocortical hormone. SEE: *menarche; pubarche.*

adrenergic (ăd-rĕn-ĕr′jĭk) [″ + ″ + Gr. *ergon,* work]. Term applied to nerve fibers that, when stimulated, release epinephrine at their endings. Includes nearly all sympathetic postganglionic fibers except those innervating sweat glands.

adrenergic neuron-blocking agents. Substances that inhibit transmission of sympathetic nerve stimuli regardless of whether alpha- or beta-adrenergic receptors are involved. SEE: *alpha-adrenergic receptor; beta-adrenergic receptor.*

adrenitis (ăd″rē-nī′tĭs) [″ + ″ + Gr. *itis,* inflammation]. Inflammation of the adrenal glands. SYN: *adrenalitis.*

adrenoceptive (ă-drē″nō-sĕp′tĭv) [″ + ″ + *recipere,* to receive]. Concerning the sites in organs or tissues that are acted upon by adrenergic transmitters.

adrenochrome (ăd″rē′nō-krōm) [″ + ″ + Gr. *chroma,* color]. A red pigment obtained by oxidation of epinephrine.

adrenocortical (ăd-rē″nō-kor′tĭ-kăl). Pert. to the adrenal cortex.

adrenocortical hormones. A group of hormones secreted by the adrenal cortex that are classified by biological activity into glucocorticoids, q.v., mineralocorticoids, q.v., androgens, q.v., estrogens, q.v., and progestins, q.v. SEE: *adrenal gland.*

adrenocorticotropic (ăd-rē″nō-kor″tĭ-kō-trŏp′ĭk) [″ + ″ + *cortex,* bark, + Gr. *tropikos,* turning]. Having a stimulating effect on the adrenal cortex.

adrenocorticotropic hormone. ABBR: ACTH. A hormone secreted by anterior lobe of the pituitary. It is essential to the growth, development, and continued function of the adrenal cortex. SYN: *corticotropin.*

adrenocorticotropin (ăd-rē″nō-kor″tĭ-kō-trŏp′ĭn). Adrenocorticotropic hormone, q.v.

adrenogenital (ăd-rē-nō-jĕn′ĭ-tăl) [″ + ″ + *genitalis,* genital]. Pert. to the adrenal glands and the genitalia.

adrenogenital syndrome. Condition caused by excess secretion of androgenic hormones by the adrenal gland or by excess medication with male hormones. In congenital forms, the female infant may be considered erroneously to be male and the male child will have accelerated growth and penile enlargement. In acquired forms, masculine secondary sex characteristics appear in the female; and there is precocious puberty in the male.

adrenogenous (ăd″rĕn-ŏj′ĕ-nŭs) [″ + ″ + Gr. *gennan,* to produce]. Originating in or produced by the adrenal gland.

adrenoleukodystrophy (ă-drē″nō-loo″kō-dĭs′trō-fē) [″ + ″ + Gr. *leukos,* white, + *dys,* bad, + *trephein,* to nourish]. A hereditary disease, transmitted as a sex-linked recessive trait, of children. There is an abnormality of the white matter of the brain and atrophy of the adrenal glands. The mental and physical deterioration progresses to dementia, aphasia, apraxia, dysarthria, and blindness. There is no treatment, except symptomatic.

adrenolytic (ăd″rĕn-ō-lĭt′ĭk) [L. *ad,* to, + *ren,* kidney, + Gr. *lysis,* a loosening]. Preventing or inhibiting the activity of adrenergic nerves. Interfering with the response of epinephrine.

adrenomegaly (ăd-rĕn″ō-mĕg′ă-lē) [″ + ″ + Gr. *megas,* large]. Enlarged adrenal gland(s).

adrenomimetic (ă-drē″nō-mĭ-mĕt′ĭk) [″ + ″ + Gr. *mimetikos,* imitating]. Sympathicomimetic, q.v.

adrenopathy (ăd″rĕn-ŏp′ă-thē) [″ + ″ + Gr. *pathos,* disease]. Any disease of the adrenal glands.

adrenopause (ăd-rĕn′ō-pawz) [″ + ″ + Gr. *pausis,* cessation]. A hypothetical age at which adrenal gland activity ceases.

adrenoprival (ăd-rĕn′ō-prī″văl) [″ + ″ + *privare,* to deprive]. Pert. to or characterized by deprivation of the function of the adrenal glands.

adrenosterone (ăd″rē-nŏs′tē-rōn). An androgenic hormone secreted by the adrenal cortex.

adrenotoxin (ăd-rē″nō-tŏk′sĭn) [″ + ″ + *toxicum,* poison]. A substance toxic to the adrenal glands.

adrenotropic (ăd-rē″nō-trŏp′ĭk) [″ + ″ + Gr. *tropikos,* turning]. Nourishing or stimulating to the adrenal glands with reference esp. to hormones that stimulate function of the adrenal glands.

ADS. *antidiuretic substance.*

adsorbate (ăd-sor′bāt). Anything that is adsorbed.

adsorbent (ăd-sor′bĕnt). A substance that leads readily to adsorption, such as activated charcoal or magnesia.

adsorption (ăd-sorp′shŭn) [L. *ad,* to, + *sorbere,* to suck in]. Adhesion by a gas or liquid to the surface of a solid.

adsternal (ăd-stĕr′năl) [″ + Gr. *sternon,* chest]. Near or toward the sternum.

adterminal (ăd-tĕr′mĭ-năl) [″ + *terminus,* boundary]. Toward extremity of any structure, as end of nerve or muscle.

adtorsion (ăd-tor′shŭn) [″ + *torsio,* twisted]. Convergent squint; inward rotation of both eyes.

adult (ă-dŭlt′) [L. *adultus,* grown up]. The fully grown and mature organism.

adulteration (ă-dŭl″tĕr-ā′shŭn) [L. *adulterare,* to pollute]. The addition or substitution of an impure or weaker, and usually cheaper, substance in a formulation or product.

adult respiratory distress syndrome (ARDS). A form of restrictive lung disease due to abnormal permeability of either the pulmonary capillaries or the alveolar epithelium. The condition is often found in patients whose lungs were initially normal but who have had some severe or systemic illness. Clinically, there is acute respiratory failure with pulmonary edema, hemorrhage into the lung tissue, hyaline membranes, and pulmonary fibrosis. The death rate is approx. 50%.

TREATMENT: Vigorous efforts to maintain the exchange of oxygen. This is done by using assisted ventilation and oxygen. Antibiotics appropriate to the infecting organism.

advance (ăd-văns′) [Fr. *avancer,* to set forth]. To carry out the surgical procedure of advancement, q.v.

advancement (ăd-văns′mĕnt) [Fr. *avancer,* to set forth]. Operation to remedy strabismus, by which the ocular muscle is severed and then attached at a point further removed from its origin.

a., capsular. Attachment of capsule of Tenon in front of its normal position.

adventitia (ăd″vĕn-tĭsh′ē-ă) [L. *adventicius,* coming from abroad]. The outermost covering of a structure or organ, such as the tunica adventitia, or outer coat of an artery.

adventitious (ăd″vĕn-tĭsh′ŭs). 1. Acquired; accidental. 2. Arising sporadically. 3. Pert. to adventitia.

adverse effects. Adverse reactions, q.v.

adverse reactions. In pharmacology and therapeutics, the development of undesired side effects or toxicity caused by the administration of drugs. Onset of such reactions may be sudden or take days to develop. Early detection by use of laboratory tests is sometimes possible in the case of drugs that might adversely affect the blood-forming organs, the liver, or kidneys. It is important that all health care personnel be alert to the possibility of a patient's developing an adverse reaction to the drug or drugs administered. SYN: *adverse effects; drug reactions.* SEE: *Drug Interactions* in *Appendix.*

adynamia (ăd″ĭ-nā′mē-ă) [Gr. *a-,* not, + *dynamis,* strength]. Weakness or loss of strength, esp. due to muscular or cerebellar disease. SYN: *asthenia; debility.*

adynamic (ăd″ĭ-năm′ĭk, ā-dī-năm′ĭk). Pert. to adynamia.

adynamic ileus. Intestinal obstruction resulting from lack of intestinal motility. This causes abdominal distention and interferes with postsurgical recovery, particularly from abdominal surgery.

A.E. *above elbow;* term used to refer to the site of amputation of an upper extremity.

Aedes (ā-ē′dēs) [Gr. *aedes,* unpleasant]. A genus of mosquitoes belonging to the family Culicidae. Many species are troublesome pests and some are transmitters of disease.

A. aegypti. A species of Aedes that transmits yellow fever and dengue.

aeluropsis (ē″lū-rŏp′sĭs) [Gr. *ailouros,* cat, + *opsis,* vision]. Condition in which the eye or palpebral fissure is slanting and narrow.

aer- (ā′ĕr) [Gr. *aer,* air]. Combining form indicating relationship to gas or air.

aerated (ā′ĕr-ā-tĕd). Containing air or gas.

aeration (ā″ĕr-ā′shŭn). 1. Act of airing. 2. Process whereby carbon dioxide is exchanged for oxygen in blood in the lungs. 3. Saturation or charging of a fluid with gases.

aerendocardia (ā-ĕr-ĕn″dō-kăr′dē-ă) [″ + *endon,* in, + *kardia,* heart]. Bubble of air in the blood within the heart.

aerenterectasia (ā″ĕr-ĕn-tĕr-ĕk-tā′zē-ă) [″ + *enteron,* intestine, + *ektasis,* stretching out]. Distention of intestine with gas.

aeriform (ā′ĕr-ĭ-form) [″ + L. *forma,* shape]. Airlike; gaseous.

aero- (ā′ĕr-ō). Combining form indicating relationship to air or gas.

Aerobacter (ā″ĕr-ō-băk′tĕr) [″ + *bakterion,* little rod]. A genus of aerobic, non-spore-bearing, gram-negative bacilli of the family Enterobacteriaceae.

A. aerogenes. Enterobacter aerogenes, q.v.

aerobe (ā'ĕr-ōb) [" + *bios,* life]. (pl. *aerobes*) A microorganism that is able to live and grow in the presence of oxygen.

a., facultative. A microorganism that prefers an environment devoid of oxygen but has adapted so that it can live and grow in the presence of oxygen.

a., obligate. A microorganism that can live and grow only in the presence of oxygen.

aerobic (ā-ĕr-ō'bĭk). 1. Living only in the presence of oxygen. 2. Concerning an organism living only in the presence of oxygen.

aerobic exercise. Exercise during which the energy needed is supplied by the oxygen inspired. Aerobic exercise is required for sustained periods of hard work and vigorous athletic activity. Opposite of anaerobic exercise, q.v.

aerobion (ā"ĕr-ō'bē-ŏn). Aerobe, q.v.

aerobiosis (ā"ĕr-ō-bī-ō'sĭs) [" + *biosis,* mode of living]. Living in an atmosphere containing oxygen.

aerocele (ā'ĕr-ō-sēl) [" + *kele,* tumor]. Distention of a cavity with gas.

aerocolpos (ā"er-ō-kŏl'pŏs) [" + *kolpos,* vagina]. Distention of the vagina with air.

aerocoly (ā"ĕr-ŏk'ō-lē) [" + *kolon,* colon]. Distention of colon with gas.

aerocystoscopy (ā"ĕr-o-sĭs-tŏs'kō-pē) [" + *kystis,* bladder, + *skopein,* to view]. Examination with a cystoscope of the bladder distended by air.

aerodermectasia (ā"ĕr-o-der"mĕk-tā'zē-ă) [Gr. *aer,* air, + *derma,* skin, + *ektasis,* stretching out]. Subcutaneous emphysema.

aerodontalgia (ā"ĕr-o-dŏnt-ăl'jē-ă) [" + *odous,* tooth, + *algos,* pain]. Pain in the teeth resulting from change in atmospheric pressure.

aerodontia (ā"ĕr-ō-dŏn'shē-ă). Branch of dentistry concerned with the effect of changes in atmospheric pressure on the teeth.

aerodynamics (ā"ĕr-ō-dī-năm'ĭks) [" + *dynamis,* force]. Science of air or gases in motion.

aeroembolism (ā"ĕr-ō-ĕm'bō-lĭzm) [" + *embolos,* plug, + *-ismos,* condition]. A condition in which nitrogen bubbles form in fluids and tissues of body during rapid ascent to high altitudes.

SYM: Boring, gnawing pain in joints; itching of skin and eyelids; unconsciousness; convulsions; paralysis. Symptoms are relieved by recompression, i.e., return to lower altitudes. Even though oxygen by mask may be available, ascents above 25,000 feet should be avoided except in planes with pressurized cabins. SEE: *bends; caisson disease.*

aeroemphysema (ā"ĕr-ō-ĕm-fĭ-zē'ma) [" + *emphysema,* an inflation]. Aeroembolism, q.v.

aerogen (ā'ĕr-o-jĕn") [" + *gennan,* to produce]. A gas-forming microorganism.

aerogenesis (ā"ĕr-ō-jĕn'ĕ-sĭs) [" + *genesis,* production]. Formation of gas.

aerogenic (ā"ĕr-ō-jĕn'ĭk). Gas forming.

aerogenous (ā"ĕr-ŏj'ĕn-ŭs). Gas forming.

aerogram (ā'ĕr-ō-grăm") [" + *gramma,* mark]. Roentgenogram of an organ after it has been inflated or filled with air or gas.

aerohydrotherapy [" + *hydor,* water, + *therapeia,* treatment]. Treatment by application of air and water.

aeromedical transportation. Air transportation of patients from a primary treatment area to a regional medical center or emergency hospital.

aerometer (ā-ĕr-ŏm'ĕ-tĕr) [" + *metron,* measure]. Device for measuring density of gases.

Aeromonas (ā"ĕr-ō-mō'năs). Genus of bacteria found in natural water sources and soil. It is a gram-negative non-spore-forming motile bacillus. Aeromonads are commonly pathogenic for cold-blooded marine animals and rarely for man.

A. hydrophilia. A type of Aeromonas that has been found to be pathogenic for man. Organisms are sensitive to gentamicin, tetracycline, kanamycin, chloramphenicol, and sodium cephalothin.

aeroneurosis (ā"ĕr-ō-nū-rō'sĭs) [Gr. *aer,* air, + *neuron,* nerve, + *osis,* condition]. A chronic functional nervous disorder affecting aviators, characterized by gastric distress, nervous irritability, insomnia, emotional instability, and increased motor activity.

aeropathy (ā-ĕr-ŏp'ă-thē) [" + *pathos,* suffering]. Morbid condition caused by a marked change in atmospheric pressure, such as mountain fever, q.v., or caisson disease, q.v.

aeroperitoneum, aeroperitonia (ā"ĕr-ō-pĕr"ĭ-tō-nē'ŭm, -tō'nē-ă) [" + *peritonaion,* peritoneum]. Distention of peritoneal cavity with gas.

aerophagia, aerophagy (ā"ĕr-ō-fā'jē-ă, ā"ĕr-ŏf'ă-jē) [" + *phagein,* to eat]. Swallowing of air.

aerophilic, aerophilous (ā"ĕr-ō-fĭl'ĭk, -of'ĭ-lŭs) [" + *philein,* to love]. Requiring air for growth and development. SYN: *aerobic.*

aerophobia (ā-ĕr-ō-fō'bē-ă) [" + *phobos,* fear]. Morbid fear of a draft or of fresh air.

aerophore (ā'ĕr-ō-for) [" + *phoros,* bearing]. A portable apparatus for inflating the lungs of stillborn or asphyxiated infants.

aerophyte (ā'ĕr-ō-fīt) [" + *phyton,* plant]. A plant or vegetative organism that derives its sustenance from air.

aeropiesotherapy (ā"ĕr-ō-pī-ē"sō-thĕr'ă-pē) [" + *piesis,* pressure, + *therapeia,* treatment]. Therapeutic use of air at either increased or decreased barometric pressure. SEE: *decompression chamber; hyperbaric oxygen.*

aeroplethysmograph (ā″ĕr-ō-plĕ-thĭz′mō-grăf) [″ + *plethysmos,* enlargement, + *graphein,* to write]. Instrument for recording respiratory volume.

aeroscope (ā″ĕr-ō-skōp′) [″ + *skopein,* to view]. Device for examining visible particles in the air.

aerosinusitis (ā″ĕr-ō-sī″nŭs-ī′tĭs) [″ + L. *sinus,* a hollow, + Gr. *itis,* inflammation]. Chronic inflammation of nasal sinuses due to changes in atmospheric pressure.

aerosis (ā″ĕr-ō′sĭs) [″ + *osis,* condition]. Accumulation of gas in tissues.

aerosol (ā′ĕr-ō-sōl) [″ + L. *solutio,* solution]. A colloidal solution that is dispensed in the form of a mist.

aerosolization (ā″ĕr-ō-sŏl″ĭ-zā′shŭn). Producing an aerosol.

aerosol therapy. The inhalation of aerosolized medicines in the treatment of pulmonary conditions such as asthma, bronchitis, and emphysema. SEE: *inhalation therapy.*

aerospace medicine. The branch of medicine concerned with the physiologic, pathologic, and psychologic problems man encounters in the environment of space.

Aerosporin (ā″ĕr-ō-spō′rĭn). Trade name for polymyxin B sulfate. SEE: *polymyxin.*

aerotaxis (ā″ĕr-ō-tăk′sĭs) [Gr. *aer,* air, + *taxis,* arrangement]. Movement of organisms away from or toward air, said of aerobic and anaerobic bacteria.

aerotherapy (ā′ĕr-ō-thĕr″ă-pē) [″ + *therapeia,* treatment]. The use of air in the treatment of disease, utilizing changes in composition and density. SEE: *aeropiesotherapy; decompression chamber; hyperbaric oxygen.*

aerothermotherapy (ā″ĕr-ō-thĕr″mō-thĕr′ă-pē) [″ + *thermos,* heat, + *therapeia,* treatment]. Therapeutic use of hot air.

aerothorax (ā″ĕr-ō-thō′răks) [″ + *thorax,* chest]. Pneumothorax, q.v.

aerotitis (ā-ĕr-ō-tī′tĭs) [″ + *ot-,* ear, + *itis,* inflammation]. Inflammation of the ear, esp. the middle ear, due to failure of the eustachian tube to remain open during sudden changes in barometric pressure, as may occur while flying, diving, or working in a pressure chamber. SYN: *barotitis.*

aerotropism (ā-ĕr-ŏt′rō-pĭzm) [″ + *trope,* a turn, + *-ismos,* condition]. The tendency of organisms, esp. bacteria and protozoa, to move toward (positive aerotropism) or away from (negative aerotropism) air.

aerourethroscope (ā″ĕr-ō-ū″rē′thrō-skōp″) [″ + *ourethra,* urethra, + *skopein,* to view]. An apparatus for visual examination of the urethra after dilatation by air.

aerourethroscopy (ā″ĕr-ō-ū″rē-thrŏs′kō-pē). Visual examination of the urethra when distended with air.

Aesculapius (ĕs″kū-lā′pē-ŭs). The Roman name for the god of medicine; son of Apollo and the nymph Coronis.

A., staff of. A staff or crude stick with a snake wound around it. Snakes were sacred to Aesculapius because it was believed that they had the power to renew their youth by shedding their old skin and growing a new one. The staff of Aesculapius is used to signify the art of healing and is used by many medical organizations. SEE: illus.; *caduceus.*

aesthetics (ĕs-thĕt′ĭks) [Gr. *aisthesis,* sensation]. The philosophy or the theory of beauty and the fine arts. These concepts are especially important in dental restorations and in plastic and cosmetic surgery. Also spelled esthetics.

afebrile (ă-fēb′rĭl) [Gr. *a-,* not, + L. *febris,* fever]. Without fever.

affect (ăf′fĕkt) [L. *affectus,* exerting influence on]. In psychology, the emotional reactions associated with an experience.

affection (ă-fĕk′shŭn). 1. Love, feeling. 2. Physical or mental disease.

affective (ă-fĕk′tĭv). Pert. to an emotion or mental state.

affective disorders. A group of disorders characterized by a disturbance of mood, accompanied by a full or partial manic or depressive syndrome that is not caused by any other physical or mental disorder.

afferent (ăf′ĕr-ĕnt) [L. *ad,* to, + *ferre,* to bear]. Carrying impulses toward a center, as when a sensory nerve carries a message toward the brain; also said of certain veins and lymphatics. Opposite of efferent, q.v.

afferent nerves. Nerves that transmit impulses from the peripheral toward the central nervous system.

affiliation (ă-fĭl-ē-ā′shŭn) [L. *affiliare,* to take to oneself as a son]. 1. Membership in a larger organization. 2. Association. In nursing education, the administrative association of two hospitals or schools of nursing. This enables nurses to obtain specialized training and experience that might not otherwise be available to them.

affinity (ă-fĭn′ĭ-tē) [L. *affinis,* neighboring]. Attraction.

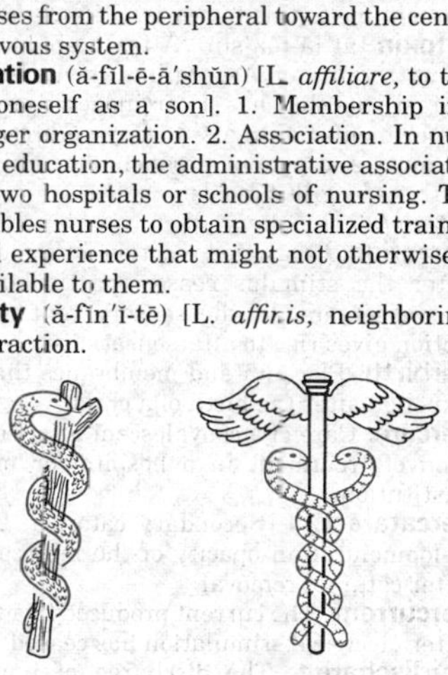

STAFF OF AESCULAPIUS CADUCEUS

a., chemical. Force causing certain atoms to combine with others to form molecules. SEE: *chemoreceptor.*

a., elective. Force causing a substance to elect one substance rather than another with which to unite.

a., selective. A., elective, q.v.

afflux (ăf'lŭks) [L. *ad,* to, + *fluere,* to flow]. Rush of blood to a part.

A-fiber. A heavily medullated, fast-conducting nerve fiber.

afibrinogenemia (ă-fī"brĭn-ō-jĕ-nē'mē-ă) [Gr. *a-,* not, + L. *fibra,* fiber, + Gr. *gennan,* to produce, + *haima,* blood]. A rare blood disease characterized by the absence or decrease of fibrinogen in the blood plasma so that the blood is incoagulable; may be congenital or acquired. (The term "hypofibrinogenemia" more accurately describes the disease process.) The acquired type is due to one of several causes that can reduce the plasma concentration of fibrinogen. This has been observed in severe trauma and burns; following extensive surgery; in obstetric complications of abruptio placentae or retention of a dead fetus; in neoplastic disease; in hepatic cirrhosis; in leukemia; in sarcoidosis; and in polycythemia vera.

TREATMENT: The clinical picture may develop suddenly. Administration of whole fresh blood and fibrinogen may prevent death from hemorrhage.

aflatoxicosis (ăf"lă-tŏk"sĭ-kō'sĭs). Poisoning caused by ingestion of peanuts or peanut products contaminated with Aspergillus flavus or other A. strains that produce aflatoxin, q.v. Farm animals and humans are susceptible to this toxicosis. SYN: *x-disease.*

aflatoxin (ăf"lă-tŏk'sĭn). A toxin produced by some strains of Aspergillus flavus and A. parasiticus that has a carcinogenic effect in experimental animals. It may be present in peanuts and peanut products contaminated with Aspergillus molds.

AFP. *alpha-fetoprotein.*

afteraction. Continued reaction for some time after the stimulus ceases, particularly in nerve centers. In the sensory centers this action gives rise to aftersensations.

afterbirth. Placenta and membranes that are expelled after the birth of a child.

aftercare. Care of a convalescent after conclusion of treatment in a hospital or mental institution.

aftercataract. 1. Secondary cataract. 2. Development of an opacity of the lens capsule after cataract removal.

aftercurrent. The current produced in a tissue after electrical stimulation has ceased.

afterdischarge. The discharge of impulses from a reflex center after stimulation of the receptor has ceased. Results in prolongation of response.

aftereffect. A response occurring sometime after the original stimulus or condition has produced its primary effect.

afterhearing. Persistence of sensation of sound after the stimulus causing the sound has ceased.

afterimage. Image that persists subjectively after the cessation of stimulus. If colors are same as object it is called positive; negative if complementary colors are seen. In the former case, the image is seen in its natural bright colors without any alteration; in the latter, the bright parts become dark, while dark parts are light.

afterimpression. Aftersensation, q.v.

aftermovement. Persistent and spontaneous contraction of a muscle after a strong contraction against resistance has ceased. This is easily demonstrated by standing and forcibly pushing the arm against a wall while standing with the frontal plane perpendicular to the wall. When this is stopped and you have moved away from the wall, the arm will involuntarily adduct and be elevated. SYN: *Kohnstamm's phenomenon.*

afterpains. Uterine cramps due to contraction of uterus, occurring during first few days after childbirth; commonly seen in multiparae. Pains more severe during nursing. The pains rarely last longer than 48 hours postpartum.

TREATMENT: Analgesics, but do not use aspirin if there is a bleeding tendency. The earlier given, the less needed.

afterperception. Perception of a sensation after cessation of stimulus.

afterpotential wave. The wave produced after the action potential wave passes along a nerve. On the recording of the electrical activity, it will be either a negative or positive wave smaller than the main spike.

aftersensation. Sensation persisting after stimulus causing it has ceased.

aftertaste. Persistence of gustatory sensations after cessation of stimulus.

aftertreatment. Secondary treatment; that following primary treatment regimen. SEE: *aftercare.*

aftervision. Afterimage, q.v.

Ag [L. *argentum*]. Chem. symb. for silver.

against medical advice. ABBR: a.m.a. Said of a patient's decision to discontinue treatment or hospitalization even though advised by competent professional personnel to continue.

agalactia (ăg"ă-lăk'shē-ă) [Gr. *a-,* not, + *gala,* milk]. Absence of milk secretion after childbirth.

agalorrhea (ă-găl"ō-rē'ă) [" + " + *rhoia,* flow]. Arrest of milk flow.

agamic (ă-găm'ĭk) [" + *gamos,* marriage]. 1.

Reproducing asexually. 2. Asexual.

agammaglobulinemia (ā-găm″ă-glŏb″ū-lĭn-ē′mē-ă) [″ + *gamma globulin* + Gr. *haima,* blood]. A rare disease characterized by the virtual absence of gamma globulin from the blood plasma with resulting loss of the ability to produce immune antibodies, and the absence of natural blood group isoantibodies from the serum; may be congenital or acquired. The sex-linked congenital form is inherited like hemophilia as a sex-linked recessive characteristic, and occurs only in male children. The non-sex-linked form occurs as an autosomal dominant characteristic. This latter form is quite rare.

agamogenesis (ăg″ă-mō-jĕn′ĕ-sĭs) [″ + *gamos,* marriage, + *genesis,* development]. 1. Asexual reproduction. 2. Parthenogenesis, q.v.

agar (ā′găr, ăg′ăr) [Malay, gelatin]. 1. Seaweed belonging to the genus Gelideum. The source of agar-agar. 2. A dried mucilaginous product obtained from certain species of algae, especially Gelideum. It is unaffected by bacterial enzymes, hence widely used as a solidifying agent for bacterial culture media; also used as a laxative because of its great increase in bulk upon absorption of water. 3. A culture medium containing agar.

agar-agar. Agar (defs. 2 and 3), q.v.

agaric (ă-găr′ĭk) [Gr. *agarikon,* a sort of fungus]. Mushroom, esp. species of the genus Agaricus.

agastria (ă-găs′trē-ă) [Gr. *a-,* not, + *gaster,* stomach]. Absence of the stomach.

agastric (ă-găst′rĭk). Lacking an alimentary canal, as in certain animals such as tapeworms.

agathanasia (ăg″ă-thă-nā′zē-ă) [Gr. *aganthos,* good, + *thanatus,* death]. The concept of death with dignity. It is concerned with omitting actions and discontinuing procedures that maintain life beyond reasonable limits. Therapy to relieve excessive pain, even though such action might shorten the terminally ill patient's life, would be embodied in this concept.

AgCl. Chem. symb. for silver chloride.

age [Fr. *age,* L. *aetas*]. 1. The time from birth to the present for a living individual as measured in units of time. 2. A particular period of life, as middle age or old age. 3. To grow old. 4. In psychology, the degree of development of an individual expressed in terms of the age of an average individual of comparable development or accomplishment.

a., achievement. ABBR: A.A. The age of a person with regard to level of acquired learning, determined by a proficiency test and expressed in terms of the chronological age of the average person showing the same level of attainment.

a., anatomical. An estimate of age as judged by the stage of development or deterioration of the body or tissue as compared with persons or tissues of known age.

a., bone. An estimate of biological age based on x-ray studies of the stage of development of ossification centers of the long bones of the extremities. SEE: *epiphysis.*

a., chronological. ABBR: C.A. Age as determined by years of existence.

a., developmental. 1. Age as judged by anatomical development. 2. Holistically, the degree of development of all aspects of the individual, i.e., mental, physical, and social.

a., emotional. Judgment of age with respect to the stage of emotional development.

a., gestational. Age of embryo or fetus as timed from the date of onset of the last menstrual period.

a., menarcheal. Elapsed time expressed in years from menarche.

a., mental. ABBR: M.A. The age of a person with regard to mental ability, determined by a series of mental tests devised by Binet and expressed in terms of the chronological age of the average person showing the same level of attainment.

a., physiological. Age as determined by body function.

age, words pert. to: adolescence; climacteric; geriatrics; maturation; menarche; menopause; puberty; senility.

aged (ājd′, ā′jĕd). 1. To have grown older or more mature. 2. Persons who have grown old. SEE: *aging.*

agenesia, agenesis (ă″jĕn-ē′sē-ă, ā-jĕn′ĕ-sĭs) [Gr. *a-,* not, + *genesis,* production]. 1. Failure of an organ or part to develop or grow. 2. Lack of potency.

agenitalism (ă-jĕn′ĭ-tăl-ĭzm) [″ + L. *genitalis,* genital, + Gr. *-ismos,* condition]. Absence of genitals.

agenosomia (ă-jĕn″ō-sō′mē-ă) [″ + *gennan,* to produce, + *soma,* body]. Condition of fetus in which the genitals are absent or poorly developed and the intestines protrude from an incompletely developed abdominal wall.

agent (ā′jĕnt) [L. *agere,* to do]. Something that causes an effect. Thus, bacteria that cause disease are said to be agents of the specific diseases they cause. A medicine would be classed as a therapeutic agent.

agent orange. A chemical defoliant mixture that contains the toxic substance dioxin. It was used in the Vietnam war.

age of consent. The age at which a minor may legally engage in voluntary sexual intercourse. Varies among states, usually between 13 and 18 years old.

agerasia (ā-jĕr-ā′sē-ă) [Gr. *a-,* not, + *geras,* old age]. Healthy, vigorous old age; youthful appearance of an old person.

ageusia, ageustia (ă-gū′sē-ă, ă-goos′tē-ă) [" + *geusis,* taste]. Absence, partial loss, or impairment of the sense of taste. SEE: *dysgeusia; hypergeusia; hypogeusia.*

ETIOL: May be due to disease of the chorda tympani or of the gustatory fibers; excessive use of condiments; effect of certain drugs; aging; or lesions involving sensory pathways or taste centers in the brain.

a., central. Ageusia due to a cerebral lesion.

a., conduction. Ageusia due to a lesion involving sensory nerves of taste.

a., peripheral. Ageusia due to a disorder of taste buds of mucous membrane of tongue.

agger (ăj′ĕr) [L.]. (pl. *aggeres*) A small elevation or eminence; a mound.

a. nasi. The ridge of the nose.

agglomerate (ă-glŏm′ĕ-rāt) [L. *ad,* to, + *glomerare,* to wind into a ball]. To congregate; to form a mass.

agglutinable (ă-gloo′tĭ-nă-bl) [L. *agglutinans,* gluing]. Capable of agglutination.

agglutinant (ă-gloo′tĭ-nănt). 1. Substance causing adhesion. 2. Causing union by adhesion, as in healing of a wound. 3. An antibody produced in the body in response to stimulation by an antigen (agglutinogen). SYN: *agglutinin.*

agglutination (ă-gloo″tĭ-nā′shŭn). 1. Clumping together, as of blood corpuscles when incompatible bloods are mixed. 2. Adhesion of surfaces of a wound.

agglutinative (ă-gloo′tĭ-nā″tĭv). Causing or capable of causing agglutination.

agglutinin (ă-gloo′tĭ-nĭn) [L. *agglutinans,* gluing]. An antibody that causes agglutination; more specifically a substance present in normal or immune serum capable of causing agglutination or clumping of specific antigens (bacteria or cells). SEE: *agglutinogen; blood groups; blood typing; isoagglutinin.*

a., anti-Rh. An agglutinin normally absent in human plasma but sometimes produced in Rh-negative mothers bearing an Rh-positive fetus or in Rh-negative individuals who have received one or more transfusions of Rh-positive blood.

a., chief. A., major, q.v.

a., cold. An agglutinin that acts only at low temperatures; present in the serum of patients with atypical pneumonia and in certain blood diseases.

a., flagellar. An agglutinin that acts only on the flagella of an organism. SYN: *a., H.*

a., group. An agglutinin that has a specific action on one species, but will agglutinate closely related species as well.

a., H. A., flagellar, q.v.

a., haupt. A., major, q.v.

a., immune. Agglutinin causing immunity, found in the blood because of either recovery from the disease or having been inoculated with the microorganism.

a., major. The immune agglutinin of which there is the largest concentration in the blood. SYN: *a., chief.*

a., minor. An immune agglutinin present in the blood in lesser concentration than the major agglutinin. SYN: *a., partial.*

a., nonspecific. Agglutinin that is found in individuals who have had a certain disease and that agglutinates organisms having no relation to the disease. Utilized in certain diagnostic tests.

a., O. An agglutinin that acts on the bodies of organisms, in contrast to flagellar agglutinins. SYN: *a., somatic.*

a., partial. A., minor, q.v.

a., somatic. A., O, q.v.

agglutinogen (ă-gloo-tĭn′ō-jĕn) [L. *agglutinans,* gluing, + Gr. *gennan,* to produce]. 1. A substance that stimulates the development of a specific agglutinin, thereby acting as an antigen. 2. A specific antigen used in agglutination tests. SEE: *blood groups.*

a.'s, A and B. Discovered by Karl Landsteiner in 1901, these two antigenic substances are found in the red blood cells of human beings and react with the alpha (anti-A) and beta (anti-B) isoagglutinins in the blood. The red corpuscles may contain A or B, both A and B, or neither A nor B agglutinogens. The four resulting blood groups are A, B, AB, and O, respectively. Blood groups are inherited according to Mendel's laws, q.v.

a.'s, M and N. These two antigenic substances are found in the red corpuscles of human beings. Anti-M and anti-N agglutinins are rarely found in normal serum. The red blood cells may contain M or N, or both M and N agglutinogens, resulting in blood types M, N, or MN, respectively.

a., Rh. A specific substance called the Rh factor, present in red cells. It was discovered in 1940 by Landsteiner and Wiener, who prepared anti-Rh serum by injecting red cells from Rhesus monkeys into rabbits or other animals. They found that the red cells of 85% of people of the white race will be agglutinated when in contact with anti-Rh. These persons are termed Rh-positive. The remaining 15% whose red cells are not agglutinated by anti-Rh are termed Rh-negative. More than 25 blood factors are known to belong to the Rh system. Their importance in blood typing and blood type incompatibility between mother and fetus makes this blood group system second in importance only to the ABO group.

agglutinogenic, agglutogenic (ă-gloo″tĭ-nō-jen′ĭk, ă-gloo″tō-jĕn′ĭk). Producing agglutinins.

agglutinoid (ă-gloo′tĭn-oyd) [L. *agglutinans,*

gluing, + Gr. *eidos,* resemblance]. An agglutinin that, through the effects of heat, age, chemicals, etc., has lost its ability to agglutinate its specific antigen although its ability to combine with its antigen remains.

agglutinophilic (ă-gloo″tĭn-ō-fĭl′ĭk) [″ + Gr. *philos,* fond]. Readily agglutinating.

agglutinophore (ă-gloo′tĭn-ō-for) [″ + Gr. *pherein,* to bear]. The active agent producing agglutination.

agglutometer (ăg″loo-tŏm′ĕ-tĕr) [″ + Gr. *metron,* measure]. Device to simplify the agglutination or Widal's test without the use of an ordinary microscope.

aggregate (ăg′rē-gāt) [L. *aggregatus,* collect]. 1. Total substances making up a mass. 2. To cluster or come together.

aggregation (ăg″rĕ-gā′shŭn). A clustering or coming together of substances.

a., cell. Clumping together of blood cells, esp. platelets or red cells.

a., familial. A cluster of the same disease in closely related families.

aggression (ă-grĕsh′ŭn) [L. *aggredi,* to approach with hostility]. 1. Angry, hateful, or destructive ideas or behavior. May be justified and real, or unrealistic and the result of disordered mental processes. In some forms of mental illness, aggression may be directed toward the self, and physical damage including suicide may result. 2. Activity performed in a forceful manner.

aging (āj′ĭng). Growing old, maturing. Progressive changes related to the passage of time. There is no precise method for determining the rate or degree of aging.

agitated depression. Depression accompanied by restlessness and increased psychomotor activity.

agitation (ăj″ĭ-tā′shŭn) [L. *agitare,* to drive]. 1. Excessive restlessness, increased mental and physical activity, esp. the latter. 2. Tremor. 3. Shaking of a container so that the contents are rapidly moved and mixed.

agitographia (ăj″ĭ-tō-grăf′ē-ă) [″ + Gr. *graphein,* to write]. Writing with excessive rapidity, with unconscious omission of words, syllables, etc.

agitophasia (ăj″ĭ-tō-fā′zē-ă) [″ + Gr. *phasis,* speech]. Excessive rapidity of speech, with slurring, omission, and distortion of sounds. Also: *agitolalia.*

aglaucopsia, aglaukopsia (ă″glaw-kŏp′sē-ă) [Gr. *a-,* not, + *glaukos,* green, + *opsis,* vision]. Green blindness; color blindness in which there is a defect in the perception of green. SEE: *color blindness.*

aglossia (ă-glŏs′ē-ă) [″ + *glossa,* tongue]. 1. Congenital absence of the tongue. 2. Lack of ability to speak.

aglossostomia (ă″glŏs-ō-stō′mē-ă) [″ + ″ + *stoma,* mouth]. Congenital absence of tongue and mouth opening.

aglutition (ă-gloo-tĭsh′ŭn) [″ + L. *glutire,* to swallow]. Difficulty in swallowing or inability to swallow.

aglycemia (ă″glī-sē′mē-ă) [″ + *glykys,* sweet, + *haima,* blood]. Lack of sugar in the blood.

aglycosuric (ă-glī″kō-sū′rĭk) [″ + ″ + *ouron,* urine]. Free from glycosuria.

agminate(d) (ăg′mĭ-nāt) [L. *agmen,* a crowd]. Aggregate; grouped in clusters.

agminated follicles. Aggregations of solitary follicles or groups of lymph nodes, principally in lower portion of small intestine. SYN: *Peyer's patches.*

agnathia (ăg-nā′thē-ă) [Gr. *a-,* not, + *gnathos,* jaw]. Absence of the lower jaw.

agnea (ăg′nē-ă) [″ + *gnosis,* knowledge]. Inability to recognize objects.

$AgNO_3$. Chem. symb. for silver nitrate.

agnogenic (ăg-nō-jĕn′ĭk) [″ + *gnosis,* knowledge, + *gennan,* to produce]. Of unknown origin or etiology.

agnosia (ăg-nō′zē-ă) [″ + *gnosis,* knowledge]. Loss of comprehension of auditory, visual, or other sensations although the sensory sphere is intact.

a., auditory. Mental inability to interpret sounds.

a., finger. Inability to identify fingers of one's own hands or of others.

a., optic. Mental inability to interpret images that are seen.

a., tactile. Inability to distinguish objects by sense of touch.

-agogue (ă-gŏg) [Gr. *agogos,* leading, inducing]. Suffix meaning a producer or leader.

agonad, agonadal (ă-gō′năd, ă-gŏn′ă-dăl) [Gr. *a-,* not, + *gone,* seed]. Lacking gonads.

agonal (ăg′ō-năl) [Gr. *agon,* a contest]. Rel. to death or agony.

agonist (ăg′ŏn-ĭst). The muscle directly engaged in contraction as distinguished from muscles that have to relax at the same time. Thus, in bending the elbow, the biceps brachii is the agonist and the triceps the antagonist, q.v.

agony (ăg′ō-nē). 1. Extreme mental or physical suffering. 2. Death struggle.

agoraphobia (ăg″ō-ră-fō′bē-ă) [Gr. *agora,* market place, + *phobos,* fear]. Great fear of being alone, or of being in public places from which escape might be difficult. Normal activities that involve being in crowds, or on a busy street or in a crowded store, are avoided. Exposure to these conditions may cause the individual to panic.

-agra [Gr. *agra,* a seizure]. Suffix indicating sudden severe pain.

agraffe (ă-grăf′) [O. Fr. *agrafer,* to hook, fasten]. An appliance for clamping together edges of a wound.

agrammatism (ă-grăm′ă-tĭzm″) [Gr. *agram-*

matos, unlettered, + *-ismos,* condition]. Inability to speak grammatical or intelligible sentences or to arrange words in grammatical sequence.

ETIOL: Cerebral disease.

agranulocyte (ă-grăn′ū-lō-sīt) [Gr. *a-,* not, + L. *granulum,* granule, + Gr. *kytos,* cell]. A nongranular leukocyte.

agranulocytic (ă-grăn-ū-lō-sĭt′ĭk). Pert. to agranulocytosis.

agranulocytosis (ă-grăn″ū-lō-sī-tō′sĭs) [″ + ″ + ″ + *osis,* condition]. An acute disease in which the white blood cell count drops to extremely low levels and neutropenia becomes pronounced. Characterized by high fever, prostration, necrotic ulcerations of the mouth, rectum, and vagina. Some cases are idiopathic; others resulting from drugs or radiation. SYN: *granulocytopenia.*

agranuloplastic (ă-grăn″ū-lō-plăs′tĭk) [″ + L. *granulum,* granule, + Gr. *plastikos,* formative]. Unable to form granular cells.

agranulosis (ă-grăn″ū-lō′sĭs). Agranulocytosis, q.v.

agraphia (ă-grăf′ē-ă) [″ + *graphein,* to write]. Loss of the ability to write. SYN: *logagraphia.* SEE: *anorthography; aphasia, motor.*

a., absolute. Complete inability to write.

a., acoustic. Inability to write words that are heard.

a., amnemonic. Inability to write sentences, although letters or words can be written.

a., atactic. A., absolute, q.v.

a., cerebral. Inability to express thoughts in writing.

a., mental. A., cerebral, q.v.

a., motor. Inability to write due to muscular incoordination.

a., optic. Inability to copy words.

a., verbal. Inability to write words although letters can be written.

agria (ăg′rē-ă) [Gr. *agrios,* wild]. Severe or extensive pustular eruption.

agromania (ăg″rō-mā′nē-ă) [Gr. *agros,* field, + *mania,* frenzy]. Unreasonable desire for solitude or solitudinous wandering. Morbid desire to live in solitude or in the country.

agrypnia (ă-grĭp′nē-ă) [Gr. *agrypnos,* sleepless]. Inability to sleep. SYN: *ahypnia; insomnia.*

agrypnocoma (ă-grĭp″nō-kō′mă) [″ + *koma,* a deep sleep]. Coma in which the individual is partially awake as if in an extreme lethargic state; may be associated with muttering, delirium, and lack of sleep.

agrypnotic (ă″grĭp-nŏt′ĭk). 1. Afflicted with insomnia. 2. Causing wakefulness.

agyria (ă-jī′rē-ă) [Gr. *a-,* not, + *gyros,* circle]. Incompletely developed convolutions of the cerebral cortex.

ague (ā′gū) [Fr. *aigu,* sharp, acute]. Originally used to indicate a chill or fever, esp. if due to malaria. Rarely used except colloquially.

ah. *hypermetropic astigmatism.*

A.H.A. *American Heart Association; American Hospital Association.*

AHF. *antihemophilic factor,* coagulation factor VIII. SEE: *coagulation factors.*

AHG. *antihemophilic globulin,* coagulation factor VIII. SEE: *coagulation factors.*

Ahlfeld's sign (ăl′fĕlts). [Friedrich Ahlfeld, Ger. obstetrician, 1843–1929] Irregular uterine contractions after the third month of pregnancy. It is a presumptive sign of pregnancy.

ahypnia (ă-hĭp′nē-ă) [Gr. *a-,* not, + *hypnos,* sleep]. Insomnia or sleeplessness. SYN: *agrypnia.*

A.I. *aortic insufficiency; artificial insemination; axioincisal.*

aichmophobia (āk″mō-fō′bē-ă) [Gr. *aichme,* point, + *phobos,* fear]. Morbid fear of being touched by pointed objects or fingers.

A.I.D. *Agency for International Development; artificial insemination by donor* (heterologous insemination).

aid (ād). Assistance provided to a person, esp. one who is sick, injured, or troubled. SEE: *first aid.*

a., hearing. A device, usually electronic, that amplifies sound to the level required to enable a hearing-impaired person to hear.

AIDS. *acquired immune deficiency syndrome.*

A.I.H. *artificial insemination by husband* (homologous insemination).

ailment. A mild illness.

ailurophobia (ā-lū″rō-fō′bē-ă) [Gr. *ailouros,* cat, + *phobos,* fear]. Morbid fear of cats.

ainhum (ān′hŭm) [African]. A fissured constriction of unknown origin causing eventual amputation of a digit. Affects usually the fourth or fifth toes and less commonly other digits of the feet or hands. It is predominately a disease of members of dark-skinned races. There is no specific treatment.

air (ār) [Gr. *aer,* air]. The invisible, tasteless, odorless mixture of gases surrounding the Earth. Air at sea level is made up of approx. 21% oxygen, 78% nitrogen, water vapor, carbon dioxide, and traces of ammonia, argon, helium, neon, krypton, xenon, and other rare gases.

a., alveolar. Air in the alveoli; that involved in the pulmonary exchange of gases between air and the blood. Its content is determined by sampling the last portion of a maximal expiration.

a., complemental. Volume of air that can be inspired over and above the tidal air, q.v., by deepest possible inspiration. SYN: *inspiratory reserve volume.*

a., dead space. The volume of air that

fills the respiratory passageways and is not available for exchange of gases with the blood.

a., functional residual. The volume of air left in the lungs at the end of a normal expiration. It is the sum of supplemental air, q.v., and residual air, q.v.

a., liquid. Air liquefied by great pressure. It produces intense cold on evaporation.

a., minimal. The small volume of air trapped in alveoli when lungs collapse with the thorax open; it is impossible to expel, even if lung is removed.

a., reserve. A., supplemental, q.v.

a., residual. The amount remaining in the lungs after the fullest possible expiration. About 1500 cc. in the adult.

a., supplemental. Volume of air that can be expired after a normal expiration by fullest possible expiration. About 1600 cc. in the adult. SYN: *expiratory reserve volume.*

a., tidal. Volume of air that flows in and out of the lungs with each normal respiration; average for adult male is about one pint (500 cc.).

air, words pert. to: "aer-" words; aspiration; atelectasis; expiration; inspiration; respiration; ventilation.

air bed. 1. Large inflated cushion used as a mattress. 2. A special bed that permits the patient actually to float on a cushion of air. SEE: *air-fluidized bed.*

air cell. Air vesicle, q.v.

air conditioning. Use of special equipment to control, esp. to lower, temperature and humidity of the air while ensuring adequate ventilation.

air conduction. The conduction of sound to the inner ear via the pathway provided by the air in the ear canal.

air curtain. A current of air directed around a patient so that air that would normally circulate around and contaminate the patient is blocked by the curtain of air. Used in isolating patients from dust-borne bacteria or allergens.

air cushion. An airtight inflatable cushion.

air embolism [L. *embolismus*]. Obstruction of a blood vessel by an air bubble.

ETIOL: Air may enter postoperatively or during hypodermic injection if syringe is not properly filled. Air should be excluded when giving an intravenous injection.

air flow, laminar. SEE: *laminar air flow.*

air-fluidized bed. A special bed consisting of a mattress filled with approx. 100 billion ceramic spheres that are suspended by a continual flow of warm air at the rate of approx. 40 cubic feet (1.13 cubic meters) per minute. This creates a surface that feels like a liquid, having a specific gravity of 1.3. The patient "floats" on the mattress with only minimal penetration. Because of the even distribution of weight, the bed is particularly useful in treating patients with burns or decubitus ulcers. Nursing care of the patient is greatly simplified because the patient can be moved by fingertip pressure.

air hunger. Shortness of breath marked by rapid, labored breathing. SEE: *dyspnea.*

airplane splint. An appliance usually used on ambulatory patients in the treatment of fractures of the humerus. It takes its name from the elevated (abducted) position in which it holds the arm suspended in air.

air pollution. Contamination of air by noxious substances, as from automobile exhaust, or industrial waste.

air sac. Air vesicle, q.v.

airsickness. Condition of giddiness, nausea, vomiting, headache, and often extreme drowsiness occurring during air flight. SEE: *seasickness.*

air splint. Type of splint used for immobilizing fractured or injured extremities. It is usually an inflatable cylinder, open at both ends, that becomes rigid when it is inflated and thus prevents the part confined in the cylinder from moving.

air swallowing. Voluntary or involuntary swallowing of air. It occurs involuntarily in infants as a result of improper feeding. In adults it occurs in neurasthenia or hysteria or when on a fluid diet. SYN: *aerophagia.*

air vesicle. Pulmonary alveolus; one of the terminal saccules of an alveolar duct where gases are exchanged in respiration.

airway. 1. Natural passageway for air to and from the lungs. 2. A device used to prevent or correct obstructed respiratory passage, esp. during anesthesia.

A.K. *above knee;* term used to refer to the site of amputation of a lower extremity.

akaryocyte (ă-kăr′ē-ō-sīt″) [Gr. *a-*, not, + *karyon,* kernel, + *kytos,* cell]. A non-nucleated cell, such as an erythrocyte.

akaryote (ă-kăr′ē-ōt) [″ + *karyon,* kernel]. Akaryocyte, q.v.

akatamathesia (ă-kăt″ă-mă-thē′zē-ă) [″ + *katamathesis,* understanding]. The mental condition of being unable to understand.

akathisia (ăk″ă-thĭ′zē-ă) [″ + *kathisis,* sitting]. Acathisia, q.v.

akee (ăk′ē, ă-kē′) [Liberian]. The tropical tree Blighia sapida. Ingestion of the unripe fruit can cause severe hypoglycemia. Also spelled ackee.

akembe (ă-kĕm′bē) [African]. An acute disease of natives of Central Africa characterized by bloody vesicles of mucous membranes with consequent melena and hematuria. Etiology is unknown.

akinesia (ă″kĭ-nē′zē-ă) [Gr. *a-*, not, + *kinesis,* movement]. Complete or partial loss of muscle movement. Also spelled acinesia.

a. algera. Akinesia with intense pain caused by any movement.

a. amnestica. Akinesia marked by failure of muscular power due to lack of use.

akinetic (ă″kĭ-nĕt′ĭk). 1. Pert. to akinesia. 2. Rel. to or characterized by amitosis.

Al. Chem. symb. for aluminum (British: aluminium).

-al [L.]. 1. Suffix indicating connection with, as in abdominal, marginal. 2. In chemistry, it indicates an aldehyde.

ala (ā′lă) [L., wing]. (pl. *alae*) 1. An expanded or winglike structure or appendage. 2. Axilla, q.v.

a. auris. Protruding portion of the external ear. SYN: *auricle; pinna.*

a. cerebelli. [NA] Winglike projection of central lobule of cerebellum. SYN: *a. lobuli centralis.*

a. cinerea. Gray triangular prominence on the floor of the fourth ventricle. The autonomic fibers of the vagus nerve arise from the cells of the nucleus of this area. SYN: *triangle of the vagus nerve; trigonum nervi vagi.*

a. cristae galli. [NA] Small projection on each side of the crista galli, q.v., of the ethmoid bone.

a. lobuli centralis. A. cerebelli, q.v.

a. major ossis sphenoidalis. [NA] Greater wing of the sphenoid bone.

a. minor ossis sphenoidalis. [NA] Lesser wing of the sphenoid bone.

a. nasi. [NA] The wing of the nose; broad portion forming the lateral wall of each nostril.

a. of ethmoid. Small projection on each side of the ethmoid bone.

a. of ilium. Broad, upper portion of the iliac bone.

a. of sacrum. Broad projection on each side of the base of the sacrum.

a. vomeris. [NA] Wing of the vomer; projection on each side of the superior border of the vomer.

alacrima (ā-lăk′rĭ-mă) [Gr. *a-*, not, + L. *lacrima,* tear]. Deficiency of or absence of tears.

alalia [″ + *lalein,* to talk]. Loss of ability to speak due to defect or paralysis of the vocal organs. Aphasia, q.v.

ETIOL: Due to organic brain disease or psychoneurosis.

alanine (ăl′ă-nēn). USP. A naturally occurring amino acid, $CH_3CH(NH_2)COOH$. It is classed as being nonessential in human nutrition.

a. aminotransferase. Glutamic-pyruvic transaminase, q.v.

alar (ā′lăr) [L. *ala,* wing]. 1. Pert. to or like a wing. 2. Axillary.

alar artery. Branch of angular artery supplying tissues of ala nasi.

alar cartilage. Cartilage forming the broad lateral wall of each nostril.

alastrim (ă-lăs′trĭm) [Portuguese *alastrar,* to spread]. Mild form of smallpox with sparse rash and low-grade fever. SYN: *variola minor.*

alate (ā′lāt) [L. *ala,* wing]. Winged.

alba [L. *albus,* white]. 1. White. 2. White substance of the brain.

albedo (ăl-bē′dō) [L.]. Whiteness. Reflection of light from a surface.

a. retinae. Retinal edema.

a. unguium. White semilunar area near nail root. SYN: *lunula.*

Albers-Schönberg disease (ăl-bārs-shĕrn′bārg). [Heinrich Ernst Albers-Schönberg, Ger. roentgenologist, 1865–1921] Excessive calcification of bones causing marblelike appearance.

Albert's disease. [Eduard Albert, Austrian surgeon, 1841–1900] Inflammation of the bursae lying over the Achilles tendon. SYN: *achillobursitis.*

albicans [L.]. (pl. *albicantia*) 1. White or whitish. 2. Corpus albicans, q.v.

a., corpus. [NA] A mass of fibrous tissue that replaces the regressing corpus luteum following rupture of the graafian follicle. It forms a white scar that gradually decreases in size and eventually disappears.

albidum (ăl′bĭ-dŭm) [L.]. White.

albiduria [L. *albidus,* white, + Gr. *ouron,* urine]. Passing of white or colorless urine of low specific gravity. SYN: *albinuria.*

albidus (ăl′bĭ-dŭs) [L.]. White.

Albini's nodules (ăl-bē′nēz). [Giuseppe Albini, It. physiologist, 1830–1911] Minute nodules on margins of mitral and tricuspid valves of the heart; sometimes seen in newborns.

albinism (ăl′bĭn-ĭzm) [L. *albus,* white, + Gr. *-ismos,* condition]. Congenital nonpathological partial or total absence of pigment in skin, hair, and eyes. Frequently accompanied by astigmatism, photophobia, and nystagmus because the choroid is not sufficiently protected from light as a result of lack of pigment.

albino (ăl-bī′nō). A person afflicted with albinism, q.v.

albinuria (ăl″bĭ-nū′rē-ă) [″ + Gr. *ouron,* urine]. Passing of white or colorless urine of low specific gravity. SYN: *albiduria.*

albocinereous (ăl″bō-sĭn-ē′rē-ŭs) [″ + *cinereus,* gray]. Pert. to both white and gray matter of brain and spinal cord.

Albright's disease. [Fuller Albright, U.S. physician, 1900–1969]. Polyostotic fibrous dysplasia, q.v., accompanied by cafe-au-lait spots and endocrine disorders, esp. precocious puberty in girls.

albuginea (ăl-bū-jĭn′ē-ă) [L. from *albus,* white]. A layer of firm, white, fibrous tissue forming the investment of an organ or part, as of the eye, testicle, ovary, or spleen. SYN: *tunica albuginea.*

a. corporum cavernosorum. A strong, very elastic, white fibrous coat, forming a sheath common to both corpora cavernosa of the penis.

a. oculi. Sclera, or tough white supporting covering of the eyeball.

a. ovarii. The layer of firm fibrous tissue lying beneath the epithelial ovarian covering.

a. testis. The thick, unyielding layer of white fibrous tissue lying under the tunica vaginalis.

albugineotomy (ăl″bū-jĭn″ē-ŏt′ō-mē) [*albuginea* + Gr. *tome,* incision]. Incision of tunica albuginea, esp. of the testis.

albugineous (ăl″bū-jĭn′ē-ŭs). Pert. to or resembling tunica albuginea.

albuginitis (ăl″bū-jĭn-ī′tĭs) [″ + Gr. *itis,* inflammation]. Inflammation of tunica albuginea.

albugo (ăl-bū′gō) [L.]. White opacity of the cornea.

albumen (ăl-bū′mĕn) [L.]. Former spelling for albumin, q.v.

albumin (ăl-bū′mĭn) [L. *albumen,* white of egg]. One of a group of simple proteins widely distributed in plant and animal tissues; it is found in the blood as serum albumin, in milk as lactalbumin, and in the white of egg as ovalbumin. It is soluble in cold water; when coagulated by heat it is no longer dissolved by cold or hot water. In the stomach coagulated albumins are made soluble by peptase, being changed at the same time into albumoses and peptones. In general, albumins from animal sources are of higher quality than those from vegetable sources, because animal proteins contain greater quantities of essential amino acids. SEE: *albumose; amino acid; peptone.*

a., acid. Compound resulting from action of acid on albumin.

a., alkali. Compound resulting from action of weak alkalies on albumin.

a., blood. A., serum, q.v.

a., circulating. Albumin present in body fluids.

a., derived. Albumin changed by chemical action; albuminate.

a., egg. White of an egg; ovalbumin.

a., human. USP. Sterile solution of serum albumin obtained from healthy blood donors. Administered intravenously to restore blood volume. Trade names are Buminate, Albuminar, and Plasbumin.

a., muscle. Form of albumin found in muscular tissue.

a., native. Any albumin normally present in an organism.

a., serum. The main protein found in the blood. SYN: *a., blood.*

a., urinary. Albumin in urine.

a., vegetable. Albumin in, or derived from, plant tissue.

albuminate (ăl-bū′mĭ-nāt). The compound formed when albumin combines with an acid or alkali (base).

albuminaturia (ăl-bū″mĭ-nă-tū′rē-ă) [L. *albumen,* white of egg, + Gr. *ouron,* urine]. Presence of albuminates in urine.

albuminiferous (ăl-bū″mĭn-ĭf′ĕ-rŭs) [″ + *ferre,* to bear]. Producing albumin.

albuminimeter (ăl-bū″mĭn-ĭm′ĕ-tĕr) [″ + Gr. *metron,* measure]. Instrument for measuring amount of albumin in urine.

albuminiparous (ăl-bū″mĭn-ĭp′ă-rŭs) [″ + *parere,* to bear]. Yielding albumin.

albuminocholia (ăl-bū″mĭ-nō-kō′lē-ă) [″ + Gr. *chole,* bile]. Albumin in the bile.

albuminogenous (ăl-bū″mĭn-ŏj′ĕ-nŭs) [″ + Gr. *gennan,* to produce]. Producing albumin.

albuminoid (ăl-bū′mĭ-noyd″) [″ + Gr. *eidos,* form]. 1. Resembling albumin. 2. A protein.

albuminolysis (ăl-bū″mĭn-ŏl′ĭ-sĭs) [″ + Gr. *lysis,* dissolution]. Proteolysis; decomposition of protein.

albuminoptysis (ăl″bū-mĭn-ŏp′tĭ-sĭs) [″ + Gr. *ptyein,* to spit]. Albumin in sputum.

albuminoreaction (ăl-bū″mĭ-nō-rē-ăk′shŭn) [″ + *re,* again, + *agere,* to act]. The presence (positive reaction) or absence (negative reaction) of albumin in the sputum. Positive reaction indicates inflammatory condition of lungs.

albuminorrhea (ăl-bū″mĭ-nō-rē′ă) [″ + Gr. *rhoia,* flow]. Presence of albumin in urine. SYN: *albuminuria,* q.v.

albuminose (ăl-bū′mĭn-ōs). 1. Albumose, q.v. 2. Albuminous, q.v.

albuminosis (ăl-bū″mĭ-nō′sĭs) [″ + Gr. *osis,* condition]. Abnormal increase of albumin in blood plasma.

albuminous (ăl-bū′mĭ-nŭs). Pert. to, resembling, or containing albumin.

albumin test. The commonest type of albumin found in urine is serum albumin. Before testing, certain precautions must be observed: The specimen of urine must be fresh. The specimen must also be clear; the safest way to ensure this is to filter it through special filter paper. Since albuminuria can be caused by many different conditions, the results of tests require careful interpretation. Quantitative methods are also available.

There are many tests for albumin, but the usual ones follow.

Acetic acid test: Over a Bunsen burner, heat the top inch (2.5 cm.) or so of a test tube filled three parts full of urine. A cloudiness will occur, which may be due to phosphate or albumin. Add 2 to 3 drops of acetic acid. If the cloud disappears it is due to phosphates; if it becomes intensified, albumin is present.

Heller's test: Pour about ½ in. (1.3 cm.) of concentrated nitric acid in a test tube, and overlay it carefully with the urine, using a pipette. If an opaque line appears at the junction of the fluids, albumin is present. The line may take a few minutes to develop. SEE: *Heller's test.*

Paper strip or tablet tests: There are several tests based on the principle that certain chemicals impregnated in paper or in tablet form will change color when exposed to protein-containing urine. Within certain limits, these tests are reliable and have the advantage of providing a result in a few seconds.

Sulfosalicylic acid test: Add 10 to 20 drops of sulfosalicylic acid to urine in a test tube. Albumin is shown as a white, cloudy precipitate. This may be carried out as a ring test, as in Heller's test.

albuminuretic [L. *albumen,* white of egg, + Gr. *ouretikos,* causing urine to flow]. Pert. to or causing albuminuria.

albuminuria (ăl-bū-mĭ-nū'rē-ă) [" + Gr. *ouron,* urine]. Presence of readily detectable amounts of serum protein, esp. serum albumin but also serum globulin and others, in the urine. It is usually a sign of renal impairment. It occurs in febrile states, malignant hypertension, congestive heart failure, nephrotic syndrome, and other kidney disorders. Its presence, however, is not always a sign of disease because it may be found in normal persons following vigorous exercise. SYN: *proteinuria.* SEE: *nephritis; nephrosis.*

a., cyclic. Presence of small amounts of albumin in the urine at regular diurnal intervals, esp. in childhood and adolescence.

a., digestive. Albuminuria following ingestion of certain foods.

a., extrarenal or accidental. Albuminuria due to contamination of urine with pus, chyle, or blood.

a., functional. Intermittent or temporary albuminuria not associated with a pathologic condition. SYN: *a., transient.*

a., intrinsic. Albuminuria resulting from intrinsic renal disease. SYN: *a., true.*

a., orthostatic. A., postural, q.v.

a., pathological. Albuminuria caused by a disease.

a., physiological. A., functional, q.v.

a., postural. Transient albuminuria in normal individuals who have remained in an erect position for a considerable length of time. SYN: *a., orthostatic.*

a., renal. Albuminuria caused by changes in epithelial cells of kidneys, making them permeable to proteins in the blood, as in all forms of nephritis.

a., toxic. Albuminuria due to toxins generated within the body or poison from outside source.

a., transient. A., functional, q.v.

a., true. A., intrinsic, q.v.

albuminuric retinitis (ăl"bū-mĭ-nū'rĭk rĕt"ĭ-nī'tĭs). Inflammation of retina associated with chronic kidney disease, characterized by hazy retina, blurred disk margin, distention of retinal arteries, retinal hemorrhages, and white patches in the fundus, esp. the stellate figure at the macula. SEE: *retinitis.*

albumoscope (ăl-bū'mō-skōp) [" + Gr. *skopein,* to view]. An instrument for determining the presence of albumin in the urine.

albumose (ăl'bū-mōs). The intermediate product produced by digestion of proteins, converted by further digestion into peptone.

albumosemia (ăl"bū-mō-sē'mē-ă) [" + Gr. *haima,* blood]. Presence of albumose in blood.

albumosuria (ăl"bū-mō-sū'rē-ă) [" + Gr. *ouron,* urine]. Presence of albumose in urine.

albus [L.]. White.

Alcaligenes (ăl"kă-lĭj'ĭ-nēz). Genus of rod-shaped, gram-negative bacteria found in the intestinal tract of man, dairy products, and soil.

A. faecalis. Species of bacteria normally found in the intestinal tract of man. Rarely becomes pathogenic.

Alcock's canal. [Thomas Alcock, London surgeon, 1784–1833] Pudendal canal; space in the external fascia of the ischiorectal fossa, above the tuberosity of the ischium, through which the internal pudendal artery, veins, and nerve pass.

alcohol (ăl'kō-hŏl) [Arabic *al-koh'l,* something subtle]. 1. A class of organic compounds formed from hydrocarbons by substituting one or more hydroxyl (OH) groups for a similar number of hydrogen atoms. 2. Ethyl alcohol, a colorless, volatile, flammable liquid of the formula C_2H_5OH. Its molecular weight is 46.07; boiling point 78.5° C. Present in fermented or distilled liquors, and is obtained, in its pure form, from grain by fermentation and fractionation distillation. The USP standard is a liquid that contains not less than 92.3% by weight of C_2H_5OH. SYN: *a., ethyl; a., grain; ethanol.*

ACTION AND USES: Used in preparing essences, tinctures, extracts; manufacturing of ether, ethylene, and other industrial products; as a rubbing compound; as an antiseptic when in 70% solution. Arrests growth of putrefactive bacteria and is, therefore, used as a preservative of biological specimens and in certain patent medicines. Used in antifreeze products because of its low freezing point. Acts as a depressant to the nervous system when taken in excessive amounts. Used I.V. to stop premature labor. SEE: *hangover.*

a., absolute. Contains 99% alcohol and not more than 1% by weight of water.

a., dehydrated. A., absolute, q.v.

a., denatured. Alcohol rendered unfit for use as a beverage or medicine by adding toxic ingredients. Used commercially as a solvent.

a., diluted. USP. Alcohol containing not less than 41% and not more than 42% by weight of ethyl alcohol. Used as a solvent. SYN: *ethanol, diluted.*

a., ethyl. Ordinary or grain alcohol. SEE: *alcohol* (def. 2).

a., grain. Ethyl alcohol. SEE: *alcohol* (def. 2).

a., methyl. CH_3OH. A colorless, volatile, flammable liquid obtained from distillation of wood. Even though its physical properties are similar to those of ethyl alcohol, it is not fit for human consumption. Poisoning with methyl alcohol can lead to blindness and death. It is used as a solvent, for fuel, as an additive for denaturing ethyl alcohol, as an antifreeze agent, and in the preparation of formaldehyde. SYN: *carbanol; methanol; a., wood.* SEE: *methyl alcohol* in *Poisons and Poisoning* in *Appendix.*

a., wood. A., methyl, q.v.

alcoholic (ăl-kō-hŏl′ĭk) [L. *alcoholicus*]. 1. Pert. to alcohol. 2. One afflicted with alcoholism, q.v.

alcoholic fermentation. The conversion of carbohydrates to alcohol through action of yeast.

alcoholic psychosis. Severe mental disorder caused by alcoholism. Included are pathological intoxication, delirium tremens, Korsakoff's psychosis, acute hallucinosis. SEE: *alcoholism, acute; delirium tremens; hallucinosis, acute alcoholic; intoxication; Korsakoff's syndrome.*

Alcoholics Anonymous. ABBR: A.A. An organization composed of alcoholics who are trying to help themselves and others abstain from alcohol by offering encouragement and discussing experiences, problems, feelings, techniques, etc. Also sponsors similar groups for families, esp. spouses, of alcoholics (Al-Anon) and for children of alcoholics (Alateen). The organization has groups in most cities in the U.S.A. and can be contacted through its listing in telephone books.

alcoholism (ăl′kō-hŏl-ĭzm) [Arabic *al-koh'l,* something subtle, + Gr. *-ismos,* condition]. Alcoholism is a chronic, progressive, and potentially fatal disease. It is characterized by tolerance and physical dependency or pathologic organ changes, or both—all the direct or indirect consequences of the alcohol ingested.

1. "Chronic and progressive" means that the physical, emotional, and social changes that develop are cumulative and progress as drinking continues.
2. "Tolerance" means brain adaptation to the presence of high concentrations of alcohol.
3. "Physical dependency" means that withdrawal symptoms occur from decreasing or ceasing consumption of alcohol.
4. The person with alcoholism cannot consistently predict on any drinking occasion the duration of the episode or the quantity that will be consumed.
5. Pathologic organ changes can be found in almost any organ, but most often involve the liver, brain, peripheral nervous system, and the gastrointestinal tract.
6. The drinking pattern is generally continuous but may be intermittent, with periods of abstinence between drinking episodes.
7. The social, emotional, and behavioral symptoms and consequences of alcoholism result from the effect of alcohol on the function of the brain. The degree to which these symptoms and signs are considered deviant will depend upon the cultural norms of the society or group in which the person lives.

(Definition prepared by the National Council on Alcoholism/American Medical Society on Alcoholism Committee on Definitions.)

ETIOL: Unknown. Psychological, physiological, and sociological factors play an important part. The exhilaration factor is often the cause of intoxication in nonalcoholic individuals. Alcoholism is an illness and should be so treated.

a., acute. Acute intoxication with temporary mental disturbances and muscular incoordination.

CAUTION: When stupor or coma is observed in a patient who is suspected of being intoxicated by alcohol, other causes such as intracranial disease, insulin shock, etc., should also be considered. Acute alcoholism can cause death.

SYM AND SIGNS: There may be motor instability (staggered gait blurred or double vision, impaired reflex action); reduced mental function; increased pulse rate; decreased blood pressure; dilated pupils; flushing of skin; drowsiness or stupor.

TREATMENT: Coma due to alcohol is a medical emergency and requires vigorous therapy. I.V. fluids, intubation to prevent aspiration of vomitus, and oxygen inhalation may be required.

a., chronic. Pathological state from habitual use of alcohol in toxic amounts.

SYM AND SIGNS: Malnutrition; vitamin deficiency; alcoholic cirrhosis of liver; gastritis; pancreatitis; and neurological disorders such as tremulousness, hallucinosis, seizures, delirium tremens.

TREATMENT: Withdrawal of alcohol, tranquilizing drugs, correction of vitamin deficiency, psychotherapy. SEE: *delirium tremens; hangover; intoxication.*

alcoholomania (ăl″kō-hŏl″ō-mā′nē-ă) [Arabic *al-koh'l*, something subtle, + Gr. *mania*, frenzy]. Abnormal craving for intoxicants.

alcoholometer (ăl″kō-hŏl-ŏm′ĕ-tĕr) [″ + Gr. *metron*, measure]. An instrument for measuring quantity of alcohol in a fluid.

alcoholophilia (ăl″kō-hŏl-ō-fĭl′ē-ă) [″ + Gr. *philein*, to love]. Morbid craving for alcohol.

alcohol syndrome, fetal. Birth defects in infants born to mothers whose chronic alcoholism persisted during the gestation period. Shortly after birth, these infants may exhibit signs of alcohol withdrawal.

alcoholuria (ăl″kō-hŏl-ū′rē-ă) [″ + Gr. *ouron*, urine]. Presence of alcohol in the urine.

aldehyde (ăl′dĕ-hīd) [*alc*ohol *dehyd*rogenatum]. 1. Oxidation product of a primary alcohol; has the characteristic group —CHO. 2. Acetaldehyde, CH_3CHO. Intermediate in yeast fermentation and alcohol metabolism. SYN: *acetic aldehyde.*

aldolase (ăl′dō-lās). An enzyme present in skeletal and heart muscle and the liver; important in converting glycogen into lactic acid. Its serum level is increased in certain muscle diseases and in viral hepatitis.

aldopentose (ăl″dō-pĕn′tōs). A five-carbon sugar with the aldehyde, —CHO, group at the end. Arabinose is an aldopentose.

aldose. A carbohydrate of the aldehyde group (—CHO).

aldosterone (ăl-dŏs′tĕr-ōn, ăl″dō-stēr′ōn). The most biologically active mineralocorticoid hormone secreted by the adrenal cortex. Functions in regulation of metabolism of sodium, chloride, and potassium. SEE: *adrenal gland.*

aldosteronism (ăl″dō-stĕr′ōn-ĭzm″). A condition in which the blood contains abnormally high levels of aldosterone. This causes retention of sodium, urinary loss of potassium, and alkalosis. The patient develops episodes of tetany, weakness, paralysis, hypertension, cardiac irregularity, polyuria, and polydipsia. Also: *hyperaldosteronism.*

a., primary. Aldosteronism due to disorders of the adrenal gland. SYN: *Conn's syndrome.*

a., secondary. Aldosteronism due to extra-adrenal disorders.

aldrin (ăl′drĭn). A derivative of chlorinated naphthalene used as an insecticide. SEE: *dieldrin* in *Poisons and Poisoning* in *Appendix.*

alemmal (ă-lĕm′ăl) [Gr. *a*-, not, + *lemma*, husk]. Without a neurilemma, as a nerve fiber.

Aleppo boil. Cutaneous leishmaniasis, caused by infection with the parasite Leishmania tropica. Characterized by one or multiple ulcerations of the skin. SYN: *Delhi boil; Oriental sore.*

alethia (ă-lē′thē-ă) [″ + *lethe*, forgetfulness]. Inability to forget; dwelling on the past.

aleukemia (ă-loo-kē′mē-ă) [″ + *leukos*, white, + *haima*, blood]. Deficiency of leukocytes in the blood. The existence of leukopenia or aleukocytosis.

aleukemic (ă″loo-kē′mĭk). Marked by aleukemia.

aleukocytosis (ă-loo″kō-sī-tō′sĭs) [″ + *leukos*, white, + *kytos*, cell, + *osis*, condition]. Absence or extreme decrease of leukocytes in the blood.

aleuron, aleurone (ăl-oo′rōn) [Gr. *aleuron*, flour]. The protein granules present in the outer layer of the endosperm of cereal grain.

Alexander-Adams operation. [William Alexander, Brit. surgeon, 1844–1919; James A. Adams, Scottish gynecologist, 1857–1930] Surgery in which the round ligaments of the uterus are shortened and their ends sutured to the exterior abdominal ring. Used in treating uterine displacement.

alexeteric (ă-lĕk″sĕ-tĕr′ĭk) [Gr. *alexeterios*, able to ward off]. Protective against infection, venom, and poison.

alexia [Gr. *a*-, not, + *lexis*, word]. Loss of the ability to read; word blindness. A form of sensory aphasia, q.v.

ETIOL: central nervous system lesion.

a., motor. Loss of the ability to read aloud while remaining able to understand what is written or printed.

a., musical. Loss of the ability to read music. It may be sensory, optic, or visual, but not motor.

a., optic or visual. Inability to understand what is written or printed.

alexic (ă-lĕks′ĭk). 1. Defensive, as an alexin. 2. Pert. to alexia.

alexin (ă-lĕks′ĭn) [Gr. *alexein*, to ward off]. Defensive substance in normal serum that, in presence of a specific sensitizer, destroys bacteria and other cells. SYN: *complement*, q.v. SEE: *immunity.*

alexipyretic (ă-lĕk″sē-pī-rĕt′ĭk) [″ + *pyretos*, fever]. 1. Reducing fever. 2. That which reduces fever. SYN: *antipyretic; febrifuge.*

alexithymia (ă-lĕk″sĭ-thī′mē-ă). Inability to verbalize feelings.

aleydigism (ă-lī′dĭg-ĭzm). Absence of function of Leydig cells, q.v., resulting in hypogonadism.

ALG. *antilymphocyte globulin.* SEE: *globulin, antilymphocyte.*

algae (ăl′jē) [L. *alga*, seaweeds]. Plants belonging to the subphylum Algae of the phylum Thallophyta, the lowest division of the plant kingdom. They are nonparasitic plants without roots, stems, or leaves; they contain chlorophyll and vary in size from microscopic forms to massive seaweeds. They live in fresh or salt water or in moist places. Some serve as food or as sources of medicinal products. Ex.: kelp and Irish moss.

algefacient (ăl″jē-fā′shĕnt) [L. *algere,* to be cold, + *faciens,* making]. 1. Cooling. 2. Agent that produces coolness or reduces fever. SYN: *refrigerant.*

algesia (ăl-jē′zē-ă) [Gr. *algesis,* sense of pain]. Supersensitiveness to pain. A form of hyperesthesia, q.v. SYN: *algesthesia.*

algesic (ăl-jē′sĭk). Painful. SYN: *algetic.*

algesichronometer (ăl-jē″zē-krō-nŏm′ĕ-tĕr) [″ + *chronos,* time + *metron,* measure]. An instrument for measuring time taken to feel pain.

algesimeter (ăl″jē-sĭm′ĕ-tĕr) [″ + *metron,* measure]. An instrument for measuring degree of sensitivity to pain. SYN: *algometer.*

algesthesia (ăl″jĕs-thē′zē-ă) [Gr. *algos,* pain, + *aisthesis,* sensation]. 1. Perception of pain. 2. Supersensitiveness to pain. A form of hyperesthesia, q.v. SYN: *algesia.*

algetic (ăl-jĕt′ĭk). Painful. SYN: *algesic.*

-algia (ăl′jē-ă) [Gr.]. Suffix signifying pain.

algicide (ăl′jĭ-sīd) [L. *alga,* seaweeds, + *caedere,* to kill]. Substance that destroys algae.

algid (ăl′jĭd). [L. *algidus,* cold]. Cold; chilly.

algid stage. Cold and cyanotic skin occurring in cholera and some other diseases.

alginate (ăl′jĭ-nāt). Any salt of alginic acid. It is derived from kelp, a type of seaweed. Used to enhance the absorptive ability of surgical dressings and as a thickening agent in foods.

alginic acid. USP. SEE: *acid, alginic.*

algiomotor (ăl″jē-ō-mō′tor) [Gr. *algos,* pain, + L. *motor,* a mover]. Causing painful contraction of muscles, particularly pain during peristalsis.

algiomuscular (ăl″jē-ō-mŭs′kū-lăr) [″ + L. *musculus,* muscle]. Algiomotor, q.v.

algogenic (ăl-gō-jĕn′ĭk). 1. [″ + *gennan,* to produce]. Causing pain. 2. [L. *algor,* cold, + Gr. *gennan,* to produce]. Lowering body temperature, esp. below normal.

algolagnia (ăl″gō-lăg′nē-ă) [Gr. *algos,* pain, + *lagneia,* lust]. Sexual satisfaction derived by experiencing pain or by inflicting pain on others.

a., active. Sadism.

a., passive. Masochism.

algolagnist (ăl-gō-lăg′nĭst). One who practices algolagnia.

algometer [″ + *metron,* measure]. Instrument for measuring degree of sensitivity to pain. SYN: *algesimeter.*

algophily (ăl-gŏf′ĭ-lē) [″ + *philein,* to love]. 1. Morbid love of pain. 2. Algolagnia, q.v.

algophobia (ăl″gō-fō′bē-ă) [″ + *phobos,* fear]. Morbid fear of pain.

algor (ăl′gor) [L., cold]. 1. A chill. 2. The sensation of cold; cold.

a. mortis. The chill of death.

algorithm (ăl′gō-rĭthm). A formula for solving a problem. In medicine, a set of steps used in diagnosing and treating a disease.

algos (ăl′gōs) [Gr.]. Pain.

algospasm (ăl′gō-spăzm) [Gr. *algos,* pain, + *spasmos,* spasm]. A painful cramp or spasm.

alible (ăl′ĭ-bl) [L. *alibilis,* nutritive]. Nutritive.

alicyclic (ăl-ĭ-sī′klĭk). Having properties of both aliphatic (open-chain) and cyclic (closed-chain) compounds, q.v.

alien (āl′yĕn). 1. Strange, foreign, or contrary. 2. A stranger, foreigner, or outsider.

alienate (āl′yĕn-āt). To isolate, estrange, or dissociate.

alienation (āl″yĕn-ā′shŭn) [L. *alienare,* to make strange]. Isolation, estrangement, or dissociation, esp. from society.

alienia (ā″lī-ē′nē-ă) [Gr. *a-,* not, + L. *lien,* spleen]. Absence of the spleen.

aliform (ăl′ĭ-form) [L. *ala,* wing, + *forma,* shape]. Wing-shaped.

aliform process. Wing of the sphenoid bone.

alignment (ă-līn′mĕnt) [Fr. *aligner,* to put in a straight line]. 1. The act of arranging in a straight line. 2. The state of being arranged in a straight line. 3. In orthopedics, the placing of portions of a fractured bone into correct anatomical position. 4. In dentistry, bringing teeth into correct position.

aliment (ăl′ĭ-mĕnt) [L. *alimentum,* nourishment]. Nutriment, food.

alimentary (ăl″ĭ-mĕn′tăr-ē) [L. *alimentum,* nourishment]. Pertaining to food or nutrition.

alimentary canal or tract. The digestive tube from the mouth to anus, including mouth or buccal cavity, pharynx, esophagus, stomach, small and large intestines, and rectum. Drugs administered orally are absorbed in the stomach or intestine by the portal vein and pass through the liver before entering the general circulation, or they may be absorbed into the lacteals and enter the bloodstream by way of the thoracic duct. SEE: *digestive system* for illus.

alimentary duct. The thoracic duct.

alimentation (ăl″ĭ-mĕn-tā′shŭn). The process of nourishing the body; it includes mastication, swallowing, digestion, absorption, and assimilation. SEE: *hyperalimentation; hypoalimentation.*

RS: absorption; anabolism; catabolism; digestion; food; metabolism.

a., artificial. Feeding, usually intravenous or by a nasal tube passed into the stomach, of patient unable to take nourishment normally.

a., forced. 1. Feeding of a patient unwilling to eat. 2. Forcing a person to eat a greater quantity than desired.

a., rectal. Feeding by means of nutrient enemas, q.v.

alimentotherapy (ăl″ĭ-mĕn″tō-thĕr′ă-pē) [L. *alimentum,* nourishment, + Gr. *therapeia,* treatment]. Treatment of disease by dietary regulation. SYN: *dietotherapy.* SEE: *dietetics.*

alinasal [L. *ala,* wing, + *nasus,* nose]. Pert. to the alae nasi or wings of the nose.

alinement (ă-līn′mĕnt) [Fr. *aligner,* to put in a straight line]. Alignment, q.v.

aliphatic (ăl″ĭ-făt′ĭk) [Gr. *aleiphar, aleiphatos,* fat, oil]. Belonging to that series of organic chemical compounds characterized by open chains of carbon atoms rather than by rings.

aliquot (ăl′ĭ-kwŏt) [L. *alius,* other, + *quot,* how many]. A portion obtained by dividing the whole into equal parts without a remainder. A portion that represents a known quantitative relationship to the whole or to other portions.

alisphenoid (ăl-ĭ-sfē′noyd) [L. *ala,* wing, + Gr. *sphen,* wedge, + *eidos,* resemblance]. Pert. to the greater wing of the sphenoid bone.

alizarin (ă-lĭz′ă-rĭn) [Arabic *ala sara,* extract]. A red dye obtained from coal tar or madder.

alkalemia (ăl″kă-lē′mē-ă) [Arabic *al-qaliy,* ashes of salt wort, + Gr. *haima,* blood]. Excessive alkalinity of the blood due to a decrease in the hydrogen ion concentration or an increase in hydroxyl ions. The blood is normally slightly alkaline (pH 7.35 to 7.45).

alkalescence (ăl″kă-lĕs′ĕns). 1. Slight alkalinity. 2. Process of becoming alkaline.

alkalescent (ăl″kă-lĕs′ĕnt). Alkaline or becoming alkaline.

alkali (ăl′kă-lī) [Arabic *al-qaliy,* ashes of salt wort]. A strong base, esp. the metallic hydroxides. Alkalies combine with acids to form salts, combine with fatty acids to form soap, neutralize acids, and turn litmus paper blue. SEE: *acid; base; pH;* words beginning with *alkal-.*

a., corrosive. Strongly corrosive metallic hydroxides most commonly of sodium, ammonium, and potassium, as well as carbonates. Because of their great combining power with water and their action on the fatty tissues, they cause rapid deep destruction. They have a tendency to gelatinize tissue, turning it a somewhat grayish color and forming a soapy, slippery surface, accompanied by pain and burning. SEE: *corrosion; corrosive poisoning.*

alkalimeter (ăl″kă-lĭm′ĕ-tĕr) [″ + Gr. *metron,* measure]. Device for measuring degree of alkalinity of a mixture.

alkalimetry (ăl″kă-lĭm′ĕ-trē). Measurement of degree of alkalinity of a mixture.

alkaline (ăl′kă-līn). Pert. to or having the reactions of an alkali.

alkaline reserve. The amount of base in the blood, principally bicarbonates, available for neutralization of fixed acids (acetoacetate, β-hydroxybutyrate, and lactate). A fall in alkaline reserve is called acidosis; a rise, alkalosis. Normally, the carbon dioxide–combining power of the venous plasma is 21–30 mEq./L. and the carbon dioxide content of whole blood is 20–25 mEq./L.

alkaline salts. SEE: *hydrogen sulfide* in *Poisons and Poisoning* in *Appendix.*

alkaline tide. The increase in alkaline reserve and occasional occurrence of alkaline urine during gastric digestion.

alkalinity (ăl″kă-lĭn′ĭ-tē). State of being alkaline. SEE: *hydrogen ion.*

alkalinize (ăl′kă-lĭn-īz″). To make alkaline. SYN: *alkalize.*

alkalinuria (ăl″kă-lĭn-ū′rē-ă) [*alkali* + Gr. *ouron,* urine]. Alkaline urine. SYN: *alkaluria.*

alkalipenia (ăl″kă-lĭ-pē′nē-ă) [″ + Gr. *penia,* poverty]. Low alkaline reserve of the body.

alkali poisoning. Ingestion of an alkali.

F.A.: Large amounts of water by mouth; diluted vinegar or lemon juice. Then olive oil or milk and egg whites by mouth. Mild stimulants to prevent shock. Tracheotomy if necessary. If esophagus is known to be injured, it is imperative to use corticosteroid therapy beginning as soon as possible. It is advisable to use a broad-spectrum antibiotic if corticosteroids are used.

TREATMENT: Morphine is useful to allay pain. Rest, heat, quiet, and adequate fluid intake are imperative.

CAUTION: Avoid emetics, strong acids, and lavage.

alkali reserve. SEE: *alkaline reserve.*

alkalitherapy (ăl″kă-lĭ-thĕr′ă-pē) [″ + Gr. *therapeia,* treatment]. Therapeutic use of alkalies. SYN: *alkalotherapy.*

alkalization (ă″kă-lĭ-zā′shŭn). Process of making alkaline.

alkalize (ăl′kă-līz). To make alkaline. SYN: *alkalinize.*

alkaloid (ăl′kă-loyd) [*alkali* + Gr. *eidos,* resemblance]. One of a group of organic alkaline substances obtained from plants. Alkaloids react with acids to form salts that are used for medical purposes.

Ex.: atropine, morphine, nicotine, quinine.

INCOMPAT: coffee (caffeine), tea (tannin).

a., synthetic. A synthetic substance similar to plant alkaloids.

alkalometry (ăl″kă-lŏm′ĕ-trē) [″ + Gr. *metron,* measure]. Determination of the alkali content of a substance.

alkalosis (ăl″kă-lō′sĭs) [″ + Gr. *osis,* condition]. Excessive alkalinity of body fluids due to accumulation of alkalies or reduction of acids. SEE: *acid-base balance.*

a., altitude. Alkalosis resulting from exposure to high altitudes. This causes respiratory alkalosis. SEE: *a., respiratory.*

a., compensated. Alkalosis in which pH of body fluids has been returned to normal. Compensatory mechanisms maintain the normal ratio of bicarbonate to carbonic acid (approx. 20:1) even though the bicarbonate level is increased.

a., hypochloremic. Metabolic alkalosis due to loss of chloride. Produced by severe vomiting.

a., hypokalemic. Metabolic alkalosis due to excess loss of potassium. May be caused by diuretic therapy.

a., metabolic. Alkalosis in which pH of body fluids is increased and serum carbon dioxide content is greater than 70 volumes % (30 mEq./L.). Commonly a result of loss of acid from excessive vomiting, but also of loss of potassium or ingestion of excessive amounts of sodium bicarbonate.

SYM: Apathy, irritability, delirium, dehydration, and occasionally tetany.

TREATMENT: Correct the primary disorder and administer sodium or potassium chloride and nonalkalinizing gels.

NURSING IMPLICATIONS: Assess the patient for symptoms of metabolic acidosis, such as decreased respiratory rate, tetany, convulsions, hyperactive reflexes, diarrhea, and nausea and vomiting. Monitor the patient's intake and output, and provide a diet high in chloride and potassium.

a., respiratory. Alkalosis in which pH of body fluids is increased but serum carbon dioxide content is less than 21 mEq./L. Caused by hyperventilation, salicylate poisoning, lesion of central nervous system, or decreased oxygen content of the air.

SYM: Lightheadedness, fainting, tetany.

TREATMENT: Discontinue use of salicylates (in salicylate poisoning); inhalation of expired CO_2 collected by breathing into a paper bag (in neurosis); correction or alleviation of central nervous system disorder or lesion. SEE: *hyperventilation.*

NURSING IMPLICATIONS: Assess the patient for symptoms of respiratory alkalosis, such as rapid respiratory rate, complaints of numbness, and any change in level of consciousness. Also provide reassurance for the patient in order to allay anxiety.

alkalotherapy (ăl″kă-lō-thĕr′ă-pē) [*alkali* + Gr. *therapeia,* treatment]. Therapeutic use of alkalies. SYN: *alkalitherapy.*

alkalotic (ăl″kă-lŏt′ĭk). Pert. to alkalosis.

alkaluria (ăl″kă-lū′rē-ă) [*alkali* + Gr. *ouron,* urine]. The condition of alkali in the urine. SYN: *alkalinuria.*

alkapton(e) (ăl-kăp′tōn) [″ + Gr. *hapto,* to bind to]. Homogentisic acid; a yellowish-red substance sometimes occurring in urine as the result of the incomplete oxidation of tyrosine and phenylalanine.

alkaptonuria (ăl″kăp-tō-nū′rē-ă) [*alkapton* + Gr. *ouron,* urine]. A rare inherited disorder characterized by the excretion of large amounts of homogentisic acid in the urine, a result of incomplete metabolism of the amino acids tyrosine and phenylalanine. Presence of the acid is indicated by the darkening of urine on standing or when alkalinated and the dark staining of diapers or other linen. SEE: *ochronosis.*

alkene (ăl′kēn). A bivalent aliphatic hydrocarbon containing one double bond; formed by removal of two hydrogen atoms.

Ex.: When the ethane molecule,

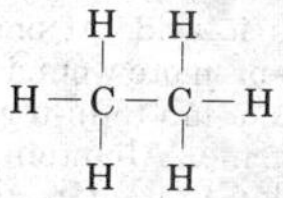

loses two hydrogen atoms it becomes ethylene,

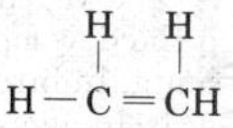

with a double bond between two carbons. These are also called unsaturated hydrocarbons.

alkyl (ăl′kĭl). A hydrocarbon molecule from which one atom of hydrogen is absent. The resulting substances are called alkyl groups or alkyl radicals.

Ex.: The methane hydrocarbon molecule,

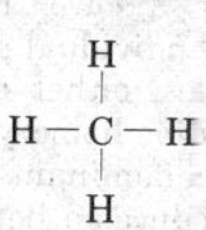

becomes an alkyl radical, in this case the methyl radical, when it loses one hydrogen molecule,

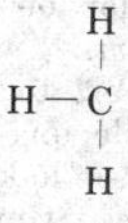

In chemical formulae, hydrocarbon radicals are abbreviated *R*.

alkylate (ăl′kĭ-lāt). Provide therapy involving the use of an alkylating agent.

alkylating agent. A substance that introduces an alkyl radical into a compound in place of a hydrogen atom.

alkylation (ăl′kĭ-lā′shŭn). A chemical process

in which an alkyl radical replaces a hydrogen atom.

all- [Gr. *allos,* other]. Prefix meaning other, different, alternate. SEE: *allo-*.

allachesthesia (ăl″ă-kĕs-thē′zē-ă) [Gr. *allache,* elsewhere, + *aisthesis,* sensation]. Perception of tactile sensation as being remote from the actual point of stimulation.

allantochorion (ă-lăn″tō-kō′rē-ŏn). Fusion of the allantois and chorion into one structure.

allantoic (ăl″ăn-tō′ĭk). Pert. to the allantois.

allantoid [Gr. *allantos,* sausage, + *eidos,* resemblance]. 1. Sausage-shaped. 2. Pert. to the allantois.

allantoin (ă-lăn′tō-ĭn). $C_4H_6N_4O_3$. A white crystalline substance occurring in allantoic and amniotic fluids and as end product of purine metabolism in mammals other than primates. Also produced synthetically by oxidation of uric acid. At one time allantoin was used to promote wound healing.

allantoinuria (ă-lăn″tō-ĭn-ū′rē-ă) [*allantoin* + Gr. *ouron,* urine]. Allantoin in the urine.

allantois (ă-lăn′tō-ĭs) [Gr. *allantos,* sausage, + *eidos,* resemblance]. An elongated bladder developing from the hindgut of the fetus in mammals, birds, and reptiles. In mammals it contributes to the development of the umbilicus and placenta. In birds and reptiles, it provides for the exchange of gases through the shell.

allayed (ā-lād′). Mitigated, q.v.

allele (ă-lēl′, ă-lĕl′) [Gr. *allelon,* of one another]. One of two or more different genes containing specific inheritable characteristics that occupy corresponding positions (loci) on paired chromosomes. A pair of alleles is usually indicated by a capital letter for the dominant and a lower case letter for the recessive. An individual possessing a pair of identical alleles, either dominant or recessive, is said to be homozygous for this gene. The union of a dominant gene and its recessive allele produces a heterozygous individual for that characteristic. More than one inheritable characteristic may be present on the same pair of genes (alleles). For example the genes for blood type A, B, and O are at the same position on alleles. SYN: *allelic gene; allelomorph.*

allelic (ă-lĕl′ĭk). Pert. to alleles.

allelic gene. Allele, q.v.

allelocatalysis (ă-lē″lō-kă-tăl′ĭ-sĭs) [″ + *katalysis,* dissolution]. Stimulation of a bacterial culture by the addition of cells of same type.

allelomorph (ă-lē′lō-morf, ă-lĕl′ō-morf) [″ + *morphe,* form]. Allele, q.v.

allelotaxis (ă-lē″lō-tăk′sĭs) [″ + *taxis,* order]. Development of a part from several embryonic structures.

Allen-Doisy test (ăl′ĕn-doy′sē). [Edgar V. Allen, U.S. anatomist, 1892–1943; Edward A. Doisy, U.S. biochemist and physiologist, b. 1893] Used to determine estrogen content. A spayed mouse is injected with the material being tested. The appearance of cornified cells on vaginal smear constitutes a positive reaction.

Allen-Doisy unit. The smallest amount of estrogen that will produce a characteristic change (appearance of cornified cells) in the vaginal epithelium of a spayed mouse. SYN: *mouse unit.*

allenthesis (ă-lĕn′thĕ-sĭs) [Gr. *allos,* other, + *en,* in, + *thesis,* a placing]. Introduction of a foreign substance into the body.

allergen (ăl′ĕr-jĕn) [Gr. *allos,* other, + *ergon,* work, + *gennan,* to produce]. Any substance that causes manifestations of allergy. It may or may not be a protein or an antigen. Among common allergens are inhalants (dusts, pollens, fungi, smoke, perfumes, odors of plastics), foods (wheat, eggs, milk, chocolate, strawberries), drugs (aspirin, antibiotics, serums), infectious agents (bacteria, viruses, fungi, animal parasites), contactants (chemicals, animals, plants, metals), and physical agents (heat, cold, light, pressure, radiations).

allergenic (ăl″ĕr-jĕn′ĭk). Producing allergy.

allergic (ă-lĕr′jĭk). Pert. to, sensitive to, or caused by an allergen.

allergization (ăl″ĕr-jĭ-zā′shŭn). Introduction of a foreign substance into the body in order to bring about a state of sensitivity.

allergy (ăl′ĕr-jē) [Gr. *allos,* other, + *ergon,* work]. An acquired hypersensitivity to a substance (allergen) that does not normally cause a reaction. It is essentially an antibody-antigen reaction but in some cases the antibody cannot be demonstrated. The reaction is due to the release of histamine or histamine-like substances from injured cells. There may be a genetic predisposition to acquire a particular allergy. The number of exposures necessary to produce enough antibodies to cause an allergy varies. An allergy may occur the second time a person is exposed to a particular allergen, or may not occur until years later when repeated exposures have produced sufficient antibodies. Manifestations most commonly involve the respiratory tract or the skin. Allergic conditions include eczema, allergic rhinitis or coryza, hay fever, bronchial asthma, urticaria (hives), and food allergy.

ETIOL: Pollen, dust, hair, fur, feathers, scales, wool, chemicals, drugs, insect bites; also specific foods such as eggs, chocolate, milk, wheat, tomatoes, citrus fruits, oatmeal, potatoes. SEE: *allergen.*

SYM: Eosinophilia frequently present; nasal congestion, tearing, sneezing, wheezing, coughing; itching rash, eruptions.

TREATMENT: Skin tests or an elimination diet, q.v., will usually identify the allergen, which should then be avoided. If an allergen cannot be avoided, its effects can be reduced by medications such as antihistamines, epinephrine, or corticosteroids. The value of desensitization, q.v., is controversial. However, if desensitization is used, it should be done year-round and not seasonally even when treating seasonal allergies.

RS: anaphylaxis; atopy; hay fever; hypersensitiveness; immunity.

allesthesia (ăl″ĕs-thē′sē-ă) [″ + *aisthesis*, sensation]. Perception of stimulus in the opposite limb from the one stimulated. SYN: *allochesthesia; allochiria.*

alliaceous (ăl″ē-ā′shŭs) [L. *allium*, garlic, + *-aceus*, of a specific kind]. Tasting like garlic or onions.

allied health professional. An individual who has received special training in one of the several fields of allied health such as nursing, laboratory, x-ray, emergency medical care, physiotherapy, or occupational therapy.

alliesthesia (ăl″ē-ĕs-thē′sē-ă) [Gr. *allios*, changed, + *aisthesis*, sensation]. The perception of an external stimulus as pleasant or unpleasant depending upon internal stimuli. A particular stimulus may be perceived as pleasant at one time and unpleasant at another.

alliteration (ă-lĭt″ĕr-ā′shŭn) [L. *ad*, to, + *litera*, letter]. A speech disorder in which words beginning with the same consonant sound are used to excess.

allo- [Gr. *allos*, other]. Prefix indicating divergence, difference from, or opposition to the normal.

alloantigen (ăl″lō-ăn′tĭ-jĕn) [″ + *anti*, against, + *gennan*, to produce]. Isoantigen, q.v.

allobiosis (ăl″ō-bī-ō′sĭs) [″ + *bios*, life]. The altered responses produced in organisms exposed to environmental or physiological changes.

allochesthesia (ăl″ō-kĕs-thē′zē-ă) [Gr. *allache*, elsewhere, + *aisthesis*, sensation]. Allesthesia, q.v.

allochezia, allochetia (ăl″ō-kē′zē-ă, ăl″ō-kē′shē-ă) [Gr. *allos*, other, + *chezein*, to defecate]. Excretion of feces through an abnormal opening.

allochiria, allocheiria (ăl″ō-kī′rē-ă) [″ + *cheir*, hand]. Allesthesia, q.v.

allochroism (ăl-ŏk′rō-ĭzm, ăl″ō-krō′ĭzm) [″ + *chroa*, color + *-ismos*, condition]. Change in color.

allochromasia (al″ō-krō-mā′sē-ă). Change in color of hair or skin.

allocinesia (ăl″ō-sĭn-ē′sē-ă) [Gr. *allos*, other, + *kinesis*, movement]. Movement on side of body opposite to the one the patient has been requested to move. SEE: *allokinesis*.

allodiploidy (ăl″ō-dĭp′loy-dē) [″ + *diploe*, fold, + *eidos*, form]. Possession of two sets of chromosomes, each from a different species. A hybrid is allodiploid.

allodynia (ăl″ō-dĭn′ē-ă). Pain resulting from unpleasant stimuli to the normal skin.

alloeroticism (ăl″ō-ē-rŏt′ĭ-sĭzm). Alloerotism, q.v.

alloerotism (ăl″ō-ĕr′ō-tĭzm) [″ + *Eros*, god of love]. Sexual urges stimulated by and directed toward another person. Opposite of autoerotism.

allogeneic, allogenic (ăl″ō-jĕ-nē′ĭk, ăl″ō-jĕn′ĭk). Having a different genetic constitution but belonging to the same species. SEE: *isogeneic.*

allograft (ăl′ō-grăft) [″ + L. *graphium*, grafting knife]. Transplant tissue obtained from the same species. The tissues that survive best are cornea, bone, artery, and cartilage. SYN: *homograft*. SEE: *autograft; heterograft.*

allokinesis (ăl″ō-kĭ-nē′sĭs) [″+ *kinesis*, movement]. Passive or reflex movement; involuntary movement.

allokinetic (ăl″ō-kĭ-nĕt′ĭk). Characterized by passive or reflex movement.

allolalia (ăl″ō-lā′lē-ă) [″ + *lalia*, talk]. 1. Speech defect or impairment, esp. due to a brain lesion. 2. A type of dysphasia in which words are spoken unintentionally, or inappropriate words are substituted for appropriate ones.

allomerism (ă-lŏm′ĕr-ĭzm) [″ + *meros*, part, + *-ismos*, condition]. Change in chemical constitution without a change in form. SEE: *allomorphism*.

allomorphism (ăl″ō-mor′fĭzm) [″ + *morphe*, form, + *-ismos*, condition]. Change in form without a change in chemical constitution. SEE: *allomerism*.

allongement (ăl-ŏnzh-mŏn′) [Fr., elongation]. Lengthening of a structure by surgical methods.

allopath (ăl′ō-păth). One who practices allopathy, q.v.

allopathy (ăl-ŏp′ă-thē) [″ + *pathos*, disease]. 1. System of treating disease by inducing a pathologic reaction that is antagonistic to the disease being treated. 2. A term erroneously used for the regular practice of medicine to differentiate it from homeopathy, q.v.

allophasis (ăl-ŏf′ă-sĭs) [Gr. *allos*, other, + *phasis*, speech]. Incoherent speech.

alloplasia (ăl″ō-plā′zē-ă) [″ + *plasis*, a molding]. Development of tissue at a location where that type of tissue would not normally occur. SYN: *heteroplasia*.

alloplasty (ăl′ō-plăs-tē) [″ + *plasis*, a molding]. 1. Plastic surgery using inert material. 2. In psychiatry, adaptation by altering the external environment rather than changing oneself. SEE: *autoplasty*.

alloploidy (ăl″ō-ploy′dē) [″ + *ploos,* fold, + *eidos,* form]. State of having two or more sets of chromosomes derived from different ancestral species.

allopolyploidy (ăl″ō-pŏl′ē-ploy-dē) [″ + *polys,* many, + *ploos,* fold, + *eidos,* form]. State of having more than two sets of chromosomes derived from different ancestral species.

allopsychic (ăl-ō-sī′kĭk) [″ + *psyche,* mind]. Pert. to mental processes in relation to the external environment.

allopsychosis [″ + ″ + *osis,* condition]. Derangement of perceptive powers.

allopurinol (ăl″ō-pū′rĭn-ŏl). USP. A drug that inhibits the enzyme xanthine oxidase. Because its action causes a reduction in both serum and urine levels of uric acid, allopurinol is used in the treatment of gout, q.v., and of renal calculi that are caused by uric acid.

Allergic response to this drug has been reported. Trade name is Zyloprim.

all-or-none law. In response to a stimulus, the heart will either contract to its greatest extent or will not contract at all. SYN: *Bowditch's law.*

allotherm (ăl′ō-thĕrm) [″ + *therme,* heat]. An animal whose body temperature varies according to the temperature of the environment. SYN: *poikilotherm.* SEE: *homothermal.*

allotoxin (ăl″ō-tŏk′sĭn) [″ + *toxikon,* poison]. Any substance within the body that neutralizes a specific toxin.

allotransplantation (ăl″ō-trăns″plăn-tā′shŭn) [″ + L. *trans,* through, + *plantare,* to plant]. Grafting or transplantation of tissue from one individual into another of the same species.

allotriogeustia (ă-lŏt″rē-ŏ-jūst′ē-ă, -gū′stē-a) [Gr. *allotrios,* strange, + *geusis,* taste]. Perverted appetite or sense of taste.

allotriophagy (ă-lŏt″rē-ŏf′ă-jē) [″ + *phagein,* to eat]. A perversion of appetite with ingestion of material not fit for food, as starch, clay, ashes, or plaster. SYN: *pica.*

allotriuria (ă-lŏt″rē-ū′rē-ă) [″ + *ouron,* urine]. Abnormal urine.

allotropic (ăl″ō-trŏp′ĭk) [Gr. *allos,* other, + *tropos,* direction]. 1. Pert. to the existence of an element in two or more distinct forms with different physical properties. 2. Altered by digestion so as to be changed in its nutritive value. 3. Indicating one who is concerned with the welfare and interests of others, i.e., not self-centered.

allotropism, allotropy (ă-lŏt′rō-pĭzm, -pē) [″ + *trope,* a turn, + *-ismos,* condition]. Existence of an element in two or more distinct forms with different physical properties.

alloxan (ăl-ŏk′săn) [*all*antoin + *ox*alic] $C_4H_2N_2O_4$. An oxidation product of uric acid. In experimental animals, it causes diabetes through the destruction of the islet cells of the pancreas.

alloy (ăl′oy, ă-loy′) [Fr. *aloyer,* to combine]. A metallic substance (e.g., brass) resulting from the fusion or mixture of two or more metals. Also, a substance (e.g., steel) formed from the fusion or mixture of a metal and a nonmetal. In dentistry, this is often an alloy containing mercury and called an amalgam.

allyl (ăl′ĭl) [L. *allium,* garlic, + Gr. *hyle,* matter]. C_3H_5. A univalent unsaturated radical. It is present in garlic and mustard.

alochia (ă-lō′kē-ă) [Gr. *a-,* not, + *lokhos,* pert. to childbirth]. Absence of lochia, the vaginal discharge following childbirth.

aloe (ăl′ō). USP. The dried juice of one of several species of plants of the genus Aloe. It is a component of compound benzoin tincture.

alogia (ă-lō′jē-ă) [Gr. *a-,* not, + *logos,* speech]. Inability to express oneself through speech.

aloin (ăl′ō-ĭn). Yellow crystalline substance obtained from aloe, q.v.

alopecia (al″ō-pē′shē-ă) [Gr. *alopekia,* fox mange]. Absence or loss of hair, esp. of the head.

ETIOL: May result from physiologic changes as a part of the aging process; effects of serious illness; drugs; endocrine disorders; certain forms of dermatitis; hereditary factors; radiation.

TREATMENT: Treatment of seborrheic dermatitis, q.v., if present. Scalp baldness may be treated by surgical transplantation of hair follicles from another part of the body to the scalp.

a. adnata. A. congenitalis, q.v.

a. areata. Loss of hair in sharply defined patches usually involving the scalp or beard. SEE: illus.

a. capitis totalis. Complete absence of hair of the scalp.

a., cicatricial. Loss of hair due to formation of scar tissue.

a., congenitalis. Baldness due to absence of hair bulbs at birth.

a. follicularis. Baldness due to inflam-

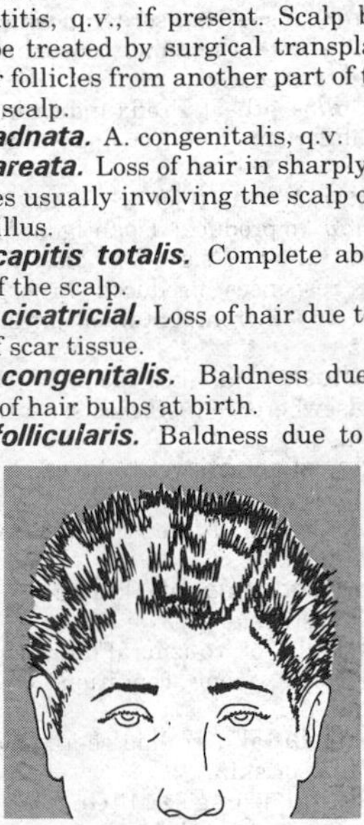

ALOPECIA AREATA

mation of the hair follicles of the scalp.

a. furfuracea. A. pityroides, q.v.

a. liminaris. Loss of hair along the hairline, both front and back, of the scalp.

a. liminaris frontalis. Loss of hair in the frontal area of the scalp of women between 15 and 20 years of age.

a., male pattern. Typical hair loss pattern of males wherein the alopecia begins in the frontal area and proceeds until only a horseshoe area of hair remains in the back and temples. This loss is dependent upon the presence of the androgenic hormone, testosterone.

a. medicamentosa. Hair loss due to administration of certain medicines, esp. those containing cytotoxic agents. SEE: *scalp tourniquet.*

a. neurotica. Loss of hair following a nervous disease or injury to nervous system, and occurring at site of injury.

a. pityroides. Loss of both scalp and body hair accompanied by desquamation of bran-like scales. SYN: *a. furfuracea.*

a. prematura. Premature baldness.

a. senilis. Baldness of old age.

a. symptomatica. Loss of hair after prolonged fevers or during the course of a disease; may result from systemic or psychogenic factors.

a. totalis. Complete loss of hair from the scalp.

a. toxica. Loss of hair thought to be due to toxins of infectious disease.

a. universalis. Complete loss of hair from all parts of body.

alpha (ăl′fă). First letter of the Greek alphabet, α. In chemistry, denotes first in a series of isomeric compounds, or position adjacent to a carboxyl group.

alpha-adrenergic blocking agent. A substance that interferes with the transmission of stimuli through pathways that normally allow sympathetic nervous excitatory stimuli to be effective. SEE: *beta-adrenergic blocking agent.*

alpha-adrenergic receptor. A site in autonomic nerve pathways wherein excitatory responses occur when adrenergic agents such as norepinephrine and epinephrine are released. SEE: *beta-adrenergic receptor.*

alpha-1 antitrypsin. An inhibitor of trypsin that may be deficient in patients who have emphysema.

alpha-fetoprotein. ABBR: AFP. An antigen present in the human fetus, and in certain pathological conditions in the adult. The amniotic fluid level can be used to evaluate fetal development. Elevated serum levels are found in adults with certain hepatic carcinomas or chemical injuries.

alpha-globulins. One of the serum globulins. SEE: *globulin, serum.*

alpha particles, rays. Radioactive, positively charged particles, 2 protons and 2 neutrons, ejected at high speeds in certain atomic disintegrations.

alpha-rhythm. In electroencephalography, rhythmical oscillations in electric potential occurring at an average rate of 10 per second. SYN: *alpha-wave.*

alpha-tocopherol. Vitamin E, q.v.

alpha-wave. Alpha-rhythm q.v.

Alport's syndrome. [Arthur Cecil Alport, S. African physician, 1880–1959] Congenital glomerulonephritis associated with deafness. Occasionally there are eye abnormalities such as cataract. Death usually occurs before middle age. There is no specific treatment for this disease.

ALS. *amyotrophic lateral sclerosis; antilymphocytic serum.*

alternans (awl-tĕr′nănz) [L *alternare*, to alternate]. Alternation.

a., pulsus. Regular heart rhythm in which strong beats alternate with weak ones.

Alternaria (awl″tĕr-nā′rē-ă). A genus of fungi of the Dematiaceae family. The fungus can cause pneumonitis. It has been implicated as the cause of pulmonary disease in wood-pulp workers.

alternating current. ABBR: A.C. An electrical current that reverses direction at regular intervals.

alternator. An electrical generator that produces alternating current.

altherm, altherm pad (ăl-thĕrm′). A device containing heat-producing chemicals for applying heat to the eye or a sinus.

alt. hor. L. *alternis horis*, every other hour.

altitude sickness. Symptoms produced by decreased oxygen in the environment. The symptoms may come on abruptly as when an airplane ascends quickly to high altitude, or slowly as in mountain climbing. The deficiency of oxygen causes headache, shortness of breath, malaise, decreased ability to concentrate, lack of judgment, light-headedness, fainting, and if severe, may cause death. The initial symptom may be euphoria so that the individual is unaware of the cause of the difficulty. Adaptation to living at high altitudes is best accomplished over a period of weeks and months. SEE: *bends.*

altricious (ăl-trĭsh′ŭs) [L. *altrix*, nourisher]. Slow in developing; requiring long nursing.

alum (ăl′ŭm) [L. *alumen*]. USP. 1. A double sulfate of aluminum and potassium or aluminum and ammonia. Strongly astringent, used topically as styptic. 2. Any of a group of double sulfates of a trivalent metal and a univalent metal.

a., ammonia. Aluminum ammonia sulfate.

a., potassium. Aluminum potassium sulfate.

alumen (ă-loo′měn) [L.]. Alum.

a. exsiccatum. Alum that has been dried or burnt; used as a dusting powder.

aluminosis (ă-loo″mĭn-ō′sĭs) [″ + Gr. *osis,* condition of]. Chronic inflammation of the lungs in alum workers due to alum particles in inspired air.

aluminum. A silver-whitish metal. SYMB: Al. At. wt. 26.9815; at. no. 13; sp. gr. 2.699.

a. acetate. A salt formed by the reaction between aluminum sulfate and lead acetate. Its aqueous solution, known as Burow's solution, is used as a local astringent.

a. ammonia sulfate. Ammonia alum; an astringent.

a. hydroxide gel. USP. A white viscous suspension containing aluminum hydroxide and hydrated aluminum oxide; an antacid especially useful in treatment of peptic ulcer.

a. potassium sulfate. Potassium alum; an astringent and styptic.

alveobronchiolitis, alveobronchitis (ăl″vē-ō-brŏng″kē-ō-lī′tĭs, -brŏng-kī′tĭs) [″ + Gr. *bronchos,* windpipe, + *itis,* inflammation]. Inflammation of the bronchioles and pulmonary alveoli; bronchopneumonia, q.v.

alveolalgia (ăl″vē-ŏ-lăl′jē-ă) [L. *alveolus,* small hollow or cavity, + Gr. *algos,* pain]. Pain in the alveolus of a tooth.

alveolar (ăl-vē′ō-lăr). Pert. to an alveolus, q.v.

alveolar air. Air in the pulmonary alveoli; that involved in the pulmonary exchange of gases. Its content is determined by sampling the last portion of a maximal expiration.

alveolar bone. Alveolar process, q.v.

alveolar-capillary block. Impaired ability of gases to pass through the pulmonary alveolar-capillary membrane.

alveolar duct. A branch of a respiratory bronchiole that leads to the alveoli of the lungs. SEE: *alveolus* for illus.

alveolar periosteum. The connective tissue between a tooth and the alveolar bone. SYN: *periodontium.*

alveolar process. The part of the mandible and maxilla containing the tooth sockets.

alveolar proteinosis. Pulmonary alveolar proteinosis, q.v.

alveolate (ăl-vē′ō-lāt). Honeycombed; pitted.

alveolectomy (ăl″vē-ŏ-lĕk′tō-mē) [L. *alveolus,* small hollow or cavity, + Gr. *ektome,* excision]. Removal of all or part of the alveolar process by surgical means.

alveoli (ăl-vē′ō-lī) [L.]. Pl. of alveolus, q.v.

a. dentales. [NA] Tooth sockets.

a. pulmonis. [NA] Air cells of the lungs.

alveolitis (ăl″vē-ŏ-lī′tĭs) [″ + Gr. *itis,* inflammation]. Inflammation of alveoli.

a., allergic. A diffuse granulomatous lung disease caused by hypersensitivity to inhalation of organic dusts. Usually occurs in those whose hobby or occupation leads to heavy exposure to dust. SYN: *pneumonitis, hypersensitivity.* SEE: *farmer's lung; bagassosis.*

alveoloclasia (ăl-vē″ō-lō-klā′sē-ă) [″ + Gr. *klasis,* fracture]. Destruction of a tooth socket.

alveolodental (ăl-vē″ō-lō-dĕn′tăl) [″ + *dens,* tooth]. Pertaining to the alveolus of the tooth and to the tooth itself.

alveololingual (ăl-vē″ō-lō-lĭng′gwăl) [″ + *lingua,* tongue]. Concerning the alveolar process and the tongue.

alveoloplasty (ăl-vē″ō-lō-plăs′tē) [″ + Gr. *plassein,* to form]. Reconstruction of the alveolus by use of plastic surgery.

alveolotomy (ăl″vē-ŏ-lŏt′ō-mē) [″ + Gr. *tome,* incision]. Surgical incision of the alveolus of a tooth.

alveolus (ăl-vē′ō-lŭs) [L., small hollow or cavity]. (pl. *alveoli*) 1. A small hollow. 2. The socket of a tooth. 3. Air cell of the lungs. SEE: illus. 4. One of the honeycombed depressions of the gastric mucous membrane. 5. A follicle of a racemose gland.

a. dentalis. Tooth socket.

a., pulmonary. One of the terminal saccules of an alveolar duct where gases are exchanged in respiration. SYN: *air vesicle; alveoli pulmonis* (pl.).

alveus (ăl′vē-ŭs) [L.]. A channel or groove.

a. hippocampi. [NA] A layer of white matter covering ventricular surface of the hippocampus.

alvine (ăl′vīn) [L. *alvus,* belly]. Pert. to the intestines or abdomen.

alvinolith (ăl-vī′nō-lĭth) [″ + Gr. *lithos,* stone]. An intestinal mass formed from calcareous salts and other matter.

alvus (ăl′vŭs) [L.]. Abdomen and viscera.

alymphia (ă-lĭm′fē-ă) [Gr. *a-,* not, + L. *lympha,* lymph]. Complete or partial deficiency of lymph.

alymphocytosis (ă-lĭm″fō-sī-tō′sĭs) [″ + ″ + Gr. *kytos,* cell, + *osis,* condition]. Decreased number or absence of lymphocytes in the blood.

alymphoplasia (ă″lĭm-fō-plā′zē-ă) [″ + ″ + Gr. *plasis,* a developing]. Failure of lymph tissue to develop.

a., thymic. A sometimes fatal disorder in which the thymus fails to develop, causing a deficiency of gamma globulin. There is deficiency of lymph tissue throughout the body.

Alzheimer's disease (ălts′hī-mĕrz). [Alois Alzheimer, Ger. neurologist, 1864–1915] A form of presenile dementia due to atrophy of frontal and occipital lobes. Usually occurs between ages 40 and 60, more often in women than men. Involves progressive, irreversible loss of memory, deterioration of intellectual

ALVEOLUS OF LUNG

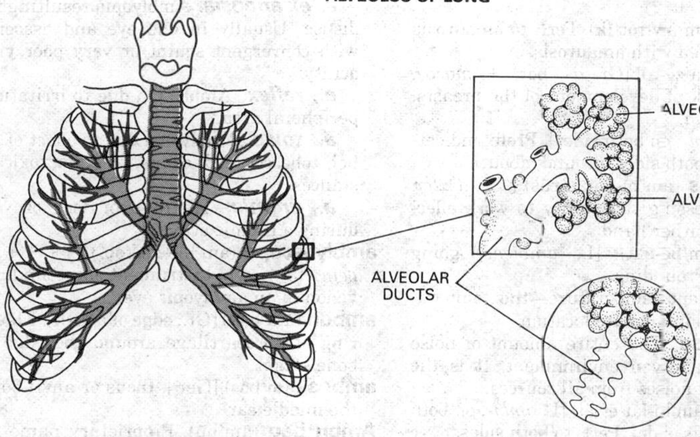

functions, apathy, speech and gait disturbances, and disorientation. Course may take from a few months to four or five years to progress to complete loss of intellectual function. SEE: *Pick's disease.*

Am. *mixed astigmatism; ametropia.* Chem. symb. for americium.

A.M.A. *American Medical Association.*

a.m.a. *against medical advice,* q.v.

amaas (ă′măs). A mild form of smallpox. SYN: *alastrim; variola minor.*

amacrine (ăm′ă-krĭn) [Gr. *a-*, not, + *makros,* long, + *is, inos,* fiber]. Lacking a long process.

amacrine cell. A modified nerve cell in the retina that has short branches (dendrites) but no long process (axon). SEE: *neuron.*

amalgam (ă-măl′găm) [Gr. *malagma,* soft mass]. Any alloy containing mercury.

a., dental. An alloy containing mercury that is used in dentistry to restore teeth.

amalgamate (ă-măl′gă-māt″). To make an amalgam.

amalgamation (ă-măl″gă-mā′shŭn). The process of mixing metallic particles with mercury to produce an amalgam. SYN: *trituration* (def. 3).

amalgamator (ă-măl′gă-mā″tor). A device that provides a mechanical means of amalgamation. This can also be done by hand using a mortar and pestle.

amanita (ăm″ă-nī′tă, -nē′tă) [Gr. *amanitai,* mushrooms]. Any of various mushrooms of the genus Amanita. Most are extremely poisonous. SEE: *Poisons and Poisoning* in *Appendix.*

amantadine hydrochloride (ă-măn′tă-dēn hī″drō-klor′īd). USP. An antiviral agent originally used for prophylaxis against certain strains of the influenza virus. Has also been used in treating Parkinson's disease. Trade name is Symmetrel.

amarthritis (ăm″ăr-thrī′tĭs) [Gr. *hama,* at same time, + *arthron,* joint, + *itis,* inflammation]. Inflammation of more than one joint at the same time. SYN: *polyarthritis.*

amasesis (ăm″ă-sē′sĭs) [Gr. *a-*, not, + *masesis,* chewing]. Inability to masticate food.

amastia (ă-măs′tē-ă) [″ + *mastos,* breast]. Lack of breast development. SYN: *amazia.*

amativeness (ăm′ă-tĭv″nĕs) [L. *amare,* to love]. 1. Sexual desire. 2. Desire to love.

amaurosis (ăm″aw-rō′sĭs) [Gr., darkening]. Complete loss of vision, esp. that in which there is no apparent pathologic condition of the eye.

a., albuminuric. Amaurosis caused by kidney disease.

a., congenital. Amaurosis present at birth.

a., diabetic. Amaurosis associated with diabetes.

a., epileptoid. Sudden blindness following an epileptic seizure and lasting up to two weeks.

a. fugax. Temporary loss of vision in one eye due to insufficient flow of blood to the retina. May last for up to 10 minutes. SYN: *blindness, transient,* q.v.

a., lead. Amaurosis caused by lead poisoning.

a. partialis fugax. Sudden transitory blindness with symptoms similar to migraine: nausea; vomiting; dizziness; and disturbances of vision.

a., reflex. Amaurosis due to reflex action caused by irritation of a remote part.

a., saburral. Amaurosis in conjunction with acute gastritis.

a., toxic. Amaurosis from optic neuritis caused by toxins that may be endogenous, such as in diabetes, or exogenous, as in alcohol or tobacco.

a., uremic. Amaurosis caused by uremic condition.

amaurotic (ăm-aw-rŏt'ĭk). Pert. to amaurosis or one afflicted with amaurosis.

amazia (ă-mā'zē-ă) [Gr. *a-*, not, + *mazos*, breast]. Lack of development of the breasts. SYN: *amastia*.

ambi- [L. *ambi-*, on both sides]. Prefix indicating both or both sides; around; about.

ambidextrous (ăm"bĭ-dĕk'strŭs) [" + *dexter*, right]. Possessing the ability to work effectively with either hand.

ambient (ăm'bē-ĕnt) [L. *ambiens*, going around]. Surrounding.

Ex.: ambient temperature—the temperature in one's immediate location.

ambient noise. The entire amount of noise present in a given environment. It is the composite of noises from all sources.

ambilateral (ăm"bĭ-lăt'ĕr-ăl) [L. *ambi-*, on both sides, + *latus*, side]. Pert. to both sides.

ambilevous (ăm-bĭ-lē'vŭs) [" + *laevus*, left-handed]. Awkward in use of either hand. SYN: *ambisinister*.

ambiopia (ăm"bē-ō'pē-ă) [" + Gr. *ops*, eye]. Double vision. SYN: *diplopia*, q.v.

ambisexual (ăm"bĭ-sĕks'ū-ăl) [" + *sexus*, sex]. Pertaining to both sexes. SEE: *bisexual*.

ambisinister (ăm"bĭ-sĭn'ĭs-tĕr) [" + *sinister*, left]. Awkward in use of either hand. SYN: *ambilevous*.

ambitendency (ăm"bĭ-tĕn'dĕn-sē) [" + *tendere*, to stretch]. Ambivalence of the will. SEE: *ambivalence*.

ambivalence (ăm-bĭv'ă-lĕns) [" + *valentia*, strength]. Coexistence of contradictory feelings about an object, person, or idea.

ambivalent (ăm-bĭv'ă-lĕnt). Relating to, or characterized by ambivalence.

ambivert (ăm'bĭ-vĕrt) [" + *vertere*, to turn]. An individual whose personality type falls between introversion and extroversion, possessing some tendencies of each.

amblyacousia (ăm"blē-ă-koo'sē-ă) [Gr. *amblys*, dull, + *akousis*, hearing]. Dullness of hearing.

amblyaphia (ăm-blē-ăf'ē-ă) [" + *haphe*, touch]. Dull sense of touch.

amblychromasia (ăm"blē-krō-mā'sē-ă) [" + *chroma*, color]. The state in which the cell nucleus stains faintly.

amblychromatic (ăm"blē-krō-măt'ĭk). Staining faintly.

amblygeustia (ăm"blē-jūs'tē-ă, ăm"blē-goos'tē-ă) [" + *geusis*, taste]. Defective or blunted taste.

amblyopia (ăm"blē-ō'pē-ă) [" + *ops*, eye]. Reduction or dimness of vision, esp. that in which there is no apparent pathologic condition of the eye.

a., crossed. Amblyopia of one eye with hemianesthesia of the opposite side of the face. Also: *a. cruciata*.

a. ex anopsia. Amblyopia resulting from disuse. Usually in one eye and associated with convergent squint or very poor visual acuity.

a., reflex. Amblyopia due to irritation of peripheral area.

a., toxic. Amblyopia due to effect of alcohol, tobacco, lead, drugs, or other toxic substances.

a., uremic. Dimness or loss of vision during a uremic attack.

amblyoscope (ăm'blē-ō-skōp") [" + " + *skopein*, to view]. Instrument for stimulating vision in an amblyopic eye.

ambon (ăm'bŏn) [Gr., edge of a dish]. Elevated ring of fibrocartilage around the edge of a bone socket.

ambos (ăm'bōs) [Ger.]. Incus or anvil bone of the middle ear.

Ambu bag (ăm'bū). Proprietary name for a ventilating bag.

ambulance [L. *ambulare*, to move about]. A vehicle for transportation of the sick and injured, it is equipped and staffed to provide medical care during transit.

ambulant, ambulatory (ăm'bū-lănt, -lă-tō"rē). Able to walk, not confined to bed.

Ambu simulator. Proprietary name for a manikin used in teaching the technique of cardiopulmonary resuscitation.

Amcill. Trade name for ampicillin, USP, q.v.

Ameba, Amoeba (ă-mē'bă). A genus of protozoa, class Sarcodina, found in soil and water; common name, ameba, q.v. Some are parasitic in man, but most of the parasitic species have been reclassified in the genus Entamoeba, q.v.

ameba, amoeba [Gr. *amoibe*, change]. (pl. *amebae, amoebae; amebas, amoebas*) A minute one-celled protozoan animal form of life found in soil and water. It constantly changes shape by sending out fingerlike processes of protoplasm (pseudopodia), by which it moves about and obtains its nourishment. It possesses an outer translucent substance called the ectoplasm; but the inner substance, endoplasm, is denser and contains a nucleus. It feeds by surrounding its food and enclosing it in the so-called food vacuole. Oxygen is absorbed from the surrounding water, and CO_2 is eliminated through the plasma membrane. Reproduction is by binary fission, in which the nucleus divides by mitosis. Some species of Entamoeba, q.v., are parasitic in man.

amebiasis (am"ĕ-bī'ă-sĭs) [" + *-iasis*, state]. Infection with amebae, esp. Entamoeba histolytica.

ETIOL: Entamoeba histolytica is acquired by ingesting food or drink containing encysted forms.

PATH: Small abscesses and, later, ulcers

of mucous membrane of colon, sometimes resulting in perforation. Liver abscesses may result from amebae being carried to liver via portal vein.

SYM: Many patients are asymptomatic. Disease is generally characterized by dysentery with diarrhea, weakness, and prostration. Nausea, vomiting, and pain may be present. One serious complication is amebic hepatitis.

DIAG: Cysts or trophozoites of E. histolytica in stools.

TREATMENT: In acute amebiasis, metronidazole (Flagyl), tetracycline, or emetine hydrochloride. Chloroquine, metronidazole, or emetine is useful in liver abscess. Repeated treatment at intervals for up to three months is necessary to assure the amebae have been eliminated.

For treatment of asymptomatic carriers of cysts, diloxanide furoate is the treatment of choice. It is available from the Parasitic Disease Drug Service, Centers for Disease Control, Atlanta, Georgia 30303, U.S.A.

a., hepatic. Infection of the liver by amebae, usually with abscess formation.

amebic (ă-mē'bĭk). Pert. to or caused by amebae.

amebic carrier state. State in which an individual harbors a form of pathogenic ameba but has no clinical signs of the disease.

amebic dysentery. Infection with Entamoeba histolytica. SEE: *amebiasis.*

amebic hepatitis. Amebic abscess of the liver.

amebicide, amebacide (ă-mē'bĭ-sīd) [Gr. *amoibe,* change, + L. *caedere,* to kill]. An agent that kills amebae.

amebiform (ă-mē'bĭ-form) [" + L. *forma,* shape]. Shaped like an ameba.

amebocyte (ă-mē'bō-sīt") [" + *kytos,* cell]. A cell showing ameboid movements.

ameboid (ă-mē'boyd) [" + *eidos,* resemblance]. Resembling an ameba.

ameboidism (ă-mē'boyd-ĭzm). 1. Ameba-like movements. 2. Denoting a condition shown by certain nerve cells.

ameboid movement. Cellular movement much like that of an amoeba. A protoplasmic pseudopod, q.v., extends and then the remaining cell contents flow into the pseudopod, which swells gradually. This type of movement allows cells such as leukocytes to move through very small openings. SEE: *diapedesis.*

ameboma (ăm"ē-bō'mă) [" + *oma,* tumor]. Tumor composed of inflammatory tissue caused by amebiasis.

ameburia (ăm"ē-bū'rē-ă) [Gr. *amoibe,* change, + *ouron,* urine]. Presence of amebae in the urine.

amelanotic (ă"mĕl-ă-nŏt'ĭk). Lacking melanin; unpigmented.

amelia (ă-mē'lē-ă) [Gr. *a-,* not, + *melos,* limb]. Congenital absence of one or more limbs.

amelification (ă-mĕl"ĭ-fĭ-kā'shŭn) [O. Fr. *amel,* enamel, + L. *facere,* to make]. Formation of dental enamel by ameloblasts.

amelioration (ă-mēl"yō-rā'shŭn) [L. *ad,* to, + *melior,* better]. Improvement; moderation of a condition.

ameloblast (ă-mĕl'ō-blăst) [O. Fr. *amel,* enamel, + Gr. *blastos,* germ]. A cell from which tooth enamel is formed.

ameloblastoma (ă-mĕl"ō-blăs-tō'mă) [" + " + *oma,* tumor]. A tumor of the jaw, esp. the lower one, arising from the enamel organ. May be partly cystic, partly solid, and may reach large size; of low-grade malignancy. SYN: *adamantinoma.*

amelodentinal [O. Fr. *amel,* enamel, + L. *dens, dent-,* tooth]. Pert. to both enamel and dentin.

amelogenesis (ăm"ĕ-lō-jĕn'ĕ-sĭs) [" + Gr. *genesis,* generation]. Formation of dental enamel.

amelus (ăm'ĕ-lŭs) [Gr. *a-,* not, + *melos,* limb]. Individual with congenitally absent arms and legs.

amenia (ă-mē'nē-ă) [Gr. *a-,* not, + *men,* month]. Amenorrhea, q.v.

amenorrhea (ă-mĕn"ō-rē'ă) [" + *men,* month, + *rhoia,* flow]. Absence or suppression of menstruation; normal before puberty, after the menopause, and during pregnancy and lactation. SYN: *amenia.* SEE: *oligomenorrhea.*

ETIOL: The most common causes of abnormal amenorrhea are congenital abnormalities of the reproductive tract; metabolic disorders (obesity, malnutrition, diabetes); systemic diseases (syphilis, tuberculosis, nephritis); emotional disorders (excitement, anorexia nervosa); endocrine disorders, esp. those involving the ovaries, pituitary, thyroid, and adrenal glands; hormonal imbalance of estrogen, progesterone, or follicle-stimulating hormones.

TREATMENT: Underlying cause should be determined and corrected. If hormone deficiencies exist, substitutional therapy is recommended.

a., dietary. Cessation of menstruation due to voluntary or involuntary (as in starvation) dietary restriction.

a., emotional. Amenorrhea resulting from shock, fright, hysteria.

a., nutritional. A., dietary, q.v.

a., pathologic. Amenorrhea due to organic disease.

a., physiologic. Amenorrhea during prepuberty, pregnancy, lactation, and postmenopause periods; not related to organic disease.

a., primary. Delay of menarche beyond

age 18.

a., secondary. Cessation of menses in a woman who has previously menstruated.

a., stress. Cessation of menstruation due to mental or physical stress.

amenorrheic (ă-mĕn″ō-rē′ĭk). Pert. to amenorrhea.

amentia (ă-mĕn′shē-ă) [L. *ab,* from, + *mens,* mind]. 1. Congenital mental deficiency; mental retardation, q.v. 2. Mental disorder characterized by confusion, disorientation, and occasionally stupor. SEE: *dementia.*

a. agitata. Form of amentia characterized by excitement, excessive motor activity, and constant hallucinations.

a. attonita. Form of amentia characterized by apathy, immobility, and semiconsciousness or stupor.

a., nevoid. Sturge-Weber syndrome; congenital syndrome characterized by port-wine nevi along distribution of trigeminal nerve; angiomas of leptomeninges and choroid; intracranial calcifications; mental retardation; epileptic seizures; and glaucoma.

a., phenylpyruvic. Mental retardation due to phenylketonuria, q.v.

Americaine. Trade name for benzocaine, USP, q.v.

americium (ăm-ĕr-ĭsh′ē-ŭm). SYMB: Am. A metallic radioactive element. At no. 95; at. wt. of longest-lived isotope 243.

ameristic (ă″mĕr-ĭs′tĭk) [Gr *a-,* not + *meristos,* divided]. Not divided into parts or fragments.

ametria (ă-mē′trē-ă) [″ + *metra,* uterus]. Congenital absence of the uterus.

ametrometer (ăm″ē-trŏm′ĕ-tĕr) [*ametropia* + Gr. *metron,* measure]. Instrument for measuring degree of ametropia, q.v.

ametropia (ă″mĕ-trō′pē-ă) [Gr. *ametros,* disproportionate, + *ops,* eye]. Imperfect refractive powers of eye, in which the principal focus does not lie on the retina. This causes hyperopia, myopia, or astigmatism, q.v.

amicrobic (ă″mī-krō′bĭk) [Gr. *a-,* not, + *mikros,* small, + *bios,* life]. 1. Lacking microbes. 2. Not caused by microbes.

amicroscopic (ă-mī″krō-skŏp′ĭk) [″ + ″ + *skopein,* to view]. Too small to be seen through a microscope. SYN: *submicroscopic.*

amidase (ăm′ĭ-dās). A deamidizing enzyme, q.v., one that catalyzes the hydrolysis of amides.

amide (ăm′ĭd). Any organic substance that contains the monovalent radical $-CONH_2$. It is usually formed by replacing the hydroxyl ($-OH$) group of the $-COOH$ by the $-NH_2$ group.

amidin (ăm′ĭ-dĭn) [Fr. *amidon,* starch]. The soluble component of starch. The insoluble constituent is amylopectin.

amido-. A prefix signifying the presence of the radical $CONH_2$.

amidulin (ă-mĭd′ū-lĭn) [Fr. *amidon,* starch]. Soluble starch.

amikacin sulfate. USP. An aminoglycoside antibiotic. Trade name is Amikin.

amimia (ă-mĭm′ē-ă) [Gr. *a-,* not, + *mimos,* mimic]. Loss of power to express ideas by signs or gestures.

a., amnesic. Amimia in which signs and gestures can be made but their meaning is not remembered.

a., ataxic. Amimia in which signs and gestures cannot be made because of nervous or muscular disorders.

amine (ă-mēn′, ăm′ĭn). Any one of a group of nitrogen-containing organic compounds that are formed when one or more of the hydrogens of ammonia have been replaced by one or more hydrocarbon radicals.

amino- (ă-mē′nō, ăm′ĭ-nō). Prefix denoting presence of an amino group (NH_2).

aminoacetic acid (ăm″ĭn-ō-ă-sē′tĭk). NH_2-CH_2COOH. A nonessential amino acid, q.v. SYN: *glycine.*

amino acid. One of a large group of organic compounds marked by presence of both an amino group (NH_2) and a carboxyl ($COOH$) group. Their basic formula is $NH_2-R-COOH$ in which R stands for any aliphatic or aromatic radical. They are amphoteric and exhibit properties marked by both the amino and carboxyl groups. They are the building blocks of which proteins are constructed, and are the end-products of protein digestion or hydrolysis.

Approximately 80 amino acids are found in nature; only 20 are necessary for human metabolism or growth but, because some are supplied by food and the others can be produced by the body, the ones that must be provided by food are called essential. These are: histidine (essential for normal adult but amount required is not known), isoleucine, leucine, lysine, methionine, cysteine, phenylalanine, tyrosine, threonine, tryptophan, and valine. The nonessential amino acids are: alanine, aspartic acid, arginine, citrulline, glutamic acid, glycine, hydroxyglutamic acid, hydroxyproline, norleucine, proline, and serine.

Arginine, while nonessential for the adult, cannot be formed quickly enough to supply the demand in infants and thus is classed as essential in early life.

Some proteins contain all the essential amino acids and are called complete proteins. Examples are milk, cheese, eggs, and meat. Proteins that do not contain all the essential amino acids are called incomplete proteins. Examples are vegetables and grains. Amino acids pass unchanged through the intestinal wall and portal vein into the blood, then through the liver into the general circulation, from which they are absorbed by the tissues according to the specific amino acid needed by that tissue to make its own protein. Amino acids if not otherwise metabolized may be converted into urea. SEE: illus.; *deaminization; digestion; protein.*

a.a., essential. In human nutrition, amino acids that are required for growth and development, and that cannot be produced by the body. They must be obtained from food.

a.a., nonessential. Amino acids that can be produced by the body and are not required in the diet.

aminoacidemia (ă-mē″nō-, ăm″ĭ-nō-ăs″ĭ-dē′mē-ă) [*amino acid* + Gr. *haima,* blood]. Excess of amino acids in the blood.

amino acid group. The NH_2 group that characterizes the amines.

aminoacidopathies (ăm″ĭ-nō-ăs″ĭ-dŏp′ă-thēz) [″ + Gr. *pathos,* disease]. Various disorders of amino acid metabolism, of which there are nearly 100, including cystinuria, alkaptonuria, and albinism.

aminoaciduria (ă-mē″nō-, ăm″ĭ-nō-ăs″ĭ-dū′rē-ă) [″ + Gr. *ouron,* urine]. Excess amino acids in the urine.

aminobenzene (ă-mē″nō-, ăm″ĭ-nō-bĕn′zēn). $C_6H_5NH_2$. The simplest aromatic amine, an oily liquid derived from benzene. Used in manufacture of dyes for medical and industrial purposes. SYN: *phenylamine.*

aminobenzoic acid. USP. $NH_2C_6H_4COOH$. A drug used as a topical ultraviolet screening agent. Trade name is Pabanol. SYN: *para-aminobenzoic acid.*

aminocaproic acid. SEE: *acid, aminocaproic.*

aminoglutethimide (ăm″ĭ-nō-gloo-tĕth′ĭ-mīd). Chemical that interferes with the production of adrenal cortical hormone. It has been used to decrease the hypersecretion of cortisol by adrenal tumors.

aminohippuric acid, sodium. USP. The sodium salt of aminohippuric acid. It is given intravenously to test renal blood flow and the excretory capacity of the renal tubules.

aminolysis (ăm″ĭ-nŏl′ĭ-sĭs) [*amine* + Gr. *lysis,* dissolution]. Metabolic transformation of amino-containing compounds by removing the amino group.

aminometradine (ăm″ĭ-nō-mĕt′ră-dēn). A nonmercurial diuretic given orally.

aminophylline (ăm-ĭ-nŏf′ĭ-lĭn, ăm″ĭ-nō-fĭl′ĭn). USP. $C_{16}H_{24}N_{10}O_4{\cdot}2H_2O$. A mixture of theophylline and ethylenediamine. Used esp. in acute asthma that has not responded to epinephrine. Used also as a stimulant to the respiratory center and heart muscle, and as

AMINO ACIDS

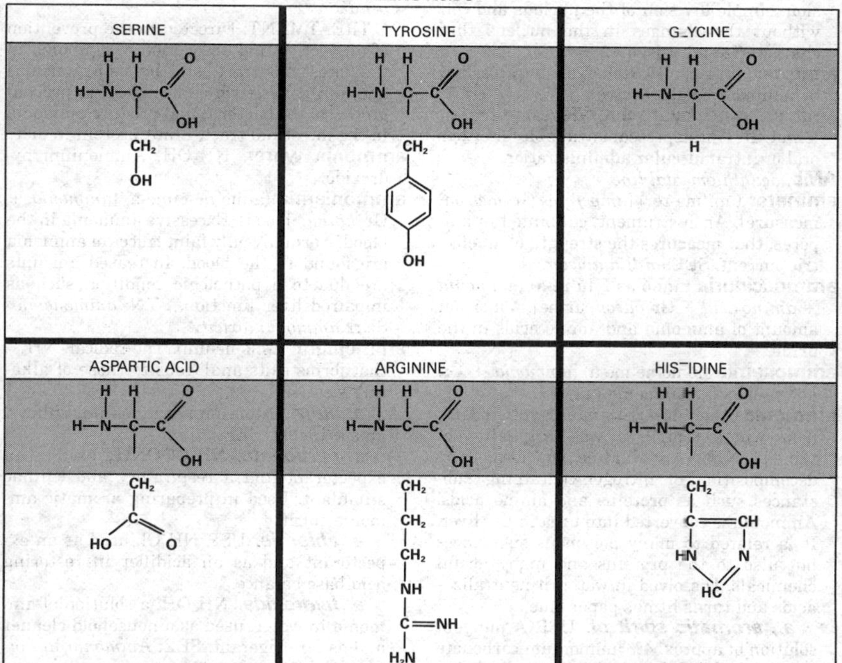

a diuretic. Trade names are Rectalad, Somophyllin, and Aminodur. SYN: *theophylline ethylenediamine.*

aminophylline poisoning. SEE: *Poisons and Poisoning* in *Appendix.*

aminopterin (ăm-ĭ-nŏp′tĕr-ĭn). A folic acid antagonist used in treatment of acute leukemia.

aminopurine (ăm″ĭ-nō-pū′rĭn). An oxidation product of purine. Includes adenine and guanine. SEE: *methyl purine; oxypurine.*

aminopyrine (ăm″ĭn-ō-pī′rēn, -rĭn). An antipyretic and analgesic drug. CAUTION: Because this drug may cause fatal agranulocytosis, it should not be used. SYN: *amidopyrine.*

aminosalicylic acid. USP. $C_7H_7NO_3$. A white or nearly white and practically odorless powder that darkens when exposed to air or light. It is an antituberculosis drug, but its effectiveness is greatly enhanced when used in combination with streptomycin and isoniazid; it is believed to delay development of bacterial resistance. SYN: *para-aminosalicylic acid.*

aminuria (ăm-ĭ-nū′rē-ă) [*amine* + Gr. *ouron,* urine]. Presence of amines in urine.

Amitid. Trade name for amitriptyline hydrochloride, USP, q.v.

amitosis (ăm″ĭ-tō′sĭs) [Gr. *a-*, not, + *mitos,* a thread, + *osis,* condition]. Direct cell division; simple division of the nucleus and cell without the changes in the nucleus that characterize mitosis, q.v.

amitotic (ăm″ĭ-tŏt′ĭk). Rel. to or characterized by amitosis. SYN: *akinetic.*

amitryptyline hydrochloride (ăm″ĭ-trĭp′tĭ-lēn). USP. Antidepressant available for either oral or intramuscular administration.

AML. *acanthiomeatal line.*

ammeter (ăm′mē-tĕr) [*ampere* + Gr. *metron,* measure]. An instrument, calibrated in amperes, that measures the strength of an electric current. SEE: *milliammeter.*

ammoaciduria (ăm″ō-ăs″ĭ-dū′rē-ă) [*ammonia* + *amino acid* + Gr. *ouron,* urine]. Abnormal amount of ammonia and amino acids in the urine.

ammonemia (ă-mō-nē′mē-ă) [*ammonia* + Gr. *haima,* blood]. Ammoniemia, q.v.

ammonia (ă-mō′nē-ă) [*Ammo,* Egyptian deity near whose temple it was originally obtained]. NH_3. An alkaline gas formed by decomposition of nitrogen-containing substances such as proteins and amino acids. Ammonia is converted into urea in the liver. It is related to many poisonous substances but also to the proteins and many useful chemicals. Dissolved in water, it neutralizes acids and turns litmus paper blue.

a., aromatic spirit of. USP. A pungent solution of approx. 4% ammonium carbonate in 70% alcohol flavored with lemon, lavender, and myristica oil. It is used to elicit reflex stimulation of respiration and as "smelling salts" to stimulate patients who have fainted.

a., blood. Ammonia in the blood. Increased values are found in liver failure. SEE: *ammoniemia.*

ammoniacal (ăm″ō-nī′ă-kăl). Having the characteristics of or pert. to ammonia.

ammonia intoxication. SEE: *ammonia toxicity.*

ammonia solution, diluted. A solution containing approx. 10 grams of ammonia per 100 ml. of water.

ammonia solution, strong. A solution containing approx. 28% ammonia in water.

ammoniated (ă-mō′nē-āt′d). Containing ammonia.

ammonia toxicity. Ammonia is produced in the intestinal tract by bacterial action. After absorption it is transported to the liver, where it is metabolized. In diseases such as cirrhosis of the liver, the ammonia absorbed may be shunted past the liver. This results in an accumulation of ammonia in the blood (ammoniemia). The resulting developments, including alterations in consciousness, neurologic changes, abnormal electroencephalogram, and a flapping tremor (asterixis), are due at least in part to ammonia toxicity. SEE: *Poisons and Poisoning* in *Appendix.*

TREATMENT: Directed to the prevention of production and absorption of ammonia in the intestinal tract; and by using enemas and antibiotics such as neomycin to prevent growth of the bacteria that produce ammonia in the intestinal tract. Limit protein in diet.

ammonia water. NH_4OH. Ammonium hydroxide.

ammoniemia (a-mō″nē-ē′mē-ă) [*ammonia* + Gr. *haima,* blood]. Excessive ammonia in the blood. Normally only faint traces of ammonia are found in the blood. Increased amounts are due to a pathologic condition such as impaired liver function. SYN: *ammonemia.* SEE: *ammonia toxicity.*

ammonium (ă-mō′nē-ŭm). The radical, NH_4^+, that forms salts analogous to those of alkaline metals.

a. alum. Aluminum ammonium sulfate, an astringent. SEE: *alum.*

a. carbonate. NH_2COONH_4, used as an expectorant and a respiratory and cardiac stimulant. Used in preparing aromatic ammonia spirit.

a. chloride. USP. NH_4Cl, used as an expectorant and as an acidifier in restoring acid-base balance.

a. hydroxide. NH_4OH, a solution of ammonia in water, used as a household cleaner and as a refrigerant. SEE: *Ammonia* in *Poisons and Poisoning* in *Appendix.*

ammoniuria (ă-mō″nē-ū′rē-ă) [″ + Gr. *ouron,* urine]. Excessive ammonia in the urine.

ammonolysis. The chemical process of removing NH_2 radicals from a compound.

ammonotelic (ă-mō″nō-tĕl′ĭk). Pert. to animals that excrete amino nitrogen in the form of ammonia. Included in this group are most aquatic vertebrates but not whales. SEE: *urea cycle; ureotelic; uricotelic.*

amnesia (ăm-nē′zē-ă) [Gr.]. A loss of memory. Often applied to episodes during which patients forget their identity, though they may conduct themselves properly enough, and following which no memory of the period persists. Such episodes are often hysterical and sometimes epileptic, while trauma, senility, alcoholism, and other organic reaction types account for a smaller number.

a., anterograde. Amnesia for events occurring after the precipitating trauma.

a., auditory. Loss of memory for the meanings of sounds or spoken words. SYN: *aphasia, auditory; deafness, word.*

a., lacunar. Loss of memory for isolated events.

a., retroanterograde. A memory disorder in which present-day events are referred to the past and vice versa.

a., retrograde. Amnesia for events occurring before the precipitating trauma.

a., tactile. Inability to distinguish objects by sense of touch. SYN: *astereognosis.*

a., transient global. Transient amnesia that occurs in otherwise healthy persons. Onset is usually sudden and may last for a few hours. Remote memory is retained even though memory for recent events is absent. Recovery is usually rapid.

a. traumatica. Amnesia caused by sudden physical injury.

a., visual. Inability to remember the appearance of objects or to be cognizant of printed words.

amnesic (ăm-nē′sĭk). Pert. to amnesia.

amnesic aphasia. Loss of memory for words.

amnestic (ăm-nĕs′tĭk). Pert. to or causing amnesia.

amniocentesis (ăm″nē-ō-sĕn-tē′sĭs) [Gr. *amnion,* lamb, + *kentesis,* puncture]. Transabdominal puncture of the amniotic sac, using a needle and syringe, in order to remove amniotic fluid. The material obtained may be studied chemically or cytologically to detect genetic and biochemical disorders or maternal-fetal blood incompatibility.

This procedure is usually performed no earlier than at 14 weeks' gestation. It is important that the analysis be done by persons who are expert in the fields of chemistry and cell culture. Cell cultures may require 30 days and if the test has to be repeated, the time required may be insufficient to allow corrective action. SEE: illus.

CAUTION: The procedure can cause abortion; and trauma to the fetus is possible.

NURSING IMPLICATIONS: Prepare the patient for what to expect during the procedure, and provide emotional support for her during the actual procedure. Monitor her vital signs and the fetal heart tones during the procedure. Assess the patient for dizziness, fainting, pain, nausea, and the onset of labor. Be aware of the development of any complications following the procedure such as fetal or maternal hemorrhage, premature labor, and signs or symptoms of infection. Inform the patient concerning complications to watch for, and instruct her to contact her physician immediately if difficulties develop.

amniochorial, amniochorionic (ăm″nē-ō-kō′rē-ăl, -kō-rē-ŏn′ĭk). Relating to both amnion and chorion.

amnioclepsis (ăm″nē-ō-klĕp′sĭs) [″ + *kleptein,* to steal]. Gradual unperceived loss of amniotic fluid.

amniogenesis (ăm″nē-ō-jĕn′ĕ-sĭs) [″ + *genesis,* generation]. Formation of the amnion.

amniography [″ + *graphein,* to write]. Roentgenography of amniotic sac after injection of a radiopaque substance into the amniotic fluid. Used in diagnosing fetal abnormalities.

amnioinfusion (ăm″nē-ō-ĭn-fū′zhŭn). Injection of solutions into the amniotic fluid. Usually done to induce abortion.

amnion (ăm′nē-ŏn) [Gr. *amnion,* lamb]. The inner of the fetal membranes, a thin, transparent sac that holds the fetus suspended in the liquor amnii or amniotic fluid, q.v. The amnion grows rapidly at the expense of the extraembryonic coelom, and by the end of the third month it fuses with the chorion, forming the amniochorionic sac. Commonly called the bag of waters. SYN: *amniotic sac.* SEE: *oligohydramnios;* words beginning with *amnio-.*

a. nodosum. Rounded or oval opaque elevations 1 to 6 mm. in diameter in the placenta that are seen in the part of the amnion in contact with the chorionic plate and near the insertion of the cord into the placenta. They are present in approx. 60% of pregnancies.

amnionitis (ăm″nē-ō-nī′tĭs) [″ + *itis,* inflammation]. Inflammation of the amnion.

amniorrhea (ăm″nē-or-rē′ă) [″ + *rhoia,* flow]. Escape of the amniotic fluid.

amniorrhexis (ăm″nē-ō-rĕk′sĭs) [″ + *rhexis,* rupture]. Rupture of the amnion.

amnioscope (ăm′nē-ō-skōp) [Gr. *amnion,* lamb, + *skopein,* to examine]. Optical device for looking inside the amniotic cavity.

a., suction. Amnioscope designed to allow suction to be applied so that it is held in place against the fetal scalp. This permits

AMNIOCENTESIS

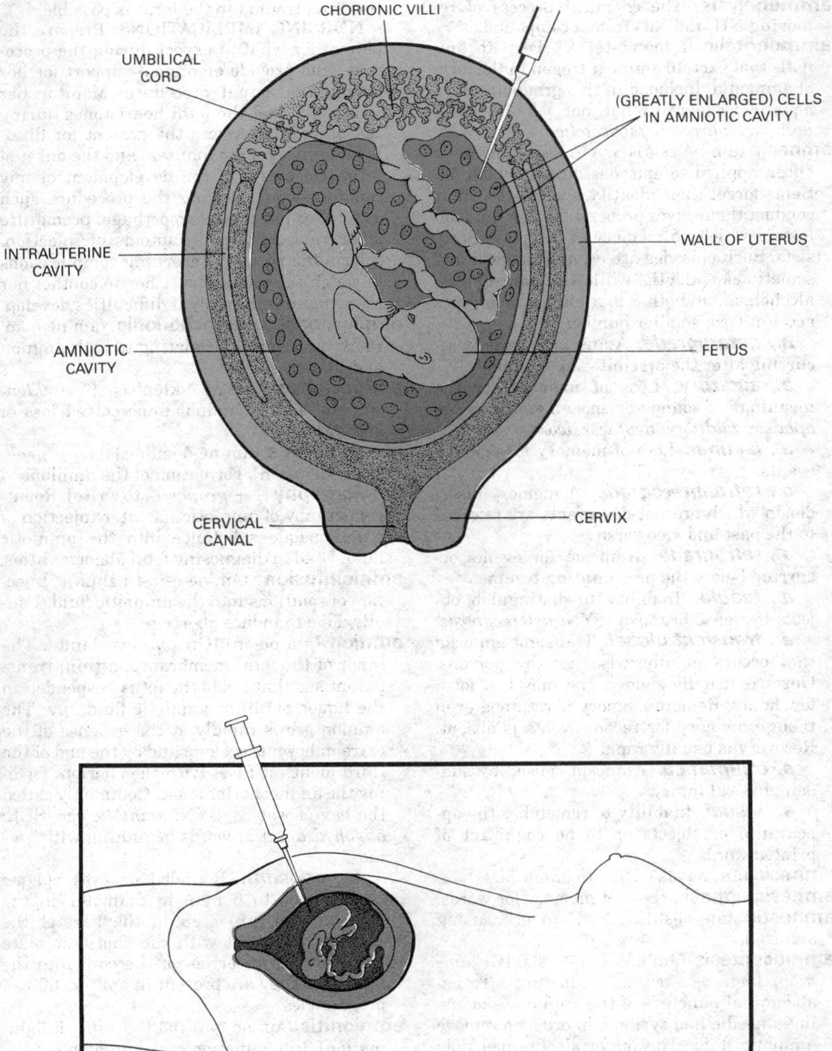

evacuation of the amniotic fluid from the area pressing against the scalp, thus leaving a clear field for sampling blood from that site.

amnioscopy. Direct visual examination of the fetus by use of an optical device that is inserted into the amniotic cavity via the abdominal wall.

amniote (ăm'nē-ōt). Any animal or group belonging to the Amniota, a major group of vertebrates, the members of which develop an amnion. Includes reptiles, birds, and mammals.

amniotic (ăm-nē-ŏt'ĭk). Pert. to the amnion.

amniotic band syndrome. A collection of fetal malformations associated with fibrous bands that appear to develop or entangle fetal parts in utero. This leads to structural malformations and deformations; and disruption of function. This condition has had a variety of synonyms including aberrant tissue bands; "Adam complex" (amniotic deformity, adhesion, mutilations); amniogenic bands; and congenital annular bands, rings, or constrictions. Defects associated with this condition include limb defects and amputations; abnormal dermal ridge patterns; simian creases; clubbed feet; craniofacial defects including cleft lip and palate; and visceral defects such as gastroschisis and omphalocele. Failure to understand the cause of this condition can lead to misdiagnosis and inappropriate family and genetic counseling.

amniotic cavity. The fluid-filled cavity of the amnion, q.v.

amniotic fluid. Liquor amnii. The liquid or albuminous fluid contained in the amnion, q.v. This fluid is transparent and almost colorless. The liquid protects the fetus from injury, helps maintain an even temperature, prevents formation of adhesions between the amnion and the skin of the fetus, and prevents conformity of the sac to the fetus. The amniotic fluid is continually being absorbed and renewed at a rapid rate. About a third of the water in the amniotic fluid is replaced each hour.

amniotic sac. Amnion, q.v.

amniotitis (ăm-nē-ō-tī'tĭs) [Gr. *amnion,* lamb, + *itis,* inflammation]. Inflammation of the amnion. SYN: *amnitis; amnionitis.*

amniotome (ăm'nē-ō-tōm) [" + Gr. *tome,* incision]. Instrument for puncturing fetal membranes.

amniotomy (ăm"nē-ŏt'ō-mē). Surgical rupture of the fetal membranes. Done to induce or expedite labor. A digital amniotome, a small pointed instrument that fits over the tip of the finger, facilitates this procedure.

NURSING IMPLICATIONS: Explain the procedure to the patient, then correctly position and drape the site, and thoroughly cleanse the perineum. When the physician has completed the amniotomy, assess the color and amount of amniotic fluid expelled. Immediately listen to the fetal heart sounds, because there is an increased risk of cord prolapse when an amniotomy is performed.

amnitis (ăm-nī'tĭs). Inflammation of the amnion. SYN: *amniotitis; amnionitis.*

amobarbital (ăm"ō-băr'bĭ-tăl). USP. $C_{11}H_{18}N_2O_3$. An odorless, white, crystalline powder. Used as a sedative.

a. sodium. $C_{11}H_{17}N_2NaO_3$. An odorless, white, granular powder. Following administration, it is absorbed and inactivated rapidly in the liver. Used as a sedative.

amodiaquine hydrochloride (ăm"ō-dī'ă-kwĭn). USP. An antimalarial drug similar in action to chloroquine. Trade name is Camoquin Hydrochloride.

amoeba (ă-mē'ba) [Gr. *amoibe,* change]. A one-celled protozoan animal form. SEE: *ameba.*

amok, amuck (ă-mŏk', ă-mŭk') [Malay, to engage furiously in battle]. A state of murderous frenzy.

amor (ā'mor) [L.]. Love, esp. sexual love.

amoralia (ă"mō-rā'lē-ă) [Gr. *a-,* not, + L. *moralis,* moral]. Condition of lacking moral sensibilities.

amorphia, amorphism (ă-mor'fē-ă, ă-mor'fĭzm) [" + *morphe,* form]. State of being without definite form.

amorphous (ă-mor'fŭs). Without definite structure.

amotio (ă-mō'shē-ō) [L. *amovere,* to move from]. A detachment.

a. retinae. Detached retina.

amoxicillin (ă-mŏks"ĭ-sĭl'ĭn). USP. A semisynthetic penicillin. Trade names include Amoxil, Polymox, Robamox, and Trimox.

Amoxil. Trade name for amoxicillin, USP, q.v.

AMP. *adenosine monophosphate,* q.v.

amperage (ăm-pĕr'ĭj). Strength of an electric current expressed in amperes.

ampere (ăm'pĕr). ABBR: amp. Unit of intensity of electric current, which is produced by 1 volt acting through resistance of 1 ohm. SEE: *electromotive force.*

ampere meter. Instrument denoting in amperes the strength of a current. SEE: *ammeter.*

amphetamine (ăm-fĕt'ă-mēn, -mĭn). A colorless liquid that volatilizes slowly at room temperature. It is a central nervous system stimulant. The preparation most commonly used is the sulfate, marketed in tablet or capsule form.

a. sulfate. USP. $(C_9H_{13}N)_2H_2SO_4$. A synthetic, white, crystalline substance that acts as a central nervous system stimulant. Used in treatment of narcolepsy and certain types of mental depression. Use of amphetamines to control appetite in treating obesity has not proven to be effective. Large doses are toxic, and prolonged use may cause drug dependence. Trade names are Benzedrine and Amphedrine.

amphetamine poisoning. SEE: *Poisons and Poisoning* in *Appendix*.

amphi- [Gr. *amphi*, on both sides]. Prefix indicating on both sides, on all sides, double. In chemistry, it denotes certain positions or configurations.

amphiarthrosis (ăm″fē-ăr-thrō′sĭs) [″ + Gr. *arthrosis*, joint]. A form of articulation in which the bony surfaces are connected by cartilage; mobility is slight, but may be exerted in all directions. The articulations of the bodies of the vertebrae are examples.

amphiaster (ăm″fē-ăs′tĕr) [″ + *aster*, star]. Double star figure formed during mitosis, q.v. SYN: *diaster*.

Amphibia (ăm-fĭb′ē-ă) [Gr *amphibios*, double life]. A class of cold-blooded animals that live on land and in water. They breathe through gills during their aquatic larval stage, but breathe through lungs in their adult stage. Includes salamanders, frogs, and toads. SEE: *metamorphosis*.

amphibious (ăm-fĭb′ē-ŭs). Able to live both on land and in water.

amphiblastula (ăm″fē-blăs′tū-lă) [Gr. *amphi*, on both sides, + *blastula*, little sprout]. A form of blastula in which the blastomeres are of unequal size. Seen in sponges.

amphiblestritis (ăm″fē-blĕs-trī′tĭs) [″ + *blestron*, fish net, + *itis*, inflammation]. Inflammation of retina. SYN: *retinitis*.

amphibolic (ăm″fĭ-bŏl′ĭk) [Gr. *amphibolia*, uncertainty]. 1. Having unknown or varying prognosis. 2. Possessing anabolic and catabolic activity.

amphicelous (ăm″fē-sē′lŭs) [Gr. *amphi*, on both sides + *koilos*, hollow]. Concave on each end, as a vertebra.

amphicentric (ăm″fē-sĕn′trĭk) [″ + *kentron*, center]. Centering or converging at both ends.

amphichroic, amphichromatic (ăm″fē-krō′ĭk, -krō-măt′ĭk) [″ + *chroma*, color]. 1. Turning red litmus paper blue, and blue, red. 2. Reacting both as an acid and an alkali. 3. Capable of exhibiting two colors.

amphicrania (ăm″fē-krā′nē-ă) [″ + *kranion*, skull]. Pain on both sides of head.

amphicreatine, amphicreatinine (ăm″fē-krē′ă-tĭn, -krē-ăt′ĭ-nĭn) [″ + *kreas*, flesh]. A leukomaine, q.v., formed in muscles.

amphicyte (ăm′fē-sīt) [″ + *kytos*, cell]. One of the cells enveloping the bodies of cerebrospinal ganglionic neurons.

amphidiarthrosis (ăm″fē-dī-ăr-thrō′sĭs) [″ + *diarthrosis*, articulation]. An articulation with amphiarthrosis and diarthrosis, such as that of the lower jaw.

amphigony (ăm-fĭg′ō-nē) [″ + *gonos*, begetting]. Sexual reproduction.

amphimixis (ăm″fē-mĭks′ĭs) [″ + *mixis*, mingling]. Mixing of maternal and paternal germ cells in reproduction, thus giving hereditary characteristics from both parents.

amphitheater (ăm″fē-thē′ă-tĕr) [″ + *theatron*, theater]. An operating room with tiers of seats around it for students and other observers.

amphitrichate, amphitrichous (ăm-fĭt′rĭ-kāt, -kŭs) [″ + *thrichos*, hair]. Having a flagellum or flagella at both ends, said of microorganisms.

ampho- [Gr. *ampho*, both]. Prefix indicating both.

amphocyte (ăm′fō-sīt) [″ + *kytos*, cell]. A cell that stains with either acid or basic stains.

amphodiplopia (ăm-fō-dĭ-plō′pē-ă) [″ + *diploos*, double, + *ops*, vision]. Double vision in each eye. SYN: *amphoterodiplopia*.

Amphojel (ăm′fō-jĕl). A trade name for aluminum hydroxide gel, USP.

ampholyte (ăm′fō-līt) [″ + *electrolyte*]. Substance that acts as a base or an acid depending upon the pH of the solution into which it is introduced.

amphopeptone (ăm″fō-pĕp′tōn). First peptone formed by tryptic digestion of protein.

amphophil, amphophilous (ăm′fō-fĭl, ăm-fŏf′ĭ-lŭs) [″ + *philos*, fond]. Having affinity for both acid and basic dyes.

amphoric (ăm-for′ĭk) [L. *amphoricus*]. Pert. to a sound as that caused by blowing across the mouth of a bottle; a resonance; a cavernous sound on percussion of a pulmonary cavity.

amphoricity (ăm″for-ĭs′ĭ-tē). The condition of producing amphoric sounds.

amphoriloquy (ăm″for-ĭl′ō-kwē) [L. *amphora*, jar, + *loqui*, to speak]. The presence of amphoric sounds in speaking.

amphorophony (ăm″for-ŏf′ō-nē) [Gr. *amphoreus*, jar, + *phone*, voice]. Amphoric voice sound.

amphoteric, amphoterous (ăm-fō-tĕr′ĭk, ăm-fŏt′ĕr-ŭs) [Gr. *amphoteros*, both]. Having the ability to react as both an acid and a base.

amphoteric compound. A compound that reacts as both an acid and a base.

amphotericin B (ăm″fō-tĕr′ĭ-sĭn). USP. An antibiotic agent obtained from a strain of Streptomyces nodosus. It is used in treatment of deep-seated mycotic infections. The drug usually is administered parenterally. Trade name is Fungizone.

amphoteric reaction. Reaction in which a compound reacts as both an acid and a base.

amphoterism (ăm-fō′tĕr-ĭzm). State of reacting as both an acid and a base.

amphoterodiplopia (ăm-fŏt″ĕr-ō-dĭ-plō′pē-ă) [″ + *diploos*, double, + *ops*, vision]. Double vision in each eye. SYN: *amphodiplopia*.

amphotonia, amphotony (ăm″fō-tō′nē-ă, ăm-fŏt′ō-nē). Hyperexcitability of both the sympathetic and parasympathetic nervous systems.

amphotonic [″ + *tonos,* tone]. Pert. to or characterized by amphotonia.

ampicillin (ămp″ĭ-sĭl′ĭn). USP. A semisynthetic penicillin; broad-spectrum antibiotic. Trade names include Alpen, Amcil, Omnipen, Penbritin, Polycillin, and Principen.

a. sodium. USP. Monosodium salt of ampicillin. Trade names include Omnipen-N, Penbritin-S, Polycillin-N, Principen/N, and Alpen-N.

amplification (ăm″plĭ-fĭ-kā′shŭn) [L. *amplificatio,* making larger]. Enlargement, magnification, expansion.

amplifier (ăm″plĭ-fī′ĕr). That which enlarges, extends, increases, or makes more powerful. In electronics, a device for increasing the electrical current or signal.

amplitude (ăm′plĭ-tūd) [L. *amplitudo*]. 1. Amount, extent, size, abundance or fullness. 2. In physics, the extent of movement, as of a pendulum or sound wave. The maximum displacement of a particle, as that of a string vibrating as measured from the mean to the extreme. 3. Magnitude of an action potential.

amplitude modulation. Modification of the amplitude esp. of a current used for muscle stimulation.

ampul, ampule (ăm′pūl) [Fr. *ampoule*]. A small glass container that can be sealed and its contents sterilized. This is a French invention for containing hypodermic solutions.

ampulla (ăm-pŭl′lă) [L., little jar]. (pl. *ampullae)* [NA] Sac-like dilatation of a canal or duct.

a. ductus deferens. An irregular and nodular dilatation of the vas deferens just before its junction with the excretory duct of the seminal vesicle.

a. of lacrimal duct. The slight dilatation of the lacrimal duct medial to the punctum.

a. of rectum. Slight dilatation of rectum proper just before continuing as anal canal. Also: *infraperitoneal portion of rectum proper.*

a. of semicircular canal. A dilatation at end of semicircular canal that houses an ampulla of a semicircular duct.

a. of semicircular ducts. Dilatation of semicircular ducts near their junction with the utricle. In their walls are the cristae ampullares.

a. of uterine tube. The dilated distal end of a uterine tube terminating in a funnel-like infundibulum.

a. of vas deferens. Ampulla ductus deferens, a dilatation at the base of the bladder near the end of the vas deferens.

a. of Vater. Papilla of Vater, q.v.

ampullitis (ăm″pŭl-lī′tĭs) [″ + Gr. *itis,* inflammation]. Inflammation of any ampulla, esp. of ductus deferens.

ampullula (ăm-pŭl′ū-lă) [dim. of L. *ampulla*]. A small dilatation, esp. of a lymph or blood vessel.

amputation (ăm″pū-tā′shŭn) [L. *amputare,* to cut around]. Removal, usually by surgery, of a limb, part, or organ.

NURSING IMPLICATIONS: In the immediate post-op period, assess the patient's vital signs and observe the stump dressing for bleeding at least every two hours. Help to prevent contracture formation by encouraging the patient to move and to do range of motion exercises as well as muscle strengthening exercises. Assist the stump to shrink by encouraging the patient to do stump conditioning exercises and by correct bandaging of the stump. Instruct the patient to massage the stump. Be willing to encourage the patient to verbalize anger and frustration, and to deal with the patient's phantom limb pain.

a., congenital. Amputation of parts of the fetus in utero, formerly believed to be caused by constricting bands but now believed to be a developmental defect.

a., double-flap. Amputation in which two flaps of soft tissue are formed to cover the end of the bone.

a. in contiguity. Amputation at a joint.

a. in continuity. Amputation elsewhere than at a joint.

a., primary. Amputation performed before inflammation sets in.

a., secondary. Amputation performed during period of suppuration.

a., spontaneous. Nonsurgical separation of an extremity or digit. SEE: *ainhum.*

a., tertiary. Amputation performed after abatement of inflammatory reaction.

amputee (ăm″pū-tē′). One who has had an amputation, esp. of the arm or leg.

A.M.T. *American Medical Technologists.*

amuck, amok (ă-mŭk′) [Malay *amok,* furious attack]. State of murderous frenzy.

amusia (ă-mū′sē-ă) [Gr. *amousos,* unmusical]. Music deafness; inability to produce or appreciate musical sounds.

a., motor. Inability to produce musical sounds.

a., sensory. Music deafness. Inability to appreciate musical sounds.

Amussat's operation (ăm′ū-săz). [Jean Z. Amussat, Fr. surgeon, 1796–1856] Surgical formation of an artificial anus, by lumbar colotomy in ascending colon.

amychophobia (ă-mī″kō-fō′bē-ă) [Gr. *amyche,* scratch, + *phobos,* fear]. Morbid fear of being scratched; fear of the claws of any animal.

amyelencephalia (ă-mī″ĕl-ĕn-sĕf-ā′lē-ă) [Gr. *a-,* not, + *myelos,* marrow, + *enkephalos,* brain]. Congenital absence of brain and spinal cord.

amyelia (ă-mī-ē'lē-ă) [" + *myelos,* marrow]. Congenital absence of spinal cord.

amyelinic (ă-mī"ĕ-lĭn'ĭk). Not possessing a myelin sheath.

amyeloneuria (ă-mī"ĕl-ō-nū'rē-ă) [" + *myelos,* marrow, + *neuron,* nerve]. Partial paralysis or impaired function of the spinal cord.

amyelotrophy (ă-mī"ĕl-ŏt'rō-fē) [" + " + *atrophia,* atrophy]. Spinal cord atrophy.

amyelus (ă-mī'ĕ-lŭs). An individual with congenital absence of the spinal cord.

amygdala (ă-mĭg'dă-lă) [L., almond]. (pl. *amygdalae*) 1. A mass of gray matter in the anterior portion of the temporal lobe. 2. Obsolete term for the tonsil.

amygdalin (ă-mĭg'dă-lĭn). A bitter-tasting glycoside derived from the pit or other seed parts of several plants including almonds and apricots. Amygdalin, from which the poisonous hydrocyanic acid can be produced by enzymatic action, is the substance known in the U.S.A. as Laetrile. Amygdalin has no therapeutic or nutritional value. SEE: *Laetrile.*

amygdaline (ă-mĭg'dă-lĭn, -lĭn) [L. *amygdalinus*]. 1. Pert. to a tonsil. 2. Pert. to or shaped like an almond. SYN: *amygdaloid.*

amygdaloid (ă-mĭg'dă-loyd) [Gr. *amygdale,* almond, + *eidos,* resemblance]. Resembling a tonsil or an almond.

amygdaloid fossa. A depression for the tonsil.

amygdaloid tubercle. A projection from the middle cornu of the lateral ventricle, marking area of the amygdaloid nucleus.

amygdalolith (ă-mĭg'dă-lō-lĭth") [" + *lithos,* stone]. Stone in a distended crypt of a tonsil.

amygdalopathy (ă-mĭg"dă-lŏp'ă-thē) [" + *pathos,* suffering]. Any disease of a tonsil.

amygdalotome (ă-mĭg'dă-lō-tōm") [" + *tome,* incision]. Instrument for excision of a tonsil.

amyl (ăm'ĭl) [L. *amylum,* starch, + Gr. *yle,* material]. C_5H_{11}. A hypothetical univalent radical, nonexistent in a free state.

a. nitrite. USP. $C_5H_{11}NO_2$, a volatile and highly flammable clear liquid. Used as a vasodilator, esp. for anginal pain.

amylaceous (ăm"ĭ-lā'shē-ŭs). Starchy.

amylase (ăm'ĭ-lās) [" + Gr. *-asis,* colloid enzyme]. A class of enzymes that split or hydrolyze starch. Those found in animals are called α-amylases; those in plants are called β-amylases. SEE: *antiamylase; enzyme; macroamylase.*

a., pancreatic. Amylopsin, q.v.

a., salivary. Ptyalin, q.v.

a., vegetable. Diastase, q.v.

amylasuria (ăm"ĭ-lās-ū'rē-ă) [" + *ouron,* urine]. Increased amount of amylase in the urine. Occurs in pancreatitis.

amylemia (ăm"ĭ-lē'mē-ă) [" + Gr. *haima,* blood]. Presence of starch in the blood.

amylin (ăm'ĭ-lĭn). The insoluble component of starch. The soluble component is amidin. SYN: *amylopectin.*

amylodextrin [" + *dexter,* right]. Soluble substance produced during the hydrolysis of starch into sugar.

amylodyspepsia (ăm"ĭ-lō-dĭs-pĕp'sē-ă) [" + Gr. *dys,* bad, + *pepsis,* digestion]. Inability to digest starchy foods.

amylogen (ăm-ĭl'ō-jĕn) [" + Gr. *gennan,* to produce]. Soluble starch.

amylogenesis (ăm"ĭ-lō-jĕn'ĕ-sĭs) [" + Gr. *genesis,* production]. The production of starch.

amylogenic (ăm"ĭ-lō-jĕn'ĭk) [" + Gr. *gennan,* to produce]. Producing starch.

amyloid (ăm'ĭ-loyd) [L. *amylum,* starch, + Gr. *eidos,* resemblance]. 1. Resembling starch; starchlike. 2. A protein-polysaccharide complex having starchlike characteristics produced and deposited in tissues during certain pathological states. It is a homogeneous, highly refractile substance staining readily with Congo red. It is associated with a variety of chronic diseases, particularly tuberculosis, osteomyelitis, leprosy, Hodgkin's disease, and carcinoma.

amyloid degeneration. Degeneration of organs or tissues from deposition of amyloid. Structures are waxy and translucent, having hyaline appearance. Liver, spleen, and kidneys most involved but any tissue may be infiltrated.

amyloid disease. Amyloidosis, q.v.

amyloid kidney. Enlarged, firm, smooth kidney usually associated with amyloid disease of spleen or liver.

SYM: Face pale, waxy skin that may be edematous. Liver and spleen may also be enlarged; not tender to pressure. Diarrhea if intestines are involved. Albumin, hyaline, and waxy casts in urine.

amyloid nephrosis. A nephrotic syndrome from myeloid degeneration of kidney.

amyloidosis (ăm"ĭ-loy-dō'sĭs) [L. *amylum,* starch, + Gr. *eidos,* resemblance, + *osis,* condition]. A metabolic disorder marked by deposition of amyloid in organs and tissue. Thought to be the result of disordered function of the reticuloendothelial system and abnormal immunoglobulin synthesis. There is no known method of preventing formation of amyloid deposits except to control the primary disease with which it is associated. SYN: *amylosis.*

a., lichen. A form of amyloidosis limited to the skin.

a., localized. Amyloidosis in which isolated amyloid tumors are formed.

a., primary. Amyloidosis not associated with a chronic disease.

a., secondary. Amyloidosis associated with a chronic disease, as tuberculosis, syphilis, Hodgkin's disease, rheumatoid arthritis, and in extensive tissue destruction. Spleen, liver, kidneys, and adrenal cortex most frequently involved.

amylolysis (ăm″ĭl-ŏl′ĭ-sĭs) [″ + Gr. *lysis*, solution]. Hydrolysis of starch into sugar in the process of digestion.

amylolytic (ăm″ĭl-ō-lĭt′ĭk). Pert. to or characterized by amylolysis.

amylolytic enzyme. An enzyme that hydrolyzes starch. SYN: *amylase*.

amylopectin (ăm″ĭl-ō-pĕk′tĭn). The insoluble component of starch. The soluble component is amidin. SYN: *amylin*.

amylophagia (ăm″ĭ-lō-fā′jē-ă) [″ + Gr. *phagein*, to eat]. Abnormal craving for starch.

amylopsin (ăm″ĭ-lŏp′sĭn) [″ + Gr. *opsis*, appearance]. Enzyme in pancreatic juice that hydrolyzes starch into achroodextrin and maltose. SYN: *amylase, pancreatic*. SEE: *digestion; duodenum; enzyme*.

amylose (ăm′ĭ-lōs) [Gr. *amylon*, starch]. A group of carbohydrates that includes starch, cellulose, and dextrin. SEE: *saccharose*.

amylosis (ăm″ĭ-lō′sĭs) [″ + *osis*, condition]. Amyloidosis, q.v.

amylosuria (ăm″ĭ-lō-sū′rē-ă) [″ + *ouron*, urine]. Amylose in the urine.

amylum (ăm′ĭ-lŭm) [L.]. Starch.

amyluria [″ + Gr. *ouron*, urine]. Starch in the urine.

amyocardia (ă-mī″ō-kăr′dē-ă) [Gr. *a-*, not, + *mys*, muscle, + *kardia*, heart]. Weakness of the heart muscle. SYN: *myasthenia cordis*.

amyoplasia (ă-mī″ō-plā′zē′ă) [″ + ″ + *plassein*, to form]. Absent muscle formation.

a. congenita. Congenital rigidity of the joints due to failure of muscle development.

amyostasia (ă-mī″ō-stā′sē-ă) [″ + ″ + *stasis*, standing]. Difficulty in standing because of lack of coordination or because of muscular tremors. SEE: *tremor*.

amyosthenia (ă-mī″ŏs-thē′nē-ă) [″ + ″ + *sthenos*, strength]. Weakness of muscles.

amyosthenic (ă-mī″ŏs-thĕn′ĭk). Pert. to muscular weakness.

amyotaxy (ă-mī″ō-tăks′ē) [″ + ″ + *taxis*, order]. Muscular ataxia.

amyotonia (ă-mī″ō-tō′nē-ă) [″ + ″ + *tonos*, tone]. Deficiency or lack of muscular tone.

a. congenita. A noninherited but sometimes familial disease characterized by absence of muscular development, with the lower extremities being the first involved. It is first seen at, or shortly after, birth. SYN: *myatonia congenita; Oppenheim's disease*.

amyotrophia, amyotrophy (ă-mī″ō-trō′fē-ă, ă-mī-ŏt′rō-fē) [″ + ″ + *trophe*, nourishment]. Muscular atrophy.

a., progressive spinal. Progressive muscular atrophy.

amyotrophic (ă-mī″ō-trŏf′ĭk). Pert. to muscular atrophy.

amyotrophic lateral sclerosis. A syndrome marked by muscular weakness and atrophy with spasticity and hyperreflexia due to degeneration of motor neurons of spinal cord, medulla, and cortex. Prognosis is very poor. If only cells of motor cranial nuclei in the medulla are involved, condition is called progressive bulbar palsy. SYN: *motor neuron disease*.

amyous (ăm′ē-ŭs) [″ + *mys*, muscle]. 1. Weak; deficient in muscular strength. 2. Without muscle.

Amytal. Trade name for amobarbital, USP, q.v.

Amytal Sodium. Trade name for amobarbital sodium, USP, q.v.

amyxia (ă-mĭks′ē-ă) [″ + *myxa*, mucus]. Absence or deficiency of mucus.

amyxorrhea (ă-mĭks-ō-rē′ă) [″ + ″ + *rhoia*, flow]. Lack of normal secretion of mucus.

An. 1. Chem. symb. for actinon. 2. *anisometropia*. 3. *anode*. 4. *antigen*.

an- [Gr.]. A negative prefix indicating without or not.

A.N.A. *American Nurses' Association*.

ana (ăn′ă). 1. [Gr.] ABBR: $\overline{aa}$. Prescription term meaning *so much of each*. 2. *antinuclear antibody*.

anabasis (ă-năb′ă-sĭs) [Gr., ascent]. Period of increased severity in a disease.

anabatic (ăn″ă-băt′ĭk). Pert. to anabasis.

anabiosis (ăn″ă-bī-ō′sĭs) [Gr. *anabiosis*, revive]. Revival after apparent death. SYN: *resuscitation*.

anabiotic (ăn-ă-bī-ŏt′ĭk). 1. Restorative. 2. Any agent that resuscitates or restores.

anabolic (ăn″ă-bŏl′ĭk) [Gr. *anabolikos*]. Promoting or pert. to anabolism.

anabolic agents. Testosterone, or a steroid hormone resembling testosterone, which stimulates anabolism (rather than catabolism) in the body.

CAUTION: Indiscriminate use of anabolic agents is inadvisable because of the undesirable side effects they may produce, particularly in women, in which case hirsutism, masculinization, and clitoral hypertrophy may occur.

anabolin (ă-năb′ō-lĭn). A product of anabolism. SYN: *anabolite*.

anabolism (ă-năb′ō-lĭzm) [Gr. *anabole*, a building up, + *-ismos*, condition]. The building up of the body substance the constructive phase of metabolism by which a cell takes from the blood the substance required for repair and growth, building it into a cytoplasm, thus converting a nonliving material into the living cytoplasm of the cell. Opposite of catabolism, the destructive phase of metabolism.

RS: assimilation; catabolism; metabolism; nutrition; synthesis.

anabolite (ă-năb'ō-līt"). Any product of anabolism. SYN: *anabolin*.

anabrosis (ăn"ă-brō'sĭs) [Gr.]. Superficial ulceration of soft tissue.

anabrotic (ăn"ă-brŏt'ĭk). 1. Pert. to or characterized by anabrosis. 2. A substance that produces anabrosis.

anacamptics (ăn"ă-kămp'tĭks) [Gr. *anakamptein*, to bend back]. Study of reflection of light or sound.

anacamptometer (ăn"ă-kămp-tŏm'ĕ-tĕr) [" + *metron*, measure]. Device for measuring intensity of deep reflexes.

anacatharsis (ăn"ă-kă-thăr'sĭs) [Gr. *anakatharsis*, upward cleansing]. Severe prolonged vomiting.

anacathartic (ăn"ă-kă-thăr'tĭk). Agent that causes vomiting. SYN: *emetic*.

anacidity (ăn"ă-sĭd'ĭ-tē) [Gr. *an-*, not, + L. *aciditas*, acid]. Abnormal deficiency of acidity, esp. of hydrochloric acid in the gastric juice.

anaclasis (ă-năk'lă-sĭs) [Gr. *anaklasis*, reflection]. 1. Refraction or reflection of light. 2. Refraction of light in the interior of the eye. 3. Reflex action. 4. Retracture for therapeutic reasons. 5. Forcible movement of a joint in order to treat fibrous ankylosis.

anaclitic (ăn"ă-klĭt'ĭk). Leaning or depending on. In psychoanalysis, pert. to the dependence of an infant on the mother figure for care.

anacrotic (ăn"ă-krŏt'ĭk) [Gr. *ana*, up, + *krotos*, stroke]. 1. Ascending or vertical upstroke of a sphygmogram. 2. Pert. to a pulse with more than one expansion of the artery. 3. Pert. to two heartbeats traced on the ascending line of a sphygmogram. SYN: *anadicrotic*. SEE: *pulse*.

anacrotic pulse. Pulse in which one or more small waves occur on ascending limb of tracing of pulse wave, as in aortic stenosis.

anacrotism (ă-năk'rō-tĭzm). Existence of a double beat on ascending line of sphygmogram. SYN: *anadicrotism*.

anacusia, anacusis, anakusis (ăn-ă-kū'sē-ă, -sĭs) [Gr. *an-*, not, + *akouein*, to hear]. Total deafness.

anadenia (ăn-ă-dē'nē-ă) [" + *aden*, gland]. 1. Absence of glands. 2. Reduced glandular function.

anadicrotic (ăn"ă-dī-krŏt'ĭk) [Gr. *ana*, up, + *dikrotos*, double beating]. 1. Pert. to a pulse with more than one artery expansion. 2. Pert. to two beats on the ascending line of a sphygmogram. SYN: *anacrotic*.

anadicrotism (ăn-ă-dĭk'rō-tĭzm). Existence of a double beat on ascending line of the sphygmogram. SYN: *anacrotism*.

anadidymus (ăn"ă-dĭd'ĭ-mŭs) [" + *didymos*, twin]. A developmental abnormality in which the lower extremities of two fetuses are joined together.

anadipsia (ăn"ă-dĭp'sē-ă) [" + *dipsa*, thirst]. Intense thirst.

anadrenalism (ăn"ă-drē'năl-ĭzm) [Gr. *an-*, not, + *adrenal* + Gr. *-ismos*, condition]. Failure of the adrenal gland to function.

anaerobe (ăn-ā'ĕr-ōb) [" + *aer*, air, + *bios*, life]. A microorganism that can live and grow in the absence of oxygen.

a., facultative. Organism that prefers an oxygen environment but is capable of living and growing in its absence.

a., obligatory. Organism that can live and grow only in absence of oxygen.

anaerobic (ăn"ă-ĕr-ō'bĭk). 1. Pert. to an anaerobe. 2. Able to live without oxygen.

anaerobic exercise. Exercise during which the energy needed is provided without utilization of inspired oxygen. This type of exercise is limited to short bursts of vigorous activity. SEE: *aerobic exercise*.

anaerobiosis (ăn-ā"ĕr-ō-bī-ō'sĭs) [" + *aer*, air, + *bios*, life, + *osis*, condition]. 1. Life in an oxygen-free atmosphere. 2. Functioning of an organ or tissue in absence of free oxygen.

anagen (ăn'ă-jĕn) [Gr. *ana*, up, + *genesis*, production]. Growing stage of hair development. SEE: *catagen; telogen*.

anagnosasthenia (ăn"ăg-nōs-ăs-thē'nē-ă) [Gr. *anagnosis*, reading, + *astheneia*, weakness]. Neurasthenia with distressing symptoms when trying to read, caused by neurosis rather than organic disease of the eye.

anakatadidymus (ăn"ă-kăt"ă-dĭd'ĭ-mŭs) [Gr. *ana*, up, + *kata*, down, + *didymos*, twin]. A congenital anomaly wherein twins are separated above and below but joined at the trunk.

anakatesthesia (ăn"ă-kăt"ĕs-thē'zē-ă) [" + " + *aisthesis*, sensation]. A sensation of hovering.

anakusis (an"ă-kū'sis) [Gr. *an-*, not, + *akouein*, to hear]. Anacusis; total deafness. SYN: *anacusia*.

anal (ā'năl) [L. *analis*]. Rel. to the anus or outer rectal opening.

anal canal. The terminal portion of the large intestine, its external aperture being the anus. This includes the internal and external sphincter muscles of the anus. The canal remains closed except during defecation and passage of flatus. It is about 1½ inches (3.8 cm.) long. SEE: illus.

analepsis (ăn"ă-lĕp'sĭs) [Gr. *analepsis*, a taking up]. Gaining strength after an illness. Restoration to health.

analeptic (ăn"ă-lĕp'tĭk) [Gr. *analeptikos*, restorative]. 1. A drug used to stimulate the central nervous system. Used esp. in treat-

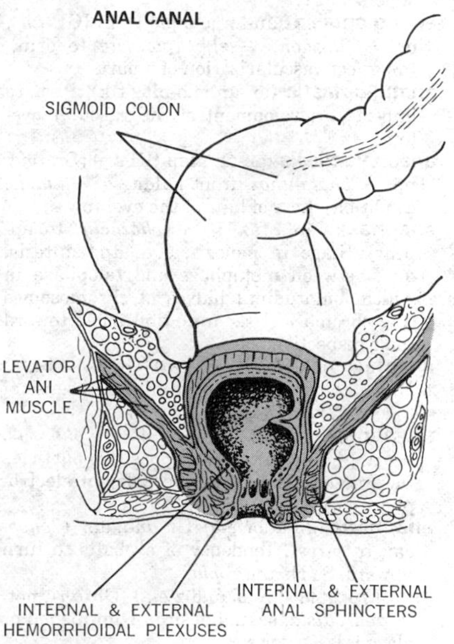

ment of poisoning by drugs that depress the central nervous system, such as the barbiturates. 2. A restorative agent.

anal erotism. Localization of libido in the anal region. SEE: *anal stage*.

analgesia (ăn-ăl-jē'zē-ă) [Gr. *an-*, not, + *algos*, pain]. Absence of normal sense of pain.

a. algera, a. dolorosa. Spontaneous pain with loss of sensitivity in a part.

a., paretic. Complete analgesia of upper limb in conjunction with partial paralysis.

analgesic (ăn"ăl-jē'sĭk). 1. Relieving pain. 2. A drug that relieves pain. SYN: *analgetic*.

analgesic nephropathy. Renal damage and impairment resulting from ingestion of a large amount of specific analgesics such as phenacetin or salicylate over an extended period of time.

analgetic (ăn"ăl-jĕt'ĭk). 1. Relieving pain. 2. A drug that relieves pain. SYN: *analgesic*.

analgia (ăn-ăl'jē-ă) [" + *algos*, pain]. State of being without pain.

analgic (ăn-ăl'jĭk). Without pain.

anal incontinence. Failure of the anal sphincter to prevent involuntary expulsion of gas, liquid, or solids from the lower bowel.

analog, analogue (ăn'ă-lŏg) [Gr. *analogos*, proportionate]. 1. One of two organs in different species that are similar in function but different in structure. 2. In chemistry, a compound that is structurally similar to another.

analogous (ă-năl'ō-gŭs). Similar in function but different in origin or structure.

analogy (ă-năl'ō-jē) [L. *analogia*, analogous]. 1. Likeness or similarity between two things that otherwise are unlike. 2. In biology, similarity in function, but difference in structure or origin. Opposite of homology.

anal personality. In Freudian psychology, a personality disorder characterized by excessive orderliness, stinginess, and obstinacy. If carried to an extreme, these qualities lead to the development of obsessive-compulsive type of behavior.

anal reflex. Contraction of anal sphincter following irritation of skin about anus. Reflex is lost in lesions of posterior columns of cord and is exaggerated in anal fissures.

anal stage. In Freudian psychology, the second phase of sexual development from infancy to childhood, in which libido is concentrated in the anal region. In order of appearance, these phases are: oral, anal, phallic, and genital.

analysand (ăn-ăl'ĭ-zănd). A patient who is being psychoanalyzed.

analysis (ă-năl'ĭ-sĭs) [Gr., a dissolving]. (pl. *analyses*) 1. Separation of anything into its constituent parts. 2. In chemistry, determination of, or separation into, its constituent parts of a substance or compound. 3. Treatment by a physician trained as a psychoanalyst.

a., chromatographic. Analysis of substances on the basis of color reaction of the constituents as they are differentially absorbed on one of a variety of materials such as filter paper.

a., colorimetric. Analysis, by adsorption, of a compound and the identification of its element by color.

a., densimetric. Analysis by determination of the specific gravity (density) of a solution, and then estimation of the amount of solids.

a., gastric. Analysis of the stomach contents to determine the concentration of free hydrochloric acid and combined (total) acid, presence or absence of lactic acid, presence or absence of occult blood, presence of pus and excessive mucus, and amount and types of bacteria.

a., qualitative. Determining the nature of the elements in a substance.

a., quantitative. Determining the quantity of each element in a substance.

a., spectrophotometric. Determination of materials in a compound by measuring amount of light they absorb in the infrared, visible, or ultraviolet regions of the spectrum.

a., volumetric. Quantitative analysis performed by the measurement of the volume of solutions or liquids.

analysis of variance. ABBR: ANOVA. A statistical technique for defining and segregating the causes of variability affecting a set of observations. Use of this technique provides a basis for analyzing the effects of various treatments or variables on the subjects or patients being investigated. In an experimental design where several samples or groups are drawn from the same population, then estimates of population variance between samples should differ from each other only by chance. ANOVA provides a method for testing the hypothesis that several random and independent samples are from a common normal population.

analyst (ăn′ă-lĭst) [Fr. *analyse*, analysis]. 1. One who analyzes. 2. A licensed practitioner of psychoanalysis. SYN: *psychoanalyst.*

analytic (ăn-ă-lĭt′ĭk) [Gr. *analytikos*]. Pert. to analysis.

analytical balance. A very sensitive scale used in chemical analysis.

analyze (ăn′ă-līz) [Fr. *analyse*, analysis]. To separate into parts or principles in order to determine the nature of the whole; examine methodically.

analyzer (ăn′ă-lī″zĕr). 1. Device used to determine the optical rotation produced when polarized light passes through a solution. 2. Any device that determines some characteristic of the object, chemical, or action being investigated. Thus there are devices for analyzing a voice; the breath for presence of certain chemicals such as alcohol; images; cells in a solution; and chemicals. SEE: *breatholyzer.*

anamnesis (ăn″ăm-nē′sĭs) [Gr. *anamnesis*, recalling]. 1. Recollection; faculty of remembering. 2. That which is remembered. 3. The past medical history of a patient. SEE: *catamnesis.*

anamnestic (ăn″ăm-nĕs′tĭk). 1. Pert. to past medical history of patient. 2. Assisting the memory.

anamniotic [Gr. *an-*, not, + *amnion*, amnion]. Without an amnion.

ananabasia (ăn-ăn″ă-bā′sē-ă) [″ + *anabasis*, an ascending]. An abulia (loss of will) in which the person seems unable to ascend heights.

ananaphylaxis (ăn-ăn″ă-fĭ-lăk′sĭs) [″ + *ana*, away from, + *phylaxis*, protection]. Prevention of anaphylaxis, q.v. Usually attained by administering repeated doses of the sensitizing substance too small to cause anaphylaxis. SYN: *antianaphylaxis; desensitization.*

ananastasia (ăn-ăn″ă-stā′sē-ă) [″ + *anastasis*, a rising up]. Loss of will power (abulia) in which the person is unable to rise from a sitting position.

anancastic (ăn″ăn-kăs′tĭk) [Gr. *anankastos*, compelled]. Pert. to obsessive-compulsive type of personality.

anangioplasia (ăn-ăn″jē-ō-plā′sē-ă) [Gr. *an-*, not, + *angeion*, vessel, + *plassein*, to form]. Imperfect vascularization of a part.

anangioplastic (ăn-ăn″jē-ō-plăs′tĭk). Pert. to imperfect development of the vascular system.

anaphalantiasis (ăn-ăf″ă-lăn-tī′ă-sĭs) [Gr. *ana*, up, + *phalanthos*, front baldness, + *-iasis*, condition]. Loss of hair of the eyebrow.

anaphase (ăn′ă-fāz) [″ + *phainein*, to appear]. Stage in meiosis, q.v., and mitosis, q.v., between metaphase and telophase in which longitudinal halves of chromosomes (the chromatids) separate and move toward their respective poles.

anaphia (ăn-ā′fē-ă, ăn-ăf′ē-ă) [Gr. *an-*, not, + *haphe*, touch]. Loss of or diminished sense of touch. SYN: *anhaphia.*

anaphoresis (ăn″ă-fō-rē′sĭs) [″ + *phoresis*, bearing]. The flow of electropositive particles toward the anode (positive pole) in electrophoresis, q.v.

anaphoria (ăn″ă-for′ē-ă) [Gr. *ana*, up, + *phorein*, to carry]. Tendency of eyeballs to turn upward. SYN: *anatropia.*

anaphrodisia (ăn-ăf″rō-dĭz′ē-ă) [Gr. *an-*, not, + *aphrodisia*, sexual desire]. Diminished or absent desire for sex.

anaphrodisiac (ăn″ăf-rō-dĭz′ē-ăk). 1. Repressing sexual desire. 2. An agent that represses sexual desire.

anaphrodite (ăn-ăf′rō-dīt). Person with impairment or absence of sexual desire.

anaphylactia (ăn″ă-fĭ-lăk′shē-ă) [Gr. *ana*, away from, backward, + *phylaxis*, protection]. Anaphylaxis, q.v.

anaphylactic (ăn″ă-fĭ-lăk′tĭk). Pert. to or characterized by anaphylaxis, q.v.

anaphylactic shock. Severe allergic (hypersensitivity) reaction resulting from injection of a substance to which an individual or animal has become sensitized. SEE: *anaphylaxis.*

SYM: Dyspnea, violent cough, chest constriction, cyanosis, fever, skin eruptions, pulse variations, convulsions, collapse.

PROG: Death may occur if emergency treatment is not given.

TREATMENT: Vasopressor agents, esp. epinephrine, corticosteroids, oxygen, artificial respiration.

anaphylactogen (ăn″ă-fĭ-lăk′tō-jĕn) [″ + *phylaxis*, protection, + *gennan*, to produce]. That which produces anaphylaxis. SYN: *allergen.*

anaphylactogenesis (ăn″ă-fĭ-lăk″tō-jĕn′ĕ-sĭs). The process of producing anaphylaxis.

anaphylactogenic (ăn″ă-fĭ-lăk″tō-jĕn′ĭk). 1. Producing anaphylaxis. 2. The agent producing anaphylactic reactions.

anaphylatoxin (ăn″ă-fĭ-lă-tŏk′sĭn). A substance composed of small polypeptides split from the C3 and C5 components of complement, q.v., during activation of complement by a specific antigen-antibody reaction.

anaphylaxis (ăn″ă-fĭ-lăk′sĭs) [″ + *phylaxis,* protection]. 1. An allergic hypersensitivity reaction of the body to a foreign protein or drug. 2. Anaphylactic shock, q.v.

Reactions that constitute anaphylactic shock occur suddenly. They include increased irritability, dyspnea, cyanosis, sometimes convulsions, unconsciousness, and death. Reactions are primarily due to contraction of smooth muscle fibers and increased permeability of capillary endothelium. Death usually results from spasm of muscles of bronchioles. Such diseases as asthma, hay fever, and urticaria (hives) are thought to be of an anaphylactic nature, being caused by the irritation of a food or by the pollen of some plants and flowers, to which the individual may have become sensitized. Sometimes marked anaphylaxis follows a blood transfusion. Serum sickness is an anaphylactic reaction that occasionally follows injection of foreign serums, esp. horse serum.

SYM: Mild anaphylaxis: fever (slight), redness of skin, itching, urticaria. Severe anaphylaxis: dyspnea, violent cough, chest constriction, cyanosis, fever, skin eruption, pulse variations, convulsions, collapse.

PROG: In mild cases, favorable; symptoms are self-limited. In severe cases, death may occur if emergency treatment is not given.

TREATMENT: Vasopressor agents, esp. epinephrine; corticosteroids; oxygen, artificial respiration.

NURSING IMPLICATIONS: Immediately establish and maintain an airway, and position the patient to facilitate breathing. Carefully assess the patient's respiratory status for any signs of increasing severity or improvement. Remain with the patient until the reaction has subsided. Promptly administer ordered medications, and chart their effect(s) carefully.

a., active. Anaphylaxis resulting from injection of an antigen.

a., heterologous. Passive anaphylaxis by transfer of serum from an animal of a different species.

a., homologous. Passive anaphylaxis by transfer of serum from an animal of the same species.

a., local. Local inflammatory reaction following repeated injections of antigenic material. SYN: *Arthus reaction.*

a., passive. Anaphylaxis induced by injection of serum from a sensitized animal into a normal one. After a few hours the latter becomes sensitized.

anaplasia (ăn″ă-plā′zē-ă) [″ + *plassein,* to form]. 1. Loss of differentiation of cells, characteristic of most malignancies. 2. Reversion of cells to a more embryonic type. SYN: *dedifferentiation.*

anaplastic (ăn″ă-plăs′tĭk) [″ + *plassein,* to form]. Pert. to anaplasia.

anapnea (ăn″ăp-nē′ă) [Gr. *anapnein,* to breathe again]. 1. Respiration. 2 Regaining the breath.

anapneic (ăn″ăp-nē′ĭk). Pert. to anapnea or relieving dyspnea.

anapophysis (ăn″ă-pŏf′ĭ-sĭs [Gr. *ana,* back, + *apophysis,* offshoot]. An accessory spinal process of a vertebra, esp. thoracic or lumbar vertebrae.

anaptic (ăn-ăp′tĭk) [Gr. *an-,* not, + *aptein,* to touch]. Pert. to or characterized by diminished or lost tactile sense.

anarithmia (ăn″ă-rĭth′mē-ă) [″ + *arithmos,* enumeration]. Form of aphasia characterized by inability to count or use numbers.

anarthria (ăn-ăr′thrē-ă) [″ + *arthron,* joint]. Loss of motor power to speak distinctly. May be a result of a neural lesion or a muscular apparatus defect.

a. centralis. Partial aphasia caused by a lesion of the central nervous system.

a. literalis. Stammering.

anasarca (ăn″ă-săr′kă) [Gr. *ana,* through, + *sarkos,* flesh]. Severe generalized edema, q.v. SYN: *dropsy.*

anasarcous (ăn″ă-săr′kŭs). Dropsical; edematous.

anaspadias (ăn″ă-spā′dē-ăs) [″ + *spadon,* a rent]. Congenital opening of urethra on dorsum of penis or opening by separation of the labia minora and a fissure of the clitoris. SYN: *epispadias.*

anastaltic (ăn″ă-stăl′tĭk) [Gr. *anastaltikos,* checking]. 1. Astringent. 2. An astringent or styptic preparation.

anastate (ăn′ă-stāt) [Gr. *anastatos,* raised up]. Any product of anabolism, q.v.

anastole (ăn-ăs′tō-lē) [Gr.]. Shrinking away or retraction of the edges of a wound.

anastomose (ă-năs′tō-mōs) [Gr. *anastomosis,* opening]. 1. To communicate directly or by means of connecting two parts together, esp. nerves or blood vessels. 2. To make such a connection surgically.

anastomosis (ă-năs″tō-mō′sĭs) [Gr., opening]. (pl. *anastomoses*) 1. A natural communication between two vessels; may be direct or by means of connecting channels. 2. The surgical or pathological connection of two tubular structures.

a., antiperistaltic. Anastomosis between two parts of the intestine such that the peristaltic flow in one part is opposite of that in the other.

a., arteriovenous. Anastomosis between an artery and a vein by which the capillary bed is bypassed.

a., crucial. An arterial anastomosis on the back of the thigh, formed by the medial femoral circumflex, inferior gluteal, lateral femoral circumflex, and first perforating arteries.

a., end-to-end. Anastomosis in which the ends of two structures are joined.

a., Galen's. The anastomosis between the superior and inferior laryngeal nerves.

a., heterocladic. Anastomosis between branches of different arteries.

a., homocladic. Anastomosis between branches of the same artery.

a., Hyrtl's. An occasional looplike anastomosis between right and left hypoglossal nerves in geniohyoid muscle.

a., intestinal. Surgical connection of two portions of the intestines. SYN: *enteroenterostomy.*

a., isoperistaltic. Anastomosis between two parts of the intestine such that the peristaltic flow in both parts is in the same direction.

a., Jacobson's. The anastomosing portion of the tympanic plexus.

a., precapillary. Anastomosis between small arteries just before they become capillaries.

a., Schmidel's. Abnormal communications between the vena cava and the portal system.

a., side-to-side. Anastomosis between two structures lying or positioned beside each other.

a., terminoterminal. Anastomosis between the peripheral end of an artery and the central end of the corresponding vein, and between the central end of the artery and peripheral end of vein.

a., ureterotubal. Anastomosis between the ureter and the fallopian tube.

a., ureteroureteral. Anastomosis between two parts of the same ureter.

anastomotic (ă-năs″tō-mŏt′ĭk). Pert. to, or marked by, anastomosis.

anatomic (ăn″ă-tŏm′ĭk) [Gr. *anatome,* dissection]. Rel. to the anatomy or structure of an organism.

anatomical snuffbox. Snuffbox, anatomical, q.v.

anatomist (ă-năt′ō-mĭst). A specialist in the field of anatomy.

anatomy (ă-năt′ō-mē) [Gr. *anatome,* dissection]. 1. The structure of an organism. 2. The branch of science dealing with the structure of organisms. 3. Dissection or cutting apart.

a., applied. Application of anatomy to diagnosis and treatment, esp. surgical treatment.

a., comparative. Comparison of homologous structures of different animals.

a., descriptive. Description of individual parts of the body. SYN: *a., systematic.*

a., developmental. Embryology of the organism from the time of egg fertilization until adulthood is attained.

a., gross. Study of structures able to be seen with the naked eye. SYN: *a., macroscopic.*

a., macroscopic. A., gross, q.v.

a., microscopic. Study of structure by use of a microscope. SYN: *histology.*

a., morbid. Study of anatomical changes that occur in diseased tissues. SYN: *a., pathological.*

a., pathological. Study of the structure of abnormal, diseased, or injured tissue.

a., radiological. Anatomical investigation based on the x-ray appearance of tissues and organs.

a., surface. Study of form and markings of the surface of the body, esp. as they relate to underlying tissues and organs.

a., systematic. A., descriptive, q.v.

a., topographic. Study of the structure and form of a portion of the body with particular emphasis on the relationships of the parts included to each other.

a., x-ray. A., radiological, q.v.

anatoxic (ăn″ă-tŏks′ĭk) [Gr. *ana,* backward, + *toxikon,* poison]. Pert. to anatoxin.

anatoxin (ăn″ă-tŏks′ĭn). A toxin, q.v., that has been treated to destroy its toxicity, but is still capable of inducing antibody formation on injection. SYN: *toxoid.*

anatricrotic (ăn″ă-trī-krŏt′ĭk) [Gr. *ana,* up, + *tresis,* three, + *krotos,* stroke]. Pert. to three beats on the ascending line of a sphygmogram.

anatricrotism (ăn″ă-trĭk′rō-tĭzm). Existence of three beats on ascending line of a sphygmogram.

anatripsis (ăn″ă-trĭp′sĭs) [Gr., friction]. Therapeutic use of rubbing or friction massage.

anatriptic (ăn″ă-trĭp′tĭk) [Gr. *anatriptos,* rubbed up]. 1. Pert to anatripsis. 2. An agent applied by rubbing.

anatropia (ăn″ă-trō′pē-ă) [Gr. *ana,* up, + *trope,* a turning]. Tendency of eyeballs to turn upward. SYN: *anaphoria.*

Anavar. Trade name for oxandrolone, USP, q.v.

anaxon(e) (ăn-ăk′sŏn) [Gr. *an-,* not, + *axon,* axis]. A nerve cell, as of the retina, having no axon.

anazoturia (ăn″ă-zō-tū′rē-ă) [″ + *zoe,* life, + *ouron,* urine]. Deficiency or lack of nitrogenous substances, esp. urea, in the urine.

Anbesol. Trade name for benzocaine, USP, q.v.

A.N.C. *Army Nurse Corps.*

AnCC. *anodal closure contraction.*

anchorage (ăng′kĕr-ĭj) [Gr. *ankyra,* anchor]. 1. Surgical fixation, as of prolapsed abdominal organs. 2. The part to which anything is fixed, as a tooth to which a bridge is fastened.

ancillary (ăn′sĭl-lăr″ē) [L. *ancillaris,* relating to a maid servant]. Something that assists another action or effect but is not essential to the accomplishment of the action.

Ancobon. Trade name for flucytosine, USP, q.v.

anconad (ăn′kō-năd) [Gr. *ankon,* elbow, + L. *ad,* to]. Toward the elbow.

anconagra (ăn″kŏn-ăg′ră) [″ + *agra,* a seizure]. Gout of the elbow.

anconal, anconeal (ăn′kō-năl, ăn-kō′nē-ăl). Pert. to the elbow.

anconal fossa, anconeal fossa. Fossa olecrani; the hollow on the distal end of the humerus in which the olecranon rests when the elbow is extended.

anconeus (ăn-kō′nē-ŭs) [Gr. *ankon,* elbow]. Short extensor muscle of forearm located on the back of the elbow. It arises from the back portion of the lateral epicondyle of the humerus, and its fibers insert on side of the olecranon and upper fourth of shaft of ulna. Extends forearm and abducts ulna in pronation of the wrist.

anconitis (ăn″kō-nī′tĭs) [″ + *itis,* inflammation]. Inflammation of the elbow joint.

Ancylostoma (ăn″sĭl-ŏs′tō-mă) [Gr. *ankylos,* crooked, + *stoma,* mouth]. A genus of nematodes of the family Ancylostomatidae whose members are intestinal parasites and include the hookworms.

A. braziliense. Species of hookworm infesting dogs and cats; may cause cutaneous larva migrans in man. SEE: *larva migrans, cutaneous.*

A. caninum. Species of hookworm infesting dogs and cats; may cause cutaneous larva migrans in man. SEE: *larva migrans, cutaneous.*

A. duodenale. Species of hookworm widely distributed in temperate regions. Commonly infests man, causing ancylostomiasis, q.v. SEE: *Necator americanus.*

Ancylostomatidae (ăn″sĭ-lŏs″tō-măt′ĭ-dē). A family of nematodes belonging to the suborder Strongylata. It includes the genera Ancylostoma and Necator, common hookworms of man.

ancylostomiasis (ăn″sĭ-lŏs-tō-mī′ă-sĭs) [Gr. *ankylos,* crooked, + *stoma,* mouth, + *-iasis,* condition]. Hookworm infestation, esp. Ancylostoma duodenale or Necator americanus. Common in tropical and semitropical areas where the effects of climate and poor sanitation bring the larvae in contact with bare skin, usually of the foot.

The hookworm eggs hatch and the larvae enter through the skin causing inflammation, itching, and sometimes allergic reactions. They pass from the skin to the venous circulation to the lungs, where they migrate to the respiratory tree. If larvae are numerous, they may cause an eosinophilic pneumonia. Larvae travel up the bronchi and are finally swallowed, thus gaining entry to the intestinal tract. Larvae mature in the intestines, where they attach to the mucous membrane and suck blood from the host. They may cause nausea, colicky pains, and diarrhea. Loss of blood leads to anemia. In children, normal mental and physical growth is retarded. SYN: *hookworm disease.*

TREATMENT: In severe cases it may be necessary to treat the severe anemia prior to ridding the patient of the parasites. Mebendazole and pyrantel pamoate are the drugs of choice for Necator infections and Ancylostoma infections.

ancyroid (ăn′sĭ-royd) [Gr. *ankyra,* anchor, + *eidos,* resemblance]. Shaped like fluke of an anchor.

Andernach's ossicles (ŏn′dĕr-nŏks). [Johann Winther von Andernach, Ger. physician, 1487–1574] Ossa suturarum; small bones found in cranial sutures. SYN: *wormian bones; sutural bones.*

Andersen's disease. [Dorothy H. Andersen, U.S. pediatrician, b. 1901] Glycogen storage disease, type IV. SEE: *glycogen storage disease.*

Andral's decubitus (ăn′drăls). [Gabriel Andral, Fr. physician, 1797–1876] Position assumed by patient of lying on sound side during beginning stages of pleurisy.

andriatrics (ăn″drē-ăt′rĭks) [Gr. *andros,* man, + *iatreia,* medical treatment]. Study of diseases of men, esp. of male genital organs. SYN: *andrology.*

andro- [Gr. *andros,* man]. A prefix signifying man, male, or masculine.

androgalactozemia (ăn″drō-găl-ăk″tō-zē′mē-ă) [″ + *gala,* milk, + *zemia,* loss]. Oozing of milk from a man's breast.

androgen (ăn′drō-jĕn) [″ + *gennan,* to produce]. Substance producing or stimulating the development of male characteristics (masculinization), such as the hormones testosterone and androsterone, q.v.

androgenic (ăn″drō-jĕn′ĭk). Causing masculinization. SYN: *andromimetic.*

androgyne (ăn′drō-jīn) [″ + *gyne,* woman]. A female pseudohermaphrodite SYN: *androgynus.*

androgynoid (ăn-drŏj′ĭ-noyd) [″ + ″ + *eidos,* resemblance]. A person possessing female gonads (ovaries) but secondary sex characteristics of a male (a female pseudohermaphrodite). Term is less commonly used for a person possessing male gonads (testes) but secondary sex characteristics of a female (a male pseudohermaphrodite).

androgynous (ăn-drŏj′ĭ-nŭs) [″ + *gyne,* woman]. 1. Resembling or pert. to an androgynoid, q.v. 2. Without definite sexual characteristics.

androgynus (ăn-drŏj′ĭ-nŭs). A female pseudohermaphrodite. SYN: *androgyne.*

android (ăn′droyd) [″ + *eidos,* resemblance]. Resembling a male; manlike.

andrology (ăn-drŏl′ō-jē) [″ + *logos,* study]. Study of diseases of men, esp. of the male genital organs. SYN: *andriatrics.*

andromimetic (ăn″drō-mĭ-mĕt′ĭk) [″ + *mimetikos,* imitative]. Causing masculinization. SYN: *androgenic.*

andromorphous (ăn″drō-mor′fŭs) [″ + *morphe,* form]. In physical structure and appearance resembling a male.

andropathy (ăn-drŏp′ă-thē) [″ + *pathos,* suffering]. Any disease peculiar to the male.

androphilic (ăn′drō-fĭl-ĭk) [″ + *philos,* fond of]. Preferring humans; said of certain parasites.

androphobia (ăn″drō-fō′bē-ă) [″ + *phobos,* fear]. Morbid fear of the male sex.

androstane (ăn′drō-stān). $C_{19}H_{32}$. A steroid hydrocarbon that is the precursor of androgenic hormones.

androsterone (ăn″drō-stēr′ōn, ăn-drŏs′tĕr-ōn). $C_{19}H_{30}O_2$, an androgenic steroid found in the urine and considered to be a metabolite of testosterone. It has been synthesized. As one of the androgens (male sex hormones), androsterone contributes to the characteristic changes of growth and development of the genitals and axillary and pubic hair, deepening of the voice, and development of the sweat glands in the male.

-ane. In chemistry, indicates a saturated hydrocarbon.

anecdotal evidence. Evidence presented to support a scientific argument that is deficient because it is based on hearsay evidence rather than a systematic collection of data.

anechoic room. A room in which the boundaries are made so that all sound produced in the room is absorbed, i.e., not reflected.

Anectine. Trade name for succinylcholine chloride, USP, q.v.

anelectrotonus (ăn″ĕl-ĕk-trŏt′ō-nŭs) [Gr. *ana,* up, + *elektron,* electric, + *tonos,* tension]. The state of diminished irritability of a nerve or muscle in region near the anode during the passage of an electric current.

Anel's operation (ă-nĕlz′). [Dominique Anel, Fr. surgeon, 1679–1730] Ligation of an artery immediately above and on proximal side of an aneurysm.

Anel's probe. A probe for the lacrimal and nasal ducts.

anemia (ă-nē′mē-ă) [Gr. *an-,* not, + *haima,* blood]. Condition in which there is a reduction in the number of circulating red blood cells per cu. mm., the amount of hemoglobin per 100 ml., or the volume of packed red cells per 100 ml. of blood. It exists when hemoglobin content is less than that required to provide the oxygen demands of the body. It is not possible to state that anemia exists when the hemoglobin is less than a specific value. If the onset of anemia is slow, the body may adjust so well that there will be no functional impairment, even though the hemoglobin may be less than 6 gm./100 ml. of blood.

Anemia is not a disease; it is a symptom of various diseases. Anemia is classified on the basis of mean corpuscular volume (MCV) as microcytic (<80), normocytic (80–94), and macrocytic (>94); on the basis of mean corpuscular hemoglobin (MCH) as hypochromic (<27), normochromic (27–32), and hyperchromic (>32); and by etiological factors.

ETIOL: Anemia may result from excessive blood loss, excessive blood cell destruction, or decreased blood cell formation. Anemia due to excessive blood loss results from acute or chronic hemorrhage. Anemia due to excessive blood cell destruction occurs in hemolytic diseases or hypersplenism. Anemia due to decreased blood formation may result from defective nucleoprotein synthesis (as in pernicious and other macrocytic anemias), deficiency of iron in the diet, inhibition of bone marrow (as in certain toxic states), loss of bone marrow, or bone marrow failure.

SYM: Pallor of skin, fingernail beds, and mucous membranes; weakness; vertigo; headache; sore tongue; drowsiness; general malaise; dyspnea; tachycardia; palpitation; angina pectoris; gastrointestinal disturbances; amenorrhea; loss of libido; slight fever.

TREATMENT: Treatment of anemia must be specific for the cause.

Anemia due to excessive blood loss: Acute blood loss: immediate measures to stop bleeding; restoration of blood volume by transfusion; measures to combat shock. Chronic blood loss: usually produces iron-deficiency anemia, see below.

Anemia due to excessive blood cell destruction: Treatment of specific hemolytic disorder.

Anemia due to decreased blood cell formation: Deficiency states: replacement therapy to combat the specific deficiency, e.g., iron, vitamin B_{12}, folic acid, ascorbic acid. Disorders of bone marrow: if anemia is due to toxic state, removal of toxic agent may result in spontaneous recovery. If anemia is idiopathic, treatment consists of transfusions as necessary, marrow-stimulating drugs, antibiotics to combat infection if necessary.

NURSING IMPLICATIONS: *Rest:* Assess patient for fatigue and plan care and activity accordingly. Patients with severe anemia are usually maintained on strict bedrest.

Skin care: For patients on bedrest—frequent position changes, massaging of skin over bony prominences, daily inspection of skin for signs of redness, dryness, or skin breakdown.

Mouth care: Assess patient daily for development of mouth lesions or ulcers. Alkaline mouthwashes are beneficial for patients who develop mouth ulcers; a tongue blade padded with gauze may be utilized instead of a toothbrush.

Diet: Encourage patients to eat by providing small portions of food and by providing them with their food preferences. If the patient has mouth lesions, oral hygiene done before meals may help to increase appetite. In addition, provide appropriate nutritional counseling for the patient's individual dietary needs.

Medications: Teach the patient about the reasons for the medications, possible side effects, and correct dosage and administration of the medication. Patients receiving iron therapy should be aware that their stools will become black, and that the medicine may cause constipation. Patients receiving liquid iron preparations should not take the medication from a silver spoon or drink milk. They should drink the medication through a straw and rinse the mouth afterwards, to help prevent staining of the teeth.

Patient education: Ensure that the patient and family understand the cause of the anemia and the rationale behind the prescribed treatment. Teaching should also include the importance of following the prescribed diet, taking prescribed medications, and continuing with periodic blood tests and medical evaluations.

a., achlorhydric. A hypochromic microcytic anemia associated with a lack of free hydrochloric acid in gastric juice.

a., addisonian. A., pernicious, q.v.

a., aplastic. Anemia caused by aplasia of bone marrow or its destruction by chemical agents (benzene, arsenic, nitrogen mustards) or physical factors (x-rays and other sources of ionizing radiation). An idiopathic form may occur.

a., blind loop. Megaloblastic anemia due to a blind loop or multiple diverticulosis of the jejunum, which becomes infected with bacteria. These organisms destroy vitamin B_{12}, thus causing anemia. May be treated surgically by removing diverticuli or blind loops or administering vitamin B_{12} and antibiotics. SEE: *a., megaloblastic.*

a., chlorotic. A microcytic hypochromic anemia occurring in adolescent girls and young women, usually associated with dietary deficiency of iron and protein. SYN: *chlorosis; green sickness.* SEE: *a., iron-deficiency.*

a., congenital hemolytic. Inherited chronic disease characterized by hemolysis of blood cells, jaundice, and splenomegaly. SYN: *icterus, hemolytic; jaundice, hemolytic.*

a., Cooley's. Anemia resulting from inheritance of a recessive trait responsible for interference with hemoglobin synthesis. SYN: *thalassemia major,* q.v.; *a., erythroblastic.*

a., crescent cell. A., sickle cell, q.v.

a., deficiency. Condition resulting from lack of an essential ingredient such as iron or vitamins in the diet, or the inability of the intestine to absorb them. SYN: *a., nutritional.*

a., drepanocytic. A., sickle cell, q.v.

a., erythroblastic. Anemia resulting from inheritance of a recessive trait responsible for interference with hemoglobin synthesis. SYN: *thalassemia major,* q.v.; *Cooley's anemia.*

a. hemolytic. Anemia resulting from hemolysis of red blood cells. Is either acquired as from the effects of toxic agents, or congenital (familial).

a., hyperchromic. Anemia in which mean corpuscular hemoglobin concentration (MCHC) is greater than normal. The red blood cells are darker staining than normal.

a., hypersplenic. Condition resulting from excessive destruction of red blood cells in the spleen.

a., hypochromic. Anemia in which there is a hemoglobin deficiency and mean corpuscular hemoglobin concentration is less than normal.

a., hypoplastic. Term that has been used to describe aplastic anemia. If anemia due to failure of formation of red blood cells is meant, then pure red blood cell aplasia is the term of choice.

a., iron-deficiency. Anemia resulting from a greater demand on the stored iron than can be supplied.

ETIOL: Inadequate iron intake, malabsorption of iron, chronic blood loss, pregnancy and lactation, intravascular hemolysis, or a combination of these factors.

Usually successfully treated with oral ferrous sulfate or ferrous gluconate and a well-balanced diet. Iron-deficiency anemia is probably the most common chronic disease of mankind. It is estimated that at least 18,000,000 people in the United States are iron-deficient.

a., Jaksch's. Infantile pseudoleukemia; enlargement of spleen and lymph nodes accompanied by progressive anemia without leukemic changes in the blood.

a., macrocytic. Anemia marked by abnormally large erythrocytes.

a., mediterranean. SEE: *thalassemia.*

a., megaloblastic. Anemia in which megaloblasts are found in the blood.

a., microcytic. Anemia with abnormally small erythrocytes.

a., myelopathic. Anemia caused by disruption, usually by metastasis, in bone marrow function.

a., normochromic. Anemia wherein the red blood cells contain the normal amount of hemoglobin.

a., normocytic. Anemia in which size and hemoglobin content of red blood cells remain normal.

a., nutritional. A., deficiency, q.v.

a. of chronic disease. Anemia associated with a variety of chronic diseases including chronic infections, cancer, rheumatoid arthritis, rheumatic fever, Hodgkin's disease, and with fractures, severe tissue injury, and in almost every condition in which there is inflammation and necrosis of tissue.

a., pernicious. A chronic macrocytic anemia characterized by achlorhydria. Occurs most commonly in 40- to 80-year-old northern Europeans of fair complexion. It has, however, been reported in other races and ethnic groups. The disease is rare in Negroes and Orientals.

ETIOL: Failure of the stomach to secrete enough intrinsic factor to ensure intestinal absorption of vitamin B_{12}, the extrinsic factor. This is due to atrophy of the glandular mucosa of the fundus of the stomach and is associated with absence of hydrochloric acid.

SYM: Weakness, sore tongue, paresthesias (tingling and numbness) of extremities, and gastrointestinal symptoms such as diarrhea, nausea, vomiting, pain; signs of cardiac failure may be present in severe anemia.

TREATMENT: Intramuscular injection of vitamin B_{12}.

a., pure red cell aplasia. Anemia due to decreased production of red cells.

a., septic. Anemia due to severe infection.

a., sickle cell. A hereditary, chronic, hemolytic anemia characterized by presence of large numbers of crescent- or sickle-shaped red blood cells in the blood. Occurs almost exclusively in blacks. Due to a variation in the hemoglobin molecule.

a., splenic. Enlargement of spleen due to portal or splenic hypertension with accompanying anemia, leukopenia, thrombocytopenia, and gastric hemorrhage. SYN: *Banti's syndrome; splenomegaly, congestive.*

a., traumatic cardiac hemolytic. Anemia caused by the rupture of the red blood cell membrane in patients who have had intracardiac plastic surgery involving placement of a prosthesis. Seen esp. in those whose aortic valve has been replaced.

anemic (ă-nē′mĭk). Pert. to anemia; deficient in red blood cells, in hemoglobin, or in volume of blood.

anemic hypoxia. Inadequate oxygenation due to reduction in amount or capability of hemoglobin to transport oxygen.

anemophobia (ăn″ĕ-mō-fō′bē-ă) [Gr. *anemos,* wind, + *phobos,* fear]. Morbid fear of drafts or of the wind.

anencephalus (ăn″ĕn-sĕf′ă-lŭs) [Gr. *an-,* not, + *enkephalos,* the brain]. Congenital absence of brain and spinal cord, the cranium being open throughout its whole extent and the vertebral canal converted into a groove.

anephrogenesis (ā-nĕf″rō-jĕn′ĕ-sĭs) [Gr. *a-,* not, + *nephros,* kidney, + *genesis,* beginning]. Congenital lack of kidneys.

anergasia (ăn″ĕr-gā′sē-ă) [Gr. *an-,* not + *ergon,* work]. Anergia; functional inactivity resulting from a structural lesion of the central nervous system.

anergastic reaction (ăn″ĕr-găs′tĭk). Disorder involving cerebral lesions or organic psychoses. Loss of memory and impairment of mental activity, function, or judgment.

anergia (ăn-ĕr′jē-ă) [″ + *ergon,* work]. Inactivity; lack of energy.

anergic (ăn-ĕr′jĭk). Sluggish; inactive. Deficient in energy; listless.

anergic stupor. Acute phase of dementia.

anergy (ăn′ĕr-jē). 1. Impaired or absent ability to react to specific antigens. 2. Anergia.

aneroid (ăn′ĕr-ŏyd) [Gr. *a-,* not, + *neron,* water, + *eidos,* form]. Operating without a fluid, as an aneroid barometer that utilizes atmospheric pressure instead of a liquid such as mercury.

anerythroplasia (ăn″ĕ-rĭth″rō-plā′zē-ă) [Gr. *an-,* not, + *erythros,* red, + *plasis,* a molding]. Absence of red blood cell formation.

anerythroplastic (ăn″ĕ-rĭth″rō-plăs′tĭk). Rel. to or characterized by anerythroplasia.

anerythropsia (ăn″ĕ-rĭ-thrŏp′sē-ă) [″ + ″ + *opsis,* vision]. Inability to distinguish red clearly.

anesthecinesia, anesthekinesia (ăn-ĕs-thē″sĭn-ē′zē-ă, -kĭ-nē′zē-ă) [″ + *aisthesis,* sensation, + *kinesis,* movement]. Sensory and motor paralysis.

anesthesia (ăn″ĕs-thē′zē-ă) [″ + *aisthesis,* sensation]. Partial or complete loss of sensation with or without loss of consciousness as result of disease, injury, or administration of an anesthetic agent, usually by injection or inhalation.

STAGES: The first stage of pharmacologically induced general anesthesia includes preliminary excitement until voluntary control is lost. Hearing is the last sense to be lost. For this reason, content of conversation of operating room staff should be guarded during this stage. The second stage consists of loss of voluntary control. In the third stage there is entire relaxation, no muscular rigidity, and deep regular breathing.

SIGNS: The signs of depth of anesthesia based upon pupillary size, eye motion, and the character of respirations as originally described for ether have been found to be unreliable and poorly correlated with the alveolar concentration of anesthetic. The type of medicines used for premedication as well as the type of anesthetic employed will influence the signs of anesthesia.

EMERGENCY MEASURES: Artificial respiration by anesthetist, injection of cardiac stimulant, inhalation of oxygen, injection of epinephrine into heart muscle. SEE: *cardiopulmonary resuscitation.*

a., audio. Anesthesia produced by sound; used by dentists to kill pain.

a., basal. The anesthetic state produced by medication prior to the administration of the principal anesthetic agent.

a., block. Regional anesthesia resulting from nerve blocking by injection of alcohol or other substance into or very near a nerve trunk. SYN: *a., conduction.*

a., bulbar. Anesthesia produced by a lesion of the pons.

a., caudal. Anesthesia produced by insertion of a needle into sacrococcygeal notch and injection of local anesthetic into the epidural space.

a., central. Pathologic anesthesia due to a lesion of the central nervous system.

a., closed. Inhalation anesthesia technique in which the gases are rebreathed. This requires appropriate treatment of the exhaled gas in order to absorb the expired carbon dioxide and to replenish the oxygen and anesthetic gas or gases.

a., conduction. A., block, q.v.

a., crossed. Anesthesia of the side opposite to the site of the lesion.

a., dissociative. A type of anesthesia characterized by catalepsy, amnesia, and marked analgesia. The patient experiences a strong feeling of dissociation from the environment.

a. dolorosa. Painfulness of a part with anesthesia of that part, as in thalamic lesions.

a., electric. Anesthesia induced by the use of an electric current.

a., endotracheal. Production of anesthesia by administering the inhaled gas via a tube that is passed through the trachea.

a., frost. A., ice, q.v.

a., general. Anesthesia that is complete and affecting the entire body with loss of consciousness when the anesthetic acts upon the brain. This type of anesthesia is usually accomplished following administration of inhalation or intravenous anesthetics. Commonly used for surgical procedures.

a., Gwathmey's. Anesthesia induced by injecting an olive oil and ether solution into the rectum.

a., hysterical. Bodily anesthesia occurring in hysteria.

a., ice. Local anesthesia produced by cooling the area. This can be accomplished by applying ice to the area or by applying a volatile liquid such as ethyl chloride to the area. Also called frost anesthesia.

a., infiltration. Local anesthesia produced by injecting the local anesthetic solution directly into the tissues, such as injection of procaine solution into the gums for dental procedures.

a., inhalation. General anesthesia produced by inhaling vapor or gas anesthetics such as ether, nitrous oxide, and methoxyflurane.

a., insufflation. Instillation of gaseous anesthetic materials into the inhaled air.

a., local. Anesthesia affecting a local area only, the anesthetic acting upon nerves or nerve tracts. SEE: *a., block; a., infiltration.*

a., mixed. General anesthesia produced by more than one drug, as nitrous oxide gas for induction followed by ether for maintenance of anesthesia.

a., neural. Injection of an anesthetic into a nerve or immediately around it (intraneural and paraneural). SYN: *a., block.*

a., neuroleptic. General anesthesia produced by the use of a neuroleptic agent such as droperidol, a narcotic analgesic, and nitrous oxide in oxygen.

a., open. Application, usually by dropping, of a volatile anesthetic agent onto a gauze held over the nose and mouth.

a., peripheral. Local anesthesia produced by blocking a nerve with an appropriate agent.

a., primary. First stage of anesthesia, q.v., before unconsciousness.

a., pudendal. A type of local anesthesia used in obstetrics. The pudendal nerve on each side, near the spinous process of the ischium, is blocked.

a., rectal. General anesthesia produced by introduction of anesthetic agent into rectum.

a., refrigeration. Anesthesia induced by lowering temperature of a part to near freezing by topical ethyl chloride spray or by immersion of the body or a part in a container of finely cracked ice.

a., regional. Nerve or field blocking, causing insensibility over a particular area. SEE: *a., block; a., infiltration.*

a., segmental. Anesthesia due to a pathological or surgically induced lesion of a nerve root.

a., sexual. Absence of sexual desire. SYN: *anaphrodisia.*

a., spinal. 1. Anesthesia resulting from disease or injury to conduction pathways of the spinal cord. 2. Anesthesia produced by injection of anesthetic into subarachnoid space of spinal cord.

a., splanchnic. Anesthesia produced by injecting an anesthetic agent into the splanchnic ganglion.

a., surgical. Depth of anesthesia at which relaxation of muscles and loss of sensation and consciousness are adequate for the performance of surgery.

a., tactile. Loss of sense of touch.

a., topical. Local anesthesia induced by application of an anesthetic directly to surface of area to be anesthetized.

a., traumatic. Loss of sensation resulting from injury to nerve.

a., twilight. State of light anesthesia. SEE: *twilight sleep.*

anesthesia, words pert. to: words beginning "anesthe-"; carbon dioxide; chloroform; cocaine; cyclopropane; ether; ethyl chloride; ethylene; halothane; labor; nitrous oxide; paraldehyde; procaine.

anesthesimeter (ăn-ĕs′thĕ-sĭm′ĕ-tĕr) [Gr. *an-*, not, + *aisthesis,* sensation, + *metron,* measure]. 1. Device that determines the quantity of anesthetic administered. 2. Device that measures the degree of loss of sensation.

anesthesiologist (ăn″ĕs-thē″zē-ŏl′ō-jĭst). A physician specializing in anesthesiology.

anesthesiology (ăn″ĕs-thē″zē-ŏl′ō-jē) [″ + ″ + *logos,* science]. Science of anesthesia.

anesthetic (ăn″ĕs-thĕt′ĭk). 1. Pert. to or producing anesthesia. 2. An agent that produces anesthesia; subdivided into general and local, according to their action. SEE: *anesthesia.*

anesthetist (ă-nĕs′thĕ-tĭst). One who administers anesthetics, esp. for general anesthesia. May be a specially trained physician or nurse.

anesthetization (ă-nĕs″thĕ-tī-zā′shŭn). Induction of anesthesia.

anesthetize (ă-nĕs′thĕ-tīz). To induce anesthesia.

anethole (ăn′ĕ-thōl). Chemical present in oil of anise and in oil of fennel. Used as a flavoring agent.

anetiologic (ăn-ē″tē-ō-lŏj′ĭk) [Gr. *an-*, not, + *aitia,* cause, + *logos,* study]. Not conforming to the principles of etiology.

anetoderma (ăn″ĕt-ō-dĕr′mă) [Gr. *anetos,* relaxed, + *derma,* skin]. Atrophy of the skin with soft fibromas forming large pendulous masses.

aneuploidy (ăn″ū-ploy′dē) [Gr. *an-*, not, + *eu,* well, + *ploos,* fold, + *eidos,* form]. Condition of having an abnormal number of chromosomes for the species indicated.

aneurine hydrochloride (ă-nū′rĭn). Thiamine hydrochloride, vitamin B_1.

aneurysm (ăn′ū-rĭzm) [Gr. *aneurysma,* a widening]. Localized abnormal dilatation of a blood vessel, usually an artery. Due to congenital defect or weakness of the wall of the vessel. SEE: illus.

ETIOL: In the aorta, arteriosclerosis accompanied by hypertension is a cause. Bacterial or mycotic infection and trauma are common causes of aneurysms in peripheral arteries.

a., aortic. Aneurysm affecting any part of the aorta.

PATH: Pressure on trachea, esophagus, veins, or nerves.

SYM: Dyspnea, cough, sputum, dysphagia, congestion of head and neck. Inequality in the right and left radial pulses.

TREATMENT: Surgery.

a., arteriovenous. Aneurysm in which artery and vein become connected by a saccule.

ETIOL: Usually traumatic, may be congenital.

SYM: Pain, expansile pulsation, bruit.

a., atherosclerotic. Aneurysm due to degeneration or weakening of the arterial wall caused by atherosclerosis.

a., berry. Small saccular congenital aneurysm of a cerebral vessel. It communicates with the vessel by a small opening. Rupture of this type of aneurysm may cause bleeding severe enough to be fatal.

a., cirsoid. A dilatation of a network of

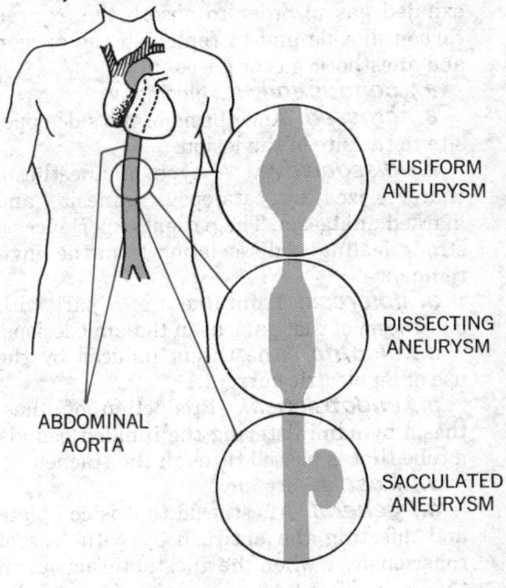

TYPES OF ANEURYSMS

vessels commonly occurring on the scalp. The mass may form a pulsating subcutaneous tumor. SYN: *a., racemose.*

a., compound. Aneurysm in which some of the layers of the vessel are ruptured and others dilated.

a., dissecting. Aneurysm in which the blood makes its way between the layers of a blood vessel wall, separating them; a result of necrosis of the medial portion of the arterial wall. SEE: illus.

a., fusiform. Aneurysm in which all the walls of a blood vessel dilate more or less equally, creating a tubular swelling. SEE: illus.

a., mycotic. Aneurysm due to bacterial infection.

a., racemose. A., cirsoid, q.v.

a., sacculated. Aneurysm due to the yielding of a weak area on one side of the vessel and not involving the entire circumference; usually due to trauma. It is attached to the artery by a narrow neck. SEE: illus.

a., varicose. Aneurysm forming a blood-filled sac between an artery and a vein.

a., venous. Aneurysm of a vein.

aneurysmal (ăn″ū-rĭz′măl) [Gr. *aneurysma,* a widening]. Pert to aneurysm.

aneurysmectomy (ăn″ū-rĭz-mĕk′tō-mē) [″ + *ektome,* excision]. Surgical removal of the sac of an aneurysm.

aneurysmoplasty (ăn″ū-rĭz′mō-plăs″tē) [″ + *plassein,* to form]. Surgical repair of an aneurysm.

aneurysmorrhaphy (ăn″ū-rĭz-mor′ă-fē) [″ + *rhaphe,* suture]. Surgical closure of the sac of an aneurysm.

aneurysmotomy (ăn″ū-rĭz-mŏt′ō-mē) [″ + *tome,* incision]. Incision of the sac of an aneurysm, allowing it to heal by granulation.

A.N.F. *American Nurses' Federation; American Nurses Foundation.*

anfractuosity (ăn-frăk″tū-ŏs′ĭ-tē) [L. *anfractus,* a winding]. A cerebral sulcus or fissure.

angel dust (PCP). "Street" or slang term for phencyclidine, q.v.

angel's trumpet [*Datura ruaveolens*]. A flowering shrub native to the southeastern U.S. Portions of the shrub are used for hallucinogenic effects. The flowers are made into a stew or tea, and the leaves are eaten. The flowers contain large quantities of the alkaloids atropine, hyoscyamine, and hyoscine. Ingestion of plant products produces intense thirst, visual disturbances, flushing, CNS hyperexcitability, sensory flooding and a delirious incoherent state. This is followed by hyperthermia, tachycardia, hypertension, visual hallucinations, disturbed consciousness, clonus, and subsequent convulsions. If condition is untreated, death may occur.

TREATMENT: gastric lavage, followed by 1 to 4 mg. of I.V. physostigmine sulfate. This dosage should reverse the acute delirious state in one or two hours, but it may need to be repeated several times for the desired effect.

angel's wing. Posterior projection of the scapula usually caused by paralysis of the serratus anterior muscle. SYN: *scapula, winged.*

Angelucci's syndrome (ăn″jĕ-loo′chēz). [Arnaldo Angelucci, It. ophthalmologist, 1854–1934] Great excitability, palpitation, and vasomotor disturbance associated with vernal conjunctivitis.

angi- (ăn′jē) [Gr. *angeion,* vessel]. Prefix meaning a blood or lymph vessel.

angiasthenia (ăn″jē-ăs-thē′nē-ă) [″ + *a-,* not, + *sthenos,* strength]. Loss of vascular tone.

angiectasia, angiectasis (ăn″jē-ĕk-tā′zē-ă, -ĕk′tă-sĭs) [″ + *ektasis,* stretching]. Dilation of a blood or lymph vessel.

angiectomy (ăn″jē-ĕk′tō-mē) [″ + *ektome,* excision]. Excision or resection of a blood vessel.

angiectopia (ăn″jē-ĕk-tō′pē-ă) [″ + *ektopos,* out of place]. Displacement of a vessel.

angiemphraxis (ăn″jē-ĕm-frăk′sĭs) [″ + *emphraxis,* stoppage]. Obstruction of a vessel.

angiitis (ăn″jē-ī′tĭs) [″ + *itis,* inflammation]. Inflammation of a blood or lymph vessel. SYN: *angitis; vasculitis.*

angina (ăn-jī′nă, ăn′jĭ-nă) [L. *angina,* quinsy, from *angere,* to choke]. 1. Angina pectoris, q.v. 2. Acute sore throat.

a. abdominis. Severe abdominal pain resulting from sclerosis of abdominal blood vessels.

a. acuta. Simple sore throat.

a., agranulocytic. Acute sore throat and ulceration of the pharynx due to agranulocytosis.

a. cruris. Angina due to obstruction of an artery, causing pain and cyanosis of the leg affected, with periodic lameness.

a. decubitus. Attacks of angina pectoris occurring while in recumbent position.

a. epiglottidea. Inflammation of the epiglottis.

a. follicularis. Inflammation of the tonsils.

a., intestinal. Abdominal pain caused by insufficient blood supply to the intestines. Usually occurs after eating.

a. laryngea. Inflammation of the larynx.

a. ludovici, a. ludwigi. A., Ludwig's, q.v.

a., Ludwig's. Submaxillary cellulitis; a deep infection of tissues of the floor of the mouth.

a. maligna. Gangrenous inflammation of the throat; septic sore throat.

a., necrotic. Angina with gangrenous patches in the mucosa of the air passages seen in scarlet fever and occasionally in diphtheria.

a. parotidea. Inflammation of the parotid glands. SYN: *mumps*.

a. pectoris. Severe pain and constriction about the heart, usually radiating to the left shoulder and down the left arm, or, rarely, from the heart to the abdomen. Pain may also radiate to the back or to the jaw. Caused by an insufficient supply of blood to the heart. SEE: illus.

SYM: Steady severe pain and feeling of pressure in region of the heart; great anxiety, fear of approaching death (angor animi), and fixation of the body; face pale, ashen, or livid; brow bathed in sweat. Dyspnea often noted; pulse variable, usually tense and quick. Blood pressure is raised during an attack. Cardiac arrhythmia may be present during angina. Attack may be of brief duration or last for a considerable period.

PROG: May be grave. Attacks may be intermittent, and with proper rest and care, recovery is possible.

TREATMENT: During attack, inhalation of amyl nitrite or use of nitroglycerin sublingually. Avoidance of excitement; physical rest.

a. pectoris vasomotoria. Angina pectoris in which symptoms are relatively mild. Pallor, cyanosis, and coldness and numbness of the extremities are characteristic.

ANGINA PECTORIS

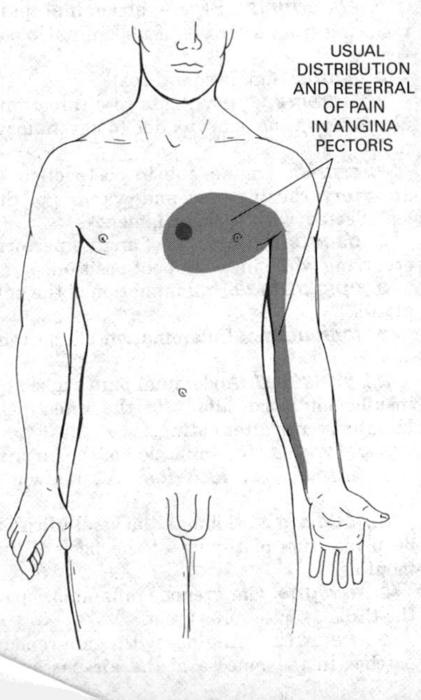

a., phlegmonous. Inflammation of the deep tissues of the throat with edema and usually suppuration.

a., Prinzmetal's. A., variant, q.v.

a. simplex. Simple sore throat. SYN: *a. acuta*.

a. streptococcus. Sore throat caused by streptococcus infection.

a. tonsillaris. Quinsy, q.v.

a. trachealis. Croup.

a., variant. Angina pectoris occurring during rest. It is not preceded by exercise or increase in heart rate. These patients have normal exercise potential when the angina is not present. Coronary artery spasm causes this condition.

a., Vincent's. Painful pseudomembranous ulceration of the mouth involving gingivae, oral mucosa, and sometimes pharynx and tonsils. Fusiform bacilli and a spirochete, Borrelia vincenti, are invariably associated with the disease but their relationship to it is not definitely established. The disease may be primarily caused by Bacillus melaninogenicus. SYN: *trench mouth*. SEE: *Vincent's angina*.

anginal (ăn′jĭ-nal). Pert. to angina.

anginiform (ăn-jĭn′ĭ-form) [L. *angina,* choking, + *forma,* having the form of]. Mimicking or resembling angina, especially angina pectoris.

anginoid (ăn′jĭ-noyd) [″ + Gr. *eidos,* resemblance]. Resembling angina, esp. angina pectoris.

anginophobia (ăn″jĭ-nō-fō′bē-ă) [″ + Gr. *phobos,* fear]. Morbid fear of an attack of angina pectoris.

anginose (ăn′jĭ-nōs) [L. *angina,* choking]. Pert. to or resembling angina.

anginous (ăn′jĭ-nŭs). Resembling angina. SYN: *anginose*.

angio- (ăn′jē-ō) [Gr. *angeion,* vessel]. A combining form denoting a seed, vessel, or something contained within a vessel.

angioataxia (ăn″jē-ō-ă-tăk′sē-ă) [″ + *ataktos,* out of order]. Variability in arterial tonus.

angioblast (ăn′jē-ō-blăst) [″ + *blastos,* germ]. 1. The earliest tissue arising from mesenchyme cells of the embryo, from which blood vessels develop. 2. A cell that participates in vessel formation.

angioblastoma (ăn″jē-ō-blăs-tō′mă) [″ + ″ + *oma,* tumor]. Tumors of particular blood vessels of the brain, or of the meninges of the brain.

angiocardiogram (ăn″jē-ō-kăr′dē-ō-grăm) [″ + *kardia,* heart, + *gramma,* writing]. Serial x-rays of the heart taken immediately after intravenous injection of a radiopaque dye.

angiocardiography (ăn″jē-ō-kăr″dē-ŏg′ră-fē)

[″ + ″ + *graphein,* to write]. Roentgenography of the heart and great vessels after intravenous injection of a radiopaque solution.

angiocardiokinetic (ăn″jē-ō-kăr″dē-ō-kī-nĕt′ĭk) [″ + ″ + *kinesis,* movement]. Causing movement (contraction or dilation) of heart and blood vessels.

angiocardiopathy (ăn″jē-ō-kăr″dē-ŏp′ă-thē) [″ + ″ + *pathos,* disease]. Disease of the blood vessels of the heart.

angiocarditis (ăn″jē-ō-kăr-dī′tĭs) [″ + ″ + *itis,* inflammation]. Inflammation of the heart and large blood vessels.

angiocavernous (ăn″jē-ō-kăv′ĕr-nŭs) [″ + L. *caverna,* cavern]. Rel. to angioma cavernosum, q.v.

angiocholecystitis (ăn″jē-ō-kō″lĕ-sĭs-tī′tĭs) [″ + *chole,* bile, + *kystis,* bladder, + *itis,* inflammation]. Inflammation of gallbladder and bile vessels.

angiocholitis (ăn″jē-ō-kō-lī′tĭs) [″ + ″ + *itis,* inflammation]. Inflammation of biliary vessels. SYN: *cholangitis.*

angiocrine (ăn′jē-ō-krĭn) [Gr. *angeion,* vessel, + *endocrine*]. Marked by vasomotor disorders resulting from disturbances of the endocrine glands.

angiodystrophia (ăn″jē-ō-dĭs-trō′fē-ă) [″ + *dys,* bad, + *trophe,* nourishment]. Faulty nutrition of vessels.

angioedema (ăn″jē-ō-ĕ-dē′mă) [″ + *oidema,* swelling]. A condition characterized by development of edematous areas of skin, mucous membranes, or viscera. It is benign and thought to be an allergic disorder, usually a food allergy. SYN: *angioneurotic edema.*

angioendothelioma (ăn″jē-ō-ĕn″dō-thē″lē-ō′mă) [″ + *endon,* within, + *thele,* nipple, + *oma,* a tumor]. (pl. *-mata* or *-mas*) A tumor consisting of endothelial cells, commonly occurring as single or multiple tumors of bone.

angiofibroma (ăn″jē-ō-fī-brō′mă) [″ + L. *fibra,* fiber, + Gr. *oma,* tumor]. (pl. *-mas* or *-mata*) A tumor consisting of fibrous tissue.

angiogenesis (ăn″jē-ō-jĕn′ĕ-sĭs) [″ + *genesis,* origin]. Development of blood vessels.

angiogenic (ăn″jē-ō-jĕn′ĭk). 1. Pert to angiogenesis. 2. Of vascular origin.

angioglioma (ăn″jē-ō-glī-ō′mă) [Gr. *angeion,* vessel, + *glia,* glue, + *oma,* tumor]. A mixed angioma and glioma.

angiogram (ăn′jē-ō-grăm) [″ + *gramma,* mark]. Serial roentgenography of a blood vessel taken in rapid sequence following the injection of a radiopaque substance into the vessel. This technique has been used to define the size and shape of various veins and arteries of organs and tissues.

a., aortic. Angiogram of aorta. Used in diagnosing aneurysms or presence of tumors that contact and deform the aorta.

a., cardiac. Angiogram of the heart. Used to determine the size and shape of the cavities of the heart and the condition of the valves.

a., cerebral. Angiogram of blood vessels of the brain.

angiograph (ăn′jē-ō-grăf″) [″ + *graphein,* to write]. A variety of sphygmograph.

angiography (ăn″jē-ŏg′ră-fē). 1. A description of blood vessels and lymphatics. 2. Roentgenography of blood vessels after injection of radiopaque substance. 3. Recording the movements of the arterial pulse by use of a sphygmograph.

a., aortic. Angiography of the aorta and its branches.

a., cardiac. Angiography of the heart and coronary arteries.

a., cerebral. Angiography of the vascular system of the brain.

a., coronary. Angiography of the coronary vessels of the heart. This can provide useful information about the adequacy of blood supply to the myocardium.

a., digital subtraction. Use of a computer technique to investigate arterial blood circulation. A reference image is obtained by use of fluoroscopy. Then a contrast medium is injected intravenously. Another film is produced from the fluoroscopic image and then the computer technique "subtracts" the image produced by surrounding tissues, and the third image is an enhanced view of the arteries.

angiohyalinosis (ăn″jē-ō-hī″ă-lĭn-ō′sĭs) [Gr. *angeion,* vessel, + *hyalos,* glass, + *osis,* condition]. Hyaline degeneration of the walls of blood vessels.

angiohypertonia (ăn″jē-ō-hī′pĕr-tō′nē-ă) [″ + *hyper,* over, + *tonos,* tension]. Spasm of blood vessels, esp. arteries. SYN: *angiospasm; vasospasm.* SEE: *hypertension.*

angiohypotonia (ăn″jē-ō-hī″pō-tō′nē-ă) [″ + *hypo,* under, + *tonos,* tension]. Angioparalysis; angioparesis; vascular dilatation. SEE: *hypotension.*

angioid (ăn′jē-oyd) [″ + *eidos,* resemblance]. Resembling a blood vessel.

angioid streaks. Dark, wavy, anastomosing striae lying beneath retinal vessels.

angiokeratoma (ăn″jē-ō-kĕr″ă-tō′mă) [″ + *keras,* horn, + *oma,* tumor]. A skin disorder occurring chiefly on feet and legs, characterized by formation of telangiectases or warty growths accompanied by thickening of the epidermis along the course of dilated capillaries.

angiokinetic (ăn″jē-ō-kī-nĕt′ĭk) [″ + *kinesis,* movement]. Pert to constriction and dilation of blood vessels. SYN: *vasomotor.*

angioleukitis (ăn″jē-ō-loo-kī′tĭs) [″ + *leukos,* white, + *itis,* inflammation]. Inflamm-

of lymphatics.

angiolipoma (ăn′jē-ō-lĭp-ō′mă) [″ + *lipos,* fat, + *oma,* tumor]. A mixed angioma and lipoma.

angiolith (ăn′jē-ō-lĭth) [″ + *lithos,* stone]. Calcareous deposit in wall of a blood vessel.

angiology (ăn″jē-ŏl′ō-jē) [″ + *logos,* science]. The science of the blood vessels and lymphatics.

angiolupoid (ăn″jē-ō-loo′poyd) [″ + L. *lupus,* wolf, + Gr. *eidos,* resemblance]. A tuberculous skin lesion consisting of small red, oval plaques.

angiolymphitis (ăn″jē-ō-lĭm-fī′tĭs) [″ + L. *lympha,* lymph, + *itis,* inflammation]. Inflammation of the lymphatics. SYN: *lymphangitis.*

angiolysis (ăn″jē-ŏl′ĭ-sĭs) [″ + *lysis,* destruction]. Obliteration of blood vessels, as in the umbilical cord when it is tied just after birth.

angioma (ăn″jē-ō′mă) [″ + *oma,* tumor]. A form of tumor, usually benign, consisting principally of blood vessels (hemangioma) or lymph vessels (lymphangioma). Considered to be remnants of fetal tissue misplaced or undergoing disordered development. SEE: *choristoma; epithelioma; hamartoma; nevus.*

a., capillary. Congenital, superficial hemangioma appearing as irregularly shaped, red discoloration of otherwise normal skin. Due to overgrowth of capillaries.

a. cavernosum. Congenital hemangioma appearing as an elevated dark-red tumor, ranging in size from a pea to that of the hand. It may pulsate; commonly involves the subcutaneous or submucous tissue and consists of blood-filled vascular spaces. It is nonmalignant, and small ones may disappear without therapy.

a., senile. Hemangioma common in elderly persons due to weakening of capillary walls; consists of a compressible mass of blood vessels. SYN: *spot, ruby.*

a., serpiginous. A skin disorder characterized by appearance of small, red, vascular dots arranged in rings; due to proliferation of capillaries.

a. simplex. A., capillary, q.v.

a., stellate. Hemangioma in which numerous telangiectatic vessels radiate from a central point. Commonly associated with hepatic disease, hypertension, and pregnancy. SYN: *spider nevus.*

a., telangiectatic. Angioma composed of abnormally dilated blood vessels.

a. venosum racemosum. Swelling associated with severe varicosities of superficial veins.

angiomalacia (ăn″jē-ō-mă-lā′sē-ă) [Gr. *angeion,* vessel, + *malakia,* softness]. Softening of blood vessel walls.

angiomatosis (ăn″jē-ō-mă-tō′sĭs) [″ + *oma,* ... + *osis,* condition]. Condition of multiple angiomas.

angiomatous (ăn″jē-ō′mă-tŭs). Resembling an angioma.

angiomegaly (ăn″jē-ō-mĕg′ă-lē) [″ + *megas,* large]: Enlargement of blood vessels, esp. in the eyelid.

angiometer (ăn″jē-ŏm′ĕ-tĕr) [″ + *metron,* measure]. Instrument for measuring tension and diameter of blood vessels.

angiomyocardiac (ăn″jē-ō-mī″ō-kăr′dē-ăk) [″ + *mys,* muscle, + *kardia,* heart]. Pert. to blood vessels and cardiac muscle.

angiomyolipoma (ăn″jē-ō-mī″ō-lĭ-pō′mă) [″ + ″ + *lipos,* fat, + *oma,* tumor]. Nonmalignant growth containing vascular, fatty, and muscular tissues.

angiomyoma (ăn″jē-ō-mī-ō′mă) [″ + ″ + *oma,* tumor]. Tumor composed of blood vessels and muscle tissue.

angiomyoneuroma (ăn″jē-ō-mī″ō-nū-rō′mă) [″ + ″ + *neuron,* nerve, + *oma,* tumor]. Painful, benign tumor of the arteriovenous anastomoses of the skin. SYN: *glomangioma.*

angiomyosarcoma (ăn″jē-ō-mī″ō-săr-kō′mă) [″ + ″ + *sarx,* flesh, + *oma,* tumor]. Tumor composed of blood vessels, muscle tissue, and connective tissue.

angioneurectomy (ăn″jē-ō-nū-rĕk′tō-mē) [″ + *neuron,* nerve, + *ektome,* excision]. Excision of vessels and nerves.

angioneuromyoma (ăn″jē-ō-nū″rō-mī-ō′mă) [″ + ″ + *mys,* muscle, + *oma,* tumor]. Glomangioma, q.v. SEE: *angiomyoneuroma.*

angioneurosis (ăn″jē-ō-nū-rō′sĭs) [″ + ″ + *osis,* condition]. Spasm or paralysis of blood vessels resulting from a disturbance of vasomotor system.

angioneurotic (ăn″jē-ō-nū-rŏt′ĭk). Pert. to angioneurosis.

angioneurotic edema. A condition characterized by development of edematous areas of skin, mucous membranes, or viscera. It is benign and thought to be an allergic disorder, usually a food allergy. Danazol has been helpful in treating this condition, but the drug should not be taken by children or by pregnant women. SYN: *angioedema; Quincke's disease.*

angioneurotomy (ăn″jē-ō-nū-rŏt′ō-mē) [″ + ″ + *tome,* incision]. Cutting of vessels and nerves.

angionoma (ăn″jē-ō-nō′mă) [Gr. *angeion,* vessel, + *nome,* ulcer]. Ulceration of a vessel.

angioparalysis (ăn″jē-ō-pă-răl′ĭ-sĭs) [″ + *paralyein,* loosen, dissolve]. Vasomotor relaxation of blood vessel tone.

angioparesis (ăn″jē-ō-pă-rē′sĭs) [″ + *paresis,* weakness]. Mild degree of angioparalysis, q.v.

angiopathology (ăn″jē-ō-pă-thŏl′ō-jē) [″ + *pathos,* suffering, + *logos,* study]. Morbid changes in diseases of the blood vessels.

angiopathy (ăn-jē-ŏp'ă-thē). Any disease of blood vessels or lymph vessels. SYN: *angiosis.*

angiophacomatosis, angiophakomatosis (ăn″jē-ō-făk″ō-mă-tō'sĭs) [″ + *phakos,* lens, + *oma,* tumor, + *osis,* condition]. Retinocerebral hemangiomatosis, Hippel's disease, q.v., or von Hippel-Lindau's disease.

angioplany (ăn'jē-ō-plăn″ē) [″ + *plane,* wandering]. Abnormal location of a blood vessel.

angioplasty (ăn'jē-ō-plăs″tē) [″ + *plassein,* to form]. Plastic surgery upon blood vessels.

angiopoiesis (ăn″jē-ō-poy-ē'sĭs) [″ + *poiein,* to make]. The process of forming vessels.

angiopoietic (ăn″jē-ō-poy-ĕt'ĭk). Pert. to or causing the formation of vessels.

angiopressure (ăn'jē-ō-prĕsh″ūr). Pressure applied to a blood vessel to arrest hemorrhage.

angiorrhaphy (ăn″jē-or'ă-fē) [″ + *rhaphe,* seam]. Suture of a vessel, esp. a blood vessel.

angiorrhexis (ăn″jē-or-ĕk'sĭs) [″ + *rhexis,* rupture]. Rupture of a vessel, esp. a blood vessel.

angiosarcoma (ăn″jē-ō-săr-kō'mă) [″ + *sarx,* flesh, + *oma,* tumor]. Malignant neoplasm originating from blood vessels. SYN: *hemangiosarcoma.*

angiosclerosis (ăn″jē-ō-sklĕ-rō'sĭs) [″ + *sklerosis,* hardening]. Hardening of the walls of the vascular system.

angioscope (ăn'jē-ō-skōp) [″ + *skopein,* to view]. A microscope for studying capillary vessels.

angioscotoma (ăn″jē-ō-skō-tō'mă) [″ + *skotoma,* darkness]. The defect produced in the visual field by the shadows of the retinal blood vessels.

angiosialitis (ăn″jē-ō-sī-ă-lī'tĭs) [″ + *sialon,* saliva, + *itis,* inflammation]. Inflammation of a salivary duct.

angiosis (ăn″jē-ō'sĭs) [Gr. *angeion,* vessel, + *osis,* condition]. Any disease of blood vessels or lymph vessels. SYN: *angiopathy.*

angiospasm (ăn'jē-ō-spăzm) [″ + *spasmos,* tension, spasm]. Spasmodic contraction of blood vessels. May cause cramping of muscles or intermittent claudication.

angiospastic (ăn″jē-ō-spăs'tĭk). Pert. to angiospasm.

angiostenosis (ăn″jē-ō-stĕ-nō'sĭs) [″ + *stenoein,* to make narrow, + *osis,* condition]. Narrowing of a vessel, esp. a blood vessel.

angiosteosis (ăn″jē-ŏs″tē-ō'sĭs) [″ + *osteon,* bone, + *osis,* condition]. Calcification of a vessel.

angiostomy (ăn″jē-ŏs'tō-mē) [″ + *stoma,* mouth]. Operation making artificial fistulous opening into a blood vessel.

angiostrophy (ăn″jē-ŏs'trō-fē) [″ + *strophe,* twist]. Twisting the cut end of a blood vessel to arrest bleeding.

angiosynizesis (ăn″jē-ō-sĭn″ĭ-zē'sĭs) [″ + *synizesis,* contraction]. Collapse of walls of a vessel and their subsequent adhesion.

angiostaxis (ăn″jē-ō-stăk'sĭs) [″ + *staxis,* trickling]. 1. Hemophilia or hemorrhagic diathesis. 2. Oozing of blood.

angiotelectasis (ăn″jē-ō-tĕl-ĕk'tă-sĭs) [″ + *telos,* end, + *ektasis,* stretching out]. Dilatation of terminal arterioles.

angiotenic (ăn″jē-ō-tĕn'ĭk) [″ + *teinen,* to stretch]. Characterized by or caused by distention of blood vessels.

angiotensin (ăn″jē-ō-tĕn'sĭn). A vasopressor substance that is formed in the body by interaction of renin and a serum globulin fraction (angiotensinogen). Formerly called angiotonin or hypertensin.

a. I. Physiologically inactive form of angiotensin; precursor of angiotensin II, q.v.

a. II. Physiologically active form of angiotensin; powerful vasopressor and stimulator of aldosterone production and secretion.

a. amide. A vasoconstrictor drug.

angiotensinogen (ăn″jē-ō-tĕn-sĭn'ō-jĕn). A serum globulin fraction formed in the liver; converted to angiotensin as a result of hydrolysis by renin.

angiotitis (ăn″jē-ō-tī'tĭs) [″ + *otos,* ear, + *itis,* inflammation]. Inflammation of blood vessels of the ear.

angiotome (ăn'jē-ō-tōm″) [Gr. *angeion,* vessel, + *tome,* incision]. Any segment of the embryonic vascular system.

angiotomy (ăn″jē-ŏt″ō-mē). Sectioning of blood vessels.

angiotonic (ăn″jē-ō-tŏn'ĭk) [″ + *tonos,* tension]. Increasing arterial tension.

angiotonin (ăn″jē-ō-tōn'ĭn). Former name for angiotensin, q.v.

angiotribe (ăn'jē-ō-trīb″) [″ + *tribein,* to crush]. Instrument for crushing the end of an artery and surrounding tissue to arrest hemorrhage. SYN: *vasotribe.*

angiotripsy (ăn'jē-ō-trĭp″sē) [″ + *tripsis,* friction]. The use of an angiotribe to arrest hemorrhage.

angiotrophic (ăn″jē-ō-trŏf'ĭk) [″ + *trophe,* nourishment]. Pert. to nutrition of blood vessels or lymph vessels.

angitis (ăn-jī'tĭs) [″ + *itis,* inflammation]. Inflammation of the blood vessels or lymph vessels. SYN: *angiitis; vasculitis.*

angle (ăng'gl) [L. *angulus*]. 1. The figure or space outlined by the diverging of two lines from a common point or by the meeting of two planes. 2. A projecting or sharp corner.

a., acromial. Angle formed by junction of lateral and posterior borders of the acromion.

a., acute. An angle less than 90°.

a., alpha. Angle formed by intersec-

of visual line with optic axis.

a., alveolar. Angle between the horizontal plane and a line drawn through the base of the nasal spine and the middle point of the alveolus of the upper jaw.

a., biorbital. Angle formed by the meeting of the axes of the orbits.

a., carrying. Angle made at the elbow by extending the long axis of the forearm and the upper arm. This obtuse angle is more pronounced in the female than in the male.

a., cerebellopontine. Angle formed by junction of the cerebellum and pons.

a., costal. Meeting point of the lower border of the false ribs with the axis of the sternum.

a., craniofacial. Angle formed by the basifacial and basicranial axes at the midpoint of the sphenoethmoidal suture.

a., facial. Angle made by lines from the nasal spine and external auditory meatus meeting between the upper middle incisor teeth.

a., flat. The angle between two lines that join at an angle of almost 180°.

a., gamma. Angle between the line of vision and the optic axis.

a., metafacial. Angle between the base of the skull and the pterygoid process.

a., obtuse. An angle greater than 90°.

a., occipital. Angle formed at the opisthion by the intersection of lines from the basion and from the lower border of the orbit.

a. of convergence. Angle between the visual axis and the median line when an object is looked at.

a. of incidence. Angle between a ray striking a surface and a line drawn perpendicular to the surface at the point of incidence.

a. of iris. Angle between the cornea and iris at the periphery of the anterior chamber of the eye.

a. of jaw. Angle formed by junction of the posterior edge of the ramus of the mandible and the lower surface of the body of the mandible.

a. of mandible. Angle of jaw, q.v.

a., ophryospinal. Angle formed at the anterior nasal spine by intersection of lines drawn from the auricular point and the glabella.

a., optic. A., visual, q.v.

a., parietal. Angle formed by the meeting of a line drawn tangent to the maximum curve of the zygomatic arch and a line drawn tangent to the end of the maximum frontal diameter of the skull. If these lines are parallel, the angle is zero; if they diverge, a negative angle is formed.

a., pontine. A., cerebellopontile, q.v.

a., pubic. Angle formed by junction of the rami of the pubes.

a., right. An angle of 90°.

a., sphenoid. Angle formed at the top of the sella turcica by intersection of lines drawn from the nasal point and the tip of the rostrum of the sphenoid.

a., sternal. Angle formed by junction of the manubrium and the body of the sternum.

a., venous. Angle formed by junction of the internal jugular and subclavian veins.

a., visual. The angle formed by lines drawn from the nodal point of the eye to the edges of the object viewed.

angophrasia (ăn″gō-frā′zē-ă) [Gr. *anchein,* to choke, + *phrasis,* utterance]. Drawling, choking speech in paralytic dementia.

angor (ăng′gor) [L., strangling]. Violent distress, as in angina pectoris.

angor animi (ăng′gor ăn′ĭ-mē) [″ + L. *animus,* soul]. The feeling that one is dying, as in angina pectoris.

angstrom unit (ŏng′strŭm). [Anders J. Ångström, Swedish physicist, 1814–1874] SYMB: Å. ABBR: A.U. An internationally adopted unit of measurement of wave length; equal to 10^{-10} meter, or 0.1 nanometer. Used especially to specify radiation wavelengths. SYN: *angstrom.*

angular (ăng′gū-lăr) [L.]. Having corners or angles.

angular artery. The artery at the inner canthus of the eye; facial artery.

angulation (ăng″ū-lā′shŭn). Abnormal formation of angles by tubular structures such as the intestine, a blood vessel, or ureter.

angulus [L.]. Angle.

anhaphia (ăn-hā′fē-ă) [Gr. *an-*, not, + *haphe,* touch]. Loss of or diminished sense of touch. SYN: *anaphia.*

anhedonia (ăn″hē-dō′nē-ă) [″ + *hedone,* pleasure]. Lack of pleasure in acts that are normally pleasurable. May be an early sign of schizophrenia.

anhedonic (ăn″hē-dŏn′ĭk). Pert. to anhedonia.

anhemolytic (ăn-hē-mō-lĭt′ĭk) [″ + *haima,* blood, + *lysis,* dissolution]. Not destructive to the blood cells.

anhepatia (ăn-hĕ-pā′shē-ă) [″ + *hepar,* liver]. Failure or deficiency of liver function.

anhepatic (ăn-hĕ-păt′ĭk). Pert. to anhepatia.

anhepatogenic (ăn-hĕp″ă-tō-jĕn′ĭk) [″ + *hepar,* liver, + *gennan,* to produce]. Not produced by or arising in the liver.

anhidrosis (ăn″hī-drō′sĭs) [″ + *hidros,* sweat]. Diminished or complete absence of secretion of sweat. May be generalized or localized, temporary or permanent, accompanying disease conditions or may be a congenital anomaly. SYN: *adiapneustia; anidrosis.*

TREATMENT: Treatment of cause or accompanying conditions. Soft, nonirritating clothing; bland, soothing ointments and lubricants for skin. Air conditioning provides comfort in most instances.

anhidrotic (ăn″hī-drŏt′ĭk). 1. Inhibiting or preventing perspiration. 2. Agent that inhibits or prevents perspiration. SYN: *anidrotic; antihidrotic; antiperspirant; antisudorific.*

anhistic, anhistous (ăn-hĭs′tĭk, -hĭs′tŭs) [″ + *histos,* tissue]. Seemingly without structure.

anhydrase (ăn″hī′drās) [″ + *hydor,* water, + *-ase,* enzyme]. Enzyme that promotes the removal of water from a chemical compound.

anhydration (ăn-hī-drā′shŭn) [″ + *hydor,* water]. 1. Removal of water from a substance. 2. Condition resulting from excessive loss of body fluid. SYN: *dehydration,* q.v.

anhydremia (ăn-hī-drē′mē-ă) [″ + ″ + *haima,* blood]. Decreased amount of plasma in the blood.

anhydride (ăn-hī′drīd) [Gr. *an-,* not, + *hydor,* water]. Compound formed by removal of water from a substance, esp. from an acid.

anhydrochloric (ăn-hī-drō-klō′rĭk) [″ + ″ + *chloros,* green]. Lacking hydrochloric acid.

anhydromyelia (ăn-hī-drō-mī-ē′lē-ă) [″ + ″ + *myelos,* marrow]. Deficiency in spinal fluid.

Anhydron. Trade name for cyclothiazide, USP, q.v.

anhydrous (ăn-hī′drŭs) [″ + *hydor,* water]. Lacking water.

anianthinopsy (ăn-ē-ăn′thĭn-ŏp″sē) [″ + *ianthinos,* violet, + *opsis,* vision]. Inability to recognize violet or purple.

anicteric (ăn″ĭk-tĕr′ĭk) [″ + *ikteros,* jaundice]. Without jaundice.

anidrosis (ăn-ĭ-drō′sĭs) [″ + *hidros,* sweat]. Anhidrosis, q.v.

anidrotic (ăn-ĭ-drŏt′ĭk). Anhidrotic, q.v.

anile (ăn′ĭl, ā′nīl) [L. *anilis,* from *anus,* an old woman]. Senile.

anileridine (ăn″ĭ-lĕr′ĭ-dēn). USP. A narcotic analgesic similar to meperidine (Demerol).

aniline (ăn′ĭ-lĭn) [Arabic *an-nil,* the indigo plant]. $C_6H_5NH_2$. The simplest aromatic amine, an oily liquid derived from benzene. Used in manufacture of dyes for medical and industrial purposes. Aniline has antipyretic action but is too toxic to use as a medicine. SYN: *aminobenzene; phenylamine.*

aniline poisoning. SEE: *Poisons and Poisoning* in *Appendix.*

anilism (ăn′ĭl-ĭzm) [″ + *-ismos,* condition]. Chronic aniline poisoning. SEE: *aniline* in *Poisons and Poisoning* in *Appendix.*

SYM: Cardiac block, weakness, intermittent pulse, vertigo, muscular depression, cyanosis.

anility (ă-nĭl′ĭ-tē) [L. *anilitas,* from *anus,* an old woman]. Senility.

anima (ăn′ĭ-mă) [L., soul]. 1. Soul. 2. According to Jung, an individual's inner self as distinguished from the external personality (persona). 3. Also according to Jung, anima refers to the feminine inner personality present in men, as opposed to animus, which refers to the masculine inner personality present in women.

animal (ăn′ĭ-măl) [L. *animalis,* living]. 1. A living organism that requires oxygen and organic foods, is incapable of photosynthesis, has limited growth, and is capable of voluntary movement and sensation. 2. Any animal other than man. 3. Pert. to or from an animal. 4. A person who is beastlike.

a., cold-blooded. An animal whose body temperature varies according to the temperature of the environment. SYN: *allotherm; poikilotherm.*

a., warm-blooded. An animal whose body temperature remains constant regardless of the temperature of the environment. SYN: *homotherm.*

animalcule (ăn″ĭ-măl′kūl) [L. *animalculum,* little animal]. Any microscopic animal organism. A protozoan.

animation (ăn-ĭ-mā′shŭn) [L. *animus,* soul]. State of being alive or active.

a., suspended. Temporary cessation of vital functions with loss of consciousness; state of apparent death.

animatism (ăn′ĭ-mă-tĭzm). Belief that everything in nature, animate and inanimate, contains a spirit or soul.

animi agitatio (ăn′ĭ-mē ă-jĭ-tā′shē-ō) [″ + *agitare,* to turn over]. Mental agitation.

animism (ăn′ĭ-mĭzm). Attribution of spiritual qualities and mental capabilities to inanimate objects.

animus [L., breath, mind, soul]. 1. An animating or energizing motive or intention. 2. A feeling of bitter hostility; grudge. 3. According to Jung, the masculine inner personality present in women. SEE: *anima.*

anion (ăn′ī-ŏn) [Gr. *ana,* up, + *ion,* going]. An ion carrying a negative charge; it is attracted by, and travels to, the anode (positive pole). Opposite of cation. Examples are acid radicals and corresponding radicals of their salts. SEE: *ion; electrolyte.*

anion gap. A concept used to estimate electrolyte (anion and cation) levels in the serum and conditions that influence them. The anion gap ranges from 8 to 18 mEq. per liter in normal patients. This is estimated by subtracting the sum of the anions chloride and bicarbonate (Cl^- + HCO_3^-) from the sum of the cations sodium and potassium (Na^+ + K^+). Because the potassium cation is low in serum, the anion gap is calculated by the formula $Na^+ - (Cl^- + HCO_3^-)$.

anionic (ăn″ī-ŏn′ĭk). Containing or pert. to anions.

anionic detergent. A chemical substance with disinfectant properties due to the presan active, negatively charged chemical group. May be natural or synthetic.

aniridia (ăn″ĭ-rĭd′ē-ă) [Gr. *an-*, not, + *iris*, rainbow, iris]. Congenital absence of all or part of the iris. SYN: *irideremia*.

anisakiasis (ăn″ĭs-să-kī′ă-sĭs). Disease of human gastrointestinal tract accompanied by intestinal colic, fever, and abscesses, caused by eating uncooked fish containing larval nematodes of the family Anisakidae.

aniseikonia (ăn-ĭs-ī-kō′nē-ă) [Gr. *anisos*, unequal, + *eikon*, image]. A condition in which the size and shape of the ocular image of one eye differs from that of the other. SYN: *anisoiconia*.

anise oil. Volatile oil obtained from distillation of the dried ripe fruit of Pimpinella anisum, or star anise, Illicium verum. It is used as a flavoring substance.

aniso- (ăn-ī′sō) [Gr. *anisos*, unequal]. Prefix meaning unequal, asymmetrical, or dissimilar.

anisoaccommodation (ăn-ī″sō-ă-kŏm″mō-dā′shŭn) [″ + L. *accommodare*, to suit]. Difference in ability of the eyes to accommodate. SEE: *accommodation*.

anisochromatic (ăn-ī″sō-krō-măt′ĭk) [″ + *chroma*, color]. Not of uniform color.

anisocoria (ăn-ī″sō-kō′rē-ă) [″ + *kore*, pupil]. Inequality of the size of the pupils; may be congenital or associated with aneurysms, head trauma, diseases of the nervous system, brain lesion, paresis, or locomotor ataxia.

anisocytosis (ăn-ī″sō-sī-tō′sĭs) [″ + *kytos*, cell, + *osis*, condition]. Condition in which there is excessive inequality in size of cells, esp. erythrocytes.

anisogamy (ăn″ī-sŏg′ă-mē) [″ + *gamos*, marriage]. Sexual fusion of two gametes of different form and size.

anisognathous (ăn″ī-sŏg′nă-thŭs) [″ + *gnathos*, jaw]. Having an upper jaw wider than the lower one.

anisohypercytosis (ăn-ī″sō-hī″pĕr-sī-tō′sĭs) [″ + *hyper*, above, + *kytos*, cell, + *osis*, condition]. Increase in number of leukocytes with altered proportion of the different varieties. Opposite of anisohypocytosis.

anisohypocytosis (ăn-ī″sō-hī″pō-sī-tō′sĭs) [″ + *hypo*, below, + *kytos*, cell, + *osis*, condition]. Decrease in number of leukocytes with altered proportion of different varieties. Opposite of anisohypercytosis.

anisoiconia (ăn-ī″sō-ī-kō′nē-ă) [″ + *eikon*, image]. Condition in which ocular image in one eye is different in size and shape from that of other. SYN: *aniseikonia*.

anisokaryosis (ăn-ī″sō-kăr″ē-ŏ′sĭs) [″ + *karyon*, nucleus, + *osis*, condition]. Unequal size of the cell nuclei.

...mastia (ăn-ī-sō-măs′tē-ă) [″ + *mastos*, ...] ...ondition in which breasts are markedly unequal.

anisomelia (ăn-ī″sō-mē′lē-ă) [″ + *melos*, limb]. Condition in which paired limbs are noticeably unequal.

anisometrope (ăn-ī″sō-mĕt′rōp) [Gr. *anisos*, unequal, + *metron*, measure, + *ops*, vision]. One afflicted with anisometropia.

anisometropia (ăn-ī″sō-mĕ-trō′pē-ă). Condition in which refractive power of the eyes is unequal.

anisometropic (ăn-ī″sō-mĕ-trŏp′ĭk). Pert. to or characterized by anisometropia.

anisonormocytosis (ăn-ī″sō-nor″mō-sī-tō′sĭs) [″ + L. *norma*, rule, + Gr. *kytos*, cell, + *osis*, condition]. Condition in which the total number of leukocytes is normal but the proportion of different types is abnormal.

anisophoria (ăn″ī-sō-fō′rē-ă) [″ + *phoros*, bearing]. Eye muscle imbalance so that the horizontal visual plane of one eye is different from that of the other.

anisopia (ăn″ī-sō′pē-ă) [″ + *ops*, vision]. Condition in which the visual power of the eyes is unequal.

anisopiesis (ăn-ī″sō-pī-ē′sĭs) [″ + *piesis*, blood pressure]. Inequality of blood pressure in different parts of the body.

anisosthenic (ăn-ī″sŏs-thĕn′ĭk) [″ + *sthenos*, strength]. Of unequal strength, said of paired muscles.

anisotonic (ăn-ī″sō-tŏn′ĭk) [″ + *tonos*, tone]. Pert. to a solution not isotonic as compared with another.

anisotropal (ăn″ī-sŏt′rō-păl) [″ + *tropos*, a turning]. 1. Not equal in every direction. 2. Unequal in power of refraction. SYN: *anisotropous*.

anisotropic (ăn-ī″sō-trŏp′ĭk). Having different optical properties in different directions, as have certain crystals; double polarizing power.

anisotropous (ăn-ī-sŏt′rō-pŭs). 1. Not equal in every direction. 2. Unequal in refractive power. SYN: *anisotropal*.

ankle (ăng′kl) [AS. *ancleow*]. 1. The joint between the leg and foot; the articulation of the tibia, fibula, and talus. The ankle is a hinge joint. 2. In popular usage, the region of this joint, including the tarsus and lower end of leg. SEE: *foot* for illus.

ankle bone. The talus, q.v.

ankle clonus. Repetitive extension-flexion movement of muscles of ankle, associated with increased muscle tonus. Commonly a symptom of corticospinal disease.

NURSING IMPLICATIONS: Keep patient's foot at a right angle to the long axis of the body. This may be accomplished by using a foot splint, and when the patient is in bed, a foot board. If the splint is removed, avoid dorsiflexion of the foot to prevent movement of the ankle, clonus, or spasm. When the involved joint is moved, it should be moved slowly and evenly. Do not grasp the extremity, but rather support it by your palms. If the joint is exercised, it should be done when the joint is warm and relaxed.

a.c. reflex. Reflex elicited by quick, vigorous dorsiflexion of the foot while the knee is held in a flexed position, resulting in repeated clonic movement of the foot so long as the foot is maintained in dorsiflexion.

ankle jerk. Contraction of calf muscles resulting in extension of the foot following a blow upon the Achilles tendon.

ankle joint. The ankle, q.v.

ankylo- (ăng'kĭ-lō) [Gr. *ankylos*, crooked]. Prefix meaning crooked, bent, a fusion or growing together of parts.

ankyloblepharon (ăng"kĭ-lō-blĕf'ăr-ŏn) [" + *blepharon*, eyelid]. Adhesion of the edges of upper and lower eyelids. SYN: *blepharosynechia.*

ankylochilia (ăng"kĭ-lō-kī'lē-a) [" + *cheilos*, lip]. Adhesion of the upper and lower lips.

ankylocolpos (ăng-kĭ-lō-kŏl'pŏs) [" + *kolpos*, vagina]. Imperforation or atresia of the vagina.

ankylodactylia (ăng-kĭ-lō-dăk-tĭl'ē-a) [" + *daktylos*, finger]. Adhesion of two or more fingers or toes.

ankyloglossia (ăng"kĭ-lō-glŏs'sē-ă) [" + *glossa*, tongue]. Abnormal shortness of frenum of tongue. SYN: *tongue-tie.*

ankylopoietic (ăng"kĭ-lō-poy-ĕt'ĭk) [Gr. *ankyle*, stiff joint, + *poiein*, to form]. 1. Indicating the presence of ankylosis. 2. Causing ankylosis.

ankyloproctia (ăng"kĭ-lō-prŏk'shē-ă) [Gr. *ankylos*, crooked, + *proktos*, anus]. Stricture or imperforation of the anus.

ankylosed. Fixed; stiffened; held by adhesions; affected with ankylosis, q.v.

ankylosis (ăng"kĭ-lō'sĭs) [Gr. *ankyle*, stiff joint, + *osis*, condition]. Immobility and fixation of a joint.

ETIOL: May be congenital (sometimes hereditary), or it may be the result of disease, trauma, or surgery.

NURSING IMPLICATIONS: If ankylosis is surgically created, maintain immobilized joint until bone has healed (usually 6 to 12 weeks); maintain correct body alignment. If nonsurgical ankylosis, maintain the joint in a functional position, utilize splints for patients with spastic muscles, and initiate passive range of motion exercises to affected joints.

a., artificial. The surgical fixation of a joint.

a., bony. The abnormal union of the bones of a joint. SYN: *a., true.*

a., dental. A condition characterized by the loss of tooth movement due to the fusion of the root cementum with the adjacent alveolar bone.

a., extracapsular. Ankylosis caused by rigidity of parts outside a joint.

a., false. A., fibrous, q.v.

a., fibrous. Ankylosis due to the formation of fibrous bands within a joint. SYN: *a., false; a., ligamentous.*

a., intracapsular. Ankylosis due to undue rigidity of structure within a joint.

a., ligamentous. A., fibrous, q.v.

a., true. A., bony, q.v.

Ankylostoma (ăng"kĭ-lŏs'tō-mă). Ancylostoma, q.v.

ankylostoma (ăng"kĭ-lŏs'tō-mă). Tonic spasm of muscles of jaw. SYN: *trismus; lockjaw.* SEE: *tetanus.*

ankylostomiasis (ăng"kĭ-lō-stō-mī'ă-sĭs). Ancylostomiasis, q.v.

ankylotia (ăng"kĭ-lō'shē-ă) [Gr. *ankylos*, crooked, + *ot-*, ear]. Stricture or imperforation of external auditory meatus of ear.

ankylotome (ăng'kĭl-ō-tōm, ăng-kĭl'ō-tōm) [" + *tome*, incision]. An instrument for cutting the frenulum of the tongue in tongue-tie.

ankylurethria (ăng"kĭl-ū-rē'thrē-ă) [" + *ourethra*, urethra]. Stricture or imperforation of the urethra.

anlage (ŏn'lō-jhă) [Ger., a laying on]. The first accumulation of cells in an embryo that constitutes the beginning of a future tissue, organ, or part. SYN: *primordium.*

annatto (ă-nō'tō) [Cariban]. Yellowish-red coloring matter obtained from the pulp of Bixa orellana, a tropical tree. The seeds are used in cooking. Also spelled anatto, annotto, arnato.

annectent (ă-nĕk'tĕnt) [L. *annectens*, tying or binding to]. Linked; connected; joined.

Annelida (ă-nĕl'ĭ-dă). The phylum that includes earthworms, leeches, and other segmented worms. Some annelids serve as intermediate hosts for parasitic worms.

annexa (ă-nĕks'ă) [L. *annectere*, to tie or bind to]. Accessory parts of a structure. SYN: *adnexa.*

annexitis (ă-nĕks-ī'tĭs) [" + Gr. *itis*, inflammation]. Inflammation of adnexa uteri. SYN: *adnexitis.*

annexopexy (ă-nĕk'sō-pĕk-sē) [" + Gr. *pexis*, putting together]. Fixation of fallopian tubes and ovary to abdominal wall. SYN: *adnexopexy.*

annular (ăn'ū-lăr) [L. *annulus*, ring]. Circular; ring-shaped.

annulorrhaphy (an"ū-lor'ă-fē) [" + Gr. *rhaphe*, seam]. Closure of a hernia ring by suture.

annulus (ăn'ū-lŭs) [L.]. (pl. *annuli*) A ring-shaped structure; a ring. Also spelled anulus, q.v.

anococcygeal (ā"nō-kŏk-sĭ'jē-al) [L. *anus*, anus, + Gr. *kokkyx*, coccyx]. Rel. to anus and coccyx.

anococcygeal body. The muscle and fibrous tissue lying between the coccyx and anus.

anococcygeal ligament. A band of fibrous tissue joining the tip of the coccyx with the external sphincter ani.

anodal (ăn-ō′dăl) [Gr. *ana,* up, + *hodos,* way]. Pert. to the anode, q.v.

anodal closure contraction. ABBR: ACC. Contraction of muscles at anode on closure of circuit.

anode (ăn′ōd) [Gr. *ana,* up, + *hodos,* way]. The positive pole of an electrical source. SEE: *cathode.*

anodmia (ăn-ŏd′mē-ă) [Gr. *an-,* not, + *odme,* stench]. Loss of the sense of smell. SYN: *anosmia.*

anodontia (ăn″ō-dŏn′shē-ă) [″ + *odous,* tooth]. Absence of teeth. SYN: *edentia.*

anodyne (ăn′ō-dīn) [″ + *odyne,* pain]. A drug that relieves pain. SYN: *analgesic; antalgesic.*

anodynia (ăn″ō-dĭn′ē-ă). Cessation or absence of pain.

anoesia (ăn″ō-ē′zē-ă) [Gr. *anoesia,* want of understanding]. Lack of power of comprehension, as in severe mental retardation. SYN: *anoia.*

anoetic (ăn″ō-ĕt′ĭk) Pert. to or afflicted with anoesia.

anoia (ă-noy′ă) [Gr. *a-,* not, + *noos,* understanding]. Anoesia, q.v.

anomaloscope (ă-nŏm′ă-lō-skōp″) [Gr. *anomalos,* irregular, + *skopein,* to examine]. Device for detecting color blindness.

anomalous (ă-nŏm′ă-lŭs) [Gr. *anomalos,* uneven]. Irregular; deviating from or contrary to normal.

anomaly (ă-nŏm′ă-lē) [Gr. *anomalia,* irregularity]. Deviation from normal. SYN: *birth defect; congenital anomaly.*

a., congenital. Intrauterine development of an organ or structure that is abnormal with reference to form, structure, or position. SYN: *birth defect.*

anomia (a-nō′mē-ă) [Gr. *a-,* not, + *onoma,* name]. Inability to remember names of objects.

anomie (ăn′ŏ-mē). A term coined by the French sociologist Emile Durkheim (1858–1917) to indicate a condition similar to alienation. The individual feels there has been a disintegration of his or her norms and values. Durkheim felt such individuals were prone to take their lives because of the anxiety, isolation, and alienation that they experience.

anonychia (ăn-ō-nĭk′ē-ă) [Gr. *an-,* not, + *onyx,* nail]. Absence of the nails.

anoopsia (ăn″ō-ŏp′sē-ă) [Gr. *ano,* upward, + *opsis,* vision]. Tendency of one eye to turn [illegible]rd. SYN: *anophoria; hyperphoria.*

[illegible]l (ā″nō-pĕr-ĭ-nē′ăl). Rel. to both the anus and perineum.

Anopheles (ă-nŏf′ĕ-lēz) [Gr. *anopheles,* harmful, useless]. A genus of mosquitoes belonging to the family Culicidae, order Diptera. It is a vector of Plasmodium, the causative agent of malaria, and may be involved in the transmission of causative agent of dengue, filariasis, and possibly other diseases.

anophoria (ăn-ō-fō′rē-ă) [Gr. *ano,* upward, + *pherein,* to bear]. Tendency of one eye to turn upward. SYN: *anoopsia; hyperphoria.*

anophthalmia (ăn-ŏf-thăl′mē-ă) [Gr. *an-,* not, + *ophthalmos,* eye]. Congenital absence of one or both eyes.

anopia (an-ō′pē-ă) [″ + *ops,* eye]. 1. Anophthalmia. 2. Anophoria.

anoplasty (ā′nō-plăs″tē) [L. *anus,* anus, + Gr. *plassein,* to form]. Plastic surgery of the anus.

Anoplura (ăn-ō-ploo′ră) [Gr. *anoplos,* unarmed, + *oura,* tail]. An order of insects composed of the sucking lice. SEE: *louse; pediculosis.*

anopsia (ăn-ŏp′sē-ă) [″ + *opsis,* sight]. 1. Hyperphoria. 2. Inability to use the vision, as in those confined in the dark, or from disuse of an eye in strabismus, or resulting from cataract, or in refractive errors.

anorchidism (ăn-or′kĭ-dĭzm″). Anorchism.

anorchism (ăn-or′kĭzm) [″ + *orchis,* testicle, + *-ismos,* condition]. Congenital absence of one or both testes. SYN: *anorchidism.*

anorectal (ā-nō-rĕk′tăl). Pert. to both the anus and rectum.

anorectic, anorectous (ăn-ō-rĕk′tĭc, -tŭs) [Gr. *anorektos,* without appetite for]. Having no appetite.

anorexia (ăn-ō-rĕk′sē-ă) [Gr. *an-,* not, + *orexis,* appetite]. Loss of appetite. Seen in depression, malaise, commencement of fevers and illnesses, also in disorders of alimentary tract, esp. of stomach, and as a result of alcoholic excesses and drug addiction, esp. cocaine. Many medicines and medical procedures have the undesired side effect of causing malaise with concurrent anorexia.

RS: acoria; ageusia; bulimia; hyperorexia; nausea; parageusia; parorexia; pica; polyphagia; pyrosis; taste.

a. nervosa. Occurs most commonly in females between the ages of 12 and 21 but may occur in older women and men.

Diagnosis is made by the following criteria: Intense fear of becoming obese. This does not diminish as weight loss progresses. The patient claims to feel fat even when emaciated. There is a weight loss of 25% of original weight. There is a refusal to maintain body weight over a minimal normal weight for age and height. There is no known physical illness to account for the weight loss.

Psychiatric therapy in a hospital is usually required if patient refuses to eat. The patient may need to be fed parenterally. SEE: *bulimia.*

anorexigenic (ăn″ō-rĕk″sĭ-jĕn′ĭk) [″ + ″ + *gennan,* to produce]. Causing loss of appetite.

anorganic (ăn″or-găn′ĭk). Inorganic, q.v.

anorgasmy (ăn-or-găz′mē) [″ + *orgasmos,* swelling]. Failure of achievement of orgasm either during sexual intercourse or masturbation.

anorthography (ăn″or-thŏg′ră-fē) [″ + *orthos,* straight, + *graphein,* to write]. Agraphia, esp. motor agraphia; loss of power to express oneself in writing. SEE: *agraphia.*

anorthopia (ăn″or-thō′pē-ă) [″ + ″ + *ops,* eye]. 1. Vision in which straight lines do not appear straight; symmetry and parallelism not properly perceived. 2. Strabismus.

anorthosis (ăn″or-thō′sĭs) [″ + ″ + *osis,* condition]. Inability to achieve penile erection.

anoscope (ā′nō-skōp) [L. *anus,* anus, + Gr. *skopein,* to view]. Speculum for examining the anus and lower rectum.

anosigmoidoscopy (ā″nō-sĭg″moy-dŏs′kō-pē) [″ + Gr. *sigmoeides,* shaped like Greek "S," + *skopein,* to view]. Direct visual examination of the anus, rectum, and colon by use of an endoscope.

anosmatic (ăn-ŏz-măt′ĭk) [Gr. *an-,* not, + *osme,* smell]. Lacking the sense of smell.

anosmia (ăn-ŏz′mē-ă). Loss of the sense of smell. SYN: *anodmia.*

anosmic, anosmous (ăn-ŏz′mĭk, -mŭs). 1. Lacking the sense of smell. 2. Odorless.

anosognosia (ăn-ō-sŏg-nō′zē-ă) [″ + ″ + *gnosis,* knowledge]. Real or pretended ignorance of the presence of disease, esp. paralysis.

anosphrasia (ăn-ŏs-frā′zē-ă) [Gr. *an-,* not, + *osphresis,* smell]. Absence of or imperfect sense of smell.

anospinal (ā″nō-spī′năl) [L. *anus* + *spina,* thorn]. Pert. to the anus and spinal cord, or to the center in the spinal cord that controls the contraction of the anal sphincter.

anostosis (ăn-ŏs-tō′sĭs) [Gr. *an-,* not, + *osteon,* bone, + *osis,* condition]. A defective formation or development of bone; failure to ossify.

anotia (ăn-ō′shē-ă) [″ + *ous,* ear]. Congenital malformation with absence of the ears.

anotropia (ăn″ō-trō′pē-ă) [Gr. *ana,* up, + *trope,* a turning]. Tendency of the eyes to turn upward and away from the visual axis.

ANOVA. Term used in statistics for *an*alysis *o*f *va*riance. SEE: *analysis of variance.*

anovaginal (ā″nō-văj′ĭ-năl). Pert. to the anus and vagina.

anovarism (ăn-ō′văr-ĭzm) [Gr. *an-,* not, + L. *ovarium,* ovary, + Gr. *-ismos,* condition]. Absence of ovaries.

anovesical (ā″nō-vĕs′ĭ-kl) [L *anus,* anus, + *vesica,* bladder]. Rel. to both anus and urinary bladder.

anovular, anovulatory (ăn-ŏv′ū-lar, ăn-ŏv′ū-lă-tō″rē) [Gr. *an-,* not, + L. *ovarium,* ovary]. Not accompanied by production of and discharge of an ovum.

anovular cycle. Menstrual cycle wherein the menstrual flow was not preceded by ovulation.

anoxemia (ăn-ŏk-sē′mē-ă) [″ + *oxygen* + Gr. *haima,* blood]. Insufficient oxygenation of the blood. SEE: *hypoxemia; respiration.*

anoxia (ăn-ŏk′sē-ă) [″ + *oxygen*]. Without oxygen. Term is often used incorrectly to indicate hypoxia, q.v.

a., altitude. Anoxia due to insufficient oxygen content of inspired air at high altitudes.

a., anemic. Anoxia due to decrease in hemoglobin concentration or number of erythrocytes in the blood.

a., anoxic. Anoxia due to disordered pulmonary mechanisms of oxygenation. May be due to reduced oxygen supply, respiratory obstruction, reduced surface area in lungs for exchange of gases (as in pneumonia) or inadequate respiratory movements.

a., hypokinetic. A., stagnant, q.v.

a., stagnant. Anoxia due to insufficient peripheral circulation, as occurs in cardiac failure, shock, arterial spasm, and thrombosis.

anoxic (ăn-ŏks′ĭk). Pert. to or caused by a general lack of oxygen, and characterized by a generally subnormal oxygen tension of the blood.

ansa (ăn′să) [L., a handle]. (pl. *ansae*) [NA] In anatomy, any structure in the form of a loop or arc.

a. cervicalis. [NA] Formerly called ansa hypoglossi. A nerve loop in the neck formed by fibers from the first three cervical nerves.

a. hypoglossi. [NA] A. cervicalis, q.v.

a. lenticularis. [NA] Tortuous fiber tract from the globus pallidus, extending around the internal capsule, to the ventral thalamic nucleus.

a. nervorum spinalium. [NA] Connecting loops of nerve fibers between the anterior spinal nerves.

a. peduncularis. [NA] Complex fiber tract from the anterior temporal lobe, extending around the internal capsule, to the mediodorsal thalamic nucleus.

a. sacralis. Nerve loop connecting the sympathetic trunk with the coccygeal ganglion.

a. subclavia. [NA] Nerve loop that passes anterior and inferior to the subclavian artery, connecting the middle and inferior cervical sympathetic ganglia.

A.N.S.I. *American National Standards Institute.*

ansiform (ăn'sĭ-form) [L. *ansa,* a handle, + *forma,* shape]. Shaped like a loop.

ant- [Gr.]. Prefix denoting opposed to, counteracting, against.

Antabuse (ăn'tă-būs"). Proprietary name for disulfiram. Administered orally in treatment of alcoholism. Ingestion of alcohol following taking of drug causes severe reactions including nausea and vomiting and may endanger the life of the patient. SEE: *Poisons and Poisoning* in *Appendix.*

antacid (ănt-ăs'ĭd) [Gr. *anti,* against, + L. *acidum,* acid]. An agent that neutralizes acidity, esp. in digestive tract.

Ex.: aluminum hydroxide; magnesium oxide.

antagonism (ăn-tăg'ō-nĭzm") [Gr. *antagonizesthai,* to struggle against]. Mutual opposition or contrary action, as between muscles or medicines.

a., bacterial. The inhibition of one bacterial organism by another.

antagonist (ăn-tăg'ō-nĭst). That which counteracts the action of something else, as a muscle or drug. Opposite of synergist.

a., narcotic. A drug that prevents or reverses the action of a narcotic. SEE: *nalorphine.*

antalgesic (ănt-ăl-jē'sĭk) [Gr. *anti,* against, + *algos,* pain]. A drug that relieves pain. SYN: *analgesic; anodyne.*

antalgic (ănt-ăl'jĭk). Antalgesic, q.v.

antalkaline (ănt-ăl'kă-līn, -lĭn) [" + *alkaline*]. An agent that neutralizes alkalinity.

antaphrodisiac (ănt"ăf-rō-dĭz'ē-ăk) [" + *aphrodisiakos,* sexual]. An agent that depresses sexual desire. SYN: *anaphrodisiac.*

antarthritic (ănt"ăr-thrĭt'ĭk) [" + *arthritikos,* gouty]. Remedy for gout and arthritis.

antasthenic (ănt"ăs-thĕn'ĭk) [" + *astheneia,* weakness]. 1. Relieving weakness; strengthening, invigorating. 2. Agent that strengthens, relieves weakness.

antasthmatic (ănt"ăz-măt'ĭk) [" + Gr. *asthma,* panting]. 1. Preventing or relieving asthma. 2. An agent that prevents or relieves an asthma attack.

antatrophic (ănt"ă-trō'fĭk) [" + *atrophia,* atrophy]. Preventing or curing atrophy.

antazoline phosphate (ăn-tăz'ō-lēn). USP. An antihistamine used in dilute solution to treat allergic conjunctivitis. A component of the trade name preparation Vasocon-A.

ante- [L.]. Prefix meaning before.

antebrachium (ăn"tē-brā'kē-ŭm) [L. *ante,* before, + *brachium,* arm]. [NA] The forearm.

antecardium (ăn"tē-kăr'dē-ŭm) [" + Gr. *kardia,* heart]. The area on the anterior surface [of th]e body overlying the heart and the lower [part of t]he thorax. SYN: *precordia; precordium.*

antecedent (ăn"tē-sē'dĕnt) [L. *antecedere,* to precede]. Something that comes before something else, a precursor.

a., plasma thromboplastin. ABBR: PTA. Blood coagulation factor XI. SYN: *Christmas factor.* SEE: *coagulation factors.*

ante cibum (ăn'tē sē'bŭm) [L.]. ABBR: a.c. Used in prescription writing to indicate *before meals.*

antecubital (ăn"tē-kū'bĭ-tăl) [" + *cubitum,* elbow]. In front of the elbow; at the bend of the elbow.

antecubital fossa. Triangular area lying anterior to and below the elbow, bounded medially by the pronator teres and laterally by the brachioradialis muscles. SYN: *cubital fossa.*

antecurvature (ăn"tē-kŭr'vă-tūr") [" + *curvatura,* bend]. Bending forward abnormally. SYN: *anteflexion.*

antefebrile (an"tē-fē'brĭl, -fē'brīl, -fĕb'rĭl) [L. *ante,* before, + *febris,* fever]. Before the development of fever. SYN: *antepyretic.*

anteflect (ăn'tē-flĕkt) [" + *flectere,* to bend]. To bend or cause to bend forward.

anteflexion (ăn"tē-flĕk'shŭn). The abnormal bending forward of part of an organ, esp. of the uterus at its body and neck. SEE: *anteversion.*

antegrade (ăn'tē-grād). Moving forward or in the same direction as the flow.

antelocation (ăn"tē-lō-kā'shŭn) [" + *locare,* to place]. Forward displacement of an organ.

antemetic (ănt"ē-mĕt'ĭk) [Gr. *anti,* against, + *emetikos,* emetic]. 1. Preventing or arresting nausea and vomiting. 2. Agent that prevents or arrests nausea and vomiting. SYN: *antiemetic.*

ante mortem (ăn'tē mor'tĕm) [L.]. Before death.

ante mortem statement. Declaration of the individual made immediately preceding death. SYN: *deathbed statement,* q.v.

antenatal (ăn"tē-nā'tăl) [" + *natus,* born]. Occurring before birth. SYN: *prenatal.*

antenatal diagnosis. Diagnostic procedures done to determine the health status of the fetus. Methods used include amniocentesis and study of the material thus obtained by microscopic examination (sex chromatin determination), cell culture, and biochemical methods; amnioscopy; amniography; and ultrasound.

antenatal surgery. Surgical procedure done on the fetus prior to delivery. This rapidly developing technique is used to ameliorate a great number of conditions. SEE: *amnioscopy; embryoscopy.*

Antepar. Trade name for piperazine citrate, USP, q.v.

antepartal; ante partum (ăn'tē păr'tăl,

-tŭm) [L.]. Before the onset of labor, used with reference to the mother.

antephialtic (ăn″tē-fē-ăl′tĭk) [Gr. *anti,* against, + *ephialtes,* nightmare]. Preventing nightmares.

antepyretic (ăn″tē-pī-rĕt′ik) [L. *ante,* before, + Gr. *pyretos,* fever]. Before the development of fever. SYN: *antefebrile.*

anterior [L.]. Before or in front of.

anterior chamber. Aqueous chamber of eye. Bounded in front by cornea, behind by iris and lens. SEE: *eye.*

anterior drawer sign. With the knee flexed to a right angle, there is increased anterior glide of the tibia in anterior cruciate ligament rupture. SEE: *posterior drawer sign.*

anterior horn cell. A large nerve cell in the anterior horn of the spinal cord. The axon of the cell is an efferent fiber innervating a muscle.

antero- [L.]. Prefix denoting anterior, front, before.

anteroexternal (ăn″tĕr-ō-ĕks-tĕr′năl) [L. *antero,* anterior, + *externus,* outside]. In anatomy, located to the front and laterally.

anterograde [″ + *gradior,* to step]. Moving frontward.

anteroinferior [″ + *inferior,* below]. In front and below.

anterointernal (ăn″tĕr-ō-ĭn-tĕr′năl) [″ + *internus,* within]. In anatomy, located to the front and to the inner side.

anterolateral [″ + *latus,* side]. In front and to one side.

anteromedian [″ + *medius,* middle]. In front and toward the center.

anteroposterior [″ + *posterior,* rear]. Passing from front to rear.

anterosuperior [″ + *superior,* above]. In front and above.

anteversion (ăn″tē-vĕr′zhŭn) [″ + *vertere,* to turn]. A tipping forward of an organ as a whole, without bending. SEE: *anteflexion.*

anteverted (an″tē-vĕrt′ĕd). Tipped forward.

anthelix (ănt′hē-lĭks, ăn′thē-lĭks) [Gr. *anti,* against, + *helix,* coil]. Curved prominence of the external ear parallel to and in front of the helix. SYN: *antihelix.*

anthelmintic, anthelminthic, antihelmintic (ănt″hĕl-mĭn′tĭk, -thĭk, ăn″tī-hĕl-mĭn′tĭk) [″ + *helmins,* worm]. An agent that destroys parasitic intestinal worms.

anthelone (ănt-hē′lōn). Urogastrone, q.v.

Anthemis (ăn′thĕm-ĭs). 1. A genus of aromatic flowering plants. 2. Camomile; chamomile; dried blossoms of Anthemis nobilis. A bitter tonic; an antispasmodic.

anthemorrhagic (ănt″hĕm-ō-răj′ĭk) [″ + *haima,* blood, + *rhegnynai,* to discharge]. Agent for preventing or arresting hemorrhage. SYN: *antihemorrhagic.*

anthocyanin (ăn″thō-sī′ă-nĭn) [Gr. *anthos,* flower, + *kyanos,* a blue substance]. Any one of a group of reddish-purple pigments occurring in flowers.

anthocyaninemia (ăn″thō-sī″ă-nĭn-ē′mē-ă) [″ + ″ + *haima,* blood]. Anthocyanin in the blood.

anthocyaninuria (ăn″thō-sī″ă-nĭn-ū′rē-ă) [″ + ″ + *ouron,* urine]. Anthocyanin in urine.

Anthomyia (ăn″thō-mī′yă) [″ + *myia,* fly]. A genus of fly of the order Diptera, related to the housefly. Larvae sometimes infest man.

A. canalicularis. A small black horsefly, whose larvae may infest the human intestine after accidental ingestion, often resulting in gastrointestinal disturbances.

anthophobia (ăn″thō-fō′bē-ă) [″ + *phobos,* fear]. Morbid dislike or fear of flowers.

anthracemia (ăn″thră-sē′mē-ă) [Gr. *anthrax,* coal, + *haima,* blood]. Presence of Bacillus anthracis in the blood.

anthracene (ăn′thră-sēn). A hydrocarbon, $C_{14}H_{10}$, obtained from distilling coal tar. Used in manufacturing dyes.

anthracia (an-thră′sē-ă) [Gr. *anthrax,* coal, carbuncle]. Presence of carbuncles.

anthracoid (ăn′thră-koyd) [″ + *eidos,* form]. Resembling or pert. to anthrax.

anthracometer (ăn″thră-kŏm′ĕ-ter) [″ + *metron,* measure]. An instrument for measuring the amount of carbon dioxide in the air.

anthraconecrosis (ăn″thră-kō-nĕ-krō′sĭs) [″ + *nekrosis,* deadness]. Gangrene in which tissue becomes dry and black.

anthracosilicosis (ăn″thră-kō-sĭl″ĭ-kō′sĭs) [″ + L. *silex,* flint, + Gr. *osis,* condition]. A form of pneumoconiosis in which carbon and silica deposits accumulate in the lungs due to breathing coal dust. SYN: *coal worker's pneumoconiosis.* SEE: *anthracosis; silicosis.*

anthracosis (ăn-thră-kō′sĭs) [″ + *osis,* condition]. Accumulation of carbon deposits in the lungs due to breathing smoke or coal dust. SYN: *black lung.*

Anthra-Derm. Trade name for anthralin, USP, q.v.

anthralin (ăn′thră-lĭn). USP. A synthetic hydrocarbon used in ointment form for treating various skin diseases including fungal infections and eczema. Trade names are Anthra-Derm and Drithocreme.

anthrax (ăn′thrăks) [Gr., coal, carbuncle]. Acute, infectious disease caused by Bacillus anthracis, usually attacking cattle, sheep, horses, and goats. Man contracts it from contact with animal hair, hides, or waste.

ETIOL: B. anthracis. Workers who handle wools, hides, and brushes are commonly affected.

SYM: Disease may attack lungs (woolsorter's disease) or the loose connective tissue, giving rise to malignant edema, necrosis of mediastinal lymph nodes and pleural sion. This is followed by respiratory distress, cyanosis, shock and coma. More commonly anthrax occurs in form of a pustule called anthrax boil or malignant pustule. This cutaneous form will exhibit redness, vesiculation and induration with central ulceration, and development of a black eschar. Rarely, the disease may occur in intestinal tract. If untreated, anthrax may be fatal.

TREATMENT: Penicillin or tetracyclines.

NURSING IMPLICATIONS: The patient should bathe daily, and receive skin care, frequent oral hygiene, and nasal care as needed. Increase fluid intake while patient is febrile, and give tepid sponge baths as needed to control hyperthermia. Encourage the patient to eat as much as can be tolerated. Maintain medical asepsis and closely observe the individual hospital policy concerning isolation.

anthropo- [Gr. *anthropos,* man]. Prefix denoting relationship to man or human life.

anthropobiology (ăn″thrō-pō-bī-ŏl′ō-jē) [″ + *bios,* life, + *logos,* study]. Study of the biology of man and the great apes.

anthropogeny (ăn″thrō-pŏj′ĕ-nē) [″ + *gennan,* to produce]. Origin and development of man.

anthropoid (ăn′thrō-poyd) [″ + *eidos,* form]. 1. Resembling man. 2. An ape.

anthropological base line. An imaginary line that passes from the lower border of the orbit to the superior margin of the external auditory meatus.

anthropology (ăn″thrō-pŏl′ō-jē) [″ + *logos,* study]. The study of man. Major divisions of the science are: physical anthropology, cultural anthropology, linguistics, and archaeology.

anthropometer (ăn″thrō-pŏm′ĕ-tĕr) [″ + *metron,* measure]. Device for measuring the human body and its parts.

anthropometry (ăn-thrō-pŏm′ĕt-rē). Science of measuring the human body. Includes craniometry, osteometry, skin fold evaluation for subcutaneous fat estimation, height and weight measurements. Usually performed by an anthropologist.

anthropomorphism (ăn″thrō-pō-mor′fĭzm) [″ + *morphe,* form, + *-ismos,* condition]. Attributing human qualities to nonhuman organisms or objects.

anthropopathy (ăn″thrō-pŏp′ă-thē) [″ + *pathos,* suffering]. Attributing human feelings to nonhumans.

anthropophagy (ăn″thrō-pŏf′ă-jē) [″ + *phagein,* to eat]. The eating of human flesh; cannibalism.

anthropophilic (ăn″thrō-pō-fĭl′ĭk) [″ + *phil-* [illegible]*in,* to love]. Preferring man, said of para- [illegible] that prefer a human host rather than [illegible]als. SYN: *androphilic.*

anthropozoonoses (ăn″thrō-pō-zō″ō-nō′sēs) [″ + *zoon,* animal, + *nosis,* disease]. Infectious diseases acquired by man from vertebrate hosts of the causative agents. Included are rabies and trichinosis.

anthysteric (ănt″hĭs-tĕr′ĭk) [Gr. *anti,* against, + *hystera,* womb]. 1. Preventing or relieving hysteria. 2. Agent that relieves hysteria. SYN: *antihysteric.*

anti- [Gr.]. Prefix meaning against.

antiadrenergic (ăn″tē-ă-drĕn-ĕr′jĭk) [Gr. *anti,* against, + L. *ad,* to, + *ren,* kidney, + Gr. *ergon,* work]. Preventing or counteracting adrenergic action.

antiagglutinin (ăn″tē-ă-gloo′tĭ-nĭn). A specific antibody opposing the action of an agglutinin.

antiamebic (ăn″tē-ă-mē′bĭk) [″ + *amoibe,* change]. A medicine used to prevent or treat amebiasis.

antiamylase (ăn″tē-ăm′ĭ-lās). Substance that opposes the action of amylase.

antianaphylaxis (ăn″tē-ăn-ă-fĭ-lăks′ĭs) [″ + *ana,* away from, + *phylaxis,* protection]. Prevention of anaphylaxis. Usually attained by administering repeated doses of the sensitizing substance too small to cause an anaphylactic reaction. SYN: *ananaphylaxis; desensitization.*

antiandrogen (ăn″tē-ăn′drō-jĕn) [″ + *androgen*]. Substance that acts to inhibit or prevent the action of androgen.

antianemic (ăn″tē-ă-nē′mĭk). Preventing or curing anemia.

antiantibody (ăn″tē-ăn′tĭ-bŏd-ē) [″ + *antibody*]. An antibody specific for, and produced in response to the administration of, another antibody.

antiantitoxin (ăn″tē-ăn″tĭ-tŏk′sin) [″ + *antitoxin*]. An antibody, produced in response to the administration of an antitoxin, that counteracts the effect of the antitoxin.

antiapoplectic (ăn″tē-ăp″ō-plĕk′tĭk). Preventing or relieving apoplexy.

antiarrhythmic (ăn″tē-ă-rĭth′mĭk) [″ + *a-,* not, + *rhythmos,* rhythm]. A drug or physical force that acts to control or prevent cardiac arrhythmias.

antiarthritic (ăn″tē-ăr-thrĭt′ĭk) [″ + *arthritikos,* gouty]. Relieving arthritis.

antibacterial (ăn″tĭ-băk-tē′rē-ăl). Destroying or stopping the growth of bacteria.

antibiosis (an″tĭ-bī-ō′sĭs) [″ + *bios,* life]. The association or relationship between two organisms wherein one is harmful to the other.

antibiotic (ăn″tĭ-bī-ŏt′ĭk). 1. Destructive to life. 2. Pert. to antibiosis. 3. Any of a variety of natural or synthetic substances that inhibit growth of or destroy microorganisms. Used extensively in treatment of infectious diseases in plants, animals, and man. SEE: *antimicrobial drugs* for table.

a., bacteriocidal or bactericidal. Antibiotic that kills microorganisms.

a., bacteriostatic. Antibiotic that inhibits growth of microorganisms.

a., broad-spectrum. Antibiotic that is effective against a wide variety of microorganisms.

antibody (ăn'tĭ-bŏd"ē). A protein substance developed in response to, and interacting specifically with, an antigen. This antigen-antibody reaction forms the basis of immunity, q.v. All antibodies belong to a special group of serum proteins, the immunoglobulins. Antibodies may be present due to previous infection, vaccination, transfer from mother to fetus in utero, or may occur without known antigenic stimulus, usually as a result of unknown, accidental exposure. In addition, the body may contain antibodies that react specifically with antigens for which there is no known history of exposure. These are termed natural antibodies. SEE: *antigen.*

a., blocking. An antibody that combines with an antigen and specifically blocks its ability to produce sensitizing reactions.

a., cross-reacting. An antibody that reacts with antigens functionally similar to its specific antigen.

a., fluorescent. An antibody reaction made visible by incorporating a fluorescent dye into the antigen-antibody reaction and examining the specimen with a microscope equipped for fluorescent microscopy.

a., maternal. An antibody produced by the mother and transferred to the fetus in utero.

a., monoclonal. SEE: *monoclonal antibodies; hybridoma.*

a., natural. An antibody present in a person without known exposure to the specific antigen, such as an anti-A antibody in a person with B blood type; may be the result of unknown, accidental exposure.

antibody-coated bacteria. Presence of antibody-coated bacteria in the urine is thought to occur in the urine only when tissue invasion has occurred. Such invasion elicits an antibody response. The antibodies are detected by use of fluorescent antibody studies. This test is used in attempting to localize the site of urinary tract infection.

antibrachium (ăn"tĭ-brā'kē-ŭm). Antebrachium; the forearm.

antibromic (ăn"tĭ-brō'mĭk) [Gr. *anti,* against, + *bromos,* smell]. 1. Deodorizing. 2. A deodorant.

anticardium (ăn"tĭ-kăr'dē-ŭm). Antecardium; the area on the anterior surface of the body overlying the heart and the lower part of the thorax. SYN: *precordia; precordium.*

anticarious (ăn"tĭ-kā'rē-ŭs) [" + *caries,* decay]. Preventing decay of teeth.

anticatarrhal (ăn"tĭ-kă-tăr'ăl) [" + L. *catarrhus,* catarrhal]. Relieving catarrh.

anticathode (ăn-tĭ-kăth'ōd) [" + *kata,* down, + *hodos,* way]. Portion of vacuum tube opposite the cathode. SYN: *target* (def. 2).

anticheirotonus (ăn"tĭ-kī-rŏt'ō-nŭs) [Gr. *anticheir,* thumb, + *tonos,* tension]. Spasmodic bending inward of thumb.

anticholagogue (ăn"tĭ-kŏl'ă-gŏg) [Gr. *anti,* against, + *chole,* bile, + *agein,* to lead forth]. Medicine used to decrease secretion of bile.

anticholinesterase (ăn"tĭ-kō-lĭn-ĕs'tĕr-ās). Substance that opposes the action of cholinesterase.

anticholinergic (ăn"tĭ-kō"lĭn-ĕr'jĭk). 1. Impeding the impulses of cholinergic, esp. parasympathetic, nerve fibers. 2. An agent that blocks parasympathetic nerve impulses. SYN: *parasympatholytic.*

anticipate (ăn-tĭs'ĭ-pāt) [L. *ante,* before, + *capere,* to take]. 1. To occur prior to the usual time of onset of a particular illness or disease, said of an event, sign, or symptom. 2. In nursing and medicine, to plan in order to be prepared for other than the routine or fully expected.

anticipatory guidance. Information concerning normal expectations of age group or disease entity in order to provide support for coping with problems before they actually arise.

anticlinal (ăn"tĭ-klī'năl) [Gr. *anti,* against, + *klinein,* to incline]. Inclined in opposite directions.

anticoagulant (ăn"tĭ-kō-ăg'ū-lănt) [" + L. *coagulans,* forming clots]. 1. Delaying or preventing blood coagulation. 2. An agent that prevents or delays blood coagulation.

a. citrate dextrose solution. USP. An anticoagulant used for storing whole blood.

a. citrate phosphate dextrose solution. USP. An anticoagulant used for storing whole blood.

a. heparin solution. USP. An anticoagulant used for storing whole blood.

a. sodium citrate solution. USP. An anticoagulant used for storing whole blood.

anticodon (ăn"tĭ-kō'dŏn). A triple arrangement of bases on transfer ribonucleic acid (tRNA) that complements the corresponding triplet on messenger ribonucleic acid (mRNA).

anticomplement (ăn"tĭ-kŏm'plĕ-mĕnt). Substance that counteracts a complement.

anticonvulsant (ăn"tĭ-kŏn-vŭl'sănt) [" + L. *convulsio,* pulling together]. 1. Preventing or relieving convulsions. 2. Agent that prevents or relieves convulsions.

anticus (ăn-tī'kŭs) [L., foremost]. Anterior. That part nearest the ventral or front surface.

anticytolysin (ăn"tĭ-sī-tŏl'ĭ-sĭn) [Gr. *anti,* against, + *kytos,* cell, + *lysis,* diss-

Substance that opposes the action of cytolysin.

anticytotoxin (ăn″tĭ-sī″tō-tŏks′ĭn) [″ + ″ + *toxikon,* poison]. A specific antibody that opposes the action of cytotoxin.

antidepressant (ăn″tĭ-dē-prĕs′sănt). Anything, medicine or other mode of therapy, that acts to prevent, cure, or alleviate mental depression.

antidiabetic (ăn″tĭ-dī″ă-bĕt′ĭk). 1. Preventing or relieving diabetes. 2. Agent that prevents or relieves diabetes.

antidiarrheal (ăn″tĭ-dī-ă-rē′ăl). Substance used to prevent or treat diarrhea.

antidinic (ăn″tĭ-dĭn′ĭk) [″ + *dinos,* dizziness]. 1. Relieving vertigo. 2. Agent that prevents or relieves vertigo.

antidiuretic (ăn″tĭ-dī-ū-rĕt′ĭk) [″ + *dia,* intensive, + *ouresis,* urination]. 1. Lessening urine secretion. 2. A drug that decreases urine secretion.

antidiuretic hormone. ABBR: ADH. Vasopressin, q.v.

antidotal (ăn″tĭ-dō′tăl). Acting as or pert. to an antidote.

antidote (ăn′tĭ-dōt) [Gr. *antidoton,* given against]. A substance that neutralizes poisons or their effects.

a., chemical. Antidote that reacts with the poison to produce a harmless chemical compound. For example, table salt precipitates silver nitrate and forms silver chloride. Chemical antidotes should be used sparingly and after their use the stomach contents should be removed by gastric lavage because they may produce serious results if allowed to remain in the stomach.

a., mechanical. Antidote that prevents absorption of the poison. Includes fats, oils, milk (casein coagulum), whites of eggs, finely divided charcoal, fuller's earth, or mineral oil. (Fats and oils are not to be used in treating phosphorus, camphor, aspidium, and cantharides poisonings.)

a., physiologic. Antidote that produces physiological effects opposite to the effects of the poison, e.g., sedatives are given for convulsants and stimulants are given for hypnotics. These should not be given without physician's definite instructions.

a., universal. Antidote that is given orally and is effective against a great number of toxic substances. There is, of course, no truly "universal antidote."

Two parts activated charcoal, one part tannic acid, and one part magnesium oxide. (The charcoal absorbs; the tannic acid precipitates metals, alkaloids, and some glucosides; and the magnesium oxide neutralizes acids.) [illegible] orally by dissolving 5 tsp. (approx. 25 [illegible] mixture in 4 oz. (120 ml.) of warm [illegible] the patient has swallowed the antidote, the stomach contents should then be removed by gastric lavage within a few minutes. Treatment may be repeated.

CAUTION: Do not use gastric lavage in patients who have ingested caustics. The stomach or esophagus may be ruptured by introduction of the tube.

antidromic (ăn″tĭ-drŏm′ĭk) [Gr. *anti,* against, + *dromos,* running]. Denoting nerve impulses traveling in the opposite direction from normal.

antidysenteric (ăn″tĭ-dĭs″ĕn-tĕr′ĭk). 1. Preventing or relieving dysentery. 2. Agent that prevents or relieves dysentery.

antidysuric (ăn″tĭ-dĭs-ū′rĭk) [″ + *dys,* painful, + *ouron,* urine]. 1. Preventing or relieving dysuria. 2. Agent that prevents or relieves dysuria.

antiemetic (ăn″tĭ-ē-mĕt′ĭk) [″ + *emetikos,* inclined to vomit]. 1. Preventing or relieving nausea and vomiting. 2. Agent that prevents or relieves nausea and vomiting.

antienzyme (ăn″tĭ-ĕn′zīm). Substance that opposes the action of an enzyme.

antiepileptic (ăn″tĭ-ĕp″ĭ-lĕp′tĭk). 1. Opposing epilepsy. 2. A medicine, procedure, or diet that combats epilepsy.

antiestrogen (ăn″tĭ-ĕs′trō-jĕn). Substance that blocks or modifies the action of estrogen.

antifebrile (ăn″tĭ-fē′brĭl, -fē′brĭl, -fĕb′rĭl) [″ + L. *febris,* fever]. 1. Reducing fever. 2. Agent that reduces fever. SYN: *antipyretic.*

antifermentative (ăn″tĭ-fĕr-mĕn′tă-tĭv). 1. Preventing or inhibiting fermentation. 2. Agent that prevents or inhibits fermentation.

antifibrinolysin (ăn″tĭ-fī″brĭ-nŏl′ĭ-sĭn) [″ + L. *fibra,* fiber, + Gr. *lysis,* dissolution]. Substance that counteracts fibrinolysis.

antifungal (ăn″tĭ-fŭng′găl). 1. Destroying or inhibiting the growth of fungi. 2. Agent that destroys or inhibits the growth of fungi.

antigalactagogue (ăn″tĭ-gă-lăk′tă-gŏg) [Gr. *anti,* against, + *gala,* milk, + *agogos,* drawing forth]. Agent that prevents or decreases the secretion of milk.

antigalactic (ăn″tĭ-gă-lăk′tĭk). 1. Preventing or diminishing the secretion of milk. 2. Agent that prevents or diminishes the secretion of milk. SYN: *antigalactagogue.*

antigen (ăn′tĭ-jĕn) [Gr. *anti,* against, + *gennan,* to produce]. A substance that induces the formation of antibodies that interact specifically with it. This antigen-antibody reaction forms the basis for immunity, q.v. An antigen may be introduced into the body or it may be formed within the body. Ex.: bacteria, toxins, foreign blood cells. SEE: *antibody.*

a.'s, histocompatibility. SEE: *histocompatibility antigens.*

a., H-Y. A histocompatibility antigen located on the cell membrane. It has a primary role in determining the sexual differentiation of the male embryo.

antigen-antibody reaction. The combination of an antigen with its specific antibody. May result in agglutination, precipitation, neutralization, complement-fixation, or increased susceptibility to phagocytosis. The antigen-antibody reaction forms the basis for immunity, q.v.

antigenic (ăn-tĭ-jĕn′ĭk). Capable of causing the production of an antibody.

antigenotherapy (ăn″tĭ-jĕn″ō-thĕr′ă-pē). Use of an antigen to stimulate antibody production in the treatment of a disease.

antiglobulin (ăn″tĭ-glŏb′ū-lĭn). Substance that opposes the action of globulin.

antigoitrogenic (ăn″tĭ-goy″trō-jĕn′ĭk) [″ + L. *guttur,* throat, + Gr. *gennan,* to produce]. Preventing the formation of a goiter.

antigonorrheic (ăn″tĭ-gŏn″ō-rē′ĭk). 1. Curing gonorrhea. 2. An agent that cures gonorrhea.

anti-G suit [″ + *G,* gravity]. Garment designed to produce uniform pressure on the lower extremities and abdomen. Normally the suit is used by aviators to help prevent pooling of blood in the lower half of the body during certain flight maneuvers. The garment has also been used in treating certain forms of internal bleeding and for severe forms of postural hypotension.

antihelix (ăn″tĭ-hē′lĭks) [″ + Gr. *helix,* coil]. Inner curved ridge of the external ear parallel to the helix.

antihemolysin (ăn″tĭ-hē-mŏl′ĭ-sĭn). A substance that opposes the action of hemolysin.

antihemophilic factor. USP. ABBR: AHF. Blood coagulation factor VIII. Trade names are Antihemophilic Globulin, Hemofil, Factorate, and Profilate. SEE: *coagulation factors.*

Antihemophilic Globulin (AHG). Trade name for antihemophilic factor (AHF), USP, q.v.

antihemorrhagic (ăn″tĭ-hĕm-ō-răj′ĭk). 1. Preventing or arresting hemorrhage. 2. Agent that prevents or arrests hemorrhage.

antihidrotic (ăn″tĭ-hī-drŏt′ĭk) [″ + *hidrotikos,* sweating]. 1. Preventing or decreasing perspiration. 2. Agent that prevents or decreases perspiration. SYN: *anhidrotic; antiperspirant; antisudorific.*

antihistamine (ăn″tĭ-hĭs′tă-mĕn, -mĭn). Drug that opposes the action of histamine.

antihistaminic (ăn″tĭ-hĭs″tă-mĭn′ĭk). 1. Opposing the action of histamine. 2. Agent that opposes the action of histamine.

antihistaminic poisoning. SEE: *Poisons and Poisoning* in *Appendix.*

antihormone (ăn″tĭ-hor′mōn). Substance that opposes the action of a hormone.

antihydropic (ăn″tĭ-hī-drŏp′ĭk) [Gr. *anti,* against, + *hydropikos,* dropsical]. 1. Relieving generalized edema. 2. Agent that relieves generalized edema.

antihypercholesterolemic (ăn″tĭ-hī″pĕr-kō-lĕs″tĕr-ŏl-ē′mĭk) [″ + *hyper,* above, + *chole,* bile, + *stereos,* solid, + *haima,* blood]. 1. Preventing or controlling elevation of the serum cholesterol level. 2. An agent that prevents or controls elevation of the serum cholesterol level.

antihypertensive (ăn″tĭ-hī′pĕr-tĕn′sĭv) [″ + ″ + L. *tensio,* tension]. 1. Preventing or controlling high blood pressure. 2. An agent that prevents or controls high blood pressure.

antihypnotic (ăn″tĭ-hĭp-nŏt′ĭk). 1. Preventing or inhibiting sleep. 2. Agent that prevents or inhibits sleep.

antihysteric (ăn″tĭ-hĭs-tĕr′ĭk). 1. Preventing or relieving hysteria. 2. Agent that prevents or relieves hysteria.

anti-icteric (ăn″tĭ-ĭk-tĕr′ĭk) [″ + *ikteros,* jaundice]. 1. Preventing or relieving jaundice. 2. Agent that prevents or relieves jaundice.

anti-immune (ăn″tĭ-ĭ-mūn′). Preventing immunity.

anti-infectious (ăn″tĭ-ĭn-fĕk′shŭs). Counteracting infection.

anti-inflammatory (ăn″tĭ-ĭn-flăm′ă-tō-rē). 1. Counteracting inflammation. 2. Agent that counteracts inflammation

anti-isolysin (ăn″tĭ-ī-sŏl′ĭ-sĭn). Substance that opposes the action of an isolysin.

antiketogenesis (ăn″tĭ-kē-tō-jĕn′ĕ-sĭs) [″ + *ketone* + Gr. *gennan,* to produce]. The prevention or inhibition of formation of ketone bodies. During starvation, diabetes, and certain other conditions, the metabolism of the ketone bodies, β-hydroxybutyric acid, acetoacetate, and acetone is decreased; thus they accumulate in the blood. Providing increased carbohydrates in the diet or intravenously will help to prevent or treat this. Carbohydrates are therefore antiketogenic. In ketonemia due to diabetes, both insulin and carbohydrates are required in order to permit the metabolism of carbohydrate to proceed at a rate that would control ketone formation.

antiketogenetic, antiketogenic (ăn″tĭ-kē″tō-jĕ-nĕt′ĭk, -jĕn′ĭk). Pert. to antiketogenesis.

antilactase (ăn″tĭ-lăk′tās) [″ + *lac,* milk, + *-ase,* enzyme]. A substance that opposes the action of lactase.

antilepsis (ăn″tĭ-lĕp′sĭs) [″ + *lepsis,* a receiving in return]. 1. Application of a remedy to a healthy part; treatment by removing something such as a body fluid, or shifting blood from the site of pathology to a healthy part of the body (revulsion), or in counterirritation. 2. Support, as of a bandage.

antileptic (ăn″tĭ-lĕp′tĭk) [Gr. *antileptikos,* able to check]. Pert. to antilepsis.

antilethargic (ăn″tĭ-lĕ-thăr′jĭk) [Gr. *anti,* against, + *lethargia,* drowsiness]. 1. Counteracting lethargy. 2. Agent that counteract lethargy.

antilipemic (ăn″tĭ-lĭ-pē′mĭk). 1. Preventing or counteracting the accumulation of fatty substances in the blood. 2. Agent that prevents or counteracts the accumulation of fatty substances in the blood.

Antilirium. Trade name for physostigmine salicylate, USP, q.v.

antilithic (ăn″tĭ-lĭth′ĭk) [″ + *lithos,* stone]. 1. Preventing or relieving calculi. 2. Agent that prevents or relieves calculi.

antilobium (ăn″tĭ-lō′bē-ŭm) [L. *ante,* before, + Gr. *lobos,* ear lobe]. Cartilaginous projection in front of the exterior meatus of the ear. SYN: *tragus.*

antiluetic (ăn″tĭ-loo-ĕt′ĭk) [Gr. *anti,* against, + L. *lues,* pestilence]. 1. Curing or relieving syphilis. 2. Agent that cures or relieves syphilis. SYN: *antisyphilitic.*

antilymphocytic serum (ăn″tĭ-lĭm″fō-sĭt′ĭk). ABBR: ALS. Serum used to reduce host rejection response to transplanted tissues. Produced by inoculating animals with certain tissues from other species.

antilysin (ăn-tĭ-lī′sĭn). Antibody that opposes the action of lysin.

antilysis (ăn-tĭl′ĭ-sĭs) [″ + *lysis,* dissolution]. Prevention or inhibition of lysis due to the action of antilysin.

antilyssic (ăn-tĭ-lĭs′ĭk) [″ + *lyssa,* frenzy]. Preventing or curing rabies. SYN: *antirabic.*

antilytic (ăn-tĭ-lĭt′ĭk). Pert. to antilysis.

antimalarial (ăn″tĭ-mă-lā′rē-ăl). 1. Preventing or relieving malaria. 2. Agent that prevents or relieves malaria. SYN: *antipaludian.*

antimere (ăn′tĭ-mēr) [″ + *meros,* a part]. One of corresponding parts of the body on opposite sides of the long axis.

antimetabolite (ăn″tĭ-mĕ-tăb′ō-līt). A substance, structurally similar to a metabolite, that opposes the action of or replaces a metabolite. It is believed that certain antibiotics are effective because they act as antimetabolites.

antimetropia (ăn″tĭ-mĕ-trō′pē-ă) [″ + *metron,* measure, + *ops,* eye]. An ocular disorder in which each eye has a different error of refraction.

Ex.: one eye may be hyperopic; the other, myopic.

antimicrobial (ăn″tĭ-mī-krō′bē-ăl). 1. Destructive to or preventing the development of microorganisms. 2. Agent that destroys or prevents the development of microorganisms.

antimicrobial drugs. Chemical substances that either kill microorganisms or prevent their growth. SEE: table.

antimicrobic (ăn″tĭ-mī-krō′bĭk) [″ + *mikros,* small, + *bios,* life]. Antimicrobial.

[illegible]timinth. Trade name for pyrantel pamoate, [illegible] q.v.

[illegible] (ăn″tĭ-mī-tŏt′ĭk). Interfering with [illegible] mitosis.

antimonial (ăn″tĭ-mō′nē-ăl). Pert. to or containing antimony.

antimony (ăn′tĭ-mō″nē). SYMB: Sb. At. wt. 121.75; at. no. 51. Stibium; a crystalline metallic element. Its compounds are used in alloys and medicines, and may form poisons.

antimony poisoning. SYM: Acrid metallic taste. Cardiac and arterial depression; sweating and vomiting about 30 minutes after ingestion. In large doses, it causes irritation of lining of alimentary tract, resembling arsenic poisioning.

F.A.: Vomiting caused by the poison may be sufficient. Gastric lavage with 1% sodium bicarbonate solution. BAL (British antilewisite) is effective esp. if the poisoning is due to a trivalent form such as tartar emetic. Otherwise treat symptomatically. SEE: *arsenic* in *Poisons and Poisoning* in *Appendix.*

antimycotic (ăn″tĭ-mī-kŏt′ĭk) [Gr. *anti,* against, + *mykes,* fungus]. Inhibiting or preventing the growth of fungi.

antinarcotic (ăn″tĭ-năr-kŏt′ĭk) [″ + *narkotikos,* benumbing]. 1. Opposing the action of a narcotic. 2. An agent that opposes the action of a narcotic.

antinatriuresis (ăn″tĭ-nā″trĭ-ū-rē′sĭs) [″ + L. *natrium,* sodium, + Gr. *ouresis,* making water]. Decreasing the excretion of sodium in the urine.

antinauseant (ăn″tĭ-naw′sē-ănt). 1. Preventing or relieving nausea. 2. Agent that prevents or relieves nausea.

antineoplastic (ăn″tĭ-nē″ō-plăs′tĭk). Preventing the development, growth, or proliferation of malignant cells. 2. Agent that prevents the development, growth, or proliferation of malignant cells.

antinephritic (ăn″tĭ-nĕ-frĭt′ĭk). 1. Preventing or relieving inflammation of the kidneys. 2. Agent that prevents or relieves inflammation of the kidneys.

antineuralgic (ăn″tĭ-nū-răl′jĭk) [″ + *neuron,* nerve, + *algos,* pain]. 1. Relieving neuralgia. 2. Agent that relieves neuralgia.

antineuritic (ăn″tĭ-nū-rĭt′ĭk). 1. Preventing or relieving inflammation of a nerve. 2. Agent that prevents or relieves inflammation of a nerve.

antinion (ăn-tĭn′ē-ŏn) [″ + *inion,* back of the neck]. The area of the skull beneath the eyebrows, opposite the inion, q.v.

antinuclear (ăn″tĭ-nū′klē-ăr). Having an affinity for or reacting with the nucleus of a cell.

antinuclear antibodies. Antibodies that react with the nuclei of cells. Found in patients with various collagen diseases.

antiodontalgic (ăn″tē-ō″dŏn-tăl′jĭk) [″ + *odous,* tooth, + *algos,* pain]. 1. Relieving toothache. 2. Agent that relieves toothache.

antiovulatory (ăn″tē-ŏv′ū-lă-tō″rē). Inhibiting

Antimicrobial Drugs

This generic list of antimicrobial drugs can only be considered as being representative of the types currently available. Some are no longer used clinically but are of historical interest.

Substance	Substance	Substance
amantadine	doxycycline	nystatin
amikacin sulfate	erythromycin	oleandomycin
p-aminosalicylic acid	ethambutol	oxacillin
amoxicillin	ethionamide	oxolinic acid
amphotericin B	flucytosine	oxytetracycline
ampicillin	furazolidone	paromomycin
bacampicillin	gentamicin	penicillin
bacitracin	glucosulfone	penicillin G benzathine
candicidin	griseofulvin	penicillin G potassium
capreomycin	haloprogin	penicillin G procaine
carbenicillin	hydroxystilbamidine	penicillin V
cefaclor	idoxuridine	phenethicillin
cefadroxil	isoniazid	phenoxymethyl penicillin
cefotaxime	kanamycin	piperacillin
cefoxitin	ketoconazole	polymyxin B
cephaloglycin	lincomycin	pyrazinamide
cephalothin	mafenide acetate	rifampin
cephapirin	methacycline	ristocetin
cephradine	methenamine mandelate	spectinomycin
chloramphenicol	methicillin	streptomycin
chlortetracycline	metronidazole	sulfacytine
cinoxacin	mezlocillin	sulfisoxazole
clindamycin	miconazole	tetracycline
clotrimazole	minocycline	ticarcillin
cloxacillin	moxalactam	tobramycin
colistimethate	nafcillin	tolnaftate
cyclacillin	nalidixic acid	trimethoprim
cycloserine	natamycin	trimethoprim-sulfamethoxazole
dapsone	neomycin	vancomycin
demeclocycline	nitrofurantoin	vidarabine
dicloxacillin	novobiocin	viomycin

or preventing ovulation.

antioxidant (ăn″tē-ŏk′sĭ-dănt). Agent that prevents or inhibits oxidation.

antioxidation (ăn″tē-ŏk″sĭ-dā′shŭn). Prevention or inhibition of oxidation.

antipaludian (ăn″tĭ-pă-loo′dē-ăn). 1. Preventing or curing malaria. 2. Agent that prevents or cures malaria. SYN: *antimalarial.*

antiparalytic (ăn″tĭ-păr-ă-lĭt′ĭk). Relieving paralysis.

antiparasitic (ăn″tĭ-păr-ă-sĭt′ĭk). 1. Destructive to parasites. 2. Agent that destroys parasites.

antipathic (ăn″tĭ-păth′ĭk) [Gr. *anti,* against, + *pathein,* to feel]. Antagonistic.

antipathy (ăn-tĭp′ă-thē). 1. Feeling of strong aversion. 2. Antagonism.

antipedicular (ăn″tĭ-pē-dĭk′ū-lăr). Effective against pediculosis, said of a medicine or procedure.

antipepsin (ăn″tĭ-pĕp′sĭn). Substance that opposes the action of pepsin

antiperiodic (ăn″tĭ-pē-rē-ŏd′ĭk) [″ + *periodos,* a circle]. Preventing regular recurrences of a disease or symptoms, as in malaria.

antiperistalsis (ăn″tĭ-pĕr″ĭ-stăl′sĭs) [″ + *peri,* around, + *stalsis,* constriction]. Reversed peristalsis; a wave of contraction in the gastrointestinal tract moving toward the oral end. In the duodenum it is associated with vomiting; in the ascending colon it occurs normally. SEE: *peristalsis.*

antiperistaltic (ăn″tĭ-pĕr″ĭ-stăl′tĭk). 1. Pert. to antiperistalsis. 2. Impeding peristalsis.

antiperspirant (ăn″tĭ-pĕr spĭ-rănt). 1. Inhibiting perspiration. 2. A substance that inhibits perspiration. SYN: *anhidrotic; antidrotic; antisudorific.*

antiphagocytic (ăn″tĭ-făg-ō-sīt′ĭk). Preventing or inhibiting phagocytosis.

antiphlogistic (ăn″tĭ-flō-jĭs′tĭk) [″ + *phlogistos,* on fire]. 1. Preventing or relieving inflammation. 2. Agent that prevents or relieves inflammation.

antiplasmin (ăn″tĭ-plăz′mĭn). Substance that opposes the action of plasmin.

antiplastic (ăn″tĭ-plăs′tĭk) [″ + *plassein,* to form]. 1. Preventing or inhibiting wound healing. 2. Agent that prevents or inhibits wound healing by preventing formation of granulation tissue.

antiplatelet (ăn″tĭ-plāt′lĕt). 1. Destructive to platelets. 2. An agent that destroys platelets.

antipodal (ăn-tĭp′ō-dăl) [Gr. *antipous,* with feet opposite]. Located at opposite positions.

antipraxia (ăn″tĭ-prăk′sē-ă). Functions or symptoms antagonistic to each other.

antiprostaglandin (ăn″tĭ-prŏs″tă-glăn′dĭn). Drug that acts to interfere with prostaglandin activity. Such drugs are used in treating arthritis and dysmenorrhea.

antiprostate (ăn″tĭ-prŏs′tāt). Anteprostate; Cowper's gland.

antiprostatitis (ăn″tĭ-prŏs″tă-tī′tĭs). Inflammation of Cowper's gland.

antiprotease (ăn″tĭ-prō′tē-ās). Substance that interferes with proteolysis.

antiprotozoal (ăn″tĭ-prō″tō-zō′ăl). Destructive to protozoa.

antipruritic (ăn″tĭ-proo-rĭt′ĭk). 1. Preventing or relieving itching. 2. Agent that prevents or relieves itching.

antipsoriatic (ăn″tĭ-sō″rē-ăt′ĭk) [″ + *psora,* itch]. 1. Preventing or relieving psoriasis. 2. Agent that prevents or relieves psoriasis.

antiputrefactive (ăn″tĭ-pū″trē-făk′tĭv). Preventing putrefaction.

antipyic (ăn-tĭ-pī′ĭk) [″ + *pyon,* pus]. Antipyogenic, q.v.

antipyogenic (ăn″tĭ-pī-ō-jĕn′ĭk) [″ + ″ + *gennan,* to produce]. 1. Preventing or inhibiting pus formation. 2. Agent that prevents or inhibits pus formation. SYN: *antipyic.*

antipyresis (ăn″tĭ-pī-rē′sĭs) [″ + *pyretos,* fever]. Use of antipyretics.

antipyretic (ăn-tĭ-pī-rĕt′ĭk). 1. Reducing fever. 2. Agent that reduces fever. SYN: *antifebrile.*

antipyrine (ăn″tĭ-pī′rēn) [″ + *pyr,* fire]. White crystalline powder, odorless and having a slightly bitter taste. An analgesic and antipyretic. Its toxicity is similar to acetanilid. It should not be used.

antipyrotic (ăn″tĭ-pī-rŏt′ĭk) [″ + *pyrotikos,* burning]. 1. Promoting the healing of burns. 2. Agent that promotes the healing of burns.

antirabic (ăn″tĭ-rā′bĭk). Preventing or curing [illegible]bies. SYN: *antilyssic.*

[illegible]**hitic** (ăn″tĭ-ră-kĭt′ĭk) [″ + *rachitis,* [illegible] 1. Helping to cure rickets. 2. Agent [illegible]rickets.

antirheumatic (ăn″tĭ-roo-măt′ĭk). 1. Preventing or relieving rheumatism. 2. Agent that prevents or relieves rheumatism.

antiricin (ăn″tĭ-rī′sĭn). Agent that opposes the action of ricin.

antiscabietic (ăn″tĭ-skā″bē-ĕt′ĭk) [Gr. *anti,* against, + L. *scabies,* itch]. 1. Preventing or relieving scabies. 2. Agent that prevents or relieves scabies.

antiscorbutic (ăn″tĭ-skor-bū′tĭk) [″ + L. *scorbutus,* scurvy]. 1. Preventing or relieving scurvy. 2. Agent that prevents or relieves scurvy.

antiseborrheic (ăn″tĭ-sĕb″ō-rē′ĭk). 1. Counteracting or effectively treating seborrhea. 2. An agent that counteracts or effectively treats seborrhea.

antisecretory (ăn″tĭ-sē-krē′tō-rē). 1. Inhibiting secretory activity of a gland or organ. 2. An agent that inhibits secretory activity of a gland or organ.

antisepsis (ăn″tĭ-sĕp′sĭs) [″ + *sepsis,* putrefaction]. The prevention of sepsis by preventing or inhibiting the growth of causative microorganisms.

antiseptic (ăn″tĭ-sĕp′tĭk). 1. Rel. to antisepsis. 2. An agent capable of producing antisepsis.

Chemically, antiseptics may be inorganic, such as the mercury preparations, or organic, such as carbolic acid (phenol). Oxidizing disinfectants liberate oxygen when in contact with pus or organic substances. When in use they should be washed away and replaced frequently to help remove pus, blood, and other substances. Different types of bacteria are sensitive to different antiseptics. SEE: *disinfectant* (table).

RS: asepsis; disinfectant; deodorant; germicide; sterilization.

antisepticism (ăn″tĭ-sĕp′tĭ-sĭzm). Therapeutic employment of antiseptic measures.

antiserum (ăn″tĭ-sē′rŭm). Serum that contains antibodies for a specific antigen; may be of human or animal origin. SYN: *serum, immune.*

a., monovalent. Antiserum containing antibodies specific for one antigen.

a., polyvalent. Antiserum containing antibodies specific for more than one antigen.

antishock garment. A special garment that can be quickly placed on a patient in shock. The device contains inflatable compartments that when filled with air compress the lower extremities and abdominal area. This compression prevents pooling of blood and fluids in the tissues. Thus the garment is quite useful in treating shock. CAUTION: This garment should not be used in treating congestive heart failure. SEE: *anti-G suit.*

antisialagogue (ăn″tĭ-sī-ăl′ă-gŏg) [Gr. *anti,* against, + *sialon,* saliva, + *agogos,* drawing forth]. An agent, as atropine, that lessens or prevents the flow of saliva.

antisialic (ăn″tĭ-sī-ăl′ĭk). 1. Inhibiting the secretion of saliva. 2. Agent that inhibits the secretion of saliva.

antisocial (ăn″tĭ-sō′shăl). Pert. to a person whose outlook and actions are socially negative and whose behavior is repeatedly in conflict with what society perceives as the norm. SEE: *asocial.*

antisocial personality disorder. SEE: *personality, antisocial.*

antispasmodic [″ + *spasmos,* convulsion]. 1. Preventing or relieving spasm. 2. Agent that prevents or relieves spasm. SEE: *spasm.*

anti-stain formulary. A formula that is effective in removing stains from various materials. An anti-stain formulary for removing stains from bed linens and other cotton fabrics is as follows:

Blood: Soak in cold water, then wash in lukewarm soap solution. For old stains, soak in 1% ammonia solution and then launder.

Chocolate or cocoa: Allow hot water to run through stained fabric; then wash in hot soap solution. Use Javelle water (a solution of potassium or sodium hypochlorite) to bleach if necessary.

Cosmetics: Nail polish, lipstick, or rouge—ordinary washing; stubborn stains remaining can be removed by acetone, followed by warm chlorine bleach.

Feces: Soak in cold water, rinse, then wash with soap and hot water. Use a brush to scrub.

Fruit stains: Stretch stained article over a basin, pour boiling water directly over the spot until it disappears. If this fails, use Javelle water, rinsing between each application.

Grass stains: Use alcohol, then wash with household baking soda and hot water. Put in the sun to bleach.

Ink (ordinary): If fresh, immerse in cold or tepid water or skimmed milk. Old ink stains respond well to lemon juice, salt, and sunlight. Whatever is used, the material should be rinsed thoroughly after using to remove all the solution.

Iodine: Soapy water, ammonia solution, and hot water rinse.

Iron rust: Use lemon juice and salt; expose to the sunlight. For firm fabrics, use strong solution of oxalic acid. Rinse very thoroughly.

Meat juices: Same as for blood.

Mercurochrome: Pour hot water through the material. Acid alcohol does very well, or equal parts of Dakin's solution and 5% acetic acid (vinegar).

Mildew: If fresh, use strong soapsuds and hang in the sunlight. If an old stain, use Javelle water, rinse thoroughly, and repeat the washing if indicated.

Paints, varnishes: Turpentine or benzol (use only in a well-ventilated area). If old stain, soak well in grease to soften, then apply turpentine or the other solutions. Chloroform dissolves lacquer paint stains. Acetone sponged on fabric removes varnish. Shellac is soluble in 50% solution of alcohol.

CAUTION: Chloroform is toxic and should be used only in a very well ventilated area.

Perspiration: Wash in strong soap solution and dry in sunlight.

Picric acid: Boil fabric in dilute sodium hydroxide solution for one-half hour and bleach in Javelle water.

Scorch: Apply hydrogen peroxide to the area, then rub well while the material is soaked in strong soap solution. Dry in sunlight.

Silver salts: If not too old, silver stains can be removed by sodium thiosulfate (photographer's hypo).

Tea or coffee: If fresh, pour boiling water through it. If old, soak in borax before pouring boiling water over it.

Urine: Soak in boiling water, then pour 5% Lysol solution over it.

antistaphylococcic (ăn″tĭ-stăf″ĭ-lō-kŏk′sĭk) [Gr. *anti,* against, + *staphyle,* bunch of grapes, + *cocci,* bacteria]. Destructive to staphylococci.

antistaphylolysin (ăn″tĭ-stăf″ĭ-lŏl′ĭ-sĭn) [″ + ″ + *lysis,* dissolution]. Substance that opposes the action of staphylolysin, a hemolysin produced by staphylococci.

antistreptococcic (ăn″tĭ-strĕp″tō-kŏk′sĭk). Destructive to streptococci.

antistreptolysin (ăn″tĭ-strĕp-tŏl′ĭ-sĭn). Antibody that opposes the action of streptolysin, a hemolysin produced by streptococci.

antisudoral (ăn″tĭ-soo′dor-ăl) [″ + L. *sudor,* sweat]. Inhibiting or preventing perspiration. SYN: *anhidrotic; antihidrotic; antiperspirant.*

antisudorific (ăn″tĭ-soo″dor-ĭf′ĭk). 1. Inhibiting or preventing perspiration. 2. An agent that prevents or inhibits perspiration. SYN: *anhidrosis; antihydrosis; antiperspirant.*

antisyphilitic (ăn″tĭ-sĭf″ĭ-lĭt′ĭk) [″ + L. *syphiliticus,* pert. to syphilis]. 1. Curing or relieving syphilis. 2. Agent that cures or relieves syphilis. SYN: *antiluetic.*

antitabetic (ăn″tĭ-tă-bĕt′ĭk) [″ + L. *tabes,* wasting away]. 1. Preventing or relieving tabes dorsalis. 2. Agent that prevents or relieves tabes dorsalis.

antithenar (ăn-tĭth′ĕn-ăr) [″ + *thenar,* palm]. The eminence on ulnar side of the palm, formed by the muscles of the little finger. SYN: *hypothenar eminence.*

antithrombotic (ăn″tĭ-thrŏm-bŏt′ĭk). Interfering with or preventing thrombosis or bl[illegible] coagulation.

antithyroid (ăn″tĭ-thī′royd) [″ + *thyreoeides,* thyroid]. 1. Preventing or inhibiting the functioning of the thyroid gland. 2. Agent that prevents or inhibits the functioning of the thyroid gland.

antitonic (ăn″tĭ-tŏn′ĭk) [″ + *tonos,* tone]. Diminishing tonicity.

antitoxic (ăn″tĭ-tŏk′sĭk) [″ + *toxikon,* poison]. Neutralizing a poison, esp. a bacterial toxin. SEE: *antitoxin.*

antitoxic serum. Serum that contains antitoxin, q.v.

antitoxigen (ăn″tĭ-tŏk′sĭ-gĕn) [″ + ″ + *gennan,* to produce]. An antigen that stimulates that production of antitoxin. SYN: *antitoxinogen.*

antitoxin (ăn″tĭ-tŏk′sĭn). An antibody produced in response to and capable of neutralizing a specific biologic toxin.

Ex.: diphtheria antitoxin, gas-gangrene antitoxin, and tetanus antitoxin, which counteract the toxins produced by the diphtheria, gas-gangrene, and tetanus bacteria. Antitoxins are used for prophylactic and therapeutic purposes. SEE: *antivenin.*

antitoxinogen (ăn″tĭ-tŏk-sĭn′ō-jĕn) [Gr. *anti,* against, + *toxikon,* poison, + *gennan,* to produce]. An antigen that stimulates production of antitoxin. SYN: *antitoxigen.*

antitragicus (ăn″tĭ-trăj′ĭ-kŭs). A small muscle in the pinna of the ear.

antitragus (ăn″tĭ-trā′gŭs) [″ + L. *tragus,* goat]. [NA] A projection on the ear of the cartilage of the auricle in front of the tail of the helix, posterior to the tragus.

antitrismus (ăn″tĭ-trĭs′mŭs) [″ + *trismos,* grinding]. A condition in which the mouth cannot close because of tonic spasm.

antitropin (ăn″tĭ-trō′pĭn). An antibody, q.v.

antitrypsin (ăn″tĭ-trĭp′sĭn). A substance that inhibits the action of trypsin.

a., alpha 1–. A low–molecular weight glycoprotein that inhibits proteolytic enzymes. Deficiency of this enzyme in the serum is associated with early-onset emphysema in adults, progressive cirrhosis of the liver in children, and respiratory distress syndrome in newborn infants.

antitrypsin deficiency. A rare inherited disease characterized by very low serum alpha 1–antitrypsin levels. This deficiency is associated with early development of emphysema because the enzyme trypsin enables the alveoli to resist enzymes released by leukocytes. Also associated with development of hepatitis in infants. This condition should be suspected in patients with early-onset emphysema and no history of smoking.

[illegible]ryptic (ăn″tĭ-trĭp′tĭk). Inhibiting the ac- [illegible] trypsin.

[illegible]lotic (ăn″tĭ-too-bĕr′kū-lŏt″ĭk). In- [illegible] pread or progress of tuberculosis in the body.

antitussive (ăn″tĭ-tŭs′ĭv) [Gr. *anti,* against, + L. *tussis,* cough]. 1. Preventing or relieving coughing. 2. An agent that prevents or relieves coughing.

a., centrally acting. An agent that depresses medullary centers, thus suppressing the cough reflex.

antiuratic (ăn″tĭ-ū-răt′ĭk) [″ + L. *uras,* urate]. 1. Preventing the precipitation of urates. 2. Substance that inhibits or prevents formation of urates.

antivaccinationist (ăn″tĭ-văk″sĭ-nā′shŭn-ĭst). One who is opposed to vaccination.

antivenene (ăn″tĭ-vĕn′ēn). Antivenin.

antivenereal (ăn″tĭ-vē-nē′rē-ăl). Preventing or curing venereal diseases.

antivenin (ăn″tĭ-vĕn′ĭn). A serum that contains antitoxin specific for an animal or insect venom. Antivenin is prepared from immunized animal sera and is used in the treatment of poisoning by animal or insect venom. SYN: *antivenene; antivenom.*

a., black widow spider. An antitoxic serum obtained from horses immunized against venom of the black widow spider (Latrodectus mactans). Specific in treatment of bites of black widow spider. Available from Merck Sharp and Dohme, West Point, PA 19486, U.S.A.

a., (crotalidae) polyvalent. USP. Antisnakebite serum obtained from serum of horses immunized against venom of four types of pit vipers: Crotalus atrox, C. adamanteus, C. terrificus, and Bothrops atrox (family Crotalidae). Specific in treatment of bites of these snakes.

antivenom (ăn″tĭ-vĕn′ŏm). Antivenin.

antivenomous (ăn″tĭ-vĕn′ō-mŭs). Opposing the action of venom.

Antivert. Trade name for meclizine hydrochloride, USP, q.v.

antiviral (ăn″tĭ-vī′răl). Opposing the action of a virus.

antivitamin. A vitamin antagonist; one of a group of substances, natural or synthetic, that opposes the action of certain vitamins.

antivivisection (ăn″tĭ-vĭv″ĭ-sĕk′shŭn). Opposition to the use of live animals in experimentation. SEE: *vivisection.*

antixenic (ăn″tĭ-zē′nĭk) [Gr. *anti,* against, + *xenos,* strange]. Pert. to living tissue reaction to any foreign substance.

antixerotic (ăn″tĭ-zē-rŏt′ĭk) [″ + *xerosis,* dryness]. Preventing dryness of the skin.

antizymotic (ăn″tĭ-zī-mŏt′ĭk) [″ + *zymosis,* fermentation]. An agent that prevents or arrests fermentation.

Ex.: alcohol; salicylic acid.

antra (ăn′tră) [L.]. Pl. of antrum, q.v.

antral (ăn′trăl). Pert. to an antrum.

antrectomy (ăn-trĕk′tō-mē) [L. *antrum,* cavity, + Gr. *ektome,* excision]. Excision of the walls of an antrum.

antritis (ăn"trī'tĭs) [" + Gr. *itis,* inflammation]. Inflammation of an antrum, esp. the maxillary sinus.

antro- [L. *antrum,* cavity]. Prefix denoting relationship to an antrum.

antroatticotomy (ăn"trō-ăt"ĭ-kŏt'ō-mē) [" + *atticus,* attic, + Gr. *tome,* incision]. Operation to open the maxillary sinus and the attic of the tympanum.

antrocele (ăn'trō-sēl) [" + Gr. *kele,* tumor]. Fluid accumulation in a cyst in the maxillary sinus.

antroduodenectomy (ăn"trō-dū"ō-dĕ-nĕk'tō-mē) [" + *duodeni,* twelve, + Gr. *ektome,* excision.] Surgical removal of the pyloric antrum and the upper portion of the duodenum.

antronasal (ăn"trō-nā'zăl) [" + *nasalis,* nasal]. Rel. to the maxillary sinus and nasal fossa.

antrophore (ăn'trō-for) [" + Gr. *phorein,* to carry]. A medicated bougie, q.v., for local treatment of any accessible cavity or canal.

antroscope (ăn'trō-skōp) [" + Gr. *skopein,* to view]. An instrument for visual examination of a cavity, esp. the maxillary sinus.

antroscopy (ăn-trŏs'kō-pē). Visual examination of a cavity, esp. the maxillary sinus, using an antroscope.

antrostomy (ăn-trŏs'tō-mē) [" + Gr. *stoma,* mouth]. Operation to form an opening in an antrum.

antrotome (ăn'trō-tōm) [" + Gr. *tome,* incision]. An instrument used to perform antrotomy.

antrotomy (ăn"trŏt'ō-mē). Cutting through an antral wall.

antrotympanic (ăn"trō-tĭm-păn'ĭk) [L. *antrum,* cavity, + Gr. *tympanon,* drum]. Rel. to the mastoid antrum and the tympanic cavity.

antrotympanitis (ăn"trō-tĭm"păn-ī'tĭs) [" + " + *itis,* inflammation]. Chronic inflammation of tympanic cavity and mastoid antrum.

antrum (ăn'trŭm) [L., cavity]. (pl. *antra*) [NA] Any nearly closed cavity or chamber, esp. in a bone.

a. auris. External acoustic meatus.

a. cariacum. The thoracic portion of the esophagus, functionally the superior portion of the stomach.

a., duodenal. The duodenal cap, a dilatation of duodenum near pylorus and seen during digestion.

a., mastoid; a. mastoideum. [NA] Cavity in the mastoid portion of the temporal bone. SYN: *a., tympanic.*

a., maxillary. The maxillary sinus; a cavity in the maxillary bone communicating with the middle meatus of the nasal cavity.

a. of Highmore. Maxillary antrum, q.v.

a., pyloric; a. pyloricum. [NA] Bulge in the pyloric portion of the stomach along the greater curvature on distention.

a., tympanic; a. tympanicum. A., mastoid, q.v.

antrum puncture. Puncture made in maxillary sinus by placing trocar through sinus wall. Instrument enters from near floor of nose 1½ inches (3.8 cm.) from external opening. Pus is then drained.

NURSING IMPLICATIONS: Irrigate antrum 24 hours after puncture. The physician may order the antrum to be irrigated with a solution such as warm normal saline. Follow hospital procedure for the irrigation. Carefully note and describe the character of drainage in the solution return.

ANTU. Alpha-naphthylthiourea, a powerful rat poison.

Antuitrin-S. Trade name for chorionic gonadotropin, USP, human, q.v.

Anturane. Trade name for su finpyrazone, USP, q.v.

anuclear (ā-nū'klē-ăr). Lacking a nucleus, said of erythrocytes.

ANUG. *acute necrotizing ulcerative gingivitis.* SEE: *trench mouth.*

anulus (ăn'ū-lŭs) [L.]. (pl. *anuli*) [NA] A ring-shaped structure; a ring. Also spelled annulus.

a. abdominalis. A. inguinalis profundus, q.v.

a. femoralis. The femoral ring; the abdominal opening of the femoral canal.

a. inguinalis profundus. The deep inguinal ring; the opening in the fascia transversalis for the ductus deferens in the male or the round ligament in the female. SYN: *a. abdominalis.*

a. inguinalis superficialis. Superficial inguinal ring; the opening in the external oblique muscle for the ductus deferens in the male and the round ligament in the female.

a. tympanicus. Tympanic ring; part of the temporal bone forming a ring at the inner end of the external auditory canal.

a. umbilicalis. The opening in the abdominal wall of a fetus through which the umbilical vessels pass.

a. urethralis. Elevated muscular ring surrounding the opening of the bladder into the urethra. SYN: *sphincter, bladder.*

anuresis (ăn-ū-rē'sĭs) [Gr. *an-,* not, + *ouresis,* urination]. Absence of urination. SEE: *anuria.*

anuretic (ăn-ū-rĕt'ĭk). Pert. to anuresis, q.v.

anuria (ăn-ū'rē-ă) [" + *ouron,* urine]. Absence of urine formation. SEE: *anuresis.*

anus (ā'nŭs) [L.]. [NA] The outlet of the rectum lying in the fold between the buttocks.

a., artificial. Opening into the bowel formed by colostomy.

a., imperforate. Condition in which the anus is closed.

a., vulvovaginal. Congenital anomaly in a female in which the anus is imperforate but there is an opening from the rectum to vagina.

anvil (ăn'vĭl) [AS. *anfilt*]. Middle ossicle of ear. SYN: *incus*. SEE: *ear* for illus.

anxietas (ăng-zī'ĕ-tăs) [L.]. Anxiety, apprehension, restlessness.

a. tibiarum. Tiredness, twitching, and unrest in legs.

anxiety (ăng-zī'ĕ-tē). A feeling of apprehension, worry, uneasiness, or dread, esp. of the future.

Everyone has been anxious at some time. Anxiety is the normal reaction to that which is threatening to one's body, lifestyle, values, or loved ones. A certain amount of anxiety is normal and stimulates the individual to purposeful action. Excess anxiety interferes with efficient functioning of the individual. SEE: *anxiety neurosis*.

anxiety disorders. A group of psychiatric disorders characterized principally by anxiety. Phobias of various types are included along with panic, obsessive-compulsive disorder, and anxiety states.

anxiety neurosis. A mental disorder characterized by excessive anxiety that is not restricted to specific situations or objects and is often associated with somatic symptoms. This disorder must be differentiated from normal anxiety, which occurs in realistically threatening situations.

Anxiety neurosis may be manifested when an individual without organic disease, during clear consciousness, complains of palpitation, heart pain, dyspepsia, constriction of the throat, bandlike pressure about head, or cold, sweaty, tremulous extremities.

anxiolytic (ăng"zī-ō-lĭt'ĭk) [L. *anxietas*, anxiety, + Gr. *lysis*, destruction]. Counteracting or diminishing anxiety. This may be done by drug, social, or psychiatric therapy.

A.O.A. *Alpha Omega Alpha*, an honorary medical fraternity in the U.S.; *American Osteopathic Association*.

A.O.C. *anodal opening contraction*.

AOD. *adult-onset diabetes mellitus*. SEE: *diabetes, non-insulin-dependent*.

A.O.R.N. *Association of Operating Room Nurses*.

aorta (ā-or'tă) [L. from Gr. *aorte*]. (pl. *aortas*, *-tae*) [NA] The main trunk of the arterial system of the body. It is about 3 cm. in diameter at its origin in the upper surface of the left ventricle. It passes upward as the ascending aorta, turns backward and to the left (arch of the aorta) at about the level of the fourth thoracic vertebra, and then passes downward as the descending aorta, which is divided into the thoracic and abdominal aorta. The latter terminates at its division into the two common iliac arteries. At the point of origin from the ventricle, the aorta contains three valves. These open when the heart beats and close when the blood flow momentarily ceases at the end of systole. SEE: illus.

The divisions of the aorta are as follows:

Ascending aorta (2 branches): Two coronary arteries (right and left) provide blood supply to the myocardium.

Aortic arch (3 branches): The innominate artery divides into the right subclavian artery, which provides blood for the right arm and other areas, and right common carotid artery, which supplies the right side of the head and neck. The left common carotid artery supplies the left side of the head and neck. The left subclavian artery provides blood for the left arm and portion of the thoracic area.

Thoracic aorta: Two or more bronchial arteries provide blood for bronchi. Four or five esophageal arteries provide blood to the esophagus. Pericardial arteries supply the pericardium. Nine pairs of intercostal arteries supply blood for intercostal areas. Mediastinal branches supply lymph glands and the posterior mediastinum. Superior phrenic arteries supply the diaphragm.

Abdominal aorta: The celiac artery supplies the stomach, liver, and spleen. The superior mesenteric artery supplies all of the small intestine except the superior portion of the duodenum. The inferior mesenteric artery supplies all of the colon and rectum except the right half of the transverse colon. Middle suprarenal branches supply the adrenal (suprarenal) glands. Renal arteries supply the kidneys, ureters, and adrenals. Testicular arteries supply testicles and ureter. Ovarian arteries (correspond to internal spermatic arteries of the male) supply the ovaries, part of ureters, and uterine tubes. Inferior phrenic arteries supply the diaphragm and esophagus. Lumbar arteries supply lumbar and psoas muscles and part of the abdominal wall musculature. The middle sacral artery supplies the sacrum and coccyx. Right and left common iliac arteries supply lower pelvic and abdominal areas and the lower extremities.

aortal (ā-or'tăl). Pert. to the aorta.

aortalgia (ā"or-tăl'jē-ă) [L. from Gr. *aorte*, aorta, + *algos*, pain]. Pain in the aortic area.

aortarctia (ā"or-tărk'shē-ă) [" + L. *arctare*, to narrow]. Aortic narrowing. SEE: *coarctation*.

aortectasia (ā"or-tĕk-tā'zē-ă) [" + *ek*, out, + *tasis*, a stretching]. Dilatation of the aorta.

aortectomy (ā"or-tĕk'tō-mē) [" + *ektome*, excision]. Excision of part of the aorta.

aortic (ā-or'tĭk). Pert. to aorta or its orifice in

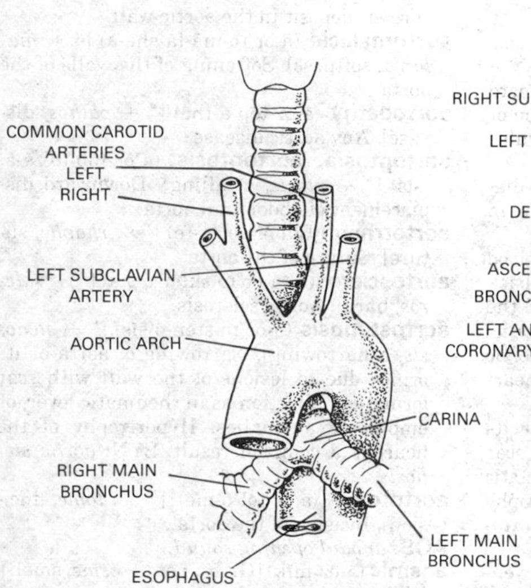

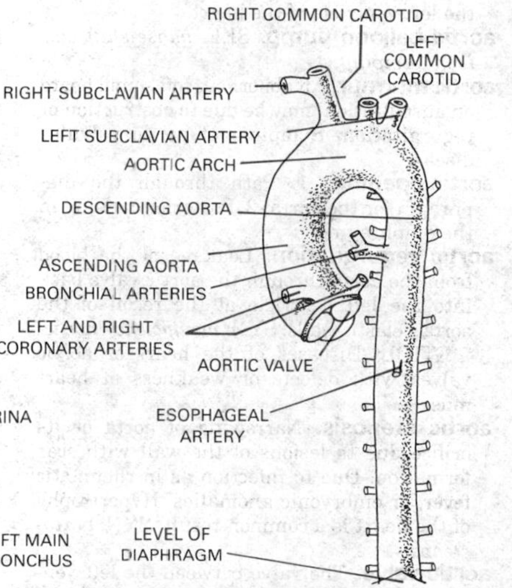

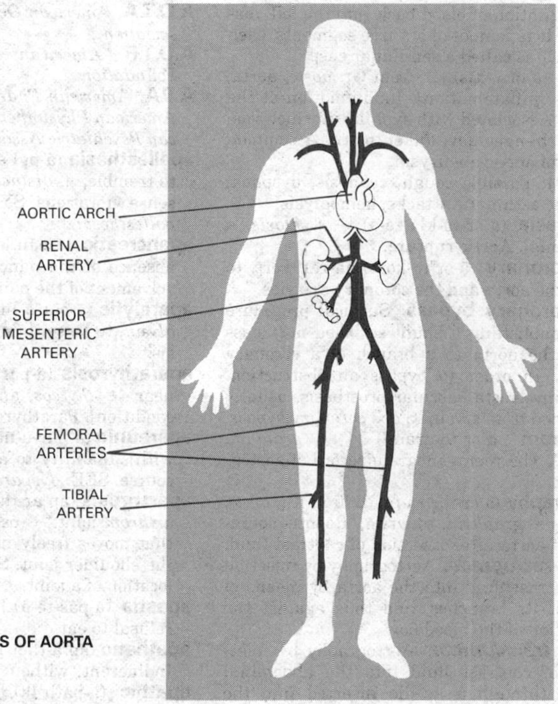

BRANCHES OF AORTA

the left ventricle of the heart.

aortic balloon pump. SEE: *phase-shift balloon pumping.*

aortic murmur. An abnormal, soft sound heard on auscultation; may be due to obstruction or regurgitation. Symptom of aortic valvular disease.

aortic opening. 1. Path through the diaphragm for the aorta. 2. Posterior opening in the diaphragm.

aortic regurgitation. Leakage of the blood from the aorta through the aortic valve back into the left ventricle at the recoil of the aorta's elastic walls. SYN: *insufficiency, aortic.*

ETIOL: Diseases of the heart or aortic valves with defects or weakness of heart muscle.

aortic stenosis. Narrowing of aorta or its orifice due to lesions of the wall with scar formation. Due to infection as in rheumatic fever, or embryonic anomalies. Hypertrophy of the heart is a common result. SYN: *aortostenosis.*

aortic valve. The valve between the left ventricle and the ascending aorta that prevents regurgitation of blood back into the left ventricle. It is composed of three segments, each of which is called a semilunar cusp.

aortitis (ā-or-tī'tĭs) [L. from Gr. *aorte,* aorta, + *itis,* inflammation]. Inflammation of the aorta. Associated with syphilis in which vascular changes have taken place. A common cause of aortic aneurysm.

SYM: Possible cough, cyanosis, dyspnea, cardiac asthmatic attacks, hemoptysis.

aortoclasia (ā″or-tō-klā'zē-ă) [″ + *klasis,* a breaking]. Aortic rupture.

aortocoronary (ā-or″tō-kor'ŏ-nā-rē). Pert. to both the aorta and the coronary arteries.

aortocoronary bypass. Surgical procedure for establishing a shunt so blood may pass from the aorta to a branch of a coronary artery in order to bypass an obstruction. This involves a vascular prosthesis, usually obtained from a vein. SYN: *coronary bypass.*

aortogram (ā-or'tō-grăm″) [″ + *gramma,* mark]. The roentgenogram record of aortography.

aortography (ā″or-tog'ră-fē) [L. from Gr. *aorte,* aorta, + *graphein,* to write]. Roentgenography of aorta after injection of contrast fluid.

a., retrograde. Aortography by injection of contrast fluid into the aorta by means of one of its branches, and thus against the direction of the blood flow.

a., translumbar. Aortography by injection of contrast fluid into the abdominal aorta through a needle inserted into the lumbar area near the level of the 12th rib.

aortoiliac (ā-or″tō-ĭl'ē-ăk). Pert. to both the aorta and the iliac arteries.

aortolith (ă-or'tō-lĭth) [″ + *lithos,* stone]. Calcareous deposit in the aortic wall.

aortomalacia (ā-or″tō-mă-lā'shē-ă) [″ + *malakia,* softness]. Softening of the walls of the aorta.

aortopathy (ā″or-tŏp'ă-thē) [″ + *pathos,* disease]. Any aortic disease.

aortoptosia, aortoptosis (ā″or-tŏp-tō'zē-ă, -sĭs) [″ + *ptosis,* a falling]. Downward displacement of abdominal aorta.

aortorrhaphy (ā″or-tor'ă-fē) [″ + *rhaphe,* suture]. Suture of the aorta.

aortosclerosis (ā-or″tō-sklĕr-ō'sĭs) [″ + *skleros,* hard]. Aortic sclerosis.

aortostenosis (ā-or″tō-stĕn-ō'sĭs) [″ + *stenosis,* a narrowing]. Narrowing of aorta or its orifice due to lesions of the wall with scar formation, infection as in rheumatic fever, or embryonic anomalies. Hypertrophy of the heart is a common result. SYN: *aortic stenosis.*

aortotomy (ā″or-tŏt'ō-mē) [″ + *tome,* incision]. Incision of the aorta.

AOS. *anodal opening sound.*

aosmic (ā-ŏz'mĭk) [Gr. *a-,* not, + *osme,* smell]. Without odor.

A.O.T.A. *American Occupational Therapy Association.*

A.O.T.F. *American Occupational Therapy Foundation.*

A.P.A. *American Pharmaceutical Association; American Physiotherapy Association; American Psychiatric Association.*

apallesthesia (ă-păl″ĕs-thē'zē-ă) [″ + *pallein,* to tremble, + *aisthesis,* feeling]. Inability to sense vibrations. SYN: *pallanesthesia.* SEE: *pallesthesia.*

apancreatic (ă-păn″krē-ăt'ĭk). 1. Caused by absence of the pancreas. 2. Pert. to noninvolvement of the pancreas.

aparalytic (ă-păr″ă-lĭt'ĭk) [Gr. *a-,* not, + *paralyein,* to loosen]. Marked by lack of paralysis.

aparathyrosis (ă-păr″ă-thī-rō'sĭs) [″ + *para,* near, + *thyreos,* an oblong shield, + *osis,* condition]. Parathyroid deficiency.

apareunia (ă″păr-ū'nē-ă) [″ + *pareunos,* lying with]. Inability to accomplish sexual intercourse. SEE: *dyspareunia.*

aparthrosis (ăp″ăr-thrō'sĭs) [Gr. *apo,* from, + *arthron,* joint, + *osis,* condition]. 1. A joint that moves freely in any direction, such as the shoulder joint. SYN: *diarthrosis.* 2. Dislocation of a joint.

apastia (ă-păs'tē-ă) [Gr., fasting]. Abnormal refusal to eat.

apathetic (ăp″ă-thĕt'ĭk) [″ + *pathos,* disease]. Indifferent; without interest. SYN: *apathic.*

apathic (ă-păth'ĭk). Indifferent. SYN: *apathetic.*

apathism (ăp'ă-thĭzm) [″ + *pathos,* disease, + *-ismos,* condition]. Slowness to react to stimuli. Opposite of erethism, q.v.

apathy (ăp'ă-thē) [Gr. *apatheia*]. Indifference; insensibility; lack of emotion.

A.P.C. *aspirin, phenacetin,* and *caffeine,* common ingredients in various headache and cold tablets. Phenacetin is no longer felt to be suitable for use in these preparations.

APE. *anterior pituitary extract.*

apeidosis (ăp"ĭ-dō'sĭs) [Gr. *apo,* away, + *eidos,* form]. Slow modification or disappearance of the clinical and histological characteristics of a disease.

apellous (ă-pĕl'ŭs) [Gr. *a-,* not, + L. *pellis,* skin]. 1. Lacking skin. 2. Lacking foreskin; circumcised.

apenteric (ăp"ĕn-tĕr'ĭk) [Gr. *apo,* from, + *enteron,* intestine]. Outside the intestine. SYN: *abenteric.*

apepsia (ă-pĕp'sē-ă) [Gr. *a-,* not, + *pepsis,* digesting]. Cessation of digestion.

apepsinia (ă"pĕp-sĭn'ē-ă). Absence of pepsin in the gastric juice.

aperient (ă-pĕr'ē-ĕnt) [L. *aperiens,* opening]. A very mild laxative.

aperistalsis (ă"pĕr-ĭ-stăl'sĭs) [Gr. *a-,* not, + *peri,* around, + *stalsis,* constriction]. Absence of peristalsis.

apéritif (ă-pĕr"ĭ-tēf') [L. *aperire,* to open]. An alcoholic beverage, such as wine, taken before a meal to stimulate the appetite.

aperitive (ă-pĕr'ĭ-tĭv). 1. Stimulating the appetite. 2. Aperient, q.v.

Apert's syndrome (ă-pārz'). [Eugene Apert, Fr. pediatrician, 1868–1940] A congenital condition marked by a peaked head and webbed fingers and toes.

apertura (ăp"ĕr-tū'ră) [L.]. (pl. *aperturae*) [NA] An opening.

aperture (ăp'ĕr-chūr"). An orifice or opening.

apex (ā'pĕks) [L., tip] (pl. *apices*) [NA] The pointed extremity of a conical structure.

a., root. The end of the root of a tooth.

apex beat. The striking of the apex of the left ventricle against the chest wall in systole. Felt in the 5th left intercostal space, approx. 3½ inches (8.9 cm.) from the middle of the sternum, about an inch (2.5 cm.) within a line drawn down from the middle of the clavicle parallel with the sternum (the mammary line). Generally may be detected by inspection or palpation; when these fail, may be localized by auscultation. If the patient is in a recumbent position, the apex beat may be detected an inch (2.5 cm.) or more higher. When the body is inclined to the left, the beat may be detected in or outside the mammary line. During forced inspiration, it may become imperceptible or be found below its usual place. During forced expiration, the beat becomes more forcible and may be found above its usual place. The patient, as a rule, should be examined in erect or sitting position while breathing quietly.

ABNORM: Deformity of chest may cause displacement in any direction.

Weak apex beat: may be noted in healthy persons at rest, in heart failure, pericardial effusion, emphysema, shock, or collapse.

Changes in force and extent: may be increased by hypertrophy of heart, excited action of heart from exercise or drugs, reflex irritation, excitement, or disease (as exophthalmic goiter).

Displacement to the left: may result from hypertrophy and dilatation of the heart (down and to the left); pneumothorax on the right; pericardial effusion (up and to left); chronic diseases of left lung and pleura associated with retraction, as fibroid phthisis and pleural adhesions; abdominal tumors and effusions (up and to left); pressure of a pleural effusion on the right side (up and to left).

Displacement to right: may be caused by chronic disease of the right lung or pleura associated with retraction; pneumothorax on the left; pressure of a pleural effusion on the left side.

Displacement downward may result from hypertrophy and dilatation of heart, chiefly the left ventricle; pressure of solid growths in upper mediastinum; aneurysm of aortic arch; enlargement of liver, causing traction through central tendon of diaphragm.

Precordial prominence: may result from deformity, enlargement of heart, pericardial effusions.

apex cardiogram. Graphic record of the movements of the chest wall produced by the apex beat.

apexigraph, apexograph (ā-pĕks'ĭ-grăf, -ō-graf) [L. *apex,* tip, + Gr. *graphein,* to write]. An instrument for determining location and size of apex of a tooth root.

apex murmur. Murmur over the apex of the heart.

Apgar score. [Virginia Apgar, U.S. anesthesiologist, 1909–1974]. System of scoring infant's physical condition one minute after birth. The heart rate, respiration, muscle tone, response to stimuli, and color are each rated 0, 1, or 2. The maximum total score is 10. Those with low scores require immediate attention if they are to survive. The test may be repeated at 5 or more minutes after birth in order to judge recovery of infants with low scores. SEE: Apgar Score table.

A.P.H.A. *American Public Health Association.*

aphacia (ă-fā'sē-ă). Aphakia, q.v.

aphacic (ă-fā'sĭk). Aphakic, q.v.

aphagia (ă-fā'jē-ă) [Gr. *a-,* not, + *phagein,* to eat]. Inability to swallow.

aphakia (ă-fā'kē-ă) [" + *phakos,* lentil]. Absence of the crystalline lens of the eye.

aphakic (ă-fā'kĭk). Pert. to aphakia.

aphalangia (ă"fă-lăn'jē-ă) [" + *phalanx,* row].

Apgar Score

Sign	Score 0	1	2
Heart rate	Absent	Slow (less than 100)	Greater than 100
Respiratory effort	Absent	Slow, irregular	Good; crying
Muscle tone	Limp	Some flexion of extremities	Active motion
Reflex irritability	No response	Grimace	Cough or sneeze
Color	Blue, pale	Body pink; extremities blue	Completely pink

Absence of fingers or toes.

aphanisis (ă-făn′ĭ-sĭs) [Gr. *aphaneia,* disappearance]. Fear or apprehension that sexual potency will be lost.

aphasia (ă-fā′zē-ă) [Gr. *a-,* not, + *phasis,* speaking]. Absence or impairment of the ability to communicate through speech, writing, or signs, due to dysfunction of brain centers. It is considered to be complete or total when both sensory and motor areas are involved. SEE: *alalia.*

a., amnesic. Loss of memory for words.

a., anomic. Inability to name objects.

a., ataxic. A., motor, q.v.

a., auditory. Inability to understand spoken words. SYN: *amnesia, auditory; deafness, word.*

a., Broca's. A., motor, q.v.

a., conduction. Aphasia due to lesion of conduction path between motor and speech centers.

a., expressive. A., motor, q.v.

a., fluent. Aphasia in which words are easily spoken but those used are incorrect and may be unrelated to the content of the other words spoken.

a., gibberish. Utterance of meaningless phrases.

a., global. Aphasia involving failure of expression and perception of language as well as other means of communication.

a., jargon. Communication that results in the use of jargon or disconnected words.

a., mixed. Combined sensory and motor aphasia.

a., motor. Aphasia in which patients know what they want to say but cannot say it. Inability to coordinate muscles controlling speech. May be complete or partial. Broca's area is disordered or diseased. SYN: *a., ataxic; a., expressive.*

a., nominal. Inability to name objects.

a., optic. Inability to call name of an object recognized by sight without the aid of sound, taste, or touch; a form of agnosia, q.v.

a., receptive. A., sensory, q.v.

a., semantic. Inability to understand meaning of words.

a., sensory. Inability to understand spoken words if auditory word center is involved (auditory aphasia) or the written word if visual word center is affected (visual aphasia). If both centers are involved, patient will not understand spoken or written word. SYN: *aphemesthesia.*

a., syntactic. Loss of proper grammatical construction.

a., traumatic. Aphasia caused by head injury.

a., visual. Inability to understand the written word. SYN: *word blindness.*

a., Wernicke's. A., sensory, q.v.

aphasic, aphasiac (ă-fā′zĭk, ă-fā′zē-ăk). Pert. to aphasia.

aphasiologist (ă-fā″zē-ŏl′ō-jĭst) [Gr. *a-,* not, + *phasis,* speaking, + *logos,* study]. Person who studies the pathology of language.

aphemesthesia (ă-fĕm″ĕs-thē′zē-ă) [″ + *pheme,* speech, + *aisthesis,* sensation]. Inability to understand words; sensory aphasia.

aphemia (ă-fē′mē-ă) [″ + *pheme,* speech]. 1. Loss of the power to speak. SYN: *aphasia, motor.* 2. Loss of the power to speak distinctly. SYN: *anarthria.*

aphephobia (af″ĕ-fō′bē-ă) [Gr. *haphe,* touch, + *phobos,* fear]. Morbid fear of being touched.

apheresis (ă-fĕr′ĕ-sĭs) [Gr. *aphairesis,* separation]. Technique of separating blood into components. These components may be further processed for special purposes such as removing toxic or unwanted substances from the blood. The technique is quite expensive.

aphonia (ă-fō′nē-ă) [″ + *phone,* voice]. Inability to produce speech sounds from larynx. Not caused by a brain lesion. May occur in chronic laryngitis.

ETIOL: Disease of vocal cords, paralysis of

laryngeal nerves, pressure on recurrent laryngeal nerve; or it may be functional due to hysteria or psychiatric causes.

a. paralytica. Aphonia resulting from paralysis of speech muscles.

a. paranoica. Obstinate silence in the mentally ill.

a., spastic. Aphonia resulting from spasm of vocal muscles, esp. that initiated by efforts to speak.

aphonogelia (ă-fō″nō-jē′lē-ă) [″ + *phone,* voice, + *gelos,* laughter]. Inability to laugh out loud.

aphose (ăf′ōz) [″ + *phos,* light]. A subjective visual perception of darkness, or of a shadow.

aphrasia (ă-frā′zē-ă) [″ + *phrasis,* speech]. Inability to speak or understand phrases.

aphrenia (ă-frē′nē-ă) [″ + *phren,* mind]. Dementia.

aphrenic, aphrenous (ă-frĕn′ĭk, -ŭs). Pert. to dementia.

aphrodisia (ăf″rō-dĭz′ē-ă) [Gr. *aphrodisios,* rel. to *Aphrodite,* goddess of love]. Sexual passion, esp. when excessive.

aphrodisiac (ăf″rō-dĭz′ē-ăk). An agent that stimulates sexual desire.

aphthae (ăf′thē) [Gr. *aphtha,* small ulcer]. Small ulcers on a mucous membrane of the mouth, as in thrush.

a., Bednar's. Whitish ulceration of the posterior hard palate in infants.

a., cachectic. Lesions formed beneath the tongue; accompanied by severe constitutional symptoms.

aphthoid (ăf′thoyd). Resembling aphthae.

aphthongia (ăf-thŏn′jē-ă) [Gr. *a-,* not, + *phthongos,* voice]. Inability to speak due to spasm of muscles controlling speech.

aphthosis (ăf-thō′sĭs) [Gr. *aphtha,* small ulcer, + *osis,* condition]. Any condition characterized by aphthae.

aphthous (ăf′thŭs) [Gr. *aphtha,* small ulcer]. Pert. to, or characterized by, aphthae.

aphylactic (ă″fĭ-lăk′tĭk) [Gr. *a-,* not, + *phylaxis,* a protecting]. Lacking immunity.

aphylaxis (ă-fĭ-lăk′sĭs). Absence of immunity.

apical (ăp′ĭ-kal, ā′pĭ-kal) [L. *apex,* tip]. Pert. to the apex of a structure.

apicectomy (ăp″ĭ-sĕk′tō-mē) [L. *apex,* tip, + Gr. *ektome,* excision]. 1. Excision of the apex of the petrous portion of the temporal bone. 2. Former term for apicoectomy, q.v.

apices (ā′pĭ-sēz, ăp′ĭ-sēz) [L.]. Pl. of apex.

apicitis (ăp-ĭ-sī′tĭs) [L. *apices,* tips, + Gr. *itis,* inflammation]. Inflammation of an apex, esp. apex of lung or tooth root.

apicoectomy (ăp-ĭ-kō-ĕk′tō-mē) [L. *apex,* tip, + Gr. *ektome,* excision]. Excision of the apex of a tooth root.

apicolocator (ă″pĭ-kō-lō′kā-tor) [″ + *locare,* to place]. Instrument for locating apex of a tooth root.

apicolysis (ăp″ĭ-kŏl′ĭ-sĭs) [″ + Gr. *lysis,* dissolution]. Artificial collapse of the apex of a lung by making an opening through the anterior chest wall.

NURSING IMPLICATIONS: Explain the procedure to the patient; during the procedure, assess the patient for symptoms of anxiety, and provide support for the patient. During and after the procedure, assess for symptoms indicative of a tension pneumothorax, such as increased pulse and respirations, cyanosis, and marked dyspnea. Also assess for symptoms of a mediastinal shift, such as cyanosis, severe dyspnea, distended neck veins, increased pulse and respiratory rate, and excessive, uncontrolled coughing.

Following the procedure, the patient is most frequently positioned on the affected side.

apicostomy (ăp″ĭ-kŏs′tō-mē) [L. *apex,* tip, + Gr. *stoma,* mouth]. Surgical removal of the mucoperiosteum and bone in order to expose the apex of the root of the tooth.

apicotomy (ăp″ĭ-kŏt′ō-mē) [L. *apex,* tip, + Gr. *tome,* incision]. Incision of an apical structure.

apinealism (ă-pĭn′ē-ăl-ĭzm) [Gr. *a-,* not, + L. *pinea,* pine cone, + Gr. *-ismos,* condition]. Absence of pineal gland.

apituitarism (ă″pĭ-tū′ĭ-tăr-ĭzm) [″ + L. *pituita,* phlegm, + *-ismos,* condition]. Loss of pituitary function or removal of pituitary body. Leads to dwarfism or pituitary cachexia. SEE: *hypophysectomy; Simmonds' disease.*

A.P.L. Trade name for chorionic gonadotropin, human, USP, q.v.

aplanatic lens (ă″plă-năt′ĭk lĕnz) [″ + *planetos,* wandering]. A lens that corrects spherical aberration.

aplasia (ă-plā′zē-ă) [″ + *plasis,* a developing]. Failure of an organ or tissue to develop normally.

a. axialis extracorticalis congenita. Congenital defect of the axon formation on the surface of the cerebral cortex.

a. cutis congenita. Defective development of localized area of skin, usually on the scalp. Area is usually covered by a thin, translucent membrane

a., gonadal. Congenital absence of gonadal tissue.

aplastic (ă-plăs′tĭk) [″ + *plastikos,* shaped]. Pert. to aplasia; having deficient or arrested development.

aplastic anemia. Anemia caused by deficient red cell production due to disorders of bone marrow.

ETIOL: Approx. half of the cases are idiopathic; most common in adolescents and young adults. Exposure to chemical and antineoplastic agents, and ionizing radiation can result in aplastic anemia. A congenital form has been described.

apnea (ăp-nē′ă) [″ + *pnoe,* breathing]. Temporary cessation of breathing. May result from reduction in stimuli to the respiratory center, as in overbreathing, in which carbon dioxide content of the blood is reduced; from failure of respiratory center to discharge impulses, as when the breath is held voluntarily; or during Cheyne-Stokes respiration.

It is a serious symptom, esp. in such conditions as arteriosclerosis, meningitis, coma, heart and kidney diseases, and also following an injury to the brain where concussion results. Sometimes Cheyne-Stokes respiration is noticed in perfectly healthy children and in the aged during profound sleep. SEE: *Cheyne-Stokes respiration; sudden infant death syndrome; sleep apnea.*

a., sleep. SEE: *sleep apnea.*

apnea alarm mattress. A mattress that is designed to sound an alarm when the infant lying on it ceases to breathe. SEE: *sudden infant death syndrome.*

apneic oxygenation. The supplying of oxygen to the upper airway of patients who are not breathing.

apneumatic (ăp″nū-măt′ĭk) [Gr. *a-,* not, + *pneuma,* air]. 1. Free of air, as in a collapsed lung. 2. Pert. to a procedure done in the absence of air.

apneumatosis (ăp″nū-mă-tō′sĭs) [″ + ″ + *osis,* condition]. Noninflation of air cells of lung; congenital atelectasis.

apneumia (ăp-nū′mē-ă) [″ + *pneumon,* lung]. Congenital absence of the lungs.

apneusis (ăp-nū′sĭs). Abnormal respiration marked by sustained inspiratory effort. Caused by surgical removal of the upper portion of the pons.

apo- (ăp′ō) [Gr. *apo,* from]. Prefix denoting separation or derivation from.

apobiosis (ăp″ō-bī-ō′sĭs) [″ + *bios,* life]. Death, esp. death of a part.

apocamnosis (ăp″ō-kăm-nō′sĭs) [Gr. *apokamnein,* to grow weary]. Weariness, easily induced fatigue.

apochromatic lens (ăp″ō-krō-măt′ĭk). A lens that corrects both spherical and chromatic aberrations.

apocope (ă-pŏk′ō-pē) [Gr. *apokope,* a cutting off]. Amputation.

apocoptic (ăp-ō-kŏp′tĭk). Pert. to or resulting from amputation.

apocrine (ăp′ō-krēn, -krīn, -krĭn) [Gr. *apo,* from, + *krinein,* to separate]. Denoting secretory cells that contribute part of their protoplasm to the material secreted. SEE: *eccrine; holocrine; merocrine.*

apocrine sweat glands. Sweat glands located in the axillae and pubic region that open into hair follicles rather than directly onto the surface of the skin as do eccrine sweat glands, q.v. They appear after puberty and are better developed in women than in men. The characteristic odor of perspiration is produced by the action of bacteria on the material secreted by the apocrine sweat glands. SEE: *sweat gland.*

apocrustic (ăp″ō-krŭs′tĭk) [Gr. *apokroustikos,* able to ward off]. 1. Astringent and repellent. 2. An astringent and repellent agent.

apodal (ă-pō′dăl) [Gr. *a-,* not, + *pous,* foot]. Lacking feet.

apodemialgia (ăp″ō-dē″mē-ăl′jē-ă) [Gr. *apodemia,* away from home, + *algos,* pain]. An abnormal desire to leave home; wanderlust. Opposite of nostalgia.

apodia (ă-pō′dē-ă) [Gr. *a-,* not, + *pous,* foot]. Congenital absence of one or both feet.

apoenzyme (ăp-ō-ĕn′zīm). The protein portion of an enzyme. SEE: *holoenzyme; prosthetic group.*

apoferritin (ăp″ō-fĕr′ĭ-tĭn). A protein that combines with iron to form ferritin. It is not found in the body except attached to iron.

apogee (ăp′ō-jē) [Gr. *apo,* from, + *gaia,* earth]. The climax or period of greatest severity of a disease.

apokamnosis (ăp″ō-kăm-nō′sĭs). Apocamnosis, q.v.

apolar (ă-pō′lăr) [Gr. *a-,* not, + *polos,* pole]. Without poles or processes. Some nerve cells are apolar.

apolepsis (ăp″ō-lĕp′sĭs) [Gr. *apolepsis,* a leaving off]. 1. Cessation of a function. 2. Retention or suppression of an excretion or secretion.

apomorphine (ăp″ō-mor′fēn) [Gr. *apo,* from, + *morphine*]. A morphine derivative prepared by removal of one molecule of water from morphine.

a. hydrochloride. A grayish white powder that becomes green on exposure to water or air. Emetic; sometimes valuable in cases of poisoning when gastric lavage cannot be employed. In small doses it may be used as an expectorant.

aponeurology (ăp″ō-nū-rŏl′ō-jē) [″ + *neuron,* nerve, tendon, + *logos,* study]. The branch of anatomy dealing with aponeuroses.

aponeurorrhaphy (ăp″ō-nū-ror′ă-fē) [″ + ″ + *rhaphe,* seam]. Suture of an aponeurosis.

aponeurosis (ăp″ō-nū-rō′sĭs) [″ + *neuron,* nerve, tendon]. (pl. *aponeuroses*) A flat fibrous sheet of connective tissue that serves to attach muscle to bone or other tissues. May sometimes serve as a fascia, q.v.

a., epicranial. Fibrous membrane connecting the occipital and frontal muscles. SYN: *galea aponeurotica.*

a., lingual. Connective tissue sheet of the tongue to which lingual muscles attach.

a., palatine. Connective tissue sheet of

the soft palate to which palatal muscles attach.

a., pharyngeal. Sheet of connective tissue lying between the mucosal and muscular layers of the pharyngeal wall. SYN: *fascia, pharyngobasilar.*

a., plantar. Sheet of connective tissue investing the muscles of the sole of the foot. SYN: *fascia, plantar.*

aponeurositis (ăp"ō-nū-rō-sī'tĭs) [" + " + *itis,* inflammation]. Inflammation of an aponeurosis.

aponeurotic (ăp"ō-nū-rŏt'ĭk) [" + *neuron,* nerve, tendon]. Pert. to an aponeurosis.

aponeurotome (ăp"ō-nū'rō-tōm) [" + " + *tome,* incision]. Surgical instrument for cutting an aponeurosis.

aponeurotomy (ăp"ō-nū-rŏt'ō-mē). Incision of an aponeurosis.

aponia (ă-pŏn'ē-ă) [Gr. *a-,* not, + *ponos,* toil, pain]. 1. Abstaining from exertion. 2. Absence of pain.

aponic (ă-pŏn'ĭk). 1. Rel. to aponia. 2. Relieving pain or fatigue.

apophyseal, apophysial (ăp"ō-fĭz'ē-ăl) [" + *physis,* growth]. Pert. to an apophysis.

apophysis (ă-pŏf'ĭ-sĭs) [Gr. *apophysis,* offshoot]. (pl. *apophyses*) [NA] A projection esp. from a bone, an outgrowth without an independent center of ossification.

Ex.: a tubercle.

a., basilar. Basilar process of the occipital bone.

a., lenticular. Lenticular process of the incus, which articulates with the stapes.

a. of Ingrassia. Smaller wing of sphenoid bone.

a. of Rau, a. raviana. Anterior process of malleus.

a., temporal. Mastoid process of the temporal bone.

apophysitis (ă-pŏf"ĭ-sī'tĭs) [" + *physis,* growth, + *itis,* inflammation]. Inflammation of an apophysis.

apoplectic (ăp"ō-plĕk'tĭk) [Gr. *apoplektikos,* crippled by stroke]. Pert. to apoplexy.

apoplectiform (ăp"ō-plĕk'tĭ-form) [Gr. *apoplexia,* stroke, + L. *forma,* appearance]. Resembling apoplexy. SYN: *apoplectoid.*

apoplectoid (ăp"ō-plĕk'toyd) [" + *eidos,* form]. Resembling apoplexy. SYN: *apoplectiform.*

apoplexia (ăp"ō-plĕk'sē-ă) [Gr. *apoplessein,* to cripple by a stroke]. Apoplexy, q.v.

a. uteri. Sudden hemorrhage from the uterus.

apoplexy (ăp'ō-plĕk"sē) [Gr. *apoplessein,* to cripple by a stroke]. 1. Copious effusion of blood into an organ, as abdominal apoplexy; pulmonary apoplexy. 2. Sudden loss of consciousness followed by paralysis caused by hemorrhage into brain, formation of an embolus or thrombus that occludes an artery, or rupture of an extracerebral artery causing subarachnoid hemorrhage. SYN: *cerebrovascular accident; stroke,* q.v.

SYM: Onset acute. Unconsciousness. Stertorous respiration due to paralysis of portion of the soft palate; expiration puffs out the cheeks and mouth. Pupils sometimes unequal, the larger one being on the side of the hemorrhage. Paralysis usually involves one side of the body, with eyeballs turned away from the affected side, skin covered with clammy sweat, surface temperature of skin is often subnormal; speech disturbances. Onset more gradual if caused by a thrombosis, q.v.

F.A.: In hospital or at home keep patient, if conscious, quiet and sitting up or lying down with head and shoulders elevated. This will help to prevent aspiration of saliva. Loosen clothing, esp. around the neck. Do not give stimulants. Apply cooling applications to head and neck.

PROG: Depends upon symptoms. Often poor.

NURSING IMPLICATIONS: *During initial attack:* Ensure maintenance of a patent airway by positioning patient in a prone position, or with head turned to the side; loosen clothing at throat. Keep patient warm and quiet.

During convalescence: Assess the patient's neurological status to detect changes in status or development of complications. Assist in determining when foods and fluids may be initiated; assess the patient's ability to swallow. Maintain good body alignment and do range of motion exercises to prevent contracture formation. Measure and record intake and output, and evaluate patient's bowel status daily. Change patient's position frequently, and have patient cough and breathe deeply to prevent respiratory complications. Take care to prevent other complications of immobilization.

Provide support and encouragement as the patient works to retrain muscles and regain lost function. Encourage any attempt to communicate with the eyes, voice, or hands. Establish a plan with the patient and family to promote patient orientation, verbal and nonverbal communication and intellectual function, and to help the patient regain lost skills in order to encourage independence.

apoptosis (ă-pŏp-tō'sĭs, ă-pō-tō'sĭs) [Gr. *apo,* from, + *ptosis,* a falling]. Disintegration of cells into membrane-bound particles that are then phagocytosed by other cells. The process may be important in limiting growth of tumors.

aporepressor (ăp"ō-rē-prĕs'or). The protein, the synthesis of which is directed by a regulator gene, that functions only when bound with specific low-molecular weight compounds called corepressors.

aposia (ă-pō'zē-ă) [Gr. *a-*, not, + *posis*, drink]. Absence of thirst. SYN: *adipsia*.

aposiopesis (ăp"ō-sī"ō-pē'sĭs) [Gr., to become silent]. Sudden cessation of speech in the middle of a sentence as if unable or unwilling to continue.

apositia (ăp"ō-sĭt'ē-ă, -sĭsh'ē-ă) [Gr. *apo*, away, + *sitos*, food]. Aversion to food.

apostasis (ă-pŏs'tă-sĭs) [Gr., departure from]. 1. The crisis or end of a disease. 2. An abscess.

apostem, apostema (ăp'ō-stĕm, -stē'mă) [Gr. *apostema*, abscess]. An abscess.

aposthia (ă-pŏs'thē-ă) [Gr. *a-*, not, + *posthe*, foreskin]. Congenital absence of the prepuce.

apotemnophilia (ăp"ō-tĕm"nō-fĕl'ē-ă) [Gr., amputation love]. A form of paraphilia characterized by the individual requesting amputation of an extremity for erotic reasons.

apothanasia (ăp"ō-thă-nā'zē-ă) [Gr. *apo*, away, + *thanatos*, death]. Prolongation of life.

apothecaries' weights and measures. An outdated and obsolete system of weights and measures formerly used by physicians and pharmacists based on 480 grains = 1 ounce and 12 ounces = 1 pound. Has been replaced by the metric system, q.v. SEE: *Weights and Measures* in *Appendix*.

apothecary (ă-pŏth'ĕ-kā-rē) [Gr. *apotheke*, storing place]. A druggist or pharmacist. In England and Ireland, one licensed by the Society of Apothecaries of London or the Apothecaries' Hall of Ireland as an authorized physician and dispenser of drugs.

apothem, apotheme (ăp'ō-thĕm, -thēm) [Gr. *apo*, from, + *thema*, deposit]. The brown precipitate that appears when vegetable decoctions or infusions are exposed to the air or are boiled a long time.

apotripsis (ăp"ō-trĭp'sĭs) [Gr. *apotribein*, to abrade]. Removal of corneal opacity.

A-poxide. Trade name for chlordiazepoxide hydrochloride, USP, q.v.

apparatus (ăp"ă-rā'tŭs, -răt'ŭs) [L. *apparare*, to prepare]. 1. A number of parts acting together in the performance of some special function. 2. A group of structures or organs that work together to perform a common function. 3. A mechanical appliance or appliances, used in operations and experiments.

a., acoustic. Auditory apparatus, the assemblage of parts essential for hearing.

a., biliary. The structures concerned with secretion and excretion of bile. Includes liver, gallbladder, and hepatic, cystic, and common bile ducts.

a., Clover's. A device used in administering ether or chloroform.

a., Fell-O'Dwyer's. An instrument for performing artificial respiration and for preventing collapse of the lung in chest operations.

a., Golgi. SEE: *Golgi apparatus*.

a., juxtaglomerular. Thickened portion of an afferent arteriole in the cortex of a kidney. Consists of modified smooth muscles that acquire a clear swollen appearance.

a., lacrimal. The tear-secreting gland and the lacrimal duct, which provides the passageway for the tears from the eye to the nasal cavity. SEE: *lacrimal apparatus* for illus.

a., respiratory. The respiratory system.

a., sound-conducting. Those parts of the acoustic apparatus that transmit sound.

a., sound-perceiving. Those parts of the acoustic apparatus that are essential for the perception of sounds.

a., urogenital. The genitourinary system.

a., vocal. The collection of organs that produce sounds and thus speech phonation.

appendage (ă-pĕn'dĭj). Anything attached or appended to a larger or major part, as a tail or a limb. SEE: *appendix*.

a., atrial. A small muscular pouch attached to each atrium of the heart.

a., auricular. A., atrial, q.v.

a.'s of the eye. The eyelid, eyelashes, eyebrow, lacrimal apparatus, and conjunctiva.

a.'s of the fetus. The amnion, chorion, and umbilical cord.

a.'s of the skin. The nails, hair, sebaceous and sweat glands.

a., uterine. The ovaries, fallopian tubes, and uterine ligaments.

appendalgia (ăp"ĕn-dăl'jē-ă) [L. *appendere*, hang to, + Gr. *algos*, pain]. Pain in lower right quadrant in region of vermiform appendix.

appendectomy (ăp"ĕn-dĕk'tō-mē) [" + Gr. *ektome*, excision]. Surgical removal of the vermiform appendix.

a., incidental. Removal of the appendix at the time of another surgical procedure in the abdominal cavity.

appendical, appendiceal (ă-pĕn'dĭ-kăl, ăp-ĕn-dĭs'ē-ăl). Pert. to an appendix.

appendical reflex. Tenderness at McBurney's point accompanied by rigidity, considered a reflex expression by way of sympathetic cerebrospinal arc.

appendicectasis (ă-pĕn"dĭ-sĕk'tă-sĭs) [L. *appendere*, hang to, + Gr. *ektasis*, a stretching]. Dilatation of the vermiform appendix.

appendicectomy (ă-pĕn"dĭ-sĕk'tō-mē) [" + Gr. *ektome*, excision]. Surgical removal of the appendix.

appendices (ă-pĕn'dĭ-sēz). Pl. of appendix, q.v.

appendicitis (ă-pĕn"dĭ-sī'tĭs) [L. *appendere*,

hang to, + Gr. *itis,* inflammation]. Inflammation of the vermiform appendix. It generally occurs in the young, most often between ages 15 and 25, and very rarely before the fifth year or after the fiftieth. It is more common in adult males than in females. The disease may be acute, subacute, or chronic. When this diagnosis is considered in the adult female, it must be differentiated from pain associated with ovulation (mittelschmerz, q.v.), ruptured ectopic pregnancy, and pelvic inflammatory disease.

a., acute. SYM: Abdominal pain, usually severe and generally throughout the abdomen, followed by nausea and vomiting; localization of pain in the right lower quadrant of abdomen with tenderness and rigidity over right rectus muscle or McBurney's point; fever usually rising within several hours, 99°–101° F. (37.2°–38.3° C.); pulse increasing with temperature; patient lying on back with right lower extremity frequently flexed to relieve muscle tension; leukocytosis present shortly after onset. In mild cases symptoms begin to subside on the second day. A well-defined abscess usually develops 24 to 72 hours after the onset of symptoms and may be palpable in the right ileocecal region.

NURSING IMPLICATIONS: *Pre-op:* Carefully assess the patient for signs and symptoms that will assist in the diagnosis of appendicitis such as: elevated temperature; nausea or vomiting; onset, intensity, and location of pain; rebound tenderness; constipation or diarrhea; and an elevated white blood cell count. The patient should be placed in a position of comfort. Prepare the patient physically and emotionally for surgery.

CAUTION: No cathartics or enemas should be administered to a patient with suspected appendicitis.

Post-op: The patient is positioned comfortably (Fowler's position if the patient had a ruptured appendix or peritonitis). Administer prescribed medications to keep the patient comfortable. Change patient's position, have patient cough and breathe deeply, and encourage early ambulation to prevent respiratory complications. Observe the dressing for presence of any bleeding or drainage. Closely monitor I.V. fluids, and measure and record the patient's intake and output.

a., chronic. May follow an acute attack leaving a cicatricial narrowing of the lumen of the appendix, or adhesions.

SYM: Gastric indigestion, frequently simulating a gastric ulcer, duodenal ulcer, or gallbladder disease. Tenderness manifested in the right lower abdomen.

TREATMENT: Surgical.

a., gangrenous. When inflammation is extreme, blood vessels are blocked in the mesentery, circulation to appendix is cut off, and diffuse peritonitis ensues.

appendicoenterostomy (ă-pĕn″dĭk-ō-ĕn″tĕr-ŏs′tō-mē) [L. *appendere,* hang to, + Gr. *enteron,* intestine, + *stoma,* mouth]. 1. Appendicostomy, q.v. 2. The establishment of an anastomosis between appendix and intestine.

appendicolithiasis (ă-pĕn″dĭ-kō″lĭ-thī′ă-sĭs) [″ + Gr. *lithos,* stone, + *-iasis,* state]. Formation of calculi in the vermiform appendix.

appendicolysis (ă-pĕn″dĭ-kŏl′ĭ-sĭs) [″ + Gr. *lysis,* a loosening]. Operation that frees appendix from adhesions. This is done by slitting the serosa at its base.

appendicopathy (ă-pĕn″dĭ-kŏp′ă-thē) [″ + Gr. *pathos,* disease]. Any disease of the vermiform appendix.

a. oxyurica. Lesion of the appendical mucosa supposedly due to oxyurids (intestinal parasitic worms).

appendicostomy (ă-pĕn′dĭ-kŏs′tō-mē) [″ + Gr. *stoma,* mouth]. Operation in which an opening is made in the vermiform appendix for the purpose of irrigating the cecum and colon.

appendicular (ăp″ĕn-dĭk′ū-lăr) [L. *appendere,* to hang to]. 1. Pert. to an appendix. SYN: *appendiceal.* 2. Pert. to the extremities, as opposed to axial, which pertains to the head and trunk.

appendix (ă-pĕn′dĭks) [L.]. (pl. *appendixes, appendices*) [NA] An appendage, esp. the appendix vermiformis. SEE: *digestive system* and *omentum* for illus. SYN: *appendage.*

a., atrial. A small muscular pouch attached to each atrium of the heart.

a., auricular. A., atrial, q.v.

a., ensiform. The lowest portion of the sternum. SYN: *a., xiphoid; xiphoid process.*

a. epididymidis. [NA] A cystic structure attached to the epididymis, a vestigial remnant of the mesonephric duct.

a. epiploica. One of numerous pouches of peritoneum, filled with fat and attached to the colon.

a. testis. [NA] Small bladderlike structure at upper end of testis, a vestigial remnant of cephalic portion of müllerian duct.

a., ventricular. Saccule, laryngeal, q.v.

a. vermiformis. [NA] A worm-shaped process projecting from the blind end of the cecum and lined with a continuation of the mucous membrane of the cecum. SYN: *processus vermiformis; vermiform appendix.*

a., vesicular. A cystic structure attached to the fimbriated end of the uterine tube. It is a vestigial remnant of the mesonephric duct.

a., xiphoid. The xiphoid process; small, lowest portion of the sternum. SYN: *a., ensiform; xiphoid process.*

apperception (ăp″ĕr-sĕp′shŭn) [L. *ad,* to, + *percipere,* to perceive]. The perception and interpretation of sensory stimuli.

apperceptive (ăp″ĕr-sĕp′tĭv). Pert. to apperception.

appestat (ăp′ĕ-stăt) [L. *appetitus,* longing for, + Gr. *states,* stand]. Area of brain (probably in the hypothalamus) that is thought to control appetite and food intake.

appetence, appetency (ăp′ĕ-tĕns, -tĕn-sē) [L. *appetere,* to strive for]. A strong appetite or desire.

appetite (ăp′ĕ-tīt) [L. *appetitus,* longing for]. Strong desire, especially for food. Appetite is differentiated from hunger in that the latter is a painful sensation caused by lack of food, whereas appetite is a pleasant sensation based on previous experience that causes one to seek food for the purpose of tasting and enjoying.

a., perverted. Desire to eat unnatural and indigestible substances such as paint or laundry starch. SYN: *pica.*

appetite, words pert. to: acoria; anorexia; apositia; bulimia; dysorexia; hyperorexia; malacia; parageusia; pica; polyphagia; taste.

appetition (ăp″ĕ-tĭsh′ŭn) [L. *appetere,* to strive for]. Desire directed toward a specific goal or object.

appetizer (ăp′ĕ-tī″zĕr). That which promotes appetite.

applanation (ăp″lă-nā′shŭn) [L. *ad,* toward, + *planare,* to flatten]. Abnormal flattening, esp. of the corneal surface.

applanometer (ăp″lă-nŏm′ĕ-tĕr) [″ + *planum,* plane, + Gr. *metron,* measure]. Device for measuring intraocular pressure. SEE: *tonometer.*

apple, Adam's. The laryngeal prominence formed by the two laminae of the thyroid cartilage.

apple packer's epistaxis. Nosebleed due to handling packing trays containing certain dyes.

apple picker's disease. Bronchitis resulting from a fungicide used on apples.

apple sorter's disease. Contact dermatitis caused by chemicals used in washing apples.

appliance (ă-plī′ăns). In dentistry, a device used to provide or facilitate a particular function, such as artificial dentures; device used to correct bite.

applicator (ăp′lĭ-kā″tor) [L. *applicare,* to attach]. Device, usually a slender rod with a pledget of cotton on the end, for making local applications.

apposition (ăp″ō-zĭ′shŭn) [L. *ad,* toward, + *ponere,* to place]. 1. Condition of being positioned side by side or fitted together. SYN: *contiguity.* 2. The adding of one substance to another one as one layer of tissue upon another. 3. Developing by means of accretion as would be the case in bone or dental cement formation.

approach (ă-prōch′). Surgical procedures for exposing an organ or tissue.

approximal (ă-prŏk′sĭ-măl) [″ + *proximus,* nearest]. Contiguous; next to.

approximate (ă-prŏk′sĭ-māt) [″ + *proximare,* to come near]. To bring close together.

apraxia (ă-prăk′sē-ă) [Gr. *a-,* not, + *praxis,* action]. 1. Inability to perform purposive movements although there is no sensory or motor impairment. 2. Inability to use objects properly.

a., akinetic. Inability to carry out spontaneous movements.

a., amnesic. Inability to produce a movement on command because the command is forgotten, although the ability to perform the movement is present.

a., developmental. A disorder of motor planning and execution occurring in developing children; thought to be due to central nervous system immaturity.

a., ideational. Misuse of objects due to inability to perceive their correct use. SYN: *a., sensory.*

a., motor. Inability to perform movements necessary to use objects properly, although the names and purposes of the objects are known and understood.

a., sensory. A., ideational, q.v.

apraxic. Pert. to or characterized by apraxia.

Apresoline. Trade name for hydralazine hydrochloride, USP, q.v.

aproctia (ă-prŏk′shē-ă) [Gr. *a-,* not, + *proktos,* anus]. Absence or imperforation of anus.

apron (ā′prŏn) [O. Fr. *naperon,* cloth]. 1. Outer garment covering front of the body for protection of clothing during surgery, during certain nursing procedures, while working with plaster of Paris, etc. 2. Part of the body resembling an apron.

a., Hottentot. Abnormally long labia minora. SYN: *velamen vulvae.*

aprosody (ă-prŏs′ō-dē) [Gr. *a-,* not, + *prosodia,* voice modulation]. Absence of normal variations of pitch, rhythm, and stress in the speech.

aprosopia (ăp″rō-sō′pē-ă) [″ + *prosopon,* face]. Congenital defect in which part or all of the face is absent.

apselaphesia (ăp″sĕl-ă-fē′zē-ă) [″ + *pselaphesis,* feeling]. Absence of tactile sense.

apsithyria (ăp″sĭ-thĭ′rē-ă) [″ + *psithyrizein,* to whisper]. Hysterical loss of voice including ability to whisper.

apsychia (ăp-sēk′ē-ă, -sī′kē-ă) [″ + *psyche,* mind]. Unconsciousness; a faint.

APT. *alum-precipitated toxoid.*

A.P.T.A. *American Physical Therapy Association.*

aptitude (ăp′tĭ-tūd). Inherent ability or skill

in learning or performing physical or mental endeavors.

aptitude test. A mental or physical (or both) test designed to evaluate skill or ability to perform certain tasks or assignments.

aptyalia, aptyalism (ăp″tē-ā′lē-ă, ăp-tē′ă-lĭzm, ă-tī′ă-lĭzm) [″ + *ptyalon,* saliva]. Absence or deficiency of secretion of saliva. SYN: *asialia; dry mouth; oligosialia; xerostomia.*

ETIOL: Disease (mumps, typhoid fever); dehydration; effect of drugs; x-ray irradiation; old age; obstruction of salivary ducts; Sjögren's syndrome, in which there is deficient secretion of lacrimal, salivary, and other glands.

apulmonism (ă-pool′mŏn-ĭzm) [Gr. *a-,* not, + L. *pulmo,* lung, + Gr. *-ismos,* condition]. Congenital absence of part or all of a lung.

apus (ā′pŭs) [″ + *pous,* foot]. A person who has apodia, congenital absence of the feet.

apyetous (ă-pī′ĕ-tŭs) [″ + *pyesis,* suppuration]. Nonsuppurative, nonpurulent. SYN: *apyous.*

apyknomorphous (ă-pĭk″nō-mor′fŭs) [″ + *pyknos,* thick, + *morphe,* form]. Not pyknomorphous; pert. to a cell that does not stain deeply because its stainable material is scattered.

apyogenous (ā-pī-ŏj′ĕn-ŭs) [″ + *pyon,* pus, + *genos,* origin]. Not due to pus.

apyous (ă-pī′ŭs). Nonsuppurative, nonpurulent. SYN: *apyetous.*

apyretic (ā-pī-rĕt′ĭk) [″ + *pyretos,* fever]. Without fever. SYN: *afebrile.*

apyrexia (ā-pī-rĕks′ē-ă) [″ + *pyrexis,* feverishness]. Absence of fever.

apyrogenetic, apyrogenic (ā″pī-rō-jĕ-nĕt′ĭk, -jĕn′ĭk) [″ + ″ + *genos,* origin]. Not causing fever.

AQ. *achievement quotient.*

aq. L. *aqua,* water.

aqua (awk′wă) [L. *aqua*]. (pl. *aquae*) Water. ABBR: a.; aq.

a. aerata. Carbonated water.

a. ammonia. NH_4OH. Ammonium hydroxide.

a. calcariae. Lime water.

a. camphorae. Camphor water.

a. destillata. Distilled water.

a. fervens. Hot water.

a. fontana. Spring water.

a. fortis. Weak nitric acid.

a. labyrinthi. The fluid in the labyrinth of the ear.

a., medicated. An aqueous solution of a volatile substance. Usually contains only a comparatively small percentage of the active drug. Many are merely water saturated with a volatile oil. They are used more as vehicles and to give odor and taste to solutions.

a. oculi. The fluid (aqueous humor) of the eye.

a. pura. Pure water.

a. purificata. Purified water.

a. regia. Nitrohydrochloric acid water (20% nitric acid and 80% hydrochloric acid). SYN: *nitromuriatic acid.*

a. rosea. Rose water.

a. sterilisata. Sterilized water.

a. tepida. Lukewarm water.

AquaMephyton. Trade name for phytonadione (vitamin K), USP, q.v.

aquanaut (ă′kwă-nawt). An individual who works underwater, esp. researchers in deep-sea environments for an extended length of time.

aquaphobia (ăk″wă-fō′bē-ă) [″ + Gr. *phobos,* fear]. Abnormal fear of water. SEE: *hydrophobia.*

Aquaphor. Trade name for petrolatum, hydrophilic, USP, q.v.

aquapuncture (ăk″wă-pŭngk′chūr) [″ + *punctura,* puncture]. Subcutaneous injection of water, as to produce counterirritation.

Aquatensen. Trade name for methyclothiazide, USP, q.v.

aquatic. 1. Pert. to water. 2. Inhabiting water.

aqueduct (ăk′wĕ-dŭkt″) [″ + *ductus,* duct]. Canal or channel. SYN: *aqueductus.*

a., cerebral. Canal in the midbrain connecting the third and fourth ventricles. SYN: *aqueductus cerebri.*

a., vestibular. Small passage reaching from the vestibule to the posterior surface of the temporal bone's petrous section. SYN: *aqueductus vestibuli.*

aqueductus (ăk″wĕ-dŭk′tŭs). [NA] A canal or channel. SYN: *aqueduct.*

a. cerebri. [NA] Canal in the midbrain connecting the third and fourth ventricles. SYN: *aqueduct, cerebral.*

a. cochleae. Canal connecting subarachnoid space and the perilymphatic space of the cochlea.

a. Fallopii. Canal for facial nerve in the temporal bone.

a. Sylvii. A. cerebri, q.v.

a. vestibuli. [NA] Small passage reaching from the vestibule to the posterior surface of the temporal bone's petrous section.

aqueous (ā′kwē-ŭs) [L. *aqua,* water]. 1. Of the nature of water; watery. 2. Aqueous humor, q.v.

aqueous chambers. Anterior and posterior chambers of the eye, which contain the aqueous humor.

aqueous humor. Transparent liquid contained in the anterior and posterior chambers of the eye. Produced by the ciliary processes, it passes from the posterior to the anterior chamber, and then to the venous system by way of the canal of Schlemm.

aquiparous (ăk-wĭp′ă-rŭs) [″ + L. *parere,* to produce]. Producing water.

AR. *achievement ratio; alarm reaction.*

Ar. Chem. symb. for argon.

ara-A. Vidarabine, USP, q.v.

arabinose (ă-răb′ĭ-nōs). Gum sugar, a pentose obtained from plants. Sometimes found in urine. SYN: *l-arabinose.*

arabinosuria (ă-răb″ĭ-nō-sū′rē-ă) [*arabinose* + Gr. *ouron,* urine]. Arabinose in the urine.

arachnid (ă-răk′nĭd). A member of the class Arachnida.

Arachnida (ă-răk′nĭ-dă) [Gr. *arachne,* spider]. A class of the Arthropoda, including the spiders, scorpions, ticks, and mites.

arachnidism (ă-răk′nĭd-ĭzm) [″ + *eidos,* form, + *-ismos,* condition of]. Systemic poisoning from spider bite. SYN: *arachnoidism.*

arachnitis (ă″răk-nī′tĭs) [″ + *itis,* inflammation]. Inflammation of the arachnoid membrane. SYN: *arachnoiditis.*

arachnodactyly (ă-răk″nō-dăk′tĭl-ē) [″ + *dactylos,* finger]. Spider fingers; a state in which fingers and sometimes toes are abnormally long, slender, and curved. SYN: *acromacria; dolichostenomelia.* SEE: *Marfan's syndrome.*

arachnoid (ă-răk′noyd) [″ + *eidos,* form]. 1. Resembling a web. 2. Arachnoid membrane; arachnoidea, q.v.

a., cranial. Arachnoidea encephali, q.v.

a., spinal. Arachnoidea spinalis, q.v.

arachnoidea (ă-răk-noyd′ē-ă). [NA] A thin, delicate membrane, the intermediate membrane that encloses the brain and spinal cord. It is separated from the pia mater, the inner membrane, by the subarachnoid space and from the dura mater, the outer membrane, by the subdural space. SYN: *arachnoid membrane.*

a. encephali. The part of the arachnoidea enclosing the brain. SYN: *arachnoid, cranial.*

a. spinalis. The part of the arachnoidea enclosing the spinal cord. SYN: *arachnoid, spinal.*

arachnoidism (ă-răk′noyd-ĭzm) [Gr. *arachne,* spider, + *eidos,* form, + *-ismos,* condition]. Systemic poisoning from spider bite. SYN: *arachnidism.* SEE: *spider, black widow.*

arachnoiditis (ă-răk″noyd-ī′tĭs) [″ + *eidos,* form, + *itis,* inflammation]. Inflammation of the arachnoid membrane. SYN: *arachnitis.*

arachnoid membrane. Arachnoidea, q.v.

arachnoid villi. Body, pacchionian, q.v.

arachnolysin (ă-răk-nŏl′ĭ-sĭn) [″ + *lysis,* dissolution]. The hemolysin present in spider venom.

arachnophobia (ă-răk″nō-fō′bē-ă) [″ + *phobos,* fear]. Morbid fear of spiders.

Aralen Hydrochloride. Trade name for chloroquine hydrochloride, USP, q.v.

Aralen Phosphate. Trade name for chloroquine phosphate, USP, q.v.

Aramine. Trade name for metaraminol bitartrate, USP, q.v.

Aran-Duchenne disease (ăr-ŏn′dū-shĕn′). SEE: *Duchenne-Aran disease.* SYN: *progressive muscular atrophy.*

araneous (ă-rā′nē-ŭs) [L. *aranea,* cobweb]. Resembling a cobweb.

Arantius' body, nodule (ăr-ăn′shē-ŭs). (pl. *Arantii*) [Julius Caesar Arantius, It. anatomist and physician, 1530–1589] Small nodule at center of each of the aortic valve cusps. SYN: *noduli valvularum aortae.*

arborescent (ăr″bor-ĕs′ĕnt) [L. *arborescere,* to become a tree]. Branching; treelike.

arborization (ăr″bor-ĭ-zā′shŭn) [L. *arbor,* a tree]. 1. Ramification; branching; esp. terminal branching of nerve fibers and capillaries. SEE: *nerve.*

arbor vitae (ăr′bor vī′tē) [L. *arbor,* tree, + *vita,* life]. 1. A treelike structure; a treelike outline seen in a section of the cerebellum. 2. A tree or shrub of the genus Thuja or Thujopsis. 3. A series of branching ridges within the cervix of the uterus. SYN: *plica palmatae.*

arboviruses (ăr″bō-vī′rŭs-ĕs) [*ar*thropod-*bo*rne *viruses*]. A large group, more than 250, of viruses that multiply in both vertebrates and arthropods such as mosquitoes and ticks. They are known to cause diseases such as yellow fever and viral encephalitis. SEE: *arenaviruses; togavirus.*

arc (ărk) [L. *arcus,* bow]. A curved line; a portion of a circle.

a., reflex. The path followed by a nerve impulse to produce a reflex action. The impulse originates in a receptor at the point of stimulation, passes through an afferent neuron or neurons to a reflex center in the brain or spinal cord, and from the center out through efferent neurons to the effector organ, where the response occurs. SEE: illus.

arcade (ăr-kād′). Any anatomic structure composed of a series of arches.

a., Flint's. The arteriovenous anastomoses at the bases of the pyramids of the kidney.

arcanum (ăr-kā′nŭm) [L. *arcanum,* a secret]. (pl. *arcana*) Secret remedy.

arcate (ăr′kāt) [L. *arcatus,* bow-shaped]. Arched, bow-shaped.

arch-, arche-, archi- [Gr. *arche,* beginning]. Prefix meaning first, principal, chief, beginning, ultimate of a kind, as in archetype.

arch [L. *arcus,* a bow]. Any anatomic structure of a curved or bow-like outline.

a., abdominothoracic. The lower boundary of the front of the thorax.

a., alveolar. Arch of the alveolar process of either jaw.

a., aortic; a. of the aorta. Proximal curved part of the aorta, at about the level of

REFLEX ARC
FOR PATELLAR REFLEX

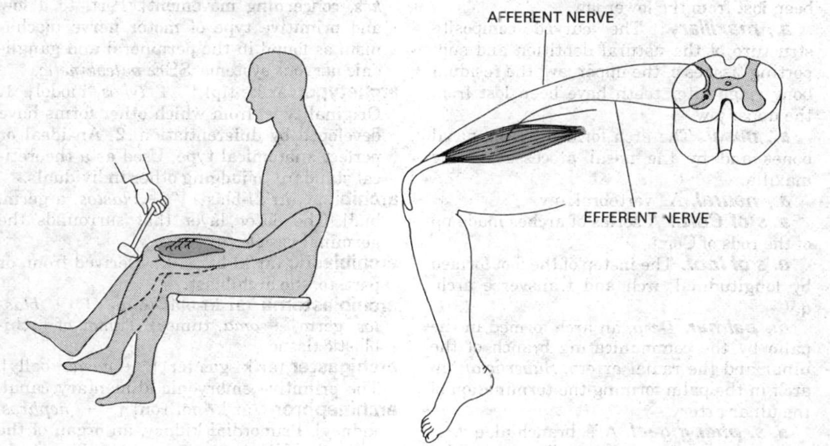

the fourth thoracic vertebra. The innominate, left common carotid, and left subclavian arteries arise from the aortic arch.

a.'s, aortic. A series of six pairs of vessels that develop in the embryo and connect the aortic sac with the dorsal aortas. During the fifth to seventh weeks, the arches undergo transformation, some persisting as functional vessels, others persisting as rudimentary structures, and some disappearing entirely.

a., axillary. An anomalous muscular slip across the axilla, between the pectoralis major and latissimus dorsi muscles. SYN: *a., Langer's; Langer's muscle.*

a.'s, branchial. A series of arches that bear the gills in lower vertebrates, and in higher vertebrates play an important role in the development of the head and neck. First is the mandibular, second, the hyoid. The third, fourth, and fifth are transitory. SYN: *a's, gill; a's, visceral.*

a., carotid. The third aortic arch, which provides the common carotid artery.

a., costal. Arch formed by the ribs.

a., crural. The inguinal ligament, which extends from the anterior superior iliac spine to pubic tubercle. SYN: *a., femoral; Poupart's ligament.*

a., deep crural. A band of fibers arching in front of sheath of femoral vessels; the downward extension of the transversalis fascia.

a., dental. An arch formed by the alveolar process and teeth on either jaw.

a., femoral. A., crural, q.v.

a., glossopalatine. The anterior pillar of the fauces, q.v.; one of two folds of mucous membrane extending from the soft palate to the sides of the tongue.

a., hemal. 1. Arch formed by the body and processes of a vertebra, a pair of ribs and the sternum, or other like parts; also the sum of all such arches. 2. In lower vertebrates, extensions from the lateral areas of the caudal vertebrae that fuse to enclose the caudal artery and vein. In man these are represented by the costal processes of the vertebrae.

a., hyoid. The second branchial arch, which gives rise to the styloid process, the stylohyoid ligament, and lesser cornu of the hyoid bone.

a., Langer's. A., axillary, q.v.

a., longitudinal. The anteroposterior arch of the foot; the medial portion is formed by calcaneus, talus, navicular, cuneiforms, and first three metatarsals; the lateral portion is formed by the calcaneus, cuboid, and fourth and fifth metatarsals.

a., mandibular. 1. The first branchial arch, from which the upper and lower jawbones and associated structures develop. It also gives rise to the malleus and incus. 2. The curved composite structure of natural dentition and supporting tissues of the lower jaw; the residual bony ridge after teeth have been lost from the lower jaw.

a., maxillary. The curved composite structure of the natural dentition and supporting tissues of the upper jaw; the residual bony ridge after teeth have been lost from the upper jaw.

a., nasal. The arch formed by the nasal bones and by the nasal processes of the maxilla.

a., neural. A., vertebral, q.v.

a.'s of Corti. A series of arches made up of the rods of Corti.

a.'s of foot. The instep of the foot formed by longitudinal arch and transverse arch, q.v.

a., palmar. *Deep,* an arch formed in the palm by the communicating branch of the ulnar and the radial artery. *Superficial,* an arch in the palm forming the termination of the ulnar artery.

a.'s, pharyngeal. A.'s, branchial, q.v.

a., pharyngopalatine. The posterior pillar of the fauces, q.v.; one of two folds of mucous membrane extending from the soft palate to the sides of the pharynx.

a., plantar. The arch formed by the external plantar artery and deep branch of the dorsalis pedis artery.

a., pubic. The arch formed by the rami of the ischia.

a., pulmonary. The fifth aortic arch on the left side. It becomes the pulmonary artery.

a., superciliary. A curved process of the frontal bone lying just above the orbit and subjacent to the eyebrow.

a., supraorbital. A bony arch formed by the upper margin of the orbit.

a., tarsal. *Inferior,* the arch of the median palpebral artery that supplies the lower eyelid. *Superior,* the arch of the median palpebral artery that supplies the upper eyelid.

a., thyrohyoid. The third branchial arch, which gives rise to the greater cornu of the hyoid bone.

a., transverse. The transverse arch of the foot formed by the navicular, cuboid, cuneiform, and metatarsal bones.

a., vertebral. The arch formed by the posterior projection of a vertebra that, with the body, encloses the vertebral foramen. SYN: *a., neural.*

a.'s, visceral. A.'s, branchial, q.v.

a., zygomatic. The arch formed by the malar and temporal bones.

archenteron (ărk-ĕn'tĕr-ŏn) [Gr. *arche,* origin, + *enteron,* intestine]. The primitive digestive cavity of the gastrula, which is lined with entoderm. Its opening to the outside is the blastopore. SYN: *gastrocoele; primary gut.*

archeokinetic (ăr"kē-ō-kĭ-nĕt'ĭk) [" + *kinetikos,* concerning movement]. Pert. to a low and primitive type of motor nerve mechanism as found in the peripheral and ganglionic nervous systems. SEE: *paleokinetic.*

archetype (ăr'kĕ-tīp) [" + *typos,* model]. 1. Original type, from which other forms have developed by differentiation. 2. An ideal or perfect anatomical type. Used as a theoretical standard in judging other individuals.

archiblast (ăr'kĭ-blăst) [" + *blastos,* a germ, bud]. The outer layer that surrounds the germinal vesicle.

archiblastic (ăr"kĭ-blăs'tĭk). Derived from, or pert. to, the archiblast.

archiblastoma (ăr"kĭ-blăs-tō'mă) [" + *blastos,* germ, + *oma,* tumor]. Tumor of archiblastic tissue.

archigaster (ăr'kĭ-găs"tĕr) [" + *gaster,* belly]. The primitive embryonic alimentary canal.

archinephron (ăr"kĭ-nĕf'rŏn) [" + *nephros,* kidney]. Primordial kidney, an organ of the embryo. SYN: *mesonephros; wolffian body.*

archineuron (ăr-kĭ-nū'rŏn) [" + *neuron,* nerve, tendon]. The central cell of the cerebral cortex, and all its processes. The nervous impulse that is transmitted to initiate physiological function originates in the archineuron.

archipallium (ăr"kĭ-păl'ē-ŭm) [" + L. *pallium,* a cloak]. Olfactory cortex, older than neopallium.

archiplasm (ăr'kĭ-plăzm) [" + *plasma,* a mold]. 1. The most primitive living substance. 2. The substance of the fertilized ovum.

archistome (ăr'kĭ-stōm) [" + *stoma,* mouth]. Invagination of blastula making a little opening into the archenteron. SYN: *blastopore.*

architectural barrier. Any limitation in the design of facilities that restricts the access of persons with disabilities and limited mobility, including those using wheelchairs.

architis (ăr-kī'tĭs) [Gr. *archos,* anus, + *itis,* inflammation]. Inflammation of the anus; proctitis.

archo- [Gr. *archos,* rectum]. Prefix denoting relationship to the rectum or anus.

archocele (ăr'kō-sēl) [" + *kele,* tumor]. Hernia of the rectum.

archocystocolposyrinx (ăr"kō-sĭs"tō-kŏl"pō-sĭr'ĭnks) [" + *kystis,* bladder, + *kolpos,* vagina, + *syrinx,* tube, fistula]. Fistula of rectum, vagina, and bladder.

archostenosis (ăr"kō-stĕ-nō'sĭs) [" + *stenosis,* a narrowing]. Stricture of the rectum.

arciform (ăr'sĭ-form) [L. *arcus,* bow, + *forma,*

shape]. Bow-shaped; shaped like an arc. SYN: *arcuate*.

arctation (ărk-tā'shŭn) [L. *arctatus*, pressing together]. Stricture of any canal opening.

arcuate (ăr'kū-āt) [L. *arcuatus*, bowed]. Bowed, shaped like an arc. SYN: *arciform*.

arcuation (ăr-kū-ā'shŭn). A bending, curvature.

arculus (ăr'kū-lŭs) [L. *arculus*, a small arch]. An arched frame to protect a part from bedclothes. SYN: *cradle*.

arcus (ăr'kŭs) [L. *arcus*, a bow]. (pl. *arcus*) An arch, q.v.

a. alveolaris mandibulae. The arch formed by the alveolar process of the mandibula.

a. alveolaris maxillae. [NA] The arch formed by the alveolar process of the maxilla.

a. dentalis. Dental arch.

a. juvenilis. Opaque ring about the periphery of the cornea similar to arcus senilis but occurring in young individuals. May be due to hypercholesterolemia, corneal irritation or inflammation, or the result of a congenital anomaly.

a. plantaris. [NA] The plantar arch.

a. senilis. Opaque white ring about periphery of the cornea, seen in aged persons. Due to deposit of fat granules in cornea or to hyaline degeneration.

ARD. *acute* (undifferentiated) *respiratory disease*.

ardanesthesia (ăr"dăn-ĕs-thē'zē-ă) [L. *ardor*, heat, + Gr. *an-*, not, + *aisthesis*, feeling]. Inability to feel heat. SYN: *thermanesthesia*.

ardent (ăr'dĕnt) [L. *ardens*, burning]. Burning; feverish.

ardor (ăr'dor) [L., heat]. Burning; great heat.

a. urinae. A burning sensation during urination.

a. veneris. Sexual desire.

area (ā'rē-ă) [L. *area*, an open space]. (pl. *areas, areae*) 1. A circumscribed space; one having definite boundaries. 2. A part of an organ that performs a specialized function.

a., acoustic. A., vestibular, q.v.

a., association. Area of the cerebral cortex that is not sensory or motor, in the usual meaning of those terms. Thought to be a region in which higher mental processes are mediated.

a., auditory. The hearing center of cerebral cortex located in the floor of the lateral fissure and surfacing on the dorsal surface of the superior temporal gyrus. It receives auditory fibers from the medial geniculate body.

a., body surface. The area covered by the skin. It is usually expressed in square meters. The surface area (S) may be calculated by multiplying 0.007184 times the weight (W) in kilograms raised to the 0.425 power and the height (H) in centimeters raised to the 0.725 power. Thus:

$$S = 0.007184 \times W^{0.425} \times H^{0.725}.$$

SEE: *rule of nines*.

a., Broca's. SEE: *Broca's area*.

a.'s, Brodmann's. The division of the cerebral cortex into 47 areas. This was originally done on the basis of cyto-architectural characteristics, but the areas are now differentiated and classified with respect to their different functions.

a. germinativa. Area of germination of the ovum.

a., Kiesselbach's. Area of anterior portion of nasal septum. Because of its abundant supply of capillaries, it is a common site of nosebleed.

a., macular. Area of the retina that functions in central vision.

a., mitral. Area over the apex of the heart, where mitral valve sounds are heard.

a., occipital. Portion of brain below the occipital bone.

a. pellucida. Clear central portion of area germinativa of the earliest stages of the embryo.

a., Rolando's. Area situated in anterior central convolution in front of fissure of Rolando in each hemisphere. Governs motor acts of the body.

a., silent. Any cortical area in the brain that upon stimulation produces no detectable motor activity or sensory phenomenon, and in which a lesion may occur without producing detectable motor or sensory abnormalities.

a., vestibular. Fundus of the internal auditory meatus. SYN: *a., acoustic*.

areata, areatus (ă"rē-ā'tă ă"rē-ā'tŭs). Occurring in circumscribed areas or patches.

areflexia (ă"rē-flĕk'sē-ă) [Gr. *a-*, not, + L. *reflectere*, to bend back]. Absence of reflexes.

arenaceous (ăr"ĕ-nā'sē-ŭs) [L. *arenaceus*, sandy]. Resembling sand or gravel. SYN: *arenoid*.

arenation (ă"rē-nā'shŭn) [L. *arena*, sand]. A sand bath or application of hot sand.

arenaviridae. Arenaviruses, q.v.

arenaviruses (ă"rē-nă-vī'rŭs-ĕs) [" + *virus*, poison]. A group of viruses once classed as causing disease by being arthropod-borne. This type of transmission is not obligatory. The principal virus in this group is lymphocytic choriomeningitis virus (LCM virus). The LCM virus rarely infects man but when it does, the disease is usually a mild form of meningitis.

arenoid (ăr'ĕ-noyd) [" + Gr. *eidos*, form]. Resembling sand or gravel. SYN: *arenaceous*.

areola (ă-rē'ō-lă) [L. *areola*, a small space]. (pl. *areolae*) 1. A small space or cavity in a tissue. 2. A circular area of different pigmentation, as around a wheal, around the nipple of the breast, or the part of the iris around the pupil.

a. mammae. [NA] The dark pigmented area surrounding the nipple.

a. papillaris. A. mammae, q.v.

a., second. A pigmented area surrounding the areola mammae during pregnancy.

a. umbilicalis. A pigmented area surrounding the umbilicus.

areolar (ă-rē'ō-lăr). Rel. to an areola.

areolar glands. Large modified sweat glands lying beneath the areola of the breast with ducts opening on its surface. They secrete a lipoid material that lubricates the nipple. SYN: *glands, Montgomery's.*

areolar tissue. Loose connective tissue that occupies the interspaces of the body.

areolitis (ăr"ē-ō-lī'tĭs) [" + Gr. *itis,* inflammation]. Inflammation of mammary areola.

areometer (ă-rē-ŏm'ĕ-tĕr) [Gr. *araios,* thin, + *metron,* a measure]. Instrument for measuring specific gravity of fluids. SYN: *hydrometer.*

arevareva (ăr-ē"vā-rā'vă) [Tahitian, skin rash]. Severe skin disease characterized by scales and accompanied by general debility. SEE: *kava.*

ETIOL: Thought to be caused by excess use of kava, an intoxicating beverage.

TREATMENT: Discontinuation of use of kava.

Arfonad. Trade name for trimethaphan camsylate, USP, q.v.

argamblyopia (ăr"găm-blē-ŏ'pē-ă) [Gr. *argos,* idle, + *amblus,* dulled, + *ops,* eye]. Reduction in vision as a result of not using the eye.

Argasidae (ăr-găs'ĭ-dī) [Gr. *argeeis,* shining]. Family of soft ticks usually infecting birds, but may attack man, causing severe pain and fever.

argema (ăr-jē'mă) [Gr. *argema,* ulcer]. White corneal ulcer.

argentaffin, argentaffine (ăr-jĕnt'ă-fĭn) [L. *argentum,* silver, + *affinis,* associated with]. Denoting cells that react with silver salts, thus giving a brown or black stain.

argentaffinoma (ăr"jĕn-tăf"ĭ-nō'mă) [" + " + Gr. *oma,* tumor]. An argentaffin cell tumor that may arise in intestinal tract, bile ducts, pancreas, bronchus, or ovary. These tumors secrete serotonin and may produce the carcinoid syndrome, q.v. SYN: *carcinoid.*

argentum (ăr-jĕn'tŭm) [L.]. SYMB: Ag. At. wt. 107.868; at. no. 47. Silver.

arginase (ăr'jĭ-nās). Enzyme of the liver that catalyzes the hydrolysis of arginine, forming urea and ornithine.

arginine (ăr'jĭ-nēn, -nĭn) [L. *argentum,* silver]. USP. $C_6H_{14}N_4O_2$. Crystalline basic amino acid obtained from decomposition of vegetable tissues, protamines, and proteins. Also prepared synthetically. It is a guanidine derivative, yielding urea and ornithine on hydrolysis. SEE: *amino acid.*

a. glutamate. The L(+)—arginine salt of L(+)—glutamic acid. It has been used in treating ammonia intoxication due to severe liver insufficiency.

a. hydrochloride. L(+)—arginine salt of hydrochloric acid. It has been used to treat ammonia intoxication due to severe liver insufficiency.

a., suberyl. A combination of suberic acid and arginine. It forms a portion of the molecule of various bufotoxins (toad poisons).

argininosuccinic acid (ăr"jĭ-nĭ"nō-sŭk-sĭn'ĭk). A compound intermediate in the synthesis of arginine. Formed from citrulline and aspartic acid.

argininosuccinicaciduria (ăr"jĭn-ĭn-ō-sŭk-sĭn"ĭk-ăs-ĭ-dū'rē-ă). Hereditary metabolic disease caused by excessive excretion, and thus deficiency, of arginosuccinase, an enzyme required to metabolize arginosuccinic acid. Clinical evidence of this defect includes mental retardation, friable tufted hair, convulsions, ataxia, liver disease, and epilepsy.

argon (ăr'gŏn) [Gr. *argos,* inactive]. SYMB: Ar. At. wt. 39.948; at. no. 18. An inert gas composing approx. 1% of the atmosphere.

Argyll Robertson pupil (ăr-gĭl' rŏb'ĕrt-sŏn). [Douglas Argyll Robertson, Scottish ophthalmologist, 1837–1909] More properly the name of a symptom often present in paralysis and locomotor ataxia (due to syphilis), in which the light reflex is absent but there is no change in the power of contraction during accommodation. Usually bilateral.

argyria, argyriasis (ăr-jĭr'ē-ă, ăr"jĭ-rī'ă-sĭs) [Gr. *argyros,* silver]. Bluish discoloration of skin and mucous membranes resulting from prolonged administration of silver. SYN: *argyrism; argyrosis.*

argyric (ăr-jĭr'ĭk). Pert. to silver.

argyrism (ăr'jĭr-ĭzm) [Gr. *argyros,* silver]. Argyria, q.v.

Argyrol (ăr'jĭ-rŏl). Trade name for mild silver protein. Used as an antiseptic in infections of the eye, nose, and throat and for urethral irrigations.

argyrophil (ăr-jĭ'rō-fĭl) [" + *philos,* fond]. Denoting cells that bind with silver salts, which can then be reduced to produce a brown or black stain.

argyrosis (ăr"jĭ-rō'sĭs) [" + *osis,* condition]. Argyria, q.v.

arhinia. Arrhinia, q.v.

arhythmia. Arrhythmia, q.v.

Arias-Stella reaction. [Javier Arias-Stella, Peruvian pathologist, b. 1924] An endometrial gland cell abnormality consisting of hyperchromatic nuclei, which may be present in normal or ectopic pregnancy. It is not a sign of endometrial adenocarcinoma.

ariboflavinosis (ă-rī"bō-flā"vĭn-ō'sĭs) [Gr. *a*-, not, + *riboflavin* + Gr. *osis*, condition]. Condition arising from a deficiency of riboflavin in the diet.

SYM: Lesions on the lips; stomatitis and, later, fissures in the angles of the mouth; seborrhea around the nose; vascularization of cornea.

TREATMENT: Riboflavin, given orally.

Aristocort. Trade name for triamcinolone, USP, q.v.

Aristocort Acetonide. Trade name for triamcinolone acetonide, USP, q.v.

Aristocort Forte Parenteral. Trade name for triamcinolone diacetate, USP, q.v.

aristogenics (ă-rĭs"tō-jĕn'ĭks) [Gr. *aristos*, best, + *gennan*, to produce]. The science that deals with the genetic and prenatal influences that affect the expression of certain characteristics in offspring. SYN: *eugenics*.

Aristospan. Trade name for triamcinolone hexacetonide, USP, q.v.

arkyochrome (ăr'kē-ō-krōm) [Gr. *arkys*, net, + *chroma*, color]. A nerve cell in which the stainable substance is arranged in a network.

arkyostichochrome (ar"kē-ō-stĭk'ō-krōm) [" + *stichos*, row, + *chroma*, color]. A nerve cell in which the stainable material is arranged both as a network and in parallel lines.

Arlidin. Trade name for nylidrin hydrochloride, USP, q.v.

arm [AS.]. 1. In anatomy, the upper extremity from shoulder to elbow. 2. In popular usage, the entire upper extremity, from shoulder to hand. SEE: illus.

a., bird. Atrophy of the forearm muscles.

a., brawny. Hard, swollen arm after removal of a breast, due to lymphedema.

a., Saturday-night. A form of paralysis of the brachial plexus, sometimes seen in intoxicated persons.

ETIOL: Sleeping in a chair, with the arm hanging over the back of the chair while the head rests on the shoulder or arm.

arm, words pert. to: axilla; "brachio-" words; brachium; forearm; humerus; radius; ulna.

A.R.M.A. *American Registry of Medical Assistants.*

armamentarium (ăr"mă-mĕn-tā'rē-ŭm) [L. *armamentum*, implement]. The total equipment of a physician or institution, such as instruments, drugs, books, supplies.

armature (ăr'mă-tūr) [L. *armatura*, equipment]. 1. In biology, a structure that serves to protect or is used to attack a predator, e.g., a stinger. 2. A part of an electrical generator, consisting of a coil of insulated wire mounted around a soft iron core.

armilla (ăr-mĭl'lă) [L., bracelet]. (pl. *armillae*) The annular ligament of the wrist.

armpit. Axilla, q.v.

Arneth, Joseph (ăr'nāt). German physician, 1873–1955.

A.'s classification of neutrophils. A classification of polymorphonuclear neutrophils based on the number of lobes (1 to 5) in the nucleus. Termed Stages 1 to 5, respectively.

A.'s formula. The normal ratio of various types of polymorphonuclear neutrophils based on the number of lobes (1 to 5) in the nucleus. The normal ratio is:

Lobes	1	2	3	4	5
%	5	35	41	17	2

Arnold, Friedrich. German anatomist, 1803–1890.

A.'s canal. Passage in the temporal bone for lesser superficial petrosal nerve.

A.'s ganglion. Otic ganglion.

A.'s nerve. Auricular branch of the vagus nerve.

Arnold-Chiari deformity (ăr'nōlt-kē'ă-rē). [Julius Arnold, Ger. pathologist, 1835–1915; Hans Chiari, Ger. pathologist, 1851–1916] A condition in which the inferior poles of the cerebellar hemispheres and the medulla protrude through the foramen magnum into the spinal canal. It is one of the causes of hydrocephalus and is usually accompanied by spina bifida and meningomyelocele.

AROM. *active range of motion.*

aroma (ă-rō'mă) [Gr. *aroma*, spice]. An agreeable odor.

aromatic (ăr"ō-măt'ĭk). 1. Having an agreeable odor. 2. Belonging to that series of organic chemical compounds in which the carbon atoms form closed rings (as in benzene) as distinguished from the aliphatic series, in which the carbon atoms form straight or branched chains.

aromatic ammonia spirit. Solution consisting of 34 gm. of ammonium carbonate in 1000 ml. diluted ammonia solution, fragrant oils, alcohol, and purified water. Used as antacid and carminative. It acts as a reflex stimulant when its vapor is inhaled.

aromatic compounds. Ring or cyclic compounds related to benzene, many having a fragrant odor.

aromatic elixir. A flavoring agent used in preparing medicines.

arrachement (ă-răsh-mŏn) [Fr., extraction]. Pulling out the capsule in a membranous cataract through a corneal incision.

arrectores pilorum (ă"rĕk-tō'rēz pĭl-ō'rŭm) [L. *arrectores*, raisers, + *pilus*, hair]. (sing.

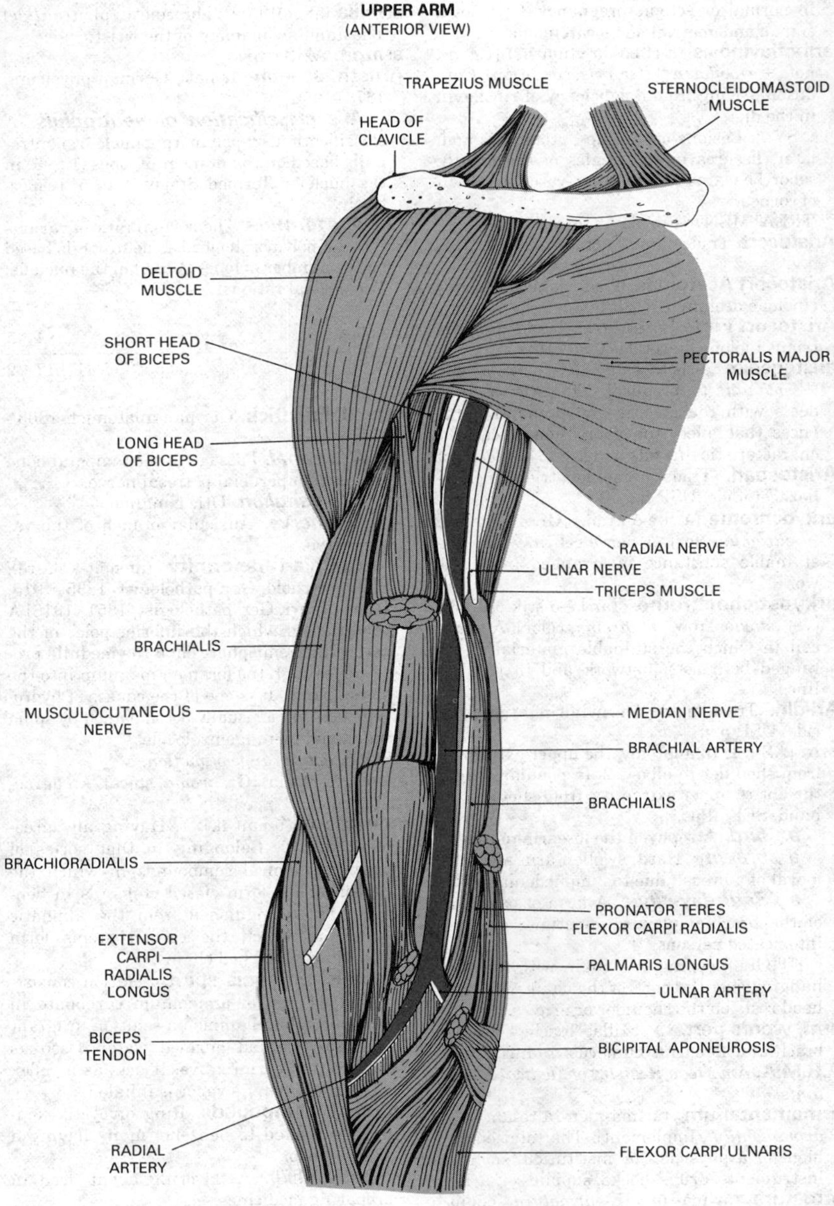
UPPER ARM
(ANTERIOR VIEW)
TRAPEZIUS MUSCLE
STERNOCLEIDOMASTOID MUSCLE
HEAD OF CLAVICLE
DELTOID MUSCLE
SHORT HEAD OF BICEPS
PECTORALIS MAJOR MUSCLE
LONG HEAD OF BICEPS
RADIAL NERVE
ULNAR NERVE
TRICEPS MUSCLE
BRACHIALIS
MUSCULOCUTANEOUS NERVE
MEDIAN NERVE
BRACHIAL ARTERY
BRACHIALIS
BRACHIORADIALIS
PRONATOR TERES
FLEXOR CARPI RADIALIS
EXTENSOR CARPI RADIALIS LONGUS
PALMARIS LONGUS
ULNAR ARTERY
BICEPS TENDON
BICIPITAL APONEUROSIS
RADIAL ARTERY
FLEXOR CARPI ULNARIS

arrector pili) Involuntary muscle fibers arising in the skin and extending down to connect with the hair follicles on the side toward which the hair slopes. Under the influence of cold or fright they contract, straighten the follicles, and raise the hairs, resulting in "gooseflesh" or cutis anserina.

arrest (ă-rĕst′). Stoppage, particularly the cessation of motion of a part normally in motion.

a., cardiac. Cessation of the heartbeat.

a., epiphysial. Arrest of growth of long bones.

a., pelvic. Condition in which the presenting part of the fetus becomes fixed in the maternal pelvis.

a., sinus. Condition in which the sinus node of the heart does not initiate impulses for heartbeat.

arrhenoblastoma (ă-rē″nō-blăs-tō′mă) [Gr. *arren,* male, + *blastos,* germ, + *oma,* tumor]. An ovarian tumor that secretes male sex hormone and thus causes secondary male sex characteristics (virilization) in the female.

arrhinia (ă-rĭn′ē-ă) [Gr. *a-,* not, + *rhis,* nose]. Congenital absence of the nose.

arrhythmia (ă-rĭth′mē-ă) [″ + *rhythmos,* rhythm]. Irregularity or loss of rhythm, esp. of the heartbeat.

a., cardiac. Irregular heart action caused by physiological or pathological disturbances in discharge of cardiac impulses from the sinoatrial node or their transmission through conductile tissue of the heart. SEE: *bradycardia; tachycardia.*

a., sinus. Cardiac irregularity characterized by an increased heart rate during inspiration and decrease in heart rate on expiration. This arrhythmia has no clinical significance except in older patients, in which case it may occur in coronary artery disease.

arrhythmic (ă-rĭth′mĭk). Pert. to or characterized by loss of rhythm.

A.R.R.T. *American Registry of Radiologic Technologists.*

arseniasis (ăr″sē-nī′ă-sĭs) [L. *arsenium,* arsenic, + *-iasis,* condition]. Chronic arsenic poisoning. SYN: *arsenicism.*

arsenic (ăr′sē-nĭk) [L. *arsenicum*]. SYMB: As. At. wt. 74.922; at. no. 33; sp. gr. 5.73. A metallic element of grayish-white color, very poisonous, used in the manufacture of dyes and medicines.

Arsenic may be present in soil, water, and air as a common environmental toxicant. Minute traces of arsenic are found in vegetables and animal forms of life and are present in eggs. Many household and garden pesticides contain various forms of arsenic. All of these are toxic if ingested or inhaled in sufficient quantity. An accumulation of arsenic in the body will cause disorders of alimentary tract, nausea, vomiting, diarrhea, dehydration, neuritis, and paralysis of wrist and ankle muscles. SEE: *Poisons and Poisoning* in *Appendix.*

a. trioxide. As_2O_3. A white powder used internally in form of a 1% solution. Previously used for a variety of conditions but is little used now. More than a few grains may be fatal. SYN: *arsenous powder; a., white.*

a., white. Arsenic trioxide, q.v.

arsenic, words pert. to acetarsone; arsphenamine; tryparsamide

arsenical (ăr-sĕn′ĭ-kăl). 1. Pert. to or containing arsenic. 2. A drug containing arsenic.

arsenic-fast. Resistant to toxic action of arsenic.

arsenicism (ăr-sĕn′ĭ-sĭzm) [L. *arsenicum,* arsenic, + Gr. *-ismos,* condition of]. Chronic arsenic poisoning. SYN: *arseniasis.*

arsenicophagy (ăr″sĕn-ĭ-kŏf′ă-jē) [″ + *phagein,* to eat]. Habitual eating of arsenic.

arsenic poisoning. Morbid condition produced by ingestion of arsenic.

SYM: In acute poisoning, may appear in a few minutes or, when taken with solid food, may not appear for many hours. Metallic taste and odor of garlic on breath, burning pain throughout gastrointestinal tract, vomiting and purging, dehydration, shock syndrome, coma, convulsions, paralysis, death.

F.A.: Lavage stomach with copious amounts of water. If this cannot be done, induce vomiting. Administer dimercaprol (British antilewisite) immediately.

TREATMENT: After first aid, maintain fluid and electrolyte balance. Morphine for pain. Treat for shock and pulmonary edema. Blood transfusion may be required because of hemolysis. SEE: *Poisons and Poisoning* in *Appendix.*

arsenionization (ăr″sĕn-ī″ŏn-ĭ-zā′shŭn). Electrolytic diffusion of arsenic ions in tissues.

arsenium (ăr-sē′nē-ŭm) [L.]. Arsenic.

arsenoblast (ăr-sĕn′ō-blăst) [Gr. *arsen,* male, + *blastos,* germ]. Male element in nucleus of impregnated ovum; a male pronucleus.

arsenoresistant (ăr-sĕn″ō-rē-zĭs′tănt) [L. *arsenium,* arsenic, + *resistere,* to withstand]. Resistant to arsenic compounds.

arsenotherapy (ăr″sē-nō-thĕr′ă-pē) [″ + Gr. *therapeia,* treatment]. Treatment with arsenic and its compounds.

arsenous (ăr′sē-nŭs) [L. *arsenium,* arsenic]. Of the nature of, or pert. to, arsenic or its compounds, esp. those containing arsenic in its lower valency. SYN: *arsenical.*

arsenous hydride. Arsine q.v.

arsenous powder. Arsenic trioxide, q.v.

arsine (ăr′sĭn). A very poisonous gas used in chemical warfare. SYN: *arsenous hydride.*

arsphenamine (ărs-fĕn′ă-mēn). A light yellow powder containing about 30% arsenic.

Formerly used in treatment of syphilis. SYN: *salvarsan.*

Artane. Trade name for trihexyphenidyl hydrochloride, USP, q.v.

artefact (ăr'tĕ-făkt) [L. *ars,* art, + *factus,* made]. 1. Anything artificially produced. 2. In histology and radiography, a structure or feature produced by the technique used and not occurring naturally. Also spelled artifact.

arterectomy (ăr"tĕ-rĕk'tō-mē) [Gr. *arteria,* artery, + *ektome,* excision]. Excision of an artery or arteries.

arteria (ăr"tē'rē-ă). (pl. *arteriae*) Artery, q.v.

arteriagra (ăr"tē-rē-ŏg'ră) [" + *agra,* a seizure]. Pain in an artery.

arterial (ăr-tē'rē-ăl). Pert. to one or more arteries.

arterial bleeding. Bleeding from an artery. Blood is bright red and comes in spurts. Arrest by applying pressure on proximal side of vessel (nearest heart).

arterial circulation. Movement of blood through the arteries. It is maintained by the pumping of the heart, elasticity and extensibility of arterial walls, peripheral resistance in the areas of small arteries, and by the quantity of blood in the body. SEE: *circulation.*

arterial varix. An enlarged and tortuous artery.

arteriasis (ăr"tĕ-rī'ă-sĭs) [" + *-iasis,* condition]. Degeneration of an artery.

arteriectasis, arteriectasia (ăr"tĕ-rē-ĕk'tă-sĭs, -ĕk-tā'zē-ă) [" + *ektasis,* a stretching out]. Arterial dilatation.

arteriectomy (ăr"tĕ-rē-ĕk'tō-mē) [" + *ektome,* excision]. Surgical removal of a part of an artery.

arterio- [Gr. *arteria,* artery]. Combining form indicating relationship to an artery.

arterioatony (ăr-tē"rē-ō-ăt'ō-nē) [" + *atonia,* languor]. Lack of tone in arterial walls.

arteriocapillary (ăr-tē"rē-ō-kăp'ĭ-lăr"ē) [" + L. *capillus,* like hair]. Pert. to both arteries and capillaries.

arteriocapillary fibrosis. Sclerosis of capillaries and arterioles.

arteriofibrosis (ăr-tē"rē-ō-fī-brō'sĭs) [" + L. *fibra,* fiber, + Gr. *osis,* condition]. Arteriocapillary fibrosis.

arteriogram (ăr-tē'rē-ō-grăm) [" + *gramma,* mark]. Roentgenogram of an artery after injection of a radiopaque dye.

arteriography (ăr"tē-rē-ŏg'ră-fē) [" + *graphein,* to write]. 1. Roentgenography of arteries after injection of a radiopaque dye. 2. Description of arteries.

arteriola (ăr-tē"rē-ō'lă) [L.]. (pl. *arteriolae*) [NA] Small artery; an arteriole.

a. macularis inferior. [NA] The inferior macular arteriole, which supplies the macula retinae of the eye.

a. macularis superior. [NA] The superior macular arteriole, which supplies the macula retinae of the eye.

a. medialis retinae. [NA] The medial arteriole of the retina.

a. nasalis retinae inferior. [NA] Inferior nasal arteriole of the retina.

a. nasalis retinae superior. [NA] Superior nasal arteriole of the retina.

a. recta. [NA] One of the small arteries of the kidney that supply the renal pyramids.

a. temporalis retinae inferior. [NA] Inferior temporal artery of the retina.

a. temporalis retinae superior. [NA] Superior temporal artery of the retina.

arteriole (ăr-tē'rē-ōl). [L. *arteriola*]. (pl. *arterioles*) A minute artery, esp. one that, at its distal end, leads into a capillary. SYN: *arteriola.*

arteriolith (ăr-tē'rē-ō-lĭth) [" + Gr. *lithos,* stone]. An arterial calculus.

arteriolitis (ăr-tĕr"ē-ō-lī'tĭs) [" + Gr. *itis,* inflammation]. Inflammation of the arteriolar wall.

arteriology (ăr-tē"rē-ŏl'ō-jē) [" + Gr. *logos,* study]. Science of arteries, usually combined with study of other vessels, as in angiology, q.v.

arteriolonecrosis (ăr-tē"rē-ō"lō-nĕ-krō'sĭs) [" + Gr. *nekros,* dead, + *osis,* condition]. Destruction of an arteriole.

arteriolosclerosis (ăr-tē"rē-ō"lō-sklĕ-rō'sĭs) [L. *arteriola,* small artery, + Gr. *sklerosis,* hardening]. Thickening of the walls of the arterioles with loss of elasticity and contractility.

arteriolosclerotic (ăr-tē"rē-ō"lō-sklĕ-rŏt'ĭk). Pert. to or characterized by arteriolosclerosis.

arteriomotor (ăr-tē"rē-ō-mō'tor) [Gr. *arteria,* artery, + L. *movere,* to move]. Causing changes in interior diameter of arteries by dilatation and constriction.

arteriomyomatosis (ăr-tē"rē-ō-mī"ō-mă-tō'sĭs) [" + *mys,* muscle, + *oma,* tumor, + *osis,* condition]. Thickening of arterial walls due to overgrowth of muscle fibers.

arterionecrosis (ăr-tē"rē-ō-nĕ-krō'sĭs) [" + *nekros,* dead, + *osis,* condition]. Arterial necrosis.

arteriopathy (ăr"tē-rē-ŏp'ă-thē) [" + *pathos,* disease]. Any disease of the arteries.

arterioplasty (ăr-tē"rē-ō-plăs'tē) [" + *plassein,* to form]. Repair or reconstruction of an artery.

arteriopressor (ăr-tē"rē-ō-prĕs'or) [" + L. *pressura,* force]. Causing increased arterial blood pressure.

arteriorrhaphy (ăr-tē"rē-or'ă-fē) [" + *rhaphe,* suture]. Arterial suture.

arteriorrhexis (ăr-tē"rē-ō-rĕk'sĭs) [" + *rhexis,* rupture]. Rupture of an artery.

arteriosclerosis (ăr-tē"rē-ō-sklĕ-rō'sĭs) [" +

sklerosis, hardening]. Term applied to a number of pathological conditions in which there is thickening, hardening, and loss of elasticity of the walls of arteries. This results in altered function of tissues and organs. Changes may occur in the intima, media, or both.

ETIOL: Cause is unknown. Aging, altered lipid metabolism, and other factors including gender, the environment, psychological, physiological, as well as genetic influences are thought to be important in determining an individual's chances of developing arteriosclerosis. Some risk factors include: hypertension; increased blood lipids, particularly cholesterol and triglycerides; obesity; cigarette smoking; diabetes mellitus; inability to cope with stress; family history of early-onset atherosclerosis; physical inactivity; and the male sex (at ages 35 to 44, the death rate for white males is 6 times that of white females).

TREATMENT: Regular exercise; diet low in saturated fatty acids; minimal use of tobacco; general moderation in all things to reduce or avoid stress; therapy for treatable diseases such as obesity, diabetes, and hypertension if any of these are present.

NURSING IMPLICATIONS: Teach the patient to avoid or decrease conditions such as anxiety and tension that can increase the severity of symptoms. Patients with arteriosclerosis should also make necessary dietary adjustments to limit cholesterol intake and to decrease weight. Advise them to stop cigarette smoking and to avoid conditions that can increase blood pressure.

Never apply external heat from hot water bottles or heating pads to an extremity with compromised blood supply. Make sure that the patient has adequate periods of rest.

a., hypertensive. Arteriosclerosis resulting from hypertension.

a., medial. Arteriosclerosis of the peripheral arteries with calcium deposits in the media. SYN: *a., Monckeberg's.*

a., Monckeberg's. A., medial, q.v.

a., nodular. Arteriosclerosis due to formation of fibrous plaques in the intima.

a. obliterans. Arteriosclerosis in which the lumen of the artery is completely occluded.

a., senile. Arteriosclerosis accompanying old age.

arteriosclerotic (ăr-tē″rē-ō-sklĕ-rŏt′ĭk). Pert. to or characterized by arteriosclerosis.

arteriospasm (ăr-tē′rē-ō-spăzm″) [Gr. *arteria,* artery, + *spasmos,* pain]. Arterial spasm.

arteriostenosis (ăr-tē″rē-ō-stĕ-nō′sĭs) [″ + *stenosis,* a narrowing]. Narrowing of the lumen of an artery, either temporary or permanent.

arteriostosis (ăr-tē″rē-ŏs-tō′sĭs) [″ + *osteon,* bone, + *osis,* condition]. Calcification of an artery.

arteriostrepsis (ăr-tē″rē-ō-strĕp′sĭs) [″ + *strepsis,* a twisting]. Twisting of divided end of an artery to arrest hemorrhage.

arteriosympathectomy (ăr-tē″rē-ō-sĭm″pă-thĕk′tō-mē) [″ + *sympatheia,* suffer with, + *ektome,* excision]. Removal of arterial sheath containing fibers of sympathetic nerve.

arteriotome (ăr-tē′rē-ō-tōm) [″ + *tome,* incision]. Knife for opening an artery.

arteriotomy (ăr″tē-rē-ŏt′ō-mē). Surgical division or opening of an artery.

arteriotony (ăr-tē″rē-ŏt′ō-nē) [″ + *tonos,* tension]. Blood pressure; intra-arterial blood tension.

arteriovenous (ăr-tē″rē-ō-vē nŭs) [″ + L. *vena,* a vein]. Rel. to both arteries and veins.

arterioversion (ăr-tē″rē-ō-vĕr′shŭn) [″ + L. *versio,* a turning]. Eversion of arterial wall to arrest hemorrhage from open end.

arterioverter (ăr-tē″rē-ō-vĕr′tĕr). An instrument for everting cut end of an artery for arresting hemorrhage.

arteritis (ăr″tē-rī′tĭs) [″ + *itis,* inflammation]. Inflammation of an artery. SEE: *endarteritis, polyarteritis.*

a., cranial. A., temporal, q.v.

a., giant cell. A., temporal, q.v.

a., granulomatous. A., temporal, q.v.

a. nodosa. Widespread inflammation of adventitia of small and medium-sized arteries with impaired function of the involved organs. SYN: *periarteritis nodosa; polyarteritis nodosa.*

a. obliterans. Inflammation of intima of artery causing occlusion of the lumen. SYN: *endarteritis obliterans.*

a., rheumatic. Inflammation of small arteries resulting from rheumatic fever.

a., rheumatoid. Inflammation of arteries resulting from rheumatoid arthritis.

a., temporal. Chronic inflammation of large arteries, usually the temporal, occipital, or ophthalmic arteries, accompanied by presence of giant cells. Causes thickening of intima with narrowing and eventual occlusion of lumen. Occurs in elderly persons. SYN: *a., cranial; a., giant cell; a., granulomatous.*

artery (ăr′tĕr-ē) [Gr. *arteria,* windpipe]. (pl. *arteries*) One of the vessels carrying blood from the heart to the tissues. The ancients believed that air circulated through them, from which supposition the name, artery, was derived.

The arteries carry the oxygenated blood from the right and left ventricles of the heart to all parts of the body. There are two major divisions, pulmonary and systemic. The pulmonary artery carries the venous blood from the right ventricle to the lungs. The systemic division begins with the aorta and carries arterial blood from the left ventricle to the various parts of the body. SEE: *aorta* and *coronary arteries* for illus.

ANAT: The arteries have three coats: the inner, tunica intima, or serous; the outer, tunica adventitia, or white fibrous; and the middle, tunica media, or yellow fibrous. SEE: *Arteries* in *Appendix*.

a., coiled. A., spiral, q.v.

a., elastic. An artery in which elastic tissue is predominant in the tunica intima and tunica media. Elastic arteries include the aorta and its larger branches (innominate, common carotid, subclavian, and common iliac)—vessels that conduct blood to the muscular arteries.

a., end. An artery whose branches do not anastomose with those of other arteries, e.g., arteries to brain and spinal cord.

a., muscular. An artery with smooth muscle tissue in its wall, esp. the tunica media, by means of which the flow of blood to tissues can be regulated through contraction and relaxation. These arteries also contract spastically when injured, thus preventing excessive loss of blood.

a., sheathed. The terminal portion of a pulp artery in the spleen. It has distinctive thickenings in its walls.

a., spiral. The coiled terminal branch of a uterine artery. It supplies the superficial two thirds of the endometrium and, in a pregnant uterus, it empties into intervillous spaces supplying blood that bathes the chorionic villi at the placental site.

a., terminal. A., end, q.v.

artery, words pert. to: adventitia; aneurysm; angina pectoris; arteriosclerosis; circulation; endarteritis; hypertonia; hypotonia; intima; lumen; media; mesarteritis; periarteritis; sclerosis.

arthragra (ăr-thrăg'ră) [Gr. *arthron,* joint, + *agra,* seizure]. Gout, q.v. SEE: *podagra.*

arthral (ăr'thrăl). Pert. to a joint.

arthralgia (ăr-thrăl'jē-ă) [" + *algos,* pain]. Pain in a joint.

a. saturnia. Joint pain resulting from lead poisoning.

arthrectomy (ăr-thrĕk'tō-mē) [" + *ektome,* excision]. Excision of a joint.

arthredema (ăr-thrĕ-dē'mă) [" + *oidema,* a swelling]. Edema of a joint.

arthrempyesis (ăr"thrĕm-pī-ē'sĭs) [" + *empyesis,* suppuration]. Suppuration in a joint.

arthresthesia (ăr"thrĕs-thē'zē-ă) [" + *aisthesis,* sensation]. Joint sensibility; the perception of articular motions.

arthritic (ăr-thrĭt'ĭk). 1. Pert. to arthritis. 2. A person afflicted with arthritis.

arthritide (ăr'thrĭ-tīd). A skin eruption caused by arthritis or gout.

arthritides (ăr-thrĭt'ĭ-dēz). Pl. of arthritis.

arthritis (ăr-thrī'tĭs) [" + *itis,* inflammation]. (pl. *arthritides*) Inflammation of a joint, usually accompanied by pain, swelling, and, frequently, changes in structure.

ETIOL: Arthritis may result from or be associated with a number of conditions including: infection (gonococcal, tuberculous, pneumococcal); rheumatic fever; ulcerative colitis; trauma; neurogenic disturbances such as tabes dorsalis; degenerative joint disease such as osteoarthritis; metabolic disturbances such as gout; neoplasms such as synovioma; hydrarthrosis; para- or periarticular conditions such as fibromyositis, myositis, or bursitis; various other conditions such as acromegaly, psoriasis, Raynaud's disease. SEE: *bursitis; rheumatism.*

a., acute secondary. Arthritis caused by osteitis. Severe pain, redness, and swelling.

a., acute suppurative. Purulent distention of synovial sac; a serious form.

a., allergic. Arthritis following ingestion of food allergens or occurring in serum sickness.

a., atrophic. A., rheumatoid, q.v.

a. deformans. A., rheumatoid, q.v.

a., degenerative. A., osteo-, q.v.

a., gonorrheal. Arthritis due to gonorrheal infection. Usually attacks knee joint; during acute stage, several joints may be affected.

TREATMENT: Penicillin, parenterally, in an appropriate dose for 10 to 14 days. If organism is resistant to penicillin, substitute appropriate antibiotic.

a., gouty. Arthritis caused by gout, q.v.

a., hypertrophic. A., osteo-, q.v.

a., juvenile rheumatoid. Rheumatoid arthritis affecting juveniles, with onset prior to age 16. Complete remission occurs in 75% of patients. SYN: *Still's disease.*

NURSING IMPLICATIONS: Assess the patient for symptoms such as redness, swelling, pain and inflammation in the joints, as well as irritability, elevated temperature, and small macular rash on trunk and extremities. Help to improve mobility of the joints by giving a warm bath before exercises, by assisting in range of motion exercises four times daily (after acute inflammation has subsided), and by applying splints at night to affected joints as ordered.

Administer all medications such as steroids and salicylates as ordered. Encourage the child to participate in activities *except* those that increase joint pain and cause undue fatigue. Recognize that the parents will need assistance in determining what they should allow the child to do, and will need support in order to encourage the child to be as independent as possible. Instruct the child and family about the disease process, its pathology, symptoms, treatment, and the expected course.

a., neurogenic. A., neurotrophic, q.v.

a., neurotrophic. Arthritis accompanying or following diseases of the nervous system. Occurs in tabes dorsalis and syringomyelia. SEE: *Charcot's joint.*

a., osteo-. A chronic disease involving the joints, esp. those bearing weight. Characterized by degeneration of articular cartilage, overgrowth of bone with lipping and spur formation, and impaired function. SYN: *a., degenerative; a., hypertrophic; degenerative joint disease.*

a., palindromic. Transient recurrent arthritis, of unknown etiology, of large joints.

a., psoriatic. A form of arthritis that may develop after psoriasis has developed. The exacerbations and remissions of arthritic symptoms parallel those of psoriasis.

a., rheumatoid. A chronic systemic disease characterized by inflammatory changes in joints and related structures that result in crippling deformities. SEE: illus.

ETIOL: The specific cause is unknown but it is generally believed that the pathological changes in the joints are related to an antigen-antibody reaction that is poorly understood. Environmental and familial factors are of doubtful importance. Onset may vary, but usually occurs in middle age.

TREATMENT: There is no specific therapy. If the condition is severe and painful, bedrest may be required for a short time. The salicylates, such as aspirin and sodium salicylate, are the most commonly used drugs in treating rheumatoid arthritis. Gold compounds, anti-inflammatory agents such as naproxen, indomethacin, and ibuprofen, and corticosteroids (for short term anti-inflammatory use only) are also used in treatment. Intra-articular injection of certain corticosteroids is useful in treating acute inflammation of synovial tissue of one or two painful joints. This local treatment is effective for up to 21 days and may be used to allow a patient to remain ambulatory. Local or systemic use of corticosteroids does not cure the basic disease process or prevent the progression of pathologic changes in the joint.

CAUTION: Long-term use of corticosteroids is contraindicated due to the development of undesired side effects.

The use of exercise and physiotherapy is important in maintaining range of motion of the affected joints. Until the inflammatory response has subsided, passive exercise is employed to prevent contractures. When in-

RHEUMATOID ARTHRITIS

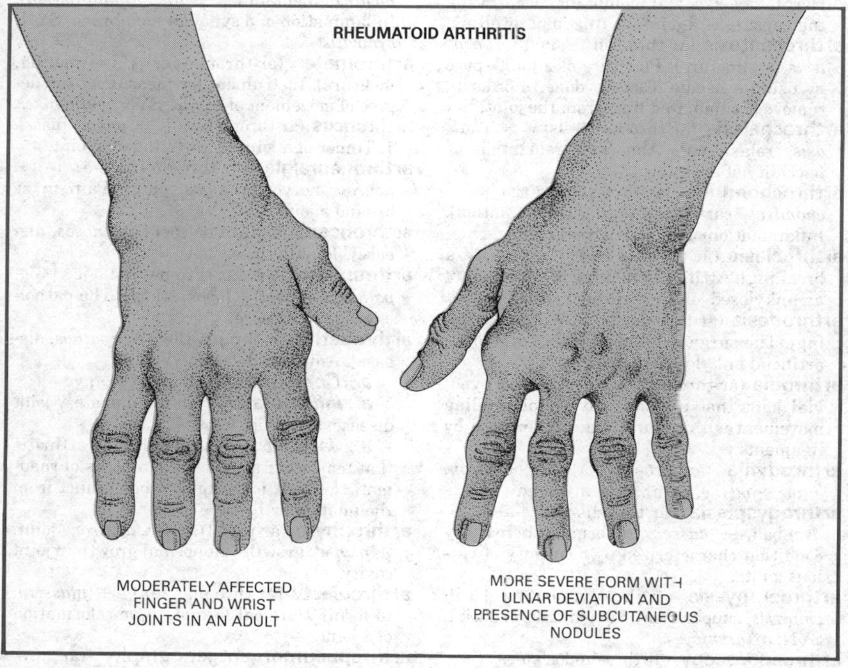

MODERATELY AFFECTED FINGER AND WRIST JOINTS IN AN ADULT

MORE SEVERE FORM WITH ULNAR DEVIATION AND PRESENCE OF SUBCUTANEOUS NODULES

flammation has subsided, active exercise is used to maintain muscle strength and range of motion. A variety of self-help devices are available for patients with severe limitation of joint movement, thus enabling these patients to remain self-sufficient. The use of surgical procedures such as arthroplasty and total hip replacement has been effective in very severe forms of rheumatoid arthritis.

a., suppurative. Inflammation of a synovial membrane with purulent effusion into the joint capsule; usually due to bacterial infection. SYN: *synovitis, purulent.*

a., syphilitic. Arthritis occurring in secondary and tertiary stages of syphilis; characterized by tenderness, swelling, and limitation of motion.

a., tuberculous. Tuberculosis of a joint.

arthritism (ăr′thrĭ-tĭzm) [Gr. *arthron,* joint, + *-ismos,* condition of]. Constitutional predisposition to the development of joint disease.

arthro- [Gr. *arthron,* joint]. Prefix pert. to joints.

arthrobacterium (ăr″thrō-băk-tē′rē-ŭm) [″ + *bakterion,* little staff]. A bacterium that reproduces by segmentation or fission.

arthrocace (ăr-thrŏk′ă-sē) [″ + *kake,* badness]. Infected cavity of a joint.

arthrocele (ăr′thrō-sēl) [″ + *kele,* tumor]. 1. Hernia of a synovial membrane, penetrating the capsule of a joint. 2. Any joint swelling.

arthrocentesis (ăr″thrō-sĕn-tē′sĭs) [″ + *kentesis,* a puncture]. Puncture of a joint space by using a needle. Usually done in order to remove accumulated fluid from the joint.

arthrochalasis (ăr″thrō-kăl′ă-sĭs) [″ + *chalasis,* relaxation]. Abnormal relaxation or flaccidity of a joint.

arthrochondritis (ăr″thrō-kŏn-drī′tĭs) [″ + *chondros,* cartilage, + *itis,* inflammation]. Inflammation of an articular cartilage.

arthroclasia (ăr″thrō-klā′zē-ă) [″ + *klasis,* a breaking]. Artificial breaking of adhesions of an ankylosed joint to provide movement.

arthrodesis (ăr-thrō-dē′sĭs) [″ + *desis,* binding]. The surgical immobilization of a joint; artificial ankylosis.

arthrodia (ăr-thrō′dē-ă) [Gr.]. A type of synovial joint that permits only simple gliding movement within narrow limits imposed by ligaments.

arthrodynia (ăr″thrō-dĭn′ē-ă) [Gr. *arthron,* joint, + *odyne,* pain]. Pain in a joint.

arthrodysplasia (ăr″thrō-dĭs-plā′zē-ă) [″ + *dys,* bad, + *plassein,* to form]. A hereditary condition characterized by deformity of various joints.

arthroempyesis (ăr″thrō-ĕm-pī-ē′sĭs) [″ + *empyesis,* suppuration]. Suppuration in a joint. SYN: *arthrempyesis.*

arthroendoscopy (ăr″thrō-ĕn-dŏs′kō-pē) [″ + *endon,* within, + *skopein,* to examine]. Inspection of interior of a joint by using an endoscope.

arthrogram (ăr′thrō-grăm) [″ + *gramma,* mark]. Visualization of a joint by x-ray study after injection of an opaque dye into the joint-space.

arthrography (ăr-thrŏg′ră-fē) [″ + *graphein,* to write]. 1. A description of the joints. 2. Roentgenography of a joint.

arthrogryposis (ăr″thrō-grĭ-pō′sĭs) [″ + *grypos,* curved, + *osis,* condition]. Fixation of a joint in a flexed or contracted position. May be due to adhesions in or around the joint.

a. multiplex congenita. Generalized fixation or ankylosis of joints that is present at birth. May be due to a variety of changes in the spinal cord, muscles, or connective tissue.

arthrokleisis (ăr″thrō-klī′sĭs) [″ + *kleisis,* a closure]. Ankylosis or fixation of a joint produced naturally or surgically.

arthrolith (ăr′thrō-lĭth) [″ + *lithos,* stone]. Calculous deposit in a joint.

arthrology (ăr-thrŏl′ō-jē) [Gr. *arthron,* joint, + *logos,* study]. The science of joints.

arthrolysis (ăr-thrŏl′ĭ-sĭs) [″ + *lysis,* a loosening]. The operation of restoring mobility to an ankylosed joint.

arthromeningitis (ăr″thrō-mĕn″ĭn-jī′tĭs) [″ + *meninx,* membrane, + *itis,* inflammation]. Inflammation of a synovial membrane. SYN: *synovitis.*

arthrometer (ăr-thrŏm′ĕ-ter) [″ + *metron,* measure]. Instrument for measuring the degree of movement of a joint. SYN: *goniometer.*

arthroncus (ăr-thrŏng′kŭs) [″ + *onkos,* mass]. 1. Tumor of a joint. 2. Swelling of a joint.

arthroneuralgia (ăr″thrō-nū-răl′jē-ă) [″ + *neuron,* nerve, + *algos,* pain]. Pain in or around a joint.

arthronosos (ăr″thrō-nō′sŏs) [″ + *nosos,* disease]. Joint disease.

arthropathology (ăr″thrō-pă-thol′ō-jē) [″ + *pathos,* disease, + *logos,* study]. The pathology of joint disease.

arthropathy (ăr-thrŏp′ă-thē) [″ + *pathos,* disease]. Any joint disease.

a., Charcot's. A., neurogenic, q.v.

a., inflammatory. An inflammatory joint disease; arthritis.

a., Jaccoud. A form of chronic arthritis that may occur after several attacks of rheumatic fever. It is thought to be distinct from rheumatoid arthritis.

arthrophyte (ăr′thrō-fīt) [Gr. *arthron,* joint, + *phyton,* growth]. Abnormal growth in joint cavity.

arthroplasty (ăr′thrō-plăs″tē) [″ + *plassein,* to form]. Surgical formation or reformation of a joint.

arthropneumoroentgenography (ăr″thrō-nū″mō-rĕnt-gĕn-ŏg′ră-fē) [″ + *pneuma,* air, + *roentgenography*]. X-raying of joint after injecting a gas such as sterile air or helium into the joint space. SEE: *arthrogram.*

arthropod (ăr′thrō-pŏd). A member of the phylum Arthropoda.

Arthropoda (ăr-thrŏp′ō-dă) [″ + *pous,* foot]. A phylum of invertebrate animals characterized by bilateral symmetry, a hard, jointed exoskeleton, segmented bodies, and jointed paired appendages. Includes the crustaceans; insects; myriapods; arachnids; and similar forms. It is the largest animal phylum, containing over 700,000 species. Many are of medical importance as causative agents of disease, as vectors, or as parasites.

arthropyosis (ăr″thrō-pī-ō′sĭs) [″ + *pyosis,* suppuration]. Suppuration of a joint.

arthrorheumatism (ăr″thrō-roo′mă-tĭzm) [″ + *rheumatismos,* flux]. Rheumatism of the joints.

arthrorrhagia (ăr″thrō-rā′jē-ă) [″ + *rhegnynai,* to burst forth]. Hemorrhage into a joint.

arthrosclerosis [Gr. *arthron,* joint, + *sklerosis,* a hardening]. Stiffening or hardening of the joints, esp. in the aged.

arthroscope (ăr′thrō-skōp) [″ + *skopein,* to examine]. An endoscope for examining interior of a joint.

arthroscopy (ăr-thrŏs′kō-pē). Direct joint visualization by means of an arthroscope.

arthrosis (ăr-thrō′sĭs) [″ + *osis,* condition]. 1. Joint. 2. Joint affection caused by trophic degeneration.

arthrospore (ăr′thrō-spor) [″ + *sporos,* a seed]. A bacterial spore formed by segmentation.

arthrosteitis (ăr″thrŏs-tē-ī′tĭs) [″ + *osteon,* bone, + *itis,* inflammation]. Inflammation of the bony structures of a joint.

arthrostomy (ăr-thrŏs′tō-mē) [″ + *stoma,* an opening]. The surgical formation of a temporary opening into a joint for drainage purposes.

arthrosynovitis (ăr″thrō-sĭn″ō-vī′tĭs) [″ + L. *synovia,* joint fluid, + Gr. *itis,* inflammation]. Inflammation of synovial membrane of a joint.

arthrotome (ăr′thrō-tōm) [″ + *tome,* incision]. Knife for making incisions into a joint.

arthrotomy (ăr-thrŏt′ō-mē). Cutting into a joint.

arthrous (ăr′thrŭs) [Gr. *arthron,* joint]. Jointed or pert. to a joint.

arthroxesis (ăr-thrŏk′sĭ-sĭs) [″ + *xesis,* scraping]. Scraping of diseased tissue from a joint.

Arthus reaction, phenomenon (ăr-toos′). [Maurice Arthus, Fr. physiologist, 1862–1945] A severe local inflammatory reaction that occurs at site of repeated injection of a nonirritating antigen (such as egg albumin) to which the animal already has precipitating antibody. It is considered an immediate hypersensitivity reaction.

artichoke factor. Chlorogenic acid, cynarin, and other substances found in artichokes that make water and some foods taste sweet if ingested within a few minutes after eating artichokes.

articular (ăr-tĭk′ū-lăr) [L. *articularis*]. Pert. to articulation.

articulate (ăr-tĭk′ū-lāt, -lăt) [L. *articulatus,* jointed]. 1. To join together as a joint. 2. In dentistry, the arrangement of teeth on a denture. 3. Clearly spoken. 4. To enunciate clearly.

articulated (ăr-tĭk′ū-lāt′d). State of articulation or of being jointed.

articulatio (ăr-tĭk″ū-lā′shē-ō) [L.]. The site of union or junction of two bones.

articulation. 1. The place of union between two or more bones; a joint. It is classified as being immovable (synarthrosis), slightly movable (amphiarthrosis), or freely movable (diarthrosis). Cartilage, or fibrous or soft tissue lines the opposing surfaces of all joints. 2. The relative position of the tongue and palate necessary to produce a given sound. 3. Enunciation of words and sentences.

a., articulator. The use of a mechanical device to simulate the action of the temporomandibular joint when placing teeth in complete dentures or partial removable dentures so that they articulate properly.

a., confluent. Speech in which syllables are run together.

a., dental. The contact relationship between upper and lower teeth when moving against each other or into or out of centric position.

articulator (ăr-tĭk′ū-lā″tor). Device used in dentistry for maintaining casts of the teeth in a precise and natural relationship.

articulo mortis (ăr-tĭk′ū-lō″ mor′tĭs) [L.]. At the time of death.

articulus (ăr-tĭk′ū-lŭs) [L.]. 1. A knuckle or a joint. 2. A segment.

artifact, artefact (ăr′tĭ-făkt, ăr′tĕ-făkt) [L. *ars,* art, + *facere,* to make]. 1. Anything artificially produced. 2. In histology and radiography, any structure or feature produced by the technique used and not occurring naturally.

artificial (ăr″tĭ-fĭsh′ăl). Not natural; formed in imitation of nature.

artificial assists. General term indicating various means of supporting bodily functions.

Ex.: artificial limb, crutch, cardiac pacemaker, or respirator.

artificial hyperemia. Bringing blood to the superficial tissues by means of counterirritation, such as may be produced by cupping or acupuncture.

artificial impregnation. Artificial insemination, q.v.

artificial insemination. ABBR: AI. Mechanical injection of viable semen into the vagina.

artificial pneumothorax. Artificial introduction of air into pleural cavity. Oxygen, nitrogen, or filtered atmospheric air is used.

artificial respiration. Maintenance of respiratory movements by artificial means.

EMERGENCY MEASURES: Call a physician immediately. Laryngeal spasm often blocks air from lungs. Passage of catheter or airway tube may be necessary. Drugs may be needed to counteract spasm and promote circulation. If such a spasm exists, attempts at artificial respiration may be useless.

IMPORTANT: It may be necessary to continue artificial respiration for hours. It should not be discontinued until the patient has revived or has been declared dead by a physician.

Keep warm with blankets; massage with friction; hot water bottles, etc. If possible, head should be directed downward to aid circulation to brain; it is desirable to turn the mouth toward the wind. Circulation must be maintained by massaging extremities toward the heart. Stimulants such as aromatic spirits of ammonia applied to nostrils intermittently and injections of drugs such as epinephrine (adrenalin) and ephedrine.

METHODS: *Mechanical methods:* These include various pressure-cycling devices designed to alter pressure within the lungs and bring about the exchange of gases.

Ex.: resuscitators; respirators (iron lungs); pulmotors; and lung motors. Also, devices for stimulation of phrenic nerves are used. SEE: *electrophrenic respiration.*

Manual methods: It is important that all efforts to institute artificial respiration be done in an orderly manner. The steps required to do this are (SEE: illus):

Step 1. Opening the airway. Head tilt–necklift and head tilt–chinlift may be used. When performing the chinlift, the fingers of one hand are placed under the lower jaw on the bony part near the chin and lifted to bring the chin forward. The fingers must not compress the soft tissue under the chin, which might obstruct the airway.

Step 2. Establishing breathlessness. Rescuer places ear over the victim's mouth and nose, looking towards the victim's chest and stomach to see if the chest rises and falls; listens for air during exhalation; and feels for patient's exhaled air on the cheek.

Step 3. Rescue breathing. Mouth to mouth, mouth to nose, or mouth to stoma (if present) are alternatives. In infants, mouth to nose and mouth will be required. Mouth to mouth:

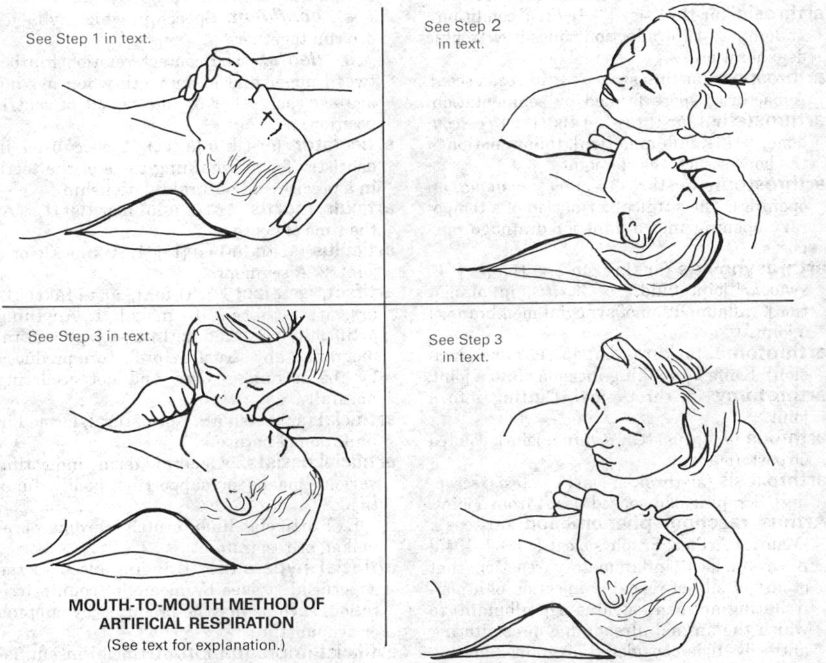
See Step 1 in text.
See Step 2 in text.
See Step 3 in text.
See Step 3 in text.

MOUTH-TO-MOUTH METHOD OF ARTIFICIAL RESPIRATION
(See text for explanation.)

The nostrils of the victim must be pinched closed to prevent air escaping. The rescuer takes a breath and with mouth open wide, places it around the victim's mouth making a seal. Rescuer then blows air into the victim's mouth, initially delivering four quick full breaths without allowing time for full lung deflation between breaths. To maintain a nonbreathing victim with a pulse, the rescuer should deliver one breath every five seconds. Rescue breathing should not be preceded by attempts to remove foreign objects from the mouth unless they are very obvious. Time is critical. If attempts to ventilate are thwarted, then the obstructed airway series should be initiated. This consists of four back blows between the shoulder blades and four abdominal thrusts between the xiphoid and the umbilicus and then an attempt to remove the foreign body. The infant and child should be done the same way; they should not be held by the ankles. SEE: *Heimlich maneuver.*

Resuscitation of conscious choking or unconscious infant: The American Heart Association recommendations for cardiopulmonary resuscitation and emergency cardiac care are provided in the table on page 140.

Choice of method depends upon the individual case. If respiration needs only to be started and maintained artificially for a limited period, as in asphyxia from such causes as gases, drowning, and electric shock, the mouth-to-mouth method is effective. If resuscitation apparatus is available, the use of O_2 and CO_2 is indicated. In cases where artificial respiration must be maintained for days, as in morphine poisoning and infantile paralysis, apparatus such as a respirator is used.

RS: asphyxia; collapse; coma; drowning; respiration; respirator; resuscitation; shock; syncope; unconsciousness.

artisan's cramp. A spasmodic affection of the muscles induced by prolonged work requiring delicate coordination and occurring only in performance of that particular work. Most apt to occur in writing, piano playing, sewing, and telegraphing.

aryepiglottic (ăr″ē-ĕp″ĭ-glŏt′ĭk) [Gr. *arytaina,* pitcher, + *epi,* upon, + *glottis,* glottis]. Pert. to the arytenoid cartilage and epiglottis.

aryl-. Prefix denoting a radical derived from an aromatic hydrocarbon.

a. group. In chemistry, a radical group of the aromatic or benzene series.

arylarsonate (ăr-ĭl-ăr′sō-nāt). Salt of arylarsonic acid.

arytenoid (ăr″ĭ-tē′noyd) [Gr. *arytaina,* ladle, + *eidos,* form]. 1. Resembling a ladle or pitcher mouth. 2. Rel. to the arytenoid cartilage, gland, ligament, or muscle.

arytenoidectomy (ăr″ĭ-tē″noyd-ĕk′tō-mē) [″ + ″ + *ektome,* excision]. Excision of arytenoid cartilage.

arytenoiditis (ăr-ĭt″ē-noy-dī′tĭs) [″ + ″ + *itis,* inflammation]. Inflammation of arytenoid cartilage or muscles.

arytenoidopexy (ăr″ĭ-tē-noy dō-pĕk″sē) [″ + ″ + *pexis,* fixation]. Surgical fixation of the arytenoid muscle or cartilage.

Arzberger's pear (ărz′bĕr-gĕrz). [Friedrich Arzberger, Austrian physicist, 1833–1905] A hollow pear-shaped device through which cool water is passed after it has been inserted into the rectum. Used in treating rectal diseases such as hemorrhoids.

AS. L. *auris sinistra,* left ear.

As. 1. *astigmatic; astigmatism.* 2. Chem. symb. for arsenic.

ASA. *acetylsalicylic acid.* SYN: *aspirin.*

asafetida, asafoetida (ăs-ă-fĕt′ĭd-ă) [L. *asa,* gum, + *foetida,* smelly]. A gum resin, obtained from the roots of Ferula asafoetida, with characteristic strong odor and garlic taste. Even though this substance is no longer used in medicine, it is of historical interest. In the early part of the 20th century it was used as a carminative and as an amulet to ward off disease. Used in Asia as a condiment and food flavoring, and as an animal repellent in veterinary medicine.

asaphia (ă-săf′ē-ă, ă-să′fē-ă) [Gr. *asapheia,* obscurity]. Inability to speak distinctly.

asbestiform (ăs-bĕs′tĭ-form) [Gr. *asbestos,* unquenchable, + L. *forma,* appearance]. Having structure similar to asbestos.

asbestos (ăs-bĕs′tŏs) [Gr. *asbestos,* unquenchable]. Fibrous, incombustible form of magnesium and calcium silicate used to make insulating materials.

asbestosis (ăs″bĕ-stō′sĭs) [″ + *osis,* condition]. Lung disease, a form of pneumonoconiosis, q.v., resulting from protracted inhalation of asbestos particles.

ascariasis (ăs″kă-rī′ă-sĭs) [Gr. *askaris,* pinworm, + *-iasis,* condition of]. Condition resulting from infestation by Ascaris lumbricoides, q.v.

ascaricide (ăs-kăr′ĭ-sīd) [″ + L. *cidus,* killing]. 1. Drug that kills ascaris worms. 2. That which kills ascaris worms.

ascarides (ăs-kăr′ĭ-dēz). Pl. of Ascaris, q.v.

Ascaris (ăs′kă-rĭs). (pl. *ascarides*) A genus of nematodes, roundworms, belonging to the superfamily Ascaridoidea. They inhabit the intestines of invertebrates.

A. lumbricoides. A species of Ascaris that lives in the human intestine. Eggs are passed with the feces and require at least two weeks' incubation in the soil before they become infective. After being swallowed, the eggs hatch and the larvae enter the venous circulation, pass to the lungs, from which they migrate up the respiratory passages and

Artificial Respiration*

Choking Infant Who Becomes Unconscious or Is Found Unconscious

Elapsed Time (Seconds) Min.	Max.	Activity and Time (Seconds)	Critical Performance	Rationale
4	10	Establish unresponsiveness. Call for help. Turn victim. (4–10 sec.)	Gently shake, tap, call out for help. Turn infant horizontal and supine.	An accurate diagnosis of unresponsiveness must be made before resuscitation begins or continues.
7	15	Open airway. Establish breathlessness. (Look, Listen, Feel) (3–5 sec.)	Tip head back; do not hyperextend. Rescuer looks toward chest with ear over mouth to look, listen and feel for breathing. Utilize head tilt–neck lift or, if needed, head tilt–chin lift.	Hyperextension of the head can collapse the trachea or cause cervical spine injury in the infant. An accurate diagnosis must be made to establish the presence of cardiopulmonary arrest or airway obstruction.
10	20	Attempt to ventilate. (3–5 sec.)	Ventilate—airway remains obstructed.	Complete airway obstruction or a foreign body is assumed.
13	25	Reattempt to ventilate. (3–5 sec.)	Reposition the head. Airway remains obstructed.	Improper head tilt is the most common cause of airway obstruction. Airway obstruction is confirmed.
15	27	Activate Emergency Medical Service System (EMSS). (2 sec.)	Second rescuer if present should activate the EMSS. Know the local EMS number.	Advanced life support (ALS) capability will be needed.
19	33	4 Back Blows (4–6 sec.)	Same as for conscious infant.	
24	39	4 Chest Thrusts (5–6 sec.)	Same as for conscious infant.	
30	47	Tongue–Jaw Lift (6–8 sec.)	Thumb in victim's mouth over tongue. Lift tongue and jaw forward with fingers wrapped around lower jaw. Remove foreign body if visualized.	Blind finger sweeps are to be avoided in the infant since the foreign body can easily be pushed back and cause further obstruction.
		Verbally indicate repeat of above sequence until effective.	Verbalize alternating the above maneuvers in rapid succession.	Persistent attempts are rapidly made in sequence in order to relieve the obstruction.

Conscious Choking Infant

Min.	Max.	Activity and Time (Seconds)	Critical Performance	Rationale
2	3	Rescuer checks for airway obstruction. (2–3 sec.)	Rescuer must identify complete obstruction by looking, listening and feeling for ventilation and for blueness of the lips.	The presence of complete airway obstruction must be properly diagnosed before proceeding with treatment.
5	8	4 Back Blows (3–5 sec.)	The infant is straddled over the rescuer's arm with the head lower than the trunk. The 4 back blows are delivered rapidly and forcefully between the shoulder blades.	Back blows when used alone may relieve the obstruction.
9	13	4 Chest Thrusts (4–5 sec.)	The infant is supported between 2 hands, turned onto the back, and the thrusts are delivered in the midsternal region in the same manner as external chest compression. The head is lower than the trunk.	The combination of back blows and chest thrusts is superior to one technique when used alone. Abdominal thrusts are not recommended in infants because of the potential injury to the abdominal organs.
		Verbally indicate repeat of above sequence until effective.	Verbalize alternating the above maneuvers in rapid sequence.	Time is of the essence. The two techniques are rapidly repeated alternately until obstruction is relieved or unconsciousness occurs.

*Reprinted by permission of the American Heart Association, Inc.

are swallowed, and reach their site of continued residence, the jejunum. The adult worms lay eggs that are passed with the feces, and a new cycle is started. Children up to the age of 12 to 14 are likely to be infected. Intestinal obstruction is a complication in children under 6 years of age.

TREATMENT: Mebendazole is the treatment of choice. Pyrantel pamoate and piperazine citrate are also effective.

ascaris. A worm of the genus Ascaris.

Aschheim-Zondek test (ăsh'hīm-tsŏn'dĕk). [Selmar Aschheim, Ger. gynecologist, 1878–1965; Bernhardt Zondek, Ger. gynecologist, 1891–1966] A test for pregnancy in which the patient's urine is injected subcutaneously into immature female mice.

Aschner's phenomenon, reflex, sign (ăsh'nĕrz). [Bernhard Aschner, Austrian gynecologist, 1883–1960] Slowing of the pulse following pressure applied to the eyeball or the carotid sinus. Sometimes used to slow the heart during attacks of supraventricular tachycardia. May also be used as a diagnostic test for angina pectoris. Slowing of the heart produced by this reflex may relieve anginal pain. SYN: *oculocardiac reflex.*

Aschoff, Ludwig (ăsh'ŏf). German pathologist, 1866–1942.

A.'s bodies. Aschoff's nodules, q.v.

A.'s cells. Large cells with basophilic cytoplasm and a large vesicular nucleus often multinucleated. Characteristic of Aschoff's nodules.

A.'s nodules. Small nodules composed of cells and leukocytes found in the interstitial tissues of the heart in rheumatic myocarditis.

asci (ăs'ī). Pl. of ascus.

ascia (ăs'ē-ă, ăs'kē-ă) [L. *ascia,* ax]. A form of spiral bandage with each turn overlapping the previous one for a third of its width.

ascites (ă-sī'tēz) [Gr. *askites*]. The accumulation of serous fluid in the peritoneal cavity. SEE: *edema.*

ETIOL: Interference in venous return as occurs in cardiac disease, obstruction of flow in vena cava or portal vein; obstruction in lymphatic drainage; disturbance in electrolyte balance as occurs in sodium retention, depletion of plasma proteins, or cirrhosis of the liver.

a. chylosus. Chyle in the ascitic fluid, usually resulting from rupture of thoracic duct.

ascitic (ă-sĭt'ĭk). Pert. to ascites.

ascitic fluid. Clear and pale straw-colored fluid occurring in ascites, sp. gr. 1.005–1.015.

Ascoli's reaction, test (ăs-kō'lēz). [Alberto Ascoli, It. serologist, 1877–1956] Precipitation test for anthrax. Used for detection of anthrax bacilli in animal hides and meat.

Ascomycetes (ăs"kō-mī-sē'tēz) [Gr. *askos,* bag, + *mykes,* fungus]. The sac fungi; the largest class of Eumycetes, the true fungi (of the phylum Thallophyta). Organisms in this group are characterized by possession of a saclike sporangium (ascus, q.v.) in which ascospores are developed. Includes the yeasts, blue molds, mildews, and truffles.

ascorbic acid (ăs-kor'bĭk) [Gr. *a-,* not, + L. *scorbutus,* scurvy]. USP. Vitamin C. It occurs naturally and can be synthesized. SEE: *acid, ascorbic; vitamin C.*

ascospore (ăs'kō-spor) [Gr. *askos,* bag, + *sporos,* seed]. A spore produced within an ascus or spore sac.

ascus (ăs'kŭs) [Gr. *askos,* bag]. (pl. *asci*) A saclike spore case within which ascospores, typically eight, are formed; characteristic of the Ascomycetes, q.v.

-ase. A suffix used in forming the name of an enzyme. It is added to the name or a part of the name of the substance upon which it acts; e.g., lipase, which acts on fats (lipids).

Asellacrin. Trade name for somatotropin (HGH), USP, q.v.

asemia, asemasia (ă-sē'mē-ă, ăs"ĭ-mā'zē-ă) [Gr. *a-,* not, + *semasia,* the giving of a sign]. Loss of previous ability to comprehend any type of symbol; a form of aphasia, q.v. May be of organic or emotional origin. Previously called asymbolia.

asepsis (ā-sĕp'sĭs) [" + *sepesthai,* to decay]. Sterile; a condition free from germs, from infection, and any form of life. SEE: *antisepsis; sterilization.*

aseptic (ā-sĕp'tĭk). Rel. to asepsis; free from septic matter.

aseptic-antiseptic [Gr. *a-,* not, + *sepsis,* decay, + *anti,* against, + *sepsis,* decay]. Both aseptic and antiseptic.

aseptic technique. Method used in surgical procedures to prevent contamination of the wound and operative site. All instruments used are sterilized, and physicians and nurses wear sterile caps, masks, and gloves.

asexual (ā-sĕk'shū-ăl) [" + L. *sexualis,* having sex]. Without sex; nonsexual.

asexualization (ā-sĕk"shū-ăl-ĭ-zā'shŭn). Sterilization by ablation of the ovaries or testes.

ash (ăsh) [AS. *aesc,* ash]. Incombustible powdery residue of a substance that has been completely incinerated.

asialia (ă"sī-ā'lē-ă, ā"sē-ā'lē-a) [" + *sialon,* spittle]. Failure to secrete or deficiency of saliva. SYN: *aptyalism.*

Asiatic cholera. An acute infectious epidemic disease. SEE: *cholera.*

asiderosis (ă"sĭd-ĕ-rō'sĭs) [" + *sideros,* iron, + *osis,* condition]. Deficiency of iron reserve in the body.

asitia (ă-sĭsh'ē-ă) [" + *sitos,* food]. 1. Aversion

to food. SEE: *anorexia*. 2. The want of food.

ASLO. *antistreptolysin-O.*

A.S.M.T. *American Society for Medical Technology.*

asocial (ā-sō′shĭl). 1. Withdrawn from society. 2. Inconsiderate of the needs of others.

asoma (ā-sō′mă) [Gr. *a*-, not, + *soma*, body]. Deformed fetus with an imperfectly formed trunk and head.

asonia (ă-sō′nē-ă) [″ + L. *sonus*, sound]. Tone deafness.

asparagine (ăs-păr′ă-jĭn). Aminosuccinic acid, a nonessential amino acid.

Asparagus (ă-spăr′ă-gŭs) [Gr. *asparagos*]. A genus of liliaceous herbs.

A. officinalis. Plant of which the tender shoots are eaten as food, and the root is used as a mild diuretic.

aspartame (ă-spăr′tām). An artificial sweetener synthesized from two amino acids, aspartic acid and phenylalanine. It is 180 times sweeter than sugar. Trade names are Equal and Nutrasweet.

aspartate aminotransferase (ă-spăr′tāt). Glutamic-oxalacetic transaminase, q.v.

aspartic acid. $COOHCHNH_2CH_2COOH$. A nonessential amino acid, q.v.; one of the products of pancreatic digestion.

aspastic (ă-spăs′tĭk) [Gr. *a*-, not, + *spastikos*, having spasms]. Nonspastic.

aspecific (ă-spē-sĭf′ĭk). Not specific.

aspect (ăs′pĕkt) [L. *aspectus*, a view]. 1. That part of a surface facing in any designated direction. 2. Appearance, looks.

aspergillin (ăs″pĕr-jĭl′ĭn). 1. A pigment produced by Aspergillus niger, q.v. 2. An inappropriate name applied to a number of antibiotic substances produced by various species of Aspergillus.

aspergillosis (ăs″pĕr-jĭl-ō′sĭs) [*aspergillus* + Gr. *osis*, condition]. Aspergillus infection in the tissues or on any mucous surface marked by inflammatory granulomatous lesions. This condition may develop in the bronchi, lungs, aural canal, skin, or the mucous membranes of the eye, nose, or urethra. It may extend through the various viscera, producing mycotic nodules in the lungs, liver, kidney, and other organs.

a., aural. A form of otomycosis, q.v.

a., pulmonary. Disease of the lungs caused by Aspergillus.

Aspergillus (ăs″pĕr-jĭl′ŭs) [L. *aspergere*, to sprinkle]. A genus of Ascomycetes, including several species of the molds, some of which are pathogenic. The principal pathogenic species is A. fumigatus, although others (A. flavus, A. nidulans, and A. niger) may be pathogenic. SEE: *aspergillosis*.

A. auricularis. A species found in the external auditory meatus. SEE: *otomycosis*.

A. barbae. A species found in mycosis of the scalp.

A. bouffardi. A species found in black mycetoma.

A. bronchialis. A species found in the bronchi of diabetic patients.

A. clavatus. A species found in soil and manure. Its cultures yield the antibacterial substance clavacin, which is too toxic for therapeutic use.

A. concentricus. A species once thought to be the cause of tinea imbricata ringworm.

A. flavus. A mold found on corn, peanuts and grain.

A. fumigatus. Found in soil and manure, this fungus is the common cause of aspergillosis in man and birds. It has been found in the ear, nose, and lungs. It yields the antibacterial substance fumigacin.

A. glaucus. A bluish mold found on dried fruit. Sometimes found in human ear infections.

A. mucoroides. A species sometimes found in the lungs.

A. nidulans. A species common in soil, causing one form of white mycetoma.

A. niger. A pathogenic form with black spores, frequently present in the external auditory meatus. Causes otomycosis.

A. ocraceus. The species that produces the characteristic odor of brewing coffee.

A. pictor. A species found in the patches of pinta.

A. repens. A species found in the external auditory canal.

aspermatic (ă-spĕr-măt′ĭk) [Gr. *a*-, not, + *sperma*, seed]. Pert. to aspermatism.

aspermatism (ă-spĕr′mă-tĭzm) [″ + ″ + *-ismos*, condition of]. 1. Absence or nonemission of semen. SYN: *aspermia*. SEE: *azoospermia*. 2. Lack of formation of sperm.

aspermatogenesis (ă-spĕr″mă-tō-jeň′ĕ-sĭs) [″ + ″ + *genesis*, production]. Nonfunction of the sperm-producing system of the testicles.

aspermia (ă-spĕr′mē-ă) [″ + *sperma*, seed]. Lack of, or failure to ejaculate, semen.

aspermous (ă-spĕr′mŭs). Pert. to aspermia. SYN: *aspermatic*.

asperous (ăs′pĕr-ŭs) [L. *asper*, rough]. Uneven; having minute elevations.

aspersion (ăs-pĕr′zhŭn) [L. *aspersio*, sprinkling]. Sprinkling an affected part with water; a form of hydrotherapy, q.v.

asphalgesia (ăs″făl-jē′zē-ă) [Gr. *asphe*-, self, + *algos*, pain]. A burning sensation sometimes felt on touching certain articles during hypnosis.

asphyctic, asphyctous (ăs-fĭk′tĭk, -tŭs) [Gr. *a*-, not, + *sphyxis*, pulse]. 1. Pert. to, or affected with, asphyxia. 2. Without pulse.

asphyxia (ăs-fĭk′sē-ă) [″ + *sphyxis*, pulse]. Condition caused by insufficient intake of oxygen.

ETIOL: *Extrinsic causes:* Choking; toxic gases; exhaust gas (principally carbon monoxide); electric shock; drugs; anesthesia; traumatic asphyxia; crushing injuries of chest; compression of chest; injury of respiratory nerves or centers; diminution of oxygenation of environment; drowning. *Intrinsic causes:* Hemorrhage into lungs or pleural cavity; foreign bodies in throat; swelling of air passages; diseases of air passages; ruptured aneurysm or abscess; edema of the lung; cardiac deficiency; tumors such as goiter; pharyngeal and retropharyngeal abscesses. *Other causes:* Paralysis of the respiratory center; anesthesia; pneumothorax; narcotic drugs; electrocution; child abuse.

SYM: In general, symptoms include dyspnea, cyanosis, rapid pulse, impairment of senses, mental disturbances; in extreme cases convulsions, unconsciousness, and death.

F.A.: Artificial respiration, q.v.

a. carbonica. Suffocation from inhalation of coal or water gas, or carbon monoxide.

a., fetal. Asphyxia occurring in a fetus; results from interference in placental circulation or from premature separation of placenta, as in abruptio placentae.

a. livida. Asphyxia in which the skin is cyanotic from lack of oxygen in blood.

a., local. Asphyxia in which a limited portion of the body is involved, such as the fingers, hands, toes, or feet due to stagnation in circulation. One of the symptoms usually associated with Raynaud's disease, q.v.

a. neonatorum. Respiratory failure in the newborn.

a. pallida. Asphyxia in which difficulty in breathing is accompanied by weak and thready pulse, pale skin, and absence of reflexes.

asphyxial (ăs-fĭk'sē-ăl). Pert. to asphyxia; asphyctic.

asphyxiant (ăs-fĭk'sē-ănt). An agent, esp. any gas, that will produce asphyxia.

asphyxiate (ăs-fĭk'sē-āt). To cause asphyxiation or asphyxia.

asphyxiation (ăs-fĭk"sē-ā'shŭn). A state of asphyxia or suffocation. Act of producing asphyxia. SEE: *asphyxia.*

aspidium (ăs-pĭd'ē-ŭm) [Gr. *aspidion,* little shield]. The root and stalk of Dryopteris flixmas (male fern) or D. marginalis (marginal fern). Used medicinally in form of oleoresin.

a. oleoresin. Extract of male fern; male fern oleoresin.

USE: As an anthelminthic in treatment of tapeworm infestation of intestines. Care should be taken that it is not administered with an oil, since absorption may occur.

aspirate (ăs'pĭ-rāt) [L. *ad,* to, + *spirare,* to breathe]. 1. Aspiration; to draw in or out by suction. 2. A sound like that of the letter *h.*

aspiration (ăs-pĭ-rā'shŭn). 1. Drawing in or out as by suction. Foreign bodies may be aspirated into the nose, throat, or lungs on inspiration. 2. The withdrawing of a fluid from a cavity by means of suction with an instrument called an aspirator. Cavities most commonly aspirated are pericardial, peritoneal, pleural and thecal (lumbar puncture). The object of aspiration is to remove fluid from an affected area such as in pleural effusion, ascites, or an abscess, or to obtain specimens such as blood from a vein or serum from the spinal canal.

EQUIP: Disinfecting solution for the skin; local anesthetic; two aspirating needles with the aspirating apparatus as indicated; utensil for receiving the fluid and a sterile receptacle for the specimen; sterile sponges, towels, basins; sterile gloves, face masks, and gowns; sterile forceps; surgical dressings as the case may require; stimulant ordered if indication arises.

NURSING IMPLICATIONS: Position patient appropriately for the body cavity to be aspirated. The patient should be draped to ensure privacy and to be kept warm. Provide support during the procedure. Carefully observe the type and amount of any drainage or material that is aspirated.

aspirator (ăs'pĭ-rā-tor). Apparatus for evacuating fluid contents of a cavity. Varieties are piston pump, compressible rubber tube, rubber bulb, and siphon, a trocar and cannula, and hypodermic needle and syringe.

aspirin (ăs'pĕr-ĭn). USP. $CH_3COOC_6H_4COOH$. A derivative of salicylic acid. It occurs as white crystals or powder. It is one of the most widely used analgesics and antipyretics. Also, because it is widely available, it is often misused, and is one of the most frequent causes of accidental poisoning in children.

aspirin poisoning. In acute poisoning, signs vary with increasing doses from mild lethargy and hyperpnea to coma and convulsions. Sweating, dehydration, hyperthermia, and restlessness may be present with moderate doses. In chronic poisoning, tinnitus, skin rash, bleeding tendency, weight loss, and mental symptoms may be present.

TREATMENT: In acute poisoning, gastric lavage or emetics. Give sodium sulfate by mouth to remove remaining salicylate. Artificial respiration with administration of oxygen may be required. For a child, if blood pressure is low, give whole blood transfusion at the rate of 10 to 15 ml./kg. body weight for 1 hour. Glucose by mouth or intravenously is indicated if hypoglycemia is present. For convulsions not due to hypoglycemia, give succinylcholine intravenously and at the same time give artificial respiration. Be certain to maintain the airway. In very severe cases, the use of exchange transfusion or hemodialysis is indicated.

SEE: *Poisons and Poisoning* in *Appendix*.

asplenia (ă-splē′nē-ă) [Gr. *a-*, not, + L. *splen*, spleen]. Absence of the spleen.

asporogenic (ăs″pō-rō-jĕn′ĭk) [″ + *sporos*, seed, + *gennan*, to produce]. Not reproducing by spores.

asporous (ă-spō′rŭs). Having no spores.

A.S.R.T. *American Society of Radiologic Technologists.*

assault (ă-sawlt′) [L. *assultus*, having assailed]. Violent physical attack on an individual. In legal medicine, the performance of a therapeutic procedure such as surgery or administration of an injection without first obtaining proper authorization.

assay (ă-sā′, ăs′ā) [O. Fr. *assai*, trial]. The analysis of a substance or mixture to determine its constituents and the relative proportion of each.

a., biological. Estimation of strength of a drug or substance by comparing its effects in test animals to a reference standard. SYN: *bioassay.*

assident (ăs′ĭ-dĕnt) [L. *assidere*, to sit by]. A term applied to symptoms to indicate they are usually but not invariably present with a certain disease.

assimilable (ă-sĭm′ĭ-lă-bl) [L. *ad*, to, + *similare*, to make like]. Capable of assimilation.

assimilate (ă-sĭm′ĭ-lāt). To absorb digested food.

assimilation (ă-sĭm″ĭ-lā′shŭn). 1. The processes whereby the products of digestion are converted to the chemical substances of the body tissues, first passing through the lacteals and blood vessels; transformation of food into living tissue. The constructive phase of metabolism, i.e., anabolism. 2. In psychology, the absorption of newly perceived information into the existing subjective conscious structure.

assisted circulation. Use of a mechanical device to augment or replace the action of the heart in pumping blood.

associated movements. Synchronous correlation of two or more muscles or muscle groups that, though not essential for the performance of some function, normally accompany it, as the swinging of arms accompanies normal walking. Associated movements are characteristically lost in cerebellar disease.

association [L. *ad*, to + *socius*, companion]. Joining or uniting; coordination with another idea or structure; relationship. In psychiatry, association refers in particular to the interrelationship of the conscious and unconscious ideas. In genetics, the occurrence together of two characteristics at a frequency greater than would be predicted by chance.

a., controlled. An idea suggested by a word uttered by the physician. SYN: *a., induced.* SEE: *association test.*

a., free. In psychoanalysis, the uninhibited and uncensored oral expression of ideas as they arise in the patient's mind.

a., induced. The idea expressed when the physician gives a stimulus word. SYN: *a., controlled.* SEE: *association test.*

association areas. Areas of the cerebral cortex that are connected to motor and sensory areas of the same side, to similar areas on the other side, and to other regions of the brain, as the thalamus. They serve to integrate the simpler motor and sensory functions.

association center. Center controlling associated movements.

association neuron. A neuron that transmits impulses from afferent to efferent neurons.

association of ideas. The linking together in a memory chain of two or more ideas, associated by some similarity, relationship, or by both having been experienced at the same time.

association test. Test in which the patient is given a word (stimulus word) and replies immediately with another word (reaction word) suggested by the first. The words chosen and the time taken in responding (association time) may be indicative of the patient's mental condition.

association time. SEE: *association test.*

assonance (ăs′ō-năns) [L. *assonans*, answering with some sound]. 1. Similarity of sounds in words or syllables. 2. Abnormal tendency to use alliteration.

Ast. *astigmatism.*

astasia (ă-stā′zē-ă) [Gr. *a-*, not, + *stasis*, stand]. Inability to stand or sit erect due to motor incoordination.

a.-abasia. A form of hysterical ataxia, q.v., with incoordination and inability to stand or walk although all leg movements can be performed while sitting or lying down.

astatine (ăs′tă-tēn, -tĭn) [Gr. *astatos*, unstable]. SYMB: At. A radioactive element. At. no. 85; at. wt. 210. May be of use in treatment of hyperthyroidism.

asteatosis (ăs″tē-ă-tō′sĭs) [Gr. *a-*, not, + *stear*, tallow, + *osis*, condition]. Any disease condition in which there is persistent scaling of the skin, suggesting scantiness or absence of sebaceous secretion.

a. cutis. A dry, fissured condition of the skin with a deficient sebaceous secretion.

ETIOL: Symptomatic form: senility or systemic disorders that give rise to trophic changes in the nervous system. Local form may be caused by frequent contact with irritants.

TREATMENT: Removal of underlying cause. Local application of oils and fats.

aster (ăs′tĕr) [Gr., star]. The stellate rays forming round the dividing centrosome during mitosis.

astereognosis (ă-stĕr″ē-ŏg-nō′sĭs) [Gr. *a-*, not, + *stereos*, solid, + *gnosis*, recognition]. Inability to recognize objects or forms by touch.

asterion (ăs-tē′rē-ŏn) [Gr., starlike]. (pl. *asteria*) A craniometric point at junction of the lambdoid, occipitomastoid, and parietomastoid sutures.

asterixis (ăs″tĕr-ĭk′sĭs) [Gr. *a-*, not, + *sterixis*, fixed position]. Abnormal muscle tremor consisting of involuntary jerking movements, esp. in the hands. Also seen in tongue and muscle groups of foot. May be due to various diseases that interfere with brain metabolism. When due to hepatic coma, asterixis is called "liver flap" or "liver tremor." SYN: *tremor, flapping*.

asternal (ā-stĕr′năl) [″ + *sternon*, chest]. 1. Not connected with the sternum. 2. Having no sternum.

asternia (ă-stĕr′nē-ă). Congenital absence of the sternum.

asteroid (ăs′tĕr-oyd) [Gr. *aster*, star, + *eidos*, shape]. Star-shaped.

asthenia (ăs-thē′nē-ă) [Gr. *asthenes*, without strength]. Lack or loss of strength; debility. Any weakness, but esp. one originating in muscular or cerebellar disease. SYN: *adynamia*.

a., neurocirculatory. A psychosomatic disorder characterized by mental and physical fatigue, dyspnea, giddiness, precordial pain and palpitation, esp. on exertion. SYN: *neurosis, cardiac*.

ETIOL: Unknown but occurs in individuals who are under conditions of stress. It is common among soldiers in combat.

TREATMENT: Removal from stress situation and psychotherapy.

asthenic (ăs-thĕn′ĭk). 1. Weak; pert. to asthenia. 2. Body habitus characterized by a narrow, shallow thorax, long thoracic cavity, and a short abdominal cavity.

asthenic personality. A personality disorder typified by low energy level, easy fatigability, lack of enthusiasm with incapacity for enjoyment, and oversensitivity to physical and emotional stress.

asthenobiosis (ăs-thĕ″nō-bī-ō′sĭs) [Gr. *asthenes*, without strength, + *bios*, life, + *osis*, condition]. Condition of reduced biological activity of an animal, resembling hibernation but not related to temperature or humidity.

asthenocoria (ăs-thē″nō-kō′rē-ă) [″ + *kore*, pupil]. A sluggish pupillary light reflex.

asthenometer (ăs″thĕ-nŏm′ĕ-ter) [″ + *metron*, measure]. An instrument for determining muscular strength or weakness.

asthenope (ăs′thĕ-nōp) [″ + *opsis*, power of sight]. An individual who is affected with asthenopia, q.v.

asthenopia (ăs″thĕ-nō′pē-ă). Weakness or tiring of eyes accompanied by pain, headache, and dimness of vision.

SYM: Pain in or around eyes; headache, usually aggravated by use of eyes for close work; fatigue; vertigo; reflex symptoms as nausea, twitching of facial muscles, migraine.

a., accommodative. Asthenopia due to strain of ciliary muscles.

a., muscular. Asthenopia caused by weakness of extrinsic ocular muscles.

a., nervous. Asthenopia of hysteric and/or neurasthenic origin.

a., photogenous. Asthenopia caused by excessive or improper illumination.

asthenopic (ăs″thĕ-nŏp′ĭk). Rel. to asthenopia.

asthenospermia (ăs″thĕ-nō-spĕr′mē-ă) [″ + *sperma*, seed]. Loss or reduction of motility of spermatozoa in semen. Associated with infertility.

asthenoxia [″ + *oxygen*]. Deficient oxygenation of waste products.

asthma (ăz′mă) [Gr., panting]. Paroxysmal dyspnea accompanied by wheezing caused by a spasm of the bronchial tubes or by swelling of their mucous membrane. No age is exempt but asthma occurs most frequently in childhood or early adulthood. The patient may assume a "hunched forward" position in an attempt to get more air. Other allergic disorders may coexist. Recurrence and severity of attacks are greatly influenced by secondary factors, by mental or physical fatigue, by exposure to fumes, by endocrine changes at various periods in life, and by emotional situations. Status asthmaticus, a continuous asthmatic state, may last for hours or days.

ETIOL: *Extrinsic causes:* Allergens inhaled in the air (pollen, mold spores, animal dander, or dust) or infections of the respiratory tract. Occasionally foods (eggs, shellfish, or chocolate) or drugs (aspirin) may precipitate an attack. *Intrinsic causes:* In some cases asthma develops in persons with allergies of unknown etiology. It may be precipitated by infection of the upper or lower respiratory tracts.

TREATMENT: Acute attacks may be relieved by a number of drugs such as epinephrine, ephedrine, cromolyn sodium, or aminophylline. For persistent asthma (status asthmaticus), the use of adrenocortical hormones may be required. Even though their use may provide dramatic relief, these hormones should be used only as long as is necessary to control the acute asthmatic attack. Prolonged use of adrenocortical hormones will lead to the development of serious side effects. The use of sedatives and expectorants is sometimes necessary. In all cases, effort should be made to control causative factors including the component of the disease due to emotional disturbance, esp. in the intrinsic group. Elimination of antigen, or countermeasures, such as immunization, desensitization, or hyposensitization, are desirable. For asthma due to infection of respiratory tract, antibiotics should be used to control infection or prevent recurrence.

NURSING IMPLICATIONS: Determine the inspiration/expiration ratio, presence of wheezing, and muscles utilized for respiration, and be aware of other symptoms indicative of respiratory distress. Place the patient in semi-Fowler's position, and administer oxygen as needed to relieve dyspnea. Remain with the patient and provide calm reassurance that the measures taken will improve breathing. Also assess for symptoms of dehydration, and in order to prevent this, encourage increased oral fluid intake to help loosen thick respiratory secretions. Administer medications (such as epinephrine, steroids, aminophylline) as ordered. Instruct the patient to do breathing exercises to increase respiratory efficiency. Instruct the patient and the family concerning what steps to take to eliminate allergens from the patient's immediate environment. Also teach them what measures to take at home to decrease the severity of or prevent future attacks.

a., bronchial. Allergic asthma. Common form of asthma due to hypersensitivity to an allergen.

a., cardiac. Asthma secondary to heart disease.

a., exercise-induced. Acute, reversible, usually self-terminating airway obstruction that develops after strenuous exercise in patients with asthma or hay fever. Very few patients will experience asthma while exercising and it is rarely sufficient to cause them to stop their activity.

a., extrinsic. Asthma due to some environmental factor, usually allergic.

a., intrinsic. Asthma assumed to be due to some endogenous cause because no external cause can be found.

a., nonatopic. A., intrinsic, q.v.

a., thymic. Asthma caused by a sudden closure of the larynx. Usually occurs in children, and is believed to result from enlargement of the thymus.

asthmatic (ăz-măt'ĭk) [L. *asthmaticus*]. Pert. to or of the nature of asthma.

astigmatic (ăs"tĭg-măt'ĭk). Pert. to or afflicted with astigmatism.

astigmatism (ă-stĭg'mă-tĭzm) [Gr. *a-*, not, + *stigma,* point, + *-ismos,* condition of]. ABBR: As. or Ast. Form of ametropia, q.v., in which the refraction of a ray of light is spread over a diffuse area rather than being sharply focused on the retina. Due to differences in curvature in various meridians of the cornea and lens of the eye.

ETIOL: Exact cause is unknown. Some types show a familial pattern.

a., compound. Astigmatism in which both horizontal and vertical curvatures are involved.

a., index. Astigmatism resulting from inequalities in refractive indices of different parts of the lens.

a., mixed. Astigmatism in which one meridian is myopic and the other hyperopic.

a., simple. Astigmatism along one meridian only.

astigmatometer (ăs"tĭg-mă-tŏm'ĕ-tĕr) [" + *stigma,* point, + *metron,* measure]. An instrument for measuring astigmatism.

astigmatoscope (ăs"tĭg-măt'ō-skōp) [" + " + *skopein,* to examine]. Instrument for detecting and measuring astigmatism.

astigmatoscopy (ă-stĭg"mă-tŏs'kō-pē). Use of the astigmatoscope.

astigmia (ă-stĭg'mē-ă). Astigmatism, q.v.

astigmometer (ăs"tĭg-mŏm'ĕ-tĕr). Astigmatometer, q.v.

astigmoscope (ăs-tĭg'mō-skōp). Astigmatoscope, q.v.

astomatous, astomous (ăs-tōm'ă-tŭs, ăs'tō-mŭs) [Gr. *a-*, not, + *stoma,* mouth]. Without a mouth or oral aperture; as certain protozoa.

astomia (ă-stō'mē-ă). Congenital absence of the mouth.

astragalectomy (ăs"trăg-ă-lĕk'tō-mē) [*astragalus* + Gr. *ektome,* excision]. Surgical removal of the talus (astragalus).

astragalus (ă-străg'ă-lŭs) [Gr. *astragalos,* ball of the ankle joint]. Obsolete term for the talus of the ankle. SEE: *talus.*

astraphobia (ăs-tră-fō'bē-ă) [Gr. *astrape,* lightning, + *phobos,* fear]. Fear of thunder and lightning.

astrict (ă-strĭkt') [L. *astringere,* to bind fast]. To contract or constrict, as the action of an astringent. To compress, as an artery in a hemorrhage.

astriction (ă-strĭk'shŭn). Action of astringent.

astringent (ă-strĭn'jĕnt) [L. *astringere,* to bind fast]. 1. Drawing together, constricting, binding. 2. An agent that has a constricting or binding effect, i.e., one that checks hemorrhages, or secretions by coagulation of proteins on a cell surface. The principal astringents are salts of metals such as lead, iron, zinc (ferric chloride, zinc oxide); permanganates; and tannic acid. SEE: *styptic*.

astro- [Gr. *astron*, star]. Prefix indicating relationship to a star, or star shaped.

astroblast (ăs'trō-blăst) [" + Gr. *blastos*, germ]. A cell that gives rise to an astrocyte. It develops from spongioblasts derived from embryonic neuroepithelium.

astroblastoma (ăs"trō-blăs-tō'mă) [" + " + *oma*, tumor]. A Grade II astrocytoma, q.v., composed of cells with abundant cytoplasm and two or three nuclei.

astrocyte (ăs'trō-sīt) [" + *kytos*, cell]. A star-shaped neuroglial cell possessing many branching processes.

astrocytoma (ăs"trō-sī-tō'mă) [" + " + *oma*, tumor]. Tumor composed of astrocytes. Classified in order of increasing malignancy as: Grade I, consisting of fibrillary or protoplasmic astrocytes; Grade II, astroblastoma, q.v.; and Grades III and IV, glioblastoma multiforme, q.v., consisting of a mixture of spongioblasts, astroblasts, and astrocytes.

astroglia (ăs-trŏg'lē-ă) [" + *glia*, glue]. Astrocytes making up neuroglial tissue.

astrokinetic motions (ăs"trō-kĭ-nĕt'ĭk) [" + *kinesis*, motion]. Pert. to movements of the centrosome.

astrophobia (ăs"trō-fō'bē-ă) [" + *phobos*, fear]. Morbid fear of stars and celestial space.

astrosphere (ăs'trō-sfēr) [" + *sphaira*, sphere]. A group of fibrils or fine rays that radiate from the centrosome (microcentrum) of the dividing cell. SYN: *aster*.

astrostatic (ăs"trō-stăt'ĭk) [" + *statikos*, standing]. Pert. to astrosphere in its resting condition.

asyllabia (ă"sĭl-ā'bē-ă) [Gr. *a-*, not, + *syllabe*, syllable]. A form of alexia, q.v., in which the patient recognizes letters but cannot form syllables or words.

asylum (ă-sī'lŭm) [L. *asylon*, sanctuary]. An institution for the care of the mentally ill, esp. those who are so severely handicapped as to be unable to care for themselves or would be a hazard to self or society if they were not institutionalized.

asymbolia (ā-, ă-sĭm-bō'lē-ă) [Gr. *a-*, not, + *symbolon*, a sign]. Inability to comprehend words, gestures, or any type of symbol. Asemia, q.v., is the more generally accepted term for this condition. SEE: *aphasia*.

asymmetry (ă-sĭm'ĕ-trē) [" + *symmetria*, symmetry]. Lack of symmetry.

asymphytous (ă-sĭm'fĭ-tŭs) [" + *symphysis*, a growing together]. Separate or distinct; not grown together.

asymptomatic (ā"sĭmp-tō-măt'ĭk) [" + *symptoma*, occurrence]. Without symptoms.

asynchronism (ă-sĭn'krō-nĭzm) [" + *syn*, together, + *chronos*, time, + *-ismos*, condition of]. 1. The failure of events to occur in time with each other as they usually do. 2. Incoordination.

asynclitism (ă-sĭn'klĭ-tĭzm) [" + *synklinein*, to lean together, + *-ismos*, condition of]. An oblique presentation of the fetal head in labor.

a., anterior. Anterior parietal presentation. SYN: *Naegele's obliquity*.

a., posterior. Posterior parietal presentation. SYN: *Litzmann's obliquity*.

asyndesis (ă-sĭn'dĕ-sĭs) [Gr *a-*, not, + *syn*, together, + *desis*, binding]. Mental defect in which related thoughts cannot be assembled to form a comprehensive concept.

asynechia (ă"sĭ-nĕk'ē-ă) [" + *synecheia*, continuity]. Lack of continuity of structure in an organ or tissue.

asynergia, asynergy (ă-sĭn-ĕr'jē-ă, ă-sĭn'ĕr-jē) [" + Gr. *synergia*, cooperation]. Lack of coordination among parts or organs normally acting in unison. In neurology, lack of coordination between muscle groups. Movements are in serial order instead of being made together. Seen in cerebellar diseases.

asynovia (ă-sĭn-ō'vē-ă) [" + *syn*, with, + *oon*, egg]. Lack, or insufficient secretion, of synovial fluid of a joint.

asyntaxia (ă"sĭn-tăk'sē-ă) [" + *syntaxis*, orderly arrangement]. Failure of proper development of the embryo.

asystematic (ă-sĭs"tĕ-măt'ĭk) [" + LL. *systema*, arrangement]. Not systematic; not limited to one system or set of organs.

asystole, asystolia (ă-sĭs'tō-lē, ă"sĭs-tō'lē-ă) [" + *systole*, contraction]. Cardiac standstill; absence of contractions of the heart.

At. Chem. symb. for astatine.

Atabrine Hydrochloride (ăt'ă-brĭn). Trade name for quinacrine hydrochloride, USP, q.v.

atactic (ă-tăk'tĭk) [Gr. *ataktos*, irregular]. Incoordinate, irregular, as muscular incoordination, esp. in aphasia. SYN: *ataxic*.

atactiform (ă-tăk'tĭ-form) [" + L. *forma*, form]. Similar to ataxia.

ataractic (ăt"ă-răk'tĭk) [Gr. *ataraktos*, quiet]. 1. Of or pert. to ataraxia. 2. A drug that produces ataraxia, q.v.; a tranquilizer.

Atarax. Trade name for hydroxyzine hydrochloride, USP, q.v.

ataraxia, ataraxy (ăt"ă-răk'sē-ă, -sē) [Gr. *ataraktos*, quiet]. A state of complete mental calm and tranquility, esp. without depression of mental faculties or clouding of consciousness.

atavism (ăt'ă-vĭzm) [L. *atavus*, ancestor, + Gr. *-ismos*, condition]. The appearance of a characteristic presumed to have been present in some remote ancestor; due to chance recombination of genes or environmental conditions favorable to their expression in the embryo.

atavistic (ăt-ă-vĭs'tĭk). Pert. to atavism.

ataxaphasia (ă-tăk"să-fā'zē-ă) [Gr. *ataxia*, lack

of order, + *phasis,* speech]. Inability to arrange words in sentences. Also spelled *ataxiaphasia.*

ataxia (ă-tăk'sē-ă) [Gr., lack of order]. Defective muscular coordination, esp. that manifested when voluntary muscular movements are attempted.

a., alcoholic. Ataxia due to a loss of proprioception, in chronic alcoholism.

a., autonomic. Incoordination between sympathetic and parasympathetic nervous systems.

a., Briquet's. Hysterical ataxia accompanied by skin and leg muscle anesthesia.

a., Brun's. Condition resulting from bilateral lesions of the frontal lobes. Stance and gait are affected and there is a tendency to fall or stagger backwards.

a., bulbar. Ataxia due to a lesion in the medulla oblongata or pons.

a., cerebellar. Ataxia due to cerebellar disease.

a., choreic. Lack of muscular coordination seen in persons with chorea.

a., Friedreich's. An inherited degenerative disease with sclerosis of the dorsal and lateral columns of the spinal cord. Accompanied by ataxia, speech impairment, lateral curvature of the spinal column, and peculiar swaying and irregular movements, with paralysis of the muscles, esp. of the lower extremities. Onset in childhood or adolescence.

a., hereditary cerebellar. Disease of late adolescence caused by atrophy of cerebellum. Characterized by ataxic gait, hesitating and explosive speech, nystagmus, and sometimes optic neuritis. SYN: *a., Marie's.*

a., hereditary spinal. A., Friedreich's, q.v.

a., hysterical. Ataxia of leg muscles due to hysteria.

a., locomotor. Degeneration of the dorsal columns of the spinal cord and sensory nerve trunks, due to infection of the central nervous system with Treponema pallidum, the causative organism of syphilis. SYN: *tabes dorsalis.*

SYM: Postural instability, esp. when eyes are closed, and a staggering wide-base gait are characteristic. Pains and paresthesias are common, esp. lightning pains, described as sharp, stabbing, and paroxysmal. Ankle and knee reflexes are diminished or lost. Other symptoms characteristic of tertiary stage of syphilis, q.v. SEE: *gait.*

TREATMENT: Penicillin. Therapy may arrest disease but complete cure is rare.

a., Marie's. A., hereditary cerebellar, q.v.

a., motor. Inability to perform coordinated muscle movements.

a., sensory. Ataxia resulting from interference in conduction of sensory responses, esp. proprioceptive impulses from muscles. Becomes aggravated when eyes are closed. SEE: *a., spinal.*

a., spinal. Ataxia due to spinal cord disease.

a., static. Loss of deep sensibility causing inability to preserve equilibrium in standing.

a.-telangiectasia. A hereditary progressive disease complex characterized by cerebellar ataxia, telangiectasia, q.v., recurrent sinopulmonary infections, and variable immunologic defects.

ataxiagram (ă-tăk'sē-ă-grăm) [Gr. *ataxia,* lack of order, + *gramma,* writing]. Ataxiagraph record or tracing.

ataxiagraph (ă-tăk'sē-ă-grăf) [" + *graphein,* to write]. Instrument for measuring the degree and direction of swaying in ataxia.

ataxiameter (ă-tăk"sē-ăm'ĕ-tĕr) [" + *metron,* measure]. Apparatus measuring ataxia.

ataxiamnesia (ă-tăk"sē-ăm-nē'zē-ă) [" + *amnesia,* forgetfulness]. Condition with ataxia and amnesia.

ataxiaphasia (ă-tăk"sē-ă-fā'zē-ă) [" + *phasis,* speech]. Inability to arrange words into sentences. Also spelled *ataxaphasia.*

ataxic, ataxial (ă-tăk'sĭk, ă-tăk'sē-ăl). Pert. to, or marked by, ataxia.

ataxophemia (ă-tăk"sō-fē'mē-ă) [" + *pheme,* speech]. Incoordination of speech muscles.

ataxophobia (ă-tăk"sō-fō'bē-ă) [" + *phobos,* fear]. Morbid dread of disorder or untidiness.

atelectasis (ăt"ĕ-lĕk'tă-sĭs) [Gr. *ateles,* imperfect, + *ektasis,* expansion]. 1. Condition in which lungs of a fetus remain unexpanded at birth. May be partial or total. 2. A collapsed or airless condition of the lung. May be caused by obstruction by foreign bodies, mucous plugs or excessive secretions, or by compression from without as by tumors, aneurysms, or enlarged lymph nodes. It sometimes is a complication following abdominal operations. A special chronic form, designated middle lobe syndrome, results from compression of the middle lobe bronchus by surrounding lymph nodes.

atelencephalia (ăt-ĕl"ĕn-sĕ-fā'lē-ă) [Gr. *ateleia,* incompleteness, + *enkephalos,* brain]. Congenital anomaly with imperfect development of the brain. Also spelled *ateloencephalia.*

atelia (ă-tē'lē-ă) [Gr. *ateleia,* incompleteness]. Imperfect or incomplete development.

ateliosis (ă-tē"lē-ō'sĭs) [Gr. *a-,* not, + *teleios,* complete, + *osis,* condition]. A form of infantilism due to pituitary insufficiency, in which growth is arrested without deformity. The voice and face may resemble those of a child.

ateliotic (ă-tē"lē-ŏt'ĭk). Pert. to or characterized by atelia.

atelo- (ăt'ĕ-lō) [Gr. *ateles,* imperfect]. Prefix denoting imperfect or incomplete.

atelocardia (ăt"ĕ-lō-kăr'dē-ă) [" + *kardia,* heart]. Congenital incomplete development of the heart.

atelocephaly (ăt"ĕ-lō-sĕf'ă-lē) [" + *kephale,* head]. Incomplete development of the head.

atelocheilia (ăt"ĕ-lō-kī'lē-ă) [" + *cheilos,* lip]. Incomplete development of the lip.

atelocheiria (ăt"ĕ-lō-kī'rē-ă) [" + *cheir,* hand]. Incomplete development of the hand.

ateloencephalia (ăt"ĕ-lō-ĕn"sĕ-fā'lē-ă). Atelencephalia.

ateloglossia (ăt"ĕ-lō-glŏs'ē-ă) [" + *glossa,* tongue]. Incomplete development of the tongue.

atelognathia (ăt"ĕ-lŏg-nā'thē-ă) [" + *gnathos,* jaw]. Incomplete development of the jaw.

atelomyelia (ăt"ĕ-lō-mī-ē'lē-ă) [" + *myelos,* marrow]. Incomplete development of the spinal cord.

atelopodia (ăt"ĕ-lō-pō'dē-ă) [Gr. *ateles,* imperfect, + *pous,* foot]. Incomplete development of the foot.

ateloprosopia (ăt"ĕ-lō-prō-sō'pē-ă) [" + *prosopon,* face]. Incomplete development of the face.

atelorrhachidia (ăt"ĕ-lō-ră-kĭd'ē-ă) [" + *rhachis,* spine]. Incomplete development of the spinal cord.

atelostomia (ăt"ĕ-lō-stō'mē-ă) [" + *stoma,* mouth]. Incomplete development of the mouth.

athelia (ă-thē'lē-ă) [Gr. *a-,* not, + *thele,* nipple]. Congenital absence of the nipples.

athermic, athermous (ă-thĕr'mĭk, -mŭs) [" + *therme,* heat]. Without fever or rise of temperature.

athermosystaltic (ă-thĕr"mō-sĭs-tăl'tĭk) [" + " + *systaltikos,* drawing together]. Not contracting due to action of heat or cold, said of skeletal muscle.

atherogenesis (ăth"ĕr-ō-jĕn'ĕ-sĭs) [Gr. *athere,* porridge, + *genesis,* generation]. The formation of atheromata in the walls of arteries.

atheroma (ăth"ĕr-ō'mă) [" + *oma,* tumor]. (pl. *atheromata*) Fatty degeneration or thickening of the walls of the larger arteries occurring in atherosclerosis, q.v. SEE: *arteriosclerosis.*

atheromatosis (ăth"ĕr-ō"mă-tō'sĭs). Generalized atheromatous disease of the arteries.

atheromatous (ăth"ĕr-ō'mă-tŭs). Pert. to atheroma.

atheronecrosis (ăth"ĕr-ō"nĕ-krō'sĭs) [" + *nekros,* dead, + *osis,* condition]. Necrosis or degeneration accompanying arteriosclerosis, q.v.

atherosclerosis (ăth"ĕr-ō"sklĕ-rō'sĭs) [" + Gr. *sklerosis,* hardness]. A form of arteriosclerosis characterized by a variable combination of changes of the intima of arteries, not arterioles, consisting of the focal accumulation of lipids, complex carbohydrates, blood and blood products, fibrous tissue and calcium deposits, and associated with changes in the media of the arteries. Atherosclerotic plaques are of two major types: one is characterized by prominent proliferation of cells with small accumulation of lipids; the other consists mostly of intracellular and extracellular lipid accumulation and a small amount of cellular proliferation.

ETIOL: Cause unknown. Risk factors include: hypertension; increased blood lipid levels, esp. cholesterol and triglycerides; obesity; cigarette smoking; diabetes mellitus; inability to cope with stress; family history of early-onset atherosclerosis; physical inactivity; and the male sex (at ages 35 to 44, the death rate for white males who have this disease is 6 times that of white females).

athetoid (ăth'ĕ-toyd) [Gr. *athetos,* not fixed, + *eidos,* resemblance]. Resembling or affected with athetosis.

athetosis (ăth-ĕ-tō'sĭs) [" + *osis,* condition]. A condition wherein there are slow, irregular, twisting, snakelike movements seen in the upper extremities, esp. in the hands and fingers, and performed involuntarily. The symptoms may be due to one of several diseases, including encephalitis and tabes dorsalis.

Types of athetosis: Athetosis with spasticity—muscle tone fluctuates between normal and hypertonic; there is frequently moderate spasticity in the proximal parts and athetosis more distally. Modified primitive spinal reflex patterns are often present.

Athetosis with tonic spasms—muscle tone fluctuates between hypotonus and hypertonus. Excessive extension or flexion is evident due to absent co-contraction. There is strong postural asymmetry and frequent spinal or hip abnormalities or deformities.

Choreoathetosis—muscle tone fluctuates either from hypotonic to normal or hypotonic to hypertonic. Co-contraction is absent, and there are extreme ranges of motion. Deformities are rare, but subluxation of the shoulder and finger joints often occurs.

Pure athetosis—this type is much rarer than others. Muscle tone fluctuates between hypotonus and normal. Deformities are rare. Twitches and jerks of muscles or individual muscle fibers are seen. Characterized by slow, writhing, involuntary movements that are more proximal than distal.

athlete's foot. A fungus infection of the foot caused by various dermatophytes, esp. Trichophyton rubrum, T. mentagrophytes, and Epidermophyton floccosum, which invade the "dead" outer layers of the skin. SYN: *dermatophytosis; ringworm; tinea pedis.*

TREATMENT: Careful attention to hygiene is important. The feet, esp. between the toes, should be carefully dried after bathing. Loose macerated skin should be gently removed and a bland drying powder applied. Shoes that provide good ventilation, and the use of socks that absorb moisture are important treatment adjuncts. Going barefoot in suitable climates will be of benefit. Severe cases should be treated with griseofulvin, but most subacute or chronic cases will respond to one of several fungicidal medications such as 2% miconazole cream, 1% clotrimazole cream or lotion, or Whitfield's tincture (3% salicylic acid, 6% benzoic acid in 70% alcohol).

athrepsia, athrepsy (ă-thrĕp'sē-ă, -sē) [Gr. *a-*, not, + *threpsis,* nourishment]. Malnutrition, marasmus, q.v.

athreptic (ă-thrĕp'tĭk). Marasmic; pert. to or afflicted with athrepsia.

athrombia (ă-thrŏm'bē-ă) [" + *thrombos,* a clot]. Defective blood clotting due to a deficiency in thrombin.

Athrombin-K. Trade name for warfarin potassium, USP, q.v.

athymia (ă-thī'mē-ă) [" + *thymos,* mind]. 1. Condition of being without feeling or emotion, seen in certain mental disorders. 2. Absence of thymus gland.

athymic (ă-thī'mĭk). Pert. to athymia.

athymism (ă-thī'mĭzm) [" + " + *-ismos,* condition of]. Absence of thymus gland or its secretions. SYN: *athymia* (def. 2).

athyrea (ă-thī'rē-ă). Athyreosis.

athyreosis (ă-thī"rē-ō'sĭs) [" + *thyreos,* shield, + *eidos,* form, + *osis,* condition]. Hypothyroidism resulting from absence or malfunction of thyroid gland due to maldevelopment, operative removal, or inactivation by irradiation or use of antithyroid agents. SYN: *athyrea; athyria; hypothyroidism.*

athyria (ă-thī'rē-ă). Athyreosis.

athyroidemia (ăth"ī-roy-, ă-thī"roy-dē'mē-ă) [" + " + " + *haima,* blood]. Absence of thyroid hormone from the blood.

athyroidism (ă-thī'roy-dĭzm) [" + " + " + *-ismos,* condition of]. Suppression of thyroid secretions, or absence of the thyroid gland; hypothyroidism.

athyrosis (ă-thī-rō'sĭs). Athyreosis.

atlantad (ăt-lăn'tăd). Toward the atlas.

atlantal (ăt-lăn'tăl). Pert. to the atlas.

atlantoaxial (ăt-lăn"tō-ăk'sē-ăl) [Gr. *atlas,* a support, + L. *axis,* a pivot]. Pertaining to the atlas, the first cervical vertebra, and the axis, the second cervical vertebra.

atlantodidymus (ăt-lăn"tō-dĭd'ĭ-mŭs) [" + *didymus,* twin]. Atlodidymus, q.v.

tlanto-occipital (ăt-lăn"tō-ŏk-sĭp'ĭ-tăl) [" + *occipitalis,* occipital]. Pertaining to the s and the occipital bones.

s (ăt'lăs) [Gr.]. [NA] The first cervical vertebra by which the head articulates with the occipital bone, so called because of Atlas, the Greek god who was supposed to support the world on his shoulders.

atloaxoid (ăt"lō-ăk'soyd) [" + L. *axis,* a pivot, + Gr. *eidos,* form]. Pert. to the atlas and axis.

atlodidymus (ăt-lō-dĭd'ĭ-mŭs) [" + Gr. *didymos,* twin]. A malformed fetus with one body and two heads.

atm. *atmosphere; atmospheric.*

atmiatrics, atmiatry (ăt-mē-ăt'rĭks, ăt-mī'ă-trē) [Gr. *atmos,* vapor, + *iatrikos,* art of healing]. Treatment of respiratory disease by medicated vapors.

atmo- [Gr. *atmos,* vapor or steam]. Prefix indicating rel. to steam or vapor.

atmosphere (ăt'mŏs-fēr) [" + *sphaira,* sphere]. 1. The gases surrounding the earth. 2. Climatic condition of a locality. 3. In physics, pressure of the air upon the earth at mean sea level, approx. 14.7 lb. to the sq. in. (101325 Pascal or 760 torr). 4. In chemistry, any gaseous medium around a body.

atmospheric (ăt"mŏs-fēr'ĭk). Pert. to the atmosphere.

at. no. *atomic number.*

ATNR. *asymmetrical tonic neck reflex.*

atocia (ăt-ō'sē-ă) [Gr. *a-*, not, + *tokos,* birth]. 1. Female sterility. 2. Nulliparity.

atom (ăt'ŏm) [Gr. *atomos,* indivisible]. The smallest part of an element that is capable of entering into a chemical reaction. The atom consists of the nucleus, which contains protons and neutrons, and of surrounding electrons. The nucleus is positively charged, and this determines the atomic number of an element. A large number of entities in the atomic nucleus have been identified, and the search for others continues. Dimensions of atoms are of the order of 10^{-8} cm. SEE: *atomic theory; electron.*

a., tagged. An atom that has been made radioactive so that its course may be followed in the body. SYN: *radioactive tracer.*

atomic (ă-tŏm'ĭk). Pert. to an atom or atoms.

atomic number. ABBR: at. no. Number of protons in the nucleus of an atom.

atomic theory. 1. Theory that all matter is composed of atoms. 2. Theories pert. to the structure, properties, and behavior of the atom.

atomic weight. ABBR: at. wt. The relative weight of an atom as compared with the standard carbon atom isotope with a mass of 12. Therefore, carbon has an at. wt. of 12; oxygen, 16; hydrogen, 1.008; and nitrogen, 14.008.

atomization (ăt"ŏm-ĭ-zā'shŭn). Converting a fluid into spray or vapor form. SEE: *nebulizer; vaporizer.*

atomize (ăt'ŏm-īz). To reduce a liquid to the

form of a spray or a vapor.

atomizer (ăt'ŏm-ī-zĕr). Apparatus for changing jet of liquid to a spray.

atonic (ă-tŏn'ĭk) [" + *tonos,* stretching]. Without normal tension or tone.

atonicity (ăt-ō-nĭs'ĭ-tē). State of being atonic, or without tone.

atony (ăt'ō-nē) [" + *tonos,* stretching]. Debility; or lack of normal tone or strength.

a., gastric. Lack of muscle tone in stomach and failure to contract normally, causing slow movement of food out of stomach. Secondary to certain diseases.

atopen (ăt'ō-pĕn) [" + *topos,* place]. An allergen, exciting cause of atopy, q.v.

atopic (ă-tŏp'ĭk). 1. Pert. to atopy. 2. Displaced; malpositioned.

atopognosis (ă-tŏp"ŏg-nō'sĭs) [" + *topos,* place, + *gnosis,* knowledge]. Inability to locate a sensation of touch or feeling.

atopy (ăt'ō-pē) [Gr. *atopia,* strangeness]. An allergy for which there was a genetic predisposition. The tendency to develop a certain type of allergy can be inherited, but not the allergy itself. The antibody produced, called reagin, which is in the immunoglobin E class, is deposited in cutaneous tissues and may enter the bloodstream; the primary reaction that appears is edema, as occurs in hay fever or rhinitis. The principal atopic manifestations are bronchial asthma, vasomotor rhinitis, and chronic urticaria. SEE: *allergy; immunity; reagin.*

atoxic [Gr. *a-,* not, + *toxikon,* poison]. Nonpoisonous.

ATP. *adenosine triphosphate.*

ATPase. *adenosinetriphosphatase.*

atraumatic (ā"traw-măt'ĭk) [Gr. *a-,* not, + *traumatikos,* relating to injury]. Not causing trauma or injury. SEE: *needle, atraumatic.*

atremia (ă-trē'mē-ă) [" + *tremein,* to tremble]. 1. Absence of trembling or tremor. 2. Inability to walk due to hysteria.

atresia (ă-trē'zē-ă) [" + *tresis,* a perforation]. Congenital absence or closure of a normal body opening or tubular structure.

a., anal; a. ani. Imperforate anus.

a., aortic. Congenital closure of the aortic valvular opening into the aorta.

a., biliary. Closure or absence of some or all of the major bile ducts.

a., duodenal. Congenital closure of a portion of the duodenum.

a., esophageal. Congenital failure of the esophageal tube to develop.

a., follicular. Normal death of the ovarian follicle following failure of the ovum to be fertilized.

a., intestinal. Congenital closure of any part of the intestine.

a., mitral. Congenital closure of the mitral valve opening.

a., prepyloric. Congenital closure of the pyloric end of the stomach.

a., pulmonary. Congenital closure of the pulmonary valve between the right ventricle and the pulmonary artery.

a., tricuspid. Congenital closure of the tricuspid valve between the right atrium and ventricle.

a., urethral. Absence or closure of the urethral orifice or canal.

a., vaginal. Congenital closure or absence of the vagina.

atresic (ă-trē'zĭk). Pert. to atresia.

atreto- (ă-trē'tō) [Gr. *atretos,* imperforate]. Prefix signifying absence of an opening.

atria (ā'trē-ă). Pl. of atrium, q.v.

atrial (ā'trē-ăl). Pert. to the atrium.

atrial fibrillation. Irregular and rapid randomized contractions of the atria working independently of the ventricles. Instead of the contraction beginning at the sinoatrial node and being conducted along the bundle of His to the ventricles, there is a rapid succession of beats at the atria. Contraction of the atrial muscle causes the waves to pass round and round in the atrium. Because of this, there is no atrial diastole or atrial heartbeat.

ETIOL: Degeneration of cardiac muscle. Occurs in late stages of mitral disease of heart, hyperthyroidism, infiltration of the atria by neoplastic tissue, and in acute rheumatic fever.

atrichia (ă-trĭk'ē-ă) [Gr. *a-,* not, + *thrix,* hair]. 1. Absence of hair. 2. Lacking cilia or flagella.

atrichosis (ă-trĭ-kō'sĭs) [" + " + *osis,* condition]. Congenital absence of hair.

atrichous (ă-trĭk'ŭs). 1. Without flagella. 2. Without hair.

atrionector (ăt"rē-ō-nĕk'tor) [L. *atrium,* corridor, + *nector,* connector] Sinoatrial node.

atrioseptopexy (ā"trē-ō-sĕp'tō-pĕk"sē) [" + *saeptum,* a partition, + Gr. *pexis,* fixation]. Plastic surgical repair of an interatrial septal defect.

atriotome (ā'trē-ō-tōm) [" + Gr. *tome,* incision]. Instrument used in surgically opening the cardiac atrium.

atrioventricular (ā"trē-ō-vĕn-trĭk'ū-lăr) [" + *ventriculus,* ventricle]. Pert. to both atrium and ventricle.

atrioventricular bundle. A bundle of modified cardiac muscle fibers that forms a part of the impulse-conducting system of the heart. It extends from the atrioventricular (A-V) node a short distance in the intraventricular septum, then divides into two branches that supply fibers to the two ventricles. SYN: *bundle of His.*

atrioventricularis communis (ā"trē-ō-vĕn-trĭk"ū-lā'rĭs kō-mū'nĭs). Persistence of the common atrioventricular canal. A congenital anomaly of the heart in which the division of the common atrioventricular canal in the embryo fails to occur. This causes atrial septal defect and atrioventricular valve incompetence.

atriplicism (ă-trĭp′lĭ-sĭzm). Poisoning due to eating one form of spinach, Atriplex littoralis.

atrium (ā′trē-ŭm) [L., corridor]. (pl. *atria*) A chamber or cavity communicating with another structure.

a. of ear. Portion of the tympanic cavity lying below the malleus; the tympanic cavity proper.

a. of heart. The upper chamber of each half of the heart. The right atrium receives deoxygenated, dark red blood from the entire body (except lungs) through the superior and inferior vena cavae and coronary sinus; the left atrium receives oxygenated red blood from the lungs through the pulmonary veins. Blood passes from the atria to the ventricles through the atrioventricular orifices. In the embryo, the atrium is a single chamber that lies between the sinus venosus and the ventricle.

a. of lungs. The space at the end of an alveolar duct that opens into the alveoli, or air sacs, of the lungs.

Atromid-S. Trade name for clofibrate, USP, q.v.

atrophia (ă-trō′fē-ă) [Gr.]. Wasting; a decrease in size of an organ or tissue. SYN: *atrophy.*

atrophic (ă-trō′fĭk). Pert. to, or marked by, atrophy.

atrophied (ăt′rō-fēd). Wasted. Afflicted with atrophy.

atrophoderma (ăt″rō-fō-dĕr′mă) [Gr. *a-*, not + *trophe,* nourishment, + *derma,* skin]. Atrophy of the skin.

atrophodermatosis (ăt-rō″fō-dĕr-mă-tō′sĭs) [″ + ″ + ″ + *osis,* condition]. Any skin disease that has cutaneous atrophy as a prominent symptom.

atrophy (ăt′rō-fē) [Gr. *atrophia*]. 1. A wasting; a decrease in size of an organ or tissue. 2. To undergo or cause atrophy.

ETIOL: May result from death and resorption of cells, diminished cellular proliferation, pressure, ischemia, malnutrition, decreased activity, or hormonal changes.

a., acute yellow. Extensive necrosis of liver cells with jaundice, mental disturbances, and cutaneous hemorrhages. A complication of hepatitis.

SYM: Early central nervous system symptoms before jaundice sets in; slow onset; some fever with nausea and vomiting; black vomit; ‑laise.

compression. Atrophy due to con‑ ‑t pressure on a part.

a., correlated. Wasting of a part following destruction of a correlated part.

a., Cruveilhier's. Atrophy of the spinal muscles.

a., healed yellow. Postnecrotic cirrhosis of the liver.

a., Hoffman's. SEE: *Werdnig-Hoffmann disease.*

a., Landouzy-Dejerine. A hereditary form of progressive muscular dystrophy with onset in childhood or adolescence. Characterized by atrophic changes in muscles of shoulder girdle and face, inability to raise arms above the head, myopathic facies, eyelids that remain partly open in sleep, and inability to whistle or purse lips. SYN: *dystrophy, Landouzy-Dejerine.*

a., muscular. Atrophy of muscle tissue, esp. due to lack of use.

a., myelopathic. Muscular atrophy resulting from a lesion of the spinal cord.

a., myotonic. Myotonia congenita, q.v.

a. of disuse. Atrophy from failure to exercise a part normally.

a., optic. Atrophy of the optic disk resulting from degeneration of the second cranial (optic) nerve.

a., pathologic. Atrophy that results from the effects of disease processes.

a., peroneal muscular. A hereditary disease characterized by atrophy of muscles supplied by peroneal nerves, progressing slowly to the muscles of hands and arms. SYN: *Charcot-Marie-Tooth disease,* q.v.

a., physiologic. Atrophy that occurs as a result of the normal aging processes in the body.

Ex.: Atrophy of embryonic structures; atrophy of childhood structures upon reaching maturity, as the thymus; atrophy of structures in cyclic phases of activity, as the corpus luteum; atrophy of structures following cessation of functional activity, as the ovary and mammary glands; and atrophy of structures with aging.

a., progressive muscular. Chronic disease marked by progressive wasting of the motor cells of the spinal cord; the muscular atrophy begins with the extremities and ultimately causes death from paralysis of muscles of respiration. SYN: *Duchenne-Aran disease.* SEE: *dystrophy, progressive muscular; sclerosis, amyotrophic lateral.*

a., Sudeck's. [P.H.M. Sudeck, Ger. surgeon, 1866–1938] Acute atrophy of a bone at the site of injury. Probably due to reflex local vasospasm.

a., trophoneurotic. Atrophy due to disease of the nerves or nerve centers supplying the affected muscles.

a., unilateral facial. Progressive atrophy of one side of the facial tissues.

a., white. Atrophy of the nerve, leaving only white connective tissue.

atropine sulfate (ăt′rō-pēn sŭl′fāt). USP. Highly poisonous salt of an alkaloid obtained from belladonna. It is a parasympatholytic agent and counteracts effects of parasympathetic stimulation.

atropine sulfate poisoning. SYM: Dryness of mouth; thirst; burning pain in throat; dry, hot, and flushed skin; hyperpyrexia; palpitations; restlessness; excitement; delirium.

F.A.: Lavage with slurry of activated charcoal or 1% tannic acid. Pilocarpine will make patient more comfortable, but barbiturates must be used for controlling excitement. SEE: *Poisons and Poisoning* in *Appendix.*

atropinism, atropism (ăt′rō-pĭn-ĭzm, -pĭzm). Atropine poisoning.

atropinization (ăt-rō″pĭn-ĭ-zā′shŭn). Administration of atropine until desired pharmacologic effect is achieved.

Atropisol. Trade name for atropine sulfate, USP, q.v.

attachment (ă-tăch′mĕnt). 1. A device or other material affixed to something else. 2. In dentistry, a wire around one tooth fixing it to a prosthetic device such as a denture.

attack (ă-tăk′) [Fr. *attaquer,* join]. 1. The onset of an illness or symptom, usually dramatic. Ex.: heart attack or an attack of gout. 2. An assault.

attendant. A paramedical hospital employee who assists in the care of patients.

attention [L. *attendere,* wait upon]. Directing or concentrating one's consciousness on only one object or an internal or external stimulus.

attention deficit disorder. The American Psychiatric Association describes this as a disease of infancy and childhood characterized by developmentally inappropriate inattention, impulsivity, and hyperactivity. The children do not persist with tasks and problems, and they have difficulty organizing and completing work. Their school work is performed impulsively and is sloppy; and is full of oversights such as omissions, insertions, and misrepresentation of easy items. The children appear not to listen or not to have heard what was said. The hyperactivity component is characterized by the children being unable to sit still and by excessive running or climbing. The activity tends to be haphazard, poorly organized, and not goal-directed. All of the symptoms vary with situation and time. Also, the condition may exist without the hyperactivity component.

The onset is usually by the age of three, and the disorder is thought to occur in the U.S.A. in 3% of prepubertal children. It is 10 times more common in boys than girls.

A variety of names have been applied to this disorder: hyperkinetic syndrome; hyperactive child syndrome; minimal brain damage; minimal brain dysfunction; minimal cerebral dysfunction.

attention reflex. Change in size of pupil when attention is suddenly fixed. SYN: *Piltz's reflex.*

attenuant (ă-tĕn′ū-ănt) [L. *attenuare,* to thin]. 1. Diluting, making thin or weak. 2. An agent that thins the blood.

attenuate (ă-tĕn′ū-āt). To render thin or make less virulent.

attenuated (ă-tĕn′ū-ăt′d) 1. Diluted. 2. Pert. to reduced virulence of pathogenic microorganism.

attenuation (ă-tĕn″ū-ā′shŭn) 1. Dilution. 2. Lessening of virulence. This may be accomplished with bacteria and viruses by heating, drying, treating with chemicals, passing through another organism, or culturing under unfavorable conditions 3. The change (decrease) in a beam of radiation as it passes through matter. 4. In acoustics, the reduction in sound intensity of the initial sound source as compared with the sound intensity at a point away from the source.

Attenuvax. Trade name for measles virus vaccine live, USP, q.v.

attic (ăt′ĭk) [L. *atticus*]. The cavity of the middle ear or the portion lying above the tympanic cavity proper. SYN: *recess, epitympanic.* SEE: *ear; tympanum*

attic disease. Chronic suppurative inflammation of the attic of the ear.

atticitis (ăt″ĭ-sī′tĭs) [L. *atticus,* attic, + Gr. *itis,* inflammation]. Inflammation of the attic of the ear.

atticoantrotomy (ăt″ĭ-kō-ăn-trŏt′ō-mē) [″ + Gr. *antron,* cave, + *tome,* incision]. Surgical opening of the attic and mastoid antrum of the ear.

atticotomy (ăt″ĭ-kŏt′ō-mē) [″ + Gr. *tome,* incision]. Surgical opening of tympanic attic of the ear.

attitude [LL. *aptitudo,* fitness]. 1. Bodily posture or position assumed, esp. with reference to position of limbs. A particular attitude is often a symptom of disease or abnormal mental state, e.g., the stereotyped position assumed by catatonics or theatric expression seen in hysteria. 2. Behavior toward a person, group, thing, or situation representative of conscious or unconscious mental views developed through cumulative experience.

a., crucifixion. Position in which body is rigid with arms at right angles to long axis of body. Seen in hysteroepilepsy and catatonia.

a., defense. Position automatically assumed to avert pain.

a., fetal. Position of the fetus with respect to maternal anatomical landmarks.

a., forced. Abnormal position due to disease or contractures.

a., frozen. Stiffness of gait, seen in amyotrophic lateral sclerosis.

a., illogical. Peculiar attitudes caused by disease, esp. hysteroepilepsy.

a., passional. Theatric or dramatic gestures and expressions of face and figure assumed by hysteric patients.

a., stereotyped. Position taken and held for a long period, seen frequently in mental diseases.

attollens (ă-tōl'ĕnz) [L.]. Raising or lifting up.

attraction (ă-trăk'shŭn) [L. *attrahere,* to draw toward]. Force, act, or process that causes bodies to approach each other.

a., capillary. The force by which liquids rise in fine tubes or through pores of loose material.

a., chemical. The tendency of atoms of one element to unite with those of another to form compounds.

a., molecular. The tendency of molecules with unlike electrical charges to attract each other. SEE: *adhesion; cohesion.*

attrition (ă-trĭsh'ŭn) [L. *attritio,* a rubbing against]. 1. Wearing away by friction or rubbing. 2. Any friction that breaks the skin. 3. A wearing away, as of teeth, in the course of normal use.

at. wt. *atomic weight.*

atypia (ā-tĭp'ē-ă) [Gr. *a-,* not, + *typos,* type]. The state of not conforming to a standard or regular type.

atypical (ā-tĭp'ĭ-kăl) [" + *typikos,* pert. to type]. Deviating from the normal; not conforming to type.

A.U. *Ångstrom unit.*

Au. Chem. symb. for gold; *Australia antigen.*

Aub-Dubois table (awb-dū-boy'). [Joseph C. Aub, U.S. physician, b. 1890; Eugene F. Dubois, U.S. physician, 1882–1959] Table of normal basal metabolic rates according to age.

audible. Capable of being heard.

audible sound. Sound containing frequency components between 15 and 15,000 Hz. (cycles per second).

audile (aw'dĭl). 1. Pert. to hearing. 2. Individual who retains more of what is heard than information received through other forms of communication. 3. In psychoanalysis, one whose mental images are auditory. SEE: *motile; visile.*

audioanesthesia (aw"dē-ō-ăn"ĕs-thē'zē-ă) [L. *audire,* to hear, + Gr. *an-,* not, + *aisthesis,* sensation]. Anesthesia or analgesia produced by sound; used by dentists to kill pain.

·diogenic (aw-dē-ō-jĕn'ĭk) [" + Gr. *genesis,* ·ration]. Originating in sound.

·am (aw'dē-ō-grăm") [" + Gr. *gramma,* ·ng]. Record of the audiometer. SEE: illus.

audiologist. A specialist in the evaluation, habilitation, and rehabilitation of persons with disorders of hearing function.

audiology (aw"dē-ŏl'ō-jē) [" + Gr. *logos,* study]. The study of hearing disorders through identification and evaluation of hearing loss, and the rehabilitation of persons with hearing loss, esp. that which cannot be improved by medical or surgical means.

audiometer (aw"dē-ŏm'ĕ-tĕr) [" + Gr. *metron,* measure]. A delicate instrument for testing hearing.

audiometry (aw"dē-ŏm'ĕ-trē). Testing of the hearing sense.

a., averaged electroencephalic. Method of testing the hearing of children who cannot be adequately tested by conventional means. The test is based on the electroencephalogram's being altered by perceived sound without the requirement of behavioral response. Thus the test may be done while an autistic, severely retarded, or hyperkinetic child is asleep or sedated. SEE: *auditory evoked response.*

audiphone (aw'dĭ-fōn) [L. *audire,* to hear, + Gr. *phone,* voice]. Instrument for conveying sound to auditory nerve through the teeth or a bone.

audition (aw-dĭ'shŭn) [L. *auditio,* hearing]. Hearing.

a., chromatic. Condition in which certain color sensations are aroused by sound stimuli.

a., colored. Condition in which color sensation is perceived when certain sounds reach the ear.

a., gustatory. Condition in which certain taste sensations are aroused by sound stimuli.

a., mental. The recollection of a sound based on previous auditory impressions.

auditive (aw'dĭ-tĭv). A person who is auditory minded, depending upon hearing rather than seeing in learning or recall.

audito-oculogyric reflex (aw"dĭt-ō-ŏk"ū-lō-jī'rĭk). The sudden turning of the head and eyes in direction of an alarming sound.

auditory (aw'dĭ-tō"rē) [L. *auditorius*]. Pert. to the sense of hearing.

auditory bulb. The membranous labyrinth and cochlea.

auditory canal. One of two canals leading to the ear. They are the external auditory meatus, leading from concha to tympanic membrane, length less than 1 inch (2.5 cm.); and the internal auditory meatus, located on posterior surface of petrous portion of temporal bone and leading from cranial cavity to inner ear, transmitting the acoustic nerve.

auditory evoked response. Response to auditory stimuli as determined by a method

AUDIOGRAM
LEFT EAR

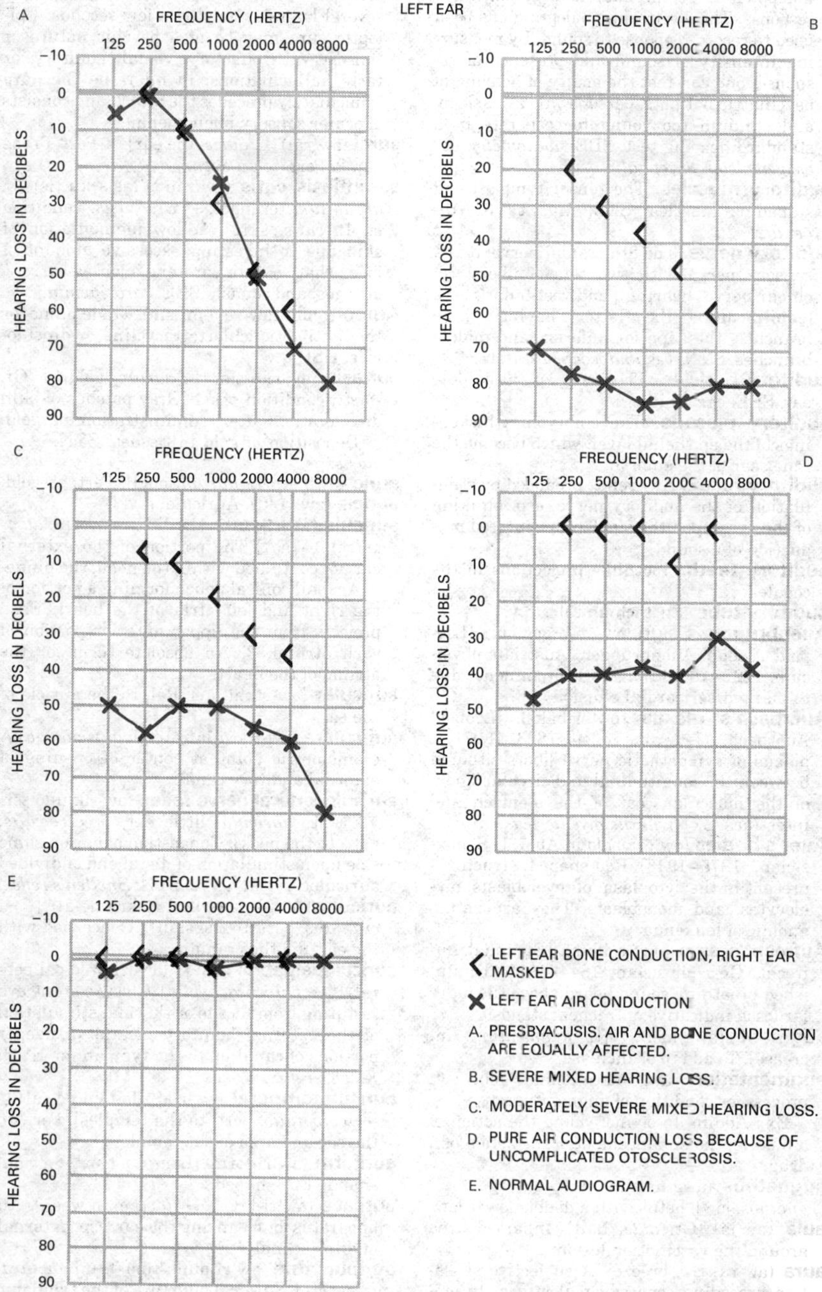

< LEFT EAR BONE CONDUCTION, RIGHT EAR MASKED

✕ LEFT EAR AIR CONDUCTION

A. PRESBYACUSIS. AIR AND BONE CONDUCTION ARE EQUALLY AFFECTED.

B. SEVERE MIXED HEARING LOSS.

C. MODERATELY SEVERE MIXED HEARING LOSS.

D. PURE AIR CONDUCTION LOSS BECAUSE OF UNCOMPLICATED OTOSCLEROSIS.

E. NORMAL AUDIOGRAM.

independent of the individual's subjective response. The electroencephalogram has been used to record response to sound. By measuring intensity of sound and presence of response, one can test the acuity of hearing of psychiatric patients, persons who are asleep, and children too young to cooperate in a standard hearing test. SEE: *audiometry, averaged electroencephalic.*

auditory muscles. The tensor tympani and stapedius muscles. SEE: *Muscles* in *Appendix.*

auditory nerve. The 8th cranial nerve; it is a sensory nerve with two sets of fibers: cochlear nerve (hearing), and vestibular nerve (equilibrium), the latter having three branches, the superior, inferior, and middle branches. SYN: *vestibulocochlear nerve.*

auditory ossicles. The bones of the middle ear. SEE: *ear* for illus.

auditory placode. The embryonic thickenings of the epithelial layer, which become the inner ear of the embryo.

auditory reflex. Any reflex produced by stimulation of the auditory nerve, esp. blinking of the eyes upon the sudden unexpected production of a sound.

auditory teeth. Toothlike projections in the cochlea.

auditory tube. Eustachian tube, q.v.

Auenbrugger's sign (ow-ĕn-broog'ĕrz). [Leopold Joseph Auenbrugger, Austrian physician, 1722–1809] Epigastric prominence due to marked pericardial effusion.

Auerbach's plexus (ow'ĕr-băks). [Leopold Auerbach, Ger. anatomist, 1828–1897] A plexus of sympathetic nerve fibers situated between the longitudinal and circular fibers of the muscular coat of the stomach and intestines. SYN: *plexus myentericus.*

Auer's bodies (ow'ĕrz). [John Auer, U.S. physician, 1875–1948] Rod-shaped structures present in the cytoplasm of myeloblasts, myelocytes, and monoblasts. They are pathognomic of leukemia.

Aufrecht's sign (owf'rĕkhts). [Emanual Aufrecht, Ger. physician, 1844–1933] Diminished breathing sound heard above the jugular fossa indicative of tracheal stenosis.

augment (awg-mĕnt') [L. *augmentum,* increase]. To add to or increase.

augmentation (awg"mĕn-tā'shŭn). The act, process, or condition of augmenting.

Ex.: Adding to or increasing the action of a muscle; the enhancement of the action of a drug.

augnathus (awg-nā'thŭs) [Gr. *au,* again, + *gnathos,* jaw]. Fetus with a double lower jaw.

la (aw'lă) [Gr. *aule,* hall]. Inflamed area und the vaccination lesion.

w'ră) [L., breeze]. A subjective sensa- preceding a paroxysmal attack. In epilepsy the aura may precede the attack by several hours or only by a few seconds. Epileptic aura may be of a psychic nature or sensory with olfactory, visual, auditory, or taste hallucinations. In migraine the aura immediately precedes the attack and consists of ocular sensory phenomena.

aural (aw'răl) [L. *auris,* the ear]. 1. Pert. to the ear. 2. Pert. to an aura.

aurantiasis cutis (aw"răn-tī'ă-sĭs kū'tĭs) [L. *aurantium,* orange, + Gr. *-iasis,* condition of; L. *cutis,* skin]. Yellow pigmentation of skin due to ingesting excessive amount of foods that contain carotene such as carrots, oranges, and squash. SEE: *carotenemia.*

Aureomycin (aw"rē-ō-mī'sĭn). Trade name for the antibiotic chlortetracycline hydrochloride, USP, q.v.

auriasis (aw-rī'ă-sĭs) [L. *aurum,* gold, + Gr. *-iasis,* condition of]. 1. Gray patches of skin discoloration after administration of gold. 2. Deposition of gold in tissues. SYN: *chrysiasis.*

auric (aw'rĭk) [L. *aurum,* gold]. Pert. to gold.

auricle (aw'rĭ-kl). Auricula, q.v.

auricula (aw-rĭk'ū-lă) [L., little ear]. (pl. *auriculae*) 1. [NA] The portion of the external ear not contained within the head; the pinna. 2. A small conical pouch forming a portion of the right and left atria of the heart. Each projects from the upper anterior portion of each atrium. 3. An obsolete term for the atrium of the heart.

auricular (aw-rĭk'ū-lăr). Rel. to the auricle of the ear.

auriculare (aw-rĭk"ū-lā'rē). (pl. *auricularia*) A craniometric point at center of opening of external auditory canal.

auriculocervical nerve reflex (aw-rĭk"ū-lō-sĕr'vĭk'l) [L. *auricula,* little ear, + *cervicalis,* pert. to the neck]. Congestion of ear on same side upon stimulation of distal end of divided auriculocervical nerve. SYN: *Snellen's reflex.*

auriculocranial (aw-rĭk"ū-lō-krā'nē-ăl) [" + *cranialis,* pert. to the skull]. Concerned with the ear and the cranium.

auriculopalpebral reflex (aw-rĭk"ū-lō-păl'pĕb-răl) [" + *palpebra,* eyelid]. Closure of the eye resulting from tactile or thermal stimulation of the external auditory meatus or deeper portions of canal up to the tympanum. SYN: *Kisch's reflex.*

auriculotemporal (aw-rĭk"ū-lō-tĕm'pō-răl) [" + *temporalis,* pert. to the temples]. Pert. to the ear and area of the temple.

auriform (aw'rĭ-form) [L. *auris,* ear, + *forma,* shape]. Ear-shaped.

aurilave (aw'rĭ-lāv) [" + *lavare,* to wash]. An apparatus for cleansing the ear, esp. external auditory canal.

auripuncture (aw'rĭ-pŭnk"tūr) [" + *punctura,* puncture]. Surgical puncture of the tympanic membrane.

auris (aw'rĭs) [L.]. The ear.

a. dextra. Right ear.

a. externa. External ear (pinna and external auditory meatus).

a. interna. Internal ear (semicircular canals, vestibule, cochlea).

a. media. Middle ear (tympanum).

a. sinistra. Left ear.

auriscalp, auriscalpium (aw'rĭ-skălp, aw"rĭ-skăl'pē-ŭm) [" + *scalpere,* to scrape]. 1. Scraping instrument used to remove foreign matter from ear. 2. Earpick.

auriscope (aw'rĭ-skōp) [" + Gr. *skopein,* to view]. Instrument for making an ear examination. SYN: *otoscope.*

aurist (aw'rĭst). Ear specialist. SYN: *otologist.*

aurotherapy (aw"rō-thĕr'ă-pē) [L. *aurum,* gold, + Gr. *therapeia,* treatment]. Treatment of disease by administration of gold salts; used in the treatment of rheumatoid arthritis.

aurum (aw'rŭm) [L.]. Gold.

auscult (aws-kŭlt'). Auscultate, q.v.

auscultate (aws'kŭl-tāt) [L. *auscultare,* listen to]. To examine by auscultation.

auscultation (aws"kŭl-tā'shŭn). Process of listening for sounds within the body, usually to sounds of thoracic or abdominal viscera, in order to detect some abnormal condition, or to detect pregnancy. The technique is also helpful in diagnosing vascular abnormalities such as arteriovenous fistulae. SEE: *percussion.*

PROCEDURE: The chest should be draped with a loose-fitting garment that can easily be moved aside to allow the stethoscope to be placed directly against the skin. When chest is covered with hair, moisten hair as otherwise it will produce friction sounds, resembling rales. Auscultate all over chest anteriorly and posteriorly, on full inspiration, full expiration, and after coughing. In comparing the two sides, auscultate symmetrical parts. Parts should be in perfect repose. Position of examiner should be as unrestrained as possible, lest sounds of examiner's own blood vessels be confused with sounds from within the subject.

a., immediate. Auscultation in which ear is applied directly to bared or thinly covered surface.

a., mediate. Auscultation in which sounds are conducted from the surface to ear through an instrument such as a stethoscope.

auscultation, words pert. to: bruit; egophony; percussion; rale; resonance, vocal; souffle.

auscultatory (aws-kŭl'tă-tō"rē). Pert. to auscultation.

auscultatory percussion. Auscultation at the same time percussion is made.

auscultoplectrum (aws-kŭl"tō-plĕk'trŭm) [L. *auscultare,* listen to, + Gr. *plektron,* hammer]. Instrument used for both auscultation and percussion.

Austin Flint murmur. [Austin Flint, U.S. physician, 1812–1886] A presystolic or late diastolic heart murmur best heard at the apex of the heart. It is present in some cases of aortic insufficiency and is thought to be due to the vibration of the mitral valve caused by the backward-flowing blood from the aorta meeting the blood flowing in from the left auricle.

Australia antigen. An antigen present in the sera of patients with viral hepatitis, but rarely present in patients with infectious hepatitis. This antigen is also found in normal populations in the tropics and southeast Asia. It was first isolated in the serum of an Australian aborigine. SYN: *hepatitis B surface antigen.*

autacoid (aw'tă-koyd) [Gr. *autos,* self, + *akos,* remedy, + *eidos,* form]. A term originally used by the British physiologists Edward Shäfer and Sharpey-Shafer as a substitute for the word *hormone.*

autarcesis (aw-tăr'sĭ-sĭs, aw"tăr-sē'sĭs) [" + *arkein,* to ward off]. Resistance to infection through natural immunity.

autarcetic (awt"ăr-sĕt'ĭk). Pert. to autarcesis.

autechoscope (aw-tĕk'ō-skōp) [" + *echos,* sound, + *skopein,* to inspect]. Instrument for self-auscultation.

autism (aw'tĭzm) [" + *-ismos,* condition of]. Mental introversion in which the attention or interest is fastened upon the patient's own ego. A self-centered mental state from which reality tends to be excluded.

a., infantile. A syndrome appearing in childhood with symptoms of self-absorption, inaccessibility, aloneness, inability to relate, highly repetitive play and rage reactions if interrupted, predilection for rhythmical movements, and many language disturbances.

ETIOL: Unknown. Some maintain that it is a form of childhood schizophrenia.

auto- [Gr. *autos,* self]. Prefix meaning self.

autoactivation (aw"tō-ăk"tĭ-vā'shŭn) [" + L. *agere,* to act]. Gland activation by its own secretion.

autoagglutination (aw"tō-ă-gloo"tĭ-nā'shŭn) [" + L. *agglutinare,* adhere to]. Blood cell agglutination of an individual by the person's own serum.

autoagglutinin (aw"tō-ă-glū'tĭ-nĭn). Substance present in an individual's blood that agglutinates that person's red blood cells.

autoallergy (aw"tō-ăl'ĕr-jē). In immunology, becoming sensitive to one's own tissues.

autoamputation (aw"tō-ăm"pū-tā'shŭn). Spontaneous amputation of a part or limb. SEE: *ainhum.*

autoanalysis (aw"tō-ă-năl'ĭ-sĭs) [" + *analyein*, break down]. Patient's own analysis of mental state underlying patient's mental disorder.

Autoanalyzer (aw"tō-ăn'ă-līz"ĕr). Trademark of an apparatus for performing analytic tests on a large number of laboratory specimens. The testing is done automatically with the specimens being tested sequentially.

autoantibody (aw"tō-ăn'tĭ-bŏd"ē) [" + *anti*, against, + AS. *bodig*, body]. Antibody acting against antigenic tissue products of the same organism in which it is formed.

autoantigen (aw"tō-ăn'tĭ-jĕn) [" + " + *gennan*, to produce]. A substance that stimulates the production of antibodies in the individual from which it was derived.

autoantitoxin (aw"tō-ăn"tĭ-tŏk'sĭn) [" + " + *toxikon*, poison]. Antitoxin produced by body itself.

autoblast (aw'tō-blăst) [" + *blastos*, germ]. Independent cell, as a protozoa.

autocatalysis (aw"tō-kă-tăl'ĭ-sĭs) [" + *katalysis*, dissolution]. Increase in the rate of a chemical reaction resulting from products that are produced in the reaction acting as catalysts. SEE: *catalyst*.

autocatharsis (aw-tō-kă-thăr'sĭs) [" + *katharsis*, a cleansing]. A form of psychotherapy in which patients in discussing their own problems gain an insight into their mental difficulties.

autochthonous (aw-tŏk'thō-nŭs) [Gr. *autos*, self, + *chthon*, earth]. 1. Found where developed, as in the case of a blood clot or a calculus. 2. Pert. to a tissue graft to a new site on the same individual.

autocinesia, autocinesis (aw"tō-sī-nē'sē-ă, -nē'sĭs) [" + *kinesis*, motion]. Voluntary movement. SYN: *autokinesis*.

autoclasis (aw"tŏk'lă-sĭs) [" + *klasis*, a breaking]. Destruction of a part from internal causes.

autoclave (aw'tō-klāv) [" + L. *clavis*, a key]. Apparatus for sterilization by steam pressure, usually at 250° F. (121° C.) for a specified length of time. SEE: *sterilization*.

autocystoplasty (aw"tō-sĭs'tō-plăs"tē) [" + *kystis*, bladder, + *plassein*, to mold]. Plastic repair of bladder with grafts from patient's own body.

autocytolysin (aw"tō-sī-tŏl'ĭ-sĭn) [" + *kytos*, cell, + *lysis*, dissolution]. Antibody found within patient's own blood plasma capable of destroying cells or tissues. SYN: *autolysin*.

autocytolysis (aw"tō-sī-tŏl'ĭ-sĭs). Self-digestion or self-destruction of cells.

autodermic (aw"tō-dĕr'mĭk) [" + *derma*, skin]. Pert. to one's own skin, esp. rel. to dermato-[illegible] with patient's own skin.

[illegible]gestion (aw"tō-dī-jĕs'chŭn) [" + L. *dis*, [illegible]t, + *gerere*, to carry]. Digestion of tissues by their own secretion, such as digestion of the stomach wall by gastric juice, which occurs in certain stomach disorders.

autodiploid (aw"tō-dĭp'loyd) [" + *diploe*, fold, + *eidos*, form]. Having two sets of chromosomes; caused by redoubling the chromosomes of the haploid cell.

autodrainage (aw"tō-drān'ĭj) [" + AS. *dreahnian*, drain]. Drainage of a cavity by sending the fluid through a channel made in patient's own tissues.

autoecholalia (aw"tō-ĕk-ō-lā'lē-ă) [" + *echo*, echo, + *lalia*, babble]. Repetition of words of one's own statements.

autoecic (aw-tē'sĭk) [" + *oikos*, house]. Pert. to parasite that goes through its entire life cycle in one organism.

autoerotism (aw"tō-ĕ-rŏt'ĭsm) [Gr. *autos*, self, + *erotikos*, rel. to love]. Sexual arousal by one's own body or sexual gratification using one's own body, as in masturbation.

autoexamination (aw"tō-ĕg-zăm"ĭ-nā'shŭn) [" + L. *examinare*, to examine]. Self-examination. SEE: *breast, self-examination of*.

autofundoscope (aw"tō-fŭn'dō-skōp) [" + L. *fundus*, bottom, + Gr. *skopein*, to examine]. Apparatus for autoexamination of retinal vessels of the eye.

autogenesis (aw-tō-jĕn'ĕ-sĭs) [" + *genesis*, production]. Abiogenesis; self-production; origination within the organism.

autogenetic, autogenic (aw-tō-jĕ-nĕt'ĭk, aw-tō-jĕn'ĭk). Pert. to self-production or autogenesis.

autogenous (aw-tŏj'ĕ-nŭs). 1. Self-producing; originating within the body. 2. Denoting a vaccine from a culture of the patient's own bacteria.

autograft (aw'tō-grăft) [" + L. *graphium*, grafting knife]. A graft transferred from one part of a patient's body to another.

autohemagglutination (aw"tō-hĕm"ă-glū"tĭ-nā'shŭn). Agglutination of one's own red cells.

autohemic (aw"tō-hē'mĭk) [" + *haima*, blood]. Done with one's own blood.

autohemolysin (aw"tō-hē-mŏl'ĭ-sĭn) [" + " + *lysis*, dissolution]. Antibody acting on corpuscles of individual in whose blood it is formed.

autohemolysis (aw"tō-hē-mŏl'ĭ-sĭs). Hemolysis of a person's blood corpuscles by the person's own serum.

autohemotherapy (aw"tō-hē"mō-thĕr'ă-pē) [" + *haima*, blood, + *therapeia*, treatment]. Treatment by withdrawal and injection intramuscularly of patient's own blood.

autohypnosis (aw"tō-hĭp-nō'sĭs). Self-induced hypnosis.

autoimmune disease (aw"tō-ĭm-mūn') [" + L. *immunis*, safe]. Disease in which the body produces disordered immunological response against itself. Normally the body's immune mechanisms are able to distinguish clearly between what is a normal substance and what is foreign. In autoimmune diseases, this system becomes defective and produces antibodies against normal parts of the body to such an extent as to cause tissue injury. Certain diseases such as hemolytic anemia, some forms of glomerulonephritis, rheumatoid arthritis, myasthenia gravis, and scleroderma are considered to be autoimmune diseases.

autoimmunity (aw″tō-ĭm-mū′nĭ-tē). The condition in which antibodies are produced against the body's own tissues. It may result in hypersensitivity reactions or autoimmune diseases.

autoimmunization (aw″tō-ĭm″ū-nĭ-zā′shŭn). The introduction of an immune response to the body's own tissue components.

autoinfection (aw″tō-ĭn-fĕk′shŭn) [Gr. *autos,* self, + L. *inficere,* to taint]. Infection produced by an agent already present in the body.

autoinfusion (aw″tō-ĭn-fū′zhŭn) [″ + L. *in,* into, + *fundere,* to pour]. Forcing blood from extremities to body core by applying Esmarch bandages, q.v.

autoinoculation (aw″tō-ĭn-ŏk″ū-lā′shŭn) [″ + L. *inoculare,* to ingraft]. Inoculation by use of organisms obtained from another part of the body.

autointoxication (aw″tō-ĭn-tŏk″sĭ-kā′shŭn) [″ + L. *in,* into, + Gr. *toxikon,* poison]. A condition caused by poisonous substances produced within the body. SYN: *toxicosis, endogenic.*

autoisolysin (aw″to-ī-sŏl′ĭ-sĭn) [″ + *isos,* equal, + *lysis,* dissolution]. An antibody that causes dissolution of cells of the subject from which it was obtained. It also causes lysis of cells of other animals of the same species.

autokeratoplasty (aw″tō-kĕr′ă-tō-plăs″tē) [″ + *keras,* harm, + *plassein,* to form]. Corneal grafting using tissue from the patient's other eye.

autokinesis (aw″tō-kĭ-nē′sĭs) [″ + *kinesis,* motion]. Voluntary movement. SYN: *autocinesia.*

autokinetic (aw″tō-kĭ-nĕt′ĭk). Being able to move voluntarily.

autolesion (aw′tō-lē″zhŭn) [″ + L. *laedere,* to wound]. Self-inflicted injury.

autologous (aw-tŏl′ō-gŭs) [″ + *logos,* proportion]. Indicating something that has its origin within an individual, esp. a factor present in tissues or fluids.

autolysate (aw-tŏl′ĭ-sāt) [″ + *lysis,* dissolution]. Specific product of autolysis.

autolysin (aw-tŏl′ĭ-sĭn). Antibody capable of destroying cells or tissue of the organism in which it is present.

autolysis (aw-tŏl′ĭ-sĭs). 1. The self-dissolution or self-digestion that occurs in tissues or cells by enzymes in the cells themselves, such as occurs after death and in some pathological conditions. 2. Hemolysis of blood cells occurring as a result of the action of an animal's own serum or plasma.

autolytic (aw″tō-lĭt′ĭk). Pert. to autolysis. SEE: *enzyme.*

automatic [Gr. *automatos,* self-acting]. Spontaneous; involuntary.

automatism (aw-tŏm′ă-tĭzm) [″ + *-ismos,* condition of]. 1. Automatic actions or behavior without conscious volition or knowledge. The subject, though amnesic, appears normal to an observer, but the real personality is latent during a secondary state or period of automatism, usually a hysterical trance. Such patients are not responsible for their acts and must not be left alone. They may carry out complicated acts without remembering having done so. 2. The spontaneous activity of cells or tissues, as the movement of cilia or the contraction of smooth muscles in tissues or organs removed from the body.

autonomic (aw-tō-nŏm′ĭk) [″ + *nomos,* law]. 1. Self-controlling; functioning independently. 2. Rel. to the autonomic nervous system.

autonomic hyperreflexia. A condition commonly seen in patients with injury to the upper spinal cord. It is caused by massive sympathetic discharge of stimuli from the autonomic nervous system. It may be triggered by distention of the bladder or colon; catheterization of or irrigation of the bladder; cystoscopy; or transurethral resection.

SYM: Sudden hypertension, bradycardia, sweating, severe headache, and gooseflesh.

TREATMENT: Ganglionic blocking agents such as mecamylamine hydrochloride, USP, or trimethaphan camsylate, USP.

autonomic nervous system. The part of the nervous system that is concerned with control of involuntary bodily functions. It regulates the function of glands, esp. the salivary, gastric, and sweat glands, and the adrenal medulla; smooth muscle tissue; and the heart. The autonomic nervous system may act on these tissues to reduce or slow activity or to initiate their function.

It is divided into the sympathetic or thoracolumbar division and the parasympathetic or craniosacral division. The *sympathetic system* is made up of the paired ganglionated sympathetic trunk; its connections (rami communicantes) with the thoracic and lumbar parts of the spinal nerve; the large and small splanchnic nerves; and certain ganglia in the abdomen (e.g., the mesenteric ganglia). The *parasympathetic system* consists of certain fibers of some cranial nerves, such as the motor fibers of the vagus, and of other fibers connected with the sacral part of the spinal cord. SEE: illus.

FUNCTIONS: Stimulating sympathetic fibers usually produces vasoconstriction in the part supplied, general rise in blood pressure, erection of the hairs, gooseflesh, pupillary dilation, secretion of small quantities of thick saliva, depression of gastrointestinal activity, and acceleration of the heart. In general, these activities occur in emergencies such as fright and are associated with the expenditure of energy as a response to the need to flee, fight, or to be frightened. They are mediated through the release of a transmitter agent, norepinephrine.

Stimulating parasympathetic nerves generally produces vasodilation of the part supplied, general fall in the blood pressure, contraction of the pupil, copious secretion of thin saliva, increased gastrointestinal activity, and slowing of the heart. SEE: *nervous system.*

autonomous (aw-tŏn′ō-mŭs). Independent of external influences.

autonomy (aw-tŏn′ō-mē) [Gr. *autos,* self, + *nomos,* law]. Functioning independently.

autopathy (aw-tŏp′ă-thē) [″ + *pathos,* disease]. A disease originating without apparent external cause.

autophagia, autophagy (aw″tō-fā′jē-ă, aw-tŏf′ă-jē) [″ + *phagein,* to eat]. 1. Biting oneself. 2. Self-consumption by a cell.

autophil (aw′tō-fĭl) [″ + *philein,* to love]. Person having a sensitive autonomic nervous system.

autophilia (aw-tō-fĭl′ē-ă). Narcissism, q.v. Self-love.

autophobia (aw″tō-fō′bē-ă) [″ + *phobos,* fear]. 1. A psychoneurotic fear of being alone. 2. Abnormal fear of being egotistical.

autophony (aw-tŏf′ō-nē) [″ + *phone,* voice]. The vibration and echolike reproduction of the patient's own voice, breath sounds, and murmurs; usually due to diseases of the middle ear and auditory tube.

autoplasmotherapy (aw″tō-plăs″mō-thĕr′ă-pē) [″ + *plasma,* a thing formed, + *therapeia,* treatment]. Treatment by injecting patient's own blood plasma.

autoplastic (aw″tō-plăs′tĭk) [″ + *plassein,* to form]. Pert. to autoplasty, q.v.

autoplasty (aw′tō-plăs″tē). 1. Plastic surgery using grafts from the patient's body. 2. In psychiatry, adaptation by altering one's self rather than changing the external environment.

autoploidy (aw″tō-ploy′dē). Autopolyploidy, q.v.

autopolyploidy (aw″tō-pŏl′ē-ploy″dē) [″ + *polys,* many, + *ploos,* fold, + *eidos,* resemblance]. The condition of having more than two complete sets of chromosomes.

autoprecipitin (aw″tō-prē-sĭp′ĭ-tĭn) [Gr. *autos,* self, + L. *praecipitare,* to cast down]. Precipitin active against serum of animal in which it was formed.

autopsia (aw-tŏp′sē-ă) [″ + *opsis,* view]. Autopsy.

autopsy (aw′tŏp-sē). Postmortem examination of the organs and tissues of a body to determine cause of death or pathological conditions. SYN: *postmortem examination.*

autopsychic (aw″tō-sī′kĭk) [″ + *psyche,* soul]. Aware of one's own personality.

autopsychosis (aw″tō-sī-kō′sĭs) [″ + *psyche,* the soul]. Mental disease in which patients' ideas about themselves are disordered.

autopyotherapy (aw″tō-pī″ō-thĕr′ă-pē) [″ + *pyon,* pus, + *therapeia,* treatment]. Treatment of disease by administration of patient's own pathological excretions.

autoradiogram. Autoradiograph, q.v. SYN: *radioautogram.*

autoradiograph (aw″tō-rā′dē-ō-grăf). The radiograph formed by radioactive materials present in the tissue or individual. This is made possible by injecting radiochemicals into the person or tissue and then exposing x-ray film by placing the individual or tissue adjacent to the film.

autoradiography. Use of autoradiographs in investigating patients. SYN: *radioautography.*

autoregulation (aw″tō-rĕg″ū-lā′shŭn). Control of an event such as blood flow through a tissue (e.g., cardiac muscle) by alteration of the tissue. Thus, if not enough blood is flowing through a tissue, certain changes occur to cause an increase; if the flow is too great, another change will cause a decrease.

autoreinfusion (aw″tō-rē″ĭn-fū′zhŭn) [″ + L. *re,* back, + *in,* into, + *fundere,* to pour]. Intravenous injection of patient's blood that has been collected from a site in which bleeding had occurred, such as the abdominal or pleural cavity.

autorrhaphy (aw-tor′ă-fē) [″ + *rhaphe,* suture]. Wound closure by using strands of tissue taken from edges of the wound.

autosensitization (aw″tō-sĕn″sĭ-tĭ-zā′shŭn). Becoming sensitized to one's own cells, fluids, or tissues.

autosepticemia (aw″tō-sĕp″tĭ-sē′mē-ă) [″ + *septos,* rotten, + *haima,* blood]. Septicemia from poisons existing within the organism.

autoserodiagnosis (aw″tō-sē″rō-dī-ăg-nō′sĭs) [″ + L. *serum,* whey, + Gr. *dia,* through, + *gnosis,* knowledge]. Diagnosis through serum from patient's blood.

autoserotherapy (aw″tō-sē″rō-thĕr′ă-pē) [″ + ″ + Gr. *therapeia,* treatment]. Treatment by hypodermic injection of patient's own blood serum.

autoserous (aw″tō-sē′rŭs). Pert. to autoserum.

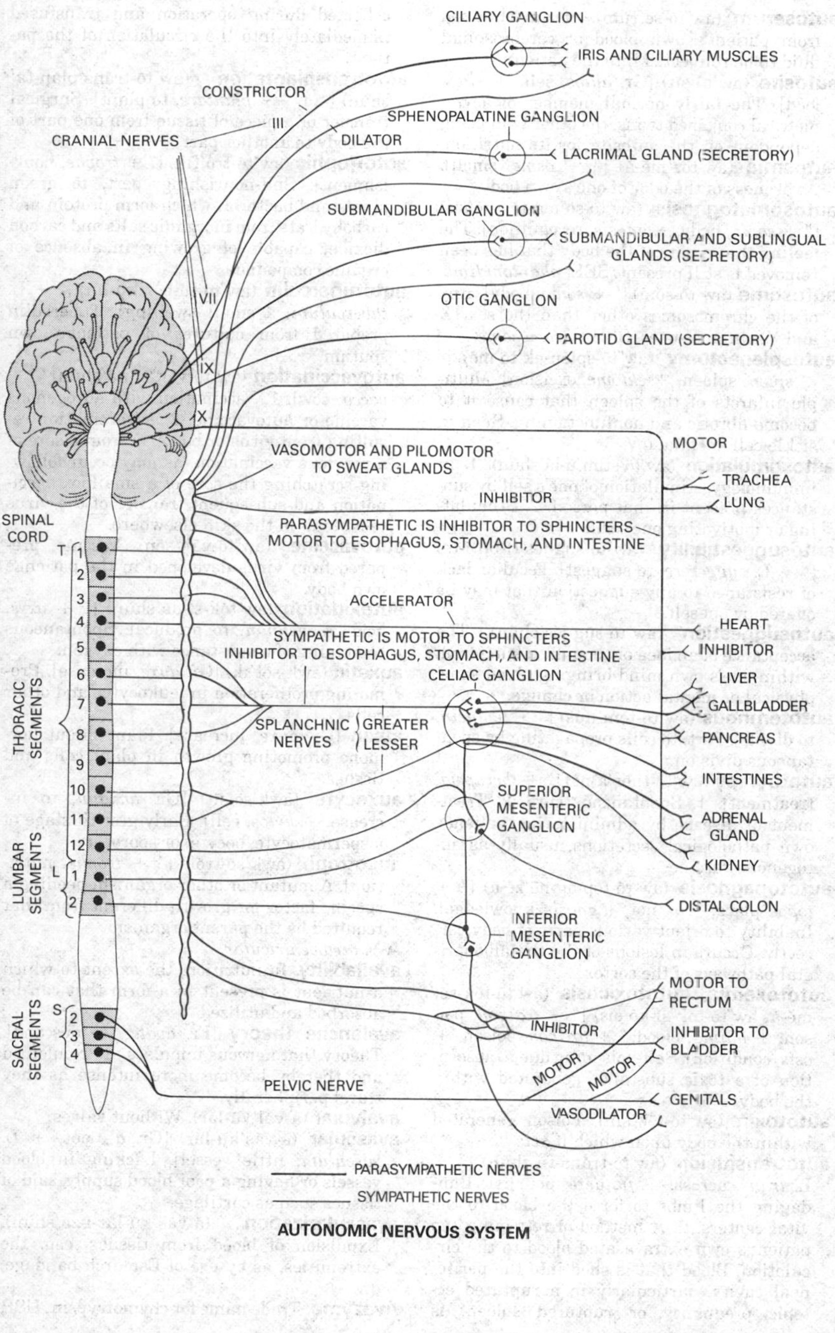
CILIARY GANGLION
IRIS AND CILIARY MUSCLES
CONSTRICTOR
III
SPHENOPALATINE GANGLION
CRANIAL NERVES
DILATOR
LACRIMAL GLAND (SECRETORY)
SUBMANDIBULAR GANGLION
SUBMANDIBULAR AND SUBLINGUAL GLANDS (SECRETORY)
VII
OTIC GANGLION
PAROTID GLAND (SECRETORY)
IX
X
MOTOR
VASOMOTOR AND PILOMOTOR TO SWEAT GLANDS
TRACHEA
INHIBITOR
LUNG
SPINAL CORD
PARASYMPATHETIC IS INHIBITOR TO SPHINCTERS
MOTOR TO ESOPHAGUS, STOMACH, AND INTESTINE
T
1
2
3
4
5
6
7
8
9
10
11
12
ACCELERATOR
HEART
SYMPATHETIC IS MOTOR TO SPHINCTERS
INHIBITOR TO ESOPHAGUS, STOMACH, AND INTESTINE
INHIBITOR
CELIAC GANGLION
LIVER
GALLBLADDER
THORACIC SEGMENTS
SPLANCHNIC NERVES
GREATER
LESSER
PANCREAS
INTESTINES
SUPERIOR MESENTERIC GANGLION
ADRENAL GLAND
LUMBAR SEGMENTS
L
1
2
KIDNEY
DISTAL COLON
INFERIOR MESENTERIC GANGLION
MOTOR TO RECTUM
S
2
3
4
SACRAL SEGMENTS
INHIBITOR
INHIBITOR TO BLADDER
MOTOR
MOTOR
PELVIC NERVE
GENITALS
VASODILATOR
PARASYMPATHETIC NERVES
SYMPATHETIC NERVES

AUTONOMIC NERVOUS SYSTEM

autoserum (aw″tō-sē′rŭm). Serum obtained from patient's own blood or cerebrospinal fluid to be reinjected into the patient.

autosite (aw′tō-sīt) [Gr. *autos,* self, + *sitos,* food]. The fairly normal member of asymmetrical conjoined twins, the other twin being dependent on the autosite for its nutrition.

autosmia (aw-tŏz′mē-ă) [″ + *osme,* smell]. Awareness of the odor of one's own body.

autosomatognosis (aw″tō-sō″mă-tŏg-nō′sĭs) [″ + *soma,* body, + *gnosis,* recognition]. The feeling that a part of the body that has been removed is still present SEE: *phantom limb.*

autosome (aw′tō-sōm) [″ + *soma,* body]. Any of the chromosomes other than the sex (X and Y) chromosomes. SEE: *chromosome.*

autosplenectomy (aw″tō-splēn-ĕk′tō-mē) [″ + *splen,* spleen, + *ektome,* excision]. Multiple infarcts of the spleen that cause it to become fibrotic and nonfunctioning. Seen in sickle cell anemia, q.v.

autostimulation (aw″tō-stĭm″ū-lā′shŭn). 1. In immunology, stimulation of one's self by substances present in that person. 2. Stimulating or motivating one's self.

autosuggestibility (aw″tō-sŭg-jĕs″tĭ-bĭl′ĭ-tē) [″ + L. *suggerere,* to suggest]. Peculiar lack of resistance to any suggestion that may be offered by oneself.

autosuggestion (aw″tō-sŭg-jĕs′chŭn). The acceptance of an idea or thought arising from within one's own mind bringing about some physical or mental action or change.

autotemnous (aw″tō-tĕm′nŭs) [″ + *temnein,* to divide]. Pert. to cells propagating by spontaneous division.

autotherapy (aw″tō-thĕr′ă-pē) [″ + *therapeia,* treatment]. 1. Spontaneous cure. 2. Treatment of disease by administering patient's own pathological secretions, usually as autogenous vaccine.

autotopagnosia (aw″tō-tŏp-ăg-nō′zē-ă) [″ + *topos,* place, + *a-,* not, + *gnosis,* knowledge]. Inability to orient various parts of body correctly. Occurs in lesions of the thalamoparietal pathways of the cortex.

autotoxemia, autotoxicosis (aw″tō-tŏk-sē′mē-ă, aw″tō-tŏk″sĭ-kō′sĭs) [″ + *toxikon,* poison, + *haima,* blood; ″ + *toxikon,* poison, + *osis,* condition]. Self-poisoning due to absorption of a toxic substance generated within the body.

autotoxin (aw″tō-tŏk′sĭn). Poison generated within the body upon which it acts.

autotransfusion (aw″tō-trăns-fū′zhŭn) [″ + L. *trans,* across, + *fundere,* pour]. 1. Bandaging the limbs to force the blood to the vital centers. 2. A method of returning the patient's own extravasated blood to the circulation. Blood that is shed into the peritoneal cavity, particularly in a ruptured ectopic pregnancy or ruptured spleen, is collected during operation and transfused immediately into the circulation of the patient.

autotransplantation (aw″tō-trăns″plăn-tā′shŭn) [″ + ″ + *plantare,* to plant]. Surgical transfer of a piece of tissue from one part of the body to another part.

autotrophic (aw″tō-trō′fĭk) [″ + *trophe,* nourishment]. Self-nourishing; pert. to green plants and bacteria, which form protein and carbohydrate from inorganic salts and carbon dioxide; capable of growing in absence of organic compounds.

autotuberculin (aw″tō-tū-bĕr′kū-lĭn) [″ + L. *tuberculum,* a small swelling]. Tuberculin prepared from cultures of patient's own sputum.

autovaccination (aw″tō-văk″sĭ-nā′shŭn) [″ + *vacca,* cow]. 1. Vaccination with autogenous vaccine or autovaccine. 2. A vaccination resulting from virus or bacteria from a sore of a previous vaccination, as may occur following scratching the sore of a smallpox vaccination and subsequent transfer of the virus to a break in the skin elsewhere.

autovaccine (aw″tō-văk′sēn) Vaccine prepared from virus developed in the patient's own body.

autoxidation (aw″tŏk-sĭ-dā′shŭn) [″ + *oxys,* acid, + *gennan,* to produce]. Spontaneous combining of a substance with oxygen.

auxetic (awk-sĕt′ĭk) [Gr. *auxe,* increase]. Promoting proliferation in leukocytes and other cells.

auxin [Gr. *auxe,* increase]. Plant-sprout hormone promoting growth in plant cells and tissues.

auxocyte (awk′sō-sīt) [Gr. *auxanu,* to increase, + *kytos,* cell]. Early growth stage of a spermatocyte, oocyte, or sporocyte.

auxotroph (awk′sō-trōf) [″ + *trophe,* nutrition]. A mutant or other organism needing a specific factor for growth different from that required by the parent organism.

A-V. *atrioventricular.*

availability. In nutrition, the extent to which a nutrient is present in a form that can be absorbed and utilized.

avalanche theory [Fr. *avaler,* to descend]. Theory that nervous impulses are reinforced and thereby become more intense as they travel peripherally.

avalvular (ă-văl′vū-lăr). Without valves.

avascular (ă-văs′kū-lăr) [Gr. *a-,* not, + L. *vasculum,* little vessel]. Lacking in blood vessels or having a poor blood supply, said of tissues such as cartilage.

avascularization (ă-văs″kū-lăr-ĭ-zā′shŭn). Expulsion of blood from tissues, esp. the extremities, as by use of Esmarch bandage, q.v.

Avazyme. Trade name for chymotrypsin, USP,

q.v.

A-V block. A heart block in which electronic impulses are impeded at the A-V node.

A-V bundle. A bundle of fibers of the impulse-conducting system of the heart. From its origin in the A-V node, it enters the interventricular septum, where it divides into two branches whose fibers pass to the right and left ventricles respectively, the fibers of each trunk becoming continuous with the Purkinje fibers of the ventricles.

Avellis' paralysis syndrome. [George Avellis, Ger. laryngologist, 1864–1916] Paralysis of half of the soft palate, pharynx, and larynx and loss of pain, heat, and cold sensations on opposite side.

Aventyl Hydrochloride. Trade name for nortriptyline hydrochloride, USP, q.v.

aversion therapy. A form of behavior in which an undesired stimulus, e.g., drinking alcohol, is presented to the patient at the same time as an unpleasant or painful stimulus. The goal is to have the individual associate the undesired stimulus with the unpleasant one and thus discontinue the former.

aviation medicine. The branch of medicine concerned with diseases and pathologic conditions resulting from, or incident to, air travel. SYN: *aerospace medicine.*

aviation physiology. The branch of physiology that deals with conditions encountered by man in high altitudes as in aircraft flights, mountain climbing, or in space vehicles. The principal factors dealt with are hypoxia, extreme temperature and radiation, effects of forces of acceleration and deceleration, weightlessness, motion sickness, enforced inactivity, and disturbance of biological rhythm.

avidin (ăv'ĭ-dĭn) [L. *avidus,* greedy]. A protein isolated from raw egg white. Said to be an inhibitor of biotin, thereby causing a deficiency in biotin. Formerly called vitamin H.

avidity. 1. Eagerness; having a strong attraction for something. 2. Concerning the ability of antibodies to bind to antigens.

avirulent (ā-vĭr'ū-lĕnt) [Gr. *a-,* not, + L. *virus,* poison]. Without virulence.

avitaminosis (ā-vī"tă-mĭ-nō'sĭs) [" + *vitamin* + *osis,* condition]. Disease due to lack of vitamins in the diet; a deficiency disease. SEE: *vitamin.*

avitaminotic (ā-vī-tăm-ĭn-ŏt'ĭk). Pert. to or affected with avitaminosis.

avivement (ă-vēv-mŏn') [Fr.]. Surgical trimming of wound edges prior to suturing them together.

Avlosulfon. Trade name for dapsone, USP, q.v.

Avogadro's law (ŏv-ō-gŏd'rōs). [Amadeo Avogadro, It. physicist, 1776–1856] Equal volumes of gases contain equal numbers of molecules, pressure and temperature being the same.

Avogadro's number. Number of molecules, 6.0225×10^{23}, in one gram–molecular weight of a compound.

avoidance (ă-voyd'ăns). The conscious or unconscious effort to escape from situations or events perceived by the individual to be threatening to personal comfort, safety, or well-being.

avoirdupois measure (ăv"ĕr-dĕ-poyz') [Fr., to have weight]. A system of weighing or measuring articles in which 7000 grains equal 1 pound. Some medicines are bought and sold by avoirdupois weight.

To find the capacity of a vessel or space in gallons, divide the contents in cubic inches by 231 for liquid gallons, or by 268.8 for dry gallons. To convert gallons to cubic inches, multiply the given number of liquid gallons by 231; then change to higher denominations if required. The dry gallon (half-peck) contains 268.8 cu. in. Six dry gallons are equal to nearly seven liquid gallons. The bushel contains 2150.42 cu. in. (35,240.0 cu. cm.) and is a cylindrical measure 18.5 in. (47 cm.) in diameter and 8 in. (20.3 cm.) deep. Measures of capacity are all cubic measures. The number of pounds in a bushel depends upon the density of the article contained therein. SEE: *apothecaries' measure; metric system; Troy weight; Weights and Measures* in *Appendix.*

avulsion (ă-vŭl'shŭn) [Gr. *a-,* not, + L. *vellere,* to pull]. A tearing away forcibly of a part or structure. If surgical repair is necessary, merely apply a sterile dressing while waiting for surgery to be done. If fingers, toes, feet, or hands are completely avulsed, they may be successfully rejoined to the body if prompt and expert care is available.

axanthopsia (ăk"săn-thŏp'sē-ă) [" + *xanthos,* yellow, + *opsis,* vision]. Yellow blindness.

axenic (ā-zĕn'ĭk) [" + *xenos,* stranger]. Germ-free, as pert. to animals, or pure, as pert. to cultures or microorganisms. Sterile.

axial (ăk'sē-ăl) [L. *axis,* axis]. Situated in or pert. to an axis.

axial line. A line running in the main axis of the body or part of it. The axial line of the hand runs through the middle digit; the axial line of the foot runs through the second digit.

axial skeleton. Head and trunk.

axifugal (ăks-ĭf'ū-găl) [" + *fugere,* to flee]. Receding from the axis. SYN: *centrifugal.*

axilemma (ăk"sĭ-lĕm'ă) [" + Gr. *lemma,* husk]. The plasma membrane of an axon.

axilla (ăk-sĭl'ă) [L. *axilla*]. (pl. *axillae*) [NA] The armpit.

axilla conformer. A splint designed to prevent adduction contractures following severe burns to the axilla region.

axillary (ăk'sĭ-lār-ē). Pert. to the axilla.

axillofemoral bypass graft (ăk″sĭl-ō-fĕm′or-ăl). The surgical establishment of a connector between the axillary artery and the common femoral arteries. A synthetic artery graft is used and implanted subcutaneously. This technique is used in treating patients with insufficient blood flow to the legs.

axio- (ăk′sē-ō) [L. *axis,* axle]. Combining form indicating relationship of the term that follows to an axis. In dentistry, the long axis of the tooth is referred to by this term.

axiobuccal (ăk″sē-ō-bŭk kăl) [L. *axis,* axle, + *bucca,* cheek]. Concerning the angle formed by the long axis of the tooth and the buccal walls of a cavity of the tooth.

axioincisal (ăk″sē-ō-ĭn-sī′zăl) [″ + *incisor,* a cutter]. Concerning the angle formed by the long axis of the tooth and the incisal walls of a cavity in the tooth.

axiolabial (ăk″sē-ō-lā′bē-ăl) [″ + *labialis,* pert. to the lips]. Concerning the angle formed by the long axis of the tooth with the labial walls of a cavity in the tooth.

axiolingual (ăk″sē-ō-lĭng′gwăl) [″ + *lingua,* tongue]. Concerning the angle formed by the long axis of the tooth and the lingual walls of a cavity in the tooth.

axiomesial (ăk″sē-ō-mē′zē-ăl) [″ + Gr. *mesos,* middle]. Concerning the angle formed by the long axis of a tooth and the mesial walls of a cavity in the tooth.

axio-occlusal (ăk″sē-ō-ŏ-klū′zăl) [″ + *occlusio,* closure]. Concerning the angle formed by the long axis of the tooth and the occlusal walls of a cavity in the tooth.

axioplasm (ăk′sē-ō-plăzm) [″ + *plasma,* a thing formed]. Neuroplasm of an axis cylinder.

axiopulpal (ăk″sē-ō-pŭl′păl) [″ + *pulpa,* pulp]. Concerning the angle formed by the long axis of a tooth and the pulpal walls of a cavity in the tooth.

axipetal (ăk-sĭp′ĕt-ăl) [L. *axis,* axis, + *petere,* to seek]. Directed toward the axis. SYN: *centripetal.*

axis [L.]. (pl. *axes*) A real or imaginary line that runs through the center of a body or about which a part revolves. 2. [NA] The second cervical vertebra or epistropheus, which bears the odontoid process (dens) about which the atlas rotates.

a., basicranial. Axis connecting the basion and gonion.

a., basifacial. Axis from subnasal point to gonion.

a., binauricular. Axis between the two auricular points.

a., celiac. Axis between the celiac artery and abdominal aorta.

a., cerebrospinal. Central nervous system.

a., frontal. Imaginary line running transversely through the center of the eyeball.

a., neural. Central nervous system.

a., optic. A line that connects the anterior and posterior poles of the eye.

a., principal. In optics, a line that passes through the optical center or nodal point of a lens perpendicular to the surface of the lens.

a., sagittal. Imaginary line running through the eyeball anteroposteriorly.

a., visual. A line passing from object of vision directly through center of cornea and lens to the fovea.

axis cylinder. An axon (def. 2), q.v.

axis traction. Traction made on the fetus in the direction of the long axis of the birth canal.

axite (ăk′sīt). Any terminal filament of an axis cylinder.

axo- [Gr. *axon,* axis]. Prefix pert. to axis or axon.

axodendrite (ăk″sō-dĕn′drīt) [″ + *dendron,* tree]. Process given off from a nerve cell axon (not an axis cylinder).

axofugal (ăk-sŏf′ū-găl) [″ + L. *fugere,* to flee]. Axifugal, q.v.

axolemma (ăk″sō-lĕm′ă) [″ + *lemma,* husk]. Axis cylinder sheath of a nerve fiber. SYN: *axilemma.*

axolysis (ăk-sŏl′ĭ-sĭs) [″ + *lysis,* dissolution]. Destruction of the axis cylinder of a nerve.

axometer (ăk-sŏm′ĕ-tĕr) [″ + *metron,* measure]. Measuring device for use in adjusting the frames of glasses so that the lenses are suitable for the optic axes of the eyes.

axon, axone (ăk′sŏn, -sōn) [Gr. *axon,* axis]. 1. A process of a neuron that conducts impulses away from the cell body. Typically, one arising from a portion of the cell devoid of Nissl granules, the axon hillock. Axons may possess either or both of two sheaths (myelin sheath and neurilemma) or neither. Axons are usually long and straight, and most end in synapses in the central nervous system or ganglia or in effector organs (e.g., motor neurons). They may give off side branches or collaterals. An axon with its sheath(s) constitutes a nerve fiber. 2. A nerve cell process that resembles an axon in structure, specifically the peripheral process of a dorsal root ganglion cell (sensory neuron) that functionally and embryologically is a dendrite, but structurally is indistinguishable from an axon. SYN: *axis cylinder.* SEE: *nerve; neuron.*

axoneme (ăk′sō-nēm) [″ + *nema,* a thread]. Axial thread of a chromosome.

axoneuron (ăk-sō-nū′rŏn) [″ + *neuron,* nerve]. A nerve cell of the cerebrospinal system.

axonometer (ăk-sō-nŏm′ĕ-tĕr) [″ + *metron,* a measure]. Device for determining the axis of astigmatism.

axonotmesis (ăk″sŏn-ŏt-mē′sĭs) [″ + *tmesis,*

incision]. Nerve injury that damages the nerve tissue without actually severing the nerve.

axon reflex. SEE: *reflex, axon.*

axopetal (ăk-sŏp'ĕ-tăl) [" + L. *petere,* to seek]. Conducted along an axon toward a cell body of a neuron.

axophage (ăk'sō-fāj) [" + *phagein,* to eat]. Glia cell found in myelin excavations in myelitis.

axoplasm (ăk'sō-plăzm) [" + *plasma,* a thing formed]. The cytoplasm (neuroplasm) of an axon that encloses the neurofibrils.

axospongium (ăk-sō-spŏn'jē-ŭm) [" + *spongos,* sponge]. The fine fibrillar network of the axon substance of a nerve cell.

Ayerza's syndrome (ō-yĕr'thŏz). [Abel Ayerza, Brazilian physician, 1861–1918] A condition characterized by dyspnea, chronic cyanosis, erythemia, enlargement of spleen and liver, and hyperplasia of bone marrow. Polycythemia usually results from pulmonary insufficiency.

Az. *azote.*

azalein (ă-ză'lē-ĭn) [L. *azalea,* azalea). A red dye.

Azapen. Trade name for methicillin sodium, USP, q.v.

azathioprine (ā"ză-thī'ō-prēn). USP. A chemical substance that is cytotoxic and is used for immunosuppression. Trade name is Imuran.

Azima battery. A projective technique using expressive media designed to uncover attitudes, motivations, and defense mechanisms of persons hospitalized for psychiatric conditions.

azo-. Prefix indicating the presence of —N:N— group in a chemical structure. This group is usually connected at either end with carbon atoms. SEE: *azo compounds.*

azo compounds. Organic substances that contain the azo group. An example is azobenzene, $C_6H_5N{:}NC_6H_5$. They are related to aniline and include important dyes and indicators. SEE: *indicator* for table.

azoic (ă-zō'ĭk) [Gr. *a-,* not, + *zoe,* life]. Containing no living organisms.

Azolid. Trade name for phenylbutazone, USP, q.v.

azoospermia (ă-zō-ō-spĕr'mē-ă) [" + *zoon,* animal, + *sperma,* seed]. Absence of spermatozoa in the semen.

Azorean disease (ā-zor'ē-ăn). A form of hereditary ataxia present in Portuguese families whose ancestors lived in the Azores. It is a degenerative disease of the nervous system. Symptoms vary but may include gait ataxia, limitation of eye movements, widespread muscle fasciculations, mild cerebellar tremor, loss of reflexes in lower limbs, and extensor plantar reflex response.

azotation (ăz"ō-tā'shŭn). Nitrogen absorption from the air.

azote (ăz'ōt) [" + *zoe,* life]. Nitrogen.

azotemia (ăz"ō-tē'mē-ă) [" – " + *haima,* blood]. Presence of nitrogenous bodies, esp. urea in increased amounts, in the blood. SEE: *uremia.*

azotenesis (ăz-ō-tĕ-nē'sĭs). Disease due to excess of nitrogen in system.

azotification (ăz-ō"tĭ-fĭ-kā'shŭn). Atmospheric nitrogen fixation.

azotized (ăz'ō-tīzd). 1. Containing nitrogen. 2. Converted into an azo compound.

Azotobacter (ă-zō"tō-băk'tĕr). Rod-shaped, gram-negative, nonpathogenic soil and water bacteria that fix atmospheric nitrogen. The single genus of the family Azotobacteraceae.

azoturia (ăz"ō-tū'rē-ă) [" + " + *ouron,* urine]. An increase in nitrogenous compounds, esp. urea, in urine.

Azulfidine. Trade name for sulfasalazine, USP, q.v.

azure lunulae (ăz'ŭr loo'nū-lē) [O. Fr. *azur,* blue, + L. *lunula,* little moon]. Blue discoloration of the base, or lunulae, of the fingernails. May be seen in patients with hepatolenticular degeneration (Wilson's disease). Blue discoloration of the entire nail may be present in argyria and following therapy with quinacrine hydrochloride.

azurophil(e) (ăz-ū'rō-fĭl) [" + Gr. *philein,* to love]. Staining readily with azure dye.

azurophilia (ăz"ū-rō-fĭl'ē-ă). Condition in which some blood cells have azurophil granules.

azygography (ăz"ĭ-gŏg'ră-fē) [Gr. *a-,* not, + *zygon,* yoke, + *graphein,* to write]. Visualization of the azygos veins by use of x-ray and radiopaque dye injected intravenously.

azygos (ăz'ĭ-gŏs) [" + *zygon,* yoke]. Occurring singly, not in pairs.

azygos vein. A single vein arising in the abdomen as a branch of the ascending lumbar vein. It passes upward through the aortic hiatus of the diaphragm into the thorax, then along the right side of the vertebral column to the level of the fourth thoracic vertebra, where it turns and enters the superior vena cava. In the thorax, it receives the hemiazygos, accessory azygos, and bronchial veins, as well as the right intercostal and subcostal veins. In cases of obstruction to the inferior vena cava, the azygous vein is the principal vein by which blood can return to the heart.

azygous (ăz'ĭ-gŭs). Single, not paired.

azymia (ă-zĭ'mē-ă) [" + *zyme,* ferment]. State of being without a ferment or enzyme.

azymic, azymous (ā-zĭ'mĭk, -mŭs, ăz'ĭ-mŭs). 1. Unfermented or unleavened. 2. Denoting the absence of an enzyme.

B

β. Beta, second letter of the Greek alphabet. SEE: *beta*.

B. 1. Chem. symb. for boron. 2. *Bacillus; Balantidium; barometric; base; bath; behavior; buccal.*

B.A. *Bachelor of Arts.*

Ba. Chem. symb. for barium.

Babbitt metal (băb'ĭt). [Isaac Babbitt, U.S. inventor, 1799–1862] Antifriction alloy of copper, antimony, and tin used occasionally in dentistry.

Babcock's operation (băb'kŏks). [William Wayne Babcock, U.S. surgeon, 1872–1963] Extirpation of the saphenous vein. Done for eradication of varicosed veins.

Babcock's test. [Stephen Moulton Babcock, U.S. surgeon, 1843–1931] Test to determine the amount of fat in milk by centrifuging equal parts of milk and sulfuric acid.

Babès-Ernst granules (bă'bāz-ĕrnst). [Victor Babès, Rumanian bacteriologist, 1854–1926; Paul Ernst, Ger. pathologist, 1859–1937] Metachromatic granules.

Babesia (bă-bē'zē-ă). [Victor Babès] A genus of the order Haemosporidia that are parasites found in the blood of cattle, sheep, horses, dogs, and other vertebrate animals. They are transmitted by ticks. They infest red blood cells, bringing about their destruction with resulting hemoglobinuria.

B. bigemina. The causative organism of Texas fever in cattle.

B. bovis. The causative organism of hemoglobinuria and jaundice (red water fever) in cattle.

babesiosis (bă-bē-zē-ō'sĭs). A rare, often severe and sometimes fatal disease of man caused by the protozoal parasite of the red blood cells, Babesia microti, and perhaps other Babesia species. The disease occurs mostly in the northeastern United States.

SYM: Fever, fatigue, and hemolytic anemia that may last briefly or for months.

DIAG: Presence of parasite in red blood cells and by serologic studies. On the blood smear it may be difficult to differentiate the parasites from the malaria organism, Plasmodium falciparum.

TREATMENT: No specific therapy.

Babinski's reflex (bă-bĭn'skēz). [Joseph Babinski, Fr. neurologist, 1857–1932] Dorsiflexion of the great toe on stimulating the sole of the foot. Normally, when the lateral aspect of the sole of the relaxed foot is stroked, the great toe is flexed. If the toe extends instead of flexes and the outer toes spread out, Babinski's reflex is present. This occurs in lesions of the pyramidal tract. Babinski's reflex is normally present in infants under the age of six months. Care must be taken to avoid interpreting voluntary extension of the toe as Babinski's reflex.

Babinski's sign. Loss of or diminished Achilles tendon reflex in sciatica.

baby [ME. *babie*]. Lay term for an infant.

b., battered. A baby or child whose body provides evidence of physical abuse such as bruises, cuts, scars, fractures, or abdominal visceral injuries that have occurred at various times in the past. SEE: *battered child syndrome*. SYN: *Caffey's syndrome*.

b., blue. Newborn child with cyanosis. This may be caused by anything that prevents proper oxygenation of the blood, esp. a congenital anomaly that permits blood to go directly from the right to the left side of the heart without going through the lungs.

b., collodion. Newborn covered with a collodion-like layer of desquamated skin. May be due to ichthyosis vulgaris.

bacampicillin hydrochloride. USP. An antibacterial drug.

bacca (băk'ă) [L.]. (pl. *baccae*) A berry.

bacciform (băk'sĭ-form) [" + *forma,* form]. Berry-shaped; coccal.

Bacid. Trade name for lactobacillus, q.v.

Bacillaceae (băs-ĭ-lā'sē-ē). A family (order Eubacteriales) of rod-shaped cells that can produce endospores. Usually gram-positive, commonly found in soil. Genera of family are Bacillus and Clostridium.

bacillar, bacillary (băs'ĭl-ăr, băs'ĭl-ă-rē). 1. Pert. to or caused by bacilli. 2. Rodlike.

bacille Calmette-Guérin (bă-sēl'). An organism of the strain Mycobacterium bovis, rendered completely avirulent by long-term cultivation on bile-glycero-potato medium. Used in BCG, q.v., vaccine in prevention of human tuberculosis. The use of this vaccine in treating certain types of cancer is experimental.

bacillemia (băs-ĭ-lē'mē-ă) [L. *bacillus,* rod, + Gr. *haima,* blood]. The presence of bacilli in the circulating blood.

bacilli (bă-sĭl'ī). Pl. of bacillus.

bacilliform (bă-sĭl'ĭ-form) [" + *forma,* form]. Resembling a bacillus in shape.

bacillophobia (băs"ĭ-lō-fō'bē-ă) [" + Gr. *phobos,* fear]. Morbid fear of bacilli.

bacillosis (băs"ĭ-lō'sĭs) [" + Gr. *osis,* infection]. Infection by bacilli.

bacilluria (băs"ĭ-lū'rē-ă) [" + Gr. *ouron,* urine]. Bacilli in the urine. SEE: *clean-catch method*.

Bacillus (bă-sĭl'ŭs) [L.]. A genus of bacteria belonging to the family Bacillaceae. All species are rod-shaped, sometimes occurring in chains. They are spore-bearing, aerobic, motile or nonmotile; most are gram-positive and nonpathogenic. One well-known species pathogenic to man is B. anthracis.

B. anthracis. An aerobic, spore-forming bacillus pathogenic to man and domestic animals, being the causative agent of anthrax, q.v.

B. subtilis. The common hay bacillus, which has a close resemblance to B. anthracis. Generally, it is considered nonpathogenic, but it occasionally causes conjunctivitis in man. It is often found as a contaminant of laboratory specimens.

bacillus. (pl. *bacilli*) 1. Any rod-shaped microorganism. 2. A rod-shaped microorganism belonging to the class Schizomycetes. SEE: *Bacillus; bacteria.*

b., abortus. Brucella abortus. Causes infectious abortion in cattle and other domestic animals. Causative agent of brucellosis (undulant fever) in man.

b., acid-fast. Bacillus not readily decolorized by acids or other means when stained.

b., Bang's. Brucella abortus. SEE: *b., abortus.*

b., Bordet-Gengou. Bordetella pertussis, formerly Haemophilus pertussis. Causative agent of whooping cough.

b. cereus. An aerobic spore-forming bacillus that may be an opportunistic invader in immunocompromised patients.

b., cholerae. Vibrio comma. Causative agent of cholera.

b., comma. Vibrio comma. Causative agent of cholera.

b., diphtheria. Corynebacterium diphtheriae. The causative agent of diphtheria.

b., Döderlein's. A large gram-positive bacillus usually present in the vagina. Considered identical with Lactobacillus acidophilus.

b., Ducrey's. Haemophilus ducreyi. The cause of soft chancre or chancroid infection of the genitalia.

b., Flexner's. Shigella flexneri. The most common cause of epidemic dysentery.

b., Friedländer's. Klebsiella pneumoniae. A cause of pneumonia.

b., gas. Clostridium perfringens. A cause of gas gangrene.

b., Hansen's. Mycobacterium leprae. Causative organism of Hansen's disease (leprosy).

b., Klebs-Loeffler. Corynebacterium diphtheriae. The cause of diphtheria.

b., Koch-Weeks. Haemophilus aegyptius. Cause of infectious conjunctivitis.

b. licheniformis. An aerobic spore-forming bacillus that occasionally causes disease in man.

b. melaninogenicus. A non-spore-forming, gram-negative bacillus that is most probably the primary cause of Vincent's angina. It may also be associated with brain and lung abscesses.

b., Morax-Axenfeld. Moraxella lacunata, a cause of conjunctivitis in man.

b., Pfeiffer's. Haemophilus influenzae.

b., Shiga. Name given to a representative dysentery bacillus first described in 1898 by Kiyoshi Shiga, a Japanese bacteriologist for whom the genus Shigella was named.

b., Sonne. Shigella sonnei. A cause of bacillary dysentery in man.

b., tubercle. Mycobacterium tuberculosis. The cause of tuberculosis in human beings.

b., typhoid. Salmonella typhi. The cause of typhoid fever.

bacitracin (băs-ĭ-trā′sĭn). USP. An antibiotic substance obtained from a strain of Bacillus subtilis. Its antibacterial actions are similar to those of penicillin, including gram-positive cocci and bacilli and some gram-negative organisms. Though available for intramuscular use, bacitracin is usually employed topically in the form of ointment due to its toxicity when used parenterally.

b., zinc. The zinc salt of bacitracin, used in topical antibacterial ointments.

back. 1. The dorsum. 2. The posterior region of the trunk from neck to pelvis.

Misuse of the back is common among those whose duties include care of the sick. Therefore, it is important to learn basic concepts in care of the back. SEE: illus. *(How to Stay on Your Feet Without Tiring Your Back).*

backache. Any pain in the back. Usually characterized by dull, continuous pain and tenderness in the muscles or their attachments in the lower lumbar, lumbosacral, or sacroiliac regions. Pain is often referred to the leg, following the distribution of the sciatic nerve.

ETIOL: Infection or abnormality in another part of the body such as uterine or prostatic disorders; disorders of the vertebral column such as intervertebral disk abnormality; local disturbances such as lumbar or sacral fractures, lumbosacral strain or sprain; structural inadequacies of supporting ligaments of the spinal column; muscle injury, spasm, myositis, or inflammation of fascial attachments; psychogenic factors.

TREATMENT: Treat specific primary cause. General treatment includes measures to allay pain and discomfort such as analgesics, preferably salicylates (codeine in severe cases), muscle relaxants, heat, whirlpool. Tender areas or trigger points may be anesthetized by local infiltration with 1% procaine or topical application of ethyl chloride spray. Special measures to relax tense muscles and improve blood flow are helpful. Orthopedic supports and strapping if necessary in special cases. Muscle re-education. Psy-

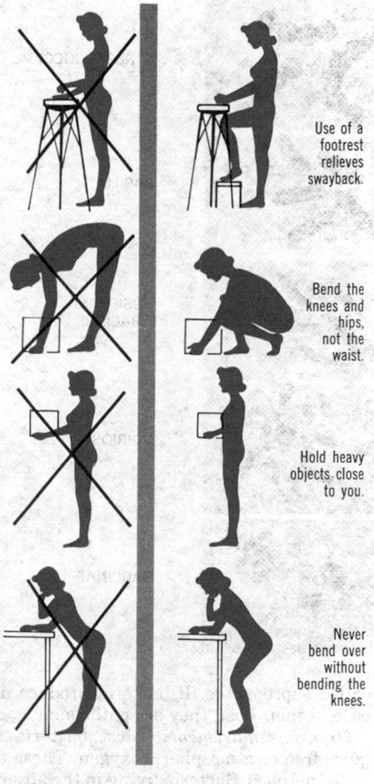
Use of a footrest relieves swayback.
Bend the knees and hips, not the waist.
Hold heavy objects close to you.
Never bend over without bending the knees.

HOW TO STAY ON YOUR FEET WITHOUT TIRING YOUR BACK

chotherapy when necessary, esp. in excessive muscle tension resulting from emotional disturbances.

backbone. The vertebral column; spinal column, q.v. SEE: *vertebra*.

backflow. Abnormal backward flow of fluids.

background radiation. Total radioactivity from cosmic rays, natural radioactive materials, and whatever other radiation may be in a specific area.

bacteremia (băk-tĕr-ē′mē-ă) [Gr. *bakterion*, rod, + *haima*, blood]. Bacteria in the blood. SEE: *sepsis*.

bacteria (băk-tē′rē-ă) [Gr. *bakterion*, rod]. (sing. *bacterium*) Any microorganism of the class Schizomycetes. Sometimes restricted to rod-shaped or nonsporulating rod-shaped microorganisms. SEE: *gram-negative; gram-positive; Gram's method*.

There are three principal forms of bacteria. *Spherical or ovoid:* When appearing singly, they are called micrococci; when in pairs, diplococci; when in irregular clusters, staphylococci; when in chains, streptococci; cocci that remain adherent after splitting successively in two or three perpendicular directions from square or cubical groups known as sarcinae. *Rod-shaped:* Known as bacilli. When the rods are somewhat oval, they are called coccobacilli; when attached end to end forming a chain, streptobacilli. *Spiral:* When the spiral organisms are rigid they are called spirilla; when flexible, spirochetes; when forming curved rods, vibrios. SEE: illus.

Most bacteria are relatively constant in form in growing cultures. But in old cultures or cultures grown under adverse environmental conditions, aberrant forms appear.

It has been estimated that each of us carries 10^{14} bacteria in and on our bodies; and that all the total population of our planet excretes in feces 10^{22} bacteria per day.

CHARACTERISTICS: *Size:* An average rod-shaped bacterium measures about 1 micrometer in diameter by 4 micrometers in length. They vary considerably in size from less than 1.0 to 0.5 micrometer in diameter to 10–20 micrometers in length in some of the longer spiral forms.

Motility: Some bacteria are incapable of movement (all cocci), but most bacilli and spiral forms exhibit independent movement. The power of locomotion depends on the possession of one or more flagella, slender whip-like appendages. Bacteria having no flagella are called atrichous; those having a flagellum at one end, monotrichous; those having flagella at each end, amphitrichous; those having a tuft at one end, lophotrichous; those having flagella protruding from all surfaces of the cell, peritrichous.

Capsules: Many bacteria possess a capsule, a layer of slimy mucoid substance that surrounds each cell. The presence of a capsule is associated with the virulence of certain pathogenic forms.

Spores: Certain species of the rod-shaped bacteria have the ability to develop an encysted or resting stage known as a spore or endospore. The size, shape, and position of the spore within the cell are characteristic of particular species. Spores are terminal if formed at the end of a cell, central if formed at the center, subterminal if formed between the center and end. Spore formation is common among the bacilli but does not usually occur in the cocci or spiral forms. Bacterial spores are remarkably resistant to heat, drying, and the action of disinfectants.

BACTERIAL FORMS

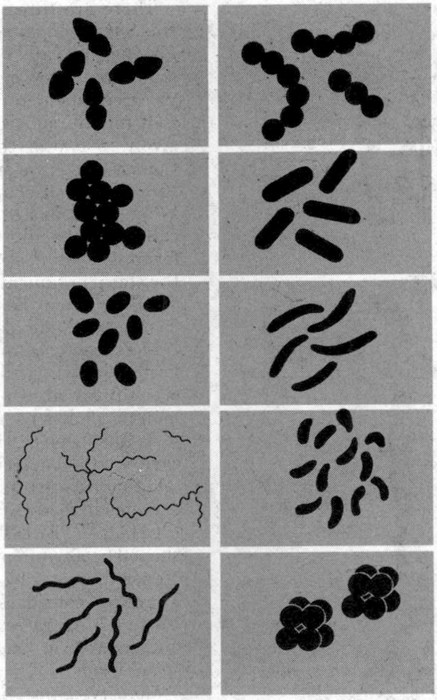

Reproduction: Binary fission is the usual mode of reproduction. Budding, branching, filamentous growth, and the development of conidia also occur.

Colony formation: A group of bacteria growing in one place is called a colony. A colony is usually composed of the descendants of a single cell. Colonies differ in shape, size, color, texture, type of margin, and other characteristics. Each species of bacteria has a characteristic type of colony formation. Sometimes a single species may produce two types of colonies: one the smooth or S-type, the other the rough or R-type. Sometimes colonies contain clear spots and have a moth-eaten appearance. Such colonies are called plaques and are thought to be due to the lytic action of bacteriophages.

Food requirements: Bacteria possess no chlorophyll, and therefore cannot carry on photosynthesis. A few can obtain their energy from inorganic substances. These are termed autotrophic and include many of the soil bacteria. The majority derive their nourishment from organic material and are termed heterotrophic. If they live on living organisms, they are called parasites; if their food is from nonliving organic matter, they are called saprophytes. If bacteria produce disease in their host, they are pathogenic.

Oxygen requirements: Most bacteria require free or atmospheric oxygen. These are called aerobes. Bacteria living in the absence of atmospheric oxygen are called anaerobes. Those showing a preference for free oxygen and yet capable of living in its absence are called facultative anaerobes; those that grow only in the absence of oxygen are called obligate anaerobes.

Temperature requirements: Most bacteria grow best at moderate temperatures. These are called mesophilic. Cold-loving bacteria, which thrive in temperatures between 0° and 30° C. (32° and 86° F.), are called psychrophilic; those that thrive in high temperatures between 40° and 70° C. (104° and 158° F.) are called thermophilic. The optimum temperature for most saprophytes is around 25° C., for most pathogens, 37° C.

ACTIVITIES: *Enzyme production:* Bacteria produce enzymes that act on complex food molecules, breaking them down into simpler materials capable of assimilation. Carbohydrases act on sugars, breaking them down to alcohol and carbon dioxide, a process called fermentation. Proteolytic enzymes bring about the decomposition of proteins with the formation of ill-smelling products, a process called putrefaction. Putrefaction is the decomposition of organic substances, esp. nitrogenous substances, in the absence of air and with resulting unpleasant odors. Decay is the gradual decomposition of organic matter exposed to air by bacteria and fungi. Bacteria are the principal agents of decay and putrefaction.

Toxin production: Many bacteria produce poisonous substances called toxins. There are two types: exotoxins, which diffuse from the bacterial cell into the surrounding medium, and endotoxins, which are liberated only when the bacterial cell dies and disintegrates. Bacteria well known for their toxin production are the diphtheria, tetanus, and botulinus organisms.

Miscellaneous: Some bacteria produce pigments; some produce light, thus appearing luminescent at night. Many chemical substances are produced as a result of bacterial activity, among them acids, gases, alcohol, aldehydes, ammonia, carbohydrates, and indol. Pathogenic forms produce hemolysins, leukocidins, coagulases, and fibrolysins. Soil bacteria play an important role in various phases of the nitrogen cycle (nitrification, nitrogen fixation, and denitrification).

METHODS OF STUDYING: Principal methods used in the study of bacteria follow:

(1) Examination of unstained bacteria in a hanging-drop preparation. Darkfield illumination is necessary to see extremely small forms.

(2) Staining methods include general stains, differential stains, stains for special bacteria, and stains for specific parts. Of the differential stains, Gram's method and staining for acid-fast bacteria are the most widely used. Bacteria fall into three groups: gram-positive bacteria (those that retain the stain); gram-negative bacteria (those that are decolorized by alcohol); and acid-fast bacteria (those that, when stained with certain dyes, retain the stain even when treated with an acid).

(3) In cultural methods, the bacteria are grown on various culture media. In synthetic media, the exact composition of the medium is known; in nonsynthetic media, the constituents are uncertain and unreliable. Media, on the basis of consistency, may be liquid (nutrient broth, milk, blood serum); liquefiable solid, which consists of liquid media made solid by addition of gelatin or agar-agar; and nonliquefiable solid (potato, carrots, starch paste).

(4) Animal inoculation.

(5) Immunological methods including immunofluorescence. This technique involves staining bacteria on smears or in tissues with fluorescein-containing reagents. After this process the preparation is rinsed to remove the unbound fluorescein and then examined with a suitable light microscope equipped with special filters and incident light source. The fluorescent-stained cells are readily apparent as yellow-green masses.

(6) Sterilization methods. Sterilization is the process of rendering any material free of living microorganisms. It may be accomplished by physical or chemical means. Physical agents employed are heat, light, ionizing radiation, and filtration. Sterilization may be accomplished in a flame; in a hot-air oven (150° to 170° C. for one hour); in streaming steam (100° C. for 20 min. or longer); by steam under pressure (10 to 15 lb or 4.5 to 6.8 kg.) in an autoclave (121° C. for 20 min.); or by ionizing radiation. Ultraviolet light is destructive to bacteria as are certain gases such as ethylene oxide, methyl bromide, and hydrogen cyanide.

Chemical agents that inhibit bacterial growth are called antiseptics and their action is described as being bacteriostatic; those that kill bacteria are called germicides or bactericides. Among disinfectants are strong acids and alkalies, metallic salts (bichloride of mercury), halogens (chlorine, iodine), oxidizing agents (hydrogen peroxide), organic compounds (phenol, formaldehyde, salicylic acid), and other substances such as boric acid. Substances used in the treatment of diseases caused by bacteria are called chemotherapeutic agents. They include the sulfonamide compounds and the antibiotics.

b., antibody-coated. Bacteria that, due to the specific antigen-antibody response they have produced in the body, become coated with those antibodies. The presence of these antibodies on bacteria may be detected by use of direct immunofluorescence.

bacterial antagonism. The action of certain bacteria in interfering with or preventing the growth and development of other microorganisms. SEE: *opportunistic infections.*

bacterial resistance. Development of resistance to a drug by an organism previously susceptible to it. This has been manifested by pathogenic organisms (as gonococci, streptococci, staphylococci, and tubercle bacilli) to various chemotherapeutic drugs, and occurs both in vitro and in vivo. It may be due to appearance of resistant mutant strains, development of alternate metabolic pathways, decomposition of the drug, or unknown factors.

bactericidal (băk″tĕr-ĭ-sī′dăl). Destructive to or destroying bacteria.

bactericide (băk-tĕr′ĭ-sīd) [Gr. *bacterion,* rod, + L. *caedere,* to kill]. An agent that destroys bacteria, but not necessarily their spores.

bacterid (băk'tĕr-ĭd). Any skin rash caused by bacterial toxins or bacteria. The bacterial infection is usually remote from the rash.

bacteriemia (băk-tĕr-ē-ē'mē-ă) [" + *haima,* blood]. Bacteremia, q.v.

bacterio- (băk-tē'rē-ō). Prefix pert. to bacteria.

bacterioagglutinin (băk-tē"rē-ō-ă-gloo'tĭ-nĭn) [" + L. *agglutinans,* gluing]. An antibody in serum that causes agglutination, or clumping, of bacteria in vitro.

bacteriocidal (băk"tĕr-ē-ō-sī'dăl). Bactericidal, q.v.

bacteriocidin (băk-tē"rē-ō-sī'dĭn) [" + L. *caedere,* to kill]. Imprecise and obsolete term for a substance in blood that kills bacteria.

bacteriocin (băk-tē'rē-ō-sĭn). Protein produced by certain bacteria that exert a lethal effect on closely related bacteria. In general, they are more potent but have a narrower range of activity than antibiotics. SEE: *colicin.*

bacteriocinogen (băk-tē"rē-ō-sĭn'ō-gĕn). A plasmid that produces bacteriocin.

bacterioclasis (băk-tē"rē-ŏk'lă-sĭs) [" + *klasis,* breaking]. The fragmentation of bacteria.

bacteriogenic (băk-tē"rē-ō-jĕn'ĭk) [" + *gennan,* to produce]. 1. Caused by bacteria. 2. Producing bacteria.

bacteriohemagglutinin (băk-tē"rē-ō-hĕm"ă-gloo'tĭ-nĭn) [" + *haima,* blood, + L. *agglutinans,* gluing]. A hemagglutinin formed in the body by bacterial action.

bacteriohemolysin (băk-tē"rē-ō-hē-mŏl'ĭ-sĭn) [" + " + *lysis,* dissolution]. A hemolysin formed in the body by bacterial action.

bacterioid (băk-tĕr'ē-oyd) [" + *eidos,* form]. Resembling bacteria.

bacteriologic, bacteriological [" + *logos,* study]. Pert. to bacteriology.

bacteriologist. An individual with academic training in the field of bacteriology..

bacteriology. Science that deals with bacteria.

bacteriolysin (băk-tē"rē-ŏl'ĭ-sĭn) [" + *lysis,* dissolution]. A substance, esp. an antibody produced within the body of an animal, that is capable of bringing about the lysis of bacteria.

bacteriolysis (băk-tē"rē-ŏl'ĭ-sĭs). The destruction or dissolution of bacteria.

bacteriolytic (băk-tē"rē-ō-lĭt'ĭk). Pert. to bacteriolysis.

bacteriophage (băk-tē'rē-ō-fāj") [Gr. *bakterion,* rod, + *phagein,* to eat]. A virus with the capability of inducing lysis of certain bacterial cells. Bacteriophages are widely distributed in nature, having been isolated from feces, sewage, and polluted surface waters. They are regarded as bacterial viruses, the phage particle consisting of a head composed of either RNA or DNA and a tail by which it attaches to host cells. SYN: *phage.*

bacteriophagia (băk-tē"rē-ō-fā'jē-ă). Destruction of bacteria by a lytic agent.

bacteriophytoma (băk-tē"rē-ō-fī-tō'mă) [" + *phyton,* plant, + *oma,* tumor]. A tumor-like growth caused by bacteria.

bacterioprecipitin (băk-tē"rē-ō-prē-sĭp'ĭ-tĭn). Precipitin produced in the body by the action of bacteria.

bacterioprotein (băk-tē"rē-ō-prō'tē-ĭn). Any of the proteins within the cells of bacteria.

bacteriopsonin (băk-tē"rē-ŏp'sō-nĭn). An opsonin, q.v., acting on bacteria.

bacteriosis (băk-tē"rē-ō'sĭs) [" + *osis,* condition]. Any disease caused by bacteria.

bacteriostasis (băk-tē"rē-ŏs'tă-sĭs) [" + *stasis,* a stopping]. The arrest of bacterial growth.

bacteriostatic (băk-tē-rē-ō-stăt'ĭk). Inhibiting or retarding bacterial growth.

bacteriotoxic (băk-tē"rē-ō-tŏk'sĭk). 1. Toxic to bacteria. 2. Due to bacterial toxins.

bacteriotoxin (băk-tē"rē-ō-tŏk'sĭn) [" + *toxikon,* poison]. Toxin specifically produced by or destructive to bacteria.

bacteriotropin (băk-tē"rē-ŏt'rō-pĭn) [" + *tropos,* a turn]. An opsonin or a substance that enhances the ability of phagocytes to engulf bacteria.

bacteristatic. Inhibiting the growth of bacteria. SEE: *bactericidal.*

Bacterium (băk-tē'rē-ŭm). A former genus designation for non-spore-forming rod-shaped bacteria without flagella. Term is no longer used in taxonomy because of lack of an identified type species. The species formerly classified as Bacterium are now assigned to other genera such as Aerobacter, Alcaligenes, Mycobacterium, Pasteurella, and Salmonella.

B. aerogenes. Aerobacter aerogenes, q.v.

B. aertrycke. Salmonella typhimurium, q.v.

B. ambiguus. Shigella ambigua.

B. cholerae suis. Salmonella choleraesuis, q.v.

B. coli. Escherichia coli, q.v.

B. paratyphi (Type A). Salmonella paratyphi.

B. paratyphi (Type B). Salmonella schottmülleri, q.v.

B. tularense. Pasteurella tularensis. SEE: *tularemia.*

B. (Eberthella) typhi. Salmonella typhi, q.v.

B. typhosum. Salmonella typhi, q.v.

bacterium. Sing. of bacteria, q.v.

bacteriuria (băk-tē"rē-ū'rē-ă) [Gr. *bakterion,* rod, + *ouron,* urine]. Presence of bacteria in the urine.

b., significant. Concentration of pathogenic bacteria in the urine of 10^5 per ml. or greater.

bacteroid (băk'tĕr-oyd) [" + *eidos,* appearance]. 1. Resembling a bacterium. 2. A structurally modified bacterium.

Bacteroides (băk-tĕr-oyd′ēz). A genus of non-spore-forming, gram-negative, anaerobic bacteria occurring normally in digestive, respiratory, and genital tracts, frequently found in necrotic tissue, and often in the blood following infections. Bacteroides are the most common bacteria in the colon. They outnumber Escherichia coli by at least 100 to 1. The species most commonly encountered is B. fragilis.

Bactocill. Trade name for oxacillin sodium.

baculiform (băk-ū′lĭ-form) [L. *baculum*, rod, + *forma*, shape]. Rod-shaped.

bag [ME. *bagge*]. A sack or pouch.

b. of waters. The amnion, q.v. The membrane enclosing the liquor amnii and the fetus. It refers sometimes to that portion of the membrane protruding into the os uteri. It is the inner embryonic membrane, the chorion being the outer envelope.

b., Politzer's. Soft rubber bag for inflation of middle ear.

bagassosis (băg-ă-sō′sĭs) [Sp. *bagazo*, husks, + Gr. *osis*, condition]. A form of hypersensitivity pneumonitis, q.v., due to inhalation of bagasse dust, the moldy, dusty fibrous waste of sugar cane after removal of the sugar-containing sap. The dust contains antigens from thermophilic actinomycetes.

baker [AS. *bacan*, cook by dry heat]. Two or more electric lamps mounted in semicircular containers used for applying heat to various parts of the body. Called electric light bakers.

Baker's cyst. [William M. Baker, Brit. surgeon, 1839–1896] Synovial cyst (pouch) arising from the synovial lining of the knee. It occurs in the popliteal fossa.

baker leg. Knock-knee; genu valgum.

BAL. *British anti-lewisite.* Trade name for dimercaprol, a compound used as an antidote in poisoning from heavy metals. SEE: *dimercaprol.*

balance (băl′ăns) [L. *bilanx*]. 1. Scale; a device for measuring weight. 2. A state of equilibrium; condition in which the intake and output of substances such as water and nutrients are approx. equal. SEE: *homeostasis.*

b., acid-base. Normal balance between acid and base production and excretion in body, resulting in a stable concentration of hydrogen ions in the body fluids.

b., analytical. A very sensitive scale used in chemistry.

b., electrolyte. Condition in which electrolytes, esp. sodium and potassium, are maintained in suitable concentrations for cellular and metabolic processes.

b., fluid. Balance between intake and excretion of fluids, esp. water, in the body.

b., nitrogen. Body state in which intake of nitrogen in protein foods is equal to nitrogen output, principally through loss of nitrogenous substances in the urine and feces.

balanic (bă-lăn′ĭk) [Gr. *balanos*, glans]. Pert. to the glans clitoridis or glans penis.

balanitis (băl-ă-nī′tĭs) [″ + *itis*, inflammation]. Inflammation of the glans penis and mucous membrane beneath it. A purulent discharge is usually present, and the prepuce is often affected.

balano- (băl′ă-nō) [Gr. *balanos*, glans]. Combining form pert. to the glans penis or the glans clitoridis.

balanoblennorrhea (băl″ă-nō-blĕn″ō-rē′ă) [″ + *blennos*, mucus, + *rhoia*, flow]. Gonorrheal inflammation of the external glans penis.

balanocele (băl′ă-nō-sēl″) [″ + *kele*, hernia]. Protrusion of the glans penis through a rupture of the prepuce.

balanoplasty (băl′ă-nō-plăs′tē) [″ + *plassein*, to form]. Plastic surgery of glans penis.

balanoposthitis (băl″ă-nō-pŏs-thī′tĭs) [″ + *posthe*, prepuce, + *itis*, inflammation]. Balanitis, q.v.

balanopreputial (băl″ă-nō-prē-pū′shē-ăl). Pert. to glans penis and prepuce.

balanorrhagia (băl″ă-nō-rā′jē-ă) [″ + *rhegnynai*, burst forth]. Hemorrhage from glans penis.

balanorrhea (băl-ăn-ō-rē′ă) [″ + *rhoia*, flow]. Balanitis with purulent discharge.

balantidial (băl-ăn-tĭd′ē-ăl). Pert. to Balantidium, a genus of protozoans.

balantidiasis (băl″ăn-tĭ-dī′ă-sĭs). Infection caused by infestation with Balantidium coli.

SYM: Abdominal pain, diarrhea, vomiting, weakness, and loss of weight.

TREATMENT: Tetracyclines, metronidazole, or paramomycin.

Balantidium (băl-ăn-tĭd′ē-ŭm) [Gr. *balantidion*, a bag]. A genus of ciliated protozoa. A number of species are found in the intestines of both vertebrates and invertebrates.

B. coli. A species of Balantidium that is the largest protozoon parasitic of man. It lives in the large intestine and is the cause of balantidiasis. It is a normal parasite of hogs.

balanus (băl′ă-nŭs) [Gr. *balanos*, glans]. The glans penis or glans clitoridis.

baldness [ME. *ballede*, without hair]. Lack of or partial loss of hair on head. SEE: *alopecia.*

Balkan frame. A framework that fits over the bed. Suspended from the frame and connected through ropes and pulleys are weights used to produce desired continuous traction while permitting freedom of motion, thus maintaining desired immobilization of the part being treated.

Balke test. [Bruno Balke, contemporary Ger.-born U.S. physician] A test to determine maximum oxygen utilization. The subject walks on a flat (0% grade) treadmill at a constant rate of 3.5 miles/hour for 2 min. The treadmill is inclined 1% each successive minute until the subject is exhausted and unable to continue. Oxygen utilization is measured throughout the test.

CAUTION: The test is not suitable for individuals who have impairment of their musculoskeletal, cardiovascular, or respiratory systems.

ball. A spherically shaped object.

b., hair. Mass of hair that has accumulated in the intestine or stomach. SYN: *trichobezoar.*

b. of foot. The padded portion at the anterior extremity of the sole of the foot.

b. of thumb. Thenar eminence of the thumb.

b. thrombus. A round blood clot, esp. one in the heart. SEE: *thrombus.*

ball-and-socket joint. Synovial joint in which one rounded bone head moves within a concavity of another bone. SYN: *enarthrosis.*

ballism, ballismus (băl'ĭzm, bă-lĭz'mŭs) [Gr. *ballismos,* jumping about]. 1. Condition characterized by jerking, twisting movements seen in chorea. 2. Obsolete term for paralysis agitans.

ballistics (bă-lĭs'tĭks) [Gr. *ballein,* to throw]. Science of the motion and trajectory of missiles such as bullets, bombs, rockets, and guided missiles.

ballistocardiograph (bă-lĭs"tō-kăr'dē-ō-grăf) [" + *kardia,* heart, + *graphein,* to write]. Mechanism for measuring and recording the impact caused by the discharge of blood from the heart at each beat and the resulting recoil. The minute movements of the body with each heart beat are recorded as they are transmitted to the special platform that supports the subject.

balloon [It. *ballone,* great ball]. To expand, dilate, or distend, as expanding a cavity by filling it with air or water in a bag.

balloon bezoar. SEE: *bezoar, balloon.*

ballooning. The distention of a cavity, as the vagina, by air, etc., for examination.

ballottable (bă-lŏt'ă-bl). Capable of showing the ballottement phenomenon. SEE: *ballottement.*

ballottement (băl-ŏt-mŏn') [Fr. *balloter,* to toss about]. A palpatory technique used in detecting or examining a floating object in the body, such as an organ or fetus. Used in examining the abdomen esp. when ascites is present. Applied particularly to a diagnostic maneuver in pregnancy. The rebound of the fetus or a fetal part, when displaced by a light tap of the examining finger through the vagina.

ball-valve action. Action of a mass, such as a pedunculated cyst or thrombus, moving to open and close the passageway of a tube or chamber and causing intermittent obstruction. Thus a ball-valve thrombus may form in the heart and cause repeated blockage of an opening connecting two chambers of the heart.

balm [Gr. *balsamon,* balsam]. 1. A balsam. 2. A soothing or healing ointment.

b. of Gilead. 1. Mecca balsam from Commiphora opobalsamum, probably Biblical myrrh. 2. Balsam fir, source of Canadian balsam. 3. Poplar bud resin.

balneology (băl-nē-ŏl'ō-jē) [L. *balneum,* bath, + Gr. *logos,* study]. The science of baths and bathing.

balneotherapy, balneotherapeutics (băl"nē-ō-thĕr'ă-pē, -thĕr"ă-pū'tĭks) [" + Gr. *therapeia,* treatment]. The use of baths in treatment of disease.

balsam (bawl'săm) [Gr. *balsamon,* balsam]. A fragrant, resinous, oily exudate from various trees and plants. Balsams are resins combined with oil. They are used in topical preparations to treat irritated skin or mucous membrane.

b. of Peru. A dark-brown, viscid, resinous liquid obtained from the bark of the tree Myroxylon perierae.

Balser's fatty necrosis (băl'zĕrs). [W. Balser, 19th-century Ger. physician] Gangrenous pancreatitis with fatty necrotic areas in interlobular tissue and sometimes in pericardial fat and bone marrow.

bamboo spine. Roentgenogram of the spine in ankylosing spondylitis resembles the stalk of the bamboo plant.

Bancroft's filariasis. [Joseph Bancroft, Brit. physician, 1836–1894] A filarial infection caused by Wuchereria bancrofti. SEE: *elephantiasis.*

band. 1. A cord or tapelike tissue that connects or holds structures together. SEE: *bundle; ligament; tract.* 2. Any appliance that encircles or binds the body or a limb. 3. Segment of a myofibril (A, I, Z).

bandage [ME. *bande,* a band]. 1. A piece of gauze or other material applied to a limb or other part of the body as a dressing. 2. To cover by wrapping with a piece of gauze or other material.

Bandages are of various types and materials and are used to hold dressings in place, apply pressure to a part, immobilize a part, obliterate cavities, give support to an injured area, and aid in checking hemorrhages. SEE: illus.

CAUTION: When bandaging, do not allow skin of one part to be held against the skin of another part or severe skin infection can result.

Types of bandages include roller, triangular, four-tailed, many-tailed (scultetus), quadrangular, elastic (elastic knit, rubber, synthetic, or combinations of these), adhesive, elastic adhesive, newer cohesive bandages under various proprietary names, impregnated bandages (plaster of Paris, waterglass [silica], starch), and stockinet. SEE: *sling*.

b., abdomen. A single wide cravat or several narrow ones that are used to hold dressing in place or to exert a moderate pressure.

b., Ace. Trade name for a woven elastic bandage available in various widths and lengths. Provides uniform support, yet permits areas such as joints to move without loosening the bandage.

b., amputation-stump. Bandage of the stump of the limb after amputation. The limb is placed on the base of the triangular bandage. The ends of the base of the triangle are joined and pinned and the point of the triangle is folded back and pinned or tied to the previously joined ends.

b., ankle. Bandage in which one loop is brought around the sole of foot and the other around the ankle and tied in front or on the side.

b., axilla. Bandage with a spica-type turn starting under the affected axilla, crossing over the shoulder of the affected side, and making the long loop under the opposite armpit.

b., back. (Triangular) Open bandage to the back. This is applied the same as the chest bandage, the point being placed above the scapula of the injured side.

b., Barton's. A double figure-of-eight bandage for the lower jaw.

b., breast. (Roller) Suspensory bandages and compresses for the breasts.

b., butterfly. Adhesive bandage used in place of sutures to hold wound edges together.

b., buttocks. T or double-T bandage or open triangle bandage for the buttocks.

b., capeline. A bandage applied to the head or shoulder or to a stump like a cap or hood.

b., chest. (Roller) Figure-of-eight (spica), many-tailed (scultetus), or triangular (open-chest) bandage for the chest.

b., circular. A bandage applied in circular turns about a part.

b., cohesive. Material that has an intense power of sticking to itself but not to other substances. Used to bandage fingers, extremities, etc., or to build up pads.

b., cravat. Triangular bandage folded to form a band around the injured part. This is done by pulling the point over toward the base, folding the base over the point, and then folding again. This makes a bandage wide enough to cover a large knee. When folded a second time, it is wide enough to make the cravat bandage of the elbow. Folded a third time, it could be used in making a figure-of-eight for the foot, ankle, hand, wrist, or head. It is an effective bandage in arresting hemorrhages and in retaining splints, and dressings. The center of the cravat should be laid against the affected part, the ends of the cravat carried around the limb and tied over the center of the base. When used to retain splints, it should be tied on the outer side of the limb and against the splint, thus preventing the knot from irritating the skin. When used to retain a dressing in the axilla, the center of the cravat should be placed under the arm and the ends carried upward and crossed over the shoulder and tied in the axillary space of the opposite side, thus forming a figure-of-eight. The cravat can also be used as a sling when only a simple support is needed.

In using cravats for ties or splints, care should be taken so that the knots do not pass over and press unduly on the surface of the limb. Knots should be placed where they are easily found and not subject to pressure; the ends should be neatly tucked in. All knots should be square or reef knots.

b., cravat elbow. Bandage in which one bends the elbow about 45° and places center of bandage over point of elbow. Then one brings one end around forearm and the other end around upper arm, pulls tight, and ties.

b., cravat, for clenched fist. Hand bandage to arrest bleeding or to produce pressure. The wrist is placed on the center of the cravat, one end is brought around over the fist and back to the starting point, and the same procedure is then repeated with the other end. The two ends are pulled tight, twisted, and carried around the fist again so that pressure is placed on the flexed fingers.

b., cravat, for fracture of clavicle. Bandage in which one first puts a soft pad 2 × 4 in. (5.1 × 10.2 cm.) in the forepart of the axilla. A sling is made by placing the point of the open bandage on the affected shoulder, the hand and wrist laid on it and directed toward the opposite shoulder, the point brought over and tucked underneath the wrist and hand. The ends are then lifted and the bandage is laid flat on the chest, the covered hand is carried up on the shoulder, the ends are brought together in the back and tied, the tightness being decided by how high the shoulder should be carried. A cravat bandage is then applied horizontally above the broad part of the elbow and tied over a pad on the opposite side of the chest. Tightening this cravat pushes out the shoulder.

b., cravat, sling. Bandage used for sup-

TYPES OF BANDAGES

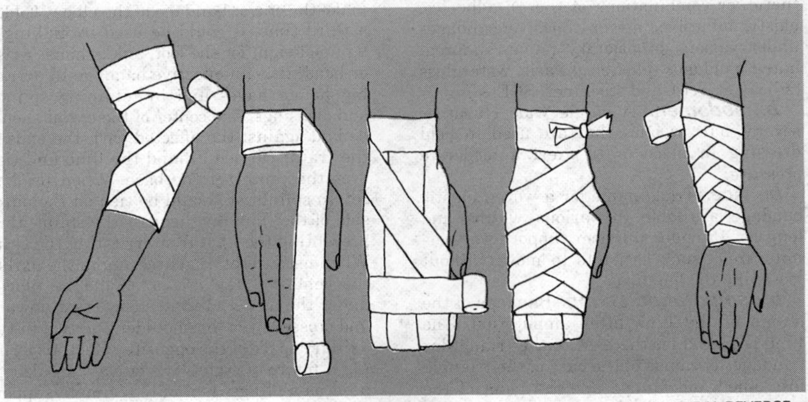

FIGURE-OF-EIGHT RECURRENT SPIRAL REVERSE

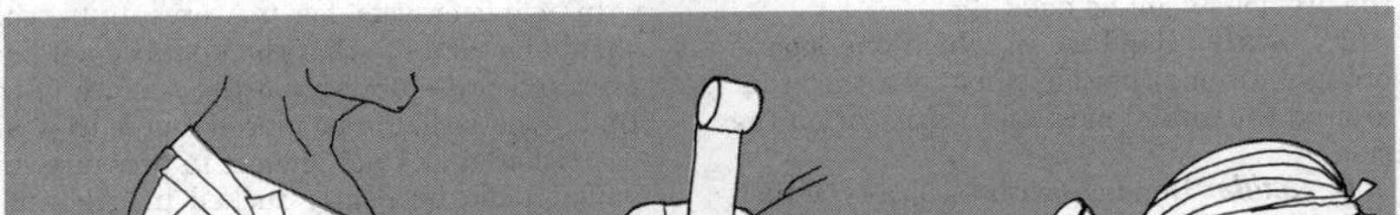

SPICA B. OF SHOULDER RECURRENT B. OF HEAD

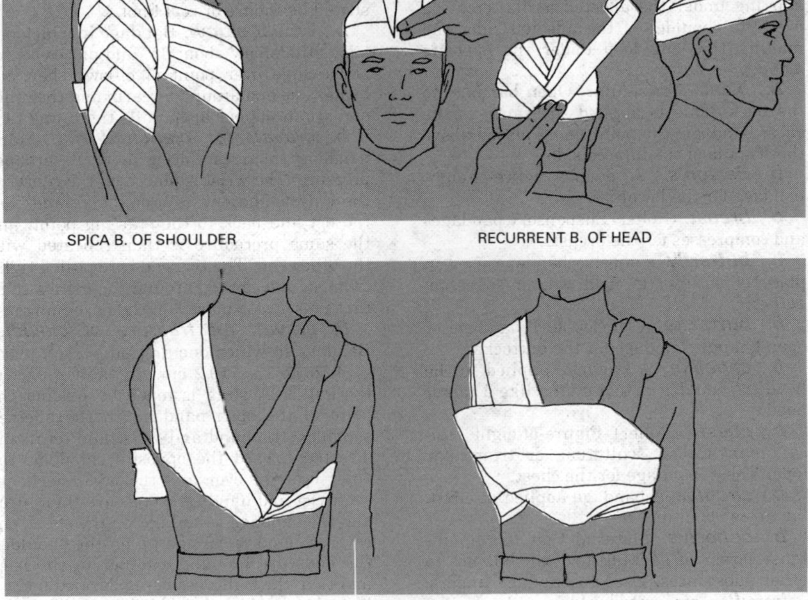

VELPEAU

TYPES OF BANDAGES

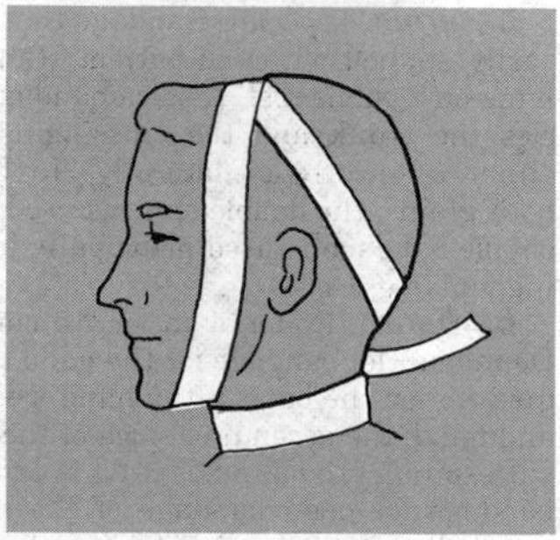

BARTON

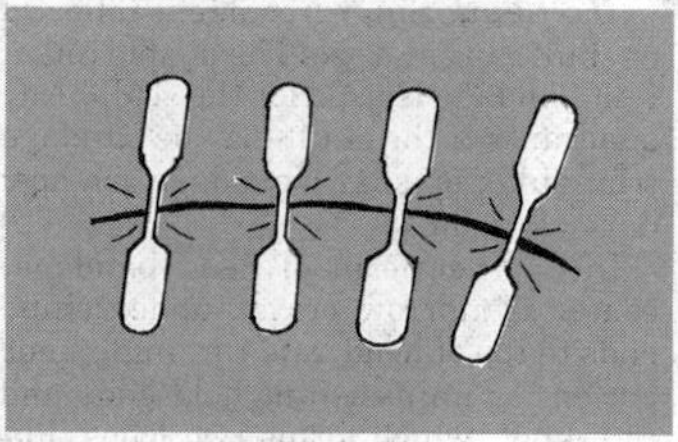

BUTTERFLY STRIPS

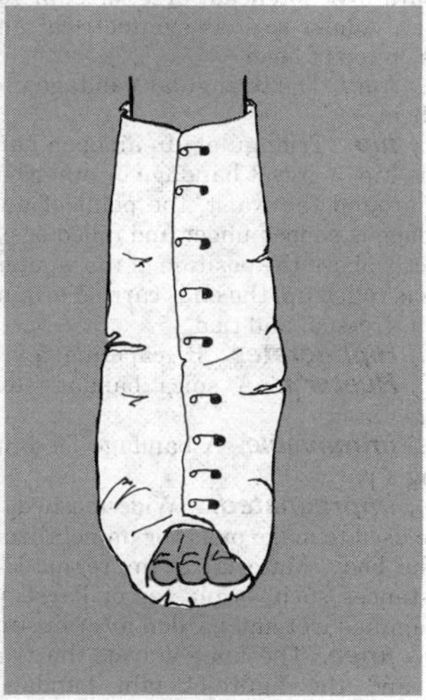

PILLOW SPLINT

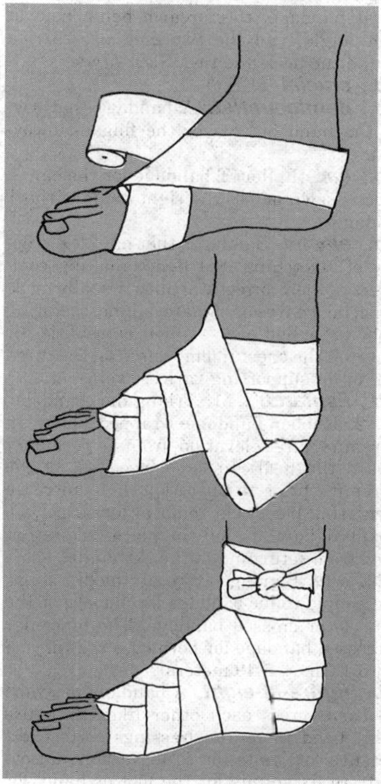

ANKLE STRAPPING

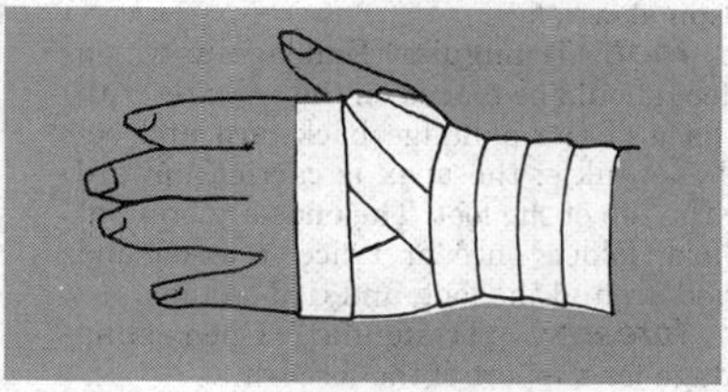

WRIST BANDAGE

port of the hand and in fracture of the upper arm. The wrist is laid upon the center of the cravat bandage, the forearm being held at right angle, and the two ends are carried around the neck and tied. SEE: *binder*.

b., crucial. SEE: *b., T.*

b., demigauntlet. A bandage that covers the hand but leaves the fingers uncovered.

b., ear. (Roller) T bandage for the ear. A piece is sewn across the right angle of the T bandage.

b., elastic. Bandages that have the property of stretching and hence making compression when correctly applied. Usually made of special weaves or of material incorporating rubber. Applied over swollen extremities or joints, on the chest in empyema, on fractured ribs, or for supporting varicose veins, etc.

b., Esmarch's. 1. Triangular bandage, q.v. 2. Rubber bandage wrapped about an extremity, after elevation, from its periphery toward the heart to force blood out of the extremity prior to operation or to increase circulating blood. On removal for surgery, a proximal band is left in place to prevent blood from returning to the extremity.

b., eye. Bandage for retaining dressings. The simple roller bandage for one eye or the monocle or crossed bandage. The binocular or crossed bandage for both eyes is 2 in. × 6 yd. (5.1 cm. × 5.49 meters).

b., figure-of-eight. A bandage in which the turns cross each other like the figure eight. Used to retain dressings or to exert pressure for joints (or to leave joint uncovered), to fix splints for the foot or hand, for the great toe, and for sprains or hemorrhage.

b., finger. Roller bandage with oblique fixation at wrist.

b., foot. (Triangular) Bandage in which the foot should be placed on the triangle with the base of the bandage backward and behind the ankle; the apex is carried upward over the top of the foot. The ends are brought forward, folded once or twice, crossed and carried around the foot, and tied on top.

b., forearm. (Triangular) Open sling bandage for support of the forearm.

b., four-tailed. A strip of cloth with each end split into two. Tails used to cover prominences such as elbow, chin, nose, knee.

b., Fricke's. Special bandage for supporting and immobilizing the scrotum.

b., Galen's. A bandage with each end split into three pieces: the middle is placed on the crown of the head; the two anterior strips are fastened at the back of the neck; the two posterior strips are on the forehead; and the two middle strips are tied under the chin.

b., Garretson's. A bandage for the lower jaw, running above the forehead and back again to cross under the occiput and ending under the chin.

b., groin. (Special) Bandage that is most easily applied with the patient standing or lying on a pelvic rest. A spica bandage encircles the trunk and the crossing is placed either anteriorly or laterally. To bandage both groins, the double spica is used. Such a double bandage is used principally in applying a plaster cast.

b., hand. (Roller, 1 in. or 2.5 cm. wide). Demigauntlet bandage for the hand to hold a dressing on the back of the hand. For thumb and hand, the ascending spica of the thumb, with spiral of the hand, is used. A triangular bandage for open bandage of the hand. A descending spica is used for the thumb and figure-of-eight bandage for amputation stump or clenched fist.

b., head. Single recurrent roller capeline or skull cap bandage. The double roller recurrent bandage is used for the scalp. Any of the quadrants of the skull may be bandaged. Use triangular or shawl bandage for open bandage of the head.

In another form of head bandage, place center of narrow cravat under chin, bring ends to top of head, and tie single knot. Have patient or an assistant hold ends and separate knot, which forms two loops. Place one low on back of head and bring the other forward over forehead, eyes, or chin as necessary. Adjust so it is symmetrical and tie ends on top of head.

b., heel. The triangular bandage used for the heel.

b., hip. (Triangular) In an open bandage of the hip, a cravat bandage or other band is tied around the waist, the point of another bandage is slipped under and rolled or pinned directly above the position of the wound. The base is rolled up, the ends carried around the thigh, crossed, and tied.

b., Hippocrates'. B., capeline, q.v.

b., Hueter's. A spica bandage for the perineum.

b., immovable. A bandage for immobilizing a part.

b., impregnated. Wide-meshed bandage used to make molds or immobilize parts of the body. Material is impregnated with substances such as plaster of Paris, which are applied wet and harden after drying.

b., knee. The knee cravat, the triangular, and the figure-of-eight bandage are used.

b., knotted. Bandage used to exert pressure on a compress or pad over a bleeding wound.

b., leg. Bandage applied by fixing the initial end by a circular or oblique fixation at the ankle or with a figure-of-eight of the foot and ankle.

b., Maissonneuve's. A plaster-of-Paris bandage made of folded cloth held in place by other bandages.

b., many-tailed. Bandage with split ends used for trunk and limbs. A piece of roller to which slips are stitched in an imbricated fashion. SEE: *b., four-tailed; b., scultetus.*

b., Martin's. Roller bandage of rubber used to make pressure on an extremity as for varicose veins, and for exsanguination, as Esmarch's bandage, q.v.

b., neck. (Roller) *Neck spica:* Bandage 2½ in. × 8 yd. (6.4 cm. × 7.3 meters). *Bandage following thyroid gland surgery:* Roller bandage 2½ in. × 9 yd. (6.4 cm. × 8.2 meters). *Adhesive plaster bandage for thyroidectomy:* Used to hold dressing on wound in place. Apply a small dressing to center of strip and then apply to back of neck. *Special bandage:* A double-loop bandage of the head and neck made by using a figure-of-eight turn.

b., oblique. A bandage applied obliquely to a limb, without reverses.

b., plaster. A bandage stiffened with a paste of plaster of Paris, which sets and becomes very hard.

b., postoperative. (Dressing) A simple divergent or convergent spica bandage.

b., pressure. A bandage for applying pressure, usually used to stop hemorrhage.

b., protective. A bandage for the purpose of covering a part or of keeping dressings in place.

b., quadrangular. A towel or large handkerchief, folded variously and applied as a bandage of head, chest, breast, or abdomen.

b., recurrent. A bandage over the end of a stump.

b., reversed. Bandage applied to a limb in such a way that the roller is inverted or half twisted at each turn so as to make it fit smoothly.

b., roller. A long strip of soft material, usually from ½ to 6 in. (1.3 to 15.2 cm.) wide and 2 to 5 yd. (1.83 to 4.57 meters) long, rolled on its short axis. When rolled from both ends to meet at center, it is called a double-headed roller.

b., rubber. A roller bandage of rubber used for pressure as in swollen parts for immobilization.

b., scultetus. Many-tailed bandage. A succession of interlocking, overlapping bands originally used to enclose a rigid support against a fractured extremity but now used without the splint or impregnated as a supporting bandage of the abdomen or lower extremity. SEE: *binder, scultetus,* for illus.

b., shoulder. Open bandage of the shoulder: Spica bandage. Shoulder and neck: Shawl bandage of both shoulders and neck.

b., spica. Bandage in which a number of figure-of-eight turns are applied, each a little higher or lower, overlapping a portion of each preceding turn so as to give an imbricated appearance. For breast, shoulder, limbs, thumb, great toe, and hernia at the groin. For support, to exert pressure, or to retain dressings.

b., spiral reverse. Technique of twisting, in its long axis, a roller bandage on itself at intervals during application to make it fit more uniformly. These reverse folds may be necessary every turn or less depending on contour of part being bandaged.

b., suspensory. A bandage for supporting any part but esp. the breast or scrotum.

b., T. Bandage shaped like the letter T. For the perineum and, in certain cases, for the head.

b., tailed. Bandage with ends split.

b., Theden's. A roller bandage applied from below upward over a graduated compress to control hemorrhage.

b., toe. Small bandage, about 2 in. (5.1 cm.) wide.

b., triangular. A 36- to 42-in. (232- to 271-cm.) square, usually muslin cut diagonally, making two triangular bandages. Frequently used in first aid. SYN: *b., Esmarch's* (def. 1). SEE: *triangular bandage* for illus.

b., Velpeau's. A special immobilizing roller bandage that incorporates the shoulder, arm, and forearm.

bandage roller. A device for rolling bandages.

Bandl's ring (băn'd'ls). [Ludwig Bandl, Ger. obstetrician, 1842–1892] Ringlike thickening and indentation at the junction of the upper and lower uterine segments that obstruct delivery of the fetus. SEE: *retraction ring.*

bandy leg. Bowleg. SYN: *genu varum.*

bank. A stored supply of body fluids or tissues for use in another individual, e.g., blood bank, eye bank, kidney bank, tissue bank.

b., sperm. Repository for storage of semen so that it may be used for artificial insemination. In some banks the specimen is frozen.

Banthine. Trade name for methantheline bromide, USP. Used as an anticholinergic.

Banting, Sir Frederick Grant. Canadian scientist, 1891–1941; co-discoverer of insulin, with Charles Herbert Best and John J. R. Macleod in 1922. Nobel laureate 1923.

Banti's syndrome (băn'tēz). [Guido Banti, It. physician, 1852–1925] A syndrome combining anemia, splenic enlargement, hemorrhages, and ultimately cirrhosis of liver. Considered secondary to portal hypertension.

bar, median. Contractures or constrictions of

vesical neck of the bladder caused by benign hypertrophy or fibrosis of the prostate. This may cause obstruction to the flow of urine from the bladder.

baragnosis (băr-ăg-nō′sĭs) [Gr. *baros*, weight, + *a-*, not, + *gnosis*, knowledge]. Inability to estimate weights. Indicative of parietal lobe lesion. Opposite of barognosis. SYN: *abarognosis*.

barber's itch. 1. An affection of the face due to infection of hair follicles and associated glands by staphylococci. Characterized by formation of papules and pustules. SYN: *folliculitis barbae*. 2. A dermatomycosis caused by a fungus, Microsporum lanosum or Trichophyton mentagrophytes, T. violaceum, or T. purpureum. SYN: *tinea barbae*.

barbital (băr′bĭ-tăl). 5,5-diethylbarbituric acid, a crystalline powder and derivative of barbituric acid. Used as a hypnotic and sedative, it is habit forming.

b., sodium. The soluble monosodium salt of barbital. Has same properties as barbital but because of greater solubility, it is more rapidly absorbed.

barbital poisoning. SEE: *barbiturates* in *Poisons and Poisoning* in *Appendix*.

barbiturates (băr-bĭt′ū-rāts, băr-bĭ-tū′rāts). A group of organic compounds derived from barbituric acid. All derivatives depress the central nervous system and depress respiration, affect heart rate, and decrease blood pressure and temperature. For sedative action, these drugs have been replaced by safer drugs such as benzodiazepines.

Ex.: Amytal, Pentothal, phenobarbital, Seconal. SEE: *Poisons and Poisoning* in *Appendix*.

barbotage (băr-bō-tŏzh′) [Fr. *barboter*, to dabble]. Repeated injection and withdrawal of fluid, as in gastric lavage, or the administration of an anesthetic into the subarachnoid space by alternate injection of anesthetic and withdrawal of cerebrospinal fluid into the syringe.

barbula hirci (băr′bū-lă hĭr′sī) [L. *barbula*, little beard, + *hircus*, goat]. 1. Hairs present on the ears. 2. Axillary hair.

baresthesia (băr-ĕs-thē′zē-ă) [Gr. *baros*, weight, + *aisthesis*, perception]. Sense of weight or pressure; pressure sense.

baresthesiometer (băr″ĕs-thē″zē-ŏm′ĕ-tĕr) [″ + ″ + *metron*, measure]. Instrument for determining sensitivity to weight or pressure.

bariatrics (băr″ē-ă′trĭks) [″ + *iatrike*, medical treatment]. Branch of medicine dealing with prevention, control, and treatment of obesity.

barium (bā′rē-ŭm). SYMB: Ba. At. wt. 137.34; at. no. 56. A soft metallic element of the alkaline earth group.

b. sulfate. USP. A radiopaque barium compound used in roentgenography of the gastrointestinal tract. Trade names are Barosperse, Esophotrast, and Baridol.

barium compounds. Compounds containing barium and suitable diluents or additives. Used to color fireworks and, in the form of insoluble barium sulfate, to visualize the hollow viscera in roentgenography. Poisoning occasionally comes from using the soluble salts in place of the insoluble sulfate. SEE: *Poisons and Poisoning* in *Appendix*.

barium enema. Use of barium sulfate as an enema to facilitate x-ray and fluoroscopic examination of the colon.

PROCEDURE: Careful preparation of the patient will greatly increase the chances of the test to produce useful information. The patient is given the following written instructions with a careful explanation to ensure compliance. 1. A minimum-residue diet must be followed for all meals for two days prior to the test. 2. Two nights prior to the test, 60 ml. (2 ounces) of milk of magnesia must be taken in 120 ml. (4 ounces) of water at bedtime. 3. On the day before the test, a clear liquid diet must be taken for all meals. 4. At 5 P.M. on the day before the test, 60 ml. (2 ounces) of castor oil must be taken. 5. At 10 P.M. on the day before the test, a cleansing enema consisting of 1500 ml. (50 ounces) of lukewarm water must be given. 6. On the day of the test, only clear liquids are allowed for meals. SEE: *diet, minimum residue*.

b.e., double contrast. A technique of barium enema x-ray study of the large intestine in which air is insufflated into the rectum and colon. This technique is thought to be much more effective in demonstrating pathologic lesions of the large intestine than is ordinary barium enema.

barium meal. Use of ingested barium sulfate to visualize the outline of the esophagus, stomach, and small intestines during x-ray or fluoroscopic examination. Also called upper G.I. series.

PROCEDURE: If the test does not follow a barium enema, the patient should receive nothing by mouth after midnight on the night preceding the test. No food or liquids should be taken by mouth until the last roentgenogram is taken. If the test is done within a few days after a barium enema examination, it is important to be sure the colon is free of barium, which could interfere with visualization of the stomach and intestines. A cleansing enema and 60 ml. (2 ounces) of milk of magnesia in 120 ml. (4 ounces) of water the evening prior to the test will remove residual barium from the colon.

barium swallow. Radiographic examination of the esophagus during and after introduction of a contrast medium consisting of barium sulfate. Structural abnormalities of the esophagus and vessels such as esophageal varices may be diagnosed by use of this technique.

barium test. Nonspecific term for any test involving use of barium sulfate as a radiopaque material for outlining anatomical areas such as the esophagus, and other portions of the intestinal tract by use of x-ray or fluorescent examination. SEE: *barium enema; barium meal.*

bark [Old Norse *börkr*]. 1. The outer cover of stems, branches, roots, and main trunks of trees and woody plants. 2. A particular kind of bark used in medicine.

Ex.: cascara sagrada, cinchona, wild cherry.

Barlow's disease. [Sir Thomas Barlow, Brit. physician, 1845–1945] A deficiency disease due to lack of vitamin C (ascorbic acid). Occurs in both breast-fed and bottle-fed babies who fail to receive adequate supplementary quantities of vitamin C. Occurs usually between 6 and 12 months of age. SEE: *scurvy, infantile.*

TREATMENT: Vitamin C. Then adequate daily intake of fruit juices (orange, grapefruit, tomato).

baro- [Gr. *baros,* weight]. Prefix indicating weight, heaviness.

barognosis (băr-ŏg-nō'sĭs) [" + *gnosis,* knowledge]. The ability to estimate weights. Opposite of baragnosis.

baroreceptor (băr"ō-rē-sĕp'tor). A sensory nerve ending that is stimulated by changes in pressure. Baroreceptors are found in the walls of the atria of the heart, vena cava, aortic arch, and carotid sinus.

baroreflexes (băr"ō-rē'flĕk-sĕs) [" + L. *reflexus,* bent back]. Reflexes mediated or activated through a group of nerves located in various blood vessels in the intrathoracic and cervical areas and in the heart and its great vessels. They are sensitive to mechanical changes produced when the pressure inside the vessel to which they are attached is altered. The response is called a baroreflex. Because the nerve groups are stimulated by mechanical rather than chemical means, they are called mechanoreceptors.

baroscope (băr'ō-skōp) [" + *skopein,* to examine]. Instrument that registers changes in the density of air.

barosinusitis (băr"ō-sī"nū-sī'tĭs) [Gr. *baros,* weight, + L. *sinus,* curve, + Gr. *itis,* inflammation]. Pain in and inflammation of one or more of the nasal sinuses due to having ascended or descended to a different altitude. This could occur while flying at a time when the outlet from a sinus is blocked. SEE: *aerotitis; barotitis.*

barospirator (băr"ō-spī'rā-tor) [" + L. *spirare,* to breathe]. Apparatus producing artificial respiration by means of air pressure variations in a closed chamber.

barotaxis (băr"ō-tăk'sĭs) [" + *taxis,* turning]. Stimulation of cells by altering the pressure of the atmosphere.

barotitis (băr"ō-tī'tĭs) [" + *otos,* ear, + *itis,* inflammation]. Inflammation of the ear due to sudden changes in barometric pressure such as occur while flying. Closure of the eustachian tube due to upper respiratory infection prevents the middle ear from adjusting to pressure changes encountered during flight. SYN: *aerotitis.*

barotrauma (băr"ō-traw'mă) [" + *trauma,* wound]. Any injury caused by a change in atmospheric pressure between a potentially closed space and the surrounding area. SEE: *aerotitis; barosinusitis; barotitis; bends; caisson disease.*

barotropism (băr-ŏt'rō-pĭzm) [" + *trope,* turning]. Barotaxis, q.v.

Barr body. [Murray L. Barr, Canadian anatomist, b. 1908] Sex chromatin mass seen within the nuclei of normal female somatic cells. According to the Lyon hypothesis, one of the two X chromosomes in each somatic cell of the female is genetically inactivated. The Barr body represents the inactivated X chromosome.

barrel chest. A chest that is rounded as in inspiration and has no apparent movement during respiration. Seen in emphysema.

barren [O. Fr. *barhaine,* unproductive]. Sterile; incapable of producing offspring.

barrier [O. Fr. *barriere*]. An obstacle, impediment, obstruction, boundary, or separation.

b., blood-brain. A barrier that exists between circulating blood and the brain, preventing certain damaging substances from reaching brain tissue and cerebrospinal fluid. It consists of either the perivascular glial membrane or the vascular endothelium or both.

Bartholin's abscess (băr'tō-lĭnz). [Casper Bartholin, Dan. anatomist, 1655–1738] An abscess that develops when Bartholin's glands become occluded in an acute inflammatory process.

Bartholin's cyst. Cyst commonly formed in chronic inflammation of Bartholin's glands, q.v. Carcinoma is rare.

Bartholin's ducts. Large ducts of the sublingual salivary gland. They parallel Wharton's duct, q.v., and open with it.

Bartholin's gland. A small compound mucus gland, situated one in each lateral wall of the vestibule of the vagina, near the vaginal opening at the base of the labia majora.

bartholinitis (băr"tō-lĭn-ī'tĭs) [*Bartholin* + Gr. *itis,* inflammation]. Inflammation of Bartholin's gland.

Barton, Clara. U.S. nurse 1821–1912. Founder

of the American National Red Cross, she aided the wounded in the Civil War. Contemporary of Florence Nightingale, q.v.

Bartonella (băr″tō-nĕl′ă). [A. L. Barton, S. Amer. physician] A genus of the family Bartonellaceae.

B. bacilliformis. Motile gram-negative bacillus; the cause of bartonellosis.

bartonellosis (băr″tō-nĕl-ō′sĭs) [*Bartonella* + Gr. *osis,* condition]. A disease caused by infection with Bartonella bacilliformis, transmitted by female sandflies (Phlebotomus). The first clinical stage is noneruptive and is called Oroya fever, a severe febrile, hemolytic anemia. The second stage is eruptive and is called verruga peruana. It is marked by the appearance of small tumors on the skin and mucous membranes. SYN: *Carrion's disease.*

TREATMENT: Responds to several antibiotics, but chloramphenicol has the added advantage of being effective against Salmonella, which may be present as a secondary infection.

Bartter's syndrome. [F. C. Bartter, U.S. physician, b. 1914] Hyperplasia of the juxtaglomerular cells of the kidney, hypokalemic alkalosis, and hyperaldosteronism without a rise in blood pressure. It usually occurs in children and may be accompanied by dwarfism. Etiology is unknown. Some cases have responded to therapy with prostaglandin inhibitors.

Baruch's law (băr′ooks). [Simon Baruch, U.S. physician, 1840–1921] Theory that water has a sedative effect when its temperature is the same as that of the skin and a stimulating effect when it is below or above the skin temperature.

bary- [Gr. *barys,* heavy]. Prefix indicating heavy, dull, hard.

baryglossia (băr-ĭ-glŏs′ē-ă) [Gr. *barys,* heavy, + *glossa,* tongue]. Slow, thick utterance of speech.

barylalia (băr-ĭ-lā′lē-ă) [″ + *lalia,* speech]. Indistinct, husky speech due to imperfect articulation.

baryphonia (băr″ĭ-fō′nē-ă) [″ + *phone,* voice]. 1. Heavy, thick quality of the voice. 2. Barylalia, q.v.

basad (bā′săd) [Gr. *basis,* base, + L. *ad,* toward]. Toward the base.

basal (bā′săl). 1. Pert. to the base. 2. Of primary importance.

basal ganglia. Four masses of gray matter located deep in the cerebral hemispheres—caudate, lentiform, and amygdaloid nuclei and the claustrum. The caudate and lentiform nuclei and the fibers of the internal capsule that separate them constitute the corpus striatum.

basal lamina. Basement lamina, q.v.; basement membrane.

basal metabolic rate. ABBR: BMR. The metabolic rate as measured under so-called basal conditions: 12 hours after eating, after a restful sleep, no exercise or activity preceding test, elimination of emotional excitement, and in a comfortable temperature. It is usually expressed in terms of Cal. (kilocalories) per square meter of body surface per hour. The use of this test is no longer justified due to the availability of better tests of thyroid function. SEE: *thyroid function tests.*

basal metabolism. The amount of energy needed for maintenance of life when the subject is at digestive, physical, and emotional rest.

basal ridge. An eminence on the lingual surface of the incisor teeth, esp. the upper ones. It is situated near the gum. SYN: *cingulum* (def. 2).

basal temperature chart. A daily chart of temperature obtained upon awakening. Some women are able to predict the time of ovulation by carefully analyzing the character and rhythm of the temperature chart. This information and other data can be used to establish that the woman is ovulating. Use of this method to control conception by predicting time of ovulation is unreliable in most cases. SEE: *conception;* illus.

base [Gr. *basis,* base]. 1. The lower part of anything; the supporting part. 2. The principal substance in a mixture. 3. Any substance that combines with hydrogen ions (protons); a hydrogen ion acceptor. Strong bases feel slippery and are corrosive to human tissues.

Ex.: sodium hydroxide (NaOH) (lye or caustic soda); potassium hydroxide (KOH) (caustic potash).

Whether an unknown chemical compound is a base or acid may be determined by the color produced when it is added to a solution containing an indicator, q.v. SYN: *alkali,* q.v. SEE: *acid; pH.*

baseball finger. Condition resulting from violent backward dislocation of the terminal phalanx onto the dorsum of the middle phalanx, as when a finger is struck on its tip when extended. SYN: *mallet finger.* SEE: *hammer finger.*

Basedow's disease (băz′ē-dōz). [Karl A. von Basedow, Ger. physician, 1799–1854] Graves' disease; exophthalmic goiter, q.v.

baseline (bās′līn). A known or initial value with which subsequent determinations of what is being measured can be compared, e.g., baseline temperature or blood pressure.

basement lamina [Gr. *basis,* base, + L. *lamina,* thin plate]. Preferred term for a thin layer of delicate noncellular material of a fine filamentous texture underlying the epithelium. Its principal component is collagen.

BASAL TEMPERATURE CHART

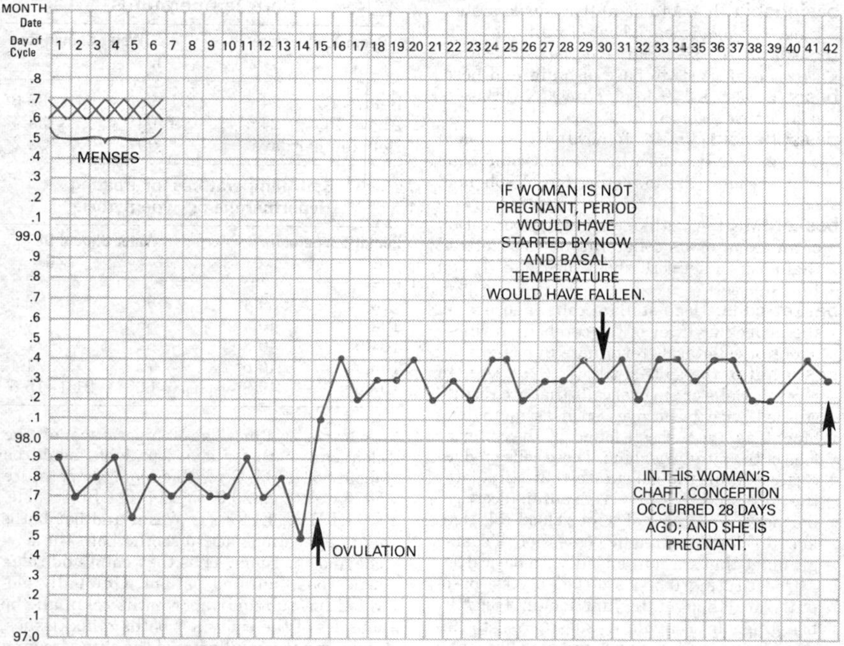

SYN: *basement membrane; hyaline membrane.*

basement membrane. Basement lamina, q.v.

baseplate (bās′plāt). Plastic substance molded to form a base. Used in constructing artificial teeth.

basi-, basio- [Gr. *basis*, base]. Prefixes denoting base or basion.

basial (bās′sē-ăl) [L. *basialis*]. Pert. to the basion.

basiarachnoiditis (bā″sē-ă-răk″noy-dī′tĭs) [Gr. *basis*, base, + *arachne*, spider, + *eidos*, form, + *itis*, inflammation]. Inflammation of the arachnoid membrane at base of brain.

basic. 1. In chemistry, possessing properties of a base. 2. Fundamental.

basicranial axis (bā″sē-krā′nē-ăl) [″ + *kranion*, skull, + *axis*, pivot]. Straight line from the basion to point of angle of mandible.

basic salt. A compound formed when only part of the hydroxide radicals of a base is replaced by the acid radical of an acid.

Basidiomycetes (bă-sĭd″ē-ō-mī-sē′tēz). One of the four major classes of true fungi of the division Eumycota. They are distinguished by the sexual spores, basidiospores, that form on a specialized structure, the basidium. Included are toadstools, mushrooms, and fungi of trees. They cause diseases of plants, and their toxins may be lethal to man when eaten. Also, the basidiospores have been implicated as a cause of allergic asthma.

basifacial axis (bā-sē-fā′shăl) [″ + L. *facies*, face. + Gr. *axis*, pivot]. Straight line from the point of angle of mandible to the subnasal point.

basihyal (bā″sē-hī′ăl) [″ + *oeides*, hyoid]. The body of the hyoid bone.

basilar (băs′ĭ-lăr) [L. *basilaris*]. Basal; pert. to a base.

basilateral (bā″sē-lăt′ĕr-ăl) [″ + L. *lateralis*, pert. to the side]. Both lateral and basilar.

basilemma (bā″sē-lĕm′ă) [Gr. *basis*, base, + *lemma*, husk]. The basement membrane.

basilic (bă-sĭl′ĭk) [L. *basilicus*]. Prominent, important.

basilic vein. Large vein on inner side of biceps of the arm just above the elbow. Usually chosen for intravenous injection or withdrawal of blood.

basiloma (băs-ĭ-lō′mă) [Gr. *basis*, base, + *oma*, tumor]. Basal cell carcinoma.

basio- [Gr. *basis*, base]. Prefix denoting base or basion.

basioccipital bone (bā″sē-ŏk-sĭp′ĭ-tăl) [″ + L. *occiput*, head]. Basilar process of occipital bone.

basion (bā′sē-ŏn). Midpoint of anterior border

of the foramen magnum.

basiphobia (bă″sē-fō′bē-ă) [Gr. *basis*, a stepping, + *phobos*, fear]. Fear of walking.

basirhinal (bā-sē-rī′năl) [Gr. *basis*, base, + *rhis*, nose]. Pert. to base of brain and nose.

basis (bā′sĭs) [L., Gr.]. (pl. *bases*) [NA] Base of a structure or organ.

basisphenoid (bā-sē-sfē′noyd) [″ + *sphen*, wedge, + *eidos*, form]. An embryonic bone that becomes the lower portion of sphenoid bone.

basket [ME.]. A netlike terminal arborization of an axon (or its collateral) of a basket cell that forms a network about the cell body of a Purkinje cell.

basket cells. Deep stellate cells (neurons) of the molecular layer of the cerebellum whose axons or collaterals terminate in baskets.

basophil(e) (bā′sō-fĭl, -fīl) [″ + *philein*, to love]. 1. Cells or parts of cells that are readily stained with basic dyes such as methylene blue. 2. A type of cell found in the anterior lobe of the pituitary gland. These cells produce corticotropin, the substance that stimulates the adrenal cortex to secrete adrenal cortical hormone. 3. A type of white blood cell (leukocyte) characterized by possession of coarse granules that stain intensely with basic dyes.

Constituting 0.5–1% of leukocytes, basophils are thought to function in blood by bringing anticoagulant substances to inflamed tissues. Increased numbers are found during the healing phase of inflammation and in chronic inflammation. SEE: *blood cell* for illus.

basophilia (bā-sō-fĭl′ē-ă). 1. A pathological condition in which basophilic erythrocytes are found in the blood. 2. Condition in which there are a high number of basophilic leukocytes in the blood.

basophilic (bā-sō-fĭl′ĭk). Pert. to the staining characteristics of various cells.

basophilism (bā-sŏf′ĭ-lĭzm). Condition characterized by excessive numbers of basophils.

b., pituitary. A clinical syndrome (Cushing's syndrome) characterized by basophilic invasion or adenoma of the pituitary gland. SYN: *Cushing's syndrome*, q.v.

basophobia (bās-ō-fō′bē-ă) [Gr. *basis*, a stepping, + *phobos*, fear]. 1. Abnormal fear of walking. 2. Emotional inability to stand or walk in the absence of muscle disease.

bass deafness. Deafness to bass notes.

Bassini's operation (bă-sē′nēz). [Edoardo Bassini, It. surgeon, 1844–1924] A specific surgical procedure for inguinal hernia.

bastard [O. Fr. *batard*]. 1. One born out of wedlock; illegitimate. 2. Not genuine; irregular.

bath [AS. *baeth*]. The medium and method of cleansing the body or any part of it, or treating it therapeutically as with air, light, vapor, or water. The temperature of the cleansing bath for a bed patient should be about 95° F. (35° C.) with a room temperature of 75° to 80° F. (23.9° to 26.7° C.). SEE: table.

Bath Temperatures

Room Temperature F.	C.	Water Should Be F.	C.
Below 76°	24.4°	94–96°	34.4–35.6°
Above 76°	24.4°	92–94°	33.3–34.4°
Hot summer days		90°	32.2°

Bath Temperatures for Treating Hyperthermia or Hyperpyrexia

Rectal Temperature F.	C.	Water Should Be F.	C.
103°	39.4°	90°	32.2°
104°	40°	86°	30°
104.5°	40.3°	82°	27.8°
105°	40.6°	76°	24.4°
105.5°	40.8°	70–60°	21.1–15.6°

THERAP. EFFECT: Warm and hot baths and applications act to soothe both the psyche and the soma. Thus they calm and relax a nervous, agitated patient. Gradually elevated hot tub and vapor baths relax all the muscles of the body. Hot baths relax tissues, including the capillaries of the skin, drawing blood from the deeper tissues, and also help to relieve pain and stimulate nerves. Cold baths and applications abstract heat and stimulate reaction, esp. if followed by brisk rubbing of the skin. Cold contracts small blood vessels when applied locally. SEE: *hydrotherapy*.

b., acid. Bath consisting of 5 oz. (150 ml.) hydrochloric acid or 1 gal. (3.8 L.) vinegar added to 30 gal. (114 L.) water.

b., air. Therapeutic use of air, warmed or vaporized, on the nude body.

b., alcohol. Application of alcohol to the patient as a stimulant and defervescent in dilute form.

b., alkaline. Eight oz. (227 gm.) of sodium bicarbonate or washing soda added to 30 gal. (114 L.) of water.

b., alum. Use of alum in washing solution as an astringent.

b., antipyretic. A bath in cool water (65° to 75° F. or 18.3° to 28.9° C.). The patient should not be cooled to the point of shivering, as this indicates excessive heat loss.

b., aromatic. Bath to which some volatile oil or perfume or some herb is added.

b., astringent. Bathing in liquid containing an astringent.

b., bed. Bath for a patient confined to bed.

NURSING IMPLICATIONS: Assemble all required equipment; ensure appropriate room temperature and that there are no drafts. Water temperature for bath should be 110–120° F. (43.3–48.1° C.). Only one body part should be washed at a time, and the part should be washed, rinsed, and dried. The patient should remain covered during the procedure. Change bath water as often as necessary. After the bath is completed, apply lotion to the skin. To complete the bath, the patient should have oral hygiene, hair combed, and a clean gown applied. The patient is expected to perform all or parts of the bath, and the nurse should bathe the patient only if the patient is unable to do so for him- or herself.

b., bland. A bath containing substances such as starch, bran, or oatmeal for the relief of skin irritation; an emollient bath.

b., blanket. Bath in which wet pack and blankets are used.

b., box. Bath in which patient's entire body except the head is completely enclosed in a box.

b., bran. Bath in which one places bran (2 to 3 lb. or 907 gm. to 1.4 kg.) in a muslin bag and soaks it in hot water 15 min., then adds bag and hot water to bath water (30 gal., 95° F., or 114 L., 35° C.), using bag as a washing-sponge.

b., brine. B., saline, q.v.

b., bubble. A bath in which the water contains many small bubbles produced mechanically as by an air pump or chemically by bubble bath preparations.

CAUTION: Perfumes used in bubble baths are frequently the cause of vaginitis, esp. in children.

b., carbon dioxide. An effervescent saline bath consisting of water, salts, and CO_2. The natural CO_2 baths are known as Nauheim baths, and approach closely CO_2 baths in their therapeutic effects.

b., cold. Bath in water at a temperature below 65° F. (18.3° C.).

b., colloid. B., emollient, q.v.

b., continuous. Bath that is administered for an extended period but seldom for longer than several hours. Used in treating hypothermia or hyperthermia, certain skin diseases, and in the past in treating some types of mental disorders, esp. agitation.

b., contrast. Bath used for hands or feet. Fill two large basins or pails of sufficient depth with water, one as hot and the other as cold as the patient can stand. Change or add hot and cold water frequently to keep temperatures same as in beginning. Put part to be treated in hot water for one minute, then into cold for a half minute, then again into hot water. Repeat for prescribed length of time, ending with cold water.

b., earth. Bathing in warmed earth or sand.

b., emollient. Bath used for irritation and inflammation of skin and after erysipelas. SEE: *b., glycerin; b., oatmeal; b., powdered borax; b., starch.*

b., foam. Tub bath in which an extract of a saponin-containing vegetable fiber has been added. Oxygen or carbon dioxide is driven through this mixture to form foam.

b., foot. Immersion of feet and legs to a depth of 4 in. (10 cm.) above ankles in water at 98° F. (36.7° C.).

b., full. Bath in which the whole body except the head is immersed in water.

b., glycerin. Bath consisting of 10 oz. (300 ml.) of glycerin added to 30 gal. (114 L.) water.

b., herb. Full bath to which is added a mixture of 1 to 2 lb. (454 to 907 gm.) of herbs such as chamomile, wild thyme, or spearmint tied in a bag and boiled with 1 gal. (3.8 L.) of water.

b., hip. B., sitz, q.v.

b., hot. Tub bath with the water covering the body to a little above the nipple level. The temperature is gradually raised from 98° F. (36.7° C.) to desired degree, usually to 108° F. (42.2° C.).

b., hot air. Exposure of entire body except head to hot air in a bath cabinet.

b., hyperthermal. Bath in which the whole body except the head is immersed in water from 105° to 120° F. (40.6° to 48.9° C.) for one to two minutes.

b., kinetotherapeutic. Bath given for underwater exercises of weak or partially paralyzed muscles.

b., lukewarm. Bath in which patient's body except head is immersed in water from 94° to 96° F. (34.4° to 35.6° C.) for 15 to 60 minutes.

b., medicated. Bath to which substances such as bran, oatmeal, starch, sodium bicarbonate, Epsom salts, pine products, tar, sulfur, potassium permanganate, and salt are added.

b., milk. Bath taken in milk for emollient or cosmetic purposes.

b., mud. The use of mud in order to apply moist heat.

b., mustard. Stimulative hot foot bath consisting of a mixture of 1 tablespoon (15 cc.) of dry mustard in a quart (946 ml.) of hot water added to a pail or large basin filled with water of 100° to 104° F. (37.8° to 40° C.). Used in rheumatic conditions and in sprains or other muscular foot pains caused by trauma.

b., Nauheim. A bath in which the body is immersed in warm water through which carbon dioxide is bubbled.

b., needle. Bath in which water is forcibly sprayed on the body in fine jet streams.

b., neutral. Bath in which no circulatory or thermic reaction occurs, temperature 92° to 97° F. (33.3° to 36.1° C.).

b., neutral sitz. Same as hot sitz bath, q.v., except temperature is 92° to 97° F. (33.3° to 36.1° C.) or for foot bath 104° to 110° F. (37.8° to 40° C.), duration 15–60 minutes.

b., oatmeal. Bath consisting of 2 to 3 lb. (907 gm. to 1.4 kg.) oatmeal added to 30 gal. (114 L.) water.

b., oxygen. Bath given by introducing oxygen into the water through a special device that is connected to an oxygen tank or by generating the oxygen by chemical means.

b., paraffin. The limb is repeatedly immersed in warm paraffin 104° to 150° F. (37.8° to 65.6° C.) and quickly withdrawn until it is encased. Paraffin may be applied with paint brush for larger joints. Used when there is need to apply topical heat to traumatized or inflamed areas.

b., powdered borax. Bath consisting of ½ lb. (227 gm.) added to 30 gal. (114 L.) water; 5 oz. (150 ml.) glycerin may be added.

b., saline. Bath given in artificial seawater made by dissolving 8 lb. (3.6 kg.) of sea salt or a mixture of 7 lb. (3.2 kg.) of sodium chloride and ½ lb. (227 gm.) of magnesium sulfate in 30 gal. (114 L.) of water. SYN: *b., salt; b., seawater.*

b., sauna. A hot, humid atmosphere created in a small enclosed area by pouring water on heated rocks.

b., seawater. B., saline, q.v.

b., sedative. A prolonged warm bath. A continuous flow of water as well as an air cushion or back rest may be used.

b., sheet. Bath given by wrapping the patient in a sheet previously dipped in water 80° to 90° F. (26.7° to 32.2° C.), and by rubbing the whole body with vigorous strokes on the sheet until all parts of the sheet feel warm.

b., shower. Water sprayed down upon the body from an overhead source.

b., sitz. Immersion of thighs, buttocks, and abdomen below the umbilicus in water. In a hot sitz bath the water is first 92° F. (33.3° C.) and then elevated to 106° F. (41.1° C.).

b., sponge. Bath in which patient is not immersed in a tub but washed with a wash cloth or sponge.

b., starch. Bath consisting of 1 lb. (454 gm.) of starch mixed into cold water, with boiling water added to make a solution of gluelike consistency, then added to 30 gal. (114 L.) of water.

b., steam. Bath given in a chamber into which steam under low pressure is allowed to escape. Best form of application is that in which subject sits in cabinet or lies in box with head outside.

CAUTION: Temperature must be controlled carefully to avoid burning the patient.

b., stimulating. Bath that increases cutaneous blood flow. SEE: *b., cold; b., mustard; b., saline.*

b., sulfur. A bath made by adding potassium sulfide (3 oz. or 85 gm.), zinc sulfate (8 tsp. or 1.3 oz.), or sulfurated lime sol. (6 oz. or 180 ml.) to 30 gal. (114 L.) water. Bath should be limited to 20 min.

b., sun. Exposure of all or part of the nude body to sunlight.

b., sweat. Bath given to induce perspiration.

b., towel. Bath given by applying towel dipped in water 60° to 70° F. (15.6° to 21.1° C.) to arms, legs, and anterior and posterior surfaces of trunk, removing towel, and drying parts.

b., vapor. Exposure of skin of body except head to vapor. Sometimes the vapor is impregnated with substances thought to possess therapeutic value, as sulfur, mercury, or camphor.

b., whirlpool. Continuous localized jets of water at a temperature of 105° to 120° F. (40.6° to 48.9° C.) agitate the water into which the body or a part of it is immersed.

bathophobia (băth″ō-fō′bē-ă) [Gr. *bathos,* deep, + *phobos,* fear]. Abnormal fear of depths. Commonly refers to fear of height or of looking down from a high place.

bathyanesthesia (băth-ē-ăn″ĕs-thē′zē-ă) [″ + *an-,* not, + *aisthesis,* perception]. Loss of deep sensibility.

bathycardia (băth″ē-kăr′dē-ă) [″ + *kardia,* heart]. Low position of the heart in the thorax due to anatomical conditions rather than disease.

bathyesthesia (băth″ē-ĕs-thē′zē-ă) [″ + *aisthesis,* sensation]. A consciousness or sensibility of parts of the body beneath the skin.

bathyhyperesthesia (băth-ē-hī″pĕr-ĕs-thē′zē-ă) [″ + *hyper,* above, + *aisthesis,* sensation]. Excessive sensitiveness of muscular tissues and deep body structures.

bathyhypesthesia (băth″ē-hīp″ĕs-thē′zē-ă) [″ + *hypo,* under, + *aisthesis,* sensation]. Impairment of sensitiveness in muscular tissues and other deep structures of body.

battered child syndrome. Physical violence inflicted upon a child by adults, usually one or both of the parents or guardians, often under circumstances that make it appear that the injury was accidental. Clinical findings: bruises, scratches, burns, hematomas, and fractures of long bones, ribs, or skull.

Poor skin hygiene and some degree of malnutrition also may be present.

DIAG: Most distinguishing feature is variation in stages of healing of bone lesions seen in roentgenogram, indicating injuries incurred at different times.

ETIOL: Most parents or guardians of abused children have a history of being so treated as a child.

PROG: Variable. Death rate is high, and surviving children often suffer from long-term physical and mental injuries, and will possibly become abusive parents.

battery [Fr. *battre*, to beat]. 1. Device for generating electrical current by chemical action. 2. A series of tests, procedures, or diagnostic examinations given to or done on a patient. 3. Assault and battery. SEE: *assault*.

Baudelocque's diameter (bōd-lŏks'). [Jean Louis Baudelocque, Sr., Fr. obstetrician, 1746–1810] Distance between the depression just beneath the last lumbar vertebra and the margin of the symphysis pubis. The external conjugate diameter of the pelvis.

Baudelocque's method. Manipulation to convert a fetal face presentation into a vertex presentation.

Baumé scales (bō-mā'). [Antoine Baumé, Fr. chemist, 1728–1805] Hydrometer scales for determination of the specific gravity of liquids.

bay (bā). An anatomical recess or depression filled with liquid.

Bayes' theorem. [Thomas Bayes, Brit. mathematician, 1702–1761] This theorem, published posthumously in 1764, is concerned with analyzing the probability that a patient may be considered to have a certain diagnosis or disease when it is known that the patient has certain attributes such as an abnormal test. It is usually known how frequently that particular attribute is present in the population considered to have the specific disease.

bayonet leg. Backward dislocation of tibia and fibula at the knee joint.

Bazin's disease (bă-zăz'). [Antoine P. E. Bazin, Fr. dermatologist, 1807–1878] Chronic skin disease occurring in young adult females. Characterized by hard cutaneous nodules that break down to form necrotic ulcers that leave atrophic scars. The disease is almost invariably preceded by tuberculosis. Nevertheless, the etiological relationship to that disease is debated. SYN: *erythema induratum*.

B cells. Types of lymphocyte that arise in the bone marrow. They are present in the blood, lymph, and connective tissue. When stimulated by certain antigens, the small B cell lymphocytes transform into large lymphocytes and some of these further differentiate into plasma cells, which are important in producing circulating antibodies. In lower animals the bursa of Fabricius is important in the development of B cells. The structure in mammals that corresponds to the bursa of Fabricius has not been identified. SYN: *B-lymphocytes*.

BCG. *bacille Calmette-Guérin*.

BCG vaccine. A form of tuberculosis vaccine. A freeze-dried preparation of a live, attenuated strain of Mycobacterium tuberculosis (bacille Calmette-Guérin) Proposed for use in adults and children for immunization against tuberculosis. The use of this vaccine in treating certain types of cancer is experimental. SEE: *bacille Calmette-Guérin*.

b.d. L. *bis die*, twice a day.

bdellometer (dĕl-ŏm'ĕ-tĕr) [Gr. *bdella*, leech, + *metron*, measure]. Mechanical substitute for a leech. SEE: *leech*.

B.E. *below elbow*, term used to refer to the site of amputation of an upper extremity; *barium enema*.

Be. Chem. symb. for beryllium.

beaded (bēd'ĕd). Referring to disjointed colonies along the inoculation line in a streak or stab.

beads, rachitic. Visible swelling where the ribs join their cartilages, seen in rickets. SYN: *rachitic rosary*.

beaker (bē'kĕr). Glass vessel with wide mouth for mixing or holding liquids.

beam. 1. In nuclear medicine and radiology, a group of atomic particles traveling a parallel course. 2. Isoelectric line of an oscilloscope.

bearing down. The expulsive effort of a parturient woman in second stage of labor. The Valsalva maneuver is utilized, causing increased pressure against the uterus by increasing intra-abdominal pressure.

beat [AS. *beatan*, to strike]. A pulsation or throb as of contraction of the heart or the passage of blood through a vessel.

b., apex. Impulse of the heart beat felt by the hand when held over the fifth intercostal space in left midclavicular line.

b., capture. Ventricular contraction responding to an impulse from the sinus that reaches the atrioventricular node at a time at which the node is nonrefractory.

b., ectopic. Heart beat beginning at a place other than sinoatrial node.

b., escaped. Heart beat that occurs after a prolonged pause.

b., forced. Extrasystole brought on by artificial heart stimulation.

b., premature. An extrasystole.

Beau's lines (bōz). [J. H. S. Beau, Fr. physician, 1806–1865] White lines across the fingernails, usually a sign of systemic disease. May be due to trauma, coronary occlusion, hypercalcemia, or skin disease. The lines are visible until the affected area of the nail has grown out and been trimmed away.

Bechterew's (also Bekhterev's) reflex (běk′ tĕr-ĕvs). [Vladimir Mikhailovich von Bechterew, Russ. neurologist, 1857–1927] 1. Contraction of facial muscles due to irritation of nasal mucosa. 2. Dilatation of pupil on exposure to light. 3. Contraction of lower abdominal muscles when skin of inner surface of thigh is stroked.

beclomethasone dipropionate. USP. A corticosteroid drug. Trade names are Vancenase and Beclovent inhaler.

bed [AS. *bedd*]. 1. A supporting structure or tissue. 2. A couch or support for the body during sleep.

MAKING AN OCCUPIED BED: CAUTION: Special drainage and irrigation tubes must be handled carefully in order not to disturb their function or placement or to cause the patient pain.

Assemble all necessary articles, placing clean linens on back of chair at bedside. Tell the patient what you are going to do; check temperature of room and adjust windows if necessary. Loosen all bedclothes; remove all but one blanket. Hang on back of chair. Remove top sheet from under remaining blanket. Place in laundry bag or fold and place on seat of chair to form receiver for dirty linens. Turn patient away from you if possible, and ensure safety by placing chair or bedrail for security. Bottom sheet is also folded in neat, flat folds to center of bed.

Place clean bottom sheet on exposed half of mattress, folding neatly to center creases. Tuck top of sheet under head of mattress, miter corner and tuck under mattress to foot of bed. Sheet must cover mattress completely. Place clean sheet with center crease to patient's back. Fold top of clean sheet and tuck securely under mattress. Assist patient to roll toward you under blanket to clean side of bed. Again insure safety. Proceed to other side of bed. Remove soiled bottom sheet and place on first piece of soiled linen on chair. Pull through clean bottom sheet and rubber sheet. Proceed as for first side, tightening sheet to avoid any wrinkles. Ask patient to raise buttocks if possible.

Remove pillows and pillow cases; replace cases with clean ones. Pull mattress to head of bed; replace pillows and adjust to patient's comfort. Place clean top sheet, wide hem to top, over blanket; draw blanket out from under sheet and replace with top of blanket well over patient's shoulders. Put on spread and turn top hem of sheet over spread at least 8 in. Remake foot of bed, allowing sufficient room for feet and toes of patient to move freely.

Remove soiled linens from room. Avoid shaking bedclothes in order to prevent spreading dust, a possible source of infection. Place patient's signal or call device in proper and convenient place, straighten room, and evaluate comfort and appearance carefully.

b., air. Bed inflated with air. Also, a special bed that literally floats the patient on a cushion of air that comes from holes in a special mattress. Used in burn cases and to prevent bedsores.

b., air-fluidized. SEE: *air-fluidized bed.*

b., capillary. A network of capillaries.

b., circular. Special bed that allows a patient to be turned end-over-end while held between two frames. This permits turning the patients without disturbing them by turning the two frames inside a circular apparatus that holds the ends of the frames. Useful in treating paralyzed or immobilized patients. Trademark: Circ-O-Lectric bed. SEE: *Circ-O-Lectric bed* for illus.

b., float. Bed in which the patient is supported either on a water mattress or on minute ceramic beads with air flowing through them. This type of bed is particularly useful in treating decubitus ulcers.

b., flotation. Bed in which the patient reclines in a hollow, flexible, mattress-shaped device that is filled with water. This enables equal distribution of pressure on the body. Used in treating and preventing decubiti.

b., fracture. Bed for patients who have fractures.

b., Gatch. Adjustable bed that provides elevation of the back and knees.

b., hydrostatic. B., water, q.v.

b., metabolic. Bed arranged to facilitate collecting the feces and urine of a patient so that metabolic rate can be calculated.

b., nail. The skin at tip of digit that lies beneath a nail.

b., open. Bed that is available for assignment to a patient.

b., recovery. Bed prepared to receive patient immediately following an operative procedure requiring anesthesia. Usually a portable bed or stretcher.

b., surgical. Bed equipped with a mechanism by which the head or the foot of the bed can be raised or lowered independently of each other.

b., tilt. SEE: *table, tilt.*

b., water. A rubber mattress filled with water. Used for prevention of bedsores. SEE: *b., flotation.*

bed blocking. Placing bedblocks under bed to raise it at head or foot.

Foot of bed raised: In shock; bleeding from lower limbs; edema of lower limbs, vulva, or scrotum; some cases of hemorrhoids; to retain enema; when weight is used on lower limbs; in reduction of inguinal hernia.

Head of bed raised: To drain abdomen or pelvis; to aid respiration; in treatment for bleeding from head, neck, or upper chest; in treatment of congestive heart failure.

bedblocks. Blocks of sturdy material, usually wood, for placement under either the two lower or upper bed legs in order to elevate the respective end of the bed.

bedbug. An insect, Cimex lectularius, the saliva of which contains an irritating substance that causes a purpuric reaction or an urticarial wheal.

TREATMENT: Antipruritic lotions containing phenol, camphor, and menthol.

CONTROL: Largely a matter of cleanliness. In heavy infestations, use appropriate insecticide, spraying furniture, mattresses, floors, baseboards, walls.

NOTE: Use of wooden frames for beds provides a nesting and breeding site for these insects.

bedfast. Unable or unwilling to leave the bed; bedridden.

bedlam. [From Hospital of St. Mary of Bethlehem, pronounced Bedlem in ME.] 1. An asylum for the insane. 2. Any place or situation characterized by a noisy uproar.

Bednar's aphthae. [Alois Bednar, physician in Vienna, 1816–1888] Infected, traumatic ulcers appearing on hard palate of infants. Usually caused by sucking infected objects.

bedpan [AS. *bedd,* bed, + *panna,* flat vessel]. A pan-shaped device placed under a bedridden patient for collecting and containing fecal and urinary excreta.

NOTE: In general, the use of a bedpan is uncomfortable and, because of the awkwardness of the position, requires more exertion on the patient's part than using a bedside toilet. Thus patients who are recovering from myocardial infarction and others should not be forced to use a bedpan if it is possible to move them from their bed to a bedside toilet.

bedrest. 1. A device for propping up patients in bed. 2. The confining of a patient to bed for rest.

bedridden. Unable or unwilling to leave the bed; bedfast.

bedsore [AS. *bedd,* bed, + *sare,* open wound]. Pressure sore; ischemic necrosis and ulceration of tissue, esp. over a bony prominence. Due to pressure from prolonged confinement in bed or from a cast or splint. The stages correspond to tissue layers. First stage consists of skin redness. The second stage shows redness, edema, and induration. In the third stage, the skin becomes necrotic, with exposure of fat. In the fourth stage, necrosis extends through the skin and fat to muscle; further fat and muscle necrosis characterize the fifth stage. In the sixth stage, bone destruction begins, progressing ultimately to osteomyelitis. SYN: *decubitus.*

Emaciated, weak, or elderly patients and those who must remain in one position because of orthopedic or similar problems are esp. likely to develop bedsores. Bedsores are located in areas over bony prominences that are thinly covered with flesh as the end of the spine, buttocks, heels, elbows, shoulder blades, and back of the head and ears in children.

PREDISPOSING CAUSES: Any factor that interferes with the circulation of the blood and mobility of the patient; prolonged fever; emaciation; obesity; paralysis; old age; poor nutrition; poorly made beds or those containing irritating bits of debris; lack of cleanliness; bruising; infrequent change of positions; cardiac diseases, nephritis, diabetes, or anemia.

TREATMENT: Prevention is easier than a cure; prophylactic measures in keeping the bed dry and clean; relieving the pressure as soon as the first signs of redness appear and reporting this occurrence to the nurse in charge or attending physician at once; use of the prescribed medication as directed by the physician. Thorough drying of skin after baths and gentle massage for stimulation of circulation; frequent change of position of patient if possible; maintenance of proper nutrition; chemical or surgical debridement of ulcers; use of sheepskin, or substitute, under vulnerable area; placing patient on special air bed, q.v., or flotation bed, q.v. Exposure to air and heat lamp are of questionable value.

bedwetting. Enuresis, q.v.

Beer's operation. [Georg Joseph Beer, Ger. ophthalmologist, 1763–1821] Flap operation for cataract or artificial pupil.

bee sting [AS. *beo,* bee, + *stingan,* to pierce]. Injury resulting from bee's venom. The stinger, which is barbed, usually remains in the wound. Pain, mottled redness, and edema result.

TREATMENT: Application of fairly strong household ammonia or baking soda paste. Remove stinger if present. If pain is severe, injection of 2% procaine solution. Antihistamines help to relieve discomfort.

NOTE: Some individuals are hypersensitive to bee venom and may suffer severe anaphylactic reactions leading to death. In such cases immediate subcutaneous or intravenous administration of epinephrine is indicated.

beeswax (bēz'wăks). Yellow wax obtained from honeycomb of bees. A purified form is used in ointments.

beeturia (bēt-ū'rē-ă). Pink to deep red col urine that sometimes follows eating of b

behavior [ME. *behaven,* to hold oneself

certain way]. 1. The manner in which one acts; the actions or reactions of individuals under specific circumstances. 2. Any response elicited from an organism.

behaviorism. A theory of conduct that regards normal and abnormal behavior as the result of conditioned reflexes quite apart from the concept of will. It does not apply to conditions resulting from structural disease.

behavior modification. Scientific analysis of behavior and its application. It is used to attempt to change in a systematic fashion maladaptive patterns of behavior. Cigarette smoking, obesity, and alcoholism are common disorders of self-control, the control of which may be possible through techniques of behavior modification.

Behçet's syndrome (bā'sĕts). [Hulusi Behçet, Turkish dermatologist, 1889–1948] A chronic recurrent disease characterized by ulceration of the mouth and genitalia, iritis, and joint pain. The joint pain usually comes later in the history of the disease than the ulcers of the mouth and genitalia. Iritis frequently is accompanied by conjunctivitis, episcleritis, keratitis, retinal thrombophlebitis, and optic atrophy. The central nervous system, heart, and intestinal tract may be involved. Onset is usually between 10 and 30 years of age, and males are affected 5 to 10 times more frequently than females. The period between attacks is irregular, but may be as short as days or as long as years. Needle punctures provoke inflammatory skin lesions, and for that reason should be avoided. Symptomatic therapy is of benefit, but there is no specific therapy for this disease of unknown etiology.

bejel (bĕj'ĕl). A nonvenereal form of syphilis endemic in Arab countries; it particularly affects children.

bel (bĕl). A unit of measurement of the intensity of sound. It is expressed as a logarithm of the ratio of two sounds of acoustic intensity, one of which is fixed or standard; the ratio is expressed in decibels, q.v.

belch [AS. *baelcan,* to eructate]. Escape of gas from the stomach through the mouth; to eructate.

belching. Raising of gas from the stomach.

ETIOL: Gastric fermentation; air swallowing; gas-containing foods.

belemnoid (bē-lĕm'noyd) [Gr. *belemnon,* dart, + *eidos,* shape]. Dart-shaped; styloid.

Bell, Sir Charles. Scottish physiologist and surgeon, 1774–1842.

B.'s law. Fact that anterior spinal nerve roots contain only motor fibers and posterior roots only sensory fibers. SYN: *Bell-Magendie's law.*

B.-Magendie's law. Bell's law, q.v.

B.'s nerve. Long thoracic nerve; nervus thoracicus longus [NA].

B.'s palsy. Unilateral facial paralysis of sudden onset. The cause is unknown but is presumed to involve swelling of the seventh (facial) nerve due to immune or viral disease, resulting in ischemia and compression of the nerve at the point where it leaves the bony tissue. Characterized by weakness of the entire half of the face followed by paralysis. The patient can not control salivation or lacrimation, and in severe cases can not close the eye on the affected side. Facial expression is distorted.

PROGNOSIS: Partial facial paralysis is invariably resolved within several months. Likelihood of complete recovery after total paralysis varies from 90% to 20%.

TREATMENT: Protection of exposed eye by temporary patching or use of methylcellulose drops. Definitive treatment is aimed at decompressing facial nerve before atrophy occurs. Corticosteroids, such as oral prednisone 60 to 80 mg./day for 1 week, which are then reduced over the second week, appear successful.

belladonna (bĕl"ă-dŏn'ă) [It., beautiful lady]. USP. An anticholinergic. Atropa belladonna, a poisonous plant with reddish flowers and shining black berries. Source of various alkaloids, including atropine and scopolamine. Used mainly for sedative and spasmolytic effects on gastrointestinal tract.

b. leaf. Powder from dried leaf and flowering top of Atropa belladonna Linné or A. belladonna acuminata. An anticholinergic agent, it is used generally in tincture form though the dry extract in tablet form may be used.

belladonna and atropine poisons. These include stramonium, hyoscyamus, scopolamine, belladonna, and atropine. SEE: *atropine* in *Poisons and Poisoning* in *Appendix.*

Bellini's tubules (bĕ-lē'nēz). [Lorenzo Bellini, It. anatomist, 1643–1704] The straight connecting tubules of the kidney.

bell-metal resonance. A metallic sound heard in pneumothorax when a coin placed on the chest wall is struck by another coin.

Bellocq's cannula (bĕl-ŏks'). [Jean J. Bellocq, Fr. surgeon, 1732–1807] An instrument for drawing in a plug through nostril and mouth to control epistaxis.

belly [AS. *baelg,* bag]. 1. The abdomen or abdominal cavity. 2. The fleshy, central portion of a muscle.

belly ache. Colic, gastralgia.

belly button. Umbilicus, q.v.; navel.

belonephobia (bĕl"ō-nĕ-fō'bē-ă) [Gr. *belone,* needle, + *phobos,* fear]. Morbid fear of sharp-pointed objects.

belonoid (bĕl'ō-noyd) [" + *eidos,* shape]. Needle-shaped.

belonoskiascopy (bĕl″ō-nō-skī-ăs′kō-pē) [″ + *skia*, shadow, + *skopein*, to see]. Subjective retinoscopy by means of shadows and movements to determine refraction.

Benadryl (bĕn′ă-drĭl). Trade name for diphenhydramine hydrochloride, USP, an antihistaminic agent.

Bence Jones protein. [Henry Bence Jones, Brit. physician, 1813–1873] Protein that occurs in urine of patients with multiple myeloma and occasionally in patients with other diseases of the reticuloendothelial system. When urine samples are heated to 50° to 60° C., a precipitate forms. This disappears when the urine is boiled and reappears when the urine cools.

Bender gestalt visual motor test. [Lauretta Bender, N.Y. psychiatrist, b. 1897] A test in which the subject copies a series of patterns. The results vary with the type of psychiatric disorder present.

Bendopa. Trade name for levodopa.

bendroflumethiazide (bĕn″drō-floo″mĕ-thī′ă-zīd). USP. A thiazide-type diuretic. Trade name is Naturetin.

bends. Painful condition in limbs and abdomen caused by bubbles of nitrogen in blood and tissues as a result of rapid reduction of air pressure. SEE: *caisson disease*.

Benedict's solution (bĕn′ĕ-dĭkts). [Stanley R. Benedict, U.S. chemist, 1844–1936] A solution used to test for presence of sugar. To 173 gm. sodium or potassium citrate and 100 gm. anhydrous sodium carbonate (dissolved in 700 ml. water) is added 17.3 gm. crystalline copper sulfate that has been dissolved in 100 ml. of water. Sufficient water is added to the mixture to make 1000 ml. SEE: *Benedict's test*.

Benedict's test. Add 8 drops of clear urine (filtered if necessary) to a test tube containing 5 ml. of Benedict's solution, q.v. Boil from 1 to 2 minutes, agitating the test tube during this time, and then allow it to cool undisturbed. Formation of red, yellow, olive green, or green precipitate indicates presence of sugar [2% or more (plus 4), 1% (plus 3), ¾% (plus 2), ½% (plus 1), respectively].

Benedikt's syndrome. [Moritz Benedikt, Austrian physician, 1835–1920] Hemiplegia with oculomotor paralysis and clonic spasm or tremor on opposite side. It is caused by lesions that damage the third nerve and involve the nucleus ruber and corticospinal tract.

Benemid. Trade name for probenecid.

benign (bē-nīn′) [L. *benignus*, mild]. Not recurrent or progressive. Opposite of malignant.

Bennett double-ring splint. Metal splint that slips on the finger and limits hyperextension of the proximal interphalangeal joint.

Bentyl. Trade name for dicyclomine hydrochloride.

bentonite (bĕn′tŏn-īt). [Fort Benton, U.S.A.] A hydrated aluminosilicate that forms a thick, slippery substance when water is added. Used as a suspending and clarifying agent. It may be heat-sterilized.

benzaldehyde (bĕn-zăl′dĕ-hīd). A pharmaceutical flavoring agent derived from oil of bitter almond.

benzalkonium chloride (bĕnz″ăl-kō′nē-ŭm klō′rīd). NF. An antimicrobial preservative. White or yellowish-white thick gel. Usually has a mild aromatic odor. In aqueous solution it has a bitter taste. Used as a detergent and germicide. Trade names are Zephiran Chloride, Roccal, and Hyamine 3500.

Benzedrine (bĕn′zĕ-drēn). Trade name for amphetamine sulfate.

benzene, benzin, benzine (bĕn′zēn, bĕn-zēn′, bĕn′zĭn) [*benz*(oin) + Gr. *ene*, suffix used in chemistry to denote unsaturated compound]. C_6H_6. A volatile liquid, immiscible with water and able to dissolve fats, that is used as a solvent. It is the simplest member of the aromatic series of hydrocarbons, and it is used in the synthesis of innumerable dyes and drugs. The phenyl radical, C_6H_6, will be recognized in the formulae for phenol, dimethylaminoazobenzene (see under azo compounds), and benzoic acid. SYN: *benzol*. SEE: *benzene* and *b. hexachloride* in *Poisons and Poisoning* in *Appendix*.

benzestrol (bĕn-zĕs′trŏl). USP. A synthetic estrogenic substance used orally.

benzethonium chloride (bĕn″zĕ-thō′nē-ŭm). USP. A synthetic quaternary ammonium detergent compound used as a disinfectant and antiseptic agent. It is incompatible with soap. Trade names are Hyamine 1622 and Phemerol Chloride.

benzidine (bĕn′zī-dīn). Compound used as a test to determine traces of blood in feces.

Prepare benzidine solution as follows: to a saturated solution of benzidine in glacial acetic acid add equal volume of 3% hydrogen peroxide and about 1 ml. of the suspected material. Appearance of a blue color indicates presence of blood.

A diet consisting of milk, crackers, and rice should be adhered to for at least 48 hours prior to the test. This permits clearing the intestinal tract of iron-containing foods so that feces can be tested for blood.

benzoate (bĕn′zō-āt). A salt of benzoic acid.

benzocaine (bĕn′zō-kān). USP. Local anesthetic, ethyl aminobenzoate, used topically. Trade name is Americaine.

benzodiazepine (bĕn″zō-dī-ăz′ĕ-pēn). A general term to describe a group of minor tranquilizing drugs with similar chemical structure and pharmaceutical activity.

benzoic acid. USP. $C_7H_6O_2$. A white crystalline material having a slight odor. Used in keratolytic ointments, and as a food preservative. Saccharin is a derivative of this acid.

benzoin (bĕn′zoyn, -zō-ĭn) [Fr. *benjoin*]. USP. A balsamic resin obtained from various species of a tree, Styrax, esp. S. benzoin or S. paralleloneuris. Used as a stimulant expectorant, as an inhalant in laryngitis and bronchitis, or as a protective coating for ulcers, etc.

benzol. Benzene.

benzonatate (bĕn-zō′nă-tāt). USP. Medicine chemically related to procaine that is used in anticough preparations. Trade name is Tessalon.

benzoylpas calcium. USP. An antibacterial drug used as a tuberculostatic.

benzoyl peroxide. USP. A keratolytic agent. Trade names are Benoxyl and Persadox.

benzthiazide (bĕnz-thī′ă-zīd). USP. A diuretic agent. Trade names are Aquatag and Exna.

benztropine mesylate (bĕnz′trō-pēn). USP. An antiparasympathomimetic agent usually used with other drugs in treating parkinsonism. Trade name is Cogentin.

benzyl. The hydrocarbon radical of benzyl alcohol and various other compounds.

b. benzoate. USP. An aromatic, clear, colorless oily liquid with a sharp, burning taste. Used as a topical scabicide. Trade name is Benylate.

benzylpenicillin procaine (bĕn″zĭl-pĕn-ĭ-sĭl′ ĭn). Penicillin G procaine.

beolocator. Device for locating and detecting hard metallic and nonmetallic objects in human tissues. When one end of the device comes in contact with the object being sought, the sound made is amplified. May be used in detecting a foreign body in the uterus, such as an I.U.D.

Bérard's aneurysm (bā-rărz′). [Auguste Bérard, Fr. surgeon, 1802–1846] An arteriovenous aneurysm in the tissues surrounding the injured vein.

Béraud's valve (bā-rōz′). [Bruno J. J. Béraud, Fr. surgeon, 1823–1865] Fold of mucous membrane of the lacrimal sac at the junction of the lacrimal duct. SYN: *Krause's valve.*

berdache (bĕr-dăsh′) [Fr.]. An individual of a definite sex, male or female, who assumes the *status* and *role* of the opposite sex and who is viewed by the community as being of one physiologic sex but as having assumed the *status* and *role* of the opposite sex. Transvestism is not synonymous with berdache, nor is homosexual behavior necessarily a component of this condition.

beriberi (bĕr′ē-bĕr′ē) [Singhalese *beri*, weakness]. A disease caused by deficiency of thiamine in diet. Characterized by peripheral neurologic, cerebral, and cardiovascular abnormalities. Early deficiency produces fatigue, irritation, poor memory, sleep disturbances, precordial pain, anorexia, abdominal discomfort, and constipation. Endemic in the Orient, Philippines and other islands of the Pacific, and formerly in rice-growing sections of the U.S. SYN: *neuritis, dietetic; neuritis, endemic.*

ETIOL: Subsistence on highly polished rice, which has lost all thiamine content through the milling process. Secondary deficiency can arise from decreased absorption, impaired absorption, or impaired utilization of thiamine.

TREATMENT: Oral or parenteral administration of thiamine; establishment of a properly balanced diet.

Berkefeld filter (bĕr′kē-fĕld). [Wilhelm Berkefeld, Ger. manufacturer, 1836–1897] A filter of diatomaceous earth designed to allow virus-size particles to pass through.

berkelium (bĕrk′lē-ŭm). [U. of California at Berkeley, where first produced] SYMB: Bk. At. wt. of best-known isotope is 247; at. no. 97. A transuranium element.

Bernard's duct (bĕr-nărz′). [Claude Bernard, Fr. physiologist, 1813–1878] An accessory pancreatic duct; ductus pancreaticus accessorius [NA].

Bernard's glandular layer. Inner layer of cells lining acini of pancreas.

Bertin, columns of (bĕr′tăn). [Exupère Joseph Bertin, Fr. anatomist, 1712–1781] Renal cortical columns supporting the blood vessels in the kidneys. The part that separates the medullary pyramids. Also called columnae renales [NA].

Bertin's ligament. Iliofemoral ligament.

berylliosis (bĕr″ĭl-lē-ō′sĭs) [*beryllium* + Gr. *osis*, condition]. Beryllium poisoning, usually of the lungs. The beryllium particles cause fibrosis and granulomata at any site whether inhaled or accidentally introduced into or under the skin.

beryllium (bĕ-rĭl′ē-ŭm) [Gr. *beryllos*, beryl]. SYMB: Be. At. wt. 9.0122; at. no. 4; sp. gr. 1.848. A metallic element.

bestiality (bĕs-tē-ăl′ĭ-tē) [L. *bestia*, beast]. Sexual intercourse with an animal. SYN: *zooerasty.*

beta (bā′tă). 1. Second letter of Gr. alphabet, written β. 2. Used as a prefix to chemical words to note isomeric variety or position in compounds of substituted groups.

beta-adrenergic blocking agent. A substance that interferes with the transmission of stimuli through pathways that normally allow sympathetic nervous inhibiting stimuli to be effective.

beta-adrenergic receptor. A site in autonomic nerve pathways wherein inhibitory responses occur when adrenergic agents such as norepinephrine and epinephrine are released.

beta cells. 1. Basophilic cells in the anterior lobe of pituitary that give a positive periodic acid stain reaction. 2. Cells of the islets of Langerhans of the pancreas that secrete insulin.

betacism (bā'tă-sĭzm) [Gr. *beta*, the letter b, + *-ismos*, condition]. Speech defect giving the *b* sound to other consonants.

Betadine. Trade name for povidone-iodine, a topical anti-infective.

betaine hydrochloride (bē'tā-ĭn) [L. *beta*, beet]. A colorless crystalline substance containing 23% hydrochloric acid. It is obtained from an alkaloid found in the beet and other plants. Used orally as a source of hydrochloric acid in treating hypochlorhydria.

beta-lactamase resistance. Term used to describe microorganisms that produce the enzyme beta-lactamase and thus have the ability to resist the action of certain types of antibiotics including penicillin. The enzyme, also called penicillinase, inactivates some but not all forms of penicillin.

Betalin S. Trade name for thiamine hydrochloride.

betamethasone (bā"tă-mĕth'ă-sōn). USP. A synthetic glucocorticoid that has the pharmaceutical actions of cortisone. Various preparations and dose forms including an ointment or cream for topical application are available. Trade name is Celestone.

Betapar. Trade name for meprednisone.

beta particles, rays. Negatively charged particles emitted by radium; more penetrating than alpha rays. Absorbed by 1 mm. lead or 0.6 mm. platinum. SEE: *electron*.

beta subunit. Glycoprotein hormones containing two different polypeptide subunits designated α and β chains. Analysis of the units of these hormones—follicle-stimulating, luteinizing, chorionic gonadotropin, and thyrotropin—enables early diagnosis of such conditions as early pregnancy and ectopic pregnancy.

betatron (bā'tă-trŏn). A circular electron accelerator that produces either high-energy electrons or x-rays.

betazole hydrochloride (bā'tă-zōl). USP. An isomer of histamine. It is used intramuscularly to attempt to stimulate gastric secretion. Contraindicated in persons who have atopic allergy. Trade name is Histalog.

bethanechol chloride (bĕ-thā'nĕ-kōl). USP. Cholinergic drug used in treating paralytic ileus and also in treating urinary retention not caused by organic disease. Trade names are Urecholine and Duvoid.

Betz cells. [Vladimir A. Betz, Russ. anatomist, 1834–1894] A form of giant pyramidal cell in the cortical motor area of the brain. The axons of these cells are included in the pyramidal tract.

bezoar (bē'zor) [Arabic *bazahr*, protecting against poison]. A hard mass of entangled material sometimes found in the stomachs and intestines of animals and man as a hairball (trichobezoar), hair and vegetable fiberball (trichophytobezoar), and foodball (phytobezoar).

b., balloon. An inflated balloon that is left in the stomach as an artificial bezoar. This experimental technique is used in treating obesity.

BFP. *biologically false positive*.

Bi. Chem. symb. for bismuth.

bi- (bī) [L. *bis*, twice]. Prefix indicating two, double, twice.

biarticular (bī"ăr-tĭk'ū-lăr) [" + *articulus*, joint]. Pert. to two joints; diarthric.

bibasic (bī-bā'sĭk) [" + Gr. *basis*, foundation]. Pert. to an acid with two hydrogen atoms replaceable by bases to form salts.

bibliomania (bĭb"lē-ō-mā'nē-ă) [Gr. *biblion*, book, + *mania*, madness]. Obsession with the collecting of books.

bibliotherapy (bĭb"lē-ō-thĕr'ă-pē) [" + *therapeia*, treatment]. A form of nonphysical and nonviolent occupational therapy wherein the patient is induced to read books. Used in treating mental illness.

bibulous (bĭb'ū-lŭs) [L. *bibulus*, from *bibere*, to drink]. Possessing the ability to absorb moisture.

bicameral (bī-kăm'ĕr-ăl) [L. *bis*, twice, + *camera*, a chamber]. Having two cavities or chambers.

bicapsular (bī-kăp'sū-lăr) [" + *capsula*, container]. Having two capsules.

bicarbonate (bī-kăr'bō-nāt). Any salt containing the HCO_3 (bicarbonate) anion. SEE: *carbonic acid*.

b., blood. Bicarbonate in the blood. The amount present is an indicator of the alkali reserve.

bicellular (bī-sĕl'ū-lăr) [" + *cellularis*, little cell]. 1. Composed of two cells. 2. Having two chambers or compartments.

biceps (bī'sĕps) [" + *caput*, head]. A muscle with two heads.

b. brachii. Muscle of the upper arm, having two heads. Flexes arm and forearm and supinates hand.

b. femoris. One of the hamstring muscles lying on posterior lateral side of thigh. Flexes knee and rotates it outward.

biceps reflex. Normal contraction of biceps muscle when tendon is percussed.

Bichat, Marie François X. (bē-shă'). French physiologist and anatomist, 1771–1802. Founder of scientific histology and pathological anatomy.

B.'s canal. The subarachnoid canal, which

extends from the third ventricle to the middle of Bichat's fissure and carries the veins of Galen.

B.'s fat ball. Mass of fat behind the buccinator muscle.

B.'s fissure. The horseshoe fissure separating the cerebrum from the cerebellum.

B.'s ligament. Lower fasciculus of the posterior sacroiliac ligament.

B.'s tunic. The tunica intima of the blood vessels.

bichloride of mercury (bī-klō'rīd). $HgCl_2$. Corrosive mercuric chloride; a crystalline salt. SEE: *mercuric chloride; mercuric chloride poisoning; mercuric chloride* in *Poisons and Poisoning* in *Appendix.*

bicipital (bī-sĭp'ĭ-tăl) [L. *biceps,* two heads]. 1. Pert. to a muscle having two heads. 2. Having two heads.

BiCNU. Trade name for carmustine, q.v.

biconcave (bī-kŏn'kāv) [L. *bis,* twice, + *concavus,* concave]. Concave on each side, esp. as a type of lens. SEE: illus.

biconvex (bī-kŏn'vĕks) [" + *convexus,* rounded raised surface]. Convex on two sides, esp. as a type of lens. SEE: illus.

bicornate, bicornis (bī-kor'nāt, -nĭs) [" + *cornutus,* horned]. Having two processes or hornlike projections.

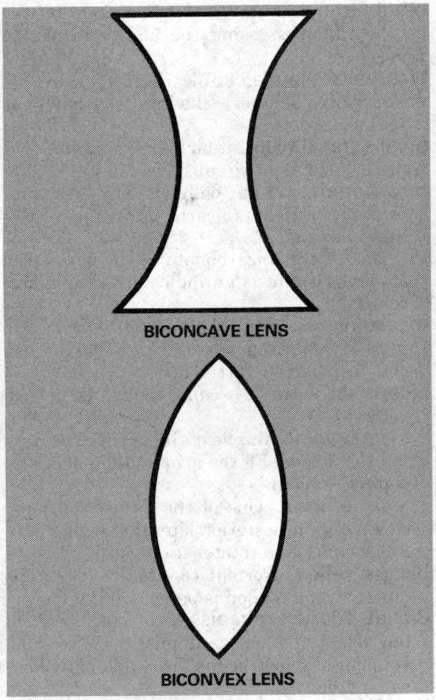

BICONCAVE LENS

BICONVEX LENS

bicornis uterus. Anomalous uterus resulting from incomplete union of the müllerian ducts. May be double or single organ with two horns.

bicoronal (bī"kō-rō'năl) [" + Gr. *korone,* crown]. Pert. to the two coronas.

bicorporate (bī-kor'pō-rāt) [" + *corpus,* body]. Having two bodies.

bicuspid (bī-kŭs'pĭd) [" + *cuspis,* point]. Having two cusps or projections or having two cusps or leaflets.

bicuspid tooth. Premolar tooth; a permanent tooth with two cusps on the grinding surface and a flattened root. There are four premolars in each jaw, two on either side between the canine and molars. SEE: *tooth.*

biscuspid valve. Valve between the left atrium and left ventricle of the heart. SYN: *mitral valve.* SEE: *heart.*

bicycle ergometer. Stationary bicycle used in determining the amount of work performed by the rider.

b.i.d. L. *bis in die,* twice daily.

bidet (bē-dā') [Fr., a small horse]. A basin designed so that one may sit astride it. There are attachments that allow a stream of water to flow over the genital and perineal area. Thus a bidet provides an excellent means of cleaning the perineum. SEE: illus.

biduous (bĭd'ū-ŭs) [L. *bis,* twice, + *dies,* a day]. Continuing for two days.

Bielschowsky disease (bē"ĕl-shō'skē). [Max Bielschowsky, Ger. neuropathologist, 1869–1940] Early juvenile type of cerebral sphingolipidosis.

bifacial (bī-fā'shē-ăl) ["+ *facies,* face]. Having similar opposite surfaces.

bifid (bī'fĭd) [" + *findere,* to cleave]. Cleft or split into two parts.

bifid spine. Congenital fissure of vertebral column. SYN: *spina bifida,* q.v.

bifid tongue. Cleft tongue.

bifocal (bī-fō'kăl) [" + *focus,* hearth]. Having two foci, as bifocal eyeglasses.

bifocal glasses. Eyeglasses that combine two lenses with different refracting powers, one for distant and one for near vision. Often prescribed for presbyopia, q.v.

bifurcate, bifurcated (bī'fŭr-kāt['d], bī-fŭr'kāt['d]) [" + *furca,* fork]. Having two branches or divisions; forked.

bifurcation (bī-fŭr-kā'shŭn). A separation into two branches; the point of forking.

bigemina (bī-jĕm'ĭ-nă) [L.]. Pl. of bigeminum.

bigeminal (bī-jĕm'ĭ-năl) [L. *bigeminum,* twin]. Double, paired.

bigeminal pulse. Pulse in which two beats follow each other in rapid succession, each group of two being separated by a longer pause. The initial beat is regarded as the normal one and is usually of greater inten-

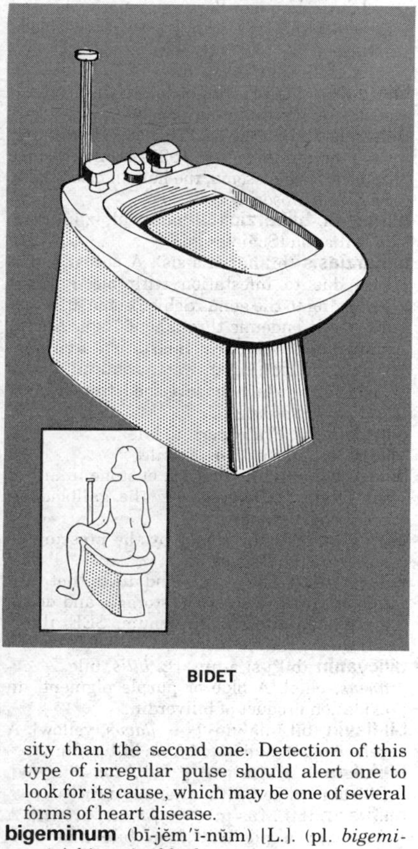

BIDET

sity than the second one. Detection of this type of irregular pulse should alert one to look for its cause, which may be one of several forms of heart disease.

bigeminum (bī-jĕm′ĭ-nŭm) [L.]. (pl. *bigemina)* A bigeminal body.

bigeminy (bī-jĕm′ĭ-nē). The condition of occurring in pairs, esp. bigeminal pulse, q.v.

bilabe (bī′lāb) [L. *bis*, twice, + *labium*, lip]. Thin, long device equipped with a hinged lower jaw. It is introduced into the bladder via the urethra for the purpose of removing small calculi from the bladder.

bilateral (bī-lăt′ĕr-ăl) [" + *latus*, side]. Pert. to, affecting, or rel. to two sides.

bilateralism (bī-lăt′ĕr-ăl-ĭzm) [" + " + Gr. *-ismos*, condition]. Bilateral symmetry, q.v.

bilateral symmetry. Symmetry of paired organs or an organism whose right and left halves are mirror images of each other or in which a median longitudinal section divides the organism into equivalent right and left halves. SYN: *bilateralism*.

bile (bīl) [L. *bilis*, bile]. A secretion of the liver. It is a thick, viscid fluid with a bitter taste that passes from the bile duct of the liver into the common bile duct and then into the duodenum as needed. The bile from the liver is straw color, while that from the gallbladder varies from yellow to brown and green.

Bile also is stored in the gallbladder, drawn upon as needed, and discharged into the duodenum. Contraction of the gallbladder is brought about by a hormone, cholecystokinin, produced by the duodenum, its secretion being stimulated by the entrance of fatty foods into the duodenum. Added to water, bile decreases surface tension, giving a foamy solution favoring the emulsification of fats and oils; this action is due to the bile salts, mainly sodium glycocholate and taurocholate.

COMP: Bile pigments (principally bilirubin, q.v., and biliverdin, q.v.) are responsible for the variety of colors observed. In addition, bile contains cholesterol, lecithin, mucin, and other organic and inorganic substances.

FUNCT: Its importance as a digestive juice is due to its emulsifying action, which facilitates the digestion of fats in the intestines by pancreatic steapsin, plus a further effect of the bile salts, which form compounds with the fatty acids and are necessary for their absorption. Bile also stimulates peristalsis. Normally the ejection of bile occurs only during duodenal digestion. Bile is both an antiseptic and a purgative. About 800 to 1000 ml./24 hr. are secreted in the normal adult. SEE: *gallbladder*.

PATH: Interference with the flow of bile produces jaundice, resulting in unabsorbed fats being found in the feces. In such instances, fats should be restricted in the diet. Gallstones also may be produced in the gallbladder when the free flow of bile from the gallbladder is impeded or when pathological conditions interfere with bile production.

TESTS: There are several methods of testing for bile in the urine.

Gmelin's Test: A depth of 1 in. (2.54 cm.) of concentrated nitric acid is carefully overlaid with the sample of urine. Bile is present when there is a play of colors at the junction of the fluids. This test also can be carried out by pouring some urine onto blotting or filter paper and then placing a drop of concentrated nitric acid on the moist paper. From the spreading edge of the drop of acid, a ring of various colors will develop in which green predominates and forms the outer band.

Iodine Test: Pour urine into a test tube to a depth of 1 in. (2.5 cm.) and carefully overlay it with dilute tincture of iodine. A bright green ring will appear at the junction of the fluids if bile is present.

RS: "bili-" words; "chol-" words; stercobilin; urobilin.

bile acids. Complex acids, of which cholic, glycocholic, and taurocholic acids are examples, and which occur as salts in bile. They give bile its foamy character, are important in the digestion of fats in the intestine, and are reabsorbed from the intestine to be used again by the liver. This circulation of bile acids is called the enterohepatic circulation. In Hay's test for bile acids, some urine is placed in a watchglass and a little powdered sulfur is sprinkled on the surface. If bile acids are present, the sulfur sinks because of the lowering of the surface tension by the bile salts.

bile ducts. Intercellular biliary passages conveying the bile from the liver to the hepatic duct, which joins the duct from the gallbladder (cystic duct) to form the common bile duct (ductus choledochus), and which enters the duodenum about 3 in. (7.6 cm.) below the pylorus. SEE: illus.; *duct, common bile; duct, cystic; duct, hepatic; gallbladder.*

bile pigments. Complex, highly colored substances found in bile derived from the red pigment (hemoglobin) of the blood and imparting brown color to intestinal contents and feces. Van den Bergh's test, q.v., is used to detect the type of bilirubin in the blood serum.

Ex.: bilirubin, biliverdin.

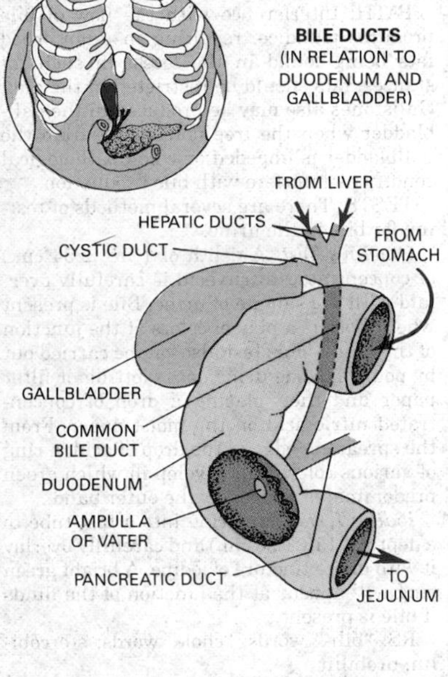

BILE DUCTS (IN RELATION TO DUODENUM AND GALLBLADDER)

bile salts. Alkali salts of bile sodium glycocholate and sodium taurocholate.

Bilharzia (bĭl-hăr′zē-ă). [Theodor M. Bilharz, Ger. helminthologist 1825–1862] Former name for Schistosoma, the human blood fluke. SEE: *Schistosoma.*

bilharzial, bilharzic (bĭl-hăr′zē-ăl, -zĭk). Pert. to Bilharzia (Schistosoma).

bilharziasis (bĭl″hăr-zī′ă-sĭs). A parasitic disease due to infestation with blood flukes belonging to the genus Schistosoma, q.v. The disease is endemic throughout Asia, Africa, and tropical America. Infestation occurs by wading or bathing in water containing cercaria, q.v., which have issued from snails. SYN: *schistosomiasis.*

bili- [L. *bilis*]. Prefix pert. to bile.

biliary (bĭl′ē-ăr-ē). Pert. to bile.

biliary calculus. Formation of stone in any of the biliary passages or in the gallbladder. SYN: *cholelithiasis.*

biliary colic. Pain caused by the pressure or passing of gallstones.

biliary tract. The organs and ducts that participate in the secretion, storage, and delivery of bile into the duodenum. SEE: illus.; *bile ducts; gallbladder; liver.*

bilicyanin (bĭl″ĭ-sī′ă-nĭn) [L. *bilis,* bile, + *cyaneus,* blue]. A blue or purple pigment, an oxidation product of biliverdin.

biliflavin (bĭl″ĭ-flā′vĭn) [″ + *flavus,* yellow]. A yellow pigment derived from biliverdin.

bilifulvin (bĭl″ĭ-fŭl′vĭn) [″ + *fulvus,* tawny]. Bilirubin mixed with other substances.

bilifuscin (bĭl″ĭ-fŭs′ĭn) [″ + *fuscus,* brown]. A dark brown pigment from bile and gallstones.

biligenesis (bĭl″ĭ-jĕn′ĕ-sĭs) [″ + Gr. *genesis,* origin]. The formation of bile.

biligenetic, biligenic (bĭl″ĭ-jĕn-ĕt′ĭk, -jĕn′ĭk) [″ + Gr. *gennan,* to produce]. Forming bile.

bilihumin (bĭl″ĭ-hū′mĭn) [″ + *humus,* earth]. A dark insoluble residue that may remain after applying solvents to bile or gallstones.

bilineurine (bĭl″ĭ-nū′rĭn) [″ + Gr. *neuron,* nerve]. Choline, q.v.

bilious (bĭl′yŭs) [L. *bilosus*]. 1. Pert. to bile. 2. Afflicted with biliousness.

bilious fever. Fever with vomiting of bile.

biliousness (bĭl′yŭs-nĕs). 1. A symptom of a disordered condition of the liver causing constipation, headache, loss of appetite, and vomiting of bile. 2. Excess of bile; bilious fever.

biliprasin (bĭl″ĭ-prā′sĭn) [″ + Gr. *prason,* green]. Green pigment similar to biliverdin and found in bile.

bilirachia (bĭl-ĭ-rā′kē-ă) [″ + Gr. *rhachis,* spine].

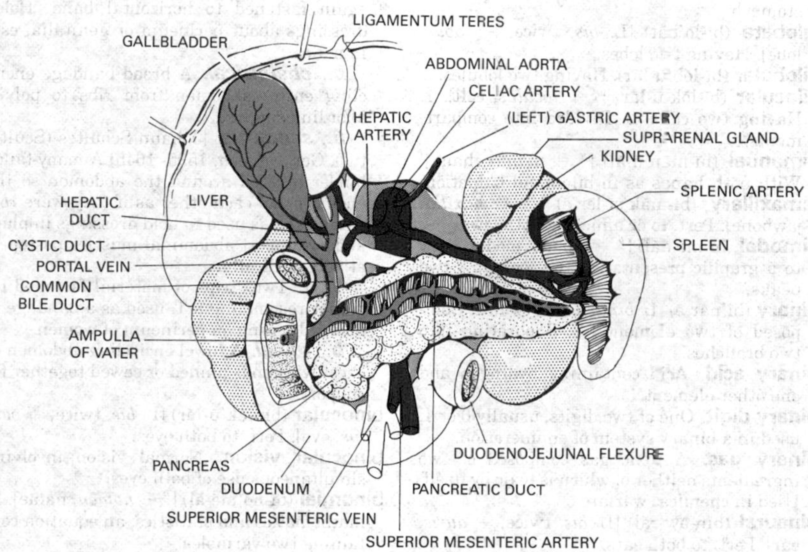

BILIARY TRACT (IN RELATION TO LIVER, PANCREAS, AND DUODENUM)

Presence of bile in the spinal fluid.

bilirubin (bĭl-ĭ-roo'bĭn) [" + *ruber,* red]. $C_{33}H_{36}O_6N_4$. The orange-colored or yellowish pigment in bile. It is carried to the liver by the blood. It is produced from hemoglobin of red blood cells by reticuloendothelial cells in bone marrow, in the spleen, and elsewhere. It is changed chemically in the liver and excreted in the bile through the duodenum. As it passes through the intestines it is converted into urobilinogen by bacterial enzymes, most of it being excreted through the feces. If urobilinogen passes into the circulation it is excreted through the urine or re-excreted in the bile. It is the accumulation of bilirubin that leads to jaundice in many cases, esp. to physiologic jaundice of the newborn.

b., direct. Bilirubin conjugated by the liver cells to form bilirubin diglucuronide, which is water-soluble.

b., indirect. Unconjugated bilirubin that is present in the blood. It is fat-soluble.

bilirubinate (bĭl-ĭ-roo'bĭn-āt). A salt of bilirubin.

bilirubinemia (bĭl"ĭ-roo-bĭn-ē'mē-ă) [" + *ruber,* red, + Gr. *haima,* blood]. Presence of bilirubin in blood. Bilirubin is normally present in small amounts. However, in certain pathological conditions in which excessive destruction of red blood cells occurs, or in which there is interference with bile excretion, the amount is increased. In the newborn infant with erythroblastosis fetalis and greatly elevated bilirubin, exchange transfusion may be required.

bilirubinuria (bĭl"ĭ-roo-bĭn-ū'rē-ă) [" + " + Gr. *ouron,* urine]. Presence of bilirubin in urine.

biliuria (bĭl-ĭ-ū'rē-ă). Presence of bile in the urine.

biliverdin (bĭl-ĭ-vĕr'dĭn) [" + Gr. *viridis,* green]. $C_{33}H_{34}O_6N_4$. A greenish pigment in bile formed by the oxidation of bilirubin.

billion [Fr. *bi,* two, + *million,* million]. 1. In the U.S.A., billion is a number equal to 1 followed by 9 zeroes (1,000,000,000 or 10^9). 2. In Europe, billion is a number equal to 1 followed by 12 zeros (10^{12}), i.e., bi million, or twice the number of zeroes in a million (10^6).

Billroth's operation(s). [C. A. Theodore Billroth, Austrian surgeon, 1829–1894]. Gastrectomy.

Billroth I: Excision of the pylorus of the stomach with anastomosis of the upper portion of the stomach to the duodenum.

Billroth II: Subtotal excision of the stomach with closure of the proximal end of the duodenum and side-to-side anastomosis of the jejunum to the remaining portion of the stomach.

bilobate (bī-lō'bāt) [L. *bis,* twice, + *lobus,* lobe]. Having two lobes.

bilobular (bī-lŏb'ū-lăr). Having two lobules.

bilocular (bī-lŏk'ū-lăr) [" + *loculus,* cell]. 1. Having two cells. 2. Divided into compartments.

bimanual (bī-măn'ū-ăl) [" + *manus,* hand]. With both hands as in bimanual palpation.

bimaxillary (bī-măk'sĭ-lĕr"ē) [" + *maxilla,* jawbone]. Pert. to or afflicting both jaws.

bimodal (bī-mō'dăl) [" + *modus,* mode]. Pert. to a graphic presentation that contains two peaks.

binary (bī'năr-ē) [L. *binarius,* of two]. 1. Composed of two elements. 2. Separating into two branches.

binary acid. Acid containing hydrogen and one other element.

binary digit. One of two digits, usually 0 or 1, used in a binary system of enumeration.

binary gas. A toxic gas composed of two ingredients neither of which is toxic by itself. Used in chemical warfare.

binaural (bĭn-aw'răl) [L. *bis,* twice, + *auris,* ear]. Pert. to both ears.

binauricular (bĭn"aw-rĭk'ū-lăr) [" + *auricula,* little ear]. Binaural; pert. to both auricles of the ear.

binder (bīnd'ĕr) [AS. *bindan,* to tie up]. A broad bandage most commonly used as an encircling support of abdomen or chest. SEE: *bandage.*

b., abdominal. A wide band fastened snugly about the abdomen for support.

b., chest. A broad band used for encircling the chest to apply heat, dressings, or pressure, and for supporting the breasts. Improved by using shoulder straps to keep the binder from slipping.

b., double-T. A horizontal band about the waist to which two vertical bands are attached in back, brought around leg, and again fastened to horizontal band. Holds dressings about perineum or genitalia, esp. in males.

b., obstetrical. A broad bandage encircling entire abdomen from ribs to pelvis, affording support.

b., scultetus. [Johann Schultes (Scultetus), Ger. surgeon, 1595–1645] A many-tailed binder applied around the abdomen so the ends overlap each other as if they were roof shingles. It is used to hold dressings in place and to support abdominal muscles postoperatively. SEE: illus.

b., T. Two strips of material fastened together resembling a T, used as a bandage to hold a dressing on perineum of women.

b., towel. A towel encircling abdomen or chest with ends pinned or sewed together for support.

binocular (bĭn-ŏk'ū-lăr) [L. *bis,* twice, + *oculus,* eye]. Pert. to both eyes.

binocular vision. Normal vision involving simultaneous use of both eyes.

binomial (bī-nō'mē-ăl) [" + *nomen,* name]. In mathematics and statistics, an equation containing two variables.

binotic (bĭn-ŏt'ĭk) [" + Gr. *ous,* ear]. Pert. to or having two ears. SYN: *binaural.*

binovular (bĭn-ŏv'ū-lăr) [" + *ovum,* egg]. Derived from or pert. to two ova. SYN: *biovular.*

binuclear, binucleate (bī-nū'klē-ăr, -āt) [" + *nucleus,* kernel]. Having two nuclei.

bio- [Gr. *bios,* life]. Prefix indicating relationship to life.

bioassay (bī"ō-ăs'ā) [" + O. Fr. *asaier,* to try]. In pharmacology, the determination of the strength of a drug or substance by comparing its effect on a live animal or an isolated organ preparation to the effect of a standard preparation.

bioastronautics (bī"ō-ăs"trō-naw'tĭks). Study of the effects of space travel on living plants and animals.

SCULTETUS BINDER

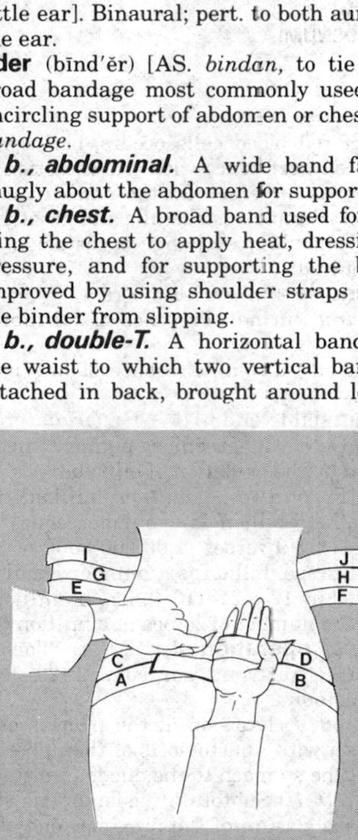

A MULTIPLE-TAIL BINDER APPLIED SEQUENTIALLY STARTING AT THE END SHOWN. EACH TAIL IS PULLED FIRM AND THEN OVERLAPPED BY THE NEXT ONE. THEY MAY BE HELD IN PLACE BY SAFETY PINS OR ADHESIVE TAPE. THIS BINDER IS UNSUITABLE FOR USE ON THE CHEST DUE TO MOVEMENT DURING BREATHING

bioavailability (bī″ō-ă-vāl″ă-bĭl′ĭ-tē). The rate and extent to which an active drug or metabolite enters the general circulation, thereby permitting access to the site of action. Bioavailability is determined either by measuring the concentration of the drug in body fluids or by the magnitude of the pharmacologic response.

biocatalyst (bī-ō-kăt′ă-lĭst) [″ + *katalyein,* to dissolve]. An enzyme; a biochemical catalyzer.

biochemical marker. Any biochemical compound such as an antigen, antibody, abnormal enzyme, or hormone that is sufficiently altered in a disease to serve as an aid in diagnosis or in predicting susceptibility to the disease.

biochemistry [″ + *chemeia,* chemistry]. The chemistry of living things; the science of the chemical changes accompanying the vital functions of plants and animals.

biochemorphology (bī″ō-kē-mor-fŏl′ō-jē) [″ + ″ + *morphe,* shape, + *logos,* study]. Science of the relationship between chemical structure and biological action.

biocide (bī′ō-sīd) [″ + L. *caedere,* to kill]. A substance, esp. a pesticide or antibiotic, capable of destroying living organisms.

bioclimatology (bī″ō-klī-mă-tŏl′ō-jē) [″ + *klima,* climate, + *logos,* study]. Study of the relationship of climate to life.

biocolloid (bī″ō-kŏl′oyd) [″ + *kollodes,* glutinous]. A colloid from animal, vegetable, or microbial tissue.

biodegradable. Susceptible to degradation by biological processes, such as bacterial or enzymatic action.

biodegradation (bī″ō-dĕg″rē-dā′shŭn). The breakdown of organic materials into simple chemicals by biochemical processes. Also called biological degradation.

biodynamics (bī″ō-dī-năm′ĭks) [Gr. *bios,* life, + *dynamis,* force]. The science of the force or energy of living matter.

bioelectronics (bī″ō-ē″lĕk-trŏn′ĭks). Study of the transfer of electrons between molecules in biological systems.

bioenergetics (bī″ō-ĕn″ĕr-jĕt′ĭks). Study of energy transfer and relationships between all living systems.

biofeedback. A training program designed to develop one's ability to control one's autonomic (involuntary) nervous system. After learning the technique, the patient may be able to control heart rate, blood pressure, and skin temperature or to relax certain muscles. The patient learns by using monitoring devices that sound a tone when changes in pulse, blood pressure, brain waves, and muscle contractions occur. Then the patient attempts to reproduce the conditions that caused the desired changes.

biogenesis (bī″ō-jĕn′ĕ-sĭs) [″ + *genesis,* origin]. Accepted theory that life can only originate from pre-existing life and never from nonliving material.

biogenetic. Pert. to biogenesis.

biogenic amines. An imprecise term for chemical substances that alter cerebral and vascular function. Included in this grouping are dopamine, epinephrine, norepinephrine, and serotonin.

biokinetics (bī″ō-kī-nĕt′ĭks) [″ + *kinetikos,* moving]. The study of growth changes and movements in developing organisms.

biologic, biological [″ + *logos,* study]. Pert. to biology.

biological degradation. The breakdown of organic materials into simple chemicals by biochemical processes.

biological rhythms. SEE: *clock, biological.*

biologicals. General term applied to medicinal compounds that are prepared from living organisms and their products. Includes serums, vaccines, antigens, and antitoxins.

biological warfare. ABBR: BW. Warfare in which disease-producing microorganisms or organic biocides are deliberately used to destroy, injure, or immobilize livestock, vegetation, or human life.

Ex.: anthrax, brucellosis, plague. SEE: *chemical warfare.*

biologic half-life. The time required to reduce the concentration of a drug in the blood, plasma, or serum by 50%. This is a measure of drug distribution and elimination. SEE: pharmacokinetics.

biologist. A specialist in biology.

biology (bī-ŏl′ō-jē) [Gr. *bios,* life, + *logos,* study]. Science of life and living things.

bioluminescence (bī″ō-loo″mĭ-nĕs′ĕns) [″ + L. *lumen,* light]. Emission of visible light from living organisms. The best known example is the cold light produced by fireflies. SEE: *luciferase.*

biolysis (bī-ŏl′ĭ-sĭs) [″ + *lysis,* dissolution]. Chemical decomposition of living tissue by the action of living organisms.

biolytic (bī-ō-lĭt′ĭk). Pert. to biolysis. Capable of destroying life.

biomass (bī′ō-măs) [″ + L. *massa,* mass]. All of the living organisms in a specified area.

biome (bī′ōm) [″ + *oma,* mass]. The totality of living organisms in a specified ecological area.

biomechanics (bī″ō-mē-kăn′ĭks). The application of mechanical forces to living organisms. Includes forces that arise from within and outside the body. SEE: *kinesiology.*

biomedical. Biological and medical; pert. to application of natural sciences to the study of medicine.

biomedical engineering. Application of the principles and practices of engineering science to biomedical research and health care.

Ex.: Development of devices such as cardiac pacemakers, hearing aids, and sophisticated artificial limbs and joints.

biometeorology (bī″ō-mē″tē-or-ŏl′ŏ-jē) [″ + *meteoros*, raised from off the ground, + *logos*, study]. Study of the effects of meteorology on all forms of life.

biometrics (bī″ō-mĕt′rĭks). Study of the application of mathematics and statistics to the analysis and solution of problems in the fields of biology and other health sciences.

biometry (bī-ŏm′ĕ-trē) [″ + *metron*, measure]. 1. Application of statistics to biological science. 2. Computation of life expectancy.

biomicroscope (bī″ō-mī′krō-skōp). A microscope used with a slit lamp for viewing segments of the living eye.

bion (bī′ŏn) [Gr. *bios*, life]. Any living organism.

bionergy (bī-ŏn′ĕr-jē) [″ + *ergon*, work]. Vital energy or life force.

bionics (bī-ŏn′ĭks). Study of biological functions and mechanisms and the application of these findings to the design of machines, esp. computers.

bionomics (bī″ō-nŏm′ĭks) [″ + *nomos*, law]. Ecology, q.v.

bionomy (bī-ŏn′ŏ-mē) The science pert. to life processes. SEE: *ecology; physiology.*

bionosis (bī-ō-nō′sĭs) [″ + *nosos*, disease]. Any disease due to pathogenic organisms.

biophagism, biophagy (bī-ŏf′ă-jĭzm, -ă-jē) [″ + *phagein*, to eat]. Absorbing or obtaining nourishment from living matter.

biophotometer (bī″ō-fō-tŏm′ĕ-tĕr) [″ + *photos*, light, + *metron*, measure]. Device for evaluating visual adaptation to the dark. Used to determine presence or absence of vitamin A deficiency.

biophysics (bī″ō-fĭz′ĭks) [″ + *physikos*, natural]. Application of physical laws to biological processes and functions.

bioplasm (bī′ō-plăzm) [″ + *plasma*, matter]. Protoplasm, q.v.; living substance.

biopsy (bī′ŏp-sē) [″ + *opsis*, vision]. Excision of a small piece of living tissue for microscopic examination. Usually performed to establish a diagnosis.

biopterin (bī-ŏp′tĕr-ĭn). The chemical, 2-amino-4-hydroxy-6-(1,2-hydroxypropyl) pteridine, important in metabolizing phenylalanine. A deficiency of this is a rare cause of phenylketonuria.

biorhythms (bī″ō-rĭth′ŭms) [″ + *rhythmos*, rhythm]. Cyclic phenomena that occur with established regularity in living organisms.

Ex.: circadian rhythms, the sleep cycle, the menstrual cycle. SEE: *clock, biological.*

bios (bī′ŏs) [Gr., life]. 1. Organic life. 2. A group of substances (including inositol, biotin, and thiamine) necessary for the most favorable growth of some yeasts.

bioscience (bī″ō-sī′ĕns) [″ + L. *scientia*, knowledge]. Biological study wherein all sciences required are utilized.

bioscopy (bī-ŏs′kō-pē) [″ + *skopein*, to examine]. Examination to determine viability or extinction of life.

biospectrometry (bī″ō-spĕk-trŏm′ĕ-trē) [″ + L. *spectrum*, image, + Gr. *metron*, measure]. Use of a spectroscope to determine the amounts and kinds of substances in tissues.

biospectroscopy (bī″ō-spĕk-trŏs′kō-pē) [″ + ″ + Gr. *skopein*, to examine]. Examination of tissue by use of a spectroscope.

biosphere (bī′ō-sfēr″) [″ + *sphaira*, ball]. That portion of the earth that supports ecological systems.

biostatics (bī″ō-stăt′ĭks) [″ + *statikos*, standing]. Science of the relationship of structure to function.

biostatistics. Vital statistics. Application of statistical processes and methods to the analysis of biological data.

biosynthesis (bī″ō-sĭn′thĕ-sĭs) [″ + *synthesis*, a putting together]. The formation of chemical compounds by a living organism.

biota (bī-ō′tă) [Gr. *bios*, life]. Combined and total animal and plant life in an area.

biotaxis, biotaxy (bī″ō-tăk′sĭs, -sē) [″ + *taxis*, arrangement]. 1. The selecting and arranging activity of living cells. 2. Systematic classification of living organisms.

Biot's breathing (bē-ōz′). [Camille Biot, 19th-century Fr. physician] Breathing characterized by several short breaths followed by long irregular periods of apnea. Seen in patients with increased intracranial pressure.

biotelemetry (bī″ō-tĕl-ĕm′ĕ-trē) [Gr. *bios*, life, + *tele*, distant, + *metron*, measure]. Recording biological events such as temperature, heart rate, ECG, and EEG in subjects remote from the investigator. This is done by using electronic devices.

biotics (bī-ŏt′ĭks) [Gr. *biotikos*, living]. The science that deals with the functions of life.

biotin (bī′ō-tĭn). A component of the vitamin B complex formerly designated as vitamin H. This water-soluble, heat-sensitive substance is essential for the activity of many enzyme systems in bacteria, animals, and presumably man. Present in many foods, but liver, kidney, milk, egg yolks, and yeast are particularly rich sources. Deficiency states have been reported in man and experimental animals when the diet contains large amounts of raw egg white. This is due to biotin being bound to a protein in the egg white that renders the biotin in the diet unavailable. Humans with biotin deficiency develop lassitude, anorexia, depression, muscle pains, hyperesthesia of the skin, and dermatitis.

biotomy (bī-ŏt′ō-mē) [Gr. *bios*, life, + *tome*,

incision]. Operation on living animals for pathological or physiological study. SYN: *vivisection*.

biotoxin (bī-ō-tŏk'sĭn) [" + *toxikon*, poison]. A toxin produced by or found in a living organism.

biotransformation. The chemical alterations that a substance undergoes in the body.

biotype (bī'ō-tīp) [" + *typos*, mark]. 1. Fundamental genetic constitution of an organism or a group of individuals possessing it. Opposed to phenotype or external appearance of an organism. 2. A genotype.

biovular twins [L. *bis*, twice, + *ovum*, egg]. Twins from two separate ova.

bipara (bĭp'ă-ră) [" + *parere*, to give birth]. A woman who has given birth for the second time to an infant or infants, alive or dead, weighing 500 gm. or more. SYN: *secundipara*.

biparasitic (bī"păr-ă-sĭt'ĭk) [" + Gr. *para*, beside, + *sitos*, food]. Pert. to a parasite living upon another parasite.

biparental (bī"pă-rĕn'tăl) [" + *parere*, to give birth]. Derived from two parents, male and female.

biparietal (bī"pă-rī'ĕ-tăl). Concerning the parietal bones or their eminences.

biparous (bĭp'ă-rŭs). Producing two ova or offspring at one time.

bipartite patella. The developing patella that matures from two centers rather than one. This usually congenital condition causes no symptoms but may be mistaken for a fracture.

biped (bī'pĕd) [" + *pes*, foot]. An animal with two feet.

bipenniform (bī-pĕn'ĭ-form) [" + *penna*, feather, + *forma*, shape]. Muscle fibers that come from each side of a tendon in the manner barbs come from the central shaft of a feather.

biperforate (bī-pĕr'fō-rāt) [" + *perforatus*, pierced with holes]. Having two openings or perforations.

biperiden (bī-pĕr'ĭ-dĕn). USP. An anticholinergic drug used in treating parkinsonism. Trade name is Akineton.

bipolar (bī-pōl'ăr) [" + *polus*, a pole]. 1. Having two poles or processes. 2. Pert. to the use of two poles in electrotherapeutic treatments. The term biterminal should be used when referring to an alternating current. 3. A two-poled nerve cell.

biramous (bī-rā'mŭs) [" + *ramus*, a branch]. Possessing two branches.

bird breeder's lung. Attacks of chills, fever, and cough with shortness of breath in persons who are closely associated with birds such as pigeons and parakeets. In some patients the onset is slow rather than acute. The symptoms are due to antigenic substances in the bird's excreta. Symptoms usually subside when exposure to the birds ceases. SYN: *pigeon breeder's disease*.

birefractive, birefringent (bī"rē-frăk'tĭv, -frĭn'jĕnt) [" + *refrangere*, to break up]. Splitting a ray of light in two. SEE: *refraction*.

birth [Old Norse *burdhr*]. Act of being born; passage of a child from the uterus.

b., complete. The instant of complete separation of the body of the infant from that of the mother, regardless of whether the cord or placenta is detached.

b., cross. Labor with fetus lying transversely across the uterus.

b., dry. Birth following premature rupture of the fetal membranes.

b., live. An infant showing one of the three evidences of life (breathing, heart action, movements of a voluntary muscle) after complete birth.

b., multiple. Birth of two or more offspring produced in the same gestation period.

b., premature. Birth of a fetus sometime after it is developed enough to survive but before reaching 5.5 lb. (2500 gm.) in weight. This weight standard applies only to Western European cultures. SEE: *prematurity*.

birth canal. The canal through which the fetus passes in birth, comprising the cervix, vagina, and vulva.

birth certificate. A legal written record of the birth of a child, required by law throughout the United States.

birth control. Prevention of implantation of the ovum, or birth, by temporary or permanent measures. Temporary birth control methods include oral steroid pills, the condom, intrauterine devices (IUD), the rhythm method, foam, the diaphragm, the cervical cap, and spermicides. Sterilization in men is performed by vasectomy and female sterilization is performed by tubal ligation. Sterilization is usually permanent but progress is being made in reversing the procedure. SEE: *contraceptive*.

birth defect. A congenital anomaly.

birth injury. Injury sustained by the neonate during the birth process.

birthmark. Nevus; a congenital discoloration of a circumscribed area of the skin, due to pigmentation or to a vascular tumor.

birth palsy. Paraplegia or hemiplegia due to birth injury.

birth rate. The number of live births in one year for each 1000 persons in the population.

bisacodyl (bĭs-ăk'ō-dĭl; bĭs"ă-kō'dĭl). USP. A cathartic drug that acts by its direct effect on the colon. May be administered orally or by rectal suppository. Trade names are Dulcolax and Theralax.

bisacromial (bĭs"ă-krō'mē-ăl) [L. *bis*, twice,

+ Gr. *akron,* point, + *omos,* shoulder]. Pert. to the two acromial processes.

bisection (bī-sĕk′shŭn) [″ + *sectio,* a cutting]. Division into two parts by cutting.

bisexual (bī-sĕks′ū-ăl) [″ + *sexus,* sex]. 1. Hermaphroditic; having imperfect genitalia of both sexes in one person. 2. An individual who is sexually attracted to others of either sex. SEE: *heterosexual; homosexual; lesbian.*

bisferious (bĭs-fĕr′ē-ŭs) [″ + *ferire,* to beat]. Having two beats; dicrotic.

bishydroxycoumarin (bĭs″hī-drŏk″sē-koo′mă-rĭn). Previously used name for dicumarol, USP, q.v.

bisiliac (bĭs-ĭl′ē-ăk) [″ + *ilium,* ilium]. Pert. to the two iliac crests or any corresponding iliac structures.

bis in die [L.]. Twice a day. ABBR: b.d.; b.i.d.

bismuth (bĭz′mŭth) [Ger. *Wismuth,* white mass]. SYMB: Bi. At. wt. 208.980; at. no. 83.

A silvery metallic element. Its compounds are used as a protective for inflamed surfaces and as an opaque medium for x-ray visualization. Its salts are used as an astringent, and in treatment of diarrhea.

b. subcarbonate. An odorless, tasteless powder used as an antacid, astringent, and protective.

INCOMPAT: Sulfides, acids, acid salts.

b. subgallate. A bright yellow powder without odor or taste. First introduced for treatment of skin diseases. General use is the same as bismuth subnitrate.

b. subnitrate. USP. Heavy white odorless powder. Used as an astringent, protective, antiseptic.

INCOMPAT: Acids, tannins, and sulfides.

bismuth poisoning. Poisoning due to ingestion of bismuth.

SYM: Metallic taste, foul breath, fever, gastrointestinal irritation, bluish line at gum margin, ulcerative process of gums and mouth, headache. Albuminuria; resembles lead poisoning with an absence of the blood changes and paralyses.

F.A.: Removal of source of bismuth; gastric lavage; high enemas; stimulants for respiration and heart if necessary; treat symptomatically.

bistoury (bĭs′tū-rē) [Fr. *bistouri,* surgical knife]. Small surgical knife used in minor operations. Special varieties are tenotomes, gum lancets, hernia knives, and lithotomy bistouries.

bisulfate (bī-sŭl′fāt). An acid sulfate in which a monovalent metal and a hydrogen ion are combined with the sulfate radical. SEE: *disulfate.*

bite (bīt) [AS. *bitan,* to bite]. 1. To cut with the teeth. 2. Puncture or tearing of the skin by the teeth, as by an animal. SEE: *bites or stings.* 3. In dentistry, the angle and manner at which the upper and lower teeth meet.

b., balanced. Balanced occlusion of the teeth.

b., close, closed. Bite in which lower incisors lie behind upper incisors.

b., end-to-end. Bite in which incisors of both jaws meet along cutting edge when jaw is closed.

b., open. Bite in which a space exists between the upper and lower incisors when the mouth is closed.

b., over. Bite in which upper incisors overlap lower ones when jaws are closed.

b., under. Condition in which lower incisors pass in front of upper incisors upon closing the mouth.

bitelock. Device used in dentistry for retaining bite rims outside the mouth in the same position they were inside the mouth.

bitemporal (bī-tĕm′pō-răl) [L. *bis,* twice, + *temporalis,* pert. to a temple]. Pert. to both temples or temporal bones.

biteplate (bīt′plāt). Dental device used to correct or diagnose malocclusion. It is worn in the palate, usually on a temporary basis.

bites or stings. Injuries in which body surfaces are torn by insects or animals, resulting in abrasions, punctures, or lacerated wounds. SEE: *dog bite; human bite; rabies; snake bite.*

SYM: May be evidence of a wound, usually surrounded by a zone of redness and swelling, often accompanied by pain, itching, or throbbing. Often become infected and may contain specific noxious materials such as bacteria, toxins, viruses, or venom.

F.A.: If it is suspected of containing poison, apply tourniquet first. Wash wound with saline solution thoroughly, apply dry sterile dressing. Administer appropriate antitetanus therapy. Treatment for shock may be needed.

Some insect bites or stings contain an acid substance resembling formic acid and consequently are relieved by topically applied alkalies, as ammonia water or baking soda paste. For intense local pain, injection of local anesthetic may be required. Systemic medication may be needed for generalized pain.

Others, such as the bee, wasp, and hornet, contain unknown organic substances for which there is no specific antidote. Remove the stinger if one is present. At the site of bites or stings by poisonous spiders, esp. the black widow, q.v., scorpions, tarantulas, and poisonous fish, a firm bandage should be applied promptly. Intravenous calcium gluconate given very slowly is specific for controlling muscle pain due to black widow spider bite. It is also effective in relieving muscular cramps due to contact with jellyfish or Portuguese man-of-war.

Sea urchin spines break off in the skin and cause irritation. Remove the spines as soon as possible; surgical methods are not usually necessary. The spines can be softened and dissolved by vinegar, and the affected area can be soaked two to three times a day. If this treatment plus wet vinegar dressings does not effect a cure, surgical intervention will be required. The spines are radiopaque and thus may be located by x-ray if they have migrated to deep tissue.

For jellyfish stings the local application of a meat tenderizer containing papain is an effective treatment. A slurry of the powder is applied as quickly as possible to the affected area. Demerol or morphine may be required for control of pain.

A sting ray injures by penetrating the skin with the barb in its tail. This causes intense pain, local swelling, nausea, vomiting, weakness, and perhaps shock. Treat symptomatically, cleanse wound thoroughly, and remove all foreign material. Soak site of wound in hot water 113° to 140° F. (45° to 60° C.) for 30 to 60 minutes. Surgical debridement and closure of wound. SEE: *black widow; scorpion; spider, brown recluse; tarantula.*

bite-wing radiograph. Dental radiograph pictures taken with the film holder held between the teeth and the film parallel to the teeth. This technique permits film to be taken of several upper and lower teeth at the same time.

Bitot's spots (bē'tōz). [Pierre A. Bitot, Fr. physician, 1822–1888] Triangular, shiny, gray spots on the conjunctiva seen in vitamin A deficiency.

bitrochanteric (bī"trō-kăn-tĕr'ĭk). Concerning both greater trochanters of the two femurs.

bitter (bĭt'ĕr) [AS. *biter,* strong]. Having a disagreeable taste.

bituminosis (bī-tū"mĭ-nō'sĭs). A form of pneumoconiosis from dust of soft coal.

biuret (bī'ū-rĕt) [L. *bis,* twice, + *urea*]. A crystalline decomposition derivative of urea.

biuret test. A method for measuring protein in the serum. The presence of biuret can be detected by the addition of sodium hydroxide and copper sulfate solutions to the sample. A rose to violet coloring indicates the presence of protein, and a pink and finally blue color indicates the presence of urea.

bivalent (bī-vā'lĕnt) [" + *valens,* powerful]. 1. Having a valence of two; having a combining power of two atoms of hydrogen. 2. In cytology, a structure consisting of two paired homologous chromosomes, each split into two sister chromatids during meiosis.

biventer (bī-vĕn'tĕr) [" + *venter,* belly]. A part or organ such as a muscle with two bellies; pert. to several muscles.

biventral (bī-vĕn'trăl). Digastric; with two bellies.

bizygomatic (bī"zī-gō-măt'ĭk). Concerning the most prominent point on each of the two zygomatic arches.

Bjerrum's screen (byĕr'oomz). [J. Bjerrum, Dan. ophthalmologist, 1827–1892] Tangent plane consisting of a large square of black cloth with a central mark for fixation, used for mapping the field of vision, esp. central and paracentral scotomata.

Bjerrum's sign. A sickle- or comet-shaped blind spot usually found in central zone of the visual field. Seen in glaucoma.

B.K. *below knee,* term used to refer to the site of amputation of a lower extremity.

Bk. Chem. symb. for berkelium.

black (blăk) [AS. *blaec*]. 1. Devoid of color or reflecting no light. 2. Marked by dark pigmentation.

black death. An acute, severe infection appearing in a bubonic or pneumonic form, caused by the bacillus Yersinia pestis. This term was applied to the condition in the Middle Ages when massive epidemics occurred in Europe. The infection is characterized by an abrupt onset with chills and fever. SEE: *plague; bubonic plague; plague, pneumonic.*

black eye. Bruising, discoloration and swelling of the eyelid and tissue around the eye due to trauma.

TREATMENT: Application of ice packs during the first 24 hrs. will inhibit swelling. Hot compresses after the first day may aid absorption of the fluids that produce discoloration.

blackhead. A plug of dried sebum in a sebaceous gland. SYN: *comedo.*

black lung. Lay term for the chronic lung disease or pneumoconiosis found in coal miners. SYN: *coal worker's pneumoconiosis.*

black measles. A severe type of measles in which the eruption is dark in color due to an effusion of blood into the skin. Also called hemorrhagic measles.

blackout. 1. Sudden loss of consciousness. This may occur while coughing, following nocturnal urination, or while swallowing in patients who have esophageal disease. SEE: *postural hypotension.* 2. Temporary loss of consciousness. In aviators, temporary or transient loss of vision or consciousness is usually due to a fall of blood pressure in the head. This is caused by the centrifugal force experienced in high-speed aircraft maneuvers. SEE: *red-out.*

black vomit. Vomit that appears black due to the presence of blood that has been in the stomach and has been acted upon by gastric juices. Usually seen in yellow fever and other conditions in which blood collects in the stomach.

blackwater fever. Hemoglobinuria following chronic falciparum malaria infection.

SYM. AND SIGNS: Sudden onset, fever, tender and enlarged liver and spleen, dark urine, epigastric pain, vomiting, jaundice, sudden shock.

black widow. A species of poisonous spider, Latrodectus mactans, found in the United States. Its bite causes severe abdominal cramps. An antivenin is available for I.V. use after an appropriate skin test. For acute pain and muscle contraction, give 10 ml. of calcium gluconate I.V. or I.M. and repeat as necessary. The very young and patients over 60 should be hospitalized if they have signs of a heavy dose of the venom. SEE: *bites or stings; spider, black widow.*

bladder (blăd′dĕr) [AS. *blaedre*]. A membranous sac or receptacle for a secretion, as the gallbladder, q.v. Commonly used to designate the urinary bladder. SEE: *b., urinary; genitourinary system; urinary tract* for illus.

b., atony of. Inability to urinate due to lack of muscular tone. It is frequently seen after traumatic deliveries or after the use of epidural anesthesia.

b., autonomous. Bladder in which there is interruption in both afferent and efferent limbs of reflex arcs. Bladder sensations absent; dribbling constant; residual urine large in amount.

b., exstrophy of. Congenital eversion of the urinary bladder. The abdominal wall fails to close and the inside of the bladder may be seen to protrude through the abdominal wall.

b., hypertonic. 1. Bladder with excessive muscular tone. 2. Increased muscular activity of the bladder.

b., irritable. State of the bladder marked by increased frequency of contraction with an associated desire to urinate.

b., nervous. Bladder condition characterized by a constant desire to urinate without the power to do so completely.

b., neurogenic. Any dysfunction of the urinary bladder from lesions of central nervous system or nerves supplying the bladder.

b., spastic. Neurogenic bladder due to complete transection of the spinal cord above the sacral segments.

b., urinary. The muscular, membranous, distensible reservoir for the urine that receives urine from the kidneys through the ureters and that discharges urine from the body through the urethra. Its function is that of a reservoir for urine SYN: *vesica urinaria* [NA].

ANAT: The lower portion, continuous with the urethra, is called the neck; its upper tip, connected with the umbilicus by the median umbilical ligament, is called the apex. The region between the two openings of the two ureters and the urethra is the trigone. The wall of the bladder consists of an inner mucous layer of transitional epithelium, a muscular coat of smooth muscle, the outer layer comprising the detrusor urinae, and a fibrous layer. On its free superior surface is a layer of peritoneum. The bladder is supported by numerous ligaments. Blood is supplied by the superior, middle, and inferior vesical arteries and numerous veins and lymphatics; and it is innervated with nerves derived from the third and fourth sacral nerve by way of the hypogastric plexus.

The bladder is situated in the anterior inferior portion of the pelvic cavity. In the female it lies in front of the anterior wall of the vagina and the uterus, and in the male it lies in front of the rectum. It has a storage capacity in health of 500 ml. (about 34 oz.) or more. In disease states it may be greatly distended. A frequent cause of distention of the bladder in elderly males is hypertrophy of the prostate gland, which surrounds the urethra and neck of the bladder. SEE: *urinary tract* for illus.

PHYS: An average of 40 to 50 oz. (about 1.2 to 1.5 L.) of urine is secreted within a 24-hour period. This value is quite dependent upon amount of fluid ingested and loss of fluid through sweat and the bowels. Inability to empty the bladder is known as retention and may call for catheterization. Sphincter muscles are part of the mechanism that controls retention within the bladder.

The force of urination is much greater in the child than in the adult because the bladder is more nearly an abdominal than pelvic organ in the child. Thus the child's abdominal muscles help to expel the urine.

PALPATION: The bladder cannot be palpated when empty. When full it appears as a tumor in the hypogastric region that, on palpation, is smooth and oval.

PERCUSSION: When containing urine, its rounded margin is easily made out by observing the tympanic sound of the intestines on one hand and dull sound of the bladder on the other.

bladder drill. Technique used in treating stress urinary incontinence in women. It consists of admitting the patient to the hospital and requiring that the urine be passed hourly. The patient charts the number of times of urination, intervals between urination, and volume of urine passed. She also notes the degree and frequency of incontinence. The intervals between urinations are gradually increased. After about 10 days the patient is discharged and instructed to continue bladder training at home. SYN: *bladder training*.

bladder training. Bladder drill, q.v.

bladder worm. A larval form of tapeworm with a rounded cyst or bladder into which a scolex is invaginated. The bladder worm of Taenia solium (pork tapeworm) encysts in muscles of pigs; that of T. saginata (beef tapeworm) in muscles of cattle. SYN: *cysticercus*.

blanch (blănch). 1. To lose color, esp. of the face, usually suddenly and in the context of being frightened or saddened. 2. To briefly scald a vegetable or nut-fruit in order to facilitate removal of the skin, peel, or covering. 3. To bleach.

bland [L. *blandus*]. Soothing, mild.

bland diet. A diet designed to buffer gastric acidity by providing meals of palatable, nonirritating foods. Content of diet includes milk, cream, prepared cereals, gelatin, soup, rice, butter, crackers, eggs, lean meats, fish, cottage cheese, custards, tapioca, cookies, and plain cake. Multivitamins may be a necessary adjunct.

IND: Gastritis, peptic ulcer, hiatus hernia.

Blandin's glands (blŏn-dănz'). [Philippe F. Blandin, Fr. surgeon, 1798–1849] Small glands deeply placed on each side of the frenulum of the tongue near the apex. SYN: *Nuhn's glands*.

blanket, hypothermia. SEE: *hypothermia blanket*.

blast. 1. [Gr. *blastos*, germ] An immature stage in cellular development; used as a word termination as in erythroblast, hematoblast, or neuroblast. 2. [AS. *bloest*, a puff of wind] A violent movement of air such as accompanies the explosion of a shell or bomb; a violent sound, as the blast of a horn.

blastema (blăs-tē'mă) [Gr. *blastema*, sprout]. Immature material from which cells and tissues are formed.

blastid (blăs'tĭd) [Gr. *blastos*, germ]. The clear space marking site of the organizing nucleus in the impregnated ovum.

blasto- [Gr. *blastos*, germ]. Prefix indicating germ or bud.

blastocele, blastocoele (blăs'tō-sēl) [" + *koilos*, hollow]. The cavity in the blastula, q.v., of the developing embryo.

blastochyle (blăs'tō-kīl) [" + *chylos*, juice]. Fluid contained in the blastocele.

blastocyst (blăs'tō-sĭst) [" + *kystis*, bag]. Stage in the development of a mammalian embryo that follows the morula. It consists of an outer layer of trophoblast to which is attached an inner cell mass. The enclosed cavity is the blastocele. The whole is called blastodermic vesicle or blastocyst. At this stage, implantation in the endometrium (lining of the uterus) occurs.

blastocyte (blăs'tō-sīt) [" + *kytos*, cell]. An undifferentiated embryonic cell.

blastocytoma (blăs-tō-sī-tō mă) [" + " + *oma*, tumor]. Blastoma, q.v.

blastoderm (blăs'tō-dĕrm) [" + *derma*, skin]. A disk of cells (germinal disk or blastodisk) that develops on the surface of the yolk in an avian or reptilian egg from which the embryo develops; also applied to the embryonic disk of mammalian embryos, a disk of cells lying between the yolk sac and the amniotic cavity from which the embryo develops. From the blastoderm, the three germ layers (ectoderm, mesoderm, and endoderm) arise.

blastodermic vesicle. A blastocyst, q.v.

blastodisk (blăs'tō-dĭsk) [" + *diskos*, disk]. Flat disk of embryonic cells on the surface of the yolk of the ovum. Formed from the blastomeres.

blastogenesis (blăs"tō-jĕn'ĕ-sĭs) [" + *genesis*, generation]. 1. Multiplication by budding. 2. Transmission of characteristics by the germ plasm.

blastokinin (blăs"tō-kī'nĭn). A globulin found in the uterine lumen of some mammals near the time of blastocyst implantation.

blastolysis (blăs-tŏl'ĭ-sĭs) [" + *lysis*, dissolution]. Lysis or destruction of a germ cell or a blastoderm.

blastoma (blăs-tō'mă) [" + *oma*, tumor]. (pl. *blastomata*) A neoplasm composed of immature, undifferentiated cells derived from the blastema of an organ or tissue.

blastomere (blăs'tō-mēr) [" + *meros*, a part]. One of the cells resulting from the cleavage of a fertilized ovum.

blastomerotomy (blăs"tō-mēr-ŏt'ō-mē) [" + " + *tome*, incision]. Destruction of blastomeres.

Blastomyces (blăst-ō-mī'sēz) [Gr. *blastos*, germ, + *mykes*, fungus]. (pl. *Blastomycetes*) A genus of yeastlike budding fungi pathogenic to man. At room temperature the genus grows as a mycelial (fungal) form and at body temperature as a yeastlike form.

B. brasiliensis. Fungus causing South American blastomycosis. This organism and disease are also called Paracoccidioides brasiliensis and paracoccidioidomycosis respectively.

B. dermatitidis. The pathogen that causes North American blastomycosis, a rare fungus infection in man.

blastomycete (blăs"tō-mī'sēt). Any organism of the genus Blastomyces.

blastomycin (blăs"tō-mī'sĭn). Sterile filtrate of soluble material obtained from a culture of Blastomyces dermatitidis. Its use as a skin test for blastomycosis is not reliable.

blastomycosis (blăs"tō-mī-kō'sĭs) [" + *mykes*, fungus, + *osis*, condition]. Infection caused by organisms of the genus Blastomyces.

b., keloidal. A skin disease (Lobo's disease) often confused with South American blastomycosis. Caused by the fungus Loboa loboi.

b., North American. A rare fungus infection caused by Blastomyces dermatitidis. Marked by inflammatory lesions of skin (cutaneous form) or lungs (pulmonary form), or a generalized invasion of skin, lungs, bones, central nervous system, kidneys, liver, and spleen (systemic form). Also called Gilchrist's disease.

b., South American. A serious infection caused by a dimorphic fungus, Paracoccidioides brasiliensis. Marked by inflammatory lesions of skin, mucous membranes, and internal organs. SYN: *paracoccidioidomycosis.*

blastopore (blăs'tō-por) [" + *poros*, passageway]. The small opening into the archenteron made by invagination of the blastula.

blastospore (blăs'tō-spor) [" + *sporos*, seed]. A spore formed by budding from a hypha, as in yeast.

blastula (blăs'tū-lă) [L.]. (pl. *blastulae*) An early stage in the development of an ovum, consisting of a hollow sphere of cells enclosing a cavity, the blastocele. In large-yolked eggs, the blastocele is reduced to a narrow slit. In mammalian development, the blastocyst or blastodermic vesicle corresponds to the blastula of lower forms.

Blatta (blăt'ă) [L.]. A genus of insects (that includes the cockroaches) of the order Orthoptera.

B. germanica. The German cockroach or croton bug.

B. orientalis. The Oriental cockroach, also known as the black beetle, a common European house pest.

bleaching powder. Chlorinated lime or calcium hypochlorite.

bleb (blĕb). Elevation of the epidermis, irregularly shaped. A blister or a bulla. May vary in size from less than a cm. to as much as 5–10 cm.; it may contain serous, seropurulent, or bloody fluid. A primary skin lesion. May occur in dermatitis herpetiformis, pemphigus, and syphilis. SEE: *bulla.*

bleeder [AS. *bledan*, to bleed]. 1. One whose ability to coagulate blood is either deficient or absent. Thus, small cuts and injuries lead to profuse bleeding. Such a person may be treated with one of several blood fractions to assist in arresting bleeding following trauma. SEE: *hemophilia.* 2. A small artery that has been cut or torn.

bleeder's disease. Hemophilia, q.v.; a congenital blood condition marked by inability of blood to coagulate. SEE: *coagulation.*

bleeding [AS. *bledan*, to bleed]. 1. Emitting blood, as from an injured vessel. 2. Process of emitting blood, as a hemorrhage or operation of letting blood.

Normally, when plasma of the blood is exposed to air, it changes to allow fibrin to form. This entangles the corpuscles and forms a blood clot. SEE: *blood, clotting of; coagulation factors; hemorrhage.*

b., arterial. Bleeding in spurts of bright red blood.

F.A.: Pressure with fingers at nearest pressure point between it and heart. Locate artery and apply digital pressure above it until bleeding stops or until the artery is ligated. SEE: table *(Arrest of Arterial Bleeding).*

b., breakthrough. Intermenstrual bleeding, esp. that which occurs during use of progestational agents.

b., occult. Inapparent bleeding, esp. that which occurs into the intestines and can be detected only by chemical tests of the feces.

b., venous. Continuous flow of dark red blood.

F.A.: May be controlled by firm continuous pressure applied directly to the bleeding site. If bleeding is from an area over soft tissues, hold a large but compact bandage against the bleeding point.

CAUTION: A tourniquet should not be used. If the bleeding is over a bony area, as in the case of a ruptured varicose vein of the leg, a coin held firmly against the vein will provide immediate control of the blood loss. The patient should then be seen by a physician as soon as possible.

bleeding time. Time required for blood to stop flowing from a small wound or pin prick. This test is done by using one of several techniques. Depending on the method used, the time may vary from 1 to 3 minutes (Duke method) or from 1 to 9 minutes (Ivy method). The Duke method consists of timing the cessation of bleeding after the ear lobe has received a standardized puncture. The Ivy method is done in a similar manner following puncture of the skin of the forearm.

blenn-, blenno- [Gr. *blennos*, mucus]. Combining form meaning mucus or pert. to it.

blennadenitis (blĕn"ăd-ĕ-nī'tĭs) [" + *aden*, gland, + *itis*, inflammation]. Inflammation of mucous glands.

blennemesis (blĕn-ĕm'ĕ-sĭs) [" + *emesis*, vomiting]. Vomiting of mucus.

blennogenic, blennogenous (blĕn"ō-jĕn'ĭk, blĕn-ŏj'ĕ-nŭs) [" + *gennan*, to produce]. Secreting mucus.

blennoid (blĕn'oyd) [" + *eidos*, form]. Like mucus; mucoid.

blennometritis (blĕn"ō-mĕ-trī'tĭs) [" + *metra*, womb, + *itis*, inflammation]. Inflammation of the uterus.

blennophthalmia (blĕn"ŏf-thăl'mē-ă) [" +

Arrest of Arterial Bleeding*

For Wounds of the Face

Artery	Course	Bone Against Which Pressure Is Applied	Spot to Apply Pressure
Temporal	Upward ½ in. (13 mm.) in front of ear	Temporal bone	Against bony prominence immediately in front of the ear or on temple
Facial	Upward across the jaw diagonally	Lower part of lower maxilla	An inch (2.5 cm.) in front of angle of lower jaw
Carotid	From outer upper edge of sternum to angle of jaw	Cervical vertebrae	Deep down and backward an inch (2.5 cm.) to the side of the prominence of the windpipe
For Wounds of the Upper Extremity			
Subclavian	Across middle of first rib to armpit	First rib behind clavicle	Deep down and backward over center of clavicle against first rib (depress the shoulder first)
Axillary	Downward across outer side of armpit to inside of humerus	Head of humerus	High up in the armpit against upper part of humerus
Brachial	Along inner side of humerus under edge of biceps muscle	Shaft of humerus	Against shaft of humerus by pulling aside and gripping biceps, pressing tips of fingers deep down against the bone
For Wounds of the Lower Extremity			
Femoral / Femoral	Down the thigh from the pelvis to the knee from a point midway between iliac spine and symphysis pubis to inner side of end of femur at knee joint	Brim of pelvis	Against brim of pelvis, midway between iliac spine and symphysis pubis
		Shaft of femur	High up on the inner side of the thigh, about 3 in. (7.6 cm.) below brim of pelvis, over the line given in the direction of the knee
Posterior Tibial	Downward to foot in hollow just behind the prominence of inner ankle	Inner side of tibia, low down above ankle	For wounds in the sole of the foot, against the tibia in center of the hollow behind the inner ankle

* Adapted from Hilda M. Gration, R.N.

ophthalmos, eye]. 1. Catarrhal conjunctivitis. 2. Gonorrheal ophthalmia.

blennorrhagia (blĕn″ō-rā′jē-ă) [″ + *rhegnynai,* to break forth]. A discharge from mucous membranes.

blennorrhea (blĕn″ō-rē′ă) [Gr. *blennos,* mucus, + *rhoia,* flow]. Any discharge from mucous membranes. SYN: *blennorrhagia.*

b., inclusion. Inflammation of conjunctiva in newborn. Caused by a filtrable virus, Chlamydia oculogenitale, that forms cytoplasmic inclusion bodies in the epithelial cells.

b. neonatorum. Gonococcal conjunctivitis in the newborn.

blennostasis (blĕn-ŏs′tă-sĭs) [″ + *stasis,* a halt]. The correction of an abnormal mucus discharge.

blennostatic. Diminishing abnormal mucus secretion.

blennothorax (blĕn″ō-thō′răks) [″ + *thorax,* chest]. Accumulation of mucus in bronchial tubes or alveoli.

blennuria (blĕn-ū′rē-ă) [″ + *ouron,* urine]. Presence of mucus in the urine.

Blenoxane. Trade name for bleomycin sulfate, USP.

bleomycin (blē-ō-mī′sĭn). Any one of a group of antitumor agents produced by Streptomyces verticellis.

b., sulfate, sterile. USP. A bleomycin used in treating various carcinomas of the skin, head, neck, and lungs, as well as testicular tumors. Trade name is Blenoxane.

blepharadenitis (blĕf″ăr-ăd-ĕ-nī′tĭs) [Gr. *blepharon,* eyelid, + *aden,* gland, + *itis,* inflammation]. Inflammation of the meibomian glands. SYN: *blepharoadenitis.*

blepharal (blĕf′ăr-ăl). Pert. to an eyelid.

blepharectomy (blĕf″ă-rĕk′tō-mē) [″ + *ektome,* excision]. Surgical excision of all or part of an eyelid.

blepharedema (blĕf″ăr-ĕ-dē′mă) [″ + *oidema,* swelling]. Edema of the eyelids causing swelling and a baggy appearance.

blepharism [″ + *-ismos,* condition]. Twitching or blinking of the eyelids.

blepharitis (blĕf″ăr-ī′tĭs) [″ + *itis,* inflammation]. Ulcerative or nonulcerative inflammation of the edges of the eyelids involving hair follicles and glands that open onto the surface.

ETIOL: In ulcerative type, bacterial infection usually by staphylococci; in nonulcerative type, cause is often unknown. May be due to allergy, exposure to dust, smoke, or irritating chemicals.

SYM: Eyelids red, tender, and sore with sticky exudate, ulcers on edges; lids may become inverted with lashes falling out and epiphora, q.v., occurring. Styes and meibomian cysts are associated with the condition.

NURSING IMPLICATIONS: Keep the scalp, eyebrows, and eyelids clean. Bathe eyelids with warm saline solution to remove any drainage or crusts. When ointment is to be applied, first cleanse eyelids, and then apply ointment to lid margins beginning at the inner and working toward the outer canthus of the eye.

b. angularis. Blepharitis in which medial angle of the eye is involved with blocking of openings of lacrimal ducts.

b. ciliaris. Inflammation affecting the ciliary margins of the eyelids.

b. marginalis. B. ciliaris, q.v.

b. parasitica. Blepharitis caused by parasites such as mites or lice.

b. squamosa. Chronic blepharitis with scaling.

b. ulcerosa. Blepharitis with ulceration.

blepharo- [Gr. *blepharon,* eyelid]. Prefix pert. to the eyelid.

blepharoadenitis (blĕf″ăr-ō-ăd″ĕ-nī′tĭs) [″ + *aden,* gland, + *itis,* inflammation]. Inflammation of meibomian glands. Also spelled blepharadenitis.

blepharoadenoma (blĕf″ăr-ō-ăd-ĕ-nō′mă) [″ + ″ + *oma,* tumor]. Adenoma or glandular tumor of eyelid.

blepharoatheroma (blĕf″ăr-ō-ăth″ĕ-rō′mă) [″ + *athere,* thick fluid, + *oma,* tumor]. Sebaceous cyst of an eyelid.

blepharochalasis (blĕf″ăr-ō-kăl′ă-sĭs) [″ + *chalasis,* relaxation]. Hypertrophy of skin of the upper eyelid due to loss of elasticity following edematous swellings such as in recurrent angioneurotic edema of lids. The skin may droop over the edge of the eyelid when the eyes are open.

blepharochromhidrosis (blĕf″ă-rō-krōm-hĭ-drō′sĭs) [″ + *chroma,* color, + *hidros,* sweat, + *osis,* condition]. Colored sweat, usually of a bluish color, from the eyelids.

blepharoclonus (blĕf″ă-rŏk′lō-nŭs) [″ + *klonos,* tumult]. Clonic spasm of the muscles that close the eyelids (orbicularis oculi).

blepharoconjunctivitis (blĕf″ă-rō-kŏn-jŭnk″tĭ-vī′tĭs) [″ + L. *conjungere,* to join together, + Gr. *itis,* inflammation]. Inflammation of eyelids and conjunctiva.

blepharodiastasis (blĕf-ă-rō-dī-ăs′tă-sĭs) [″ + *diastasis,* separation]. Excessive separation of eyelids, causing eye to open wide.

blepharoncus (blĕf″ă-rŏn′kŭs] [″ + *onkos,* tumor]. Tumor of the eyelid.

blepharopachynsis (blĕf″ă-rō-pă-kĭn′sĭs) [″ + *pachynsis,* thickening]. Abnormal thickening of the eyelid.

blepharophimosis (blĕf″ă-rō-fī-mō′sĭs] [″ + *phimosis,* narrowing]. Narrowing of slit between eyelids at external angle of eye due to angle being covered by vertical fold of skin.

blepharoplast (blĕf′ă-rō-plăst). A minute mass of chromatin in a cell forming the base of a flagellum. Morphologically it is identical to a centriole. SYN: *basal body.*

blepharoplasty (blĕf′ă-rō-plăs″tē). Plastic surgery upon the eyelid.

blepharoplegia (blĕf″ă-rō-plē′jē-ă) [Gr. *blepharon,* eyelid, + *plege,* a stroke]. Paralysis of an eyelid.

blepharoptosis (blĕf″ă-rō-tō′sĭs) [″ + *ptosis,* a falling]. Drooping of the upper eyelid.

blepharopyorrhea (blĕf″ă-rō-pī-ō-rē′ă) [″ + *pyon,* pus, + *rhoia,* flow]. Purulent material flowing from the eyelid.

blepharorrhaphy (blĕf″ă-ror′ă-fē) [″ + *rhaphe,* seam]. Reducing length of or obliterating palpebral fissure by stitching margins of eyelids. May be required to prevent damage to the cornea. SYN: *tarsorrhaphy.*

blepharorrhea (blĕf″ă-rō-rē′ă) [″ + *rhoia*, flow]. Discharge from the eyelid.

blepharospasm (blĕf′ă-rō-spăsm) [″ + *spasmos*, spasm]. A twitching or spasmodic contraction of the orbicularis oculi muscle due to habit spasm, eyestrain, or nervous irritability.

blepharosphincterectomy (blĕf″ă-rō-sfĭnk″tĕr-ĕk′tō-mē) [″ + *sphinkter*, a constrictor, + *ektome*, excision]. Excision of part of the orbicularis palpebrarum to relieve pressure of eyelid on cornea.

blepharostat (blĕf′ă-rō-stăt) [″ + *histanai*, cause to stand]. Device for separating the eyelids during an operation.

blepharostenosis (blĕf″ă-rō-stĕn-ō′sĭs) [″ + *stenosis*, a narrowing]. Narrowing of the palpebral slit through inability to open the eye normally.

blepharosynechia (blĕf″ă-rō-sĭ-nē′kē-ă) [″ + *synecheia*, a holding together]. Adhesion of the edges of the upper and lower eyelids. SYN: *ankyloblepharon*.

blepharotomy (blĕf-ă-rŏt′ō-mē) [″ + *tome*, incision]. Surgical incision of eyelid.

blepsopathia (blĕp″sō-păth′ē-ă) [Gr. *blepsis*, sight, + *pathos*, disease]. Neurasthenia caused by excessive eyestrain.

blind [AS.]. Without the sense of sight.

blindness. Amaurosis; loss of sight.

b., amnesic color. Inability to remember names of colors seen.

b., color. Absence of or defect in the perception of color. SEE: *color blindness*.

b., cortical. Blindness resulting from a lesion of visual area of cerebral cortex.

b., day. Inability to see in daylight; hemeralopia.

b., eclipse. Blindness due to burning the macula while viewing an eclipse without using protective lenses.

b., hysterical. Partial or total blindness associated with attacks of hysteria and occurring in absence of any organic defect.

b., letter. Inability to understand the meaning of letters; a form of aphasia.

b., night. Nyctalopia; inability to see at night.

b., psychic. Sight without recognition due to brain lesion.

b., snow. Blindness resulting from glare of sunlight upon the snow. May result in photophobia and conjunctivitis, the latter resulting from effects of ultraviolet rays. Usually temporary.

b., transient. Temporary blindness in one or both eyes. The onset is usually sudden. May be caused in both eyes by any condition that temporarily interferes with maintenance of blood pressure in the ophthalmic arteries, such as migraine; carotid artery insufficiency; temporal arteritis; retinal artery spasm caused by hypertensive encephalopathy, uremia, or eclampsia; optic neuritis; glaucoma; and hysteria. SYN: *amaurosis fugax*.

b., word. Inability to understand written or printed words.

blindness, words pert. to: ablepsia; acatamathesia; achloropsia; "achro-" words; acritochromacy; aglaukopsia; amaurosis; amaurotic; aphemesthesia; axanthopsia; blind spot; braille; hemeralopia; hemiachromatopsia; hemianopia; meropia; nyctamblyopia; nyctalopia; nyctotyphlosis; Optacon; tritanopia; typhlology; xanthocyanopia.

blind spot. Physiological scotoma situated 15° to outside of visual fixation point; corresponds to point where optic nerve enters the eye (optic disk), a region devoid of rods and cones. SYN: *optic disk*.

blink. To open and close eyes quickly, may be voluntary or involuntary.

blink reflex. Automatic closing of the eyes in response to a sudden movement of an object toward the eyes.

blister [MD. *bluyster*, a swelling]. 1. A collection of fluid below or within the epidermis. 2. To form a blister.

TREATMENT: Mild antiseptic, protective dressing; if extremely painful because of pressure, may be aseptically punctured and then treated as a wound.

b., blood. Small subcutaneous or intracutaneous extravasation of blood due to rupture of blood vessels.

TREATMENT: Apply antiseptic and a firm dressing with moderate pressure to aid in stopping extravasation and hasten absorption. In some cases it is desirable to puncture aseptically and aspirate.

b., fever. Herpes simplex of lip.

b., fly. Blister produced by application of cantharides to the skin.

bloated (blōt′ĕd) [AS. *bloat*]. Swollen or distended beyond normal size as by serum, water, or gas.

block [MD. *blok*, trunk of a tree]. 1. An obstruction or stoppage. 2. A method of regional anesthesia used to stop the passage of sensory impulses in a nerve, nerve trunk, dorsal root of a spinal nerve, or spinal cord, thus depriving a patient of sensation in the area involved. SEE: *anesthesia*. 3. To obstruct any passageway or opening.

b., air. A leakage of air from the respiratory passageways and its accumulation in connective tissues of the lungs, there forming an obstruction to the normal flow of air.

b., atrioventricular. A heart block in which impulses are impeded at the A-V node. SYN: *A-V block*.

b., ear. Blockage of auditory tube to the middle ear. May result from trauma, i-tion, or an accumulation of cerumen.

b., field. Regional anesthesia in which a limited operative area is walled off by an anesthetic.

b., heart. Interferences with the heart's contraction, causing dissociation of the atrial and ventricular rhythms. Due to failure of the contractile impulses to pass through the conductile tissue (atrioventricular node and bundle of His). SEE: *heart block*.

b., neuromuscular. A disturbance in transmission of impulses from motor endplate to a muscle. May be caused by an excess or deficiency of acetylcholine or by drugs that act to simulate the action of an excess or deficiency of acetylcholine.

b., paravertebral. Infiltration of stellate ganglion with a local anesthetic.

b., sinoatrial. Heart block in which there is interference in the passage of impulses between the sinus node and the atria.

b., spinal. Blockage in the flow of cerebrospinal fluid within the spinal canal.

b., ventricular. Interference in the flow of cerebrospinal fluid between the ventricles or from the ventricles through the foramina to the subarachnoid space.

blockade (blŏk-ād'). Prevention of the action of something, such as the effect of a drug or of a body function.

blocking. 1. Obstructing; the arrest of passage through. 2. In psychoanalysis, a sudden break in free association as a defense against unpleasant ideas.

blocking factors. Substances present in the serum of tumor-bearing animals that are capable of blocking the ability of immune lymphocytes to kill tumor cells.

blood [AS. *blod*]. The cell-containing fluid that circulates through the heart, arteries, veins, and capillaries carrying nourishment, electrolytes, hormones, vitamins, antibodies, heat, and oxygen to the tissues and taking away waste matter and carbon dioxide.

FUNCT: Nutrition and respiration of tissues that are located far from the food and air supplies; transportation of waste from the tissues to the excretory organs; chemical and thermal regulation and coordination of the body; defense against infection through the action of antibodies, q.v., and phagocytes, q.v.

COMP: Human blood is composed of fluid (plasma) in which are suspended red and white corpuscles, platelets, and fat globules and a great variety of chemical substances including carbohydrates, proteins, hormones, and gases such as oxygen, carbon dioxide, and nitrogen. Blood consists of approx. 22% olids and 78% water. SEE: *blood cell* for s.

pressed in metric units, an adult weighing 70 kg. has a blood volume of about 5 L. or 70 ml./kg. of body weight. The blood specific gravity varies from 1.048 to 1.066, the corpuscles being heavier and plasma lighter than this. Blood is of slightly higher specific gravity in men than in women. Specific gravity is higher after exercise and at night.

In passing through the lungs the blood gives up carbon dioxide; after leaving the heart it is carried to the tissues as arterial blood, and then returned to the heart. It moves in the aorta at an average speed of 30 cm./second, and it makes the circuit of the vascular system in about 20 seconds. It constitutes approximately 7 to 8% of the body weight. The pH of the blood is from 7.35 to 7.45. SEE: *blood count; circulation; corpuscle; plasma; platelet*.

FORMATION: Red blood cells are produced at the rate of approx. 2,400,000 each second. This is necessitated by the fact that each red blood cell lives for approx. 120 days.

CHARACTERISTICS: Blood has a distinctive, somewhat metallic, odor. Arterial blood is bright red or scarlet and usually pulsates as it issues from a cut artery. Venous blood is dark red or crimson and flows steadily as it comes from a cut vein.

b., clotting of. The process whereby blood changes into a jelly-like, nonfluid mass. A brief description of the clotting of blood follows; a more detailed account is presented at coagulation, q.v. Blood plasma normally contains the protein fibrinogen. Thrombin is formed from elements present in the blood when blood is exposed to air, foreign substances, or juices from injured tissues. Thrombin converts fibrinogen into the insoluble fibrin, an elastic stringy substance that forms a meshwork in which the corpuscles are caught. Calcium deficiency causes tendency to slow clotting. SEE: *coagulation*.

b., cord. A specimen of blood obtained from the umbilical cord vein or artery of the fetus.

b., defibrinated. Whole blood from which fibrin was separated during the clotting process. If whole blood is stirred, the stringy elastic fibrin comes out on the stirrer; it can be washed until white. The remaining thick, red blood can no longer clot and is called defibrinated blood. If it is centrifuged, the clear liquid that now appears in the upper half of the centrifuged tube is called serum; this differs from plasma chiefly in that it does not contain fibrinogen (the precursor of fibrin). The corpuscles are in the lower portion of the tube.

b., occult. The presence of blood in such small quantities that it is not apparent to the eye. Thus blood may be present in feces but of such color and consistency as to be unnoticed by the patient. Usually detected only by chemical tests or by microscopic or spectroscopic examination. SEE: *benzidin test.*

b., sludged. Blood in which red corpuscles have massed together in the smaller blood vessels, and block or slow the blood flowing through the vessels.

RS: erythrocyte; leukocyte.

b., unit of. Approximately one pint (473 ml.) of blood. The usual amount available for use in transfusion.

b., vessels. The veins, arteries, and capillaries.

blood bank. The place where whole blood and certain derived components are processed, typed, and stored until needed for transfusion. Blood is mixed with sodium citrate, physiological saline solution, and glucose, and is stored at 4° C. (39° F.). Banked blood should be used as soon as possible because the longer it is stored, the fewer red blood cells survive in usable form. Ninety percent of the red cells survive up to 14 days of storage, but only 70% remain after 24 days.

blood-brain barrier. A barrier membrane between circulating blood and the brain, preventing certain damaging substances from reaching brain tissue and cerebrospinal fluid. SEE: *membrane, glial.*

blood cell. Minute body in the blood. There are several principal types: erythrocytes or red blood corpuscles, leukocytes or white blood corpuscles, and platelets. SEE: illus.; *blood.*

blood cell casts. Masses of red cells molded by the renal tubules, the blood originating from the glomeruli. Abnormal microscopic body in the urine composed of coagulated serum covered with red blood cells.

blood clot. Coagulated mass of blood. SYN: *coagulum.* SEE: *blood, clotting of.*

blood component. One of the components forming the blood. Blood may be transfused in its whole state or one of its components may be administered. The following are blood components:

Cryoprecipitated antihemophilic factor (AHF). A concentrate prepared from thawed plasma. Used in treating hemophiliacs. Each concentrate contains approx. 100 U. of AHF and approx. 300 mg. of fibrinogen, the clotting factor in the blood.

Fibrinogen. The clotting factor in the blood. Used in treating bleeding due to hypofibrinogenemia. The cryoprecipitated AHF concentrate contains approx. 300 mg. of fibrinogen.

Granulocyte cells. White blood cells; mature granular leukocytes. This blood component is experimentally used in patients with leukemia or in the chemotherapy of cancer

TYPES OF CELLS PRESENT IN BLOOD

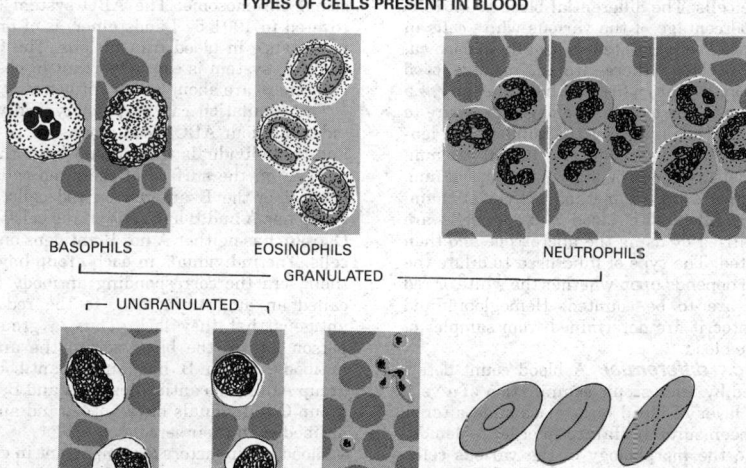

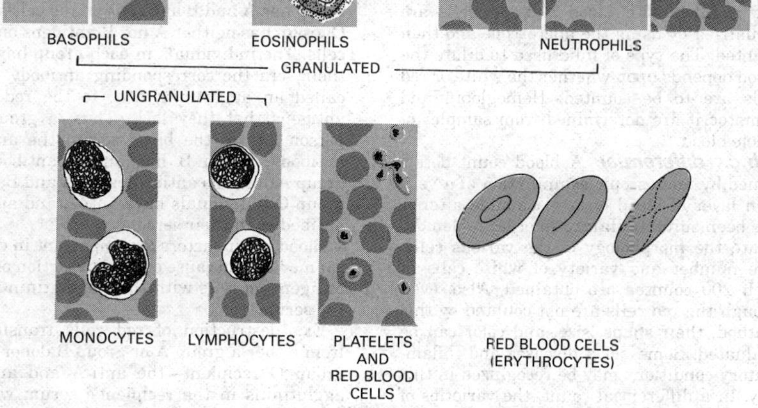

patients.

Packed frozen red cells. Whole blood from which the plasma has been removed, and that has been frozen in a solution of glycerol, glucose, fructose, and sodium ethylenediamine tetraacetic acid. The cells are thawed just before transfusion. The advantage of this technique is that the blood can be stored in a frozen state at −80° C for as long as a year.

Packed red cells. Blood from which the plasma has been removed. Used for patients who need red cells but do not need plasma. Use of this component reduces overload of the circulatory system and the risk of undesired antigenic response to the infused blood.

Plasma. Blood from which the cellular material has been removed. The use of plasma as a blood component has decreased due to the risk of viral hepatitis transmission.

Plasma protein fraction. A solution of the proteins of liquid human plasma. Used in treating shock caused by hemorrhage, trauma, infections, burns, or surgery.

Plasma concentrate. One unit, 10 to 30 ml., is obtained from one unit of platelet-rich plasma. Used in treating thrombocytopenia.

blood corpuscles. The solid or cellular elements in the blood. SYN: *blood cell*. SEE: *erythrocyte; leukocyte*.

blood count. Enumeration of the red corpuscles and the leukocytes per cu. mm. of whole blood. A blood count indicates the number of these cells. The differential blood count tells the percentage of the various white cells in each 100 cells counted. Normally in each cu. mm. of blood there are an average of 5 million erythrocytes in the male and 4.5 million in the female. Prolonged exposure to high altitude increases the number. The leukocytes average 5,000 to 10,000/cu. mm. Platelets average 150,000 to 400,000/cu. mm. by direct counting method. A special chamber is filled with blood and the cells are visualized by using the microscope and then counted. The type of fluid used to dilute the blood depends upon whether the white or red cells are to be counted. Hemoglobin and hematocrit are determined from samples of whole blood.

b.c., differential. A blood count determined by microscopic examination of a very thin layer of blood on a glass slide after it has been suitably stained in order to demonstrate the morphology of the various cells. The number and variety of white cells in each 200 counted are obtained. Also, even though the red cells are not counted by this method, their shape, size, and color can be valuated. Some blood diseases and inflam- tory conditions may be recognized in this In a differential count, the varieties of ukocytes and their percentages normally should be: neutrophils (segmented), 40–60%; eosinophils, 1–3%; basophils, 0.5–1%; lymphocytes, 20–40%; monocytes, 4–8%.

blood crossmatching. The process of mixing a sample of the donor's red blood cells with the recipient's serum (major crossmatching), and mixing a sample of the recipient's blood with the donor's serum (minor crossmatching). This is done before transfusion to determine compatibility of blood.

blood donor. One who gives blood to be used for transfusion.

blood dust. Minute colorless bodies in the blood, particles of the blood corpuscle. SYN: *hemoconia*.

blood gas analysis. Chemical analysis of the blood for the concentration of oxygen and carbon dioxide. This may be done on arterial or venous blood; the specimen may be obtained from an arm vein or by use of a catheter extending from a peripheral vein to the heart. The blood sample is usually collected in a heparinized vacuum tube with care being taken to assure that the specimen is not exposed to air.

blood groups. A genetically determined system of antigens located on the surface of the erythrocyte. There are at least 14 human blood group systems; each system is determined by a series of two or more genes that are allelic or closely linked on a single autosomal chromosome. The ABO system (discovered in 1901 by Landsteiner) is of prime importance in blood transfusions. The Rhesus (Rh) system is esp. important in obstetrics. There are about 30 Rh antigens.

The population can be phenotypically divided into four ABO blood groups: A, B, AB, and O. Individuals in A group have the A antigen on the surface of their red cells; B group has the B antigen on red cells; AB group has A and B antigens on red cells; and O group has neither A nor B antigens on red cells. The individuals in each group have in their sera the corresponding antibody, also called an agglutinin, q.v., to the red cell antigens that they lack. Thus, a group A person has in the blood serum the anti-B antibody; group B has anti-A antibodies; group AB has no antibodies for A and B; and group O individuals have anti-A and anti-B antibodies in their sera.

Blood group factors are important in clinical medicine because of the interaction of the antigens on cells with their agglutinin(s) in the serum.

Ex.: destruction of red cells transfused from either a group A or group B donor to a group O recipient—the anti-A and anti-B agglutinins in the recipient's serum would react with the A or B antigens on the donor's red cells.

Analysis of blood groups is important in identifying blood stains for medicolegal purposes; for genetic and anthropological studies, and in determining the probability of fatherhood in disputes involving claimed or disclaimed paternity. SEE: *Rh blood factor.*

bloodless. Without blood.

bloodletting. Removal of blood from the body as a therapeutic measure, usually by venipuncture. This technique is used in treating hemochromatosis, polycythemia vera, and in infants born with elevated hematocrits.

blood platelets. Small, colorless bodies in circulating blood, averaging about 3 microns in diameter. They tend to agglutinate into small clusters in shed blood. Platelets may originate from giant bone marrow cells (megakaryocytes). They play an important role in clotting through release of thrombokinase, which, in the presence of calcium, reacts with prothrombin to form thrombin.

The normal number in circulating blood in adults is about 150,000 to 400,000/cu. mm. Reduction below normal is called thrombocytopenia. In certain forms of hemophilia, blood platelets are abnormally stable and fail to release thrombokinase, thus increasing coagulation time.

blood poisoning. A vague term usually used to indicate the presence of large numbers of bacteria in the circulating blood. SEE: *pyemia; septicemia; toxemia.*

blood pressure. As popularly used, the pressure, determined indirectly, existing in the large arteries at the height of the pulse wave; the systolic intra-arterial pressure. More generally, the pressure exerted by the blood on the wall of any vessel. This pressure reaches its highest values in the left ventricle during systole. It decreases in the arterial system as the distance from the heart increases, and is lower in capillaries than in the arteries. The systolic arterial blood pressure rises during activity or excitement and falls during sleep. In the normal, relaxed, sitting adult, it may be as low as 100 and as high as 140 mm. of mercury (Hg).

The following findings are considered abnormal: systolic pressure persistently above 140; diastolic pressure persistently above 100; pulse pressure constantly greater than 50. Blood pressure varies with age, sex, altitude, muscular development, and according to states of mental and physical stress and fatigue. Usually it is lower in women than in men, low in childhood, and higher in elderly individuals. SEE: *b.p., normal.*

RS: diastole; hypertension; hypotension; pulse pressure; systole.

b.p., central. Blood pressure in the heart chambers, in a great vein, or close to the heart. If determined in a vein, it is termed central venous blood pressure; if in the aorta or a similar large artery close to the heart, it is designated central arterial blood pressure.

b.p., diastolic. Blood pressure during the relaxation phase between heart beats, normally about 80 mm. Hg It is dependent primarily upon the elasticity of the arteries and peripheral resistance, which in turn is dependent upon caliber of arterioles and capillaries.

b.p., direct measurement of. Determining the blood pressure in one of several arteries. Done by placing a sterile needle or small catheter inside an artery and having the blood pressure transmitted through that system to a suitable recorder. As the blood pressure fluctuates, the changes are recorded graphically.

b.p., indirect measurement of. A simple external method for measuring blood pressure.

Palpatory method: The same arm, usually the right, should be used each time the pressure is measured. The arm should be raised to heart level if the patient is sitting, or kept parallel to the body if the patient is recumbent. The patient's arm should be relaxed and supported in a resting position. Exertion during the examination could result in a higher blood pressure reading. Either a mercury-gravity or aneroid-manometer type of blood pressure apparatus may be used. The blood compression cuff should be the width and length appropriate for the size of the subject's arm: narrow (2.5 to 6 cm.) for infants and children and wide (13 cm.) for adults. The inflatable bag encased in the cuff should be 20% wider than one third the circumference of the limb used. The deflated cuff is placed evenly and snugly around the upper arm so that its lower edge is about one inch above the point of the brachial artery where the bell of the stethoscope will be applied. While feeling the radial pulse, inflate the cuff until the pressure is about 30 mm. above the point where the radial pulse was no longer felt. Deflate the cuff slowly and record as accurately as possible the pressure at which the pulse returns to the radial artery. Systolic blood pressure is determined by this method; diastolic blood pressure cannot be determined by this method.

Auscultatory method: Begin as above. After inflating the cuff until the pressure is about 30 mm. above the point where the radial pulse disappears, place the bell of the stethoscope over the brachial artery just below the blood pressure cuff. Then deflate the cuff slowly, about 2 to 3 mm. of Hg per heart beat. The first sound heard from the ar is recorded as the systolic pressure. The point at which sounds are no longer heard is recorded as the diastolic pressure. For convenience the blood pressure is recorded as figures separated by a slant. The systolic value is recorded first.

Ex.: 120/80 indicates systolic pressure of 120 and diastolic of 80.

Sounds heard over the brachial artery change in quality at some point prior to the point the sounds completely disappear. Some physicians consider this the diastolic pressure. This value should be noted when recording the blood pressure by placing it between the systolic pressure and the pressure noted when the sound disappears. Thus, 120/90/80 would indicate a systolic pressure of 120 with a first diastolic pressure of 90 and a second diastolic pressure of 80. The latter pressure would be the point of disappearance of all sounds from the artery. When the values are so recorded, the physician may use either of the last two figures as the diastolic pressure. When the change in sound and the disappearance of all sound coincide, the result should be written as follows: 120/80/80.

Doppler method: A technique used to determine blood pressure in newborn infants and anyone in whom the sounds normally heard are difficult to hear. The changes in arterial pressure are determined by use of ultrasound.

b.p., mean. Half of the sum of systolic and diastolic values. For a normal person in good health, about 100 mm. Hg.

b.p., negative. Blood pressure is less than atmospheric pressure as in the great veins near the heart.

b.p., normal. In healthy young persons, 100 to 140 mm. Hg and 60 to 90 mm. diastolic. Loss of resilience in the vascular tree and physiological changes of age must be considered when levels above 140 mm. are obtained in apparently healthy, older persons.

b.p., systolic. The greatest force caused by the contraction of the left ventricle of the heart.

blood pressure monitor. A device that automatically obtains and usually records the blood pressure at certain intervals. The apparatus may use the direct or indirect method of determining pressure. In some models, an alarm or light signal is activated if the pressure rises or falls to abnormal levels.

bloodshot. Local congestion of the smaller blood vessels of a part, as when the vessels of the conjunctiva are dilated and visible.

blood shunting. A condition in which blood, going through an abnormal pathway or ...s, does not travel its normal route. May ... when an arteriovenous fistula forms or in congenital anomalies of the heart in which the blood passes from the right atrium or ventricle directly to the left atrium or ventricle respectively, through a defect in the wall (septum) that normally separates the atria and ventricles.

blood smear. Drop of blood spread thin on a slide for purpose of examination.

PROCEDURE: Clean glass with alcohol, rinse in warm water, and wipe clean with lint-free towel or lens paper. Slide must be grease-free. Place a small drop of blood on the slide. Bring the end of another slide (spreader slide) against first slide at a 45° angle and pull it back against drop of blood so that the drop will spread between the point of contact of the two slides. Then push spreader slide forward against the first slide and the blood will form an even smear. The smear must be thin. Dry slide by waving in air. Do not heat.

STAIN: A common method follows: Cover the blood smear with Wright's stain. Allow to stand 2 min. Add an equal amount of distilled water or buffer solution, mixing uniformly. Let stand 5 min. Gently wash off stain. Allow to dry. If permanent slide is desired, mount with balsam or methacrylate.

bloodstream. The blood that flows through the circulatory system of an organism.

blood sugar. Sugar in the form of glucose, normally 60 to 100 mg./100 ml. of blood. It rises after a meal to as much as 150 mg./100 ml. of blood but this may vary. SEE: *glucose.*

blood test. A test to determine the chemical, physical, or serological characteristics of the blood or some portion of it.

blood transfusion. Transfer of blood of one person into blood vessels of another. In direct or immediate transfusion, the blood is transferred via a tube directly from the donor to the recipient. In indirect or mediate transfusion, the blood is collected in a receptacle from the donor before transfusion.

NURSING IMPLICATIONS: Take special care to check accurately the patient's blood type against the blood type on the bag of blood to be administered. Blood is not compatible with most I.V. solutions and should never be administered with any solution except physiological saline solution. Obtain and record the patient's temperature and pulse rate prior to administration of blood. Blood should be double-checked for correct type by two people before infusion is started. Once the blood transfusion has begun, remain with the patient for the first 15 minutes to assess for any adverse reactions. If any signs of incompatibility such as hives, chest pain, back pains, shortness of breath, chills, or overall aching feeling should occur, immediately stop the infusion, keep the vein patent by infusing physiological saline, and notify the physician immediately. Take the patient's vital signs every 30 minutes during the transfusions, and if incompatibility is suspected, also obtain a urine specimen.

Blood should run at a rate to deliver the prescribed volume in no longer than 2 to 2½ hours. Blood should be refrigerated until used. Sometimes special conditions require warming the blood just prior to administering it.

blood typing. The method used to determine various factors when blood is tested according to blood group systems such as ABO, MN, or Rh-Hr.

blood urea nitrogen. ABBR: BUN. Nitrogen in the blood in the form of urea. The normal concentration is 9 to 25 mg./ml. The level of urea in the blood provides a rough estimate of kidney function. An increase in the blood urea nitrogen level usually indicates decreased renal function.

blood vessels. The veins, arteries, and capillaries.

blood warmer. Device for warming banked blood to body temperature prior to using it for transfusion.

bloody sweat. Excretion of blood or blood pigment through the sweat gland. SYN: *hemathidrosis*.

bloody weeping. Hemorrhage from conjunctiva.

blotch. A blemish, spot, or area of discoloration on the skin.

blowfly. One of a number of genera of flies belonging to the family Calliphoridae. Most are scavengers, their larvae living in decaying flesh or meat although occasionally they may live in decaying or suppurating tissue. However, one species, the screw-worm fly, Callitroga hominivorax, attacks living tissue, laying its eggs in the nostrils or open wounds of the host domestic animals or man, giving rise to myiasis, q.v.

blowpipe. A tube through which a gas or current of air is passed under pressure, being directed upon a flame. It is employed to concentrate and intensify the heat of the flame.

blue [O. Fr. *bleu*]. 1. A primary color of the spectrum; sky color; azure. 2. Cyanotic.

blue baby. SEE: *baby, blue*.

bluebottle flies. Flies of the family Calliphoridae. They breed in dung or the flesh of dead animals.

Blumberg's sign (blŭm'bĕrgs). [Jacob Moritz Blumberg, Ger. surgeon and gynecologist, 1873–1955] The occurrence of a sharp acute pain when the examiner presses his or her hand over McBurney's point and then releases the hand pressure suddenly. This sign is indicative of peritoneal inflammation. SYN: *rebound tenderness*.

Blumenbach's clivus (bloo'mĕn-bawks). [Johann F. Blumenbach, Ger. physiologist and anthropologist, 1752–1840] Sloping part of sphenoid bone behind posterior clinoid processes.

blush [AS. *blyscan*, to be red]. Redness of the face and neck due to vasodilation caused by emotion or heat. Blushing may also be associated with certain diseases, including carcinoid syndrome, pheochromocytoma, and Zollinger-Ellison syndrome.

B-lymphocytes. B cells, q.v.

Blyth's test (blīths). [Alexander W. Blyth, Brit. physician, 1846–1921] A test for the detection of lead in drinking water. In the presence of lead a white precipitate forms on the addition of a small amount of alcoholic tincture of cochineal to the water to be tested.

B.M.A. *British Medical Association.*

B.M.R. *basal metabolic rate.*

B.M.S. *Bachelor of Medical Science.*

BNA. *Basle Nomina Anatomica*, an anatomical nomenclature adopted by the German Anatomical Society in 1895, at Basel, Switzerland. It includes some 4500 terms. Has more recently been revised as NA terms. SEE: *Nomina Anatomica*.

Boas' point (bō'āz). [Ismar I. Boas, Ger. physician, 1858–1938] A tender spot left of the 12th dorsal vertebra in patients with gastric ulcer.

Bochdalek's ganglion (bŏk'dăl-ĕks). [Victor Bochdalek, Czech. anatomist, 1801–1883] Ganglion of plexus of dental nerve in the maxilla above the canine tooth.

Bodo (bō'dō). A genus of the Bodonidae, flagellate protozoa often found in stale feces or urine and sometimes in the urinary bladder. Nonpathogenic.

body [AS. *bodig*]. 1. Soma; the physical part of man as distinguished from mind and spirit. 2. The trunk. 3. The principal mass of any structure. 4. The largest or most important part of any organ.

EXAM: The nude body is examined and both sides compared. Physical examination is made by inspection, palpation, manipulation, mensuration, auscultation, q.v., and use of the sense of smell. Physical examination should also include observation of the body as the person walks and goes through the various ranges of motions of the trunk, neck, and extremities. Chemical and microscopic examination may be made of the blood, sputum, feces, urine, cerebrospinal fluids, and other fluids of the body. X-ray is also used and checked with clinical findings.

b., acetone. Ketone bodies. One of a number of substances that increase in th- blood as a result of faulty fat metab-

Among them are β-hydroxybutyric acid, acetoacetic acid, and acetone. They are increased in persons with untreated or inadequately controlled diabetes mellitus and are the primary cause of acidosis. They may also occur in other metabolic disturbances.

b., amygdaloid. Almond-shaped gray matter in the lateral wall and roof of the third ventricle of the brain.

b., aortic. One of two small bodies that are located in the arch of the aorta and contain the endings of the aortic nerve. They respond to oxygen concentration in the blood and to changes in blood pressure.

b., asbestosis. The minute bodies formed by the deposition of various salts and minerals around an asbestos particle. These may be found in the sputum, lung, or feces.

b.'s, Aschoff. Microscopic foci of fibrinoid degeneration and granulomatous inflammation found in interstitial tissues of the heart in rheumatic fever.

b., Barr. The sex chromatin mass that represents the genetically inactivated X chromosome found in somatic cells of normal females. SEE: *Barr body.*

b., basal. A small granule usually present at the base of a flagellum or a cilium in protozoa. SYN: *granule, basal.*

b., carotid. A flat structure at the bifurcation of the common carotid artery. Contains cells that respond to changes in concentration of oxygen in the blood and to changes in blood pressure, thus aiding in regulating circulation.

b., chromaffin. One of a number of bodies composed principally of chromaffin cells, q.v., that lie serially arranged along both sides of the dorsal aorta and in the kidney, liver, and gonads. They are ectodermal in origin, having the same origin as cells of the sympathetic ganglia. SYN: *paraganglia.*

b.'s, chromophilous. Large granular bodies in nerve cells, demonstrated by selective staining. SYN: *b.'s, Nissl; granules, Nissl.*

b., ciliary. Thickened part of the vascular tunic of the eye between the base of the iris and the anterior part of the choroid. Consists of three zones: ciliary disk, ciliary crown, and ciliary muscle. SEE: *eye* for illus.

b., coccygeal. An arteriovenous anastomosis at the tip of the coccyx formed by the middle sacral artery. Also called glomus coccygeum [NA].

b.'s, Donovan. The common name for the causative organism. Calymmatobacterium granulomatis, of granuloma inguinale, q.v.

b., foreign. An object present at a site ...e it would not normally or naturally be ...t.

b., geniculate, lateral. One of two bodies forming elevations on the lateral portion of the posterior part of the thalamus. Each is the termination of afferent fibers from the retina, which it receives through the optic nerves and tracts.

b., geniculate, medial. One of two bodies lying in the posterior part of the dorsal thalamus. Each receives fibers from the acoustic center of the medulla and from the inferior colliculus through the brachium.

b., Hensen's. A modified Golgi net found in the hair cells of the organ of Corti.

b., inclusion. Nonliving substances in the protoplasm of a cell. Seen in disease caused by virus infections.

b., ketone. One of a number of substances that increase in the blood as a result of faulty fat metabolism. Among them are β-hydroxybutyric acid, acetoacetic acid, and acetone. They increase in persons with untreated or inadequately controlled diabetes mellitus and are the primary cause of acidosis. They may also occur in other metabolic disturbances.

b.'s, Leishman-Donovan. Small bodies found in the spleen and liver of victims of kala-azar or dum-dum fever. Now known to be Leishmania donovani, causative organism of the disease. They are found both within and outside of living cells and in circulating blood.

b., malpighian. 1. A renal corpuscle consisting of a glomerulus enclosed in Bowman's capsule. 2. A lymph nodule found in the spleen.

b., mammillary. A rounded body of gray matter found in the diencephalon. It forms a rounded eminence projecting into the anterior portion of the interpeduncular fossa. Their nuclei constitute an important relay station for olfactory impulses.

b., medullary. The deeper white matter of the cerebellum enclosed within the cortex.

b.'s, Negri. Inclusion bodies found in the cells of the central nervous system of animals infected with rabies. They are acidophilic masses appearing in large ganglion cells or in cells of the brain, esp. those of the hippocampus and cerebellum. Their presence is considered conclusive proof of rabies.

b.'s, Nissl. Large granular bodies in nerve cells, demonstrated by selective staining. They are absent in the axon and axon hillock. They show changes under various physiological conditions and in pathological conditions may dissolve and disappear (chromatolysis). SYN: *b., chromophilous; granules, Nissl.*

b., olivary. A rounded mass located in the anterolateral portion of the medulla oblongata. Consists of a convoluted sheet of gray matter enclosing white matter. SYN: *oliva.*

b., pacchionian. Arachnoid granulation. Numerous small ovoid or villus-like projections of the arachnoid membrane of the brain. They may project into the superior sagittal sinus as arachnoid villi or they may press against the outer dura and grow into the inner plate of the cranium, forming ovoid depressions. SYN: *arachnoid villi; granulation, arachnoidal.*

b., perineal. The mass of tissue that separates the anus from the vestibule and the lower part of the vagina. SEE: *perineum* for illus.

b., pineal. A glandlike structure in the brain, shaped like a pine cone, and located in a pocket near the splenium of the corpus collosum. It appears to be the major site of melatonin biosynthesis in most mammals and in man, but the effect of melatonin on the body and the exact function of the pineal body remain unknown. SYN: *pineal gland.*

b., pituitary. The hypophysis; pituitary gland, q.v.

b., polar. A small cell produced in oogenesis resulting from the divisions of the primary and secondary oocytes.

b., postbranchial. One of two bodies that develop from the posterior wall of the 4th pharyngeal pouch. They become incorporated into the thyroid gland. SYN: *ultimobranchial body.*

b., psammoma. A laminated calcareous body seen in certain types of tumors, sometimes associated with chronic inflammation.

b.'s, quadrigeminal. Four rounded projections from the roof of the midbrain. SYN: *colliculus superior et inferior* [NA].

b., restiform. The inferior cerebellar peduncles. Two bands of fibers that connect the medulla with the cerebellum.

b., striate. The corpus striatum, composed of the cordate and lenticular nucleoli of the brain.

b., trachoma. Mass of cells present as an inclusion body in the conjunctival epithelial cells of individuals with trachoma.

b., vertebral. A short column of bone forming the weight-supporting portion of a vertebra. From its dorsolateral surfaces project the roots of the arch of a vertebra.

b., vitreous. A jelly-like substance within the eye that fills the space between the lens and the retina. It is colorless, structureless, and transparent.

b., wolffian. The mesonephros or middle kidney of the embryo.

body cavities. The thorax, abdomen, and pelvis.

body composition. Quantitation of the various components of the body, esp. of the fat, water, and muscle. Determination of the specific gravity of the body is done to estimate the percent fat. This may be calculated by various methods, including underwater weighing, which determines the density of the individual; use of radioactive potassium, ^{40}K; measuring the total body water by dilution of tritium; and use of various anthropometric measurements such as height, weight, and skin fold thickness at various sites. The obese person has a lower body density than does the lean person, because the specific gravity of fat tissue is less than that of muscle tissue. The fat content for young men will vary from about 5 to 27% and for women from about 18 to 35%.

body fluids. Total body water in humans varies from 50% of the body weight in obese individuals to 70% in the non-obese. The principal compartments for body fluids are intracellular and extracellular. A much smaller segment, the transcellular, includes fluid in the tracheobronchial tree, the gastrointestinal tract, the bladder, cerebrospinal fluid, and the aqueous humor of the eye. The chemical composition of fluids in the various compartments is carefully regulated. SEE: *acid-base balance.*

body image. The subjective image or picture people have of their physical appearance based on their own observations and the reaction of others.

body language. The unconscious use of posture, gestures, or other forms of nonverbal expression in communication. SEE: *kinesics.*

body mechanics. Application of kinesiology to use of the body in daily life activities and to the prevention and correction of problems related to posture.

body section radiography. Radiological examination of specific layers of the body, blurring out intervening anatomical structures.

body snatching. Robbing a grave of its body. Done in the past to obtain bodies for anatomical study in medical schools.

body surface area. The surface area of the body expressed in square meters. This may be calculated when the height and weight of a subject are known by using a standard formula. Body surface area is an important measure in calculating pediatric dosages, in the management of burn patients, and in determining radiation doses. SEE: *area, body surface; burns; rule of nines.*

body type. Classification of the human body according to muscle and fat distribution. SEE: *ectomorph; endomorph; mesomorph; somatotype.*

Boeck's sarcoid (běks). [Caesar P. M. Boeck, Norwegian physician, 1845–1917] Former name for sarcoidosis, a disease of unknow[n] etiology characterized by widespread [gran]lomatous lesions that may affect or tissue of the body. The liver is frequently affected, as are the skin, lungs, lymph nodes, spleen, eyes, and small bones of the hands and feet.

Boerhaave syndrome (boor'hă-vĕ). [H. Boerhaave, Dutch physician, 1668–1738] Complete, spontaneous rupture of the esophagus usually associated with violent retching or vomiting. SEE: *Mallory-Weiss syndrome.*

boil [AS. *byl,* a swelling]. A furuncle, an acute circumscribed inflammation of the subcutaneous layers of the skin, gland, or hair follicle. The deeper tissue inflammation is so severe that blood clots in the vessels and forms a "core." This is the cause of the acuteness of the pain; the "core" is ultimately expelled or reabsorbed. Boils are most commonly due to tissue invasion by staphylococci.

TREATMENT: Protect from irritation; apply moist heat intermittently. Keep skin scrupulously clean and avoid injury or trauma to involved region. Bedrest may be necessary in severe cases. After lesions are fluctuant, surgical incision and drainage may be desirable. The area around draining abscesses should be protected by an antibiotic ointment to prevent new lesions on surrounding areas. If lesions are large and located on the face, an appropriate antibiotic should be used systemically to prevent possible complications such as meningitis or septicemia.

boiling. Process of vaporization of a liquid. Boiling water destroys most microorganisms (but may not kill spores and some viruses); toughens and hardens albumin in eggs; toughens, i.e., denatures, fibrin and dissolves tissues in meat; bursts starch granules; and softens cellulose in cereals and vegetables.

boiling point. The degree of heat required to bring a liquid to a boil, which varies according to the chemicals present in different liquids. Water boils at 212° F. (100° C.) under ordinary conditions at sea level. To kill most vegetable forms of microorganisms, water should be boiled 30 minutes. Aeration (pouring from one vessel to another) will overcome the flat taste of boiled water.

bolometer (bō-lŏm'ĕ-tĕr) [Gr. *bole,* a ray, + *metron,* measure]. 1. Device for measuring the force of the heart beat apart from blood pressure. 2. An instrument for gauging minute degrees of radiant heat.

bolus (bō'lŭs) [L., from Gr. *bolos,* a lump]. 1. ...mass of masticated food ready to be swal-...d. 2. A rounded preparation of medicine ...al ingestion. 3. A concentrated mass of ...nostic substance given intravenously, ... an opaque contrast medium, or an ...us medication. 4. Tissue equivalent ...iation therapy to increase the dose ...r to equalize the dose to a curved surface.

b., alimentary. The mass of masticated food in the esophagus that is ready to be passed into the stomach.

bombesin (bŏm'bĕ-sĭn). A neuropeptide present in the gut and brain tissue of man. It is also present in increased concentrations in cell cultures of small cell carcinomas of the lung.

bond. A force that binds ions or atoms together. It is represented by a line drawn from one molecule or atom to another as in H—O—H.

bonding, mother-infant. The very important emotional and physical attachment, i.e., bond, between infant and mother that is initiated in the first hour or two after normal delivery of a baby who has not been dulled by anesthetic agents or drugs. It is believed that the stronger this bond, the greater the chances of a mentally healthy infant-mother relationship in both the short- and long-term period following childbirth. Because of this it is further believed that initial contact between mother and infant should be in the delivery room and that this contact should be for as long as possible in the first hours after birth.

bone [AS. *ban,* bone]. 1. Osseous tissue, a specialized form of dense connective tissue consisting of bone cells (osteocytes) embedded in a matrix made up of calcified intercellular substance. SEE: illus. 2. An individual unit of the skeleton. SYN: *os.* SEE: illus.; *cell* for illus.

Bones provide shape and support for the body of vertebrates. They also serve as storage sites for mineral salts; and play an important role in providing in the marrow a site for the formation of blood cells. Bone consists of about 50% water and 50% solid matter, the solids being chiefly cartilage hardened by impregnation with inorganic salts, esp. carbonate and phosphate of lime. The proportion of lime in bone gradually increases, and in old age there is such a large proportion that the bones are brittle and break easily. They surround and protect some vital organs, and give points of attachment for the muscles, serving as levers and making movement possible. The outer surface is less porous than the inner and is called the compact tissue; the more porous portion is called cancellous tissue. The compact tissue is tunneled by a central canal containing marrow and fine branching canals. Small blood vessels and lymphatics for the maintenance and repair of bone tissue run in these canals. This is known as the haversian system. The exterior covering of the bone, or periosteum, serves to extend the blood supply to the bone. According to their shape, bones are classified as flat, irregular, long, and short.

BONE

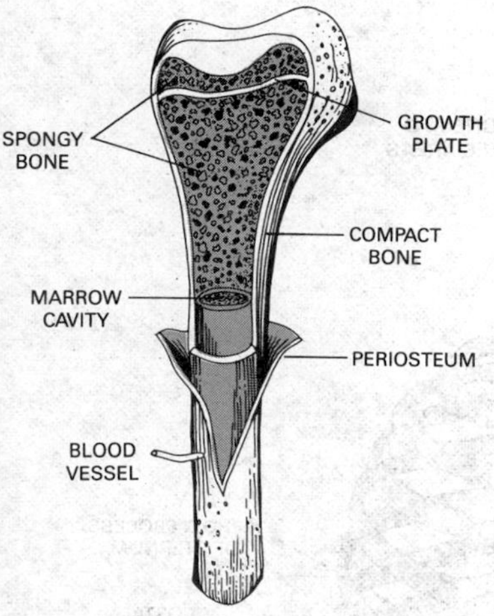

SECTION OF SHAFT OF A LONG BONE

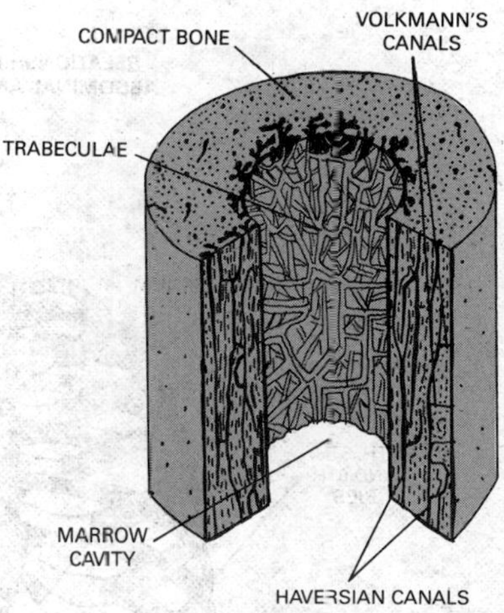

For depressions, openings, and cavities in bones: SEE: *antrum* (nearly enclosed cavity); *canal; fissure* (slitlike opening); *foramen* (opening for blood vessels and nerves); *fossa* (concavity); *groove; meatus* (tubelike passage or opening; canal); *sinus* (air cavity within a bone; or groove lodging a blood sinus); *sulcus* (groove).

For processes (enlargements or protrusions) of bones: SEE: *crest* (a ridge); *condyle* (rounded process for articulation); *head* (rounded end of a bone separated from body by a constricted region, the neck); *spine* (pointed process); *trochanter* (very large process); *tubercle* (small rounded process); *tuberosity* (large rounded process).

For names of principal bones: SEE: *skeleton*.

b., ankle. The astragalus or talus, q.v.

b., breast. The sternum, q.v.

b., brittle. Abnormal brittleness of bones.

b., cancellous. A spongy bone in which the matrix forms connecting bars and plates, partially enclosing many intercommunicating spaces filled with bone marrow.

b., cartilage. Endochondral bone that develops from cartilage.

b., cavalry. A localized bony formation in adductor magnus femoris, sometimes seen in horseback riders. SYN: *riders' bone.*

b., collar. The clavicle.

b., compact. Dense hard bone with microscopic spaces.

b., cotyloid. Bone that during development forms a part of medial portion of the acetabulum. It fuses with the pubis.

b., cranial. A bone of the cranium or brain case.

b., dermal. Membrane bone.

b., endochondral. B., cartilage, q.v.

b., incarial. The interparietal bone, part of the occipital bone.

b., incisive. Part of maxilla bearing the incisor teeth.

b., innominate. Hip bone, composed of the ilium, ischium, and pubis.

b., intracartilaginous Cartilage or endochondral bone.

b., ivory. B., marble, q.v.

b., marble. Abnormally calcified bones with spotted appearance in a roentgenogram. SYN: *b., ivory.* SEE: *Albers-Schönberg disease; osteopetrosis.*

b., membrane. The bone that develops within a connective tissue membrane.

b., perichondrial. Bone formed beneath the perichondrium.

b., periosteal. Bone formed by osteoblasts of the periosteum.

b., ping pong. The thin shell of osseous tissue covering a giant cell sarcoma in a bone.

b., replacement. Any bone that develops within cartilage.

b., sesamoid. A type of short b
curring in the hands and feet and

RELATIONSHIP OF BONES TO ABDOMINAL AND PELVIC AREAS

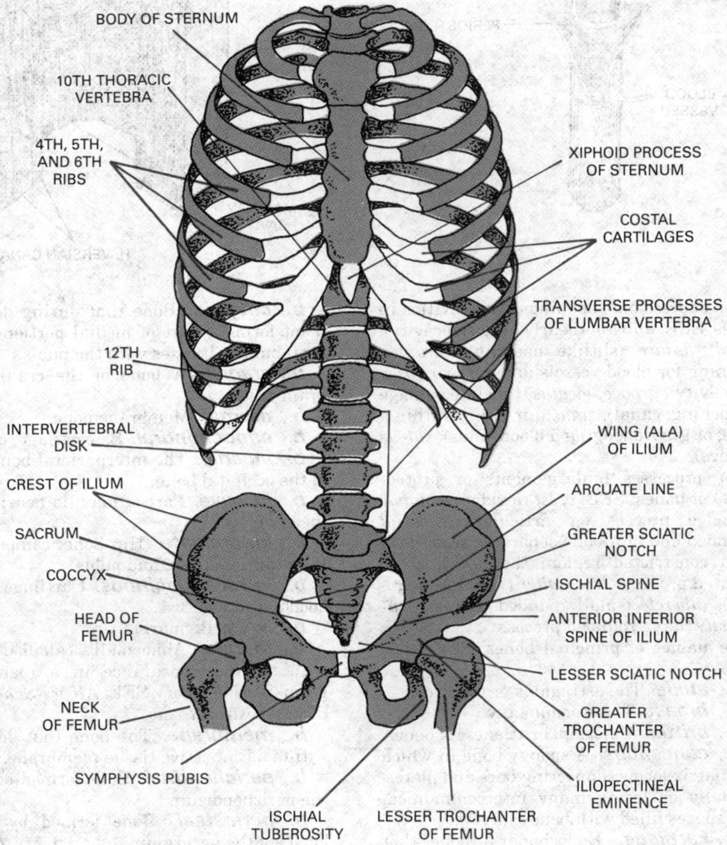

in tendons or joint capsules.

b., spongy. B., cancellous, q.v.

b., sutural. B., wormian, q.v.

b., thigh. The femur.

b., wormian. A small, irregularly shaped bone often found in the sutures of the cranium. SYN: *b., sutural.*

bone age. An estimate of biological age based on x-ray studies of the stage of development of ossification centers of the long bones of the extremities. SEE: *epiphysis.*

bone cell. A nucleated cell occupying a separate lacuna of bone. SEE: *osteoblast; osteoclast.*

bone cyst. A cystic bone tumor.

bone graft. A piece of bone taken from an animal (foreign) or from some bone of the patient that is used to take the place of a removed bone or bony defect. SEE: *graft; prosthesis.*

bonelet. A small bone; ossicle.

bone marrow. The soft organic material that fills the cavities of the bone. SEE: *marrow.*

bone marrow transplant. Transplantation of bone marrow from one individual to another. Used in treating aplastic anemia and immunodeficient patients. Transplantation of bone marrow has helped to produce prolonged remission in certain types of acute leukemia.

Bonine (bō'nēn). Trade name for meclizine hydrochloride, USP, an agent used for prevention and treatment of motion sickness and vomiting.

bony. Resembling or of the nature of bone. SYN: *osseous.*

booster (boo'stěr). An additional dose of an immunizing agent to increase the protection afforded by the original series of injections. The booster is given some months or years after the initial immunization.

boot. A special shoe or bandage for covering the foot, ankle, and lower leg.

borate (bō'rāt). Any basic salt of boric acid. SEE: *Poisons and Poisoning* in *Appendix.*

borated. Anything to which borax has been added.

borax (bor'ăks) [L., from Arabic, from Persian *burah*]. Sodium borate. Its chief use is as a detergent and water softener; also a weak antiseptic.

borborygmus (bor"bō-rĭg'mŭs) [Gr. *borborygmos,* rumbling in the bowels]. (pl. *borborygmi*) A gurgling, splashing sound normally heard over the large intestine; caused by passage of gas through the intestine.

PATH: Its absence may indicate paralytic ileus, or obstruction of the bowels due to torsion, volvulus, or strangulated hernia.

border (bor'děr). The outer part or edge; boundary.

b., striated. A modified layer of the surface protoplasm of columnar epithelial cells lining the intestine. It consists of regular, perpendicular striations consisting of minute protoplasmic processes.

border brush. A brushlike structure found on the free surface of epithelial cells in the proximal convoluted portion of a renal tubule. The microvilli that form the border greatly increase the exposed surface area of the cell.

Bordetella (bor"dě-těl'lă). [Jules Bordet, Belg. physician, bacteriologist, and physiologist, 1870–1961] A genus of Brucellaceae bacteria that are hemolytic gram-negative coccobacilli. Some species are parasitic and pathogenic in warm-blooded animals, including humans.

B. pertussis. The causative agent of whooping cough. First isolated by Bordet and Gengou. Formerly called Hemophilus pertussis.

Bordet-Gengou bacillus (bor-dā'zhōn-goo'). [Jules Bordet; Octave Gengou, Fr. bacteriologist, 1875–1957] Bordetella pertussis, the causative agent of whooping cough.

boredom. Feeling of tiredness or depression because of lack of activity or challenging and meaningful stimuli.

boric acid. H_3BO_3. An odorless white crystalline powder containing boron, it is obtained by condensation and evaporation from certain mineral salts. It is used as a mild antiseptic solution, esp. for the eyes, mouth, and bladder.

boric acid poisoning. Boric acid is highly poisonous when taken internally.

SYM: Nausea, vomiting, diarrhea.

TREATMENT: Wash out stomach. Give saline cathartic and large volumes of water. Oxygen and plasma or blood transfusions as necessary. SEE: *Poisons and Poisoning* in *Appendix.*

borism. Symptoms caused by internal use of borax or boron compounds. Includes dry skin, eruptions, and gastric disturbances.

Bornholm disease (born'hōm). [named for the Danish island Bornholm] An epidemic disease caused by coxsackie B virus. Characterized by sudden onset of pain in chest and fever. SYN: *pleurodynia, epidemic.*

boroglycerin (bor"ō-glĭs'ĕr-ĭn). $C_3H_5BO_3$. A compound formed when boric acid and glycerin are heated together.

boroglycerol (bor"ō-glĭs'ĕr-ŏl). Boroglycerin, q.v.

boron [*bor*ax + carb*on*]. A nonmetallic element, found only as a compound such as boric acid or borax, q.v. SYMB: B. At. wt. 10.81; at. no. 5.

Borrelia (bor-rē'lē-ă). A genus of bacteri- some of which are causative agents f- lapsing fevers in man.

B. duttonii. Causative agent for tick-borne relapsing fever in Central and South America.

B. recurrentis. Causative agent of louse-borne relapsing fever.

B. vincentii. A parasite of the human oral cavity, occurring in conjunction with a fusiform bacillus in necrotizing ulcerative gingivitis and stomatitis. SEE: *angina, Vincent's.*

boss [O. Fr. *boce,* a swelling]. A round circumscribed swelling or growth. Thus a boss is present when a tumor becomes large enough to produce swelling.

bosselated (bŏs'ĕ-lāt-ĕd). Marked by numerous bosses.

Boston arm. A particular type of prosthesis for persons who have had an arm amputated above the elbow. The arm, which operates by means of a small battery-driven motor, obeys signals received from electric energy produced by movement of the remaining muscle groups. This allows control of elbow function with respect to direction and strength of motion.

Botallo's duct (bō-tăl'ōz). [Leonardo Botallo, It. anatomist, 1530–1600] Ductus arteriosus, q.v.

botfly (bŏt'flī). (pl. *botflies*) Insect belonging to the order Diptera of the family Oestridae. Parasitic to mammals, esp. horses and sheep. Human infestation is rare.

botryoid (bŏt'rē-oyd) [Gr. *botrys,* bunch of grapes, + *eidos,* appearance]. Resembling a bunch of grapes. SYN: *staphyline.*

botuliform (bŏt-ū'lĭ-form) [L. *botulus,* sausage, + *forma,* shape]. Shaped like a sausage.

botulin (bŏt'chū-lĭn). The neurotoxin responsible for botulism, q.v. It is not destroyed by the action of gastric or intestinal secretions.

botulinic acid. A toxin found in putrid sausage.

botulism (bŏt'ū-lĭzm) [" – Gr. *-ismos,* condition]. A severe form of food poisoning from food containing the botulinus toxin produced by Clostridium botulinum. This organism is found in the soil and in the intestinal tract of domestic animals. Cases of human botulism are usually associated with development of the bacteria under anaerobic conditions in raw, improperly canned or otherwise preserved foods, esp. meats (as ham and sausage) and nonacid vegetables (as string beans). The toxin is a powerful exotoxin. It ... ermolabile, losing its toxic properties ... exposed to temperature of 80° C. (176° ... 30 min. or boiling at 100° C. (212° F.) ... nin. The toxin has a selective action ... ntral nervous system. In fatal cases, ... nd respiratory paralysis occur ... volvement of the medullary cen- ... ality rate in the United States is 20–35%.

SYM: Fatigue, weakness, dizziness, blurred or double vision, headache, and digestive complaints, as nausea, vomiting, diarrhea, and abdominal pain. Progresses to paralysis of the central nervous system and of the cardiac and respiratory systems.

TREATMENT: It is important to administer polyvalent antiserum (Types A, B, and E) as soon as the condition is suspected and prior to the onset of neurological symptoms. Do not withhold treatment while waiting for results of laboratory tests. SEE: *botulinum toxin* in *Poisons and Poisoning* in *Appendix.*

b., infant. An infectious form of botulism first recognized in 1976. Most cases occur in infants less than one year of age.

SYM: Constipation, lethargy, listlessness, poor feeding, ptosis, loss of head control, difficulty in swallowing, hypotonia, generalized weakness, and respiratory insufficiency.

The disease may be mild or severe. It is thought to cause 5% of the cases of sudden infant death syndrome (SIDS).

TREATMENT: Careful supportive care.

bouba (boo'bă). Yaws, q.v.

Bouchut's respiration (boo-shooz'). [Jean A. E. Bouchut, Fr. physician, 1818–1891] Respiration in which expiration is longer than inspiration, seen in children with bronchopneumonia and asthma.

Bouchut's tubes. A set of tubes used for intubation of the larynx.

bougie (boo'zhē) [Fr. *bougie,* candle]. A slender, flexible instrument for exploring and dilating tubal organs, esp. the male urethra.

bouillon (boo-, bool-yŏn') [Fr.]. Clear broth made from meat. Used in foods and as a culture medium for bacteria.

bouquet (boo-kā') [Fr., nosegay]. A cluster or bunch of structures, esp. of blood vessels.

bourdonnement (boor-dōn-mŏn') [Fr.]. A humming sound.

boutonnière (boo-tŏn-yār') [Fr., buttonhole]. 1. Incision through perineum behind an impervious stricture. 2. A buttonhole-like opening in a membrane.

boutonnière deformity. Contractures of hand musculature characterized by proximal interphalangeal joint flexion and distal interphalangeal joint hyperextension.

boutons terminaux (boo-tŏn' tĕr-mĭ-nō') [Fr., terminal buttons]. Bulblike expansions at the tip of axons that come into synaptic contact with the cell bodies of other neurons.

bovine (bō'vīn) [L. *bovinus*]. Pert. to cattle.

bowel [O. Fr. *boel,* intestine]. The intestine.

bowel movement. Evacuation of feces. Number of bowel movements varies in normal individuals, some having a movement after each meal, others one in the morning and one at night, and still others only one in several days. Thus, to say that the healthy person must have at least one bowel movement a day in order to maintain health is unreasonable and not based on factual evidence. CAUTION: Persistent change in bowel habits may be a sign of a malignant growth in the lower gastrointestinal tract and for that reason should be investigated thoroughly. SYN: *defecation*.

bowleg (bō'lĕg). A bending outward of the lower limb. SYN: *bandy leg; genu varum*. SEE: *rickets*.

Bowman's capsule (bō'măns). [Sir William Bowman, Brit. physician, 1816–1892] The renal or malpighian corpuscle. It consists of a visceral layer closely applied to the glomerulus and an outer parietal layer. It functions as a filter in the formation of urine. SEE: *kidney* for illus.

Bowman's glands. The olfactory glands. Branched tubuloalveolar glands located in the lamina propria of the olfactory membrane. The glands produce mucus that keeps the olfactory surface moist.

Bowman's membrane. Thin homogeneous membrane separating corneal epithelium from corneal substance. SYN: *lamina, anterior elastic*.

boxing. In dentistry, the building up of vertical walls, usually in wax, around the impression to produce the desired size and form of the base of the cast, and to preserve certain landmarks of the impression.

box-note. In emphysema, a hollow sound heard on percussion.

box splint. Splint for fractures below the knee.

Boyer's bursa (bwă-yăz'). [Baron Alexis de Boyer, Fr. surgeon, 1757–1833] A bursa anterior to the thyrohyoid membrane.

Boyer's cyst. A painless and gradual enlargement of the subhyoid bursa.

Boyle's law. [Robert Boyle, Brit. physicist, 1627–1691] Law stating that at a constant temperature, the volume of a gas varies inversely with the pressure. SEE: *Charles' law; Gay-Lussac's law*.

Bozeman-Fritsch catheter (bōz'măn-frĭtch). [Nathan Bozeman, U.S. surgeon, 1825–1905; and Heinrich Fritsch, Ger. gynecologist, 1844–1915] Double-lumen uterine catheter with several openings at tip.

B.P. *blood pressure; British Pharmacopoeia*.

b.p. *boiling point*.

Br. 1. *Brucella*. 2. Chem. symb. for bromine.

brace (brās). 1. Any one of a great variety of devices, usually used in orthopedics, for holding joints or limbs in place. 2. Colloquial term for temporary dental prostheses used to align or reposition teeth.

brachia (brā'kē-ă). Pl. of brachium.

brachial (brā'kē-ăl) [L. *brachiolis*]. Pert. to the arm.

brachial artery. Main artery of arm. Continuation of the axillary artery on the inside of the arm. SEE: illus.

brachialgia (brā"kē-ăl'jē-ă) [" + Gr. *algos*, pain]. Intense pain in the arm.

brachialis (brā"kē-ăl'ĭs) [L. *brachialis*, brachial]. A muscle of the arm lying immediately under the biceps brachii.

brachial plexus. Network of lower cervical and upper dorsal spinal nerves supplying the arm, forearm, and hand. SEE: *Nerve Plexuses* in *Appendix*.

brachial veins. The veins that accompany the brachial artery.

brachiocephalic (brā"kē-ō-sĕ-făl'ĭk) [L. *brachium*, arm, + Gr. *kephale*, head]. Pert. to arm and head.

brachiocrural (brā"kē-ō-kroo'răl) [" + L. *cruralis*, pert. to the leg]. Pert. to arm and thigh.

brachiocubital (brā"kē-ō-kū'bĭ-tăl) [" + L. *cubitus*, forearm]. Pert. to the arm and forearm.

brachiocyllosis (brā"kē-ō-sĭl-ō'sĭs) [" + *kyllosis*, a crooking]. Abnormal curvature of the arm.

brachioradialis (brā"kē-ō-rā'dē-ă'lĭs) [" + *radialis*, radius]. A muscle lying on the lateral side of the forearm. SEE: *Muscles* in *Appendix*.

brachium (brā'kē-ŭm) [L., arm, from Gr. *brakhion*, shorter, hence "upper arm" as opposed to longer forearm]. (pl. *brachia*) [NA] 1. The upper arm from shoulder to elbow. 2. Anatomical structure resembling an arm.

b. conjunctivum. The superior cerebellar peduncle. SEE: *peduncle, cerebellar, superior*.

b. pontis. The middle cerebellar peduncle. SEE: *peduncle, cerebellar, middle*.

brachy- [Gr. *brachys*, short]. Prefix for short.

brachybasia (brăk-ē-bā'sē-ă) [" + *basis*, walking]. A slow shuffling gait seen in partial paraplegia. SEE: *gait*.

brachycardia (brăk-ē-kăr'dē-ă) [" + *kardia*, heart]. Slowness of heart action. SYN: *bradycardia*.

brachycephalic, brachycephalous (brăk"ē-sĕ-făl'ĭk, -sef'ă-lŭs) [Gr. *brachys*, short, + *kephale*, head]. Having a cephalic index of 81.0 to 85.4. This is considered to be a short head, but is not necessarly abnormal, as this index falls within the standard range of variation among humans.

brachycheilia (brăk"ē-kī'lē-ă) [" + *cheilos*, lip]. Condition of having abnormally short lip or lips.

brachydactylia (brăk"ē-dăk-tĭl'ē-ă) [" + *daktylos*, finger]. Abnormal shortness of the fingers and toes.

brachygnathia (brăk-ĭg-nā'thē-ă) [" + *gna-*

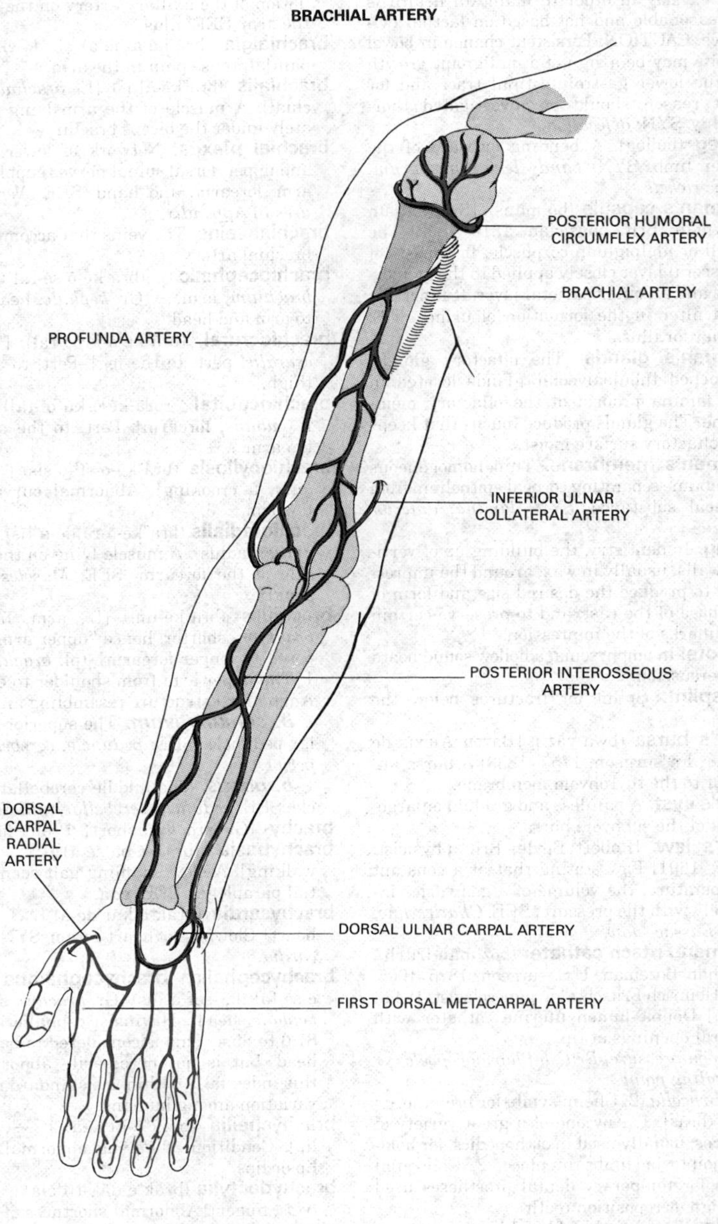
BRACHIAL ARTERY
POSTERIOR HUMORAL CIRCUMFLEX ARTERY
BRACHIAL ARTERY
PROFUNDA ARTERY
INFERIOR ULNAR COLLATERAL ARTERY
POSTERIOR INTEROSSEOUS ARTERY
DORSAL CARPAL RADIAL ARTERY
DORSAL ULNAR CARPAL ARTERY
FIRST DORSAL METACARPAL ARTERY

thos, jaw]. Abnormal shortness of the lower jaw.

brachymetropia (brăk"ē-mĕ-trō'pē-ă) [" + *metron,* measure, + *opsis,* sight]. Myopia; nearsightedness.

brachymorphic (brăk"ē-mor'fĭk) [" + *morphe,* form]. Shorter and broader than usual, with reference to body type.

brachyphalangia (brăk"ē-fă-lăn'jē-ă) [" + *phalanx,* closely knit row]. Shortness of a bone or bones of a finger or toe.

brachystasis (bră-kĭs'tă-sĭs) [" + *stasis,* standstill]. Condition in which a muscle does not relax upon contracting but maintains its shortened state.

brachytherapy (brăk"ē-thĕr'ă-pē) [" + *therapeia,* treatment]. In radiation therapy, the use of implants of radioactive materials such as radium, cesium, iridium, or gold at the site. It is in contrast to teletherapy.

Bradford frame. [Edward H. Bradford, U.S. orthopedic surgeon, 1848–1926] An oblong frame, about 7 × 3 feet (2.13 × 0.91 meters), made of 1 in. (2.5 cm.) pipe covered with canvas strips that run from one side of the frame to the other and are movable. Used for patients with fractures or disease of the hip or spine, thus permitting the patient to urinate and defecate without moving the spine or changing position.

brady- [Gr. *bradys,* slow]. Prefix indicating slow.

bradyacusia (brăd"ē-ă-koo'sē-ă) [" + *akouein,* to hear]. Dullness of hearing.

bradyarrhythmia (brăd"ē-ă-rĭth'mē-ă) [" + *a-,* not, + *rhythmos,* rhythm]. Slow and irregular heart rate.

bradycardia (brăd"ē-kăr'dē-ă) [" + *kardia,* heart]. A slow heart beat characterized by a pulse rate that is under 60 beats per minute. SEE: *arrhythmia; tachycardia.*

b., sinus. A slow sinus rhythm with an atrial rate below 60 beats per minute in an adult or below 70 beats per minute in a child.

bradycrotic (brăd"ē-krŏt'ĭk) [" + *krotos,* pulsation]. Pert. to slowness of pulse.

bradydiastole (brăd"ē-dī-ăs'tō-lē) [" + *diastole,* dilatation]. Prolongation of the diastolic pause, as in myocardial lesions.

bradyecoia (brăd"ē-ē-koy'ă) [Gr. *bradyekoos,* slow of hearing]. Partial deafness.

bradyesthesia (brăd"ē-ĕs-thē'zē-ă) [" + *aisthesis,* perception]. Slowness of perception.

bradyglossia (brăd"ē-glŏs'ē-ă) [" + *glossa,* tongue]. Abnormal slowness of speech. SYN: *bradylalia; bradyphrasia.*

bradykinesia (brăd"ē-kĭ-nē'sē-ă) [" + *kinesis,* motion]. Extreme slowness of movement.

bradykinin (brăd"ē-kī'nĭn) A plasma kinin. SEE: *kinin.*

bradylalia (brăd"ē-lā'lē-ă) [" + *lalein,* to talk]. Slowness of speech. SYN: *bradyglossia; bradyphrasia.* SEE: *speech.*

bradylexia (brăd"ē-lĕks'ē-ă) [Gr. *bradys,* slow, + *lexis,* word]. Abnormal slowness of reading not attributable to lack of intelligence. SEE: *dyslexia.*

bradylogia (brăd"ē-lō'jē-ă) [' + *logos,* word]. Slow speech due to mental impairment.

bradyphagia (brăd"ē-fā'jē-ă) [" + *phagein,* to eat]. Abnormal slowness in eating.

bradyphrasia (brăd"ē-frā'zē-ă) [" + *phrasis,* utterance]. Slowness of speech; seen in some types of mental disease.

bradypnea (brăd"ĭp-nē'ă, brăd"ĭ-nē'ă) [" + *pnoe,* breathing]. Abnormally slow breathing.

bradyrhythmia (brăd"ē-rĭth'mē-ă) [" + *rhythmos,* rhythm]. 1. Slowness of heart or pulse rate. 2. In electroencephalography, slowness of brain waves (1 to 6 per sec.).

bradyspermatism (brăd-ē-spĕr'mă-tĭzm) [" + *sperma,* semen + *-ismos,* condition]. Abnormally slow ejaculation of semen.

bradysphygmia (brăd"ē-sfĭg'mē-ă) [" + *sphygmos,* pulse]. Abnormally slow pulse.

bradystalsis (brăd"ē-stăl'sĭs) [" + *stalsis,* constriction]. Abnormal slowness of peristalsis.

bradytachycardia (brăd"ē-tăk"ē-kăr'dē-ă) [" + *tachys,* swift, + *kardia,* heart]. Increased heart rate alternating with slow rate. SEE: *sick sinus syndrome.*

bradytocia (brăd"ē-tō'sē-ă) [" + *tokos,* childbirth]. Slow parturition.

bradyuria (brăd"ē-ū'rē-ă) [" + *ouron,* urine]. Slowness in passing urine.

braille (brāl). [Louis Braille, blind Fr. educator, 1809–1852] A system of reading and writing that enables the blind to see by using their sense of touch. Raised dots, which represent numerals and letters of the alphabet, can be identified by the fingers. SEE: *Optacon; Braille Alphabet* in *Appendix.*

brain (brān) [AS. *braegen*]. A large soft mass of nerve tissue contained within the cranium. Cranial portion of the central nervous system. SYN: *encephalon.*

ANAT: The brain is composed of neurons (nerve cells) and neuroglia or supporting cells. The brain consists of gray and white matter. Gray matter is composed principally of nerve cell bodies and is concentrated in the cerebral cortex and the nuclei and basal ganglia. White matter is composed of nerve cell processes, which form tracts connecting various parts of the brain with each other.

The brain consists of five parts: the cerebrum, cerebellum, pons varolii, medulla oblongata, and midbrain. The weight of the brain and spinal cord is about 1350 to 1400 gm., of which 2% is the cord. The cerebrum represents about 85% of the weight of the brain. *Lobes:* Frontal, parietal, occipital, temporal, insula. *Glands:* Pituitary, pineal. *Membranes:* Meninges, consisting of the dura mater (external), arachnoid (middle), and pia mater (internal). *Nerves:* Cranial. SEE: *Nerves, cranial,* in *Appendix; cranial nerves* for illus.

Subdivisions of the brain are (1) diencephalon, q.v., including the epithalamus, thalamus, and hypothalamus (optic chiasma, hypophysis, tuber cinereum, and maxillary bodies); (2) myelencephalon, q.v., including the corpora quadrigemina, tegmentum, crura cerebri, and the medulla oblongata; (3) metencephalon, q.v., including the cerebellum and pons; (4) telencephalon, q.v., including the rhinencephalon, corpora striata, and cerebrum (cerebral cortex).

Ventricles: The cavities of the brain are the first and second lateral ventricles, which lie in the cerebral hemispheres, the third ventricle of the diencephalon, and the fourth ventricle of the medulla. The first and second communicate with the third by the interventricular foramina, the third with the fourth by the cerebral canal (aqueduct of Sylvius), the fourth with the subarachnoid spaces by the two foramina of Luschka and the foramen of Magendie. The ventricles are filled with cerebrospinal fluid, which is formed by the choroid plexuses in the walls and roofs of the ventricles. SEE: illus.

PHYS: The brain is the primary center for regulating and coordinating body activities. Sensory impulses are received through afferent nerves; these register as sensations, which are the basis for perception. It is the seat of consciousness, thought, memory, reason, judgment, and emotion. Motor impulses are discharged through efferent nerves to muscles and glands initiating activities. Through reflex centers automatic control of body activities is maintained. The most important reflex centers are the cardiac, vasomotor, and respiratory centers, which regulate circulation and respiration. SEE: *central nervous system; spinal cord.*

brain death. Cessation of brain function. Criteria for concluding that the brain has died include: lack of response to stimuli; absence of all reflexes; absent respirations; isoelectric electroencephalogram for at least 30 minutes that will not change in response to sound or pain stimuli. The patient may be kept alive by life-support devices, but death is the inevitable outcome.

CAUTION: Some drugs, including barbiturates, methaqualone, diazepam, mecloqualone, meprobamate, and trichloroethylene can produce short periods of isoelectric encephalograms.

brain edema. An increase in brain volume due to an increase in its water content. It is caused by a variety of conditions but the mechanisms are several, including increased permeability of brain capillary endothelial cells; swelling of brain cells associated with hypoxia or water intoxication; and interstitial edema resulting from obstructive hydrocephalus. SYN: *brain swelling.*

brain fever. Meningitis.

Brain's reflex. [W. Russell Brain, physician, 1895–1966] Extension of flexed arm on assuming quadripedal posture.

brain sand. Laminated bodies consisting principally of phosphates, carbonates of calcium, and magnesium found in the pineal body.

brain scan. Use of radioactive isotopes injected into the circulation to detect abnormalities in structure and function of the brain.

brain stem. The stemlike part of the brain that connects the cerebral hemispheres with the spinal cord. Comprises the medulla oblongata, the pons, and the midbrain.

brainstorm. 1. Sudden idea. 2. Temporary outburst of mental excitement; often maniacal, esp. in paranoia.

brain swelling. Brain edema, q.v.

brain tumor. Term usually used inexactly to describe any intracranial mass—neoplastic, cystic, inflammatory (abscess), or syphilitic. Except for the latter, the usual therapy is surgical. SEE: *neoplasm; tumor.*

SYM: The general symptoms are those due to an increase in intracranial pressure such as headache, changes in the retina such as choked disk recognized by ophthalmoscopic examinations, and vomiting (without nausea). Mental changes (esp. dullness), epileptiform convulsions, and giddiness are often general but may be localized signs. In addition, history and cranial x-ray pictures are of great value. The injection of air into the ventricles prior to x-ray examination is known as pneumoventriculography.

Neoplasms of the brain do not metastasize to other parts of the body. They contain almost no blood vessels and may produce pain or other sensations. The most malignant ones in childhood are gliomas, q.v.

brainwashing. Intense psychological indoctrination, usually political, for the purpose of displacing the individual's previous thoughts and attitudes with those selected by the regime or person inflicting the indoctrination.

bran. The outer coating or husk of cereal grains, such as wheat or oats, produced as a by-product of milling these grains. Because some of the cellulose in bran is indigestible, it may be used to add bulk to the diet and thus be of assistance in preventing and treating constipation. SEE: *fiber, dietary.*

BRAIN

LATERAL ASPECT

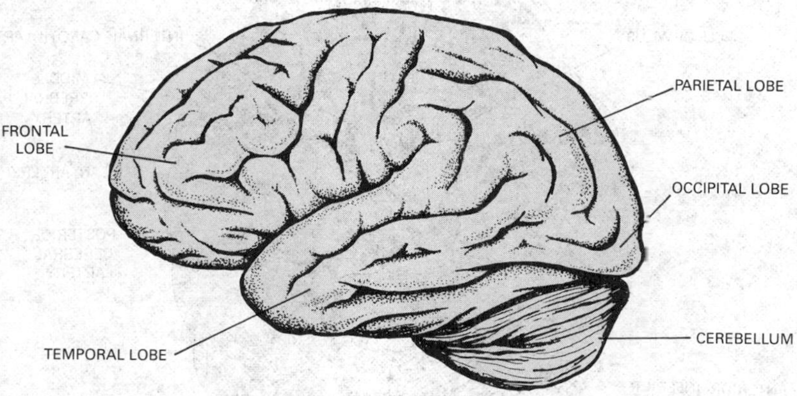

MEDIAL ASPECT

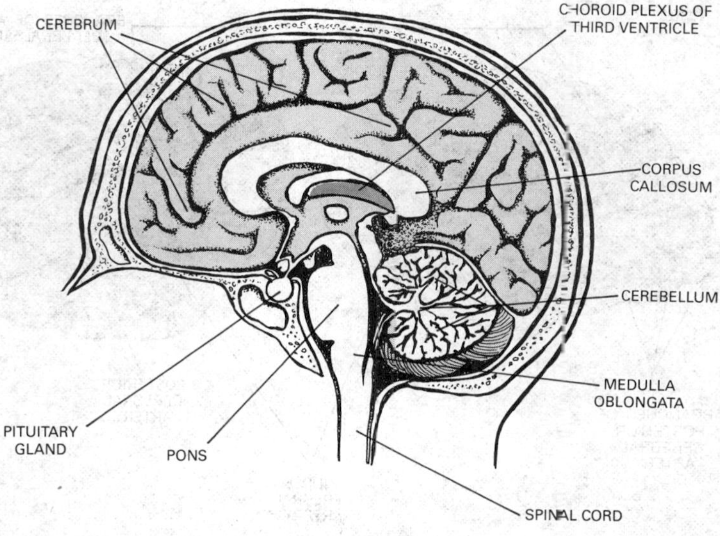

VASCULAR ANATOMY OF BRAIN

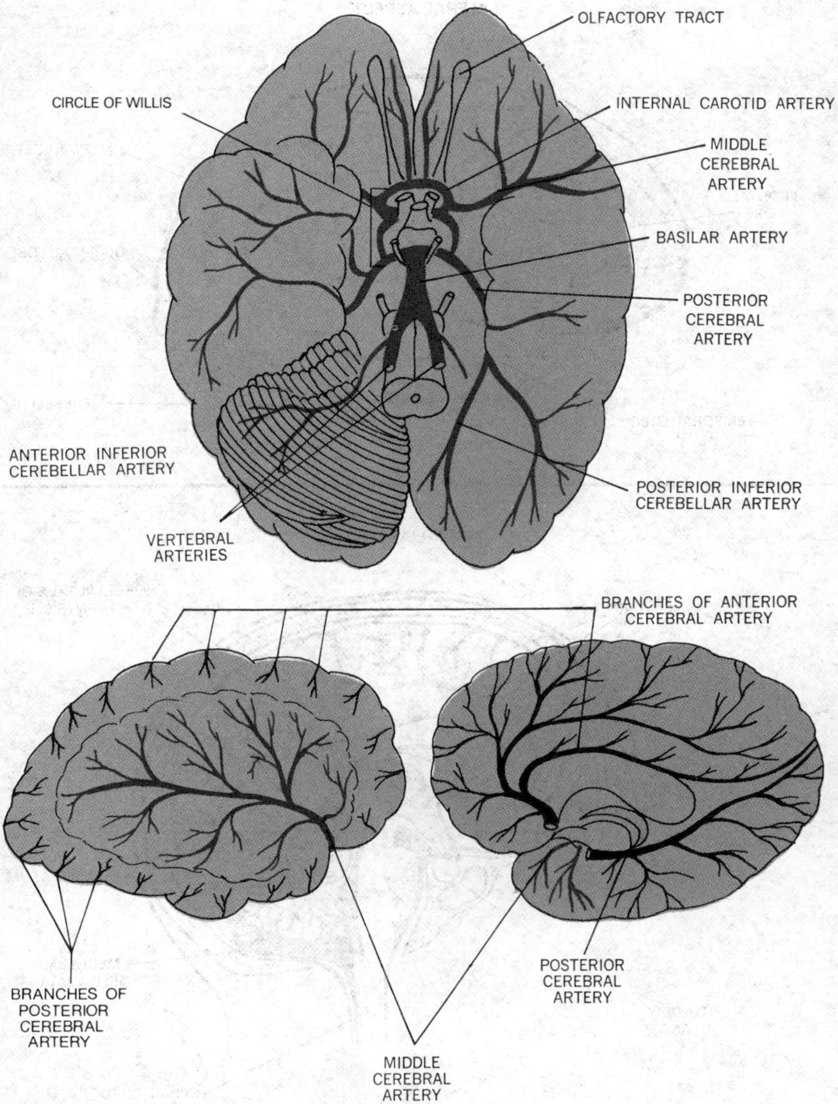
OLFACTORY TRACT
CIRCLE OF WILLIS
INTERNAL CAROTID ARTERY
MIDDLE CEREBRAL ARTERY
BASILAR ARTERY
POSTERIOR CEREBRAL ARTERY
ANTERIOR INFERIOR CEREBELLAR ARTERY
POSTERIOR INFERIOR CEREBELLAR ARTERY
VERTEBRAL ARTERIES
BRANCHES OF ANTERIOR CEREBRAL ARTERY
BRANCHES OF POSTERIOR CEREBRAL ARTERY
POSTERIOR CEREBRAL ARTERY
MIDDLE CEREBRAL ARTERY

branch. In anatomy, a subdivision arising from a main or larger portion, esp. of an artery, vein, nerve, or lymphatic vessel.

branchial (brăng'kē-ăl) [L. *branchia,* gills]. Pert. to or resembling gills of a fish or a homologous structure in higher animals.

branchial arches. Five pairs of arched structures that form the lateral and ventral walls of the pharynx of the embryo. They are partially separated from each other externally by the branchial clefts and internally by the pharyngeal pouches. The fifth arch is rudimentary. They play an important role in the formation of structures of the face and neck. The first is the mandibular arch, the second the hyoid arch. SYN: *visceral arches.*

branchial clefts. A series of openings between the embryonic branchial arches. They become functional gill slits in fish.

branchial grooves. A series of furrows separating the embryonic branchial arches. They are homologous to the branchial clefts of fish and amphibians.

branchial muscles. Muscles that develop from the mesoderm of the embryonic branchial arches. Include most muscles of face and neck.

branchiogenic, branchiogenous (brăng"kē-ō-jĕn'ĭk, brăng"kē-ŏj'ĕ-nŭs) [L. *branchia,* gills, + Gr. *gennan,* to generate]. Having origin in a branchial cleft.

branchioma (brăng"kē-ō'mă) [" + Gr. *oma,* tumor]. A tumor derived from the branchial epithelium.

branchiomeric (brăng"kē-ō-mĕr'ĭk) [" + Gr. *meros,* part]. Of or pert. to the branchial arches.

Brandt-Andrews maneuver. Technique for expressing the placenta from the uterus during the third stage of labor. One hand puts gentle traction on the cord while the other is used to press the anterior surface of the uterus backward. SEE: *Credé's method.*

brandy. An alcoholic liquid obtained by the distillation of fermented fruit, esp. grapes, usually containing 50% ethyl alcohol by volume. Used medically as a tonic, peripheral vasodilator, and as a sedative.

Branhamella (Neisseria) catarrhalis (brăn"hă-mĕl'ă). A species of Neisseria that is usually nonpathogenic but occasionally causes bacterial endocarditis.

brash. A burning sensation in the stomach sometimes accompanied by belching of sour fluid. SYN: *heartburn; pyrosis.*

brass poisoning. Poisoning due to the inhalation of fumes of zinc and zinc oxide with destruction of tissue in the respiratory passage. Rarely fatal.

SYM: Dryness and burning in respiratory tract; cough; headache; chills.

TREATMENT: Entirely symptomatic. Inhalations of humidified air make patient more comfortable.

brawny induration. Pathological hardening and thickening of tissues.

Braxton Hicks sign. [John Braxton Hicks, Brit. gynecologist, 1825–1897] Intermittent painless uterine contractions that may occur every 10 to 20 minutes. They occur after the third month of pregnancy. These contractions do not represent true labor pains but are often so interpreted. The sign is not present in every pregnancy. Also called Hicks sign.

break. 1. In orthopedics, a fracture. 2. To interrupt continuity in a tissue or electric circuit or channel of flow or communication.

breakbone fever. An acute febrile disease characterized by sudden onset, with headache, fever, prostration, joint and muscle pain, lymphadenopathy, and a rash that appears simultaneously with a second temperature rise following an afebrile period. Causative agent is a Group B arbovirus. SYN: *dengue.*

breast [AS. *breost*]. 1. The upper anterior aspect of the chest. 2. Mammary gland, a compound alveolar gland consisting of 15 to 20 lobes of glandular tissue separated from each other by interlobular septa. Each lobe is drained by a lactiferous duct that opens on the tip of the nipple. The mammary gland secretes milk used for nourishment of the infant. SEE: *infant feeding; lactiferous glands; milk;* illus.

DEVELOP: During puberty, estrogens from the ovary stimulate growth and development of the duct system. During pregnancy, progesterone secreted by the corpus luteum and placenta acts synergistically with estrogens to bring the alveoli to complete development. Following parturition, prolactin (luteotrophin) in conjunction with adrenal corticoids initiates lactation, and oxytocin from the posterior pituitary induces ejection of milk. Sucking or milking reflexly stimulates both milk secretion and discharge of milk.

CHANGES IN PREGNANCY: First 6 to 12 weeks, there is fullness and tenderness, erectile tissues develop in nipples, nodules are felt, pigment is deposited around the nipple (primary areola) (in blondes the areolae and nipples become darker pink and in brunettes they become dark brown and in some cases even black), and a few drops of fluid may be squeezed out. Next 16 to 20 weeks, the secondary areola shows small whitish spots in pigmentation due to hypertrophy of the sebaceous glands, the so-called glands of Montgomery.

NURSING IMPLICATIONS: *Preventive care:* Most complications of the breast during the puerperal period will not occur if proper care is given. Early treatment of soreness, cracks, and fissures is accomplished by use of a sterile nipple shield while the baby

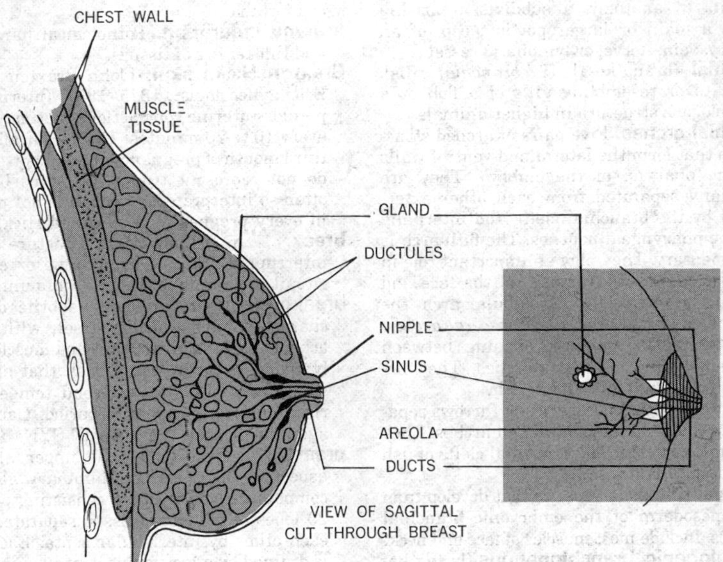

VIEW OF SAGITTAL CUT THROUGH BREAST

nurses. Antiseptic oil or ointment may be used.

The infant will begin nursing for several minutes' duration from either breast. Gradually the time is increased according to the tolerance of the mother's nipples. When lactation is well established, it takes the infant 10 to 15 minutes to empty the breast. Breast engorgement usually occurs on the third to fourth day postpartum. Treatment includes increasing the amount of time the baby spends nursing (to relieve the engorgement), decreasing the amount of time between feedings, and massaging the breasts prior to each feeding to soften them and to bring the milk out into the ducts so the infant will not have to suck vigorously to get the milk flow started. The trauma that occurs to nipples in the establishment of lactation occurs primarily during the "latching on" phase with its relatively high degree of negative pressure. Once the infant is nursing, it is counterproductive to detach the infant before the breast is emptied. If the breast is so full that the infant is unable to grasp the nipple, hot packs and massage should be used, with manual expression of the milk as necessary. A well-fitting brassiere should be worn when the mother is not nursing.

Care of the nipples: Keep nipples clean and dry. Nipples should be washed with warm water prior to each feeding. After each nursing period, a bland cream or ointment such as lanolin should be applied. Airing of the nipples between feedings is also helpful. The breast should be properly supported with a well-fitting brassiere that pulls upward and inward. Also instruct the mother in the correct technique for self-examination of the breast.

b., chicken. Deformity in which the chest protrudes, caused by rickets or obstructed respiration in infancy. SYN: *pigeon breast.*

b., self-examination of. A technique that enables a woman to detect changes in her breasts. The examination should be done after the menstrual period, as normal physiologic changes that may confuse results occur in the premenstrual period. This method of self-examination is esp. useful in the early detection of breast cancer.

The use of all available means to diagnose and treat breast cancer without delay cannot be overemphasized. It is the most common type of cancer in women. In 1984, it is estimated that over 100,000 new cases of breast cancer were diagnosed and an estimated one third of that number died of it, making cancer of the breast the leading cause of death due to malignancy in women. Every person caring for female patients should be familiar with the method of self-examination of the breast. Women esp. should know this technique in order to be able to examine themselves as well as to instruct others.

Self-examination of the breast should be done once a month soon after the completion of the menstrual period and on a monthly basis after menopause. If any abnormality, a lump, or thickening is discovered, see your physician immediately.

Technique: (SEE: illus.) 1. Stand before a mirror. Inspect both breasts for anything unusual, such as any discharge from the nipples, puckering, dimpling, or scaling of the skin.

The next two steps are designed to emphasize any change in the shape or contour of your breasts. As you do them, you should be able to feel your chest muscles tighten. 2. Watching closely in the mirror, clasp your hands behind your head and press hands forward. 3. Next, press hands firmly on hips and bow slightly toward the mirror as your pull your shoulders and elbows forward.

Some women do the next part of the exam in the shower. Fingers glide over soapy skin, making it easy to concentrate on the texture underneath. 4. Raise your left arm. Use three or four fingers of your right hand to explore your left breast firmly, carefully, and thoroughly. Beginning at the outer edge, press the flat part of your fingers in small circles, moving the circles slowly around the breast. Gradually work toward the nipple. Be sure to cover the entire breast. Pay special attention to the area between the breast and the armpit, including the armpit itself. Feel for any unusual lump or mass under the skin. 5. Gently squeeze the nipple and look for a discharge. Repeat the exam on your right breast.

6. Other women do steps 4 and 5 lying down. If you wish to, lie flat on your back, left arm over your head and a pillow or folded towel under your left shoulder. This position flattens the breast and makes it easier to examine. Use the same circular motion described earlier. Repeat on your right breast.

You might want to try both positions—standing and lying down—to see which is most comfortable for you. However, the most importance choice is the decision to do breast examination each month.

breast pump. A manual or electric pump used to draw milk from the female breast.

breath (brĕth) [AS. *braeth,* odor]. The air inhaled and exhaled in act of respiration.

DIAG: *Foul odor (os fetor)*: May indicate neglect of mouth or teeth; improper diet; constipation; mouth breathing; lack of exercise; use of drugs, alcohol, or tobacco. It also depends upon the food ingested and may indicate stomatitis, necrosis of jaw, caries of teeth, tonsillitis, diphtheria, gangrene and abscess of the lungs, fetid bronchitis, bronchiectasis, pyothorax, catarrh, diabetes, kidney disease, and other disorders. Mouthwashes and gargles are ineffective in removing the odor if os fetor is due to systemic causes or ingestion of food such as garlic. *Urinous odor:* Indicates uremia. *Sweetish odor* (that of ripe apples): Found in diabetes mellitus, esp. during coma. This sweet odor is due to the excretion of acetone in the breath. This condition develops quickly in infants and children who have gone several hours without food.

Rattling and shortness of breath: Edema; presence of fluids in the air passages. *Sighing breath:* Air hunger; occurs in internal hemorrhage. Therefore be alert to the development of this symptom following abdominal surgery and in typhoid fever.

breathing. Act of inhaling and exhaling air. SEE: *chest; respiration.*

b., asthmatic. Harsh breathing with a prolonged wheezing expiration heard all over the chest.

b., bronchial. Harsh breathing with a prolonged high-pitched expiration that sometimes has a tubular quality. Heard in consolidation of lung tissue.

b., cog-wheel. Respiratory murmur, not continuous but broken into waves, not indicative of any special disease but frequently observed in bronchitis and in incipient phthisis.

b., continuous positive-pressure. A method of mechanically assisted pulmonary ventilation. A device administers air or oxygen to the lungs under a continuous pressure that never returns to zero. SYN: *ventilation, continuous positive-pressure.*

b., intermittent positive-pressure. Mechanical method for assisting pulmonary ventilation employing a device that administers air or oxygen for the inflation of the lungs under positive pressure. Exhalation is usually passive. SYN: *ventilation, intermittent positive-pressure.*

b., shallow. A type of breathing that occurs in acute pulmonary disease. Noted when chest walls are thick, in the old and feeble, in emphysema, in pleural effusion, in incipient phthisis, in painful affections of the chest such as pleurodynia and early pleurisy, and in pulmonary edema.

breatholyzer (brĕth'ō-lī-zĕr). Apparatus used to analyze specific contents of expired air. One such device is used to test for presence of alcohol in expired air in order to determine whether or not a person is legally intoxicated.

breech [AS. *brec,* buttocks]. The nates, or buttocks.

breech presentation. A common abnormality of delivery where the fetal buttocks present rather than the head. SEE: *presentation,*

BREAST SELF-EXAMINATION

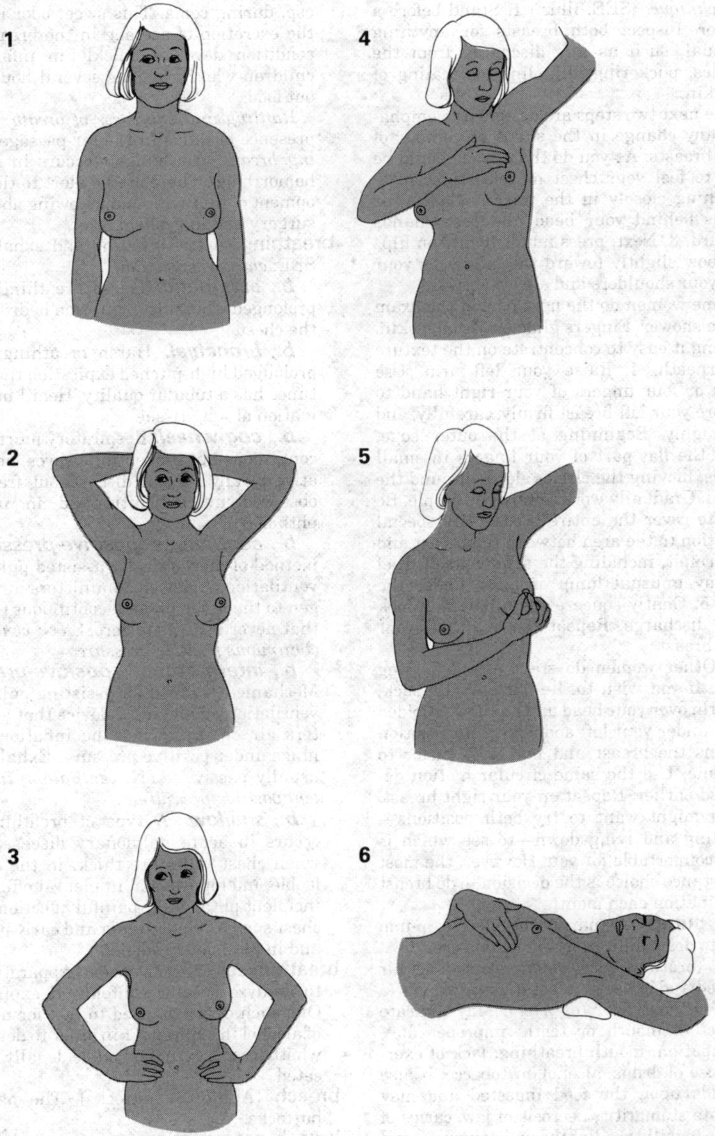

breech.

breeze. A movement of air.

bregma (brĕg'mă) [Gr., front of head]. (pl. *bregmata*) That point on the skull where the coronal and sagittal sutures join. The anterior fontanel in the fetus and young infant.

bregmatic. Pert. to the bregma.

bregmocardiac reflex (brĕg"mō-kăr'dē-ăk) [Gr. *bregma*, front of head, + *kardia*, heart]. Reduced heart rate following pressure on posterior fontanel.

brei (brī) [Gr., pulp]. Tissue that has been finely ground to a pulp in which the cells are intact; used in biochemical research.

Breisky's disease (brī'skēz). [August Breisky, Ger. gynecologist, 1832–1889] Atrophic disease affecting the female external genitalia, seen most often in older women. Characterized by severe itching and a white marblelike appearance of the skin, frequently with excoriations. Without medical intervention, the skin may undergo malignant degeneration. SYN: *kraurosis vulvae; leukoplakia vulvae.*

Brenner's tumor. [Fritz Brenner, Ger. pathologist, 1877–1969]. A benign fibroepithelioma of the ovary.

Breokinase. Trade name for urokinase.

Brethine. Trade name for terbutaline sulfate.

brevicollis (brĕv"ĭ-kŏl'ĭs) [L. *brevis*, short, + *collum*, neck]. Shortness of the neck.

brevilineal (brĕv-ĭ-lĭn'ē-ăl) [L. *brevis*, short, + *linea*, line]. Shorter and broader than usual, with reference to body type. SYN: *brachymorphic.*

Brevital Sodium. Trade name for methohexital sodium.

Bricanyl. Trade name for terbutaline sulfate.

bridge (brĭj) [AS. *brycg*]. 1. Narrow band of tissue. 2. Dental plate replacing missing teeth that is attached to adjacent teeth for support.

b. of nose. The upper portion of the external nose formed by the junction of the nasal bones.

bridgework (brĭj'work). A partial denture held in place by attachments other than clasps.

b., fixed. Partial plates held by crowns or inlays cemented to the natural teeth.

b., removable. Partial plates held by clasps that permit their removal.

bridle (brī'dl). In anatomy, a frenum.

Bright's disease. [Richard Bright, Brit. physician, 1789–1858] A vague and obsolete descriptive term for disease of the kidneys. Usually refers to nonsuppurative inflammatory or degenerative kidney diseases characterized by proteinuria and hematuria and sometimes by edema, hypertension, and nitrogen retention. SEE: *nephritis.*

brim. 1. An edge or margin. 2. Brim of pelvis. Superior aperture of the lesser or true pelvis; the inlet. Formed by the iliopectineal line of the innominate bone and the sacral promontory. Oval-shaped in the female; heart-shaped in the male.

brisement (brēz-mŏn') [Fr., crushing]. Breaking, by forcible means, of anything, as of an ankylosis.

Brissaud's reflex (brĭs-sōz'). [Edouard Brissaud, Fr. physician, 1852–1909] Contraction of tensor fascia latae muscle following stroking or tickling of sole of foot. A component of the extensor plantar response.

Bristamycin. Trade name for erythromycin stearate.

British antilewisite. ABBR: BAL. Trade name for dimercaprol, a compound used as an antidote in poisoning due to heavy metals such as arsenic, gold, and mercury.

British Pharmacopoeia. ABBR: B.P. The standard reference on drugs and their preparations used in Great Britain.

British thermal unit. ABBR: BTU. Amount of heat necessary to raise the temperature of 1 lb. of water from 39° F. to 40° F. One BTU is equal to 252 calories or 1,055 joules.

brittle diabetes. Diabetes in which regulation of the insulin dosage is difficult because of the unpredictable variation in insulin sensitivity and a tendency to ketosis. This type of diabetes is particularly prone to be present in individuals whose diabetes developed during childhood.

broach (brōch) [ME. *broche*, pointed rod]. 1. A dental instrument used for enlarging a root canal or for removing the pulp. 2. Technique of preparing the intramedullary canal of a bone by using a cutting device. This is done in preparation for a prosthetic replacement.

Broadbent's sign. [Sir William Henry Broadbent, Brit. physician, 1835–1907] A visible retraction of the left side and back in the region of the 11th and 12th ribs synchronous with the cardiac systole in adhesive pericarditis.

Broca's area (brō'kăs). [Pierre Paul Broca, Fr. surgeon, 1824–1880] Area of the left hemisphere of the brain at the posterior end of the inferior frontal gyrus. It contains the motor speech area and controls movements of tongue, lips, and vocal cords. Loss of speech may follow hemorrhage into this area. SYN: *motor speech area.* SEE: *aphasia, motor.*

Brodie's abscess. [Sir Benjamin Collins Brodie, Brit. surgeon, 1783–1862] An abscess of the head of a bone, esp. of the head of the tibia.

ETIOL: It is usually of tubercular origin or from subacute staphylococcal infection.

SYM: May be aching pains in area, followed by slight swelling and tenderness on movement. Symptoms less acute but similar to osteomyelitis.

brom-, bromo- [Gr. *bromos*, stench]. Prefixes

indicating presence of bromine.

bromelains (brō′mĕ-lāns). Proteolytic enzyme present in the pineapple plant. Is effective as a meat tenderizer. The enzyme will clot milk. Trade name is Ananase.

bromide (brō′mīd) [Gr. *bromos,* stench]. A binary compound of bromine combined with an element or a radical. It is a central nervous system depressant, and overdosage can cause serious mental disturbance.

bromide poisoning. Poisoning due to an overdose of bromide.

SYM: Prompt vomiting; drowsiness; irritability; ataxia; vertigo; confusion; mania; hallucinations; coma; skin rashes (bromide acne); and neurological disturbances.

F.A.: Large doses of sodium chloride or ammonium chloride by any route. Give saline cathartic. SEE: *Poisons and Poisoning* in *Appendix.*

bromidrosiphobia (brō″mĭd-rō-sĭ-fō′bē-ă) [″ + *hidros,* sweat, + *phobos,* fear]. Abnormal fear of personal odors, accompanied by hallucinations.

bromidrosis, bromhidrosis (brō″mĭ-drō′sĭs). Sweat that is fetid or offensive due to bacterial decomposition. It occurs mostly on feet, groins, and axillae.

NURSING IMPLICATIONS: Daily periodic cleansing with soap and water, use of deodorants, and frequent changes of clothing as needed.

RS: anhidrosis; chromidrosis; uridrosis.

bromine (brō′mēn, -mĭn) [Gr *bromos,* stench]. Liquid nonmetallic element. It is obtained from natural brines from wells and sea water. Its compounds are used in medicine and photography. SYMB: Br. At. wt. 79.904; at. no. 35. SEE: *bromide.*

bromism, brominism (brō′mĭzm, brō′mĭn-ĭzm) [″ + *-ismos,* state of]. Poisoning resulting from prolonged use of bromides. SEE: *bromides* in *Poisons and Poisoning* in *Appendix.*

bromocriptine mesylate (brō″mō-krĭp′tēn). USP. An ergot derivative that suppresses secretion of prolactin. It has been used to stimulate ovulation in the galactorrhea-amenorrhea syndrome. It is used experimentally in treating acromegaly Trade name is Parlodel.

bromoderma (brō″mō-dĕr′mă) [″ + *derma,* skin]. Acne-like eruption due to allergic sensitivity to bromides.

bromodiphenhydramine hydrochloride (brō″mō-dī″fĕn-hī′dră-mēn). USP. An antihistamine; also has sedative properties. Trade name is Ambodryl Hydrochloride.

bromoiodism (brō″mō-ī′ō-dĭzm) [″ + *ioeides,* violet colored, + *-ismos,* state of]. Poisoning from bromine and iodine or their compounds.

bromomania (brō″mō-mā′nē-ă) [″ + *mania,* insanity]. Mental disorder caused by chronic misuse of bromides.

bromomenorrhea (brō″mō-mĕn-ō-rē′ă) [″ + *men,* month, + *rhoia,* flow]. Menstrual discharge characterized by an offensive odor.

bromopnea (brōm″ŏp-nē′ă) [″ + *pnoe,* breath]. Offensive breath; halitosis.

brompheniramine maleate (brōm″fĕn-ĭr′ă-mēn). USP. An antihistamine. Trade name is Dimetane.

Brompton's cocktail. [Brompton Chest Hospital, England] A mixture of cocaine, morphine, and antiemetics used to alleviate pain and induce euphoria, esp. in patients with cancer.

bronchadenitis (brŏng″kăd-ē-nī′tĭs) [Gr. *bronchos,* windpipe, + *aden,* gland, + *itis,* inflammation]. Inflammation of bronchial glands.

bronchi (brŏng′kī) [L.]. (sing. *bronchus*) [NA] The two main branches leading from the trachea to the lungs, providing the passageway for air movement. The trachea divides opposite the 3rd dorsal vertebra into the right and left main bronchi. The point of division is called the carina tracheae [NA] and is the site where foreign bodies too large to enter either bronchus would rest after passing through the trachea. The right bronchus is shorter and more vertical than the left one. After entering the lung each bronchus divides further and terminates in bronchioles. SEE: illus.

b., foreign bodies in. The presence of any foreign material in the bronchi may cause various diseases, large objects leading to collapse of the lung. Beans, nuts, or seeds may cause pneumonia, bronchitis, or lung abscess.

SYM: Immediate choking and gagging. Later, symptoms of bronchitis, atelectasis, pneumonia, or lung abscess. Small metal bodies may produce no symptoms.

PROG: Good if removed before complications occur. Better in case of metallic objects than in those consisting of vegetable matter.

TREATMENT: Removal through bronchoscope.

bronchi, words pert. to: alveobronchitis, "bronch-" words; mesobronchitis; rales.

bronchial (brŏng′kē-ăl). Pert. to the bronchi or bronchioles.

bronchial crises. Paroxysms of coughing in locomotor ataxia.

bronchial glands. Mucous or mixed glands in the bronchi or bronchioles.

bronchial tree. Bronchi and bronchial tubes.

bronchial tubes. The smaller divisions of the bronchi.

bronchial washing. Irrigation of one or both bronchi in order to collect cells for cytologic study or to help cleanse the bronchi.

bronchiarctia (brŏng″kē-ărk′shē-ă) [L. *bronchus,* bronchus, + *arctare,* to compress]. Bronchial tube stenosis. SYN: *bronchiostenosis.*

bronchiectasis (brŏng″kē-ĕk′tă-sĭs) [″ + Gr. *ektasis,* dilatation]. Chronic dilatation of a bronchus or bronchi, with a secondary infection that usually involves the lower portion of the lung. Dilatation may be in an isolated segment or spread throughout the bronchi.

ETIOL: Acquired or congenital, on one or both sides of chest. Acquired bronchiectasis usually secondary to obstruction or infections, as bronchopneumonia, chronic bronchitis, tuberculosis, whooping cough.

SYM: Cough, dyspnea, expectoration of foul secretion, esp. in the morning or when changing position. On standing, sputum separates into three layers: a bottom one that is thick and contains pus cells; a middle layer of greenish fluid; and an upper layer of froth.

TREATMENT: Antibiotics for treatment and prophylaxis, and postural drainage. Resection of affected areas in selected patients. Aerosols for bronchodilation in bronchospasm. SEE: *postural drainage.*

NURSING IMPLICATIONS: Carefully assess the patient for presence of increasing severity of respiratory distress. Oral fluid intake should be increased, and a humidifier or vaporizer used to help thin thick secretions. Teach and encourage the patient to cough and breathe deeply; have chest physical therapy and postural drainage done as ordered. Suctioning should be done to remove secretions if and when the patient is unable to clear airway spontaneously. Patient should understand reasons for use of medications such as antibiotics, bronchodilators, and expectorants. Also instruct the patient to avoid or eliminate irritants such as dust, smoke, and other bronchial irritants. The patient should understand the need for rest and a high-protein diet until the disease has subsided.

bronchiloquy (brŏng-kĭl′ō-kwē) [″ + *loqui,* to speak]. Unusual vocal resonance over a bronchus covered with consolidated lung tissue.

bronchiocele (brŏng′kē-ō-sēl) [″ + Gr. *kele,* tumor]. Circumscribed dilatation of a bronchus.

bronchiogenic (brŏng″kē-ō-jĕn′ĭk) [″ + Gr. *gennan,* to originate]. Having origin in the bronchi.

bronchiole (brŏng′kē-ōl) [L. *bronchiolus,* air passage]. (pl. *bronchioles*) One of the smaller subdivisions of the bronchial tubes.

b., respiratory. The last division of the bronchial tree. They are branches of terminal bronchioles and continue to the alveolar ducts that lead to the alveoli.

b., terminal. Next to the last subdivision of a bronchiole, leading to the respiratory bronchioles.

bronchiolectasis (brŏng″kē-ō-lĕk′tă-sĭs) [″ + Gr. *ektasis,* dilatation]. Dilatation of the

TRACHEA AND BRONCHI
(SEEN FROM THE FRONT)

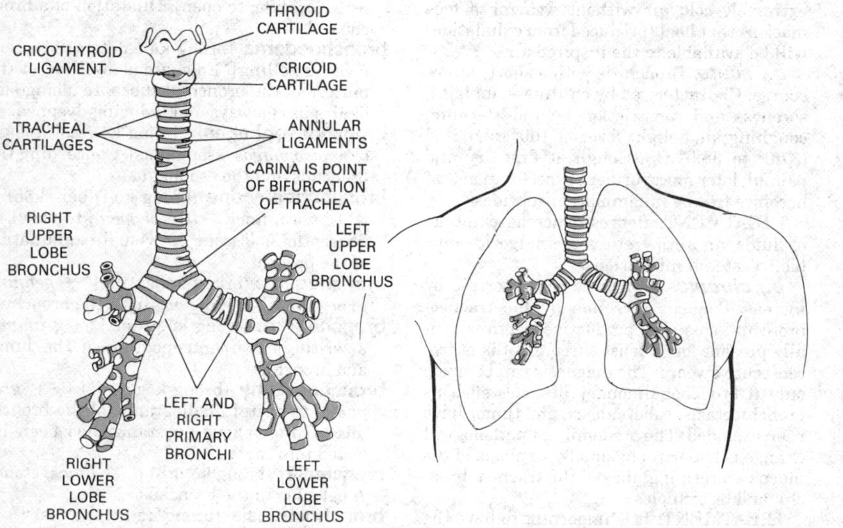

bronchioles; capillary bronchiectasis.

bronchiolitis (brŏng″kē-ō-lī′tĭs) [″ + Gr. *itis,* inflammation]. Inflammation of the bronchioles.

b. exudativa. A form of bronchiolitis with fibrinous exudation and grayish sputum; often associated with asthma.

b., vesicular. Bronchopneumonia, q.v.

bronchiolus (brŏng-kē′ō-lŭs) [L.]. (pl. *bronchioli*) [NA] Bronchiole; one of the smaller subdivisions of the bronchial tubes.

bronchiospasm (brŏng′kē-ō-spăzm) [L. *bronchus,* bronchus, + Gr. *spasmos,* fit]. Spasmodic contraction of the bronchial tubes.

bronchiostenosis (brŏng″kē-ō-stĕn-ō′sĭs) [″ + Gr. *stenosis,* a narrowing]. Narrowing of the bronchial tubes. SYN: *bronchiarctia.*

bronchitis (brŏng-kī′tĭs) [″ + Gr. *itis,* inflammation]. Inflammation of mucous membrane of the bronchial tubes.

ETIOL: Infectious agents such as viruses, esp. influenza virus, or pyogenic organisms such as various species of Streptococcus, Pneumococcus, Staphylococcus, and Hemophilus. Infection often preceded by the common cold. Predisposing factors are exposure, chilling, fatigue, and malnutrition. Acute bronchial irritation may also be caused by various physical and chemical agents such as dusts and fumes. Allergic factors may be of importance.

NOTE: Even though the pathway of air to the bronchi and lungs is capable of warming inspired cold air, there are limits beyond which this system fails. Thus it is inadvisable to let anyone sleep in an area that is extremely cold or to exercise vigorously in extremely cold air without wearing a face mask so that heat (produced from exhalation) will be available to the inspired air.

b., acute. Bronchitis with a short, severe course. Characterized by chilliness, malaise, soreness and constriction behind sternum, coughing, and slight fever of 100° to 102° F. (37.8° to 38.9° C.). Cough at first dry and painful, later mucopurulent expectoration that becomes free as inflammation subsides.

TREATMENT: Bedrest, increased intake of fluids, an antipyretic and analgesic, antibiotics, steam inhalations.

b., chronic. Bronchitis characterized by increased mucus secretion by the tracheobronchial tree. The productive cough is usually present for at least three months of two consecutive years. The diagnosis can be made only if bronchopulmonary diseases such as bronchiectasis, tuberculosis, and tumor have been excluded. The predominant pathological change is hypertrophy and hyperplasia of the mucus-secreting glands of the trachea, bronchi, and bronchioles.

TREATMENT: It is important to have the patient who smokes stop smoking. Change of climate and occupation may be indicated but may be impossible due to social and economic circumstances. If infection is present, appropriate antibiotics should be administered.

b., plastic. Bronchitis characterized by violent cough and paroxysms of dyspnea in which casts of the bronchial tubes are expectorated.

b., putrid. Chronic form of bronchitis with foul-smelling sputum.

b., vegetal. Bronchitis resulting from lodging of foods of vegetable origin in the bronchus.

bronchium (brŏng′kē-ŭm) [L. *bronchus*]. (pl. *bronchia*) One of the subdivisions of the bronchus, smaller than the bronchus and larger than the bronchioles.

broncho-, bronch- [Gr. *bronchos,* windpipe]. Prefix rel. to the bronchi.

bronchoadenitis (brŏng″kō-ăd″ē-nī′tĭs) [″ + *aden,* gland, + *itis,* inflammation]. Bronchadenitis; inflammation of the bronchial glands.

bronchoalveolar (brŏn″kō-ăl-vē′ō-lăr) [″ + L. *alveolus,* small hollow]. Concerning the bronchi and alveoli.

bronchoblennorrhea (brŏng″kō-blĕn″ō-rē′ă) [″ + *blennos,* mucus, + *rhoia,* flow]. Chronic bronchitis in which sputum is copious and thin.

bronchocele (brŏng′kō-sēl) [″ + *kele,* tumor]. A localized dilatation of a bronchus.

bronchoconstriction (brŏng″kō-kŏn-strĭk′shŭn) [″ + L. *constringere,* to draw together]. Constriction of the bronchial tubes.

bronchodilatation (brŏng″kō-dĭl-ă-tā′shŭn) [″ + L. *dilatare,* to open]. Dilatation of a bronchus.

bronchoedema (brŏng″kō-ē-dē′mă) [″ + *oidema,* swelling]. Edematous swelling of the mucosa of the bronchial tubes, reducing size of air passageways and inducing dyspnea.

bronchoesophageal (brŏng″kō-ē-sŏf″ă-jē′ăl) [″ + *oisophagos,* esophagus]. Concerning the bronchus and the esophagus.

bronchofiberscope (brŏng″kō-fī′bĕr-skōp) [″ + L. *fibra,* fiber, + Gr. *skopein,* to view]. A fiberoptic endoscope for visual examination of the bronchi.

bronchogenic (brŏng-kō-jĕn′ĭk) [″ + *gennan,* to originate]. Having origin in the bronchus.

bronchogram (brŏng′kō-grăm) [″ + *gramma,* a writing]. A roentgenogram of the lungs and bronchi.

bronchography (brŏng-kŏg′ră-fē) [″ + *graphein,* to write]. Radiography of the bronchi after a radiopaque substance has been injected into them.

broncholith (brŏng′kō-lĭth) [″ + *lithos,* stone]. A calculus in the bronchus.

broncholithiasis (brŏng″kō-lĭth-ī′ă-sĭs) [″ +

lithos, stone, + *-iasis,* state]. Bronchial inflammation or obstruction caused by calculi in the bronchi.

bronchomotor (brŏng″kō-mō′tor) [″ + L. *motus,* moving]. Causing change of caliber of the bronchi.

bronchomycosis (brŏng″kō-mī-kō′sĭs) [″ + *mykes,* fungus, + *osis,* condition]. Any fungus infection of the bronchi or bronchial tubes, usually caused by fungi of the genus Candida.

bronchopathy (brŏng-kŏp′ă-thē) [″ + *pathos,* disease]. Any pathological condition involving the bronchi or bronchioles.

bronchophony (brŏng-kŏf′ō-nē) [″ + *phone,* voice]. The voice as heard over a normal bronchus through the stethoscope.

bronchoplasty (brŏng′kō-plăs″tē) [″ + *plassein,* to form]. Surgical repair of a bronchial defect.

bronchoplegia (brŏng″kō-plē′jē-ă) [″ + *plege,* stroke]. Paralysis of the muscles of the walls of the bronchial tubes.

bronchopleural (brŏng″kō-ploor′ăl) [″ + *pleura,* side, rib]. Pert. to the bronchi and the pleural cavity.

bronchopneumonia (brŏng″kō-nū-mō′nē-ă) [″ + *pneumonia,* lung inflammation]. Inflammation of the terminal bronchioles and alveoli. SEE: *pneumonia.*

ETIOL: May be caused by various types of pneumococci; Group A hemolytic streptococcus; Klebsiella pneumoniae; various staphylococci; and Francisella tularensis. May also be caused by other pathogenic bacteria and viruses, rickettsias, and fungi.

SYM: Cough and expectoration; respiration short and shallow from 50 to 75 breaths/minute. Cyanosis may ensue. Nostrils dilate with each inspiration, and in children the temperature reaches 103° to 105° F. (39.4° to 40.6° C.). Before death, the temperature may go as high as 108° F. (42.2° C.) with a pulse of 140. Duration of the fever, 2 to 3 weeks. Improvement may be followed by increased severity as new patches form.

In the aged, many of these symptoms are absent. There is a slight cough and little sputum, and fever of 100° to 101° F. (37.8° to 38.3° C.) may or may not be in evidence. Weakness, sore throat, chills, and chest pain may be present. The elderly and bedridden are esp. susceptible.

PROG: Depends principally upon time at which treatment is initiated, recovery generally occurring more quickly in those treated during the first three days. Also prognosis more favorable for those under 50; unfavorable for the very young and very old. Mortality greatly reduced by use of antibiotics.

COMPLICATIONS: Lung abscess, atelectasis, empyema, pericarditis, and paralytic ileus.

TREATMENT: Bedrest, increased intake of fluids, analgesics for pain, antibiotics, soft diet, oxygen for cyanosis. Treatment of shock if it occurs.

NURSING IMPLICATIONS: Carefully monitor the patient for any changes in the type and amount of respiratory distress, particularly frequency and type of cough, dyspnea, and chest pain. Restlessness and apprehension are also symptoms of respiratory distress and should be closely noted. Also work to promote lung expansion and aeration through turning and changing the patient's position frequently, and having the patient cough and breathe deeply 3–10 times each hour. The use of spirometry, which allows the patient to know the values obtained, provides incentive. The patient may receive humidifed oxygen, and guidelines for care of the patient receiving oxygen therapy should be followed.

Early ambulation is helpful, but the patient must be allowed to rest and encouraged not to become overly fatigued.

The patient should have good oral hygiene, may need or prefer small, frequent feedings (to decrease the possibility of abdominal distention), and will need increased protein in addition to good nutrition in order to assist with the resolution of the pneumonia and to promote healing. Hyperthermia is prevented through environmental temperature control, antipyretic administration as ordered, and tepid sponge baths in addition to increased oral fluids (unless contraindicated).

bronchopulmonary (brŏng″kō-pŭl′mō-nă-rē) [Gr. *bronchos,* windpipe, + L. *pulmonarius,* pert. to lung]. Pert. to bronchi and lungs.

bronchopulmonary lavage. Washing out or irrigation of the bronchi and bronchioles in order to remove tenacious secretions.

bronchorrhagia (brŏng″kor-ā′jē-ă) [″ + *rhegnynai,* to break forth]. Bronchial hemorrhage.

bronchorrhaphy (brŏng-kor′ă-fē) [″ + *rhaphe,* suture]. Suturing of a wound of the bronchus.

bronchorrhea (brŏng-kō-rē′ă) [″ + *rhoia,* flow]. Abnormal secretion from the bronchial mucous membrane, sometimes very offensive.

bronchorrhoncus (brŏng″kor-ŏn′kŭs) [″ + *rhonchos,* snore]. A bronchial rale.

bronchoscope (brŏng′kō-skōp) [″ + *skopein,* to see]. An endoscope designed to pass through the trachea to allow visual inspection of the tracheobronchial tree. The device is also designed to permit the passage of an instrument that can be used to obtain tissue for biopsy or to remove a foreign body from the tracheobronchial tree.

bronchoscopy (brŏng-kŏs′kō-pē). Examination of the bronchi through a bronchoscope.

bronchosinusitis (brŏng″kō-sī″nŭs-ī′tĭs) [″ + L. *sinus,* a hollow, + Gr. *itis,* inflammation]. Infection of bronchi and sinus at the same time.

bronchospasm (brŏng′kō-spăzm) [″ + *spasmos,* a spasm]. Spasm of the bronchus.

bronchospirochetosis (brŏng″kō-spī″rō-kē-tō′sĭs) [″ + *speira,* coil, + *chaite,* wavy hair, + *osis,* condition]. Hemorrhagic bronchitis; bronchopulmonary spirochetosis resulting from spirochetes.

bronchospirometer (brŏng″kō-spī-rŏm′ĕ-tĕr) [″ + L. *spirare,* to breathe, + Gr. *metron,* measure]. An instrument for determining the volume of air inspired from one lung and for collecting air for analysis.

bronchostaxis (brŏng″kō-stăk′sĭs) [″ + *staxis,* dripping]. Hemorrhage from the walls of a bronchus.

bronchostenosis (brŏng″kō-stĕn-ō′sĭs) [″ + *stenosis,* a narrowing]. Stenosis of a bronchus.

bronchostomy (brŏng-kŏs′tō-mē) [″ + *stoma,* mouth]. Surgical formation of an opening into a bronchus.

bronchotomy (brŏng-kŏt′ō-mē) [″ + *tome,* incision]. Surgical incision of a bronchus, the larynx, or trachea.

bronchotracheal (brŏng″kō-trā′kē-ăl) [″ + *trachea,* rough]. Pert. to both bronchi and trachea.

bronchovesicular (brŏng″kō-vē-sĭk′ū-lăr) [″ + L. *vesicula,* small bladder.]. Pert. to bronchial tubes and alveoli with special reference to sounds intermediate between bronchial or tracheal sounds and alveolar sounds.

bronchus (brŏng′kŭs) [Gr. *bronchos,* windpipe]. (pl. *bronchi*) One of the two large branches of the trachea. The trachea proper terminates at the level of the 4th dorsal vertebra. SEE: *bronchi.*

Bronkaid Mist. Trade name for epinephrine, USP.

Bronkephrine. Trade name for ethylnorepinephrine hydrochloride, USP.

Bronkosol. Trade name for isoetharine.

brontophobia (brŏn″tō-fō′bē-ă) [Gr. *bronte,* thunder, + *phobos,* fear]. Abnormal fear of thunder.

bronzed skin. Seen in chronic adrenocortical insufficiency, i.e., Addison's disease. Also seen in hemochromatosis, some cases of diabetes mellitus, and cirrhosis of the liver.

brood capsule. Cystlike bodies that develop within a hydatid cyst of Echinococcus granulosus.

broth [ME.]. 1. A nutrient drink made from meat, such as bouillon, usually served hot. 2. A liquid medium made from meat. It is used in making bacterial culture media.

brow. The forehead.

brownian movement (brow′nē-ăn). [Robert Brown, Brit. botanist, 1773–1858] Oscillatory movement of particles resulting from chance bombardment by molecules moving at high velocities.

Brown-Séquard's paralysis (brown′sā-kărz′). [Charles E. Brown-Séquard, Fr. physician, 1818–1894] Reflex flaccid paraplegia occurring during some urinary tract affections.

Brown-Séquard's syndrome. Hemisection of the spinal cord with the following neurological changes: 1. Paralysis on the same side as the lesion, loss of position and vibratory sense, and ataxia. 2. Loss of pain and temperature sensitivity on the side opposite the lesion.

brow presentation. Condition in which the brow or face of the infant comes first on presentation in labor; makes vaginal delivery almost impossible. Cesarean section is frequently needed if the presentation cannot be altered. SEE: *presentations of fetus* for illus.

Brucella (broo-sĕl′ă). [Sir David Bruce, Brit. bacteriologist, 1855–1931] A genus of bacteria. It is nonmotile, aerobic, gram-negative, and pathogenic to man, and it causes undulant fever and abortion in cattle, hogs, and goats. SEE: *brucellosis.*

brucellar. Pert. to Brucella.

brucellin (broo-sĕl′ĭn). An extract of a suspension of any species of Brucella. Injected intradermally, it may be of assistance in diagnosing brucellosis.

brucellosis (broo″sĕl-ō′sĭs) [*Brucella* + Gr. *osis,* condition]. A widespread infectious febrile disease affecting principally cattle, swine, and goats, but sometimes affecting other animals, including man. It is caused by bacteria of the genus Brucella, three species being involved: B. melitensis and B. suis, the cause of brucellosis in goats and swine respectively, and B. abortus, the cause of contagious abortion in cattle and other domestic animals. In man it is called brucellosis or Malta fever, q.v., and is caused by any of the three species.

Bruch's membrane (brooks). [Karl W. L. Bruch, Ger. anatomist, 1819–1884] A glassy membrane of the uvea of the eye lying between the choroid membrane and the pigmented epithelium of the retina. SYN: *lamina basalis of the choroid; vitreous lamella.*

brucine (broo′sēn, broo′sĭn). [J. Bruce, African traveler, 1730–1794] A poisonous alkaloid from Strychnos nux vomica and other Strychnos species. Similar to but less powerful than strychnine, q.v.

Bruck's disease (brooks). [Alfred Bruck, Ger. physician, b. 1865] A rare disease characterized by muscle atrophy and skeletal disorders such as multiple fractures and ankyloses.

bruise (brooz) [O. Fr. *bruiser,* to break]. An injury with diffuse effusion into subcutaneous tissue and in which skin is discolored but not broken. A contusion, q.v. SEE: *Wounds* in *Appendix.*

b. of head, chest, and abdomen. May be associated with internal injuries.

SYM: Pain, swelling, tenderness, discoloration.

NURSING IMPLICATIONS: Collect data regarding the exact cause and location of the injury. Assess for possible additional injuries dependent on the specific location of the original injury. Cleanse skin abrasions thoroughly. A frequent (hourly) neurological exam should be done on any patient who has or may have sustained a head injury.

bruissement (broo-ēs-mŏn') [Fr., droning noise]. A purring sound heard upon auscultation.

bruit (brwē, broot') [Fr., noise]. An adventitious sound of venous or arterial origin heard on auscultation.

b., placental. A purring or blowing noise originating in the pregnant uterus due to fetal circulation of blood. It is synchronous with the maternal pulse.

Brunner's glands (brŭn'ĕrz). [Johann C. Brunner, Swiss anatomist, 1653–1727] Compound glands of the duodenum and upper jejunum. They are embedded in the submucous tissue and lined with columnar epithelium. They are similar to the pyloric glands of stomach. They secrete a clear, alkaline mucinous solution. SYN: *glands, duodenal.*

brush border. Hollow microvilli on the free surface of specialized cells in the renal tubules and intestinal epithelium.

Brushfield spots. [T. Brushfield, Brit. physician, 1858–1937] Gray or pale yellow spots sometimes present at the periphery of the iris of children with Down's syndrome, q.v.

brushing. A technique of tactile stimulation using small, electrically rotated brushes over selected dermatomes to elicit muscular responses in the rehabilitation of persons with central nervous system damage.

bruxism (brŭk'sĭzm) [Gr. *brychein,* to grind the teeth, + *-ismos,* condition]. Grinding of the teeth, esp. during sleep.

Bryant's traction. Traction applied to the lower leg with the force pulling vertically. Used esp. in treating fractures of the femur in children.

Bryrel. Trade name for piperazine citrate.

B.S. *Bachelor of Science; Bachelor of Surgery.*

BSE. *breast self-examination.* SEE: *breast* for illus.

BTU. *British thermal unit.*

bubo (boo'bō) [Gr. *boubon,* groin, swollen gland]. (pl. *buboes*) An inflamed, swollen or enlarged lymph node often exhibiting suppuration, occurring commonly after infective disease due to absorption of infective material. Nodes most commonly affected are those of the groin and axilla.

b., axillary. Bubo in the axilla or armpit.

b., indolent. Bubo in which suppuration does not occur.

b., inguinal. Bubo in the region of the groin.

b., pestilential. Bubo occurring in bubonic plague.

b., venereal. Bubo resulting from a venereal disease. SEE: *lymphogranuloma venereum.*

bubonadenitis (boo-bŏn-ăd-ē-nī'tĭs) [" + *aden,* gland, + *itis,* inflammation]. Inflammation of an inguinal gland.

bubonic plague [" + L. *plaga,* stroke, wound]. An acute, infectious disease associated with a high fatality rate. Called the black death in the Middle Ages. SEE: *plague.*

ETIOL: Caused by Yersinia pestis, usually from infected rats and ground squirrels, which is transmitted to human beings by bite of the rat flea. It is characterized by enlargement of lymphatic glands and severe toxic symptoms, accompanied by intense adenitis or pneumonia.

bucardia (bū-kăr'dē-ă) [Gr. *bous,* ox, + *kardia,* heart]. Severe hypertrophy of the heart. Cor bovinum.

bucca (bŭk'ă) [L., cheek]. (pl. *buccae*) [NA] The cheek; fleshy portion of side of face.

buccal (bŭk'ăl). Pert. to the cheek or mouth.

buccal cavity. The mouth.

buccal fat pad. The corpus adiposum or sucking pad, q.v., an encapsulated mass of fat lying superficial to the buccinator muscle. It is well developed in infants and is thought to aid in the act of sucking.

buccal glands. Small saliva-secreting glands situated in the mucous membranes of the mouth.

buccinatolabialis (bŭk"sĭn-ă-tō-lā"bē-ā'lĭs) [L. *buccinator,* trumpeter, + *labialis,* pert. to the lips]. The buccinator and orbicularis oris considered as a single muscle.

buccinator (bŭk'sĭn-ā-tor). The muscle of the cheek. SEE: *Muscles* in *Appendix.*

buccoaxiocervical (bŭk"kō-ăk"sē-ō-sĕr'vĭ-kăl). The angle formed by the intersection of the buccal, axial, and cervical walls of a cavity in a tooth.

buccocervical (bŭk"kō-sĕr vĭ-kăl). Concerning the buccal surface and cervical margin of a tooth.

buccoclusal (bŭk"kō-kloo'săl). Concerning the buccal and occlusal surfaces of a tooth.

buccodistal (bŭk"kō-dĭs'tăl). Concerning the buccal and distal surfaces of a tooth.

buccogingival (bŭk"kō-jĭn'jĭ-văl). Concerning the buccal and gingival surfaces of a tooth.

buccolabial (bŭk″kō-lā′bē-ăl). Concerning the buccal and labial surfaces of a tooth.

buccolingual (bŭk″kō-lĭng′gwăl). Concerning the buccal and lingual surfaces of a tooth.

buccomesial (bŭk″kō-mē′zē-ăl). Concerning the buccal and mesial surfaces of a tooth.

buccopharyngeal (bŭk″kō-fă-rĭn′jē-ăl). Concerning the mouth and pharynx.

buccopulpal (bŭk″kō-pŭl′păl). Concerning the buccal and pulpal surfaces of a tooth.

buccoversion (bŭk″kō-vĕr′zhŭn) [L. *bucca,* cheek, + *versio,* turning]. A tooth that twists in a buccal direction.

buccula (bŭk′ū-lă) [L., a little cheek]. A fold of redundant fatty tissue under the chin. Known as a double chin.

Buck's extension. [Gurdon Buck, U.S. surgeon, 1807–1877] An apparatus consisting of a weight and pulley for applying extension to a limb by attaching it so force will be applied in the long axis of the extremity.

Buck's traction. Traction of the lower extremity applied in line with the long axis of the leg. The force is applied to adhesive tape attached to the skin.

Bucky diaphragm. [Gustav P. Bucky, Ger.-born U.S. roentgenologist, 1880–1963] A grid that is suspended immediately beneath the x-ray table. It is constructed so that the effects of backscatter and secondary radiation are eliminated when x-ray photographs of dense structures are taken.

buclizine hydrochloride (bū′klĭ-zēn). An antihistamine used to treat motion sickness. Trade name is Vibazine.

bucnemia (bŭk-nē′mē-ă) [Gr. *bous,* ox, + *kneme,* leg]. Tense inflammatory swelling of the leg.

bud [ME. *budde,* to swell]. 1. In anatomy, a small structure resembling a bud of a plant. 2. In embryology, a small protuberance or outgrowth that is the anlage or primordium of an organ or structure.

b., taste. An ovoid body embedded in the stratified epithelium of the tongue and also found sparingly on the epiglottis and soft palate. Buds contain the sensory receptors for taste. SEE: *taste cells.*

b., tooth. The earliest form of tooth development.

budding. A method of asexual reproduction in which a budlike process grows from the side or end of the parent and develops into a new organism, which in some cases remains attached and in others separates and lives an independent existence. It is common in lower animals (sponges, coelenterates) and plants (yeasts, molds).

Buerger's disease (bŭr′gĕrz). [Leo Buerger, U.S. physician, 1879–1943] A chronic recurring inflammatory vascular occlusive disease, chiefly of the peripheral arteries and veins of the extremities. Although a rare condition, the incidence is high among young Jewish males. SYN: *thromboangiitis obliterans.*

SYM: Paresthesia of the foot or pain confined to one toe. Easy fatiguability. Cramps in legs but not to be confused with those occurring in the aged. Legs give out, esp. when walking. Ulceration or moist gangrene may set in; amputation may be necessary.

TREATMENT: Absolute and continued abstinence from tobacco in all forms is extremely important. Avoid excessive use of affected limb, exposure to temperature extremes, trauma, use of drugs that diminish blood supply to extremities, and fungus infections. If gangrene, pain, or ulceration is present, complete bedrest is advised. For arterial spasm, blocking of the sympathetic nervous system by injection of various drugs or by sympathectomy may be done.

bufa-, bufo- (bū′fă, bū′fō) [L. *bufo,* toad]. Combining form indicating origin from or association with toads.

buffalo hump. Deposition of excess fat in lower midcervical and upper thoracic area of the back. Usually due to excessive adrenocortical hormone production or therapy.

buffer (bŭf′ĕr) [ME. *buffe,* to deaden shock of]. 1. A substance, esp. a salt of the blood, tending to preserve original hydrogen-ion concentration of its solution, upon adding an acid or base. 2. A substance tending to offset reaction of an agent administered in conjunction with it.

b., blood. Buffer present in the blood. The principal buffers are carbonic acid, carbonates and bicarbonates, monobasic and dibasic phosphates, and proteins. Hemoglobin is an important protein buffer.

buffy coat. Light stratum of a blood clot seen when the blood is centrifuged or allowed to stand in a test tube. The red blood cells settle to the bottom and, between the plasma and the red blood cells, there is a light-colored layer that contains mostly white blood cells.

bug. A lay term applied loosely to any small insect or arthropod; more specifically a member of the order Hemiptera, which includes the squash bug, chinch bug, and bedbug. They have sucking mouth parts, incomplete metamorphosis, and two pairs of wings, the fore pair being half membranous. The following bugs are of medical importance.

b., assassin. A member of the family Reduviidae. Many are predaceous; others are blood-sucking. Pantastrongulus, Triatoma, and Rhodnius are vectors of trypanosome diseases (Chagas' disease) in man. SEE: *trypanosomiasis.*

b., bed. A member of the family Cimicidae, esp. of the genus Cimex. SEE: *bedbug.*

b., kissing. Several species of the family Reduviidae. Melanolestes picipes is the common kissing bug, or black corsair.

b., red. The larvae of mites of the family Trombiculidae, commonly called chiggers, q.v.

bulb [L. *bulbus,* bulbous root; Gr. *bolbos*]. Any rounded or globular structure.

b., aortic. Dilated portion of the truncus arteriosus in the embryo that gives rise to the roots of the aorta and pulmonary arteries.

b., duodenal. Upper duodenal area just beyond pylorus.

b., hair. The expanded portion at the lower end of the hair root.

b. of the eye. The eyeball, q.v.

b. of the urethra. The posterior portion of the corpus spongiosum found between the two crura of the penis.

b. of the vestibule. The vaginal bulb or bulbus vestibuli, q.v.

b., olfactory. The anterior enlargement of the olfactory tract.

b., terminal, of Krause. An encapsulated sensory nerve ending similar in structure to the corpuscles of Pacini. SYN: *corpuscle of Golgi-Manzoni.*

bulbar. Pert. to or shaped like a bulb.

bulbar paralysis. Paralysis due to changes in motor centers of the oblongata. SEE: *paralysis.*

bulbiform (bŭl′bĭ-form) [″ + *forma,* shape]. Shaped like a bulb.

bulbitis (bŭl-bī′tĭs) [″ + Gr. *itis,* inflammation]. Inflammation of the urethra in its bulbous portion.

bulbocavernosus (bŭl″bō-kăv″ĕr-nō′sŭs) [″ + *cavernosus,* hollow]. A muscle ensheathing the bulb of the penis in the male or covering the bulbus vestibuli in the female.

bulboid (bŭl′boyd) [″ + Gr. *eidos,* resemblance]. Shaped like a bulb.

bulbomimic reflex (bŭl″bō-mĭm′ĭk) [″ + Gr. *mimikos,* imitator]. Contraction of facial muscles following pressure on eyeball.

bulbonuclear (bŭl″bō-nū′klē-ăr) [″ + *nucleus,* kernel]. Pert. to the nuclei in the medulla oblongata.

bulbospongiosum (bŭl″bō-spŏn″jē-ō′sŭm). One of the three voluntary muscles of the penis. It acts to empty the canal of the urethra after urination; and to assist in erection of the corpus cavernosum urethrae. The anterior fibers contribute to penile erection by contracting to compress the deep dorsal vein of the penis.

bulbospongiosum reflex. Contraction of bulbospongiosus muscle on percussing dorsum of penis.

bulbourethral glands (bŭl″bō-ū-rē′thrăl) [″ + Gr. *ourethra,* uretha]. Cowper's glands. Two small glands about the size of a pea, one on each side of the prostate gland, each with a duct about 1 in. (2.5 cm.) long, terminating in the wall of the urethra. They secrete a viscid fluid forming part of the seminal fluid. SEE: *prostate; urethra.*

bulbous (bŭl′bŭs) [L. *bulbus*). Bulb-shaped; swollen; terminating in an enlargement.

bulbus [L.; Gr. *bolbos*]. Bulb, q.v.

b. corpus spongiosum. Bulb of the urethra. A bulbous swelling of the corpus spongiosum penis at the base of the penis.

b. vestibuli. [NA] Two oval masses of erectile tissue lying beneath the vestibule and resting on the urogenital diaphragm. They are homologous to the bulbus spongiosum penis of the male.

bulimia (bū-lĭm′ē-ă) [L.]. 1 Excessive and insatiable appetite. 2. A neurotic disorder esp. of young adolescents and young women characterized by bouts of overeating followed by voluntary vomiting, fasting, or induced diarrhea. SYN: *bulimarexic.* SEE: *anorexia nervosa.*

bulimic. Pert. to bulimia.

bulla (bŭl′lă) [L., a bubble]. (pl. *bullae*) A large blister or skin vesicle filled with fluid; a bleb, q.v. SEE: *pompholyx.*

b. ethmoidalis. [NA] A rounded projection into the middle meatus of the nose underneath the middle turbinated bone, formed by an anterior ethmoid cell.

b. ossea. The dilated portion of the bony external meatus of the ear. SEE: *pompholyx.*

bullet wound. Puncture wound from a bullet. SEE: *wound, bullet; Wounds* in *Appendix.*

bullous (bŭl′ŭs) [L. *bulla,* bubble]. Having the nature of a bulla, q.v.

BUN. *blood urea nitrogen.*

bundle. A group of fibers. SYN: *fasciculus,* q.v.; *fasciola.*

b., Arnold's. The frontopontile tract. It passes from the cerebral cortex of the frontal lobe through the internal capsule and cerebral peduncle to the pons.

b., atrioventricular. A bundle of fibers of the impulse-conducting system of the heart. From its origin in the A-V node, it enters the interventricular septum, where it divides into two branches whose fibers pass to the right and left ventricles respectively, the fibers of each trunk becoming continuous with the Purkinje fibers of the ventricles. SYN: *A-V bundle; bundle of His.* SEE: *heart block.*

b. of His. B., atrioventricular, q.v.

b. of Türck. The temporopontile tract. Fibers pass from the cerebral cortex of temporal lobe and terminate in the pons.

b., Schultze's. Comma-shaped path of fibers in middle of spinal cord's fasciculus cuneatus.

bundle branch block. A defect in the heart's electrical conduction system wherein there is failure of conduction down one of the main branches of the bundle of His. SEE: *heart block*.

bunion (bŭn'yŭn). Inflammation and thickening of the bursa of the joint of the great toe, usually associated with marked enlargement of the joint and lateral displacement of the toe.

ETIOL: Caused by wearing tight-fitting shoes that force toes together.

Bunsen burner (bŭn'sĕn). [Robert W. E. von Bunsen, Ger. chemist, 1811–1899] A gas burner with an adjustment by which the air holes at the bottom of the tube can be closed or opened. If the holes are closed, the flame burns yellow and gives light but a relatively small amount of heat. By adjusting the air intake, a blue flame is produced. This is the hottest, most efficient and smokeless flame that can be produced by the burner.

buphthalmia, buphthalmos (būf-thăl'mē-ă, -mōs) [Gr. *bous,* ox, + *ophthalmos,* eye]. Condition of infantile glaucoma resulting in uniform enlargement of eye, particularly the cornea. Disease may stop spontaneously or continue until it produces blindness. SEE: *hydrophthalmos*.

TREATMENT: Iridectomy, sclerotomy, miotics.

bur, burr (bŭr). A device that rotates at high speed and is so designed and held in a special tool to enable dentist to cut by grinding the tooth, bone, or previous restorations.

Burdach's tracts (boor'dăks). [Karl F. Burdach, Ger. physiologist, 1776–1847] Continuation of the dorsolateral column of the spinal cord into the medulla oblongata. SYN: *cuneate fasciculus*.

buret, burette (bū-rĕt') [Fr.]. A special hollow glass tube usually with a stopcock at the lower end. It is marked so that the amount of liquid released through the outlet will be known. Used in chemical analysis to measure the amount of liquid reagent used.

Burkitt's lymphoma. [D. P. Burkitt, contemporary Ugandan physician] A highly undifferentiated lymphoblastic lymphoma that involves sites other than the lymph nodes and reticuloendothelial system. It is rare in the United States and most common in Central Africa, where the distribution suggests that climatic factors, such as insect vectors, are determinants. There is a strong association of this disease with the Epstein-Barr virus.

burn [AS. *baernan,* to burn]. Tissue injury resulting from excessive exposure to thermal, chemical, electrical, or radioactive agents. The effects vary according to the type, duration, and intensity of the agent and part of body involved. The effects may be local, resulting in cell injury or death, or both local and systemic, involving primary shock (that occurring immediately after the injury and rarely fatal) or secondary shock (that developing insidiously following severe burns and often fatal). Burns are usually classified as:

First degree (minimal depth in skin): Superficial burns, damage being limited to outer layer of the epidermis. Characterized by erythema, hyperemia, tenderness, and pain. No vesiculation.

Second degree (superficial to deep partial thickness of skin): Burns in which damage extends through the epidermis and into the dermis but not of sufficient extent to interfere with regeneration of epidermis. If secondary infection results, the damage from a second-degree burn may be equivalent to that of a third degree. Vesicles usually present.

Third degree (full thickness of skin including tissue beneath skin): Burns in which both epidermis and dermis are destroyed with damage extending into underlying tissues. Tissues may be charred or coagulated. SEE: illus.

TREATMENT: Emergency treatment of burns that cover less than half of the body should be cooling of the burned portion by immersion in water of approx. 50° F. (10° C.). This will bring about almost immediate relief of pain and will aid subsequent healing of the wound. If facilities for immersion are not available, cold compresses may be used. Treatment varies with type of burn and extent of body involved. Therapy for all burns involves asepsis and proper care of wounds, establishing and maintaining the airway, relief from pain, prevention or control of infection if it occurs, prevention or relief of shock, maintenance of water and electrolyte balance, and proper nutrition, esp. to correct hypoproteinemia, which usually accompanies burns. The treatment of shock takes precedence over local therapy. Loss of water and heat from the local burned area due to evaporation is greatly increased. Thus maintenance of fluid and caloric intake is essential.

In severe burns shock is always present and may cause death. Morphine is administered immediately, followed by intravenous injections of whole blood and of salt and water solutions to prevent shock. When pain has eased, charred clothing is removed and burned area is gently washed with a sterile normal saline solution. Treatment may be by use of pressure dressings or by open technique. Experimentation with techniques such as an air bed, which keeps the body suspended on a layer of air, and use of topical silver nitrate are in progress and show promise. Also, the use of split-thickness skin

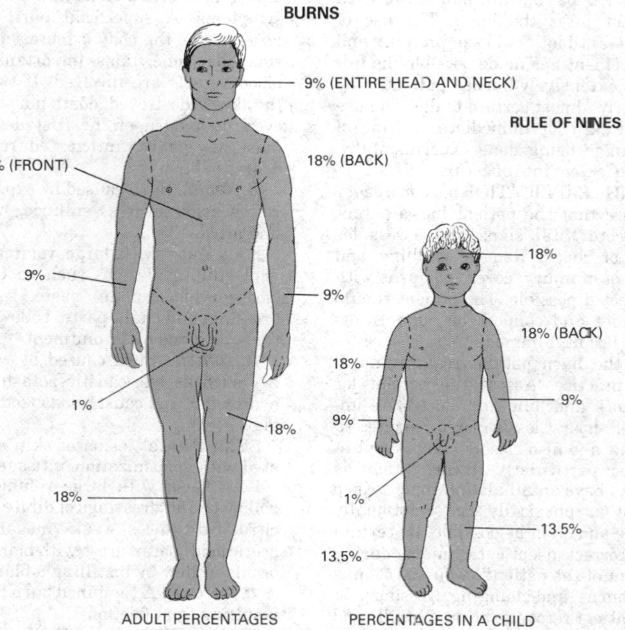
BURNS
RULE OF NINES
9% (ENTIRE HEAD AND NECK)
18% (FRONT)
18% (BACK)
9%
9%
1%
18%
18%
ADULT PERCENTAGES
18%
18% (BACK)
18%
9%
9%
1%
13.5%
13.5%
PERCENTAGES IN A CHILD

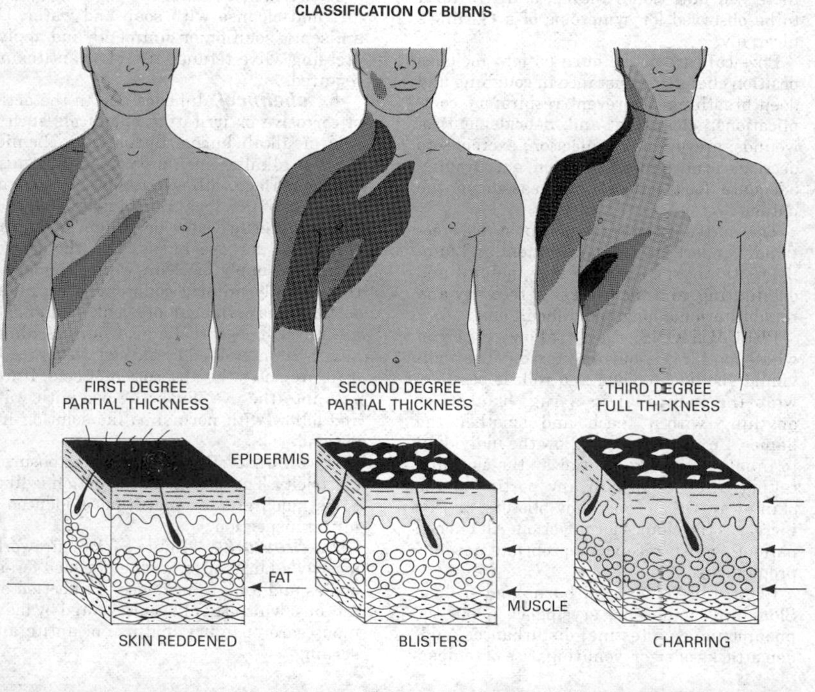
CLASSIFICATION OF BURNS
FIRST DEGREE
PARTIAL THICKNESS
SECOND DEGREE
PARTIAL THICKNESS
THIRD DEGREE
FULL THICKNESS
EPIDERMIS
FAT
MUSCLE
SKIN REDDENED
BLISTERS
CHARRING

grafts from the patient are now being used much sooner after the burn. The use of appropriate antibiotics, blood protein, and fluid replacement has made possible the full recovery of extensively burned patients who were formerly almost certain to die. The use of artificial skin for immediate grafting of burned skin is being done experimentally. SEE: *Burn Centers* in *Appendix*.

NURSING IMPLICATIONS: *Emergency care:* Ensure that the patient has a patent airway; record vital signs and assess for symptoms of shock. Remove clothing and assess extent of injury; cover the burns with a clean sheet if possible. The patient should be kept quiet and comfortable, and transported to a hospital immediately.

Care of the burn patient requires much skill and practice. Assess the patient for signs of shock and fluid and electrolyte imbalance every hour. Closely monitor and record urine output and also closely assess respiratory status, particularly if the patient is suspected to have an inhalation injury. Keep the patient as physically and emotionally comfortable and quiet as possible. Be certain to follow correct aseptic technique during debridement of the patient's wounds, cleansing of the burns, and changing dressings.

As the patient recovers, he or she will need increased nutritional intake, and will need to be observed for symptoms of a Curling's ulcer, q.v.

Physical care of the burn patient includes position changes; assistance in coughing and deep breathing to prevent respiratory complications; cleansing and debridement of wounds; prevention of infection; exercises to decrease contracture formation; encouraging adequate food intake; and reassuring the patient.

The nurse must provide constant emotional support for the burn patient and family, as the burns are extremely painful and debilitating, and the process of recovery and rehabilitation a long and difficult one.

PRECAUTIONS: Never allow a person whose clothing is burning to run. The individual should lie down and roll. If possible, wrap the individual in a rug, blanket, or anything within reach and smother the flames. Be careful not to allow the individual to inhale the smoke. Cut away the clothing, taking care not to pull any portion of the skin away. Do not open any blisters, as this increases the chance for infection. All burned patients must receive appropriate tetanus prophylaxis.

COMPLICATIONS (in burns and scalds): Sloughing, gangrene, erysipelas, nephritis, pneumonia, or intestinal disturbances. Sudden attacks of rigor, vomiting, rise of temperature, and convulsions are all suspicious symptoms. A superficial burn covering a large part of the body is more serious than a small, deep one, unless important nerves and blood vessels are involved. If two thirds of the skin is destroyed, death may be expected, even in a burn of the first degree. Shock must always be anticipated regardless of degree of burn.

b., acid. Burn caused by exposure to corrosive acids such as sulfuric, hydrochloric, and nitric.

F.A.: Wash with large volumes of water; apply dilute alkalies such as baking soda (sodium bicarbonate) paste, soap solution dressing, and chalk paste. Follow by application of a bland oil or ointment.

b., alkali. Burn caused by caustic alkalies such as lye, caustic potash (potassium hydroxide), and caustic soda (sodium hydroxide).

SYM: Painful lesion of skin often associated with gelatinization of tissue.

F.A.: Wash with large volumes of water. Follow by wet dressings of dilute acid such as citrus fruit juices, weak vinegar, and dilute acetic acid. Later, dress with bland ointments or oils. Follow by instilling a bland oil.

b., brush. A combined burn and abrasion resulting from friction.

TREATMENT: Carefully brush away loose dirt and cleanse with soap and water. Use antiseptic solution or ointments and apply a dressing. Give tetanus toxoid or antitoxin if required.

b., chemical. Injuries due to the action of corrosive or irritating chemicals such as acid or alkali burns. Burns from chemical acids or alkalies should be treated by flushing the surface with water, thereby removing all traces of the drug. Do not delay irrigation because sterile water or saline is unavailable, even for eye burns. Use the nearest available supply of clean water. Remember that usually an acid counteracts an alkali, so that weak vinegar or weak ammonia is always safe. A carbolic acid burn is almost always counteracted by alcohol. Never use oil as it promotes the absorption of acid. If lime gets into the eye, flush the eye with water and follow with normal saline solution irrigation.

b., electric. Burn caused by exposure to electricity. The extent of destruction is likely to be much greater than that evidenced by initial inspection.

b., fireworks. Injury from fireworks; usually a burn, often with embedded foreign bodies and a high incidence of infection and tetanus, which should be prevented by meticulous care of injury and use of antitetanus serum.

b., flash. A burn resulting from an explosive blast such as occurs from ignition of highly imflammable fluids, or in war from a high-explosive shell or a nuclear blast.

b., gunpowder. Burn resulting from exploding gunpowder. It is often followed by tetanus, which should be prevented by administration of antitetanus serum and meticulous care of injury.

b. of eye. Burn of eyeball due to contact with chemical, thermal, electrical, or radioactive agents.

F.A.: Wash immediately with the nearest available supply of water. Do not delay because water is not sterile or cool. Irrigation may need to be continued for hours if burn is due to lye.

b., radiation. Burn resulting from overexposure to radiant energy as from roentgen rays, radium emanations, sunlight, or nuclear blast.

b., respiratory. Burn in which the respiratory tract is injured, as from inhalation of hot gases.

b., thermal. Burn resulting from contact with fire, hot objects, or fluids.

b., x-ray. SEE: *b., radiation.*

Burnett's syndrome. [Charles Burnett, U.S. physician, b. 1901] Milk-alkali syndrome, q.v.

burning foot syndrome. A sensation of burning of the sole of the foot. Occurs in certain vitamin deficiencies and in patients with chronic renal failure, due to build-up of toxic waste products.

burnisher (bĕr'nĭsh-ĕr). A smooth-headed dental instrument used to polish a tooth or dental appliance.

Buro-sol Concentrate. Trade name for aluminum acetate topical solution.

Burow's solution. [Karl A. Burow, Ger. surgeon, 1809–1874] Solution of aluminum acetate. Used in dermatology as a drying agent for weeping skin lesions.

burr. SEE: *bur.*

burrow (bŭr'rō). A tunnel made in the skin by the itch mite, Sarcoptes scabiei.

burrowing. The formation of a subcutaneous tunnel made by a parasite or of a fistula or sinus containing pus.

bursa (bŭr'să) [Gr., a leather sack]. (pl. *bursae*) 1. A padlike sac or cavity found in connecting tissue usually in the vicinity of joints. It is lined with synovial membrane and contains a fluid, synovia, that acts to reduce friction between tendon and bone, tendon and ligament, or between other structures where friction is likely to occur. 2. A blind sac or cavity.

b., Achilles. Bursa located between the tendon of Achilles and the calcaneus.

b., adventitious. Bursa not usually present but that develops in response to friction or pressure.

b., olecranon. Bursa at the elbow joint lying between olecranon process and the skin.

b., omental. The lesser peritoneal cavity; the cavity of the great omentum. It communicates with the greater or true peritoneal cavity via the vestibule and epiploic foramen.

b., patellar. One of several bursae located in the region of the patella. Includes the suprapatellar, infrapatellar, and prepatellar bursae. Some communicate with the cavity of the knee joint.

b., pharyngeal. A small, median, blind sac found in lower portion of the pharyngeal tonsil.

b., subacromial. A large bursa lying between the acromion and coracoacromial ligament above and the insertion of the supraspinatus muscle below.

bursae (bŭr'sē). Pl. of bursa, q.v.

bursal (bŭr'săl). Pert. to a bursa.

bursalis (bŭr-săl'ĭs) [L., pert. to a bursa]. Obturator internus muscle.

bursalogy (bŭr-săl'ō-jē) [Gr. *bursa,* a leather sack, + *logos,* study]. Anatomy, pathology, and physiology of bursae.

bursectomy (bŭr-sĕk'tō-mē) [" + *ektome,* excision]. Excision of a bursa.

bursitis (bŭr-sī'tĭs) [" + *itis,* inflammation]. Inflammation of a bursa, esp. those located between bony prominences and muscle or tendon, as the shoulder and knee. Common forms include painful shoulder (SEE: *bursa, subacromial*), miner's or tennis elbow (SEE: *bursa, olecranon*), housemaid's knee (prepatellar bursitis), and bunion, q.v.

TREATMENT: Rest and immobilization of affected part during acute stage. Active mobilization as soon as acute symptoms subside will help to prevent adhesions. Analgesics, heat, and diathermy are helpful. Injection of local anesthetics or cortisone into bursa may be required. In chronic bursitis, surgical removal of calcification may be necessary.

bursolith (bŭr'sō-lĭth) [" + *lithos,* stone]. A calculus formed in a bursa.

bursopathy (bŭr-sŏp'ă-thē) [" + *pathos,* disease]. Any pathological condition of a bursa.

bursotomy (bŭr-sŏt'ō-mē) [" + *tome,* incision]. Incision of a bursa.

bursula (bŭr'sū-lă) [L., little sack]. A small bursa.

b. testium. The scrotum.

Burton's line (bŭr'tŏns). [Henry Burton, Brit. physician, 1799–1849] A blue line along the margin of the gums visible in chronic lead poisoning.

busulfan (bū-sŭl'făn). USP An antineoplastic agent used in treating chronic granulocytic leukemia. Trade name is Myleran.

butacaine sulfate (bū′tă-kān). USP. A topical local anesthetic. Trade name is Butyn Sulfate.

butamben (bū-tăm′bĕn). USP. An anesthetic agent that is used topically. It is poorly and slowly absorbed and thus does not cause systemic toxicity. Name previously was butyl aminobenzoate. Trade name is Butesin.

butane (bū′tān). C_4H_{10}. A gaseous, inflammable hydrocarbon derived from petroleum.

Butazolidin (bū″tă-zŏl′ĭ-dĭn). Trade name for phenylbutazone, USP, used in treatment of acute rheumatic disease. It has a potent anti-inflammatory action.

Butisol Sodium (bū′tĭ-sōl sō′dē-ŭm). Trade name for butabarbital sodium, USP, a sedative and hypnotic.

butt [ME. *butte,* end]. To join two square-ended objects together.

butterfly. 1. Anything shaped like a butterfly. 2. An adhesive bandage used in place of sutures to hold wound edges together. SEE: illus.

butterfly rash. Skin rash of both cheeks joined by an extension across the bridge of the nose. Seen in systemic lupus erythematosus, esp. after the patient's face has been exposed to sunlight. Also seen in seborrheic dermatitis, tuberous sclerosis, q.v., and dermatomyositis, q.v. SEE: *lupus erythematosus; butterfly* for illus.

buttocks (bŭt′ŭks) [AS. *buttuc,* end]. The external prominences posterior to the hips. Formed by the gluteal muscles and underlying structures. SYN: *nates.*

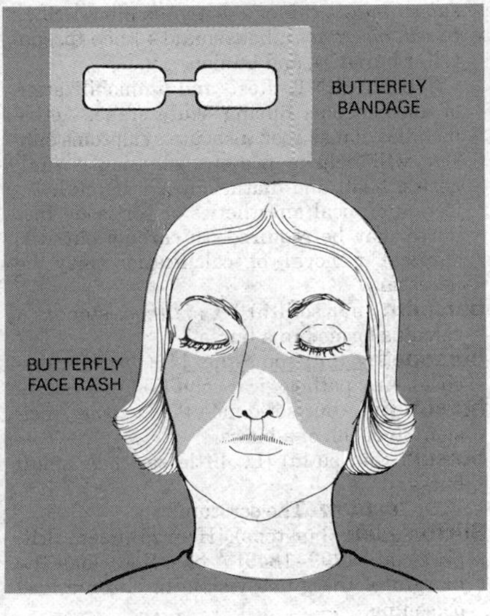

BUTTERFLY

button (bŭt′n). 1. An anatomical or pathological structure that resembles a button. 2. A medical device shaped like a button.

buttonhole. A straight cut through the wall of a cavity.

button suture. Suture in which threads are passed through buttons on the surface and tied to prevent thread from cutting through or into underlying tissue.

butyl aminobenzoate (bū′tĭl ăm″ĭ-nō-bĕn′zō-āt). Name previously used for butamben, USP, q.v.

butylene (bū′tĭ-lēn). A hydrocarbon gas, C_4H_8.

butyraceous (bū″tĭ-rā′shŭs) [L. *butyrum,* butter]. Containing or resembling butter.

butyrate (bū′tĭ-rāt). A salt of butyric acid.

butyric acid (bū-tĭr′ĭk) [L. *butyrum,* butter]. C_3H_7COOH. A fatty acid derived from butter but rare in most fats. It is a viscid liquid with a rancid odor. Used in disinfectants, emulsifying agents, and pharmaceuticals.

butyrin (bū′tĭr-ĭn). A soft yellowish semiliquid fat that is present in butter.

butyroid (bū′tĭ-royd) [″ + *eidos,* appearance]. Having the appearance or consistency of butter.

butyrometer (bū″tĭ-rŏm′ĕ-tĕr) [″ + *metron,* measure]. Device for estimating amount of butterfat in milk.

butyrophenone (bū″tĭ-rō-fē′nōn). A class of chemicals some of which are useful in treating mental disorders. One, haloperidol, USP, is particularly useful in treating Gilles de la Tourette's syndrome.

butyrous (būt′ĭ-rŭs). Of butterlike consistency.

bypass. A means of circumvention; a shunt. It is surgically possible to install an alternate route for the blood to bypass an obstruction if a main or vital artery such as the abdominal aorta or a coronary artery becomes obstructed. The various procedures are named according to the arteries involved.

Ex.: coronary artery, aortoiliac, or femoropopliteal bypasses. The heart itself may be bypassed by providing an extracorporeal device to pump blood while a surgical procedure is being done on the heart.

bysma (bĭs′mă) [Gr., plug]. A plug or tampon.

byssinosis (bĭs″ĭ-nō′sĭs) [Gr. *byssos,* cotton, + *osis,* condition]. Pneumoconiosis of cotton, flax, and hemp workers. Characterized by wheezing and tightness in the chest, caused by the inhalation of dust and foreign materials contained therein, including bacteria, mold, and fungi. The disease does not occur in textile workers who work with cotton after it is bleached. Symptoms are usually more pronounced at the beginning of each work week than later on. SEE: *pneumoconiosis.*

byssocausis (bĭs″ō-kaw′sĭs) [″ + *kausis,* burning]. Cauterization by moxa; moxibustion, q.v.

byssoid (bĭs′oyd) [″ + *eidos,* form]. Consisting of a filamentous fringe, the filaments being of unequal length.

C

C. 1. Chem. symb. for carbon. 2. *kilocalorie* (when capitalized) and *calorie* (if not capitalized); *Celsius* (scale or thermometer); *centigrade;* L. *centum,* one hundred; *circa,* about, or approximate date; *clonus; closure; compound; congius* (gallon); L. *cum,* with.

C^{14}. Radioactive carbon.

Ca. 1. Chem. symb. for calcium. 2. *cathode.*

Cabot's ring bodies (kăb'ŏts). [Richard C. Cabot, U.S. physician, 1868–1939] Blue-staining threadlike inclusions in the red blood cells in severe anemia. They may appear as rings, figure-of-eights, or twisted. Their origin is unknown.

cac-, caci-, caco- [Gr. *kakos,* bad]. Prefix denoting bad or diseased.

CaC_2. Calcium carbide.

cacanthrax (kăk-ăn'thrăks) [" + *anthrax,* carbuncle]. Anthrax.

cacao (kă-kā'ō, kă-kaw'ō) [Mex.-Sp. from Nahuatl *cacahuatl,* cacao beans]. 1. Seed of Theobroma cacao used to prepare cacao butter (theobroma oil), chocolate, and cocoa. 2. A reddish to brown powder prepared from the roasted ripe seeds of Theobroma cacao Linné (family Sterculiaceae) and having a chocolate odor and taste. Used in a syrup base, as a flavoring vehicle for certain medications.

cachectic (kă-kĕk'tĭk) [Gr. *kakos,* bad, + *hexis,* condition]. Pert. to cachexia.

cachet (kă-shā') [Fr., a seal]. Two concave pieces of wafer (rice paper) between which medicine is placed. The margins of the wafer are sealed together. Used for administering medicines with an unpleasant taste. It is swallowed whole.

cachexia (kă-kĕks'ē-ă) [Gr. *kakos,* bad, + *hexis,* condition]. A state of ill health, malnutrition, and wasting. It may occur in many chronic diseases, certain malignancies, and advanced pulmonary tuberculosis.

c., cancerous. Cachexia caused by a cancerous condition.

c. hypophysiopriva. Symptoms resulting from total loss of function of the pituitary gland.

c., lymphatic. Cachexia caused by Hodgkin's disease of the lymph nodes.

c., malarial. Cachexia due to chronic malaria.

c., pituitary. Group of symptoms caused by atrophy of pituitary gland, including emaciation, premature aging, atrophy of genitals with loss of secondary sex characteristics, and lowering of basal metabolic rate. SYN: *Simmond's disease.*

c., strumipriva. Cachexia due to removal of the thyroid gland.

cachinnation (kăk-ĭ-nā'shŭn) [L. *cachinare,* to laugh aloud]. Excessive hysterical laughter.

$CaCl_2$. Calcium chloride; a bleaching powder.

caco-, cac-, caci- [Gr. *kakos,* bad]. Prefix denoting bad or diseased.

$CaCO_3$. Calcium carbonate; chalk.

CaC_2O_4. Calcium oxalate.

cacochylia (kăk-ō-kī'lē-ă) [" + *chylos,* juice, chyle]. Impaired digestion.

cacodylate (kăk'ō-dĭl-āt). A salt of cacodylic acid.

cacoethes (kăk"ō-ē'thēz) [' + *ethos,* character]. Any bad habit, propensity, or disorder.

cacogenesis (kăk"ō-jĕn'ĕ-sĭs) [" + *genesis,* development]. Any abnormal development or growth.

cacogenic (kăk"ō-jĕn'ĭk). Pert. to cacogenesis.

cacogeusia (kăk"ō-gū'sē-ă) " + *geusis,* taste]. The presence of an abhorrent, obnoxious taste in the mouth.

cacoplastic (kăk"ō-plăs'tĭk) [" + *plastikos,* formed]. 1. Pert. to or causing morbid growth. 2. Incapable of normal development or formation.

cacorhythmic (kăk"ō-rĭth'mĭk) [" + *rhythmos,* rhythm]. Showing irregularity of rhythm.

cacosmia (kă-kŏz'mē-ă) [" + *osme,* smell]. 1. An unpleasant odor. 2. Subjective perception of a disagreeable odor. SYN: *kakosmia.* SEE: *olfactory hallucination; parosmia.*

cacotrophy (kăk-ŏt'rō-fē) [" + *trophe,* nourishment]. Malnutrition.

cacumen (kăk-ū'mĕn) [L. *cacumen,* summit]. (pl. *cacumina*) 1. The anterior portion of the superior vermis of the cerebellum. SYN: *culmen.* 2. The top or apex of a plant.

cadaver (kă-dăv'ĕr) [L., corpse]. (pl. *cadavera*) A dead body; a corpse. Term usually applied to a body used for dissection.

cadaveric (kă-dăv'ĕr-ĭk). Pert. to a dead body.

cadaverine (kă-dăv'ĕr-ĭn) [L. *cadaver,* corpse]. A malodorous substance, pentamethylenediamine, produced by the bacterial decomposition of proteins. May occur in the urine in cystinuria.

cadaverous (kă-dăv'ĕr-ŭs). Resembling, esp. having the color or appearance of, a corpse.

cadence (kā'dĕns) [L. *cadere,* to fall]. Rhythmic movement or beat as in marching or dancing.

cadmiosis (kăd-mē-ō'sĭs). A form of pneumoconiosis, q.v., due to inhalation of and tissue reaction to cadmium dust.

cadmium (kăd'mē-ŭm) [Gr. *cadmia,* earth]. A metallic element present in zinc ores. It is a soft, bluish-white metal and is used industrially in electroplating and in atomic reactors. Its salts are poisonous. SYMB: Cd. At. wt. 112.40; at. no. 48; sp. gr. 8.65. SEE: *Poisons* *and Poisoning* in *Appendix.*

caduca (kă-dū′kă) [L. *caducus,* falling off]. Thickened membrane of the uterus; the decidua of the uterus.

caduceus (kă-dū′sē-ŭs) [L., a herald's wand]. In mythology, the wand or staff carried by Hermes or Mercury, having two serpents entwined around it and surmounted by two wings. Used as the medical insignia of certain groups such as the U.S. Army Medical Corps. Even though it is sometimes used to symbolize the medical profession, the staff of Aesculapius, q.v., Roman god of medicine, is usually considered to be the more appropriate symbol. SEE: *Aesculapius* for illus.

caelotherapy (sē″lō-thĕr′ă-pē) [L. *caelum,* heaven, + Gr. *therapeia,* treatment]. Therapy utilizing religion or religious symbols.

café au lait spot. Spots of patchy pigmentation of skin, usually light brown in color, that are characteristic of neurofibromatosis, q.v., but are also found in some normal individuals.

Cafergot. Trade name for a combination of caffeine and ergotamine tartrate.

caffeine (kăf′ēn, kă-fēn′). USP. $C_8H_{10}N_4O_2$. An alkaloid present in coffee and tea. It is a central nervous system stimulant and a diuretic. The amount of caffeine received when coffee, decaffeinated coffee, tea, and cola drinks are ingested varies with respect to the strength of the preparation of brewed coffee or tea as well as the size of the container used for dispensing these beverages. A careful investigation of home-prepared coffee and tea in the Toronto, Canada, area indicated the range of caffeine in percolated coffee was 195–1170 mg./ml.: for instant coffee 102–554; for decaffeinated instant coffee 2–8; and for tea 43–400. The caffeine in cola drinks has been found to range from 40 to 164 mg./ml.

c. and sodium benzoate. A mixture of equal parts of caffeine and sodium benzoate. Used as a CNS stimulant.

c. and sodium salicylate. A mixture of caffeine with sodium salicylate, containing about 52% caffeine. Combines action of caffeine, q.v., and salicylate. SEE: *salicylate, sodium.*

c., citrated. A mixture of equal parts of caffeine and citric acid. Used as a CNS stimulant.

caffeine poisoning. SEE: *aminophylline* in *Poisons and Poisoning* in *Appendix.*

caffeinism (kăf′ēn-ĭzm). Toxic effects of chronic excessive use of caffeine.

SYM: Sudden flushing of the face, palpitation of the heart, trembling, general depression, anxiety, insomnia, and nervousness.

Caffey, John (kăf′fē). U.S. pediatrician, 1895–1966.

C.'s disease. Infantile cortical hyperostosis.

C.'s syndrome. Battered child syndrome, q.v., first described in 1946.

cage, thoracic. The soft tissue and bones enclosing the thorax.

cainotophobia (kī-nō″tō-fō′bē-ă) [Gr. *kainotes,* novelty, + *phobos,* fear]. Fear of novelty. SYN: *cenotophobia.*

caisson disease (kā′sŏn) [Fr. *caisse,* a box]. A condition that develops in divers subjected to rapid reduction of air pressure after coming to the surface following exposure to compressed air. The cause is nitrogen bubbles in the tissue spaces and small blood vessels. Symptoms appear when a diver is exposed to a depth of 33 feet (10.1 meters) or greater for sufficient time for the tissues to be saturated with nitrogen, and then ascends to the surface rapidly; or when an aviator ascends rapidly in an unpressurized aircraft from sea level to 18,000 feet (5486 meters) or higher.

SYM: Deep boring, usually constant pain in joints; itching or burning of the skin; burning sensation in lungs and coughing; and a variety of neurological signs.

TREATMENT: Recompression and then slow decompression. This is done in a special hyperbaric chamber. SYN: *decompression illness.* SEE: *bends.*

caked breast. Accumulation of milk in the secreting ducts of the breast following delivery. SEE: *breast.*

Cal. *large Calorie.* Also abbr. C. One large Calorie is equal to 1000 calories. A large Calorie may be noted by capitalizing the initial letter of the word or by using kilocalorie (abbr. kcal.).

cal. *small calorie.* Also abbr. c. When a small calorie is indicated the initial letter should not be capitalized, to differentiate from a kilocalorie or large Calorie. SEE: *Cal.*

calage (kăl-ăzh′) [Fr., wedging]. Propping of body by means of pillows to prevent movement of the viscera. This is done to relieve seasickness.

calamine (kăl′ă-mīn). USP. A pink powder, containing zinc oxide with small amt. of ferric oxide. Used externally in various skin conditions as a protective and astringent, as an ointment, or as a lotion.

calamus scriptorius [L.]. Inferior portion of the floor of the fourth ventricle of the brain. It is shaped like a pen and lies between the restiform bodies.

calcaneal, calcanean (kăl-kā′nē-ąl, -ăn) [L. *calcaneus,* heel bone]. Pert. to the calcaneus, the heel bone.

calcaneoapophysitis (kăl-kā′nē-ō-ă-pŏf″ĕ-zī′tĭs) [″ + Gr. *apophysis,* offshoot, + *itis,* inflammation]. Pain and inflammation of the posterior portion of the calcaneus at the place of insertion of the Achilles tendon.

calcaneocuboid (kăl-kā″nē-ō-kū′boyd) [″ + Gr. *kubos,* cube, + *eidos,* resemblance]. Concerning the calcaneum and cuboid bone.

calcaneodynia (kăl-kā″nē-ō-dĭn′ē-ă) [″ + Gr. *odyne,* pain]. Pain in the heel.

calcaneofibular (kăl-kā″nē-ō-fĭb′ū-lăr) [″ + *fibula,* pin]. Concerning the calcaneum and fibula.

calcaneonavicular (kăl-kā″nē-ō-nă-vĭk′ū-lăr) [″ + *navicula,* boat]. Concerning the calcaneum and navicular bone.

calcaneoscaphoid (kăl-kā″nē-ō-skā′foyd) [″ + Gr. *skaphe,* skiff, + *eidos,* resemblance]. Concerning the calcaneum and scaphoid bone.

calcaneotibial (kăl-kā″nē-ō-tĭb′ē-ăl) [″ + *tibia,* shinbone]. Concerning the calcaneum and tibia.

calcaneum (kăl-kā′nē-ŭm) [L. *calcaneus,* heel bone]. (pl. *calcanea*) Calcaneus.

calcaneus (kăl-kā′nē-ŭs) [L.]. (pl. *calcanei*) 1. [NA] The heel bone, or os calcis. It articulates with the cuboid bone and with the astragalus. 2. Talipes calcaneus.

calcanodynia (kăl″kăn-ō-dĭn′ē-ă) [″ + Gr. *odyne,* pain]. Pain in the heel when standing or walking; calcaneodynia.

calcar (kăl′kăr) [L., a spur]. A spurlike process.

c. avis. [NA] Lower of two elevations on inner wall of posterior horn of lateral ventricle of brain. SYN: *hippocampus minor.*

c. femorale. A bony spur that strengthens the femoral neck.

c. pedis. The heel.

calcareous (kăl-kā′rē-ŭs) [L. *calcarius*]. Of the nature of lime; chalky.

calcarine (kăl′kăr-ĭn) [L. *calcar,* spur]. Spur-shaped.

calcariuria (kăl-kăr″ē-ū′rē-ă) [L. *calcarius,* containing lime, + Gr. *ouron,* urine]. Presence of calcium lime salts in the urine.

calcaroid (kăl′kăr-oyd) [L. *calcar,* spur, + Gr. *eidos,* appearance]. Deposit in brain tissue that resembles calcification.

calcemia (kăl-sē′mē-ă) [L. *calx,* lime, + Gr. *haima,* blood]. Increased calcium in the blood.

calcic (kăl′sĭk) [L. *calcarius*]. Pert. to calcium or lime.

calcicosis (kăl″sĭ-kō′sĭs) [L. *calx,* lime, + Gr. *osis,* infection]. Pneumoconiosis caused by inhaling dust from limestone (marble).

calciferol (kăl-sĭf′ĕr-ŏl). Vitamin D_2. A synthetic vitamin D, it has the most vitamin D activity of those substances derived from ergosterol. It is used for prophylaxis and treatment of vitamin D deficiency, rickets, and hypocalcemic tetany. SYN: *ergocalciferol.*

calciferous (kăl-sĭf′ĕr-ŭs) [″ + *ferre,* to carry]. Containing calcium, chalk, or lime.

calcific (kăl-sĭf′ĭk) [″ + *facere,* to make]. Forming or composed of lime.

calcification (kăl″sĭ-fĭ-kā′shŭn). Process in which organic tissue becomes hardened by the deposition of lime salts in the tissues.

c., arterial. Deposition of calcium in walls of arteries.

c., metastatic. Calcification of soft tissue with transference of calcium from bone, as in osteomalacia and disease of the parathyroid glands.

calcific tendinitis. Deposition of calcium in chronically inflamed tendon, esp. the tendons of the shoulder.

calcigerous (kăl-sĭj′ĕr-ŭs) [″ + *gerere,* to bear]. Containing calcium or lime salts.

Calcimar. Trade name for calcitonin.

calcination (kăl″sĭ-nā′shŭn) [L. *calcinare,* to char]. Drying by roasting to produce a powder.

calcine (kăl′sĭn). To expel water and volatile materials by heating to a high temperature. Lime is formed from limestone in this manner by the removal of carbon dioxide.

calcinosis (kăl″sĭ-nō′sĭs) [L. *calx,* lime, + Gr. *osis,* condition]. Condition marked by abnormal deposition of lime salts in tissues.

c. circumscripta. Subcutaneous calcification.

calcipectic (kăl″sĭ-pĕk′tĭk) [″ + Gr. *pexis,* fixation]. Pert. to calcipexis, q.v.

calcipenia (kăl″sĭ-pē′nē-ă) [″ + Gr. *penia,* poverty]. Calcium deficiency in body tissues and fluids.

calcipexis, calcipexy (kăl″sĭ-pĕk′sĭs, -pĕk′sē) [″ + Gr. *pexis,* fixation]. The fixation of calcium in body tissues.

calciphylaxis (kăl″sĭ-fĭ-lăk′sĭs) [″ + Gr. *phylaxis,* a guarding]. A state of induced tissue sensitivity characterized by calcification of tissue when challenged by an appropriate stimulus.

calciprivia (kăl″sĭ-prĭv′ē-ă) [″ + *privus,* without]. Deficiency or absence of calcium.

calcitonin (kăl″sĭ-tō′nĭn). A hormone from the thyroid gland in man. It is important in bone and calcium metabolism. In other mammals, it is produced by the ultimobranchial bodies, which become fused with the thyroid. For that reason it formerly was designated thyrocalcitonin.

calcium (kăl′sē-ŭm) [L. *calx,* lime]. Silver-white metallic element, a major component of limestone. SYMB: Ca. At. wt. 40.08; at. no. 20.

Lime, CaO, is its oxide. Calcium phosphate constitutes 75% of the body ash and about 85% of mineral matter in bones. SEE: "*calci-*" words.

FUNCT: Calcium must be carried by the blood in solution in order to be available for bone growth and metabolism. Unless certain activating substances, such as vitamin D, are present, increased calcium intake does not affect the tissues or blood calcium. The secretions of the parathyroid glands are a factor in the utilization of calcium, making it possible for the blood to carry dissolved calcium. Several factors influence absorption of calcium from the gastrointestinal tract: quantities of bread, rice, oatmeal, and corn in the diet decrease absorption of calcium and phosphorus; and the normal alkalinity of the small intestines promotes the formation of insoluble calcium salts.

Calcium is of great importance in blood coagulation; it gives firmness and rigidity to bones and teeth; it is important in acid-base balance; it is essential for lactation; it is important in activating enzymes; it is essential for the function of nerves and muscles, including the myocardium, and for maintaining the permeability of membranes.

Calcium is taken into the body as a constituent of various foods. While much of it may prove insoluble and escape absorption, some of it passes through the intestine into the blood, where it can be measured by chemical tests. Its level in the serum is normally 8.5 to 10.5 mg./dl. Low blood calcium causes tetany with muscular twitching, spasms, and convulsions. Blood deprived of its calcium will not clot; and it is essential for the curdling of milk.

Calcium is deposited in the bones but can be mobilized again to keep the blood level constant when there is a period of insufficient intake. At any given time the body of an adult contains about 700 gm. of calcium phosphate; of this, 120 gm. are the element calcium. Ordinarily an adult takes in 0.8 gm. of calcium per day. During pregnancy, 1.3 gm. of calcium a day will be required.

SOURCES: *Excellent.* Beans; cauliflower; chard; cheese; cream; egg yolk; kale; milk; molasses; rhubarb. *Good:* Almonds; beets; bran; cabbage; carrots; celery; chocolate; dates; figs; kohlrabi; lemons; lettuce; oranges; oysters; parsnips; pineapples; raspberries; rutabagas; shellfish; spinach; turnips; walnuts; watercress.

DEFICIENCY: Symptoms are brittle bones, poor development of bones and teeth, dental caries, rickets, tetany, heart atony, hyperirritability, excessive bleeding. Laboratory error and variation may be the causes of inaccurate or inconsistent values in evaluating the calcium level.

c. carbonate, precipitated. $CaCO_3$. USP. Precipitated chalk. A fine, white, tasteless and odorless powder. Used as an antacid and as an antidote to corrosive acid poisoning.

c. chloride. $CaCl_2$. USP. A very deliquescent salt occurring as translucent crystals having a sharp saline taste. It is used to raise the calcium content of the blood in disorders resulting from lack of sufficient calcium, such as in hypocalcemic tetany. Used in solution and administered intravenously.

INCOMPAT: Ephedrine.

c. cyclamate. A non-nutritious sweetening agent. SEE: *cyclamate.*

c. disodium edetate. A substance used to bind certain metallic ions in the body. Used in treating poisoning due to those metals.

c. gluconate. USP. A granular or white powder without odor or taste. Its actions and uses are the same as calcium chloride. Except it is more pleasant to taste and nonirritating when administered orally or intramuscularly in a 10% solution.

c. glycerophosphate. Calcium salt of glycerophosphoric acid. Used as a dietary supplement and in formulating drugs.

c. hydroxide. USP. $Ca(OH)_2$. A white powder used in preparing calcium hydroxide solution, which is used as an astringent applied to the skin and mucous membranes. In solution it is called lime water. SYN: *lime, slaked.*

c. lactate. USP. A white, odorless and nearly tasteless powder, less irritating than the chloride. Used orally or parenterally as an alternative to calcium gluconate.

c. levulinate. USP. Soluble white powder used when intravenous administration of calcium is required.

c. mandelate. Calcium salt of mandelic acid. Used in treating urinary tract infections.

c. oxalate. A calcium-containing substance that is present in urine in crystalline form. It is a constituent of some renal calculi.

c. oxide. A corrosive and easily pulverized mineral occurring as a hard white or grayish-white mass. Used as a germicide and disinfectant.

c. pantothenate. USP. One of the B complex vitamins. SEE: *vitamin B complex.*

c. phosphate, precipitated. A white, amorphous powder used as an antacid in treatment of gastric hyperacidity.

c. saccharin. A non-nutritious sweetening agent. SEE: *saccharin.*

c. sulfate. A white powder that absorbs water. Used in making plaster of Paris, q.v.

c., total serum. The sum of the diffusible and nondiffusible calcium in the blood serum.

c. tungstate. Fluorescent material used for imaging in radiology; used in intensifying screens.

calcium antagonists. Calcium channel blockers, q.v.

calcium channel blockers. A group of drugs that act by slowing the influx of calcium ions into muscle cells. This results in decreased arterial resistance and decreased myocardial oxygen demand. These drugs are, therefore, valuable in treating angina pectoris due to coronary artery spasm, and chronic effort-associated angina. These drugs can cause hypotension; thus it is important to monitor blood pressure during the initial treatment period. SYN: *calcium antagonists.*

Calcium Disodium Versenate. Trade name for edetate calcium disodium.

calciuria (kăl″sē-ū′rē-ă) [″ + Gr. *ouron,* urine]. Presence of calcium in the urine.

calcophorous (kăl-kōf′or-ŭs) [″ + Gr. *phoros,* bearing]. Containing or producing lime or any salts of calcium.

calcospherite (kăl″kō-sfē′rīt) [″ + Gr. *sphaira,* sphere]. One of many small calcareous bodies found in tumors, nervous tissue, the thyroid, and prostate.

calculary (kăl′kū-lā-rē) [L. *calculus,* pebble]. Pert. to a calculus.

calculi (kăl′kū-lī). Pl. of calculus, q.v.

calculifragous (kăl″kū-lĭf′ră-gŭs) [″ + *frangere,* to break]. Breaking of calculi.

calculogenesis (kăl″kū-lō-jĕn′ĕ-sĭs) [″ + Gr. *genesis,* origin]. Formation of calculi.

calculosis (kăl″kū-lō′sĭs) [″ + *osis,* condition]. Formation of or tendency to form calculi.

calculous (kăl′kū-lŭs). Like a calculus.

calculus (kăl′kū-lŭs) [L., pebble]. (pl. *calculi*) Commonly called stone; any abnormal concretion within the animal body. A calculus is usually composed of mineral salts. These pathological concretions can occur in the kidneys, ureter, bladder, or urethra, and are usually formed of crystalline urinary salts held together by viscid organic matter. SEE: *gallstone; kidney stone.*

ETIOL: Abnormal function of the parathyroid glands; disordered uric acid metabolism as in gout; excess intake of milk and alkali. The cause of most kidney stones is unknown.

c., biliary. Cholelithiasis, q.v.; gallstones, q.v., composed almost entirely of excessive blood pigment with calcium deposits in some. SEE: *gallbladder.*

c., hemic. Calculus formed of coagulated blood.

c., pancreatic. Calculus in the pancreas, q.v., formed of calcium carbonate with other salts and inorganic materials.

c., renal. Calculus in the kidney. SYN: *nephrolithiasis.*

SYM: Blockage of flow of urine from kidney if the ureter is blocked by the stone; sudden, severe, and paroxysmal renal colic; ureteral stricture; various degrees of inflammation.

PROG: Serious if allowed to continue untreated.

TREATMENT: Relief of pain, force fluids unless passage is completely blocked by the calculus. Medicines that are designed to relax smooth muscle help in passing the stone and relieving pain. If the stone is preventing urine flow or if the stone continues to grow and cause infection, surgery must be performed.

c., salivary. Calculus in salivary duct. Usually affects duct of submandibular gland.

SYM: Obstructs flow of saliva, causing severe pain and swelling of gland, esp. while eating.

TREATMENT: Removal of stone by surgery.

c., urinary. Calculus in any part of the urinary system.

SYM: Sudden stoppage of flow of urine with sharp pain due to obstruction, and, if firmly impacted, complete retention of urine.

TREATMENT: Removal of calculus by surgical means or special techniques involving the use of instruments introduced through the urethra into the bladder and ureter.

c., vesical. Calculus in the bladder.

SYM: Increased frequency of urination, pain, and diurnal hematuria increased by exercise all are consistent with this condition.

PROG: Stone is usually small enough to pass through urethra.

TREATMENT: The use of an analgesic and an antispasmodic if necessary; adequate fluid intake. Special urological or surgical procedure if stone is large or impacted.

calculus, words pert. to: "calcu-" words; "chol-" words; gravel; "lith-" words.

calefacient (kăl″ĕ-fā′shĕnt) [L. *calere,* to be warm, + *facere,* to make]. Conveying or that which conveys a sense of warmth when applied to a part of the body.

calf (kăf) [AS. *cealf*]. The fleshy muscular back part of the leg below the knee formed by the gastrocnemius and soleus muscles.

caliber (kăl′ĭ-bĕr) [Fr. *calibre,* diameter of bore of gun]. The diameter of any orifice, canal, or tube.

calibration (kăl-ĭ-brā′shŭn). 1. The determination of the accuracy of an instrument by comparing the information or measurement provided with that of a known standard or an instrument known to be accurate. 2. Measuring the size of anything, esp. the diameter of vessels or the caliber of an orifice.

calibrator (kăl′ĭ-brā-tor). 1 Instrument for measuring the size of tubes or orifices. 2. Device for dilating tubes.

caliceal (kăl″ĭ-sē′ăl) [Gr. *kalyx,* cup]. Concerning a calix.

calicectasis (kăl″ĭ-sĕk′tă-sĭs) [″ + *ektasis,* dilatation]. Dilatation of the renal calyx.

calices. Pl. of calix, q.v.

caliculus (kă-lĭk'ū-lŭs) [L., small cup.] A cup-shaped structure.

c. gustatorius. [NA] A taste bud. SEE: *taste buds.*

c. ophthalmicus. [NA] The optic cup.

caliectasis (kăl"ē-ĕk'tă-sĭs) [Gr. *kalyx,* cup, + *ektasis,* dilatation]. Dilatation of the renal calyx. SYN: *calicectasis.*

californium (kăl"ĭ-for'nē-ŭm). [Named for California, the state and university where it was first discovered in 1950] A chemical element prepared by bombardment of curium with alpha particles. It has properties similar to dysprosium. SYMB: Cf. At. wt. 251; at. no. 98.

caligo (kă-lī'gō) [L., darkness]. Dimness of vision.

caliper(s) (kăl'ĭ-pĕr) [Fr. *calibre,* diameter of bore of gun]. Instrument for measuring diameters of solids such as those of chest or pelvis.

calisthenics (kăl"ĭs-thĕn'ĭks) [Gr. *kalos,* beautiful, + *sthenos,* strength]. An exercise program that emphasizes development of gracefulness, suppleness, and range of motion and the strength required for such movement.

calix (kā'lĭks) [Gr. *kalyx,* cup]. (pl. *calices*) [NA] Any cuplike organ or cavity. SYN: *calyx.*

Calliphora vomitoria (kă-lĭf'ĕr-ă). Common blowfly, whose larvae sometimes cause myiasis disorders.

callisection [L. *callus,* hardened, insensitive, + *sectio,* a cutting]. Vivisection under anesthesia.

callomania (kăl"ō-mā'nē-ă) [Gr. *kalos,* beautiful, + *mania,* madness]. Belief in one's own beauty; a delusion of the insane.

callosal (kă-lō'săl) [L. *callus,* hardened skin]. Pert. to the corpus callosum.

callosity, callositas (kă-lŏs'ĭ-tē, -ĭ-tăs) [L. *callosus,* hard]. Circumscribed thickening and hypertrophy of the horny layer of the skin. May be oval or elongated, grayish or brownish, slightly elevated, with smooth burnished surfaces; they appear on flexor surfaces of hands and feet. Caused by friction, pressure, or other irritation. SYN: *callus.*

TREATMENT: Temporary removal by salicylic acid or careful shaving. Permanent removal only by removal of cause.

callosomarginal (kă-lō"sō-măr'jĭ-năl) [L. *callus,* hardened skin, + *margo,* margin]. Pert. to the corpus callosum and marginal gyrus, marking sulcus between them.

callosum (kă-lō'sŭm) [L. *callosus,* hard]. The great commissure of the brain between the cerebral hemispheres. SYN: *corpus callosum.*

callous (kăl'ŭs). Hard, like a callus.

callus (kăl'ŭs) [L., hardened skin]. 1. Hypertrophied thickening of circumscribed area of horny layer of skin. SYN: *callosity.* 2. The osseous material woven between ends of a fractured bone that is ultimately replaced by true bone in the healing process. SEE: *porosis.*

c., definitive. The exudate, found between two ends of a fractured bone, that develops into true bone.

c., provisional. Temporary deposit between ends of a fractured bone that is resorbed when true bone develops.

calmative (kă'-, kăl'mă-tĭv). 1. Sedative; soothing. 2. An agent that acts as a sedative.

Calmette's reaction (kăl-mĕtz'). [Albert Leon Charles Calmette, Fr. bacteriologist, 1863–1933] Ophthalmic reaction, q.v.

calomel (kăl'ō-mĕl) [Gr. *kalos,* beautiful, + *melas,* black]. Mercurous chloride.

calor (kā'lor) [L., heat]. 1. Heat. 2. Moderate heat of fever. It is one of the four classic signs of inflammation. The others are rubor (redness), tumor (swelling), and dolor (pain).

calorescence (kăl"or-ĕs'ĕns). In physics, the conversion of invisible nonluminous rays of heat to incandescent rays.

Calori's bursa (kăl-ō'rēz). [Luigi Calori, It. anatomist, 1807–1896] Bursa found between arch of aorta and trachea.

caloric (kă-lor'ĭk) [L. *calor,* heat]. Rel. to heat or to a calorie.

caloricity (kăl"or-ĭs'ĭ-tē). Power of developing and maintaining body heat.

calorie (kăl'ō-rē) [L. *calor,* heat]. A unit of heat. A calorie may be equated to work or to other units of heat measurement. To convert small calories to joules multiply by 4.186.

c., gram. C., small.

c., kilogram. C., large.

c., large. ABBR: C., Cal., or kcal. The amount of heat needed to change temperature of one kilogram of water from 14.5° C to 15.5° C. Commonly employed in metabolic studies. When writing of human nutrition the large or kilogram calorie is used. It is always capitalized in order to distinguish it from a small calorie. SYN: *c., kilogram.*

c., small. ABBR: c., cal. The amount of heat needed to change temperature of one gram of water one degree centigrade. SYN: *c., gram; microcalorie.*

calorifacient (kă-lor"ĭ-fā'shĕnt) [L. *calor,* heat, + *faciens,* making]. Producing heat.

calorific (kăl"ō-rĭf'ĭk). Producing heat.

calorigenic (kă-lor"ĭ-jĕn'ĭk) [" + Gr. *gennan,* to produce]. Pert. to production of heat or energy.

calorimeter (kăl"ō-rĭm'ĕ-tĕr) [" + Gr. *metron,* measure]. Instrument for determining the amount of heat exchanged in a chemical reaction or by the animal body in specific conditions.

c., bomb. Apparatus for determination of potential energy of foods. Heat produced in combustion is measured by the amount of heat absorbed by a known quantity of water in which the calorimeter is immersed.

c., respiration. Apparatus for determination of heat production produced from exchange of respiratory gases.

calorimetry (kăl″ō-rĭm′ĕ-trē). Determination of heat loss or gain.

caloripuncture (kăl″ō-rĭ-pŭnk′tūr). Use of heated needles in cauterization by puncture. SYN: *ignipuncture.*

calory. Calorie.

calvaria (kăl-vā′rē-ă) [L., human skull]. [NA] The domelike superior portion of the cranium, composed of the superior portions of the frontal, parietal, and occipital bones. Also called skull cap; cranium, q.v.; skull.

Calvé-Perthes disease (kăl-vā′pĕr′tās). [Jacques Calvé, Fr. orthopedist, 1875–1954; Georg C. Perthes, Ger. surgeon, 1869–1927] A disorder characterized by aseptic necrosis of the epiphysis of the head of the femur.

calvities (kăl-vĭsh′ē-ēz) [L. *calvus,* bald]. Baldness; alopecia, q.v.

calx (kălks) [L.]. 1. Lime. 2. [NA] The heel.

c. chlorinata. Chlorinated lime. Used as a deodorant and disinfectant.

c. sulfurata. Sulfurated lime. Used as a depilatory.

c. usta, c. viva. Burnt lime; quicklime.

calyces. Pl. of calyx.

calyciform (kă-lĭs′ĭ-form) [Gr. *kalyx,* cup, + L. *forma,* shape]. Cup-shaped.

Calymmatobacterium granulomatis (kă-lĭm″mă-tō-băk-tē′rē-ŭm). The organism, a gram-negative bacillus, that causes granulum inguinale, q.v. SYN: *Donovan body.*

calyx (kā′lĭx) [Gr. *kalyx,* cup]. (pl. *calyces*) Any

Recommended Daily Caloric and Protein Allowances*[†1]

Designed for the maintenance of good nutrition of practically all healthy people in the U.S.A.

	Age (years) from to	Weight kg.	Weight lb.	Height cm.	Height in.	Energy kcal.[2]	Protein g.
INFANTS	0.0–0.5	6	13	60	24	kg. × 115	kg. × 2.2
	0.5–1.0	9	20	71	28	kg. × 105	kg. × 2.0
CHILDREN	1–3	13	29	90	35	1300	23
	4–6	20	44	112	44	1700	30
	7–10	28	62	132	52	2400	34
MALES	11–14	45	99	157	62	2700	45
	15–18	66	145	176	69	2800	56
	19–22	70	154	177	70	2900	56
	23–50	70	154	177	70	2700	56
	51+	70	154	177	70	2400	56
FEMALES	11–14	46	101	157	62	2200	46
	15–18	55	120	163	64	2100	46
	19–22	55	120	163	64	2100	44
	23–50	55	120	163	64	2000	44
	51+	55	120	163	64	1800	44
PREGNANT						+300	+30
LACTATING						+500	+20

*Adapted from Recommended Daily Dietary Allowances, Food and Nutrition Board, National Academy of Sciences, National Research Council, Washington, D.C. Revised 1980.

†For complete table, SEE: *Appendix.*

[1]The allowances are intended to provide for individual variations among most normal persons as they live in the United States under usual environmental stresses. Diets should be based on a variety of common foods in order to provide other nutrients for which human requirements have been less well defined.

[2]Kilojoules (KJ) = 4.186 × kcal.

cuplike organ or cavity. SYN: *calix* [NA].

camera (kăm'ĕr-ă) [L., vault]. In anatomy, a chamber or cavity.

c. anterior bulbi. [NA] The anterior chamber of the eye between the cornea and the iris.

c. posterior bulbi. [NA] Posterior chamber of the eye between the iris and the lens.

camisole (kăm'ĭ-sōl) [Fr., little shirt]. A straitjacket.

camomile. The flowering heads of the plant Anthemis nobilis. Used in bitters to improve appetite and digestion. Also spelled chamomile.

Camoquin Hydrochloride. Trade name for amodiaquine hydrochloride.

camphor (kăm'for) [Malay *kapur,* chalk]. USP. A gum obtained from an evergreen tree native to China and Japan.

ACTION AND USES: Topically, as 0.1% preparation, as an antipruritic.

camphorated. Combined with or containing camphor.

camphorated oil. Liniment containing camphor.

camphoromania (kăm-for-ō-mā'nē-ă) [" + Gr. *mania,* madness]. Abnormal craving for camphor.

camphor poisoning. SEE: *Poisons and Poisoning* in *Appendix.*

campimeter (kămp-ĭm'ĕ-tĕr) [L. *campus,* field, + Gr. *metron,* measure]. Device for measuring field of vision.

campimetry (kămp-ĭm'ĕ-trē). Measurement of field of vision. SYN: *perimetry* (def. 2).

camposspasm (kăm'pō-spăzm). Camptocormia.

camptocormia (kămp"tō-kor'mē-ă) [Gr. *kamptos,* bent, + *kormos,* trunk]. Deformity characterized by habitual flexion of trunk forward when individual is erect. SYN: *camptospasm.*

camptodactylia (kămp"tō-dăk-tĭl'ē-ă) [" + *dactylos,* finger]. Permanent flexion of fingers or toes.

camptomelic dwarfism. A condition in which infants have craniofacial anomalies, defects of the ribs, and scapular hypoplasia. The cause is unknown and death usually occurs in the neonatal period.

camptospasm (kămp'tō-spăzm) [" + *spasmos,* spasm]. Camptocormia.

Campylobacter (kăm'pĭ-lō-băk'tĕr) [Gr. *kampylos,* curved, + *bakterion,* little rod]. A genus of bacteria consisting of gram-negative, non-spore-forming, spirally curved motile rods. One or both ends of the cell have a single polar flagellum.

C. fetus. Species with several subspecies that can cause disease in man as well as animals.

C. jejuni. A subspecies of C. fetus that was formerly called Vibrio fetus. It can cause an acute enteric disease characterized by diarrhea, abdominal pain, malaise, fever, nausea, and vomiting. The disease is usually self-limiting. Treatment consists of fluid and electrolyte replacement and treatment with the antibiotic to which the organism is sensitive.

canal (kă-năl') [L. *canalis,* channel]. A narrow tube, channel, or passageway. SEE: *duct; foramen; groove; space.*

c., adductor. A triangular space lying beneath the sartorius muscle and between the adductor longus and the vastus medialis muscles. It extends from the apex of the femoral triangle to the popliteal space and transmits the femoral vessels and the saphenous nerve. Also called Hunter's canal.

c., Alcock's. Canalis pudendalis [NA]. A canal on the pelvic surface of the obturator internus muscle formed by the obturator fascia. It transmits the pudendal vessels and nerve. SYN: *c., pudendal.*

c., alimentary. The digestive tract from mouth through the intestine.

c.'s, alveolar. Canales alveolares [NA]. Canals in the maxilla that transmit the posterior superior alveolar blood vessels and nerves to the upper teeth. SYN: *c.'s, dental.*

c., alveolar, inferior. C., mandibular.

c., anal. Canalis analis [NA]. The terminal portion of the rectum opening at the anus.

c., auditory, external. The external auditory meatus; transmits sound waves.

c., auditory, internal. A canal in the petrous portion of the temporal bone that transmits the acoustic and facial nerves and the acoustic artery.

c., birth. Parturient canal; passageway through which the fetus passes in parturition. Specifically the cervix, vagina, and vulva.

c., carotid. Canalis caroticus [NA]. A canal in the petrous portion of the temporal bone that transmits the interior carotid artery and the interior carotid plexus of sympathetic nerves.

c., central. Canalis centralis [NA]. A small canal lying in the center of the spinal cord extending from the fourth ventricle to the conus medullaris. Contains cerebrospinal fluid.

c., cervical. Canalis cervicis uteri [NA]. Canal in the cervix of the uterus extending from the internal to external os.

c., cochlear, spiral. Canalis spiralis cochleae [NA]. A part of the bony labyrinth of the ear. A spiral tube about 30 mm. long making two and three-quarters turns about a central bony axis, the modiolus. Contains the scala tympani, scala vestibuli, and cochlear duct.

c., condylar. Canalis condylaris [NA]. A canal in the occipital bone that transmits emissary vein from the transverse sinus. Opens anterior to the occipital condyle.

c., craniopharyngeal. A canal in the sphenoid bone of a fetus that contains the stalk of Rathke's pouch.

c.'s, dental. Alveolar canals.

c.'s, ethmoidal. Two grooves running transversely across the lateral mass of the ethmoid bone to the cribiform plate that lie between ethmoid and frontal bones. The anterior ethmoidal canal transmits the anterior ethmoidal vessels and the nasociliary nerve; the posterior ethmoidal canal transmits the posterior ethmoidal vessels and nerve.

c., facial. Canalis facialis [NA]. A canal in the internal acoustic meatus of the temporal bone that transmits the facial nerve.

c., femoral. Canalis femoralis [NA]. The medial division of the femoral sheath. It is a short compartment about 1.5 cm. long lying behind the inguinal ligament. Contains some lymphatic vessels and a lymph node.

c., gastric. A longitudinal groove on the inner surface of the stomach following the lesser curvature. Extends from esophagus to pylorus.

c., haversian. Minute canals found in compact bone that contain blood and lymph vessels, nerves, and sometimes marrow. Each is surrounded by lamellae of bone comprising a haversian system. SEE: *bone.*

c., hyaloid. Canalis hyaloideus [NA]. A canal in the vitreous body of the eye extending from the optic papilla to the posterior surface of the lens. It serves as a lymph channel. In the fetus it transmits the hyaline artery to the lens.

c., hypoglossal. Canalis hypoglossi [NA]. Canal in the occipital bone that transmits the hypoglossal nerve and a branch of the posterior meningeal artery.

c., incisive. Canalis incisivus [NA]. A short canal in the maxillary bone leading from the incisive fossa in the roof of the mouth to the floor of the nasal cavity. Transmits nasopalatine nerve and branches of the greater palatine arteries to the nasal fossa.

c., infraorbital. Canalis infraorbitalis [NA]. Canal in the maxilla lying in the floor of the orbit that transmits the infraorbital nerve and artery. It terminates anteriorly at the infraorbital foramen.

c., inguinal. Canalis inguinalis [NA]. A narrrow, somewhat elongated opening in the lower lateral portion of the abdominal wall, extending from the abdominal (internal) inguinal ring to the subcutaneous (external) inguinal ring. It is an oblique passageway about 1½ in. (3.8 cm.) long and serves in the male to transmit the spermatic cord and the ilioinguinal nerve and in the female the round ligament of the uterus and the ilioinguinal nerve. It forms a channel through which an indirect inguinal hernia descends.

c., intestinal. The alimentary canal from stomach to anus.

c., lacrimal. The lacrimal duct.

c., mandibular. Canalis mandibulae [NA]. Canal in the mandible that transmits the inferior alveolar blood vessels and nerve to the teeth.

c., maxillary. C.'s, alveolar.

c., medullary. The marrow cavity of long bones.

c., nasolacrimal. Canal lying between the lacrimal bone and the inferior nasal conchae. Contains the nasolacrimal duct.

c., Nuck's. In the female, a persistent peritoneal pouch that accompanies the round ligament of the uterus through the inguinal canal.

c., nutritive. An opening on the surface of compact bone through which blood vessels gain access to the medullary cavity of long bones.

c., obturator. An opening in the obturator membrane of the hip bone that transmits the obturator vessels and nerve.

c., optic. Optic foramen through which the optic nerve passes.

c., pharyngeal. Canal between sphenoid and palatine bones for transmission of branches of sphenopalatine vessels.

c., portal. The connective tissue (continuation of Glisson's capsule) and its contained vessels (interlobular branches of hepatic artery, portal vein, and bile duct and lymphatic vessel) located between adjoining liver lobules.

c., pterygoid. Canalis pterygoideus [NA]. Canal of the sphenoid bone transmitting pterygoid vessels, artery, and nerve.

c., pterygopalatine. Canalis palatinus major [NA]. Canal lying between maxillary and palatine bones that transmits descending palatine nerves and artery.

c., pudendal. C., Alcock's.

c., pulp. The central cavity of a tooth filled with pulp. Contains blood vessels and sensory nerve endings.

c., root. The passageway in the root of a tooth. The nerve and blood supply pass through the canal.

c., sacral. Canalis sacralis [NA]. Cavity within the sacrum, a continuation of the vertebral canal.

c., Schlemm's. A space or series of spaces at the junction of the sclera and the cornea of the eye into which aqueous humor is drained from the anterior chamber through the pectinate villi.

c.'s, semicircular, bony. Canals located in the bony labyrinth of the internal ear and enclosing the three semicircular ducts (superior, posterior, and lateral) that open into the vestibule. They are enclosed within the petrous portion of the temporal bone.

c.'s, semicircular, membranous. Semicircular ducts. SEE: *duct, semicircular.*

c., spinal. C., vertebral.

c., spiral, cochlear. C., cochlear, spiral.

c., spiral, of the modiolus. Canalis spiralis modioli [NA]. A series of irregular spaces that follow the course of the attached margin of the osseous spiral lamina to the modiolus. They provide for the transmission of filaments of the cochlear nerve and blood vessels. The spiral ganglion lies in the spiral canal.

c., uterine. The cavity of the uterus.

c., uterocervical. The cavity of the cervix of the uterus.

c., uterovaginal. The combined cavity of the uterus and vagina.

c., vaginal. The cavity of the vagina.

c., vertebral. Canalis vertebralis [NA]. The cavity formed by the foramina of the vertebral column. It contains the spinal cord and its meninges.

c.'s, Volkmann's. Small canals found in bone through which blood vessels pass from the periosteum. They connect with the blood vessels of haversian canals or the marrow cavity.

canalicular (kăn″ă-lĭk′ū-lăr) [L. *canalicularis*]. Pert. to a canaliculus.

canaliculus (kăn″ă-lĭk′ū-lŭs) [L.]. (pl. *canaliculi*) A small channel or canal.

canalis (kă-nā′lĭs) [L.]. (pl. *canales*) Canal.

canalization (kăn″ăl-ī-zā′shŭn). Formation of channels in tissue.

canavanine (kă-năv′ă-nĭn). An amino acid originally isolated from soybean meal. SEE: *soybean.*

cancellated (kăn′sĕ-lāt″ĕd) [L. *cancellus*, lattice]. Reticulated; latticelike structure.

cancelli (kăn-sĕl′ī). Pl. of cancellus. Reticulations forming spongy tissue of bones.

cancellous (kăn′sĕl-ŭs) [L. *cancellus*, lattice]. Having a reticular or latticework structure, as the spongy tissue of bone.

cancellus (kăn-sĕl′ŭs) [L.]. (pl. *cancelli*) An osseous plate of which cancellous bone is composed; any structure arranged as a lattice.

cancer (kăn′sĕr) [L., crab, creeping ulcer]. A malignant tumor. Cancer comprises a broad group of malignant neoplasms that are divided into two categories: carcinoma, q.v., and sarcoma, q.v. Carcinomas have their origin in epithelial tissues while sarcomas develop from connective tissues and those structures that had their origin in mesodermal tissues. Cancer is invasive and tends to metastasize to new sites. It spreads directly into surrounding tissues and also may be disseminated through the lymphatic and circulatory systems.

Cancer incidence and deaths in the U.S.A. by site and sex are shown in the accompanying table based on projections from incidence data in 1981. The American Cancer Society estimates that 700,000 new cases of cancer were diagnosed in 1978 and 390,000 persons died of cancer in that year; this is 1070 per day or one death from cancer each 80 seconds. It was estimated that 117,000 deaths from cancer in 1978 could have been prevented by earlier diagnosis and treatment. In the last 40 years in the U.S.A., the cancer death rate has declined in women and increased in men. It was estimated that 55 of each 100 cancer deaths in 1978 would be men. However, many types of cancer can be effectively treated and cured. An estimated 233,000 Americans, or about one third of all people who developed cancer in 1978, will be alive at least five years after treatment.

ETIOL: Exact cause of cancer in human beings is unknown. Unregulated, disorganized proliferation of cell growth may be caused by various forms of chronic irritation. Certain agents, carcinogens, q.v., have been discovered to cause cancer. Some forms of cancer in animals are apparently caused by viruses.

SYM: The important warning signals of cancer are unusual bleeding or discharge from any internal or external body site; a lump or thickening in any area but esp. the breast; a sore that does not heal; a change in bowel or bladder habits; hoarseness or persistent cough; indigestion or difficulty in swallowing; change in size or shape or appearance of a wart or mole; unexplained loss of weight. These are the major signs of cancer and once any one of them is observed in oneself or in a patient it should be brought to a physician's attention without delay.

DIAG: Depending on the site, diagnosis is made by various means, the most important being biopsy, q.v., use of devices for visualization of hollow organs, roentgenography including computerized axial tomography (CAT), ultrasound, cytology such as the Papanicolaou test, q.v., and palpation for lumps. Some of these techniques and devices will demonstrate an increase in the size or change in the shape of an organ but such alteration may be due to either a benign or malignant growth.

TREATMENT: Surgery, chemotherapy, q.v., radium and x-rays are recognized effective methods of treatment of patients with cancer. Application of proper method or a combina-

1984 ESTIMATED CANCER INCIDENCE BY SITE AND SEX

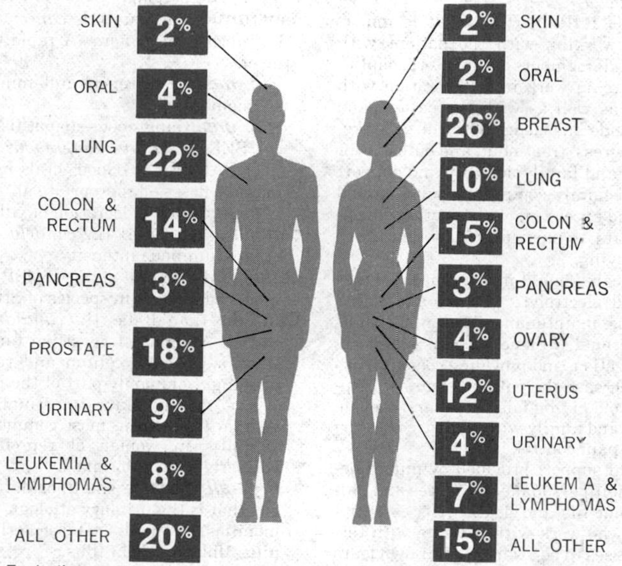

Excluding non-melanoma skin cancer and carcinoma in situ of uterine cervix.

1984 ESTIMATED CANCER DEATHS BY SITE AND SEX

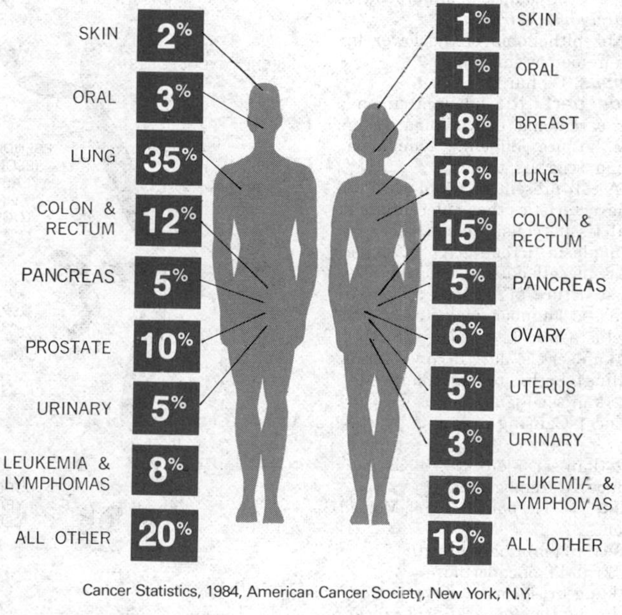

Cancer Statistics, 1984, American Cancer Society, New York, N.Y.

tion of methods is necessary for effective therapy. Therefore, *early diagnosis is the most important factor.*

NURSING IMPLICATIONS: It is important when working with the patient with cancer that all members of the interdisciplinary health team work in collaboration with each other as well as with the patient and family. Provide knowledge of the disease process, its progress, treatment, and outcome for the patient and family. Identify and support patient and family coping mechanisms and allow for and encourage verbalization of feelings and fears, in particular with relation to death and dying.

Physical care should include maintenance of fluid and electrolyte balance and nutritional status, maintenance of elimination as well as personal hygiene, decreasing effects of immobilization, and providing comfort. Also strive to decrease the patient's fears of helplessness, avoid giving false hope, and provide the patient and family with realistic reassurance about pain control.

Emotional support provided by nurses depends on their personal experiences and philosophy about life and death. It is essential for nurses who work with patients with terminal illnesses to be aware of their own fears and feelings related to death and dying.

c., black. Cancer with dark pigmentation.

c., hard. Cancer composed of fibrous tissue. SYN: *carcinoma, scirrhous.*

c., lip. An epithelioma of the lower lip usually seen in men or smokers.

c., scirrhous. C., hard.

cancer, words pert. to: adenocarcinoma; brain tumor; carcinoma; epithelioma; Hodgkin's disease; hospice; leukemia; lymphoma; polyp; sarcoma; scirrhus; tumor.

cancer cell. A cell present in neoplasm that possesses characteristics that differentiate it from normal tissue cells. Among such are degree of anaplasia, irregularity in shape, indistinctness of cell outline, nuclear size, changes in structure of nucleus and cytoplasm, increased number of mitoses, and ability to metastasize.

cancericidal (kăn″sĕr-ĭ-sī′dăl) [L. *cancer,* crab, + *cidus,* killing]. Lethal to malignant cells.

cancerigenic (kăn″sĕr-ĭ-jĕn′ĭk) [″ + Gr. *gennan,* to produce]. Causing cancer. SYN: *carcinogenic.*

cancerogenic (kăn″sĕr-ō-jĕn′ĭk) [″ + Gr. *gennan,* to produce]. Carcinogenic.

cancerophobia [″ + Gr. *phobos,* fear]. Morbid fear of cancer.

cancerous. Pert. to malignant growth.

cancra (kăng′kră). Pl. of cancrum.

cancriform (kăng′krĭ-form) [″ + *forma,* appearance]. Having the appearance of cancer.

cancroid (kăng′kroyd) [″ + Gr. *eidos,* appearance]. 1. Like a cancer. 2. A type of keloid, q.v. 3. Epithelioma, q.v.

cancrum (kăng′krŭm) [L. *cancer,* crab, creeping ulcer]. (pl. *cancra*) A rapidly spreading ulcer.

c. nasi. Gangrenous inflammation of nasal membranes.

c. oris. Gangrenous stomatitis, q.v.; noma, q.v. SEE: *stomatitis, gangrenous.*

TREATMENT: Good oral hygiene and massive doses of appropriate antibiotic.

c. pudendi. Ulceration of vulva.

candela (kăn-dĕl′ă) [L. *candela,* candle]. A unit of luminous intensity.

candicidin (kăn″dĭ-sī′dĭn). USP. Antibiotic produced by certain species of Streptomyces.

Candida (kăn′dĭ-dă) [L. *candidus,* glowing white]. A genus of yeastlike fungi that develop a pseudomycelium and reproduce by budding. Commonly part of the normal flora of the mouth, skin, intestinal tract, and vagina. One of the most common causes of vaginitis in women of reproductive age. Formerly called Monilia.

C. albicans. A small, oval, budding fungus that is the primary etiologic organism of moniliasis (candidiasis). Formerly called Monilia albicans. SEE: illus.

CANDIDA ALBICANS

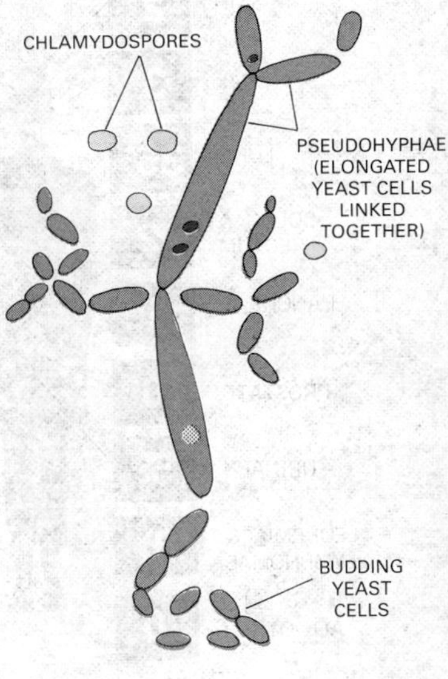

candidiasis (kăn″dĭ-dī′ă-sĭs). Infection of the skin or mucous membrane with any species of Candida, but chiefly Candida albicans, q.v. Usually localized in skin, nails, mouth, vagina, bronchi, or lungs, but may invade the bloodstream. SYN: *moniliasis.*

candle [L. *candela*]. A solid mass of combustible material such as tallow or wax in which a wick is imbedded. When the wick is lit, the wax burns slowly to produce heat and light. Candles are used in bacteriology, where they are placed lighted in an airtight jar and allowed to extinguish themselves. In so doing, an atmosphere containing approximately 10% carbon dioxide is produced. This CO_2 concentration is required for culturing certain organisms, particularly Neisseria gonorrhoeae.

candy striper. A volunteer nurse's aide. So named because of the red and white striped uniform worn.

cane. A slender stick held in the hand and used for support during walking.

canescent (kă-nĕs′ĕnt) [L. *canus,* gray]. Grayish in color.

cane sugar. Sucrose. Table sugar obtained from sugar cane. SEE: *saccharose.*

canine (kā′nīn) [L. *caninus,* pert. to a dog]. 1. Pert. to a dog. 2. A canine tooth; the four teeth, also known as the eyeteeth (upper and lower), between the incisors and molars. SEE: *dentition* for illus.

canities (kăn-ĭsh′ē-ēz) [L., gray hair]. Congenital (rare) or acquired whiteness of the hair. The acquired form may develop rapidly or slowly and be partial or complete. SYN: *achromatrichia.*

c. unguium. Gray or white streaks in nails. SYN: *leukonychia.*

canker (kăng′kĕr) [L. *cancer,* crab, creeping ulcer]. Ulceration of the mouth and lips. SEE: *stomatitis, aphthous.*

cannabis (kăn′ă-bĭs) [Gr. *kannabis,* hemp]. The dried flowering tops of the Cannabis sativa (hemp) plant. Tetrahydrocannabinols present produce euphoric effects when ingested or smoked. Cannabis preparations are being used experimentally to alleviate symptoms of severe glaucoma. SYN: *marijuana.* SEE: *hashish.*

cannula (kăn′ū-lă) [L., a small reed]. A tube or sheath enclosing a trocar, the tube allowing the escape of fluid after withdrawal of the trocar from the body.

cannulate (kăn′ū-lāt). To introduce a cannula through a passageway.

canthal (kăn′thăl) [Gr. *kanthos,* angle]. Pert. to a canthus.

cantharidal (kăn-thăr′ĭ-dăl) [Gr. *kantharis,* beetle, + *eidos,* form]. Pert. to or containing cantharides.

cantharides (kăn-thăr′ĭ-dēz). (sing. *cantharis*) Dried insects of the species Cantharis vesicatoria. Formerly used externally as a counterirritant and vesicant, and internally for its supposed aphrodisiac effect. Its use has been entirely discontinued. Poisonous if taken internally in large doses. SYN: *Spanish fly.*

Cantharis (kăn′thă-rĭs). (pl. *Cantharides*) A genus of beetles, C. vesicatoria, known as Spanish fly. SEE: *cantharides.*

canthectomy (kăn-thĕk′tō-mē) [Gr. *kanthos,* canthus, + *ektome,* excision]. Excision of a canthus.

canthi (kăn′thī). Pl. of canthus.

canthitis (kăn-thī′tĭs) [″ + *itis,* inflammation]. Inflammation of a canthus.

cantholysis (kăn-thŏl′ĭ-sĭs) [″ + *lysis,* a loosening]. Incision of a canthus of an eye to widen the palpebral slit.

canthoplasty (kăn′thō-plăs″tē) [″ + *plassein,* to form]. Plastic surgery of canthus of the eye. Enlargement of palpebral fissure by division of the external canthus.

canthorrhaphy (kăn-thor′ă-fē) [″ + *rhaphe,* suture]. Suturing of a canthus.

canthotomy (kăn-thŏt′ō-mē) [″ + *tome,* incision]. Surgical division of a canthus.

canthus (kăn′thŭs) [Gr. *kanthos,* corner of the eye]. (pl. *canthi*) The angle at either end of the slit between the eyelids; the external canthus or commissura palpebrarum lateralis [NA], and the internal canthus or commissura palpebrarum medialis [NA].

Cantil. Trade name for mepenzolate bromide.

CaO. Calcium oxide, quicklime, calx.

$Ca(OH)_2$. Calcium hydroxide; slaked lime.

cap (kăp) [LL. *cappa,* hood]. 1. A covering. SYN: *tegmentum.* 2. First part of the duodenum. SYN: *pyloric cap.*

c., cradle. Seborrhea of the scalp seen in infants.

c., knee. Bone in front of the knee. SYN: *patella.*

capacitance (kă-păs′ĭ-tăns) [L. *capacitas,* holding]. 1. The state of being able to store an electric charge. 2. The ratio of the charge transferred from one to the other of a pair of conductors to the potential difference between the conductors.

capacitation (kă-păs″ĭ-tā′shŭn) [L. *capacitas,* holding]. Making something have the capacity to evolve, e.g., the process of the sperm becoming capable of fertilization.

capacitor (kă-păs′ĭ-tor). Electronic device for storing electric charges.

capacity. 1. The potential ability to contain, or to hold the power to do something. 2. Cubic content. 3. Ability to perform mentally. 4. A measure of the electric output of a generator.

CAPD. *continuous ambulatory peritoneal dialysis.* SEE: *peritoneal dialysis.*

capeline (kăp′ĕ-lĭn) [Fr., a hat]. A bandage

used for the head, or the stump of an amputated limb. SEE: *bandage, head.*

capillarectasia (kăp″ĭ-lăr′ĕk-tā′sē-ă) [L. *capillaris,* hairlike, + Gr. *ektasis,* dilatation]. Dilatation of capillary vessels.

Capillaria (căp″ĭ-lăr′ē-ă). A genus of parasitic nematodes.

C. philippinensis. Species of roundworm discovered in the Philippines. It causes severe diarrhea, malabsorption, and enteric protein loss in man; mortality is high.

capillariasis (kăp″ĭ-lă-rī′ă-sĭs) [*Capillaria* + Gr. *-iasis,* condition]. A disease, first described in 1968, due to infestation of the small bowel with the roundworm Capillaria philippinensis. Reported from northern Luzon in the Philippine Islands.

TREATMENT: Thiabendazole.

capillaries (kăp′ĭ-lă″rēz). Pl. of capillary.

capillariography (kăp″ĭ-lăr″ē-ŏg′ră-fē) [L. *capillaris,* hairlike, + Gr. *graphein,* to write]. Radiographic examination of the capillaries after injection of a contrast medium.

capillaritis (kăp″ĭ-lăr-ī′tĭs) [″ + Gr. *itis,* inflammation]. Inflammation of the capillaries. SYN: *telangiitis.*

capillarity (kăp″ĭ-lăr′ĭ-tē). A surface tension effect, seen by the elevation or depression of a liquid at the point of contact with a solid, as in capillary tubes. SYN: *capillary attraction.*

capillaropathy (kăp″ĭ-lăr-ŏp′ă-thē) [″ + Gr. *pathos,* disease]. Capillary disorders or disease.

capillaroscopy (kăp″ĭ-lăr-ŏs′kō-pē) [″ + Gr. *skopein,* to examine]. Examination of capillaries for diagnostic purposes.

capillary (kăp′ĭ-lăr″ē) [L. *capillaris,* hairlike]. (pl. *capillaries*) 1. Any of the minute blood vessels, averaging 0.008 mm. in diameter, carrying blood and forming the capillary system. Capillaries connect the smallest arteries (arterioles) with the smallest veins (venules). 2. Pert. to a hair; hairlike.

c.'s, arterial. The very small vessels that are the terminal branches of the arterioles or metarterioles.

c.'s, bile. Intercellular biliary passageways that convey bile from liver cells to the interlobular bile ducts.

c.'s, blood. Minute blood vessels that convey blood from the arterioles to the venules. They form an anastomosing network that brings the blood into intimate relationship with the tissue cells. Their wall consists of a single layer of squamous cells called endothelium through which blood and oxygen diffuse to the tissue; and products of metabolic activity enter the bloodstream. They average about 8 microns in diameter, but are capable of being constricted so as to have almost no lumen at all.

c.'s, lymphatic. The smallest lymphatic vessels. They are thin-walled tubes forming a dense network in most tissues of the body. They differ from blood capillaries in that they are generally slightly larger in diameter and end blindly but anastomose freely with other lymphatics. They collect interstitial fluid, thus the composition of the lymph will vary with respect to the tissue being drained. Intestinal lymphatics will contain fatty materials during digestion; those from the liver will contain proteins. Lymph capillaries unite to form larger lymphatic vessels, which drain into lymph nodes, which are drained by efferent lymph vessels, which flow into the venous blood system at the junction of the internal jugular and subclavian veins.

c.'s, venous. The minute vessels that convey blood from a capillary network into the small veins or venules.

capillary attraction. Capillarity, q.v.

capillary permeability. The ability of substances to diffuse through capillary walls into the tissue spaces. It is influenced by hypoxia, adrenal cortical hormone, and the concentration of calcium ions in the blood.

capillus (kă-pĭl′ŭs) [L., a hair]. (pl. *capilli*) 1. A hair, esp. of the head. 2. A filament. 3. A hair's breadth.

capital [L. *capitalis*]. Pert. to the head.

capitate (kăp′ĭ-tāt) [L. *caput,* head]. Head-shaped; having a rounded extremity.

capitation fee (kăp″ĭ-tā′shŭn). Amount paid a physician annually from each patient in a medical group plan.

capitatum (kăp″ĭ-tā′tŭm). Os capitatum [NA]. Third bone in distal row of carpus, i.e., the wrist. SYN: *os magnum.*

capitellum (kăp″ĭ-tĕl′ŭm) [L., small head]. The round eminence at lower end of the humerus articulating with radius; its radial head. SYN: *capitulum humeri* [NA].

capitula [L.]. Pl. of capitulum.

capitular (kă-pĭt′ū-lăr). Pert. to a capitulum.

capitulum (kă-pĭt′ū-lŭm, kă-pĭch′ū-lŭm) [L., small head]. (pl. *capitula*) [NA] A small, rounded articular end of a bone.

c. fibulae. The proximal extremity or head of the fibula; articulates with tibia.

c. humeri. [NA] Rounded prominence at distal end of humerus. Articulates with the radius. SYN: *capitellum.*

c. mallei. In the middle ear, the head or large rounded extremity of the malleus; bears facet for the incus.

c. stapedis. The head of the stapes; articulated with lenticular process of incus of the middle ear.

capnophilic (kăp-nō-fĭl′ĭk) [Gr. *kapnos,* smoke, + *philein,* to love]. Describing bacteria that grow best in an atmosphere containing carbon dioxide.

capotement (kă-pōt-mŏn′) [Fr.]. A splashing sound that may be heard when the dilated stomach contains air and fluid.

Capoten. Trade name for captopril, q.v.

capping (kăp′ĭng). 1. Placing a protective substance over the exposed pulp of a tooth. 2. In immunology, the aggregation of living B-lymphocytes that have reacted with fluorescein-labeled anti-immune globulin cells to form a polar cap.

capreomycin sulfate. USP. A tuberculostatic drug. Trade name is Capastat Sulfate.

capsicum (kăp′sĭ-kŭm). Cayenne pepper; dried ripe fruit of capsicum. Used as a carminative, stimulant, and rubefacient.

capsid (kăp′sĭd). The protein covering around the central core of a virus particle. The capsid, which develops from protein units called protomers, protects the nucleic acid in the core of the virus particle from the destructive enzymes in biological fluids and promotes attachment of the virus to susceptible cells.

capsitis (kăp-sī′tĭs) [L. *capsa*, box, + Gr. *itis*, inflammation]. Capsulitis of crystalline lens.

capsomer (kăp′sō-mĕr) [″ + Gr. *meros*, part]. The short ribbons of protein that make up a portion of the capsid viral particle.

capsula [L., little box]. (pl. *capsulae*) [NA] A sheath or continuous enclosure around an organ or structure.

c. articularis. [NA] Capsule of a joint.

c. bulbi. Tenon's capsule, q.v.

c. fibrosa perivascularis. Glisson's capsule.

c. glomeruli. [NA] Bowman's capsule; malpighian capsule.

c. lentis. [NA] Crystalline lens capsule of the eye.

capsulae (căp′sū-lē) [L.]. Pl. of capsula, q.v.

capsular. Pert. to a capsule.

capsulation. Enclosure in a capsule.

capsule [L. *capsula*, little box]. 1. Capsula, q.v. 2. A special container made of gelatin. Size is for a single dose of a drug; the enclosure prevents the patient from tasting the drug.

c., articular. A two-layered sleeve or covering for a synovial joint. The inner layer is synovial and the outer is fibrous.

c., auditory. Embryonic cartilaginous capsule enclosing the developing ear.

c., bacterial. The membrane that surrounds some bacterial cells. It is a loose gel-like structure that, in pathogenic bacteria, helps to protect against phagocytosis.

c., Bowman's. The glomerular capsule of the kidneys.

c., cartilage. The layer of matrix that forms the innermost portion of the wall of a lacuna enclosing a single cell or a group of cartilage cells. It is basophilic.

c., Glisson's. An outer capsule of fibrous tissue in which is invested the liver, its ducts and vessels. SYN: *capsula fibrosa perivascularis* [NA].

c., glomerular. Bowman's capsule, q.v.

c., joint. The fibrous tissues enclosing a joint.

c., lens. A transparent structureless membrane that surrounds and encloses the lens of the eye.

c., nasal; c., optic; c., otic. Cartilaginous capsules that develop in the embryonic skull to enclose each of the paired sense organs—nasal cavity, eyes, and ears, respectively.

c. of the kidney. Fat-containing connective tissue surrounding the kidney.

c. of Tenon. A thin fibrous sac enveloping the eyeball, forming a socket in which it rotates.

c., renal. Fibrous capsule surrounding the kidney.

c., suprarenal. A tough connective tissue capsule that encloses the adrenal gland.

capsulectomy (kăp″sū-lĕk′tō-mē) [L. *capsula*, little box, + Gr. *ektome*, excision]. Surgical removal of a capsule.

capsulitis (kăp″sū-lī′tĭs) [″ + Gr. *itis*, inflammation]. Inflammation of a capsule.

capsulociliary (kăp″sū-lō-sĭl′ē-ĕr-ē) [″ + *ciliaris*, pert. to the eyelashes]. Pert. to capsule of lens and ciliary structures.

capsulolenticular (kăp″sū-lō-lĕn-tĭk′ū-lăr) [″ + *lenticularis*, pert. to a lens]. Concerning the capsule of the eye and the lens.

capsuloplasty (kăp′sū-lō-plăs″tē) [″ + Gr. *plassein*, to mold]. Plastic surgery of a capsule, esp. one of a joint.

capsulorrhaphy (kăp″sū-lor′ă-fē) [″ + Gr. *rhaphe*, suture]. Suture of a joint capsule or of a tear in a capsule.

capsulotome (kăp′sū-lō-tōm″) [″ + Gr. *tome*, incision]. Instrument for incising the capsule of the crystalline lens.

capsulotomy (kăp″sū-lŏt′ō-mē). Cutting of the capsule of crystalline lens.

captopril. A drug that blocks the conversion of angiotensin I to angiotensin II. It is used in diagnosing renovascular hypertension that can be alleviated by surgery, and in treating the vascular and renal crises that may occur in scleroderma. Trade name is Capoten.

caput (kā′pŭt, kăp′ŭt) [L.]. (pl. *cap′ita*) [NA] 1. The head. 2. The chief extremity of an organ.

c. gallinaginis. Round protuberance on the urethral floor. SYN: *colliculus seminalis* [NA].

c. medusae. Plexus of dilated veins about the umbilicus seen in one form of cirrhosis of the liver (Cruveilhier-Baumgarten syndrome) indicating portal vein obstruction. It may be seen in newborns.

c. succedaneum. Swelling produced on the presenting part of the fetal head during labor. It may be mistaken for the bag-of-waters. It recedes within 2 to 3 days.

ETIOL: Effusion of serum into cellular tissue of exposed scalp through venous interference from pressure.

caramel (kăr′ă-mĕl, kăr′mĕl). NF. Flavoring and coloring agent made by heating sugar or glucose to 180–200° C. until it forms a uniform dark brown, thick mass. The sweet taste is destroyed by this process.

carbachol (kăr′bă-kŏl). USP. Drug with action similar to acetylcholine. Used to produce miosis during eye surgery. Trade names are Miostat and Isopto Carbachol.

carbamazepine (kăr-bă-măz′ĕ-pēn). Drug used for treatment of trigeminal neuralgia and temporal lobe epilepsy. Trade name is Tegretol.

carbamide (kăr′bă-mīd, kăr-băm′īd). $CO(NH)_2$. Urea in an anhydrous, sterile powder form.

carbaminohemoglobin (kăr-băm″ĭ-nō-hē″mō-glō′bĭn). Chemical combination of carbon dioxide and hemoglobin.

carbarsone (kăr′băr-sōn). USP. A white, crystalline, odorless powder; contains about 28% arsenic, having a chemical structure resembling tryparsamide. Used as an antiamebic agent. Trade name is Carb-O-Sep.

carbenicillin indanyl sodium (kăr″bĕn-ĭ-sĭl′ĭn). USP. A semisynthetic antibiotic of the penicillin group.

carbidopa (kăr″bĭ-dō′pă). USP. Drug used with levodopa in treating parkinsonism.

carbinoxamine maleate (kăr″bĭn-ŏk′să-mēn). USP. An antihistamine that acts by blocking histamine receptors. Trade name is Clistin.

Carbocaine. Trade name for mepivacaine hydrochloride.

carbohydrase (kăr″bō-hī′drās). One of a group of enzymes (such as amylase and lactase) that hydrolyze carbohydrates.

carbohydrate (kăr″bō-hī′drāt) [L. *carbo*, carbon, + Gr. *hydor*, water]. A group of chemical substances, including sugars, glycogen, starches, dextrins, and celluloses, that contain only carbon, oxygen, and hydrogen. Usually the ratio of hydrogen to oxygen is 2:1. It is estimated that glucose and its polymers (including starch and cellulose) represent the most abundant organic chemical compounds on earth, surpassing in quantity even the great stores of fuel hydrocarbons beneath the earth's crust.

Carbohydrates are one of the three classes of nutrients. Green plants utilize the sun's energy to combine carbon dioxide and water to form carbohydrates. Most plant carbohydrates (celluloses) are unavailable for direct metabolism by vertebrates. However, the bacteria present in some vertebrates' intestinal tracts break down cellulose to molecules that can be absorbed. Man's intestinal tract lacks the enzyme that splits cellulose into sugar molecules, but humans do split starch into maltose by means of their salivary and pancreatic amylase enzymes.

CLASSIFICATION: Carbohydrates are grouped according to the number of carbon atoms they contain and how many of the basic types are combined into larger molecules. The most common simple sugars, monosaccharides, contain five or six carbon atoms and are called pentoses and hexoses, respectively. Two monosaccharides linked together are called a disaccharide. A series or chain of monosaccharides or disaccharides is called a polysaccharide. Ribose is the most important pentose; glucose, fructose, and galactose are the most important hexoses in human metabolism. The disaccharide sugars present in the diet are maltose (2 D-glucose molecules), sucrose or cane sugar (glucose + fructose), and lactose or milk sugar (D-glucose and D-galactose). These sugars are split and eventually converted to glucose by the action of enzymes. The two important polysaccharides are starch and glycogen, the latter of which is called animal starch. The basic monosaccharide building-block for both of these large polymers is glucose. Dietary starch and glycogen are metabolized first to glucose and then to CO_2 and water in the human.

COMP: All carbohydrates contain only carbon, hydrogen, and oxygen molecules.

FUNCT: Carbohydrates are a basic source of energy. They are stored in the body as glycogen in virtually all tissues but principally in the liver and muscles. From these sites it can be mobilized, making these stores an important source of reserve energy.

DIGESTION AND ABSORPTION: Cooked but not raw starch is broken down by salivary amylase to disaccharide. Both cooked and raw starch are split in the small intestine by pancreatic amylase. Disaccharides cannot be absorbed until they have been separated into glucose molecules by enzymes present in the brush border of cells lining the intestinal tract. Glucose and galactose are the actively absorbed sugars. Fructose is absorbed by diffusion.

METABOLISM: Although very complex at the molecular level, the metabolism of carbohydrates can be explained as follows. Carbohydrates are absorbed in the form of glucose, galactose, or fructose. These monosaccharides are available for direct utilization in energy production or they may be stored after conversion to glycogen. The glycogen is available for metabolism to glucose

Digestion of Carbohydrates

Enzyme	Found in	Carbohydrates	End product
Sucrase (invertase)	Intestine	Sucrose	Glucose and fructose
Maltases	Intestine and mucosal cells of intestine	Maltose	Two D-glucose
Lactase	Intestine	Lactose	D-Glucose and D-galactose
Salivary amylase	Saliva (mouth)	Cooked starch, glycogen, and dextrins	Maltose
Pancreatic amylase	Pancreas	Raw and cooked starch and glycogen	Maltose

Classification of Important Carbohydrates

Classification	Examples	Some Properties
Monosaccharides $(C_6H_{10}O_5)\cdot H_2O$ or $C_6H_{12}O_6$	Glucose Fructose	Crystalline, sweet, very soluble, readily absorbed
Disaccharides $(C_6H_{10}O_5)_2\cdot H_2O$ or $C_{12}H_{22}O_{11}$ hydrolyzed to simple sugars	Sucrose Lactose Maltose	} Crystalline, sweet, soluble, digestible Present in milk
Polysaccharides $(C_6H_{10}O_5)_n$ composed of many molecules of simple sugars (Since polysaccharides can be composed of various numbers of monosaccharides and disaccharides, n refers to an unknown number of these groups.)	Starch Dextrin Cellulose Glycogen	Amorphous, little or no flavor, less soluble. Vary in solubility and digestibility.

whenever there is need for reserve energy.

SOURCES: Carbohydrates are present in food in digestible and indigestible forms. Those that can be utilized are an important source of energy. Those that can't be utilized, usually some form of cellulose, are beneficial in adding bulk to the diet. Whole grains, vegetables, legumes (peas and beans), tubers (potatoes), fruits, honey, and refined sugar are all excellent sources of carbohydrate. Calories derived from sugar and candy have been termed empty calories because these foods lack essential amino acids, vitamins, and minerals.

NUTRITION: Carbohydrates contain 4.1 Cal./gm. and are esp. useful as a source of energy. As indicated, however, some forms are virtually devoid of dietary essentials other than calories.

carbohydrate loading. Dietary manipulation for the purpose of enhancing amount of glycogen stored in muscle tissue. Used by athletes prior to high-intensity endurance events such as competing in a marathon foot race. Phase I is begun seven days prior to competition. It depletes glycogen from specific muscles used in the event by exercising to exhaustion while participating in the sport for which one is preparing. The glycogen exhaustion is maintained by a high-fat, high-protein diet for three days. It is important that 100 grams of carbohydrate be included in this phase in order to prevent ketosis, q.v. Phase II consists of a high-carbohydrate diet of at least 1000 to 2000 kcal. for three days. This is called the supersaturation phase because the goal is to enhance glycogen storage. Synthesis of glycogen is facilitated by the extended period of depletion in Phase I. Carbohydrates used should be complex ones, e.g., those present in grain-derived food such as bread and pasta, rather than simple carbohydrate–containing items such as candy and soft drinks. Phase III is during the day of the event. Any type of food may be eaten up to 4 to 6 hours prior to competition. Food eaten from that time up to the time of competition is a matter of individual preference.

carbolic acid [L. *carbo,* carbon, + *oleum,* oil]. Obsolete name for phenol, q.v.

carbolism (kăr′bŏl-ĭzm). Poisoning by carbolic acid. SEE: *phenol.*

carbolize (kăr′bŏl-īz). To add or mix with carbolic acid.

carboluria (kăr″bō-lū′rē-ă) [′ + *oleum,* oil, + Gr. *ouron,* urine]. Phenol in the urine.

carbomycin (kăr-bō-mī′sĭn). An antibiotic obtained from Streptomyces halstedii. Effective against gram-positive bacteria and certain viruses.

carbon [L. *carbo,* coal]. SYMB: C. At. wt. 12.0111; at. no. 6. This nonmetallic element is the characteristic constituent of organic compounds.

Carbon occurs in two pure forms, diamond and graphite, and in impure form in charcoal, coke, and soot. Its compounds are constituents of all living tissue. Carbon combines with hydrogen, nitrogen, and oxygen to form the basis of all organic matter. Organic carbon compounds provide energy in foods.

carbon-14. ABBR: ^{14}C. Radioactive isotope of carbon with a half-life of 5600 yrs. It is used as a tracer in metabolic studies and in archeology to date materials containing carbon.

carbonate (kăr'bŏn-āt) [L. *carbo,* carbon]. Any salt of carbonic acid.

c. of soda. Sodium carbonate used commercially in crude form, as washing soda. The free alkali present is irritating and in strong concentrations has the effect of sodium hydroxide, q.v.

carbon dioxide. USP. CO_2. A colorless gas, heavier than air, generally produced in the combustion or decomposition of carbon or its compounds. It is the final metabolic product of carbon compounds present in food. The body eliminates CO_2 through the lungs, in urine, and in perspiration. It is also given off by decomposition of vegetable or animal matter or formed by alcoholic fermentation as in rising bread. It is necessary to all plant life and is absorbed directly from the air.

In small quantities (up to about 5%) in inspired air, it stimulates respiration; in greater quantities, it produces an uncomfortable degree of mental activity with confusion. Although not supposed to be poisonous, it will cause death by suffocation. Great amounts are added to the atmosphere daily but, because it is used by green plants, the air content is kept down to about 0.03%. Approx. one sq. meter of leaf surface can absorb the carbon dioxide from 2500 L. of air in one hour. It is estimated an acre of trees uses 4½ tons (4,082 kg.) of CO_2 a year. SEE: *carbon dioxide solid therapy.*

carbon dioxide combining power. This test, done on blood serum, is a determination of the amount of carbon dioxide that the blood serum can hold in chemical combination. It is a test of the buffer capacity of the blood.

The blood serum CO_2 determination is used to help measure the degree of acidosis or alkalosis. Carbon dioxide in solution forms a weak acid (H_2CO_3), and the amount of this acid that the blood serum can take up is a measure of its reserve power to prevent the occurrence of acidosis. The normal amount is 50–70 ml./dl. of blood (usually expressed as 50–70 volumes %). Values below 50 indicate acidosis, above 70 alkalosis.

carbon dioxide inhalation. CO_2 (5 to 7½%), mixed with oxygen for inhalation, stimulates breathing the same way as increased CO_2 production during exercise. Inhalation of oxygen and CO_2 is used as an accessory during artificial respiration and as a continuation of resuscitation after spontaneous breathing has returned. Also used to stimulate respiration in patients with pulmonary diseases.

carbon dioxide poisoning. CO_2 gas is most commonly used in carbonated drinks. Commercially it is used in its solidified form to make dry ice. Poisoning is rarely fatal unless the patient is in a closed space. It is a profound respiratory stimulant.

SYM: Extremely deep breathing; sensation of pressure in the head; ringing in ears; acid taste in mouth; slight burning in nose. Within a short time, respiration almost ceases and patient becomes unconscious.

TREATMENT: Remove to fresh air, administer artificial respiration, oxygen inhalation.

carbon dioxide solid therapy. Solid carbon dioxide (CO_2 snow) is used for therapeutic refrigeration. Solid CO_2 has a temperature of $-80°$ C. Application to skin 1–2 seconds causes superficial frostbite, 4–5 seconds a blister, 10–15 seconds superficial necrosis, 15–45 seconds ulceration. Used mostly for removal of certain nevi and warts, occasionally for telangiectasia.

carbon dioxide test. The alkaline reserve in the plasma is indicated by the volume percentage of CO_2 in the blood. Acidosis shows a concentration below 50 ml./dl. of blood, while in coma it is as low as 20.

carbonemia (kăr"bō-nē'mē-ă) [L. *carbo,* coal, + Gr. *haima,* blood]. Excess accumulation of carbonic acid in the blood.

carbonic. Pert. to carbon.

c. acid. H_2CO_3. Acid resulting from mixture of carbon dioxide and water.

c. anhydrase. An enzyme that catalyzes union of H_2O and CO_2 to form carbonic acid or reverse action. Present in red blood cells.

carbonize (kăr'bŏn-īz). To char or convert into charcoal.

carbon monoxide. CO. An insidious poisonous gas. It is a colorless, tasteless, odorless gas that gives no warning of its presence; it is widely distributed as the result of imperfect combustion and oxidation. It is found in the exhaust gas from all internal combustion engines used in most motor-powered vehicles. It is present in illuminating gas and results from the inefficient and incomplete combustion of coal. It is found in sewers,

Toxic Symptoms of Carbon Monoxide*

Carbon Monoxide Concentration		
Percent CO in Air	Parts Per Million	Response
0.005	50	No apparent toxic symptoms
0.01	100	Can be tolerated for several hrs. without symptoms
0.02	200	Possible mild frontal headache in 2–3 hrs.
0.08	800	Headache, dizziness, and nausea in 45 min.; collapse and possible unconsciousness in 2 hrs.
0.16	1600	Headache, dizziness, and nausea in 20 min.; collapse and possible death in 2 hrs.
0.32	3200	Headache and dizziness in 5–10 min.; unconsciousness and possible death in 10–15 mins.
0.64	6400	Headache and dizziness in 1–2 min.; possible death in 10–15 min.
1.28	12,800	Immediate unconsciousness; possible death in 1–3 min.

*Adapted from Hamilton, A. and Hardy, H.: *Industrial Toxicology,* edition 3, Publishing Sciences Group, Littleton, Mass., 1974.

cellars, and mines.

Smoking tobacco increases the CO content of the blood and thus interferes with the transport of oxygen in the blood. This in turn also decreases the individual's ability to see at night.

carbon monoxide poisoning. Poisoning can occur from small amounts of CO inhaled over a long period of time or from large amounts inhaled in a short time. For example, riding in a closed automobile or parking in an automobile with motor running may cause death from the inhalation of these noxious fumes from leaking exhausts and exhaust heaters. Another cause of death is the operation of a gasoline motor in an enclosed area such as a closed garage or basement. Poisoning from CO is produced as a result of a chemical combination of this gas with the hemoglobin of the blood, thus preventing the blood from carrying oxygen to the tissues. Since this combination is relatively stable, patients may need prolonged periods of oxygen administration in addition to artificial respiration.

The affinity of CO for hemoglobin is more than 200 times as great as that of oxygen. Therefore exposure to CO causes a marked reduction in the ability of the blood to transport oxygen. SEE: *Poisons and Poisoning* in *Appendix.*

SYM: The symptoms of CO poisoning are somewhat variable. Respiration is deep and difficult. Carboxyhemoglobin, which is the substance formed when carbon monoxide combines with hemoglobin, is cherry red in color. Thus the tissues and skin of individuals with CO poisoning and a carboxyhemoglobin level of 30 percent or greater are much pinker than normal. Their appearance has been described as "cherry red." The pulse may be slowed initially but it soon becomes increased. There may be pounding of the heart; dizziness is frequent; muscular function may be so weakened as to cause inability to stand. There may be ringing in the ears, throbbing in the temples, headache, faintness and nausea, and dilated pupils. A patient who is breathing when found usually recovers when brought into the fresh air and given stimulants. SEE: table.

TREATMENT: Immediately remove the person from exposure to CO. Administer 100% oxygen, under pressure (hyperbaric) if possible. Use artificial respiration if indicated. Keep the patient absolutely quiet and immobile in order to reduce the body's oxygen requirements. If cerebral edema develops, give 50 ml. of 50% glucose I.V.; and prednisone 1 mg./kg. I.V. every 4 hours as needed. A sedative such as diazepam may be needed if patient becomes excited during recovery.

COMPLICATIONS: When such patients recover they often have some nervous system involvement including various types of paralysis, blindness, interference with sensation, muscular spasms, or twitchings for an indefinite period of time. Most of these complications disappear in time, but occasionally they remain permanently.

carbon tetrachloride (tĕt″ră-klō′rīd). CCl_4. A clear, colorless liquid with ethereal odor resembling chloroform; not flammable. Although having narcotic and anesthetic properties resembling chloroform, it is too toxic to be suitable as an anesthetic. In general, this substance is too toxic for any medical use. Inhalation of a small quantity has been known to produce death. The mechanism of injury is acute atrophy of the liver and kidney.

carbon tetrachloride poisoning. Toxic effects due to prolonged inhalation.

SYM: Irritation of eyes, nose, and throat; headache; nausea; anorexia; weakness; abdominal pain.

F.A.: Remove clothes contaminated with carbon tetrachloride. Oxygen inhalation and artificial respiration. Lavage with saline solution. Leave saline cathartic in stomach.

SEE: *Poisons and Poisoning* in *Appendix*.

carbonuria (kăr″bō-nū′rē-ă) [L. *carbo,* carbon, + Gr. *ouron,* urine]. The presence or excretion of carbon compounds in the urine.

carbonyl (kăr′bŏn-ĭl) [″ + Gr. *hyle,* matter]. The divalent radical CO, characteristic of aldehydes and ketones.

carboxyhemoglobin (kăr-bŏk″sē-hē″mō-glō′bĭn) [″ + Gr. *oxys,* acid, + *haima,* blood, + L. *globus,* sphere]. Compound formed by carbon monoxide and hemoglobin in poisoning by carbon monoxide.

carboxyl (kăr-bŏk′sĭl). The characteristic group (COOH) of organic carboxylic acids, e.g., formic acid (HCOOH), acetic acid (CH_2COOH).

carboxylase (kăr-bŏk′sĭ-lās). An enzyme that catalyzes the removal of the carboxyl group (COOH) from amino acids; an enzyme found in brewer's yeast that catalyzes the decarboxylation of pyruvic acid with the production of acetaldehyde and carbon dioxide. In the body, this requires the presence of vitamin B_1 (thiamine), which acts as a coenzyme.

carboxylic acids. A group of organic acids that contain the carboxylic acid, –COOH group.

carboxylmethylcellulose sodium. USP. Chemical used as a pharmaceutic aid and as a food additive.

carbuncle, carbunculus (kăr′bŭng″k'l, kăr-bŭng′kū-lŭs) [L. *carbunculus,* small glowing ember]. A circumscribed inflammation of the skin and deeper tissues that terminates in a slough and suppuration and is accompanied by marked constitutional symptoms.

ETIOL: Staphylococci. Predisposing factors the same as in furuncle, q.v. Diabetics are particularly susceptible.

SYM: It is characterized by a painful node, at first covered by tight reddened skin that later becomes thin and perforates, discharging pus through several openings. Also fever, leukocytosis, and sometimes prostration. Most commonly found on nape of neck, on upper back or on buttocks.

TREATMENT: Antibiotics given systemically are usually effective. Incision and drainage when lesion is about to point or come to a head. Keep covered with warm compresses to promote blood supply to the area.

NURSING IMPLICATIONS: Use sterile technique when changing dressings. The dressings should be changed frequently to facilitate drainage and promote healing. All contaminated equipment should be disinfected, and all soiled dressings disposed of properly.

carbuncular. Pert. to a carbuncle.

carbunculosis (kăr-bŭng″kū-lō′sĭs) [″ + Gr. *osis,* condition]. Appearance of several carbuncles in succession.

carbutamide (kăr-bū′tă-mīd). An oral hypoglycemic agent.

carcass (kăr′kăs). A dead body. Usually applied to nonhuman bodies.

carcinelcosis (kăr″sĭ-nĕl-kō′sĭs) [Gr. *karkinos,* crab, + *helkosis,* ulceration]. An ulcer of a cancerous nature.

carcinoembryonic antigens (kăr″sĭn-ō-ĕm″brē-ŏn′ĭk). ABBR: CEA. Antigens originally isolated from colon tumors; they were thought erroneously to be specific for those tumors. Now used to monitor the course of cancer therapy. If the previously elevated CEA level returns to normal after surgery, removal of the colonic tumor is thought to be complete.

carcinogen (kăr′sĭn-, kăr-sĭn′ō-jĕn). Any substance or agent that produces or incites cancer.

carcinogenesis (kăr″sĭ-nō-jĕn′ĕ-sĭs) [″ + *genesis,* production]. The production or origin of cancer.

carcinogenic (kăr″sĭ-nō-jĕn′ĭk). Producing cancer.

carcinoid (kăr′sĭ-noyd) [″ + *eidos,* resemblance]. A tumor derived from the argentaffin cells in the intestinal tract, bile ducts, pancreas, bronchus, or ovary. These tumors secrete serotonin (5-hydroxy-tryptamine) and other vasoactive substances.

carcinoid syndrome. A syndrome produced by metastatic carcinoid tumors that secrete excessive amounts of vasoactive substances such as serotonin, bradykinin, histamine, and prostaglandins.

SYM: Include one or more of the following: brief episodes of flushing, esp. of the face and neck; tachycardia; facial and periorbital edema; hypotension; intermittent abdominal pain with diarrhea; valvular lesions of the heart; loss of weight; hypoproteinemia; signs of pellagra. The latter symptom is due to the body's available tryptophan, which is the precursor of serotonin, being used for serotonin production instead of for manufacture of niacin and protein.

TREATMENT: Symptoms usually develop only after the tumor has metastasized; nevertheless, surgical removal of accessible tumors is indicated. High-protein diet with niacin supplement. Serotonin antagonist for control of diarrhea and malabsorption. Cortisone may be helpful in controlling inanition.

carcinolysis (kăr″sĭ-nŏl′ĭ-sĭs) [Gr. *karkinos,* crab, + *lysis,* destruction]. Destruction of carcinoma cells.

carcinolytic (kăr″sĭ-nō-lĭt′ĭk). Destructive to cancer cells.

carcinoma (kăr″sĭ-nō′mă) [″ + *oma,* tumor]. A new growth or malignant tumor that occurs in epithelial tissue. These neoplasms tend to infiltrate and give rise to metastases. It may affect almost any organ or part of the body and spread by direct extension or through lymphatics or the bloodstream. Etiology is unknown. SYN: *cancer.*

c., alveolar cell. A type of carcinoma of the lung.

c., basal cell. An epidermoid carcinoma common on face of elderly. It has a low degree of malignancy. It gives rise to the typical rodent ulcer.

c., bronchogenic. Carcinoma of the lung that arises from the epithelial lining of the bronchi.

c., chorionic. A tumor containing cells characteristic of the chorion of the embryo. Occurs in the testis, ovary, and other parts of the body. SYN: *choriocarcinoma.*

c., cylindrical. A carcinoma of glands usually of entodermal origin including adenocarcinoma and carcinoma simplex. Cells are nearly cylindrical in shape.

c., embryonal. Malignant teratoma.

c., epidermoid. A tumor on a surface such as the skin. Usually of two types: one a wartlike growth, slow-growing, mildly malignant; the other a flat and rapidly infiltrating neoplasm.

c., giant cell. Carcinoma characterized by presence of giant cells.

c., glandular. Carcinoma of cells of the secreting variety. SEE: *adenocarcinoma.*

c. in situ. ABBR: CIS. Malignant cell changes in the epithelial tissue that do not extend beyond the basement membrane.

c., lipomatous. Carcinoma of fatty tissue.

c., medullary. Carcinoma that is soft because of the predominance of cells and in which there is little fibrous tissue.

c., melanotic. Carcinoma containing melanin.

c., mucinous. Carcinoma in which the glandular tissue secretes mucin.

c., oat cell. A poorly differentiated tumor of the bronchus that contains small oat-shaped cells.

c., scirrhous. A form of cylindrical carcinoma with a firm, hard structure.

c., squamous-cell. A form of epidermoid carcinoma principally of squamous cells.

carcinomatophobia (kăr″sĭ-nō″mă-tō-fō′bē-ă) [Gr. *karkinos,* crab, + *oma,* tumor, + *phobos,* fear]. Morbid fear of carcinoma.

carcinomatosis (kăr″sĭ-nō″mă-tō′sĭs) [″ + ″ + *osis,* condition]. The condition of having widespread dissemination of carcinoma in the body.

carcinophilia (kăr″sĭ-nō-fĭl′ē-ă) [″ + *philos,* love]. Having affinity for cancer cells.

carcinosarcoma (kăr″sĭ-nō-săr-kō′mă) [″ + *sarx,* flesh, + *oma,* tumor]. A malignant tumor containing the elements of both carcinoma and sarcoma.

c., embryonal. Wilms tumor, q.v.

carcinosis (kăr″sĭ-nō′sĭs) [″ + *osis,* condition]. Carcinomatosis, q.v.

cardamom, cardamon [Gr. *kardamomon*]. Dried ripe fruit of an herb, Elettaria repens or E. cardomomum, used as an aromatic and carminative.

Cardarelli's sign (kăr″dă-rĕl′lēz). [Antonio Cardarelli, It. physician, 1831–1926] Tugging of the trachea to one side; may be present with aneurysm of the aorta.

cardia (kăr′dē-ă) [Gr. *kardia,* heart]. Upper orifice of stomach connecting with the esophagus.

cardiac (kăr′dē-ăk) [L. *cardiacus*]. 1. Pert. to the heart. 2. Pert. to the cardia.

cardiac arrest. Sudden cessation of functional circulation. SEE: *cardiopulmonary resuscitation.*

cardiac arrhythmia. SEE: *arrhythmia.*

cardiac atrophy. Fatty degeneration of the heart.

cardiac catheterization. Passage of a tiny plastic tube into the heart through a blood vessel. Samples of blood are withdrawn for testing; blood pressure and cardiac output are measured. Used in diagnosis of heart disorders and anomalies.

NURSING IMPLICATIONS: Prepare the patient physicially and emotionally for the procedure.

Post-catheterization: Take vital signs (including apical pulse taken for one full minute) every 15 minutes for the first hour or two after the procedure. Also maintain the pressure dressing and keep the extremity that was cannulated in an extended position. The patient continues bedrest as ordered (usually for 12–24 hours post-catheterization). Check the dressing for bleeding, and be alert for the patient complaining that the dressing is getting increasingly tight, because this may indicate hematoma formation. Also assess the neurovascular status of the extremity, particularly distal to the site where the extremity was cannulated.

cardiac compensation. The ability of the heart through its reserve power to compensate for impaired functioning of its valves.

cardiac cycle. The period from the beginning of one beat of the heart to the beginning of the succeeding beat, including the *systole*, contraction of the atria and ventricles propelling the blood onward, and the *diastole*, the period during which the cavities are being refilled with blood. The atria contract immediately before the ventricles. The ordinary cycle lasts 0.8 second with the heart beating approx. 60 to 85 times a minute in the adult at rest. The atrial systole lasts 0.1 second; the ventricular systole 0.3 second, and the diastole 0.4 second; thus even though the heart seems to be working continuously, it actually rests for a good portion of each cardiac cycle.

RS: circulation; diastole; heart; systole.

cardiac failure. Condition resulting from inability of the heart to pump sufficient blood to meet the needs of the body. SEE: *heart failure.*

cardiac hypertrophy. Enlargement of the heart. SEE: *heart, hypertrophy of.*

cardiac insufficiency. Inadequate cardiac output due to failure of the heart to function properly, as in valvular deficiency.

cardiac massage. SEE: *cardiopulmonary resuscitation.*

cardiac output. The amount of blood discharged from the left or right ventricle per minute. For an average adult at rest, cardiac output is approx. 3.0 L. per square meter of body surface area each minute. SYN: *volume, minute.*

cardiac plexus. Plexus cardiacus [NA]. The nerve plexus at the base of the heart made up of branches of the vagus nerves and sympathetic trunks. Afferent nerves from this plexus provide the nerve supply to the heart.

cardiac reflex. A reflex in which the response is a change in cardiac rate. Stimulation of sensory nerve endings in the wall of the carotid sinus by increased arterial blood pressure reflexly slows the heart (Marey's law); stimulation of vagus fibers in the right side of the heart by increased venous return reflexly increases heart rate (Bainbridge's reflex).

cardiac reserve. The capacity of the heart to increase cardiac output and raise blood pressure above basal pressure to meet body requirements.

cardialgia (kăr″dē-ăl′jē-ă) [Gr. *kardia*, heart, + *algos*, pain]. Pain at the pit of the stomach or region of the heart, usually occurring in paroxysms.

cardiaortic (kăr″dē-ā-or′tĭk) [″ + *aorte*, aorta]. Pert. to the heart and the aorta.

cardiasthenia (kăr″dē-ăs-thē′nē-ă) [″ + *astheneia*, weakness]. Type of neurasthenia with predominance of cardiac symptoms.

cardiasthma (kăr″dē-ăz′mă) [″ + *asthma*, panting]. Dyspnea due to heart disease.

cardiectasia, cardiectasis (kăr″dē-ĕk-tā′sē-ă, -ĕk′tă-sĭs) [″ + *ektasis*, dilatation]. Dilatation of the heart.

cardiectomy (kăr″dē-ĕk′tō-mē) [″ + *ektome*, excision]. Excision of the cardiac end of the stomach.

Cardilate. Trade name for erythrityl tetranitrate.

cardinal [LL. *cardinalis*, important]. Of primary importance, as in cardinal symptoms: temperature, pulse, respiration.

cardio- [Gr. *kardia*, heart]. Prefix pert. to the heart.

cardioaccelerator (kăr″dē-ō-ăk-sĕl′ĕr-ā-tor) [″ + L. *accelerare*, to hasten]. That which increases the rate of the heart beat.

cardioactive (kăr″dē-ō-ăk′tĭv) [″ + L. *activus*, acting]. Acting upon the heart.

cardioangiography (kăr″dē-ō-ăn″jē-ŏg′ră-fē) [″ + *angeion*, vessel, + *graphein*, to write]. Angiocardiography, q.v.

cardioangiology (kăr″dē-ō-ăn″jē-ŏl′ō-jē) [″ + ″ + *logos*, study]. The science of the heart and blood vessels.

cardioaortic (kăr″dē-ō-ā-or′tĭk) [″ + *aorte*, aorta]. Pert. to the heart and the aortic artery.

cardiocatheterization (kăr″dē-ō-kăth″ĕ-tĕr-ĭ-zā′shŭn). Cardiac catheterization, q.v.

cardiocele (kăr′dē-ō-sēl) [″ + *kele*, tumor]. A herniation or protrusion of the heart through an opening in the diaphragm, or through a wound.

cardiocentesis (kăr″dē-ō-sĕn-tē′sĭs) [″ + *kentesis*, puncture]. Surgical incision or puncture of the heart.

cardiochalasia (kăr″dē-ō-kă-lā′zē-ă) [″ + *chalasis*, relaxation]. Relaxation of the muscles of the cardiac sphincter of the stomach.

cardiocirrhosis (kăr″dē-ō-sĭr-rō′sĭs) [″ + *kirrhos*, orange-yellow, + *osis*, condition]. Cirrhosis of the liver, and heart disease.

cardiodiaphragmatic (kăr″dē-ō-dī″ă-frăg-măt′

ĭk). Concerning the heart and the diaphragm.

cardiodilator (kăr″dē-ō-dī′lā-tor) [″ + L. *dilatare,* to enlarge]. Device for dilating the cardia of the gastroesophageal junction.

cardiodynamics (kăr″dē-ō-dī-năm′ĭks). Science of forces involved in propulsion of blood from heart to tissues and back to heart.

cardiodynia (kăr″dē-ō-dĭn′ē-ă) [Gr. *kardia,* heart, + *odyne,* pain]. Pain in the region of the heart.

cardiogenesis (kăr″dē-ō-jĕn′ĕ-sĭs) [″ + *genesis,* origin]. Formation and growth of the embryonic heart.

cardiogenic (kăr″dē-ō-jĕn′ĭk) [″ + *gennan,* to produce]. Having origin in the heart itself.

cardiogenic shock. Failure to maintain blood supply to the circulatory system and tissues because of inadequate cardiac output. SEE: *shock.*

cardiogram (kăr′dē-ō-grăm″) [″ + *gramma,* mark]. A graph, on special paper, of the electrical activity of the heart muscle. Made with an electrocardiograph machine. SYN: *electrocardiogram.*

cardiograph (kăr′dē-ō-grăf″) [″ + *graphein,* to write]. A device for registering the electrical activity of the heart muscle.

cardiographic (kăr″dē-ō-grăf′ĭk). Pert. to cardiography.

cardiography (kăr″dē-ŏg′ră-fē). The recording and study of the electrical activity of the heart.

cardiohepatic (kăr″dē-ō-hĕ-păt′ĭk) [″ + *hepatos,* liver]. Pert. to heart and liver.

cardiohepatomegaly (kăr″dē-ō-hĕp″ă-tō-mĕg′ă-lē) [″ + ″ + *megas,* large]. Enlargement of the heart and liver.

cardioinhibitory (kăr″dē-ō-ĭn-hĭb′ĭ-tō-rē) [″ + L. *inhibere,* to check]. Inhibiting action of the heart.

cardiokinetic (kăr″dē-ō-kĭ-nĕt′ĭk) [″ + *kinesis,* motion]. Pert. to that which excites heart action.

cardiolipin (kăr″dē-ō-lĭp′ĭn) [″ + *lipos,* fat]. An extract of beef hearts that contains phosphorylated polysaccharide esters of fatty acids. It is used in certain tests for syphilis.

cardiolith (kăr′dē-ō-lĭth″) [″ + *lithos,* stone]. A concretion or calculus in the heart.

cardiologist (kăr-dē-ŏl′ō-jĭst) [″ + *logos,* study]. A physician specializing in treatment of heart disease.

cardiology (kăr-dē-ŏl′ō-jē). The study of the heart.

cardiolysin (kăr″dē-ŏl′ĭ-sĭn) [″ + *lysis,* loosening]. A lysin acting on heart muscle.

cardiolysis (kăr-dē-ŏl′ĭ-sĭs). Operation for separation of adhesions constricting the heart in adhesive mediastinopericarditis. Involves resection of the ribs and sternum over the pericardium.

cardiomalacia (kăr″dē-ō-mă-lā′shē-ă) [Gr. *kardia,* heart, + *malakia,* softening]. Softening of the heart muscle.

cardiomegaly (kăr″dē-ō-mĕg′ă-lē) [″ + *megas,* large]. Hypertrophy of the heart. SYN: *megacardia.*

cardiomotility (kăr″dē-ō-mō-tĭl′ĭ-tē) [″ + L. *motilis,* moving]. The ability of the heart to move.

cardiomyoliposis (kăr″dē-ō-mī″ō-lĭp-ō′sĭs) [″ + *mys,* muscle, + *lipos,* fat, + *osis,* condition]. Fatty degeneration of the heart.

cardiomyopathy (kăr″dē-ō-mī-ŏp′ă-thē) [″ + ″ + *pathos,* disease]. Disease of the heart muscles. Usually refers to disease of obscure etiology.

c., alcoholic. Disease of the heart muscle due to alcohol consumption.

cardiomyopexy (kăr″dē-ō-mī′ō-pĕk″sē) [″ + ″ + *pexis,* fixation]. Surgical fixation of a vascular tissue such as pectoral muscle to the cardiac muscle and pericardium in order to improve blood supply to the myocardium.

cardionecrosis (kăr″dē-ō-nē-krō′sĭs) [″ + *nekros,* dead, + *osis,* condition]. Necrosis of the heart tissue.

cardionecteur, cardionector (kăr″dē-ō-nĕk′tĕr) [″ + L. *nector,* joiner]. The system that regulates heart beat: the sinoatrial node in which the stimulus for atrial contraction arises; the bundle of His, which transmits the impulse from the atrium to the atrioventricular node, which governs ventricular contraction.

cardionephric (kăr″dē-ō-nĕf′rĭk) [″ + *nephros,* kidney]. Pert. to heart and kidney.

cardioneural (kăr″dē-ō-nū′răl) [″ + *neuron,* nerve]. Pert. to nervous control of the heart.

cardioneurosis (kăr″dē-ō-nū-rō′sĭs) [″ + ″ + *osis,* condition]. Functional neurosis with cardiac symptoms.

cardiopathy (kăr″dē-ŏp′ă-thē) [″ + *pathos,* disease]. Any disease of the heart.

cardiopericarditis (kăr″dē-ō-pĕr″ĭ-kăr-dī′tĭs) [″ + *peri,* around, + *kardia,* heart, + *itis,* inflammation]. Inflamed myocardium and pericardium.

cardiophobia (kăr″dē-ō-fō′bē-ă) [″ + *phobos,* fear]. Morbid fear of heart disease.

cardiophone (kăr′dē-ō-fōn) [″ + *phone,* voice]. Device, esp. a stethoscope, for listening to sound of the heart.

cardioplasty (kăr″dē-ō-plăs′tē) [″ + *plassein,* to form]. Operation on the cardiac sphincter of the stomach to relieve cardiospasm.

cardioplegia (kăr″dē-ō-plē′jē-ă) [″ + *plege,* stroke]. Paralysis of the heart.

cardiopneumatic (kăr″dē-ō-nū-măt′ĭk) [″ + *pneuma,* breath]. Pert. to the heart and the lungs.

cardiopneumograph (kăr′dē-ō-nū′mō-grăf) [″ + ″ + *graphein,* to write]. Device for recording motion of heart and lungs.

cardioptosis (kăr″dē-ŏp-tō′sĭs) [″ + *ptosis,* falling]. Prolapse of the heart.

cardiopulmonary (kăr″dē-ō-pŭl′mō-nĕr-ē) [″ + L. *pulmo,* lung]. Pert. to both heart and lungs.

cardiopulmonary arrest. Sudden cessation of functional ventilation and circulation. SEE: *cardiopulmonary resuscitation.*

cardiopulmonary resuscitation. The American Heart Association recommends the following:

IF UNCONSCIOUS: Be certain there is an adequate airway. Elevate head and push jaw up. Then clear vomitus, false teeth, or other matter from mouth and pharynx.

IF NOT BREATHING SEE: *resuscitation, oral.*

IF PULSE IS ABSENT: If the pupils are dilated and there is a deathlike appearance, massage the heart by using the following *closed chest* (i.e., not surgical) *compression method:* Press on the sternum with sufficient force to depress it 1½ to 2 in. (3.8 to 5.1 cm.). Do this once per second. At the same time continue mouth-to-mouth resuscitation. Continue both mouth-to-mouth resuscitation and intermittent chest compression until spontaneous pulse and respiration return. If one person is doing the resuscitation, alternate two quick inflations with 15 chest compressions. If there are two operators, do these maneuvers at the rate of one inflation for every fifth chest compression.

cardiopuncture [″ + L. *punctura,* piercing]. Surgical puncture of the heart. SYN: *cardiocentesis.*

cardiopyloric (kăr″dē-ō-pī-lor′ĭk) [″ + *pyloros,* gatekeeper]. Pert. to the cardiac and pyloric ends of the stomach.

cardiorenal (kăr″dē-ō-rē′năl) [Gr. *kardia,* heart, + L. *renalis,* pert. to kidney]. Pert. to both heart and kidneys.

cardiorrhaphy (kăr″dē-or′ă-fē) [″ + *rhaphe,* a suture]. Suturing of the heart muscle.

cardiorrhexis (kăr″dē-ō-rĕk′sĭs) [″ + *rhexis,* rupture]. Rupture of the heart.

cardiosclerosis (kăr″dē-ō-sklĕ-rō′sĭs) [″ + *sklerosis,* hardening]. Hardening of the cardiac tissues and arteries.

cardioscope (kăr′dē-ō-skōp) [″ + *skopein,* to examine]. Instrument for examining the interior of the heart.

cardioscopy (kăr″dē-ŏs′kō-pē). Examination of the interior of the heart through the use of a cardioscope.

cardiospasm (kăr′dē-ō-spăzm) [″ + *spasmos,* spasm]. Disordered motor function of the distal end of the esophagus and failure of the esophageal orifice (cardia) of the stomach to relax. Thus, the word is a misnomer in that failure of relaxation (achalasia) and absence of esophageal motility (aperistalsis) are the pathological processes involved.

ETIOL: Due to absence or injury of ganglion cells in Auerbach's plexus.

SYM: Substernal fullness, dysphagia, regurgitation, esp. at night.

TREATMENT: Bland semisolid foods warmed to body temperature are of some help, but dilatation of the esophageal sphincter will allow the esophagus to drain by force of gravity. It may be possible to do this mechanically; if not, surgical myotomy may be required.

cardiosphygmograph (kăr″dē-ō-sfĭg′mō-grăf) [″ + *sphygmos,* throb, + *graphein,* to write]. Instrument for graphically recording movements of the heart and pulse.

cardiostenosis (kăr″dē-ō-stĕn-ō′sĭs) [″ + *stenosis,* narrowing]. Heart constriction and its development.

cardiosymphysis (kăr″dē-ō-sĭm′fĭ-sĭs) [″ + *symphysis,* growing together]. Mediastinopericarditis.

cardiotachometer (kăr″dē-ō-tăk-ŏm′ĕ-tĕr) [Gr. *kardia,* heart, + *tachos,* speed, + *metron,* measure]. An instrument for measuring the total number of heart beats over a long period of time.

cardiotherapy (kăr″dē-ō-thĕr′ă-pē) [″ + *therapeia,* treatment]. The treatment of cardiac diseases.

cardiothyrotoxicosis (kăr″dē-ō-thī″rō-tŏk″sĭ-kō′sĭs) [″ + *thyreos,* shield, + *toxikon,* poison, + *osis,* condition]. Heart disease due to disease of the thyroid gland, usually hyperthyroidism.

cardiotomy (kăr″dē-ŏt′ō-mē) [″ + *tome,* incision]. Incision of the heart.

cardiotonic (kăr″dē-ō-tŏn′ĭk) [″ + *tonos,* tone]. Increasing tonicity of the heart. Various drugs, including digitalis, are cardiotonic. SEE: *inotropic.*

cardiotoxic (kăr″dē-ō-tŏk′sĭk) [″ + *toxikon,* poisoning]. Exercising a poisonous effect upon the heart.

cardiovalvulitis (kăr″dē-ō-văl″vū-lī′tĭs) [″ + L. *valvula,* valve, + Gr. *itis,* inflammation]. Inflammation of valves of the heart.

cardiovalvulotome (kăr″dē-ō-văl′vū-lō-tōm″) [″ + ″ + Gr. *tome,* incision]. An instrument for excising part of a valve, esp. the mitral valve.

cardiovascular (kăr″dē-ō-văs′kū-lăr) [″ + L. *vasculum,* small vessel]. Pert. to the heart and blood vessels.

cardiovascular reflex. 1. Sympathetic increase in heart rate when increased pressure in, or distention of, great veins occurs. 2. Reflex vasoconstriction resulting from reduced venous pressure.

cardiovasology (kăr″dē-ō-văs-ŏl′ō-jē) [″ + L. *vas,* vessel, + Gr. *logos,* study]. Science of the heart and blood vessels. SYN: *cardio-angiology.*

cardioversion (kăr′dē-ō-vĕr″zhŭn) [″ + L. *versio,* a turning]. Conversion of a pathological cardiac rhythm (arrhythmia), such as ventricular fibrillation, to normal sinus rhythm. Usually accomplished by use of a device called a cardioverter, which administers countershocks to the heart through electrodes placed on the chest wall.

CAUTION: Cardioversion should not be used in sinus tachycardia or arrhythmias (other than ventricular fibrillation) caused by digitalis toxicity. It should be used only in emergency situations when potassium administration and other measures have failed. The cardioverter may induce lethal ventricular fibrillation unresponsive to further electrical shocks.

cardioverter (kăr′dē-ō-vĕr″tĕr) Electrical device used to administer electrical shocks to the heart when electrodes are placed on the chest wall. Useful in emergency treatment of cardiac arrhythmias such as ventricular tachycardia. Changing the arrhythmia to normal sinus rhythm is called cardioversion, q.v.

carditis (kăr-dī′tĭs) [″ + *itis,* inflammation]. Inflammation of the heart muscles. Usually involves two of the following: pericardium, myocardium, or endocardium.

c., Coxsackie. Carditis or pericarditis that may occur in infections with enteroviruses of the Coxsackie groups, and also echovirus groups.

Cardrase. Trade name for ethoxzolamide.

caries (kār′ēz, kār′ĭ-ēz) [L., rottenness]. Gradual decay and disintegration of soft, or bony tissue, or a tooth. If the decay is allowed to progress, the surrounding tissue will become inflamed and an abscess will form.

Ex.: chronic abscess; tuberculosis; and bacterial invasion of teeth. In caries, the bone disintegrates by pieces, while in necrosis large masses of bone are discharged. Deficiency of vitamins C and D has a direct influence upon caries of the teeth.

c., arrested. The state in which a carious lesion appears not to progress between dental examinations.

c., bottle mouth. Extensive caries and discoloration of the teeth that can be observed in young children from 19 months to 4 years old who have had prolonged bottle feedings.

c., dental. Decay of the teeth. A progressive decalcification of the enamel and dentin of a tooth. The etiological factors are not fully known but attention to diet by minimizing intake of refined carbohydrates and good dental hygiene prevent growth of bacteria that play a role in promoting the develop-

DENTAL CARIES

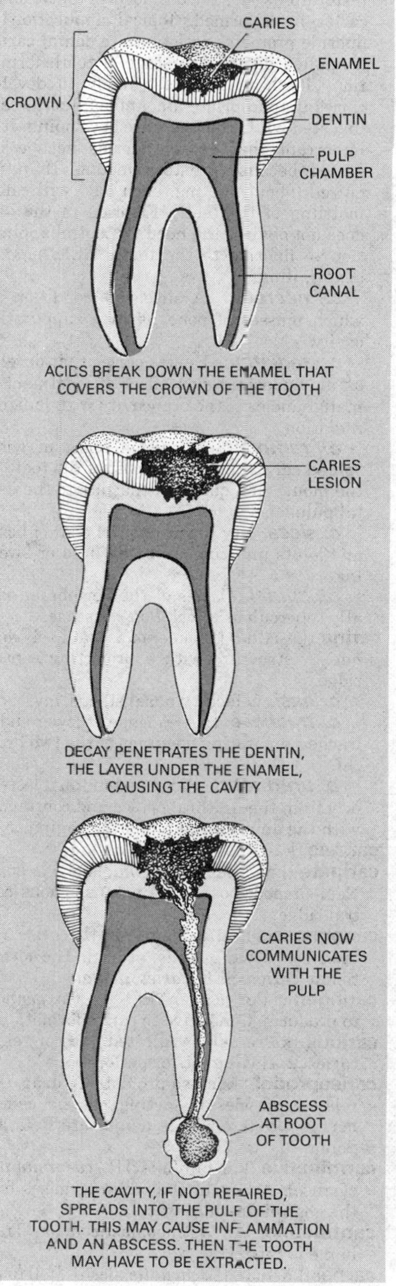

ACIDS BREAK DOWN THE ENAMEL THAT COVERS THE CROWN OF THE TOOTH

DECAY PENETRATES THE DENTIN, THE LAYER UNDER THE ENAMEL, CAUSING THE CAVITY

THE CAVITY, IF NOT REPAIRED, SPREADS INTO THE PULP OF THE TOOTH. THIS MAY CAUSE INFLAMMATION AND AN ABSCESS. THEN THE TOOTH MAY HAVE TO BE EXTRACTED.

ment of caries. Early detection and dental restorations offer the best form of control once caries have formed. Topical application of fluoride promotes resistance to dental caries if applied during the stage of tooth formation. Teeth will be less likely to develop caries if appropriate amounts of fluoride are ingested while the teeth are developing. It is important that excess fluoride not be ingested because greater amounts than required (about one mg. each day) will cause mottling of the teeth. Fluoride in the diet does not obviate the need for topical application of fluoride to the teeth. SEE: *plaque, dental;* illus.

c., necrotic. A diseased condition in which masses of bone lie in a suppurative cavity.

c., radiation. Dental caries that develop as an undesired side effect of treatment of malignancies of the oral cavity with ionizing radiation.

c., rampant. A sudden onset of widespread caries that affect most of the teeth in the mouth and quickly penetrate to the dental pulp.

c. sicca. Dry tuberculosis of ends of bones and joints unaccompanied by fluid or swelling.

c., spinal. Caries of the vertebrae, usually tuberculous. SYN: *Pott's disease.*

carina (kă-rī′nă) [L., keel of a boat]. (pl. *carinae*) A structure with a projecting central ridge.

c. nasi. Olfactory nasal sulcus, q.v.

c. tracheae. [NA] A ridge at lower end of trachea separating openings of the two bronchi.

c. urethralis. Ridge extending posteriorly from the urethral orifice and continuous with the anterior column of the vagina.

carinae (kă-rī′nē) [L.]. Pl. of carina.

carinate (kăr′ĭ-nāt) [L. *carina,* keel of a boat]. Keel-shaped; possessing a conspicuous central ridge.

cariogenesis (kār″ē-ō-jĕn′ĕ-sĭs) [L. *caries,* rottenness, + Gr. *genesis,* origin]. The formation of caries. SEE: *caries, dental.*

cariogenic (kā″rē-ō-jĕn′ĭk) [″ + Gr. *gennan,* to produce]. Conducive to caries formation.

carious (kā′rē-ŭs). 1. Affected with or rel. to caries. 2. Having pits or perforations.

carisoprodol (kăr″ī-sō-prō′dŏl). A drug that relaxes muscles by acting on the central nervous system. Trade names are Rela and Soma.

carminative (kăr-mĭn′ă-tĭv) [L. *carminativus,* cleanse]. An agent that relieves gases from the gastrointestinal tract.

carmustine. An antineoplastic drug. Trade name is BiCNU.

carnal (kăr′năl) [L. *carnalis,* flesh]. Rel. to the desires and appetites of the flesh; sensual.

carnal knowledge. A phrase used in medicolegal cases to denote sexual intercourse; usually between an adult and a child.

carneous (kăr′nē-ŭs) [L. *carneus,* fleshy]. Fleshy.

carnification (kăr″nĭ-fĭ-kā′shŭn) [″ + *facere,* to make]. Alteration of tissues, esp. the change of pulmonary tissue to a form resembling skeletal muscle.

carnitine (kăr′nĭ-tĭn). A chemical, γ-trimethylamine-β-hydroxybutyrate, that is important in metabolizing palmitic and stearic acids. It has been used therapeutically in treating myopathy due to carnitine deficiency.

carnivore (kăr′nĭ-vor). An animal that primarily eats meat, particularly an animal of the order Carnivora, which includes cats, dogs, and bears.

carnivorous (kăr-nĭv′ō-rŭs) [L. *carnivorus*]. Flesh eating.

carnophobia (kăr″nō-fō′bē-ă) [″ + Gr. *phobos,* fear]. Abnormal aversion to meat.

carnose (kăr′nōs). Having the consistency of or resembling flesh.

carnosine (kăr′nō-sĭn). A chemical substance, β-alanylhistidine, present in muscle. Its function is unknown.

carnosity (kăr-nŏs′ĭ-tē) [L. *carnositas,* fleshiness]. An excrescence resembling flesh; a fleshy growth.

carotenase (kăr-ŏt′ĕ-nās) [Gr. *karoton,* carrot]. An enzyme that converts carotene into vitamin A. SYN: *carotinase.*

carotene (kăr′ō-tēn) [Gr. *karoton*]. A yellow crystalline pigment present in various plant and animal tissues. It is abundant in yellow vegetables (carrots, squash, corn). Carotene, which exists in several forms, is the precursor of vitamin A. It is stored in the liver and converted to vitamin A in the liver.

carotenemia (kăr″ō-tĕ-nē′mē-ă) [″ + *haima,* blood]. Carotene in the blood characterized by yellowing of the skin (pseudojaundice). Carotenemia can be distinguished from true jaundice by the lack of yellow discoloration of the conjunctivae in carotenemia. SYN: *carotenosis.*

carotenoid (kă-rŏt′ĕ-noyd) [″ + *eidos,* form]. 1. One of a group of pigments (as carotene, q.v.) ranging in color from light yellow to purple, widely distributed in plants and animals. 2. Resembling carotene.

carotenosis [″ + *osis,* condition]. Carotenemia, q.v.

carotic (kă-rŏt′ĭk) [Gr. *karos,* deep sleep]. 1. Carotid. 2. Resembling stupor; stupefying.

caroticotympanic (kă-rŏt″ĭ-kō-tĭm-păn′ĭk). Concerning the carotid canal and the tympanic cavity, i.e., middle ear.

carotid (kă-rŏt′ĭd) [Gr. *karos,* deep sleep]. 1. Pert. to the right and left common carotid arteries, both of which arise from the aorta, and are the principal blood supply to the head and neck. Each of these two arteries divides to form external and internal carotid arteries. 2. Pert. to any carotid part, as carotid sinus.

carotid body. A flat structure at the bifurcation of the common carotid artery. Contains cells that respond to changes in concentration of oxygen in the blood and to changes in blood pressure.

carotid sinus. A dilated area at the bifurcation of the common carotid artery that is richly supplied with sensory nerve endings of the sinus branch of the vagus nerve. These, when stimulated by distention of the vessel wall brought about by a rise in blood pressure, bring about reflex vasodilation and a slowing of the heart rate.

carotidynia (kăr-ŏt″ĭ-dĭn′ē-ă) [″ + *odyne,* pain]. Pain elicited by pressure on the common carotid artery. Also spelled carotodynia.

carotin [Gr. *karoton,* carrot]. Carotene.

carotinase. Carotenase.

carotinemia. Carotenemia.

carpal [Gr. *karpalis*]. Pert. to the carpus or wrist.

carpale (kăr-pā′lē) [Gr. *karpos*]. Any wrist bone.

carpal tunnel. The canal in the wrist bounded by osteofibrous material through which the flexor tendons and the median nerve pass.

carpal tunnel syndrome. Soreness, tenderness, and weakness of the muscles of the thumb caused by pressure on the median nerve at the point at which it goes through the carpal tunnel of the wrist.

TREATMENT: Surgical relief of tension if conservative therapy fails.

carpectomy (kăr-pĕk′tō-mē) [″ + *ektome,* excision]. Excision of the carpus or portion of it.

carphenazine maleate (kăr-fĕn′ă-zēn). USP. A tranquilizer of the phenothiazine class. Trade name is Proketazine.

carphologia, carphology (kăr-fō-lō′jē-ă, -fŏl′ō-jē) [Gr. *karphos,* dry twig, + *legein,* to pluck]. Involuntary picking at bedclothes, seen esp. in febrile or exhaustive delirium of the low muttering type. A grave symptom in cases of extreme exhaustion or approaching death. SYN: *floccillation.*

carpo- [Gr. *karpos*]. Prefix pert. to the carpus.

carpometacarpal [″ + *meta,* beyond, + *karpos,* wrist]. Pert. to both carpus and metacarpus.

carpopedal (kăr″pō-pĕd′ăl) [″ + L. *ped,* foot]. Pert. to both the wrist and the foot.

carpopedal spasm. Spasm of the hands and feet, sometimes seen in laryngismus stridulus, q.v., and in the hyperventilation syndrome. SEE: *tetany.*

carpoptosis (kăr″pŏp-tō′sĭs) [″ + *ptosis,* a falling]. Wrist drop.

carpus (kăr′pŭs) [L.] [NA] The eight bones of the wrist joint. SEE: *skeleton; wrist.*

carrageen, carragheen (kăr′ă-gēn). Irish moss. Dried red alga, Chondrus crispus, from which the substance carrageenan, or carragheenan, is obtained. It is used as a demulcent and thickening agent in medicines and foods.

Carrel-Dakin treatment (kăr-ĕl′dā′kĭn). [Alexis Carrel, Fr.-U.S. surgeon, 1873–1944; Henry D. Dakin, U.S. chemist, 1880–1952] Method of wound irrigation first utilized in 1915. The wound is intermittently irrigated with Dakin's solution, q.v.

carrier [O. Fr. *carier,* to bear]. 1. A person who harbors a specific pathogenic organism in the absence of discernible symptoms or signs of the disease and who is potentially capable of spreading the organism to others. 2. That which carries anything, as an insect such as a fly that passively carries infectious organisms. 3. A substance that, when combined with another substance (transport substance), is capable of passing through cell membranes as occurs in active transport mechanisms. SEE: *fomes; microorganisms; vector.* SEE: *communicable disease* for table. 4. A heterozygote; one who carries a recessive gene together with its normal allele.

CLASSIFICATION: *Infection by animal carriers:* Some microorganisms may be carried from animal to man by direct contact, indirect transfer, or by intermediary hosts.

Airborne infection: Pathogenic organisms in the respiratory tract, discharged from the mouth or nose, may be borne on the air and settle on food, clothing, walls, and floors, and if they are of the type that resists drying for a long period, they may remain virulent until transmitted to another person. Coughing, sneezing, and expectorating may be responsible for droplet infection.

Contact infection: This is the result of transmission from person to person as in kissing, coming in contact with those afflicted with communicable diseases or with utensils handled by one with an infection.

Food-borne infection: Bacteria may be transported by food. Root and salad vegetables may carry bacteria from the soil or from manure used as fertilizer. Cooking provides safeguards by destroying microorganisms on food.

Human carriers: Some parasites may live in or upon the body of persons who themselves do not suffer from the parasites but may carry them to others. Carriers may be asymptomatic contact carriers (those who never show symptoms), incubationary carriers (those in whom the infection is starting but has not completed the incubation period), and convalescent carriers (those who have recovered but still harbor the organism causing their disease).

Insect vectors: An insect may act as a physical carrier, as the tick that may transmit the organism causing Rocky Mountain spotted fever, or one may act as an active intermediate host, such as the Anopheles mosquito, which transmits malaria.

Prenatal infection: This is the result of the fetus being infected from the mother's bloodstream or from contiguity with the maternal membranes.

Soil-borne infection: Soil-borne, spore-forming organisms commonly enter the body through wounds as in tetanus and gas gangrene.

Water-borne infection: Organisms producing typhoid, dysentery, cholera, and amebic infections may be carried through a water supply or water in public pools used for bathing. These organisms may pass into the water from the feces of an infected person and be communicated to others.

c., active. One who harbors a pathogenic organism for a considerable period following recovery from disease due to the organism.

c., convalescent. One who harbors an infective organism during recovery from the disease caused by the organism.

c., genetic. A person whose chromosomes contain a pathologic mutant gene that may be transmitted to offspring. In some cases such as Tay-Sachs disease, this can be detected prenatally by a laboratory test done on amniotic fluid.

c., healthy. One who harbors an infectious organism but does not succumb to the disease.

c., incubatory. One who harbors and spreads an infectious organism during the incubation period of a disease.

c., intermittent. One who is capable of spreading infectious organisms at intervals.

c., passive. C., healthy.

carrier-free (kăr'ē-ĕr-frē). A radioactive isotope that is not attached to a carrier.

Carrion's disease (kăr-ē-ōnz'). [Daniel A. Carrion, a Peruvian student who lost his life after voluntarily taking an injection, 1850–1885] An infectious disease occurring in the valleys of the Andes Mountains in Peru, Chile, Bolivia, and Colombia. It appears in an acute febrile anemic stage followed in several weeks by a nodular skin eruption. Caused by Bartonella bacilliformis transmitted by the sandfly. SYN: *bartonellosis.*

car sickness. Sickness induced by riding in cars. A form of motion sickness, q.v.

cartilage (kăr'tĭ-lĭj) [L. *cartilago,* gristle]. A specialized type of dense connective tissue consisting of cells embedded in a ground substance or matrix. The matrix is firm and compact, rendering it capable of withstanding considerable pressure or tension. Cartilage has a bluish-white or gray color and is semi-opaque; it has no nerve or blood supply of its own. The cells lie in cavities called lacunae. They may be single or in groups of two, three, or four.

Cartilage constitutes a part of the skeleton in adults, occurring in the costal cartilages of the ribs, the nasal septum, in the external ear and lining the eustachian tube, in the wall of the larynx, in the trachea and bronchi, between bodies of the vertebrae, and covering the articular surfaces of bones. It forms the major portion of the embryonic skeleton, providing a model in which most bones develop.

c., articular. Hyaline cartilage covering the articular surfaces of bones.

c., costal. Cartilage connecting the true ribs and the sternum.

c., fibrous. Cartilage containing visible collagenic fibers. SYN: *fibrocartilage.*

c., hyaline. A bluish-white glassy translucent cartilage. The matrix appears homogeneous although it contains collagenous fibers forming a fine network. The walls of the lucunae stain intensely with basic dyes. Hyaline cartilage is flexible and slightly elastic. Its surface is covered by the perichondrium except on articular surfaces. Found in articular cartilage, in costal cartilages, in septum of the nose, in larynx and trachea.

c., semilunar. One of the interarticular cartilages of the knee joint.

c., thyroid. The largest cartilage of the larynx, a shield-shaped cartilage that forms the prominence known as the Adam's apple.

c., yellow. A network of yellow elastic fibers, holding cartilage cells, and pervading intercellular substance. Found in the epiglottis, the external ear, and the auditory tube. It strengthens them and maintains their shape.

cartilage, words pert. to: "cartilag-" words; "chondr-" words; cricoid.

cartilaginification (kăr"tĭ-lă-jĭn"ĭ-fĭ-kā'shŭn) [" + *facere,* to make]. Cartilage formation or chondrification; the development of cartilage from undifferentiated tissue.

cartilaginoid (kăr"tĭ-lăj'ĭ-noyd) [" + Gr. *eidos,* form]. Resembling cartilage.

cartilaginous (kăr"tĭ-lăj'ĭ-nŭs). Pert. to or consisting of cartilage.

cartilago (kăr"tĭ-lă'gō) [L.]. (pl. *cartilagines*) [NA] Cartilage.

caruncle (kăr'ŭng-kl) [L. *caruncula,* small flesh]. A small fleshy growth.

c., lacrimal. Caruncula lacrimalis [NA]. Caruncle found on the conjunctiva near the inner canthus. A small reddish elevation at the medial angle of the eye.

c., urethral. A small, red, papillary growth, highly vascular, sometimes found in the urinary meatus in females. It is characterized by pain on urination and is very sensitive to friction.

caruncula (kăr-ŭng'kū-lă) [L.]. (pl. *carunculae*) [NA] A tiny, fleshy protuberance. SYN: *caruncle*.

c. hymenales. [NA] Small irregular nodules representing remains of the hymen.

cary-, caryo- [Gr. *karyon*, nucleus]. A combining form meaning nucleus. SEE: words beginning with *kary-*, *karyo-*.

cascade (kăs-kād'). The continuation of a process through a series of steps; each step initiates the next step until the final step is reached. The action may or may not become cumulative as each step progresses. SEE: *citric acid cycle*.

cascara sagrada (kăs-kăr'ă să-gră'dă). USP. The dried bark of Rhamnus purshiana, a small tree grown on western U.S. coast, and in parts of South America. The main ingredient in aromatic cascara sagrada fluid extract, a cathartic.

case [L. *casus*, happening]. 1. An occurrence of disease; incorrectly used to refer to a patient. 2. An enclosing structure.

c., brain. The cranium.

caseate (kā'sē-āt) [L. *caseus*, cheese]. To undergo cheesy degeneration, as in certain necroses.

caseation (kā"sē-ā'shŭn). 1. Process of conversion of necrotic tissue into a granular amorphous mass resembling cheese. 2. Precipitation of casein during coagulation of milk.

case history. The complete medical, family, social, and psychiatric history of a patient up to the time of admission for the present illness.

casein (kā'sē-ĭn) [L. *caseus*, cheese]. The principal protein in milk; it is present in milk curds. It supplies all of the amino acids necessary for growth and development. When coagulated by rennin or acid, it becomes one of the principal ingredients of cheese. SEE: *caseinogen*.

caseinogen (kā-sē-ĭn'ō-jĕn) [" + Gr. *gennan*, to produce]. The principal protein, from which casein is derived, in milk. It is the substance in solution, and casein is the result of its precipitation. Its conversion into casein is the essential process in the curdling of milk.

caseous (kā'sē-ŭs). 1. Resembling cheese. 2. Pert. to transformation of tissues into a cheesy mass.

$CaSO_4$. Calcium sulfate.

Casoni's reaction (kă-sō'nēz). [Tomaso Casoni, It. physician, 1880–1933] Appearance of a wheal surrounded by an erythematous zone following intradermal injection of sterile hydatid fluid. A test for presence of hydatid cysts resulting from infection with Echinococcus granulosus.

cassette (kă-sĕt') [Fr., little box]. A flat, lightproof box with an intensifying screen in it, for holding x-ray film or a case for film or magnetic tape.

cast [ME. *casten*, to carry]. 1. A solid mold of a part, usually applied in situ for immobilization as in fractures, dislocations, and other severe injuries. Most often made of plaster of Paris, sodium silicate, starch, or dextrin that is rubbed into crinoline, then soaked in water, carefully applied to the immobilized part, and allowed to harden. SEE: illus. 2. In dentistry, a positive copy of tissues of the jaw over which denture bases may be made. 3. Pliable or fibrous material shed in various pathological conditions, the product of effusion. It is molded to the shape of the part in which it has been accumulated. According to source, casts are classified as bronchial, intestinal, nasal, esophageal, renal, tracheal, urethral, and vaginal; as to constituents, classified as bloody, fatty, fibrinous, granular, hyaline, mucous, and waxy.

c., blood. A urinary cast composed principally of red blood cells.

c., body. Cast used to immobilize the spine. It may extend from the thorax to the groin.

c., bronchial. A cast seen in sputum of patients with asthma and some with bronchitis.

c., epithelial. A cast containing cells from inner lining of uriniferous tubules. Seen in acute nephritis.

c., fatty. Any cast made up of fat globules.

c., fibrinous. Yellowish-brown cast seen in acute nephritis.

c., granular. Dark urinary cast of granular substance; usually a degenerative form of a hyaline or waxy cast.

c., hyaline. Urinary cast made up of homogenous protein.

c., pseudo-. Epithelial cells swollen and held in groups, resembling casts. Alkaline urine has a tendency to dissolve casts.

c., pus. Leukocyte cast found in urine in suppuration of kidney.

c., urinary. Cast found in the urine formed from protein precipitates in the renal tubules.

c., uterine. Cast from the uterus passed in exfoliative endometritis or membranous dysmenorrhea.

c., waxy. Light yellowish, well-defined urinary cast with tendency to split transversely, found in some cases of amyloid degeneration and advanced nephritis.

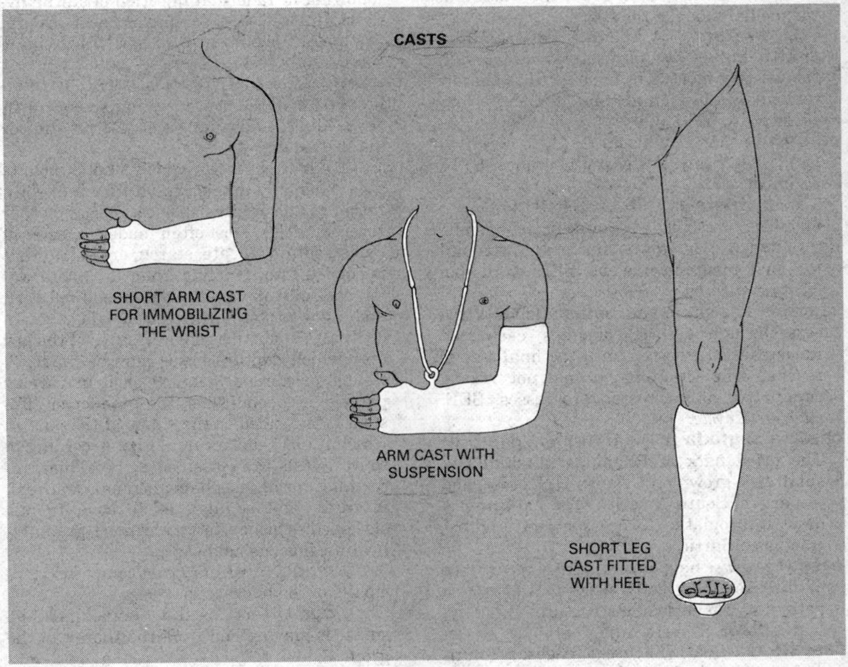

Castellani's paint (kăs-tĕl-ăn′ēz). [Aldo Castellani, It. physician, 1878–1971] Paint used as a disinfectant for skin and in treatment of fungus infections of the skin. Composed of phenol, resorcinol, basic fuchsin, boric acid, and acetone.

Castle's intrinsic factor [William Bosworth Castle, U.S. physician and educator, b. 1897] A substance secreted by the stomach, essential for the absorption of cyanocobalamin (vitamin B_{12}; extrinsic factor). Absence of intrinsic factor causes pernicious anemia.

castor oil. USP. A fixed oil expressed from the seed of the plant Ricinus communis. Used externally as an emollient and internally as a cathartic. In the digestive tract it is hydrolyzed to ricinoleic acid, which acts as an irritant type of laxative. Trade name is Neoloid.

castrate (kăs′trāt) [L. *castrare*, to prune]. 1. To remove the testicles or ovaries. SEE: *spay.* 2. One who has been castrated.

castrated. Rendered incapable of reproduction by removal of the testicles or ovaries.

castration (kăs-trā′shŭn). 1. Excision of the testicles or ovaries. 2. Destruction or inactivation of the gonad.

c., female. Removal of the ovaries. SYN: *oophorectomy; spaying.*

c., male. Removal of the testes. SYN: *orchiectomy.*

c., parasitic. Destruction of the gonads by parasitic organisms early in life. It may result from direct infestation of the gonad or indirectly from effects of infestation in other parts of the body.

castration complex. Morbid fear of castration.

casualty (kăz′ū-ăl-tē) [L. *casualis*, accidental]. 1. Accident causing injury or death. 2. Person injured or killed in an accident. 3. Serviceman captured, missing, injured, or killed.

casuistics (kăz-ū-ĭs′tĭks) [L. *casus*, chance]. 1. Analysis of records of clinical cases in order to establish the general characteristics of a disease. 2. The determination of right and wrong in moral questions by application of ethical principles to a particular case.

CAT. Computerized axial tomography.

cat. Any member of the Felidae family, including lions, leopards, wildcats, and esp. the domesticated cat, Felis catus. SEE: *cat bite fever; cat scratch disease.*

cata- [Gr. *kata*, down]. Prefix indicating down or downward, against, or according to.

catabasis (kă-tăb′ă-sĭs) [Gr. *kata*, down, + *basis*, going]. The decline of a disease.

catabatic (kăt-ă-băt'ĭk). Pert. to catabasis, q.v.
catabolic (kăt"ă-bŏl'ĭk). Pert. to catabolism.
catabolin (kă-tăb'ō-lĭn). Catabolite.
catabolism (kă-tăb'ō-lĭzm) [Gr. *katabole,* a casting down, + *-ismos,* condition]. The destructive phase of metabolism, the opposite of anabolism. Catabolism includes all the processes in which complex substances are converted into simpler substances, usually with the release of energy. SEE: *anabolism; metabolism.*
catabolite (kă-tăb'ō-līt). Any product of catabolism. SYN: *catabolin.*
catacrotic (kăt"ă-krŏt'ĭk) [" + *krotos,* beat]. Indicating the downstroke of pulse tracing interrupted by an upstroke.
catacrotism (kă-tăk'rō-tĭzm) [" + " + *-ismos,* condition]. A pulse with one or more secondary expansions of the artery following the main beat.
catadicrotic (kăt"ă-dī-krŏt'ĭk) [" + *dis,* twice, + *krotos,* beat]. Manifesting one or more secondary expansions of a pulse on the descending limb of the tracing.
catadicrotism (kăt"ă-dī'krō-tĭzm) [" + " + " + *-ismos,* condition]. Two minor expansions following the main beat of an artery.
catadioptric (kăt"ă-dī-ŏp'trĭk) [" + *diopsesthai,* to see through]. Pert. to refraction and reflection of light simultaneously.
catagen (kăt'ă-jĕn) [" + *gennan,* to produce]. Intermediate phase of hair-growth cycle that falls after the growth or anagen stage and before the resting or telogen phase.
catagenesis (kăt"ă-jĕn'ĕ-sĭs) [" + *genesis,* production]. Retrogression or involution.
catalase (kăt'ă-lās). An enzyme present in almost all cells. It catalyzes the decomposition of hydrogen peroxide to water and oxygen.
catalepsy (kăt'ă-lĕp"sē) [Gr. *kata,* down, + *lepsis,* seizure]. A condition seen in psychotic patients wherein there is generalized diminished responsiveness usually characterized by a trancelike state. Doctors and nurses should keep in mind that even though the patient is in a trance, conversations may be heard. Therefore one's actions toward and talk about such patients should be no different than if they were not in a cataleptic state.
cataleptic. Pert. to catalepsy.
cataleptiform (kăt-ă-lĕp'tĭ-form) [" + *lepsis,* seizure, + L. *forma,* shape]. Having the form of catalepsy.
cataleptoid (kăt"ă-lĕp'toyd) [" + " + *eidos,* resemblance]. Resembling or simulating catalepsy.
catalysis (kă-tăl'ĭ-sĭs) [Gr. *katalysis,* dissolution]. The speeding up of the rate of a chemical reaction by a catalyst, q.v.
catalyst (kăt'ă-lĭst). A substance that speeds up the rate of a chemical reaction without itself being permanently altered in the reaction. Catalysts are effective in small quantities and are not used up in the reaction, i.e., they can be recovered unchanged.

Ex.: hydrochloric acid, which catalyzes the hydrolysis of sucrose; ptyalin, which catalyzes the hydrolysis of starch. SYN: *catalyzer.*
catalytic (kăt-ăl-ĭt'ĭk) [Gr. *katalysis,* dissolution]. Pert. to catalysis, q.v.
catalyze (kăt'ă-līz) [Gr. *katalysis,* dissolution]. To cause catalysis.
catalyzer (kăt'ă-lī-zĕr). A catalyst, q.v.
catamenia (kăt-ă-mē'nē-ă) [Gr. *katamenia*]. Periodic discharge of menstrual blood from the uterus. SYN: *menses; menstruation.*
catamenial (kăt"ă-mĕn'ē-ăl). Pert. to the menses or catamenia.
catamnesis (kăt-ăm-nē'sĭs) [Gr. *kata,* down, + *mneme,* memory]. A patient's medical history, after treatment; follow-up history. SEE: *anamnesis.*
cataphasia (kăt-ă-fā'zē-ă) [" + *phasis,* speech]. A speech disorder causing an involuntary repetition of the same word.
cataphora (kă-tăf'ō-ră) [Gr. *kataphora*]. Lethargy with short remissions.
cataphoresis (kăt"ă-fō-rē'sĭs) [Gr. *kata,* down, + *phoresis,* being carried]. The transmission of electronegative ions or drugs into the body tissues or through a membrane by use of an electric current.
cataphoria (kăt"ă-fō'rē-ă) [" + *pherein,* to bear]. Tendency of visual axes to incline below the horizontal plane.
cataphoric. Pert. to cataphora or cataphoresis.
cataphrenia (kăt"ă-frē'nē-ă) [" + *phren,* mind]. A type of dementia that usually resolves in recovery.
cataphylaxis (kăt"ă-fĭ-lăk'sĭs) [" + *phylaxis,* guard]. The process of carrying antibodies and leukocytes to the site of an infection.
cataplasia, cataplasis (kăt"ă-plā'zē-ă, kă-tăp'lă-sĭs) [" + *plassein,* to form]. Atrophic change in tissues or cells.
cataplasm (kăt'ă-plăzm) [L. *cataplasma*]. A poultice, q.v.
cataplectic (kăt-ă-plĕk'tĭk) [" + *plexis,* stroke]. Pert. to cataplexy.
cataplexy, cataplexia (kăt'ă-plĕks-ē, kăt-ă-plĕk'sē-ă). A form of sudden emotional shock, or stroke, without loss of consciousness, accompanied by loss of muscular tone, causing the patient to fall to the floor.

ETIOL: May be the result of intense emotion or the sudden onset of a disease, or rarely, a part of a narcoleptic attack.
Catapres. Trade name for clonidine hydrochloride.
cataract (kăt'ă-răkt) [L. *cataracta*]. Opacity of lens of eye or its capsule or both. Varieties

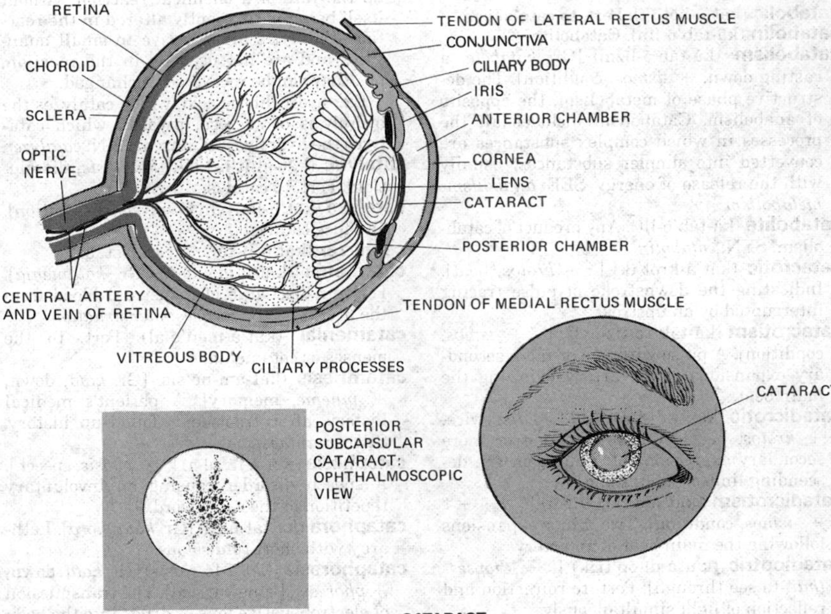

CATARACT

are capsular, polar, lamellar, nuclear, cortical, morgagnian, congenital, infantile, traumatic, diabetic, senile. SEE: illus.

STAGES: Incipient stage (spoke-shaped opacities, cloudlike opacities, opacity of cortex or nucleus). Stage of swelling or immature stage (swollen lens, shallow anterior chamber). Mature stage (lens shrinks due to loss of fluid and becomes opaque, anterior chamber regains its normal depth, no shadow thrown by iris or lens with focal illumination). Hypermature stage (lens becomes either solid and shrunken or soft and liquid).

ETIOL: Common form is result of the aging process; other forms may be congenital or caused by infection or injury.

TREATMENT: Surgical removal of lens except in presence of associated inflammation. Corrective eyeglasses, contact lenses; or more recently, the use of an artificial lens implanted in the eye has been used. SEE: *phacoemulsification*.

NURSING IMPLICATIONS: *Pre-op:* Prepare patient for postoperative need to have eyes bandaged.

Post-op: Modern surgical technology does not require rigid adherence to the practice of immobilization of the head. Care should be taken to prevent increases in intraocular pressure, so the patient should be instructed not to sneeze, cough, or bend from the waist. Rapid movements should be avoided. The patient may turn to the unoperated side (if a unilateral repair). The patient should be oriented to the environment and the nurse should spend time talking with the patient at intervals to decrease the effects of sensory deprivation. All persons entering the room should be certain the patient knows they are in the room in order to prevent startling the patient. The patient should receive analgesics as needed, and be out of bed as allowed by the physician.

Check the operative site for any drainage or symptoms of infection. Instruct the patient and family in the correct technique for administration of eye drops, as well as the need for an eye shield or eyeglasses for protection as ordered by the physician.

c., capsular. Cataract of opacity of the capsule.

c., lenticular. Cataract occurring in the lens.

c., morgagnian. A fluid cataract with a hard nucleus.

c., overripe. Stage following a mature cataract in which lens solidifies and shrinks or becomes soft.

c., ripe. Mature cataract.

c., senile. Cataract of old persons.

cataractogenic (kăt"ă-răk"tō-jĕn'ĭk) [L. *cataracta,* cataract, + Gr. *gennan,* to produce]. The causation of or formation of a cataract.

catarrh (kă-tăr') [Gr. *katarrhein,* to flow down]. Term formerly applied to inflammation of mucous membranes, esp. of head and throat.

c., dry. Severe spells of coughing with little or no expectoration. Generally seen in the old in association with emphysema or asthma.

catarrhal (kă-tăr'ăl). Of the nature of or pert. to catarrh.

catastalsis (kăt-ă-stăl'sĭs) [Gr. *kata,* down, + *stalsis,* contraction]. Movement of a contraction wave of the stomach downward, not preceded by a wave of inhibition.

catatonia (kăt-ă-tō'nē-ă) [" + *tonos,* tension]. 1. A phase of schizophrenia in which the patient is unresponsive. The tendency to assume and remain in a fixed posture and inability to move or talk are characteristic of this phase. 2. Stupor.

catatonic. Stuporous; pert. to catatonia.

catatricrotic (kăt"ă-trī-krŏt'ĭk) [" + *treis,* three, + *krotos,* beat]. Manifesting a third impulse in the descending stroke of the sphygmogram.

catatricrotism (kăt"ă-trī'krō-tĭzm). Condition in which the pulse shows a third impulse in the descending stroke of a pulse tracing.

catatropia (kăt"ă-trō'pē-ă) [" + *tropos,* turning]. Having both eyes turned downward.

cat bite fever. An infectious disease caused by Pasteurella multocida transmitted by the bite of a cat. Characterized by abscess formation at the site of the bite. Not to be confused with cat scratch disease, q.v.

TREATMENT: Meticulous wound cleansing. Generously applied antiseptic to all parts of bite. Consider cautery and debridement. Antirabies treatment when indicated. Sterile dressings. SEE: *bites or stings.*

catchment area. Geographical area defining the portion of a population served by a designated medical facility.

catecholamines (kăt"ĕ-kōl'ă-mēns). Biologically active amines, epinephrine and norepinephrine, derived from the amino acid tyrosine. They have marked effect on the nervous and cardiovascular systems, metabolic rate, temperature, and smooth muscle. SEE: *serotonin.*

catelectrotonus (kăt"ē-lĕk-trŏt'ō-nŭs) [" + *elektron,* amber, + *tonos,* tension]. The state of increased excitability produced in a nerve or muscle in the region near the cathode during the passage of an electric current.

catenating (kăt'ĕn-āt"ĭng) [L. *catena,* chain]. 1. Concerning a disease that is linked with another. 2. Formation of a series of symptoms. SEE: *concatenation.*

catenoid (kăt'ĕ-noyd) [" + Gr. *eidos,* resemblance]. Chainlike; pert. to protozoan colonies whose individuals are joined end-to-end.

caterpillar sting. More than 50 species of butterfly and moth larvae possess urticating hairs that contain a toxin. Contact with these hairs can cause numbness and swelling of the infected area, severe radiating pain, localized swelling, enlarged regional lymph nodes, nausea, and vomiting. Even though shock and convulsions may occur, no deaths have been reported. The disease is self-limiting. The larva of the flannel moth, Megalopyge opercularis, known as the puss caterpillar or *woolly worm,* is frequently the cause of this sting, particularly in the southern U.S.A.

catgut. Sheep's intestine twisted for use as an absorbable ligature.

catharsis (kă-thăr'sĭs) [Gr. *katharsis,* purification]. 1. Purgative action of the bowels. 2. The freudian method of freeing the mind by recalling from the patient's memory an event or experience that was the exciting cause of a psychoneurosis. SEE: *abreaction.*

cathartic (kă-thăr'tĭk) [Gr. *kathartikos,* purging]. An active purgative, producing bowel movements.

Ex.: cascara sagrada; castor oil. SEE: *purgative.*

cathepsins (kă-thĕp'sĭns). Enzymes, particularly those involved in protein metabolism.

cathepsis (kă-thĕp'sĭs) [Gr. *kathepsis,* boiling down]. In living tissues, synthesis or hydrolysis of proteins; in dead tissues, autolysis of proteins.

catheresis (kăth-ĕ-rē'sĭs) [Gr. *kathairesis,* destruction]. 1. Weakness resulting from medication. 2. Weak action.

catheter (kăth'ĕ-tĕr) [Gr. *katheter,* something

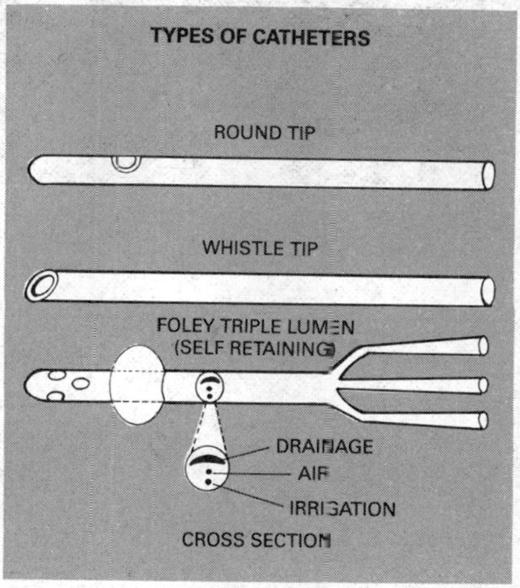

inserted]. A tube passed through the body for evacuating or injecting fluids into body cavities. Made of elastic, elastic web, rubber, glass, metal, or plastic. SEE: illus.

c., cardiac. A long, fine catheter esp. designed for passage through the lumen of a blood vessel into the chambers of the heart. SEE: *cardiac catheterization*.

c., double-channel. Catheter providing for inflow and outflow.

c., elbowed. Catheter that has an acute bend near the beak. Used in patients with enlarged prostate. SYN: *c., prostatic*.

c., eustachian. Catheter passed into eustachian tube through nasal passages.

c., female. A short catheter, about 5 in. (12.7 cm.) in length, used to pass into the bladder of the female.

c., Foley. A urinary tract catheter that has a balloon attachment at one end. After the catheter is inserted the balloon is filled with sterile water. Thus the catheter is prevented from leaving the bladder until the balloon is emptied.

c., indwelling. Any catheter that is allowed to remain in place in the bladder.

c., Karman. Catheter used for suction curettage of the uterus.

c., male. Catheter used to pass into the bladder of the male. Catheter is 12 to 13 in. (30.5 to 33 cm.) long.

c., prostatic. Catheter, 15 to 16 in. (38 to 40.6 cm.) long, with a short elbowed tip designed to pass prostatic obstruction. SYN: *c., elbowed*.

c., self-retaining. Catheter that can be retained at will, effecting bladder drainage.

c., suprapubic. A urinary catheter closed drainage system. It is inserted through the skin, about 2.5 cm. above the symphysis pubis, into the distended bladder. This is usually done under general anesthesia. If it is to remain in place, it is sutured to the abdominal skin.

c., vertebrated. Catheter in sections to be fitted together, so that it is flexible.

c., winged. Catheter with little flaps at each side of beak to aid in retaining it in the bladder.

catheter fever. Reactionary rise in temperature caused by a urinary tract infection following passage of a catheter or urethral bougie.

catheterization (kăth″ĕ-tĕr-ĭ-zā′shŭn) [Gr. *katheterismos*]. Use or passage of a catheter.

c., cardiac. The passage of a catheter into the heart through an arm vein and blood vessels leading into the heart for the purpose of obtaining cardiac blood samples, detecting abnormalities, and determining intracardiac

URINARY CATHETERIZATION

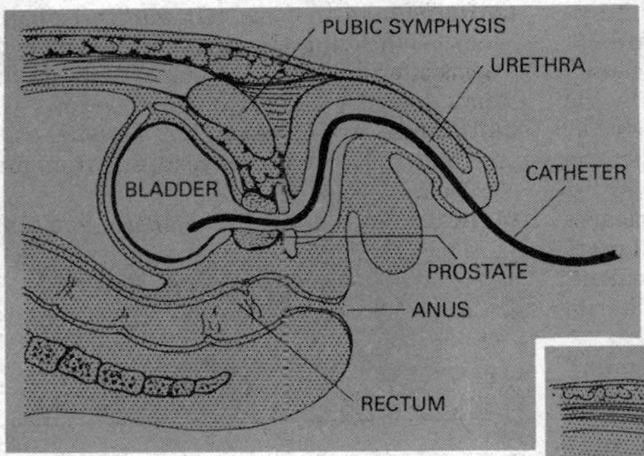

MALE

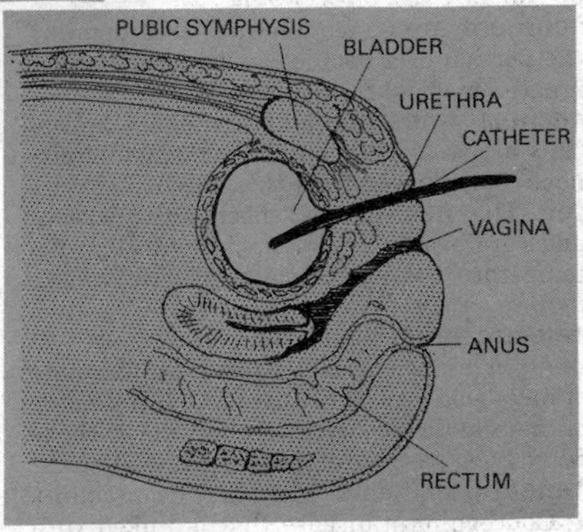

FEMALE

pressure. SEE: *cardiac catheterization.*

c., urinary bladder. Introduction of a catheter through the urethra into the bladder for withdrawal of urine. SEE: illus.

NURSING IMPLICATIONS: Explain procedure and reason for catheterization to the patient. Assemble necessary equipment, and properly position and drape the patient. Follow hospital procedure for insertion of the catheter. Maintain sterile technique. After insertion of an indwelling catheter, connect it to a closed straight drainage system. Document the procedure results and the patient's response in the nurse's progress notes.

FOR FEMALE: Patient should be in a supine position with knees flexed and apart, and with the feet flat against each other (frog position). Pillows may be placed under the head and shoulders to relax abdominal muscles.

FOR MALE: Patient should be in a supine position with legs extended. Care should be taken following the procedure to return the prepuce to its normal position to prevent any subsequent swelling.

catheterize (kăth'ĕ-tĕr-īz). To pass or introduce a catheter into a part, usually indicating catheterization of bladder.

cathexis (kă-thĕk'sĭs) [Gr. *kathexis,* retention]. The emotional or mental energy used in concentrating on an object or idea.

cathodal (kăth'ō-dăl) [Gr. *kathodos,* downward path]. Pert. to the cathode.

cathode (kăth'ōd). ABBR: ca. 1. The negative electrode from which electrons are emitted. Opposite of the anode or positive pole. 2. In a vacuum tube, the electrode that serves as the source of the electron stream.

cathode stream. Negatively charged electrons sent out as particles from the cathode in discharges through the vacuum. They move in a straight line and, upon hitting solid matter, produce roentgen rays.

cathodic (kă-thŏd'ĭk). 1. Pert. to a cathode. 2. Proceeding outwardly or efferently as applied to a nerve impulse.

Cathomycin. Trade name for the antibiotic novobiocin.

cation (kăt'ī-ŏn) [Gr. *kation,* descending]. An ion with a positive charge of electricity. It is attracted by and travels to the cathode (negative pole). Opposite of anion. SEE: *ion.*

catlin (kăt'lĭn). Surgical knife with double edges.

catoptric (kă-tŏp'trĭk) [Gr. *katoptrikos,* reflecting]. Pert. to reflected light or mirrors.

catoptrophobia (kăt"ŏp-trō-fō'bē-ă) [Gr. *katoptron,* mirror, + *phobos,* fear]. Morbid fear of mirrors or of breaking them.

CAT scan. Computerized axial tomography scan. Use of a computer to produce, from x-ray data, a cross-sectional view of the anatomical part being investigated. SEE: *tomography, computerized axial.*

cat scratch disease. A febrile disease characterized by lymphadenitis, thought to be transmitted by cats. A few days after a minor scratch a pustule develops at the site. Regional lymphadenopathy develops within 2 weeks. Fever, malaise, headache and anorexia accompany the lymphadenopathy.

ETIOL: The causative organism is unknown.

TREATMENT: Tetracycline therapy may shorten the course, but spontaneous remission usually occurs within 4 weeks.

PROG: Excellent.

cat's eye pupil. A slitlike pupil.

cat's eye reflex. SEE: *reflex, cat's eye.*

cauda (kaw'dă) [L.]. (pl. *caudae*) [NA] A tail or tail-like structure.

c. epididymidis. [NA] The inferior portion of the epididymis that is continuous with the ductus deferens.

c. equina. [NA] The terminal portion of the spinal cord and the roots of the spinal nerves below the first lumbar nerve.

c. helicis. [NA] A pointed process extending inferiorly from the helix of the auricular cartilage of the ear.

c. pancreatis. [NA] The tail of the pancreas.

c. striati. Tail-like posterior extremity of the corpus stratium.

caudad (kaw'dăd) [L. *cauda,* tail, + *ad,* toward]. Toward the tail; in a posterior direction.

caudal (kawd'ăl) [L. *caudalis*]. 1. Pert. to any tail-like structure. 2. Inferior in position.

caudate (kaw'dāt) [L. *caudatus*]. Possessing a tail.

caudation (kaw-dā'shŭn) [L. *cauda,* tail]. 1. A lengthened or elongated clitoris. 2. Having a tail or tails.

caudocephalad (kaw-dō-sĕf'ă-lăd) [" + Gr. *kephale,* head, + L. *ad,* toward]. Moving from the tail-end toward the head.

caul (kawl) [O. Fr. *cale,* a small cap]. 1. Membranes or portions of the amnion covering head of fetus at birth. 2. The great omentum.

cauliflower ear. Lay term for malformation of ear due to trauma, as seen in boxers. Thickening of the ear is due to accumulation of fluid and blood clots in the tissue after repeated injury. Plastic surgery may restore the ear to a normal shape.

caumesthesia (kaw"mĕs-thē'zē-ă) [Gr. *kauma,* burn, + *aisthesis,* sensation]. A sense of heat when surrounding temperature is normal.

causalgia (kaw-săl'jē-ă) [" + *algos,* pain]. Intense burning pain accompanied by trophic skin changes, due to injury of nerve fibers.

cause [L. *causa*]. That which brings about a particular condition, result, or effect.

c., antecedent. An event or condition that predisposes to a condition.

c., determining. The final event or condition that brings about a cause.

c., predisposing. That which favors the development of a disease or condition.

c., proximate. An event or condition that immediately precedes and causes a disease.

c., remote. An event or condition that is not immediate in its effect but is a factor in predisposing to the development of a disease or condition.

c., ultimate. The remote event or condition that initiated a train of events that resulted in the development of the disease.

caustic (kaw′stĭk) [Gr. *kaustikos,* capable of burning]. 1. Corrosive and burning; destructive to living tissue. 2. An agent, particularly an alkali, that will destroy living tissue.

Ex.: silver nitrate, potassium hydroxide, nitric acid.

cauterant (kaw′tĕr-ănt) [Gr. *kauter,* a burner]. 1. Escharotic; caustic 2. A caustic agent.

cauterization (kaw″tĕr-ī-zā′shŭn) [Gr. *kauteriazein,* to burn]. Cautery; destruction of tissue with a caustic, an electric current, a hot iron, or by freezing.

RS: chemocautery; electrocautery; galvanocautery; moxibustion.

c., chemical. Cauterization by the use of chemical agents, esp. caustic substances.

c., electrical. Cauterization by platinum wires heated to incandescence by an electric current. SYN: *electrocautery; galvanocautery.*

cauterize (kaw′tĕr-īz). To burn with a cautery, or to apply one.

cautery (kaw′tĕr-ē) [Gr. *kauter,* a burner]. A means of destroying tissue by electricity, freezing, heat, or corrosive chemicals. Used in potentially infected wounds; to destroy excess granulation tissue. Thermocautery consists of red-hot or white-hot object, usually piece of wire or pointed metallic instrument, heated in a flame or with electricity (galvanocautery, electrocautery).

cava (kā′vă). 1. A hollow area or a body cavity. 2. Vena cava.

caval (kā′văl). Pert. to the vena cava.

cavalry bone. Rider's bone; bony deposit in the adductor muscles of the thigh.

cavern (kăv′ĕrn). A cavity caused by a disease process.

cavernitis (kăv″ĕr-nī′tĭs) [L. *caverna,* hollow, + Gr. *itis,* inflammation]. Inflammation of the corpus cavernosum of the penis.

cavernoma (kăv″ĕr-nō′mă) [″ + Gr. *oma,* tumor]. A cavernous angioma. SEE: *hemangioma.*

cavernositis (kăv″ĕr-nō-sī′tĭs) [″ + Gr. *itis,* inflammation]. Inflammation of the corpus cavernosum.

cavernous (kăv′ĕr-nŭs) [L. *caverna,* a hollow]. Containing hollow spaces.

cavitary (kăv′ĭ-tā″rē). Pertaining to a cavity.

cavitation [L. *cavitas,* a cavity]. Formation of a cavity. May occur as a normal process as in the formation of the amnion in human development or pathologically as in the development of cavities in lung tissue in pulmonary tuberculosis.

cavitis (kā-vī′tĭs) [″ + Gr. *itis,* inflammation]. Inflammation of a vena cava.

cavity (kăv′ĭ-tē) [L. *cavitas,* hollow]. A hollow space, such as a body organ or the hole in a tooth produced by caries.

c., abdominal. The cavity of the peritoneum between the diaphragm and pelvis, containing all the abdominal organs.

c., alveolar. A tooth socket.

c., amniotic. Fluid-filled cavity around the developing embryo.

c., articular. The synovial cavity of a joint.

c., body. In vertebrates, the space between the body wall and the visceral organs. SYN: *coelom.*

c., buccal. The cavity of the mouth.

c., cotyloid. The acetabulum.

c., cranial. The cavity of the skull, which contains the brain.

c., glenoid. A shallow concavity on the lateral surface of the head of the scapula that receives the head of the humerus.

c., oral. The mouth or buccal cavity. Includes the vestibule and oral cavity proper.

c., pelvic. The cavity of the pelvis. Includes the major pelvic cavity, which lies between the iliac fossa and above the iliopectineal lines, and the minor pelvic cavity, which lies below the iliopectineal lines or the inlet of the pelvis.

c., pericardial. The space between the epicardium (visceral pericardium) and the parietal pericardium.

c., peritoneal. The potential space between the parietal peritoneum lining the body wall and the visceral peritoneum forming surface layer of visceral organs.

c., peritoneal, lesser. The omental bursa.

c., pleural. The potential space between the parietal pleura and visceral pleura.

c., pulp. Cavity in a tooth containing the dental pulp and nerve termination.

c., Rosenmüller's. Cavity on either side of the openings of the eustachian tube.

c., serous. A space between two layers of serous membrane.

Ex.: pleural, pericardial, and peritoneal cavities.

c., splanchnic. One of the cavities of the body containing important organs such as the cranial, thoracic, and abdominal cavities.

SYN: *visceral cavity.*

c., tympanic. Cavity of the middle ear.

c., uterine. Cavity of the body of the uterus.

cavity classification. Any method of arranging the cavities or lesions of teeth into groups that can be recognized and described. Carious lesions are usually named for the surface of the tooth affected (labial, buccal, or occlusal), the type of tooth surface involved (pit and fissure or smooth surface), and by an accepted numbering designation.

cavity preparation. An artificial cavity prepared in the tooth for the purpose of restoring the tooth by use of appropriate dental materials; a dental cavity refers to a carious lesion unless it modifies preparation.

cavum (kā'vŭm) [L. *cavus,* a hollow]. [NA] A cavity or space.

c. abdominis. [NA] The abdominal cavity.

c. conchae. [NA] The inferior portion of the cavity of the auricle of the ear. It leads to the external acoustic meatus.

c. mediastinale. The mediastinum.

c. medullare. [NA] The medullary cavity of a long bone.

c. oris. [NA] The oral cavity.

c. pelvis. [NA] The pelvic cavity.

c. trigeminale. The space between the two layers of the dura mater of the brain in which the trigeminale ganglion is located. SYN: *space, Meckel's.*

c. tympani. [NA] The middle ear cavity.

c. uteri. [NA] The cavity of the uterus.

cavus (kā'vŭs) [L., hollow]. Condition of exaggerated height of arch of foot. SYN: *talipes cavus.*

cayenne pepper (kī-ĕn', kā-ĕn'). Capsicum, q.v.

C bar. Curved part of a hand splint that maintains the thumb web space.

C.B.C. *complete blood count.*

C.C. *chief complaint; Commission Certified,* with reference to certification of stains by the Biological Stain Commission.

cc. *cubic centimeter.*

CCl_3•CHO. Chloral.

CCl_4. Carbon tetrachloride.

CCNU. Code name for a chemotherapeutic agent used in treating certain neoplastic conditions. Also called *lomustine.*

C.C.U. *coronary care unit.*

Cd. Chem. symb. for cadmium.

CDC. *Centers for Disease Control.*

Ce. Chem. symb. for cerium.

cebocephalus (sē"bō-sĕf'ă-lŭs) [Gr. *kebos,* monkey, + *kephale,* head]. Fetus with a monkey-like head.

cecal (sē'kăl) [L. *caecalis,* pert. to blindness]. 1. Pert. to cecum. 2. Blind, terminating in a closed extremity.

cecectomy (sē-sĕk'tō-mē) [L. *caecum,* blindness, + Gr. *ektome,* excision]. Surgical removal of the cecum.

cecitis (sē-sī'tĭs) [" + Gr. *itis,* inflammation]. Inflammation of the cecum.

cecocolopexy (sē"kō-kō'lō-pĕk'sē) [" + Gr. *kolon,* colon, + *pexis,* fixation]. Surgical fixation of the colon and the cecum.

cecocolostomy (sē"kō-kō-lŏs'tō-mē) [" + " + *stoma,* mouth]. Colostomy consisting of joining of the cecum to the colon.

cecoileostomy (sē"kō-ĭl"ē-ŏs'tō-mē) [" + *ileum,* ileum, + Gr. *stoma,* opening]. Surgical formation of anastomosis between the cecum and the ileum.

Cecon. Trade name for ascorbic acid.

cecopexy (sē'kō-pĕk"sē) [" + Gr. *pexis,* fixation]. Surgical fixation of the cecum to the abdominal wall.

cecoplication (sē"kō-plĭ-kā'shŭn) [" + *plica,* fold]. Reduction of a dilated cecum by making a fold in its wall.

cecoptosis (sē"kŏp-tō'sĭs) [" + Gr. *ptosis,* a dropping]. Falling displacement of the cecum.

cecosigmoidostomy (sē"kō-sĭg"moyd-ŏs'tō-mē) [" + Gr. *sigmoeides,* shaped like Gr. letter S, + *stoma,* opening]. Surgical formation of a communication between the cecum and sigmoid.

cecostomy (sē-kŏs'tō-mē) [" + Gr. *stoma,* opening]. Surgical formation of an artificial opening into the cecum.

cecotomy (sē-kŏt'ō-mē) [" + Gr. *tome,* incision]. Incision into the cecum.

cecum (sē'kŭm) [L. *caecum,* blindness]. A blind pouch or cul-de-sac that forms the first portion of the large intestine, located below the entrance of the ileum at the ileocecal valve. It averages about 6 cm. in length and 7.5 cm. in width. At its lower end is the vermiform appendix. SEE: *abdominal quadrants* for illus.

Cedilanid. Trade name for lanatoside C.

Cedilanid-D. Trade name for deslanoside.

Cefadyl. Trade name for cephapirin sodium.

cefamandole nafate. USP. An antibacterial drug. Trade name is Mandol.

cefotoxin sodium. USP. An antibacterial drug.

Celbenin. Trade name for methicillin sodium.

-cele [Gr. *kele,* hernia]. Suffix indicating a swelling or tumor.

Celestone. Trade name for betamethasone.

celiac (sē'lē-ăk) [Gr. *koilia,* belly]. Rel. to the abdominal regions.

celiac artery. The first branch of the abdominal aorta. Branches supply the stomach, liver, spleen, duodenum, and pancreas.

celiac disease. Intestinal malabsorption syndrome characterized by diarrhea, malnutrition, bleeding tendency, and hypocalcemia.

TREATMENT: Gluten-free diet that may have to be continued for an indefinite period.

celiac plexus. Sympathetic plexus lying near the origin of celiac artery. SEE: *Nerve Plexuses* in *Appendix*.

celiectomy (sē″lē-ĕk′tō-mē) [″ + *ektome,* excision]. 1. Surgical removal of an abdominal organ. 2. Excision of celiac branches of vagus nerve.

celiocentesis (sē″lē-ō-sĕn-tē′sĭs) [″ + *kentesis,* puncture]. Puncture of the abdomen.

celiocolpotomy (sē″lē-ō-kōl-pŏt′ō-mē) [″ + *kolpos,* vagina, + *tome,* incision]. Surgical incision of the vagina through the abdominal wall.

celioenterotomy (sē″lē-ō-ĕn″tĕr-ŏt′ō-mē) [″ + *enteron,* intestine, + *tome,* incision]. Incision in the abdominal wall to gain access to the intestines.

celiogastrostomy (sē″lē-ō-găs-trŏs′tō-mē) [″ + *gaster,* stomach, + *stoma,* opening]. Incision in the abdominal wall for making a gastric fistula. SYN: *laparogastrostomy.*

celiogastrotomy (sē″lē-ō-găs-trŏt′ō-mē) [Gr. *koilia,* belly, + *gaster,* stomach, + *tome,* incision]. Incision into the stomach through the abdominal wall.

celiohysterectomy (sē″lē-ō-hĭs-tĕr-ĕk′tō-mē) [″ + *hystera,* uterus, + *ektome,* excision]. Removal of uterus through the abdomen.

celiohysterotomy (sē″lē-ō-hĭs″tĕr-ŏt′ō-mē) [″ + ″ + *tome,* incision]. Opening into the uterus through an abdominal incision.

celioma (sē-lē-ō′mă) [″ + *oma,* tumor]. An abdominal tumor.

celiomyalgia (sē″lē-ō-mī-ăl′gē-ă) [″ + *mys,* muscle, + *algos,* pain]. Rheumatic pain in muscles of the abdomen.

celiomyomectomy (sē″lē-ō-mī″ō-mĕk′tō-mē) [″ + ″ + *oma,* tumor, + *ektome,* excision]. Cutting of muscular tissue via an abdominal incision.

celiomyomotomy (sē″lē-ō-mī″ō-mŏt′ō-mē) [″ + ″ + ″ + *tome,* incision]. Incision of muscles of the abdomen.

celiomyositis (sē″lē-ō-mī″ō-sī′tĭs) [″ + ″ + *itis,* inflammation]. Inflammation of muscles of the abdomen.

celioparacentesis (sē″lē-ō-păr″ă-sĕn-tē′sĭs) [″ + *para,* beside, + *kentesis,* puncture]. Puncture of the abdomen for purposes of tapping or drainage.

celiopathy (sē″lē-ŏp′ă-thē) [″ + *pathos,* disease]. Any disease of the abdomen.

celiorrhaphy (sē″lē-or′ă-fē) [″ + *rhaphe,* suture]. Suture of wound in the abdominal wall. SYN: *laparorrhaphy.*

celiosalpingectomy (sē″lē-ō-săl″pĭn-jĕk′tō-mē) [″ + *salpinx,* tube, + *ektome,* excision]. Removal of the fallopian tubes through an abdominal incision.

celioscope (sē′lē-ō-skōp) [″ + *skopein,* to examine]. An endoscope for visual examination of a body cavity.

celioscopy (sē″lē-ŏs′kō-pē). Examination of a body cavity through a celioscope.

celiotomy (sē″lē-ŏt′ō-mē) [″ + *tome,* incision]. Surgical incision into the abdominal cavity.

c., vaginal. Incision into the abdomen through the vagina.

celitis (sē-lī′tĭs) [″ + *itis,* inflammation]. Abdominal inflammation. SYN: *peritonitis.*

cell [L. *cella,* a chamber]. 1. A small enclosed or partly enclosed cavity such as an air cell. 2. A mass of protoplasm containing a nucleus or nuclear material. It is the unit of structure of all animals and plants. SEE: illus.

Cells and the products of cells comprise all the tissues of the body. All functional activities of the body are carried on by cells, and the structure and form of a cell are closely correlated with its functions. Cells arise only from pre-existing cells, new cells arising by cell division. Growth and development result from the increase in numbers of cells and the differentiation of cells into different types of tissues. Specialized germ cells, the spermatozoa and ova, contain in their nuclei the genes for hereditary characteristics.

Meiosis, q.v., is one type of cell division, in which two successive divisions of the nucleus of germ cells produce cells that contain half the number of chromosomes present in somatic cells. *Mitosis,* q.v., is the other type of cell division, in which each daughter cell contains the same number of chromosomes as the parent cell. SEE: *cell division* for illus.

Cell inclusions or paraplastic bodies include food substances (fat droplets, glycogen and protein granules); chromophilic substance (Nissl bodies); pigment granules (melanin); crystals of various substances; and secretory granules. Also present in the cytoplasm are submicroscopic bodies, once called microsomes, demonstrated by differential centrifugation. They are small fragments of the endoplasmic reticulum and contain particles of ribonucleoprotein (ribosomes). Thus, microsomes should be called ribosomes. Ribosomes are important in protein synthesis within the cell.

STRUCTURE: When a typical cell is killed, fixed, and stained, it exhibits a centrally located nucleus surrounded by cytoplasm.

Nucleus: The nucleus possesses a nuclear membrane that encloses clear karyoplasm. One or more densely staining bodies, the nucleoli, usually are present.

Cytoplasm: This includes the cell protoplasm lying outside the nucleus. Its outermost layer constitutes the cell membrane, which forms the limiting membrane of the cell. Within the ground substance of the cytoplasm is the ergastoplasm (granular en-

THE CELL

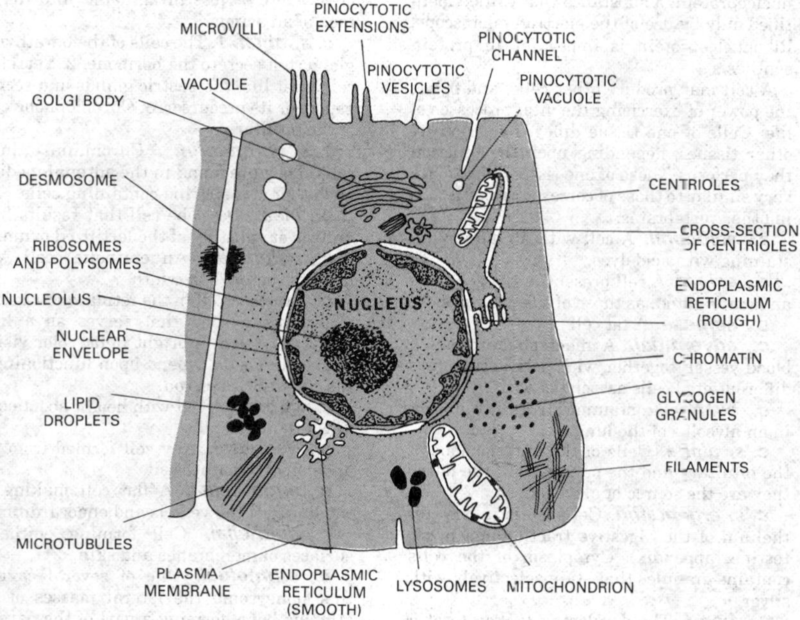
MICROVILLI
PINOCYTOTIC EXTENSIONS
PINOCYTOTIC CHANNEL
PINOCYTOTIC VESICLES
PINOCYTOTIC VACUOLE
VACUOLE
GOLGI BODY
DESMOSOME
CENTRIOLES
CROSS-SECTION OF CENTRIOLES
RIBOSOMES AND POLYSOMES
NUCLEUS
NUCLEOLUS
ENDOPLASMIC RETICULUM (ROUGH)
NUCLEAR ENVELOPE
CHROMATIN
LIPID DROPLETS
GLYCOGEN GRANULES
FILAMENTS
MICROTUBULES
PLASMA MEMBRANE
ENDOPLASMIC RETICULUM (SMOOTH)
LYSOSOMES
MITOCHONDRION

TYPES OF HUMAN CELLS

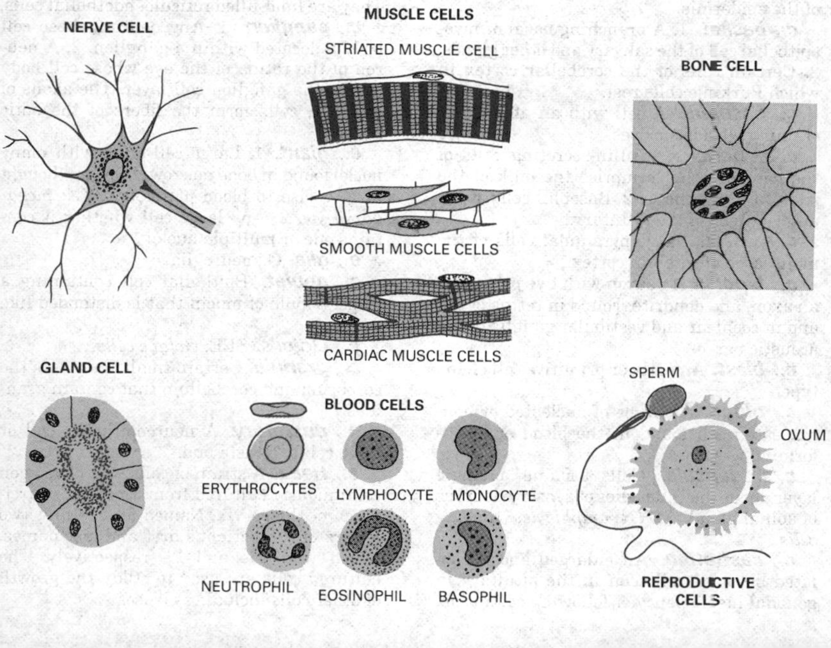
MUSCLE CELLS
NERVE CELL
STRIATED MUSCLE CELL
BONE CELL
SMOOTH MUSCLE CELLS
CARDIAC MUSCLE CELLS
GLAND CELL
BLOOD CELLS
ERYTHROCYTES
LYMPHOCYTE
MONOCYTE
NEUTROPHIL
EOSINOPHIL
BASOPHIL
SPERM
OVUM
REPRODUCTIVE CELLS

doplasmic reticulum), which contains ribonucleoprotein, a substance that can be identified only by use of the electron microscope. Ribonucleoprotein is important in protein synthesis.

A cell may produce other cells, and it has the power of exercising the vital processes of life. Cells of one tissue differ from those of other tissues, depending upon the function they perform. Those of one tissue in man are very similar to those of corresponding tissues in other vertebrates.

c., acidophil. A cell with an affinity for staining with acid dyes.

c., acinar. A cell present in the acinus of an acinar gland, as those of the pancreas.

c., adipose. A fat cell.

c., adventitial. A macrophage along a blood vessel, together with perivascular undifferentiated cells associated with it.

c., air. A cell containing air such as present in an alveolus of the lung.

c.'s, alpha. Cells of the anterior lobe of the pituitary and the pancreas. In the latter they are the source of glucagon.

c.'s, argentaffin. Cells found in the epithelium of the digestive tract (stomach, intestine, appendix). Cytoplasm of the cells contains granules that stain selectively with silver.

c., band. The developing leukocyte at a stage at which the nucleus is not segmented.

c., basal. A type of cell in the basal layer of the epidermis.

c., basket. 1. A branching basal or myoepithelial cell of the salivary and other glands. 2. Certain cells of the cerebellar cortex in which Purkinje cells rest.

c., basophil. A cell with an affinity for staining with basic dyes.

c.'s, beta. 1. Insulin-secreting cells of the pancreas that comprise the bulk of the islets of Langerhans. 2. Basophil cells of the anterior lobe of the pituitary.

c.'s, Betz. Large pyramidal cells of the motor area of cerebral cortex.

c., bipolar. A neuron with two processes, an axon, and dendrite. Found in retina of eye and in cochlear and vestibular ganglia of the acoustic nerve.

c., blast. An early or primitive cell of any type.

c., blood. Any type of nucleated or non-nucleated cell found in the blood or blood-forming tissues.

c.'s, capsule. Cells forming a single layer about the cell bodies of sensory neurons of spinal ganglia. SYN: *amphicytes; satellite cells.*

c., castration. An enlarged and vacuolated basophil cell seen in the pituitary in gonadal insufficiency or following castration.

c., centroacinar. A duct cell of the pancreas more or less invaginated into the lumen of an acinus.

c.'s, chief. 1. The cells of the parathyroid gland that secrete the hormone. 2. Secretory cells that line the gastric glands and secrete pepsin or its precursor. 3. Chromophobe cells of the pituitary.

c.'s, chromaffin. Chromium-staining cells. They are found in the adrenal medulla and other epinephrine-containing cells.

c., cleavage. The cell that results from mitosis or splitting of the fertilized ovum.

c., columnar. An epithelial cell with height greater than width.

c., cone. A cell in the retina whose scleral end forms a cone that serves as a light receptor. Vision in bright light, color vision, and acute vision depend upon functioning of the cones. SEE: *c., rod.*

c., cuboid. A cell with height about equal to width and depth.

c., daughter. Any cell formed from the division of a mother cell.

c., endothelial. A flat cell making up the lining of the vessels and endocardium.

c., epithelial. Cell forming epithelial surfaces of membranes and skin.

c., ethmoidal. One of several cavities that honeycomb the lateral masses of the ethmoid bone, forming a part of the paranasal air sinuses. SYN: *ethmoid sinus.*

c.'s, foam. Cells that contain vacuoles. They are lipid-filled reticuloendothelial cells.

c., ganglion. 1. Any neuron whose cell body is located within a ganglion. 2. A neuron of the retina of the eye whose cell body lies in the ganglion cell layer. The axons of ganglion cells form the fibers of the optic nerve.

c., giant. 1. Large cell often with many nuclei found in bone marrow. They are thought to give rise to blood platelets. SYN: *megakaryocyte.* 2. Any large cell whether it contains one or multiple nuclei.

c., glia. C., neuroglia.

c., goblet. Epithelial cell containing a large globule of mucin that is distended like a goblet.

c., Golgi's. SEE: *Golgi's cells.*

c., granule. Certain small neurons of the cerebrum and cerebellum that contain granules.

c., gustatory. A neuroepithelial cell or taste cell of a taste bud.

c., HeLa. A strain of cells that have been continuously cultured from a patient's carcinoma of the cervix. Named for the first two letters of the patient's first and last names, which were He and La respectively. The cultured cells are used to study the growth of other cells including viruses.

c., horizontal. A neuron of the inner nuclear layer of the retina. The axons of these cells run horizontally and serve to connect various parts of the retina.

c.'s, Hürthle. Large eosinophil-staining cells occasionally present in the thyroid gland.

c., hybridoma. SEE: *hybridoma cell.*

c., interstitial. One of the many cells found in connective tissue of the ovary and the seminiferous tubules of the testes, accounting for their internal secretion.

c.'s, islet. Cells of the islet of Langerhans of the pancreas.

c., juxtaglomerular. Cell of the juxtaglomerular apparatus of the kidney. These granulated cells are thought to produce renin.

c., Kupffer. A fixed phagocytic cell found in the sinusoids of the liver.

c., L.E. Abbreviation for *lupus erythematosus,* q.v., cell. A mature neutrophilic polymorphonuclear leukocyte characteristic of lupus erythematosus. SEE: *L. E. cell.*

c., Leydig's. The interstitial cells of the testes.

c., littoral. A macrophage found in the sinuses of lymphatic tissue.

c., lutein. A cell of the corpus luteum of the ovary that contains fatty granules of a yellowish color. Granulose lutein cells are hypertrophied follicle cells; these lutein (paralutein) cells develop from the theca interna.

c., mast. A cell found in connective tissue of vertebrates that contains heparin and histamine.

c.'s, mastoid. The air cells in the mastoid process of the temporal bone.

c.'s, microglia. Neuroglial cells of mesodermal origin present in the brain and spinal cord.

c., mother. Any type of cell that divides and gives rise to two or more cells. The latter are called daughter cells.

c., mucous. A cell that secretes mucus found in mucus-secreting glands.

c., myeloma. The cell present in the bone marrow of patients with multiple myeloma.

c., nerve. The special cell of nerves that have processes extending from the cell body. One process, the axon, transmits nerve impulses, and the others, dendrites, receive impulses and transmit them to the cell body.

c.'s, neuroglia. Non-nerve cells of the supporting tissue of the central nervous system and the retina of the eye. Includes astrocytes, oligodendrocytes, and microglia.

c., Niemann-Pick. A foamy, lipid-filled cell present in the spleen and bone marrow in Niemann-Pick's disease.

c., olfactory. A special cell of the olfactory mucosa that has a combined neuroepithelial function.

c., oxyntic. Parietal cell of the stomach. In the human, hydrochloric acid, q.v., is formed in these cells.

c., parent. C., mother.

c.'s, phalangeal. Cells that support the hair cells of the organ of Corti. They form several rows of outer phalangeal cells (Deiter's cells) and a single row of inner phalangeal cells.

c., pigment. Any cell that normally contains pigment granules.

c.'s, plasma. Cells derived from lymphoid elements. They are found in lymphoid tissue and the cellular connective tissue of the intestinal tract. They are important in antibody production.

c., prickle. A cell possessing spinelike protoplasmic processes that connect with similar processes of adjoining cells. Found in the stratum germinativum of the epidermis.

c.'s, primordial. The original germ cells that in the embryo migrate to the gonadal ridge, where they form all of the germ cells.

c., Purkinje's. Cell of the cerebral cortex of the brain with dendrites extending into the molecular layer and axons that go to the white matter of the cerebellum.

c., pus. A leukocyte present in pus. Cells of this type are often degenerated or necrotic.

c., pyramidal. A nerve cell of the cerebral cortex.

c., red. The erythrocyte of the blood, the principal purpose of which is to transport oxygen to the cells of the body. The hemoglobin that the red cell contains is oxygenated in the lungs and the oxygen is released to the tissues throughout the body.

c., reticular. The undifferentiated cell of the spleen, bone marrow, and lymphatic tissue that has the potential to develop into one of several types of connective tissue cells or into macrophages.

c.'s, reticuloendothelial. Reticular or endothelial cells of the reticuloendothelial system, q.v.

c., Rieder. Myeloblast that may be present in acute leukemia, possessing a lobulated or double nucleus.

c., rod. A cell in the retina of the eye whose scleral end is long and narrow, forming a rod, a sensory element of the eye. Rods are stimulated by dim light. SEE: *c., cone.*

c., rosette. Nuclear material surrounded by phagocytes. These cells occur frequently in blood in which L.E. cells are present. The rosette cell is not diagnostic of lupus erythematosus. SEE: *L.E. cell.*

c., Rouget. Cells with branching processes that, in a frog, surround the walls of a capillary. They are capable of contracting upon stimulation.

c.'s, satellite. 1. Flat epithelium-like cells

forming the inner portion of a double-layered capsule that covers a neuron. 2. Neuroglial cells enclosing the cell bodies of neurons in spinal ganglia.

c., segmented. A segmented neutrophil, i.e., one with a nucleus of two or more lobes connected together by slender filaments.

c., sensory. A cell that when stimulated gives rise to nerve impulses that are conveyed to the central nervous system.

c.'s, septal. Cells attached to or in the septa of the lungs. They function in some animals as macrophages.

c., Sertoli. A supporting tissue cell of the seminiferous tubules of the testicle. Spermatids attach to these cells until they become mature spermatozoa.

c., sickle. An abnormal erythrocyte shaped like a sickle. SEE: *anemia, sickle cell.*

c., signet-ring. A vacuolated cell with the nucleus off center. Mucus-secreting adenocarcinomas usually contain these cells.

c., somatic. A body cell rather than a germ cell.

c., spider. An astrocyte.

c., squamous. Flat scalelike epithelial cell.

c., stellate. A star-shaped cell with processes extending out from it.

c., Sternberg-Reed; c., Reed-Sternberg. A giant multinucleated cell seen in Hodgkin's disease.

c., stipple. A red blood cell that contains small basophilic-staining dots. Seen in lead poisoning, malaria, severe anemia, and leukemia.

c., sympathicotrophic. Large epithelial cells occurring in groups in the hilus of the ovary. Thought to be chromaffin cells.

c., sympathochromaffin. Chromaffin cells of ectodermal origin present in the fetal adrenal gland. Sympathetic and medullary cells arise from them.

c., target. An erythrocyte with a rounded, central area surrounded by a clear ring lightly stained, and this in turn surrounded by a dense ring of peripheral protoplasm. Present in certain blood disorders.

c., tart. Phagocytes that have ingested unaltered nuclei of cells. These nuclei are observed unchanged within the phagocytic cell.

c., taste. Cell of a taste bud.

c., totipotent. Undifferentiated embryonic cell that has the potential for developing into any type of cell.

c., Türk's irritation. A cell resembling a plasma cell, found in cases of severe anemia or chronic infection.

c., visual. A rod or cone cell of the retina.

c., wandering. A macrophage capable of ameboid movement.

c., white. Any one of the leukocytes of the blood.

c.'s, zymogenic. Chief cells or enzyme-producing cells of the gastric glands.

cell culture. The growth of cells in vitro, q.v., for experimental purposes. The cells proliferate but do not organize into tissue.

cell division. The fission of a cell. SEE: *meiosis; mitosis;* illus.

cell growth cycle. The order of physical and biochemical events that occur during growth of cells. In tissue culture studies, the cyclic changes are divided into specific periods or phases: the DNA synthesis or S period; the G-2 period or gap; the M or mitotic period; and the G-1 period.

cell mass. In embryology, the mass of cells that develops into an organ or structure.

cell membrane. The membrane that encloses the cell. Composed of proteins, lipids, and carbohydrates.

cellobiose (sĕl″ō-bī′ōs). A disaccharide resulting from the hydrolysis of cellulose.

cellophane (sĕl′ō-fān). Thin, transparent, waterproof sheet of cellulose acetate. Used as a dialysis membrane.

cell organelle. Any of the structures in the cytoplasm of a cell. Includes the cell membrane, mitochondria, endoplasmic reticulum, Golgi complex, ribosomes, lysosomes, nucleus, and centriole. SEE: *organelle* for illus.

cell receptor. SEE: *receptor.*

cellula (sĕl′ū-lă) [L., little cell]. (pl. *cellulae*) [NA] 1. A minute cell. 2. A small compartment.

cellular (sĕl′ū-lăr). Pert. to, composed of, or derived from cells.

cellulase (sĕl′ū-lās). An enzyme that converts cellulose to cellobiose. Present in some microorganisms and marine life.

cellulicidal (sĕl″ū-lĭ-sī′dăl) [″ + *caedere,* to kill]. Destructive to cells.

cellulifugal (sĕl″ū-lĭf′ū-găl) [″ + *fugere,* to flee]. Extending or moving away from a cell.

cellulipetal (sĕl″ū-lĭp′ĭ-tăl) [″ + *petere,* to seek]. Extending or moving toward a cell.

cellulitis (sĕl-ū-lī′tĭs) [″ + Gr. *itis,* inflammation]. Inflammation of cellular or connective tissue, spreading as in erysipelas. An infection in or close to the skin is usually localized by the body defense mechanisms. However, if inflammation spreads through the tissue, the process is called cellulitis.

c., pelvic. Inflammation of the parametrium, q.v. May occur in puerperal fever or septic conditions of the uterus and appendages. SYN: *parametritis.*

cellulofibrous (sĕl″ū-lō-fī′brŭs) [″ + *fibra,* fiber]. Both cellular and fibrous.

celluloneuritis (sĕl″ū-lō-nū-rī′tĭs) [″ + Gr. *neuron,* nerve, + *itis,* inflammation]. Inflam-

CELL DIVISION

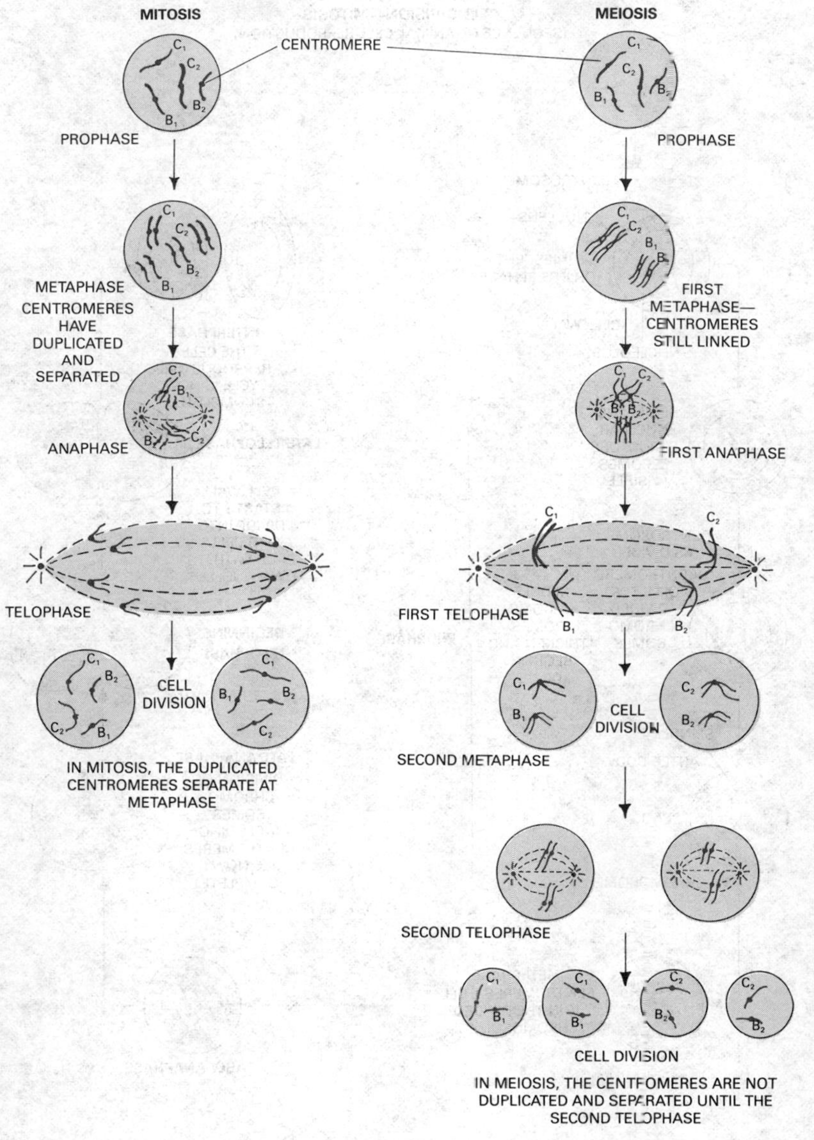
MITOSIS
MEIOSIS
CENTROMERE
C1
C2
B1
B2
PROPHASE
METAPHASE
CENTROMERES HAVE DUPLICATED AND SEPARATED
ANAPHASE
TELOPHASE
CELL DIVISION
IN MITOSIS, THE DUPLICATED CENTROMERES SEPARATE AT METAPHASE
FIRST METAPHASE—CENTROMERES STILL LINKED
FIRST ANAPHASE
FIRST TELOPHASE
SECOND METAPHASE
SECOND TELOPHASE
IN MEIOSIS, THE CENTROMERES ARE NOT DUPLICATED AND SEPARATED UNTIL THE SECOND TELOPHASE

CELL DIVISION—MITOSIS
(SEQUENCE OF ANIMAL CELL REPRODUCTION)

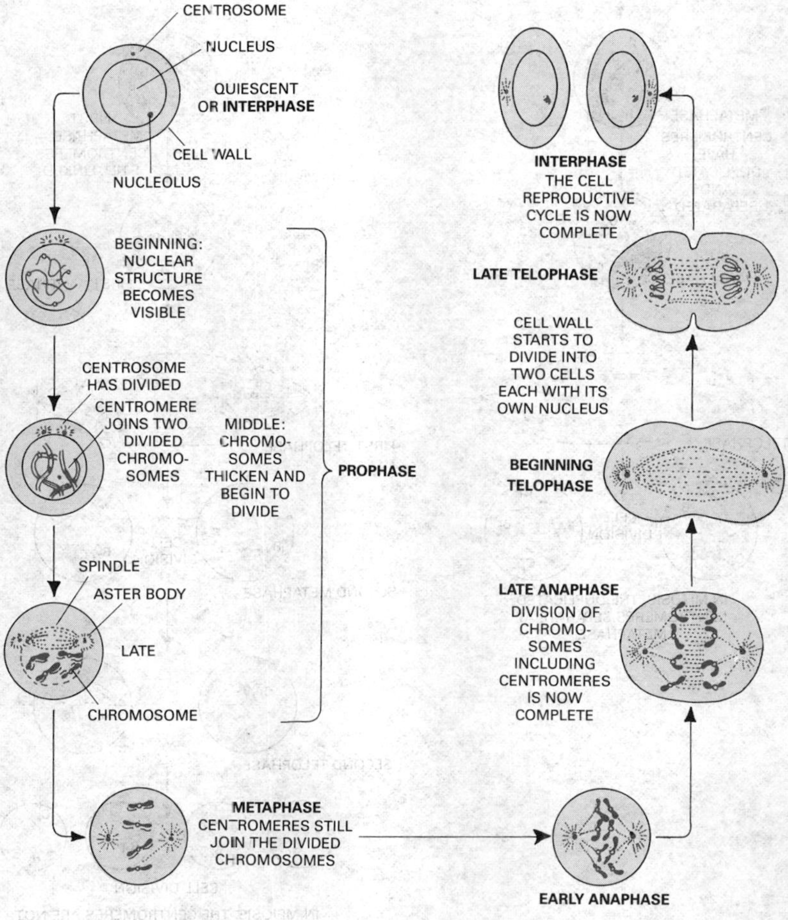
CENTROSOME
NUCLEUS
QUIESCENT OR INTERPHASE
CELL WALL
NUCLEOLUS
BEGINNING: NUCLEAR STRUCTURE BECOMES VISIBLE
CENTROSOME HAS DIVIDED
CENTROMERE JOINS TWO DIVIDED CHROMO- SOMES
MIDDLE: CHROMO- SOMES THICKEN AND BEGIN TO DIVIDE
PROPHASE
SPINDLE
ASTER BODY
LATE
CHROMOSOME
METAPHASE
CENTROMERES STILL JOIN THE DIVIDED CHROMOSOMES
EARLY ANAPHASE
LATE ANAPHASE
DIVISION OF CHROMO- SOMES INCLUDING CENTROMERES IS NOW COMPLETE
BEGINNING TELOPHASE
CELL WALL STARTS TO DIVIDE INTO TWO CELLS EACH WITH ITS OWN NUCLEUS
LATE TELOPHASE
INTERPHASE
THE CELL REPRODUCTIVE CYCLE IS NOW COMPLETE

mation of nerve cells.

c., acute anterior. Acute anterior poliomyelitis.

cellulose (sĕl'ū-lōs) [L. *cellula,* little cell]. Plant fiber; a fibrous form of carbohydrate, $(C_6H_{10}O_5)_n$, constituting the supporting framework of plants. It is composed of a great number of glucose units. When ingested, it stimulates peristalsis and aids in intestinal elimination. When ingested by humans cellulose provides no nutrient value because it is not chemically changed or absorbed in digestion; it remains a polysaccharide, q.v.

Some foods that contain cellulose are: apples, apricots, asparagus, beans, beets, bran flakes, broccoli, cabbage, celery, mushrooms, oatmeal, onions, oranges, parsnips, prunes, spinach, turnips, wheat flakes, whole grains, whole wheat bread. SEE: *fiber, dietary.*

c., oxidized. USP. Cellulose that has been oxidized by nitrogen dioxide and is made to resemble cotton or gauze. Used to arrest bleeding by direct application to site of hemorrhage.

c. sodium, carboxymethyl. USP. A hydrophilic cellulose derivative used as a bulk-forming type of laxative. It is also used as a food additive for the purpose of thickening various types of prepared foods. ABBR: CMC.

cellulotoxic (sĕl"ū-lō-tŏk'sĭk) [" + Gr. *toxikon,* poison]. 1. Poisonous to cells. 2. Caused by cell toxins.

cell wall. Cell membrane. Plant cells are enclosed by a wall that contains cellulose. This membrane actively and passively regulates the flow of all substances in and out of the cell.

celology (sē-lŏl'ō-jē) [Gr. *kele,* hernia, + *logos,* study]. The surgical study of hernias.

celom, celoma (sē'lŏm, sē-lō'mă) [Gr. *koiloma,* a hollow]. The coelom, q.v.

Celontin. Trade name for methsuximide.

celoschisis (sē-lŏs'kĭ-sĭs) [Gr. *koilia,* belly, + *schisis,* fissure]. Congenital fissure of the abdominal wall.

celoscope (sē'lō-skōp) [" + *skopein,* to examine]. Device for visual examination of a body cavity.

celosomia (sē-lō-sō'mē-ă) [" + *soma,* body]. Congenital fissure of sternum with herniation of fetal viscera.

celozoic [" + *zoon,* animal]. Inhabiting the intestinal cavity of the body, said of parasitic protozoa.

Celsius scale (sĕl'sē-ŭs). [Anders Celsius, Swedish astronomer, 1701–1744] A temperature scale on which the boiling point of water is 100° and the melting point of ice is 0°. This is the official scientific name of the temperature scale that is also known as centigrade. SEE: *Miscellaneous Units of Measurement* in *Appendix.*

cement (sē-mĕnt'). 1. Any material that when prepared in the appropriate manner hardens into a firm mass. 2. The process of causing two objects to stick together as would be the case in using an adhesive to join a gold inlay to the cavity of a tooth. 3. The material used to make one substance adhere to another.

cementicle (sē-mĕn'tĭ-kl). Small calcified area in the periodontal membrane of the root of a tooth.

cementitis (sē"mĕn-tī'tĭs) [L. *cementum,* cement, – Gr. *itis,* inflammation]. Inflammation of the dental cementum.

cementoblast (sē-mĕn'tō-blăst) [" + Gr. *blastos,* germ]. A cell of the inner layer of the dental sac of a developing tooth. It deposits cementum, q.v., upon the dentin of the root.

cementoclasia (sē-mĕn"tō-klā'sē-ă) [" + Gr. *klasis,* breaking]. Decay of the cementum of a tooth root.

cementoclast (sē-mĕn'tō-klăst). A multinucleated cell of great size associated with the removal of cementum during root resorption, more correctly referred to as an odontoclast.

cementoma (sē"mĕn-tō'mă) [" + Gr. *oma,* tumor]. A tumor having its origin in the substantia ossea.

cementum (sē-mĕn'tŭm) [L.]. [NA] Thin layer of modified bone formed by cementoblasts and deposited upon the dentin of the root of a tooth; the substantia ossea. To it is attached the alveolar periosteum or periodontal membrane, which binds the tooth to its socket

cenesthesia (sĕ"nĕs-thē'zē-ă) [Gr. *koinos,* common, + *aisthesis,* feeling]. The normal feeling of being alive and aware.

cenesthesic, cenesthetic. Pert. to cenesthesia.

cenesthopathia, cenesthopathy (sē-nĕs-, sĕn-ĕs-thō-păth'ē-ă, -thŏp'ă-thē) [" + " + *pathos,* disease]. Malaise or a general feeling of ill-being. Not referable to a specific part of the body.

Cenolate. Trade name for ascorbic acid.

cenosis (sĕn-ō', sē-nō'sĭs) [Gr. *kenos,* empty, + *osis,* condition]. A morbid discharge.

cenosite (sĕn'ō-, sē'nō-sīt) [Gr. *koinos,* common, + *sitos,* food]. A microorganism not depending for life upon its host, but parasitic in character.

cenotic (sĕn-ŏt', sē-nŏt'ĭk) [Gr. *kenos,* empty]. Pert. to cenosis.

cenotophobia (sĕn"ō-, sē"nō-tō-fō'bē-ă) [Gr. *kainotes,* novelty, + *phobos,* fear]. Morbid aversion to new things and new ideas. SYN: *cainotophobia.*

cenotype (sē'nō-, sĕn'ō-tīp) [" + *typos,* a type]. An original type; term used in ontogeny and cytology.

censor (sĕn'sĕr) [L. *censor,* judge]. In psychoanalysis, a psychic inhibition that prevents abhorrent unconscious thoughts or impulses from seeking objective expression unless in a form unrecognized at the conscious level.

center (sĕn′tĕr) [L. *centrum*, center]. 1. Middle point of a body. 2. A group of nerve cells within the central nervous system that controls a specific activity or function.

c., apneustic. A center in the brain stem that regulates breathing.

c., auditory. Center for hearing in the anterior gyri of the transverse temporal gyri. SEE: *area, auditory.*

c., autonomic. A center in the brain or spinal cord that regulates any of the activities under the control of the autonomic nervous system. There are a few cortical centers but most are located in the hypothalamus, medulla oblongata, and spinal cord.

c., Broca's. Center in the inferior frontal gyrus that controls motor aspects of speech. SYN: *c., speech*. SEE: *Broca's area.*

c., cardioaccelerator. A center in the medulla oblongata that gives rise to impulses that speed up the heart rate. Impulses reach the heart by way of sympathetic fibers.

c., cardioinhibitory. A center in the medulla oblongata containing neurons whose axons, parasympathetic fibers, pass by way of the vagus nerves to the heart. Impulses from this center cause the heart rate to slow down.

c., chondrification. A center of cartilage formation.

c., ciliospinal. A center in the spinal cord from which arise sympathetic impulses that dilate the pupils of the eyes.

c.'s, defecation. Two centers, a medullary center located in the medulla oblongata and a spinal center located in second to fourth sacral segments of the spinal cord. The anospinal centers control the sphincter reflexes for the process of defecation.

c., deglutition. A center in the medulla oblongata on the floor of the fourth ventricle that controls swallowing.

c., epiotic. Ossification center of mastoid process.

c., germinal. An area in lymph node tissue that responds in a specific manner to antigenic stimulation.

c., gustatory. Cerebral center that is supposed to control taste. SYN: *taste area.*

c.'s, heat-regulating. Two centers, a heat loss center and a heat-production center, located in the hypothalamus. They regulate body temperature.

c., higher. 1. A center in the cerebrum from which impulses based on conscious sensations, wishes, or desires are initiated. 2. A center in any portion of the brain, in contrast to one in the cord.

c., lower. Center in the brain, stem or spinal cord.

c., medullary. An area in the brain stem that regulates respiratory activity.

c., micturition. Center controlling reflexes of urinary bladder. Located in second to fourth and fourth to sixth sacral segments of the cord; higher centers are present in medulla oblongata, hypothalamus, and cerebrum.

c., motor cortical. The area in the frontal lobe, the origin of impulses for voluntary movements.

c., nerve. One of many centers in cerebrospinal or ganglionic systems originating or controlling vital function.

c., ossification. Spot where ossification begins in bones.

c., pneumotaxic. Center in the pons that rhythmically inhibits inspiration.

c.'s, psychocortical. Centers of cerebral cortex concerned with voluntary muscular movements.

c., reflex. A region within the brain or spinal cord where connections (synapses) are made between afferent and efferent neurons of a reflex arc.

c., respiratory. A region in the medulla oblongata that controls respiratory movements. It consists of inspiratory, expiratory, and pneumotaxic centers.

c., speech. Center in the inferior frontal gyrus that controls motor aspects of speech.

c., taste. C., gustatory.

c., temperature. C., thermoregulatory.

c., thermoregulatory. Temperature-regulating centers in the hypothalamus.

c., trophic. One of many centers located in cerebrospinal and sympathetic systems presiding over nutrition.

c., vasoconstrictor. A center in the medulla that brings about the constriction of blood vessels.

c., vasodilator. A center located in the medulla oblongata that brings about vasodilation of blood vessels.

c., vasomotor. A center through which the diameter of blood vessels is controlled; the vasoconstrictor and vasodilator centers.

c., visual. Center in occipital lobe that controls sight.

c., Wernicke's. An area in the dominant hemisphere of the brain that functions to recall, recognize, and interpret words and other sounds in the process of using language.

c., word. An area in the dominant hemisphere of the brain that functions to recognize and perceive spoken or written words.

Centers for Disease Control. ABBR: CDC. Division of the U.S. Public Health Service, in Atlanta, Georgia, for investigation and control of various diseases, esp. those that have epidemic potential.

centesis (sĕn-tē′sĭs) [Gr. *kentesis*, puncture]. Puncture of a cavity.

centigrade (sĕn′tĭ-grād) [L. *centum*, a hundred, + *gradus*, a step]. ABBR: C. 1. Having 100 degrees. 2. Pert. to a thermometer divided into 100°. The boiling point of water is 100° and the freezing point is 0°. The official scientific name for the centigrade scale is Celsius. SEE: *thermometer*.

centigram (sĕn′tĭ-grăm) [" + Gr. *gramma*, a small weight]. A measure of weight; the hundredth part of a gram; 0.15432 gr. SEE: *metric system; Metric System* in *Appendix*.

centiliter (sĕn′tĭ-lē-tĕr) [" + Gr. *litra*, measure of wt.]. One-hundredth part of a liter (1 liter equals approx. 33 fluid ounces); 10 ml. SEE: *metric system*.

centimeter (sĕn′tĭ-mē-tĕr) [" + Gr. *metron*, measure]. ABBR: cm. Unit of length in metric system, q.v. One-hundredth part of a meter. To convert centimeters to inches, multiply by 0.3937. To convert inches to centimeters, multiply by 2.54.

centinormal (sĕn″tĭ-nor′măl) [" + *norma*, rule]. One-hundredth part of the normal, as the strength of a solution.

centipede (sĕn′tĭ-pēd″) [" + *pes*, foot]. An arthropod of the subclass Chilopoda characterized by an elongated flattened body of many segments, each with a pair of jointed legs. The first pair of appendages are hooklike claws bearing openings of ducts from poison glands. The bites of large tropical centipedes may cause severe local and sometimes general symptoms but they are rarely fatal.

centipoise (sĕn′tĭ-poyz). A unit of viscosity one one-hundredth of a poise. SEE: *poise*.

centrad (sĕn′trăd) [Gr. *kentron*, center, + L. *ad*, toward]. Toward the center.

central (sĕn′trăl). Situated at, or rel. to, a center.

central core disease. A rare form of benign familial polymyopathy characterized by hypotonia, delay in walking, and muscle weakness that does not progress. When stained in certain ways and studied microscopically, there is a central area of the muscle fibers that does not stain; thus, the name.

central nervous system. ABBR: CNS. Brain and spinal cord, with their nerves and end-organs that control voluntary acts. Includes parts of the brain governing consciousness and mental activities; parts of brain, spinal cord, and their sensory and motor nerve fibers controlling skeletal muscles; and end organs of the body wall. SEE: *autonomic, parasympathetic,* and *sympathetic nervous systems; brain* and *cranial nerves* for illus.

COMP: Nerve tissue that forms the brain, spinal cord, and the nerves from both. Tissue is made up of gray and white matter. Gray matter is composed of cells of nervous tissue, while the white matter is composed of nerve fibers from the cells. White matter in the brain and cord carries messages or impulses from the body or outside world to the cells or gray matter.

central venous pressure. ABBR: CVP. The pressure within the superior vena cava; it reflects the pressure under which the blood is returned to the right atrium. The normal range is between 5 and 10 cm. H_2O (2 to 8 mm. Hg). A high CVP indicates circulatory overload (as in congestive heart failure) whereas a low CVP indicates reduced blood volume (as in hemorrhage or fluid loss). CVP can be estimated by examination of the cervical veins or dorsal veins of the hand, if the neck and hand are at the level of the heart.

centraphose (sĕn′tră-fōz) [Gr. *kentron*, center, + *a-*, not, + *phos*, light]. A subjective sensation of darkness or light originating in the optic brain centers. SYN: *centrophose; chromophose*.

Centrax. Trade name for prazepam.

centre. Center.

centriciput (sĕn-trĭs′ĭ-pŭt) [" + L. *caput*, head]. The central part of the upper surface of the skull between the occiput and sinciput.

centrifugal (sĕn-trĭf′ū-găl) [" + L. *fugere*, to flee]. Receding from the center. SYN: *axifugal*. SEE: *centrifuge*.

centrifugal force. The force that impels a thing, or parts of it, outward from the center of rotation. SEE: *centrifuge*.

centrifuge (sĕn′trĭ-fūj). A device that spins test tubes at high speeds. Thus, centrifugal force, q.v., causes the heavy particles in the liquid in the tubes to settle to the bottom and the lighter liquid to go to the top. When unclotted blood is centrifuged the plasma goes to the top and the heavy red cells go to the bottom of the tube. The white blood cells are heavier than the plasma but lighter than the red blood cells. Therefore they form a thin layer between the red blood cells and the plasma.

centrilobular (sĕn″trĭ-lŏb′ū-lăr). Concerning the center of a lobule.

centriole (sĕn′trē-ōl). A minute organelle consisting of a hollow cylinder closed at one end and open at the other, found in the cell center or attraction sphere of a cell. Preceding mitosis it divides, forming two daughter centrioles (diplosomes). During mitosis the centrioles migrate to opposite poles of the cell and each forms the center of the aster to which the spindle fibers are attached: SEE: *mitosis*.

centripetal (sĕn-trĭp′ĕ-tăl) [" + L. *petere*, to seek]. Directed toward the axis. SYN: *axipetal*.

centrocyte (sěn′trō-sīt) [″ + *kytos,* cell]. A cell having single and double hematoxylin-stainable granules of varying size in its protoplasm.

centrodesmus (sěn-trō-děz′mŭs) [Gr. *kentron,* center, + *desmos,* a band]. The matter connecting the two centrosomes in a nucleus during mitosis.

centrolecithal (sěn″trō-lěs′ĭ-thăl) [″ + *lekithos,* yoke]. Pert. to an egg, esp. an ovum, with the yolk centrally located.

centromere (sěn′trō-mēr) [″ + *meros,* part]. A constricted region of a chromosome that divides the chromosome into two arms.

centrophose (sěn′trō-fōz) [″ + *phos,* light]. A subjective sensation of a light or dark spot having its origin in the optic brain centers. SYN: *centraphose.* SEE: *chromophose.*

centrosclerosis (sěn″trō-sklě-rō′sĭs) [″ + *sklerosis,* a hardening]. Filling of the bone marrow space with bone tissue.

centrosome (sěn′trō-sōm) [″ + *soma,* body]. A region of the cytoplasm of a cell usually lying near the nucleus, containing in its center one or two centricles, the diplosome. SEE: *mitosis.*

centrosphere (sěn′trō-sfēr) [″ + *sphaira,* sphere]. The cytoplasm of the centrosome.

centrostaltic (sěn″trō-stăl′tĭk) [″ + *stellein,* send forth]. Pert. to a center of motion.

centrum (sěn′trŭm) [L.]. (pl. *centra*) 1. Any center, esp. an anatomical one. 2. Body of a vertebra.

c. semiovale. A mass of white matter at center of each cerebral hemisphere.

c. tendineum. Central tendon of the diaphragm.

cephalad (sěf′ă-lăd) [Gr. *kephale,* head, + L. *ad,* toward]. Toward the head.

cephalalgia (sěf-ă-lăl′jē-ă) [″ + *algos,* pain]. Headache, pain in the head. A symptom of numerous diseases and disorders. SEE: *headache.*

cephalalgic (sěf-ăl-ăl′jĭk). Of the nature of cephalalgia.

cephalea (sěf-ă-lē′ă) [Gr. *kephale,* head]. Cephalalgia.

cephaledema (sěf″ăl-ē-dē′mă) [″ + *oidema,* swelling]. Edema of the head.

cephalexin (sěf″ă-lěk′sĭn). USP. An analogue of the antibiotic cephalosporin. Effective against gram-positive and gram-negative organisms. Trade name is Keflex.

cephalhematocele (sěf″ăl-hē-măt′ō-sēl) [″ + *haima,* blood, + *kele,* tumor]. A bloody tumor communicating with the dural sinuses.

cephalhematoma (sěf″ăl-hē″mă-tō′mă) [″ + ″ + *oma,* tumor]. A subcutaneous swelling containing blood, often found on the head of a baby several days after birth when delivery was accompanied by use of forceps. The swelling disappears within two to three months.

cephalic (sě-făl′ĭk) [L. *cephalicus*]. 1. Cranial; pert. to the head. 2. Superior in position.

cephalic index. An arbitrary measure of cranial capacity. Derived from the division of the maximal length of the head into the value of the maximal breadth multiplied by 100.

cephalin (sěf′ă-lĭn) [Gr. *kephale,* head]. A phospholipid, resembling lecithin, present in the brain of mammals.

cephalitis (sěf″ăl-ī′tĭs) [″ + *itis,* inflammation]. Encephalitis.

cephalocaudal pattern of development. Principle of maturation that motor development, control, and coordination progress from the head to the feet.

cephalocele (sěf′ă-lō-sēl) [″ + *kele,* hernia]. Protrusion of the brain from the cranial cavity.

cephalocentesis (sěf″ă-lō-sěn-tē′sĭs) [″ + *kentesis,* puncture]. Surgical puncture of cranium.

cephalodynia (sěf″ă-lō-dĭn′ē-ă) [″ + *odyne,* pain]. Pain in the head. SYN: *cephalalgia; headache.*

cephaloglycin (sěf″ă-lō-glī′sĭn). USP. An analogue of the antibiotic cephalosporin. Trade name is Kafocin.

cephalogyric (sěf″ă-lō-jī′rĭk) [″ + *gyros,* a turn]. Of or pert. to rotation of the head.

cephalohemometer (sěf″ă-lō-hē-mŏm′ē-tĕr) [″ + *haima,* blood, + *metron,* measure]. Instrument for determining changes in intracranial blood pressure.

cephalomenia (sěf″ă-lō-mē′nē-ă) [″ + *men,* month]. Vicarious menstruation from the nose or head.

cephalomeningitis (sěf″ă-lō-měn″ĭn-jī′tĭs) [″ + *meninx,* membrane, + *itis,* inflammation]. Inflammation of the cerebral meninges.

cephalometer (sěf-ă-lŏm′ē-tĕr) [″ + *metron,* measure]. Device for measuring the head.

cephalometry (sěf″ă-lŏm′ĕ-trē). Measurement of the head.

cephalomotor (sěf″ă-lō-mō′tor) [Gr. *kephale,* head, + L. *motus,* motion]. Pert. to movements of the head.

cephalone (sěf′ă-lōn) [″ + *on,* being]. A mentally retarded individual with a large head.

cephalonia (sěf″ă-lō′nē-ă). A condition marked by mental retardation and enlargement of the head.

cephalopathy (sěf″ă-lŏp′ă-thē) [″ + *pathos,* disease]. Any disease of the head or brain.

cephalopelvic (sěf″ă-lō-pěl′vĭk). Concerning the fetal head and the maternal pelvis; esp. the size of the pelvic outlet through which the fetal head will pass during delivery.

cephaloplegia (sěf″ă-lō-plē′jē-ă) [″ + *plege,* stroke]. Paralysis of muscles about head or, less accurately, face.

cephalorhachidian (sĕf″ă-lō-ră-kĭd′ē-ăn) [″ + *rhachis,* spine]. Pert. to the head and spine.

cephaloridine (sĕf″ă-lor′ĭ-dēn). USP. An analogue of the antibiotic cephalosporin C. Trade name is Loridine.

cephaloscope (sĕf′ă-lō-skōp) [″ + *skopein,* to examine]. Device for auscultation of the head.

cephalosporin (sĕf″ă-lō-spor′ĭn). General term for a group of antibiotic derivatives of cephalosporin C. Cephalosporin C is obtained from the fungus Cephalosporium.

cephalothin sodium (sĕf′ă-lō-thĭn″). USP. A semisynthetic analogue of the antibiotic cephalosporin C. Trade name is Keflin.

cephalothoracic (sĕf″ă-lō-thō-răs′ĭk) [″ + *thorakos,* chest]. Concerning the head and the thorax.

cephalothoracopagus (sĕf″ă-lō-thō″ră-kŏp′ă-gŭs) [″ + ″ + *pagos,* thing fixed]. A double fetus joined at head and thorax.

cephalotome (sĕf′ă-lō-tōm) [″ + *tome,* incision]. Instrument for cutting the head of the fetus.

cephalotomy (sĕf-ă-lŏt′ō-mē). Cutting the fetal head to facilitate delivery.

cephalotrypesis (sĕf″ă-lō-trĭp-ē′sĭs) [″ + *trypesis,* a boring]. Removing a portion of bone from the skull. SYN: *trephination.*

cephapirin sodium (sĕf-ă-pī′rĭn). USP. An antibiotic similar to cephalothin. Trade name is Cefadyl.

Cephulac. Trade name for lactulose.

ceptor (sĕp′tor) [L. *receptor,* receiver]. General term for a nerve ending that, upon being stimulated, passes the stimulus on to the cell to which the ceptor is attached.

c., chemical. Ceptor that initiates chemical reactions in the body.

c., contact. Ceptor that receives stimuli contributed by direct physical contact.

c., distance. Ceptor that perceives stimuli remote from the immediate environment.

cera (sē′ră) [L.]. Wax.

c. alba. White wax.

c. flava. Yellow wax.

ceramics, dental [Gr. *keramos,* potters' clay]. The use of porcelain or porcelain-type materials in dental work.

ceramide (sĕr′ă-mīd). A class of lipids that do not contain glycerol. They are derived from a sphingosine. Glycosphingolipids, q.v., and sphingomyelins, q.v., are derived from ceramides.

c. oligosaccharides. A class of glycosphingolipids.

ceramodontia (sē-răm″ō-dŏn′shē-ă) [Gr. *keramos,* potters' clay, + *odous,* tooth]. Dental ceramics.

cerate ceratum (sē′rāt) [L. *ceratum*]. A medicinal formulation for topical use containing wax and of such consistency that it may be spread easily at ordinary temperature upon muslin or similar material with a spatula, and yet not so soft as to liquefy and run when applied to the skin. Rarely prescribed.

ceratocele (sĕr′ă-tō-sēl) [Gr. *keras,* horn, + *kele,* hernia]. Hernia of Descemet's membrane through outer layer of the cornea. SYN: *keratocele.*

ceratotome (sē-răt′ō-tōm) [″ + *tome,* incision]. A knife for division of the cornea.

cercaria (sĕr-kā′rē-ă) [Gr. *kerkos,* tail]. (pl. *cercariae*) A free-swimming stage in the development of a fluke or trematode. Cercariae develop within sporocysts or redia that parasitize snails or bivalve mollusks. They emerge from the mollusk and either enter their final host directly or encyst in an intermediate host that is eaten by the final host. In the latter case, the encysted tailless form is known as a metacercaria SEE: *fluke; trematode.*

cerclage (sār-klŏzh′) [Fr., hooping]. Encircling tissues with a ligature, wire, or loop.

Cercomonas (sĕr-kŏm′ō-năs) [Gr. *kerkos,* tail, + *monas,* unit]. A genus of free-living, coprozoic, flagellate protozoa. May be present in stale specimens of feces or urine. Not pathogenic.

cercomoniasis (sĕr″kō-mō-nī′ă-sĭs). Infestation with Cercomonas intestinalis.

cercus (sĕr′kŭs) [L., tail]. (pl. *cerci*) A hairlike structure.

cerea flexibilitas (sē′rē-ă flĕk″sĭ-bĭl′ĭ-tăs) [L. *cera,* wax + *flexibilitas,* flexibility]. A cataleptic state in which limbs retain any position in which they are placed. Characteristic of catatonic patients. SEE *catalepsy.*

cereals [L. *cerealis,* of grain]. Edible seeds or grains.

COMP: The composition of all cereals is of a similar character. The carbohydrates are the principal nutrient present and protein is next. Cereals contain 70 to 80% carbohydrate in the form of starch; and 8 to 15% protein. Vitamin B complex is abundant in wheat germ. There is a small amount of sodium chloride with potash and phosphorus predominating. Magnesium is abundant. Iron is found in the germ and outer layer. Water is low and some of the cellulose is lost in milling. The whole grain contains about 1% fat.

cerebellar (sĕr-ĕ-bĕl′ăr) [L., little brain]. Pert. to the cerebellum.

cerebellifugal (sĕr″ĕ-bĕl-ĭ-fū′găl) [″ + *fugere,* to flee]. Extending or proceeding from the cerebellum.

cerebellipetal (sĕr″ĕ-bĕl-lĭp′ĭ-tăl) [″ + *petere,* to seek]. Extending toward the cerebellum.

cerebellitis (sĕr″ĕ-bĕl-ī′tĭs) [″ + Gr. *itis,* inflammation]. Inflammation of the cerebellum.

cerebellospinal (sĕr″ĕ-bĕl-ō-spī′năl) [″ + *spina,* a thorn]. Pert. to cerebellum and spinal cord.

Comparison of Food Value of Principal Cereals* in Their Raw Unenriched Flour Form

	Cal. per 100 gm.	Protein gm.	Carbohydrate gm.	Fat gm.	Fiber gm.	Calcium mg.	Phosphorus mg.	Potassium mg.	Sodium mg.
Barley	349	8.2	78.8	1.0	0.5	16	2	160	3
Corn	368	7.8	76.8	2.6	0.8	6	164	—	1
Oatmeal	390	14.2	68.2	7.4	1.2	53	405	352	2
Rice	363	6.7	80.4	0.4	0.3	24	94	92	5
Rye	357	9.4	77.9	1.0	0.4	22	185	156	1
Wheat	365	11.8	74.5	1.2	0.4	20	97	95	2

*Adapted from USDA Handbook #8, 1963.

cerebellum (sĕr-ĕ-bĕl'ŭm) [L.]. [NA] A portion of the brain forming the largest portion of the rhombencephalon. It lies dorsal to the pons and medulla oblongata, overhanging the latter. It consists of two lateral cerebellar hemispheres and a narrow medial portion, the vermis. It is connected to the brain stem by three pair of fiber bundles, the inferior, middle, and superior peduncles. The cerebellum is involved in synergic control of skeletal muscles and plays an important role in the coordination of voluntary muscular movements. It receives afferent impulses and discharges efferent impulses but does not serve as a reflex center in the usual sense; however it may reinforce some reflexes and inhibit others.

cerebral (sĕr'ĕ-brăl, sĕ-rē'brăl) [L. *cerebrum*, brain]. Pert. to the cerebrum.

cerebral anoxia. Lack of oxygen supply to the brain. Usually due to cardiopulmonary arrest, q.v. If nothing is done to treat this condition, irreversible anoxic damage to the brain will begin after 4 to 6 minutes and sooner in some cases. If basic resuscitation measures are begun before the end of this period, the onset of cerebral death may be postponed. SEE: *cardiopulmonary resuscitation.*

cerebral hemorrhage. The result of rupture of a sclerosed or diseased blood vessel in the brain. Often associated with high blood pressure.

RS: apoplexy; hemiplegia; stroke.

cerebral palsy. SEE: *palsy cerebral.*

cerebration (sĕr"ĕ-brā'shŭn) [L. *cerebratio*, brain activity]. Mental action of the brain.

cerebrifugal (sĕr"ĕ-brĭf'ū-găl) [L. *cerebrum*, brain, + *fugere*, to flee]. Away from the brain; pert. to efferent nerve fibers.

cerebripetal (sĕr"ĕ-brĭp'ĕ-tăl) [" + *petere*, to seek]. Proceeding toward the cerebrum, as nerve fibers or impulses.

cerebritis (sĕr"ĕ-brī'tĭs) [" + Gr. *itis*, inflammation]. Inflammation of the brain, esp. the cerebrum.

cerebroid (sĕr'ĕ-broyd) [" + Gr. *eidos*, resemblance]. Resembling brain tissue.

cerebromalacia (sĕr"ĕ-brō"mă-lā'shē-ă) [" + Gr. *malakia*, softening]. Softening of the brain, esp. of the cerebrum.

cerebromedullary (sĕr"ĕ-brō-mĕd'ū-lā-rĕ). Pert. to the brain and spinal cord. SYN: *cerebrospinal.*

cerebromeningitis (sĕr"ĕ-brō-mĕn"ĭn-jī'tĭs) [" + Gr. *meninx*, membrane, + *itis*, inflammation]. Inflammation of the cerebrum and its membranes.

cerebropathy (sĕr-ĕ-brŏp'ă-thē) [" + Gr. *pathos*, disease]. Any disease of the brain, esp. the cerebrum.

cerebrophysiology (sĕr"ĕ-brō-fĭz-ē-ŏl'ō-jē) [" + Gr. *physis*, nature, + *logos*, study]. Physiology of the brain.

cerebropontile (sĕr"ĕ-brō-pŏn'tĭl) [" + *pons*, bridge]. Pert. to the cerebrum and pons varolii.

cerebropsychosis (sĕr"ĕ-brō"sī-kō'sĭs) [" + *psychosis*, life]. Any mental disorder due to cerebral lesion.

cerebrosclerosis (sĕr"ĕ-brō"sklĕ-rō'sĭs) [" + Gr. *sklerosis*, hardening]. Hardening of the brain, esp. of the cerebrum.

cerebroscope (sĕr-ē'brō-skōp) [" + Gr. *skopein*, to examine]. An ophthalmoscope used in diagnosing diseases of the brain.

cerebroscopic (sĕr-ĕ"brō-skŏp'ĭk). Pert. to cerebroscopy.

cerebroscopy (sĕr-ĕ-brŏs'kō-pē) [" + Gr. *skopein*, to examine]. Diagnostic use of the ophthalmoscope in diseases of the brain.

cerebrose (sĕr'ĕ-brōs). $C_6H_{12}O_6$. A compound (brain sugar) derived from brain tissue.

cerebroside (sĕr'ĕ-brō-sīd"). A lipid or fatty substance present in nerve and other tissues.

cerebrosidosis (sĕr"ĕ-brō"sī-dō'sĭs). Form of lipoidosis with kerasin in the fatty cells. SEE: *Gaucher's disease.*

cerebrosis (sĕr"ĕ-brō'sĭs) [L. *cerebrum*, brain, + Gr. *osis*, condition]. Any brain disease.

cerebrospinal (sĕr"ĕ-brō-spī'năl) [" + *spina*, thorn]. Referring to the brain and spinal cord, as the cerebrospinal axis.

cerebrospinal axis. The central nervous system.

cerebrospinal fever. Inflammation of the meninges of the brain and spinal cord; sometimes called spotted fever because of rash on the body. SYN: *meningitis*.

cerebrospinal fluid. A water cushion protecting the brain and spinal cord from physical impact. Usually shrinking or expanding of the cranial contents is quickly balanced by increase or decrease of this fluid.

FORMATION: The fluid is formed by the choroid plexuses of the lateral and third ventricles, that of the lateral ventricles passing through the foramen of Monro to the third, and through the aqueduct of Sylvius to the fourth ventricle. Here it may escape through the central foramen of Magendie, or the lateral foramen of Luschke into the cisterna magna, and so over the brain and cord surfaces, occupying the subarachnoid spaces. It is absorbed by the arachnoid villi and through the perineural lymph spaces of both brain and cord.

CHARACTERISTICS: The fluid is watery, clear, and colorless. Normally the initial pressure of spinal fluid in a recumbent adult, as determined by spinal puncture, is equivalent to 70 to 180 ml. of water. Amount in normal adult is 100 to 140 ml. Sp. gr.: 1.003 to 1.008. Total cell count in adults is 0–10/ml.; in children 0–20/ml. (cells should be counted at once); total protein 20–45 mg./dl.; and glucose 0–75 mg./dl. Its concentration and alkaline reserve are similar to that of the blood. It does not clot on standing. Although the choroid plexuses can reflect certain blood constituents (e.g., iodides), changes in blood sugar, chloride, or urea will manifest themselves quickly in the fluid as well. Otherwise, changes take place largely subsequent to secretion. Turbidity suggests an excessive cell count, if due to red blood cells. Centrifugation will show a red deposit.

Formation of a web after a clear fluid has been allowed to stand is characteristic of tuberculous meningitis (rarely other inflammatory reactions). Cerebrospinal fluid usually shows a yellowish discoloration when containing blood from the subarachnoid spaces (in contrast to blood from trauma of puncture), although for a few days the cells may not be entirely disintegrated. A similar appearance may result from a spinal block above the point of puncture, the fluid spontaneously coagulating due to an excessive albumin content. Total protein is increased in infections (as meningitis, brain abscess, tabes dorsalis), various types of hemorrhage or thrombosis, virus diseases (as encephalitis, anterior poliomyelitis, lymphocytic meningitis), and conditions such as chronic alcoholism. Cell count increases esp. in tuberculous meningitis, epidemic encephalitis, lymphocytic choriomeningitis, poliomyelitis (several days after onset), syphilis of central nervous system, and certain types of tumors of the spinal cord or brain. SEE: *lumbar puncture*.

cerebrospinal ganglia. Sensory ganglia on the roots of cranial and spinal nerves.

cerebrospinal nerves. The cranial nerves, q.v., and spinal nerves, q.v.

cerebrospinal puncture. A puncture for the collection of cerebrospinal fluid. It may be collected from spaces around the spinal cord (lumbar puncture), from the cisterna magna (cisternal puncture), or in infants with open fontanelles (by ventricular puncture).

cerebrosuria (sĕr″ē-brō-sū′rē-ă) [L. *cerebrum*, brain, + Gr. *ouron*, urine]. Cerebrose in the urine.

cerebrotomy (sĕr″ē-brŏt′ō-mē) [″ + Gr. *tome*, incision]. 1. Incision of the brain to evacuate an abscess. 2. Dissection of the brain.

cerebrovascular (sĕr″ē-brō-văs′kū-lăr) [″ + *vasculum*, vessel]. Pert. to the blood vessels of the brain, esp. to pathological changes.

cerebrovascular accident. A general term most commonly applied to cerebrovascular conditions that accompany either ischemic or hemorrhagic lesions. These conditions are usually secondary to atherosclerotic disease, hypertension, or a combination of both. Also called apoplexy, stroke, "a shock," or CVA.

cerebrum (sĕr′ē-brŭm, sĕr-ē brŭm) [L.]. The largest part of the brain, consisting of two hemispheres separated by a deep longitudinal fissure. The hemispheres are united by three commissures—the corpus callosum and the anterior and posterior hippocampal commissures. The surface of each hemisphere is thrown into numerous folds or convolutions called gyri separated by furrows called fissures or sulci.

EMBRYOLOGY: The cerebrum develops from the telencephalon, the most anterior portion of the prosencephalon or forebrain.

STRUCTURE: Each cerebral hemisphere consists of three primary portions—the rhinencephalon or olfactory lobe, the corpus striatum, and the pallium or cerebral cortex. The cortex is a layer of gray matter that covers the surface of each hemisphere. The part covering the rhinencephalon (phylogenetically the oldest) is called archipallium; the larger nonolfactory cortex is called neopallium. Within the cerebrum are two cavities, the lateral ventricles (right and left), and the rostral portion of the third ventricle. The white matter or medullary substance of each hemisphere consists of three kinds of fibers: commissural fibers, which pass from one hemisphere to the other; projection fibers, which convey impulses to and from the cortex; and association fibers, which connect various parts of the cortex within one hemisphere.

Basal ganglia: Masses of gray matter deeply embedded within each hemisphere. They are the caudate, lentiform, and amygdaloid nuclei and the claustrum. *Fissures and sulci:* Lateral cerebral fissure (of Sylvius), central sulcus (of Rolando), parieto-occipital fissure, calcarine fissure, cingulate sulcus, collateral fissure, sulcus circularis, longitudinal cerebral fissure. *Gyri:* Superior, middle, and inferior frontal gyri; anterior and posterior central gyri; superior, middle, and inferior temporal gyri; cingulate, lingual, fusiform, and hippocampal gyri. *Lobes:* Principal lobes are frontal, parietal, occipital, temporal, and central (insula or island of Reil).

FUNCT: The cerebrum is concerned with sensations or the interpretation of sensory impulses; and all voluntary muscular activities. It is the seat of consciousness and the center of the higher mental faculties such as memory, learning, reasoning, judgment, intelligence, and the emotions.

On the basis of function, several areas have been identified and located. Among them are motor projection areas, which give rise to fibers carrying efferent impulses to effector organs, the skeletal muscles; sensory projection areas, which receive impulses from sense organs or sensory receptors by way of the brain stem, including the somesthetic (visual, auditory, gustatory, and olfactory) areas; and association areas, which are concerned with the higher mental faculties.

Cerespan. Trade name for papaverine hydrochloride.

cerium (sē'rē-ŭm) [L.]. A metallic element obtained from the rare earths. It is used as a sulfate in quantitative analysis. SYMB: Ce. At. wt. 140.12; at. no. 58.

ceroid (sē'royd). A fatty pigment present in various tissues.

ceroma (sē-rō'mă) [L. *cera,* wax, + Gr. *oma,* tumor]. A waxy tumor that has undergone amyloid degeneration.

ceroplasty (sē'rō-plăs"tē [" + Gr. *plassein,* to mold]. Manufacture of anatomical models and pathological specimens in wax.

certifiable (sĕr"tĭ-fī'ă-b'l). 1. Pert. to infectious diseases that must be reported or registered with the health authorities. 2. In forensic medicine, a term applied to a mentally incompetent individual who requires the care of a guardian or institution.

certification (sĕr"tĭ-fĭ-kā'shŭn). 1. A legal document prepared by an official body that indicates a person or institution has met certain standards; or that the person has completed a prescribed course of instruction or training. 2. The completion of a form indicating the cause of death. 3. The legal process based on medical evidence of declaring a person insane or mentally incompetent due to senility. SEE: *commitment.*

ceruloplasmin (sĕ-roo"lō-plăz'mĭn). A glycoprotein, blue in color, to which the majority of the copper in the blood is attached. It is decreased in Wilson's disease, q.v.

cerumen (sĕ-roo'mĕn) [L. *cera,* wax]. The waxlike, soft brown secretion found in the external canal of the ear.

ceruminal (sĕ-roo'mĭ-năl). Pert. to the cerumen.

ceruminolysis (sĕ-roo"mĭ-nŏl'ĭ-sĭs). The dissolution or disintegration of cerumen in the external ear canal.

ceruminolytic agent (sĕ-roo"mĭ-nō-lĭt'ĭk). An agent that dissolves cerumen in the external ear canal. Obstruction of the ear canal with cerumen can cause itching, pain, and temporary conductive hearing loss. Removal of the obstruction manually with a blunt curet or loop or by irrigation should be the first approach to treatment. Cerumen solvents are not always recommended because they often do not solve the problem and they frequently cause maceration of skin of the canal and allergic reactions.

ceruminosis (sĕ-roo"mĭ-nō'sĭs) [" + Gr. *osis,* condition]. Excessive secretion of cerumen.

ceruminous (sĕ-roo'mĭ-nŭs). Pert. to cerumen.

ceruminous glands. Modified sweat glands in the skin lining the external auditory canal that secrete cerumen.

ceruse (sē'roos) [L. *cerussa*]. The basic carbonate of lead; white lead formerly used in paint.

cervical (sĕr'vĭ-kăl) [L. *cervicalis*]. 1. Of, pert. to, or in the region of the neck. 2. Pert. to the cervix of an organ, as the cervix uteri.

cervical cap. A device made of a flexible material that is shaped to provide a covering for the uterine cervix. Used to prevent conception.

cervical nerves. The first eight spinal nerves. SEE: *skeleton; spinal nerves.*

cervical plexus. A plexus formed by loops joining the anterior rami of the first four cervical nerves. It receives communicating rami from the sympathetic ganglia. SEE: *Nerve Plexuses* in *Appendix.*

cervical ribs. SEE: *rib, cervical.*

cervical spondylosis. Degenerative arthritis, osteoarthritis, of the cervical vertebrae and related tissues. If severe, it may cause pressure on nerve roots with subsequent pain or paresthesia in the arms.

cervical vertebrae. First seven bones of the spinal column. SEE: *skeleton.*

cervicectomy (sĕr"vĭ-sĕk'tō-mē) [L. *cervix,* neck, + Gr. *ektome,* excision]. Removal of the cervix uteri.

cervices. Pl. of cervix.

cervicitis (sĕr-vĭ-sī'tĭs) [" + Gr. *itis,* inflammation]. Inflammation of the cervix uteri.

cervico- (sĕr'vĭ-kō) [L. *cervix*]. Prefix pert. to the neck or to the neck of an organ.

cervicobrachial (sĕr"vĭ-kō-brā'kē-ăl) [" + Gr. *brachion,* arm]. Pert. to the neck and arm.

cervicocolpitis (sĕr"vĭ-kō-kŏl-pī'tĭs) [" + Gr. *kolpos,* vagina, + *itis,* inflammation]. Inflammation of the cervix and vagina.

cervicodynia (sĕr"vĭ-kō-dĭn'ē-ă) [" + Gr. *odyne,* pain]. A pain or cramp of the neck; cervical neuralgia.

cervicofacial (sĕr"vĭ-kō-fā'shē-ăl) [" + *facies,* face]. Pert. to the neck and face.

cervicovaginitis (sĕr"vĭ-kō-văj"ĭ-nī'tĭs) [" + *vagina,* sheath, + Gr. *itis,* inflammation]. Inflammation of the cervix of the uterus and the vagina.

cervicovesical (sĕr"vĭ-kō-vĕs'ĭ-kăl) [" + *vesica,* bladder]. Pert. to the cervix uteri and bladder.

cervix (sĕr'vĭks) [L.]. (pl. *cervices*) [NA] The neck or a part of an organ resembling a neck. SEE: words beginning with *cervico-*.

c. uteri. Neck of the uterus. The lower part from the internal os outward to the external os. It is rounded and conical in shape, and a portion protrudes into the vagina. It is about 1 in. (2.5 cm.) long, penetrated by the cervical canal, through which the fetus and menstrual flow escape. It may be torn in childbirth, esp. in the primigravida.

Deeper tears may occur in manual dilatation and use of forceps; breech presentation also may be a cause. Laceration may be single, bilateral, stellate, or incomplete. Tears are repaired by suturing in order to prevent hemorrhage and later complications.

c. vesicae. Neck of the bladder.

c.e.s. *central excitatory state.*

cesarean hysterectomy (sē-sār'ē-ăn) [L. *caesarea,* cut]. Cesarean section, q.v., immediately followed by hysterectomy.

cesarean section. Removal of the fetus by means of an incision into the uterus, usually by way of the abdominal wall. May be performed by extraperitoneal or intraperitoneal abdominal route. There are several varieties of cesarean section, differing mainly in the technique employed. The most frequent indication for cesarean section is fetopelvic (also called cephalopelvic) disproportion. Either the fetus is too large to be delivered through the pelvic outlet, the pelvis is abnormally small, or there is a combination of these factors. Some physicians feel that a breech presentation of the fetus is best handled by cesarean section. It is not necessarily true that once a patient has had a cesarean section that all subsequent deliveries must be done in this manner.

c.s., cervical. Surgical removal of the fetus, placenta, and membranes through an incision in the portion of the uterus just above the cervix.

c.s., classic. Cesarean section where the fetus, placenta, and membranes are removed surgically by an incision through the abdominal and uterine walls.

c.s., extraperitoneal. Surgical removal of the fetus, placenta, and membranes through an incision into the lowest portion of the anterior aspect of the uterus. This approach does not entail entering the peritoneal cavity.

c.s., postmortem. Surgical removal of the fetus from the uterus immediately after maternal death.

cesarotomy (sēz"ă-rŏt'ō-mē) [" + Gr. *tome,* incision]. Cesarean section, q.v.

cesium (sē'zē-ŭm) [L. *caesius,* sky blue]. A metallic element. It has a number of isotopes, radioactive isotope ^{137}Cs being used therapeutically for irradiation of cancerous tissue. SYMB: Cs. At. wt. 132.905; at. no. 55.

Cestan-Chenais syndrome (sĕs-tăn'shĕn-ā'). [Raymond Cestan, Fr. neurologist, 1872–1934; Louis J. Chenais, Fr. physician, 1872–1950] A neurological disorder produced by a lesion of the pontobulbar area of the brain.

Cestoda (sĕs-tōd'ă) [Gr. *kestos,* girdle]. A subclass of the class Cestoidea, phylum Platyhelminthes, which includes the tapeworms, having a scolex and a chain of segments (proglottids).

Ex.: Taenia. Intestinal parasites of man and other vertebrates.

cestode (sĕs'tōd) [" + *eidos,* form]. A tapeworm; a member of the Cestoda family.

cestodiasis (sĕs"tō-dī'ă-sĭs) [" + " + *-iasis,* condition]. Infestation with tapeworms. SEE: *Cestoda; tapeworm.*

cestoid (sĕs'toyd) [" + *eidos,* form]. Like a tapeworm.

Cestoidea (sĕs-toy'dē-ă). A class of flatworms of the phylum Platyhelminthes. Includes the tapeworms.

Cetacort. Trade name for hydrocortisone.

Cetamide. Trade name for sulfacetamide sodium 10%.

Cetane. Trade name for ascorbic acid.

Cetraria (sē-trā'rē-ă). 1. A genus of lichens, chiefly found in northern latitudes. 2. C. islandica, or Iceland moss, a lichen used in treating bowel disorders.

cetylpyridinium chloride USP. An anti-infective agent used topically and as a preservative in the manufacture of drugs. Trade names are Ceepryn and Cepacol.

Cevalin. Trade name for sodium ascorbate.

Ce-Vi-Sol. Trade name for ascorbic acid.

CF. *Christmas factor; citrovorum factor.*

Cf. Chem. symb. for californium.

C.F.T. *complement fixation test.*

C.G.S. *centimeter-gram-second,* a name given to a system of units for length, weight, and time.

CH_4. Methane; marsh gas.

C_2H_2. Acetylene.

C_2H_4. Ethylene.

C_6H_6. Benzene.

Chaddock's reflexes (chăd'ŏks). [Charles G. Chaddock, U.S. neurologist, 1861–1936] 1. Extension of great toe when the outer edge of the dorsum of the foot is stroked. Present in disease of the corticospinal tract. 2. Flexion of wrist and fanning of fingers when tendon of palmaris longus muscle is pressed.

chafe (chāf) [O. Fr. *chaufer,* to warm]. To injure by rubbing or friction.

chafing (chāf'ĭng). A superficial inflammation that develops when skin is subjected to friction from clothing or adjacent skin as may occur at the axilla, groin, anal region, or between digits of hands and feet or at the neck or wrists. Erythema, maceration, and sometimes fissuring occur. Bacterial or mycotic infection may result secondarily. SYN: *erythema intertrigo.*

Chagas' disease (chăg'ăs). [Carlos Chagas, Braz. physician, 1879–1934] Disease caused by Trypanosoma cruzi and transmitted by the biting reduviid bug. Characterized by fever, lymphadenopathy, hepatosplenomegaly, and facial edema. Chronic cases may be mild or asymptomatic, or may be accompanied by myocardiopathy, megaesophagus, and megacolon, with fatal outcome. In Brazil and Argentina, the disease is often severe; in Chile the disease is mild. SYN: *trypanosomiasis, American.*

chain (chān) [O. Fr. *chaine,* chain]. 1. A related series of events or things. 2. In bacteriology, bacterial organisms strung together. 3. In chemistry, the linkage of atoms together in a straight line or in a circle or ring. The ring or straight-line structures may have side chains branching off from the main compound.

c., food. SEE: *food chain.*

chaining (chān'ĭng). A behavioral therapy process whereby reinforcement is given for behaviors related to established behavior. Also: *chained reinforcement.*

chalasia (kă-lā'zē-ă) [Gr. *chalasis,* relaxation]. Relaxation of sphincters.

chalazion (kă-lā'zē-ŏn) [Gr. *khalaza,* hailstone]. (pl. *chalazia, -zions*) Small, hard tumor analogous to sebaceous cyst developing on the eyelids, formed by distention of a meibomian gland with secretion. SYN: *meibomian cyst.* SEE: *steatoma.*

chalcosis (kăl-kō'sĭs) [Gr. *chalkos,* copper, + *osis,* condition]. 1. Chronic poisoning from copper. 2. Copper deposits in lungs and tissues.

chalice cell (chăl'ĭs) [L. *calix,* cup]. Crateriform shell remaining after mucus has been discharged from an epithelial cell. SYN: *goblet cell; cell, mucous.*

chalicosis (kăl-ĭ-kō'sĭs) [Gr. *chalix,* limestone, + *osis,* condition]. Pneumoconiosis associated with the inhalation of dust produced by stone cutting.

chalinoplasty (kăl'ĭ-nō-plăs"tē) [Gr. *chalinos,* corner of mouth, + *plassein,* to mold]. Plastic surgery of the mouth and lips, esp. of corners of the mouth.

challenge (chăl'ĕnj). In immunology, administration of a specific antigen to an individual known to be sensitive to that antigen in order to produce an immune response.

chalone (kăl'ōn) [Gr. *chalan,* to relax]. A poorly defined substance that acts to regulate certain intracellular activity, including cell division.

chalybeate (kă-lĭb'ē-āt) [Gr. *chalyps,* steel]. 1. Pert. to or composed of iron; ferruginous. 2. Agent containing iron.

chamber (chām'bĕr) [Gr. *kamara,* vault]. Compartment or closed space.

c., anterior. The space between the cornea and iris of the eye.

c., aqueous. Anterior and posterior chambers of the eye, containing the aqueous humor.

c., hyperbaric. An airtight enclosure strong enough to withstand high internal pressure. Used to expose animals, humans, or an entire surgical team to increased air pressure. Used to treat gas gangrene, bends, and for certain surgical procedures.

c., low pressure. Chamber designed to simulate high altitudes by exposing humans or animals to low atmospheric pressure. Such studies are essential for simulated flights into the atmosphere and space.

c., posterior. Space behind the iris, anterior to the lens of the eye.

c., vitreous. Cavity behind the lens in the eye containing the vitreous humor.

chamomile, camomile (kăm'ĕ-mĭl) [Gr. *khamaemelon,* earth apple]. Flowers of the Anthemis yielding a bluish volatile oil and a bitter infusion.

chancre (shăng'kĕr) [Fr., ulcer]. A hard, syphilitic primary ulcer, the first sign of syphilis, appearing approx. two to three weeks after infection.

CAUTION: During the chancre stage, the condition is highly contagious and the chancre itself contains many spirochetes. Discovery of these organisms in the chancre is the basis for the positive darkfield test for syphilis. Syphilis may occur, however, without a chancre developing. SEE: *syphilis.*

SYM: Begins as a painless erosion or papule that ulcerates superficially. Generally single; sometimes multiple. Has a scooped-out appearance due to level or sloping edges that are adherent. It has a shining red or raw floor with some deposit. Induration constant. Slightly purulent secretion. Heals without leaving scar. May appear at almost any site including mouth, penis, urethra, hand, toe, eyelid, conjunctiva, vagina, or cervix.

c., hard. Primary lesion of syphilis. SYN: *hunterian chancre.* SEE: *chancre; syphilis.*

c., simple. A nonsyphilitic venereal ulcer. SYN: *chancroid; c., soft.*

c., soft. C., simple, q.v.

c., true. The primary lesion of syphilis, q.v. SEE: *chancre.*

chancroid (shăng′kroyd) [″ + Gr. *eidos,* form]. A highly infectious nonsyphilitic venereal ulcer. It is caused by Hemophilus ducreyi (also called Ducrey's bacillus), a gram-negative bacillus. SYN: *chancre, simple.*

INCUBAT: Approx. three to five days.

SYM: Begins with pustule or ulcer, multiple, abrupt edges, rough floor, yellow exudate, purulent secretion, sensitive and inflamed. Scar remains. Rapid progress. May affect the penis, urethra, vulva, or anus. Multiple lesions may develop by autoinoculation. Types include transient, phagedenic, giant, and serpiginous.

TREATMENT: Sulfonamides, tetracyclines, or chloramphenicol.

chancrous (shăng′krŭs). Pert. to or of the nature of chancre.

change of life. The menopause, q.v.; climacteric, q.v.

chapped (chăpt) [ME. *chappen*]. Inflamed, roughened, fissured, as from exposure to cold.

character (kăr′ăk-tĕr). 1. The total qualities, esp. those of the personality, thought, and morality as evidenced from the individual's speech, writings, and actions, that distinguish one person from another. 2. The feature or characteristic of an organism or individual that results from the expression of the genetic information received, i.e., inherited, from the parents.

c., acquired. A trait or quality that was not inherited but is the result of environmental influence.

c., anal. Personality type that is the result of the persistence of the anal or excretory stage of development into adulthood. Such persons are frequently compulsive with respect to neatness, obstinancy, and frugality. Though not a precise definition of a mental disorder, the term “anal character” is useful in describing the behavior of affected individuals.

c., dominant. In genetics, a trait that is manifest even though it was present in only one gene.

c., primary sex. An inherited trait directly concerned with the reproductive tract.

c., recessive. In genetics, a trait that does not develop or appear unless it was present in the genes received from both parents.

c., secondary sex. Trait peculiar to either sex but not concerned with the reproductive tract. Voice quality, facial hair, and body fat distribution are examples.

c., sex-conditioned. A genetic trait carried by both sexes but expressed or inhibited by the sex of the individual.

c., sex-limited. A trait present in only one sex even though the gene responsible is present in both sexes.

c., sex-linked. A trait transmitted only on the sex-determining chromosome.

characteristic (kăr″ăk-tĕr-ĭs′tĭk). 1. The trait or character that is typical of an organism or individual. 2. In logarithmic expressions, the number to the left of the decimal point, as distinguished from the mantissa, which is the number to the right of the decimal point.

characteristic radiation. X radiation produced by the shifting of electrons within an atom to another orbit.

charbon (shăr-bŏn′) [Fr., coal]. Infection with Bacillus anthracis. SYN: *anthrax.*

charcoal (chăr′kōl) [ME. *charcole*]. Activated charcoal, USP, very fine powder prepared from soft charred wood.

ACTION AND USES: Internally for adsorption of gastrointestinal gas and for adsorption of poisonous alkaloids that have been swallowed.

Charcot's joint (shăr-kōz′). [Jean M. Charcot, Fr. neurologist, 1825–1893] A type of diseased joint associated with tabes dorsalis, syringomyelia, or other conditions involving disease or injury to the spinal cord, characterized by hypermobility. Decalcification of bone on joint surfaces occurs accompanied by overgrowth of bone about margins. Pain is usually absent although there are exceptions. Deformity and instability of the joint are characteristic.

Charcot-Leyden crystals (shăr-kō′lī′dĕn). [Charcot; Ernest V. von Leyden, Ger. physician, 1832–1910] Colorless, hexagonal, double-pointed and often needlelike crystals found in the sputum in asthma and bronchial bronchitis or in the feces in ulcerative cases of the intestine, esp. amebiasis.

Charcot-Marie-Tooth disease. [Charcot; Pierre Marie, Fr. neurologist, 1853–1940; Howard Tooth, Brit. physician, 1856–1926] A form of progressive neural muscular atrophy, a disease with hereditary tendencies characterized by progressive weakness of distal muscles of the arms and feet. The muscles atrophy, reflexes are lost, foot drop develops, and there is loss of cutaneous sensations. Usually develops in childhood but may occur in adults; more common in males. Its cause is unknown. SYN: *atrophy, peroneal muscular.*

Charcot's triad. The combination of nystagmus, intention tremor, and scanning speech. It is frequently associated with multiple sclerosis.

charlatan (shăr'lă-tăn) [It. *ciarlatano*]. A pretender to special knowledge or ability, as in medicine. SYN: *quack.*

charlatanry (shăr'lă-tăn-rē). Undue pretension to knowledge or skill that is not possessed. SYN: *quackery.*

Charles' law (shărl). [Jacques A. C. Charles, Fr. physicist, 1746–1823] At constant pressure, a given amount of gas will expand its volume in direct proportion to the absolute temperature. SYN: *Gay-Lussac's law.* SEE: *Boyle's law.*

charleyhorse. Pain and tenderness in the fibromuscular tissue of the thighs usually due to muscle strain or tear. Characterized by sudden onset and aggravation upon movement. SYN: *fibromyositis.*

F.A.: Relief can be obtained from rest, local applications of cold, gentle massage, and aspirin.

chart [L. *charta,* paper]. 1. A simple form or sheet of paper for recording the course of a patient's illness. Includes records of temperature, pulse, respiratory rate, blood pressure, urinary and fecal output, and doctors' and nurses' notes. 2. To record on a graph the sequence of events such as vital signs. SEE: *charting.* 3. The complete clinical record of a patient, including physical and psychosocial state of health as well as results of diagnostic tests. Plans for meeting the needs of the patient are also included. SEE: *problem-oriented medical record.*

c., dental. A diagrammatic representation of the teeth of the mouth on which the clinical and radiographic findings can be recorded, often including the restorations present, decayed surfaces, missing teeth, and periodontal conditions.

charta (kăr'tă) [L.]. Preparation intended principally for external application, made either by saturating paper with medicinal substances or by applying the latter to the surface of the paper by the addition of some adhesive liquid.

charting. The process of making a tabulated record of the progress of the patient during the hospital stay. A clinical record. Record information about the patient and the treatment. The physician needs detailed information that the nurse or others may contribute through observation of and contact with the patient. These notes, containing details of the patient's reactions and progress, aid the physician in making a diagnosis. Almost any member of the professional health-care team may be responsible for providing and recording information concerning the patient's therapy, course, and progress. Verbal reports are not sufficient; they take time and may be misunderstood. NOTE: Procedures for charting may be different for various hospitals. The system specified by each hospital should be used. Written documentation is considered legal evidence. It must be clear, concise, and legible. Slang should not be used. SEE: *Charting* in *Appendix.*

GENERAL RECORDS: *Blood pressure:* Record is usually kept on sheet with temperature, pulse, and respiration record. *Diet:* If patient is on regular diet, it is sufficient to chart breakfast, dinner, and supper but, when on any other diet, chart exactly what the patient is given at each meal and the amount of food actually eaten. The amount of liquids taken (not "Water p.r.n."); hours of giving; kind of diet (full, light, soft, liquid, special); appetite. *Discharge or death:* Discharge or death of patient with hour and date of same and the name of the individual who ordered discharge or who pronounced the patient dead.

Fluids: Hours of giving; kind; amount. *Heat:* Chart by whose order heat is applied to an unconscious patient, and who executed the order. *Infant feeding:* The formula should be charted the first time; afterwards, amount given, and, if regurgitated, approximate the amount. *Laboratory:* Hour; kind of specimen; by whom taken; by whom ordered (not necessary in case of routine urine specimen on admission).

Dressings: Change of dressings on wounds and the amount and character of drainage (remark "Specimen Saved" if this has been done); hour; by whom; stitches or drains removed; patient's reaction if pained or shocked by dressing. *Drugs:* Any unfavorable reaction from drugs or treatments. Chart time when drugs or treatments are administered. All medicines, treatments, preparation, etc., are to be charted by the nurse who administers them whether in charge of the patient or not. Confine name of medicine, dose and route of administration, and frequency to the prescribed column. When administering soluble salts or medicines dispensed in liquid form, state dose actually administered, not the amount of solution. Any prominent or unusual therapeutic action or idiosyncrasy resulting from a drug should be recorded.

Nursing care: Hour; baths and shampoos; alcohol rubs and decubitus dressing; special mouth care; sitting up for first time; out of bed for first time; walking for first time; narcotics (treatments are also charted, but as treatments). *Operations:* Name of operation; preparation; preoperative medication if given by nurse or in ward; hour of going to O.R.; hour of going to and leaving recovery room, or intensive care unit (ICU); hour of return to room; condition on return to room; hour of recovery from anesthetic; condition every half hour for next three or four hours, depending on state patient is in and severity of operation. Recovery room or ICU staff members will record treatment and condition while patient is in their care.

Personal care: Baths, personal hygiene, and patient's reactions to these. For women, record menstruation and type of menstrual protection used. *Physician:* Record physician's visit. Physician's orders must be recorded as well as the time they are written and carried out. *Physiotherapy:* Hour of going for treatment and hour of return; condition of patient. *Postoperative:* Changing position of postoperative patients should be recorded under "Remarks." Record passive and active exercise of patient. *Specimens:* Record the taking of specimens of blood, exudates, transudates, etc., for examination. The result will be shown by the report of the pathologist. *Surgical preparations:* The nurse who does surgical preparations will sign his or her name after "Preliminary preparation of field of operation." Observe the same rule for narcotics.

Symptoms: Accurate description of all symptoms, i.e., character of pulse and respiration, mental state, description of pain, and nature of any discharge, etc. The remarks should be appropriate and well chosen. Subjective as well as objective symptoms should be recorded. *Time:* Everything relating to the patient's progress should be charted as it occurs. Record the hour with all statements on charts. Record on the first line of the sheet the day, date of admission, whether the patient walked in or was admitted by ambulance, and condition of patient. Four-hour graphic charts are kept for all surgical and obstetrical cases the first three days (usually at 8, 12, and 4, around the clock); and for all patients whose temperature is above normal. The temperature, pulse, and respirations of all other patients are charted appropriately according to the institution.

Treatments: Hour of giving; nature of treatment; by whom given; patient's reaction. *X-ray:* Hour; to x-ray room or portable at bedside; return from x-ray room; condition of patient.

Visits of clergyman (specially important in case of Roman Catholic patients): Hour; name of clergyman; rite performed.

Miscellaneous: Any sudden or marked change in patient's condition; notification of patient's relatives and clergyman. Special charts are also provided for certain purposes such as the temperature, pulse, and respiration chart; anesthesia chart generally kept by the anesthetist; blood-pressure chart used in conditions apt to affect the blood pressure; intake and output charts used in all patients with fluid and electrolyte imbalance; and laboratory records usually filed with the patient's chart. If any laboratory records have been made and not filed with the chart, their existence should be noted on the clinical chart at the time made and also upon the final page of the chart.

PHYSICAL SYMPTOMS: *Appetite:* Good, poor, special likes or dislikes. *Convulsions:* Type, duration, consciousness lost; note fecal or urinary incontinence; was patient injured during convulsion or in fall that came with convulsion; aura. *Defecation:* (see Excretions; Feces; Urine in this entry). *Diaphoresis* (perspiration): State whether slight, moderate, or profuse. *Emesis:* Amount, color, odor, consistency of the vomitus, and manner of ejecting. (See Vomiting in this entry.)

Enemas: Results and unusual appearances, distention before or after, describe results fully. Note whether or not flatus was expelled with the return of the enema. Chart the solution, strength, and amount used. Also douches and irrigations.

Excretions: Time, character, and other facts. *Feces:* Enema or natural movement; amount; consistency; color; abnormal odor; abnormal constituents. Defecation accompanied by pain or tenesmus.

General appearance: Color; posture; rash; mood; mental state. *Hemorrhages, discharges, etc.:* Description, etc. When unusual, save specimens for examination. *Nausea:* Accompanied by vomiting; following certain foods, drugs, or treatments. *Nerves:* All symptoms of nervousness, excitability, etc. *Pain:* Location; time of onset; character; sharp, dull, burning, grinding, throbbing; duration (constant, how long); intermittent; intervals.

Pathological conditions: Vomiting, convulsions, etc. Record time of onset, duration, severity, general appearance of patient before, during, and after the attack. In convulsions it is important to record the localization of the convulsive motion if present, and whether or not the patient was incontinent; and if the patient fell, what, if any, injury was sustained and what treatment was provided. T.P.R. immediately after, and what was done to relieve condition. Explanation as to the cause if known. *Pulse:* Rate: beats per minute. Character: full, bounding, weak, thready, faint. Rhythm: regular, irregular, intermittent. *Respiration:* Rate per minute. Character: deep, shallow, difficult, easy, labored, quiet, stertorous, Cheyne-Stokes. Rhythm: regular, irregular, gasping.

Sleep: Hours of sleeping during the day as well as the night. If impossible to estimate accurately, approximate it and note that it is an approximation. Time and amount. Sleepwalking, nightmares, or talking in sleep should be recorded. *Temperature:* Indicate whether taken by mouth, rectum, or axilla; degree; following chill or treatment. If temperature is quite high and patient does not appear to have fever of that extent, take temperature again but remain at bedside to be sure patient is not placing thermometer against some hot object.

T.P.R.: Temperature, pulse, and respiration taken as ordered. The nurse charts the T.P.R. and general condition of the patient before going to the operating room, and the pulse and respiration with general condition upon return from the operating room. *Unconsciousness or coma:* Time of onset; conditions associated with or that caused onset; appearance of patient while in coma; medicines or treatment given while in coma; duration. *Unusual conditions:* Chart these such as appearance of blood, twitching, convulsions, coma, drowsiness, lethargy, unconsciousness.

Urine: State time of voiding, amount, color and appearance, whether voided or per catheter. Note time of beginning 24-hour specimen collection, when bladder is emptied for the purpose, this specimen is sent to laboratory for qualitative test. Note time of completion of collecting a 24-hour specimen; note amount on chart and on laboratory label. Send specimen to the laboratory for all patients remaining in the hospital over night. Check may be used in the urine column when patient uses lavatory or defecates. At all other times the amount of urine is to be charted (totaled every 12 hours and total charted also). Record if urination is accompanied by pain or burning; any abnormal appearance; specimen to laboratory.

Vomiting: Cause; forcible or projectile; vomitus amount, color, odor, consistency, any unusual constituents.

MENTAL SYMPTOMS: Calmness; cheerfulness; delirium (kind); depression (degree); apparent effect of visitors, etc.; delusions and on what subjects; hallucinations; illusions and on what subjects; temper fits; willingness to cooperate; worry.

Visitors: Reaction to visitors and mood change after visitors depart. Especially important in depressed and psychiatric patients.

c., dental. The recording on a chart the clinical findings within the mouth; while examining each tooth and probing the gingival sulcus, the noting of the restorations present, missing teeth, periodontal pocket depth, and conditions of all soft tissues.

chartula (kăr′tū-lă) [L., small piece of paper]. A paper folded to form a receptacle containing a dose of medicinal substance.

chasma (kăz′mă) [Gr., a cleft]. An opening, gap, or wide cleft.

chaude-pisse (shōd-pēs′) [Fr.]. A burning sensation during urination, esp. in acute gonorrhea.

chauffage (shō-fŏzh′) [O. Fr. *chaufer,* to heat]. Treatment with a heated cautery at low temperature applied over a body part about ¼ in. (6 mm.) from it.

chaulmoogra oil, chaulmugra, chaulmaugra (chŏl-moo′grŭ, chŏl-mŏ′grŭ) [Bengali *caulmugra*]. A vegetable oil used in treatment of leprosy and some dermatoses. Though generally replaced by sulfones in treatment of leprosy, chaulmoogra oil is still used in endemic areas because of its availability and low cost.

Chaussier's areola (shō-sē-āz′). [François Chaussier, Fr. physician, 1746–1828] Indurated tissue around the lesion of a malignant pustule.

chavicine (chăv′ĭ-sēn). A yellow, oily ingredient of black pepper.

Ch.B. *Bachelor of Surgery;* used mostly in the United Kingdom.

CHD. *coronary heart disease.*

check [O. Fr. *eschec*]. 1. To slow down or arrest the course of. 2. To verify.

check bite. A sheet of hard wax that is used to make an impression of teeth to check articulation.

check-up. General term for visit to a physician for a physical examination.

Chediak-Higashi syndrome (shē′dē-ăk-hē-gă′shē). [A. Chediak and O. Higashi, contemporary Cuban and Japanese physicians, respectively] A lethal metabolic disorder, inherited as an autosomal recessive, in which neutrophils contain peroxidase-positive inclusion bodies. Partial albinism, photophobia, and pale optic fundi are clinical features. Children usually die by the age of 5 to 10 of a lymphoma-like disease.

cheek [AS. *ceace*]. Side of face forming lateral wall of mouth below eye. SYN: *bucca.*

cheekbone. The malar bone, q.v.; os zygomaticum [NA]; zygomatic bone.

cheek retractor. Device that encloses the cheek at the angle of the mouth for properly exposing operating field.

cheilectomy (kī-lĕk′tō-mē) [Gr. *cheilos,* lip, + *ektome,* excision]. 1. Surgical removal of abnormal bone around a joint in order to facilitate joint mobility. 2. Surgical removal of a lip.

cheilectropion (kī″lĕk-trō′pē-ŏn) [″ + *ektrope,* a turning aside]. Eversion of the lip.

cheilitis (kī-lī′tĭs) [″ + *itis,* inflammation]. Inflammation of the lip.

c. actinica. Irritation of lips resulting from exposure to sunlight.

c. exfoliativa. Seborrheic dermatitis of the lips.

c. glandularis. Disorder of the lips resulting from hypertrophy of mucous glands and their ducts. SYN: *myxadenitis labialis.*

c. venenata. Dermatitis of the lips resulting from chemical irritants present in lipsticks, lip cream, and various other materials.

cheilognathopalatoschisis (kī″lō-nā″thō-păl-ă-tŏs′kĭ-sĭs) [″ + *gnathos,* jaw, + L. *palatum,* palate, + Gr. *schisis,* cleft]. Developmental anomaly in which there is a cleft in the hard and soft palate, upper jaw, and lip.

cheilophagia (kī″lō-fā′jē-ă) [″ + *phagein,* to eat]. Habit of biting one's own lip.

cheiloplasty (kī′lō-plăs″tē) [″ + *plassein,* to form]. Plastic operation upon the lips.

cheilorrhaphy (kī-lor′ă-fē) [″ + *rhaphe,* suture]. Surgical repair of a cleft lip.

cheirology (kī-rŏl′ō-jē) [″ + *logos,* study]. Communication by use of the hands and fingers. SYN: *dactylology.*

cheiloschisis (kī-lŏs′kĭ-sĭs) [″ + *schisis,* cleft]. Harelip.

cheilosis (kī-lō′sĭs) [″ + *osis,* condition]. Morbid condition of lips with reddened appearance and fissures at the angles, seen frequently in deficiency of vitamin B complex, esp. riboflavin.

cheilostomatoplasty (kī″lō-stō-măt′ō-plăs″tē) [″ + *stoma,* mouth, + *plassein,* to form]. Plastic surgery and restoration of mouth.

cheilotomy, chilotomy (kī-lŏt′ō-mē) [″ + *tome,* incision]. Excision of part of the lip.

cheirognostic (kī″rŏg-nŏs′tĭk) [Gr. *cheir,* hand, + *gnostikos,* knowing). 1. Able to distinguish left from right side of body. 2. Able to perceive which side of the body is being stimulated.

cheirospasm (kī′rō-spăsm) [″ + Gr. *spasmos,* spasm]. Writer's cramp; spasm of the muscles of the hand.

chelate (kē′lāt) [Gr. *chele,* claw]. 1. In chemistry, to combine with a ring structure much as a claw would grasp an object, said of the ion of a metal. 2. In toxicology, to use a compound to enclose or grasp a toxic substance and make it nonactive and thus nontoxic.

chelating agent. A drug that is used to chelate, q.v., substances, esp. toxic chemicals in the body.

chelation (kē-lā′shŭn) [Gr. *chele,* claw]. Combining of metallic ions with certain heterocyclic ring structures so that the ion is held by chemical bonds from each of the participating rings. When this structure is diagrammed it appears that the metallic ion is being held by a claw. Calcium disodium edetate, q.v., is a chelating agent.

cheloid (kē′loyd) [Gr. *kele,* tumor, + *eidos,* form]. Keloid.

chemabrasion (kēm-ă-brā′shŭn). Use of a chemical to destroy superficial layers of skin. Technique may be used to treat scars, tattoos, or abnormal pigmentation. SYN: *chemexfoliation.*

chemexfoliation (kēm′ĕks-fō′lē-ā″shŭn). Chemabrasion, q.v.

chemical [Gr. *chemeia,* chemistry]. Pert. to chemistry.

Chemical Abstract Service. ABBR: CAS. A branch of the American Chemical Society that maintains a registry of chemicals, active ingredients used in drugs, and food additives. Each chemical is assigned a permanent CAS number through which current data can be traced.

chemical bond. SEE: *bond, chemical.*

chemical change. A change in which a substance breaks up or combines with other substances to make new substances with new properties or characteristics.

Ex.: oxygen and hydrogen combine to form water. Sodium (a metal) and chlorine (a gas) combine to form sodium chloride, or common salt. Oxygen combines with hemoglobin when the hemoglobin in the blood comes into contact with the oxygen in the air in the alveoli of the lungs to form oxyhemoglobin. The difference can be seen by comparing the bright scarlet color of the arterial blood containing oxyhemoglobin with the bluish color of the venous blood containing reduced hemoglobin.

chemical compound. 1. A substance consisting of two or more chemical elements in definite proportions and in chemical combination and for which a chemical formula can be written, as in water (H_2O) or salt (NaCl). 2. A substance that can be separated by chemical means into simpler substances.

chemical element. 1. Element. 2. Any chemical compound or substance composed of chemical elements. SEE table; *Physical Constants of the Elements* in *Appendix.*

chemical reflex. Any reflex action initiated by a chemical stimulus.

chemical warfare. The tactics and technique of conducting warfare by use of toxic chemical agents and the deliberate introduction of disease-producing organisms into populations of people, animals, or plants. The chemicals include nerve gases; agents that cause temporary blindness, paralysis, hallucinations, or deafness; eye and lung irritants; mustard gas; defoliants; and herbicides. SEE:

Selected Chemical Substances and Their Common Names

Common or Latin Names	Chemical Names
Aqua fortis	Nitric acid
Aqua regia	Nitrohydrochloric acid
Blue vitriol	Copper sulfate
Caustic potash	Potassium hydroxide
Chalk	Calcium carbonate
Common Salt	Sodium chloride
Copperas or Green vitriol	Ferrous sulfate
Cream of tartar	Potassium bitartrate
Dry alum	Aluminum and Potassium sulfate
Epsom salts	Magnesium sulfate
Glauber's salts	Sodium sulfate
Grape sugar	Glucose
Laughing gas	Nitrous oxide
Lime	Calcium oxide
Lunar caustic	Silver nitrate
Muriate of lime	Calcium chloride
Niter or Saltpeter	Potassium nitrate
Oil of vitriol	Sulfuric acid
Rust of iron	Iron oxide
Sal ammoniac	Ammonium chloride
Salt of tartar	Potassium carbonate
Slaked lime	Calcium hydroxide
Soda, baking	Sodium bicarbonate
Spirits of Hartshorn	Ammonia
Spirits of salt	Hydrochloric acid
Stucco or Plaster of Paris	Calcium sulfate
Verdigris	Basic copper acetate
Vinegar	Acetic acid (diluted)
Water	Hydrogen oxide
White vitriol	Zinc sulfate

biological warfare.

chemiluminescence (kĕm″ĭ-loo″mĭ-nĕs′ĕns). Cold light or light produced as a result of a chemical reaction and without the production of heat, e.g., the light produced by certain bacteria, fungi, and fireflies. SEE: *luciferase.*

chemise (shĕ-mēz′) [LL. *camisa,* linen shirt]. Surgical dressing consisting of a square bandage tied around a catheter passing through the center of the bandage.

chemist (kĕm′ĭst). One trained in chemistry.

chemistry [Gr. *chemeia,* chemistry]. The science that deals with the molecular and atomic structure of matter and of the composition of substances—their formation, decomposition, and the various transformations that they may undergo.

c., analytical. Chemistry concerned with the detection of the presence of chemical substances (qualitative analysis) or the determination of the amounts of substances present (quantitative analysis) in a compound.

c., biological. The chemistry of living things, involving all the chemical processes that take place within an organism, such as the digestion of food, anabolism, and catabolism. SYN: *biochemistry.*

c., general. The study of the entire field of chemistry with emphasis on fundamental concepts or laws.

c., inorganic. The chemistry of compounds not containing carbon.

c., nuclear. Radiochemistry or the study of changes that take place within the nucleus of an atom, esp. when the nucleus is bombarded by electrons, neutrons, or other subatomic particles.

c., organic. The chemistry of carbon compounds.

c., pathological. The study of chemical changes induced by disease processes, e.g., changes in the chemistry of organs and tissues; blood; secretions; or excretions.

c., pharmaceutical. The chemistry of medicines, their composition, synthesis, analysis, storage, and actions.

c., physical. Theoretical chemistry or that concerned with fundamental laws underlying chemical changes and the expression of these laws mathematically.

c., physiological. The study of the chemical nature of living matter and the changes occurring in the metabolic activities of plants and animals.

chemobiotic (kē″mō-bī-ŏt′ĭk). Combination of an antibiotic with a chemotherapeutic agent.

chemocautery (kĕm″ō-kaw′tĕr-ē) [Gr. *chemeia,* chemistry, + *kauterion,* branding iron]. Cauterization by chemical agents.

chemoceptor (kĕm′ō-sĕp-tĕr). A chemoreceptor, q.v.

chemocoagulation (kē″mō-kō-ăg″ū-lā′shŭn) [″ + L. *coaglutio,* coagulation]. Coagulation brought about by chemical agents.

chemodectoma (kē″mō-dĕk-tō′mă) [″ + *dektikos,* receptive, + *oma,* tumor]. Tumor of the chemoreceptor system.

chemoluminescence (kē″mō-loo″mĭ-nĕs′ĕns). A chemical reaction that produces light. SYN: *chemiluminescence.* SEE: *luciferase.*

chemolysis (kē-mŏl′ĭ-sĭs) [″ + *lysis,* dissolution]. Destruction by chemical action.

chemonucleolysis (kēm″ō-nū-klē-ŏl′ĭ-sĭs). Method of dissolving a herniated nucleus pulposus, q.v., by injection of the enzyme chymopapain into it.

chemopallidectomy (kē″mō-păl″ĭ-dĕk′tō-mē) [″ + L. *pallidum,* globus pallidus, + Gr. *ektome,* excision]. Destruction of a portion of the globus pallidus of the brain by use of a chemical.

chemoprophylaxis (kē″mō-prō″fĭ-lăk′sĭs). Use of a drug or chemical to prevent a disease, e.g., the taking of an appropriate medicine to prevent malaria.

chemopsychiatry (kē″mō-sī-kī′ă-trē). Use of drugs in treating psychiatric illnesses.

chemoreceptor (kē″mō-rē-sĕp′tor) [″ + L. *recipere,* to receive]. A sense organ or sensory nerve ending (as in a taste bud) that is stimulated by and reacts to certain chemical stimuli and that is located outside of the central nervous system. Chemoreceptors are found in the large arteries of the thorax and neck (carotid and aortic bodies), the taste buds, and in the olfactory cells of the nose. SEE: *carotid body; taste buds.*

chemoreflex (kē″mō-rē′flĕks) [″ + L. *reflectere,* to bend back]. Reflex resulting from chemical stimulus.

chemoresistance (kē″mō-rē-zĭs′tăns). Specific resistance of a body cell or microorganism to the effect of a drug.

chemosensitive (kē″mō-sĕn′sĭ-tĭv). Reacting to the action of a chemical or change in chemical composition.

chemosensory (kē″mō-sĕn′sō-rē). Detection of a chemical by sensory means, esp. by odor detection.

chemoserotherapy (kē″mō-sē″rō-thĕr′ă-pē). Combined use of a drug and serum in treating disease.

chemosis (kē-mō′sĭs) [Gr. *cheme,* cockleshell, + *osis,* condition]. Edema of conjunctiva about the cornea.

chemosmosis (kē″mŏs-mō′sĭs). Chemical reaction through a semipermeable membrane.

chemosterilant (kē″mō-stĕr′ĭ-lănt). 1. Chemical that kills microorganisms. 2. Chemical that produces sterility, usually of the male, in organisms such as insects.

chemosurgery. Destruction of tissue by use of chemical compounds.

chemosynthesis (kē″mō-sĭn′thĕ-sĭs). The formation of a chemical compound from other chemicals or agents. In biological systems, this involves metabolism.

chemotactic (kē″mō-tăk′tĭk). Pert. to chemotaxis.

chemotaxis (kē″mō-tăk′sĭs) [Gr. *chemeia,* chemistry, + *taxis,* arrangement]. Attraction and repulsion of living protoplasm to a chemical stimulus. SYN: *chemotropism.*

chemothalamectomy (kē′mō-thăl-ă-mĕk′tō-mē). Chemical destruction of a part of the thalamus of the brain.

chemotherapeutic index. The ratio of the toxicity of a drug, expressed as maximum tolerated dose/kg. of body weight to the minimal curative dose/kg. of body weight. This index is utilized in judging the safety and effectiveness of drugs used in treating parasitic conditions.

chemotherapy (kē″mō-thĕr′ă-pē) [″ + *therapeia,* treatment]. In the treatment of disease, the application of chemical reagents that have a specific and toxic effect upon the disease-causing microorganism.

chemotic (kē-mŏt′ĭk). Pert. to chemosis.

chemotropism (kē-mŏt′rō-pĭzm) [″ + *tropos,* a turning]. Ability or impulse to progress or turn in a certain direction due to the influence of certain chemical stimuli, as the root of a plant toward its food supply.

chenodeoxycholic acid. An experimental drug that is given orally to dissolve cholesterol gallstones.

chenopodium oil (kĕn-ō-pō′dē-ŭm) [Gr. *chen,* goose, + *pous,* foot]. Oil of American wormseed. A pale-yellow, volatile oil with pungent, irritating odor.

ACTION AND USES: Antihelmintic against hookworm.

cherophobia (kē″rō-fō′bē-ă) [Gr. *chairein,* to rejoice, + *phobos,* fear]. Morbid fear of and aversion to gaiety.

cherry-red spot. A red spot in each retina. Seen in Tay-Sachs disease, q.v.

cherubism (chĕr′ū-bĭzm). Cherubic appearance of the face of a child due to infiltration of the jaw, esp. the mandible, with masses of vascular fibrous tissue containing giant cells.

chest [AS. *cest,* a box]. The thorax.

MENSURATION: The object of measuring the chest is to determine the comparative bulk of the two sides and the amount of expansion and retraction accompanying inspiration and expiration of the two sides. The points of measurement are between the spinous processes behind and the median line in front on the level of the 6th costosternal articulation. The right side is from half an inch to an inch (1.3 to 2.5 cm.) larger than the left. When a pleural cavity is distended with air or fluid, the measurement of the affected side may exceed that of the healthy side by 2 or 3 inches (5.6 to 7.6 cm); after removal of the fluid there may be an equal diminution in the measurement of the affected side, as compared with the healthy one. In unilateral emphysema, the total difference between the fullest inspiration and fullest expiration on the affected side will scarcely exceed 1⁄16 of an inch (1.6 mm.), while on the other side there may be a difference of 2 or 3 in. (5.6 to 7.6 cm.).

PALPATION: Serves to detect any thoracic tenderness, edema, friction fremitus, or rales. Edema of chest walls is recognized by pitting when pressure is made with finger; it may be observed in empyema and in certain types of heart failure.

The friction sound of pleurisy and harsh, sonorous rales can be detected sometimes by palpation. Thoracic tenderness is observed in pleurisy, pneumonia associated with pleurisy; pleurodynia, intercostal neuralgia (confined to certain spots); fracture of the ribs; and in contusion and inflammation of the pleural surfaces.

PERCUSSION: Place finger being used as a pleximeter firmly against chest and preferably parallel to ribs. Make finger that is used as plexor strike the one on chest perpendicularly, fix forearm, and use no more force than can be obtained from a gentle swing of the wrist. Percuss all parts of chest anteriorly and posteriorly, during both inspiration and expiration. In comparing sides be sure to percuss corresponding parts.

Normal resonance: On the right side, pulmonary resonance extends from half an inch to an inch (1.3 to 2.5 cm) above the clavicle, downward to upper border of 6th rib in front, and to a line drawn through the 10th spinous process posteriorly. On the left side, pulmonary resonance extends from a half inch to an inch (1.3 to 2.5 cm.) above the clavicle downward within the mammary line to the 10th rib, and posteriorly to a line drawn through the 10th spinous process.

Cracked pot sound: Modified tympany can be simulated by percussing over the cheek when mouth is partially open. May be heard normally over the chest of a crying infant. In the adult it usually indicates a cavity that has a free communication with a bronchus. Best detected by keeping ear near open mouth of patient while percussing.

Dullness or flatness: Recognized in tuberculous condition, pneumonic consolidation, pleural effusions of all kinds; collapse of lung, congestion and edema of lung, enlargement of liver or spleen (at base), and neoplastic growths in the lung. It is important to determine the extent of movement of the diaphragm. To do this have the patient hold breath in deep inspiration while in a sitting position. Then quickly percuss the chest on both sides posteriorly to find and mark the lowest point of pulmonary resonance. Repeat this while the patient holds breath following complete expiration. On both sides of the chest the top and bottom marks should be from ¾ to 2½ in. (2 to 6 cm.) apart. The top line on the right is usually a cm. or two higher than the left due to the presence of the liver below the right diaphragm. Diseases that interfere with aeration of the lungs or that paralyze the diaphragm will cause the normal movement of the diaphragm to be altered.

Hyperresonance: Observed in pneumothorax, tuberculous or bronchiectatic cavities, emphysema, lowered pulmonary tension in the initial stage of pneumonia and above a pleural effusion (Skoda's resonance), flatulent distention of the stomach or colon frequently observed over the left base.

Tympanitic note: A hollow drumlike sound, like that normally obtained by percussing the larynx or empty stomach. The conditions mentioned under Hyperresonance are also capable of producing tympany.

Pitch: Depends largely upon the volume of air, tension of walls of cavity, and upon size of opening that communicates with the cavity. The less the air the greater the tension, and the smaller the opening the higher will be the pitch of the note. In beginning tuberculous consolidation, the note over the affected apex is higher pitched. It must be remembered that normally the note over the right apex is higher pitched than that over the left.

RS: breathing; fremitus; resonance; respiration; "thoraco-" words.

c., emphysematous. Chest characteristic of advanced emphysema. The thorax is short and round; the anterior-posterior diameter is often as long as the transverse diameter; ribs are horizontal; the angle formed by divergence of the costal margin from the sternum is very obtuse or quite obliterated. Often termed barrel-shaped.

c., flail. A condition of the chest wall due to multiple fractures of the rib cage; it moves paradoxically, i.e., in with inspiration and out during expiration.

c., flat. Deformity of chest in which the anterior-posterior diameter is short, the thorax long and flat, and ribs oblique. The scapula is prominent; spaces above and below clavicles are depressed. Angle formed by divergence of the costal margins from the sternum is very acute.

c., pigeon. Condition of the chest in which sides are considerably flattened and sternum prominent. The sternal ends of the ribs are enlarged or beaded and this characteristic has given rise to the term rachitic rosary. Often a circular construction of the thorax at level of the xiphoid cartilage. Due to obstruction of infantile respiration or to rickets.

chestnut, horse. The inedible seed pod of the horse chestnut or buckeye tree (Aesculus hippocastanum). The nut contains a glucoside, aesculin, that is toxic. The young twigs and sprouts of A. hippocastanum are also toxic. Symptoms of aesculin poisoning include muscle twitching, weakness, incoordination, dilated pupils, vomiting, diarrhea, stupor, and paralysis. Other species of chestnuts are edible.

chest prominences and depressions. An unnatural prominence or depression is often observed over the lower part of the sternum and is generally congenital. The term funnel breast or shoemaker's breast (because it may result from pressure of tools) has been applied to the sternal depression. The correct term is pectus excavatum.

A unilateral or local depression may be caused by consolidation, cavity, or pleurisy with fibrous adhesions.

A unilateral or local prominence may be due to pleurisy with effusion; pneumothorax, hydrothorax, hemothorax; aneurysm or tumor; compensatory emphysema resulting from impairment of the opposite lung; cardiac enlargements (left side); enlargements of abdominal organs, esp. liver and spleen.

chest P.T. *chest physical therapy.*

chest regions. Anterior, posterior and lateral. *Anterior divisions* (R. and L.): clavicular, infraclavicular, and supraclavicular, mammary and inframammary, upper and lower sternal. *Posterior divisions* (R. and L.): scapular, infrascapular, interscapular, and suprascapular. *Lateral divisions:* Axillary and infra-axillary.

chest thump. A sharp blow to the chest in the precordial area. Done to attempt restoration of normal heartbeat in patients with cardiac arrest or ventricular tachycardia.

Cheyne-Stokes respiration (chān'stōks'). [John Cheyne, Scot. physician, 1777–1836; William Stokes, Irish physician, 1804–1878] A common and bizarre breathing pattern characterized by a period of apnea lasting 10 to 60 seconds followed by gradually increasing depth and frequency of respirations. It accompanies depression of frontal lobe and diencephalic dysfunction. Postulated to be due to an abnormality in the neurologic respiration center. This condition may be present as a normal finding in children. SEE: *respiration, Cheyne-Stokes* for illus.

Chiari's deformity (kē-ăr'ēz). SEE: *Arnold-Chiari deformity.*

Chiari-Frommel syndrome (kē-ăr'ē-frŏm'mĕl). [H. Chiari, Austrian pathologist, 1851–1916; R. Frommel] Persistent lactation and amenorrhea following childbirth. It is due to the continued secretion of prolactin and decreased gonadotropin production. A pituitary adenoma may or may not be present.

chiasm, chiasma (kī'ăzm, kī-ăz'mă) [Gr. *khiasma,* cross]. A crossing or decussation.

c., optic. An incomplete crossing of the optic fibers (the outer fibers not crossing each other); the point of crossing of the fibers of the optic nerves.

chickenpox. An acute viral disease with mild constitutional symptoms (headache, fever, malaise) followed by an eruption appearing in crops and characterized by macules, papules, vesicles, and crusting. Chickenpox and herpes zoster are different manifestations of infection with the same virus. SYN: *varicella,* q.v.

chief complaint(s). The symptom or group of symptoms that represents the primary reason(s) for the patient's seeking health care.

chiggers (chĭg'ĕrs). Redbugs. The six-legged larvae of mites of the family Trombiculidae, order Acarina of the class Arachnida. They are parasitic on insects, various vertebrates, and man. Eggs are laid on the ground and hatch in about 12 days, after which they attach to host at first opportunity. They attach themselves to the surface of the skin and inject a salivary secretion that dissolves the surrounding tissue, producing a wheal with intense itching and severe dermatitis. A tubular structure, a stylostome, is developed that is used in ingesting the semidigested tissue debris. The mites do not feed on blood. The most common species attacking humans in North America is Trombicula alfreddugesi. The irritation is the result of sensitization to the injected saliva. To prevent being infested when exposed, wear clothes that are tight at the neck and arms and stuff pant legs into shoes with high tops. Certain chemical compounds such as diethyltoluamide (Off) will repel chiggers. SEE: *Tunga.*

TREATMENT: Proprietary preparations are available that, when applied to the affected area, asphyxiate the mite. One of these Kwell, contains hexachlorohexane. Benzyl benzoate ointment and gamma benzene hexachloride are also effective.

chigo, chigre (chē'gō, chē'grā) [Sp.]. A jigger

or sand flea.

chilblain (chĭl'blān) [AS. *cele,* cold, + *blegen,* to puff]. Inflammation, itching, and swelling of the feet, toes, or fingers caused by mild frostbite. SYN: *frostbite; kibe; pernio.*

SYM: Reddish, violaceous plaques or patches on hands and feet, occasionally the ears. Persistent, giving rise to smarting, burning, itching, esp. when parts become warm. In severe types frostbite corresponds to second-degree burns, showing vesicles, bullae, ulcer, and necrosis.

NURSING IMPLICATIONS: If circulation is not restored, parts involved should be *gradually* warmed by placing in *tepid* water or by encircling them with warm hands. *Affected parts should not be massaged.* Patient should be placed in a warm (not hot) environment and encouraged to drink warm, nutritious drinks (not alcoholic beverages). A bed cradle may be used to protect the body from abrasion of bedclothes.

TREATMENT: Analgesics; antibiotics; anticoagulants and vasodilators are used to attempt to prevent loss of blood supply to the affected area. SEE: *windchill factor.*

child [AS. *cild,* child]. Any human between infancy and puberty. SEE: *pediatrics.*

child abuse. Emotional, physical, or sexual injury to a child. Also seen after instances of severe disruption in the process of parental attachment. May be due to positive action or omission on the part of those responsible for the care of the child. SEE: *battered child syndrome.*

childbed. Period during and immediately subsequent to parturition. SYN: *puerperium.*

childbed fever. Puerperal sepsis.

childbirth. The process of giving birth to a child. SYN: *labor; parturition.*

c., natural. The delivery of a fetus without the use of analgesics, sedatives, or anesthesia. Termed natural because this method was the only approach to childbirth prior to the development of obstetrical techniques. Natural childbirth is accomplished in the modern world by having the woman, and often the spouse, go through a training period months prior to actual delivery. This training is called psychoprophylactic preparation for childbirth. More recently, natural childbirth has come to include a more noninterventionist approach, with less reliance on technology and a greater reliance on emotional support during labor and delivery, as appropriate. SEE: *Lamaze; psychoprophylactic childbirth.*

child neglect. Failure by those responsible for caring for a child to provide for the child's nutritional, emotional, and physical needs.

chilectropion (kī"lĕk-trō'pē-ŏn) [Gr. *cheilos,* lip, + *ektrope,* turning out]. Eversion of the lip. SYN: *cheilectropion.*

chilitis (kī-lī'tĭs) [" + *itis,* inflammation]. Inflammation of the lips. SYN: *cheilitis,* q.v.

chill (chĭl) [AS. *cele,* cold]. An attack of shivering accompanied by the sensation of coldness and pallor of the skin produced by involuntary contraction of many muscle groups. It may be due to a disturbance in the temperature-regulating centers of the hypothalamus. Chills accompany various diseases, esp. malaria and pneumococcal pneumonia, and are coarse or fine, diffuse, or trembling. SEE: *windchill factor.*

ETIOL: Infections or diseases (as malaria, pneumococcal pneumonia, bacteremia); parasites in blood; bacterial vaccines; and transfusion reactions. Postoperative chills or chills in puerperium are indicative of infection.

SYM: A real chill is ushered in by extreme sensation of cold; shivering; chattering of the teeth and, in extreme cases, a marked tremor of the entire body followed by a rapidly rising temperature.

NURSING IMPLICATIONS: Make patient comfortable by applying blankets and putting in a warm (not hot) environment. Provide warm drinks when patient is able to tolerate them or when permitted by physician. Take patient's temperature and then retake it 20–30 minutes after the chill has subsided. Record the duration and severity of the chill.

c., nervous. A tremor accompanied by a chilly sensation but not with fever. It may follow severe pain or extreme nervousness. It usually passes quickly and seldom is serious.

chilo-, cheilo- [Gr. *cheilos,* lip]. Prefix denoting relationship to the lip.

chiloangioscopy (kī"lō-ăn"jē-ŏs'kō-pē) [" + *angeion,* vessel, + *skopein,* to examine]. Microscopic examination of the circulation in the lip.

Chilomastix mesnili (kī"lō-măs'tĭks mĕs-nĭl'ē). A species of Mastigophora. A protozoon that is considered a presumptive parasite in the intestines.

chimera (kī-mē'ră). In human biology, the mixing of the blood (and blast cells) of embryos of double-egg twins so that even though each twin originally had a different blood group, each now has a mixed group.

chimney sweeps' cancer. Epithelioma of the scrotum. Due to chronic irritation by coal soot. SEE: *cancer.*

chimpanzee (chĭm-păn'zē). An intelligent ape native to parts of Africa. Because of its similarity to man, it is used in experimental medicine.

chin [AS. *cin,* chin]. Point of the lower jaw; region below lower lip. SYN: *mentum* [NA].

China clay. Kaolin, q.v.

Chinese restaurant syndrome. A group of transient symptoms that some persons develop after eating food containing a considerable amt. of monosodium glutamate.

SYM: Burning sensation, headache, facial pressure, perspiration, and chest pain.

chin jerk. Reflex contraction of muscles of mastication on suddenly depressing the jaw.

chin reflex. Clonic movement resulting from percussing or stroking lower jaw.

chip. A small fragment of something.

chiragra (kī-răg'ră) [Gr. *cheir,* hand, + *agra,* seizure]. Pain in the hand.

chiralgia (kī-răl'jē-ă) [" + *algos,* pain]. Pain in the hand of nontraumatic or neuralgic origin.

c. paresthetica. Numbness and pain in the hand, esp. in the region supplied by the radial nerve.

chirismus (kī-rĭs'mŭs). Spasm of hand muscles.

chirognostic (kī"rŏg-nŏs'tĭk) [" + *gnostikos,* knowing]. Having the ability to distinguish the right from the left, or the side of the body being stimulated.

chirokinesthesia (kī"rō-kĭn"ĕs-thē'zē-ă) [" + *kinesis,* movement, + *aisthesis,* sensation]. Subjective perception of motions of the hand.

chiromegaly (kī"rō-mĕg'ă-lē) [" + *megas,* large]. Enlargement of the hands, wrists, or ankles.

chiroplasty (kī'rō-plăs"tē) [" + *plassein,* to form]. A plastic operation on the hand.

chiropodist (kī-rŏp'ō-dĭst, kī-) [" + *pous,* foot]. One who practices chiropody. SYN: *podiatrist.*

chiropody (kī-rŏp'ō-dē). Treatment of disorders of the feet.

chiropractic (kī"rō-prăk'tĭk) [Gr. *cheir,* hand, + *prattein,* to do]. System of health care based on the premise that the relationship between structure and function in the human body is a significant health factor and that such relationships between the spinal column and the nervous system are significant, since the normal transmission and expression of nerve energy are essential to the restoration and maintenance of health. (Adapted from definition supplied by the American Chiropractic Association.)

chiropractor. A person certified and licensed to practice chiropractic care.

chirospasm (kī'rō-spăzm) [" + *spasmos,* spasm]. Spasmodic affection of muscles of hand; writer's cramp.

chirurgery, chirurgia (kī-rŭr'jĕr-ē, kī-rŭr'gē-ă). Surgery, q.v.

chisel (chĭs'l). A beveled-edge steel cutting instrument used in dentistry and orthopedics.

chi-square (kī-skwār). A statistical test to determine the similarity of the number of occurrences being investigated to the expected occurrences. The symbol for chi-square is χ^2.

chitin (kī'tĭn) [Gr. *chiton,* tunic]. A white, horny substance in outer covering of body of invertebrates such as crabs. Also occurs in some fungi.

chitinous (kī'tĭ-nŭs). Pert. to or composed of chitin.

Chlamydia (klă-mĭd'ē-ă) [Gr. *chlamys,* cloak]. A genus of microorganisms that cause a wide variety of diseases in man and animals, including ornithosis (parrot fever), lymphogranuloma venereum, trachoma, related diseases such as inclusion conjunctivitis and sometimes nonspecific urethritis. Although these organisms were formerly considered to be viruses, the evidence indicates they resemble bacteria, esp. rickettsiae, much more than viruses. The genus can be divided into two species: Chlamydia trachomatis, group A; and C. psittaci, group B.

chloasma (klō-ăz'mă) [Gr. *chloazein,* to be green]. Pigmentary skin discolorations, usually those occurring in yellowish-brown patches or spots.

SYM: Areas rounded or oval with ill-defined margins; light yellow to black. In those due to external factors, pigmentation develops only at site of irritation or beyond.

c. gravidarum. Brownish pigmentation of the face, often occurring in pregnancy. It usually disappears after delivery. Also seen in some persons who take progestational agents for birth control. SYN: *mask of pregnancy.*

c., idiopathic. Chloasma caused by external agents such as sun, heat, mechanical means, and x-rays.

c., symptomatic. Chloasma caused by various diseases, as syphilis or cancer.

c. traumaticum. Skin discolorations from traumatic agents.

c. uterinum. Chloasma of pregnancy and other uterine conditions.

chloracne (klor-ăk'nē). A generalized acneiform dermatitis that may occur in persons exposed to chemicals containing chlorine.

chloral (klō'răl) [Gr. *chloros,* green]. 1. An oily liquid having a bitter taste. 2. Chloral hydrate.

chloral hydrate. USP. Colorless, transparent crystals having aromatic, slightly acrid odor, and having a caustic, faintly bitter taste; soluble in alcohol and water. Trade names are Noctec and S K Chloral Hydrate.

ACTION AND USES: As a sedative and hypnotic. Most commonly used to induce sleep as it allows almost normal sleep pattern in most patients.

chloral hydrate poisoning. Depresses and eventually paralyzes the central nervous system. Can be toxic to the liver. There may be nausea and vomiting due to gastric irritation. Pulse is feeble, respirations are shallow and irregular; lassitude; weakness; dizziness; sleep.

F.A.: Gastric lavage with coffee or tea. Central nervous system stimulants by mouth, injection, or rectum. Artificial respiration, Trendelenburg position, I.V. glucose. SEE: *Poisons and Poisoning* in *Appendix*.

chlorambucil (klō-răm'bū-sĭl). USP. A cytotoxic agent used in treating chronic lymphocytic leukemia, Hodgkin's disease, and certain lymphomas. Trade name is Leukeran.

chloramines (klō'ră-mīns). Organic chlorine compounds that decompose slowly, liberating chlorine. Used extensively in dairies, food manufacturing establishments, and as a germicide.

Ex.: chloramine-T; dichloramine-T.

chloramphenicol (klō"răm-fĕn'ĭ-kōl). USP. An antibiotic originally isolated from Streptomyces venezuelae. It is now made synthetically. It is a broad-spectrum agent and is especially useful in typhoid fever (in which it is the antibiotic of choice) and other infections caused by Salmonellae, and in rickettsial infections. Trade names are Chloromycetin and Chloroptic.

CAUTION: Certain blood dyscrasias may follow the use of chloramphenicol, esp. in neonates; consequently it should not be used indiscriminately or for minor infections. If used for prolonged periods, careful blood checks should be made. Be sure to read the literature that comes with each package of this medicine prior to deciding to use it rather than another antibiotic. SEE: *gray syndrome of the newborn*.

chlorate (klō'rāt). A salt of chloric acid. SEE: *potassium chlorate; Poisons and Poisoning* in *Appendix*.

chlorbutanol. Chlorobutanol, q.v.

chlorbutol. Chlorobutanol, q.v.

chlorcyclizine hydrochloride. Official name for the hydrochloride of 1-(p-chloro-α-phenylbenzyl)-4-methylpiperazine, an antihistamine. Trade name is Perazil.

chlordane (klor'dān). A poisonous substance used as an insecticide. SEE: *Poisons and Poisoning* in *Appendix*.

chlordantoin (klor-dăn'tō-ĭn). A topical antifungal preparation.

chlordiazepoxide hydrochloride (klor"dī-ăz"ĕ-pŏk'sīd). USP. A benzodiazepine derivative used in treating anxiety, alcohol withdrawal syndrome, and as a premedication in anesthesia. Trade names are A-poxide, Chlordiazachel, Librium, and Murcil.

chloremia (klō-rē'mē-ă) [Gr. *chloros*, green, + *haima*, blood]. Increased chloride in the blood.

chlorhexidene gluconate (klor-hĕk'sĭ-dēn). An anti-infective agent. Trade name is Hibiclens.

chlorhydria (klor-hī'drē-ă) [" + *hydor*, water]. Excess of hydrochloric acid in the stomach.

chloride (klō'rīd) [Gr. *chloros*, green]. A binary compound of chlorine; a salt of hydrochloric acid. Blood serum contains 100–110 mEq./L. (350–390 mg./dl.), principally as sodium chloride. Chloride levels are elevated in nephritis, eclampsia, anemia, and cardiac disease; decreased in fevers, diabetes, and pneumonia.

chloridemia (klō"rĭ-dē'mē-ă) [" + *haima*, blood]. Chlorides in the blood.

chloride poisoning. SEE: *barium salts* in *Poisons and Poisoning* in *Appendix*.

chloride test, urine. To a test tube half filled with urine add a drop or two of nitric acid, which holds the phosphates in solution. Then a 3% solution of silver nitrate is added to the specimen, drop by drop, until about six drops have been added. This forms a curdled white precipitate at once. The test should be compared with a known normal specimen of urine. Diminished chlorides are found in chronic nephritis, early stages of pneumonia, malignant disease, and in gastritis. Chlorides are increased in a diet rich in salt, in rickets, and in hepatic cirrhosis.

chloriduria (klō"rĭ-dū'rē-ă) [" + *ouron*, urine]. Excess of chlorides in urine.

chlorinated (klō'rĭn-ā-tĕd). Impregnated with chlorine.

chlorinated lime. Calcium hypochlorite and calcium chloride; widely used in solution as a bleach and as an antiseptic.

chlorination (klō"rĭ-nā'shŭn). Treatment of water by addition of chlorine and its compounds for the killing of bacteria. For effective disinfection, a concentration of 0.5 to 1 part of chlorine per million parts of water is necessary.

chlorine (klō'rēn) [Gr. *chloros*, green]. SYMB: Cl. At. wt. 35.453; at. no. 17. A highly irritating gas destructive to the mucous membranes of the respiratory passages. It is very poisonous and excessive inhalation may cause death. Chlorine is an active bleaching agent and germicide. Both of these effects are due to its oxidizing powers. It is used extensively in the disinfection of water supplies and in treatment of sewage.

FUNCT: Chlorine is found combined with sodium in the blood and exercises some influence upon metabolism, helps to maintain osmotic pressure, and aids in the regulation and stimulation of muscular action. The body fluids contain 0.85% salt solution. The inorganic salts keep in solution proteins of the blood, milk, and other secretions. Chlorine is present in the hydrochloric acid of the gastric juice. It aids digestion, activates enzymes, and is essential to normal gastric secretion.

chlorine preparations. Preparations used for disinfecting. Compounds (hypochlorites), as Dakin's solution or Javelle water, are very effective in their germicidal power. As a disinfecting agent in washing dishes and utensils used by infected patients, 1/10 of 1% solution should be used; the dishes should then be washed well in soap and hot water and rinsed well, or boiled and then washed well after the boiling.

For disinfection of the stools of patients, 5% or even stronger solutions may be used for ½ hour or longer. The utensil is set aside and covered while the solution functions. Dakin's solution is nonirritating and is used as a wound disinfectant, but it must be carefully prepared daily by the laboratory and used only when fresh.

chlorite (klō'rīt). A salt of chlorous acid; used as a disinfectant and bleaching agent.

chlormerodrin Hg 197 injection (klor-mĕr'ō-drĭn). USP. A radioactive drug used in testing renal function.

chlormerodrin Hg 203 injection. USP. A radioactive drug used in testing renal function.

chloroazodin (klor-ō-ăz'ō-dĭn). α, α'-Azobis [chloroformamidine], an antibacterial preparation of chlorine used as a topical antiseptic.

chlorobutanol (klō-rō-bū'tă-nŏl). Colorless crystals with camphor odor and taste. SYN: *chlorbutanol; chlorbutol.*

USES: Antiseptic and local anesthetic used in dentistry, and as a preservative in many pharmaceuticals.

INCOMPAT: Decomposed by alkalies and should not be mixed with borax or carbonates. Soluble in ether, chloroform, and volatile oils.

chloroform (klō'rō-form) [Gr. *chloros,* green, + L. *forma,* form]. $CHCl_3$. A heavy, clear, colorless liquid with strong etherlike odor, formed by the action of chlorinated lime on methyl alcohol. At one time chloroform was administered by inhalation to produce anesthesia; but this usage is obsolete.

chloroformism (klō'rō-form"ĭzm). The habit of inhaling chloroform for pleasure.

chloroleukemia (klō"rō-loo-kē'mē-ă) [" + *leukos,* white, + *haima,* blood]. Leukemia with chlorosis.

chloroma (klō-rō'mă) [" + *oma,* growth]. A greenish sarcoma of the periosteum of cranial bones; green cancer.

Chloromycetin (klō"rō-mī-sē'tĭn). Trade name for chloramphenicol, USP, q.v.

chloropenia (klō"rō-pē'nē-ă) [" + *penia,* poverty]. Deficiency in chlorine. SYN: *hypochloremia.*

chloropenic (klō"rō-pēn'ĭk). Deficient in chlorine.

chlorophane (klō'rō-fān) [" + *phainein,* to show]. A green-yellow pigment in the retina.

chlorophenothane (klō"rō-fĕn'ō-thān). An insecticide, better known as DDT, q.v., that is quite effective but should not be used because of its toxicity.

chlorophyll, chlorophyl (klō'rō-fĭl) [" + *phyllon,* leaf]. The green pigment in plants that accomplishes photosynthesis. Essential in the utilization of that energy is combining carbon dioxide (CO_2) and carbohydrate according to the following scheme: $6\ CO_2 + 6\ H_2O + \text{light} \rightarrow C_6H_{12}O_6 + 6\ O_2$. Thus the primary source of energy in our planet is the light absorbed by chlorophyll. Four forms of chlorophyll (a, b, c, and d) occur in nature.

chloropia, chloropsia (klō-rō'pē-ă, klō-rŏp'sē-ă) [" + *opsis,* vision]. Vision defect in which all things appear green.

chloroplast, chloroplastid (klō'rō-plăst, klō"rō-plăs'tĭd) [" + *plastos* formed]. Small, round, green bodies found in the cells of leaves and stem of plants that are important in the process of photosynthesis. They possess a stroma and contain four pigments: chlorophyll a, chlorophyll b, carotene, and xanthophyll.

chloroprivic (klō"rō-prĭv'ĭk) [" + L. *privare,* to deprive of]. Lack of, or due to loss of, chlorides.

chloroprocaine hydrochloride (klō"rō-prō'kān). USP. A local anesthetic more potent and less toxic than procaine. Trade names are Nesacaine and Nesacaine-CE.

Chloroptic. Trade name for chloramphenicol.

chloroquine hydrochloride (klō'rō-kwĭn). USP. $C_{18}H_{26}ClN_3 \cdot 2H_3PO_4$. A white crystalline powder used for its antimicrobial action, esp. in the treatment of malaria. It is useful also in amebic dysentery complicated by liver abscess and in treating lupus erythematosus. Trade name for chloroquine phosphate, USP, is Aralen Phosphate; trade name for chloroquine hydrochloride, USP is Aralen Hydrochloride.

chlorosis (klō-rō'sĭs) [" + *osis,* condition]. A form of iron-deficiency anemia. SEE: *anemia, iron deficiency.*

chlorothiazide sodium (klō"rō-thī'ă-zīd). USP. An effective diuretic. Administered orally. Trade name is Sodium Diuril.

chlorothymol (klō"rō-thī'mŏl). A phenol-derived germicide.

chlorotic (klō-rŏt'ĭk). Of the nature of or afflicted with chlorosis.

chlorotrianisene (klō"rō-trī-ăn'ĭ-sēn). USP. A synthetic estrogen that is about one eighth as potent as diethylstilbestrol. It is little used because it accumulates in fat tissue. Trade name is Tace.

chlorpheniramine maleate (klor"fĕn-ĭr'ă-mēn). USP. An antihistamine that may be used orally or by injection. Trade name is

Chlor-Trimeton.

chlorphenoxamine hydrochloride (klor″fĕn-ŏk′să-mēn). USP. Drug used in treating parkinsonism. Trade name is Phenoxene.

chlorpromazine (klor-prō′mă-zēn). USP. A tranquilizing agent, it is used primarily in its hydrochloride form in major and minor psychotic states. Trade name for chlorpromazine hydrochloride is Thorazine.

chlorpromazine poisoning. SEE: *Poisons and Poisoning* in *Appendix*.

chlorpropamide (klor-prō′pă-mīd). USP. An oral hypoglycemic agent of the sulfonylurea class. Trade name is Diabinese.

CAUTION: This drug should be used only in patients with diabetes of the insulin-independent type who, if weight reduction and dietary control fail, cannot be treated with diet alone and who are unwilling or unable to take insulin.

chlorprothixene (klor-prō-thĭks′ēn). USP. Drug used in treating mental illness. Trade name is Taractan.

chlorquinaldol (klor-kwĭn′ăl-dŏl). A hydroxyquinoline useful in treating amebiasis. Because of possible neurotoxicity, it is not the treatment of choice.

chlortetracycline hydrochloride (klor″tĕt-ră-sī′klēn). A golden-colored antibiotic isolated from a strain of Streptomyces aureofaciens. It is a broad-spectrum antibiotic, inhibiting growth of or destroying some strains of streptococci, staphylococci, pneumococci, rickettsiae, and viruses. Trade name is Aureomycin.

chlorthalidone (klor-thăl′ĭ-dōn). USP. An effective diuretic. Trade name is Hygroton.

Chlor-Trimeton. Trade name for chlorpheniramine maleate.

chlorzoxazone (klor-zŏk′să-zōn). A muscle relaxant. Trade name is Paraflex.

Ch.M. *chirurgiae magister,* Master of Surgery.

choana (kō′ă-nă) [Gr. *choane,* funnel]. (pl. *choanae*) A funnel-shaped opening, esp. one of the posterior nares, the communicating passageways between the nasal fossae and the pharynx.

choanoid (kō′ăn-oyd) [″ + *eidos,* shape]. Shaped like a funnel.

choke [ME. *choken*]. To prevent respiration by compression or obstruction of the larynx or trachea.

choked disk. Edema of the optic disk. SEE: *papilledema*.

chokes. Respiratory symptoms such as substernal distress, paroxysmal cough, tachypnea, or asphyxia, which may occur in decompression illness, esp. in cases of aeroembolism resulting from exposure to pressure lower than atmospheric. SEE: *caisson disease*.

choke-saver. Commercial name for a curved tweezer-like forceps, usually made of plastic, for inserting into the throat of a person choking. The device is used to grasp and remove the food from the obstructed airway. SEE: *Heimlich maneuver*.

choking [ME. *choken,* to suffocate]. Obstruction within respiratory passage or constriction about the neck, interfering with breathing and circulation of brain. May also result from spasm of the larynx induced by an irritating gas. SEE: *Emergency Measures* listed below for *choking on food; Heimlich maneuver.*

SYM: Face purple; eyes protrude; arms thrown about; coughing; constriction and injury about neck; cyanosis; dizziness; unconsciousness.

choking on food. Inadequately chewed food may be inhaled inadvertently. Most commonly involved is a piece of meat or other solid food. The usual result is panic accompanied by inability to speak, cyanosis, and fainting. Lay persons in the vicinity may assume the patient is having a heart attack.

EMERGENCY MEASURES: By using the fingers or curved forceps, reach into the throat, dislodge the obstruction, and remove it. It may be possible to forcibly eject the food by quickly and forcibly compressing the abdomen and lower chest (the Heimlich maneuver). This maneuver consists of (1) wrapping your arms around the victim's waist from behind; (2) making a fist with one hand and placing it against the victim's abdomen between the navel and rib cage; (3) clasping your fist with your free hand and pressing in with a quick forceful upward thrust. Repeat several times if necessary. This will produce sudden air pressure on the object. If an object is lodged in the throat and breathing is possible, interference should be limited until professional aid is available. Tracheotomy may be needed. SEE: *Heimlich maneuver*.

cholagogue (kō′lă-gŏg) [Gr. *chole,* bile, + *agein,* to lead forth]. An agent that increases the flow of bile into the intestine, i.e., a choleretic, or cholecystagogue.

Cholan-DH. Trade name for dehydrocholic acid.

cholangiectasis (kō-lăn″jē-ĕk′tă-sĭs) [″ + *angeion,* vessel, + *ektasis,* dilatation]. Dilation of bile ducts.

cholangiocarcinoma (kō-lăn″jē-ō-kăr″sĭ-nō′mă) [″ + ″ + *karkinos,* crab, + *oma,* tumor]. Malignancy of the bile ducts.

cholangioenterostomy (kō-lăn″jē-ō-ĕn″tĕr-ŏs′tō-mē) [″ + ″ + *enteron,* intestine, + *stoma,* opening]. Surgically produced communication between a bile duct and the intestine.

cholangiogastrostomy (kō-lăn″jē-ō-găs-trŏs′tō-mē) [″ + ″ + *gaster,* stomach, + *stoma,* mouth]. Surgical formation of a communication between the bile duct and stomach.

cholangiography (kō-lăn″jē-ŏg′ră-fē) [″ + ″ + *graphein,* to write]. X-ray examination of the bile ducts.

cholangiole (kō-lăn′jē-ōl) [″ + ″ + *ole,* dim. suffix]. The small terminal portion of the bile duct.

cholangiolitis (kō-lăn″jē-ō-lī′tĭs) [″ + ″ + ″ + Gr. *itis,* inflammation]. Inflammation of the bile ducts. This occurs in various forms of hepatitis.

cholangioma (kō-lăn-jē-ō′mă) [″ + *angeion,* vessel, + *oma,* tumor]. A tumor of the biliary ducts.

cholangiostomy (kō″lăn-jē-ŏs′tō-mē) [″ + ″ + *stoma,* mouth]. The surgical formation of a fistula into the gallbladder.

cholangiotomy (kō″lăn-jē-ŏt′ō-mē) [″ + ″ + *tome,* incision]. Incision of an intrahepatic bile duct for removal of gallstones.

cholangitis (kō″lăn-jī′tĭs) [″ + *angeion,* vessel, + *itis,* inflammation]. Inflammation of the bile ducts.

cholanopoiesis (kō″lă-nō-poy-ē′sĭs) [Gr. *chole,* bile, + *ano,* upward, + *poiesis,* making]. Synthesis of cholic acid in the liver.

cholate (kō′lāt). Any salt or ester of cholic acid.

cholecalciferol (ko″lē-kăl-sĭf′ĕr-ŏl). USP. Vitamin D_3; an antirachitic, oil-soluble vitamin occurring as white, odorless crystals.

cholecyst (kō′lē-sĭst) [″ + *kystis,* bladder]. The gallbladder.

cholecystagogue (kō″lē-sĭs′tă-gŏg) [″ + ″ + *agogos,* leader]. Drug or action that causes emptying of the gallbladder.

cholecystalgia (kō″lē-sĭs-tăl′jē-ă) [″ + ″ + *algos,* pain]. Biliary colic.

cholecystangiography (kō″lē-sĭs″tăn-jē-ŏg′ră-fē) [″ + ″ + *angeion,* vessel, + *graphein,* to write]. Radiographic examination of the gallbladder and biliary ducts after injection of a contrast medium.

cholecystectasia (kō″lē-sĭs-tĕk-tā′zē-ă) [″ + ″ + *ektasis,* dilatation]. Dilatation of the gallbladder.

cholecystectomy (kō″lē-sĭs-tĕk′tō-mē) [″ + ″ + *ektome,* excision]. Excision of a gallbladder.

NURSING IMPLICATIONS: Place patient in semi-Fowler's position to facilitate drainage. Assess dressing and drainage tube for bleeding frequently. Ensure that tube is securely fastened to patient. Check vital signs frequently (every 2 to 4 hours) for the first 24 hours post-op. Observe color of skin and sclerae for evidence of jaundice. Encourage patient to change positions and cough and breathe deeply to prevent post-op complications. Assess for symptoms indicative of hemorrhage or shock. Observe and record amount and type of drainage and check for obstruction of drainage tube. Maintain patient on a low-fat diet.

cholecystenterorrhaphy (kō″lē-sĭs-tĕn″tĕr-or′ă-fē) [″ + ″ + *enteron,* intestine, + *rhaphe,* suture]. Suture of gallbladder to intestinal wall.

cholecystenterostomy (kō″lē-sĭs-tĕn″tĕr-ŏs′tō-mē) [″ + ″ + *enteron,* intestine, + *stoma,* opening]. Surgical establishment of a connection between the gallbladder and the small intestine.

cholecystic (kō″lē-sĭs′tĭk). Pert. to the gallbladder.

cholecystitis (kō″lē-sĭs-tī′tĭs) [Gr. *chole,* bile, + *kystis,* bladder, + *itis,* inflammation]. Inflammation of the gallbladder. It may be acute or chronic.

ETIOL: Acute cholecystitis is nearly always caused by gallstones. Other causes may be bacteria or chemical irritants. Chronic cholecystitis may occur with or without stones. However, not all patients with gallstones experience cholecystitis.

SYM: In acute cholecystitis there is fever, gradually developing or sudden pain in upper abdomen, nausea, vomiting, visible jaundice in about 25% of patients. Frequently pain is referred to back or right shoulder. Approx. 10% of patients do not have pain. In chronic cholecystitis symptoms are usually less severe than in acute cholecystitis, but recurring stones may or may not be present.

TREATMENT: In acute cholecystitis, cholecystectomy; if this is not possible, draining of gallbladder (cholecystostomy) followed by cholecystectomy at a later date. In chronic cholecystitis, cholecystectomy if stones are present. If there are no stones, antispasmodics, laxatives, rest, and sedation if necessary, and further study to determine cause.

NURSING IMPLICATIONS: Assess patient for nausea, vomiting, increased pulse and respiratory rate, flatulence, right upper quadrant pain, and food intolerance. If surgery is to be performed, prepare the patient physically and emotionally for surgery. Nutrition education includes instruction concerning avoidance of fatty foods and decreased calories for weight reduction.

cholecystnephrostomy (kō″lē-sĭst″nē-frŏs′tō-mē) [″ + *kystis,* bladder, + *nephros,* kidney, + *stoma,* mouth]. Making a surgical anastomosis of the gallbladder into the renal pelvis.

cholecystocolostomy (kō″lē-sĭs″tō-kō-lŏs′tō-mē) [″ + ″ + *kolon,* colon, + *stoma,* mouth]. Making a surgical passage from the gallbladder to colon.

cholecystocolotomy (kō″lē-sĭs″tō-kō-lŏt′ō-mē) [″ + ″ + ″ + *tome,* incision]. Surgical incision into the gallbladder and colon.

cholecystoduodenostomy (kō″lē-sĭs″tō-dū″ō-dē-nŏs′tō-mē) [″ + ″ + L. *duodeni,* twelve,

+ Gr. *stoma*, mouth]. Surgical formation of a passage from the gallbladder to duodenum.

cholecystogastrostomy (kō"lē-sĭs"tō-găs-trŏs'tō-mē) [" + " + *gaster*, belly, + *stoma*, mouth]. Surgical formation of a passage from the gallbladder to the stomach.

cholecystogram (kō"lē-sĭs'tō-grăm) [" + " + *gramma*, mark]. An x-ray picture of the gallbladder.

cholecystography (kō"lē-sĭs-tŏg'ră-fē) [" + " + *graphein*, to write]. Examination of the gallbladder by x-ray study.

cholecystoileostomy (kō"lē-sĭs"tō-ĭl-ē-ŏs'tō-mē) [" + *kystis*, bladder + L. *ileum*, ileum, + Gr. *stoma*, mouth]. Forming a communication between the gallbladder and ileum.

cholecystojejunostomy (kō"lē-sĭs"tō-jē-jū-nŏs'tō-mē) [" + " + L. *jejunum*, empty, + Gr. *stoma*, mouth]. Forming a communication between the gallbladder and jejunum.

cholecystokinin (kō"lē-sĭs"tō-kī'nĭn) [" + " + *kinein*, to move]. A hormone secreted into the blood by the mucosa of the upper small intestine. It stimulates gallbladder contraction and pancreatic enzyme secretion. At one time it was believed that pancreozymin and cholecystokinin were separate hormones, but they are not.

cholecystolithiasis (kō"lē-sĭs"tō-lĭ-thī'ă-sĭs) [" + " + *lithos*, stone, + *-iasis*, condition]. Gallstones in the gallbladder.

cholecystolithotripsy (kō"lē-sĭs"tō-lĭth'ō-trĭp"sē) [" + " + " + *tripsis*, a rubbing]. Crushing of a gallstone in the unopened gallbladder.

cholecystomy (kō"lē-sĭs'tō-mē) [Gr. *chole*, bile, + *kystis*, bladder, + *tome*, incision]. Cholecystotomy.

cholecystopathy (kō"lē-sĭs-tŏp'ă-thē) [" + " + *pathos*, disease]. Any gallbladder affection.

cholecystopexy (kō"lē-sĭs'tō-pĕk"sē) [" + " + *pexis*, fixation]. Suturing the gallbladder to the abdominal wall.

cholecystoptosis (kō"lē-sĭs-tō-tō'sĭs) [" + " + *ptosis*, fall]. Downward displacement of the gallbladder.

cholecystorrhaphy (kō"lē-sĭs-tor'ă-fē) [" + *kystis*, bladder, + *rhaphe*, suture]. Suturing of the gallbladder.

cholecystostomy (kō"lē-sĭs-tŏs'tō-mē) [" + " + *stoma*, opening]. Surgical formation of an opening into the gallbladder through the abdominal wall.

cholecystotomy (kō"lē-sĭs-tŏt'ō-mē) [" + " + *tome*, incision]. Incision of the gallbladder through the abdominal wall for removal of gallstones.

choledochal (kō-lē-dŏk'ăl) [" + *dochos*, receptacle]. Rel. or pert. to the common bile duct.

choledochectasia (kō-lĕd"ō-kĕk-tā'zē-ă) [" + " + *ektasis*, distention]. Distention of the common bile duct.

choledochectomy (kō-lĕd"ō-kĕk'tō-mē) [" + " + *ektome*, excision]. Excision of a portion of the common bile duct.

choledochitis (kō"lē-dō-kī'tĭs) [" + " + *itis*, inflammation]. Inflammation of the common bile duct.

choledochoduodenostomy (kō-lĕd"ō-kō-dū-ō-dē-nŏs'tō-mē) [" + " + L. *duodeni*, twelve, + Gr. *stoma*, opening]. Surgical communication between the common bile duct and duodenum.

choledochoenterostomy (kō-lĕd"ō-kō-ĕn-tĕr-ŏs'tō-mē) [" + " + *enteron*, intestine, + *stoma*, opening]. Surgical passage between the common bile duct and intestine.

choledochography (kō-lĕd"ō-kŏg'ră-fē) [" + *dochos*, receptacle, + *graphein*, to write]. X-ray examination of the bile duct following administration of a radiopaque substance.

choledochojejunostomy (kō-lĕd"ō-kō-jē-jū-nŏs'tō-mē) [" + " + L. *jejunum*, empty, + Gr. *stoma*, mouth]. Surgical joining of the common bile duct to the jejunum of the small intestine.

choledocholith (kō-lĕd'ō-kō-lĭth") [" + " + *lithos*, stone]. Calculus, or stone, in the common bile duct.

choledocholithiasis (kō-lĕd"ō-kō-lĭ-thī'ă-sĭs) [" + " + *lithos*, stone, + *-iasis*, condition]. Calculi in the common bile duct.

choledocholithotomy (kō-lĕd"ō-kō-lĭth-ŏt'ō-mē) [" + " + " + *tome*, incision]. Removal of a gallstone through an incision of the bile duct.

choledocholithotripsy (kō-lĕd'ō-kō-lĭth"ō-trĭp-sē) [" + " + " + *tripsis*, a crushing]. Crushing of a gallstone in the common bile duct.

choledochoplasty (kō-lĕd'ō-kō-plăs"tē) [Gr. *chole*, bile, + *dochos*, receptacle, + *plassein*, to form]. Operation for repair of the common bile duct.

choledochorrhaphy (kō-lĕd"ō-kor'ă-fē) [" + " + *rhaphe*, suture]. Suturing the severed ends of the common bile duct.

choledochostomy (kō-lĕd"ō-kŏs'tō-mē) [" + " + *stoma*, mouth]. Surgical formation of an opening into the common bile duct through the abdominal wall.

choledochotomy (kō"lĕd-ō-kŏt'ō-mē) [" + " + *tome*, incision]. Surgical incision of the common bile duct.

choledochus (kō-lĕd'ō-kŭs) [" + *dochos*, receptacle]. The common bile duct. SYN: *ductus choledochus* [NA].

Choledyl. Trade name for oxtriphylline.

choleic (kō-lē'ĭk). Cholic; pert. to the bile.

cholelith (kō'lē-lĭth) [" + *lithos*, stone]. A biliary concretion of gallstone.

cholelithiasis (kō"lē-lĭ-thī'ă-sĭs) [" + " + *-iasis*, condition]. Formation or presence of calculi or bilestones in the gallbladder or common duct. The stones may or may not cause symptoms.

SYM: Digestive disturbances; heaviness in right hypochondrium; tenderness on pressure over gallbladder. Gallstone colic when a stone obstructs the bile duct. Pain may radiate to back and right shoulder. Colic usually manifest when stomach is empty. Jaundice if flow of bile is obstructed. Pain may be associated with vomiting and sweating. If distended, the gallbladder is palpable.

TREATMENT: Cholecystectomy; in very poor-risk patients, cholecystostomy.

cholelithic (kō″lē-lĭth′ĭk). Pert. to or caused by biliary calculus.

cholelithotomy (kō″lē-lĭ-thŏt′ō-mē) [″ + *lithos,* stone, + *tome,* incision]. Removal of gallstones through a surgical incision.

cholelithotripsy, cholelithotrity (kō″lē-lĭth′ō-trĭp-sē, kō″lē-lĭ-thŏt′rĭ-tē) [″ + ″ + *tripsis,* a crushing]. Crushing of a biliary calculus.

cholemesis (kō-lĕm′ĕ-sĭs) [″ + *emein,* to vomit]. Bile in the vomitus.

cholemia (kō-lē′mē-ă) [″ + *haima,* blood]. Bile or its pigments in the blood.

cholepathia (kō″lē-păth′ē-ă) [″ + *pathos,* disease]. Disease of the bile duct.

c. spastica. Spasmodic contraction of biliary ducts.

choleperitoneum (kō″lē-pĕr″ĭ-tō-nē′ŭm) [″ + *peri,* around, + *teinein,* to stretch]. Bile in the peritoneum.

cholepoiesis (kō″lē-poy-ē′sĭs) [″ + *poiein,* to make]. The formation of bile.

cholera (kŏl′ĕr-ă) [L. *cholera,* bilious diarrhea]. An acute infection involving the entire small bowel, characterized by profuse watery diarrhea and vomiting, which produces severe loss of fluids and electrolytes, muscular cramps, oliguria, dehydration, and collapse. SYN: *Asiatic cholera.*

ETIOL: Causative organism Vibrio cholerae (also called Vibrio comma, cholera bacillus, comma bacillus, Koch's bacillus), which is a short, curved, motile, gram-negative rod producing a potent endotoxin that interferes with cellular metabolism. It is a mucolytic enzyme. Transmission is through water, milk, or other foods contaminated with excreta of patients or carriers.

INCUBAT: A few hours to four to five days.

SYM: Four stages are usually described as follows:

Invasion: At the conclusion of the incubation period there is malaise, headache, diarrhea, and anorexia. Headache and slight fever are present. May last a few days and then subside. Under such circumstances, may be termed cholerine. Sometimes this stage is missing entirely.

Evacuation: Purging, violent vomiting, and muscular cramps. Stools loose, copious, and watery, and present a typical rice-water appearance. Sometimes there are particles of blood and mucus. Vomiting is severe and persistent; the material expelled may also resemble rice water. Muscular cramps commonly start in extremities; involve calves of legs; and later even arms, hands, feet, and trunk. Thirst is unquenchable, and hiccough sometimes develops. Signs of depression soon terminate in collapse. Duration of this stage, 2 to 12 hours, seldom more.

Stage of Collapse: Almost complete arrest of circulation; eyes sunken; cheeks hollow; nose pinched; skin dry and wrinkled; body surface cold and covered with clammy sweat; breath cool; temperature in axilla 85–95° F. (29.4–35° C.), while in the rectum it may be 103° F. (39.4° C.) or more. Respirations quickened, pulse weak, systolic blood pressure decreased; urine output diminished or absent; diarrhea and cramps may continue. The mind usually is clear until shortly prior to death, when coma develops Stage lasts from few hours to one or two days, and generally ends in death. Cause of death is dehydration and electrolyte imbalance.

Stage of Reaction: Sometimes, even when death seems imminent, surface temperature begins to rise, vomiting ceases, bowel evacuations become less frequent and more feculent, and convalescence is established. Complete recovery may ensue in from one to two weeks. Occasionally, typhoid symptoms set in, temperature goes to 106–107° F. (41.1–41.7° C.), and outcome is fatal. Sometimes in this stage, an erythemal eruption or one of the urticarial type appears, particularly on extremities. Such eruptions have no special significance.

TREATMENT: Vigorous replacement of fluid and electrolytes by intravenous administration of a 2 to 1 mixture of normal saline and ⅙ molar sodium lactate. If patient is in shock give 100 ml./kg. body weight and less if shock is not present. The fluid should be given rapidly until blood pressure returns to normal. Children will require additional potassium. Fluids also should be given *ad lib* by mouth. Tetracycline given early in the disease is effective in killing the causative organism.

PROPHYLAXIS: Proper sanitation and cholera vaccine. Following the initial two or three injections, booster doses should be administered every six months if the person remains in an endemic area.

c. sicca. A term sometimes applied to a fulminating variety of cholera that occurs without vomiting or diarrhea.

choleragen (kŏl′ĕr-ă-gĕn). The potent enterotoxin produced by Vibrio cholerae. It acts on the mucosal cells of the small bowel to cause increased secretion of chloride and bicarbonate into the intestine.

cholerase (kŏl'ĕr-ās). The special bacteriolytic enzyme of Vibrio cholerae.

choleresis (kŏl-ĕr-ē'sĭs, kō-lĕr'ĕ-sĭs) [Gr. *chole,* bile, + *hairesis,* removal]. The secretion of bile by the liver.

choleretic (kŏl-ĕr-ĕt'ĭk). 1. Stimulating excretion of bile by the liver. 2. Any agent that increases excretion of bile by the liver.

choleric (kŏl'ĕr-ĭk). Irritable; quick-tempered without apparent cause.

choleriform (kŏl-ĕr'ĭ-form) [L. *cholera* + *forma,* shape]. Resembling cholera.

cholerigenous, cholerigenic (kŏl-ĕr-ĭj'ĕn-ŭs, kŏl"ĕr-ĭ-jĕn'ĭk) [" + Gr. *gennan,* to produce]. Giving rise to cholera.

cholerine (kŏl'ĕr-ĭn). A mild form or initial stages of Asiatic cholera.

choleroid (kŏl'ĕr-oyd) [" + Gr. *eidos,* form]. Having a resemblance to cholera.

choleromania (kŏl"ĕr-ō-mā'nē-ă) [" + Gr. *mania,* madness]. Madness occasionally seen in cholera.

cholerophobia (kŏl"ĕr-ō-fō'bē-ă) [" + Gr. *phobos,* fear]. Morbid fear of acquiring cholera.

cholestasia (kō"lē-stā'zē-ă) [Gr. *chole,* bile, + *stasis,* stoppage]. Arrest of the bile excretion.

cholestatic. Pert. to or caused by cholestasia.

cholesteatoma (kō"lē-stē"ă-tō'mă) [" + *steatos,* fat, + *oma,* tumor]. An epithelial pocket or cyst-like sac filled with keratin debris. Can occur in the meninges, central nervous system, and bones of skull, but is most common in the middle ear and mastoid area. The cystic process, which is filled with a combination of epithelial cells and cholesterol, most commonly enlarges to occlude the middle ear. Enzymes formed within the sac cause erosion of adjacent bones, including the ossicles, and destroy them. Cholesteatomas are divided into congenital, primary acquired, and secondary acquired.

cholesteremia, cholesterolemia (kō-lĕs"tĕ-rē'mē-ă, kō-lĕs"tĕr-ŏl-ē'mē-ă) [" + *stereos,* solid, + *haima,* blood]. The presence of excess cholesterol in the blood. SYN: *hypercholesterolemia.*

cholesterin (kō-lĕs'tĕr-ĭn). Cholesterol, q.v.

cholesterinemia (kō-lĕs'tĕr-ĭn-ē'mē-ă). Cholesteremia.

cholesterinuria (kō-lĕs"tĕr-ĭn-ū'rē-ă) [" + *stereos,* solid, + *ouron,* urine]. Presence of cholesterol in the urine.

cholesterohydrothorax (kō-lĕs"tĕr-ō-hī"drō-thō'răks) [" + " + *hydor,* water, + *thorax,* chest]. An effusion in the pleural cavity of fluid that contains cholesterol.

cholesterol (kō-lĕs'tĕr-ŏl) [" + *stereos,* solid]. $C_{27}H_{45}OH$. A monohydric alcohol. A sterol widely distributed in animal tissues and occurring in the yolk of eggs, various oils, fats, nerve tissue of the brain and spinal cord, the liver, kidneys, and adrenal glands. It can be synthesized in the liver and is a normal constituent of bile. It is the principal constituent of most gallstones. It is important in metabolism, serving as a precursor of various steroid hormones, e.g., sex hormones, adrenal corticoids. SEE: *lipoproteins.*

cholesteroluria (kō-lĕs"tĕr-ŏl-ū'rē-ă) [" + " + *ouron,* urine]. Presence of cholesterol in urine.

cholesterosis (kō-lĕs-tĕr-ō'sĭs) [" + " + *osis,* condition]. Cholesterol deposition in excessive amounts.

cholestyramine resin (kō"lē-stī'ră-mĭn). USP. An ion-exchange resin used to treat itching associated with jaundice. It acts by lowering the level of bile acids in the serum. Trade name is Questran.

choletelin (kō-lĕt'ĕl-ĭn) [" + *telos,* end]. Yellow pigment that is the oxidation product of bilirubin.

choletherapy (kō"lē-thĕr'ă-pē) [" + *therapeia,* treatment]. Use of bile salts as a medicine.

choleuria (kō"lē-ū'rē-ă) [" + *ouron,* urine]. Bile in urine.

choleverdin (kō"lē-vĕr'dĭn) [" + L. *viridis,* green]. Green pigment appearing in gallstones and in urine in jaundice. SYN: *biliverdin.*

cholic acid (kō'lĭk). The sodium salt of conjugated taurocholic or glycocholic acid.

choline (kō'lĭn, -lēn) [Gr. *chole,* bile]. $C_5H_{15}NO_2$. An amine, widely distributed in plant and animal tissues. It is a constituent of lecithin and other phospholipids. It is essential in normal fat and carbohydrate metabolism. A deficiency leads to lipoidosis of the liver. It is also involved in protein metabolism, serving as a methylating agent, and it is a precursor of acetylcholine.

cholinergic (kō"lĭn-ĕr'jĭk) [" + *ergon,* work]. 1. Nerve endings that liberate acetylcholine. 2. An agent that produces the effect of acetylcholine.

cholinergic fibers. They include all preganglionic fibers, all postganglionic parasympathetic fibers, postganglionic sympathetic fibers to the sweat glands, and efferent fibers to skeletal muscle.

cholinesterase (kō"lĭn-ĕs'tĕr-ās). Any enzyme that catalyzes the hydrolysis of choline esters, such as acetylcholinesterase, which catalyzes the breakdown of acetylcholine to acetic acid and choline. Cholinesterases are inhibited by physostigmine (eserine).

cholinoceptive (kō"lĭn-ō-sĕp'tĭv) [" + L. *receptor,* receiver]. Concerning sites on cells that are acted on by cholinergic transmitters.

cholinolytic (kō"lĭn-ō-lĭt'ĭk) [" + *lysis,* dissolution]. A drug or chemical that blocks the action of acetylcholine.

cholinomimetic (kō"lĭ-nō-mĭ-mĕt'ĭk) [" + *mimetikos*, imitating]. Acting in the same way as acetylcholine.
cholochrome (kō'lō-krōm) [" + *chroma*, color]. Any bile pigment.
chologenic (kō"lō-jĕn'ĭk) [" + *gennan*, to produce]. Producing or stimulating the production of bile.
cholohemothorax (kō"lō-hĕm"ō-thō'răks) [" + *haima*, blood, + *thorax*, chest]. Presence of bile and blood in the thorax.
chololith (kŏl'ō-lĭth) [" + *lithos*, stone]. A gallstone; biliary calculus.
chololithiasis (kŏl"ō-lĭth-ī'ăs-ĭs) [" + " + *-iasis*, state]. Presence of concretions in the gallbladder. SYN: *cholelithiasis*.
cholorrhea (kŏl"ō-rē'ă) [" + *rhoia*, flow]. Excessive secretion of bile.
Choloxin. Trade name for dextrothyroxine sodium.
choluria (kō-lū'rē-ă) [" + *ouron*, urine]. Bile salts in the urine.
chondral (kŏn'drăl) [Gr. *chondros*, cartilage]. Pert. to cartilage.
chondralgia (kŏn-drăl'jē-ă) [" + *algos*, pain]. Pain in or around a cartilage.
chondralloplasia (kŏn"drăl-ō-plā'zē-ă) [" + *allos*, other, + *plassein*, to form]. Presence of cartilage in abnormal places.
chondrectomy (kŏn-drĕk'tō-mē) [" + *ektome*, excision]. Surgical excision of a cartilage.
chondric (kŏn'drĭk) [Gr. *chondros*, cartilage]. Pert. to cartilage.
chondrification (kŏn-drĭ-fĭ-kā'shŭn) [" + L. *facere*, to make]. Conversion into cartilage.
chondrigen (kŏn'drĭ-jĕn) [" + *gennan*, to produce]. Basal substance of cartilage and corneal tissue, which turns into chondrin on boiling. Also spelled *chondrogen*.
chondrin (kŏn'drĭn) [Gr. *chondros*, cartilage]. Gelatinlike matter obtained by boiling cartilage.
chondritis (kŏn-drī'tĭs) [" + *itis*, inflammation]. Inflammation of cartilage.
chondroadenoma (kŏn"drō-ăd-ē-nō'mă) [" + *aden*, gland, + *oma*, tumor]. Cartilaginous tissue in an adenoma.
chondroangioma (kŏn"drō-ăn-jē-ō'ma) [" + *angeion*, vessel, + *oma*, tumor]. Cartilaginous elements in an angioma.
chondroblast (kŏn'drō-blăst) [" + *blastos*, germ]. A cell that forms cartilage.
chondroblastoma (kŏn"drō-blăs-tō'mă) [" + " + *oma*, tumor]. A benign neoplasm in which the cells resemble cartilage cells and the tumor appears to be cartilage.
chondrocalcinosis (kŏn"drō-kăl"sĭn-ō'sĭs) [" + L. *calx*, lime, + Gr. *osis*, condition]. Pseudogout; chronic recurrent arthritis clinically similar to gout. The crystals found in synovial fluid are calcium pyrophosphate dihydrate and not urate crystals. The most commonly involved joint is the knee.
chondroclast (kŏn'drō-klăst) [" + *klastos*, broken into bits]. A giant cell involved in the absorption of cartilage.
chondrocostal (kŏn"drō-kŏs'tăl) [" + L. *costa*, rib]. Pert. to the ribs and costal cartilages.
chondrocranium (kŏn-drō-krā'nē-ŭm) [" + *kranion*, head]. The cartilaginous embryonic cranium before ossification.
chondrocyte (kŏn'drō-sīt) [" + *kytos*, cell]. A cartilage cell.
chondrodermatitis nodularis chronica helicis. Growth of nodules on the helix of the ear.
chondrodynia (kŏn"drō-dĭn'ē-ă) [" + *odyne*, pain]. Pain in or about a cartilage.
chondrodysplasia (kŏn"drō-dĭs-plā'zē-ă) [" + Gr. *dys*, + *plasis*, a molding]. Disease, usually hereditary, resulting in disordered growth. Characterized by multiple exostoses of growth of the epiphyses, esp. of the long bones, metacarpals, and phalanges. SYN: *dyschondroplasia; Ollier's disease*.
chondrodystrophy (kŏn"drō-dĭs'trō-fē) [" + " + *trophe*, nourishment]. Achondroplasia, q.v.
chondroendothelioma (kŏn"drō-ĕn"dō-thē"lē-ō-mă) [" + *endon*, within, + *thele*, nipple, + *oma*, tumor]. An endothelioma that contains cartilage.
chondroepiphysitis (kŏn"drō-ĕp"ĭ-fĭz-ī'tĭs) [" + *epiphysis*, a growing on, + *itis*, inflammation]. Inflammation of the epiphyseal portion of the bone and the attached cartilage.
chondrofibroma (kŏn"drō-fī-brō'mă) [" + L. *fibra*, fiber, + Gr. *oma*, tumor]. A mixed tumor with elements of chondroma and fibroma.
chondrogen (kŏn'drō-jĕn) [Gr. *chondros*, cartilage, + *gennan*, to produce]. Basal substance of cartilage and corneal tissue, which turns into chondrin on boiling. Also spelled *chondrigen*.
chondrogenesis (kŏn"drō-jĕn'ĕ-sĭs) [" + *genesis*, production]. Formation of cartilage.
chondrogenic (kŏn"drō-jĕn'ĭk). Forming cartilage.
chondroid (kŏn'droyd) [" + *eidos*, resemblance]. Resembling cartilage; cartilaginous.
chondroitin (kŏn-drō'ĭ-tĭn). Substance present in connective tissue, including the cornea and cartilage.
chondrolipoma (kŏn-drō-lĭp-ō'mă) [" + *lipos*, fat, + *oma*, tumor]. Cartilaginous and fatty tissue tumor.
chondrology (kŏn-drŏl'ō-jē) [" + *logos*, study]. The science of cartilages.
chondrolysis (kŏn-drŏl'ĭ-sĭs) [" + *lysis*, dissolution]. The breaking down and absorption of cartilage.
chondroma (kŏn-drō'mă) [" + *oma*, tumor]. A cartilaginous tumor of slow growth. It may

occur any place where there is cartilage. It causes no pain.

chondromalacia (kŏn-drō-măl-ā'shē-ă) [" + *malakia,* softness]. Softness of the articular cartilage, usually involving the patella.

chondromatosis (kŏn"drō-mă-tō'sĭs) [" + *oma,* tumor, + *osis,* condition]. Formation of multiple chondromas of the hands and feet.

chondromatous (kŏn-drŏm'ă-tŭs) [" + *oma,* tumor]. Pert. to chondroma, or tumor of a cartilage.

chondromucin (kŏn"drō-mū'sĭn). Chondromucoid, q.v.

chondromucoid (kŏn"drō-mū'koyd) [" + L. *mucus,* mucus, + Gr. *eidos,* form]. A basophilic glycoprotein present in interstitial substance of cartilage.

chondromucoprotein (kŏn"drō-mū"kō-prō'tē-ĭn) [" + " + *protos,* first]. The ground substance, i.e., the fluid or solid material that occupies the space between the cells and fibers of cartilage.

chondromyoma (kŏn"drō-mī-ō'mă) [" + *mys,* muscle, + *oma,* tumor]. Myoma and cartilaginous neoplasm combined.

chondromyxoma (kŏn"drō-mĭks-ō'mă) [" + *myxa,* mucus, + *oma,* tumor]. Chondroma with myxomatous elements.

chondromyxosarcoma (kŏn-drō-mĭk"sō-săr-kō'mă) [" + " + *sarx,* flesh, + *oma,* tumor]. A cartilaginous and sarcomatous tumor.

chondro-osseus (kŏn"drō-ŏs'ē-ŭs) [" + L. *osseus,* bony]. Composed of cartilage and bone.

chondro-osteodystrophy (kŏn"drō-ŏs"tē-ō-dĭs'trō-fē) [" + *osteon,* bone, + *dys,* bad, + *trophe,* nourishment]. Developmental deformity of the epiphyses. This produces dwarfism, kyphosis, and pigeon breast.

chondropathology (kŏn"drō-pă-thŏl'ō-jē) [Gr. *chondros,* cartilage, + *pathos,* disease, + *logos,* study]. Pathology of disease of cartilages.

chondropathy (kŏn-drŏp'ăth-ē). Any disease of cartilage.

chondroplasia (kŏn"drō-plā'zē-ă) [" + *plassein,* to mold]. Formation of cartilage.

chondroplast (kŏn'drō-plăst). A cell that forms cartilage. SYN: *chondroblast.*

chondroplasty (kŏn'drō-plăs"tē) [" + *plassein,* to mold]. Plastic or reparative surgery on cartilage.

chondroporosis (kŏn"drō-pō-rō'sĭs) [" + *poros,* passage]. The porous condition of pathological or normal cartilage during ossification.

chondroproteins (kŏn-drō-prō'tē-ĭns) [" + *protos,* first]. A group of glucoproteins found in cartilage, tendons, and connective tissue.

chondrosarcoma (kŏn-drō-săr-kō'mă) [" + *sarx,* flesh, + *oma,* tumor]. Cartilaginous sarcoma.

chondrosin (kŏn'drō-sĭn). Material produced when chondroitin sulfate is hydrolyzed.

chondrosis (kŏn-drō'sĭs) [" + *osis,* condition]. The development of cartilage.

chondrosternal (kŏn"drō-stĕr'năl) [" + *sternon,* chest]. Pert. to sternal cartilage.

chondrosternoplasty (kŏn"drō-stĕr'nō-plăs"tē) [" + " + *plassein,* to mold]. Surgical correction of a deformed sternum.

chondrotome (kŏn'drō-tōm) [" + *tome,* incision]. Device for cutting cartilage.

chondrotomy (kŏn-drŏt'ō-mē). Dissection or surgical division of cartilage.

chondroxiphoid (kŏn"drō-zī'foyd) [" + *xiphos,* sword, + *eidos,* resemblance]. Concerning the sternum and the xiphoid process.

Chondrus [L., cartilage]. A genus of red algae that includes Chondrus crispus, the source of carrageenin, a mucilaginous substance used as an emulsifying agent. Commonly called Irish moss or carrageen.

Chopart's amputation (shō-părz'). [François Chopart, Fr. surgeon, 1743–1795] Disarticulation at the midtarsal joint.

chorda (kor'dă) [Gr. *chorde,* cord]. (pl. *chordae*) A cord or tendon.

c. dorsalis. The notochord.

c. gubernaculum. An embryonic structure forming a part of the gubernaculum testis in the male and the round ligament in the female.

c. obliqua. The oblique ligament, an oblique cord that connects the shafts of the radius and ulna. Extends from the lateral side of the tubercle of the ulna to a point just below the radial tuberosity.

c. tympani. [NA] A branch of the facial nerve that leaves the cranium through the stylomastoid foramen, traverses the tympanic cavity and joins a branch of the lingual nerve. Efferent fibers innervate the submandibular and sublingual glands; afferent fibers convey taste impulses from anterior two thirds of the tongue.

c. umbilicalis. Umbilical cord connecting fetus and placenta.

c. vocalis. Vocal folds of the larynx.

c. Willisii. One of several fibrous cords across the superior longitudinal sinus of the brain.

chordae tendineae (kor'dē tĕn-dĭn'ē-ē). [NA] Small tendinous cords that connect the free edges of the atrioventricular valves to the papillary muscles.

chordal (kor'dăl). Pert. to a chorda, esp. the notochord.

Chordata (kor-dā'tă) [LL., notochord]. A phylum of the animal kingdom including all animals that have a notochord during their development. Includes all vertebrates.

chordee (kor-dē') [Fr., corded]. Painful downward curvature of the penis on erection.

Occurs in congenital anomaly (hypospadia) or in urethral infection such as gonorrhea. SEE: *Peyronie's disease.*

chorditis (kor-dī'tĭs) [Gr. *chorde,* cord, + *itis,* inflammation]. Inflammation of the spermatic or vocal cord.

c. nodosa. Formation of small whitish nodules on one or both vocal cords in individuals who misuse their voice.

SYM: Hoarseness, inability of singers to register tones properly.

TREATMENT: Voice rest. Surgical removal of nodules if they do not respond to conservative therapy.

chordoma (kor-dō'mă) [" + *oma,* tumor]. Rare tumor that occurs any place along the vertebral column. Composed of embryonic nerve tissue and vacuolated physaliform cells. The neoplasm may cause death because of the damage of the expanding tissue and the surgical inaccessibility of the tumor.

chordotomy (kor-dŏt'ō-mē) [" + *tome,* incision]. Division of any cord to relieve pain.

chorea (kō-rē'ă) [Gr. *choreia,* dance]. A nervous condition marked by involuntary muscular twitching of the limbs or facial muscles.

c., acute. Sydenham's chorea, q.v.

c., Bergeron's. SEE: *c., electric.* SYN: *Dubini's disease.*

c., chronic. C., Huntington's. SYN: *chronic progressive hereditary chorea.*

c., electric. A rare form of chorea characterized by sudden involuntary contraction of a group of muscles. This causes violent movements as if the patient had been stimulated by an electric current.

c., epidemic. Dancing mania; uncontrolled dancing. Manifest in the 14th century in Europe. SYN: *choreomania; choromania; dancing mania.*

c. gravidarum. A form of Sydenham's chorea seen in some pregnant women, usually in those who have had chorea before, esp. in their first pregnancy. SEE: *c., Sydenham's.*

c., Henoch's. A form of progressive electric chorea.

c., hereditary. Huntington's chorea, q.v.

c., Huntington's. An inherited disease of the central nervous system that usually has its onset between 30 and 50 years of age. The patient has progressive dementia with bizarre involuntary movements characteristic of chorea. The disease slowly progresses and death is usually due to an intercurrent infection. The chorea may be controlled by phenothiazines; but there is no effective therapy for the mental deterioration.

c., hyoscine. Movements simulating chorea and sometimes accompanied by delirium, seen in acute hyoscine intoxication.

c., mimetic. Chorea due to imitative movements.

c. minor. C., Sydenham's.

c., posthemiplegic. Chorea affecting partially paralyzed muscles subsequent to a hemiplegic attack.

c., senile. Mild, usually benign disorder of the elderly marked by chorea-like movements but not associated with mental disorder.

c., Sydenham's. A disease, usually of childhood, commonly occurring between five and 15 years of age or during pregnancy; more females than males are affected. Usually associated with rheumatic fever. Characterized by involuntary purposeless contractions of the muscles of the trunk and extremities; anxiety; impairment of memory and sometimes of speech. SYN: *c. minor; Saint Vitus' dance.*

PROG: Recovery usually in course of 6 to 10 weeks. Relapses not infrequent, esp. in pregnancy. A possible sequel is chronic chorea. Rare complication is death from heart disease.

TREATMENT: Rest of body and mind. The child should remain in school unless the chorea is so severe as to make this inadvisable. Protection against injury in severe cases. Sedation may be needed if chorea is severe.

choreal (kō-rē'al, kō'rē-ăl). Pert. to chorea.

choreic (kō-rē'ĭk). Pert. to or of nature of chorea.

choreiform (kō-rē'ĭ-form) [Gr. *choreia,* dance, + L. *forma,* form]. Of the nature of chorea.

choreoathetoid (kō"rē-ō-ăth'ĕ-toyd) [" + *athetos,* not fixed, + *eidos,* resemblance]. Concerning choreoathetosis, q.v.

choreoathetosis (kō"rē-ō-ăth"ĕ-tō'sĭs) [" + " + *osis,* condition]. Type of athetosis frequently seen in cerebral palsy, characterized by extreme range of motion, jerky involuntary movement more proximal than distal, and fluctuating muscle tone from hypotonia to hypertonia.

choreomania (kō"rē-ō-mā'nē-ă) [" + *mania,* madness]. Dancing mania. Seen in the Middle Ages. SYN: *chorea, epidemic; choromania.*

choreophrasia (kō-rē"ō-frā'zē-ă) [" + *a-,* not, + *phrasis,* speech]. Condition in which meaningless words and phrases are repeated.

chorioadenoma (kō"rē-ō-ăd"ĕn-ō'mă) [Gr. *chorion,* outer membrane enclosing an embryo, + *aden,* gland, + *oma,* tumor]. Adenoma of the chorion.

c. destruens. A type of hydatidiform mole in which the chorionic villi penetrate the myometrium.

chorioallantois (kō"rē-ō-ă-lăn'tō-ĭs). In embryology, the membrane formed by the union of the chorion and allantois. In the human embryo, this develops to form the placenta.

chorioamnionitis (kō″rē-ō-ăm″nē-ō-nī′tĭs) [″ + *amnion,* lamb, + *itis,* inflammation]. Inflammation of the membranes that cover the fetus.

chorioangioma (kō″rē-ō-ăn-jē-ō′mă) [″ + *angeion,* vessel, + *oma,* tumor]. A vascular tumor of the chorion.

choriocapillaris (kō″rē-ō-kăp-ĭl-lā′rĭs) [Gr. *choroeides,* resembling a membrane, + L. *capillaris,* hairlike]. Capillary layer of choroid.

choriocarcinoma (kō″rē-ō-kăr″sĭ-nō′mă) [Gr. *chorion,* chorion, + *karkinoma,* cancer]. An extremely rare, very malignant neoplasm, usually of the uterus but sometimes at site of ectopic pregnancy. Though actual cause is unknown, it may occur following hydatid mole, a normal pregnancy, or abortion.

TREATMENT: The response of this cancer to methotrexate, USP, therapy may be dramatic. Complete remissions for over 10 years have been observed.

choriocele (kō′rē-ō-sēl) [Gr. *choroeides,* resembling a membrane, + *kele,* hernia]. A protrusion of the choroid coat of the eye through a defective sclera.

chorioepithelioma (kō″rē-ō-ĕp″ĭ-thē″lē-ō′mă). Choriocarcinoma.

choriogenesis (kō″rē-ō-jĕn′ĕ-sĭs) [Gr. *chorion,* chorion, + *genesis,* origin]. Formation of the chorion.

chorioid (kō′rē-oyd). Choroid.

chorioma (kō″rē-ō′mă) [″ + *oma,* tumor]. (pl. *choriomata*) A tumor of the chorion. There are a number of types including chorioadenoma, choriocarcinoma, q.v., and syncytioma.

choriomeningitis (kō″rē-ō-mĕn″ĭn-jī′tĭs) [″ + *meninx,* membrane, + *itis,* inflammation]. Cerebral meningitis with cellular infiltration of the meninges.

c., lymphocytic. An acute central nervous system disease of viral origin characterized by grippelike symptoms (fever, malaise, headache) sometimes followed by acute septic meningitis.

chorion (kō′rē-ŏn) [Gr.]. An extraembryonic membrane that, in early development, forms the outer wall of the blastocyst. It is formed from the trophoblast and its inner lining of mesoderm. From it develop chorionic villi, which establish an intimate connection with the endometrium, giving rise to the placenta. SEE: *placenta* and *umbilical cord* for illus.; *trophoblast*.

c. frondosum. The outer surface of the chorion. Its villi contact the decidua basalis. This is the placental portion of the chorion.

c. laeve. The smooth, nonvillous portion of the chorion.

chorionepithelioma (kō″rē-ŏn-ĕp″ĭ-thē″lē-ō′mă) [″ + *epi,* on, + *thele,* nipple, + *oma,* tumor]. Choriocarcinoma, q.v.

chorionic (kō-rē-ŏn′ĭk). Pert. to the chorion.

chorionic plate. In the placenta, that portion of the chorion attached to the uterus.

chorionic villi. The vascular projections from the chorion.

chorionitis (kō″rē-ŏn-ī′tĭs) [″ + *itis,* inflammation]. Inflammation of the chorion.

chorioretinal (kō″rē-ō-rĕt′ĭ-năl). Concerning the choroid and the retina of the eye.

chorioretinitis (kō″rē-ō-rĕt″ĭn-ī′tĭs) [Gr. *chorioeides,* skinlike, + L. *rete,* network, + Gr. *itis,* inflammation]. Inflammation of choroid and retina.

chorista (kō-rĭs′tă) [Gr. *choristos,* separated]. An error of development in which tissues have grown in a displaced position.

choristoma (kō-rĭs-tō′mă) [″ + *oma,* tumor]. A neoplasm due to overdevelopment of embryonic rudiments.

choroid (kō′royd) [Gr. *chorioeides,* skinlike]. Dark brown vascular coat of the eye between the sclera and retina, extending from ora serrata to optic nerve. Consists of blood vessels united by connective tissue containing pigmented cells and is made up of five layers: suprachoroid; layer of large vessels; layer of medium-sized vessels; layer of capillaries; lamina vitrea (homogeneous membrane placed next to pigmentary layer of retina). It is a part of the uvea or vascular tunic of the eye.

choroideremia (kō-roy-dĕr-ē′mē-ă) [″ + *eremia,* destitution]. A hereditary primary choroidal degeneration transmitted as an X-linked trait. In males, the earliest symptom is night blindness followed by constricted visual field and eventual blindness. In females, the condition is nonprogressive and vision is usually normal.

choroiditis (kō″royd-ī′tĭs) [″ + *itis,* inflammation]. Inflammation of the choroid.

c., anterior. Choroiditis in which outlets of exudation are at the choroidal periphery.

c., areolar. Choroiditis in which inflammation spreads from around the macula lutea.

c., central. Choroiditis in which exudation is limited to the macula.

c., diffuse. Choroiditis in which the fundus is covered with spots.

c., exudative. Choroiditis in which the choroid is covered with patches of inflammation.

c. guttata senilis. C., Tay's.

c., metastatic. Choroiditis due to embolism.

c., suppurative. Choroiditis in which suppuration occurs.

c., Tay's. A familial condition characterized by degeneration of the choroid, esp. in the region about the macula lutea. Occurs in aged persons.

choroidocyclitis (kō-roy″dō-sĭk-lī′tĭs) [Gr. *chorioeides*, skinlike, + *kyklos*, a circle, + *itis*, inflammation]. Inflammation of the choroid coat and ciliary processes.

choroidoiritis (kō-royd″ō-ī-rī′tĭs) [″ + *iris*, iris, + *itis*, inflammation]. Inflammation of the choroid coat and iris.

choroidopathy (kō″roy-dŏp′ă-thē) [″ + *pathos*, disease]. Any disease of the choroid.

choroidoretinitis (kō-royd″ō-rĕt″ĭn-ī′tĭs) [″ + L. *rete*, network, + Gr. *itis*, inflammation]. Inflammation of the choroid and retina.

choromania (kō″rō-mā′nē-ă) [Gr. *choros*, dance, + *mania*, madness]. Dance mania; a form of chorea.

Christian Science. A system of religious teaching based on Christian Scientists' interpretation of Scripture. Founded in 1866 by Mary Baker Eddy. The system emphasizes full healing of disease by mental and spiritual means because a major belief is that cause and effect are mental.

Christian-Weber disease. [Henry A. Christian, U.S. physician, 1876–1951; Frederick P. Weber, Brit. physician, 1863–1962] Nodular, nonsuppurating panniculitis accompanied by fever.

Christmas disease. [*Christmas*, name of the first patient with the disease who was studied] A form of hemophilia in males resulting from plasma thromboplastin component (PTC or Factor IX) deficiency. Transmitted as an X-linked trait. SYN: *hemophilia B*.

Christmas factor. Plasma thromboplastin component (PTC); ABBR: CF. A thromboplastin activator present in blood plasma.

chromaffin (krō-măf′ĭn) [Gr. *chroma*, color, + L. *affinis*, having affinity for]. 1. Staining readily with chromium salts. 2. Denoting pigmented cells forming medulla of the adrenal glands and the paraganglia.

chromaffin cells. Cells such as those of the adrenal medulla that contain granules that stain brown when cells are stained with a fluid containing potassium bichromate.

chromaffinoma (krō″măf-ĭ-nō′mă) [″ + ″ + Gr. *oma*, tumor]. A chromaffin cell tumor. SYN: *paraganglioma*.

chromaffinopathy (krō″măf-ĭn-ŏp′ă-thē) [″ + ″ + Gr. *pathos*, disease]. Any disease of chromaffin tissue.

chromaffin reaction. The turning brown of cytoplasmic granules containing epinephrine when subjected to stains containing chromium salts. Such granules stain green with ferric chloride, yellow with iodine, and brown with osmic acid.

chromaffin system. The mass of tissue forming paraganglia and medulla of suprarenal glands, which secretes adrenalin and stains readily with chromium salts. Similar tissue is found in the organs of Zuckerkandl, and in the liver, testes, ovary, and heart. SEE: *adrenal gland*.

chromaphil (krō′mă-fĭl) [″ + *philein*, to love]. Pert. to a histological element or cell that stains readily with chromium salts. SYN: *chromaffin*.

chromate (krō′māt) [Gr. *chromatos*, color]. A salt of chromic acid. SEE: *potassium chromate*.

chromatic (krō-măt′ĭk). Pert. to color.

chromatid (krō′mă-tĭd) The two halves into which a chromosome is longitudinally divided during mitosis and meiosis. They are held together at the centromere and migrate to opposite poles of the dividing cell at anaphase.

chromatin (krō′mă-tĭn) [Gr. *chroma*, color]. A deeply staining substance present in the nucleus of a cell that contains the genetic material. It is a deoxyribonucleic acid attached to a protein structure base.

chromatin-negative. Lacking the sex chromatin; characteristic of nuclei in cells of normal human males. SEE: *Barr body*.

chromatinolysis (krō″mă-tĭn-ŏl′ĭ-sĭs) [″ + *lysis*, dissolution]. 1. Destruction of chromatin. 2. The emptying of a cell, bacterial or other, by lysis.

chromatinorrhexis (krō″mă-tĭn-or-rĕk′sĭs) [″ + *rhexis*, rupture]. Splitting of chromatin.

chromatin-positive. Having the sex chromatin (the Barr body, q.v.); characteristic of nuclei in cells of normal human females.

chromatism (krō′mă-tĭzm) [″ + *-ismos*, condition]. 1. Unnatural pigmentation. 2. Chromatic aberration.

chromatogenous (krō″mă-tŏj′ĕn-ŭs) [″ + *gennan*, to produce]. Causing pigmentation or color.

chromatogram (krō-măt′ō-grăm) [″ + *gramma*, mark]. Record produced by chromatography.

chromatography (krō″mă-tŏg′ră-fē) [″ + *graphein*, to write]. A method of separating two or more chemical compounds in solution by virtue of their being removed from the solution at different rates when percolated down a column of a powdered absorbent or passed across the surface of an absorbent paper.

c., adsorption. Chromatography accomplished by applying the material to be tested to one end of a sheet or column containing a solid. As the material moves, the various constituents adhere to the surface of the particles of the solid at different distances from the starting point in accordance with their chemical characteristics.

c., column. A form of adsorption chromatography wherein the adsorptive material is packed into a column.

c., gas. Chromatography wherein the gases to be separated from each other are adsorbed as they pass over the appropriate solids.

c., gas-liquid. ABBR: GLC. Chromatographic analysis wherein a gas moves over a liquid, and chemical substances are separated by their different adsorption rates on the liquid.

c., paper. Chromatography in which paper strips are used as the porous solid medium.

c., partition. Chromatography in which substances in solution are separated by being exposed to two immiscible solvents. The immobile solvent is located between the spaces of an inert material such as starch, cellulose, or silica. The substances move with the mobile solvent as it passes down the column at a rate governed by their partition coefficient.

c., thin layer. ABBR: TLC. Chromatography involving the differential adsorption of substances as they pass through a thin layer or sheet of cellulose or some other inert compound.

chromatoid (krō'mă-toyd) [Gr. *chroma,* color, + *eidos,* resemblance]. Staining in the same manner as chromatin.

chromatokinesis (krō"mă-tō-kī-nē'sĭs) [" + *kinesis,* movement]. The movement of chromatin during the division of a cell.

chromatolysis (krō"mă-tŏl'ĭ-sĭs) [" + *lysis,* dissolution]. Dissolution of chromophil substance (Nissl's bodies) in neurons in certain pathological conditions, or following injury to the cell body or axon.

chromatometer (krō-mă-tŏm'ĕt-ĕr) [" + *metron,* measure]. A scale of colors for testing color perception.

chromatophil, chromatophilic (krō'mă-tō-fĭl", krō"mă-tō-fĭl'ĭk) [" + *philein,* to love]. Staining easily.

chromatophore (krō-măt'ō-for) [" + *phoros,* bearing]. A pigment-bearing cell.

chromatopsia (krō"mă-tŏp'sē-ă) [" + *opsis,* vision]. Abnormally colored vision.

chromatoptometry (krō"măt-ŏp-tŏm'ĕ-trē) [" + *optos,* visible, + *metron,* measure]. Measurement of color perception.

chromatosis (krō"mă-tō'sĭs) [" + *osis,* condition]. 1. Pigmentation. 2. The pathological deposition of pigment in any part of the body where it is not normally present or excessive deposition where it is present.

chromaturia (krō-mă-tū'rē-ă) [" + *ouron,* urine]. Abnormal color of the urine.

chromesthesia (krō"mĕs-thē'zē-ă) [" + *aisthesis,* perception]. The association of color sensations with words, taste, smell, or sounds.

chromicize (krō'mĭ-sīz). To impregnate with chromium or its salts.

chromidiosis (krō-mĭd-ē-ō'sĭs). Movement of chromatin and nuclear substance from nucleus to the cytoplasm of the cell.

chromidium (krō-mĭd'ē-ŭm) [" + *-idion,* a dim. termination]. (pl. *chromidia*) An extranuclear granule seen in the cytoplasm of a cell.

chromidrosis, chromhidrosis (krō"mĭd-rō'sĭs) [" + *hidros,* sweat]. Excretion of colored sweat. Red sweat may be due to an exudation of blood into the sweat glands or to microorganisms in those glands.

ETIOL: May be due to ingestion or absorption of certain substances, as pigment-producing bacteria. May be caused by certain disorders of metabolism.

SYM: Localized in eyelids, breasts, axillae, genitocrural regions; occasionally on hands and limbs. It is grayish, bluish, violaceous, brownish; it collects on skin, giving a greasy, powdery appearance to parts.

TREATMENT: Relief of underlying condition.

RS: anhidrosis; bromidrosis; hidrosis; hyperhidrosis; uridrosis.

chromium (krō'mē-ŭm) [L., color]. SYMB: Cr. At. wt. 51.996; at. no. 24. A very hard, metallic element.

chromium poisoning. SYM: A disagreeable taste in the mouth, pain, diarrhea, collapse, and cramping. If fatal, death is due to uremia.

TREATMENT: Chalk, magnesia, and other weak alkalies to neutralize its acid effects. Wash out stomach and give cathartics, analgesics for pain.

chromoblast (krō'mō-blăst) [Gr. *chroma,* color, + *blastos,* germ]. An embryonic cell that becomes a pigment cell.

chromocenter (krō'mō-sĕn"tĕr) [" + *kentros,* middle]. Irregular clumps of chromatin material seen in the nuclei of cells that are not dividing. SYN: *karyosome.*

chromocrinia (krō"mō-krĭn'ē-ă) [" + *krinein,* to separate]. The secretion or excretion of pigmented matter.

chromocystoscopy (krō"mō-sĭs-tŏs'kō-pē) [" + *kystis,* bladder, + *skopein,* to examine]. Determination of functional activity of kidneys and bladder by use of dyes.

chromocyte (krō'mō-sīt) [" + *kytos,* cell]. Any colored cell.

chromocytometer (krō"mō-sī-tŏm'ĕt-ĕr) [" + " + *metron,* measure]. Instrument for determining the hemoglobin in red blood corpuscles.

chromodacryorrhea (krō"mō-dăk"rē-ō-rē'ă) [" + *dacryon,* tear, + *rhoia,* flow]. Flow of blood-stained tears.

chromogen (krō'mō-jĕn) [" + *gennan,* to produce]. Any principle that may be changed into coloring matter.

chromogenesis (krō"mō-jĕn'ĕ-sĭs) [" + *gene-*

sis, production]. Production of pigment.

chromogenic (krō″mō-jĕn′ĭk). Pigment-producing.

chromolipoid (krō″mō-lĭp′oyd) [″ + *lipos*, fat, + *eidos*, appearance]. Any lipoid that is pigmented. SYN: *lipochrome.*

chromolysis (krō-mŏl′ĭ-sĭs) [″ + *lysis*, dissolution]. Dissolution of chromophil substance (Nissl bodies) in neurons in certain pathological conditions, or following injury to the cell body or axon. SYN: *chromatolysis.*

chromomere (krō′mō-mēr) [Gr. *chroma*, color, + *meros*, part]. 1. One of a series of chromatin granules found in a chromosome. 2. A highly refractile purple granule that forms the central portion of a blood platelet.

chromometer (krō-mŏm′ĕ-tĕr) [″ + *metron*, measure]. Device for determining the pigment in a substance. SYN: *colorimeter.*

chromometry (krō-mŏm′ĕt-rē). The estimation of coloring matter in the substance examined.

chromomycosis (krō″mō-mī-kō′sĭs) [″ + *myxa*, mucus, + *osis*, condition]. A chronic fungal infection of the skin marked by itching and warty plaques on the skin and subcutaneous swellings of feet, legs, and other exposed areas. Various fungi have been implicated, including Phialophora verrucosa, P. pedrosoi, P. compacta, and Cladosporium carrionii. Some of these are also called Fonsecaea pedrosoi and F. compacta. SYN: *chromoblastomycosis; dermatitis verrucosa.*

chromoparic (krō-mō-păr′ĭk) [″ + L. *parere*, to produce]. Producing color. Usually refers to bacteria that color their immediate surroundings. SYN: *chromogenic.*

chromopexic, chromopectic (krō″mō-pĕk′sĭk, -pĕk′tĭk) [″ + *pexis*, fixation]. Pert. to fixation of coloring matter, as the liver function in forming bilirubin.

chromophane (krō′mō-fān) [″ + *phainein*, to show]. Retinal pigment.

chromophil(e) (krō′mō-fĭl, -fīl) [″ + *philein*, to love]. 1. Any structure that stains easily. 2. One of two types of cells present in pars distalis of the pituitary gland. It is considered a secretory cell.

chromophilic, chromophilous (krō-mō-fĭl′ĭk, krō-mŏf′ĭl-ŭs). Staining readily.

chromophobe (krō′mō-fōb) [″ + *phobos*, fear]. Any cell or tissue that stains either poorly or not at all. A type of cell found in pars distalis of the pituitary gland.

chromophobia (krō″mō-fō′bē-ă). Condition of staining poorly.

chromophobic (krō-mō-fō′bĭk). Resistant to staining.

chromophore (krō′mō-for) [″ + *pherein*, to bear]. Any chemical that when present in a cell that has been prepared properly displays color.

chromophoric (krō″mō-for′ĭk) [″ + *pherein*, to bear]. Pert. to or bearing color.

chromophose (krō′mō-fōz) [″ + *phos*, light]. A subjective sensation of a spot of color in the eye. SYN: *centraphose; centrophose.*

chromophytosis (krō″mō-fī-tō′sĭs) [″ + *phyton*, plant, + *osis*, condition]. Tinea versicolor, q.v.

chromoplasm (krō′mō-plăzm) [″ + *plasma*, something formed]. Chromatin, q.v.

chromoplastid [″ + *plastos*, formed]. Colored plastids other than chloroplasts present in plant cells.

chromoprotein (krō″mō-prō′tē-ĭn) [″ + *protos*, first]. One of a group of conjugated proteins consisting of a protein combined with hematin or another colored, metal-containing, prosthetic group.

Ex.: hemoglobin; hemocyanin; chlorophyll; flavoproteins; cytochromes.

chromopsia [″ + *opsis*, vision]. Chromatopsia; colored vision.

chromoptometer (krō″mŏp-tŏm′ĕ-tĕr) [″ + *opsis*, sight, + *metron*, measure]. Instrument for determining keenness of color vision.

chromoradiometer [″ + L. *radius*, ray, + Gr. *metron*, measure]. An instrument for measuring penetrative power of roentgen rays.

chromoscope (krō′mō-skōp) [″ + *skopein*, to examine]. Instrument for determining color perception.

chromoscopy (krō-mŏs′kō-pē). Examination for color vision.

chromosome (krō′mō-sōm) [Gr. *chroma*, color, + *soma*, body]. A linear thread in the nucleus of a cell. It contains the DNA, which transmits genetic information. Chromosomes stain deeply with basic dyes and are esp. conspicuous during mitosis. They contain the genes or hereditary determiners. The normal number of chromosomes is constant for each species, being 46 in man (23 pairs in all somatic cells). These constitute the diploid number. In the formation of the gametes (ovum and spermatozoon) the number is reduced to one half (haploid number), i.e., the ovum and sperm each contain 23, or one of each of the 23 pairs. Of these, 22 are considered autosomes and one is the sex chromosome (X or Y). At time of fertilization, the chromosomes from the sperm unite with the chromosomes from the ovum. This random union determines the sex of the embryo. The female sex chromosome from the ovum may contribute only an X to the embryo. The male sex chromosome may contribute an X or a Y to join with the chromosome derived from the ovum. Thus the embryo may have XX in its sex chromosome, in which case a female would develop; or XY, in which case a male would develop. SEE: *Barr body; gene; heredity; karyotype;* illus.

KARYOTYPE OF PAIRS OF HUMAN CHROMOSOMES OF MALE AND FEMALE

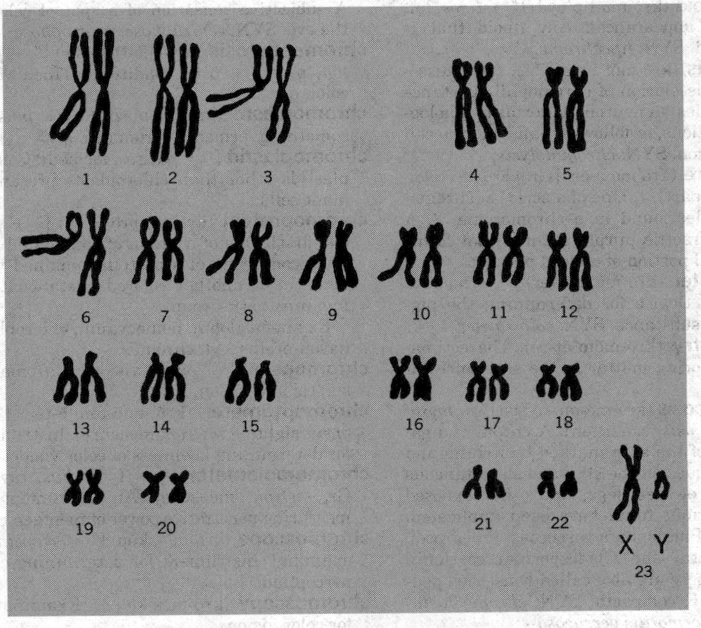

MALE

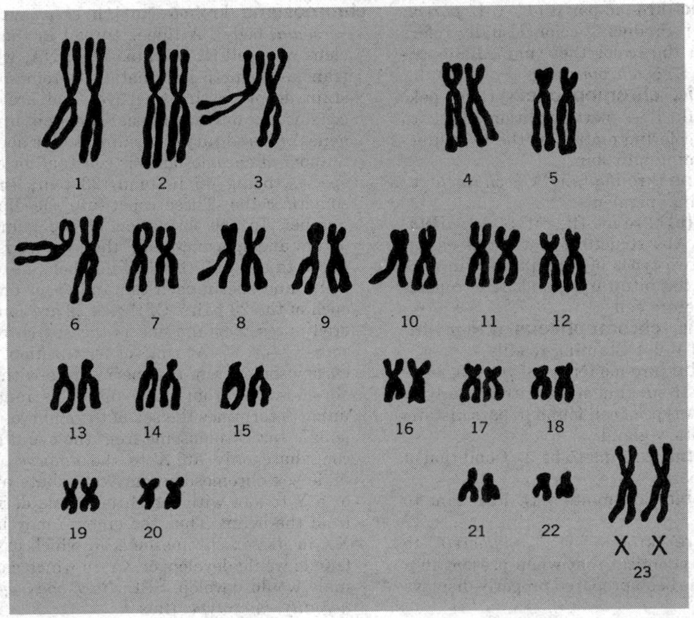

FEMALE

c., accessory. An unpaired sex chromosome. SEE: *c., sex.*

c.'s, banded. Special staining of chromosomes delineates bands of various width on the regions or loci of the chromosomes. This facilitates analyzing and investigating chromosomes.

c., bivalent. A double chromosome resulting from the conjugation of two homologous chromosomes in synapsis, which occurs during the first meiotic division.

c.'s, giant. Extremely large chromosomes seen in the salivary glands and in other organs and tissues of insects.

c., Philadelphia; c., Ph[1]. An abnormality of chromosome 22 (see illus.) characterized by a shortening of its long arms. This anomaly is found in many patients with chronic leukemia.

c., sex. One of two chromosomes, the X and Y chromosomes, that are concerned with the determination of sex in humans and carry the genes for sex-linked characters.

c., somatic. An autosome.

c., X. One of a pair of female-determining chromosomes (XX) present in the somatic cells of all human females. Characteristics transmitted on the X chromosome are said to be X-linked or sex-linked.

c., Y. The male member of a pair of human chromosomes (XY) present in the somatic cells of all human males. The only characteristic that is thought to be on the Y chromosome is the trait for hairy ears.

chromotherapy (krō″mō-thĕr′ă-pē) [Gr. *chroma,* color, + *therapeia,* treatment]. The use of colored light in the treatment of disease.

chromotoxic (krō″mō-tŏk′sĭk) [″ + *toxikon,* poison]. Caused by toxic action on the hemoglobin.

chromotrichia (krō″mō-trĭk′ē-ă) [″ + *thrix,* hair]. Coloration of the hair.

chromotropic (krō″mō-trŏp′ĭk) [″ + *tropikos,* turning]. 1. Being attracted to color. 2. Attracting color.

chromoureteroscopy (krō″mō-ū-rē″tĕr-ŏs′kō-pē) [″ + *oureter,* ureter, + *skopein,* to examine]. Inspecting orifices of ureters after giving a substance to dye the urine.

chronaxie (krō′năk-sē) [Gr. *chronos,* time, + *axia,* value]. A number expressing the sensitiveness of a nerve to electrical stimulation. It is the minimum duration, measured in milliseconds, during which a current of prescribed strength must pass through a motor nerve in order to cause contraction in the associated muscle; the strength of direct current (the rheobasic voltage) that will just suffice if given an indefinite time is first determined, and exactly double this strength is taken for the final determinations.

chronaximeter (krō″năk-sĭm′ĕt-ĕr) [″ + ″ + *metron,* measure]. Device for measuring chronaxie.

chronic [Gr. *chronos,* time]. 1. Long, drawn out; of long duration. 2. Designating a disease showing little change or of slow progression. Opposite of acute.

chronic bacterial prostatitis. ABBR: CBP. Inflammation of the prostate due to longstanding bacterial infection. Clinical symptoms of fever, pain, and dysuria may be relatively mild as compared to acute infection. Therapy depends upon the causative organism and in addition to antibiotics may involve treatment of prostatic hypertrophy.

chronic granulomatous disease. Congenital disease, characterized by polymorphonuclear leukocytes that are able to ingest but unable to kill certain bacteria. Twenty percent of cases reported are in girls. Evidence for X-linked, i.e., sex-linked, inheritance is present in most boys but not in girls with the disease. Carrier females rarely experience severe bacterial infections. Death is due to chronic and recurrent infections. SEE: *nitroblue tetrazolium test.*

TREATMENT: There is no specific therapy. Prolonged antibiotic therapy is helpful in preventing infection. Bone marrow transplantation has been tried experimentally.

chronicity (krŏn-ĭs′ĭt-ē). State of being chronic.

chronic obstructive lung disease. ABBR: COLD. Disease process that causes decreased ability of the lungs to perform their function of ventilation. Diagnostic criteria include history of persistent dyspnea on exertion with or without chronic cough and less than one-half normal predicted maximum breathing capacity. Diseases that cause this are chronic bronchitis, pulmonary emphysema, chronic asthma, and chronic bronchiolitis. Also called chronic obstructive pulmonary disease. SEE: *emphysema.*

chronobiology (krŏn″ō-bī-ŏl′ō-jē) [Gr. *chronos,* time, + *bios,* life, + *logos,* study]. Study of the timing characteristics of life processes to attempt to describe the factors that influence biological rhythms. SEE: *circadian; clock, biological.*

chronognosis (krŏn″ŏg-nō′sĭs) [″ + *gnosis,* knowledge]. Subjective realization of the passage of time.

chronograph (krŏn′ō-grăf) [″ + *graphein,* to write]. Device for recording short intervals of time.

chronological (krŏn″ō-lŏj′ĭ-kăl) [″ + *logos,* study]. Occurring in natural sequence according to time.

chronoscope (krŏn′ō-skōp) [″ + *skopein,* to examine]. Device for measuring extremely short intervals of time.

chronotaraxis (krō-nō-tăr-ăk′sĭs) [″ + *tar-*

axis, without order]. Being unable to orient one's self with respect to time.

chronotropic (krŏn″ō-trŏp′ĭk) [″ + *tropikos,* turning]. Influencing rate of occurrence of an event, such as the heartbeat. SEE: *inotropic.*

chronotropism [″ + ″ + *-ismos,* condition]. Interference with periodic events such as the heartbeat.

c., negative. Modifying rate by decreasing it.

c., positive. Modifying rate by increasing it.

Chronulac. Trade name for lactulose.

chrysarobin (krĭs″ă-rō′bĭn) [Gr. *chrysos,* gold, + Brazilian *araraba,* bark]. A mixture of neutral principles obtained from goa powder, which is deposited in the wood of Araroba, a leguminous tree of South America. It is used topically, as an ointment, for treatment of certain skin disorders.

chrysiasis (krĭ-sī′ă-sĭs). Deposition of gold in living tissues as in gold therapy. SYN: *aurantiasis.*

chrysoderma (krĭs″ō-dĕr′mă) [″ + *derma,* skin]. Discoloration of the skin due to deposition of gold.

chrysotherapy (krĭs″ō-thĕr′ă-pē) [″ + *therapeia,* treatment]. Use of gold compounds as a medicine. This practice is still employed in treating rheumatoid arthritis.

Chvostek's sign (vōs′tĕks). [Franz Chvostek, Austrian surgeon, 1835–1884] Spasm of facial muscles following a tap on one side of the face over the area of the facial nerve. Seen in tetany, q.v.

chylangioma (kī″lăn-jē-ō′mă) [Gr. *chylos,* juice, + *angeion,* vessel, + *oma,* tumor]. Tumor of intestinal lymph vessels containing chyle.

chyle (kīl) [Gr. *chylos,* juice]. The milklike, alkaline contents of the lacteals and lymphatic vessels of the intestine, consisting of the products of digestion and principally absorbed fats. It is carried by the lymphatic vessels to the cisterna chyli and then by way of the thoracic duct to the left subclavian vein, where it enters the bloodstream. A large quantity is formed in 24 hours.

RS: achylia; cisterna chyli; oligochylia; receptaculum chyli; secretion.

chylemia (kī-lē′mē-ă) [″ + *haima,* blood]. Chyle in the peripheral circulation.

chylifacient (kī″lĭ-fā′shĕnt) [″ + L. *facere,* to make]. Forming chyle.

chylifaction, chylification (kī-lĭ-făk′shŭn, kī-lĭ-fĭ-kā′shŭn). The formation of chyle.

chylifactive (kī-lĭ-făk′tĭv). Forming chyle; chylifacient.

chyliferous (kī-lĭf′ĕr-ŭs) [″ + L. *ferre,* to carry]. Carrying chyle.

chyliform (kī′lĭ-form) [″ + L. *forma,* shape]. Resembling chyle.

chylocele (kī′lō-sēl) [″ + *kele,* tumor]. Distention of the tunica vaginalis testis with infused chyle.

chyloderma (kī″lō-dĕr′mă) [″ + *derma,* skin]. Lymph accumulated in the enlarged lymphatic vessels and thickened skin of the scrotum. SYN: *elephantiasis, scrotal.*

chylology (kī-lŏl′ō-jē) [″ + *logos,* study]. The study of chyle.

chylomediastinum (kī″lō-mē″dē-ăs-tī′nŭm) [″ + L. *mediastinum,* median]. Chyle in the mediastinum.

chylomicron (kī″lō-mī′krŏn) [″ + *mikros,* small]. Small particle of fat in the blood after digestion and absorption of fat in food. Perceptible under a microscope.

chylopericardium (kī″lō-pĕr″ĭ-kăr′dē-ŭm) [″ + L. *peri,* around, + Gr. *kardia,* heart]. Chyle in the pericardium.

chyloperitoneum (kī″lō-pĕr″ĭ-tō-nē′ŭm) [″ + *peritonaion,* peritoneum]. Effused chyle in peritoneal cavity.

chylophoric (kī″lō-for′ĭk) [″ + *phoros,* bearing]. Conveying chyle; chyliferous.

chylopneumothorax (kī″lō-nū″mō-thō′răks) [″ + *pneumon,* lung, + *thorax,* chest]. Chyle and air in the pleural space.

chylopoiesis (kī″lō-poy-ē′sĭs) [″ + *poiesis,* production]. Formation of chyle and its absorption by lacteals in the intestines. SYN: *chylification.*

chylorrhea (kī″lō-rē′ă) [Gr. *chylos,* juice, + *rhoia,* flow]. Escape of chyle due to rupture of the thoracic duct.

chylothorax [″ + *thorax,* chest]. Chyle in pleural cavities.

chylous (kī′lŭs). Pert. to or of the nature of chyle.

chyluria (kī-lū′rē-ă) [″ + *ouron,* urine]. Presence of chyle or fat globules in the urine.

chymase (kī′mās). An enzyme in gastric juice that accelerates the action of the pancreatic enzymes.

chyme (kīm) [Gr. *chymos,* juice]. The mixture of partly digested food and digestive secretions found in the stomach and small intestine during digestion of a meal. It is a varicolored, thick, but nearly liquid mass. SEE: *oligochymia.*

chymopapain (kī-mō-pă′pā-ĭn). An enzyme related to papain that is used to treat herniated nucleus pulposus.

chymosin (kī′mō-sĭn) [Gr. *chymos,* juice]. Rennin.

chymotrypsin (kī″mō-trĭp′sĭn) [″ + *tryein,* to rub, + *pepsis,* digestion]. A proteolytic enzyme present in the intestine that, with trypsin, hydrolyzes proteins to peptones or further. It is secreted by the pancreas. Trade names are Avazyme and Enzeon.

C.I. *chemotherapeutic index* (parasitology); *color index.*

Ci. *curie.*

cib. Abbr. for L. *cibus,* food.

cibisotome (sĭ-bĭs′ō-tōm) [Gr. *kibisis,* pouch, + *tome,* incision]. Instrument for incision of capsule of the lens.

cibophobia (sī″bō-fō′bē-ă) [L. *cibus,* food, + Gr. *phobos,* fear]. A morbid aversion to or fear of food.

cicatricial (sĭk″ă-trĭsh′ăl) [L. *cicatrix,* scar]. Pert. to a cicatrix, q.v.

cicatricotomy (sĭk″ă-trĭk-ŏt′ō-mē) [″ + Gr. *tome,* incision]. Incision of a cicatrix or scar.

cicatrix (sĭk′ă-trĭks, sĭk-ā′trĭks) [L.]. A scar left by a healed wound. Lack of color is due to absence of pigmentation. Cicatricial tissue is less elastic than normal tissue, hence it usually presents a contracted appearance. SEE: *keloid.*

cicatrizant (sĭk-ăt′rĭ-zănt) [L. *cicatrix,* scar]. Favoring or causing, or an agent that aids in, cicatrization.

cicatrization (sĭk″ă-trĭ-zā′shŭn). Healing by scar formation. SEE: *intention.*

cicatrize (sĭk′ă-trīz). To heal by scar tissue.

cicutism (sĭk′ū-tĭzm). Poisoning resulting from ingestion of Cicuta maculata or C. virosa, water hemlock.

ciguatera (sē″gwă-tā′ră) [Sp. Amer. from W. Indies *cigua,* sea snail]. A form of fish poisoning due to eating fish normally considered to be safe to eat such as sea bass, grouper, or snapper. Why the fish are toxic at one time and not another is unknown. Clinically there is tingling about the lips, tongue, and throat with nausea, vomiting, diarrhea, weakness, and numbness. There is no specific therapy but treatment of respiratory paralysis may be required. Gastric lavage is indicated if vomiting has not occurred. Mortality is less than 10%.

ciguatoxin (sē″gwă-tŏk′sĭn). The toxic substance that causes ciguatera. The structure is unknown, but the toxin has anticholinesterase activity.

cilia (sĭl′ē-ă) [L.]. (sing. *cilium*) 1. [NA] Eyelashes. 2. Hairlike processes projecting from epithelial cells, as in the bronchi, that propel mucus, pus, and dust particles. SEE: illus.

ciliariscope (sĭl″ē-ă′rĭ-skōp) [L. *ciliaris,* pert. to eyelash, + Gr. *skopein,* to examine]. Instrument for examination of the ciliary region of the eye.

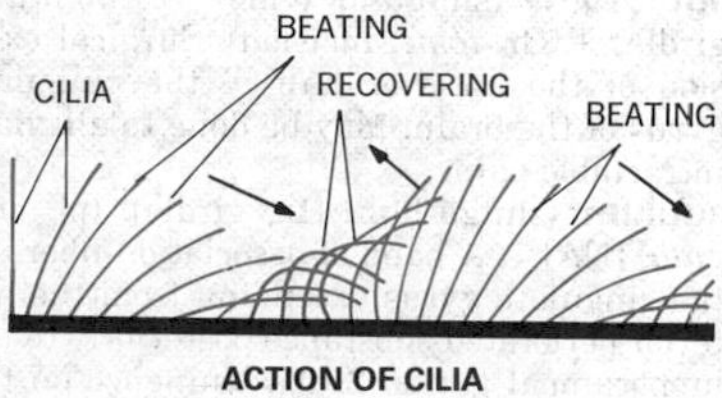

ACTION OF CILIA

ciliarotomy (sĭl″ē-ă-rŏt′ō-mē) [″ + Gr. *tome,* incision]. Surgical section of the ciliary zone in glaucoma.

ciliary (sĭl′ē-ĕr″ē) [L. *ciliaris,* pert. to eyelash]. Pert. to any hairlike processes, esp. to the eyelashes, and to eye structures such as the ciliary body.

ciliary apparatus. Ciliary body, q.v.

ciliary arteries. Branches of the ophthalmic artery that supply the choroid layer.

ciliary body. Thickened part of vascular tunic of the eye between the base of the iris and the anterior part of the choroid. SYN: *ciliary apparatus.* SEE: *eye* for illus.

ciliary ganglion. A ganglion lying in the posterior part of the orbit. Receives preganglionic fibers through the oculomotor nerve from the Edinger-Westphal nucleus of the midbrain. From it six short ciliary nerves pass to the eyeball. Postganglionic fibers innervate the ciliary muscle, sphincter of the iris, and the smooth muscles of blood vessels of these structures, and also the cornea.

ciliary glands. A form of sweat glands of the eyelid. SEE: *glands, Moll's.*

ciliary muscle. Smooth muscle forming a part of the ciliary body of the eye. Contraction pulls the choroid forward, lessening tension on fibers of the zonula (suspensory ligament), thereby allowing the lens, which is elastic, to assume a more spherical shape; thus accommodation for near vision is accomplished.

ciliary nerves, long. Two or three branches of the nasal nerves supplying the ciliary muscle, iris, and cornea.

ciliary nerves, short. Several branches of the ciliary ganglion supplying the ciliary muscle, iris, and tunics of the eyeball.

ciliary processes. About 70 folds arranged meridionally so as to form a circle. They have the same structure as the rest of the choroid and secrete nutrient fluids that nourish neighboring parts, as cornea, lens, vitreous body. They also serve as points of attachment for the suspensory ligament of the lens.

ciliary reflex. Normal contraction of pupil in accommodation of vision from distant to near.

Ciliata (sĭl″ē-ă′tă). A class of Protozoa characterized by the presence of cilia.

ciliate (sĭl′ē-āt) [L. *cilia,* eyelashes]. Ciliated.

ciliated (sĭl′ē-ā-tĕd]. Possessing cilia.

ciliated epithelium. Epithelium with hairlike processes on the surface. They wave actively only in one direction. Present in the respiratory tract and fallopian tubes.

ciliectomy (sĭl″ē-ĕk′tō-mē) [″ + Gr. *ektome,* excision]. Excision of a portion of the ciliary body or ciliary border of the eyelid.

ciliogenesis (sĭl″ē-ō-jĕn′ĕ-sĭs). Formation of cilia.

ciliospinal (sĭl″ē-ō-spī′năl) [″ + *spinalis*, pert. to a spine]. Pert. to the ciliary body and spinal cord.

ciliospinal center. Spinal cord center that controls dilation of the pupil.

ciliospinal reflex. Dilation of the pupil following stimulation of the skin of the neck by pinching or scratching the skin.

ciliostatic (sĭl″ē-ō-stăt′ĭk) [″ + Gr. *statos*, placed]. Interfering with or preventing movement of the cilia.

ciliotomy (sĭl″ē-ŏt′ō-mē) [″ + Gr. *tome*, incision]. Surgical cutting of the ciliary nerve.

cilium (sĭl′ē-ŭm) [L.]. [NA] Sing. of cilia.

cillosis (sĭl-ō′sĭs) [L.]. Spasmodic twitching of the eyelid.

cimbia (sĭm′bē-ă) [L.]. Slender band of white fibers crossing the ventral surface of a cerebral peduncle.

cimetidine. A drug that is a histamine H_2 receptor antagonist; represents a new class of pharmacological agents. It inhibits gastric secretions and is indicated for treatment of gastric and duodenal ulcers. Trade name is Tagamet. SEE: *peptic ulcer*.

Cimex lectularius (sī′mĕks lĕk-tū-lā′rē-ŭs). The bedbug. An insect belonging to the order Hemiptera. SEE: *bedbug*. SYN: *Acantha lectularia*.

cimicosis (sĭm″ĭ-kō′sĭs). Itching due to the bite of a bedbug.

cinchona (sĭn-kō′nă, -chō′nă) [Sp. *cinchon*, Countess of Cinchon]. The dried bark of the tree cinchona, the source of quinine. SEE: *quinine*.

cinchonism (sĭn′kŏn-ĭzm) [″ + Gr. *-ismos*, condition]. Poisoning from cinchona or its alkaloids. SYN: *quininism*.

cinchophen (sĭn′kō-fĕn). Light yellow powder with slightly bitter taste. It frequently produces serious side effects, e.g., a fatal form of hepatitis. At one time it was used in treating gout, but it is seldom used in contemporary medical therapy.

cinchophen poisoning. SYM: Gastric irritation; nausea; vomiting; belching; heartburn; vertigo; weakness; diarrhea; itching; rash; jaundice; stupor. When chronic, it is often associated with profound liver damage. Individuals with gallbladder disease or inflammation or cirrhosis of the liver and those who are undernourished or suffering from alcoholism are esp. susceptible.

F.A.: Largely symptomatic. Wash out stomach; give large quantities of fluids and saline catharsis.

cinclisis (sĭn′klĭ-sĭs) [Gr. *kinklisis*, a wagging]. Swift spasmodic movement of any part of the body.

cincture sensation (sĭnk′chūr) [L. *cinctura*, girdle]. Sensation of a tight girdle about the waist. SYN: *zonesthesia*.

cineangiocardiography (sĭn″ē-ăn″jē-ō-kăr″dē-ŏg′ră-fē) [Gr. *kinesis*, movement, + *angeion*, vessel, + *kardia*, heart, + *graphein*, to write]. Continuous photographic record of the blood vessels by use of fluoroscopy. A radiopaque agent is injected just prior to the study.

c., radionuclide. The use of a scintillation camera to record and project the image of a radioisotope as it travels through the heart and great vessels.

cinecystourethrogram (sĭn-ē-sĭs″tō-ū-rē′thrō-grăm). Motion picture record of radiological investigation of the urinary bladder and urethra when they are filled with and are emptying themselves of a radiopaque medium.

cinefluorography (sĭn″ē-floo″or-ŏg′ră-fē). Motion pictures of images produced by fluoroscopic examination.

cinematics (sĭn″ē-măt′ĭks) [Gr. *kinema*, motion]. Science of motion; kinematics.

cinematoradiography (sĭn″ē-măt-ō-rā″dē-ŏg′ră-fē) [″ + L. *radius*, ray, + Gr. *graphein*, to write]. Radiography of an organ in motion.

cinemicrography (sĭn″ē-mī-krŏg′ră-fē) [Gr. *kinesis*, motion, + *mikros*, small, + *graphein*, to write]. Motion picture record of the object seen through the use of a microscope.

cineplastics (sĭn″ē-plăs′tĭks) [″ + *plassein*, to form]. Formation of muscles in a stump after amputation so that it is possible to impart motion and direction to an artificial limb.

cineraceous (sĭn-ē-rā′shŭs) [L. *cinis*, ashes]. Like ashes.

cineradiography (sĭn″ē-rā″dē-ŏg′ră-fē) [Gr. *kinesis*, motion, + L. *radius*, ray, + Gr. *graphein*, to write]. Motion picture record of images produced during fluoroscopic examination.

cinerea (sĭn-ē′rē-ă) [L. *cinereus*, ashen-hued]. Gray matter of the brain or spinal cord.

cinereal (sĭn-ē′rē-ăl). Pert. to the cinerea.

cineritious (sĭn″ĕr-ĭsh′ŭs) [L. *cineritius*, ashen]. Ashen-gray color.

cinesi- [Gr. *kinesis*, motion]. Prefix rel. to motion. SEE: words beginning with *kinesi-*.

cineurography (sĭn″ē-ū-rŏg′ră-fē) [Gr. *kinesis*, motion, + *ouron*, urine, + *graphein*, to write]. Use of cineradiography to obtain motion picture of the urinary tract.

cingulotomy (sĭn′gū-lŏt″ō-mē) [L. *cingulum*, girdle, + Gr. *tome*, incision]. Surgical excision of the anterior half of the cingulate gyrus of the brain. May be done to alleviate intractable pain.

cingulum (sĭn′gū-lŭm) [L., girdle]. (pl. *cingula*) [NA] 1. A band of association fibers in the cingulate gyrus extending from the anterior perforated substance posteriorly to the hippocampal gyrus. 2. An eminence on the lingual surface of the incisor teeth, esp. the upper ones. It is situated near the gum. SYN:

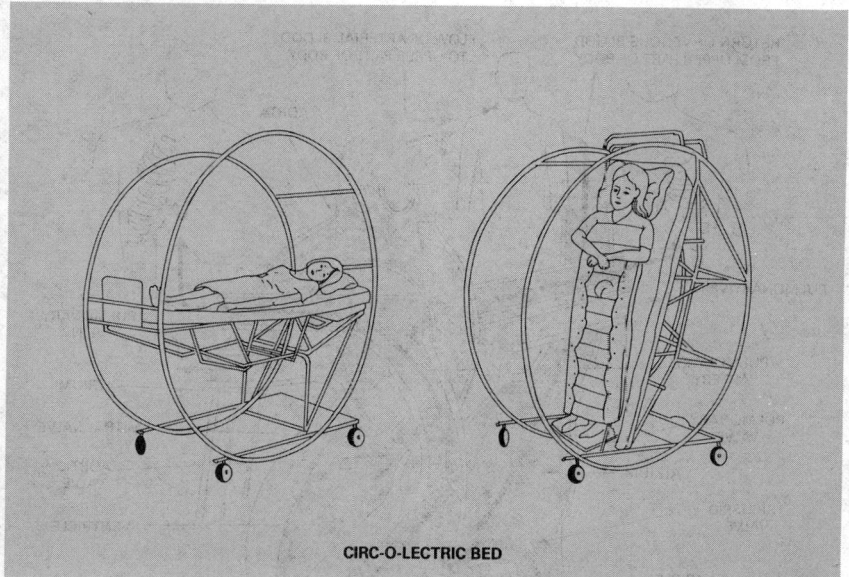

CIRC-O-LECTRIC BED

basal ridge.

cinoxacin. USP. An antibacterial drug. Trade name is Cinobac.

CinQuin. Trade name for quinidine sulfate.

cion (sī'ŏn) [Gr. *kion,* pillar]. The uvula.

circa (sĭr'kă) [L.]. ABBR: c. About. Used before dates or figures that are approximate.

circadian (sĭr"kă-dē'ăn, sĭr-kā'dē-ăn) [L. *circa,* about, + *dies,* day]. Pert. to events that occur at approximately 24-hour intervals, such as certain physiological phenomena. SEE: *clock, biological.*

circinate (sĕr'sĭ-nāt) [L. *circinatus,* made round]. Circular.

circle [L. *circulus,* a little ring]. Any ring-shaped structure.

c. of diffusion. One or more circles on projection plane of an image not in focus of the lens of the eye.

c. of Willis. Union of the anterior and posterior cerebral arteries (branches of the carotid), forming an anastomosis at the base of the brain. SEE: *Willis' circle* for illus.

Circ-O-Lectric bed. A bed designed to allow the patient's position to be changed from supine to prone by rotating the bed through 180° by use of electromechanical rotation. SEE: illus.

circuit (sĕr'kĭt) [L. *circuire,* to go around]. 1. Course or path of an electric current. 2. The path followed by a fluid circulating in a system of tubes or cavities. 3. The path followed by nerve impulses in a reflex arc from sensory receptor to effector organ.

circular [L. *circularis*]. 1. Shaped like a circle. 2. Recurrent.

circulation [L. *circulatio*]. Movement in a regular or circular course.

c., bile salts. Circulation of the sodium glycocholate and taurocholate found in hepatic bile, which pass with it into the duodenum and then into the intestine, where they are absorbed along with the fats.

c., blood. Circulation in which the blood leaving the left ventricle enters the aorta, from which it is pumped into the various large arteries. It thus reaches the coronary arteries of the heart itself and the arteries of the head, body wall, abdominal viscera, and extremities. Passing through the various capillary systems, it is gathered into veins, of which there are two collecting systems: (1) Most veins empty their blood into the superior and inferior venae cavae. (2) The veins from the stomach, pancreas, spleen, and intestine unite to form the portal vein, which runs to the liver. In the latter, it breaks up into a new capillary system, which drains through the hepatic veins into the vena cava inferior. The combined blood of the venae cavae and the coronary veins enters the right atrium, passes through the right ventricle, and is forced out into the pulmonary artery. The pulmonary capillary system drains by way of the pulmonary veins into the left atrium and thence into the left ventricle.

c., collateral. Circulation that is established through an anastomosis between two

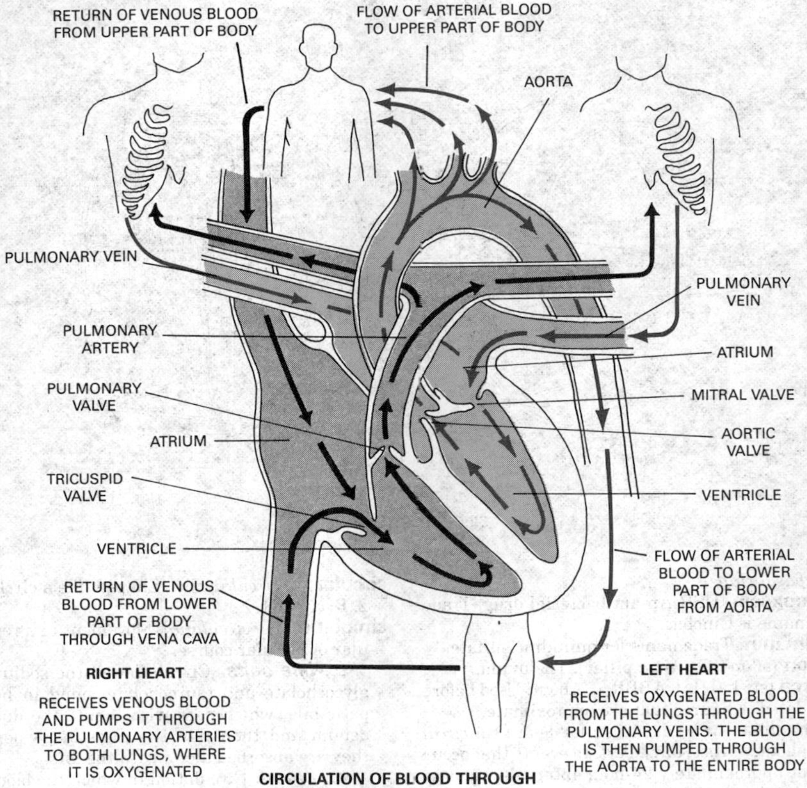

CIRCULATION OF BLOOD THROUGH HEART AND MAJOR VESSELS

vessels supplying or draining two adjacent vascular areas. This enables the blood to bypass an obstruction in the larger vessel that supplies or drains the two areas or will enable blood to flow to or from a tissue even though the principal vessel involved may be obstructed.

c., coronary. Circulation through the muscular tissue of the heart. Blood leaves the aorta through the right and left coronary arteries, which supply the myocardium. Blood passes through capillaries and is collected in veins, most of which empty into the coronary sinus, which opens into the right atrium. A few of the small veins open directly into the atria and ventricles. SEE: illus.

c., extracorporeal. Circulation of blood outside the body. This may be through an artificial kidney or a heart-lung device.

c., fetal. Circulation through the fetus. Blood, oxygenated in the placenta, passes through the umbilical vein and ductus venosus to the inferior vena cava and thence to the right atrium of the fetus, from which it may follow one of two courses—through the foramen ovale to the left atrium and then through the aorta to the tissues, or through the right ventricle, pulmonary artery, and ductus arteriosus to the aorta and then to the tissues. In either case the blood bypasses the lungs, which are not functioning before birth. Blood is returned to the placenta through the umbilical arteries, which are continuations of the hypogastric arteries. At birth or shortly after, the ductus arteriosus and the foramen ovale close, establishing normal circulation. Failure of either to occur may give rise to a blue baby. SEE: *fetal circulation* for illus.; *ductus arteriosus, patent*.

c., lymph. Lymph is formed from the tissue fluid that fills the tissue spaces of the body. It is collected into lymph capillaries, which carry the lymph to the larger lymph vessels. These converge to form one of two main trunks, the right lymphatic duct and the thoracic duct. The right lymphatic duct drains the right side of the head, neck, and trunk and right upper extremity; the thoracic duct drains all the remaining portion of the body. It has its origin at the cisterna chyli, which receives the lymphatics from the abdominal organs. It courses upward through the diaphragm and thorax and empties into the left subclavian artery near its junction with the left interior jugular vein. The right lymphatic duct empties into the right subclavian vein. Along the course of lymph vessels there are lymph nodes, which function as filtering structures. They filter out bacteria and particulate substances, thus preventing their entrance into the bloodstream. Lymph flow is maintained by difference in pressure at the two ends of the system. Important accessory factors aiding the flow of lymph are breathing movements and muscular activities.

c., portal. Circulation in which blood from the systemic arteries is supplied to the abdominal organs and is collected into the portal vein, through which the blood enters the liver. It passes into sinusoids, which lead to central veins of the lobules and eventually to the hepatic veins, which empty into the inferior vena cava. A portal system also exists in the circulation between the hypothalamus and the hypophysis (anterior pituitary). The hypothalamus releases hormone-releasing factors into the blood, where they are carried to the hypophysis and the appropriate hormone released.

c., pulmonary. Circulation in which the venous blood that is received into the right atrium passes through the tricuspid valve into the right ventricle. From there it passes into the pulmonary artery, which divides into two branches, one going to each lung. (This is the only instance in which an artery contains venous or dark blood deficient in oxygen.) The artery branches in the lung into capillaries, and here, by means of the hemoglobin in the red corpuscles, the blood takes up oxygen from the inspired air. Red arterial blood returns to the heart by the four pulmonary veins, two from each lung, entering the left atrium. (This is the only instance in which veins contain fully oxygenated blood.)

c., systemic. General circulation through the whole body except the lungs.

c., venous. Circulation of the blood via the veins.

circulation rate. The minute volume or output of the heart per minute. In an average size adult with a pulse rate of 70, the amount is about three liters per square meter of body surface each minute.

circulation time. The time required by a particle of blood to make the complete circuit of both the systemic and pulmonary systems. Circulation time is determined by injecting a substance into a vein and timing its reappearance in arteries at the point of injection. This procedure necessitates that the blood with the contained substance passes through veins to the heart and through the right atrium and ventricle, through the pulmonary circuit to the lungs, and back through the left atrium and ventricle, and then out through the aorta and arteries to the place where detected. Dyes such as fluorescein and methylene blue or substances such as potassium ferrocyanide or histamine have been used as tracers. Average circulation time is 18 to 24 seconds.

Circulation time is reduced in anemia and hyperthyroidism; increased in hypertension, myxedema, and cardiac failure. Circulation time may also be measured by injecting into a vein a substance that can be detected by the sense of taste when it is transported to the tongue. The normal circulation time from an arm vein to the tongue is 10 to 16 seconds. In the aorta, the blood flows at a speed of approx. 30 cm. per second.

circulatory. Pert. to circulation.

circulatory collapse. Shock, q.v.

circulatory failure. Failure of the cardiovascular system to provide body tissues with an adequate amount of blood for proper functioning. It may be caused by cardiac failure or peripheral circulatory failure, as occurs in shock, in which there is general peripheral vasodilation with "pooling" of blood in the expanded vascular space, resulting in decreased venous return.

circulatory overload. State of increased blood volume, usually due to transfusions that increase the venous pressure, esp. in patients with heart disease. This can result in heart failure, pulmonary edema, and cyanosis.

circulatory system. The cardiovascular system consisting of the heart and blood vessels (arteries, arterioles, capillaries, venules, veins, and sinuses) and the lymphatic system. SEE: *blood; chest; heart.*

INSPECTION: Inspection detects any abnormal centers of pulsation; the apex beat and its position, force, and extent; and any unnatural prominence over the precordial region. SEE: *abdominal examination; apex beat; chest; heart; lung; pulsation; pulse.*

circulus (sĕr′kū-lŭs) [L.]. Circle or ring.

circum- [L.]. Prefix meaning around, as circumduction.

circumarticular (sĕr″kŭm-ăr-tĭk′ū-lăr) [L.

circum, around, + *articulus,* small joint]. Surrounding a joint. SYN: *periarthric.*

circumcision (sĕr″kŭm-sĭ′zhŭn) [L. *circumcisio,* a cutting around]. Surgical removal of the end of the prepuce of the penis. Circumcision is usually done at the request of the parents. There are very few medical indications for this procedure.

NURSING IMPLICATIONS: The area should be kept clean and assessed for bleeding every hour for the first two hours after the procedure. Sterile petroleum gauze is usually applied to the penis after circumcision, and this is usually left in place for 24 hours, and is replaced if it comes dislodged before that time period is up. The infant should not be positioned on the abdomen for the first few hours following the procedure.

c., ritual. The religious rite performed by the Jews and Muslims at the time of removal of the prepuce.

circumclusion (sĕr″kŭm-klū′zhŭn) [L. *circumcludere,* to shut in]. Acupressure by use of a pin under an artery and a wire loop over it, attached to each end of the pin.

circumcorneal (sĕr″kŭm-kor′nē-ăl) [L. *circum,* around, + *corneus,* horny]. Around the cornea.

circumduction (sĕr″kŭm-dŭk′shŭn) [″ + *ducere,* to lead]. 1. The action or swing of a limb, such as the arm, in such a manner that it describes a cone-shaped figure, the apex of the cone being formed by the joint at the proximal end, while the complete circle is formed by the free distal end of the limb. 2. Circular movement of the eye.

circumference (sĕr-kŭm′fĕr-ĕns) [″ + *ferre,* to bear]. The perimeter of an object or body.

circumferential (sĕr″kŭm-fĕr-ĕn′shăl). 1. Encircling. 2. Concerning the periphery or circumference of an object or body.

circumflex (sĕr′kŭm-flĕks) [″ + *flectere,* to bend]. Winding around, as a vessel.

circuminsular (sĕr″kŭm-ĭn′sū-lăr) [″ + *insula,* island]. Surrounding the island of Reil in the cerebral cortex.

circumlental (sĕr″kŭm-lĕn′tăl) [″ + *lens,* lens]. Situated around the lens of the eye.

circumnuclear (sĕr″kŭm-nū′klē-ăr) [″ + *nucleus,* kernel]. Surrounding the nucleus.

circumocular (sĕr″kŭm-ŏk′ū-lăr) [″ + *oculus,* eye]. Surrounding the eye.

circumoral (sĕr″kŭm-ō′răl) [L. *circum,* around, + *os,* mouth]. Encircling the mouth.

circumoral pallor. White area around the mouth contrasting vividly with color of face, seen esp. in scarlet fever.

circumorbital (sĕr″kŭm-or′bĭt-ăl) [″ + *orbita,* orbit]. Around an orbit.

circumpolarization (sĕr″kŭm-pō″lăr-ī-zā′shŭn) [″ + *polaris,* polar]. The rotation of a ray of polarized light.

circumrenal (sĕr″kŭm-rē′năl) [″ + *renalis,* pert. to kidney]. Around or about the kidney.

circumscribed (sĕr′kŭm-skrībd) [″ + *scribere,* to write]. Limited in space by that which is drawn around or confines an area.

circumstantiality (sĕr″kŭm-stăn″shē-ăl′ĭ-tē) [L. *circum,* around, + *stare,* to stand]. The mention of irrelevant facts and details in conversation. Usually a symptom of mental disorder.

circumvallate (sĕr″kŭm-văl′āt) [″ + *vallare,* to wall]. Surrounded by a wall or raised structure.

circumvallate papillae. V-shaped row of papillae at base of tongue.

circumvascular (sĕr″kŭm-văs′kū-lăr) [″ + *vasculum,* vessel]. Perivascular; around a blood vessel.

cirrhosis (sĭ-rō′sĭs) [Gr. *kirrhos,* orange yellow, + *osis,* condition]. A chronic disease of the liver characterized by formation of dense perilobular connective tissue, degenerative changes in parenchymal cells, alteration in structure of the cords of liver lobules, fatty and cellular infiltration, and sometimes development of areas of regeneration. In addition to the clinical signs and symptoms inherent in the cause of the cirrhosis, those due to cirrhosis are the result of loss of functioning liver cells and increased resistance to flow of blood through the liver (portal hypertension). When severe enough, this leads to ammonia toxicity, q.v.

ETIOL: May be due to various factors such as nutritional deficiency (lack of proteins, choline, or methionine), poisons (including alcohol, carbon tetrachloride, phosphorus), or previous inflammation caused by a virus or bacteria. SEE: *liver.*

TREATMENT: Therapy depends upon the cause and severity of the disease.

c., alcoholic. Cirrhosis occurring in persons who are chronic alcoholics. Approx. 20% of chronic alcoholics develop cirrhosis.

c., atrophic. Cirrhosis in which the liver is decreased in size.

c., biliary. Cirrhosis marked by prolonged jaundice due to chronic retention of bile and inflammation of bile ducts. SEE: *c., obstructive biliary; c., primary biliary.*

c., cardiac. Congestive cirrhosis resulting from passive congestion of the liver due to congestive heart failure.

c., fatty. Cirrhosis with fatty infiltration of the liver cells.

c., hypertrophic. Cirrhosis in which the connective tissue hyperplasia causes the liver to be greatly enlarged.

c., infantile. Cirrhosis occurring in childhood resulting from protein malnutrition. SEE: *kwashiorkor.*

c., macronodular. Cirrhosis characterized by large irregular regenerating nodules and broad bands of fibrous tissue. These areas contain portal spaces and terminal hepatic veins. Seen following viral and idiopathic hepatitis. Formerly termed postnecrotic or posthepatic cirrhosis.

c., metabolic. Cirrhosis due to metabolic disease such as hemochromatosis, glycogen storage disease, or Wilson's disease.

c., micronodular. Cirrhosis characterized by thin bands of fibrotic tissue and small nodules of regeneration. Previously termed portal or Laennec's cirrhosis. SYN: *c., alcoholic.*

c., obstructive biliary. Cirrhosis resulting from obstruction of the common duct by a stone, tumor, etc.

c., primary biliary. A rare, progressive form of cirrhosis characterized by enlargement of the liver, jaundice, and pruritus.

c., syphilitic. Cirrhosis occurring in tertiary syphilis, in which gummas form in the liver and, on healing, cause coarse lobulation.

c., toxic. Cirrhosis resulting from toxic substances as in poisoning by carbon tetrachloride or phosphorus.

c., zooparasitic. Cirrhosis resulting from infestation with animal parasites, esp. blood flukes of the genus Schistosoma, or liver flukes, Clonorchis sinensis.

cirrhotic (sĭ-rŏt′ĭk). Pert. to or affected with cirrhosis.

cirsectomy (sĕr-sĕk′tō-mē) [Gr. *kirsos,* varix, + *ektome,* excision]. Excision of a portion of a varicose vein.

cirsoid (sĕr′soyd) [″ + *eidos,* resemblance]. Resembling a varix. SYN: *varicose.*

cirsomphalos (sĕr-sŏm′fă-lŏs) [″ + *omphalos,* navel]. Varicose veins around the navel.

cirsotome (sĕr′sō-tōm) [″ + *tome,* incision]. Instrument for cutting varicose veins.

cirsotomy (sĕr-sŏt′ō-mē). Treatment of a varicosity by multiple incisions.

C.I.S. *central inhibitory state.*

cis (sĭs) [L., on the same side]. In organic chemistry, a form of isomerism in which similar atoms or radicals are on the same side. In genetics, a prefix meaning the location of two or more genes on the same chromosome of a homologous pair.

cisplatin (sĭs′plă-tĭn). An antineoplastic chemical used in treating testicular tumors and ovarian cancer. The drug's nephrotoxicity may be almost eliminated by ensuring a diuresis of 150 ml./hr. when the drug is administered. Trade name is Platinol.

cissa (sĭs′ă) [Gr. *kissa*]. Pica. Abnormal craving to eat inedible materials.

cistern (sĭs′tĕrn). A reservoir for storage of fluid.

cisterna [L.]. (pl. *cisternae*) [NA] A reservoir or cavity.

c. chyli. [NA] A dilated sac into which empties the intestinal, two lumbar, and two descending lymphatic trunks; the origin of the thoracic duct. SYN: *receptaculum chyli.*

c. subarachnoidalis. [NA] A wide space in the cranial cavity between the arachnoid and the pia mater. It contains cerebrospinal fluid.

cisternal (sĭs-tĕr′năl). Concerning a cavity filled with fluid.

cisternal puncture. A spinal puncture with a hollow needle between the cervical vertebrae, through the dura mater into the cisterna at the base of the brain.

PURPOSE: To inject a drug or a serum as in cerebral meningitis or cerebral syphilis; to remove spinal fluid for diagnostic purposes, or to reduce intracranial pressure. Should be used as a source of spinal fluid only if fluid cannot be obtained by lumbar puncture. SEE: *cerebrospinal fluid; spinal puncture.*

cisvestitism (sĭs-vĕs′tĭ-tĭzm) [L. *cis,* on the same side, + *vestitus,* dressed, + Gr. *-ismos,* condition]. Wearing of clothes appropriate to one's sex but suitable for a calling or profession other than one's own.

Ex.: a civilian who dresses in a uniform of the armed services.

Citanest. Trade name for prilocaine hydrochloride.

Citelli's syndrome (chē-tĕl′ēz). [Salvatore Citelli, It. laryngologist, 1875–1947] Insomnia or drowsiness, and lack of concentration associated with intelligence disorders, seen in children with infected adenoids or sphenoid sinusitis.

citrate (sĭt′rāt, sī′trāt). Compound of citric acid and a base.

citrated (sĭt′rāt-ĕd). Combined or mixed with citric acid or a citrate.

citrate solution. Solution used to prevent clotting of the blood. Its use permits whole blood to be stored in a refrigerator until it is needed for transfusion.

citric acid. USP. $C_6H_8O_7{\cdot}H_2O$. A tribasic acid present in the juice of many fruits, esp. citrus fruits. SEE: *acid, citric.*

citric acid cycle. A complicated series of reactions in the body involving the oxidative metabolism of pyruvic acid and liberation of energy. It is the main pathway of terminal oxidation in the process of which not only carbohydrates but proteins and fats are utilized. SYN: *Krebs cycle; tricarboxylic acid cycle.* SEE: *Krebs cycle* for illus.

citronella (sĭt″rŏn-ĕl′ă). Volatile oil obtained from Cymbopogon citratus, lemon grass. Used in perfumes and as an insect repellant. It contains geraniol and citronellal.

citrovorum factor. Folic acid, q.v.

citrulline (sĭt-rŭl'lĭn). An amino acid, $C_6H_{13}N_3O_3$, formed from ornithine. It is present in watermelons.

citrullinemia (sĭt-rŭl"lĭ-nē'mē-ă). A type of aminoaciduria accompanied by increased amounts of citrulline in the blood, urine, and spinal fluid. Clinically, there will be ammonia intoxication, liver disease, vomiting, mental retardation, convulsions, and failure to thrive.

citrullinuria (sĭt-rŭl"lĭ-nū'rē-ă). Increased amount of citrulline in the urine.

Cl. 1. Chem. symb. for chlorine. 2. *chloride; clavicle; Clostridium.*

cladosporiosis (klăd"ō-spō-rē-ō'sĭs) [Gr. *klados*, branch, + *sporos*, seed, + *osis*, condition]. A general term for an infection, usually of the central nervous system, due to the fungus Cladosporium.

Cladosporium. A genus of fungi. The condition tinea nigra is caused by either C. werneckii or C. mansonii.

clairvoyance (klār-voy'ăns) [Fr.]. Alleged ability to be aware of events that occur at a distance without receiving any sort of sensory information concerning the event.

clamp (klămp) [MD. *klampe*, metal clasp]. Device used in surgery to grasp, join, compress, or support an organ, tissue, or vessel.

clang [L. *clangere*, to peal]. A loud, metallic sound.

clap. Colloquial term for gonorrhea.

clapotage, clapotement (klă"pō-tăzh', klă-pŏt-maw') [Fr.]. Any splashing sound in succussion of a dilated stomach.

clapping (klăp'ĭng). Percussion of the chest to loosen secretions. The hand is used in a cupped position. Also called cupping or tapping.

Clapton's lines. Green lines on dental margin of gums in copper poisoning.

clarificant (klăr-ĭf'ĭk-ănt) [L. *clarus*, clear, + *facere*, to make]. Any agent that clears the turbidity of a liquid.

clarification (klăr"ĭ-fĭ-kā'shŭn). Making a solution free of turbidity.

Clarke, Jacob A.L. British anatomist, 1817–1880.

C.'s bodies. Alveolar sarcomatous intranuclear bodies of breast.

C.'s column. The dorsal nucleus of the spinal cord.

Clarke-Hadfield syndrome. [Cecil Clarke; Geoffrey Hadfield, Brit. pathologist, b. 1899] Infantilism caused by pancreatic insufficiency. A child suffering from this syndrome is underweight and fails to grow.

Clark's rule. A method of calculating pediatric drug dosages. The weight of the child in pounds is multiplied by the adult dose and the result is divided by 150. The weight of the child can also be divided by 150 to obtain the appropriate fraction of the adult dose. SEE: *dosage.*

clasmatocyte (klăz-măt'ō-sīt) [Gr. *klasma*, fragment, + *kytos*, cell]. A large, wandering, uninucleated cell with many branches. A fixed macrophage of loose connective tissue. It is capable of ingesting particulate material and has the property of selectively storing certain dyes in colloidal solution. In inflammatory conditions it becomes actively ameboid and is important in providing protection against local invasion by bacteria, which it ingests. SYN: *histiocyte; tissue macrophage.*

clasmatodendrosis (klăz-măt"ō-dĕn-drō'sĭs) [" + *dendron*, tree, + *osis*, condition]. A breaking up of astrocytic protoplasmic expansions.

clasmatosis (klăz"mă-tō'sĭs) [" + *osis*, condition]. Crumbling into small bits; fragmentation, as of cells.

clasp (klăsp). Device for holding an object or tissue.

clasp-knife rigidity. Spastic action in a joint in cerebral palsies. Passive flexion of the joint causes increased resistance of the extensors. This gives way abruptly if the pressure to produce flexion is continued.

class [L. *classis*, division]. 1. In biology, a taxonomic group of clearly defined animals or plants classified below a phylum and above an order. 2. In statistics, a group of variables that fall within certain value limits.

classification (klăs"ĭ-fĭ-kā'shŭn). The orderly separation of a group of similar organisms, animals, or individuals into classes according to traits or characteristics that are common to each class or group. The animal kingdom is divided as: kingdom, subkingdom, phylum, class, order, family (including species), and genus. The plant kingdom is divided as: kingdom, division, class, natural order, and genus. The names of class categories are Latinized. SEE: *taxonomy.*

clastic (klăs'tĭk) [Gr. *klastos*, broken]. Causing division into parts.

clastothrix (klăs'tō-thrĭks) [" + *thrix*, hair]. Splitting of the hair. SYN: *trichorrhexis nodosa.*

Claude's syndrome (klawdz). [Henri Claude, Fr. psychiatrist, 1869–1945] Paralysis of the third cranial nerve, contralateral ataxia and tremor. Caused by a lesion in the red nucleus of the brain.

claudication (klaw-dĭ-kā'shŭn) [L. *claudicare*, to limp]. Lameness; limping.

c., intermittent. A severe pain in calf muscles occurring during walking but that subsides with rest. It results from inadequate blood supply, which may be due to arterial spasm, atherosclerosis, arteriosclerosis, or an occlusion.

c., venous. Claudication resulting from inadequate venous drainage.

Claudius' cell (klaw'dē-ŭs). [Friedrich Claudius, Austrian anatomist, 1822–1869] Large columnar cells external to the organ of Corti.

Claudius' fossa. Small depression in posterior part of pelvis, on either side, in which lies the ovary.

claustrophilia (klaws-trō-fĭl'ē-ă) [L. *claustrum,* a barrier, + Gr. *philein,* to love]. Dread of being in an open space; a morbid desire to be shut in with doors and windows closed.

claustrophobia (klaws-trō-fō'bē-ă) [" + Gr. *phobos,* fear]. Fear of being confined in any space, as in a locked room. Opposite of agoraphobia.

claustrum (klŏs'trŭm) [L.]. 1. A barrier. 2. Thin layer of gray matter separating the external capsule from the island of Reil.

clausura (klaw-sū'ră) [L.]. Atresia of a passage.

clava (klā'vă) [L., club]. (pl. *clavae*) An elevation on dorsal surface of the medulla oblongata caused by the underlying nucleus gracilis, the superior extremity of the fasciculus gracilis.

clavate (klā'vāt). Club-shaped.

clavicle (klăv'ĭ-k'l) [L. *clavicula,* little key]. The collarbone; a bone, curved like the letter f, that articulates with the sternum and the scapula.

c., dislocation of. *Forward, sternal end:* TREATMENT: Place knee against spine and draw shoulders back; apply clavicle bandage with pad on dislocated end of bone.

Outer extremity: Bone upon upper surface of acromion or upon anterior part of spine of the scapula.

SYM: Prominence upon surface of acromion that disappears when arm is raised. Shoulders flattened, arm hanging close to trunk.

TREATMENT: Raise shoulder, draw backward; place pad in axilla, bringing elbow close to side; secure arm and forearm to chest with pad in axilla; pressure by pad and gutta percha plate on projecting clavicle strapped in place.

c., fracture of. SYM: Swelling, pain, protuberance with sharp depression over the injured bone. Patient holds the immobile arm by supporting it at the elbow.

F.A.: Place ball of cloth or one or two handkerchiefs, tightly rolled, under armpit. Apply arm sling; bandage elbow to side, hand and forearm extending across the chest. Or lay patient on back on the floor with rolled-up blanket under shoulders until medical aid arrives. This position keeps shoulders back and prevents broken ends of bone from rubbing.

TREATMENT: Have assistant draw arms and shoulders backward. Raise shoulders and support in upward, backward, and outward direction. Maintain position by clavicle strap or figure-of-eight wrap between the shoulders and over the back.

clavicotomy (klăv"ĭ-kŏt'ō-mē) [" + Gr. *tome,* incision]. Surgical division of the clavicle.

clavicular (klă-vĭk'ū-lăr). Pert. to the clavicle.

clavus (klā'vŭs) [L., nail]. 1. A corn or callosity. 2. A sharp pain in the head described as feeling like a nail being driven into it.

clawfoot. A deformity of the foot characterized by excessively high longitudinal arch, usually accompanied by dorsal contracture of toes. SYN: *pes cavus.*

clawhand. A hand characterized by hyperextension of the proximal phalanges of the digits and extreme flexion of middle and distal phalanges. Usually the result of injury to ulnar and median nerves. SYN: *main en griffe.*

claw toe. A toe with dorsal flexion of 1st phalanx and plantar flexion of 2nd and 3rd phalanges. SYN: *hammertoe.*

Clayton gas. Sulfur dioxide; used to fumigate ships.

clean-catch method. Procedure for obtaining a urine specimen in order to obtain a sample for culture that will have minimal chance of being contaminated. For females, while the labia are held apart, the periurethral area is cleaned with a mild soap or antibacterial solution, rinsed with copious amounts of plain water, and then, with the labia still held apart, the urine is passed and the specimen is collected in a sterile container. It is preferable that the sample be obtained after the urine flow is well established, i.e., a midstream specimen. For males, cleanse the urethral meatus and obtain the midstream specimen in a sterile container. If the male is uncircumsized, be certain that the foreskin is retracted prior to cleansing the penis.

cleaning, ultrasonic. Use of high-frequency vibrations to clean instruments.

clean room. A type of controlled environment facility in which all incoming air passes through a filter capable of removing 99.97% of all particles 0.3 microns and larger. The temperature, pressure, and humidity in the room are controlled Clean rooms are used in research and in controlling infections, especially for persons who may not have normally functioning immune systems.

Ex.: Individuals who have been treated with drugs that prevent immune response as part of the therapeutic preparation for transplantation of an organ.

In very rare instances a child is born without the ability to develop the immune system. Such children are kept in a clean room while waiting for specific therapy such as bone marrow transplantation. Alternatively, these children may be kept in a suit that completely isolates them from physical contact with the environment but allows them to be mobile. The suit, sometimes called a "space bubble," is attached to filtering devices needed to screen the air supplied to the child.

clearance. The elimination of a substance from the blood plasma by the kidneys. SEE: *renal clearance test.*

clearing agent. Substance that makes tissues prepared for microscopic examination more transparent.

cleavage (klē'vĕj) [AS. *cleofian,* to cleave]. 1. Splitting a complex molecule into two or more simpler ones. 2. Cell division following the fertilization of an egg. SYN: *segmentation.*

cleavage cell. The blastomere.

cleavage lines. Lines indicating the prevailing direction of fibers in the corium of the skin. In a living subject or fresh cadaver, a puncture wound does not remain round but becomes elliptical in the direction of the fibers. Lines in general run obliquely. This is important to the surgeon because an incision parallel to these lines will heal with much less scarring than one across the lines. SYN: *Langer's lines.* SEE: *Langer's lines* for illus.

cleft (klĕft) [ME. *clift,* crevice]. 1. A fissure or elongated opening. 2. Divided or split.

c., branchial. An opening between the branchial arches of an embryo. In lower vertebrates it becomes a gill cleft.

c., facial. An anomaly resulting from failure of facial processes of embryo to fuse. Common ones are oblique facial cleft, an open nasolacrimal furrow extending from eye to lower portion of nose that is sometimes continuous with a cleft in upper lip, and transverse facial cleft, which extends laterally from the angle of the mouth.

cleft cheek. Transverse facial cleft. SYN: *macrostomia.*

cleft foot. A bipartite foot resulting from failure of a digit and its corresponding metatarsal to develop.

cleft hand. A bipartite hand resulting from failure of a digit and its corresponding metacarpal to develop.

cleft lip. Harelip. A congenital cleft or separation of the upper lip. May be associated with cleft palate.

cleft palate. A congenital fissure in the roof of the mouth forming a communicating passageway between mouth and nasal cavities. May be unilateral or bilateral and complete or incomplete.

cleft sternum. A congenital fissure of the breastbone.

cleft tongue. A bifid tongue; one with a separated tip.

cleido- (klī'dō) [Gr. *kleis,* used for closing]. Prefix pert. to the clavicle.

cleidocostal (klī"dō-kŏs'tăl) [" + L. *costa,* rib. Concerning the clavicle and the ribs.

cleidorrhexis (klī"dō-rĕk'sĭs) [" + *rhexis,* rupture]. Fracture or bending of the clavicles of the fetus for delivery.

cleidotomy (klī-dŏt'ō-mē) [" + *tome,* incision]. Dividing a fetal clavicle to facilitate delivery.

clemastine fumarate (klĕm'ăs-tēn). USP. An antihistamine drug. Trade names are Tavist and Tavegyl.

clenching (klĕnch'ĭng). With the teeth in contact, forcible, repeated contraction of the jaw muscles. This causes pulsating and bilateral contractions of the temporalis and pterygomassetric muscles. This may be done consciously, subconsciously while awake, or during sleep. SEE: *bruxism.*

cleptomania (klĕp"tō-mā'nē-ă). Kleptomania. Impulsive stealing in which the motive is not related to the intrinsic value of the stolen article. There is often deep regret following the act.

click (klĭk). 1. An abrupt and brief sound heard in listening to the heart sounds. 2. Any brief sound but esp. one heard during a joint movement.

clidinium bromide (klĭ-dĭn'ē-ŭm). USP. A drug used in treating peptic ulcers and other conditions wherein it is desirable to inhibit the action of the parasympathetic nervous system. Trade name is Quarzan.

client. The patient of a health care professional.

climacteric (klī-măk'tĕr-ĭk, klī-măk-tĕr'ĭk) [Gr. *klimakter,* a rung of a ladder]. The period that marks the cessation of a woman's reproductive ability (female climacteric or menopause); a corresponding period of lessening of sexual activity in the male (male climacteric).

climatology, medical [Gr. *klima,* sloping surface of the earth, + *logos,* study]. Branch of meteorology that includes the study of climate and its relationship to disease. SEE: *bioclimatology.*

climatotherapy (klī"măt-ō-thĕr'ăp-ē) [" + *therapeia,* treatment]. Treatment of disease by having patient move to a more favorable climate.

climax (klī'măks) [Gr. *klimax,* ladder]. 1. Period of greatest intensity. 2. The sexual orgasm, q.v.

clindamycin hydrochloride (klĭn"dă-mī'sĭn). USP. An antibiotic effective against gram-positive cocci. At one time it was thought to have the side effect of causing colitis. It is now believed that the colitis that may develop during therapy with clindamycin is due to resistant strains of Clostridium difficile.

clinic (klĭn′ĭk) [Gr. *klinikos,* pert. to a bed]. 1. Medical and dental instruction in which patients are observed directly, symptoms noted, and treatments discussed. 2. A center for physical examination and treatment of ambulant patients who are not hospitalized. 3. A place where individuals gather together with patients for the study of disease. 4. A place where preliminary diagnosis is made and treatment given, as an x-ray clinic, a dental clinic, or child-guidance clinic.

clinical. 1. Founded on actual observation and treatment of patients as distinguished from data or facts obtained by experimentation or pathology. 2. Pert. to a clinic.

clinical analysis. The chemical analysis and study of body fluids, excreta, and tissues in the diagnosis and treatment of disease.

clinical judgment. The exercise of the clinician's experience and knowledge in diagnosing and treating illness and disease.

clinical pathology. Division of pathology that utilizes clinical analysis and other laboratory procedures in the diagnosis and treatment of disease.

clinical thermometer. Glass or electronic instrument that measures body temperature. The glass, nondisposable type may be disinfected by first cleansing with cotton and soap solution, using a rotary motion downward to bulb end. This removes adherent mucus, which coagulates in some disinfectants, thereby retaining organisms. Rinse thoroughly in tepid, not hot, water and submerge in 70% alcohol for 10 minutes. Rinse before use. SEE: *thermometer.*

clinical trial. A carefully designed and executed investigation of the effects of a drug administered to human subjects. The goal is to define the clinical efficacy and pharmacologic effects (toxicity, side effects, incompatibilities, or interactions) of the substance. The U.S. government requires strict testing of all new drugs prior to their approval for use as therapeutic agents. SEE: *double-blind technique; randomization.*

clinician (klĭn-ĭsh′ăn) [Gr. *klinikos,* pert. to a bed]. A physician or dentist with expertise in clinical practice as distinguished from one specializing in research.

c., nurse. A nurse practitioner or clinician is a registered nurse with preparation in a specialized educational program. This preparation at present may be in the context of a formal continuing education program, a baccalaureate nursing program, or an advanced-degree nursing program. It is envisioned that in the future a nurse practitioner or clinician will be academically prepared at the baccalaureate or higher degree level. This preparation enables the nurse practitioner to provide nursing care as a primary health care provider in a variety of settings. Primary care provides health care to individual patients or groups of patients in order to maintain their health status and to prevent serious illness or disability. In any health care setting, the focus is mainly on the maintenance of wellness, the prevention of illness, and dealing with acute or chronic health problems. (Adapted from definition provided by the American Nurses' Association.)

clinicopathologic (klĭn″ĭ-kō-pă″thō-lŏj′ĭk). Concerning the clinical and pathological manifestations of a disease.

clinicopathologic conference. ABBR: CPC. A teaching conference in which the clinical findings are presented to a physician previously unfamiliar with the case, who then attempts to diagnose the disease that would explain the clinical findings. The exact diagnosis is then presented by the pathologist, who has either examined the tissue removed at surgery or has done the autopsy.

clinocephaly (klī″nō-sĕf′ă-lē) [Gr. *klinein,* to bend, + *kephale,* head]. Congenital flatness or saddleshape of the top of the head. Caused by bilateral premature closure of the sphenoparietal sutures.

clinodactyly (klī″nō-dăk′tĭ-lē) [″ + *daktylos,* finger]. Permanent medial or lateral deflection of one or more fingers.

clinoid (klī′noyd) [Gr. *kline,* bed, + *eidos,* appearance]. Resembling a bed in shape.

clinoid processes. Three pairs of prominences on upper surface of sphenoid bone.

clinometer (klī-nŏm′ĕ-tĕr) [Gr. *klinein,* to slope, + *metron,* measure]. Instrument for estimation of torsional deviation of eyes. Used to measure ocular muscle paralysis. SYN: *clinoscope.*

clinoscope (klī′nō-skōp) [″ + *skopein,* to examine]. Instrument for measuring the weakness of ocular muscles.

clinostatism (klī′no-stăt″ĭzm). The recumbent position.

clip. A metallic instrument for holding tissue or other material together.

cliseometer (klĭs″ē-ŏm′ĕt-ĕr) [Gr. *klisis,* inclination, + *metron,* measure]. Device for measuring the inclination that the pelvis makes with the spinal column.

Clistin. Trade name for carbinoxamine maleate.

clithrophobia (klĭth″rō-fō′bē-ă) [Gr. *kleithria,* keyhole, + *phobos,* fear]. Morbid fear of being locked in.

clition (klĭt′ē-ōn) [Gr. *kleitys,* slope]. A craniometric point in center of highest part of the clivus on the sphenoid bone.

clitoridectomy (klī″tō-rĭd-ĕk′tō-mē) [Gr. *klei-*

toris, clitoris, + *ektome*, excision]. Excision of clitoris.

clitoriditis (klĭ″tō-rĭd-ī′tĭs) [″ + *itis*, inflammation]. Inflammation of the clitoris.

clitoridotomy (klĭ″tō-rĭd-ŏt′ō-mē) [″ + *tome*, incision]. Incision of the clitoris; female circumcision.

clitoris (klī′tō-rĭs, klĭt′ō-rĭs) [Gr. *kleitoris*]. One of the structures of the female genitalia. It is a small erectile body located beneath the anterior labial commissure and partially hidden by the anterior portion of the labia minora. It is homologous to the penis of the male.

STRUCTURE: It consists of three parts: a body, two crura, and a glans. The body, about an inch (2.5 cm.) in length, consists of two fused corpora cavernosa. It extends from the pubic arch above to the glans below. The two crura are continuations of the corpora cavernosa and serve to attach them to the inferior rami of the pubic bones. They are covered by the ischiocavernosus muscles. The glans, which forms the free distal end, is a small rounded tubercle composed of erectile tissue. It is highly sensitive. The glans is usually covered by a hoodlike prepuce and its ventral surface is attached to the frenulum of the labia.

clitoris crises. Involuntary attack of sexual excitement in women with tabes dorsalis.

clitorism (klī′tō-rĭzm). 1. The counterpart of priapism. A long-continued, painful condition in the female with recurring erection of the clitoris. 2. Enlargement of the clitoris.

clitoritis (klĭ″tō-rī′tĭs). Inflammation of the clitoris. SYN: *clitoriditis*.

clitoromegaly (klĭ″tō-rō-mĕg′ă-lē) [″ + *megas*, large]. Enlargement of the clitoris. May be caused by an endocrine disease, or by use of anabolic steroids by female athletes.

clivus (klī′vŭs) [L., a slope]. A surface that slopes, as the sphenoid bone.

c. blumenbachii. The slope at the base of the skull.

clo. A unit for thermal insulation of clothing. The amount of insulation necessary to maintain comfort in a sitting-resting subject in a normally ventilated room (air movement at the rate of 10 cm./second) at a temperature of 70° F. (21° C.) with relative humidity of less than 50%.

cloaca (klō-ā′kă) [L. *cloaca*, a sewer]. 1. Cavity lined with endoderm at the posterior end of the body that serves as a common passageway for urinary, digestive, and reproductive ducts. Present in adult birds, reptiles, and amphibia, and in the embryos of all vertebrates. 2. An opening in the sheath covering necrosed bone.

clock [LL. *clocca*]. Device for measuring time.

c., biological. An internal system in organisms that regulates behavior in a rhythmic manner. Functions such as growth, feeding, the wake-sleep cycle, the menstrual cycle, and reproduction coincide with certain external events such as day and night, the tides, and the seasons. Biological clocks appear to be set by environmental conditions in some animals, but if they are isolated from their environment they continue to function according to the usual rhythm. A gradual change in environment does produce a gradual change in the timing of the biological clocks.

clofazimine (klō-fă′zĭ-mēn). A drug used in treating patients with leprosy who are resistant to the sulfones. Only available from the U.S. Public Health Service Hospital, Carville, Louisiana 70721, U.S.A.

clofibrate (klō-fī′brāt). USP. Drug used to reduce plasma concentration of lipids. Used in treating hyperlipoproteinemias, q.v., types III, IV, and V. Trade name is Atromid-S.

Clomid. Trade name for clomiphene citrate.

clomiphene citrate (klō′mĭ-fēn). USP. A nonsteroidal agent used to stimulate ovulation in women who have potentially functioning pituitary and ovarian systems. Women treated with this medicine who become pregnant have an increased incidence of multiple births. Trade name is Clomid.

clonal (klōn′ăl). Concerning a clone, q.v.

clonazepam (klō-năz′ĕ-păm). USP. An anticonvulsant drug. Trade name is Clonopin.

clone (klōn) [Gr. *klon*, a cutting used for propagation]. 1. In microbiology, the asexual progeny of a single cell. 2. A group of plants propagated from one seedling or stock. The members of the group are identical in character but do not reproduce from seed. 3. In tissue culture, a group of cells descended from a single cell.

clonic (klŏn′ĭk) [Gr. *klonos*, turmoil]. Pert. to clonus; alternate contraction and relaxation of muscles.

clonicity (klŏn-ĭs′ĭ-tē). Condition of being clonic.

clonicotonic (klŏn″ĭ-kō-tŏn′ĭk) [Gr. *klonos*, turmoil, + *tonikos*, tonic]. Both clonic and tonic, as some forms of muscular spasm.

clonic spasm. Spasm marked by muscular rigidity and then relaxation.

clonidine hydrochloride (klō′nĭ-dēn). An antihypertensive drug. Trade name is Catapres.

clonism, clonismus (klŏn′ĭzm, klō-nĭz′mŭs) [″ + *-ismos*, condition of]. Condition of being affected with clonic spasms, or a succession of them.

clonograph (klŏn′ō-grăf). Device for recording spasmodic contractions and movements.

Clonopin. Trade name for clonazepam.

clonorchiasis (klō″nor-kī′ă-sĭs). A disease of the Orient due to the Chinese liver fluke,

Clonorchis sinensis, which infects the bile ducts of man. Infection occurs when one eats uncooked freshwater fish containing encysted larvae. The early symptoms are loss of appetite and diarrhea; later there may be signs of cirrhosis of the liver. The disease may be prevented by thoroughly cooking fish, or by freezing it at −10° C. (14° F.) for a minimum of 5 days. The disease rarely causes death, but it may last for 30 years. Treatment with chloroquine phosphate is beneficial but not curative. Praziquantel has been used experimentally.

Clonorchis sinensis (klō-nor'kĭs sī-nĕn'sĭs). The trematode fluke, Chinese liver fluke. An important cause of disease, esp. in the Orient. SEE: *clonorchiasis.*

clonospasm (klŏn'ō-spăzm) [" + *spasmos,* spasm]. Rapid alternation of muscular contraction and relaxation. The rate is much slower than a tremor. In upper motor neuron paralysis, sharp flexion of the ankle often produces ankle clonus.

clonus (klō'nŭs). Spasmodic alternation of muscular contraction and relaxation. Opposite of tonus.

Cloquet's canal (klō-kāz'). [Jules Germain Cloquet, Fr. surgeon, 1790–1883] An irregular passage (hyaloid) through the center of the vitreous body in the fetus.

Clostridium (klō-strĭd'ē-ŭm) [Gr. *kloster,* spindle]. A genus of bacteria belonging to the family Bacillaceae. They are anaerobic, spore-forming rods and are widely distributed in nature; over 250 species are recognized. They are common in the soil and in the intestinal tract of man and animals and are frequently found in wound infections. Several are pathogenic in man, being the primary causative agents for gas gangrene.

C. botulinum. Species that grows in improperly processed food. Produces a powerful toxin, the cause of botulism, q.v.

C. chauvoei. Causative organism for blackleg or symptomatic anthrax in cattle.

C. difficile. Species of bacteria, the toxin from which causes enterocolitis. Several antibiotics were at one time thought to cause a particular type of colitis. It was later demonstrated that C. difficile was the true cause.

C. histolyticum. A proteolytic organism found in feces and soil, isolated from necrotic war wounds and found in some cases of gas gangrene.

C. novyi. Species found in many cases of gas gangrene.

C. perfringens. Most common causative agent of gas gangrene. SYN: *gas bacillus.*

C. septicum. Species found in cases of gangrene in man, cattle, hogs, and other domestic animals.

C. sporogenes. Species frequently associated with other organisms in mixed gangrenous infections. It is nonpathogenic.

C. tetani. The causative organism of tetanus or lockjaw. Produces a powerful exotoxin, a portion of which affects nerve tissue, another portion is hemolytic.

C. welchii. C. perfringens.

closure (klō'shŭr). Shutting or bringing together as in suturing together the edges of a laceration type of wound.

clot (klŏt) [AS. *clott,* lump]. 1. A thrombus; a coagulum, as of blood or lymph. SEE: *blood, clotting of; coagulation factors; thrombosis.* 2. To coagulate.

c., agony. Clot formed in the heart when death ensues from prolonged heart failure.

c., antemortem. Clot formed in the heart or its cavities before death.

c., blood. A coagulum formed of blood.

c., chicken fat. A yellow-colored blood clot appearing to contain no erythrocytes.

c., currant jelly. A clot of fibrin of reddish color and jellylike consistency.

c., distal. Clot formed in a vessel on distal side of a ligature.

c., external. Clot formed outside a blood vessel.

c., heart. A clot within the heart.

c., internal. Clot formed by coagulation of blood within a vessel.

c., laminated. Clot formed in a succession of layers filling an aneurysm.

c., muscle. Clot formed in muscle tissue.

c., passive. Clot formed in the sac of an aneurysm.

c., plastic. Clot formed from the intima of an artery at the point of ligation.

c., postmortem. Clot formed in the heart or blood vessel after death.

c., proximal. Clot formed on the proximal side of a ligature.

c., stratified. Clot consisting of layers of different colors.

clothes louse. A body louse. SYN: *Pediculus humanus corporis.* SEE: *pediculosis corporis.*

clothing [AS. *clath,* cloth]. Wearing apparel. Used both functionally and decoratively. From the medical standpoint, clothes serve to conserve heat or to protect the body.

Ex.: gloves, sunhelmets, and shoes. Air spaces in a fabric conserve heat. It is texture, not the material alone, that conserves heat. Woolen fabrics lose in warmth when the material is matted down and the air spaces are destroyed. Wool and silk absorb more moisture than other fabrics but silk loses it more readily. Cotton and linen come next but linen loses moisture more quickly than cotton. Knitted fabrics absorb and dry more readily than woven fabrics of the same material. Temperature inside an individual's hat may vary from 13° to 20° F. (7° to 11° C.)

warmer than the outside temperature. Body heat is increased when moisture from wet garments cannot escape.

clotrimazole (klō-trĭm′ă-zōl). USP. An antifungal drug that is also used in treating vulvovaginal candidiasis. Intravaginal use occasionally causes burning, redness, and itching in either the patient, her sex partner, or both. Trade names are Gyne-Lotrimin, Mycelex G, and Lotrimin.

clotting. The formation of a jellylike substance from blood shed at the site of an injury to a blood vessel. This action usually halts blood flow from the wound. SEE: *coagulation.*

clouding of consciousness. A state of mental confusion characterized by insufficiency of perception and impaired attention and resulting in loss of orientation of time and place, amnesia, and ill-adjusted reactions. Occurs in toxic, febrile, and other deliria as well as in cases where insufficient oxygen is being supplied to the brain. SEE: *consciousness.*

cloudy swelling. Microscopic appearance of tissues that have degenerated and become swollen.

cloven spine. Congenital defect of spinal canal walls caused by lack of union between laminae of the vertebrae. SYN: *spina bifida.*

clove oil [L. *clavus,* a nail or spike]. A volatile oil distilled from the dried flower buds of the clove tree, Eugenia caryophyllus.

ACTION AND USES: Antiseptic and aromatic. Also used to relieve pain in teeth. It is applied directly to the area.

clownism (klown′ĭzm). Grotesque actions and attitudes, esp. those in certain hysterical states or in epilepsy.

cloxacillin sodium (klŏks″ă-sĭl′ĭn). USP. A penicillinase-resistant antibiotic. Trade names are Cloxapen and Tegopen.

Cloxapen. Trade name for cloxacillin sodium.

clubbing (klŭb′ĭng). A condition that affects the fingers and toes in many diseases of varying etiologies. The most outstanding feature of clubbing is a lateral and longitudinal curvature of the nails accompanied by soft tissue enlargement; presenting a bulbous, shiny appearance. Most commonly found in diseases of the lung, infective endocarditis, steatorrhea, and occasionally as a familial condition not associated with pathology. SEE: illus.

clubfoot. Nontraumatic congenital foot deformity. SEE: *talipes.*

clubhand. Deformity of the hand resembling clubfoot. SYN: *talipomanus.*

clump (klŭmp) [AS. *clympre,* a lump]. 1. A mass of bacteria in solution. May be caused by an agglutination reaction. 2. To gather together.

clumping [AS. *clympre,* a lump]. Thick grouping of microorganisms in a culture when specific immune serum is added. SYN: *agglutination.*

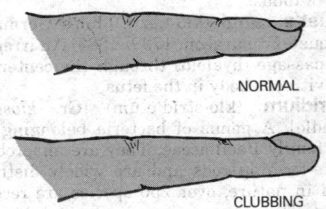

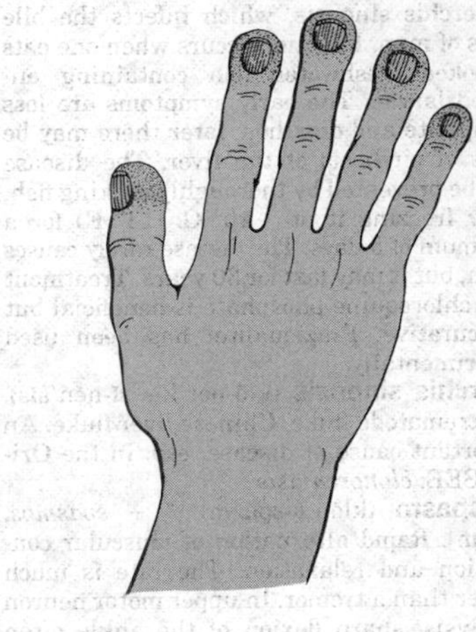

CLUBBING

NORMAL

CLUBBING

clunes (kloo′nēz) [L. pl. of *clunis,* buttock]. [NA] The buttocks; nates.

cluster headache. A headache similar to migraine, occurring as often as two or three times each night over a period of weeks and usually 2–3 hours after falling asleep. After this cluster of headaches, the patient may be free of symptoms for weeks or months. Even though the headache may recur in association with stress, overwork, or emotional trauma, the etiology is unknown. SYN: *headache, histamine.*

SYM: The headaches come on abruptly and are characterized by intense throbbing pain behind the nostril and one eye. The eye and nose water, the skin over the throbbing area becomes red, and the pupil of the eye may become constricted. An attack rarely lasts longer than two hours.

TREATMENT: Ergotamine tartrate is useful for both treatment and prophylaxis.

cluttering (klŭt′ĕr-ĭng). A speech defect characterized by omission of letters or syllables.

Clutton's joint. [Henry Hugh Clutton, Brit. surgeon, 1850–1909] Hydroarthrosis of the knee joint often associated with interstitial keratitis, seen in congenital syphilis.

clysis (klī'sĭs) [Gr. *klyzein,* to cleanse]. (pl. *clyses*) Injection of fluid into the body other than orally. This may be done by injecting the fluid into tissue spaces, the rectum, or the abdominal cavity. Technique is used to inject fluids parenterally in situations where venipuncture is not possible.

clysma (klĭs'mă) [Gr. *klysma,* a drenching]. An enema.

clyster (klĭs'tĕr) [Gr. *klyster,* syringe]. An enema; a clysma.

C.M. *chirurgiae magister,* Master in Surgery.

Cm. Chem. symb. for curium.

cm. *centimeter.*

c/m. *counts per minute.*

cm^2. *square centimeter.*

cm^3. *cubic centimeter.*

C.M.A. *Canadian Medical Association.*

CMI. *cell-mediated immunity.*

c/min. *counts per minute.*

c.mm. *cubic millimeter.*

CN. *cyanogen.*

C.N.A. *Canadian Nurses' Association.*

cnemial (nē'mē-ăl). Pert. to the leg, esp. the shin.

cnemis (nē'mĭs) [Gr. *knemis,* legging]. Shin, lower leg, tibia.

cnemitis (nē-mī'tĭs) [" + *itis,* inflammation]. Inflammation of the tibia.

cnemoscoliosis (nē"mō-skō"lē-ō'sĭs) [" + *skoliosis,* curvature]. Lateral bending of the leg.

C.N.M. *certified nurse-midwife.*

CNS. *central nervous system.*

CO. Chem. formula for carbon monoxide.

CO_2. Chem. formula for carbon dioxide.

CO_2 therapy. 1. Therapeutic application of low temperatures with solid carbon dioxide. SEE: *cryotherapy; hypothermia* (def. 2). 2. Inhalation of carbon dioxide to stimulate breathing.

Co. Chem. symb. for cobalt.

CoA. Coenzyme A, q.v.

coacervate (kō-ăs'ĕr-vāt) [L. *coacervatus,* heaped up]. The formation of an aggregate in a solution that is about to emulsify or in an emulsion that is demulsifying.

coadaptation (kō"ăd-ăp-tā'shŭn). Mutual adaptation of two independent organisms, organs, or persons.

coadunation (kō"ăd-ū-nā'shŭn) [L. *co-,* together, + *ad,* to, + *unus,* one]. Union or junction of dissimilar substances in one mass.

coagglutination (kō"ă-gloo"tĭn-ā'shŭn) [L. *coagulare,* to curdle]. Clumping by an antigen and the homologous antibody of the corpuscles of another organism.

coagula (kō-ăg'ū-lă) [L]. Pl. of coagulum.

coagulability (kō-ăg"ū-lă-bĭl'ĭ-tē). The condition of being capable of forming clots, esp. blood clots.

coagulable (kō-ăg'ū-lă-b'l). Capable of clotting; apt to clot.

coagulant (kō-ăg'ū-lănt) [L. *coagulans,* congealing]. 1. That which causes a fluid to coagulate. 2. Causing coagulation.

coagulase (kō-ăg'ū-lāz) [L. *coagulum,* blood clot]. Any enzyme, such as thrombin, that causes coagulation.

coagulate (kō-ăg'ū-lāt) [L. *coagulare,* to congeal]. To solidify or to change from a fluid state to a semisolid mass.

coagulated. Clotted or curdled.

coagulated proteins. Derived (insoluble) proteins, resulting from the action of alcohol on protein, or heat on protein solutions.

coagulation (kō-ăg"ū-lā'shŭn) [L. *coagulatio,* clotting]. The process of clotting. Coagulation depends upon the presence of several substances. Some of the most important are prothrombin, thrombin, thromboplastin (thrombokinase), calcium in ionic form, and fibrinogen. Prothrombin is converted to thrombin by the action of thromboplastin in the presence of calcium ions. Thrombin then acts on the soluble fibrinogen of the plasma, converting it to insoluble fibrin. The fibrin forms a meshwork of fibers in which the corpuscles of the blood become entangled, thus forming a clot. Shrinkage of the fibrin causes the exudation of plasma–minus–fibrinogen, which constitutes blood serum. When blood is shed through an injured vessel, thromboplastin is liberated from the injured tissues and from degenerating blood platelets. This initiates the clotting mechanism. In schematic and quite simplified form, the clotting process is as follows:

$$\text{prothrombin} + \text{thromboplastin} + \text{calcium ions} \rightarrow \text{thrombin}$$

$$\text{thrombin} + \text{fibrinogen} \rightarrow \text{fibrin.}$$

Clotting is retarded by cold; smooth surfaces; substances that combine with calcium such as EDTA (ethylenediamine tetraacetic acid); neutral salts such as magnesium or sodium sulfate; and by certain substances of biological origin such as hirudin, heparin, snake venoms, cysteine, and dicumarol. Clotting is hastened by warming; providing a rough surface; or by use of a chemical substance such as adrenalin, thrombin, or thromboplastin.

coagulation factors. A great number of terms have been applied to the various factors involved in the coagulation process. The generally accepted terms for the factors as well as their Roman numeral designation are provided here. In the past, Factor VI, called accelerin, was used but is no longer employed.

Factor I, fibrinogen. *Factor II,* prothrombin. *Factor III,* tissue factor. *Factor IV,* calcium ions. *Factor V,* an unstable protein substance with a molecular weight estimated to be 290,000. *Factor VII,* proconvertin or serum prothrombin conversion accelerator. *Factor VIII,* antihemophilic factor. *Factor IX,* plasma thromboplastin component or Christmas factor. *Factor X,* Stuart factor of Prower factor. *Factor XI,* plasma thromboplastin antecedent. *Factor XII,* Hageman or glass factor. *Factor XIII,* fibrin stabilizing factor.

coagulation time. The time required for a small amount of blood to coagulate. This can be determined by collecting blood in a small test tube and noting elapsed time from moment blood is shed to time it coagulates or by collecting blood in a small capillary tube and breaking off small pieces of the tube at 30-second intervals. Coagulation is indicated by the appearance of fine threads of fibrin between the broken ends of the tube. Normal time, using the capillary tube method, is 6 to 17 minutes.

coagulative (kō-ăg′ū-lā″tĭv). Causing coagulation.

coagulometer (kō-ăg″ū-lŏm′ĕt-ĕr) [L. *coagulare,* to congeal, + Gr. *metron,* measure]. Device for measuring the blood's coagulation time.

coagulopathy (kō-ăg″ū-lŏp′ă-thē) [″ + Gr. *pathos,* disease]. Defect in the blood clotting mechanism. SEE: *coagulation.*

c., consumption. Disseminated intravascular clotting.

coagulum (kō-ăg′ū-lŭm) [L.]. (pl. *coagula*) 1. A blood clot. 2. A curd.

coalesce (kō-ăl-ĕs′) [L. *coalescere*]. To fuse; run or grow together.

coalescence (kō-ă-lĕs′ĕns). Fusion or growing together of two or more parts of bodies.

coal tar. USP. A tar that is produced in the destructive distillation of bituminous coal. Used as an ingredient of ointments for treating eczema and other skin diseases.

coal worker's pneumoconiosis. Form of pneumoconiosis in which carbon and silica accumulate in the lungs due to breathing coal dust. SYN: *black lung.*

coapt (kō′ăpt) [L. *coaptare,* to fit together]. To bring together, as in suturing a laceration.

coaptation (kō″ăp-tā′shŭn) [L. *coaptare,* to fit together]. The adjustment of separate parts to each other, as the edges of fractures.

coarctate (kō-ărk′tāt) [L. *coarctare,* to tighten]. To press or pressed together.

coarctation (kō″ărk-tā′shŭn). 1. Compression of the walls of a vessel. 2. Shriveling. 3. A stricture.

c. of aorta. Localized malformation resulting in narrowing of the aorta.

coarctotomy (kō″ărk-tŏt′ō-mē) [″ + Gr. *tome,* incision]. Cutting or division of a stricture.

coat [L. *cotta,* a tunic]. A covering or a layer in the wall of a tubular structure, as the inner coat (tunica intima), middle coat (tunica media), and outer coat (tunica adventitia) of an artery.

Coats' disease. [George Coats, Brit. ophthalmologist, 1876–1915] Development of large white masses deep in the blood vessels of the retina. This term is now used to describe at least 6 separate retinal disorders.

cobalamin (kō-băl′ă-mĭn). Chemical that contains cobalt and is contained in all of the several B_{12} vitamins. SEE: *cyanocobalamin.*

cobalamin concentrate. USP. Medicine containing 500 mg. of cobalamin in each gram. Used in treating vitamin B_{12} deficiency.

cobalt (kō′bălt). SYMB: Co. At. wt. 59.933; at. no. 27; sp. gr. 8.9. A gray, hard, ductile metal. Cobalt deficiency causes anemia in ruminants but it has not been demonstrated in man. Cobalt is an essential element in vitamin B_{12}. Even though cobalt stimulates production of red blood cells, its use as a therapeutic agent is not advised. Overdose of cobalt in children may use death. In adults it may cause anorexia, nausea, vomiting, deafness, and thyroid hyperplasia with resultant compression of the trachea.

cobalt-57. Radioactive isotope of cobalt with a half-life of 272 days.

cobalt-60. Radioactive isotope of cobalt. Used as a source of beta and gamma rays in treating malignancies. It has a half-life of 5.27 years.

cobra (kō′bră). Any one of a group of poisonous snakes native to parts of Africa, Asia, and India. They all have the ability to expand their neck into a flattened hood.

cobra venom solution. Minute quantities of cobra venom in sterile physiological salt solution.

COBS. *cesarean-obtained barrier-sustained;* in reference to animals delivered sterilely by cesarean section and maintained in a germ-free environment.

coca (kō′kă). Dried leaves of the shrub Erythroxylon coca, from which several alkaloids including cocaine are obtained.

cocaine hydrochloride (kō-kān′, kō′kān). USP. The hydrochloride of an alkaloid obtained from the shrub Erythroxylon coca, native to Bolivia and Peru. The plant is cultivated extensively in South America. Cocaine is classed as a drug of abuse when used for nonmedical purposes. It does not produce physiological dependence but a psychological dependence may develop in those who use it over extended periods of time. "Street" names for cocaine include snow; coke; lady; jam; flake; nose candy; and heaven-leaf.

USE: a topical anesthetic applied to mucous membranes.

cocaine hydrochloride poisoning. SYM: Initially a stimulation of the nervous system with excitement, incoherent talking, restlessness or hallucinations followed by profound depression, nausea, dizziness, tingling of hands and feet, fever, alterations of pulse, increased respiration, dilated pupils; occasionally convulsions, collapse, and death from respiratory arrest.

TREATMENT: For acute cocaine poisoning, administer diazepam or a barbiturate intravenously. If cocaine was administered subcutaneously or intramuscularly, its absorption can be slowed by using a tourniquet or by applying ice packs to the injection site. Artificial respiration and oxygen may be needed. If patient survives for three hours prognosis is good.

CAUTION: Do not administer morphine or opium derivatives.

cocainism (kō'kān-ĭzm). The habitual use of cocaine. SEE: *cocaine hydrochloride poisoning.*

cocainization (kō"kān-ĭ-zā'shŭn). Inducing analgesia by use of cocaine.

cocainomania (kō"kān-ō-mā'nē-ă). Intense desire for cocaine and its effects.

cocarboxylase (kō"kăr-bŏk'sĭ-lās). Thiamine pyrophosphate, q.v.

cocarcinogen (kō-kăr'sĭ-nō-jĕn"). Something, either a chemical or environmental factor, that enhances the action of a carcinogen, the end result of which is the development of a malignancy.

coccal (kŏk'ăl). Concerning or caused by cocci.

cocci (kŏk'sī). Pl. of coccus.

Coccidia (kŏk-sĭd'ē-ă) [Gr. *kokkos,* berry]. An order of protozoa belonging to the class Sporozoa. All are intracellular parasites usually infecting epithelial cells of the intestine and associated glands. They are principally parasites of lower animals and cause great economic loss due to their toxic effect upon domestic and game animals. Only one species, Isospora hominis, infects humans. The geographic area of infestation is largely confined to the Far East.

coccidian (kŏk-sĭd'ē-ăn). 1. Concerning Coccidia. 2. Any member of the order Coccidia.

Coccidioides. A genus of fungi with but a single species, Coccidioides immitis, that is pathogenic for man. SEE: *coccidioidomycosis.*

coccidioidin (kŏk"sĭd-ē-oy'dĭn). USP. An antigenic substance prepared from Coccidioides immitis. Used as a skin test in diagnosing coccidioidomycosis.

coccidioidomycosis (kŏk-sĭd"ĭ-oyd-ō-mī-kō'sĭs) [" + *eidos,* form, + *mykes,* fungus, + *osis,* condition]. A coccidioidal granuloma. Exists in two forms: primary coccidioidomycosis, which is an acute self-limiting disease involving only the respiratory organs, and progressive coccidioidomycosis, a chronic, diffuse, granulomatous disease that may involve almost any part of the body. SYN: *desert rheumatism; granuloma, coccidioidal; valley fever.*

ETIOL: Caused by a pathogenic fungus, Coccidioides immitis.

PROG: For the primary type, favorable; for the progressive type, grave, often fatal.

TREATMENT: None is needed in the primary form of the disease. Amphotericin B is the only effective drug for the progressive granulomatous form.

coccidiosis (kŏk-sĭd-ē-ō'sĭs) [" + *osis,* condition]. Pathogenic condition resulting from infestation with coccidia. SEE: *Coccidia.*

coccobacilli (kŏk"ō-bă-sĭl'ī). Bacilli that are short and thick and somewhat ovoid in form. SEE: *bacteria* for illustration.

coccobacteria (kŏk"ō-băk-tē'rē-ă). 1. Spherical-shaped bacteria. 2. Any kind of cocci.

coccogenous (kŏk-ŏj'ĕn-ŭs) [Gr. *kokkos,* berry, + *gennan,* to produce]. Produced by cocci.

coccoid (kŏk'oyd) [" + *eidos,* appearance]. Resembling a micrococcus.

coccus (kŏk'ŭs) [Gr. *kokkos,* berry]. (pl. *cocci*) A type of bacteria that is spherical or ovoid in form. When cocci appear singly they are designated micrococci; in pairs, diplococci; in clusters like bunches of grapes, staphylococci; in chains, streptococci; in cubical packets of eight, sarcinae. Many are pathogenic, causing such diseases as septic sore throat, erysipelas, scarlet fever, rheumatic fever, pneumonia, gonorrhea, meningitis, and puerperal fever. SEE: *bacteria.*

coccyalgia, coccydynia (kŏk"sē-ăl'jē-ă, kŏk"sē-dĭn'ē-ă) [Gr. *kokkyx,* coccyx, + *algos,* pain; " + *odyne,* pain]. Pain in the coccyx.

coccygeal (kŏk-sĭj'ē-ăl). Pert. to or in the region of the coccyx.

coccygeal body. Small arteriovenous anastomosis at the level of the coccyx. It is associated with the median sacral artery.

coccygeal nerves. Lowest of spinal nerves; pair of nerves arising from the coccygeal section of the spinal cord and entering into the pudendal plexus.

coccygectomy (kŏk"sĭ-jĕk'tō-mē) [" + *ektome,* excision]. Excision of the coccyx.

coccygeus (kŏk-sĭj'ē-ŭs). Concerning the coccyx.

coccygodynia (kŏk-sĭ-gō-dĭn'ē-ă) [" + *odyne,* pain]. Pain in the coccygeal region. SYN: *coccyalgia; coccydynia.*

coccyx (kŏk'sĭks) [Gr. *kokkyx,* coccyx]. Small bone at the base of the spinal column in man, formed by four fused rudimentary vertebrae. Usually ankylosed and articulating with the sacrum above.

cochineal (kŏch′ĭn-ēl) [L. *coccinus,* scarlet]. Dried female insect of Coccus cacti, used as a dye in laboratory work.

cochlea (kŏk′lē-ă) [Gr. *kokhlos,* land snail]. A winding cone-shaped tube forming a portion of the inner ear. It contains the organ of Corti, the receptor for hearing.

The cochlea is coiled, resembling a snail shell, winding two and three-quarters turns about a central bony axis, the modiolus. Projecting outward from the modiolus is a thin bony plate, the spinal lamina, that partially divides the cochlear canal into an upper passageway, the scala vestibuli, and a lower one, the scala tympani. Lying between the two scalae is the cochlear duct, in the floor of which lies the spiral organ (of Corti). The base of the cochlea adjoins the vestibule. At the cupola or tip, the two scalae are joined at the helicotrema. SEE: illus.

cochlear (kŏk′lē-ăr). Pert. to the cochlea.

cochleare (kŏk″lē-ā′rē) [L., spoon]. Latin word used in writing prescriptions. Indicates a spoon or spoonful.

cochleariform (kŏk″lē-ăr′ĭ-form) [″ + L. *forma,* shape]. Spoon-shaped.

cochlear nerve. The division of the vestibulocochlear nerve (8th cranial nerve) that supplies the cochlea. SEE: *vestibulocochlear nerve.*

cochleitis (kŏk″lē-ī′tĭs) [Gr. *kokhlos,* land snail, + *itis,* inflammation]. Inflammation of the cochlea. SYN: *cochlitis.*

cochleo-orbicular reflex (kŏk″lē-ō-or-bĭk′ū-lăr). Contraction of orbicularis palpebrarum muscle resulting from sudden noise being produced near ear. SYN: *cochleopalpebral reflex.*

cochleopalpebral reflex (kŏk″lē-ō-păl′pĕ-brăl). Contraction of orbicularis palpebrarum muscle resulting from sudden noise being produced near ear. SYN: *cochleo-orbicular reflex.*

cochleovestibular (kŏk″lē-ō-vĕs-tĭb′ū-lăr) [″ + L. *vestibulum,* vestibule]. Pert. to the cochlea and vestibule of the ear.

cochlitis (kŏk-lī′tĭs) [″ + *itis,* inflammation]. Cochleitis; inflammation of the cochlea.

cockroach [Sp. *cucaracha*]. Blatta orientalis. A common insect belonging to the order Orthoptera that infests homes and eating places. They are swift-running omnivorous insects averaging about 2 cm. in length. Through their dual contact with filth and food, they may mechanically transmit bacteria, protozoan cysts, and helminth ova. Com-

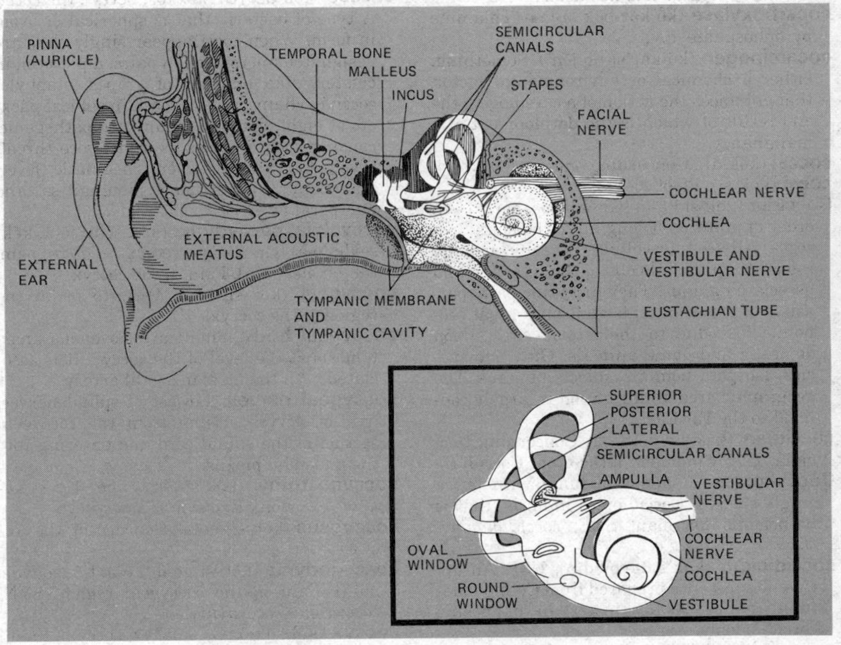

COCHLEA (IN RELATION TO THE INNER AND OUTER AUDITORY APPARATUS)

mon genera are Blatta, Blatella, and Periplaneta.

cocktail (kŏk'tāl). Any beverage containing several ingredients.

c., lytic. Term that originated in France; a mixture of analgesic and phenothiazine derivatives used in anesthesia as a premedication.

cock-up splint. A static splint designed to maintain the wrist in either wrist extension or dorsal flexion.

cock-up toe. Toe deformity with dorsiflexion of the metatarsophalangeal joint and flexion of the interphalangeal and distal interphalangeal joints.

cocoa butter. Theobroma oil. The fat obtained from the roasted seed of Theobroma cocoa.

USES: As a base in suppositories and as a topical skin lubricant.

coconsciousness (kō-kŏn'shŭs-nĕs). Conscious states of which we are unaware because they are not in the focus of attention but are at the fringe of consciousness.

cocontraction (kō"kŏn-trăk'shŭn). Muscular state in which antagonist muscles act in coordination for the purpose of holding a limb straight.

Coco-Quinine. Trade name for quinine sulfate.

coctolabile (kŏk"tō-lā'bĭl) [L. *coctus,* cooked, + *labilis,* perishable]. Something that is altered or destroyed when heated to the temperature of boiling water.

coctoprecipitin (kŏk"tō-prē-sĭp'ĭt-ĭn) [" + *praecipitare,* to cast down]. A precipitin produced by injecting a serum that has been boiled.

coctostabile (kŏk"tō-stā'bĭl) [" + *stabilis,* resisting]. Incapable of being altered or destroyed by heating to the temperature of boiling water.

code (kōd). 1. A collection or rules and regulations or specifications. 2. A set of symbols for communicating information, or for concealing the information from those not familiar with the true meaning of the symbols. 3. A form of coded message used in transmitting information in a hospital especially when the information is broadcast over a public address system, e.g., "code blue" or "code 9" could be used to indicate a particular type of emergency to an emergency care team.

c., genetic. The instructions present in living cells that specify and control the synthesis of polypeptides and proteins from amino acids. These instructions are contained in 64 nucleotide triplet sequences, called codons, 61 of which specify the 20 amino acids present in proteins, and 3 of which serve to halt the addition of amino acids to a polypeptide being synthesized. These 3 triplets are called termination codons. The genetic code is present in viruses, bacteria, plants, and animals.

c., triplet. In DNA, the nucleotide containing three bases, the information coded in which controls the sequence of amino acids in forming a protein.

codeine (kō'dēn) [Gr. *kodeia,* poppyhead]. An alkaloid obtained from opium, or synthetically from morphine as methylmorphine.

ACTION AND USES: Analgesic or hypnotic sedative with effects resembling morphine. Used commonly for its effectiveness in suppressing coughs.

c. phosphate. USP. Phosphate of the alkaloid codeine, used because of its free solubility in water. Much weaker than morphine.

c. sulfate. The sulfate of the alkaloid codeine. Used the same as codeine.

codeine poisoning. Poisoning due to an acute overdose of codeine.

SYM: The most serious effects are depression of the central nervous system including those centers that control respiration and heart rate. If the dose is sufficient, death may be the outcome.

TREATMENT: Similar to treatment for morphine poisoning, q.v.

INCOMPAT: Ferrous iodide, Lugol's solution.

cod liver oil. A fixed oil obtained from the fresh livers of the codfish. The official oil is standardized for its vitamin A and D content.

ACTION AND USES: Formerly widely used in cases of nutritional deficiency to supply vitamins A and D. Esp. used for prophylaxis of rickets in infants. Rarely used now due to the availability of more efficient and more palatable agents.

INCOMPAT: Light and air, both of which cause the oil to become rancid.

codon (kō'dŏn). A sequence of three bases in a strand of DNA that provides the genetic code for a specific amino acid.

Codroxomin. Trade name for hydroxocobalamin.

coefficient (kō"ĕ-fĭsh'ĕnt) [L. *co-,* together, + *efficere,* to produce]. 1. In chemistry, a numerical figure put before a chemical formula or compound to indicate the number of molecules of that substance taking part in the chemical reaction. 2. An expression of a ratio between two different quantities, or the effect produced by varying certain factors.

c. of absorption. Volume of gas absorbed by a unit volume of a liquid at 0° C. and a pressure of 760 mm. Hg.

c., isotonic. Number indicating the amount of salt to be added to distilled water to prevent the destruction of erythrocytes when the salt solution is added to the blood.

Coelenterata (sē-lĕn"tĕr-ā'tă) [Gr. *koilos,* hollow, + *enteron,* intestine]. A phylum of invertebrates that includes corals, hydras, jellyfish, and sea anemones. Contact with some species can result in sting injuries. SEE: *bites and stings*.

coelom (sē'lŏm) [Gr. *koiloma*, a cavity]. The cavity in an embryo between the split layers of lateral mesoderm. In mammals, it develops into the pleural, peritoneal, and pericardial cavities.

c., extraembryonic. In man, the cavity in the developing blastocyst that lies between the mesoderm of the chorion and the mesoderm covering the amniotic cavity and yolk sac.

coenocyte (sē'nō-sīt, sĕn'ō-sīt) [Gr. *koinos*, common, + *kytos*, cell]. A multinucleated mass of protoplasm; a mass of protoplasm in which cell membranes are lacking between the nuclei. SYN: *syncytium*.

coenzyme (kō-ĕn'zīm) [L. *co-*, together, + Gr. *en*, in, + *zyme*, leaven]. Enzyme activators. A diffusible, heat-stable substance of low molecular weight that, when combined with an inactive protein called apoenzyme, forms an active compound or a complete enzyme called holoenzyme.

Ex.: adenylic acid, riboflavin, and coenzymes I and II.

coenzyme A. An enzyme important to a variety of biological processes. It is a precursor for biosynthesis of fatty acids and sterols and is an acetylating agent. SYN: *acetyl CoA*.

coetaneous (kō"ē-tā'nē-ŭs) [" + *aetas*, age]. Having the same age or date.

coexcitation (kō-ĕk-sī-tā'shŭn) [" + *excitare*, to arouse]. Simultaneous excitation of two parts or bodies.

cofactor (kō'făk-tor). A factor acting in conjunction with another. In general, it is necessary that the cofactor be present for the other factor to be active.

coferment (kō-fĕr'mĕnt) [" + *fermentum*, leaven]. A coenzyme.

coffee-ground vomitus. Vomit similar to coffee grounds in pigment and consistency, occurring as a result of the presence of blood in the vomitus.

Cogan's syndrome (kō'găns). [David G. Cogan, U.S. ophthalmologist, b. 1908] Interstitial keratitis associated with tinnitus, vertigo, and usually deafness.

Cogentin. Trade name for benztropine mesylate.

cognition (kŏg-nĭsh'ŭn) [L. *cognoscere*, to know]. Awareness with perception, reasoning, intuition, and memory; the mental process by which knowledge is acquired.

cogwheel respiration. Repeated sudden brief interruptions of inspiration and expiration.

coherent (kō-hĕr'ĕnt) [L. *cohaerere*, to stick together]. 1. Sticking together, as parts of bodies or fluids. 2. Consistent; making a logical whole.

cohesion (kō-hē'zhŭn). The property of adhering.

cohesive (kō-hē'sĭv). Adhesive; sticky.

Cohnheim's areas (kōn'hīmz). [Julius Friedrich Cohnheim, Ger. pathologist, 1839–1884] Irregular groups of fibrils seen in a cross section of a striated muscle fiber.

Cohnheim's theory. Theory that tumors result from embryonal cells not utilized for fetal development.

coil (koyl). 1. A continuous material such as tubing, rope, or a spring arranged in a spiral, loop, or circle. 2. Popular term for a type of intrauterine contraceptive device.

coilonychia (koy"lō-nĭk'ē-ă) [Gr. *koilos*, hollow, + *onyx*, nail]. Koilonychia. Dystrophy of the fingernails in which they are thin and concave with raised edges. Sometimes associated with iron-deficiency anemia.

coin counting. A sliding movement of tips of thumb and index finger over each other in paralysis agitans.

coin test. Test for pneumothorax. A coin placed on the chest over the suspected area is struck with another coin. A metallic ringing sound is heard if a cavity containing air is underneath.

coital (kō'ĭ-tăl). Pert. to sexual intercourse.

coition (kō-ĭsh'ŭn) [L. *coire*, to come together]. Coitus; sexual intercourse.

coitophobia (kō"ĭ-tō-fō'bē-ă) [" + Gr. *phobos*, fear]. Morbid fear of sexual intercourse.

coitus (kō'ĭ-tŭs). Sexual intercourse between man and woman by insertion of the penis into the vagina. SYN: *coition; copulation; sexual intercourse*.

c. à la vache. Coitus from behind with the female in the knee-chest position.

c. interruptus. Coitus with withdrawal of the penis from the vagina before seminal emission occurs.

c. reservatus. Coitus with intentional suppression of ejaculation.

c. Saxonius. Coitus with manual pressure on the urethra at the underside of the penis or in the perineum to block the emission of semen at the time of ejaculation. This may be done by the female partner to prevent premature ejaculation. SYN: *squeeze technique*.

col (kŏl). The nonkeratinized, depressed gingival tissue that lies between adjacent teeth; it extends labiolingually between the interdental papillae below the interproximal contact of the teeth.

Cola (kō'lă) [W. African *kola*]. A genus of tropical trees that produce the kola nut. An extract of the kola nut is used in pharmaceutical preparations and as a main ingredient in some carbonated beverages.

Colace. Trade name for docusate sodium.
colalgia (kō-lăl'jē-ă) [Gr. *kolon*, colon, + *algos*, pain]. Pain in the colon.
colation (kō-lā'shŭn) [L. *colare*, to strain]. Straining, filtering.
colauxe (kŏl-ăwk'sē) [Gr. *kolon*, colon, + *auxe*, increase]. Distention of the colon.
colchicine (kŏl'chĭ-sĭn). USP. Medicine used in treating an acute attack of gout. Because the drug stimulates smooth muscles, diarrhea may be an undesired side effect.
COLD. *chronic obstructive lung disease.* SEE: *COPD.*
cold [AS. *ceald*, cold]. 1. A general term for coryza or inflammation of the respiratory mucous membranes known as the common cold. 2. Lacking heat or warmth; having a low temperature. Opposite of heat.

c., chest. Cold with inflammation of the bronchial mucous membranes. SYN: *bronchitis.*

c., common. Acute catarrhal inflammation of any or all parts of the respiratory tract from the nasal mucosa to the nasal sinuses, throat, larynx, trachea, and bronchi. It is highly contagious. Incubation period is from 12 to 72 hours. Lasting immunity does not develop. Even though the common cold does not cause death, its economic importance is vast because it is the greatest cause of absenteeism in industry and schools. SYN: *acute coryza.*

ETIOL: May be due to any one of a considerable number of viruses including rhinoviruses and coronaviruses.

SYM: Congestion of nasal mucosa with partial or complete occlusion of nostrils; continuous watery discharge with more or less continuous sniffling and blowing of nose. Also sneezing, lacrimation, irritated nasopharynx, chilliness, and malaise. Fever in adults is rare; if fever is present, influenza or other cause of the infection must be suspected. Symptoms are usually resolved within 2 to 10 days.

TREATMENT: Treatment is mainly for the relief of symptoms. Spraying with ephedrine hydrochloride, use of phenylephrine (Neosynephrine) spray or drops, or inhalation of benzedrine or menthol relieves nasal congestion. Analgesics are useful to relieve aching. Preparations containing codeine will usually relieve a cough but should not be used when the cough is productive. An expectorant containing either iodinated glycerol or potassium iodide–saturated solution may relieve cough. Antihistamines in persons with nasal allergy sometimes are effective in controlling the nasal secretions. Bedrest is recommended for febrile patients. There is no evidence that high doses of vitamin C are of benefit in treating the common cold; but some studies have shown a reduced period of disability in persons who took as much as 8 grams of vitamin C on the first day of disease. Analgesics such as aspirin may be of benefit in treating the malaise. There is no effective vaccine. Interferon and an interferon-inducer have been used experimentally. Antibiotics are of use only if there is secondary bacterial infection.

CONTAGIOUSNESS: The virus may be present in the nasal secretions for a week or longer after the onset of symptoms.

cold agglutinin. A red blood cell agglutinin that acts at only relatively low temperatures (ranging from 0° to 20° C.). This agglutinin occurs as part of the disease process in some cases of viral and mycoplasmal infections.
cold agglutinin disease. Term applied to a group of disorders characterized by hemolytic anemia, obstruction of the microcirculation, or both. Due to agglutination of red blood cells by the cold agglutinin. In some this is caused by a transient infectious disease, and in others, the cause is idiopathic. The latter occurs mostly in women over the age of 50.
cold cream. USP. A water-in-oil emulsion ointment base used topically on the skin.
cold pack. Wrapping of a patient or an area in towels dipped in cold water before application. Usually used to reduce fever, pain, swelling, or inflammation.
cold pressor test. Test that measures the response of the blood pressure to the immersion of one hand in ice water. An excessive increase in pressure indicates a latent hypertensive state. Also called *Hines and Brown test.*
cold sore. Herpes simplex of lips and face.
colectomy (kō-lĕk'tō-mē) [Gr. *kolon*, colon, + *ektome*, excision]. Excision of part or of all of the colon.
coleocystitis (kō"lē-ō-sĭs-tī'tĭs) [Gr. *koleos*, sheath, + *kystis*, bladder, + *itis*, inflammation]. Inflammation of the vagina and bladder. SYN: *colpocystitis.*
coleoptosis (kō"lē-ŏp-tō'sĭs) [" + *ptosis*, falling]. Prolapse of the wall of the vagina.
coleotomy (kō"lē-ŏt'ō-mē) [" + *tome*, incision]. Incision into the pericardium or into the vagina. SYN: *colpotomy.*
colestipol hydrochloride (kō-lĕs'tĭ-pōl). An ion-exchange resin similar in action to cholestyramine, q.v.
colibacillemia (kō"lĭ-băs-ĭl-lē'mē-ă) [Gr. *kolon*, colon, + L. *bacillus*, little rod, + Gr. *haima*, blood]. Colon bacillus in the blood.
colibacillosis (kō"lĭ-băs-ĭ-lō'sĭs) [" + " + Gr. *osis*, condition]. Infection with the colon bacillus.
colibacilluria (kō-lĭ-băs-ĭl-ū'rē-ă) [" + " + Gr. *ouron*, urine]. Presence of Escherichia coli in the urine.

colibacillus (kō″lĭ-bă-sĭl′ŭs) [″ + L. *bacillus,* little rod]. The colon bacillus, Escherichia coli.

colic (kŏl′ĭk) [Gr. *kolikos,* pert. to the colon]. 1. Spasm in any hollow or tubular soft organ accompanied by pain. 2. Pert. to colon. SEE: *cholecystalgia; tormina.*

c., biliary. Colic in bile ducts usually associated with a gallstone.

c., infantile. Colic occurring in infants, principally during the first few months.

c., intestinal. Colic in which pain may occur throughout the abdomen.

c., lead. Severe abdominal colic associated with lead poisoning. Lead line may be found on gums and basic stippling in red blood cells.

c., menstrual. Abdominal pain at the time of menstruation. SYN: *dysmenorrhea.*

c., renal. Pain in region of one of the kidneys and toward the thigh. Pain radiates from kidney region around and over abdomen into the groin. It accompanies the passage of calculus.

c., uterine. Severe abdominal pain arising in uterus, usually during the menstrual period.

colica (kŏl′ĭ-kă) [L.]. Colic.

colicin (kŏl′ĭ-sĭn). A bacteriocin produced by some strains of Escherichia coli that is lethal to other E. coli. Since its original discovery in 1925, approximately 20 colicins have been described, and some are produced by bacteria other than E. coli. All colicins are now called bacteriocins, q.v.

colicky (kŏl′ĭk-ē). Concerning colic or affected by it.

colicolitis (kō″lĭ-kō-lī′tĭs) [Gr. *kolon,* colon, + *kolon,* colon, + *itis,* inflammation]. Colitis due to Escherichia coli.

colicoplegia (kō″lĭ-kō-plē′jē-ă) [″ + *plege,* stroke]. Colic and paralysis due to lead poisoning.

colicystitis (kō″lĭ-sĭs-tī′tĭs) [″ + *kystis,* bladder, + *itis,* inflammation]. Inflammation of bladder resulting from infection with Escherichia coli.

colicystopyelitis (kō-lĭ-sĭs″tō-pī″ĕ-lī′tĭs) [″ + ″ + *pyelos,* pelvis, + *itis,* inflammation]. Inflammation of bladder and pelvis of kidney caused by Escherichia coli.

coliform (kō′lĭ-form) [″ + L. *forma,* form]. 1. Sieve form; cribriform. 2. Pert. to a group of bacteria that includes Aerobacter aerogenes and Escherichia coli. Their presence in water, esp. that of E. coli, is presumptive evidence of fecal contamination.

colilysin (kō-lĭl′ĭ-sĭn) [″ + *lysis,* dissolution]. A hemolysin formed by Escherichia coli.

colinephritis (kō″lĭ-nē-frī′tĭs) [″ + *nephros,* kidney, + *itis,* inflammation]. Nephritis caused by the colon bacillus, Escherichia coli.

coliplication (kō″lĭ-plĭ-kā′shŭn) [″ + L. *plica,* fold]. Operation for correcting a dilated colon.

colipuncture (kō′lĭ-pŭnk″chūr) [″ + L. *punctura,* a piercing]. Puncture of the colon to relieve distention. SYN: *colocentesis.*

colipyuria (kō″lĭ-pī-ū′rē-ă) [″ + *pyon,* pus, + *ouron,* urine]. Pus in urine due to Escherichia coli.

colisepsis [″ + *sepsis,* putrefaction]. Infection caused by the colon bacillus.

colistimethate sodium, sterile (kō-lĭs″tĭ-mĕth′āt). USP. A form of colistin, q.v., suitable for use intramuscularly or intravenously. Trade name is Coly-Mycin M Parenteral.

colistin sulfate (kō-lĭs′tĭn). USP. Polymyxin E. An antibiotic effective against some of the gram-negative bacteria, esp. Pseudomonas, that are resistant to other antibiotics. Trade name is Coly-Mycin S.

colitis (kō-lī′tĭs) [″ + *itis,* inflammation]. Inflammation of the colon.

c., mucous. Colon, irritable, q.v.

c., ulcerative. Ulceration of mucosa of colon.

SYM: Passage of offensive watery stools with mucus and pus. Abdominal pain, tenderness, or colic. Intermittent or irregular fever. Hemorrhage and perforation may occur.

colitoxemia (kō″lĭ-tŏk-sē′mē-ă) [Gr. *kolon,* colon, + *toxikon,* poison, + *haima,* blood]. Toxemia caused by the colon bacillus, Escherichia coli.

colitoxicosis (kō″lĭ-tŏk″sĭ-kō′sĭs) [″ + ″ + *osis,* condition]. Systemic poisoning caused by the colon bacillus, Escherichia coli.

colitoxin (kō″lĭ-tŏk′sĭn) [″ + *toxikon,* poison]. A toxin produced by the colon bacillus.

coliuria (kō″lĭ-ū′rē-ă) [″ + *ouron,* urine]. Presence of Escherichia coli in the urine. SYN: *colibacilluria.*

colla (kŏl′lă). Pl. of collum, q.v.

collagen (kŏl′ă-jĕn) [Gr. *kolla,* glue, + *gennan,* to produce]. A fibrous insoluble protein found in the connective tissue, including skin, bone, ligaments, and cartilage. Collagen represents about 30% of the total body protein.

collagenase (kŏl-lăj′ĕ-nās) [″ + ″ + *-ase,* enzyme]. An enzyme that induces changes in collagen to cause its degradation.

collagenation (kŏl-lăj″ĕ-nā′shŭn). Presence of collagen in cartilage.

collagen vascular diseases. A group of diseases of the blood vessels that share anatomical and pathological features. The etiology of these diseases is unknown; thus they are grouped together on the basis of common clinical signs and symptoms. Generalized inflammation of connective tissue and blood vessels is usually seen, and in some cases fibrinoid deposition in connective tissue fibers and blood vessels is present.

Diseases currently included in this category are: cutaneous and systemic lupus erythematosus; progressive systemic sclerosis; scleroderma; polymyositis and dermatomyositis; polymalgia rheumatica; and polyarteritis.

collagenic (kŏl″ă-jĕn′ĭk). Producing or containing collagen.

collagenoblast (kŏl-lăj′ĕ-nō-blăst) [″ + ″ + *blastos,* germ]. A fibroblast-derived cell that when mature produces collagen.

collagenolysis (kŏl″ă-jĕn-ŏl′ĭ-sĭs) [″ + ″ + *lysis,* dissolution]. The degradation or destruction of collagen.

collagenosis (kŏl-lăj″ĕ-nō′sĭs) [″ + ″ + *osis,* condition]. A collagen disease, q.v.

collapse [L. *collapsus,* fallen to pieces]. 1. An abnormal retraction of the walls of an organ. 2. A sudden exhaustion, prostration, or weakness due to decreased circulation of the blood.

SYM: Similar to those of hemorrhage. The peripheral arteries are depleted of blood, and the veins, esp. in the splanchnic region, are congested; apathy; extreme pallor; cold, clammy perspiration; thin, rapid pulse; fall of blood pressure; unconsciousness.

NURSING IMPLICATIONS: Lower the head of the bed or place patient in Trendelenburg position. Assess vital signs for symptoms of shock; administer I.V. fluids as ordered. Keep patient warm but not hot. Remain with the patient and provide reassurance that he or she is being cared for appropriately.

c. of lung. An airless state of all or part of a lung. Normal in fetus. Artificially induced by pneumothorax; thoracoplasty; or avulsion of phrenic nerve. May occur spontaneously due to rupture of a bleb on the pleural surface of the lung.

collapsing. Falling into extreme and sudden prostration resembling shock.

collapsing pulse. Pulse of aortic insufficiency or regurgitation. SYN: *Corrigan's pulse; water-hammer pulse.*

collapsotherapy (kō-lăp″sō-thĕr′ă-pē) [L. *collapsus,* fallen to pieces, + Gr. *therapeia,* treatment]. Treatment of pulmonary affections by unilateral pneumothorax and immobilization of affected lung.

collar (kŏl′ăr) [L. *collum,* neck]. 1. A band worn round the neck. 2. Structure or marking formed like a neckband.

c. of Venus. Mottled appearance of the skin of the neck occasionally seen in syphilis. SYN: *melanoleukoderma colli; venereal collar.*

collarbone. The clavicle, q.v.

collateral (kō-lăt′ĕr-ăl) [L. *con,* together, + *lateralis,* pert. to a side]. 1. Accompanying, side by side as in a small side branch of a blood vessel or nerve. 2. Subordinate or accessory.

collateral circulation. Circulation of small anastomosing vessels, esp. when a main artery is obstructed.

collateral eminence. An elevation in the floor of the lateral ventricle.

collateral fissure. A fissure on the median surface of the cerebral hemisphere.

collateral ganglia. Ganglia of the sympathetic division of the autonomic nervous system, located near origins of the celiac and mesenteric arteries. These include the celiac and mesenteric ganglia. SYN: *prevertebral ganglia.*

collaterals. Pl. of collateral.

collateral trigone. The angle between the diverging inferior and posterior horns of the lateral ventricle.

collecting tubules. Small ducts that receive urine from several renal tubules. Several tubules join together to provide a passage for the urine to larger straight collecting tubules (papillary ducts of Bellini) that open into the pelvis of the kidney.

Colles' fascia (kŏl′ēz). [Abraham Colles, Ir. surgeon, 1773–1843] Inner layer of superficial fascia of perineum.

Colles' fracture. The transverse fracture of the distal end of the radius (just above wrist) with displacement of hand backward and outward.

NURSING IMPLICATIONS: The nurse (in E.R.) assesses patient for pain, swelling, and any obvious deformity of the distal forearm, observes the extremity above the fracture site, and palpates the extremity to determine the presence of pulse and sensation distal to the fracture. Skin color and temperature distal to the fracture site are also evaluated. The extremity is usually immobilized with a temporary splint, and the patient sent for an X-ray of the affected extremity.

colliculectomy (kŏl-lĭk″ū-lĕk′tō-mē) [L. *colliculus,* mound, + Gr. *ektome,* excision]. Removal of the colliculus seminalis.

colliculitis (kŏl-lĭk″ū-lī′tĭs) [″ + Gr. *itis,* inflammation]. Inflammation of the colliculus seminalis.

colliculus (kŏl-lĭk′ū-lŭs) [L.]. (pl. *colliculi*) A little eminence.

c. bulbi; c. bulbi intermedius. Erectile tissue encircling the male urethra at the entrance to the bulb.

c. cervicalis. The crest on the posterior wall of the female urethra.

c. inferior. [NA] One of two elevations forming the lower portion of the corpora quadrigemina of the midbrain.

c. seminalis. [NA] An oval enlargement on the crista urethralis, an elevation in the floor of the prostatic portion of the urethra. On its sides are the openings of the ejaculatory ducts and numerous ducts of the prostate gland. SYN: *c. urethralis*.

c. superior. [NA] One of two elevations forming the upper portion of the corpora quadrigemina of the midbrain.

c. urethralis. C. seminalis.

collimation (kŏl″ĭ-mā′shŭn) [L. *collineare*, to align]. The process of making parallel. Thus, x-ray machines are fitted with a collimator to insure that the rays are parallel and not diffuse.

colliquation (kŏl″ĭ-kwā′shŭn) [L. *con*, together, + *liquare*, to melt]. 1. Abnormal discharge of a body fluid. 2. Softening of tissues to liquefaction. 3. A wasting.

colliquative (kō-lĭk′wă-tĭv). Pert. to a liquid and excessive discharge, as a colliquative diarrhea.

collodion (kō-lō′dē-ŏn) [Gr. *kollodes*, resembling glue]. USP. A preparation containing pyroxylin (gunpowder) dissolved thoroughly in ether and alcohol. It is a viscous liquid having an odor of ether and is highly flammable. When applied, it dries to form a strong, thin, transparent film and is useful in sealing the edge of a dressing, esp. on the scalp.

c., flexible. A preparation of collodion containing camphor and castor oil. It is more elastic than collodion in ether and alcohol.

c., salicylic acid. Flexible collodion with salicylic acid. Used as a keratolytic agent.

colloid (kŏl′oyd) [Gr. *kollodes*, glutinous]. 1. A type of solution. A gluelike substance such as a protein or starch whose particles (molecules or aggregates of molecules) when dispersed in a solvent to the greatest possible degree remain uniformly distributed and fail to form a true solution. 2. The size of a microscopic colloid; particles ranging from 10^{-9} to 10^{-11} meters (1 to 100 nanometers). 3. A homogeneous gelatinous substance found within the follicles of the thyroid gland and containing the thyroid secretion.

c., thyroid. Semifluid, jellylike substance filling the follicles of the thyroid gland. It contains the thyroid hormone.

colloidal (kŏl-loyd′ăl). Pert. to a colloid.

colloidal dispersion. A mixture containing colloid particles that fail to settle out and are held in suspension. They are common in animal and plant tissues, the protoplasm of cells being a colloidal mixture. Particles of colloidal dispersions are too large to pass through cell membranes and such dispersions usually appear cloudy.

colloid chemistry. The application of chemistry to systems and substances, and the problems of emulsions, mists, foams, and suspensions.

colloid cyst. A sac containing a jellylike liquid.

colloid degeneration. Mucoid degeneration seen in the protoplasm of epithelial cells.

colloidin (kŏl-loy′dĭn). A jellylike substance seen in colloid degeneration.

colloidoclasia (kŏl-oyd″ō-klā′sē-ă) [″ + *klasis*, fracture]. An alteration in the equilibrium of body colloids producing anaphylactic shock. Resulting from entrance into the bloodstream of unaltered colloids such as proteins.

colloidopexy (kŏl-oyd′ō-pĕk″sē) [″ + *pexis*, fixation]. Fixation of colloids during metabolism.

colloid suspension. A mixture holding particles in suspension, the forms of which change with the forces acting upon them, such as milk, fat, etc.

colloma (kō-lō′mă) [Gr. *kolla*, glue, + *oma*, tumor]. A colloid degeneration of a cancer.

collonema (kŏl″ō-nē′mă) [″ + *nema*, yarn]. A tumor, esp. a lipoma, that has undergone mucoid degeneration.

collopexia (kŏl″ō-pĕk′sē-ă) [L. *collum*, neck, + Gr. *pexis*, fixation]. Fixation of the cervix uteri.

collum (kŏl′lŭm) [L.]. (pl. *colla*) 1. The necklike part of an organ. 2. The neck.

collyrium (kō-lĭr′ē-ŭm) [Gr. *kollyrion*, eye salve]. An eyewash or lotion for the eye.

coloboma (kŏl″ō-bō′mă) [Gr. *koloboma*, a mutilation]. A lesion or defect of the eye, usually a fissure or cleft of the iris, ciliary body, or choroid. May be congenital, pathological, or surgical. Sometimes the eyelid is involved.

colocecostomy (kō″lō-sē-kŏs′tō-mē) [Gr. *kolon*, colon, + L. *caecum*, blindness, + Gr. *stoma*, mouth]. Surgical joining of the colon to the cecum of the small intestine.

colocentesis (kō″lō-sĕn-tē′sĭs) [″ + *kentesis*, puncture]. Surgical puncture of the colon to relieve distention.

colocholecystostomy (kō″lō-kō″lē-sĭs-tŏs′tō-mē) [″ + *chole*, bile, + *kystis*, bladder, + *stoma*, opening]. Surgical formation of a communication between colon and gallbladder. SYN: *cholecystocolostomy*.

coloclysis, coloclyster (kō-lŏk′lĭ-sĭs, kō″lō-klĭs′tĕr) [″ + *klysis*, washing]. A colonic enema.

colocolostomy (kō″lō-kō-lŏs′tō-mē) [″ + *kolon*, colon, + *stoma*, mouth]. Formation of a connection between two portions of the colon.

colocutaneous (kō″lō-kū-tā′nē-ŭs) [″ + L. *cutis*, skin]. 1. Concerning the colon and the skin. 2. A pathological, or surgically made connection between the colon and the skin. SEE: *colostomy*.

colocynth (kŏl′ō-sĭnth) [Gr. *kolokynthe*, fruit of Citrullus colocynthis]. Dried pulp of unripe colocynth fruit.

ACTION AND USES: A type of cathartic

COLON AND RECTUM

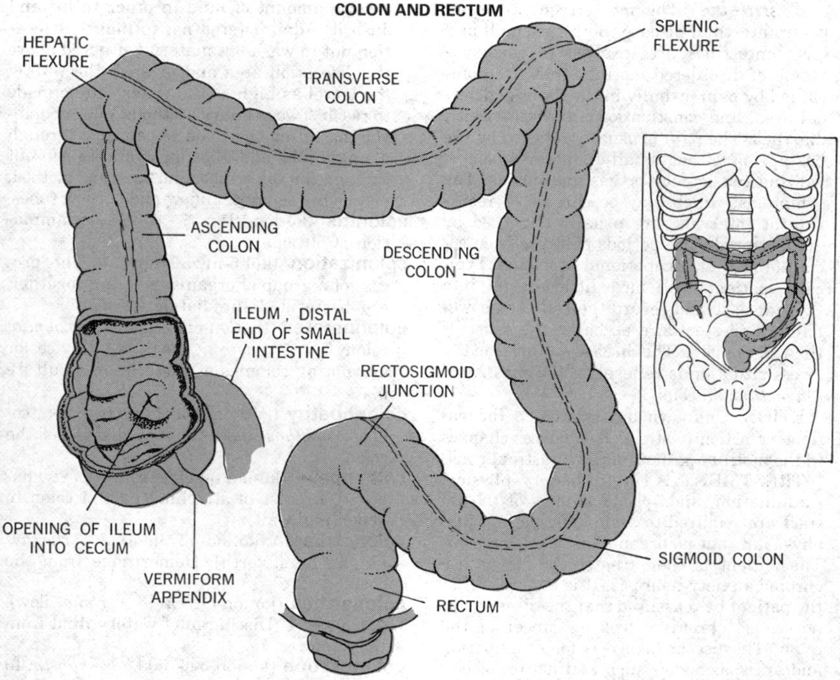

that has such drastic action that it should not be used.

coloenteritis (kō″lō-ĕn″tĕr-ī′tĭs) [Gr. *kolon,* colon, + *enteron,* intestine, + *itis,* inflammation]. Inflammation of mucous membrane of small and large intestines.

colofixation (kō″lō-fĭk-sā′shŭn). Suspension of the colon in the treatment of ptosis.

Cologel. Trade name for methylcellulose.

colon [L.; Gr. *kolon*]. [NA] The large intestine from the end of the ileum to the rectum, about 59 inches (1.5 meters) long. Divided into the ascending, transverse, descending, and the sigmoid or pelvic colon. Beginning at the cecum, the first part of the large intestine, the ascending colon, passes upward to the right colic or hepatic flexure, where it turns as the transverse colon passing ventral to the liver and stomach. On reaching the spleen, it turns downward (left colic or splenic flexure) and continues as the descending colon to the brim of the pelvis, where it is continuous with the sigmoid colon, and extends to the rectum. SEE: illus.

FUNCT: *Mechanical:* Mixing the intestinal contents. *Chemical:* No digestive enzymes are secreted in the colon, but an alkaline fluid aids in the completion of digestion begun in the small intestine. Those products of bacterial action that are absorbed into the bloodstream are carried by the portal circulation to the liver before they enter into the general circulation. There is also a great deal of water absorbed in the colon rather than in the small intestine. The fluids of the body are conserved in this way and, in spite of the large volumes of secretions added to the food during its progress through the alimentary canal, the contents of the colon are gradually dehydrated until they assume the consistency of normal feces or even become quite hard. SEE: *absorption; defecation.*

c., bacteria of. Escherichia coli is the most important but not the most common bacterium that normally inhabits the colon. It is outnumbered by the gram-negative anaerobic Bacteroides bacilli by at least 100 to 1. Whatever digestion takes place in the colon results from bacterial action. A large number of fermentative bacteria are found in the middle portion of the colon. Putrefying bacteria are found in the lower part of the colon. These may produce toxic products, such as indol, skatol; however, if absorbed, such products undergo detoxification in the liver.

c., irritable. The most frequently seen gastrointestinal disease. Both the small and large intestines are involved in this syndrome of disordered motility that is accompanied by pain, usually in the lower abdominal area, and constipation alternating with diarrhea. The pain is usually relieved by the passage of either small-diameter stools of varying consistency or gas and mucus. The symptoms, which may be chronic or recurring at intervals, are usually triggered by anxiety-producing periods of stress from social, family, or occupational problems. Typically, patients will have little insight into their disease and regard their altered bowel habits and stool size as being the cause of their discomfort. The disease subsides as the stress situation is relieved. SYN: *spastic colon; colitis, mucous.*

ETIOL: Unknown but related to the patient's reaction to stress that induces changes in the motility pattern of the intestinal tract.

TREATMENT: A careful history, physical examination, and special studies of the GI tract are required to assure the patient and physician that no organic disease is present. The patient is then treated for his or her chronic anxiety neurosis. It is essential that the patient be reassured that the disease will not cause chronic colitis or cancer of the colon. The use of laxatives for constipation and antispasmodics such as tincture of belladonna for abdominal cramps may be of assistance, but may prevent the patient from learning to recognize the importance of the gastrointestinal signs and symptoms.

NOTE: This disease will not cause malignancy of the GI tract, but it is important to periodically review the patient for such pathologic changes because presence of this syndrome does not mean the individual is free of the potential of developing malignancies in any body site.

c., toxic dilatation of. Marked dilatation of the colon, esp. the transverse colon, occurring as a complication of a primary disease of the colon. Clinically there are tachycardia, fever, and leukocytosis. There may or may not be abdominal tenderness, a palpable abdominal mass, mental confusion, cramping, and change in number of bowel movements each day. The condition may occur as a complication of ulcerative colitis, Crohn's disease, or amebic colitis.

colon, words pert. to: anus; appendix; cecum; cholecystocolostomy; colalgia; colic; colitis; "colo-" words; diverticulitis; intestines; jejunum; megacolon; peristalsis; rectum.

colonalgia (kō″lŏn-ăl′jē-ă) [Gr. *kolon,* colon, + *algos,* pain]. Pain in the colon.

colonic (kō-lŏn′ĭk). Pert. to the colon.

colonic irrigation. Injection into the colon of a large amount of fluid in order to fill and flush it. Administered not to induce defecation but to wash out material situated above the defecation area and to wash the wall of the bowel as high as the water can be made to reach. Two primary methods: one tube, involving filling the colon to capacity through a single tube and allowing liquid to run out through the same tube; and two-tube method, employing separate inflow and outflow tubes.

colonitis (kō-lŏn-ī′tĭs) [″ + *itis,* inflammation]. Colitis.

colonization (kŏl″ō-nī-zā′shŭn). 1. The process of a group of organisms living together, esp. bacteria. 2. Innidiation, q.v.

colonometer (kŏl″ŏn-ŏm′ĕ-tĕr) [L. *colonia,* colony, + Gr. *metron,* measure]. Device for estimating colonies of bacteria on a culture plate.

colonopathy (kō″lō-nŏp′ă-thē) [Gr. *kolon,* colon, + *pathos,* disease]. Any disease of the colon.

colonopexy (kō-lŏn′ō-pĕk″sē) [″ + *pexis,* fixation]. Process of attaching part of colon to abdominal wall.

colonorrhagia (kō″lŏn-ō-rā′jē-ă) [″ + *rhegnynai,* to burst forth]. Hemorrhage from the colon.

colonorrhea (kō″lŏn-ō-rē′ă) [″ + *rhoia,* flow]. 1. Colitis. 2. Discharge of watery fluid from the colon.

colonoscope (kō-lŏn′ō-skōp) [″ + *skopein,* to examine]. Instrument for examination of the colon. SEE: *sigmoidoscope.*

colonoscopy (kō″lŏn-ŏs′kō-pē). Examination of the upper portion of the rectum with an elongated speculum or a colonoscope.

colony (kŏl′ō-nē) [L. *colonia*]. A growth of microorganisms in a culture. Usually considered to have grown from a single organism.

colony counter. Apparatus for counting bacterial colonies in a culture plate.

colony-stimulating factor. A protein present in human serum that stimulates the growth of bone-marrow granulocytes in vitro.

colopexostomy (kō″lō-pĕks-ŏs′tō-mē) [Gr. *kolon,* colon, + *pexis,* fixation, + *stoma,* mouth]. Resection of the colon and fixation to abdominal wall to establish an artificial anus.

colopexotomy (kō″lō-pĕks-ŏt′ō-mē) [″ + ″ + *tome,* incision]. Incision and fixation of colon.

colopexy, colopexia (kō′lō-pĕk″sē, -pĕks′ē-ă). Fixation of the sigmoid or cecum to the abdominal wall by suture.

coloplication (kō″lō-plī-kā′shŭn) [″ + L. *plica,* fold]. Making a fold in the colon to reduce its lumen.

coloproctectomy (kō″lō-prŏk-tĕk′tō-mē) [″ + *proktos,* anus, + *ektome,* excision]. Surgical removal of the rectum and colon.

coloproctitis [″ + ″ + *itis,* inflammation]. Colonic and rectal inflammation. SYN: *colo-*

rectitis.

coloproctostomy (kō"lō-prŏk-tŏs'tō-mē) [" + " + *stoma,* opening]. Making a communication between a segment of colon and the rectum.

coloptosia (kō"lŏp-tō'sē-ă) [" + *ptosis,* dropping]. Prolapse of the colon, esp. of the transverse colon.

coloptosis (kō-lŏp-tō'sĭs). A downward displacement of the colon.

colopuncture (kō'lō-pŭnk-chūr) [" + L. *punctura,* piercing]. Surgical puncture of the colon to relieve distention. SYN: *colocentesis.*

color [L.]. A visible quality, distinct from form, and light and shade.

color, words pert. to: achromate; achromoderma; "achro-" words; alba; albedo; albicans; albinism; allochroism; allochromasia; anerythropsia; anisochromatic; aurantiasis; auric; carotene; carotenemia; "chrom-" words; isochromatic; melanin; nigrities; pigmentation; rubefacient; rubiginous; rubor; vermilion border; versicolor; xanthic.

color blindness. Absence of or defect in the perception of colors. The most frequently used class of color blindness is based on the perception of red, green, and blue (termed the 1st, 2nd, and 3rd color factors, respectively). If there is a defect in the perception of one of these colors, a color will be perceived as if it were composed only of the other two colors. Based on the color or colors for which there is defective perception, a person may suffer from red, green, or blue blindness. Color blindness in which all colors are perceived as gray is termed monochromasia.

color deficient. A preferred term for color blindness, inability to identify one or more of the primary colors. Children may become unduly alarmed by hearing the words color blindness; thus, color deficient, which is technically correct, is preferred.

colorectitis (kō"lō-rĕk-tī'tĭs) [Gr. *kolon,* colon, + L. *rectum,* straight, + Gr. *itis,* inflammation]. Inflammation of colon and rectum. SYN: *coloproctitis.*

colorectostomy (kō"lō-rĕk-tōs'tŏ-mē) [" + " + Gr. *stoma,* opening]. Formation of passage between colon and rectum.

colorectum (kŏl"ō-rĕk'tŭm). The colon and rectum.

color gustation. A sense of color aroused by stimulation of taste receptors.

color hearing. A sense of color caused by a sound.

colorimeter (kŭl"or-ĭm'ĕ-tĕr) [L. *color,* color, + Gr. *metron,* measure]. Instrument for measuring intensity of color in a substance or fluid, esp. one for determining the amount of hemoglobin in the blood.

color index. An outmoded method of expressing the amount of hemoglobin present in each red cell.

colorrhaphy (kō-lor'ă-fē) [Gr. *kolon,* colon, + *rhaphe,* suture]. Suture of the colon.

coloscopy (kō-lŏs'kō-pē). Visual examination of the colon by use of a sigmoidoscope.

colosigmoidostomy (kō"lō-sĭg"moy-dŏs'tō-mē) [" + *sigmoeides,* shaped like Gr. "S," + *stoma,* mouth]. Surgical joining of the descending colon to the pelvic colon.

colostomy (kō-lŏs'tō-mē) [Gr. *kolon,* colon, + *stoma,* mouth]. The opening of some portion of the colon onto the abdominal surface. Performed when it is impossible for the feces to pass through the colon and out the anus due to a pathological condition. Temporary colostomies are done to divert the fecal flow from an inflamed area or from an operative area. SEE: illus.; *ostomy* for colostomy care.

NURSING IMPLICATIONS: Cleanse the site with sterile solution as ordered. All fecal material should be removed and care taken to prevent excoriation of the skin around the stoma. After cleansing, the the skin should be dried and the colostomy drainage bag applied. The karaya adhesive ring (or other type of appliance) should fit close to the stoma to ensure a firm seal, and to prevent leakage. This procedure is repeated as often as needed and as necessary when the appliance is loosened. If reusable bags are used, the bag may be emptied without being removed.

Colostomy irrigations may be ordered. The procedure is similar to colon irrigations, except a soft rubber catheter is used to administer the irrigation. Hospital procedure should be followed.

Instruct the patient to avoid certain foods such as cabbage, cauliflower, broccoli, green beans, nuts, and food with seeds. Offer encouragement to the patient and family when teaching them proper care of the colostomy. This is a difficult adjustment for them. Encourage the patient and family to verbalize their fears and concerns, and offer support. Also put the patient in touch with the local chapter of the Ostomy Association.

c., double barrel. A temporary colostomy in which there are two openings into the colon; one distal and one proximal. Elimination occurs through the proximal stoma thus allowing the distal length of the colon to rest and heal as in colitis, q.v. When healing is complete, the two ends are rejoined and normal function resumes.

c., terminal. Colostomy wherein the proximal cut end of the colon is formed into a stoma and the distal colon is either resected or closed.

c., wet. 1. Colostomy in the right side of the colon or in the ileum. The drainage from

COLOSTOMY SITES

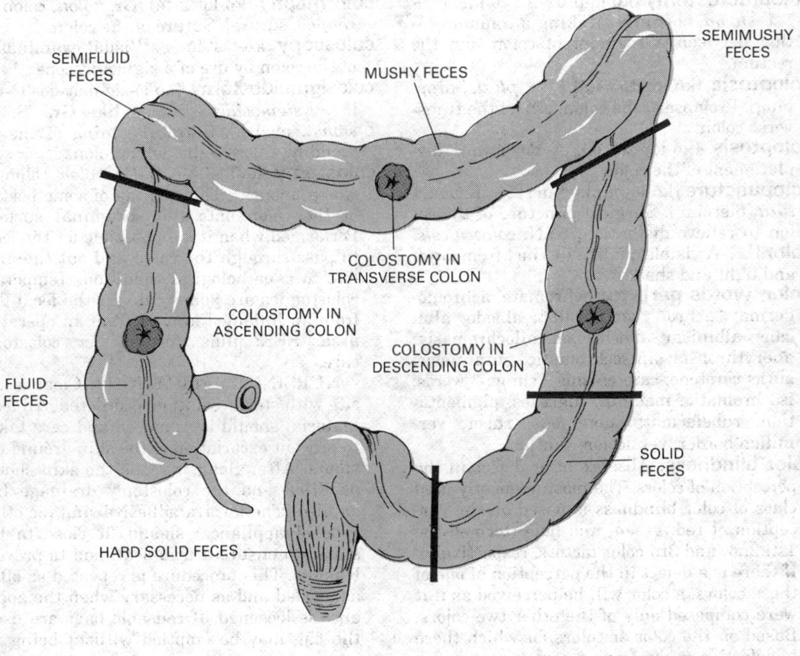

this type of colostomy is liquid. 2. Colostomy in the left colon distal to the point where the ureters have been anastomosed. Thus the urine and fecal material are excreted through the same stoma.

colostrorrhea (kō-lŏs″trō-rē′ă) [L. *colostrum*, colostrum, + Gr. *rhoia*, flow]. Abnormal secretion of colostrum.

colostrum [L.]. Breast fluid that may be secreted from the second trimester of pregnancy onward, but is most particularly noted in the first 2 to 3 days after birth and before the onset of true lactation. This thin yellowish fluid contains a great quantity of proteins and calories in addition to antibodies and lymphocytes.

colotomy (kō-lŏt′ō-mē) [Gr. *kolon*, colon, + *tome*, incision]. Incision of colon.

colovaginal (kō″lō-văj′ĭ-năl). Concerning the colon and vagina or communication between the two.

colovesical (kō″lō-vĕs′ĭ-kăl). Concerning the colon and the urinary bladder or communication between the two.

colpalgia (kŏl-păl′jē-ă) [Gr. *kolpos*, vagina, + *algos*, pain]. Vaginal pain.

colpatresia (kŏl-pă-trē′zē-ă) [″ + *a-*, not, + *tresis*, a perforation]. Occlusion or pathological closure of the vagina; vaginal atresia.

colpectasia (kŏl-pĕk-tā′sē-ă) [″ + *ektasis*, distention]. Dilatation of the vagina.

colpectomy (kŏl-pĕk′tō-mē) [″ + *ektome*, excision]. Surgical removal of the vagina.

colpeurynter (kŏl′pū-rĭn″tĕr) [″ + *eurynein*, to dilate]. A bag for dilatation of the vagina.

colpeurysis (kŏl-pū′rĭs-ĭs). Dilatation of the vagina by surgery.

colpitis (kŏl-pī′tĭs) [″ + *itis*, inflammation]. Inflammation of the vagina. SEE: *vaginitis*.

colpocele (kŏl′pō-sēl) [″ + *kele*, hernia]. Hernia into the vagina.

colpoceliotomy (kŏl″pō-sē″lē-ŏt′ō-mē) [″ + *koilia*, belly, + *tome*, incision]. Entering the abdomen surgically through the vagina.

colpocleisis (kŏl″pō-klī′sĭs) [″ + *kleisis*, a closure]. Operation of occluding the vagina.

colpocystitis (kŏl″pō-sĭs-tī′tĭs) [″ + *kystis*, bladder, + *itis*, inflammation]. Inflammation of vagina and bladder.

colpocystocele (kŏl″pō-sĭs′tō-sēl) [″ + *kystis*, bladder, + *kele*, hernia]. Prolapse of the bladder into the vagina.

colpocystoplasty (kŏl″pō-sĭs′tō-plăs″tē) [″ + ″ + *plassein*, to form]. Surgical treatment of vesicovaginal fistula.

colpocystosyrinx (kŏl″pō-sĭs-tō-sĭr′ĭnks) [″ + ″ + *syrinx*, fistula]. Fistula between the bladder and vagina.

colpocystotomy (kŏl″pō-sĭs-tŏt′ō-mē) [″ + ″ + *tome,* incision]. Cutting into the bladder through the vagina.

NURSING IMPLICATIONS: Measure and record intake and output; carefully assess patient for bladder distention. If the patient has a retention catheter, it should be irrigated as ordered to insure patency. Irrigations over the vulva may be ordered to help keep the patient clean and comfortable. The perineum should be dried thoroughly after the irrigations.

colpocytology (kŏl″pō-sī-tŏl′ō-jē) [″ + *kytos,* cell, + *logos,* study]. Study of the cells shed by the vaginal mucosa.

colpodynia (kŏl″pō-dĭn′ē-ă) [Gr. *kolpos,* vagina, + *odyne,* pain]. Pain in the vagina. SYN: *colpalgia.*

colpohyperplasia (kŏl″pō-hī-pĕr-plā′zē-ă) [″ + *hyper,* over, + *plasis,* a forming]. Excessive growth of mucous membrane of the vagina.

c. cystica. Infectious inflammation of the vaginal walls characterized by the production of small blebs.

colpomicroscope (kŏl″pō-mī′krō-skōp) [″ + *mikros,* small, + *skopein,* to view]. Optical device for very high power magnification of the vaginal mucosa and the cervix.

colpomyomectomy (kŏl″pō-mī″ō-mĕk′tō-mē) [″ + *mys,* muscle, + *oma,* tumor, + *ektome,* excision]. Removal of a fibroid tumor of the uterus through the vagina.

colpomyomotomy (kŏl″pō-mī″ō-mŏt′ō-mē) [″ + ″ + ″ + *tome,* incision]. Incision of the uterus through the vagina for removal of a tumor.

colpoperineoplasty (kŏl″pō-pĕr″ĭn-ē′ō-plăs″tē) [″ + *perinaion,* perineum, + *plassein,* to form]. Plastic surgery on vagina and perineum.

colpoperineorrhaphy (kŏl″pō-pĕr″ĭn-ē-or′ră-fē) [″ + ″ + *rhaphe,* suture]. Operation for mending perineal tears in the vagina.

colpopexy (kŏl′pō-pĕk″sē) [″ + *pexis,* fixation]. Suture of a relaxed and prolapsed vagina to the abdominal wall.

colpoplasty (kŏl′pō-plăs″tē) [″ + *plassein,* to form]. Plastic surgery of the vagina.

colpoptosis (kŏl″pŏp-tō′sĭs) [″ + *ptosis,* a falling]. Prolapse of the vagina.

colporrhagia (kŏl″pō-rā′jē-ă) [″ + *rhegnynai,* to burst forth]. Excessive vaginal discharge; vaginal hemorrhage.

colporrhaphy (kŏl-por′ă-fē) [″ + *rhaphe,* suture]. Suture of the vagina.

colporrhexis (kŏl″pō-rĕk′sĭs) [″ + *rhexis,* rupture]. Laceration or rupture of the vaginal walls.

colposcope (kŏl′pō-skōp) [″ + *skopein,* to examine]. An instrument used for examination of the tissues of the vagina and cervix by means of a magnifying lens.

colposcopy (kŏl-pŏs′kō-pē). The examination of vaginal and cervical tissues by using a colposcope. Colposcopy is used in selecting sites of abnormal epithelium for biopsy in patients with abnormal Pap smears. It is helpful in defining tumor extension and for evaluating benign lesions. It has also proved to be valuable in postpubertal vaginal examination of diethylstilbestrol-exposed offspring.

colpospasm, colpospasmus (kŏl′pō-spăzm, kŏl″pō-spăz′mŭs) [Gr. *kolpos,* vagina, + *spasmos,* spasm]. Spasm of the vagina.

colpostat (kŏl′pō-stăt) [″ + L. *stare,* to stand]. Device for holding an instrument, such as a radium applicator, in place in the vagina.

colpostenosis (kŏl″pō-stĕn-ō′sĭs) [″ + *stenosis,* narrowing]. Stenosis or narrowing of the vagina.

colpostenotomy (kŏl″pō-stĕn-ŏt′ō-mē) [″ + ″ + *tome,* incision]. A cutting operation for dilating the lumen in stricture of the vagina.

colpotherm (kŏl′pō-thĕrm) [″ + *therme,* heat]. Electrical heating device introduced into the vagina.

colpotomy (kŏl-pŏt′ō-mē) [″ + *tome,* incision]. Incision into the wall of the vagina.

colpoureterocystotomy (kŏl″pō-ū-rē″tĕr-ō-sĭs-tŏt′ō-mē) [″ + *oureter,* ureter, + *kystis,* bladder, + *tome,* incision]. Exposure of the ureteral orifices by incision through the walls of the vagina and bladder.

colpoureterotomy (kŏl″pō-ū-rē″tĕr-ŏt′ō-mē) [″ + ″ + *tome,* incision]. Incision of the ureter through the vagina.

colpoxerosis (kŏl″pō-zē-rō′sĭs) [″ + *xerosis,* dryness]. Abnormal dryness of the vaginal mucosa.

columbium. Former name for niobium, q.v.

columella (kŏl″ū-mĕl′lă) [L., small column]. 1. A little column. 2. In bacteriology, portion of the sporangiophore upon which are borne the spores.

c. cochleae. The modiolus of the cochlea.

c. nasi. The anterior part of the septum of the nose; a turbinate bone.

column (kŏl′ŭm) [L. *columna,* pillar]. A cylindrical supporting structure.

c., anal. Vertical folds in the anal canal.

c., anterior. The anterior portion of the gray matter on each side of the spinal cord. With reference to white matter, the posterior funiculus.

c., Clarke's. A group of large cells in the medial portion of the base of the posterior gray column of the spinal cord.

c., fornix. A column of the fornix, two arched bands of fibers that form the anterior portion of the fornix. Fibers lead to mammillary body.

c., gray. Gray matter in the anterior and posterior horns of the spinal cord.

c., lateral. A column in lateral portion of gray matter of spinal cord. Contains cell bodies of preganglionic neurons of sympathetic nervous system. The lateral funiculus or the white matter between roots of spinal nerves.

c. of Burdach. The fasciculus cuneatus, q.v.

c. of Goll. The fasciculus gracilis, q.v.

c. of Gowers. Tract of ascending fibers anterior to the direct cerebellar column and on the lateral surface of the spinal cord.

c. of Morgagni. One of several vertical ridges in mucous membrane at junction of anus and rectum.

c., posterior. The posterior horn of the gray matter of the spinal cord. It consists of an expanded portion or caput connected by a narrower cervix to the main portion of gray matter. The posterior funiculus of the white matter.

c., rectal. C., anal, q.v.

c., renal. A column of Bertin, cortical material of the kidney that extends centrally, separating the pyramids.

c., spinal. The line of vertebrae from the head to the pelvis, making up the bony flexible case for the spinal cord. SYN: *vertebral column.*

c., vertebral. The portion of the axial skeleton consisting of vertebrae (7 cervical, 12 thoracic, 5 lumbar, a sacrum and coccyx) joined together by intervertebral disks. It forms the main supporting axis of the body, encloses and protects the spinal cord, and serves for attachment of the appendicular skeleton and muscles for moving the various bodily parts. SYN: *spinal column.*

c., vesicular. Line of ganglion cells on inner side of posterior column.

columna (kō-lŭm′nă) [L.]. (pl. *columnae*) [NA] A column or pillar.

c. carnea. A muscular projection within the cardiac ventricles. SYN: *trabecula carnea cordis.*

c. nasi. Nasal septum.

c. rugarum vaginae. Folds of mucous membrane of the vagina that are arranged in a columnar fashion. SYN: *c. vaginalis.*

c. vaginalis. C. rugarum vaginae, q.v.

columnar layer. Retinal rod-and-cone layer.

columning (kŏl′ŭm-ĭng). Introduction of tampons in vagina to support the prolapsed uterus.

Coly-Mycin M. Trade name for colistin sodium.

Coly-Mycin S Oral. Trade name for colistin sulfate.

coma (kō′mă) [L.; Gr. *koma,* a deep sleep]. An abnormal deep stupor occurring in illness, as a result of it, or due to an injury. The patient cannot be aroused by external stimuli. More than 50% of cases are a result of trauma to the head or circulatory accidents in the brain caused by hypertension, arteriosclerosis, thrombosis, tumor, abscess formation, or insufficient flow of blood to the brain. Other frequent causes of coma are acute infections of the brain or meninges; acute infections and bacterial intoxications as in fevers, botulism, and other infectious diseases; effects of drugs (alcohol, atropine, barbiturates, chloral, hyoscine, paraldehyde, and phenols); trauma as in accidents, hemorrhage, and electrocution; gases or fumes such as carbon dioxide or carbon monoxide; extreme temperature; neurosis such as in malingering. SEE: *Glasgow coma scale.*

F.A.: Should be strictly limited. Patient should not be moved other than to position the head in order to help the airway clear. Movement without competent supervision may be dangerous. The shirt collar should be loosened.

TREATMENT: In certain types of poisoning, gastric lavage is indicated. Insulin injection for diabetic coma may be given unless the coma is caused by too much insulin.

CAUTION: If there is a question of whether the coma is due to an overdose of insulin or diabetic coma, it is safe to give glucose intravenously; administration of insulin might be disastrous.

Urine should be examined for albumin, sugar, narcotics and acetone. In uremic coma, stimulate diuresis. In coma due to hysteria, the patient requires careful nursing care and observation but no specific therapy is indicated.

NURSING IMPLICATIONS: Nursing care for patients in a coma, regardless of the cause, includes: maintaining a patent airway; monitoring vital signs; performing a neurologic assessment every four hours; assessing the patient's level of consciousness; and maintaining fluid and electrolyte balance. Also maintain the patient's skin integrity, provide passive range of motion exercises, protect the patient's eyes from corneal irritation, and prevent the complications of immobilization. It is important to keep in mind that the level of coma may permit the patient to be aware of the surroundings and to hear all that is said. SEE: *shock.*

c., alcoholic. Coma due to alcohol.

c., apoplectic. Coma due to intracranial vascular accident; so-called shock or stroke. One side of body and one or more of the extremities may be paralyzed. No fever at first but one pupil may be larger than the other. Coma usually indicates increased intracranial pressure. SEE: *apoplexy; stroke.*

Diagnosis of Diabetic and Hypoglycemic Coma

	Diabetic Coma	Hypoglycemic Coma
Onset	Gradual	Often sudden
History	Often of acute infection in a diabetic or insufficient insulin intake. Previous history of diabetes may be absent.	Recent insulin injection, inadequate meal, or excessive exercise after insulin
Skin	Flushed, dry	Pale, sweating
Tongue	Dry or furred	Moist
Breath	Smell of acetone	Acetone odor rare
Thirst	Intense	Absent
Respiration	Deep (air hunger) (Kussmaul)	Shallow
Vomiting	Common	Rare
Pulse	Rapid, feeble	Full and bounding
Eyeball Tension	Low	Normal
Urine	Sugar and acetone present	No sugar or acetone, unless bladder has not been emptied for some hours
Blood Sugar	Raised (over 200 mg./dl.)	Subnormal (20–50 mg./dl.)
Blood Pressure	Low	Normal
Abdominal Pain	Common and often acute	Absent

c., diabetic. Coma occurring in diabetes, due to lack of insulin, which causes metabolic changes with excess production of acetone bodies, q.v., and metabolic acidosis. Paralysis not present. SEE: table.

SYM: Sweet breath. Hyperglycemia is present, and eyeballs may be soft due to dehydration.

TREATMENT: Correct use of insulin has prevented diabetic coma to a large extent but an overdose may induce hypoglycemic coma. Thus, do not give insulin until the diagnosis of diabetic coma is made. Examine urine hourly for dextrose; if urine is sugar-free, more dextrose must be given.

c., hepatic. Coma due to liver failure. SEE: *hepatic coma.*

c., hypoglycemic. Unconsciousness due to a decreased level of blood glucose. This may be due to a disease of the pancreas, an overdose of insulin, or starvation.

c., irreversible. Coma from which the patient cannot recover. SYN: *brain death.*

c., Kussmaul's. The coma, acidosis, and deep breathing seen in diabetic coma.

c., uremic. The result of disturbed kidney metabolism, causing autointoxication through the retention of metabolic end products that would normally be excreted by the kidneys. Interference with the acid-base balance develops.

SYM: In general, respiration stertorous, face livid; skin dry and may be covered with "uremic frost," which is a collection of urea excreted in the sweat; hard and rapid pulse; blood pressure elevated; sphincters relaxed according to cause; urinous odor on breath; urine scanty and containing many casts and albumin. Complete retention may occur.

c., vigil. Coma in which the patient's eyes are open wide, and they are in a vacant stare; face is expressionless; but patient is unconscious. May occur in typhus or typhoid fever.

coma scale. SEE: *Glasgow coma scale.*

comatose (kō′mă-tōs). In a condition of coma.

combustion (kŏm-bŭst′yŭn). 1. Burning. 2. In metabolism, the oxidation of food with production of heat.

comedo (kŏm′ē-dō) [L. *comedere,* to eat up]. (pl. *comedones, comedos*) Blackhead. Discolored dried sebum plugging an excretory duct of the skin.

ETIOL: Either increased activity of sebaceous glands or material secreted is unable to escape through a too-narrow opening.

SYM: Commonly affects the face, back, and ears; chronic, frequently associated with seborrheic dermatitis or acne; usually during adolescence.

PROG: Obstinate and persistent, but amenable to treatment.

TREATMENT: Aside from careful and gentle removal of plugs, treatment is essentially that of acne, q.v.

comes (kō′mēz) [L., companion]. (pl. *comites*) A blood vessel that accompanies a nerve or another blood vessel.

Comfolax. Trade name for docusate sodium.

comma bacillus. Vibrio comma, the causative organism of cholera. Named for its shape.

comma tract of Schultz. The fasciculus

interfascicularis, a tract of descending fibers located between the fasciculus cuneatus and fasciculus gracilis in the posterior funiculus of the spinal cord.

commensal (kŏ-mĕn'săl) [L. *com-*, together, + *mensa*, table]. One of two or more organisms that live in an intimate, nonparasitic relationship. SYN: *symbion; symbiont*. SEE: *symbiosis*.

commensalism (kŏ-mĕn'săl-ĭzm"). The symbiotic relationship of two organisms of different species in which neither is harmful to the other and one gains some benefit such as protection or nourishment.

Ex.: nonpathogenic bacteria in human intestine.

comminute (kŏm'ĭ-nūt) [L. *com-*, together, + *minuere*, to crumble]. To break into pieces.

comminuted fracture. A fracture wherein the bone is splintered or crushed.

comminution (kŏm"ĭ-nū'shŭn) [L. *comminutio*, crumbling]. Reducing a solid body to varying sizes by grating, pulverizing, slicing, granulating, and by other processes. SEE: *attenuation*.

commissura (kŏm"mĭ-sū'ră) [L.]. (pl. *commissurae*) A commissure.

commissural (kŏm-mĭs'ū-răl). Pert. to a commissure.

commissure (kŏm'ĭ-shūr) [L. *commissura*, a joining together]. 1. A transverse band of nerve fibers passing over the midline in the central nervous system. 2. The coming together of two structures, as the lips, eyelids, or nymphae.

c., anterior cerebral. A band of white fibers that passes through lamina terminalis connecting the two cerebral hemispheres.

c., anterior gray. A commissure in spinal cord lying anterior to central canal.

c., anterior white. A commissure in spinal cord lying anterior to central canal and anterior to the anterior gray commissure.

c. of fornix. A band of fibers connecting the two crura.

c., posterior, of brain. A commissure just above the midbrain containing fibers that connect the superior colliculi.

c., posterior, of spinal cord. A gray commissure connecting two halves of spinal cord. It lies posterior to the central canal.

commissurorrhaphy (kŏm"ĭ-shūr-or'ă-fē) [" + Gr. *rhaphe*, suture]. Surgical procedure of joining the parts of a commissure together in order to decrease the size of the opening.

commissurotomy (kŏm"ĭ-shūr-ŏt'ō-mē) [" + Gr. *tome*, incision]. Surgical incision of any commissure. May be used in treating mitral stenosis in order to increase the size of the mitral orifice. This is done by incising the adhesions that cause the leaves of the valve to stick together. Commissurotomy may also be used in treating certain psychiatric conditions by incising the anterior commissure of the brain.

commitment (kŏ-mĭt'mĕnt). The legal procedure for hospitalization of a patient who may not be competent to make that decision or who does not choose to be hospitalized. Usually done in connection with patients with mental illness, but may be used to hospitalize patients with certain contagious diseases. SEE: *certification*.

common bile duct. Duct carrying bile to the duodenum and receiving it from the cystic duct of the gallbladder and the hepatic ducts. SEE: *biliary tract* for illus.

commotio (kŏ-mō'shē-ō) [L. *commotio*, a disturbance]. A concussion, esp. cerebral.

c. retinae. Retinal concussion, usually a result of trauma to the eyeball.

c. spinalis. Concussion of the spine.

commune (kŏm'yoon). A group of people with common goals and beliefs who live in the same area, usually in one or more small homes or residences. Some communes are committed to the concept of holistic medicine.

communicable disease. 1. A disease that may be transmitted directly or indirectly from one individual to another. 2. One due to an infectious agent or toxic products produced by it. SEE: table.

communicable disease, words pert. to: agent; carrier; contagion; endemic; epidemic; host, intermediate; immunity; incidence; incubation; infection; isolation; microbe; microorganism; prevalence; quarantine; transmissible; vector.

communicans (kŏ-mū'nĕ-kănz) [L. *communicare*, to connect with]. One of a number of communicating nerves or arteries.

communis (kŏ-mū'nĭs) [L.]. 1. Common, nonspecific. 2. In anatomy, something such as a vessel that supplies several branches.

community medicine. Health care for all members of a community with particular emphasis on preventive medicine and public health.

Comolli's sign (kō-mŏl'lēz). [Antonio Comolli, It. pathologist, b. 1879] A triangular swelling corresponding to the outline of the fractured scapula.

compact [L. *compactus*, joined together]. Closely and tightly packed together. Dense; solid.

compact bone. Hard or dense bone, which forms the superficial layer of all bones, in contrast to spongy or cancellous bone found chiefly in the ends of long bones.

compaction (kŏm-păk'shŭn). Simultaneous engagement of the presenting parts of twins in the pelvis so that labor can not progress.

comparative anatomy. Human anatomy

Method of Transmission of Some Common Communicable Diseases

Disease	How Agent Leaves the Bodies of the Sick	How Organisms May Be Transmitted	Method of Entry into the Body
Cholera	Excreta from intestinal tract	As in typhoid fever	As in typhoid fever
Diphtheria	Sputum and discharges from nose and throat Skin lesions	Direct contact Droplet infection from patient coughing Hands of nurse Articles used by and about patient	Through mouth to throat or nose to throat
Gonococcal disease	Lesions Discharges from infected mucous membranes	Direct contact as in sexual intercourse Towels, bathtubs, toilets, etc. Hands of infected persons soiled with their own discharges Hands of attendant	Directly onto mucous membrane Through breaks in membrane
Hepatitis, Infectious Viral or Serum	Excreta from intestinal tract or from blood or serum	Direct contact with feces of patient Direct contact with equipment contaminated by blood from the patient	Oral route or by inoculation when viral contaminated equipment such as needles and syringes is used
Hookworm	Feces	Direct contact with soil polluted with feces Eggs in feces hatch in sandy soil Feces may also contaminate food	Larvae enter through breaks in skin, especially skin of feet, and after devious passage through the body settle in the intestine
Influenza	As in pneumonia	As in pneumonia	As in pneumonia
Leprosy	Uncertain, may be from lesions Bacilli found in nodules that may break down, forming lesions	Uncertain, probably via feces	Uncertain, probably via mouth
Measles (Rubella)	As in streptococcal sore throat	As in streptococcal sore throat	As in streptococcal sore throat
Meningitis, meningococcal	Discharges from nose and throat	Direct contact Hands of nurse or attendant Articles used by and about patient Flies	Mouth and nose
Mumps	Discharges from infected glands and mouth	Direct contact with persons affected	Mouth and nose

Method of Transmission of Some Common Communicable Diseases (*cont.*)

Disease	How Agent Leaves the Bodies of the Sick	How Organisms May Be Transmitted	Method of Entry into the Body
Ophthalmia neonatorum (gonococcal infection of eyes of newborn)	Purulent discharges from the eye	Direct contact with infected areas as vagina of infected mother during birth Other infected babies Hands of doctor or nurse Linens, etc.	Directly on the conjunctiva
Pneumonia	Sputum and discharges from nose and throat	Direct contact Hands of nurse Articles used by and about patient	Through mouth and nose to lungs
Poliomyelitis	Discharges from nose and throat, and via feces	Direct contact Hands of nurse or attendant Rarely in milk	Through mouth and nose
Rubeola	Secretions from nose and throat	Droplet spread from nose or throat by direct contact with nasal or throat secretions. Airborne spread is possible.	Through mouth and nose
Smallpox	Discharges from nose and throat Skin lesions	Direct contact Hands of nurse Articles used by and about patient	Thought to be through mucous membrane of respiratory tract
Streptococcal sore throat	Discharges from nose and throat Skin lesions	Direct contact Hands of nurse Articles used by and about patient	Through mouth and nose
Syphilis	Infected tissues Lesions Blood Transfer through placenta to fetus	Direct contact Kissing or sexual intercourse Contaminated needles and syringes	Directly into blood and tissues through breaks in skin or membrane Contaminated needles and syringes
Tetanus	Excreta from infected herbivorous animals and man	Soil, especially that with manure or feces in it Dust, etc. Articles used about stables	Directly into bloodstream through wounds (Organism is an anaerobe and prefers deep, incised wound.)
Trachoma	Discharges from infected eyes	Direct contact Hands, towels, handkerchiefs, possibly clothing	Directly on conjunctiva

Method of Transmission of Some Common Communicable Diseases (*cont.*)

Disease	How Agent Leaves the Bodies of the Sick	How Organisms May Be Transmitted	Method of Entry into the Body
Tuberculosis, Bovine		Milk from infected cow	As in Tuberculosis, Human
Tuberculosis, Human	Sputum Lesions Feces	Direct contact such as kissing Droplet infection from person coughing with mouth uncovered Sputum from mouth to fingers, thence to food and other things Soiled dressings	Through mouth to lungs and intestines From intestines via lymph channels to lymph vessels and to tissues
Typhoid fever	Feces and urine	Direct contact Hands of nurse or attendant Linen and all articles used by and about patient Hands of carriers soiled by their own feces Water polluted by excreta Food grown in or washed with such water Milk diluted with contaminated water Flies	Through mouth in infected food or water and thence to intestinal tract
Whooping cough	Discharges from respiratory tract	Direct contact with persons affected	Mouth and nose

compared with that of animals.

compartmental syndrome. Any condition in which a structure such as a nerve or tendon is being constricted in a space, e.g., *carpal tunnel syndrome.* The sheath or tendon may due to disease or inflammation be enlarged and no longer able to move freely in the compartment.

compatibility [L. *compati,* to sympathize with]. 1. State of suitability to be mixed or taken together without unfavorable results, as drugs. 2. The ability of two individuals or groups to live together without undue strife or tension.

compatible. Not opposed to; able to mix with another substance without undesired changes.

Compazine. Trade name for prochlorperazine maleate.

compensating. Making up for a deficiency.

compensation [L. *cum,* with, + *pensare,* to weigh]. 1. Making up for a defect, as cardiac circulation competent to meet demands made upon it regardless of valvular defect. 2. In psychoanalysis, a psychic mechanism best described by an example. The individual handicapped by a physical deformity or variation or by a character defect may escape the consciousness or revelation of the inferiority by accomplishment resulting from compensatory ambition. More simply, the short man may strut or the incompetent brag. Sublimation, q.v., is often similar, but varies in that the substitution of a higher social goal gratifies the infrasocial drive by replacement, rather than going to the opposite extreme in a merely camouflaging manner.

c., failure of. Inability of heart muscle to cope with cardiac output required. It indicates a diseased heart muscle.

ETIOL: Diseased myocardium; back pressure, due to mitral regurgitation; mitral or aortic stenosis; or aortic regurgitation.

competence (kŏm′pĕ-tĕns). In psychiatry, having the ability to manage one's affairs, and by inference, not to be insane. Usually stated as being mentally competent.

competition (kŏm″pĕ-tĭsh′ŭn). The simultaneous attempt of similar substances to attach to a receptor site or an enzyme or cell wall.

complaint (kŏm-plānt′). Verbalization or otherwise communication of the principal reason the patient is seeking medical assistance.

complement (kŏm′plĕ-mĕnt) [L. *complere,* to complete]. A series of enzymatic proteins in normal serum that, in the presence of a specific sensitizer, destroy bacteria and other cells. There are 14 components that combine with the antigen-antibody complex to effect cell lysis. Once activated the components are involved in a great number of immune defense mechanisms including anaphylaxis, leukocyte chemotaxis, and phagocytosis. SYN: *alexin.* SEE: *antibody; antigen; immunity.*

complemental, complementary. Supplying something that is lacking.

c. air. Amount of air that can be inspired over and above the tidal air by the deepest inspiration. SEE: *air.*

c. colors. Any two spectral colors that, when blended, produce white light.

complement fixation. The action of a complement on an antigen that in turn has been acted on by its antibody. During the uniting of antigen, antibody, and complement, the complement is rendered inactive or destroyed. This process is known as fixation of complement. The process is the basis of the Wassermann and Kolmer tests for syphilis.

complementoid (kŏm″plĕ-mĕn′toyd) [L. *complere,* to complete, + Gr. *eidos,* form]. A complement, the lysis-causing power of which has been destroyed.

complementophil (kŏm″plĕ-mĕnt′ō-fĭl) [″ + Gr. *philein,* to love]. Having the power to combine with a complement.

complex [L. *complexus,* woven together]. 1. All the ideas, feelings, and sensations connected with a subject. 2. Intricate. 3. An atrial or ventricular systole as it appears on an electrocardiograph tracing. 4. A subconscious idea (or group of ideas) that has become associated with a repressed wish or emotional experience and that may influence behavior although the person may not have any appreciation of the connection between the repressed thoughts or actions.

In freudian theory, a grouping of ideas with an emotional background. These may be harmless, and the individual fully aware of them, e.g., an artist sees every object with a view to a possible picture and is said to have established a complex for art. Often, however, the complex is aroused by some painful emotional reaction such as fright or excessive grief that, instead of being allowed a natural outlet, becomes unconsciously repressed and later manifests itself in some abnormality of mind or behavior. According to Freud, the best method of determining the complex is through the medium of psychoanalysis. SEE: *Electra complex; Oedipus complex.*

c., castration. Morbid fear of being castrated.

c., Electra. Excessive love of her father by an adult female. SEE: *Electra complex.*

c., Ghon. The primary lesion in tuberculosis, consisting of the affected area of the lung and a corresponding lymph node. These usually heal and become calcified.

c., Golgi. An organelle present in most cells but larger in secretory cells. Enclosed are vacuoles, sacs, and secretory material. This complex is vital to the cell's function. SEE: *Golgi apparatus; organelle* for illus.

c., inferiority. A state of mind in which one feels inferior to others.

c., Oedipus. Excessive love of his mother by an adult male, usually accompanied by hostility toward father. SEE: *Oedipus complex.*

c., superiority. Exaggerated conviction of one's own superiority; also pretense of being superior to compensate for a supposed inferiority.

complexion (kŏm-plĕk′shŭn). The color and appearance of the facial skin.

complexus (kŏm-plĕk′sŭs) [L.]. Semispinalis capitis muscle.

compliance (kŏm-plī′ăns). 1. The property of altering size and shape in response to application of force, weight, or release from such force. Thus the lung and thoracic cage of a child may have a high degree of compliance as compared to that of an elderly adult. 2. Cooperative performance in relation to prescriptive therapy.

complication [L. *cum,* with, + *plicare,* to fold]. An added difficulty; a complex state. A disease or accident superimposed upon another without being specifically related, yet affecting or modifying the prognosis of the original disease, e.g., pneumonia is a complication of measles and is the cause of many deaths from that disease.

component. A constituent part.

component blood therapy. Use of a specific blood component such as plasma or washed red cells instead of an entire unit of whole blood. This practice reduces the chances for adverse reaction to whole blood transfusion while permitting the desired and essential ingredient of blood to be administered.

compos mentis (kŏm″pŭs mĕn′tĭs) [L.]. Of sound mind; sane.

compound [L. *componere,* to place together]. 1. A substance composed of two or more units or parts combined in definite proportions by weight and having specific properties of its own. Compounds are formed in plants and animals and are of two types, organic and inorganic. 2. Made up of more than one part.

c., dental. A nonelastic molding or impression material used in dentistry that softens when heated and solidifies without chemical change when cooled, i.e., a thermoplastic material.

c., inorganic. One of many compounds that, in general, contains no carbon.

c., organic. A compound containing carbon, such as carbohydrates, proteins, and fats.

compound astigmatism. Myopia of both vertical and horizontal meridians.

compound fracture. Fracture of bone where broken end of bone has penetrated the skin.

compound microscope. A microscope consisting of two or more lenses.

compress [L. *compressus,* squeezed together]. 1. (kŏm′prĕs) Cloth, wet or dry, folded and applied firmly to a part. 2. (kŏm-prĕs′) To press together into smaller space. 3. To close by squeezing together, as a wound.

c., chest. Application of two pieces of linen of sufficient size to fit the entire chest from the clavicles down to the umbilicus.

c., cold. Soft, absorbent cloth, several layers thick, dipped in cold water, slightly wrung out, applied to given part. To maintain constant temperature, compress is frequently renewed or ice bag or rubber coil through which ice water is circulating is placed on it. Duration of application is usually 30 to 60 minutes.

c., forehead. A soft, moist towel renewed at least every two minutes.

c., hot. Soft, absorbent cloth folded into several layers, dipped in hot water 107 to 115° F. (41.7 to 46.1° C.), barely wrung out and placed on part to be treated; covered with a piece of flannel large enough to overlap the linen slightly. Temperature is maintained at constant level by renewing compress or by rubber coil through which hot water 107 to 115° F. (41.7 to 46.1° C.) is circulated.

c., wet. Application of two or more folds of soft cloth wrung out of water at prescribed temperatures and covered with flannel.

compressed spectral array. ABBR: CSA. Graphical display of recorded material from a series of data such as from an electroencephalogram so that sequential tracings are displayed one above another. This permits instantaneous visual comparison of alterations in the electrical activity of the brain. Thus the data that would require hundreds of feet of chart paper for conventional EEG recording may, by use of this method, be displayed on a single sheet of paper.

compression (kŏm-prĕsh′ŭn) [L. *compressio,* a compression]. A squeezing together; state of being pressed together.

c., cerebral. Pressure on the brain produced by increased intracranial fluids, embolism, thrombosis, tumors, and skull fractures. More serious than concussion, q.v.

SYM: Deep unconsciousness; full, bounding pulse; deep, stertorous, slow respirations; flushed face; high blood pressure; pupils varying in size. Temperature may rise and there may be retention or incontinence of urine and feces.

DANGER SIGNALS: Coma; Cheyne-Stokes respiration; rise in temperature; quickening of pulse.

NURSING IMPLICATIONS: Assess patient closely for: symptoms of increased intracranial pressure, respiratory distress, convulsions, bleeding from the ears or nose, or drainage of cerebrospinal fluid from the ears (which may indicate a fracture). Observe for any alterations in sensory, motor, or mental status. Pupillary size, equality, and ability to react to light are all observed for and recorded as frequently as indicated. Maintain seizure precautions. SEE: *coma.*

c., digital. Compression of blood vessels by means of the fingers in order to stop hemorrhage.

c., myelitis. Compression caused by pressure on the spinal cord, often due to a tumor.

compression gloves. Any type of glove made of stretch material so that pressure is maintained against the fingers and hands. This helps to reduce edema.

compressor. 1. Instrument for making pressure on a part. 2. A muscle that compresses a part, as the compressor hemispherium bulbi, which compresses the bulb of the urethra.

compulsion (kŏm-pŭl′shŭn) [L. *compulsio,* compulsion]. Repetitive stereotyped act performed to relieve fear connected with obsession; dictated by the patient's subconscious against the subject's wishes and, if denied, causing uneasiness.

compulsion neurosis. Obsession or psychoneurosis that compels one to perform an absurd act or to say something silly. SYN: *obsessional neurosis.*

compulsive (kŏm-pŭl′sĭv). Pert. to or characterized by compulsion.

compulsive ideas. An idea that continues against one's will to suggest the commitment of an overt act that would normally be against one's better judgment.

compulsory (kŏm-pŭl'sor-ē). Compelling action against one's will.

computerized axial tomography. ABBR: CAT. SEE: *tomography, computerized axial.* SYN: *CAT scan.*

con- [L.]. Prefix meaning together with.

conarium (kō-nā'rē-ŭm) [L.]. The pineal body of the brain.

conation (kō-nā'shŭn) [L. *conatio*, an attempt]. The desire or impulse, arising from inside oneself, to act.

conative (kŏn'ă-tĭv). Pert. to the strivings and desires of a person as demonstrated by behavior and actions.

concanavilin A (kŏn"kă-năv'ĭ-lĭn). A lectin, q.v., derived from the Jack bean, that stimulates proliferation of certain types of cells, esp. T-cell lymphocytes but not B cells. SEE: *phytohemagglutinin.*

concatenation (kŏn-kăt"ĭ-nā'shŭn) [L. *con*, together, + *catena*, chain]. A group of events or effects acting in concert or occurring at the same time.

Concato's disease (kŏn-kō'tōs). [Luigi M. Concato, It. physician, 1825–1882] Polyserositis.

concave (kŏn'kāv, kŏn-kāv') [" + *cavus*, hollow]. Having a spherically depressed or hollow surface.

concavity (kŏn-kăv'ĭ-tē). A surface with curved, bowl-like sides.

concavoconcave (kŏn-kā"vō-kŏn'kāv) [" + *cavus*, hollow, + *con*, with, + *cavus*, hollow]. Concave on opposing sides.

concavoconvex (kŏn-kā"vō-kŏn'vĕks) [" + " + *convexus*, vaulted]. Concave on one side and convex on opposite surface. SEE: *convex.*

conceive (kŏn-sēv') [L. *concipere*, to take to oneself]. 1. To become pregnant. 2. To form a mental image or to bring into mind; to form an idea.

concentration (kŏn-sĕn-trā'shŭn) [L. *con*, together with, + *centrum*, center]. 1. Increase in strength of a fluid by evaporation. 2. Medicine strengthened by evaporation. 3. Fixation of mind on one subject to exclusion of all other thoughts.

c., hydrogen ion. Concentration of hydrogen ions in a solution; the symbol is pH, q.v.

concentric (kŏn-sĕn'trĭk) [" + *centrum*, center]. Having a common center.

concept (kŏn'sĕpt) [L. *conceptum*, something understood]. An idea.

conception (kŏn-sĕp'shŭn). 1. The mental process of forming an idea. 2. The union of the male sperm and the ovum of the female; fertilization. With a cycle of 28 days, menstruation normally lasts five days followed by a period of repair and proliferation of the lining of the uterus (endometrium) for about a week. Until ovulation occurs, the female is sterile. In general, ovulation occurs about 12 to 14 days prior to the beginning of the next menstrual period. Thus sexual intercourse during the middle of the menstrual cycle is most likely to result in conception. During this period, the ovum is discharged from the follicle and makes its way through the fallopian tube to the uterus. If fertilization does not occur during this time, the ovum disintegrates and for the remaining portion of the menstrual cycle (the 10 days preceding menstruation) conception is less likely to occur.

However, one of the most variable events known in human biology is the menstrual cycle. It is therefore quite difficult, and in many cases impossible, to predict optimum time of conception or the reverse by attempting to calculate ovulation time from the time the last menstrual period occurred. Also, sperm survival time in the female reproductive tract is variable. SEE: *basal temperature chart; contraception.*

conceptus (kŏn-sĕp'tŭs). The products of conception.

concha (kŏng'kă) [Gr. *konche*, shell]. (pl. *conchae*) 1. The outer ear or the pinna. 2. One of the three nasal conchae. SEE: *c., nasal.*

c. auriculae. [NA] A concavity on the median surface of the auricle of the ear, divided by a ridge into the upper cymba conchae and a lower cavum conchae. The latter leads to the exterior auditory meatus.

c. bullosa. Distention of turbinate bone due to cyst formation.

c., nasal. One of the three scroll-like bones that project medially from the lateral wall of the nasal cavity; a turbinate bone. The superior and middle conchae are processes of lateral mass of the ethmoid bone; the inferior concha is a face bone. Each overlies a meatus.

c. sphenoidalis. [NA] In a fetal skull, one of two curved plates located on anterior portion of body of sphenoid bone. Forms part of roof of nasal cavity.

conchitis (kŏng-kī'tĭs) [" + *itis*, inflammation]. Inflammation of any concha.

conchoidal (kŏng-koy'dăl) [" + *eidos*, shape]. Having the shape of a shell.

conchoscope (kŏng'kō-skōp) [" + *skopein*, to examine]. Instrument for examination of the nasal cavity.

conchotome (kŏng'kō-tōm) [" + *tome*, incision]. Device for excision of middle turbinate bone.

conchotomy (kŏng-kŏt'ō-mē). Surgical incision of a nasal concha.

concoction (kŏn-kŏk'shŭn) [L. *con*, with, + *coquere*, to cook]. Mixture of two medicinal substances usually done with the aid of heat.

concomitant (kŏn-kŏm'ĭ-tănt) [" + *comes*,

companion]. Accessory; taking place at the same time.

concordance (kŏn-kor'dăns). In twins, the equal representation of a genetic trait in each.

concrement (kŏn'krē-mĕnt) [L. *concrementum*]. A concretion as of protein and other substances. If infiltrated with calcium salts, it is termed a calculus.

concrescence (kŏn-krĕs'ĕns) [L. *con*, with, + *crescere*, to grow]. The union of separate parts; coalescence.

concrete (kŏn'krēt, kŏn-krēt') [L. *concretus*, solid]. Condensed, hardened, or solidified.

concretio cordis (kŏn-krē'shē-ō kor'dĭs). Obliteration of the pericardial space due to chronic constrictive pericarditis.

concretion (kŏn-krē'shŭn) [" + *crescere*, to grow]. A calculus.

concubitus (kŏn-kū'bĭ-tŭs) [L.]. Coitus, sexual intercourse.

concussion (kŏn-kŭsh'ŭn) [L. *concussus*, shaken violently]. 1. An injury resulting from impact with an object. 2. Loss of function either partial or complete as that resulting from a blow or fall.

c. of brain. Cerebral concussion. A common result of a blow to the head or fall on the end of spine with force sufficient to be transmitted upward. This usually causes unconsciousness, either temporary or prolonged. Return of consciousness may be gradual. Patient may suddenly draw up knees and vomit.

SYM: Vary with location and extent of injury from transient dizziness to various paralyses, or unconsciousness; unequal pupils, shock. If uncomplicated, patient regains consciousness in a short period of time. Period of reaction, accompanied by vomiting, temperature 99° to 100° F. (37.2 to 37.8° C.), rapid pulse, flushed face, restlessness, headache, cerebral irritation, lasts for 12 to 24 hours.

F.A.: Keep patient quietly lying down with head and shoulders slightly elevated. Do not give stimulants. Transportation should be delayed if possible. Sedatives are generally contraindicated. Cool applications to head and neck are soothing. Reassure patient if conscious. Warm extremities if cold. Report any adverse symptoms, such as bleeding, or alteration in pupil size or reaction, at once. Darkened room best.

CAUTION: Do not give morphine. SEE: *contusion; transportation of injured*.

c. of labyrinth. Deafness resulting from a blow to the head or ear.

c., spinal. Loss of function in spinal cord resulting from a blow or severe jarring.

condensation (kŏn"dĕn-sā'shŭn) [" + *densare*, to make thick]. 1. Making more dense or compact. 2. Changing a liquid to a solid or a gas to a liquid. 3. In psychoanalysis, the union of ideas to form a new mental pattern. 4. In chemistry, a type of reaction in which two or more molecules of the same substance react with each other and form a new and heavier substance with different chemical properties. 5. A mechanical process used in dentistry to remove excess mercury from amalgam or to form a dense gold foil restoration; it improves the physical properties of the material used and forces it to adapt more perfectly to the cavity preparation.

condenser (kŏn-dĕn'sĕr). Device for solidifying vapors and liquids. SEE: *capacitance*.

c., electrical. Device for storing of electricity by using two conducting surfaces and a nonconductor.

condiment (kŏn'dĭ-mĕnt) [L. *condire*, to pickle]. Appetizing ingredient added to food.

CLASSIFICATION: *Aromatic:* vanilla; cinnamon; cloves, chervil; parsley; bay leaf, etc. *Acrid or peppery:* pepper; ginger; allspice, etc. *Alliaceous or allylic:* onion, mustard; horseradish. *Acid:* vinegar; capers; gherkins; citron. *Animal origin:* caviar; anchovies. *Miscellaneous:* salt; sugar; truffles.

In general, condiments have little nutritional value. Sugar is an exception. They are extremely useful in making food more appetizing.

ACTION: They are appetizers and stimulate the secretion of saliva and intestinal juices.

conditioned reflex. Reflex acquired as a result of training and repetition.

conditioning (kŏn-dĭsh'ŭn-ĭng). 1. Improving the physical capability of a person by an exercise program. 2. In psychology, the use of a special and different stimulus in conjunction with a familiar stimulus. After a sufficient period of time in which the two stimuli have been simultaneously presented, the special stimulus alone will cause the response that could originally be produced only by the familiar stimulus. The late Russian physiologist, Ivan Pavlov, used dogs to demonstrate that the strange stimulus, ringing of a bell, could cause the animal to salivate if the test was done after a period of *conditioning* during which the bell and the familiar stimulus, food, were presented simultaneously. SYN: *classical conditioning*.

c., operant. The learning of a particular action or type of behavior that is followed by a reward. This technique was publicized by the contemporary Harvard psychologist, B. F. Skinner, who trained animals to activate (by pecking, in the case of a pigeon, or pressing a bar, in the case of a rat) an apparatus that released a pellet of food.

condom (kŏn'dŭm) [L. *condus*, a receptacle].

A thin, flexible sheath worn over the penis. It is used during sexual intercourse to prevent sperm from entering the vagina and to help prevent venereal disease.

conductance (kŏn-dŭk′tăns) [L. *conducere,* to lead]. The conducting ability of a body or a circuit for electricity. The best conductor is that which offers the least resistance, such as gold, silver, and copper. When expressed as a numerical value, conductance is the reciprocal of resistance. The unit is the ohm.

conduction (kŏn-dŭk′shŭn). 1. The process whereby a state of excitation affects successive portions of a tissue or cell, so that the disturbance is transmitted to remote points. Conduction occurs not only in the fibers of the nervous system but also in muscle fibers. 2. The transfer of electrons, ions, heat, or sound waves through a conductor or conducting medium.

c., bone. Sound conduction through cranial bones.

conductivity (kŏn″dŭk-tĭv′ĭ-tē). The specific electric conducting ability of a substance. Conductivity is the reciprocal of unit resistance or resistivity. The unit is the ohm/cm. Specific conductivity is sometimes expressed as a percentage. In such cases, the conductivity is given as a percentage of the conductivity of pure copper under certain standard conditions.

conductor (kŏn-dŭk′tor). 1. Medium transmitting a force. 2. A guide directing a surgical knife or probe.

conduit (kŏn′doo-ĭt). A channel or aqueduct, esp. an artificial one surgically constructed.

c., ileal. Attachment of one or both ureters to one end of an isolated loop of ileum; the other end is attached to an opening in the abdominal wall.

condylar (kŏn′dĭ-lăr) [Gr. *kondylos,* knuckle]. Pert. to a condyle.

condylarthrosis (kŏn″dĭl-ăr-thrō′sĭs) [″ + *arthrosis,* a joint]. A form of diarthrosis, q.v.; an ovoid head in an elliptical cavity.

condyle (kŏn′dīl) [Gr. *kondylos,* knuckle]. (pl. *condyles*) A rounded protuberance at the end of a bone forming an articulation.

condylectomy (kŏn″dĭ-lĕk′tō-mē) [″ + *ektome,* excision]. Excision of a condyle.

condylion (kŏn-dĭl′ē-ŏn) [Gr. *kondylion,* knob]. A point on either the lateral or medial surface of the mandibular condyle.

condyloid (kŏn′dĭ-loyd) [Gr. *kondylos,* knuckle, + *eidos,* appearance]. Pert. to or resembling a condyle.

condyloid process. Articular process on ramus of mandible consisting of a capitulum and neck. Articulates with mandibular fossa of temporal bone.

condyloid tubercle. A tubercle on capitulum of condyloid process of the mandible for attachment of temporomandibular ligament.

condyloma (kŏn″dĭ-lō′mă) [Gr. *kondyloma,* wart]. A wartlike growth of the skin, usually seen on the external genitalia or near the anus. There are two types, a pointed variety, and a broad flat form usually of syphilitic origin.

c. acuminatum. An ordinary wart in the genital and perianal areas. It is caused by a virus and may be spread by one area containing a wart inoculating an area that it contacts. The spread of a wart from one labium to the other by auto-inoculation is possible. The wart is usually of a venereal origin.

c. latum. A mucous patch on the vulva or anus, coated with gray exudate, flattened in form, with delimited area, characteristic of syphilis.

condylomatous (kŏn″dĭ-lō′mă-tŭs). Pert. to a condyloma.

condylotomy (kŏn″dĭ-lŏt′ō-mē) [Gr. *kondylos,* knuckle, + *tome,* incision]. Division without removal of a condyle.

condylus (kŏn′dĭ-lŭs). (pl. *condyli*) Condyle.

cone (kōn) [Gr. *konos,* cone]. 1. A three-dimensional figure with circular base with sides sloping to a point above. May be solid or hollow. 2. In the outer layer of the retina (the layer closest to the front of the eye), the flask-shaped cells that receive visual stimuli. SEE: *rods.*

c., ocular. Cone of light in eye with point on the retina.

c., retinal. The specialized cone-shaped cells of the retina of the eye. These cells, along with the retinal rods, are light-sensitive. The cones receive color stimuli.

cone of light. Triangular areas of reflected light on the membrana tympani extending downward from the umbo.

conexus (kō-nĕk′sŭs) [L.]. A connecting structure.

confabulation (kŏn-făb″ū-lā′shŭn) [L. *confabulari,* to talk together]. In psychoanalysis, the verbal relating of imaginary experiences to fill in gaps in the memory.

confectio, confection (kŏn-fĕk′shē-ō, -shŭn) [L. *conficere,* to prepare]. Sugarlike soft solids in which one or more medicinal substances are incorporated with the object of affording an agreeable form for their administration and a convenient method for their preservation. Not often prescribed, and not official.

configuration (kŏn-fĭg″ū-rā′shŭn). 1. The shape and appearance of anything. 2. In chemistry, the position of atoms in a molecule.

confinement (kŏn-fīn′mĕnt) [O. Fr. *confiner,* to restrain in a place]. The period of childbirth.

conflict (kŏn′flĭkt) [L. *confligere,* to contend].

1. Opposing action of incompatibles. 2. In psychiatry, the conscious or unconscious struggle between two opposing desires or courses of action. A technical term applied to a state in which social goals dictate behavior contrary to more primitive (often subconscious) desires.

confluence of sinuses. The union of the sagittal sinus with the transverse sinuses.

confluent (kŏn'floo-ĕnt) [L. *confluere,* to run together]. Running together, as when the pustules in smallpox merge.

conformation (kŏn"for-mā'shŭn). The form or shape of a part, body, material, or molecule.

confrontation (kŏn"frŭn-tā'shŭn) [L. *con,* together with, + *frons,* face]. 1. The examination of two patients together, one with a disease and the other from whom the disease was supposed to be contracted. 2. A method employed in determining extent of visual fields in which that of the patient is compared with that of the examiner. 3. In counseling, a feedback procedure in which patient's behavior and apparent feelings are presented in an attempt to facilitate better understanding of his or her actions.

confusion (kŏn-fū'zhŭn). Not being aware of or oriented with respect to time, place, or self.

congelation (kŏn"jĕ-lā'shŭn) [L. *congelare,* to freeze]. Freezing, or a frostbite.

congener (kŏn'jĕn-ĕr) [L. *con,* together, + *genus,* race]. 1. Two or more muscles with the same function. 2. Something that by structure, function, or origin is similar to another. In the production of alcoholic beverages by fermentation, chemical substances termed congeners are also produced. These chemicals, over a hundred of which are known, impart aroma and flavor to the alcoholic compound. The precise role of these congeners in producing toxic effects is unknown.

congenerous (kŏn-jĕn'ĕr-ŭs). Possessing the same function, as synergistic muscles.

congenital (kŏn-jĕn'ĭ-tăl) [L. *congenitus,* born together]. Present at birth.

congenital anomaly. An abnormality present at birth.

congested (kŏn-jĕs'tĕd) [L. *congerere,* to heap together]. Containing an abnormal amount of blood.

congestion. The presence of an excessive amount of blood or tissue fluid in an organ or in tissue. SYN: *hyperemia.*

c., active. Congestion resulting from increased flow of blood to a part or dilatation of blood vessels.

c., passive. Hyperemia resulting from interference with flow of blood from capillaries into venules. May also result from myocardial insufficiency.

congestive (kŏn-jĕs'tĭv). Pert. to congestion.

congius (kŏn'jē-ŭs) [L.]. (pl. *congii*) A gallon.

conglobate (kŏn'glō-bāt) [L. *con,* together, + *globare,* to make round]. In one mass, as lymph glands.

conglobation (kŏn"glō-bā'shŭn). Aggregation of particles in a rounded mass.

conglomerate (kŏn-glŏm'ĕr-āt) [" + *glomerare,* to heap]. 1. An aggregation in one mass. 2. Clustered; heaped together.

conglutin (kŏn-gloo'tĭn) [L. *conglutinare,* to glue together]. A protein resembling casein found in peas, beans, and almonds.

conglutinant (kŏn-gloo'tĭ-nănt). Promoting adhesion, as of the edges of a wound.

conglutinate (kŏn-gloo'tĭ-nāt). Having the quality of adhesiveness.

conglutination (kŏn-gloo"tĭn-ā'shŭn). 1. Coalescence, adhesion. 2. Reaction, such as agglutination.

coniasis (kō-nī'ă-sĭs) [Gr. *konis,* dust, + *-iasis,* condition]. Dust-like calculi in gallbladder and bile ducts.

conidia (kō-nĭd'ē-ă). (sing. *conidium*) Asexual spores of fungi.

conidiophore (kŏn-ĭd'ē-ō-for) [" + *phoros,* bearing]. The stalk supporting conidia.

coniofibrosis (kō'nē-ō-fī-brō'sĭs) [Gr. *konis,* dust, + L. *fibra,* fiber, + Gr. *osis,* condition]. Pneumoconiosis produced by dust such as that from asbestos or silica. This causes fibrosis to develop in the lung.

coniology (kō-nē-ŏl'ŏ-jē) [" + *logos,* study of]. The study of dust and its effects.

coniosis (kō"nē-ō'sĭs) [" + *osis,* condition]. Any condition caused by inhalation of dust.

coniosporosis (kō"nē-ō-spō-rō'sĭs) [" + *sporos,* seed, + *osis,* condition]. Hypersensitivity reaction consisting of asthma and pneumonitis caused by breathing the spores of Cryptostroma corticale or Coniosporium corticale. These fungi grow under the bark of some types of trees. Workers who strip the bark from these trees may develop this condition.

conization (kŏn"ĭ-zā'shŭn) [Gr. *konos,* cone]. Excision of a cone of tissue, as of the mucous membrane of the cervix.

conjugata (kŏn"jū-gā'tă) [L. *conjugatus,* yoked together]. [NA] Diameter of pelvis, measured from center of the promontory of the sacrum to the back of the symphysis pubis. SYN: *conjugate.*

c. vera. Conjugate. SYN: *conjugate, true.*

conjugate (kŏn'jū-gāt). 1. Paired or joined. 2. An important diameter of the pelvis, measured from the center of the promontory of the sacrum to the back of the symphysis pubis. In obstetrics, the diagonal conjugate is measured and the true conjugate is estimated. SYN: *c. diameter.* SEE: *c., diagonal; c., external.*

c. deviation. Deviation of both eyes to

either side.

c., diagonal. Diameter measured from the lower edge of the symphysis to the promontory of the sacrum, which can be determined during life, whereas the true conjugate cannot be measured. The true conjugate is estimated by deducting 1.5 to 2.0 cm. from the length of the diagonal conjugate. It is about ½ to ¾ in. (1.3 to 1.9 cm.) longer than the true conjugate, or about 5 in. (12.7 cm.).

c. diameter. Conjugate.

c., external. Diameter measured from the spine of the last lumbar vertebra to the front of the pubes (this is done by using calipers); it is normally about 8 in. (20.3 cm.).

c., true. Conjugate. SYN: *conjugata vera.*

conjugation (kŏn″jū-gā′shŭn). A coupling together. In biology, the union of two unicellular organisms accompanied by an interchange of nuclear material as in Paramecium.

conjunctiva (kŏn″jŭnk-tī′vă, kŏn-jŭnk′tĭ-vă) [L. *conjungere,* to join together]. Mucous membrane that lines eyelids and is reflected onto eyeball.

DIVISIONS: Palpebral conjunctiva covers undersurface of lids; bulbar conjunctiva coats anterior portion of eyeball; fornix conjunctiva is the transition portion forming fold between lid and globe.

INSPECTION: Palpebral and ocular portions should be examined. Color and degree of moisture and presence of foreign bodies should be observed; also petechial hemorrhages and inflammation.

PATH: Conditions are trachoma, pannus, and discoloration. Yellowish discoloration is seen in jaundice and pale conjunctivae observed in anemias.

conjunctival reflex. Closure of eyelids when conjunctiva is touched or threatened.

conjunctivitis (kŏn-jŭnk″tĭ-vī′tĭs) [″ + Gr. *itis,* inflammation]. Inflammation of conjunctiva.

TREATMENT: Directed against the specific type of infection.

c., actinic. Conjunctivitis resulting from exposure to ultraviolet (actinic) rays.

c., acute contagious. Pinkeye, q.v.

c., angular, of Morax-Axenfeld. Conjunctivitis affecting the inner angle of the conjunctivae.

c., catarrhal. Conjunctivitis due to a variety of causes such as foreign bodies, various bacteria, or irritation from heat, cold, or chemicals.

c., epidemic hemorrhagic. Virus infection with sudden pain in the eye. This progresses to swollen eyelids, hyperemia of the conjunctiva, and later subconjunctival hemorrhage. The disease, which is self-limiting and for which there is no specific therapy, usually affects both eyes. Several viral agents can cause this disease. Included are picornavirus, enterovirus 70, adenovirus 11, and coxsackievirus A24.

c., follicular. Type of conjunctivitis characterized by pinkish round bodies in retrotarsal fold.

c., gonorrheal. A severe, acute form of purulent conjunctivitis caused by the gonococcus Neisseria gonorrhea. SEE: *ophthalmia neonatorum.*

c., granular. Acute contagious inflammatory conjunctivitis with granular elevations on the lids that ulcerate and cicatrize. SYN: *trachoma.*

c., inclusion. Acute purulent inflammation of the conjunctivae caused by Chlamydia trachomatis. The neonate is infected as it passes through the mother's genital tract. The adult may be infected while swimming or from a sex partner.

c., membranous. Acute conjunctivitis characterized by a false membrane with or without infiltration.

c. of newborn. Ophthalmia neonatorum, q.v.

c., phlyctenular. An allergenic form of conjunctivitis commonly seen in children. Characterized by nodules that may ulcerate.

c., purulent. Form of conjunctivitis due to organisms producing purulence, esp. gonococci.

c., vernal. Conjunctivitis beginning in the spring. Most probably due to allergy.

conjunctivoma (kŏn-jŭnk″tĭ-vō′mă) [L. *conjungere,* to join together, + Gr. *oma,* tumor]. A tumor of the conjunctiva.

conjunctivoplasty (kŏn″jŭnk-tī′vō-plăs″tē) [″ + Gr. *plassein,* to form]. Removal of part of cornea, but replacing with flaps from the conjunctiva.

connective [L. *connectere,* to bind together]. Pert. to that which connects or binds together.

connective diseases. A group of diseases of connective tissue that share anatomical and pathological features. The etiology of these diseases is unknown; thus they are grouped together on the basis of common clinical signs and symptoms. Generalized inflammation of connective tissue and blood vessels is usually seen, and in some cases fibrinoid deposition in connective tissue fibers and blood vessels is present. SYN: *collagen diseases.*

Diseases currently included in this category are: cutaneous and systemic lupus erythematosus; scleroderma; polymyositis and dermatomyositis; and polyarteritis.

connective tissue. Tissue that supports and connects other tissues and tissues and parts. The cells of connective tissue are comparatively few in number, the bulk of the tissue consisting of intercellular substance or matrix, the nature of which gives each type of connective tissue its particular properties. Connective tissues are highly vascular with the exception of cartilage. Connective tissue proper includes the following types: mucous, fibrous (areolar, white fibrous, yellow fibrous, or elastic), reticular, and adipose. Dense connective tissue includes cartilage and bone (osseous tissue).

Conn's syndrome. [J. W. Conn, contemporary U.S. physician] Primary hyperaldosteronism; the symptoms and clinical condition include muscle weakness, polyuria, hypertension, hypokalemia, and alkalosis associated with an abnormally high rate of secretion of aldosterone by the adrenal cortex.

conoid (kō'noyd) [Gr. *konos,* cone, + *eidos,* shape]. Resembling a cone; conical.

conoid ligament. Lower and inner portion of coracoclavicular ligament.

conoid tubercle. Eminence on inferior surface of clavicle to which is attached the conoid ligament.

consanguinity (kŏn″săn-gwĭn'ĭ-tē) [L. *consanguinitas,* kinship]. Relationship by blood, i.e., being descended from a common ancestor.

conscious (kŏn'shŭs) [L. *conscius,* aware]. Being aware and having perception; awake. SEE: *coma.*

consciousness. A state of awareness. It implies an orientation to time, place, and person, i.e., the individual knows approximately the date, the nature of the environment, name, and other pertinent personal data. The content of consciousness is a composite of memories and the comprehension of external reality; the emotional status and the individual's goals also enter. It is, then, a large part of what is described as "personality" in its largest sense.

Consciousness varies its intensity and extent from minute to minute. In crises, vivid ideational association may lead to an exaggerated state of awareness. In states of relaxed contentment, it lessens, to disappear completely in sleep. This differs from the pathological condition of coma, in which the patient cannot be aroused.

In so-called pathological sleep (i.e., encephalitis lethargica) and in stupor, though aroused, the patient is unable to postpone again lapsing into dullness, whereas, up to a point, normal sleep can be adequately combated by the demands of reality. Stupor is produced largely by the factors resulting in coma; the personality is relatively intact but "hazy." However, there are conditions in which a real personality change manifests itself. Clouding of consciousness may simulate the dullness but usually not the other characteristics of stupor. On the contrary, such patients may impress one as being alert.

Alteration of consciousness and attention; impaired orientation and recent memory are characteristic of delirium. A quiet delirium may not easily reveal itself, even in certain states of automatism in which one finds evidence of the "real personality"; there may appear on casual examination little to arouse suspicion, yet brutal acts or total absence of memory may indicate major abnormalities.

Again, in somnambulistic (sleepwalking) states, experiences may register but cannot be recalled after return to a normal state. Consciousness, on the other hand, may erroneously appear to be present in so-called "coma vigil" because the eyes are open and expression may be alert. SEE: *c., levels of.*

c., clouding of. A phase of delirium in which the patient's consciousness is cloudy or not clear.

Clouding of consciousness may be diagnosed from the appearance of the patient in catatonic stupor and it may be difficult to realize the patient is quite lucid and that experiences are being registered accurately and can be later recalled. In true clouding, stimuli usually fail to register.

c., cosmic. The inner reaches of consciousness in which there is recognition of knowledge or facts independent of physical influence.

c., disintegration of. Cause of most mental disorders not resulting from organic conditions. Produced by the contents of the unconscious gradually disrupting the conscious.

c., levels of. The state of consciousness may vary from fully alert to coma. It is important to use a standardized system of describing the state rather than vague terms such as semiconscious, semicomatose, or semistuporous.

Alert wakefulness: The patient clearly appreciates the environment and responds quickly and appropriately to visual, auditory, and other sensory stimuli.

Drowsy: The patient doesn't fully appreciate the environment and responds to stimuli appropriately but with delay and slowness. May be roused by verbal stimuli but may ignore some of them. Patient is capable of verbal response unless aphasia, aphonia, or anarthria is present. Lethargy and obtundation are also descriptive of the drowsy state.

Stupor: Patient aroused by intense stimuli only. Loud noise may elicit a nonspecific reaction. Motor response and reflex reactions are usually preserved unless the patient is paralyzed.

Coma. Patient does not perceive the environment and intense stimuli produce a rudimentary response if any at all. The presence of reflex reactions depends on the location of the lesion(s) in the nervous system.

consensual (kŏn-sĕn′shū-ăl) [L. *consensus,* agreement]. Reflex stimulation of one part or side as the result of excitation of another part or opposite side.

consensual light index. When one eye is exposed to an intensity of light different from that to which the other is exposed, both pupils will react.

consensual light reflex. Pupillary reflex (def. 3), q.v.

consensual reflex. Any reflex occurring on opposite side of body from point of stimulation.

consenting adult. An adult who consents to participate in social or sexual activity that might be or formerly was regarded as abnormal, e.g., sadomasochistic sexual activity, or homosexual acts.

conservative (kŏn-sĕr′vă-tĭv) [L. *conservare,* to preserve]. Pert. to utilization of a simple rather than a radical method of either medical or surgical therapy.

consolidation (kŏn-sŏl-ĭ-dā′shŭn) [L. *consolidare,* to make firm]. The act of becoming solid. Esp. used in connection with the solidification of the lungs due to pathological engorgement of the lung tissues as occurs in acute pneumonia.

constant (kŏn′stănt) [L. *constans,* standing together]. 1. Unchanging. 2. A condition, fact, or situation that does not change.

constellation (kŏn″stĕl-lā′shŭn) [L. *con,* together, + *stella,* star]. Ideas arising from unrepressed emotions.

constipation (kŏn″stĭ-pā′shŭn) [L. *constipare,* to press together]. Difficult defecation; infrequent defecation with passage of unduly hard and dry fecal material; sluggish action of the bowels.

NOTE: It is virtually impossible to state how frequently the bowels should move in order to be classed as "normal." The range of variation in healthy individuals can vary from two to three bowel movements per day to two per week.

CAUTION: A continuous change in frequency of bowel movements may be a sign of serious intestinal or colonic disease. A change in bowel habits should be discussed with a physician.

CAUSES: Predisposing: No regular bowel movements from childhood; worry, anxiety, fear, sedentary life. Direct: Failure to establish definite and regular times for bowel movements; improper diet; intestinal obstruction; tumors; excessive use of laxatives; weakness of intestinal musculature (atony) or excessive tonicity (spasticity); use of certain drugs; presence of anal lesions. It is also a concomitant in some types of insanity.

GENERAL CORRECTIVE MEASURES: Plenty of fresh vegetables, fruits, milk, and an abundance of water. Attempt to establish regular bowel, exercise, and eating habits.

c., atonic. Constipation due to weakness of muscles of colon and rectum.

c., obstructive. Constipation due to an obstruction in the intestines. Surgical aid may be needed. Preoperative diet should contain low-residue and no gas-forming foods.

c., spastic. Constipation due to excessive tonicity of the intestinal wall, esp. the colon.

constitution [L. *constituere,* to establish]. The physical makeup and functional habits of the body.

constitutional. Pert. to the body as a whole.

constitutional disease. 1. Disease that affects the entire body rather than a specific part. 2. Disease that is dependent upon an individual's hereditary makeup, such as hemophilia.

constriction [L. *con,* together, + *stringere,* to draw]. 1. A binding or squeezing of a part. 2. The narrowing of a vessel or opening, as constriction of blood vessels or the pupil of the eye.

constrictor. 1. That which binds or restricts a part. 2. A muscle that constricts a vessel, opening, or passageway, as the constrictors of the faucial isthmus and pharynx, the circular fibers of the iris, intestine, and blood vessels.

constructive metabolism. The building-up or anabolic process. SEE: *anabolism; catabolism.*

consultant [L. *consultare,* to counsel]. A consulting health care worker, such as nurse, physician, pharmacist, or psychologist who acts in an advisory capacity.

consultation. In a specific patient, diagnosis and proposed treatment by two or more health care workers at one time.

consumption (kŏn-sŭmp′shŭn) [L. *consumere,* to waste away]. 1. Tuberculosis. 2. Wasting. 3. The using up of anything.

consumption-coagulopathy. Clinical condition of altered blood coagulation wherein depletion of the clotting factors I, II, V, VII, and platelets occurs. A pathological state secondary to a variety of diseases. SYN: *disseminated intravascular coagulation.*

consumptive. Pert. to or afflicted with tuberculosis.

contact [L. *con,* with, + *tangere,* to touch]. 1. Mutual touching or apposition of two bodies. 2. One who has been recently exposed to a contagious disease.

c., complete. When entire proximal surface of a tooth touches entire surface of an adjoining tooth, proximally.

c., direct. Transmission of a contagious disease by a healthy person coming in contact with a person who is a carrier of or has the disease.

c., indirect. The spread of a contagious disease by some medium other than directly touching an infected person.

c., mediate. C., indirect, q.v.

c., proximal; c., proximate. Touching of teeth on their adjacent surfaces.

contactant (kŏn-tăk′tănt). A substance that produces an allergic or sensitivity response when in direct contact with the skin.

contact dermatitis. Inflammation of the skin due to coming in contact with an irritating or sensitizing chemical.

contact lens. Device made of various materials, either rigid or flexible, that fit over the cornea or part of the cornea in order to alter the refractive ability of the lens of the eye.

c.l., bifocal. Contact lens that contains two corrections in the same lens.

c.l., hard. Contact lens made of rigid, translucent materials.

c.l., soft. Contact lens made of flexible, translucent materials.

contact surface. Proximal surface of a tooth.

contagion (kŏn-tā′jŭn) [L. *contingere,* to touch]. 1. The process of transferring a specific disease either by direct or indirect contact. 2. A contagious disease. 3. Any virus or bacterium that causes a contagious disease. SEE: *virulent; virus.*

contagious (kŏn-tā′jŭs). Communicable; transmitted readily from one person to another either directly or indirectly, with reference to the organism that causes a disease.

contagious pustular dermatitis. A cutaneous disease of sheep and goats transmitted to man by direct contact. The lesion on man is usually solitary and on the hands, arms, or face. This maculopapular area may progress to a pustule up to 3 cm. in diameter and may last 3 to 6 weeks. The etiological agent is a type of poxvirus. There is no specific treatment. SYN: *human orf.*

contagium (kŏn-tā′jē-ŭm) [L.]. The agent causing infection or contagion.

containers, care and handling of. Contamination of the container in which a specimen is to be placed may render the results of the examination futile and therefore interfere with the diagnosis. Care must be taken to avoid contamination of any container used for the collection of specimens. Use of sterile disposable containers for collecting specimens is recommended.

Sterilization of glassware: This is accomplished by hot air or dry heat, boiling water, flowing steam, steam under pressure, certain gases, and the use of germicidal chemicals.

Labels: All containers should be labeled with the name of the patient, room number, and the name of the attending physician. Labels should be placed on the container, not on the lid. Request forms, sometimes used as labels, are made up to suit the individual laboratory or hospital. Provision is made for recording necessary data as indicated, including date when specimen was taken, under what circumstances, for what substances the examination is to be done, and any other information desired.

Time: If the required specimen cannot be furnished at once, make a note of what is needed; inform the patient, the supervisor, and any other nurse who may attend the patient in your absence.

Charting: Note on the chart all specimens sent to the laboratory, when sent, and any other data that seem pertinent such as the appearance of the specimen or unusual occurrences while obtaining it.

Care of specimen: Cover immediately after depositing in the container; check label or request form. Make sure that the container is intact and that there is no danger of spilling while in transit.

contaminant (kŏn-tăm′ĭ-nănt). Substance or organism that causes contamination.

contaminate (kŏn-tăm′ĭ-nāt) [L. *contaminare,* to render impure]. 1. To soil, stain, or pollute. 2. To render unfit for use through introduction of a substance that is harmful or injurious. 3. To make impure or unclean. 4. To deposit a radioactive substance in any place where it is not supposed to be.

contamination. 1. The act of contaminating, esp. introduction of disease germs or infectious material into or on normally sterile objects. 2. In psychiatry, the fusion and condensation of words so that they run together when spoken.

content. That which is contained in something.

contiguity (kŏn″tĭ-gū′ĭ-tē) [L. *contiguus,* touching]. Contact or closely associated.

c., amputation in. Amputation through a joint.

c., law of. If two ideas occur in association, they are apt to be repeated.

c., solution of. Dislocation or displacement of two normally contiguous parts.

continence (kŏn′tĭ-nĕns) [L. *continere,* to hold together]. Self-restraint, used esp. in connection with refraining from sexual indulgence. Also used in reference to the ability to control urination and defecation. SEE: *incontinence.*

continent (kŏn′tĭ-nĕnt). 1. Capable of controlling urination and defecation. 2. Not yielding to sexual desire. SEE: *continence.*

continued (kŏn-tĭn′ūd). Uninterrupted.

continuity (kŏn″tĭ-nū′ĭ-tē) [L. *continuus,* continued]. The state of being continuous or intimately united.

c., amputation in. Amputation through a long bone.

c., solution of. Division of normally continuous parts by fracture, rupture, laceration, incision.

continuous (kŏn-tĭn′ū-ŭs) [L. *continere,* to hold together]. Without break, cessation, or interruption.

continuous spectrum. An unbroken series of wavelengths, either visible or invisible. Also an unbroken range of radiations of different wavelengths in any portion of the invisible spectrum.

contortion (kŏn-tor′shŭn) [L. *contorquere,* to twist together]. A twisting into an unusual shape.

contour (kŏn′toor) [It. *contornare,* to go around]. Outline or surface configuration of a part.

contoured (kŏn′toord). Having an irregular, undulating surface resembling a relief map, said of bacterial colonies.

contra- [L.]. Prefix indicating opposite or against, as contraindication.

contra-aperture [L. *contra,* against, + *apertura,* opening]. A second opening made in an abscess.

contraception (kŏn″tră-sĕp′shŭn) [″ + *conceptio,* a conceiving]. The prevention of conception, q.v. SEE: *contraceptive.*

contraceptive (kŏn″tră-sĕp′tĭv). Any process, device, or method that prevents conception. Categories of contraceptives include steroids; chemical; physical or barrier; combinations of physical or barrier and chemical; "natural"; abstinence; and permanent.

STEROIDS: *Oral contraceptives,* colloquially termed "the pill," consist of chemicals that are quite similar to natural hormones (estrogen or progesterone). They act by preventing ovulation. When taken according to the instructions, these pills are almost 100% effective. Long-acting *injectable* or *implanted* steroid contraceptives are undergoing clinical trials. Diethylstilbestrol is used as a *"morning after"* contraceptive, esp. in cases of rape or incest.

CHEMICAL: *Spermicides* in the form of foam, cream, jelly, spermicide-impregnated sponge, or suppositories are placed in the vagina prior to intercourse. They may be used alone or in combination with a barrier contraceptive. They act by killing the sperm. *Douching* after intercourse is not effective enough in preventing conception to be thought of as a method of contraception.

PHYSICAL OR BARRIER: *IUD's,* or intrauterine contraceptive devices, are plastic or metal objects placed inside the uterus. They are thought to act by preventing the fertilized egg from attaching itself to the lining of the uterus. Their effectiveness is only slightly lower than that of oral contraceptives. *Diaphragms* are made of a dome-shaped piece of rubber with a flexible spring circling the edge. They are available in various sizes and are inserted into the vagina so as to cover the cervix. A diaphragm must be used in conjunction with a chemical spermicide, which is used prior to positioning the diaphragm. A specially fitted *cervical cap* is also available as a barrier-type contraceptive. There is also a *sponge* impregnated with a contraceptive cream or jelly. These are placed in the vagina up to several hours prior to intercourse. The male partner can use a *condom,* a flexible tube-shaped barrier placed over the erect penis so that the ejaculate is contained in the tube and is not deposited in the vagina. Condoms may be made of rubber or animal membranes, are available in dry as well as wet-lubricated forms, and are manufactured in various colors. Used properly, the condom is a reliable means of contraception. It is more effective as a means of contraception if combined with a chemical spermicide. Condoms also help prevent spread of venereal disease by providing a physical barrier.

NATURAL: *Ovulation methods* involve abstaining from intercourse for a specified number of days before, during, and after ovulation. Rhythm is based on calculating the fertile period by the calendar. In practice, this method has a high rate of failure. Other methods include determining ovulation by charting the woman's basal temperature (SEE: *basal temperature chart*) as well as judging the time of ovulation by observing cyclical changes in the cervical mucus. *Withdrawal,* which is the removal of the penis from the vagina just prior to ejaculation, is a method available for use by men. In practice, it is subject to a high failure rate because sperm may be contained in the pre-ejaculatory fluid from the penis.

PERMANENT: For women: *Tubal ligation* involves surgical division of the fallopian tubes and ligating the cut ends. This procedure does not interfere with the subsequent enjoyment of sexual intercourse. This form of sterilization is effective but virtually irreversible. For men: *Vasectomy* consists of cutting the vas deferens and tying each end so that the sperm can no longer travel from the testicle to the urethra. The procedure has to be done bilaterally and the ejaculate tested for several months postoperatively to be certain sperm are not present. Until two successive tests reveal absence of sperm, the method should not be regarded as having been successful. Attempts to reverse this surgical procedure have been successful only in a small percentage of cases. Vasectomy does not interfere with the normal enjoyment of sexual intercourse.

contract (kŏn-trăkt') [L. *contrahere,* to draw together]. 1. To draw together, reduce in size, or shorten. 2. To acquire through infection, as to contract a disease.

contractile (kŏn-trăk'tĭl). Able to contract or shorten.

contractility (kŏn-trăk-tĭl'ĭ-tē). Having the ability to contract or shorten.

contraction (kŏn-trăk'shŭn). A shortening or tightening, as that of a muscle, or a reduction in size; a shrinking.

c., Braxton Hicks. SEE: *Braxton Hicks sign.*

c., carpopedal. Contraction of the flexor muscles of the hands and feet due to tetany hypocalcemia, or hyperventilation.

c., Dupuytren's. [Baron G. Dupuytren, Fr. surgeon, 1777–1835] Contracture of palmar fascia causing the ring and little fingers to bend into the palm so that they cannot be extended. SEE: *contracture, Dupuytren's,* for illus.

c., isometric. Muscular contraction in which the muscle does not change its length.

c., isotonic. Muscular contraction in which the muscle maintains constant tension by changing its length during the action.

c., postural. The unconscious contraction of muscles that maintain posture.

c., tetanic. Continuous contraction of muscles.

c., tonic. Spasmodic contraction of a muscle for an extended period of time.

contracture (kŏn-trăk'chūr) [L. *contractura*]. 1. Permanent contraction of a muscle due to spasm or paralysis. 2. A condition of fixed high resistance to the passive stretch of a muscle, as may result from fibrosis of tissues surrounding a joint.

c., Dupuytren's. Flexion deformity of hands and fingers due to contraction of the palmar fascia. SEE: illus.

c., functional. Decrease of a contracture during anesthesia or sleep.

c., ischemic. Contraction of a muscle in which the muscle tissue has been replaced by fibrous tissue due to injury.

c., physiological. A temporary condition in which tension and shortening of a muscle are maintained for a considerable time although there is no tetanus. May be induced by heat, action of drugs, or acids.

c., Volkmann's. Pronation and flexion of the hand, with atrophy of the muscles of the forearm. Results from circulatory impairment due to pressure from a cast, constricting dressings, or injury to the radial artery. This can be prevented by being alert to signs

DUPUYTREN'S CONTRACTURE

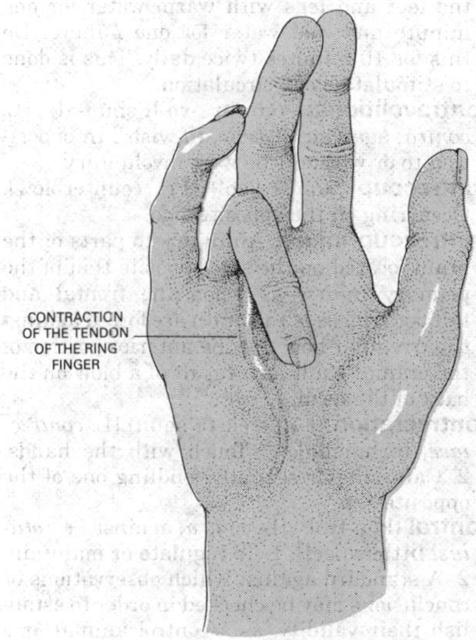

of coldness, pallor, cyanosis, pain, and swelling of the part below the injury or constriction and removal of the cause.

contrafissura (kŏn″tră-fĭ-shū'ră) [L. *contra,* against, + *fissura,* fissure]. A skull fracture at a point opposite from where the blow was received.

contraindication (kŏn″tră-ĭn-dĭ-kā'shŭn) [″ + *indicare,* to point out]. Any symptom or circumstance indicating the inappropriateness of a form of treatment otherwise advisable.

contralateral (kŏn″tră-lăt'ĕr-ăl) [″ + *latus,* side]. Originating in, or affecting, the opposite side of the body. Opposed to homolateral and ipsilateral.

contralateral reflexes. 1. Passive flexion of one part following flexion of another. 2. Passive flexion of one leg causing similar movement of opposite leg.

contrast (kŏn'trăst). In radiography, the difference between adjacent densities on a radiograph resulting from the part radiographed and film characteristics.

contrast medium. A radiopaque substance used to provide during x-ray study a contrast in density between the tissue or organ being filmed and the medium. Thus barium sulfate will when swallowed help to demonstrate the outline of the intestinal tract as x-ray films are taken during the passage of that particular contrast medium.

contrast sprays. Spray administered by having patient sit on side of bathtub, spraying the feet and legs with warm water for one minute and cold water for one minute. Do this for 10 minutes twice daily. This is done to stimulate blood circulation.

contravolitional (kŏn″tră-vō-lĭ′shŭn-ăl) [L. *contra*, against, + *velle*, to wish]. In opposition to or without the will; involuntary.

contrecoup (kŏn-tr-koo′) [Fr., counterblow]. Occurring on the opposite side.

contrecoup injury. An injury to parts of the brain located on the side opposite that of the primary injury, as when the frontal and temporal lobes of the brain are forced against the irregular bones of the anterior portion of the cranial vault as a result of a blow on the back of the head.

contrectation (kŏn″trĕk-tā′shŭn) [L. *contrectare*, to handle]. 1. Touch with the hands. 2. Caressing or sexually fondling one of the opposite sex.

control (kŏn-trōl′) [L. *contra*, against, + *rotulus*, little wheel]. 1. To regulate or maintain. 2. A standard against which observations or conclusions may be checked in order to establish their validity, as a control animal, one that has not been exposed to the treatment or condition being studied in the other animals.

controlled substance act. The Comprehensive Drug Abuse Prevention and Control Act. A law enacted in 1971 designed to control the distribution and use of all depressant and stimulant drugs and other drugs of abuse or potential abuse as may be designated by the Drug Enforcement Administration of the Department of Justice.

Labels of drugs included in this list include a large "C" followed by a Roman numeral designation. Alternatively the Roman numeral is within the large "C".

The act specifies record-keeping by the pharmacist, the format for prescription writing, and limits the amount of a drug that can be legally dispensed. This and whether refills are allowed varies with the nature of the drug. Centrally acting drugs such as narcotics, stimulants, and certain sedatives are divided into five classes called schedules I through V. Schedule I drugs are experimental. Prescriptions for Schedule II drugs may not be refilled. Prescriptions for Schedule III and IV drugs may be refilled up to 5 times within 6 months of the time the initial prescription was written. Schedule V drugs are restricted only to the extent that all nonscheduled prescription drugs are regulated.

contrude (kŏn-trood′) [L. *con*, with, + *trudere*, to thrust]. 1. Abnormal lingual curve or line of dental arch. 2. To crowd together, as the teeth.

contrusion (kŏn-troo′zhŭn). Having the teeth crowded.

contuse (kŏn-tooz′) [L. *contundere*, to bruise]. To bruise.

contusion (kŏn-too′zhŭn). An injury in which the skin is not broken; a bruise.

SYM: Pain, swelling, and discoloration.

F.A.: Apply cold applications. Follow with firm bandage to prevent swelling. Twenty-four to 48 hours later, application of heat is desirable, followed by gentle massage. SEE: *concussion*.

conus (kō′nŭs) [Gr. *konos*]. 1. A cone. 2. Posterior staphyloma of myopic eye.

c. arteriosus. [NA] Right cardiac ventricle's upper rounded anterior angle, where pulmonary artery arises.

c. medullaris. [NA] Conical portion of lower spinal cord.

convalescence (kŏn″văl-ĕs′ĕns) [L. *convalescere*, to become strong]. The period of recovery after the termination of a disease or an operation.

convalescent. 1. Getting well. 2. One who is recovering from a disease or operation.

convalescent diet. A diet suitable for the condition from which the patient is recovering. SEE: *soft diet*.

convection (kŏn-vĕk′shŭn) [L. *convehere*, to convey]. The transference of heat by means of currents in liquids or gases.

convergence (kŏn-vĕr′jĕns) [L. *con*, with, + *vergere*, to incline]. 1. The moving of two or more objects toward the same point. 2. In reflex activity, the coming together of several axons or afferent fibers upon one or a few motor neurons; the condition whereby impulses from several sensory receptors converge upon the same motor center, resulting in a limited and specific response. 3. Visual lines directed to a nearby point.

convergent (kŏn-vĕr′jĕnt). Tending toward a common point.

conversion (kŏn-vĕr′zhŭn) [L. *convertere*, to turn round]. Change from one state to another. In obstetrics, the change in position of a fetus in the uterus in order to facilitate delivery. SEE: *version*.

conversion reaction. A conversion type of hysterical neurosis in which there is loss of or alteration in physical functioning suggesting a physical disorder but instead representing the expression of a psychological conflict or need. The disturbance is not under voluntary control and cannot be explained by a disease process; it is not limited to pain or sexual dysfunction.

conversion symptom. A term for a repressed emotion that becomes manifest through a physical symptom; seen in hyste-

VISUAL CONVERGENCE

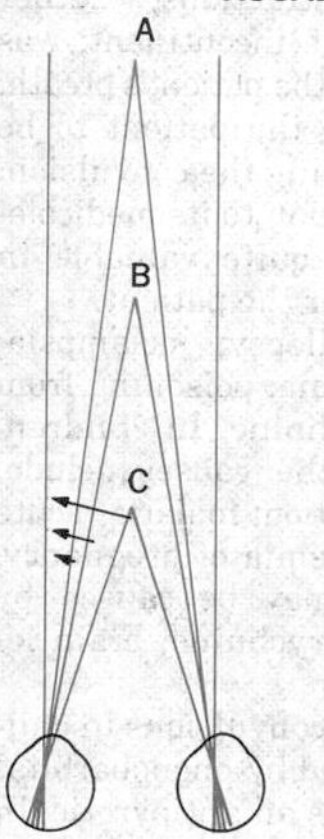

When an object is brought from a distant position (A) to an intermediate position (B), or to a near position (C), the eyes are rotated medially to make the lines of vision meet at the object. The closer the object, the greater the degree of convergence as measured by the angles indicated by arrows.

ria.

convex (kŏn′vĕks, kŏn-vĕks′) [L. *convexus,* vaulted, arched]. Curved evenly; resembling the segment of a sphere.

convexoconcave (kŏn-vĕk″sō-kŏn′kāv, -kŏn-kāv′) [″ + *concavus,* vaulted hollow]. Concave on one side and convex on opposite surface. SYN: *concavoconvex.*

convexoconvex [″ + *convexus,* arched]. Convex on two opposite faces.

convolute (kŏn′vō-loot) [L. *convolvere,* to roll together]. Rolled, as a scroll.

convoluted. Convolute, rolled.

convoluted tubule. In the kidney, the proximal convoluted tubule, which lies between Bowman's capsule and the loop of Henle; the distal convoluted tubule, which lies between the loop of Henle and the collecting duct.

convolution (kŏn″vō-loo′shŭn) [L. *convolvere,* to roll together]. 1. A turn, fold, or coil of anything that is convoluted. 2. In anatomy, a gyrus, one of the many folds on the surface of the cerebral hemispheres. They are separated by grooves (sulci or fissures). SEE: *gyrus.*

c., angular. A gyrus forming posterior portion of inferior parietal lobule.

c.'s, annectant. The four gyri connecting the convolutions on upper surface of occipital lobe with parietal and temporosphenoidal lobes.

c., anterior choroid. Gyrus choroides.

c., anterior orbital. A convolution that lies in front of the orbital sulcus.

c., Arnold's. Gyri posteriores inferiores.

c., ascending frontal. A convolution forming anterior boundary of fissure of Rolando.

c., ascending parietal. A convolution parallel to ascending frontal convolution, separated from it by fissure of Rolando, except at extremities, where they are generally united.

c., Broca's. The inferior, or third, frontal convolution.

c.'s, cerebral. Convolutions of the cerebrum.

c., collosal. Gyrus fornicatus.

c., cuneate. Gyral isthmus.

c., dentate. A small, notched gyrus, rudimentary in man, situated in dentate fissure.

c.'s, exterior olfactory. Small projections forming outer boundary of the olfactory grooves.

c., hippocampal. Uncinate gyrus.

c., inferior frontal. The lower and outer part of frontal lobe.

c., inferior occipital. A small convolution lying between middle and inferior occipital fissures.

c., insular. One of a group of small convolutions forming the island of Reil, entirely concealed by the operculum.

c.'s, intestinal. The coils of the intestines.

c., marginal. Convolution beginning in front of locus perforatus anterior and bounding longitudinal fissure on mesial aspect of the hemisphere.

c., middle frontal. Convolution continuous posterior with ascending frontal convolution and extending forward over anterior end of hemisphere to its orbital surface.

c., middle occipital. A convolution between the first and third occipital convolutions.

c., middle temporosphenoidal. A small gyrus continuous with the middle occipital or angular gyrus.

c.'s, occipitotemporal. Two small convolutions on lower surface of temporosphenoidal lobe.

c. of the corpus callosum. Gyrus fornicatus, q.v.

c. of the sylvian fissure. The convolution that bounds the fissure of Sylvius.

c., olfactory. Olfactory lobe.

c.'s, orbital. Small gyri on orbital surface of frontal lobe.

c.'s, parietal. Ascending parietal convolution and superior parietal convolution.

c., posterior orbital. A small convolution on posterior and outer side of orbital sulcus, and continuous with inferior frontal convolution.

c., second frontal. A convolution on the frontal lobes, lying posteriorly between the superior and inferior frontal sulci. SYN: *c., middle frontal.*

c., superior frontal. A convolution that bounds great longitudinal fissure, arising posterior from upper end of ascending frontal convolution.

c., superior occipital. Upper of the three convolutions on superior surface of occipital lobe.

c., superior parietal. Portion of parietal lobe limited anteriorly by upper part of the fissure of Rolando, posteriorly by exterior parieto-occipital fissure, and inferiorly by intraparietal sulcus.

c., superior temporosphenoidal. Upper of three convolutions forming temporosphenoidal lobe. It lies just below and is parallel with sylvian fissure.

c., supramarginal. The anterior portion of interior parietal lobule behind inferior extremity of intraparietal fissure (sulcus), below which it joins the ascending parietal convolution.

c., transverse orbital. The gyrus occupying posterior portion of inferior surface of frontal lobe, at anterior extremity of fissure of Sylvius.

c., uncinate. A convolution extending from near the posterior extremity of the occipital lobe to apex of the temporosphenoidal.

convulsant (kŏn-vŭl'sănt) [L. *convellere,* to pull together]. 1. An agent that produces a convulsion. 2. Causing onset of a convulsion.

convulsant poisons. Toxic substances that cause the person affected to experience convulsions. The common ones are strychnine and other drugs of the nux vomica group, and various infrequently used drugs, such as picrotoxin.

SYM: These produce a sense of suffocation, dyspnea, and then muscular rigidity; there are powerful tetanic contractions that may be very painful. These spasms may be brought on by trivial stimuli, such as touching the patient, or they may come on at varying intervals of from 3 to 30 minutes and may last from one to five minutes. Trismus, cyanosis, and tachycardia are frequent accompaniments. Death results from asphyxia or exhaustion.

TREATMENT: Appropriate therapy will depend upon substance that caused the convulsion. General measures for emptying the stomach or attempting to neutralize the drug may be indicated. Sedatives may be ordered by the physician. Oxygen and artificial respiration may be indicated.

convulsion (kŏn-vŭl'shŭn). Paroxysms of involuntary muscular contractions and relaxations.

NOTE: It is important for the person who observes the convulsion to record on the chart the following: time of onset; duration; whether or not convulsion started in a certain area of the body or became generalized from the start; type of contractions; whether or not the patient became incontinent; was there an abnormal odor to the patient's breath; did the convulsion cause the patient to be injured or strike head during the convulsion. This information, in addition to its medicolegal importance, will be quite valuable in diagnosis and in caring for the patient.

ETIOL: General: epilepsy; eclampsia; meningitis; tetanus; uremia; poisoning from camphor, cyanides, strychnine. In children, the cause is often fever. Other causes include: rickets; syphilis; malnutrition; malaria; acute infectious disease; or toxemia of pregnancy. In adults, convulsions may be caused by epilepsy; heat cramps; strychnine; brain lesions; or food poisoning.

TREATMENT: Febrile convulsions in children are usually controlled by phenobarbital with or without aspirin as an antipyretic. In adults, the cause must first be found. Keep patient from injuring self. Soft pad between teeth to avoid biting tongue or cheeks. If fever is present, tepid or cool bath. Sedatives or anesthesia may be advised by physician. Aftercare: rest in bed; absolute quiet; careful diagnosis without unduly disturbing patient. SEE: *febrile convulsions*.

c., clonic. Convulsion having intermittent contractions, muscles being alternately contracted and relaxed.

c., febrile. Convulsion associated with fever, esp. in children between the ages of 6 months and 2 to 3 years. Three to 5 percent of children have febrile convulsions. Most febrile convulsions represent a symptom of an acute febrile illness. Nevertheless the child should be examined for the possibility of another cause such as tetany, epilepsy, lead encephalopathy, cerebral concussion, cerebral hemorrhage or tumor, hypoglycemia, or poisoning with a convulsant drug.

c., hysterical. Convulsion caused by hysteria.

c., mimetic. A spasm of facial muscles.

c., oscillating. Convulsion involving separate bundles of muscle fibers that contract alternately.

c., puerperal. Eclamptic convulsion in pregnant or puerperal woman.

c., salaam. Nodding spasm.

c., tonic. Convulsion in which the contractions are maintained for a time, as in tetany.

c., toxic. Convulsion caused by action of a toxin on nervous system.

c., uremic. Convulsion caused by uremic condition.

convulsion, words pert. to: anticonvulsive; apoplexy; athetosis; chill; chorea; coma; consciousness; electroconvulsive therapy; epilepsy; hysteria; ictus; mimetic; paroxysm;

rabies; strychnine; tetanus; tic; tremor.

convulsive (kŏn-vŭl′sĭv). Pert. to convulsions.

convulsive reflex. Incoordinate contraction of muscles in a convulsive manner.

convulsive tic. Spasm of face.

cooking [L. *coquere,* to cook]. The process of heating foods in order to prepare them for eating. Cooking makes most foods more palatable, easier to masticate, improves their digestibility, and destroys or inactivates harmful organisms or toxins that may be present. Cooking releases the aromatic substances and extractives that contribute odors and taste to foods. These odors help to stimulate the appetite.

CAUTION: Not all toxic substances are inactivated by heat. Most microorganisms and parasites are destroyed in the ordinary process of cooking, but some require a higher degree of heat and longer cooking to effect this result. Pork has to be cooked completely throughout in order to kill the encysted larvae of Trichinella. SEE: *trichinosis.*

ACTION: *On protein:* Soluble proteins become coagulated. *On soluble substances:* These, including heat-labile vitamins, are often inactivated by boiling, and even mineral substances and starches, though insoluble to a certain extent, may suffer loss in this process. *On starch:* The starch granules now swell and are changed from insoluble (raw) starch to soluble starch capable of being converted into sugar in the process of digestion and of being assimilated in the system.

Cooley's anemia. [Thomas Cooley, U.S. pediatrician, 1871–1945] Anemia resulting from inheritance of a recessive trait responsible for interference with the rate of hemoglobin synthesis. SYN: *thalassemia major.*

Coombs' test. [R. R. A. Coombs, contemporary Brit. immunologist, b. 1921] A test for antiglobulins in the red cell; used in diagnosing various hemolytic anemias.

coordination (kō-or″dĭn-ā′shŭn) [L. *co-,* same, + *ordinare,* to arrange]. The working together of various muscles for the production of a certain movement. More generally, the working together of different systems of the body in a given process, as the coordination between the system of glands and involuntary muscles in digestion.

COPD. *chronic obstructive pulmonary disease.* SEE: *COLD.*

cope (kōp) [ME. *caupen,* to contend with]. The ability to deal with effectively and handle the stresses to which one is subjected.

coping. Adjusting or adapting successfully to a challenge. The psychological method by which an individual accomplishes this is called the coping mechanism.

copodyskinesia (kō″pō-dĭs″kĭn-ē′sē-ă) [Gr. *kopos,* fatigue, + *dys,* difficult, + *kinesis,* motion]. Fatigue of or difficulty in moving a group of muscles used in working. May be out of proportion to that which would be expected from the amount of work done, in which case it is called occupational neurosis.

copolymer (kō-pŏl′ĭ-mĕr). A polymer composed of two different kinds of monomers.

copper [L. *cuprum*]. SYMB: Cu. At. wt. 63.54; at. no. 29; sp. gr. 8.96. A metal, small quantities of which are utilized by the body. Its salts are irritant poisons. SEE: *Poisons and Poisoning* in *Appendix; Wilson's disease.*

FUNCT.: The total body content of copper is 100 to 150 mg.; the amount ingested each day is less than 2 mg. Copper is an essential component of several enzyme systems. It is present in the liver, and is excreted by the kidneys and in the bile.

DEFICIENCY SYM: Anemia; weakness; impaired respiration and growth; and poor utilization of iron.

SOURCES: Found in many vegetable and animal tissues.

copperas (kŏp′ĕr-ăs). $FeSO_4 \cdot 7H_2O$. Pale bluish-green crystals of ferrous sulfate. Used as disinfectant and deodorizer. SYN: *ferrous sulfate; green vitriol.*

copperhead. A poisonous snake, Agkistrodon contortrix, common in the southern United States. SEE: *snakebite; snake, poisonous.*

copper sulfate. $CuSO_4 \cdot 5H_2O$. Blue vitriol. Deep-blue shiny crystals or granular powder. Astringent when used in proper dilution. Also used as an algicide.

copper sulfate poisoning. SYM: A disagreeable coppery metallic taste with tightness in the throat, nausea and vomiting, thirst, abdominal pains, cramps, and suppression of urine.

F.A.: Wash out stomach, give egg whites raw or beaten. Give demulcent drinks.

copremesis (kŏp-rĕm′ĕ-sĭs) [Gr. *kopros,* dung, + *emesis,* vomiting]. The vomiting of fecal material.

coproantibody (kŏp″rō-ăn′tĭ-bŏd″ē). Any one of a group of antibodies in the feces to various enteric bacteria. They are of the IgA type. Their ability to protect the host has not been shown.

coprolagnia (kŏp″rō-lăg′nē-ă) [″ + *lagneia,* lust]. An erotic satisfaction at the sight or odor of excreta.

coprolalia (kŏp″rō-lā′lē-ă) [″ + *lalia,* babble]. A morbid desire to use sacrilegious or obscene words in ordinary conversation. Seen in some forms of severe mental disorder.

coprolith (kŏp′rō-lĭth) [″ + *lithos,* stone]. Hard, inspissated feces.

coprology (kŏp-rŏl′ō-jē) [″ + *logos,* study of]. Study of the feces. SYN: *scatology.*

coproma (kŏp-rō′mă). Stercoma, q.v.

coprophagy (kŏp-rŏf′ă-jē) [″ + *phagein,* to

eat]. The eating of excrement. SYN: *rhypophagy; scatophagy.*

coprophilia (kŏp"rō-fĭl'ē-ă) [" + *philein,* to love]. Abnormal interest in feces; a perversion in adults.

coprophilic. Term applied to organisms that normally live in fecal material.

coprophobia (kŏp"rō-fō'bē-ă) [" + *phobos,* fear]. A morbid disgust at defecation and feces.

coproporphyria (kŏp"rō-por-fĭr'ē-ă) [" + *porphyra,* purple]. An inherited form of porphyria in which an excess amount of coproporphyrin is excreted in the feces.

coproporphyrin (kŏp"rō-por'fĭr-ĭn). A porphyrin present in urine and feces. Coproporphyrins I and II are normally present in minute and equal amounts, but quantities are altered in certain diseases as poliomyelitis, infectious hepatitis, and in lead poisoning.

coproporphyrinuria (kŏp"rō-por"fĭr-ĭn-ū'rē-ă). Excess coproporphyrin in the urine.

coprostanol (kŏp"rō-stā'nōl). A derivative of cholesterol present in feces, usually the result of bacterial action in the large intestine.

coprozoa (kŏp"rō-zō'ă) [" + *zoon,* animal]. Protozoa in fecal matter outside of the intestine.

coprozoic (kŏp"rō-zō'ĭk). Pert. to coprozoa; found in feces or fecal matter.

copula (kŏp'ū-lă) [L., link]. 1. Any connecting part. 2. A median elevation on floor of embryonic pharynx representing future root of the tongue; copula linguae.

copulation (kŏp"ū-lā'shŭn) [L. *copulatio*]. Sexual intercourse. SYN: *coition; coitus; concubitus.*

cor (kor) [L.]. [NA] The heart.

c. pulmonale. SEE: *cor pulmonale.*

coracoacromial (kor"ă-kō-ă-krō'mē-ăl) [Gr. *korax,* raven, + *akron,* point, + *omos,* shoulder]. Pert. to acromial and coracoid processes.

coracoid (kor'ă-koyd) [" + *eidos,* appearance]. Resembling, in shape, a crow's beak.

coracoid process. Process on upper anterior surface of scapula.

cord [Gr. *khorde*]. 1. A stringlike structure. 2. The umbilical cord. 3. A firm elongated structure consistent with a thrombosed vein, esp. one in the extremities, where it may be detected by palpation.

c., spermatic. Cord by which the testis is connected to the abdominal inguinal ring. It consists of the ductus deferens, blood vessels, lymphatics, and nerves supplying the testis and epididymis. These are enclosed in the cremasteric fascia, which forms an investing sheath.

c., spinal. That portion of the central nervous system contained in the spinal canal. The center of the cord consists of gray matter, which is composed of nerve cells, dendrites, and their processes. The white matter is arranged in tracts outside the gray matter. It consists of medullated nerve fibers that are going to and from the brain, connecting various layers of gray matter in the cord, and leaving and entering the spinal column. The cord serves as a conducting pathway for sensory impulses to the brain and motor impulses from the brain. It also serves as a reflex center for many reflex acts. SYN: *medulla spinalis* [NA].

c., umbilical. The cord that connects the circulatory system of the fetus to the placenta.

cordal (kor'dăl). Concerning a cord, e.g., spinal or vocal cord.

cordate (kor'dāt) [L. *cor,* heart]. Shaped like a heart.

cord bladder. Distention of the bladder without discomfort.

SYM: Tending to void frequently and dribbling after urination.

ETIOL: Lesion affecting the posterior roots of the spinal column at the level of bladder innervation above the sacral level.

cordectomy (kor-dĕk'tō-mē) [Gr. *khorde,* cord, + *ektome,* excision]. Surgical removal of a cord.

cordiform (kor'dĭ-form) [L. *cor,* heart, + *forma,* shape]. Shaped like a heart.

corditis (kor-dī'tĭs) [Gr. *khorde,* cord, + *itis,* inflammation]. Inflammation of the spermatic cord. SYN: *funiculitis.*

cordopexy (kor'dō-pĕk"sē) [" + *pexis,* fixation]. Operative fixation of an anatomical cord, esp. the vocal cords.

cordotomy (kor-dŏt'ō-mē) [" + *tome,* incision]. Spinal cord section of lateral pathways to relieve pain. SYN: *chordotomy.*

Cordran. Trade name for flurandrenolide.

core (kor). The center of a structure.

coreclisis (kor"ē-klī'sĭs) [Gr. *kore,* pupil of the eye, + *kleisis,* closure]. Occlusion of the pupil. SYN: *iridencleisis.*

corectasia, corectasis (kor-ĕk-tā'zē-ă, -ĕk'tă-sĭs) [" + *ektasis,* dilatation]. Dilatation of the pupil of the eye resulting from disease.

corectome (kō-rĕk'tōm) [" + *ektome,* excision]. Instrument used for cutting or removing the iris. SYN: *iridectome.*

corectomy (kō-rĕk'tō-mē). Surgical removal of the iris. SYN: *iridectomy.*

corectopia (kor-ĕk-tō'pē-ă) [" + *ek,* out of, + *topos,* place]. Having the pupil to one side of the center of the iris.

coredialysis (kō"rē-dī-ăl'ĭ-sĭs) [" + *dialysis,* separation]. Separation of outer border of iris from its ciliary attachment.

corediastasis (kor"ē-dī-ăs'tă-sĭs) [" + *diastasis,* a standing apart]. Dilatation of pupil.

corelysis (kor-ĕl'ĭ-sĭs) [" + *lysis,* destruction].

Obliteration of pupil because of adhesions of iris to cornea.

coremorphosis (kor″ē-mor-fō′sĭs) [″ + *morphe,* form, + *osis,* condition]. Establishment of an artificial pupil.

coreometer (kō″rē-ŏm′ĕ-tĕr) [″ + *metron,* measure]. Instrument for measurement of the pupil.

coreometry (kō″rē-ŏm′ĕ-trē). Measurement of the pupil of the eye.

coreoplasty (kō′rē-ō-plăs″tē) [″ + *plassein,* to form]. Any operation for forming an artificial pupil.

corepressor (kō″rē-prĕs′sor). The substance capable of activating the repressor produced by a regulator gene.

corestenoma (kor″ē-stĕn-ō′mă) [″ + *stenoma,* contraction]. Narrowing of pupil.

c. congenitum. Partial congenital obliteration of pupil by outgrowths from the iris that form a partial gridlike covering over the pupil.

core temperature. The body's temperature in deep structures such as the liver or heart, as opposed to the peripheral areas.

coretomedialysis (kor″ĕt-ō-mē-dē-ăl′ĭ-sĭs) [″ + *tome,* incision, + *dialysis,* division]. Making of an artificial pupil through the iris. SYN: *iridodialysis.*

coretomy (kō-rĕt′ō-mē) [″ + *tome,* incision]. Any incision of the iris. SYN: *iridotomy.*

Cori cycle (kō′rē). [Carl F. Cori, U.S. pharmacologist and biochemist, b. 1896; Gerty T. Cori, U.S. biochemist, 1896–1957] In carbohydrate metabolism, the breakdown of muscle glycogen, with formation of lactic acid, which enters the bloodstream, is converted to liver glycogen, which in turn breaks down into glucose, which is carried to muscles where it is reconverted to muscle glycogen.

corium (kō′rē-ŭm) [L., skin]. (pl. *coria*) [NA] The layer of the skin lying immediately under the epidermis; the true skin. Consists of two layers, papillary and reticular. It is composed of loose connective tissue in which are numerous capillaries, lymphatics, and nerve endings. In it lie hair follicles, sebaceous glands, sweat glands and their ducts, and smooth muscle fibers. SYN: *cutis vera; dermis.*

corm (korm) [Gr. *kormos,* a trimmed tree trunk]. A short bulb-shaped, underground stem of a plant such as the cochicum.

corn [L. *cornu,* horn]. Horny induration and thickening of the skin, hard or soft, according to location. SYN: *clavus.*

ETIOL: Pressure or friction or both from ill-fitting shoes.

SYM: Hard corns on exposed surfaces have a horny core of conical shape extending down into the derma, causing pain and irritation. Soft corns that occur between the toes are kept soft by moisture and maceration. This may lead to inflammation beneath the corn. Infection with pyogenic organisms results in suppuration.

TREATMENT: Remove cause by use of properly fitting shoes of soft leather and proper shape. Materials made from spongelike substances for absorbing energy and thus preventing friction are available for lining shoes or bandaging the area of the foot being abraded. Local application of a keratolytic agent for removal of corn. Corn pads to relieve pressure. Services of a chiropodist may be necessary. Special care to patients with diabetes or a circulatory condition.

cornea (kor′nē-ă) [L. *corneus,* horny]. [NA] The clear, transparent anterior portion of the fibrous coat of the eye comprising about one sixth of its surface. Its curvature being greater than that of the remainder of the bulb enables it to function as an important refractive medium. It is continuous at its periphery with the sclera. It is composed of five layers: layer of epithelium; Bowman's membrane (anterior limiting membrane); substantia propria corneae [NA]; Descemets' membrane; and a layer of endothelium.

cornea, words pert. to: abrasio corneae; anterior chamber; arcus senilis; "cera-" words; chemosis; circumcorneal; "kerat-" words; macula cornea; megalocornea; microcornea; nebula; pannus; phlyctenula; rhytidosis; staphyloma; synechia.

corneal. Pert. to the cornea.

corneal impression. Obtaining of antigen material by pressing a swab or slide against the cornea. Used in doing certain tests for rabies.

corneal reflex. Closure of eyelids resulting from direct corneal irritation.

corneitis (kor″nē-ī′tĭs) [L. *corneus,* horny, + Gr. *itis,* inflammation]. Inflammation of the cornea. SYN: *keratitis.*

Cornell Medical Index. A lengthy all-inclusive self-administered history form developed at Cornell University Medical School.

corneoblepharon (kor″nē-ō-blĕf′ă-rŏn) [″ + Gr. *blepharon,* eyelid]. Adhesion of the eyelid to the cornea.

corneoiritis (kor″nē-ō-ī-rī′tĭs) [L. *corneus,* horny, + Gr. *iris,* iris, + *itis,* inflammation]. Inflammation of iris and cornea.

corneomandibular reflex (kor″nē-ō-măn-dĭb′ū-lăr). Deflexion of mandible toward opposite side when cornea is irritated while mouth is open and relaxed.

corneosclera (kor″nē-ō-sklē′ră) [L. *corneus,* horny, + *skleros,* hard]. The cornea and sclera considered together comprising the tunica fibrosa [NA] or fibrous coat of the eye.

corneous (kor′nē-ŭs) [L. *corneus*]. Horny; hornlike.

corneous layer. Horny outer layer of the epidermis. SYN: *stratum corneum* [NA].

corneum (kor′nē-ŭm) [L., horny]. Horny layer of the skin. SYN: *stratum corneum.* SEE: *stratum* for illus.

corniculate (kor-nĭk′ū-lāt). Containing small horn-shaped projections.

corniculum (kor-nĭk′ū-lŭm) [L., little horn]. A small, hornlike process.

cornification (kor″nĭ-fĭ-kā′shŭn) [″ + *facere,* to make]. The process by which squamous epithelial cells are converted into hard horny material as in the corneum of the skin or in structures such as horns, hair, and feathers that are derived from epithelium.

cornified (kor′nĭ-fīd). Changed into horny tissue.

cornu (kor′nū) [L., horn]. (pl. *cornua*) [NA] Any projection like a horn.

c. ammonis. Hippocampus major of brain.

c. anterius. [NA] The anterior horn of the lateral ventricle.

c. coccygeum. [NA] Two upward projecting processes that articulate with the sacrum.

c. cutaneum. Hornlike excrescence on skin.

c. inferius. [NA] The inferior horn of the lateral ventricle.

c. of the hyoid. The greater and lesser horns of the hyoid bones, q.v.

c. of the sacrum. Two small processes projecting inferiorly on either side of the sacral hiatus leading into the sacral canal.

c. posterius. [NA] The posterior horn of the lateral ventricle.

cornua (kor′nū-ă). Pl. of cornu.

cornual (kor′nū-ăl). Pert. to a cornu.

corona (kŏ-rō′nă) [Gr. *korone,* crown]. [NA] Any structure resembling a crown.

c. capitis. Crown of head.

c. ciliaris. [NA] Circular figure on inner surface of ciliary body.

c. dentis. [NA] Crown of a tooth.

c. glandis. [NA] Posterior border of glans penis.

c. radiata. 1. [NA] Ascending and descending fibers of the internal capsule that, above the corpus callosum, extend in all directions to the cerebral cortex. Many of the fibers arise in the thalamus. 2. A thin mass of follicle cells that adhere firmly to the zona pellucida of the human ovum following ovulation.

c. veneris. Syphilitic blotches on forehead that parallel the hairline.

coronal (kō-rō′năl). Pert. to a corona.

coronal plane. Plane dividing the body into front and back portions.

coronal suture. Suture that joins the parietal and frontal bones of the cranium.

coronary (kor′ō-nă-rē) [L. *coronarius,* pert. to a crown or circle]. Encircling, as the blood vessels that supply blood directly to the heart muscle. Loosely used to refer to the heart. Coronary pain is usually dull and heavy; typically the patient describes the pain as being viselike or producing a feeling of compression or squeezing of the chest.

coronary angiography. Radiographic examination of the coronary arteries after injection of a contrast agent.

coronary arteries. 1. One of a pair of arteries that supply blood to the myocardium of the heart. They arise within the right and left aortic sinuses at base of the aorta. Decreased flow of blood through these arteries induces attacks of angina pectoris, q.v. 2. The cervical branch of the uterine artery.

coronary artery disease. ABBR: CAD. Narrowing of the coronary arteries sufficiently to prevent adequate blood supply to the myocardium. The narrowing is usually caused by arteriosclerosis; and it may progress to the point where the heart muscle is damaged due to lack of blood supply. SEE: *angina pectoris; coronary bypass;* illus.

coronary bypass. A shunt, established surgically, that permits blood to travel from the aorta to a branch of the coronary artery at a point past an obstruction. Used in treating coronary artery disease. SYN: *aortocoronary bypass.*

coronary care unit. A specially equipped area of a hospital for providing intensive nursing and medical care for patients who have acute coronary thrombosis.

coronary heart disease. ABBR: CHD. Myocardial damage due to insufficient blood supply. The disease is caused by pathological changes in the coronary arteries sufficient to interfere with adequate blood flow.

coronary occlusion. Closing off of a coronary artery. SYN: *coronary thrombosis.*

coronary plexus. A network of autonomic nerve fibers that lies close to base of heart.

coronary sinus. The vessel cavity or passage that receives the cardiac veins from the heart. It opens into right atrium.

coronary thrombosis. Occlusion of one or more of the coronary arteries of the heart.

coronaviruses (kor″ō-nă-vī′rŭs-ĕs) [L. *corona,* crown, + *virus,* poison]. A group of viruses that are morphologically similar, ether-sensitive, and probably composed of RNA, that are responsible for some but not all common colds. So named because their microscopic appearance is that of a virus particle surrounded by a crown.

coroner (kor′ŏ-nĕr) [L. *corona,* crown]. An official (originally, English crown officer) who investigates and holds inquests concerning those dead from unknown or violent causes. The coroner may or may not be a physician,

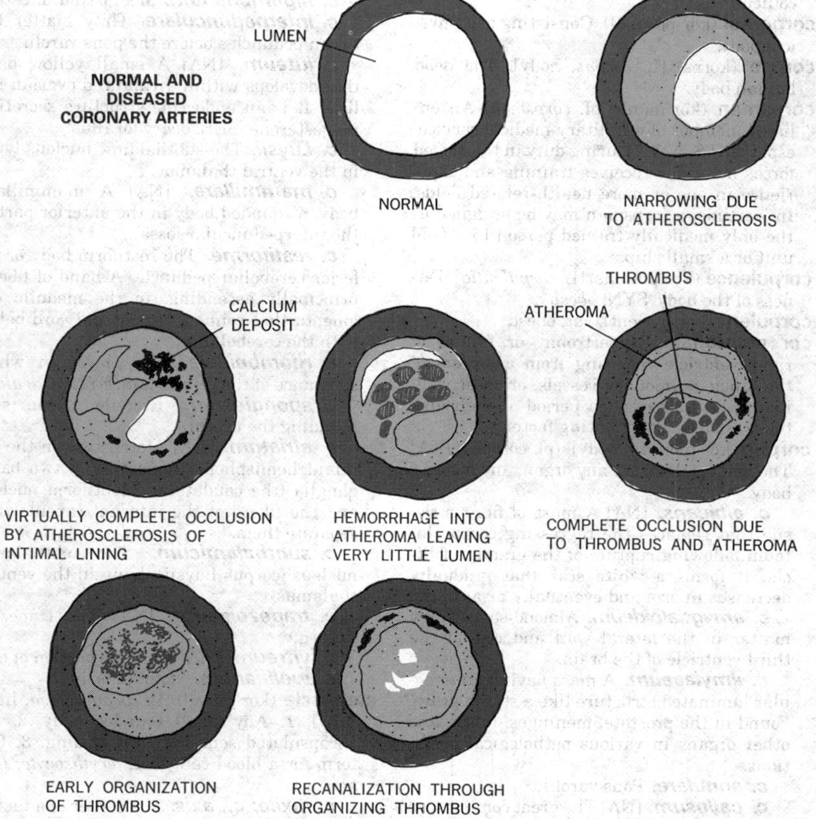

depending upon the law in each state.

coronoid (kor′ō-noyd) [Gr. *korone*, something curved, kind of crown, + *eidos*, appearance]. Shaped like a crown.

coronoidectomy (kor″ō-noy-dĕk′tō-mē) [″ + ″ + *ektome*, excision]. Excision of the coronoid process of the mandible of the jaw.

coronoid fossa. An oval depression on anterior surface of distal end of humerus. Receives coronoid process of ulna.

coronoid process. 1. A process on proximal end of ulna. Forms anterior portion of semilunar notch. 2. A process on the anterior upper end of the ramus of the mandible that serves for attachment of the temporalis muscle.

coroparelcysis (kor″ō-păr-ĕl′sĭ-sĭs) [Gr. *kore*, pupil, + *parelkein*, to draw aside]. Surgically bringing the pupil to one side in central corneal opacity so that it lies under a transparent area.

coroscopy (kō-rŏs′kō-pē) [″ + *skopein*, to examine]. Shadow test to determine refractive error of an eye. SYN: *skiascopy*.

corotomy (kō-rŏt′ō-mē) [″ + *tome*, incision]. Surgical incision of the iris. Iridotomy, q.v.

corpora (kor′pō-ră). Pl. of corpus, q.v.

c. Arantii. Tubercle found in center of semilunar valves of heart.

c. arenacea. Psammoma bodies found in the pineal body. SYN: *brain sand*.

c. cavernosa penis. [NA] Two columns of erectile tissue on dorsum of the penis.

c. olivaria. Two oval masses behind pyramids of the oblongata.

c. paraaortica. Organs of Zuckerkandl, q.v.

c. quadrigemina. The superior portion

of the midbrain consisting of two pairs of rounded bodies, the superior and inferior colliculi.

corporeal (kor-pō'rē-ăl). Consisting of a physical body.

corpse (korps) [L. *corpus,* body]. The dead human body.

corpsman (kor'măn). (pl. *corpsmen*) An enlisted member of a military medical service, esp. the U.S. Navy. During duty in the armed forces he or she receives training and experience in one or more health-related fields. In wartime, a corpsman may be assigned as the only medically trained person to a field unit or a small ship.

corpulence (kor'pū-lĕns) [L. *corpulentia*]. Fatness of the body. SYN: *obesity.*

corpulent (kor'pū-lĕnt). Fat; obese.

cor pulmonale. Hypertrophy or failure of right ventricle resulting from disorders of the lungs, pulmonary vessels, or chest wall. Living for an extended period at high altitudes is also a contributing factor.

corpus (kor'pŭs) [L., body]. (pl. *corpora*) [NA] The principal part of any organ; any mass or body.

c. albicans. [NA] A mass of fibrous tissue that replaces the regressing corpus luteum following rupture of the graafian follicle. It forms a white scar that gradually decreases in size and eventually disappears.

c. amygdaloideum. Almond-shaped gray matter in the lateral wall and roof of the third ventricle of the brain.

c. amylaceum. A mass having an irregular laminated structure like a starch grain. Found in the prostate, meninges, lungs, and other organs in various pathological conditions.

c. annulare. Pons varolii.

c. callosum. [NA] The great commissure of the brain between the cerebral hemispheres.

c. cavernosum. Any erectile tissue, esp. the erectile bodies of the penis, clitoris, male or female urethra, bulb of the vestibule, or the nasal conchae.

c. cerebellum. The two lateral portions of the cerebellum exclusive of the central flocculonodular node.

c. ciliare. [NA] Ciliary body.

c. dentale. Gray layer in white substance of the cerebellum. SYN: *c. rhomboidale.*

c. fimbriatum. White layer edging the lower cornu of the lateral ventricle.

c. flavum. A waxy body seen in the central nervous system.

c. fornicis. [NA] The body of the fornix.

c. geniculatum. The medial or lateral geniculate body, q.v.; a mass of gray matter lying in the thalamus.

c. hemorrhagicum. Blood clot formed in the cavity left by rupture of the graafian follicle.

c. highmorianum. Mediastinum testis.

c. interpedunculare. Gray matter between peduncles before the pons varolii.

c. luteum. [NA] A small yellow body that develops within a ruptured ovarian follicle. It is an endocrine structure secreting progesterone. SEE: *ovary* for illus.

c. Luysii. The subthalamic nucleus lying in the ventral thalamus.

c. mammillare. [NA] A mammillary body; a rounded body in the anterior part of the interpeduncular fossa.

c. restiforme. The restiform body or inferior cerebellar peduncle. A band of fibers, principally ascending, in the medulla oblongata that connects the spinal cord below with the cerebellum.

c. rhomboidale. Gray layer in white substance of the cerebellum. SYN: *c. dentale.*

c. spongiosum. Erectile tissue surrounding the urethra.

c. striatum. [NA] A structure in the cerebral hemispheres consisting of two basal ganglia (the caudate and lentiform nuclei), and the fibers of the internal capsule that separate them.

c. subthalamicum. The subthalamic nucleus (corpus Luysii), lying in the ventral thalamus.

c. trapezoideum. [NA] The trapezoid body, q.v.

c. vitreum. [NA] Vitreous portion of eye.

c. wolffianum. Wolffian body.

corpuscle (kor'pŭs-ĕl) [L. *corpusculum,* little body]. 1. Any small rounded body. 2. An encapsulated sensory nerve ending. 3. Old term for a blood cell. SEE: *erythrocyte; leukocyte.*

c., axile; c., axis. The center of a tactile corpuscle.

c., blood. An erythrocyte or leukocyte.

c., bone. A bone cell.

c., cancroid. Characteristic nodule in cutaneous epithelioma.

c., cartilage. A cell characteristic of cartilage.

c., chromophil. Tiny body found in cytoplasm of a nerve cell. SYN: *Nissl body.*

c.'s, chyle. Corpuscles seen in chyle.

c., colloid. Corpus amylaceum.

c., colostrum. A cell containing phagocytosed fat globules present in milk secreted the first few days after parturition. SYN: *colostrum body.*

c.'s, corneal. Connective tissue corpuscles found in fibrous tissue of cornea.

c.'s, Drysdale's. Transparent cells found in the fluid of certain ovarian cysts.

c., genital. Encapsulated sensory nerve endings resembling pacinian corpuscles present in skin of external genitalia and nipple.

c., ghost. A decolorized red blood cell. SYN: *achromatocyte; phantom corpuscle.*

c.'s, Gierke's. Particles seen in the thymus gland. SYN: *Hassall's corpuscles.*

c.'s, Gluge's. Particles seen in diseased nervous tissue.

c.'s, Golgi-Mazzoni. Tactile corpuscles in the skin of the finger tips.

c.'s, Hassall's. Corpuscles found in the thymus gland. SYN: *c.'s, Gierke's.*

c.'s, Krause's. Sensory encapsulated nerve endings in mucosa of genitalia, mouth, nose, and eyes.

c., lymph. A lymphocyte.

c., malpighian. 1. A renal corpuscle consisting of a glomerulus and Bowman's capsule, which encloses it. 2. A malpighian body of the spleen.

c.'s, Mazzoni's. Nerve endings resembling Krause's corpuscles.

c., Meissner's. An encapsulated touch receptor found in connective tissue immediately underlying the epidermis of the skin, esp. on palmar and volar surfaces of hands and feet. SYN: *c., tactile.*

c., milk. Fat-filled globules present in milk. They represent the distal ends of mammary gland cells that are broken off in apocrine secretion.

c., pacinian. A large, ovoid, sensory end-organ consisting of concentric layers or lamellae of connective tissue surrounding a nerve ending. They are present in tendons, intermuscular septa, connective tissue membranes, and sometimes internal organs, and function as proprioceptive receptors and as receptors of deep pressure.

c., phantom. A decolorized red blood cell. SYN: *c., ghost.*

c., Purkinje's. SEE: *Purkinje cells.*

c., red. An erythrocyte.

c., renal. A glomerulus and the capsule (Bowman's capsule) that surrounds it. It is located at the proximal end of a renal tubule. SYN: *c., malpighian.*

c., reticulated. Erythrocytes that when properly stained show filamentous reticulations.

c., splenic. A nodule of lymphatic tissue present in the spleen.

c., tactile. A sensory end-organ that responds to touch, as Meissner's corpuscle, q.v.

c., terminal. A nerve ending. SEE: *nerve.*

c., thymic. Corpuscles found in the thymus.

c., Wagner's tactile. A sensory end-organ that responds to touch, as Meissner's corpuscle, q.v.

c., white. A leukocyte.

corpuscular (kor-pŭs'kū-lăr). Pert. to corpuscles.

corpusculum (kŏr-pŭs'kū-lŭm) [L., little body]. (pl. *corpuscula*) [NA] Corpuscle.

corrective (kŏ-rĕk'tĭv) [L. *corrigere,* to correct]. 1. A drug that modifies action of another. 2. Pert. to such a drug.

correlation (kor"ĕ-lā'shŭn) [L. *com-,* together, + *relatio,* relation]. 1. The processes by which the various activities of the body, esp. nervous impulses, occur in proper relation to each other. 2. In statistics, the degree to which one variable increases or decreases with respect to another variable. The positive correlation is greatest when the coefficient of correlation is plus 1.0; the negative correlation is maximum when the coefficient is minus one; the correlation is least when the value is zero. A variable can have a positive or negative correlation with another variable.

correspondence. The act or state of corresponding, i.e., occurring in proper relationship to other phenomena.

c., retinal. Condition occurring in normal vision in which images formed on the maculae or other points of the retinas of the two eyes are mentally blended and seen as a single image.

corresponding. Agreeing with, matching, or fitting.

corresponding points of retina. Identical points; points on the retinas of the two eyes that when stimulated give rise to a single image.

Corrigan's pulse (kor'ĭ-găns). [Sir Dominic J. Corrigan, Ir. physician, 1802–1880] A full bounding pulse that appears to be completely empty between beats. Associated with aortic insufficiency. SYN: *waterhammer pulse.*

corrosion (kŏ-rō'zhŭn) [L. *corrodere,* to corrode]. Slow disintegration or wearing away of something by a destructive agent.

corrosive (kŏ-rō'sĭv). Producing corrosion.

corrosive alkalies. Corrosive hydroxides most commonly of sodium, ammonium, and potassium, as well as carbonates. Because of their great combining power with water and their action on the fatty tissues, they cause rapid deep destruction. They have a tendency to gelatinize tissue, turning it a somewhat grayish color and forming a soapy, slippery surface, accompanied by pain and burning.

corrosive poisoning. Poisoning by strong acids, alkalies, strong antiseptics including bichloride of mercury, carbolic acid (phenol), lysol, cresol compounds, tincture of iodine, and arsenic compounds. These are destructive and cause disintegration similar to that caused by burns. If they are swallowed, any part of alimentary canal may be affected. Tissues involved are altered, easily perforated, or destroyed. Death comes very shortly from shock or swelling of throat and pharynx, which causes choking, or by closure of esophagus, causing slow starvation. SEE: individual poisons in *Poisons and Poisoning* in *Appendix*.

SYM: Intense burning about mouth, throat, pharynx, and abdomen; abdominal cramping, retching, nausea, vomiting, and often collapse. There may be bloody vomitus (hematemesis) and diarrhea; the stools are watery, mucoid, bloody, and possibly stained with the poison or its products, resulting from its action on the contents of the alimentary tract. Stains about the lips, cheeks, tongue, mouth, or pharynx are often characteristic brown; stains on mucous membranes may be violet-colored or black. Carbolic acid or phenol leaves a white or gray stain resembling boiled meat; hydrochloric acid stains are grayish; nitric acid leaves a yellow stain; sulfuric acid leaves tan or dark burns.

TREATMENT: Immediate treatment preferably in a hospital is mandatory. It is also important to attempt to discover the chemical substance ingested; for this reason save all materials such as bottles, food, jars or containers that may help to answer this question. This is essential when the patient is either comatose or an infant. In treating corrosive poisoning, DO NOT INDUCE VOMITING; DO NOT ATTEMPT GASTRIC LAVAGE; and DO NOT ATTEMPT TO NEUTRALIZE THE CORROSIVE SUBSTANCE. Vomiting will increase the severity of damage to the esophagus by having the corrosive substance again come in contact with it. Attempting gastric lavage may result in perforating either the esophagus or stomach. Immediately dilute the corrosive substance by having patient drink milk or water. If trachea has been damaged tracheostomy may be needed. Opiates will be needed to control pain. For esophageal burns begin broad-spectrum antibiotics and corticosteroid therapy. Intravenous fluids will be required if esophageal or gastric damage prevents ingestion of liquids. Long-range therapy will be directed toward preventing or treating esophageal scars and strictures.

corrugator (kor′ū-gā″tor) [L. *con,* together, + *rugare,* to wrinkle]. A muscle that lies above the orbit arising medially from frontal bone and having its insertion on skin of medial half of the eyebrows. It draws the brow medially and inferiorly.

Cortef. Trade name for hydrocortisone.

Cortef Acetate. Trade name for hydrocortisone acetate.

Cortenema. Trade name for hydrocortisone retention enema.

cortex (kor′tĕks) [L., rind]. (pl. *cortices*) 1. [NA] The outer layer of an organ as distinguished from the inner medulla as in the adrenal gland, kidney, ovary, lymph node, thymus, and cerebrum and cerebellum of the brain. 2. The outer layer of a structure as a hair or the lens of the eye. 3. The outer superficial portion of the stem or root of a plant.

c., adrenal. The outer layer of the adrenal gland; secretes mineralocorticoids, androgens, and glucocorticoids.

c., cerebellar. The surface layer of the cerebellum consisting of three layers: outer or molecular, middle, and inner or granular layer. Purkinje's cells are present in the middle layer.

c., cerebral. The thin, convoluted surface layer of gray matter of the cerebral hemispheres, consisting principally of cell bodies of neurons arranged in five layers. There are also numerous fibers.

c., interpretive. The temporal cortex where memories of the past may be evoked by electric stimulation.

c., renal. SEE: *kidney.*

c., temporal. Outer layer of brain behind the temples.

Corti, Alfonso (kor′tē). Italian anatomist, 1822–1888.

C., canal of. A triangular-shaped canal extending the entire length of the organ of Corti. Its walls are formed by the external and internal pillar cells.

C.'s membrane. A delicate film of gelatinous consistency that covers the cochlear duct of the inner ear. SEE: *C., organ of.*

C., organ of. An elongated spiral structure running the entire length of the cochlea in the floor of the cochlear duct and resting on the basilar membrane. It is the end-organ of hearing and contains hair cells, supporting cells, and neuroepithelial receptors stimulated by sound waves. SEE: *C.'s membrane.*

cortiadrenal (kor″tē-ăd-rē′năl) [L. *cortex,* rind, + *ad,* toward, + *ren,* kidney]. Pert. to cortex of adrenal gland.

cortical (kor′tĭ-kăl). Pert. to a cortex.

corticate (kor′tĭ-kāt). Possessing a cortex or bark.

corticectomy (kor″tĭ-sĕk′tō-mē) [″ + Gr. *ektome,* excision]. Surgical removal of a portion of the cerebral cortex.

cortices (kor″tĭ-sēz′). Pl. of cortex.

corticifugal (kor″tĭ-sĭf′ū-găl) [L. *cortex,* rind, + *fugere,* to flee]. Conducting impulses away from the outer surface or cortex; particularly denoting axons of pyramidal cells of the cerebral cortex. SYN: *corticoefferent.*

corticipetal (kor″tĭ-sĭp′ĕ-tăl) [″ + *petere,* to seek]. Conducting impulses toward the outer surface, or cortex; particularly denoting fibers of the thalamic radiation conveying impulses to sensory areas of cerebral cortex.

SYN: *corticoafferent.*

corticoadrenal (kor″tĭ-kō-ăd-rē′năl) [″ + *ad,* toward, + *ren,* kidney]. Pert. to cortex of adrenal gland.

corticoafferent (kor″tĭ-kō-ăf′fĕr-ĕnt) [″ + *adferre,* to bear to]. Conducting impulses toward the outer surface or cortex; conveying impulses to sensory areas of the cerebral cortex. SYN: *corticipetal.*

corticobulbar (kor″tĭ-kō-bŭl′băr) [″ + *bulbus,* bulb]. Pert. to the cerebral cortex and upper portion of the brain stem, as corticobulbar tract.

corticoefferent (kor″tĭ-kō-ĕf′ĕr-ĕnt) [″ + *efferre,* to bring out of]. Conducting impulses away from the outer surface or cortex; particularly denoting axons of pyramidal cells of the cerebral cortex. SYN: *corticifugal.*

corticoid (kor′tĭ-koyd) [″ + Gr. *eidos,* form]. Any of a number of hormonal steroid substances obtained from the cortex of the adrenal gland. SYN: *corticosteroid.*

corticopeduncular (kor″tĭ-kō-pē-dŭng′kū-lăr) [″ + *pedunculus,* little foot]. Pert. to cortex and cerebral peduncles.

corticopleuritis (kor″tĭ-kō-ploo-rī′tĭs) [″ + Gr. *pleura,* rib, + *itis,* inflammation]. Inflammation of the outer parts of the pleura.

corticopontine (kor″tĭ-kō-pŏn′tīn) [″ + *pons,* bridge]. Concerning or connecting the cerebral cortex and the pons of the brain.

corticospinal (kor″tĭ-kō-spī′năl) [″ + *spina,* thorn]. Pert. to cerebral cortex and spinal cord. SYN: *spinocortical.*

corticosteroid (kor″tĭ-kō-stēr′oyd). Any of a number of hormonal steroid substances obtained from the cortex of the adrenal gland. They are classified according to their biological activity as glucocorticoids, mineralocorticoids, and androgen. Adrenal corticosteroids do not initiate cellular and enzymatic activity, but permit many biochemical reactions to proceed at optimal rates.

corticosterone (kor″tĭ-kŏs′tē-rōn). A hormone of the adrenal cortex. Corticosterone influences carbohydrate, potassium and sodium metabolism. It is essential for normal absorption of glucose, the formation of glycogen in the liver and tissues, and the normal utilization of carbohydrates by the tissues. SEE: *adrenocorticotropic hormones.*

corticothalamic (kor″tĭ-kō-thă-lăm′ĭk) [″ + Gr. *thalamos,* chamber]. Concerning or connecting the cerebral cortex and the thalamus of the brain.

corticotrophic, corticotropic (kor″tĭ-kō-trŏf′ĭk, -trŏp′ĭk) [″ + Gr. *trophe,* nourishment; ″ + Gr. *trope,* a turn]. Pert. to corticotrophin.

corticotrophin, corticotropin (kor″tĭ-kō-trō′fĭn, -trō′pĭn). The adrenocorticotrophic factor or principle in the anterior lobe of the pituitary gland. Stimulates adrenal cortex to secrete steroid hormones. Trade names are Acthar and Corticotrophin Gel ACTH. Trade name for corticotrophin zinc hydroxide is Cortrophin Zinc ACTH. SYN: *ACTH.*

corticotrophin releasing factor. A substance present in the hypothalamus that controls secretion of adrenocorticotrophin.

cortin (kor′tĭn) [L. *cortex,* rind]. An extract of the cortex of the adrenal gland; contains a mixture of the active steroid agents such as corticosterone.

cortisol (kor′tĭ-sŏl). An adrenocortical hormone, usually referred to pharmaceutically as hydrocortisone. Closely related to cortisone, q.v., in physiological effects.

cortisone (kor′tĭ-sōn). A hormone isolated from the cortex of the adrenal gland and also prepared synthetically. It is closely related to cortisol, and is largely inactive in man until it is converted to cortisol. It is important for its regulatory action in metabolism of fats, carbohydrates, sodium, potassium, and proteins. Also used as an anti-inflammatory agent. Trade name for cortisone acetate, USP, is Cortone Acetate.

Cortone Acetate. Trade name for cortisone acetate.

Cortril. Trade name for hydrocortisone.

Cortril Acetate-AS. Trade name for hydrocortisone acetate.

Cortrophin Gel ACTH. Trade name for corticotropin (injection), repository.

Cortrophin Zinc ACTH. Trade name for corticotropin zinc hydroxide.

Cortrosyn. Trade name for cosyntropin.

coruscation (kō-rŭs-kā′shŭn) [L. *coruscare,* to glitter]. The subjective sensation of flashes of light before the eyes.

corybantism (kor″ĭ-băn′tĭzm) [Gr. *Korybas,* a priest of Cybele who accompanied the goddess, during her travels, with music and wild dancing, + *-ismos,* condition]. Wild delirium, terrifying hallucinations, and muscular spasms, none of which are conducive to sleep.

Corynebacterium (kō-rī″nē-băk-tē′rē-ŭm) [Gr. *coryne,* a club, + *bacterion,* a small rod]. A genus of the family Corynebacteriaceae. The bacteria are rod-shaped, gram-positive, and non-motile. Though many of the species are pathogens in domestic animals, birds, reptiles, and plants, the most important is the species, C. diphtheriae, q.v., pathogenic in man.

C. diphtheriae. The causative agent of diphtheria in man. SYN: *Klebs-Loeffler bacillus.* SEE: *diphtheria.*

C. vaginale. An organism that may cause vaginitis. It was also known as Hemophilus vaginalis. The currently accepted name is Gardnerella vaginalis, q.v.

coryza (kō-rī′ză) [Gr. *koryza,* catarrh]. An acute catarrhal inflammation of the nasal mucous membrane accompanied by profuse nasal discharge. SEE: *cold.*

cosensitize (kō-sĕn′sĭ-tīz) [L. *con,* with, + *sensitivus,* sensitive]. To sensitize to more than one infection.

Cosmegen. Trade name for dactinomycin.

cosmetic (kŏz-mĕt′ĭk). 1. Preparation such as powder or cream for improving appearance. 2. Serving to preserve or promote appearance.

cosmetic surgery. Surgical procedures, usually plastic surgery, directed toward preserving appearance or correcting ugly scars or burns.

cosmic (kŏz′mĭk) [Gr. *kosmos,* order, the universe]. Pert. to the universe as a whole.

costa (kŏs′tă) [L.]. (pl. *costae*) [NA] Rib.

c. fluctuans. A floating rib.

c. spuria. [NA] A false rib.

c. vera. [NA] A true rib.

costal (kŏs′tăl). Pert. to a rib.

costal cartilage. A cartilage that connects the end of a true rib with the sternum or the end of a rib with the costal cartilage above.

costalgia (kŏs-tăl′jē-ă) [L. *costa,* rib, + Gr. *algos,* pain]. Pain in a rib or in the intercostal spaces as in intercostal neuralgia.

costal pit. Cup-shaped depression at distal end of transverse process of a thoracic vertebra for articulation with tubercle of rib.

costectomy (kŏs-tĕk′tō-mē) [″ + Gr. *ektome,* excision]. Operation of excising or resecting a rib.

costive (kŏs′tĭv) [L. *constipare,* to press together]. Constipated.

costiveness (kŏs′tĭv-nĕs). Constipation.

costocervical (kŏs″tō-sĕr′vĭ-kăl). Concerning the ribs and the neck.

costochondral (kŏs″tō-kŏn′drăl) [L. *costa,* rib, + Gr. *chondros,* cartilage]. Pert. to a rib and its cartilage.

costoclavicular (kŏs″tō-klă-vĭk′ū-lăr) [″ + *clavicula,* a little key]. Pert. to ribs and clavicle.

costocoracoid (kŏs″tō-kor′ă-koyd) [″ + Gr. *korax,* crow, + *eidos,* form]. Pert. to ribs and coracoid process of scapula.

costopneumopexy (kŏs″tō-nū′mō-pĕk″sē) [″ + Gr. *pneumon,* lung, + *pexis,* fixation]. Anchoring a lung to a rib.

costosternal (kŏs″tō-stĕr′năl) [″ + Gr. *sternon,* chest]. Pert. to a rib and the sternum.

costosternoplasty (kŏs″tō-stĕr′nō-plăs″tē) [″ + ″ + *plassein,* to form]. Surgical repair of funnel chest. A portion of a rib is used to support the sternum.

costotome (kŏs′tō-tōm) [″ + Gr. *tome,* incision]. Knife or shears for cutting through a rib or cartilage.

costotomy (kŏs-tŏt′ō-mē). 1. Incision or division of a rib or part of one. 2. Excision of a rib. SYN: *costectomy.*

costotransverse (kŏs″tō-trăns-vĕrs′) [″ + *transvertere,* to turn across]. Pert. to the ribs and transverse processes of articulating vertebrae.

costovertebral (kŏs″tō-vĕr′tĕ-brăl) [″ + *vertebra,* joint]. Pert. to a rib and a vertebra.

costoxiphoid (kŏs″tō-zĭ′foyd) [″ + Gr. *xiphos,* sword, + *eidos,* resemblance]. Concerning or connecting the ribs and the xiphoid process of the sternum.

cosyntropin (kō-sĭn-trō′pĭn). Synthetic corticotropin used to test for adrenal insufficiency. The medicine is given intramuscularly or intravenously and the plasma cortisol is determined in order to judge the adequacy of response. Trade name is Cortrosyn.

C.O.T.A. *certified occupational therapy assistant.*

Cotazym. Trade name for pancrelipase.

cotton [ME. *cotoun,* from Arabic *qutn,* cotton]. A soft, white, fibrous material obtained from the fibers enclosing the seeds of various plants of the Malvaceae, esp. those of the genus Gossypium.

c., purified. USP. Cotton fibers from which the oil has been completely removed, enhancing ability to absorb liquids.

c., styptic. Cotton impregnated with an astringent.

cotton-wool spot. The appearance of the retina in certain conditions including hypertension and other diseases.

co-twin (kō-twĭn). Either one of twins.

cotyledon (kŏt″ĭ-lē′dŏn) [Gr. *kotyledon,* hollow of a cup]. 1. Mass of villi on chorionic surface of the placenta. 2. Any of rounded portions into which the placenta's uterine surface is divided. 3. Seed leaf of a plant embryo.

cotyloid (kŏt′ĭ-loyd) [Gr. *kotyloeides,* cup-shaped]. Shaped like a cup.

cotyloid cavity. The acetabulum or socket receiving the head of the femur.

couching (kow′chĭng) [Fr. *coucher,* to lay down]. Obsolete method for displacement of the lens downward as a means of treating cataract.

cough (kawf) [ME. *coughen*]. A forceful and sometimes violent expiratory effort preceded by a preliminary inspiration. The glottis is partially closed, the accessory muscles of expiration are brought into action, and the air is noisily expelled.

A cough may be due to a variety of conditions, as can be seen below. There is no one course of therapy. Each disease is evaluated and treated accordingly. It is usually inadvisable to suppress completely coughs due to inflammation of the respiratory tract. This is particularly true if sputum is produced as a result of coughing. SEE: *expectoration.*

c., aneurysmal. Cough that is brassy and clanging, heard in patients suffering from aneurysm.

c., asthmatic. Cough that is more like an attack of dyspnea.

c., brassy. Cough heard in patients in whom there is pressure on the left recurrent laryngeal nerve, as in aortic aneurysm.

c., bronchial. Cough heard in patients with bronchiectasis, q.v. May be provoked by change of posture, as getting up in the morning. Sputum has a fetid odor, is copious, and is dirty gray. Cough heard in bronchitis, q.v., in earlier stages is hacking and irritating; in later stages looser and easier. Sputum is thin frothy mucus.

c., diphtherial. Cough heard in laryngeal diphtheria; noisy and brassy, with stridulous breathing.

c., dry. Cough unaccompanied by moisture.

c., ear. A reflex cough induced by irritation in the ear that stimulates Arnold's nerve (ramus auricularis nervi vagi).

c., effective. Cough in which sputum or any exudate is expectorated. SYN: *c., productive.*

c., hacking. A series of repeated efforts, as occurs in the early stages of pulmonary tuberculosis.

c., harsh. A metallic cough occurring in laryngitis.

c., moist. A loose cough accompanied by production of mucus or exudate.

c., paroxysmal. Cough occurring in whooping cough and bronchiectasis.

c., productive. Cough in which mucus or an exudate is expectorated. SYN: *c., effective.*

c., pulmonary. Cough that is hard and painful, seen in pneumonia. Hacking and irritating in early stages of tuberculosis; in later stages, frequent and paroxysmal. SEE: *sputum.*

c., reflex. Cough due to irritation from the middle ear, pharynx, stomach, or intestine. It may occur singly or coupled, or may be hacking in character.

c., uterine. A reflex cough resulting from irritation of female organs, esp. the uterus.

c., whooping. 1. Pertussis. 2. The paroxysmal cough ending in a whooping inspiration that occurs in pertussis.

coulomb (koo'lŏm, -lōm). [Charles A. de Coulomb, Fr. physicist, 1736–1806] ABBR: C. Unit of electrical quantity. It is the quantity of electricity that flows across a surface when a steady current of one ampere flows for one second.

Coumadin. Trade name for warfarin sodium.

count. The computation obtained by determining the number of units of the object being counted per unit of volume. Types of counts include: bacteria count, various blood cell counts, platelet count, reticulocyte count, differential count of white blood cells, and parasite count.

counter (kown'tĕr). Device for counting anything.

c., Coulter. Device for automatically counting the blood cells.

c., Geiger. Device for detecting and counting ionizing radiation.

c., scintillation. Device for detecting and counting radiation. Flashes of light are produced when radiation is detected.

counteract (kown"tĕr-ăkt'). To act against or in opposition to.

counteraction (kown"tĕr-ăk'shŭn). That action of a drug or chemical agent having an action opposing that of another agent.

countercurrent exchanger. The exchange of chemicals between two countercurrent streams separated by a membrane. This permits the fluid leaving one side of the membrane to be similar to the composition of the fluid entering the other end of the other stream.

counterextension (kown"tĕr-ĕks-tĕn'shŭn) [L. *contra,* against, + *extendere,* to extend]. Back pull or resistance to extension on a limb.

counterimmunoelectrophoresis (kown"tĕr-ĭm"ū-nō-ē-lĕk"trō-fō-rē'sĭs) [" + *immunis,* safe, + Gr. *elektron,* amber, + *phoresis,* bearing]. Process in which antigens and antibodies are placed in separate wells and an electric current is passed through the diffusion medium. Antigens migrate to the anode and antibodies to the cathode. If the antigen and antibody correspond to each other, they will upon meeting in the diffusion medium precipitate and form a precipitin band or line.

counterincision (kown"tĕr-ĭn-sĭzh'ŭn) [" + *incisio,* incision]. A second incision made either to promote drainage or to relieve the stress on a wound as it is sutured.

counterirritant (kown"tĕr-ĭr'ĭ-tănt) [" + *irritare,* to excite]. An agent such as mustard plaster that is applied locally to produce inflammatory reaction for the purpose of affecting some other part, usually adjacent to or underlying the surface irritated. There are three degrees of irritation produced by the following classes of agents: rubefacients, which redden the skin, the 1st degree; vesicants, q.v., which produce a blister or vesicle, the 2nd degree; and escharotics, which form an eschar or slough or cause death of tissue, the 3rd degree. SEE: *acupuncture; escharotic; moxibustion; plaster, mustard.*

counterirritation (kown"tĕr-ĭr"ĭ-tā'shŭn). Superficial irritation that relieves some other irritation of deeper structures.

counteropening (kown"tĕr-ō'pĕn-ĭng) [L. *contra,* against, + AS. *open,* open]. A second opening, as in an abscess that is not draining satisfactorily from the first incision.

counterpressure instrument. An instrument that provides counter-retraction to offset that exerted by exit of needle.

counterpulsation, intra-aortic balloon. ABBR: IABC. The use of a balloon attached to a catheter inserted through the femoral artery into the descending thoracic aorta for producing alternating inflation and deflation during diastole and systole respectively. This permits lowering resistance to aortic blood flow during diastole and increasing resistance during diastole. The result is to decrease the work of the heart and to increase flow of blood to the coronary arteries. The inflation of the balloon is accomplished by using helium. This method is useful for treating shock.

counterpuncture [" + *punctura,* puncture]. Counteropening. An additional opening made to help drainage, as an abscess.

countershock. The application of an electric current to the heart directly or indirectly in order to alter a disturbance in cardiac rhythm.

counterstain (kown'tĕr-stān). Application of a different stain to tissues that have already been prepared for microscopic examination by having been stained. The added stain helps to contrast the tissues originally stained.

countertraction (kown"tĕr-trăk'shŭn). Application of traction so the force opposes the traction already established. Used in reducing fractures.

countertransference (kown"tĕr-trăns-fĕr'ĕns). In psychoanalytic theory, the development by the analyst of an emotional (i.e., transference) relationship with the patient. The therapist may in this situation lack objectivity.

coup de soleil (kū-dă-sō-lā') [Fr.]. Sunstroke.

coupling (kŭp'lĭng). In cardiology, the regular occurrence of premature systole just after a normal systolic beat.

course, courses (kors, kor'sĕs) [L. *cursus,* a flowing]. Colloquial term for menstruation.

Courvoisier's law (koor-vwă'zē-āz). [Ludwig Courvoisier, Fr. surgeon, 1843–1918] Law pert. to dilatation of gallbladder. Disease processes that cause sudden blockage of the common bile duct, e.g., a stone, do not usually cause dilatation of the gallbladder. When the duct is obstructed slowly, as would be the case in infiltration of tissue around the duct (as in cancer), dilatation of the gallbladder is usually present.

couvade (koo-văd'). The custom in some primitive cultures of the father remaining in bed as if ill during the time the mother is confined for childbirth.

covalence, covalent (kō-văl'ĕns, -ĕnt). The sharing of electrons between two atoms, which bonds the atoms; pert. to such sharing of electrons.

covariance (kō-vā'rē-ăns). In statistics, the expected value of the product of the deviations of corresponding values of two variables from their respective means.

covariant (kō-vā'rē-ănt). In mathematics, pert. to variation of one variable with another so that a specified relationship is unchanged.

cover. To provide protection, esp. in the sense of assisting the body to protect against that which would normally not require such help or cover.

Ex.: The adrenal gland is normally capable of responding to stress by increasing the secretion of adrenal cortical hormones but, if a patient has received adrenocortical hormones for some time and then discontinues them, the adrenal will for a period of time be unable to respond adequately to stress such as a surgical procedure or trauma. In that case, artificial hormones would have to be given until the stress is over. Thus the patient would be covered by receiving adrenocortical hormones in the period of stress.

coverglass, coverslip. Thin glass disk to cover a tissue or bacterial specimen to be examined microscopically.

Cowden's disease. [Cowden, family name of first patient described] Hamartoma, multiple, q.v.

Cowling's rule. A method for calculation of pediatric drug dosages. The age of the child at the next birthday is divided by 24. However, the most safe and accurate methods of pediatric dosage calculation include the weight and body surface area or both of the patient. SEE: *Clark's rule; Young's rule.*

Cowper's glands. [William Cowper, Brit. anatomist, 1666–1709] A pair of compound tubular glands about the size of a pea beneath the bulb of the male urethra, and emptying a mucous secretion into it. They are small round bodies, yellow in color. They correspond to the Bartholin glands, q.v., in the female. SYN: *bulbourethral glands.*

cowperitis (kow"pĕr-ī'tĭs) [*Cowper* + Gr. *itis,* inflammation]. Inflammation of Cowper's glands.

cowpox (kow'poks). Vaccinia; pustular eruption on teats and bag of a cow in form of bluish vesicles, similar to smallpox. When given to humans, usually by vaccination, some degree of immunity against smallpox is obtained. SYN: *vaccinia.* SEE: *Jenner, Edward.*

coxa (kŏk'să) [L.]. (pl. *coxae*) [NA] Hip or hip joint.

c. plana. Aseptic necrosis of the upper end of the epiphysis of the head of the femur. SYN: *osteochondritis deformans juvenile.*

c. valga. Deformity produced when angle of the head of the femur with the shaft is increased above 120°. Opposed to coxa vara.

c. vara. A deformity produced by decrease in the angle made by the head of the femur with the shaft. Normally it should be 120°; but in coxa vara it may be 80–90°. Coxa vara occurs in rickets or may result from bone injury.

coxalgia (kŏk-săl'jē-ă) [L. *coxa,* hip, + Gr. *algos,* pain]. 1. Pain in the hip. SYN: *coxodynia.* 2. Hip joint disease. SYN: *coxitis.*

coxarthrosis (kŏks"ărth-rō'sĭs) [" + Gr. *arthron,* joint, + *osis,* condition]. Term used in foreign literature to indicate arthritis of the hip.

Coxiella (kŏk"sē-ĕl'lă). [Harold R. Cox, U.S. bacteriologist, b. 1907] A genus of bacteria related to rickettsiae.

C. burnetii. [Cox; Sir Frank Macfarlane Burnet, Australian Nobelist, b. 1899] Causative organism of Q fever, q.v.

coxitis (kŏk-sī'tĭs) [L. *coxa,* hip, + Gr. *itis,* inflammation]. Hip joint disease. SYN: *coxalgia* (def. 2).

coxodynia (kŏk"sō-dĭn'ē-ă) [" + Gr. *odyne,* pain]. Pain in the hip joint. SYN: *coxalgia* (def. 1).

coxofemoral (kŏk"sō-fĕm'ŏ-răl) [" + *femur,* thigh]. Pert. to the hip and femur.

coxotuberculosis (kŏk"sō-tū-bĕr"kū-lō'sĭs) [" + *tuberculum,* a little swelling, + *osis,* diseased condition]. Tuberculous condition of the hip joint.

coxsackievirus (kŏk-săk'ē-vī"rŭs) [*Coxsackie,* a city in N.Y., + L. *virus,* poison]. A group of viruses, the first of which was isolated in 1948 from two children in Coxsackie, N.Y. There are 23 group A and 6 group B coxsackieviruses. Most coxsackievirus infections in man are mild, but the viruses do produce a variety of illnesses including aseptic meningitis, herpangina, epidemic pleurodynia, epidemic hemorrhagic conjunctivitis, acute upper respiratory infection, and myocarditis of the newborn. It is also possible that coxsackie infection during the first trimester of pregnancy is causally related to increased incidence of congenital heart lesions in newborns. SEE: *picornaviruses.*

cozymase (kō-zī'măs). Nicotinamide-adenine dinucleotide. ABBR: NAD.

C.P. *candle power; cerebral palsy; chemically pure.*

C.P.A. *Canadian Physiotherapy Association.*

CPAP. *continuous positive air pressure.*

CPK. *creatine phosphokinase.*

c.p.m. *counts per minute* of ionizing emissions from a radioactive material.

CPPV. *continuous positive pressure ventilation.*

CPR. *cardiopulmonary resuscitation.*

C.P.S. *cycles per second.*

CR. *conditioned reflex.*

C.R. 1. *crown-rump;* the axis for measurement of a fetus. 2. *central ray;* the center of a divergent x-ray beam.

Cr. Chem. symb. for chromium.

crab louse. Phthirus inguinalis and Phthirus pubis. Louse that infests the pubic region and other hairy areas of the body. SEE: *pediculosis.*

cracked pot sound. Percussion sound resembling that heard when striking a cracked pot, indicative of a pulmonary cavity.

cradle [AS. *cradel*]. Frame for keeping bedclothes from pressing on a wound or fractured part. SYN: *arculus.*

cradle cap. Seborrheic dermatitis of the newborn usually appearing on the scalp, face, and head. Thick, yellowish, crusted lesions will develop on the scalp, and scaling, papules, or fissuring will appear behind the ears and on the face. SEE: *seborrhea.*

TREATMENT: Mild shampoo daily; corticosteroid cream to the affected area twice daily.

cramp [ME. *crampe*]. A spasmodic, esp. a tonic, contraction of one or many muscles, usually painful. In certain occupations, the attempted use of muscle groups habitually employed may lead to a so-called professional cramp, though other motor formulae are easily executed by the affected muscles. In writer's cramp, the attempt to write induces painful spasm of the hand muscles (similarly telegrapher's, watchmaker's, or seamstress's cramp). SEE: *heat cramps; systremma; writer's cramp.*

SYM: Excruciating pain, hard and contracted lumps of muscle.

TREATMENT: Depends upon cause and location. In muscular cramps try to extend muscle, compress it, and apply heat and massage.

cranial (krā'nē-ăl) [L. *cranialis*]. Pert. to the cranium.

cranial bones. Bones that comprise the cranium or brain case.

cranial nerves. Twelve pair of nerves that have their origin in the brain. In addition to the 12 pair of cranial nerves, there is a small combined efferent and afferent nerve that goes from the olfactory area of the brain to the nasal septum. This nerve, which is thought by some anatomists to be the first cranial nerve, is called terminal nerve. SEE: illus.

DIAG: Lesions of the cranial nerves give rise to the following manifestations (lesions are described as if one of each pair of nerves were diseased): *First* (Olfactory): Loss or disturbance of the sense of smell. *Second* (Optic): Blindness of various types, depending upon the exact location of the lesion. *Third* (Oculomotor): Ptosis (drooping) of eyelid, deviation of the eyeball outward, dilatation of the pupil, double vision. *Fourth*

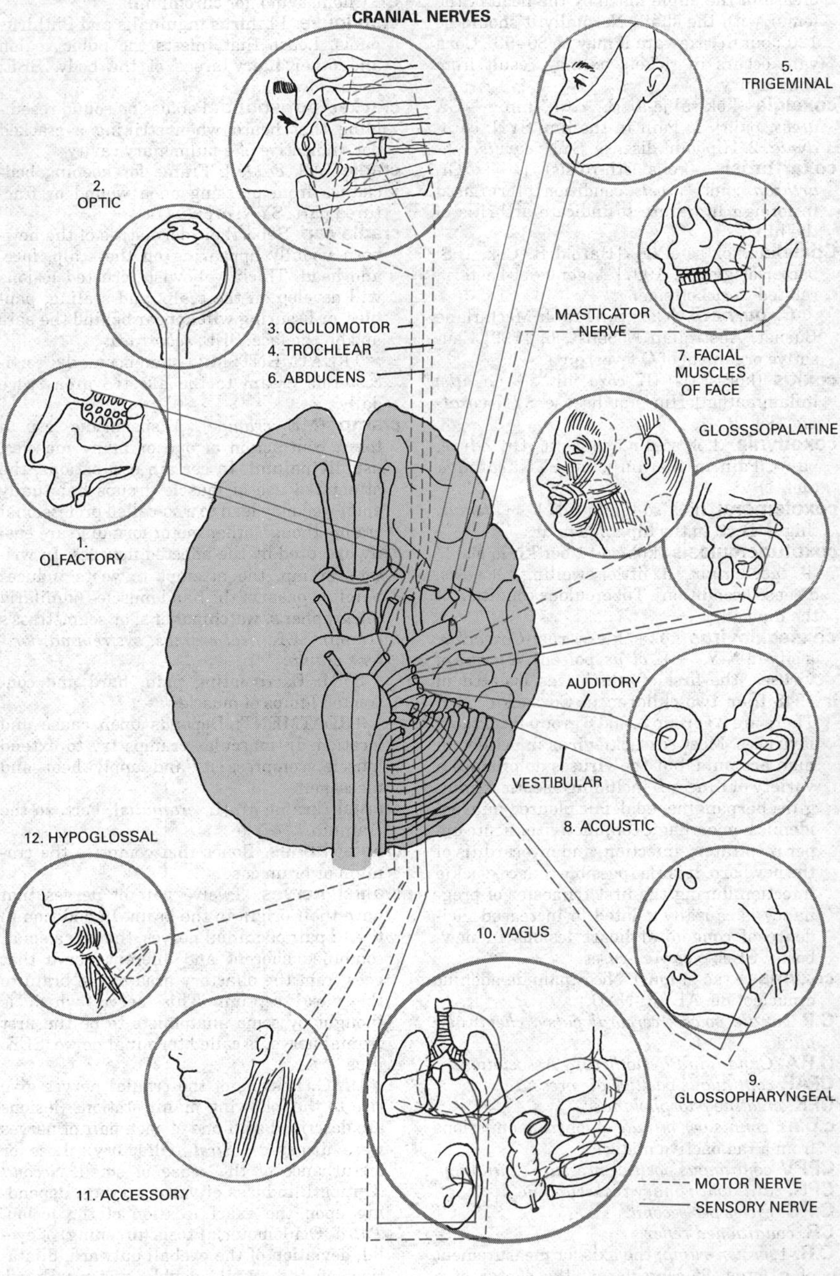
CRANIAL NERVES
1. OLFACTORY
2. OPTIC
3. OCULOMOTOR
4. TROCHLEAR
6. ABDUCENS
5. TRIGEMINAL
MASTICATOR NERVE
7. FACIAL
MUSCLES OF FACE
GLOSSSOPALATINE
AUDITORY
VESTIBULAR
8. ACOUSTIC
9. GLOSSOPHARYNGEAL
10. VAGUS
11. ACCESSORY
12. HYPOGLOSSAL
MOTOR NERVE
SENSORY NERVE

(Trochlear): Rotation of the eyeball upward and outward, double vision. *Fifth* (Trigeminal): Sensory root: Pain or loss of sensation in face, forehead, temple, and eye. Motor root: Deviation of the jaw toward paralyzed side, difficulty in chewing. *Sixth* (Abducens): Deviation of the eye outward, double vision. *Seventh* (Facial): Paralysis of all the muscles on one side of the face; inability to wrinkle the forehead, to close the eye, to whistle; deviation of the mouth toward the sound side. *Eighth* (Vestibulocochlear): Deafness or ringing in the ears; dizziness; nausea and vomiting; reeling. *Ninth* (Glossopharyngeal): Disturbance of taste; difficulty in swallowing. *Tenth* (Vagus): Disease of the vagus nerve is usually limited to one or more of its divisions. Paralysis of the main trunk on one side causes hoarseness and difficulty in swallowing and talking. The commonest disease of the vagus is of its left recurrent branch, which causes hoarseness as its principal manifestation. *Eleventh* (Spinal Accessory): Drooping of the shoulder; inability to rotate the head away from affected side. *Twelfth* (Hypoglossal): Paralysis of one side of the tongue; deviation of tongue toward paralyzed side; thick speech.

craniectomy (krā-nē-ĕk'tō-mē) [Gr. *kranion,* skull, + *ektome,* excision]. Opening of skull and removal of a portion of it.

NURSING IMPLICATIONS: Vital signs, esp. blood pressure, should be taken every 15 minutes for the first 12 hours post-op, then every half hour for the next 12 hours, then as ordered. The patient will need continuous assessment for the first 24 hours post-op. Any changes in blood pressure, pulse, respirations, temperature, or evidence of paralysis, or changes in motor, sensory, or mental status should be reported immediately.

cranio- [Gr. *kranion,* L. *cranium,* skull]. Prefix pert. to the skull or cranium.

cranioacromial (krā"nē-ō-ă-krō'mē-ăl) [Gr. *kranion,* skull, + *akron,* extremity]. Rel. to the cranium and the acromion.

craniocele (krā'nē-ō-sēl) [" + *kele,* hernia]. Protrusion of the brain from the skull. SEE: *encephalocele.*

craniocerebral (krā"nē-ō-sĕr-ē'brăl) [" + L. *cerebrum,* brain]. Rel. to skull and brain.

cranioclasis (krā"nē-ŏk'lă-sĭs) [" + *klasis,* fracture]. Crushing of the fetal head to permit delivery.

cranioclast (krā'nē-ō-klăst) [" + *klastos,* broken]. Instrument for crushing fetal skull to facilitate delivery, esp. of a dead or deformed fetus.

cranioclasty (krā'nē-ō-klăs"tē). Crushing of fetal head in dystocia.

craniocleidodysostosis (krā"nē-ō-klī"dō-dĭs-ŏs-tō'sĭs) [" + *kleis,* clavicle, + *dys,* bad, + *osteon,* bone, + *osis,* condition]. A congenital condition that involves defective ossification of bones of head, face, and clavicles.

craniodidymus (krā"nē-ō-dĭd'ĭ-mŭs) [" + *didymos,* twin]. Congenitally deformed fetus with two heads.

craniofacial (krā"nē-ō-fā'shăl). Concerning the head and face.

craniograph (krā'nē-ō-grăf) [" + *graphein,* to write]. Device for making graphs of the skull.

craniology (krā"nē-ŏl'ō-jē) [" + *logos,* study]. The study of the skull, its size, and shape, esp. in reference to variation seen in different population groups.

craniomalacia (krā-nē-ō-mă-lā'shē-ă) [" + *malakia,* softening]. Softening of the skull bones.

craniometer (krā-nē-ŏm'ĕ-tĕr) [" + *metron,* measure]. Instrument for making cranial measurements.

craniometric points. Any prominences or marks on skull for defining the configuration of the cranium; for use in craniometry.

craniometry (krā-nē-ŏm'ĕ-trē) [" + *metron,* measure]. Study of the skull and measurement of its bones.

craniopagus (krā-nē-ŏp'ă-gŭs) [" + *pagos,* a fixed or solid thing]. Twins joined at the skulls.

craniopharyngeal (krā"nē-ō-făr-ĭn'jē-ăl) [Gr. *kranion,* skull, + *pharynx,* pharynx]. Pert. to cranium and pharynx.

craniopharyngioma (krā"nē-ō-făr-ĭn-jē-ō'mă) [" + " + *oma,* tumor]. Tumor of portion of the hypophysis cerebri.

cranioplasty (krā'nē-ō-plăs-tē) [" + *plassein,* to form]. Plastic operation on skull.

craniopuncture (krā'nē-ō-pŭnk"chūr) [" + L. *punctura,* puncture]. Puncture of the skull.

craniorhachischisis (krā"nē-ō-ră-kĭs'kĭ-sĭs) [" + *rhachis,* spine, + *schizein,* to split]. Congenital fissure of skull and spine.

craniosacral (krā"nē-ō-sā'krăl). Concerning the skull and the sacrum.

cranioschisis (krā"nē-ŏs'kĭ-sĭs) [" + *schizein,* to split]. Congenital fissure of the skull.

craniosclerosis (krā"nē-ō-sklē-rō'sĭs) [" + *skleros,* hard, + *osis,* condition]. Abnormal thickening of the skull bones. This is usually associated with rickets.

cranioscopy (krā"nē-ŏs'kō-pē) [" + *skopein,* to view]. Examination of the skull.

craniospinal (krā'nē-ō-spī'năl). Concerning the skull and the spine.

craniostenosis (krā"nē-ō-stē-nō'sĭs) [" + *stenosis,* narrowing]. Contracted skull due to premature closure of the cranial sutures.

craniostosis (krā-nē-ŏs-tō'sĭs) [Gr. *kranion,* skull, + *osteon,* bone, + *osis,* condition]. Congenital ossification of cranial sutures.

craniosynostosis (krā"nē-ō-sĭn"ŏs-tō'sĭs) [" + *syn,* together, + *osteon,* bone, + *osis,* condition]. Premature closure of the skull sutures.

craniotabes (krā″nē-ō-tā′bēz) [″ + L. *tabes,* a wasting]. In infancy, abnormal softening of the skull bones. Those in the occipital region become almost paper thin.

ETIOL: Marasmus, rickets, or syphilis.

craniotome (krā′nē-ō-tōm) [″ + *tome,* incision]. Device for forcibly perforating and dividing fetal skull in labor in order to allow labor to continue. This is done in cases where the fetus has died in utero.

craniotomy (krā-nē-ŏt′ō-mē). 1. Breaking up fetal skull to facilitate delivery in difficult parturition. 2. Incision through the cranium.

craniotonoscopy (krā″nē-ō-tō-nŏs′kō-pē) [″ + *tonos,* tone, + *skopein,* to examine]. Auscultatory percussion of cranium.

craniotympanic (krā″nē-ō-tĭm-păn′ĭk) [″ + *tympanon,* kettle-drum]. Pert. to skull and middle ear.

cranium (krā′nē-ŭm) [L.]. (pl. *crania*) That portion of the skull that encloses the brain; consists of single frontal, occipital, sphenoid, and ethmoid bones and the paired temporal and parietal bones. SEE: *skeleton.*

crapulent, crapulous [L. *crapula,* excessive drinking]. Rel. to excessive drinking and eating; intoxication.

crater (krā′tĕr). A circular depression with an elevated area at the periphery.

crateriform (krā-tĕr′ĭ-form) [Gr. *krater,* bowl, + L. *forma,* shape]. In bacteriology, colonies that are saucer-shaped, craterlike, or goblet-shaped.

cravat bandage (kră-văt′) [Fr. *cravate,* a necktie]. Triangular bandage folded to form a band around the injured part. SEE: *bandage.*

crazy bone. Colloquial term for the olecranon, q.v.

C-reactive protein. A globulin that in the presence of calcium ions precipitates the C substance, q.v., of pneumococcal cells. C-reactive protein is an abnormal protein detectable in blood only during the active phase of certain acute illnesses, esp. rheumatic fever.

cream of tartar. $KHC_4H_4O_6$. Potassium bitartrate. Used in baking powder.

crease (krēs) [ME. *crest,* crest]. A line produced by a fold.

c., gluteofemoral. The crease that bounds the inferior border of the buttocks.

creatinase (krē-ăt′ĭn-ās) [Gr. *kreas,* flesh, + *-ase,* enzyme]. An enzyme that decomposes creatinine.

creatine (krē′ă-tĭn) [Gr. *kreas,* flesh]. $NH{:}C(NH_2)N(CH_3){\cdot}CH_2COOH + H_2O$. Methylglycocyamine, a colorless, crystalline substance that can be isolated from various animal organs and body fluids. It combines readily with phosphate to form phosphocreatine (creatine phosphate), which serves as a source of high-energy phosphate released in the anaerobic phase of muscle contraction. Found esp. in muscle juice and in blood. Creatine may be present in a greater quantity in the urine of women than men. Creatine excretion is increased in pregnancy and decreased in hypothyroidism.

creatinemia (krē″ă-tĭn-ē′mē-ă) [″ + *haima,* blood]. Excess of creatine in circulating blood.

creatine phosphokinase. ABBR: CPK. Enzyme present in skeletal and cardiac muscle and the brain. Catalyzes the reversible transfer of high-energy phosphate between creatine and phosphocreatine and between adenosine diphosphate (ADP) and adenosine triphosphate (ATP). Serum CPK is increased 10 to 25 times the normal level in the first few hours following myocardial infarction. The level returns to normal within two to four days. CPK serum levels are also increased in progressive muscular dystrophy and following trauma to skeletal muscle. It is not elevated in liver disease or pulmonary infarction.

creatinine (krē-ăt′ĭn-ĭn) [Gr. *kreas,* flesh]. $C_4H_7ON_3$. 1-methylglycocyamidine, the end product of creatine metabolism. It also can be isolated as colorless crystals from animal material. It is one of the nonprotein constituents of blood, and increased quantities of it are found in advanced stages of renal disease. It is a normal, alkaline constituent of urine and blood. About 0.02 gm./kg. of body weight is excreted by the kidneys per day.

creatinuria (krē-ă″tĭn-ū′rē-ă) [″ + *ouron,* urine]. Excess concentration of creatinine in urine.

creatorrhea (krē″ă-tō-rē′ă) [″ + *rhoia,* flow]. The presence of undigested muscle fibers in the feces, seen in some cases of pancreatic disease.

Credé's method (krā-dāz′). [Karl S. F. Credé, Ger. gynecologist, 1819–1892] 1. The means whereby the placenta is expelled by downward pressure on the uterus through the abdominal wall with the thumb on the posterior surface of the fundus uteri and the flat of the hand on the anterior surface, the pressure being applied in the direction of the birth canal. This may cause inversion of the uterus if done improperly. 2. For treatment of the eyes of the newborn, the use of 1% silver nitrate solution instilled into the eyes immediately after birth for the prevention of ophthalmia neonatorum (gonorrheal ophthalmia), q.v. 3. For emptying a flaccid bladder, pressure is placed over the symphysis pubis to expel the urine periodically.

cremains [contraction of *cre*mated *remains*]. That which remains after the body has been prepared for burial by cremation.

cremaster (krē-măs′tĕr) [L., to suspend]. One

of the fascia-like muscles suspending and enveloping the testicles and spermatic cord.

cremasteric (krē-măs′tĕr-ĭk). Pert. to the cremaster muscle.

cremasteric fascia. One of the coverings of the spermatic cord.

cremasteric reflex. Retraction of testis when skin is stroked on front inner side of thigh.

cremate (krē′māt) [L. *crematio,* a burning]. To dispose of the body of a dead person by burning. The ashes may or may not be buried.

crematorium (krē″mă-tō′rē-ŭm) [L.]. A place for the burning of corpses.

crenate (krē′nāt) [L. *crenatus*]. Notched or scalloped, as crenated condition of blood corpuscles.

crenation (krē-nā′shŭn). The conversion of normally round red corpuscles into shrunken, knobbed, starry forms, as when blood is mixed with salt solution of 5% strength. SEE: *plasmolysis.*

crenocyte (krē′nō-sīt). Crenated red blood cell.

creosote (krē′ō-sōt) [Gr. *kreas,* flesh, + *sozein,* to preserve]. A mixture of phenols obtained from wood tar. Used as a disinfectant and as a preserver of wood.

crepitant (krĕp′ĭ-tănt) [L. *crepitare*]. Crackling; having or making a crackling sound.

crepitation (krĕp-ĭ-tā′shŭn). 1. A crackling sound heard in certain diseases, as the rale heard in pneumonia. 2. A grating sound heard on movement of ends of a broken bone.

crepitus (krĕp′ĭ-tŭs) [L.]. 1. The noise of gas discharged from the intestines. 2. Crepitation.

c. redux. Rale indicating approaching recovery in pneumonia.

crepuscular (krē-pŭs′kū-lăr) [L. *crepusculum,* twilight]. Pert. to twilight; used to describe twilight mental state.

crescent (krĕs′ĕnt) [L. *crescens*]. Shaped like a sickle or the new moon.

c., articular. A crescent-shaped cartilage present in certain joints as the menisci of the knee joint.

c. of Giannuzzi. A crescent-shaped group of serous cells lying at the base of or along the side of a mucous alveolus of a salivary gland.

c., myopic. Grayish patch in fundus of eye due to atrophy of choroid.

crescent bodies. Achromocytes, q.v.

crescentic (krĕs-ĕn′tĭk). Sickle-shaped.

Crescormon. Trade name for somatropin.

cresol (krē′sŏl). Yellowish-brown liquid obtained from coal tar and containing not more than 5% of phenol.

USE: A disinfectant in a 1 to 5% solution for articles or areas that do not come in direct contact with food.

cresomania, croesomania (krē″sō-mā′nē-ă). [Croesus, wealthy king of Lydia, 6th-century B.C.] Hallucination of possessing great wealth.

crest [L. *crista,* crest]. A ridge or an elongated prominence, esp. one on a bone.

c., alveolar. The most coronal portion of the bone surrounding the tooth; the continuous upper ridge of bone of the alveolar process, which is usually the first bone lost as a result of periodontal disease.

CREST syndrome [*C*alcinosis, *R*aynaud's phenomenon, *E*sophageal dysfunction, *S*clerodactyly, *T*elangiectasia]. Scleroderma, q.v. SYN: *progressive systemic sclerosis.*

cretin (krē′tĭn) [Fr.]. One afflicted with congenital myxedema due to lack of thyroid secretion. Characterized by lack of growth and mental development; the patient rarely if ever exceeds the mental age of 10. The skin is rough and dry, and the hair coarse, dry, and brittle. Teeth erupt slowly and are of poor quality and irregularly placed. The tongue is large and apt to protrude from a mouth that constantly drools saliva. A cretin child is characteristically potbellied, swaybacked, and prone to umbilical hernia. SEE: *cretinism.*

cretinism (krē′tĭn-ĭzm) [″ + Gr. *-ismos,* condition]. Congenital condition due to lack of thyroid secretion, characterized by arrested physical and mental development, dystrophy of the bones and soft parts, and lowered basal metabolism. The acquired form of this disease is myxedema, q.v.

ETIOL: A congenital deficiency in secretion of the thyroid hormones.

SYM: Myxedema, and impaired mental ability.

TREATMENT: Appropriate thyroid preparation.

cretinoid (krē′tĭ-noyd) [″ + Gr. *eidos,* resemblance]. Having the symptoms of cretinism, or resembling a cretin, due to a congenital condition.

cretinous (krē′tĭ-nŭs). Pert. to a cretin or to cretinism.

crevice (krĕv′ĭs) [Fr. *crever,* to break]. A small fissure or crack.

c., gingival. The fissure produced by the marginal gingiva with the tooth surface.

crevicular (krĕv-ĭk′ū-lăr). Pert. to the gingival crevice.

CRF. *corticotrophin-releasing factor,* esp. the substance present in extract of the hypothalamus that brings about the release of ACTH from the anterior pituitary.

crib (krĭb) [AS. *cribbe,* manger]. 1. A framework around a denture or a natural tooth to serve as a brace or supporting structure. 2. A small bed with long legs and high sides for an infant or young child.

cribbing (krĭb′ĭng). Aerophagia; swallowing air.

crib death. The completely unexpected and unexplained death of an apparently well, or virtually well, infant. The most common cause of death between the second week and first year of life. The distribution is worldwide and its occurrence over the years has been constant. Occurs more frequently in the third and fourth months of life, in premature infants, in males, and in infants living in poverty. More cases occur in winter than in summer, and almost all infants die in their sleep. A variety of measures have been utilized in an attempt to predict the onset of apnea, which is thought to occur prior to death. Thus an apnea alarm device has been used to monitor the infant, so that emergency resuscitation may be instituted shortly after the onset of apnea. SYN: *sudden infant death syndrome.*

ETIOL: The cause is uncertain. In 10% to 15% of cases, autopsies show an unsuspected cardiovascular or CNS anomaly, or evidence of overwhelming infection. Other findings are minimal but suggest that an agonal episode of motor activity had occurred and was accompanied by increased negative intrathoracic pressure.

cribrate (krĭb′rāt) [L. *cribratus*]. Profusely pitted or perforated like a sieve.

cribration (krĭb-rā′shŭn). The state of being perforated.

cribriform (krĭb′rĭ-form) [L. *cribum,* a sieve, + *forma,* form]. Sievelike.

cribriform fascia. The portion of deep fascia that covers the fossa ovalis of the thigh.

cribriform plate. The thin, perforated, medial portion of the horizontal plate of the ethmoid bone.

cricoarytenoid (krī″kō-ă-rĭt′ĕn-oyd) [Gr. *krikos,* ring, + *arytaina,* pitcher, + *eidos,* form]. Extending between the cricoid and arytenoid cartilages.

cricoderma (krī-kō-dĕr′mă) [″ + *derma,* skin]. Ring-shaped infiltrations in center of indurations on the skin.

cricoid (krī′koyd) [″ + *eidos,* form]. Shaped like a signet ring.

cricoid cartilage. The lowermost cartilage of the larynx. It is shaped like a signet ring, the broad portion or lamina being posterior, the anterior portion forming the arch.

cricoidectomy (krī″koyd-ĕk′tō-mē) [″ + ″ + *ektome,* excision]. Excision of cricoid cartilage.

cricoidynia (krī-koy-dĭn′ē-ă) [″ + ″ + *odyne,* pain]. Pain in cricoid cartilage.

cricopharyngeal (krī″kō-făr-ĭn′jē-ăl) [″ + *pharynx,* gullet]. Pert. to the cricoid cartilage and pharynx.

cricothyroid (krī-kō-thī′royd) [″ + *thyreos,* shield, + *eidos,* form]. Pert. to the thyroid and cricoid cartilages.

cricothyrotomy (krī″kō-thī-rŏt′ō-mē) [″ + ″ + *tome,* incision]. Division of the cricoid and thyroid cartilage.

cricotomy (krī-kŏt′ō-mē) [″ + *tome,* incision]. Division of the cricoid cartilage.

cricotracheotomy (krī″kō-trā″kē-ŏt′ō-mē) [″ + *tracheia,* windpipe, + *tome,* incision]. Division of the cricoid cartilage and upper trachea in closure of the glottis.

cri du chat syndrome (krē-dū-shă). A hereditary congenital anomaly so-named because the infant's cry resembles the cry of a cat. Characterized by mental retardation, microcephaly, dwarfism, epicanthal folds, and laryngeal defect. Due to a deletion of the short arm of chromosome 4 or 5 of the B group.

Crigler-Najjar syndrome (krēg′lĕr-nă′hār). [John F. Crigler, U.S. physician, b. 1919; Victor A. Najjar, U.S. physician, b. 1914] A familial form of congenital hyperbilirubinemia associated with brain damage and resembling kernicterus. The syndrome is caused by an enzyme deficiency in the liver and faulty bilirubin conjugation. Transmitted as an autosomal recessive trait; death usually occurs within 15 months after birth.

criminal [L. *crimen,* crime]. 1. Pert. to crime. 2. A person who has committed or been convicted of a crime.

criminology (krĭm″ĭ-nŏl′ō-jē). Scientific study of criminals and their relation to society.

crinogenic (krĭn″ō-jĕn′ĭk) [Gr. *krinein,* to secrete, + *gennan,* to produce]. Producing or stimulating secretion.

crisis (krī′sĭs) [Gr. *krisis,* turning point]. (pl. *crises*) 1. The turning point of a disease; a very critical period often marked by a long sleep and profuse perspiration. 2. The term used for the sudden descent of a high temperature to normal or below; generally occurs within 24 hours. 3. Sharp paroxysms of pain occurring over the course of a few days in certain diseases. 4. In counseling, an unstable period in a person's life characterized by inability to adapt to a change resulting from a precipitating event.

c., abdominal. General term for severe abdominal pain due to many possible causes.

c., addisonian. Acute failure of the adrenal gland.

c., celiac. Rapid onset of malnutrition in celiac disease with severe watery diarrhea, vomiting, dehydration, and acidosis. Vigorous antibiotic and nutritional therapy is required.

c., Dietl's. Sudden, severe attack of gastric pain, chills, fever, nausea, and general collapse. In cases of floating kidney, the ureter becomes kinked and urine is obstructed, producing symptoms of renal colic.

c., salt-losing. Acute vomiting, dehydration, hypotension, and sudden death as a result of acute loss of sodium. May be caused by adrenal hyperplasia, salt-losing nephritis, or gastrointestinal disease.

c., sickle cell. Severe abdominal pain due to sickle cell anemia.

c., tabetic. Abdominal pain due to syphilis.

c., thyroid. Sudden increase in severity of symptoms of thyrotoxicosis; marked by fever and extreme tachycardia. Outcome occasionally fatal. SYN: *thyroid storm*, q.v.

c., true. Temperature drop accompanied by a fall in the pulse rate.

crisis intervention. Problem-solving activity intended to correct or prevent the continuation of a crisis; as in poison control centers, or suicide prevention services. Usually these activities are mediated through telephone services manned by professional or paraprofessional workers in the medical and social fields. SEE: *Poison Control Centers* in *Appendix*.

crispation (krĭs-pā′shŭn) [L. *crispare,* to curl]. Mild involuntary muscle-twitching that causes a sensation of creeping of the skin.

crista (krĭs′tă) [L.]. (pl. *cristae*) 1. [NA] A crest or ridge. 2. A projection, sometimes branched, of the inner wall of a mitochondrion into its fluid-filled cavity.

c. ampullaris. [NA] A localized thickening of the membrane lining the ampullae of the semicircular canals; it is covered with neuroepithelium containing auditory cells.

c. galli. [NA] A ridge on the ethmoid bone to which the falx cerebri is attached.

c. lacrimalis posterior. [NA] A vertical ridge on the lateral surface of the lacrimal bone.

c. spiralis. A ridge on the spiral lamina of the cochlea, q.v.

criterion (krī-tē′rē-ŏn) [Gr. *kriterion,* a means for judging]. (pl. *criteria*) Standard or attribute for judging a condition or establishing a diagnosis.

critical (krĭt′ĭ-kăl) [Gr. *kritikos,* critical]. 1. Pert. to a crisis. 2. Dangerous.

CRNA. *certified registered nurse anesthetist.*

crocodile tears. 1. Excess tear production that occurs when salivary glands are stimulated during eating in patients with incomplete recovery from facial paralysis. 2. Tears produced as an insincere display of grief or concern. So named because crocodiles allegedly weep after eating their victims.

Crohn's disease (krōnz). [Burrill B. Crohn, U.S. gastroenterologist, b. 1884] Regional ileitis; regional enteritis. SEE: *ileitis, regional.*

cromolyn sodium (krō′mō-lĭn). Disodium cromoglycate, a medicine unrelated to steroids or epinephrine that is quite useful in treating airway obstruction associated with asthma. This medicine is used in children and young adults as maintenance therapy. It is of no benefit in treating acute attacks of asthma. Trade name is Intal.

Crookes' dark space. [Sir William Crookes, Brit. physicist, 1832–1919] Nonluminous region enveloping outline of the cathode in a discharge tube. SEE: *cathode*.

Crookes' tube. An early form of vacuum discharge tube used for the study of cathode rays.

cross [L. *crux*]. 1. Any structure or figure in the shape of a cross. 2. In genetics, the mating or the offspring of the mating of two individuals of different strains, varieties, or species.

crossbirth. Presentation of the fetus where the long axis of the fetus is at right angles to that of the mother and requires version.

cross bite. A form of dental malocclusion in the buccolingual direction.

crossbreeding. Mating of individuals of different breeds or strains.

cross-bridges. In the fine structure of muscles, the thick and thin elements of the A bands of the myofibrils intermix to form dark bands.

cross-dress. To dress in clothing appropriate for one of the opposite sex.

crossed. Passing from one side to the other, as crossed pyramidal tract, in which nerve fibers cross from one side of the medulla to the other.

crossed reflexes. 1. Passive flexion of one part following flexion of another. 2. Passive flexion of one leg causing similar movement of opposite leg.

cross education. Contralateral facilitation or changes resulting from exercise.

cross-eye. Manifest inward deviation of the visual axis of one eye toward that of the other eye when looking at an object. SYN: *esotropia*. SEE: *squint; strabismus*.

cross-fertilization. The fusion of male and female gametes from different individuals.

crossing over. In genetics, the mutual interchange of blocks of genes between two homologous chromosomes. It occurs during synapsis in meiosis.

crossmatching. Test to establish blood compatibility before transfusion. SEE: *blood groups*.

crossover. The result of the reciprocal exchange of genetic material between chromosomes.

Crotalus (krŏt′ă-lŭs) [Gr. *krotalon,* rattle]. A genus of snakes that includes most rattlesnakes. All are highly poisonous.

crotamiton (krō″tă-mī′tŏn). USP. An effective scabicide. Eurax is the trade name for a preparation of which crotamiton is a component.

crotaphion (krō-tăf'ē-ŏn) [Gr. *krotaphos,* the temple]. Tip of greater wing of sphenoid bone.

crotonism (krō'tŏn-ĭzm). Poisoning from croton oil.

croton oil (krō'tŏn) [Gr. *kroton,* castor oil plant seed]. Oleum tiglii; a fixed oil expressed from the seed of the croton plant, Croton tiglium.

ACTION: Drastic cathartic, externally as a rubefacient. This chemical has no place in medicine and should not be used.

croton oil poisoning. SYM: Severe burning pain in mouth and stomach; vomiting; marked diarrhea; and shock. Skin cold and clammy; face pinched; pulse rapid and small; collapse follows.

TREATMENT: Aspirate stomach or administer an emetic. If patient is fully conscious, give soothing drinks such as milk or whites of eggs; then saline cathartic. Stimulate; apply external heat. Atropine, belladonna, or morphine to relieve cramping. Intravenous fluids may be required to maintain hydration, but a local poison control center should first be consulted.

croup (croop). Childhood disease characterized by a resonant barking cough, suffocative and difficult breathing, laryngeal spasm, and sometimes by the formation of a membrane.

c., catarrhal. Acute catarrhal laryngitis.

c., diphtheritic. Diphtheria of the larynx.

c., membranous. Inflammation of larynx with exudation forming a false membrane. SYN: *laryngitis, croupous.*

ETIOL: Several viruses may cause this disease. These include parainfluenza, respiratory syncytial, and various influenza viruses.

SYM: Those of laryngitis; loss of voice; noisy, difficult, and stridulous breathing; weak, rapid pulse; livid skin, fever moderate.

PROG: Grave, unless tracheostomy has been performed. The illness usually subsides in three to four days.

TREATMENT: Humidification of the air by whatever means is available such as vaporizers or steam. Antibiotics and corticosteroids are of no proven benefit. If hypoxia is present, inhalation of 40% concentration of well-humidified oxygen is indicated. This is best accomplished by use of a face mask. SEE: *carpopedal spasm; steam tent.*

c., spasmodic. Catarrhal laryngitis without formation of false membrane, but with spasm of the glottis. Occurs in children.

SYM: Difficult breathing, metallic cough, reddened and swollen epiglottis with tenacious mucus.

PROG: Favorable.

TREATMENT: Heat applied to throat; inhalation of steam.

croupous (kroo'pŭs). Pert. to croup or having a fibrinous exudation.

Crouzon's disease (kroo-zŏnz'). [Octave Crouzon, Fr. neurologist, 1874–1938] Congenital disease characterized by hypertelorism (widely spaced eyes), craniofacial dysostosis, exophthalmos, optic atrophy, and divergent squint.

crowing (krō'ĭng). A noisy, harsh sound on inspiration.

crown [L. *corona,* wreath]. The top or highest part of an organ, tooth, or other structure, as the top of the head. Corona [NA].

crowning [L. *corona,* wreath]. Stage in delivery when fetal head presents at the vulva. Crowning occurs when the largest diameter of the infant's head comes through the vulvar opening.

crownwork. Artificial crown for a tooth.

CRP. *C-reactive protein.*

CRTT. *certified respiratory therapy technician.*

crucial (kroo'shăl) [L. *crucialis*]. 1. Cross-shaped. 2. Decisive; of supreme importance; critical.

cruciate (kroo'shē-āt). Cross-shaped, as in the cruciate ligaments of the knee.

crucible (kroo'sĭ-b'l) [L. *crucibulum*]. A dish or container for substances that are being melted, burned, or dehydrated while exposed to high temperatures.

cruciform (kroo'sĭ-form) [L. *crux,* cross, + *forma,* shape]. Shaped like a cross.

crude (krood) [L. *crudus,* raw]. Raw, unrefined, or in a natural state.

crura (kroo'ră) [L., legs]. (sing. *crus*) A pair of elongated masses or diverging bands, resembling legs.

c. cerebelli. Cerebellar peduncles.

c. cerebri. Pair of bands joining cerebrum to medulla and pons.

c. of diaphragm. Two pillars connecting spinal column and diaphragm.

c. of the fornix. Arches made by division of the fornicate extremities.

crural (kroo'răl) [L. *cruralis*] Pert. to the leg or thigh; femoral.

crural arch. Femoral arch.

crural hernia. Femoral hernia.

crural nerve. Femoral nerve. SEE: *Nerves* in *Appendix.*

crural palsies. Palsies of the nerves of the legs (e.g., 12th thoracic, 1st to 5th lumbar, and 1st to 3rd sacral spinal nerves).

crus (krŭs) [L.]. (pl. *crura*) [NA]. 1. The leg. 2. Any structure resembling the leg.

c. cerebri. [NA] Either of the two peduncles connecting the cerebrum with the pons.

crush syndrome. Renal failure (edema, oliguria) following severe local injuries, esp. those involving crushing of the lower extremities.

crust [L. *crusta*]. 1. A scab. A secondary lesion; dry serous or seropurulent, brown, yellow, red, or green exudations on a free surface. Seen in eczema, seborrhea, syphilis, impetigo, favus, and ringworm of the scalp. 2. An outer covering or coat.

crusta [L.]. (pl. *crustae*) Crust.

crutch [AS. *crycc*]. 1. A device for aiding a lame, weak, or injured person in walking. Usually a long staff with padded crescent-shaped portion at the top for placing under the armpit. A great variety of crutches and devices that serve the same purpose are available: the most common is the axillary; various forms of walkers that provide a mobile stable platform that the patient holds on to while walking; forearm crutch that provides points of contact between the hand and the forearm; the shelf crutch, an adapted forearm crutch, that permits a person who can't bear weight on the hands to use a crutch; three-or four-legged cane for the person with poor balance who needs mild support. It is important that the patient be instructed as to the proper use of a crutch, as nerve lesions can result from improper use. 2. In psychoanalysis, the use of some affliction that may be real or imaginary to explain personal inadequacy or failure.

Crutchfield tongs. [W. Gayle Crutchfield, U.S. surgeon, b. 1900] Device for inserting into each side of the skull. Traction is then applied parallel to the long axis of the cervical spine by applying traction to the device.

crutch paralysis. Paralysis or weakness of the muscles of the arm(s) as a result of compression of the nerves of the brachial plexus or radial nerve by the head of the crutch. It is important that crutches be fitted so that the weight of the body is borne by the hands and arms, and not by the head of the crutch as it is forced into the axilla.

Cruveilhier-Baumgarten syndrome (kroo-väl-yă'bŏm'găr-tĕn). [Jean Cruveilhier, Fr. pathologist, 1791–1874; P. Clemens von Baumgarten, Ger. pathologist, 1848–1928] Cirrhosis of the liver caused by patency of the umbilical or paraumbilical veins and the resultant collateral circulation. It is associated with prominent periumbilical veins, portal hypertension, liver atrophy, and splenomegaly.

cry (krī). Production of inarticulate sounds, with or without weeping, which may be sudden, loud, or quiet as in a sob. These sounds are made in response to a variety of stimuli: fright, fear, pain, apprehension, sadness, glee, or joy. SEE: *cry reflex*.

c., cephalic. Sudden shrill cry by an infant. May be indicative of cerebral disease.

c., epileptic. Sudden, loud cry that may accompany the onset of an epileptic seizure.

c., hydrocephalic. An involuntary night cry by a child with acute tuberculous meningitis or acute-onset hydrocephalus.

c., night. Any sudden outcry at night. May be caused by onset of acute joint pain.

cryalgesia (krī-ăl-jē'zē-ă) [Gr. *kryos*, cold, + *algos*, pain]. Pain from the application of cold.

cryanesthesia (krī-ăn-ĕs-thē'zē-ă) [" + *an-*, not, + *aisthesis*, sensation]. Loss of sense of cold.

cryesthesia (krī-ĕs-thē'zē-ă) [" + *aisthesis*, sensation]. Sensitiveness to the cold.

crymodynia (krī"mō-dĭn'ē-ă) [Gr. *krymos*, frost, + *odyne*, pain]. Pain from cold, esp. rheumatic pain aggravated by cold or damp weather.

crymophilic (krī"mō-fĭl'ĭk) [" + *philein*, to love]. Showing preference for cold, as in psychrophilic bacteria. SYN: *cryophilic*.

crymophylactic (krī"mō-fī-lăk'tĭk) [" + *phylaxis*, protective]. Resistant to cold.

crymotherapy (krī"mō-thĕr'ă-pē) [" + *therapeia*, treatment]. The use of cold in treating disease. SYN: *cryotherapy*.

cryoaerotherapy (krī"ō-ā"ĕr-ō-thĕr'ă-pē) [Gr. *kryos*, cold, + *aer*, air, + *therapeia*, treatment]. Cold air bath in which, by degrees, the patient is accustomed to freezing temperature.

cryobank (krī'ō-bănk). Storage of biological tissues at very low temperatures.

cryobiology (krī"ō-bī-ŏl'ō-jē) [" + *bios*, life, + *logos*, study]. Study of effect of cold on biological systems.

cryocautery (krī"ō-kaw'tĕr-ē) [" + *kauter*, a burner]. Device for application of cold sufficient to kill tissue.

cryoextraction (krī"ō-ĕks-trăk'shŭn). Use of a cooling probe introduced into the lens of the eye to produce an ice ball limited to the lens. The ice ball, which includes the lens, is then removed. Used in treating cataracts.

cryofibrinogen (krī"ō-fī-brĭn'ō-jĕn). An abnormal fibrinogen that precipitates when cooled and dissolves when reheated to body temperature.

cryogen (krī'ō-jĕn) [" + *gennan*, to produce]. Substance that produces low temperatures.

cryogenic (krī"ō-jĕn'ĭk). Producing or pert. to low temperatures.

cryoglobulin (krī"ō-glŏb'ū-lĭn) [" + L. *globulus*, globule]. An abnormal protein, globulin, that precipitates when cooled and dissolves when reheated to body temperature.

cryoglobulinemia (krī"ō-glŏb"ū-lĭn-ē'mē-ă) [" + " + Gr. *haima*, blood]. Presence in the blood of an abnormal protein that forms gels at low temperatures. Found in association with pathological conditions such as multiple myeloma, leukemia, and certain forms of pneumonia.

cryohypophysectomy (krī″ō-hī″pō-fĭz-ĕk′tō-mē) [Gr. *kryos*, cold, + *hypo*, under, + *physis*, growth, + *ektome*, excision]. Destruction of the hypophysis by use of cold.

cryometer (krī-ŏm′ĕ-tĕr) [″ + *metron*, measure]. A thermometer for measuring very low temperatures.

cryophilic (krī″ō-fĭl′ĭk) [″ + *philein*, to love]. Showing preference for cold, as in psychrophilic bacteria. SYN: *crymophilic; psychrophilic.*

cryoprecipitate (krī″ō-prē-sĭp′ĭ-tāt). The precipitate formed when serum from patients with rheumatoid arthritis, glomerulonephritis, systemic lupus erythematosus and other chronic diseases in which immune complexes are pathogenic is stored at 4° C. The joint fluid from rheumatoid arthritis patients will also form a precipitate when so stored.

cryopreservation. Preservation of biological materials, such as tissue, fluids, blood, or plasma at very low temperatures. This enables the tissue to be used in another individual at a later time, as it remains viable after thawing. The technique is used to preserve human semen for artificial insemination.

cryoprobe (krī′ō-prōb). Device for applying cold to a tissue. Liquid nitrogen is the coolant frequently used. SEE: *cryoextraction.*

cryoprotectants. Drugs that permit cells to survive freezing and thawing.

cryoprotective (krī″ō-prō-tĕk′tĭv). Pert. to a chemical that protects cells from the effect of cold.

cryoprotein (krī″ō-prō′tē-ĭn). Any protein that precipitates when cooled below body temperature. SEE: *cryofibrinogen; cryoglobulin.*

cryospray (krī′ō-sprā). Spraying of liquid nitrogen on tissues in order to destroy them.

cryostat (krī′ō-stăt). Device for maintaining very low temperatures.

cryosurgery (krī″ō-sĕr′jĕr-ē) [″ + ME. *surgerie*, surgery]. Technique of exposing tissues to extreme cold in order to produce well-demarcated areas of cell injury and destruction. The tissue is usually cooled to below −20° C. Used in malignant tumors, to control pain, to produce lesions in the brain, and to control bleeding. The cold is usually produced by use of a probe through which liquid nitrogen circulates.

cryothalamotomy (krī″ō-thăl″ă-mŏt′ō-mē) [″ + L. *thalamus*, inner chamber, + Gr. *tome*, incision]. Destruction of a portion of the brain by cooling the end of a slender probe placed in the thalamus. This is usually done by circulating liquid nitrogen through the hollow stylus. Has been used in the treatment of parkinsonism.

cryotherapy (krī-ō-thĕr′ă-pē) [″ + *therapeia*, treatment]. The therapeutic use of cold.

cryotolerant (krī″ō-tŏl′ĕr-ănt) [″ + L. *tolerare*, to bear]. Able to tolerate very low temperatures.

crypt (krĭpt) [Gr. *kryptos*, hidden]. 1. A small sac or cavity extending into an epithelial surface. 2. A tubular gland, esp. one of the intestine.

c., anal. One of a number of small indentations lying immediately behind junction of anal skin and rectal mucosa.

c. of iris. An irregular excavation on anterior surface of the iris near pupillary and ciliary margins.

c. of Lieberkühn. A tubular gland of the intestine that secretes intestinal juice. Its wall is composed of columnar epithelium containing argentaffin cells and, at the base of the gland, cells of Paneth. They open between bases of the villi.

c., synoviparous. A saclike extension of the synovial cavity into the capsule of a joint. Sometimes they become blind sacs.

c., tonsillar. A deep invagination of the surface-stratified epithelium into substance of the lingual or palatine tonsils. It is surrounded by lymph nodules and may be branched.

cryptanamnesia (krĭpt″ăn-ăm-nē′zē-ă) [″ + *an-*, not, + *amnesia*, forgetfulness]. Subconscious memory. SYN: *cryptomnesia.*

cryptectomy (krĭp-tĕk′tō-mē) [″ + *ektome*, excision]. Excision of a crypt.

cryptesthesia (krĭp-tĕs-thē′zē-ă) [″ + *aisthesis*, sensation]. Subconscious awareness of facts or occurrences other than through the senses or through rational thinking, such as intuition or clairvoyance.

cryptic (krĭp′tĭk) [Gr. *kryptikos*, hidden]. 1. Having a hidden meaning; occult. 2. Tending to hide or disguise.

cryptitis (krĭp-tī′tĭs) [Gr. *kryptos*, hidden, + *itis*, inflammation]. Inflammation of a crypt or follicle, esp. an anal crypt.

cryptocephalus (krĭp″tō-sĕf′ă-lŭs) [″ + *kephale*, head]. Congenital deformity in which the head is inapparent.

cryptococcosis (krĭp″tō-kŏk-ō′sĭs) [″ + *kokkos*, berry, + *osis*, condition]. A systemic fungus infection that may involve any organ of the body, lungs, or skin, but having a marked predilection for the brain and its meninges. SYN: *torulosis.*

ETIOL: Cryptococcus neoformans (Torula histolytica), a fungus.

SYM: Development of single or multiple abscesses. In the cerebral type there is headache, dizziness, vertigo, stiffness of neck muscles; in final stages, coma and respiratory failure. Often mistaken for brain tumor.

PROG: Poor; in cerebral and meningeal forms usually fatal.

TREATMENT: Amphotericin B is somewhat beneficial in certain cases.

Cryptococcus (krĭp″tō-kŏk′ŭs). A genus of pathogenic yeastlike fungi. The causative agent of cryptococcosis. Former term was Torula.

cryptodidymus (krĭp-tō-dĭd′ĭ-mŭs) [″ + *didymos,* twin]. A congenital anomaly in which one fetus is concealed within another.

cryptogenic (krĭp″tō-jĕn′ĭk) [″ + *gennan,* to produce]. Of unknown or indeterminate origin.

cryptogenic infection. The invasion of bacteria without outward evidence of entry into the body. SEE: *infection.*

cryptolith (krĭp′tō-lĭth) [″ + *lithos,* stone]. A concretion in a glandular follicle.

cryptomenorrhea (krĭp″tō-mĕn″ō-rē′ă) [″ + *men,* month, + *rhoia,* flow]. Monthly subjective symptoms of menses without flow of blood. May be caused by an imperforate hymen.

cryptomerorachischisis (krĭp″tō-mē″rō-ră-kĭs′kĭ-sĭs) [″ + *meros,* part, + *rhachis,* spine, + *schisis,* cleavage]. Spina bifida occulta without a tumor but with bony deficiency.

cryptomnesia (krĭp-tŏm-nē′zē-ă) [″ + *mnesis,* memory]. Subconscious memory. SYN: *cryptanamnesia.*

cryptophthalmus (krĭp″tŏf-thăl′mŭs) [″ + *ophthalmos,* eye]. Complete congenital adhesion of eyelids to globe of eye.

cryptoplasmic (krĭp″tō-plăz′mĭk) [″ + *plasma,* matter]. Having existence in a concealed form.

cryptopodia (krĭp″tō-pō′dē-ă) [Gr. *kryptos,* hidden, + *pous,* foot]. Fibromata of feet so diffuse as to resemble pads.

cryptopyic (krĭp″tō-pī′ĭk) [″ + *pyon,* pus]. Having concealed suppuration, as a pyemia without apparent etiology.

cryptorchid, cryptorchis (krĭpt-or′kĭd, -or′kĭs) [″ + *orchis,* testis]. An individual with testicles that have not descended into the scrotum.

cryptorchidectomy (krĭpt″or-kĭ-dĕk′tō-mē) [″ + ″ + *ektome,* excision]. Operation for correction of an undescended testicle.

cryptorchidism, cryptorchism (krĭpt-or′kĭd-ĭzm, -kĭzm) [″ + *orchis,* testis, + *-ismos,* condition of]. Failure of testicles to descend into scrotum.

cryptorrhea (krĭp-tō-rē′ă) [″ + *rhoia,* flow]. Excessive secretion of a ductless gland.

cryptorrhetic, cryptorrheic (krĭp″tō-rĕt′ĭk, -rē′ĭk). Pert. to the internal secretions.

cryptoscope (krĭp′tō-skōp) [″ + *skopein,* to examine]. Fluoroscope.

cryptotoxic (krĭp″tō-tŏk′sĭk) [″ + *toxikon,* poison]. Having unknown toxic properties.

cryptoxanthin (krĭp″tō-zăn′thĭn). A substance present in a variety of foods, e.g., eggs and corn, that can be converted to vitamin A in the body.

cry reflex. 1. Normal ability of an infant to cry. Not usually present in premature infants. 2. Spontaneous crying by infants during sleep. Due to some painful disease such as tuberculosis of the joints.

crystal (krĭs′tăl) [Gr. *krystallos,* ice]. A solid body in which the atoms are arranged in a definite symmetrical pattern and having faces lying at definite angles to each other as crystals formed from salts or water.

c.'s, Charcot-Leyden. Protein-containing crystals found in diseased tissues wherein eosinophils are being destroyed. Present in sputum from asthma patients, leukemic bloods, and pleural effusions containing large numbers of eosinophils.

c.'s, Charcot-Neumann. Spermin crystals found in semen and some animal tissues.

c.'s, Charcot-Robin. A type of crystal formed in blood in leukemia.

c.'s of hemin. Yellowish or brown crystals that appear when dried blood or hemoglobin is heated after adding a few drops of acetic acid and salt. They are crystals of hemin, the hydrochloride of heme. Their presence constitutes a delicate and reliable test for blood.

c.'s, spermin. Crystals composed of spermine phosphate and seen in prostatic fluid on addition of a drop of ammonium phosphate solution.

crystallin (krĭs′tăl-ĭn). Globulin of the crystalline lens.

crystalline (krĭs′tă-lĭn). Resembling crystal.

crystalline deposits. Acid group includes the urates, oxalates, carbonates, and sulfates. The alkaline group includes the phosphates and cholesterin ammonium urate.

crystalline lens. The lens of the eye in the capsule behind the pupil. It separates the aqueous from the vitreous humor. It is transparent and refracts the rays of transmitted light to bring them to focus on the retina.

crystallization (krĭs″tă-lĭ-ză′shŭn) [Gr. *krystallos,* ice]. The formation of crystals.

crystallography (krĭs″tă-lŏg′ră-fē) [″ + *graphein,* to write]. Study of crystals. Useful in investigating renal calculi.

crystalloid [″ + *eidos,* form]. 1. Like a crystal. 2. A substance capable of crystallization, which in solution can be diffused through animal membranes. Opposite of colloid.

crystalloiditis (krĭs″tăl-oyd-ī′tĭs) [″ + ″ + *itis,* inflammation]. Inflammation of crystalline lens.

crystallophobia [Gr. *krystallos,* ice, + *phobos,* fear]. Abnormal fear of glass or objects made of glass.

crystalluria (krĭs-tă-lū′rē-ă) [″ + *ouron,* urine]. The appearance of crystals in the urine. May occur following the administration of sulfonamides. Their formation can be prevented by administration of adequate amounts of alkali.

Crystodigin. Trade name for digitoxin.

CS. *cesarean section.*

Cs. Chem. symb. for cesium.

c-section. *cesarean section,* q.v.

C.S.F. *cerebrospinal fluid.*

CS gas. A gas, orthochlorobenzalmalonitrile, used in riot control. Named after its two inventers, Corson and Stoughton.

C substance. A complex carbohydrate present in the cell wall of pneumococcal cells. SEE: *C-reactive protein.*

Ctenocephalides (tĕn-ō-sĕf-ăl′ĭ-dēz) [Gr. *ktenodes,* like a cockle, + *kephale,* head]. A genus of fleas belonging to the order Siphonaptera. Common species are Ct. canis and Ct. felis, the dog flea and cat flea, respectively. The adults feed on their hosts while larvae live on dried blood and feces of adult fleas. Adults may attack man and other animals. They serve as intermediate host of the dog tapeworm, Dipylidium caninum, and may transmit other helminth and protozoan infections.

c-terminal. In chemical nomenclature, the alpha carboxyl group of the last amino acid.

CTZ. *chemoreceptor trigger zone.* A zone in the medulla that is sensitive to certain chemical stimuli. Stimulation of this zone will produce an effect such as nausea.

Cu. Chem. symb. for L. *cuprum,* copper.

cubic measure. A unit or a system of units used to measure volume or capacity. SEE: *Cubic Measure* in *Weights and Measures* in *Appendix.*

cubital (kū′bĭ-tăl) [L. *cubitum,* elbow]. Pert. to the ulna or to the forearm.

cubital fossa. Triangular area lying anterior to and below the elbow, bounded medially by the pronator teres and laterally by the brachioradialis muscle. SYN: *antecubital fossa.*

cubitus (kū′bĭ-tŭs) [L]. [NA] Elbow; forearm; ulna.

c. valgus. A deformity of the arm in which the forearm deviates laterally. May be congenital or due to injury or disease. In females, slight cubitus valgus is normal and is one of the secondary sex characteristics.

c. varus. A deformity of the arm in which the forearm deviates medially.

cuboid (kū′boyd) [Gr. *kubos,* cube, + *eidos,* resemblance]. Like a cube.

cuboid bone. Outer bone of tarsal or instep bones articulating posteriorly with the 4th and 5th metatarsals.

cu. cm. *cubic centimeter.*

cucurbit (kū-kĕr′bĭt) [L. *cucurbita,* gourd]. Cupping glass. SEE: *cupping.*

cue. In psychology, a stimulus or set of stimuli to which a person has learned to respond.

cued speech. A language for the deaf that combines lip reading with cues provided by the hands. The use of this technique permits the deaf person to understand a greater variety of words and the mechanics of language than either sign language or lip reading alone.

cuff (kŭf) [ME. *cuffe,* glove]. Anatomical structure encircling a part.

cuffed endotracheal tube. An airway catheter used to provide an airway through the trachea and at the same time prevent aspiration of foreign material into the bronchus. This is accomplished by an inflatable cuff that surrounds the tube. The cuff is inflated after the tube is placed in the trachea.

cuffing (kŭf′ĭng). A collection of inflammatory cells in the shape of a ring around small blood vessels.

cuirass (kwē-răs′) [Fr. *cuirasse,* breastplate]. A firm bandage around the chest.

cul-de-sac (kŭl″dĭ-săk′) [Fr., bottom of the sack]. 1. A blind pouch or cavity. 2. The rectouterine pouch or pouch of Douglas, an extension of the peritoneal cavity, which lies between the rectum and posterior wall of uterus.

culdocentesis (kŭl″dō-sĕn-tē′sĭs) [″ + Gr. *kentesis,* puncture]. Obtaining material from the posterior vaginal cul-de-sac by aspiration or surgical incision through the vaginal wall. Procedure is done for therapeutic or diagnostic reasons.

culdoscope (kŭl′dō-skōp). An endoscope used in performing a culdoscopic examination.

culdoscopy (kŭl-dŏs′kō-pē). Examination of the viscera of the pelvic cavity of the female after introduction of an endoscope through the wall of the posterior fornix of the vagina.

-cule, -cle [L.]. Suffix indicating little, as molecule, corpuscle.

Culex (kū′lĕks) [L., gnat]. A genus of small to medium-sized mosquitoes of cosmopolitan distribution. Some species are vectors of disease organisms.

C. pipiens. The common house mosquito. Serves as a vector of Wuchereria bancrofti, the causative agent of filariasis.

C. quinquefasciatus. Mosquito common in the tropics and subtropics; the most important intermediate host of Wuchereria bancrofti.

Culicidae (kū-lĭs′ĭ-dē). A family of insects belonging to the order Diptera. Includes the mosquitoes.

culicide (kū′lĭ-sīd) [L. *culex,* gnat, + *caedere,* to kill]. An agent that destroys gnats and mosquitoes.

culicifuge (kū-lĭs′ĭ-fūj) [L. *culex,* gnat, + *fugere,* to flee]. An agent to repel mosquito attacks.

Cullen's sign (kŭl′ĕnz). [Thomas S. Cullen,

U.S. gynecologist, 1863–1953] Bluish discoloration of the periumbilical skin due to intraperitoneal hemorrhage. This may be caused by ruptured ectopic pregnancy or acute pancreatitis.

culmen (kŭl'mĕn) [L., summit]. (pl. *culmina*) 1. Top or summit of a thing. 2. [NA] Most prominent part of the vermis superior of the cerebellum. Near its anterior extremity.

cult [L. *cultus*, care]. 1. A system of therapy, usually unorthodox, that has not been approved by accepted methods of scientific analysis. 2. Obsessive commitment to an ideal or principle, or to an individual personifying that ideal.

cultivation (kŭl"tĭ-vā'shŭn) [L. *cultivare*, to cultivate]. The propagation of living organisms, esp. growing microorganisms in an artificial medium.

cultural (kŭl'tū-răl) [L. *cultura*, tillage]. Pert. to cultures of microorganisms.

culture (kŭl'tūr). 1. The propagation of microorganisms or of living tissue cells in special media that are conducive to their growth. 2. The man-made part of the environment; man's symbols, ideas, values, traditions, institutions, and technology.

c., blood. Culture used in the diagnosis of specific infectious diseases. Test consists of withdrawing blood from a vein under sterile precautions, placing it in or upon suitable culture media, and determining whether or not bacteria grow in the media. If organisms do grow, they are identified by bacteriological methods.

c., cell. An in vitro growth of cells.

c., contaminated. A culture whereupon bacteria from a foreign source have infiltrated the original bacteria being grown.

c., continuous flow. Bacterial culture in which a fresh flow of culture media is maintained. This allows the bacteria to maintain their growth rate.

c., gelatin. A culture of bacteria on a gelatin medium.

c., hanging block. A thin slice of agar seeded on its surface with bacteria, and then inverted on a cover slip and sealed in the concavity of a hollow glass slide.

c., hanging drop. A culture accomplished by inoculating the bacterium into a drop on a cover glass and mounting upside down over the depression on a concave slide.

c., negative. A culture made from suspected matter that fails to reveal the suspected organism.

c., positive. A culture that reveals the suspected organism.

c., pure. The culture of a single form of microorganism uncontaminated by other organisms.

c., slant. Culture in which the medium is placed in a tube that is slanted to allow greater surface for growth of the inoculum of bacteria.

c., stab. A bacterial culture made by thrusting into the culture medium a point inoculated with the matter under examination.

c., stock. A permanent culture from which transfers may be made.

c., streak. Spreading of the bacteria inoculum by drawing a wire containing the inoculum across the surface of the medium.

c., tissue. The growing of tissue cells in artificial nutrient media.

c., type. Standard strains of bacteria that are maintained in a suitable storage area. These permit bacteriologists to compare known strains with unknown or partially identified strains.

culture medium. A substance on which microorganisms may grow. Those most commonly used are broths, gelatin, and agar, which contain the same basic ingredients.

culture shock. The emotional trauma of being exposed to the culture, mores, and customs of a culture vastly different from the one to which one has been accustomed.

cu. mm. *cubic millimeter.*

cumulative (kū'mū-lă-tĭv) [L. *cumulus*, a heap]. Increasing in effect by successive additions; the total is usually greater than the sum of all the additions.

cumulative drug action. The action of small but repeated doses of drugs that are not immediately eliminated from the body. They tend to accumulate in the system and can produce symptoms of poisoning.

Ex.: lead, silver, and mercurial preparations.

cumulus (kū'mū-lŭs) [L., a little mound]. A small elevation; a heap of cells.

c. oophorus. A solid mass of follicular cells that surrounds the developing ovarian follicle. It projects into the antrum of the graafian follicle. SYN: *discus proligerus.*

cuneate (kū'nē-āt) [L. *cuneus*, wedge]. Wedge-shaped.

cuneate fasciculus. Continuation of postero-external column of cord into the medulla. SYN: *c. funiculus.*

cuneate funiculus. Cuneate fasciculus, q.v.

cuneate nucleus. Gray matter at end of cuneate fasciculus.

cuneiform (kū-nē'ĭ-form) [" + *forma*, shape]. Wedge-shaped.

cuneiform bones. Bones of the internal, middle, and external tarsus.

cuneiform cartilage. One of two small pieces of yellow elastic cartilage that lies in the aryepiglottic fold of the larynx immediately anterior to the arytenoid cartilage.

cuneo- (kū'nē-ō) [L. *cuneus*, wedge]. Prefix

rel. to a wedge.

cuneocuboid (kū″nē-ō-kū′boyd) [″ + Gr. *kubos*, cube, + *eidos*, shape]. Pert. to cuboid and cuneiform bones.

cuneohysterectomy (kū″nē-ō-hĭs″tĕr-ĕk′tō-mē) [″ + Gr. *hystera*, uterus, + *ektome*, excision]. Excision of a wedge of tissue from the posterior surface of the cervix uteri to correct abnormal anteflexion.

cuneus (kū′nē-ŭs) [L., wedge]. (pl. *cunei*) Wedge-shaped lobule of brain on mesial surface of occipital lobe.

cuniculus (kū-nĭk′ū-lŭs) [L., an underground passage]. (pl. *cuniculi*) Burrow in epidermis made by the itch mite.

cunnilinguist (kŭn-ĭ-lĭn′gwĭst) [L. *cunnus*, pudenda, + *lingua*, tongue]. One who practices cunnilingus, q.v.

cunnilingus (kŭn-ĭ-lĭn′gŭs). Sexual activity in which the mouth and tongue are used to stimulate the female genitalia. SEE: *fellatio*.

cunnus (kŭn′ŭs) [L.]. The vulva, q.v.; pudenda.

cup [LL. *cuppa*, drinking vessel]. 1. Small drinking vessel. 2. A cupping glass. SEE: *cupping*. 3. An athletic supporter (jockey strap) reinforced with a piece of firm material to cover the male genitalia. Worn to protect the penis and testicles during vigorous and contact sports. 4. Either of the two cup-shaped halves of a brassiere that fits over a breast. 5. A method of producing counterirritation. SEE: *cupping*.

c., favus. A cup-shaped crust that develops in certain fungus infections. SEE: *favus*.

c., glaucomatous. A depression in the optic disk occurring in late stages of glaucoma.

c., optic. In the embryo, a double-layered cuplike structure connected to the diencephalon by a tubular optic stalk. It gives rise to the sensory and pigmented layers of the retina.

c., physiologic. A slight concavity in the center of the optic disk.

cup arthroplasty of hip. Surgical technique for remodeling the femoral head and acetabulum and then covering the head with a metal cup (Vitallium). The cup prevents the raw bone surfaces from growing together. Used in treating arthritis of the hip. In older patients, total hip replacement, q.v., is usually the treatment of choice.

Cupid's bow. The normal bow-shape of the upper lip of the mouth.

cupola, cupula (kū′pō-lă, -pū-lă) [L. *cupula*, little tub]. 1. The little dome at the apex of the cochlea and spiral canal of the ear. 2. The portion of costal pleura that extends superiorly into the root of the neck. It is dome shaped and accommodates the apex of the lung.

cupping. Application to the skin of a glass vessel, from which air has been exhausted by heat, or of a special suction apparatus in order to draw blood to the surface. This is done to produce counterirritation. SEE: *leech*; *moxibustion*.

cupric (kū′prĭk). Concerning divalent copper, Cu^{++}, in solution.

cupric sulfate. Copper sulfate, blue vitriol.

cuprous (kū′prŭs). Concerning monovalent copper, Cu^{+}, in a compound.

cuprum (kū′prŭm) [L.]. Copper, q.v. ABBR: Cu.

cupruresis (kū″proo-rē′sĭs) [L. *cuprum*, copper, + Gr. *ouresis*, to void urine]. Excretion of copper in the urine.

curare (kū-, koo-răr′ē) [phonetic equivalent of Carib Indian name for extracts of plants used as arrow poisons]. One of several different resinous substances obtained from extracts of South American trees including species of chondrodendron. The pharmacologically active ingredient of curare used medically is the alkaloid D-tubocurarine. This drug is used to facilitate skeletal muscle relaxation during anesthesia. SEE: *tubocurarine chloride*.

curarization (kū″răr-ī-zā′shŭn). Condition following introduction of a purified form of curare: eyelids heavy; nystagmus; husky voice; weak jaw and throat muscles; inability to raise head, arms, and legs. Employed to lessen severity of convulsions produced by pentylenetetrazol and electric shock therapy and relaxation of muscles as in tetanus.

curative (kū′ră-tĭv) [L. *curare*, to take care of]. Having healing or remedial properties.

curd [ME]. Milk coagulum, comprised mainly of casein.

cure [L. *cura*, care]. 1. Course of treatment to restore health. 2. Restoration to health.

curet, curette (kū-rĕt′) [Fr. *curette*, a cleanser]. A spoon-shaped scraping instrument for removing foreign matter from a cavity.

curettage (kū″rĕ-tăzh′) [Fr.]. Scraping of a cavity. SYN: *curettement*.

c., uterine. Scraping with a curette to remove contents of uterus as is done following inevitable or incomplete abortion, to produce abortion, to obtain specimens for use in diagnosis, and to remove growths, such as polyps.

NURSING IMPLICATIONS: The procedure should be explained to the patient, and any questions answered. Physical preparation for the procedure should be completed. The patient should be properly placed in lithotomy position for the procedure. Asepsis should be maintained during the procedure. Postoperatively, a perineal pad count is done to determine the extent of uterine bleeding—excess bleeding should be reported to the physician. Administer analgesics as ordered and needed to keep the patient comfortable.

c., suction. Vacuum aspiration, q.v.

curettement (kū-rĕt′mĕnt) [Fr.]. Curettage, q.v.

Curie (kūr′ē, kū-rē′). 1. Marie, Polish-born Fr. chemist, 1867–1934; discovered radioactivity of thorium; discovered polonium and radium, and isolated radium from pitchblende. Awarded Nobel Prize in physics in 1903 with her husband, and in chemistry in 1911. 2. Pierre, Fr. chemist, 1859–1906. He and his wife were awarded the Nobel Prize in 1903.

curie. [Marie Curie] ABBR: Ci. The standard unit of quantity of radon, being the amt. in equilibrium with 1 gm. of radium element. This quantity decays at the rate of 3.7×10^{10} disintegrations per second.

curiegram (kū′rē-grăm) [*curie* + Gr. *gramma*, writing]. A photogram made by radium rays.

curietherapy (kū″rē-thĕr′ă-pē) [″ + Gr. *therapeia*, treatment]. Radium therapy.

curium (kū′rē-ŭm). [Pierre and Marie Curie] SYMB: Cm. At. wt. of the longest-lived isotope, 247; at. no. 96. A transuranium element.

curled. In bacteriology, said of parallel chains in wavy strands, such as in anthrax colonies.

Curling's ulcer (kŭr′lĭngz). [Thomas Curling, Brit. physician, 1811–1888] Acute peptic ulcer that sometimes occurs following a severe burn. A form of stress ulcer, q.v.

currant jelly clot. Soft red postmortem blood clot in heart and vessels.

current [L. *currere*, to run]. A flow, as of water or the transference of electrical impulses.

c., alternating. A current that periodically flows in opposite directions. Alternating current waves may be either sinusoidal or nonsinusoidal. The alternating current wave used most commonly therapeutically is the sinusoidal.

c., direct. A current that flows in one direction only. When used medically it is called the galvanic current.

curriculum (kŭ-rĭk′ū-lŭm) [L.]. A course of study in a special field or covering a specific time.

Curschmann's spirals (koorsh′mănz). [Heinrich Curschmann, Ger. physician, 1846–1910] Coiled spirals of mucus occasionally seen in sputum of asthma patients, etc. SEE: *sputum.*

curse (kĕrs). 1. To attempt to inflict injury by appeal to a malevolent supernatural power. 2. Injury assumed to have been inflicted by a malevolent supernatural power.

c., Ondine's. [*Ondine*, character in Greek mythology] 1. Primary alveolar hypoventilation due to reduced responsiveness of the respiratory center to carbon dioxide. 2. Loss of autonomic respiratory function due to a lesion in the cervical portion of the spinal cord.

curvature [L. *curvatura*, a slope]. A normal or abnormal bending or sloping away; a curve.

c., angular. A sharp bending of the vertebral column.

curvature of spine. One of four normal curves or flexures of the vertebral column as seen in profile: cervical, thoracic, lumbar, and sacral. Abnormal curvatures may occur as a result of maldevelopment or disease processes. SEE: *kyphosis; lordosis; scoliosis.*

curve [L. *curvus*]. A bend.

c. of Carus. An arc corresponding to the pelvic axis.

c. of Spee. The curve established by viewing the occlusal alignment of teeth, beginning with the tip of the lower canine and extending back along the buccal cusps of the natural premolar and molar teeth to the ramus of the mandible.

curvi- [L. *curvus*, curve]. Combining form meaning curved.

curvilinear. Concerning or pertaining to a curved line.

Cushing, Harvey (koosh′ĭng). U.S. surgeon, 1869–1939.

C.'s disease. Cushing's syndrome, q.v., in which the hypersecretion of glucocorticoids is secondary to hypersecretion of adrenocorticotrophic hormone from the pituitary.

C.'s syndrome. A syndrome resulting from hypersecretion of the adrenal cortex in which there is excessive production of glucocorticoids. May be caused by a tumor of the adrenal gland or excess stimulation of that gland as a result of hyperfunction of the anterior pituitary. Prolonged administration of large doses of adrenocortical hormones will also cause this syndrome. Symptoms are protein loss, adiposity, fatigue and weakness, osteoporosis, amenorrhea, impotence, capillary fragility, edema, excess hair growth, diabetes mellitus, skin discoloration and turgidity (plethora), and purplish striae of skin.

cushingoid (koosh′ĭng-oyd). Resembling Cushing's syndrome.

cushion. In anatomy, a mass of connective tissue, usually adipose, that acts to prevent undue pressure upon underlying tissues or structures.

cusp (kŭsp) [L. *cuspis*, point]. 1. Point of the crown of a tooth. 2. One of the leaflike divisions or parts of the valves of the heart. SEE: *bicuspid valve; semilunar cusps; tricuspid valve.*

cuspid (kŭs′pĭd). The canine teeth. SEE: *dentition* for illus.

cuspidate (kŭs′pĭ-dāt) [L. *cuspidatus*]. Having cusps.

custom. A generally accepted practice or behavior by a particular group of people or a social group.

cutaneous (kū-tā′nē-ŭs) [L. *cutis*, skin]. Pert. to the skin. SYN: *dermal; integumentary.*

cutaneous nerves. Nerves that provide sensory pathways for stimuli to the skin. SEE: *Nerves* in *Appendix.*

cutaneous respiration. The transpiration of gases through the skin.

cutdown (kŭt′down). A surgical procedure for locating a vein or artery to permit intravenous or intra-arterial administration of fluids or drugs. Required in patients with vascular collapse due to shock or other causes.

cuticle (kū′tĭ-k′l) [L. *cuticula*, little skin]. 1. A layer of solid or semisolid substance that covers the free surface of a layer of epithelial cells. It may be of a horny or chitinous consistency; sometimes it is calcified; the enamel of a tooth, and the capsule of the lens of the eye are considered cuticles. 2. The epidermis of the skin.

cuticula (kū-tĭk′ū-lă) [L.]. Cuticle.

c. dentis. A skinlike membrane that may cover the teeth after they have erupted. The membrane is easily removed by a dentist. SYN: *Nasmyth's membrane.*

cuticularization (kū-tĭk″ū-lăr-ī-zā′shŭn). Growth of skin over a sore or wound.

cutie pie. A colloquial term for a portable instrument that is used to determine the level of radiation in a given area.

cutin (kū′tĭn) [L. *cutis*, skin]. A wax that combines with cellulose to form the cuticle of plants.

cutireaction (kū″tē-rē-ăk′shŭn). Inflammatory or irritative reaction appearing on the skin; skin reaction.

c., von Pirquet's. Reaction of skin after inoculation with tuberculosis toxins.

cutis (kū′tĭs) [L.]. [NA] The skin; consisting of the epidermis and the corium (dermis), and resting upon the subcutaneous tissue.

c. anserina. Gooseflesh caused by erection of skin papillae, as from cold, shock, fright, or fear.

c. aurantiasis. Yellow discoloration of the skin resulting from ingesting excessive quantities of vegetables, such as carrots, containing carotenoid pigments. SEE: *carotenemia.*

c. hyperelastica. A congenital or familial condition characterized by excessive elasticity of the skin, loose-jointedness, easy bruisability, and development of pseudotumors at joints. SYN: *Ehlers-Danlos syndrome.*

c. laxa. Congenital hereditary disorder characterized by dermatolysis or hypertrophy of the skin and subcutaneous tissue.

c. marmorata. Transitory purplish discoloration of skin on exposure to cold.

c. pendula. C. laxa, q.v.

c. testacea. Condition characterized by formation of plates of greasy material on trunk and extremities. SYN: *seborrhea.*

c. unctosa. Excessive secretion of sebaceous glands. SEE: *seborrhea.*

c. vera. The corium, q.v.; deep layer of skin, the dermis, q.v.

c. verticis gyrata. Looseness and hypertrophy of the scalp skin, which may hang in folds.

cutization (kū-tī-zā′shŭn). Skinlike condition of a mucous membrane as result of continued exposure.

cut throat. Laceration of throat. Seriousness of injury depends upon angle of thrust of cutting object and location, and the amount of tissue damage.

F.A.: Send for doctor. Have subject lying down, head and shoulders raised. If trachea is severed, keep open and free from clot. Compress bleeding points with sterile cloths. Reassure such patients, keep their lips moist, do not leave them for an instant. Artificial respiration if necessary.

cuvette (kŭv-ĕt′) [Fr. *cuve*, a tub]. Small transparent glass container, esp. one used to hold liquids that are to be examined photometrically.

CVA. *cerebrovascular accident.*

CVP. *central venous pressure.*

cyanemia (sī″ăn-ē′mē-ă) [Gr. *kyanos*, dark blue, + *haima*, blood]. Blue color of blood.

cyanephidrosis (sī″ăn-ĕf″ĭ-drō′sĭs) [″ + *ephidrosis*, sweating]. Bluish sweat.

cyanhemoglobin (sī″ăn-hē″mō-glō′bĭn). Hemoglobin combined with cyanide. The blood containing this is cherry-red.

cyanhidrosis (sī-ăn-hī-drō′sĭs) [″ + *hidrosis*, sweat]. Exuding bluish sweat.

cyanide (sī′ă-nīd″). A compound containing the radical —CN, as potassium cyanide (KCN), sodium cyanide (NaCN).

cyanide poisoning. Cyanides are among the most common and most deadly poisons known. They stop cellular respiration by inhibiting the action of cytochrome oxidase, carbonic anhydrase, and other enzyme systems. The seeds of certain stone fruits, such as apricots, jetberry bush and toyon, and seeds of fruits of some members of the apple family contain chemicals that upon digestion yield cyanide. This occurs only if the seeds are broken. The fatal dose for a small child varies from 5 to 25 seeds. SEE: *Poisons and Poisoning* in *Appendix.*

SYM: Start within a few seconds, rarely longer than two minutes. The patient utters a cry, becomes unconscious, and falls. Respiration is first rapid and convulsive, later slow and gasping. Death usually comes within five minutes. When smaller doses are taken, there is an acrid taste, a choking feeling, anxiety, dizziness, confusion, and headache. Convulsions with frothing of the mouth. Often incontinence. Pulse rapid, feeble, and irregular.

F.A.: Must be very prompt. Have victim inhale amyl nitrate immediately for 15 to 30 seconds. Do this every 2 to 3 minutes. While this is being done, give I.V. sodium nitrate 0.3 gm. in 10 ml. of water at rate of 2.5 to 5 ml. per minute. As soon as this is completed, administer through the same needle 25 to 50 ml. of 50% solution of sodium thiosulfate. Immediate artificial respiration with 100% oxygen is required also. In one hour, repeat half doses of medicines listed above. External heat, epinephrine for collapse, and keep the patient in a recumbent position.

cyanmethemoglobin (sī"ăn-mĕt"hē-mō-glō'bĭn). Combination of cyanide and methemoglobin.

cyano- [Gr. *kyanos*, dark blue]. Combining form meaning dark blue.

cyanoacrylate adhesives. Monomers of N-alkyl cyanoacrylate that have been used as a tissue adhesive. This use is limited by the toxicity of the glue. Commercially available versions are called "superglue."

CAUTION: Superglue will cause tissues such as the skin covering fingers to form a firm adhesion. When this happens while using "superglue," the bond may have to be removed surgically.

cyanocobalamin (sī"ăn-ō-kō-băl'ă-mĭn). USP. A component of the vitamin B complex. It is essential for blood formation. Used in treating pernicious anemia. Trade names are Berubigen, Betalin 12, Crystallin, Rubramin PC, and Bevatine 12. SYN: *vitamin* B_{12}.

cyanoderma (sī"ă-nō-dĕr'mă) [" + *derma*, skin]. Blue discoloration of skin. SYN: *cyanosis*.

cyanogen (sī-ăn'ō-jĕn) [" + *gennan*, to produce]. 1. The radical CN. 2. A poisonous gas, CN — CN.

cyanomycosis (sī"ăn-ō-mī-kō'sĭs) [" + *mykes*, fungus, + *osis*, condition]. Development of blue pus due to Micrococcus pyocyaneus.

cyanopathy (sī"ăn-ŏp'ă-thē) [" + *pathos*, disease]. Blue discoloration of skin. SYN: *cyanosis*.

cyanophil (sī-ăn'ō-fĭl) [" + *philein*, to love]. Blue-staining substance of plants and animals.

cyanophilous (sī-ăn-ŏf'ĭl-ŭs). Having an affinity for a blue dye or stain.

cyanopia, cyanopsia (sī-ăn-ō'pē-ă, -ŏp'sē-ă) [" + *opsis*, vision]. Vision in which all objects appear to be blue.

cyanosed. Affected with cyanosis.

cyanosis (sī-ă-nō'sĭs) [" + *osis*, condition]. Slightly bluish, grayish, slatelike, or dark purple discoloration of the skin due to presence of abnormal amounts of reduced hemoglobin in the blood. May not appear in patients with severe anemia even though their blood is poorly oxygenated because there is not enough reduced hemoglobin present to cause the blue color to be visible.

ETIOL: Deficiency of oxygen and excess of carbon dioxide in blood caused by gas or any condition interfering with entrance of air into the respiratory tract; overdoses of certain drugs; or any form of asphyxiation.

TREATMENT: Remove cause. Artificial respiration together with oxygen inhalation or oxygen plus carbon dioxide in patients with chronic lung disease. Stimulants; heat and massage are valuable adjuncts. SEE: *asphyxia; unconsciousness*.

c., congenital. Cyanosis usually associated with stenosis of the pulmonary orifice, an imperfect ventricular septum, or a patulous foramen ovale or ductus arteriosus. SEE: *tetralogy of Fallot*.

c., delayed. C., tardive.

c., enterogenous. Cyanosis induced by intestinal absorption of toxins or by certain drugs. SEE: *methemoglobinemia*.

c. retinae. Bluish appearance of retina seen in congenital heart disease, polycythemia, and in certain poisonings, such as dinitrobenzol.

c., tardive. Cyanosis resulting from an interatrial or interventricular septal defect.

cyanotic (sī-ăn-ŏt'ĭk). Of the nature of, affected with, or pert. to cyanosis.

cyanuria (sī"ă-nū'rē-ă). The voiding of blue urine.

cybernetics (sī"bĕr-nĕt'ĭks) [Gr. *kybernetes*, helmsman]. The science of control and communication in biological, electronic, and mechanical systems. This includes analysis of feedback mechanisms that serve to govern or modify the actions of various systems.

cycad (sī'kăd). A variety of plants including Cycas revoluta and C. circinalis, from which cycasin has been isolated.

cycasin (sī'kă-sĭn). Toxic substance present in cycad plants. The chemical may be important in inducing cancer in some lower animals.

cyclacillin (sī-klă-sĭl'ĭn). USP. An antibacterial drug. Trade name is Cyclapen-W.

cyclamate (sī klă-māt). A salt of cyclamic acid that is used as a non-nutritive artificial sweetener. It is about 30 times as sweet as sugar. Its general use has been restricted because of the chemical's toxic effect on lower animals.

cyclandelate (sī-klăn'dĕ-lāt). A vasodilator of unproven value. Trade name is Cyclospasmol.

cyclarthrosis (sī-klăr-thrō'sĭs) [Gr. *kyklos*, circle, + *arthron*, joint, + *osis*, condition]. A lateral ginglymus or pivot joint, which makes rotation possible.

cycle (sī′kl) [Gr. *kyklos,* circle]. A series of movements or events; a sequence usually recurring at regular intervals.

c., cardiac. The series of consecutive movements through which the heart passes in performing one heartbeat; it includes contraction or systole, relaxation or diastole, and a short rest pause called the diastasis cordis. A complete cycle corresponds to one pulse beat, which requires a variable length of time depending upon the heart rate.

c., Cori. A series of reactions that accounts for the disposal of lactate formed during muscular activity, i.e., muscle glycogen to lactic acid to liver glycogen to blood glucose to muscle glycogen.

c., gastric. Progression of peristaltic waves over the stomach wall.

c., genesial. 1. The period from puberty to menopause. 2. The period of sexual maturity.

c., glycolytic. The successive steps by which glucose is broken down in living tissue.

c., Krebs. A series of reactions occurring in muscle cells and possibly all tissues in which pyruvic acid (or two-carbon derivatives of carbohydrate, fat, or protein) formed anaerobically are converted through a series of interrelated oxidation-reduction and other reactions to carbon dioxide and water, with the release of energy principally utilized in the formation of adenosine triphosphate (ATP). It is considered to be the final common pathway for the oxidation of and interconversions between the three primary classes of foods. SYN: *citric acid cycle; tricarboxylic acid cycle (TCA).* SEE: *Krebs cycle* for illus.

c., menstrual. A series of periodically recurring changes in the hormonal status of women and in the endometrium of the uterus culminating in menstruation, q.v.

cyclectomy (sī-klĕk′tō-mē) [Gr. *kyklos,* circle, + *ektome,* excision]. 1. Excision of a portion of the ciliary body or muscle. 2. Excision of the ciliary border of the eyelids.

cyclic (sī′klĭk). Periodic; occurring in cycles.

cyclic AMP. A cyclic nucleotide participating in the activities of many hormones, including catecholamines, ACTH, and vasopressin. SYN: *adenosine 3′,5′-cyclic monophosphate.*

cyclic AMP synthetase. Adenylate cyclase, q.v.

cyclicotomy (sĭk″lĭ-kŏt′ō-mē) [″ + *tome,* incision]. Cutting of the ciliary muscle.

cyclic vomiting. Periodic and recurring attacks of vomiting occurring in persons of a nervous temperament. The condition is usually associated with acidosis. SEE: *nausea; vomiting.*

SYM: Dizziness, loss of appetite, headache, nausea may occur. Patient then vomits about every half hour for 1 to 2 days. Great thirst, slight rise of temperature, rapid pulse, prostration.

NURSING IMPLICATIONS: Monitor vital signs, maintain fluid and electrolyte balance, administer medications as ordered for relief of headache and nausea and vomiting, and provide frequent oral hygiene. A calm, stress-free environment should be provided.

cyclitis (sĭk-lī′tĭs) [″ + *itis,* inflammation]. Inflammation of the ciliary body.

SYM: Tenderness in ciliary region, swelling of upper lid, circumcorneal injection, deposits on Descemet's membrane, reduced or hazy vision, increased or decreased tension. Pain in or about the eye, worse at night and on pressure. Its course is rapid, and progressively unfavorable.

COMPLICATIONS: Iritis, choroiditis, scleritis, glaucoma.

TREATMENT: Local: atropine, heat, protection from light. General: salicylates, induced diaphoresis, rest; treat underlying cause if possible.

c., plastic. Ciliary body inflammation accompanied by that of entire uveal tract, giving rise to a fibrinous exudate in anterior chamber and vitreous.

c., purulent. Suppurative inflammation of ciliary body and iris.

c., serous. Simple inflammation without iritis.

cyclizine hydrochloride. USP. Antihistamine used in treating and preventing motion sickness. Trade name is Marezine hydrochloride.

cyclo- [Gr. *kyklos,* circle]. 1. A combining form meaning circular or pert. to a cycle. 2. A combining form pert. to the ciliary body of the eye.

cyclobenzaprine hydrochloride (sī″klō-bĕn′ză-prēn). USP. A muscle relaxant drug. Trade name is Flexeril.

cycloceratitis (sī″klō-sĕr″ă-tī′tĭs). Inflammation of cornea and ciliary body. SYN: *cyclokeratitis.*

cyclochoroiditis (sī″klō-kō″royd-ī′tĭs) [″ + *chorioeides,* skinlike, + *itis,* inflammation]. Inflammation of ciliary body and choroid coat of eye.

cyclodialysis (sī″klō-dī-ăl′ĭ-sĭs) [″ + *dialysis,* dissolution]. Operation performed in certain types of glaucoma to produce communication between anterior chamber and suprachoroidal space for the escape of aqueous humor.

cycloguanil pamoate (sī-klō-gwăn′ĭl). An antimalarial that is available in the U.S.A. only for investigational use.

Cyclogyl. Trade name for cyclopentolate hydrochloride.

cycloid (sī'kloyd) [" + *eidos,* form]. 1. Resembling a circle. 2. Denoting a ring of atoms. 3. Extreme variations of mood from elation to melancholia. SEE: *cyclothymia.*

cyclokeratitis (sī"klō-kĕr-ă-tī'tĭs) [" + *keras,* cornea, + *itis,* inflammation]. Inflammation of cornea and ciliary body.

cyclomethycaine sulfate (sī"klō-mĕth'ĭ-kān). USP. A local and topical anesthetic. It is relatively effective when used on the mucous membranes of the mouth, nose, eye, and bronchi. Trade name is Surfacaine.

Cyclopar. Trade name for tetracycline hydrochloride.

cyclopentamine hydrochloride (sī"klō-pĕn'tă-mēn). USP. A vasoconstrictor drug. Trade name is Clopane Hydrochloride.

cyclopentolate hydrochloride (sī"klō-pĕn'tō-lāt). Moderately long-acting drug used as a cycloplegic and mydriatic. Trade name is Cyclogyl.

cyclophoria (sī"klō-fō'rē-ă) [" + *phoros,* bearing]. Rotation of eyeball due to weakness of oblique muscles. SYN: *periphoria.*

cyclophosphamide (sī"klō-fŏs'fă-mīd). USP. An effective antineoplastic agent that has also been used as an immunosuppressive agent in organ transplantation. Trade name is Cytoxan.

cyclopia (sī-klō'pē-ă) [Gr. *kyklos,* circle, + *ops,* eye]. Condition of being a cyclops, q.v.

cycloplegia (sī"klŏ-plē'jē-ă) [" + *plege,* a stroke]. Paralysis of ciliary muscle.

cycloplegic (sī-klŏ-plē'jĭk). Producing cycloplegia.

cyclopropane (sī"klŏ-prō'pān). C_3H_6. A gaseous anesthetic agent, colorless, slightly heavier than air, with a not unpleasant odor. Administered with 70 to 95% oxygen, it produces unconsciousness in 1 to 2 minutes. Fire and explosion must be guarded against.

cyclops (sī'klŏps). A fetal malformation with one eye.

cycloserine (sī"klō-sĕr'ĕn). USP. A broad-spectrum antibiotic that has been used in combination with other drugs in treating tuberculosis. It is contraindicated in patients with epilepsy and in those with depression or anxiety. Trade name is Seromycin.

cyclosis (sī-klō'sĭs) [Gr. *kyklosis,* circulation]. A streaming movement of protoplasm such as is seen in certain plant and animal cells.

Cyclospasmol. Trade name for cyclandelate.

cyclothiazide (sī"klō-thī'ă-zīd). USP. A diuretic of the benzothiazide group. The drug also acts to lower blood pressure in hypertensive patients. Trade names are Anhydron and Fluidil.

cyclothymia (sī"klŏ-thī'mē-ă) [" + *thymos,* mind]. In psychiatry, mild fluctuations of the manic-depressive type. They may be so mild as to be almost normal.

cyclotomy (sī-klŏt'ō-mē) [" + *tome,* incision]. Surgical incision of the ciliary muscle of the eye.

cyclotron (sī'klō-trŏn). A particle accelerator in which the particle is rotated between the ends of a magnet, gaining speed with each rotation.

cyclotropia (sī"klō-trō'pē-ă). Permanent cyclophoria, i.e., deviation of the anterior-posterior axis of the eye away from the axis necessary to produce visual fusion.

cycrimine hydrochloride (sī'krĭ-mĭn). USP. Drug used in treating parkinsonism. Trade name is Pagitane Hydrochloride.

cyesis (sī-ē'sĭs) [Gr. *kyesis*]. Pregnancy.

cylicotomy (sĭl"ĭ-kŏt'ō-mē) [Gr. *kylix,* cup, + *tome,* incision]. Cutting of ciliary muscle.

cylinder (sĭl'ĭn-dĕr) [Gr. *kylindros*]. A hollow, tube-shaped body.

c.'s, crossed. Two cylindrical lenses at right angles to each other. Used in diagnosing astigmatism.

c.'s, urinary. Cylindrically shaped casts in the urine.

cylindroadenoma (sĭ-lĭn"drō-ăd"ē-nō'mă) [Gr. *kylindros,* cylinder, + *aden,* gland, + *oma,* tumor]. An adenoma containing cylindrical masses of hyaline material.

cylindroid (sĭl-ĭn'droyd) [" + *eidos,* shape]. 1. Cylinder-shaped. 2. A mucous, spurious cast in urine Recognized by their twists and turns, varying markedly in diameter in different places, most frequently pointed at the ends and frequently crossing an entire field. They do not usually have cellular intrusions.

cylindroma (sĭl"ĭn-drō'mă) [" + *oma,* tumor]. Malignant tumor containing a collection of cells forming cylinders.

cylindruria (sĭl"ĭn-drū'rē-ă) [" + *ouron,* urine]. Presence of cylindroids in the urine.

cyllosis (sĭl-ō'sĭs) [Gr. *kyllosis*]. Clubfoot.

cymbocephalic (sĭm"bō-sĕ-făl'ĭk) [Gr. *kymbe,* boat, + *kephale,* head]. Having a boat-shaped head.

cynanthropy (sĭn-ăn'thrō-pē) [Gr. *kyon,* dog, + *anthropos,* man]. Insanity in which the patient behaves like a dog.

cynic spasm [Gr. *kynikos,* doglike]. Spasm of facial muscles causing a grin or snarl like a dog. SYN: *risus sardonicus.*

cynobex (sī'nō-bĕks) [Gr. *kyon,* dog, + *bex,* cough]. Dry, barking cough.

cynophobia (sī"nō-fō'bē-ă) [" + *phobos,* fear]. 1. Unreasonable fear of dogs. 2. Morbid fear of rabies. SYN: *lyssophobia* (def. 2).

cypridophobia (sĭp"rĭ-dō-fō'bē-ă) [Gr. *Kypris,* Venus, + *phobos,* fear]. 1. Morbid fear of venereal disease. 2. Abnormal fear of the sexual act. 3. False belief of having a venereal disease.

cypriphobia (sĭp-rĭ-fō'bē-ă). Morbid aversion to and fear of coitus.

cyproheptadine hydrochloride (sī″prō-hĕp′tā-dēn). USP. An anti-allergy drug that is also used in postgastrectomy dumping syndrome. Trade name is Periactin.

cyrtometer (sĭr-tŏm′ĕ-tĕr) [Gr. *kyrtos*, bent, + *metron*, measure]. Instrument for measuring circumference of chest and comparison of chest curves. Also used to measure other curved portions of the body.

cyrtosis (sĭr-tō′sĭs) [″ + *osis*, condition]. Having any abnormal curvature of the spine. SEE: *kyphosis*.

cyst (sĭst) [Gr. *kystis*, bladder, sac]. 1. A closed sac or pouch, with a definite wall, that contains fluid, semifluid, or solid material. It is usually an abnormal structure resulting from developmental anomalies, obstruction of ducts, or from parasitic infection. 2. In biology, a structure formed by, and enclosing, certain organisms, in which they become inactive, as the cyst of certain protozoans or of the metacercariae of flukes. It may serve as a reproductive structure, as in hydatid cysts.

c., adventitious. Cyst formed around a foreign body.

c., alveolar. Dilation and rupture of pulmonary alveoli to form air cysts.

c., blood. Bloody tumor. SYN: *hematoma*.

c., blue dome. A cyst close to the surface of the breast. The blue color is due to bleeding into the cyst.

c., branchial. C., cervical.

c., cervical. A closed epithelial sac derived from a branchial groove of its corresponding pharyngeal pouch.

c., chocolate. Ovarian cyst with darkly pigmented gelatinous content.

c., colloid. Cyst with gelatinous contents.

c., congenital. Cyst present at birth resulting from abnormal development, as a dermoid cyst, imperfect closure of a structure as in spina bifida; or nonclosure of embryonic clefts, ducts, or tubules, such as cervical cysts.

c., daughter. Cyst growing out of the walls of another cyst.

c., dentigerous. Cyst containing teeth. SYN: *odontoma, follicular*. SEE: *c., dermoid*.

c., dermoid. Cyst containing elements of hair, teeth, or skin. It occurs commonly in the ovary or testes and contains derivatives of all three germ layers.

c., distention. Cyst formed in a natural enclosed cavity as a follicular cyst of the ovary.

c., echinococcus. C., hydatid, q.v.

c., epidermal. 1. Cyst that forms in skin due to the blockage of a pilosebaceous follicle. 2. Cyst that contains epidermis.

c., extravasation. Cyst arising from hemorrhage into tissues.

c., exudation. Cyst caused by trapping of an exudate in a closed area.

c., follicular. Cyst arising from a follicle, as a follicular cyst of the thyroid gland or ovary.

c., Gartner's. Cyst developing from a vestigial mesonephric duct (Gartner's duct) in a female.

c., hydatid. Cyst formed by the growth of the larval form of the Echinococcus granulosus, usually in the liver.

c., implantation. Cyst resulting from displacement of portions of the epidermis as may occur in injuries.

c., intraligamentary. Cystic formation between the layers of the broad ligament.

c., involutional. Cyst occurring in the normal involution of an organ or structure, as in the mammary gland.

c., keratin. Cyst containing keratin.

c., meibomian. Tumor or cyst produced by inflammation of a meibomian gland of the eyelid. SYN: *chalazion*.

c., mucoid. Cyst containing mucoid material that has formed from degenerating connective tissue. Usually occurs over a distal joint of the finger.

c., mucous. Retention cyst composed of mucus.

c., nabothian. Cystic formation caused by closure of the ducts of the nabothian glands in the cervix uteri as a result of healing of an erosion.

c., odontogenic. Cyst associated with the teeth as a dentigerous or radicular cyst.

c., ovarian. Cystic formation in the ovary. SEE: *ovary*.

c., parasitic. Cyst enclosing the larval form of certain parasites as the cysticercus or hydatid of tapeworms or the larva of certain nematodes, i.e., Trichinella.

c., parovarian. Cystic formation of the parovarium.

c., pilonidal. An elongated closed sac lined with stratified epithelium usually containing hair, occurs in midline over sacral area of back. SYN: *pilonidal sinus*.

c., porencephalic. An anomalous cavity of the brain that communicates with the ventricular system.

c., proliferative. Cyst lined with epithelium that proliferates, forming projections that extend into the cavity of the cyst.

c., radicular. A granulomatous cyst located alongside the root of a tooth.

c., retention. Cyst retaining the secretion of a gland, as in a mucous or sebaceous cyst.

c., sebaceous. Cyst of a sebaceous gland.

c., seminal. Cyst of the epididymis, ductus deferens, or other sperm-carrying ducts that contain semen.

c., suprasellar. A cyst of the hypophyseal stalk just above the floor of the sella turcica. Its wall is frequently calcified or ossified.

c., tubo-ovarian. An ovarian cyst that ruptures into the lumen of an adherent uterine tube.

c., unilocular. Cyst containing only one cavity.

c., vaginal. Cystic formation in the vagina.

c., vitelline. Congenital cyst of the gastrointestinal canal. Lined with ciliated epithelium, it is the remains of the omphalomesenteric duct.

cyst, words pert. to: encysted; endocyst; hydrocyst; hydroma; steatoma.

cystadenocarcinoma (sĭs-tăd″ē-nō-kăr″sĭ-nō′mă) [Gr. *kystis*, bladder, + *aden*, gland, + *karkinos*, crab, + *oma*, tumor]. Glandular malignancy that forms cysts as it grows.

cystadenoma (sĭst″ăd-ĕn-ō′mă) [″ + ″ + *oma*, tumor]. An adenoma containing cysts. Cystoma blended with adenoma.

c., pseudomucinous. Cyst filled with a thick, viscid fluid and lined with tall epithelial cells.

c., serous. Cyst filled with a clear serous fluid and lined with cuboidal epithelial cells.

cystalgia (sĭs-tăl′jē-ă) [″ + *algos*, pain]. Pain in the bladder.

cystathionine (sĭs″tă-thī′ō-nĭn). An intermediate compound in the metabolism of methionine to cysteine.

cystathioninuria (sĭs″tă-thī″ō-nĭ-nū′rē-ă). Hereditary disease caused by a deficiency of the enzyme important in metabolizing cystathionine. Clinically there are mental retardation, thrombocytopenia, and acidosis.

cystauxe (sĭs-tŏk′sē) [″ + *auxe*, increase]. Enlargement or thickening of the urinary bladder.

cystectasy (sĭs-tĕk′tă-sē) [″ + *ektasis*, dilatation]. 1. An operation for extracting calculus from the bladder by dividing the membranous portion of the urethra, and then dilating the neck of the bladder. 2. Dilatation of bladder.

cystectomy (sĭs-tĕk′tō-mē) [″ + *ektome*, excision]. 1. Removal of a cyst. 2. Excision of the cystic duct and the gallbladder, or just the cystic duct. 3. Excision of the urinary bladder or a part of it.

cysteic acid. Acid produced by the oxidation of cysteine. Further oxidation produces taurine.

cysteine hydrochloride (sĭs′tē-ĭn, sĭs-tē′ĭn). USP. A sulfur-containing amino acid, $HSCH_2CH(NH_2)COOH$, which is contained in many proteins. Valuable as a source of sulfur in metabolism.

cystelcosis (sĭs″tĕl-kō′sĭs) [″ + *helkosis*, ulceration]. Ulceration of the urinary bladder.

cystic (sĭs′tĭk) [Gr. *kystis*, bladder]. 1. Of or pert. to a cyst. 2. Pert. to the gallbladder. 3. Pert. to the urinary bladder.

cystic duct. The duct of the gallbladder. It unites with the hepatic duct from the liver to form the common bile duct. SEE: *biliary tract* for illus.

cysticercoid (sĭs″tĭ-sĕr′koyd) [″ + *kerkos*, tail, + *eidos*, appearance]. The larval encysted form of a tapeworm. It differs from a cysticercus in having a much reduced bladder.

cysticercosis (sĭs″tĭ-sĕr-kō′sĭs) [″ + ″ + *osis*, condition]. Infestation with cysticerci.

cysticercus (sĭs″tĭ-sĕr′kŭs). (pl. *cysticerci*) The encysted larval form of a tapeworm, consisting of a rounded cyst or bladder into which the scolex is invaginated. SYN: *bladder worm.*

c. cellulosae. The bladder worm that is the larva of the pork tapeworm, Taenia solium.

cystic fibrosis. An inherited disease of exocrine glands affecting the pancreas, respiratory system, and sweat glands. Usually begins in infancy and is characterized by chronic respiratory infection, pancreatic insufficiency, and heat intolerance. The etiology and primary defect of cystic fibrosis is unknown. Prognosis is poor, as there is no cure, but the advent of effective antibiotics has prolonged the life span of many patients. SYN: *fibrocystic disease of pancreas; mucoviscidosis.*

cysticotomy (sĭs″tĭ-kŏt′ō-mē) [″ + *tome*, incision]. Incision of cystic bile duct. SYN: *choledochotomy.*

cystiform (sĭs′tĭ-form) [″ + L. *forma*, form]. Having the form of a cyst.

cystigerous (sĭs-tĭj′ĕr-ŭs) [″ + L. *gerere*, to bear]. Containing cysts.

cystine (sĭs′tēn) [Gr. *kystis*, bladder]. $C_6H_{12}N_2S_2O_4$. A sulfur-containing amino acid, which is produced by the action of acids on proteins that contain this compound. It is an important source of sulfur in metabolism.

cystinemia (sĭs″tĭ-nē′mē-ă) [*cystine* + Gr. *haima*, blood]. The presence of cystine in blood.

cystinosis (sĭs′tĭ-nō′sĭs) [″ + Gr. *osis*, condition]. An inherited disease of cystine metabolism resulting in abnormal deposition of cystine in body tissues. The cause is disordered proximal renal tubular function. Clinically, failure to grow is accompanied by the development of rickets, corneal opacities, acidosis, and deposition of cystine in tissues. SYN: *cystine storage disease.*

cystinuria (sĭs″tĭ-nū′rē-ă) [″ + *ouron*, urine]. 1. The presence of cystine in urine. 2. A hereditary, metabolic disorder characterized by excretion of large amounts of cystine, lysine, arginine, and ornithine in the urine. Results in the development of recurrent urinary calculi.

cystistaxia (sĭs″tĭ-stăk′sē-ă) [Gr. *kystis*, bladder, + *staxis*, dripping]. Blood oozing from the mucous membrane of the bladder.

cystitis (sĭs-tī′tĭs) [″ + *itis*, inflammation]. Inflammation of the bladder usually occurring secondary to ascending urinary tract infections. Associated organs (kidney, prostate, urethra) may be involved. May be acute or chronic.

SYM: *Acute:* Frequent and painful urination. *Chronic:* Secondary to some other lesion with possibly pyuria as only symptom.

TREATMENT: Antibiotics are useful in treating the infection but more definitive therapy will be required if the basic cause is a renal calculus or a structural defect in the urinary tract such as obstruction.

cystitome (sĭs′tĭ-tōm) [″ + *tome*, incision]. Instrument for incision into sac of crystalline lens.

cystitomy (sĭs-tĭt′ō-mē). 1. Incision of capsule of crystalline lens. 2. Incision into the gallbladder. SYN: *cholecystotomy.*

cysto-, cyst- [Gr. *kystis*, bladder]. Prefix pert. to the urinary bladder or a cyst.

cystoadenoma (sĭs″tō-ăd″ĕ-nō′mă) [″ + *aden*, gland, + *oma*, tumor]. A tumor containing cystic and adenomatous elements.

cystocarcinoma (sĭs″tō-kăr″sĭ-nō′mă) [″ + *karkinos*, ulcer, + *oma*, tumor]. Glandular tumor distended with fluid secretion of the gland.

cystocele (sĭs′tō-sēl) [″ + *kele*, hernia]. A bladder hernia that protrudes into the vagina. Injury to the vesicovaginal fascia during delivery may allow the bladder to pouch into the vagina, causing a cystocele. SYN: *vesicocele.*

cystocolostomy (sĭs″tō-kō-lŏs′tō-mē) [″ + *kolon*, colon, + *stoma*, mouth]. Formation of communication between the gallbladder and colon.

cystodiaphanoscopy (sĭs″tō-dī″ă-făn-ŏs′kō-pē) [″ + *dia*, through, + *phanein*, to shine, + *skopein*, to examine]. Transillumination of abdomen by an electric light in bladder.

cystodynia (sĭs″tō-dĭn′ē-ă) [″ + *odyne*, pain]. Pain in the urinary bladder. SYN: *cystalgia.*

cystoelytroplasty (sĭs″tō-ē-lĭt′rō-plăs-tē) [″ + *elytron*, sheath, + *plassein*, to form]. Repair of a vesicovaginal fistula.

cystoepiplocele (sĭs″tō-ĕ-pĭp′lō-sēl) [″ + *epiploon*, omentum, + *kele*, hernia]. Herniation of a portion of the bladder and the omentum.

cystoepithelioma (sĭs″tō-ĕp″ĭ-thē″lē-ō′mă) [″ + *epi*, upon, + *thele*, nipple, + *oma*, tumor]. Epithelioma in stage of cystic degeneration.

cystofibroma (sĭs″tō-fī-brō′mă) [″ + L. *fibra*, fiber, + Gr. *oma*, tumor]. Fibrous tumor containing cysts.

cystogastrostomy (sĭs″tō-găs-trŏs′tō-mē) [″ + *gaster*, stomach, + *stoma*, mouth]. Joining an adjacent cyst, usually of the pancreas, to the stomach.

cystogram (sĭs′tō-grăm) [″ + *gramma*, mark]. A roentgenogram of the bladder.

cystography (sĭs-tŏg′ră-fē) [″ + *graphein*, to write]. Taking roentgenograms of the bladder by using a radiopaque dye injected into the bladder.

cystoid (sĭs′toyd) [″ + *eidos*, appearance]. Resembling a cyst.

cystojejunostomy (sĭs″tō-jē-jū-nŏs′tō-mē) [″ + L. *jejunum*, empty, + Gr. *stoma*, mouth]. Joining of an adjacent cyst to the jejunum.

cystolith (sĭs′tō-lĭth) [″ + *lithos*, stone]. A vesical calculus.

cystolithectomy (sĭs-tō-lĭ-thĕk′tō-mē) [″ + *lithos*, stone, + *ektome*, excision]. Excision of a stone from the bladder.

cystolithiasis (sĭs-tō-lĭ-thī′ă-sĭs) [Gr. *kystis*, bladder, + *lithos*, stone, + *-iasis*, condition]. Formation of calculi in the bladder.

cystolithic (sĭs″tō-lĭth′ĭk). Pert. to a vesical calculus.

cystolutein (sĭs″tō-loo′tē-ĭn) [″ + L. *luteus*, yellow]. Yellow pigment found in some ovarian cysts.

cystoma (sĭs-tō′mă) [″ + *oma*, tumor]. (pl. *cystomata, cystomas*) A cystic tumor; a growth containing cysts.

cystometer (sĭs-tŏm′ĕ-tĕr) [″ + *metron*, measure]. Device for estimating the capacity of the bladder and its changing pressure reactions.

cystometrography (sĭs″tō-mĕ-trŏg′ră-fē) [″ + ″ + *graphein*, to write]. Graphic record of the pressure in the bladder at varying stages of filling.

cystomorphous (sĭs″tō-mor′fŭs) [″ + *morphe*, form]. Cystlike; cystoid.

cystopexy (sĭs′tō-pĕk″sē) [″ + *pexis*, fixation]. Surgical fixation of bladder to wall of abdomen.

cystoplasty (sĭs′tō-plăs″tē) [″ + *plassein*, to form]. Plastic operation upon the bladder.

cystoplegia (sĭs″tō-plē′jē-ă) [″ + *plege*, stroke]. Paralysis of the bladder.

cystoproctostomy (sĭs″tō-prŏk-tŏs′tō-mē) [″ + *proktos*, rectum, + *stoma*, mouth]. Surgical formation of a connection between the urinary bladder and the rectum.

cystoptosia, cystoptosis (sĭs″tŏp-tō′sē-ă, -sĭs) [″ + *ptosis*, a dropping]. Prolapse into the urethra of the vesical mucous membrane.

cystopyelitis (sĭs″tō-pī-ĕ-lī′tĭs) [″ + *pyelos*, pelvis, + *itis*, inflammation]. Inflammation of both the urinary bladder and the renal pelvis.

cystopyelonephritis (sĭs″tō-pī″ĕ-lō-nĕf-rī′tĭs) [″ + ″ + *nephros*, kidney, + *itis*, inflammation]. Cystitis combined with pyelitis.

cystoradiography (sĭs″tō-rā″dē-ŏg′ră-fē) [″ + L. *radius*, ray, + Gr. *graphein*, to write]. Radiography of the gallbladder or urinary bladder.

cystorectostomy (sĭs″tō-rĕk-tŏs′tō-mē) [″ + L. *rectum*, straight, + Gr. *stoma*, mouthlike opening]. Establishment of a surgical communication between the bladder and rectum.

cystorrhagia (sĭs″tō-rā′jē-ă) [″ + *rhegnynai*, to burst forth]. Hemorrhage from the urinary bladder.

cystorrhaphy (sĭst-or′ă-fē) [″ + *rhaphe*, suture]. Surgical suture of the bladder.

cystorrhea (sĭs″tō-rē′ă) [″ + *rhoia*, flow]. A discharge of mucus from the urinary bladder.

cystosarcoma (sĭs″tō-săr-kō′mă) [″ + *sarx*, flesh, + *oma*, tumor]. Sarcoma containing cysts or cystic formations.

cystoscope (sĭst′ō-skōp) [″ + *skopein*, to examine]. Instrument for interior examination of bladder and ureter. It is introduced through the urethra into the bladder.

cystoscopy (sĭs-tŏs′kō-pē) [″ + *skopein*, to examine]. Examination of the bladder with the cystoscope.

cystospasm (sĭs′tō-spăzm) [Gr. *kystis*, bladder, + *spasmos*, spasm]. Spasmodic contractions of the urinary bladder.

cystostomy (sĭs-tŏs′tō-mē) [″ + *stoma*, mouthlike opening]. Surgical incision into the bladder to establish a temporary opening.

cystotome (sĭs′tō-tōm) [″ + *tome*, incision]. Instrument for incision of bladder.

cystotomy (sĭs-tŏt′ō-mē) [″ + *tome*, incision]. Incision of bladder.

cystotrachelotomy (sĭs″tō-trā″kē-lŏt′ō-mē) [″ + *trachelos*, neck, + *tome*, incision]. Incision into neck of bladder.

cystoureteritis (sĭs″tō-ū-rē″tĕr-ī′tĭs) [″ + *oureter*, ureter, + *itis*, inflammation]. Inflammation of ureter and urinary bladder.

cystoureterogram (sĭs″tō-ū-rē′tĕr-ō-grăm) [″ + ″ + *gramma*, mark]. Roentgenographic study of the bladder and ureter.

cystourethritis (sĭs″tō-ū″rē-thrī′tĭs) [″ + *ourethra*, urethra, + *itis*, inflammation]. Inflammation of the urinary bladder and the urethra.

cystourethrocele (sĭs″tō-ū-rē′thrō-sēl) [″ + ″ + *kele*, hernia]. Prolapse of the bladder and urethra of the female.

cystourethrography (sĭs″tō-ū-rē-thrŏg′ră-fē) [″ + ″ + *graphein*, to write]. X-ray examination of the bladder and urethra by use of radiopaque contrast media.

c., chain. Examination in which a sterile beaded radiopaque chain is introduced, by means of a special catheter, into the bladder so that one end of the chain is in the bladder and the other extends outside via the urethra. This exam is useful in demonstrating anatomical relationships, esp. in female patients with persistent urinary incontinence.

c., voiding. Cystourethrography done prior to, during, and after voiding.

cystourethroscope (sĭs″tō-ū-rē′thrō-skōp) [″ + *ourethra*, urethra, + *skopein*, to examine]. Device for examining the posterior urethra and urinary bladder.

cystovesiculography (sĭs″tō-vĕ-sĭk-ū-lŏg′ră-fē). Roentgenographic examination of the bladder and seminal vesicles.

cytarabine (sī-tăr′ă-bēn). USP. Drug originally developed as an antileukemic agent and now used in treating herpesvirus hominis infections that cause either keratitis or encephalitis. Trade name is Cytosar-U. SYN: *cytosine arabinoside; ara-C*. SEE: *ara-A*.

cytase (sī′tās) [Gr. *kytos*, cell, + *-ase*, enzyme]. Term used by Metchnikoff for the enzyme complement.

-cyte (sīt) [Gr. *kytos*, cell]. Suffix denoting cell.

cytidine (sī′tĭ-dĭn). A nucleoside that is one of the four main riboside components of ribonucleic acid. It consists of a cytosine and D-ribose.

cyto-, cyt- [Gr. *kytos*, cell]. Prefix denoting the cell.

cytoanalyzer (sī″tō-ăn″ă-lī′zĕr). Device for detecting malignant cells in microscopic preparations or in fluids. The technique has not been perfected.

cytoarchitectonic (sī″tō-ărk″ĭ-tĕk-tŏn′ĭk) [″ + *architektonike*, architecture]. Pert. to structure and arrangement of cells.

cytobiology (sī″tō-bī-ŏl′ō-jē) [″ + *bios*, life, + *logos*, study of]. Biology of cells.

cytobiotaxis (sī″tō-bī-ō-tăk′sĭs) [″ + ″ + *taxis*, arrangement]. The influence of cells upon other living cells. SYN: *cytoclesis*.

cytoblast (sī′tō-blăst) [″ + *blastos*, germ]. A cell nucleus. SEE: *cyton*.

cytocentrum (sī″tō-sĕn′trŭm) [″ + *kentron*, center]. Minute body in cytoplasm of cell close to nucleus. SYN: *centrosome*. SEE: *sphere, attraction*.

cytocerastic (sī′tō-sē-răs′tĭk) [″ + *kerastos*, mixed]. Pert. to cells changing to a higher form. SYN: *cytokerastic*.

cytochalasin B (sī″tō-kăl′ă-sĭn). A substance that destroys the contractile microfilaments in cells. This fragments cells and permits the fragments to be investigated.

cytochemism (sī″tō-kĕm′ĭzm) [″ + *chemeia*, chemistry, + *-ismos*, condition]. Reaction of body cells to chemical substances.

cytochemistry (sī″tō-kĕm′ĭs-trē). The chemistry of the living cell.

cytochrome (sī′tō-krōm) [″ + *chroma*, color]. A pigment widely distributed in animals and plants. It plays an important role in cellular respiration. It is a mixture of three hemochromogens designated cytochromes A, B, and C.

cytochrome oxidase. An enzyme of importance in biological oxidations, functioning in the transfer of electrons from cytochromes to oxygen, thus activating oxygen, which unites with hydrogen to form water.

cytochrome P-450. A protein similar to hemoglobin in the microsomes of liver cells and in organs such as the ovary, adrenal gland, testes, and placenta that produces steroids. Important in catalyzing the metabolism of steroid hormones and fatty acids and in the detoxification of a variety of chemical substances.

cytochylema (sī″tō-kī-lē′mă) [Gr. *kytos,* cell, + *chylos,* juice]. The more fluid constituent of cell protoplasm. SYN: *hyaloplasm.*

cytocidal (sī″tō-sī′dăl) [″ + L. *caedere,* to kill]. Lethal to cells.

cytocide (sī′tō-sīd). An agent that kills cells.

cytoclasis (sī″tŏk′lă-sĭs) [″ + *klasis,* destruction]. Destruction of cells.

cytoclastic [″ + *klasis,* destruction]. Destructive to cells.

cytoclesis (sī″tō-klē′sĭs) [″ + *klesis,* a call]. The influence of living cells upon other cells. SYN: *cytobiotaxis.*

cytodendrite (sī″tō-dĕn′drīt) [″ + *dendron,* tree]. A dendrite given off from the body of a nerve cell.

cytodiagnosis (sī″tō-dī″ăg-nō′sĭs) [″ + *dia,* through, + *gignoskein,* to know]. Diagnosis of pathogenic conditions by the study of cells present in exudates, fluids, etc.

cytodieresis (sī″tō-dī-ĕr′ĕ-sĭs) [″ + *diairesis,* division]. Cell division.

cytodistal (sī″tō-dĭs′tăl) [″ + *distare,* to be distant]. Pert. to a neoplasm remote from the cell of origin.

cytogenesis (sī″tō-jĕn′ĕs-ĭs) [″ + *genesis,* origin]. Origin and development of the cell.

cytogenetics (sī″tō-jĕ-nĕt′ĭks). The study of cytology in relation to genetics, esp. the study of chromosomal behavior in mitosis and meiosis. Modern cytogenetics has led to the identification of chromosomes as bearers of the genes and deoxyribonucleic acid (DNA) as the key molecule of the gene.

cytogenic (sī-tō-jĕn′ĭk) [″ + *gennan,* to produce]. Producing cells or promoting the production of cells.

cytogenous (sī-tŏj′ĕn-ŭs) [″ + *gennan,* to produce]. Producing cells.

cytogeny (sī-tŏj′ĕ-nē) [″ + *genesis,* beginning]. The formation and development of the cell.

cytoglycopenia (sī″tō-glī-kō-pē′nē-ă) [″ + *glykys,* sweet, + *penia,* poverty]. Deficient glucose of blood cells. Also spelled cytoglucopenia.

cytohistogenesis (sī″tō-hĭs″tō-jĕn′ĕ-sĭs) [″ + *histos,* web, + *genesis,* origin]. The structural development of cells.

cytohyaloplasm (sī″tō-hī′ăl-ō-plăzm) [″ + *hyalos,* glass, + LL. *plasma,* a form]. Fibrillary network of protoplasm. SYN: *hyaloplasm.*

cytoid (sī′toyd) [″ + *eidos,* form]. Resembling a cell.

cytoinhibition (sī″tō-ĭn″hĭ-bĭsh′ŭn) [″ + L. *inhibere,* to restrain]. Phagocytic cell action that prevents the destruction of ingested bacteria by the cell.

cytokalipenia (sī″tō-kăl-ĭ-pē′nē-ă) [″ + L. *kalium,* potassium, + Gr. *penia,* poverty]. A potassium deficiency in body or blood cells.

cytokerastic (sī″tō-kĕ-răs′tĭk) [″ + *kerastos,* mixed]. Pert. to cellular development from a lower to a higher form.

cytokinesis (sī″tō-kĭ-nē′sĭs) [″ + *kinesis,* movement]. The separation of the cytoplasm into two parts, which occurs in the latter stages of mitosis or cell division. SYN: *cytodieresis.*

cytology (sī-tŏl′ō-jē) [″ + *logos,* study of]. The science that deals with the formation, structure, and function of cells.

cytolymph (sī′tō-lĭmf) [″ + L. *lympha,* lymph]. Matrix of cytoplasm of cells. SYN: *cytochylema; hyaloplasm.*

cytolysin (sī-tŏl′ĭ-sĭn) [″ + *lysis,* dissolution]. An antibody that causes disintegration of cells.

cytolysis (sī-tŏl′ĭ-sis). Dissolution or destruction of living cells. Hemolysis is the term used in case of red blood corpuscles, and bacteriolysis for bacteria.

cytomegalic inclusion disease. A disease, esp. of the neonatal period, characterized by variable severity in which an asymptomatic infection may leave no sequelae to a disease with fever, hepatosplenomegaly, microcephaly, and, in neonates, mental or motor retardation and perhaps death. Due to infection with cytomegalovirus, which can occur congenitally, postnatally, or later in life. The virus can produce a latent infection that may be subsequently activated by pregnancy, multiple blood transfusions, or following immunosuppression therapy.

TREATMENT: There is no specific therapy.

cytomegalovirus (sī″tō-mĕg″ă-lō-vī′rŭs). One of a group of species-specific herpesviruses. The human cytomegalovirus inhabits the salivary glands and causes cytomegalic inclusion disease, q.v.

Cytomel. Trade name for liothyronine sodium.

cytometaplasia (sī″tō-mĕt″ă-plā′zē-ă) [Gr. *kytos,* cell, + *metaplasis,* change]. Change of form or function of cells.

cytometer (sī-tŏm′ĕ-ter) [″ + *metron,* measure]. Instrument for counting and measuring cells.

cytometry (sī-tŏm'ĕ-trē). The counting and measuring of cells.

cytomicrosome (sī-tō-mī'krō-sōm) [" + *mikros,* small, + *soma,* body]. One of the minute granules in the protoplasm (cytoplasm) of the cell.

cytomitome (sī"tō-mī'tōm) [" + *mitos,* thread]. Any part of the network of the cytoplasm.

cytomorphology (sī"tō-mor-fŏl'ō-jē) [" + *morphe,* form, + *logos,* study of]. The study of the structure of cells.

cytomorphosis (sī"tō-mor-fō'sĭs) [" + " + *osis,* condition]. The cellular transformations that a cell undergoes during its life.

cyton (sī'tŏn) [Gr. *kytos,* cell]. 1. A cell. 2. The body of a nerve cell. SYN: *perikaryon.*

cytopathic (sī"tō-păth'ĭk) [" + *pathos,* disease]. 1. Concerning pathological changes in a cell. 2. Concerning the ability of an agent, esp. a virus, to injure or destroy a cell.

cytopathogenic effect (sī"tō-păth"ō-jĕn'ĭk) [" + *pathos,* disease, + *gennan,* to produce]. In tissue culture, the morphologic changes seen in the cultured cells due to the effect of some pathogenic agent such as a virus.

cytopathology (sī"tō-păth-ŏl'ō-jē) [" + " + *logos,* study]. Study of the cellular changes in disease.

cytopenia [" + *penia,* lack]. Diminution of cellular elements in blood or other tissues.

cytophagocytosis (sī"tō-făg"ō-sī-tō'sĭs) [" + *phagein,* to eat, + *kytos,* cell, + *osis,* condition]. Destruction of other cells by phagocytes. SYN: *cytophagy.*

cytophagous (sī-tŏf'ă-gŭs). Devouring or destructive of cells.

cytophagy (sī-tŏf'ă-jē). Cell destruction by phagocytes. SYN: *cytophagocytosis.*

cytophilic (sī-tō-fĭl'ĭk) [" + *philein,* to love]. Having an affinity for or attracted by cells, e.g., antibodies.

cytophotometry (sī"tō-fō-tŏm'ĕ-trē). The use of an electronic device for analyzing the physical size of cells and detecting the amount of certain types of chemicals in single cells. This is done by fixing and staining cells with fluorescent materials that combine with specific constituents of cells in proportion to the amount present. SYN: *cell-flow system analysis.*

cytophylaxis (sī"tō-fī-lăk'sĭs) [" + *phylaxis,* guarding against]. The protection of cells against lysis.

cytophyletic (sī"tō-fī-lĕt'ĭk) [" + *phyle,* tribe]. Pert. to genealogy of cells.

cytophysics (sī"tō-fĭz'ĭks) [" + *physike,* (study of) nature]. The physics of cellular activity.

cytophysiology (sī"tō-fĭz-ē-ŏl'ō-jē) [" + *physis,* nature, + *logos,* study]. Physiology of the cell.

cytopipette (sī"tō-pī'pĕt). A pipette for obtaining specimens of cells, esp. from body fluids or cavities.

cytoplasm (sī'tō-plăzm) [" + LL. *plasma,* a form, from Gr. *plassein,* to mold, spread out]. The protoplasm of a cell outside the nucleus.

cytoplast (sī'tō-plăst). The cytoplasm of a cell body as distinguished from the contents of the nucleus.

cytoplastin [Gr. *kytos,* cell]. The plastin substance of the cytoplasm.

cytoproximal (sī"tō-prŏk'sĭ-măl) [" + L. *proximus,* nearest]. Pert. to the portion of an axon nearest to the cell body from which it originates.

cytoreticulum (sī"tō-rĕ-tĭk'ū-lŭm) [" + L. *reticulum,* network]. The fibrillar network supporting fluid of protoplasm.

cytorrhyctes (sī"tō-rĭk'tēz) [" + *oryssein,* to dig]. Inclusion bodies in cells. They are composed of virus elementary bodies. They were once thought to be of protozoal origin.

Cytosar-U. Trade name for cytarabine.

cytoscopy (sī-tŏs'kō-pē) [" + *skopein,* to examine]. Microscopic examination of cells for purposes of diagnosis.

cytosine (sī'tō-sĭn). A pyrimidine base, $C_4H_5N_3O$, which is a component of ribonucleic and deoxyribonucleic acids.

c. arabinoside. Drug originally developed as an antileukemic agent and now used in treating herpesvirus hominis infections that cause either keratitis or encephalitis. SYN: *cytarabine.*

cytoskeleton (sī"tō-skĕl'ĕ-tŏn). The internal structural framework of a cell.

cytosol (sī'tō-sŏl). The soluble portion of a cell, which contains no particles. SEE: *cytoplasm.*

cytosome (sī'tō-sōm) [" + *soma,* body]. The portion of a cell exclusive of the nucleus.

cytospongium (sī"tō-spŭn'jē-ŭm) [" + *sphongos,* sponge]. The fibrillar network of the cytoplasm of a cell. SYN: *spongioplasm.*

cytost (sī'tōst) [Gr. *kytos,* cell]. A specific toxin given off by an injured or destroyed cell.

cytostasis (sī-tŏs'tă-sĭs) [" + *stasis,* stoppage]. Stasis of white blood corpuscles, as in incipient stage of inflammation.

cytostatic (sī"tō-stăt'ĭk) [" + *stasis,* stoppage]. Preventing the growth and proliferation of cells.

cytostome (sī'tō-stōm) [" + *stoma,* mouth]. The mouth opening of one-celled organisms.

cytotactic (sī"tō-tăk'tĭk). Pert. to cytotaxia.

cytotaxia, cytotaxis (sī-tō-tăk'sē-ă, -sĭs) [" + *taxis,* arrangement]. Attraction or repulsion of cells for each other.

cytotherapy [" + *therapeia,* treatment]. 1. Treatment by use of glandular extracts; organotherapy. 2. Use of cytotoxic or cytolytic substances or serums in treating disease.

cytothesis (sī-tŏth'ĕ-sĭs) [" + *thesis,* a placing]. Restoration or repair of injured cells.

cytotoxic (sī"tō-tŏks'ĭk). Destructive to cells.

cytotoxic agents. Chemicals that destroy cells or prevent their multiplication. They are a group of compounds developed for use in cancer chemotherapy. The ideal agent for such use should destroy the fast-growing cancer cells without injuring the normal cells of the body.

cytotoxin (sī"tō-tŏk'sĭn) [" + *toxikon*, poison]. An antibody or toxin that attacks the cells of particular organs. SEE: *endotoxin; erythrotoxin; exotoxin; leukocidin; lysis; neurotoxin.*

cytotrophoblast (sī"tō-trō'fō-blăst) [" + *trophe*, nourishment, + *blastos*, germ]. The thin inner layer of the trophoblast composed of cuboidal cells, the outer layer being the syntrophoblast. SYN: *layer, Langhans'.*

cytotropic (sī"tō-trŏp'ĭk, -trōp'ĭk) [" + *trope*, a turn]. Having an affinity for cells.

cytotropism (sī-tŏt'rō-pĭzm) [" + *trope*, a turn, + *-ismos*, condition]. The attraction of cells for certain chemicals, drugs, viruses, bacteria, or physical conditions such as heat or cold.

Cytoxan (sī-tŏk'săn). Trade name for cyclophosphamide, q.v.

cytozoic (sī"tō-zō'ĭk) [" + *zoon*, animal]. Living within or attached to a cell, as certain protozoa.

cytozoon (sī-tō-zō'ŏn). A protozoon that lives as an intracellular parasite.

cytula (sĭ'tū-lă) [L., small cell]. The impregnated ovum.

cyturia (sĭ-tū'rē-ă) [Gr. *kytos*, cell, + *ouron*, urine]. Presence of any kind of cells in the urine.

Czermak's spaces (chār'măks). [Johann N. Czermak, Bohemian physician, 1828–1873] The interglobular spaces in dentin due to failure of calcification.

D

δ. Delta, q.v., fourth letter of the Greek alphabet.

D. 1. L. *da*, give; *date; daughter; deciduous;* L. *detur*, let it be given; *died; diopter; divorced; doctor.* 2. Chem. symb. for deuterium.

D-. In chemistry, a symbol used as a prefix and written as a small capital letter to indicate the structure of certain organic compounds with asymmetric carbon atoms. If the asymmetric carbon is represented as

|
HCO·H
|

the name of the compound is preceded by D-. If it is represented as

|
HO·CH
|

the compound's name would be preceded by L-.

In other chemical nomenclature, a small letter *d*- or *l*- indicates the direction of rotation of a polarized light shown through a solution of the compound. When the plane of the light is rotated to the right, i.e., dextrorotatory, the compound's name is preceded by *d*-. If the light is rotated to the left, i.e., levorotatory, the name is preceded by *l*-.

If a D-compound that has an asymmetric carbon is also capable of rotating light and does so dextrorotatory, its name is preceded by D(+); if levorotatory, D(−). If the asymmetric carbon is of the L- form and is dextrorotatory, its name is prefixed by L(+); if levorotatory, the name is preceded by L(−).

d. *density;* L. *dexter* or *dextro*, right; L. *dies*, day; *distal; dorsal; duration.*

daboia, daboya (dă-boy'ă). Indian name for Russell's viper, a large poisonous snake of India, Burma, and Thailand. Venom of Russell's viper is used to enhance the action of certain blood coagulation factors.

dacarbazine (dă-kăr'bă-zēn). An alkylating agent used in treating neoplasms including malignant melanoma and Hodgkin's disease. Trade name is DTIC-Dome.

dacnomania (dăk"nō-mā'nē-ă) [Gr. *daknein*, to bite, + *mania*, insanity]. An irrational impulse to kill.

dacryadenalgia (dăk"rē-ăd-ĕn-ăl'jē-ă) [Gr. *dakryon*, tear, + *aden*, gland, + *algos*, pain]. Pain in a lacrimal gland. SYN: *dacryoadenalgia.*

dacryadenitis (dăk"rē-ăd-ĕ-nī'tĭs) [" + " + *itis*, inflammation]. Inflammation of a lacrimal gland.

dacryadenoscirrhus (dăk"rē-ăd"ĕn-ō-skĭr'us) [" + " + *skirrhos*, hardening]. Induration of a lacrimal gland.

dacryagogatresia (dăk"rē-ă-gŏg"ă-trē'sē-ă) [Gr. *dakryon*, tear, + *agogos*, leading, + *a*-, not, + *tresis*, perforate]. Occlusion of a tear duct.

dacryagogue (dăk'rē-ă-gŏg). An agent that stimulates the secretion of tears.

dacrycystalgia (dăk"rē-sĭs-tăl'jē-ă) [" + *kystis*, cyst, + *algos*, pain]. Pain in a lacrimal gland. SYN: *dacryocystalgia.*

dacryelcosis (dăk"rē-ĕl-kō'sĭs) [" + *helkosis*, ulceration]. Ulceration of the lacrimal apparatus.

dacryoadenalgia (dăk"rē-ō-ăd"ĕn-ăl'jē-ă) [" + *aden*, gland, + *algos*, pain]. Pain in a lacrimal gland. SYN: *dacryadenalgia.*

dacryoadenectomy (dăk"rē-ō-ăd"ĕ-nĕk'tō-mē) [" + " + *ektome*, excision]. Surgical removal of the lacrimal gland.

dacryoadenitis (dăk"rē-ō-ăd"ĕn-ī'tĭs) [" + " + *itis*, inflammation]. Inflammation of lacrimal gland. It is rare; seen as complication in epidemic parotitis (mumps of lacrimal gland) and present in Mikulicz's disease. May be acute or chronic.

dacryoblennorrhea (dăk"rē-ō-blĕn"ō-rē'ă) [" + *blenna*, mucus, + *rhoia*, flow]. Discharge of mucus from a lacrimal sac, and chronic inflammation of the sac.

dacryocele (dăk'rē-ō-sēl) [" + *kele*, hernia]. Protrusion of a lacrimal sac.

dacryocyst (dăk'rē-ō-sĭst) [" + *kystis*, cyst]. The lacrimal sac.

dacryocystalgia (dăk"rē-ō-sĭs-tăl'jē-ă) [" + " + *algos*, pain]. Pain in the lacrimal sac.

dacryocystectomy (dăk"rē-ō-sĭs-tĕk'tō-mē) [" + *kystis*, cyst, + *ektome*, excision]. The excision of membranes of the lacrimal sac.

dacryocystitis (dăk"rē-ō-sĭs-tī'tĭs) [" + " + *itis*, inflammation]. Inflammation of the tear sac involving mucous membrane of the lacrimal sac with submucous membrane, which later extends to connective tissue, surrounding it with resulting cellulitis. Usually secondary to prolonged obstruction of the nasolacrimal duct.

SYM: Profuse tearing (epiphora); redness and swelling in area of sac, which may also extend to lids and conjunctiva; pain, esp. on pressure over the lacrimal sac; overflow of tears.

TREATMENT: Hot compresses; application of ophthalmic antibiotic preparations; oral antibiotics; incision and drainage if fluctuant; attempt to restore permeability of duct with probe when acute symptoms have subsided; in chronic cases extirpate sac or do intranasal operation (dacryocystorhinostomy).

dacryocystoblennorrhea (dăk"rē-ō-sĭs"tō-blĕn-ō-rē'ă) [" + " + *blenna*, mucus, + *rhoia*, flow]. Chronic inflammation of and discharge from the lacrimal sac.

dacryocystocele (dăk"rē-ō-sĭs'tō-sēl) [Gr. *dakryon*, tear, + *kystis*, cyst, + *kele*, hernia]. Herniated protrusion of lacrimal sac.

dacryocystography (dăk"rē-ō-sĭs-tŏg'ră-fē) [" + " + *graphein*, to write]. Radiographic examination of the nasolacrimal drainage system after introduction of a contrast agent.

dacryocystoptosis (dăk"rē-ō-sĭs-tŏp-tō'sĭs) [" + " + *ptosis*, a falling]. Prolapse of the lacrimal sac.

dacryocystorhinostenosis (dăk"rē-ō-sĭs"tō-rī-nō-stĕ-nō'sĭs) [" + " + *rhis*, nose, + *stenosis*, narrowing]. Narrowing or obliteration of the canal connecting the lacrimal sac with the nasal cavity. Test for patency is done by placing a weak sugar solution in the conjunctival space. If the duct is patent, the patient will report a sweet taste in the mouth.

dacryocystorhinostomy (dăk"rē-ō-sĭs"tō-rī-nŏs'tō-mē) [" + " + " + *stoma*, opening]. Surgical connecting of lumen of tear sac with nasal cavity.

dacryocystorhinotomy (dăk"rē-ō-sĭs"tō-rī-nŏt'ō-mē) [" + " + " + *tome*, incision]. Surgical probing of the duct leading from the lacrimal sac into the nose.

dacryocystosyringotomy (dăk"rē-ō-sĭs"tō-sĭr"ĭn-gŏt'ō-mē) [" + *kystis*, cyst, + *syrinx*, tube, + *tome*, incision]. Making an opening between the lacrimal sac and the nasal cavity.

dacryocystotome (dăk"rē-ō-sĭs'tō-tōm) [" + " + *tome*, incision]. Device for incision of lacrimal sac.

dacryocystotomy (dăk"rē-ō-sĭs-tŏt'ō-mē). Incision of the lacrimal sac.

dacryogenic. Promoting the shedding of tears.

dacryohelcosis (dăk"rē-ō-hĕl-kō'sĭs) [" + *helcosis*, ulceration]. Ulceration of the lacrimal sac or duct.

dacryohemorrhea (dăk"rē-ō-hĕm"ō-rē'ă) [" + *haima*, blood, + *rhoia*, flow]. Discharge of bloody tears.

dacryolin (dăk'rē-ō-lĭn) [Gr. *dakryon*, tear]. An albuminous matter in tears.

dacryolith, dacryolite [' + *lithos*, stone]. Concretion in lacrimal passages.

dacryolithiasis (dăk"rē-ō-lĭ-thī'ă-sĭs) [" + *lithiasis*, formation of stones]. Presence of stones or calculi in the lacrimal apparatus.

dacryoma (dăk"rē-ō'mă) [" + *oma*, tumor]. 1. A lacrimal tumor. 2. A tumor-like swelling due to obstruction of the lacrimal duct.

dacryon (dăk'rē-ŏn) [Gr. *dakryon*]. The lacrimal point of juncture of the lacrimal, frontal, and upper maxillary bones.

dacryops (dăk'rē-ŏps) [" + *ops*, eye]. Constant flow of tears; dacryorrhea.

dacryopyorrhea (dăk"rē-ō-pī"ō-rē'ă) [" + *pyon*, pus, + *rhoia*, discharge]. Discharge of pus from lacrimal duct.

dacryopyosis [" + *pyosis*, suppuration]. Suppuration in the lacrimal sac or duct.

dacryorrhea (dăk"rē-ō-rē'ă) [" + *rhoia*, flow]. Excessive flow of tears.

dacryosolenitis (dăk"rē-ō-sō-lĕn-ī'tĭs) [" + *solen*, duct, + *itis*, inflammation]. Inflammation of a lacrimal or nasal duct.

dacryostenosis (dăk"rē-ō-stĕn-ō'sĭs) [" + *stenosis*, narrowing]. Stricture of a lacrimal or nasal duct.

dacryosyrinx (dăk"rē-ō-sĭ'rĭnks) [" + *syrinx*, tube]. A lacrimal fistula.

dactinomycin. An antibiotic of the actinomycin complex used as an antineoplastic agent. Trade name is Cosmegen.

dactyl (dăk'tĭl) [Gr. *daktylos*, finger]. A finger or toe; a digit of the hand or foot.

dactyledema (dăk"tĭl-ĕ-dē'mă) [" + *oidema*, swelling]. Edema of the fingers or toes.

dactylion. Adhesions between or union of fingers or toes.

dactylitis [" + *itis*, inflammation]. Chronic inflammation of bones of fingers and toes in very young children.

ETIOL: Usually tuberculous or syphilitic.

d., sickle cell. Painful swelling of the feet and hands during the first several years of life of children with sickle cell anemia, q.v.

dactylocampsodynia (dăk"tĭ-lō-kămp"sō-dĭn'ē-ă) [" + *kampsis*, bend, + *odyne*, pain]. Painful contraction of one or more fingers.

dactylogram [" + *gramma*, mark]. A fingerprint.

dactylography [" + *graphein*, to write]. 1. The study of fingerprints. 2. The act of using a machine for blind deaf-mutes to convey the signs of speech by touch.

dactylogryposis (dăk"tĭ-lō-grĭ-pō'sĭs) [" + *gryposis*, curve]. Permanent contraction of the fingers.

dactylology (dăk-tĭl-ŏl'ō-jē) [" + *logos*, study]. Representing words by signs made with the fingers. SYN: *sign language*.

dactylolysis (dăk"tĭ-lŏl'ĭ-sĭs) [" + *lysis*, dissolution]. Spontaneous dropping off of fingers or toes. Seen in leprosy and ainhum and sometimes in utero when a hair firmly wrapped around a digit will cause amputation of the finger or toe.

dactylomegaly (dăk"tĭ-lō-mĕg'ă-lē) [" + *megas*, large]. Abnormally large size of fingers and toes.

dactyloscopy (dăk"tĭ-lŏs'kō-pē) [" + *skopein*, to examine]. Examination of fingerprints for purpose of identification.

dactylospasm (dăk'tĭ-lō-spăzm) [" + *spasmos*, spasm]. Cramp of a finger or toe.

dactylus (dăk'tĭ-lŭs) [Gr. *daktylos*]. A toe or finger.

daily living skills. SEE: *activities of daily living*.

dairy food substitute. Foods resembling existing dairy foods in taste and appearance but different in composition from the dairy food for which they are substituted.

Dakin's solution (dā'kĭns). [Henry D. Dakin, U.S. chemist, 1880–1952] A solution for cleansing wounds, developed during World War I. A very dilute neutral solution (0.45 to 0.5%) of sodium hypochlorite and 0.4% boric acid.

Dale reaction. [Sir Henry H. Dale, 1875–1969, Brit. scientist and in 1936 Nobel prize winner] A test that demonstrates the ability of muscle tissues from an animal that has been made anaphylactic to contract when reexposed to the antigen. Either guinea pig uterine muscle or intestines are used. The test is very specific, as unrelated antigens will not cause the sensitized muscle to contract. Werner Schultz demonstrated the same phenomenon independent of Dale's work. SYN: *Schultz reaction*.

Dalmane. Trade name for flurazepam hydrochloride.

dalton (dawl'tŏn). An arbitrary unit of mass equal to $\frac{1}{12}$ the mass of carbon-12 or 1.657×10^{-24} gram.

Dalton, John. British chemist, 1766–1844.

D.-Henry law. [Joseph Henry, U.S. physicist, 1797–1878] When a mixture of gases is in equilibrium with a liquid, each gas will dissolve in the liquid in proportion to its partial pressure in the gas.

D.'s law. In a mixture of gases, the total pressure is equal to the sum of the partial pressures of each gas.

daltonism (dawl'tŏn-ĭzm). [John Dalton] Color blindness to perception of red and green.

dam. A thin sheet of rubber used in dentistry and surgery to isolate a part from the surrounding tissues and fluids. Frequently a rubber dam is used as a surgical drain.

damp. 1. Moist, humid. 2. A noxious gas in a mine.

d., after. A gaseous mixture formed by the explosion of methane and air in a mine; contains large percentage of carbon dioxide, nitrogen, and carbon monoxide.

d., black. An atmosphere formed by the slow absorption of oxygen and the giving off of carbon dioxide by the coal in a mine.

d., cold. Vapor charged with carbon dioxide.

d., fire. Methane, CH_4, found in coal mines.

d., white. Carbon monoxide.

damping. The steady diminution of the amplitude of successive vibrations as of an electric wave or current.

danazol (dă'nă-zōl). USP. Drug that suppresses the action of the anterior pituitary. It is used in treating endometriosis. Trade name is Danocrine.

dance, Saint Vitus'. A disease characterized by involuntary and irregular jerkings and movements in diverse groups of muscles. SEE: *chorea*.

Dance's sign. [Jean B. H. Dance, Fr. physician, 1797–1832] Slight retraction in the right iliac region in some cases of intussusception.

dancing disease. In Europe during the Middle Ages, epidemic dancing mania supposed to have been caused by the bite of the tarantula. SEE: *tarantism*.

dancing mania. Epidemic chorea.

D. and C. *dilation* of the cervix and *curettage* of the uterus; a gynecologic procedure.

dander (dăn'dĕr). Small scales from the hair or feathers of animals that may cause allergy in sensitive individuals.

dandruff. Normal exfoliation of the epidermis of the scalp in the form of dry, white scales. May be worse in diseased condition. Sometimes due to seborrhea, q.v.

dandy fever. Dengue, q.v. An acute, epidemic, febrile disease occuring in tropical areas.

Dandy-Walker syndrome (dăn'dē-wawk'ĕr). [Walter E. Dandy, U.S. neurosurgeon, 1886–1946; Arthur E. Walker, U.S. surgeon, b. 1907] Congenital hydrocephalus caused by blockage of the foramina of Magendie and Luschka, through which the cerebral spinal fluid passes.

Dane particles. [David S. Dane, contemporary Brit. virologist] Spheres 42 nanometers in diameter present in the serum of patients with hepatitis B. They contain hepatitis B surface (HB_sAg) and core (HB_cAg) antigens. They are composed of viruses and appear to be infectious. The blood of patients with hepatitis B infection has been found to have 10^7 Dane particles per ml.

Danocrine. Trade name for danazol, USP.

danthron (dăn'thrŏn). USP. A cathartic that helps to produce soft or semifluid stools. Trade names are Dorbane and Istizin.

Dantrium. Trade name for dantrolene sodium.

dantrolene sodium (dăn'trō-lēn). A muscle relaxant used to relieve spasticity. Trade name is Dantrium.

Danysz phenomenon. A phenomenon that provides an example of the reversibility of precipitation of complexes of antibodies and antigens. When a specified amount of diphtheria toxin is added all at once to an antitoxin serum, the mixture is nontoxic; but if the same quantity of toxin is added in portions at about 30-minute intervals, the mixture is toxic.

dapsone (dăp'sōn). USP. An antibacterial sulfone that is the drug of choice for treatment of all forms of leprosy. Also used in treatment of dermatitis herpetiformis. Frequent blood studies must be done on patients receiving this drug for prolonged periods, as hemolysis, leukopenia, and methemoglobinemia can occur. Trade name is Avlosulfon.

Daranide. Trade name for dichlorphenamide.

Daraprim. Trade name for pyrimethamine.

Darbid. Trade name for isopropamide iodide.

Daricon. Trade name for oxyphencyclimine hydrochloride.

Darier's disease (dăr-ē-āz'). [J. F. Darier, Fr. dermatologist, 1856–1938] A rare hereditary condition characterized by verrucous papular growths that coalesce into plaques of various sizes on the scalp, face, neck, trunk, and axillae. SYN: *keratosis follicularis*.

Darling's disease (dăr'lĭngz). [Samuel Taylor Darling, U.S. physician, 1872–1925] Histoplasmosis.

dartoid (dăr'toyd) [Gr. *dartos*, skinned, + *eidos*, form]. Resembling the tunica dartos in its slow, involuntary contractions.

dartos [Gr.]. The muscular, contractile tissue beneath the skin of the scrotum. SYN: *tunica dartos* [NA].

dartos muscle reflex. Wormlike contraction of dartos muscle following sudden cold application to perineum.

dartrous [Gr. *dartos*, skinned]. Of the nature of herpes; herpetic.

Darvon. Trade name for propoxyphene hydrochloride.

Darvon-N. Trade name for propoxyphene napsylate.

darwinian ear. [Charles Robert Darwin, Brit. naturalist, 1809–1882] An exaggeration of darwinian tubercle, q.v.

darwinian tubercle. A blunt point projecting from upper part of the helix of the ear.

darwinism (dăr'wĭ-nĭzm). The theory of biological evolution, q.v., through natural selection, q.v.

dasymeter (dăs-ĭm'ĕ-tĕr). Device for estimating density of gases.

Datril. Trade name for acetaminophen.

Datura (dā-tū'ră). A genus of plants, one member of which, Datura stramonium, contains constituents of hyoscyamine and scopolamine, which have anticholinergic properties.

daughter (daw'tĕr). 1. A decay product. 2. A product of cell division, as a daughter cell or daughter nucleus. 3. One's female child.

daunorubicin hydrochloride. USP. An antibiotic drug used as an antitumor agent in treating acute leukemia. Trade name is Cerubidine.

Davidsohn's sign. [Hermann Davidsohn, Prussian physician, 1842–1911] The lessening or absence of pupillary light reflex when an electric light is held in the closed mouth. Indicates presence of a tumor or fluid in the maxillary sinus.

day blindness. Inability to see well in a bright light.

day-care center. A place for the care of preschool children both of whose parents are employed or for some other reason are unable to care for their child during normal working hours.

dB, db. *decibel*.

D.C. *Doctor of Chiropractic; direct current.*

D.D.S. *Doctor of Dental Surgery.* SEE: *D.M.D.*

DDST. *Denver Developmental Screening Test.*

DDT. Dichloro-diphenyltrichloroethane; now called chlorophenothane. A powerful insecticide effective against a wide variety of insects, esp. the flea, fly, louse, mosquito, bedbug, cockroach, Japanese beetle, and European corn borer. However, many species develop resistant populations, and birds and fish that feed on affected insects suffer toxic effects. The United States in 1972 banned the use of DDT for all but essential public health use and for a few minor uses to protect crops for which there were no effective alternatives.

When ingested orally, it may cause acute poisoning. Symptoms are vomiting, numbness and partial paralysis of limbs, anorexia, tremors, and depression, resulting in death. SEE: *Poisons and Poisoning* in *Appendix*.

de- [L. *de*, from]. Prefix indicating down or from.

deacidification [" + *acidus*, sour, + *facere*, to make]. Neutralization of acidity.

deactivation [" + *activus*, acting]. The process of becoming inactive.

dead [AS. *dead*]. Without life or life processes. SEE: *death*.

deaf [AS. *deaf*]. 1. Partially or completely lacking the sense of hearing. 2. Unwillingness to listen; heedless.

deafferentation (dē-ăf"ĕr-ĕn-tā'shŭn). Cutting the afferent nerve supply.

deaf-mute. A person who is unable to hear or speak.

deaf-mutism. The state of being both deaf and unable to speak.

deafness [AS.]. Complete or partial loss of ability to hear. Some deaf persons will experience the hallucination of hearing music. This is not due to insanity.

ETIOL: May occur from several causes such as injury or disease of that part of the cortex controlling the center for hearing; disease of the middle ear or the eighth cranial nerve; toxic effects of certain drugs; hysteria without any abnormality of the ear or brain; injury of the ear from loud noises such as the firing of a gun at close range; an abnormal mental state producing auditory aphasia or psychic deafness, q.v.; or congenital defects.

Some forms of conduction deafness may be remedied by a fenestration operation or stapes mobilization. SEE: *otosclerosis*.

d., aviator's. A temporary or permanent nerve deafness found in a moderate percentage of aviators. This form of deafness is caused by prolonged exposure to loud noise levels.

d., bass. Inability to hear low-frequency tones.

d., central. Deafness resulting from lesions of auditory tracts of the brain or auditory centers of the cerebral cortex.

d., cerebral. Deafness due to brain lesion.

d., ceruminous. Deafness due to plugs of cerumen (ear wax).

d., conduction. Deafness resulting from any condition that prevents sound waves from being transmitted to the auditory receptors. May result from wax obstructing the external auditory meatus, inflammation of the middle ear, ankylosis of ear bones, or fixation of footplate of stirrup. SEE: *otosclerosis*.

d., cortical. Deafness due to disease of the cortical centers without a lesion.

d., nerve. Deafness due to a lesion of the auditory nerve or central neural pathways.

d., occupational. Deafness caused by working in places where noise levels are quite high. Persons working in such an environment should wear devices to protect the hearing sense from the noise.

d., perceptive. Deafness resulting from lesions involving sensory receptors of the cochlea or fibers of the acoustic nerve, or a combination.

d., psychic. Condition in which auditory sensations are perceived but not comprehended.

d., tone. Inability to distinguish musical sounds.

d., word. Condition in which sounds are heard but interpretation of the words is impossible. A form of aphasia, q.v.

dealbation (dē-ăl-bā'shŭn) [L. *de*, from, + *albare*, to whiten]. Bleaching.

deamidase (dē-ăm'ĭ-dās). An enzyme that splits amides to form carboxylic acid and ammonia.

deamidization (dē-ăm"ĭ-dĭ-zā'shŭn). The removal of an amide group by hydrolysis.

deaminase. An enzyme that causes the removal of an amino group from organic compounds.

deamination, deaminization. Loss of the NH_2 radical from amino compounds. Alanine can be deaminized to give ammonia and pyruvic acid: $CH_3CH(NH_2)COOH + O = CH_3CO{\bullet}COOH + NH_3$. Deaminization may be simple, oxidative, or hydrolytic. Oxidizing enzymes are called deaminizing enzymes when the oxidation is accompanied by splitting off of amino groups.

deaquation (dē"ă-kwā'shŭn) [" + *aqua*, water]. Dehydration; removal of water from anything.

dearterialization (dē"ăr'tēr"ē-ăl-ī-zā'shŭn) [" + Gr. *arteria*, artery]. Changing character of arterial into venous blood; deoxygenation.

dearticulation (dē"ăr-tĭk"ū-lā'shŭn). Dislocation of a joint.

death [AS. *death*]. Permanent cessation of all vital functions. The following definitions of death have also been considered: (1) Total irreversible cessation of: cerebral function, spontaneous function of the respiratory system, and spontaneous function of the circulatory system. (2) The final and irreversible cessation of perceptible heart beat and respiration. Conversely, as long as any heart beat or respiration can be perceived, either with or without mechanical or electrical aids, and regardless of how the heart beat and respiration were maintained, death has not occurred.

Conditions such as cardiac standstill or complete lack of renal function have meant certain death at one time. But the use of cardiac pacemakers, artificial hearts and kidneys, heart transplants, and kidney transplants has made this definition of death untenable.

NURSING IMPLICATIONS: When death has occurred in a hospital or other institution for care of the sick, the patient's name, hour of death, and name of the ward should be written on a piece of paper and attached to the body or otherwise identified according to the custom of the institution. It is important that the "laying out" be completed before the commencement of rigor mortis. If a physician is not present at the time of death, inform the next of kin at once because no preparation of the body may be begun until the doctor has officially pronounced the patient dead. The private duty nurse may be asked to continue on duty for several hours. In any case, the nurse should not leave until assured everything in the room is in order and no further service is necessary. SEE: *life*.

SIGNS: The principal sign of death is cessation of the heart's action. Other indications are absence of reflexes, cessation of electrical activity in the brain as determined by EEG, manifestations of rigor mortis, q.v., and a mottled discoloration of the body, esp. over all parts where there is pressure. In case of an emergency, the usual symptoms of death often are found to be unreliable. Attempts at resuscitation should continue to be made indefinitely. No harm can be done in attempting to resuscitate one who seems to be deceased; successes are numerous.

Determining time lapse since death occurred: Take the rectal temperature. In general the body loses one degree of Fahrenheit temperature each hour following death. Of course, the rate of heat loss varies with temperature of the surrounding air, water, or snow.

d., black. Former name for bubonic plague.

d., brain. Brain death, q.v.

d., crib. Sudden infant death syndrome q.v.

d., fetal. Death of a fetus in utero.

d., functional. Central nervous system death with vital functions being artificially supported.

d., local. Gangrene or necrosis of a part.

d., molecular. Death of cell life.

death, words pert. to: agonal; ante mortem; autopsy; demise; euthanasia; in articulo mortis; in extremis; lethal; "necr-" words; posthumous; post mortem; putrefaction; rigor mortis; suicide.

deathbed. 1. The bed on which a person dies. 2. The final hours preceding death.

deathbed statement. A declaration made at the time immediately preceding death. Such a statement, if made with the consciousness and belief that death is impending, may be held in law as equally binding with a statement made under oath. SYN: *antemortem statement.*

death rate. The number of deaths occurring per 1000 of the population in a given area within a specified time. SYN: *mortality.*

death rattle. A sound heard in the throat of the dying. Caused by the accumulation of mucus in the throat due to absence of the cough reflex. The breath moving through the mucus makes the "rattle" sound.

"death with dignity." A concept resulting from the fact that it is possible to maintain metabolic functions in persons who will or may eventually remain in a coma for the remainder of their lives. In order to prevent this prolongation of life, a patient, or the family if the patient is unconscious, may sign this statement: "I request that I be allowed to die and not be kept alive by artificial means or heroic measures. I ask also that drugs be mercifully administered to me to alleviate terminal suffering even if they may hasten the moment of death."

debilitant [L. *debilis,* weak]. 1. A remedy used to reduce excitement. 2. That which weakens.

debilitate. To produce weakness or debility.

debility. Weakness of tonicity in functions or organs of the body.

débouchement (dā-boosh-mŏn') [Fr.]. Opening or emptying into another part.

Debove's membrane (dĕ-bōvz'). [Georges Maurice Debove, Fr. physician, 1845–1920] Layer of connective tissue cells between the epithelium and basement tissue of respiratory and intestinal epithelia.

débride (dā-brēd') [Fr.]. To perform the action of debridement.

débridement (dā-brēd-mŏn') [Fr.]. The removal of foreign material and dead or damaged tissue, esp. in a wound.

debris (dĕ-brē') [Fr., remains]. The remains of broken down or damaged cells or tissue.

debrisoquin (dĕb-rĭs'ō-kwĭn). An antihypertensive medicine not generally available in the U.S.A.

debt (dĕt). Deficit.

d., oxygen. After strenuous, i.e., anaerobic, physical activity, the oxygen required, in addition to that required while resting, in the recovery period to oxidize the excess lactic acid produced and to replenish the depleted stores of adenosine triphosphate and phosphocreatinase.

deca-, dec- [Gr. *deka*]. Prefix indicating ten.

Decaderm. Trade name for dexamethasone.

Decadron. Trade name for dexamethasone.

Decadron-LA. Trade name for dexamethasone acetate.

Deca-Durabolin. Trade name for nandrolone decanoate.

decagram (dĕk'ă"grăm) [" + *gramma,* weight]. A weight of 10 grams.

decalcification (dē"kăl-sĭ-fĭ-kā'shŭn) [L. *de,* from, + *calx,* lime, + *facere,* to make]. The removal of, or the withdrawal of, lime salts from bone or teeth.

decalcify. To soften bone by removal of calcium or its salts by acids.

decaliter (dĕk'ă-lē"tĕr) [Gr. *deka,* ten, + Fr. *litre,* liter]. A measure of 10 liters, equivalent to about 10.57 quarts. SEE: *deciliter.*

decalvant (dē-kăl'vănt) [L. *decalvare,* to make bald]. Destroying hair or making bald.

decameter (dĕk'ă-mē-tĕr) [Gr. *deka,* ten, + *metron,* measure]. A measure of 10 meters; 393.71 in.

decamethonium bromide (dĕk"ă-mē-thō'nē-ŭm). USP. A neuromuscular blocking agent that relaxes muscles. Used in anesthesia and to prevent muscle trauma during electroshock therapy. Trade name is Syncurine.

CAUTION: An overdose may be lethal due to prolonged apnea and cardiac collapse. This drug should be used only by those familiar with its pharmacology and where facilities and staff for respiratory and cardiovascular resuscitation are immediately available.

decannulation (dē-kăn"nū-lā'shŭn). The removal of a cannula.

decanormal (dĕk"ă-nor'măl) [" + L. *norma,*

rule]. Pert. to a solution 10 times as strong as a normal one. It contains 10 gm. equivalent weights of the substance per liter. SEE: *normal.*

decant (dē-kănt′) [L. *de,* from, + *canthus,* rim of a vessel]. To pour off liquid so the sediment remains in the bottom of the container.

decantation. The gentle pouring off of a liquid from its sediment.

decapitation (dē-kăp″ĭ-tā′shŭn) [″ + *caput,* head]. 1. The separation of the head from the body; beheading. 2. Separating the head from the shaft of a bone. SYN: *detruncation.*

decapsulation [″ + *capsula,* little box]. Removal of a capsule of an organ.

decarboxylase (dē″kăr-bŏk′sĭ-lās). An enzyme that catalyzes the release of carbon dioxide from compounds such as amino acids.

decarboxylation, decarboxylization (dē″kăr-bŏks-ĭ-lā′shŭn, -ĭl″ĭ-zā′shŭn). A chemical reaction whereby the carboxyl group, —COOH, is removed from an organic compound.

Decaspray. Trade name for dexamethasone.

decavitamin capsules or tablets (dĕk″ă-vī′tă-mĭn). USP. A vitamin preparation that contains vitamins A, D, and C; calcium pantothenate; folic acid; niacin amide; pyridoxine hydrochloride (vitamin B_6); riboflavin; thiamine hydrochloride (vitamin B_1); a suitable form of alpha tocopherol (vitamin E); and cyanocobalamin (vitamin B_{12}).

decay (dē-kā′) [″ + *cadere,* to fall]. 1. Gradual loss of vigor with physical and mental deterioration as in aging. SEE: *senility.* 2. To waste away. 3. Decomposition of organic matter by the action of microorganisms. SEE: *cementoclasia.* 4. Disintegration of radioactive substances.

deceleration (dē-sĕl″ĕ-rā′shŭn). Decrease in velocity.

decerebrate (dē-sĕr′ĕ-brāt) [″ + *cerebrum,* brain]. 1. To eliminate cerebral function by decerebration. 2. A person or animal who has been subjected to decerebration.

decerebrate posture. The posture present in an individual with decerebrate rigidity. The extremities are stiff and extended, and the head is retracted.

decerebrate rigidity. SEE: *rigidity, decerebrate.*

decerebration (dē-sĕr-ĕ-brā′shŭn). Removal of the brain or cutting the spinal cord at the level of the brain stem. SEE: *pithing.*

dechlorination, dechloridation [″ + Gr. *chloros,* green]. Reduction in the amount of chlorides in the body by reduction of or withdrawal of salt in the diet.

decholesterolization (dē″kō-lĕs″tĕr-ŏl-ī-zā′shŭn) [″ + *chole,* bile, + *stereos,* solid]. Reduction of cholesterol in the blood.

Decholin. Trade name for dehydrocholic acid.

deci- [L. *decimus,* tenth]. Prefix indicating one tenth.

decibel (dĕs′ĭ-bĕl) [L. *decimus,* tenth, + *bel,* unit of sound]. The unit for expressing, logarithmically, the difference in two powers, usually between electric or acoustic energy signals.

decidophobia [*decide* + Gr. *phobos,* fear]. Fear of making a decision.

decidua (dē-sĭd′ū-ă) [L. *deciduus,* falling off]. The name given to the endometrium or lining of the uterus during pregnancy, and the tissue around the ectopically located fertilized ovum, e.g., in the fallopian tube or peritoneal cavity. The gland structures of the endometrium and the interstitial cells undergo marked hypertrophy. The decidua divides itself into an outer or compact layer and an inner spongy layer.

d. basalis. [NA] That part of the decidua that unites with the chorion to form the placenta. SYN: *d. serotina.*

d. capsularis. [NA] That part of the decidua that surrounds the chorionic sac. SYN: *d. reflexa.*

d. menstrualis. The layer of the uterine endometrium that is shed during menstruation.

d. parietalis. [NA] The endometrium during pregnancy except at the site of the implanted blastocyst. SYN: *d. vera.*

d. reflexa. D. capsularis.

d. serotina. D. basalis.

d. vera. D. parietalis.

decidual (dē-sĭd′ū-ăl). Pert. to or resembling the decidua.

deciduation (dē-sĭd″ū-ā′shŭn). The loss of the decidua during menstruation.

deciduitis (dē-sĭd″ū-ī′tĭs) [″ + Gr. *itis,* inflammation]. Inflammation of the decidua.

deciduoma (dē-sĭd″ū-ō′mă) [″ + Gr. *oma,* tumor]. A uterine tumor containing decidual tissue. Thought to arise from portions of decidua retained within the uterus following an abortion.

d., benign. The more or less normal invasion of the uterine musculature by the syncytium, which disappears after the gestation is completed.

d., Loeb's. Decidual tissue produced within the uterus of experimental animals as a result of mechanical or hormonal stimulation.

d., malignant. A tumor consisting of syncytial and Langhans cells, which have a tendency to invade the general system by means of the bloodstream. Specific therapy with methotrexate may cause a complete remission. SYN: *choriocarcinoma; chorioepithelioma.*

ETIOL: This tumor may arise following a full-term pregnancy, an ectopic pregnancy, an abortion, a miscarriage, and particularly a vesicular mole.

DIAG: May be made by histological study, aided by the symptoms and the Aschheim-Zondek test, which remains strongly positive during the presence of this type of tumor.

TREATMENT: Chemotherapy with the folic acid antagonist methotrexate (USP).

deciduomatosis (dē-sĭd″ū-ō-mă-tō′sĭs) [″ + Gr. *oma,* tumor, + *osis,* condition]. Excessive and irregular formation of decidual tissue in the nonpregnant state.

deciduosarcoma [″ + Gr. *sarx,* flesh, + *oma,* tumor]. A tumor of the chorion. SYN: *choriocarcinoma; chorioepithelioma.*

deciduous (dē-sĭd′ū-ŭs) [L. *deciduus*]. Falling off; subject to being shed.

deciduous teeth. The milk teeth or temporary teeth, 10 in each jaw: 4 incisors, 2 canines, and 4 molars. They usually appear at 6 months and are lost by the end of 6 years. Those of the lower jaw appear before the upper ones, as follows: Lower central incisors at 5 to 9 months; upper incisors at 8 to 12 months; lower lateral incisors and first molars at 12 to 15 months; canines at 18 to 24 months; second molars at 24 to 30 months. SEE: *dentition.*

decigram (dĕs′ĭ-grăm) [L. *decimus,* tenth, + Gr. *gramma,* weight]. One tenth of a gram.

deciliter (dĕs′ĭ-lē-tĕr) [″ + Fr. *litre*]. ABBR: dl. A unit of volume in the SI system of measurement that is equal to 0.1 liter or 100 milliliters.

decimeter (dĕs′ĭ-mē″tĕr) [″ + Gr. *metron,* measure]. One tenth of a meter.

decinormal (dĕs″ĭ-nor′măl) [″ + *norma,* rule]. Having one tenth the strength of a normal solution. SEE: *normal.*

decipara (dĕs″ĭ-păr′ă) [″ + *parere,* to bear]. A woman who has given birth for the tenth time to an infant or infants, alive or dead, weighing 500 grams or more. SYN: *para X.*

Declaration of Geneva. A statement adopted in 1948 by the Second General Assembly of the World Medical Association. Some medical schools use it at graduation exercises.

"At the time of being admitted as Member of the Medical Profession I solemnly pledge myself to consecrate my life to the service of humanity. I will give to my teachers the respect and gratitude which is their due; I will practice my profession with conscience and dignity; The health of my patient will be my first consideration; I will respect the secrets which are confided in me; I will maintain by all the means in my power, the honor and the noble traditions of the medical profession; my colleagues will be my brothers; I will not permit considerations of religion, nationality, race, party politics or social standing to intervene between my duty and my patient; I will maintain the utmost respect for human life, from the time of conception; even under threat, I will not use my medical knowledge contrary to the laws of humanity. I make these promises solemnly, freely and upon my honor." SEE: *Hippocratic oath; Nightingale Pledge; Prayer of Maimonides.*

Declaration of Hawaii. The General Assembly of the World Psychiatric Association has laid down the following ethical guidelines for psychiatrists all over the world. These guidelines were unanimously adopted by the association in 1976.

(1) The aim of psychiatry is to promote health and personal autonomy and growth. To the best of his or her ability, consistent with accepted scientific and ethical principles, the psychiatrist shall serve the best interests of the patient and be also concerned for the common good and a just allocation of health resources.

To fulfill these aims requires continuous research and continual education of health care personnel, patients, and the public.

(2) Every patient must be offered the best therapy available and be treated with the solicitude and respect due to the dignity of all human beings and to their autonomy over their own lives and health.

The psychiatrist is responsible for treatment given by the staff members and owes them qualified supervision and education. Whenever there is a need, or whenever a reasonable request is forthcoming from the patient, the psychiatrist should seek the help or the opinion of a more experienced colleague.

(3) A therapeutic relationship between patient and psychiatrist is founded on mutual agreement. It requires trust, confidentiality, openness, cooperation, and mutual responsibility. Such a relationship may not be possible to establish with some severely ill patients. In that case, as in the treatment of children, contact should be established with a person close to the patient and acceptable to him or her.

If and when a relationship is established for purposes other than therapeutic, such as in forensic psychiatry, its nature must be thoroughly explained to the person concerned.

(4) The psychiatrist should inform the patient of the nature of the condition, of the proposed diagnostic and therapeutic procedures, including possible alternatives, and of the prognosis. This information must be offered in a considerate way and the patient be given the opportunity to choose between appropriate and available methods.

(5) No procedure must be performed or treatment given against or independent of a

patient's own will, unless the patient lacks capacity to express his or her own wishes or, owing to psychiatric illness, cannot see what is in his or her best interest or, for the same reason, is a severe threat to others.

In these cases compulsory treatment may or should be given, provided that it is done in the patient's best interests and over a reasonable period of time, a retroactive informed consent can be presumed, and, whenever possible, consent has been obtained from someone close to the patient.

(6) As soon as the above conditions for compulsory treatment no longer apply the patient must be released, unless he or she voluntarily consents to further treatment.

Whenever there is compulsory treatment or detention there must be an independent and neutral body of appeal for regular inquiry into these cases. Every patient must be informed of its existence and be permitted to appeal to it, personally or through a representative, without interference by the hospital staff or by anyone else.

(7) The psychiatrist must never use the possibilities of the profession for maltreatment of individuals or groups, and should be concerned never to let inappropriate personal desires, feelings, or prejudices interfere with the treatment.

The psychiatrist must not participate in compulsory psychiatric treatment in the absence of psychiatric illness. If the patient or some third party demands actions contrary to scientific or ethical principles the psychiatrist must refuse to cooperate. When, for any reason, either the wishes or the best interests of the patient cannot be promoted he or she must be so informed.

(8) Whatever the psychiatrist has been told by the patient, or has noted during examination or treatment, must be kept confidential unless the patient releases the psychiatrist from professional secrecy, or else vital common values or the patient's best interest makes disclosure imperative. In these cases, however, the patient must be immediately informed of the breach of secrecy.

(9) To increase and propagate psychiatric knowledge and skill requires participation of the patients. Informed consent must, however, be obtained before presenting a patient to a class and, if possible, also when a case history is published, and all reasonable measures be taken to preserve the anonymity and to safeguard the personal reputation of the subject.

In clinical research, as in therapy, every subject must be offered the best available treatment. His or her participation must be voluntary, after full information has been given of the aims, procedures, risks, and inconveniences of the project, and there must always be a reasonable relationship between calculated risks or inconveniences and the benefit of the study.

For children and other patients who cannot themselves give informed consent this should be obtained from someone close to them.

(10) Every patient or research subject is free to withdraw for any reason at any time from any voluntary treatment and from any teaching or research program in which he or she participates. This withdrawal, as well as any refusal to enter a program, must never influence the psychiatrist's efforts to help the patient or subject.

The psychiatrist should stop all therapeutic, teaching, or research programs that may evolve contrary to the principles of this Declaration. SEE: *Declaration of Geneva; Hippocratic oath; Nightingale pledge; Prayer of Maimonides.*

declination (dĕk″lĭ-nā′shŭn). Cyclophoria, q.v.

declinator (dĕk′lĭn-ā″tor) [L. *declinare,* to turn aside]. Instrument used during trephining for holding apart the dura mater.

decline (dē-klīn′). 1. Progressive decrease. 2. Declining period of a disease.

declivis cerebelli (dē-klīv′ĭs sĕr-ĕ-bĕl′ī) [L.]. Sloping posterior portion of the monticulus of the superior vermis of the cerebellum.

decoction (dē-kŏk′shŭn) [L. *de,* down, + *coquere,* to boil]. A liquid medicinal preparation made by boiling vegetable substances with water. When the strength and method of preparation are not otherwise specified, it is made by boiling five parts of the coarsely comminuted drug for 15 minutes with enough water to make 100 parts. There are no official decoctions.

decollation (dē′kŏl-ā′shŭn) [″ + *collum,* neck]. Decapitation, esp. of the fetus during labor. SYN: *detruncation.*

décollement (dā-kōl-mŏn′) [Fr., ungluing]. Separation of two adherent structures.

decoloration (dē-kŭl″or-ā′shŭn). Loss or removal of color or pigment.

decompensation [L. *de,* from, + *compensare,* to make good again]. 1. Failure of heart to maintain adequate circulation. 2. In psychology, failure of defense system mechanism such as occurs in relapses of mental patients.

decomplementize. Removal of complement.

decomposition (dē-kŏm-pō-zĭsh′ŭn) [″ + *componere,* to put together]. 1. The putrefactive process; decay. 2. Reducing a compound body to its simpler constituents. SEE: *fermentation; resolution.*

d., double. A chemical change in which the molecules of two interacting compounds exchange a portion of their constituents.

d., hydrolytic. Chemical change in substances due to addition of a molecule of water.

d., simple. A chemical change by which a molecule of a single compound breaks into its simpler constituents or substitutes the entire molecule of another body for one of these constituents.

decompress. 1. To pass from a state of stress to tranquillity. 2. To relieve pressure, esp. that produced by air or gas.

decompression [" + *compressio,* a squeezing together]. 1. The removal of pressure, as from gas in the intestinal tract. SEE: *Wangensteen's method.* 2. The slow reduction or removal of pressure on deep-sea divers and caisson workers to prevent development of nitrogen bubbles in the tissue spaces.

d., explosive. In aviators or divers, decompression resulting from an extremely rapid rate of change from one pressure to a much lesser pressure. This may occur if a high-altitude aircraft suddenly loses its cabin pressurization or if a diver ascends quite rapidly. Either of these causes violent expansion of body gases.

decompression chamber. A tank in which patients suffering from decompression sickness are placed. After entry into the chamber, the barometric pressure is increased to the level that relieves the patient's symptoms, and then very slowly decreased until pressure is equal to outside pressure.

decompression illness. A condition that develops in divers subjected to rapid reduction of air pressure after coming to the surface following exposure to compressed air. The cause is nitrogen bubbles in the tissue spaces. SYN: *caisson disease.* SEE: *bends.*

decongestant. 1. Reducing congestion or swelling. 2. An agent that reduces congestion, esp. nasal.

decontamination. The process of rendering an object, person, or area free of a contaminating substance such as bacteria, poison gas, or a radioactive substance.

decorticate posture. Characteristic posture of a patient with a lesion at or above the upper brainstem. The patient is rigidly still with arms flexed, fists clenched, and the legs extended.

decortication [" + *cortex,* bark]. The removal of the surface layer of an organ or structure, as the removal of a portion of the cortex of the brain from the underlying white portion.

d., pulmonary. Removal of the pleura of the lung or a portion of the surface lung tissue.

d., renal. Removal of capsule of the kidney.

decrement (dĕk'rē-mĕnt) [L. *decrementum,* decrease]. The period in the course of a febrile disease when the fever subsides.

decrepitate (dē-krĕp'ĭ-tāt) [L. *decrepitare,* to crackle]. To cause decrepitation or a crackling noise.

decrepitation. A crackling noise.

decrepitude (dē-krĕp'ĭ-tūd). State of general feebleness and decline that sometimes accompanies old age; weak; infirm.

decrudescence (dē-kroo-dĕs'ĕns). Decrease in the severity of the symptoms of disease.

decubation (dē-kū-bā'shŭn) [L. *de,* down, + *cumbere,* to lie]. 1. The act of lying down. 2. The recovery stage of an infectious disease.

decubital. Pert. to a bedsore.

decubitus (dē-kū'bĭ-tŭs) [L., a lying down]. 1. A bedsore. 2. A patient's position in bed.

d., acute. A severe, sometimes fatal, bedsore that can occur on the affected side in hemiplegia.

d., Andral's. Position assumed by patient of lying on sound side during early stages of pleurisy.

d., dorsal. Lying on the back.

d., lateral. Lying on the side.

d., ventral. Lying on the stomach.

decubitus ulcer. Ulcer resulting from pressure to an area of the body from a bed or chair. The sacral iliac spines, heels, and trochanters are most prone to decubitus ulcer formation.

NURSING IMPLICATIONS: The nurse should work to prevent decubiti through frequent inspection of the skin for redness and signs of skin breakdown. Good skin care, especially over bone prominences, and turning and position changes every two hours, passive range of motion exercises, early ambulation, provision of nutritious meals, and use of a water mattress or lamb's wool are all needed. It is important that special beds and mattresses used in treating or preventing decubiti be kept in proper working order. In the event of decubiti development, the above measures should be continued. In addition, the decubiti should be thoroughly cleansed and debrided, and ordered treatments should be carried out. Direct application of sugar to decubiti has been found to be of assistance in promoting healing.

decurrent (dē-kŭr'ĕnt) [L. *decurrere,* to run down]. Traveling or extending down from above.

decussate (dē-kŭs'āt) [L. *decussare,* to make an X]. 1. To cross, or crossed, as in the form of the letter x. 2. Interlacing or crossing of parts.

decussation. 1. A crossing of structures in form of an x. 2. The place of crossing. SYN: *chiasma.*

d. of pyramids. Crossing of fibers of pyramids of the medulla oblongata from one pyramid to the other.

d., optic. The crossing of the fibers of the

optic nerves; the optic chiasma.

decussorium (dē-kŭs-ō'rē-ŭm). Instrument for depression of the dura following trephining.

dedifferentiation. 1. The return of parts to a homogeneous state. 2. Process by which mature differentiated cells or tissues are sites of origin of immature elements of the same type, as in some cancers.

dedolation (dĕd"ō-lā'shŭn). 1. Removal of a thin shaving of skin using an oblique slicing cut. 2. The feeling that the limbs have been bruised.

deduction (dē-dŭk'shŭn). Reasoning from the general to the particular.

deep [AS. *deop*]. Below the surface.

deep reflexes. Reflexes within, or fractional stretch reflexes. Opposed to superficial or skin reflexes.

deer fly. A biting fly, Chrysops discalis, that transmits the causative organism of deer fly fever, a form of tularemia.

deer fly fever. An acute plague-like infectious disease caused by Francisella tularensis. Transmitted to man by the bite of an infected tick or other bloodsucking insect; direct contact with infected animals; by eating inadequately cooked meat or by drinking water that contains the organism. SYN: *tularemia.*

SYM: From 1 to 10 days but averaging 3 days after infection, headache, chilliness, vomiting, aching pains, and fever develop. Site of infection develops into an ulcer. Glands at elbow or in armpit become enlarged, tender, and painful; later may develop into an abscess. Sweating, loss of weight, and debility.

TREATMENT: Streptomycin and tetracyclines are effective.

DEF. *decayed, extracted,* and *filled* teeth.

defatted [" + AS. *faelt,* to fatten]. Freed from or deprived of fat.

defecalgesiophobia (dĕf"ĕ-kăl"jē-sē-ō-fō'bē-ă) [L. *defaecare,* to remove dregs, + Gr. *algesis,* pain, + *phobos,* fear]. Fear of defecating because of pain.

defecation (dĕf-ĕ-kā'shŭn) [L. *defaecare,* to remove dregs]. Evacuation of the bowels. The bulk of the feces depends upon the amount and composition of food ingested. One does not, however, have to eat in order to have bowel movements. A large quantity of cellular material is desquamated from the epithelial lining of the intestinal tract each day. The food residues, reaching the rectum, cause the urge to defecate. The sensation is related to periodic increase of pressure within the rectum and contracture of its musculature. The expulsion of a fecal mass is accompanied by coordinated action of the following mechanisms: involuntary contraction of the circular muscle of the rectum behind the bowel mass followed by contraction of the longitudinal muscle; relaxation of the internal (involuntary) and external (voluntary) sphincter ani; voluntary closure of the glottis, fixation of the chest, and contraction of the abdominal muscles, causing an increase in intra-abdominal pressure. SEE: *constipation; feces; stool.*

defect (dē'fĕkt). A flaw or imperfection.

d., congenital. Imperfection present at birth.

d., filling. Interruption of the contour of the inner surface of the stomach or intestine revealed by roentgenography.

d., septal. A defect in one or more of the septa between the heart chambers.

defective [L. *defectus,* a failure]. 1. Not perfect. 2. A person deficient in one or more physical, mental, or moral powers.

defeminization (dē-fĕm"ĭ-nĭ-zā'shŭn). The loss of female sexual characteristics.

defense [L. *defendre,* to repel]. 1. Resistance to disease. 2. Acting to protect one's self from harm or injury.

defense mechanism. 1. Any reaction, whether general or cellular, that serves to protect against something harmful, as in immune reactions. Any defense mechanism occurring in excess can be pathological. 2. In psychoanalysis, a method of unconscious behavior used to resolve or conceal conflicts or anxieties. Ex.: compensation; denial; projection.

defense reflex. Retraction or tension in defense against an action or threatened action.

defensive. Defending; a means of protecting from injury.

defensive medicine. To practice medicine as if each patient is a potential malpractice suit. This is done by ordering an inordinate number of laboratory and test procedures.

deferens (dĕf'ĕr-ĕnz) [L. *deferens,* carrying away]. Deferent.

deferent (dĕf'ĕr-ĕnt). Conveying anything away from or downward. SEE: *afferent; efferent.*

deferentectomy (dĕf-ĕr-ĕn-tĕk'tō-mē) [" + Gr. *ektome,* excision]. Cutting of a ductus deferens.

deferential (dĕf-ĕr-ĕn'shăl) [L. *deferre,* to bring to]. Pert. to or accompanying the ductus deferens.

deferentitis (dĕf"ĕr-ĕn-tī'tĭs) [" + Gr. *itis,* inflammation]. Inflammation of the ductus deferens.

deferoxamine mesylate (dĕ-fĕr-ŏks'ă-mēn). USP. A drug with a very high affinity for iron. It is used parenterally to reduce the iron stored in the body in patients with hemochromatosis, acute iron poisoning, or abnormal storage of iron due to multiple blood transfusions. Trade name is Desferal.

deferred shock. Delayed onset of symptoms of shock.

defervescence [L. *defervescere,* to become calm]. The period that marks the subsidence of fever to normal temperature.

defibrillation. Stopping fibrillation of the heart through the use of drugs or by physical means. SEE: *cardioversion; defibrillation, electrical.*

d., electrical. Stopping fibrillation of the heart by using an electrical device that applies countershocks to the heart through electrodes placed on the chest wall. It is hoped that this countershock will allow the heart's normal pacemaker to take over. The electrical "dose" required for defibrillation is less for light-weight individuals than for larger persons. SEE: *cardioversion; cardioverter.*

defibrillator (dē-fĭb″rĭ-lā′tor). Electric device that produces defibrillation of the heart.

defibrination, defibrinization [L. *de,* from, + *fibra,* fiber]. Process of being deprived of fibrin. SEE: *coagulation.*

deficiency (dē-fĭsh′ĕn-sē) [L. *deficere,* to lack]. A lack; less than the normal amount.

deficiency disease. Condition due to a deficiency of a substance essential in body metabolism. The deficiency may be due to either inadequate intake, digestion, absorption, or utilization. It may also be due to excess loss through excretion or to an intestinal parasite such as hookworm or tapeworm.

Ex.: Night blindness and keratomalacia due to lack of vitamin A; beriberi or polyneuritis due to lack of thiamine; pellagra due to lack of niacin; scurvy due to lack of vitamin C; rickets and osteomalacia due to lack of vitamin D; pernicious anemia due to lack of gastric intrinsic factor and vitamin B_{12}.

deficit (dĕf′ĭ-sĭt). A deficiency or lack, e.g., muscular or mental deficit.

definition [L. *definire,* to limit]. 1. The precise determination of the limits of anything, esp. a disease process. 2. The detail with which images are recorded on radiographic film or screens.

definitive. Clear and final; without question.

deflection (dē-flĕk′shŭn). To turn away from a previous or usual course.

defloration (dĕf″lō-rā′shŭn) [L. *de,* from, + *flos, flor-,* flower]. Rupture of the hymen during coitus, by accident, surgically, or through vaginal examination. Not many females have a hymen that is of such size or consistency as to require its surgical rupture. SEE: *hymen; virginity.*

deflorescence. Disappearance of an eruption of the skin.

defluvium (dē-floo′vē-ŭm) [L.]. Falling out.

d. capillorum. Loss of hair.

defluxio (dē-flŭk′sē-ō) [L.]. A flowing down.

d. capillorum. A falling out of hair.

d. ciliorum. A falling out of eyelashes.

defluxion (dē-flŭk′shŭn). A flowing down; copious discharge or loss of any kind.

deformability (dē-form″ă-bĭl′ĭ-tē). Capable of being deformed.

deformation [L. *de,* from, + *forma,* form]. The act of deforming; a disfiguration.

deformity. An alteration in the natural form of a part or organ. Distortion of any part or general disfigurement of the body. It may be acquired or congenital. If present after injury, usually implies presence of fracture, dislocation, or both. May be due to extensive swelling, extravasation of blood, or rupture of muscles.

d., anterior. Abnormal anterior convexity of the spine. SYN: *lordosis.*

d., gunstock. Deformity in which the forearm when extended makes an angle with the arm because of displacement of the axis of the extended arm.

ETIOL: Condylar fracture at the elbow.

d., Madelung's. Distortion of the radius at its lower end with ulnar displacement backward.

d., mutilans. SEE: *mutilans deformity.*

d., seal fin. Lateral deviation of the fingers in rheumatoid arthritis.

d., silverfork. The peculiar deformity seen in Colles' fracture of the forearm. SEE: *Colles' fracture.*

d., Sprengel's. Congenital upward displacement of the scapula.

d., Velpeau's. D., silverfork.

d., Volkmann's. Congenital tibiotarsal dislocation.

defundation [″ + *fundus,* base]. Excision of the uterine fundus.

defurfuration (dē″fĕr-fū-rā′shŭn) [″ + *furfur,* bran]. Shedding of epidermis in scales; branny desquamation. May occur in various skin conditions including seborrheic dermatitis (dandruff), psoriasis, ichthyosis, and eczema.

deg. *degeneration; degree.*

deganglionate (dē-găn′glē-ŏn-āt″) [″ + Gr. *ganglion,* knot]. To deprive of ganglia.

degenerate [L. *degenerare,* to fall from one's ancestral quality]. 1. To deteriorate. 2. Characterized by deterioration.

degeneration [L. *degeneratio*]. Deterioration or impairment of an organ or part in structure of cells and the substances of which they are a part. Opposed to regeneration.

d., Abercrombie's. D., amyloid.

d., adipose. D., fatty.

d., albuminoid. D., amyloid.

d., amyloid. Degeneration resulting from deposition of amyloid between cells in various organs and tissues, esp. affecting blood vessels. Seen in wasting diseases.

d., ascending. Nerve fiber degeneration progressing to the center from the periphery.

d., bacony. D., amyloid.

d., calcareous. Infiltration of lime salts into tissues.

d., caseous. Cheesy alteration of tissues

seen in tuberculosis.

d., cloudy swelling. A condition in which protein substances in cells become cloudy, the cells increasing in size with minute droplets of protein substances. This may occur in any inflamed tissue.

d., colloid. Jellylike disorganization of tissues.

d., congenital macular. Various forms of congenital degeneration of the macula of the eye.

d., cystic. Cyst formation accompanying degeneration.

d., descending. Nerve fiber degeneration progressing toward the periphery from the original lesion.

d., fatty. Deposition of abnormal amounts of fat in cells, or the replacement or infiltration of tissues by fat cells.

d., fibroid. Change of membranous tissue into that of a fibrous nature.

d., gray. Degeneration in white nerve tissue due to chronic inflammation, assuming a gray color.

d., hepatolenticular. A hereditary syndrome transmitted as an autosomal recessive trait in which a decrease of ceruloplasmin, q.v., permits accumulation of copper in various organs (brain, liver, kidney, and cornea) associated with increased intestinal absorption of copper. A pigmented ring (Kayser-Fleischer ring) at the outer margin of the cornea is pathognomonic. Syndrome is characterized by degenerative changes in the brain, cirrhosis of the liver, splenomegaly, tremor, muscular rigidity, involuntary movements, spastic contractures, psychic disturbances, dysphagia, and progressive weakness and emaciation. SYN: *Wilson's disease.*

d., hyaline. A form of degeneration in which the tissues assume a homogeneous and glassy appearance. Caused by hyaline deposits replacing musculoelastic elements of blood vessels with a firm, transparent substance that causes loss of elasticity. It is responsible for hardening of the arteries and is often followed by calcification or deposit of lime salts in dead tissue. Calcification also may result in concretions.

d., hydropic. Pathological change in cells characterized by the appearance of water droplets in the cytoplasm.

d., lardaceous. D., amyloid.

d., lipoidal. Deposition of fat droplets in cells.

d., macular. Degeneration of the macula of the eye.

d., mucoid. Deposition of mucus in the connective tissues.

d., mucous. Deposition of mucous or mucoid substance in the connective tissue of organs, or epithelial cells.

d., myxomatous. D., mucoid.

d., Nissl. Nerve cell degeneration after division of the axon.

d., parenchymatous. D., cloudy swelling.

d., pigmentary. Degeneration in which affected cells develop an abnormal color.

d., polypoid. Formation of polyp-like growths on mucous membrane.

d., secondary. D., wallerian.

d., senile. Bodily and mental changes of the aged.

d., spongy. Familial demyelination of the deep layers of the cerebral cortex. The affected area has a spongy appearance. Symptoms include mental retardation, enlarged head, muscular flaccidity, and blindness. Death usually occurs prior to 18 months of age.

d., subacute combined, of spinal cord. Degeneration of the posterior and lateral columns of the spinal column. Clinically, paresthesia, sensory ataxia, and sometimes spastic paraplegia are present. The disease is the result of pernicious anemia.

d., vitreous. D., hyaline.

d., wallerian. Nerve fiber degeneration after separation from its nutritive center.

d., waxy. D., amyloid.

d., Zenker's. Amyloid degeneration in muscular tissue.

degeneration, words pert. to: amylosis; "ather-" words; athetoid; atrophic; cacogenic; caseation; catalysis; colloid; sarcomatosis; steatosis.

degenerative. Pert. to or accompanied by degeneration.

deglutible (dē-gloo'tĭ-bl) [L. *deglutire,* to swallow]. Capable of being swallowed.

deglutition (dē"gloo-tĭsh'ŭn). The act of swallowing.

deglutitive. Pert. to deglutition.

degradation (dĕg"rĕ-dā'shŭn) [LL. *degradare,* to go down a step]. Physical, metabolic, or chemical change to a less complex form. Thus foods are physically degraded during chewing, and then chemically degraded from complete compounds, such as proteins and starches, to amino acids and sugars respectively. SEE: *biodegradation.*

degree (dē-grē'). 1. A unit of measurement on a scale. 2. A unit of angular measure. 3. A stage of severity of a disease. 4. A status of academic attainment granted by the institution in which the individual studied.

degustation (dē"gŭs-tā'shŭn) [L. *degustatio*]. The sense of taste; the function or act of tasting.

dehiscence (dē-hĭs'ĕns) [L. *dehiscere,* to gape]. A bursting open, as of a graafian follicle or a wound, esp. a surgical abdominal wound.

NURSING IMPLICATIONS: In surgical

dehiscence, notify the surgeon immediately. Cover the wound with a sterile towel or dressing moistened with warm sterile physiological saline solution. Have the patient decrease the tension on abdominal muscles by slightly flexing the knees. Keep the patient calm and quiet, and reassure the patient that the wound will be cared for. Advise the patient that surgery will be required, and prepare the patient for surgery.

dehumanization (dē-hū″măn-ī-zā′shŭn) [L. *de,* from, + *humanus,* human]. Loss of human qualities, as occurs in persons who are psychotic or in previously normal individuals subjected to torture or mental stress imposed by others as could occur in prisoners.

dehumidifier (dē″hū-mĭd′ĭ-fī″ĕr). Device for removing moisture from the air.

dehydrate [L. *de,* from, + Gr. *hydor,* water]. 1. In chemistry, to deprive of, lose, or become free of water. 2. The loss of or deprivation of water from the body or tissues. To become dry.

dehydration (dē″hī-drā′shŭn). 1. Removal of water from a substance. 2. Condition resulting from excessive loss of body fluid. Occurs when output of fluid exceeds fluid intake. May result from fluid deprivation, excessive loss of fluid, reduction in total quantity of electrolytes, or injection of hypertonic solutions.

dehydroandrosterone (dē-hī″drō-ăn-drō-stēr′ōn, -drŏs′tĕr-ōn). Previously used name for dehydroepiandrosterone, q.v.

dehydrocholesterol (dē-hī″drō-kō-lĕs′tĕr-ŏl). A sterol found in the skin and other tissues that after activation by radiation forms vitamin D.

dehydrocholic acid. USP. A bile salt that stimulates production of bile from the liver. Trade names are Cholan D-H, Decholin, Dilabil, and Ketochol.

dehydrocorticosterone (dē-hī″drō-kor-tĭ-kōs′tĕr-ōn). 11-dehydrocorticosterone (Kendall's compound A). $C_{21}H_{28}O_4$. A physiologically active steroid isolated from the adrenal cortex. It is important in water and salt metabolism. SEE: *adrenal gland.*

dehydroepiandrosterone (dē-hī″drō-ĕp″ē-ăn-drŏs′tĕr-ōn). An androgenic substance, $C_{19}H_{28}O_2$, present in urine. It has about one fifth the potency of androsterone.

dehydrogenase (dē-hī-drŏj′ĕ-nās). An enzyme that catalyzes the oxidation of a specific substance causing it to give up its hydrogen.

dehydrogenate (dē-hī′drō-jĕn-āt). To remove hydrogen from a chemical compound.

dehydroisoandrosterone (dĕ-hī″drō-ī″sō-ăn-drŏs′tĕr-ōn). A 17-ketosteroid excreted in normal male urine. It possesses androgenic activity.

deinstitutionalization. A planned program for placing hospitalized psychiatric patients in the community by way of halfway houses, residential hotels, group homes, and boarding houses.

deionization (dē-ī″ŏn-ī-zā′shŭn). Removal of ions from a substance, thus producing a substance free of minerals.

Deiters' cells (dī′tĕrz). [Otto F. C. Deiters, Ger. anatomist, 1834–1863] 1. Supporting cells in organ of Corti. 2. Neuroglia cells.

Deiters' nucleus. Collection of cells behind the acoustic nucleus.

Deiters' process. Axis cylinder process or neuraxon.

déjà entendu (dā′zhă ŏn-tŏn-doo′) [Fr., already heard]. Recognition of something previously understood.

déjà vu (dā′zhă voo) [Fr., already seen]. The impression that something seen or some situation being experienced for the first time has been previously seen or experienced.

dejecta (dē-jĕk′tă) [L. *dejectio,* dejection]. Feces; intestinal waste.

dejection, dejecture (dē-jĕk′shŭn, -tūr). 1. A cast-down feeling or mental depression. 2. Defecation or act of defecation.

Dejerine, Joseph J. (dā″zhĕr-ēn′). French neurologist, 1849–1917.

D.'s disease. Interstitial neuritis of infants.

D.-Sottas atrophy. [Jules Sottas, Fr. neurologist, b. 1866] Progressive and hypertrophic interstitial neuritis of infants.

D.'s syndrome. Condition where deep sensation is depressed but tactile sense is normal, caused by lesion of long root fibers of posterior column.

dekaliter. A unit of volume in the SI system of measurement that is equal to 10 liters. SEE: *decaliter; deciliter.*

delacrimation (dē-lăk″rĭ-mā′shŭn) [L. *de,* from, + *lacrima,* tear]. Excessive flow of tears. SEE: *epiphora.*

delactation (dē″lăk-tā′shŭn) [″ + *lactare,* to suckle]. Weaning or cessation of lactation.

Delalutin. Trade name for hydroxyprogesterone caproate.

delamination [″ + *lamina,* plate]. The division into layers, esp. that of a blastoderm into two layers—epiblast and hypoblast.

Delatestryl. Trade name for testosterone enanthate.

de-lead (dē-lĕd′). To remove lead from the body or a tissue.

deleterious (dĕl″ĕ-tē′rē-ŭs) [Gr. *deleterios*]. Harmful.

deletion (dē-lē′shŭn). In cytogenetics, the loss of genetic material from a chromosome.

Delhi boil. Aleppo boil, q.v.

deligation (dĕl-ī-gā′shŭn) [L. *deligare,* to tie up]. The application of ligatures or binder.

delimitation [L. *de,* from, + *limitare,* to limit].

Determination of limits of an area or organ in diagnosis.

delinquent (dē-lĭn'kwĕnt). One whose behavior is criminal or antisocial.

deliquesce (dĕl″ĭ-kwĕs') [L. *deliquescere,* to melt away]. To cause liquefaction or moistening.

deliquescence (dĕl″ĭ-kwĕs'ĕns). The process of becoming liquefied or moist as the result of absorption of water from the air. Ordinary table salt has this property.

deliquescent (dĕl″ĭ-kwĕs'ĕnt). Pert. to a substance that absorbs water from the atmosphere.

délire de toucher (dā-lēr' dŭ too-shā'). [Fr.]. An abnormal desire to touch or feel things.

deliriant, delirifacient (dē-lĭr'ē-ănt, dē-lĭr″ĭ-fā'shĭ-ĕnt) [L. *delirare,* to be deranged]. An agent that will produce delirium, e.g., atropine or hyoscine.

delirium (dē-lĭr'ē-ŭm) [L.]. A state of mental confusion and excitement characterized by disorientation for time and place, usually with illusions and hallucinations. The mind wanders and speech is incoherent, and the patient is in a state of continual aimless physical activity. There are many forms of delirium, depending on the cause, which may be fever, shock, exhaustion, anxiety, or drug overdose.

RS: alcoholism; carphologia; dipsomania; restraint.

d., acute. Delirium developing suddenly and speedily, resulting in recovery or death.

d., alcoholic. D. tremens.

d., chronic. Delirium of chronic psychoses without febrile characteristics.

d. constantium. Delirium of patients with reiteration of fixed idea.

d. cordis. Atrial fibrillation.

d. epilepticum. Delirium following an epileptic attack or appearing instead of an attack.

d., febrile. Delirium occurring with fever.

d. hystericum. Delirium of hysteria.

d., lingual. Delirium in which meaningless sounds are muttered constantly.

d. mussitans. Excitement causing lingual delirium.

d. of negation. Delirium in which patient thinks body parts are missing.

d. of persecution. Delirium in which patient feels persecuted by surrounding persons.

d., partial. Delirium reacting on only a portion of the mental faculties, causing only some of the patient's actions to be unreasonable.

d., toxic. Delirium produced by presence of toxins in the body.

d., traumatic. Delirium following injury or shock.

d. tremens. ABBR: DT's. A psychic disorder involving anxiety, and visual and auditory hallucinations found in habitual and excessive users of alcoholic beverages. Usually seen during withdrawal from alcohol. SEE: *alcoholism; hangover.*

SYM: Hallucinations such as seeing snakes or monsters or hearing noises. Patient may be quiet and paranoid, but usually is excited, trembling, perspiring, anxious, and talking or yelling incoherently.

F.A.: Close observation; sedatives; quiet, darkened environment; fluids in large quantities.

NURSING IMPLICATIONS: Maintain hydration through oral and I.V. fluids, and provide a high-protein diet. Closely monitor the patient; someone should stay with the patient. Provide proper environmental lighting to decrease visual hallucinations. Carefully assess the patient's hepatic, cardiovascular, and respiratory status, since cirrhosis, congestive heart failure, and pneumonia may be complications of delirium tremens. Although not ideal, restraints may be needed to maintain safety. Be patient, tactful, and understanding.

CAUTION: This syndrome is a true medical emergency that should be treated aggressively due to the possibility of death. Also, it is important to be certain there is not a coexisting disease such as head trauma with concussion, or an acute infectious disease; or that the signs and symptoms are not due to some toxic substance other than ethanol.

delitescence (dĕl″ĭ-tĕs'ĕns) [L. *delitescens,* hiding]. 1. An unusually complete and speedy resolution of an inflammation. 2. The latent period prior to development of symptoms following poisoning.

deliver [L. *deliberare,* to free completely]. 1. To aid in childbirth. 2. To remove or extract, as a tumor from a cystic enclosure or a cataract.

delivery. Expulsion of the child with placenta and membranes from the mother at birth. SEE: *labor.*

d., abdominal. Delivery of the child by cesarean section.

d., forceps. Delivery of the child by the use of instruments.

d., postmortem. Delivery of the child either by the abdominal or vaginal route after death of the mother.

d., precipitate. Delivery that occurs under nonaseptic conditions and when the physician is not present. In the true sense, it is one that follows a rapid labor, regardless of who is present.

NOTE: Watch the patient carefully. A multipara needs more careful watching than a primipara. Nevertheless, it may occur in a primipara.

Do not wait for the head to be visible in a multipara if she is having frequent hard contractions, particularly if she is bearing down. Have a physician see her immediately. In a primipara it is fairly safe to wait in the majority of cases until a small portion of the head is seen at the vaginal orifice during a contraction before putting the patient up for delivery. Remember to watch the primipara or multipara who has received an analgesic, since precipitation can occur with little or no warning. This means watching for bulging of the perineum during the contractions by viewing the vulva and not taking it for granted that because the patient is fairly quiet no progress in labor is being made.

d., premature. Delivery of a fetus before full term.

d., spontaneous. Delivery of the child without external aid.

d., vaginal. Delivery of an infant through the birth canal.

dellen (dĕl'ĕn). A transient depression in the corneal surface of the eye. May be due to swelling of adjacent tissue or from wearing contact lenses.

delomorphous (dĕl"ō-mor'fŭs) [Gr. *delos,* evident, + *morphe,* form]. Having definite form and shape.

delomorphous cells. Granular cells that stain easily. Found next to basement membrane in the stomach and glands in the cardiac region.

delousing (dē-lows'ĭng) [L. *de,* from, + AS. *lus,* louse]. Ridding the body of lice. SEE: *louse.*

delta. 1. Δ or δ, the fourth letter of the Greek alphabet. 2. A triangular space.

Delta-Cortef. Trade name for prednisolone.

deltacortisone (dĕl"tă-kor'tĭ-sōn). Prednisone, q.v., a steroid hormone with glucocorticoid activity.

delta fornicis (dĕl'tă for'nĭ-sĭs) [L.]. A triangular surface on lower side of fornix.

Deltasone. Trade name for prednisone.

deltoid [Gr. *delta,* letter d, + *eidos,* resemblance]. Shaped like the Greek letter delta (Δ); triangular.

deltoid ligament. Internal lateral ligament of ankle joint.

deltoid muscle. The musculus deltoideus, which covers the shoulder prominence.

deltoid ridge. Ridge on humerus where deltoid muscle is attached.

delusion (dē-loo'zhŭn) [L. *deludere,* to cheat]. A false belief brought about without appropriate external stimulation and inconsistent with the individual's own knowledge and experience. Seen most often in psychoses, where patients cannot separate delusion from reality. Differs from hallucination, q.v., in that the latter involves the false excitation of one or more of the senses. The most important delusions are those that cause patients to harm others or themselves.

Ex.: fear of being poisoned causing the patient to refuse food; delusions leading to suicide or inflicting injury upon self; false beliefs such as having been guilty of an unpardonable sin; delusions of persecution.

d., depressive. Delusion causing a saddened state.

d., expansive. Unreasonable conviction of one's own power, or importance; seen in manic patients.

d., fixed. Delusion that remains unaltered.

d., fleeting. A type of delusion that comes and goes.

d., nihilistic. Delusion that causes the victim to believe that everything has ceased to exist.

d. of grandeur. A false sense of possessing wealth or power. SYN: *megalomania.*

d. of negation. D., nihilistic.

d. of persecution. Delusion in which patients feel everyone around them is against them.

d., reference. Delusion that causes the victim to read a meaning not intended in the acts or words of others, often an interpretation of slight or ridicule.

d., systematized. Logical correlation with false reasoning and deduction.

d., unsystematized. Delusion without any correlation between ideas and surroundings.

delusional. Pert. to a delusion.

demarcation (dē"măr-kā'shŭn) [L. *demarcare,* to limit]. Setting a limit or boundary.

demecarium bromide (dĕm"ē-kā'rē-ŭm). USP. An anticholinesterase agent used in treating glaucoma. Trade name is Humorsol.

demeclocycline hydrochloride (dĕm"ĕ-klō-sī'klēn). USP. A tetracycline-type antibiotic. Trade name is Declomycin.

dement [L. *dementare,* to make insane]. One afflicted with dementia.

demented. Of unsound mind.

dementia (dē-mĕn'shē-ă) [L. *dementare,* to make insane]. Irrecoverable deteriorative mental state with absence or reduction of intellectual faculties, due to organic brain disease.

d., alcoholic. Dementia in terminal portion of chronic alcoholic state.

d., apoplectic. Dementia following cerebral hemorrhage or tumors.

d., epileptic. Dementia seen in some cases of long-continued epilepsy.

d., organic. Dementia caused by lesions of nerve centers.

d. paralytica. A form of neurosyphilis

characterized by sudden onset with deterioration of memory and concentration and irritability. Behavior deteriorates, and emotional instability develops. Neurasthenia, depression, and delusions of grandeur with lack of insight may be present.

d. paranoides. Dementia with paranoid tendencies. SYN: *paranoid schizophrenia.*

d., postfebrile. Dementia following severe cases of infectious diseases.

d., presenile. Dementia beginning in middle age, usually resulting from cerebral arteriosclerosis. Symptoms are apathy, loss of memory, and disturbances of speech and gait.

d., primary. Dementia occurring by itself, without relationship to another form of psychosis.

d., secondary. Dementia occurring after a primary mental disease, such as mania.

d., senile. Dementia occurring in the aged. Characterized by progressive mental deterioration with loss of memory, esp. for recent events, with occasional intercurrent attacks of excitement.

d., syphilitic. Dementia caused by lesion of syphilis.

d., tabetic. Dementia that may occur following tabes dorsalis.

d., terminal. Dementia following another form of mental disease. SEE: *d., secondary.*

d., toxic. Dementia due to excessive use of a drug.

Demerol (děm'ĕr-ŏl). Trade name for meperidine hydrochloride, a white, odorless, crystalline compound, soluble in water, having a neutral reaction and an analgesic effect similar to morphine.

CAUTION: Continued use will lead to addiction.

demi- [L. *dimidius,* half]. Prefix indicating half.

demibain (děm'ĭ-băn) [Fr., half bath]. Half a bath; sitz bath.

demic (děm'ĭk) [Gr. *demos,* people]. Concerning the living body of man.

demilune (děm'ĭ-loon) [L. *dimidius,* half, + *luna,* moon]. A crescent-shaped group of serous cells that form a caplike structure over a mucous alveolus. They are present in mixed glands, esp. the submandibular gland.

demineralization [L. *de,* from, + *minare,* to mine]. Loss of mineral salts, esp. from the bones.

demise (dĕ-mīz') [L. *dimittere,* to dismiss]. Destruction or death.

demodectic (děm-ō-děk'tĭk). Concerning or caused by the mite Demodex.

Demodex [Gr. *demos,* fat, + *dex,* worm]. Genus of mites and ticks of the class Arachnida and order Acarina.

D. folliculorum. The hair follicle or face mite, an elongated wormlike organism that infests hair follicles and sebaceous glands of various mammals including man.

demography (dē-mŏg'ră-fē) [Gr. *demos,* people, + *graphein,* to write]. The statistical and quantitative study of characteristics of human populations. Size, growth, density, age and sex distribution, and vital statistics are included in the data collected.

demorphinization (dē-mor"fĭn-ī-zā'shŭn). Gradual decrease in the dose of morphine being used by one addicted to that drug.

demotivate. To cause loss of incentive or motivation.

Demours' membrane (dē-mūr'). [Pierre Demours, Fr. ophthalmologist, 1702–1795] A fine membrane between the endothelial layer of the cornea and the substantia propria. SYN: *Descemet's membrane.*

demucosation (dē"mū-kō-sā'shŭn) [L. *demucosatio*]. Removal of mucosa of any part of body.

demulcent [L. *demulcens,* stroking softly]. An agent that will soothe the part or soften the skin to which applied. The term is usually restricted to agents acting on mucous membrane.

Ex.: glycerin, honey, lanolin, olive oil.

Demulen. Trade name for combination of estrogen with progestogen.

de Musset's sign. SEE: *Musset's sign.*

demutization (dē"mū-tī-zā'shŭn) [L. *de,* from, + *mutus,* mute]. Overcoming mutism by teaching the patient to speak or use sign language.

demyelinate (dē-mī'ĕ-lĭn-āt) [" + Gr. *myelos,* marrow]. Destruction or removal of the myelin sheath of nerve tissue. Seen in Guillain-Barré syndrome, q.v.

demyelination (dē-mī"ĕ-lī-nā'shŭn). Removal of the myelin sheath of a nerve.

denarcotize (dē-năr'kō-tīz). To withdraw narcotic from an addicted person.

denaturation (dē-nā"chŭr-ā'shŭn). Adding a substance to alcohol that makes it toxic and unfit for human consumption but usually does not interfere with its use for other purposes.

denatured [" + *natura,* nature]. The destruction of the usual nature of a substance, as the addition of methanol to alcohol renders it unfit for consumption.

denatured protein. A protein that has been treated in some manner that caused it to lose some of its physical and chemical properties. Cooking egg white denatures the albumin present.

dendraxon (děn-drăk'sŏn) [Gr. *dendron,* tree, + *axon,* axle]. The terminal filaments of the neuraxon of a nerve cell.

dendric (děn'drĭk). Pert. to or possessing a

dendron.

Dendrid. Trade name for idoxuridine (IDU).

dendriform (dĕn'drĭ-form) [" + L. *forma*, shape]. Branching, or like a tree in shape.

dendrite (dĕn'drīt) [Gr. *dendrites*, pert. to a tree]. A branched protoplasmic process of a neuron that conducts impulses to the cell body. There are usually several to a cell. They form synaptic connections with other neurons. SYN: *dendron; neurodendrite*. SEE: illus.

d., extracapsular. Dendrites of neurons of autonomic ganglia that pierce the capsule surrounding the cell and extend for considerable distances from the cell body.

d., intracapsular. Dendrites of neurons of autonomic ganglia that ramify beneath the capsule, forming a network about the cell body.

dendritic. Treelike in form.

dendritic calculus. A renal stone molded in the form of the pelvis and calyces.

dendroid (dĕn'droyd) [" + *eidos*, form]. 1. Dendriform, pert. to dendrites. 2. Arborescent, treelike.

dendron (dĕn'drŏn) [Gr. *dendron*, tree]. A dendrite; a protoplasmic branch from a nerve cell. SYN: *neurodendrite*.

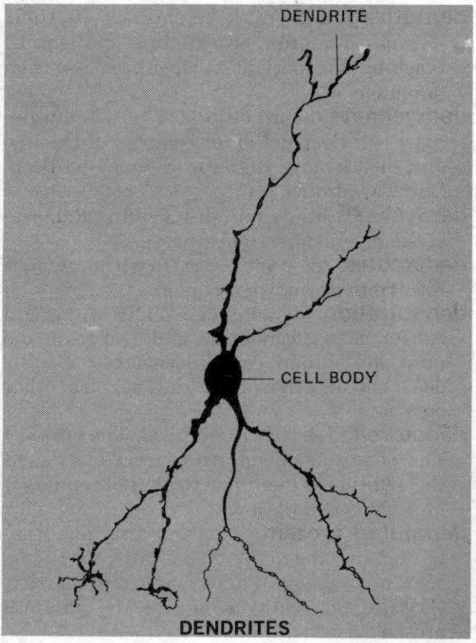

dendrophagocytosis (dĕn"drō-făg-ō-sī-tō'sĭs) [" + *phagein*, to eat, + *kytos*, cell, + *osis*, condition]. The absorption of portions of astrocytes by microglia cells.

denervated [L. *de*, from, + Gr. *neuron*, nerve]. 1. Excision, incision, or blocking of a nerve supply. 2. A condition in which the nerve supply is blocked or cut off.

dengue (dăng'gā, -gē) [Sp.]. An acute febrile disease characterized by sudden onset, with headache, fever, prostration, joint and muscle pain, lymphadenopathy, and a rash that appears simultaneously with a second temperature rise following an afebrile period. SYN: *breakbone fever*.

ETIOL: Group B arbovirus transmitted by the mosquito. Incubation period is 3 to 15 days, usually 5 to 6 days.

SYM: Two fever periods with intermissions; eruptions similar to measles; severe pain in muscles and joints.

TREATMENT: No specific treatment. Analgesic and sedative agents. Mosquito control for prophylaxis.

denial (dĕ-nī'ăl). Refusal to admit the reality of, or to acknowledge the presence or existence of something. A defense mechanism.

denidation (dĕn"ī-dā'shŭn) [L. *de*, from, + *nidus*, nest]. Normal removal of the superficial mucosal surface of the lining of the uterus during menstruation.

dens (dĕnz) [L.]. (pl. *dentes*) [NA] 1. A tooth. SEE: *dentition* for illus. 2. The odontoid process of the axis. A process on the body of the axis that serves as a pivot for the rotation of the atlas.

d. bicuspidus. D. premolaris.

d. caninus. (pl. *dentes canini*) [NA] The canine tooth.

d. deciduus. (pl. *dentes decidui*) [NA] Milk tooth, first tooth.

d. incisivus. (pl. *dentes incisivi*) [NA] Incisor tooth.

d. molaris. (pl. *dentes molares*) [NA] Molar tooth, grinder.

d. permanens. (pl. *dentes permanentes*) [NA] One of the 32 teeth making up the so-called permanent teeth.

d. premolaris. (pl. *dentes premolares*) [NA] One of the premolar teeth.

d. sapientiae. A wisdom tooth; late tooth; third molar. SYN: *d. serotinus*.

d. serotinus. [NA] A wisdom tooth; third molar.

densimeter (dĕn-sĭm'ĕ-tĕr) [L. *densus*, thick, + Gr. *metron*, measure]. Instrument for measuring densities. In radiology, an instrument that measures the density of a radiograph.

densitometer (dĕn"sĭ-tŏm'ĕ-tĕr). A special densimeter for measuring bacterial growth and effect of antiseptics and bacteriophages upon it.

densitometry (dĕn″sĭ-tŏm′ĕ-trē). 1. Determination of the density of a substance. 2. Determining ionizing radiation.

density [L. *densitas,* thickness]. 1. Relative weight of a substance compared with a reference standard. SEE: *specific gravity.* 2. The quality of being dense. 3. The degree of blackness on a radiograph or the relationship between the light given and the light passing through a radiograph.

dental. Pert. to the teeth.

dental arch. The arch formed by the cutting and chewing surfaces of the teeth.

dental caries. Decay of the teeth. SEE: *caries; fluoridation.*

dental chart. A diagrammatic representation of the teeth of the mouth on which the clinical and radiographic findings can be recorded. It often includes the restorations present, decayed surfaces, missing teeth, and periodontal conditions.

dental consonant. A consonant pronounced with the tongue at or near the front upper teeth. Term used in speech therapy.

dental curve. The curve or bow of the line of the teeth in the jaw. The different portions of the curve are described as follows: *alignment curve,* the line passing through the center of the teeth from the middle line through the last molar; *buccal curve,* the curve extending from the cuspid to the 3rd molar; *compensating curve,* the occlusal line of bicuspids and molars; *labial curve,* the curve extending from cuspid to cuspid.

dental disk. A thin circular piece of paper, cloth, or other substance charged with abrasive powder for cutting or polishing teeth and fillings.

dental dysfunction. Malfunctioning of the parts of the dental structure.

dental engine. A machine operated with foot power or by an electric or a water motor to give a swift rotary motion to drills, burs, and burnishers.

dental engineering. Use of the principles of engineering in dentistry.

dental floss. Waxed or unwaxed thread used for cleaning and removing plaque between the teeth and testing for defects in the teeth.

dental formula. A brief method of expressing the dentition of mammals in which the numbers of the teeth are given in the form of a fraction, each portion of which represents one quadrant; the numbers of the upper teeth forming the numerator, and those of the lower teeth the denominator.

The first number listed represents the incisors, the second is for the canine, the third premolar, and the fourth molar. The dental formula of the right half of the mouth of man is:

$$\frac{2-1-2-3}{2-1-2-3}$$

dental geriatrics. The scientific study and treatment of dental conditions of the aged.

dentalgia (dĕn-tăl′jē-ă) [L. *dens,* tooth, + Gr. *algos,* pain]. Toothache.

dental handpiece. An instrument designed to hold the rotary instruments used in dentistry to remove tooth structure or to smooth and polish restorative materials; it may be powered by foot pedal, electric motor, and air or water turbines.

dental hygienist. A trained person who professionally cleans teeth and, usually in schools or institutions, offers instruction on general care of the teeth.

dental index. A system of numbers for indicating comparative size of the teeth.

dental instruments. A variety of steel instruments with points or cutting surfaces at either or both ends, which can be sharpened, sterilized, and used in the special procedures of dentistry.

dental materials. The various types of colloids, plastics, resins, and metal alloys used in dentistry to take impressions, restore teeth, or duplicate the dentition; the science or department devoted to research and instruction in the use of restorative materials in dentistry.

dental plaque. A gummy mass of microorganisms that grows on the crowns and spreads along the roots of teeth. It usually is too small to be seen and is both colorless and transparent. Dental plaques are the forerunners of dental caries and periodontal disease. They may be prevented by proper daily self-care of the teeth, including careful use of dental floss, and periodic prophylaxis by a dentist or dental hygienist. SEE: *caries; periodontitis; pyorrhea alveolans.*

dental prosthesis. An artificial part used in the mouth to replace missing structural tissue or teeth. SYN: *denture.*

dental pulp. The embryonic connective tissue that is vascular, well innervated, and occupies the central space within the tooth and its roots.

dental tape. Waxed or unwaxed thin tape used for cleaning and removing plaque between the teeth.

dentaphone (dĕn′tă-fōn) [″ + Gr. *phone,* sound]. Device for conveying sound through the teeth.

dentate (dĕn′tāt) [L. *dentatus,* toothed]. Notched; having short triangular divisions of the margin; toothed.

dentes [L.]. Teeth. Pl. of dens.

dentia (dĕn′shē-ă) [L.]. Process of eruption of teeth.

d. praecox. Premature eruption of teeth.

d. tarda. Delayed eruption of teeth.

dentibuccal (dĕn-tĭ-bŭk′l) [L. *dens,* tooth, + *bucca,* cheek]. Pert. to both the cheek and teeth.

denticle (dĕn′tĭ-kl) [L. *denticulus,* little tooth]. 1. A small toothlike projection. 2. A small tooth.

denticulate [L. *denticulatus,* small toothed]. Finely toothed or serrated.

denticulate body. Corpus dentatum of the cerebellum.

dentification [L. *dens,* tooth, + *facere,* to make]. Conversion into dental structure.

dentiform [″ + *forma,* shape]. Toothlike.

dentifrice (dĕn′tĭ-frĭs) [″ + *fricare,* to rub]. A powder or other substance for cleaning teeth.

dentigerous (dĕn-tĭj′ĕr-ŭs) [″ + *gerere,* to bear]. Having or containing teeth.

dentilabial (dĕn-tĭ-lā′bē-ăl) [″ + *labium,* lip]. Pert. to both teeth and lips.

dentilingual (dĕn-tĭ-lĭn′gwăl) [″ + *lingua,* tongue]. Pert. to both teeth and tongue.

dentimeter (dĕn-tĭm′ĕ-tĕr) [″ + Gr. *metron,* measure]. Device for measuring teeth.

dentin (dĕn′tĭn) [L. *dens,* tooth]. The main, or osseous, tissues of a tooth surrounding the pulp cavity.

dentinal. Pert. to dentin.

dentinification [″ + *facere,* to make]. An old term meaning the formation of dentin. SYN: *dentinogenesis.*

dentinitis [″ + Gr. *itis,* inflammation]. Inflammation of dentin.

dentinoblast (dĕn′tĭn-ō-blăst) [″ + Gr. *blastos,* germ]. An old term meaning a dentin-forming cell. SYN: *odontoblast.*

dentinogenesis (dĕn″tĭn-ō-jĕn′ĕ-sĭs) [″ + *gennan,* to produce]. Formation of dentin in development of a tooth.

d. imperfecta. Hereditary aplasia or hypoplasia of the enamel and dentin of a tooth.

dentinoid [″ + Gr. *eidos,* form]. Resembling dentin.

dentinoma [″ + Gr. *oma,* tumor]. A tumor comprised of tissues that give origin to the teeth; consisting mainly of dentin.

dentinosteoid (dĕn″tĭn-ŏs′tē-oyd) [″ + Gr. *osteon,* bone, + *eidos,* form]. A tumor composed of dentin and bone.

dentinum (dĕn′tĭ-nŭm). Dentin.

dentiparous (dĕn-tĭp′ă-rŭs) [″ + *parere,* to bear]. Pert. to development and formation of teeth.

dentist [L. *dens,* tooth]. An authorized practitioner of dentistry.

dentistry. 1. That branch of medicine that deals with the care of the teeth and associated structures of the oral cavity. It is concerned with the prevention, diagnosis, and treatment of diseases of the teeth and gums. 2. The art or profession of a dentist. SYN: *odontology.*

d., esthetic. Repair and restoration or replacement of carious or broken teeth.

d., four-handed. The concept and practice of extensive utilization of a chairside dental assistant to facilitate and enhance the productivity of the dentist.

d., forensic. The area of dentistry particularly related to jurisprudence; most often seen as the identification of unknown persons by the details of their dentition and tooth restorations.

d., geriatric. The area of dentistry devoted to the dental health care of the aged.

d., operative. Branch of dentistry dealing with restorative dental operations on the mouth.

d., prosthodontic. The art of replacing defective or missing teeth through the use of artificial appliances such as bridges, crowns, and dentures.

d., public health. The area of dentistry that seeks to improve the dental health of communities by epidemiological studies, research in preventive methods, and better distribution, management, and utilization of dentists.

dentition [L. *dentitio*]. 1. The type, number, and arrangement of teeth in the dental arch. SEE: illus.; *teeth* for illus.

d., permanent. The eruption of the permanent teeth (32) beginning at about the age of six years in humans. Completed by the 15th year with the exception of wisdom teeth, which appear between the 17th and 25th years. The order of eruption follows: The incisors are followed by the bicuspids and the canines; then the second molars are followed by the third molars. The appearance of the first molars is highly variable, but in some instances they may be the first permanent teeth to appear. SEE: *teeth.*

d., primary. Eruption of 20 deciduous or milk teeth in humans. The order of eruption follows: Two lower central incisors, 5 to 9 months; two upper central incisors, 8 to 12 months; two upper lateral incisors, 10 to 12 months; two lower lateral incisors, 12 to 15 months; four anterior molars, 12 to 15 months; four canines, 18 to 24 months; four posterior molars, 24 to 30 months.

dentoalveolar (dĕn″tō-ăl-vē′ō-lăr) [L. *dens,* tooth, + *alveolus,* small hollow]. Pert. to alveolus of a tooth and to the tooth itself.

dentoalveolitis (dĕn″to-ăl″vē-ō-lī′tĭs) [″ + ″ + Gr. *itis,* inflammation]. A purulent inflammation of the tooth socket linings characterized by looseness of the teeth and shrinkage of the gum. SYN: *pyorrhea alveolaris.*

dentofacial (dĕn″tō-fā′shăl). Concerning the teeth and face.

dentoid [″ + Gr. *eidos,* form]. Dentiform; odontoid; tooth-shaped.

dentoidin. An old term for the organic ground

DENTITION

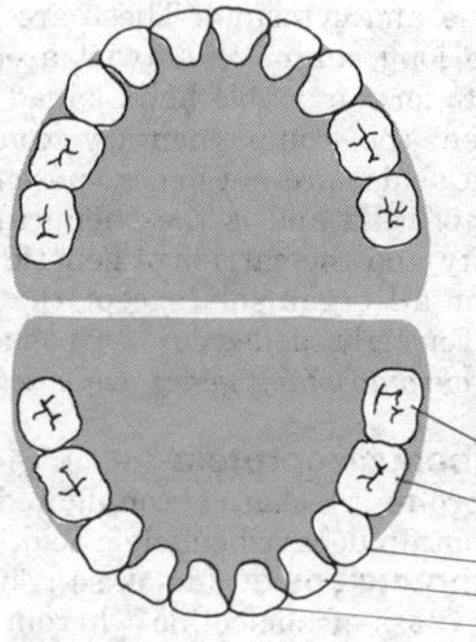

CHILD

ERUPTION OF DECIDUOUS (MILK) TEETH

UPPER	ERUPTION
CENTRAL INCISOR	8–10 MO.
LATERAL INCISOR	8–10 MO.
(CUSPID) CANINE	16–20 MO.
FIRST MOLAR	15–21 MO.
SECOND MOLAR	20–24 MO.
LOWER	
SECOND MOLAR	20–24 MO.
FIRST MOLAR	15–21 MO.
(CUSPID) CANINE	15–21 MO.
LATERAL INCISOR	15–21 MO.
CENTRAL INCISOR	6– 9 MO.

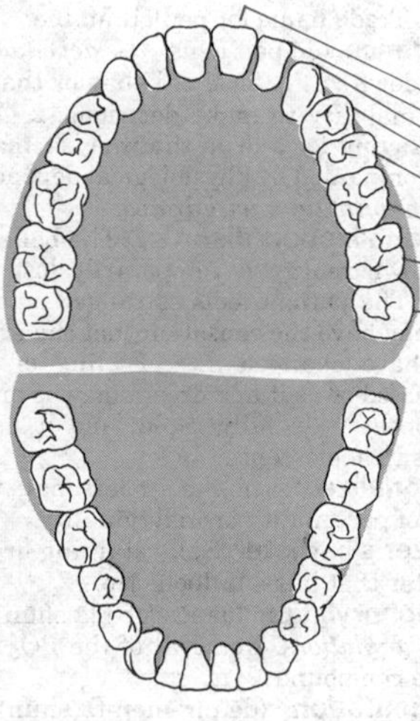

ADULT

ERUPTION OF PERMANENT TEETH

UPPER	COMPLETED BY
CENTRAL INCISOR	7th YR.
LATERAL INCISOR	8th YR.
(CUSPID) CANINE	11–12 YR.
FIRST PREMOLAR (BICUSPID)	9th YR.
SECOND PREMOLAR (BICUSPID)	10th YR.
FIRST MOLAR	6th YR.
SECOND MOLAR	12–13 YR.
THIRD MOLAR	17–25 YR.
LOWER	
THIRD MOLAR	17–25 YR.
SECOND MOLAR	12–13 YR.
SECOND PREMOLAR (BICUSPID)	10th YR.
FIRST PREMOLAR (BICUSPID)	9th YR.
FIRST MOLAR	6th YR.
(CUSPID) CANINE	11–12 YR.
LATERAL INCISOR	8th YR.
CENTRAL INCISOR	7th YR.

substance of dentin. SYN: *predentin*.

dentulous (dĕn′tū-lŭs). Having one's natural teeth. SEE: *edentulous*.

denture (dĕn′chūr). A complete set of artificial teeth set in appropriate plastic materials to substitute for the natural dentition and related tissues.

NURSING IMPLICATIONS: Dentures should be cleansed after each meal. They should be gently brushed with warm water, scrubbed with moderate pressure, and soaked in a warm acidic solution. Solutions and mixtures accepted by the American Dental Association are: 1. Ammonia water 28% (use 2 ml. in 30 ml. of water); 2. Trisodium phosphate (600 mg. in 30 ml. water); 3. Sodium hypochlorite (bleach) (2 ml. in 120 ml. water). Store dentures in an opaque, covered container. Remove dentures from comatose or moribund patients as well as prior to any surgical procedure.

d., full. Denture that replaces all of the teeth in both jaws.

d., immediate. A complete set of artificial teeth to be inserted immediately after removal (extraction) of natural teeth.

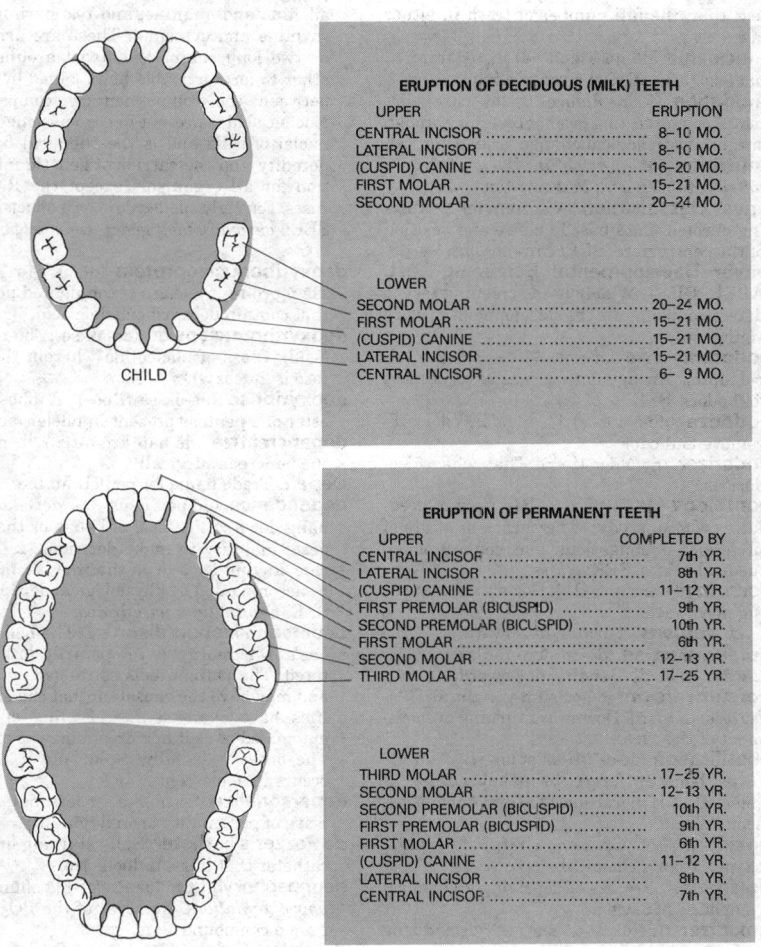

d., partial. A dental appliance replacing less than the full number of teeth in either jaw.

denucleated (dē-nū'klē-āt"ĕd) [L. *de,* from, + *nucleus,* kernel]. Deprived of a nucleus.

denudation [L. *denudare,* to lay bare]. Removal of a protecting layer or covering through surgery, pathological change, or trauma.

denutrition (dē"nū-trĭsh'ŭn) [L. *de,* from, + *nutrire,* to nourish]. Malnutrition.

Denver classification. A system for classifying chromosomes based on size and position of the centromere. SEE: *chromosome.*

Denver Developmental Screening Test. ABBR: DDST. Widely used screening test to detect problems in the development of very young children.

deodorant (dē-ō'dor-ănt) [" + *odorare,* to perfume]. An agent that masks or absorbs foul odors. SEE: *odor.*

deodorize (dē-ō'dor-īz) [" + *odor,* odor]. To remove foul odor.

deodorizer (dē-ō'dor-īz-ĕr). That which deodorizes.

deontology (dē"ŏn-tŏl'ō-jē) [Gr. *deonta,* needful, + *logos,* study]. The theory or study of professional obligations and commitments; medical ethics. SEE: *ethics.*

deorsum (dē-or'sŭm) [L.]. Downward or turning downward.

d. vergens. Turning downward.

deorsumduction (dē-or"sŭm-dŭk'shŭn) [" + *ducere,* to lead]. Bending downward.

deorsumversion (dē-or"sŭm-vĕr'zhŭn) [" + *vertere,* to turn]. Downward turning or movement of the eyes.

deossification (dē-ŏs"ĭ-fĭ-kā'shŭn) [L. *de,* from, + *os,* bone, + *facere,* to make]. Loss of or removal of mineral matter from bone or osseous tissue.

deoxidate [" + Gr. *oxys,* sharp]. To remove oxygen from a chemical.

deoxidation. Process of depriving a chemical compound of oxygen.

deoxidizer (dē-ŏk'sĭ-dī-zĕr). A deoxidizing agent.

deoxycholic acid (dē-ŏk"sē-kō'lĭk). $C_{24}H_{40}O_4$, a crystalline acid found in bile.

deoxycorticosterone (dē-ŏk"sē-kor"tē-kŏs'tĕr-ōn). A hormone from the adrenal gland. It acts principally on salt and water metabolism.

deoxygenation (dē-ŏk"sĭ-jĕn-ā'shŭn). Removal of oxygen from a chemical compound or tissue.

deoxyribonuclease (dē-ŏk"sē-rī"bō-nū'klē-ās). ABBR: DNase. An enzyme that hydrolyzes and thus depolymerizes deoxyribonucleic acid (DNA).

deoxyribonucleic acid (dē-ŏk"sē-rī"bō-nū-klē'ĭk). ABBR: DNA. A complex protein of high molecular weight consisting of deoxyribose, phosphoric acid, and four bases (two purines, adenine and guanine, and two pyrimidines, thymine and cytosine). These are arranged as two long chains that twist around each other to form a double helix joined by bonds between the complementary components. Nucleic acid is present in chromosomes of the nuclei of cells and is the chemical basis of heredity and the carrier of genetic information for all organisms except the RNA viruses. Formerly spelled desoxyribonucleic acid. SEE: *chromosome; gene; ribonucleic acid; virus.*

deoxyribonucleoprotein (dē-ŏk"sē-rī"bō-nū"klē-ō-prō'tē-ĭn). Class of conjugated proteins that contain deoxyribonucleic acid.

deoxyribonucleoside (dē-ŏk"sē-rī"bō-nū'klē-ō-sīd). Class of nucleotide wherein the pentose is 2-deoxy-D-ribose.

deoxyribose (dē-ŏk"sē-rī'bōs). A phosphoric ester of a pentose present in nucleic acid.

depancreatize (dē-păn'krē-ă-tīz). To remove the pancreas surgically.

Depen. Trade name for penicillamine.

dependence (dē-pĕn'dĕns) [L. *dependere,* to hang down]. 1. A form of behavior that suggests inability to make decisions. 2. A psychic craving for a drug that may or may not be accompanied by physiological dependency. SEE: *habituation; withdrawal.*

depersonalization disorder. The belief that one's own reality is temporarily lost or altered. The patient feels estranged or unreal and may have the sensation that the extremities have changed size. Feeling of being automated or as if in a dream may be present. The onset is usually rapid; and it usually occurs in adolescence.

depersonalize. To make impersonal; to deprive of personality or individuality.

de Pezzer's catheter. Self-retaining urethral catheter that has a bulbous tip.

dephosphorylation (dē-fŏs"for-ĭ-lā'shŭn) [" + *phosphorylation*]. Removal of the PO_3 group from a compound.

depigmentation (dē"pĭg-mĕn-tā'shŭn). Removal of pigment, esp. from the skin, by use of chemical or physical means.

depilate (dĕp'ĭl-āt) [L. *depilare,* to deprive of hair]. To remove hair.

depilation (dĕp"ĭl-ā'shŭn). The process of hair removal. SEE: *epilation.*

depilatory. An agent used for the removal of hair.

deplete (dē-plēt') [L. *depletus,* emptied]. To empty; to produce depletion.

depletion (dē-plē'shŭn). Removal of substances from the body such as blood, fluids, iron, fat, protein.

deplumation (dē"ploo-mā'shŭn) [L. *de,* from, + *pluma,* feather]. Loss of eyelashes as result of disease.

depolarization (dē-pō″lăr-ī-zā′shŭn) [″ + *polus,* pole]. The process of reducing to a nonpolarized condition; neutralization of polarity.

depolymerization (dē-pŏl″ĭ-mĕr-ī-zā′shŭn). The breakdown or splitting of polymers into their basic building blocks or monomers.

Ex.: the glucose monomer may be polymerized to form the large glycogen polymer and then broken down, i.e., depolymerized, to form glucose.

Depo-Medrol. Trade name for methylprednisolone acetate.

Depo-Provera. Trade name for medroxyprogesterone acetate.

deposit (dē-pŏz′ĭt) [L. *depositus,* having put aside]. 1. Sediment; precipitate. 2. Matter collected in any part of an organism.

depot (dē′pō, dĕp′ō) [Fr. *depot,* fr. L. *depositum*]. A place of storage, esp. in the body, such as fat depot.

depravation (dĕp″ră-vā′shŭn) [L. *depravare,* completely destroyed]. Pathological deterioration of function or secretion.

depressant [L. *depressus,* pressed down]. An agent that will depress a body function or nerve activity, such as sedative medicines.

d., cardiac. Depressant that decreases heart rate and contractility.

d., cerebral. Depressant that lessens brain activity, making the patient dull and less active. Large doses may produce sleep.

d., motor. Depressant that lessens contractions of involuntary muscles.

d., respiratory. A drug that lessens frequency and depth of breathing.

d., secretory. Agent causing decreased glandular secretions.

depressed (dĕ-prĕst′). 1. Below the normal level, as when fragments of bone are forced below their normal level and that of surrounding portions of bone. 2. Low in spirits; dejected. 3. Decreased level of function. SEE: *depression.*

depression (dē-prĕsh′ŭn) [L. *depressio,* a pressing down]. 1. A hollow or lowered region. 2. The lowering of a part, such as the mandible. 3. The decrease of a vital function such as respiration. 4. Mental depression characterized by altered mood. There is loss of interest in all usually pleasurable outlets such as food, sex, work, friends, hobbies, or entertainment. Diagnostic criteria include presence of at least four of the following every day for at least two weeks: 1. Poor appetite or significant weight loss; or increased weight gain. 2. Insomnia or hypersomnia. 3. Psychomotor agitation or retardation. 4. Loss of interest or pleasure in usual activities, or decreased sex drive. 5. Loss of energy, or fatigue. 6. Feelings of worthlessness, self-reproach, or excessive or inappropriate guilt. 7. Complaints of or evidence of diminished ability to think or concentrate. 8. Recurrent thoughts of death, suicidal ideation, wish to be dead, or attempted suicide. SEE: *depression, situational; grief reaction.*

d., bipolar. Depression in which disorders of both mood and elation are alternately present.

d., endogenous. Mental depression without apparent cause.

d., situational or reactive. Mental depression usually self-limiting, following severe life disappointments such as a death in the family, loss of a job, or a personal financial catastrophe.

d., unipolar. Mental depression characterized by mind shifts from a normal baseline to a depressed state.

depressomotor (dē-prĕs′ō-mō″tor) [″ + *motor,* mover]. A drug that diminishes muscular movements by lessening the impulses for motion sent from the brain or spinal cord.

depressor [L.]. Instrument for depressing a part.

d., tongue. Device used to depress and displace the tongue in order to facilitate visual examination of the throat.

depressor fibers. Muscles that depress or draw down a part.

depressor nerve. A nerve, the stimulation of which lessens or inhibits the activity of an organ or tissue.

depressor reflex. More or less transient stimulation of depressor fibers.

deprivation (dĕp″rĭ-vā′shŭn) [L. *de,* from, + *privare,* to remove]. Loss or absence of necessary parts or functions.

d., emotional. Isolation of an individual, esp. an infant, from normal emotional stimuli. In infants, this produces impairment of mental and physical development.

d., sensory. A situation or environment wherein the usual sensory stimuli, such as noise and light, as well as human contact are absent or, in the case of noise, masked by a continuous dull noise. Persons exposed partially or completely to such an environment include astronauts, patients in artificial respirators, and patients with temporary loss of a sense (as in bandaging of both eyes). Prolonged exposure to lack of sensory stimuli may cause hallucinations and other signs and symptoms of mental disorder.

depth [ME. *depthe*]. Richness; intensity; quality of being deep.

depth dose. Actual amount of radiation exposure at a specific point below the surface of the body.

depth perception. Perception of spatial relationships; three-dimensional perception.

depth psychology. Psychology of unconscious behavior. Opposed to psychology of conscious behavior.

depulization (dē-pūl″ĭ-zā′shŭn) [L. *de,* from, + *pulex,* flea]. Destruction of fleas, including those that carry the plague bacillus.

depurant (dĕp′ū-rănt) [L. *depurare,* to purify]. 1. A medicine that helps to purify by promoting the removal of waste material from the body. 2. Removal of waste material.

depuration. Process of freeing from impurities.

depurative. Having cleansing properties.

depurator. An agent that purifies.

de Quervain's disease. Tenosynovitis due to relative narrowness of the tendon sheath of the abductor pollicus longus and the extensor pollicus brevis.

deradelphus (dĕr-ă-dĕl′fŭs) [Gr. *dere,* neck, + *adelphos,* brother]. Malformed twins, fused above the thorax and having one head, but separated below the chest as two bodies.

deradenitis (dĕr″ăd-ĕn-ī′tĭs) [″ + *aden,* gland, + *itis,* inflammation]. Inflammation of a lymph gland of the neck.

deradenoncus (dĕr″ăd-ĕn-ŏnk′ŭs) [″ + *onkos,* tumor]. Swelling or tumor of a neck gland.

derangement (dē-rānj′mĕnt) [Fr. *deranger,* unbalance]. Disorder of the mental functions, esp. those involving the intellect.

Dercum's disease (dĕr′kŭms). [Francis X. Dercum, U.S. neurologist, 1856–1931] Scattered areas of painful cutaneous nodules or fat accumulations in menopausal women. SYN: *adiposis dolorosa.*

dereism (dē′rē-ĭzm) [L. *de,* from, + *res,* thing]. In psychiatry, activity and thought based on fantasy and wishes rather than logic or reason.

dereistic (dē″rē-ĭs′tĭk) [″ + *res,* thing]. Pert. to overexercise of the imagination to the extent of ignoring reality, as seen in day dreaming. SEE: *autism.*

derencephalus (dĕr″ĕn-sĕf′ă-lŭs) [Gr. *dere,* neck, + *enkephalos,* brain]. Congenitally deformed fetus with a rudimentary skull and bifid cervical vertebrae.

derivation (dĕr″ĭ-vā′shŭn) [L. *derivare,* to draw off]. The source or origin of a substance.

derivative (dĕ-rĭv′ă-tĭv). 1. That which is not original or fundamental. 2. Anything derived from another body or substance. 3. That which produces derivation. 4. In embryology, that which develops from a preceding structure, as the derivatives of the germ layers.

derm, derma [Gr. *derma,* skin]. The cutis vera, or true skin.

dermabrasion (dĕrm′ă-brā″zhŭn) [″ + L. *abrasio,* wearing away]. A surgical procedure for removal of acne scars, nevi, tattoos, or fine wrinkles on the skin by using sandpaper or mechanical methods on the frozen epidermis. Procedure is dangerous and should not be used indiscriminately.

Dermacentor (dĕr″mă-sĕn′tor). A genus of ticks belonging to the order Acarina, family Ixodidae.

D. andersoni. The wood tick, a species of ticks that is parasitic on man or other mammals during some part of its life cycle. May transmit causative agents of Rocky Mountain spotted fever, scrub typhus, tularemia, anaplasmosis, brucellosis, Q fever, and several forms of virus encephalomyelitis. Also causes tick paralysis.

D. variabilis. A species of ticks similar to D. andersoni. In central and eastern United States, it is the main vector for Rocky Mountain spotted fever. Parasitic to dogs, horses, cattle, rabbits, and man.

Dermacort. Trade name for hydrocortisone.

dermad [Gr. *derma,* skin, + L. *ad,* toward]. Toward the skin; externally.

dermadrome (dĕr′mă-drōm). Skin manifestation of a systemic disease.

dermal. Rel. to the skin or derma. SYN: *cutaneous; integumentary.*

dermalaxia (dĕr″mă-lăk′sē-ă) [″ + *malaxis,* softening]. Morbid relaxation or softness of the skin.

dermalgia (dĕr-măl′jē-ă) [″ + *algos,* pain]. Pain localized in the skin.

dermamyiasis (dĕr-mă-mī-ī′ă-sĭs) [″ + *myia,* fly, + *-iasis,* condition]. Skin disease caused by invasion of larvae of dipterous insects.

dermapostasis (dĕr″mă-pŏs′tă-sĭs) [″ + *apostasis,* a falling away]. Abscess formation accompanying a skin disease.

dermat-, dermato- [Gr. *dermatos*]. Prefixes indicating relationship to skin.

dermatalgia (dĕr″mă-tăl′jē-ă) [″ + *algos,* pain]. Paresthesia with localized pain in the skin. SYN: *dermalgia.*

dermatatrophia (dĕrm″ăt-ă-trō′fē-ă) [″ + *atrophia,* atrophy]. Atrophy of the skin.

dermatauxe (dĕr-mă-tŏk′sē) [″ + *auxe,* increase]. Hypertrophy of the skin.

dermatitis (dĕr″mă-tī′tĭs) [Gr. *dermatos,* skin, + *itis,* inflammation]. Inflammation of skin evidenced by itching, redness, and various skin lesions.

ETIOL: May be due to one of several causes: skin irritants such as poison ivy, corrosives, acids, and alkalies or hypersusceptibility on part of patient to conditions that would not cause skin irritation in persons who were not hypersusceptible.

TREATMENT: Remove primary cause if due to systemic effect. If caused by local agent, remove irritant by washing with soap and water. Dress with calamine lotion or bland oils or ointment.

d., actinic. Reaction of skin to sunlight or other sources of photochemical activity such as x-rays or ultraviolet light.

d. aestivalis. Hot weather dermatitis.

d., allergic. Inflammation believed to be due to an allergy. SEE: *allergen; allergy.*

d., atopic. Dermatitis of unknown etiology characterized by itching and scratching in an individual with inherently irritable skin. There may be allergic, hereditary, or psychological components. The disease rarely occurs prior to two months of age and may occur initially quite late in life. In about 70% of all cases there is a family history of the disease. About 3% of all infants have atopic dermatitis. The symptoms are made worse by contact with wool, climatic changes, and excessive exposure to soap, water, and oils. The skin lesion in infants consists of swollen papules that are itchy and become exudative and crusty due to the scratching. Secondary infection and lymphadenopathy are common. About half of the infantile cases clear up by 18 months of age. The lesions in children and adults are similar to those of infancy but lichenification is present.

TREATMENT: Avoidance of soaps and ointments. Bathing should be kept to a minimum, but bath oils may help to prevent drying of skin. Use of soft-textured clothing that does not contain wool. Fingernails should be kept short to decrease damage from scratching. Antihistamines may help to reduce itching at night. Avoid heavy exercise because of its induction of perspiration. Use a nonlipid softening lotion followed by a cortisone or hydrocortisone lotion in a propylene glycol base twice daily. Oral antibiotics may be needed for a brief period to control secondary infection.

d., berlock. Dermatitis occurring upon sequential exposure to sunlight after application of perfumes or other toiletries that contain bergamot oil in their formulation.

d. calorica. Inflammation due to heat or cold, as in sunburn.

d., cercarial. Dermatitis resulting from infestation with the cercaria of blood flukes belonging to the genus Schistosoma. SYN: *schistosome dermatitis; swimmer's itch.*

d., contact. Inflammation and irritation of the skin due to contact with an irritating substance. Usually due to a combination of reduced ability of the skin to resist injury and exposure to a material in strong concentration such as soap or chemical. Some individuals are sensitive to such apparently innocuous compounds as perfumes and deodorants.

TREATMENT: Remove patient from offending material and treat skin as indicated. SYN: *d. venenata.*

d., cosmetic. Dermatitis caused by an ingredient in a cosmetic preparation. A form of contact dermatitis.

d., exfoliative. Chronic inflammation of the skin commonly involving whole surface and characterized by redness and abundant flaky desquamation. Most cases are of unknown etiology.

SYM: May be primary with constitutional symptoms (fever, debility, and gastrointestinal upset), with sudden eruption, pink turning dark red, followed by thin, flaky, loosely adherent, grayish or brownish scales, tender skin, tension, and stiffness. In secondary type it follows certain scaly diseases of the skin (eczema, seborrheic dermatitis, psoriasis). Pigmentation (slate or mahogany color) is frequent. In extensive eruptions the patient may become depressed due to the cosmetic implications of the condition.

TREATMENT: Attention to general health. Locally, soothing oily applications. Corticosteroid and antibiotic therapy.

d. herpetiformis. Chronic inflammatory disease characterized by erythematous, papular, vesicular, bullous, or pustular lesions with tendency to grouping and with intense itching and burning.

ETIOL: Direct cause unknown. Occurs mostly in adult males though no age is exempt. Some patients have associated asymptomatic gluten-sensitive enteropathy. HLA-B-8 antigen is frequently associated with this disease.

SYM: Lesions develop suddenly and spread peripherally. Disease is variable and erratic, and attack may be prolonged for weeks or months. Secondary infection may follow trauma to the inflamed areas.

TREATMENT: Oral dapsone will provide substantial relief of symptoms in a few days. Also sulfapyridine may be used.

d. hiemalis. Dermatitis occurring in cold weather.

d. infectiosa eczematoides. Pustular eruption during or following a pyogenic disease.

d. medicamentosa. Drug eruption.

ETIOL: Idiosyncrasy or sensitization to the drug in question. Cosmetics, arsenic, iodides, bromides, phenobarbital, and antibiotics are some of the offending agents.

SYM: With exception of bromine and iodine, the eruption is not characteristic and may resemble almost any condition or disease.

TREATMENT: Removal of cause.

d. multiformis. Form of dermatitis with lesions of a pustular nature.

d. papillaris capillitii. Formation on scalp and neck of surface elevations interspersed with pustules and ending in scarlike elevations resembling keloids.

d., poison ivy. Dermatitis resulting from ivy poisoning. SYN: *d., rhus.* SEE: *poison ivy* *dermatitis.*

d., primary. Skin eruption that is a direct, rather than an allergic, response.

d., radiation. Dermatitis due to radiation exposure.

d., rhus. A contact dermatitis caused by substances present in certain plants. SEE: *poison ivy dermatitis; toxicodendron.*

d. seborrheica. Acute or subacute inflammatory skin disease of unknown etiology beginning on the scalp, characterized by rounded, irregular, or circinate lesions covered with yellowish or brownish-gray greasy scales. SYN: *alopecia furfuracea; pityriasis capitis; seborrhea corporis; seborrhea sicca.*

SYM: On the scalp, it may be dry with abundant grayish branny scales, or oozing and crusted, constituting eczema capitis, and may spread to forehead and postauricular regions. On the forehead it shows scaly and infiltrated lesions with dark red bases, some itching, localized loss of hair. On eyebrows and eyelashes dry, dirty white scales, itching. On nasolabial folds or vermilion border of lips inflammation with itching. On sternal region, greasy and unctuous to the touch. May appear in interscapular, axillary, and genitocrural regions also.

TREATMENT: When limited to scalp, frequent shampooing and use of mild keratolytic agents. Selenium-containing shampoos have been helpful. Generalized seborrheic dermatitis requires careful attention including scrupulous skin hygiene, keeping skin as dry as possible, dusting powders. Topical and systemic cortisone preparations may be required.

d., stasis. Eczema of the legs with edema, pigmentation, and sometimes chronic inflammation. Usually due to impaired circulation.

d. venenata. Any inflammation caused by local action of various animal, vegetable, or mineral substances on the surface of the skin.

ETIOL: Drugs, acids, alkalies, plants (poison ivy, oak, or sumac). Runs an acute course with recurrence on reexposure to the sensitizing agent.

SYM: Vary from simple hyperemia to gangrene and sloughing. Majority are erythematous, limited to part touched by irritant, becoming papular, vesicular, or pustular with burning or itching.

TREATMENT: Apply local drying solutions such as aluminum acetate. Calamine lotion is helpful in drying the lesions and for control of itching. In severe cases, the use of topical and systemic cortisone may be needed.

d. verrucosa. Chronic fungal infection of the skin characterized by the formation of wartlike nodules. These may enlarge and form papillomatous structures that sometimes ulcerate. SYN: *chromoblastomycosis,* q.v.

ETIOL: May be due to one of several fungi including Hormodendrum pedrosoi or Phialophora verrucosa.

d., x-ray. Skin inflammation due to effects of x-rays.

dermatoautoplasty (dĕr″mă-tō-aw′tō-plăs″tē) [Gr. *dermatos,* skin, + *autos,* self, + *plassein,* to form]. Grafting of skin taken from some portion of the patient's own body.

Dermatobia (dĕr″mă-tō′bē-ă) [″ + *bios,* life]. A genus of botflies belonging to the order Diptera of the family Oestridae.

D. hominis. A species of botflies, found in parts of tropical America, whose larvae infest man and cattle. The eggs are transported by mosquitoes.

dermatobiasis (dĕr″mă-tō-bī′ă-sĭs). Infestation by the larvae of Dermatobia hominis, the eggs of which are carried to the skin by mosquitoes. The larvae then hatch and bore into the skin while the mosquito feeds. Marble-like boils form at the site of infestation.

dermatocele (dĕr′mă-tō-sēl″) [″ + *kele,* hernia]. Tendency of hypertrophied skin and subcutaneous tissue to hang loosely in folds. SYN: *dermatolysis.*

d. lipomatosis. A pedunculated lipoma with cystic degeneration.

dermatocelidosis (dĕr″mă-tō-sĕl″ĭ-dō′sĭs) [″ + *kelis,* spot, + *osis,* condition]. Freckles; a macular eruption. SYN: *dermatokelidosis.*

dermatocellulitis (dĕr″mă-tō-sĕl″ū-lī′tĭs) [″ + L. *cellula,* little cell, + Gr. *itis,* inflammation]. Inflammation of subcutaneous connective tissue.

dermatoconiosis (dĕr″mă-tō-kō″nē-ō′sĭs) [″ + *konia,* dust]. Any irritation of the skin caused by dust, esp. one due to occupational exposure.

dermatocyst (dĕr′mă-tō-sĭst) [″ + *kystis,* cyst]. A skin cyst.

dermatodynia (dĕr″mă-tō-dĭn′ē-ă) [″ + *odyne,* pain]. Pain in the skin. SYN: *dermatalgia.*

dermatofibroma [″ + L. *fibra,* fiber, + Gr. *oma,* tumor]. A nonmalignant skin fibroma. SEE: *dimple sign.*

dermatofibrosarcoma (dĕr″mă-tō-fī″brō-săr-kō′mă) [″ + ″ + Gr. *sarx,* flesh, + *oma,* tumor]. Fibrosarcoma of the skin.

dermatogen (dĕr-măt′ō-jĕn) [″ + *gennan,* to produce]. Antigen from a skin disease.

dermatogenous (dĕr″mă-tŏj′ĕn-ŭs). Producing skin or disease of skin.

dermatoglyphics (dĕr″mă-tō-glĭf′ĭks) [″ + *glyphe,* a carving]. Study of surface markings of the skin, esp. those of hands and feet. Useful in identification and genetic studies. SEE: *fingerprint* for illus.

dermatographia, dermatography. A form

of urticaria due to physical allergy.

dermatoheteroplasty (dĕr″mă-tō-hĕt′ĕr-ō-plăs″tē) [″ + *heteros,* other, + *plassein,* to mold]. Skin grafting from an individual of a different species.

dermatokelidosis (dĕr″mă-tō-kĕl″ĭ-dō′sĭs) [″ + *kelidoun,* to stain]. A macular eruption; freckle.

dermatologist (dĕr″mă-tŏl′ō-jĭst) [Gr. *dermatos,* skin, + *logos,* study]. A physician who specializes in treating diseases of the skin.

dermatology (dĕr″mă-tŏl′ō-jē). The science of the skin and its diseases.

dermatolysis (dĕr″mă-tŏl′ĭ-sĭs) [″ + *lysis,* a loosening]. Tendency of hypertrophied skin and subcutaneous tissue to hang in folds. Loose skin. SYN: *cutis laxa; cutis pendula; pachydermatocele* (def. 1).

dermatoma (dĕr″mă-tō′mă) [″ + *oma,* tumor]. Circumscribed thickening of skin.

dermatome (dĕr′mă-tōm) [Gr. *derma,* skin, + *tome,* incision]. 1. Instrument for incising the skin or for cutting thin slices for transplantation of skin. 2. A segmental skin area innervated by various spinal cord segments. SEE: illus. 3. The lateral portion of the somite of an embryo, which gives rise to the dermis of the skin; the cutis plate.

dermatomere (dĕr′mă-tō-mēr) [Gr. *dermatos,* skin, + *meros,* part]. A segment of embryonic integument.

dermatomucosomyositis (dĕr″mă-tō-mū-kō″sō-mī-ō-sī′tĭs) [″ + L. *mucosa,* mucous membrane, + Gr. *mys,* muscle, + *itis,* inflammation]. Inflammation involving mucosa and muscles.

dermatomycosis (dĕr″mă-tō-mī-kō′sĭs) [″ + *mykes,* fungus, + *osis,* condition]. (pl. *dermatomycoses*) A skin infection caused by certain fungi of the genera Trichophyton, Epidermophyton, and Microsporum.

dermatomyoma [″ + *mys,* muscle, + *oma,* tumor]. Myoma of the skin.

dermatomyositis (dĕr″mă-tō-mī″ō-sī′tĭs) [″ + ″ + *itis,* inflammation]. A disease of connective tissue. An acute, subacute, or chronic disease of unknown etiology. Characterized by edema, dermatitis, and inflammation of the muscles.

SYM: Fever, malaise, general weakness, weakness of the pelvic and shoulder girdle muscles; skin and mucosal lesions often present. About one third of patients will have dysphagia.

TREATMENT: Symptomatic: bedrest, physiotherapy, salicylates. Adrenocortical steroids are helpful in most cases.

NURSING IMPLICATIONS: Careful turning is needed along with frequent position changes. Maintenance of correct body alignment, massage, graduated exercises, and resistance exercises are beneficial in preventing or treating muscle atrophy and contractures. Warm baths and moist heat applications are helpful in relief of stiffness. Mouth lesions may be irrigated with warm saline solution as needed.

dermatoneurosis [″ + *neuron,* nerve, + *osis,* condition]. Skin disease of nervous origin. SEE: *neurodermatitis.*

dermatopathia [″ + *pathos,* disease]. Any disease of the skin.

dermatopathology [″ + ″ + *logos,* study]. Study of diseases of the skin.

dermatopathy. Any skin disease. SYN: *dermatopathia.*

dermatophiliasis (dĕr″mă-tō-fĭ-lī′ă-sĭs). 1. Infestation with Tunga penetrans, a pathogenic actinomycetes. 2. Dermatophilosis.

dermatophilosis (dĕr″mă-tō-fĭ-lō′sĭs). An actinomycotic infection that occurs in certain hooved animals and rarely in man.

dermatophobia [″ + *phobos,* fear]. Abnormal fear of having a skin disease.

dermatophylaxis (dĕr′mă-tō-fĭ-lăk′sĭs) [″ + *phylaxis,* protection]. Protecting the skin from infection.

dermatophyte (dĕr′mă-tō-fīt) [″ + *phyton,* plant]. A fungal parasite that grows in or on the skin. They rarely penetrate deeper than the epidermis or its appendages—hair and nails. They cause such skin diseases as favus, tinea, ringworm, and eczema. Important dermatophytes include the genera Microsporum, Trichophyton, and Epidermophyton.

dermatophytid (dĕr″mă-tŏf′ĭ-tĭd). A toxic rash or eruption occurring in dermatomycosis.

dermatophytosis (dĕr″mă-tō-fī-tō′sĭs) [″ + *phyton,* plant, + *osis,* condition]. A fungus infection of the skin of the hands and feet, esp. between the toes. SYN: *athlete's foot; ringworm of feet; tinea pedis.*

dermatoplastic [″ + *plassein,* to form]. Pert. to skin grafting.

dermatoplasty (dĕr′mă-tō-plăs″tē). Transplanting living skin to cover cutaneous defects caused by injury, operation, or disease.

NURSING IMPLICATIONS: Nursing measures are directed toward protection of the graft site from dislodgement, from trauma or infection; and promotion of healing of the donor site. As with any patient who has skin grafting, good nutrition is essential.

dermatorrhagia (dĕr″mă-tō-rā′jē-ă) [Gr. *dermatos,* skin, + *rhegnynai,* to burst forth]. Hemorrhage into or from the skin.

dermatorrhea (dĕr″mă-tō-rē′ă) [″ + *rhoia,* flow]. Excessive secretion of sebaceous glands.

dermatosclerosis (dĕr″mă-tō-sklĕr-ō′sĭs) [″ + *sklerosis,* hardening]. A progressive collagen disease of the skin that manifests as a diffuse leathery induration of the skin frequently followed by atrophy and pigmentation. The localized form is known as morphea. Involve-

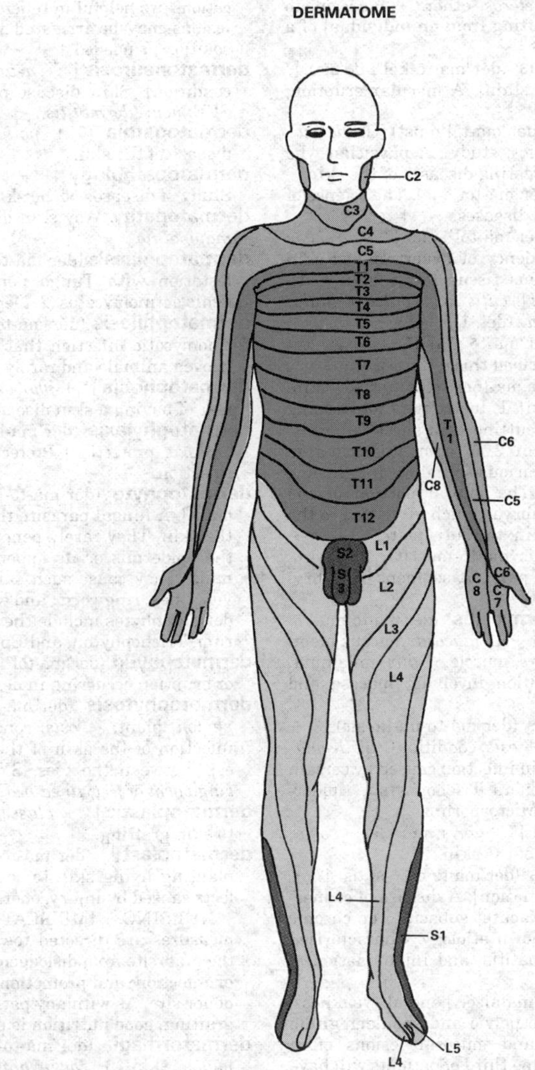
DERMATOME
C2
C3
C4
C5
T1
T2
T3
T4
T5
T6
T7
T8
T9
T10
T11
T12
T 1
C6
C8
C5
S2
S 3
L1
L2
C 8
C6
C 7
L3
L4
L4
S1
L5
L4
CERVICAL (C)
THORACIC (T)
LUMBAR (L)
SACRAL (S)

ment of internal organs is to be expected. SYN: *scleroderma.*

dermatoscopy (dĕr″mă-tŏs′kō-pē) [″ + *skopein,* to examine]. Examination of the skin with a high-powered lens or microscope.

dermatosis (dĕr″mă-tō′sĭs) [″ + *osis,* condition]. (pl. *dermatoses*) Any disease of the skin in which inflammation is not necessarily a feature. Not a synonym for dermatitis.

d. papulosa nigra. Eruption consisting of many tiny tumors or milia on skin of face. Greatest incidence is among blacks.

d., progressive pigmentary. Reddish papules principally on legs; eruption is slowly progressive.

dermatosome (dĕr′mă-tō-sōm) [″ + *soma,* body]. Section of equatorial plate in mitosis.

dermatotherapy [″ + *therapeia,* treatment]. Treatment of skin diseases.

dermatotome (dĕr′mă-tō-tōm″) [″ + *tome,* incision]. 1. One of the fetal skin segments. 2. A knife for incising the skin or small lesions. SYN: *dermatome* (def. 1).

dermatotropic (dĕr″mă-tō-trŏp′ĭk) [″ + *trope,* a turning]. Acting preferentially on the skin.

dermatoxerasia (dĕr″mă-tō-zē-rā′zē-ă) [″ + *xerasia,* dryness]. Roughening of skin. SYN: *xeroderma.*

dermatozoon [″ + *zoon,* animal]. An animal parasite of the skin.

dermatozoonosis (dĕr″mă-tō-zō″ō-nō′sĭs) [″ + ″ + *nosos,* disease]. Any skin disease caused by an animal parasite.

dermatrophia (dĕr-mă-trō′fē-ă) [″ + *atrophia,* atrophy]. Atrophy of the skin.

dermic (dĕr′mĭk) [Gr. *derma,* skin]. Pert. to the skin.

dermis (dĕr′mĭs) [L.]. The skin; cutis vera or true skin. SYN: *corium* [NA].

dermoblast [Gr. *derma,* skin, + *blastos,* germ]. Part of mesoblastic layer, developing into the corium.

dermographia, dermography (dĕr-mō-grăf′ē-ă, -mŏg′ră-fē) [″ + *graphein,* to write]. A form of urticaria due to allergy.

dermoid (dĕr′moyd) [″ + *eidos,* form]. 1. Resembling the skin. 2. A dermoid cyst.

dermoid cyst. An ovarian teratoma. A nonmalignant cystic tumor in which are found elements derived from the ectoderm, such as hair, teeth, or skin. These tumors occur frequently in the ovary but may develop in other organs such as the lungs.

dermoidectomy (dĕr″moyd-ĕk′tō-mē) [″ + ″ + *ektome,* excision]. Excision of a dermoid cyst.

dermolipoma (dĕr″mō-lĭ-pō′mă). 1. Growth of yellow fatty tissue beneath the bulbar conjunctiva. 2. Lipoma of the skin.

dermomycosis (dĕr″mō-mī-kō′sĭs) [″ + *mykes,* fungus, + *osis,* condition]. A skin disease produced by a vegetable parasite. SYN: *dermatomycosis.*

dermonosology (dĕr″mō-nō-sŏl′ō-jē) [″ + *nosos,* disease, + *logos,* study]. The science of classification of skin diseases.

dermopathy (dĕr-mŏp′ă-thē) [″ + *pathos,* disease]. Any skin disease.

dermophlebitis (dĕr″mō-flĕ-bī′tĭs) [″ + *phleps,* vein, + *itis,* inflammation]. Inflammation of superficial veins and surrounding skin.

dermophyte (dĕr′mō-fīt) [″ + *phyton,* plant]. A vegetable skin parasite. SYN: *dermatophyte.*

dermoskeleton [″ + *skeleton*]. Apparent external covering of the body; the hair, nails, and teeth in man. SYN: *exoskeleton.*

dermosynovitis (dĕr″mō-sĭn-ō-vī′tĭs) [″ + L. *synovia,* joint fluid, + Gr. *itis,* inflammation]. Inflammation of the skin overlying an inflamed bursa or tendon.

dermotropic (dĕr″mō-trŏp′ĭk) [″ + *trope,* a turning]. Acting esp. on the skin.

dermovascular (dĕr″mō-văs′kū-lăr) [″ + *vas,* vessel]. Concerning the skin and its blood vessels.

derodidymus (dĕr″ō-dĭd′ĭ-mŭs) [Gr. *dere,* neck, + *didymos,* double]. A malformed fetus with two necks and heads but a single body and normal limbs. SYN: *dicephalus.*

DES. *diethylstilbestrol,* q.v.

desalination. Partial or complete removal of salts from a substance, as from seawater or brackish water so that it is suitable for agricultural or household purposes.

desaturation [L. *de,* from, + *saturare,* to fill]. A process whereby a saturated organic compound is converted into an unsaturated one, as when stearic acid, $CH_3(CH_2)_{16}COOH$, is changed into oleic acid, $CH_3(CH_2)_7CH{:}CH(CH_2)_7COOH$. The product has different physical and chemical properties after this transformation. SEE: *saturated hydrocarbon.*

Desault's apparatus (dĕ-sōz′). [Pierre J. Desault, Fr. surgeon, 1744–1795] Bandage used for fracture of clavicle. SEE: *bandage.*

descemetitis (dĕs″ĕ-mĕ-tī′tĭs). Inflammation of Descemet's membrane on the corneal posterior surface. SYN: *cyclitis, serous.*

Descemet's membrane (dĕs-ĕ-māz′). [Jean Descemet, Fr. anatomist, 1732–1810] A fine membrane between the endothelial layer of the cornea and the substantia propia.

descemetocele (dĕs″ĕ-mĕt′ō-sēl). Protrusion of Descemet's membrane.

descendens (dē-sĕn′dĕns) [L. *de,* from, + *scendere,* to climb]. Descending; a descending structure.

d. hypoglossi. A branch of the hypoglossal nerve given off at the point where it curves around the occipital artery, which passes down obliquely across the sheath of the carotid vessels (sometimes within it) to form a loop just below the middle of the neck with branches of the 2nd and 3rd cervical nerves.

descensus (dē-sĕn'sŭs) [L.]. Process of falling, descent.

d. testis. Normal passage of the testicle from the abdominal cavity down into the scrotum. Occurs during last few months of fetal life. SYN: *migration of testicle.*

d. uteri. Defective pelvic floor allowing the uterus or part of the uterus to protrude out of the vagina. SYN: *procidentia; prolapse of uterus.*

VARIETIES: First degree: where the cervix uteri reaches down to the vaginal introitus. Second degree: where the cervix uteri protrudes out of the vagina. Third degree: where the entire uterus lies outside of the vagina.

ETIOL: This condition may be congenital or acquired, although it is most usually acquired. The etiological factors are congenital weakness of the uterine supports and injury to the pelvic floor or uterine supports during childbirth.

SYM: The condition is most often seen following instrumental deliveries or where the patient has been allowed to bear down before the cervix is fully dilated. Frequently associated with this is a prolapse of the anterior and posterior vaginal walls, as seen in cystocele and rectocele. In the early stages there are dragging sensations in the lower abdomen, backache while standing and on exertion, sensation of weight and bearing down in the perineum, frequency of urination and incontinence of urine in cases associated with cystocele. In the later stages a protrusion or a swelling at the vulva is noticed on standing or straining, and leukorrhea is present. In procidentia there is frequently pain on walking, inability to urinate unless the mass is reduced, and quite commonly cystitis.

TREATMENT: The treatment depends upon the age of the patient, the degree of prolapse, and the associated pathology. Where conservation is desired, the use of the pessary is clearly indicated, or conservative surgery (round ligament shortening and pelvic floor repair) may suffice. In the elderly patient, where the uterus is pathological, a hysterectomy (abdominal or vaginal) accompanied by vaginal plastic procedure is indicated.

d. ventriculi. Downward displacement of the stomach. SYN: *gastroptosis.*

DES daughters. Daughters of mothers who received diethylstilbestrol (DES) during pregnancy. SEE: *DES syndrome; diethylstilbestrol.*

desensitization. 1. Prevention of anaphylaxis. Usually attained by administering repeated doses of the sensitizing substance too small to cause anaphylaxis. However, if desensitization is used, it should be done year-round and not seasonally even when treating seasonal allergies. SYN: *antianaphylaxis.* 2. In psychiatry, the alleviation of an emotionally upsetting life situation.

desensitize [L. *de,* from, + *sentire,* to perceive]. 1. To deprive of or lessen sensitivity by nerve section or blocking. 2. To abate anaphylactic sensitiveness by administration of the specific antigen in low dosage.

desert fever, desert rheumatism. Coccidioidomycosis, q.v.

desexualize (dē-sĕks'ū-ăl-īz) [" + *sexus,* sex]. To castrate; to remove sexual traits.

Desferal. Trade name for deferoxamine mesylate.

desferrioxamine (dĕs-fĕr'ē-ŏks'ă-mēn). Deferoxamine, q.v.

desiccant (dĕs'ĭ-kănt). Causing desiccation or dryness.

desiccate (dĕs'ĭ-kāt) [L. *desiccare,* to dry up]. To dry.

desiccation (dĕs"ĭ-kā'shŭn). The process of drying up. SEE: *electrodesiccation.*

desipramine hydrochloride (dĕs-ĭp'ră-mēn). USP. An antidepressant. Trade names are Norpramin and Pertofrane.

deslanoside (dĕs-lăn'ō-sīd). USP. A cardiac glycoside, obtained from digitalis leaf, that has the same action as lanatoside C. Trade name is Cedilanid-D.

desmalgia (dĕs-măl'jē-ă) [Gr. *desmos,* band, + *algos,* pain]. Pain in a ligament.

desmectasia, desmectasis (dĕs-mĕk-tā'zē-ă, -mĕk'tă-sĭs) [" + *ektasis,* dilatation]. Stretching of a ligament.

desmepithelium (dĕs-mĕp-ĭ-thē'lē-ŭm) [" + *epi,* upon, + *thele,* nipple]. The epithelial lining of vessels and synovial cavities.

desmitis (dĕs-mī'tĭs) [" + *itis,* inflammation]. Inflammation of a ligament.

desmo- [Gr. *desmos*]. Prefix indicating a band, a ligament.

desmocranium (dĕs"mō-krā'nē-ŭm) [" + L. *cranium*]. In the embryo, the earliest form of the skull.

desmocyte (dĕs'mō-sīt) [" + *kytos,* cell]. A supporting tissue cell. SYN: *fibroblast; fibrocyte.*

desmocytoma (dĕs"mō-sī-tō'mă) [" + " + *oma,* tumor]. A tumor formed of desmocytes; a sarcoma.

desmodynia [" + *odyne,* pain]. Pain in a ligament.

desmoenzyme. An intracellular enzyme.

desmogenous (dĕs-mŏj'ĕ-nŭs) [" + *gennan,* to produce]. Of connective tissue origin.

desmography (dĕs-mŏg'ră-fē) [" + *graphein,* to write]. A description of or treatise on ligaments.

desmoid (dĕs'moyd) [" + *eidos,* form]. 1. Tendonlike; fibroid. 2. A very tough and firm fibroma.

desmology (dĕs-mŏl'ō-jē) [" + *logos*, science]. Science of tendons and ligaments.

desmoma [" + *oma*, tumor]. A tumor of the connective tissue.

desmoneoplasm (dĕs"mō-nē'ō-plăzm) [" + *neos*, new, + *plasma*, matter]. A connective tissue tumor.

desmopathy (dĕs-mŏp'ă-thē) [" + *pathos*, disease]. Any disease affecting ligaments.

desmoplasia (dĕs-mō-plā'zē-ă) [" + Gr. *plassein*, to form]. An abnormal tendency to form fibrous tissue or adhesive bands.

desmoplastic [" + *plassein*, to form]. Causing or forming adhesions.

desmopyknosis (dĕs"mō-pĭk-nō'sĭs) [" + *pyknosis*, condensation]. Surgical procedure for shortening of round ligaments by attaching them by loops to the anterior uterine wall.

desmorrhexis (dĕs-mō-rĕk'sĭs) [" + *rhexis*, rupture]. Rupture of a ligament.

desmosis (dĕs-mō'sĭs) [" + *osis*, condition]. Any disease of the connective tissue.

desmosome (dĕs'mō-sōm) [" + *soma*, body]. A small thickening in an intercellular bridge.

desmotomy (dĕs-mŏt'ō-mē) [" + *tome*, incision]. Dissection of ligament.

desoximetasone (dĕs-ŏk"sē-mĕt'ă-sōn). USP. A corticosteroid used topically. Trade name is Topicort.

desoxy-. Prefix meaning deoxidized or a reduced form of. SEE: words beginning with *deoxy-*.

desoxycorticosterone (dĕs-ŏk"sē-kor-tĭ-kŏs'tĕr-ōn). An active steroid hormone produced by the adrenal cortex. It plays an important role in the regulation of water and salt metabolism.

d. acetate. USP. An acetate ester of desoxycorticosterone and the form in which the hormone is usually administered in its therapeutic use. It may be injected intramuscularly or used buccally. Trade names are Doca Acetate and Percorten Acetate.

desoxyribonucleic acid (dĕs"ŏk-sē-rĭb"ō-nū'klē-ĭk). Former spelling for deoxyribonucleic acid, q.v.

despumation (dĕs"pū-mā'shŭn) [L. *de*, from, + *spuma*, froth]. Separation of froth or scum from a liquid.

desquamate (dĕs'kwă-māt) [L. *desquamare*, to remove scales]. To shred or scale off the surface epithelium.

desquamation (dĕs"kwă-mā'shŭn). Shedding of the epidermis.

d., furfuraceous. Shedding of branlike scales.

desquamative (dĕs-kwŏm'ă-tĭv). Of the nature of desquamation, or pert. to or causing it. SYN: *keratolytic*.

DES syndrome. The occurrence of neoplasms of the vagina in young women whose mothers received diethylstilbestrol early in their pregnancy.

destructive [L. *destructus*, destroyed]. Causing ruin or destruction. Opposite of constructive.

destructive lesion. A pathological change such as an infection, tumor, or injury that causes the death of tissue or an organ.

desudation (dē-sū-dā'shŭn) [L. *de*, from, + *sudare*, to perspire]. Excessive sweating often followed by slight pustular eruption.

desulfhydrase (dē"sŭlf-hī'drās). An enzyme that cleaves cysteine into hydrogen sulfide, ammonia, and pyruvic acid

desynchronosis (dē-sĭn"krō-nō'sĭs) [" + Gr. *synkhronos*, same time]. The time difference between that of a person's present location and that to which the person is accustomed. This causes an upset of the individual's internal biological clock. Occurs in persons traveling across a number of time zones in a short period of time. Lay term for this condition is "jet lag."

DET. *diethyltryptamine*.

det. L. *detur*, let it be given.

detachment [O. Fr. *destachier*, to unfasten]. To become separate.

d., retinal. The pathological condition where the retina or a part of it becomes separated from the choroid.

detail. In radiology, the sharpness with which an image is presented on a radiograph.

detector [L. *detectus*, uncovered]. Device for determining the presence of something.

d., lie. A polygraph, an instrument for determining minor physical changes assumed to occur under the stress of lying or any other emotion. Variations in respiratory rhythm, pulse rate, blood pressure, and sweating of hands are measured. Increased perspiration lessens resistance to passage of electrical current. The test has popular appeal among law enforcement departments but results obtained are presumptive and not absolute.

d., radiation. Instrument used to detect the presence of radiation.

detergent [L. *detergere*, to cleanse]. 1. A medicine that purges or cleanses; cleansing. 2. A cleaning or wetting agent prepared synthetically from a variety of chemicals. These are classed as anionic if they have a negative electrical charge or cationic if they have a positive charge. SEE: *soap*.

deterioration [L. *deteriorare*, to deteriorate]. Retrogression; said of impairment of mental or physical functions.

determinant (dē-tĕr'mĭ-nănt) [L. *determinare*, to limit]. That which determines the character of anything.

determination [L. *determinatus,* limiting]. Establishing the nature or precise identity of a substance, organism, or event.

determinism (dē-tĕr′mĭn-ĭzm) [″ + Gr. *-ismos,* condition of]. The theory that all human action is the result of predetermined and inevitable physical, psychological, or environmental conditions that are uninfluenced by the will of the individual.

detersive [L. *detergere,* to cleanse]. Detergent; cleansing or purging.

det. in dup. [L. *detur in duplo*]. Let twice as much be given.

detonation (dĕ″tō-nā′shŭn) [L. *detonare,* to thunder loudly]. A violent noise caused by an explosive combustion.

detortion, detorsion (dē-tor′shŭn). 1. Surgical therapy for torsion of a testicle, ureter, or volvulus of the bowel. 2. Correction of any bodily curvature or deformity.

detoxicate (dē-tŏk′sĭ-kāt) [L. *de,* from, + Gr. *toxikon,* poison]. To remove the toxic principle of a substance. SYN: *detoxify.*

detoxification [L. *de,* from, + Gr. *toxikon,* poison, + L. *facere,* to make]. 1. Reduction of the toxic properties of a poisonous substance. SEE: *biotransformation.* 2. Process of removing the physiological effects of a drug or substance from an addicted individual.

detoxify (dē-tŏk′sĭ-fī). 1. To remove the toxic quality of a substance. 2. Treatment of a toxic overdose of any medicine but esp. of the toxic state produced by drugs of abuse or acute alcoholism.

detrition (dē-trĭsh′ŭn) [ML. *detritio*]. The wearing away of a part, esp. through friction, as that of the teeth.

detritus (dē-trī′tŭs) [L., wearing away]. Any broken down, degenerative, or carious matter produced by disintegration.

detruncation (dē″trŭn-kā′shŭn) [L. *de,* from, + *truncus,* trunk]. Decapitation, esp. of a fetus. SYN: *decollation.*

detrusor urinae (dē-trū′sor ū-rī′nē) [L.]. External longitudinal layer of muscular coat of bladder.

detumescence (dē″tū-mĕs′ĕns) [L. *de,* down, + *tumescere,* to swell]. 1. Subsidence of a swelling. 2. Subsidence of erectile tissue of genital organs (penis and clitoris) following erection.

deutencephalon (dūt-ĕn-sĕf′ă-lŏn) [Gr. *deuteros,* second, + *enkephalos,* brain]. The interbrain. SYN: *diencephalon; thalamencephalon.*

deuteranomalopia (doo″tĕr-ă-nŏm″ă-lō′pē-ă) [″ + *anomalos,* irregular, + *ops,* eye]. Partial color blindness in which the primary colors are perceived but green is poorly appreciated.

deuteranopia, deuteranopsia (dū″tĕr-ăn-ō′pē-ă, -ŏp′sē-ă) [″ + *anopia,* blindness]. Green blindness; color blindness in which there is a defect in the perception of green. SEE: *color blindness.*

deuterate (dū′tĕr-āt). To combine with deuterium.

deuterium (dū-tē′rē-ŭm) [Gr. *deuteros,* second]. SYMB: H^2 or D. Heavy hydrogen; the mass two isotope of hydrogen.

d. oxide. An isotope of water in which hydrogen has been displaced by its isotope, deuterium. Its properties differ from ordinary water in that it has a higher freezing and boiling point and in the fact that it is incapable of supporting life. SYN: *heavy water.*

deutero-, deuter-, deuto- [Gr. *deuteros,* second]. Prefix indicating second or secondary.

deuteron (dū′tĕr-ŏn). SYMB: d. The nucleus of deuterium or heavy hydrogen.

deuteropathia, deuteropathy [Gr. *deuteros,* second, + *pathos,* disease]. A disease associated with or secondary to another disease.

deuteroplasm [″ + *plasma,* matter]. The reserve food supply in the yolk or ovum.

deutoscolex (dū″tō-skō′lĕks) [″ + *skolex,* worm]. Secondary daughter cysts that develop on the inner wall of a hydatid cyst.

devasation (dē″văs-ā′shŭn) [L. *de,* from, + *vasa,* vessel]. Destruction of blood vessels.

devascularization (dē-văs″kū-lăr-ĭ-zā′shŭn) [″ + *vascularis,* pert. to a vessel]. 1. Loss or draining of blood from a part. 2. Decrease in the blood supply to a part of the body.

developer. In radiology, the solution used to make the latent image visible on the radiographic film.

development [O. Fr. *desveloper,* to unwrap]. Growth to full size or maturity, as in the progress of an egg to the adult state.

RS: aplasia; apposition; chorista; dysplasia.

d., psychomotor and physical, of infant. SEE: *psychomotor and physical development of the infant.*

developmental. Pert. to development.

deviance [L. *deviare,* to turn aside]. Away from the accepted norm.

deviant. Something (or someone) that is variant when compared with the norm or an accepted standard.

d., sex. One whose sexual behavior is considered to be abnormal or socially unacceptable. SEE: *paraphilia.*

deviant behavior. Actions that are considered to be abnormal.

deviate (dē′vē-āt″) [L. *deviare,* to turn aside]. 1. To move steadily away from a designated norm. 2. An individual whose attitude or behavior differs from the norm.

deviation (dē-vē-ā′shŭn). Going out of the way; departure from normal.

d., axis. A change in the direction of the major electrical axis of the heart as determined by the electrocardiogram.

d., conjugate. Deviation of face and eyes to the same side.

d., minimum. The smallest deviation that a prism can produce.

d., standard. In statistics, the measure of variability from the central tendency of any frequency curve.

device (dĭ-vīs') [O. Fr. *devis,* contrivance]. An apparatus, machine, or shaped object constructed to perform a specific function.

d., intrauterine contraceptive. Device made in a variety of shapes and from several different materials, including plastic or copper, and placed in the uterus to prevent conception. ABBR: I.U.C.D. or I.U.D.

devil's grip. Epidemic pleurodynia.

deviometer (dē"vē-ŏm'ĕ-tĕr) [L. *de,* from, + *via,* way, + Gr. *metron,* measure]. Device for estimating degree of strabismus.

devisceration (dē-vĭs"ĕr-ā'shŭn) [" + *viscus,* internal organ]. Removal of viscera. SYN: *evisceration.*

devitalization [" + *vita,* life]. 1. Destruction or loss of vitality. 2. Anesthetizing sensitive pulp of a tooth; known as killing the nerve.

devolution (dĕv"ō-loo'shŭn) [L. *devolvere,* to roll down]. Any destructive process in which organic substances are broken down into simple compounds; degradation. SYN: *catabolism.*

dew cure. Walking with bare feet in grass wet with dew. A form of hydrotherapy that is of questionable therapeutic value. SYN: *kneippism.*

dew point. Temperature at which dew begins to form as the moisture in the air condenses.

dexamethasone (dĕk"să-mĕth'ă-sōn). USP. A synthetic glucocorticoid drug. Trade names are Decadron and SK-Dexamethasone.

dexbrompheniramine maleate (dĕks"brŏm-fĕn-ĭr'ă-mēn). USP. An antihistamine.

dexchlorpheniramine maleate (dĕks"klor-fĕn-ĭr'ă-mēn). USP. An antihistamine. Trade name is Polaramine.

dexter (dĕks'tĕr) [L.]. On the right side. SEE: *sinistral.*

dextrad (dĕks'trăd) [L. *dexter,* right, + *ad,* toward]. 1. Toward the right side. 2. A right-handed person.

dextral (dĕks'trăl). Pert. to the right side.

dextrality (dĕks-trăl'ĭ-tē). Right-handedness. SEE: *sinistrality.*

dextran (dĕks'trăn) [L. *dexter,* right]. $C_6H_{10}O_5$. A monodextrin, it is a plasma expander and is used in emergency situations to treat shock by increasing blood volume.

dextrase (dĕks'trās). An enzyme that splits dextrose and converts it into lactic acid.

dextraural (dĕks-traw'răl) [L. *dexter,* right, + *auris,* ear]. Hearing better with the right ear.

dextriferron (dĕks"trĭ-fĕr'ŏn). Ferric hydroxide, used in treating iron-deficiency anemia.

dextrin (dĕks'trĭn) [L. *dexter,* right]. A yellowish-white powder that forms mucilaginous solutions in water and can be prepared by the action of heat or acid on starch. It is a carbohydrate of the formula $(C_6H_{10}O_5)_{11}$. In digestion, it is a soluble or gummy matter into which starch is converted by diastase; it is the result of the first chemical change in the digestion of starch.

dextrinuria (dĕks"trĭn-ū'rē-ă) [" + Gr. *ouron,* urine]. Dextrin in the urine.

dextro- [L. *dexter,* right]. Prefix indicating to the right.

dextroamphetamine sulfate (dĕks"trō-ăm-fĕt'ă-mēn sŭl'fāt). USP. A compound related to amphetamine sulfate (i.e., an isomer of amphetamine). Sometimes written d-amphetamine sulfate or dextro-amphetamine sulfate. Used as a central nervous system stimulant in treatment of mild depression. The drug is of benefit in treating abnormally hyperactive children, but concomitant psychotherapy and parent counseling are essential. Continued use of this drug in children depresses their growth; thus growth should be carefully monitored. The drug has no place in the long-term treatment of obesity. Prolonged use can cause psychological dependence. Trade name is Dexedrine. The "street" name is "speed."

dextrocardia (dĕks"trō-kăr'dē-ă) [" + Gr. *kardia,* heart]. Having the heart on the right side of the body.

dextrocardiogram [" + " + *gramma,* a writing]. A cardiogram representing action of the right ventricle.

dextrocular (dĕks-trŏk'ū-lăr) [" + *oculus,* eye]. Having a stronger right eye than left.

dextrocularity (dĕks"trŏk-ū-lăr'ĭ-tē). The condition of having the right eye stronger than the left.

dextroduction [" + *ducere,* to lead]. The movement of visual axis to the right.

dextrogastria [" + Gr. *gaster,* belly]. Having the stomach on the right side of the body.

dextroglucose (dĕks"trō-glū'kōs). Dextrose.

dextrogyrate (dĕks"trō-jī'rāt) [" + *gyrare,* to turn]. To turn to the right. Bending of light rays to the right.

dextrogyre (dĕks'trō-jīr). A substance turning to the right.

dextromanual [" + *manus,* hand]. Right-handed.

dextromethorphan (dĕk"strō-mĕth'or-făn). USP. A cough suppressant. A great number of cough medicines include this drug in their formula.

dextropedal (dĕks-trŏp'ĕ-dăl) [" + *pes, ped-,* foot]. Having greater dexterity in using the right leg than the left one.

dextrophobia [" + Gr. *phobos,* fear]. Abnormal aversion to objects on right side of body.

dextroposition (dĕks″trō-pō-zĭsh′ŭn). Displaced to the right.

dextropropoxyphene (dĕk″strō-prō-pŏk′sē-fĕn). Propoxyphene, q.v., an analgesic that can cause addiction.

dextrorotatory (dĕks″trō-rō′tă-tor-ē) [″ + *rotare,* to turn]. Turning rays of light to the right.

dextrose (dĕks′trōs). USP. $C_6H_{12}O_6$. A simple sugar of the monosaccharose group; a crystalline solid that can be made by the action of acids on starches. It is very soluble in water, is an important constituent of corn syrup and honey, and is an example of one kind of carbohydrate, q.v. The most important of the monosaccharide group. It is usually associated with levulose. Its presence in the urine in large amounts is most probably a result of diabetes. However, its presence may be associated with brain injuries, cirrhosis of the liver, normal pregnancies, and as a result of the administration of epinephrine or thyroxine. It is formed in the digestive tract by the action of enzymes on carbohydrates. It occurs naturally in plants and in the body fluids of animals. SYN: *glucose; grape sugar.*

RS: diabetes; glycosuria; hyperglycemia; hypoglycemia; monosaccharoses.

dextrose and sodium chloride injection. A sterile solution of dextrose, salt, and water for use intravenously. It contains no antimicrobial agents.

dextrosinistral (dĕks″trō-sĭn′ĭs-trăl) [L. *dexter,* right, + *sinister,* left]. From right to left.

dextrosuria (dĕks-trō-sū′rē-ă). Dextrose in the urine.

dextrothyroxine sodium (dĕks″trō-thī-rŏk′sĭn). USP. A thyroxine-like drug used in treating type II hyperlipoproteinemia. Trade name is Choloxin.

dextrotropic, dextrotropous (dĕks″trō-trŏp′ĭk, -trō′pŭs) [″ + Gr. *tropos,* a turning]. Turning to the right.

dextroversion [″ + *vertere,* to turn]. Turned or located toward the right.

dezymotize (dē-zī′mō-tīz) [L. *de,* from, + Gr. *zyme,* leaven]. To free of ferments or germs.

DFP. *diiopropyl fluorophosphate.* SEE: *isoflurophate.*

dg. *decigram.*

DHE-45. Trade name for dihydroergotamine mesylate.

dhobie itch (dō′bē) [Hindi, laundryboy]. Tropical name for form of tinea cruris more intense than that observed in temperate zones.

di- [Gr. *dis,* twice]. Prefix indicating twice, double, or two.

diabetes (dī″ă-bē′tēz) [Gr. *diabetes,* passing through]. A general term for diseases characterized by excessive urination. Usually refers to diabetes mellitus, q.v.

d., bronze. A disease of iron metabolism characterized by enlargement of the liver, pigmentation of the skin so that it takes a bronzed hue, diabetes mellitus, and frequently cardiac failure. It is a rare condition seen ten times as frequently in males as females. The majority of cases develop after the fourth decade. SYN: *hemochromatosis.*

d. insipidus. Polyuria and polydipsia caused by inadequate secretion of vasopressin, the antidiuretic hormone, by the neurohypophysis (main portion of the posterior lobe of the pituitary gland). More common in the young.

SYM: Urine output of 5 to 10 liters/24 hours is common. Sp. gr. usually 1.001 to 1.005 and free of sugar and albumin. Thirst, weakness, dry skin.

ETIOL: In almost half of all cases, the cause is unknown. Trauma to the head that causes damage to the pituitary or a tumor in that area causes the remainder of cases.

PROG: Essentially chronic.

TREATMENT: Eradication of causative factor if determined. When not due to specific injury of the pituitary, the disease is easily controlled by use of vasopressin replacement therapy. This may be given by injection or nasal spray.

d. mellitus. A disorder of carbohydrate metabolism, characterized by hyperglycemia and glycosuria and resulting from inadequate production or utilization of insulin. SEE: *coma, diabetic.*

ETIOL: Basic cause is still unknown but direct cause is failure of beta cells of the pancreas to secrete an adequate amount of insulin. In most instances diabetes mellitus is the result of a genetic disorder, but it may also result from a deficiency of beta cells caused by inflammation, malignant invasion of the pancreas, or surgery. In the absence of insulin, glycogenesis and glycolysis are adversely affected. It is currently thought that insulin acts primarily at the cell membrane, facilitating transport of glucose into cells.

SYM: Principal symptoms are elevated blood sugar (hyperglycemia), sugar in urine (glycosuria), excessive urine production (polyuria), excessive thirst (polydipsia), and increase in food intake (polyphagia). Urine sp. gr. 1.020 to 1.040; sugar excessive; urine contains diacetic acid, beta-hydroxybutyric acid, acetone when disease process is in advanced stage. More common in women and after the age of 40. Increased thirst; frequent urination; itching, frequently about the genitals. Fasting blood sugar raised above normal range of 90 to 120 mg./dl. of blood; boils and carbuncles; vascular changes may be present. Loss of weight; emaciation; weakness; and debility. When severe diabetes is allowed to progress without proper treatment, coma ensues with weakness and sweet (acetone) odor of breath; nausea, headache, vomiting, dyspnea, sense of intoxication, delirium, and deep coma resulting in death.

COMPLICATIONS: Diabetic acidosis due to excessive production of ketone bodies; low resistance to infections, esp. those involving extemities; and ulceration of lower extremities; increase in incidence of toxemia in pregnancy; cardiovascular and renal disorders; disturbances in electrolyte balance; eye disorders such as blindness.

PROG: Diabetes is a chronic, incurable disease but symptoms can be ameliorated and life prolonged by proper therapy. The isolation and eventual production of insulin in 1921 by Canadian physicians Banting and Best made it possible to allow persons with the disease to lead a normal life.

TREATMENT: Consists of diet, insulin, exercise, and hygienic measures. At first the patient should be placed on a well-balanced diet adequate in all basic essentials: carbohydrates, proteins, fats, vitamins, minerals, and fluids. In many patients this may be all that is required. It is important that obese persons with this disease be placed on a diet that will enable them to lose weight. Control of diabetes is much more difficult in an obese person. Blood sugar determinations may need to be made at frequent intervals. Long-term blood glucose regulation may be objectively assessed by determining the glycosylated hemoglobin (hemoglobin A_{1c}) in blood. SEE: *hemoglobin A_{1c}*.

NOTE: Blood sugar and glucose are considered to be the same.

When a patient is given an adequate diet and glucose still appears in the urine, use of insulin may be necessary. Its use is not required in every case and may be dangerous if not properly given. Drugs have been given by mouth for the control of mild cases of diabetes. These have been used with success mostly in middle-aged and older patients who still have some beta cell function.

Diet: A balanced diet of approximately 1000 to 1200 Calories may be prescribed. The diet is modified according to the weight of the patient. This should be increased promptly if levels of glucose in the blood are brought within normal limits. The age, weight, and type of work or physical activity in which the patient is engaged are important in planning a diet. Standardized diets have been worked out in which the necessary proportions of carbohydrates, proteins, and fats are outlined. The diets vary from 1200 to 3000 Calories. Frequent feedings (5–6/24 hours) rather than the standard three meals are preferred. The older the patient, as a rule, the smaller the proportion of fat in the diet.

NURSING IMPLICATIONS: Carefully assess the patient for symptoms indicative of insulin shock or diabetic acidosis. Do urine analysis for glucose and ketones daily or more often if indicated. Administer insulin or oral hypoglycemic agents as ordered; know the action, peak, onset and duration of action for each specific type of insulin you administer. Explain dietary restrictions to the patient, in addition to the need for a steady, consistent level of exercise on a daily basis.

Patients with diabetes must understand their disease, its possible complications, and treatment. Be certain that the patient understands the need for good hygiene, proper care of the feet, dosage and administration of insulin or oral agent, technique for urine analysis for glucose and ketones, and the signs of insulin shock and diabetic acidosis, and what to do if either of these conditions should develop.

Materials are available that diabetic patients can use to test their own urine and blood for glucose. Supervision is advisable while patients are learning to use those techniques.

d.m., brittle. Unpredictable variation in a patient's glucose tolerance. This type of diabetes is particularly prone to be present in individuals whose diabetes developed during childhood. SEE: *d.m., insulin-dependent, Type I.*

d.m., chemical. A stage of diabetes mellitus in which the various tests for altered glucose metabolism other than the fasting blood glucose level are abnormal but there are no obvious clinical signs or symptoms of diabetes.

d.m., endocrine. Diabetes mellitus associated with certain diseases of the pituitary, thyroid, or adrenal glands.

d.m., iatrogenic. Diabetes mellitus brought on by administration of drugs such as corticosteroids, certain diuretics, or birth control pills.

d.m., insulin-dependent, Type I. Diabetes mellitus that usually has its onset prior to the age of 25 years, where the essential abnormality is related to absolute insulin deficiency. This form usually is quite difficult to regulate. SYN: *juvenile-onset diabetes*. SEE: table.

d.m., latent. Diabetes mellitus that manifests itself during times of stress such as pregnancy, infectious disease, obesity, or trauma. Previous to the stress, no clinical or laboratory findings of diabetes are present. There is a very strong chance that such individuals will eventually develop overt diabetes mellitus.

d.m., non-insulin-dependent, Type II. A group of forms of diabetes mellitus that occur predominantly in adults. The insulin produced is sufficient to prevent ketoacidosis but insufficient to meet the total needs of the body. The non-obese patients with this form of diabetes can usually be controlled by diet and oral hypoglycemic agents. Occasionally insulin therapy is required. The obese patients with this form of diabetes can be controlled by reduction in overfeeding. SEE: table.

d., pancreatic. Diabetes associated with disease of the pancreas.

d., phlorizin. Glycosuria caused by administration of phlorizin.

d., renal. Renal glycosuria; condition characterized by a low renal threshold for sugar. Glucose tolerance is normal and diabetic symptoms are lacking.

d., true. D. mellitus.

diabetic (dī-ă-bĕt′ĭk). Pert. to diabetes.

diabetic acidosis. SEE: *acidosis, diabetic.*

diabetic center. Area in the floor of the fourth ventricle of the brain.

diabetic coma. Loss of consciousness due to severe diabetes mellitus that has not been treated or to treatment that has not been adequately regulated. SEE: *coma, diabetic.*

diabetic ear. Otitis media diabetica.

diabetic neuritis. Multiple neuritis of diabetes.

diabetic tabes. Diabetes with neuritic pains in leg and loss of patellar tendon reflex.

diabetogenic (dī″ă-bĕt″ō-jĕn′ĭk) [″ + *gennan,* to produce]. Causing diabetes.

diabetogenous (dī″ă-bē-tŏj′ĕn-ŭs). Caused by diabetes.

Diabinese. Trade name for chlorpropamide.

diabrosis (dī″ă-brō′sĭs) [Gr., eating through]. A corrosion causing perforation of a vessel or organ.

diabrotic (dī-ă-brŏt′ĭk). 1. Corrosive. 2. An escharotic or corrosive.

diacele (dī′ă-sēl) [Gr. *dia,* between, + *koilia,* a hollow]. The third ventricle of the brain.

diacetate (dī-ăs′ĕ-tāt). A salt of diacetic acid.

diacetemia (dī-ăs″ĕ-tē′mē-ă). Presence of diacetic acid in the blood.

diacetic acid (dī″ă-sĕt′ĭk). Acetoacetic acid, found in acidosis and in the urine of the diabetic. It is similar to acetone and is found in serious diabetes and in any condition that produces starvation and excessive fat metabolism, such as persistent vomiting.

diacetonuria, diaceturia (dī-ăs″ĕ-tō-nū′rē-ă, dī-ăs″ĕ-tū′rē-ă). Diacetic acid in urine.

diacetylmorphine (dī″ă-sē″tĭl-mor′fēn). Heroin.

diacid (dī-ăs′ĭd) [Gr. *dis,* twice, + L. *acidus,* soured]. Having two atoms of hydrogen replaceable with a base.

diaclasia (dī-ă-klā′zē-ă) [Gr. *dia,* through, + *klan,* to break]. A fracture, esp. breaking a bone before surgery.

Comparison of Type I Insulin-Dependent Diabetes Mellitus and Type II Non-Insulin-Dependent Diabetes Mellitus

	Type I	Type II
Age at onset	usually under 25	usually over 40
Type of onset	abrupt	gradual
HLA association	positive	negative
Insulin in blood	little to none	some usually present
Islet cell antibodies	present at onset	absent
Symptoms	polyuria, polydipsia, polyphagia, weight loss, ketoacidosis	polyuria, polydipsia, pruritus, peripheral neuropathy
Control	insulin and diet	diet (sometimes only diet control), hypoglycemic agents, sometimes insulin
Vascular and neural changes	eventually develop	will usually develop
Stability of condition	fluctuates, difficult to control	fairly stable, usually easy to control

diaclast (dī'ă-klăst) [" + *klan,* to break]. Device for perforating the fetal skull.

diacrinous (dī-ăk'rĭn-ŭs) [Gr. *diakrinein,* to separate]. Pert. to cells that secrete outwardly rather than into circulation. SYN: *exocrine.*

diacrisis (dī-ăk'rĭ-sĭs) [Gr. *diakrisis,* separation]. 1. A change in the character of a secretion. 2. Any disease having an altered secretion. 3. A critical discharge or excretion in a disease.

diacritic, diacritical [Gr. *dia,* through, + *krinein,* to judge]. Diagnostic; said of symptoms.

diaderm [Gr. *dia,* through, + *derma,* skin]. Blastoderm composed of ectoderm and entoderm, and containing between them the segmentation cavity.

diadochokinesia (dī-ăd"ō-kō-kĭn-ē'zē-ă) [Gr. *diadokos,* succeeding, + *kinesis,* motion]. Ability to make antagonistic movements, as pronation and supination of the hands in quick succession. SEE: *disdiadochokinesia.*

Diafen. Trade name for diphenylpyraline hydrochloride.

diagnose (dī'ăg-nōs) [Gr. *diagignoskein,* to discern]. To determine the cause and nature of a pathological condition; to recognize a disease.

diagnosis (dī"ăg-nō'sĭs). (pl. *diagnoses*) 1. The term denoting name of the disease or syndrome a person has or is believed to have. 2. The use of scientific and skillful methods to establish the cause and nature of a person's illness. This is done by evaluating the history of the disease process; the signs and symptoms present; laboratory data; special tests such as x-ray pictures and electrocardiograms. The value of establishing a diagnosis is to provide a logical basis for treatment and prognosis.

d., antenatal. Diagnostic procedures done to determine the health status of the fetus. Methods used include amniocentesis and study of the material obtained by microscopic (sex chromatin determination), cell culture, and biochemical methods and by amnioscopy, amniography, and ultrasound.

d. by exclusion. Establishing a diagnosis by eliminating other possibilities.

d., clinical. Diagnosis determined by symptoms alone. They may be objective (visible symptoms); subjective (those of internal or mental origin); and cardinal (those pert. to respiration, pulse, and temperature). Most diseases have a symptom or symptoms in common with some other disease.

d., cytological. Diagnosis based on cells present in body tissues or exudates.

d., differential. Comparison of symptoms of two similar diseases to determine from which the patient is suffering.

d., nursing. SEE: *nursing diagnosis.*

d., pathological. Diagnosis based on structural lesions present.

d., physical. Diagnosis by external examination only.

d., serological. Diagnosis made by using a serological test such as that for syphilis or typhoid.

diagnosis, words pert. to: abdomen; auscultation; blood; breathing; chest; colic; coma; constipation; convulsion; cough; examination; eye; face; fatigue; feces; fever; gait; gums; headache; infection; inflammation; inspection; nail; nausea; pain; pallor; palpation; palpitation; percussion; perspiration; position; pulse; pus; reflexes; respiration; skin; sputum; syncope; teeth; temperature; tongue; unconsciousness; urine; vertigo; vomiting.

diagnostic. Pert to a diagnosis.

diagnostician (dī"ăg-nŏs-tĭsh'ŭn) [Gr. *diagignoskein,* to discern]. One skilled in diagnosis.

diakinesis (dī"ă-kĭ-nē'sĭs) [Gr. *dia,* through, + *kinesis,* motion]. In cell division, the final stage in prophase of meiosis. At this time the homologous chromosomes shorten and thicken.

dial (dī'ăl) [L. *dialis,* daily, fr. *dies,* day]. A graduated circular face similar to a clockface upon which some measurement is indicated by a pointer that moves as the entity (pressure, temperature, or heat) being measured changes.

d., astigmatic. Black lines of uniform width drawn across a circular dial as if they were connecting opposing numbers on the face of a clock. Used in testing for astigmatism.

dialy- [Gr. *dia,* through, + *lysis,* dissolution]. Prefix meaning to separate.

dialysance (dī"ă-lī'săns). In kidney dialysis, the minute rate of net exchange of a substance between blood and dialysis fluid per unit blood-bath concentration gradient.

dialysate (dī-ăl'ĭ-săt). A liquid that has been dialyzed. In renal failure, dialysate refers to the fluid used to remove or deliver compounds or electrolytes that the failing kidney cannot excrete or retain in the proper concentrations.

dialysis (dī-ăl'ĭ-sĭs) [Gr. *dia,* through, + *lysis,* dissolution]. 1. The passage of a solute through a membrane. 2. Process of diffusing blood across a semipermeable membrane to remove toxic materials and to maintain fluid, electrolyte, and acid-base balance in cases of impaired kidney function or absence of the kidneys. SEE: *hemodialysis.*

d., continuous ambulatory peritoneal. ABBR: CAPD. A type of maintenance dialysis that utilizes an implanted peritoneal catheter. Fluid is drained into and from the peritoneal cavity by gravity. CAPD is an alternative to chronic hemodialysis and is considerably less expensive.

d., peritoneal. Dialysis in which the lining of the peritoneal cavity is used as the dialysis membrane. Dialysing fluid introduced into the peritoneal cavity is allowed to remain there for an hour or two and is then removed. The procedure may be repeated as often as indicated. Care must be taken to prevent the development of peritonitis. This is done by using strict sterile technique.

d., renal. Dialysis of blood in order to remove liquid and chemicals that the kidneys would normally remove if they were present and functioning.

dialysis acidosis. Metabolic acidosis due to prolonged hemodialysis wherein the pH of the dialysis bath has been inadvertently reduced by the action of contaminating bacteria.

dialytic. Belonging to or resembling the process of dialysis.

dialyzable (dī-ă-līz'ă-b'l). Capable of dialysis.

dialyze (dī'ă-līz). To make a dialysis or to have made one.

dialyzer (dī'ă-līz"ĕr) [Gr. *dia,* through, + *lysis,* dissolution]. Apparatus used in performing dialysis.

diamagnetic [" + *magnes,* magnet]. 1. Repelled by a magnet. 2. Assuming a position at right angles to the lines of force of a magnetic field.

diameter (dī-ăm'ĕ-tĕr) [" + *metron,* a measure]. The distance from any point on the periphery of a surface, body, or space to the opposite point.

d., anteroposterior, of pelvic cavity. The distance between the middle of the symphysis pubis and the upper border of the 3rd sacral vertebra. It is usually 13.5 cm.

d., anteroposterior, of pelvic inlet. The distance from the posterior surface of the symphysis pubis to the promontory of the sacrum (about 11 cm. in the adult female). SYN: *true conjugate d. of pelvic inlet.*

d., anteroposterior, of pelvic outlet. Distance between the tip of the coccyx and the lower edge of the symphysis pubis.

d., biparietal. Transverse distance between parietal eminences on each side (about 9.25 cm.).

d., bitemporal. Distance between the temporal bones (about 8 cm.).

d., bitrochanteric. Distance between the highest points of the greater trochanters.

d., bizygomatic. Greatest transverse distance between most prominent points of the zygomatic arches.

d., cervicobregmatic. Distance between anterior fontanel and junction of the neck with floor of the mouth.

d., diagonal conjugate, of pelvis. The distance from the upper part of the symphysis pubis to the most distant part of the brim of the pelvis.

d., external conjugate. Anteroposterior diameter of the pelvic inlet measured externally; distance from the skin over the upper part of symphysis pubis to the skin over a point corresponding to the sacral promontory.

d., frontomental. Distance from top of the forehead to point of the chin.

d., interspinous. Distance between the two anterior superior spines of the ilia.

d., mentobregmatic. Distance from chin to middle of anterior fontanel.

d., obstetric, of pelvic inlet. Shortest distance between sacrum and symphysis. This diameter is shorter than the true conjugate.

d., occipitofrontal. The distance from the posterior fontanel to the root of the nose.

d., occipitomental. Greatest distance between the most prominent portion of the occiput and point of chin (about 13.5 cm.).

d. of fetal skull. Important diameters at full term are suboccipitobregmatic, 3.75 in. (9.5 cm.); cervicobregmatic, 3.75 in. (9.5 cm.); frontomental, 3.2 in. (8.1 cm.); occipitomental, 5 in. (12.7 cm.); supraoccipitomental, 5.5 in. (14 cm.); occipitofrontal, 4.5 in. (11.4 cm.); suboccipitofrontal, 4 in. (10.2 cm.); biparietal, 3.75 in. (9.5 cm.); bitemporal, 3.2 in. (8.1 cm.)

d. of pelvis. *Anteroposterior:* the distance between the sacrovertebral angle and the symphysis pubis. *Bi-ischial:* between the ischial spines. *Conjugata diagonalis:* between the sacrovertebral angle and the symphysis pubis. *Conjugata vera:* the true conjugate between the sacrovertebral angle and the middle of the posterior aspect of the symphysis pubis (about 1.5 cm. less than the diagonal conjugate). *Intercristus:* between the crests of the ilium. *Interspinous:* between the spines of the ilium. *Intertrochanteric:* between the greater trochanters when the hips are extended and the legs are held together. *Internal conjugate:* between the promontory of the sacrum and the upper edge of the symphysis pubis. *Pelvic:* any diameter of the pelvis found by measuring a straight line between any two points. SEE: *pelvis.*

diamid(e) (dī-ăm'ĭd, -īd) [L. *di,* two, + *amide*]. A compound that contains two amine groups. Sometimes used incorrectly to indicate a diamine or hydrazine.

diamidine (dī-ăm'ĭ-dēn). Any chemical compound that contains two amidine, $C(NH)NH_2$, groups.

diamine (dī-ăm'ĭn, -ēn). A chemical compound with two amino, $—NH_2$, groups.

diaminuria (dī-ăm"ĭ-nū'rē-ă). Presence of diamines in the urine.

Diamox. Trade name for acetazolamide, a diuretic.

Dianabol. Trade name for methandrostenolone.

dianoetic (dī″ă-nō-ĕt′ĭk) [Gr. *dia,* through, + *nous,* mind]. Pert. to intellectual function, particularly logic and orderly analysis.

diapason (dī″ă-pā′sŭn) [″ + *pason,* all]. A diagnostic tuning fork used to determine the degree of deafness.

diapause (dī′ă-pawz) [″ + *pausis,* pause]. The state of metabolic inactivity that some plants, seeds, eggs, and insect forms assume in order to survive adverse conditions such as winter.

diapedesis (dī″ă-pĕd-ē′sĭs) [″ + *pedan,* to leap]. Passage of blood cells, esp. leukocytes, by ameboid movements through the unruptured wall of a capillary vessel.

diaphane (dī′ă-fān) [Gr. *dia,* through, + *phainein,* to appear]. A very small electric light utilized in transillumination.

diaphanometer (dī″ă-făn-ŏm′ĕ-tĕr) [″ + ″ + *metron,* measure]. A device for estimating the amount of solids in a fluid by its transparency.

diaphanometry (dī″ă-făn-ŏm′ĕt-rē). Determination of translucency of a fluid, as the urine.

diaphanoscope (dī-ă-făn′ō-skōp) [″ + *phainein,* to appear, + *skopein,* to examine]. Device for transillumination of body cavities.

diaphanoscopy (dī″ă-făn-ŏs′kō-pē). Examination by the diaphanoscope; transillumination.

diaphemetric (dī″ă-fē-mĕt′rĭk) [″ + *haphe,* touch, + *metron,* measure]. Pert. to degree of tactile sensibility.

diaphorase (dī-ăf′ō-rās). The flavoprotein catalyst of the reoxidation of nicotinamide-adenine dinucleotide (NAD) or nicotinamide-adenine dinucleotide phosphate (NADP) by mitochondrial electron transport chain.

diaphoresis (dī″ă-fō-rē′sĭs) [″ + *pherein,* to carry]. Profuse sweating.

diaphoretic (dī″ă-fō-rĕt′ĭk) [″ + *pherein,* to carry]. 1. A sudorific or an agent that increases perspiration. The term sudorific is usually confined to those active agents that cause drops of perspiration to collect on the skin, such as camphor, opium, or pilocarpine. Heat may also be included as such an agent. 2. A patient who is sweating profusely.

diaphragm (dī′ă-frăm) [Gr. *diaphragma,* a partition]. 1. Thin membrane such as one used for dialysis. 2. In microscopy, an apparatus located beneath the opening in the stage by means of which the amount of light passing through the object can be regulated. 3. A rubber or plastic cup that fits over the cervix uteri and is used for contraceptive purposes. SEE: illus.; *contraceptive.* 4. A musculomembranous wall separating the abdomen from the thoracic cavity with its convexity upward. It contracts with each inspiration, flattening out downward, permitting the descent of the bases of the lungs. It relaxes with each expiration, elevating it and restoring its inverted basin shape. The deeper the inspiration, the lower the descent of the diaphragm; the greater the expiration, the higher it rises.

CONTRACEPTIVE DIAPHRAGM

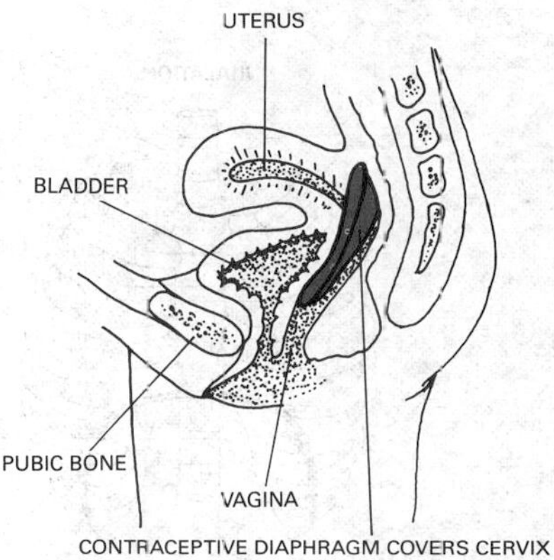

Its origin is at a level with the 6th ribs or intercostal spaces anteriorly and the 11th or 12th ribs posteriorly. The right half rises higher than the left. The lower surface is in relation to the suprarenal bodies of the kidney, liver, spleen, and cardiac end of the stomach. It aids in defecation and parturition by its ability to cause an increase in intra-abdominal pressure while the person attempts to exhale with the glottis closed. It becomes spasmodic in hiccoughs and sneezing. SEE: illus.; *Boerhaave's syndrome; phrenic; "phren-" words; Valsalva's maneuver.*

d., Bucky. A grid suspended immediately beneath the x-ray table and above the film tray, so constructed that the effects of backscatter and secondary radiation are eliminated when x-ray photographs of dense structures are taken.

d., hernia of. Congenital or traumatic protrusion of abdominal contents through the diaphragm.

d., pelvic. The musculofascial layer forming the lower boundary of the abdominopelvic cavity. It is funnel-shaped and is

MOVEMENT OF RIB CAGE AND DIAPHRAGM DURING RESPIRATION

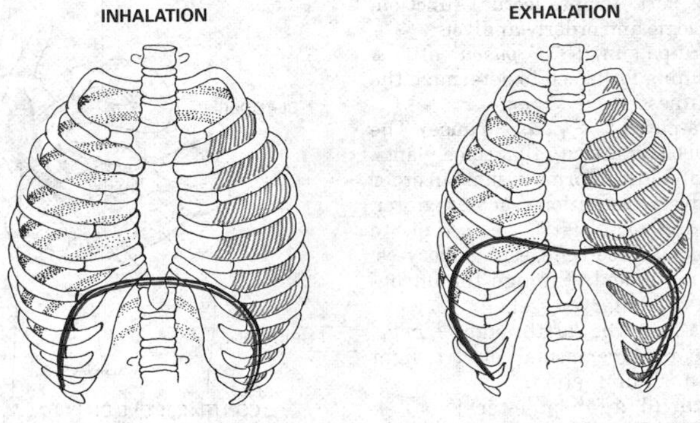

THE DIAPHRAGM HAS DESCENDED, AND THE RIB CAGE HAS MOVED UP AND OUT TO ALLOW THE LUNGS TO EXPAND

THE DIAPHRAGM HAS ASCENDED, AND THE RIB CAGE HAS MOVED DOWN AND IN AS THE LUNGS CONTRACT

pierced in the midline by the urethra, vagina, and rectum. Consists of a muscular layer made up of the paired levator ani and coccygeus muscles. The fascial layer consists of two portions, the parietal and visceral layers, the former being made up of the peritoneum continuous with the connective tissue sheaths of the psoas and iliac muscles; the visceral layer is split from the parietal layer at the white line passing downward and inward to form the upper sheath of the levator ani muscles; the anterior part of this layer unites the bladder with the posterior wall of the pubes. The middle portion splits into three parts: the vesical layer, investing bladder and urethra; the rectovaginal layer, forming the rectovaginal septum; the rectal layer, investing the rectum. The posterior part is the base of the broad ligament, where it sheaths the uterine arteries and supports the cervix.

d., urogenital. Urogenital trigone, or triangular ligament. A musculofascial sheath that lies between the ischiopubic rami. It lies superficial to the pelvic diaphragm and in the male surrounds the membranous urethra; in the female, it surrounds the vagina.

diaphragmalgia (dī″ă-frăg-măl′jē-ă) [Gr. *diaphragma*, a partition, + *algos*, pain]. Pain in the diaphragm.

diaphragmatic. Pert. to the diaphragm.

diaphragmatocele (dī″ă-frăg-măt′ō-sēl) [″ + *kele*, hernia]. Hernia of the diaphragm.

diaphragmitis (dī″ă-frăg-mī′tĭs) [″ + *itis*, inflammation]. Inflammation of the diaphragm.

diaphragmodynia [″ + *odyne*, pain]. Pain in the diaphragm.

diaphyseal (dī″ă-fĭz′ē-ăl). Part of or affecting the shaft of a long bone.

diaphysectomy [Gr. *diaphysis*, a growing through, + *ektome*, excision]. Removal of part of the shaft of a long bone.

diaphysis (dī-ăf′ĭ-sĭs). [NA] The shaft or middle part of a long cylindrical bone. SEE: *apophysis; epiphysis.*

diaphysitis (dī″ă-fĭ-zī′tĭs) [Gr. *diaphysis*, a growing through, + *itis*, inflammation]. Inflammation of shaft of a long bone.

Diapid. Trade name for lypressin.

diaplexus [Gr. *dia*, through, + L. *plexus*, braid]. Choroid plexus of the third ventricle.

diapophysis (dī-ă-pŏf′ĭ-sĭs) [″ + *apophysis*, outgrowth]. An upper articular surface of transverse process of a vertebra.

diarrhea (dī-ă-rē′ă) [″ + *rhein*, to flow]. Frequent passage of unformed watery bowel movements. It is a frequent symptom of gastrointestinal disturbances.

ETIOL: Diet; inflammation or irritation of the mucosa of the intestines; gastrointestinal infections; certain drugs; psychogenic factors.

NURSING IMPLICATIONS: Assess patient for symptoms of dehydration, such as poor skin turgor, dry mucous membranes, decreased tear formation, warm, dry skin, elevated temperature, and decreased urine output. (In addition, note presence of depressed fontanel in infants.) Monitor intake and output, and administer oral and I.V. fluids as ordered. Encourage proper handwashing and body hygiene. Apply powder, cornstarch, or ointment to the perineum to prevent skin excoriation. Administer antidiarrheal medications as prescribed.

d., acute. Diarrhea characterized by sudden onset.

TREATMENT: Strong tea; whey; rice milk; arrowroot; corn flour; blackberry brandy; adsorbents, as aluminum hydroxide. Gradual return to ordinary diet. These are more or less home remedies that act as demulcents or astringents for the irritated intestinal mucosa. They are often effective but severe cases of diarrhea may require additional therapy specifically directed to the etiology of the disease. Also in severe cases fluid- and electrolyte-replacement therapy may be needed. Agents that reduce intestinal activity, such as antispasmodics and paregoric, may provide distinct symptomatic relief.

d., dysenteric. Diarrhea due to dysentery, q.v., characterized by mucous or bloody stools.

d., emotional. Diarrhea caused by emotional stress.

d., epidemic, in newborn. Contagious diarrhea in newborn caused by pathogenic strains of Escherichia coli, occurring in epidemics in hospitals.

d., fatty. Diarrhea with stools containing undigested fat particles.

d., infantile. Diarrhea in children under two years. Dysentery, q.v.

SYM: Dry skin, high temperature, thirst, pains, increase in frequency and amount of stools with change of color and consistency.

d., lienteric. Watery stools with undigested food particles.

d., membranous. Diarrhea with passage of pieces of intestinal mucosa.

d., mucous. Diarrhea with mucus in stools.

d., purulent. Presence of pus in stools, a result of intestinal ulceration.

d., simple. Variety of diarrhea in which stools contain only normal excreta.

d., summer. Diarrhea occurring in children during summer heat.

d., travelers'. Diarrhea experienced by travelers. The cause of some cases is enteropathogenic strains of E. coli. There is no effective method of prophylaxis except to attempt to avoid eating uncooked food or drinking beverages that could be contaminated. In general, the disease is self-limiting and usually lasts 3 to 4 days. Symptomatic therapy for tenesmus, fluid loss, vomiting, and malaise is indicated. If diarrhea persists without signs of severe systemic disease, the use of paregoric or diphenoxylate will be of benefit. Diphenoxylate with atropine (trade name: Lomotil) is contraindicated in children under 2 yrs. of age.

diarthric (dī-ăr'thrĭk) [Gr. *dis,* two, + *arthron,* joint]. Pert. to two or more joints.

diarthrosis [Gr. *diarthrosis,* a movable articulation]. An articulation in which opposing bones move freely; a hinge joint.

diarticular [Gr. *dis,* two, + L. *articulus,* joint]. Pert. to two joints. Specifically, pert. to the temporomandibular joints, where the mandible articulates in two places with the skull.

diaschisis (dī-ăs'kĭ-sĭs) [Gr. *dia,* apart, + *schizein,* to split]. Condition where disturbance or injury to one part of central nervous system causes alteration in function of some distant part.

diascope (dī'ă-skōp) [" + *skopein,* to examine]. A glass plate held against the skin for examining superficial lesions.

Diasone Sodium Enterab. Trade name for sulfoxone sodium.

diastalsis (dī-ă-stăl'sĭs) [" + *stalsis,* contraction]. A wave of inhibition before a downward contraction in the intestine. Similar to peristalsis.

diastaltic. 1. Pert. to diastalsis. 2. Denoting reflex action.

diastase (dī'ăs-tās) [Gr. *diastasis,* a separation]. A specific enzyme or ferment in plant cells, such as in sprouting grains and malt and in the digestive juice that converts starch into sugar.

diastasis (dī-ăs'tă-sĭs) [Gr.]. 1. In surgery, injury to a bone involving separation of an epiphysis. 2. In cardiac physiology, the last part of diastole. It follows the period of most rapid diastolic filling of the ventricles, consists of a period of retarded inflow of blood from atria into ventricles, lasts (in man under average conditions) about 0.2 seconds, and is immediately followed by atrial systole.

d. recti. A lateral separation of the two halves of the musculus rectus dominis. A benign condition when it occurs in pregnant women.

diastema (dī"ă-stē'mă) [Gr. *diastema,* an interval or space]. (pl. *diastemata*) 1. A fissure. 2. A space between two adjacent teeth.

diastematocrania (dī"ă-stĕm"ă-tō-krā'nē-ă) [" + *kranion,* cranium]. Congenital sagittal fissure of the skull.

diastematomyelia (dī"ă-stĕm"ă-tō-mī-ē'lē-ă) [" + *myelos,* marrow]. Congenital fissure of the spinal cord, frequently associated with spina bifida, q.v.

diastematopyelia (dī″ă-stĕm″ă-tō-pī-ē′lē-ă) [″ + *pyelos,* pelvis]. Congenital median slit of the pelvis.
diaster [Gr. *dis,* two, + *aster,* star]. Double star figure formed during mitosis, q.v. SYN: *amphiaster.*
diastole (dī-ăs′tō-lē) [Gr. *diastellein,* to expand]. The normal period in the heart cycle during which the muscle fibers lengthen, the heart dilates, and the cavities fill with blood; diastole of the atria occurs before that of the ventricles. Roughly, the period of relaxation alternating with systole or contraction. SEE: *heart; murmur; pulse; systole.*
diastolic (dī-ăs-tŏl′ĭk). Pert. to diastole.
diastolic pressure. The point of least pressure in the arterial vascular system. The failure of the diastolic pressure to drop in proportion to the systolic pressure is a danger sign.
diataxia [Gr. *dis,* two, + *ataxia,* lack of order]. Bilateral ataxia.
diatela, diatele (dī-ă-tē′lă, -tēl′) [Gr. *dia,* between, + L. *tela,* web]. Membranous roof of third ventricle.
diaterma [″ + *terma,* end]. Portion of the floor of the third ventricle.
diathermal (dī″ă-thĕr′măl) [″ + *therme,* heat]. Ability to absorb heat rays.
diathermanous. Diathermal.
diathermia [Gr. *dia,* through, + *therme,* heat]. Diathermy.
diathermic. Of the nature of diathermy or of its results.
diathermy (dī′ă-thĕr″mē) [Gr. *dia,* through, + *therme,* heat]. The therapeutic use of a high-frequency current to generate heat within some part of the body. The frequency is greater than the maximum frequency for neuromuscular response and ranges from several hundred thousand to millions of cycles per second. Used to increase blood flow to specific areas. Should not be used in acute stage of recovery from trauma.
d., medical. The generation of heat within the body by the application of high-frequency oscillatory current for warming, but not damaging, tissues.
d., short-wave. Treatment by use of wavelengths of 3 to 30 meters.
d., surgical. Diathermy of high frequency for electrocoagulation or cauterization.
diathesis (dī-ăth′ĕ-sĭs) [Gr. *diatithenai,* to dispose]. Constitutional predisposition to a certain disease, condition, or group of diseases. Can be allergic, hemorrhagic, or rheumatic diatheses.
diathetic. Pert. to diathesis.
diatom (dī′ă-tŏm) [Gr. *diatemnein,* to cut through]. One of a group of unicellular microscopic algae. They possess a siliceous, or calcium-containing, cell wall.
diatomic. 1. Containing two atoms; said of molecules. 2. Bivalent.
diatrizoate meglumine (dī″ă-trī-zō′āt). USP. A radiopaque substance used intra-arterially to visualize the arterial vesicle and veins of the heart and brain; and great vessels such as the aorta. Also used to visualize the kidneys and bladder. Trade names are Cardiografin, Hypaque Meglumine, and Reno-M.
diatrizoate sodium. USP. A radiopaque substance used to visualize various body organs such as the kidney, bladder, uterus, and tubes.
diaxon, diaxone [Gr. *dis,* two, + *axon,* axis]. A neuron having two axons.
diazepam (dī-ăz′ĕ-păm). USP. An anti-anxiety and sedative drug that is used extensively in the United States. It is effective in treating status epilepticus and acute cocaine poisoning. Trade name is Valium.
diazo-. Prefix used in chemistry to note that a compound contains the $-N=N-$ group.
diazo reaction. A deep red color in urine produced by the action of p-diazobenzenesulfonic acid and ammonia on aromatic substances found in the urine in certain conditions.
diazotize (dī-ăz′ō-tīz). In chemistry, conversion of NH_2 groups into diazo, $-N=N-$, groups.
diazoxide (dī-ăz-ŏk′sīd). USP. Drug used in treating acute hypertension emergencies to produce lowering of the blood pressure; and in treating hypoglycemia due to hyperinsulinism. Trade names are Hyperstat (I.V. only) and Proglycem (oral).
dibasic (dī-bā′sĭk) [″ + *basis,* base]. Containing in each molecule two atoms of hydrogen replaceable by a base; said of acid.
Dibenzyline. Trade name for phenoxybenzamine hydrochloride.
diblastula (dī-blăs′tū-lă) [″ + *blastos,* sprout]. A blastula containing the ectoderm and entoderm.
Dibothriocephalus (dī-bŏth″rē-ō-sĕf′ăl-ŭs). Former name for the genus Diphyllobothrium.
dibucaine hydrochloride. USP. A local anesthetic similar to cocaine in action when applied topically and similar to procaine and cocaine when injected. Trade name is Nupercaine Hydrochloride.
DIC. *disseminated intravascular coagulation.*
dicalcic, dicalcium (dī-kăl′sĭk) [″ + L. *calx,* lime]. Containing two atoms of calcium in a molecule.
dicalcium phosphate (dī-kăl′sē-ŭm fŏs′făt). Dibasic calcium phosphate. Used as a source of calcium to supplement the diet.
dicentric (dī-sĕn′trĭk). Having two centers or two centromeres.

dicephalus (dī-sĕf'ă-lŭs) [" + *kephale,* head]. Congenitally deformed fetus with two heads.

dichloramine-T (dī-klor'ă-mēn). White powder containing about 28% chlorine.

ACTION AND USES: Germicide and disinfectant.

2,4-dichlorophenoxyacetic acid. A toxic substance previously used as a weed killer. ABBR: 2,4-D. SEE: *Poisons and Poisoning* in *Appendix.*

dichlorphenamide (dī"klor-fĕn'ă-mīd). USP. A carbonic anhydrase inhibitor used in treating glaucoma. Trade names are Daranide and Oratrol.

dichorionic (dī"kō-rē-ŏn'ĭk). Having two chorions. This may occur in two-egg (dizygotic) twins.

dichotomy, dichotomization (dī-kŏt'ō-mē, dī-kŏt"ō-mī-zā'shŭn) [Gr. *dicha,* twofold, + *tome,* incision]. 1. Bifurcation of a vein. 2. Cutting or dividing into two parts.

dichroic (dī-krō'ĭk). Pert. to dichroism.

dichroism (dī'krō-ĭzm) [Gr. *dis,* two, + *chroa,* color]. Property of a substance appearing to be one color by direct light and another by transmitted light.

dichromate (dī-krō'māt). A chemical that contains the Cr_2O_7 group.

dichromatic. Being able to see only two colors.

dichromatism (dī-krō'mă-tĭzm). Ability to distinguish only two primary colors.

dichromatopsia (dī"krō-mă-tŏp'sē-ă) [" + *chroma,* color, + *opsis,* sight]. Ability to distinguish only two primary colors.

dichromic. 1. Containing two atoms of chromium. 2. Seeing only two colors.

dichromophil [" + *chroma,* color, + *philein,* to love]. Double staining with both acid and basic dyes.

dichromophilism (dī"krō-mŏf'ĭl-ĭzm) [" + " + " + *-ismos,* condition of]. Having the capacity for double staining.

Dick method. [George F. Dick, 1881–1967, and Gladys H. Dick, 1881–1963, U.S. physicians] A toxin-antitoxin injection for the prevention of scarlet fever.

Dick test. A test for susceptibility or immunity to scarlet fever. The erythrogenic toxin from Streptococci is injected intracutaneously. In a negative reaction, there may occur some slight inflammatory changes due to irritation by proteins in fluid administered. In a manner somewhat similar to the Schick testing for diphtheria, a person's susceptibility to scarlet fever may be ascertained by the injection of a standardized toxin of the β-hemolytic streptococcus. A positive (susceptible) reaction in the form of erythema appears in about 12 to 24 hours. Patients convalescing from scarlet fever invariably give a negative reaction. SEE: *Schick test.*

dicloxacillin sodium (dī-klŏks"ă-sĭl'ĭn). USP. A semisynthetic penicillin useful in treating penicillinase-resistant staphylococci. Trade names are Dycill and Dynapen.

Dicodid. Trade name for hydrocodone bitartrate.

dicoelus (dī-sē'lŭs) [" + *koilos,* hollow]. 1. Concave or hollowed out on two sides. 2. Containing two cavities.

dicophane (dī'kō-fān). A powerful insecticide now rarely used because of its toxicity. SYN: *chlorophenothane; DDT.*

dicoria (dī-kō'rē-ă) [" + *kore,* pupil]. Double pupil in each eye.

dicoumarin (dī-koo'mă-rĭn). Dicumarol, q.v.

dicrotic (dī-krŏt'ĭk) [Gr. *dikrotos,* beating double]. Having one heartbeat for two arterial pulsations; rel. to a double pulse.

dicrotic notch. In a pulse tracing, a notch on the descending limb.

dicrotic wave. A positive wave following the dicrotic notch.

dicrotism (dī'krŏt-ĭzm) [" + *-ismos,* condition of]. The state of being dicrotic.

dictyoma (dĭk"tē-ō'mă) [Gr. *diktyon,* net, + *oma,* tumor]. A tumor of the ciliary epithelium. Also spelled diktyoma.

dictyosome (dĭk'tē-ō-sōm) [" + *soma,* body]. Cytoplasmic body similar to the Golgi apparatus. It is thought to be a dispersed element of the Golgi apparatus.

Dicumarol (dī-koo'mă-rŏl). Trade name for bishydroxycoumarin, USP, an anticoagulant that decreases activity of prothrombin in the blood plasma and hence increases prothrombin time. Used in prophylaxis and treatment of intravascular clotting, in postoperative thrombophlebitis, pulmonary embolism, acute peripheral embolism and thrombosis, and recurrent idiopathic thrombophlebitis. Used also in management of acute coronary thrombosis. Frequently an adjunct to heparin, q.v. The dose is determined by periodically testing the prothrombin time. If heparin is being given, it is important that three to four hours elapse between the last dose of heparin and the time the blood is drawn for the prothrombin test.

CONTRA: Subacute bacterial endocarditis, recent brain, spinal, or eye surgery, purpura and blood dyscrasias, in vitamin K deficiency, and in absence of prothrombin determination. The drug is excreted in the mother's milk. Thus, breast-fed infants whose mothers are receiving Dicumarol should be carefully observed for bleeding tendency. In cases of hemorrhage due to this drug, stop the drug immediately and give vitamin K intravenously; whole fresh blood may be needed. SEE: *vitamin K.*

dicyclic (dī-sī'klĭk). 1. Having or concerning two cycles. 2. In chemistry, containing two cyclic ring structures.

dicyclomine hydrochloride (dī-sī′klō-mēn). USP. An anticholinergic drug used as an antispasmodic. Trade name is Bentyl.

didactic (dī-dăk′tĭk) [Gr. *didaktikos*]. Concerning instruction by lectures and by use of texts as opposed to clinical or bedside teaching of medicine.

didactylism (dī-dăk′tĭ-lĭzm) [Gr. *dis,* two, + *daktylos,* finger]. The congenital condition of having only two digits on a hand or foot.

didelphic (dī-dĕl′fĭk) [″ + *delphys,* uterus]. Having or pert. to a double uterus.

didymalgia, didymodynia (dĭd-ĭ-măl′jē-ă, dĭd″ĭ-mō-dĭn′ē-ă) [Gr. *didymos,* twin, + *algos,* pain]. Pain in a testicle.

didymitis (dĭd-ĭ-mī′tĭs) [″ + *itis,* inflammation]. Inflammation of a testicle. SYN: *orchitis.*

didymus (dĭd′ĭ-mŭs) [Gr. *didymos,* twin, testis]. 1. A twin. 2. A congenital abnormality involving joined twins. 3. A testicle.

diechoscope (dī-ĕk′ō-skōp) [Gr. *dis,* two, + *echo,* echo, + *skopein,* to examine]. A stethoscope for simultaneous auscultation from two different sites.

diecious (dī-ē′shŭs) [″ + *oikos,* house]. Having sexually distinct males and females, esp. in botany.

dieldrin (dī-ĕl′drĭn). A chlorinated hydrocarbon used as an insecticide. It is toxic to man and marine and terrestrial animals. SEE: *Poisons and Poisoning* in *Appendix.*

dielectric [Gr. *dia,* through, + *elektron,* amber]. An insulating substance offering great resistance to passage of electricity by conduction.

diembryony (dī-ĕm′brē-ŏn″ē). The development of two embryos in a single egg.

diencephalon (dī″ĕn-sĕf′ă-lŏn) [Gr. *dis,* two, + *enkephalos,* brain]. Second portion of the brain or that lying between the telencephalon and mesencephalon. It includes the epithalamus, thalamus, metathalamus, and hypothalamus. SYN: *thalamencephalon.*

dienestrol (dī″ēn-ĕs′trŏl). USP. A nonsteroid, synthetic estrogen used for estrogen therapy.

Dientamoeba (dī″ĕn-tă-mē′bă). A genus of parasitic protozoa characterized by possession of two similar nuclei. They belong to the class Sarcodina.

D. fragilis. A species of parasitic amebae inhabiting the intestine of man. There is strong evidence that it may sometimes be pathogenic, producing symptoms such as intestinal colic and diarrhea.

dieresis (dī-ĕr′ĕ-sĭs) [Gr. *diairesis,* a division]. 1. Breaking up or dispersion of things normally joined, as by an ulcer. 2. Mechanical separation of parts by surgical means.

dieretic. Pert. to dieresis; dissolvable or separable.

diet [Gr. *diaita,* way of living]. 1. Liquid and solid food substances regularly consumed in the course of normal living. 2. A prescribed allowance of food adapted for a particular state of health or disease, as a diet prescribed for use by a diabetic. 3. To cause to eat or drink sparingly in accordance with prescribed rules.

d., balanced. Diet adequate in energy-providing substances (carbohydrates and fats), tissue-building compounds (proteins), inorganic chemicals (water and mineral salts), agents that regulate or catalyze metabolic processes (vitamins), and substances for certain physiological processes, such as bulk for promoting peristaltic movements of the digestive tract.

d., minimum residue. Diet used for short periods of time to insure a minimum of solid material in the intestinal tract. Foods allowed include one glass of milk per day; clear fluids and juices; lean meat; noodles; and refined cereals.

d., reduction. Diet that reduces the caloric content sufficiently to cause weight loss. Normal metabolism must be preserved, as must bulk, mineral, protein, vitamin, and water requirements. The energy value of ingested foods should be 600 to 1500 Cal. below maintenance levels for the individual's weight.

diet, words pert. to: bland diet; calcium (high and low) diet; elimination diet; fat (low) diet; feeding; fluid diet; liquid diet; roughage diet; salt-free diet; Sippy diet; soft diet.

dietary (dī′ĕ-tā″rē). 1. Pert. to diet. 2. A system of dieting. 3. A regulated food allowance.

dietary fiber. SEE: *fiber, dietary.*

dietetic (dī-ĕ-tĕt′ĭk). 1. Pert. to diet or its regulation. 2. Food specially prepared for restrictive diets.

dietetics [Gr. *diaitetikos*]. The science of applying nutritional data to the regulation of the diet of healthy and sick individuals. Some fundamental principles and facts of this science will be summarized here. SEE: *Dietetics* in *Appendix.*

CONSERVATION OF ENERGY: In order to obtain metabolic balance, there must be as much caloric value (energy and heat) in the food as will equal the amount of work done by the subject or patient plus the heat constantly lost. The number of calories in daily food must in the long run equal the energy required for basic metabolic needs plus additional energy output resulting from muscular work and added heat losses. Thus a subject whose basal rate is 1000 Calories (kilogram calories) per 24 hours may during the day do work and lose heat, adding about 1500 Calories to the energy output; he or she must, therefore, obtain 2500 Calories.

One gm. of fat yields approx. 9 Cal. One

gm. of carbohydrate or protein yields about 4 Cal.

NOTE: To convert Calories to kilojoules, multiply Calories (kilocalories) times 4.186.

CONSERVATION OF MATTER: Everything that leaves the body, whether exhaled as carbon dioxide and water or excreted as urea and minerals, must be replaced in the food. Thus, a person excreting 10 gm. of nitrogen daily must receive 10 gm. of it in his or her diet, for the element can neither be created nor destroyed. This metabolic balance may be monitored by the use of careful chemical analysis of all that is eaten and excreted.

DIFFICULTY OF SOME ORGANIC SYNTHESES: The power of the body to build tissue is limited, and for a given purpose, only certain raw materials can be used. Thus, proteins are made up of carbon, hydrogen, oxygen, and nitrogen, but eating charcoal and inhaling the gases would not enable one to make tissue protein. For instance, hemoglobin cannot be synthesized unless the body is supplied with proteins containing one of the essential building blocks, the pyrrole ring, for this complex molecule. This group occurs in the amino acids tryptophan, proline, and hydroxyproline; proteins that do not contain these amino acids therefore are insufficient for needs of the body.

SUMMARY: A diet should contain water, carbohydrates, fats, proteins, minerals, roughage (indigestible residue), and vitamins.

diethazine hydrochloride (dī-ĕth'ă-zēn). An anticholinergic used in treating parkinsonism.

diethylcarbamazine citrate (dī-ĕth"ĭl-kăr-băm'ă-zēn). USP. Medicine used in treating filarial infections. Trade names are Hetrazan, Banocide, and Filarabits.

diethylpropion hydrochloride (dī-ĕth"ĭl-prō'pē-ŏn). USP. An adrenergic drug with actions similar to those of the amphetamines. Trade names are Tenuate and Tepanil.

diethylstilbestrol (dī-ĕth"ĭl-stĭl"bĕs'trŏl). USP. ABBR: DES. A synthetic preparation possessing estrogenic properties. It is several times more potent than natural estrogens and may be given orally. It is used therapeutically in the treatment of menopausal disturbances and other disorders due to estrogen deficiencies.

CAUTION: Should not be administered during pregnancy. Such use has been found to be related to subsequent vaginal malignancies in the daughters of mothers who were so treated. SEE: *DES daughters; DES syndrome.*

diethyltoluamide (dī-ĕth"ĭl-tŏl-ū'ă-mīd). USP. An effective insect repellant, esp. for repelling arthropods.

diethyltryptamine (dī-ĕth"ĭl-trĭp'tă-mĭn). A hallucinogenic agent that at low dose levels has effects similar to LSD.

dietitian (dī-ĕ-tĭsh'ăn) [Gr. *diaita*, way of living]. An individual whose training and experience is in the area of nutrition, and who has the ability to apply that information to the regulation of diet in the healthy and sick.

Dietl's crisis (dē't'ls). [Joseph Dietl, Pol. physician, 1804–1878] Renal colic resulting from kinking and partial obstruction of the ureter, accompanied by scanty bloodstained urine.

dietotherapy (dī"ĕ-tō-thĕr'ă-pē). Use of the sciences of dietetics and nutrition in treating disease.

Dieulafoy's triad (dyū-lă-fwăhz'). [Georges Dieulafoy, Fr. physician, 1839–1911] Tenderness, muscular contraction, and skin hyperesthesia at McBurney's point in acute appendicitis.

differential (dĭf"ĕr-ĕn'shăl) [L. *differre*, to carry apart]. Marked by differences.

differential blood count. Determination of the number of each variety of leukocytes in one cubic milliliter of blood. SEE: *blood count, differential.*

differential diagnosis. Diagnosis based on comparison of symptoms of two or more similar diseases to determine which the patient is suffering from. SEE: *diagnosis.*

differentiation. 1. Acquisition of functions different from those of the original type. 2. The distinguishing of one disease from another.

diffraction (dĭ-frăk'shŭn) [L. *diffringere*, to break to pieces]. The change that occurs in light when it passes through crystals, prisms, or parallel bars in a grating, in which the rays are deflected and, thus, appear to be turned aside. This produces dark or colored bands or lines or other phenomena. Term is also applied to similar phenomena in sound and electricity.

diffusate (dĭf'ū-sāt) [L. *dis*, apart, + *fundere*, to pour]. In the process of dialysis, that portion of a liquid that passes through a membrane and that contains crystalloid matter in solution. SYN: *dialysate.*

diffuse (dĭ-fūs'). Spreading, scattered, spread.

diffusible (dĭ-fūz'ĭ-bl). Capable of being diffused.

diffusion (dĭ-fū'zhŭn) [" + *fundere*, to pour]. 1. Absorption of a liquid such as the absorption by cells of water from lymph when the percentage of salt is less in lymph than in the cells. When the percentage is greater in the lymph than in the cells, water is withdrawn from the latter. SEE: *osmosis.* 2. A process whereby various gases interpenetrate and become mixed as a result of the incessant motion of their molecules. Similarly, if aqueous solutions of different materi-

DIFFUSION

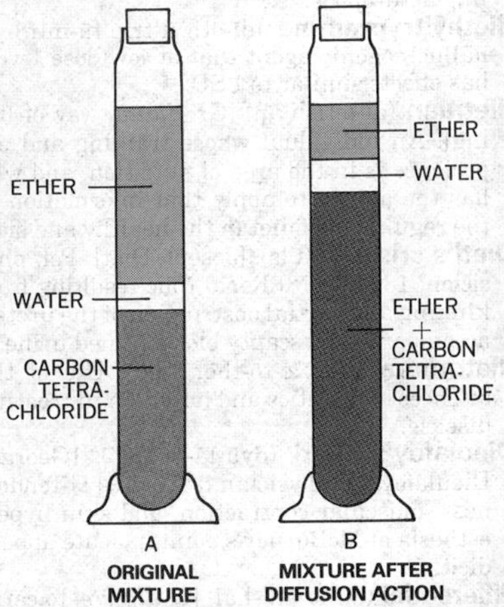

A: At the beginning of the experiment, a thin layer of water separates a large volume of ether from an equal volume of the much heavier carbon tetrachloride. B: Three weeks later, the layers are still distinct, but the lowest layer has visibly increased in volume at the expense of the uppermost layer. Ether has passed through the water into the carbon tetrachloride.

als stand in contact, mixing occurs on standing even if the solutions are separated by thin membranes. SEE: illus. 3. The tendency of molecules of a substance (gaseous, liquid, or solid) to move from a region of high concentration to one of lower concentration.

digastric (dī-găs′trĭk) [Gr. *dis,* twice, + *gaster,* belly]. Having two bellies; said of certain muscles.

digenesis [″ + *genesis,* production]. Reproduction in which alternate generations are asexual.

Digenetica (dī-jĕ-nĕt′ĭ-kă). An order of parasitic flatworms belonging to the class Trematoda and characterized by having an asexual generation, living usually in molluscs, alternating with a sexual generation living in vertebrates as their final host. It includes all the flukes parasitic in man. These include four groups of flukes. SEE: *fluke.*

digest [L. *dis,* apart, + *gerere,* to carry]. 1. To undergo digestion. As in the process involved in changing food from a solid physical form to a soft, moisturized mass that is then acted upon in the intestinal tract by chemicals, including enzymes. SEE: *metabolism.* 2. To make a condensation of a subject.

digestant. 1. An agent that will digest food or aid in digestion, such as pepsin or pancreatin. 2. A preparation made from the digestive glands or lining membrane of the stomach, classified according to the foods it digests, such as carbohydrate or protein.

digestible. That which is capable of being digested.

digestion [L. *digestio,* a taking apart]. The process by which food is broken down mechanically and chemically in the gastrointestinal tract and converted into absorbable forms. Salt, the simplest sugars (such as glucose), crystalloids in general, and water can be absorbed unchanged, but starches, fats, and proteins for the most part are not absorbable until split into smaller molecules by the process of digestion. Even the sugar sucrose (a disaccharide) must first be split into two simple hexoses, glucose and fructose, in order to be absorbed. The chemical actions are chiefly hydrolytic; they are brought about by a variety of enzymes, each of which acts in an acid or alkaline or neutral juice according to its peculiar properties.

The higher molecular weight carbohydrates are converted into monosaccharides, q.v. Proteins, through successive stages of action of peptones and polypeptides, ultimately are converted into amino acids and fats into fatty acids and glycerine. In the stomach the soluble casein of milk is converted into insoluble paracasein, resulting in its coagulation or clotting. This is brought about by the enzyme pepsin. An enzyme, lipase, is able to attack fats in emulsified form. It liberates, for instance, butyric acid from the fats in milk. This chemical causes the characteristic odor of vomitus. The chemical actions are facilitated by the churning wave-like motions, i.e., peristalsis, of the stomach walls. When the chyme is ready to leave the stomach, the pylorus opens from time to time and the chyme is quickly propelled into the duodenum. SEE: table.

d., artificial. Digestion outside the living organism by a ferment.

d., duodenal. The chyme, which is usually acid as it comes from the stomach, is made alkaline and the fats it contains are emulsified by the action of bile. Enzymes adapted to these new conditions are supplied by the pancreatic juice, which enters by two ducts, and by the intestinal juice, which comes from small glands in the wall of the intestine itself. The hydrolysis of starches, fats, and proteins is carried to its physiological completion here and in the remainder of the small intestine.

d., extracellular. Digestion occurring outside the body of the cell.

d., gastric. Portion of the digestive process taking place in the stomach.

d., intestinal. Hydrolytic processes continue here and absorption of the products is active. From the ileum, the food residues

Action of Digestive Enzymes on Foods

Food Component	Enzyme	Secretion	Site of Action
Protein	Pepsin Trypsin	Gastric juice, acid Pancreatic juice, alkaline	Stomach Small intestine
Fats	Lipase	Pancreatic juice	Small intestine
	Salivary amylase	Saliva, alkaline	Mouth and to some small extent in stomach
Carbohydrates	Pancreatic amylase Invertase	Pancreatic juice, alkaline Succus entericus	Small intestine Small intestine

Action of Digestive Secretions on Proteins, Fats, and Carbohydrates

Secretion	Proteins	Fats	Carbohydrates
Saliva			Cooked starch into maltose
Gastric Juice	Curdles milk Proteins into peptones		
Pancreatic Juice	Peptones to simpler substances	Fats to fatty acids and glycerol	Raw and cooked starch into maltose Sugars into simpler forms
Bile		Emulsifies fats	
Intestinal Juice	Completes the change of peptones into amino acids		Completes the change of all sugars into the simplest form. NOTE: Disaccharides are hydrolyzed to monosaccharides in the mucosal cells lining the small intestine.

pass in a nearly liquid state through a small opening into the ascending colon. A sphincter muscle prevents backflow. True digestive processes in the colon are slight, but there is normally much bacterial action (the products of which are mostly absorbed) and reabsorption of water. The remaining substances, now colored by pigments that entered with bile and changed to a firm consistency by the loss of water, pass on through the transverse colon, the descending colon, and the sigmoid flexure into the rectum. They are retained in the rectum by the action of sphincters until defecation occurs. SEE: *absorption*.

d., intracellular. Metabolic processes within cells.

d., oral. Portion of the digestive process taking place in the mouth. This is the physical process of chewing food and the chemical process of starch-splitting by the enzyme ptyalin, which is present in the saliva.

d., pancreatic. Portion of digestive process influenced by pancreatic juice.

d., salivary. Digestive action by the saliva. SEE: *salivary digestion*.

d., secondary. Cellular assimilation of nutritive material.

digestive (dī-jĕs′tĭv). Pert. to digestion.

digestive juice. One of several secretions that aid in processes of digestion.

digestive system. All the organs and glands associated with ingestion and digestion of

DIGESTIVE SYSTEM

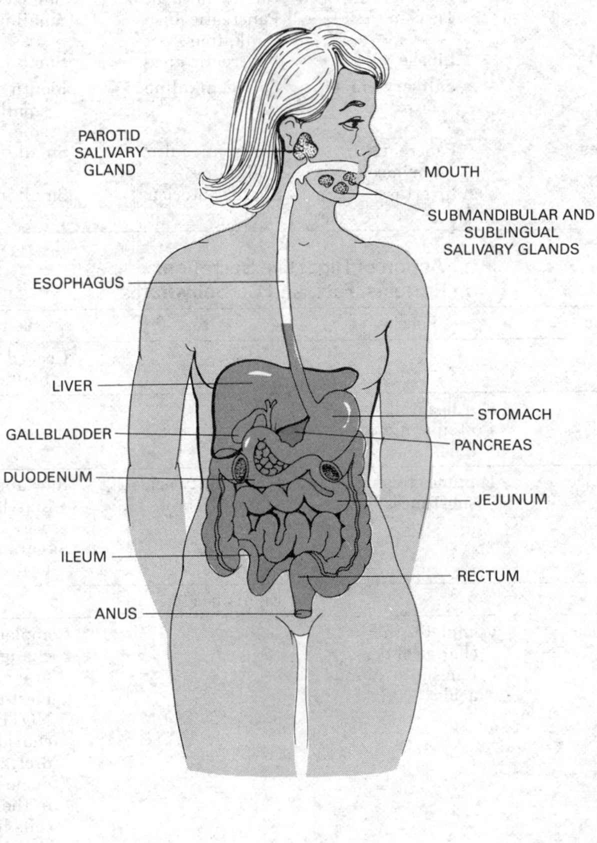

food; the tract from the mouth to the anus. SEE: illus.

digit (dĭj′ĭt) [L. *digitus,* finger]. (pl. *digits*) A finger or toe.

digital (dĭj-ĭ-tăl). Pert. to or resembling a finger or toe.

digital amniotome. A small apparatus that fits over the tip of the index finger. A small knife-like projection at the end of the device is used to puncture the bag of waters prior to delivery of the fetus. This usually expedites progression of labor.

digital subtraction angiography. Angiography, digital subtraction, q.v.

digitalis (dĭj″ĭ-tăl′ĭs) [L. *digitus,* finger]. USP. Foxglove. The dried leaves of Digitalis purpurea used in powdered form in tablets or capsules. Cardiotonic glycosides, esp. digitoxin and digoxin, are obtained from various species of the Digitalis plant. Trade name is Digiglusin. SEE: *Poisons and Poisoning* in *Appendix.*

ACTION AND USES: Digitalis glycosides increase the force of myocardial contraction, increase the refractory period of the atrioventricular (A-V) node, and to a lesser degree affect the sinoatrial (S-A) node. This enables the heart to pump more blood, i.e., to increase cardiac output. Digitalis is indicated in congestive heart failure, and its use causes diuresis and general amelioration of this condition. It is usually necessary to continue the drug after the heart failure is controlled. Digitalis is also used in atrial fibrillation and flutter and in paroxysmal atrial tachycardia.

CONTRA: Digitalis is not indicated in sinus tachycardia or premature systoles in the absence of heart failure. Its use in shock caused by infections is of no benefit and may be harmful. It should not be used in ventricular fibrillation or if the patient is allergic to digitalis.

PRECAUTIONS: Potassium depletion, which may accompany diuresis, sensitizes the myocardium to digitalis and may permit toxicity to develop with what would otherwise be the usual dose. Patients with acute myocardial infarction, severe pulmonary disease, or far-advanced heart failure may be more sensitive to digitalis and thus prone to develop arrhythmia. Calcium affects the heart in a manner similar to digitalis; its use in a digitalized patient may produce serious arrhythmias. In myxedema, digitalis requirements are decreased because excretion rate of the drug is decreased. Patients with incomplete A-V block, esp. those with Stokes-Adams attacks, may develop complete heart block if given digitalis. Because renal insufficiency delays the excretion of digitalis, the dose must be adjusted accordingly in those patients.

digitalis poisoning. Toxicity that may develop acutely or chronically from the cumulative effect of digitalis. Patients on digitalis therapy must know how to take their pulse and be aware of the signs and symptoms of heart block or other adverse effects. They should also include a potassium-containing food in their daily diet.

SYM: Digestive disturbances such as nausea and vomiting, irregular pulse, diarrhea, and yellow vision. Frequently distressing headache. Cardiac irregularities are common, esp. slowing of heart with ventricular extrasystoles or partial heart block.

F.A.: Evacuate stomach and discontinue digitalis and diuretics. Because these patients are usually chronically ill, special care is necessary in their management.

digitalization (dĭj″ĭ-tăl-ĭ-zā′shŭn). Subjection of an organism to the action of digitalis.

digital reflex. Sudden flexion of terminal phalanx of a finger or thumb when nail is suddenly tapped.

digitate [L. *digitus,* finger]. Having fingerlike impressions or processes.

digitation (dĭj-ĭ-tā′shŭn). A fingerlike process.

digiti (dĭj′ĭ-tī). Pl. of digitus.

digitiform (dĭj′ĭ-tĭ-form). Similar to a finger.

digitoxin (dĭj-ĭ-tŏk′sĭn). USP. A cardiotoxic glycoside obtained from various species of the Digitalis plant. A heart stimulant, administered orally or parenterally. SEE: *digitalis.* Trade names are Crystodigin and Purodigin.

digitus [L]. (pl. *digiti*) A finger or toe.

diglossia (dī-glŏs′ē-ă) [Gr. *dis,* double + *glossa,* tongue]. Having a double tongue.

digoxin (dĭ-jŏk′sĭn). USP. A cardiotonic glycoside obtained from Digitalis lanata. A heart stimulant administered orally or parenterally. Trade name is Lanoxin.

diglyceride (dī-glĭs′ĕr-īd). Glyceride combined with two fatty acid molecules. SEE: *triglyceride.*

dignathus (dĭg-nā′thŭs) [″ + *gnathos,* jaw]. A congenital deformity in which there are two jaws.

dihydric (dī-hī′drĭk). A compound containing two hydrogen atoms.

dihydrocodeinone bitartrate (dī-hī″drō-kō′dē-ĭ-nōn). An opioid analgesic that is used in combination with a number of other drugs.

dihydroergotamine mesylate (dī-hī″drō-ĕr-gŏt′ă-mēn). USP. A vasoconstrictor used in treating migraine. Trade name is DHE-45.

dihydrosphingosine. A long-chain amino alcohol present in sphingolipids:

$$CH_3(CH_2)_{12}-CH=CH-\underset{}{\overset{OH}{\overset{|}{C}}}-\overset{NH_2}{\overset{|}{C}}-CH_2OH$$

SEE: *sphingolipids; sphingosine.*

dihydrotachysterol (dī-hī″drō-tăk-ĭs′tĕr-ŏl). USP. A hydrogenated tachysterol; a steroid, obtained by irradiation of ergosterol. Aids absorption of calcium from digestive tract in hypoparathyroidism. Trade name is Hytakerol.

dihydrotheelin (dī-hī″drō-thē′ĕl-ĭn). $C_{18}H_{24}O_2$, a crystalline steroid, produced by the ovary, possessing estrogenic properties. Large quantities are found in the urine of pregnant women and mares, and in the urine of stallions, the latter two serving as sources of the commercial product. It is effective when given subcutaneously or intramuscularly but not when administered orally. It is converted to estrone in the body. SYN: *estradiol.*

dihydroxyaluminum aminoacetate (dī″hī-drŏk″sē-ă-lū′mĭ-nŭm). An antacid used in treating gastric hyperacidity. Trade name is Robalate.

dihydroxyaluminum sodium carbonate. A gastric antacid. Trade name is Rolaids.

dihydroxycholecalciferol (dī″hī-drŏk″sē-kō″lē-kăl-sĭf′ĕ-rōl). A group of compounds considered to be hormones because of their ability to influence absorption and metabolism of calcium. One of these, 1,25-$(OH)_2$ cholecalciferol, or calciferol, is thought to be the active form of vitamin D, q.v. Previously used name for calciferol.

dihydroxymorphinone hydrochloride (dī″hī-drŏk″sē-mor′fī-nōn). An opioid analgesic. Trade name is Numorphan.

3,4-dihydroxyphenylalanine (dī-hī-drŏk″sē-fĕn″ĭl-ăl′ă-nēn). Dopa, q.v.

dihysteria (dī″hĭs-tĕr′ē-ă) [Gr. *dis*, double, + *hystera*, the uterus]. State of having a double uterus.

diiodohydroxyquin (dī″ī-ō″dō-hī-drŏk′sē-kwĭn). Previously used name for iodoquinol, USP.

diisopropylphosphorofluoridate. A strong miotic used in treating glaucoma. Trade name is Floropryl.

CAUTION: If used in large doses, may cause bronchial constriction and cardiospasm. The antidote is atropine sulfate.

diktyoma (dĭk-tē-ō′mă) [Gr. *diktyon*, net, + *oma*, tumor]. A tumor of the ciliary epithelium. SYN: *dictyoma*.

dilaceration (dī″lăs-ĕr-ā′shŭn) [L. *dilacerare*, to tear apart]. A tearing apart, as of a cataract. SEE: *discission*.

Dilantin (dī-lăn′tĭn). Trade name for phenytoin sodium, USP. Previously termed diphenylhydantoin sodium. A derivative of glyceryl urea. An anticonvulsant used esp. in the treatment of epilepsy.

dilatant (dī-lā′tănt) [L *dilatare*, to enlarge]. Anything that causes dilation.

dilatation (dĭl-ă-tā′shŭn). 1. Expansion of an organ or vessel. 2. Expansion of an orifice with a dilator.

d., digital. Dilatation of an opening or a cavity by use of the fingers.

d., heart. Abnormal increase in the size of the cavities of the heart, a common result of valvular disease or hypertension.

d., stomach. Condition in which the stomach is extremely dilated. Acute dilatation of the stomach or acute gastromesenteric ileus may occur as a postoperative or postpartum condition and usually results from obstruction of the duodenum.

dilation. 1. Expansion of an orifice with a dilator. 2. Expansion of an organ, orifice, or vessel. SYN: *dilatation*.

dilation and curettage. ABBR: D and C. A surgical procedure that expands the cervical canal of the uterus (dilation) so that the surface lining of the uterine wall can be scraped (curettage).

dilator (dī-lā′tor) [L. *dilatare*, to expand]. Instrument for dilating muscles, stretching cavities or openings.

d., Barnes'. Rubber bag that is filled with fluid for dilatation of the cervix uteri.

d., Bossi's. A multiple-pronged instrument that dilates by separation of the prongs. Used for dilation of the cervix uteri.

d., Goodell's. Similar to the Bossi except that it has three prongs.

d., gynecologic. An instrument for dilating the cervix uteri.

d., Hegar's. Graduated metal sounds that are inserted into the cervical canal and cause a graded dilatation.

d., tent. Small cone made of seaweed, sponge, or tree roots that is inserted into the uterine canal dry and, on absorbing moisture, expands to cause a slow dilatation. SEE: *laminaria digitata*.

d., vaginal. A glass, plastic, or metal device for dilating the vagina.

Dilaudid Hydrochloride. Trade name for hydromorphone hydrochloride.

dildo, dildoe. An artificial penis-shaped device used intravaginally to produce sexual pleasure.

diluent (dĭl′ū-ĕnt) [L. *diluere*, to wash away]. An agent that dilutes the substance or solution to which it is added.

dilution (dī-loo′shŭn). 1. Process of rendering a substance attenuated or diluted. 2. A diluted substance.

Dilyn. Trade name for guaifenesin.

dim. Reduced light or action of decreasing light present.

dimenhydrinate (dī″mĕn-hī′drĭn-āt). USP. A drug occurring as an odorless crystalline white powder. It is used to prevent or treat motion sickness and to control nausea, vomiting, and dizziness in other conditions. Trade names are Dommanate, Dramamine, and Eldodram.

dimension (dī-mĕn′shŭn). The measure of anything. It is expressed in commonly recognized and accepted units.

dimer (dī′mĕr). 1. In chemistry, esp. polymer chemistry, the combination of two identical molecules to form a single compound. 2. In virology, a capsomer containing two subunits.

dimercaprol (dī-mĕr-kăp′rōl). USP. $C_3H_8OS_2$. A compound, 2,3-dimercaptopropanol, used as an antidote in poisoning from heavy metals such as arsenic, gold, and mercury. It occurs as a colorless liquid with a disagreeable odor. Mixed with benzyl benzoate and oil, it is administered intramuscularly. Trade name is BAL in Oil.

Dimetane. Trade name for brompheniramine maleate.

dimethicone (dī-mĕth′ĭ-kōn). A silicone oil used to protect the skin against water-soluble irritants.

dimethindene maleate (dī″mĕth-ĭn′dēn). USP. An antihistamine. Trade names are Forhistal Maleate and Triten.

dimethisoquin hydrochloride (dī″mē-thī′sō-kwĭn). USP. A topical anesthetic agent. Trade name is Quotane.

dimethisterone (dī″mĕth-ĭs′tĕr-ōn). A progestational agent.

dimethylamine (dī-mĕth″ĭl-ăm′ĭn). A malodorous product of decaying materials that contain proteins.

***p*-dimethylaminoazobenzene** (dī-mĕth″ĭl-ăm″ĭ-nō-ăz″ō-bĕn′zēn). A carcinogenic dye, butter yellow.

dimethyl phthalate (dī-mĕth″ĭl-thăl′āt). An insect repellant.

dimethyl sulfoxide (dī-mĕth′ĭl sŭlf-ŏks′ĭd). ABBR: DMSO. A solvent used to facilitate absorption of medicines through the skin. It is a colorless liquid with little odor, but when it is applied to the skin, the patient will notice a garlic-like taste sensation. It has been used in treating interstitial cystitis and in treating certain sports injuries.

dimethyltryptamine (dī-mĕth″ĭl-trĭp′tă-mēn). An agent that in low doses has hallucinogenic action similar to LSD.

dimetria (dī-mē′trē-ă) [Gr. *dis,* double, + *metra,* uterus]. A double uterus.

dimorphous (dī-mor′fŭs) [″ + *morphe,* form]. Occurring in two different forms.

dimple sign. Sign used to differentiate a benign lesion, dermatofibroma, from malignant nodular melanoma, which it may mimic. Upon application of lateral pressure with the thumb and index finger, the dermatofibroma will dimple or become indented; melanomas, melanocytic nevi, and normal skin protrude above the initial plane.

dimpling. The formation of slight depressions in the flesh due to retraction of the subcutaneous tissue. Occurs in certain carcinomas, such as cancer of the breast. SEE: *peau d'orange.*

dineuric (dī-nū′rĭk) [″ + *neuron,* nerve]. Having two axis-cylinder processes.

dinical (dĭn′ĭ-kl) [Gr. *dinos,* vertigo]. Pert. to giddiness or vertigo or to their relief.

2,4-dinitrophenol (dī-nī″trō-fē′nŏl). An isomeric compound formerly used in making dyes. It is very toxic, and is used only as a reagent. SEE: *Poisons and Poisoning* in *Appendix.*

Dinoflagellata (dī″nō-flăj″ĕ-lā′tă) [″ + *flagellum,* whip]. An order of minute marine protozoa that have been associated with a red discoloration of seawater known as "red tide." They are toxic to fish.

dinoprost tromethamine (dī′nō-prŏst). A drug that causes uterine contractions and may be used to induce abortion during the very early stage of pregnancy. SYN: *prostaglandin* F_{2a}.

dinucleotide (dī-nū′klē-ō-tīd). The product of cleaving a polynucleotide.

Dioctophyma (dī-ŏk″tō-fī′mă). A genus of roundworm that is found in dogs but rarely in man.

dioctyl calcium sulfosuccinate (dī-ŏk′tĭl). A stool softener. Previously used name for docusate calcium.

dioctyl sodium sulfosuccinate. Previously used name for docusate sodium, q.v.

Diodrast (dī′ō-drăst). Trade name for iodopyracet, a radiopaque medium used in x-ray studies, esp. of the urinary tract.

diopter, dioptre [Gr. *dia,* through, + *optos,* visible]. Refractive power of lens with focal distance of 1 meter, used as unit of measurement in refraction.

dioptometer (dī″ŏp-tŏm′ĕ-tĕr) [″ + ″ + *metron,* measure]. Device for measuring ocular refraction.

dioptometry (dī″ŏp-tŏm′ĕ-trē). The determination of refraction and accommodation of the eye.

dioptral (dī-ŏp′trăl). Pert. to a diopter.

dioptric (dī-ŏp′trĭk). Pert. to refraction of light.

dioptrics. The science of refraction of light.

diovulatory (dī-ŏv′ū-lā-tō″rē). Production of two ova in the same ovarian cycle.

dioxide (dī-ŏk′sīd) [Gr. *dis,* two, + *oxys,* sharp]. A compound having two oxygen atoms per molecule.

dioxybenzone (dī-ŏks″ĭ-bĕn′zōn). USP. Chemical for protecting skin from the sun.

dipeptid(e) (dī-pĕp′tĭd, -tīd) [″ + *peptein,* to digest]. A derived protein obtained by hydrolysis of proteins or condensation of amino acids.

dipeptidase (dī-pĕp′tĭ-dās). An enzyme that catalyzes the hydrolysis of dipeptides to amino acids.

diperodon (dī-pĕr′ō-dŏn). USP. A local anesthetic.

Dipetalonema perstans (dī-pĕt″ă-lō-nē′mă). A species of filaria that infests wild or domestic animals and occasionally man. In man, the adult worm migrates to the subcutaneous tissue and produces a nodule. The adult worm may, rarely, be seen beneath the conjunctiva.

diphallus (dī-făl′ŭs) [″ + *phallos,* penis]. A condition in which there is either a complete or incomplete doubling of the penis or clitoris.

diphasic (dī-fā′zĭk) [″ + *phasis,* a phase]. Having two phases.

diphemanil methylsulfate (dī-fē′mă-nĭl). USP. An anticholinergic drug used in treating gastric hyperacidity. Trade name is Prantal.

diphenadione (dī-fĕn″ă-dī′ōn). USP. An anticoagulant. Trade name is Dipaxin.

diphenhydramine hydrochloride (dī″fĕn-hī′dră-mēn hī-drō-klō′rīd). USP. An antihistaminic agent. It is an odorless, white, crystalline powder. Trade name is Benadryl.

diphenoxylate hydrochloride (dī″fĕn-ŏk′sĭ-lāt). A smooth muscle relaxant used in combination with atropine in treating diarrhea.

diphenylhydantoin sodium (dī-fĕn″ĭl-hī-dăn′

tō-ĭn). A white odorless powder, freely soluble in water. An anticonvulsant used esp. in the treatment of epilepsy. The official name is phenytoin. Trade name is Dilantin.

diphenylpyraline hydrochloride (dī-fĕn″ĭl-pī′ră-lēn). An antihistamine. Trade names are Diafen and Hispril.

diphonia (dī-fō′nē-ă) [Gr. *dis,* two, + *phone,* voice]. Simultaneous production of two different voice tones.

2,3-diphosphoglycerate. ABBR: 2,3-DPG. An organic phosphate in red blood cells that alters the affinity of hemoglobin for oxygen. Blood cells stored in a blood bank lose 2,3-diphosphoglycerate but once they are infused, the substance is resynthesized or reactivated.

diphtheria (dĭf-thē′rē-ă) [Gr. *diphthera,* membrane]. An acute infectious disease characterized by the formation of a false membrane on any mucous surface and occasionally on the skin. Usually accompanied by great prostration. SEE: *antitoxin; Klebs-Loeffler bacillus; Schick test; toxin-antitoxin.*

ETIOL: Causative organism Corynebacterium diphtheriae, a gram-positive nonmotile, non-spore-forming, club-shaped bacillus. In stained smears, the bacilli are usually arranged at sharp angles with each other. This gives the characteristic Chinese-letter appearance. The disease is rare under one year of age. The vast majority of cases occur before the age of 10, but older children and adults are not exempt. Both sexes are equally susceptible. Esp. prevalent in fall and winter months. Transmission through direct contact with a human carrier, or as a result of exposure through contact with articles that have been contaminated by the diphtheria patient.

INCUBAT: Two to five days, occasionally longer.

SYM: Onset gradual. Usually slight headache and malaise. Temperature 100° to 101° F. (37.8° to 38.3° C.) and sore throat with presence of yellowish-white or grayish membrane adherent to tonsils or pharyngeal walls. Cervical adenitis may develop early in severe types. In nasal diphtheria, fever is a much more evident symptom. Adenitis often is severe, with serous discharge from nostrils, which may be blood tinged. Strong fetid odor of breath common. Myocarditis and late neuritis are commonly present.

DIFF. DIAG: Tonsillitis; scarlet fever; acute pharyngitis; streptococcus sore throat; peritonsillar abscess; infectious mononucleosis; Vincent's angina; acute moniliasis; and staphylococcus infections in the respiratory tract following chemotherapy. Examination of a smear from infected area is advisable, but cultures should be obtained in every instance for the purpose of confirming the diagnosis. In the laryngeal type, edema of the glottis, foreign bodies, and retropharyngeal abscess need to be considered.

PROG: Favorable when antitoxin in sufficient amounts is administered within three days from time of onset. If it is given on the first day, death hardly ever occurs. In laryngeal diphtheria, intubation or rarely tracheotomy may be necessary as well as an adequate dose of diphtheria antitoxin. Age is an important factor, with death more frequent in very young or very old patients than in intermediate age group. When therapy is not given promptly, the incidence of nerve damage is quite high. If the patient survives, the myocarditis and neuritis will completely resolve.

ACTIVE IMMUNIZATION: Not all individuals are susceptible to diphtheria, and this factor may be determined by means of the Schick test, q.v. Therefore, it is advisable to use this test in adults before administering either toxin-antitoxin or toxoid. Routine immunization should begin at age three months, diphtheria toxoid being administered in combination with pertussis vaccine and tetanus toxoid; this is then followed by booster doses. Diphtheria toxoid, following a subcutaneous test for hypersensitivity, is used for immunization of adults.

GENERAL MEASURES: Strict bedrest during acute and convalescent stages of disease. In cases with myocardial involvement, prolonged rest in bed may be as important as the early administration of diphtheria antitoxin.

TREATMENT: Specific treatment consists of diphtheria antitoxin after determination of lack of sensitivity to horse serum. No interference with diphtheria membrane is advisable. Gargles should not be used, although cleansing mouthwashes are permissible. On the other hand, the use of suction in nasal cases is sometimes of distinct advantage. A liquid diet (consisting of plenty of water, fruit juices, and nourishing broths) or a soft diet is recommended. In the acute stage, stimulants should not be administered. In fact, they are more likely to do harm than good. Surgical interference is sometimes a necessity in laryngeal diphtheria. Intubation is always to be preferred to tracheotomy, provided an experienced operator is available and hospitalization, which will make possible any attention required within a moment's notice, is provided. For myocarditis, there is no specific therapy. Digitalis and quinidine should be only for arrythmias with rapid ventricular rate.

d., cutaneous. Diphtheritic lesions of the skin, usually limited to the site of infection.

d., laryngeal. Considered to be a complication of diphtheria. Results from extension of the membrane from the pharynx with gradual occlusion of the airway. Signs are restlessness, use of accessory respiration muscles, and development of cyanosis. If this is not remedied effectively, death results.

d., surgical. Diphtheric membrane formation on wounds.

diphtheria antitoxin. USP. The antitoxin used in treating diphtheria.

diphtherial. Pert. to diphtheria.

diphtheriaphor (dĭf-thē'rē-ă-for) [Gr. *diphthera,* membrane, + *pherein,* to carry]. A diphtheria carrier or vector.

diphtheria toxin for Schick test. USP. The toxin used for determining immunity to diphtheria. SEE: *Schick test.*

diphtheria toxoid. USP. Immunizing agent for diphtheria.

diphtheric, diphtheritic (dĭf-thē'rĭk, dĭf-thĕr-ĭt'ĭk). Pert. to diphtheria.

diphtherin (dĭf'thē-rĭn). The toxin of diphtheria, from Corynebacterium diphtheriae.

diphtheroid (dĭf'thĕ-royd) [" + *eidos,* appearance]. 1. Resembling diphtheria or the bacteria that cause diphtheria. 2. The formation of a false or pseudomembrane not due to the diphtheria bacillus.

diphtherotoxin (dĭf"thĕr-ō-tŏk'sĭn) [" + *toxikon,* poison]. The specific toxin of the diphtheria bacillus.

diphthongia (dĭf-thŏn'jē-ă) [Gr. *dis,* two, + *phthongos,* voice]. The simultaneous utterance of two vocal sounds of different pitch in pathological conditions of the larynx.

Diphyllobothrium (dī-fĭl"ō-bŏth'rē-ŭm) [" + *phyllon,* leaf, + *bothrion,* pit]. A genus of tapeworms belonging to the order Pseudophyllidea and characterized by possession of a scolex possessing two slitlike grooves or bothria. Formerly called Dibothriocephalus.

D. cordatum. The heart-shaped tapeworm, a small species infesting dogs and seals in Greenland, formerly known as D. mansoni. The plerocercoids are occasionally found in man.

D. erinacei. A species infesting dogs, cats, and other carnivores. Larval stages are occasionally found in man.

D. latum. The broad or fish tapeworm. The adult lives in the intestine of fish-eating mammals and man. It is the largest human tapeworm and may reach a length of 50 to 60 feet or 15.2 to 18.3 meters (average 20 feet or 6.1 meters). The eggs develop into ciliated larvae called coracidia, which are eaten by certain species of copepods, in which each becomes an oncosphere, which develops into a procercoid. Further development occurs in a fish, where it develops into a wormlike plerocercoid or sparganum larva. Infection of the final host occurs after eating raw or improperly cooked fish. Infection can be prevented by thoroughly cooking all freshwater fish, or by keeping the fish frozen at −10° C (14° F) for 48 hours prior to eating.

SYM: Pathological effects are abdominal pain, loss of weight, digestive disorders, progressive weakness, and a severe type of anemia that is clinically identical with pernicious anemia.

TREATMENT: Niclosamide. The therapy may need to be repeated if examination of the stools indicates presence of infection after three months of treatment.

diphyodont (dĭf'ē-ō-dŏnt) [" + *phyein,* to produce, + *odous,* tooth]. Having two sets of teeth, as man.

diplacusis (dĭp"lă-kū'sĭs) [" + *akousis,* hearing]. Variety of disturbed perception of pitch characterized by hearing two tones for every sound produced.

diplegia (dī-plē'jē-ă) [Gr. *dis,* twice, + *plege,* a stroke]. Paralysis of similar parts on both sides of the body.

d., infantile. Birth palsy.

d., spastic. Congenital spastic stiffness of the limbs.

diplegic (dī-plē'jĭk). Pert. to diplegia.

diploalbuminuria (dĭp"lō-ăl-bū"mĭn-ū'rē-ă) [Gr. *diplous,* double, + L. *albumen,* white of egg, + Gr. *ouron,* urine]. Coexistence of physiologic and pathologic albuminuria.

diplobacillus [" + L. *bacillus,* a little stick]. A double bacillus, two being linked end to end.

diplobacterium [" + *bakterion,* little rod]. An organism made up of two adherent bacteria.

diploblastic (dĭp"lō-blăs'tĭk) [" + *blastos,* germ]. The ectoderm and endoderm having two germ layers.

diplocardia [" + *kardia,* heart]. Having the two lateral halves of the heart partially separated by a groove.

diplocephaly (dĭp"lō-sĕf'ă-lē) [" + *kephale,* head]. Having two heads.

diplococcemia (dĭp"lō-kŏk-sē'mē-ă) [" + *kokkos,* berry, + *haima,* blood]. Diplococci in the blood.

diplococci (dĭp"lō-kŏk'sē, -kŏk'ī). Pl. of diplococcus. SEE: *bacteria* for illus.

Diplococcus (dĭp-lō-kŏk'ŭs) [" + *kokkus,* berry]. A genus of bacteria belonging to the family Lactobacillaceae. They are gram-positive organisms occurring in pairs.

D. pneumoniae. A species of bacteria, oval or spherical in shape, gram positive and nonmotile. They possess a capsule. The species is made up of a number of distinct strains of which more than 80 serological types have been isolated. It is the causative agent of certain types of pneumonia, esp.

lobar pneumonia, and is associated with other infectious diseases such as cerebrospinal meningitis, otitis media, and septicemia. SYN: *pneumococcus; Streptococcus pneumoniae.*

diplococcus (dĭp″lō-kŏk′ŭs). (pl. *diplococci*) Any of various spherical bacteria appearing in pairs, esp. of the genus Diplococcus. SEE: *bacteria* for illus.

diplocoria (dĭp″lō-kō′rē-ă) [″ + *kore,* pupil]. Double pupil in the eye.

diploë (dĭp′lō-ē) [Gr. *diploe,* fold]. Spongy tissue between the two layers of compact bone of the skull.

diploetic, diploic. Pert. to the diploë.

diplogenesis [Gr. *diplous,* double, + *genesis,* production]. Having two parts or producing two substances; production of double fetus or the doubling of some fetal parts.

diploid (dĭp′loyd) [″ + *eidos,* form]. Having two sets of chromosomes. Said of somatic cells, which contain twice the number of chromosomes present in the egg or sperm. SEE: *chromosome; meiosis; mitosis.*

diplokaryon (dĭp″lō-kăr′ē-ŏn) [″ + *karyon,* nucleus]. A nucleus containing twice the diploid number of chromosomes.

diplomellituria (dĭp″lō-mĕl″ĭ-tūr′ē-ă) [″ + *meli,* honey, + *ouron,* urine]. Condition in which diabetic and nondiabetic glycosuria occur either simultaneously or alternately in the same individual.

diplomyelia (dĭp″lō-mī-ē′lē-ă) [″ + *myelos,* marrow]. Condition in certain types of spina bifida in which the spinal cord appears to be doubled due to a lengthwise fissure.

diploneural [″ + *neuron,* nerve]. Having two nerves from different origins, as certain muscles.

diplopagus (dĭp-lŏp′ă-gŭs) [″ + *pagos,* a thing fixed]. Conjoined twins that share some organs.

diplophonia (dĭp-lō-fō′nē-ă) [″ + *phone,* voice]. Having two different voice tones at the same time. SYN: *diphonia.*

diplopia (dĭp-lō′pē-ă) [″ + *ope,* sight]. Double vision. May be monocular.

d., binocular. Double vision occurring when both eyes are used but not in focus. Seen in disease of the eyeballs, cranial nerve affections, and disease of the cerebellum, cerebrum, and meninges.

d., crossed. Binocular vision in which the images are reversed.

d., direct. D., homonymous.

d., heteronymous. D., crossed.

d., homonymous. Double vision in which right-hand image appears on right side and left-hand image on left side. SEE: *d., crossed.*

d., monocular. Double vision with one eye.

d., unocular. D., monocular.

d., vertical. Diplopia with one of two images higher than the other.

diplopiometer (dĭp-lō″pē-ŏm′ĕ-tĕr) [Gr. *diplous,* double, + *ope,* sight, + *metron,* measure]. Device for estimating double vision.

diploscope [″ + *skopein,* to examine]. Device for study of binocular vision.

diplosomatia, diplosomia (dĭp″lō-sō-mā′shē-ă, dip″lō-sō′mē-ă) [″ + *soma,* body]. Twins joined at one or more points.

diplotene (dĭp′lō-tēn). In cell division, the stage of the first meiotic prophase. The homologous pairs of chromatids begin to separate.

dipole (dī′pōl). 1. Two equal and opposite charges separated by a distance. 2. In chemistry, one portion of the molecule has a certain charge and the other portion has an equal and opposite charge.

dipping. 1. Palpation of the liver by a quick depression movement of the fingers while the hand is held flat on the abdomen. 2. The act of immersing an object in a solution, esp. applied to the dipping of cattle or dogs for the control of ticks.

Diprosone. Trade name for betamethasone dipropionate.

diprosopus (dĭp-rō-sōp′ŭs) [Gr. *dis,* twice, + *prosopon,* face]. A malformed fetus characterized by a double face.

dipsesis (dĭp-sē′sĭs) [Gr., a thirst]. Extreme thirst or craving for abnormal liquids.

dipsogen (dĭp′sō-jĕn). An agent that induces thirst.

dipsomania (dĭp″sō-mā′nē-ă) [Gr. *dipsa,* thirst, + *mania,* madness]. A morbid and uncontrollable craving for alcoholic beverages. SEE: *alcoholism.*

dipsophobia (dĭp-sō-fō′bē-ă) [″ + *phobos,* fear]. Morbid fear of drinking.

dipsosis (dĭp-sō′sĭs) [″ + *osis,* condition]. Abnormal thirst.

dipsotherapy (dĭp″sō-thĕr′ă-pē) [″ + *therapeia,* treatment]. Limitation of water intake as a means of treatment.

dipstick (dĭp′stĭk). A chemical-impregnated paper strip used for analysis of urine samples.

Diptera (dĭp′tĕr-ă) [Gr. *dipteros,* having two wings]. An order of insects characterized by having sucking or piercing mouth parts, one pair of wings, and complete metamorphosis. It includes the flies, gnats, midges, and mosquitoes. It contains many species involved in the transmission of pathogenic organisms, as in malaria.

dipterous (dĭp′tĕr-ŭs). Having two wings; characteristic of the order Diptera.

dipygus (dī-pī′gŭs) [Gr. *dis,* two, + *pyge,* rump]. A congenitally deformed fetus with a double pelvis.

dipylidiasis (dĭp″ĭ-lĭ-dī′ă-sĭs). Infestation with the tapeworm, Dipylidium caninum.

Dipylidium (dĭp″ĭ-lĭd′ē-ŭm) [Gr. *dipylos,* having two entrances]. A genus of tapeworms belonging to the family Dipyliidae that infests dogs and cats.

D. caninum. A species of Dipylidium, a common parasite of dogs and cats. Occasionally human infestation may occur through the accidental ingestion of lice or fleas, which serve as the intermediate host.

direct [L. *diregere,* to direct]. Immediate; uninterrupted; straight.

direct current. ABBR: DC or dc. An electric current flowing continuously in one direction only. SEE: *electric shock.*

directionality. Ability to perceive one's position in relationship with the environment; sense of direction. Problems with directionality are frequently found in children with learning disabilities or suspected minimal brain dysfunction.

direct light reflex. Prompt contraction of sphincter of iris when light entering through pupil strikes retina of eye.

director. Grooved device for guiding a knife in surgery.

direct reflex. Reflex in which response occurs on same side as the stimulus.

dirigomotor (dĭr″ĭ-gō-mō′tor) [L. *dirigere,* to direct, + *motor,* mover]. Controlling or directing muscular activity.

Dirofilaria (dī″rō-fĭ-lā′rē-ă). A genus of filaria.

D. immitis. Heartworm, a species of filaria that occurs in dogs, but may infest man.

dis-. 1. [L. *dis,* apart] Prefix indicating free of, to undo. 2. [Gr. *dis,* twice] Prefix meaning double or twice.

disability (dĭs″ă-bĭl′ĭ-tē). Lack of ability to perform mental or physical tasks that one can normally do. The term is used in legal medicine to apply esp. to the loss of mental or physical powers as a result of injury or disease. SEE: *handicap.*

d., developmental. Term used for conditions due to congenital abnormality, trauma, deprivation, or diseases that interrupt or delay the sequence and rate of normal growth, development, and maturation.

disaccharidase (dī-săk′ă-rĭ-dās). A group of enzymes that split disaccharides into monosaccharides.

disaccharide (dī-săk′ĭ-rĭd) [Gr. *dis,* twice, + *sakkharon,* sugar]. A carbohydrate composed of two monosaccharides. SEE: *carbohydrate.*

disarticulation [L. *dis,* apart, + *articulus,* joint]. Amputation through a joint.

disassimilation [″ + *ad,* to, + *similare,* to make like]. Changing assimilated material into less complex compounds for the production of energy.

disc [Gr. *diskos,* quoit]. A flat, round, platelike structure. SEE: *disk.*

discharge (dĭs-chărj′, dĭs′chărj) [ME. *dischargen,* to discharge]. 1. The escape (esp. by violence) of pent up or accumulated energy or of explosive material. 2. The flowing away of a secretion or excretion of pus, feces, urine, etc. 3. The material thus ejected.

d., cerebrocortical. The violent action of an injured or malfunctioning portion of the cerebral cortex that gives rise to an epileptic paroxysm.

d., convective. Discharge from a high potential source in the form of electrical energy passing through the air to the patient.

d., disruptive. A passage of current through an insulating medium due to the breakdown of the medium under electrostatic stress.

d., lochial. Uterine excretion following childbirth. SEE: *lochia.*

discharging. The emission of or the flowing out of material as the discharge of pus from a lesion. Excreting.

discharging lesion. A lesion of a nerve center in the brain suddenly discharging motor impulses.

dischronation [L. *dis,* apart, + Gr. *chronos,* time]. Lack of a sense of relativity in the consciousness of time.

discission (dĭs-sĭzh′ŭn) [″ + *scindere,* to cut]. Rupture of the capsule of the crystalline lens in operation for cataract.

discitis (dĭs-kī′tĭs) [Gr. *diskos,* disk, + *itis,* inflammation]. Diskitis.

disclosing agent. A diagnostic aid used in dentistry to reveal areas of the teeth that are not being cleaned adequately. The dye is erythrosine sodium, USP, and is applied to the teeth in a 2% solution or by a tablet that is chewed by the patient.

discoblastic [″ + *blastos,* germ]. Pert. to discoid segmentation of yolk in an impregnated ovum.

discoblastula (dĭs″kō-blăs′tū-lă). A modified blastula found in highly telolecithal eggs, as in birds in which the blastomeres form a cellular cap (germinal disk or blastoderm) that is separated from the yolk by a space, the blastocoele.

discogenic (dĭs″kō-jĕn′ĭk) [″ + *gennan,* to produce]. Caused by an intervertebral disk.

discography (dĭs-kŏg′ră-fē). Use of a contrast medium injected into the intervertebral disk in order to examine it by x-ray.

discoid. Like a disk.

discoplacenta [Gr. *diskos,* disk, + *plakous,* a flat cake]. A disklike placenta.

discordance (dĭs-kor′dăns). In genetics, the expression of a trait in only one of a twin pair. SEE: *concordance.*

discrete (dĭs-krēt′) [L. *discretus,* separated]. Separate; said of certain eruptions on the skin. SEE: *confluent.*

discrimination [L. *discriminare*, to divide]. The process of distinguishing or differentiating.

d., one-point. The ability to locate specifically a point of pressure on the surface of the skin.

d., tonal. The ability to distinguish one tone from another. This is dependent upon the integrity of the transverse fibers of the basilar membrane of the organ of Corti.

d., two-point. The ability to localize two points of pressure on the surface of the skin and to identify them as discrete sensations. SYN: *tactile discrimination.*

discus [Gr. *diskos*, quoit]. (pl. *discuses* or *disci*) [NA] A disk.

d. articularis. [NA] An interarticular fibrocartilage; an articular disk.

d. proligerus. The cumulus oophorus.

disdiaclast (dĭs-dī′ă-klăst) [Gr. *dis*, twice, + *diaklan*, to break through]. A doubly refracting element in the tissues of striated muscles.

disdiadochokinesia (dĭs-dī″ă-dō″kō-kĭ-nē′zē-ă) [L. *dis*, apart, + Gr. *diadochos*, succeeding, + *kinesis*, motion]. Inability to make finely coordinated movements of a part in opposite directions, as when quickly supinating and pronating the hand. SEE: *diadochokinesia.*

disease (dĭ-zēz′) [Fr. *des*, from, + *aise*, ease]. Literally the lack of ease; a pathological condition of the body that presents a group of symptoms peculiar to it and that sets the condition apart as an abnormal entity differing from other normal or pathological body states. SYN: *dyscrasia.*

d., acute. Disease having a rapid onset and of relatively short duration.

d., anticipated. A disease that may be predicted to occur in individuals with a certain genetic, physical, or environmental predisposition.

d., autoimmune. Disease in which the body produces disordered immunological response against itself. Normally the body's immune mechanisms are able to distinguish clearly between what is a normal substance and what is foreign. In autoimmune diseases, this system becomes defective and produces antibodies against normal parts of the body to such an extent as to cause tissue injury. Certain diseases such as hemolytic anemia, some forms of glomerulonephritis, rheumatoid arthritis, myasthenia gravis, and scleroderma are considered to be autoimmune diseases.

d., chronic. A disease having a slow onset and lasting for a long period of time.

d., chronic granulomatous. A genetically determined defect in the ability of polymorphonuclear leukocytes to kill certain bacteria. Clinically, suppurative lymphadenitis, dermatitis, pulmonary disease, and hepatosplenomegaly are present. A rare disease that occurs mostly in male infants and children. Despite vigorous appropriate antibiotic therapy, death occurs in a short time.

d., collagen. SEE: *collagen disease.*

d., communicable. A disease, the causative organism of which is transmissible from one person to another either directly or indirectly through a carrier or vector.

d., complicating. A disease that occurs during the course of another disease.

d., congenital. Disease that is present at birth. May be due to hereditary factors, prenatal infection, injury, or the effect of a drug the mother took during pregnancy.

d., constitutional. 1. Disease due to an individual's hereditary makeup. 2. A disease involving the body as a whole in contrast to one involving specific organs. SEE: *diathesis.*

d., contagious. An infectious disease readily transmitted from one person to another.

d., cystine storage. An inherited disease of cystine metabolism resulting in abnormal deposition of cystine in body tissues. The cause is disordered proximal renal tubular function. Clinically, the child fails to grow, and develops rickets, corneal opacities, and acidosis. SYN: *cystinosis.*

d., deficiency. A disease resulting from inadequate intake or absorption of essential dietary factors such as vitamins or minerals.

d., degenerative. A disease resulting from degenerative changes that occur in tissues and organs, characteristic of old age.

d., degenerative joint. Osteoarthritis, q.v.

d., demyelinating. Disturbance of nerve cells due to destruction of their myelin sheaths.

d., endemic. A disease that is present more or less continuously or recurs in a community.

d., epidemic. Disease that attacks a large number of individuals in a community at the same time.

d., epizootic. An epidemic that affects animals of a particular area in a short period of time.

d., extrapyramidal. Any one of several degenerative diseases of the nervous system that involve the extrapyramidal system and the basal ganglion of the brain. The symptoms include tremors, chorea, athetosis, and dystonia. Parkinsonism, q.v., is a form of extrapyramidal disease.

d., familial. A disease that occurs in several individuals of the same family.

d., focal. Disease located at a specific and distinct area such as the tonsils, adenoids, or in a boil.

d., functional. A disease in which no anatomical changes can be observed to account for the symptoms present.

d., glycogen storage. SEE: *glycogen storage disease.*

d., heavy chain. A group of diseases involving serum immunoglobulins. The globulins contain heavy chain subunits. If the immunoglobulin A (IgA) is affected, then abdominal lymphoma and malabsorption occur. When immunoglobulin G (IgG) is affected, there are lymphadenopathy, weakness, weight loss, and repeated bacterial infections. If immunoglobulin M (IgM) is involved, the lymphadenopathy affects the abdominal lymph nodes, the liver, and the spleen. Bence Jones proteinuria occurs.

d., hemolytic, of the newborn. Erythroblastosis fetalis, q.v.

d., hemorrhagic, of the newborn. Bleeding tendency in the newborn characterized by melena, purpura, and prothrombin deficiency. The disease is self-limiting.

d., hereditary. Disease due to hereditary factors transmitted from parent to offspring.

d., hookworm. SEE: *ancylostomiasis; Necator americanus.*

d., hypokinetic. Physical and mental illness produced by lack of or by insufficient exercise.

d., iatrogenic. A disease caused by medical or surgical intervention. The implication is that the disease would not have occurred if the individual had not sought medical care.

d., idiopathic. Disease for which no causative factor can be recognized.

d., infectious. Disease resulting from the presence of a pathogenic organism in the body.

d., intercurrent. A disease that occurs during the course of another unrelated disease.

d., iron storage. Hemochromatosis, q.v.

d., malignant. 1. Cancer. 2. Disease, including cancer but not limited to that, in which the progress is extremely rapid and generally threatening or resulting in death within a short time.

d., mediterranean. SEE: *thalassemia.*

d., metabolic. Disease due to abnormality of the body chemistry. The abnormality may be due to underproduction of a needed substance, such as insulin in diabetes, or overproduction, such as thyroid hormone in thyrotoxicosis.

d., motor neuron. One of several types of diseases of the motor neurons: progressive muscular atrophy, progressive bulbar palsy, and amyotrophic lateral sclerosis. These diseases are characterized by degeneration of anterior horn cells of the spinal cord, the motor cranial nerve nuclei, and the pyramidal tracts. They occur principally in males. In the U.S.A., amyotrophic lateral sclerosis is known to the laity as Lou Gehrig's disease. He was a well-known athlete whose baseball career and life were prematurely ended as a result of this disease.

d., occupational. Disease resulting from factors associated with the occupation in which the patient is engaged.

d., organic. Disease resulting from recognizable anatomical changes in an organ or tissue of the body.

d., pandemic. An epidemic disease that is extremely widespread, involving the entire world.

d., parasitic. Disease resulting from the growth and development of parasitic organisms (plants or animals) in or upon the body.

d., periodontal. SEE: *periodontitis.*

d., psychosomatic. Psychological factors contribute to the initiation or exacerbation of a physical illness. Conditions that are in the general category of psychosomatic disorders are obesity, tension headache, some types of asthma, neurodermatitis, peptic ulcer, some attacks of angina pectoris, and frequency of urination.

NOTE: It is not possible for a human being to be consciously sick without there being some interplay between the emotions and the bodily functions.

d., secondary. A disease that occurs as the result of another disease, e.g., the disease of obesity may cause secondary diseases of the joints and muscles of the lower extremities due to the increased trauma incident to transporting and supporting the added weight.

d., self-limited. A disease that even if untreated eventually goes away

d., sporadic. Disease in which only occasional cases occur; not epidemic or endemic.

d., storage. Disorder involving abnormal deposition of a substance in body tissues. SEE: *glycogen storage disease; Wilson's disease.*

d., subacute. Disease in which symptoms are less pronounced but more prolonged than in an acute disease; intermediate between acute and chronic disease.

d., systemic. A generalized disease rather than a localized or focal one.

d., thyrotoxic heart. Disease due to increased activity of the thyroid gland, characterized by cardiac enlargement, atrial fibrillation, and heart failure. SEE: *thyrotoxicosis.*

d., venereal. ABBR: V.D. Disease usually acquired through sexual relations. Includes syphilis, gonorrhea, granuloma inguinale, herpes genitalis, Chlamydia trachomatis infections, trichomoniasis, anogenital warts, scabies, pediculosis pubis, enteric infections due to anal-oral contacts, lymphogranuloma venereum, and chancroid. SEE: *sexually transmitted diseases.*

disengagement [Fr.]. The emergence of the fetal head from within the maternal pelvis.

disequilibrium (dĭs-ē″kwĭ-lĭb′rē-ŭm) [L. *dis,* apart, + *aequus,* equal, + *libra,* balance]. An unequal and unstable equilibrium.

dish, Petri. SEE: *Petri dish.*

disinfect (dĭs-ĭn-fĕkt′) [″ + *inficere,* to corrupt]. To free from infection by physical or chemical means.

disinfectant. A chemical that prevents infection by killing bacteria. Common disinfectants are the halogens: chlorine, fluorine, iodine; salts of heavy metals: mercuric chloride (bichloride of mercury), silver nitrate; acids: sulphuric acid, boric acid; alkalies: chloride of lime; organic compounds: formaldehyde, alcohol 70%, iodoform, organic acids, phenol (carbolic acid), cresols, benzoic and salicylic acids and their sodium salts; miscellaneous substances: thymol, hydrogen peroxide, potassium permanganate, ethylene oxide. An agent that frees from infection. Term is usually applied to a chemical or physical agent that kills vegetative forms of microorganisms.

disinfection. The application of disinfectants. It is not possible to insure 100% disinfection of a room unless the entire room and its contents are treated with a gaseous agent such as ethylene oxide. Disinfestation, or the killing of vermin by chemicals and their vapors, however, is possible. SEE: Methods of Disinfection table.

d., concurrent. Prompt disinfection and suitable disposal of infected excreta during the entire course of a disease.

d. of blankets and woolens. May be steam-disinfected or soaked for two hours in 5% carbolic acid solution and then washed and rinsed thoroughly. Cotton goods may also be so treated or boiled before washing. Materials that might be harmed by conventional methods of disinfection may be treated in a chamber with ethylene oxide gas.

d. of excreta. Should be soaked in 5% carbolic acid solution for one hour before disposal. All infected excreta should be burned. Sputum may be treated as excreta if impossible to burn.

d. of field of operation. A safe rule is to make the disinfection too extensive. Thus, in operations upon large wounds of the scalp and in all operations on the skull and its contents, the entire scalp must be shaved and disinfected. SEE: illus.

In operations upon the breast, the axilla and half of the chest must be prepared. If glands of the neck are involved, the entire neck must be included in field of operation.

In amputation of foot and lower third of the leg, the disinfection must extend as far as the knee, and in all higher amputations it should include the whole limb and corresponding side of pelvis.

In all abdominal operations below the umbilicus, the pubic area must be shaved and the surface disinfection must include the whole anterior surface and both sides as far as the breasts.

In operations on the stomach, liver, and bile ducts, the field extends from the pubic area to the breasts. A general warm bath with liberal use of tincture of green soap should precede disinfection of the field of operation in all abdominal and pelvic operations, including hernia and varicocele.

In operations upon parts of the body difficult to disinfect as scalp, palm of hand, and sole of foot, it is advisable to scrub with hot water and tincture of green soap and then rinse. Use either 70% solution of alcohol, povidone, USP, benzalkonium chloride, or other suitable disinfectant. Alcohol is useful in hand and surface disinfection.

CAUTION: The mucous membranes are active, absorbing surfaces so that the use of solutions of carbolic acid, mercuric bichloride, and other potent antiseptics is prohibited in these areas. The free use of any of these agents in the vagina, uterus, or rectum has frequently resulted in serious poisoning and in some instances death.

In operations in the oral cavity, such as excision of superior or inferior maxilla, and amputation of tongue, the employment of a disinfecting solution is preceded by thorough cleansing of the teeth and the mucous membrane is swabbed with hydrogen peroxide.

In operations upon the rectum, the procedure in common use consists of shaving perianal area and giving cleansing enemas.

Vaginal disinfection is preceded by shaving and disinfection of the external genitals. After a thorough cleansing with warm water and tincture of green soap, a douche of warm water with a suitable disinfectant is recommended.

Catheterization should always be preceded by disinfection of the meatus with green soap and rinsing the area thoroughly with sterile water.

The external ear canal should be mechanically cleansed of wax, dirt, or blood clots, and then carefully disinfected by a low-pressure stream of warm hydrogen peroxide, until it is absolutely clean. This should not be done if the eardrum has been ruptured.

d., terminal. Disinfection of the room and infected materials and the end of the

DISINFECTION OF FIELDS OF OPERATION

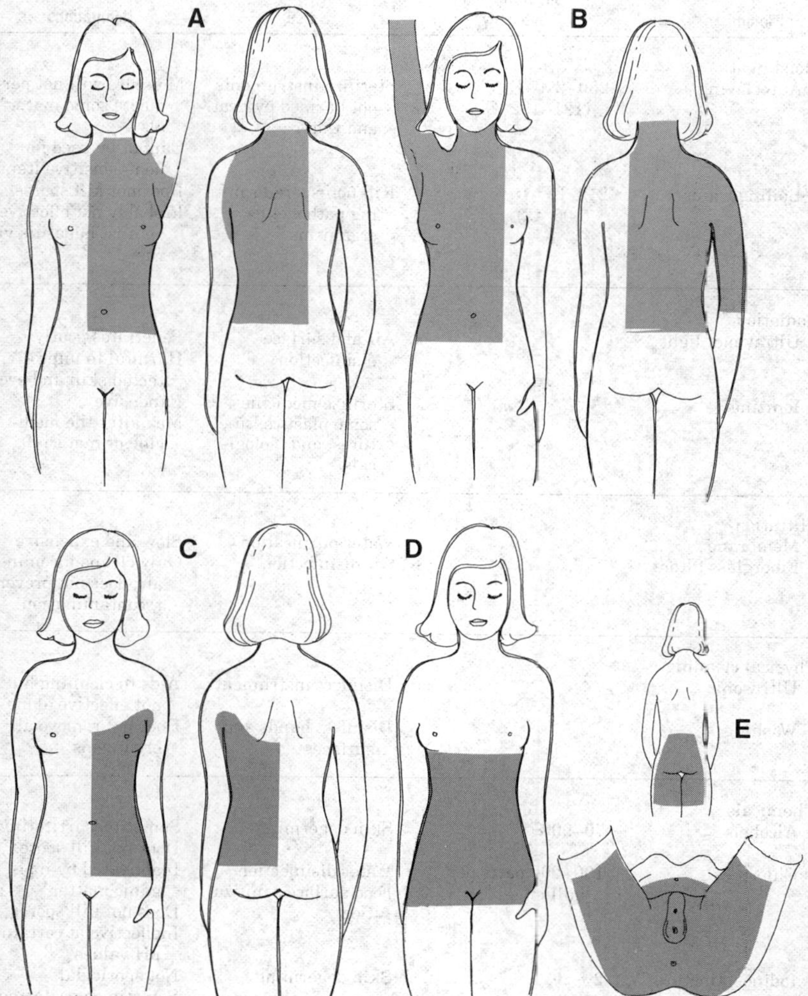

A - LEFT MASTECTOMY

B - RIGHT MASTECTOMY

C - LEFT NEPHROTOMY

D - ABDOMINAL SURGERY

E - PERINEAL SURGERY

Methods of Disinfection*

Method	Concentration or Intensity	Use	Limitations
Moist heat			
Autoclaving	250–270° F. (121–132° C.)	Sterilize instruments not harmed by heat and water	Moisture will not permeate some materials Cannot be used for heat-sensitive items
Boiling water	212° F. (100° C.)	Kill non-spore-forming pathogenic organisms	Does not kill spores Probably not effective against hepatitis virus
Radiation			
Ultraviolet light		Air and surface disinfection	Penetrates poorly Harmful to unprotected skin and eyes
Ionizing		Sterilize medicines, some plastics, sutures, and biologicals	Expensive May alter the medicine or material.
Filtration			
Membrane		Water purification	Slow and expensive
Fiberglass filters		Air disinfection	Only cleans incoming air; does not prevent recontamination
Physical cleaning			
Ultrasonic		Disinfect instruments	Aids in cleaning but not effective alone
Washing		Disinfect hands and surfaces	Does not remove all organisms
Chemicals			
Alcohols	70–90%	Skin degerming	Sometimes irritating Does not kill spores
Chlorines	100–200 parts per million	Water disinfection Food surface sanitization	Inactivated by inorganic matter Does not kill spores Ineffective at certain pH values
Iodines, tincture	2%	Skin degerming	Not sporicidal Sometimes irritating
Iodines, iodophors	74–450 parts per million	General disinfectant	Not sporicidal
Phenols	1–4%	General disinfectant	Ineffective against some bacteria May be irritating or corrosive

*Adapted from Benarde, M. A. (ed.): *Disinfection: A Treatise*. Marcel Dekker, Inc., New York, 1970.

Methods of Disinfection* (*Continued*)

Method	Concentration or Intensity	Use	Limitations
Quaternary ammonia compounds, tincture	0.1%	Skin degerming	Neutralized by soap Not sporicidal
Quaternary ammonia compounds, aqueous	Diluted one part to 750 parts	General disinfectant	May be incompatible with some water Ineffective against some bacteria
Mercurials	0.1%	Skin degerming	Slow acting May be irritating
Formaldehyde (formalin)	5%	Drastic disinfection	Irritating, corrosive
Glutaraldehyde	2%	Instrument sterilization	Irritates mucous membranes Unstable
Germicidal soaps (hexachlorophene)	2–3%	Skin degerming	Bacteriostatic rather than bactericidal
Gaseous			
Ethylene oxide	450 mg./liter of air	Sterilization of heat-sensitive materials or those that must be kept dry	Temperature, time, humidity critical Treated materials need to air for varying periods of time (depending on composition) following treatment
Formaldehyde gas		Fumigation Sterilization of heat-sensitive materials	Irritating, corrosive

infectious stage of a disease.

disinfestation (dĭs″ĭn-fĕs-tā′shŭn) [L. *dis,* apart, + *infestare,* to strike at]. The process of killing infesting insects or parasites.

disinhibition (dĭs″ĭn-hĭ-bĭsh′ŭn). Abolition of or countering inhibition.

disinsected. Freed of insects.

disinsertion. Detachment of the retina at its periphery.

disintegration [″ + *integer,* entire]. The product of catabolism; the falling apart of the constituents of a substance.

disjoint. To disarticulate or to separate bones from their natural positions in a joint.

disjunction (dĭs-jŭnk′shŭn). Chromosome separation at the anaphase of the first meiotic division.

disk [Gr. *diskos,* a disk]. A flat, round, plate-like structure.

d., anisotropic. A dark, shining, highly refractile disk forming a part of the striation of the myofibril of a striated muscle fiber. SYN: *Q disk.*

d., articular. The biconcave oval disk of fibrous connective tissue that separates the two joint cavities of the temporomandibular joint on each side.

d., Bowman's. Disk-like segment of a striated muscle fiber.

d., choked. A swollen optic disk due to inflammation or edema. SYN: *papilledema.*

d., dental. A thin circular paper or other materials carrying polishing or cutting materials; it is driven by a dental engine and utilized in a variety of procedures with natural or artificial teeth.

d., embryonic. An oval disk of cells in the blastocyst of a mammal from which the embryo proper develops. Its lower layer, the endoderm, forms the roof of the yolk sac. Its upper layer, the ectoderm, forms the floor of the amniotic cavity. The primitive streak develops on the upper surface of the disk.

d., epiphyseal. Disklike epiphysis at ends of vertebral centrum.

d., germinal. A disk of cells on the surface of the yolk of a teloblastic egg from which the embryo develops. SYN: *blasto-*

derm.

d., intervertebral. The fibrocartilaginous tissue between the vertebral bodies.

d., M. A thin line lying in the center of Hensen's disk.

d., Merkel's. Tiny expanded end of a sensory nerve fiber found in epidermis and in epithelial root sheath of a hair. SYN: *tactile disk.*

d., optic. Area of the retina where optic nerve enters it. SEE: *blind spot.*

d., proligerous. D., germinal.

d., Q. The anistropic or A disk of a striated muscle myofibril.

d., slipped. Lay term for herniated intervertebral disk.

d., tactile. D., Merkel's.

d., Z. The intermediate disk of a striated muscle fiber. SEE: *striated muscle.*

diskectomy (dĭs-kĕk'tō-mē). Surgical removal of a herniated intervertebral disk.

diskiform (dĭs'kĭ-form). Shaped like a dish or disk.

diskitis (dĭsk-ī'tĭs) [Gr. *diskos,* disk, + *itis,* inflammation]. Inflammation of a disk, esp. an interarticular cartilage. SYN: *meniscitis.*

dislocation [L. *dis,* apart, + *locare,* to place]. The displacement of any part, esp. the temporary displacement of a bone from its normal position in a joint.

d., closed. D., simple.

d., complete. A dislocation that completely separates the surfaces of a joint.

d., complicated. A dislocation associated with other major injuries.

d., compound. Dislocation in which the joint communicates with the external air.

d., congenital. Dislocation existing from or before birth.

d., consecutive. Dislocation in which the luxated bone has changed its position since its first displacement.

d., divergent. Dislocation in which the ulna and radius are dislocated separately.

d., habitual. Dislocation that often recurs after replacement.

d., incomplete. A subluxation; a slight displacement.

d., metacarpophalangeal joint. Dislocation of finger. This is usually complicated by an interposition of tendons or other structures. When reduced, it tends to slip out immediately. In many instances, manipulating of this region only tends to make it more difficult for a subsequent reduction; therefore, immobilize the disturbed area with well-placed and padded splints of hand and wrist. Send patient to doctor promptly.

d., Monteggia's. Dislocation of hip joint in which head of femur is near anterosuperior spine of the ilium.

d., Nelaton's. Dislocation of the ankle in which the talus is forced up between the end of the tibia and the fibula.

d., old. A dislocation in which no reduction has been accomplished even after many days, weeks, or months.

d., partial. D., incomplete.

d., pathologic. Dislocation that results from paralysis or disease of joint or supporting tissues.

d., primitive. Dislocation in which the bones remain as originally displaced.

d., recent. Dislocation seen shortly after it occurred.

d., simple. Dislocation in which the joint is not penetrated by a wound.

d., slipped. D., herniated.

d., subastragalar. Separation of the calcaneum and the scaphoid from the talus.

d., traumatic. Dislocation due to injury or violence.

dismember. To remove an extremity or a portion of it.

dismutase (dĭs-mū'tās). An enzyme that acts on two molecules of the same substance. One of these is oxidized and the other reduced, thereby producing two new compounds.

d., superoxide. An enzyme present in aerobic but not in strictly anaerobic bacteria. It functions to destroy the poisonous highly reactive free-radical form of O_2, superoxide (O_2^-), formed by flavoenzymes. Thus, aerobic bacteria are protected from the lethal effect of superoxide by the action of this enzyme.

disodium edetate (dī-sō'dē-ŭm). A chelating agent, disodium, dihydrogen, ethylene diamine tetra-acetate dihydrate. It is used in treating hypercalcemia.

disomus (dī-sō'mŭs) [Gr. *dis,* twice, + *soma,* body]. A malformed fetus with a double trunk.

Disonate. Trade name for docusate sodium.

disopyramide phosphate (dī-sō-pēr'ă-mīd). USP. Drug used in treating cardiac arrhythmias. Trade name is Norpace.

disorder. Pathological condition of the mind or body.

disorganization [L. *dis,* apart, + Gr. *organon,* a unified organ]. Alteration in an organic part, causing it to lose most or all of its distinctive characteristics.

disorientation (dĭs"ō-rē-ĕn-tā'shŭn) [" + *oriens,* arising]. Inability to estimate direction or location, or to be cognizant of time or of persons.

disparate points (dĭs'păr-ăt, dĭs-păr'ăt) [L. *disparare,* to separate]. Points on the two retinas that are not corresponding or identical, causing objects to appear double.

dispensary [L. *dispensare,* to give out]. Place or clinic for dispensation of medicines and treatment.

dispensatory (dĭs-pĕn'să-tō-rē) [L. *dispensatorium*]. Publication, in book form, of the description and composition of medicines.

dispense (dĭs-pĕns'). To prepare or deliver medicines.

dispersate (dĭs'pŭr-sāt). Suspension of finely divided particles in a liquid.

disperse (dĭs-pĕrs') [L. *dis,* apart, + *spargere,* to scatter]. 1. To scatter, esp. applied to the scattering of light rays. 2. To dissipate or effect the disappearance of, as of a tumor or the particles of a colloidal system.

dispersion (dĭs-pĕr'zhŭn). 1. Act of dispersing. 2. That which is dispersed.

d., coarse. Mechanical suspension.

d., colloidal. Colloid solution.

d., medium. Liquid in which a colloid is dispersed.

d., molecular. A true solution.

dispersoid. A colloid in which the dispersed phase is great.

dispersonalization (dĭs-pĕr"sŏn-ăl-ī-zā'shŭn). Mental state in which the individual denies the existence of his or her personality or parts of the body.

dispireme (dī-spī'rēm) [Gr. *dis,* twice, + *speirema,* coil]. Stage that succeeds the diaster and precedes division of the cell body when threads of the daughter cell are convoluted.

displacement [Fr. *deplacer,* to lay aside]. 1. Removal from the normal or usual position or place. 2. Adding to a fluid one of greater density causing the first fluid to be dispersed. 3. Transference of emotion from the original idea it was associated with to a different idea, thus allowing the patient to avoid acknowledging the original source.

disposition [L. *disponere,* to arrange]. A natural tendency or aptitude exhibited by an individual or group of individuals. This may be manifested toward acquiring a certain disease, presumably due to hereditary factors. SEE: *diathesis.*

disproportion (dĭs"prō-por'shŭn). One entity being of a size different from that considered to be normal.

d., cephalopelvic. In obstetrics, the head of the fetus is larger than the pelvic outlet.

dissect (dĭ-sĕkt', dī-sĕkt') [L. *dissecare,* to cut up]. To separate tissues and parts of a cadaver for anatomical study.

dissection (dĭ-, dī-sĕk'shŭn). The cutting of parts for purpose of separation and studying of the same.

disseminated [L. *dis,* apart, + *seminare,* to sow]. Scattered or distributed over a considerable area, esp. applied to disease organisms; scattered throughout an organ or the body.

disseminated intravascular coagulation. ABBR: DIC. A pathological form of coagulation that is diffuse rather than localized, as would be the case in normal coagulation. The process damages rather than protects the area involved; and several clotting factors are consumed to such extent that generalized bleeding may occur. The disease occurs in association with incomplete abortion, and following certain surgical procedures, esp. those involving the lung, brain, or prostate.

TREATMENT: Treat the primary illness, administer heparin, and provide appropriate therapy including whole blood if necessary.

dissipation (dĭs-ĭ-pā'shŭn) [L. *dissipare,* to scatter]. 1. Dispersion of matter. 2. Act of being wasteful and living a dissolute life, esp. drinking alcoholic beverages to excess.

dissociation (dĭs-sō"sē-ā'shŭn) [L. *dis,* apart, + *sociatio,* union]. Separation, as the separation by heat of a complex compound into simpler molecules.

d., atrioventricular. Dissociation that occurs when independent pacemakers of the atria and ventricles of the heart are not in harmony.

d., microbic. A change in the morphology of a cultured microbial colony due to mutation or selection.

d. of personality. Split in consciousness resulting in two different phases of personality, neither being aware of the words, acts, and feelings of the other. SEE: *dual personality; multiple personality; vigilambulism.*

d., psychological. Disunion of mind (which the person is not aware.

Ex.: dual personalities, fugues, somn/ bulism, selective amnesia.

dissolution [L. *dissolvere,* to dissolve]. 1. [2. Pathological resolution or breakin the integrity of an anatomical entity a

dissolve (dĭ-zŏlv') [L. *dissolvere,* to To cause absorption of a solid in liquid. power

dissolvent (dĭ-zŏl'vĕnt). 1. Havi being to dissolve. 2. That which is ca dissolved. solution.

dissolving. To cause to enter ord or dis-

dissonance (dĭs'ō-năns). 1nds, particu- agreement. 2. Unpleasar larly musical ones. ity of thought,

d., cognitive. Inco philosophy, or actions. re, to be distant].

distad (dĭs'tăd) [L. Away from the cent re, to be distant]. Far-

distal (dĭs'tăl) [L. d r, from a medial line, or thest from the ce Opposed to proximal. In from the trunk stal refers to teeth farther dental usage, of the given arch. from the mid e between two objects.

distance. Sp

d., foc Distance from the optical center of a lens to the focal point.

d., interocclusal. Distance between the occlusal surfaces of opposed teeth when the mandible is at rest.

d., interocular. Distance between two eyes. SEE: *hypertelorism*.

d., target-skin. Distance between the source of radiation and the skin.

distemper (dĭs-tĕm′pĕr). In veterinary medicine, a virus infection of animals.

distend [L. *distendere*, to stretch out]. 1. To stretch out. 2. To become inflated.

distensibility (dĭs-tĕn″sĭ-bĭl′ĭ-tē). The property of being distensible.

distention. The state of being distended.

distichiasis (dĭs″tĭ-kī′ă-sĭs) [Gr. *distichia*, a double row]. Two rows of eyelashes, one or both of which are directed inward toward the eye.

distill (dĭs-tĭl′) [L. *destillare*, to drop from]. Vaporizing by heat and condensing and collecting the volatilized products.

distillate (dĭs′tĭl-āt, dĭs-tĭl′āt). That which has been derived from the distillation process.

distillation. Condensation of a vapor that has been obtained from a liquid heated to the volatilization point, as the condensation of steam from boiling water. Distillation is used for the purification of water and for other purposes. Distilled water should be stored in covered containers because it readily takes up impurities from the atmosphere.

d., destructive. The process of decomposing complex organic compounds by heat in the absence of air and condensing the vapor of the liquid products.

d., dry. Distillation of solids without adding liquids.

d., fractional. Separation of liquids based upon the difference in their boiling points.

…tobuccal (dĭs″tō-bŭk′ăl) [L. *distare*, to be …tant, + *bucca*, cheek]. Pert. to the distal … buccal walls of bicuspid and molar teeth.

…usion (dĭs″tō-kloo′zhŭn). Condition in … the lower teeth meet the upper teeth … he normal position.

Dis…, Distomum (dĭs′tō-mă, -mŭm) [Gr. *dis*, … *stoma*, mouth]. Former name of genus …atode worms. Its members have been pl… many new genera.

distome. …ke with two suckers, an oral and a vent… …cker or acetabulum.

distomia (dī-…ē-ă) [″ + *stoma*, mouth]. Congenitally …ed fetus with two mouths.

distomiasis (dĭs…ī′ă-sĭs). Infestation with flukes that may …t the intestine, liver, bile ducts, gallbladd… …lood vessels, or lungs.

disto-occlusal (dĭs″tō-…oo′zăl). Concerning the distal and occlusal …faces of a tooth.

distortion [L. *dis*, apart, + …rsio, a twisting]. 1. A twisting or bending ou… regular shape. 2. A writhing or twisting mov…ment as of the muscles of the face. 3. A defor…ity in which the part or structure is altered …n shape. 4. In ophthalmology, visual perception of an image that does not provide a true picture. This is due to astigmatism or to retinal abnormalities. 5. In psychiatry, the process of modifying unconscious mental elements so that they can enter consciousness without being censored. 6. In radiology, the difference in size and shape of a radiographic image as compared to the actual part examined.

distractibility. A condition of mental wandering in which the thoughts are attracted by extraneous conditions or influenced by a dissociation of consciousness.

distraction (dĭs-trăk′shŭn) [L. *dis*, apart, + *tractio*, a drawing]. 1. State of mental confusion or derangement. 2. Separation of the surfaces of a joint by extension without injury or dislocation of the parts.

distraught (dĭs-trawt′) [L. *distrahere*, to perplex]. The mental state of being in doubt, deeply troubled, and having conflicting thoughts. Patient may be frantic and have need to be continuously occupied.

distress (dĭs-trĕs′) [L. *distringere*, to draw apart]. Physical or mental trouble or suffering.

distribution [L. *dis*, apart, + *tribuere*, to allot]. 1. The dividing and spreading of anything, esp. blood vessels and nerves, to tissues. 2. The presence of entities at various sites or in particular patterns throughout the body such as hair, fat, or nutrients.

districhiasis (dĭs-trĭk-ī′ă-sĭs) [Gr. *dis*, double, + *thrix*, hair]. Two hairs growing from the same hair follicle.

distrix (dĭs′trĭks). The splitting of ends of the hairs.

disturbance. 1. Interruption of the normal sequence or continuity. 2. A departure from the considered norm.

d., emotional. Mental disorder.

disulfate (dī-sŭl′fāt). A compound containing two sulfate radicals. SEE: *bisulfate*.

disulfiram (dī-sŭl′fĭ-răm). USP. A drug administered orally to treat alcoholism. Trade name is Antabuse.

CAUTION: The reaction to use of alcohol while this drug is being administered may cause such severe reactions as respiratory depression, shock, acute congestive heart failure, myocardial infarction, unconsciousness, convulsions, and sudden death.

disulfiram poisoning. SEE: *Antabuse* in *Poisons and Poisoning* in *Appendix*.

dithiazanine iodide (dī″thī-ăz′ă-nēn). An antihelminthic.

Dittrich's plugs (dĭt′rĭks). [Franz Dittrich, Ger. pathologist, 1815–1859] Small particles in fetid sputum composed of pus, detritus, bacteria, and fat globules.

diurese (dī″ū-rēs′). To cause diuresis.

diuresis (dī″ū-rē′sĭs) [Gr. *diourein*, to urinate]. Secretion and passage of large amounts of urine. This occurs in diabetes mellitus. It can be an early sign of chronic interstitial nephritis. May also be due to hysteria, result of fear and anxiety, ingestion of large quantities of liquids, diabetes insipidus, or the action of drugs that have the ability to cause diuresis. SEE: *diuretic.*

diuretic (dī″ū-rĕt′ĭk). Increasing or an agent that increases the secretion of urine. Diuretics act in two ways: by increasing glomerular filtration or by decreasing reabsorption from the tubules. An increase in blood flow in the renal vessels increases urine formation by increasing glomerular filtration-pressure and by increasing the number of glomeruli functioning. Diuretics act on the kidney cells, increasing permeability, and also on the circulation to the kidneys. Cold applications have a diuretic action by contracting superficial vessels and raising blood pressure. SEE: *diuresis.*

Diuril (dī′ū-rĭl). Trade name for chlorothiazide, a diuretic agent.

diurnal [L. *dies,* day]. 1. Daily. 2. Happening in the daytime or pert. to it. SEE: *nocturnal.*

divagation (dī-vă-gā′shŭn) [L. *divagari,* to wander about]. Disconnected and incoherent speech.

divalent (dī-vā′lĕnt). A molecule with an electric charge of two; bivalent.

divergence (dī-vĕr′jĕns) [L. *divergere,* to turn aside]. Separation from a common center, esp. that of the eyes.

divergent. Radiating in different directions.

diver's paralysis. Occupational disease due to returning too suddenly to normal atmosphere after working under high air pressure. SYN: *bends; caisson disease.*

diverticula (dī″vĕr-tĭk′ū-lă) [L. *devertere,* to turn aside]. Pl. of diverticulum.

diverticulectomy (dī″vĕr-tĭk″ū-lĕk′tō-mē) [″ + Gr. *ektome,* excision]. Surgical removal of a diverticulum.

diverticulitis (dī″vĕr-tĭk″ū-lī′tĭs) [″ + Gr. *itis,* inflammation]. Inflammation of a diverticulum or of diverticula in the intestinal tract, esp. in the colon, causing stagnation of feces in little distended sacs of the colon (diverticula) and pain.

d., acute. SYM: Similar to appendicitis: inflammation of peritoneum, formation of an abscess, and, finally, gangrene accompanied by perforation may ensue.

d., chronic. SYM: Constipation growing worse, mucus in stools, griping abdominal pains at intervals. Wall of bowels may thicken, which may produce chronic intestinal obstruction.

diverticulosis (dī″vĕr-tĭk″ū-lō′sĭs) [″ + Gr. *osis,* condition]. Diverticula in the colon without inflammation or symptoms. Only a small percentage of persons with diverticulosis go on to develop diverticulitis.

diverticulum (dī″vĕr-tĭk′ū-lŭm) [L. *devertere,* to turn aside]. (pl. *diverticula*) A sac or pouch in the walls of a canal or organ. SEE: illus.

d., false. Diverticulum without muscular coats in wall or pouch. This type of diverticulum is acquired.

d., Meckel's. Diverticulum caused by continued existence of the omphalomesenteric duct. Its occurrence is fairly common. Usually located on ileum close to ileocecal valve.

d. of colon. Outpocketing of the colon. These are asymptomatic and cause difficulty when they become inflamed.

d. of duodenum. Diverticulum commonly located near entrance of common and pancreatic ducts.

d. of jejunum. Diverticulum usually marked by severe pain in upper abdomen, followed occasionally by massive hemorrhage from intestine.

d. of stomach. Diverticulum of wall of stomach.

d., true. Diverticula involving all the coats of muscle in the pouch wall. Usually congenital.

diving reflex. Submersion of the face and nose of animals, including man, in water produces a complex cardiovascular reflex that constricts blood flow except to the brain; decreases cardiac output and rate; and produces stable or slightly increased arterial blood pressure. The reflex enables aquatic animals to remain submerged for long periods because it reduces their oxygen requirements. In man, the reflex has been used to treat paroxysmal atrial tachycardia.

division (dĭ-vĭzh′ŭn) [L. *dividere,* to divide]. 1. A separation into parts. 2. That which separates, as anatomical boundary, partition, or wall.

divulsion (dĭ-vŭl′shŭn) [L. *dis,* apart, + *vellere,* to pluck]. Forcibly pulling apart.

divulsor (dĭ-vŭl′sor) [L. *dis,* apart, + *vellere,* to pluck]. Device for dilatation of a part, esp. the urethra.

d., pterygium. Instrument for separating corneal portion of the pterygium.

d., tendon. Device for separating tendon from surrounding tissue.

Dix, Dorothea Lynde. A Massachusetts schoolteacher (1802–1887) who crusaded for prison reform and for care of the menta' 'll. She was responsible for founding m pitals in the U.S., Canada, and s eign countries. During the Ci organized the nursing service armies.

dizygotic twins (dī″zī-gŏt′ *zygon,* yoke]. Twins w two ova. SYN: *frate* *zygotic twins.*

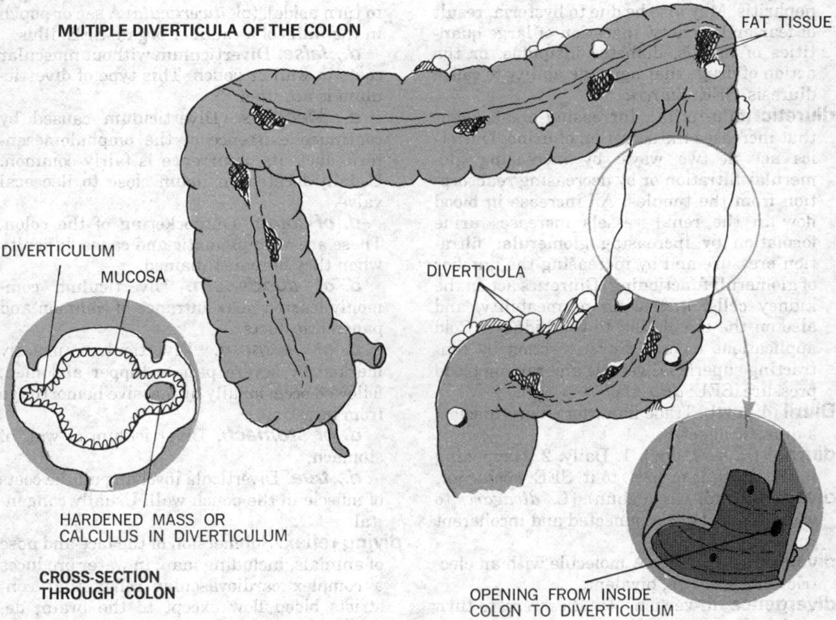

dizziness [AS. *dysig,* foolish]. A sensation of whirling or feeling a tendency to fall. SYN: *giddiness*. SEE: *vertigo.*

dl. *deciliter.*

D.M.D. *Doctor of Dental Medicine.*

DMF Index. The total number of decayed, missing, and filled teeth.

DMSO. *dimethyl sulfoxide,* q.v.

DMT. *dimethyltryptamine,* q.v.

DNA. *deoxyribonucleic acid.*

D.O. *Doctor of Osteopathy.*

DOA. *dead on arrival.*

Dobell's solution (dō'bĕlz). [Horace B. Dobell, Brit. physician, 1828–1917] Carbolic acid, borax, sodium bicarbonate, glycerine, and water in solution.

Dobie's globule (dō'bēz). [William M. Dobie, Brit. physician, 1828–1915] A very tiny spherical body in the light band of a striated muscle fiber.

Doca Acetate. Trade name for desoxycorticosterone acetate.

doctor [L. *docere,* to teach]. 1. The recipient of an advanced degree, such as doctor of medicine (M.D.); doctor of philosophy (Ph.D.); doctor of science (D.Sc.); doctor of science in nursing (D.S.N.); doctor of dental medicine ...M.D.); or doctor of divinity (D.D.). 2. One ... graduating from a medical, veter- ...al school, successfully passes an examination and is licensed by a state government to practice medicine, veterinary medicine, or dentistry.

Because of the great variety of doctoral degrees, the use of the word doctor is sometimes confusing. This may be remedied when writing or speaking of those who possess an M.D. degree by using the word physician.

doctrine (dŏk'trĭn). The system of principles taught or advocated.

docusate calcium (dŏk'ū-sāt). USP. A stool softener. Trade name is Surfak.

docusate sodium. USP. A stool softener. Trade names are Colace, Modane Soft, and Doxinate.

Dodex. Trade name for cyanocobalamin.

dog bite. Lacerated or punctured wound by a dog. The dog should be observed for 10 days to determine the presence of rabies.

CAUTION: The physically handicapped and infants should not be left alone with dogs, esp. large ones. Dogs known to be gentle pets have been known to kill infants living in the same household.

NURSING IMPLICATIONS: Report dog bites to the public health department. Thoroughly cleanse wound, and make sure that the patient receives routine tetanus prophylaxis.

TREATMENT: Immediate and thorough

cleansing of bite wounds with strong soap (20% solution of medicinal soap). Appropriate antirabies therapy if the animal is known to have rabies. SEE: *rabies.*

Döhle's bodies (dē'lēz). [Paul Döhle, Ger. pathologist, 1855–1928] Leukocyte inclusions in the periphery of neutrophils. These are present in association with burns, infections, trauma, and neoplastic diseases.

dol. Symb. for degree of pain intensity registered on the dolorimeter.

Dolene. Trade name for propoxyphene hydrochloride.

dolichocephalic (dŏl"ĭ-kō-sĭ-făl'ĭk) [Gr. *dolichos,* long, + *kephale,* head]. Having a skull with a long anteroposterior diameter.

dolichocolon (dŏl"ĭ-kō-kō'lŏn) [" + *kolon,* colon]. Abnormally long colon.

dolichofacial (dŏl"ĭ-kō-fā'shăl). Pertaining to a long face.

dolichohieric (dŏl"ĭ-kō-hī-ĕr'ĭk) [" + *hieron,* sacred]. Having a long, slender sacrum.

dolichomorphic (dŏl"ĭ-kō-mor'fĭk) [" + *morphe,* form]. Pertaining to a body type that is long and slender. SEE: *ectomorph.*

dolichopellic, dolichopelvic (dŏl"ĭ-kō-pĕl'ĭk, -pĕl'vĭk) [" + *pyelos,* an oblong trough]. Having an abnormally long or narrow pelvis.

dolichosigmoid (dŏl"ĭ-kō-sĭg'moyd) [" + *sigmoeides,* sigmoid]. Having an abnormally long sigmoid flexure of the colon.

dolichuranic (dŏl"ĭk-ū-răn'ĭk) [" + *ouranos,* palate]. Concerning a long alveolar arch of the maxilla.

Dolophine Hydrochloride. Trade name for methadone hydrochloride.

dolor (dō'lor) [L.]. (pl. *dolores*) Pain. One of the principal indications of inflammation. The others are rubor (redness), tumor (swelling), and calor (heat).

dolorific (dō"lor-ĭf'ĭk) [L. *dolor,* pain]. Causing pain.

dolorimeter (dō"lor-ĭm'ĭ-tĕr) [" + Gr. *metron,* measure]. Device for measuring degree of pain.

dolorogenic [" + Gr. *gennan,* to produce]. Causing pain.

domatophobia (dō-măt-ō-fō'bē-ă) [Gr. *doma,* house, + *phobos,* fear]. Abnormal aversion to being in a house; a form of claustrophobia.

domiciliary (dŏm"ĭ-sĭl'ē-ār"ē) [L. *domus,* house]. Pert. to or carried on in a house.

dominance [L. *dominans,* ruling]. 1. Genetic quality through which one of an allelic pair of hereditary factors has the capacity to suppress the expression of the other so that the first prevails in the heterozygote. 2. Often used to refer to the preferred hand or side of the body, as in right-hand dominance.

dominant. In genetics, a trait or characteristic that will be expressed in the offspring even though it is carried on only one of the homologous chromosomes. SEE: *recessive.*

Donath-Landsteiner phenomenon (dō'năth-lănd'stī-nĕr). [Julius Donath, Viennese physician, 1870–1950; Karl Landsteiner, Austrian-born U.S. physician, 1868–1943] A test for paroxysmal hemoglobinuria. Blood from the patient is cooled to 5° C. and a cold hemolysin in the plasma combines with the red blood cells if the patient has the illness. Upon warming, the sensitized red cells are hemolyzed by the complement normally present.

donee (dō-nē') [L. *donare,* to give]. One who receives something, such as a blood transfusion, from a donor.

Donnan's equilibrium (dŏn'ănz). [Frederick G. Donnan, Brit. chemist, 1870–1956] Condition where an equilibrium is established between two solutions separated by a semipermeable membrane so that the sum of the anions and cations on one side is equal to that on the other side.

donor. 1. One who furnishes blood, tissue, or an organ to be used in another person. 2. In chemistry, a compound that frees part of itself to unite with another compound called an acceptor, q.v.

d., universal. One whose blood is of Group O, and whose blood is therefore usually compatible with most other blood types. In actual practice this compatibility rarely occurs because of the many factors other than the major blood antigens (A, B, AB) that determine blood compatibility.

donor card. A document used by a person who wishes to make an anatomical gift, at the time of his or her death, of an organ needed for transplantation. SEE: illus; *transplantation.*

Donovan body. [Charles Donovan, Ir. physician, 1863–1951] The common name for the causative organism, Calymmatobacterium granulomatosis, of granuloma inguinale. SEE: *Donovania granulomatosis.*

Donovania granulomatosis (dŏn-ō-vā'nē-ă). A contagious bacterial disease that is nonfatal, chronic and progressive, autoinoculable, and affects the skin and mucous membrane of the genital and anal area. The initial lesion, a small nodule, vesicle, or papule, slowly spreads and develops into a large granuloma that ulcerates and may form scars. If untreated, there may be extensive destruction of the genital organs. SYN: *donovanosis; granloma inguinale; granuloma venereum.*

ETIOL: Infection with Calymmatobacterium granulomatosis.

TREATMENT: Tetracycline, trimethoprim-sulfamethoxazole, streptomycin, and chloramphenicol are effective.

dopa. A chemical substance, 3,4-dihydroxyphenylalanine, produced by the oxidation of

UNIFORM DONOR CARD

OF ______________________________

Print or type name of donor

In the hope that I may help others, I hereby make this anatomical gift, if medically acceptable, to take effect upon my death. The words and marks below indicate my desires.

I give: (a) _____ any needed organs or parts

(b) _____ only the following organs or parts

____

Specify the organ(s) or part(s)

for the purposes of transplantation, therapy, medical research or education;

(c) _____ my body for anatomical study if needed.

Limitations or special wishes, if any: ______________________________

Signed by the donor and the following two witnesses in the presence of each other:

______________________________ ______________________________

Signature of Donor — Date of Birth of Donor

______________________________ ______________________________

Date Signed — City & State

______________________________ ______________________________

Witness — Witness

This is a legal document under the Uniform Anatomical Gift Act or similar laws.

tyrosine to tyrosinase. It is a precursor of catecholamines and melanin.

dopamine hydrochloride (dō′pă-mēn). A catecholamine synthesized by the adrenal gland. It is the immediate precursor in the synthesis of norepinephrine. Dopamine hydrochloride acts to increase blood pressure, esp. systolic pressure, and to increase urinary output. It is used in the treatment of shock. Trade names are Intropin and Dopastet.

dopaminergic (dō″pă-mēn-ĕr′jĭk). 1. Caused by dopamine. 2. Concerning tissues that are influenced by dopamine.

dopa-oxidase (dō″pă-ŏk′sĭ-dās). Enzyme in some epithelial cells that converts dopa to melanin.

Dopar. Trade name for levodopa.

doping. In athletic medicine, administration of a drug that is designed to improve the competitor's performance. The existence of a drug that safely accomplishes this has not been demonstrated.

Doppler effect (dŏp′lĕr). The apparent frequency of waves, such as sound, varies with change in distance between the source and the receiver. The frequency seems to increase as the distance decreases and to decrease as the distance is increased.

doraphobia (dō″ră-fō′bē-ă) [Gr. *dora,* hide, + *phobos,* fear]. Abnormal aversion to touching the hair or fur of animals.

Dorello's canal. A bony canal in tip of temporal bone enclosing the abducens nerve.

Dorendorf's sign. [Hans Dorendorf, Ger. physician, b. 1866] A filling up or fullness of the supraclavicular groove in aneurysm of the aortic arch.

dornase (dor′nās). Short for deoxyribonuclease.

d., pancreatic. Dornase prepared from beef pancreas. Used to loosen thick pulmonary secretions.

dorsa [L.]. Pl. of dorsum.

dorsabdominal [L. *dorsum,* back, + *abdomen,* belly]. Pert. to the back and abdomen.

dorsad [″ + *ad,* toward]. Toward the back.

dorsal [L. *dorsum,* back]. 1. Pert. to the back. 2. Indicating a position toward a rear part. Opposed to ventral.

dorsal cord stimulation. Procedure for relieving pain by electric stimulation of the spinal cord through electrodes sutured to the posterior spinal cord.

dorsal elevated position. Position where patient is on his or her back with head and shoulders elevated at an angle of 30° or more.

dorsalgia (dōr-săl′jē-ă) [″ + Gr. *algos,* pain]. Pain in the back. SYN: *notalgia; rachialgia.*

dorsal inertia posture. Position in which patient rests on the back and shows a tendency to turn to either side or to slip down in bed if head of bed is elevated. This may be seen in great weakness, acute infectious diseases such as typhoid, mental apathy, and muscular weakness.

dorsalis (dor-sā′lĭs) [L.]. Dorsal, i.e., pertaining to the back.

dorsal nerves. Nerves emerging from the dorsal vertebrae.

dorsal recumbent position. Similar to dorsal elevated position except the extremities are moderately flexed and rotated outward, the soles of the feet rest upon the bed or table, or the legs may be extended. With legs not flexed, this position is used for examination of chest, abdomen, and lower limbs. With legs flexed, it is used in giving douches, for bathing, for catheterizing, and for applying abdominal compresses. The patient may be placed in this position for bimanual palpation or for vaginal examinations and repair of perineal lesions following parturition.

dorsal reflex. Irritation of the skin over the erector spinal muscles, causing contraction of muscles of the back.

dorsal rigid posture. Position in which both legs (or the right one only) are drawn up. Observed in peritonitis, meningitis, ascites, and tympanites. The right leg is drawn up in appendicitis, pelvic inflammation, renal calculus in right ureter, psoas abscess, or peritonitis on the right side.

dorsal slit. A surgical method of making the foreskin of the penis easily retractable. The foreskin is cut in the dorsal midline but not far enough to extend into the mucous membrane next to the glans.

dorsal vertebrae. Twelve bones of the spinal column between the cervical and lumbar vertebrae.

dorsi-, dorso-, dors- [L.]. Combining form indicating back.

dorsiduct [L. *dorsum,* back, + *ducere,* to lead]. To draw toward the back or backward.

dorsiduction. Drawing toward the back.

dorsiflect (dor′sĭ-flĕkt) [″ + *flectere,* to bend]. To bend backward.

dorsiflexion. Movement of a part at a joint so as to bend the part toward the dorsum or posterior aspect of the body. Thus dorsiflexion of the foot indicates movement of the foot backward at the ankle. Dorsiflexion of the toes indicates moving the toes away from the sole of the foot. When the hand is overextended and bent backward, it is dorsiflexed. Opposite of plantar flexion.

dorsimesad (dor″sĭ-mĕs′ăd). In the direction of the dorsimeson.

dorsimeson (dor-sĭ-mĕs′ŏn) [″ + Gr. *meson,* middle]. The median plane of the back.

dorsispinal (dor″sĭ-spī′năl) [″ + *spina,* thorn]. Pert. to the back and spine.

dorsocephalad (dor″sō-sĕf′á-lăd) [″ + Gr

kephale, head, + L. *ad,* toward]. Situated toward the back of the head.

dorsodynia (dor″sō-dĭn′ē-ă) [″ + Gr. *odyne,* pain]. Pain in the muscles of upper part of back.

dorsolateral (dor″sō-lăt′ĕr-ăl). Concerning the back and the side.

dorsosacral [″ + *sacrum,* sacred bone]. Pert. to lower back.

dorsosacral position. Position in which patient is upon the back as in the dorsal recumbent position, q.v., except that thighs are flexed upon abdomen and legs upon thighs, which are abducted. Leg holders are used to support legs in position. Used for gynecological examinations and treatments, in plastic operations of genital tract, in vaginal hysterectomy, and in diagnosis and treatment of diseases of urethra and bladder. SYN: *lithotomy position.* SEE: *position* for illus.

dorsoventral (dor″sō-vĕn′trăl). Concerning the back and frontal surfaces of the body.

dorsum [L.]. (pl. *dorsa*) The back or posterior surface of a part.

dosage [Gr. *dosis,* a giving]. Determination of the amount, frequency, and number of doses of medication or radiation for a patient.

d. calculation for children. There is no absolutely reliable formula for calculating the dose of a medicine an infant or child should receive. Several rules for calculating a child's dose are given here, but those that use body surface area are most accurate.

Young's rule for children:

for children from 1 to 12 years:

Formula:

$$\frac{\text{Age in yr.}}{\text{Age} + 12} \times \text{Adult dose} = \text{Child's dose.}$$

Ex.: The adult dose of a substance is 500 mg. How much should a 4-year-old child receive?

$$\frac{4}{4 + 12} \times 500 = 125$$

The child should receive 125 mg.

Body surface area: The surface area in square meters is divided by 1.7 and multiplied by the adult dose.

Ex.: A child of 0.4 sq. meters of surface area who needs a drug for which the adult dose is 500 mg.:

$$\frac{0.4}{1.7} \times 500 = 117$$

Thus the dose would be 117 mg. Obviously, medicines are not packaged in 117-mg. doses; so either 100 mg. or 125 mg. could be safely given. If the medicine were in liquid form, the dose could be easily determined by using the same formula. SEE: *body surface area.*

dose (dōs) [Gr. *dosis,* a giving]. Amount of a medicinal preparation or of radiation to be administered at one time.

d., absorbed. The dose of ionizing radiation imparted to a tissue or target.

d., air. The intensity of radiation measured in air at the target.

d., bolus. A medicine given intravenously at a controlled but rapid rate.

d., booster. SEE: *booster.*

d., cumulative. 1. Total dose of radiation resulting from repeated exposures. 2. The summation of dose of a drug present in the body after repeated medication. This takes into account the medicine excreted or biotransformed that is, therefore, no longer effective.

d., curative. The dose required to cure an illness or disease.

d., divided. Fractional portions administered at short intervals.

d., erythema. Smallest amount of x-rays that will produce erythema within two weeks following treatment.

d., fatal. The dose that kills. SEE: LD_{50}.

d., infective. The amount of infectious organisms, esp. bacteria and viruses, that will cause disease.

d., lethal. A fatal dose.

d., maintenance. Dose required to maintain the desired effect.

d., maximum. Largest dose it is safe to administer.

d., median curative. Dose that cures the disease in half of the persons treated.

d., median infective. The infective dose that causes disease in half of those given that dose.

d., minimum. Smallest dose that will be effective.

d., skin. Radiation dose to the skin including secondary radiation from backscatter, i.e., radiation reflected from the surroundings.

d., therapeutic. Dose required to produce the desired effect.

d., threshold. SEE: *erythema dose.*

d., tissue tolerance. The largest dose, esp. of radiation, that will not harm tissues.

d., toxic. Dose that causes signs and symptoms of drug toxicity.

dose response curve. A graph in which the degree of the effect of a drug or chemical is charted at specific doses. Connecting these points as the dose is increased produces the curve of response with respect to the dose administered.

dosimeter (dō-sĭm′ĭ-tĕr) [″ + *metron,* measure]. Device for measuring x-ray output.

dosimetric (dō″sĭ-mĕt′rĭk). Pert to dosimetry.

dosimetry (dō-sĭm′ĕt-rē) [″ + *metron,* measure]. Measurement of doses.

dot. A small speck.

d., Trantas. [Alexio Trantas, Gr. ophthalmologist, b. 1867] Chalky concretions in the conjunctiva around the limbus of the eye. Seen in vernal conjunctivitis.

dotage [ME. *doten,* to be silly]. Senility; feeblemindedness of very old age.

double (dŭb'l) [L. *duplus,* twofold]. Combining two things or qualities.

double-blind technique. A method of scientific investigation in which neither the subject nor the investigator working with the subject or analyzing data knows what treatment, if any, the subject is receiving. At the completion of the experiment, the "code" is broken and data are analyzed with respect to the various treatments used. This method attempts to eliminate observer and subject bias.

double consciousness. Expression of two phases of personality.

double personality. A split in consciousness, neither personality being aware of acts and words of other. SEE: *dual personality; multiple personality.*

double touch. Exploration with a finger in one cavity and thumb in another.

double uterus. Dihysteria, q.v. SYN: *uterus didelphys.*

double vision. Seeing two images of an object at the same time. SYN: *diplopia.*

douche (doosh) [Fr.]. A current of vapor or stream of hot or cold water directed against a part. Douches may be made of plain water or medicated. The douche may be for the purpose of personal hygiene or for the treatment of a local condition.

d., air. Air current directed on body for therapeutic purposes. Usually directed to the tympanum for opening the eustachian tube.

d., alternating. D., Scotch.

d., astringent. Douche containing substances such as alum or zinc sulfate for shrinking the mucous membrane.

d., circular. Needle spray or application of water to body through horizontal jets the size of a needle from a number of small rows of sprays so placed that the water is projected against the skin of bather from four directions simultaneously.

d., cleansing. An external or perineal douche for cleansing genitalia following defecation or following operations such as hemorrhoidectomy, curettage, rectal surgery, circumcision, or perineorrhaphy. Mild antiseptic or disinfectant solution, 98° to 104° F. (36.7° to 40° C.), poured or sprayed over the parts, followed by gentle drying and inspection for cleanliness.

d., deodorizing. Douche used to deodorize the vagina and vaginal secretions when they have an offensive odor.

d., high. Douche in which the bag is at least 4 ft. (121.92 cm.) above the hips of the patient.

d., jet. Douche applied to the body in a solid stream from the douche hose.

d., low. Douche in which the bag is 1 to 1½ feet (31 to 46 cm.) above the hips of the patient.

d., medicated. Douche containing a medicinal substance for the treatment of local conditions.

d., neutral. Douche given at average surface temperature of body—90° to 97° F. (32.2° to 36.1° C.).

d., perineal. Spray projected upward from a bidet, q.v., placed just above the floor; patient sits on the seat of the bidet and receives douche upon perineum.

d., Scotch. Douche consisting of alternating hot and cold jets of water against local area of skin.

d., vaginal. Douche of vagina used for deodorant, antiseptic, stimulating, or hemostatic purposes. Temperature of solutions: antiseptic or deodorant douche, 105° to 112° F. (40.6° to 44.4° C.); stimulating or hemostatic douche, 118° to 120° F. (47.8° to 48.9° C.). Solution should flow slowly with little pressure, the douche solution container being elevated up to two feet (61 cm.) above patient's pelvis. Quantity generally 2 to 3 qt. (2 or 3 L.) of solution unless otherwise ordered.

NOTE: The vagina, like many other areas of the body, has the ability to cleanse itself. Thus there is very little reason for a normal, healthy woman to use a vaginal douche. Douching can upset the balance of the vaginal flora and change vaginal pH, thus predisposing the woman to vaginitis. There is no evidence that a postcoital vaginal douche is effective as a contraceptive.

Douglas' cul-de-sac, pouch. [James Douglas, Scot. anatomist, 1675–1742] Peritoneal sac that lies behind uterus and in front of rectum.

Douglas' fold. The arcuate line of the sheath of the rectus abdominalis muscle.

douglasitis (dŭg-lăs-ī'tĭs). Inflammation of the cul-de-sac of Douglas.

dowel [ME. *dowle,* peg]. Metal pin for fastening an artificial crown to a tooth root.

down. 1. Lanugo, the fine hairs of the skin of the newborn. 2. The fine soft feathers of the young of some birds; and the small feathers underneath the large feathers of adult birds, particularly waterfowl. Used in clothing to protect from the cold.

Down's syndrome. [J. Langdon Down, Brit. physician, 1828–1896] Preferred term for mongolism, a variety of congenital moderate-to-severe mental retardation. Marked by sloping forehead, small ear canals, presence of epicanthal folds causing an Oriental appearance of eyes, gray or very light yellow spots at periphery of iris (Brushfield's spots), short broad hand with a single palmar crease (simian crease), a flat nose or absent bridge, low-set ears, and generally dwarfed physique. SYN: *trisomy 21; trisomy* G.

Women who are at high risk of giving birth to a child with Down's syndrome are those over 40; those who have had a previous child with the syndrome; and those who themselves have Down's syndrome (pregnancy is rare in this condition). In addition, there is a high risk of having a child with Down's syndrome when there is parental mosaicism with a 21 trisomic cell population.

Down's syndrome may be diagnosed antenatally by use of several techniques. SEE: *amniocentesis*.

ETIOL: Patients with Down's syndrome have an extra chromosome, usually number 21 or 22.

doxapram hydrochloride (dŏk'să-prăm). USP. A respiratory stimulant. Trade name is Dopram.

Doxinate. Trade name for docusate sodium.

doxorubicin hydrochloride (dŏk″sō-rū'bĭ-sĭn). USP. An antineoplastic antibiotic agent. Trade name is Adriamycin.

doxycycline (dŏk″sē-sī'klēn). USP. A broad-spectrum antibiotic of the tetracycline group. Trade name is Vibramycin.

doxylamine succinate (dŏk-sĭl'ă-mēn). USP. An antihistamine. Trade names are Decapryn Succinate and Unisom.

Doyère's eminence (dwă-yārz'). [Louis Doyère, Fr. physiologist, 1811–1863] Elevation where a nerve filament enters a muscle.

D.P. *Doctor of Pharmacy; Doctor of Podiatry.*

D.P.H. *Diploma in Public Health.*

D.P.T. Vaccine for diphtheria, pertussis, and tetanus. Used in the immunization program for infants and children.

DR. *reaction of degeneration.*

dr. *drachm; dram.*

drachm (drăm) [Gr. *drachme,* a Gr. unit of weight]. ABBR: dr. A unit of weight in apothecaries' system. SYMB: ʒ. SYN: *dram,* q.v.

dracontiasis (drăk″ŏn-tī'ă-sĭs) [Gr. *drakontion,* little dragon]. Dracunculiasis.

dracunculiasis (dră-kŭng″kū-lī'ă-sĭs). Infestation with the nematode Dracunculus medinensis.

dracunculosis (dră-kŭng″kū-lō'sĭs). Dracunculiasis.

Dracunculus (dră-kŭng'kū-lŭs). A genus of parasitic nematodes.

D. medinensis. The guinea worm or "fiery serpent." A species of nematode that is a common human parasite, esp. in Africa and India. Infection of the human occurs when water containing infected crustacea of the genus Cyclops is swallowed. The larvae are liberated in the stomach or duodenum, then migrate through the viscera and become adults. The adult female after mating burrows under the skin of the leg. Larvae are discharged into environment through the ulcer caused by the worm, esp. when legs are in water. The infection may be prevented by boiling suspect water, or by treating it with chlorine, or by filtering it to remove the infected Cyclops.

TREATMENT: The head of the adult worm can be seen in the ulcer. Slow traction on the worm will remove it. Use of thiabendazole or niridazole is also effective.

draft, draught. A dose of liquid medicine intended to be taken in a single dose.

drag. Street language for clothing of one sex worn by a person, often a homosexual, of the opposite sex.

drain (drān) [AS. *dreahnian,* to draw off]. 1. Exit or tube for discharge of a morbid matter. 2. To draw off a fluid.

d., capillary. Drawing off by capillary attraction.

d., cigarette. Drain made by covering a small strip of gauze with rubber.

d., Mikulicz's. Single layer of gauze pushed into the wound cavity, to which is added thick gauze wicks that project from the cavity.

d., nonabsorbable. Drain made from horsehair, gauze, rubber, glass, or metal. Types are abdominal, antrum, perineal, and suprapubic.

d., Penrose. A cigarette drain made with a piece of small rubber tubing through which gauze has been pulled.

drainage (drān'ĭj). The free flow or withdrawal of fluids from a wound or cavity, as pus from a cavity or wound. SEE: *autodrainage; drain.*

d., capillary. Drainage by method of capillary attraction.

d., closed. Drainage of a wound or body space so that the air is excluded.

d., closed sterile. A sterile tube draining a body site such as the abdominal cavity or pleural space that is designed to prevent the entry of air and bacteria into the tubing or the area being drained.

d., funnel. Drainage with glass funnels.

d., negative pressure. Drainage in which negative pressure is maintained in the tube. Used in treating pneumothorax and in certain types of drains or catheters in the intestinal tract.

d., open. Drainage of a wound or body cavity so that air is not excluded from the area of the cavity.

d., postural. Drainage for the nasal area, bronchi, and sinuses. The patient is placed in a position in which gravity will allow drainage. SEE: *postural drainage* for illus.

d., suction. SEE: *d., negative pressure.*

d., tidal. A method, controlled mechanically, of filling the bladder with solution by gravity and periodically emptying the bladder by siphonage. Usually used when the patient lacks control of the bladder as in injuries or lesions of the spinal cord.

drainage tube. Device for allowing escape of pus, serum, blood, or other fluids from a wound or abscess.

drained weight. The actual weight of food that has been allowed to drain in order to remove the liquids in which it has been prepared.

dram [Gr. *drachme*]. ABBR: dr. A unit of weight in apothecaries' system. SYMB: ʒ. SYN: *drachm.*

d., fluid. A teaspoonful or ⅛ of a fluid ounce or 57.1 gr. of distilled water, the equivalent of 3.7 ml. In Great Britain, 54.8 gr. of distilled water or 3.5 ml.

Dramamine (drăm′ă-mēn). Trade name for dimenhydrinate, the chlorotheophylline salt of the antihistaminic agent diphenhydramine. Dramamine has a depressant effect on hyperstimulated labryinthine function, and is used to treat or prevent nausea, vomiting, vertigo, and motion sickness.

dramatism [Gr. *drama,* acting, + *-ismos,* state of]. Dramatic behavior and lofty speech seen in psychological disturbances.

drapetomania (drăp″ĕt-ō-mā′nē-ă) [Gr. *drapetes,* runaway, + *mania,* madness]. Insane impulse to wander from home.

drastic [Gr. *drastikos,* effective]. 1. Acting strongly. 2. A very active cathartic, usually producing many explosive bowel movements accompanied by pain and tenesmus. The use of this type of cathartic is not advisable.

draught (drăft) [ME. *draught,* a pulling]. 1. A drink. 2. Drawing liquid into the mouth. 3. Breeze produced by wind or fan. 4. A liquid medicinal dose to be taken all at once.

drawer sign. Sign diagnostic of rupture of the cruciate ligament(s) of the knee. The knee is flexed to a right angle and the examiner attempts to pull the lower leg away from the patient, pulling parallel to the long axis of the upper leg. There will be an increased glide, anterior or posterior of the tibia, if rupture is present of the anterior or posterior cruciate ligament respectively.

draw sheet. Historically, the term draw sheet was given to a long roll or bolt of muslin that was stretched across the width of the bed with the free end initially placed under the patient's buttocks. When this became soiled, it was drawn from under the patient and rolled up on the opposite side of the cot or bed, allowing the patient to lie on a clean section of the roll of muslin.

The draw sheet is used to protect the bottom sheet and mattress from drainage and soilage, and it is easier to change, for both the patient and nurse, than the entire bed. When a draw sheet is folded and placed under a patient to use for lifting and turning, it is called a lift sheet. In many hospitals, draw sheets have been replaced by paper and plastic pads that resemble disposable diapers.

dream [AS. *dream,* joy]. Occurrence of ideas, emotions, and sensations during sleep. Some dreams may be recalled upon awakening, others may not be. SEE: *R.E.M.; sleep.*

drench. A dose of medicine that is administered to an animal by pouring into its mouth.

drepanocyte (drĕp′ă-nō-sīt) [Gr. *drepane,* sickle, + *kytos,* cell]. Sickle or crescent cell.

drepanocytemia (drĕp″ă-nō-sī-tē′mē-ă) [″ + ″ + *haima,* blood]. Sickle-cell anemia.

drepanocytic (drĕp″ă-nō-sĭt′ĭk). Pert. to or resembling a sickle cell.

dressing [O. Fr. *dresser,* to prepare]. Covering, protective or supportive, for diseased or injured parts.

NURSING IMPLICATIONS: Assemble needed equipment and wash hands thoroughly. Follow strict aseptic technique during dressing changes. Dispose of discarded dressings properly. Wash hands following the procedure. Carefully note the presence of any drainage on the dressing or around the incision. Also note the condition of the suture line for presence of any erythema or edema.

RS: bandage; compress.

d., absorbent. Gauze, sterilized gauze, absorbent cotton.

d., antiseptic. Dressing consisting of gauze permeated with an antiseptic solution.

d., dry. Dressing consisting of dry gauze, absorbent cotton, or other dry material.

d., fixed. Dressing permeated with starch, silicate of soda, or plaster of Paris. When this dressing dries, it provides fixation of the part so treated.

d., hot moist. The most common form is a hot normal saline solution, as hot as can be borne by the bare forearm of the nurse. The sterile towel is unfolded and the gauze dressing is dropped into it. Then immerse the center of the towel in solution and wring out by turning the dry ends in opposite directions. The dressing is applied with sterile forceps directly to the wound. Sometimes a dry sterile towel is used over it to keep the dressing in place. Heat is best maintained by infrared lamp.

CAUTION: Do not burn the patient.

d., non-adherent. Dressing that has little or no tendency to adhere to dried secretions from the wound.

d., occlusive. Dressing that seals a wound completely to prevent infection from

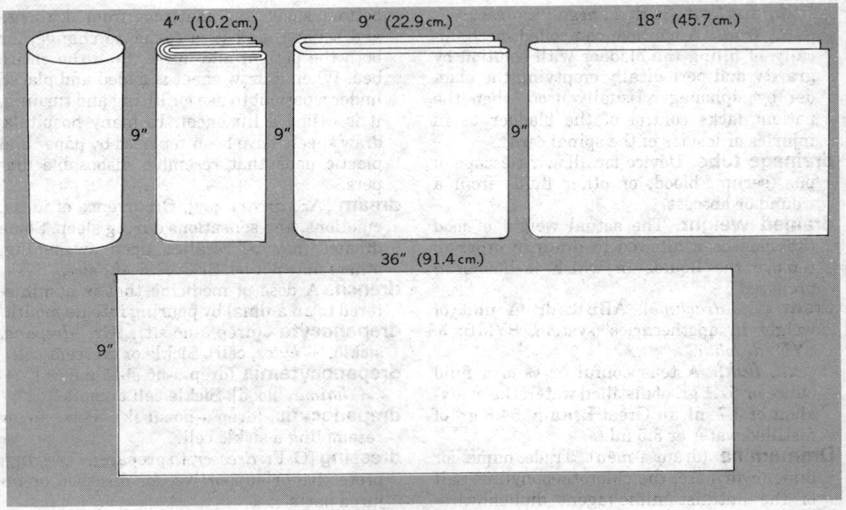

UNIVERSAL DRESSING

A universal dressing may easily be made by beginning with 9 × 36 in. (22.9 × 91.4 cm.) absorbent gauze several layers thick. This is folded across three times and finally rolled. It is then placed in a suitable container and sterilized. When needed, it may be used as a roll, as a 9 × 4 in. (22.9 × 10.2 cm.) flat bandage, as a 9 in. (22.9 cm.) square bandage, or as a 9 × 28 in. (22.9 × 45.7 cm.) dressing. Completely unfolded, it is suitable as a large burn dressing; folded, it may be used as a cervical collar.

without and to prevent moisture from within from escaping through the dressing.

d., pressure. Dressing that is used to apply pressure to the wound. May be used following skin grafting.

d., protective. Dressing applied for the purpose of preventing injury or infection to the part so treated.

d., universal. A large flat bandage that may be folded several times to make a relatively large dressing or folded several more times to make a smaller and thicker bandage. This process can be continued until the unit is suitable for use as a cervical collar. The bandage is easily made and stored. SEE: illus.

d., water. Dressing consisting of gauze, cotton, or similar dressing material that is kept wet by the application of sterilized water.

drill. Device for rotating a sharp and shaped cutting instrument. Used for preparing teeth for restoration and in orthopedics.

Drinker respirator. [Philip Drinker, U.S. engineer in industrial hygiene, 1894–1972] Apparatus in which alternating positive and negative air pressure upon the patient's thoracic area, by allowing the air in the otherwise immobile lung to be alternately filled with air and emptied, acts to produce artificial respiration. Commonly called the iron lung.

drip [ME. *drippen*, to drip]. 1. To fall in drops. 2. To instill a liquid slowly, drop by drop.

d., intravenous. Slow injection of a suitable solution a drop at a time, intravenously.

d., Murphy. Slow rectal instillation of a fluid drop by drop.

d., nasal. Method of administering fluid slowly to dehydrated babies by means of a catheter with one end placed through the nose into the esophagus.

d., postnasal. A condition due to chronic sinusitis in which a discharge flows from the postnasal region into the pharynx.

drive (drīv) [AS. *drifan*]. The force or impulse to act.

Drolban. Trade name for dromostanolone propionate.

dromomania (drō″mō-mā′nē-ă) [Gr. *dromos*, a running, + *mania*, madness]. Insane impulse to wander.

dromostanolone propionate (drō″mō-stăn′ō-lōn). USP. An antineoplastic drug. Trade name is Drolban.

dromotropic [″ + *tropikos*, a turning]. Pert.

to supposed fibers in cardiac nerves that influence conductivity of muscles.

drop [AS. *dropa*]. 1. A minute spherical mass of liquid. 2. Failure of a part to maintain its normal position. Usually due to paralysis or injury.

d., culture. A bacterial culture in a drop of culture medium.

d.'s, ear. Medication administered by drops placed in the external canal of the ear.

d.'s, eye. Medication placed in conjunctival sac.

d., foot. Condition in which toes drag and foot hangs, caused by paralysis of the anterior tibial muscles.

d., hanging. Application of a drop of solution to a small glass coverslip. This is then inverted over a glass slide with a depression in it. The contents of the suspended solution can be examined microscopically.

d.'s, nose. Medication instilled in or sprayed into the nasal cavity.

d. wrist. Paralysis of extensor muscles causing hand to hang down from forearm.

droperidol (drō-pĕr'ĭ-dŏl). USP. A drug used for premedication for surgery. It is neuroleptic, sedative, and tranquilizing. Trade name is Inapsine.

droplet. Very small drop.

droplet infection. Infection conveyed by means of infective particles, as when carried in a spray from the nose or mouth. Usual mode of infection for common cold.

dropper. A tube, usually narrowed at one end for dispensing drops of liquid. If water is so dispensed, about 20 drops will equal one milliliter. SEE: *d., medicine*.

d., medicine. According to USP XX, a medicine dropper consists of a tube made of glass or other suitable transparent material that generally is fitted with a collapsible bulb and, while varying in capacity, is constricted at the delivery end to a round opening having an external diameter of 3 mm. The dropper, when held vertically, delivers water in drops each of which weighs between 45 mg. and 55 mg.

In using a medicine dropper, one should keep in mind that few medicinal liquids have the same surface and flow characteristics as water, and therefore the size of drops varies materially from one preparation to another.

Where accuracy of dosage is important, a dropper that has been calibrated esp. for the preparation with which it is supplied should be employed. The volume error incurred in measuring any liquid by means of a calibrated dropper should not exceed 15%, under normal use conditions.

dropsy (drŏp'sē) [Gr. *hydor*, water]. Obsolete term for generalized edema.

Drosophila (drō-sŏf'ĭ-lă). A genus of flies belonging to the order Diptera. Includes the common fruit flies.

D. melanogaster. A genus of fruit flies used extensively in the study of genetics. The development of the chromosome theory of heredity was largely the outcome of research on this species.

drowning [ME. *dr(o)unen*, to drown]. Asphyxiation due to immersion in liquid. This may also result from a spasm of the glottis, which allows neither air nor water to pass into the lungs (dry drowning). An acute asphyxial reaction to ingested water or liquid followed by laryngeal relaxation and flooding of the respiratory tract with water is another mechanism of drowning (wet drowning). Drowning can occasionally result from vagally induced cardiac arrest after immersion in extremely cold water.

NOTE: Delayed death due to hypoxia can occur 15 min. to 3 days after immersion. It is imperative that resuscitated patients be kept in the hospital for observation until this possibility can be excluded.

SYM: Unconsciousness, cessation of respiration, cyanosis, depending upon duration of submersion. Due to action of the epiglottis, there is very little, if any, water in the lung.

F.A.: Artificial respiration at once. Do not waste time trying to get water out of lungs. If available, use oxygen or oxygen–carbon dioxide mixtures with resuscitation. May have to be kept up for several hours. Cardiac resuscitation may also be required. SEE: *drownproofing*.

NOTE: Prolonged immersion does not necessarily mean that resuscitation will result in a brain-damaged individual. This is esp. true if the individual has been immersed in very cold water.

RS: artificial respiration; asphyxia; shock; syncope; unconsciousness.

drownproofing. A method of staying afloat by using a minimum amount of energy. May be kept up for hours even by nonswimmers, whereas only the most fit and expert of swimmers could stay afloat for more than 30 minutes. Details of the drownproofing technique may be obtained from local chapters of the American Red Cross. SEE: illus.

TECHNIQUE: 1. *Rest:* Take a deep breath and sink vertically beneath the surface, relax your arms and legs, keep chin down and allow fingertips to brush against knees. Keep neck relaxed and back of head above the surface. 2. *Get set:* Gently raise arms to a crossed position with back of wrists touching forehead. At the same time step forward with one leg and backward with the other. 3. *Lift head, exhale:* Without moving your arms and legs from the previous position, raise your

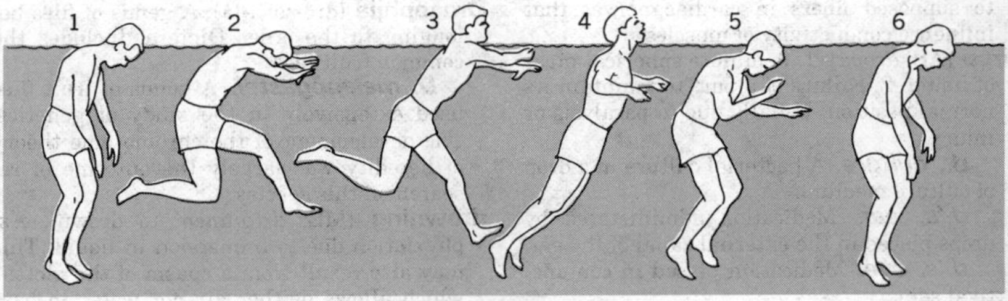

DROWNPROOFING TECHNIQUE

1, Rest. 2, Get set. 3, Lift head, exhale. 4, Stroke and kick, inhale. 5, Head down, press. 6, Rest.

head quickly but smoothly to the vertical and exhale through your nose. 4. *Stroke and kick, inhale:* To support your head above the surface while you inhale through your mouth, gently sweep the arms outward and downward and step downward with both feet. 5. *Head down, press:* As you drop beneath the surface, put your head down and press downward with your arms and hands to arrest your descent. 6. *Rest:* Important to relax completely as in the first step for six to ten seconds.

Dr.P.H. *Doctor of Public Health.*

drug [O. Fr. *drogue,* chemical material]. Any substance that when taken into the living organism may modify one or more of its functions.

drug abuse. The use or overuse, usually by self-administration, of any drug in a manner that deviates from the prescribed pattern.

drug action. Function of a drug in various body systems.

Local: When the drug is applied locally or directly to a tissue or organ, it may combine with the cells' albumin to form an albuminate. This action may be (1) astringent when the drug cannot act because the albuminate does not dissolve, (2) corrosive when the drug is strong enough to destroy cells, or (3) irritating when too much of the drug combines with cells to impair them.

General or systemic action: This occurs when the drug enters the bloodstream by absorption or direct injection, affecting tissues and organs not near the site of entry. Systemic action may be (1) Specific when specific in the cure of a certain disease; (2) Substitutive or replacement when it supplies substances deficient in the body; (3) Physical when some of the constituents of a cell are dissolved by the action of the drug in the bloodstream; (4) Chemical when the drug or some of its principles combine with the constituents of cells or organs to form a new chemical combination; (5) Salt action by osmosis, q.v., caused by dilution of salt (also acids, sugars, and alkalies) in the stomach or intestines by fluid withdrawn from the blood and tissues, or by diffusion, q.v., when water is absorbed by cells from the lymph; (6) Selective, action produced by drugs that only affect certain tissues or organs; (7) Synergistic, the stimulating of the action of one drug by another drug; (8) Antagonistic, counteraction of one drug by another; (9) Physiological, the effect of a drug similar to that which the body normally produces; (10) Therapeutic, the effect upon diseased organs or tissues; (11) Side action, creating an effect not primarily desired; (12) Empiric, an effect produced but not proved by clinical or laboratory tests to be effective; (13) Toxicological, a toxic or undesired effect generally from result of an overdose or long-term usage.

Cumulative: The effect of drugs that are slowly excreted or absorbed so that with repeated doses an accumulation of the drug in the body produces a toxic effect. Such drugs should not be administered continuously.

Incompatible: Ill effects produced by two or more drugs antagonistic to each other. SEE: *Drug Interactions* in *Appendix*.

RS: active principle; antidote; biotransformation; dosage; dose response curve; double-blind test; names of individual drugs; names of poisons; prescription writing.

drug addiction. A condition caused by excessive or continued use of habit-forming drugs. Illicit drugs may or may not contain the kind and amount of drug the user thought was purchased. For this reason a user may have a serious reaction (even death) to the unknown substance present in the material.

SYM: The symptom pattern may be changed according to the drug used. In general there may be a change in personality, loss of appetite, dulled appetite, disturbance in normal sleep-rhythm, generally a weight loss. The addict may be dull, sleepy, and incoordinated in movement, having the appearance of intoxication. The eyes often tearing and bloodshot; a watery fluid at times dripping from the nose. When intramuscular or intravenous injection is used there may be scars, hardening and swelling of the arm tissues. Serum hepatitis may occur when narcotic addicts use dirty needles and syringes for administering drugs to themselves or fellow addicts. SEE: *hepatitis*.

drug administration. *Acids:* When acids are administered orally they should be given well diluted through a glass tube or by stomach tube because they are corrosive to the enamel and dentin of the teeth. They should be given with much water and the drinking tube should be placed well back in the mouth to prevent the fluid coming in contact with the teeth before passing into the throat. Hydrochloric acid is one preparation that should always be given using this technique.

Habit-forming drugs: These should be given as ordered by the physician.

Horse serum: When injections containing it are administered, information should be obtained as to whether the patient has ever received horse serum and what reaction there was at that time to it. If the patient is allergic to horse serum, a test for sensitivity should always be done by injecting a few drops of the greatly diluted material containing horse serum hypodermically, and within a short time a reaction will occur. A small spot appears at the site of the injection if the patient has a tendency toward an unfavorable reaction. The physician will provide instructions for desensitizing a person allergic to horse serum.

Insulin: When this is administered, it should be given hypodermically or intravenously according to the instructions of the attending physician. The type of insulin, dosage, and frequency of dosage vary greatly with each patient.

Laxatives: These are best given in the evening because it usually takes 6 or 8 hours for them to produce an effect. Saline purgatives are usually given well diluted on an empty stomach in the morning. Other purgatives usually are given as ordered and needed.

Mouthwash: Stock solutions used for mouthwash should be diluted one half or more before being given to the patient. Only enough for the immediate mouth washing should be given to the patient at a particular time.

Oxygen: The most commonly used method for administration of oxygen consists of inserting a catheter into a nostril or into each nostril. Oxygen may also be given from a tank by means of a mask over the patient's nose and mouth, or the patient may be placed in an oxygen tent, an oxygen chamber, or room. The last two methods are not only expensive but also extremely dangerous and must be used cautiously, as the danger from fire hazard is very great. Oxygen given by catheter should be hydrated by bubbling through water prior to passage into the nose. Dry oxygen will cause severe irritation of the nasal and respiratory mucosa.

Saline purgatives: Should always be given to the patient when the stomach is empty, preferably in the morning.

Sleeping pills: All such preparations should be given from one-half to one hour before sleep is desired. All procedures should be taken care of before the medicament is given in order that nothing shall disturb the patient after the drug is administered.

Vaccines: If the vaccines are alum-precipitated or alumina absorbed, the preferred route of administration is intramuscular. Typhoid booster injections are given intracutaneously, and all other fluid preparations are given subcutaneously.

drug dependence. A psychic (and sometimes physical) state resulting from interaction of a living organism and a drug. Characterized by behavioral and other responses that include a compulsion to take the drug on a continuous or periodic basis in order to experience its psychic effects or to avoid the discomfort of its absence. Tolerance may or may not be present and a person may be dependent on more than one drug.

drug eruption. Dermatitis medicamentosa.

drug-fast. Resistance, as of bacteria, to action of a drug or drugs.

drug fever. Fever caused by the administration of a drug. Almost any drug has the ability to produce in some individuals this undesired side-effect.

druggist (drŭg'ĭst). Pharmacist.

drug handling. Carefully read the label or other printed instruction issued with medicine. Measure the ordered doses (quantities) accurately and never guess. A measuring glass or spoon should be used, marked in milliliters, ounces, or both. When giving a dose of medicine, be sure to whom it has to be given, what has to be given, when it has to be given, and the amount to be given. Do not leave the bedside until you see the patient actually swallow medicines intended to be taken orally.

NOTE: The cover must never be left off the container because a necessary property may evaporate, the drug may become dangerously concentrated, or the medicine may absorb moisture from the air and become difficult to handle or dilute. The drug storage compart-

Comparison of Toxic and Allergic Drug Reactions

Differences may be indistinct. Shock from drug overdose may be no different from allergic shock.

	Toxic	Allergic
Incidence	May occur with any drug	Occurs infrequently
Dosage	Usually high	Therapeutic
Reaction time	May occur with first dose, or may be due to cumulative effect	Usually only upon re-exposure, but some drugs cross-react with chemicals of similar structure
Symptoms	May be similar to pharmacological action of drug	Not related to pharmacological action of drug
Associated disorders	None	Asthma, hay fever

ment must be kept locked.

drug interaction. The pharmacological interaction of drugs taken concurrently. The result may be antagonism, synergism, or may be lethal in some cases. It is important for the patient and physician to be aware of the potential interaction of drugs that are prescribed as well as those that the patient may be self-administering. SEE: *Drug Interactions* in *Appendix*.

drug rashes. Rashes produced in some patients by application or ingestion of drugs. In general, drug rashes are not specific for certain drugs. Therefore the following should be used only as a rough guide.

Antibiotics: erythema. *Antipyrine:* papular, erythematous rash, sometimes accompanied by edema and much irritation. *Arsenic:* papular or erythematous rash, sometimes urticarial. Prolonged use may produce pigmentation of skin. *Belladonna:* erythematous rash, usually accompanied by intense itching. *Bromides:* usually like acne vulgaris; sometimes erythema. *Chloral:* papular erythema. *Iodides:* usually papular erythema, sometimes with acnelike pustules. *Phenolphthalein:* macular rash, sometimes purpuric. *Quinine:* very irritable erythema or urticaria. *Salicylate:* erythematous rash, possibly morbilliform.

drug reaction. Adverse and undesired reaction to a substance taken for its pharmacological effects. An estimated 15% of hospitalized patients will develop toxic or allergic drug reactions. SEE: table.

drug receptors. The part or parts of a cell that interact with a drug or drugs. The proteins in cells in the form of enzymes are the most important class of drug receptors. Chemotherapeutic agents used in treating malignancies react with nucleic acid receptors. Some anesthetic agents react with lipid receptors on the cell membrane.

drugs, words pert. to: ampule; analeptic; analgesic; anesthetic; antacid; anthelmintic; antiarthritic; antidiuretic; antiemetic; antipyretic; antiseptic; antispasmodic; carminative; cathartic; convulsant; decoction; demulcent; depressant; diaphoretic; digestant; diuretic; ecbolic; elixir; emetic; expectorant; ferment; glucoside; half-life; hematinic; hemostatic; hormone; hypnotics; laxative; Medic Alert; medicine; oil; ointment; oxytocic; pharmacology; pharmacopeia; pill; purgative; rubefacient; sedative; solution; stimulant; synergism; tablet; tincture; tonic; troche; vaccine; vasoconstrictor; vasodilator; vermicide.

drum. The ear drum of tympanic cavity; the tympanum or cavity of the middle ear.

drunkenness [AS. *drinean,* to drink]. Alcoholic intoxication. In legal medicine, intoxication or being "under-the-influence" of alcohol is defined according to the concentration of alcohol in the blood or exhaled air. The precise concentration used to define legal intoxication varies between states. Clinically, a blood level of 0.3% to 0.4% of ethyl alcohol is classed as marked intoxication. A level of 0.4% to 0.5% is consistent with alcoholic stupor, and a level over 0.5% is sufficient to cause alcoholic coma.

drusen (droo′zĕn) [Ger. *Druse,* weathered ore]. Small, hyaline, globular pathological growths formed on optic papilla or on Descemet's membrane.

dry eye. In certain conditions there is insufficient lubrication in the eye and the conjunctiva becomes much less moist than normal. This produces pain and discomfort in the eyes. This may occur in any condition that causes scars of the cornea, such as erythema multiforme, trachoma, or corneal burns; Sjögren's syndrome; lagophthalmos; Riley-Day syndrome; absence of lacrimal gland; paralysis of the facial or trigeminal nerves; medication with atropine; deep anesthesia; and debilitating diseases. Suitable prepared water-soluble polymers are effective in treating this condition.

dry ice. Solidified carbon dioxide used for commercial refrigeration. Also used in the form of a pencil-shaped block for treating certain skin lesions such as warts by freezing. The temperature of solid carbon dioxide is −78.5° C. For this reason it is extremely important to use thick cloth gloves when handling it. Momentary skin contact with dry ice can cause severe frostbite and blisters.

dry measure. A measure of volume for dry commodities. SEE: *Weights and Measures* in *Appendix*.

Drysdale's corpuscles (drīz'dālz). [Thomas M. Drysdale, U.S. gynecologist, 1831–1904] Non-nucleated granular cells present in the fluid of certain ovarian cysts.

DTIC-Dome. Trade name for dacarbazine.

dt's. *delirium tremens.*

dualism (dū'ă-lĭzm) [L. *duo,* two, + Gr. *-ismos,* condition]. 1. The condition of being double or twofold. 2. The theory that the human individual consists of two entities, mind and matter, that are independent of each other. 3. The theory that various blood cells arise from two types of stem cells: myeloblasts giving rise to the myeloid elements, and lymphoblasts giving rise to the lymphoid elements.

dual personality. A form of multiple personality seen in hysteria and schizophrenia that results in the expression of two different phases of personality at various intervals, neither personality as a rule being aware of the words, acts, and feelings of the other. When this occurs in schizophrenia the individual psychic function is split off from the personality as a whole and becomes autonomous. This may be unrelated to and contradictory of the main personality. SEE: *dissociation of personality; multiple personality; vigilambulism.*

duazomycin (dū-ăz"ō-mī'sĭn). An antineoplastic agent.

Dubini's disease (dū-bē'nēz). [Angelo Dubini, It. physician, 1813–1902] Rapid rhythmic contractions of a group or groups of muscles. SYN: *chorea, electric; spasmus Dubini.*

Dubin-Johnson syndrome. [Isadore Dubin, U.S. pathologist, b. 1913; F. B. Johnson, contemporary U.S. physician] Inherited defect of bile metabolism that causes retention of conjugated bilirubin in hepatic cells. The patient is mildly jaundiced.

duboisine (dū-bŏy'sēn). Alkaloid derivative of plant Duboisea myoporoides. It is a form of hyoscyamine used as a mydriatic.

Dubowitz tool or score. [Lilly and Victor Dubowitz, contemporary physicians] A method of estimating the gestational age of an infant based on 21 strictly defined clinical signs. This method provides the correct gestational age ± 2 weeks in 95% of infants.

Duchenne, Guillaume B. A. (dū-shĕn'). French neurologist, 1806–1875.

D.'s disease. Degeneration of the posterior roots and column of the spinal cord and of the brain stem. Characterized by attacks of pain, progressive ataxia, loss of reflexes, functional disorders of the bladder, larynx, and gastrointestinal system, and impotence. Develops in conjunction with syphilis and most frequently affects middle-aged males. SYN: *tabes dorsalis.*

D.'s muscular dystrophy. Pseudohypertrophic muscular dystrophy characterized by weakness and pseudohypertrophy of the affected muscles. The disease begins in childhood, is progressive, and affects the shoulder and pelvic girdle muscles. The disease, mostly of males, is transmitted as a sex-linked recessive trait. Death usually occurs at an early age.

D.'s paralysis. Bulbar paralysis.

Duchenne-Aran disease (dū-shĕn'ăr-ăn'). [Duchenne; F. A. Aran, Fr. physician, 1817–1861] Progressive spinal muscular atrophy, characterized by chronic progressive wasting of muscles with subsequent weakness and paralysis. The upper extremity is most commonly involved. Caused by degeneration of the anterior horn cells of the spinal cord. Occasionally the bulbar nuclei of the brain are involved. A variety of conditions may lead to the development of this disease: infections, avitaminosis, or toxins.

Duchenne-Erb paralysis (dū-shĕn'ayrb). [Duchenne; W. H. Erb, Ger. internist, 1840–1921] Paralysis of muscles supplied by nerves from the upper brachial plexus

Ducrey's bacillus (dū-krāz'). [Augusto Ducrey, It. dermatologist, 1860–1940] Small, rod-shaped organism found in pairs, the cause of chancroid or soft chancre.

duct [L. *ducere,* to lead]. 1. A narrow tubular vessel or channel, esp. one serving to convey secretions from a gland. 2. A narrow enclosed channel containing a fluid, as the semicircular duct of the ear.

d., accessory pancreatic. Duct of the pancreas leading into the pancreatic duct or the duodenum near the mouth of the common bile duct.

d., alveolar. A branch of a respiratory bronchiole that leads to the alveolar sacs of the lungs.

d., Bartholin's. The major duct of the sublingual gland.

d.'s, biliary. The canals that carry bile. The intrahepatic ducts include the bile canaliculi and interlobular ducts; the extrahepatic ducts include the hepatic, cystic, and common bile ducts. SYN: *bile ducts.*

d., cochlear. Canal of the cochlea.

d., common bile. Duct formed by the confluence of the hepatic and cystic ducts. Conveys bile to the duodenum opening at the papilla of Vater. SYN: *ductus choledochus* [NA].

d., cystic. Excretory duct of the gallbladder.

d., efferent. Any duct conveying secretion from a gland.

d., ejaculatory. Duct that conveys semen into urethra.

d., endolymphatic. In the embryo, a tubular projection of the otocyst ending in a blind extremity, the endolymph sac. In the adult, it connects the endolymphatic sac with the utricle and saccule.

d., excretory. Any duct that conveys a product from an organ as the excretory duct of a salivary gland.

d., galactophorous. Duct carrying milk in lobes of mammary glands.

d., Gartner's. A remnant of the wolffian duct extending from the parovarium through the broad ligament into the vagina.

d.'s, hepatic. Ducts that receive bile from right and left lobes of liver and carry it to the common bile duct. SYN: *ductus hepaticus dexter* [NA]; *ductus hepaticus sinister* [NA].

d., interlobular. A duct passing between lobules within a gland, e.g., one of the ducts carrying bile.

d., lacrimal. One of two short ducts, inferior and superior, that convey tears from the lacrimal lake to the lacrimal sac. Their openings are on the margins of the upper and lower eyelids. SYN: *canal, lacrimal.*

d.'s, lactiferous. A group of 15 to 20 ducts that drain the lobes of the mammary gland. Each opens in a slight depression in the tip of the nipple.

d., Leydig's. D., mesonephric.

d., lymphatic. One of two main ducts conveying lymph to the bloodstream: the left lymphatic duct (thoracic duct) and the right lymphatic duct. SEE: *lymphatic drainage* for illus.

d., lymphatic, left. D., thoracic.

d., lymphatic, right. The duct that drains lymph from the right side of the body above the diaphragm. Discharges into the right innominate vein. Smaller than the left lymphatic duct.

d., mammary. D., lactiferous.

d., mesonephric. The duct that, in the embryo, connects the mesonephros with the cloaca. In the male, it develops into the reproductive ducts (ductus epididymidis, ductus deferens, seminal vesicle, and ejaculatory duct). In the female, it gives rise to the duct of the epoophoron, a rudimentary structure. SYN: *wolffian duct.*

d., metanephric. Ureter.

d., milk. D., lactiferous.

d.'s, müllerian. Bilateral ducts in the embryo that form the uterus, vagina, and fallopian tubes. SYN: *Müller's ducts.*

d., nasolacrimal. The duct that conveys tears from the lacrimal sac to the nasal cavity. It opens beneath the inferior nasal concha.

d. of the epoophoron. Gartner's duct, q.v.

d. of Santorini. Accessory pancreatic duct.

d. of Wirsung. D., pancreatic.

d., omphalomesenteric. D., vitelline.

d., pancreatic. Duct that conveys pancreatic juice to the duodenum. SYN: *d. of Wirsung.*

d., papillary. Any one of the large collecting tubules of the kidney.

d., paramesonephric. The genital canal in the embryo. In the female, it develops into the oviducts, uterus, and vagina; in the male, it degenerates to form the appendix testis.

d.'s, paraurethral. D.'s, Skene's.

d., parotid. Duct through which secretions from the parotid gland enter into mouth. SYN: *d., Stensen's.*

d.'s, prostatic. About 20 ducts that discharge prostatic secretion into the urethra. SYN: *ductus prostatici* [NA].

d.'s of Rivinus. Five to 15 ducts (the minor sublingual ducts) that drain the posterior portion of the sublingual gland.

d., salivary. Any of the ducts that drain a salivary gland.

d., secretory. The smaller canals of a gland.

d., segmental. A pair of embryonic tubes located between visceral and parietal layers of mesoblast on each side of the body.

d.'s, semicircular. Three membranous tubes forming a part of the membranous labyrinth of the inner ear. They lie within the semicircular canals and bear corresponding names: anterior, posterior, and lateral.

d., seminal. Any of the ducts that convey semen, specifically the ductus deferens and the ejaculatory duct.

d.'s, Skene's. Two slender ducts of Skene's glands that open on either side of the urethral orifice in the female. SYN: *d.'s, paraurethral.*

d., spermatic. Excretory duct of the testicle that later joins the duct of the seminal vesicle to become the ejaculatory duct. SYN: *ductus deferens* [NA]; *vas deferens.*

d., Stensen's. D., parotid.

d., striated. A class of ducts contained within the lobules of glands, esp. salivary glands, that contain radially appearing striations within the cells, denoting the presence of mitochondria.

d.'s, sublingual. The excretory ducts of the sublingual gland. SEE: *d., Bartholin's.*

d., submandibular. Duct of the submandibular gland. It opens on a papilla at the side of the frenulum of the tongue.

d., tear. A duct that conveys tears. Includes excretory ducts of lacrimal glands, and lacrimal and nasolacrimal ducts.

d., testicular. D., spermatic.

d., thoracic. The left lymphatic duct. Drains the left side of the body above the diaphragm and all of the body below the diaphragm. Discharges into the left innominate vein.

d., umbilical. D., vitelline.

d., utriculosaccular. A narrow tube emanating from the utricle and opening into the endolymphatic duct.

d., vitelline. The narrow duct that, in the embryo, connects the yolk sac (umbilical vesicle) with the intestine. SYN: *d., umbilical; yolk stalk.*

d., Wharton's. The duct of the submandibular gland. SYN: *d., submandibular.*

d., wolffian. SEE: *wolffian duct.*

ductile (dŭk'tĭl) [L. *ductilis,* fr. *ducere,* to lead]. Capable of being elongated without breaking.

ductless [L. *ducere,* to lead, + AS. *loessa,* less]. Having no duct, secreting only internally.

ductless glands. Glands without ducts; they secrete internally one or more hormones that have a specific action upon the body. SEE: *endocrine gland; exocrine.*

ductule (dŭk'tūl). A very small duct.

d., aberrant. One of a group of small tubules associated with the epididymis. They end blindly, representing the vestigial remains of the caudal group of mesonephric tubules.

ductulus (dŭk'tū-lŭs). Ductule, or small duct.

ductus (dŭk'tŭs). (pl. *ductus*) [NA] Duct, q.v.

d. arteriosus. [NA] A channel of communication between the main pulmonary artery and the aorta of the fetus.

d. arteriosus, patent. Persistence of a communication between the main pulmonary artery and the aorta, after birth.

The condition of patent and persistent ductus arteriosus in preterm infants has been successfully treated by using drugs that inhibit prostaglandin synthesis, such as indomethacin.

d. choledochus. [NA] The common bile duct.

d. cochlearis. [NA] The cochlear duct. SYN: *scala media.*

d. communis. A duct about 3 in. (7.6 cm.) long formed by union of the cystic and hepatic ducts. Carries the bile to the intestine.

d. deferens. [NA] Excretory duct of the testicle. Conveys sperm from the epididymis to the ejaculatory duct. SYN: *vas deferens.*

d., efferent. One of a group of 12 to 14 small tubes that constitute the efferent ducts of the testis. They lie within the epididymis and connect the rete testis with the ductus epididymis. Their coiled portions constitute the lobulus epididymis.

d. epoophori longitudinalis. The caudal part of the mesonephric duct. It normally degenerates but may persist in the female. SYN: *duct of the epoophoron.*

d. hemithoracicus. [NA] Ascending branch of the thoracic duct, opening either into the right lymphatic duct or close to the angle of union of the right subclavian and right internal jugular veins.

d. hepaticus dexter. [NA] Duct issuing from the right lobe of the liver and uniting with the ductus hepaticus sinister to form the hepatic duct. Drains the right and caudate lobes.

d. hepaticus sinister. [NA] Duct that unites with the ductus hepaticus dexter to form the hepatic duct. Drains the left and caudate lobes.

d. prostatici. [NA] Ducts for secretion of prostate into the urethra.

d. reuniens. The endolymph-containing canal of the inner ear that connects the saccule with the cochlear duct. SYN: *Hensen's canal.*

d., sacculo-utricularis. Small tube connecting the saccule of the internal ear with the utricle.

d. venosus. [NA] The smaller, shorter, and posterior of two branches into which the umbilical vein divides after entering the abdomen. Empties into the inferior vena cava.

Duffy system. A blood group consisting of two antigens determined by allelic genes. SEE: *blood groups.*

duipara (doo-ĭp'ă-ră) [L. *duo,* two, + *parere,* to bear]. A female pregnant for the second time. SYN: *secundipara.*

Duke method. SEE: *bleeding time.*

dulcite (dŭl'sīt) [L. *dulcis,* sweet]. $C_6H_{14}O_6$. A sugar found in certain plants.

Dulcolax. Trade name for bisacodyl.

dull [ME. *dul*]. 1. Not resonant on percussion. 2. Not mentally alert.

dullness, dulness. 1. Lack of normal resonance on percussion. 2. State of being dull.

dumb [AS.]. Lacking the power or faculty to speak. SYN: *mute.*

dumbness. Muteness.

dumping syndrome. A syndrome characterized by sweating and weakness after eating. Occurs in patients who have had gastric resections. Exact cause is unknown but rapid emptying (i.e., dumping of the stomach contents) into the small intestine is associated with the symptoms. It is often ameliorated by a regimen of small meals at frequent intervals.

duodenal (dū-ō-dē'năl, dū-ŏd'ĕ-năl) [L. *duodeni,* twelve]. Pert. to the duodenum.

duodenal bulb. Area of duodenum just beyond the pylorus.

duodenal delay. Delay in the movement of food through the duodenum due to conditions such as inflammation of lower portion of the intestine, which reflexly inhibits duodenal movements.

duodenal ulcer. Damaged mucous membrane, usually accompanied by suppuration. Sometimes a sore that bleeds is present. This creates danger of perforation. A duodenal ulcer heals slowly due to constant passage of irritating fluids, enzymes, and food over it. SEE: *peptic ulcer.*

duodenectasis (dū"ō-dĕn-ĕk'tă-sĭs) [" + Gr. *ektasis,* expansion]. Chronic dilatation of the duodenum.

duodenectomy (dū"ō-dĕn-ĕk'tō-mē) [" + Gr. *ektome,* excision]. Excision of part or all of the duodenum.

duodenitis (dū"ŏd-ĕ-nī'tĭs) [" + Gr. *itis,* inflammation]. Inflammation of the duodenum.

duodenocholecystostomy (dū"ō-dē"nō-kō-lĭ-sĭs-tŏs'tō-mē) [" + Gr. *chole,* bile, + *kystis,* bladder, + *stoma,* mouth]. Formation by surgical means of a fistula between the duodenum and gallbladder. SYN: *duodenocystostomy.*

duodenocholedochotomy (dū"ō-dē"nō-kō-lĕd-ō-kŏt'ō-mē) [" + Gr. *choledochos,* bile duct, + *tome,* incision]. Surgical incision of the duodenum to reach the gallbladder.

duodenocystostomy (dū"ō-dē"nō-sĭs-tŏs'tō-mē). Duodenocholecystostomy.

duodenoenterostomy (dū"ō-dē"nō-ĕn"tĕr-ŏs'tō-mē) [" + Gr. *enteron,* intestine, + *stoma,* opening]. Formation of passage between the duodenum and intestine.

duodenogram (dū-ŏd'ĕ-nō-grăm)) [" + Gr. *gramma,* a writing]. A roentgenogram of the duodenum.

duodenohepatic (dū-ŏd"ĕ-nō"hĕ-păt'ĭk) [" + Gr. *hepatos,* liver]. Pert. to duodenum and liver.

duodenoileostomy (dū"ō-dē"nō-ĭl"ē-ŏs'tō-mē). Surgical establishment of a communication between the duodenum and ileum.

duodenojejunostomy (dū"ō-dē"nō-jĕ-joo-nŏs'tō-mē) [" + *jejunum,* empty, + Gr. *stoma,* opening]. Making a passage between the duodenum and jejunum.

duodenorrhaphy (dū"ō-dĕ-nor'ă-fē) [" + Gr. *rhaphe,* suture]. Suturing the duodenum.

duodenoscopy (dū"ŏd-ĕ-nŏs'kō-pē) [" + Gr. *skopein,* to examine]. Inspection of the duodenum with an endoscope.

duodenostomy (dū"ŏd-ĕ-nŏs'tō-mē) [" + Gr. *stoma,* opening]. Surgical formation of a permanent opening into the duodenum through the wall of the abdomen.

duodenotomy (dū"ŏd-ĕ-nŏt'ō-mē) [" + Gr. *tome,* incision]. An incision into the duodenum.

duodenum (dū"ō-dē'nŭm, dū-ŏd'ĕ-nŭm) [L. *duodeni,* twelve]. [NA] The first part of the small intestine, connecting with the pylorus of the stomach and extending to the jejunum. The duodenum receives hepatic and pancreatic secretions through the same duct (duct of Wirsung). It is 8 to 11 in. (20 to 28 cm.) long, the average length being 10 in. (25 cm.). Brunner's glands and Lieberkühn's glands are found in the duodenum. Chyle is formed here. It is a crucial section of the alimentary canal. In it occurs the mixing of acid chyme from the stomach, bile from the liver and gallbladder, pancreatic juice, and intestinal juices secreted by the glands of Brunner and Lieberkühn. The nerve supply comes from the celiac plexus. Pancreaticoduodenal branches of the hepatic and superior mesenteric arteries and the right gastric artery supply blood. SEE: *abdominal quadrants* and *digestive system* for illus.

ACTION: The entry of acid chyme into the duodenum brings about discharge of bile from the gallbladder and the secretion of pancreatic juice by the pancreas. These enter through the duct of Wirsung. Bile salts alkalinize the chyme and emulsify the fats. Through the action of pancreatic enzymes, the following changes occur: steapsin (pancreatic lipase) hydrolyzes neutral fats to fatty acids and glycerol; amylopsin (pancreatic amylase) hydrolyzes starch to maltose; maltase hydrolyzes maltose to glucose. Three proteolytic enzymes (trypsin, chymotrypsin, and peptidase) act on proteins, hydrolyzing them to proteoses, peptones, and amino acids.

Secretory phenomena: At least two substances are secreted by the duodenum. One of these, secretin, q.v., stimulates the pancreas to increase production of its juice. The other, cholecystokinin, causes the gallbladder to contract and force its contents through the bile duct, then to the duct of Wirsung and then into the duodenum. In addition, nervous mechanisms contribute to the coordination that exists here, regulating the rate of discharge of chyme from the stomach, varying both quality and quantity of the various secretions, and determining the rate of passage through the duodenum.

Motor phenomena: The first part of the duodenum (pars superior, duodenal cap, duodenal bulb) is the small portion immediately following the pylorus of the stomach. It is regularly full of material and consequently visible in roentgenograms as a spade-shaped shadow. The next part (pars descendens) is that into which the common bile duct (ductus choledochus) and pancreatic ducts open. Movement through it and through the pars inferior and the pars ascendens is so rapid that they are normally inconspicuous on x-ray film. Throughout the duodenum the mucosa is thrown into folds (plicae circulares). The folds are permanent and inactive. The villi, which stud the surface of the folds as well as the spaces between them, exhibit waving and thrusting movements.

RS: bile; Brunner's glands; choledochoduodenostomy; digestion; duodenal ulcer; enzyme; gallbladder; gastric juice; intestine; Lieberkühn crypts; liver; pancreas; pancreatic juice; succus entericus.

duplication, duplicature [L. *duplicare,* to double]. A doubling or folding, or state of being folded.

duplicitas (dū-plĭs′ĭ-tăs). Fetal abnormality in which the cephalic or the pelvic end is doubled.

dupp (dŭp). In cardiac auscultation, the expression for the second heart sound heard over the apex. This sound is shorter and of higher pitch than *lubb,* the first heart sound.

Dupuytren, Baron G. (dū-pwē-trăn′). French surgeon, 1777–1835.

D.'s contracture. Contracture of palmar fascia causing the ring and little fingers to bend into the palm so that they cannot be extended. SEE: *contracture, Dupuytren's,* for illus.

D.'s fracture. Fracture dislocation of the ankle. The talus is displaced upward.

dura (dū′ră) [L. *durus,* hard]. Dura mater.

Durabolin. Trade name for nandrolone phenpropionate.

Duracillin. Trade name for penicillin G procaine.

dural (dū′răl) [L. *durus,* hard]. Pert. to the dura.

dura mater [L., hard mother]. The outer membrane covering the spinal cord (dura mater spinalis [NA]) and brain (dura mater cerebri [NA] or dura mater encephali [NA]). SEE: *pia mater; tentorium cerebelli.*

duramatral. Pert. to the dura. SYN: *dural.*

Durand-Nicolas-Favre disease. Lymphogranuloma venereum, q.v.

duraplasty [″ + Gr. *plassein,* to form]. Plastic repair of the dura mater.

Duraquin. Trade name for quinidine gluconate.

durematoma (dū″rĕm-ă-tō′mă) [″ + Gr. *haima,* blood, + *oma,* tumor]. Accumulation of blood between arachnoid and dura.

duritis (dū-rī′tĭs) [″ + Gr. *itis,* inflammation]. Inflammation of the dura. SYN: *pachymeningitis.*

duroarachnitis (dū″rō-ăr″ăk-nī′tĭs) [″ + Gr. *arachne,* spider, + *itis,* inflammation]. Inflammation of dura and arachnoid membrane.

Duroziez' murmur (dū-rō″zē-āz′). [Paul Louis Duroziez, Fr. physician, 1826–1897] The systolic and diastolic murmur heard over a large artery when pressure is applied to the area just distal to the stethoscope.

dust. Minute, fine particles of earth; any powder.

d., blood. Hemoconia, q.v.

d., ear. Fine calcareous bodies found in the gelatinous substance of the otolithic membrane of the ear; otoconia or otoliths.

dust cells. Reticuloendothelial cells in the walls of the alveoli of the lungs that ingest or destroy dust particles.

dusting powder. Any fine powder for dusting on skin.

d.p., absorbable. USP. Powder prepared from cornstarch. It is used as a lubricant for surgical gloves.

Duverney's gland (dū-vĕr-nāz′). [Joseph G. Duverney, Fr. anatomist, 1648–1730] The vulvovaginal gland.

Duverney's fracture. Fracture of the ilium.

Duvoid. Trade name for bethanechol chloride.

D.V.M. *Doctor of Veterinary Medicine.*

dwarf [AS. *dweorg,* dwarf]. An abnormally short or undersized person.

d., achondroplastic. Type of dwarfism characterized by normal trunk but shortened extremities, a large head, and prominent buttocks.

d., asexual. Dwarf with deficient sexual development.

d., hypophyseal. Dwarf whose condition resulted from hypofunction of the anterior lobe of the hypophysis.

d., infantile. Dwarf with marked physical, mental, and sexual underdevelopment.

d., Levi-Lorain. An hypophyseal or pituitary dwarf.

d., micromelic. Dwarf with very small

limbs.

d., ovarian. An undersized female due to absence or underdevelopment of the ovaries.

d., phocomelic. Dwarf with abnormally short diaphyses of either pair of extremities or of all four.

d., physiologic. A person normally developed except for stature.

d., pituitary. D., hypophyseal.

d., primordial. Dwarf in whom there is a selective deficiency of growth hormone but with otherwise normal endocrine function.

d., rachitic. Dwarf whose condition is due to rickets.

d., renal. Dwarf whose condition is due to renal osteodystrophy.

d., thanatophoric. Type of dwarfism caused by generalized failure of endochondral bone formation. Characterized by large head, prominent forehead, hypertelorism, saddle nose, and short limbs extending straight out from trunk. Most of these infants die soon after birth.

dwarfism. Condition of being abnormally small. May be hereditary or a result of endocrine dysfunction, deficiency diseases, renal insufficiency, diseases of the skeleton, or other causes.

Dy. Chem. symb. for dysprosium.

dyad [Gr. *duas,* pair]. 1. A pair. 2. A pair of chromosomes formed by the division of a tetrad in meiosis. A dyad represents a single chromosome split precociously for a subsequent division. 3. In chemistry, a bivalent element or radical.

dyadic. Pertaining to the social interaction between two people.

Dycill. Trade name for dicloxacillin sodium.

Dyclone. Trade name for dyclonine hydrochloride.

dyclonine hydrochloride (dī'klō-nēn). USP. A topical anesthetic used in otolaryngology. Trade name is Dyclone.

dydrogesterone (dī″drō-jĕs'tĕr-ōn). USP. A progestational agent.

dye. Any substance that is of itself colored or that is used to impart color to another material such as a thin slice of tissue prepared for microscopic examination. Dyes may also be employed in manufacturing test reagents used in medical laboratories.

dynamia (dī-năm'ē-ă) [Gr. *dynamis,* power]. Vital energy or ability to combat disease.

dynamic (dī-năm'ĭk). Pert. to vital force or inherent power. Opposed to static.

dynamics. The science of bodies in motion and their forces.

dynamic splint. A splint fabricated with moving parts to allow mobility by providing forces that substitute for weak or absent muscle strength.

dynamogenesis (dī″nă-mō-jĕn'ĕ-sĭs) [″ + *genesis,* growth]. The capacity to call forth increased energy.

dynamogenic [″ + *gennan,* to produce]. Pert. to, or caused by, an increase of energy.

dynamograph (dī-năm'ō-grăf) [″ + *graphein,* to write]. Device for recording muscular strength.

dynamometer (dī″nă-mŏm'ĕ-tĕr) [″ + *metron,* measure]. 1. A device for measuring muscular strength. 2. A device for determining the magnifying power of a lens.

dynamoneure (dī-năm'ō-nūr) [″ + *neuron,* nerve]. A motor spinal nerve cell.

dynamoscope (dī-năm'ō-skōp) [″ + *skopein,* to examine]. Instrument for auscultation of muscles.

dynamoscopy (dī-năm-ŏs'kō-pē). 1. Auscultation of muscles. 2. Visual evaluation of the function of an organ or system.

Dynapen. Trade name for dicloxacillin sodium.

dyne (dīn) [Gr. *dynamis,* power]. Force needed for imparting an acceleration of one cm. per second to a one-gram mass.

dyphylline (dī-fĭl'ĭn). A medicine used in treating asthma. There is little evidence that it is effective.

Dyrenium. Trade name for triamterene.

dys- [Gr.]. Prefix meaning bad, difficult, painful.

dysacousia, dysacusis, dysacousma (dĭs″ă-koo'zē-ă, -koo'sĭs, -kooz'mă) [Gr. *dys,* bad, + *akousis,* hearing]. 1. Discomfort caused by loud noises. 2. Difficulty in hearing.

dysadrenalism (dĭs″ăd-rē'năl-ĭzm). Disordered function or disease of the adrenal gland.

dysalbumose (dĭs-ăl'bū-mōs) [″ + *albumen,* white of egg]. A variety of albumose insoluble in water or hydrochloric acid.

dysantigraphia (dĭs″ăn-tĭ-grăf'ē-ă) [″ + *anti,* against, + *graphein,* to write]. Inability to copy writing or printed letters.

dysaphia (dĭs-ă'fē-ă) [″ + *haphe,* touch]. Dullness of the sense of touch.

dysarthria (dĭs-ăr'thrē-ă) [″ + *arthroun,* to utter distinctly]. Difficult and defective speech due to impairment of the tongue or other muscles essential to speech.

dysarthrosis [″ + *arthrosis,* joint]. Joint malformation or deformity.

dysautonomia (dĭs″aw-tō-nō'mē-ă) [″ + *autonomia,* freedom to use own laws]. A rare hereditary disease involving the autonomic nervous system characterized by mental retardation, motor incoordination, vomiting, frequent infections, and convulsions. It is seen almost exclusively in Ashkenazi Jews.

dysbarism (dĭs'băr-ĭzm) [″ + *barys,* heavy, + *-ismos,* condition]. Symptom complex following exposure of body to less-than-atmospheric pressure in air flight or altitude chamber. When occurring in severe form, sometimes called decompression sickness or bends.

dysbasia (dĭs-bā'zē-ă) [" + *basis,* a step]. Difficulty in walking, esp. when due to disease of the brain or spinal cord.

dysbolism (dĭs'bō-lĭzm) [" + *ballein,* to change]. Disordered metabolism.

dysbulia (dĭs-bū'lē-ă) [" + *boule,* will]. 1. Inability to fix the attention; difficulty experienced in thinking; mind weariness. 2. Weak and uncertain willpower.

dyscalculia (dĭs"kăl-kū'lē-ă). Inability to solve mathematical problems due to brain disease or injury.

dyscephaly (dĭs-sĕf'ă-lē). Malformation of the head and facial bones.

dyschezia (dĭs-kē'zē-ă) [" + *chezein,* go to defecate]. Painful or difficult bowel movements.

dyschiria (dĭs-kī'rē-ă) [" + *cheir,* hand]. Inability to tell which side of the body has been touched. If referred to the wrong side it is called allochiria, q.v., or allesthesia, q.v. If referred to both sides it is called synchiria, q.v. SYN: *achiria.*

dyscholia (dĭs-kō'lē-ă) [Gr. *dys,* bad + *chole,* bile]. Any pathological condition of the bile.

dyschondroplasia (dĭs"kŏn-drō-plā'zē-ă) [" + *chondros,* cartilage, + *plassein,* to form]. Disease, usually hereditary, resulting in disordered growth. Characterized by multiple exostoses of growth of the epiphyses, esp. of the long bones, metacarpals, and phalanges. SYN: *chondroplasia; Ollier's disease.*

dyschroa, dyschroia (dĭs-krō'ă, dis-kroy'ă) [" + *chroia,* complexion]. Discolored skin, esp. of the face; poor or bad complexion.

dyschromatopsia (dĭs"krō-mă-tŏp'sē-ă) [" + *chroma,* color, + *opsis,* vision]. Imperfect color vision.

dyschromia. Discoloration, as of the skin.

dyschronism (dĭs-krō'nĭzm) [" + *chronos,* time]. 1. Disturbed time relation, esp. that which occurs when one is transported from one time zone to one that is 5 to 10 hours ahead of or behind the original. This leads to disturbances of biological rhythms. 2. Separate as to time.

dyscinesia (dĭs-sī-nē'zē-ă). Impairment in ability to perform voluntary movement. SYN: *dyskinesia.*

dyscoria (dĭs-kō'rē-ă) [" + *kore,* pupil]. Abnormal form or shape of the pupil.

dyscrasia (dĭs-krā'zē-ă) [Gr. *dyskrasia,* bad temperament]. An old term meaning abnormal mixture of the four humors. The word is now used as a synonym for disease.

dyscrasic (dĭs-krā'sĭk). Pert. to dyscrasia.

dyscrinism (dĭs-krī'nĭzm) [Gr. *dys,* bad, + *krinein,* to secrete, + *-ismos,* condition of]. Any disorder of secretions, esp. of an endocrine gland.

dysdiadochokinesia (dĭs"dī-ăd"ō-kō-kĭ-nē'sē-ă) [" + *diadochos,* succeeding, + *kinesis,* movement]. Inability to quickly substitute antagonistic motor impulses to produce antagonistic muscular movements.

dysembryoplasia (dĭs-ĕm"brē-ō-plā'sē-ă) [" + *embryon,* embryo, + *plassein,* to form]. Fetal malformation occurring during growth of the embryo.

dysemia [" + *haima,* blood]. Any blood disease.

dysenteric (dĭs"ĕn-tĕr'ĭk). Pert. to dysentery.

dysentery (dĭs'ĕn-tĕr"ē) [" + *enteron,* intestine]. A term applied to a number of intestinal disorders, esp. of the colon, characterized by inflammation of the mucous membrane.

ETIOL: Bacterial or viral infection; infestation by protozoa or parasitic worms; chemical irritants.

SYM: Abdominal pain, tenesmus, diarrhea with passage of mucus or blood.

d., amebic. Dysentery due to amebas.

d., bacillary. An acute infectious disease caused by bacteria of the genus Shigella, esp. Sh. dysenteriae, Sh. boydii, Sh. flexneri, and Sh. sonnei. It may occur sporadically or in epidemics. In addition to intestinal symptoms, a severe toxemia may occur due to exo- and endotoxins produced by the organisms.

d., balantidial. Dysentery caused by the ciliate protozoan, Balantidium coli.

d., malignant. A form of dysentery in which symptoms are very pronounced and progress rapidly, usually terminating fatally.

d., viral. Dysentery caused by virus.

dyserethesia (dĭs"ĕr-ē-thē'zē-ă) [" + *erethizein,* to irritate]. Impaired response to stimuli.

dysergasia (dĭs"ĕr-gā'zē-ă) [" + *ergon,* work]. Inability to function properly. In psychiatry, a behavior disorder characterized by disorientation, hallucinations, dream states, and delirium. May sometimes be due to toxic conditions such as uremia or alcohol intoxication.

dysergastic (dĭs-ĕr-găs'tĭk). Pert. to dysergasia.

dysergastic reaction. Hallucinations, fears, disorientation, dream states, and other mental disorders resulting from poor circulation and metabolism of the brain.

dysergia (dĭs-ĕr'jē-ă) [" + *ergon,* work]. Lack of coordination in muscular voluntary movements.

dysesthesia (dĭs"ĕs-thē'zē-ă) [" + *aisthesis,* sensation]. 1. Sensations on the skin, such as of the pricks of pins and needles, or of crawling. SYN: *formication.* 2. Impairment of a sensitivity, esp. of touch. 3. Painfulness of any sensation that is not normally painful.

d., auditory. Abnormal discomfort from loud noises. SYN: *dysacusia.*

d. pedis. Severe itching and burning of the plantar surface of the feet and toes. May occur as a reaction to heparin therapy.

dysfunction (dĭs-fŭnk′shŭn) [″ + L. *functio,* a performance]. Abnormal, inadequate, or impaired function of an organ or part.

dysgalactia [″ + *gala,* milk]. Defective milk secretion.

dysgammaglobulinemia. Disproportion in the concentration of immunoglobulins in the blood. May be congenital or acquired.

dysgenesis (dĭs-jĕn′ĕ-sĭs) [Gr. *dys,* bad, + *genesis,* creation]. Defective or abnormal development, particularly in the embryo.

d., gonadal. Congenital endocrine disorder caused by failure of the ovaries to respond to pituitary hormone (gonadotropin) stimulation. Clinically there is amenorrhea, failure of sexual maturation, and usually short stature. About a third of these patients have webbing of the neck and may have cubitus valgus. Intelligence may be impaired. SYN: *Turner's syndrome.*

ETIOL: Due to a defect in or absence of the second sex chromosome.

dysgenic [″ + *gennan,* to produce]. Pert. to dysgenesis.

dysgenitalism [″ + L. *genitalia,* organs of reproduction, + Gr. *-ismos,* state of]. Condition caused by abnormal genital development.

dysgerminoma (dĭs″jĕr-mĭn-ō′mă) [″ + L. *germen,* a sprout, + Gr. *oma,* tumor]. A malignant neoplasm of the ovary.

dysgeusia (dĭs-gū′zē-ă) [″ + *geusis,* taste]. Impairment or perversion of the gustatory sense such that normal tastes are interpreted as being unpleasant or completely different from the characteristic taste of a particular food or chemical compound. SEE: *hypogeusia, idiopathic.*

dysglandular [″ + L. *glans,* acorn]. Abnormal functioning of glands, esp. those of internal secretion.

dysglobulinemia (dĭs-glŏb″ū-lĭn-ē′mē-ă) [″ + L. *globulus,* globule, + Gr. *haima,* blood]. Abnormality of the amount or quality of blood globulins.

dysgnathia (dĭs-nā′thē-ă) [″ + *gnathos,* jaw]. Abnormality of the mandible and maxilla.

dysgnosia (dĭs-nō′sē-ă) [Gr. *dysgnosia,* difficulty of knowing]. Any anomaly of intellect. SYN: *dysthymia* (def. 2).

dysgonesis (dĭs″gō-nē′sĭs) [Gr. *dys,* bad, + *gone,* seed]. 1. Functional disorder of the genital organs. 2. Poor growth of bacterial culture.

dysgonic. Bacterial cultures of sparse growth.

dysgraphia (dĭs-grăf′ē-ă) [″ + *graphein,* to write]. 1. Inability to write properly. Usually the result of a brain lesion. 2. Writer's cramp.

dyshematopoiesia (dĭs-hĕm″ă-tō-poy-ē′sē-ă) [″ + *haima,* blood, + *poiein,* to make]. Imperfect blood formation.

dyshidria (dĭs-hĭd′rē-ă) [″ + *hidros,* sweat]. Dyshidrosis.

dyshidrosis (dĭs-hī-drō′sĭs) [″ + ″ + *osis,* condition]. 1. Disorder of the sweating apparatus. 2. A recurrent vesicular eruption on skin of hands and feet marked by intense itching. SYN: *pompholyx.*

TREATMENT: The control of sweating or proper absorption of perspiration will be of benefit. For the feet, wearing absorbent socks, well-ventilated shoes, and application of substances that reduce sweating will help to control symptoms. Individuals who do not wear shoes are rarely found to have this disorder. Acute attacks will respond to treatment with a corticosteroid in an ointment combined with diiodohydroxyquin. This is applied at night with an occlusive dressing.

dysidrosis (dĭs-ī-drō′sĭs). Dyshidrosis, q.v.

dyskaryosis (dĭs-kăr″ē-ō′sĭs). Abnormality of the nucleus of a cell.

dyskeratosis (dĭs″kĕr-ă-tō′sĭs) [″ + *keras,* horn, + *osis,* condition]. 1. Epithelial alterations in which a certain number of isolated malpighian cells become differentiated. 2. Any alteration in the keratinization of the epithelial cells of the epidermis. Characteristic of many skin disorders.

dyskinesia (dĭs″kī-nē′sē-ă) [″ + *kinesis,* movement]. Defect in voluntary movement.

d. algera. Condition in which active movement is painful if done quickly but not if slow movement. Due to hysteria.

d. intermittens. Limb disability occurring intermittently.

d., tardive. Slow, rhythmical, automatic stereotyped movements, either generalized or in single muscle groups. These occur as an undesired effect of therapy with certain psychotropic drugs, esp. the phenothiazines.

d., uterine. Pain in the uterus on movement.

dyskinetic. Concerning dyskinesia.

dyslalia (dĭs-lā′lē-ă) [Gr. *dys,* bad, + *lalein,* to talk]. Impairment of speech due to defect of speech organs.

dyslexia (dĭs-lĕk′sē-ă) [″ + *lexis,* diction]. A condition in which an individual with normal vision is unable to interpret written language. Exact cause is unknown, but thought to be due to a CNS defect in ability to organize graphic symbols. SEE: *alexia.*

dyslochia (dĭs-lō′kē-ă) [″ + *lochia,* lochia]. Disordered or premature cessation of lochial discharge.

dyslogia (dĭs-lō′jē-ă) [″ + *logos,* understanding]. Difficulty in expression of ideas.

dysmasesis (dĭs″mă-sē′sĭs) [″ + *masesis,* mastication]. Difficulty in masticating.

dysmaturity. Condition in which infants weigh

less than would be expected for the known length of the gestational period. These infants are sometimes referred to as being small-for-date.

dysmegalopsia [" + *megas,* big, + *opsis,* vision]. Inability to visualize correctly the size of objects; they appear larger than they really are.

dysmelia (dĭs-mē'lē-ă) [" + *melos,* limb]. Congenital deformity or absence of a portion of one or more limbs.

dysmenorrhea (dĭs"mĕn-ō-rē'ă) [" + *men,* month, + *rhein,* to flow]. Pain in association with menstruation. One of the most frequent gynecologic disorders. It is classified into *primary,* q.v., and *secondary,* q.v. It is estimated that about 50% of menstruating women experience this disorder and that about 10% of these are incapacitated for several days each period. This disorder is the greatest single cause of absence from school and work among menstrual-age women. In the U.S.A., it is estimated that this illness causes the loss of 140,000,000 work hours each year.

d., congestive. Condition caused by pelvic congestion.

d., inflammatory. Condition caused by pelvic inflammation.

d., membranous. A severe spasmodic dysmenorrhea that is accompanied by the passage of a cast or partial cast of the uterine cavity.

d., neurotic. Form caused by neurosis.

d., primary. SYM: The pain usually begins just before or at the onset of menstruation. The pain is spasmodic and located in the lower abdomen, but it may also radiate to the back and thighs. Also included in some but not all individuals are nausea, vomiting, diarrhea, low back pain, headache, dizziness, and in severe cases, syncope and collapse. These symptoms may last from a few hours to several days but seldom persist for more than 3 days; in primary dysmenorrhea, these symptoms tend to decrease or disappear after the individual has experienced childbirth the first time, and to decrease with age.

DIAG: A cramping, labor-like pain that starts just prior to or at the time of the onset of menstruation. The first attack occurs with or shortly after menarche and occurs subsequently only if preceded by ovulation; pelvic examination is normal. It is essential that secondary dysmenorrhea be ruled out.

ETIOL: The exact cause is unknown, but uterine ischemia due to increased production of prostaglandins with increased contractility of the muscles of the uterus (i.e., the myometrium) is felt to be the principal mechanism. As in any disease or symptom, the individual's reaction to and tolerance of pain will influence the extent of the disability experienced. Primary dysmenorrhea is not a behavioral or psychologic disorder.

TREATMENT: Oral contraceptives and antiprostaglandin drugs including aspirin; mefenamic acid (trade name is Ponstel) or ibuprofen (trade name is Motrin); or naproxen (trade names are Anaprox and Naprosyn). One of these medicines should be taken in the appropriate dose 3 to 4 times a day and with milk to lessen the chance of gastric irritation.

d., secondary. This condition frequently causes pain quite similar to that of the primary form of dysmenorrhea, but it usually begins some years after menarche. A history of the occurrence of pain in association with pelvic inflammatory disease, or use of an IUD, or endometriosis, or fertility problems suggests the diagnosis of secondary dysmenorrhea.

TREATMENT: Therapy for the underlying disease and in the meantime use of the antiprostaglandin drugs. These drugs are especially useful when the disorder is due to the presence of an IUD.

d., spasmodic. Dysmenorrhea caused by uterine contractions of spasmodic form.

dysmetria (dĭs-mē'trē-ă) [Gr. *dys,* bad, + *metron,* measure]. An inability to fix the range of a movement in muscular activity. Rapid and brusque movements are made with more force than necessary. Seen in cerebellar affections.

RS: adiadochokinesis; asynergia; gait.

dysmetropsia [" + " + *opsis,* vision]. Inability to visualize correctly the size and shape of things.

dysmimia (dĭs-mĭm'ē-ă) [" + *mimia,* imitation]. 1. Inability to express oneself by gestures or signs. 2. Inability to imitate.

dysmnesia (dĭs-nē'zē-ă) [" + *mneme,* memory]. Any impairment of memory.

dysmorphophobia (dĭs"mor-fō-fō'bē-ă) [Gr. *dysmorphas,* deformed, + *phobos,* fear]. Morbid fear of deformity.

dysmorphosis (dĭs"mor-fō'sĭs) [" + *osis,* condition]. Not normal in form.

dysmyotonia (dĭs"mī-ō-tō'nē-ă) [Gr. *dys,* bad, + *mys,* muscle, + *tonos,* tone]. Muscle atony; abnormal muscle tonicity.

dysodontiasis (dĭs"ō-dŏn-tī'ă-sĭs) [" + *odous,* tooth, + *-iasis,* process]. Painful or difficult dentition.

dysontogenesis (dĭs"ŏn-tō-jĕn'ĕ-sĭs) [" + *on,* being, + *gennan,* to produce]. Defective development of an organism, esp. of an embryo.

dysontogenetic. Pert to dysontogenesis.

dysopia, dysopsia (dĭs-ō'pē-ă, -ŏp'sē-ă) [" + *opsis,* vision]. Defective vision.

dysorexia (dĭs"ō-rĕk'sē-ă) [" + *orexis,* appetite]. Perverted or lessened appetite.

dysosmia (dĭs-ŏz′mē-ă) [″ + *osme,* smell]. Distortion of normal smell perception.

dysostosis (dĭs″ŏs-tō′sĭs) [″ + *osteon,* bone, + *osis,* condition]. Defective ossification.

d., cleidocranial. A congenital ossification of the skull with partial atrophy of clavicles.

d., craniocerebral. A hereditary disease characterized by ocular hypertelorism, exophthalmos, strabismus, widening of the skull, high forehead, beaked nose, and hypoplasia of the maxilla.

d., mandibulofacial. Hypoplasia of the facial bones; downward sloping of the palpebral tissues; defects of the ear; macrostomia; and a fish-face appearance. It occurs in two forms that are thought to be autosomal dominants.

dysoxia (dĭs-ŏk′sē-ă). The ultimate utilization of oxygen is at the tissue level. This general term indicates that the mitochondria of the cell are unable to utilize oxygen properly. In such conditions, the metabolism of oxygen is abnormal even though the supply of oxygen is adequate.

dysoxidizable [″ + L. *oxidum,* oxide]. Not easy to oxidize.

dyspancreatism [″ + *pankreas,* pancreas, + *-ismos,* condition of]. Impaired pancreatic function.

dyspareunia (dĭs″pă-rū′nē-ă) [Gr. *dyspareunos,* unhappily mated as bedfellows]. Occurrence of pain during sexual intercourse.

dyspepsia (dĭs-pĕp′sē-ă) [″ + *peptein,* to digest]. Imperfect or painful digestion. Not a disease in itself but symptomatic of other diseases or disorders. Characterized by vague abdominal discomfort, a sense of fullness after eating, eructation, heartburn, nausea and vomiting, and loss of appetite. These symptoms may occur irregularly and in different patterns from time to time. The symptoms are increased in times of stress. SYN: *indigestion.*

d., acid. Dyspepsia due to excessive acidity of the stomach.

d., alcoholic. Dyspepsia caused by excessive use of alcoholic beverages.

d., biliary. Form of dyspepsia in which there is insufficient quantity or quality of bile secretion.

d., cardiac. Form of dyspepsia occurring during heart disease.

d., gastric. Dyspepsia caused by faulty stomach function.

d., gastrointestinal. Dyspepsia caused by faulty function of stomach and intestines.

d., hepatic. Dyspepsia caused by liver disease.

d., hysterical. Dyspepsia present during hysterical attacks.

dyspeptic (dĭs-pĕp′tĭk). 1. Affected with or pert. to dyspepsia. 2. One afflicted with dyspepsia.

dyspermasia [Gr. *dys,* bad, + *sperma,* seed]. Dyspermia.

dyspermatism. Dyspermia.

dyspermia. Difficult or painful emission of sperm during coitus.

dysphagia (dĭs-fā′jē-ă) [″ + *phagein,* to eat]. Inability to swallow or difficulty in swallowing. SEE: *achalasia; cardiospasm.*

d. constricta. Dysphagia due to narrowing of the pharynx or esophagus.

d. lusoria. Dysphagia caused by pressure exerted on the esophagus by an anomaly of the right subclavian artery.

d. paralytica. Dysphagia due to paralysis of muscles of deglutition and esophagus.

d. spastic. Dysphagia resulting from a spasm of pharyngeal or esophageal muscles.

dysphagy (dĭs′fă-jē). Dysphagia.

dysphasia (dĭs-fā′zē-ă) [″ + *phasis,* speech]. Impairment of speech resulting from a brain lesion.

dysphemia (dĭs-fē′mē-ă) [″ + *pheme,* speech]. Stammering or a speech problem of psychoneurotic origin.

dysphonia (dĭs-fō′nē-ă) [″ + *phone,* voice]. Difficulty in speaking; hoarseness.

d. clericorum. Hoarseness due to public speaking.

d. puberum. Change of voice in boys at time of puberty.

dysphoria (dĭs-fō′rē-ă) [Gr. *dysphoria,* excessive anguish]. Exaggerated feeling of depression and unrest without apparent cause.

dysphrasia (dĭs-frā′zē-ă) [Gr. *dys,* bad, + *phrasis,* speech]. Impairment of speech due to a brain lesion. SYN: *dysphasia.*

dysphylaxia (dĭs-fĭ-lăk′sē-ă) [″ + *phylaxis,* watching]. Waking too early from sleep.

dyspigmentation (dĭs″pĭg-mĕn-tā′shŭn). Abnormality of the skin or hair pigment.

dyspituitarism (dĭs″pĭ-tū′ĭ-tăr-ĭzm) [″ + L. *pituita,* mucus, + Gr. *-ismos,* condition]. Condition due to disorder of the pituitary body.

dysplasia [″ + *plassein,* to form]. Abnormal development of tissue. SYN: *alloplasia; heteroplasia.*

d., anhidrotic. A congenital condition marked by absent or deficient sweat glands, intolerance of heat, and abnormal development of teeth and nails.

d., cervical. Abnormal changes in the tissues covering the cervix uteri.

d., chondroectodermal. Condition marked by defective development of bones, nails, teeth, and hair and by congenital heart disease. SYN: *Ellis-van Creveld syndrome.*

d., hereditary ectodermal. Hereditary defect marked by few or absence of sweat glands and hair follicles, smooth shiny skin, abnormalities or absence of teeth, nail deformities, cataracts or alterations of cornea, absence of mammary glands, concave face, prominent eyebrows, conjunctivitis, deficient hair growth, and mental retardation.

d., monostotic fibrous. Replacement of bone by fibrous tissue. Marked by pain usually in tibia or femur. Cause is unknown.

d., polyostotic fibrous. Replacement of bone by avascular fibrous tissue. Marked by difficulty in walking and multiple bone deformities and fractures. Usually commences in childhood. Cause is unknown.

dyspnea (dĭsp-nē'ă, dĭsp'nē-ă) [" + *pnoe,* breathing]. Air hunger resulting in labored or difficult breathing, sometimes accompanied by pain. Normal when due to vigorous work or athletic activity.

ETIOL: Insufficient oxygenation of the blood resulting from disturbances in the lungs, low oxygen pressure of air, circulatory disturbances, hemoglobin deficiency. Other causes may be acidosis, excessive CO_2 content of blood, lesions of the respiratory center, emotional excitation, hyperexcitability of Hering-Breuer reflex, cardiac asthma, and orthopnea. It may be a subjective feeling.

SYM: Audible labored breathing, distressed anxious expression, dilated nostrils, protrusion of abdomen and expanded chest, gasping, marked cyanosis.

NURSING IMPLICATIONS: Assess the alleviating and aggravating factors. Do a complete respiratory assessment to identify additional symptoms of respiratory distress that the patient may have. Place patient in a high Fowler's position, or the position of comfort, whichever the patient prefers. Administer oxygen and medications as ordered. Remain with the patient until breathing becomes less labored and anxiety has decreased.

d., cardiac. Dyspnea due to cardiac insufficiency, as in acute myocardial infarction.

d., expiratory. Dyspnea as in asthma and bronchitis; wheezing and painful expiration. Secretions in respiratory tract cause the sound.

d., inspiratory. Dyspnea due to interference in passage of air to the lungs.

dyspneic (dĭsp-nē'ĭk). Affected with or due to dyspnea.

dyspragia (dĭs-prā'jē-ă). Dyspraxia.

dyspraxia (dĭs-prăk'sē-ă) [Gr. *dyspraxia,* ill success]. Difficulty or pain in performing any function. SYN: *dyspragia.*

dysprosium (dĭs-prō'sē-ŭm) A metallic element of the yttrium group of rare earths. SYMB: Dy. At. wt. 162.50; at. no. 66.

dysraphia, dysraphism (dĭs-rā'fē-ă, -fĭzm) [Gr. *dys,* bad, + *rhaphe,* a seam]. In the embryo, failure of raphe formation or failure of fusion of parts that normally fuse.

d., spinal. A general term applied to failure of fusion of parts along the dorsal midline. May involve any of the following structures: skin, vertebrae, skull, meninges, brain and spinal cord.

dysrhythmia (dĭs-rĭth'mē-ă) [" + *rhythmos,* rhythm]. Abnormal, disordered, or disturbed rhythm.

dysstasia [" + *stasis,* standing]. Difficulty in standing.

dysstatic. Exhibiting difficulty in standing.

dyssynergia [" + *synergia,* cooperation]. Failure of muscular coordination. SYN: *ataxia.*

dystaxia (dĭs-tăk'sē-ă) [" + *taxis,* arrangement]. Partial ataxia.

dystectia (dĭs-tĕk'shē-ă) [" + L. *tectum,* roof]. In the embryo, failure of closure of the neural tube. Thus deformities such as spina bifida or meningocele are produced.

dysteleology (dĭs"tē-lē-ŏl'ō-jē) [" + *telos,* end, + *logos,* knowledge]. Study of rudimentary organs that have no apparent useful purpose to life or organism.

dysthymia (dĭs-thĭm'ē-ă) [" + *thymos,* mind] 1. Any condition caused by defective function of the thymus gland. 2. Any anomaly of intellect. 3 Mental depression.

dysthyreosis (dĭs"thī-rē-ō'sĭs) [" + *thyreos,* shield, + *osis,* condition]. Impaired functional activity of thyroid gland. SYN: *dysthyroidism.*

dysthyroidism (dĭs-thī'roy-dĭzm) [" + " + *eidos,* form, + *-ismos,* condition]. Imperfect development and function of the thyroid gland.

dystocia (dĭs-tō'sē-ă) [" + *tokos,* birth]. Difficult labor. May be produced by either the passenger (the fetus) or the small size of the pelvic outlet.

FETAL CAUSES: Usually large babies. Other factors are: malpositions of the fetus (transverse presentation, face, brow, breech, or compound presentations); abnormalities of the fetus (hydrocephalus, tumors of the neck or abdomen, hydrops); multiple pregnancy (interlocked twins).

MATERNAL CAUSES: *Uterus:* Primary and secondary uterine inertia; congenital anomalies of the uterus (bicornuate uterus); tumors of the uterus (fibroids, carcinoma of the cervix); abnormal fixation of the uterus by previous operation. *Bony pelvis:* Contracted pelvis; generally contracted pelvis; flat and generally contracted pelvis; funnel pelvis; exostoses of the pelvic bones; tumors of the pelvic bones. *Cervix uteri:* Bandl's contraction ring; rigid cervix that will not dilate; stenosis and stricture preventing dilatation. *Ovary:* Ovarian cysts that block the pelvis. *Vagina and vulva:* Cysts; tumors; atresias and stenoses.

DIAG: Can generally be made by vaginal examination and external pelvimetry before the patient goes into labor.

TREATMENT: Varies according to the condition present that causes the dystocia. The goal is correction of the abnormality in order to allow the fetus to pass. If this is not possible, operative delivery is necessary. SEE: *cesarean section.*

dystonia (dĭs-tō'nē-ă) [Gr. *dys,* bad, + *tonos,* tone]. Impaired or disordered tonicity, esp. muscle tone.

d. musculum deformans. A symptom characterized by distorted twisting or movement of a part or all of the body. May be caused by toxic or infectious diseases of the nervous system, or its cause may be unknown. It is important that the patient not be treated as if the disease were due to hysteria or mental illness. Treatment usually is successful but exacerbations may occur.

dystonic. Pert. to dystonia or hyper- or hypotonicity of tissues.

dystopia (dĭs-tō'pē-ă) [" + *topos,* place]. Malposition; displacement of any organ.

d. canthorum. Lateral displacement of the inner canthi of the eyes.

dystopic (dĭs-tŏp'ĭk). Not in place.

dystopy (dĭs'tō-pē) [" + *topos,* place]. Dystopia.

dystrophia (dĭs-trō'fē-ă) [" + *trephein,* to nourish]. Disorder caused by defective nutrition or metabolism. SYN: *dystrophy.*

dystrophic (dĭs-trŏf'ĭk). Pert. to dystrophia.

dystrophoneurosis (dĭs-trŏf"ō-nū-rō'sĭs) [" + *trephein,* to nourish, + *neuron,* nerve, + *osis,* condition]. 1. Defective nutrition caused by a nervous disease. 2. Any nervous disorder caused by faulty nutrition.

dystrophy (dĭs'trō-fē). Disorder caused by defective nutrition or metabolism. SYN: *dystrophia.*

d., adiposogenital. A condition characterized by a peculiar type of obesity and hypogenitalism due to a disturbance in the hypothalamus, which controls food intake, and of the pituitary, which controls gonadal develpment. SYN: *Fröhlich's syndrome.*

d., Landouzy-Dejerine. A hereditary form of progressive muscular dystrophy with onset in childhood or adolescence. Characterized by atrophic changes in muscles of shoulder girdle and face, inability to raise arms above the head, myopathic facies, eyelids that remain partly open in sleep, and inability to whistle or purse lips. SYN: *atrophy, Landouzy-Dejerine.*

d., progressive muscular. A familial disease characterized by progressive atrophy and wasting of muscles. Onset is usually at an early age and it occurs more frequently in males than females. Its cause is thought to be a genetic defect in muscle metabolism.

d., pseudohypertrophic muscular. A hereditary disease usually beginning in childhood in which muscular ability is lost. At first there is muscular pseudohypertrophy followed by atrophy.

dystrypsia (dĭs-trĭp'sē-ă) [Gr. *dys,* bad, + *tripsis,* rubbing]. Impaired secretion of pancreas.

dysuria (dĭs-ū'rē-ă) [" + *ouron,* urine]. Painful or difficult urination, symptomatic of numerous conditions. Dysuria may be indicative of cystitis; urethritis; infection anywhere in the urinary tract; urethral stricture; hypertrophied, cancerous, or ulcerated prostate in the male; prolapse of uterus in the female; pelvic peritonitis and abscess; metritis; cancer of the cervix; dysmenorrhea; or psychological abnormalities. May also be caused by certain medications, esp. opiates and medicines used to prevent motion sickness. Pain and burning may also be caused by concentrated acid urine.

dysuriac. One affected with dysuria.

dyszooamylia (dĭs-zō"ō-ăm-ĭl'ē-ă) [" + *zoon,* animal, + *amylon,* starch]. Failure of liver to transform dextrose into glycogen.

dyszoospermia (dĭs"zō-ō-spĕrm'ē-ă) [" + " + *sperma,* seed]. Imperfect formation of spermatozoa.

E

E. *emmetropia; energy; Escherichia; eye.*
E_1. *estrone.*
E_2. *estradiol.*
E_3. *estriol.*
e. *electric charge; electron;* L. *ex,* from.
ea. *each.*
ead. L. *eadem,* the same.
Eales' disease (ēlz). [Henry Eales, Brit. physician, 1852–1913] Recurrent hemorrhages into the retina and vitreous, most commonly seen in males in the second and third decades of life. The cause is unknown.
ear [AS. *ear*]. Organ of hearing. Consisting of external, middle, and internal ear. SEE: illus.; *hearing, functional test for; labyrinth* for additional illus.

EXAM: Hearing ability may be estimated by asking the individual to repeat phrases or answer questions that the examiner states while facing away from the patient. For accuracy, however, the hearing should be tested by using an accurately calibrated audiometer. This is esp. true if the test of hearing acuity is done on an individual who works in a noisy environment. Comparing subsequent tests of hearing with the original or baseline record will permit determining the effect, if any, of the noisy work environment on the individual's hearing.

Also examine for color, size, and shape of ear; discharge from middle or inner ear; tenderness upon pressure in front or back of ear; inflammation or bulging of drum; perforations or scars of drum. Deafness may indicate wax in the external ear canals, disorders of the 8th (vestibulocochlear) nerve, disease of the middle ear, or the toxic effect of drugs. Pallor of ears, tongue, and gums indicates shock or anemia. Ringing in ears may be noted in cerebral hyperemia and anemia, in disease of ear, Ménière's disease, and after use of certain drugs such as quinine or salicylic acid. SEE: *hearing, sensorineural.*

e., Blainville's. Congenital asymmetry of the ears.

e., Cagot. An ear without a lower lobe.

e., cauliflower. A deformity consisting of a thickening of the external ear resulting from trauma that caused a hematoma. Commonly seen in boxers.

e., external. Portion of the ear consist-

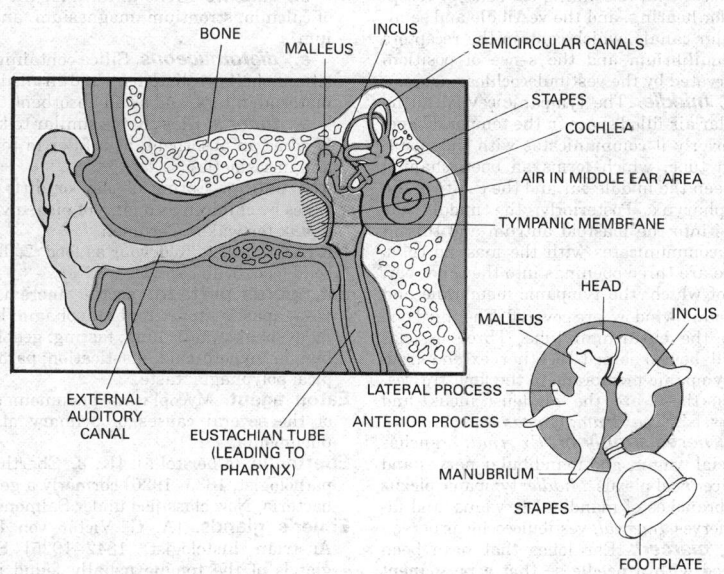

EXTERNAL AND INNER EAR

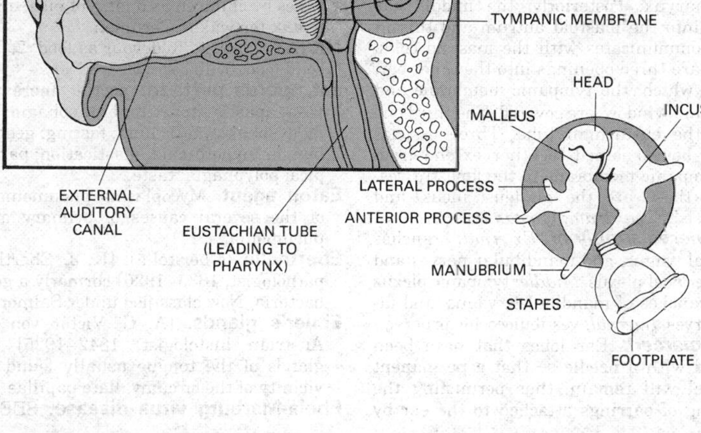

ing of the auricle and external auditory canal, and separated from the middle ear by the tympanic membrane or eardrum.

e., foreign bodies in. These are usually insects, pebbles, beans, or peas.

SYM: Pain, ringing, or buzzing in the ear. If due to a live insect, there is usually a great noise.

TREATMENT: Do not attempt to lure insects from the ear canal with a bright light; they may be stimulated to crawl deeper. Drop in bland oil and float insect out. In case of a solid foreign body, oil or water should not be used because they might either push the object further in the ear or cause it to swell and become firmly embedded. Such foreign bodies in the ear do not constitute an emergency and should be left untreated until seen by a physician.

Water sometimes enters the ears of swimmers and will not flow out spontaneously. Usually this can be dislodged by a sudden tap on the side of the head above the ear, or by introducing a long wisp of cotton, which will draw out the water by capillary action. Also a few drops of 70% alcohol instilled in the canal will hasten evaporation of the so-called trapped water. Occasionally this sensation of water in the ear is not due to water but to swelling of the cerumen, q.v. In such instances a physician should be consulted.

e., internal. Portion of the ear consisting of the cochlea, containing the sensory receptors for hearing, and the vestibule and semicircular canals, which contain the receptors for equilibrium and the sense of position. Innervated by the vestibulocochlear nerve.

e., middle. The tympanic cavity, an irregular air-filled space in the temporal bone. Anteriorly it communicates with the eustachian tube, which forms an open channel between the middle ear and the cavity of the nasopharynx. Posteriorly, the middle ear opens into the mastoid antrum and this in turn communicates with the mastoid cells. There are three openings into the inner ear, two of which, the tympanic membrane and the round window, are covered. The third one is to the eustachian tube. Three ossicles (small bones) joined together extend from the tympanic membrane to the fenestra vestibuli; these are the malleus, incus, and stapes. SEE: *eardrum; tympanum.*

e., nerve supply of. *External:* branches of facial, vagus, and mandibular nerves and from cervical plexus. *Middle:* tympanic plexus and branches of mandibular, vagus, and facial nerves. *Internal:* vestibulocochlear nerve.

e., pierced. Ear lobes that have been pierced with a needle so that a permanent channel will remain, thus permitting the wearing of earrings attached to the ear by use of a connector through the channel.

ear, words pert. to: acoustic meatus; acoustic nerve; aditus ad antrum; angiotitis; annulus tympanicus; antihelix; antitragus; antrotympanitis; auditory; auricula; "auris-" words; binaural; cavum tympani; cerumen; cochlea; concha; crista ampullaris; cupola; deafness; endolymph; epitympanum; eustachian; foreign bodies; helix; hydrotis; incus; labyrinth; labyrinthitis; malleus; ossicle; "ot-" or "oto-" words; pinna; scala; socioacusis; tinnitus aurium; tympanum; "utri-" words; vestibule of ear.

earache. Pain in the ear. SYN: *otalgia; otodynia.*

ear bones. The ossicles of the tympanic cavity: malleus, incus, and stapes. SEE: *ear* for illus.

eardrum (ēr′drŭm). The cavity in the middle ear. SYN: *tympanum.*

ear dust. Calcareous concretions in the membranous labyrinth. SYN: *otoconia; otolith.*

ear oximeter. A device that determines the oxygen content of the blood flowing through the ear.

ear plug. A device for preventing sound from entering the ear by occluding the external auditory canal.

CAUTION: Should not be used while swimming because it may interfere with pressure equalization.

earth. The soil on the surface of the world.

e., alkaline. General term for the oxides of calcium, strontium, magnesium, and barium.

e., diatomaceous. Silica containing fossilized shells of diatoms. Used in insulating material, filters, and as an absorbent.

e., fuller's. Clay that is similar to kaolin. Used as an absorbent, as a filler in textiles, and in cosmetics.

earth eating. Eating of clay or dirt; sometimes by children as a form of pica, q.v.

earwax (ēr′wăks). Cerumen.

eat [AS. *etan*]. 1. To devour as food. 2. To take solid food. 3. To corrode.

eat, words pert. to: acoria; anorexia nervosa; apastia; appetite; bradyphagia; bulimia; dysphagia; fastidium; fasting; geophagia; hunger; hyperorexia; mastication; parorexia; pica; polyphagia; taste.

Eaton agent. Mycoplasma pneumoniae, one of the several causes of primary atypical pneumonia.

Eberthella (ā″bĕr-tĕl′ă). [K. J. Eberth, Ger. pathologist, 1835–1926] Formerly a genus of bacteria. Now classified under Salmonella.

Ebner's glands. [A. G. Victor von Ebner, Austrian histologist, 1842–1925] Serous glands of the tongue usually found in the vicinity of the circumvallate papillae.

Ebola-Marburg virus disease. SEE: *Mar-*

burg virus disease.

ebonation (ē″bō-nā′shŭn) [L. *e,* out, + AS. *ban,* bone]. Removal of bony fragments from a wound.

Ebstein's anomaly (ĕb′stīnz). [Wilhelm Ebstein, Ger. physician, 1836–1912] A congenital condition of the heart, symptoms of which are fatigue, palpitation and dyspnea, resulting from downward displacement of the tricuspid valve from the annulus fibrosus.

ebullism (ĕb′ū-lĭzm) [L. *ebullire,* to boil over]. Formation of water vapor in body tissue, which occurs when the body is exposed to extreme reduction in barometric pressure.

eburnation (ĕb″ūr-nā′shŭn) [L. *eburnus,* made of ivory]. Changes in bone causing it to become dense and hard like ivory.

eburneous (ē-bŭr′nē-ŭs). Resembling ivory; ivory-colored.

EBV. *Epstein-Barr virus.* SEE: *mononucleosis, infectious.*

ecaudate (ē-kaw′dāt) [L. *e,* without, + *cauda,* tail]. Without a tail.

ecbolic (ĕk-bŏl′ĭk) [Gr. *ekbolikos,* throwing out]. 1. Hastening uterine evacuation by causing contractions of the uterine muscles. 2. Any agent producing or hastening labor or abortion. SYN: *oxytocic.*

ECC. *external cardiac compression.* SEE: *cardiopulmonary resuscitation.*

eccentric (ĕk-sĕn′trĭk) [Gr. *ek,* out, + *kentron,* center]. 1. Proceeding away from a center. 2. Peripheral.

eccentro-osteochondrodysplasia (ĕk-sĕn″trō-ŏs″tē-ō-kŏn″drō-dĭs-plā′zhē-ă) [Gr. *ekkentros,* from the center, + *osteon,* bone, + *chondros,* cartilage, + *dys,* bad, + *plassein,* to form]. A pathological condition of bones caused by imperfect bone formation. Ossification occurs in eccentric centers instead of one common center.

eccentropiesis (ĕk-sĕn″trō-pī-ē′sĭs) [″ + *piesis,* pressure]. Pressure from within exerted outward.

ecchondroma (ĕk-ŏn-drō′mă) [Gr. *ek,* out, + *chondros,* cartilage, + *oma,* tumor]. A chondroma or cartilaginous tumor.

ecchondrotome (ĕk-ŏn′drō-tōm) [″ + ″ + *tome,* incision]. Knife for excision of cartilage.

ecchymoma (ĕk-ĭ-mō′mă) [″ + *chymos,* juice, + *oma,* tumor]. A swelling resulting from the accumulation of blood in subcutaneous tissues such as occurs following a bruise.

ecchymosis (ĕk-ĭ-mō′sĭs) [″ + ″ + *osis,* condition]. (pl. *ecchymoses*) A form of macula appearing in large irregularly formed hemorrhagic areas of the skin. The color is blue-black changing to greenish brown or yellow.

ETIOL: Extravasation of blood into skin or mucous membrane.

ecchymotic (ĕk-ĭ-mŏt′ĭk) [″ + *chymos,* juice]. Resembling or rel. to an ecchymosis.

eccrine (ĕk′rĭn) [Gr. *ekkrinein,* to secrete]. Pert. to secretion, esp. of sweat. SEE: *endocrine; exocrine.*

eccrine sweat glands. Glands distributed over the entire skin surface that, because they secrete sweat, are important in regulating body heat. The total number of glands is from two to five million. There are over 400/sq. cm. on the palms and about 80/sq. cm. on the thighs. SEE: *sweat glands* for illus; *apocrine sweat glands; sweat glands.*

eccritic (ĕk-krĭt′ĭk) [Gr. *ekkritikos*]. Promoting or that which promotes excretion.

eccyclomastopathy (ĕk-sī′klō-măs-tŏp′ă-thē) [Gr. *ek,* out, + *kyklos,* circle, + *mastos,* breast, + *pathos,* disease] A mass of lesions of the breast made up of connective tissue and epithelial cells.

eccyesis (ĕk″sī-ē′sĭs) [″ + *kyesis,* pregnancy]. Extrauterine or ectopic pregnancy.

ecdemomania (ĕk″dē-mō-mā′nē-ă) [Gr. *ekdemos,* journeying, + *mania,* madness]. Wanderlust; abnormal desire to wander. SYN: *drapetomania; dromomania.*

ecderon (ĕk′dĕ-rŏn) [Gr. *ek,* out, + *deros,* skin]. Epidermis or outer portion of skin as distinguished from enderon, q.v., or inner portion.

ecdysis (ĕk′dĭ-sĭs) [Gr. *ekdysis,* getting out]. (pl. *ecdyses*) 1. The shedding or sloughing off of the epidermis of the skin. SYN: *desquamation.* 2. The shedding of the outer covering of the body as occurs in certain animals such as insects, crustaceans, and snakes. SYN: *molt.*

ECG, ecg. *electrocardiogram.*

echeosis (ĕk″ē-ō′sĭs) [Gr. *eche,* loud sound, + *osis,* condition]. Mental disturbance caused by noise.

echidnase (ē-kĭd′nās) [Gr. *echidna,* viper]. An enzyme present in the venom of viper snakes. It produces inflammation.

echidnin (ē-kĭd′nĭn). 1. The venom of poisonous snakes. 2. The active principle present in snake venom.

Echidnophaga (ĕk″ĭd-nŏf′ă-gă). A genus of fleas belonging to the family Pulicidae.

E. gallinacea. The sticktight flea, an important flea pest of poultry. It collects in clusters on the heads of poultry and in the ears of mammals. It may infest humans, esp. children.

echinate (ĕk′ĭ-nāt) [Gr. *echinos,* hedgehog]. 1. Spiny. 2. In agar streak, a growth with pitted or toothed margins along the inoculation line; in stab cultures, coiled growth with pointed outgrowths. SYN: *echinulate.*

echinococcosis (ē-kī″nō-kŏk-ō′sĭs, ĕk″ĭ-nō-kŏk-ō′sĭs) [″ + *kokkos,* berry, + *osis,* condition]. Infestation with Echinococcus.

echinococcotomy (ē-kī″nō-kŏk-ŏt′ō-mē) [″ +

" + *tome,* incision]. Operation for evacuation of an echinococcus cyst.

Echinococcus (ĕ-kī"nō-kŏk'ŭs). (pl. *Echinococci*) A genus of tapeworms. They are minute forms consisting of a scolex and three or four proglottids.

E. granulosus. A species of tapeworms that infests dogs and other carnivores. Its larva, called a hydatid, develops in other mammals, including man, and causes the formation of hydatid cysts in the liver or lungs. SEE: *hydatid.*

E. hydatidosus. Variety of Echinococcus characterized by development of daughter cysts from the mother cyst. SEE: *hydatid.*

echinosis (ĕk"ĭ-nō'sĭs) [Gr. *echinos,* hedgehog, + *osis,* condition]. Crenated red blood cells that are irregular in shape.

Echinostoma (ĕk"ĭ-nŏs'tō-mă) [" + *stoma,* mouth]. A genus of flukes characterized by a spiny body and the presence of a collar of spines near the anterior end. They are found in the intestines of many vertebrates, esp. aquatic birds. They occasionally occur as accidental parasites in man.

echinulate (ĕ-kĭn'ū-lāt). A bacterial growth having pointed processes or spines. SYN: *echinate.*

echo (ĕk'ō) [Gr. *ekho*]. A reverberating sound produced when sound waves are reflected back to their source.

e., amphoric. Amphoric sound sometimes heard in auscultation of chest. SEE: *chest.*

echo acousia. Subjective echoes of sounds just normally heard.

echocardiogram (ĕk"ō-kăr'dē-ō-grăm"). The graphic record produced by echocardiography, q.v.

echocardiography (ĕk"ō-kăr"dē-ŏg'ră-fē). A noninvasive diagnostic method that uses ultrasound, q.v., to visualize internal cardiac structures. All cardiac valves can be visualized, and the dimensions of each ventricle and the left atrium can be measured.

echoencephalogram (ĕk"ō-ĕn-sĕf'ă-lō-grăm"). Recording of the ultrasonic echoes of the brain. Esp. useful in diagnosing conditions that cause a shift in the midline structures of the brain.

echogram (ĕk'ō-grăm). The record made by echography.

echography (ĕk-ŏg'ră-fē) [" + *graphein,* to write]. The use of ultrasonic technique to produce a photograph of the echo produced when sound waves are reflected from tissues of different density. SEE: *ultrasonography.*

echokinesia (ĕk"ō-kĭn-ē'sē-ă) [" + *kinesis,* movement]. Involuntary repetition of another's gestures.

echolalia (ĕk-ō-lā'lē-ă) [" + *lalia,* talk, babble]. An involuntary parrotlike repetition of words spoken by others, often accompanied by twitching of muscles. Frequently seen in catatonic schizophrenia.

echomimia (ĕk"ō-mĭm'ē-ă) [" + *mimesis,* imitation]. The imitation of the actions of others as seen in schizophrenia. SYN: *echopraxia.*

echomotism (ĕk"ō-mō'tĭzm) [" + L. *motus,* moving]. Imitation of movements.

echopathy (ĕ-kŏp'ă-thē) [" + *pathos,* disease]. A neurosis in which there is pathological repetition of another's actions and words.

echophotony (ĕk"ō-fŏt'ō-nē) [" + *phos,* light, + *tonos,* tone]. Mental association of certain sounds with particular colors.

echophrasia (ĕk"ō-frā'sē-ă) [" + *phrasis,* speech]. Echolalia.

echopraxia (ĕk"ō-prăk'sē-ă) [" + *prassein,* to perform]. Imitation without meaning of motions made by others. SYN: *echomimia; echomotism.*

echo sign. Repetition of closing word of a sentence, a sign of epilepsy or other brain conditions.

echothiophate iodide (ĕk"ō-thī'ō-fāt). USP. A cholinergic drug used topically in the eye for treatment of glaucoma. Trade names are Echodide and Phospholine Iodide.

ECHO virus. One of the viruses belonging to the group originally known as *E*nteric *C*ytopathogenic *H*uman *O*rphan group. They are associated with nonbacterial viral meningitis, enteritis, pleurodynia, acute respiratory infection, and myocarditis. More than 30 viruses were assigned to this group initially. Later, some of these were reclassified. Thus types 10 and 28 were removed from the ECHO group and are now classed as reovirus 1 and rhinovirus 1, respectively.

Eck's fistula (ĕks). [N. V. Eck, Russian physiologist, 1847–1908] Artificial communication between the portal vein and the inferior vena cava; used in experimental surgery in animals.

eclabium (ĕk-lā'bē-ŭm) [Gr. *ek,* out, + L. *labium,* lip]. Eversion of a lip.

eclampsia (ĕ-klămp'sē-ă) [" + *lampein,* to shine]. Coma and convulsive seizures between the 20th week of pregnancy and the end of the first week postpartum. Develops in 1 out of 200 patients with pre-eclampsia, q.v., and is usually fatal if untreated.

ETIOL: Unknown. Occurs more often in primigravidae. Pre-existing hypertension and glomerulonephritis contribute to cause.

PATH: Seen most frequently in the kidney, liver, brain, and placenta. The kidney shows degenerated tubal nephritis; the tubal epithelium shows cloudy swelling, fatty degeneration, and coagulation necrosis. The liver is enlarged and mottled. There are portal vein thrombosis and degeneration of the periphery of the lobules with subcapsular hemorrhages. The brain shows edema, hyperemia, thrombosis, and hemorrhages. In the placenta, there are infarcts, thromboses, and hemorrhages. There is also retinal edema.

SYM: Edema of the legs and feet, puffiness of the face, hypertension and albuminuria. Severe headaches, dizziness, spots before the eyes, epigastric pain and nausea, convulsions (beginning with fixation of the eyeballs, rolling of the eyes, twitchings of the face, arms, and hands; the paroxysms then involve the entire body), and coma. There may be one or many convulsions. The pulse is rapid and bounding, the temperature usually rises to 103° or 104° F. (39.4 or 40° C.) and the blood pressure may be quite elevated. The patient may remain in coma until death.

TREATMENT: Prophylaxis is of primary importance. Good prenatal care with careful and frequent observation and recording of the patient's blood pressure, urine output, and weight. Institute appropriate therapy as soon as there are any abnormal findings, and terminate pregnancy if unsuccessful in reducing the signs of danger.

CAUTION: The routine use of diuretics in pregnancy is contraindicated because diuretics are of no benefit and may do considerable harm by masking signs and symptoms that would alert the patient and the physician to the onset of eclampsia.

Convulsions: Prevent the patient from doing herself bodily harm (restrain her in bed, protect the tongue by keeping the teeth separated). Give magnesium sulfate intravenously, 4 gm. in 10 min. and then 1 gm. each hr. if urinary output is maintained. I.V. diazepam may be necessary to control seizures. Constant monitoring of blood pressure, pulse, respirations, reflexes, urinary output, and I.V. fluid intake is necessary.

Delivery: Delivery is not indicated until the patient has reached a stable condition; usually within 4 to 6 hours. If the patient is in active labor, the most conservative methods should be followed. Cesarean section should not be done unless there is some other obstetrical reason. If medical management effects no improvement, then labor must be instituted by administration of an oxytocic agent. Local rather than general anesthesia is preferred.

NURSING IMPLICATIONS: Monitor patient continuously. Record vital signs and fetal heart tones every 1 to 2 hours; measure intake and output, decrease environmental stimuli (quiet environment and bedrest with siderails up). Take seizure precautions. Observe the patient for signs of impending labor. Provide the woman with calm reassurance. Notify the physician immediately if there is any change in the condition of either the fetus or the mother.

eclamptic. Rel. to, or of the nature of, eclampsia.

eclamptogenic (ĕk-lămp″tō-jĕn′ĭk) [Gr. *ek,* out, + *lampein,* to shine, + *gennan,* to produce]. Causing convulsions.

eclectic (ĕk-lĕk′tĭk) [Gr. *eklektikos,* selecting]. Selecting from various sources what seems to be the best.

eclecticism (ĕk-lĕk′tĭ-sĭzm) [″ + *-ismos,* state of]. A former system of medicine treating disease through specific remedies for individual signs or symptoms rather than for distinct diseases. Remedies principally botanical.

eclectic system of medicine. A system employing a selected method, as indigenous plants or specifics according to patient's symptoms rather than for specific diagnostic entities.

ecmnesia (ĕk-nē′zē-ă) [Gr. *ek,* out, + *mnesis,* memory]. Inability to remember recent events, as seen in senility. The memory of before and after events is not affected.

ecocide (ĕk″ō-sīd′) [Gr. *oikos,* house, + L. *caedere,* to kill]. Willful destruction of some portion of the environment.

E. coli. Escherichia coli, q.v.

ecology (ē-kŏl′ō-jē) [Gr. *oikos,* house, + *logos,* study of]. Science of the relations and interactions of the totality of organisms to their environment, including the relations and interactions of organisms to each other in that environment. SYN: *bionomics.*

Econochlor. Trade name for chloramphenicol.

Econopred. Trade name for prednisolone acetate (suspensions).

Economo's disease. [Constatin Von Economo, Austrian neurologist, 1876–1931] SEE: *encephalitis lethargica.*

écorché (ā″kor-shā′) [Fr.]. A representation of an animal or human form without skin so that the muscles are clearly seen.

ecosphere (ĕk′ō-sfēr″) [Gr. *oikos,* house, + L. *sphera,* ball]. Portions of the universe habitable by living organisms and plant life.

ecostate (ē-kŏs′tāt) [L. *e,* without, + *costa,* rib]. Without ribs.

ecosystem (ĕk′ō-sĭs″tĕm). The smallest ecology unit. The living organisms and plants and their environment in a defined area.

Ecotrin. Trade name for aspirin.

écouvillonage (ā-koo″vē-yō-nŏzh′) [Fr. *ecouvillon,* a stiff brush or swab]. The cleansing and application of remedies to a cavity by means of a brush or swab.

ecphoria (ĕk-for′ē-ă) [Gr. *ek,* out of, + *pherein,* to bear]. An engram or the reestablishment of a memory trace or engram.

écrasement (ā-krăz-mŏn′) [Fr.]. Excision by means of an écraseur.

écraseur (ā-kră-zĕr′) [Fr., crusher]. A wire

loop used for excisions.

ecstasy (ĕk′stă-sē) [Gr. *ekstasis,* a standing out]. An exhilarated, trancelike condition or state of exalted delight.

ecstrophy (ĕk′strō-fē) [Gr. *ekstrophe,* a turning out]. Turning an organ inside out. SYN: *exstrophy.*

ECT. *electroconvulsive therapy.*

ectad [Gr. *ektos,* outside, + L. *ad,* toward]. Toward the surface; outward; externally.

ectal. External, outer, on the surface.

ectasia, ectasis (ĕk-tā′sē-ă, ĕk′tă-sĭs) [Gr. *ek,* out, + *teinein,* to stretch]. Dilatation of any tubular vessel.

e., hypostatic. Dilatation of a blood vessel from the pooling of blood in dependent parts, esp. the legs.

ectasia iridis. Smallness of the pupil of the eye caused by displacement of the iris.

ectasia ventriculi paradoxa. Hourglass stomach.

ectatic. Distensible or capable of being stretched.

ectental [Gr. *ektos,* without, + *entos,* within]. Pert. to entoderm and ectoderm.

ectental line. Point of entodermal and ectodermal junction in the gastrula.

ectethmoid (ĕk-tĕth′moyd) [″ + *ethmos,* sieve, + *eidos,* form]. Lateral mass of the ethmoid bone.

ecthyma (ĕk-thī′mă) [Gr. *ek,* out, + *thyein,* to rush]. An infection of the skin. Usually a result of neglected treatment of impetigo, q.v. It is marked by shallow lesions with adherent crusts or scabs. May be followed by pigmentation and scarring. Treatment is the same as that for impetigo, q.v.

ectiris (ĕk-tī′rĭs) [Gr. *ektos,* outside, + *iris,* iris]. The external portion of the iris.

ecto- [Gr. *ektos,* outside]. Prefix meaning outside.

ectoantigen (ĕk″tō-ăn′tĭ-gĕn) [″ + *anti,* against, + *gennan,* to produce]. An antigen assumed to have its origin in ectoplasm of bacterial cells or one loosely attached to the surface of bacteria and capable of being separated from the bacterial cell.

ectoblast (ĕk′tō-blăst) [″ + *blastos,* germ]. 1. Ectoderm. 2. Any outer membrane; as a cell wall.

ectocardia (ĕk-tō-kăr′dē-ă) [″ + *kardia,* heart]. Displacement of the heart.

ectocervical (ĕk″tō-sĕr′vĭ-kăl). Concerning the ectocervix.

ectocervix (ĕk″tō-sĕr′vĭks). The portion of the canal of uterine cervix that is lined with squamous epithelium.

ectochoroidea (ĕk″tō-kō-roy′dē-ă) [″ + *khorioeides,* choroid]. Outer layer of choroid coat of the eye.

ectocinerea (ĕk″tō-sĭn-ē′rē-ă) [″ + L. *cinereus,* ashen]. The outer gray matter of the brain.

ectocolostomy (ĕk″tō-kŏ-lŏs′tō-mē) [″ + *kolon,* colon, + *stoma,* opening]. Formation through the abdominal wall of an opening into the colon.

ectocondyle (ĕk″tō-kŏn′dīl) [″ + *kondylos,* knuckle]. The outer condyle of the bone.

ectocornea (ĕk-tō-kor′nē-ă) [″ + L. *corneus,* horny]. External layer of the cornea.

ectocuneiform (ĕk-tō-kū′nē-ĭ-form) [″ + L. *cuneus,* wedge, + *forma,* form]. External cuneiform bone.

ectocytic (ĕk″tō-sī′tĭk) [″ + *kytos,* cell]. Outside of the cell.

ectodactylism (ĕk″tō-dăk′tĭl-ĭzm) [″ + *daktylos,* finger, + *ismos,* state of]. Lack of a digit or digits.

ectoderm (ĕk′tō-dĕrm) [″ + *derma,* skin]. The outer layer of cells in a developing embryo. From it are developed skin structures, teeth and glands of mouth, the nervous system, organs of special sense, the pineal, and part of pituitary and suprarenal glands. SYN: *epiblast.* SEE: *entoderm; mesoderm.*

ectodermal. Rel. to the ectoderm.

ectodermatosis, ectodermosis (ĕk″tō-dĕr″mă-tō′sĭs, -dĕr-mō′sĭs) [″ + *derma,* skin, + *osis,* diseased condition]. Illness resulting from congenital maldevelopment of ectodermal structures.

e. erosiva pluriorificialis. A form of erythema multiforme characterized by fever, chills, profuse salivation, small blisters on tongue, lips, and cheeks, and erythematous lesions on the hands. This rare disease occurs in children and young persons.

ectodermic. Pert. to the ectoderm. SYN: *ectodermal.*

ectodermoidal (ĕk″tō-dĕr-moyd′ăl) [Gr. *ektos,* outside, + *derma,* skin, + *eidos,* form]. Pert. to or resembling the ectoderm.

ectoentad (ĕk″tō-ĕn′tăd) [″ + *entos,* within]. From without inward.

ectoenzyme (ĕk″tō-ĕn′zīm) [″ + *en-,* in, + *zyme,* leaven]. An extracellular enzyme, or one that acts outside of the cell that secretes it.

ectogenous (ĕk-tŏj′ĕ-nŭs) [″ + *gennan,* to produce]. 1. Having its origin outside of a body or structure, as infection. 2. Ability to grow outside of the body, as a parasite.

ectoglia (ĕk-tŏg′lē-ă) [″ + *glia,* glue]. Superficial embryonic layer in beginning of stratification of the medullary tube of the embryo.

ectoglobular (ĕk″tō-glŏb′ū-lăr) [″ + L. *globulus,* globule]. Not within blood cells or globular bodies.

ectogony (ĕk-tŏg′ō-nē) [″ + *gone,* seed]. Influence of the embryo on the mother.

ectolecithal (ĕk″tō-lĕs′ĭ-thăl) [″ + *lekithos,* yolk]. Pert. to ovum having food yolk placed near the surface.

ectomere (ĕk'tō-mēr) [" + *meros,* part]. One of the blastomeres forming the ectoderm.

ectomesoblast (ĕk"tō-mĕs'ō-blăst) [" + *mesos,* middle, + *blastos,* germ]. Cells from which the ectoblast and mesoblast will develop.

ectomorph (ĕk'tō-morf) [" + *morphe,* form]. Body build characterized by predominance of tissues derived from the ectoderm. Characterized by linearity of body build with sparse muscular development. SEE: *endomorph; mesomorph; somatotype.*

ectomy (ĕk'tō-mē) [Gr. *ektome*]. Excision of any organ or gland.

ectonuclear (ĕk-tō-nū'klē-ăr) [Gr. *ektos,* outside, + L. *nucleus,* kernel]. Occurring outside a cell nucleus.

ectopagus (ĕk-tŏp'ă-gŭs) [" + *pagos,* something fixed]. An abnormal fetus consisting of twins fused at the thorax.

ectoparasite (ĕk"tō-păr'ă-sīt") [" + Gr. *parasitos,* parasite]. A parasite that lives on the outer surface of the body, as fleas, lice, or ticks.

ectoperitonitis (ĕk"tō-pĕr"ĭ-tō-nī'tĭs) [" + *peritonaion,* peritoneum, + *itis,* inflammation]. Inflammation of the parietal layer of peritoneum (layer lining the abdominal wall).

ectophyte (ĕk'tō-fīt) [" + *phyton,* plant]. A parasite of vegetable origin growing on the skin.

ectopia (ĕk-tō'pē-ă) [Gr. *ektopos,* displaced]. Malposition or displacement, esp. congenital, of an organ or structure.

e. cordis. Malposition of the heart in which it lies outside the thoracic cavity.

e. lentis. Displacement of the crystalline lens of the eye.

e. pupillae. Displacement of the pupil. SYN: *corectopia.*

e. renis. Displacement of the kidney.

e. testis. Displacement of the testis.

e. vesicae. Displacement of the bladder, esp. exstrophy of the bladder.

e., visceral. An umbilical hernia.

ectopic (ĕk-tŏp'ik). In an abnormal position. Opposite of entopic.

ectopic beat. Electrical stimulation of cardiac contraction beginning at a point other than the sinoatrial node.

ectopic pregnancy. Implantation of the fertilized ovum outside of the uterine cavity. There is usually a poorly developed decidual reaction in the uterus. SEE: *pregnancy, ectopic,* for illus.

LOCATIONS: *Abdominal:* In the free abdominal cavity and attached to one of the abdominal viscera. *Interstitial:* In the interstitial portion of the tube. *Ovarian:* In the ovary. The ovarian and primary abdominal types are very rare. *Tubal:* In the fallopian tube, the type most frequently encountered. The pregnancy may be situated in the interstitial, ampullar, or isthmic portion of the tube, the isthmic type being the most common.

ETIOL: Most commonly associated with inflammatory conditions of the tube and other conditions that mechanically interfere with the downward passage of the ovum, such as diverticula, polypi in the tubal lumen, and peritoneal adhesions. Any variety of pregnancy or any combination of varieties may occur (uterine plus ectopic, bilateral ectopic).

SYM: Amenorrhea; tenderness, soreness, pain on affected side; pallor, weak pulse, signs of shock or hemorrhage; pain may be reflected to shoulder; perhaps bluish discoloration of umbilicus.

Unruptured: Amenorrhea may or may not be present; vague pains in the abdomen usually on one side; irregular hemorrhage. The diagnosis at this stage can be made by the usual biological tests for pregnancy.

Ruptured: Without a severe hemorrhage: there is severe pain in the lower abdomen with repeated fainting spells. Diagnosis is made by transvaginal needle puncture of the peritoneal cavity. This will reveal free blood. If bleeding is severe and surgical therapy is not instituted without delay, death may result.

DIFF. DIAG: Ectopic pregnancy must be differentiated from appendicitis, uterine pregnancy, acute salpingitis, twisting of the pedicle of an ovarian cyst or pedunculated fibroid tumor, and hemorrhage from a ruptured graafian follicle or corpus luteum cyst.

TREATMENT: Once the diagnosis of ectopic pregnancy is made, operative treatment is indicated. In those cases where there is profound shock from hemorrhage, the patient should be supported by blood transfusion and saline infusions before major surgery is attempted.

ectopic rhythm. Any cardiac rhythm that is abnormal or irregular.

ectopic secretion (ĕk-tŏp'ĭk). The secretion of hormones by tumors arising from tissues that do not normally secrete the hormone or hormones.

ectoplasm [Gr. *ektos,* outside, + *plasma,* a thing formed]. The outermost layer of cell protoplasm.

ectoplasmic. Pert. to ectoplasm. SYN: *ectoplastic.*

ectoplast (ĕk'tō-plăst) [" + *plastikos,* formed]. Cell membrane.

ectoplastic. Formed at the periphery. SYN: *ectoplasmic.*

ectopotomy (ĕk-tō-pŏt'ō-mē) [Gr. *ektopos,*

displaced, + *tome,* incision]. Removal of the fetus in ectopic pregnancy.

ectopterygoid (ĕk″tō-tĕr′ĭ-goyd) [Gr. *ektos,* outside, + *pteryx,* wing, + *eidos,* form]. External or lateral pterygoid muscle. Acts to bring jaw forward.

ectopy (ĕk′tō-pē) [Gr. *ektopos,* displaced]. Displacement. SYN: *ectopia.*

ectoretina (ĕk″tō-rĕt′ĭ-nă) [Gr. *ektos,* outside, + L. *rete,* net]. Outer layer of retina.

ectostosis (ĕk-tŏs-tō′sĭs) [″ + *osteon,* bone, + *osis,* condition]. Formation of bone beneath the periosteum.

ectothrix (ĕk′tō-thrĭks) [″ + *thrix,* hair]. Any fungus that produces arthrospores on the hair shafts.

Ectotrichophyton (ĕk″ō-trī-kŏf′ĭ-tŏn) [″ + *thrix,* hair, + *phyton,* plant]. Former name for Trichophyton megalosporon ectothrix, a genus of parasitic fungi causing tinea or ringworm of the hair.

ectozoon (ĕk-tō-zō′ŏn) [″ + *zoon,* animal]. Parasitic animal that infests the outer integument of the body.

ectro- [Gr. *ektrosis,* abortion]. Combining form meaning congenital absence of a part.

ectrodactylism (ĕk″trō-dăk′tĭl-ĭzm) [″ + *daktylos,* finger, + *-ismos,* state of]. Congenital absence of all or part of a digit.

ectrogeny (ĕk-trŏj′ĕ-nē) [″ + *gennan,* to produce]. Congenital absence of a part of the body.

ectromelia (ĕk″trō-mē′lē-ă) [″ + *melos,* limb]. Hypoplasia of the long bones of the limbs.

ectromelus (ĕk-trŏm′ĕ-lŭs) [″ + *melos,* limb]. Individual with ectromelia.

ectropic (ĕk-trō′pĭk) [Gr. *ek,* out, + *trope,* turning]. Pert. to complete or partial eversion of a part, generally the eyelid.

ectropion (ĕk-trō′pē-ŏn). Eversion of an edge or margin, as the edge of an eyelid.

ETIOL: Old age; relaxation of skin; cicatrix following trauma; infection; palsy of facial nerve.

ectropionize. To evert or cause an eversion.

ectrosyndactyly (ĕk″trō-sĭn-dăk′tĭ-lē) [″ + *syn,* together, + *dactylos,* finger]. Congenital absence of one or more fingers; the remaining fingers are fused together.

eczema (ĕk′zĕ-mă) [Gr. *ekzein,* to boil out]. Acute or chronic cutaneous inflammatory condition with erythema, papules, vesicles, pustules, scales, crusts, or scabs alone or in combination. They may be dry or with watery discharge, with thickening, infiltration, and more or less itching or burning. Eczema is more the description of a symptom than of a disease. This word has become synonymous with dermatitis caused by a number of external and internal factors acting singly or in combination. It has therefore no specific connotation, particularly with respect to etiology. SEE: *allergy; dermatitis.*

ETIOL: No class, age, or sex is exempt, but those with thin, dry skins are more susceptible. The lesions are not infectious. Two classes of causes: external or exciting (irritation, allergic contact, reaction to exposure to certain microorganisms, occupational and nonoccupational, chemical); and constitutional or predisposing. The latter includes eczema caused by genetic and psychological factors.

SYM: Primary type characterized by erythematous, papular, vesicular, or pustular lesions. In secondary type, the lesions evolve from primary variety. Invasion by pathogenic organisms may cause suppuration.

PROG: Chronic, amenable to treatment but prone to relapse and recurrence.

NURSING IMPLICATIONS: Institute measures to decrease scratching, such as application of hand mitts, or cutting the nails very short. Cleanse the skin with water (soap is often irritating), and apply creams as ordered. Keep the involved areas as clean and dry as possible to decrease chances of infection. Allergens that aggravate the condition should be eliminated from the diet and the environment.

TREATMENT: Depends upon the etiology and will therefore be highly individualized according to the causative agent, organism, or condition.

e., erythematous. Dry, pinkish, ill-defined patches with itching and burning; slight swelling with tendency to spread and coalesce; branny scaling; roughness and dryness of skin. May become generalized.

e. fissum. Form of eczema with painful fissures.

e. herpeticum. Massive crops of vesicles that become pustular, occurring when infection with herpes simplex virus takes place in a person, usually an infant, with pre-existing eczema. SYN: *Kaposi's varicelliform eruption.*

e. hypertrophicum. Eczema with a permanent enlargement of papillae of the skin or with skin growths.

e., lichenoid. Eczema with a thickened condition of the skin.

e. marginatum. Eczema caused by ringworm. SYN: *tinea cruris.*

e., nummular. Lesions are coin- or oval-shaped.

e., pustular. Includes many forms: follicular, impetiginous, or consecutive types including eczema rubrum (red, glazed surface with little oozing), eczema madidans (raw, red, and covered with moisture), eczema crustosum (more or less crusting with exudate), eczema fissum (thick, dry, inelastic skin with cracks and fissures), squamous eczema (chronic on soles, legs, scalp; multiple circumscribed infiltrated patches with thin, dry scales), eczema sclerosum (marked thickening, elephantiasis-like papillary hypertrophy resulting in rough, horny, verrucose patches on legs, soles, and palms with fissuring), furrowed eczema (slightly erythematous skin, harsh and dry, with innumerable cracks on outer epidermal layer).

e., seborrheic. Form marked by excessive secretion from the sebaceous glands. SYN: *seborrhea.*

e. vaccinatum. Generalized vaccinial lesions or local lesions elsewhere than at vaccination site in persons who have eczema and have been vaccinated. Also may occur as result of accidental contact with a recently vaccinated parent or sibling. SYN: *Kaposi's varicelliform eruption.*

eczematous (ĕk-zĕm'ă-tŭs). Marked by or resembling eczema.

ED. *effective dose; erythema dose.*

ED_{50}. The median effective dose; the dose that produces the desired effect in 50% of subjects tested.

EDC. *expected date of confinement.*

Edecrin. Trade name for ethacrynic acid.

edema (ĕ-dē'mă) [Gr. *oidema,* swelling]. (pl. *edemas* or *edemata*) A local or generalized condition in which the body tissues contain an excessive amount of tissue fluid. Generalized edema is sometimes called dropsy, q.v., or anasarca, q.v. Spelled oedema in Great Britain.

ETIOL: May result from increased permeability of the capillary walls; increased capillary pressure due to venous obstruction or heart failure; lymphatic obstruction; disturbances in renal functioning; reduction of plasma proteins; inflammatory conditions; fluid and electrolyte disturbances, particularly those causing sodium retention; malnutrition; starvation; chemical substances such as bacterial toxins, venoms, caustic substances, and histamine. May occur by diffusion, q.v., osmosis, q.v., or dialysis, q.v.

TREATMENT: Bedrest desirable. Salt intake restricted; may be moderate or severe restriction depending upon degree of edema. Fluid intake restricted; may be as low as 600 ml. in 24 hours. This prescription may be relaxed when free diuresis has been attained. Diuretics are effective when renal function is good and edema mild and when underlying abnormality of cardiac function, capillary pressure, or salt retention is being corrected simultaneously. One of a variety of effective diuretics may be used. Diuretics are contraindicated in the true nephritic edema of acute diffuse glomerulonephritis. They are often useless in cardiac edema associated with advanced renal insufficiency. The diet in edema should be adequate in protein, high in calories, rich in vitamins, and low in salt. When diuresis appears, the patient may resume a normal diet.

e., acute circumscribed. Form of edema with localized swelling, usually on the face.

e., angioneurotic. Large areas of swelling of subcutaneous tissues, mucous membranes, and occasionally viscera. May be due to allergic sensitivity to drugs, food, or physical agents such as cold or wind, but in many cases the cause is unknown. SYN: *angioedema.*

e., blue. Hysteric paralysis inducing a swollen, bluish condition of a limb.

e., brain. Swelling of brain tissue due to accumulation of fluid. May be caused by a tumor, toxic chemicals, or infections.

e. bullosum vesicae. Form of edema affecting the bladder.

e., cardiac. Accumulation of fluid in body tissues due to congestive heart failure. It is most apparent in the dependent portion of the body.

e., cerebral. Brain edema, q.v.

e., dependent. Edema or swelling of that part of the body lower than the heart. Thus, the legs are more edematous than are the upper arms.

e., inflammatory. Edema due to inflammation.

e., malignant. Edema characterized by a rapid course and speedy destruction of tissue.

e. neonatorum. Edema in newborn, esp. premature infants. Condition is usually transitory, involving hands, face, feet, and genitalia, and it rarely becomes generalized.

e. of glottis. An infiltration of the submucosa of the larynx with cough, loss of voice, and feeling of suffocation.

e., pitting. Edema, usually of the skin of the extremities, that when pressed firmly with a finger will maintain the depression produced by the finger.

e., pulmonary. Accumulation of fluid in the lungs due to left-sided failure of the heart, i.e., more blood is supplied to the pulmonary circulation than is removed.

e., purulent. Edema caused by purulent infiltration.

e., salt. Form of edema caused by increase of salt in the diet.

edema, words pert. to: angioneurotic edema; cephaledema; chemosis; nephritis; phlegmasia alba dolens; urticaria bullosa.

edematogenic (ĕ-dĕm"ă-tō-jĕn'ĭk). Causing edema.

edematous (ĕ-dĕm'ăt-ŭs) [Gr. *oidema,* swelling]. Pert. to, or affected with, edema.

edentia (ē-dĕn'shē-ă) [L. *e,* without, + *dens,* tooth]. Absence of teeth.

edentulous (ē-děnt′ū-lŭs). Without teeth.

edetate, calcium disodium (ĕd′ĕ-tāt). USP. The disodium salt of ethylenediaminetetraacetic acid. A chelating agent used in diagnosing and treating lead poisoning. Trade names are Calcium Disodium Versenate and Versene CA.

edible (ĕd′ĭ-bl) [L. *edere,* to eat]. Suitable for food; fit to eat, nonpoisonous.

edrophonium chloride (ĕd″rō-fō′nē-ŭm). USP. A cholinergic drug. Trade name is Tensilon. SEE: *edrophonium test.*

edrophonium test. Use of edrophonium chloride to test for the presence of myasthenia gravis. The appropriate dose is injected intravenously; if there is no effect, then a larger dose is given within 45 seconds. A positive test demonstrates brief improvement in strength unaccompanied by lingual fasciculation. The test may also be used to test for an overdose of a cholinergic drug. An excessive dose of cholinergic drug produces weakness that closely resembles myasthenia. A very small dose of edrophonium chloride given intravenously will make the weakness worse if it is due to cholinergic drug overdose and will improve the weakness if it is due to myasthenia gravis.

CAUTION: The test should not be done unless facilities for respiratory resuscitation are immediately available.

EDTA. *ethylenediaminetetraacetic acid.*

eduction (ē-dŭk′shŭn) [L. *e,* out, + *ducere,* to lead]. Emergence from a particular state or condition. Thus, coming out of the effects of general anesthesia is an example of eduction. SEE: *induction* (def. 4).

edulcorant (ē-dŭl′kō-rănt) [″ + *dulcorare,* to sweeten]. Sweetening.

edulcorate (ē-dŭl′kō-rāt). 1. To sweeten. 2. To wash out salts or acids.

EEE. *eastern equine encephalitis.*

EEG. *electroencephalogram.*

E.E.N.T. *eye, ear, nose, and throat.*

EFA. *essential fatty acids.*

E-Ferol. Trade name for vitamin E.

effacement (ĕ-fās′mĕnt). In obstetrics, during the normal progress of delivery, the dilation of the cervix, enlarging the cross-sectional area of the canal to permit passage of the fetus.

effect (ĕ-fĕkt′). Result of an action or force.

e., additive. A therapeutic effect of a combination of two or more drugs that is greater than the sum of the individual drug effects.

e., cumulative. Drug effect that is apparent only after a number of doses have been given. Caused by excretion or metabolic degradation of only a fraction of each dose given. Sometimes it is therapeutically desirable although this type of effect is usually avoided.

effectiveness (ē-fĕk′tĭv-nĕs). The ability to cause the expected or intended effect or result.

effector [L. *effectus,* accomplishing]. One of the nerve endings having the efferent process end in a gland or muscle cell. The terminal arborizations of efferent or motor nerves. Also applied to effector organs (muscles and glands).

effector organ. A structure, specifically muscles and glands, that when stimulated produces an effect.

effeminate. Pert. to the state or condition of a male having the physical characteristics of a female.

effemination (ĕ-fĕm″ĭ-nā′shŭn) [L. *effeminare,* to make feminine]. The production of female physical characteristics in a male. SYN: *femininization.*

efferent [L. *ex,* away from, + *ferre,* to carry]. Carrying away from a central organ or section, as efferent nerves, which conduct impulses from the brain or spinal cord to the periphery, efferent lymph vessels, which convey lymph from lymph nodes, and efferent arterioles, which carry blood from glomeruli of the kidney. Opposite of afferent, q.v.

efferent nerves. Nerves that carry impulses having the following effects: motor, causing contraction of muscles; secretory, causing glands to secrete; and inhibitory, causing some organs to become quiescent. SYN: *motor nerves.*

effervesce (ĕf″ĕr-vĕs′) [L. *effervescere,* to boil up]. To boil or form bubbles on the surface of a liquid.

effervescence (ĕf-ĕr-vĕs′ĕns). Formation of bubbles of gas rising to surface of fluid.

effervescent. Bubbling. Rising in little bubbles of gas.

effleurage (ĕf-loor-ăzh′) [Fr. *effleurer,* to touch lightly]. Deep or gentle stroking in massage.

efflorescence (ĕf-flor-ĕs′ĕns) [L. *efflorescere,* to bloom]. A rash; a redness of the skin. SYN: *exanthem.*

efflorescent. Becoming powdery or drying from loss of water of crystallization.

effluent (ĕf′loo-ĕnt) [L. *effluere,* to flow out]. 1. A flowing out. 2. Fluid material discharged from a sewage treatment plant or an industrial plant.

effluvium (ĕf-loo′vē-ŭm). (pl. *effluvia*) A malodorous exhalation, particularly one that is toxic.

effort syndrome. Neurocirculatory asthenia, q.v.

effuse (ĕ-fūs′) [L. *ex,* out, + *fundere,* to pour]. Thin, widely spreading. Applied to a bacterial growth that forms a very delicate film over a surface.

effusion (ĕ-fū′zhŭn). Escape of fluid into a

part, as the pleural cavity, such as pyothorax (pus), hydrothorax (serum), hemothorax (blood), chylothorax (lymph), pneumothorax (air), hydropneumothorax (serum and air), and pyopneumothorax (pus and air).

Efudex. Trade name for fluorouracil.

egersis (ē-gĕr'sĭs) [Gr., a waking]. Extreme or abnormal wakefulness; extreme alertness.

egesta (ē-jĕs'tă) [L. *e,* out, + *gerere,* to bear]. Waste matter eliminated from the body, esp. excrement.

egg [AS. *aeg*]. 1. The female sex cell or ovum, applied esp. to a fertilized ovum that is passed from the body and develops outside, as in fowls. 2. The mammalian ovum.

eglandulous (ē-glănd'ū-lŭs) [" + *glandula,* glandule]. Without glands.

ego (ē'gō, ĕg'ō) [L. *ego,* I]. In psychoanalysis, one of the three major divisions in the model of the psychic apparatus. The others are id and superego. The ego possesses consciousness and memory and serves to mediate between the primitive instinctual or animal drives (the id), internal social prohibitions (the superego), and reality. Thus the ego allows one to adapt to what might otherwise be a very unpleasant situation. The psychiatric use of the term should not be confused with its common usage in the sense of self-love or selfishness. SEE: *id; superego.*

egocentric (ē"gō-sĕn'trĭk) [L. *ego,* I, + *centrum,* center]. Pert. to a withdrawal from the external world with concentration upon inner self.

ego-dystonic (ē"gō-dĭs-tŏn'ĭk) [" + Gr. *dys,* bad, + *tonos,* tension]. Pert. to something that is repulsive to the individual's self-image.

egoism (ē'gō-ĭzm). An inflated estimate of one's value or effectiveness.

egomania (ē"gō-mā'nē-ă) [" + Gr. *mania,* madness]. Abnormal self-esteem and self-interest.

egophony (ē-gŏf'ō-nē) [Gr. *aix,* goat, + *phone,* voice]. A nasal sound, somewhat like the bleat of a goat, heard in auscultation of the chest when the subject speaks in a normal tone. Present in persons with pleural effusion.

ego-syntonic (ē"gō-sĭn-tŏn'ĭk) [" + Gr. *syn,* together, + *tonos,* tension]. Pert. to something that is consistent with the individual's self-image.

egotism (ē'gō-tĭzm). 1. The tendency to regard oneself more highly than is warranted by the facts, and to boast of one's abilities or achievements. 2. An inflated sense of self-importance; conceit. SEE: *egoism.*

egotropic (ē"gō-trŏp'ĭk) [L. *ego,* I, + Gr. *tropos,* a turning]. Interested chiefly in one's self; self-centered.

Ehlers-Danlos syndrome (ā'lĕrz-dăn'lŏs). [E. Ehlers, Danish dermatologist, 1863–1937; H. A. Danlos, Fr. dermatologist, 1844–1912] An inherited disorder of the elastic connective tissue. The characteristic soft velvety skin is fragile and hyperelastic and bruises easily. Hyperextensibility of joints, visceral malformations, atrophic scars, pseudotumors, and calcified subcutaneous cysts are present.

ETIOL: Unknown.

TREATMENT: No specific therapy.

PROG: Patients may be uncomfortable and inconvenienced by their disease but the outlook for life is good.

Ehrenritter's ganglion (ār ĕn-rĭt"ĕrs). [Johann Ehrenritter, late eighteenth century Austrian anatomist] The superior ganglion of the glossopharyngeal nerve.

Ehrlich's side-chain theory (ār'lĭks). [Paul Ehrlich, Ger. bacteriologist, 1854–1915] A theory proposed to explain immune reactions wherein the antigen-antibody reaction is compared to a chemical structure with side chains or chemical receptors. The body cells, through these chemical receptors, combine with antigens that eventually are released as circulating antibodies.

eidetic (ī-dĕt'ĭk) [Gr. *eidos,* form]. Rel. to or having the ability of total visual recall of anything previously seen.

eidoptometry (ī-dŏp-tŏm'ĕ-trē) [Gr. *eidos,* form, + *optein,* to see, + *metron,* measure]. Determination of ability to perceive form visually.

eighth cranial nerve. The acoustic nerve. SYN: *vestibulocochlear nerve.*

Eikenella corrodens (ī"kĕn-ĕl'ă). A gram-negative rod normally present in the mouth.

eikonometry (ī"kō-nŏm'ĕ-trē) [Gr. *eikon,* image, + *metron,* measure]. 1. Determination of distance of an object by measuring the image produced by a lens of known focus. 2. Optical instrument used in detecting presence of aniseikonia.

eiloid (ī'loyd) [Gr. *eilein,* to coil, + *eidos,* appearance]. Having a coil-like structure.

Eimeria (ī-mē'rē-ă). A genus of sporozoan parasites belonging to the class Telosporidea, subclass Coccidia. They are intracellular parasites living in the epithelial cells of vertebrates and invertebrates. They rarely are parasitic to man.

E. hominis. A species that has been found in empyema in man.

einsteinium (īn-stīn'ē-ŭm). [Albert Einstein, German-born U.S. physicist, 1879–1955] SYMB: Es. At. wt. 254.0881; at. no. 99. A radioactive element.

Eisenmenger's complex. [Victor Eisenmenger, Ger. physician, 1864–1932] Congenital cyanotic heart defect consisting of ventricular septal defect, dextroposition of the aorta, pulmonary hypertension with pulmonary artery enlargement and hypertrophy of the right ventricle.

eisodic (ī-sŏd'ĭk) [Gr. *eis,* into, + *hodos,* way]. Centripetal or afferent, as nerve fibers of a reflex arc.

ejaculatio (ē-jăk"ū-lā'shē-ō) [L.]. Sudden expelling; ejaculation.

e. praecox. Premature ejaculation. Inability to prevent ejaculation of semen at the beginning of copulation or prior to it.

ejaculation (ē-jăk"ū-lā'shŭn) [L. *ejaculari,* to throw out]. Ejection of the seminal fluid from the male urethra.

PHYS: Ejaculation consists of two phases: (1) the passage of semen and the secretions of the accessory organs (bulbourethral and prostate glands and seminal vesicles) into the urethra and (2) the expulsion of the seminal fluid from the urethra. The former is brought about by contraction of the smooth muscle of the ductus deferens and the increased secretory activity of the glands; the latter by the rhythmical contractions of the bulbocavernosus and ischiocavernosus muscles and the levator ani. The prostate discharges its secretions before those of the seminal vesicle. The sensations associated with ejaculation constitute the male orgasm.

Ejaculation is a reflex phenomenon. Afferent impulses arising principally from stimulation of the glans penis pass to the spinal cord by way of the internal pudendal nerves. Efferent impulses arising from a reflex center located in the upper lumbar region of the cord pass through sympathetic fibers in the hypogastric nerves and plexus to the ductus deferens and seminal vesicles. Other impulses arising from the 3rd and 4th sacral segments pass through the internal pudendal nerves to the ischiocavernous and bulbocavernous muscles. Erection of the penis usually precedes ejaculation. Ejaculation occurs normally during copulation, masturbation, or as a nocturnal emission. The seminal fluid normally contains 60 to 150 million sperm/ml. The volume of the ejaculation is from 2 to 5 ml. SEE: *semen.*

RS: coitus; excitation; orgasm.

e., retrograde. Ejaculation in which the seminal fluid is discharged into the bladder rather than to the outside through the urethra. A condition usually present after prostatectomy.

ejaculatory. Pert. to ejaculation.

ejaculatory duct. The terminal portion of the seminal duct formed by the union of the ductus deferens and the excretory duct of the seminal vesicle.

ejecta (ē-jĕk'tă) [L. *ejectus,* thrown out, ejected]. Material, esp. waste material, excreted by the body. SYN: *dejecta; egesta.*

ejection (ē-jĕk'shŭn). Removal of something, esp. a sudden removal.

e., ventricular. Forceful expulsion of blood from the ventricles of the heart.

EKG. Abbr. for Ger. *elektrokardiogramm.* SEE: *ECG.*

ekphorize (ĕk'fō-rīz) [Gr. *ek,* out, + *phorein,* to bear]. In psychiatry, to bring back the effect of a psychic experience in an attempt to experience it again in memory. SEE: *engram.*

elaboration (ē-lăb"ō-rā'shŭn). The process of metabolizing food so that it may be utilized by the body.

elaiopathy (ē"lā-ŏp'ă-thē) [Gr. *elaion,* oil, + *pathos,* disease]. Swelling of joints caused by contusion and followed by fatty deposits. SYN: *eleopathy.*

elastase (ē-lăs'tās). A pancreatic enzyme that in the presence of trypsin cleaves amino acids from proteins.

elastic (ē-lăs'tĭk) [Gr. *elastikos,* elastic]. Capable of being stretched and returning to its original state; having elasticity.

elastic bandage. Bandage that can be stretched to exert continuous pressure.

elastic cartilage. Yellow cartilage such as is found in the epiglottis, pharynx, external ears, and auditory tube.

elasticity (ē"lăs-tĭs'ĭ-tē). The quality of returning to original size and shape after compression or stretching.

elastic skin. Rare condition in which there is unusual elastic state of the skin.

elastic stocking. Stocking worn to apply pressure to the extremity, aiding the return of blood from the extremity to the heart through the deep veins.

elastic tissue. Connective tissue supplied with elastic fibers as found in the middle coat of arteries.

elastin (ē-lăs'tĭn). A protein substance forming the principal constituent of yellow elastic tissue, comprising about 30% of this tissue.

elastinase (ē-lăs'tĭn-ās) [Gr. *elastikos,* elastic]. An enzyme that dissolves elastin.

elastofibroma (ē-lăs"tō-fī-brō'mă) [" + L. *fibra,* fiber, + Gr. *oma,* tumor]. A benign soft tissue tumor that contains elastic and fibrous elements.

elastoid (ē-lăs'toyd) [" + *eidos,* form]. Pert. to a substance formed by hyaline degeneration.

elastoma (ē"lăs-tō'mă) [" + *oma,* tumor]. A chronic disease of the skin; pseudoxanthoma.

elastomer (ē-lăs'tō-mĕr) [" + *meros,* a part]. A polymeric substance that has elastic properties similar to rubber.

elastometer (ē"lăs-tŏm'ĕ-tĕr) [" + *metron,* measure]. Device for measuring elasticity.

elastometry. The measurement of elasticity of tissues.

elastorrhexis (ē-lăs"tō-rĕk'sĭs) [" + *rhexis,*

rupture]. Rupture of elastic tissue.

elastose (ē-lăs′tōs). A peptone resulting from gastric digestion of elastin.

elastosis (ē″lăs-tō′sĭs) [″ + *osis,* condition]. Any disease of elastic tissues.

elation (ē-lā′shŭn) [L. *elatus,* borne out of]. Joyful emotion. It is of pathological origin when out of accord with patient's actual circumstances.

Elavil. Trade name for amitriptyline hydrochloride.

elbow (ĕl′bō) [AS. *eln,* forearm, + *boga,* bend]. Joint of arm and forearm. SEE: illus.

e., tennis. A strain of the lateral forearm muscles near their origin on the lateral epicondyle of the humerus. SYN: *epicondylitis, lateral humeral.*

elbow conformer. A splint applied to prevent flexion contractures following burns to the upper extremity. The device is fabricated to conform to the anterior arm. Pressure is applied to the olecranon process by a soft, cupped pad.

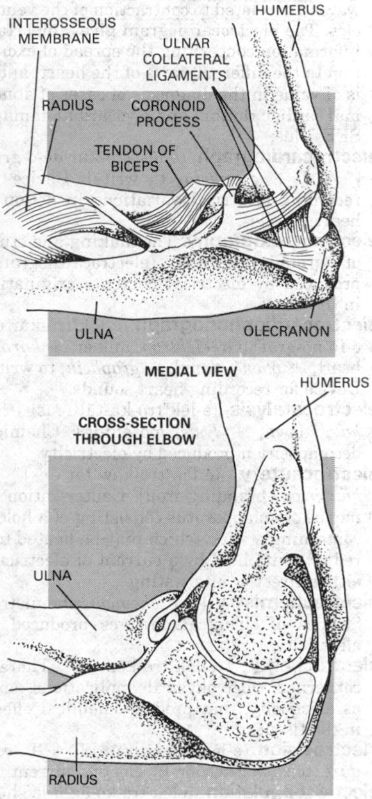

ELBOW JOINT

elbow jerk. Involuntary bending of elbow caused by striking tendon of biceps or triceps muscle.

elbow joint. Joint between arm and the forearm. Includes the humeroulnar, humeroradial, and proximal radioulnar articulations.

elbow reflex. Sharp extension of forearm resulting from tapping of triceps tendon while arm is held loosely in bent position.

Eldecort. Trade name for hydrocortisone.

Eldodram. Trade name for dimenhydrinate.

Eldopaque. Trade name for hydroquinone.

Eldoquin. Trade name for hydroquinone.

elective therapy. A treatment or surgical procedure not requiring immediate attention and therefore planned for the patient's convenience.

Electra complex. [Gr. Elektra, Agamemnon's daughter, who helped assassinate her mother because of love for her father, whom the former had slain] In psychoanalysis, a group of symptoms due to suppressed sexual love of daughter for father. SEE: *Jocasta complex; Oedipus complex.*

electric [Gr. *elektron,* amber]. Pert to, caused by, or resembling electricity.

electricity A form of energy that exhibits magnetic, chemical, mechanical, and thermal effects. Electricity is formed from the interactions of positive and negative charges. SEE: *electromotive force.*

e., frictional. Generation of static electricity by rubbing two articles together.

e., galvanic. Electricity generated by chemical action.

e., induced. Electricity generated in a body from another body close by without contact.

e., magnetic. Electricity induced by means of a magnetic device.

e., negative. Electric charge caused by an excess of electrons negatively charged.

e., positive. Electric charge caused by loss of negative electrons.

e., static. Electricity generated by friction of certain materials.

electric light baker. Device for warming a part, as in arthritis. SEE: *baker.*

electric shock. Injury from electricity, which varies according to type and strength of current, length of contact, and location of contact. Electric shocks vary from trivial burns to complete charring and destruction of skin; or unconsciousness from paralysis of the respiratory center, fibrillation of the heart, or both.

Whether or not an electric shock will cause death is influenced by the pathway the current takes through the body, the amount of current, and the skin resistance. Thus a very small amount of electric energy applied directly to the heart may be enough to cause the heart to cease activity. Conversely, a very large amount of electric energy may be unable to penetrate the dry calloused skin of the fingers and hands and thus be harmless.

An effective current greater than 15 milliamperes for alternating current and 75 milliamperes for direct current causes muscle tissue to contract. The hand exposed to a sufficient electric current is unable to release its grip. The chest muscles will be paralyzed and respiration will cease if sufficient current passes across the thorax.

Emergency insulation: Protection against such currents may be made with dry nonconductors such as folded newspapers, magazines, cardboard, wood, rubber, or clothing. These may be used to move patient from the contact or to remove wire from patient. It is always preferable to turn off the current if possible. If patient is in water, remember that it is electrically charged and special precautions must be taken. On a humid or rainy day, ordinary insulators may contain sufficient moisture to conduct electricity. Make sure insulators are dry.

High-tension currents, such as those used about x-ray equipment or in conducting currents for long distances or for special industrial locations, cannot be insulated by such means. Such currents may penetrate or pass through rubber, paper, or strips of wood. A safe procedure is to ascertain the source of current and have it shut off; otherwise, multiple tragedies could result.

SYM: Burns, loss of consciousness.

F.A.: Carefully free victim from source of current with nonconductors or shut off current. Prolonged artificial respiration may be necessary. SEE: *cardiopulmonary resuscitation; resuscitation; shock.*

electrify [Gr. *elektron,* amber, + L. *facere,* to make]. To charge a body with electricity.

electrization. The act of charging or treating by use of electricity.

electro-, electr- [Gr. *elektron,* amber]. Prefix indicating relationship to electricity.

electroaffinity (ē-lĕk″trō-ă-fĭn′ĭ-tē). Measure of the capability of ions to retain their charge.

electroanalgesia (ē-lĕk″trō-ăn″ăl-jē′zē-ă) [″ + *analgesia,* want of feeling]. Producing relief from pain by using low-intensity electrical currents applied locally or through implanted electrodes.

electroanalysis (ē-lĕk″trō-ă-năl′ĭ-sĭs). Use of electricity in making a chemical analysis.

electroanesthesia (ē-lĕk″trō-ăn″ĕs-thē′zē-ă) [″ + *an-,* not, + *aisthesis,* sensation]. 1. Local anesthesia induced by an anesthetizing substance injected into tissues by electricity. 2. General anesthesia produced by a device that passes electricity of a certain frequency, amplitude, and wave form through the brain. Has been used experimentally in both the U.S.S.R. and U.S.A.

electrobiology (ē-lĕk″trō-bī-ŏl′ō-jē) [″ + *bios,* life, + *logos,* study of]. Science of electric phenomena in the living body.

electrobioscopy (ē-lĕk″trō-bī-ŏs′kō-pē) [″ + *bios,* life, + *skopein,* to examine]. Electric test to determine if life is present.

electrocardiogram (ē-lĕk″trō-kăr′dē-ō-grăm″) [″ + *kardia,* heart, + *gramma,* writing]. ABBR: ECG. A record of the electrical activity of the heart; shows certain waves called P, Q, R, S, and T waves. Sometimes a U wave is seen. The first or P wave is caused by the depolarization of the atrial muscle tissues, whose electrical changes in turn caused atrial contraction. The Q, R, S, and T waves are related to contraction of the ventricles. The electrocardiogram gives important information concerning the spread of excitation to the different parts of the heart, and it is of value in the diagnosis of cases of abnormal cardiac rhythm and myocardial damage. SEE: illus.

electrocardiograph (ē-lĕk″trō-kăr′dē-ō-grăf) [″ + ″ + *graphein,* to write]. Device for recording electrical variations in action of heart muscles.

electrocardiography. The making and study of graphic records (electrocardiograms) produced by electrical currents originating in the heart.

electrocardiophonograph (ē-lĕk″trō-kăr″dē-ō-fō′nō-grăf) [Gr. *elektron,* amber, + *kardia,* heart, + *phone,* sound, + *graphein,* to write]. Device for recording heart sounds.

electrocatalysis (ē-lĕk″trō-kă-tăl′ĭ-sĭs) [″ + *kata,* down, + *lysis,* loosening]. Chemical decomposition produced by electricity.

electrocautery (ē-lĕk″trō-kaw′tĕr-ē) [″ + *kauterion,* branding iron]. Cauterization by means of an apparatus consisting of a holder containing a wire, which may be heated to a red or white heat by a current of electricity, either direct or alternating.

electrochemistry [″ + *chemeia,* chemistry]. Science of chemical changes produced by electricity.

electrochemy (ē-lĕk′trō-kĕm-ē). Therapy concerned with physical applications, such as electricity, that produce chemical effects in the tissues.

electrocision (ē-lĕk″trō-sĭzh′ŭn) [″ + L. *caedare,* to cut]. Excision by electric current.

electrocoagulation (ē-lĕk″trō-kō-ăg″ū-lā′shŭn) [″ + L. *coagulare,* to thicken]. Coagulation of tissue by means of a high-frequency electric current. The heat producing the coagu-

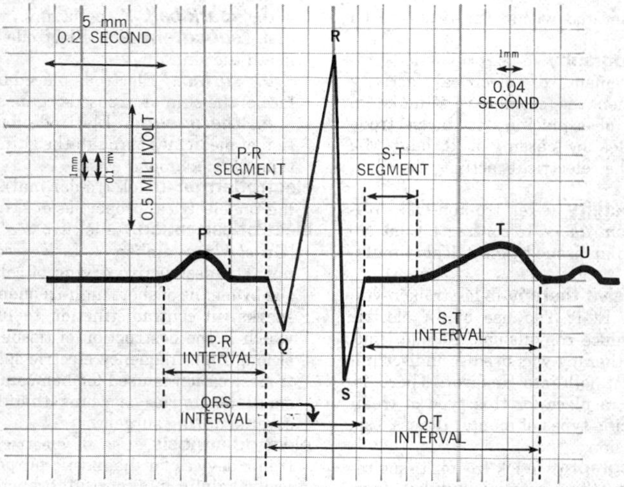

QRST COMPLEX OF ELECTROCARDIOGRAM

ELECTROCARDIOGRAM LEADS

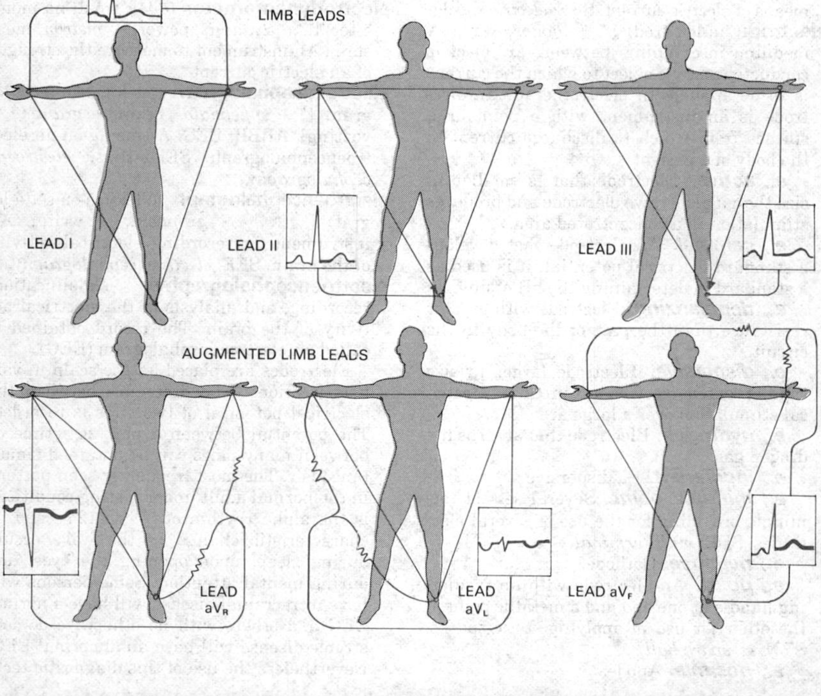

lation is generated within the tissue to be destroyed.

electrocochleography (ē-lĕk″trō-kŏk-lē-ŏg′ră-fē). Measurement of electrical activity produced when the cochlea is stimulated. Technique involves placing a needle electrode on the cochlea by passing it through the eardrum. The electrical activity is then recorded.

electrocontractility (ē-lĕk″trō-kŏn-trăk-tĭl′ĭ-tē) [″ + L. *contrahere,* to contract]. Contraction of muscular tissue by electrical stimulation.

electroconvulsive therapy (ē-lĕk″trō-kŏn-vŭl′sĭv). ABBR: ECT. The use of an electric shock to produce convulsions. At one time, this form of therapy was used so indiscriminately that it fell into disfavor. There is, nevertheless, a place for this type of treatment in specific types of mental illness, esp. acute depression.

electrocorticography (ē-lĕk″trō-kor″tĭ-kŏg′ră-fē). Recording the electrical impulses from the brain by placing electrodes directly on the cerebral cortex.

electrocryptectomy (ē-lĕk″trō-krĭp-tĕk′tō-mē) [″ + *kryptos,* concealed, + *ektome,* excision]. Destruction of tonsillar crypts by diathermy.

electrocution (ē-lĕk″trō-kū′shŭn) [″ + L. *acutus,* sharpened]. The destruction of life by means of electric current. SEE: *electric shock.*

electrode (ē-lĕk′trōd) [″ + *hodos,* way]. A medium intervening between an electric conductor and the object to which the current is to be applied. In electrotherapy an electrode is an instrument with a point or a surface from which to discharge current to the body of a patient.

e., active. Electrode that is smaller in size than a dispersive electrode and produces stimulation in a concentrated area.

e., calomel. An electrode that develops a standard electrical potential. It is used as a standard in determining the pH of fluids.

e., depolarizing. Electrode with greater resistance than the part of the body in the circuit.

e., dispersive. Electrode larger in size than an active electrode. It produces electrical stimulation over a large area.

e., hydrogen. Electrode that absorbs hydrogen gas.

e., indifferent. E., dispersive.

e., multiple point. Several sets of terminals providing for the use of several electrodes. SEE: *multiterminal.*

e., negative. Cathode.

e., point. An electrode with an insulating handle at one end and a metallic point at the other for use in applying static sparks. SYN: *e., spark ball.*

e., positive. Anode.

e., spark ball. E., point, q.v.

e., subcutaneous. Electrode placed beneath the skin.

e., surface. Electrode placed on the surface of the skin or exposed organ.

e., therapeutic. Electrode for introduction of medicines through the skin by ionization. SEE: *iontophoresis.*

electrodermal (ē-lĕk″trō-dĕr′măl). Concerning the electrical properties of skin.

electrodesiccation (ē-lĕk″trō-dĕs″ĭ-kā′shŭn) [Gr. *elektron,* amber, + L. *desiccare,* to dry up]. The destructive drying of cells and tissue by means of short high-frequency electric sparks, in contradistinction to fulguration, which is the destruction of tissue by means of long high-frequency electric sparks. Electrodesiccation is used for hemostasis of very small capillaries or veins that have been severed during surgery.

electrodiagnosis. Use of electric and electronic devices for diagnostic purposes. Their use is helpful in almost all branches of medicine, but particularly in investigating function of the heart, nerves and muscles.

electrodialysis (ē-lĕk″trō-dī-ăl′ĭ-sĭs) [″ + *dia-,* apart, + *lysis,* dissolving]. (pl. *electrodialyses*) A method of separating electrolytes from colloids by passing a current through a solution containing both.

electrodynamometer (ē-lĕk″trō-dī″nă-mŏm′ĕ-tĕr) [″ + *dynamis,* power, + *metron,* measure]. An instrument to measure the strength of an electric current.

electroencephalogram (ē-lĕk″trō-ĕn-sĕf′ă-lō-grăm) [″ + *enkephalos,* brain, + *gramma,* a writing]. ABBR: EEG. A tracing on an electroencephalograph. SEE: illus.; *electroencephalography.*

electroencephalograph (ē-lĕk-trō-ĕn-sĕf′ă-lō-grăf) [″ + ″ + *graphein,* to write]. An instrument for recording electrical activity of the brain. SEE: *electroencephalography.*

electroencephalography. Amplification, recording, and analysis of the electrical activity of the brain. The record obtained is called an electroencephalogram (EEG).

Electrodes are placed on the scalp in various locations. The difference between the electrical potential of two sites is recorded. The potential between a pair at a time or between many pairs can be obtained simultaneously. The most frequently seen pattern in the normal adult under resting conditions is the alpha rhythm of 8½ to 12/second. A characteristic change in the wave occurs during sleep, upon opening the eyes, and during mental attention. Some persons who have intracranial disease will have a normal EEG and others with no otherwise demonstrable disease will have an abnormal EEG. Nevertheless the use of this diagnostic tech-

NORMAL AND ABNORMAL ELECTROENCEPHALOGRAM WAVE PATTERNS

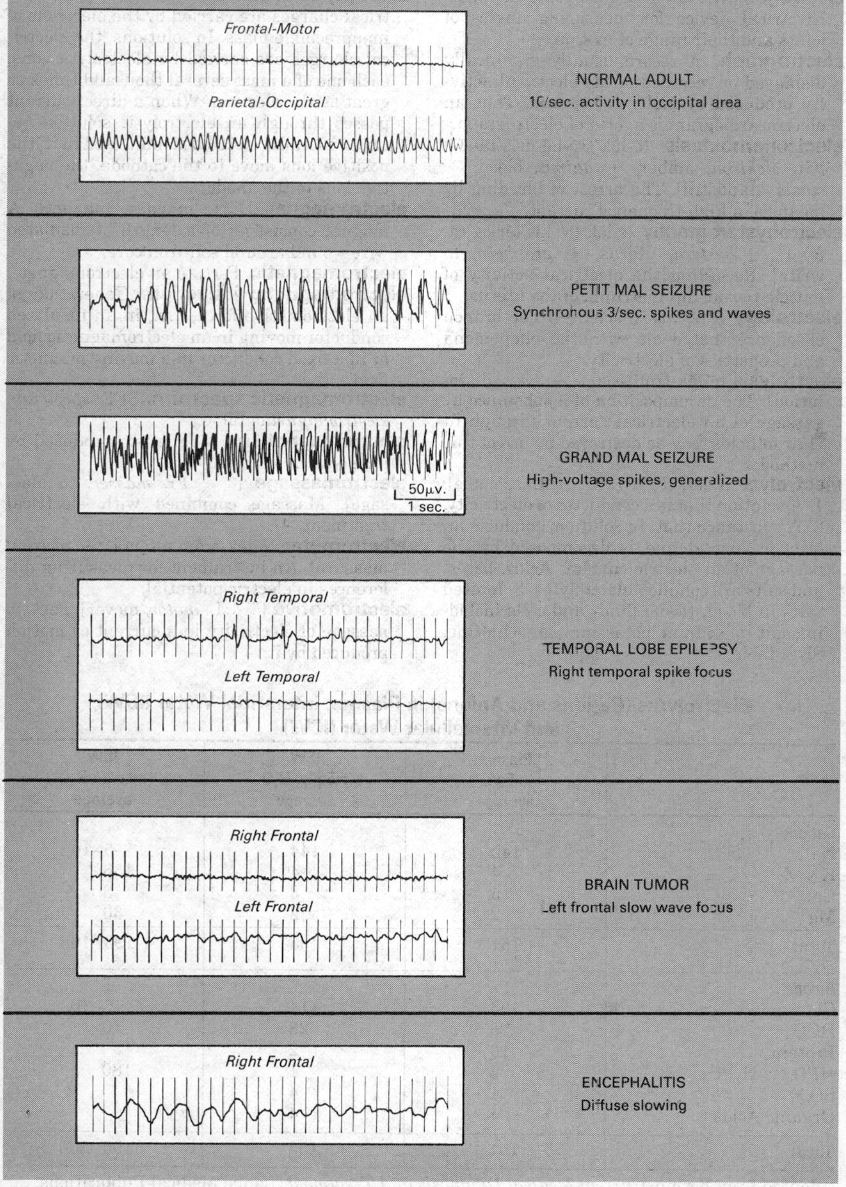

*Reprinted with permission from The Merck Manual, 13th ed., Merck & Co., Inc., 1977, pp 1408–1409.

nique has proved to be very helpful in studying epilepsy and convulsive disorders and in localizing lesions in the cerebrum. SEE: *rhythm, alpha; rhythm, beta; wave, theta.*

electrogoniometer (ē-lĕk″trō-gō″nē-ŏm′ĕ-tĕr). Electrical device for measuring angles of joints and their range of motion.

electrograph. A record usually graphically displayed or recorded of the electrical activity produced by biological tissues. Thus an electrocardiogram is a form of electrograph.

electrohemostasis (ē-lĕk″trō-hē-mŏs′tă-sĭs) [Gr. *elektron,* amber, + *haima,* blood, + *stasis,* standstill]. The arrest of bleeding by means of a high-frequency current.

electrohysterography (ē-lĕk″trō-hĭs″tĕr-ŏg′ră-fē) [″ + *hystera,* uterus, + *graphein,* to write]. Recording the electrical activity of muscle tissue, myometrium, of the uterus.

electrology [″ + *logos,* science]. The branch of science that deals with the phenomena and properties of electricity.

electrolysis (ē″lĕk-trŏl′ĭ-sĭs) [″ + *lysis,* dissolution]. The decomposition of a substance by passage of an electrical current through it. Hair follicles may be destroyed by use of this method.

electrolyte (ē-lĕk′trō-līt) [″ + *lytos,* soluble]. 1. A solution that is a conductor of electricity. 2. A substance that, in solution, conducts an electric current and is decomposed by the passage of an electric current. Acids, bases, and salts are common electrolytes. 3. Ionized salts in blood, tissue fluids and cells including salts of sodium, potassium, and chlorine. SEE: table.

e., amphoteric. A solution that produces both hydrogen (H^+) and hydroxyl (OH^-) ions.

electrolytic (ē-lĕk″trō-lĭt′ĭk). Caused by or rel. to electrolysis.

electrolytic conduction. In metals, the electrical charges are carried by the electrons of inappreciable mass. In solutions, the electrical charges are carried by electrolytic ions, each one of a mass several thousand times as great as the electron. When a direct current passes through an electrolytic solution between metallic electrodes immersed in it, the positive ions move to the cathode, the negative ions to the anode.

electromagnet [″ + *magnes,* magnet]. A magnet consisting of a length of insulated wire wound around soft iron core.

electromagnetic. Pert. to an electromagnet.

electromagnetic induction. Generation of an electromotive force, q.v., in an insulated conductor moving in an electromagnetic field or in a fixed conductor in a moving magnetic field.

electromagnetic spectrum. SEE: *spectrum, electromagnetic;* table.

electromagnetism. Magnetism produced by an electrical current.

electromassage [″ + Fr. *masser,* to massage]. Massage combined with electrical treatment.

electrometer (ē-lĕk-trŏm′ĕ-tĕr) [″ + *metron,* measure]. An instrument for measuring differences in electric potential.

electromotive [″ + L. *motor,* mover]. Pert. to passage of electricity in a current or motion produced by it.

Electrolytes (Cations and Anions) in Plasma, Interstitial Water (ISW), and Intercellular Water (ICW)

	Plasma mEq/L average	ISW mEq/kg H_2O average	ICW mEq/kg H_2O average
Cations			
Na^+	140	144	5–10
K^+	4	4	155
Ca^{2+}	5	3	3
Mg^{2+}	2	2	30
Total	151	153	193–198
Anions			
Cl^-	103	114	5–10
HCO_3^-	26	28	10
$Protein^-$	16	2	
HPO_4^{2-}; $H_2PO_4^-$	2	1	180
SO_4^{2-}	1	4	
Organic Acids	4	4	
Total	151	153	195–200

Adapted from Krupp, *Current Medical Diagnosis and Treatment,* Lange Medical Publications, 1982.

Electromagnetic Spectrum

Frequency Hz (cycles per second)	Character of Radiation	Wavelength Cm	
10^{23}			
	Cosmic Rays	10^{-12}	
10^{22}			
		10^{-11}	
10^{21}			
	Gamma Rays	10^{-10}	
10^{20}			
		10^{-9}	
10^{19}			
	X-Rays	10^{-8}	
10^{18}			
		10^{-7}	
10^{17}			
		10^{-6}	
10^{16}	Ultraviolet Radiation		
		10^{-5}	
10^{15}	Visible Light		
		10^{-4}	
10^{14}			
	Infrared Radiation	10^{-3}	
10^{13}			
		10^{-2}	
10^{12}	Submillimeter Waves		
		10^{-1}	
10^{11}			
		1.0	
10^{10}	Microwaves (Radar)		
		10	
10^{9}			UHF (ultra high frequency)
		10^{2}	
10^{8}	Television and FM Radio		VHF (very high frequency)
		10^{3}	
10^{7}	Short Wave Radio		HF (high frequency)
		10^{4}	
10^{6}	AM Radio		MF (medium frequency)
		10^{5}	
10^{5}			LF (low frequency)
	Maritime Communications	10^{6}	
10^{4}			VLF (very low frequency)

Adapted from Scientific Encyclopedia, Van Nostrand Reinhold Co., fifth ed., 1976.

electromotive force. ABBR: EMF. The effect of differences of potential that, on the closing of a circuit, causes a flow of electricity from one place to another, giving rise to an electric current. The strength of an electric current is directly proportional to the impressed electromotive force and inversely proportional to the resistance in the case of direct current and to the impedance in the case of alternating current. Electromotive force is measured in volts or in some convenient multiple or fraction of a volt. Microvolt, millivolt and kilovolt are, respectively, one-millionth volt, one-thousandth volt, and 1000 volts.

In order to understand the terms used to define electricity, a somewhat simple analogy can be made between water flowing through a pipe and electricity flowing through a wire. The *amount* of electricity, measured in *amperes,* can be compared to the *amount* of water flowing; the *pressure* of electricity, measured in *volts* and called *electromotive force,* can be compared to the *pressure* forcing the water through the pipe; the *resistance* to the flow of electricity, measured in *ohms,* can be compared to the *resistance* to the flow of water through a pipe. Obviously, as the size of the pipe increases, the resistance decreases.

The relationship of the strength of electric current to electromotive force (volts) and the resistance (ohms) to the flow of electricity in a circuit is expressed by the formula:

$$I = \frac{E}{R}$$

I (current expressed in amperes); E (volts); and R (resistance expressed in ohms). This formula expresses Ohm's law, q.v.

electromyogram (ē-lĕk″trō-mī′ō-grăm) [Gr. *elektron,* amber, + *mys,* muscle, + *gramma,* writing]. A graphic record of the contraction of a muscle as a result of electrical stimula-

tion.

electromyography (ē-lĕk″trō-mī-ŏg′ră-fē) [″ + ″ + *graphein,* to write]. The preparation, study of, and interpretation of electromyograms.

electron [Gr. *elektron,* amber]. An extremely minute charge of negative electricity that revolves about the central core or nucleus of an atom. Its mass is about 1/1840 that of a hydrogen atom, or 9.11×10^{-28} grams. When emitted from radioactive substances, electrons are known as beta particles or rays.

electronarcosis (ē-lĕk″trō-năr-kō′sĭs). The induction of narcosis or unconsciousness by the application of electricity to the brain.

electron-dense. In electron microscopy, pert. to tissue of a density that prevents penetration by electrons.

electronegative [″ + L. *negare,* to deny]. Condition of being charged with negative electricity, which results in the attraction of bodies positively charged and the repulsion of bodies negatively charged.

electroneurolysis (ē-lĕk″trō-nū-rŏl′ĭ-sĭs). Destruction of a nerve by use of an electric needle device.

electronic. Pert. to electrons.

electronization [Gr. *elektron,* amber]. The use of radiation to restore electrical equilibrium to diseased cells.

electron microscope. SEE: *microscope, electron; microscope, scanning electron.*

electron volt. The energy acquired by an electron as it passes through a potential of 1 volt.

electronystagmography (ē-lĕk″trō-nĭs″tăg-mŏg′ră-fē) [″ + *nystagmos,* drowsiness, + *graphein,* to write]. A method of recording nystagmus activity by detecting the electrical activity of the extraocular muscles. SEE: *nystagmus.*

electro-oculogram (ē-lĕk″trō-ŏk′ū-lō-grăm″). Recording of the electrical currents produced by eye movements. SEE: *electroretinogram.*

electropathology (ē-lĕk″trō-pă-thŏl′ō-jē) [″ + *pathos,* suffering, + *logos,* study of]. Determining electrical reaction of muscles and nerves as means of diagnosis.

electrophoresis (ē-lĕk″trō-for-ē′sĭs) [″ + *phoresis,* bearing]. The movement of charged colloidal particles through the medium in which they are dispersed as a result of changes in electrical potential. Electrophoretic methods are useful in the analysis of protein mixtures as protein particles move with different velocities dependent principally on the number of charges carried by the particle. SEE: *diathermy; iontophoresis; phoresis.*

electrophorus (ē-lĕk″trŏf′ō-rŭs) [″ + *phorein,* to bear]. An instrument for obtaining static electricity by means of induction.

electrophrenic (ē-lĕk″trō-frĕn′ĭk). Pert. to stimulation of the phrenic nerve by electricity.

electrophrenic respiration. Application of intermittent electrical stimuli to cutaneous electrodes over the phrenic nerves in the neck to rhythmically stimulate respiration. Used in the patient whose respiratory center has been damaged.

electrophysiology (ē-lĕk″trō-fĭz″ē-ŏl′ō-gē) [″ + *physis,* nature, + *logos,* study of]. A branch of physiology that deals with the relationships of body functions to electrical phenomena such as the effects of electrical stimulation upon the tissues, the production of electrical currents by organs and tissues, and the therapeutic use of electrical currents.

electropositive [″ + L. *positivus,* emphatic]. The condition of being subject to repulsion by bodies positively electrified and to attraction by bodies negatively electrified.

electropuncture [″ + L. *punctura,* a piercing]. Piercing tissues with an electric needle.

electroradiometer (ē-lĕk″trō-rā-dē-ŏm′ē-tĕr) [″ + L. *radius,* ray, + Gr. *metron,* measure]. An electroscope for differentiation of radiant energy.

electroresection (ē-lĕk″trō-rē-sĕk′shŭn). Removal of tissue by use of an electrical device such as a cautery.

electroretinogram (ē-lĕk″trō-rĕt′ĭ-nō-grăm). ABBR: ERG. A record of the action currents of the retina produced by visual or light stimuli.

electroscission (ē-lĕk″trō-sĭ′zhŭn) [″ + L. *scindere,* to cut]. Division of tissues by electrocautery.

electroscope (ē-lĕk′trō-skōp) [″ + *skopein,* to see]. An instrument that detects intensity of radiation.

electroshock. Shock produced by an electric current.

electroshock therapy. The induction of convulsive seizures by the passing of an electric current through the brain. Used in the treatment of acute depression.

electrosleep. Sleep production as a result of the passage of mild electrical impulses through parts of the brain. Has been used experimentally in treating insomnia and mental illness.

electrostatic [Gr. *elektron,* amber, + *statikos,* causing to stand]. Pert. to static electricity.

electrostatic generator. A device that generates static electricity.

electrostatic unit. Any unit of electrical measurement based on the attraction or repulsion of a static charge as distinguished from an electromagnetic unit, which is defined in terms of the attraction or repulsion of magnetic poles.

electrostimulation (ē-lĕk″trō-stĭm″ū-lā′shŭn).

Use of electrical current to stimulate a tissue, such as muscle or bone. In the latter case, the stimulation is used experimentally to facilitate and hasten healing of fractures.

electrosurgery (ē-lĕk″trō-sŭr′jĕ-rē) [″ + L. *chirurgia,* surgery]. Surgical procedures wherein electricity is required either in the actual surgical apparatus or in the application of electrical cautery.

electrosynthesis (ē-lĕk″trō-sĭn′thĕ-sĭs). Use of electricity to synthesize chemical compounds.

electrotaxis (ē-lĕk″trō-tăk′sĭs) [″ + *taxis,* arrangement]. The movement of a cell or an organism toward or away from an electrical stimulus.

electrothanasia (ē-lĕk″trō-thă-nā′zē-ă) [″ + *thanatos,* death]. Death resulting from electric shock; electrocution.

electrotherapeutics (ē-lĕk″trō-thĕr-ă-pū′tĭks) [″ + *therapeutike,* treatment]. The use of electricity in the treatment of disease. SYN: *electrotherapy.*

electrotherapist (ē-lĕk″trō-thĕr′ă-pĭst) [″ + *therapeia,* treatment]. An individual who has had special training and has acquired skill in the therapeutic use of electricity. The term is sometimes used incorrectly to designate anyone who administers electrical treatments.

electrotherapy. Use of electricity in treating disease. SYN: *electrotherapeutics.*

electrothermotherapy (ē-lĕk″trō-thĕr″mō-thĕr′ă-pē) [″ + ″ + *therapeia,* treatment]. The production of heat within the living tissues for therapeutic purposes by means of bodily resistance to the passing of an electric current.

electrotome (ē-lĕk′trŏ-tōm) [″ + *tome,* incision]. An electrocautery device used for surgical procedures.

electrotonic (ē-lĕk″trō-tŏn′ĭk) [″ + *tonos,* tension]. Of or pert. to electrotonus.

electrotonus (ē-lĕk-trŏt′ō-nŭs). The change in the irritability of a nerve or muscle during the passage of an electric current.

electrotropism (ē-lĕk-trŏt′rō-pĭzm) [″ + *trope,* a turning, + *-ismos,* condition of]. Reaction of cells to an electrical current.

electrovalence (ē-lĕk″trō-vā′lĕns). The ionic linkage between atoms in which each accepts or donates electrons so that each atom ends up with a completed electron shell.

electroversion (ē-lĕk″trō-vĕr′zhŭn). SEE: *cardioversion.*

electuary (ē-lĕk′tū-ă-rē) [Gr. *ekleikhein,* to lick up]. Medicinal substance mixed with honey or sugar to form a paste suitable for oral consumption.

eleidin (ĕ-lē′ĭ-dĭn) [Gr. *elaion,* oil]. An acidophil substance present in the stratum lucidum of the epidermis.

element [L. *elementum,* a rudiment]. In modern chemistry, a substance that cannot be separated into substances different from itself by ordinary chemical processes. Elements exist in a free and in a combined state. More than 100 have been identified. SEE: *Elements* in *Appendix.*

Some of the elements found in the human body are oxygen, aluminum, carbon, cobalt, hydrogen, nitrogen, calcium, phosphorus, potassium, sulfur, sodium, chlorine, magnesium, iron, fluorine, iodine, copper, manganese, and zinc.

e.'s, trace. Chemical elements present in the body or in the diet in extremely small amounts. Some are absolutely necessary for metabolism.

element, words pert. to: atom; atomic; chemical change; chemical compound; electron; mineral compounds; neutron; nucleus; oxidation; oxide; radical; radioactive; valence.

eleoma (ĕl″ē-ō′mă) [Gr. *elaion,* oil, + *oma,* tumor]. A swelling in tissue produced by the injection of oil.

eleopathy (ĕl″ē-ŏp′ă-thē) [″ + *pathos,* disease]. Swelling of joints as a result of fatty deposits. SYN: *elaiopathy.*

eleoptene (ĕl-ē-ŏp′tēn) [″ + *ptenos,* fleeting]. The most volatile component of a volatile oil.

eleosaccharum (ĕl″ē-ō-săk′ă-rŭm) [″ + *sakcharon,* sugar]. A mixture of powdered sugar with a volatile oil.

eleotherapy (ĕl″ē-ō-thĕr′ă-pē) [Gr. *elaion,* oil, + *therapeia,* treatment]. The use of oil for therapeutic purposes.

elephantiasis (ĕl″ĕ-făn-tī′ă-sĭs) [Gr. *elephas,* elephant, + *-iasis,* condition]. A chronic infectious condition characterized by pronounced hypertrophy of the skin and subcutaneous tissues resulting from obstruction of the lymphatic vessels. The lower extremities and the scrotum are parts most frequently involved. SYN: *pachydermatosis.*

ETIOL: Elephantiasis may be congenital (Milroy's disease) or the result of metastatic invasion of the lymph nodes by tumor cells. Inflammatory elephantiasis results from filariasis or local infection of the lymph nodes. Elephantiasis caused by infection of the lymphatics by Wuchereria bancrofti is common in tropical countries.

e. arabum. Elephantiasis.

e., scrotal. Elephantiasis that is mainly located in the scrotum. SYN: *chyloderma.*

elevation (ĕl″ĕ-vā′shŭn). A raised area that protrudes above the surrounding area.

e.'s, tactile. Small raised areas of palms and soles that contain a cluster of nerve endings.

elevator [L. *elevare,* to lift]. 1. Curved retractor for holding lid away from the globe of the eye. 2. Retractor for raising depressed bones by levers or screws.

eleventh cranial nerve. Motor nerve made up of a cranial and a spinal part that supplies the trapezius and sternomastoid muscles and pharynx. Accessory portion joins the vagus, to which it supplies motor and some of its cardioinhibitory fibers. SYN: *accessory nerve; spinal accessory nerve.*

eliminant (ē-lĭm'ĭ-nănt) [L. *e,* out, + *limen,* threshold]. 1. Effecting evacuation. 2. Agent aiding in elimination.

eliminate (ē-lĭm'ĭ-nāt). To expel; to rid the body of waste material.

elimination. 1. Excretion of waste products by the skin, kidneys, and intestines. 2. Leave out, omit, remove.

elimination diet. A diet used to determine which foods cause an allergic response. The patient starts with a very few foods and if none of these causes sensitivity, one food is added to the diet. If that causes no reactions, then another food is added, etc. Offending foods discovered by this technique are then eliminated from the diet.

elimination, words pert. to: absorption; constipation; defecation; dejecta; egesta; ejecta; enema; evacuate; feces; flatus; stool.

elinguation (ē"lĭn-gwā'shŭn) [" + *lingua,* tongue]. The operation of removing the tongue from the oral cavity.

ELISA. *enzyme-linked immunoabsorbent assay.*

elixir (ē-lĭk'sĕr) [Arabic *al-iksir,* philosopher's stone]. A sweetened, aromatic, hydro-alcoholic liquid used in the compounding of oral medicines. Elixirs constitute one of the most commonly used types of medicinal preparation taken orally in liquid form.

Elixophyllin. Trade name for theophylline.

ellipsis (ē-lĭp'sĭs) [Gr., a leaving out]. In psychiatric therapy, the patient's omitting important words or ideas during treatment.

ellipsoid (ē-lĭp'soyd). Spindle-shaped.

elliptocyte (ē-lĭp'tō-sīt). Oval-shaped red cells. About 15% of red cells are normally oval shaped, but in anemia and hereditary elliptocytosis, the percentage is increased. In birds, reptiles, and some other animals, the red cells are normally elliptocytes.

elliptocytosis (ē-lĭp"tō-sī-tō'sĭs). Condition of increased number of elliptocytes. This occurs in some forms of anemia.

e., hereditary. A benign inherited condition in which the red cells are oval or elliptically shaped. This inherited curiosity occurs in about one in each 2000 births.

Ellis-van Creveld syndrome. A congenital syndrome consisting of polydactyly, chondrodysplasia with acromelic dwarfism, hydrotic ectodermal dysplasia, and congenital heart defects. It is thought to be transmitted as an autosomal trait. SYN: *dysplasia, chondroectodermal.*

elongation (ē"lŏng-gā'shŭn). The condition of being extended, or the process of extending.

elope. Pert. to a patient, to depart from a hospital, esp. a psychiatric hospital, without permission.

eluate (ĕl'ū-āt). The material washed out by elution.

eluent (ē-lū'ĕnt). The solvent or dissolving substance used in elution.

elution (ē-lū'shŭn) [L. *e,* out, + *luere,* to wash]. In chemistry, separation of one material from another by washing. If a material contains water-soluble and water-insoluble materials, the passage of water, the eluent, through the mixture will remove that portion of the material that is water soluble, the eluate, and leave the water-insoluble residue.

elutriation (ē-lū-trē-ā'shŭn) [L. *elutriare,* to cleanse]. The separation of insoluble particles from finer ones by decanting the fluid.

emaciate (ē-mā'sē-āt) [L. *emaciare,* to grow thin]. To cause to become excessively lean.

emaciated. Excessively lean.

emaciation. State of being extremely lean.

ETIOL: Malnutrition; diseases of gastrointestinal canal. If rapid: marasmus, Addison's disease, tuberculosis, anorexia nervosa, cancer, diabetes, suppuration, hyperthyroidism, chronic diarrhea, stricture of esophagus, pyloric obstruction, parasites, loss of sleep, exophthalmic goiter, starvation. SEE: *anorexia; marasmus; tabes; wasting.*

emaculation (ĕm-ăk"ū-lā'shŭn) [L. *emaculare,* to remove spots]. Removal of spots from the skin.

emailloid (ā-mī'loyd) [Fr. *email,* enamel, + Gr. *eidos,* form]. Tumor having its origin in tooth enamel.

emanation [L. *e,* out, + *manare,* to flow]. 1. Something given off; radiation; emission. 2. A gaseous product of radioactive disintegration.

e., actinium. Emanation given off by actinium. SYN: *actinon.*

e., radium. A radioactive gas given off by radium. SYN: *radon.*

e., thorium. Radioactive gas given off by thorium. SYN: *thoron.*

emasculation (ē-măs"kū-lā'shŭn) [L. *emasculare,* to castrate]. 1. Castration. 2. Excision of the entire male genitalia. 3. Figuratively, making powerless or ineffective.

embalming (ĕm-băm'ĭng) [L. *im-,* put on, + *balsamum,* balsam]. Use of antiseptics and preservatives in and on the dead body in order to prepare it for burial. This prevents premature biodegradation of the body.

embarrass (ĕm-băr'ăs). To interfere with or compromise function.

Embden-Meyerhof pathway. [G. G. Embden, Ger. chemist, 1874–1933; O. Meyerhof, Ger. biochemist, 1884–1951] A series of metabolic and enzymatic changes that occur in many plants and animals when glucose, glycogen, or starch is metabolized anaerobically to produce lactic acid. In the process, energy in the form of adenosine triphosphate (ATP) is produced. This is the principal means of producing energy in mammals, including man.

embedding [" + AS. *bedd,* to bed]. In histology, the process by which a piece of tissue is placed in a firm medium such as paraffin in order to support it and keep it intact during the subsequent cutting into thin sections for microscopic examination.

embolalia, embololalia (ĕm"bō-lā'lē-ă, ĕm" bō-lō-lā'lē-ă) [Gr. *embolos,* thrown in, + *lalia,* babble]. Meaningless language of the insane. SYN: *embolophrasia.*

embole (ĕm'bō-lē) [Gr. *embolus,* a throwing in]. 1. Reduction of a dislocation. 2. Formation of the gastrula by invagination. SYN: *emboly.*

embolectomy (ĕm"bō-lĕk'tō-mē) [" + *ektome,* excision]. Removal of an embolus from a vessel. This may be done surgically or by use of enzymes that dissolve the clot. The latter method is used in treating acute myocardial infarction and other areas where blood flow is obstructed by a blood clot.

embolic. Pert. to or caused by embolism.

emboliform [" + L. *forma,* form]. 1. Resembling a nucleus. 2. Wedge-shaped, as the nucleus emboliformis.

embolism (ĕm'bō-lĭzm) [" + *-ismos,* condition]. Obstruction of a blood vessel by foreign substances or a blood clot. Diagnosis depends upon predisposing factors. Arteriosclerosis favors a diagnosis of thrombosis while atrial fibrillation, bacterial endocarditis, or thrombophlebitis points to embolism. Embolism is usually due to blood clots.

RS: embolus, thrombosis, thrombus.

e., air. Embolism caused by air bubble. SEE: *air.*

e., fat. Embolism caused by globules of fat obstructing blood vessels.

e., pulmonary. Obstruction of the pulmonary artery or one of its branches. Usually caused by an embolus from thrombosis in lower extremities. SEE: illus.

NURSING IMPLICATIONS: Observe the patient for shortness of breath, weakness, cyanosis, pallor, and substernal pain. Intervene to prevent stasis by ensuring that a patient at risk for the development of emboli wears elastic stockings; does exercises to improve venous return; and ambulates early after surgery. Patients on bedrest should increase their oral intake of fluids to prevent development of hemoconcentration. Women with a history of emboli should be instructed not to take oral contraceptives.

EMBOLISM

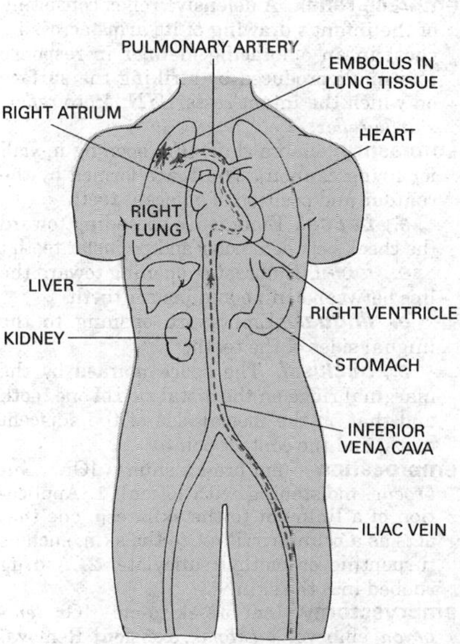

PATH OF BLOOD CLOT FROM LEG VEIN TO THE LUNG

e., pyemic. Embolism caused by purulent matter.

embolophrasia (ĕm"bō-lō-frā'zē-ă) [" + *phrasis,* utterance]. Meaningless speech. SYN: *embolalia.*

embolus (ĕm'bō-lŭs) [Gr. *embolos,* plug]. (pl. *emboli*) A mass of undissolved matter present in a blood or lymphatic vessel brought there by the blood or lymph current. Emboli may be solid, liquid, or gaseous. Other emboli may consist of bits of tissue, tumor cells, globules of fat, air bubbles, clumps of bacteria, and foreign bodies. Emboli may arise within the body or they may gain entrance from without. Occlusion of vessels from emboli usually results in the development of infarcts, q.v. SEE: *thrombosis; thrombus.*

e., air. An air bubble in the veins, right atrium or ventricle, or capillaries.

e., coronary. Embolus in one of the coronary arteries, which may be a complication of arteriosclerosis and cause angina pectoris.

e., pulmonary. Embolus in pulmonary artery or one of its branches.

emboly (ĕm'bō-lē) [Gr. *emboie,* a throwing in]. Formation of the gastrula by invagination. SYN: *embole.*

embolysis (ĕm-bŏl'ĭ-sĭs). The dissolution of an embolus, esp. one due to a blood clot.

embrace reflex. A defensive reflex consisting of the infant's drawing of its arms across its chest in an embracing manner in response to stimuli produced by striking the surface on which the infant rests. SYN: *Moro reflex; startle reflex.*

embrasure (ĕm-brā'zhŭr) [Fr., opening in wall for firing cannon]. The space formed by the contour and position of adjacent teeth.

e., buccal. Embrasure spreading toward the cheek between molar and premolar teeth.

e., labial. Embrasure opening toward the lips between canine and incisor teeth.

e., lingual. Embrasure opening to the lingual sides of the teeth.

e., occlusal. The space marked by the marginal ridge on the distal side of one tooth and that on the mesial side of the adjacent tooth, and the contact points.

embrocation (ĕm"brō-kā'shŭn) [Gr. *embroche,* moistening with lotion]. 1. Application of a liniment to the skin, esp. one that acts as a counterirritant to the skin, such as turpentine or methyl salicylate. 2. A drug rubbed into the skin.

embryectomy (ĕm"brē-ĕk'tō-mē) [Gr. *embryon,* embryo, + *ektome,* excision]. Removal of an extrauterine embryo.

embryo (ĕm'brē-ō) [Gr. *embryon*]. 1. The young of any organism in an early stage of development. 2. Stage in prenatal development of a mammal between the ovum and the fetus. In humans, stage of development between the 2nd and 8th weeks inclusive. SEE: illus.

DEVELOP: *Zygote:* (1st week): Following fertilization, cells multiply (cleavage), which results in formation of a morula, which in turn develops into a blastocyst consisting of a trophoblast and inner cell mass. Two cavities (amniotic cavity and yolk sac) arise within the inner cell mass. These are separated by the embryonic disk, which gives rise to the three germ layers (ectoderm, mesoderm, and endoderm), these developing into the embryo proper. The blastocyst wall of trophoblast gives rise to auxiliary structures. The zygote enters the uterus and implantation occurs.

Embryo (2nd through 8th weeks): The embryo increases in length from about 1.5 mm. to 23 mm. The germ layers of the embryonic disk give rise to the principal organ systems and the embryo begins to show the human form. During this period of organogenesis, the embryo is particularly sensitive to the effect of toxic chemicals.

Fetus (3rd to 9th month): The alimentary canal, liver, pancreas, and lungs develop from endoderm. Muscle, all connective tissues, blood, lymphatic tissue and the epithelium of blood vessels, body cavities, kidney, gonads, and suprarenal cortex develop from mesoderm. The epidermis, nervous tissue, hypophysis, and the epithelium of the organs, nasal cavity, mouth, salivary glands, bladder, and urethra develop from ectoderm.

embryocardia (ĕm"brē-ō-kăr'dē-ă) [Gr. *embryon,* embryo, + *kardia,* heart]. Heart action in which first and second sounds are equal and resemble the fetal heart sounds. A sign of cardiac distress.

embryoctony (ĕm"brē-ŏk'tō-nē) [" + *kteinein,* to kill]. Destroying the fetus in utero, as in cases where delivery is impossible, or during abortion. SEE: *craniotomy.*

embryogenetic, embryogenic [" + *gennan,* to originate]. Pert. to or giving rise to an embryo.

embryogeny (ĕm"brē-ŏj'ĕ-nē). The growth and development of an embryo.

embryography [" + *graphein,* to write]. A treatise on the embryo.

embryology [" + *logos,* study]. The science that deals with the origin and development of an individual organism.

embryoma (ĕm-brē-ō'mă) [" + *oma,* tumor]. A tumor consisting of derivatives of the embryonic germ layers but lacking in organization.

embryonal (ĕm'brē-ō-năl). Pert. to or resembling an embryo.

embryonic (ĕm"brē-ŏn'ĭk) [Gr. *embryon,* embryo]. Pert. to or in condition of an embryo.

embryonization. Reversion of a cell or tissue to an embryonic structure.

embryonoid (ĕm'brē-ō-noyd) [" + *eidos,* form]. Having the appearance of an embryo.

embryopathy (ĕm"brē-ŏp'ă-thē) [" + *pathos,* disease]. Any pathological condition in the embryo.

embryoplastic [" + *plassein,* to form]. Having a part in the formation of an embryo; said of cells.

embryoscopy. Direct visualization of the fetus or embryo in the uterus by inserting the light source and image-detecting portion of a fetoscope into the amniotic cavity through a small incision in the abdominal wall. Use of this technique permits visualization of the fetus, photography of the fetus, surgical correction of certain types of congenital defects, as well as obtaining specimens of amniotic fluid for analysis of chemical and cellular materials.

embryotocia (ĕm"brē-ō-tō'sē-ă) [" + *tokos,* birth]. Abortion.

embryotome (ĕm'brē-ō-tōm") [" + *tome,* incision]. Instrument used in dismemberment of fetus in utero.

embryotomy (ĕm"brē-ŏt'ō-mē). The dissection of a fetus to aid delivery.

embryotoxon (ĕm"brē-ō-tŏks'ŏn) [" + *toxon,* bow]. Congenital marginal opacity of the

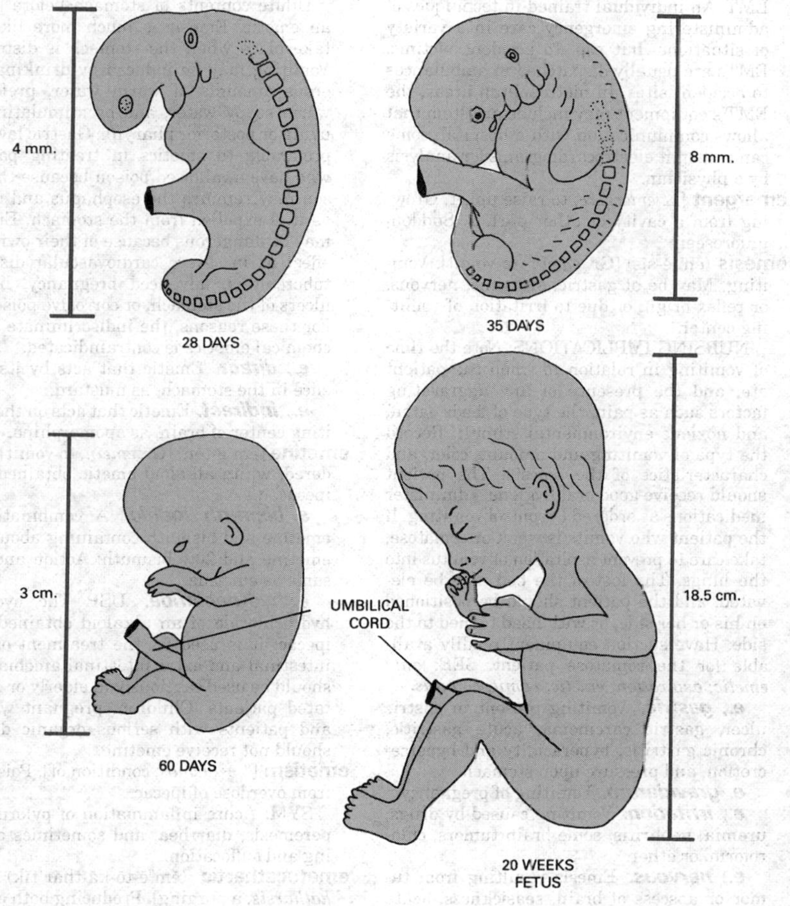

STAGES OF DEVELOPMENT OF HUMAN EMBRYO

cornea. SYN: *arcus juvenilis.*

embryotroph (ĕm′brē-ō-trōf) [″ + *trophe,* nourishment]. A fluid resulting from the enzyme action of the trophoblasts upon the neighboring maternal tissue that nourishes the embryo from the time of implantation into the uterus.

embryotrophy (ĕm″brē-ŏt′rō-fē). Nutrition of the fetus.

embryulcia (ĕm″brē-ŭl′sē-ă) [″ + *elkein,* to draw]. Forcible removal of the fetus by instruments, as in embryotomy.

embryulcus (ĕm″brē-ŭl′kŭs) [Gr. *embryoulkos*]. Instrument for extracting a dead fetus from the uterus.

emedullate (ē-mĕd′ū-lāt) [L. *e,* out, + *medulla,* marrow]. To remove the marrow from a bone.

emergency [L. *emergere,* to raise up]. 1. A sudden change in a patient's condition such that immediate medical or surgical intervention is required. 2. An unexpected serious occurrence that may cause a great number of injuries. They usually require immediate attention. SEE: *Emergencies* in *Appendix.*

emergency, words pert. to: artificial respiration; asphyxia; bites or stings; burn; choking; convulsion; drowning; fainting; foreign bodies; poison control center; poisoning; radiation accidents, emergency handling of; shock.

emergency medical technician. ABBR:

EMT. An individual trained in techniques of administering emergency care in a variety of situations, but esp. to accident victims. EMTs are usually dispatched in ambulances to accident sites. In metropolitan areas, the EMT's equipment may include a system that allows communication with a hospital; some can transmit electrocardiograms for analysis by a physician.

emergent [L. *emergere,* to raise up]. 1. Growing from a cavity or other part. 2. Sudden, unforeseen.

emesis (ĕm'ĕ-sĭs) [Gr. *emein,* to vomit]. Vomiting. May be of gastric, systemic, nervous, or reflex origin or due to irritation of vomiting center.

NURSING IMPLICATIONS: Note the time of vomiting in relation to when the patient ate, and the presence of any aggravating factors such as pain, the type of foods eaten, and noxious environmental stimuli. Record the type of vomiting and amount, color, and characteristics of the emesis. The patient should receive good oral hygiene; administer medications as ordered to control vomiting. If the patient who vomits is weak or comatose, take care to prevent aspiration of vomitus into the lungs. The foot of the bed may be elevated, and the patient should be positioned on his or her side, or with head turned to the side. Have suction equipment readily available for the comatose patient. SEE: *antemetic; aspiration; emetic; vomit; vomitus.*

e., gastric. Vomiting present in gastric ulcer, gastric carcinoma, acute gastritis, chronic gastritis, hyperacidity and hypersecretion, and pressure upon stomach.

e. gravidarum. Vomiting of pregnancy.

e., irritation. Vomiting caused by drugs, uremia, nephritis, some brain tumors, chloroform, or ether.

e., nervous. Emesis resulting from tumor or abscess of brain, seasickness, acute myelitis, meningitis, anemia and hyperemia of brain, concussion and contusion of brain, fracture of skull, Ménière's disease, or migraine.

e., reflex. Emesis caused by irritation of fauces and pharynx, coughing, removal of viscous secretion from nasopharynx, unpleasant odors and sights, shock, nervousness, anticipation, anxiety, hysteria, morning sickness, gastric crisis of tabes, or hiccoughs.

emetic (ĕ-mĕt'ĭk) [Gr. *emein,* to vomit]. An agent that produces vomiting. Emetics may induce vomiting by their local effect, as copper sulfate, zinc sulfate, mustard, and ipecac in small doses diluted in water; or by their effect on the central nervous system, such as is produced by apomorphine hydrochloride given parenterally. SEE: *vomiting; vomitus.*

Dilute contents of stomach before giving an emetic. Emesis is much more likely to take place when the stomach is distended. Vomiting may be induced by drinking generous amounts of warm water, preferably warm soapy water, and by stimulating the uvula or posterior pharynx. Gastric lavage is preferable to emetics in treating patients who have swallowed poison because the poison may reinjure the esophagus and mouth as it is expelled from the stomach. Emetics may be dangerous because of their own toxic effect as in severe cardiovascular diseases, tuberculosis, advanced pregnancy, hernia, ulcers of the stomach, or corrosive poisoning. For these reasons, the indiscriminate use of chemical emetics is contraindicated.

e., direct. Emetic that acts by its presence in the stomach, as mustard.

e., indirect. Emetic that acts on the vomiting center of brain, as apomorphine.

emetine (ĕm'ĕ-tēn) [Gr. *emein,* to vomit]. Powdered, white alkaloid emetic obtained from ipecac, q.v.

e. bismuth iodide. A combination of emetine and bismuth containing about 20% emetine and 20% bismuth. Action and uses same as emetine.

e. hydrochloride. USP. The hydrated hydrochloride of an alkaloid obtained from ipecac. It is used for the treatment of both intestinal and extra-intestinal amebiasis. It should be used cautiously in elderly or debilitated patients. Children, pregnant women, and patients with serious organic disease should not receive emetine.

emetism [" + *-ismos,* condition of]. Poisoning from overdose of ipecac.

SYM: Acute inflammation of pylorus, hyperemesis, diarrhea, and sometimes coughing and suffocation.

emetocathartic (ĕm"ĕ-tō-kă-thăr'tĭk) [" + *katharsis,* a purging]. Producing both emesis and catharsis.

emetology (ĕm"ĕ-tŏl'ō-jē) [" + *logos,* study of]. Study of anatomy of vomiting organs and physiology of vomiting.

E.M.F. *electromotive force; erythrocyte maturation factor.*

EMG. *electromyogram,* q.v.

emigration [L. *e,* out, + *migrare,* to move]. Passage of white blood corpuscles through the walls of capillaries and veins during inflammation.

eminence [" + *minere,* to hang on]. A prominence or projection, esp. of a bone.

e., arcuate. A rounded eminence on upper surface of petrous portion of temporal bone. SYN: *jugum petrosum.*

e., articular, of the temporal bone. A rounded eminence forming the anterior boundary of the glenoid fossa.

e., auditory. A collection of gray matter on the floor of 4th ventricle of the brain at its lower part, forming the deep origin of the auditory nerve.

e., bicipital. A tuberosity for insertion of biceps muscle on radius.

e., blastodermic. An elevated mass of cells of a developing ovum forming the blastoderm.

e., canine. A vertical ridge on the external surface of the maxilla.

e., collateral. Eminence between middle and posterior horns in lateral ventricle of brain.

e., frontal. A rounded prominence on either side of the median line and a little below center of the frontal bone.

e., germinal. A mass of follicle cells that surround the ovum. SYN: *cumulus oophorus.*

e., hypothenar. Eminence on ulnar side of palm, formed by muscles of little finger.

e., iliopectineal. Eminence on upper aspect of pubic bone above the acetabulum, marking the junction of bone with the ilium.

e., intercondyloid. A process on the head of the tibia lying between the two condyles.

e., mamillary. Projection of inner pillars of fornix. SYN: *corpus mamillare* [NA].

e., median. Anterior bodies of medulla oblongata separated by anterior median fissure.

e., nasal. A prominence on vertical portion of frontal bone above the nasal notch and between the two superciliary ridges.

e., occipital. Protuberance on occipital bone.

e. of Doyère. Slight elevation of muscular fiber corresponding to entrance of a nerve fiber into the muscle.

e., olivary. Oval projection at upper part of medulla oblongata above extremity of lateral column. SYN: *oliva* [NA]; *olivary body.*

e., parietal. The marked convexity on outer surface of parietal bone.

e.'s, portal. The small median lobes on the lower surface of the liver.

e., pyramidal. An elevation on the mastoid wall of the tympanic cavity. It contains a cavity in which lies the stapedius muscle. SYN: *pyramid of tympanum.*

e., thenar. Eminence formed by muscles below the thumb on the palm of the hand.

eminentia (ĕm″ĭn-ĕn′shē-ă) [L.]. (pl. *eminentiae*) An eminence.

emiocytosis (ē″mē-ō-sī-tō′sĭs) [L. *emit,* to send forth, + Gr. *kytos,* cell, + *osis,* condition]. The process of movement of intracellular material to the outside. Granules join the cell membrane, which ruptures to allow the substance to be free in the intracellular fluid. SEE: *endocytosis.*

emissary (ĕm′ĭ-să-rē) [L. *e,* out, + *mittere,* to send]. 1. Providing an outlet. 2. An outlet.

emissary veins. Small veins that pierce the skull and carry blood from the sinuses within the skull to the veins without.

emissio (ē-mĭs′sē-ō) [L.]. A discharge; emission.

emission (ē-mĭsh′ŭn) [L. *e,* out, + *mittere,* to send]. An issuance or discharge; the sending forth or discharge, such as of an atomic particle, exhalation, or of a light or heat wave.

e., nocturnal. Involuntary discharge of semen during sleep. SYN: *wet dream.*

emmenagogue (ĕm-ĕn′ă-gŏg) [Gr. *emmena,* menses, + *agogos,* leading]. A substance that promotes or assists the flow of menstrual fluid. SEE: *ecbolic.*

e., direct. That which has a direct effect on the reproductive tract, such as a hormone.

e., indirect. An agent that alters the menstrual function by changing the primary disorder in the general state of health.

emmenia (ĕ-mē′nē-ă) [Gr. *emmena*]. The menstrual flow.

emmenic. Pert. to the menses.

emmeniopathy (ĕ-mē″nē-ŏp′ă-thē) [Gr. *emmena,* menses, + *pathos,* disease]. Any disorder of menstruation.

emmenology (ĕm″ĕn-ŏl′ō-jē) [″ + *logos,* science]. Science of menstruation.

emmetrope (ĕm′ĕ-trōp) [Gr. *emmetros,* in due measure, + *opsis,* sight]. One endowed with normal vision.

emmetropia (ĕm″ĕ-trō′pē-ă). Normal condition of the eye in refraction in which, when the eye is at rest, parallel rays focus exactly on the retina. SEE: illus.; *astigmatism; myopia.*

emmetropic. Normal vision. SEE: *hypermetropic; myopic.*

Emmet's operation. [Thomas A. Emmet, U.S. gynecologist, 1828–1919] 1. Uterine trachelorrhaphy, i.e., suture of torn uterine cervix. 2. Suturing of a lacerated perineum. 3. Converting a sessile submucous tumor of the uterus into a pedunculated one. 4. Operation for prolapse of uterus.

emollient (ē-mŏl′yĕnt) [L. *e,* out, + *mollire,* to soften]. An agent that will soften and soothe the part when applied locally. The term is usually confined to agents affecting the surface of the body. SEE: *demulcent.*

Ex.: ointment of rose water; olive oil; petrolatum.

emotion (ē-mō′shŭn) [L. *emovere,* to stir up]. 1. Passions or sensibilities characterized by physical changes in the body such as alteration in heart rate and respiratory activity, vasomotor reactions, and changes in muscle tone. 2. A mental state or feeling such as fear, hate, love, anger, grief, or joy arising as a subjective rather than as a conscious mental effort. These constitute the drive that

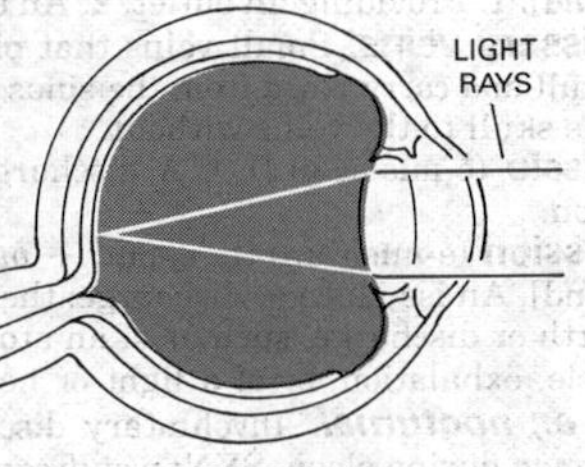

EMMETROPIA
LIGHT RAYS FOCUS ON RETINA

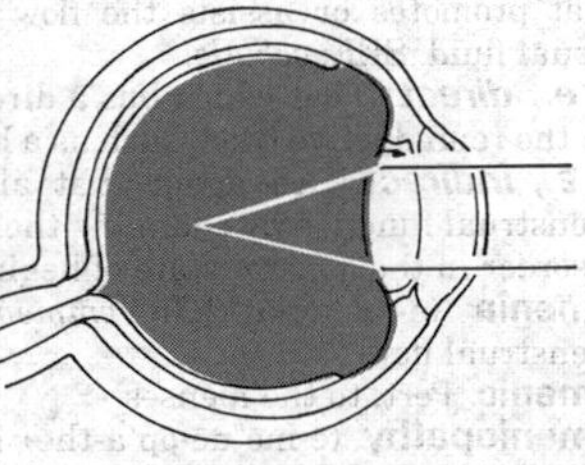

MYOPIA
LIGHT RAYS FOCUS
IN FRONT OF RETINA

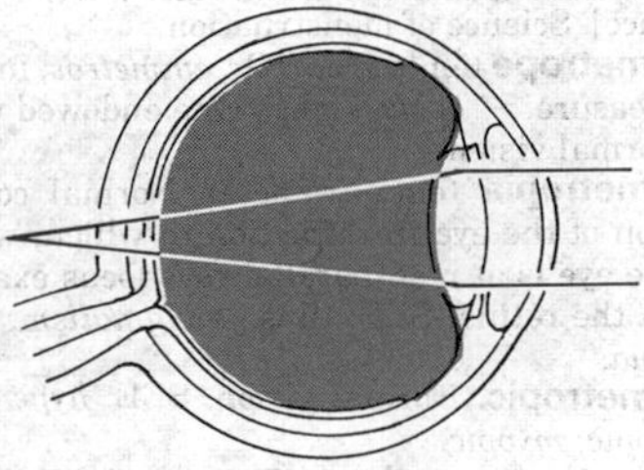

HYPEROPIA
LIGHT RAYS FOCUS PAST RETINA

brings about the emotional or mental adjustment necessary to satisfy instinctive needs. Physiological changes invariably accompany alteration in the emotions but such change may not be apparent to either the person experiencing the emotion or an observer.

Frustration is normally associated with displeasure and intensification of perception of personal need; the process of gratification is accompanied by pleasurable feeling that persists for a variable period in less intense form.

Anxiety or fear arises when one doubts one's ability to meet a situation adequately. Neutralization consists of flight from danger or a struggle (fight) to remove the threat. Civilized people may find a goal unattainable because their conditioned (moral) reactions regard the goal as socially objectionable or they may even deny the goal entirely. Thus conflicts arise and the stage is set for the onset of psychogenic disease.

DISORDERS: Emotions are not felt in the same way by healthy persons as by those suffering from mental disease. In schizophrenia there is a decrease of pleasure, hate, love, and other emotions. There is loss of ability to feel and express emotions such as love or hate. The patients are said to be blunted. The emotions they do show are not in harmony with their ideas. For example, they may smile while describing tortures and terrors.

Unhappiness is marked in manic depressive psychosis. It varies in degree and may lead to suicide. In the excited stage undue happiness is marked. SEE: *anhedonia*.

emotion, words pert. to: anhedonia; anxiety; anxiety neurosis; catharsis; conflict; depression; empathy; disease, psychosomatic; exaltation; fear; frustration; love; mania; manic-depressive; phobia; sympathy.

emotional [L. *emovere*, to stir up]. Rel. to any of the emotions.

emotional need. Each of us has inner needs with respect to the emotions of love, fear, anxiety, sadness, loneliness, and anger. These needs may be understood and handled by the healthy individual, but are especially difficult to cope with during illness or mental stress. The medical care team needs to be alert to the possibility that the patient's needs in these areas need to be managed and treated. This is best done by demonstrating empathy for the patient and being close by when needed. In times of stress and anxiety, the therapy of holding the aged patient's hand has remarkable therapeutic effects. SEE: *TLC*.

emotivity (ē″mō-tĭv′ĭ-tē). One's capability for emotional response.

empasm, empasma (ĕm′păzm, ĕm-păs′mă) [Gr. *en*, in, + *passein*, to sprinkle]. A powder, usually perfumed, for external application to the body.

empathic [″ + *pathos*, feeling]. Pert. to, or characterized by, empathy.

empathy (ĕm′pă-thē). Objective awareness of and insight into the feelings, emotions, and behavior of another person and their meaning and significance. Not the same as sympathy, which is usually nonobjective and noncritical.

emperipolesis (ĕm-pĕr″ĭ-pō-lē′sĭs) [Gr. *en*, into, + *peripolesis*, a going about]. Penetration by lymphocytes of another cell.

emphractic (ĕm-frăk′tĭk) [Gr. *emphraxis*, an obstruction]. 1. Obstructive, as clogging of pores of skin. 2. Anything that obstructs a function.

emphraxis (ĕm-frăk′sĭs) [Gr.]. A stoppage or

obstruction; an infarction.

emphysatherapy (ĕm″fĭz-ă-thĕr′ă-pē) [Gr. *emphysan,* to inflate, + *therapeia,* treatment]. Injection of gas into a cavity for therapeutic purposes.

emphysema (ĕm″fĭ-sē′mă) [Gr. *emphysan,* to inflate]. 1. Pathological distention of tissues by gas or air in the interstices. 2. A chronic pulmonary disease characterized by increase beyond the normal in the size of air spaces distal to the terminal bronchiole with destructive changes in their walls. SYN: *chronic obstructive pulmonary disease; pulmonary emphysema.*

DIAG: Precise diagnosis of emphysema is difficult to establish. Clinically the patient may have breathlessness that may be present only during exertion. Cough with production of sputum usually indicates the presence of chronic bronchitis.

NURSING IMPLICATIONS: Maintain a patent airway by eliminating all bronchial irritants such as smoke from the environment. Encourage the patient to increase oral fluid intake to assist in liquefaction of thick secretions. Administer medications ordered to decrease bronchospasm. Administer inhalation therapy and postural drainage as needed.

Help to prevent respiratory infections through such interventions as encouraging good pulmonary hygiene, avoidance of contact with persons with respiratory infections, and by correct administration of ordered antibiotics. Good nutrition is essential; teach the patient that eating frequent and smaller meals may prevent increased intra-abdominal pressure, and thus ease respirations.

Also teach the patient breathing exercises such as diaphragmatic breathing to increase respiratory efficiency.

TREATMENT: Patient should avoid contact with atmospheric pollution, esp. that caused by cigarette smoke. Bronchodilators, mucolytic agents, weight reduction if patient is obese, antibiotics for infections, and the use of oxygen therapy only if clearly needed to prevent hypoxia.

emphysematous (ĕm″fĭ-sĕm′ă-tŭs). Affected with or pert. to emphysema.

empiric (ĕm-pĭr′ĭk) [Gr. *empeirikos,* skilled, experienced]. 1. Based on experience. SEE: *empirical.* 2. A practitioner whose skill or art is based upon what has been learned through experience.

empirical (ĕm-pĭr′ĭk-ăl). Based on experience rather than on scientific principles.

empiricism (ĕm-pĭr′ĭs-ĭzm) [Gr. *empeirikos,* skilled, experienced, + *-ismos,* condition of]. 1. Experience, not theory, as basis of medical science. 2. Quackery.

Empirin. Trade name for aspirin.

emplastic (ĕm-plăs′tĭk) [Gr. *emplastikos,* clogging]. 1. A constipating medicine. 2. Adhesive or able to be used as a plaster.

emplastrum [L.]. (pl. *emplastra*) A plaster or preparation for external application; adheres to the skin when applied. SEE: *plaster.*

emprosthotonos (ĕm″prŏs-thŏt′ō-nŏs) [Gr. *emprosthen,* forward, + *tonos,* tension]. A form of spasm in which the body is flexed forward. Sometimes seen in tetanus and strychnine poisoning. Opposite of opisthotonos.

empty-sella syndrome. On lateral x-ray of the skull, the sella turcica, which normally contains the pituitary gland, is found to be empty. Clinically, the patients may show no endocrine abnormality or may have signs of decreased pituitary function. The only treatment needed is to provide hormonal replacement in those who demonstrate hypopituitarism. In autopsy studies, the condition of empty-sella has been found in about 5% of presumably normal persons.

emptysis (ĕmp′tĭ-sĭs) [Gr., a spitting]. Expectoration of blood or blood-stained mucus. SYN: *hemoptysis.*

empyema (ĕm″pī-ē′mă) [Gr.]. Pus in a body cavity, esp. in the pleural cavity (pyothorax). Usually result of a primary infection in the lungs.

SYM: Chills, fever, and sweating. Skin is gray, malar flushed, appetite poor with marked malaise, pain in chest, cough, and emaciation. Dyspnea may ensue.

TREATMENT: Antibiotic therapy, aspiration of pleural fluid. Treatment of primary condition. Surgical drainage may be necessary.

NURSING IMPLICATIONS: Assess the patient for symptoms of respiratory distress. Position the patient sitting up, inclined to the affected side to facilitate drainage, then have patient lean to the opposite side to aid in lung expansion. If the patient has chest tubes in place, correctly position and secure drainage bottles, observe for fluctuations of fluid or bubbling in the bottles, and record the amount and type of drainage. Hemostats should be at the bedside in the event that a bottle should break; Vaseline gauze should be at the bedside in the event that the tube comes dislodged.

The patient with empyema should have an increased fluid intake and a high-protein diet. Breathing exercises should be done at least once a day to help promote lung expansion.

e., interlobular. Form of empyema with pus between lobes of lung.

e. necessitatis. Form of empyema in which pus can escape spontaneously.

e., pulsating. Form of empyema with cardiac beats causing pulsation of chest wall.

empyesis (ĕm″pī-ē′sĭs) [Gr., suppuration]. 1. Any skin eruption characterized by pustules. 2. Any accumulation of pus. 3. Hypopyon, accumulation of pus in the anterior chamber of the eye.

empyocele (ĕm′pī-ō-sēl) [Gr. *empyein,* to suppurate, + *kele,* tumor]. A collection of pus in a sacculated cavity, esp. in the scrotum; a suppurating hydrocele.

empyreuma (ĕm″pī-roo′mă) [Gr., a live coal]. The characteristic odor of animal or vegetable material being burned in a closed container.

EMT. *emergency medical technician.*

emulsification (ē-mŭl″sĭ-fĭ-kā′shŭn) [L. *emulsio,* emulsion, + *facere,* to make.]. 1. Process of making an emulsion. 2. The breaking down of large fat globules in the intestine to smaller, uniformly distributed particles, accomplished largely through the action of bile acids, which lower surface tension.

emulsifier. Anything used to make an emulsion.

emulsify (ē-mŭl′sĭ-fī). To form into an emulsion.

emulsion [L. *emulsio*]. 1. A mixture of two liquids not mutually soluble. If they are thoroughly shaken, one will divide into globules and is called the discontinuous or dispersed phase; the other is then the continuous phase. Milk is an emulsion in which butterfat is the discontinuous phase and the liquid portion the continuous phase. 2. In radiology, that part of the radiographic film that is sensitive to radiation and contains the image after development.

emulsoid (ē-mŭl′soyd) [″ + Gr. *eidos,* form]. A colloid in an aqueous solution in which the colloid has a marked attraction for water to the extent that the dispersoid, q.v., contains large quantities of water. SYN: *hydrophilic lyophilic colloid.*

Ex.: protoplasm, starch, soap, gelatin, and egg white.

emunctory (ē-mŭnk′tō-rē) [L. *emungere,* to cleanse]. 1. Pert. to organ or duct having an excretory function. 2. An excretory duct, as the pores of skin.

E.N.A. *extractable nuclear antigen.*

enamel (ĕn-ăm′ĕl) [O. Fr. *esmail,* enamel]. The hard, white, dense substance forming a covering for the crown of the teeth. It is the hardest substance in the body. SYN: *enamelum* [NA].

e., mottled. Condition in which the enamel acquires a mottled appearance as a result of the ingestion of excessive amounts of fluorides in water or foods.

enamel organ. A cup-shaped structure that forms on the dental lamina of an embryo. It produces the enamel and serves as a mold for the remainder of the tooth.

enamelum. [NA] Enamel.

enanthem, enanthema (ĕn-ăn′thĕm, -ăn-thē′mă) [Gr. *en,* in, + *anthema,* blossoming]. Eruption of mucous membrane. SEE: *exanthem; Koplik's spots; rash.*

enanthematous (ĕn″ăn-thĕm′ă-tŭs). Of the nature of an enanthema.

enanthesis (ĕn″ăn-thē′sĭs) [Gr. *en,* in, + *anthein,* to bloom]. A skin eruption caused by systemic disease such as typhoid fever or syphilis.

enanthrope (ĕn-ăn′thrōp) [″ + *anthropos,* man]. 1. Any disease originating in the body. 2. An auto-infection.

enantiobiosis (ĕn-ăn″tē-ō-bī-ō′sĭs) [Gr. *enantios,* opposite, + *bios,* life]. The condition in which associated organisms are antagonistic to each other. SEE: *symbiosis.*

enantiomorph (ĕn-ăn′tē-ō-morf″). One of a pair of isomers, each of which is a mirror image of the other. They may be identical in chemical characteristics, but in solution one rotates a beam of polarized light in the opposite direction of the other. The isomers are called dextro if they rotate light to the right, and levo if they rotate light to the left.

enantiopathy (ĕn-ăn″tē-ŏp′ă-thē) [″ + *pathos,* disease]. Treatment of one disease by using another disease that produces changes or symptoms antagonistic to it.

enarthritis (ĕn″ăr-thrī′tĭs) [Gr. *en,* in, + *arthron,* joint, + *itis,* inflammation]. Inflammation of a ball-and-socket joint.

enarthrosis (ĕn″ăr-thrō′sĭs) [″ + *arthron,* joint, + *osis,* condition]. (pl. *enarthroses*) A ball-and-socket joint such as the hip joint. A form of diarthrosis.

en bloc (ĕn blŏk) [Fr., as a whole]. In surgery, to remove as a whole or as a lump.

encanthis (ĕn-kăn′thĭs) [Gr. *en,* in, + *kanthos,* angle of the eye]. An excrescence or new growth at the inner angle of the eye.

encapsulation [″ + *capsula,* a little box]. 1. Enclosure in a sheath not normal to the part. 2. The process of the formation of a capsule or a sheath about a structure.

encatarrhaphy (ĕn″kăt-ăr′ă-fē) [Gr. *enkatarrhaptein,* to sew in]. Insertion of an organ or tissue into a part where it is not normally found.

enceinte (ŏn-sănt′) [Fr.]. Pregnant.

encephalalgia (ĕn-sĕf″ăl-ăl′jē-ă) [Gr. *enkephalos,* brain, + *algos,* pain]. Deep-seated head pain. SYN: *cephalalgia.*

encephalatrophy (ĕn-sĕf″ă-lăt′rō-fē) [″ + *a-,* not, + *trophe,* nourishment]. Cerebral atrophy.

encephalic (ĕn″sĕf-ăl′ĭk) [Gr. *enkephalos,* brain]. Pert. to the brain or its cavity.

encephalitis (ĕn-sĕf″ă-lī′tĭs) [″ + *itis,* inflammation]. Inflammation of the brain.

ETIOL: It may be a specific disease entity caused by an arthropod-borne (arbor) virus, or it may occur as a sequela of influenza, measles, German measles, chickenpox, herpesvirus infection, smallpox, vaccinia, or other diseases.

NURSING IMPLICATIONS: Assess the patient for symptoms of increased intracranial pressure such as projectile vomiting, change in level of consciousness, unreactive or slowly reactive pupils, decreased pulse rate, and increased blood pressure. Maintain a patent airway, adequate fluid balance and nutritional status. Take seizure precautions; and monitor intake and output.

e., acute disseminated. E., postinfection, q.v.

e., cortical. Encephalitis of brain cortex only.

e., epidemic. Any form of encephalitis that occurs as an epidemic.

e., equine. A mosquito-borne type of viral encephalitis originally isolated as an encephalitis affecting horses.

e., equine, eastern. Primarily a viral disease of birds and wild animals, transmitted to horses and man by mosquitoes. More severe than other types of encephalitis. Outbreaks have occurred in the eastern and Gulf Coast states.

e., equine, western. A mild type of viral encephalitis that has occurred in western United States and Canada.

e., hemorrhagic. Herpes encephalitis where there is hemorrhage along with brain inflammation.

e., herpes. Encephalitis due to infection with herpes simplex virus. Though rare, it is frequently fatal. It has been successfully treated with an antiviral agent.

e. hyperplastica. Acute encephalitis without suppuration.

e., infantile. Brain inflammation in the young that may cause cerebral palsy.

***e., Japanese* (B type).** Similar to St. Louis encephalitis, it is caused by a different strain of mosquito-borne virus. Occurs in summer and fall.

e., lead. Encephalitis due to lead poisoning.

e. lethargica. A disease of the nervous system thought to be caused by a virus. Characterized by lethargy, oculomotor paralysis, clonic and choreiform movements, rigidity, delirium, stupor, coma, and reversal of sleep rhythm. The disease first appeared pandemically in 1916 to 1917, and is now considered extinct. SYN: *Economo's disease.*

e., meningo-. Encephalitis combined with meningitis.

e. neonatorum. A form of encephalitis occurring within the first several weeks of life.

e. periaxialis. Inflammation of the white matter of the cerebrum, occurring mainly in the young.

e., postinfection. Encephalitis occurring following a smallpox vaccination or one of the common communicable diseases, as chickenpox.

e., postvaccinal. Acute encephalitis following vaccination.

e., purulent. Encephalitis characterized by abscesses in the brain.

e., Russian spring-summer. Encephalitis due to a tick-borne virus. It may also be transmitted to man by drinking goat milk.

e., St. Louis. A mosquito-borne virus disease that first occurred epidemically in the summer of 1933 in and around St. Louis, a city in the U.S.A. Now endemic in the U.S.A., Trinidad, Jamaica, Panama, and Brazil. Occurs most frequently during summer and early fall.

e., toxic. Encephalitis resulting from metal poisonings, as lead poisoning.

encephalocele (ĕn-sĕf′ă-lō-sēl) [Gr. *enkephalos,* brain, + *kele,* hernia]. Protrusion of the brain through a cranial fissure. SYN: *hydrencephalocele.*

encephalocystocele (ĕn-sĕf″ă-lō-sĭs′tō-sēl) [″ + *kystis,* sac, + *kele,* hernia]. Hernia of the brain. The hernia sac is filled with cerebrospinal fluid.

encephalogram (ĕn-sĕf′ă-lō-grăm) [″ + *gramma,* a writing]. Roentgenogram of the brain. Usually done with air injected into the ventricles in order to provide contrast in the picture.

encephalography (ĕn-sĕf″ă-lŏg′ră-fē) [″ + *graphein,* to write]. X-ray examination of the head, esp. examination following the introduction of air into the ventricles through a lumbar or cisternal puncture.

encephaloid (ĕn-sĕf′ă-loyd) [″ + *eidos,* form]. 1. Resembling the cerebral substance. 2. A malignant neoplasm of brainlike texture.

encephalolith (ĕn-sĕf′ă-lō-lĭth) [″ + *lithos,* stone]. A calculus of the brain.

encephaloma (ĕn-sĕf″ă-lō′mă) [″ + *oma,* tumor]. Tumor of the brain.

encephalomalacia (ĕn-sĕf″ă-lō-mă-lā′sē-ă) [″ + *malakia,* softening]. Cerebral softening.

encephalomeningitis (ĕn-sĕf″ă-lō-mĕn″ĭn-jī′tĭs) [″ + *meninx,* membrane, + *itis,* inflammation]. Inflammation of the brain and its membranes.

encephalomeningocele (ĕn-sĕf″ă-lō-mĕ-nĭng′gō-sēl) [″ + ″ + *kele,* hernia]. Protrusion of membranes and brain substance through the cranium.

encephalomere (ĕn-sĕf′ă-lō-mēr″) [″ + *meros,* part]. A primitive segment of the embryonic brain. SYN: *neuromere.*

encephalometer (ĕn-sĕf″ă-lŏm′ĕ-tĕr) [″ + *metron,* measure]. An instrument for measuring the cranium and locating brain regions.

encephalomyelitis (ĕn-sĕf″ă-lō-mī-ĕl-ī′tĭs) [″ + *myelos,* marrow, + *itis,* inflammation]. An acute inflammation of the brain and spinal cord.

e., acute disseminated. Acute disorder of the brain and spinal cord due to causes such as vaccination or acute exanthema. SYN: *e., postinfectious.*

e., benign myalgic. An epidemic disease of unknown etiology. It usually occurs in young institutionalized persons. There are the usual symptoms of encephalitis but few physical signs. It may be confused with poliomyelitis. SYN: *Icelandic disease.*

e., equine. Virus disease of horses that may be communicated to man. Includes eastern and western equine encephalitis.

e., postinfectious. E., acute disseminated, q.v.

e., postvaccinal. Encephalomyelitis following smallpox vaccination.

encephalomyeloneuropathy (ĕn-sĕf″ă-lō-mī″ĕ-lō-nū-rŏp′ă-thē). Any disease involving the brain, spinal cord, and nerves.

encephalomyelopathy (ĕn-sĕf″ă-lō-mī″ĕl-ŏp′ă-thē) [″ + ″ + *pathos,* disease]. Any disease of brain and spinal cord.

encephalomyeloradiculitis (ĕn-sĕf′ă-lō-mī″ĕ-lō-ră-dĭk″ū-lī′tĭs). Inflammation of the brain, spinal cord, and nerve roots.

encephalomyocarditis (ĕn-sĕf′ă-lō-mī″ō-kăr-dī′tĭs). Any disease involving the brain and the cardiac muscle.

encephalon (ĕn-sĕf′ă-lŏn) [Gr. *enkephalos,* brain]. [NA] The brain, including the cerebrum, cerebellum, medulla oblongata, pons, diencephalon, and midbrain.

encephalopathy (ĕn-sĕf″ă-lŏp′ă-thē) [″ + *pathos,* disease]. Any dysfunction of the brain.

encephalopuncture (ĕn-sĕf″ă-lō-punk′tūr) [″ + L. *punctura,* a piercing]. Puncture into the brain substance.

encephalopyosis (ĕn-sĕf″ă-lō-pī-ō′sĭs) [″ + *pyosis,* suppuration]. Abscess of the brain.

encephalorrhagia (ĕn-sĕf″ă-lō-rā′jē-ă) [″ + *rhegnynai,* to burst forth]. Cerebral hemorrhage. SEE: *hemorrhage, cerebral.*

encephalosclerosis (ĕn-sĕf″ă-lō-sklĕ-rō′sĭs) [″ + *sklerosis,* hardening]. Hardening of the brain.

encephalosis [″ + *osis,* diseased condition]. A degenerative process of the brain.

encephalospinal [″ + L. *spina,* thorn, spine]. Pert. to brain and spinal cord.

encephalotome (ĕn-sĕf′ă-lō-tŏm) [Gr. *enkephalos,* brain, + *tome,* incision]. Instrument for incising brain tissue.

encephalotomy (ĕn-sĕf″ă-lŏt′ō-mē). 1. Brain dissection. 2. Surgical destruction of the brain of a fetus to facilitate delivery.

enchondroma (ĕn″kŏn-drō′mă) [Gr. *en,* in, + *chondros,* cartilage, + *oma,* tumor]. A benign cartilaginous tumor occurring generally where cartilage is absent or within a bone where it expands the diaphysis. SYN: *enchondrosis.*

enchondrosarcoma (ĕn-kŏn″drō-săr-kō′mă) [″ + ″ + *sarx,* flesh, + *oma,* tumor]. Sarcoma made up of cartilaginous tissue.

enchondrosis (ĕn-kŏn-drō′sĭs) [″ + ″ + *osis,* diseased condition]. A benign cartilaginous outgrowth from bone or cartilaginous tissue. SYN: *enchondroma.*

enclave (ĕn′klāv) [Fr. *enclaver,* to enclose]. A mass of tissue that becomes enclosed by tissue of another kind.

enclitic (ĕn-klĭt′ĭk) [Gr. *enklinein,* to lean on]. Having the planes of the fetal head inclined to those of the maternal pelvis.

encolpitis (ĕn-kŏl-pī′tĭs) [Gr. *en,* in, + *kolpos,* vagina, + *itis,* inflammation]. Inflamed condition of the vaginal mucosa. SYN: *endocolpitis.*

encopresis (ĕn-kō-prē′sĭs) [″ + *kopros,* excrement]. A condition associated with constipation and fecal retention. Watery colonic contents bypass the hard fecal masses and pass through the rectum. This is often confused with diarrhea.

encranial [″ + *kranion,* cranium]. Intracranial or within the cranium.

encyesis (ĕn″sī-ē′sĭs) [″ + *kyesis,* pregnancy]. Normal uterine pregnancy.

encysted (ĕn-sĭst′ĕd) [″ + *kystis,* bladder, pouch]. Surrounded by membrane; encapsulated. SYN: *saccate.*

end [AS. *ende*]. A termination; extremity.

endadelphos (ĕnd″ă-dĕl′fŏs) [Gr. *endon,* within, + *adelphos,* brother]. A congenitally deformed fetus, the twin of which is enclosed in the body or in a cyst on the fetus.

Endamoeba (ĕn″dă-mē′bă). Entamoeba.

endangeitis, endangiitis (ĕnd″ăn-jē-ī′tĭs) [Gr. *endon,* within, + *angeion,* vessel, + *itis,* inflammation]. Inflammation of the endangium or inner coat of blood vessels.

endangium (ĕn-dăn′jē-ŭm) [″ + *angeion,* vessel]. Innermost coat or intima of blood vessels.

endaortitis (ĕnd″ā-or-tī-tĭs) [″ + *aorte,* aorta, + *itis,* inflammation]. Inflammation of inner coat of the aorta.

endarterectomy (ĕnd″ăr-tĕr-ĕk′tō-mē). Surgical removal of the lining of an artery. This is done on almost any major artery that is diseased or blocked, such as carotid, femoral, or popliteal arteries.

endarterial (ĕnd″ăr-tē′rē-ăl) [″ + *arteria,* artery]. 1. Pert. to the inner portion of an artery. 2. Within an artery.

endarteritis (ĕnd-ăr-tĕr-ī'tĭs) [" + " + *itis,* inflammation]. Inflammation of innermost coat (intima) of an artery resulting from syphilis, trauma, pyogenic bacteria, or infective thrombi.

e., acute. Rare inflammation of large arteries.

e., chronic. Degeneration of arterial coats in the aging. SYN: *atheroma.*

e. deformans. Thickening of intima or replacement with atheromatous or calcareous deposits.

e. obliterans. Chronic progressive thickening of intima leading to stenosis or obstruction of lumen.

e. syphilitic. Endarteritis caused by syphilis.

end-artery. An artery that does not communicate with other arteries.

endbrain. Telencephalon.

end-bud. The terminal of a sensory nerve. SYN: *end-bulb.*

end-bulb. The terminal portion of a sensory nerve. SYN: *end-bud.*

e. of Krause. An encapsulated nerve ending found in the skin and mucous membranes.

endemic [Gr. *en,* in, + *demos,* people]. A disease that occurs continuously in a particular population, but has low mortality, as measles. Used in contrast to epidemic.

endemoepidemic (ĕn-dĕm"ō-ĕp-ĭ-dĕm'ĭk) [" + " + *epi,* on, among, + *demos,* people]. Endemic, but becoming epidemic periodically.

Endep. Trade name for amitriptyline hydrochloride.

endergonic (ĕnd"ĕr-gŏn'ĭk) [Gr. *endon,* within, + *ergon,* work]. Pert. to chemical reactions that require energy in order to occur.

endermatic, endermic [Gr. *endon,* within, + *derma,* skin]. Administration of medicine by absorption through the skin.

endermosis [" + " + *osis,* condition]. 1. Administration of medicines through the skin. 2. Herpetic affection of any mucous membrane.

end-feet. Terminal buttons; the enlarged ends of nerve fibers that terminate adjacent to the dendrite of another nerve cell.

ending. The finish or final portion of a tissue or cell.

endoaneurysmorrhaphy (ĕn"dō-ăn"ū-rĭs-mor'ăf-ē) [Gr. *endon,* within, + *aneurysma,* aneurysm, + *rhaphe,* suture]. Opening an aneurysmal sac and suturing its orifice.

endoangiitis (ĕn"dō-ăn-jē-ī'tĭs) [" + *angeion,* vessel, + *itis,* inflammation]. Inflammation of the inner coat of blood vessels. SYN: *endangiitis; endoarteritis; endophlebitis.*

endoantitoxin (ĕn"dō-ăn-tē-tŏk'sĭn) [" + *anti,* against, + *toxikon,* poison]. An antitoxin within a cell.

endoappendicitis (ĕn"dō-ă-pĕn"dĭ-sī'tĭs) [" + L. *appendere,* to hang, + Gr. *itis,* inflammation]. Inflammation of mucosa of the vermiform appendix.

endoarteritis (ĕn"dō-ăr"tĕr-ī'tĭs) [" + *arteria,* artery, + *itis,* inflammation]. Inflammation of the innermost coat of an artery from syphilis, trauma, bacteria, or infective thrombi.

endoauscultation (ĕn"dō-ăws"kŭl-tā'shŭn) [" + L. *auscultare,* to listen to]. Auscultation by esophageal tube passed into the stomach or by a tube passed into the heart.

endobiotic (ĕn"dō-bī-ŏt'ĭk) [" + *bios,* life]. Pert. to an organism living parasitically in the host.

endoblast (ĕn'dō-blăst) [" + *blastos,* germ]. 1. The nucleus cell. 2. Inner layer of the blastoderm. SYN: *endoderm; hypoblast.*

endobronchitis (ĕn"dō-brŏng-kī'tĭs). Inflammation of the smaller bronchi

endocardiac, endocardial [" + *kardia,* heart]. Within the heart or arising from the endocardium.

endocarditis (ĕn"dō-kăr-dī'tĭs) [" + " + *itis,* inflammation]. Inflammation of the lining membrane of the heart. It is usually confined to the external lining of the valve, sometimes to the lining membrane of its chambers. May be due to invasion of microorganisms or an abnormal immunological reaction.

NURSING IMPLICATIONS: During the acute phase, it is essential to maintain the patient on bedrest and provide a calm, quiet environment. Take vital signs, including apical pulse rate, every 2 to 4 hours (or more frequently if ordered). You may place the patient in Fowler's position with arms supported on pillows at sides to help relieve dyspnea. Administer antibiotics as ordered. When patient begins activity or ambulation, take pulse before and after the activity to determine the effects of the stress on the heart muscle. Teach the patient the importance of taking prescribed prophylactic antibiotics.

TREATMENT: Antibiotic therapy for at least one month. The type of antibiotic used will be determined by the bacterial organisms involved.

e., acute bacterial. Endocarditis that begins abruptly and progresses rapidly. Usually caused by virulent organisms such as staphylococci or pneumococci.

e., atypical verrucous. Nonbacterial endocarditis in which the accumulation of debris on the endocardium is associated with various wasting diseases.

e., bacterial. SEE: *e., acute bacterial.*

e., chronic. E., ulcerative.

e., infective. Endocarditis due to microorganisms.

e., Libman-Sacks. Nonbacterial endocarditis. SEE: *e., atypical verrucous.*

e., malignant. A fatal type of endocarditis that is usually secondary to suppurative inflammation elsewhere. SEE: *e., ulcerative.*

e., mural. Endocarditis of the lining of the heart chambers but not including the heart valve.

e., rheumatic. Endocarditis that occurs following rheumatic fever.

e., subacute bacterial. A condition usually caused by colonization of the Streptococcus viridans group (mainly S. salivarius, S. mitis, S. bovis, S. fecalis, S. sanguis) in an abnormal heart or in valves damaged previously by rheumatic fever.

e., syphilitic. Endocarditis due to syphilis having extended from aortic involvement to the aortic valves.

e., tuberculous. Endocarditis involving the heart valves; caused by the tubercle bacillus.

e., ulcerative. A rapidly destructive form of acute bacterial endocarditis characterized by necrosis or ulceration of the valves and the deposition of colonies of micrococci. Usually fatal.

e., valvular. Endocarditis affecting only the covering of the valves and not the lining of the heart chambers.

e., vegetative. Endocarditis associated with fibrinous clots on ulcerated valvular surfaces.

e., verrucous. Nonbacterial endocarditis occurring frequently in lupus erythematosus.

e. viridans. E., subacute bacterial.

endocardium [Gr. *endon,* within, + *kardia,* heart]. [NA] Serous lining membrane of inner surface and cavities of the heart. It is continuous with the intima or interior coat of arteries.

endocervical (ĕn″dō-sĕr′vĭ-kăl) [″ + L. *cervix,* neck]. Pert. to the endocervix.

endocervicitis (ĕn″dō-sĕr″vĭ-sī′tĭs) [″ + ″ + Gr. *itis,* inflammation]. Inflammation of mucous lining of the cervix uteri. Usually chronic, due to infection, and accompanied by cervical erosion.

SYM: White or yellow mucoid discharge.

TREATMENT: Electrocauterization of cervical lesion. An antibiotic for local application may be prescribed.

endocervix (ĕn″dō-sĕr′vĭks) [″ + L. *cervix,* neck]. The lining of the canal of the cervix uteri.

endochondral (ĕn″dō-kŏn′drăl) [″ + *chondros,* cartilage]. Within a cartilage.

endochorion (ĕn″dō-kō′rē-ŏn) [″ + *chorion,* chorion]. The inner chorion; vascular layer of allantois.

endocolitis (ĕn″dō-kō-lī′tĭs) [″ + *kolon,* colon, + *itis,* inflammation]. Inflammation of the mucosa of colon. SEE: *colitis.*

endocolpitis (ĕn″dō-kŏl-pī′tĭs) [″ + *kolpos,* vagina, + *itis,* inflammation]. Inflammation of the vaginal mucosa. SYN: *encolpitis.*

endocorpuscular (ĕn″dō-kor-pŭs′kū-lăr) [″ + L. *corpusculum,* small body (corpuscle)]. Within a corpuscle.

endocranial (ĕn″dō-krā′nē-ăl) [″ + *kranion,* cranium]. 1. Intracranial or within the cranium. 2. Pert. to the endocranium.

endocranitis (ĕn″dō-krā-nī′tĭs) [″ + ″ + *itis,* inflammation]. Inflammation of endocranium.

endocranium (ĕn″dō-krā′nē-ŭm). The dura mater of the brain, which forms the lining membrane of the cranium.

endocrinasthenia (ĕn″dō-krĭn″ăs-thē′nē-ă) [Gr. *endon,* within, + *krinein,* to secrete, + *astheneia,* weakness]. Neurasthenia due to dysfunction of the endocrine system.

endocrine (ĕn′dō-krīn, -krĭn, -krēn) [″ + *krinein,* to secrete]. 1. An internal secretion. 2. Pert. to a gland that secretes directly into the bloodstream.

endocrine gland. A ductless gland that produces an internal secretion discharged into the blood or lymph and circulated to all parts of the body. Hormones, the active principles of the glands, produce effects on tissues more or less remote from their place of origin. In addition to their endocrine function, some glands also produce an external secretion.

The endocrine glands include hypophysis (pituitary gland), thyroid gland (the thymus and pineal body have not been shown to produce any hormones), parathyroid glands, adrenal (suprarenal) glands, islands of Langerhans of the pancreas, and the gonads (ovaries and testes). Other structures such as the gastrointestinal mucosa and the placenta have an endocrine function. SEE: illus.; table.

The hormones secreted by the ductless glands may have a specific effect on an organ or tissue or a general effect on the entire body, as in the case of the thyroid hormone, which affects the rate of metabolism. Among the physiological processes affected by hormones are rate of metabolism and the metabolism of specific substances, growth and developmental processes, the secretory activity of other endocrine glands, the development and functioning of the reproductive organs, sexual characteristics and libido, the development of personality and higher nervous functions, the ability of the body to meet conditions of stress, resistance to disease.

Endocrine dysfunction may result from hyposecretion, in which an inadequate amount

ENDOCRINE SYSTEM

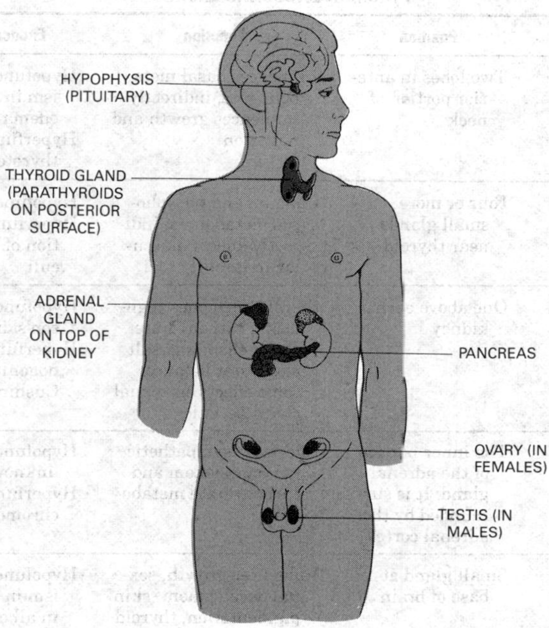

of the hormone(s) is secreted, or hypersecretion, in which excessive amounts of hormones are produced. Secretion of endocrine glands may be under nervous control, under control of chemical substances in the blood, or, in some cases, under control of other hormones. Many pathological conditions are the result of or associated with the malfunctioning of the endocrine glands.

endocrino- [Gr. *endon*, within, + *krinein*, to secrete]. Combining form for endocrine.

endocrinology (ĕn″dō-krĭn-ŏl′ō-jē) [″ + ″ + *logos*, study of]. The science of the endocrine, or ductless glands, and their functions.

endocrinopathic. Of the nature of endocrinopathy.

endocrinopathy (ĕn″dō-krĭn-ŏp′ă-thē) [″ + ″ + *pathos*, disease]. Any disease resulting from disorder of an endocrine gland or glands.

endocrinotherapy (ĕn″dō-krĭn″ō-thĕr′ă-pē) [″ + ″ + *therapeia*, treatment]. Treatment with endocrine preparations.

endocyst (ĕn′dō-sĭst) [″ + *kystis*, bladder, pouch]. The innermost layer of any hydatid cyst.

endocystitis (ĕn″dō-sĭs-tī′tĭs) [″ + ″ + *itis*, inflammation]. Inflammation of mucous membrane of bladder. SEE: *cystitis*.

endocytosis. A method of ingestion of a foreign substance by a cell. The cell wall invaginates in to form a space for the material and then the opening closes to trap the material inside the cell. SEE: *phagocytosis; pinocytosis; exocytosis; emiocytosis*.

endoderm (ĕn′dō-dĕrm) [″ + *derma*, skin]. Inner layer of cells of an embryo. SYN: *entoderm; hypoblast*.

endodermal. Pert to the entoderm. SYN: *entodermal*.

Endodermophyton (ĕn″dō-dĕr-mŏf′ĭ-tŏn) [″ + *derma*, skin, + *phyton*, a growth]. Former name of a genus of parasitic fungi growing in the epidermis of the skin. Now included in the genus Trichophyton.

endodiascope (ĕn″dō-dī′ă-skōp) [″ + *dia*, through, + *skopein*, to examine]. X-ray tube that may be placed within a cavity of the body for radiological examination and radiation therapy.

endodiascopy (ĕn″dō-dī-ăs′kō-pē). X-ray examination of a body cavity with an endodiascope.

endodontia (ĕn″dō-dŏn′shē-ă) [″ + *odous*, tooth]. Endodontics.

endodontics (ĕn″dō-dŏn′tĭks). A branch of dentistry concerned with diagnosis, treatment, and prevention of diseases of the dental pulp and its surrounding tissues.

Principal Endocrine Glands

Name	Position	Function	Endocrine Disorders
Thyroid	Two lobes in anterior portion of neck	Influences basal metabolic rate; indirectly influences growth and nutrition	Hypofunction—Cretinism in young; myxedema in adult; goiter Hyperfunction—Goiter; thyrotoxicosis
Parathyroid	Four or more small glands near thyroid	Calcium and phosphorus metabolism; indirectly affects muscular irritability	Hypofunction—Tetany Hyperfunction—Resorption of bone; renal calculi
Adrenal Cortex	One above each kidney	Steroid hormones regulating carbohydrate metabolism and salt and water balance; some effects on sexual characteristics	Hypofunction—Addison's disease Hyperfunction—Adrenogenital syndrome; Cushing's syndrome
Adrenal Medulla	The inner portion of the adrenal gland. It is surrounded by the adrenal cortex	Effects on sympathetic nervous system and carbohydrate metabolism	Hypofunction—Almost unknown Hyperfunction—Pheochromocytoma
Anterior Pituitary	Small gland at base of brain	Influences growth, sexual development, skin pigmentation, thyroid function, adrenocortical function through effects on other endocrine glands (except for growth factor, which acts directly on cells)	Hypofunction—Dwarfism in child; decrease in all other endocrine gland functions except parathyroids Hyperfunction—Acromegaly in adult; diabetes, gigantism in child
Posterior Pituitary	Attached to anterior pituitary	Oxytocic factor influencing some aspects of uterine contraction Antidiuretic factor influencing absorption of water by kidney tubule	Unknown Hypofunction—Diabetes insipidus
Testes and Ovaries	Testes—in the scrotum Ovaries—in the pelvic cavity	Development of secondary sex characteristics; some effect on metabolism	Hypofunction—Lack of sex development or regression in adult Hyperfunction—Abnormal sex development
Pancreas (endocrine portion)	Abdominal cavity. Head adjacent to duodenum; tail close to spleen and kidney	Secretes insulin and glucagon, which regulate carbohydrate metabolism	Hypofunction—Diabetes mellitus Hyperfunction—If a tumor produces excess insulin, hypoglycemia; if excess glucagon, diabetes mellitus

endodontist. A specialist in the practice of endodontics.
endodontitis (ĕn″dō-dŏn-tī′tĭs) [″ + *odous,* tooth, + *itis,* inflammation]. Inflammation of the dental pulp. SYN: *pulpitis.*
endodontium. Obsolete term for pulp of a tooth. SEE: *pulp.*
endodontologist. An endodontist.
endodontology. Endodontics.
endoectothrix (ĕn″dō-ĕk′tō-thrĭks) [″ + *ektos,* outside, + *thrix,* hair]. Any fungus growth on and in the hair.
endoenteritis (ĕn″dō-ĕn″tĕr-ī′tĭs) [″ + *enteron,* intestine, + *itis,* inflammation]. Inflammation of mucous membrane of intestines.
endoenzyme (ĕn″dō-ĕn′zīm) [″ + *en,* in, + *zyme,* leaven]. An intracellular enzyme.
endogamy (ĕn-dŏg′ă-mē) [″ + *gamos,* marriage]. 1. The custom or tribal restriction of marriage within a tribe or group. 2. In biology, reproduction by joining together gametes descended from the same ancestral cell.
endogastric (ĕn″dō-găs′trĭk) [″ + *gaster,* belly]. Pert. to the stomach's interior.
endogastritis (ĕn″dō-găs-trī′tĭs) [″ + ″ + *itis,* inflammation]. Inflammation of the lining membrane of the stomach.
endogenic (ĕn″dō-jĕn′ĭk) [″ + *gennan,* to produce]. Having origin within the organism. SYN: *endogenous.*
endogenous (ĕn-dŏj′ĕ-nŭs). 1. Produced or arising from within a cell or organism. 2. Concerning spore formation within the bacteria cell. SYN: *endogenic.*
endogenous opiate-like substance. SEE: *endorphins; enkephalins; opiate receptor.*
endogeny (ĕn-dŏj′ĕ-nē). Formation of growth within the cell.
endoglobar, endoglobular (ĕn″dō-glōb′ăr, ĕn″dō-glŏb′ū-lăr) [Gr. *endon,* within, + L. *globulus,* a globule]. Within the blood corpuscles.
endointoxication (ĕn″dō-ĭn-tŏk″sĭ-kā′shŭn) [″ + L. *in,* into, + Gr. *toxikon,* poison]. Poisoning due to an endogenous toxin.
endolabyrinthitis (ĕn″dō-lăb″ĭ-rĭn-thī′tĭs) [″ + *labyrinthos,* labyrinth, + *itis,* inflammation]. Inflamed condition of the membranous labyrinth.
endolaryngeal (ĕn″dō-lă-rĭn′jē-ăl) [″ + *larynx,* larynx]. Within the larynx.
Endolimax nana (ĕn″dō-lī′măks nă′nă) [″ + *leimax,* meadow]. A species of ameba inhabiting the intestine of man, monkeys, and other mammals. It is usually nonpathogenic in man and is found in the intestines of healthy persons.
endolumbar [″ + L. *lumbus,* loin]. In the lumbar portion of the spinal cord.
endolymph (ĕn′dō-lĭmf) [″ + L. *lympha,* clear fluid]. Pale transparent fluid within the labyrinth of the ear.
endolymphatic. Rel. to the endolymph.
endolymphatic duct. A slender duct extending from posterior surface of the saccule of the inner ear. It ends blindly in the petrous portion of temporal bone as a dilated pouch, the endolymphatic sac.
endolysin (ĕn-dŏl′ĭ-sĭn) [″ + *lysis,* a loosening]. Bacterial substance within a leukocyte that destroys bacteria.
endolysis. Disintegration of cell cytoplasm.
endomastoiditis (ĕn″dō-măs″toy-dī′tĭs) [″ + *mastos,* breast, + *eidos,* form, + *itis,* inflammation]. Inflammation of mucosa lining the mastoid cavity and cells.
endometer (ĕn-dŏm′ĕ-tĕr). Electronic device used to determine the length of a tooth's root canal.
endometrectomy (ĕn″dō-mē-trĕk′tō-mē) [″ + *metra,* uterus, + *ektome,* excision]. Excision of uterine mucosa. SEE: *curettage.*
endometrial (ĕn″dō-mē′trē-ăl) [″ + *metra,* uterus]. Pert. to the lining of the uterus.
endometrial cyst. An ovarian cyst or tumor lined with endometrial tissue. Usually seen in ovarian endometriosis.
endometrial dating. Microscopic examination of a suitable, stained specimen from the endometrium of the uterus in order to establish the number of days to the next menstrual period. The dating is on the basis of an ideal 28-day cycle. Thus, day 8 indicates menstruation is 20 days away and day 23 that it is 5 days away. This system was devised by Doctor John Rock, a physician at Harvard University, to enable gynecologists to visualize endometria being discussed without having to provide detailed descriptions of the material studied.
endometrial jet washing. Collection of fluid that has been used to irrigate the uterine cavity. Cells present in the fluid are examined for evidence of malignancy. Method is used as a screening test for endometrial carcinoma.
endometrioma (ĕn″dō-mē″trē-ō′mă) [Gr. *endon,* within, + *metra,* uterus, + *oma,* tumor]. A tumor containing shreds of ectopic endometrium; found most frequently in the ovary, cul-de-sac, rectovaginal septum, and the peritoneal surface of the posterior portion of the uterus.
endometriosis (ĕn″dō-mē″trē-ō′sĭs) [″ + ″ + *osis,* condition]. Ectopic endometrium located in various sites throughout the pelvis or in the abdominal wall. SEE: illus.
e., direct. Invasion of the myometrium by the mucous membrane lining the uterus.
e., implantation. E., peritoneal.
e., internal. E., direct.
e., metastatic. Extraperitoneal lesions in circumstances resembling metastatic pel-

SITES OF OCCURRENCE OF ENDOMETRIOSIS

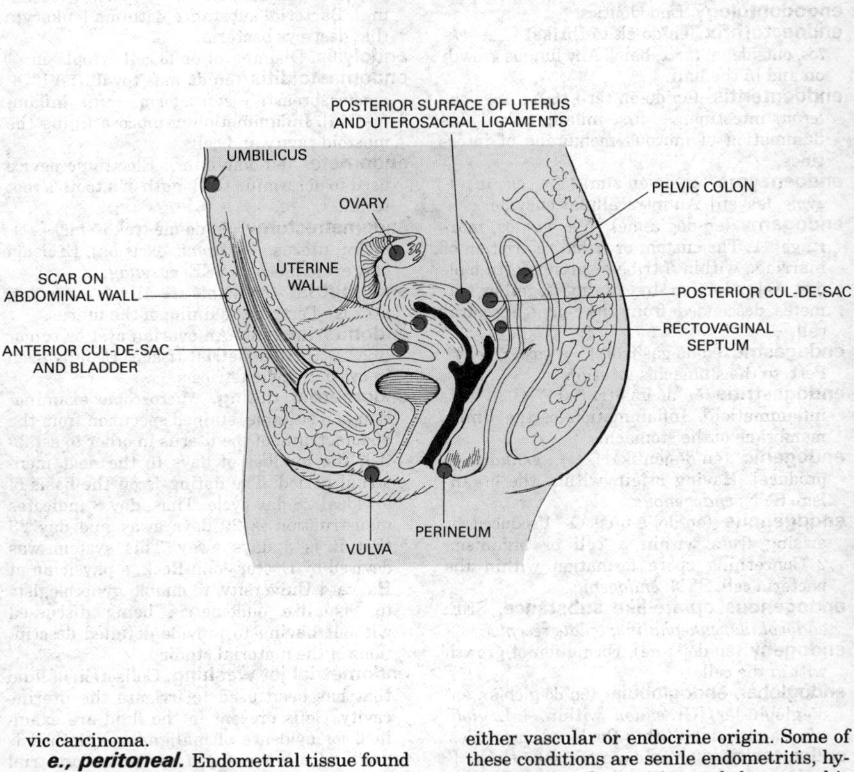

vic carcinoma.

e., peritoneal. Endometrial tissue found throughout the pelvis.

e., primary. E., direct.

e., transplantation. Endometriosis taking place within abdominal incision scar following pelvic surgery.

endometritis (ĕn″dō-mē-trī′tĭs) [″ + ″ + *itis,* inflammation]. Inflammation of the endometrium.

ETIOL: Produced by bacterial invasion. May be acute, subacute, or chronic, the acute cases most commonly resulting from infection by staphylococci, E. coli bacilli, or gonococci; trauma; septic abortion. The subacute and chronic types are the result of repeated acute attacks. Occasionally the chronic type may be due to infection with the tubercle bacillus. There are many other conditions that are labeled as endometritis but are of either vascular or endocrine origin. Some of these conditions are senile endometritis, hyperplastic endometritis, and hypertrophic endometritis.

SYM: In acute cases the symptoms are usually low back and low abdominal pain, dysmenorrhea, menorrhagia, sterility, and constipation. In chronic endometritis, there is scant serosanguineous vaginal discharge. A positive diagnosis cannot be made without a curettage and a histological study of the recovered material. SEE: *cervix uteri; endometrium; uterus.*

e., cervical. Inflammation of the inner portion of the cervix uteri.

e., decidual. Inflammation of the mucous membrane of a gravid uterus.

e. dissecans. Endometritis accompanied by development of ulcers and shedding of the mucous membrane.

e., puerperal. Acute endometritis following childbirth.

endometrium (ĕn-dō-mē'trē-ŭm) [Gr. *endon,* within, + *metra,* uterus]. [NA] The mucous membrane lining the inner surface of the uterus. Histologically it consists of a surface epithelium made up of a single layer of columnar cells, a few of which bear cilia. Invaginations of the epithelium form simple, branched tubular glands that extend to the myometrium. The glands are separated by connective tissue resembling mesenchyme, which forms the stroma. There is no submucosa, the mucosa lying closely attached to the myometrium.

The endometrium is supplied by two types of arteries: straight arteries, which supply the deeper third or basal layer of the endometrium, and spiral arteries, which supply the spongy and compact layers. They penetrate between the glands and form a subepithelial capillary plexus. These arteries show marked changes in response to hormonal stimulation during the menstrual cycle. Beginning with menarche and ending at menopause, the uterine endometrium passes through cyclic changes that constitute the menstrual cycle, q.v. These changes are related to the development and maturation of the graafian follicle in the ovary, the discharge of the ovum, and the subsequent development of the corpus luteum in the ovary.

Following fertilization of the ovum, the endometrium serves as nesting place and implantation occurs. The endometrium fuses with the developing chorion of the embryo and at birth there is a splitting off and shedding of the uterine lining or decidua. During pregnancy, the decidua basalis, the endometrium lying between the chorionic vesicle and myometrium, develops into the maternal portion of the placenta, q.v.

The endometrial lining is shed if the ovum is not fertilized or if the fertilized ovum does not implant. When this is completed, the cycle begins again. SEE: *ovary* for illus.

endometry (ĕn-dŏm'ĕ-trē) [Gr. *endon,* within, + *metron,* measure]. Measurement of the interior of a cavity or organ.

endomorph (ĕn"dō-morf') [" + *morphe,* form]. Body build characterized by predominance of tissues derived from the endoderm. SEE: *ectomorph; mesomorph; somatotype.*

endomyocarditis (ĕn"dō-mī-ō-kăr-dī'tĭs) [" + *mys,* muscle, + *kardia,* heart, + *itis,* inflammation]. Inflammation of the endocardium and myocardium.

endomysium (ĕn"dō-mĭs'ē-ŭm) [" + *mys,* muscle]. A thin sheath of connective tissue consisting principally of reticular fibers that invests each striated muscle fiber and binds the fibers together within a fasciculus.

endoneuritis [" + *neuron,* nerve, + *itis,* inflammation]. Inflammation of the endoneurium.

endoneurium (ĕn"dō-nū'rē-ŭm). A delicate connective tissue sheath that surrounds nerve fibers within a fasciculus. SYN: *Henle's sheath.*

endonuclease (ĕn"dō-nū'klē-ās). Enzyme that cleaves the ends of polynucleotides.

endoparasite (ĕn"dō-păr'ă-sīt) [" + *parasitos,* parasite]. Any parasite living within its host.

endopathy (ĕn"dŏp'ă-thē) [" + *pathos,* disease]. Any endogenous disease.

endopelvic (ĕn"dō-pĕl'vĭk) [" + L. *pelvis,* basin]. Within the pelvis.

endopelvic fasciae. The downward continuation of the parietal peritoneum of the abdomen to form the pelvic fasciae, which are very important to the support of the pelvic viscera.

endopeptidase (ĕn"dō-pĕp'tĭ-dās). A proteolytic enzyme that cleaves peptides in their centers more than from their ends.

endopericarditis (ĕn"dō-pĕr"ĭ-kăr-dī'tĭs) [" + *peri,* around, + *kardia,* heart, + *itis,* inflammation]. Endocarditis complicated by pericarditis.

endoperimyocarditis (ĕn"dō-pĕr"ĭ-mī"ō-kăr-dī'tĭs) [" + " + *mys,* muscle, + *kardia,* heart, + *itis,* inflammation]. Inflammation of the pericardium, myocardium, and endocardium.

endoperitonitis (ĕn"dō-pĕr"ĭ-tō-nī'tĭs) [" + *peritonaion,* peritoneum, + *itis,* inflammation]. Inflammation of the peritoneum.

endophasia (ĕn'dō-fā'zē-ă) [" + *phasis,* utterance]. Formation of words by the lips without producing sound.

endophlebitis (ĕn"dō-flē-bī'tĭs) [" + *phleps,* vein, + *itis,* inflammation]. Inflammation of the inner coat or membrane of a vein.

e. obliterans. Endophlebitis causing obliteration of a vein.

e. portalis. Inflammation of the portal vein.

endophthalmitis (ĕn"dŏf-thăl-mī'tĭs) [" + *ophthalmos,* eye, + *itis,* inflammation]. Inflammation of the inside of the eye that may or may not be limited to a particular chamber, i.e., anterior or posterior.

endoplasm [" + *plasma,* matter formed]. The central, more fluid portion of the cytoplasm of a cell. Opposed to ectoplasm.

endoplasmic reticulum. A connecting network of microcanals or tubules that course through the nucleus of the cell and cytoplasm, and sometimes to the cell exterior. They have been visualized by the use of the electron microscope. One form with ribosome particles attached is called granular or rough-surfaced endoplasmic reticulum; another form that is free of ribosomes is called agranular or smooth-surfaced endoplasmic reticulum. These structures are essential to the metabolic functions of cells. SEE: *cell* for illus.; *ribosome*.

end-organ. The expanded end of a nerve fiber in a peripheral structure.

e., neuromuscular. Spindle-shaped bundle of specialized muscle fibers in which sensory nerve fibers terminate in muscles.

e., neurotendinous. Specialized tendon fasciculi in which sensory nerve fibers terminate in tendons. SYN: *tendon spindle*.

e., sensory. An encapsulated termination of a nerve fiber that serves as a receptor. SEE: *receptor, sensory*.

endorhinitis (ĕn″dō-rī-nī′tĭs) [Gr. *endon,* within, + *rhis,* nose, + *itis,* inflammation]. Inflammation of the mucous membranes of the nose. SYN: *coryza*.

endorphins (ĕn-dor′fĭns, ĕn′dor-fĭns). Chemical substances, polypeptides, produced in the brain. They act as opiates and produce analgesia by binding to opiate receptor sites involved in pain perception. The threshold for pain is therefore increased by this action. The most active of these compounds is β-endorphin. SYN: *endogenous opiate-like substance*. SEE: *enkephalins; opiate receptor*.

endorrhachis (ĕn″dō-rā′kĭs) [″ + *rhachis,* spine]. Membrane lining of the spinal canal.

endosalpingitis (ĕn″dō-săl″pĭn-jī′tĭs) [″ + *salpinx,* trumpet, + *itis,* inflammation]. Inflammation of lining of fallopian tubes.

endosalpingoma (ĕn″dō-săl″pĭn-gō′mă). Adenomyoma of the uterine tube.

endosalpinx (ĕn″dō-săl′pĭnks) [″ + *salpinx,* tube]. The mucous membrane lining the uterine tube.

endoscope (ĕn′dō-skōp) [″ + *skopein,* to examine]. A device consisting of a tube and optical system for observing the inside of a hollow organ or cavity. This may be done through a natural body opening or through a small incision.

endoscopy (ĕn-dŏs′kō-pē). Inspection of body organs or cavities by use of the endoscope.

endosepsis (ĕn″dō-sĕp′sĭs) [″ + *sepsis,* decay]. Septicemia having its origin within the body.

endoskeleton [″ + *skeleton,* skeleton]. Internal bony framework of the body. Opposite of exoskeleton.

endosmometer (ĕn″dŏs-mŏm′ĕ-tĕr) [″ + *osmos,* a thrusting, + *metron,* measure]. Device for estimating passage by osmosis of a substance through a membrane or tissue.

endosmosis (ĕn″dŏs-mō′sĭs) [″ + ″ + *osis,* condition]. Osmosis in which flow of water is from the outside liquid to the solution within a membranous cell.

endospore [″ + *sporos,* a seed]. A thick-walled spore within a bacterium.

endosteitis (ĕn″dŏs-tē-ī′tĭs) [″ + *osteon,* bone, + *itis,* inflammation]. Inflammation of the endosteum or of medullary cavity of a bone. SYN: *endostitis*.

endosteoma (ĕn-dŏs″tē-ō′mă) [″ + ″ + *oma,* tumor]. A tumor in the medullary cavity of a bone.

endosteum (ĕn-dŏs′tē-ŭm) [″ + *osteon,* bone]. Membrane lining the medullary cavity of a bone.

endostitis (ĕn″dŏs-tī′tĭs) [″ + ″ + *itis,* inflammation]. Inflammation of the endosteum or the medullary cavity of a bone. SYN: *endosteitis*.

endostoma (ĕn-dŏs-tō′mă) [″ + ″ + *oma,* tumor]. Osseous tumor within a bone.

endostosis (ĕn″dŏs-tō′sĭs) [″ + ″ + *osis,* condition]. The development of an endostoma.

endotendineum (ĕn″dō-tĕn-dĭn′ē-ŭm) [″ + L. *tendo,* tendon]. The connective tissue in tendons between the bundles of fibers.

endothelial (ĕn″dŏ-thē′lē-ăl) [Gr. *endon,* within, + *thele,* nipple]. Pert. to or consisting of endothelium.

endotheliocyte (ĕn″dŏ-thē′lē-ō-sīt″) [″ + ″ + *kytos,* cell]. A large phagocytic wandering cell of circulating blood and tissue.

endotheliocytosis (ĕn″dŏ-thē″lē-ō-sī-tō′sĭs) [″ + ″ + ″ + *osis,* condition]. Abnormal increase in endothelial cells.

endotheliolysin (ĕn″dŏ-thē-lē-ŏl′ĭ-sĭn) [″ + *thele,* nipple, + *lysis,* dissolution]. An antibody found in snake venom that dissolves endothelial cells.

endotheliolytic (ĕn″dŏ-thē-lē-ō-lĭt′ĭk). Capable of destroying endothelial tissue.

endothelioma (ĕn″dŏ-thē-lē-ō′mă) [″ + *thele,* nipple, + *oma,* tumor]. Malignant growth of lining cells of the blood vessels.

endotheliomyoma (ĕn″dŏ-thē″lē-ō-mī-ō′mă) [″ + ″ + *mys,* muscle, + *oma,* tumor]. Muscular tumor with elements of endothelium.

endotheliomyxoma (ĕn″dŏ-thē″lē-ō-mĭks-ō′mă) [″ + ″ + *myxa,* mucus, + *oma,* tumor]. Myxoma with element from endothelium.

endotheliosis (ĕn″dō-thē″lē-ō′sĭs). Increased growth of endothelium.

endotheliotoxin (ĕn″dō-thē-lē-ō-tŏks′ĭn) [″ + ″ + *toxikon,* poison]. A specific toxin that acts on endothelial capillary cells and causes hemorrhages.

endothelium (ĕn″dŏ-thē′lē-ŭm) [″ + *thele,* nipple]. [NA] A form of squamous epithelium consisting of flat cells that line the blood and lymphatic vessels, the heart, and various other body cavities. It is derived from mesoderm.

endothermal, endothermic [Gr. *endon,* within, + *therme,* heat]. 1. Storing up potential energy or heat. 2. Absorbing heat. 3. Absorption of heat during chemical reactions.

endothermy (ĕn′dō-thĕr″mē). Elevation of temperature of deep body tissue in response to high-frequency current.

endothrix (ĕn′dō-thrĭks) [″ + *thrix,* hair]. Any fungus growing inside the hair shaft.

endothyropexy (ĕn″dō-thī′rō-pĕks″ē) [″ + *thyreos,* shield, + *pexis,* fixation]. Surgery involving displacement of the thyroid gland and fixing it to the side of the neck.

endotoscope (ĕn-dō′tō-skōp) [″ + *ous,* ear, + *skopein,* to examine]. An ear speculum. SYN: *otoscope.*

endotoxemia (ĕn″dō-tōks-ē′mē-ă). Toxemia due to the presence of endotoxins in the blood.

endotoxicosis (ĕn″dō-tŏk″sĭ-kō′sĭs) [Gr. *endon,* within, + *toxikon,* poison, + *osis,* condition]. Poisoning due to an endotoxin.

endotoxin. Bacterial toxin confined within the body of a bacterium, freed only when the bacterium is broken down. SEE: *cytotoxin; enterotoxin; erythrotoxin; exotoxin; neurotoxin.*

endotoxin shock. Shock due to release of endotoxins from bacteria.

endotracheal tube, cuffed. Tube used to provide an airway through the trachea and at the same time prevent aspiration of foreign material into the bronchus. This is accomplished by an inflatable cuff that surrounds the tube. It is inflated after the tube is placed in the trachea.

endotracheitis (ĕn″dō-trā-kē-ī′tĭs) [″ + *tracheia,* trachea, + *itis,* inflammation]. Inflammation of the tracheal mucosa.

endotrachelitis (ĕn″dō-trā-kĕl-ī′tĭs) [″ + *trachelos,* neck, + *itis,* inflammation]. Inflammation of the endocervical tissues of the uterine cervix. SYN: *endocervicitis.*

endovasculitis (ĕn″dō-văs″kū-lī′tĭs) [″ + L. *vasculum,* vessel, + Gr. *itis,* inflammation]. Inflammation of the endangium or inner coat of a blood vessel. SYN: *endangeitis.*

endovenous (ĕn″dō-vē′nŭs) [″ + L. *vena,* vein]. Within a vein. SYN: *intravenous.*

endplate. The terminal mass of a nerve fiber ending on a muscle cell.

e., motor. An ending in a striated muscle fiber. SYN: *myoneural junction.*

end product. The final material or substance left at the completion of a series of reactions, either chemical or physical.

end result. The ultimate or final result.

Enduron. Trade name for methyclothiazide.

endyma (ĕn′dĭm-ă) [Gr., a garment]. Membranous lining of cerebral ventricles and central canal of spinal cord. SYN: *ependyma.*

enema (ĕn′ĕ-mă) [Gr.]. 1. Introduction of solutions into the rectum and colon. This is done to stimulate bowel activity and to cause emptying of the lower intestine; to introduce food or medicine for therapeutic purposes; to give anesthesia; or to aid in roentgenography. 2. Solution introduced into the rectum.

e., antispasmodic. Enema used to counteract spasms.

e., barium. Administration of barium sulfate in solution as a diagnostic aid in x-ray examination of colon.

e., carminative. Enema given to relieve distention caused by flatus and to stimulate peristalsis.

e., cleansing. Enema to empty the lower intestine or the colon. Use 15 to 60 ml. for an infant, 240 to 360 ml. for a child, and 960 to 1930 ml. (approx. 1 to 2 L.) for an adult.

NURSING IMPLICATIONS: Explain procedure to the patient and ensure privacy. Assemble all needed equipment, position the patient properly, and drape to ensure privacy. Follow hospital procedure for administration of enema. Be sure that during enema, the container is no more than 18 inches above the rectum, and that the solution is at the correct temperature. Clear tubing of air. Lubricate tip of rectal tube and insert into rectum. Fluid should flow into the rectum slowly. Coach the patient to breathe slowly and deeply during the procedure to help relax abdominal muscles. When the procedure is completed, position patient on a bed pan or assist to the bathroom. Chart the amount, type and consistency of return from enema.

e., double-contrast. An enema of barium or other radiopaque material that is injected and evacuated. This is followed by injection of air. Roentgenograms of the lower intestinal tract are then taken.

e., emollient. Enema given to soothe and protect the intestinal mucosa by making a coating over membranes, to allay local pain and irritation, and to act as a vehicle for the rectal administration of drugs. It should be given at a temperature of about 105° F. (40.6° C.). The record must show if the patient felt relieved and to what extent and if the solution was retained.

e., high. Enema designed to reach most of the colon. Rubber tube is inserted into rectum to carry water as far as possible.

e., lubricating. An enema administered after an operation for hemorrhoids in order to soften the feces and lubricate the anal canal. When there is an impaction of feces, a lubricating enema may be given, followed in two hours by a cleansing enema. Either olive oil, 4 to 6 oz. (120 to 180 ml.), warmed, may be given, or warmed cottonseed oil in the same quantities. The patient should remain in a prone position with hips elevated for half an hour following the enema in order to help retain the oil, thus aiding it in passing higher into the colon.

e., medicinal. An enema to which some

drug or medication has been added on order of the attending physician. It may be given to medicate diseased conditions of the rectum, sigmoid, or colon; or for absorption of a medicine for its systemic effects. It is necessary that this enema be retained and absorbed.

e., nutrient. Enema containing predigested foods for the purpose of giving sustenance to a patient unable to be fed otherwise. SYN: *nutritive enema*.

e., one-two-three. Mixture of 1 oz. (30 ml.) magnesium sulfate, 2 oz. (60 ml.) glycerine, and 3 oz. (90 ml.) hot water. This mixture must be given with a small tube because of the small quantity and the action desired. The results following the injection are more satisfactory if given very carefully with assistance to help the patient retain it.

e., physiological salt solution. A normal salt solution is five grams or one teaspoon of salt to a pint (473 ml.) of water. The distention made by this enema excites peristalsis and evacuation. There is no harm in retaining this enema. Often ordered to be retained in treating dehydration.

e., retention. An enema that may be used to provide nourishment or medication. This enema must be formulated from constituents that will not stimulate the nerve endings and reflexly promote peristalsis. It necessarily must consist of a small amt. of solution, usually 100 to 240 ml.

NURSING IMPLICATIONS: Inform the patient of the purpose of this procedure so that full cooperation can be attained. The rectum and lower bowel must first be cleansed well and all irritation from evacuation should subside before you administer the enema, or the purpose will not be accomplished. Place patient on left side with knees flexed. Insert the rectal tube high (6 inches or 15 cm. or more). Expel air from the tubing before it is inserted. Unless absolutely necessary, once inserted, the tube should not be moved until the procedure is completed. The fluid should run in slowly, stopping at intervals, to aid retention. If the patient experiences the least desire to expel the solution, fluid should be stopped until the desire to evacuate is passed. Withdraw the tube quickly, and place pressure on the buttocks (compressing them together) for a minute or two to prevent evacuation.

e., saline. Enema consisting of normal saline solution or magnesium sulfate in warm water.

e., soapsuds. Use prepared soapsuds or if liquid soap is used, 30 ml. to 1000 ml. of water is the right proportion. Strong soapsuds should not be used because of the danger of injuring intestinal mucosa. Mild white soaps, such as castile, are best.

enema, words pert. to: clysis; coloclyster; colonic irrigation; enteroclysis; medication routes, rectal; rectal feeding; rectum.

energetics (ĕn″ĕr-jĕt′ĭks). Science of study of energy esp. in relation to human use of energy in the form of food and the expenditure of energy in doing work or athletic exercise.

energy (ĕn′ĕr-jē) [Gr. *energeia*]. The capacity of a system for doing work or its equivalent in the strict physical sense. Energy is manifested in various forms: motion (kinetic energy), position (potential energy), light, heat, ionizing radiation, or sound. SEE: *calorie*.

Changes in energy may be physical or chemical or both. Movement of a part of the body shortens and thickens the muscles involved and changes the position and size of cells temporarily, but the intake of oxygen in the blood combined with sugar and fat creates a chemical change and produces heat (energy) and waste products within the cells, which in turn produce fatigue. SEE: *calorie*.

e., conservation of. The theory that energy cannot be created or destroyed, but is transformed into other forms.

e., latent. Energy that exists but is not being used.

e., radiant. That form of energy that is transmitted through space without the support of a sensible medium. Radio waves, infrared waves, visible rays, ultraviolet waves, x-rays, gamma rays and cosmic rays are energy in this form. SEE: *electromagnetic spectrum* for table.

energy, words pert. to: kinetic; metabolism; radiant; unit.

enervation [L. *enervatio*]. 1. Deficient in nervous strength; weakness. 2. Resection or removal of a nerve.

enflagellation (ĕn″flăj-ĕl-lā′shŭn). Production and development of flagella.

enflurane (ĕn′floo-rān). USP. An anesthetic agent. Trade name is Ethrane.

ENG. *electronystagmography.*

engagement. In obstetrics, the entrance of the fetal head or the part being presented into the superior pelvic strait. SYN: *lightening*. SEE: *labor*.

Engelmann's disk. [Theodor W. Engelmann, Ger. physiologist, 1843–1909] A narrow zone of transparent material lying on each side of the intermediate disk in the isotropic or I disk of a striated muscle fiber.

englobe [Gr. *en*, in, + L. *globus*, a ball]. To absorb within a spherical body, as the ingestion of bacteria by the phagocytes.

engorged (ĕn-gorjd′) [O. Fr. *engorgier*, to obstruct, to devour]. Distended, as with blood or fluids.

engorgement. Vascular congestion; disten-

tion.

engram (ĕn'grăm) [Gr. *engramm*]. A durable mark or trace. The protoplasmic change left by a stimulus in neural tissue.

enhancement (ĕn-hăns'mĕnt). Increasing the effect of ionizing radiation on tissues by use of oxygen or other chemicals.

enissophobia (ĕn-ĭs"ō-fō'bē-ă) [Gr. *enissein,* to reproach, + *phobos,* fear]. Fear of criticism, esp. for having committed a sin.

enkatarrhaphy (ĕn"kă-tăr'ăf-ē) [Gr. *enkatarrhaptein,* to sew in]. Burying of structure by suturing adjacent tissue over it.

enkephalins (ĕn-kĕf'ă-lĭns). Chemical substances, polypeptides, produced in the brain. They act as opiates and produce analgesia by binding to opiate receptor sites involved in pain perception. The threshold for pain is therefore increased by this action. It is possible that enkephalins have a role in explaining the withdrawal signs of narcotic addiction. SYN: *endogenous opiate-like substance.* SEE: *endorphins; opiate receptor.*

enlargement (ĕn-lărj'mĕnt). An increase in size of anything, esp. of an organ or tissue.

enol (ē'nŏl). A form that a ketone may take by a method known as tautomerism. A substance changes from the enol form to the ketone form by the oscillation of a hydrogen atom from the enol form to the ketone form.

enolase (ē'nō-lās). An enzyme present in muscle tissue that converts phosphoglyceric acid to phosphopyruvic acid.

enology (ē-nŏl'ō-jē) [Gr. *oinos,* wine, + *logos,* study]. The science of production and evaluation of wine. Also spelled oenology.

enomania (ē"nō-mā'nē-ă) [" + *mania,* madness]. Craving for alcoholic beverages.

enophthalmos (ĕn"ŏf-thăl'mŭs) [Gr. *en,* in, + *ophthalmos,* eye]. Recession of eyeball into orbit. Opposite of exophthalmos.

enosimania (ĕn"ŏs-ĭ-mā'nē-ă) [Gr. *enosis,* a quaking, + *mania,* madness]. A mental state characterized by excessive and irrational terror.

enostosis (ĕn"ŏs-tō'sĭs) [Gr. *en,* in, + *osteon,* bone, + *osis,* condition]. An osseous tumor within the cavity of a bone.

Enovid, Enovid-E. Trade names for estrogen with progestogen.

enriched. The addition of something extra. For example, the addition of vitamins or minerals to a food in order to *enrich* it.

ensiform (ĕn'sĭ-form) [L. *ensis,* sword, + *forma,* form]. Swordlike structure.

ensisternum (ĕn"sĭs-tĕr'nŭm) [" + Gr. *sternon,* sternum]. The lowest portion of the sternum. SYN: *xiphoid process.*

enstrophe (ĕn'strō-fē) [Gr. *en,* in, + *strephein,* to turn]. Inversion; a turning inward, esp. of eyelids.

E.N.T. *ear, nose, and throat.*

entad (ĕn'tăd) [" + L. *ad,* toward]. Toward the inside; inwardly.

ental (ĕn'tăl) [Gr. *entos,* within]. Pert. to the interior; inside, central.

entamebiasis (ĕn"tă-mē-bī'ă-sĭs) [" + *amoibe,* change]. Infestation with Entamoeba.

Entamoeba (ĕn"tă-mē'bă). A genus of parasitic ameba, several of which are found in the human digestive tract.

E. buccalis. E. gingivalis.

E. coli. Species normally found in the human intestinal tract. Nonpathogenic to man.

E. gingivalis. Nonpathogenic species that inhabits the mouth.

E. histolytica. A pathogenic species of ameba, the cause of amebic dysentery and tropical liver abscess. SEE: *amebiasis.*

E. kartulisi. Species found in the pus of necrotic bone abscesses.

E. tetragena. Species now considered identical with E. histolytica.

E. undulans. A species found in the intestine.

enteradenitis (ĕn"tĕr-ăd"ĕ-nī'tĭs) [Gr. *enteron,* intestine, + *aden,* gland, + *itis,* inflammation]. Inflammation of intestinal glands.

enteral (ĕn'tĕr-ăl) [Gr. *enteron,* intestine]. Within or by way of the intestine.

enteralgia (ĕn"tĕr-ăl'jē-ă) [" + *algos,* pain]. Neuralgia or pain in the intestines. Intestinal cramps or colic.

enterectasia (ĕn"tĕr-ĕk-tā'sē-ă) [" + *ektasis,* dilatation]. Dilatation of the small intestines.

enterectomy (ĕn"tĕr-ĕk'tō-mē) [" + *ektome,* excision]. Excision of a portion of the intestines.

enterelcosis (ĕn"tĕr-ĕl-kō'sĭs) [" + *helkosis,* ulceration]. Intestinal ulceration.

enteric (ĕn-tĕr'ĭk) [Gr. *enteron,* intestine]. Pert. to the small intestine.

enteric-coated. A type of drug formulation where tablets or capsules are coated with a special compound that will not dissolve until the pill or tablet is exposed to the fluids in the small intestine.

enteric fever. Typhoid fever, q.v.

enteritis (ĕn"tĕr-ī'tĭs) [" + *itis,* inflammation]. Inflammation of the intestines, more particularly of the mucous and submucous tissues of the small intestines.

entero-, enter- [Gr. *enteron,* intestine]. Prefix denoting some relationship to the intestines.

enteroanastomosis (ĕn"tĕr-ō-ăn-ăs"tō-mō'sĭs) [" + *anastomosis,* opening]. Intestinal anastomosis.

enteroantigen (ĕn"tĕr-ō-ăn'tĭ-jĕn) [" + *anti,* against, + *gennan,* to form]. An antigen derived from the intestines.

enteroapokleisis (ĕn"tĕr-ō-ăp"ō-klī'sĭs) [" +

apokleisis, a shutting out]. Operation for exclusion of a part of the intestine.

Enterobacter. A group of enteric bacilli of the family Enterobacteriaceae that occur in soil, dairy products, water, sewage, and the intestinal tracts of man and animals. They are often secondary pathogens, or opportunistic infections.

E. aerogenes. A species of Enterobacter. It occurs normally in the intestine of man and other animals and is found in decayed matter, on grains and plants. The organism is important in causing urinary tract infections and intestinal disease when antibiotic therapy causes elimination of other organisms. Formerly called Aerobacter aerogenes.

Enterobacteriaceae (ĕn″tĕr-ō-băk-tē″rē-ā′sē-ē). A family of gram-negative, non-spore-forming rods. Some of the genera are intestinal pathogens. Included in the family are Shigella, Salmonella, Escherichia, Klebsiella, Proteus, and Yersinia.

enterobacteriotherapy (ĕn″tĕr-ō-băk-tē″rē-ō-thĕr′ă-pē) [″ + *bakterion,* little rod, + *therapeia,* treatment]. Use of vaccines containing intestinal bacteria.

enterobiasis (ĕn″tĕr-ō-bī′ă-sĭs) [Gr. *enteron,* intestine, + *bios,* life]. Infestation with pinworms (Enterobius vermicularis). SYN: *oxyuriasis.*

enterobiliary (ĕn″tĕr-ō-bĭl′ē-ār-ē) [″ + L. *bilis,* bile]. Pert. to the intestines and the bile passages.

Enterobius (ĕn″tĕr-ō′bē-ŭs) [″ + *bios,* life]. A genus of parasitic nematode worms, formerly Oxyuris vermicularis.

E. vermicularis. A species of nematode worms, the adult form of which inhabits the large intestine in humans. The genital organs and bladder may become infected in females, causing cystitis due to the bacteria that the female worm carries. Infestations are characterized by irritation of the anal region and allergic reaction of the neighboring skin accompanied by intense itching, which may result in loss of sleep, excessive irritability, and a secondary infection of the area around the anus as a result of the scratching. Distribution is worldwide. Female worms average 8 to 13 mm. in length and males 2 to 5 mm. SYN: *pinworm.*

DIAG: Finding adult worms in feces or on the anus; or by applying transparent, pressure-sensitive tape to the perianal area and then examining the tape microscopically for eggs. This latter test is more likely to be positive in the morning prior to bathing.

TREATMENT: Pyrantel pamoate, mebendazole, and pyrivinium pamoate are effective.

enterocele (ĕn′tĕr-ō-sēl) [″ + *kele,* hernia]. 1. A hernia of the intestine through the vagina. 2. Posterior vaginal hernia.

enterocentesis (ĕn″tĕr-ō-sĕn-tē′sĭs) [″ + *kentesis,* puncture]. Puncture of intestine to withdraw gas or fluids.

enterocholecystostomy (ĕn″tĕr-ō-kō″lē-sĭs-tŏs′tō-mē) [″ + *chole,* bile, + *kystis,* a bladder, + *stoma,* opening]. Making an opening between the gallbladder and small intestine. SYN: *cholecystenterostomy.*

enterocholecystotomy (ĕn″tĕr-ō-kō″lē-sĭs-tŏt′ō-mē) [″ + ″ + ″ + *tome,* incision]. Incision of both gallbladder and intestine.

enterocinesia (ĕn″tĕr-ō-sĭn-ē′sē-ă) [″ + *kinesis,* movement]. Intestinal movement. SYN: *peristalsis.*

enterocinetic (ĕn″tĕr-ō-sĭn-ĕt′ĭk). Pert. to or promoting peristalsis.

enteroclysis (ĕn″tĕr-ŏk′lĭ-sĭs) [″ + *klysis,* a washing out]. 1. Injection of a nutrient or medicinal liquid into bowel. 2. Irrigation of colon with large amt. of fluid intended to fill the colon completely and flush it. SEE: *enema.*

enterococcus (ĕn″tĕr-ō-kŏk′ŭs). Any species of streptococcus inhabiting the human intestine.

enterocoele (ĕn′tĕr-ō-sēl) [″ + *koilia,* hollow]. The abdominal cavity.

enterocolectomy (ĕn″tĕr-ō-kō-lĕk′tō-mē) [″ + *kolon,* colon, + *ektome,* excision]. Surgical removal of the terminal ileum, cecum, and ascending colon.

enterocolitis (ĕn″tĕr-ō-kō-lī′tĭs) [″ + ″ + *itis,* inflammation]. Inflammation of intestines and colon. This serious condition may be so acute as to require immediate treatment of shock, regulation of electrolyte balance, and antibiotics if ordered by physician.

enterocolostomy (ĕn″tĕr-ō-kō-lŏs′tō-mē) [″ + ″ + *stoma,* mouth]. Surgical joining of the small intestine to the colon.

enterocrinin (ĕn″tĕr-ŏk′rĭ-nĭn) [″ + *krinein,* to separate]. Hormone from animal intestines that aids digestion by stimulating the secretion of intestinal juice by the intestinal glands.

enterocutaneous (ĕn″tĕr-ō-kū-tā′nē-ŭs). Communication between the skin and the intestine.

enterocyst (ĕn′tĕr-ō-sĭst) [Gr. *enteron,* intestine, + *kystis,* bladder]. A benign cyst of the intestinal wall.

enterocystocele (ĕn″tĕr-ō-sĭs′tō-sēl) [″ + *kele,* hernia]. Hernia of the bladder wall and intestine.

enterocystoma (ĕn″tĕr-ō-sĭs-tō′mă) [″ + ″ + *oma,* tumor]. Cystic tumor of the intestinal wall.

enterocystoplasty (ĕn″tĕr-ō-sĭs″tō-plăs′tē) [″ + ″ + *plastos,* formed]. A plastic surgical procedure involving the use of a portion of intestine to enlarge the bladder.

enterodynia (ĕn″tĕr-ō-dĭn′ē-ă) [″ + *odyne,* pain]. Pain in the intestine. SYN: *enteralgia.*
enteroenterostomy (ĕn″tĕr-ō-ĕn″tĕr-ŏs′tō-mē) [″ + *enteron,* intestine, + *stoma,* opening]. Formation of a communication between two intestinal segments that are not continuous.
enteroepiplocele (ĕn″tĕr-ō-ē-pĭp′lō-sēl) [″ + *epiploon,* omentum, + *kele,* hernia]. Hernia of small intestine and omentum.
enterogastritis (ĕn″tĕr-ō-găs-trī′tĭs) [″ + *gaster,* belly, + *itis,* inflammation]. Inflammation of stomach (gastritis) and intestines (enteritis).
enterogastrone (ĕn″tĕr-ō-găs′trōn). A hormone secreted by the intestinal mucosa that, by depressing gastric motility and secretion, controls the release of food from the stomach into the duodenum. A meal high in fat content will cause greater secretion of this hormone than will a normal feeding.
enterogenous (ĕn″tĕr-ŏj′ĕ-nŭs) [″ + *gennan,* to produce]. Originating in the small intestines.
enterogram [″ + *gramma,* mark]. Tracing or graph of intestinal movements.
enterography [″ + *graphein,* to write]. 1. A description of the intestines. 2. Making of an enterogram.
enterohepatic (ĕn″tĕr-ō-hĕ-păt′ĭk) [″ + *hepar,* liver]. Pert. to intestines and the liver.
enterohepatitis (ĕn″tĕr-ō-hĕp-ă-tī′tĭs) [″ + ″ + *itis,* inflammation]. Inflamed condition of intestine and liver.
enterohydrocele (ĕn″tĕr-ō-hī′drō-sēl) [″ + *hydor,* water, + *kele,* hernia]. Hydrocele with loop of intestine in the sac.
enteroidea (ĕn″tĕr-oy′dē-ă) [″ + *eidos,* form]. The intestinal fevers; those caused by intestinal bacilli including typhoid fever.
enterokinase (ĕn″tĕr-ō-kī′nās) [″ + *kinesis,* movement]. A substance or hormone occurring in the mucosa of the duodenum, necessary for the activation of the trypsinogen of the pancreatic juice that is converted into trypsin. One of the enzymes of the succus entericus, it has no fat-splitting properties.

RS: enzyme; trypsin; trypsinogen.

enterokinesia. Peristalsis, q.v.
enterolith (ĕn′tĕr-ō-lĭth) [″ + *lithos,* stone]. An intestinal concretion.
enterolithiasis (ĕn″tĕr-ō-lĭ-thī′ă-sĭs). The formation or existence of intestinal calculi.
enterology [″ + *logos,* study]. The study of the intestinal tract.
enterolysis (ĕn″tĕr-ŏl′ĭ-sĭs) [″ + *lysis,* dissolution]. Surgical therapy of intestinal adhesions.
enteromegalia, enteromegaly (ĕn″tĕr-ō-mĕ-gā′lē-ă, ĕn″tĕr-ō-mĕg′ă-lē) [″ + *megas,* large]. Abnormal enlargement of the intestines. SYN: *megacolon.*
Enteromonas hominis (ĕn″tĕr-ŏm′ō-năs hŏm′ĭn-ĭs). A minute flagellated, protozoan parasite that lives in the intestine of man. It is rare and considered nonpathogenic.
enteromycosis (ĕn″tĕr-ō-mī-kō′sĭs) [″ + *mykes,* fungus, + *osis,* diseased condition]. Disease of intestine resulting from bacteria or fungi.
enteromyiasis (ĕn″tĕr-ō-mī-ī′ă-sĭs) [″ + *myia,* fly]. Disease caused by the presence of maggots (the larvae of flies) in the intestines.
enteron (ĕn′tĕr-ŏn) [Gr.]. The alimentary canal.
enteroneuritis (ĕn″tĕr-ō-nū-rī′tĭs) [″ + *neuron,* nerve, + *itis,* inflammation]. Inflammation of nerves of the intestines.
enteroparesis (ĕn″tĕr-ō-păr′ē-sĭs) [″ + *paresis,* relaxation]. Reduced peristalsis of the intestines followed by dilation of the walls.
enteropathogen (ĕn″tĕr-ō-păth′ō-jĕn) [″ + *pathos,* disease, + *gennan,* to produce]. Any microorganism that causes intestinal disease.
enteropathy (ĕn″tĕr-ŏp′ă-thē) [″ + *pathos,* disease]. Any intestinal disease.
enteropeptidase (ĕn″tĕr-ō-pĕp′tĭ-dās). Enterokinase, q.v.
enteropexy (ĕn′tĕr-ō-pĕks″ē) [″ + *pexis,* fixation]. Fixation of the intestine to the abdominal wall or to another portion of the intestine.
enteroplasty (ĕn′tĕr-ō-plăs″tē) [″ + *plassein,* to form]. Plastic operation on intestines. SEE: *laparotomy.*
enteroplegia (ĕn″tĕr-ō-plē′jē-ă) [″ + *plege,* stroke]. Paralysis of intestines. SEE: *paralytic ileus.*
enteroplex (ĕn′tĕr-ō-plĕks) [″ + *plexis,* a weaving]. Instrument for joining cut edges of intestines.
enteroplexy. Union of divided parts of the intestine.
enteroproctia (ĕn″tĕr-ō-prŏk′shē-ă) [″ + *proktos,* anus]. The condition of having an artificial anus.
enteroptosis (ĕn″tĕr-ŏp-tō′sĭs) [″ + *ptosis,* a dropping]. Prolapse of the intestine or abdominal organs.
enterorrhaphy (ĕn″tĕr-or′ă-fē) [″ + *rhaphe,* suture]. The stitching of an intestinal wound or of the intestines to some other structure.
enterorrhexis (ĕn″tĕr-ō-rĕks′ĭs) [″ + *rhexis,* rupture]. Rupture of the intestine.
enteroscope (ĕn′tĕr-ō-skōp″) [″ + *skopein,* to examine]. A device for visually examining the inside of the intestines.
enterosepsis (ĕn″tĕr-ō-sĕp′sĭs) [″ + *sepsis,* decay]. Intestinal toxemia; sepsis developed from the intestinal contents. SYN: *enterotoxism.*
enterospasm (ĕn′tĕr-ō-spăzm) [Gr. *enteron,* intestine, + *spasmos,* spasm]. Intermittent painful contractions of the intestines.
enterostasis (ĕn″tĕr-ō-stā′sĭs) [″ + *stasis,* a

standing]. Cessation of or delay in the passage of food through the intestine.

enterostenosis (ĕn″tĕr-ō-stĕ-nō′sĭs) [″ + *stenosis,* a narrowing]. Narrowing or stricture of the intestine.

enterostomal therapist. Individual trained to assist patients who have had an ostomy in learning the proper methods of caring for their ostomy sites.

enterostomy (ĕn″tĕr-ŏs′tō-mē) [″ + *stoma,* opening]. Surgical formation of a permanent opening into the intestine through the abdominal wall.

enterotome (ĕn′tĕr-ō-tōm) [″ + *tome,* incision]. Instrument for incision of intestines.

enterotomy (ĕn-tĕr-ŏt′ō-mē). Incision or dissection of the intestines.

enterotoxemia (ĕn″tĕr-ō-tŏk-sē′mē-ă). Condition in which toxins are absorbed from the intestine and are circulating in the blood.

enterotoxigenic (ĕn″tĕr-ō-tŏk″sĭ-jĕn′ĭk). Producing enterotoxins, as in enterotoxigenic strains of the bacillus E. coli. These bacilli are important in causing "travelers' diarrhea."

enterotoxin (ĕn″tĕr-ō-tŏk′sĭn) [″ + *toxikon,* poison]. 1. A toxin produced in or originating in the intestinal contents. 2. A toxin specific for the cells of the mucosa. 3. A toxin produced by certain species of bacteria that produces symptoms characteristic of food poisoning.

enterotoxism. Absorption of toxins from the intestinal contents.

enterotropic [″ + *trope,* a turning]. Affecting or attracted by the intestines.

enterovirus. A group of viruses that originally included the viruses polio, coxsackie, and ECHO, which infected the human gastrointestinal tract. Now enteroviruses are classed as a genus of picornaviruses.

enterozoic (ĕn″tĕr-ō-zō′ĭk) [″ + *zoon,* animal]. Pert. to parasites inhabiting the intestines.

enterozoon (ĕn″tĕr-ō-zō′ŏn). (pl. *enterozoa*) Any intestinal animal parasite.

entheomania (ĕn″thē-ō-mā′nē-ă) [Gr. *entheos,* inspired, + *mania,* madness]. Religious insanity.

enthesis (ĕn′thĕ-sĭs) [Gr., a putting in]. The use of metallic or other inert substances to substitute for or replace lost tissue.

enthetic (ĕn-thĕt′ĭk). 1. Pert. to enthesis, q.v. 2. Introduced from outside. SYN: *exogenous.*

enthlasis (ĕn′thlă-sĭs) [Gr., dent caused by pressure]. Depressed fracture of the skull containing bone fragments, i.e., comminuted.

entity (ĕn′tĭ-tē) [L. *ens,* being]. 1. A thing existing independently, containing in itself all the conditions necessary to individuality. 2. That which forms a complete whole, denoting a distinct condition or disease.

ento- [Gr. *entos,* within]. Prefix indicating within, inside.

entoblast (ĕn′tō-blăst) [″ + *blastos,* germ]. 1. The entoderm, q.v., or hypoblast. 2. The cell nucleolus.

entocele (ĕn′tō-sēl) [″ + *kele,* hernia]. 1. Internal hernia. 2. Displacement of a part inwardly.

entochondrostosis (ĕn″tō-kŏn″drŏs-tō′sĭs) [″ + *chondros,* cartilage, + *osis,* condition]. The development of bone within cartilage.

entochoroidea (ĕn″tō-kō-roy′dē-ă) [″ + *chorioeides,* choroid]. The inner layer of the choroid; coat of the eye.

entocineria (ĕn″tō-sĭn-ē′rē-ă) [″ + L. *cinereus,* ashen]. The internal gray matter of nerve centers, esp. of the brain.

entocone (ĕn′tō-kōn) [″ + *konos,* cone]. The inner posterior cusp of an upper molar tooth.

entocornea (ĕn″tō-kor′nē-ă) [″ + L. *corneus,* horny]. Posterior or inner lining membrane of cornea. SYN: *Descemet's membrane.*

entocyte (ĕn′tō-sīt) [″ + *kytos,* cell]. Interior part of a cell within the ectoplasm. SYN: *endoplasm.*

entoderm (ĕn′tō-dĕrm) [″ + *derma,* skin]. Inner layer of cells in the blastoderm, q.v. Innermost of the three primary germ layers of a developing embryo. It gives rise to the epithelium of the digestive tract and its associated glands, the respiratory organs, bladder, vagina, and urethra. SYN: *endoderm; hypoblast.*

entoectad (ĕn″tō-ĕk′tăd) [″ + *ektos,* without, + L. *ad,* toward]. Proceeding from within outward.

entome (ĕn′tōm) [Gr. *en,* in, + *tome,* incision]. Knife for division of urethral stricture.

entomion (ĕn-tō′mē-ŏn) [Gr. *entome,* notch]. The tip of mastoid angle of the parietal bone.

entomology (ĕn″tō-mŏl′ō-jē) [Gr. *entomon,* insect, + *logos,* science]. The study of insects.

e., medical. That branch of entomology that deals with insects and their relationship to disease, esp. to disease of humans.

entophyte (ĕn′tō-fīt) [Gr. *entos,* within, + *phyton,* plant]. Any vegetable parasite living within the body.

entopic [Gr. *en,* in, + *topos,* place]. Normally situated; in a normal place. Opposite of ectopic.

entoptic (ĕn-tŏp′tĭk) [Gr. *entos,* within, + *optikos,* seeing]. Pert. to the interior of the eye.

entoptic phenomena. Visual phenomena arising from within the eye, characterized by seeing floating bodies, circles of light, black spots, and transient flashes of light. May be due to individuals seeing their own blood cells move through the retinal vessels, or floaters, which are small specks of tissue floating in the vitreous fluid. SEE: *photopsia; muscae volitantes.*

entoretina (ĕn″tō-rĕt′ĭ-nă) [″ + L. *rete,* a net]. Internal layer of the retina.

entotic (ĕn-tō′tĭk, ĕn-tŏt′ĭk) [″ + *ous,* ear]. Pert. to interior of ear or to perception of sound as a result of condition of the auditory apparatus.

entozoon (ĕn″tō-zō′ŏn) [″ + *zoon,* animal]. (pl. *entozoa*) Any animal parasite living within the body of another animal.

entrain. To alter the biological rhythm of an organism so that it assumes a cycle different from a 24-hour one.

entropion (ĕn-trō′pē-ŏn) [Gr. *en,* in, + *trepein,* to turn]. Inversion or turning inward of an edge, esp. the margin of the lower eyelid.

e., cicatricial. An inversion resulting from scar tissue on the inner surface of the lid.

e., spastic. An inversion resulting from a spasm of the orbicularis oculi muscles.

entropionize (ĕn-trō′pē-ō-nīz). To invert or correct by turning in.

entropy (ĕn′trŏ-pē) [Ger. *Entropie*]. That portion of energy within a system that cannot be utilized for mechanical work but is available for internal use.

enucleate (ē-nū′klē-āt) [L. *enucleare,* to remove the kernel of]. 1. To remove a part or a mass in its entirety. 2. To destroy or take out the nucleus of a cell. 3. To remove the eyeball surgically. 4. To remove a cataract surgically.

enucleation (ē-nū″klē-ā′shŭn). Removal of an entire mass or part without rupture, esp. pert. to a tumor or the eyeball.

enucleator (ĕ-nū′klē-ā-tor). Instrument for separating a tumor mass, as a myoma.

enuresis (ĕn″ū-rē′sĭs) [Gr. *enourein,* to void urine]. Involuntary urination. May be complete or partial, diurnal or nocturnal, dependent upon pathological or functional causes, or it may be voluntary as representative of a behavior pattern. Children, for instance, may feel neglected or feel a desire for attention and attempt to center attention upon themselves by deliberately wetting the bed. Urinary control is usually established after the second year, although incontinence may be reestablished due to disease of the urinary tract or to neurological disease.

Children suffering from enuresis may be shy and sensitive or sometimes gloomy. These nervous manifestations may result from their reaction to the condition or they may be a part of the behavior pattern of which the enuresis is a symptom.

ETIOL: Enuresis may result from urethral irritation. Fecal incontinence is sometimes associated with it. Excessive water drinking may contribute to enuresis. There may be a neurological basis caused by injury to the spinal cord or it may be associated with various diseases such as either diabetes insipidus and mellitus, epilepsy, or mental deficiency. Cystitis may be present.

NURSING IMPLICATIONS: Assess patient for fever, flank pain, urinary frequency or urgency, dysuria, and pus or mucus in urine, because enuresis may be indicative of a urinary tract infection, esp. in children. Show empathic understanding, since enuresis is embarrassing and frustrating to the child and family. The child should have a decreased fluid intake in the evening and should void immediately before going to bed; the parents should waken the child and take him or her to the bathroom to void before they go to bed.

e., diurnal. Urinary incontinence during the day. Its etiology is usually of a pathological nature. It may be caused by muscular contractions brought about by laughing, coughing, or crying. Often persists for long periods of time, esp. after protracted illness. It occurs more commonly in females.

e., nocturnal. Urinary incontinence during the night. It is irregular and unaccompanied by urgency or frequency. Incontinence may cease for several weeks only to return. This type is more common in boys than in girls.

Fluid should be restricted late in day and diurnal voidings should be spaced at more than ordinary intervals. The child may be awakened once or twice in the night and, when fully awake, robed and walked to the bathroom. As improvement is noticed the number of awakenings may be lessened. The foot of the bed may also be elevated. Electronic devices that awaken the child the moment the bed is wet are available.

TREATMENT: When no organic disease is present the use of imipramine as a temporary adjunct may be helpful. This is usually given in a dose of 10 to 50 mg. orally at bedtime; but the effectiveness may decrease with continued administration. The bladder may be trained to hold larger amounts of urine. This procedure has decreased the rate of occurrence of enuresis.

CAUTION: Imipramine is not recommended for children under six years of age. Blood counts should be taken at least monthly during therapy to detect the possible side effect of agranulocytosis.

envelope (ĕn′vĕ-lōp). A covering, or container.

e., nuclear. A double membrane-layer of lipids and proteins surrounding the nucleus of a cell.

envenomation (ĕn-vĕn″ō-mā′shŭn). The introduction of poisonous venoms into the body by means of a bite or sting.

environment [O. Fr. *en-,* in, + *viron,* circle]. The surroundings, conditions, or influences that affect an organism or the cells within an organism.

envy. To be unhappy about or to wish to possess the qualities or physical belongings of someone else.

enzootic (ĕn″zō-ŏt′ĭk) [Gr. *en,* in, + *zoon,* animal]. An endemic disease limited to a small number of animals.

enzygotic (ĕn″zī-gŏt′ĭk) [Gr. *en,* in, + *zygon,* yoke]. Developed from the same ovum.

enzygotic twins. Twins developed from one ovum. SYN: *monozygotic twins.* SEE: *dizygotic twins.*

enzyme (ĕn′zīm) [″ + *zyme,* leaven]. An organic catalyst produced by living cells but capable of acting independently. Enzymes are complex proteins that are capable of inducing chemical changes in other substances without being changed themselves. Enzymes are present in digestive juices, where they act upon food substances, causing them to break down into simpler compounds. They are capable of accelerating the speed of chemical reactions. SEE: table.

ACTION: The reactions effected by the digestive enzymes are chiefly decompositions of a hydrolytic nature, but enzymes are equally important in the synthetic reactions of assimilation.

Each hydrolytic enzyme has been given a name indicating the substance upon which it acts with the addition of the suffix *-ase.* Lipases indicate fat-splitting enzymes; amylases, starch-splitting ones; and proteases, protein-splitting enzymes. Some of them take a qualifying adjective, as salivary or pancreatic enzymes. Some of the best-known enzymes such as rennin, pepsin, trypsin, and thrombin do not end in *-ase* because they were named before this method of nomenclature was instituted.

The substance acted upon by an enzyme is

Summary of the Main Enzymatic Processes in Digestion

Site	Secretion	Enzyme	Substrate	Degree of Digestion	Products of Digestion
Mouth	Saliva	Ptyalin	Raw starch	Slight	Dextrins, maltose
Stomach	Gastric juice	Pepsins	Protein	Incomplete	Proteoses, peptones
		Gelatinase	Gelatin	Complete	Liquefied gelatin
		Lipase	Triglycerides	Very slight	Fatty acids, glycerol
Intestine	Pancreatic juice	Trypsin Chymotrypsin Carboxypeptidase	Proteins Proteoses Peptones Peptides	Nearly complete	Amino acids
		Steapsin	Fats	Nearly complete	Insoluble fatty acids, glycerol
		Amylopsin	Raw and cooked starch	Nearly complete	Dextrins, maltose
Intestine	Intestinal juice and intestinal mucosa	Erepsin	Ordinary peptides	Nearly complete	Amino acids
		Amylase	Starch	Nearly complete	Dextrins, maltose
		Enterokinase	Trypsinogen		Trypsin
		Maltase	Maltose	Complete	Glucose
		Lactase	Lactose	Complete	Glucose, galactose
		Sucrase	Sucrose	Usually complete	Glucose, fructose
		Nucleosidases (in mucosa)	Nucleosides	Usually complete	Purine bases, carbohydrates

called the substrate. Proenzyme or zymogen is the name given to precursors of an enzyme. The more common groups of digestive tract enzymes are: hydrolytic; fat-, protein-, starch-, and sugar-splitting enzymes; coagulating enzymes or those that cause clotting, such as thrombin; oxidases or oxidizing enzymes; deamidizing enzymes, those that are important in removing amines or amino groups during oxidation; reductases or reducing enzymes; splitting enzymes; and joining enzymes.

Enzymes are specific in their action; they will act only upon a certain substance or a group of closely related chemical substances and no other. Each enzyme has an optimum temperature at which it acts with greatest efficiency; each is influenced by the reaction of the medium in which it acts, there being an optimum degree of acidity or alkalinity.

Enzyme activity can be retarded or inhibited by temperature extremes, presence of salts of heavy metals (copper, mercury), dehydration, and ultraviolet radiation.

Enzymes sometimes require the presence of additional substances to make them active. Nonspecific substances that activate enzymes are called activators (Ex.: HCl for pepsin). Specific substances that act selectively with certain enzymes only are called coenzymes (Ex.: enterokinase for trypsinogen). Several hundred enzymes have been identified but as many as a thousand are thought to be present in mammals.

e., activating. An enzyme that catalyzes the attaching of an amino acid to the appropriate transfer ribonucleic acid.

e.'s, allosteric. Enzymes that can have their activity modified by binding certain types of effectors, called allosteric effectors, to a non-active site on the enzyme.

e., amylolytic. Enzyme that catalyzes the conversion of starch to sugar.

e., autolytic. Enzyme that produces autolysis or cell digestion.

e., bacterial. Enzyme developed by bacteria.

e.'s, branching. Enzymes, glycosyltransferases, that transfer a carbohydrate unit from one molecule to another.

e., coagulating. Enzyme that catalyzes the conversion of soluble proteins into insoluble ones. SYN: *coagulase.*

e., deamidizing. Enzyme that divides amino acids into ammonia compounds.

e., debranching. An enzyme, dextrin-1-6-glucosidase, that removes a carbohydrate unit from molecules that contain short carbohydrate units attached as side chains.

e., decarboxylating. Enzyme that separates CO_2 from organic acids, such as carboxylase.

e., digestive. Enzyme that is involved in digestive processes in the alimentary canal.

e., extracellular. Enzyme that produces its effects outside the cell that produces it.

e., fermenting. Enzyme produced by bacteria or yeasts that brings about the fermentation of substances, esp. carbohydrates.

e., glycolytic. Enzyme that catalyzes the oxidation of sugar.

e., hydrolytic. Enzyme that catalyzes hydrolysis.

e., inhibitory. An enzyme that blocks a chemical reaction.

e., inorganic. A metallic colloidal solution, acting somewhat like an enzyme.

e., intracellular. An enzyme that acts within the cell that produces it.

e., inverting. Enzyme that catalyzes the hydrolysis of sucrose.

e., lipolytic. Enzyme that catalyzes the hydrolysis of fats. SYN: *lipase.*

e., mucolytic. An enzyme that depolymerizes mucus by splitting mucoproteins. They are called mucinases. Examples are lysozyme and hyluronidase.

e., oxidizing. Enzyme that catalyzes oxidative reactions. SYN: *oxidase.*

e., proteolytic. Enzyme that catalyzes conversion of proteins into peptides.

e., redox. Any enzyme that catalyzes oxidation-reduction reactions.

e., reducing. Enzyme that removes oxygen. SYN: *reductase.*

e., respiratory. Enzyme that acts within tissue cells catalyzing oxidative reactions with the release of energy, such as cytochromes, and flavoproteins.

e., splitting. Any enzyme that acts to facilitate removal of part of a molecule.

e., steatolytic. E., lipolytic, q.v.

e., transferring. Any enzyme that facilitates the moving of one molecule to another compound. SYN: *transferase.*

e., uricolytic. Enzyme that catalyzes conversion of uric acid into urea.

e., yellow. One of a group of flavoproteins involved in cellular oxidations.

enzyme induction. The adaptive increase in the number of molecules of a specific enzyme secondary either to an increase in its rate of synthesis or a decrease in its rate of degradation.

enzyme-linked immunoabsorbent assay. ABBR: ELISA. A rapid enzyme immunoassay method in which either an antibody or an antigen can be coupled to an enzyme. The resulting complex will retain both immunological and enzymatic activity. Use of this method provides for detection of either an antigen or an antibody. Certain bacterial antigens and antibodies as well as hormones can be detected by use of the ELISA method.

These assays are quite sensitive and specific as compared with the radioimmune assay (RIA) tests, and have the advantage of not requiring radioisotopes and the expensive counting apparatus.

enzymology (ĕn″zī-mŏl′ō-jē). The study of enzymes and their actions.

enzymolysis (ĕn-zīm-ŏl′ĭ-sĭs) [Gr. *en,* in, + *zyme,* leaven, + *lysis,* dissolution]. Chemical change or disintegration due to an enzyme.

enzymopathy (ĕn″zī-mŏp′ă-thē). Any disease in which an enzyme deficiency is involved.

enzymopenia (ĕn-zī″mō-pē′nē-ă). Deficiency of an enzyme.

enzymuria (ĕn″zī-mū′rē-ă) [″ + ″ + *ouron,* urine]. Presence of enzymes in the urine.

eonism (ē′ō-nĭzm). [Chevalier d'Eon, Fr. political adventurer, 1728–1810] Male transvestism.

eosin (ē′ō-sĭn) [Gr. *eos,* dawn (rose-colored)]. 1. A dye derived from action of bromine on fluorescein, $C_{20}H_8Br_4O_5$. An acid dye much used for staining tissues for microscopic examination. SYN: *tetrabromfluorescein.* 2. Any of several similar dyes. 3. Rosy-red; dawn-colored.

eosinoblast (ē″ō-sĭn′ō-blăst) [″ + *blastos,* germ]. A bone marrow cell that develops into a myelocyte. SYN: *myeloblast.*

eosinopenia (ē″ō-sĭn-ō-pē′nē-ă) [″ + *penia,* poverty]. Abnormally small number of eosinophilic cells in the peripheral blood.

eosinophil (ē″ō-sĭn′ō-fĭl) [″ + *philein,* to love]. A cell or cellular structure that stains readily with the acid stain eosin. Specifically refers to a granular leukocyte. SEE: *blood cell* for illus.

eosinophile (ē″ō-sĭn′ō-fĭl). 1. Eosinophilic. 2. Eosinophil.

eosinophilia (ē″ō-sĭn-ō-fĭl′ē-ă) [Gr. *eos,* dawn, + *philein,* to love]. 1. Accumulation of unusual number of eosinophils in the blood. 2. Condition of staining readily with eosin.

eosinophilic (ē″ō-sĭn-ō-fĭl′ĭk). Readily stainable with eosin.

eosinophilic leukocytes. Spherical cells having a diameter of 9 to 14 microns, found in blood and sometimes in connective tissues. The nucleus is polymorphic, usually having two lobes connected by a thin strand. The cytoplasm contains numerous coarse, highly refractile granules that stain intensely with eosin or other acid stains. They constitute 1% to 3% of the white cell count. Eosinophilic leukocytes originate in the red bone marrow. Their function is not well established. They are ameboid but do not exhibit phagocytic activity. They increase in number in certain diseases such as asthma and in certain infestations with animal parasites. They decrease in number in circulating blood following the administration of ACTH or cortisone.

eosinophilous (ē″ō-sĭn-ŏf′ĭ-lŭs) [″ + *philein,* to love]. 1. Easily stainable with eosin. 2. Having eosinophilia.

eosinotactic (ē″ō-sĭn-ō-tăk′tĭk) [″ + *taktikos,* arranged]. Attraction or repulsion of eosinophil cells.

epactal (ē-păk′tăl) [Gr. *epaktos,* added to]. Supernumerary.

eparterial (ĕp″ăr-tē′rē-ăl) [Gr. *epi,* over, upon, + *arteria,* artery]. Located over or above an artery.

epaxial (ĕp-ăk′sē-ăl) [″ + L. *axis,* axis]. Situated above or behind any axis.

epencephalon (ĕp″ĕn-sĕf′ă-lŏn) [″ + *enkephalos,* brain]. The anterior portion of the embryonic hindbrain (rhombencephalon) from which arise the pons and cerebellum. SYN: *metencephalon.*

ependyma (ĕp-ĕn′dĭ-mă) [Gr. *ependyma,* an upper garment, wrap]. [NA] Membrane lining the cerebral ventricles and central canal of spinal cord.

e. medullae spinalis. The spinal portion of the ependyma.

e. ventriculorum cerebral. The ventricular portion of the ependyma.

ependymal (ĕp-ĕn′dĭ-măl). Pert. to the ependyma.

ependymal cells. Cells of the developing neural tube that give rise to the ependyma. They arise from spongioblasts derived from the neural epithelium.

ependymal layer. The innermost of three layers that form the neural tube of an embryo.

ependymitis (ĕp″ĕn-dĭ-mī′tĭs) [″ + *itis,* inflammation]. Inflammation of the ependyma.

ependymoblast (ĕp-ĕn′dĭ-mō-blăst) [″ + *blastos,* germ]. An embryonic ependymal cell or ependymocyte.

ependymocyte (ĕp-ĕn′dĭ-mō-sīt) [″ + *kytos,* cell]. An ependymal cell.

ependymoma (ĕp-ĕn″dĭ-mō′mă) [″ + *oma,* tumor]. A tumor arising from fetal inclusion of ependymal elements.

ephebiatrics (ĕ-fē-bē-ăt′rĭks) [Gr. *epi,* at, + *hebe,* youth, + *iatrikos,* medical]. A branch of medicine dealing with adolescents.

ephebic (ĕ-fē′bĭk) [Gr. *ephebikos*]. Pert. to adolescence.

ephebology (ĕf-ē-bŏl′ō-jē) [″ + ″ + *logos,* study of]. The study of puberty and its changes.

ephedrine (ĕ-fĕd′rĭn, ĕf′ĕ-drēn). An alkaloid originally obtained from species of Ephedra; first isolated by Nagai in 1887. In ancient Chinese medicine it was used as a diaphoretic and antipyretic. It was not until recent times, however, that its action was studied and its valuable therapeutic properties made known. It is a sympathomimetic drug. It is usually produced synthetically. Action is similar to that of epinephrine. Its effects, although less powerful, are more prolonged, and it exerts an action when given orally, whereas epinephrine is effective only by injection. Ephedrine orally (or by injection) dilates the bronchial muscles, contracts the nasal mucosa, and raises the blood pressure. Chiefly used for its bronchodilator effect in asthma, and for its constricting effects on the nasal mucosa in hay fever.

INCOMPAT: Calcium chloride; iodine; tannic acid.

e. hydrochloride. A more soluble salt of the alkaloid, having the same action and uses as ephedrine.

e. sulfate. USP. The sulfate of ephedrine. It occurs as fine white crystals or as a powder. Its action and uses are the same as those for ephedrine. Trade name is Isofedrol.

ephelis (ĕf-ē'lĭs) [Gr. *ephelis,* freckle]. (pl. *ephelides*) Freckle.

ephemeral (ĕ-fĕm'ĕr-ăl) [Gr. *epi,* on, + *hemera,* day]. Of brief duration.

ephidrosis (ĕf"ĭ-drō'sĭs) [Gr., a sweating]. Abnormal amt. of sweating.

e. cruenta. Sweat containing blood.

e. tincta. Colored sweat. SYN: *chromidrosis.*

epi-, ep- [Gr.]. Prefix meaning upon, over, at, in addition to, after.

epiandrosterone (ĕp"ē-ăn-drŏs'tĕr-ōn). An androgenic hormone normally present in the urine.

epiblast (ĕp'ĭ-blăst) [Gr. *epi,* upon, + *blastos,* germ]. Outer layer of cells of the blastoderm. SYN: *ectoderm.*

epiblastic (ĕp-ĭ-blăs'tĭk). Pert. to the epiblast.

epiblepharon (ĕp"ĭ-blĕf'ă-rŏn) [" + Gr. *blepharon,* eyelid]. A fold of skin passes across the margin of either the upper or lower eyelid so that the eyelashes are pressed against the eye.

epibole, epiboly (ĕ-pĭb'ŏ-lē) [Gr. *epibole,* cover]. Inclusion of the hypoblast within the epiblast, due to swifter growth of the latter. SEE: *emboly.*

epibulbar (ĕp"ĭ-bŭl'băr). Lying upon the bulb of any structure; more specifically, located upon the eyeball.

epicanthus [Gr. *epi,* upon, + *kanthos,* canthus]. A vertical fold of skin extending from the root of the nose to the median end of the eyebrow, covering the inner canthus and caruncle. It is a characteristic of certain ethnic groups and may occur as a congenital anomaly in others.

epicardia (ĕp"ĭ-kărd'ē-ă) [" + *kardia,* heart]. The abdominal portion of the esophagus extending from the diaphragm to the stomach, about 2 cm. in length.

epicardium. [NA] The inner or visceral layer of the pericardium, q.v., which forms a serous membrane forming the outermost layer of the wall of the heart.

epichordal (ĕp"ĭ-kord'ăl) [" + *khorde,* cord]. Located dorsad to the notochord.

epichorion (ĕp"ĭ-kō'rē-ŏn) [" + *chorion*]. The portion of the decidua of the placenta that covers the ovum.

epicomus (ē-pĭk'ō-mŭs) [" + *kome,* hair]. A congenital malformation consisting of a parasitic twin or head attached to the summit or vertex of the skull.

epicondylalgia (ĕp"ĭ-kŏn-dĭ-lăl'jē-ă) [" + *kondylos,* condyle, + *algos,* pain]. Pain in the elbow joint in the region of the epicondyles.

epicondyle (ĕp-ĭ-kŏn'dīl) [" + *kondylos,* condyle]. The eminence at the articular end of a bone above a condyle.

epicondylitis (ĕp"ĭ-kŏn"dĭ-lī'tĭs) [" + " + *itis,* inflammation]. Inflammation of the epicondyle of the humerus and surrounding tissues.

e., lateral humeral. Tennis elbow, q.v.

epicranium [" + *kranion,* cranium]. Soft parts covering the cranium.

epicranius (ĕp"ĭ-krā'nē-ŭs). Occipitofrontal muscle and scalp.

epicrisis (ĕp'ĭ-krī"sĭs) [" + *krisis,* crisis]. A secondary crisis following the initial critical stage of a disease.

epicritic (ĕp-ĭ-krĭt'ĭk) [Gr. *epikritikos,* judging]. 1. Pert. to extreme sensibility, such as that of the skin when it discriminates between degrees of sensation caused by touch or temperature. 2. Pert. to an epicrisis. 3. Something such as pain or itching that is well localized.

epicystitis [Gr. *epi,* upon, + *kystis,* bladder, + *itis,* inflammation]. Inflammation of cellular tissue above the bladder.

epicystotomy (ĕp"ĭ-sĭs-tŏt'ō-mē) [" + " + *tome,* incision]. Opening above the symphysis pubis into the bladder.

epicyte (ĕp'ĭ-sīt) [" + *kytos,* cell]. 1. An epithelial cell. 2. A cell membrane.

epidemic (ĕp"ĭ-dĕm'ĭk) [" + *demos,* people]. Appearance of an infectious disease or condition that attacks many people at the same time in the same geographical area. SEE: *endemic; epizootic.*

epidemic acute nonbacterial gastroenteritis. A disease that occurs in outbreaks mostly in children and usually in the winter rather than the summer as do the outbreaks of bacterial gastroenteritis. The disease usually lasts one to two days and is self-limiting. Symptoms include nausea, vomiting, diarrhea, mild fever, and abdominal pain. The causative organism, the virus termed Norwalk agent, has been identified but not isolated. SEE: *Norwalk agent.* SYN: *winter vomiting disease.*

epidemiologic (ĕp"ĭ-dē-mē-ō-lŏj'ĭk) [" + *demos,* people, + *logos,* study]. Pert. to the study of epidemics.

epidemiologist (ĕp″ĭ-dē-mē-ŏl′ō-jĭst). A specialist in the field of epidemiology.

epidemiology (ĕp″ĭ-dē-mē-ŏl′ō-jē). Science concerned with defining and explaining the interrelationships of factors that determine disease frequency and distribution.

epidermal, epidermic [″ + *derma,* skin]. Pert. to the epidermis.

epidermatoplasty (ĕp″ĭ-dĕr-măt′ō-plăs-tē) [″ + ″ + *plassein,* to mold]. Grafting with pieces of epidermis with the underlying layer of the corium.

epidermic (ĕp-ĭ-dĕr′mĭk) [″ + *derma,* skin]. Pert. to the external layer of the skin or epidermis.

epidermis (ĕp″ĭ-dĕr′mĭs) [″ + *derma,* skin]. Cuticle, or outer layer of skin. It is nonvascular and is formed from within outward. It consists of four layers or strata: stratum germinativum (stratum mucosum, malpighian layer), the innermost layer; stratum granulosum epidermis [NA], located immediately above the stratum germinativum; stratum lucidum [NA], the clear layer; stratum corneum [NA], the outermost layer of the epidermis.

epidermitis (ĕp″ĭ-dĕr-mī′tĭs) [″ + ″ + *itis,* inflammation]. Inflammation of the superficial layers of the skin.

epidermization (ĕp″ĭ-dĕr″mĭ-zā′shŭn). 1. Skin grafting. 2. Conversion of deeper germinative layer of cells into outer layer of epidermis.

epidermodysplasia verruciformis (ĕp″ĭ-dĕr″mō-dĭs-plā′sē-ă). Generalized warts of the skin.

epidermoid (ĕp″ĭ-dĕr′moyd) [Gr. *epi,* upon, + *derma,* skin, + *eidos,* form]. 1. Resembling or pert. to the epidermis. 2. A tumor arising from aberrant epidermal cells. SYN: *cholesteatoma.*

epidermolysis (ĕp″ĭ-dĕr-mŏl′ĭ-sĭs) [″ + ″ + *lysis,* loosening]. Loosening of the epidermis.

e. bullosa. A genetically transmitted form characterized by formation of deep-seated bullae appearing after irritation or rubbing of a part.

epidermoma (ĕp″ĭ-dĕr-mō′mă) [″ + ″ + *oma,* growth]. An excrescence on the skin.

epidermomycosis (ĕp-ĭ-dĕr″mō-mī-kō′sĭs) [″ + ″ + *mykes,* fungus, + *osis,* condition]. Skin disease caused by a fungus.

Epidermophyton (ĕp″ĭ-dĕr-mŏf′ĭ-tŏn) [″ + ″ + *phyton,* plant]. A genus of fungi, similar to Trichophyton but affecting the skin and nails instead of the hair.

E. floccosum. The causative agent of certain types of tinea, esp. tinea pedis (athlete's foot), tinea cruris, tinea unguium, and tinea corporis.

epidermophytosis (ĕp″ĭ-dĕr-mō-fī-tō′sĭs) [″ + ″ + ″ + *osis,* condition]. Infection by a species of Epidermophyton.

epidermosis (ĕp″ĭ-dĕr-mō′sĭs) [″ + ″ + *osis,* condition]. Any disease affecting the skin, esp. the epidermis.

epididymectomy (ĕp″ĭ-dĭd″ĭ-mĕk′tō-mē) [″ + *didymos,* testis, + *ektome,* excision]. Removal of the epididymis.

epididymis (ĕp″ĭ-dĭd′ĭ-mĭs). (pl. *epididymides*) A small oblong body resting upon and beside the posterior surface of the testes, consisting of a convoluted tube 13 to 20 ft. (3.97 to 6.1 meters) long, enveloped in the tunica vaginalis, ending in the ductus deferens. It consists of the head (caput or globus major), which contains 12 to 14 efferent ducts of the testis, the body, and the tail (cauda or globus minor). It constitutes the first part of the excretory duct of each testis. The epididymis is supplied by the internal spermatic, deferential, and external spermatic arteries; it is drained by corresponding veins. SEE: illus.

epididymitis (ĕp″ĭ-dĭd″ĭ-mī′tĭs) [″ + *didymos,* testis, + *itis,* inflammation]. Inflammation of the epididymis.

ETIOL: May be complication of gonorrhea, syphilis, tuberculosis, mumps, prostatitis, urethritis, prostatectomy, or following prolonged use of indwelling catheter.

SYM: Fever and chills, pain in inguinal region, swollen epididymis.

TREATMENT: Bedrest, support of scrotum, and appropriate antibiotic.

epididymodeferentectomy (ĕp″ĭ-dĭd″ĭ-mō-dĕf″ĕr-ĕn-tĕk′tō-mē) [″ + ″ + L. *deferens,* carrying away, + Gr. *ektome,* excision]. Excision of epididymis and ductus deferens.

epididymodeferential (ĕp″ĭ-dĭd″ĭ-mō-dĕf″ĕr-ĕn′shăl). Concerning both the epididymis and ductus deferens.

epididymography (ĕp″ĭ-dĭd″ĭ-mŏg′ră-fē) [″ + ″ + *graphein,* to write]. Radiographic examination of the epididymus after the introduction of a contrast agent.

epididymoorchitis (ĕp″ĭ-dĭd″ĭm-ō-or-kī′tĭs) [″ + *didymos,* testis, + *orchis,* testis, + *itis,* inflammation]. Epididymitis with orchitis, q.v.

epididymotomy (ĕp″ĭ-dĭd″ĭ-mŏt′ō-mē) [″ + ″ + *tome,* incision]. Incision into the epididymis.

epididymovasostomy (ĕp-ĭ-dĭd″ĭ-mō-văs-ŏs′tō-mē) [″ + ″ + L. *vas,* vessel, + Gr. *stoma,* mouth]. Anastomosing between the epididymis and the vas.

epididymovesiculography (ĕp″ĭ-dĭd″ĭ-mō-vĕ-sĭk″ū-lŏg′ră-fē). Radiographic examination of the epididymus and seminal vesicle after introduction of a contrast agent.

epidural [Gr. *epi,* upon, + L. *durus,* hard]. Located over or upon the dura.

epidural space. Space outside of dura mater

EPIDIDYMIS

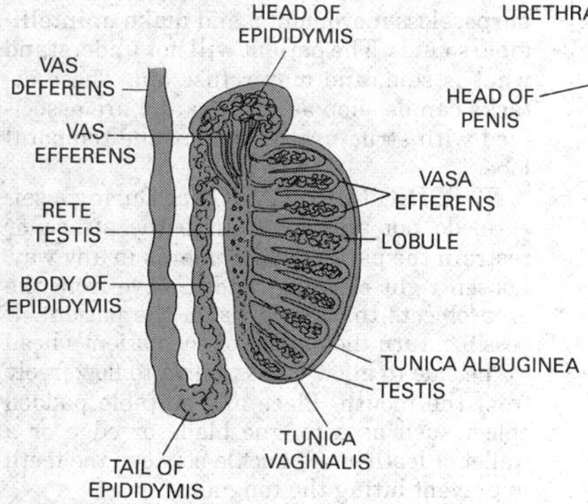

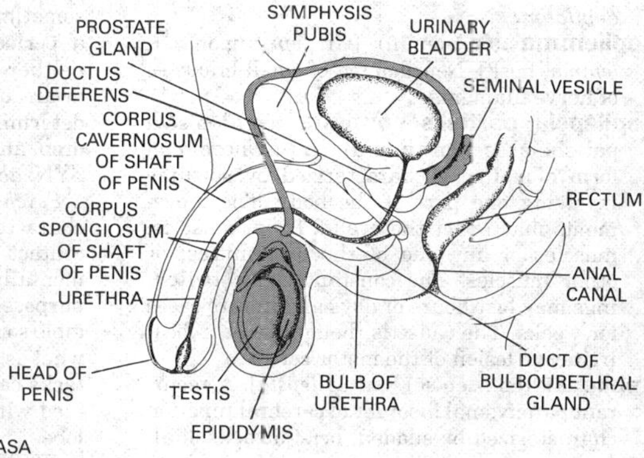

of brain and spinal cord.

epifascial (ĕp″ĭ-făsh′ē-ăl). On or upon a fascia.

epifolliculitis (ĕp″ĭ-fŏl-lĭk″ū-lī′tĭs) [″ + L. *folliculus,* follicle, + Gr. *itis,* inflammation]. Inflammation of hair follicles of the scalp.

epigaster [″ + *gaster,* belly]. Embryonic structure that develops into the large intestine. SYN: *hindgut.*

epigastralgia (ĕp″ĭ-găs-trăl′jē-ă) [″ + ″ + *algos,* pain]. Pain in the epigastrium.

epigastric. Pert. to the epigastrium. SEE: *precordium.*

epigastric reflex. Contraction of the upper portion of the rectus abdominis muscle when skin of the epigastric region is scratched.

epigastrium (ĕp″ĭ-găs′trē-ŭm) [″ + *gaster,* belly]. Region over the pit of the stomach. SEE: *Auenbrugger's sign.*

epigastrocele (ĕp″ĭ-găs′trō-sēl) [″ + ″ + *kele,* hernia]. Hernia in the epigastrium.

epigastrorrhaphy (ĕp″ĭ-găs-tror′ă-fē) [″ + ″ + *rhaphe,* suture]. Suture of an abdominal wound in the epigastric area.

epigenesis (ĕp″ĭ-jĕn′ĕ-sĭs) [″ + *genesis,* formation]. In embryology, the theory that parts of an organism arise by a process of progressive development from simple to complex structures through the utilization of cells as building units.

epiglottidean (ĕp″ĭ-glŏ-tĭd′ē-ăn) [″ + *glottis,* glottis]. Pert. to the epiglottis.

epiglottidectomy (ĕp″ĭ-glŏt″ĭd-ĕk′tō-mē) [″ + ″ + *ektome,* excision]. Excision of the epiglottis.

epiglottiditis (ĕp″ĭ-glŏt″tĭd-ī′tĭs) [″ + ″ + *itis,* inflammation]. Inflammation of the epiglottis. SYN: *epiglottitis.*

epiglottis (ĕp″ĭ-glŏt′ĭs) [Gr.]. (pl. *epiglottides*) [NA] A thin, leaf-shaped structure located immediately posterior to the root of the tongue. It covers the entrance of the larynx when the individual swallows, thus preventing food or liquids from entering the airway. SEE: *larynx* for illus.

epiglottitis (ĕp″ĭ-glŏt-ī′tĭs) [″ + *itis,* inflammation]. Inflammation of the epiglottis. Appears most commonly in young children. If untreated, may be so severe as to cause death.

SYM: Sore throat, fever, croupy cough, drooling, cyanosis, and even coma.

TREATMENT: Establishment of airway by tracheostomy if necessary. Administration of appropriate antibiotic.

epihyal (ĕp-ĭ-hī′ăl). Pert. to the arch of the hyoid.

epilate (ĕp′ĭ-lāt) [L. *e,* out, + *pilus,* hair]. To extract the hair by the roots.

epilating. Depilating; extracting a hair.

epilation (ĕp-ĭ-lā′shŭn). Extraction of hair. SYN: *depilation; electrolysis.*

epilatory (ĕ-pĭl′ă-tor-ē). Pert. to removal of

hairs, or that which removes them. SYN: *depilatory.*

epilemma (ĕp-ĭ-lĕm′ă) [Gr. *epi,* upon, + *lemma,* husk]. Neurilemma of small branches of nerve filaments.

epilepsia partialis continua (ĕp″ĭ-lĕp′sē-a păr-shē-ăl′ĭs cŏn-tĭn′ū-ă) [L.]. Uncommon form of epilepsy characterized by seizures involving one part of the body. The movements may affect the eyelid, facial muscles, muscles of any one of the extremities, or other muscles. The constant clonic twitchings may last hours or days and in rare cases for weeks. The cause is thought to be a focal irritative lesion of the motor cortex.

epilepsy (ĕp′ĭ-lĕp″sē) [Gr. *epilepsia*]. A recurrent paroxysmal disorder of cerebral function characterized by sudden, brief attacks of altered consciousness, motor activity, or sensory phenomena. Convulsive seizures are the most common form of attacks, but any recurrent seizure pattern is considered epilepsy.

Epilepsy is usually classified by the type of seizure the person has. The previous system of classification described seizures as grand mal, petit mal, or psychomotor. A new *International Classification System* describes seizures in relation to the area of the brain involved. The new system divides seizures into two main groups: partial and generalized. The more familiar names for seizures are listed below, but information on the new classification system can be obtained from the Epilepsy Foundation of America, 1828 L Street NW, Washington D.C. 20036.

ETIOL: Idiopathic epilepsy accounts for 75% of this disease in adults. This type may be due to a microscopic brain lesion occurring during birth or other trauma, or may be due to unexplained metabolic disturbances. Symptomatic epilepsy may be associated with other disorders such as: hyperpyrexia, CNS infections, metabolic disturbances, ingestion of toxic agents, brain lesions or defects, or cerebral trauma.

SYM: The symptoms of epilepsy vary according to the type of cerebral dysfunction. In some cases the only symptom of a seizure is a fleeting interruption of consciousness, a twitching limb, an aching stomach, or occasionally a headache.

Grand mal seizures are what most people think comprises epilepsy. They are generalized, and affect the entire brain. A sensation of sinking or rising in the epigastrium, the aura, is the start of a seizure. The seizure proceeds with loss of consciousness; falling; and tonic then clonic contractions of the muscles. Urinary and fecal incontinence may occur. The attack usually lasts 2 to 5 minutes.

Petit mal attacks are brief and general seizures with a 10 to 30 second loss of consciousness, eye or muscle flutterings, and sometimes loss of muscle tone. There may be a period of unconsciousness so brief that neither the patient nor observers would be aware of it. These seizures are genetically determined, occur predominantly in children, and rarely begin after the age of twenty. SYN: *absence seizures.*

Psychomotor attacks are focal seizures characterized by a 1 to 2 minute loss of contact with surroundings. The patient is mentally confused, may stagger, perform purposeless movements, and make unintelligible sounds. The patient will not understand what is said, and may refuse aid. These attacks can develop at any age and are associated with structural lesions in the temporal lobe.

NURSING IMPLICATIONS: During a seizure, do not attempt to stop the attack or restrain the patient's movements in any way. Loosen tight clothing, and remove from the area objects that could harm the patient. If possible, turn the patient or the patient's head to the side to allow excess saliva to flow freely from the mouth. Place any suitable padded object such as a tongue blade or edge or a wallet or leather belt buckle between the teeth to prevent biting the tongue.

Carefully observe the patient during a seizure; note the onset, extent, and duration of the seizure, body parts involved, the specific type of seizure activity, the level of consciousness of the patient during the seizure, cyanosis, or incontinence. Assist the patient in identification of what may trigger the seizure, or of a warning aura. The patient must understand the importance of regularly taking prescribed medications, of keeping follow-up appointments, of having necessary blood work done. The patient with epilepsy should wear a Medic Alert bracelet.

TREATMENT: Several anticonvulsant drugs are available, and alone or in combinations, they can help control seizures.

e., idiopathic. Presence of epilepsy without known cause.

e., jacksonian. Epilepsy in which convulsions start in certain groups of muscles or one side of the body, usually in an extremity, and then sometimes spreading throughout the whole body.

e., myoclonic. A slowly progressive, hereditary epilepsy in which clonic contractions of muscles, esp. those of the extremities, occur between seizures.

e., nocturnal. Epilepsy that occurs only during sleep. Symptoms similar to grand mal.

e., photogenic. Epileptic seizures induced by intermittent flash of lights into the eye.

e., reflex. Epilepsy in which attacks are induced by sensory stimuli.

e., sleep. Spasmodic uncontrollable desire to sleep. SYN: *narcolepsy.*

e., temporal lobe. Impaired consciousness in association with psychic changes such as automatic behavior, impaired judgment, and antisocial acts. There are no seizures, but loss of consciousness may occur. The cause is disease of the temporal lobe of the brain.

e., traumatic. Epilepsy caused by trauma to the brain.

e., uncinate. Epilepsy due to a lesion of the uncinate gyrus of the temporal lobe. Preceded by aura of smell.

epileptic (ĕp″ĭ-lĕp′tĭk) [Gr. *epileptikos*]. 1. Concerning epilepsy. 2. Individual suffering from epileptic attacks.

epileptiform (ĕp″ĭ-lĕp′tĭ-form) [Gr. *epilepsia,* epilepsy, + L. *forma,* form]. Having the form of epilepsy.

epileptogenic, epileptogenous (ĕp″ĭ-lĕp-tō-jĕn′ĭk, -tŏj′ĕ-nŭs) [″ + *gennan,* to produce]. Giving rise to epileptoid convulsions.

epileptoid [″ + *eidos,* resemblance]. Resembling epilepsy. SYN: *epileptiform.*

epileptology [″ + *logos,* study]. Study of epilepsy.

epiloia (ĕp″ĭ-lŏy′ă). A syndrome consisting of progressive mental deficiency, adenoma sebaceum, convulsions, hypertrophic sclerosis of the brain, tumors in the kidneys, and nodules on floor of lateral ventricle. SYN: *tuberous sclerosis.*

epimandibular (ĕp″ĭ-măn-dĭb′ū-lăr) [Gr. *epi,* upon, above, + L. *mandibulum,* jaw]. Located upon the lower jaw.

epimer (ĕp′ĭ-mĕr). One of a pair of isomers that differ only in the position of the H— and OH— attached to one asymmetric carbon atom.

epimere (ĕp′ĭ-mēr) [Gr. *epi,* upon, + *meros,* apart]. In embryology, the dorsal muscle-forming portion of the somite.

epimerite (ĕp″ĭ-mĕr′īt) [″ + *meros,* part]. An organelle of certain protozoa by which they attach themselves to epithelial cells.

epimorphosis (ĕp″ĭ-mor′fō-sĭs) [″ + *morphoun,* to give shape, + *osis,* condition]. Regeneration of a part of an organism by growth at the cut surface.

epimysium (ĕp″ĭ-mĭz′ē-ŭm) [″ + *mys,* muscle]. Outermost sheath of connective tissue that surrounds a skeletal muscle. Consists of irregularly distributed collagenous, reticular, and elastic fibers, connective tissue cells, and fat cells. SYN: *perimysium externum.*

epinephrine (ĕp″ĭ-nĕf′rĭn) [″ + *nephros,* kidney]. USP. $C_9H_{13}NO_3$. A hormone secreted by the adrenal medulla in response to splanchnic stimulation. This substance and norepinephrine are the two active hormones produced by the adrenal medulla. Epinephrine, which has been synthesized, is also produced by tissues other than the adrenal. It is employed therapeutically as a vasoconstrictor, cardiac stimulant, and to relax bronchioles. Its effects are similar to those brought about by stimulation of the sympathetic division of the autonomic nervous system. Used to check local hemorrhage and to relieve asthmatic attacks. Also to prolong action of local anesthetics by constricting blood vessels to prevent rapid absorption. Trade names are Adrenaline, Primatene Mist, Bronkaid Mist, and Sus-Phrine. SYN: *adrenaline.*

INCOMPAT: Light; heat; air; iron salts; and alkalies.

e. bitartrate. USP. $C_9H_{13}NO_3C_4H_6O_6$. A white or grayish-white crystalline powder. It is a sympathomimetic agent used for topical application to the eye. Trade names are Adrenate, Medihaler-Epi, Asmatane Mist, Lyophrin, and Suprarenin.

epinephrinemia (ĕp″ĭ-nĕf″rĭ-nē′mē-ă) [″ + ″ + *haima,* blood]. Epinephrine in the blood.

epinephritis (ĕp″ĭ-nĕf-rī′tĭs) [″ + *nephros,* kidney, + *itis,* inflammation]. Inflammation of an adrenal gland.

epinephroma (ĕp-ĭ-nĕ-frō′mă) [″ + ″ + *oma,* tumor]. A lipomatoid tumor of the kidney. SYN: *hypernephroma.*

epineural (ĕp″ĭ-nū′răl) [″ + *neuron,* nerve]. Located upon a neural arch.

epineurium (ĕp″ĭ-nū′rē-ŭm). The general connective tissue sheath of a nerve. SEE: *nerve.*

epiotic (ĕp″ē-ŏt′ĭk) [″ + *ous,* ear]. Located above the ear.

epiotic center. Ossification center of temporal bone forming upper and posterior part of the auditory capsule.

epipastic (ĕp″ĭ-păs′tĭk) [″ + *passein,* to sprinkle]. Resembling a dusting powder.

epipharynx (ĕp″ĭ-făr′ĭnks) [″ + *pharynx,* pharynx]. Nasal portion of pharynx. SYN: *rhinopharynx.*

epiphenomenon (ĕp″ĭ-fē-nŏm′ĕ-nŏn) [″ + *phainomenon,* phenomenon]. An exceptional symptom or occurrence in a disease that is not related to the usual course of the disease.

epiphora (ĕ-pĭf′ō-ră) [Gr., downpour]. Abnormal overflow of tears down the cheek due to excess secretion of tears or to obstruction of the lacrimal duct.

epiphylaxis (ĕp″ĭ-fĭ-lăks′ĭs) [Gr. *epi,* upon, + *phylaxis,* protection]. Increase of defensive powers of the body.

epiphyseal (ĕp″ĭ-fĭz′ē-ăl) [″ + *physis,* growth]. Pert. to or of the nature of an epiphysis. Also spelled epiphysial.

epiphyseolysis (ĕp″ĭ-fĭz″ē-ŏl′ĭ-sĭs) [″ + ″ + *lysis,* loosening]. Separation of an epiphysis. Also spelled epiphysiolysis.

epiphyseopathy (ĕp″ĭ-fĭz-ē-ŏp′ă-thē) [″ + ″ + *pathos,* disease]. Any disease of an epiphysis or of the pineal gland. Also spelled epiphysiopathy.

epiphysial (ĕp″ĭ-fĭz′ē-ăl). Of the nature of or concerning an epiphysis. Also spelled epiphyseal.

epiphysis (ĕ-pĭf′ĭ-sĭs) [Gr., a growing upon]. (pl. *epiphyses*) [NA] 1. In the developing infant and child, a secondary bone-forming (ossification) center separated from a parent bone in early life by cartilage. As growth proceeds and at a different time for each epiphysis, it becomes a part of the larger (or parent) bone. It is possible to judge the biological age of a child from the development of these ossification centers as shown in x-rays. 2. A center for ossification at each extremity of long bones. SEE: *diaphysis.*

epiphysitis (ĕ-pĭf″ĭ-sī′tĭs) [″ + *itis,* inflammation]. Inflammation of an epiphysis, esp. that at the hip, knee, and shoulder in infants.

epipial (ĕp″ĭ-pī′ăl) [″ + L. *pia,* tender]. Situated above or upon the pia mater.

epiplocele (ĕ-pĭp′lō-sēl) [Gr. *epiploon,* omentum, + *kele,* hernia]. Hernia containing omentum.

epiploenterocele (ĕ-pĭp″lō-ĕn′tĕr-ō-sēl) [″ + *enteron,* intestine, + *kele,* hernia]. Hernia consisting of omentum and intestine.

epiploic (ĕp″ĭ-plō′ĭk) [Gr. *epiploon,* omentum]. Pert. to the omentum.

epiploic foramen. The opening between the greater and lesser peritoneal cavities.

epiploitis (ĕ-pĭp″lō-ī′tĭs) [″ + *itis,* inflammation]. Inflammation of the omentum.

epiplomerocele (ĕ-pĭp″lō-mē′rō-sēl) [″ + *meros,* thigh, + *kele,* hernia]. Femoral hernia containing omentum.

epiplomphalocele (ĕ-pĭp″lŏm-făl′ō-sēl) [″ + *omphalos,* navel, + *kele,* hernia]. Umbilical hernia with omentum protruding.

epiploon (ĕ-pĭp′lō-ŏn) [Gr., omentum]. The omentum, esp. the greater omentum. SYN: *omentum.*

epiplopexy (ĕ-pĭp′lō-pĕks″ē) [″ + *pexis,* fixation]. Suturing of omentum to the anterior abdominal wall.

epiplosarcomphalocele (ĕ-pĭp″lō-săr″kŏm-făl′ō-sēl) [″ + *sarx,* flesh, + *omphalos,* navel, + *kele,* hernia]. An umbilical hernia with protruding omentum. SYN: *epiplomphalocele.*

epiploscheocele (ĕ-pĭp″lŏs-kē′ō-sēl) [″ + *oscheon,* scrotum, + *kele,* hernia]. Omental hernia into the scrotum.

epipygus (ĕp″ĭ-pī′gŭs) [Gr. *epi,* upon, + *pyge,* buttocks]. A developmental anomaly in which an accessory limb is attached to the buttocks.

episclera (ĕp″ĭ-sklē′ră) [″ + *skleros,* hard]. Outermost superficial layer of the sclera of the eye.

episcleral (ĕp″ĭ-sklē′răl). 1. Pert. to the episclera. 2. Overlying the sclera of the eye.

episcleritis (ĕp″ĭ-sklē-rī′tĭs) [″ + *skleros,* hard, + *itis,* inflammation]. Inflammation of the subconjunctival layers of the sclera.

episioelytrorrhaphy (ĕ-pĭs″ē-ō-ĕl″ĭ-tror′ă-fē) [″ + *elytron,* vagina, + *rhaphe,* suture]. Surgical narrowing of vagina and vulva.

episioperineoplasty (ĕ-pĭz″ē-ō-pĕr″ĭ-nē′ō-plăs″tē) [″ + *perinaion,* perineum, + Gr. *plassein,* to form]. Plastic surgery of the perineum and vulva.

episioperineorrhaphy (ĕ-pĭs″ĭ-ō-pĕr″ĭ-nē-or′ă-fē) [″ + ″ + *rhaphe,* suture]. Suturing the vulva and perineum for the support of a prolapse of the uterus.

NURSING IMPLICATIONS: Give perineal care as needed, and teach the patient the correct perineal hygiene of wiping from front to back. Anesthetic sprays or creams may be ordered, and local heat applications through use of a heat lamp, warm soaks, or sitz baths may be ordered and should be administered for pain relief. Inspect the perineum at intervals to assess for symptoms of infection or hematoma formation.

episioplasty (ĕ-pĭs″ē-ō-plăs′tē) [″ + *plassein,* to form]. Plastic surgery on the vulva.

episiorrhaphy (ĕ-pĭs″ē-or′ă-fē) [″ + *rhaphe,* suture]. Suture of a lacerated perineum.

episiostenosis (ĕ-pĭs″ē-ō-stĕ-nō′sĭs) [″ + *stenosis,* narrowing]. Narrowing of the vulvar slit.

episiotomy (ĕ-pĭs″ē-ŏt′ō-mē) [″ + *tome,* incision]. Incision of perineum at end of second stage of labor to avoid laceration of perineum and to facilitate delivery.

episome (ĕp′ĭ-sōm). A term previously used to describe bacterial elements, certain plasmids, that could replicate either autonomously or in association with the chromosome.

epispadias (ĕp″ĭ-spā′dē-ăs) [Gr. *epi,* upon, + *spadon,* a rent]. Congenital opening of urethra on dorsum of penis or opening by separation of the labia minora and a fissure of the clitoris. SYN: *anaspadias.*

episplenitis (ĕp″ĭ-splĕ-nī′tĭs) [″ + *splen,* spleen, + *itis,* inflammation]. Inflammation of the splenic capsule.

epistasis (ĕ-pĭs′tă-sĭs) [Gr., stoppage]. 1. A film that forms on urine that has been allowed to stand. 2. The suppression of any discharge. SEE: *hypostasis.*

epistaxis (ĕp″ĭ-stăk′sĭs) [Gr.]. Hemorrhage from nose; nosebleed.

ETIOL: May occur secondary to local infections (vestibulitis, rhinitis, sinusitis); systemic infections (scarlet fever, typhoid); drying of nasal mucous membrane; trauma (including picking the nose); arteriosclerosis; hypertension; and bleeding tendencies associated with anemias.

TREATMENT: Lie quietly propped up in bed, cold compresses, epinephrine locally, and if necessary, followed by cautery of bleeding vessel, then nasal packing if indicated.

NURSING IMPLICATIONS: Attempt to stop bleeding by seating the patient so head is above heart level, or by compressing side of nose against nasal septum for 5 to 10 minutes. Pressure across the upper lip or cold cloths placed over the nose and on the nape of the neck may also help to stop the bleeding. Instruct the patient not to breathe through or blow the nose.

episternal (ĕp″ĭ-stĕr′năl) [Gr. *epi,* upon, + *sternon,* chest]. Situated above the sternum.

episternum. Upper portion of the sternum. SYN: *manubrium sterni.*

epistropheus (ĕp″ĭ-strō′fē-ŭs). (pl. *epistrophei)* Former term for axis of the second cervical vertebra.

epitendineum (ĕp″ĭ-tĕn-dĭn′ē-ŭm) [″ + L. *tendere,* to stretch]. The fibrous sheath enveloping a tendon.

epitenon (ĕp-ĭ-tĕn′ŏn) [″ + *tenon,* tendon]. The connective tissue holding a tendon within its sheaths. SYN: *epitendineum.*

epithalamus (ĕp″ĭ-thăl′ă-mŭs) [″ + *thalamos,* chamber]. [NA] The uppermost portion of the diencephalon of the brain. It includes the pineal body, trigonum habenulae, habenula, and the habenular commissure.

epithalaxia (ĕp″ĭ-thă-lăk′sē-ă) [″ + *thele,* nipple, + *allaxis,* exchange]. Desquamation of epithelial cells, esp. of lining of the intestine.

epithelia [″ + *thele,* nipple]. (pl. of *epithelium)* Epithelial layer of cells. SEE: *epithelium.*

epithelial (ĕp″ĭ-thē′lē-ăl). Pert. to or composed of epithelium.

epithelial cancer. Carcinoma composed of epithelial cells. SYN: *epithelioma.*

epithelial casts. Aggregations of renal epithelium with cells filled with granules or fat droplets. They often preserve their original form in the epithelial tubes.

epithelial cells. Cells that are irregular in shape, having a single nucleus. Frequently two or three are joined together.

epithelialization (ĕp″ĭ-thē″lē-ăl-ī-zā′shŭn). The growth of skin over a wound.

epithelial tissue. Those cells that form the outer surface of the body, and line the body cavities and the principal tubes and passageways leading to the exterior. They form the secreting portions of glands and their ducts and important parts of certain sense organs. The cells of epithelial tissues lie closely approximated to each other and contain very little intercellular substance. They are arranged in one or a few layers and are devoid of blood vessels. SEE: *tissue.*

epitheliitis (ĕp″ĭ-thē″lē-ī′tĭs). Overgrowth and inflammation of the mucosal epithelium following injury such as could be caused by ionizing radiation.

epithelioblastoma (ĕp″ĭ-thē″lē-ō-blăs-tō′mă) [″ + *thele,* nipple, + *blastos,* germ, + *oma,* tumor]. Epithelial cell tumor.

epitheliogenic, epitheliogenetic (ĕp″ĭ-thē″lē-ō-jĕn′ĭk, -jĕ-nĕt′ĭk) [″ + ″ + *gennan,* to produce]. Caused by epithelial proliferation.

epithelioglandular (ĕp″ĭ-thē″lē-ō-glăn′dū-lăr). Concerning the epithelial cells of a gland.

epithelioid (ĕp″ĭ-thē′lē-oyd) [″ + ″ + *eidos,* form]. Resembling epithelium.

epitheliolysin (ĕp″ĭ-thē-lē-ŏl′ĭ-sĭn) [″ + ″ + *lysis,* dissolution]. A specific lysin formed in blood serum of an animal in which epithelial cells of an animal of a different species were injected. Epitheliolysin destroys the cells of an animal of the same species as that from which the epithelial cells were derived.

epitheliolysis (ĕp″ĭ-thē-lē-ŏl′ĭ-sĭs). Death of epithelial tissue. The destruction or dissolving of epithelial cells by an epitheliolysin.

epithelioma (ĕp″ĭ-thē-lē-ō′mă) [″ + *thele,* nipple, + *oma,* tumor]. A malignant tumor consisting principally of epithelial cells; a carcinoma. A tumor originating in the epidermis of the skin or in a mucous membrane.

e. adamantinum. A tumor of the jaw arising from the enamel organ. Of low-grade malignancy; may be solid or partly cystic. SYN: *adamantinoma.*

e. adenoides cysticum. A basal cell carcinoma of low malignancy occurring on the surface of the body, esp. the face. Characterized by formation of cysts. SYN: *acanthoma.*

e., basal cell. Epithelioma derived from cells in the basal layer of the epidermis (stratum germinativum).

e., deep-seated. Epithelioma that involves lymphatic glands with irregular rounded ulcers occurring after several months.

e. molluscum. An infective skin disease caused by a virus; characterized by umbilicated lesions on the skin. SYN: *molluscum contagiosum,* q.v.

epitheliomatous (ĕp″ĭ-thē-lē-ō′mă-tŭs). Pert. to epithelioma.

epitheliosis (ĕp″ĭ-thē″lē-ō′sĭs) [″ + *thele,* nipple, + *osis,* condition]. Trachomatous proliferation of the conjunctival epithelium.

epithelium (ĕp″ĭ-thē′lē-ŭm) [″ + *thele,* nipple]. (pl. *epithelia)* [NA] The layer of cells forming the epidermis of the skin and the surface layer of mucous and serous membranes. The cells rest on a basement membrane and lie closely approximated to each other with little intercellular material between them. The epithelium may be simple, consisting of a single layer, or it may be stratified, consisting of several layers. Cells comprising the epithelium may be flat (squamous), cube-shaped (cuboidal) or cylindrical (columnar). Modified forms of epithelium include ciliated, pseudostratified, glandular, and neuroepithelium. The epithelium may include goblet cells, which secrete mucus. Stratified squamous epithelium may be keratinized for a protective function or abnormally in pathologic response. Squamous epithelium is classified as endothelium, which lines the blood vessels and the heart, and mesothelium, which lines the serous cavities. Epithelium serves the general functions of protection, absorption, secretion, and specialized functions such as movement of substances through ducts, production of germ cells, and reception of stimuli. Its ability to regenerate is excellent; and it may replace itself as frequently as every 24 hours.

e., attachment. The epithelial layer that extends downward from the bottom of the gingival sulcus along the tooth and attaches to it.

e., ciliated. Epithelial cells with fine hairlike protuberances, called cilia, on their free border. These cells are able to sweep particles in a certain direction.

e., columnar. Epithelium composed of cells shaped like pillars.

e., cuboidal. Epithelium consisting of cube-shaped or prismatic cells with height approx. equal to width.

e., germinal. The epithelium that covers the surface of the genital ridge of the urogenital folds of an embryo. It gives rise to seminiferous tubules of the testes and the surface layer of the ovary. It was once thought to give rise to the germ cells (spermatozoa and ova).

e., glandular. Epithelium consisting of cells that secrete.

e., laminated. E., stratified.

e., mesenchymal. Epithelium of the squamous type that lines the subarachnoid and subdural cavities, the chambers of the eye, and the perilymphatic spaces of the ear.

e., pavement. Epithelium of flat, platelike cells in a single layer.

e., pigmented. Epithelium containing pigment granules.

e., pseudostratified. Epithelium in which the bases of cells rest on the basement membrane but the distal ends of some do not reach the surface. Nuclei of the cells lie at different levels, giving the appearance of stratification.

e., reduced enamel. The combined epithelial layers of the enamel organ, which form a protective layer over the enamel crown as it erupts, and then become the primary attachment epithelium surrounding the tooth.

e., squamous. E., pavement.

e., stratified. Epithelium with the cells in layers.

e., sulcular. The nonkeratinized epithelium that lines the gingival sulcus.

e., transitional. A form of stratified epithelium in which the cells have the ability to adjust themselves to mechanical changes such as stretching and contracting. Found only in the urinary system (pelvis and kidney, ureter, bladder, and a part of the urethra).

epitope (ĕp′ĭ-tōp). Any component of an antigen molecule that functions as an antigenic determinant by permitting the attachment of certain antibodies. SEE: *paratope*.

epitrichial layer. Periderm, q.v.

epitrichium (ĕp″ĭ-trĭk′ē-ŭm) [Gr. *epi*, upon, + *trichion*, hair]. Superficial layers of the epidermis of the fetus. SYN: *periderm*.

epitrochlea (ĕp″ĭ-trŏk′lē-ă) [″ + *trochalia*, pulley]. The inner condyle of the humerus.

epitrochlear (ĕp″ĭ-trŏk′lē-ăr). Pert. to the inner condyle of the humerus.

epiturbinate (ĕp″ĭ-tĕr′bĭn-āt) [″ + L. *turbo*, top]. The tissue upon or covering the turbinate bone.

epitympanum (ĕp″ĭ-tĭm′pă-nŭm) [″ + *tympanon*, drum]. Attic of the middle ear; area above the drum membrane.

epizoic (ĕp″ĭ-zō′ĭk) [″ + *zoon*, animal]. Living as a parasite on the exterior of an animal.

epizoicide (ĕp″ĭ-zō′ĭ-sīd) [″ + ″ + L. *caedere*, to kill]. That which destroys epizoa.

epizoon (ĕp″ĭ-zō′ŏn) [″ + *zoon*, animal]. (pl. *epizoa*) An animal organism living as a parasite on the exterior of the host animal.

epizootic. Any disease of animals that attacks many animals in the same area.

eponychium (ĕp″ō-nĭk′ē-ŭm) [″ + *onyx*, nail]. 1. The horny embryonic structure from which the nail develops. 2. Perionychium [NA].

eponym (ĕp′ō-nĭm) [Gr. *eponymos*, named after]. A name for anything (diseases, organs, functions, places) adapted from the name of a particular person.

epoophorectomy (ĕp″ō-ō-fō-rĕk′tō-mē) [Gr. *epi*, upon, + *oophoron*, ovary, + *ektome*, excision]. Removal of the parovarium.

epoophoron (ĕp″ō-ŏf′ō-rŏn). A rudimentary structure located in the mesosalpinx. Consisting of a longitudinal duct (duct of Gartner) and ten to fifteen transverse ducts, it is the remains of the upper portion of the mesonephros and is the homologue of the head of the epididymis in the male. SYN: *Rosenmüller's body; parovarium*.

epoxy (ē-pŏk′sē). General term for polymers that contain molecules wherein oxygen is attached to two different carbon atoms. They are widely used as adhesives.

Eprolin. Trade name for vitamin E.

Epsilan-M. Trade name for vitamin E.

epsilon-amino-caproic acid. A synthetic substance used to correct an overdose of certain fibrinolytic agents. Also useful in treating excessive bleeding due to increased fibrinolytic activity in the blood.

epsom salt (ĕp'sŭm). Magnesium sulfate.

EPSP. *excitatory postsynaptic potential.*

Epstein-Barr virus. [M. A. Epstein, Y. M. Barr] ABBR: EBV. A virus discovered in 1964. It is believed to be the causative agent in infectious mononucleosis. In South African children, it is associated with Burkitt's lymphoma; and in Asian populations with nasopharyngeal carcinoma. Why the virus has these different and varied associations in different geographical areas is unknown.

Epstein's pearls. In newborn infants, whitish-yellow accumulation of epithelial cells, or retention cysts on the hard palate. They are harmless and disappear within a few weeks.

epulis (ĕp-ū'lĭs) [Gr. *epoulis,* a gumboil]. (pl. *epulides*) A fibrous sarcomatous tumor having its origin in the periosteum of the lower jaw.

epuloid (ĕp'ū-loyd) [" + *eidos,* form]. 1. Like an epulis. 2. Tumor of the jaw or gum resembling an epulis.

epulosis (ĕp"ū-lō'sĭs) [Gr. *epoulosis*]. Cicatrization; a cicatrix.

epulotic (ĕp"ū-lŏt'ĭk) [Gr. *epoulotikos*]. Promoting cicatrization.

Equanil. Trade name for meprobamate.

equation [L. *aequare,* to make equal]. 1. State of being equal. 2. In chemistry, a symbolic representation of a chemical reaction.

equator [L. *aequator*]. Line encircling a round body and equidistant from both poles.

e. oculi. An imaginary line encircling the bulb of the eye midway between anterior and posterior poles.

e. of cell. The boundary of a plane through which the division of a cell occurs.

e. of crystalline lens; e. lentis. Line that marks the junction of the anterior and posterior surfaces. To it are attached the fibers of the suspensory ligament.

equatorial. Pert. to an equator.

equatorial plate. Mass of chromosomes at equator of the nuclear spindle during karyokinesis.

equi- [L. *aequus,* equal]. Prefix meaning equal.

equilibrating (ē-kwĭl'ĭ-brāt-ĭng) [L. *aequilibris,* in perfect balance]. Maintaining equilibrium.

equilibration. The process of modifying the masticatory forces or occlusal surfaces of teeth to produce simultaneous occlusal contacts between upper and lower teeth, and to equalize the stress of occlusal forces of the supporting tissues of the teeth.

equilibrium [L. *aequus,* equal, + *libra,* balance]. State of balance. Condition in which contending forces are equal.

e., nitrogenous. Condition in which the nitrogen excreted equals the nitrogen intake.

e., physiological. Having egesta equal to the ingesta.

equilin (ĕk'wĭl-ĭn) [L. *equus,* horse]. Crystalline estrogenic hormone derived from pregnant mares' urine.

equine (ē'kwīn) [L. *equus,* a horse]. Concerning or originating from a horse.

equinovarus (ē-kwī"nō-vā'rŭs) [L. *equinus,* equine, + *varus,* bent inward]. A form of clubfoot with a combination pes equinus and pes varus, i.e., walking without touching the heel to the ground and with the sole turned inward.

equipotential (ē"kwĭ-pō-tĕn'shăl) [L. *aequus,* equal, + *potentia,* ability]. Having the same electrical charge or physical strength.

equivalence (ē-kwĭv'ă-lĕns) [" + *valere,* to be worth]. Quality of being equivalent.

equivalent (ē-kwĭv'a-lĕnt). 1. Equal in power, force, or value. 2. Amount of weight of any element needed to replace a fixed weight of another body.

equivalent weight. The weight of a chemical element that is equivalent to and will replace in a chemical reaction a hydrogen atom (1.008 grams).

E.R. *external resistance.*

Er. Chem. symb. for erbium.

erasion (ē-rā'zhŭn) [L. *e,* out, + *radere,* to scrape]. Laying open a diseased part and scraping away diseased tissue.

Erben's reflex (ĕrb'ĕnz). [Siegmund Erben, Austrian physician, b. 1863] Retardation of pulse when head and trunk are forcibly bent forward.

erbium (ĕr'bē-ŭm). A rare metallic element. SYMB: Er. At. wt. 167.26; at. no. 68; sp. gr. 9.051.

Erb's paralysis. [Wilhelm H. Erb, Ger. neurologist, 1840–1921] Paralysis of group of muscles of shoulder and upper arm involving cervical roots of 5th and 6th spinal nerves. The arm hangs limp, the hand rotates inward, and normal movements are lost.

Erb's point. The point on the side of the neck 2 to 3 cm. above the clavicle and in front of the transverse process of the sixth cervical vertebra. Electrical stimulation over this area causes various arm muscles to contract.

erectile (ē-rĕk'tīl) [L. *erigere,* to erect]. Able to become erect.

erectile tissue. Vascular tissue that, when filled with blood, becomes erect or rigid, as the clitoris, penis, or nipples.

erection. The state of swelling, hardness, and stiffness observed in the penis and to a lesser extent in the clitoris of the female, generally due to sexual excitement. Caused by engorgement with blood of the corpora cavernosa and the corpus spongiosum of the penis and the corpus cavernosa clitoridis of the female.

Erection is necessary in the male for the natural intromission of the penis into the vagina of the female and for the emission of semen. The blood withdraws from the penis after ejaculation and the erection is reduced. Erection of the penis may occur as the result of sexual excitement, during sleep, or due to physical stimulation of the penis. Abnormal persistent erection of the penis not due to sexual excitement, but due to certain disease states, is called priapism, q.v. SEE: *nocturnal emission.*

erector [L. *erigere,* to erect]. A muscle that raises a part.

erector spinae reflex. Irritation of the skin over the erector spinae muscles causing contraction of muscles of the back. SYN: *dorsal reflex; lumbar reflex.*

eremophobia (ĕr″ĕm-ō-fō′bē-ă) [Gr. *eremos,* solitary, + *phobos,* fear]. Dread of being alone.

erepsin (ē-rĕp′sĭn). Term applied to a peptide-splitting enzyme found in the succus entericus (intestinal juice). The peptide-splitting action is due to the action of several peptidases that act on peptides that have escaped pancreatic digestion. This action converts polypeptides to amino acids.

erethism (ĕr′ĕ-thĭzm) [Gr. *erethismos,* irritation]. Excessive excitement or irritation to stimuli. Opposite of apathism.

e. mercurialis. Mental illness occurring as a result of chronic mercury poisoning.

erethismic (ĕr″ĕ-thĭz′mĭk). Pert. to or causing erethism. SYN: *erethitic.*

erethisophrenia (ĕr″ĕ-thĭ-zō-frē′nē-ă) [″ + *phren,* mind]. Unusual mental excitability.

erethistic (ĕr″ĕ-thĭs′tĭk) [Gr. *erethismos,* irritation]. Erethismic, exciting.

erethitic (ĕr″ĕ-thĭt′ĭk). Causing erethism; irritable, excited.

ereuthrophobia (ĕr″ū-thrō-fō′bē-ă) [Gr. *erythros,* red, + *phobos,* fear]. Pathological fear of blushing. SYN: *erythrophobia.*

ERG. *electroretinogram.*

erg [Gr. *ergon,* work]. In physics, the amount of work done when a force of 1 dyne acts through a distance of 1 cm. One erg is roughly 1/980 gram-centimeter. That is, to raise a load of 1 gm. against gravity the distance of 1 cm. requires that a force of 980 dynes operate through a distance of 1 cm. and hence that 980 ergs of work be done.

ergasiomania (ĕr-gā″sē-ō-mā′nē-ă) [Gr. *ergasia,* work, + *mania,* madness]. An abnormal desire to be busy at work.

ergasiophobia (ĕr-gā″sē-ō-fō′bē-ă) [″ + *phobos,* fear]. Abnormal dislike for work of any kind or for assuming responsibility.

ergasthenia (ĕr″găs-thē′nē-ă) [Gr. *ergon,* work, + *astheneia,* weakness]. A symptom, condition, or weakness due to overwork.

ergastic (ĕr-găs′tĭk) [Gr. *ergastikos*]. Possessing potential energy.

ergocalciferol (ĕr-gō-kăl-sĭf′ĕr-ŏl). USP. Vitamin D_2, an activated product of ergosterol. Primarily used in prophylaxis and treatment of vitamin D deficiency. Trade names are Deltalin and Drisdol. Previously used names are Oleovitamin D, synthetic; and Calciferol.

ergogenic (ĕr″gō-jĕn′ĭk) [Gr. *ergon,* work, + *gennan,* to produce]. To increase work, esp. to increase potential for work output.

ergograph (ĕr′gō-grăf) [″ + *graphein,* to write]. An apparatus for recording the contractions of muscles and measuring the amount of work done.

Ergomar. Trade name for ergotamine tartrate.

ergometer (ĕr-gŏm′ĕ-tĕr) [″ + *metron,* measure]. An apparatus for measuring the amount of work done by a human or animal subject.

e., bicycle. Stationary bicycle used in determining the amount of work performed by the rider.

ergonomics (ĕr″gō-nŏm′ĭks) [″ + *nomikos,* law]. The science that is concerned with the problem of how to fit a job to man's anatomical, physiological, and psychological characteristics in such a way as to enhance human efficiency and well-being.

ergonovine maleate (ĕr″gō-nō′vĭn). USP. An ergot derivative used in treating migraine, and in obstetrics to stimulate contractions of the uterus. Trade name is Ergotrate Maleate.

ergophobia (ĕr″gō-fō′bē-ă) [″ + *phobos,* fear]. Morbid dread of working.

ergophore (ĕr′gō-for) [″ + *pherein,* to bear]. That part of an antigen on which the specific properties of the substance depend. SYN: *toxophore.*

ergostat (ĕr′gō-stăt) [″ + *statos,* standing]. A machine for measuring work done by a contracting muscle.

Ergostate. Trade name for ergotamine tartrate.

ergosterol (ĕr-gŏs′tĕr-ŏl). A sterol found in plant and animal tissues. It is converted to vitamin D_2 by irradiation.

ergot (ĕr′gŏt). A drug obtained from Claviceps purpurea, a fungus that grows parasitically on rye. Several valuable alkaloids, as ergotamine, q.v., are obtained from ergot.

ergotamine (ĕr-gŏt′ă-mēn). $C_{33}H_{35}O_5N_5$. A crystalline alkaloid derived from ergot.

e. tartrate. USP. A white crystalline substance that stimulates smooth muscle of blood vessels and the uterus, inducing vasoconstriction and uterine contractions. Used in the treatment of migraine. Trade names are Ergomar, Ergostate, and Gynergen.

ergotherapy (ĕr″gō-thĕr′ă-pē) [″ + *therapeia,* treatment]. Work used as a treatment of disease.

ergotism (ĕr′gŏ-tĭzm). Poisoning resulting from excessive use of ergot or from eating food made from rye or wheat infected with the fungus Claviceps purpurea. May be acute or chronic. SEE: *ergot poisoning.*

ergot poisoning. May result from eating bread made with grain contaminated with the Claviceps purpurea fungus; or by taking overdoses of the drug.

SYM: Appear several hours after ingestion. Vomiting, burning, and cramping in abdomen; great thirst; profound weakness; diarrhea; slow weak pulse; anesthesia, tingling, and twitching in extremities; dilated pupils; occasionally convulsions; anuria. If patient survives, generalized gangrene, particularly of the extremities, may develop.

F.A.: Slurry of activated charcoal by mouth followed by emesis or gastric lavage and instillation of a saline cathartic, external heat. SEE: *Poisons and Poisoning* in *Appendix.*

ergotrate (ĕr′gō-trāt). An active principle isolated from ergot.

Ergotrate Maleate. Trade name for ergonovine maleate.

ergotropic [Gr. *ergon,* work, + *tropos,* a turning]. Pert. to ergotropy.

ergotropy (ĕr-gŏt′rō-pē). Injection of nonspecific proteins to increase body resistance.

Eristalis (ĕr-ĭs′tă-lĭs). A genus of flies belonging to the family Syrphidae. The larva, called rat-tailed maggot (E. tenax), may cause intestinal myiasis in man.

erode (ē-rōd′) [L. *erodere*]. 1. To wear away. 2. To eat away by ulceration.

erogenous (ĕr-ŏj′ĕ-nŭs) [Gr. *eros,* love, + *gennan,* to produce]. Causing sexual excitement. SYN: *erotogenic.*

erogenous zone. Any part of the body, touching or stroking of which can cause sexual excitement. SEE: *zone, erogenous.*

erosion (ē-rō′shŭn) [L. *erodere,* to gnaw away]. An eating away of tissue. External or internal destruction of a surface layer by physical or inflammatory processes.

e., dental. The wearing away of the surface layer (enamel) of a tooth.

e. of cervix uteri. The alteration of the epithelium on a portion of the cervix as a result of irritation by infection.

SYM: In the early stages, the epithelium shows necrosis, which nature tries to heal by a downgrowth of epithelium from the endocervical canal. If this is accomplished by a single layer of tissue having a grossly granular appearance, it is called a simple granular erosion. If the growth is excessive and shows papillary tufts, it is called a papillary erosion. Histologically, the papillary erosion shows many glands of the branching racemose type whose epithelium is the mucus-bearing cell with the nucleus at the base. In the healing process, squamous epithelium grows over the eroded area with the following results: the squamous cells take the place of the tissue beneath it completely, giving a complete healing, or the glands fill with squamous plugs and remain in that state, or the mouths of the glands are occluded by the squamous cells and cysts are formed (nabothian cysts). In the congenital type of erosion, the portio is covered by high columnar epithelium. SEE: *Papanicolaou test.*

TREATMENT: Prophylaxis, proper care of the cervix following delivery. Cauterization of the early erosion with electrocautery is usually curative.

erosive (ē-rō′sĭv). 1. Able to produce erosion. 2. An agent that erodes tissues or structures.

erotic (ĕ-rŏt′ĭk) [Gr. *erotikos*]. Pert. to sexual passion.

eroticism (ĕ-rŏt′ĭ-sĭzm) [″ + *-ismos,* condition]. Sexual desire.

e., allo-. Eroticism directed to an external object rather than to self.

e., anal. Sensations of pleasure experienced through defecation during a stage in the development of children. In psychiatry, fixation of the libido at the anal-erotic developmental stage.

e., auto-. 1. Self-gratification of the sexual instinct. Usually by manual stimulation of erogenous areas, esp. the penis or clitoris. SEE: *masturbation; urolagnia.* 2. Self-admiration combined with sexual emotion, such as that obtained from viewing one's naked body or one's genitals.

e., oral. 1. In psychiatry, fixation of the libido to the oral phase of development. 2. Sexual pleasure derived from use of the mouth.

erotism (ĕr′ō-tĭzm). Eroticism.

erotogenic (ĕ-rŏ″tō-jĕn′ĭk) [Gr. *eros,* love, + *gennan,* to produce]. Producing sexual excitement. SEE: *zone, erogenous.*

erotology (ĕr″ō-tŏl′ō-jē) [″ + *logos,* study]. The study of love and its manifestations.

erotomania (ĕ-rō″tō-, ĕ-rŏt″ō-mā′nē-ă) [″ + *mania,* madness]. Pathological exaggeration of sexual behavior.

erotopathia (ĕ-rō″tō-, ĕ-rŏt″ō-păth′ē-ă) [″ + *pathos,* disease]. Any abnormal sex impulse.

erotophobia (ĕ-rō″tō-, ĕ-rŏt″ō-fō′bē-ă) [″ + *phobos,* fear]. Aversion to sexual love or its manifestations.

erratic [L. *errare,* to wander]. Wandering, having an unpredictable or fluctuating course or pattern. SYN: *eccentric.*

errhine (ĕr′īn) [Gr. *en,* in, + *rhis,* nose]. 1. Causing increased nasal discharge. 2. An agent that increases nasal secretion or discharge.

erubescence [L. *erubescere,* to grow red].

Reddening of the skin; a blush.

eructation (ĕ-rŭk-tā'shŭn) [L. *eructare*]. Producing gas from the stomach, usually with a characteristic sound; belching.

eruption (ē-rŭp'shŭn) [L. *eruptio*, a breaking out]. 1. Breaking out and becoming visible, esp. applied to the appearance of a skin lesion or rash accompanying a disease such as measles or scarlet fever. 2. The appearance of a lesion such as redness or spotting on the skin or mucous membrane. 3. The breaking through of a tooth through the gum; the cutting of a tooth.

e., creeping. A skin lesion characterized by a tortuous elevated red line that progresses at one end while fading out at the other. It is caused by the migration of the larvae of certain nematodes, esp. Ancylostoma braziliense and A. canis, which occur as accidental invaders of man. SYN: *larva migrans*.

e., drug. Skin reaction resulting from the ingestion of certain drugs such as iodides. SYN: *dermatitis medicamentosa*.

e., serum. Eruption that occurs following the injection of a serum. May be accompanied by chills and fever.

eruptive. Pert. to breaking out.

erysipelas (ĕr"ĭ-sĭp'ĕ-lăs) [Gr. *erythros*, red, + *pella*, skin]. Acute febrile disease with localized inflammation and redness of skin and subcutaneous tissue accompanied by systemic disturbance.

ETIOL: Streptococcus pyogenes.

SYM: Fever; chills; nausea; vomiting; painful and warm skin; face and head lesions that are hot and red usually seen within 24 to 48 hours. Bullae may develop.

TREATMENT: Penicillin or erythromycin. Cool magnesium sulfate solution compresses for skin. Aspirin for pain.

PROG: Excellent with treatment. If untreated, nephritis, abscesses, and septicemia may develop.

erysipelatous (ĕr"ĭ-sĭ-pĕl'ă-tŭs). Of the nature of or pert. to erysipelas.

erysipeloid (ĕr-ĭ-sĭp'ĕ-loyd) [" + " + *eidos*, form]. An infective dermatitis resembling erysipelas usually limited to the hands and characterized by hyperemia, edema, and occasionally systemic complications.

ETIOL: Caused by Erysipelothrix rhusiopathiae, usually acquired by handling shellfish, poultry, or meat.

TREATMENT: Penicillin, cephalosporin, or clindamycin.

Erysipelothrix (ĕr"ĭ-sĭ-pĕl'ŏ-thrĭks) [" + " + *thrix*, hair]. A genus of bacteria belonging to the family Corynebacteriaceae. They are branching filamentous, rod-shaped, nonmotile organisms.

E. insidiosa. The causative agent of swine erysipelas and erysipeloid in man.

erysipelotoxin (ĕr"ĭ-sĭp"ĕ-lō-tŏk'sĭn). The toxin produced by Streptococcus pyogenes, the causative agent of erysipelas.

erysiphake (ĕr-ĭs'ĭ-fāk). A small spoon-shaped device used in cataract surgery to remove the lens by suction.

erythema (ĕr"ĭ-thē'mă) [Gr., redness]. A form of macula showing diffused redness over the skin.

ETIOL: Caused by capillary congestion, usually due to dilatation of the superficial capillaries as a result of some nervous mechanism within the body, inflammation, or some external influence such as heat, exposure to sunlight, or cold.

e. ab igne. Localized erythema due to exposure to heat.

e. annulare. Erythema that is ring-shaped.

e. congestivum. Erythema with congestive state of skin.

e., diffuse. Erythema that is widely spread over body.

e. hyperaemicum. Erythema caused by heat or cold (erythema caloricum, chilblain), sun (erythema solare), artificial heat as from hot water bottle or electric pad (erythema ab igne).

e. induratum. Chronic vasculitis of the skin occurring in young adult females. Characterized by hard cutaneous nodules that break down to form necrotic ulcers and leave atrophic scars. SYN: *Bazin's disease*.

e. infectiosum. Contagious form of erythema with rose-colored eruption.

e. intertrigo. Chafing of opposing surfaces with erythema and often with maceration and abrasion. SYN: *chafing*.

e. marginatum. A form of erythema multiforme in which the center of the area fades, leaving elevated edges.

e. multiforme. A macular eruption with dark red papules or tubercles. Usually on extremities appearing in successive eruptions of short duration. No itching, burning, or rheumatic pains. May appear in separate rings, concentric rings, disk-shaped patches, distributed elevations, and figured arrangements.

e. nodosum. Red and painful nodules on legs, associated with rheumatism. Also caused by certain drugs and food poisoning.

e., punctate. Erythema occurring in minute points, as scarlet fever rash.

e. toxicum. A benign, self-limited occurrence of firm, yellow-white papules or pustules from 1 to 2 mm. in size that are present in about 50% of full-term infants. The cause is unknown, and the lesions disappear without need for treatment.

e. venenatum. Form caused by contact

with a toxic substance.

erythematic, erythematous (ĕr″ĭ-thē-măt′ĭk, ĕr″ĭ-thĕm′ă-tŭs) [Gr. *erythema,* redness]. Pert. to or marked by erythema.

erythemogenic (ĕr″ĭ-thē″mō-jĕn′ĭk) [″ + *gennan,* to produce]. Pert. to erythema.

erythralgia (ĕr″ĭ-thrăl′jē-ă) [″ + *algos,* pain]. A condition of painful redness of the skin. SYN: *erythromelalgia.*

erythrasma (ĕr″ĭ-thrăz′mă). Reddish-brown eruption in patches in the axillae and groin caused by Corynebacterium minitissimum.

erythredema (ĕ-rĭth″rē-dē′mă) [″ + *oidema,* swelling]. An infantile disease characterized by lesions of the skin on the hands and feet, swelling of the extremities, digestive disturbances and itching. It is frequently followed by arthritis involving multiple joints and with muscle weakness. Its cause is unknown but mercury may be an etiological agent. SYN: *acrodynia.*

erythremia (ĕr″ĭ-thrē′mē-ă) [″ + *haima,* blood]. Polycythemia vera, q.v.

erythrism (ĕ-rĭth′rĭzm) [″ + *-ismos,* condition of]. Redness of the hair and beard with ruddy complexion.

erythristic (ĕr″ĭ-thrĭs′tĭk). Having a ruddy complexion and red hair.

erythrityl tetranitrate (ĕ-rĭth′rĭ-tĭl). USP. Drug used to dilate the coronary arteries. Used in treating angina pectoris. Trade name is Cardilate.

erythro- [Gr. *erythros*]. Prefix meaning red.

erythroblast (ĕ-rĭth′rō-blăst) [″ + *blastos,* germ]. Any form of nucleated red corpuscles. The earliest stages in the development are pronormoblast, basophilic normoblast, polychromatic normoblast, and orthochromatic normoblast. Nucleated red cells are not normally seen in the circulating blood. Erythroblasts contain hemoglobin. In the embryo they are found in blood islands of the yolk sac, body mesenchyma, liver, spleen, and lymph nodes; after the third month they are restricted to the bone marrow.

erythroblastemia (ĕ-rĭth″rō-blăs-tē′mē-ă) [″ + ″ + *haima,* blood]. An excessive number of erythroblasts in the blood.

erythroblastic. Pert. to erythroblasts.

erythroblastoma (ĕ-rĭth″rō-blăs-tō′mă) [″ + *blastos,* germ, + *oma,* tumor]. A tumor (myeloma) with cells resembling megaloblasts.

erythroblastosis (ĕ-rĭth″rō-blăs-tō′sĭs) [″ + ″ + *osis,* condition]. A condition marked by the presence of erythroblasts in the blood.

e. fetalis. A hemolytic disease of the newborn characterized by anemia, jaundice, enlargement of the liver and spleen, and generalized edema (hydrops fetalis). SEE: *hemolytic disease of the newborn.*

erythrochloropia (ĕ-rĭth″rō-klor-ō′pē-ă) [Gr. *erythros,* red, + *chloros,* green, + *ops,* eye]. Partial color blindness with ability to see red and green, but not blue and yellow.

erythrochromia (ĕ-rĭth″rō-krō′mē-ă) [″ + *chroma,* color]. Hemorrhagic red pigmentation of the spinal fluid.

Erythrocin Lactobionate-I.V. Trade name for erythromycin lactobionate for injection.

erythroclasis (ĕr″ĕ-thrŏk′lă-sĭs). The splitting up of red blood cells.

erythroclastic (ĕ-rĭth″rō-klăs′tĭk) [″ + *klasis,* a breaking]. Destructive to red blood cells.

erythrocyanosis (ĕ-rĭth-rō-sī″ă-nō′sĭs) [″ + *kyanos,* blue, + *osis,* condition]. Red or bluish discoloration on the skin with swelling, itching, and burning.

erythrocyte (ĕ-rĭth′rō-sīt) [″ + *kytos,* cell]. A mature red blood cell or corpuscle. Each is a non-nucleated, biconcave disk averaging 7.7 microns in diameter. The body of the cell consists of a spongelike stroma containing a respiratory pigment, hemoglobin, enclosed in a cell membrane of proteins in combination with lipoid substances. Hemoglobin is a conjugated protein consisting of a colored iron-containing portion (hematin) and a simple protein (globin). It combines readily with oxygen to form an unstable compound (oxyhemoglobin). The total surface area of the red cells of an average adult is 3820 square meters or about 2000 times greater than the total body surface area. SEE: *blood cell* for illus.

NUMBER: In a normal person, the number of erythrocytes averages about 5,000,000 per cu. mm. (5,500,000 for males, 4,500,000 for females). The total number in an average-sized person is about 35 trillion. The number per cu. mm. varies with age (being higher in infants), time of day (being lower during sleep), activity and environmental temperature (increasing in both conditions), and altitude. Persons living at altitudes of 10,000 ft. (3,048 m.) or more may have a red cell count of 8,000,000/cu. mm. or more.

If an individual has a normal blood volume of 5 L. (70 ml./kg. of body weight), 5,000,000 red blood cells/cu. mm. of blood, and the erythrocytes have an average life span of 120 days, then the body needs to produce 2,400,000 red blood cells per second in order to maintain this concentration of blood.

PHYS: The primary function of the red blood cells is to carry oxygen and carbon dioxide but they also play a role in the regulation of the acid-base balance of the blood and in the formation of bile pigments, which are derived from decomposition products of hemoglobin.

DEVELOP: Red cell formation (erythropoiesis) in the adult takes place in the red bone marrow, principally in the vertebrae, ribs, sternum, diploë of cranial bones, and proximal ends of the humerus and femur. They arise from large nucleated stem-cells (promegaloblasts), which give rise to pronormoblasts, in which hemoglobin appears. These give rise to normoblasts, which extrude their nuclei. Red cells at this stage possess a fine reticular network and are known as reticulocytes. This reticular structure is lost before the cells enter circulation as mature erythrocytes. The proper formation of erythrocytes depends upon several factors, among them healthy condition of the bone marrow, dietary substances such as iron, cobalt, and copper, all essential for the formation of hemoglobin, plus essential amino acids and certain vitamins, esp. B_{12} and folic acid (pteroylglutamic acid).

The average length of life of a red blood cell is 120 days. Cells are continuously dying, disintegrating, and being replaced. The cellular debris is picked up by the cells of the reticuloendothelial system, esp. those of the spleen, liver, and bone marrow. Hemoglobin is broken down, and proteins and iron are stored and utilized in the formation of new erythrocytes. The iron-containing portion (hematin) gives rise to bilirubin, which is excreted in the bile as one of the bile pigments.

VARIETIES: On microscopic examination erythrocytes may reveal variations in the following respects: size (anisocytosis); shape (poikilocytosis); staining reaction (achromia, hypochromia, hyperchromia, polychromatophilia); structure (possession of bodies such as Cabot's rings, Howell-Jolly bodies, Heinz bodies; parasites such as malaria; a reticular network; or nuclei); and number (anemia, polycythemia).

e., achromatic. An erythrocyte from which the hemoglobin has been dissolved; a colorless corpuscle.

e., basophilic. Erythrocyte in which cytoplasm stains blue, indicating the presence of basophilic material. May be diffuse (basophilic material uniformly distributed) or punctate (material appearing as pin point dots).

e., crenated. Erythrocyte with a serrated or indented edge, usually the result of withdrawal of water from the cell as occurs when cells are placed in hypertonic solutions.

e., immature. An erythroblast; any immature erythrocyte.

e., orthochromatic. Erythrocyte that stains with acid stains only, cytoplasm appearing pink.

e., polychromatic. Erythrocyte that does not stain uniformly.

erythrocyte sedimentation rate. SEE: *sedimentation rate.*

erythrocythemia (ĕ-rĭth″rō-sī-thē′mē-ă) [Gr. *erythros,* red, + *kytos,* cell, + *haima,* blood]. Enormous increase in circulating red blood cells. SEE: *erythremia; polycythemia vera.*

erythrocytolysin (ĕ-rĭth″rō-sī-tŏl′ĭ-sĭn). Anything that hemolyzes red blood cells.

erythrocytolysis (ĕ-rĭth″rō-sī-tŏl′ĭ-sĭs) [″ + ″ + *lysis,* dissolution]. Dissolution of red blood corpuscles with the escape of hemoglobin.

erythrocytometer (ĕ-rĭth″rō-sī-tŏm′ĕ-tĕr) [″ + ″ + *metron,* measure]. Instrument for counting red blood cells.

erythrocytoopsonin (ĕ-rĭth″rō-sī″tō-ŏp-sō′nĭn) [″ + ″ + *opsonein,* to prepare food for]. A substance opsonic for red corpuscles.

erythrocytopenia (ĕ-rĭth″rō-sī″tō-pē′nē-ă) [″ + ″ + *penia,* poverty]. Decreased amount of red blood cells in the body. SYN: *erythropenia.*

erythrocytopoiesis (ĕ-rĭth″rō-sī″tō-poy-ē′sĭs) [″ + ″ + *poiesis,* making]. Formation of red blood cells; erythropoiesis.

erythrocytorrhexis (ĕ-rĭth″rō-sī″tō-rĕk′sĭs) [″ + ″ + *rhexis,* rupture]. The breaking up of red blood cells with particles or fragments of the cell escaping into the plasma. SYN: *plasmorrhexis.*

erythrocytoschisis (ĕ-rĭth″rō-sī-tŏs′kĭ-sĭs) [″ + ″ + *schisis,* division]. The breaking up of red blood cells into small disk-like particles resembling blood platelets.

erythrocytosis (ĕ-rĭth″rō-sī-tō′sĭs) [″ + ″ + *osis,* increasing condition]. Abnormal increase in the number of red blood cells in circulation, secondary to many disorders.

erythroderma (ĕ-rĭth″rō-dĕr′mă) [″ + *derma,* skin]. Abnormal redness of skin, usually pert. to widespread areas of erythema. SYN: *erythrodermia.*

e. desquamativum. A disease, resembling seborrhea, of breast-fed infants. Characterized by redness of skin and development of scales.

e. ichthyosiforme congenitum. A congenital condition characterized by thickening and redness of the skin; may resemble ichthyosis or lichen.

e., maculopapular. A condition of the skin characterized by redness and eruption of macules and papules.

e. squamosum. An eruption of the skin consisting of groups of papules covered by scales. SYN: *parapsoriasis.*

erythrodermia (ĕ-rĭth″rō-dĕr′mē-ă). Erythroderma.

erythrodextrin (ĕ-rĭth″rō-dĕx′trĭn) [″ + L. *dexter,* right]. Dextrin formed by hydrolysis of starch. When iodine is mixed with it, a red color is produced. SEE: *achroodextrin.*

erythrodontia (ĕ-rĭth″rō-dŏn′shē-ă) [″ + *odous,* tooth]. Reddish-brown staining of the teeth.

erythrogenesis (ĕ-rĭth″rō-jĕn′ĕ-sĭs) [″ + *genesis,* development]. The development of red blood cells.

erythroid (ĕr'ĭ-throyd) [" + *eidos,* form]. 1. Of a reddish color. 2. Concerning the red blood cells.

erythrokeratodermia (ĕ-rĭth"rō-kĕr"ă-tō-dĕr'mē-ă) [" + *keras,* horn, + *derma,* skin]. Reddening and hardening of the skin.

erythrokinetics (ĕ-rĭth"rō-kĭ-nĕt'ĭks) [" + *kinesis,* motion]. The quantitative description of the rate of production of red blood cells and their life-span.

erythroleukemia (ĕ-rĭth"rō-loo-kē'mē-ă) [Gr. *erythros,* red, + *leukos,* white, + *haima,* blood]. Malignant growth of both the red- and white-blood-cell-forming tissues. Rapid and progressive disorder accompanied by severe anemia and many abnormal white and red cells in the blood. Changes similar to those of pernicious anemia and myelocytic leukemia.

erythroleukosis (ĕ-rĭth"rō-loo-kō'sĭs) [" + " + *osis,* condition]. Abnormal increase of red cells and granulocytes.

erythrolysin (ĕr"ĭ-thrŏl'ĭ-sĭn) [" + *lysis,* dissolution]. An agent causing erythrolysis. SYN: *erythrocytolysin; hemolysin.* SEE: *lysin.*

erythrolysis. Dissolution of red blood corpuscles. SYN: *erythrocytolysis.*

erythromania (ĕ-rĭth"rō-mā'nē-ă) [" + *mania,* madness]. Uncontrolled blushing.

erythromelalgia (ĕ-rĭth"rō-mĕl-ăl'jē-ă) [" + *melos,* limb, + *algos,* pain]. A condition affecting the extremities, esp. the feet, characterized by burning and throbbing sensations, which come and go.

erythromelia (ĕ-rĭth"rō-mē'lē-ă) [" + *melos,* limb]. Erythema of extensor surfaces of extremities but without pain.

erythromycin (ĕ-rĭth"rō-mī'sĭn) [" + *mykes,* fungus]. USP. An antibiotic from Streptomyces erythreus. It is effective orally against many gram-positive and some gram-negative organisms. Trade names are Erythrocin, Ethyl Succinate, E.E.S., Pediamycin, E-Mycin E, and Wyamycin E.

erythron (ĕr'ĭ-thrŏn) [Gr. *erythros,* red]. The concept of blood as a body system including the circulating red cells and the organ from which they arise.

erythroneocytosis (ĕ-rĭth"rō-nē"ō-sī-tō'sĭs) [" + *neos,* new, + *kytos,* cell, + *osis,* condition]. Presence of immature red blood cells in the peripheral blood.

erythronoclastic (ĕ-rĭth"rō-nō-klăs'tĭk) [" + *klan,* to break]. Destructive to the erythron.

erythroparasite (ĕ-rĭth"rō-păr'ă-sīt) [" + *parasitos,* parasite]. A red blood cell parasite.

erythropathy (ĕr"ĭ-thrŏp'ă-thē) [" + *pathos,* disease]. Disease of the red blood cells.

erythropenia (ĕ-rĭth"rō-pē'nē-ă) [" + *penia,* poverty]. Deficiency in number of red blood cells.

erythrophage (ĕ-rĭth'rō-fāj) [" + *phagein,* to eat]. A phagocyte that destroys red blood cells.

erythrophagia. Destruction of red blood cells by phagocytes.

erythrophile, erythrophilous (ĕ-rĭth'rō-fĭl, ĕr"ĭ-thrŏf'ĭ-lŭs) [" + *philein,* to love]. Readily staining red.

erythrophobia (ĕ-rĭth"rō-fō'bē-ă) [" + *phobos,* fear]. 1. Abnormal dread of blushing or fear of being diffident or of being embarrassed. 2. A morbid fear of, or aversion to, anything colored red.

erythrophose (ĕ-rĭth'rō-fōz) [" + *phos,* light]. Any red subjective perception of a bright spot. SEE: *phose.*

erythrophthisis (ĕ-rĭth"rō-thī'sĭs) [" + *phthisis,* wasting]. Serious damage to the restorative power of the red corpuscles.

erythropia, erythropsia (ĕr"ĭ-thrō'pē-ă, -thrŏp'sē-ă) [" + *opsis,* vision]. Condition in which objects appear to be red.

erythroplasia (ĕ-rĭth"rō-plā'zē-ă) [" + *plasis,* molding, forming]. A condition characterized by the appearance of erythematous lesions of the mucous membranes.

e. of Queyrat. A rare precancerous dermatosis of the genital mucosa that occurs predominantly in uncircumcised men. Treatment with fluorouracil is usually effective.

erythropoiesis (ĕ-rĭth"rō-poy-ē'sĭs) [" + *poiesis,* making]. The formation of red blood cells.

erythropoietic (ĕ-rĭth"rō-poy-ĕt'ĭk). Pert. to red blood cells.

erythropoietin (ĕ-rĭth"rō-poy'ĕ-tĭn). A hormone that stimulates red blood cell production. It is an alpha-globulin that is either formed in or released by the kidney as well as by other tissues.

erythroprosopalgia (e-rĭth"rō-prō-sō-păl'jē-ă) [" + *prosopon,* face, + *algos,* pain]. A neuropathy characterized by redness and pain in the face.

erythropsia (ĕr-ĭ-thrŏp'sē-ă) [" + *opsis,* vision]. Perversion of color vision in which all objects look red.

erythropsin (ĕ-rĭth-rŏp'sĭn) [" + *opsis,* vision]. Pigment in the external portion of the rods of the retina. SYN: *rhodopsin.*

erythrorrhexis (ĕ-rĭth"rō-rĕks'ĭs) [" + *rhexis,* rupture]. Rupture of a red cell and escape of its plasma. SYN: *erythrocytorrhexis; plasmorrhexis.*

erythrosine sodium. USP. A dye used as a dental disclosing agent. Applied to the teeth in a 2% solution or in soluble tablets, which are chewed. SEE: *disclosing agent.*

erythrosis (ĕr-ĭ-thrō'sĭs) [" + *osis,* condition]. A reddish-purple discoloration of the skin and mucous membranes in polycythemia.

erythrostasis (ĕ-rĭth"rō-stā'sĭs) [" + *stasis,* standing still]. Accumulation of red blood cells in vessels due to blood flow having ceased. SEE: *sludged blood.*

erythrotoxin (ĕ-rĭth″rō-tŏk′sĭn) [″ + *toxikon,* poison]. An exotoxin that attacks red blood cells.

erythruria (ĕr-ĭ-thrū′rē-ă) [″ + *ouron,* urine]. Red color of the urine.

Es. Chem. symb. for einsteinium.

escape [O. Fr. *escaper*]. 1. To escape from confinement; leak or seep out. 2. The act of attaining freedom.

e., vagal. Occurrence of a ventricular contraction when the normal rhythmical beat of the heart has been stopped or inhibited by stimulation of the vagus nerve.

e., ventricular. Occurrence of single or repeated ventricular contractions from impulses arising in the atrioventricular node rather than the sinoauricular node. SYN: *extrasystole, nodal.*

escape beat. SEE: *beat, escape.*

eschar (ĕs′kăr) [Gr. *eschara,* scab]. A slough, esp. one following a cauterization or burn. SEE: *escharotic.*

escharotic (ĕs-kăr-ŏt′ĭk) [Gr. *escharotikos*]. Agent used to destroy tissue and to cause sloughing, which produces what is known as an eschar. Escharotics may be acids, alkalies, metallic salts, phenol or carbolic acid, carbon dioxide, or electric cautery.

escharotomy (ĕs-kăr-ŏt′ō-mē) [Gr. *eschara,* scab, + *tome,* incision]. Removal of the eschar formed on the skin and underlying tissue of severely burned areas. Procedure is particularly helpful in restoring circulation to the extremities of patients in which the eschar forms a tight swollen band around the circumference of the limb.

Escherich's reflex (ĕsh′ĕr-ĭks). [Theodor Escherich, Ger. physician, 1857–1911] Pursing or muscular contraction of lips resulting from irritation of mucosa of lips.

Escherichia (ĕsh-ĕr-ĭk′ē-ă). A genus of bacteria belonging to the family Enterobacteriaceae, tribe Eschericheae. They are common inhabitants of the alimentary canal of man and other animals.

E. coli. The colon bacillus. Short, plump, gram-negative, non-spore-forming motile bacilli almost constantly present in the alimentary canal of humans and other animals. They are normally nonpathogenic in the intestinal tract. Outside the body and under certain conditions, particularly in the urinary tract, E. coli is responsible for infections in other systems and for enteritis in infants. Certain enteropathogenic strains are a principal cause of traveler's diarrhea. The presence of the bacilli in milk or water is an indicator of fecal contamination.

eschrolalia (ĕs-krō-lā′lē-ă) [Gr. *aischros,* indecent, + *lalia,* babble]. Meaningless utterance of obscene words. SYN: *coprolalia.*

escorcin (ĕs-kor′sĭn). A stain derived from escalin. It is used to stain and identify defects or injury of the cornea of the eye.

esculent (ĕs′kū-lĕnt). Suitable for use as food.

escutcheon (ĕs-kŭch′ăn) [L. *scutum,* a shield]. The pattern of pubic hair growth. It is different in the male and female.

eserine (ĕs′ĕr-ĭn) [*esere,* African name for the Calabar bean]. Physostigmine, q.v.

Eserine Salicylate. Trade name for physostigmine salicylate.

ESF. *erythropoietic stimulating factor.* SEE: *erythropoietin.*

Esidrix. Trade name for hydrochlorothiazide.

Eskabarb. Trade name for phenobarbital.

Eskalith. Trade name for lithium carbonate.

Esmarch's bandage (ĕs′mărks). [Johannes F. A. von Esmarch, Ger. surgeon, 1823–1908] 1. A triangular bandage. 2. A rubber bandage used to control bleeding. Before the surgery is begun, the bandage is applied tightly to the limb, commencing at the distal end and reaching above the site of operation, where a rubber tourniquet is firmly applied. The bandage is then removed. This renders the surgical area virtually bloodless.

CAUTION: Tourniquet must not be applied so tightly as to cause nerve damage and it must be removed in time to prevent injury caused by lack of blood flow to the distal tissues. SEE: *bandage.*

esodic (ē-sŏd′ĭk) [Gr. *es,* toward, + *hodos,* way]. Pert. to sensory nerves conducting impulses toward the brain and spinal cord. SYN: *afferent; centripetal.*

esoethmoiditis (ĕs″ō-ĕth″moy-dī′tĭs) [Gr. *eso,* inward, + *ethmos,* sieve, + *eidos,* form, + *itis,* inflammation]. Inflammation of membrane of ethmoid cells.

esogastritis (ĕs″ō-găs-trī′tĭs) [″ + *gaster,* belly, + *itis,* inflammation]. Inflammation of the gastric mucous membrane.

esophagalgia (ē-sŏf-ă-găl′jē-ă) [Gr. *oisophagos,* esophagus, + *algos,* pain]. Pain in the esophagus.

esophageal (ē-sŏf″ă-jē′ăl). Pert. to the esophagus.

esophageal web. Thin membranous structures that include mucosal and submucosal coats across the esophagus. They may be congenital or may follow trauma, inflammation, or ulceration of the esophagus. SEE: *Plummer-Vinson syndrome.*

esophagectasia, esophagectasis (ē-sŏf″ă-jĕk-tā′sē-ă, -jĕk′tă-sĭs) [″ + *ektasis,* distention]. Dilatation of the esophagus.

esophagectomy (ē-sŏf″ă-jĕk′tō-mē) [″ + *ektome,* excision]. Excision of a part of the esophagus.

esophagismus (ē-sŏf-ă-jĭs′mŭs) [″ + *-ismos,* condition]. Esophageal spasm.

esophagitis (ē-sŏf-ă-jī'tĭs) [" + *itis,* inflammation]. Inflammation of the esophagus.

esophagobronchial (ē-sŏf"ă-gō-brŏng'kē-ăl) [" + *bronchos,* windpipe]. Concerning the esophagus and the bronchus.

esophagocele (ē-sŏf'ă-gō-sēl) [" + *kele,* hernia]. Hernia of the esophagus.

esophagodynia (ē-sŏf"ă-gō-dĭn'ē-ă) [Gr. *oisophagos,* esophagus, + *odyne,* pain]. Pain in the esophagus.

esophagoenterostomy (ē-sŏf"ă-gō-ĕn-tĕr-ŏs'tō-mē) [" + *enteron,* intestine, + *stoma,* mouth]. Formation of communication between the esophagus and intestine following excision of stomach.

esophagogastrectomy (ē-sŏf"ă-gō-găs-trĕk'tō-mē) [" + *gaster,* belly, + *ektome,* excision]. Surgical removal of all or part of the stomach and esophagus.

esophagogastroanastomosis (ē-sŏf"ă-gō-găs"trō-ă-năs"tō-mō'sĭs) [" + " + *anastomosis,* opening]. Joining the esophagus to the stomach.

esophagogastroplasty (ē-sŏf"ă-gō-găs'trō-plăs"tē) [" + " + *plassein,* to form]. Plastic repair of the esophagus and the stomach.

esophagogastroscopy (ē-sŏf"ă-gō-găs-trŏs'kō-pē) [" + " + *skopein,* to examine]. Inspection of esophagus and stomach by using a type of endoscope.

esophagogastrostomy (ē-sŏf"ă-gō-găs-trŏs'tō-mē) [" + " + *stoma,* mouth]. Formation of a communication between the esophagus and stomach.

esophagojejunostomy (ē-sŏf"ă-gō-jĕ-jū-nŏs'tō-mē) [" + L. *jejunum,* empty, + Gr. *stoma,* mouth]. Surgical anastomosis of a free end of the jejunum to the esophagus. This provides a bypass for food in cases of esophageal stricture.

esophagomalacia (ē-sŏf"ă-gō-mă-lā'sē-ă) [Gr. *oisophagos,* esophagus, + *malakia,* softness]. Softening of the esophageal walls.

esophagomycosis (ē-sŏf"ă-gō-mī-kō'sĭs) [" + *mykes,* fungus, + *osis,* condition]. Bacterial or fungus disease of esophagus.

esophagomyotomy (ē-sŏf"ă-gō-mī-ŏt'ō-mē) [" + *mys,* muscle, + *tome,* incision]. Cutting of the muscular coat of the esophagus. May be used in treating stenosis of the lower esophagus.

esophagoplasty (ē-sŏf'ă-gō-plăs"tē) [" + *plassein,* to form]. Repair of the esophagus by a plastic operation.

esophagoplication (ē-sŏf"ă-gō-plī-kā'shŭn) [" + L. *abplicare,* to fold]. The surgical procedure of reducing dilation of the esophagus by taking tucks in its walls.

esophagoptosia, esophagoptosis (ē-sŏf"ă-gŏp-tō'sē-ă, -sĭs) [" + *ptosis,* a falling]. Relaxation and prolapse of the esophagus.

esophagoscope (ē-sŏf'ă-gō-skōp) [" + *skopein,* to examine]. A type of endoscope for examination of the esophagus.

esophagospasm (ē-sŏf'ă-gō-spăzm") [" + *spasmos,* spasm]. Spasm of the esophagus.

esophagostenosis (ē-sŏf"ă-gō-stĕn-ō'sĭs) [" + *stenosis,* contraction]. Stricture or narrowing of the esophagus.

esophagostomy (ē-sŏf-ă-gŏs'tō-mē) [" + *stoma,* opening]. Surgical formation of an opening into the esophagus

esophagotome (ē-sŏf'ă-gō-tōm) [" + *tome,* incision]. Instrument for forming an esophageal fistula.

esophagotomy (ē-sŏf-ă-gŏt'ō-mē). Surgical incision into the esophagus SEE: *achalasia; cardiospasm; dysphagia.*

esophagotracheal (ē-sŏf"ă-gō-trā'kē-ăl). Concerning the esophagus and the trachea, or a communication between the two.

esophagus (ē-sŏf'ă-gŭs) [Gr *oisophagos*]. (pl. *esophagi*) [NA] A muscular canal extending from the pharynx to the stomach. This vital structure is essential for carrying swallowed foods and liquids from the mouth to the stomach. Length about 9 to 9.75 in. (23 to 25 cm.)

e., foreign bodies in. The patient may complain of pain or an uncomfortable feeling deep in the chest.

A physician should always be called. Foreign bodies are ordinarily not dangerous and usually pass through the alimentary tract in a few days without danger. However, it may be dangerous to give cathartics or enemas. These patients should always be under the care of a physician. SEE: *Heimlich maneuver.*

F.A.: The article often can be dislodged by making the patient vomit by using the finger to stimulate the oral pharynx or back part of the throat.

esophoria (ĕs-ō-fō'rē-ă) [Gr *eso,* inward, + *phorein,* to bear]. Tendency of visual lines to converge. Inward turning or amount of inward turning of the eye. Opposite of exophoria. SYN: *esotropia.* SEE: *heterotropia.*

esosphenoiditis (ĕs"ō-sfē-noyd-ī'tĭs) [" + *sphen,* wedge, + *eidos,* form, + *itis,* inflammation]. Osteomyelitis of the sphenoid bone.

esotropia (ĕs-ō-trō'pē-ă) [" + *tropos,* turning]. Marked turning inward of eye, crossed eyes. SYN: *esophoria.*

ESP. *extrasensory perception.*

ESR. *electron spin resistance, erythrocyte sedimentation rate.*

-ess [O. Fr. *-esse*]. Suffix noting female sex.

essence [L. *essentia,* being or quality]. 1. The spirit or principle of anything. 2. An alcoholic solution of volatile oil.

essential [L. *essentialis*]. 1. Pert. to an essence. 2. Indispensable. 3. Independent of a local morbid condition, having no obvious external cause. SEE: *idiopathic*.

EST. *electroshock therapy*. SEE: *electroconvulsive therapy*.

ester [L. *aether*, ether]. In organic chemistry, a compound formed by the combination of an organic acid with an alcohol. Water is eliminated in this reaction.

Ex.: Ethyl acetate is an ester formed by combining acetic acid with ethyl alcohol. Esters are commonly liquids with characteristic fruity or flowery odors.

esterase (ĕs′tĕr-ās). Generic term for an enzyme that catalyzes the hydrolysis of esters.

esterification (ĕs-tĕr″ĭ-fĭ-kā′shŭn). Combination of an organic acid with an alcohol to form an ester.

esterize. To convert into an ester.

esthematology (ĕs″thĕm-ă-tŏl′ō-jē) [Gr. *aisthema*, sensation, + *logos*, science]. Science of the sense organs and their function.

esthesia (ĕs-thē′zē-ă) [Gr. *aisthesis*, sensation]. 1. Perception, feeling, sensation. 2. Any disease that affects sensation or perception.

esthesiology (ĕs-thē″zē-ŏl′ō-jē) [″ + *logos*, science]. Science of sensory phenomena. SYN: *esthematology*.

esthesiomania (ĕs-thē″zē-ō-mā′nē-ă) [″ + *mania*, madness]. Insanity with sensory hallucinations and perverted moral sensibilities.

esthesiometer (ĕs-thē-zē-ŏm′ĕ-tĕr) [″ + *metron*, measure]. Device for measuring tactile sensibility. Also spelled aesthesiometer.

esthesioneurosis (ĕs-thē″zē-ō-nū-rō′sĭs) [″ + *neuron*, nerve, + *osis*, condition]. Any sensory impairment.

esthesiophysiology (ĕs-thē″sē-ō-fĭs-ē-ŏl′ō-jē) [″ + *physis*, nature, + *logos*, study]. Physiology of the sense organs.

esthesioscopy (ĕs-thē″zē-ŏs′kō-pē) [″ + *skopein*, to examine]. Testing tactile and other forms of sensibility.

estheticokinetic (ĕs-thĕt″ĭ-kō-kĭn-ĕt′ĭk) [″ + *kinesis*, motion]. Being both sensory and motor.

esthetics (ĕs-thĕt′ĭks). Aesthetics, q.v.

esthiomene (ĕs″thē-ŏm′ĕ-nē) [Gr. *esthiomenos*, eating]. A chronic hypertrophic ulcerative vulvovaginitis. A complication of lymphogranuloma venereum.

Estinyl. Trade name for ethinyl estradiol.

estival (ĕs′tĭ-văl) [L. *aestivus*]. Rel. to or occurring in summer.

estivoautumnal [″ + *autumnalis*, pert. to autumn]. Pert. to summer and autumn, formerly applied to a type of malaria.

Estrace. Trade name for estradiol.

estradiol (ĕs-tră-dī′ŏl). USP. $C_{18}H_{24}O_2$, a steroid produced by the ovary and possessing estrogenic properties. Large quantities are found in the urine of pregnant women and mares and in the urine of stallions, the latter two serving as sources of the commercial product. Estradiol is effective when given subcutaneously or intramuscularly but not when administered orally. It is converted to estrone in the body. Trade names are Estrace and Progynon. SEE: *estrogen*.

e. dipropionate. An ester of estradiol.

estrin (ĕs′trĭn). Estrogen.

estrinization (ĕs″trĭn-ĭ-zā′shŭn). Production of vaginal epithelial changes characteristic of estrogen stimulation.

estriol (ĕs′trē-ŏl). USP. $C_{18}H_{24}O_3$ Estrogenic hormone considered to be the metabolic product of estrone and estradiol. It is found in the urine of the female.

estrogen (ĕs′trō-jĕn) [Gr. *oistros*, mad desire, + *gennan*, to produce]. Any natural or artificial substance that induces estrogenic activity; more specifically the estrogenic hormones, estradiol and estrone, produced by the ovary; the female sex hormones. Estrogens are responsible for the development of secondary sexual characteristics and for cyclic changes in the vaginal epithelium and endothelium of the uterus. Natural estrogens include estradiol, estrone, and their metabolic product, estriol. When used therapeutically, estrogens are usually given in the form of a conjugate such as ethinyl estradiol, conjugated estrogens, USP, q.v., or the synthetic estrogenic substance, diethylstilbestrol. These preparations are effective when given by mouth.

Estrogens provide a satisfactory replacement hormone for the treatment of menopause. It is important to observe closely patients treated this way for any malignant changes in the breast or endometrium. Estrogen should be administered intermittently and in the lowest effective dose.

e.′s, conjugated. USP. Estrogenic substances, principally estrone and equilin, excreted by pregnant mares. Trade names are Premarin and Sodestrin.

estrogenic (ĕs-trō-jĕn′ĭk). Causing estrus; acting to produce the effects of an estrogen.

estrone (ĕs′trōn). USP. $C_{18}H_{22}O_2$. An estrogenic hormone found in the urine of pregnant women and mares. It is also prepared synthetically. Used in the treatment of estrogen deficiencies. It is less active than estradiol but more active than estriol. Trade name is Theelin.

estropipate. USP. Estrogen. Previously used name was piperazine estrone citrate. Trade name is Ogen.

estrual (ĕs′troo-ăl) [Gr. *oistros*, mad desire]. Pert. to estrus of animals.

estruation. The sexually fertile period in animals; the so-called period of heat.

estrus, oestrus [Gr. *oistros*, mad desire]. The cyclic period of sexual activity in female mammals, other than human females, called heat, characterized by congestion of and secretion by the uterine mucosa, proliferation of vaginal epithelium, swelling of the vulva, ovulation, and acceptance of the male by the female.

estrus cycle. The cycle from the beginning of one estrus period to the beginning of the next. Includes proestrus, estrus, and metestrus followed by a short period of quiescence called diestrus.

estuarium (ĕs″tū-ā′rē-ŭm) [L.]. Vapor bath.

état criblé (ā-tă′ krēb-lā′) [Fr., sievelike state]. Multiple irregular perforations of Peyer's patches of the intestines. These patches are characteristic of typhoid fever.

état mamelonné (ā-tă′ mă-mĕl-ŏn-ā′) [Fr., knobby state]. Condition of gastric mucosa in chronic inflammation with nodular projections.

ethacrynic acid. USP. A diuretic drug. Trade name is Edecrin.

ethambutol hydrochloride (ĕ-thăm′bū-tōl). USP. A drug used in treating tuberculosis. It is used in combination with isoniazid. Trade name is Myambutol.

Ethamide. Trade name for ethoxzolamide.

ethamivan (ĕth-ăm′ĭ-văn″). Drug used to stimulate respiration. It is no longer commercially available in the U.S.A.

ethanol (ĕth′ă-nŏl). Ethyl alcohol. SEE: *alcohol.*

ethaverine hydrochloride (ĕth″ă-vĕr′ēn). Drug used to produce coronary artery relaxation. Its use is of questionable value.

ethchlorvynol (ĕth-klor′vĭ-nŏl). USP. A sedative hypnotic drug that may produce addiction. Trade name is Placidyl.

ethene (ĕth-ēn′). Ethylene, $CH_2=CH_2$.

ether [Gr. *aither,* air]. Any organic compound in which an oxygen atom links together with carbon chains. The ether used for anesthesia is diethyl ether, $C_4H_{10}O$. As an anesthetic it causes postoperative nausea and profuse salivation.

ether anesthesia. $C_4H_{10}O$. Ethyl oxide or diethyl ether, the common ether previously used in anesthesia. It is rarely used now.

CAUTION: Ether is highly flammable and should be handled with great care. Also, it should not be stored once the can is opened because toxic products form when ether is exposed to light.

NURSING IMPLICATIONS: Observe the patient's level of consciousness, take vital signs, and observe for nausea and vomiting as the patient recovers from the effects of the anesthesia. Position the patient on side or with head turned to the side to decrease chance of aspiration if the patient vomits. Cold compresses may be placed on the head. Rectal irrigations or insertion of a rectal tube may be ordered to relieve gas pressure.

ether asphyxia. Suffocation during ether anesthetization. SEE: *resuscitation.*

ether bed. Bed prepared to receive patient immediately following an operative procedure requiring anesthesia.

ethereal (ĕ-thē′rē-ăl) [Gr. *aither,* air]. Pert. to or made with ether.

etherization (ē″thĕr-ĭ-zā′shŭn). Administration of ether to induce anesthesia.

etherize (ē′thĕr-īz). To anesthetize by use of ether.

etheromania (ē″thĕr-ō-mā′nē-ă) [″ + *mania,* madness]. Addiction to use of ether.

ethics [Gr. *ethos,* moral custom]. A system of moral principles or standards governing conduct.

e., dental. A system of principles governing dental practice; a moral obligation to render the best possible quality of dental service to the patient and to maintain an honest relationship with other members of the profession and mankind in general.

e., medical. A system of principles governing medical conduct. It deals with the relationship of a physician to the patient, the patient's family, fellow physicians, and society at large.

e., nursing. A system of principles governing conduct of a nurse. It deals with the relationship of a nurse to the patient, the patient's family, associates and fellow nurses, and society at large.

ethinamate (ĕ-thĭn′ă-māt). USP. A mild sedative and hypnotic drug. Trade name is Valmid.

ethinyl estradiol (ĕth′ĭ-nĭl). USP. Trade names are Estinyl and Feminone. SEE: *estradiol.*

ethionamide (ĕ-thī″ŏn-ăm′īd). USP. A drug used in treating tuberculosis. It is used in combination with other drugs. Trade name is Trecator-SC.

ethionine (ĕ-thī′ō-nĭn). A progestational agent used in some oral contraceptives.

ethmocarditis (ĕth″mō-kăr-dī′tĭs) [Gr. *ethmos,* sieve, + *kardia,* heart, + *itis,* inflammation]. Inflammation of cardiac connective tissue.

ethmoid (ĕth′moyd) [″ + *eidos,* form]. Sievelike; cribriform.

ethmoid bone. Sievelike spongy bone that forms a roof for the nasal fossae and part of the floor of the anterior fossa of the skull. It contains a number of thin-walled cellular cavities, the ethmoidal cells, which are arranged in three groups. They open into the nasal cavity.

ethmoid sinus. Air cells or space inside the ethmoid bone, opening into nasal cavity.

ethmoidal. Pert. to the ethmoid bone or sinuses.

ethmoidectomy (ĕth-moy-dĕk′tō-mē) [″ + *ei-*

dos, form, + *ektome,* excision]. Excision of ethmoid cells that open into nasal cavity.

ethmoiditis (ĕth″moy-dī′tĭs) [″ + ″ + *itis,* inflammation]. Inflammation of ethmoidal cells. May be acute or chronic.

SYM: Headache, acute pain between eyes, nasal discharge.

ethnic (ĕth′nĭk) [Gr. *ethnikos,* of a nation]. Concerning groups of people within a cultural system who desire or are given special status based on traits such as religion, culture, language, or appearance.

ethnobiology (ĕth″nō-bī-ŏl′ō-jē) [Gr. *ethnos,* race, + *bios,* life, + *logos,* science]. Study of the biological characteristics of various races.

ethnography (ĕth-nŏg′ră-fē) [″ + *graphein,* to write]. The study of the culture of a single society. Data are gathered during a period of residence with the group by direct observation. SEE: *anthropology.*

ethnology (ĕth-nŏl′ō-jē) [″ + *logos,* science]. The comparative study of cultures using ethnographic data. SEE: *anthropology.*

ethology (ĕ-, ē-thŏl′ō-jē) [Gr. *ethos,* manners, habits, + *logos,* science]. Scientific study of customs and behavior of animals in their natural habitat

ethopropazine hydrochloride (ĕth″ō-prō′pă-zēn). USP. An autonomic nervous system blocking agent used in treating parkinsonism. Trade name is Prasidol.

ethosuximide (ĕth″ō-sŭk′sĭ-mīd). USP. An anticonvulsant drug. Trade name is Zarontin.

ethotoin (ĕ-thō′tō-ĭn). An anticonvulsant that, because of its moderate effectiveness, is little used. Trade name is Peganone.

ethoxzolamide (ĕth″ŏks-zōl′ă-mīd). USP. A carbonic anhydrase inhibitor used in treating glaucoma. Trade names are Cardrase and Ethamide.

ethyl (ĕth′ĭl) [Gr. *aither,* air, + *hyle,* matter]. In organic chemistry, the radical C_2H_5, which is contained in a great number of compounds, including ethyl ether, ethyl alcohol, and ethyl acetate.

e. acetate. $CH_3COOC_2H_5$. A colorless flammable liquid used as a solvent.

e. alcohol. C_2H_5OH. Grain alcohol. SEE: *alcohol; Poisons and Poisoning* in *Appendix.*

e. aminobenzoate. Benzocaine, a topical anesthetic.

e. biscoumacetate. An anticoagulant drug.

e. chaulmoograte. The ethyl esters of the fatty acids of chaulmoogra oil. Used in the treatment of leprosy.

e. chloride. USP. C_2H_5Cl. A very volatile liquid with a pleasant odor. When sprayed on the skin, it evaporates so quickly that the tissue is cooled immediately. Because of this property, the skin is anesthetized.

USES: Local anesthetic in minor surgery. It is a topical anesthetic and is used only for very short periods of anesthesia.

e., vanillin. A flavoring agent.

ethylamine (ĕth″ĭl-ăm′ĭn). $CH_3CH_2NH_2$. An amine formed in the decomposition of certain proteins.

ethylcellulose (ĕth″ĭl-sĕl′ū-lōs). An ether of cellulose. It is used in preparing drugs.

ethylene (ĕth′ĭl-ēn). CH_2CH_2. A colorless gas prepared from alcohol by dehydration. Present in illuminating gas. It is colorless and has a sweetish taste but a pungent, foul odor. It is lighter than air and diffusible when liberated. It is flammable and explosive.

e. glycol. $C_2H_6O_2$. The simplest glycol; a colorless alcohol used as an antifreeze. SEE: *Poisons and Poisoning* in *Appendix.*

e. oxide. A chemical, C_2H_4O, that in its gaseous state is used to sterilize materials that can't withstand heat or steam. Also used as a fumigant.

ethylene anesthesia. Since ethylene is a rather weak anesthetic, it usually is given in a combination of oxygen 20%, cyclopropane 10%, and ethylene 70%.

PHYS. EFFECTS: Ethylene causes less alteration in the blood gases than nitrous oxide. Ethylene alone causes very little muscular relaxation; the blood pressure may rise and respiration is not depressed. Analgesia results before loss of hearing or before complete unconsciousness. Nausea and vomiting seldom persist as long as 24 hr., but generally disappear before consciousness has returned.

ADVAN: Slightly stimulating to cardiac and respiratory systems. It is not irritating to mucous glands and kidneys. It has a short period of induction and makes possible a very rapid recovery. There is an absence of cyanosis and a minimum of emesis.

DISADVAN: It has an objectionable smell; it is highly flammable and explosive; many lives have been lost because someone was careless and a spark was emitted from some immediate source.

PRECAUTIONS: Ethylene should be stored where there is adequate ventilation. It should be administered away from fire, electric appliances, or x-ray apparatus. To prevent sparks, all lights should be turned on before bringing the tanks into the room. Furniture should never be dragged into the room or rolled into the room while the anesthetic is being given. The humidity of the room should be controlled during the administration of this anesthetic. Nylon clothing or undergarments should not be worn by anyone in the room; friction from the material may generate static electricity.

Ethylene does not combine as readily with

air as do other anesthetics but floats around as clouds. The vapor rises in a cloudlike form and any gust of air may carry it out of the room; a devastating explosion will result if someone on the outside is smoking or if the fumes contact an electrical spark.

Ethylene always is stored in red tanks; oxygen in green tanks; nitrous oxide in blue tanks; carbon dioxide in gray tanks.

ethylenediamine (ĕth″ĭ-lēn-dī′ă-mēn). USP. Drug used as a solvent for theophylline; it is therefore present in aminophylline injection.

ethylmorphine (ĕth″ĭl-mor′fēn). A drug similar to codeine, used as an anti-cough preparation.

ethylnorepinephrine hydrochloride (ĕth″ĭl-nor-ĕp″ĭ-nĕf′rĭn). USP. An adrenergic drug used in treating asthma. Trade name is Bronkephrine.

ethynodiol diacetate (ĕ-thī″nō-dī′ŏl). USP. A progestational drug.

ethynyl (ĕth″ĭ-nĭl). An organic radical, H≡C—.

etiocholanolone (ē″tē-ō-kō-lăn′ō-lōn). A steroid produced by testosterone catabolism. It is excreted in the urine.

etiologic, etiological (ē″tē-ō-lŏj′ĭk, -ĭ-kăl) [Gr. *aitia,* cause, + *logos,* study]. Pert. to the cause or causes of disease.

etiology (ē″tē-ŏl′ō-jē). The study of the causes of disease.

etiotropic (ē″tē-ō-trŏp′ĭk) [Gr. *aita,* cause, + *tropos,* turning]. Directed against the cause of a disease, said of a drug or treatment that destroys or inactivates the causal agent of a disease. Opposite of nosotropic.

etymology (ĕt″ĭ-mŏl′ō-jē) [Gr. *etymologia*]. The science of the origin and development of words. Most medical words are derived from Latin and Greek, but many of those from the Greek have reached us through the Latin, being modified by that language. Generally when two Greek words are used to form one word, they are connected by the letter "o." Many medical words have been formed from one or more roots, forms used or adapted from the Latin or Greek, and many of them are modified either by a prefix or a suffix, or both. A knowledge of important Latin or Greek roots and prefixes will reveal the meaning of a great many other words. SEE: *Prefixes and Suffixes* in *Appendix.*

Eu. Chem. symb. for europium.

eu- [Gr. *eus,* good]. Prefix meaning healthy, normal, good, well.

Eubacteriales (ū″băk-tē-rē-ā′lēz) [Gr. *eus,* good, + *bakterion,* little rod]. An order of bacteria that includes many of the microorganisms pathogenic to man.

Eubacterium (ū″băk-tē′rē-ŭm). Genus of bacteria that is a member of the order Eubacteriales.

eubiotics (ū″bī-ŏt′ĭks) [″ + *bios,* life]. The science of healthy and hygienic living.

eubolism (ū′bŏl-ĭzm). Normal metabolism.

eucalyptol (ū″kă-lĭp′tŏl) [″ + *kalyptein,* to cover]. A substance obtained from oil of eucalyptus. Has an aromatic odor and has been used in expectorants.

eucalyptus oil (ū-kă-lĭp′tŭs). Oil distilled from fresh leaves of the plant. Used as an expectorant.

eucapnia (ū-kăp′nē-ă) [″ + *kapnos,* smoke]. Presence of normal amounts of carbon dioxide in the blood.

eucatropine hydrochloride (ū-kăt′rō-pēn). USP. An anticholinergic used as a mydriatic. It is applied topically to the eye.

euchlorhydria (ū″klor-hī′drē-ă). Presence of the normal amount of free hydrochloric acid in the gastric juice.

eucholia (ū-kō′lē-ă) [″ + *chole,* bile]. Normal condition of bile regarding its constituents and amount secreted.

euchromatin (ū-krō′mă-tĭn) [″ + *chroma,* color]. Chromatin that is rich in nucleic acid and is genetically active. SEE: *heterochromatin.*

euchylia (ū-kī′lē-ă) [″ + *chylos,* chyle]. Normal condition of the chyle.

eucrasia (ū-krā′sē-ă) [″ + *krasis,* mixture]. Condition of normal health; state of the body in which all activities are in normal balance.

eudiaphoresis (ū″dī-ă-fō-rē′sĭs) [″ + *dia,* through, + *pherein,* to carry]. Normal secretion of perspiration.

eudiometer (ū″dē-ŏm′ĕ-tĕr) [Gr. *eudia,* good weather, + *metron,* measure]. An instrument for testing purity of air and making analysis of gases.

euesthesia (ū-ĕs-thē′sē-ă) [Gr. *eus,* good, + *aisthesis,* sensation]. Having normal senses.

eugenics (ū-jĕn′ĭks) [″ + *gennan,* to produce]. The science that deals with the genetic and prenatal influences that affect the expression of certain characteristics in offspring. SYN: *aristogenics.*

eugenol (ū′jĕn-ŏl). USP. A material obtained from clove oil and other sources. A topical analgesic used in dentistry. It is also mixed with zinc oxide to form a material that will harden sufficiently to be used as a temporary dental filling.

euglobulin (ū-glŏb′ū-lĭn). A true globulin, or one that is insoluble in distilled water and soluble in dilute salt solution. SEE: *pseudoglobulin.*

eugonic (ū-gŏn′ĭk) [Gr. *eus,* good, + *gone,* seed]. Pert. to a luxuriant growth of bacteria.

eukaryon (ū-kăr′ē-ŏn) [″ + *karyon,* nucleus]. The nucleus of a eukaryote cell.

eukaryote (ū-kăr′ē-ōt). An organism in which the cell nucleus is surrounded by a membrane. SEE: *prokaryote.*

eukinesia (ū-kĭn-ē'sē-ă) [" + *kinesis,* motion]. Normal power of movement.

Eulenburg's disease (oyl'ĕn-bŭrgz). [Albert Eulenburg, Ger. neurologist, 1840–1917] Myotonia congenita. SYN: *Thomsen's disease; paramyotonia congenita.*

Eumycetes (ū"mī-sē'tēz) [" + *mykes,* fungus]. A class of Thallophyta including all the true fungi.

eunoia (ū-noy'ă) [" + *nous,* mind]. Soundness of mind.

eunuch (ū'nŭk) [Gr. *eune,* bed, + *echein,* to guard]. Castrated male; one who has had his testicles removed, esp. before puberty so that secondary sexual characteristics do not develop. Absence of the male hormone produces certain symptoms, such as a female type of voice and loss of hair on the face. In Middle Eastern and Eastern countries, eunuchs were employed to guard the women of a harem.

eunuchism (ū'nŭk-ĭzm) [" + " + *-ismos,* condition]. Condition resulting from complete lack of male hormone. This may be due to atrophy or removal of testicles.

e., pituitary. Condition produced by failure of the anterior lobe of the pituitary to secrete gonadotrophic hormones; secondary hypogonadism.

eunuchoid (ū'nŭ-koyd) [" + " + *eidos,* form]. Having the characteristics of a eunuch such as retarded development of sex organs, absence of beard and bodily hair, high-pitched voice, and striking lack of muscular development.

eunuchoidism (ū'nŭk-oyd-ĭzm) [" + " + " + *-ismos,* condition]. Deficient production of male hormone, androgen, by the testes.

eupancreatism (ū-păn'krē-ă-tĭzm) [Gr. *eus,* good, + *pankreas,* pancreas, + *-ismos,* condition]. Normal condition of the pancreas.

eupepsia [" + *pepsis,* digestion]. Normal digestion as distinguished from dyspepsia.

eupeptic. Pert. to good digestion.

euphonia (ū-fōn'ē-ă) [" + *phone,* voice]. Having a normal clear voice.

euphoria (ū-for'ē-ă) [" + *phoros,* bearing]. 1. A condition of good health. 2. In psychiatry, an exaggerated feeling of well-being; mild elation.

euplastic (ū-plăs'tĭk) [" + *plastikos,* formed]. Healing quickly and well.

euploidy (ū-ploy'dē) [" + *ploos,* fold, + *eidos,* form]. In genetics, the state of having complete sets of chromosomes.

eupnea (ūp-nē'ă) [" + *pnein,* to breathe]. Normal breathing as distinguished from dyspnea and apnea.

eupraxia (ū-prăks'ē-ă) [" + *prassein,* to do]. Normal capacity to execute a motor pattern. SEE: *paralysis.*

eupraxic (ū-prăks'ĭk). Contributing to proper functioning.

europium (ŭ-rō'pē-ŭm). A rare element of the lanthanide series. SYMB: Eu. At. no. 63; at. wt. 151.96.

Eurotium (ū-rō'shē-ŭm) [Gr. *euros,* mold]. A genus of molds.

eury- (ū'rē) [Gr. *eurys,* wide]. A prefix indicating broad.

eurycephalic (ū"rē-sĕ-făl'ĭk) [" + *kephale,* head]. Having a broad or wide head.

eustachian (ū-stā'kē-ăn, -shĕn). [Bartolommeo Eustachio, It. anatomist, 1524–1574]. Pert. to the auditory tube. SEE: *ear; eustachian tube.*

eustachian catheter. Instrument for insertion into eustachian tube.

eustachianography. Radiographic examination of the eustachian tube and middle ear after the introduction of a contrast agent.

eustachian tube. The auditory tube, extending from the middle ear to the pharynx, 3 to 4 cm. long and lined with mucous membrane. Occlusion of the tube leads to the development of otitis media. SEE: *politzerization.* SYN: *otopharyngeal tube.*

eustachian valve. Valve at the entrance of the inferior vena cava.

eustachitis (ū"stā-kī'tĭs). Inflammation of the eustachian tube.

eusystole (ū-sĭs'tō-lē) [Gr. *eus,* good, + *systellein,* to draw together]. A state of the systole of the heart that is normal in time and force.

eutectic (ū-tĕk'tĭk) [Gr. *eutektos*]. Easily melted.

eutectic mixture. A mixture of two or more substances that has a melting point lower than that of any of its constituents.

euthanasia (ū-thă-nā'zē-ă) [Gr. *eus,* good, + *thanatos,* death]. 1. Dying easily, quietly, and painlessly. 2. The act of willfully ending life in individuals with an incurable disease.

euthenics (ū-thĕn'ĭks) [Gr. *euthenia,* well-being]. The science of improvement of a population through modification of the environment.

Eutheria. Mammals with a true placenta.

Euthroid. Trade name for liotrix.

euthyroid (ū-thī'royd). Normal thyroid gland function.

eutocia (ū-tō'sē-ă) [Gr. *eus,* good, + *tokos,* birth]. Normal or natural labor and childbirth.

Eutonyl. Trade name for pargyline hydrochloride.

Eutrombicula (ū"trŏm-bĭk'ū-lă). A genus of mites.

eutrophication (ū-trŏf"ĭ-kā'shŭn) [Gr. *eutrophein,* to thrive]. Alteration of the environment by increasing the nutrients required by one species to the disadvantage of other species in the ecosystem.

ev, eV, EV. *electron volt.*

evacuant (ē-văk'ū-ănt) [L. *evacuans,* making

empty]. Drug that stimulates the bowels to move.

evacuate [L. *evacuatio,* emptying]. 1. To discharge, esp. from the bowels; to empty the uterus. 2. To move patients from place or site of accident or catastrophe to a hospital or shelter.

evacuation (ē-văk″ū-ā′shŭn). 1. Act of emptying, esp. the bowels. 2. The material discharged from the bowels; stool. 3. Removal of air from a closed container; the production of a vacuum. 4. Act of moving people to a safe place, esp. from a disaster or a war-torn area.

evacuator (ē-văk′ū-ā-tor). Device for emptying, as of the bowels, or for irrigating the bladder and removing calculi.

evaginate (ē-văj′ĭ-nāt) [L. *evaginare,* to unsheath]. Pert. to protrusion of some part or organ from its normal place.

evagination (ē-văj-ĭ-nā′shŭn). 1. Emergence from a sheath. 2. Protrusion of an organ or part. SEE: *invagination.*

evaluation. The judgment of anything; but in medicine, consideration of the health and physical and mental capability and potential of a patient or of one considered to be healthy.

evanescent (ĕv″ă-nĕs′ĕnt) [L. *evanescere,* to vanish]. Not permanent; of brief duration; passing gradually.

Evans blue. [Herbert M. Evans, U.S. anatomist, 1882–1971] USP. A diazo dye occurring as a bluish-green powder, very soluble in water. It is used intravenously as a diagnostic agent.

Evans syndrome. An autoimmune disease characterized by thrombocytopenia and hemolytic anemia.

evaporation [L. *e,* out, + *vaporare,* to steam]. 1. Change from liquid form to vapor. 2. Loss in volume due to conversion of a liquid into a vapor.

eventration (ē″vĕn-trā′shŭn) [L. *e,* out, + *venter,* belly]. 1. Partial protrusion of the abdominal contents through an opening in the abdominal wall. 2. Removal of contents of the abdominal cavity.

eversion (ē-vĕr′zhŭn) [″ + *vertere,* to turn]. Turning outward. SEE: *chilectropion.*

evidement (ā-vĕd-mŏn′) [Fr., a scooping out]. Scraping away diseased tissue.

evil [AS. *yfel*]. Disease or illness.

eviration (ē″vī-rā′shŭn) [L. *e,* out, + *vir,* man]. 1. Castration. 2. In psychiatry, delusion in a male who thinks he has become a woman.

evisceration (ē-vĭs″ĕr-ā′shŭn) [″ + *viscera,* viscera]. 1. Removal of the viscera or of the contents of a cavity. 2. Spilling out of abdominal contents resulting from wound dehiscence.

NURSING IMPLICATIONS: Contact physician immediately. Cover the wound with a sterile towel moistened with sterile physiological saline (warm). Tension on the abdomen may be decreased by having the patient flex knees slightly, and be placed in Fowler's position. Reassure the patient that he or she is all right and will be helped. Inform the patient of the need for surgery, and prepare the patient for surgery.

evisceroneurotomy (ē-vĭs″ĕr-ō-nū-rŏt′ō-mē) [″ + ″ + Gr. *neuron,* nerve, + *tome,* incision]. Scleral evisceration of the eye with division of optic nerve.

evocation (ĕv″ō-kā′shŭn) [″ + *vocare,* to call]. To create anew by memory recall or by imagination.

evoked response. Method of testing the function of certain sense organs, even if the subject is unconscious or uncooperative. A patient who is thought to be deaf can be exposed to sound. If the hearing pathway is intact, the electroencephalograph will record that the sound stimulus did indeed reach the brain. SEE: *auditory evoked response.*

evolution (ĕv″ō-lū′shŭn) [L. *e,* out, + *volvere,* to roll]. A process of orderly and gradual change or development. More generally, any orderly and gradual process of modification whereby a system, whether physical, chemical, social, or intellectual, becomes more highly organized.

e., theory of. The theory that all species of plants and animals, including man, have come into existence by gradual continuous change from earlier forms. SEE: *natural selection.*

evulsion (ē-vŭl′shŭn) [″ + *vellere,* to pluck]. 1. Tearing away of a part or new growth. 2. Forcible extraction as of teeth.

Ewing's tumor or sarcoma (ū′ĭngz). [James Ewing, U.S. pathologist, 1866–1943] A diffuse endothelioma or endothelial myeloma forming a fusiform swelling on a long bone.

ex- [L., Gr. *ex,* out]. Prefix indicating out, away from, completely.

exacerbation (ĕks-ăs″ĕr-bā′shŭn) [″ + *acerbus,* harsh]. Aggravation of symptoms or increase in the severity of a disease.

exaltation [L. *exaltare,* to lift up]. A mental state characterized by feelings of grandeur, excessive joy, elation, and optimism; an abnormal feeling of personal well-being or self-importance.

examination [L. *examinare,* to examine]. The act or process of inspection of the body and its systems to determine the presence or absence of disease. Terms employed indicate type of examination: physical, bimanual, digital, oral, rectal, OB (obstetrical), roentgenological, cystoscopic.

Local physical examination includes specific parts and organs. Four procedures utilized are inspection, palpation, percussion, and auscultation. Laboratory examination includes urinalysis, blood tests, cultures, and various special means of visualizing body spaces and organs and their functions. SEE: *abdominal examination.*

exangia (ĕks-ăn′jē-ă) [Gr. *ex,* out, + *angeion,* vessel]. Any dilatation of a blood vessel, as an aneurysm or varix.

exanthem (ĕks-ăn′thĕm) [Gr. *exanthema,* eruption]. (pl. *exanthems*) Any eruption of the skin accompanied by inflammation, such as measles, scarlatina, erysipelas.

e. subitum. An acute disease of infants. Probably due to a virus. Marked by high fever for three or four days and sometimes convulsions at the onset. A diffuse maculopapular rash usually appears just at the time the fever suddenly subsides. Treatment is symptomatic. SYN: *roseola infantum.* SEE: *convulsion.*

exanthema (ĕks-ăn-thē′mă) [Gr.] (pl. *exanthemas, -mata*) Exanthem.

exanthematous (ĕks″ăn-thĕm′ă-tŭs). Pert. to an eruption or rash.

exanthrope (ĕks′ăn-thrōp) [Gr. *ex,* out, + *anthropos,* man]. A cause or source of a disease originating outside the body.

exarticulation (ĕks″ăr-tĭk-ū-lā′shŭn) [L. *ex, out,* + *articulus,* joint]. 1. Amputation of a limb through a joint. 2. Excision of a part of a joint.

excavation (ĕks″kă-vā′shŭn) [″ + *cavus,* hollow]. 1. A hollow or depression. 2. Formation of a cavity.

e., atrophic. A hollow or cupped appearance of the optic nerve head as seen by use of the ophthalmoscope.

e., dental. The preparation of a cavity in a tooth prior to filling.

e. of optic nerve. A slight depression in the center of the optic papilla or disk from which retinal vessels emerge. Depression is total in glaucoma as a result of high intraocular pressure.

e., rectouterine. The rectouterine pouch or pouch of Douglas.

excavator (ĕks′kă-vā″tor). Instrument for removing tissue or bone. It may be spoon-shaped if used on soft tissue and spoon-shaped with sharp edges if used in dentistry.

excerebration (ĕk″sĕr-ĕ-brā′shŭn) [″ + *cerebrum,* brain]. Removal of the brain, esp. that of the dead fetus in order to facilitate delivery.

exchange transfusion. Transfusion and withdrawal of small amounts of blood repeated until blood volume is almost entirely exchanged. Used in infants born with hemolytic disease and in patients with uremia.

excipient (ĕk-sĭp′ē-ĕnt) [L. *excipiens,* excepting]. Any substance added to a medicine to permit it to be formed into the proper shape and consistency; the vehicle for the drug.

excise (ĕk-sīz′) [L. *ex,* out, + *caedere,* to cut]. To cut out or remove surgically.

excision (ĕk-sĭ′zhŭn) [L. *excisio*]. An act of cutting away or taking out.

excitability [L. *excitare,* to arouse]. Sensitiveness to being stimulated.

e., independent. Power of a muscle to respond to a stimulus without intervention of motor nerves.

e., muscle. The property of a muscle fiber to be excited to contract. This is a function of the chemical state of the nerve membrane and the time since a previous stimulus was applied.

e., nerve. The property of a nerve to produce an action potential. This is a function of the permeability of the nerve membrane. The membrane is influenced by physical, chemical, and electrical forces. Also, the intensity of electrical stimuli will influence the ability of the nerve to be excited.

e., reflex. Sensitiveness to reflex irritation.

excitant (ĕk-sīt′ănt). An agent that will excite a special function of the body; subdivided, according to action, as motor, cerebral, etc. Amphetamine, cocaine, and strychnine are examples of excitants.

excitation [L. *excitatio*]. 1. The act of exciting. 2. Condition of being stimulated or excited.

e., direct. Stimulation of a muscle by placing an electrode in it or physically stimulating it.

e., indirect. Stimulation of a muscle via its nerve.

excitation wave. The wave of irritability originating in the sinoatrial node that sweeps over the conductile tissue of the heart and induces contraction of the atria and ventricles.

exciting. Causing excitement.

excitoglandular (ĕk-sīt″ō-glăn′dū-lăr) [L. *excitare,* to arouse, + *glans,* kernel]. Increasing glandular function.

excitometabolic (ĕk-sīt″ō-mĕt″ă-bŏl′ĭk) [″ + Gr. *metabole,* change]. Inducing metabolic changes.

excitomotor (ĕk-sīt″ō-mō′tor) [″ + *motor,* moving]. Increasing rapidity of muscular activity.

excitomuscular (ĕk-sīt″ō-mŭs′kū-lăr) [″ + Gr. *mys,* muscle]. Causing muscular activity.

excitor (ĕk-sī′tor) [L. *excitare,* to arouse]. That which incites to greater activity. SYN: *stimulant.*

excitosecretory (ĕk-sīt″ō-sē′krĕ-tor-ē) [″ + *secretio,* a hiding]. Tending to bring about secretion.

excitovascular (ĕk-sī″tō-văs′kū-lăr) [″ + *vascularis,* pert. to a vessel]. Increasing circulation activity.

exclave (ĕks′klāv) [Gr. *ex,* out, + L. *clavis,*

key]. A detached portion of an organ, an accessory gland such as a spleen or pancreas.

exclusion (ĕks-kloo'zhŭn) [L. *exclusio*, fr. *ex*, out, + *claudere*, to shut]. To shut off or remove from the main part.

excochleation (ĕks-kŏk-lē-ā'shŭn) [L. *ex*, out, + *cochlea*, spoon]. Scraping out or curetting the contents of a cavity.

excoriation (ĕks-kō-rē-ā'shŭn) [" + *corium*, skin]. Abrasion of the epidermis or of the coating of any organ of the body by trauma, chemicals, burns, or other causes.

excrement (ĕks'krĕ-mĕnt) [L. *excrementum*]. Waste material passed out of the body, esp. feces. SEE: *excretion*.

excrementitious (ĕks"krĕ-mĕn-tĭsh'ŭs). Of the nature of excrement.

excrescence (ĕks-krĕs'ĕns) [L. *ex*, out, + *crescere*, to grow]. Any outgrowth from the surface of a part.

excreta (ĕks-krē'tă) [L.]. Waste matter excreted from the body, including feces, urine, and perspiration. In some diseases, the excreta of the patient contains infectious material. This must be disinfected and handled carefully by hospital personnel.

Pads made of absorbent materials should be placed under the patient who has involuntary discharges. When disposed of, the pads should be placed in sturdy plastic bags. In handling all infected discharges, the nurse should wear rubber gloves and a face mask.

DISINFECTION: When using the following disinfecting materials, be certain they do not come in contact with skin or eyes.

Phenol: A 5% solution to be used in quantity at least equal to the amount of the material to be disinfected.

Chlorinated lime: Dissolve in the proportion of 4 oz. (120 ml.) to one gal. (3.8 L.) of water. One qt. (946 ml.) of this solution for disinfection of each liquid discharge. For solid fecal matter a stronger solution or a larger quantity of this solution will be required.

excrete (ĕks-krēt') [L. *excretus*, sifted out]. To expel or eliminate waste material from the body, blood, or organs.

excretin (ĕks'krē-tĭn). A crystalline substance derived from the feces. A fraction of the hormone secretin, which stimulates pancreatic secretion.

excretion (ĕks-krē'shŭn) [L. *excretio*]. 1. Waste matter, excreta. 2. The elimination of waste products from the body.

ORGANS: *Intestines:* indigestible residue, water, and bacteria. *Kidneys:* water, nitrogenous substances (urea, uric acid, creatine, creatinine), mineral salts. *Respiratory system:* carbon dioxide, water vapor, and other gases. *Skin:* small amt. through perspiration of water, salts, minute quantities of urea. Its excretory function is stimulated by kidney inactivity. In renal failure, diaphoretics, hot packs, and warm blankets stimulate skin, thus helping to avoid uremic coma.

excretion, words pert. to: defecation; dejecta; diarrhea; elimination excrement; excreta; expectoration; feces; hydragogue; incontinence; lung; perspiration; pore; respiration; skin; sputum; stool; sweat; urine; void; vomit; vomiting; vomitus.

excretory (ĕks'krē-tō-rē) [L. *excretus*, sifted out]. Pert. to or bringing about excretion.

excursion (ĕks-kŭr'zhŭn) [L. *excursio*]. 1. Wandering from the usual course. 2. Extent of movement of a part such as the extremities or eyes.

excurvation (ĕks"kŭr-vā'shŭn) [Gr. *ex*, out, + L. *curvus*, bend]. A curvature outward.

excystation (ĕk"sĭs-tā'shŭn) [" + *kystis*, cyst]. Pert. esp. to the escape of certain organisms (parasitic worms or protozoa) from an enclosing cyst wall or envelope. Process that occurs in the life cycle of an intestinal parasite after encysted form is ingested.

exencephalia (ĕks"ĕn-sĕf-ā'ē-ă) [" + *enkephalos*, brain]. A congenital anomaly in which the brain is located outside the skull. A term for encephalocele, hydrencephalocele, and meningocele.

exenteration (ĕks-ĕn"tĕr-ā'shŭn) [" + *enteron*, intestine]. Evisceration.

exercise [L. *exercitus*, having drilled]. Performed activity of the muscles, voluntary or otherwise, esp. to maintain fitness. SEE: table.

e., active. A form of bodily movement that the patient performs by voluntary contraction and relaxation of muscles.

e., assistive. A form of bodily movement that the patient performs by voluntary contraction and relaxation of muscles with the aid of a therapist.

e., blowing. Exercise in which the patient blows into a tube connected to a bottle with water in it. That bottle is attached to another bottle so that the air pressure produced forces water from one bottle into the other. This increases intrabronchial pressure, which tends to aid in expansion of the lung. It is by this means that obliteration of an empyema cavity is facilitated. SEE: *empyema*.

e., Buerger's postural. Exercise used for circulatory disturbances of the extremities.

e., corrective. Use of specific exercises to correct deficiencies caused by trauma or inactivity.

e., crawling. Exercise devised for treatment of scoliosis, q.v., essentially for children. SEE: *patterning*.

e., free. Bodily movement that is carried through by patient with no external assis-

Exercise: Energy Required*

Calories Required per Hour of Exercise	Activity
80	Sitting quietly, reading
200	Golf with use of powered cart
250	Walking 3 miles/hr. (4.83 km./hr.); housework; light industry; cycling 6 miles/hr. (9.7 km./hr.)
330	Heavy housework; walking 3.5 miles/hr. (5.6 km./hr.); cycling 6 miles/hr. (9.7 km./hr.); golf, carrying own bag; tennis, doubles; ballet exercises
400	Walking 5 miles/hr. (8 km./hr.); cycling 10 miles/hr. (16.1 km./hr.); tennis, singles; water skiing
500	Manual labor; gardening; shoveling
660	Running 5.5 miles/hr. (8.9 km./hr.); cycling 13 miles/hr. (20.9 km./hr.); climbing stairs; heavy manual work
1020	Running 8 miles/hr. (12.9 km./hr.); climbing stairs with 30-pound (13.61 kg.) load

*These estimates are approximate and can serve only as a general guide. They are based on an average person who weighs 160 pounds (72.58 kg.).

Energy requirements for swimming are not provided because of the variables such as temperature of the water, whether the water is fresh or salt, buoyancy of the individual, and whether the water is calm or not.

tance.

e., isokinetic. Contraction of a muscle during which the force exerted while the muscle shortens is maximal.

e., isometric. Active contraction where the force is exerted against stable resistance, thereby not shortening muscle length.

e., isotonic. Active muscle contraction where the force exerted remains constant and muscle length is decreased.

e., Kegel. [Arnold Kegel, contemporary U.S. physician] An exercise for strengthening the pubococcygeal levator ani muscles. Basically, the patient tightens those muscles that would be used in attempting to prevent defecation or urination. Dr. Kegel placed a bulb in the vagina and attached it to a manometer. The patient could while doing the exercises observe the pressure increase and decrease as the muscles were contracted and relaxed. Increase in the strength of the muscles helps to control urinary and fecal incontinence and to enhance the pleasure derived from sexual intercourse.

e., muscle-setting. Contracting and relaxing a skeletal muscle or group of muscles without moving the part or changing the muscle length. SYN: *e., static*.

e., passive. Form of bodily movement that is carried through by the therapist without the assistance or resistance of the patient.

e., range of motion. Movements of joints through their full range of motion. Can be used to prevent loss of this ability or to regain the full range of motion after an injury or fracture. SEE: illus.

e., resistive. Form of supervised bodily movement, with or without apparatus, that offers resistance to muscle action.

e., static. Alternate contraction and relaxation of a skeletal muscle or group of muscles without movement of the joint. SYN: *e., muscle-setting*.

e., therapeutic. Scientific supervision of bodily movement, with or without apparatus, for purpose of restoring normal function to diseased or injured tissues.

exercise bone. Bony growth that develops in a muscle because of overexercise.

exercise electrocardiogram. Electrocardiogram taken during graded increases in rate of exercise. SEE: *stress test*.

exercise prescription. An exercise schedule usually for the purpose of increasing the state of physical fitness of a previously sedentary individual who has recently had a serious illness such as myocardial infarction, or who is physically fit and wants to know the amount, frequency, and kind of exercise to take in order to develop and maintain a state of fitness. The actual prescription is individualized, taking into account the age, health status, availability of facilities, and the need of adequate supervision, particularly in the case of persons who have or have

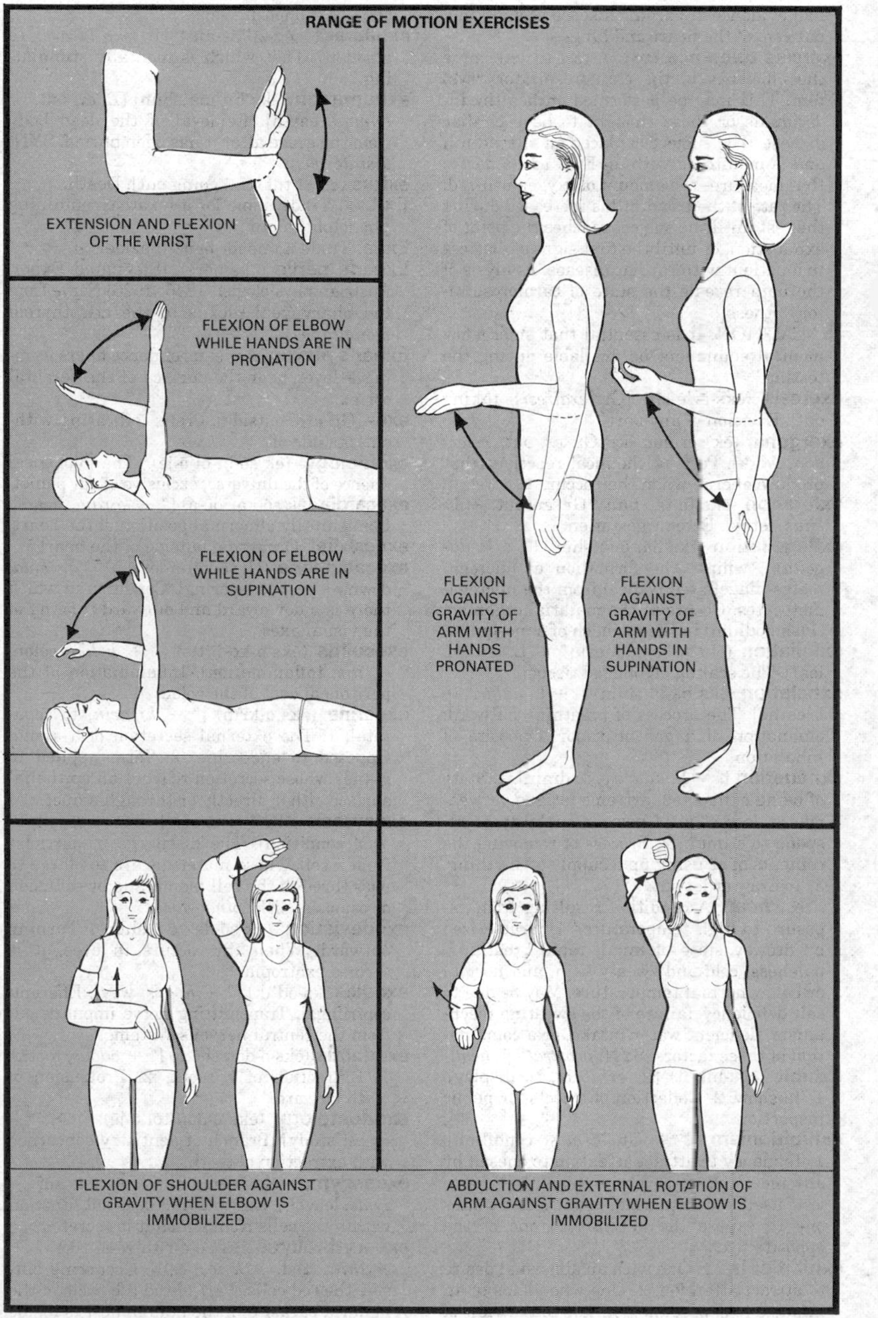
RANGE OF MOTION EXERCISES
EXTENSION AND FLEXION OF THE WRIST
FLEXION OF ELBOW WHILE HANDS ARE IN PRONATION
FLEXION OF ELBOW WHILE HANDS ARE IN SUPINATION
FLEXION AGAINST GRAVITY OF ARM WITH HANDS PRONATED
FLEXION AGAINST GRAVITY OF ARM WITH HANDS IN SUPINATION
FLEXION OF SHOULDER AGAINST GRAVITY WHEN ELBOW IS IMMOBILIZED
ABDUCTION AND EXTERNAL ROTATION OF ARM AGAINST GRAVITY WHEN ELBOW IS IMMOBILIZED

had evidence of chronic disease of any kind, but esp. of the heart and lungs.

exercise tolerance test. A test to determine the efficiency of the cardiorespiratory system. This may be performed on healthy individuals or those thought to have cardiac disease. The subject is placed on a treadmill and is monitored with an ECG and a device that measures the amount of oxygen utilized. The rate of the treadmill is increased during the test until the subject reaches the point of exhaustion, or until the first signs of distress in a patient with cardiac disease. Analysis of the data reveals the state of cardiorespiratory fitness.

CAUTION: It is essential that emergency medical equipment be available during the testing.

exeresis (ĕks-ĕr'ĕ-sĭs) [Gr. *exairesis,* taking out]. Excision of any part.

exergonic (ĕk″sĕr-gŏn'ĭk) [Gr. *ex,* out, + *ergon,* work]. Pert. to chemical reactions that produce energy when they occur.

exfetation (ĕks-fē-tā'shŭn) [Gr. *ex,* out, + L. *fetus,* fetus]. Ectopic gestation.

exflagellation (ĕks″flăj-ĕ-lā'shŭn) [″ + L. *flagellum,* whip]. The formation of microgametes (flagellated bodies) from the microgametocytes. Occurs in the malarial organism (Plasmodium) in the stomach of a mosquito.

exfoliation (ĕks″fō-lē-ā'shŭn) [″ + L. *folium,* leaf]. The scaling off of dead tissue.

exhalation (ĕks″hă-lā'shŭn) [″ + L. *halare,* to breathe]. The process of breathing outward; emanation of a gas or vapor. Opposite of inhalation.

exhaustion [″ + L. *haurire,* to drain]. 1. State of being exhausted, extreme fatigue, or weariness; loss of vital powers; inability to respond to stimuli. 2. Process of removing the contents of or using up a supply of anything. 3. To draw or let out.

e., heat. A condition resulting from exposure to high temperatures. Characterized by drowsy state of mind, rapid breathing, paleness, cold and sweaty skin, and normal or below normal temperature. May be due to salt deficiency, failure of the sweating mechanism, deficient water intake, or a combination of these factors. SYN: *prostration, heat.*

exhibit (ĕgs-hĭb'ĭt) [L. *exhibere,* to display]. 1. To show. 2. Collection of objects for public inspection.

exhibitionism [″ + Gr. *-ismos,* condition]. 1. Tendency to attract attention to oneself by any means. 2. A psychoneurosis that manifests itself in an abnormal impulse that causes one to expose the genitals to one of the opposite sex.

exhibitionist. 1. One with an abnormal desire to attract attention. 2. One who yields to an impulse to expose the genitals to the view of one of the opposite sex.

exhilarant (ĕg-zĭl'ăr-ănt) [L. *exhilarare,* to gladden]. That which is mentally stimulating.

exhumation (ĕks″hū-mā'shŭn) [L. *ex,* out, + *humus,* earth]. Removal of the dead body from the grave after it has been buried. SYN: *disinterment.*

exitus (ĕk'sĭ-tŭs) [L., going out]. Death.

Ex-Lax. Trade name for a laxative containing phenolphthalein.

Exna. Trade name for benzthiazide.

Exner's nerve (ĕks'nĕrz). [Siegmund Exner, Austrian physiologist, 1846–1926] Nerve from the pharyngeal plexus to the cricothyroid membranes.

Exner's plexus. A plexus of nerve fibers forming a layer near the surface of the cerebral cortex.

exo- [Gr. *exo,* outside]. Prefix indicating without; outside of.

exobiology (ĕk″sō-bī-ŏl'ō-jē). The biological science of the universe, exclusive of our planet.

exocardia (ĕk″sō-kăr'dē-ă) [″ + *kardia,* heart]. Congenitally abnormal position of the heart.

exocardial. Occurring outside of the heart.

exocataphoria (ĕks″ō-kăt-ă-for'ē-ă) [″ + *kata,* down, + *phoros,* bearing]. Condition in which there is a downward and outward turning of the visual axes.

exocolitis (ĕks″ō-kō-lī'tĭs) [″ + *kolon,* colon, + *itis,* inflammation]. Inflammation of the peritoneal coat of the colon.

exocrine (ĕks'ō-krĭn) [″ + *krinein,* to separate]. 1. The external secretion of a gland. Opposed to endocrine. 2. Term applied to glands whose secretion reaches an epithelial surface either directly or through a duct.

exocytosis (ĕks″ō-sī-tō'sĭs) [″ + *kytos,* cell, + *osis,* condition]. The discharge of particles from a cell. These materials are too large to pass through the cell membrane by diffusion or osmosis. SEE: *pinocytosis.*

exodeviation (ĕk″sō-dē″vē-ā'shŭn). Turning outward. When this occurs in eyes, it is termed exotropia.

exodic (ĕks-ŏd'ĭk) [″ + *hodos,* way]. Efferent, centrifugal. Transmitting nerve impulses out from the central nervous system.

exodontia (ĕks-ō-dŏn'shē-ă) [″ + *odous,* tooth]. 1. Extraction of a tooth. 2. Protrusion of teeth forward.

exodontology (ĕks″ō-dŏn-tŏl'ō-jē) [″ + ″ + *logos,* study]. Branch of dentistry concerned with extraction of teeth.

exoenzyme (ĕk-sō-ĕn'zīm) [″ + *en,* in, + *zyme,* leaven]. Enzyme that does not function within the cells from which it is secreted.

exoerythrocytic (ĕk″sō-ĕ-rĭth″rō-sĭ'tĭk) [″ + *erythros,* red, + *kytos,* cell]. Occurring outside the red cells. Part of the life cycle of the malaria parasite in the human host is inside the red cell; the rest is outside, i.e., exoerythrocytic.

exogamy (ĕks-ŏg'ă-mē) [" + *gamos*, marriage]. 1. Marriage outside of a particular group. 2. In biology, conjugation between protozoan gametes of different ancestry.

exogastritis (ĕks"ō-găs-trī'tĭs) [" + *gaster*, belly, + *itis*, inflammation]. Inflammation of the peritoneal coat of stomach.

exogenous (ĕks-ŏj'ĕ-nŭs) [" + *gennan*, to produce]. Originating outside an organ or part.

exohysteropexy (ĕks"ō-hĭs"tĕr-ō-pĕks'ē) [" + *hystera*, uterus, + *pexis*, fixation]. Fixation of the uterus by implanting the fundus into the abdominal wall.

exometritis (ĕks"ō-mē-trī'tĭs) [" + *metra*, womb, + *itis*, inflammation]. Inflammation of the peritoneal coat of the uterus.

exomphalos (ĕks-ŏm'fă-lŭs) [Gr. *ex*, out, + *omphalos*, navel]. 1. Umbilical protrusion. 2. Umbilical hernia.

exopathic (ĕk"sō-păth'ĭk) [Gr. *exo*, outside, + *pathos*, disease]. Pert. to a disease originating outside of the body.

exophoria (ĕks"ō-fō'rē-ă) [" + *phoros*, bearing]. Tendency of visual axes to diverge outward. Opposite of esophoria.

exophthalmia (ĕks"ŏf-thăl'mē-ă) [" + *ophthalmos*, eye]. Abnormal protrusion of the eyeball. SYN: *exophthalmos*.

e. cachectica. Exophthalmic goiter.

e. fungosa. Late state of glioma retinae.

exophthalmic (ĕks"ŏf-thăl'mĭk). Pert. to protrusion of the eyeball.

exophthalmic goiter. A condition marked by protrusion of the eyeballs, increased heart action, enlargement of the thyroid gland, weight loss, nervousness. SYN: *thyrotoxicosis*. SEE: *hyperthyroidism*.

exophthalmometer (ĕk"sŏf-thăl-mŏm'ĕ-tĕr). Device for measuring the degree of protrusion of the eyeballs.

exophthalmos, exophthalmus (ĕks"ŏf-thăl'mŏs, -mŭs). Abnormal protrusion of eyeball. May be due to thyrotoxicosis, tumor of the orbit, orbital cellulitis, leukemia, or aneurysm.

e., pulsating. Exophthalmos accompanied by pulsation and bruit due to an aneurysm behind the eye.

exoplasm (ĕk'sō-plăzm) [" + *plasma*, matter]. Outer protoplasm of a cell. SYN: *ectoplasm*.

exoserosis (ĕks"ō-sĕr-ō'sĭs) [" + *serum*, whey, + Gr. *osis*, condition]. An oozing of serum or discharging of an exudate.

exoskeleton (ĕk"sō-skĕl'ĕ-tŏn) [" + *skeleton*, skeleton]. 1. The hard outer covering of certain invertebrates such as the molluscs and arthropods. Composed of chitin, calcareous material, or both. 2. In vertebrates, the hard outer covering such as the shell of a turtle, or more specifically, the hard parts of the body surface derived principally from the ectoderm. These include such structures as hair, hooves, horns, nails, feathers, and scales.

exosmosis (ĕks"ŏs-mō'sĭs) [" + *osmos*, a thrusting, + *osis*, condition]. Diffusion of a fluid from within outward, as from a blood vessel.

exosplenopexy (ĕks"ō-splĕn'ō-pĕks-ē) [" + *splen*, spleen, + *pexis*, fixation]. Suturing the spleen to opening in the abdominal wall.

exostosis (ĕks"ŏs-tō'sĭs) [" + *osteon*, bone]. (pl. *exostoses*) A bony growth that arises from the surface of a bone, often involving the ossification of muscular attachments. SYN: *hyperostosis; osteoma; osteoncus*.

e. bursata. An exostosis arising from the epiphysis of a bone and covered with cartilage and a synovial sac.

e. cartilaginea. Exostosis consisting of cartilage underlying the periosteum.

e., dental. Exostosis on the root of a tooth.

e., multiple osteocartilaginous. A hereditary disorder of growth characterized by the development of multiple exostoses, usually located on the diaphyses of long bones near the epiphyseal lines. Results in irregularities of growth of the epiphyses and often secondary deformities.

exoteric (ĕks"ō-tĕr'ĭk) [Gr. *exoterikos*, outer]. Pert. to causes developing outside the body. SYN: *exopathic*.

exothermal, exothermic [Gr. *exo*, outside, + *therme*, heat]. Chemical reaction with production of heat.

exothymopexy (ĕks"ō-thī'mō-pĕks"ē) [" + *thymos*, thymus, + *pexis*, fixation]. Suturing of an enlarged thymus gland to the sternum.

exothyropexy (ĕks"ō-thī'rō-pĕks"ē). Suture of the thyroid and external fixation to induce atrophy.

exotic (ĕg-zŏt'ĭk) [Gr. *exotikos*]. Not native; originating in another part of the world.

exotoxin (ĕks"ō-tŏks'ĭn) [Gr. *exo*, outside, + *toxikon*, poison]. A toxin produced by a microorganism and excreted into its surrounding medium. It can usually be recovered from the liquid medium in which the toxin-producing organisms have developed. Exotoxins usually are unstable, being sensitive to the effects of chemicals, light, and heat. Exotoxins are produced by certain bacteria, including diphtheria and tetanus organisms. Exotoxins differ with regard to the particular tissues of the host that may be affected.

RS: cytotoxin; endotoxin; erythrotoxin; leukocidin; leukotoxic; neurotoxin.

exotropia (ĕks"ō-trō'pē-ă) [" + *tropos*, turning]. Divergent strabismus; abnormal turning of one or both eyes outward.

expander (ĕk-spăn′dĕr) [L. *expandere,* to spread out]. That which increases the size, volume, or amount of something. SEE: *plasma volume expander.*

expansion (ĕks-păn′shŭn) [L. *expandere,* to spread out]. Increase of volume; spreading out.

expansive delusion. Overvaluation of one's power and wealth, accompanied by a feeling of well-being. These beliefs are not consistent with reality. SEE: *megalomania.*

expectant [Gr. *ex,* out, + L. *spectare,* to watch]. Waiting.

expectation. Hoping, anticipation.

expected date of confinement. ABBR: EDC. The predicted date of childbirth. SEE: *Pregnancy Table for Expected Date of Delivery.*

expectorant (ĕk-spĕk′tō-rănt) [Gr. *ex,* out, + L. *pectus,* breast]. An agent that facilitates the removal of the secretions of the bronchopulmonary mucous membrane. Expectorants are classed as sedative or stimulating. Ammonium carbonate, ammonium chloride, and ipecac are considered expectorants.

expectoration (ĕk-spĕk″tō-rā′shŭn). Expulsion of mucus or phlegm from the throat or lungs. It may be mucous, mucopurulent, serous, or frothy. In pneumonia, it is viscid and tenacious, sticks to anything, and is rusty in appearance. In bronchitis, it is frothy, often streaked with blood, and greenish-yellow because of pus. In advanced tuberculosis, it varies from small amt. of frothy fluid to abundant offensive greenish-yellow sputum often streaked with blood. SEE: *sputum.*

expel (ĕks-pĕl′) [L. *expellere*]. To drive out.

experiment [L. *experimentum,* to test]. The scientific procedure used to test the validity of a hypothesis, to gain further evidence or knowledge, or to test the usefulness of a drug or type of therapy that has not been tried previously.

expiration (ĕks″pĭ-rā′shŭn) [Gr. *ex,* out, + L. *spirare,* to breathe]. 1. The expulsion of air from the lungs in breathing. Its sound is the shortest breath sound heard. In general, if the duration of expiration is longer than inspiration, a pathological condition such as emphysema or asthma is present. Muscles used in expiration are the internal intercostal muscles, musculus rectus abdominis [NA], musculus transversus abdominis [NA], the triangularis sterni, and possibly the iliocostalis, serratus posterior inferior, and quadratus lumborum. SEE: *diaphragm* for illus.; *inspiration; respiration.* 2. Death.

e., active. Expiration accomplished as a result of muscular activity, as in forced respiration. The muscles used in respiration are the muscles of the abdominal wall (external and internal oblique, rectus, and transversus abdominis); the internal intercostals, serratus posterior inferior, platysma, and quadratus lumborum.

e., passive. Expiration during quiet respiration in which no muscular effort is required. It is brought about by the elasticity of the lung, recoil of the elastic tissues of the chest such as the costal cartilages, and the weight of the thoracic wall.

expiratory (ĕks-pī′ră-tor″ē). Pert. to expiration.

expiratory center. The part of the respiratory center in the medulla controlling expiratory movements.

expire. 1. To breathe out or exhale. 2. To die.

explant (ĕks-plănt′) [″ + L. *planta,* sprout]. To remove a piece of living tissue from the body and transfer to an artificial culture medium for growth as in tissue culture. Opposite of implant.

explode (ĕks-plōd′) [L. *explodere,* fr. *ex,* out, + *plaudere,* to clap the hands]. To burst or to have rapid onset such as an epidemic; or sudden decompression of a cavity, boil, or object. Explosive decompression occurs when the pressure in the cabin of an airplane flying at high altitude is suddenly decreased.

exploration [L. *explorare,* to search out]. Examination of an organ or part by various means.

exploratory. Pert. to an exploration.

explorer. An instrument used in exploration, esp. a device used to locate foreign bodies or to define passageways in body sinuses or cavities.

e., dental. A sharp-pointed instrument used to detect unsound enamel, carious lesions, or imperfect margins of restorations in teeth.

explosive speech. Sudden and explosive utterance. SEE: *speech.*

exponent (ĕks′pō-nĕnt). The mathematical method of indicating the power to which the entity symbolized is to be raised. It is placed as a superscript; e.g., 10^2 or x^2 indicates 10 and x are to be squared or multiplied by themselves. The exponent can have any numerical value and may be positive or negative. SEE: *Scientific Notation* in *Appendix.*

expose. 1. To open up as in surgically opening the abdominal cavity. 2. To be without heat or shelter. 3. To have been in contact with an infected person or agent. 4. To display one's genitalia publicly, esp. when members of the opposite sex are present. Colloquially, this is termed "flashing."

express [L. *expressare*]. To squeeze out.

expression. 1. Expelling anything by pressure. 2. Facial disclosure of feeling or a physical state. SYN: *facies.* SEE: *face.*

expressivity. The extent to which a heritable trait is manifest in the individual carrying the gene.

expulsion rate. In gynecology, the rate of spontaneous expulsion of an intrauterine contraceptive device (IUD) in the group of women who use them. Usually expressed with respect to the time elapsed following implantation.

expulsive [L. *expellere,* to drive out]. Having a tendency to expel.

exsanguinate (ĕks-săn'gwĭn-āt) [Gr. *ex,* out, + *sanguis,* blood]. Loss of blood to the point where life can no longer be sustained.

exsanguination (ĕk-săn"gwĭn-ā'shŭn). The process of expressing blood from a part.

exsanguine (ĕks-săn'gwĭn). Anemic; bloodless.

exsection (ĕk-sĕk'shŭn) [L. *exsectus,* having cut]. Excision.

Exsel. Trade name for selenium sulfide.

exsiccant (ĕk-sĭk'ănt) [L. *exsiccare,* to dry out]. 1. Absorbing or drying up a discharge. 2. An agent that absorbs moisture. 3. A dusting or drying powder.

exsiccation (ĕk"sĭ-kā'shŭn). 1. To make dry. 2. In chemistry, removing the water from compounds or solutions. SYN: *desiccation.*

exsiccative (ĕk-sĭk'kă-tĭv). Causing to dry up or that which dries. SYN: *desiccative.*

exsomatize (ĕk-sō'mă-tīz) [Gr. *ex,* out, + *soma,* body]. To remove from the body.

exsorption (ĕk-sorp'shŭn). Movement of material including cells and electrolytes from the blood to the lumen of the intestines. In pathological conditions such as intestinal obstruction, this process may cause a great increase in pressure inside the area of the intestinal tract affected.

exstrophy (ĕks'trō-fē) [" + *strephein,* to turn]. A congenital turning inside out of an organ. SYN: *eversion.*

e. of bladder. A congenital malformation in which the lower portion of the abdominal wall and anterior wall of the bladder are missing and the bladder is everted through the opening. SYN: *ectopia vesicae.*

exsufflation (ĕk"sŭ-flā'shŭn) [" + *sufflatio,* blown up]. Forceful expulsion of air from a cavity by artificial means, such as use of a mechanical exsufflator.

ext. L. *extractum,* extract.

extemporaneous [LL. *extemporaneus*]. Not prepared according to formula but devised for the occasion.

extended care facility. A medical care institution for patients who require long-term custodial or medical care, esp. for a chronic disease or a disease requiring prolonged rehabilitation therapy.

extended family. A family consisting of members of the immediate family plus grandparents and other relatives.

extender (ĕk-stĕn'dĕr) [Gr. *ex,* out, + L. *tendere,* to stretch]. That which causes an increase in the time something lasts or has an effect. The time required for absorption of some medicines given intramuscularly may be increased by injecting them with a substance such as an oil, which has that effect.

extension (ĕks-tĕn'shŭn) [L. *extensio*]. 1. The movement by which both ends of any part are pulled apart. A movement that brings the members of a limb into or toward a straight condition. Opposite of flexion. 2. The application of a pull (traction) to a fractured or dislocated limb.

e., Buck's. A method of producing traction by applying adhesive tape or flannel-backed adhesive tape to the skin and keeping it in smooth close contact by means of circular bandaging of the part to which it is applied. The adhesive strips are placed longitudinal to the arm or leg, the superior ends being about 1 in. (2.5 cm.) from the fracture site. Weights sufficient to produce the required extension are fastened to the inferior end of the adhesive strips by means of a rope that is run over a pulley to permit free motion.

extensor [L.]. A muscle that extends a part.

exterior [L.]. Outside of; external.

exteriorize. 1. To expose a part temporarily in surgery. 2. In psychiatry, the process of turning one's interests outward.

extern(e) (ĕks'tĕrn) [L. *externus,* outside]. A medical student, living outside of a hospital, who assists in the medical and surgical care of patients. SEE: *intern.*

external. Exterior; lateral; opposite of medial or internal.

externalia (ĕks"tĕr-nā'lē-ă) [L. *exter,* outside, + *genitalis,* genital]. External genitals.

externalize (ĕks-tĕr'nă-līz). 1. In surgery, to provide exposure to the outside. 2. In psychiatry, to direct one's inner conflicts to the outside rather than keeping them hidden inside.

exteroceptive (ĕks"tĕr-ō-sĕp'tĭv) [L. *externus,* outside, + *receptus,* having received]. Pert. to end organs receiving impressions from without.

exteroceptor (ĕks"tĕr-ō-sĕp'tor). A sense organ, as the eye, adapted for the reception of stimuli from outside the body.

exterofective (ĕks"tĕr-ō-fĕk'tĭv) [" + *facere,* to make]. Pert. to responses to stimuli mediated by the central nervous system and somatic nerves in contrast to those mediated through the autonomic nervous system.

extima (ĕks'tĭ-mă) [L., outermost]. The outer layer.

extinction [L. *exstinctus,* having extinguished]. 1. The process of extinguishing or putting out. 2. The complete inhibition of a conditioned reflex as a result of failure to reinforce it.

extinguish (ĕks-tĭng'gwĭsh) [L. *extinguere,* to render extinct]. To abolish, esp. to remove a reflex. This may be done by surgical, psychological, or pharmacologic means depending upon the type of reflex involved.

extirpation (ĕks-tĭr-pā'shŭn) [L. *extirpare,* to root out]. Excision of a part; taking out by the roots.

extorsion (ĕks-tor'shŭn) [Gr. *ex,* out, + L. *torsio,* twisting]. Rotation of an organ or limb outward.

extra- [L. *extra,* outside]. Prefix meaning outside of, in addition to, beyond.

extra-articular [" + *articulus,* joint]. Outside a joint.

extracapsular (ĕks"tră-kăp'sū-lăr). Outside a capsule, e.g., a joint capsule or the capsule of the lens of the eye.

extracellular (ĕks"tră-sĕl'ū-lăr). Outside the cell.

extracorporeal (ĕks"tră-kor-por'ē-ăl) [" + *corpus,* body]. Outside of the body.

extracorticospinal (ĕks"tră-kor"tĭ-kō-spī'năl). Outside the corticospinal tract of the central nervous system.

extracranial (ĕks"tră-krā'nē-ăl). Outside the skull.

extract (ĕks-trăkt', ĕks'trăkt) [L. *extractum*]. 1. To pull out or remove forcibly, as to extract a tooth. 2. A solid or semisolid preparation made by extracting the soluble portion of a compound by using water or alcohol and evaporating the solution. 3. Active principle of a drug obtained by distillation or chemical processes.

e., alcoholic. Extract in which alcohol acts as the solvent.

e., aqueous. Extract in which water is the solvent.

e., aromatic fluid. Extract made from an aromatic powder.

e., compound. Extract prepared from more than one drug or substance.

e., ethereal. Extract using ether as the vehicle.

e., fluid. Extract made into a solution from a vegetable drug that contains medicinal components.

e., powdered. A dried crushed extract.

e., soft. Extract of the consistency of honey.

e., solid. Extract made by evaporating the fluid part of a solution.

extractable nuclear antigen. ABBR: E.N.A. An antigen present in the cells of patients with certain types of connective tissue disorders. Corticosteroids are very helpful in treating patients with high concentrations of extractable nuclear antigen.

extraction [L. *extractum,* drawing out]. 1. Pulling out, as a tooth. 2. The removing of the active portion of a drug from its vehicle.

extractive (ĕks-trăk'tĭv). That which was extracted or removed in the process of extraction.

extractor. Instrument for removing foreign bodies. Varieties include esophageal, throat, shot, tympanum, tissue.

e., tissue. Needles, trocars, or pointed instruments with a form of barb for extracting soft tissue for examination.

e., tube. Device for removing an intubation tube from trachea.

extractum (ĕks-trăk'tŭm) [L., a drawing out]. (pl. *extracta)* ABBR: ext. Solid or semisolid preparations produced by evaporating solutions of vegetable principles. The official extracts are either powders or soft solids. The majority can be obtained in powdered form and many physicians prefer them that way. Extracts are usually about five times the strength of the crude drug. SEE: *fluidextract.*

extracystic (ĕks"tră-sĭs'tĭk) [L. *extra,* outside, + Gr. *kystis,* bladder]. Outside of or unrelated to a bladder or cystic tumor.

extradural (ĕks-tră-dū'răl) [" + *durus,* hard]. 1. On outer side of the dura mater. 2. Unconnected with the dura mater.

extraembryonic (ĕks"tră-ĕm"brē-ŏn'ĭk) [" + Gr. *embryon,* embryo]. Apart and outside of the embryo, e.g., the amnion.

extragenital (ĕks"tră-jĕn'ĭ-tăl) [" + *genitalis,* genital]. Outside of or unrelated to the genital organs.

extrahepatic (ĕks"tră-hĕ-păt'ĭk) [L. *extra,* outside, + Gr. *hepatos,* liver]. Outside of or unrelated to the liver.

extraligamentous [" + *ligare,* to bind]. Outside of or unrelated to a ligament.

extramalleolus (ĕks"tră-măl-lē'ō-lŭs) [" + *malleolus,* little hammer]. The external or lateral malleolus of the ankle.

extramarginal (ĕks"tră-măr'jĭ-năl) [" + *margo,* margin]. Pert. to subliminal consciousness.

extramastoiditis (ĕks"tră-măs"toyd-ī'tĭs) [" + Gr. *mastos,* breast, + *eidos,* form, + *itis,* inflammation]. Inflammation of outside tissues contiguous to the mastoid process.

extramedullary (ĕks"tră-mĕd'ū-lă-rē) [" + *medulla,* marrow]. Outside or unrelated to any medulla, esp. the medulla oblongata.

extramural (ĕks"tră-mū'răl) [" + *murus,* wall]. Outside the wall of the organ or vessel.

extraneous (ĕks-trā'nē-ŭs) [L. *extraneus,* external]. Outside and unrelated to an organism.

extranuclear [L. *extra,* outside, + *nucleus,* kernel]. Outside of a nucleus.

extraocular (ĕks"tră-ŏk'ū-lăr) [" + *oculus,* eye]. Outside the eye, as in extraocular eye muscles.

extrapolar [" + *polus,* pole]. Outside instead of between poles, as the electrodes of a battery.

extrapyramidal (ĕks″tră-pĭ-răm′ĭ-dăl). Outside the pyramidal tracts of the central nervous system.

extrapyramidal syndrome. Any one of several degenerative diseases of the nervous system that involve the extrapyramidal system and the basal ganglion of the brain. The symptoms include tremors, chorea, athetosis, and dystonia. Parkinsonism, q.v., is an extrapyramidal syndrome.

extrapyramidal system. SEE: *system, extrapyramidal.*

extrasensory. Pert. to forms of perception not dependent upon the five primary senses, as thought transference.

extrasensory perception. ABBR: ESP. Perception, esp. of another person's thoughts or actions not received by use of the senses.

extrasystole (ĕks″tră-sĭs′tō-lē) [″ + Gr. *systole,* contraction]. Premature contraction of the heart. In humans, it is the result of some factor that initiates an impulse in the impulse-conducting system. It may occur in either the presence or absence of organic heart disease. It may be of reflex origin, being initiated by stimuli from almost any part of the body, or it may be of central origin. It may be induced experimentally by stimulating the heart at any time except during the absolute refractory period.

e., atrial. Premature contraction of the atrium at some point outside the S-A node.

e., nodal. Extrasystole occurring as a result of the origin of an impulse in the A-V node.

e., ventricular. Extrasystole that occurs after the normal contraction of the ventricle has ceased. Usually followed by a long compensatory pause.

extratubal (ĕks″tră-tū′băl). Outside a tube, esp. the uterine tube.

extrauterine (ĕks″tră-ū′tĕr-ĭn) [″ + *uterus,* womb]. Outside the uterus.

extravaginal (ĕks″tră-văj′ĭ-năl) [″ + *vagina,* vagina]. Outside the vagina.

extravasate (ĕks-trăv′ă-sāt) [″ + *vas,* vessel]. 1. To escape from a vessel into the tissues, said of serum, blood, or lymph. 2. Fluids escaping from vessels.

extravasation (ĕks-trăv″ă-sā′shŭn). The escape of fluids into the surrounding tissue. SYN: *suffusion.*

extravascular (ĕks″tră-văs′kū-lăr) [″ + *vasculum,* vessel]. Outside a vessel.

extraventricular [″ + *ventriculus,* little belly]. Outside of any ventricle, esp. one of the heart.

extremital (ĕks-trĕm′ĭ-tăl) [L. *extremus,* outermost]. Pert. to an extremity. SYN: *distal.*

extremity. 1. The terminal part of anything. 2. An arm or leg.

e., lower. The lower limb including the hip, thigh, leg, ankle, and foot.

e., upper. The upper limb including the shoulder, arm, forearm, wrist, and hand.

extrinsic (ĕks-trĭn′sĭk) [LL. *extrinsecus,* outer]. From, or coming from, without.

extrinsic muscles. ABBR: e.m. Those muscles partly attached to the trunk and partly to a limb. Those muscles outside an organ that control the position of that organ, such as e. m. of eye or e. m. of tongue.

extrospection (ĕks″trō-spĕk′shŭn) [L. *extra,* outside, + *spectare,* to look]. Continual inspection by the patient of his or her skin for evidence of dirt. Associated with mysophobia, compulsive fear of dirt.

extroversion (ĕks″trō-vĕr′zhŭn) [″ + *vertere,* to turn]. 1. Eversion; turning inside out. 2. The direction of attention and energy outward from the self. SEE: *introversion.*

extrovert. A personality-reaction type; one who is interested mainly in external objects and actions. The extreme pathological extrovert reaction is seen in manic-depressive psychosis. Opposite of introvert.

extrude (ĕks-trūd′) [L. *extrudere,* to squeeze out]. To push out of a normal position or situation.

extrusion (ĕks-troo′zhŭn). 1. Occupying an abnormal external position. 2. In dentistry, position of a tooth when pushed forward from line of occlusion.

extubation (ĕks″tū-bā′shŭn) [Gr. *ex,* out, + L. *tuba,* tube]. Removal of a tube, as a laryngeal tube.

exuberant (ĕg-zū′bĕr-ănt) [L. *exuberare,* to be very fruitful]. 1. Excessive as in the increased and excessive growth of a tissue or bacterial culture. 2. Joyful, happy.

exudate (ĕks′ū-dāt) [L. *exsudare,* to sweat out.]. Accumulation of a fluid in a cavity, or matter that penetrates through vessel walls into adjoining tissue, or the production of pus or serum.

In comparison with a transudate, there are more cells, protein, and solid material in an exudate. Exudates may be classified as catarrhal, fibrinous, hemorrhagic, diphtheritic, purulent, and serous, the fluids being different in various affections. A fibrinous exudate may wall off a cavity, resulting in adhesions following surgery, as in empyema and appendicitis. Inflammatory processes tend to wall off the injured area to localize the inflammation and to prevent its spread. SEE: *empyema; exudation; infection; inflammation; pus; resorption; transudate.*

exudation (ĕks″ū-dā′shŭn). Morbid oozing of fluids, usually the result of inflammatory conditions. SEE: *exudate.*

exudative (ĕks′ū-dā″tĭv). Having the property of exudation.

exude (ĕg-zūd′, ĕk-sūd′) [L. *exsudare,* to sweat

out]. To pass off slowly through the tissues; said of a semisolid or fluid.

exumbilication (ĕks″ŭm-bĭl″ĭ-kā′shŭn) [Gr. *ex*, out, + L. *umbilicus*, navel]. Protrusion of navel. SYN: *exomphalos*.

exuviae (ĕks-ū′vē-ē) [L.]. Material cast off or shed.

eye [AS. *eage*]. Organ of vision. SEE: illus.

ANAT: Composed of three coats. From inside the eye out they are retina, sensory for light; uvea (choroid, ciliary body, and iris); sclera and cornea, serve as protection for the delicate retina. These layers enclose two cavities, the more anterior or ocular chamber being the space lying in front of the lens. It is divided by the iris into an anterior chamber and a posterior chamber, both of which are filled with a watery aqueous humor. The cavity behind the lens is much larger and filled with a jelly-like vitreous body. The lens

ANATOMY OF EYE

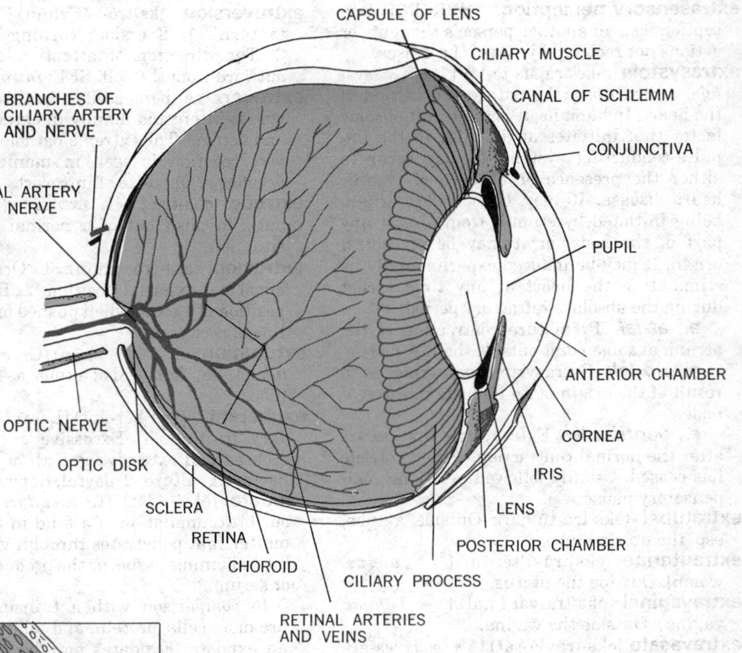

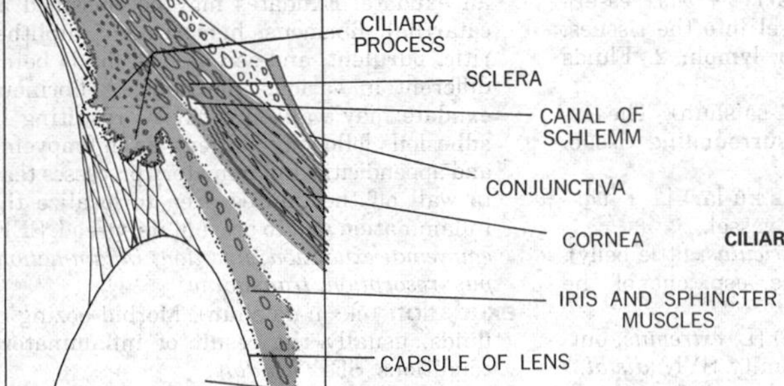

CILIARY APPARATUS

is suspended behind the iris by the ciliary zonule. Anteriorly, the cornea is covered by the conjunctiva, which continues and forms the inner layer of the eyelids. Movements of the eyeball are brought about by six muscles: the superior, inferior, medial and external rectus muscles, and the superior and inferior oblique muscles.

Nerve supply: 2nd or optic nerve. *Eye muscles:* 3rd or oculomotor, 4th or trochlear, and 6th or abducens. *Lid muscles:* facial to orbicularis oculi and oculomotor to levator palpebrae. Sensory fibers to orbit furnished by ophthalmic and maxillary fibers of the 5th or trigeminal. Sympathetic postganglionic fibers are derived from the carotid plexus, their cell bodies lying in the superior cervical ganglion. They supply the dilator muscle of the iris, lacrimal gland, and smooth muscle fibers in the eyelid; parasympathetic fibers from the ciliary ganglion pass to the ciliary muscle and constrictor muscles of the iris.

FUNCT: Light entering the eye passes through the cornea, then through the pupil, an opening in the iris, and on through the crystalline lens and the vitreous body to the retina. The aqueous humor, lens, and vitreous body constitute the refracting media of the eye. Through changes in the curvature of the lens brought about by its elasticity and contraction of the ciliary muscles, light rays are focused on the retina, where they stimulate the rods and cones, the sensory receptors. The cones are concerned with color vision and the rods with vision in dim light. Sensory impulses are conveyed over the optic nerve to the brain where, in the visual area of the cerebral cortex located in the occipital lobe, they register as visual sensations. The amount of light entering the eye is regulated by the pupil, its size being controlled by the dilator and constrictor muscles of the iris.

DIAG: Following trauma to the head and in certain disease states, the size, shape, motion, and reactions of the pupils provide extremely important diagnostic information.

Contracted pupils: May denote irritative lesions of the 3rd nerve in early stages of some types of anesthesia or during alcoholic excitement, or may result from therapeutic dose of an opiate such as morphine. Contraction of one pupil indicates irritative lesion of the opposite side of the brain, situated at the 3rd nerve nuclei, or a paralysis of the sympathetic nerve fibers due to a lesion somewhere in their course.

Dilated pupils: May result from taking the medicines belladonna or atropine, or from irritation of the sympathetic nerve fibers. May occur during attacks of dyspnea in the last stages of anesthesia. Dilation of one

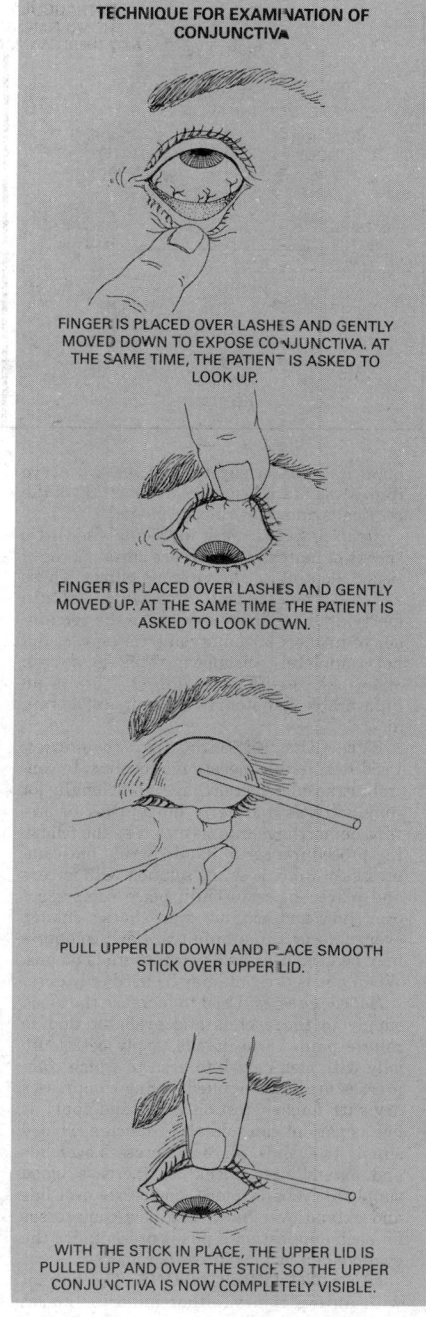

TECHNIQUE FOR EXAMINATION OF CONJUNCTIVA

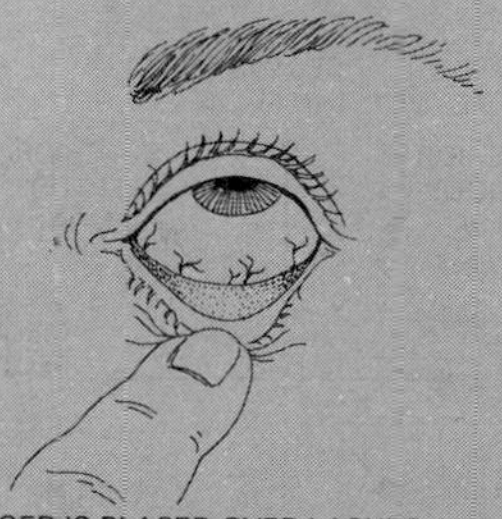

FINGER IS PLACED OVER LASHES AND GENTLY MOVED DOWN TO EXPOSE CONJUNCTIVA. AT THE SAME TIME, THE PATIENT IS ASKED TO LOOK UP.

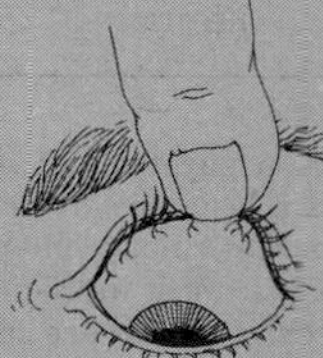

FINGER IS PLACED OVER LASHES AND GENTLY MOVED UP. AT THE SAME TIME THE PATIENT IS ASKED TO LOOK DOWN.

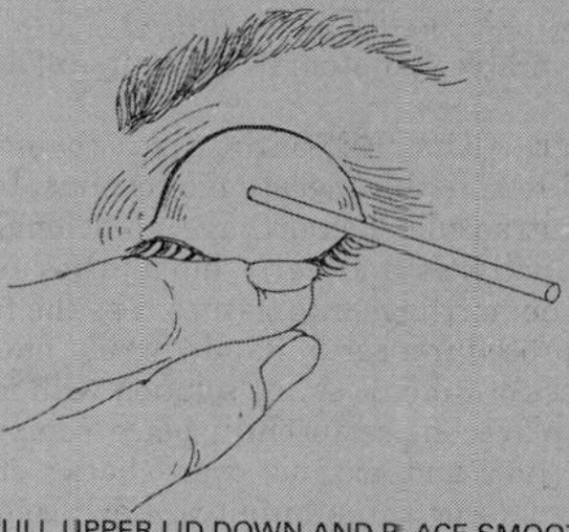

PULL UPPER LID DOWN AND PLACE SMOOTH STICK OVER UPPER LID.

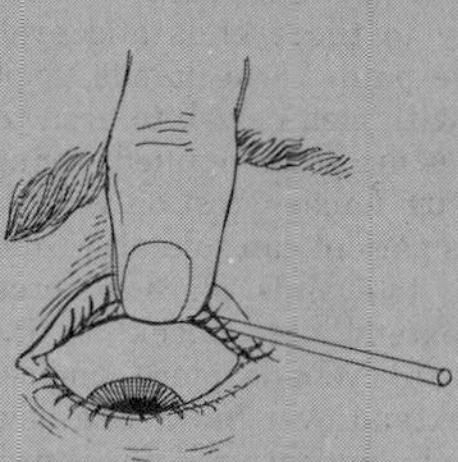

WITH THE STICK IN PLACE, THE UPPER LID IS PULLED UP AND OVER THE STICK SO THE UPPER CONJUNCTIVA IS NOW COMPLETELY VISIBLE.

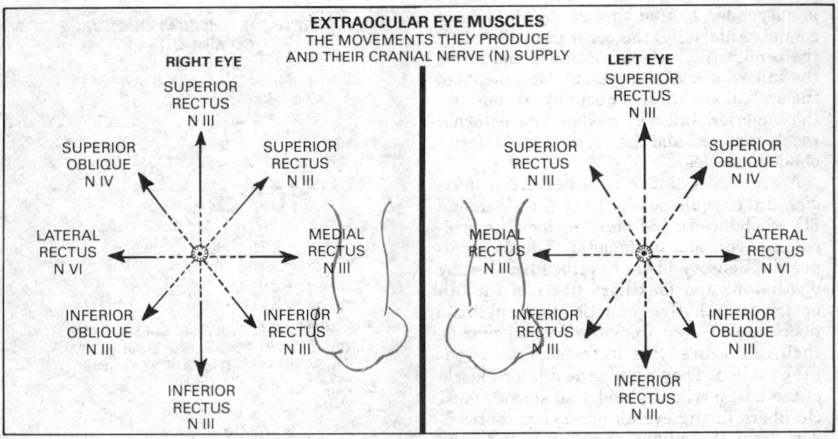

pupil indicates a paralysis of the 3rd nerve from some brain lesion or an irritation of the cervical sympathetic nerve fibers.

Floating specks: Most individuals see little specks of material, which are small pieces of tissue, floating in the vitreous humor. These are called muscae volitantes, which is Latin for flying flies. These specks are the remainder of intraocular embryonic tissue that did not completely disappear. This is not an abnormal condition. *Squinting:* This is an unfavorable symptom in the course of a brain disease.

EYE COMPRESSES: *Cold compresses:* Used to relieve congestion of eyelids; to control intraocular hemorrhage; occasionally for conjunctivitis and early lid injuries to prevent hemorrhage into tissues. Use the following procedure: scrub hands, wring out compresses of isotonic saline solution with forceps and place on ice to chill; place compresses over lids and extend over cheek; change every two or three minutes. Each compress may be used over and over if there is no pus. When pus is present, may be used only once.

Hot compresses: Used to increase the blood supply to the eyelids and eyeballs, and to relieve pain. Scrub hands, apply petroleum jelly with clean swab to area to which compresses are to be applied; wring compresses dry with forceps, test on wrist, and apply as hot as patient can tolerate. To increase blood supply to eyelids, place compresses over lids and extend over cheek; to increase blood supply to eyeballs, place compresses over lids and extend over brow. Use new compresses for each application if pus is present; dry the eyelid when last compress is removed.

NURSING IMPLICATIONS: The patient with an eye injury, either minor or major, will fear blindness. It is therefore essential that he or she be reassured. The visual acuity should be tested at once. If the globe has been penetrated, do not apply a patch to the eye but use a suitable shield. Do not attempt to remove a penetrating foreign body. Withhold all medicines, esp. corticosteroids, until the patient has been seen by a physician.

e., aphakic. An eye from which the crystalline lens has been removed.

e., black. Ecchymosis of the tissues surrounding the eye.

e., crossed. Strabismus with deviation of the visual axis of one eye toward that of the other eye.

e., dark-adapted. An eye that has become adjusted for viewing objects in dim light; one adapted for scotopic or rod vision. Depends upon the regeneration of a light-sensitive substance, visual purple.

e., dominant. The eye to which a person unconsciously gives preference as a source of stimuli for visual sensations. The dominant eye is usually used in sighting a gun or in using a monocular microscope.

e., dry. Dry eye, q.v.

e., exciting. In sympathetic ophthalmia, the damaged eye, which is the source of sympathogenic influences.

e., fixating. In strabismus, the eye that is directed toward the object of vision.

e., foreign body in. Manifested by pain, lacrimation, spasm of the eye; later there is redness, swelling, and occasionally headache. Infection may be carried into the eye, resulting in an ulcer of the cornea. Metal produces a chemical effect as it disintegrates, an action that affects the eyeball. The x-ray is sometimes used to detect any tiny particles of metal, and the electromagnet to assist in removing them. Sympathetic ophthalmia, q.v., the transference of inflammation from an injury of one eye to the normal eye, may be produced by wounds that pierce the eyeball. Loss of vision in both eyes may result if the affected eye is not removed.

F.A.: Tearing often washes dust from the eye, or bringing the upper lid over the lower and directing the patient to roll the eye often deposits the dust on the margin of the lower lid.

Great care is necessary in removing larger particles. This should be done in a quiet, well-lighted place with clean, preferably sterile, materials. Follow by instillation of 1 or 2 drops of a bland oil into the eye. A mild antiseptic such as 5 to 10% mild silver proteinate is desirable. If the eye is inflamed, use repeated hot compresses.

If for any reason the patient cannot be taken care of at once, the eye should be bandaged to keep it closed and thus avoid scratching the conjunctiva. There should be no delay in having the speck removed, as serious injury to the eyeball or to the vision may result. In general, the longer the foreign body remains in the eye, the deeper it becomes embedded.

e., light-adapted. An eye that has become adjusted to viewing objects in bright light; one adapted for phototic or cone vision; one in which visual purple has been bleached.

e., pink-. Acute contagious conjunctivitis. SEE: *pink-eye.*

e., squinting. The eye that deviates from the object of fixation in strabismus.

e., sympathizing. In sympathetic ophthalmia, the uninjured eye, which responds to sympathogenic influences.

eyeball. The globe of the eye. It has three humors: aqueous, lens or crystalline, and vitreous. Tension and position of the globe in relationship to orbit should be noted.

PATH: *Exophthalmos:* If the protrusion is bilateral, the condition may be due to goiter. The eye may appear to protrude in fright, asthma, and spasmodic croup. It is noted in thrombosis of superior longitudinal sinus, cardiac atrophy, laryngeal stenosis, and paralysis of ocular movements. One or both may be affected by hemorrhage in orbit, aneurysm, exostosis, or tumor of orbit, or enlarged lacrimal glands. *Enophthalmos:* Bilateral or unilateral recession of eyeball.

eye bank. An organization that collects and stores corneas for transplantation.

eyebrow. The arch over the eye; also its covering, esp. the hairs.

eye closure reflex. Contraction of orbicularis palpebrarum with closure of lids resulting from percussion above supraorbital nerve. SYN: *McCarthy's reflex; supraorbital reflex.*

eye contact. The meeting of the eyes of two persons; to look directly into the eyes of another.

eyecup. 1 The optic vesicle, evagination of the embryonic brain from which the retina develops. 2. A small cup that fits over the eye, used for bathing the surface of the eye.

eye drops. Any medicinal substance intended to be dropped in liquid form onto the conjunctiva.

CAUTION: Many medicines are not absorbed from the conjunctiva; they may be readily absorbed from the nasolacrimal duct. For this reason, esp. in children, it is advisable to close off the duct by applying pressure to the inner canthus of the eye for a few minutes after each instillation. This is of particular importance when using drugs such as belladonna to which young children are especially sensitive.

eyeglass. A glass lens used to aid the defective eye in seeing.

eyeground. Fundus of eye, seen with ophthalmoscope.

eyelash. A stiff hair on the margin of the eyelid. SYN: *cilium.*

eyelid. One of two movable protective folds that when closed cover the anterior surface of the eyeball. They are separated by the palpebral fissure. The upper (palpebrae superior) is the larger and more movable. It is raised by contraction of the levator palpebrae superioris muscle. Angles formed by the lids at inner and outer ends are known as the canthi. The cilia, or eyelashes, arise from the edges of the eyelids. The posterior surface is lined by the conjunctiva, a mucous membrane.

e., drooping. Ptosis of the eyelid.

e., fused. A congenital anomaly resulting from failure of the fetal eyelids to separate.

eye muscle imbalance. Pathological condition of the extraocular muscles of one or both eyes. This causes the eyes to be misaligned in one or more axes. SEE: *eye, crossed; esophoria; exophoria.*

eyepiece (ī′pēs). The portion of an optical device such as a microscope closest to the viewer's eye.

eyestrain. Tiredness of the eye due to overuse.

eyewash. Any suitable liquid material used to wash the eye. Ex.: sterile physiological saline or sterile water.

F

F. 1. *Fahrenheit; field of vision; folic acid; formula; function; Fusiformis.* 2. Chem. symb. for fluorine.

F_1. In genetics, the first filial generation, the offspring of a cross between two unrelated individuals.

F_2. The second filial generation or the offspring of a cross between two individuals of the F_1 generation.

FA., F.A. *fatty acid; filterable agent; first aid; fluorescent antibody.*

F.A.A.N. *Fellow of the American Academy of Nursing.*

fabella (fă-bĕl′lă) [L., little bean]. (pl. *fabellae*) Fibrocartilage or bones that sometimes develop in the head of the gastrocnemius muscle.

fabism (fā′bĭzm) [L. *faba*, bean, + Gr. *-ismos*, condition]. Favism, q.v.

fabrication (făb″rĭ-kā′shŭn) [L. *fabricatus*, having built]. A deliberately false statement told as if it were true. Present in Korsakoff's syndrome, q.v.

Fabry's disease (fă′brēz). [J. Fabry, Ger. physician, 1860–1930] An inherited metabolic disease wherein a glycolipid, ceramidetrihexoside, accumulates in the organs and tissues. The excessive amounts present in the kidneys and other organs impair their function. The disease has been treated experimentally by intravenous administration of the enzyme essential to the metabolism of the specific glycolipid.

F.A.C.D. *Fellow of the American College of Dentists.*

face [L. *facies*]. Anterior part of the head from forehead to chin and extending laterally to but not including the ears; the visage or countenance. SEE: illus.

ANAT: There are 14 bones in the face. Arteries include branches from the left common carotid, the right common carotid, and branches from the circle of Willis. The veins include exterior and interior jugular.

DIAG: The following conditions affect the features: mouth breathing, chronic alcoholism, narcotic drug use, abdominal diseases, pain, fear, mental depression, fatigue, facial hemiplegia, cretinism, myxedema, congenital syphilis, exophthalmic goiter, paralysis agitans, encephalitis lethargica, locomotor ataxia, acromegaly, Down's syndrome, acute

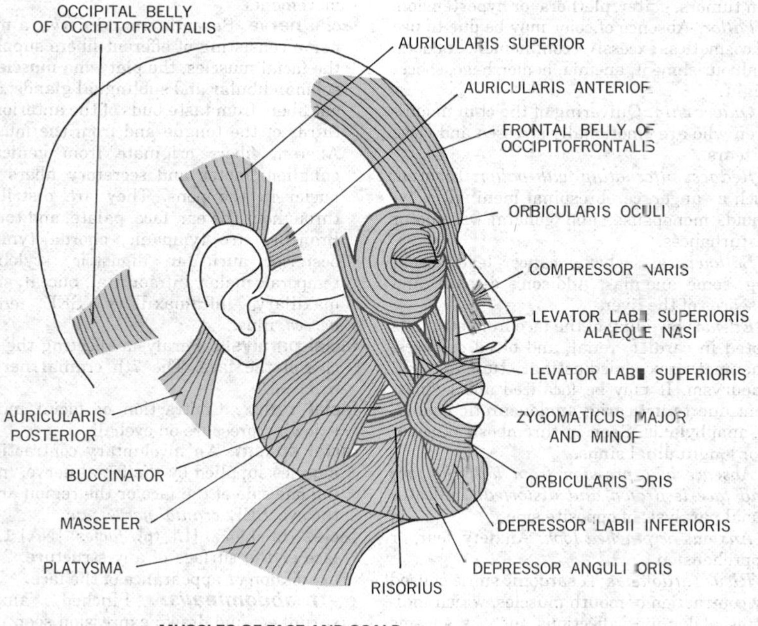

MUSCLES OF FACE AND SCALP

diffuse peritonitis, dyspnea, hysteria, late stages of pulmonary tuberculosis, lobar pneumonia, renal diseases, typhoid fever, hippocratic facies.

Brownish-yellow spots: Commonly called liver spots. Seen in pregnancy, malignancies of liver or uterus, and in exophthalmic goiter. Cosmetics and facial irritants, sunburn, and exposure to weather are also factors. Occur in many diseases including Addison's disease, diabetes, hemochromatosis, pellagra, acanthosis nigricans. Also occur in arsenic poisoning.

Depigmentation: Vitiligo, and scars.

Yellowish discoloration: Jaundice due to presence of excess of bile pigments in the blood. Carotenemia may cause a yellowish discoloration.

Cyanosis: Deficient oxygenation of the blood, which may be due to acquired or congenital malformations of the heart, to asthma, whooping cough, pulmonary tuberculosis, croup, obstruction of trachea, aneurysm, tumor, asphyxia, drug poisoning, emphysema, or dilation of right side of the heart.

Flushing (hyperemia): May be permanent or evanescent. If due to emotions or sunburn, it will be temporary. Permanent flushing may be due to febrile diseases, pulmonary tuberculosis, convulsions, alcoholism, ovarian tumors, goiter, plethora, or hypertension.

Pallor: Absence of color may be due to use of cosmetics, excessive confinement indoors, malnourishment, anemia, hemorrhage, shock, fright.

Quiver chin: Quivering of the chin in children who are emotionally stressed and close to tears.

Redness alternating with pallor: Emotion such as anger, cerebrospinal meningitis, typhoid, menopause, and general vasomotor disturbances.

Sallowness: Cachexia, cancer, lead poisoning, some anemias, Addison's disease, and diseases of the liver.

Edema: Swelling of the face from edema is noted in cardiac, renal, and blood diseases, pneumothorax, mediastinal tumors, and aneurysm. It may be localized and evanescent due to urticaria, angioneurotic edema, or anaphylaxis. Seen in thrombosis of superior longitudinal sinus.

Absence of expression from half the face and face is drawn and distorted: Indicates facial paralysis of opposite side.

Anxious or pinched look: Anxiety, fear, or apprehension.

Risus sardonicus: A sardonic smile caused by contraction of mouth muscles, which indicates abdominal affections such as spasms and peritonitis.

Spasms: May be intermittent, continuous, bilateral, or unilateral. May be due to dental disorders or diseases of skin, nose, or eyes. May be mimic or habit spasms; choreic, winking spasms; convulsive tic; blepharospasm. Closure of eyelids caused by spasm of orbicular muscles due to affection of the nerve supply, the eye muscles, or to eye diseases. Spasm of eyelids, chin, upper lips, or muscles of face seen in early stages of meningitis. Tonic spasms due to tetanus, spasms following paralysis, hysteria, and tic douloureux.

RS: anemia; argyria; Bell's palsy; chloasma; cranial nerves; cyanosis; edema; exophthalmic goiter; expression; eye; eyelid; facial; facies; flush; forehead; hyperemia; jaundice; jaw; lip; mouth; nose; poisoning; risus sardonicus; sallow; skeleton; skin; skull; spasm; tic; vitiligo.

f., moon. Full, round face seen in Cushing's syndrome, q.v. May also be a side effect of corticosteroid therapy.

facet, facette (făs′ĕt) [Fr. *facette,* small face]. A small, smooth area on a bone or other hard surface.

facetectomy (făs″ĕ-tĕk′tō-mē) [″ + Gr. *ektome,* excision]. Surgical removal of the auricular facet of a vertebra.

facial [L. *facialis*]. Pert. to the face.

facial center. Brain center causing facial movements.

facial nerve. Seventh cranial nerve, a mixed nerve consisting of efferent fibers supplying the facial muscles, the platysma muscle, the submandibular and sublingual glands; afferent fibers from taste buds of the anterior two thirds of the tongue and from the muscles. Afferent fibers originate from geniculate ganglion; motor and secretory fibers from nuclei in the pons. They are distributed throughout the ear, face, palate, and tongue. Branches are tympanic, chorda tympani, posterior auricular, digastric, stylohyoid, temporal, malar, infraorbital, buccal, supramaxillary, inframaxillary. SEE: *cranial nerves;* illus.

facial paralysis. Paralysis affecting the muscles of the face. The 7th cranial nerve is involved.

facial reflex. Contraction of facial muscles following pressure on eyeball.

facial spasm. An involuntary contraction of muscles supplied by the facial nerve, involving one side of the face or the region around the eye. SEE: *cranial nerves; tic.*

facies (fā′shē-ēz) [L]. (pl. *facies*) [NA] 1. The face or the surface of any structure. 2. The expression or appearance of the face.

f. abdominalis. Pinched, anxious, shrunken, and drawn expression seen in abdominal problems.

f., adenoid. Dull, lethargic appearance

SUPERFICIAL BRANCHES OF FACIAL NERVE (7th CRANIAL)

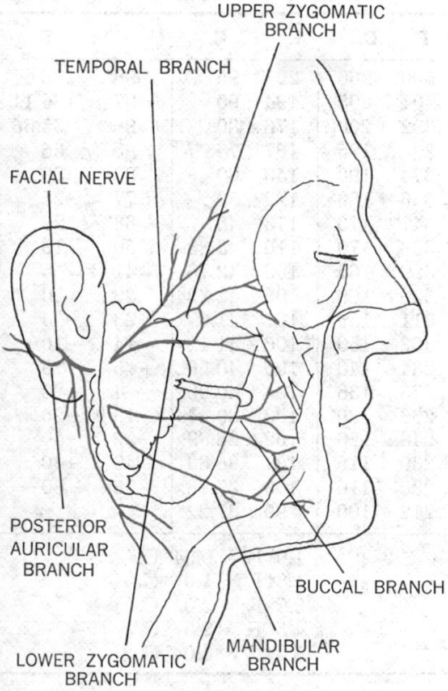

with open mouth. May be due to hypertrophy of adenoids, or chronic mouth breathing.

f. aortica. Expression seen in aortic valve insufficiency with bluish sclerae, sunken cheeks, and sallow face.

f. hepatica. Facies seen in liver disease. Skin is sallow, conjunctivae yellow, and eyeballs sunken.

f. hippocratica. Facies seen in those dying from long-continued illness or from cholera. Cheeks and temples hollow, eyes sunken, complexion leaden, and lips relaxed.

f. leontina. Lion-like face seen in certain forms of leprosy.

f., mask-like. Expressionless face with little or no animation seen in parkinsonism.

f. mitralis. Facies seen in mitral insufficiency. Capillaries more or less visible, cheeks pink, more or less cyanotic.

f., myopathic. Facies due to muscular relaxation. Lids drop and lips protrude.

f., parkinsonian. A mask-like face, and infrequent eye blinking. The individual can move the face, but in repose, the face is expressionless. Characteristic of parkinsonism.

f., typhoid. Dusky complexion, injected conjunctivae, and dull expression seen in early course of typhoid.

facilitation (fă-sĭl″ĭ-tā′shŭn) [L. *facilis,* easy]. Hastening of an action or process, esp. the energy of a nerve impulse being added to that of other impulses activated at the same time. In neuromuscular rehabilitation, used as a generic term to refer to various techniques to elicit muscular contraction through reflex activation.

facing [L. *facies,* face]. An inlay that forms the outer surface of a tooth.

faciobrachial (fā″shē-ō-brā′kē-ăl) [″ + Gr. *brachion,* arm]. Pert. to the face and arm, esp. to juvenile muscular dystrophy.

faciocephalalgia (fā″shē-ō-sĕf″ă-lăl′jē-ă) [″ + Gr. *kephale,* head, + *algos,* pain]. Neuralgia of the face and head.

faciocervical (fā″shē-ō-sĕr′vĭ-kăl) [″ + *cervix,* neck]. Pert. to the face and neck, esp. to progressive dystrophy of facial muscles.

faciolingual (fā″shē-ō-lĭn′gwăl) [″ + *lingua,* tongue]. Pert. to the face and the tongue, esp. a paralysis of them.

facioplasty (fā″shē-ō-plăs′tē) [″ + Gr. *plassein,* to form]. Plastic surgery of the face.

facioplegia (fā″shē-ō-plē′jē-ă) [″ + Gr. *plege,* stroke]. Facial paralysis. SYN: *prosopoplegia.*

facioscapulohumeral (fā″shē-ō-skăp″ū-lō-hū′mĕr-ăl) [″ + *scapula,* shoulder blade, + *humerus,* shoulder]. Pert. to the face, the scapula, and the upper arm.

F.A.C.O.G. *Fellow of the American College of Obstetricians and Gynecologists.*

F.A.C.P. *Fellow of the American College of Physicians.*

F.A.C.S. *Fellow of the American College of Surgeons.*

F.A.C.S.M. *Fellow of the American College of Sports Medicine.*

factitial (făk-tĭsh′ăl). Artificially produced, not natural. A factitial fever may be produced by the patient's artificially heating the thermometer. This is done while the patient thinks he or she is unobserved by the staff.

factitious (făk-tĭsh′ŭs) [L. *facticius,* made by art]. Something produced artificially; not natural.

factitious disorders. Disorders that are not real, genuine, or natural. The symptoms, physical and psychological, are produced by the individual and are under voluntary control. These symptoms and the behavior are used to pursue goals that are involuntarily adopted. The goal is to assume the role of patient and to stay in a hospital. This is attained by a variety of means such as taking anticoagulants, feigning right lower quadrant pain with nausea and vomiting, dizziness, fainting, fever of unknown origin, and massive hemoptysis. Mental symptoms may include memory loss hallucinations, and uncooperativeness. These patients have a severe personality disturbance. SEE: *Münchhausen syndrome.*

factor [L., maker]. 1. A contributing cause in any action. 2. In genetics, a gene. 3. An essential element such as a vitamin or immunoglobulin.

f., accessory food. A substance in food that does not serve as a source of energy for the user but is essential for normal growth and development or metabolic activities; a vitamin.

f., antianemic. A substance stored in the liver that is essential for the normal development of red blood cells in the bone marrow. It is formed in the stomach and intestine by the interaction of an extrinsic factor, vitamin B_{12}, and an intrinsic factor present in gastric juice. It is used in the treatment of pernicious anemia.

f., antihemophilic. SEE: *antihemophilic factor.*

f.'s, coagulation. Blood components that are essential to the clotting process. They are designated by Roman numerals; if activated, an "a" is added to the numeral. SEE: *coagulation factors.*

f., lethal. A gene or an abnormality in genetic composition that causes death of a zygote or of an individual before the reproductive age.

f., milk. A substance present in certain strains of mammary cancer–prone mice that is transferred to offspring through milk from the mammary glands. It is capable of inducing the development of mammary cancer in suckling mice exposed to the factor.

f., proliferation inhibiting. A lymphokine that inhibits cell division in tissue culture.

f., Rh. An antigen present on the surface of erythrocytes. SEE: *Rh blood group.*

Factorate. Trade name for antihemophilic factor (AHF).

facultative (făk′ŭl-tā″tĭv) [L. *facultas,* capability]. 1. Having the capacity to do something that is not compulsory. 2. In biology and particularly bacteriology, having the ability to live under certain conditions. Thus, a microorganism may be facultative with respect to oxygen and be able to live with or without oxygen.

faculty. A normal mental attribute or sense; ability to function.

FAD. *flavin adenine dinucleotide.*

fagopyrism (făg-ō-pīr′ĭzm, -ŏp′ĭ-rĭzm) [L. *fagopyrum,* buckwheat]. Buckwheat poisoning.

Fahrenheit scale (făr′ĕn-hīt″). [Gabriel D. Fahrenheit, Ger. physicist, 1686–1736] A temperature scale with the freezing point of water at 32° and the boiling point at 212°. Indicated by F. SEE: *Celsius scale; Kelvin scale; thermometer; Miscellaneous Units of Measurement* in *Appendix.*

Fahrenheit and Celsius Scales

F.	C.	F.	C.	F.	C.
500°	260°	203°	95°	98°	36.67°
401	205	194	90	97	36.11
392	200	176	80	96	35.56
383	195	167	75	95	35
374	190	140	60	86	30
356	180	122	50	77	25
347	175	113	45	68	20
338	170	110	43.33	50	10
329	165	109	42.78	41	5
320	160	108	42.22	32	0
311	155	107	41.67	23	− 5
302	150	106	41.11	14	−10
284	140	105	40.56	+ 5	−15
275	135	104	40.00	− 4	−20
266	130	103	39.44	−13	−25
248	120	102	38.89	−22	−30
239	115	101	38.33	−40	−40
230	110	100	37.78	−76	−60
212	100	99	37.22		

1.0° F. = 0.54° C.
1.8° F. = 1.0 ° C.
3.6° F. = 2.0 ° C.
4.5° F. = 2.5 ° C.
5.4° F. = 3.0 ° C.

failure (fāl′yĕr). To not be able to function, esp. to have lost or to lose that which was once present, as in failing eyesight or hearing.

f., heart. Condition in which the heart is not able to perform adequately its function of pumping blood. This may be temporary or chronic.

f., kidney or renal. Condition in which the kidneys are not able to perform adequately their functions. This may be partial, temporary, chronic, acute, or complete.

f., respiratory. Condition in which the lungs are unable to perform adequately their function of moving air into and carbon dioxide out of the lungs. This may be due to disease of the lung tissue, or paralysis or weakness of the respiratory muscles.

faint [O. Fr. *faindre,* to feign]. 1. To feel weak as though about to lose consciousness. 2. Weak. 3. Syncope: loss of consciousness due to cerebral anemia or insufficient blood to the brain.

SYM: Prior to onset patient may be pale, weak, dizzy, have cold perspiration and uncomfortable abdominal sensation. Patient may fall to the ground unconscious. Pulse is usually weak, rapid, and often irregular.

F.A.: It is important to have the person in a horizontal position, preferably with the head low in order to facilitate blood flow to the brain. At the same time, be certain there is a clear airway. Be certain the clothing is loose, esp. if a tight collar was being worn. Fainting usually is of short duration and is counteracted by the individual's being in a supine position. Nevertheless it is important to attempt to establish the cause of the faint prior to dismissing the episode as being of no consequence. If recovery from fainting is not prompt, then it is important to move the patient to a hospital.

RS: apoplexy; asphyxia; coma; shock; swoon, syncope; unconsciousness.

faintness. 1. A sensation of impending loss of consciousness. 2. A sensation due to lack of food.

faith healing. Healing accomplished by supplication to a divine being or power without medical or chemical aid. Although this area is open to fraudulent practice, the medical community cannot completely eliminate the psychosomatic aspects of illness that may be affected in this manner.

falcate (făl'kāt) [L. *falx,* sickle]. Sickle-shaped.

falces (făl'sēz) [L.]. Pl. of falx.

falcial (făl'shăl). Pert. to the falx.

falciform (făl'sĭ-form) [L. *falx,* sickle, + *forma,* form]. Sickle-shaped.

falciform ligament. The triangular ligament attached to sides of the sacrum and coccyx by its base.

falciform ligament of liver. A wide, sickle-shaped reflection of the peritoneum that serves as a principal attachment of the liver to the diaphragm, and serves to separate the right from the left lobes of the liver. Its broad attachment extends from the posterior, superior portion of the liver to the anterior convex portion, which is connected to the internal surface of the right rectus abdominis muscle.

falciform process. That portion of the falciform ligament along the inner margin of the ramus of the ischium.

falcular. 1. Sickle-shaped. 2. Pert. to the falx cerebelli.

fallectomy (făl-ĕk'tō-mē). Cutting away part of the fallopian tube.

falling drop. 1. A metallic tinkle heard over the normal stomach and bowel when inflated. 2. The same sound heard over large cavities containing fluid and air, as in hydropneumothorax.

fallopian canal (fă-lō'pē-ăn). [Gabriele Falloppio, It. anatomist, 1523–1562] Canal in petrous bone. The facial nerve passes through this canal.

fallopian ligament. Round ligament of the uterus.

fallopian tube. The tube or duct that extends laterally from the lateral angle of the fundal end of the uterus and terminates near the ovary. It serves to convey the ovum from the ovary to the uterus and spermatozoa from the uterus toward the ovary. Medially each tube opens into the uterus; distally each opens into the peritoneal cavity. Each lies in the superior border of the broad ligament.

ANAT: The narrow region near the uterus, the isthmus, continues laterally as a wider ampulla. The latter expands to form the terminal funnel-shaped infundibulum, at the bottom of which lies a small opening, the ostium, through which the ovum enters the oviduct. Surrounding each ostium are a number of fingerlike processes called fimbria extending towards the ovary. Each tube averages about 4½ in. (11.4 cm.) in length and ¼ in. (6 mm.) in diameter. Its wall consists of three layers: mucosa, muscular layer, and serosa. The epithelium of the mucosa consists of ciliated and nonciliated cells. Ciliary action aids in the movement of the ovum toward the uterus. The muscular layer consists of an inner circular and an outer longitudinal layer of smooth muscle. The serosa consists of connective tissue underlying the outermost layer of peritoneum. The blood supply is derived from branches of the uterine and ovarian arteries. The nerve supply is from the pelvic, ovarian, and uterine nerve plexuses, sending fibers to the tubes. SYN: *oviduct; uterine tube.* SEE: *uterus; genitalia, female,* for illus.

Fallot, tetralogy of (făl-ō'). [Etienne L. A. Fallot, Fr. physician, 1850–1911] A congenital condition characterized by defect in the interventricular septum, stenosis of the pulmonary artery, dextroposition of the aorta, and hypertrophy of the right ventricle. Modern surgical therapy has made it possible to treat this condition effectively.

fallotomy (făl-ŏt'ō-mē). Division of the fallopian tubes. SYN: *salpingotomy.*

fallout. Settling of radioactive fission products from the atmosphere after release of such materials into the air after explosion of an atomic bomb or device; or from a radiation accident such as could occur at any installation using radioactive materials.

false [L. *falsus*]. That which is untrue or incorrect.

false-negative (făwls'nĕg'ă-tĭv). A test or procedure that indicates the abnormality or disease being investigated is not present when in fact it is. SEE: *false-positive.*

false-positive (făwls'pŏs'ĭ-tĭv). A test or procedure that indicates the abnormality or disease being investigated is present when in fact it is not. SEE: *false-negative.*

false ribs. The lower five pairs of ribs that do

not unite directly with the sternum. SEE: *rib; vertebrae.*

falsification (făwl″sĭ-fĭ-kā′shŭn). The act of writing or stating that which is not true.

f., retrospective. Deliberate or unconscious alteration of memory for past events or situations. A mental mechanism for ego-preservation.

falx [L.]. (pl. *falces*) [NA] Any sickle-shaped structure.

f. cerebelli. [NA] A fold of the dura mater that forms a vertical partition between the hemispheres of the cerebellum.

f. cerebri. [NA] A fold of the dura mater that lies in the longitudinal fissure and separates the two cerebral hemispheres.

f. inguinalis. [NA] The conjoined or conjoint tendon that forms the origin of the transversus abdominis and internal oblique muscles.

f. ligmentosa. The broad ligament of the liver. SYN: *falciform ligament of liver.*

fames (fā′mēz) [L.]. Hunger.

familial [L. *familia,* family]. Pert. to or common to the same family; e.g., a disease occurring more frequently in a family than would be expected by chance.

familial Mediterranean fever. An inherited autosomal recessive disorder that is seen most commonly in Middle Eastern ethnic groups but has appeared in family clusters in persons of Irish or Italian descent. The attacks, which almost always include fever, first appear between the ages of 5 and 15. Included in the syndrome are some but not necessarily all of the following: abdominal pain resembling peritonitis, chest pain of pleural or pericardial origin, erysipelas-like redness near the ankle, and joint involvement. Duration and frequency of attacks are unpredictable. Some of the patients develop amyloidosis. Otherwise, the prognosis is favorable even though there is no specific therapy.

familial periodic paralysis. A rare familial disease in which attacks of flaccid paralysis, often at time of awakening, occur. This condition is usually associated with hypokalemia, but is sometimes present even though the blood potassium level is normal or elevated. The condition may, in affected individuals, be precipitated by administration of glucose.

family. 1. A group of individuals who have descended from a common ancestor. 2. In biological classification, the division between an order and a genus.

family planning. The planning and spacing of conception of children according to the wishes of the couple rather than to chance. This is accomplished by practicing some form of birth control.

family practice. Comprehensive medical care with particular emphasis on the family unit, in which the physician's continuing responsibility for health care is not limited by the patient's age or sex nor by a particular organ system or disease entity.

Family practice is the specialty which builds upon a core of knowledge derived from other disciplines, drawing most heavily on Internal Medicine, Pediatrics, Obstetrics and Gynecology, Surgery and Psychiatry, and which establishes a cohesive unit, combining the behavioral sciences with the traditional biological and clinical sciences. The core of knowledge encompassed by the discipline of Family Practice prepares the family physician for a unique role in patient management, problem solving, counseling and as a personal physician who coordinates total health care delivery. (Definition supplied by The American Academy of Family Physicians.)

Fanconi's syndrome. [Guido Fanconi, Swiss pediatrician, b. 1882] 1. Congenital hypoplastic anemia. 2. Aminoaciduria associated with rickets, q.v., due to failure of the proximal renal tubules or to dysfunction of the deamination process. Symptoms include rickets, polyuria, and growth failure. Dietary therapy is of some help but the patients usually die prior to puberty.

fang [AS., to plunder]. 1. A sharp-pointed tooth. 2. The root of a tooth.

fango (făn′gō) [Italian, mud]. Mud obtained from thermal springs in Battaglia, Italy. Used in treating rheumatism and gout.

Fannia (făn′ē-ă). A genus of small house flies.

fantast (făn′tăst) [Gr. *phantasia,* imagination]. A daydreamer.

fantasy (făn′tă-sē) [Gr. *phantasia,* imagination]. The mechanism of creating in one's mind that which is unreal and may be disordered and weird.

F.A.O.T.A. *Fellow of the American Occupational Therapy Association.*

farad (făr′ăd). [Michael Faraday, Brit. physicist, 1791–1867] A unit of electrical capacity. The capacity of a condenser that, charged with 1 coulomb, gives a difference of potential of 1 volt. This unit is so large that one-millionth part of it has been adopted as a practical unit called a microfarad.

faraday (făr′ă-dā). The amount of electrical charge associated with one gram equivalent of an electrochemical reaction. Equal to approx. 96,000 coulombs. SEE: *coulomb; farad.*

faradic. Pert. to induced electricity.

faradism. The therapeutic use of an interrupted current to stimulate muscles and nerves. Such a current is derived from the secondary or induction coil.

faradization. 1. The treatment of nerves or

muscles with faradic current. 2. The condition of nerves or muscles so treated.

faradotherapy. Treatment of disease by faradic current.

farcy (făr′sē) [L. *farcire,* to stuff]. A chronic form of glanders, q.v.

f., button. Farcy marked by dermal tubercular nodules.

farina (fă-rē′nă) [L.]. Finely ground meal commonly made from wheat or other grain. Used as cereal and flour.

farinaceous (făr″ĭ-nā′shŭs). 1. Starchy. 2. Pert. to flour.

farmer's lung. A form of hypersensitivity alveolitis caused by exposure to moldy hay that has fermented. Actinomyces micropolyspora faeni and Thermoactinomyces vulgaris are the causative microorganisms. SEE: *alveolitis, hypersensitivity; bagassosis.*

farpoint. The farthest point of vision at which objects can be seen distinctly with eyes in complete relaxation.

Farre's tubercles (fărz). [John R. Farre, Brit. physician, 1775–1862] Carcinomatous masses on surface of the liver.

farsighted. Pert. to farsightedness.

farsightedness. An error of refraction in which, with accommodation completely relaxed, parallel rays come to a focus behind the retina. Individuals affected can see distant objects clearly, but cannot see near objects in proper focus. SYN: *hyperopia.*

fascia (făsh′ē-ă) [L., a band]. (pl. *fasciae*) [NA] A fibrous membrane covering, supporting, and separating muscles. It also unites the skin with underlying tissue. Fascia may be superficial, a nearly subcutaneous covering permitting free movement of the skin, or it may be deep, enveloping and binding muscles.

f., Abernethy's. A layer of areolar tissue separating the external iliac artery from the iliac fascia over the psoas muscle.

f., anal. Fascia of connective tissue covering levator ani muscle from the perineal aspect.

f., aponeurotic. Thick fascia that provides attachment for a muscle.

f., Buck's. A fascial covering of the penis, derived from Colles' fascia.

f., cervical, deep. Fascia of the neck covering the muscles, vessels, and nerves.

f., cervical, superficial. Fascia of the neck just inside the skin.

f., Cloquet's. Femoral fascia.

f., Colles'. Inner layer of the perineal fascia.

f., cremasteric. Fascia covering the cremaster muscle of the spermatic cord.

f., cribriform. The fascia of the thigh covering the saphenous opening.

f., crural. Deep fascia of the leg.

f., deep. The connective tissue covering for all of the body. It is just below the superficial fascia and skin.

f., dentate. Gray matter in the cerebral dentate convolution. SYN: *gyrus, dentate.*

f., endothoracic. Fascia that separates the pleura of the lung from the inside of the thoracic cavity and the diaphragm.

f., extrapleural. Endothoracic fascia.

f., infundibuliform. Funnel-shaped fascia, derived from the interior abdominal wall, encasing the spermatic cord and testis.

f., intercolumnar. Fascia derived from the external abdominal ring sheathing the spermatic cord and testis.

f. lata. [NA] Wide fascia encasing thigh muscles.

f., lumbodorsal. Deep investing membrane covering deep muscles of the trunk and back.

f., pectineal. Pubic section of fascia lata.

f., pelvic. Fascial tissues of extreme importance in the maintenance of normal strength in the pelvic floor. SEE: *diaphragm, pelvic.*

f., pharyngobasilar. Sheet of connective tissue lying between the mucosal and muscular layers of the pharyngeal wall. SYN: *aponeurosis, pharyngeal.*

f., plantar. Sheet of connective tissue investing the muscles of the sole of the foot. SYN: *aponeurosis, plantar.*

f., Scarpa's. The deep layer of the superficial fascia of the abdomen.

f., superficial. The connective tissue layer just below the skin.

f., thyrolaryngeal. Fascia covering the thyroid gland.

f. transversalis. Fascia located between the perineum and transversalis muscle. It lines the abdominal cavity.

fasciae (făsh′ē-ē). Pl. of fascia.

fascial (făsh′ē-ăl) [L. *fascia,* band]. Pert. to or of the nature of fascia.

fascial reflex. Muscular contraction resulting from percussing facial fascia.

fasciaplasty (făsh′ē-ă-plăs″tē) [″ + Gr. *plassein,* to form]. Plastic surgery of fascia.

fascicle (făs′ĭ-kl) [L. *fasciculus,* little bundle]. A fasciculus.

fascicular (fă-sĭk′ū-lăr). 1. Arranged like a bundle of rods. 2. Pert. to a fasciculus.

fasciculation (fă-sĭk″ū-lā′shŭn). 1. Formation of fascicles. 2. Involuntary contraction or twitching of muscle fibers. These can be seen under the skin. 3. Spontaneous contractions of muscle fibers without causing movement at a joint. A biolelectric potential caused by deterioration of anterior horn cells.

fasciculus (fă-sĭk′ū-lŭs). (pl. *fasciculi*) [NA] A small bundle, esp. of nerve or muscle fibers. More specifically a division of a funiculus of the spinal cord consisting of fibers of one or more tracts. Sometimes the term is used as a synonym for tract. SYN: *fasciola.*

f. cuneatus. A triangular-shaped bundle of nerve fibers lying in the dorsal funiculus of the spinal cord. Its fibers enter the cord through the dorsal roots of spinal nerves and terminate in the medulla. SYN: *column of Burdach.*

f., dorsolateral. Tract, dorsolateral, q.v.

f., fundamental. Portion of anterior column of the spinal cord continuing into the medulla oblongata.

f. gracilis. A bundle of nerve fibers lying in the dorsal funiculus of the spinal cord medial to the fasciculus cuneatus. Conducts sensory impulses from the periphery to the medulla. SYN: *column of Goll.*

f., longitudinal, dorsal. A bundle of association fibers connecting the frontal lobe with the occipital and temporal lobes.

f., longitudinal, inferior. A bundle of association fibers connecting the occipital and temporal lobes of the brain.

f., longitudinal, medial. A bundle of fibers running from the spinal cord to the upper portion of the midbrain.

f., longitudinal, posterior. Nerve fiber bundle running between corpora quadrigemina and nuclei of 4th and 6th nerves.

f., unciform. Fibers within sylvian fissure connecting frontal and temporosphenoid lobes. SYN: *uncinate fasciculus.*

fasciectomy (făsh″ē-ĕk′tō-mē) [L. *fascia,* band, + Gr. *ektome,* excision]. Excision of strips of fascia.

fasciitis (făs″ē-ī′tĭs). Inflammation of any fascia.

fasciodesis (făsh″ē-ŏd′ĕ-sĭs) [″ + Gr. *desis,* binding]. Operation of attaching a fascia to a tendon or another fascia.

Fasciola (fă-sī′ō-lă) [L. *fasciola,* a band]. A genus of flukes belonging to the class Trematoda.

F. hepatica. A species of flukes infesting the liver and bile ducts of cattle, sheep, and other herbivores; the common liver fluke. An occasional parasite of man. Intermediate hosts are snails belonging to the genus Lymnaea.

fasciola (fă-sī′ō-lă, fă-sē′ō-lă) [L., a band]. (pl. *fasciolae*) A bundle of nerve or muscle fibers.

f. cinerea. Upper portion of dentate fascia.

fasciolar (fă-sē′ō-lăr). Pert. to the fasciola cinerea.

fasciolopsiasis (făs″ē-ō-lŏp-sī′ă-sĭs). Infection of the body with a genus of trematode worms, Fasciolopsis buski. It is contracted by ingesting plants grown in water infested by the intermediate host, snails. SYN: *distomiasis.*

SYM: Diarrhea, abdominal pain, anasarca, and eosinophilia.

TREATMENT: Tetrachlorethylene.

Fasciolopsis buski (făs″ē-ō-lŏp′sĭs). A fluke that infests the intestinal tract of certain mammals including man. Symptoms include vomiting, anorexia, and diarrhea alternating with constipation. The number of flukes present may be sufficient to cause intestinal obstruction. The disease occurs in Asia, including central and south China. SEE: *fasciolopsiasis.*

fascioplasty (făsh′ē-ō-plăs″tē) [″ + Gr. *plassein,* to form]. Plastic operation on a fascia.

fasciorrhaphy (făsh-ē-or′ă-fē) [″ + Gr. *rhaphe,* suture]. Suturing a fascia.

fasciotomy (făsh-ē-ŏt′ō-mē) [″ + Gr. *tome,* incision]. Surgical incision and division of a fascia.

fascitis (fă-sī′tĭs) [″ + Gr. *itis,* inflammation]. Inflamed condition of a fascia.

fast. 1. [AS. *faest,* fixed] Resistant to the effects or action of a chemical substance. 2. [AS. *faestan,* to hold fast] Abstention from food.

f., acid. Term applied to bacteria, esp. the Mycobacteria, that after staining are not decolorized when treated with acid.

fastidium (făs-tĭd′ē-ŭm) [L., aversion]. Aversion to food or to eating. Sometimes seen in hysteria but not as the result of delusions.

fastigium (făs-tĭj′ē-ŭm) [L., ridge]. 1. The highest point. The full period of development of acute, infectious diseases when the temperature reaches the maximum or stadium and all symptoms have developed. 2. The most posterior portion of the 4th ventricle formed by the junction of the anterior and posterior medullary vela projecting into the medullary substance of the cerebellum.

fasting [AS. *faestan,* to hold fast]. Going without food. Energy requirements of body metabolism during fasting are supplied by the oxidization of fats, which, if glucose is not supplied, results in the products of incomplete fat combustion such as fatty acids, diacetic acid, and acetone, producing ketosis and a mild acidosis. This condition occurs quickly in children as they have little glycogen reserve. CAUTION: Unsupervised fasting in order to lose weight can cause death.

fastness [AS. *faest,* fixed]. Ability of bacteria to resist stains or destructive agents.

fat [AS. *faett*]. 1. Adipose tissue of the body, which serves as an energy reserve. SEE: *obesity.* 2. Grease, oil. 3. In chemistry, triglyceride ester of fatty acids; one of a group of organic compounds closely associated in nature with the phosphatides, cerebrosides, and sterols. The term lipid, q.v., is applied in general to a fat or fatlike substance. Fats are insoluble in water but soluble in ether, chloroform, benzene, and other fat solvents. Upon hydrolysis, fats break down into fatty acids and glycerol (an alcohol). Fats are hydrolyzed by the action of acids, alkalies, lipases (fat-splitting enzymes) and superheated steam.

CHEM. STRUCTURE: In the fat molecule, one molecule of glycerol is combined with three of fatty acids. Three fatty acids, oleic acid ($C_{18}H_{34}O_2$), stearic acid ($C_{18}H_{36}O_2$), and palmitic acid ($C_{18}H_{32}O_2$), comprise the bulk of fatty acids present in neutral fats found in body tissues. According to the fatty acid with which the glycerol is combined, corresponding fats are triolein, tristearin, and tripalmitin. These three fats are the principal fats present in foods.

PHYS: Fats serve as a source of energy. Subcutaneous fat also provides an insulating layer that inhibits heat loss. Fat acts to support and protect certain organs such as the eye and kidney; provides a concentrated reserve of food; provides essential fatty acids necessary for normal growth and development; and in foods is a vehicle for natural fat-soluble vitamins. In conjunction with carbohydrates, fats serve as protein sparers. They are an important constituent of cell structure, forming an integral part of the cell membrane. When properly distributed, fat gives a pleasing contour to the body.

DIGESTION AND ABSORPTION: In the stomach, emulsified fats such as cream or egg yolk are acted on by gastric lipase; however, most fats undergo digestion in the intestine, where they are acted on by a pancreatic lipase, steapsin, which hydrolyzes them to fatty acids and glycerol. Although containing no lipolytic enzymes, bile is essential for the digestion of fats. It aids in the emulsification of fats and has a hydrotropic action, i.e., renders substances such as fatty acids, which are normally insoluble in water, readily soluble in the intestinal juices. Bile salts also act as specific activators of the pancreatic lipase. Bile salts react with fatty acids, forming water-soluble, diffusible soaps that facilitate the emulsification of fats. Glycerol and fatty acids enter the epithelial cells, where they recombine to form neutral fats, most of which enter the lacteals. The fats are carried by the lymph through lymph vessels to the thoracic duct, from which they enter the bloodstream. After a meal rich in fats, the mesenteric lymph vessels are filled with a milklike fluid, the chyle, containing finely emulsified fat particles called chylomicrons.

METABOLISM: Absorbed fats are utilized in the following ways: oxidized with the release of energy; deposited in adipose tissue as storage fat; incorporated in the cells of tissues as an integral part of the protoplasm; desaturated and stored in the liver; excreted in the secretions of the mammary and sweat glands and in the feces.

Intermediary metabolism: In the oxidation of fat to carbon dioxide and water, several intermediary substances (ketones) are formed. The principal ones are acetoacetic acid, beta-hydroxybutyric acid, and acetone. Excessive production of ketone bodies, which occurs when fats are incompletely oxidized, is called ketosis. This especially occurs when there is an interference in carbohydrate metabolism, as in diabetes. Ketosis also occurs in starvation, in certain fevers, toxemias of pregnancy, and hyperthyroidism. Ketosis results in acidosis.

SOURCES: In addition to fat being absorbed from the intestine, body fat may arise from the conversion of carbohydrates (glucose) or proteins into fat. Fatty acids cannot be converted directly to glucose in the body, but a portion of the molecule of fatty acids of certain length can be utilized as carbohydrate.

NUTRITION: Fats have a high caloric value, yielding about 9 Cal. per gm. as compared with about 4 Cal. for carbohydrates and proteins. The average diet of 3000 Cal. may derive 40% of the caloric value from fats. Nutritionists and epidemiologists feel that decreasing fat in the diet to 30% would decrease the risk of developing cancer, esp. of the colon, breast, and prostate. In addition to their nutritive values, fats improve the taste and odor of foods, provide a feeling of satiety, and because of their high caloric content are of special importance in high-caloric diets.

CONTRA: Fat intake should be reduced in certain diseases such as hepatitis and in low-caloric diets.

RS: bile; fatty acid; gallbladder; glycerin; ketone; ketosis; lipase; liver.

f., neutral. Compounds of the higher fatty acids (palmitic, stearic, and oleic) with glycerol. They are the common fats of animal and plant tissues.

fat, words pert. to: absorption; acid; "adip-" words; anorexia nervosa; body composition; caloric excess; calorie; cholesterol; chondrolipoma; diet; digestion; energy; fasting; fatty acid; food; food requirements; fuel value; glucose; hydrogenation; ketogenic diet; ketone; ketosis; "lip-" words; obesity; palmitic acid; palmitin; reduction diet; steapsin; stearin; stearrhea.

fatal (fāt'l) [L. *fatalis*]. 1. Inevitable. 2. Causing death.

fatigability (făt″ĭ-gă-bĭl'ĭ-tē). Condition of becoming easily tired or exhausted.

fatigue (fă-tēg') [L. *fatigare,* to tire]. 1. A feeling of tiredness or weariness resulting from continued activity. 2. The state or condition of an organ or tissue in which its response to stimulation is reduced or lost as a result of overactivity. 3. To bring about a condition of fatigue.

Fatigue may be the result of excessive activity, which results in the accumulation of metabolic waste products such as lactic acid; malnutrition (deficiency of carbohydrates, proteins, minerals, or vitamins); circulatory disturbances such as heart disease or anemia, which interfere with the supply of oxygen and energy materials to tissues; respiratory disturbances, which interfere with the supply of oxygen to tissues; infectious diseases, in which toxic products are produced or body metabolism altered; endocrine disturbances such as occur in diabetes, hyperinsulinism, and menopause; psychogenic factors such as emotional conflicts, frustration, anxiety, neurosis, boredom; physical factor such as being crippled. Environmental noise and vibration contribute to the development of fatigue.

f., acute. Fatigue with sudden onset such as occurs following excessive exertion; relieved by rest.

f., chronic. Long-continued fatigue not relieved by rest. Indicative of disease such as tuberculosis or diabetes or other conditions of altered body metabolism.

f., muscular. The reduced capacity of a muscle to perform work as a result of repeated contractions. Fatigue may be partial or complete.

fatty (făt'ē). Of, or pert. to, fats or fatty substances; adipose. SEE: *fat; heart; obesity.*

fatty acid. A hydrocarbon in which one of the hydrogen atoms has been replaced by a carboxyl (COOH) group; a monobasic aliphatic acid made up of an alkyl radical attached to a carboxyl group.

Saturated fatty acids have single bonds in their carbon chain with the general formula $C_nH_{2n}O_2$. They include acetic, butyric, caproic, caprylic, capric, lauric, formic, myristic, palmitic, and stearic acids. Unsaturated fatty acids have one or more double or triple bonds in the carbon chain. They include those of the oleic series (oleic, tiglic, hypogeic, and palmitoleic) and the linoleic or linolic series (linoleic, linolenic, clupanodonic, arachidonic, hydrocarpic, and chaulmoogric acids). Fatty acids are insoluble in water. This would prevent their being absorbed from the intestines were it not for the action of bile salts on the fatty acids to enable them to be absorbed.

f.a., essential. The unsaturated fatty acids (linoleic, linolenic, and arachidonic) cannot be synthesized in the body and have been considered to be essential to maintain health. SEE: *digestion.*

fatty casts. Casts seen in the urine sediments. They are usually abnormal and consist of a mass of fat globules.

fatty degeneration. A change involving the deposition of fat in the cytoplasm of cells.

fauces (fŏ'sēz) [L.]. [NA] The constricted opening leading from the mouth and the oral pharynx. It is bounded by the soft palate, base of the tongue, and the palatine arches. The anterior pillars of the fauces are known as the glossopalatine arch, and the posterior pillars as the pharyngopalatine arch. SEE: *fossa.*

faucial (fŏ'shăl) [L. *fauces,* throat]. Pert. to the fauces.

faucial reflex. Gagging or vomiting resulting from irritation of fauces.

faucitis (fŏ-sī'tĭs) [" + Gr. *itis,* inflammation]. Inflammation of the fauces.

fauna (faw'nă) [L. *Faunus,* mythical deity of herdsmen]. All of the animals, including microscopic forms, in the area considered. SEE: *flora.*

faveolate (fā-vē'ō-lāt) [L. *faveolus,* little honeycomb]. Honeycombed. SYN: *alveolate.*

faveolus (fā-vē'ō-lŭs) [L., little honeycomb]. A depression or small pit, esp. on the skin. SYN: *foveola.*

favism (fā'vĭzm) [It. *fava,* bean, + Gr. *-ismos,* condition]. A hereditary condition common in Sicily and Sardinia resulting from sensitivity to a species of bean, Vicia faba. It is characterized by fever, acute hemolytic anemia, vomiting, diarrhea, and may lead to prostration and coma. It is caused by ingestion of the beans or inhalation of the pollen of the plant by persons who have an inherited deficiency of the enzyme glucose-6-phosphate dehydrogenase.

favus (fā'vŭs) [L., honeycomb]. Fungal skin disease characterized by pinhead to pea-sized, saucer-shaped, yellowish crust (scutulum) over hair follicles and accompanied by musty odor and itching. It may spread all over the body. SEE: *scutulum.*

F.D. *fatal dose; focal distance.*

F.D.A. *Food and Drug Administration.*

Fe. Chem. symb. for L. *ferrum,* iron.

fear [AS. *faer*]. Fright, dread. Primitively, the emotional reaction to an environmental threat; it now also presents itself frequently as an indicator of inner problems. Fear is met clinically in anxiety neuroses, anxious psychotogenic conditions such as depression, and in toxic deliria (delirium tremens). At the somatic level, hyperthyroidism and hyperadrenalism may strongly simulate the fear state. SEE: *emotion; Phobias* in *Appendix.*

febricide (fĕb'rĭ-sīd) [L. *febris,* fever, + *cidus,* killing]. Destructive to fever. SYN: *antipyretic.*

febrifacient (fĕb-rĭ-fā'sē-ĕnt) [L. *febris,* fever,

+ *facere,* to make]. Producing fever.

febrific (fĕ-brĭf'ĭk). Producing or conveying fever.

febrifugal (fĕb-rĭf'ū-găl) [" + *fugare,* to put to flight]. Reducing fever.

febrifuge (fĕb'rĭ-fūj). That which reduces fever. SYN: *antipyretic.*

febrile (fē'brĭl, fē'brīl, fĕb'rĭl) [L. *febris,* fever]. Feverish; pert. to a fever. SEE: *fever.*

febrile convulsions. About three to five percent of children will experience a convulsion associated with fever. Most will have this in the period between six months and two to three years of age. Febrile convulsions are rare after age six to eight. Boys are more susceptible to this type convulsion than girls. It is important to do a complete history and physical examination including neurological appraisal in order to be certain the convulsion does indeed represent only the symptom of an acute febrile illness.

TREATMENT: Appropriate therapy for reduction of the elevated body temperature, and a sedative dose of phenobarbital, 3 mg./kg. of body weight. It is important that the measures to reduce the temperature not be so vigorous as to cause hypothermia. The application of cool compresses with gentle flow of air over the body will suffice. A hypothermia blanket is also suitable for use. Ice water baths, and vigorous fanning of the child as alcohol is applied will most probably produce hypothermia and should not be used. In the past, the recommendation has been made that a child who has experienced a single febrile convulsion should have daily anticonvulsant therapy for a two- to four-year period. The efficacy and advisability of this have not been proved.

febrile state. A term used to describe constitutional symptoms that accompany a rise in temperature. Pulse and respiration usually rise with headache, pains, malaise, loss of appetite, concentrated and diminished urine, constipation, restlessness, insomnia, irritability.

febriphobia (fĕb"rĭ-fō'bē-ă) [" + Gr. *phobos,* fear]. Anxiety or fear induced by a rise in body temperature.

febris (fē'brĭs) [L.]. Fever.

f. enterica. Typhoid fever.

f. flava. Yellow fever.

f. undulans. Brucellosis.

fecal (fē'kăl) [L. *faeces,* refuse]. Pert. to, or of the nature of, feces.

fecal vomit. Feces in vomitus. Occurs in strangulated hernia or intestinal obstruction preventing anal outlet.

fecalith (fē'kă-lĭth) [" + Gr. *lithos,* stone]. A fecal concretion. SYN: *coprolith.*

fecaloid (fē'kă-loyd) [" + Gr. *eidos,* form]. Resembling feces.

fecaloma (fē"kăl-ō'mă) [" + Gr. *oma,* tumor]. A large mass of accumulated feces in the rectum resembling a tumor. SYN: *scatoma; stercoroma.*

fecaluria (fē"kăl-ū'rē-ă) [" + Gr. *ouron,* urine]. Fecal matter in the urine.

feces (fē'sēz) [L. *faeces*]. Stools; excreta; dejecta; excrement. Body waste such as food residue, bacteria, epithelium, and mucus, discharged from the bowels by way of the anus. SYN: *stool.*

COMP: The total weight of the stool in a healthy adult male on a normal diet will be 100 to 200 gm. daily. Of this, 65% will be water and the remainder dry matter. Excreted nitrogen will be less than 1.7 gm. daily. The stool is composed of residue of food including undigested cellulose; water; secretions from intestinal glands, stomach, and liver; indole; skatole; cholesterol; mucus and epithelial cells; purine bases; pigment; microorganisms; inorganic salts; and sometimes foreign substances. The normal reaction is neutral or slightly alkaline. The stools of infants usually are acid.

DIAG: Inspection should include color, form, odor, and the presence of any observable foreign substances.

Color: May be indicative of various disorders. *Black* or *tarry* stools can indicate bleeding or hemorrhage into the gastrointestinal tract. Tarry is used to describe stools containing digested blood. May also follow the use of drugs such as bismuth, iron, tannin, manganese, or charcoal. *Bloody:* May indicate hemorrhoids, cancer of the rectum, ulcers, fissures, abraded rectal membrane from dry feces, eroded rectal polypus, acute proctitis, foreign bodies, colitis, intussusception or strangulated hernia in children, cancer of the colon, typhoid fever, or phosphorus poisoning. *Clay-colored:* May denote impaired bile formation or obstruction, phosphorus poisoning, or yellow atrophy of the liver. *Green:* In general, this indicates in children and infants that the bowel contents have passed quickly through the intestinal tract.

Form and Consistency: Normally soft and formed. Hard, nodular, or scybalous in constipation. Fluid or mushy in diarrhea. Consistently flattened or ribbonlike in rectal obstruction or spastic colitis. Greasy in jaundice.

Mucus: Amount should be noted. Present in both abnormal as well as normal circumstances. May occur as superficial gelatinous streaks or blobs; mixed with the stool and only apparent on making a thin paste with water; mixed with blood as in dysentery; composing almost the entire stool, sometimes as firm bands or cords.

Odor: This varies with disease and dietary

differences. It is most marked on a meat diet. Variations such as sour, pungent, or putrid occur in different diseases. *Offensive odor:* In jaundice, acute indigestion, enteritis, typhoid fever, and occasionally in constipation. *Putrid odor:* May be the result of syphilitic or carcinomatous ulceration of the rectum or gangrenous dysentery. *Sour odor:* Normal stools of infants.

Parasites: The presence of various intestinal parasites can be determined by examination of the feces. Gross examination may reveal the presence of nematodes (roundworms) or tapeworms; however, microscopic examination is necessary to determine the presence of protozoa, helminth ova, or larvae. In examination of feces, stools are collected in clean dry containers. For microscopic examination, representative bits of feces or mucus are emulsified in saline solution on a clean slide, then spread evenly, and covered with a coverglass. Enterobiasis (pinworms) is best diagnosed by examination of scrapings or contact slides from the anal and perianal regions.

feces, words pert. to: anus; colon; constipation; defecation; elimination; enema; excreta; excretion; impaction; intestine; meconium; melanorrhea; melena; rectum; scatology; sigmoid; steatorrhea; stool.

Fechner's law (fĕk'nĕrz). [Gustav T. Fechner, Ger. philosopher, 1801–1887] A theory stating that the magnitudes of sensation produced by given stimuli form an arithmetical progression, the stimuli forming a geometrical progression.

$Fe(C_3H_5O_3)_2$. Ferrous lactate; lactate of iron.

$FeCl_2$. Ferrous chloride.

$FeCl_3$. Ferric chloride.

$FeCO_3$. Ferrous carbonate.

fecula (fĕk'ū-lă) [L. *faecula,* dregs]. 1. Sediment. 2. Starch.

feculent (fĕk'ū-lĕnt) [L. *faeculentus*]. Having sediment.

fecundate (fē'kŭn-dāt) [L. *fecundare,* to bear fruit]. To fertilize or impregnate or render fertile.

fecundation (fē"kŭn-dā'shŭn). Impregnation; fertilization.

f., artificial. Impregnation by injecting the seminal fluid into the uterus by mechanical means. SYN: *artificial insemination.*

fecundity (fē-kŭn'dĭ-tē). Ability to produce offspring; fertility.

feedback. The return of some output to the place of origin by the system that receives it.

To a certain degree, blood pressure and blood sugar are regulated by feedback mechanisms. Feedback may be negative or positive. Thus a positive feedback signal indicates that more blood glucose needs to be made available when blood sugar level falls. Conversely, there will be a negative feedback signal when the blood sugar level rises to normal, indicating that production of blood sugar should be reduced or stopped.

feeding [AS. *fedan,* to give food to]. Taking or giving nourishment.

f., artificial. 1. Providing a liquid food preparation through a tube passed into the stomach or the rectum. Also through gastrostomy or duodenostomy. SEE: *hyperalimentation.* 2. Feeding of a baby with food other than mother's milk.

f., breast. Feeding of an infant at the breast.

f., forcible. Forcing food to a patient who cannot or will not take nourishment.

f., intravenous. Administration of fluids and nutrients through a vein.

f., rectal. Type rarely used, because little nourishment can be absorbed through colon. Normal saline often used with glucose, making a 5 to 10% solution by adding 15 to 30 gm. of sugar to 10 oz. (300 ml.) of normal saline.

f., tube. Feeding through a tube that extends through the mouth or nostril and into the stomach. Indicated for patients who cannot swallow or masticate food, but who have functioning GI tracts. The nasal method is most often used, and requires a much smaller tube and little more dexterity but less likely to be successfully resisted. A tube lubricated with glycerin is gently passed into pharynx and, avoiding the larynx, it is passed into the stomach. Entry into the larynx may produce struggling and cyanosis.

CAUTION: Prior to feedings be certain tube is in stomach and not in the bronchus. This can be determined by aspirating the tube and observing for gastric contents or by listening to the end of the tube. If air comes out of the tube with each expiration, the tube is not in the stomach. If proper placement of the tube is in doubt, careful instillation of a very small amount of sterile water will help to demonstrate the location of the tube. If the tube is in the bronchus, the air will cause the water to return or bubble during expiration. Foods or nutritional substances as ordered by the physician are fed slowly.

feeling [AS. *felan,* to feel]. The conscious phase of nervous activity. The emotions are centrally stimulated feelings and those sensations peripherally produced by excitation of peripheral nerves, including those of the special senses.

Feen-A-Mint. Trade name for phenolphthalein.

Feer's disease (fārz). [Emil Feer, Swiss pediatrician, 1864–1955] Acrodynia, q.v.

feet [AS. *fet*]. (sing. *foot*) The pedal extremities of the legs. SEE: *foot.*

Fehling's solution (fā'lĭngz). [Hermann von Fehling, Ger. chemist, 1812–1885] A solution used for detecting the presence of sugar in urine. It consists of equal parts of Solutions A and B prepared as follows: Solution A (copper solution): dissolve 34.66 gm. of copper sulfate crystals in an amount of water to make 500 ml. Solution B (alkaline tartrate solution): dissolve 173 gm. of crystallized potassium sodium tartrate and 50 gm. of sodium hydroxide in an amount of water to make 500 ml. Mix equal portions of Solutions A and B just before using. This mixture is then added to the urine sample and the liquid is boiled. If sugar is present, a red precipitate of cuprous oxide is formed.

Feingold diet (fīn'gōld). [Benjamin Feingold, U.S. pediatrician, 1900–1982] A diet in which all foods containing artificial coloring, flavoring, and preserving materials are excluded. Used in treating hyperactive children.

fel (fĕl) [L.]. Bile.

feline (fē'līn) [L. *feles,* cat]. Concerning cats.

fellatio (fĕl-ā'shē-ō) [L. *fellare,* to suck]. Oral stimulation of the penis. SEE: *cunnilingus.*

felon (fĕl'ŏn) [ME. *feloun,* malignant]. Infection or abscess of soft tissue of terminal joint of a finger. SYN: *whitlow.*

feltwork. 1. Fibrous network. 2. A plexus of nerve fibrils.

Felty's syndrome (fĕl'tēz). [A. R. Felty, U.S. physician, b. 1895] Splenomegaly, lymphadenopathy, and rheumatoid arthritis in adults.

female [L. *femella,* little woman]. 1. An individual of the sex that produces ova or bears young. 2. Characteristics of this sex. SEE: *genitalia, female.*

feminine (fĕm'ĭ-nĭn). Concerning or being of the female sex.

feminism [L. *femininus*]. The development of female secondary sexual characteristics in the male. SEE: *gynecomastia.*

feminization. The normal development of female secondary sexual characteristics, or the pathologic development of these in the male.

f., testicular. An apparent female where genetic sex is male. Caused by the inability of the tissues to respond to the male hormone produced by the testicles. External genitalia are rudimentary, and the testicles may be in the abdomen.

Feminone. Trade name for ethinyl estradiol.

femoral (fĕm'or-ăl) [L. *femoralis*]. Pert. to the thigh bone or femur.

femoral artery. Artery that begins at the external iliac artery and terminates behind the knee as the popliteal artery on the inner side of the femur. SYN: *arteria femoralis* [NA].

femoral reflex. Extension of knee and flexion of foot resulting from irritation of skin over upper anterior third of thigh.

femoral vein. Continuation of the popliteal vein upward toward the external iliac vein. SYN: *vena femoralis* [NA].

femorocele (fĕm'ō-rō-sēl") [L. *femur,* thigh, + Gr. *kele,* hernia]. Femoral hernia.

femorotibial (fĕm"ō-rō-tĭb'ē-ăl) [" + *tibia,* pipe]. Rel. to the femur and tibia.

femto- [Danish *femten,* fifteen]. In metric system nomenclature, a prefix indicating that the entity following is to be multiplied by 10^{-15}. Thus a femtogram is 10^{-15} gram. SEE: *Metric System* in *Appendix.*

femur (fē'mŭr) [L.]. [NA] The thigh bone. It extends from the hip to the knee and is the longest and strongest bone in the skeleton. SEE: illus.

RS: calcar femorale; cavalry bone; femoral; trochanter.

RIGHT FEMUR
(FRONT VIEW)

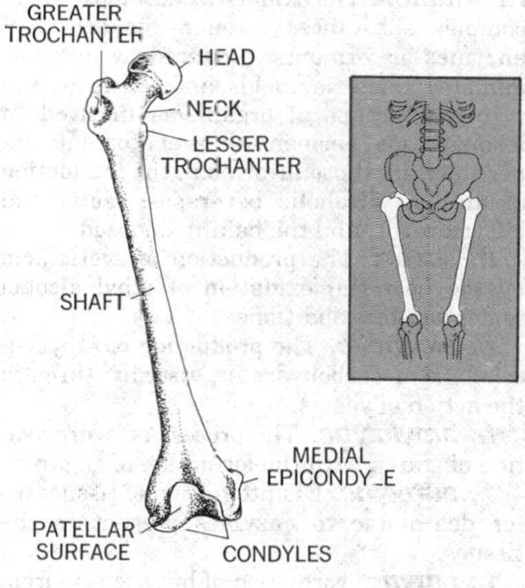

fenestra (fĕn-ĕs'tră) [L., window]. (pl. *fenestrae*) 1. An aperture frequently closed by a membrane. 2. An open area, as in the blade of a forceps.

f. cochleae. [NA] The opening leading into the cochlea. It is closed by a membrane, the secondary tympanic membrane.

f. rotunda. Window, cochlear, q.v.; window, round, q.v.

f. vestibuli. [NA] An oval opening on the inner wall of the middle ear or tympanum leading to the vestibule, into which the base of the stapes fits.

fenestrated (fĕn'ĕs-trāt"ĕd) [L. *fenestra,* window]. Having openings.

fenestration. 1. Condition of having a fenestra. 2. An operation in which an artificial opening is made into the labyrinth of the ear.

Performed in cases of otosclerosis, to treat the associated deafness.

fenfluramine hydrochloride (fĕn-floor′ă-mēn). An adrenergic agent. Trade name is Pondimin.

fenoprofen calcium (fĕn-ō-prō′fĕn). USP. An anti-inflammatory analgesic agent. Trade name is Nalfon.

fentanyl citrate (fĕn′tă-nĭl). USP. A potent synthetic analgesic. Trade name is Sublimaze.

Feosol. Trade name for ferrous sulfate.

Feostat. Trade name for ferrous fumarate.

Fergon. Trade name for ferrous gluconate.

ferment (fĕr-mĕnt′, fĕr′mĕnt) [L. *fermentum*]. 1. To decompose. 2. A substance capable of producing fermentation in other substances. 3. A catalytic agent that is capable of inducing fermentation in substances with which it comes in contact.

RS: enzyme; pancreatin; papain; steapsin; trypsin; trypsinogen; tyrosinase; yeast.

fermentation. The oxidative decomposition of complex substances through the action of enzymes or ferments, produced by microorganisms. Bacteria, molds, and yeasts are the principal groups of organisms involved in fermentation. Fermentations of economic importance are those involved in the production of alcohol, alcoholic beverages, lactic and butyric acids, and the baking of bread.

f., acetic. The production of acetic acid by the bacterial oxidation of ethyl alcohol under aerobic conditions.

f., alcoholic. The production of ethyl alcohol from carbohydrates, usually through the action of yeasts.

f., amylolytic. The process of hydrolyzation of starch with the formation of sugar.

f., autolytic. Disintegration of tissues after death due to enzymes present in the tissues.

f., butyric. Formation of butyric acid from bacterial action on carbohydrates under anaerobic conditions.

f., citric acid. Formation of citric acid from action of molds on carbohydrates.

f., invertin. Fermentation that converts cane sugar into dextrose and levulose.

f., lactic. Formation of lactic acid from carbohydrates by action of bacteria. The genera Streptococcus and Lactobacillus are the forms usually involved. Bacterial action is responsible for the souring of milk.

f., oxalic acid. Formation of oxalic acid from carbohydrates from the action of certain molds, esp. Aspergillus.

f., propionic acid. Formation of propionic acid from carbohydrates from action of certain bacteria.

f., viscous. Production of gelatinous material by different forms of bacilli.

fermentum (fĕr-mĕn′tŭm) [L]. Yeast; a ferment.

fermium (fĕr′mē-ŭm). [Enrico Fermi, 1901–1954, winner of the Nobel Prize in physics in 1938] Radioactive element. SYMB: Fm. At. wt. 257; at. no. 100.

fern [AS. *fearn*]. A flowerless plant belonging to the class Filicinae of the division Tracheophyta. At one time a substance derived from male ferns was used in treating certain kinds of intestinal parasites.

fern pattern, ferning. The palm leaf pattern visible by microscope that cervical mucus assumes when placed in a thin layer on a glass slide and allowed to dry. This occurs only during certain stages of the menstrual cycle. The pattern, caused by crystallization of the mucus as it dries, is dependent upon the concentration of electrolytes present, esp. sodium chloride. Usually seen at midcycle in normal menstruating women; therefore it may be helpful in determining time of ovulation in women who have difficulty becoming pregnant. The mucus has a beaded pattern at other times in the cycle and during pregnancy.

Fero-Gradumet. Trade name for ferrous sulfate.

-ferous [L. *ferre*, to bear]. Suffix meaning producing.

ferrated (fĕr-āt′ĕd) [L. *ferrum*, iron]. Combined with iron or containing iron.

ferri-, ferro- [L. *ferrum*, iron]. Prefix used to indicate presence of iron.

ferric. 1. Pert. to or containing iron. SYN: *ferruginous*. 2. Denoting a compound containing iron in its trivalent form (F^{+++}).

f. ammonium citrate. Thin, garnet-red crystals, containing about 17% iron. Used in hypochromic anemia.

f. chloride. $FeCl_3$. Used principally in form of tincture as an astringent application to throat and as a hematinic.

ferrin. An iron-containing compound isolated from liver tissue.

ferritin (fĕr′ĭ-tĭn). An iron-phosphorus-protein complex containing about 23% iron. It is formed in the intestinal mucosa by the union of ferric iron with a protein, apoferritin. Ferritin is the form in which iron is stored in the tissues, principally in the reticuloendothelial cells of the liver, spleen, and bone marrow.

ferrokinetics (fĕr″rō-kĭ-nĕt′ĭks) [″ + Gr. *kinesis*, movement]. Consideration of the absorption, utilization, storage, and excretion of iron.

ferropexia (fĕr-ō-pĕks′ē-ă). Iron fixation.

ferroprotein (fĕr″ō-prō′tē-ĭn). A protein combined with an iron-containing radical. Ferroproteins are important oxygen-transferring enzymes (e.g., Warburg's enzyme, cytochrome, oxidase).

ferrotherapy (fĕr″ō-thĕr′ă-pē) [″ + Gr. *therapeia,* treatment]. Use of iron in treating anemia.

ferrous (fĕr′ŭs) [L. *ferrum,* iron]. 1. Pert. to iron. SYN: *ferruginous.* 2. Denoting a compound containing iron with a valence of two (F^{++}).

f. fumarate. USP. $C_4H_2FeO_4$. An iron preparation used to treat anemias. Trade names are Feostat, Ferranol, and Fumasorb.

f. gluconate. Occurs as a yellowish powder or granules. Used as a hematinic. Trade name is Fergon.

f. sulfate. USP. $FeSO_4$. Iron sulfate. Pale, bluish-green crystals, that are taken orally as a hematinic. Incompatible with alkalies, chlorides, tannic acid, and oxidizing agents. Trade names are Feosol, Fero-Gradumet, and Mol-Iron.

ferruginous (fĕr-ū′jĭ-nŭs) [L. *ferrugo,* iron rust]. 1. Pert. to or containing iron. 2. Of the color of iron rust.

ferrule (fĕr′ūl) [L. *viriola,* little bracelet]. A band or ring of metal applied to the end of the root or crown of a tooth in order to strengthen it.

ferrum (fĕr′ŭm) [L., iron]. SYMB: Fe. Iron.

fertile (fĕr′tĭl) [L. *fertilis*]. Capable of reproduction.

fertility (fĕr-tĭl′ĭ-tē). Quality of being productive or fertile.

fertilization [L. *fertilis,* reproductive]. 1. Fecundation; union of an ovum with the spermatozoon of the male, the male sex cell being carried in the seminal discharge. This usually takes place in the fallopian tube. Viable spermatozoa have been found in the tube 48 hours after the last coitus. After the ovum is fertilized, cell division begins. The fertilized ovum then enters the uterus, where it may implant for continued nurture and development. 2. In botany, the union of the male and female gametes. In higher plants, when the pollen tube enters the ovule, two gametes emerge, one uniting with the egg to form the zygote, from which the embryo develops; the other uniting with two endosperm nuclei to form a primary endosperm cell, from which the endosperm (reserve food) develops. SEE:

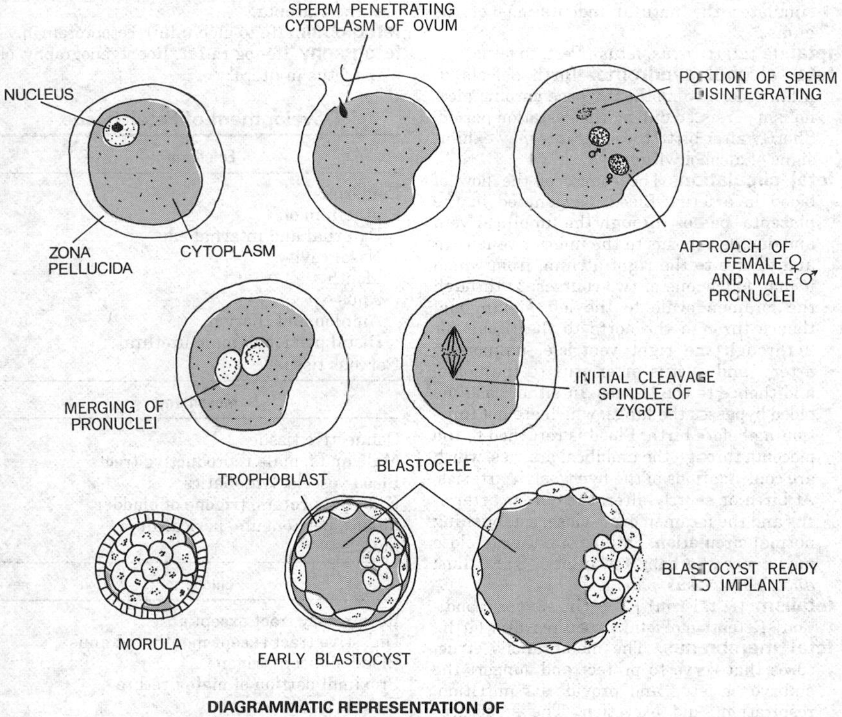

DIAGRAMMATIC REPRESENTATION OF OVUM AND EVENTS OF FERTILIZATION

illus.

RS: coitus; conception; contraceptive; impregnation; ovum; spermatozoa; sterile; sterility.

fertilizin (fĕr″tĭ-lī′zĭn). A substance, possibly a glycoprotein, extracted from starfish or sea urchin eggs that causes agglutination of the sperm of the same species. It probably aids in fertilization by fixing sperm to the egg membrane. It is complementary to antifertilizin, a substance extracted from sperm that agglutinates eggs.

fervescence (fĕr-vĕs′ĕns) [L. *fervescere,* to grow hot]. Increase of fever.

fester (fĕs′tĕr) [L. *fistula,* ulcer]. To become inflamed and suppurate.

festinant (fĕs′tĭ-nănt). Increasing in speed, accelerating.

festination (fĕs″tĭ-nā′shŭn) [L. *festinatio*]. Abnormal and involuntary increase in speed of walking in an attempt to catch up with the displaced center of gravity due to the patient's leaning forward. Seen in certain neurological diseases.

festoon (fĕs-toon′) [L. *festus,* festal]. A carving in the base material of a denture that simulates the natural indentations of the gums.

fetal (fē′tăl) [L. *fetus,* fetus]. Pert. to fetus.

fetal alcohol syndrome. Birth defects in infants born to mothers whose chronic alcoholism persisted during the gestation period. Shortly after birth these infants may exhibit signs of alcohol withdrawal.

fetal circulation. The course of the flow of blood in a fetus. Blood, oxygenated in the placenta, passes through the umbilical vein and ductus venosus to the inferior vena cava and thence to the right atrium, from which it may follow one of two courses: 1) through the foramen ovale to the left atrium and thence through the aorta to the tissues or 2) through the right ventricle, pulmonary artery, and ductus arteriosus to the aorta, and thence to the tissues. In either case the blood bypasses the lungs, which are not functioning before birth. Blood is returned to the placenta through the umbilical arteries, which are continuations of the hypogastric arteries. At birth or shortly after, the ductus arteriosus and the foramen ovale close, establishing normal circulation. Failure of either to close may cause the baby to be blue. SEE: illus; *ductus arteriosus, patent.*

fetalism (fē′tăl-ĭzm) [″ + Gr. *-ismos,* condition]. Retention of fetal structures after birth.

fetal membranes. The membranous structures that serve to protect and support the embryo or fetus and provide its nutrition, respiration, and excretion. The structures are the yolk sac, allantois, amnion, chorion, decidua, and placenta.

feticide (fē′tĭ-sīd) [″ + *cidus,* kill]. Destruction of fetal life. SEE: *infanticide.*

fetid (fē′tĭd) [L. *fetidus,* stink]. Rank or foul in odor.

fetish (fē′tĭsh) [Portug. *feitico,* charm, sorcery]. 1. An object, such as an idol or charm, that is thought to have mysterious, magical, and supernatural power. 2. In psychiatry, the love object of a person who suffers from fetishism, q.v.

fetishism (fē′tĭsh-, fĕt′ĭsh-ĭzm) [″ + Gr. *-ismos,* condition]. 1. Belief in some object as possessing power or capable of being a stimulus. 2. Substitution for a normal love object (a person) of parts or possessions of such a one. Libido gratification from contact with articles of dress, or a braid of hair. 3. A form of mental illness in which sexual stimulus is found at the sight of a shoe, glove or other article of apparel, or of some part of the body such as the hair, esp. the pubic hair. To the masochist such symbols are indicative of domination.

fetochorionic (fē″tō-kor-ē-ŏn′ĭk) [L. *fetus,* fetus, + Gr. *chorion,* membrane]. Pert. to the fetus and the chorion or chorionic membrane of the placenta.

fetoglobulin (fē″tō-glŏb′ū-lĭn). Fetoprotein, q.v.

fetography (fē-tŏg′ră-fē). Roentgenography of the fetus in utero.

Development of Fetal Tissue

Ectoderm
Epidermis
Epithelium of:
External and internal ear
Nasal cavity
Mouth
Anus
Amnion and chorion
Distal portion of male urethra
Nervous tissue
Mesoderm
Connective tissues
Male and female reproductive tracts
Blood vessels, lymphatics
Kidneys, ureters, trigone of bladder
Pleura, peritoneum, pericardium
Muscles
Entoderm
Respiratory tract except nose
Digestive tract except mouth and anus
Bladder except trigone
Proximal portion of male urethra
Female urethra

fetology (fē-tŏl′ō-jē) [″ + Gr. *logos,* study].

FETAL CIRCULATION

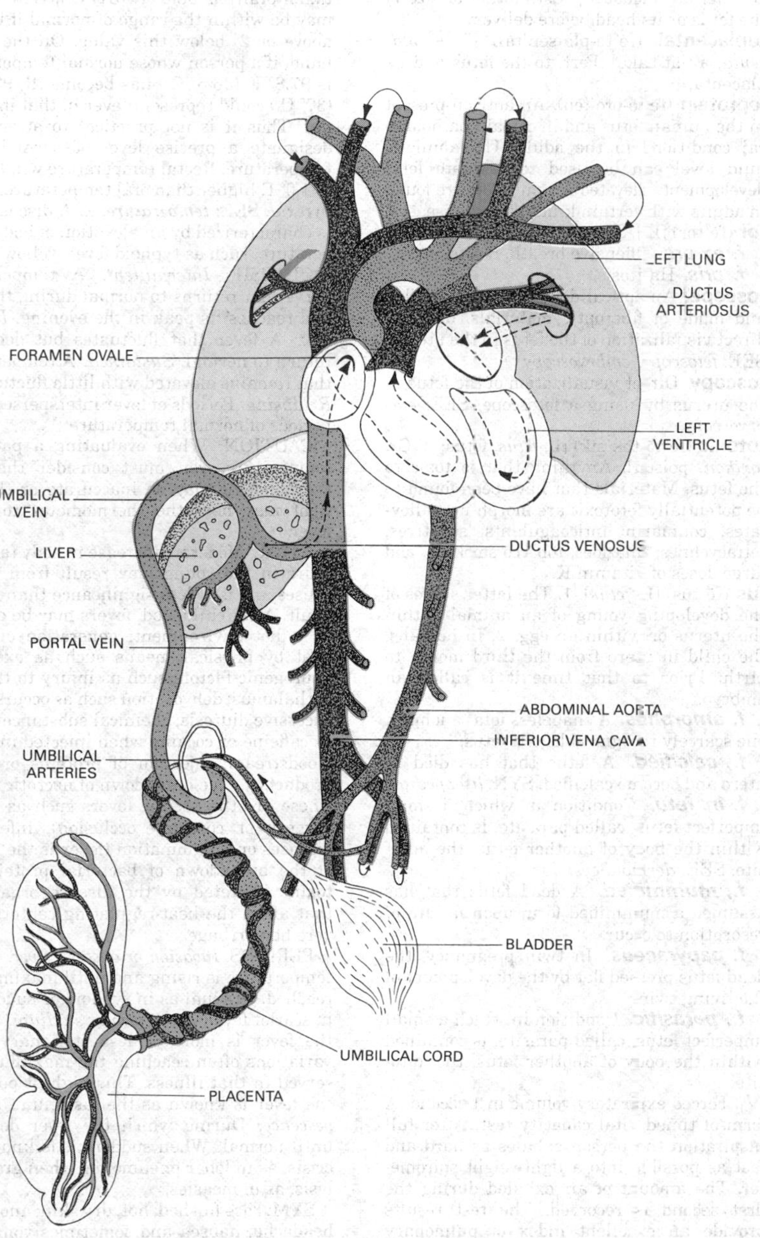
LEFT LUNG
DUCTUS ARTERIOSUS
FORAMEN OVALE
LEFT VENTRICLE
UMBILICAL VEIN
LIVER
DUCTUS VENOSUS
PORTAL VEIN
ABDOMINAL AORTA
INFERIOR VENA CAVA
UMBILICAL ARTERIES
BLADDER
UMBILICAL CORD
PLACENTA

Study of the fetus.

fetometry (fē-tŏm'ĕ-trē) [L. *fetus*, fetus, + Gr. *metron*, measure]. Estimation of size of the fetus or its head before delivery.

fetoplacental (fē"tō-plă-sĕn'tăl) [" + *placenta*, a flat cake]. Pert. to the fetus and its placenta.

fetoprotein (fē"tō-prō'tēn). An antigen present in the human fetus and in certain pathological conditions in the adult. The amniotic fluid level can be used to evaluate fetal development. Elevated serum levels are found in adults with certain kinds of liver diseases.

fetor (fē'tor) [L.]. Stench; an offensive odor.

f. ex ore. Offensive breath, halitosis.

f. oris. Halitosis.

fetoscope. An optical device, usually flexible and made of fiberoptic materials, used for direct visualization of the fetus in the uterus. SEE: *fetoscopy; embryoscopy.*

fetoscopy. Direct visualization of the fetus in the uterus by using a fetoscope. SEE: *embryoscopy.*

fetotoxic (fē"tō-tŏk'sĭk) [L. *fetus*, fetus, + Gr. *toxikon*, poison]. Anything that is toxic to the fetus. Materials that have been found to be potentially fetotoxic are morphine, salicylates, coumarin anticoagulants, sedatives, tetracyclines, thiazides, tobacco smoking, and large doses of vitamin K.

fetus (fē'tŭs) [L. *fetus*]. 1. The latter stages of the developing young of an animal within the uterus or within an egg. 2. In humans, the child in utero from the third month to birth. Prior to that time it is called an embryo.

f. amorphus. A shapeless fetal anomaly, one scarcely recognizable as a fetus.

f., calcified. A fetus that has died in utero and become calcified. SYN: *lithopedion.*

f. in fetu. Condition in which a small imperfect fetus, called parasite, is contained within the body of another fetus, the autosite. SEE: *dermoid cyst.*

f., mummified. A dead fetus that has assumed a mummified form upon failure of resorption to occur.

f. papyraceus. In twin pregnancy, the dead fetus pressed flat by the development of the living twin.

f., parasitic. Condition in which a small imperfect fetus, called parasite, is contained within the body of another fetus, the autosite.

FEV_1. Forced expiratory volume in 1 second. A form of timed vital capacity test. After full inspiration the person exhales as hard and fast as possible into a lightweight spirometer. The amount of air exhaled during the first second is recorded. The test results provide an excellent index of pulmonary function.

fever [L. *febris*]. 1. Elevation of temperature above the normal. The normal temperature taken orally is 98.6° F. (37° C.). However, it may be within the range of normal if it is 1° above or 2° below this value. On the other hand, if a person whose normal temperature is 97.8° F. (36.5° C.) has become ill, 98.6° F. (37° C.) could represent fever in that individual. Thus it is not practical to attempt to designate a precise level of normal body temperature. Rectal temperature will be 0.5° to 1.0° F. higher than oral temperature. SYN: *pyrexia.* SEE: *temperature.* 2. A disease that is characterized by an elevation of body temperature, such as typhoid fever, yellow fever.

CLASSIF: *Intermittent:* A temperature curve that returns to normal during the day and reaches its peak in the evening. *Remittent:* A fever that fluctuates but does not return to normal. *Sustained:* A temperature that remains elevated with little fluctuation. *Relapsing:* Periods of fever interspersed with periods of normal temperature.

CAUTION: When evaluating a patient's temperature, you must consider that the thermometer may be inaccurate or the patient may heat the thermometer to feign fever.

ETIOL: Moderate increase in body temperature in the young may result from minor causes and is of less significance than in the adult. After childhood, fevers may be caused by a hot environment; generation of body heat by physical means such as exercise; neurogenic factors such as injury to the hypothalamus; dehydration such as occurs after excessive diuresis; chemical substances such as caffeine or cocaine when injected into the bloodstream; injection of proteins or their products, or the breakdown of necrotic tissue (these are the aseptic fevers such as follow surgery or coronary occlusion); infectious diseases or inflammation (fever is the result of the breakdown of bacterial proteins or toxins liberated by the disease organisms that affect the heat-regulating centers); severe hemorrhage.

PERIODS: *Invasion or onset of fever:* While temperature is rising and until maximum is reached. Gradual as in typhoid or sudden as in scarlet fever. *Fastigium or stadium:* When the fever is more or less stationary with variations often reaching the maximum observed in that illness. This highest point in the fever is known as the fastigium. *Defervescence:* During which the fever declines until normal. When sudden, it is known as crisis, as in lobar pneumonia; when gradual, lysis, as in measles.

SYM: Face flushed; hot, dry skin; anorexia; headache; nausea and sometimes vomiting; constipation and sometimes diarrhea; aching all over; scant, highly colored urine. Delirium is possible if temperature is over 105° F. (40.5° C.) or in some cases with less fever. Convulsions may follow, esp. in children; coma. SEE: *convulsion*.

f., childbed. An infection of the birth canal following trauma from childbirth. SYN: *puerperal sepsis*.

f., continuous. A sustained fever as in scarlet fever, typhus, or pneumonia in which there is slight diurnal variation.

f., drug. Fever caused by the administration of a drug. Almost any drug has the ability to produce this undesired side effect in some individuals.

f., induced. Fever artificially produced to favorably modify the course of a disease as in central nervous system syphilis. Sustained fever of 105° F. (40.5° C.), or even higher, maintained for 6 to 8 or 10 hours may be induced by the use of medical diathermy or injection of malarial parasites.

f., intermittent. Fever that comes and goes.

f. of unknown origin. ABBR: FUO. An illness of at least three weeks' duration with fever exceeding 38.3° C. on several occasions and diagnosis has not been established after one week of hospital investigation. The main causes are systemic and localized infections, neoplasms, or collagen-vascular diseases such as rheumatoid arthritis, disseminated lupus erythematosus, and polyarteritis nodosa. Less common causes are granulomatous disease, inflammatory disease of the bowel, pulmonary embolization, drug fever, cirrhosis of the liver, and rare disease such as Whipple's disease. Some cases remain undiagnosed.

f., periodic. Familial Mediterranean fever. An inherited disease of unknown etiology of Sephardic Jews, Armenians, and Arabs. Symptoms are intermittent attacks of fever, abdominal pain, and pleurisy. Joint changes are similar to those of rheumatoid arthritis. Renal failure due to amyloidosis sometimes occurs. There is no known therapy.

f., relapsing. Any one of a group of acute infectious diseases caused by a variety of Borrelia. There are alternating periods of fever and normal temperature, the typical temperature curve being a characteristic of the disease. SEE: *relapsing fever*.

f., remittent. Fever that never falls to a normal temperature but shows some diurnal variation.

f., septic. Fever due to septic matter in the body. SEE: *septicemia*.

fever, words pert. to: ague; antifebrile; apyrexia; calor; chill; crisis; dengue; fastigium; febrifacient; febrifuge; febrile convulsions; FUO; heat; infection; inflammation; influenza; lysis; malaria; pulse; "pyr-" words; quartan; quintan; quotidian; respiration; sepsis; suppuration; temperature.

fever blister. Area of inflammation of the lips or mucous membrane of the mouth. Caused by herpes simplex virus, usually type I. SYN: *fever sore*.

F.F.D. *focal film distance*. Distance from the focal spot of the x-ray tube to the film.

FH_4. *5,6,7,8-tetrahydrofolic acid*, folacin, the active form of folic acid.

fiat (fī′ăt) [L.]. Let there be made, a term used in writing prescriptions.

fiber [L. *fibra*]. 1. Threadlike or filmlike element, as a nerve fiber. A neuron or the axonal portion of a neuron. 2. An elongated threadlike structure; a fiber may be cellular in composition as nerve fiber or muscle fiber, or may be a cellular product as collagen fiber, elastic fiber, oxytalan fiber, or reticular fiber.

RS: chondrofibroma; cilia; cimbia; cingulum; "fibr-" words; filament; filum.

f., accelerator. Fiber nerve pathway causing increased heart rate upon stimulation.

f., afferent. Fiber carrying incoming impulses to nerve cells.

f., dietary. Components of food that are resistant to chemical digestion. Includes portions of food that are made up of cellulose, hemicellulose, lignin, and pectin. These substances add bulk to the diet by absorbing large amounts of water, and are used in diets to produce a large bulky bowel movement. Foods rich in fiber include whole grain foods, bran flakes, fruits, leafy vegetables, root vegetables and their skins, and prunes, which also contain the laxative substance diphenylisatin. SYN: *roughage*.

Diets high in fiber may help to prevent diverticula of the intestinal tract, may help to lower blood cholesterol and possibly prevent cancer of the intestinal tract. Some diabetic individuals on low insulin doses have been able to further lower their insulin requirements by following a diet high in fiber and carbohydrates and low in sucrose.

f., efferent. Fiber carrying outgoing impulses.

f., inhibitory. Fiber nerve pathway causing slower heart action upon stimulation.

f., medullated. Nerve fiber in which axis cylinder is sheathed in myelin.

f., nerve. The part of a nerve cell that carries impulses. SEE: *nerve*.

f., nonmedullated. Nerve fiber in which there is no myelin sheath between axis cylinder and neurilemma. SYN: *f., unmyelinated*.

f.'s, Purkinje. Atypical muscle fibers lying beneath the endocardium that form the impulse-conducting system of the heart.

f., unmyelinated. F., nonmedullated, q.v.

fibercolonoscope (fī″bĕr-kō-lŏn′ō-skōp). Fiberoptic endoscope for examining the colon.

fibergastroscope (fī″bĕr-găs′trō-skōp). Fiberoptic endoscope for examining the stomach.

fiber-illuminated (fī′bĕr-ĭl-loo″mĭn-ā″tĕd). Transmission of light to an object by use of fiberoptic bundles.

fiberoptic. A flexible material made of glass or plastic that transmits light along its course by reflecting it from the side or wall of the fiber. Use of this principle permits transmission of light and therefore visual images around corners. Devices utilizing fiberoptic materials are quite useful in endoscopic examinations.

fiberscope (fī′bĕr-skōp). A flexible endoscope that uses fiberoptic, q.v., materials for visualization.

fibra (fī′bră) [L.]. [NA] (pl. *fibrae*) A fiber.

fibralbumin (fī″brăl-bū′mĭn) [″+ *albumen*, white of egg]. Globulin.

fibremia (fī-brē′mē-ă) [″ + Gr. *haima*, blood]. Fibrin formed in the blood, causing embolism or thrombosis. SYN: *inosemia*.

fibril (fī′brĭl) [L. *fibrilla*]. A small fiber. A very small filamentous structure, often the component of a cell or a fiber.

f., muscle. An extremely minute fibril found within the cytoplasm of smooth muscle cells and in the sarcoplasm of striated and cardiac muscle fibers. SYN: *myofibril*.

f., nerve. Delicate fibril found in the cell body and processes of a neuron. SYN: *neurofibril*.

fibrilla (fī-brĭl′ă) [L.]. (pl. *fibrillae*) A fibril or small fiber.

fibrillar, fibrillary. Pert. to, or consisting of, fibrils.

fibrillated (fī′brĭ-lāt′d) [L. *fibrilla*, little fiber]. Composed of minute fibers. SYN: *fibrillar; fibrous*.

fibrillation (fī″brĭl-ā′shŭn). 1. The formation of fibrils. 2. Quivering or spontaneous contraction of individual muscle fibers. 3. An abnormal bioelectric potential occurring in neuropathies and myopathies.

f., atrial. Extremely rapid, incomplete contractions of the atria resulting in fine, rapid, irregular, and uncoordinated movements.

f., ventricular. A condition similar to atrial fibrillation, resulting in rapid, tremulous, and ineffectual contractions of the ventricles. May result from mechanical injury to the heart, occlusion of coronary vessels, effects of certain drugs such as excess of digitalis or chloroform, and electrical stimuli.

fibrillogenesis (fī-brĭl″ō-jĕn′ĕ-sĭs). Formation of fibrils.

fibrillolysis (fī″brĭl-ŏl′ĭ-sĭs) [″ + Gr. *lysis*, dissolution]. Dissolution of fibrils.

fibrillolytic (fī″brĭl-ō-lĭt′ĭk). Dissolving fibrils.

fibrin (fī′brĭn) [L. *fibra*, fiber]. A whitish, filamentous protein formed by the action of thrombin on fibrinogen. The conversion of fibrinogen, a hydrosol, into fibrin, a hydrogel, is the basis for the clotting of the blood. The fibrin is deposited as fine interlacing filaments in which are entangled red and white blood cells and platelets, the whole forming a coagulum or clot.

RS: blood clot; coagulation; fibrinogen; prothrombin; thrombin.

f. foam. A spongelike substance prepared from human fibrin. When impregnated with thrombin, it is used in surgery as a hemostatic agent. It is esp. useful in neurosurgery and in injuries to parenchymatous organs. It is slowly absorbed.

fibrinocellular (fī″brĭ-nō-sĕl′ū-lăr). Composed of fibrin and cells, as in certain exudates.

fibrinogen (fī-brĭn′ō-jĕn) [″ + Gr. *gennan*, to produce]. A protein present in the blood plasma that through the action of thrombin in the presence of calcium ions is converted into fibrin; this is essential for clotting of blood. Also called factor I. SEE: *blood, clotting of; coagulation; factors, coagulation*.

fibrinogenic, fibrinogenous. Producing fibrin.

fibrinogenolysis (fī″brĭ-nō-jĕ-nŏl′ĭ-sĭs) [″ + ″ + *lysis*, dissolution]. Decomposition or dissolution of fibrin.

fibrinogenopenia (fī-brĭn″ō-jĕn″ō-pē′nē-ă) [″ + Gr. *gennan*, to produce, + *penia*, poverty]. Reduction in the amount of fibrinogen in the blood, usually the result of a liver disorder.

fibrinoid (fī′brĭ-noyd) [″ + Gr. *eidos*, form]. Resembling fibrin.

fibrinoid change. Alteration in connective tissues in response to immune reactions. The tissue becomes swollen, homogenous, and bandlike in appearance.

fibrinoid material. A fibrinous substance that develops in the placenta, increasing in quantity as the placenta becomes older. Its origin is attributed to the degenerating decidua and trophoblast. It forms an incomplete layer in the chorion and decidua basalis and also occurs in the form of small irregular patches on the surface of the chorionic villi. In late pregnancy, the material may have a striated or canalized appearance, to which the term canalized fibrinoid is applied.

fibrinokinase (fī″brĭ-nō-kī′nās). An enzyme present in animal tissues. It activates plasminogen.

fibrinolysin (fī″brĭn-ŏl′ĭ-sĭn) [L. *fibra*, fibrin, + Gr. *lysis*, dissolution]. The substance, also called plasmin, formed from plasminogen. Its function is to dissolve fibrin. SEE: *fibrinolysis*.

fibrinolysis (fī″brĭn-ŏl′ĭ-sĭs). Dissolution of fibrin by fibrinolysin. Caused by the action of a proteolytic enzyme system. This system is continually active in the body, but its action is greatly increased by various stress stimuli such as intense exercise, anoxia, hypoglycemia, or bacterial infections.

fibrinolytic (fī″brĭn-ō-lĭt′ĭk). Pert. to the splitting up of fibrin.

fibrinopenia (fī″brĭn-ō-pē′nē-ă) [″ + Gr. *penia,* poverty]. Fibrin and fibrinogen deficiency in the blood.

fibrinopeptide (fī″brĭ-nō-pĕp′tīd). The substance removed from fibrinogen during blood coagulation.

fibrinoplastic (fī″brĭn-ō-plăs′tĭk) [″ + Gr. *plassein,* to form]. Concerning fibroplastin.

fibrinopurulent (fī″brĭ-nō-pū′roo-lĕnt) [″ + *purulentus,* festering]. Consisting of pus and fibrin.

fibrinoscopy (fī-brĭ-nŏs′kō-pē) [″ + Gr. *skopein,* to examine]. The diagnosis of disease by physical and chemical examination of the fibrin of blood clots and exudates. SYN: *inoscopy.*

fibrinosis (fī-brĭ-nō′sĭs) [″ + Gr. *osis,* condition]. Excess of fibrin in the blood.

fibrinous (fī′brĭn-ŭs) [L. *fibra,* fiber]. Pert. to, of the nature of, or containing fibrin.

fibrinuria (fī-brĭn-ū′rē-ă) [″ + Gr. *ouron,* urine]. Passage of fibrin in the urine.

fibro- [L. *fibra*]. Prefix indicating relationship to fibers or fibrous tissues.

fibroadenia (fī″brō-ă-dē′nē-ă) [″ + Gr. *aden,* gland]. Fibrous degeneration of glandular tissue.

fibroadenoma (fī″brō-ăd″ĕ-nō′mă) [″ + ″ + *oma,* tumor]. Adenoma with fibrous tissue forming a dense stroma.

fibroadipose [″ + *adeps,* fat]. Being fibrous and fatty.

fibroangioma [″ + Gr. *angeion,* vessel, + *oma,* tumor]. A fibrous tissue angioma.

fibroareolar (fī″brō-ă-rē′ō-lăr) [″ + *areola,* little space]. With fibrous tissue and areolar arrangement.

fibroblast (fī′brō-blăst) [″ + Gr. *blastos,* germ]. Any cell or corpuscle from which connective tissue is developed. SYN: *desmocyte; fibrocyte.*

fibroblastoma (fī″brō-blăs-tō′mă) [″ + ″ + *oma,* tumor]. Tumor of connective tissue or fibroplastic cells.

fibrobronchitis (fī″brō-brŏn-kī′tĭs) [″ + Gr. *bronchia,* air tubes, + *itis,* inflammation]. Croupous or fibrinous bronchitis.

fibrocalcific (fī″brō-kăl-sĭf′ĭk). Partially calcified fibrous material.

fibrocarcinoma (fī″brō-kăr″sĭ-nō′mă) [″ + Gr. *karkinos,* cancer, + *oma,* tumor]. A carcinoma in which the trabeculae are resistant and thickened with granular degeneration of the cells.

fibrocartilage (fī″brō-kăr′tĭ-lĭj) [″ + *cartilago,* gristle]. A type of cartilage in which the matrix contains thick bundles of white or collagenous fibers. Found in the intervertebral disks.

fibrocellular (fī″brō-sĕl′ū-lăr) [″ + *cellula,* little cell]. Both fibrous and cellular. SYN: *fibroareolar.*

fibrochondritis (fī″brō-kŏn-drī′tĭs) [″ + Gr. *chondros,* cartilage, + *itis,* inflammation]. Inflammation of fibrocartilage.

fibrochondroma (fī″brō-kŏn-drō′mă) [″ + ″ + *oma,* tumor]. Tumor of fibrous tissue and cartilage.

fibroclast (fī′brō-klăst) [″ + Gr. *klastos,* broken]. A fibroblast-like cell capable of breaking down collagen fibers and responsible for the rapid turnover and remodeling of collagen in the temporomandibular ligament, symphysis pubis ligament, and other active areas.

fibrocyst (fī′brō-sĭst) [″ + Gr. *kystis,* cyst]. A fibrous tumor that has undergone cystic degeneration or one that has accumulated fluid in the interspaces.

fibrocystic (fī″brō-sĭs′tĭk). 1. Consisting of fibrocysts. 2. Fibrous with cystic degeneration.

fibrocystic disease of the breast. A nonspecific diagnosis for a condition in which there are palpable lumps in the breasts, usually associated with pain and tenderness, that fluctuate with the menstrual cycle and that become progressively worse until menopause. At least 50% of women of reproductive age have palpably irregular breasts.

fibrocystic disease of pancreas. Cystic fibrosis, q.v.

fibrocystoma (fī″brō-sĭs-tō′mă) [″ + Gr. *kystis,* cyst, + *oma,* tumor] Fibroma combined with cystoma.

fibrocyte (fī′brō-sīt) [″ + *kytos,* cell]. A fibroblast.

fibrodysplasia (fī″brō-dĭs-plā′sē-ă) [″ + Gr. *dys,* bad, + *plassein,* to form]. Fibrous dysplasia.

fibroelastic (fī″brō-ē-lăs′tĭk) [″ + Gr. *elastikos,* elastic]. Pert. to connective tissue containing both white nonelastic collagenous fibers and yellow elastic fibers.

fibroelastosis (fī″brō-ē″lăs-tō′sĭs). Overgrowth of fibroelastic tissue.

f., endocardial. Fibroelastosis of the endocardium, leading to cardiac failure.

fibroenchondroma (fī″brō-ĕn″kŏn-drō′mă) [″ + Gr. *en,* in, + *chondros,* cartilage, + *oma,* tumor]. An enchondroma containing fibrous elements.

fibroepithelioma (fī″brō-ĕp″ĭ-thē″lē-ō′mă) [″ + Gr. *epi,* upon, + *thele,* nipple, + *oma,* tumor]. A new growth containing fibrous and epithelial elements.

fibroglia (fī-brŏg′lē-ă) [″ + Gr. *glia,* glue]. Supporting tissue of fibroblasts.

fibroglioma (fī-brō-glī-ō′mă) [″ + Gr. *glia,* glue, + *oma,* tumor]. A fibroma partly glioma.

fibroid (fī′broyd) [″ + Gr. *eidos,* form]. 1. Containing or resembling fibers. SEE: *degeneration.* 2. A colloquial term for fibroma, esp. fibroma of the uterus.

f., interstitial. Tumor in muscular wall of uterus that may grow inward and form a polypoid fibroid, or outward and become a subperitoneal fibroid.

f., uterine. Fibroid in uterus. SEE: *fibroma, uterine.*

fibroidectomy (fī-broyd-ĕk′tō-mē) [″ + ″ + *ektome,* excision]. Surgical removal of a fibroid tumor.

fibrolipoma (fī″brō-lī-pō′mă) [″ + Gr. *lipos,* fat, + *oma,* tumor]. A lipoma having excessive fibrous tissue.

fibroma (fī-brō′mă) [″ + Gr. *oma,* tumor]. (pl. *fibromata*) A fibrous, encapsulated, connective tissue tumor. A fibroma is irregular in shape, slow in growth, and has a firm consistency. Pressure or cystic degeneration may cause pain. May be found in the periosteum. May affect the jaws, the occiput, pelvis, vertebrae, ribs, long bones, and sternum.

f., intramural. Tumor located in muscle tissue of the uterus between the peritoneal coat and endometrium.

f. of breast. A benign, nonulcerative, and painless tumor of the breast.

f., submucous. Fibroma encroaching upon endometrial cavity; sessile or pedunculated.

f., subserous. Fibroma lying beneath peritoneal coat of uterus, often pedunculated.

f., uterine. A fibroid tumor of the uterus.

PATH: A benign tumor varying in size from a few millimeters in diameter to a size large enough to fill the entire abdominal cavity. May be single or multiple. These tumors are completely encapsulated by a fibrous connective tissue capsule in which the blood vessels that supply the tumor are found. They are subjected to numerous benign degenerations such as necrobiotic changes (red and gray degeneration), hyaline changes, telangiectatic and lymphangiectatic changes, calcareous degeneration, fatty degeneration, and infection. Occasionally, a fibroid will show sarcomatous degeneration.

SYM: Fibromata rarely cause symptoms before the age of 30. Although the cardinal symptoms of fibromata are supposed to be dysmenorrhea, menorrhagia, and leukorrhea, these symptoms are found infrequently and the symptomatology is directly related to the location of the tumors in the uterus. Thus tumors that encroach upon the bladder region cause frequency and dysuria; those pressing on the rectum cause rectal tenesmus; those that encroach upon the endometrium cause menorrhagia and dysmenorrhea, and very large subserous growths may be absolutely symptomless. SEE: *dysmenorrhea; dysuria; menorrhagia; tenesmus.*

TREATMENT: Fibromata producing no symptoms should be left in place and the patient kept under observation. If unusually rapid growth is evidenced, they should be removed. Also, if pregnancy is a possibility, tumors of such size as to interfere with childbearing should be removed.

fibromatosis (fī″brō-mă-tō′sĭs) [L. *fibra,* fiber, + Gr. *oma,* tumor, + *osis,* condition]. The simultaneous development of many fibromas. SYN: *fibrosis.*

f. gingivae. An inherited condition wherein there is hypertrophy of the gums prior to the time of eruption of the teeth. Hypertrichosis is usually present.

f., palmar. Dupuytren's contracture, q.v.

fibromatous (fī-brō′mă-tŭs). Pert. to, or of the nature of, a fibroma.

fibromectomy (fī″brō-mĕk′tō-mē) [″ + Gr. *oma,* tumor, + *ektome,* excision]. Removal of a fibroid tumor.

fibromembranous (fī″brō-mĕm′bră-nŭs) [″ + *membrana,* web]. Having both fibrous and membranous tissue.

fibromuscular (fī″brō-mŭs′kū-lăr) [″ + *musculus,* muscle]. Consisting of muscle and connective tissue.

fibromyitis (fī″brō-mī-ī′tĭs) [″ + Gr. *mys,* muscle, + *itis,* inflammation]. Inflammation of the muscular system followed by fibrous degeneration of muscular fibers and atrophy.

fibromyoma (fī″brō-mī-ō′mă) [″ + ″ + *oma,* tumor]. 1. Fibrous tissue myoma. 2. A fibroid tumor of the uterus that contains more fibrous than muscle tissue.

fibromyomectomy (fī″brō-mī″ō-mĕk′tō-mē) [″ + ″ + *ektome,* excision]. Removal of a fibromyoma from the uterus, leaving that organ in place.

fibromyositis (fī″brō-mī″ō-sī′tĭs) [″ + *mys,* muscle, + *itis,* inflammation]. A group of common nonspecific illnesses characterized by pain, tenderness, and stiffness of joints, capsules, and adjacent structures. SEE: *charleyhorse.*

fibromyotomy (fī″brō-mī-ŏt′ō-mē) [″ + ″ + *tome,* incision]. Opening of a fibroid tumor.

fibromyxoma (fī″brō-mĭk-sō′mă) [″ + Gr. *myxa,* mucus, + *oma,* tumor]. A fibroma that has undergone partial myxomatous degeneration.

fibromyxosarcoma (fī″brō-mĭk″sō-săr-kō′mă) [″ + ″ + *sarkos,* flesh, + *oma,* tumor]. 1. A sarcoma containing fibrous and myxoid tissue. 2. A sarcoma that has undergone mucoid degeneration.

fibroneuroma (fī″brō-nū-rō′mă) [″ + Gr. *neuron,* nerve, + *oma,* tumor]. A mixed neuroma and fibroma. SYN: *neurofibroma.*

fibro-osteoma (fī″brō-ŏs-tē-ō′mă) [″ + Gr. *osteon,* bone, + *oma,* tumor]. Tumor containing bony and fibrous elements. SYN: *osteofibroma.*

fibropapilloma (fī″brō-păp-ĭ-lō′mă) [″ + *papilla,* nipple, + Gr. *oma,* tumor]. A mixed fibroma and papilloma sometimes occurring in the bladder.

fibroplasia (fī″brō-plā′sē-ă) [″ + Gr. *plasis,* a molding]. The development of fibrous tissue, as in wound healing.

f., retrolental. Rentrolental fibroplasia, q.v.

fibroplastic (fī″brō-plăs′tĭk) [″ + Gr. *plassein,* to form]. Giving formation to fibrous tissue.

fibroplastin (fī″brō-plăs′tĭn). A globulin in blood serum and other body fluids. SYN: *paraglobulin.*

fibropurulent (fī″brō-pūr′ū-lĕnt) [″ + *purulentus,* festering]. Pus containing flakes of fibrous tissue.

fibrosarcoma (fī″brō-săr-kō′mă) [L. *fibra,* fiber, + Gr. *sarkos,* flesh, + *oma,* tumor]. A spindle-celled sarcoma containing much connective tissue.

fibrose (fī′brōs). To form or produce fibrous tissue.

fibroserous (fī″brō-sē′rŭs) [″ + *serosus,* serous]. Containing fibrous and serosal elements. The pericardium is such a tissue.

fibrosis (fī-brō′sĭs) [″ + Gr. *osis,* condition]. Abnormal formation of fibrous tissue.

f., arteriocapillary. Arteriolar and capillary fibroid degeneration.

f., diffuse interstitial pulmonary. Hamman-Rich syndrome, q.v.

f. of lungs. Formation of scar tissue in connective tissue framework of lungs following inflammation or pneumonia and in pulmonary tuberculosis.

f., postfibrinosis. Development of fibrosis in a tissue in which fibrin has been deposited.

f., proliferative. Formation of new fibrous tissue from connective tissue cells.

f., pulmonary. Fibrosis of the lung following any pulmonary disease.

f., retroperitoneal. Fibrosis, of unknown etiology, of the retroperitoneal area. It may progress to cause obstruction of the great blood vessels and ureters.

f. uteri. Diffuse growth of fibrous tissue throughout the uterus.

fibrositis (fī-brō-sī′tĭs) [″ + Gr. *itis,* inflammation]. Nonsuppurative inflammation of white fibrous connective tissue anywhere in the body, but esp. of locomotor system. SYN: *rheumatism, muscular.*

fibrothorax (fī″brō-thō′răks) [″ + Gr. *thorax,* chest]. Fibrosis that causes the two pleural surfaces of the lung to adhere to each other.

fibrotic (fī-brŏt′ĭk). Marked by or pert. to fibrosis.

fibrous (fī′brŭs) [L. *fibra,* fiber]. Composed of or containing fibers.

fibula (fĭb′ū-lă) [L., pin]. [NA] The outer and smaller bone of the leg from the ankle to the knee, articulating above with the tibia and below with the tibia and talus. One of longest and thinnest bones of the body.

fibular. Pert. to the fibula.

fibulocalcaneal (fĭb″ū-lō-kăl-kā′nē-ăl) [″ + *calcaneus,* pert. to the heel]. Pert. to the fibula and calcaneus or os calcis.

ficin (fī′sĭn) [L. *ficus,* fig]. Sap from the fig tree. It contains an enzyme that is capable of hydrolysing proteins.

F.I.C.S. *Fellow of the International College of Surgeons.*

field [AS *feld*]. A specific area in relationship to an object.

f., auditory. The space or distance within the limit of hearing.

f., high-power. The portion of the object seen when the high magnification lenses of the microscope are used.

f., low-power. The portion of the object seen when the low magnification lenses of the microscope are used.

f. of vision. That portion of space that the fixed eye can see. SEE: *perimetry.*

fifth cranial nerve. A large mixed nerve arising superficially from the side of the pons near its superior border. It is attached to the brain stem by two roots: a large sensory root and a small motor root. SYN: *trigeminal nerve.*

fifth ventricle. Space separating the two layers of the septum pellucidum of the brain.

FIGLU, FIGlu. *formiminoglutamic acid.*

FIGLU excretion test. Test for folic acid deficiency. When histidine is administered to a patient with folic acid deficiency, there will be an increase in the formiminoglutamic (FIGLU) acid in the urine.

figurate (fĭg′ū-rāt) [L. *figuratum,* figured]. Skin lesions that have a certain form, such as geographic, annular, or circular.

figure [L. *figura*]. 1. A body, form, shape, or outline. 2. A number.

figure-ground discrimination. The ability to perceive visually the outline of an object from visually competing background stimuli. This ability is often impaired following central nervous system damage.

fila (fī′lă) [L. *filum,* thread]. Pl. of filum.

filaceous (fī-lā′shŭs). Composed of filaments.

filament [L. *filamentum*]. 1. A fine thread. 2. A thread-like coil of tungsten found in the x-ray tube that is the source of electrons.

f., axial. A fine filament forming the central axis of the tail of a spermatozoon.

filamentous. Made up of long, interwoven or irregularly placed threadlike structures.

filar (fī′lăr) [L. *filum*, thread]. Filamentous.

Filaria (fĭl-ā′rē-ă) [L. *filum*, thread]. Term formerly applied to a genus of nematodes belonging to the superfamily Filarioidea.

F. bancrofti. Wuchereria bancrofti.

F. loa. Loa loa.

F. medinensis. Dracunculus medinensis.

F. sanguinis hominis. Wuchereria bancrofti.

filaria (fĭl-ā′rē-ă) [L. *filum*, thread]. A long filiform nematode belonging to the superfamily Filarioidea. The adults live in vertebrates. In man they may be found in the lymphatic vessels and lymphatic organs, circulatory system, connective tissues, subcutaneous tissues, and serous cavities. Typically, the female produces larvae called microfilariae, which may be sheathed or sheathless. These reach the peripheral blood or lymphatic vessels, where they may be ingested by a blood-sucking arthropod (mosquitoes, gnats, flies). In the intermediate host, they transform into rhabditoid larvae, which metamorphose into infective filariform larvae. These migrate to the proboscis and are deposited in or on the skin of the vertebrate host.

filarial (fĭ-lā′rē-ăl). Pert. to or caused by filariae.

filariasis (fĭl-ă-rī′ă-sĭs) [″ + Gr. *-iasis*, condition]. A chronic disease due to one of the filariae species.

filaricidal (fĭ-lăr″ĭ-sīd′ăl) [″ + *caedere*, to kill]. Pert. to that which is destructive to Filaria.

Filarioidea (fĭ-lăr″ē-oy′dē-ă). A superfamily of filarial nematodes that parasitize many animal species, including man. SEE: *filariasis*.

file (fīl). A metal device with a roughened surface. It is used for shaping bones and teeth.

filial generation. In genetics, the first offspring of a specific mating or crossmating. This is abbreviated F_1. Descendants resulting from F_1 matings are known as the F_2 or second filial generation.

filiform (fĭl′ĭ-form) [″ + *forma*, form]. In biology, pert. to a growth that is uniform along the inoculation line in stab or streak cultures. 2. Hairlike, filamentous.

fillet (fĭl′ĕt) [Fr. *filet*, a band]. 1. A loop of thread, cord, or tape used for providing traction or suspension of tissue during surgery. 2. Bundles of sensory fibers in the medulla, pons, and brain.

filling (fĭl′ĭng) [AS. *fyllan*, to fill]. 1. The material for insertion in a prepared tooth cavity; usually amalgam. 2. The operation of filling tooth cavities.

film. 1. A thin skin, membrane, or covering. 2. A thin sheet of material, usually cellulose, coated with a light-sensitive emulsion used in taking photographs. 3. In microscopy, a thin layer of blood or other material spread on a slide or coverslip.

f., bite-wing. Roentgenogram taken with a part of the film holder held between the teeth and the film parallel to the teeth. This technique permits films to be taken of several upper and lower teeth at the same time.

f., spot. An x-ray film of a small anatomical area.

f., x-ray. A special photographic film that is sensitive to x-rays.

film badge. A badge containing film that is sensitive to x-rays. Used to determine the cumulative exposure to x-rays of persons who work in radiology.

filopressure (fī′lō-prĕ″shūr) [L. *filum*, thread, + *pressura*, pressure]. Pressure on a blood vessel caused by a ligature.

filovaricosis (fī″lō-văr-ĭ-kō′sĭs) [″ + *varix*, a dilated vein, + Gr. *osis*, condition]. Dilatation or thickening of the axis cylinder of a nerve fiber.

filter [L. *filtrare*, to strain through]. 1. To pass a liquid through any porous substance that prevents particles larger than a certain size to pass through. 2. Device for filtering liquids, light rays, or radiations. SEE: *absorption; osmosis*.

f. bed. Large-scale filter to purify the water supply.

f., Berkefeld. A diatomaceous earth filter designed to remove bacteria from solutions passed through it, but allow virus-sized particles to pass through into the filtrate.

f., infrared. Cell of water and red glass that confines radiation to spectral region from 600 to 1400 mμ, red glass alone from 600 to 4000 mμ.

f., Kitasato's. Suction variety of filter using porcelain dilator.

f., membrane. Filter made from biologically inert cellulose esters, polyethylene, or other porous materials.

f., Millipore. Trademark name of a filter with controlled pore size that separates particles above specific sizes from the solutions that flow through.

f., Pasteur-Chamberland. Filter of unglazed porcelain capable of retaining bacteria and some viruses. Either pressure or suction is required to force or draw the liquid through the filter.

f., umbrella. Filter placed in a blood vessel in order to prevent emboli from passing that point. Has been used in the vena cava to prevent emboli in the veins from reaching the lungs.

f., Wood's. A glass screen allowing passage of ultraviolet rays and absorbing rays of visual light. Used in diagnosing certain dermatological conditions, esp. tinea capitis.

filterable [L. *filtrare,* to strain through]. Capable of passing through the pores of a porcelain filter, through which bacteria cannot pass.

filtrate (fĭl'trāt). The fluid that has been passed through a filter. The residue is the precipitate.

f., glomerular. The fluid that passes from the blood through the capillary walls of the glomeruli of the kidney. It is a protein-free plasma from which urine is formed.

filtration (fĭl-trā'shŭn). The process of removing particles from a solution by allowing the liquid portion to pass through a membrane or other partial barrier. This barrier contains holes or spaces through which the liquid may pass but which are too small to permit the solid particles to pass. SEE: *filter.*

filtration of roentgen rays. The absorption of some of the relatively longer wavelengths of roentgen radiation by placing some absorbing medium in the path of the rays such as aluminum, copper, or zinc.

filtrum [L.]. A filter.

filum (fī'lŭm) [L.]. (pl. *fila*) [NA] A thread-like structure.

f. coronaria. A fibrous band extending from the base of the medial cusp of the tricuspid valve to the aortic annulus.

f. terminale. [NA] A long, slender filament at the end of the spinal cord.

fimbria (fĭm'brē-ă) [L., fringe]. (pl. *fimbriae*) Any structure resembling fringe or border.

f. ovarica. The longest fringelike extremity of the fallopian tubes; extending from the infundibulum close to the ovary.

f. tubae. Fringelike portion at abdominal end of the fallopian tubes.

fimbriate (fĭm'brē-āt"). 1. Having fingerlike projections. 2. Fringed.

fimbriated [L. *fimbria,* fringe]. Fringed.

fimbriocele (fĭm'brē-ō-sēl") [" + Gr. *kele,* hernia]. Hernia including the fimbriated portion of the oviduct.

fine motor skills. Skills pertaining to the synergy of small muscles, primarily in the hand, and related to manual dexterity and coordination.

finger [AS.]. One of the five digits of the hand.

f., baseball. Condition resulting from violent backward dislocation of the terminal phalanx onto the dorsum of the middle phalanx, as when a finger is struck on its tip when extended. SEE: *f., hammer.*

f., clubbed. Enlarged terminal phalanx of the finger.

f., dislocation of. Dislocations of a finger occur only at a joint. If there has been a crushing injury, assume that a fracture is present until an x-ray has been made. Dislocations of a finger usually are easily diagnosed and quite easily reduced. They may be caused by blows, falls, and similar accidents.

First, be certain there is no fracture. Then treat the dislocation by asking the patient to steady and support his or her own wrist (or having somebody else to do so) for countertraction. Take hold of the finger beyond the dislocated muscles and tendons and, with the free hand, slip the dislocated bone into place. Apply a splint from the tip of the finger well into the palm of the hand. This may be made of plastic, tongue depressors, or heavy cardboard.

NOTE: Do not under any circumstances attempt to reduce a dislocation of the thumb joint nearest to the palm of the hand until x-ray examination has ruled out the possibility of fracture.

f., hammer. Permanent flexion of the terminal phalanx of the finger; due to damage of the extensor tendon.

f., mallet. F., hammer, q.v.

f., webbed. Condition in which some or all of the fingers are congenitally fused. Syndactylism.

finger, words pert. to: acroataxia; acrodynia; arachnodactyly; camptodactylia; dactyl; dactylus; digit; nail; phalanx.

finger cot. A protective covering for a finger. Usually made of plastic, rubber, or metal so that an injured finger may be protected from trauma during the healing process.

finger ladder. A device that is attached to the wall and in which notches are cut along an inclined line. The patient "walks" up this notched ladder by placing the fingertips in the notches. This permits stretching of the flexion and abduction muscles of the shoulder and increases the range of motion of the joints of the arms and hands.

fingerprint. An imprint made by the cutaneous ridges of the fleshy portion of the distal end of a finger. Fingerprints are used for purposes of identification as they are individually unique. SEE: illus.

finger-stall. A protective covering for the finger. It may be made of rubber, plastic, metal, or leather. SYN: *finger cot.*

finite. Having limits or boundaries.

FiO_2. *fraction of inspired oxygen.*

fire [AS. *fyr*]. 1. Flame producing heat. 2. Fever.

f., St. Anthony's. Former term for erysipelas.

fire emergencies. If a person's clothing catches fire, he or she should be rolled in a rug or blanket to smother flames. Running only fans the flames. It may be necessary to trip a burning person in order to prevent his or her running about. If an individual is out-

FINGERPRINTS

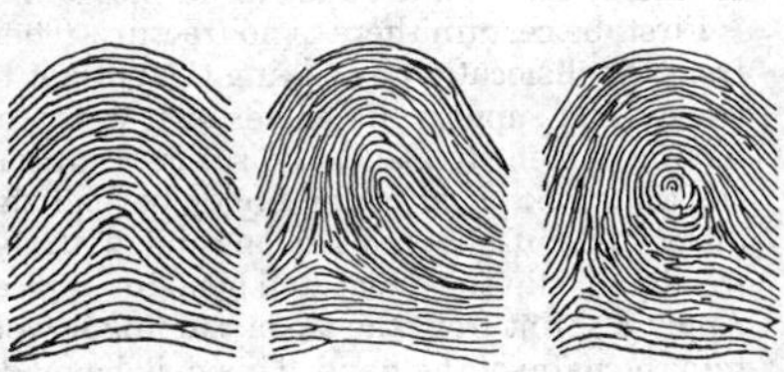

DERMATOGLYPHIC AREAS OF THE HAND

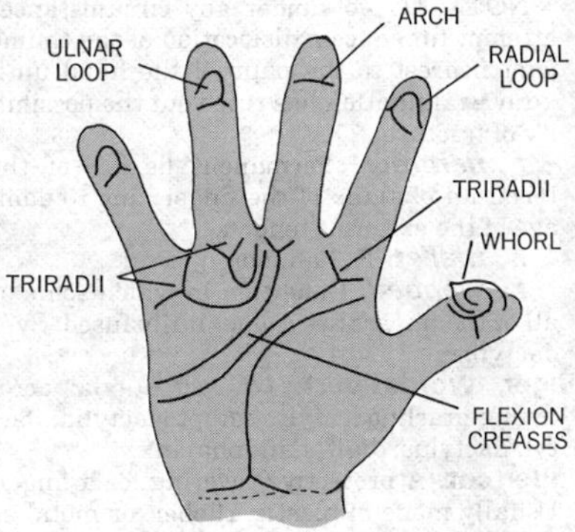

doors, rolling in the dirt will smother flames.

If the victim is trapped in a burning building, the occupied room should have doors and windows closed to prevent cross breezes from increasing the fire. The window should be opened only if the patient is to be rescued through the window. Do not open any door more than a few inches to ascertain possibility of escape. A burst of flame or hot air may push door in and asphyxiate anyone in the room. Wet cloths or towels should be held over mouth and nostrils to keep out smoke and gases. SEE: *burn; flames; gases; transportation.*

first aid. The administration of emergency assistance to individuals who have been injured or otherwise disabled, prior to the arrival of a doctor or transportation to a hospital or doctor's office. First aid should never be the substitution for definitive medical care. SEE: *cardiopulmonary resuscitation; Medical Emergencies* in *Appendix.*

RS: artificial respiration; bites or stings; burn; choking; coma; convulsion; dislocation; drowning; electric shock; fainting; fish poisoning; flames, inhalation of; food poisoning; foreign bodies; fracture; freezing; frostbite; fumes; insect bites and stings; laceration; poison; poison control center; poisoning; radiation accidents, emergency handling of; radioactive patient; shock; snakebite; unconsciousness.

first cranial nerves. Nerves supplying the nasal olfactory mucosa. Consists of delicate bundles of unmyelinated fibers, the filia olfactoria, which pass through the cribriform plate and terminate in the olfactory glomeruli of the olfactory bulb. The filia are the central processes of bipolar receptor neurons of olfactory mucous membrane. SYN: *olfactory nerves.*

first intention healing. Healing that takes place when wound edges are held or sutured together without granulation tissue having been formed. SEE: *healing.*

Fishberg concentration test (fĭsh'bĕrg). [A. M. Fishberg, U.S. physician, b. 1898] A test of the ability of the kidneys to concentrate, i.e., produce a urine of high specific gravity.

fish poisoning. A form of food poisoning caused by eating certain fish. Some fish are inherently poisonous; others become poisonous through decomposition, through infection, by feeding on other poisonous forms, or by poisonous metabolic substances produced during the spawning season. SEE: *ciguatera.*

SYM: When poisoning is due to a toxin, the principal signs are vomiting and muscular paralysis. These occur within thirty minutes to four hours after eating the fish. Convulsions may occur along with diarrhea, abdominal cramps, and shock.

TREATMENT: Removal of toxic fish from stomach by gastric lavage, emetics, and then cathartics. Treat convulsions with appropriate sedative and treat shock with fluid replacement, whole blood, and plasma expanders.

fishskin disease. A disease of the skin characterized by increase of the horny layer and deficiency of the skin secretions. SYN: *ichthyosis.*

fission (fĭsh'ŭn) [L. *fissio*]. 1. Splitting into two or more parts. 2. A method of asexual reproduction seen in bacteria, protozoa, and other lower forms of life in which the cell or the body divides into two or more parts, each of which develops into a complete individual. 3. Bombarding or splitting the nucleus of a heavy atom to release energy and neutrons.

fissiparous (fĭ-sĭp'ă-rŭs) [L. *fissus,* cleft, + *parere,* to bring forth]. Reproducing by fission.

fissura (fĭs-ū'ră) [L.]. (pl. *fissurae*) [NA] Fissure. SYN: *cleft; sulcus.*

fissural (fĭsh'ū-răl). Pert. to a fissure.

fissure (fĭsh'ūr) [L. *fissura*]. 1. A groove or natural division, cleft or slit, deep furrow in the brain, liver, spinal cord, and other organs. 2. Ulcer or cracklike sore. 3. A break in the enamel of a tooth.

f., anal. A linear ulcer on the margin of the anus.

f., auricular. Fissure of petrous portion of the temporal bone.

f., branchial. SEE: *branchial clefts.*

f., Broca's. Fissure encircling the third left frontal convolution of the brain.

f., Burdach's. Fissure connecting lateral surface of insula and inner surface of operculum of the brain.

f., calcarine. Fissure extending from the cerebrum's occipital end to the occipital fissure.

f., callosomarginal. A conspicuous sulcus in mesial surface of cerebral hemisphere running above and concentric with the curved upper surface of the corpus callosum.

f., central. F., Rolando's.

f., Clevenger's. Inferior temporal sulcus.

f., collateral. Fissure on the inferior surface of cerebral hemisphere separating subcalcarine and subcollateral gyri.

f.'s, Henle's. Connective tissue areas between the muscular fibers of heart.

f., hippocampal. Fissure of brain extending from posterior part of corpus callosum to the tip of temporal lobe.

f., inferior orbital. A fissure at the apex of the orbit through which pass the infraorbital blood vessels and maxillary branch of the trigeminal nerve.

f., interparietal. Intraparietal sulcus.

f., longitudinal. A fissure on the lower surface of the liver.

f., occipitoparietal. The fissure between the occipital and parietal lobes of the brain.

f. of Bichat. A fissure below the corpus callosum in the cerebellum.

f. of Sylvius. A fissure separating the frontal and parietal lobes from the temporal lobe of the brain.

f., palpebral. Opening separating the upper and lower eyelids.

f., portal. The opening into the liver on its undersurface; continues into the liver as the portal canal.

f., Rolando's. Fissure separating frontal and parietal lobes.

f., sphenoidal. Fissure separating the wings and body of the sphenoid.

f., transverse. 1. The fissure between the cerebellum and cerebrum of the brain. 2. A fissure on lower surface of the liver that serves as the hilum transmitting vessels and ducts to the liver.

f., umbilical. Anterior portion of liver's longitudinal fissure, which contains the round ligament, the obliterated umbilical vein.

f., Wernicke's. Fissure dividing the temporal and parietal lobes from the occipital lobe.

f., zygal. A transverse cerebral sulcus that connects two parallel sulci. The three sulci are in the form of an H.

fistula (fĭs'tū-lă) [L., *fistula,* pipe]. An abnormal tubelike passage from a normal cavity or tube to a free surface or to another cavity. May be due to congenital incomplete closure of parts or may result from abscesses, injuries, or inflammatory processes.

f., anal. Fistula near the anus.

f., arteriovenous. Direct communication between an artery and vein.

f., biliary. Fistula through which bile is discharged after a biliary operation.

f., blind. Fistula open at only one end.

f., branchial. An open branchial cleft.

f., cervical. 1. An abnormal opening into the cervix uteri. 2. An opening in the neck leading to the pharynx, resulting from incomplete closure of the brachial clefts.

f., complete. Fistula with both external and internal openings.

f., craniosinus. Communication between the intracranial space and a paranasal sinus.

f., enterovaginal. Fistula between the bowel and vagina.

f., fecal. Fistula in which there is a discharge of feces through the opening.

f., gastric. Direct communication between the stomach and the skin over the abdomen.

f., horseshoe. Perianal fistula in which the tract goes around the rectum and communicates with the skin at one or more points.

f., incomplete. A fistula that has only one opening and that is to the skin, i.e., it does not communicate with an internal cavity or organ.

f., metroperitoneal. Fistula between uterine and peritoneal cavities.

f., parotid. Fistula from the parotid gland to the skin surface.

f., perineovaginal. Opening from the vagina through the perineum.

f., pulmonary arteriovenous, congenital. Direct communication within the lung of a pulmonary artery with a pulmonary vein. This congenital condition allows blood to bypass the oxygenation process in the lungs.

f., rectovaginal. Opening beween the rectum and vagina.

f., thyroglossal. A midline fistula just above the thyroid that connects the openings in the skin to a persistent embryonic thyroglossal duct.

f., umbilical. A direct communication between the umbilicus and the gut. Usually due to the failure of closure of the urachal duct.

f., ureterovaginal. Opening between the ureter and vagina.

f., vesicouterine. Opening between the uterus and bladder.

f., vesicovaginal. Opening from the bladder into the vagina.

fistulatome (fĭs′tū-lă-tōm″) [″ + Gr. *tome,* incision]. Instrument for incising a fistula.

fistulectomy (fĭs″tū-lĕk′tō-mē) [″ + Gr. *ektome,* excision]. Excision of a fistula.

fistulization (fĭs″tū-lī-zā′shŭn) [L. *fistula,* pipe]. Becoming fistulous.

fistuloenterostomy (fĭs″tū-lō-ĕn-tĕr-ŏs′tō-mē) [″ + Gr. *enteron,* intestine, + *stoma,* opening]. Operative closure of a biliary fistula and formation of new passage of bile into the intestine.

fistulous (fĭs′tū-lŭs). Pert. to, or containing, a fistula.

fit (fĭt) [AS. *fitt*]. 1. A sudden attack, convulsion, or paroxysm. SEE: *convulsion.* 2. Modification of one structure to that of another, as in dental restoration.

fix. 1. To stain microscopic specimens for examination. 2. Slang for obtaining a dose of a drug of abuse.

fixation [L. *fixatio*]. 1. The act of holding or fastening in a fixed position. Immobilizing, making rigid. 2. The condition of being fixed. 3. A phase of Freudian psychosexual development in which the libido is arrested at an inferior or presexual level. 4. SEE: *fix* (def. 1).

f., complement. The action of a complement, a constituent of fresh blood serum, on an antigen, which in turn has been acted on by its antibody. During the uniting of antigen, antibody, and complement, the complement is rendered inactive or destroyed. This process is known as fixation of complement and is the basis of the Wassermann and Kolmer tests for syphilis. SEE: *complement.*

f., field of. The widest limits of vision in all directions within which the eyes can fixate.

f. of eyes. The movement of the eyes for the most acute vision in which they are directed toward an object so that the visual axes meet and the image of the object falls on corresponding points of each retina.

fixation point. The fovea or the point on the retina where the visual axes (lines) meet the point of clearest vision.

fixative (fĭk′să-tĭv) [L. *fixus,* fastened]. 1. A substance that serves to make firm or fixed. 2. A substance used to harden and preserve pathological specimens.

fixed eruption. Skin lesions that appear in response to exposure to a drug. The eruption reappears at approx. the same site when the drug is again administered. Discontinuation of the medication is indicated.

fixing. In histology, rapid killing of tissue elements so that their normal living form is preserved. This is done to permit accurate and undistorted microscopic visualization of the tissues.

Fl. *fluid.*

flaccid (flăk′sĭd) [L. *flaccidus,* flabby]. Relaxed, flabby, having defective or absent muscular tone.

flaccid paralysis. Paralysis in which there is loss of muscle tone, loss of or reduction of tendon reflexes, atrophy and degeneration of muscles, and reaction of degeneration. Due to lesions of lower motor neurons of spinal cord.

flagella (flă-jĕl′ă) [L.]. Pl. of flagellum.

flagellant (flăj′ĕ-lănt) [L. *flagellum,* whip]. 1. Pert. to flagellum. 2. Pert. to stroking in massage. 3. One who practices flagellation.

flagellate (flăj′ĕ-lāt). 1. With one or more flagella. 2. A protozoon with one or more flagella.

flagellation (flăj″ĕ-lā′shŭn). 1. Whipping. 2. Massage by strokes. 3. Applying electricity by tapping the body. 4. A form of sexual aberration in which the libido is stimulated by whipping oneself, being whipped, or whipping someone else.

flagelliform (flă-jĕl′ĭ-form) [″ + *forma,* shape]. Shaped like a flagellum.

flagellum (flă-jĕl′ŭm) [L., whip]. (pl. *flagella*) A hairlike, motile process on the extremity of a bacterium or protozoon.

Flagyl. Trade name for metronidazole.

flail chest. A condition of the chest wall due to multiple fractures of the rib cage; it moves paradoxically in with inspiration and out during expiration.

flail joint. A joint with excessive mobility usually due to paralysis of the muscles that control it.

flames, inhalation of. SYM: Intense irritation of nose, throat, pharynx, windpipe, and lungs with choking, coughing, interference with respiration, and intense swelling of the throat. Breathing is markedly limited. Shock is a common result.

TREATMENT: Be prepared to vigorously treat pulmonary edema by limiting fluid intake to the minimum required to maintain adequate urine output. Bronchospasm is treated with aminophylline given I.V. slowly or isoproterenol aerosol mist. Administration of oxygen; occasionally tracheotomy is necessary. SEE: *burn; fire; gases.*

flange (flănj). A border that projects above the main structure. In dentistry, the part of an artificial denture that extends from the imbedded teeth to the border of the denture.

flank [O. Fr. *flanc*]. The part of the body

between ribs and upper border of ilium. Also loosely used to refer to the outer side of the thigh, hip, and buttock. SEE: *latus*.

flap [Dutch *flappen,* to strike]. 1. A mass of partially detached tissue used in plastic surgery of an adjacent area or in covering the end of a bone after resection. 2. An uncontrolled movement seen in some diseases. SEE: *asterixis*.

f., amputation. A flap of skin used to cover the end of a part left after an amputation.

f., extraction. Removal of cataract so as to make a flap in the cornea.

f., island. A skin flap in which the edges are free but the center is attached and contains the vascular supply.

f., jump. A skin flap moved from place to place by successively cutting one end and attaching it to a new site.

f., pedicle. A flap made by suturing the edges to form a tube. Then one end of the tube is cut and sutured to another site. By use of the jump flap technique, such a flap may be moved, in several stages, a great distance.

f., skin. A flap containing only skin.

f., sliding. Horizontal movement of a flap to cover a nearby raw area.

f., tube. A long pedicle flap. SEE: *f., pedicle*.

flare. A flush or spreading area of redness that surrounds a line made by drawing a pointed instrument across the skin. It is the second reaction in the triple response, q.v., of skin to injury and is due to dilatation of the arterioles.

flash. 1. Hot flash. SEE: *hot flashes*. 2. Excess material from a mold.

flashbacks. The return of imagery and hallucinations after the immediate effects of hallucinogens have worn off. These may occur for an extended period. They may be of a frightening or threatening form but may consist only of perceptual distortion.

flash method. Means of pasteurizing milk by rapidly raising temperature of milk to 178°F. (80.1° C.), maintaining it there for a few minutes, and rapidly chilling it until the temperature is 40° F. (4.4° C.)

flash point. The temperature at which a substance will burst into flame spontaneously.

flask [LL. *flasco*]. A small bottle with a narrow neck.

flatfoot. Abnormal flatness of sole and arch of foot. This condition may exist without causing symptoms or interfering with normal function of the foot. The inner longitudinal and anterior transverse metatarsal arches are those that may be depressed. It may be acute, subacute, or chronic. SYN: *pes planus; splayfoot*.

f., spasmodic. Flatfoot where the foot is held everted by spasmodic contraction of the peroneal muscle.

flatness. Resonance heard on percussion over solid organs or when there is fluid in the thoracic cavity.

flatulence (flăt'ū-lĕns) [L. *flatulentus*]. Excessive gas in the stomach and intestines. SEE: *distention; gastrointestinal decompression; paralytic ileus; Wangensteen's method*.

NURSING IMPLICATIONS: Evaluate patient for abdominal distention and presence and location of "gas pains." Encourage the patient to be out of bed and ambulatory.

flatulent (flăt'ū-lĕnt). Affected with or caused by gas in the alimentary tract.

flatus (flā'tŭs) [L., a blowing]. 1. Gas in the digestive tract. 2. Expelling of gas from any body orifice. SEE: *borborygmus; eructation*.

f., vaginal. Expulsion of air from the vagina.

flatus tube. A rectal tube to facilitate expulsion of flatus. It is used in cases of severe distention and before a saline enema.

NURSING IMPLICATIONS: Gas in the lower bowel may be relieved by a rectal tube—the tube is lubricated and inserted for 20 minutes. The tube may be reinserted every four hours. Hot water bottle or heating pad applied to the abdomen may also be ordered.

flatworm. A worm belonging to the phylum Platyhelminthes.

flavedo (flă-vē'dō) [L.]. Yellowness, as of the skin; sallowness; jaundice.

flavescent (flă-vĕs'ĕnt). Yellowish.

flavin (flā'vĭn). One of a group of natural water-soluble pigments occurring in milk, yeasts, bacteria, and some plants. All contain the flavin or isoalloxazine nucleus and are yellow in color. Present in riboflavin and in Warburg's yellow enzyme.

flavism (flā'vĭzm) [L. *flavus,* yellow, + Gr. *-ismos,* condition]. Having a yellow tinge.

flavivirus (flă"vē-vī'rŭs). A genus of Togaviridae. They were previously called group B arboviruses. Viruses that cause yellow fever, certain types of encephalitis, and dengue are species in this genus.

flavo- [L. *flavus,* yellow]. Prefix indicating yellow.

Flavobacterium. A genus of rod-shaped bacteria belonging to the Achromobacteraceae. They are found in soil and water and produce an orange-yellow pigment in cultures. Flavobacterium meningosepticum is especially virulent for the premature infant, in whom it causes meningitis. The fatality rate is quite high.

flavone (flā'vōn). The chemical from which the natural colors of many vegetables are derived.

flavoprotein. One of a group of conjugated proteins that constitute the yellow enzymes essential in cellular respiration.

flavor (flā'vor). 1. The quality of a substance that affects the sense of taste. It may also stimulate the sense of smell. 2. A material that is added to a food or medicine to improve its taste.

Flaxedil. Trade name for gallamine triethiodide.

flaxseed. Seed of Linum usitatis simum. SYN: *linseed.*

fl. dr. *fluidram.*

flea (flē) [AS. *flea*]. Any insect of the order Siphonaptera. Fleas are wingless, suck blood, and have legs adapted for jumping. Usually they are parasitic on warm-blooded animals including man. Fleas of the genus Xenopsylla transmit the bacillus of plague (Pasteurella pestis) from rats to humans. Fleas may transmit other diseases such as tularemia, endemic typhus, and brucellosis. They serve as intermediate hosts for the cat and dog tapeworms.

f., cat. Ctenocephalides felis.

f., chigger. Tungra penetrans. SYN: *chigger; jigger; sand flea.*

f., dog. Ctenocephalides canis.

f., human. Pulex irritans.

f., rat. Xenopsylla cheopis.

flea bites. Hemorrhagic puncta surrounded by erythematous and urticarial patches as the result of the injection of flea saliva.

TREATMENT: Ice applied to the site will decrease the pain. Application of a corticosteroid cream may decrease the inflammatory response.

PREVENTION: Treat the skin with an insect repellent available in form of a powder, spray, or oil for topical use.

flea infestation. A home with dogs or cats may become infested with fleas. It is possible to kill the flea population by treating the house for 24 hrs. by using naphthalene. This substance is available in flake form for use as a moth repellent. The flakes are spread on newspapers in the middle of each room, and the house is closed for 24 hrs.

CAUTION: It is essential to disconnect all electrical equipment in the house prior to this procedure because an electrical spark could cause the fumes to explode. Any plants, pets, or humans could suffer adverse effects if they remain in the house during the treatment period. The house should be thoroughly ventilated after the treatment period in order to remove the fumes.

fleam (flēm) [Fr. *flieme*]. Lancet used in venesection.

Flechsig's areas (flĕk'zĭgz). [Paul E. Flechsig, Ger. neurologist, 1847–1929] Anterior, lateral, and posterior areas of each lateral half of the medulla.

fleece of Stilling. Meshwork of white fibers that surrounds the dentate nucleus of the cerebellum.

Fleet Bisacodyl. Trade name for bisacodyl.

Fleet Enema. Trade name for sodium biphosphate.

Fleet Mineral Oil Enema. Trade name for mineral oil.

Fleming, Sir Alexander (flĕm'ĭng). Scottish physician, 1881–1955, who in 1945, along with Ernst B. Chain and Sir Howard W. Florey, was awarded the Nobel Prize in medicine and physiology for the discovery of penicillin.

flesh [AS. *flaesc*]. The soft tissues of the animal body, esp. the muscles. SEE: *carnivorous; meat.*

f., examination of animal. Examine for color, consistency, proportion of fat, odor, and, after cooking, its taste. In general, it should be neither very pale nor dark purple; it should be marbled and of firm and elastic consistency; it should be free from odor; touching the flesh should not moisten the finger.

NOTE: *Yellow:* May be produced by food eaten by animal. In disease, due to animals having been jaundiced. *Brown:* Rare except in old meat undergoing decomposition. *Dark Purple:* May indicate animal died a natural death or suffered from acute fever, tuberculosis, or rinderpest. Avoid. *Dark Reddish-Brown:* May indicate animal was hunted or overdriven; poisoned, drowned, or suffocated. Avoid. *Scarlet:* Rare. Indicates arsenic or carbon monoxide poisoning. *Redness:* Indicates that animal may have been poisoned or the meat frozen. *Green or Violet:* Indicates the beginning of dangerous putrefaction. *Saffron:* Indicates artificial coloring of smoked pork. *Brilliant Red:* Due to poisonous bacteria. *Gray:* Usually in sausages. Due to bacteria. *Phosphorescent:* Not due to putrefaction. Usually found in fish and shellfish. Increased by heat. Sometimes in meat, esp. veal, caused by bacteria, and generally transmitted from fish kept in the same place with meat. *White:* Rare except in calves. Found in certain diseases. Avoid.

f., goose. Cutis anserina.

f., proud. Excessive granular tissue in a wound or ulcer.

Fletcher factor. A blood clotting factor, prekallikrein.

fletcherism. [Horace Fletcher, U.S. dietitian, 1849–1919] Taking small amounts of food at a time with excessive mastication.

flex [L. *flexus*, bent]. To bend upon itself, as a muscle.

flexibilitas cerea (flĕks"ĭ-bĭl'ĭ-tās sē'rē-ă) [L.]. A cataleptic state in which limbs retain any position in which they are placed. Characteristic of catatonic patients. SEE: *catalepsy.*

flexibility [L. *flexus,* bent]. Quality of being bent without breaking; adaptability. SYN: *pliability.*

flexible. Capable of being bent without breaking.

flexile (flĕks'ĭl) [L. *flexus,* bent]. Pliant, flexible.

flexion (flĕk'shŭn) [L. *flexio*]. The act of bending or condition of being bent in contrast to extension. SEE: *antecurvature.*

flexor (flĕks'or) [L.]. A muscle that bends a part in a generally proximal direction. Opposed to extensor.

flexura (flĕk-shoo'ră) [L.]. Flexure.

flexure (flĕk'shĕr) [L. *flexura*]. A bend.

f., colic, left. The bend in the colon at which point the transverse colon becomes the descending colon.

f., colic, right. The bend at the transition point where the ascending colon becomes the transverse colon.

f., dorsal. The convex curve in the thoracic area of the spine.

f., duodenojejunal. Curve at meeting point of jejunum and duodenum.

f., hepatic. The right flexure of the colon. The bend in the large intestine forming the junction of the ascending with the transverse colon.

f., sigmoid. The s-like loop (in left iliac fossa) of the descending colon as it joins the rectum. SEE: *colon.*

f., splenic. The left flexure of the colon. The bend at junction of transverse with descending colon.

flicker. The visual sensation of alternating intervals of brightness caused by interruptions in light stimuli.

flicker phenomenon. When an intermittent light stimulus is seen, there is a rate that will produce the sensation that the light is continuous.

flight of ideas. In psychoanalysis, continuous but fragmentary stream of talk. The general train of thought can be followed but direction is frequently changed, often by chance stimuli from the environment. May be seen in acute manic states.

flint disease. Pneumoconiosis associated with the inhalation of dust produced by stone cutting. SYN: *chalicosis.*

floaters (flō'tĕrs) [AS. *flotian,* float]. Translucent specks of various sizes and shapes that float across the visual field. These are due to small bits of protein or cells floating in the vitreous. The great majority of people have these benign materials in their eyes. SEE: *muscae volitantes.*

floating [AS. *flota,* a raft]. Moving about; out of normal location.

floating kidney. Kidney movable from its normal bed of fat.

floating ribs. The 11th and 12th ribs, which do not articulate with the sternum.

floats. Glass capsules containing labels to float in an exposed liquid to designate its nature.

floccillation, floccitation flŏk"sĭ-lā'shŭn, -tā'shŭn) [L. *floccilatio*]. Semiconscious picking at bedclothes in fevers and stupors. SYN: *carphologia; carphology.*

floccose (flŏk'ōs) [L. *floccosus,* full of wool tufts]. In biology, pert. to a growth made up of short and densely but irregularly interwoven filaments.

floccular (flŏk'ū-lăr) [L. *flocculus,* little tuft]. Pert. to the flocculus of the cerebellum.

flocculation (flŏk"ū-lā'shŭn) The gathering together of the fine dispersed particles in a solution into larger, usually visible particles.

flocculence (flŏk'ū-lĕns"). State of being flocculent or resembling shreds or tufts of cotton.

flocculent (flŏk'ū-lĕnt). Resembling the white portion of floating island or a fluid or culture containing whitish shreds of mucus.

flocculoreaction (flŏk"ū-lō-rē-ăk'shŭn) [" + *re,* again, + *agere,* to act]. Flocculation of a serum reaction.

flocculus (flŏk'ū-lŭs) [L., little tuft]. (pl. *flocculi*) 1. A small tuft of wool-like fibers. 2. [NA] A lobe below and behind the middle peduncle of the cerebrum on each side of the median fissure.

flooding (flŭd'ĭng). 1. Colloquial term for excessive amount of menstrual flow. 2. In treating phobias, repeated exposure to the disturbing ideas, situations or conditions until these conditions no longer produce anxiety.

Flood's ligament. [Valentine Flood, Ir. surgeon, 1800–1847] A band of ligaments attached to the lower part of the lesser tuberosity of the humerus.

floor [AS. *flor*]. The surface that forms the lower limit of a cavity or space, as the floor of the cranial cavity, fourth ventricle, mouth, nasal fossa, or pelvis.

flora [L. *flos,* flower]. 1. Plant life as distinguished from animal life. 2. Plant life occurring or adapted for living in a specific environment. Thus one speaks of the intestinal, vaginal, or skin flora. SEE: *fauna.*

florid [L. *floridus,* blossoming]. Having a bright deep-red color. Used to describe skin coloration.

Florinef Acetate. Trade name for fludrocortisone acetate.

Floropryl. Trade name for isoflurophate.

floss. To use dental floss or tape to remove plaque and calculus from the otherwise inaccessible dental surfaces between teeth.

f., dental. A waxed or unwaxed tape or thread used to clean and remove plaque between the teeth and below the gumline.

flour [L. *flos,* flower]. Finely ground meal obtained from wheat or other grain; any soft fine powder. SEE: *Foods* in *Appendix.*

flow [AS. *flowan,* to flow]. 1. Action of flowing with respect to time. 2. The act of moving or running freely.

flower [L. *flos,* flower]. That part of a plant that comprises the organs of reproduction such as the anthemis, arnica, and matricaria. A complete flower includes a calyx, corolla, stamens, which produce pollen, and a pistil, which produces the ovule.

flowmeter. Device for measuring the flow of a gas or liquid. Used esp. in monitoring flow of anesthetic gases.

floxuridine (flŏks-ŭr'ĭ-dēn). USP. An antimetabolite used in treating certain forms of cancer. Trade name is FUDR.

fl. oz. *fluid ounce,* 29.57 milliliters.

flu (floo). Influenza.

flucticuli (flŭk-tĭk'ū-lī) [L., little waves]. (sing. *flucticulus*) Wavelike markings on lateral wall of third ventricle.

fluctuant (flŭk'chū-ănt). Varying, or unstable. SEE: *fluctuation.*

fluctuation [L. *fluctuatio*]. 1. A variation from one course to another. 2. A wavy impulse felt in palpation and produced by vibration of body fluid.

DIAG: If fluctuation is felt over the lower abdomen, ascites usually is present. May be caused by peritoneal hemorrhage. If it is confined to limited portion of abdomen, tuberculous peritonitis may be implicated; over central portion, bladder distention; in lower abdomen in women, an ovarian cyst or pregnancy; in right hypochondrium, a hydatid cyst, abscess of liver, distended gallbladder; over left hypochondrium, cysts or abscess; above umbilicus, dilated colon or stomach partly filled with fluid and gas.

flucytosine (flū-sī'tō-sēn"). An antifungal drug. It is usually used with amphotericin B in order to decrease the emergence of resistant strains of yeasts and fungi. Trade name is Ancobon.

fludrocortisone (floo"drō-kor'tĭ-sōn). A synthetic corticosteroid.

f. acetate. A corticosteroid drug. Trade name is Florinef Acetate.

fluid [L. *fluidus*]. A nonsolid, liquid, or gaseous substance. SEE: *secretion.*

f., allantoic. The fluid present in the allantoic sac.

f., amniotic. A clear yellowish fluid that fills the fetal membranes in pregnancy. Spec. grav. approx. 1.006. It is composed of albumin, salts (chiefly urea), and water, and suspended in it are lanugo, epidermal cells, vernix caseosa, and meconium. It is derived from the amnion. Its chief function is protection for the fetus. SEE: *amnion; meconium.*

f., cerebrospinal. Fluid found in central canal of spinal cord, in the ventricles of the brain, and in the subarachnoid space about the brain and spinal cord. It is formed by the choroid plexuses of the ventricles.

f., extracellular. Tissue fluid or fluid occupying spaces between the tissue cells.

f., extravascular. All the body fluids outside the blood vessels. Includes tissue fluid, fluids within the serous and synovial cavities, the cerebrospinal fluid, and lymph.

f., interstitial. F., extracellular.

f., intracellular. The fluid contained within cells and comprising about 50% of body weight.

f., intraocular. The fluid within the anterior and posterior chambers of the eye.

f., seminal. Semen.

f., serous. Fluid in the serous cavities.

f., spinal. Cerebrospinal fluid present in the spinal canal of the spinal cord.

f., synovial. The fluid contained within synovial cavities, bursae, and tendon sheaths. SYN: *synovia.*

fluid balance. Regulation of amount of water in the body. The balance is upset when fluids are lost by vomiting, diarrhea, bleeding, or when dehydration occurs. Treatment of fluid imbalance depends upon the cause, the kind and quantity of fluids lost, and the state of renal function.

fluid diet. Diet for those either unable to tolerate solid food or for patients whose gastrointestinal tract needs to be free of solid matter.

fluid repair. Solution in water of electrolytes and usually glucose, given intravenously to correct or repair fluid and electrolyte imbalance.

fluid retention. Failure to eliminate fluid from the body because of renal, cardiac, or metabolic disease, or combinations of these disorders. Retention of salt is another cause of fluid retention. Excess salt in the body requires retention of water to maintain the proper chemical and physical properties of body fluids. A low-sodium diet is indicated in fluid retention. The use of diuretics will depend upon the functional state of the kidneys.

fluidextract, fluidextractum [L. *fluidus,* fluid, + *extractum,* extract]. Solution of the soluble constituents of vegetable drugs of such strength that each cc. or ml. represents 1 gm. of the drug. Fluidextracts contain alcohol as a solvent or preservative, and many of these form precipitates when water is added.

f., aromatic cascara. USP. Liquid preparation of cascara sagrada, magnesium oxide, glycyrrhiza extract, saccharin, anise oil, coriander oil, methyl salicylate, alcohol, and water. Used as a cathartic.

f., glycyrrhiza. A liquid preparation of glycyrrhiza.

f., ipecac. A fluid preparation of the powdered rhizome and roots of Cephaelis ipecacuanha or C. acuminata. It is used as an emetic and expectorant.

fluidounce. Measure of apothecaries' fluid volume, equal to eight fluidrams or 29.57 ml. SYMB: f℥.

fluidram. Apothecaries' measure of fluid volume, equal to 3.697 ml. SYMB: fʒ.

fluke (flook) [AS. *floc*, flatfish]. A parasitic worm belonging to the class Trematoda, phylum Platyhelminthes. Those parasitic in man belong to the order Digenea. Most flukes have complex life cycles that include asexual generations that live in a mollusc (snail or bivalve). Stages of a typical fluke include adult, egg, miracidium, sporocyst, redia, cercaria, and metacercaria.

f., blood. A schistosome; flukes of the genus Schistosoma, S. haematobium, S. mansoni, and S. japonicum. Adults live principally in the mesenteric and pelvic veins. They cause schistosomiasis and schistosome dermatitis (swimmer's itch).

f., intestinal. Species of intestinal flukes infesting man include Gastrodiscoides hominis, Fasciolopsis buski, Heterophyes heterophyes, Metagonimus yokogawai.

f., liver. Species living in the liver and bile ducts. Those infesting man include Clonorchis sinensis, Fasciola hepatica, Dicrocoelium dendriticum, and Opisthorchis felineus.

f., lung. Fluke that infests lung tissue. Only one species is common in man, namely Paragonimus westermani.

flumethasone pivalate (floo-měth'ă-sōn). USP. A synthetic corticosteroid. Trade name is Locorten.

flumina pilorum (floo'mĭ-nă pī-lō'rŭm) [L., rivers of hair]. [NA] The curved lines along which the hairs of the body are arranged, esp. in the fetus; hairs lying in same direction.

fluocinolone acetonide (floo-ō-sĭn'ō-lōn). USP. A synthetic corticosteroid. Trade names are Fluonid and Synalar.

Fluogen. Trade name for influenza virus vaccine, trivalent.

Fluonid. Trade name for fluocinolone acetonide.

fluor albus (floo'or ăl'bŭs) [L., white flow]. White discharge from the uterus or vagina. SYN: *leukorrhea.*

fluorescein sodium (floo"ō-rěs'ē-ĭn). USP. A red crystalline powder. Used chiefly for diagnostic purposes and for detecting foreign bodies in or lesions of the cornea of the eye. Trade names are Fluor-I-Strip A.T., Fluorescite, Ful-Glow, and Funduscein.

fluorescence (floo"ō-rěs'ěnts). Property of certain substances to emit light when exposed to certain types of light radiation. Usually ultraviolet, first noted in fluorspar; caused by absorption of certain wavelengths and simultaneous emission of a longer wavelength that terminates simultaneously with the cessation of the incident exciting radiation.

fluorescent (floo-ō-rěs'ěnt). 1. In biology, having one color by transmitted light and another by reflected light. 2. Luminous when exposed to other light rays.

fluorescent antibody. ABBR: FA. An antibody that has been stained or marked by a fluorescent material. Use of the fluorescent antibody technique permits rapid diagnosis of various kinds of infections.

fluorescent screen. 1. A sheet of cardboard, paper, or glass coated with a material that fluoresces visibly, such as calcium tungstate. It is used as the chief part of a fluoroscope when roentgen rays, radium rays, or electrons impinge upon it. 2. A sheet of cardboard, paper, or glass, coated with anthracene or other fluorescing materials to observe ultraviolet radiations. SYN: *intensifying screen.*

fluorescent treponemal antibody-absorption test. ABBR: FTA-ABS. Test for syphilis using fluorescent antibody q.v., technique.

Fluorescite. Trade name for fluorescein sodium, USP.

fluoridation (floo"or-ĭ-dā'shŭn). The addition of fluorides to a water supply as a means of preventing a high rate of dental caries.

The development of dental caries in the deciduous and permanent teeth can be decreased by providing fluoride either as a supplement in the drinking water, by topical application to the teeth, or by daily medication with fluoride. There are several important considerations: fluoride in excess daily dose will cause discoloration of the teeth if the fluoride is ingested while the teeth are developing, i.e., from birth to 8 or 10 years; fluoride taken after the age of 8 to 10 will have little effect on the prevention of dental caries.

The rate of loss of teeth in individuals receiving fluoride from infancy will be only one quarter that of persons who received no fluoride. The most certain and effective method of administering fluoride is by providing drinking water that contains one part per million, 1 mg./1000 ml., of fluoride. This will assure a daily dose of fluoride of 0.25 to 0.50 mg. per day. CAUTION: Children drinking water that is fluoricated should not be given supplemental fluoride medication.

fluoride (floo'ō-rīd). A compound of fluorine with a radical; a salt of hydrofluoric acid.

f., stannous. A compound applied topically to the teeth to prevent dental caries.

Contains at least 71% stannous tin and approx. 25% fluoride.

fluoride dental treatment. The application of a fluoride solution or gel to the teeth as a means of controlling or preventing caries.

fluoride poisoning. SEE: *Poisons and Poisoning* in *Appendix.*

fluorine (floo'ō-rēn, floor'ēn). SYMB: F. At. wt. 18.9984; at. no. 9. Gaseous chemical element. Fluorine is found in the soil in combination with calcium. It seems absolutely necessary to plant life. In animal life, it helps to form the bones and teeth. It is found in cow's milk, egg yolk, and brain.

Fluor-I-Strip-A.T. Trade name for fluorescein sodium, USP.

fluoroacetate (floo″or-ō-ăs'ĕ-tāt). A salt of fluoroacetic acid. SEE: *Poisons and Poisoning* in *Appendix.*

fluorometer (floo-or-ŏm'ĕ-tĕr). 1. Device for determining the amount of radiation produced by x-rays. 2. Device for adjusting a fluoroscope in order to establish better the location of the target and to produce an undistorted image or shadow.

fluorometholone (floor″ō-mĕth'ō-lōn). USP. A synthetic corticosteroid. Trade names are Oxylone and FML Liquifilm.

Fluoroplex. Trade name for fluorouracil.

fluoroscope (floo'or-ō-skōp). A device consisting of a fluorescent screen suitably mounted, either separately or in conjunction with a roentgen tube, by means of which the shadows of objects interposed between the tube and the screen are made visible.

fluoroscopy. The use of a fluoroscope for medical diagnosis or for testing various materials by roentgen rays. SYN: *photoscopy.*

fluorosis (floo-or-ō'sĭs). Chronic fluorine poisoning, sometimes marked by mottling of tooth enamel. Often results from too much fluoride in drinking water.

fluorouracil (floor″ō-ŭr'ă-sĭl). USP. An antimetabolite used in treating certain forms of cancer. Trade names are Adrucil, 5-FU, Efudex, and Fluoroplex.

fluoxymesterone (floo-ŏk″sē-mĕs'tĕr-ōn). USP. An anabolic and androgenic hormone. Trade names are Ora-Testryl and Halotestin.

fluphenazine enanthate (floo-fĕn'ă-zēn). USP. A phenothiazine-type tranquilizer. Trade name is Prolixin Enanthate.

fluprednisolone (floo″prĕd-nĭs'ō-lōn). A corticosteroid drug. Trade name is Alphadrol.

flurandrenolide (floor″ăn-drĕn'ō-lĭd). USP. A corticosteroid drug. Trade name is Cordran.

flurazepam hydrochloride (floor-ăz'ĕ-păm). A sedative-hypnotic drug. Trade name is Dalmane.

flurogestone acetate (floor″ō-jĕs'tōn). A progestational drug.

flurothyl (floor'ō-thĭl). USP. A central nervous system stimulant.

fluroxene (floor-ŏks'ēn). An anesthetic agent administered by inhalation. CAUTION: It may be flammable and explosive.

flush [ME. *flusshen,* to fly up]. 1. Sudden redness of the skin. 2. Irrigating of a cavity with water.

f., hectic. Redness of the cheeks seen in some chronic affections such as pulmonary tuberculosis and resulting from a rise of temperature.

f., hot. Flush accompanied with sensation of heat; common in neuroses, psychoneuroses, and during menopause.

f., malar. A bright-colored flush over the malar area and cheekbones. May be associated with any febrile disease.

flutter [AS. *floterian,* to fly about]. A tremulous movement, esp. of the heart as atrial and ventricular flutter.

f., atrial. Condition in which contractions of the atrium become extremely rapid (200 to 400 per min.). In pure flutter, a regular rhythm is maintained; in impure flutter, the rhythm is irregular.

f., diaphragmatic. Rapid contractions of the diaphragm. They may occur intermittently or be present for an extended period. The cause is unknown.

f., mediastinal. Abnormal side-to-side motion of the mediastinum during respiration.

f., ventricular. Ventricular contractions of the heart at a rate of 250 or more.

flutter-fibrillation. Atrial fibrillation of the heart that resembles fibrillation and flutter.

flux [L. *fluxus,* a flow]. 1. An excessive flow or discharge from an organ or cavity of the body. 2. Discharge from the bowels.

fly [AS. *fleoge*]. An insect belonging to the order Diptera, characterized by possessing sucking mouth parts, one pair of wings, and incomplete metamorphosis, such as the May fly, house fly, or dragonfly. Term is sometimes applied to insects belonging to other orders. SEE: *Diptera.*

f., black. A fly of the genus Simulium.

f., blow. Flies of the family Calliphoridae. They breed in dung or the flesh of dead animals. SYN: *bluebottle flies.* SEE: *Calliphora vomitoria.*

f., bot. Botfly.

f., flesh. The Sarcophagidae.

f., house. Musca domestica.

f., sand. Phlebotomus.

f., screwworm. A fly belonging to the families Calliphoridae and Sarcophagidae.

f., Spanish. Cantharides.

f., tsetse. Glossina palpalis; fly that transmits African sleeping sickness or trypanosomiasis.

f., warble. Dermatobia.

Fm. Chem. symb. for fermium.

f.m. L. *fiat mistura,* make a mixture. An abbreviation used in prescription writing.

foam (fōm) [AS. *fam*]. A mixture of finely divided gas bubbles interspersed in a liquid.

foam stability test. Procedure for determining the presence or absence of surface-active material in the amniotic fluid. The surfactant is usually deficient in respiratory distress syndrome, q.v. Concentration of the surfactant is determined by placing varying dilutions of amniotic fluid in tubes containing saline and alcohol. The tubes are agitated. Those tubes that produce no bubbles are classed as negative and those with a great number of bubbles are positive.

focal [L. *focus,* hearth]. Pert. to a focus.

focal infection. Infection occurring near a focus, such as the cavity of a tooth.

focal lesion. A limited central lesion.

focal spot. Area on the x-ray tube target that is bombarded with electrons to produce X radiation.

foci (fō'sī) [L.]. Pl. of focus.

focus [L., hearth]. (pl. *foci*) 1. The point of convergence of light rays or waves of sound. 2. The starting point of a disease process.

f., real. Point at which convergent rays intersect.

f., virtual. The point at which divergent rays would intersect if prolonged backward.

fog. Droplets suspended in a gas, as water droplets in air.

fogging. 1. A method of testing vision, used particularly in testing astigmatism and in postcycloplegic examination. 2. Method of intense application of an insecticide. The solution is nebulized and appears in the air as a fog. 3. Unwanted density on the radiographic film resulting from exposure to secondary radiation, light, chemicals, or heat.

fold [AS. *fealdan,* to fold]. A ridge; a doubling back. SYN: *plica.*

f., amniotic. Folded edge of the amniotic membrane where it rises over and finally encloses the embryo of birds, reptiles, and some mammals.

f., aryepiglottic. The ridge-like lateral walls of the entrance to the larynx.

f., circular. A large fold that extends into the lumen of the small intestine.

f., costocolic. Ligament arising from the peritoneum that attaches the splenic flexure of the colon to the diaphragm.

f., Douglas'. A fold of peritoneum extending on each side to the base of the broad ligament. This forms the rectouterine space, called Douglas' pouch.

f.'s, gastric. The folds of mucosa, mostly longitudinal, in the empty stomach.

f., genital. Fold of skin in the embryo on each side of the genital tubercle that develops into the labia minora in the female.

f., gluteal. The linear crease in the skin that separates the buttocks from the thighs.

f., lacrimal. A valve-like fold in the lower part of the nasolacrimal duct.

f., mesouterine. Fold of peritoneum supporting the uterus.

f., mucosal. A fold of mucosal tissue.

f., nail. The folded-in epidermal tissue surrounding the sides and base of nails.

f., palmate. The ridges on the cervical canal of the uterus.

f., semilunar, of conjunctiva. Fold of conjunctiva at the inner angle of the eye.

f., transverse, of rectum. Transverse mucosal folds of the rectum. SYN: *valves of Houston.*

f., ventricular; f., vestibular. The false vocal cord.

f., vestigial. The ligament of the left superior vena cava. SYN: *Marshall's fold.*

f., vocal. F., ventricular, q.v.

folia (fō'lē-ă) [L.]. Pl. of folium.

foliaceous (fō-lē-ā'shē-ŭs) [L. *folia,* leaves]. Resembling or pert. to a leaf.

folic acid (fō'lĭk). USP. $C_{19}H_{19}N_7O_6$. A member of the vitamin B complex. Used in treatment of sprue. Found naturally in green plant tissue, liver, and yeast. Also called pteroylglutamic acid. Trade name is Folvite.

CAUTION: Folic acid should not be used in treatment of pernicious anemia because it does not protect patients against the development of changes in the central nervous system that accompany this type of anemia.

folie (fō-lē') [Fr.]. Mania; psychosis.

f. à deux. Occurrence of psychosis, usually of the paranoid type at the same time in two closely associated persons. Rarely more than two persons are involved.

f. du doute. Abnormal doubts about ordinary acts and beliefs; inability to decide upon definite course of action or conduct.

f. du pourquoi. Unreasonable and unrelenting questioning.

f. gemellaire. Psychosis occurring in both twins.

folinic acid. The active form of folic acid. Used in counteracting the effects of folic acid antagonists, and in treating anemia due to folic acid deficiency. Trade name is Calcium Folinate.

folium (fō'lē-ŭm) [L., leaf]. (pl. *folia*) Thin, broad, leaflike structure.

f. vermis. [NA] A fold on the posterior part of the upper surface of the vermis of the cerebellum.

follicle [L. *folliculus,* little bag]. A small secretory sac or cavity.

f., aggregated. An aggregation of solitary nodules or groups of lymph nodules found chiefly in the ileum near its junction with the colon. They are circular or oval, about 1 cm. wide and 2 to 3 cm. long. They lie in the mucosa and submucosa and always occur on the side of the intestine opposite to the attachment of mesentery. In typhoid fever, they undergo hyperplasia and often become ulcerated. SYN: *Peyer's patch*.

f., atretic. An ovarian follicle that has undergone degeneration or involution.

f., dental. The connective tissue structure that encloses the developing tooth within the substance of the jaw prior to tooth eruption. The dental sac and its contents.

f., gastric. The glands in the gastric mucosa of the stomach.

f., graafian. The complete development of the primary oocyte in the cortex of the ovary to the stage where the ovum is fully developed. SEE: *graafian follicle; ovary; ovum* for illus.

f., growing. A developing follicle of the ovary.

f., hair. An invagination of the epidermis from which a hair develops.

f., lymphatic. The densely packed collection of lymphocytes and lymphoblasts that make up the cortex of lymph glands.

f., nabothian. Dilated cyst of the glands of the cervix uteri.

f., ovarian. A spherical structure in the cortex of the ovary consisting of an oogonium or an oocyte and its surrounding epithelial (follicular) cells. Follicles are of three types: primary, consisting of an oogonium and a single layer of follicular cells; growing, in which the follicle cells proliferate, forming several layers, and the first maturation division occurs; vesicular, or graafian follicle, which possesses a cavity (antrum) containing the follicular fluid (liquor folliculi). The oocyte lies in the cumulus oophorus, a mass of cells on the inner surface. The cells lining the follicle constitute the stratum granulosum. The follicle is a secretory structure producing estrogen and progesterone. SEE: *corpus luteum*.

f., primordial. The follicle of the ovary, which consists of the ovum enclosed in a single layer of cells.

f., sebaceous. Oil gland of the skin.

f., solitary. A single lymph nodule of the intestine.

f., thyroid. Spherical or ovoid structure found in the thyroid gland lined with a single layer of cuboidal epithelial cells, which secrete the thyroid hormone. The follicles are filled with colloid, a viscid substance rich in iodine.

f., vesicular. Follicle containing a cavity; a mature ovarian or graafian follicle.

follicle-stimulating hormone. ABBR: FSH. Hormone produced by the anterior pituitary. It stimulates growth of the follicle in the ovary and spermatogenesis in the testis.

follicular. Pert. to a follicle or follicles.

follicular tonsillitis. Inflammation of follicles on surface of the tonsil, which become filled with pus.

follicular tumor. A sebaceous cyst.

folliculitis (fō-lĭk″ū-lī′tĭs) [L. *folliculus*, little bag, + Gr. *itis*, inflammation]. Inflammation of a follicle or follicles.

f. barbae. Ringworm of the beard.

f. decalvans. Purulent follicular inflammation of the scalp resulting in irregular alopecia and scarring.

ETIOL: Cause unknown. Believed to be caused by staphylococci. Affects mostly males between 2nd and 4th decades.

SYM: Initial inflammatory papule or pustule at mouth of follicle pierced by a hair is followed by crusting and desiccation, when it drops off along with loosened hair. Bald patches with slight depressed whitish center surrounded by inflamed margin. Extends peripherally.

PATH: Sebaceous gland atrophy and flattened papillae.

PROG: Baldness is permanent although extension may be arrested.

TREATMENT: Externally, topical antibiotics or corticosteroids and frequent shampoos.

f., keloidal. Chronic dermatitis with production of hard papules that join together to form keloid tissue.

folliculoma (fō-lĭk″ū-lō′mă) [″ + Gr. *oma*, tumor]. A tumor of the ovary originating in a graafian follicle in which the cells resemble the cells of the stratum granulosum.

folliculose (fō-lĭk′ū-lōs). Composed of follicles.

folliculosis (fō-lĭk″ū-lō′sĭs) [″ + Gr. *osis*, condition]. Presence of an abnormal quantity of lymph follicles.

folliculus (fō-lĭk′ū-lŭs) [L.]. (pl. *folliculi*) [NA] A follicle.

Follutein. Trade name for chorionic gonadotropin.

Folvite. Trade name for folic acid.

fomentation (fō″mĕn-tā′shŭn) [L. *fomentatio*]. A hot, wet application for the relief of pain or inflammation. SEE: *dressing, hot moist; stupe*.

fomes (fō′mēz) [L., tinder]. (pl. *fomites*) Any substance that adheres to and transmits infectious material.

fomites (fō′mĭ-tēz). Pl. of fomes.

Fontana's spaces (fŏn-tă′năz). [Felice Fontana, It. scientist, 1730–1805] Spaces between the processes of ligamentum pectinatum of the iris. These convey the aqueous humor.

fontanel, fontanelle (fŏn″tă-nĕl′) [Fr. *fontanelle*, little fountain]. An unossified space or

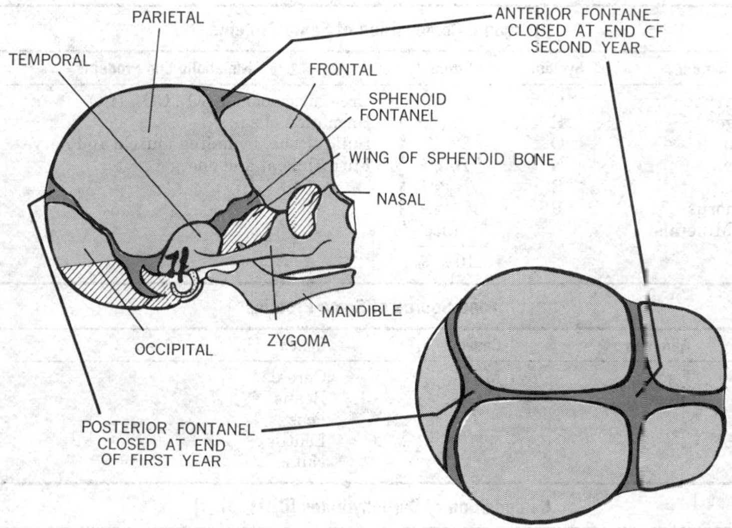

FONTANELS OF INFANT'S SKULL AND BONES OF SKULL

soft spot lying between the cranial bones of the skull of a fetus. SEE: illus.

f., anterior. Fontanel at the junction of the coronal, frontal, and sagittal sutures.

f., posterior. Fontanel at the junction of the sagittal and lambdoid sutures.

fonticulus (fŏn-tĭk′ū-lŭs) [L., little fountain]. [NA] Fontanel.

food [AS. *foda*]. (pl. *foods*) Any material that provides the nutritive requirements of an organism to maintain growth and physical well-being. SEE: *Foods* in *Appendix*.

COURSE: *Alimentary canal:* Foods enter the mouth and in the buccal area are reduced to a pulp or semifluid mass through the processes of mastication and insalivation (the mixing of food with saliva). Swallowing or deglutition then occurs. In swallowing, the food mass or bolus passes into the pharynx and then through the esophagus to the stomach, the entrance to which is controlled by the cardiac sphincter.

Stomach: In the stomach the food is stored and mixed with gastric juice. This action combined with the gastric acidity kills many of the microorganisms present in food. After it attains a certain fluid consistency, it passes through the pyloric sphincter into the small intestine.

Small intestine: In the first portion or duodenum, the intestinal contents (now called chyme) are mixed with bile secreted by the liver and with pancreatic juice, both of which enter through the opening of the common bile duct. In the next two portions, the jejunum and ileum, the chyme is mixed with the intestinal juice secreted by the intestinal glands or crypts of Lieberkühn. In the small intestine, digestion is completed and the end products of digestion (simple sugars, amino acids, fatty acids and glycerol) are absorbed into the capillaries and lacteals of the intestinal mucosa.

Large intestine: Remaining material passes from the small intestine into the large intestine (colon) through the ileocecal valve located at the junction of the ascending colon and the cecum, a blind pouch that terminates in the vermiform appendix. The material continues through the colon (ascending, transverse, descending, and sigmoid) to the rectum, from which it is discharged as feces through the anal canal at the anus, or anal orifice. In the large intestine, the major portion of the water of the intestinal contents is absorbed. Digestive changes are limited to the action of bacteria, which brings about putrefaction and fermentation of incompletely digested foods.

f., contamination of. Food may be the

Source and Analysis of Some Foods

Organic Composition of Some Proteins

Element	Symbol	Percent	Metabolic End Products
Carbon	C	53 %	Urea, uric acid, H_2SO_4, CO_2, H_2O
Hydrogen	H	7 %	Formation of salts
Oxygen	O	22 %	Build tissue, including muscle and nerve
Nitrogen	N	16 %	Furnish heat and energy
Sulfur	S	½%	
Phosphorus	P	½%	
Other Minerals		trace	
		100 %	

Food Source of Some Proteins

Albumen	Casein	Gluten
Eggs	Milk	Cereals
Meat	Cheese	Beans
		Peas
		Lentils
		Nuts

Composition of Carbohydrates $[C_n(H_2O)_{n-1}]$

Element	Symbol	Percent	Metabolic End Products
Carbon	C	76%	CO_2 and H_2O
Hydrogen	H	12%	Energy
Oxygen	O	12%	
		100%	

Examples of Carbohydrates in Food

Glucose	Sucrose	Cellulose, Glycogen, and Starch
$C_6H_{12}O_6$	$C_{12}H_{22}O_{11}$	$(C_6H_{10}O_5)_n$

Carbohydrates and fats are sources of heat and energy, but neither can take the place of proteins, the only food source of nitrogen. Carbohydrates consist principally of sugars, starch, and cellulose.

Composition of Some Fats

Element	Symbol	Percent	Metabolic End Products
Carbon	C	45%	CO_2 and H_2O
Hydrogen	H	6%	Produce heat and energy but do not build
Oxygen	O	49%	tissues or cells
		100%	

Origin of Fats

Animal	Oils	Nuts	Fruits
Butter, Oleomargarine, Eggs, Lard, Cooking Oils, Meat, Dairy Products	Cottonseed, Corn, Sunflower, Safflower	Peanuts	Palm, Olive

Additional Dietary Requirements

Water, Minerals (Iodine, Iron, Magnesium, Calcium, Copper, Chromium, Cobalt, Zinc, Selenium, Manganese, and Molybdenum), Vitamins

cause of illness because it may act as the carrier of pathogenic organisms such as those that cause enteritis (Salmonella) or tuberculosis, parasites such as those that cause trichinosis, or certain types of worms (roundworms, tapeworms).

f., convenience. Food in which one or more steps in preparation have been completed before the product is offered for retail sale. Examples include frozen vegetables, bake mixes, and heat-and-serve types of food.

f., dietetic. Food that has been modified in nutrient content in some way in order to be used in special diets, esp. for diabetics.

f., enriched. Foods in which the vitamin and mineral content has been increased either by addition or by irradiation.

f., nutrient substances of. Substances that in the body serve as a source of energy or provide material for the growth and repair of tissue. Foods are organic substances (proteins, carbohydrates, fats) present in animal and plant tissues. The term "food" is commonly used to refer to any substance taken into the body that serves a nutrient function. Thus any discussion of food would include vitamins, minerals, water, and trace elements (zinc, chromium, cobalt, magnesium, manganese, molybdenum, selenium).

f., textured. Food products manufactured from a variety of nutritional components. In texture they may resemble conventional protein-source foods such as meat or poultry.

food additives. Substances or a mixture of substances other than basic foodstuff that are present in a food as a result of any aspect of production, processing, storage, or packaging. Accidental contaminants are not considered to be food additives.

food adulterant. A substance that makes food impure or inferior, such as toxic organisms, filth, pesticide residues, radioactive fallout, any poisonous or deleterious substance, or any substance added to increase bulk or weight in a food product.

food allergies. Allergic reactions resulting from ingestion of foods to which a person has become sensitized. One may become sensitive to almost any food. However, certain foods such as milk, eggs, wheat, shellfish, chocolate, and oranges are frequent offenders.

SYM: Urticaria (hives), certain eczemas, nausea, vomiting, diarrhea, and intestinal cramps. A syndrome (angioneurotic edema) characterized by a transient swelling of various parts of the body and spasm of the intestine may result.

Food and Drug Administration. ABBR: FDA. In the U.S.A., an official regulatory body for foods, drugs, cosmetics, and medical devices. It is a part of the U.S. Department of Health and Human Services.

food ball. Gastric stone made up of fruit and vegetable skins, seeds, and fibers. SYN: *phytobezoar.*

food chain. The sequential transfer of food energy from green plants to animals that eat plants, then to animals that eat the plant-eating animals; e.g., cows eat plants, other animals including man eat the meat of cows. Interruption of the chain at any point may produce an ecological disaster.

food exchanges. Commonly used foods grouped according to similarities in composition so that such foods may be used interchangeably in diet planning.

food poisoning. An imprecise term indicating an illness resulting from the ingestion of foods containing poisonous substances. True food poisoning includes mushroom poisoning, shellfish poisoning, poisoning resulting from foods contaminated with poisonous insecticides or toxic substances such as lead or mercury, and milk sickness (due to milk from cows that have fed on certain poisonous plants). Also, occasionally poisoning resulting from eating foods that have undergone putrefaction or decomposition or poisoning from bacteria.

food requirements. It is assumed that an average healthy man (154 lb. or 70 kg.) performing light to moderate muscular work requires 2700 Cal./day and an average healthy woman (128 lbs. or 58 kg.) requires 2000 Cal./day. This would be supplied in part by protein but mostly by fat and carbohydrates. Persons in sedentary occupations require fewer calories. In general, adults require 1 gm. of protein per day for each kilogram of their ideal weight.

A diet made up of ordinary foods and supplying the necessary amounts of protein and energy undoubtedly supplies an abundance of mineral matter. The assumption is usually made that, provided a woman is engaged in some moderately active occupation, she requires fewer calories each day because of her comparatively smaller build. Calculated on the basis of food energy required per kilogram of body weight, children and pregnant women require more food than other adults.

The criteria for an adequate diet are difficult to define because food habits vary from one area to another as well as from individual to individual. There is no single diet or individual food that is essential for life or health. Also, it is not possible to state that the ideal diet, with respect to assuring maximum growth and development, would be the one that would assure maximum longevity. SEE: *Dietetics* in *Appendix*.

foot [AS. *fot*]. 1. The terminal portion of the lower extremity. The bones of the foot include the tarsus, metatarsus, and phalanges. SEE: illus.; *skeleton*. 2. A unit of measurement containing 12 in. (30.48 cm.). ABBR: ft.

f., arches of. Four arches: internal longitudinal, outer longitudinal, and two transverse arches.

f., athlete's. A fungus infection of the foot.

f., cleft. Condition in which a cleft extends between the digits to the metatarsal region, usually due to a missing digit.

f., contracted. A deformity of the foot characterized by an excessively high longitudinal arch and dorsal contracture of toes.

f., flat. Abnormal flatness of sole and arch of foot. This condition may exist without causing symptoms or interfering with normal function of the foot. The inner longitudinal and anterior transverse metatarsal arches are those that may be depressed. It may be acute, subacute, or chronic. SYN: *pes planus*.

BONES OF FOOT AND ANKLE

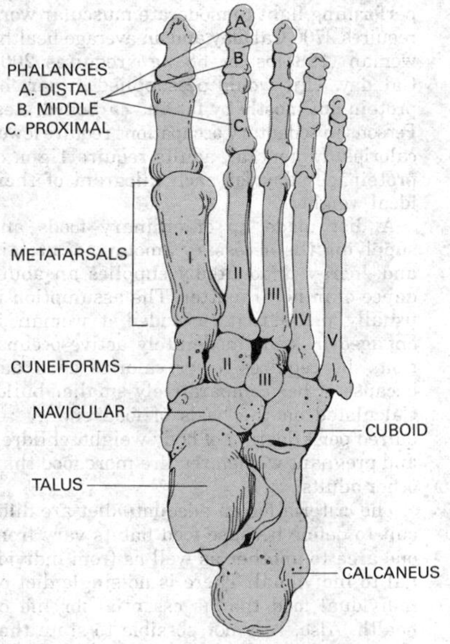

f., immersion. Condition of foot resulting from prolonged immersion of the feet in water.

f., Madura. Bone hypertrophy and degeneration, frequently followed by suppuration or gangrene.

f., march. Spontaneous fracture of one of the metatarsal bones of the foot.

f., splay. Flatfoot accompanied by extreme eversion of the foot.

f., trench. Degeneration of the skin of the feet due to prolonged exposure to moisture. The condition may be prevented by being certain that clean, dry socks are worn at all times. The feet do not have to be exposed to cold to develop this condition.

f., weak. Condition resulting from weakened muscles or from faulty walking habits. Results in chronic eversion of the foot.

foot and mouth disease. A viral disease of cattle and horses that is rarely transmitted to man.

SYM: In humans, fever, headache, malaise with dryness and burning sensation of the mouth. Vesicles develop on the lips, tongue, mouth, palms, and soles.

TREATMENT: Symptomatic. Full recovery occurs in 2 to 3 weeks.

foot board. A board or similar material placed at the foot end of the patient's bed. It extends up above the mattress and, when used properly, will help to prevent footdrop. The patient should be positioned in bed so that when the legs are fully extended, the soles of the feet just touch the board.

foot-candle. An amount of light equivalent to 1 lumen, q.v., per square foot.

footdrop. Plantar flexion of the foot due to weakness or paralysis of the anterior muscles of the lower leg. This may occur in any patient who is in bed continuously, esp. if comatose. A foot board should be used to prevent footdrop.

footling presentation. Presentation of feet foremost in labor.

footplate. The flat part of the stapes, a bone in the middle ear.

foot pound. The amount of energy required to lift one pound of mass a vertical distance of one foot.

footprint. An impression of the foot, esp. an ink impression used for identification of infants.

forage (fō-rŏzh′) [Fr., boring]. Creating a channel through an enlarged prostate by use of an electric cautery. This technique may be used in other tissues.

foramen (for-ā′mĕn) [L.]. (pl. *foramina*) [NA] A passage or opening; an orifice, a communication between two cavities of an organ, or a hole in a bone for passage of vessels or nerves.

f., apical. The opening in the end of the root of the tooth through which the blood, lymphatic, and nerve supply to the dental pulp passes.

f., condyloid, anterior. The opening above the condyle of the occipital bone. The twelfth cranial nerve passes through it.

f., condyloid, posterior. The opening behind the condyle of the occipital bone. A small vein passes through it.

f., epiploic. The opening connecting the peritoneal cavity to its lesser sac.

f., ethmoidal. Openings in the medial wall of the orbit. The ethmoidal nerve and artery pass through these openings.

f., external auditory. The external auditory meatus through which sound waves travel in order to reach the tympanic membrane and the inner ear.

f., incisive. Small openings sometimes present in the incisive fossa of the hard palate.

f., internal auditory. The opening in the petrous portion of the sphenoid bone through which the seventh and eighth cranial nerves pass.

f., interventricular. The opening between the third and fourth ventricles of the brain.

f., intervertebral. Opening between adjacent articulated vertebrae for passage of nerves to and from spinal cord.

f., jugular. The opening in the base of the skull through which pass the sigmoid and inferior petrosal sinus, and the ninth, tenth, and eleventh cranial nerves.

f., Magendie's. SEE: *Magendie's foramen.*

f. magnum. Opening of the occipital bone through which passes the spinal cord from the brain.

f., mastoid. Opening in the mastoid part of the temporal bone. A small vein passes through it.

f., obturator. Large oval foramen below acetabulum bounded by the pubis and ischium. SEE: *Magendie's foramen.*

f. of Monro. Opening between the third and lateral ventricles of the brain.

f. of Vesalius. An opening sometimes present in the sphenoid bone, medial to the foramen ovale. A vein from the cavernous sinus passes through it.

f. of Winslow. F., epiploic, q.v.

f., olfactory. An opening in the ethmoid bone for passage of the olfactory nerves.

f., optic. The opening in the lesser wing of the sphenoid bone. The optic nerve and artery pass through it.

f. ovale. 1. An opening between the two atria of the heart in the fetus. The opening closes shortly before or after birth in most cases. If it remains open, it is possible to repair the defect surgically. 2. Oval opening in posterior margin of great sphenoidal wing, for inferior maxillary nerve and small meningeal artery.

f., palatine. F., incisive, q.v.

f. rotundum. Opening in the great wing of the sphenoid bone through which the maxillary branch of the trigeminal nerve passes.

f., sacral, anterior. One of the openings on the anterior aspect of the sacrum through which pass the anterior primary branches of the sacral nerve.

f., sacral, posterior. One of the openings on the posterior aspect of the sacrum through which pass the posterior primary branches of the sacral nerve.

f., Scarpa's. An opening behind the upper medial incisor tooth through which passes the nasopalatine nerve. This opening is not always present.

f., sphenopalatine. Opening between the palatine and sphenoid bones. It provides a passage from the pterygopalatine fossa to the nasal cavity for the sphenopalatine artery and nasal nerves.

f., sciatic, greater. Opening bounded by the hip bone, sacrum, and the sacrotuberous ligament.

f., sciatic, lesser. Opening bounded by the hip bone, sacrum, and sacrospinous ligament.

f., spinous. Opening in the spine of the sphenoid bone through which passes the middle meningeal artery.

f., supraorbital. An opening that is sometimes present above the superior border of the orbit. The supraorbital nerve and vessels pass through it.

f., thebesian. One of the openings leading directly into the atria and ventricles of the heart. Very small thebesian veins empty into these openings.

f., transverse. Opening in the transverse process of a cervical vertebra.

f., vena caval. Opening in the diaphragm through which pass the vena cava and branches of the right vagus nerve.

f., vertebral. The large opening between the neural arch and the body of the vertebra.

f., Weitbrecht's. Opening in the articular capsule of the shoulder joint.

f., zygomatic-orbital. One or more small openings on the outer surface of the zygomatic bone. The zygomatic nerve passes through it.

Forbes' disease. Glycogen storage disease, type III, q.v.

force. Strength; any external energy or power that produces a change in motion of the body.

f., catabolic. Energy produced by metabolism of food.

f., electromotive. ABBR: EMF. The energy that causes flow of electricity in a conductor. The energy is measured in volts.

f., reserve. The energy available above that required for normal functioning of the heart.

f., unit of. Arbitrary definition of a certain amount of force. For example, a dyne is the amount of force acting continuously on a mass of one gram that will accelerate the mass one cm. per second per second.

forceps (for′sĕps) [L.]. Pincers for holding, seizing, or extracting. There are many distinct types of forceps, varying according to the operation for which they are intended.

f., alligator. Sturdy toothed forceps with a double clamp.

f., artery. Forceps for holding ends of an artery in order to perform ligation.

f., bone. Forceps used for cutting bone and for removal of bone fragments.

f., capsule. Forceps for removal of the lens of the eye in membranous cataract.

f., Chamberlen. The original obstetric forceps named after the inventor Peter Chamberlen (1560–1631) or his son Peter (1601–1683). They kept their development secret until Hugh Chamberlen (1664–1726) disclosed it.

f., clamp. Any forceps with an automatic lock.

f., dental. Forceps of varying shapes for grasping teeth during extraction procedures.

f., dressing. Forceps for general use in dressing wounds, removal of dead tissue and drainage tubes.

f., Halsted's. F., mosquito, q.v.

f., mosquito. A very small, delicately pointed hemostat. SYN: *f., Halsted's.*

f., needle. Forceps for grasping and holding a needle.

f., obstetric. Forceps used to extract the fetal head from the pelvis during delivery. They serve the dual purpose of allowing withdrawal force to be applied to the fetal head and protecting the head during the passage.

f., rongeur. Forceps used for cutting bone.

f., tissue. Forceps with tiny teeth for grasping delicate tissues.

f., towel. Forceps for clipping towels to the site of the operative wound.

forcipate (for′sĭ-pāt) [L. *forceps,* tongs]. Shaped like forceps.

forcipressure [″ + *pressura,* pressure]. Arresting hemorrhage by pressure on an artery with forceps.

Fordyce's disease (for′dī-sēs). [John Fordyce, U.S. dermatologist, 1858–1925] Enlarged ectopic sebaceous glands in the mucosa of the mouth and genitals. They appear as small yellow spots, called Fordyce's spots. They are asymptomatic and present in the majority of people.

Fordyce-Fox disease (for′dīs-fŏks′). [John Fordyce; G. H. Fox, New York dermatologist, 1846–1925] A disease similar to prickly heat in which itchy follicular papules are present in the axillae, areola of the breast, umbilicus, pubic area, or labia majora.

Fordyce's spots. SEE: *Fordyce's disease.*

fore- [AS.]. Prefix meaning before or in front of.

forearm [AS. *fore,* in front, + *arm,* arm]. The portion of the arm between the elbow and wrist.

forebrain [″ + *bregen,* brain]. Anterior portion of the brain of the embryo. SYN: *prosencephalon.*

forefinger. The first or index finger.

forefoot. The part of the foot in front of the tarsometatarsal joint.

foregut [″ + *gut,* a pouring]. First part of the embryonic digestive tube from which pharynx, esophagus, stomach, and duodenum are formed. SYN: *protogaster.*

forehead [AS. *forheafod*]. The anterior part of the head below the hairline and above the eyes. SYN: *frons.*

foreign bodies. Slivers, cinders, dirt, or small objects that lodge in the skin, ears, eyes, or nose, or internally. They frequently lead to infection. If not removed, they lead to unsightly marks or tattooing of the skin and inflammation of the tissue involved.

F.A.: *In skin:* Carefully clean the areas involved. Foreign material can be removed carefully piece by piece or by vigorous swabbing with gauze or brush and a soapy solution. Follow with an antiseptic dressing.

In attempting to remove a small foreign body, first cleanse the area with mild soap and warm water. Sterilize a clean needle by heating it to a dull or bright red color in a flame; this can be done with a single match. Inasmuch as both ends of the needle get hot, it is wise to hold the far end in a nonconductor of heat such as folds of paper or stick it in a cork or in the edge of a small book. Allow it to cool and disregard black deposit on the needle; it is sterile carbon and will not interfere with the procedure. Introduce the needle at right angles to the direction of sliver and lift it out. Most persons attempt to stick the needle in direction of the foreign body and consequently have to thrust many times before they manage to lift the sliver out. When it is removed, apply an antiseptic and cover wound with a sterile dressing. Tetanus antitoxin or a tetanus booster may be required depending on the depth of the wound and the history of immunization.

In the ear: Water should not be introduced if any vegetable matter is in the ear because it may cause the foreign body to be pushed further into the ear or cause it to swell and become firmly embedded. Place a globule of ordinary glue on the end of a match stick or an applicator; gently introduce it until it touches the foreign body and then remove gently.

If an insect is in the ear, the patient may experience loud buzzing, pain, and dizziness. Flood ear with warm oil or water, letting insect float out.

In wounds: Foreign bodies are often present in wounds. Generally these should be left undisturbed if a surgeon is available within a short time. If the foreign body is large, it might be embedded in large blood vessels, or muscles. Removing it might result in much loss of blood or might cause breaking off of splinters, particles of rust or dirt. Within a few moments, blood and the natural reaction of swelling would tend to fill in the wound and cover this foreign material, making it exceedingly difficult for the physician to care for the patient. Therefore it is much wiser to leave a large foreign body in position and obtain the services of a physician promptly.

forensic (for-ĕn′sĭk) [L. *forensis,* public]. Pert. to the law; legal.

forensic medicine. Medicine in relation to the law; as in autopsy proceedings, or the determination of time of death or cause of death, or in the determination of sanity. Also, the legal aspects of medical ethics and standards.

foreplay. Fondling of the sex partner in order to produce mutual sexual arousal and pleasure prior to intercourse.

forepleasure [AS. *fore,* in front, + L. *placere,* to please]. Sexual pleasure preceding orgasm.

foreskin [″ + O. Norse *skinn,* skin]. Prepuce, q.v., or loose skin at and covering the end of the penis or clitoris, like a hood. Excision of the prepuce constitutes circumcision. Smegma praeputii, q.v., is secreted by Tyson's glands and collects under foreskin. SEE: *circumcision.*

NURSING IMPLICATIONS: In infants, see that the prepuce is not adherent or interfering with urination. Retract foreskin daily so that there is no interference with urination and to prevent formation of adhesions. Teach parents to clean area properly with mild soap and water daily and whenever diaper is changed. Report abnormalities to the physician.

forewaters (for′wăt-ĕrz). The thin mucus secretion discharged from the vagina during pregnancy. It is produced by the uterine glands, and is considered to be normal.

fork. An elongated instrument that splits at the end to form two or more prongs.

f., tuning. Device that when struck at the forked end vibrates and thus can be heard and felt. It is used in testing the sensations of hearing, including bone conductions and vibration. A fork that vibrates at 256 cycles per second is suitable for use in these tests.

form. The distinctive size, shape, and external appearance of anything.

-form [L. *forma*]. Suffix meaning having the form of.

formaldehyde (for-măl′dĕ-hīd) HCOH. A colorless, pungent, irritant gas commonly made by oxidation of methyl alcohol; the simplest member of the group of aldehydes. It is used as a preservative as an aqueous solution of 37% formaldehyde. This chemical has been shown to be carcinogenic in certain animals.

ACTION AND USES: A disinfectant, preservative, or fumigant. A 10% solution is useful as an astringent. A 1% or 2% solution is used for cleansing dishes, instruments, or fabrics. Formaldehyde is a powerful disinfectant, esp. in the form of gas because of its penetrating power, but it is active only in the presence of an abundance of moisture. The solution is germicidal in the strength of 1 to 2%, but the action may be delayed 20 to 30 minutes. It hardens tissues and is often used in histology for tissue preservation. It has a similar hardening effect on the living skin; it is very irritating to mucous membranes and produces reddening, inflammation, and necrosis if applied repeatedly or continuously. It is sometimes used in soap for disinfection of the hands. A 10% solution is used for sterilizing feces, urine, and sputum; 5 to 10% for clothing and towels. SEE: *aldehyde; fumigation.*

formaldehyde poisoning. SYM: Local irritation of eyes, nose, mouth, throat, respiratory and gastrointestinal tracts, and central nervous system, causing vertigo, stupor, abdominal pain, convulsions, unconsciousness, renal damage. SEE: *Poisons and Poisoning* in *Appendix.*

F.A.: Administration of 0.2% ammonia water changes formaldehyde into methenamine. This should be given with large amounts of milk, water and egg white. Then use gastric lavage or induce vomiting. After that leave milk in stomach. Morphine may be needed for pain. Treat acidosis with sodium bicarbonate. Shock and respiratory distress should be treated as needed.

formalin (for′mă-lĭn). Aqueous solution of 37% formaldehyde. SEE: *aldehyde.*

formate (for′māt). A salt of formic acid.

formatio (for-mā′shē-ō) [L.] (pl. *formationes*) [NA] A structure with definite arrangement and shape.

f. reticularis. Dorsal part of the medulla oblongata.

formation. 1. A structure, shape, or figure. 2. The giving of form or shape to, or the development of, a structure.

f., reticular. A reticular structure formed of gray matter and interlacing fibers of white matter found in the medulla oblongata between the pyramids and the floor of the 4th ventricle. It is also present in the spinal cord, midbrain, and pons. Fibers from this structure are believed to be able to activate the cortex of the brain independently of specific sensory or other neural systems. Thus reticular formation is part of the reticular activating or alerting system.

forme fruste (form froost) [Fr., defaced]. (pl. *formes frustes*) An aborted form of disease arrested before running its course. Thus the disease appears in an atypical and indefinite form.

formic [L. *formica,* ant]. Pert. to ants, or to formic acid.

formic acid. HCOOH. A clear, pungent liquid obtained from the oxidation of formaldehyde or wood alcohol. Originally it was obtained from the distillation of the bodies of red ants. It is the cause of the pain and swelling resulting from the bites or stings of certain insects.

formic aldehyde. Formaldehyde.

formication. A sensation as of insects creeping upon the body; a form of paresthesia. One of the more common side effects of cocaine withdrawal.

formic ether. Volatile anesthetic liquid ethyl formate.

formiciasis (for″mĭs-ī′ă-sĭs) [L. *formica,* ant, + Gr. *-iasis,* condition]. Irritation caused by ant bites.

formilase (for′mĭ-lās). An enzyme that catalyzes conversion of acetic acid to formic acid.

formiminoglutamic acid. ABBR: FIGLU. A chemical intermediate in the metabolism of histidine to glutamic acid. Folacin, FH_4, is an essential coenzyme for this reaction. If there is a deficiency of folic acid, then excess amounts of formiminoglutamic acid will appear in the urine.

formol (for′mŏl). Formaldehyde solution. SEE: *formalin.*

formula [L., a little form]. (pl. *formulas, -lae*) 1. A rule prescribing ingredients and proportions for the preparation of a compound. 2. In chemistry, an expression by symbols of the constitution of a molecule consisting of letters, each denoting one atom of one elementary substance, with figures written as subscripts denoting the number of atoms present.

Ex.: water consists of two molecules of the element hydrogen and one of oxygen. The formula is H_2O. It may also be written HOH or H—O—H.

Collections of atoms that constitute a group by themselves (radical) are often separated by periods or parentheses, and in this case figures prefixed or appended to the parentheses or placed before an expression contained within periods apply to all the symbols embraced by the parentheses or periods. In all other cases, a figure prefixed to a symbolical expression for a molecule, like a coefficient in an algebraic formula, is understood to be a multiplier of all the symbols following.

f., Arneth's. Method of estimating number of immature leukocytes by means of an elaborate differential blood count, based upon their shape and number of lobes in the nucleus. It is seldom used.

f., chemical. SEE: *formula* (def. 2).

f., dental. Formula showing the number and arrangement of the teeth. For human permanent teeth:

$$\frac{2—1—2—3 \quad \text{(right upper jaw)}}{2—1—2—3 \quad \text{(right lower jaw)}}$$

In this formula the numerators indicate the number in the maxilla and the denominators those in the mandible; the incisor, canine, premolar, and molar are listed in order, respectively. Thus if one upper incisor were missing that portion of the formula would be written

$$\frac{1}{2}$$

If a lower molar were missing, the notation would be

$$\frac{3}{2}$$

f., empirical. The formula of a compound that shows the atoms and their numbers in a molecule, as H_2O.

f., molecular. The chemical formula indicating the elements and number of each present but providing no information concerning the two- or three-dimensional arrangement of the chemical elements in the formula. For example, the organic carboxylic acid radical —COOH may also be written

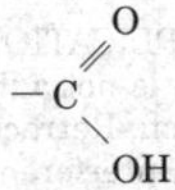

The latter provides some information about the arrangement of the elements in the radical. SEE: *f., spatial.*

f., official. Formula in a pharmacopeia.

f., spatial or stereochemical. A method of depicting chemical formulae so that the elements and their number are known as well as the position of the elements in space in relation to each other.

f., structural. The formula of a compound that shows the relationship of the atoms to each other in a molecule. The atoms are shown joined by valence bonds, e.g., H—O—H.

formulary [L. *formula*, a little form]. A book of formulas.

F., National. ABBR: NF. A book previously issued by the American Pharmaceutical Association. Now published by the U.S. Pharmacopeial Convention, Inc. It provides standards and specifications for drugs.

formyl. The radical of formic acid, HCO.

fornicate 1. [L. *fornicatus*] Arched or vaultlike. 2. [L. *fornicari*] To have sexual intercourse with a partner to whom one is not married.

fornication. Sexual intercourse between unmarried partners.

fornices (for'nĭ-sēz) [L.]. Pl. of fornix.

fornicolumn [L. *fornix*, arch, + *columna*, column]. The anterior pillar of the fornix.

fornicommissure (for-nĭ-kŏm'ĭ-sūr) [" + *commissura*, a joining together]. The commissure or body of the fornix uteri.

fornix [L., arch]. (pl. *fornices*) [NA] 1. A fibrous vaulted band connecting the cerebral lobes. 2. Any body with vaultlike or arched shape.

f. conjunctivae. [NA] Loose fold connecting palpebral and bulbar conjunctivae.

f. uteri. Anterior and posterior spaces into which the upper vagina is divided. These recesses are formed by protrusion of the cervix uteri into the vagina.

f. vaginae. [NA] F. uteri.

Fort Bragg fever. [Fort Bragg, North Carolina, U.S.A., a U.S. military base] Pretibial fever, q.v.

fortification spectrum. Appearance of dark patch with zigzag outline in visual field causing a temporary blindness in that portion of the eye. SYN: *teichopsia.*

Foshay's test. [Lee Foshay, U.S. physician, 1896–1961] The intradermal injection of a suspension of killed Francisella tularensis, the causative agent of tularemia. The appearance of an area of erythema at the injection site is considered a positive reaction.

fossa (fŏs'ă) [L.]. (pl. *fossae*) [NA] A furrow or shallow depression.

f., amygdaloid. Depression containing the tonsil.

f., articular, of mandible. The depression on the inferior surface of the temporal bone that accepts the condyle of the mandible. SYN: *f., glenoid; f., mandibular; f., articular, of temporal bone.*

f., articular, of temporal bone. F., articular, of mandible, q.v.

f., axillary. The armpit; axilla.

f., canine. The wide, shallow depression on the external surface of the maxilla superolateral to the canine tooth. It serves as the origin of the levator anguli oris muscle.

f., cerebral. Any one of several depressions on the inside floor of the cranium.

f., Claudius'. Triangular area harboring the ovary.

f., condylar. The depression behind the occipital epicondyle.

f., coronoid. The depression on the anterior surface of the lower end of the humerus. During full flexion of the forearm, the coronoid process of the ulna fits into the depression.

f., cranial. F., cerebral, q.v.

f., digastric. Depression behind the lower margin of the mandible at the side of the symphysis menti. The anterior belly of the digastric muscle attaches here.

f., epigastric. The pit of the inside of the stomach.

f., ethmoid. The groove in the cribriform plate of the ethmoid bone. The olfactory bulb of the brain occupies the depression. SYN: *olfactory groove.*

f., glenoid. The depression on the scapula that provides space for articulation with the head of the humerus.

f., hyaloid. The depression on the anterior surface of the vitreous body of the eye. The lens is located there.

f., hypophyseal. The deep depression in the sphenoid bone in which the pituitary gland rests. SYN: *sella turcica.*

f., iliac. One of the concavities of the iliac bones of the pelvis.

f., incisive. The depression on the anterior surface of the body of the maxilla medial to the root of the canine incisor tooth.

f., infratemporal. The irregular space below and medial to the zygomatic arch, posterior to the maxilla and medial to the upper part of the ramus of the mandible.

f., interpeduncular. The deep groove in the anterior surface of the midbrain, between the cerebral peduncles. The third cranial nerve emerges here.

f., ischiorectal. The space on either side of the lower end of the rectum and anal canal. It is bounded laterally by the obturator internus muscle and the tuberosity of the ischium medially by the levator ani and coccygeus muscles, and posteriorly by the gluteus maximus muscle.

f., lacrimal. Hollow of frontal bone holding the lacrimal gland.

f., mandibular. The depression in the temporal bone. The condyle of the mandible fits into this fossa.

f., mastoid. Small triangular area between the posterior wall of the acoustic meatus and the posterior root of the zygomatic process of the temporal bone.

f., nasal. The cavity between the anterior

opening to the nose and the nasopharynx.

f., navicular. Fossa between the vulva and fourchette.

f. ovalis. Opening in thigh through which the large saphenous vein passes.

f. ovalis cordis. [NA] Remnant of embryonic foramen ovale in right cardiac atrium.

f., ovarian. A depression in the parietal peritoneum of the pelvis in which rests the ovary.

f., pituitary. F., hypophyseal, q.v.

f., Rosenmüller's. Depression in the pharynx posterior to opening of eustachian tube.

f., subpyramidal. The depression in the inferior wall of the middle ear. It is inferior to the round window and posterior to the pyramid.

f., supraspinous. The concave triangular area above the spinous process of the posterior surface of the clavicle.

f. supratonsillaris. [NA] Space between anterior and posterior pillars of the fauces above the tonsil.

f., temporal. The depression on the side of the skull below the temporal lines. It is deep to the zygomatic arch and is continuous with the infratemporal fossa.

fossae (fŏs'ē) [L.]. Pl. of fossa.

fossette (fŏ-sĕt') [Fr.]. 1. A small depression or fossa. 2. A small, but deep, corneal ulcer.

fossula (fŏs'ū-lă). Small fossa.

Fothergill's disease (fŏth'ĕr-gĭlz). [John Fothergill, Brit. physician, 1712–1780] 1. Scarlatina angiosa, an ulcerative sore throat present in severe scarlet fever. 2. Trigeminal neuralgia.

foulage (foo-lŏzh') [Fr.]. Massage by kneading with pressure on the muscles.

fourchet, fourchette (foor-shĕt') [Fr. *fourchette,* a fork]. A tense band or transverse fold of mucous membrane at the posterior commissure of the vagina, connecting the posterior ends of the labia minora. The fossa navicularis, a more or less deep cul-de-sac anterior to the fourchette, separates it from the hymen. It disappears after defloration or parturition, leaving a more open vulva below and behind. SYN: *frenulum labiorum pudendi* [NA].

fourth cranial nerve. A small mixed nerve making its exit from the dorsal surface of the midbrain. It contains efferent motor fibers to the superior oblique muscle of the eye and afferent sensory fibers conveying proprioceptive impulses from the same muscle. SYN: *trochlear nerve.*

fovea (fō'vē-ă) [L.]. (pl. *foveae*) [NA] A pit or cuplike depression. SEE: *fossa.*

f. centralis retinae. [NA] Pit in the middle of macula lutea.

foveate (fō'vē-āt) [L. *foveatus*]. Pitted; having depressions.

foveation (fō″vē-ā'shŭn). Pitting, as in smallpox.

foveola (fō-vē'ō-lă) [L., little pit]. (pl. *foveolae*) A minute pit or depression.

Fowler's position. [George R. Fowler, U.S. surgeon, 1848–1906] A semi-sitting position. The head of an adjustable bed can be elevated to the desired height to produce angulation of the body, usually 45° to 60°. A wedge support can be used to elevate the head and back of the patient, if an adjustable bed is not available. The position is used to facilitate breathing and drainage, and for the comfort of the patient, particularly for eating or talking while restricted to bed.

Fowler's solution. [Thomas Fowler, Brit. physician, 1736–1801] An arsenical solution containing 0.95 to 1.5 gm. of arsenic trioxide for each 100 ml. of solution. SYN: *potassium arsenite solution.*

Fox-Fordyce disease (fŏks-for'dīs). SEE: *Fordyce-Fox disease.*

foxglove (fŏks'glŏv). Common name for the plant Digitalis purpurea, from which the drug digitalis is obtained. Foxglove was mentioned in the writings of Welsh physicians in 1250 and later by William Withering in a book published in 1785.

Fr. Chem. symb. for francium.

fraction [L. *fractio,* act of breaking]. In biological chemistry, the separable part of a substance such as blood or plasma.

f. of inspired oxygen. ABBR: FiO_2. The concentration of oxygen in the inspired air, esp. that supplied as supplemental oxygen by mask or catheter. Concentrations of oxygen greater than 50% are toxic if administered for other than brief periods.

fractional. Pert. to a fraction or a portion of a whole.

fractional test meal. Fractional examination of stomach contents. The method for collection and examination of stomach contents follows: First the residual contents are removed and then the test meal given; after the meal, samples are removed every 15 min. for 2 hours, examined, and submitted for chemical tests. Free hydrochloric acid, bile, blood, starch, mucus, and the total of acids are analyzed. Free hydrochloric and total acids are normally present in small amounts. In peptic ulcers there is a high acid curve. There is a low curve in carcinoma, and an absence of acid in pernicious anemia.

fracture [L. *fractura,* break]. 1. A sudden breaking of a bone. 2. A broken bone. SEE: illus.

CAUSES: In certain diseases and conditions bones break spontaneously without trauma, as in osteomalacia, syphilis, and osteomyelitis.

TYPES OF FRACTURES AND TERMINOLOGY

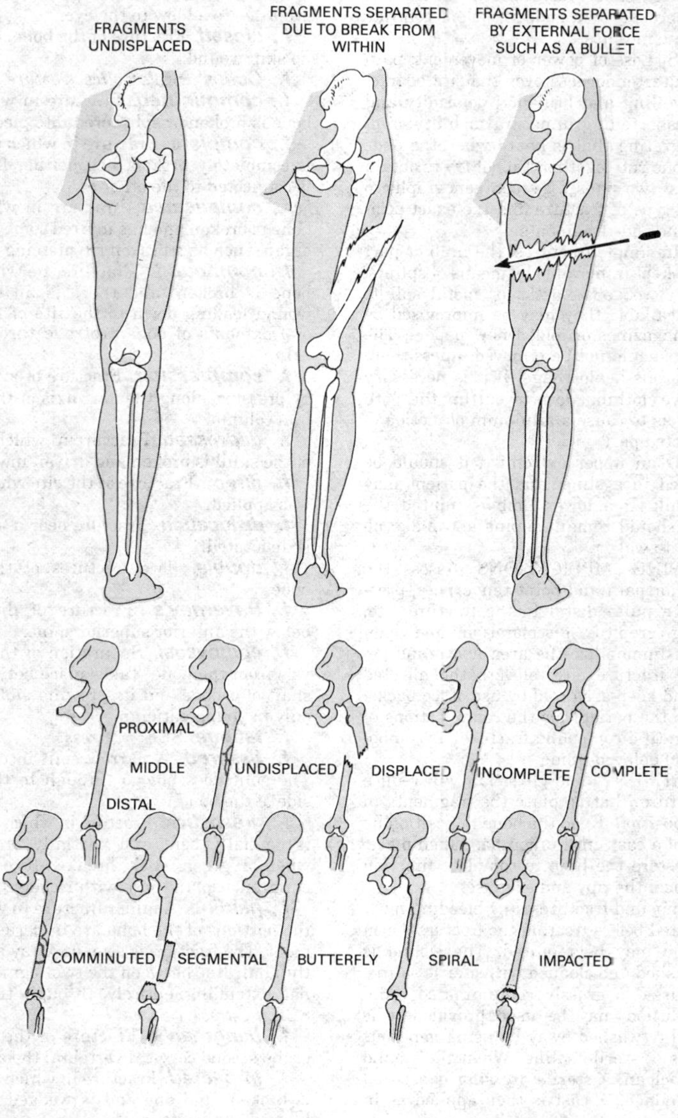

Direct violence: The bone is broken directly at the spot where the force was applied, as in fracture of the tibia by being run over. *Indirect violence:* The bone is fractured by a force applied at a distance from the site of fracture and transmitted to the fractured bone, as fracture of the clavicle by falling on the outstretched hand. *Muscular contraction:* The bone is broken by a sudden violent contraction of the muscles.

SIGNS: Loss of power of movement; pain with acute tenderness over the site of fracture; swelling and bruising; deformity and possible shortening; unnatural mobility; crepitus or grating that is heard when the ends of the bone rub together. Do not try to obtain these last two signs. Use roentgenography to find the type of fracture and the exact position of the bone fragments.

F.A.: In simple fractures, the limb or part must be kept immovable by means of splints. If proper wooden, plastic, or metal splints are unavailable they may be improvised by using magazines or folded newspapers. The clothing should not be removed unless there is dangerous hemorrhage. If it is necessary to remove clothing, do so by cutting the cloth away so as to cause a minimum of motion of the affected part.

If it is an upper extremity, it should be supported in a sling, and the patient may then walk. If a lower limb is injured the patient should remain supine and make no attempt to walk.

NURSING IMPLICATIONS: Assess the patient for pain and point tenderness, presence of a pulse distal to the fracture site, swelling, crepitus, discoloration, and open wounds. Immobilize the area above and below the fracture site, elevate the affected area, and keep area cold by use of ice packs. Observe the patient for the complications of infection (if a compound fracture), fat embolism, and delayed union.

TREATMENT: The physician will reduce the fracture, that is, place the fragments in proper position. Keep the bone in position by means of a cast until union has taken place. Then restore the limb to complete function by physical therapy and exercise.

In compound fractures, any bleeding must be arrested before treating the fracture. Open reduction may be required. The wound is then washed and cleaned with sterile saline. If the area is grossly contaminated, mild soap solution may be used provided it is thoroughly washed away by using generous amounts of sterile saline. When the wound is quite clean, a sterile dressing is secured by a bandage. A cast is then applied as in simple fractures.

A weak electric current applied to fractured bones has been found to promote healing.

RS: buttonhole fracture; cerclage; extension; greenstick fracture; malunion; splint.

f., avulsion. Tearing of a piece of bone away from the main bone by the force of muscular contraction.

f., blow-out. Fracture of the wall of the orbit due to a blow to the eye.

f., closed. Fracture of the bone, but with no skin wound.

f., Colles'. SEE: *Colles' fracture.*

f., comminuted. Fracture in which the bone is broken or splintered into pieces.

f., complete. Fracture in which the bone is completely broken, i.e., neither fragment is connected to the other.

f., complicated. Fracture in which the bone is broken and has injured some internal organ, such as a broken rib piercing a lung.

f., compound. Fracture in which the bone is broken, and there is an external wound leading down to the site of fracture; or fragments of bone protrude through the skin.

f., compression. Fracture of a vertebra by pressure along the long axis of the vertebral column.

f., depressed. Fracture in which a piece of the skull is broken and driven inwards.

f., direct. Fracture at the site where force was applied.

f., dislocation. Fracture near a joint that is dislocated.

f., double. Two fractures of the same bone.

f., Duverney's. Fracture of ilium just below the anterior superior spine.

f., epiphyseal. Separation of the epiphysis from the bone. Takes place between the shaft of a bone and its growing end. Occurs only in young patients.

f., fatigue. SEE: *f., stress.*

f., fissured. A narrow split in the bone. The split does not go through to the other side of the bone.

f., greenstick. Fracture in which the bone is partially bent and partially broken, as when a green stick breaks. It occurs in children, esp. in those with rickets.

f., hairline. A minor fracture in which all the portions of the bone are in perfect alignment. The fracture is seen on x-ray as a very thin hair line between the two segments, but not extending entirely through the bone. SEE: *f., stress.*

f., hangman's. Fracture of the pedicles of the second cervical vertebra, the axis.

f., impacted. Fracture in which the bone is broken, and one end is wedged into the interior of the other.

f., incomplete. Fracture in which the

line of fracture does not include the whole bone. SEE: *f., stress.*

f., indirect. Fracture distant to the place where the force was applied.

f., intrauterine. Fracture of a bone in the fetus while it is in utero.

f., lead pipe. Fracture in which the bone is compressed and bent so that one side of the fracture bulges and on the other side there is a slight crack.

f., open. Fracture in which there is an open wound present at the fracture site. SYN: *f., compound.*

f., pathologic. Fracture of a diseased or weakened bone produced by a force that would not have fractured a healthy bone. The underlying disease may be metastases from the primary cancer, cancer of the bone, or osteoporosis.

f., pretrochanteric. Fracture that passes through the greater trochanter of the femur.

f., ping-pong. A depressed fracture of the skull that resembles the indentation that can be made by pressing firmly on a ping-pong ball.

f., Pott's. Fracture of the lower end of the fibula with outward displacement of the ankle and foot. The medial malleolus of the fibula may or may not be fractured.

f., Smith's. Colles' fracture, q.v.

f., spiral. An oblique fracture.

f., spontaneous. F., pathological, q.v.

f., stellate. Fracture in which cracks emerge from the central point.

f., stress. A fine hairline fracture that appears without evidence of soft tissue injury. These are difficult to diagnose by x-ray and may not become visible until 3–4 weeks after the onset of symptoms. This type of fracture may occur in runners who are running too much, too fast, with improper shoes, and on hard surfaces.

f., transcervical. Fracture through the neck of the femur.

f., transverse. Fracture in which the fracture line is at right angles to the long axis of the bone.

fracture dislocation. Fracture near a joint that is dislocated.

fragilitas (frā-jĭl′ĭ-tăs) [L.]. Fragility.

f. crinium. Brittleness, as of the hair, showing splitting and breaking of the shaft. Cause unknown.

f. ossium. Brittleness of bones.

f. unguium. Abnormal brittleness of nails.

fragility. State of brittleness.

f., capillary. Breaking down of capillaries with hemorrhage into almost any site but most noticeably in the skin.

f., erythrocyte. Increased tendency of the red blood cells to rupture when the salt content of the blood is decreased.

f. of blood. Tendency of red blood cells to rupture. This is determined by subjecting the cells in laboratory tests to different concentrations of saline.

If red blood cells are placed in distilled water, they swell rapidly and burst because they normally are suspended in a solution of much greater osmotic pressure. This phenomenon is called hemolysis. If they are suspended in a solution of normal saline, the cells retain their normal shape and do not burst. If they are placed in successively weaker solutions of saline, a point is reached at which some of the cells burst and liberate their hemoglobin within a given length of time, while others do not (partial hemolysis). Finally, at a given dilution, all of the cells have burst within the allotted time, which is usually two hours. The cells of normal blood begin to hemolyze in about 0.44%, and complete hemolysis occurs in about 0.35% saline solution.

fragment (frăg′mĕnt). A part broken off a larger entity.

fragmentation [L. *fragmentum,* detached part]. Breaking up into fragments.

frambesia (frăm-bē′zē-ă) [Fr. *framboise,* raspberry]. An infectious tropical disease caused by a spirochete, Treponema pertenue. SYN: *yaws.*

frambesioma (frăm-bē-zē-ō′mă) [″ + Gr. *oma,* swelling]. Primary lesion of yaws in the form of a protruding nodule. This mother yaw appears at the site of inoculation of the causative agent, Treponema pertenue.

frame. A supporting structure.

f., Balkan. A framework that fits over the bed. Suspended from the frame and connected through ropes and pulleys are weights used to produce desired continuous traction while permitting freedom of motion, thus maintaining desired immobilization of the part being treated.

f., Bradford. [Edward H. Bradford, U.S. orthopedic surgeon, 1848–1926] An oblong frame, about 7 × 3 feet (2.13 × 0.91 meters), made of 1 in. (2.5 cm.) pipe covered with canvas strips that run from one side of the frame to the other and that are movable. Used for patients with fractures or disease of the hip or spine, thus permitting the patient to urinate and defecate without moving the spine or changing position.

f., quadriplegic standing. Device for supporting a patient with all four extremities paralyzed.

f., Stryker. A device that supports two rectangular pieces of lightweight but strong material so that one side is on the anterior surface of the patient and the other is on the posterior surface. Thus the patient is held firmly between the pieces of material as if part of a sandwich. The device may be rotated around the patient's long axis. This permits turning the patient without his or her assistance. After a turn is completed, the uppermost portion of the frame can be moved away from the patient. SEE: *Stryker frame* for illus.

f., trial. An eyeglass frame for holding trial lenses while the person is being fitted for glasses.

framework. The basic system or design of anything.

Franceschetti's syndrome (frăn″chĕs-kĕt′ēz). [Adolph Franceschetti, Swiss ophthalmologist, b. 1896] Mandibulofacial dysostosis with hypoplasia of the facial bones, downward angulation of the palpebral fissures, macrostomia, ear defects, and defectively formed extremities. SYN: *Treacher-Collins syndrome.*

Franciscella tularensis (frăn″sĭ-sĕl′ă too″lă-rĕn′sĭs). [Edward Francis, Tulare County, California] A short, nonmotile, encapsulate, non-spore-forming, gram-negative organism that causes tularemia, q.v., in man. Formerly classed as Pasteurella tularensis or Bacterium tularense.

francium (frăn′sē-ŭm). [Named for France, the country in which it was discovered] SYMB: Fr. At. no. 87. The at. wt. of the most stable isotope is 233. A radioactive metallic element occurring as a natural isotope.

frank. Obvious, esp. in reference to a clinical sign or condition such as blood in the urine, sputum, or feces.

Frankenhäuser's ganglion (frăng′kĕn-hoy″zĕrs). [Ferdinand Frankenhäuser, 19th-century Ger. gynecologist] A nerve ganglion sometimes found in lateral walls of the cervix uteri.

Frankfort horizontal plane. A cephalometric plane joining the anthropometric landmarks of porion and orbitale; the reproducible position of the head when the upper margin of the ear openings and lower margin of the orbit of eye are horizontal.

Franklin glasses. [Benjamin Franklin, U.S. statesman and inventor, 1706–1790] Bifocal spectacles.

fraternal twins. Two offspring that have developed in the uterus at the same time, but are the result of independent fertilization of two ova. SYN: *dizygotic twins.* SEE: *monozygotic twins.*

fratricide (frăt′rĭ-sīd″) [L. *fratricidium*]. Murder of one's brother or sister.

Fraunhofer's lines (frown′hōf-ĕrz). [Joseph von Fraunhofer, Ger. optician, 1787–1826] Absorption bands or lines seen in a spectrum, caused by the absorption of groups of light rays in their passage through solids, liquids, or gases.

F.R.C.P. *Fellow of the Royal College of Physicians.*

F.R.C.P.(C.). *Fellow of the Royal College of Physicians of Canada.*

F.R.C.S. *Fellow of the Royal College of Surgeons.*

F.R.C.S.(C.). *Fellow of the Royal College of Surgeons of Canada.*

freckle (frĕk′l) [O. Norse *freknur*]. Small local brownish or yellowish pigmentation of the skin due to an accumulation of melanin. SYN: *ephelis; lentigo.*

ETIOL: Exposure to sun in majority of individuals stimulates melanin production.

f., Hutchinson's. A noninvasive malignant melanoma.

free association. 1. Trend of thoughts when not under mental restraint or direction. 2. The procedure in psychoanalysis that requires the patient to speak aloud his thought flow, word for word, without censorship.

free medical clinics. Clinics that are established by the community rather than a hospital and provide free medical care. They are unusual in that their purpose is to deal with illnesses and conditions that are both medical and social.

freeze-drying. Preservation of tissue by rapidly freezing the specimen and then dehydrating it in a high vacuum. SYN: *lyophilization.*

freezing [AS. *freosan*]. 1. Passing from liquid to solid state because of loss of heat. 2. To become stiff, rigid, and inflexible from cold. Frigidity of a limb can result from exposure to cold. Most common in the debilitated, the exhausted, and those alcoholics who fall asleep in a location exposed to extreme cold.

SYM: Paleness, cyanosis, coldness. Unconsciousness usually develops.

F.A.: Protect part with a cradle and apply dry heat at room temperature. Alternatively, the patient may be placed in tepid bath water. Sudden applications of heat are undesirable. SEE: *frostbite; windchill factor.*

freezing mixtures. For ice bags, 5 oz. (150 ml.) each of ammonium chloride and potassium nitrate, and one part water.

freezing point. Temperature at which liquids freeze.

Freiberg's infraction (frī′bĕrgz). [A. H. Freiberg, U.S. surgeon, 1868–1940] Osteochondritis of the head of the second metatarsal bone of the foot.

fremitus (frĕm′ĭ-tŭs) [L.]. Vibratory tremors, esp. those felt through the chest wall by palpation. Varieties are vocal or tactile, friction, hydatid, rhonchal or bronchial, cavernous or succussion, pleural, pericardial, tussive, thrills. SEE: *palpation; thrill.*

f., tactile. The vibration or thrill felt while the patient is speaking and the hand is held against the chest.

f., tussive. Vibrations felt when the hand is held against the chest when the patient coughs.

f., vocal. Vibrations of the voice transmitted to the ear on auscultation of the chest of a person speaking. In determining the vocal fremitus, observe the following precautions: Palpate symmetrical parts of the chest, making firm pressure. When comparing, use the same pressure on both sides. Apply hands as nearly parallel to ribs as possible; remember the fremitus normally increases over the right apex. It is decreased in pleural effusions (air, pus, blood, serum, or lymph); emphysema; pulmonary collapse from an obstructed bronchus; pulmonary edema; and morbid growths of the lung.

frenal (frē'năl) [L. *fraenum,* bridle]. Pert. to the frenum.

French scale. A system used to indicate the outer diameter of catheters and sounds. Each unit on the scale is approx. equivalent to ⅓ mm.; thus a 21 French sound is 7 mm. in diameter.

frenectomy (frē-nĕk'tō-mē) [" + Gr. *ektome,* excision]. Surgically cutting of any frenum, usually the frenum of the tongue.

frenosecretory (frē"nō-sē'krĕ-tor-ē) [L. *fraenum,* bridle, + *secernere,* to secrete]. Exercising an inhibitory power over secretions.

frenotomy (frē-nŏt'ō-mē) [" + Gr. *tome,* incision]. Division of any frenum, esp. for tongue-tie.

frenuloplasty (frĕn'ū-lō-plăs"tē) [" + Gr. *plassein,* to form]. Surgical correction of an abnormally attached frenulum.

frenulum (frĕn'ū-lŭm) [L., a little bridle]. (pl. *frenula*) 1. [NA] A small frenum. SYN: *vinculum.* 2. A small fold of white matter on the upper surface of the anterior medullary velum extending to corpora quadrigemina.

f. clitoridis. [NA] The union of inner parts of the labia minora on undersurface of the clitoris, q.v.

f. labiorum pudendi. [NA] Fold of membrane connecting the posterior ends of the labia minora.

f. linguae. [NA] A fold of mucous membrane that extends from the floor of the mouth to the inferior surface of the tongue along its midline.

f. of ileocecal valve. Prolongation of the two lips of the ileocolic valve around the inner wall of the colon.

f. of the lips, labialis oris. A fold of mucous membrane extending from the middle of the inner surface of the lip to the alveolar mucosa; seen in both upper and lower jaws.

f. of tongue. Frenulum that attaches the lower side of the tongue to the floor of the buccal cavity.

f. preputii. [NA] Frenulum that unites the foreskin (prepuce) to the glans penis.

frenum (frē'nŭm) [L. *fraenum,* bridle]. (pl. *frena*) A fold of mucous membrane that connects two parts, one more or less movable, and serves to check the movement of this part. SEE: *frenulum.*

frenzy (frĕn'zē) [ME. *frenesie*]. A state of violent mental agitation; maniacal excitement. SEE: *panic.*

frequency [L. *frequens,* often]. 1. The number of repetitions of a phenomenon in a certain period of time or within a distinct population as the frequency of heart beat, frequency of sound vibrations or frequency of a disease entity. SEE: *incidence.* 2. The rate of oscillation or alternation in an alternating current circuit, in contradistinction to periodicity in the interruptions or regular variations of current in a direct current circuit. Frequency is computed on the basis of a complete cycle, a complete cycle being one in which the current rises from zero to a positive maximum, returns to zero, and descends to an opposite negative minimum and returns to zero.

fretum (frē'tŭm) [L.]. A constriction.

Freud, Sigmund (froyd). [Sigmund Freud, Austrian neurologist, 1856–1939] A famous neurologist and psychoanalyst whose teachings stress the following theories:

1. Of the existence of a subconscious mind.

2. That emotional processes have the attribute of quantity and can be displaced from one idea to another.

3. That the child experiences a rich sexual life and from this are derived the later stages of narcissism, homosexuality, or heterosexuality.

4. That dreams are fulfillments of wishes that find no realization in waking hours; theories are also formulated with regard to the importance of sex in dreams.

5. That forgetting, misplacing articles, and slips of the tongue or pen are the outward manifestation of repression.

RS: abreaction; complex; consciousness; heterosexuality; homosexuality; narcissism; Oedipus complex; psychoanalysis; subconsciousness.

freudian (froy'dē-ăn). Pert. to Sigmund Freud's theories of unconscious or repressed libido or past sex experiences or desires as the cause of various neuroses, the cure for which is the restoration of such conditions to consciousness through psychoanalysis. SEE: *Freud, Sigmund.*

Freund's adjuvant (froynds). [J. Freund, Hungarian-born scientist, 1890–1960] Mixture of killed microorganisms, usually Mycobacteria, in an oil and water emulsion. The material is administered to induce antibody formation. Because the oil retards absorption of the mixture, the antibody response is much greater than if the killed microorganisms were administered alone.

friable (frī'ă-b'l) [L. *friabilis*]. Easily broken or pulverized.

friction [L. *frictio*]. Rubbing. In massage, strong circular manipulations always followed by centripetal stroking. In hydrotherapy, friction is used in drying patients after tonic baths, and in shampoos and drip sheet rubs.

f., dry. Friction using no liquid.

f., moist. Friction using a liquid or oil.

frictional electricity. Electricity produced by friction. SEE: *electricity, static.*

friction rub. The distinct sound heard when two dry surfaces are rubbed together. If the sound is loud enough, the condition producing the sound can also be felt.

f.r., pericardial. Friction rub that may be present in pericarditis, particularly when the disease process first starts.

Friedländer's bacillus (frēd'lĕn-dĕrz). [Carl F. Friedländer, Ger. physician, 1847–1887] Klebsiella pneumoniae, a species of bacteria that causes pneumonia and is a secondary invader in bronchitis or sinusitis.

Friedländer's disease. Endarteritis obliterans, inflammation of the artery sufficient to cause complete closure of the lumen.

Friedman's test (frēd'mănz). [Maurice H. Friedman, U.S. physiologist, b. 1903] Pregnancy test. The injection of the urine of a woman suspected of pregnancy into an unmated female rabbit will cause the formation of corpora lutea and corpora hemorrhagica in the rabbit at the end of two days if the woman is pregnant. Tests that are less difficult to perform are now available.

Friedreich's ataxia (frēd'rĭks). [Nikolaus Friedreich, Ger. neurologist, 1825–1882] An inherited degenerative disease with sclerosis of the dorsal and lateral columns of the spinal cord. Accompanied by ataxia, speech impairment, lateral curvature of the spinal column, and peculiar swaying and irregular movements, with paralysis of the muscles, esp. of the lower extremities. Onset occurs in childhood or early adolescence. SYN: *ataxia, hereditary spinal.*

Friedreich's sign. 1. Sudden collapse of the cervical veins that were previously distended at each diastole. Caused by an adherent pericardium. 2. Lowering of the pitch of the percussion note that occurs over an area of cavitation during inspiration.

Fried's rule. To determine the child's dose of a medicine, multiply the child's age in months times the adult dose and divide by 150.

fright [AS. *fryhto*]. Extreme sudden fear.

f., precordial. Nausea and fear felt before the onset of manic-depressive illness.

fright neuroses. Traumatic hysteria.

frigid (frĭj'ĭd) [L. *frigidus*]. 1. Cold. 2. Irresponsive to emotion, applied esp. to the inability on the part of a woman to feel sexual desire. SEE: *impotence.*

frigidity (frĭ-jĭd'ĭ-tē). Inhibited sexual excitement during sexual activity. In males, this manifests as partial or complete failure to attain or maintain erection until completion of the sex act.

In females, there is partial or complete failure to attain or maintain the vaginal lubrication-swelling response of sexual excitement until completion of the sex act.

frigolabile (frĭg"ō-lā'bĭl) [L. *frigor,* cold, + *labilis,* unstable]. Capable of being destroyed by low temperature.

frigorific (frĭg"ō-rĭf'ĭk) [L. *frigorificus*]. Generating cold.

frigorism [L. *frigor,* cold, + Gr. *-ismos,* condition]. A condition caused by long exposure to cold.

frigostabile (frĭg"ō-stā'bl) [" + *stabilis,* firm]. Incapable of being destroyed by low temperature.

frigotherapy (frĭg"ō-thĕr'ă-pē) [" + Gr. *therapeia,* treatment]. The use of cold in treatment of disease. SYN: *cryotherapy.*

frit (frĭt) [It. *fritta,* fry]. 1. The material from which glass or the glazed portion of pottery is made. 2. A similar material for making the glaze of artificial teeth.

frog belly. Flaccid abdomen in children afflicted by rickets, and atony of abdominal cells resulting from dyspepsia, accompanied by flatulence.

frog face. Flatness of face resulting from intranasal disease.

Fröhlich's syndrome (frā'lĭks). [Alfred Fröhlich, Austrian neurologist, 1871–1953] A condition characterized by obesity and sexual infantilism, atrophy or hypoplasia of the gonads, and altered secondary sex characteristics. Due to disturbance of the hypothalamus and hypophysis, usually secondary to a neoplasm. SYN: *adiposogenital dystrophy.*

Froin's syndrome (frō-ănz'). [Georges Froin, Fr. physician, b. 1874] Yellow cerebrospinal fluid that rapidly coagulates. It contains an excess of lymphocytes and protein, particularly globulin.

frolement (frōl-mōn') [Fr.]. 1. Very light friction with the hand in massage. SEE: *massage.* 2. A sound resembling rustling heard in auscultation.

Froment's sign (frō-măz'). [Jules Froment, Fr. physician, b. 1878] Flexion of the distal phalanx of the thumb when a sheet of paper is held between the thumb and index finger. An indication of ulnar nerve palsy.

Frommann's lines (frŏm'ănz). [Carl Frommann, Ger. anatomist, 1831–1892] Transverse lines in the axis cylinder of medullated nerve fibers. Demonstrated by staining with silver nitrate.

frons (frŏnz) [L.]. [NA] The forehead.

frontad [L. *frons, front-,* brow, + *ad,* toward]. Toward the frontal aspect.

frontal [L. *frontalis*]. 1. Anterior. 2. Pert. to the forehead bone.

frontal bone. Forehead bone.

frontal lobe. Four main convolutions in front of the central sulcus of the cerebrum.

frontal plane. A plane parallel with the long axis of the body and at right angles to the median sagittal plane.

frontal sinuses. A pair of hollow spaces in the frontal bone lying above the orbits. They are lined with mucous membrane, contain air, and communicate with the middle nasal meatus by means of the nasofrontal duct.

fronto- [L. *frons,* brow]. Prefix indicating anterior position or relationship with the forehead.

frontomalar (frŏn″tō-mā′lăr) [″ + *mala,* cheek]. Rel. to the frontal and malar bones.

frontomaxillary (frŏn″tō-măx′ĭ-lār″ē) [″ + *maxilla,* jaw]. Rel. to the frontal bone and maxillary bones.

frontoparietal (frŏn″tō-pă-rī′ĕ-tăl) [″ + *parietalis,* pert. to a wall]. Pert. to the frontal and parietal bones.

frontotemporal [″ + *tempora,* the temples]. Pert. to frontal and temporal bones.

front-tap reflex. Contraction of gastrocnemius muscles resulting from percussing the stretched muscles of the extended leg.

frost [AS.]. Frozen vapor deposit.

f., urea. Deposit of urea crystals on the skin from evaporation of sweat in a patient whose kidneys are severely impaired, such as in uremia.

frostbite. Freezing or effect of freezing of a part of the body. Exposed areas such as ears, cheeks, nose, fingers, and toes are usually affected.

SYM: Tingling, redness followed by paleness and numbness of affected area. It is of three degrees: transitory hyperemia following numbness; formation of vesicles; and gangrene.

F.A.: Do not rub part with snow. Slow rewarming or rapid rewarming in water at 103° to 105° F. (39.4° to 40.6° C.). Rapid rewarming is used if it is certain that the vascular tissues are not injured. Stimulate with orally administered hot fluids such as tea, coffee, or beef bouillon. Patient should not be allowed to smoke. Artificial respiration if unconscious. Patients have been known to recover without loss of fingers or toes even though amputation seemed inevitable.

frost-itch. Itching of skin provoked by cold temperatures. SYN: *pruritus hiemalis.*

frottage (frō-tŏzh′) [Fr., rubbing]. 1. A condition of hyperesthesia sexualis inducing an irresistible impulse of pressing against someone in a crowd, thus producing an orgasm. 2. Massage technique using rubbing.

frotteur (frō-tĕr′) [Fr. *frottage,* rubbing]. One who practices frottage.

frozen section. The cutting of a thin piece of tissue from a frozen specimen. This permits rapid examination under the microscope. A technique used while the patient is still anesthetized. The surgeon's further action will be influenced by the results of this rapid test.

F.R.S. *Fellow of the Royal Society.*

fructofuranose (frŭk″tō-fū′rā-nōs). The furanose form of fructose.

fructokinase (frŭk″tō-kī′nās). Enzyme that catalyzes transfer of high-energy phosphate from a donor to fructose.

fructose (frŭk′tōs) [L. *fructus,* fruit]. USP. Levulose; fruit sugar. A monosaccharide and a hexose, having the same empirical formula as glucose, $C_6H_{12}O_6$, and found in corn syrup, honey, fruit juices, and in the syrup resulting from the inversion of sucrose, an invert sugar. May be utilized as glucose is in providing a source of energy or may be stored in the body after being converted to glycogen. SEE: *disaccharide.*

fructose intolerance. Inability to metabolize the carbohydrate fructose due to a hereditary absence or deficiency of the enzyme aldolase. Ingestion of fructose leads to hypoglycemia, nausea, vomiting, sweating, trembling, dizziness and occasionally convulsions and coma. Rarely, death will occur.

DIAG: Fall in blood glucose following I.V. administration of fructose.

TREATMENT: Acute attacks are treated by administering glucose. For long-term therapy, all foods containing fructose, which is present in sweet fruits and sugar cane, and sucrose and sorbitol, the latter used as a sweetening agent in foods and drugs, must be eliminated from the diet.

fructosemia (frŭk″tō-sē′mē-ă) [″ + Gr. *haima,* blood]. Presence of fructose in the blood.

fructoside (frŭk′tō-sīd). A carbohydrate that upon hydrolysis yields fructose.

fructosuria (frŭk″tō-sū′rē-ă) [″ + Gr. *ouron,* urine]. Fructose in the urine.

fruit [L. *fructus,* fruit]. A ripened ovary of seed-bearing plants and the surrounding tissue as the pod of a bean, nut, grain, or berry. The edible product of a plant consisting of ripened seeds and the enveloping tissue. Fruits in general tend to add bulk to the diet. This quality, as well as their containing specific laxative substances in some cases, makes fruits quite helpful in treating constipation.

COMP: Carbohydrates in the form of fruit sugars are the chief nutritive value of fruits. Seventy-five percent of it is a mixture of dextrose and levulose. Good source of vitamins, minerals and iodine.

Pectose bodies: The principle in fruits that causes them to jell. Pectose is found in unripe fruit; pectin is found in ripe fruit or fruit that has been cooked in a weak acid solution.

Principal acids: Acetic in wine and vinegar. Citric in lemons, oranges, limes, and citron. Malic in apples, pears, apricots, peaches, currants, and gooseberries. Oxalic in rhubarb, sorrel, and cranberries. Tartaric in grapes, pineapples, and tamarinds. Salicylic in currants, cranberries, cherries, plums, grapes, and crabapples.

Combined acids: Citric and malic in raspberries, strawberries, gooseberries, and cherries. Citric, malic, and oxalic in cranberries.

frumentaceous (froo-mĕn-tā'shŭs) [L. *frumentum,* grain]. Resembling or belonging to grain.

frustration [L. *frustratus,* disappointed]. 1. The failure of libido to find adequate outlet. 2. The condition that results from the thwarting or prevention of acts that if performed would bring satisfaction or gratification of physical or personality needs.

FSH. *follicle-stimulating hormone.* Secreted by the anterior lobe of the hypophysis.

FSH-RF. *follicle-stimulating hormone releasing factor.*

ft. L. *fiat* or *fiant,* let there be made; *florentium,* former name for promethium; *foot.*

FTA-ABS. *fluorescent treponemal antibody-absorption test for syphilis.*

5-FU. Trade name for fluorouracil.

fuchsin (fook'sĭn). A red dye that can be prepared in an acid or basic form.

fucose (fū'kōs). A mucopolysaccharide present in blood group substances and in human milk.

fucosidosis (fū"kō-sĭ-dō'sĭs). Hereditary disease resulting from absence of the enzyme required to metabolize fucosidase. Clinically, neurological deterioration begins shortly after a period of normal early development. Heart disease, thick skin, and hyperhidrosis develop. This is followed by death at an early age.

-fuge [L. *fugare,* to put to flight]. Suffix meaning to expel or drive away.

fugitive (fū'jĭ-tĭv) [L. *fugitivus*]. 1. Temporary, transient. 2. Wandering; pert. to inconstant symptoms.

fugue (fūg) [L. *fuga,* flight]. A dissociative reaction in hysterical neurosis. The person acts normal during the fugue but will have no memory for what happened, when recovery occurs.

f., psychogenic. Sudden, unexpected travel away from one's home or place of work with inability to recall one's past. The individual may partially or completely assume a new identity. The condition is not due to organic brain disease. The condition may follow severe mental stress such as marital quarrels or a natural disaster. It is usually of short duration but can last for months. Recovery is the usual outcome without recurrences.

fulgurant (fŭl'gū-rănt) [L. *fulgurans*]. Severe and sudden coming and going like a flash of light, as a shooting pain.

fulgurating [L. *fulgurare,* to lighten]. Pert. to fulguration.

fulguration (fŭl-gū-rā'shŭn). Destruction of tissue by means of long high-frequency electric sparks. SEE: *electrodesiccation.*

fulling [O. Fr. *fauler,* to fill]. A movement in massage; kneading with the limb held between the hands, rolling it backward and forward.

full term. In obstetrics, an infant born during the time between completion of 38 to 41 weeks of gestation. SYN: *infant, term.*

fulminant (fool'-, fŭl'mĭ-nănt) [L. *fulminans*]. Coming in lightninglike flashes of pain, as in tabes dorsalis. SYN: *fulgurant.*

fulminating. Occurring with very great rapidity, said of certain pains. SYN: *fulgurant.*

Fulvicin P/G. Trade name for griseofulvin ultramicrosize.

Fulvicin-U/F. Trade name for griseofulvin microsize.

fumarase (fū'mă-rās). An enzyme present in many plants and animals. It catalyzes the production of L-malic acid from fumaric acid.

fumaric acid. One of the organic acids in the citric acid cycle for the metabolism of the acetate produced from fats, carbohydrates, and proteins.

fumes [L. *fumus,* smoke]. Vapors, esp. those having irritating qualities.

f., nitric acid. Used in various chemical processes. Poisoning is produced by the action of the corrosive fumes on the respiratory tract.

SYM: Choking, gasping, swelling of mucous membranes, tightness in chest, pulmonary edema, cough, and shock. Symptoms may last for one week or more.

TREATMENT: Immediately remove the patient from the fumes, then maintain good ventilation of lungs. Therapy for shock and pulmonary edema. Administration of oxygen under pressure using a mask may be required along with analgesics for anxiety. Remove clothes if they are contaminated. Cortisone may be helpful in diminishing inflammatory response in lungs.

fumigant (fū'mĭ-gănt) [L. *fumigare,* to make

smoke]. An agent used in disinfecting a room. The substance used produces fumes that are lethal to insects and rodents. Chemicals used include hydrogen cyanide gas, acrylonitrile, carbon tetrachloride, ethylene oxide, and methyl bromide.

fumigation (fū″mĭ-gā′shŭn). 1. The use of poisonous fumes or gases to destroy living organisms, esp. rats, mice, insects, and other vermin. Fumigants are relatively ineffective against bacteria and viruses; consequently the practice of terminal disinfection of the sick room, formerly a common practice, has been discontinued. 2. The disinfection of rooms by gases.

fuming [L. *fumus,* smoke]. Having a visible vapor.

function (fŭng′shŭn) [L. *functio,* performance]. 1. The action performed by any structure. In a living organism this may pertain to a cell or a part of a cell, tissue, organ, or system of organs. 2. The act of carrying on or performing a special activity. Normal function is the normal action of an organ. Abnormal activity or the failure of an organ to perform its activity is the basis of disease or disease processes. Structural changes in an organ constitute pathological changes and are common causes of malfunctioning, although an organ may act abnormally in the absence of observable structural changes.

function, words pert. to: absorption; anabolism; assimilation; catabolism; digestion; excretion; malfunction; metabolism; secretion.

functional. 1. Pert. to function. 2. A word applied to disturbances of function in a variety of ways. The disturbance of function of one organ by structural change in another is at times termed functional, but incorrectly so because it represents organic change. Disturbances of function resulting from unfortunate conditioning of the organism to an external situation may more suitably be called functional, although this conditioning may be purely structural.

functional disease. General term for inorganic disease or one in which changes of an organ are not in evidence; a disturbance of any organ's functions.

functional overlay. The emotional response to physical illness. This may take the form of a conversion or hysterical response, affective overreaction, prolonged symptoms of physical illness after signs of the illness have subsided, or combinations of these reactions. Functional overlay may appear to be the primary disease and require skillful diagnosis to determine the actual cause of illness.

functional psychosis. Disorder exhibited in psychosis in which no pathology of the central nervous system is apparent.

functioning tumor. A tumor that is capable of synthesizing the same product as the normal tissues from which it arises, esp. endocrine or nonendocrine tumors that produce hormones.

funda (fŭn′dă) [L., sling]. A four-tailed bandage.

fundal (fŭn′dăl) [L. *fundus,* base]. Pert. to a fundus.

fundament (fŭn′dă-mĕnt) [L. *fundamentum*]. 1. A foundation. 2. The anus.

fundectomy (fŭn-dĕk′tō-mē) [L. *fundus,* base, + Gr. *ektome,* excision]. Removal of the fundus of any organ.

fundic (fŭn′dĭk). Pert. to a fundus.

fundiform (fŭn′dĭ-form) [L. *fundus,* sling, + *forma,* shape]. Sling-shaped or looped.

fundoplication (fŭn″dō-plĭ-kā′shŭn). Surgical reduction of the size of the opening into the fundus of the stomach and suturing the previously removed end of the esophagus to it. Used in treating reflux of gastric contents into the esophagus.

fundus [L., base]. (pl. *fundi*) [NA] 1. The larger part, base or body of a hollow organ. 2. The portion of an organ most remote from its opening.

f. oculi. Posterior inner part of eye as seen with ophthalmoscope.

f. of bladder. The base of the urinary bladder, the portion closest to the rectum.

f. of gallbladder. The lower dilated portion of the gallbladder.

f. of stomach. The uppermost portion of the stomach, posterior and lateral to the entrance of the esophagus.

f. tympani. The floor of the tympanic cavity close to the jugular fossa. It contains the bulb of the internal jugular vein.

f. uteri. The body of the uterus above the openings of the fallopian tubes.

funduscope (fŭn′dŭs-skōp) [″ + Gr. *skopein,* to examine]. Device, an ophthalmoscope, for examining the fundus of the eye.

fundusectomy (fŭn″dŭs-ĕk′tō-mē) [″ + Gr. *ektome,* excision]. Excision of the fundus of the stomach. SYN: *cardiectomy.*

fungal (fŭng′găl). Caused by fungus or pert. to fungus.

fungal septicemia. Presence of pathogenic fungi in the blood. May be seen as a complication of parenteral hyperalimentation. SYN: *fungemia.*

fungate (fŭng′gāt) [L. *fungus* mushroom]. To grow like a fungus.

fungating (fŭn′gāt-ĭng). Growing rapidly like a fungus, applied to certain tumors.

fungemia (fŭn-jē′mē-ă) [″ + Gr. *haima,* blood]. Presence of fungi in the blood. SYN: *fungal septicemia.*

Fungi (fŭn′jī) [L. *fungus,* mushroom]. A division of plantlike organisms that includes molds and yeasts. Fungi grow as single cells as in yeast or as multicellular filamentous colonies as in molds and mushrooms. They do not contain chlorophyll and thus are dependent upon a saprophytic or parasitic existence. True fungi have a plant body composed of hyphae. Included are the algal fungi (Phycomycetes), sac fungi (Ascomycetes), club fungi (Basidiomycetes), and imperfect fungi (Fungi Imperfecti or Deuteromycetes). Many forms are pathogenic to plants and animals.

fungi. Pl. of fungus.

fungicide (fŭn'jĭ-sīd) [L. *fungi,* mushrooms, + *cidus,* killing]. An agent that kills fungi and their spores.

fungiform (fŭn'jĭ-form) [" + *forma,* shape]. Fungus-shaped.

fungiform papillae. Small rounded eminences on middle and anterior parts of dorsum and esp. along sides of tongue.

fungistasis (fŭn-jĭ-stā'sĭs) [" + Gr. *stasis,* a halting]. A condition in which the growth of fungi is inhibited.

fungistat (fŭn'jĭ-stăt) [" + Gr. *statikos,* standing]. An agent that inhibits the growth of fungi.

fungistatic. Inhibiting the growth of fungi.

fungitoxic (fŭn"jĭ-tŏk'sĭk). A toxic effect on fungi.

fungoid (fŭn'goyd) [" + Gr. *eidos,* form]. Having the appearance of a fungus.

fungosity (fŭn-gŏs'ĭ-tē). A soft, spongy funguslike growth.

fungous (fŭn'gŭs). Fungus.

fungus (fŭn'gŭs) [L., mushroom]. (pl. *fungi*) 1. A vegetable cellular organism that subsists on organic matter. 2. A plantlike organism belonging to the division Fungi. 3. A spongelike morbid growth on the body that resembles fungi. SEE: *actinomycosis.*

funic (fū'nĭk) [L. *funis,* cord]. Pert. to the umbilical cord.

funic souffle. The purring sound heard over the pregnant uterus and having the same rate as the fetal heartbeat. That sound is from blood rushing through vessels in the umbilical cord.

funicle (fū'nĭ-kl) [L. *funiculus,* little cord]. A small, threadlike structure. SYN: *funiculus.*

funicular (fū-nĭk'ū-lăr). Pert. to the spermatic or umbilical cord.

funicular process. That part of the tunica vaginalis that covers the spermatic cord.

funiculitis (fū-nĭk"ū-lī'tĭs) [" + Gr. *itis,* inflammation]. Inflammation of the spermatic cord.

funiculopexy (fū-nĭk'ū-lō-pĕks"ē) [" + Gr. *pexis,* fixation]. Suturing the spermatic cord to the tissues in cases of undescended testicle.

funiculus (fū-nĭk'ū-lŭs) [L., little cord]. (pl. *funiculi*) 1. [NA] Any small structure resembling a cord. 2. A division of the white matter of the spinal cord consisting of fasciculi or fiber tracts lying peripherally to the gray matter. Differentiated into dorsal, lateral, and ventral funiculi.

funiform (fū'nĭ-form) [L. *funis,* cord, + *forma,* shape]. Cordlike.

funis (fū'nĭs) [L., cord]. 1. A cordlike structure, such as the spermatic cord or the umbilical cord.

funnel [L. *fundere,* to pour]. Conical, wide-open-mouthed device for pouring through its open tube at end into another vessel.

funnel breast, funnel chest. Congenital anomaly consisting of sternal depression of chest walls so that the chest is funnel-shaped.

funny bone. The internal condyle of the humerus. So termed because pressure applied over this area stimulates the ulnar nerve and produces a distinct sensation.

F.U.O. *fever of unknown origin.*

Furacin. Trade name for nitrofurazone.

Furadantin. Trade name for nitrofurantoin.

Furantoin. Trade name for nitrofurantoin.

furcal [L. *furca,* fork]. Forked.

furcation (fŭr-kā'shŭn). The anatomical area of a multirooted tooth where the roots divide. Also: *furca.*

furcula (fŭr'kū-lă) [L., little fork]. The hypobranchial eminence, an elevation in the floor of the embryonic pharynx at the level of the 3rd and 4th branchial arches. It gives rise to the epiglottis and the aryepiglottic folds.

furfur [L., bran]. (pl. *furfures*) Dandruff scales.

furfuraceous (fŭr-fū-rā'shŭs). Scaly or resembling scales.

furibund (fū'rĭ-bŭnd) [L. *furibundus*]. Maniacal; raging, as in certain types of insanity.

furor [L., rage]. Extremely violent outbursts of anger, often without provocation.

f. femininus. Nymphomania, q.v.

furosemide (fū-rō'sĕ-mīd). USP. An oral diuretic.

furred [O. Fr. *forre,* lining]. Said of the tongue on which a dustlike deposit has formed.

furrow [AS. *furh*]. A groove.

f., atrioventricular. The groove demarcating the atria of the heart from the ventricles.

f., digital. Any one of several transverse lines on the palmar surface of the fingers across the joints.

f., gluteal. The vertical groove on the skin between the buttocks.

furuncle (fū'rŭng-kl) [L. *furunculus*]. A boil. SYN: *furunculus.*

furuncular (fū-rŭng'kū-lăr). Pert. to a boil.

furunculoid (fū-rŭng'kū-loyd) [" + Gr. *eidos,* form]. Resembling a furuncle or boil. SYN: *furunculous.*

furunculosis (fū-rŭng"kū-lō'sĭs) [" + Gr. *osis,*

condition]. A condition resulting from boils.

furunculous. Pert. to or of the nature of a boil or boils.

furunculus (fū-rŭng′kū-lŭs) [L., a boil]. (pl. *furunculi*) Boil, furuncle. Acute, deep-seated phlegmonous inflammation formed in the skin usually ending in suppuration and necrosis.

ETIOL: Staphylococcal infection of follicular or sebaceous glands.

SYM: Neck, axillae, face, buttocks, and breasts are common sites of predilection. Begins in hair follicle or sudoriparous gland as a subcutaneous swelling or acuminate pustule around a hair shaft. The skin is smooth and shining with pain and tenderness. The lesion may come to a head or become boggy and fluctuant, or regression may take place before suppuration, resulting in disappearance by absorption. Lesion ruptures spontaneously or following incision, discharging necrotic tissue and pus. Healing follows.

TREATMENT: Moist heat, incision on pointing of lesion, and appropriate systemic antibiotic.

Fusarium (fū-ză′rē-ŭm) [L. *fusus*, spindle]. A genus of fungi.

fuscin (fŭs′ĭn) [L. *fuscus*, brown]. A brown pigment, a melanin, present in the outermost layer (pigmented epithelium) of the retina.

fuse (fūz) [L. *fusus*, poured]. 1. A safety device comprising a strip of wire of easily fusible (meltable) metal, the conductance of which is predetermined. The metal fuses and breaks circuit when excess of current passes through. 2. To unite or blend together as the coherence of adjacent body structures.

fusible (fū′zĭ-b'l). Capable of being melted.

fusiform (fū′zĭ-form) [L. *fusus*, spindle, + *forma*, shape]. Tapering at both ends; spindle-shaped.

fusimotor (fū″sĭ-mō′tor). Concerning the motor innervation of the intrafusal muscle fibers arising from the gamma efferent neurons of the anterior gray matter of the spinal cord.

fusion (fū′shŭn) [L. *fusio*]. Meeting and joining together through liquefaction by heat. The process of fusing or uniting.

f., diaphyseal-epiphyseal. Surgical obliteration of the epiphyseal line of a bone so that epiphysis and diaphysis are joined.

f., nuclear. Joining of the nucleus of two atoms to form a larger nucleus. This occurs when temperatures reach millions of degrees. A large amount of energy is produced.

f., spinal. Surgical fusion of two or more vertebrae. SYN: *spondylosyndesis*.

fusocellular [L. *fusus*, spindle, + *cellulus*, little cell]. Spindle celled.

fustigation (fŭs″tĭ-gā′shŭn) [L. *fustigatio*]. In massage, beating with light rods.

fututrix (fū-tū′trĭks). A female who practices tribadism, q.v.

F wave. Flutter waves in atrial fibrillation. Detectable on the ECG at 300–350/minute.

FWB. *full weight bearing.*

G

γ. Third letter of Greek alphabet; gamma is the anglicized equivalent. Symbol for microgram and immunoglobulin.
G. The Newtonian constant of gravitation.
g. 1. The force of gravity exerted upon a body during acceleration or deceleration. 2. *gingival.* 3. *gram.* 4. *gender.*
Ga. Chem. symb. for gallium.
GABA. *gamma-aminobutyric acid.*
gadfly. A fly belonging to the family Tabanidae, q.v., that lays eggs under the skin of its victim, causing swellings simulating a boil. Multiple furuncles appear with hatching of larva. SEE: *botfly.*
gadolinium (găd″ō-lĭn′ē-ŭm). A very rare element. SYMB: Gd. At. wt. 157.25; at. no. 64.
Gaffkya (găf′kē-ă). [Georg T. A. Gaffky, Ger. bacteriologist, 1850–1918] A genus of bacteria of the family Micrococcaceae.
G. tetragena. A species occurring normally in the upper respiratory tract of man that occasionally causes arthritis, meningitis, pneumonia, soft-tissue abscesses, or endocarditis.
gag. 1. Device for keeping the jaws open during surgery. 2. To retch or cause to retch.
gage (gāj). Gauge.
gag reflex. Gagging and vomiting resulting from irritation of fauces.
gain. To increase something such as weight, strength, or health.
g., secondary. In psychiatry, gain obtained from an illness by the patient. This may be the receipt of special attention or money as could be the case if disability payments were received from an employer or insurer.
Gaisböck's syndrome (gīs′bĕks). [Felix Gaisböck, Ger. physician, 1869–1955] Abnormal number of red corpuscles in blood without other signs and symptoms characteristic of polycythemia vera.
gait (gāt) [ME. *gait,* passage]. Manner of walking.
g., ataxic. Gait characterized by staggering and unsteadiness.
g., cerebellar. A staggering movement seen in cerebellar disease.
g., double step. Gait in which alternate steps are of a different length or at a different rate.
g., drag-to. Gait in which the feet are dragged to the crutches rather than lifted.
g., equine. Gait characterized by high steps; characteristic of peroneal paralysis.
g., festinating. Gait in which patients walk on toes as though pushed. Starts slowly, increases, and may continue until the patients grasp some object in order to stop.
g., gluteal. Leaning of the trunk to the affected side while walking. Caused by paralysis of the gluteus medius muscle.
g., helicopod. Gait in which the feet or foot describes a half circle with each step. Sometimes seen in hysteria.
g., hemiplegic. Gait in which patients abduct the paralyzed limb, swing it around, and bring it forward so the foot comes to the ground in front of them.
g., scissor. Gait in which legs cross in walking.
g., spastic. A stiff movement, toes seeming to catch and drag, legs held together, hips and knee joints slightly flexed. Seen in spastic paraplegia, sclerosis of lateral pyramidal columns of cord, tumor of spinal cord, and arachnoiditis.
g., steppage. Gait in which foot and toes are lifted high, heel brought down first. Seen in peripheral neuritis, late stages of diabetes, alcoholism, and chronic arsenical poisoning.
g., swing-through. Gait in which the crutches are advanced and the legs are swung between and past them.
g., swing-to. Gait in which the crutches are advanced and the legs are advanced to the crutches.
g., tabetic. The high-stepping ataxic walk in which the feet slap the ground. It is caused by tabes dorsalis.
g., three-point. Gait in which the crutches and the affected leg are advanced, then the other leg is advanced.
g., two-point. Gait in which the right foot and left crutch are advanced, then the left foot and right crutch are moved forward.
g., waddling. Gait in which feet are wide apart and walk resembles that of a duck. Seen in coxa vara and double congenital displacement of hip when lordosis is present.
galact-, galacto- [Gr. *gala,* milk]. Combining forms pert. to milk.
galactacrasia (gă-lăk″tă-krā′zē-ă) [″ + *akrasia,* bad mixture]. An abnormal composition of milk from the breast.
galactagogue (gă-lăk′tă-gŏg) [″ + *agogos,* leading]. Agent that promotes the flow of milk.
galactan (gă-lăk′tăn). A complex carbohydrate that forms galactose upon hydrolysis.
galactase. An enzyme or proteolytic ferment of milk.
galactemia (gă-lăk-tē′mē-ă) [″ + *haima,* blood]. Milky condition of the blood.
galactic (gă-lăk′tĭk). Pert. to flow of milk.
galactidrosis (gă-lăk″tĭ-drō′sĭs) [″ + *hidros,*

sweat]. A milk-like sweat.

galactischia (găl″ăk-tĭsk′ē-ă) [″ + *ischein,* to suppress]. Suppression of the secretion and flow of milk.

galactoblast (gă-lăk′tō-blăst) [″ + *blastos,* germ]. Body found in mammary acini; contains fat globules.

galactocele (gă-lăk′tō-sēl) [″ + *kele,* hernia]. 1. A tumor caused by occlusion of a milk duct. 2. Hydrocele containing a milk-like liquid.

galactoid. Resembling milk.

galactokinase (gă-lăk″tō-kī′nās). Enzyme that catalyzes transfer of high-energy phosphate groups from a donor to D-galactose. D-galactose-1-phosphate is produced by this reaction.

galactolipin [″ + *lipos,* fat]. A phosphorus-free lipid combined with galactose; a cerebroside.

galactoma (găl-ăk-tō′mă) [″ + *oma,* tumor]. Cystic tumor of female breast. SYN: *galactocele* (def. 1).

galactometer [″ + *metron,* measure]. Device for measuring the specific gravity of milk. SYN: *lactometer.*

galactopexic (găl-ăk-tō-pěk′sĭk) [″ + *pexis,* fixation]. Holding galactose.

galactopexy (gă-lăk′tō-pěk″sē). The fixation of galactose by the liver.

galactophagous (găl″ăk-tŏf′ă-gŭs) [″ + *phagein,* to eat]. Feeding upon milk.

galactophlysis (găl″ăk-tŏf′lĭ-sĭs) [″ + *phlysis,* eruption]. Eruption of vesicles containing milk-like contents.

galactophore (găl-ăk′tō-for) [″ + *pherein,* to bear]. A milk duct.

galactophoritis (găl-ăk″tō-for-ī′tĭs) [″ + ″ + *itis,* inflammation]. Inflammation of a milk duct.

galactophorous (găl″ăk-tŏf′or-ŭs). Giving milk.

galactophthisis (găl″ăk-tŏf′thĭ-sĭs) [Gr. *gala,* milk, + *phthisis,* a wasting]. Debility and emaciation as a result of excessive or prolonged milk secretion.

galactophygous (găl-ăk-tŏf′ĭ-gŭs) [″ + *phyge,* flight]. Arresting flow of milk.

galactoplania (gă-lăk″tō-plā′nē-ă) [″ + *plane,* wandering]. Secretion of milk in some part of the body other than the mammary gland.

galactopoietic (gă-lăk″tō-poy-ět′ĭk) [″ + *poiein,* to make]. 1. Having to do with the production of milk. 2. A substance that promotes the secretion of milk.

galactopyra (gă-lăk″tō-pī′ră) [″ + *pyr,* fire]. Milk fever.

galactorrhea (gă-lăk″tō-rē′ă) [″ + *rhoia,* flow]. 1. Continuation of lactation or flow of milk at intervals after cessation of nursing. 2. Excessive flow of milk.

galactosamine (gă-lăk″tō-săm′ĭn). Galactose containing an amine group on the second carbon.

galactose (gă-lăk′tōs). $C_6H_{12}O_6$. A monosaccharide or simple hexose sugar. Galactose is an isomer of glucose and is formed, along with glucose, in the hydrolysis of lactose. It is dextrorotatory and reduces alkaline copper solutions such as Fehling's solution. It is a component of cerebrosides. Galactose is readily absorbed in the digestive tract; in the liver it is converted into glycogen.

galactosemia (gă-lăk″tō-sē′mē-ă). An inborn error of metabolism inherited as an autosomal recessive trait characterized by inability to convert galactose to glucose. It is due to congenital absence of the enzyme that is required for conversion of galactose to glucose and its derivatives. This enzyme is galactose 1-phosphate uridyl transferase. Diagnosis is confirmed by testing the newborn's urine for noncarbohydrate reducing substances. The infant with galactosemia will fail to thrive within a week after birth due to anorexia, vomiting, and diarrhea unless galactose and lactose are removed from the diet. If untreated, the disease may progress to starvation and death. Untreated children who do survive usually fail to grow and are mentally retarded, and have cataracts.

Galactosemia can be diagnosed in utero by amniocentesis. If a pregnant woman is a known carrier, it is advisable that she exclude lactose and galactose from her diet.

galactosidase (gă-lăk″tō-sī′dās). Enzyme that catalyzes the metabolism of galactosides.

galactosides (gă-lăk′tō-sīds). Carbohydrates that contain galactose.

galactosis (găl″ăk-tō′sĭs) [″ + *osis,* condition]. The secretion of milk.

galactostasis (găl″ăk-tŏs′tă-sĭs) [″ + *stasis,* a stopping]. Cessation or checking of milk secretion.

galactosuria (găl-ăk″tō-sū′rē-ă) [″ + *ouron,* urine]. Galactose in the urine.

galactotherapy (gă-lăk″tō-thĕr′ă-pē) [″ + *therapeia,* treatment]. 1. Treatment of a nursing infant by drugs administered to the mother. 2. Therapeutic use of milk, as a milk diet. SYN: *lactotherapy.*

galactotoxin (gă-lăk″tō-tŏks′ĭn) [″ + *toxikon,* poison]. A toxic substance in milk produced by bacteria.

galactotoxism (gă-lăk″tō-tŏk′sĭzm). Poisoning due to drinking milk that contains toxic substances.

galactotrophy (găl″ăk-tŏt′rō-fē) [″ + *trophe,* nourishment]. Feeding with nothing but milk.

galactoxism (găl″ăk-tŏks′ĭzm) [″ + *toxikon,* poison, + *-ismos,* state of]. Poisoning by milk containing toxic substances. SYN: *galactotoxism.*

galactozymase (gă-lăk″tō-zī′mās) [″ + *zyme,*

leaven]. A starch-hydrolyzing enzyme in milk.

galacturia (găl-ăk-tū'rē-ă) [" + *ouron*, urine]. The passing of milky urine. SYN: *chyluria*.

galea (gā'lē-ă) [L. *galea*, helmet]. 1. [NA] A helmetlike structure. 2. A type of head bandage.

g. aponeurotica. The aponeurosis of the scalp. It connects the anterior and posterior bellies of the occipitofrontalis muscle.

galeanthropy (gā"lē-ăn'thrō-pē) [Gr. *gale*, cat, + *anthropos*, man]. A delusion that one has become transformed into a cat.

Galen, Claudius. A noted Greek physician and medical writer, circa 130–200 A.D., residing in Rome, where he was physician to Marcus Aurelius. Recognized as the authority on medicine through the Middle Ages. Called the father of experimental physiology.

G.'s veins. The veins running through the tela chorioidea formed by the joining of the terminal and choroid veins and forming the vena cerebri magna, which empties into the straight sinus of the brain.

galena (gă-lē'nă). Lead sulfide ore.

galenic (gă-lĕn'ĭk). Pert. to Galen or his teachings.

galenicals, galenics (gă-lĕn'ĭ-kăls, -ĭks). 1. Herb and vegetable medicines. 2. Crude drugs and medicinals as distinguished from pure active principles contained in them. 3. A medicine prepared according to an official formula.

galeophilia (găl"ē-ō-fĭl'ē-ă) [Gr. *gale*, cat, + *philein*, to love]. Fondness for cats.

galeophobia (găl"ē-ō-fō'bē-ă) [" + *phobos*, fear]. Abnormal aversion to cats.

galeropia, galeropsia (găl-ĕr-ō'pē-ă, -ŏp'sē-ă) [Gr. *galeros*, cheerful, + *opsis*, vision]. Unusual clearness of vision.

gall [AS. *gealla*, sore place]. 1. An excoriation. 2. The bitter secretion of the liver stored in the gallbladder; bile. It has no enzymes, but it assists in the emulsifying of fats. It also stimulates the intestines and multiplies the action of the pancreatic juice threefold. It is discharged through the cystic duct into the duodenum.

RS: bile ducts; calculus; "chol-" words; colic, biliary; cystic duct.

gallamine triethiodide (găl'ă-mīn trī"ē-thī'ō-dīd). USP. A drug that inhibits transmission of nerve impulses across the myoneural junction of voluntary muscles. Trade name is Flaxedil.

gallate (găl'lāt). A salt of gallic acid.

gallbladder [AS. *gealla*, sore place, + *blaedre*, bladder]. Pear-shaped sac on undersurface of right lobe of liver holding bile from the liver until discharged through cystic duct; 3 to 4 in. (7.6 to 10.2 cm.) long, 1 in. (2.54 cm.) greatest diameter; capacity 50 to 75 ml. concentrated bile equivalent to 1½ pt. (710 ml.) liver bile. In addition to its function as a storage site for bile, the gallbladder acts to concentrate the bile by removing water content.

gall duct [" + L. *ductus*, a passage]. Tube carrying bile from the liver and gallbladder. SYN: *bile duct*.

gallium (găl'ē-ŭm) [L. *Gallia*, Gaul]. A rare metal, small amounts of which are found in bauxite and zinc blends. SYMB: Ga. At. wt. 69.72; at. no. 31.

gallon [Med. L. *galleta*, jug]. Four liquid measure quarts; 231 cubic inches or 3.79 liters. In England the Imperial liquid gallon is 277.4 cubic inches or 4.55 liters.

gallop rhythm. An abnormal third or fourth heart sound in a tachycardia of 100 or more beats per minute. The sound resembles that produced by a galloping horse and is indicative of serious heart disease.

gallstone [AS. *gealla*, sore place + *stan*, stone]. Concretion formed in the gall bladder or bile ducts. Traditionally gallstones have been classified according to their composition. This information was then used to demonstrate the cause of the stone formation. This is no longer considered valid. Generally the core of all gallstones contains a mixture of cholesterol, bilirubin and protein.

SYM: Stone may remain dormant and give little distress unless inflammation and distention of the gallbladder take place or unless it enters and is unable to pass through the biliary ducts, when colic ensues. The pain may radiate to the back and right shoulder, usually several hours after eating and when the stomach is empty. Flatulence is a common symptom. Jaundice is usually absent.

TREATMENT: Analgesics, meperidine being the drug of choice, under a physician's directions. Morphine is thought to increase spasm of the sphincter of Oddi and thus is not used for pain relief.

RS: bilifuscin; calculus; cholelithiasis.

Galton's whistle. [Sir Francis Galton, Brit. scientist, 1822–1911] A whistle used to test the hearing.

galvanic. [Luigi Galvani, It. physiologist, 1737–1798] Pert. to galvanism.

galvanic battery. A series of cells, giving a combined effect of all the units, and generating electricity by chemical reaction.

galvanic cell. One of a series of cells generating electricity through chemical reaction.

galvanic current. Direct electric current, usually from a battery.

galvanism. [Luigi Galvani] Therapeutic use of direct current of electricity.

galvanization (găl"văn-ī-zā'shŭn). Employment of a galvanic current as a therapeutic measure.

galvanocautery (găl″vă-nō-kaw′tĕr-ē) [*galvanism* + Gr. *kauterion,* cautery]. Cauterization of tissue by means of an electric current. SEE: *electrocautery.*

galvanocontractility (găl″vă-nō-kŏn″trăk-tĭl′ĭ-tē) [″ + L. *contractus,* drawn together]. Capability of a muscle to contract under a galvanic stimulation.

galvanofaradization (găl″vă-nō-făr″ă-dĭ-zā′shŭn). Combined use of continuous and interrupted electrical current in treating a nerve or a muscle.

galvanometer (găl″vă-nŏm′ĕ-tĕr) [″ + Gr. *metron,* measure]. An instrument that measures current by electromagnetic action. SYN: *rheometer* (def. 1).

galvanopalpation (găl″vă-nō-păl-pā′shŭn) [″ + L. *palpare,* to touch]. A method of measuring tactile sensibility of the nerves of the skin by use of electric current.

galvanopuncture (găl″vă-nō-pŭng′chūr) [″ + L. *punctura,* puncture]. Introduction of needles to complete a galvanic current.

galvanoscope (găl-văn′ō-skōp) [″ + Gr. *skopein,* to examine]. Instrument that shows the presence and direction of a galvanic current.

galvanosurgery (găl″vă-nō-sĕr′jĕr-ē) [″ + Gr. *cheir,* hand, + *ergon,* work]. Use of galvanism in surgery.

galvanotaxis (găl″vă-nō-tăk′sĭs) [″ + Gr. *taxis,* arrangement]. The tendency of a living organism to arrange itself in a medium so that its axis bears a certain relationship to the direction of the electric current in the medium.

galvanotherapeutics, galvanotherapy (găl″vă-nō-thĕr″ă-pū′tĭks, -thĕr′ă-pē) [″ + Gr. *therapeia,* treatment]. Treatment by means of electricity. SYN: *electrotherapy.*

galvanothermy (găl″văn-ō-thĕrm′ē) [″ + Gr. *therme,* heat]. Treatment by the heat from a galvanic battery.

galvanotonus (găl-văn-ŏt′ō-nŭs) [″ + Gr. *tonos,* tension]. Tonic contractions caused by a galvanic current.

galvanotropism (găl″văn-ŏt′rō-pĭzm) [″ + Gr. *tropos,* a turn]. The tendency of an organism to grow, turn, or move in relationship with an electric current.

Gamastan. Trade name for immune globulin.

Gamene. Trade name for gamma benzene hexachloride (or lindane).

gamete (găm′ēt) [Gr. *gamein,* to marry]. A mature male or female reproductive cell; the spermatozoon or ovum. SEE: *chromosome; meiosis.*

RS: conception; fertilization; gene; ovum; spermatozoon.

gametic (găm-ĕt′ĭk). Pert. to gametes.

gametocide (găm′ĕ-tō-sīd″) [″ + L. *caedere,* to kill]. An agent destructive to gametes or gametocytes, particularly those of malaria.

gametocyte (gă-mē′tō-sīt) [″ + *kytos,* cell]. A stage of the malaria protozoon that reproduces in the blood of the Anopheles mosquito.

gametogenesis (găm″ĕt-ō-jĕn′ĕ-sĭs) [″ + *genesis,* production]. Development of gametes: oogenesis or spermatogenesis.

gametogony (găm″ĕ-tŏg′ō-nē). The phase in the life cycle of the malarial parasite (Plasmodium) in which male and female gametocytes, which infect the mosquito, are formed.

gametophyte (găm′ĕ-tō-fīt) [″ + *phyton,* plant]. In plants, the sexual or gamete-producing generation that alternates with the asexual or spore-producing generation.

gamic (găm′ĭk) [Gr. *gamein,* to marry]. Sexual, esp. as applied to eggs that develop only after fertilization in contrast to those that develop without fertilization. SEE: *parthenogenesis.*

gamma. 1. Third letter of the Gr. alphabet, γ. 2. In chemistry it is used to designate the third of a series, as the third carbon atom in an aliphatic chain. 3. One microgram; or one thousandth of a milligram (0.001 mg.); one millionth of a gram.

gamma benzene hexachloride (găm′ă bĕn′zēn hĕk″să-klor′īd). An insecticide used in treating scabies. Trade names are Gamene and Kwell. SYN: *lindane.*

gammacism. Inability to pronounce correctly g and k sounds.

Gammagee. Trade name for serum globulin.

gamma globulin. A protein formed in the blood. Ability to resist infection is related to concentration of such proteins. SEE: *immunoglobulin.*

Gammar. Trade name for serum globulin.

gamma rays. Electromagnetic waves of extremely short wavelength emitted by radioactive substances. They are thought to be of the same nature as x-rays. They have greater penetrating power than alpha or beta rays. SEE: *ray.*

gammopathy (găm-ŏp′ă-thē). A disease in which there is an increase in serum immunoglobulin as in myeloma; but Bence Jones protein is not present in the urine.

Gamna nodules. [Carlos Gamna, It. physician, b. 1896] Nodules in the spleen that stain yellow or brown. Present in certain varieties of splenic enlargement.

Gamna's disease. A type of splenomegaly characterized by slow, progressive enlargement of the spleen and the presence of Gamna's nodules.

gamo- [Gr. *gamos,* marriage]. Combining form indicating relationship to marriage or sexual union.

gamogenesis (găm″ō-jĕn′ĕ-sĭs) [″ + *genesis,* production]. Sexual reproduction.

gamont (găm′ŏnt) [″ + *on,* being]. A sexual form of certain protozoa. SEE: *gametocyte.*

gamophobia (găm″ō-fō′bē-ă) [″ + *phobos,* fear]. Neurotic fear of marriage.

gampsodactylia (gămp″sō-dăk-tĭl′ē-ă) [Gr. *gampsos,* curved, + *daktylos,* digit]. Deformity of the toes causing them to resemble claws. SYN: *clawfoot.*

ganglia (găng′glē-ă). Plural form of ganglion.

ganglial (găng′lē-ăl) [Gr. *ganglion,* knot]. Pert. to a ganglion. SYN: *ganglionic.*

gangliated (găng′lē-ā-tĕd). 1. Having ganglia. 2. Intermixed.

gangliectomy (găng″glē-ĕk′tō-mē) [″ + *ektome,* excision]. Excision of a ganglion.

gangliform (găng′lĭ-form) [″ + L. *forma,* shape]. Formed like a ganglion.

gangliitis (găng″glē-ī′tĭs) [″ + *itis,* inflammation]. Inflammation of a ganglion.

ganglioblast (găng′glē-ō-blăst″) [″ + *blastos,* germ]. An embryonic ganglion cell.

gangliocyte (găng′glē-ō-sīt″) [″ + *kytos,* cell]. A ganglion cell.

gangliocytoma (găng″glē-ō-sī-tō′mă) [″ + ″ + *oma,* tumor]. Ganglioneuroma.

ganglioglioma (găng″glē-ō-glī-ō′mă) [″ + *glia,* glue, + *oma,* tumor]. A ganglion-cell glioma.

ganglioglioneuroma (găng″glē-ō-glī″ō-nū-rō′mă) [″ + ″ + *neuron,* nerve, + *oma,* tumor]. Ganglion cells, glia cells, and nerve fibers in a nerve tumor.

ganglioma (găng-lē-ō′mă) [″ + *oma,* tumor]. 1. Tumor of a lymphatic gland. 2. A swelling of lymphoid tissue.

ganglion (găng′lē-ŏn) [Gr.]. (pl. *ganglia* or *ganglions*) 1. A mass of nervous tissue composed principally of nerve-cell bodies and lying outside the brain or spinal cord. Ex.: the chain of ganglia that form the main sympathetic trunks; the dorsal root ganglion of a spinal nerve. 2. Cystic tumors developing on a tendon or aponeurosis; sometimes occur on the back of the wrist.

g., abdominal. Any one of the abdominal ganglia.

g., anterior cerebral. Corpus striatum. Corpus striatum and corpus lenticulare considered together.

g., aorticorenal. A ganglion lying near the lower border of the celiac ganglion. It is located near the origin of the renal artery.

g., Arnold's auricular. Tiny ganglion located beneath the foramen ovale of the ear. SYN: *g., otic.*

g., auricular. G., Arnold's auricular.

g., autonomic. A ganglion of the autonomic division of the nervous system.

g., basal. Mass of gray matter beneath the 3rd ventricle. Consisting of the caudate, lentiform, and amygdaloid nuclei and the claustrum.

g., basal optic. Mass of gray matter beneath the 3rd ventricle.

g., cardiac. Tiny ganglion toward which converge the fibers of superficial cardiac plexus. It lies on the right side of the ligamentum arteriosus. SYN: *Wrisberg's ganglion.*

g., carotid. Ganglion formed by filamentous threads from the carotid plexus beneath the carotid artery.

g., celiac. One of a pair of prevertebral or collateral ganglia located near the origin of the celiac artery. They form a part of the celiac plexus.

g., cephalic. One of the parasympathetic ganglia in the head: otic, pterygopalatine, and submandibular ganglia.

g., cerebral. Main cerebral nerve centers.

g., cervical. Three pairs of ganglia (superior, middle, inferior) located in the neck region. They are the ganglia of the cervical portion of the sympathetic trunk.

g., cervicothoracic. G., stellate, q.v.

g., cervicouterine. Ganglion near the uterine cervix. SYN: *g., Frankenhäuser's.*

g., ciliary. Tiny ganglion located in the rear portion of the orbit. SYN: *g., lenticular; g., ophthalmic.*

g., coccygeal. A ganglion located in the coccygeal plexus and forming the lower termination of the two sympathetic trunks; sometimes absent.

g., collateral. One of several ganglia of th sympathetic nervous system. They are in the mesenteric nervous plexuses near the abdominal aorta.

g., Corti's. Ganglion on the cochlear nerve.

g., dorsal root. A ganglion located on the dorsal root of a spinal nerve. Contains the cell bodies of sensory neurons. SYN: *g., spinal.*

g., false. An enlargement on a nerve that does not contain a ganglion.

g., Frankenhäuser's. Cervical ganglion of the uterus.

g., gasserian. G., trigeminal, q.v.

g., geniculate. A ganglion on the pars intermedia, the sensory root of the facial nerve. It lies in the anterior border of the anterior geniculum of the facial nerve.

g., inferior mesenteric. A prevertebral sympathetic ganglion located in the inferior mesenteric plexus near the origin of the inferior mesenteric artery.

g., intervertebral. G., spinal.

g., jugular. A ganglion located on the root of the vagus nerve and lying in upper portion of jugular foramen.

g., lateral. One of a chain of ganglia forming the main sympathetic trunk.

g., lenticular. G., ciliary.

g., lumbar. Ganglia usually occurring in fours in the lumbar portion of the sympathetic trunk.

g., lymphatic. Lymph nodes.

g., nodose. Ganglion of the trunk of the vagus nerve. Located immediately below the jugular ganglion. It makes connections with the spinal accessory nerve, hypoglossal nerve, and the superior cervical ganglion of the sympathetic trunk.

g., ophthalmic. G., ciliary.

g., otic. A small ganglion located deep in the zygomatic fossa immediately below the foramen ovale. It lies medial to the mandibular nerve. It supplies postganglionic parasympathetic fibers to the parotid gland. SYN: *g., Arnold's auricular.*

g., parasympathetic. Ganglia on the cholinergic nerves of the sympathetic nervous system.

g., petrous. Ganglion located on lower margin of temporal bone's petrous portion.

g., pharyngeal. Ganglion in contact with the glossopharyngeal nerve.

g., phrenic. One of a group of ganglia joining the phrenic plexus.

g., pterygopalatine. G., sphenopalatine, q.v.

g., renal. One of a group of ganglia joining the renal plexus.

g., sacral. Four small ganglia located in the sacral portion of the sympathetic trunk. They lie on the anterior surface of the sacrum and are connected to the spinal nerves by gray rami.

g., Scarpa's. G., vestibular, q.v.

g., semilunar. G., trigeminal, q.v.

g., sensory. Ganglia of the peripheral nervous system. They transmit sensory stimuli.

g., simple. Cystic tumor in a tendon sheath.

g., sphenopalatine. A ganglion associated with the great superficial petrosal nerve (branch of facial) and the maxillary nerve. It transmits both sympathetic and parasympathetic fibers to the nasal mucosa, palate, pharynx and orbit.

g., spinal. Ganglionic enlargement of spinal nerves' dorsal roots. SYN: *g., dorsal root.*

g., spiral. A long, coiled ganglion in the cochlea of the ear. It contains bipolar cells, the peripheral processes of which terminate in the organ of Corti. The central processes form the cochlear portion of the acoustic nerve and terminate in the cochlear nuclei of the medulla.

g., stellate. Ganglion formed by joining of the inferior cervical ganglion with the first thoracic sympathetic ganglion.

g., submandibular. A ganglion lying between the mylohyoideus and hyoglossus muscles and suspended from the lingual nerve by two small branches. Peripheral fibers pass to the submandibular, sublingual, lingual, and adjacent salivary glands.

g., superior mesenteric. A prevertebral ganglion of the sympathetic nervous system. It lies close to the celiac ganglion and with it forms a part of the celiac plexus. It lies close to the base of the superior mesenteric artery.

g., suprarenal. Ganglion situated in the suprarenal plexus.

g., sympathetic. Ganglia of the thoracolumbar (sympathetic) division of the autonomic nervous system. Include vertebral or lateral ganglia (those forming the sympathetic trunk) and prevertebral or collateral ganglia, more peripherally located.

g., temporal. Tiny ganglion joining the anterior branches of the superior cervical ganglion.

g., terminal. A ganglion of the autonomic division of the nervous system that lies close to or within the organ innervated.

g., thoracic. One of 11 or 12 ganglia of the thoracic area of the sympathetic trunk.

g., trigeminal. Ganglion on the sensory portion of the fifth cranial nerve.

g., tympanic. An enlargement on the tympanic portion of the glossopharyngeal nerve.

g., vestibular. A bilobed ganglion located on the vestibular branch of the acoustic nerve at the base of the internal acoustic meatus. Its peripheral fibers arise in the maculae of the sacculus and utriculus and the cristae of the ampullae of the semicircular ducts.

g., Wrisberg's. Collection of autonomic nerve cells in the superficial cardiac plexus.

g., wrist. G., simple.

ganglionated. Having or consisting of ganglia.

ganglionectomy (găng″lē-ō-nĕk′tō-mē) [″ + *ektome,* excision]. Excision of a ganglion.

ganglioneuroma (găng″lē-ō-nū-rō′mă) [″ + *neuron,* nerve, + *oma,* tumor]. A neuroma containing ganglion cells.

ganglionic (găng-lē-ŏn′ĭk). Pert. to or of the nature of a ganglion.

ganglionic blockade. Blocking the transmission of stimuli in autonomic ganglia. Pharmacologically, this is done by the use of drugs that occupy receptor sites for acetylcholine; and by stabilizing the postsynaptic membranes against the actions of acetylcholine liberated from presynaptic nerve endings. The usual effects of drugs that cause ganglionic blockade are: vasodilatation of arterioles with increased peripheral blood flow; hypotension; dilation of veins with pooling of blood in tissues, decreased venous return, and decreased cardiac output; tachycardia;

mydriasis; cycloplegia; reduced tone and motility of the gastrointestinal tract with consequent constipation; urinary retention; dry mouth; and decreased sweating. Ganglionic blocking drugs are little used in treating hypertension, but are used in treating autonomic hyperreflexia, and to produce controlled hypotension during certain types of surgery. Two drugs used for ganglionic blocking are mecamylamine hydrochloride, USP; and trimethaphan camsylate, USP.

ganglionitis (găng"lē-ŏn-ī'tĭs) [" + *itis,* inflammation]. Inflamed condition of a ganglion.

ganglionostomy (găng"glē-ō-nŏs'tō-mē) [" + *stoma,* mouth]. Surgical incision of a simple ganglion, q.v.

ganglioplegia (găng"glē-ō-plē'jē-ă) [" + *plege,* stroke]. Failure of nervous stimuli to be transmitted by a ganglion. SEE: *ganglionic blockade.*

ganglioside (găng'glē-ō-sīd). A particular class of glycosphingolipid present in nerve tissue and in the spleen.

gangliosidosis (găng"glē-ō-sī-dō'sĭs). (pl. *gangliosidoses*) Accumulation of abnormal amounts of specific gangliosides in the nervous system.

gangosa (găng-gō'să) [Sp. *gangosa,* muffled voice]. Ulceration of the nose and hard palate, regarded as a late stage of yaws.

gangrene (găng'grēn) [Gr. *gangraina,* an eating sore]. A necrosis, or death, of tissue, usually due to deficient or absent blood supply. SEE: *necrosis.*

ETIOL: Usually results from obstruction of the blood supply to an organ or tissue. May result from inflammatory processes, injury, or degenerative changes such as arteriosclerosis. It is commonly a sequela of boils, frostbite, crushing injuries, or diseases such as diabetes mellitus and Raynaud's disease. Emboli in large arteries in almost any part of the body will cause gangrene of the area distal to that point. The part that dies is known as a slough if the soft tissues are involved or a sequestrum if it is a bone that dies. The dead matter must be removed before healing can take place.

g., angioneurotic. State resulting from thrombotic arteries and veins.

g., diabetic. Condition arising in some diabetics as a result of vascular pathology.

g., dry. Condition that results when the part that dies has little blood and remains aseptic. The arteries but not the veins are obstructed. The tissues dry and drop off, the process continuing for weeks or months.

SYM: Pain in early stages. The part is cold and black and begins to atrophy. The most distal parts are generally affected first, the necrosis then spreading upward. Usually seen in arteriosclerosis associated with diabetes.

g., embolic. Gangrenous condition arising subsequent to an embolic obstruction.

g., gas. Gangrene in a wound infected by a gas bacillus, the most common etiologic agent being Clostridium perfringens.

TREATMENT: Antibiotics, clostridial antitoxin. In some cases, surgical intervention may be necessary.

g., humid. G., moist.

g., idiopathic. Gangrene of unknown etiology.

g., inflammatory. Gangrene associated with acute infections and inflammation.

g., moist. Gangrene that is wet as a result of tissue necrosis and bacterial infection.

SYM: The part is hot and red; later it is cold and bluish, commencing to slough. It spreads rapidly and there is an offensive odor. Death may result in a few days.

g., primary. Gangrene developing in a part without previous inflammation.

g., secondary. Gangrene developing subsequent to local inflammation.

g., symmetric. Gangrene on opposite sides of the body in corresponding parts. Usually the result of vasomotor disturbances. Characteristic of Raynaud's and Buerger's disease.

g., traumatic. Gangrene resulting from extensive injuries.

gangrenous. Of the nature of gangrene.

ganoblast (găn'ō-blăst) [Gr. *ganos,* brightness, + *blastos,* cell]. The cell that forms enamel of a tooth. SYN: *ameloblast.*

Ganphen. Trade name for promethazine hydrochloride.

Ganser's syndrome (găn'zĕrz). [Sigbert J. M. Ganser, Ger. psychiatrist, 1853–1931] Factitious disorder, q.v.

Gantanol. Trade name for sulfamethoxazole.

Gantrisin. Trade name for sulfisoxazole.

gap [Old Norse *gap,* chasm]. An opening or a break; an interruption in continuity.

g., auscultatory. A period of silence that sometimes occurs in the determination of blood pressure by the auscultatory method. The exact cause is unknown, but it may occur in patients with hypertension or aortic stenosis. SEE: *blood pressure.*

Garamycin. Trade name for gentamicin sulfate.

Garamycin Ophthalmic. Trade name for gentamicin sulfate.

Gardnerella vaginalis. [Herman Gardner, contemporary U.S. physician] A bacterium that may cause vaginitis in otherwise healthy women. Formerly called Hemophilus vaginalis or Corynebacterium vaginale.

Gardnerella vaginalis vaginitis. Vaginitis due to the bacterium Gardnerella vaginalis (formerly termed either Hemophilus vaginalis or Corynebacterium vaginale). The bacilli are usually gram-negative but may be gram-variable in old cultures. The disease is most probably sexually transmitted. Diagnosis is best made clinically rather than microbiologically in that Gardnerella are often found in healthy, asymptomatic individuals. Clinically, there is a characteristic malodorous discharge, elevated vaginal pH, and wet preparation of vaginal epithelial cells that are heavily stippled with bacteria. These are called "clue cells." This disease may be due to the combined action of Gardnerella vaginalis and anaerobic bacteria rather than the former alone.

TREATMENT: metronidazole.

Gardner's syndrome. [Eldon J. Gardner, 20th-century U.S. geneticist] Familial polyposis of the colon associated with a high risk of developing carcinoma of the colon. Also present are multiple osteomas and soft-tissue tumors of the skin. The condition is inherited as an autosomal dominant trait.

gargarism (găr'găr-ĭzm) [Gr. *gargarisma*]. A gargle or throat wash.

gargle [L. *gurgulio,* windpipe]. 1. A wash for the throat. 2. To wash out the mouth and throat by tipping the head back, allowing the fluid to accumulate in the back of the throat while agitating it by the forceful expiration of air.

gargoylism (găr'goyl-ĭsm). A condition, usually congenital, characterized by dwarfism, kyphosis, and other skeletal abnormalities, disturbances in lipoid metabolism, and usually mental deficiency. SYN: *Hurler's syndrome; lipochondrodystrophy.*

garlic [AS. *gar,* spear, + *leac,* the leek]. An edible, strongly flavored bulb of Allium sativum used mainly for seasoning. The active principle of garlic is allyl sulfide. Garlic may have medicinal properties.

Garré's disease (găr-āz'). [Carl Garré, Swiss surgeon, 1858–1928] Chronic sclerosing osteitis or osteomyelitis due to pyogenic cocci.

Gartner's duct. [Hermann T. Gartner, Danish surgeon and anatomist, 1785–1827] A small duct lying parallel to the uterine tube. It is a vestigial structure representing the persistent mesonephric duct. SYN: *duct of the epoophoron; ductus epoophori longitudinalis* [NA].

G.A.S. *general adaptation syndrome.* SEE: *stress.*

gas. One of the basic forms of matter. The molecules are free and move swiftly in all directions. Thus a gas not only takes the shape of the containing vessel but expands and fills the vessel no matter what its volume. Among the common important gases are oxygen; nitrogen; hydrogen; helium; sewer gas, which contains carbon monoxide; carbon dioxide; the anesthetic gases; ammonia; and the poisonous war gases. Liquids and solids when heated often give off fumes that may be poisonous; among the more common are the mineral acids, ammonia water, mercury and its compounds, cyanides, and zinc-containing metals. SEE: *anesthesia; g.'s, war.*

g., binary. Toxic nerve gas formed when two relatively harmless components are mixed. Devised for use in chemical warfare. SEE: *g.'s, war.*

g.'s, blood. The principal gases found in the blood are oxygen, nitrogen, and carbon dioxide. They may be dissolved in the plasma or they may exist in loose chemical combination with other compounds, as oxygen combined with hemoglobin.

g., Clayton. SEE: *Clayton gas.*

g., coal. A flammable, explosive, and toxic gas produced from the distillation of coal; it is used for heating and lighting. The principal constituents are methane, carbon monoxide, and hydrogen.

g.'s, digestive tract. Among the gases in the digestive tract are oxygen, nitrogen, hydrogen, carbon dioxide, methane, and in decomposition of proteins, hydrogen sulfide, indole, and skatole.

g., illuminating. A mixture of various combustible gases including hydrogen and carbon monoxide. Its poisonous effects are largely due to carbon monoxide, q.v.

g., inert. Gas such as helium, argon, neon, or krypton, which reacts little if at all with other substances.

g., laughing. Nitrous oxide, N_2O, which has analgesic and anesthetic properties and is commonly used for minor operations and some dental procedures.

g., lewisite. A poisonous gas that contains arsenic and has the odor of geraniums.

SYM: Similar to those of vesicant gas but come on at once and as a rule are not so severe. Arsenic can be recovered from the serum of the blisters and symptoms of arsenic poisoning may occur.

TREATMENT: Similar to that for vesicant gas. SEE: *g., vesicant; g.'s, war.*

g., lung irritant. A gas causing irritation of lungs, such as chlorine or phosgene.

SYM: Burning sensation of the eyes, nose, and throat; bronchitis and pneumonia. Sometimes followed by pulmonary edema and probably death.

TREATMENT: Remove patient from exposure and apply respirator. If the patient was exposed to phosgene (which has the odor of musty hay), the symptoms may be delayed and the patient may collapse later. It is important, therefore, to provide complete rest, remove patient on a stretcher, and provide warmth. Oxygen may be required in large quantities over a fairly long period. SEE: *g.'s, war.*

g., marsh. Methane.

g., mustard. Dichlorethyl sulfide. Poisonous gas used in warfare. SEE: *g., vesicant; g.'s, war.*

g., nerve. A gas that acts by interfering with or preventing transmission of nerve impulses. SEE: *g.'s, war.*

g., nose irritant. Diphenylchloroarsine, an irritant smoke.

SYM: Intense pain in the nose, throat, and air passages; sneezing followed by headache and aching in teeth and jaws; acute mental depression; and sometimes vomiting.

TREATMENT: Patients must be reassured that no permanent harm is done and should be warned against removing respirator in spite of the fact that the symptoms may get worse after donning it. Nasal douching with warm sodium bicarbonate is helpful. SEE: *g.'s, war.*

g., sewer. Gas produced by decaying matter in sewage. It is toxic and usually flammable, and explosive.

g., suffocating. Any of several war gases, such as phosgene, or diphosgene, made from chlorine compounds. It causes irritation of bronchi and lungs, resulting in pulmonary edema. SEE: *g., lung irritant; g.'s, war.*

g., tear. A gas such as bromoacetone that irritates the conjunctiva and produces a flow of tears.

TREATMENT: As a rule, none is necessary. When the victim is removed from the contaminated area, the symptoms tend to subside gradually. Irrigating the eyes with large amounts of clear water or physiological saline will hasten recovery.

g., toxic. Hydrocyanic acid type gas. Any harmful gas.

g., vesicant. A type of gas that attacks the skin in every part of the body, causing blisters. Clothing and boots become contaminated and a source of danger. Mustard and lewisite gas are examples.

SYM: Symptoms do not appear at once; may be six hours or longer before the patient is aware of anything being wrong. Pain in the eyes, lacrimation, and discharge may be the first evidence. The eyelids swell and the patient is unable to see. There is a diffuse redness of the skin followed by blistering and ulceration.

TREATMENT: Decontamination is essential and must be thorough. Bathe eyes freely with normal saline or plain water; a drop or two of castor oil will prevent lids sticking; no bandage should be worn. The patient should be scrubbed, if possible, under a hot or warm shower for 10 minutes. If, in spite of these precautionary measures, blisters arise, they should be treated with a mild antiseptic and a protective dressing.

PROG: Healing is very slow, but generally complete if correct treatment is promptly begun.

g., vomiting. Gas that induces emesis, specifically chloropicrin.

g.'s, war. Any chemical substances, whether solid, liquid, or vapor, used to produce poisonous gases with irritant effects. They can be classified as lacrimators, sternutators (sneeze-causing), lung irritants, vesicants, and those that act as a systemic poison such as nerve gas. Some gases have multiple effects.

Gases are known as persistent or nonpersistent, i.e., those that diffuse and are dispersed fairly rapidly and those that linger and evaporate slowly.

It is of great importance that persons rendering first aid should avoid becoming casualties. Precautions must be taken. Masks must be worn by rescuers as well as being fitted to the patients. Strict discipline must be maintained during gas raids in order to avoid panic. If gas training has been thorough and if organization is good, much may be done to lessen the effect and maintain good morale.

Decontamination centers are essential and nurses must understand that thorough decontamination of clothing, boots, and ambulances is vital, and they should make themselves familiar with the necessary procedures. It is also important to remove all contaminated clothing prior to bringing the patient into the hospital emergency room. If this precaution is not taken, the unaffected persons in the area may become casualties.

gas bacillus. Term for Clostridium perfringens.

gas distention. Distention resulting from abnormal gaseous accumulation in the abdominal cavity. It may be acute, chronic, local, or general, and may involve the abdominal wall, or intra-abdominal viscera in addition to the cavity. A preoperative enema may prevent gas formation. Gas can develop postoperatively as a complication of surgery. It is usually limited to the lower part of the small intestine and all of the large intestine.

TREATMENT: No cold fluids. Change of posture insertion of a rectal tube. Enema only as advised by surgeon.

gaseous. Of the nature or form of gas.

gas excretions. Carbon dioxide, which is excreted through the lungs as a result of normal metabolic processes. The amount produced increases as physical activity increases.

gas gangrene. Gangrene, q.v., caused by Clostridium perfringens.

gasoline. A product of the destructive distillation of petroleum. Commercial gasolines may contain toxic additives such as tetraethyl lead or tricresyl phosphate.

CAUTION: The practice of using one's mouth to produce suction on a tube in order to siphon gasoline from a gas tank is dangerous because of the possibility of inhaling or swallowing this toxic substance.

gasoline poisoning. SYM: Giddiness; headache; intoxication; nervous disturbance; muscular tremors; difficulty in respiration; paralyses; convulsions; cyanosis; unconsciousness; pulmonary hemorrhage. Usually no local disturbance of stomach unless the gasoline has been swallowed.

F.A.: Fresh air, inhalation of oxygen and carbon dioxide; artificial respiration when necessary. Otherwise treat symptoms. If clothing and skin have been grossly contaminated, all precautions to prevent sparks and open flames must be taken. Gasoline is highly flammable and when mixed with air is also explosive.

gasometric (găs″ō-mĕt′rĭk). Pert. to measurement of gases.

gasometry (găs-ŏm′ĕ-trē). Estimation of amount of gas present in a mixture.

gasp [Old Norse *geispa*]. To catch the breath; to inhale and exhale with quick, difficult breaths; the act of gasping.

gas pains. Abdominal pain produced by distention by gas of all or part of the intestinal tract. May be a sign of postsurgical paralytic ileus. SEE: *flatulence*.

gasserectomy (găs″ĕr-ĕk′tō-mē). Excision of the gasserian ganglion. SEE: *ganglion, gasserian*.

gaster-, gastero-, gastro- [Gr. *gaster*, belly]. Combining forms indicating stomach or the region of the stomach.

gasteralgia (găs-tĕr-ăl′jē-ă) [″ + *algos*, pain]. Gastralgia.

Gasterophilus (găs″tĕr-ŏf′ĭ-lŭs). A genus of botflies belonging to the family Oestridae, order of Diptera. The larvae infest horses.

G. hemorrhoidalis. A species that infests horses.

G. intestinalis. Botflies that infest the stomachs of horses.

G. nasalis. The chin fly. Eggs are laid on shafts of hair on the lower lip and jaw of horses.

gastorrhagia (găs-tor-ā′jē-ă) [″ + *rhegnynai*, to burst forth]. Gastrorrhagia.

gastradenitis (găs″trăd-ĕn-ī′tĭs) [″ + *aden*, gland, + *itis*, inflammation]. Inflammation of the stomach glands.

gastralgia (găs-trăl′jē-ă) [″ + *algos*, pain]. Pain in the stomach from any cause.

gastralgokenosis (găs-trăl″gō-kĕn-ō′sĭs) [″ + *algos*, pain, + *kenosis*, emptiness]. Gastric pain due to emptiness of stomach; hunger pangs due to hunger contractions; powerful peristaltic contractions that sweep over the stomach.

gastratrophia (găs″tră-trō′fē-ă) [″ + *atrophia*, atrophy]. Atrophy of the stomach.

gastrectasia, gastrectasis [″ + *ektasis*, dilatation]. Dilatation of the stomach. May be acute or chronic.

ETIOL: Obstruction of pylorus; atony, overeating, omental hernia, periduodenal adhesions.

SYM: *Acute:* Severe, sudden pain accompanied by collapse. Small rapid pulse, temperature subnormal, upper abdominal pain resembling angina pectoris. Distended and tympanic abdomen. Vomiting of fluids and eructation of gas. *Chronic:* Vomiting of food taken several days before. Vomitus is sour and contains fatty acids, mucus, and bacteria.

gastrectomy (găs-trĕk′tō-mē) [″ + *ektome*, excision]. Surgical removal of a part or the whole of the stomach.

gastric (găs′trĭk) [Gr. *gaster*, stomach]. Pert. to the stomach. SEE: *digestion; stomach*.

gastric analysis. Analysis to determine quality of secretion, amount of free and combined hydrochloric acid, absence or presence of blood, bile, bacteria, fatty acids. The test is particularly helpful in suspected cases of gastric bleeding, gastric carcinoma, or pernicious anemia.

gastric digestion. The phase of digestion that occurs in the stomach. The stomach serves as a temporary storage and mixing place for food. The semisolid mass of food known as chyme is mixed with the salivary juices, and certain other substances are added from the stomach, including hydrochloric acid, mucus, pepsin and some lipase.

CHEM. ASPECTS: During the meal, stimuli from the brain are carried to the stomach by way of the vagi; they result from the sensations of sight, smell, and taste. In addition, the stretching of the stomach wall stimulates the gastric glands. This causes the hormone gastrin to be discharged from the pyloric region into the blood. The circulating gastrin reaches the gastric glands and causes them to secrete.

The following changes occur in the food while in the stomach. Pepsin acts on proteins of high molecular weight, hydrolyzing them to proteoses and peptones. Pepsin also coagulates milk. Hydrochloric acid is essential for the activity of pepsin. It also dissolves collagen, splits nucleoproteins, hydrolyzes disaccharides, and is responsible for the antiseptic action of the gastric juice. Gastric lipase acts on emulsified fats, reducing them to fatty acids and glycerol. SEE: *digestion.*

MOTOR ASPECTS: After the initial relaxation, the stomach increases its pressure upon its contents. The cardiac sphincter closes firmly to prevent regurgitation into the esophagus. The pyloric part of the stomach begins to exhibit wavelets of contraction that travel toward the pylorus. They become deeper, and their focus of origin shifts in the direction of the cardia. At first the pylorus, like the cardia, remains firmly closed and the wavelets result only in mixing and in facilitating the chemical comminution and solution. Now the pylorus begins to open occasionally, allowing the acid chyme to spurt at intervals into the duodenum. The further course of the chyme is described under *digestion, duodenal.* How quickly the chyme leaves the stomach is influenced by the amount of the feeding, its osmotic character and the amount of fat present. In general, a high-fat-content meal will leave the stomach at a slower rate than a low-fat meal.

gastric glands. Cardiac, fundic or oxyntic, and pyloric excretory glands of the stomach. These are tubular glands lying in the mucosa of the wall. The general result of gastric digestion is the reduction of the ingested mass to a mushy, gray mixture called acid chyme. Gastric glands contain zymogenic, or peptic cells, which secrete pepsinogen, the inactive form of pepsin; parietal border, or oxyntic cells, which secrete hydrochloric acid; and mucous cells found in the neck of the gland, which secrete mucin.

gastricism (găs′trĭ-sĭzm) [Gr. *gaster,* stomach, + *-ismos,* condition]. Any disease of the stomach.

gastric juice. The digestive juice of the gastric glands of the stomach. It is a thin colorless fluid containing pepsin, hydrochloric acid, mucin, small quantities of inorganic salts, and the intrinsic factor of the antianemic principle. It is strongly acid, having a pH of 0.9 to 1.5, its total acidity being equivalent to 10 to 50 ml. of tenth-normal (10%) hydrochloric acid; free HCl is from 0 to 30 ml. of tenth-normal HCl. The amount secreted in 24 hours varies greatly. The mixture of acid and pepsin has effects that neither substance has alone, and acts upon some proteins with remarkable speed. There is also a lipase that can release butyric fat from butterfat and this gives the characteristic odor to vomitus.

DIAG: *Achlorhydria:* Pernicious anemia is the most common cause of this finding in persons who do not have gastric cancer. *Carcinoma:* Boas-Oppler bacilli, sarcinae, blood, and sometimes tumor cells are present; frequently no hydrochloric acid is found. *Hyperacidity:* May indicate gastric ulcer. *Lactic acid:* Present in carcinoma. *Pus cells:* Indicate severe inflammation of the stomach. *Red cells:* Same significance as pus cells plus evidence of hemorrhage.

RS: digestion; gastric analysis; hydrochloric acid; hyperchlorhydria; hypochlorhydria; stomach.

gastric lavage. Washing out of the stomach. Used to empty stomach when contents are irritating, as in prolonged postanesthetic vomiting and in some cases of regurgitant vomiting in acute intestinal obstruction. Also to clean cavity before an operation is performed upon it; to remove poison in cases in which this method of treatment is indicated; and to remove a test meal.

METHOD: Prop patient up in bed if possible. A rubber sheet and towel are placed around the neck and arranged to protect clothing in front. The apparatus required is an esophageal tube with plastic or glass connection; a length of rubber tubing and a funnel; several pints of solution and a solution thermometer; glycerine to lubricate tube; a towel and container for vomitus (patient may hold this); a vessel for measuring amount of returned fluid; a container for stomach contents; and sodium bicarbonate solution, 4 gm. to a pint (473 ml.) of water prepared at a temperature of 100° F. (37.8° C.).

Explain the procedure to the patient if the patient is capable of understanding. Clean the patient's mouth and ask him or her to swallow the lubricated tube that is placed in the mouth. Encourage the patient to control the desire to retch. As the tube is swallowed, gently help to pass it along. When a special mark on the tube is on a level with the patient's lips, the tube should be in the stomach, and the funnel is attached to the glass connection by a short length of rubber tubing and is then inverted to empty the stomach of its contents. If nothing is seen, the tube should be passed farther in until it is in the stomach.

CAUTION: Prior to attempting to instill liquids into the stomach via the tube, be certain that end of tube is in stomach and not in bronchus. If proper placement of the tube is in doubt, careful instillation of a very small amount of sterile water will help to demonstrate the location of the tube. If the tube is in the bronchus, the air will cause the water to return during expiration. Foods or nutritional substances as ordered by the physician are fed slowly.

If possible, collect stomach contents in vessel provided. Then pinch the tube below funnel and fill the funnel with solution, expel air from the tube by pinching and rubbing it upward toward the funnel. Let fluid run in very slowly, using from ½ to 1 pt. (237 to 473 ml.) at a time; invert funnel and let this run out; repeat until all fluid has been used or until it returns clear. When the treatment is finished, pinch tube and withdraw it quickly, giving patient a mouthwash immediately, and then place soiled tube in a basin of tepid water. The siphoned gastric contents should be examined, and the amount of returned solution measured and inspected for blood, bile, and mucus. If necessary, it should be saved for the doctor's inspection or labeled and specimen sent to laboratory if so ordered.

gastricsin (găs-trĭk'sĭn). A proteolytic enzyme present in gastric secretions.

gastric ulcer. An ulcer of the stomach. SYN: *peptic ulcer.*

gastrin. A group of hormones secreted by the mucosa of the pyloric area of the stomach in various species of animals, including man. The hormones are released into gastric venous blood, from which it flows into the liver and into the general circulation. When the hormones reach the glands of the stomach, gastric acid secretion is stimulated. Gastrins also affect the secretory activity of the gallbladder, pancreas, and small intestine. Gastrins are released in response to meat extracts, ethyl alcohol in about 10% concentration, and by distention of the antrum of the stomach.

gastrinoma (găs"trĭn-ō'mă). The tumor associated with Zollinger-Ellison syndrome, q.v.

gastritis (găs-trī'tĭs) [" + *itis,* inflammation]. Inflammation of the stomach. Characterized by epigastric pain or tenderness, nausea, vomiting, and systemic electrolyte changes if vomiting persists. The mucosa may be atrophic or hypertrophic.

ETIOL: Generally unknown. May result from infection, excessive indulgence in alcoholic beverages, dietary indiscretions. Pain in the region of the stomach may be due to causes other than gastritis, such as cancer. Gastritis may be due to an excess or a deficiency of hydrochloric acid.

g., acute. SYM: Moderate fever; anorexia, coated tongue; intense pain in epigastrium; persistent vomiting; thirst; prostration.

TREATMENT: Symptomatic, because the process heals spontaneously. If massive bleeding persists, surgery may be required.

g., atrophic. Chronic gastritis with atrophied mucosa and glands.

g., chronic. SYM: Usually asymptomatic but one or more of the following may be present: mild nausea and anorexia; sense of distention or fullness after eating a small meal; bad taste in mouth; pain over epigastrium may be mild or acute.

TREATMENT: Antispasmodics, antacids, reassurance and sedatives.

g., giant hypertrophic. Gastritis with excessive proliferation of the folds of mucosa of the stomach.

g., hypertrophic. Gastritis combined with glandular hypertrophy and infiltration.

g., toxic. Gastritis due to any toxic agent, including poisons, or corrosive chemicals.

gastro- [Gr. *gaster,* stomach]. Used as a combining form to denote the stomach.

gastroanastomosis (găs"trō-ăn-ăs"tō-mō'sĭs) [" + *anastomosis,* outlet]. Formation of passage between the pyloric and cardiac ends of the stomach for relief of hourglass contraction.

gastrocamera (găs"trō-kăm'ĕ-ră). A camera small enough to be swallowed. Used to photograph the inside of the stomach.

gastrocardiac (găs"trō-kăr'dē-ăk) [" + *kardia,* heart]. Concerning the stomach and the heart.

gastrocele (găs'trō-sēl) [" + *kele,* hernia]. Hernia of the stomach.

gastrocnemius (găs"trŏk-nē'mē-ŭs) [" + *kneme,* leg]. The large muscle of the posterior portion of the lower leg. It is the most superficial of the calf muscles. Extends foot and helps to flex knee upon thigh.

gastrocolic (găs"trō-kŏl'ĭk) [" + *kolon,* colon]. Pert. to stomach and colon.

gastrocolic omentum. The greater omentum. SYN: *epiploon.*

gastrocolic reflex. Peristaltic wave in colon induced by entrance of food into fasting stomach.

gastrocolitis (găs"trō-kō-lī'tĭs) [" + " + *itis,* inflammation]. Inflammation of the stomach and colon.

gastrocoloptosis (găs"trō-kŏl"ŏp-tō'sĭs) [" + " + *ptosis,* dropping]. Downward prolapse of stomach and colon.

gastrocolostomy (găs"trō-kŏl-ŏs'tō-mē) [" + " + *stoma,* opening]. Establishment of a permanent passage between the stomach and colon.

gastrocolotomy (găs"trō-kō-lŏt'ō-mē) [" + " + *tome,* incision]. Incision into stomach and colon.

gastrocolpotomy (găs"trō-kŏl-pŏt'ō-mē) [" + *kolpos,* vagina, + *tome,* incision]. An incision through the abdominal wall into upper part of the vagina.

gastrocutaneous (găs"trō-kū-tā'nē-ŭs) [" + *cutis,* skin]. Concerning the stomach and skin, or a communication between the two.

gastrodialysis (găs"trō-dī-ăl'ĭ-sĭs) [" + *dia,* through, + *lysis,* dissolution]. 1. Dialysis, i.e., washing out, of the stomach in order to help clear both the stomach and the blood of toxic materials that are secreted into the stomach. 2. Sloughing of the mucosa of the stomach.

gastrodiaphane (găs″trō-dī′ă-fān) [″ + *dia,* through, + *phainein,* to show]. Device for electrically illuminating stomach interior, making its outlines visible through the abdomen.

gastrodiaphanoscopy (găs″trō-dī-ăf″ă-nŏs′kō-pē) [″ + ″ + ″ + *skopein,* to examine]. Examination of interior of the stomach by rendering its walls translucent by an electric light, introduced through the esophagus into the stomach.

gastrodiaphany (găs″trō-dī-ăf′ă-nē). Transillumination of the stomach. SEE: *gastrodiaphanoscopy.*

gastrodidymus (găs″trō-dĭd′ĭ-mŭs) [″ + *didymos,* twin]. Congenitally deformed twins united by a common abdominal cavity.

gastrodisciasis (găs″trō-dĭs-kī′ă-sĭs). Infestation by a fluke, Gastrodiscoides hominis.

Gastrodiscoides (găs″trō-dĭs-koy′dēz). A genus of flukes belonging to family Gastrodiscidae, suborder Amphistomata.

G. hominis. A species of flukes commonly infesting hogs but occasionally found in man.

gastroduodenal (găs″trō-dū″ō-dēn′ăl) [Gr. *gaster,* stomach, + L. *duodeni,* twelve]. Rel. to the stomach and duodenum.

gastroduodenitis (găs″trō-dū-ŏd″ĕn-ī′tĭs) [″ + ″ + Gr. *itis,* inflammation]. Inflammation of stomach and duodenum.

gastroduodenoscopy (găs″trō-dū″ō-dĕ-nŏs′kō-pē) [″ + ″ + *skopein,* to examine]. Use of an endoscope for visual examination of the stomach and duodenum.

gastroduodenostomy (găs″trō-dū″ō-dĕn-ŏs′tō-mē) [″ + ″ + Gr. *stoma,* mouth]. Formation of an artificial opening between the stomach and duodenum.

gastrodynia (găs″trō-dĭn′ē-ă) [″ + *odyne,* pain]. Pain in the stomach. SYN: *gastralgia.*

gastroenteralgia (găs″trō-ĕn″tĕr-ăl′jē-ă) [″ + *enteron,* intestine, + *algos,* pain]. Pain in stomach and intestines.

gastroenteric (găs″trō-ĕn-tĕr′ĭk). Pert. to stomach and intestines or to a condition involving both.

gastroenteritis (găs″trō-ĕn-tĕr-ī′tĭs) [″ + *enteron,* intestine, + *itis,* inflammation]. Inflammation of the stomach and intestinal tract.

gastroenteroanastomosis (găs″trō-ĕn″tĕr-ō-ă-năs″tō-mō′sĭs). Surgically joining the stomach to the small intestine.

gastroenterocolitis (găs″trō-ĕn″tĕr-ō-kŏl-ī′tĭs) [″ + ″ + *kolon,* colon, + *itis,* inflammation]. Inflammation of the stomach, small intestine, and colon.

gastroenterocolostomy (găs″trō-ĕn″tĕr-ō-kō-lŏs′tō-mē) [″ + ″ + ″ + *stoma,* opening]. Creation of a passage between the stomach, small intestine, and colon.

gastroenterology (găs″trō-ĕn″tĕr-ŏl′ō-jē) [″ + ″ + *logos,* study]. The branch of medical science concerned with study of the physiology and pathology of the stomach, intestines, and related structures such as the esophagus, liver, gallbladder, and pancreas.

gastroenteropathy (găs″trō-ĕn″tĕr-ŏp′ă-thē). Any disease of the gastrointestinal tract.

gastroenteroptosis (găs″trō-ĕn″tĕr-ŏp-tō′sĭs) [″ + ″ + *ptosis,* a dropping]. Prolapse of stomach and intestines.

gastroenterostomy (găs″trō-ĕn-tĕr-ŏs′tō-mē) [″ + *enteron,* intestine, + *stoma,* opening]. Surgical anastomosis between the stomach and small bowel. This operation is required for patients who are suffering from carcinoma or cicatricial stricture of the pyloric orifice of the stomach.

gastroenterotomy (găs″trō-ĕn″tĕr-ŏt′ō-mē) [″ + ″ + *tome,* incision]. Incision of stomach and intestine through abdominal wall.

gastroepiploic (găs″trō-ĕp″ĭ-plō′ĭk) [″ + *epiploon,* omentum]. Pert. to stomach and greater omentum.

gastroesophageal (găs″trō-ĕ-sŏf″ă-jē′ăl) [″ + *oisophagos,* esophagus]. Concerning the stomach and esophagus.

gastroesophagitis (găs″trō-ē-sŏf″ă-jī′tĭs) [″ + ″ + *itis,* inflammation]. Inflammation of stomach and esophagus.

gastroesophagostomy (găs″trō-ē-sŏf″ă-gŏs′tō-mē) [″ + ″ + *tome,* incision]. Formation of passage from the esophagus into the stomach.

gastrofiberscope (găs″trō-fī′bĕr-skōp). A flexible endoscope, utilizing fiber optics, for visual examination of the stomach.

gastrogastrostomy (găs″trō-găs-trŏs′tō-mē) [″ + ″ + *stoma,* opening]. Surgical formation of passage in persistent hourglass contraction of the stomach between the two gastric pouches. SYN: *gastroanastomosis.*

gastrogavage (găs″trō-gă-văzh′) [″ + Fr. *gavage,* cramming]. Artificial feeding through an opening into the stomach or a tube passed into the stomach.

gastrogenic (găs″trō-jĕn′ĭk) [Gr. *gaster,* stomach, + *gennan,* to produce]. Having its origin in the stomach.

gastrohelcosis (găs″trō-hĕl-kō′sĭs) [″ + *helkos,* ulcer]. Ulcer of the stomach.

gastrohepatic [″ + *hepar,* liver]. Pert. to stomach and liver.

gastrohepatitis (găs″trō-hĕp-ă-tī′tĭs) [″ + ″ + *itis,* inflammation]. Combination of gastritis and hepatitis.

gastroileac (găs-trō-ĭl′ē-ăk) [″ + L. *ileum,* groin]. Pert. to stomach and ileum.

gastroileac reflex. Physiologic relaxation of ileocecal valve resulting from food in stomach.

gastroileitis (găs″trō-ĭl-ē-ī′tĭs). Inflammation of the stomach and ileum.

gastroileostomy (găs″trō-ĭl-ē-ŏs′tō-mē). Surgical anastomosis between the stomach and ileum.

gastrointestinal [″ + L. *intestinalis,* intestine]. Pert. to stomach and intestine.

gastrointestinal bleeding. Bleeding from the gastrointestinal tract. This is an important sign. It requires prompt therapy, and its cause must be determined.

gastrointestinal decompression. Drainage of gases from the intestinal tract by use of suction through a tube inserted through the nostrils and into the digestive tract. SEE: *Wangensteen's method.*

gastrojejunostomy (găs-trō-jĕ-jū-nŏs′tō-mē) [″ + L. *jejunum,* empty, + Gr. *stoma,* opening]. Surgical anastomosis between the stomach and jejunum.

gastrolienal (găs″trō-lī′ĕn-ăl) [″ + L. *lien,* spleen]. Concerning the stomach and spleen.

gastrolith (găs′trō-lĭth) [″ + *lithos,* stone]. A calculus in the stomach.

gastrolithiasis (găs″trō-lĭth-ī′ă-sĭs) [″ + *lithos,* stone]. Formation of calculi in the stomach.

gastrology (găs-trŏl′ō-jē) [″ + *logos,* study]. Study of function and diseases of the stomach.

gastrolysis (găs-trŏl′ĭ-sĭs) [″ + *lysis,* loosening]. Surgical breaking of adhesions between stomach and adjoining structures.

gastromalacia (găs-trō-mă-lā′shē-ă) [″ + *malakia,* softening]. Softening of the stomach walls.

gastromegaly (găs″trō-mĕg′ă-lē) [″+ *megas,* large]. Enlargement of the stomach.

gastromycosis (găs″trō-mī-kō′sĭs) [″ + *mykes,* fungus, + *osis,* condition]. Disease of the stomach due to fungi.

gastromyotomy (găs″trō-mī-ŏt′ō-mē) [″ + *mys,* muscle, + *tome,* incision]. Incision of circular muscle fibers of the stomach.

gastromyxorrhea (găs″trō-mĭks″ō-rē′ă) [″+ *myxa,* mucus, + *rhoia,* flow]. Excessive secretion of gastric mucus.

gastronephritis (găs″trō-nĕ-frī′tĭs) [″ + *nephros,* kidney, + *itis,* inflammation]. Inflammation of the stomach and kidney at same time.

gastropancreatitis (găs″trō-păn″krē-ă-tī′tĭs) [″ + *pan,* all, + *kreas,* flesh, + *itis,* inflammation]. Inflammation of the stomach and pancreas at same time.

gastroparalysis (găs″trō-păr-ăl′ĭ-sĭs) [″ + *para,* beyond, + *lyein,* to loosen]. Paralysis of the stomach.

gastropathy (găs-trŏp′ă-thē) [″ + *pathos,* disease]. Any disorder of the stomach.

gastropexy, gastropexis (găs′trō-pĕk″sē, -sĭs) [″ + *pexis,* fixation]. Suturing of the stomach to the abdominal walls for correction of displacement.

gastrophrenic (găs″trō-frĕn′ĭk) [Gr. *gaster,* stomach, + *phren,* diaphragm]. Rel. to the stomach and diaphragm.

gastroplasty (găs′trō-plăs″tē) [″ + *plassein,* to form]. Plastic surgery on the stomach.

gastroplegia (găs″trō-plē′jē-ă) [″ + *plege,* stroke]. Paralysis of the stomach.

gastroplication (găs″trō-plī-kā′shŭn) [″ + L. *plicare,* to fold]. Stitching the walls of the stomach to reduce dilatation.

gastroptosis (găs″trō-tō′sĭs) [″ + *ptosis,* falling]. Downward displacement of the stomach. This rarely if ever causes symptoms or illness.

gastropulmonary (găs″trō-pŭl′mō-năr-ē) [″ + L. *pulmo,* lung]. Concerning the stomach and the lungs.

gastropylorectomy (găs″trō-pī″lor-ĕk′tō-mē) [″ + *pyloros,* pylorus, + *ektome,* excision]. Excision of stomach at pyloric end.

gastropyloric. Rel. to stomach and pylorus.

gastroradiculitis (găs″trō-ră-dĭk″ū-lī′tĭs) [″ + L. *radix,* root, + Gr. *itis,* inflammation]. Inflammation of the posterior spinal nerve roots, the sensory fibers of which supply the stomach.

gastrorrhagia (găs″trō-rā′jē-ă) [″ + *rhegnynai,* to burst forth]. Hemorrhage from the stomach.

gastrorrhaphy (găs-tror′ă-fē) [″ + *rhaphe,* suture]. 1. Suture of an injured stomach wall. 2. Gastroplication.

gastrorrhea (găs-trō-rē′ă) [″ + *rhoia,* flow]. An excessive secretion of gastric juice.

gastroschisis (găs-trŏs′kĭ-sĭs) [″ + *schisis,* cleft]. A congenital fissure that remains open in the wall of the abdomen.

gastroscope (găs′trō-skōp) [″ + *skopein,* to examine]. An endoscope for inspecting the stomach's interior.

gastroscopy (găs-trŏs′kō-pē). Examination of the stomach and abdominal cavity by a gastroscope.

gastrospasm (găs′trō-spăzm) [″ + *spasmos,* spasm]. A spasm of the stomach.

gastrosplenic (găs″trō-splĕn′ĭk) [″ + *splen,* spleen]. Of or pert. to stomach and spleen.

gastrostaxis (găs″trō-stăk′sĭs) [″ + *staxis,* trickling]. Oozing of blood from the mucosa of the stomach.

gastrostenosis (găs″trō-stĕn-ō′sĭs) [″ + *stenosis,* narrowing]. Contracted state of the stomach.

g. cardiaca. Stenosis of cardiac orifice of the stomach.

g. pylorica. Stenosis of pylorus of the stomach.

gastrostogavage (găs-trŏs″tō-gă-văzh′) [″ + *stoma,* opening, + Fr. *gaver,* to stuff]. Feeding by means of a tube leading from outside the body into the stomach through a gastric fistula. SEE: *gavage.*

gastrostolavage (găs-trŏs″tō-lă-văzh′) [″ + Fr. *lavage,* fr. L. *lavare,* to wash]. Irrigation of the stomach through a gastric fistula, or surgically constructed gastrostomy.

gastrostoma (găs-trŏs′tō-mă) [″ + *stoma,* opening]. A fistula of the stomach.

gastrostomy (găs-trŏs′tō-mē). Surgical creation of a gastric fistula through the abdominal wall. It is necessary in carcinoma and in some cases of cicatricial stricture of the esophagus for the purpose of introducing food into the stomach.

NURSING IMPLICATIONS: Keep the skin around the gastrostomy tube clean and dry, and protect the skin from excoriating gastric secretions. After feedings, flush the tube with water to prevent clogging. Teach the patient and family correct technique for care and feeding through the gastrostomy tube. Oral hygiene should be done at least once a day.

gastrosuccorrhea (găs″trō-sŭk″or-ē′ă) [″ + L. *succus,* juice, + Gr. *rhoia,* flow]. An excessive secretion of gastric juice with increased acidity. SYN: *hypersecretion.*

gastrotherapy (găs″trō-thĕr′ă-pē) [″ + *therapeia,* treatment]. Treatment of gastric diseases.

gastrothoracopagus (găs″trō-thō″ră-kŏp′ă-gŭs) [″ + *thorax,* chest, + *pagos,* thing fixed]. Congenitally deformed twins joined at the stomach and thorax.

gastrotome (găs′trō-tōm) [″ + *tome,* incision]. Instrument for incising stomach or abdomen.

gastrotomy (găs-trŏt′ō-mē) [″ + *tome,* incision]. Gastric or abdominal incision.

gastrotonometer (găs″trō-tō-nŏm′ĕ-tĕr) [″ + *tonos,* tension, + *metron,* measure]. Instrument for measuring intragastric pressure by insufflation of air or carbonic acid gas.

gastrotropic (găs″trō-trŏp′ĭk) [″ + *tropos,* turning]. Attracted to or affecting the stomach.

gastrotympanites (găs″trō-tĭm″pă-nī′tēz) [″ + *tympanites,* distention]. Distention of the stomach by gas or air.

gastrula (găs′troo-lă). [L., little belly]. Stage in embryonic development following the blastula in which the embryo assumes a two-layered condition. The outer layer is the ectoderm or epiblast; the inner layer, the endoderm or hypoblast. The latter lines a cavity, the gastrocoele or archenteron, that opens to the outside through an opening, the blastopore.

gastrulation (găs″troo-lā′shŭn). The development of the gastrula in the embryo.

Gatch bed. [Willis D. Gatch, U.S. surgeon, 1878–1961] A bed in which the patient can be raised and held in a half-sitting position.

gate theory. The hypothesis that painful stimuli may be prevented from reaching higher levels of the central nervous system by stimulation of larger sensory nerves. This is one of the proposed explanations of the action of acupuncture.

gatism (gā′tĭzm) [Fr. *gâter,* to spoil]. Vesical or rectal incontinence.

Gaucher, Philippe C. E. (gō-shā′). French physician, 1854–1918.

G.'s cells. Large reticuloendothelial cells seen in Gaucher's disease, q.v. They contain a small, eccentrically placed nucleus, and kerasin.

G.'s disease. A rare chronic congenital disorder of lipid metabolism. Fatty substances called glycosphingolipids accumulate in the reticuloendothelial cells. Associated with enlarged spleen, increased skin pigmentation, and bone lesions. SYN: *lipoidosis, cerebroside.*

gauge (gāj). 1. Device for measuring size, capacity, amount, or power of an object or substance. 2. A standard of measurement.

Gaultheria Oil. Trade name for a compound that contains methyl salicylate.

Gault's reflex (gawlts). Contraction of orbicularis palpebrarum muscle to produce a blinking of the eye following a loud noise close to the ear. The reflex is tested in cases of suspected malingering to feign deafness. SEE: *malingerer.*

gauntlet (gawnt′lĕt) [Fr. *gant,* glove]. A glove-like bandage that fits the hand and fingers.

gauss (gows). [Johann Karl F. Gauss, Ger. physicist, 1777–1855] The unit of intensity of a magnetic flux.

Gauss' sign (gows). [Carl J. Gauss, Ger. gynecologist, 1875–1957] Unusual mobility of the uterus in the early weeks of pregnancy.

gauze (gawz) [O. Fr. *gaze,* gauze]. Thin, loosely woven muslin or similar material used for bandages and surgical sponges.

g., absorbent. USP. Gauze made of specified amounts of cotton and rayon, or all cotton. It has been sterilized.

g., antiseptic. Gauze containing an antiseptic substance.

g., aseptic. A gauze that is sterilized. Often packaged in an aseptic container, usually paper, and ready for use.

g., petrolatum. USP. Absorbent gauze saturated with petrolatum. It has been sterilized.

gavage (gă-văzh′) [Fr. *gaver,* to stuff]. Feeding with a stomach tube or with a tube passed through the nares, pharynx, and esophagus into the stomach. The food is in liquid or semiliquid form at a temperature of about 100° F. (37.8°C.). SEE: *gastrostogavage.*

Gavard's muscle (gă-văr′). [Hyacinthe

Gavard, Fr. anatomist, 1753–1802] The oblique muscular fibers of the stomach's coat.

Gay's glands. [Alexander H. Gay, Russian anatomist, 1842–1907] Large sebaceous circumanal glands.

Gay-Lussac's law (gā″lū-săks′). [Joseph L. Gay-Lussac, Fr. naturalist, 1778–1850] Law stating that if pressure remains constant, the volume of a gas will vary directly with change in the absolute temperature. SYN: *Charles' law.* SEE: *Boyle's law.*

gaze (gāz). To look or stare intently in one direction.

Gd. Chem. symb. for gadolinium.

Ge. Chem. symb for germanium.

Gee, Samuel J. (gē). London physician, 1839–1911.

G.'s disease. Infantile nontropical sprue. Also called *Gee-Herter disease; Gee-Herter-Heubner disease.*

G.-Thaysen disease. Adult form of nontropical sprue.

gegenhalten (gā″gĕn-hălt′ĕn) [Ger.]. In cerebral cortical disease, involuntary resistance to passive movement.

Geigel's reflex (gī′gĕlz). [Richard Geigel, Ger. physician, 1859–1930] Reflex in females wherein there is a contraction of muscular fibers, adjacent to the superior portion of Poupart's ligaments, when the inner anterior aspect of the upper thigh is stroked. Corresponds to the cremasteric reflex, q.v., in males.

Geiger counter (gī′gĕr). [Hans Geiger, Ger. physicist in England, 1882–1945] An instrument for detecting ionizing radiation.

gel (jĕl) [L. *gelare,* to congeal]. A semisolid condition of a precipitated or coagulated colloid; jelly; a jellylike colloid. It contains a large amount of water.

g., aluminum hydroxide. USP. A white, viscous suspension of aluminum hydroxide used as an antacid.

gelasmus (jĕ-lăs′mŭs) [Gr. *gelasma,* a laugh]. 1. Spasmodic laughter of the insane. 2. Hysterical laughter.

gelate (jĕl′āt). To cause formation of a gel.

gelatin (jĕl′ă-tĭn) [L. *gelatina,* gelatin]. A derived protein obtained by the hydrolysis of collagen present in the connective tissues of the skin, bones, and joints of animals.

USES: As a food, in preparation of pharmaceuticals, and as a medium for culture of bacteria.

g., nutrient. Bacterial culture medium composed of broth and gelatin.

gelatinase. An enzyme present in bacteria, molds, and yeast that liquefies gelatin.

gelatin culture. Gelatinous base used for bacterial growth.

gelatiniferous (jĕl″ăt-ĭn-ĭf′ĕr-ŭs) [″ + *ferre,* to bear]. Producing gelatin.

gelatinize (jĕl-ăt′ĭn-īz) [L. *gelatina,* gelatin]. To convert into gelatin.

gelatinoid (jĕl-ăt′ĭn-oyd) [″ + Gr. *eidos,* form]. Resembling gelatin.

gelatinolytic (jĕl-ăt″ĭn-ō-lĭt′ĭk) [″ + Gr. *lysis,* dissolution]. Dissolution or splitting up of gelatin.

gelatinous (jĕl-ăt′ĭn-ŭs). Containing or of the consistency of gelatin.

gelatin sponge, absorbable. USP. Gelatin in the form of a sterile absorbable sponge. Used as a hemostat to control oozing of blood from minute vessels. Trade name is Gelfoam.

CAUTION: This material may seem to be effective when used at a time when blood pressure is decreased as could be the condition during surgery, but may fail as the patient becomes normotensive.

gelation (jĕl-ā′shŭn). The transformation of a colloid from a sol into a gel.

Gelfoam. Trade name for absorbable gelatin sponge that acts as a hemostat.

Gellé's test (zhĕl-āz′). [Marie Ernst Gellé, Fr. physician, 1834–1923] A tuning fork is connected with a rubber tube inserted in the ear. Pressure or suction in the tube is produced by an attached bulb. If ear is normal, vibrations are felt.

gelose (jĕ′lōs) [L. *gelare,* to congeal]. 1. Gelatinous element of agar, $(C_6H_{10}O_5)_n$. 2. Bacterial culture medium.

gelosis (jĕl-ō′sĭs). A hard lump that is so firm as to appear frozen. Occurs esp. in muscle tissue.

gelotherapy (jĕl″ō-thĕr′ă-pē) [Gr. *gelos,* laughter, + *therapeia,* treatment]. Inducing hilarity in treatment of certain forms of mental illness.

gelotripsy (jĕl′ō-trĭp″sē) [L. *gelare,* to congeal, + Gr. *tripsis,* a rubbing]. The massaging away of indurated swellings.

-gels. A word termination to indicate colloids in a solid state.

gemellipara (jĕm″ĕl-lĭp′ă-ră) [L. *gemelli,* twins, + *parere,* to produce]. One who has borne twins.

gemellology (gĕm″ĕl-ŏl′ō-jē) [L. *gemellus,* twin, + Gr. *logos,* study]. Study of twins.

gemellus (jĕm-ĕl′ŭs) [L., twin]. (pl. *gemelli*) Either of two muscles inserted in the obturator internus tendon.

geminate (jĕm′ĭ-nāt) [L. *geminatus,* paired]. In pairs.

gemination (jĕm-ĭ-nā′shŭn). 1. Development of two teeth or two crowns within a single root. 2. A doubling.

gemistocyte (jĕm-ĭs′tō-sīt) [Gr. *gemistos,* laden, full, + *kytos,* cell]. In the central nervous system, an astrocyte that is swollen and has an eccentric nucleus. Seen adjacent to areas of edema or infarct.

gemma (jĕm′mă) [L., bud]. 1. A small budlike

reproductive structure produced by lower forms of life. 2. Any small budlike structure such as a taste bud or end bulb.

gemmation (jĕm-mā′shŭn) [L. *gemmare,* to bud]. Cell reproduction by budding. Budlike processes or daughter cells, each containing chromatin, separate from the mother cell from which the bud is projected.

gemmule (jĕm′ūl) [L. *gemmula,* little bud]. 1. A gemma. 2. One of numerous minute processes present on the dendrites of a neuron.

gena (jē′nă) [L.]. The side of the face; cheek.

genal (jē′năl). Pert. to the cheek. SYN: *buccal.*

gender [L. *genus,* kind]. The sex of an individual, i.e., male or female.

gender identity. The sex classification of an individual.

g.i., mistaken. Assignment of incorrect sex to a newborn. This may lead to the individual's having a gender role opposite of the chromosomal sex.

gender role. The behavior and appearance of an individual with respect to the cultural classifications male and female. Gender role may, due to congenital or developmental abnormalities, be in contrast to the chromosomal sex.

gene (jēn) [Gr. *gennan,* to produce]. (pl. *genes*) The basic unit of heredity. Each gene occupies a certain location on a chromosome. They are self-producing, ultramicroscopic structures capable under certain circumstances of giving rise to a new character, such a change being called a mutation. Hereditary traits are controlled by pairs of genes in the same position on a pair of chromosomes. These gene pairs, or alleles, may both be dominant or both be recessive in their expression of that trait. In either of those cases the individual is said to be homozygous for the trait controlled by that gene pair. If the gene pair (alleles) consists of one dominant and one recessive gene, the individual is heterozygous for the trait controlled by that gene pair. SEE: *chromosome; DNA; RNA.*

g.'s, allelic. Pairs of genes located at the same site on chromosome pairs.

g.'s, complementary. Non-allelic, independent genes neither of which will express its effect without the presence of the other.

g., dominant. A gene that will express its effect without assistance from its allele.

g., histocompatibility. A gene that controls the specificity of the antigenic response of tissues. SEE: *HLA antigens.*

g., holandric. A gene located in the nonhomologous portion of the Y chromosome of males.

g., inhibiting. A gene that prevents the expression of another gene.

g., lethal. A gene that, when in a homozygous condition, brings about an effect that results in the death of an individual, usually in utero.

g., modifying. A gene that influences or alters the effect of another gene.

g., mutant. An altered gene that permanently functions in a different manner than it did prior to the alteration.

g., operator. It is postulated that certain genes have a role in controlling the actions of other genes. Such a gene is called an operon or operator gene.

g., pleiotropic. A gene that has multiple effects.

g., recessive. A gene that expresses its effect only when the gene is present in both chromosomes. Simplistically, a "double dose" is required.

g., regulator. Gene that can control some specific activity of another gene.

g., sex-linked. A gene contained within the X or Y chromosome.

g., structural. Gene that determines the structure of polypeptide chains by controlling the sequence of amino acids.

g., X-linked. A gene located on the X chromosome. The X and Y chromosomes determine sex.

genera. Pl. of genus.

general adaptation syndrome. ABBR: G.A.S. Syndrome described by Hans Selye, a contemporary Canadian physician, as the total organism's nonspecific response to stress, q.v. The response occurs in the following three stages: (1) Alarm reaction, wherein the body recognizes the stressor and the pituitary-adrenocortical system responds by producing the hormones essential to either flight or fight. In this stage heart rate increases, blood sugar is elevated, pupils dilate, and digestion slows. (2) Resistance or adaptive stage, in which the body begins to repair the effect of the arousal. The acute stress symptoms diminish or disappear. If, however, the stress continues, adaptation fails in its attempts to maintain the defense. (3) Exhaustion stage occurs when the body can no longer respond to the stress. As a consequence, one or several of a great variety of diseases such as emotional disturbances, cardiovascular and renal diseases, and certain types of asthma may develop. SEE: *stress.*

generalize [L. *generalis*]. 1. To become or render nonspecific. 2. To become systemic, as a local disease.

generation (jĕn″ĕr-ā′shŭn) [L. *generare,* to beget]. 1. An act of forming a new organism. 2. A group of animals or plants the same distance removed from an ancestor, as the first filial (F_1) generation. SEE: *filial generation.* 3. The average period of time between the birth of parents and the birth of their children. This could be 16 to 20 years in some cultures and 20 to 25 years in others. Also the time would be different if only female parents were considered in computing this average unless all marriages occurred between persons of the same age. 4. The production of an electric current.

g., alternate. A mode of reproduction in which sexual generation alternates with an asexual generation, characteristic of all plants above the Thallophytes. It also occurs in some of the lower animals.

g., asexual. Reproduction that occurs without the union of sexual elements or gametes, such as reproduction by fission or spore production.

g., filial. The offspring of a given mating or cross; F_1.

g., parental. In genetics, the generation in which a specific study is begun.

g., sexual. Reproduction by the union of male and female cells.

generative (jĕn′ĕr-ă-tĭv). Concerned in reproduction of or affecting the species.

generator (gĕn′ĕr-ā″tor). That which produces something, esp. a device that produces heat, electricity, or impulses.

g., pulse. Device that produces stimuli intermittently; thus a cardiac pacemaker requires this type of generator.

generic (jĕn-ĕr′ĭk) [L. *genus,* kind]. 1. General. 2. Pert. to a genus. 3. Distinctive.

generic name. The nonproprietary name of a drug or pharmaceutical preparation.

genesiology (jĕn-ē-zē-ŏl′ō-jē) [Gr. *genesis,* generation, + *logos,* science]. The science of reproduction.

genesis (jĕn′ĕ-sĭs). 1. Act of reproducing; generation. 2. The origin of anything.

gene splicing. In genetic molecular biology, the substitution of a portion of DNA is spliced into the DNA of another gene.

genetic (jĕn-ĕt′ĭk). Pert. to reproduction.

genetic code. The information system in living cells that determines the amino acid sequence in polypeptides. By this action all of the genetic information transmitted to an offspring is specified. The code is universal in that it applies to all living things.

genetic counseling. The application of what is known about human genetics in providing advice to those concerned about the possibility of their offspring being free of hereditary abnormality.

genetic engineering. The synthesis, alteration, or repair of genetic material by synthetic means.

geneticist (jĕn-ĕt′ĭ-sĭst) [Gr. *gennan,* to produce]. One who specializes in genetics.

genetics. The study of heredity and its variation.

g., biochemical. Science of the biochemistry of genes and chemical influences on the gene.

g., clinical. Clinical investigation of the importance of genetics in health and disease.

g., molecular. Study of genetics at the molecular level in contrast with the study of entire genes, or chromosomes. SEE: *gene splicing.*

genetopathy (jĕn-ĕ-tŏp′ă-thē) [Gr. *genesis,* generation, + *pathos,* disease]. Disease affecting reproductive function.

genetotrophic (jĕ-nĕt″ō-trŏf′ĭk). Concerning genetics and nutrition.

genetous (jĕ-nĕt′ŭs). Congenital.

Geneva Convention. In 1864 the major military powers met in Geneva, Switzerland, to establish regulations concerning the status of those wounded in military action on land. The result was that the sick and wounded and all those involved in their care including physicians, nurses, corpsmen, ambulance drivers, and chaplains were declared to be neutral and, therefore, would not be the target of military action. These provisions were expanded in 1868 to include naval military action. There is, unfortunately, much evidence that warring nations have not always abided by the provisions of this Convention.

genial (jē′nē-ăl) [Gr. *geneion,* chin]. Rel. to the chin.

genic (jĕn′ĭk) [Gr. *gennan,* to produce]. Rel. to or caused by genes.

-genic. Suffix indicating generation or production.

genicular (jĕ-nĭk′ū-lăr). Concerning the knee.

geniculate (jĕn-ĭk′ū-lāt) [L. *geniculare,* to bend the knee]. 1. Bent as a knee. 2. Pert. to the ganglion or geniculum of the facial nerve.

geniculate otalgia. Pain transmitted from the facial nerve to the ear.

geniculocalcarine tract. Radiation, optic, q.v.

geniculum (jĕn-ĭk′ū-lŭm) [L. *geniculum,* little knee]. A structure resembling a knot, or a knee. Indicates an abrupt bend or angle in a small structure.

genion (jē′nē-ŏn) [Gr. *geneion,* chin]. Apex of the spina mentalis.

genioplasty (jē′nē-ō-plăs″tē) [″ + *plassein,* to form]. Plastic surgery of the chin or cheek.

genital (jĕn′ĭ-tăl) [L. *genitalis,* belonging to birth]. Pert. to the genitals.

genital herpes. SEE: *herpes genitalis.*

genitalia, genitals (jĕn-ĭ-tāl′ē-ă, jĕn′ĭ-tăls). Organs of generation; reproductive organs.

g., female. Organs concerned with reproduction in the female sex. The external genitalia collectively are termed the vulva or pudendum and include the mons veneris, labia majora, labia minora, clitoris, fourchet, fossa navicularis, vestibule, vestibular bulb,

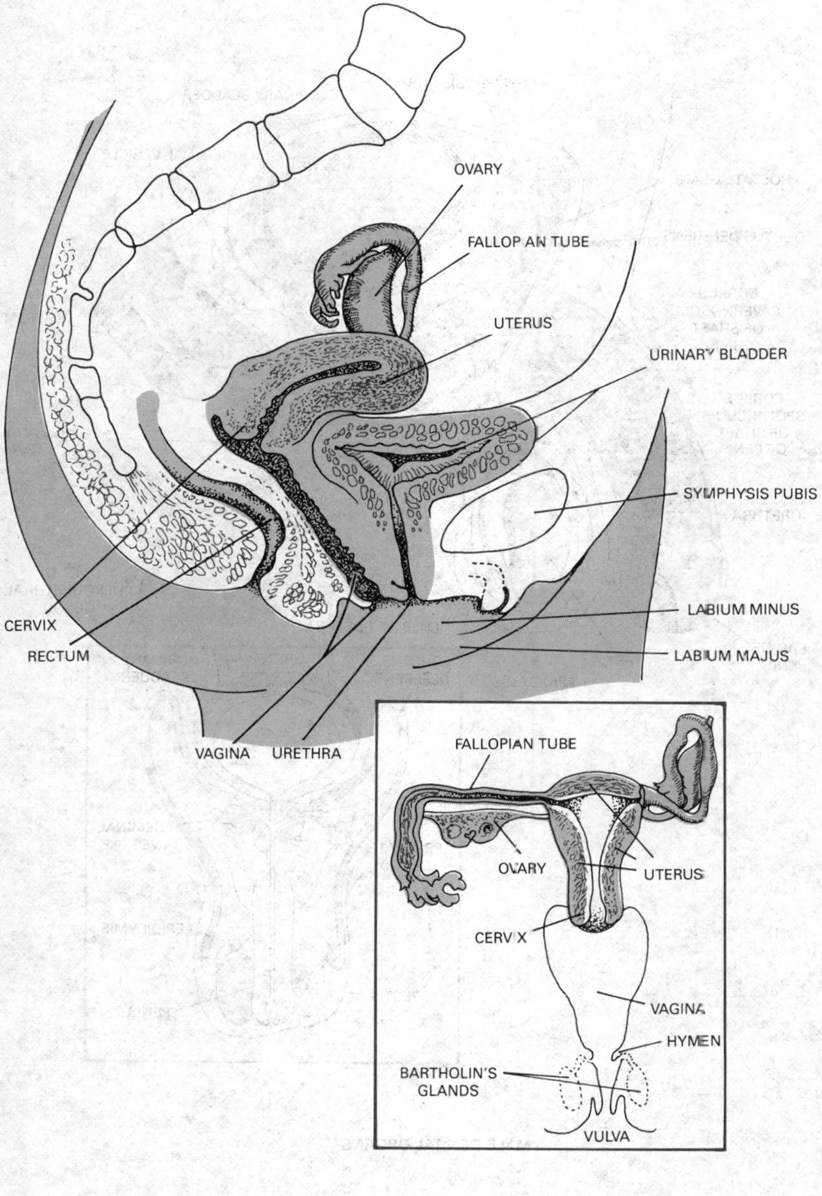

FEMALE GENITAL ORGANS

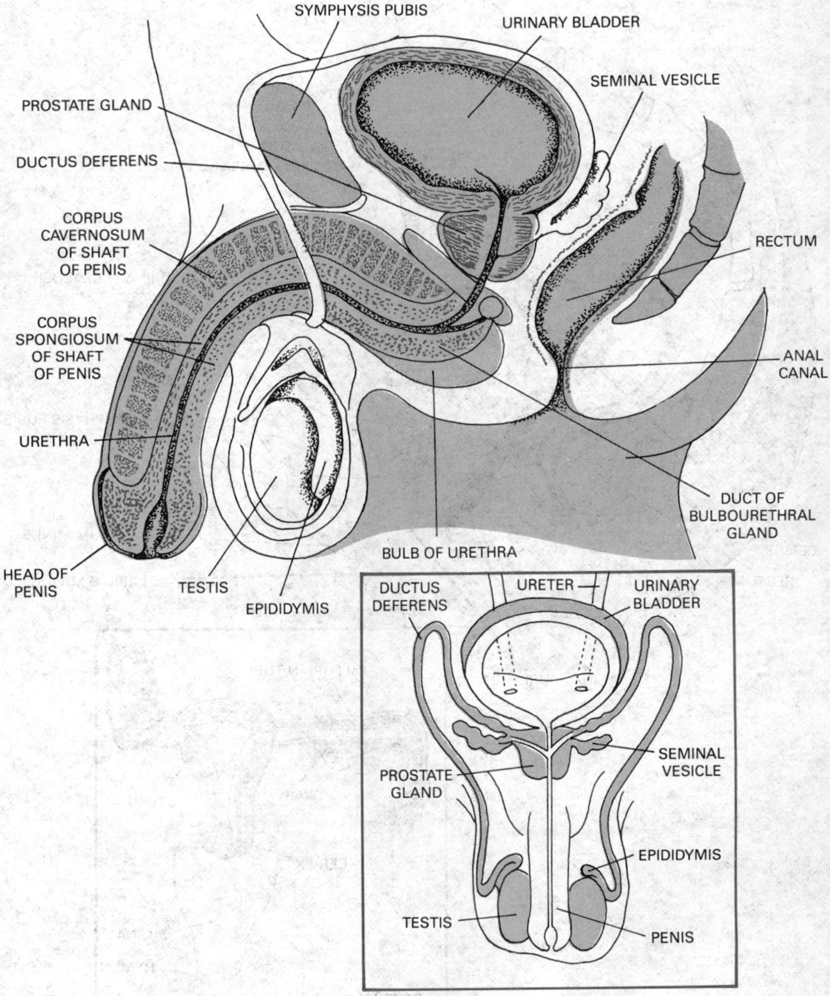
SYMPHYSIS PUBIS
URINARY BLADDER
SEMINAL VESICLE
PROSTATE GLAND
DUCTUS DEFERENS
CORPUS CAVERNOSUM OF SHAFT OF PENIS
RECTUM
CORPUS SPONGIOSUM OF SHAFT OF PENIS
ANAL CANAL
URETHRA
DUCT OF BULBOURETHRAL GLAND
BULB OF URETHRA
HEAD OF PENIS
TESTIS
EPIDIDYMIS
DUCTUS DEFERENS
URETER
URINARY BLADDER
SEMINAL VESICLE
PROSTATE GLAND
EPIDIDYMIS
TESTIS
PENIS

MALE GENITAL ORGANS

Skene's glands, glands of Bartholin, hymen and vaginal introitus, and perineum. The internal genitalia are the two ovaries, fallopian tubes, uterus, and vagina. SEE: illus.

g., male. Reproductive organs of the male sex. Two bulbourethral (Cowper's) glands, two ejaculatory ducts, two glandular organs producing spermatozoa (the testes or gonads), penis with urethra, two seminal ducts (vasa deferentes or ductus deferentes), two seminal vesicles, two spermatic cords, scrotum, and prostate gland. SEE: illus.; *penis; prostate.*

genitocrural (jĕn″ĭ-tō-kroo′răl). Concerning the genitalia and the leg.

genitofemoral (jĕn″ĭ-tō-fĕm′or-ăl). Genitocrural, q.v.

genitoplasty (jĕn′ĭ-tō-plăs″tē) [L. *genitalis,* genital, + Gr. *plassein,* to form]. Reparative surgery on the genital organs.

genitourinary (jĕn″ĭ-tō-ūr′ĭ-năr-ē) [″ + Gr. *ouron,* urine]. Pert. to the genitals and the urinary organs.

genitourinary system. Organs and parts concerned with the kidneys, urinary bladder, and organs of generation and their accessories.

genius (jēn′yŭs). 1. The distinctive or inherent character of a disease. 2. An individual with exceptional physical, mental, or creative power.

genocide (jĕn′ō-sīd″) [Gr. *genos,* race, + L. *caedere,* to kill]. Willful and planned murder of a particular social or ethnic group.

genodermatosis (jĕn″ō-dĕr-mă-tō′sĭs) [Gr. *gennan,* to produce, + *derma,* skin, + *osis,* condition]. Any genetically determined disease of the skin.

genome (jē′nōm). The haploid chromosome complement; the complete set of chromosomes.

Genoptic. Trade name for gentamicin sulfate, USP.

genotype (jĕn′ō-tīp) [″ + *typos,* type]. 1. Basic combination of genes of an organism. 2. A type species of a genus. SEE: *phenotype.*

gentamicin (jĕn″tă-mī′sĭn). An antibiotic derived from the fungi of the genus Micromonospora.

g. sulfate. USP. An antibiotic obtained from the actinomycetes Micromonospora purpurea. Trade names are Garamycin and Genoptic.

gentian (jĕn′shŭn). Dried rhizome roots of the plant Gentiana lutea.

g. violet. USP. $C_{25}H_{30}ClN_3$. A dye derived from coal tar. Widely used as a stain in histology, cytology, and bacteriology. Used therapeutically as a topical anti-infective. Its chemical name is hexamethylpararosaniline chloride.

gentianophil(e) (jĕn′shăn-ō-fĭl). Easily and readily staining with gentian violet.

gentianophobic (jĕn″shăn-ō-fō′bĭk). Not staining very well with gentian violet.

Gentran 40 and 75. Trade names for dextran.

genu (jē′nū) [L.]. (pl. *genua*) [NA] 1. The knee. 2. Any structure of angular form resembling a bent knee.

g. extrorsum. G. varum.

g. introrsum. G. valgum.

g. recurvatum. Hyperextension at the knee joint.

g. valgum. Knock-knee; a condition where knees are very close to each other and the ankles are apart.

g. varum. Bowleg; a condition of curving out of the legs.

genua (jĕn′ū-ă). Pl. of genu.

genuclast (jĕn′ū-klăst) [″ + Gr. *klan,* to break]. Instrument for breaking knee-joint adhesions.

genucubital (jĕn″ū-kū′bĭ-tăl) [″ + *cubitus,* elbow]. Pert. to the elbows and knees.

genucubital position. Knee-elbow position. Position with the patient on the knees, thighs upright, body resting on elbows, head down on hands. Employed when not possible to use the knee-chest position.

genupectoral (jĕn″ū-pĕk′tor-ăl) [″ + *pectus,* breast]. Pert. to the chest and knees.

genupectoral position. Knee-chest position. A position assumed by the female patient in which the patient is supported upon her knees and chest. This position is used for purposes of examination and treatment. SEE: *knee-chest position; position* for illus.

genus (jē′nŭs) [L. *genus,* kind]. (pl. *genera*) In biology, the taxonomic division between the species and the family.

genyantralgia (jĕn″ē-ăn-trăl′jē-ă) [Gr. *genys,* jaw, + *antron,* cave, + *algos,* pain]. Pain in the antrum of Highmore or frontal nasal sinuses.

genyantritis (jĕn″ē-ăn-trī′tĭs) [″ + ″ + *itis,* inflammation]. Inflammation of the antrum of Highmore or frontal nasal sinuses.

genyplasty (jĕn′ĭ-plăs″tē) [″ + *plassein,* to form]. Any plastic operation on the jaw.

geobiology (jē″ō-bī-ŏl′ō-jē) [Gr. *geo,* earth, + *bios,* life, + *logos,* study]. Study of terrestrial life.

Geocillin. Trade name for carbenicillin indanyl sodium.

geode (jē′ōd) [Gr. *geodes,* earthlike]. A dilated lymph space.

geographic tongue. Condition of tongue marked by numerous denuded patches on dorsal surface coalescing into freeform shapes similar to geographic presentations or maps. SYN: *glossitis areata exfoliativa.*

geomedicine (jē″ō-mĕd′ĭ-sĭn) [Gr. *geo,* earth, + L. *medecina,* medicine]. Study of the influence of geography and thus climate on health.

Geopen. Trade name for carbenicillin disodium, USP.

geophagia, geophagism, geophagy (jē-ō-fā′jē-ă, -ŏf′ă-jĭzm, -ŏf′ă-jē) [″ + *phagein,* to eat]. A condition in which the patient eats inedible substances, as chalk, clay or earth. SYN: *geotragia.* SEE: *pica.*

geotaxis (jē″ō-tăk′sĭs) [″ + *taxis,* arrangement]. Geotropism, q.v.

geotragia (jē″ō-trā′jē-ă) [″ + *trogein,* to chew]. Earth eating. SYN: *geophagia.*

geotrichosis (jē″ō-trī-kō′sĭs). Infection by a fungus, Geotrichum, that usually attacks the lungs. Symptoms resemble those of chronic bronchitis or tuberculosis. May also infect the mouth or intestine.

Geotrichum (jē-ŏt′rĭ-kŭm). A genus of fungi belonging to the family Eremascaceae; the causative agent of geotrichosis.

geotropism (jē″ŏt′rō-pĭzm) [″ + *tropos,* a turning]. The influence of gravity on living organisms.

gephyrophobia (jē-fī″rō-fō′bē-ă) [Gr. *gephyra,* bridge, + *phobos,* fear]. Aversion to bodies of water, to crossing on bridges over water, or to traveling on boats.

geratology (jĕr″ă-tŏl′ō-jē). Gerontology, q.v.

Gerdy's fibers (zhĕr′dēz). [Pierre N. Gerdy, Fr. physician, 1797–1856] The superficial transverse ligament of the palm.

geriatrics (jĕr″ē-ăt′rĭks) [Gr. *geras,* old age, + *iatrike,* medical treatment]. The study of all aspects of aging including the physiological, pathological, psychological, economic, and sociological problems of the elderly. SYN: *gerontology.*

Gerlach's valve (gĕr′lăks). [Joseph von Gerlach, Ger. anatomist, 1820–1896] An inconstant valve present at the opening of the vermiform process (appendix) into the cecum.

Gerlier's disease (zhĕr-lē-āz′). [Felix Gerlier, Swiss physician, 1840–1914] A transitory disease of unknown etiology of the nervous system. Characterized by vertigo, paralysis, and visual disturbances. Usually occurs in farm workers exposed to cattle.

germ [L. *germen,* sprout, fetus]. 1. A microorganism, esp. one that causes disease. 2. The first rudiment of an organism.

g., dental. The embryonic structure that gives rise to the tooth; it consists of the enamel organ, dental papilla, and dental sac. SYN: *tooth bud.*

g., hair. The rudimentary structure from which a hair develops. Consists of an ingrowth of epidermal cells called hair peg that pushes into the corium.

g., wheat. The vitamin-rich embryo of the wheat seed or kernel. It contains vitamin E, thiamine, riboflavin, and other vitamins.

germanium (jĕr-mā′nē-ŭm) [L. *Germania,* Germany]. A grayish-white metallic element of the silicon group. SYMB: Ge. At. wt. 72.59; at. no. 32; sp. gr. 5.323 (25° C.).

German measles. Acute contagious disease with rash of short duration, resembling measles and scarlet fever. General signs and symptoms are mild, and in adults the rash may be the only symptom noticed. Swelling and tenderness of the posterior auricular and posterior cervical lymph nodes occurs in the prodromal stage. The rash is sometimes accompanied by fever, malaise, joint pain, and mild coryza.

DIAG: Serological tests on serum collected during the acute and convalescent stages. A fourfold increase in the antibody titer is diagnostic.

The disease is important because of the effect it may have on the fetus if it occurs in the first trimester of pregnancy. The risk of the fetus so exposed being born with a severe congenital defect is quite high. Women who are pregnant and have not had a proven case of rubella should be protected from this disease. At one time immune serum globulin was thought to provide sufficient protection to warrant its use. The antibody titer against rubella virus present in the original immune globulin was much lower than that in those currently available. Thus an immune serum globulin with a known high titer of antibody against rubella virus should be given to women who are pregnant and are known not to have had rubella.

COMPLICATIONS: Encephalitis occurs at the rate of 1 per 1000 to 2000 cases. It usually begins 3 to 7 days after the rash. Bronchopneumonia or bronchiolitis due to measles virus may occur early in the disease. About 15% of patients develop secondary bacterial infections such as cervical adenitis, purulent otitis, and pneumonia.

CAUTION: Pregnant women should not be given rubella virus vaccine. SYN: *rubella.*

germ cell. An ovum or spermatozoon.

germ epithelium. Ridge of epithelium in the embryo from which the sexual portions of the body are derived.

germicidal (jĕrm″ĭ-sī′dăl) [L. *germen,* sprout, + *caedere,* to kill]. 1. Destructive to germs. 2. Pert. to an agent destructive to germs.

germicide (jĕr′mĭ-sīd). A substance that destroys microorganisms. Bacteria and spores may be killed by boiling for 30 minutes, by dry heat at 160° to 170° C. for an hour, and by steam at 121° C. for 20 minutes. SEE: *antiseptics; disinfectant.*

germinal [L. *germen,* sprout]. Pert. to a germ or reproductive cells (egg or sperm), or to germination.

germinal center. A light area of lymphocytopoietic cells that occupies the center of lymphatic nodules of the spleen, tonsils, and lymph nodes.

germinal disk. A disk of cells on the surface of the yolk of a teloblastic egg from which the embryo develops. SYN: *blastoderm.*

germinal epithelium. 1. The epithelium that covers the surface of the genital ridge of an embryo. 2. The epithelium that covers the surface of a mature mammalian ovary.

germinal vesicle. Purkinje vesicle, q.v.

germination [L. *germinare,* to sprout]. 1. Development of an impregnated ovum into an embryo. 2. The sprouting of the spore or seed of a plant.

germinoma (jĕr″mĭ-nō′mă). Neoplasm arising from germ cells in the testis or ovary.

germ layers. Three primary cell layers in the embryo from which the organs and tissues develop. They are the ectoderm, mesoderm, and endoderm.

germ plasm. The reproductive tissues.

germ theory. Theory that certain diseases are the result of the presence of pathologic microorganisms in the body.

gerocomia (jĕr″ō-kō′mē-ă) [Gr. *geron,* old man, + *komein,* to care for]. The medical care of the elderly.

geroderma, gerodermia (jĕr-ō-dĕr′mă, -mē-ă) [″ + *derma,* skin]. An appearance of senility brought about by premature loss of hair, wrinkling of the skin, and general atrophy.

gerodontology (jĕr″ō-dŏn-tŏl′ō-jē). Branch of dentistry that deals with dental problems of the aged.

geromarasmus (jĕr″ō-măr-ăs′mŭs) [″ + *marasmos,* a wasting]. Emaciation that accompanies extreme old age.

geromorphism (jĕr″ō-mor′fĭzm) [″ + *morphe,* form, + *-ismos,* state of]. Appearance of age in youth.

gerontal (jĕ-rŏn′tăl) [Gr. *geron,* old man]. Pert. to an old man or to the aged. SYN: *senile.*

gerontology (jĕ-rŏn-tŏl′ō-jē) [″ + *logos,* study of]. Geriatrics.

gerontophilia (jĕr″ŏn-tō-fĭl′ē-ă) [″ + *philein,* to love]. Fondness or love for old people.

gerontopia (jĕr″ŏn-tō′pē-ă) [″ + *opsis,* vision]. Change in vision of elderly persons, by which they go back to the sight of their youth. This may be an early sign of beginning cataract. SYN: *senopia.*

gerontotherapeutics (jĕr-ŏn″tō-thĕr″ă-pū′tĭks) [″ + *therapeia,* treatment]. Therapy of the aged, the goal of which is to prevent or slow the onset of senescence.

gerontoxon (jĕ-rŏn-tŏks′ŏn) [″ + *toxon,* bow]. Degenerative circle about corneal exterior surface seen in the aged. SYN: *arcus senilis.*

Gerota's capsule (gā-rō′tăz). [Dimitru Gerota, Rumanian anatomist, 1867–1939] The perirenal fascia.

gestagen (jĕs′tă-jĕn). That which produces progestational effects. This general term is usually applied to natural or synthetic steroid hormones used to alter reproductive physiology.

gestalt (gĕs-tawlt′) [Ger. *Gestalt,* form]. The concept that the configuration of objects and experience is present as a whole formation that cannot be analyzed by breaking it into its component parts.

gestation (jĕs-tā′shŭn) [L. *gestare,* to bear]. In mammals, the length of time from conception to birth. The average gestation time is a species-specific trait. In humans, the average length, as calculated from the first day of the last normal menstrual period, is 280 days, with a normal range of 259 days (37 weeks) to 287 days (41 weeks). Infants born prior to the 37th week are classed as premature, and those born after the 41st week are postmature. SEE: *pregnancy.*

g., abdominal. Ectopic gestation in which the product of conception develops in the peritoneal cavity.

g., cornual. Gestation in an ill-developed cornu of a bicornuate uterus.

g., ectopic. Gestation in which the fetus develops outside the uterus.

g., interstitial. Tubal gestation in which the ovum is developed in a portion of the fallopian tube that traverses the wall of the uterus.

g., ovarian. A form of ectopic gestation in the ovary.

g., plural. Gestation in which there is more than one embryo.

g., prolonged. Gestation prolonged beyond the usual period.

g., secondary. Gestation in which the ovum becomes dislodged from the original seat of implantation and continues to develop in a new situation.

g., secondary abdominal. Extrauterine gestation in which the fetus, originally situated in oviduct or elsewhere, has developed in the abdominal cavity.

g., tubal. Ectopic gestation in which the product of conception grows in the fallopian tube.

g., tuboabdominal. Extrauterine gestation in which the fetal sac is formed partly of the abdominal extremity of the oviduct and partly of plastic exudation in the area.

g., tubo-ovarian. Extrauterine gestation in which the fetal sac is made up of the ovary and the abdominal end of the fallopian tube.

g., uterotubal. Gestation in which the ovum develops partially in the uterine end of the fallopian tube and partially within the cavity of the uterus.

gestational age. The estimated age of a fetus

expressed in weeks, calculated from the first day of the last normal menstrual period.

gestation sac. The amnion and its contents.

gestation time. The duration of a normal pregnancy for a particular species. SEE: *pregnancy table.*

gestosis (jĕs-tō'sĭs) [L. *gestare,* to bear, + Gr. *osis,* condition]. Any disorder of pregnancy.

geumaphobia (gū"mă-fō'bē-ă) [Gr. *geuma,* taste, + *phobos,* fear]. Abnormal dislike or fear of tastes.

GFR. *glomerular filtration rate.*

GH. *growth hormone.*

Ghon's primary lesion, tubercle (gănz). [Anton Ghon, Czechoslovakian pathologist, 1866–1936] A small, sharply defined shadow in roentgenographic film of the lung seen in certain cases of pulmonary tuberculosis in children. It is usually the primary lesion of tuberculosis in children.

ghost corpuscle. Depigmented red blood corpuscle. SYN: *phantom corpuscle.*

GH-RH. *growth hormone–releasing hormones.*

GI. *gastrointestinal.*

Giannuzzi's cells (jăn-noot'sēz). [Guiseppe Giannuzzi, It. anatomist, 1839–1876] Crescent-shaped groups of serous cells found in the mixed salivary glands. They appear as darkly staining cells forming a caplike structure on the alveoli.

giant [Gr. *gigas,* giant]. An individual or structure much larger than normal.

giant cell. Cell of large size with several nuclei, appearing to be made up of many cells, but not clearly outlined. Found in both kinds of marrow, esp. in red marrow and spleen. Also found in tissues that are healing, around foreign bodies, and in the inflammatory reaction to tuberculosis. SYN: *megakaryocyte.*

giant cell tumor. 1. A tumor of bone that probably arises from connective tissue of the bone marrow. Histologically, it contains a vascular reticulum of stromal cells and multinucleated giant cells. It may or may not be malignant. 2. A yellow giant cell tumor of a tendon sheath. 3. Epulis. 4. Chondroblastoma.

giantism (jī'ăn-tĭzm). Excessive development of the size of a body or its parts. SYN: *gigantism.*

Giardia (jē-ăr'dē-ă). [Alfred Giard, Fr. biologist, 1846–1908] A genus of protozoa possessing flagella. They inhabit the small intestine of man and other animals; are pear-shaped; and have two nuclei and four pairs of flagella. They attach themselves to the cells of the intestinal mucosa, from which they absorb their nourishment.

G. lamblia. Species of Giardia found in man. They were formerly considered nonpathogenic but evidence indicates that they interfere with the absorption of fats. The most frequently observed symptoms of infection with G. lamblia are diarrhea, cramps, nausea, weakness, weight loss, abdominal distention, greasy stools, belching, and vomiting. Onset of the symptoms begins about two weeks after exposure and the disease will persist for two to three months. There is no known chemoprophylaxis for giardiasis, but treatment with metronidazole or quinacrine is highly effective. SYN: *Lamblia intestinalis.*

giardiasis (jī"ăr-dī'ă-sĭs). Infection with Giardia lamblia. SYN: *lambliasis.*

Gibbon's hydrocele (gĭb'ŏns). [Q. V. Gibbon, U.S. surgeon, 1813–1894] A hydrocele and large hernia combined.

gibbosity (gĭ-bŏs'ĭ-tē) [LL. *gebbosus,* humped]. 1. Condition of having a humpback. 2. A hump or gibbus, as the deformity of Pott's disease.

gibbous (gĭb'ŭs). Humped; protuberant or humpbacked.

gibbus (gĭb'ŭs) [L. *gibbosus*]. Hunchback, gibbous.

Gibney's boot, bandage (gĭb'nēz). [Virgil P. Gibney, New York surgeon, 1847–1927] A basket-weave bandage made of adhesive tape, used in treating ankle sprain, or to support the ankle.

Gibson's murmur (gĭb'sŭnz). [George A. Gibson, Edinburgh physician, 1854–1913] A continuous cardiac murmur that increases in systole. It is heard best at the left of the sternum in the first and second intercostal spaces. It occurs in patients with patent ductus arteriosus.

giddiness [AS. *gydig,* insane]. A lightheaded sensation. SYN: *dizziness.* SEE: *vertigo.*

Giemsa's stain (gēm'zăs). [Gustav Giemsa, Ger. chemist, 1867–1948] A stain for staining blood smears. Used for differential leukocyte counts and for the detection of parasitic microorganisms.

Gierke's disease (gēr'kĕz). [Edgar O. K. von Gierke, Ger. pathologist, 1877–1945] Glycogen storage disease, Type I, q.v.

Gifford's reflex (gĭf'fords). [Harold Gifford, U.S. oculist, 1858–1929] Pupillary contraction resulting from endeavoring forcibly to close eyelids that are held apart.

giga (jĭg'ă, jī'gă). In measuring nomenclature, a prefix indicating that the entity following is to be multiplied by 10^9. SEE: *Metric System* in *Appendix.*

gigantism (jī'găn-tĭzm) [Gr. *gigas,* giant, + *-ismos,* state of]. Excessive development of the body or of a part. SYN: *giantism.*

g., acromegalic. Gigantism in which overgrowth of the bones of the hands, feet, and face is present. Due to excessive production of the pituitary growth hormone after full skeletal growth has been attained.

g., eunuchoid. Gigantism accompanied by eunuchoid features and sexual insufficiency.

g., normal. Gigantism of the body in which the bodily proportions and sexual development are normal. Usually the result of hypersecretion of growth hormone.

gigantoblast (jī-găn'tō-blăst) [" + *blastos,* germ]. A very large nucleated red corpuscle.

gigantocyte (jī-găn'tō-sīt) [" + *kytos,* cell]. 1. A giant cell. 2. A very large erythrocyte.

gigantosoma (jī-găn"tō-sō'mă) [" + *soma,* body]. Abnormal size of the body. SYN: *giantism; gigantism.*

Gigli's saw (jēl'yēz). [Leonardo Gigli, It. gynecologist, 1863–1908] A wire saw originally used to cut the symphysis pubis to facilitate delivery of a fetus. Now used in removing part of the skull in craniotomy.

Gilbert's disease (zhēl-bārz'). [Nicolas A. Gilbert, Fr. physician, 1858–1927] A hereditary disease due either to a deficiency of the enzyme glucuronyl transferase, excess bilirubin production, or a hemolytic disorder. The disease causes no symptoms but an excess of unconjugated bilirubin is present in the urine. SYN: *familial nonhemolytic jaundice.*

Gilchrist's disease (gĭl'krĭsts). [Thomas C. Gilchrist, U.S. dermatologist, 1862–1927] Blastomycosis, North American, q.v.

Gilles de la Tourette's syndrome. [Georges Gilles de la Tourette, Fr. neurologist, 1857–1904] A rare disease of unknown etiology that begins in childhood and may continue throughout life. It is now thought to be a neurological rather than a psychiatric disease. The disease, which affects boys three times more frequently than girls, is estimated to affect 0.1 to 0.5 per thousand in the U.S.A. There are a variety of symptoms, including lack of muscle coordination, involuntary purposeless movements, tics, and incoherent grunts and barks that may represent stifled obscenities. Some of the victims will at the time of puberty begin to experience attacks of coprolalia and involuntary swearing. This aspect of the disease complicates social adjustment.

PROGNOSIS: All forms of therapy have in the past been of little help. Recently, however, certain drugs including haloperidol have allowed dramatic improvement in some patients.

Gimbernat's ligament (hĭm-bĕr-năts'). [Antonio de Gimbernat, Sp. surgeon, 1734–1790] Pectineal portion of the inguinal ligament. Its lateral free edge forms the medial portion of the femoral ring.

gingiva (jĭn-jī'vă, jĭn'jĭ-vă) [L.]. The gum; the tissue that surrounds the necks of the teeth and covers the alveolar processes of the maxilla and mandible.

g., alveolar. The part of the gums that covers the alveolar process of the teeth.

g., attached. The gingiva lying between the free gingival groove and the mucogingival line. It is firmly attached by lamina propria to underlying periosteum, bone, and tooth.

g., free. The unattached portion of the gingiva. It forms part of the wall of the fissure surrounding the anatomic crown of a tooth.

g., labial. Gingiva covering labial surfaces of the teeth.

g., lingual. Gingiva covering lingual surface of the teeth.

g., marginal. The crest of the free gingiva surrounding the tooth like a collar. It is about one mm. wide and forms the soft tissue portion of the gingival sulcus.

gingival (jĭn'jĭ-văl) [L. *gingiva,* gum]. Rel. to the gums.

gingivalgia (jĭn"jĭ-văl'jē-ă) [" + Gr. *algos,* pain]. Pain in the gums.

gingivally (jĭn'jĭ-văl"lē). Toward the gums.

gingivectomy (jĭn"jĭ-vĕk'tō-mē) [" + Gr. *ektome,* excision]. Excision of diseased gum tissue in periodontal pathologies. SYN: *ulectomy.*

gingivitis (jĭn-jĭ-vī'tĭs) [" + Gr. *itis,* inflammation]. Inflammation of the gums characterized by redness, swelling, and tendency to bleed. SYN: *ulitis.*

ETIOL: May be local due to improper dental hygiene, poorly fitting dentures or appliances, poor occlusion. It may accompany generalized stomatitis associated with mouth and upper respiratory infections. May also occur in deficiency diseases such as scurvy, blood dyscrasias, or metallic poisoning.

g., expulsive. Osteoperiostitis of a tooth in which the tooth is expelled from its socket.

g. gravidum. Gingivitis of pregnancy. Characterized by generalized hypertrophy of the gums that may progress to the state of tumor formation.

g., interstitial. Inflammation of the gums and alveolar processes that precedes pyorrhea.

g., necrotizing acute. Fusospirillosis, q.v.

g., phagedenic. A rapidly spreading ulceration of the gums accompanied by extensive ulceration and sloughing of tissue.

g., Vincent's. An ulcerative necrotizing inflammation. Both fusobacteria and spirochetes are found in the lesions.

TREATMENT: Hydrogen peroxide mouthwash twice daily, penicillin or tetracycline or metronidazole. SYN: *trench mouth; stomatitis, Vincent's.*

gingivoglossitis (jĭn″jĭ-vō-glŏs-sī′tĭs) [″ + Gr. *glossa,* tongue, + *itis,* inflammation]. Inflammation of the gums and tongue. SYN: *stomatitis.*

gingivolabial (jĭn″jĭ-vō-lā′bē-ăl). Concerning the gums and the lips.

gingivoplasty (jĭn′jĭ-vō-plăs″tē) [″ + Gr. *plassein,* to form]. Surgical correction of the gingival margin.

gingivosis (jĭn″jĭ-vō′sĭs) [″ + Gr. *osis,* condition]. Chronic gingivitis characterized by degeneration and atrophy of the gum tissue.

gingivostomatitis (jĭn″jĭ-vō-stō″mă-tī′tĭs) [″ + Gr. *stoma,* mouth, + *itis,* inflammation]. Inflammation of the gingival tissue and the mucosa of the mouth.

g., acute necrotizing ulcerative. ABBR: ANUG. Severe stomatitis with ulceration and necrosis of the oral mucosa and the gingival tissue. SYN: *trench mouth; Vincent's angina.*

g., herpetic. Inflammation of the gingival tissue and oral mucosa due to infection with herpes simplex virus.

ginglyform (jĭng′lĭ-form) [Gr. *ginglymos,* hinge, + L. *forma,* shape]. In the form of a hinged joint. SYN: *ginglymoid.*

ginglymoarthrodial (jĭng″lĭ-mō-ăr-thrō′dē-ăl) [″ + *arthrodia,* gliding joint]. Pert. to a joint that is both hinged and arthrodial. SEE: *arthrodia.*

ginglymoid (jĭng′lĭ-moyd) [″ + *eidos,* form]. Pert. to or shaped like a hinged joint.

ginglymus (jĭng′lĭ-mŭs) [Gr. *ginglymos,* hinge]. A hinge joint; diarthrosis. SEE: *joint.*

ginseng (jĭn′sĕng) [Chinese *jin-tsan,* life of man]. The root of the Chinese or American ginseng. It is used therapeutically by some cultures as an aphrodisiac or stimulant. There is no medical evidence to support such use.

Giraldés' organ (hĭr-ăl-dās′). [Joachim A. C. C. Giraldés, Portuguese surgeon in Paris, 1808–1875] A vestige of the wolffian body at posterior side of the testicle. SYN: *paradidymis.*

girdle [AS. *gyrdel,* girdle]. 1. A zone or belt; cingulum, the waist. 2. A structure that resembles a circular belt or band.

g., pelvic. The portion of the lower extremities to which the lower limbs are attached. Composed of the two innominate or hip bones.

g., shoulder. The portion of the upper extremities to which the upper limbs are attached. Composed of the two clavicles and two scapulae.

girdle pain. Zonesthesia, q.v.

girdle symptom. A symptom in tabes as of a tight girdle, such as a feeling of constriction about the chest; also found in compression of the cord due to collapse of the vertebrae as in Pott's disease.

Gitaligin. Trade name for gitalin.

gitalin (jĭt′ă-lĭn). A cardiac glycoside extracted from digitalis. Trade name is Gitaligin.

gitter cell. A honeycombed cell packed with a number of lipoid granules. SYN: *microglia,* q.v.

giving-up. The state, in either the patient or those providing the care, of feeling the situation, condition, or illness is one in which the course and prognosis are inevitably dismal. This leads to the feeling of complete hopelessness and despair. Quite obviously the act of giving up is inappropriate in any situation but particularly when there is a chance that the diagnosis is incorrect. SEE: *grief reaction; helplessness; hopelessness.*

gizzard (gĭz′ărd). The very strong muscular stomach of certain birds. Food is mixed with gastric juice and macerated with the aid of small stones, called grit, that are ingested and remain in the gizzard.

glabella [L. *glaber,* smooth]. The smooth surface of the frontal bone lying between the superciliary arches; the portion directly above the root of the nose.

glabrate [L. *glaber,* smooth]. 1. Bald. 2. Smooth.

glabrous [L. *glaber,* smooth]. 1. Bald. 2. Smooth. SYN: *glabrate.*

glacial (glā′shăl) [L. *glacialis,* icy]. Glassy; resembling ice.

gladiate (glā′dē-āt) [L. *gladius,* sword]. Sword-shaped. SYN: *ensiform; xiphoid.*

gladiolus (glă-dī′ō-lŭs) [L. *gladiolus,* little sword]. The intermediate and principal segment of the sternum, q.v.

glairy. Viscous; albuminous; mucoid.

gland [L. *glans,* acorn]. 1. A secretory organ or structure. 2. A cell or a group of cells that have the ability to manufacture a secretion that is discharged and used in some other part of the body.

On the basis of complexity of structure, glands may be simple (consisting of one or a few secreting units) or compound (consisting of many secreting units whose secretions leave the gland by a common duct). Simple tubular glands may be straight, coiled, or branched. Glands consisting of one cell are called unicellular, those of more than one cell multicellular.

On the basis of their secretion, glands are mucous (those producing a viscous slimy secretion); serous (those producing a clear watery secretion); or mixed (those producing both).

On the basis of the presence or absence of ducts, glands are exocrine (those that possess ducts that carry the secretions to an epithelial surface) and endocrine (those without ducts and whose secretions enter the blood or lymph). The latter are gonads or sex glands and pineal, pituitary, thyroid, parathyroid, thymus, and adrenal glands.

On the basis of the shape of the secreting units, glands are tubular (secreting portion elongated with a narrow lumen) or saccular (secreting portion in the form of a sac or flask). If the lumen of the secreting portion is wide, it is termed an alveolus; if narrow, an acinus. Glands composed of these types of units are termed alveolar and acinar respectively.

On the basis of the manner by which secretion is accomplished, glands are merocrine (secretion forms within cells and is passed through cell membranes into excretory ducts); apocrine (secretion forms in apical ends of cells, which break off and form a part of the secretion) such as the mammary gland; and holocrine (entire cell with its contents is extruded as the secretion) such as sebaceous glands. SEE: *cell* for illus.

g., absorbent. Any one of the lymphatic glands.

g., accessory. A small gland functioning as an accessory to another gland of similar structure some distance removed.

g., acinotubular. A gland structurally midway between an acinous and a tubular gland.

g., acinous. A gland whose secreting units are composed of saclike structures each possessing a narrow lumen.

g., adrenal. An endocrine gland lying above each kidney.

g.'s, aggregate. Lymphatic glands in patch formation found mainly in ileum. SYN: *Peyer's patches.*

g.'s, albuminous. Digestive tract glands secreting a fluid containing albumin.

g.'s, anal. Glands in the region of the anus.

g., apocrine. A gland whose cells lose some of their cytoplasmic contents in the formation of secretion. Examples include the mammary glands and some sweat glands. SEE: *eccrine sweat glands.*

g.'s, areolar. Large sebaceous and rudimentary milk glands present in the areola surrounding the nipple of the female breast. SYN: *Montgomery's glands.*

g.'s, auricular. External otic lymph nodes.

g.'s, axillary. Axillary lymph nodes.

g.'s, Bartholin's. Numerous glands that open into the vestibule of the vagina. Homologous to bulbourethral glands of the male.

g.'s, Blandin's. Tiny racemose glands that secrete mucus and saliva. Located near the tip of the undersurface of the tongue.

g.'s, Bowman's. Simple branched tubular glands present in the olfactory mucosa of the nasal cavity.

g.'s, brachial. Lymph glands in the arm and forearm.

g.'s, bronchial. Mixed glands lying in the submucosa of the bronchi and bronchial tubes.

g.'s, Bruch's. Conjunctival lymph nodes in lower lids.

g.'s, Brunner's. Glands in the duodenal submucosa secreting intestinal juice.

g.'s, buccal. Acinous glands in the cheek tissue.

g., bulbourethal. One of two small glands above the bulb of corpus spongiosum, whose secretion forms part of seminal fluid. SYN: *Cowper's glands.*

g.'s, cardiac. Glands of the stomach near the cardiac orifice of the esophagus.

g., carotid. Tiny gland at bifurcation of the common carotid artery. SYN: *carotid body.*

g., celiac. Several lymph nodes anterior to the abdominal aorta.

g.'s, ceruminous. Glands in the external auditory canal that excrete cerumen.

g.'s, cervical. Lymph glands situated in the neck.

g.'s, ciliary. G.'s, Moll's.

g.'s, circumanal. G.'s anal.

g.'s, Cobelli's. Glands in the esophageal mucosa.

g., coccygeal. G., Luschka's.

g., compound. A gland consisting of a number of branching duct systems that open into the main excretory duct.

g., compound tubular. Gland composed of numerous minute tubules leading to a lone duct.

g., conglobate. G., lymph.

g., Cowper's. G., bulbourethral.

g.'s, cutaneous. Glands of the skin, esp. the sebaceous and sudoriferous glands. Includes modified forms such as the ciliary, ceruminous, anal, preputial, areolar, and meibomian glands.

g., cytogenic. A gland whose product is living cells, such as the testis or ovary.

g., ductless. A gland that lacks an excretory duct. SEE: *endocrine gland.*

g.'s, duodenal. G.'s Brunner's.

g., Ebner's. Serous glands of the tongue located in the region of the vallate papillae, their ducts opening into the furrows surrounding the papillae.

g., eccrine. A simple sweat gland of the skin. SEE: *eccrine sweat gland; g., apocrine.*

g., endocrine. An organ or structure that secretes a hormone that is absorbed into the blood or lymph; a ductless gland. The principal endocrine glands are the pituitary, ovary, adrenal, pancreas, placenta, thyroid, and testes, q.v. SEE: *endocrine gland.*

g.'s, female. Bartholin's, nabothian, Skene's, uterine, and mammary glands; the ovaries and glans clitoridis.

g.'s, Frankel's. Tiny glands located below the margin of the vocal cords.

g., fundic. Glands of the body and fundus of the stomach; gastric glands, which secrete gastric juice.

g., gastric. Any one of three different types of glands in the mucosa of the stomach: cardiac in the superior area; oxyntic in the fundus; and pyloric in the distal portion.

g.'s, Gay's. Multiple sweat glands developed to a great extent in the perianal area.

g., genal. Gland in buccal submucosa.

g.'s, genital. Ovaries in female and testes in male.

g.'s, hair. Sebaceous glands opening into each hair follicle.

g.'s, haversian. Glands that secrete synovial fluid.

g.'s, hematopoietic. Glands that participate in blood production.

g.'s, hemolymph. Modified glands that contain blood and lymph sinuses and that probably participate in the formation of the leukocytes and the destruction of red blood corpuscles.

g.'s, hepatic. Lymph nodes located in front of the portal vein.

g., holocrine. SEE: *holocrine*.

g.'s, inguinal. Lymph nodes in the inguinal region.

g., interscapular. Embryonic lymphatic tissue.

g., interstitial. Gland in connective tissue of seminiferous tubules of testes that produces internal secretions. SYN: *Leydig's cells*.

g.'s, intestinal. Simple or branched tubular glands of the intestine that secrete the succus entericus. Include Brunner's glands and crypts of Lieberkühn.

g.'s, jugular. G.'s, cervical.

g.'s, Krause's. Small glands in the conjunctiva of the eyelids.

g.'s, labial. Multiple acinous glands between the mucosa of the lips and the opening on the inner lip.

g., lacrimal. A compound tubuloalveolar gland, located in the roof of the orbit, that secretes tears.

g.'s, lactiferous. G., mammary.

g.'s, Lieberkühn's. Tiny tubular glands on the intestinal mucosa.

g., lingual. Glands of the tongue; includes the anterior lingual glands (glands of Nuhn), posterior lingual glands (glands of von Ebner), and mucous glands at the root of the tongue.

g.'s, Littré's. Tiny mucous glands in the urethral mucosa in the cavernous portion.

g.'s, lumbar. Lymphatics located behind the peritoneal region and the lower section of the diaphragmatic posterior part.

g., Luschka's. Gland located near the coccygeal tip.

g., lymph; g., lymphatic. Nodule of lymphatic tissue, found along the path of a lymphatic vessel.

g., mammary. A compound alveolar gland that secretes milk. In the human female, they are made up of lobes and lobules bound together by areolar tissue. The main ducts are 15 to 20 in number and are known as lactiferous ducts, each one discharging through a separate orifice on the surface of the nipple. The dilatations of the ducts form reservoirs for the milk during lactation, q.v. The pink or dark-colored skin around the nipple is called the areola, q.v.

g.'s, meibomian. G.'s, tarsal.

g., merocrine. A gland in which the cells remain intact in the process of the elaboration and discharge of their secretion. SEE: *eccrine sweat glands*.

g.'s, Mery's. G., bulbourethral.

g., mixed. A gland that has both endocrine and exocrine function. An example is the pancreas.

g.'s, Moll's. Modified sweat glands in the eyelid.

g.'s, Montgomery's. G.'s, areolar.

g.'s, Morgagni's. G.'s, Littré's.

g.'s, muciparous. Glands that secrete mucus.

g.'s, nabothian. Dilated mucous glands in the uterine cervix.

g.'s, odoriferous. Glands exuding odoriferous materials, as those around the prepuce or anus.

g.'s of Zeis. Large sebaceous glands found in the eyelids. They are associated with the follicles of the eyelashes.

g.'s, olfactory. Glands in the olfactory mucous membranes.

g.'s, oxyntic. Gastric glands usually found in the abdominal cardiac region.

g.'s, palatine. Mucous glands in the tissue of the palate.

g., palpebral. G.'s, tarsal.

g., parathyroid. One of the several small endocrine glands about 6 mm. long by 3 to 4 mm. broad on the back of, and at lower edge of the thyroid gland, or embedded within its substance. These glands secrete parathyroid hormone, which regulates calcium and phosphorus metabolism.

g.'s, paraurethral. Small rudimentary glands that open on either side of the posterior portion of the urethral orifice in the female. SYN: *g.'s, Skene's*.

g., parotid. Largest salivary gland, located in front of the ear. It is a compound tubuloacinous serous gland.

g., peptic. G., gastric, q.v.

g.'s, Peyer's. G.'s, aggregate.

g., pineal. Tiny glandular body of conical shape located between two superior quadrigeminal bodies. Connected with the thalamus but not a part of the brain.

g., pituitary. A small, gray, rounded body attached to the base of the brain by the infundibular stalk, a downward extension of the floor of the third ventricle. It averages 1.3 × 1.0 × 0.5 cm. in size and about 0.6 gm. in weight. SYN: *hypophysis*.

g.'s, preputial. G.'s, Tyson's.

g., prostate. A gland that surrounds the neck of the bladder and, in the male, the urethra. It is partly glandular, with ducts opening into the prostatic portion of the urethra, and partly muscular. It secretes a thin, opalescent, slightly alkaline fluid that forms part of semen. Consists of a median lobe and two lateral lobes. About 2 × 4 × 3 cm., and weighing about 20 gm., it is enclosed in a fibrous capsule containing smooth muscle fiber in its inner layer. Muscular fibers separate glandular tissue and encircle the urethra.

g.'s, pyloric. Gastric glands near the pylorus that secrete gastric juice.

g., racemose. G., acinous.

g.'s, Rivini's. G.'s, sublingual.

g., saccular. G., acinous.

g., salivary. Any gland secreting saliva, as parotid, sublingual, submandibular and buccal glands.

g., sebaceous. A simple or branched alveolar gland that secretes sebum. They are found in the skin. Their ducts usually open into hair follicles.

g., sentinel. SEE: *rods, signal*.

g., seromucous. A mixed serous and mucous gland.

g.'s, serous. G.'s, albuminous.

g., sex. The ovary or testis.

g.'s, Skene's. Glands lying just inside of and on the posterior aspect of the urethra in the female. When the margins of the urethra are drawn apart and the mucous membrane gently everted, the two small openings of Skene's glands, one on each side of the floor of the urethra, become visible. Trauma frequently causes a gaping of the urethra, exposing the glands; and in acute gonorrhea, they are almost always infected.

g.'s, solitary. G.'s, intestinal.

g.'s, sublingual. Tiny salivary glands situated on either side of the tongue.

g., submandibular. The mixed serous-mucous salivary glands that lie below the mandible.

g.'s, sudoriferous. Glands, situated in the skin, that secrete perspiration. SYN: *sweat glands*.

g., suprarenal. G., adrenal.

g.'s, sweat. G.'s, sudoriferous. SEE: *sweat glands* for illus.

g.'s, synovial. Glands that secrete synovial fluid. SYN: *g.'s, haversian*.

g., target. Any gland affected by the action or secretion of another gland, e.g., the thyroid is a target gland of the pituitary.

g.'s, tarsal. Glands situated in the eyelid. They secrete sebaceous substance that keeps the lids from adhering to each other. SYN: *meibomian gland*.

g., thymus. The thymus body or thymus, q.v.

g., thyroid. A ductless gland located in the base of the neck on both sides of the lower part of the larynx and upper part of the trachea. It consists of two lateral lobes connected by an isthmus. Sometimes a third medial or pyramidal lobe extends upward from the isthmus. Histologically it consists of a large number of closed vesicles called follicles that contain the thyroglobulin, which, in turn, contains various active substances such as thyroxine. The thyroid gland is enlarged in goiter and it may appear to pulsate due to the increased blood supply.

g.'s, tracheal. Acinous glands of the tracheal mucosa.

g., tubular. A gland whose terminal secreting portions are narrow tubes.

g.'s, Tyson's. Tiny sebaceous glands found on the inner surface of the prepuce and on the glans of the penis.

g.'s, urethral. G.'s, Littré's.

g.'s, vaginal. Acinous glands in the vaginal mucosa. These are found only in the uppermost portion near the cervix. The major portion of the vaginal mucosa is devoid of glands.

g.'s, vestibular. Glands of the vaginal vestibule. They include the minor vestibular glands and the major vestibular glands (glands of Bartholin).

g.'s, vulvovaginal. G.'s, Bartholin's.

g.'s, Waldeyer's. Glands in the eyelid.

g.'s, Weber's. Glands in the tongue mucosa.

g., Zuckerkandl's. Tiny yellowish lobe occasionally seen between geniohyoid muscles. An accessory thyroid gland.

gland, words pert. to: "aden-" words; "adreno-" words; endocrine; holocrine; name of each gland; seborrhea; "sial-" words.

glanders (glăn'dĕrz). Contagious infection caused by Pseudomonas mallei in horses, donkeys, and mules. It is communicable to man.

SYM: Fever, inflammation of the skin and mucous membranes, esp. those of the nasal cavity, with formation of ulcers and abscesses. Small subcutaneous nodules develop, which break down, giving rise to ulcers. Beginning as small areas, these tend to spread and coalesce and finally involve large areas that exude a viscid, mucopurulent discharge with a foul odor. May occur in acute or chronic form. In the acute septicemic form, prognosis is grave. It is almost invariably fatal.

TREATMENT: Experience with the disease is limited but sulfadiazine is the recommended therapy.

glandilemma (glăn″dĭ-lĕm′ă) [L. *glans,* acorn, + Gr. *lemma,* sheath]. The outer covering or capsule of a gland.

glandula (glăn′dū-lă). (pl. *glandulae*) A small gland. SYN: *glandule.*

glandular [L. *glandula,* little acorn]. Pert. to or of the nature of a gland.

glandular therapy. Treatment of disease with endocrine glands or their extracts. SYN: *organotherapy.*

glandule (glăn′dūl). A small gland. SYN: *glandula.*

glans [L. *glans,* acorn]. (pl. *glandes*) A gland.

g. clitoridis. [NA] The head of the clitoris. SEE: *clitoris.*

g. penis. [NA] Bulbous end of the penis. SEE: *penis.*

Glanzmann's thrombasthenia (glănz′mănz). [Edward Glanzmann, Swiss pediatrician, 1887–1959] A rare congenital abnormality of blood platelets. It is characterized by easy bruising, and epistaxis that sometimes requires blood transfusions. The bleeding is prolonged, clot retraction is diminished, and platelets do not aggregate during blood coagulation or after addition of ADP (adenosine diphosphate). The only therapy is platelet transfusions.

glare [ME. *glaren,* to gleam]. A condition causing temporary blurring of vision with possible permanent injury to retina. Caused by intense light (visible radiation) emanating from highly reflecting objects such as sunlight reflected from water or snow or projected by automobile headlight or by a therapeutic lamp.

glaserian artery (glā-sē′rē-ăn). [Johann Heinrich Glaser, Swiss anatomist, 1629–1675] A branch of the internal maxillary artery, it supplies the tympanum. SYN: *tympanic artery.*

glaserian fissure. A narrow slit posterior to the mandibular fossa of the temporal bone. The chorda tympani nerve passes through it. SYN: *petrotympanic fissure.*

Glasgow coma scale. A scale for evaluating and quantitating the degree of coma by determining the best motor, verbal, and eye-opening response to standardized stimuli. Coma is diagnosed by absence of motor and verbal response and eye-opening. A score of 7 or less is classed as coma when this scale is used. A score of 9 or greater excludes the diagnosis of coma. For details of scoring a response, SEE: table.

glass [AS. *glaes*]. A hard, brittle, amorphous, transparent material composed of silica and various bases.

g., polarized. A medium that permits the exiting light waves to vibrate in only one direction.

g., safety. A type of laminated glass that meets specific requirements concerning the force necessary to break it and is so designed that it breaks without shattering. Its use in automobiles reduces the risk of injury involving broken glass.

g., tempered. Glass that has been treated with heat so that the force required to break it is increased in comparison with ordinary glass.

g., ultraviolet transmitting. Glass designed to admit ultraviolet radiation through it. The glass is designed to transmit about half of the solar radiation, between the wavelengths of 290 and 320 nanometers.

glasses [AS. *glaes,* glass]. 1. Transparent refractive device worn to correct refraction errors in the patient's eyes. 2. Device worn to protect eyes from glare or particles in the air.

g., bifocal. Glasses in which the refracting power of the lower portion differs from that in the upper portion, the lower portion being used for viewing near objects or reading, the upper portion for distant objects. SYN: *Franklin glasses.*

g., safety. Glasses using heat-treated glass or impact-resistant plastic lenses. Their use serves to protect the eyes from dangerous slivers of glass that are produced when ordinary lenses are broken in an accident. Use of glass of this kind in manufacturing lenses for eyeglasses is mandatory in the U.S.A.

g., sun. Glasses with tinted lenses for decreasing the intensity of light seen through them.

g., trifocal. Glasses with three different corrections in each lens: one each for near, intermediate, and far vision.

glassy. Hyaline; vitreous. Descriptive term to indicate a tissue that looks like glass and is smooth and shiny.

Glauber's salt (glō′bĕrz). [Johann Rudolf Glauber, Ger. physician, 1604–1668] Sodium sulfate.

glaucoma (glaw-kō′mă) [L., cataract]. Disease of eye characterized by increase in intraocular pressure, which results in atrophy of optic nerve and blindness. There are two types: primary, which occurs without known cause, and secondary, in which there is an increase in intraocular pressure as a result of other eye disease. The acute type often is attended by acute pain. The chronic type has an insid-

Glasgow Coma Scale*

Eye Opening	Points	Best Verbal Response	Points	Best Motor Response	Points
Spontaneous Indicates arousal mechanisms in brain stem are active	4	*Oriented* Patient knows who and where he or she is, and the year, season, and month	5	*Obeys Commands* Do not class a grasp reflex or change in posture as a response	6
To Sound Eyes open to any sound stimulus	3	*Confused* Responses to questions indicate varying degrees of confusion and disorientation	4	*Localized* Moves a limb to attempt to remove stimulus	5
To Pain Apply stimulus to limbs, not to face	2			*Flexor: Normal* Entire shoulder or arm is flexed in response to painful stimuli	4
Never	1	*Inappropriate* Speech is intelligible but sustained conversation is not possible	3	*Flexion: Abnormal* Slow stereotyped assumption of decorticate rigidity posture in response to painful stimuli	3
		Incomprehensible Unintelligible sounds such as moans and groans are made	2	*Extension* Abnormal with adduction and internal rotations of the shoulder and pronation of the forearm	2
		None	1	*None* Be certain that a lack of response is not due to a spinal cord injury	1

This scale, originally described in 1974 and further discussed in 1979 by Teasdale and his associates, is widely used in assessing head injury patients, both at the time of the injury and as the patient is followed. The score is recorded every 2–3 days.

*Adapted from Teasdale, G., and Jennett, B., Lancet II, 1974, p. 81, and Teasdale, G., et al. Acta Neurochirurgica Suppl. 28, 1979, pp. 13–16.

ious onset. Normal tonometer reading is 13 to 22. An early sign of glaucoma is subjective complaint that lights appear to have halos around them.

ETIOL: Failure of removal, i.e., drainage, of aqueous humor from the eye at a rate to keep up with its production in the anterior chamber. Thus, narrowing or closure of the filtration angle that interferes with drainage of aqueous through the canal of Schlemm will cause an accumulation of intraocular fluid followed by increased intraocular pressure. But, glaucoma may develop even though the filtration angle is normal and the canal of Schlemm appears to be functioning; the cause of this form of glaucoma is not known.

NURSING IMPLICATIONS: Patients with glaucoma need to know and understand that the disease can be controlled, but not cured. Teach them to avoid situations that increase intraocular pressure, such as upper respiratory infections, and vigorous physical activity, such as heavy lifting and pulling. Instruct them not to wear tight constricting clothing, and to avoid emotional upset. Stress the importance of maintaining regular bowel habits, periodic medical check-ups, regular use of the eyes (reading and watching television), and wearing a Medic Alert tag.

TREATMENT: *Nonoperative:* Miotics (eserine, pilocarpine); phospholine iodide. Experimental studies indicate that marijuana, q.v., alleviates the symptoms of severe glaucoma. Control of associated disorders such as diabetes. *Operative:* Paracentesis of cornea; iridectomy (broad peripheral); cyclodialysis; anterior sclerotomy; sclerotomy with inclusion of iris, as iridotasis or iridocleisis; sclerectomy. SEE *ciliarotomy.*

g. absolutum. Glaucoma where the eye is completely blind; cornea is insensitive; anterior chamber shallow; excavated optic disk; eye is as hard as stone; extremely painful.

g., congenital. G., infantile, q.v.

g., chronic. Glaucoma where the tonometer indicates intraocular pressure reading of up to 45 or 50; enlargement of anterior ciliary veins; cornea is clear; dilated pupil; pain; poor vision during attacks; visual field may be normal; cupping of the optic disk is not present in the early stages.

g., infantile. Glaucoma due to increased intraocular tension occurring in infancy and producing uniform enlargement of eye.

g., juvenile. Glaucoma in children and young adults.

g., narrow angle. Glaucoma caused by a shallow anterior chamber and thus a narrow filtration angle through which the aqueous humor normally passes. Because the rate of movement of the aqueous is impaired, increased intraocular tension develops. SYN: *g., closed angle.*

g., open angle. Any form of glaucoma in which the filtration angle is normal.

g., simplex. Glaucoma where intraocular pressure is not high; contracted visual field; glaucomatous cupping; blindness; no acute attacks.

glaucomatous (glaw-kō'mă-tŭs). Pert. to glaucoma.

GLC. *gas-liquid chromatography.* SEE: *chromatography, gas-liquid.*

gleet (glēt). A mucous discharge from the urethra in chronic gonorrhea.

Glénard's disease (glā-närz'). [Frantz Glénard, Fr. physician, 1848–1920] Prolapse of one or more of the internal organs. SYN: *enteroptosis; splanchnoptosia.*

glenohumeral (glē"nō-hū'mĕr-ăl) [Gr. *glene,* socket, + L. *humerus,* humerus]. Pert. to the humerus and the glenoid cavity.

glenohumeral ligaments. Three ligaments in the shoulder.

glenoid (glē'noyd) [" + *eidos,* form]. Having the appearance of a socket.

glenoid cavity. The socket that receives the head of the humerus below the acromion at the junction of the superior and axillary borders.

glenoid fossa. The fossa of the temporal bone that receives the condyle or capitulum of the mandible. SYN: *fossa, articular; fossa, mandibular; fossa of temporal bone.*

glenoid lip. A rim of fibrous tissue around the margin of the glenoid socket.

glia (glī'ă) [Gr. *glia,* glue]. The neuroglia, q.v.; the non-nervous or supporting tissue of the brain and spinal cord.

glia cells. Neuroglia cells. Includes astrocytes, oligodendroglia (oligoglia), and microglia. SEE: *cell; neuroglia.*

gliacyte (glī'ă-sīt) [" + *kytos,* cell]. A neuroglia cell.

gliadin (glī'ă-dĭn). A protein separable from the gluten of wheat. It is deficient in the essential amino acid lysine. The sticky mass that results when wheat flour and water are mixed is due to gliadin.

glial (glī'ăl). Concerning glia or neuroglia.

gliarase (glī'ă-rās) [Gr. *glia,* glue]. Astrocytic mass with incomplete fission of cytoplasm.

glide. 1. To move in a smooth, virtually frictionless manner. 2. Movement in a smooth, virtually frictionless manner.

g., mandibular. The movement of the mandible in any direction as the teeth come into contact.

glioblastoma (glī"ō-blăs-tō'mă) [" + *blastos,* germ, + *oma,* tumor]. A neuroglia cell tumor. SYN: *glioma.*

g. multiforme. A neoplasm of the central nervous system, esp. the cerebrum, consisting of a variety of cellular types.

gliococcus (glī"ō-kŏk'ŭs) [" + *kokkos,* berry]. A micrococcus encompassed in a gelatinous mass.

gliocyte (glī'ō-sīt) [" + *kytos,* cell]. A neuroglia cell. SYN: *gliacyte.*

gliocytoma (glī-ō-sī-tō'mă) [" + " + *oma,* tumor]. A neuroglia cell tumor.

gliogenous (glī-ŏj'ĕ-nŭs) [" + *gennan,* to produce]. Of the nature of neuroglia.

glioma (glī-ō'mă) [" + *oma,* tumor]. (pl. *gliomata*) 1. A sarcoma of neuroglial origin. 2. Neoplasm or a tumor composed of neuroglia cells. SYN: *neuroglioma.*

g. retinae. Malignant tumor of retina; occurs in children; metastasizes late. SEE: *pseudoglioma.*

gliomatosis (glī"ō-mă-tō'sĭs) [" + " + *osis,* condition]. Formation of a glioma, esp. a large one.

gliomatous (glī-ō'mă-tŭs). Affected with or of the nature of a glioma.

gliomyoma (glī"ō-mī-ō'mă) [" + *mys,* muscle, + *oma,* tumor]. A mixed glioma and myoma.

glioneuroma (glī"ō-nū-rō'mă) [" + *neuron,* nerve, + *oma,* tumor]. A tumor having the characteristics of glioma and neuroma.

gliosarcoma [" + *sarx,* flesh, + *oma,* tumor]. Glioma combined with fusiform cells of sarcoma.

gliosis (glī-ō'sĭs) [" + *osis,* condition]. Proliferation of neuroglial tissue in the central nervous system.
gliosome (glī'ō-sōm) [" + *soma,* body]. One of the rounded bodies seen in neuroglia cells.
gliotoxin (glī"ō-tŏk'sĭn). An antibiotic obtained from several different fungi, esp. Trichoderma.
glissonian cirrhosis. Inflammation of peritoneal coat of the liver. SYN: *perihepatitis.*
glissonitis. Inflammation of Glisson's capsule.
Glisson, Francis (glĭs'ŭn). British physician and anatomist, 1597–1677.

G.'s capsule. The outer capsule of fibrous tissue investing the liver.

G.'s disease. Rickets, q.v.

globi (glō'bī) [L.]. Plural of globus.
globin (glō'bĭn) [L. *globus,* globe]. 1. A protein constituent of hemoglobin. 2. One of a particular group of proteins.
globoid (glō'boyd) [" + Gr. *eidos,* form]. Resembling a globe. SYN: *spheroid.*
globular (glŏb'ū-lăr) [L. *globus,* a globe]. Resembling a globe or globule; spherical.
globule (glŏb'ūl) [L. *globulus,* globule]. Any small, rounded body.
globulin (glŏb'ū-lĭn) [L. *globulus,* globule]. One of a group of simple proteins insoluble in pure water but soluble in neutral solutions of salts of strong acids. Examples include serum globulin; fibrinogen; myosinogen; lactoglobulin.

g., Ac. Accelerator globulin; a globulin present in blood serum that speeds up the conversion of prothrombin to thrombin in the presence of thromboplastin and calcium ions.

g., antihemophilic. A clotting component present in the plasma that is essential for the normal agglutination and disintegration of blood platelets. It is deficient in the blood of hemophiliacs. SEE: *hemophilia.*

g., antilymphocyte. Globulin from a person who has become immunized to lymphocytes. Used as an immunosuppressant.

g., gamma. That fraction of serum globulin with which most of the immune antibodies are associated. Most of the antibodies to viruses, bacterial agglutinogens, exotoxins, and injected foreign proteins are contained in the gamma globulin fraction. SEE: *immunoglobulin.*

g., immune. USP. A sterile, nonpyrogenic solution of globulins normally present in human blood. It is used in passive immunization of nonimmune persons exposed to infectious hepatitis, poliomyelitis, mumps, rubella, rubeola, and varicella. Previously used name: immune serum globulin, human. Trade names are Gamastan, Gammagee, Gammar, Immu-G, Immuglobulin, and Gamimune.

g., $Rh_o(D)$ immune. A sterile nonpyrogenic solution of globulins derived from human blood plasma that contains antibodies to the erythrocyte factor $Rh_o(D)$. It is used to prevent development of $Rh_o(D)$ antibodies in $Rh_o(D)$-negative mothers following a miscarriage, therapeutic abortion, or delivery of an $Rh_o(D)$-positive fetus or child. This is of benefit in preventing the development of erythroblastosis fetalis, q.v., in the next pregnancy.

g., serum. Globulins present in blood plasma or serum; the fraction of the blood serum with which antibodies are associated. By electrophoresis, they can be separated into alpha, beta, and gamma globulins, which differ in their isoelectric points.

globulinuria (glŏb"ū-lĭn-ū'rē-ă) [L. *globulus,* globule, + Gr. *ouron,* urine]. Globulin in the urine.
globulose (glŏb'ū-lōs) [L. *globulus,* globule]. Albumose or protein produced by the digestion of globulins.
globus [L.]. A globe or sphere.

g. hystericus. A lump in the throat in hysteria and other neuroses. SYN: *spheresthesia.*

g. major. Head of epididymis.

g. minor. Lower end of epididymis.

g. pallidus. [NA] Pale section within the lenticular nucleus of the brain. SEE: *paleostriatum.*

glomangioma (glō-măn"jē-ō'mă) [L. *glomus,* a ball, + Gr. *angeion,* vessel, + *oma,* tumor]. A benign tumor that develops from an arteriovenous glomus (cluster of blood cells) of the skin.
glomectomy (glō-mĕk'tō-mē). Surgical removal of any glomus.
glomerate (glŏm'ĕr-āt) [L. *glomerare,* to wind into a ball]. Conglomerate, clustered, grouped.
glomerular (glō-mĕr'ū-lăr) [L. *glomerulus,* little ball]. Pert. to a glomerulus; clustered.
glomerular disease. A large group of diseases that have basic pathological involvement of the glomerulus. They may be classified by clinical severity, by histologic changes in the kidney, or by etiology. Etiologic factors include *primary glomerular disease;* disease secondary to *systemic disease* such as lupus erythematosus or polyarteritis; *infectious disease* such as streptococcal infection, malaria, syphilis, or schistosomiasis; *metabolic disease* such as diabetes or amyloidosis; *toxins* such as mercury, gold, snake venom; or *serum sickness;* and *hypersensitivity* to drugs. SEE: *kidney; nephritis; nephrotic syndrome.*

Clinical findings are those associated with the primary dysfunction and pathological changes in the glomerulus, which include proteinuria and hypertension. If protein loss exceeds 5 grams a day, the nephrotic syndrome, q.v., will develop.

glomeruli (glō-mĕr'ū-lī) [L. *glomerulus,* little ball]. (sing. *glomerulus*) 1. Small structures in the malpighian body of the kidney made up of capillary blood vessels in a cluster and enveloped in a thin wall. 2. Plexuses of capillaries. Twisted secretory parts of sweat glands.

glomerulitis (glō-mĕr"ū-lī'tĭs) [" + Gr. *itis,* inflammation]. Inflammation of glomeruli, esp. of the renal glomeruli.

glomerulonephritis (glō-mĕr"ū-lō-nĕ-frī'tĭs) [" + Gr. *nephros,* kidney, + *itis,* inflammation]. A form of nephritis in which the lesions involve primarily the glomeruli. May be acute, subacute, or chronic. This condition frequently follows infections, esp. those of the upper respiratory tract due to particular strains of streptococci. It may also be caused by systemic lupus erythematosus, subacute bacterial endocarditis, cryoglobulinemia, various forms of vasculitis including polyarteritis nodosa, Henoch-Schönlein purpura, and visceral abscess. Characterized by hematuria, proteinuria, red-cell casts, edema, and hypertension. Investigation of serum complement and renal biopsy will facilitate diagnosis and help to predict the prognosis.

NURSING IMPLICATIONS: Assess the patient for symptoms of glomerulonephritis such as hematuria, mild edema, anorexia, irritability, flank pain, constipation, decreased urine output, dizziness, drowsiness, blurred vision, and hypertension.

Overall nursing care for the patient with glomerulonephritis includes observations for changes in amount of edema, daily weighing, measuring and recording intake and output, taking vital signs every two to four hours, and searching for signs of skin breakdown. The patient will need proper skin care and turning, as well as instruction in dietary and fluid restriction. In addition, the patient will need diversional activities, encouragement, and emotional support.

glomerulopathy (glō-mĕr"ū-lŏp'ă-thē). Any disease of the glomerulus of the kidney.

glomerulosclerosis (glō-mĕr"ū-lō-sklē-rō'sĭs). Fibrosis of the renal glomeruli.

g., diabetic. A type of glomerulosclerosis seen in some cases of diabetes mellitus. Eosinophilic material is present in various parts of the glomerulus. SYN: *g., intercapillary.*

g., intercapillary. G., diabetic, q.v.

glomerulus (glō-mĕr'ū-lŭs) [L]. (pl. *glomeruli*) 1. A small, rounded mass or spherical structure. 2. One of the small structures in the malpighian body of the kidney made up of capillary blood vessels in a cluster and enveloped in a thin wall. SEE: *kidney* for illus.

g., olfactory. A rounded body found in the olfactory bulb, formed by the numerous terminal branches of the dendrites of a mitral cell intertwining with the terminal fibers of several olfactory receptor cells.

glomoid (glō'moyd). Similar in appearance to a glomus.

glomus (glō'mŭs) [L., a ball]. A small, round swelling made up of tiny blood vessels and found in stroma containing many nerve fibers.

g. caroticum. [NA] A flat structure at the bifurcation of the common carotid body. Contains cells that respond to changes in concentration of oxygen in the blood and to changes in blood pressure.

g. choroideum. [NA] An enlargement of the choroid plexus at its entrance into the lateral ventricle.

g. coccygeum. [NA] The coccygeal body.

glossa [Gr. *glossa,* tongue]. The tongue.

glossal. Rel. to the tongue.

glossalgia (glŏs-săl'jē-ă) [" + *algos,* pain]. Pain in the tongue. SYN: *glossodynia.*

glossectomy (glŏs-ĕk'tō-mē) [" + *ektome,* excision]. Partial or complete excision of tongue. SYN: *elinguation.*

Glossina (glŏs-sī'nă). A genus of flies called tsetse flies. Includes about 20 species of bloodsucking flies that are confined principally to central and southern Africa. They transmit the trypanosomes (Trypanosoma gambiense, T. rhodesiense), the causative agents of sleeping sickness in man, and other trypanosomes that infect wild and domestic animals. Important species are Glossina palpalis, G. morsitans, G. tachinoides, and G. swynnertoni. SEE: *sleeping sickness; Trypanosoma.*

glossitis (glŏs-sī'tĭs) [" + *itis,* inflammation]. Inflammation of the tongue.

g., acute. Glossitis associated with stomatitis, q.v. The tongue is covered with ulcers and is tender and painful. Another form affects the parenchyma of tongue and is characterized by edema, which may spread to surrounding structures, producing asphyxia and necessitating tracheotomy operation.

SYM: Tongue is painful; saliva thick and viscid, rendering swallowing difficult. Marked malaise, and often a rise in temperature.

TREATMENT: Oral cleanliness with frequent antiseptic mouthwashes. Anesthetic oral solution for pain. Bland or liquid diet.

g. areata exfoliativa. Condition of tongue marked by numerous denuded patches on the dorsal surface coalescing into free-form shapes similar to geographic areas on a map. SYN: *geographic tongue.*

g. desiccans. A painful, raw, and fissured tongue.

g., median rhomboidal. An inflammatory area, somewhat diamond shaped, found on the dorsum of the tongue anterior to the vallate papillae.

g., Moeller's. A chronic superficial inflammation of the tongue characterized by burning or pain and increased sensitivity to hot and spicy foods. SYN: *glossodynia exfoliativa.*

g. parasitica. Black or hairy tongue, characterized by the appearance on the dorsum of the tongue of a dark, furlike patch consisting of hypertrophied filiform papillae, pigment, and shed epithelial cells. SYN: *glossophytia.*

glosso- [Gr. *glossa,* tongue]. Prefix pert. to the tongue.

glossocele (glŏs′sō-sēl) [″ + *kele,* swelling]. Swelling and protrusion of the tongue as a result of disease or malformation.

glossodynamometer (glŏs″sō-dī″nă-mŏm′ĕ-tĕr) [″ + *dynamis,* power, + *metron,* measure]. Device for measuring contractile power of the tongue muscles.

glossodynia (glŏs″ō-dĭn′ē-ă) [″ + *odyne,* pain]. Pain in the tongue. SYN: *glossalgia.*

g. exfoliativa. A chronic superficial inflammation of the tongue characterized by burning or pain and increased sensitivity to hot and spicy foods. SYN: *glossitis, Moeller's.*

glossoepiglottic (glŏs″ō-ĕp-ĭ-glŏt′ĭk) [″ + *epi,* upon, + *glottis,* back of tongue]. Pert. to the ligament between the base of tongue and epiglottis.

glossoepiglottidean (glŏs″ō-ĕp-ĭ-glŏ-tĭd′ē-ăn). Rel. to the tongue and epiglottis.

glossoepiglottidean folds. Three mucous membrane folds from base of tongue to the epiglottis. SYN: *plicae epiglotticae.*

glossoepiglottidean ligament. Elastic band from base of tongue to the epiglottis in middle glossoepiglottidean fold.

glossograph (glŏs′ō-grăf) [″ + *graphein,* to write]. An instrument for recording the tongue's movements in speaking.

glossohyal (glŏs″ō-hī′ăl) [″ + *hyoeides,* U-shaped]. Rel. to tongue and hyoid bone. SYN: *hyoglossal.*

glossokinesthetic (glŏs″ō-kĭn″ĕs-thĕt′ĭk) [″ + *kinesis,* movement, + *aisthetikos,* perceptive]. Pert. to movements of the tongue, esp. those in speech.

glossolabial (glŏs″ō-lā′bē-ăl) [″ + L. *labium,* lip]. Pert. to the tongue and lips.

glossolalia (glŏs″ō-lā′lē-ă) [″ + *lalia,* babble]. Repetition of senseless remarks not related to the subject or situation involved.

glossology (glŏ-sŏl′ō-jē) [″ + *logos,* study]. Study of the tongue and its diseases. SYN: *glottology.*

glossolysis (glŏ-sŏl′ĭ-sĭs) [″ + *lysis,* loosening]. Paralysis of tongue. SYN: *glossoplegia.*

glossopalatine (glŏs″ō-păl′ă-tīn) Pert. to the tongue and the palate.

glossopathy (glŏ-sŏp′ă-thē) [″ + *pathos,* disease]. Disease of the tongue.

glossopharyngeal (glŏs″ō-fă-rĭn′jē-ăl) [″ + *pharynx,* pharynx]. Rel. to tongue and pharynx.

glossopharyngeal nerve. Ninth cranial nerve. Function: Special sensory (taste), visceral sensory, and motor. Origin: By several roots from the medulla oblongata. Distribution: Pharynx, ear, meninges, posterior third of tongue, parotid gland. Branches: Carotid, tympanic, pharyngeal, lingual, tonsillar, and sinus nerve of Hering. SEE: illus.

glossophytia (glŏs″ō-fĭ′tē-ă) [Gr. *glossa,* tongue, + *phyton,* plant]. Black or hairy tongue, characterized by the appearance on the dorsum of the tongue of a dark furlike patch consisting of hypertrophied filiform papillae, pigment, and shed epithelial cells. SYN: *hyperkeratosis linguae; black tongue; hairy tongue.*

glossoplasty (glŏs′ō-plăs″tē) [″ + *plassein,* to form]. Reparative surgery of the tongue.

glossoplegia (glŏs″ō-plē′jē-ă) [″ + *plege,* stroke]. Paralysis of tongue, usually unilateral. SYN: *glossolysis.*

ETIOL: Cerebral hemorrhage, disease, or injury that involves the hypoglossal nerve.

glossoptosis (glŏs″ŏp-tō′sĭs) [″ + *ptosis,* a dropping]. A dropping of the tongue downward out of normal position.

glossopyrosis (glŏs″ō-pī-rō′sĭs) [″ + *pyrosis,* a burning]. A burning sensation of the tongue.

glossorrhaphy (glŏ-sor′ă-fē) [″ + *rhaphe,* suture]. Suture of wound of the tongue.

glossoscopy (glŏ-sŏs′kō-pē) [″ + *skopein,* to examine]. Inspection of the tongue.

glossospasm (glŏs′ō-spăzm) [″ + *spasmos,* spasm]. Spasmodic contraction of muscles of the tongue.

glossotomy (glŏ-sŏt′ō-mē) [″ + *tome,* incision]. Incision of tongue.

glossotrichia (glŏs″ō-trĭk′ē-ă) [″ + *thrix,* hair]. Hairy tongue due to greatly elongated filiform papillae that give the tongue a hairy appearance.

glossy. Smooth and shining.

glossy skin. Shiny appearance of the skin due to atrophy or injury to nerves.

glottic [Gr. *glottis,* back of tongue]. Of or pert. to the tongue, or the glottis.

glottis (glŏt′ĭs) [Gr. *glottis,* back of tongue]. (pl. *glottises* or *glottides*) [NA] The sound-producing apparatus of the larynx consisting of the two vocal folds and the intervening space, the rima glottidis. A leaf-shaped lid of fibrocartilage (the epiglottis) protects this opening.

g., edema of. The accumulation of fluid in the tissues lining the larynx. It may result from irritation of the larynx from improper use of the voice, excessive use of tobacco or

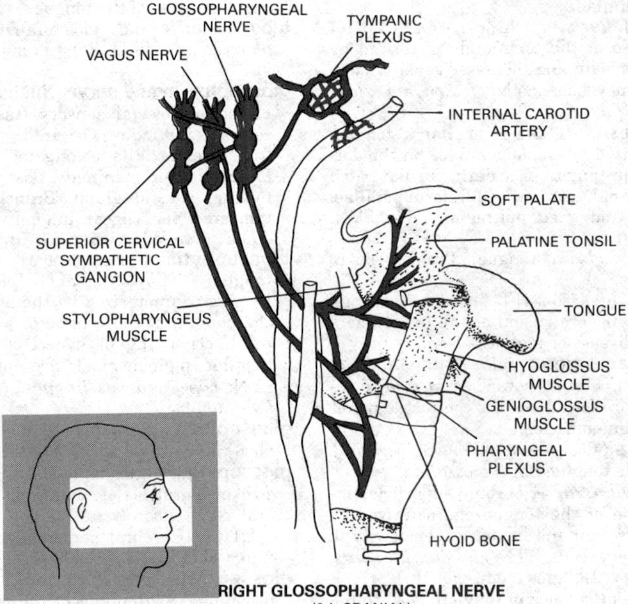

RIGHT GLOSSOPHARYNGEAL NERVE
(9th CRANIAL)

alcohol, chemical fumes, acute infections, or more serious conditions such as tuberculous or syphilitic laryngitis.

SYM: Hoarseness, and later complete aphonia, extreme dyspnea at first on inspiration but later on expiration also. Stridulous respiration; barking cough when epiglottis is involved.

glottitis (glŏ-tī'tĭs) [" + *itis,* inflammation]. Inflammation of the tongue. SYN: *glossitis.*

glottology (glŏ-tŏl'ō-jē) [" + *logos,* study]. The study of the tongue and its diseases. SYN: *glossology.*

glucagon (gloo'kă-gŏn). USP. A polypeptide hormone that has the property of increasing the concentration of glucose in the blood. It is obtained from pork and beef pancreas glands. Glucagon is secreted by the alpha cells of the human pancreas. Parenteral administration of glucagon produces relaxation of the smooth muscle of the stomach, duodenum, small bowel, and colon.

glucagonoma (glū"kă-gŏn-ō'mă). A malignant tumor of the alpha cells of the islets of Langerhans of the pancreas. Principal signs and symptoms include weight loss, diabetes mellitus, skin rash, glossitis, elevated serum glucagon levels, and anemia. Treatment is surgical.

gluciphore (gloo'sĭ-for). Glucophore.

glucocerebroside (gloo"kō-sĕr'ĕ-brō-sīd"). Cerebroside with the carbohydrate glucose contained in the molecule. Present in tissues in Gaucher's disease.

glucocorticoid (gloo"kō-kort'ĭ-koyd) [" + L. *cortex,* cortex, + Gr. *eidos,* form]. A general classification of adrenal cortical hormones that are primarily active in protecting against stress and in affecting protein and carbohydrate metabolism. SEE: *mineralocorticoid.*

glucofuranose (gloo"kō-fū'ră-nōs). The form of glucose containing the furanose ring.

glucogenesis (gloo"kō-jĕn'ĕ-sĭs). Formation of glucose from glycogen.

glucohemia (gloo"kō-hē'mē-ă) [" + *haima,* blood]. Sugar in the blood. SYN: *glycosemia.*

glucokinase (gloo"kō-kī'nās). An enzyme in the liver and pancreas. In the presence of ATP, it catalyzes the conversion of glucose to glucose 6-phosphate.

glucokinetic (gloo"kō-kī-nĕt'ĭk). Acting to maintain the blood glucose level.

gluconeogenesis (gloo"kō-nē"ō-jĕn'ĕ-sĭs) [Gr. *gleukos,* sweet (new wine), + *neos,* new, + *genesis,* origin]. The formation of glycogen from noncarbohydrate sources such as amino or fatty acids. It occurs in the liver under such conditions as low carbohydrate intake or starvation. SYN: *glyconeogenesis.*

glucophore (gloo'kō-for) [" + *phorein,* to carry].

The portion of a chemical compound that imparts a sweet taste to the substance.

glucoprotein (gloo″kō-prō′tē-ĭn). Glycoprotein.

glucopyranose (gloo″kō-pī′ră-nōs). The form of glucose containing the six-carbon pyran ring.

glucosamine (gloo″kō-săm′ēn). An aminosaccharide present in chitin and mucus.

glucose (gloo′kōs) [Gr. *gleukos,* sweet (new wine)]. 1. A sugar. In medicine, the word is used to indicate the sugar dextrose. This is also called d-glucose. 2. An intermediate in metabolism of carbohydrates in the body. Formed during digestion.

Glucose is the most important carbohydrate in body metabolism. It is formed during digestion from the hydrolysis of di- and polysaccharides, esp. starch, and absorbed from the intestines into the blood of the portal vein. In its passage through the liver, excess glucose is converted into glycogen (glycogenesis). The concentration of sugar in the blood is approximately 0.1% (100 mg./dl.), the amount being maintained at a fairly constant level (80 to 120 mg./dl.) through the action of insulin produced by the islets of Langerhans of the pancreas. Failure of the pancreas to produce adequate insulin results in hyperglycemia, in which the blood sugar (glucose) level may rise to 200 mg./dl. or higher. When above the renal threshold (about 160 to 180 mg./dl.), glucose appears in the urine (glycosuria). This is a symptom of diabetes. Overproduction of insulin or injection of insulin as in insulin shock treatment reduces the blood sugar below normal, a condition known as hypoglycemia, q.v.

In the tissue, glucose may be converted into glycogen, utilized to form fat, or oxidized to carbon dioxide and water. Free glucose is not used in the tissues until phosphorylated by ATP (adenosine triphosphate). This occurs through the action of an enzyme, hexokinase, with the resultant production of glucose-6-phosphate. Through a complex series of reactions involving several enzymes, the action of certain hormones, and the formation of several intermediate products including lactic and pyruvic acids, oxidation to carbon and water is brought about. Hormones of the anterior lobe of the hypophysis, the adrenal gland (cortex and medulla), thyroid, and the gonads play a role in carbohydrate metabolism.

When the blood sugar is below normal, fat stores are metabolized. Incomplete metabolism of fats leads to the formation of ketone bodies, also a symptom of diabetes. Blood sugar acts as a protein sparer, q.v. Nervous tissue is esp. dependent upon glucose as its source of energy, the brain being able to oxidize glucose directly. SEE: *carbohydrate.*

g., blood level of. The glucose found in the blood stream has a dual origin. First, glucose is present normally in both the whole blood and plasma; secondly, the greater percentage of the normal glucose concentration has an exogenous origin—that is, from the food intake. The normal glucose concentration in the blood is 80 to 120 mg./dl. Increased concentration is associated with the following conditions: acromegaly; adrenal tumors; increased intracranial pressure; diabetes mellitus; hemochromatosis; hyperthyroidism; hyperpituitarism; hyperadrenalism. Decreased concentration is associated with Addison's disease; adenoma or carcinoma of islets of Langerhans; cretinism; hyperinsulinism; hypopituitarism; hypothyroidism; insulin shock; muscular dystrophy; myxedema.

g., liquid. A liquid obtained from the incomplete hydrolysis of starch. It is a thick syrupy liquid, sweet in taste, containing d-glucose (dextrose), dextrins, and other carbohydrates. It is used for nutritive purposes and in various pharmaceutical and food preparations.

glucose-6-phosphate dehydrogenase. An enzyme present in the liver and kidney that is important in converting glycerol to glucose. ABBR: G6PD. SEE: *favism.*

Hemolytic anemia is produced when persons who have a hereditary deficiency of glucose-6-phosphate dehydrogenase are given certain drugs.

glucose tolerance test. A test done by giving a certain amount of glucose to the patient orally or intravenously. Blood samples are drawn at specified intervals and the blood glucose determined in each sample. By this means, the ability of the patient to metabolize glucose can be determined. In suspected cases of hyperinsulinism, the test is prolonged to six hours with samples of blood being drawn hourly and analyzed for sugar content. If the blood-sugar level continues to drop after three hours, falling below 80 mg./dl., hyperinsulinism is indicated although other conditions may produce a deficiency in blood sugar (hypoglycemia).

A dose of oral cortisone 8½ hours and 2½ hours prior to giving the glucose is sometimes administered. This is called the oral cortisone glucose tolerance test. The cortisone increases the demand for insulin and thus reveals deficiency in insulin response.

glucosidase (gloo-kō′sĭ-dās). An enzyme that catalyzes the hydrolysis of a glucoside.

glucoside (gloo′kō-sīd) [Gr. *gleukos,* sweet (new wine)]. A glycoside that upon hydrolysis yields a sugar, glucose, and one or two additional products. Glucosides are numerous and widely distributed in plants. Many glucosides have medicinal properties; for example, digitalin and strophanthin, present in digitalis and strophanthus respectively, have a specific effect upon the heart. SEE: *glycoside*.

glucosin (gloo′kō-sĭn). Any one of a series of bases derived by action of ammonia on glucose.

glucosulfone sodium (gloo″kō-sŭl′fōn). A derivative of dapsone used in treating leprosy.

glucosuria (gloo″kō-sū′rē-ă) [″ + *ouron*, urine]. Abnormal amount of sugar in the urine. SYN: *glycosuria*.

glucuronic acid. An important acid, $CHO(CHOH)_4COOH$, in human metabolism by virtue of its detoxifying action. It combines with certain toxic substances and renders them harmless.

β-glucuronidase (gloo″kū-rŏn′ĭ-dās). An enzyme that splits glycosidic linkages in glucuronides. It is involved in cell division.

glucuronide (gloo-kū′rŏn-īd). The combination of glucuronic acid with phenol, alcohol, or any acid containing the carboxyl, COOH, group.

glue ear. A descriptive term for chronic accumulation of a high-viscosity fluid in the middle ear. Occurs principally in children 5 to 8 years old. It causes deafness, which can be treated by removal of the exudate.

glue-sniffing. Inhaling the vapor from types of glue or solvents that contain toxic chemicals such as benzene, toluene, or xylene. This produces an altered state of consciousness and has occasionally caused death.

Gluge's corpuscles (gloo′gēz). [Gottlieb Gluge, Ger. pathologist, 1812–1898] Granular cells containing fat droplets, usually found in degenerating nervous tissue.

glutamate (gloo′tă-māt). Salt of glutamic acid.

glutamic acid (gloo-tăm′ĭk) [L. *gluten*, glue, + *am*monium]. $COOH(CH_2)_2CH(NH_2)COOH$. An amino acid formed in the hydrolysis of proteins. It is the only amino acid metabolized by the brain.

glutamic-oxaloacetic transaminase. ABBR: GOT, or SGOT for serum glutamic-oxaloacetic transaminase. Enzyme that is involved in the transfer of the amino group of glutamic acid to oxaloacetic acid to form α-ketoglutaric acid and aspartic acid. When cells of either the liver or heart are injured, this enzyme's blood level is increased, thus providing a chemical indicator of hepatitis or myocardial tissue damage. SYN: *aspartate aminotransferase*.

glutamic-pyruvic transaminase. ABBR: GPT, or SGPT for serum glutamic-pyruvic transaminase. Enzyme that is involved in the transfer of the amino group of glutamic acid to pyruvic acid to form α-ketoglutaric acid and L-alanine. When cells of either the liver or heart are injured, this enzyme's blood level is increased, thus providing a chemical indicator of hepatitis or myocardial tissue damage. SYN: *alanine aminotransferase*.

glutaminase (gloo-tăm′ĭ-nās). An enzyme that catalyzes the breakdown of glutamine into glutamic acid and ammonia.

glutamine (gloo′tă-mĭn, -mēn″). The monoamide of aminoglutaric acid. It is present in the juices of many plants and is essential in the hydrolysis of proteins.

γ-glutamyl transpeptidase. A tissue enzyme that is elevated in many conditions involving hepatic damage including alcohol-induced hepatic injury; in patients with renal disease, pancreatitis, diabetes mellitus, coronary artery disease, and carcinoma of the prostate; and in individuals taking phenytoin and barbiturates.

glutaral (gloo′tă-răl). USP. A solution of glutaraldehyde in sterile water.

glutaraldehyde (gloo″tă-răl′dĕ-hīd). A sterilizing agent effective against all microorganisms including viruses and spores.

glutathione (gloo-tă-thī′ōn) [″ + Gr. *theion*, sulfur]. A tripeptide of glutamic acid, cysteine, and glycine. Found in small quantities in active animal tissues; takes up and gives off hydrogen; fundamentally important in cellular respiration.

g., reduced. The form of glutaraldehyde present in red blood cells. It detoxifies hydrogen peroxide that forms either spontaneously or after drug administration, thus protecting red cells from injury due to hydrogen peroxide.

gluteal (gloo′tē-ăl) [Gr. *gloutos*, buttock]. Pert. to the buttocks.

gluteal fold. Crease between the thigh and the buttocks. SEE: *rump*.

gluteal reflex. Contraction of gluteal muscles from stimulation of their skin.

glutelin (gloo′tĕ-lĭn) [L. *gluten*, glue]. A simple protein found in grain seeds, soluble in alkalies and dilute acids but not in neutral solutions. SEE: *protein*.

gluten [L., glue]. Vegetable albumin, a protein that can be prepared from wheat and other grain.

gluten enteropathy. Adult celiac disease; a condition associated with malabsorption of food from the intestinal tract. The symptoms of diarrhea and malnutrition are usually controlled by eliminating gluten from the diet. SEE: *gluten-free diet*.

gluten-free diet. Elimination of gluten from the diet by avoiding all products containing wheat, rye, oats, or barley. Gluten is present in a large number of foods where thickening sauces are used; thus it is essential that the diet be discussed with a dietitian.

glutethimide (gloo-tĕth′ĭ-mīd). USP. A hypnotic drug. Trade name is Doriden.

glutin. The viscid portion of wheat gluten. SYN: *gliadin.*

glutinous (gloo'tĭn-ŭs) [L. *glutinosus,* glue]. Adhesive; sticky.

glutitis [Gr. *gloutos,* buttock, + *itis,* inflammation]. Inflammation of the muscles of the buttocks.

glycase (glī'kās) [Gr. *glykys,* sweet]. The enzyme that converts maltose into dextrose. SEE: *enzyme.*

glycemia (glī-sē'mē-ă) [" + *haima,* blood]. Sugar or glucose in the blood. SYN: *glycosemia.*

glyceraldehyde (glĭs"ĕr-ăl'dĕ-hīd). An aldose, $CH_2OHCHOHCH_2$, produced by the metabolism of fructose in the liver.

glyceride (glĭs'ĕr-īd) [Gr. *glykys,* sweet]. An ester of glycerin compounded with an acid.

glycerin (glĭs'ĕr-ĭn). USP. $C_3H_8O_3$. A trihydric alcohol, trihydroxy-propane, present in chemical combination in all fats. It is a syrupy colorless liquid, soluble in all proportions in water and alcohol. It is made commercially by the hydrolysis of fats, esp. during the manufacture of soap. Used extensively as a solvent, as a preservative, and as an emollient in various skin diseases. Given orally, it is effective in reducing intracranial pressure; and preoperatively to reduce intraocular pressure in glaucoma. Trade names are Glyrol, Ophthalgan, and Osmoglyn.

glycerite (glĭs'ĕr-īt) [L. *glyceritum*]. A medicine mixed in a glycerin solution.

glycerol (glĭs'ĕr-ŏl) [Gr. *glykys,* sweet]. Glycerin.

glyceryl (glĭs'ĕr-ĭl). The trivalent radical C_3H_5 of glycerol.

g. monostearate. An emulsifying agent used in preparing creams and ointments.

g. triacetate. A water-soluble ester of glycerin. It is used as a solvent and plasticizer. SYN: *triacetin.*

g. trinitrate. Nitroglycerin, USP. A valuable medicine used in treating angina pectoris or in preventing an attack if given prior to exercise.

NOTE: Tablets should be stored in tightly sealed, dark containers to prevent loss of potency.

glyceryl trinitrate. Previously used name for nitroglycerin.

glycine (glī'sēn, -sĭn) [Gr. *glykys,* sweet]. NH_2CH_2COOH. A nonessential amino acid, q.v. SYN: *glycocin; aminoacetic acid.*

glyco-, glyc- (glī-kō) [Gr. *glykys,* sweet]. Prefix used in chemical compounds to indicate relationship to sugar or the presence of glycerol or similar substance.

glycobiarsol (glī"kō-bī-ăr'sŏl). USP. An amebicide.

glycocalyx (glī"kō-kăl'ĭks). A thin layer of material that covers the surface of some cells such as muscle cells, fibroblasts, pericytes, and epithelial cells.

glycocholate (glī"kō-kŏl'āt). A salt of glycocholic acid.

glycocholic acid. The combination of glycine with the bile constituent cholic acid.

glycocin. Glycine.

glycoclastic (glī"kō-klăs'tĭk) [" + *klan,* to break]. Pert. to the hydrolysis and digestion of sugars.

glycocoll (glī'kō-kŏl) [" + *kolla,* glue]. Glycine.

glycogen (glī'kŏ-jĕn) [" + *gennan,* to produce]. $C_6H_{10}O_{5x}$. A polysaccharide commonly called animal starch, a whitish powder that can be prepared from mammalian liver and muscle and other animal tissues. Formation of glycogen from carbohydrate sources is called glycogenesis, from noncarbohydrate sources glyconeogenesis. The conversion of glycogen to glucose is called glycogenolysis. Glycogen is the form in which carbohydrate is stored in the animal body for future conversion into sugar and for subsequent use in performing muscular work or for liberating heat. SEE: *glycogen storage disease; glyconeogenesis.*

Glycogen usually is formed from sugar. It is converted when needed by the tissues into glucose. It is utilized by muscles and, with their contraction, breaks down into lactic acid. Oxygen is then needed to convert lactic acid back into glycogen, at which time some of the lactic acid is burned, producing carbonic acid and heat. Sugar from the blood takes the place of the lactic acid consumed.

glycogenase (glī-kō'jĕn-ās). An enzyme in the liver that hydrolyzes glycogen. Its end product is dextrose.

glycogenesis (glī"kō-jĕn'ĕ-sĭs) [" + *genesis,* formation]. The formation of glycogen from glucose.

glycogenetic. Pert. to the formation of glycogen.

glycogenic. Rel. to glycogen.

glycogenolysis (glī"kō-jĕn-ŏl'ĭ-sĭs) [" + *gennan,* to produce, + *lysis,* dissolution]. Conversion of glycogen into glucose in body tissues.

glycogenolytic (glī"kō-jĕn"ō-lĭt'ĭk) [" + " + *lysis,* dissolution]. Pert. to the hydrolysis of glycogen.

glycogenosis (glī"kŏ-jĕn-ō'sĭs) [" + " + *osis,* diseased condition]. Abnormal accumulation of normal or abnormal forms of glycogen in tissue. The so-called glycogen storage diseases are grouped into various types according to the enzyme deficiency responsible.

glycogen storage disease. Any one of several diseases characterized by abnormal storage and accumulation of glycogen in tissues, esp. the liver.

g. s. d., Type I. Gierke's disease, q.v.

g. s. d., Type II. Disease due to a defect in α-1,4-glucosidase in the heart. SYN: *Pompe's disease.*

g. s. d., Type III. Deficiency of two debranching enzymes in liver and muscle tissues. SYN: *Forbes' disease.*

g. s. d., Type IV. Defect of the branching enzymes. Present are liver and spleen enlargement, hepatic failure, followed by death. SYN: *Andersen's disease.*

g. s. d., Type V. McArdle's disease, q.v.

g. s. d., Type VI. Deficiency of liver phosphorylase, characterized by growth retardation, hepatomegaly, hypoglycemia, and acidosis. SYN: *Hers' disease.*

g. s. d., Type VII. Deficiency of phosphofructokinase, characterized by weakness and cramping of muscles following exercise.

g. s. d., Type VIII. Due to an unknown enzyme deficiency, it is characterized by hepatomegaly, ataxia, nystagmus, spasticity, and death.

g. s. d., Type IX. Deficiency of liver phosphorylase kinase, characterized by hepatomegaly. The onset is in childhood, but the symptoms may disappear during adolescence.

g. s. d., Type X. Deficiency of kinase, causing liver and muscle symptoms that are mild.

glycogeusia (glī"kō-jū'sē-ă) [Gr. *glykys,* sweet, + *geusis,* taste]. A sweet taste.

glycohemia (glī"kō-hē'mē-ă) [" + *haima,* blood]. Abnormal amount of sugar in the blood. SYN: *glycosemia.*

glycol (glī'kōl, -kŏl) [" + *alcohol*]. Any one of the dihydric alcohols related to ethylene glycol, $C_2H_4(OH)_2$.

glycolic acid. A fatty acid formed by the reduction of oxalic acid. It is present in unripe grapes.

glycolipid(e) (glī"kō-lĭp'ĭd) [" + *lipos,* fat]. Compound of fatty acids with a carbohydrate, containing nitrogen, but no phosphoric acid. Found in myelin sheath of nerves.

glycolysis (glī-kŏl'ĭ-sĭs) [" + *lysis,* dissolution]. Hydrolysis of sugar by an enzyme in the body.

glycolytic. Pert. to hydrolyzing sugar.

glycolytic enzyme. An enzyme that catalyzes the hydrolysis of sugars.

glycometabolic (glī"kō-mĕt-ă-bŏl'ĭk) [" + *metabole,* change]. Rel. to metabolism of sugar.

glycometabolism (glī"kō-mĕ-tăb'ŏ-lĭzm). Utilization of sugar, q.v., by the body. SEE: *metabolism.*

glyconeogenesis (glī"kō-nē"ō-jĕn'ĕ-sis) [" + *neos,* new, + *genesis,* formation]. The formation of glycogen from noncarbohydrates, such as fat or amino acids from protein. SYN: *gluconeogenesis.*

glyconucleoprotein (glī"kō-nū"klē-ō-prō'tē-ĭn) [" + L. *nucleus,* kernel, + Gr. *protos,* first]. A nucleoprotein so named to emphasize the presence of sugar units in the substance.

glycopenia (glī-kō-pē'nē-ă) [" + *penia,* poverty]. Abnormally low level of blood glucose; hypoglycemia.

glycopexic (glī"kō-pĕks'ĭk) [" + *pexis,* fixation]. Pert. to the fixing or storing of sugar.

glycopexis (glī"kō-pĕk'sĭs). The storing of glycogen in the liver.

glycophilia (glī"kō-fĭl'ē-ă) [" + *philein,* to love]. A condition in which there is a marked tendency to hyperglycemia.

glycopolyuria (glī"kō-pŏl"ē-ū'rē-ă) [" + *polys,* much, + *ouron,* urine]. Diabetes mellitus with moderately increased sugar in the urine but greatly increased uric acid.

glycoprival, glycoprivous (glī"kō-prī'văl, -vŭs) [" + L. *privus,* deprived of]. Lacking in or without carbohydrates.

glycoprotein (glī"kō-prō'tē-ĭn) [" + *protos,* first]. A compound consisting of a carbohydrate and protein.

gycoptyalism (glī"kō-tī'ăl-ĭzm) [" + *ptyalon,* saliva, + *-ismos,* state of]. Excretion of glucose in the saliva. SYN: *melitoptyalism.*

glycopyrrolate (glī"kō-pĭr'rō-lāt). USP. An anticholinergic drug. Trade name is Robinul.

glycorrhachia (glī-kō-rā'kē-ă) [" + *rhachis,* spine]. Sugar in the cerebrospinal fluid.

glycorrhea (glī"kō-rē'ă) [" + *rhoia,* flow]. Discharge of sugar from the body as in urine.

glycosecretory (glī"kō-sē-krē'tō-rē) [" + L. *secretus,* separate]. Pert. to or determining the formation of glycogen.

glycosemia (glī-kō-sē'mē-ă) [" + *haima,* blood]. Abnormal amount of sugar in the blood.

glycosialia (glī"kō-sī-ăl'ē-ă) [" + *sialon,* saliva]. Sugar in the saliva.

glycosialorrhea (glī"kō-sī"ăl-ō-rē'ă) [" + " + *rhoia,* flow]. Excessive secretion of saliva containing glucose.

glycoside. A substance derived from plants that upon hydrolysis yields a sugar and one or more additional products. Depending on the sugar formed, glycosides are designated glucosides or galactosides. SEE: *glucoside.*

glycosphingolipids (glī"kō-sfĭng"ō-lĭp'ĭds). A group of carbohydrate-containing fatty acid derivatives of ceramide, q.v. Three classes of these lipids are cerebrosides, gangliosides, and ceramide oligosaccharides. When the enzymes essential to the metabolism of these compounds are absent, the glycosphingolipids accumulate, particularly in the nervous system. Death is the usual outcome.

glycostatic (glī"kō-stăt'ĭk) [Gr. *glykys,* sweet, + *statikos,* standing]. Acting to maintain the level of sugar in the body.

glycosuria (glī"kō-sū'rē-ă) [" + *ouron,* urine]. The presence of glucose in the urine. Traces of sugar, particularly glucose, may occur in normal urine but are not detected by ordinary qualitative methods. In routine urinalyses the presence of a reducing sugar is suspicious of diabetes mellitus. It is found when the blood sugar level exceeds the renal threshold (about 170 mg./dl. of blood). Fasting level of blood glucose is usually between 80 and 120 mg./dl. of blood.

Glycosuria may result from pancreatic (insulin) insufficiency; disorders of the endocrine glands, esp. the hypophysis, adrenals, thyroid, or ovaries; excessive carbohydrate intake; excessive glycogenolysis; or reduction of renal threshold. SYN: *glycuresis*.

g., alimentary. Glycosuria following ingestion of large amounts of starches or sugars.

g., diabetic. Glycosuria resulting from hyposecretion of insulin.

g., emotional. Glycosuria resulting from emotional states such as worry or anxiety.

g., phloridzin. Glycosuria resulting from the injection of phloridzin, which reduces the renal threshold for glucose.

g., pituitary. Glycosuria resulting from dysfunction of the anterior pituitary.

g., renal. Glycosuria occurring when glucose is persistent and not accompanied by hyperglycemia. It occurs when the renal threshold for glucose is decreased.

glycosyl (glī'kō-sĭl). The radical obtained when a certain OH group is detached from a saccharide.

glycosylated hemoglobin. SEE: *hemoglobin* A_{1c}; TREATMENT under *diabetes mellitus*.

glycotropic (glī"kō-trŏp'ĭk) [" + *tropos*, a turning]. Acting to antagonize insulin, or to increase the blood sugar level.

glycuresis (glī"kū-rē'sĭs) [" + *ouresis*, urination]. Presence of glucose in the urine. SYN: *glycosuria*.

glycuronuria (glĭ-kū"rō-nū'rē-ă). Glycuronic acid in the urine.

glycylglycine (glĭs"ĭl-glĭs'ĭn). The simplest form of a polypeptide.

glycyltryptophan (glĭs"ĭl-trĭp'tō-făn). A dipeptide of glycine and tryptophan.

glycyrrhiza (glĭs-ĭ-rī'ză) [" + *rhiza*, root]. NF. The dried root of Glycyrrhiza glabra, known commercially as Spanish licorice. Used as an ingredient of glycyrrhiza fluidextract and glycyrrhiza syrup, both of which are used as flavoring agents in compounding medicine. This substance has a weak cortisone-like action. SEE: *licorice*.

glyoxalase (glē-ŏk'să-lās). An enzyme that catalyzes the conversion of methylglyoxal to lactic acid by the addition of water.

glyoxylic acid. An acid produced by the action of glycine oxidase on glycine or sarcosine.

Glysennid. Trade name for sennosides A and B.

gm. *gram*.

G.M.L. *glabellomeatal line*. Imaginary line through the glabella and the external auditory meatus.

gnashing. Grinding the teeth. SEE: *bruxism*.

gnat (năt). Any of a number of small insects belonging to the order Diptera, suborder Orthorrhapha. Term applied generally to insects smaller than mosquitoes. Includes black flies, midges, and sandflies.

g., buffalo. A small dipterous insect belonging to the genus Simulium, q.v.

gnathalgia (năth-ăl'jē-ă) [Gr. *gnathos*, jaw, + *algos*, pain]. Pain in the jaw. SYN: *gnathodynia*.

gnathic (năth'ĭk) [Gr. *gnathos*, jaw]. Pert. to an alveolar process or to the jaw.

gnathion (năth'ē-ŏn). Lowest point of middle line of lower jaw; a craniometric point.

gnathitis (năth-ī'tĭs) [" + *itis*, inflammation]. Inflammation of the jaw or adjacent soft parts.

gnatho- (năth'ō) [Gr. *gnathos*, jaw]. Prefix pert. to jaw or cheek.

gnathocephalus (năth"ō-sĕf'ă-lŭs) [" + *kephale*, head]. A malformed fetus in which the head consists principally of the jaws.

gnathodynamometer (năth"ō-dī"nă-mŏm'ĕ-tĕr) [" + *dynamis*, power, + *metron*, measure]. Device for measuring biting force.

gnathodynia (năth"ō-dĭn'ē-ă) [" + *odyne*, pain]. Pain in the jaw. SYN: *gnathalgia*.

gnathoplasty (năth'ō-plăs"tē) [" + *plassein*, to form]. Reparative surgery of jaws or cheek.

gnathoschisis (năth-ŏs'kĭ-sĭs) [" + *schizein*, to split]. Congenital jaw cleft.

Gnathostoma (năth-ŏs'tō-mă) [" + *stoma*, mouth]. A genus of nematode worms that infest the stomach walls of domestic and wild animals. They occasionally accidentally infest man.

gnathostomiasis (năth"ō-stō-mī'ă-sĭs). Infestation with Gnathostoma.

gnosia (nō'sē-ă) [Gr. *gnosis*, knowledge]. The perceptive faculty of recognizing persons, things, and forms.

gnotobiotics (nō"tō-bī-ŏt'ĭks) [Gr. *gnotos*, known, + *bios*, life]. Study of animals that have been raised in germ-controlled or germ-free surroundings.

GnRH. *gonadotropin-releasing hormone*.

goblet cell. A type of secretory cell found in the epithelium of the intestinal and respiratory tracts; a unicellular gland that secretes mucus. Mucin droplets accumulate in the distal end of the cell, forming a large ovoid mass that causes the cell to become swollen and distorted in shape. The free surface of the cell finally ruptures and liberates the mucus. SYN: *cell, mucous; chalice cell*. SEE: *cell; gland; mucus; secretion*.

goggle-eyed. Having abnormally protruding eyes. SYN: *exophthalmic*.

goiter (goy′tĕr) [L. *guttur*, throat]. An enlargement of the thyroid gland. SYN: *struma*.

ETIOL: May be due to lack of iodine in diet, thyroiditis, inflammation from infection, tumors, or hyper- or hypofunction of the thyroid gland.

g., aberrant. Supernumerary thyroid enlargement.

g., acute. A goiter that grows rapidly.

g., adenomatous. Thyroid enlargement due to growth of encapsulated adenomata.

g., colloid. Goiter in which there is a great increase of follicular contents.

g., congenital. Goiter present at birth.

g., cystic. A goiter in which a cyst or a number of cysts are formed. May result from the degeneration of tissue or liquefaction within an adenoma.

g., diffuse. Goiter in which the thyroid tissue is diffuse in contrast to its nodular form as in adenomatous goiter.

g., diver. A movable goiter, located sometimes below and at other times above the sternal notch.

g., endemic. Goiter development in certain geographic localities, esp. those in which iodine is deficient in food and water.

g., exophthalmic. Goiter with exophthalmos. SYN: *Graves' disease; hyperthyroidism; thyrotoxicosis*.

ETIOL: Unknown. Occurs in constitutionally predisposed individuals. Incidence is higher in females.

SYM: Bulging eyeballs, i.e., exophthalmos, generally present, enlarged thyroid, tremor of fingers and muscles of hands, tachycardia, increased metabolism, vomiting and diarrhea, profuse perspiration, nervous irritability, skin eruptions, emaciation, anemia, hyperglycemia. Goiters are more prevalent in fresh water and lake countries and less so on the sea coast, due to the lack of iodine in fresh water. Iodine, iodized salt, and antithyroid drugs are used in treating the disease. SEE: *thyroid storm*.

DIAG: The disease is diagnosed by using laboratory tests that measure the levels of various thyroid hormones in the serum, or the ability of the thyroid gland to take up radioactive iodine.

g., fibrous. Goiter with hyperplastic capsule and struma of the thyroid gland.

g., follicular. G., parenchymatous.

g., hyperplastic. G., parenchymatous.

g., intrathoracic. Goiter in which a portion of the thyroid tissue lies within the thoracic cavity.

g., lingual. Hypertrophied mass forming a tumor at the posterior portion of the dorsum of the tongue.

g., nodular. Enlarged thyroid that contains nodules.

g., parenchymatous. Goiter characterized by multiplication of cells lining the follicles or alveoli. There is usually a reduction in colloid and the follicular cavities assume various sizes and are often obliterated by infoldings of their walls. Fibrous tissue may increase markedly. Iodine content of gland is low. Goiter usually of a diffuse nature.

g., perivascular. Goiter surrounding a large blood vessel.

g., retrovascular. Goiter development behind a large blood vessel.

g., simple. Thyroid gland hyperplasia unaccompanied by constitutional symptoms.

g., substernal. Enlargement of lower part of thyroid isthmus.

g., suffocative. Goiter that causes shortness of breath due to pressure.

g., toxic. Exophthalmic goiter or goiter in which there is an excessive production of the thyroid hormone. SEE: *goiter, exophthalmic*.

g., vascular. Goiter due to distention of blood vessels of thyroid gland.

goitrogens (goy′trō-jĕns) [L. *guttur*, throat, + *gennan*, to produce]. Substances that cause goiters. These occur in nature in certain foods including turnips, rutabaga, and cabbage.

gold. SYMB: Au (from L. *aurum*, shining down). At. wt. 196.967; at. no. 79; sp. gr. 19.32. A metallic element, yellow in color. Its salts are used in early rheumatoid arthritis and in nondisseminated lupus erythematosus. Radioactive gold, Au-198 injection, is used in treatment of certain types of cancer and as an aid in outlining certain organs, as in liver scanning. SEE: *scanning*.

G. Au-198 Injection. USP. A sterile colloidal solution of radioactive gold (^{198}Au).

g. sodium thiomalate. USP. A water-soluble gold preparation. Trade name is Myochrysine.

goldbeater's skin. A strong, thin membrane prepared from the cecum of the ox. It has been used as a surgical dressing.

Goldblatt kidney. [Harry Goldblatt, Cleveland physician, b. 1891] Kidney of a dog that has been deprived of part of its blood supply in order to induce hypertension experimentally. This condition may occur in man due to vascular disease.

Golgi apparatus (gōl′jē). [Camillo Golgi, It. histologist, 1844–1926] A lamellar membranous structure near the nucleus of almost all cells. It contains curved parallel series of flattened saccules that are often expanded at their ends. The structure is best seen by electron microscopy. In secretory cells the apparatus functions to concentrate and package the secretory product. Its function in other cells, though apparently important, is poorly understood.

Golgi's cells. Multipolar nerve cells in the cerebral cortex and posterior horns of spinal cord. The two types are: Type I, those that possess long axons, and Type II, those that possess short axons.

Golgi's corpuscle. A sensory nerve ending or receptor found in tendons or aponeuroses; an end-organ of muscle sense. SYN: *organ, Golgi's.*

Goll's tract (gōlz). [Friedrich Goll, Swiss anatomist, 1829–1904] Tract in the posterior white column of the spinal cord. SYN: *fasciculus gracilis* [NA].

gomphosis (gŏm-fō'sĭs) [Gr., bolting together]. [NA] A conical process fitting into a socket in an immovable joint.

Ex.: a tooth in its bony socket in the alveolus.

gonad (gō'năd, gŏn'ăd) [Gr. *gone,* seed]. 1. The embryonic sex gland before differentiation into definitive testis or ovary. 2. A generic term referring to both the female sex glands, or ovaries, and the male sex glands, or testes. Each forms the cells necessary for human reproduction, spermatozoa from the testes, ova from the ovaries.

INTERNAL SECRETIONS: *Female:* The vesicular follicles of the ovaries secrete estrogen, which is important in regulating and controlling female reproductive function including the development of secondary sex characteristics. The corpus luteum produces progesterone, which helps to prepare the lining of the uterus (endometrium) to receive and assist in the implantation of the fertilized ovum. *Male:* The interstitial cells of the testes secrete the androgen testosterone, which stimulates metabolism, increases muscular strength, and influences the development of secondary sex characteristics.

Hormones from both sexes have been isolated and standardized and are used in the treatment of conditions arising from an insufficiency of these hormones. SEE: *estrogen; ovary; testicle; testosterone.*

gonadal (gō'năd-ăl). Pert. to a gonad. SYN: *gonadial.*

gonadal dysgenesis. Congenital endocrine disorder caused by failure of the ovaries to respond to pituitary hormone (gonadotropin) stimulation. Clinically there is amenorrhea, failure of sexual maturation, and usually short stature. About a third of these patients have webbing of the neck and many have marked cubitus valgus, q.v. Intelligence may be impaired. These patients usually have only 45 chromosomes, the second X chromosome being absent. SYN: *Turner's syndrome.*

gonadectomy (gŏn-ă-dĕk'tō-mē) [Gr. *gonos,* genitals, + *ektome,* excision]. Excision of a testis or ovary.

gonadial (gō-năd'ē-ăl). Pert. to a reproductive gland. SYN: *gonadal.*

gonadopathy (gŏn"ă-dŏp'ă-thē) [" + *pathos,* disease]. Any disease of the sexual glands.

gonadotherapy (gŏn"ă-dō-thĕr'ă-pē) [" + *therapeia,* treatment]. Treatment by injection of extracts containing testicular or ovarian hormones.

gonadotrope (gō-năd'ō-trōp) [" + *trope,* turning]. 1. A person whose body constitution is dominated by gonadal hormones. 2. A gonadotrophic hormone.

gonadotrophic (gŏn"ă-dō-trŏf'ĭk) [" + *trophe,* nourishment]. Rel. to stimulation of the gonads.

gonadotrophic hormones. Gonadotropins, q.v., or gonad-stimulating hormones.

gonadotropin (gŏn"ă-dō-trō'pĭn). A gonad-stimulating hormone.

g.'s, anterior pituitary. Hormones produced by the anterior lobe of the hypophysis. Include the follicle-stimulating hormone (FSH) and luteinizing hormone (LH). In the male this is called the interstitial cell–stimulating hormone (ICSH).

g., chorionic. Gonadotropins produced by the chorionic villi of the placenta. They are present in the blood and urine of pregnant women and in the blood of pregnant mares. Their presence in urine is the basis of the Aschheim-Zondeck, Friedman, and other pregnancy tests. SYN: *hormone, anterior pituitary.*

gonadotropin-releasing hormone. The releasing hormone produced in the hypothalamus. It acts on the pituitary to cause release of the gonadotropic hormones.

gonaduct (gŏn'ă-dŭkt) [" + L. *ductus,* canal]. The seminal duct or the oviduct.

gonalgia (gō-năl'jē-ă) [Gr. *gony,* knee, + *algos,* pain]. Pain in the knee

gonangiectomy (gŏn"ăn-jē-ĕk'tō-mē) [Gr. *gone,* seed, + *angeion,* vessel, + *ektome,* excision]. Excision of the vas deferens or a part of it. SYN: *vasectomy.*

gonarthritis (gŏn"ăr-thrī'tĭs) [Gr. *gony,* knee, + *arthron,* joint, + *itis,* inflammation]. Inflammation of knee joint.

gonarthromeningitis (gŏn-ăr"thrō-mĕn-ĭn-jī'tĭs) [" + " + *meninx,* membrane, + *itis,* inflammation]. Synovitis of the knee joint.

gonarthrotomy (gŏn"ăr-thrŏt'ō-mē) [" + " + *tome,* incision]. Incision of knee joint.

gonatocele (gŏn-ăt'ō-sēl) [" + *kele,* tumor, swelling]. White swelling; tumor of the knee.

gonecyst, gonecystis (gŏn'ĕ-sĭst, gŏn-ĕ-sĭs'tĭs) [Gr. *gone,* seed, + *kystis,* a bladder]. A seminal vesicle.

gonecystitis (gŏn"ĕ-sĭs-tī'tĭs) [" + " + *itis,*

inflammation]. Inflammation of seminal vesicles.

gonecystolith (gŏn″ē-sĭs′tō-lĭth) [″ + ″ + *lithos*, stone]. A concretion or calculus in a seminal vesicle.

Gongylonema (gŏn″jĭ-lō-nē′mă) [Gr. *gongylos*, round, + *nema*, thread]. A genus of nematode worms belonging to the suborder Spirurata. They are parasitic in the wall of the esophagus and stomach of domestic animals. Occasionally, they are accidental parasites in man. G. pulchrum is the species most frequently involved.

goniometer (gō″nē-ŏm′ĕ-ter) [Gr. *gonia*, angle, + *metron*, measure]. Apparatus to measure joint movements and angles. Recording electrogoniometers are available.

g., finger. Device for measuring the range of motion of a finger, arm, or leg.

gonion (gō′nē-ŏn) [Gr. *gonia*, angle]. Point of angle of the mandible or lower jaw.

goniopuncture (gō″nē-ō-pŭnk′tūr). Surgical procedure for allowing aqueous humor to drain from the eye. Used in treating glaucoma.

gonioscope (gō′nē-ō-skōp) [″ + *skopein*, to examine]. An instrument for inspecting the angle of the anterior chamber of the eye and for determining ocular motility and rotation.

goniosynechia (gō′nē-ō-sĭ-nĕk′ē-ă). Adhesion of the iris to the cornea of the eye.

goniotomy (gō″nē-ŏt′ō-mē) [″ + *tome*, incision]. Surgical procedure for removing obstructions to the free flow of aqueous humor into the canal of Schlemm of the eye.

gono-, gon- (gŏn′ō) [Gr. *gonos*, genitals]. Prefix meaning generation, genitals, offspring, semen.

gonocide (gŏn′ō-sīd) [″ + L. *caedere*, to kill]. Destructive to the gonococcus.

gonococcal (gŏn″ō-kŏk′ăl) [″ + *kokkos*, berry]. Rel. to or caused by gonococci.

gonococcemia (gŏn″ō-kŏk-sē′mē-ă) [″ + ″ + *haima*, blood]. Gonococci in the blood. SYN: *gonohemia*.

gonococci (gŏn″ō-kŏk′sī). Pl. of gonococcus.

gonococcic (gŏn″ō-kŏk′sĭk) [″ + *kokkos*, berry]. Pert. to the gonococcus.

gonococcic smears. Stains used are Gram's method and methylene blue. Gonococci appear in pairs and tetrads. They are gram-negative and intracellular.

gonococcide (gŏn″ō-kŏk′sīd) [″ + ″ + L. *caedere*, to kill]. An agent that kills gonococci.

gonococcocide (gŏn″ō-kŏk′ō-sīd). Gonococcide.

gonococcus (gŏn″ō-kŏk′ŭs) [Gr. *gonos*, genitals, + *kokkos*, berry]. (pl. *gonococci*) The organism causing gonorrhea, a member of the species Neisseria gonorrhoeae. It is an intracellular diplococcus and tends to occur in pairs. It is classified as a gram-negative bacterium and may be found in or on the genitals, in the blood, the joints, the heart, the eye, urine, feces, and in boils. SEE: *gonorrhea*.

gonocyte (gŏn′ō-sīt) [″ + *kytos*, cell]. The primitive reproductive cell.

gonohemia (gŏn″ō-hē′mē-ă) [″ + *haima*, blood]. Gonococcal septicemia. SYN: *gonococcemia*.

gonophore (gŏn′ō-for) [″ + *phorein*, to carry]. Any structure that stores up, transports, or activates sex cells such as the spermatic duct, seminal vesicle, oviduct, or uterus.

gonorrhea (gŏn″ō-rē′ă) [″ + *rhoia*, flow]. A specific, contagious, catarrhal inflammation of the genital mucous membrane of either sex. The disease also may affect other structures of the body such as the heart, conjunctiva, oral mucosa, rectum, or joints. In the female the parts involved may be the urethra, vulva, vulvovaginal glands, vagina, endocervix, Skene's glands, Bartholin's glands, or fallopian tubes.

ETIOL: Infection by the gonococcus, Neisseria gonorrhoeae.

SYM: *Male:* Yellow mucopurulent discharge from the penis resulting from inflammation of the urethra. May become deep seated and affect the prostate. Slow, difficult, and painful urination, and sometimes painful induration of the penis.

CAUTION: It was previously thought that gonorrhea in the male was always symptomatic. This is not true, and suspected cases should always have cultures for the gonococcus. To be certain the patient is cured, the infected sites should be cultured one and two weeks after completion of treatment.

NOTE: In either sex, it is important to obtain a serological test for syphilis prior to starting antibiotic therapy. Penicillin therapy may mask a case of syphilis. Also it is important to test all sexual contacts of the patient for presence of gonorrhea and syphilis.

Female: Gonorrhea in the female may be asymptomatic and even when symptoms are present they may not be uncomfortable enough to cause the patient to seek medical care. Symptoms include one or more of the following: urethral or vaginal discharge; painful or frequent urination; lower abdominal pain; tenderness in the area of Bartholin's and Skene's glands; acute pelvic inflammatory disease.

DIAG: Gram's stain of the urethral discharge is almost 100% accurate in diagnosing gonorrhea in the male. This is not true for the female. The material for diagnosis in the female should be obtained from multiple sites including the cervix, vaginal vault, and urethra, and by milking of Bartholin's and

Skene's glands. The material should be inoculated without delay on Thayer-Martin medium.

PROG: The inflammation may clear up without serious results, or it may become chronic (involving deeper tissues and producing urethral stricture) or produce complications (prostatitis, epididymitis, orchitis, cystitis, arthritis, and endocarditis). No case of acute gonorrhea in the female should be considered as cured until three successive negative smears from the cervix and Bartholin's and Skene's glands are obtained, at least two of which should be examined immediately after a menstrual period.

NURSING IMPLICATIONS: Instruct the patient to take antibiotics as prescribed, to have moist heat applied or sitz baths done as ordered, and to refrain from sexual intercourse until the disease has been properly treated. The patient should also know that his or her sexual contacts should receive treatment. Discuss prevention of future infections. Wear gloves when obtaining cultures or specimens from persons suspected of having gonorrhea.

PROPHYLAXIS: Use of condoms during sexual activity or avoidance of contact with infected persons; immediate penicillin as a preventive following contact. In newborn, instillation of one drop of 1% silver nitrate in each eye. If the mother has gonorrhea, both she and the infant should be treated with parenteral pencillin. SEE: *ophthalmia neonatorum.*

TREATMENT: Penicillin is specific and is regarded as the drug of choice except in cases due to penicillinase-producing strains of Neisseria gonorrhoeae (PPNG). In those individuals, the drug of choice is spectinomycin I.M. or cefoxitin I.M. with oral probenecid. Local therapy may be required for eradication of foci of infection in the female, involving such structures as Skene's duct, Bartholin's glands, and the cervix.

gonorrheal. Of the nature of or pert. to gonorrhea.

gonorrheal arthritis. Arthritis or rheumatism resulting from gonorrheal infection.

Gonyaulax catanella (gŏn″ē-aw′lăks). A species of plankton that makes certain shellfish that eat them toxic. It is also one of the causes of "red tide" when present in massive numbers in the ocean. This has occurred in certain beaches of North America. Shellfish present in such water contain the toxin present in the plankton.

gonycampsis (gŏn″ĭ-kămp′sĭs) [Gr. *gony,* knee, + *kampsis,* bending]. Abnormal curvature of the knee.

gonycrotesis (gŏn″ĭ-krō-tē′sĭs) [″ + *krotesis,* knocking]. Knock-knee, genu valgum.

gonyectyposis (gŏn″ē-ĕk-tĭ-pō′sĭs) [″ + *ektyposis,* modeling in relief]. Bowlegs. SYN: *genu varum.*

gonyocele (gŏn′ē-ō-sēl) [″ + *kele,* swelling]. Tuberculous synovitis of the knee.

gonyoncus (gŏn″ē-ŏn′kŭs) [″ + *onkos,* tumor]. Tumor of the knee.

gonzo. Slang for bizarre, eccentric, or wild behavior.

Goodell's sign. [William Goodell, U.S. gynecologist, 1829–1894] Softening of the cervix in pregnancy.

Goodpasture's syndrome. [E. W. Goodpasture] Progressive glomerulonephritis, hemoptysis, and hemosiderosis. It is a rare disease. Death is usually due to renal failure.

Good Samaritan Law. Legal stipulation for protection of the physician and others who give first aid in an emergency situation. The necessity for such legislation arose when physicians who assisted in giving emergency care were later accused of malpractice by the victim.

goose flesh. A skin reaction caused by erection of skin papillae from cold or shock due to contraction of the arrector pili muscles. This causes transient roughness of the skin. SYN: *cutis anserina; piloerection.*

Gordon's reflex. [Alfred Gordon, U.S. neurologist, 1874–1953] Extension of great toe when sudden pressure is made on deep flexor muscles of calf of leg. It is present in pyramidal tract disease. SEE: *Babinski's reflex.*

gorget (gor′jĕt) [Fr. *gorge,* throat, because of shape of instrument]. An instrument grooved to protect soft tissues from injury on point of the knife.

Gossypium (gŏ-sĭp′ē-ŭm) [L.]. A genus of perennial shrub of the Malvaceae family. Widely grown because of cotton fiber derived from the covering of seeds. Bark of some species is diuretic, emmenagogic, and oxytocic. SEE: *cotton; gossypol.*

gossypol. A toxic chemical present in cotton seed. It has been used experimentally as an infertility agent in the male.

GOT. *glutamic-oxaloacetic transaminase.* SYN: *aspartate aminotransferase.*

gouge (gowj). Instrument for cutting away hard tissue of bone.

goundou (goon′doo). Bilateral hyperostosis of the nasal bones. Seen in West Africans who have or had yaws.

gout (gowt) [L. *gutta,* drop]. Hereditary metabolic disease that is a form of acute arthritis and is marked by inflammation of the joints. Joints affected may be at any location but gout usually begins in the knee or foot.

ETIOL: Excessive uric acid in blood and deposits of urates of sodium in and around joints. Several different metabolic abnormalities may cause hyperuricemia.

SYM: Most persons with hyperuricemia are asymptomatic. When an attack of acute gouty arthritis does develop, it usually begins at night with moderate pain that increases in intensity to the point where no body position provides relief.

TREATMENT: Acute gout responds to colchicine. Long-term therapy is directed to preventing hyperuricemia. This is accomplished by giving uricosuric drugs such as probenecid or allopurinol. Patients with gout have a tendency to form uric acid kidney stones. To help prevent this, fluids should be forced at the rate of 3 liters each day. Because salicylates interact to interfere with the uricosuric action of either probenecid or allopurinol, they should be avoided.

NURSING IMPLICATIONS: The patient is usually on bedrest for the first 24 hours, and with the affected joints elevated during the acute phase. Administer analgesics as ordered, and apply compresses (hot or cold) as ordered for pain relief. Encourage oral fluid intake, and instruct the patient concerning a low-purine diet.

DIET: Should be well balanced and devoid of purine-rich foods.

g., abarticular. Gout that involves structures other than the joints.

g., chronic. Persistent form of gout.

g., tophaceous. Gout marked by the development of tophi (deposits of sodium urate) in the joints, the external ear, and about the fingernails.

gouty. Of the nature of or rel. to gout.

gouty diathesis. Predisposition to gout.

Gowers' tract (gow'ĕrz). [Sir William R. Gowers, Brit. neurologist, 1845–1915] Tract formed of fibers from posterior roots of lateral tract of the spinal cord reaching the cerebellum by way of the superior peduncle.

G.P. *general practitioner.*

G6PD. *glucose-6-phosphate dehydrogenase.*

GPT. *glutamic-pyruvic transaminase.* SYN: *alanine aminotransferase.*

gr. *grain.*

graafian follicle (grăf'ē-ăn). [Regnier de Graaf, Dutch physician and anatomist, 1641–1673] A mature vesicular follicle of the ovary. Beginning with puberty and continuing until the menopause, except during pregnancy, a graafian follicle develops at approx. monthly intervals. Each follicle contains a nearly mature ovum (an oocyte) that, upon rupture of the follicle, is discharged from the ovary, a process called ovulation. Ovulation occurs usually about the 13th day of the menstrual cycle, dated from the first day of the menstrual period. Within the ruptured graafian follicle, the corpus luteum develops. Both the follicle and the corpus luteum are glands of internal secretion, the former secreting estrogens, and the latter, estrogen and progesterone. SEE: *ovum* for illus.

gracile (grăs'ĭl) [L. *gracilis,* delicate]. Slender; slight.

gracile nucleus. Mass of medullary gray matter terminating the funiculus gracilis.

gracilis (grăs'ĭ-lĭs) [L., slender]. A long slender muscle on the medial aspect of the thigh.

gradatim (grā-dā'tĭm) [L.]. Gradually or by degrees.

Gradenigo's syndrome (gră-dĕn-ē'gōz). [Giuseppe Gradenigo, It. physician, 1859–1926] Suppurative otitis media with abducens nerve paralysis and pain in temporal region.

gradient (grā'dē-ĕnt). A slope or grade; an increase or decrease of varying degrees or the curve that represents such.

g., axial. A gradient of physiological or metabolic activity exhibited by embryos and many adult animals, the principal one of which follows the main axis of the body, being highest at the anterior end and lowest at the posterior end.

graduate (grăd'ū-āt, -ăt) [L. *gradus,* a step]. 1. A vessel marked by lines for measuring liquids. 2. One who has been awarded an academic or professional degree from a college or university.

graduated. Marked by a series of lines indicating degrees of measurement, weight, or volume.

graduated tenotomy. Partial surgical division of tendon of an eye muscle.

Graefe's sign (grā'fēz). [Albrecht von Graefe, Ger. ophthalmologist, 1828–1870] Failure of the upper lid to follow a downward movement of the eyeball when the patient changes his or her vision from looking up to looking down. Seen in Graves' disease (hyperthyroidism) with exophthalmos.

graft (grăft) [L. *graphium,* grafting knife]. 1. Tissue that is transplanted or implanted in a part of the body to repair a defect. Homograft involves grafting material from another individual of the same species. Heterograft indicates the grafted tissue or organ was obtained from a species different from the recipient. 2. The process of placing tissue at a different site than from where it was derived to repair a defect.

RS: allograft; autograft; transplantation; zoografting.

g., allograft, allogeneic. Graft from a genetically nonidentical donor of the same species as the recipient.

g., autodermic. G., autogenous.

g., autogenous. Graft taken from another part of the patient's body.

g., autologous. G., autogenous.

g., avascular. Graft in which vascular

infiltration does not occur.

g., bone. A piece of bone generally taken from the tibia and inserted elsewhere in the body to replace another osseous structure. Banks for storage of bone have been established.

g., cable. Nerve graft made up of bundles of segments from an unimportant nerve.

g., cadaver. Grafting tissue, including skin, cornea, or bone, obtained from a body immediately after death.

g., delayed. A skin graft that is partially elevated and then replaced so that it may be moved later to another site.

g., dermal. A split-skin or full-thickness skin graft. The graft will grow hair and have active sweat and sebum glands.

g., fascia. Use of fascia usually removed from the fascia lata for repairing defects in other tissues.

g., fascicular. Nerve graft with each bundle of nerves being separately sutured.

g., free. Graft that is completely separated from its original site and then transferred.

g., full-thickness. Graft of the entire layer of skin without the subcutaneous fat.

g., heterodermic. Graft in which the donor is of another species.

g., heteroplastic. Graft taken from another person.

g., homologous. Graft in which the donor is of the same species as the recipient.

g., isologous. Graft in which the donor and recipient are genetically identical, i.e., are usually identical twins.

g., lamellar. Very thin corneal graft used to replace surface layer of opaque corneal tissue.

g., nerve. Transplantation of a healthy nerve to replace a segment of a damaged nerve.

g., Ollier-Thiersch. Wide, thin strips of skin used to cover a wound.

g., omental. Use of a portion of the omentum to cover or repair a defect in a hollow viscus, or to cover a suture line in an abdominal organ.

g., ovarian. Implantation of a section of an ovary into the muscles of the abdominal wall.

g., pedicle. A skin graft that is left attached at one end until the free end has begun to receive nourishment from the new site.

g., periosteum. Application of a piece of bone and its periosteum to another site.

g., pinch. A graft consisting of small bits of skin.

g., postmortem. Tissue taken from a body after death and stored under proper conditions to be used later on a patient requiring a graft of such tissue.

g., rope. G., cable, q.v.

g., sieve. Graft in which a section of skin is removed except for small, regularly spaced areas that remain. The removed portion is used at the new site. The small remaining areas will grow to cover the entire area at the donor site.

g., skin. Removal of small sections of skin to a clean, raw surface such as a large superficial burn.

g., split-skin. Grafts of a part of the skin thickness.

g., sponge. Small piece of sponge placed over an ulcerating part to stimulate epidermal growth.

g., thick-split. Grafts of about half or more of the thickness of the skin.

g., Thiersch's. Graft in which only epidermis and small amount of dermis are used.

g., Wolfe's. Graft in which the whole thickness of the skin is used.

g., zooplastic. Graft taken from an animal.

grafting. Implantation of skin or tissue from a healthy site to an injured site.

graft-versus-host reaction. The pathological reaction between the host and tissue grafted. Occurs when the host's immune response is deficient because of immunosuppressive therapy.

Graham's law (grā'ămz). [Thomas Graham, Brit. chemist, 1805–1869] The rate of diffusion of a gas is inversely proportional to the square root of its density.

grain [L. *granum*]. 1. The seed or seedlike fruit of many members of the grass family, esp. corn, wheat, oats, and other cereals. 2. A weight; 0.065 of a gram. ABBR: gr. 3. Direction of fibers or layers.

gram. A unit of weight (mass) of the metric system. It equals approx. the weight of a cubic centimeter or a milliliter of water. It is equal to 15.432 grains or 0.03527 ounce (avoirdupois). One thousand grams equal one kilogram. ABBR: gm.; g. SEE: table.

gram-equivalent. In chemistry, the weight in grams of a substance that will react with one gram of hydrogen.

gramicidin (grăm"ĭ-sī'dĭn). USP. One of the antibiotics produced by Bacillus brevis.

grammeter. A unit of work energy equivalent to that expended in raising a weight of one gram vertically a height of one meter.

Gram's method. [Hans C. J. Gram, Danish physician, 1853–1938] A method for staining bacteria. It is of importance in the identification of bacteria.

PROCEDURE: Prepare a film on a slide, dry, and fix with heat. Stain with aniline gentian violet or ammonium oxalate crystal violet one minute. Rinse in water, then im-

Gram Conversion into Ounces (Avoirdupois)*

Gm.	Oz.	Gm.	Oz.	Gm.	Oz.	Gm.	Oz.
1	0.03	30	1.06	59	2.08	88	3.10
2	0.07	31	1.09	60	2.12	89	3.14
3	0.11	32	1.13	61	2.15	90	3.17
4	0.14	33	1.16	62	2.18	91	3.21
5	0.18	34	1.20	63	2.22	92	3.24
6	0.21	35	1.23	64	2.26	93	3.28
7	0.25	36	1.27	65	2.29	94	3.31
8	0.28	37	1.30	66	2.33	95	3.35
9	0.32	38	1.34	67	2.36	96	3.38
10	0.35	39	1.37	68	2.40	97	3.42
11	0.39	40	1.41	69	2.43	98	3.46
12	0.42	41	1.44	70	2.47	99	3.49
13	0.45	42	1.48	71	2.50	100	3.53
14	0.49	43	1.51	72	2.54	125	4.41
15	0.53	44	1.55	73	2.57	150	5.30
16	0.56	45	1.59	74	2.61	175	6.18
17	0.60	46	1.62	75	2.64	200	7.05
18	0.63	47	1.65	76	2.68	250	8.82
19	0.67	48	1.69	77	2.71	300	10.58
20	0.70	49	1.73	78	2.75	350	12.34
21	0.74	50	1.76	79	2.79	400	14.11
22	0.77	51	1.80	80	2.82	450	15.87
23	0.81	52	1.83	81	2.85	454	16.00
24	0.84	53	1.87	82	2.89	500	17.64
25	0.88	54	1.90	83	2.93	600	21.16
26	0.91	55	1.94	84	2.96	700	24.69
27	0.95	56	1.97	85	3.00	800	28.22
28	0.99	57	2.01	86	3.03	900	30.75
29	1.02	58	2.04	87	3.07	1000	35.27

* One gram is equal to 0.03527 ounce (avoirdupois)

merse in Gram's iodine solution for one minute. Rinse off iodine solution and decolorize in 95% ethyl alcohol or acetone. Counterstain with dilute carbolfuchsin or safranine for 30 seconds. Rinse with water, blot dry, and examine. Gram-positive bacteria will retain the violet stain and gram-negative bacteria will adopt the red counterstain.

NOTE: In order to provide a simple means of checking on the accuracy of the staining materials, a small amount of material from between one's teeth can be placed on the slide at the opposite end from that of the specimen being examined. Gram-negative and gram-positive organisms are always present in the mouth. Thus that end of the slide is examined first. If both types of organisms are seen, proceed to examine the specimen.

gram molecule. The weight in grams of a substance equal to its molecular weight. SYN: *mole*.

gram-negative. Losing the stain and taking the color of the red counterstain in Gram's method of staining. A primary characteristic of certain microorganisms. SEE: *Gram's method;* table.

gram-positive. Retaining the color of the gentian violet stain in Gram's method of staining. SEE: *Gram's method;* table.

Grancher's disease (grăn-shăz′). [Jacques J. Grancher, Fr. physician, 1843–1907] Pneumonia with splenization, q.v., of the lung. SYN: *splenopneumonia*.

Grancher's sign. Raised pitch of expiratory murmur in pulmonary consolidation.

grandiose (grăn′dē-ōs). In psychiatry, concerning one's unrealistic and exaggerated concept of self-worth, importance, wealth, and ability.

grand mal (grăn măl) [Fr., great evil]. A form of epileptic attack with or without coma. SEE: *epilepsy*.

granular [L. *granulum*, little grain]. Of the nature of granules. Roughened by prominences like those of seeds.

granular cast. Coarse or fine granule, short and plump, sometimes yellowish, similar to hyaline cast. Soluble in acetic acid. Seen in inflammatory and degenerative nephropathies. SEE: *cast*.

Some of the Gram-negative Bacteria

Genus	Species	Colloquial or Old Names	Disease Caused in Man
Pseudomonas	P. mallei	Bacillus mallei or the glanders bacillus	Glanders
	P. aeruginosa	Bacillus pyocyaneus	Suppuration ("blue pus")
Vibrio	V. comma	Comma bacillus	Cholera
Neisseria	N. meningitidis	Meningococcus	Cerebrospinal meningitis
	N. gonorrhoeae	Gonococcus	Gonorrhea
	N. catarrhalis	Micrococcus catarrhalis	Nasopharyngeal catarrh
Proteus	P. vulgaris	Bacillus proteus	Suppuration
Escherichia	E. coli	Bacillus coli	Occasionally suppuration, cystitis, and pyelitis
Klebsiella	K. pneumoniae	Pneumobacillus or Bacillus mucosus capsulatus	Occasionally pneumonia
Legionella	L. pneumophila		Pneumonia
Salmonella	S. typhosa	Typhoid bacillus	Typhoid fever
	S. paratyphi (A&B) S. enteritidis S. typhimurium	Bacillus paratyphosus, etc. (Salmonella group)	Paratyphoid fever, gastroenteritis (food poisoning)
Shigella	S. dysenteriae	The dysentery bacilli	Bacillary dysentery
Yersinia	Y. pestis	Pasteurella pestis; plague bacillus	Plague
Hemophilus	H. influenzae	Pfeiffer's bacillus	Meningitis, conjunctivitis, and influenza
Bordetella	B. pertussis	Bordet-Gengou bacillus	Whooping cough
Brucella	Br. melitensis	Micrococcus melitensis	Brucellosis
	Br. abortus	Bang's bacillus	
	Br. suis		

granulatio (grăn″ū-lā′shē-ō) [L.]. A granule.

granulation. 1. Formation of granules or state or condition of being granular. 2. Fleshy projections formed on the surface of a gaping wound that is not healing by first intention or indirect union. Each granulation represents the outgrowth of new capillaries by budding from the existing capillaries and then joining up into capillary loops supported by cells that will later become fibrous scar tissue. Granulations bring a rich blood supply to the healing surface.

g., arachnoidal. Villus-like projections of the subarachnoid layer of the meninges that project into the superior sagittal sinus and other venous sinuses of the brain. Through them cerebrospinal fluid reenters the bloodstream. SYN: *pacchionian bodies.*

g., exuberant. An excessive mass of granulation tissue formed in the healing of a

The Chief Gram-positive Bacteria

Genus	Species	Colloquial or Old Names	Disease Caused in Man
Corynebacterium	C. diphtheriae	Diphtheria bacillus Klebs-Löeffler bacillus	Diphtheria
Streptococcus	Str. pyogenes		Suppuration, scarlet fever, septicemia
	Str. viridans	Str. mitis	Subacute bacterial endocarditis
Staphylococcus	Staph. aureus		Suppuration, pyemia, gastroenteritis, pneumonia, osteomyelitis, toxic shock syndrome, scalded skin syndrome
	Staph. epidermidis	Staph. albus	Endocarditis
Sarcina	Sarcina lutea		Rarely suppuration
Bacillus	B. anthracis	Anthrax bacillus	Anthrax
	B. subtilis	Hay bacillus	Eye infections (rarely)
Clostridium	Cl. tetani	Tetanus bacillus	Tetanus
	Cl. botulinum	Bacillus botulinus	Botulism
	Cl. perfringens	Cl. welchii	Gas gangrene
Diplococcus	D. pneumoniae	Streptococcus pneumoniae	Lobar and broncho-pneumonia; other infections
Gardnerella	G. vaginalis	Haemophilus vaginalis Corynebacterium vaginale	Vaginitis

wound or ulcer; proud flesh.

granule (grăn′ūl) [L. *granulum,* little grain]. 1. A small, grainlike body. 2. In histology, a minute mass in a cell that has an outline but no apparent structure.

g., acidophil. Granules that stain readily with acid dyes.

g., agminated. Small round or angular particle of disintegrated red blood corpuscle in the blood.

g., albuminous. Cytoplasmic granule in many normal cells. Not affected by ether or chloroform, but disappears from view when acetic acid is added.

g., alpha. Albuminous granule in leukocytes. Coarse, eosinophil, and highly refractive. SYN: *g., eosinophil; g., oxyphil.*

g., Altmann's. Mitochondria.

g., amphophil. Granule that stains with both acid and basic dyes. SYN: *g., beta.*

g., azurophil. Granule that takes a stain with azure dyes easily. Found in lymphocytes and monocytes; small and red or reddish-purple in color. They are inconstant in number, being present in about 30% of the cells.

g., basal. A small, deeply staining granule, found in certain protozoa, from which the flagellum arises. SYN: *blepharoplast.*

g.'s, basophil. Cellular granules that stain with a basic dye.

g., beta. An azurophil granule found in beta cells of the hypophysis or islets of Langerhans of the pancreas. SYN: *g., amphophil.*

g., chromatin. Small masses of deeply staining substance suspended within the meshes of the linin network of the nucleus of a cell.

g., chromophil. A granule of chromophil

substance present in the cytoplasm of neurons. SYN: *g., Nissl.*

g.'s, cone. The nuclei of the cones, sensory cells of the retina. They form the outer zone of the outer nuclear layer of the retina.

g.'s, delta. Small granules in the delta cells of the pancreas.

g., eosinophil. G., alpha.

g., epsilon. Neutrophil granule in polymorphonuclear leukocytes of the blood.

g., glycogen. Minute particles of glycogen seen in liver cells following fixation.

g.'s, hyperchromatin. Granules that stain with azure dye.

g., iodophil. Granules found in polymorphonuclear leukocytes and seen in various acute infectious diseases. Stain easily with iodine.

g.'s, juxtaglomerular. Secretory granules in the juxtaglomerular cells of the glomerulus of the kidney.

g., Kölliker's interstitial. Granule in the sarcoplasm of a striated muscle fiber.

g., metachromatic. Granules found in protoplasm of numerous bacteria; irregular in size. Stains deeply.

g.'s, Much's. Granules sometimes seen in sputum from patients with tuberculosis. They do not stain with acid-fast stain but do take gram stain. These particles are probably degenerated tubercle bacilli.

g.'s, neutrophil. Granules such as those found in neutrophil leukocytes, which stain with both basic and acid dyes, assuming a neutral tint.

g., Nissl. A chromophil granule found in the cell bodies of neurons. SYN: *Nissl bodies.*

g., oxyphil. G., alpha.

g., pigment. Granules of coloring matter seen in pigment cells.

g., Plehn's. Basophilic granule seen in the conjugating form of Plasmodium vivax.

g., protein. Protein particles of minute size in cells.

g., rod. Nucleus of the rod visual cell found in the external nuclear layer of the retina connected with the rods.

g., Schüffner's. Polychrome methylene blue–staining granule found in parasitized erythrocytes of tertian malaria; coarse and red.

g.'s, secretory. G.'s, zymogen.

g., seminal. Minute particles in semen, supposed to derive from disintegrated nuclei in nutritive cells from seminiferous tubules.

g.'s, thread. Filamentous mitochondria.

g.'s, zymogen. Granules present in gland cells, esp. the secretory cells of the pancreas, the chief cells of the gastric glands, and serous cells of the salivary glands. They are the precursors of the enzymes secreted. SYN: *g.'s, secretory.*

granulitis (grăn-ū-lī'tĭs) [L. *granulum,* little grain, + Gr. *itis,* inflammation]. Acute miliary tuberculosis.

granuloadipose (grăn"ū-lō-ăd'ĭ-pōs). Fatty degeneration with the presence of fatty granules.

granuloblast (grăn'ū-lō-blăst) [" + Gr. *blastos,* germ]. Mother cell of a granulocyte. A myeloblast found in bone marrow.

granulocyte (grăn'ū-lō-sīt") [" + Gr. *kytos,* cell]. A granular leukocyte; a polymorphonuclear leukocyte (neutrophil, eosinophil, or basophil).

granulocytopenia (grăn"ū-lō-sī"tō-pē'nē-ă) [" + " + *penia,* poverty]. Abnormal reduction of granulocytes in the blood. SYN: *granulopenia.*

granulocytopoiesis (grăn"ū-lō-sī"tō-poy-ē'sĭs) [" + " + *poiein,* to form]. The formation of granulocytes.

granulocytosis (grăn"ū-lō-sī-tō'sĭs) [" + " + *osis,* condition]. Abnormal increase in the number of granulocytes in the blood.

granuloma [" + Gr. *oma,* tumor]. A granular tumor or growth, usually of lymphoid and epitheloid cells. It occurs in various infectious diseases such as leprosy, cutaneous leishmaniasis, yaws, and syphilis.

g. annulare. A condition of the skin characterized by development of reddish nodules arranged in the form of a circle.

g., apical. G., dental.

g., benign, of thyroid. A lymphadenoma of the thyroid.

g., coccidioidal. A chronic, generalized granulomatous disease caused by the fungus Coccidioides immitis. SEE: *coccidioidomycosis.*

g., dental. Granuloma developing at the root of a tooth. May contain epithelial nests or colonies of bacteria.

g., eosinophilic. A form of xanthomatosis, q.v., accompanied by eosinophilia and formation of cysts on bone.

g. fissuratum. A circumscribed, firm, fissured, fibrotic tumor caused by chronic irritation. It may occur where a hard object such as dentures or the ear pieces of glasses rub against the labioalveolar fold or the retroauricular fold respectively. The tumor is not malignant and disappears when the irritating object is removed.

g., foreign body. Chronic inflammation around foreign bodies such as sutures, talc, splinters, or gravel.

g. fungoides. Mycosis fungoides.

g., infectious. Any infectious disease in which granulomas are formed, such as tuberculosis or syphilis. Granulomas are also formed in mycoses, protozoan infections, and in certain metazoal diseases.

g. inguinale. A granulomatous ulcerative disease in which the initial lesion commonly appears in the genital area as a painless nodule.

ETIOL: A short gram-negative bacillus, Calymmatobacterium granulomatis. These microorganisms are commonly called Donovan bodies, q.v.

TREATMENT: Gentamicin, tetracyclines, or ampicillin. When treatment is completed the patient should be followed for six months to determine if syphilis was contracted along with the granuloma.

g. iridis. Granuloma that develops on the iris.

g., lipoid. Granuloma that contains fatty tissue or cholesterol.

g., lipophagic. A granuloma in which the macrophages have phagocytosed the surrounding fat cells.

g., Majocchi's. G., trichophytic, q.v.

g., malignant. Lymphogranulomatosis; Hodgkin's disease.

g., paracoccidioidal. Paracoccidioidomycosis.

g. pyogenicum. Granuloma containing pyogenic organisms that develop at the site of a wound. They may also occur at the tip of the fingers along the sides of the nails or beneath the free edge of the nail. They bleed easily and are usually painful to touch. SYN: *septic granuloma.*

g., swimming pool. Chronic skin infection with Mycobacterium balnei. This organism may be present in unchlorinated swimming pools.

g., telangiectaticum. A very vascular granuloma at any site, but esp. in the nasal mucosa or pharynx.

g., trichophytic. Granulomas of the skin of the follicles and follicular areas of the legs. Caused by fungi, usually Trichophyton rubrum.

granulomatosis (grăn″ū-lō″mă-tō′sĭs) [L. *granulum,* little grain, + Gr. *oma,* tumor, + *osis,* diseased condition]. The development of multiple granulomas.

g. siderotica. Iron-containing granulomata of the lungs.

g., Wegener's. Rare disease of unknown etiology characterized by widespread granulomatous lesions of the bronchi, necrotizing arteriolitis, and glomerulonephritis.

granulomatous (grăn″ū-lŏm′ă-tŭs). Containing granulomas.

granulopenia (grăn″ū-lō-pē′nē-ă) [″ + Gr. *penia,* poverty]. Abnormal decrease of granulocytes in the blood. SYN: *granulocytopenia.*

granuloplasm (grăn′ū-lō-plăzm). Granular cytoplasm.

granuloplastic (grăn″ū-lō-plăs′tĭk) [″ + Gr. *plassein,* to form]. Developing granules.

granulopoiesis (grăn″ū-lō-poy-ē′sĭs) [″ + Gr. *poiein,* to make]. The formation of granulocytes.

granulopotent (grăn″ū-lō-pō′tĕnt) [″ + *potentia,* power]. Potentially capable of forming granules.

granulosa (grăn″ū-lō′să). Layer of cells in the theca of the graafian follicle.

granulosa cell tumor. Tumor of the ovary. The cells resemble those of the primordial follicle. The neoplasm is associated with feminization.

granulosa-theca cell tumor. Tumor of the ovary in which the cells are derived from the graafian follicle. The tumor is associated with signs of feminization.

granulose (grăn′ū-lōs). The soluble portion of starch. It is converted into sugar by hydrolysis.

granulosis (grăn″ū-lō′sĭs) [″ + Gr. *osis,* condition]. A mass of minute granules.

g. rubra nasi. Disease of the skin of the nose.

ETIOL: Inflammatory infiltration about the nose with slightly elevated papules and dilated sweat glands.

SYM: Moist erythematous patch on numerous macules.

granum (grā′nŭm) [L.]. Grain.

grapes. 1. The fruit of the genus Vitis. Contains acid potassium tartrate. Acidity decreases with the age of the grape and sugar increases. The sugar is nearly all glucose and is more abundant than in any other fruit. Raisins (sweet dried grapes) contain more sugar and less water. 2. Structure or growth resembling a grape or bunch of grapes.

grape sugar. Dextrose.

graph (grăf). A visual presentation of statistical, clinical, or experimental data represented by a relationship between 2 sets of numbers or variables on an abscissa (y) (vertical) axis and the ordinate (x) (horizontal) axis. 2. Any visual representation of a numerical relationship.

-graph [Gr. *graphos,* written]. Suffix indicating the instrument used in recording data.

graphesthesia (grăf″ĕs-thē′zē-ă) [″ + *aisthesis,* perception]. The ability by which outlines, numbers, words, or symbols traced or written upon the skin are recognized.

graphite (grăf′īt) [Gr. *graphein,* to write]. A soft form of carbon.

grapho- [Gr. *graphein,* to write]. Prefix meaning to write.

graphology (grăf-ŏl′ō-jē) [″ + *logos,* study]. Examination of handwriting in diseases of the nerves as a means of diagnosis or as a means of analyzing personality.

graphomotor (grăf″ō-mō′tor) [″ + L. *motor,* mover]. Pert. to movements involved in writing.

graphophobia (grăf″ō-fō′bē-ă) [″ + *phobos,* fear]. Abnormal fear of writing.

graphorrhea (grăf″ō-rē′ă) [″ + *rhoia,* flow]. Writing of many meaningless words and phrases.

graphospasm (grăf′ō-spăzm) [″ + *spasmos,* spasm]. Writer's cramp.

GRAS List. Indicates food additives *generally recognized as safe* by the U.S. Food and Drug Administration. SEE: *food additives.*

grasp. Specific types of prehension involving the fingers or the palmar surface or both. Types of grasp include: cylindrical, as in holding a cylinder, where the fingers and palmar surface are in opposition, and ball grasp, as in holding a spherical object, where the fingers, thumb and palmar surface surround an object. Related terms: prehension, pinch, hook.

grattage (gră-tăzh′) [Fr., a scraping]. Removal of morbid growths by rubbing with a brush or harsh sponge.

grave [L. *gravis,* heavy]. Serious; dangerous; severe.

grave wax. Waxlike matter on flesh caused by exposure to moisture with exclusion of air, as a body in the water or underground. SYN: *adipocere.*

gravel [Fr. *gravelle,* coarse sand]. Crystalline dust or concretions of crystals from the kidneys. Generally made up of phosphates, calcium, oxalate, and uric acid.

Graves' disease. [Robert J. Graves, Irish physician, 1797–1853] Exophthalmic goiter. SEE: *goiter, exophthalmic.*

gravid (grăv′ĭd) [L. *gravida,* pregnant]. Pregnant; heavy with child.

gravida (grăv′ĭ-dă) [L.]. A pregnant woman.

gravidism [″ + Gr. *-ismos,* state of]. State of being pregnant.

graviditas (gră-vĭd′ĭ-tăs). Pregnancy.

gravidity (gră-vĭd′ĭ-tē) [L. *gravida,* pregnant]. Pregnancy.

gravidocardiac (grăv″ĭd-ō-kăr′dē-ăk) [″ + Gr. *kardia,* heart]. Pert. to cardiac disorders resulting from pregnancy.

gravimetric (grăv″ĭ-mĕt′rĭk) [L. *gravis,* heavy, + Gr. *metron,* measure]. Determined by weight.

gravistatic (grăv″ĭ-stăt′ĭk) [″ + Gr. *statikos,* causing to stand]. Resulting from gravitation, as in a form of gravistatic pulmonary congestion.

gravitation [L. *gravitas,* weight]. Force and movement tending to draw every particle of matter together, esp. the attraction of the earth for bodies at a distance from its center.

gravity. Property of possessing weight. The force of the earth's gravitational attraction.

g., specific. ABBR: sp. gr. Weight of a substance compared with an equal volume of water. Water is used as a standard and considered to have a specific gravity of one (1.000).

Gravlee jet washer. Proprietary device for irrigating the endometrial cavity with sterile isotonic saline and then removing the solution and the dislodged cells. The cells are stained and examined for evidence of malignancy.

gray. Color without hue between extremes of black and white.

gray matter. Nervous tissues of a grayish color in which myelinated nerve fibers do not predominate. It contains large numbers of cell bodies of neurons. The term is generally applied to the gray portions of the central nervous system, which include the cerebral cortex, basal ganglia, and nuclei of the brain, and the gray columns of the spinal cord, which form an H-shaped region surrounded by white matter. Sympathetic ganglia and nerves may also be gray. SYN: *substantia grisea* [NA].

gray syndrome of the newborn. The appearance of vomiting, lack of sucking response, irregular and rapid respiration, abdominal distention, and cyanosis in newborn infants treated at birth with chloramphenicol. Flaccidity and an ashen-gray color are present within 24 hours. Death occurs in about 40% of the patients, most frequently in the fifth day of life.

CAUTION: Children less than one month of age being treated with chloramphenicol should receive no more than 25 mg./kg. of body weight each day.

green. A color intermediate between blue and yellow, afforded by rays of wavelength between 492 and 575 nanometers. SEE: words beginning with *chloro-*.

g., brilliant. A derivative of malachite green. Used in staining bacteria.

g., indocyanine. A dye used intravenously to determine blood volume.

g., malachite. A dye used as a stain and antiseptic.

green blindness. A type of color blindness in which green colors cannot be distinguished. SYN: *aglaucopsia.*

Greenfield's disease. [J. Godwin Greenfield, Brit. neuropathologist, 1884–1958] Metachromatic leukodystrophy, q.v.

green soap. USP. A potassium soap made by the saponification of suitable vegetable oils excluding coconut oil, palm kernel oil, without the removal of glycerin.

green soap tincture. Green soap to which lavender oil and alcohol have been added.

greenstick fracture. Fracture involving only part of the thickness of a bone. SEE: *fracture; Fractures* in *Appendix.*

green vitriol. Ferrous sulfate. SYN: *copperas.*

greffotome (grĕf′ō-tōm) [Fr *greffe,* graft, +

Gr. *tome*, incision]. Instrument for making tissue grafts.

grenz rays [Ger. *Grenze*, boundary]. Roentgen rays with an average wavelength of two angstroms. SEE: *ray*.

grid. 1. A chart with an abscissa (y) (vertical) axis and ordinate (x) (horizontal) axis to plot graphs upon. 2. A device made of parallel lead pieces used to screen scattered radiation when taking an x-ray.

grief reaction. The emotional reaction that follows the loss of a love-object. Somatic symptoms include easy fatigability, hollow or empty feelings in the chest and abdomen, sighing hyperventilation, anorexia, insomnia, and the feeling of having a lump in the throat. Psychological symptoms begin with an initial stage of shock and disbelief accompanied by an inner awareness of mental discomfort, sorrow, and regret. These may be followed by tears, sobbing, and cries of pain. The duration of the reaction is variable but may last for over a year.

griffe des orteils (grēf dāz or-tā') [Fr.]. Muscular atrophy of foot with contraction. SYN: *clawfoot*.

Grifulvin V. Trade name for griseofulvin microsize.

grinder (grīn'dĕr) [AS. *grindan*, to gnash]. A molar tooth. SYN: *dens molaris* [NA].

grinders' disease. Chronic lung disease due to dust inhalation. SYN: *pneumoconiosis; siderosis*.

grinding. Forceful rubbing together as in chewing. SEE: *bruxism*.

g., selective. Altering and correcting the occlusion of teeth by grinding in accordance with what is required.

grip, grippe (grĭp) [Fr. *gripper*, to seize]. Acute infectious disease marked by fever, prostration, pains in head and back, and upper respiratory tract symptoms such as cough and nasal congestion. SYN: *influenza*.

gripes (grīps) [AS. *gripan*, to grasp]. Intermittent severe pains in bowels. SYN: *colic*.

griping. An acute intermittent cramp-like pain, esp. in the abdomen.

Grisactin. Trade name for griseofulvin microsize.

griseofulvin. An antifungal antibiotic for oral administration. Especially effective in ringworm. Trade names for griseofulvin are Fulvicin-U/F, Gris-PEG, and Grifulvin V.

Gris-PEG. Trade name for griseofulvin.

gristle (grĭs'ĕl) [AS.]. Cartilage.

grits. Coarsely ground corn. It may be prepared as a thick mush or it can be poured into a mold, allowed to set and solidify, and then sliced and fried.

grocers' itch. Eczema of the hands due to irritation from handling flour and sugar. SEE: *eczema*.

groin [AS. *grynde*, abyss]. The depression between the thigh and trunk. The inguinal region.

groove [MD. *groeve*, ditch]. Long narrow channel, depression, or furrow. SYN: *sulcus*.

g., bicipital. Groove for the long tendon of the triceps located on the anterior surface of the humerus. SYN: *g., intertubercular*.

g., branchial. A groove in the embryo that is lined with ectoderm and lies between two branchial arches. SEE: *branchial arches; branchial grooves*.

g., carotid. A broad groove on the inner surface of the sphenoid bone lateral to the body. It lodges the carotid artery and the cavernous sinus.

g., costal. A groove on the lower internal border of a rib. It lodges the intercostal vessels and nerve. SYN: *g., subcostal*.

g., costovertebral. A broad groove that extends along each side of the vertebrae. It lodges the sacrospinalis muscle and its subdivisions. SYN: *g., vertebral*.

g., Harrison's. A groove or line extending laterally from the xiphoid process of the sternum. It marks the attachment of the diaphragm to the costal margins. Seen in severe rickets in children.

g., infraorbital. A groove on the orbital surface of the maxilla that transmits the infraorbital vessels and nerve.

g., intertubercular. G., bicipital.

g., labial. A groove that develops in each of the primitive jaws. It gives rise to the vestibule separating the lips from the gums.

g., lacrimal. 1. A groove on the posterior surface of the frontal process of the maxilla. 2. A groove on the anterior surface of the posterior lacrimal crest of the lacrimal bone. The two grooves lodge the lacrimal sac.

g., laryngotracheal. A groove along the ventral surface of the anterior portion of the embryonic gut that gives rise to the respiratory organs.

g., malleolar. A groove on the anterior surface of the distal end of the tibia that lodges tendons of the tibialis posterior and flexor digitorum longus musculi.

g., medullary. G., neural.

g., musculospiral. G., radial.

g., mylohyoid. Groove on the inner surface of the mandible that runs obliquely forward and downward and lodges the mylohyoid nerve and artery. In the embryo it lodges Meckel's cartilage.

g., nasolacrimal. A groove extending from the inner angle of the eye to the primitive olfactory sac in the embryo. It separates the maxillary and lateral nasal processes; its epithelial lining gives rise to the nasolacrimal duct.

g., nasopalatine. A groove on the vomer

that lodges the nasopalatine nerve and vessels.

g., neural. A longitudinal groove on the dorsal surface of the embryo lying between the neural folds. Upon closure of the folds to form the neural tube, the groove becomes the cavity of the neural tube, eventually giving rise to the ventricles of the brain and the central canal of the spinal cord.

g., obturator. A groove at the superior and posterior angle of the obturator foramen through which pass the obturator vessels and nerve.

g., olfactory. A shallow groove on the superior surface of the cribriform plate of the ethmoid on each side of the crista galli. It lodges the olfactory bulb.

g., palatine. One of a number of grooves on the inferior surface on the palatine process of the maxilla. They lodge the palatine vessels and nerves.

g., peroneal. 1. A shallow groove on the lateral aspect of the calcaneus. 2. A deep groove on the inferior surface of the cuboid bone. Each transmits the tendon of the peroneus longus muscle.

g., pharyngeal. G., branchial.

g., primitive. In the embryo, a shallow groove in the primitive streak of the blastoderm, bordered by the primitive folds.

g., pterygopalatine. A groove on the maxillary surface of the perpendicular portion of the palatine bone that, with corresponding grooves on the maxilla and pterygoid process of the sphenoid, transmits the palatine nerve and descending palatine artery.

g., radial. A broad, shallow groove running in a spiral direction on the posterior surface of the humerus. It transmits the radial nerve and the profunda branchi artery. SYN: *g., musculospiral.*

g., rhombic. One of seven transverse grooves in the floor of the developing rhombencephalon. They separate the neuromeres.

g., sagittal. A shallow groove on the inner surface of the parietal bones that lodges the superior sagittal sinus. SYN: *sagittal sulcus.*

g., sigmoid. Groove on the inner surface of the mastoid portion of the temporal bone. It transmits the transverse sinus.

g., subcostal. G., costal.

g., tympanic. A groove at the bottom of the exterior auditory meatus that receives the inferior portion of the tympanic membrane.

g., urethral. A groove on the caudal surface of the genital tubercle or phallus bordered by the urethral folds. The latter close, transforming the groove into the cavernous urethra.

g., vertebral. G., costovertebral.

g., visceral. G., branchial.

gross (grōs) [L. *grossus,* thick]. 1. Visible to the naked eye. 2. Consisting of large particles or components; coarse or large. 3. Having an insensitiveness or lack of social refinement.

gross anatomy. Study of organs and parts seen without the aid of a microscope.

gross lesion. Lesion visible to the eye without the aid of a microscope.

gross motor skills. Skills pertaining to the synergy of large muscle groups, as in balancing, running, and throwing.

ground. 1. Basic substance or foundation; reduced to a powder; pulverized. 2. In electronics, the negative or earth pole that has zero electrical potential.

ground bundle. A bundle of nerve fibers that immediately surrounds the gray matter of the spinal cord. It is divided into three regions, the anterior, lateral, and posterior bundles, which lie in the corresponding funiculi. These consist principally of short descending fibers.

ground itch. Inflammation of the skin resulting from the invasion of the larvae of hookworms (Ancylostoma or Necator). SYN: *ancylostomiasis.* SEE: *larva migrans.*

ground substance. The fluid, semifluid, or solid material that occupies the intercellular spaces in fibrous connective tissue, cartilage, or bone. SYN: *matrix.*

group [It. *gruppo,* knot]. A number of similar objects or structures taken or considered together; thus bacteria with similar metabolic characteristics are considered together as a group. Atomic molecules and compounds with similar structures or properties are classified within certain groups.

g., alcohol. The hydroxyl, $-OH$, group, which imparts alcoholic characteristics to organic compounds. These may be in three forms: primary, $-CH_2OH$; secondary, $=CHOH$; and tertiary, $\equiv COH$.

g., azo. The group $-N=N-$.

g., coli-aerogenes. Coliform bacteria.

g., colon-typhoid-dysentery. Collective term for Escherichia, Salmonella, and Shigella bacteria.

g., peptide. The $-CONH-$ radical.

g., prosthetic. 1. In a conjugated protein, the nonprotein portion of the molecule. 2. The nonprotein component of a coenzyme.

g., saccharide. The monosaccharide unit, $C_6H_{10}O_5$, which is a component of higher polysaccharides.

grouping. Classification of individual traits according to a shared characteristic.

g., blood. Classification of blood of different individuals according to agglutinating and hemolyzing qualities before making a blood transfusion. SEE: *blood groups; blood transfusion.*

grouping serum. A serum used for determining the blood group to which unknown cells belong. The grouping serums commonly used are human serums secured from donors and rabbit antiserums prepared commercially.

group therapy. A form of simultaneous psychotherapy involving two or more patients and one or more psychotherapists.

group-transfer. An oxidation-reduction chemical reaction involving the exchange of chemical groups. A transferase enzyme is required.

growing pains. An imprecise term indicating ill-defined pain in the musculoskeletal system of young persons. There is no evidence that the pain is related to rapid growth.

growth [AS. *growan,* to grow]. The progressive development or increase in size of a living thing. This may be normal as in growth of an embryo or child or pathological as in a cyst or benign or malignant tumor.

METHODS: By the synthesis of new protoplasm and multiplication of cells or by the manufacture and deposition of organic substances such as fatty acids inside cells.

TYPES: (1) General *body growth* is seen in the increase in the physical size of the body and increase in the total weight of the muscles and various internal organs. Growth is usually slow and steady but has a marked acceleration just after birth and at the time of puberty (the growth spurt).

(2) *Organs of the lymphoid type,* such as the thymus and the lymph nodes, grow fastest early in life, reach their peak of development at the age of about 12, and then regress.

(3) *The neural type of organ,* such as the brain, cord, eye, and meninges, grows in childhood but is close to its adult size by the age of 8 years. This size is maintained without regression.

(4) *The genital type of growth* is seen in the testes, ovaries, and other genitourinary structures. Their growth is the slowest of these four types in infancy, but at puberty they grow faster and cause the striking changes in appearance that comprise the secondary sex characteristics.

Not all of the organs of the body are included in the above four types. Some structures, such as the mammary glands, have several cycles of growth and regression in a lifetime.

growth hormone. Hormone that is liberated by the anterior pituitary and important in regulating growth. SYN: *somatotropin.*

gruel [L. *grutum,* meal]. Any cereal boiled in water.

grumose, grumous (groo'mōs, -mŭs) [L. *grumus,* heap]. 1. Made up of coarse granular bodies in the center. 2. Lumpy, clotted.

Grünfelder's reflex (groon'fĕld-ĕrs). Fanlike spreading of toes with upward flexion of great toe resulting from pressure over posterior fontanel.

gryposis (grĭ-pō'sĭs) [G. *gryposis,* a crooking]. Abnormal curvature of any part of the body but esp. the nails.

GSR. *galvanic skin response.*

G-suit. A coverall-type garment designed for use by aviators. The suit contains compartments that inflate and bring pressure on the legs and abdomen so as to prevent blood from pooling there. In aviators this helps to prevent unconsciousness caused by positive acceleration. The suit has been used in medicine to treat postural hypotension.

gt. L. *gutta,* a drop.

gtt. L. *guttae,* drops.

GU. *genitourinary.*

guaiacol (gwī'ă-kōl). *o*-Methoxyphenol. A substance similar to phenol obtained by fractional distillation of creosote or by synthetic means. Used as antiseptic and germicide, intestinal antiseptic, and expectorant.

guaifenesin (gwī-fĕn'ĕ-sĭn). USP. An expectorant. Trade name is Robitussin.

guanase (gwăn'ās) [Sp. *guano,* from Quechua *huanu,* dung]. An enzyme in a number of glands; it converts guanine into xanthine.

guanethidine (gwăn-ĕth'ĭ-dēn). A drug that depresses the function of postganglionic adrenergic nerves. Thus sympathetic nerve activity is inhibited. Guanethidine is used in treating hypertension.

g. sulfate. USP. An adrenergic blocking agent used in treating hypertension.

guanidine (gwăn'ĭ-dēn). A crystalline organic compound, $NH{:}C(NH_2)_2$, found among the decomposition products of proteins.

guanidinemia (gwăn"ĭd-ĕn-ē'mē-ă) [*guanidine* + Gr. *haima,* blood]. Guanidine in the blood.

guanidoacetic acid. A chemical formed in the liver, kidney, and other tissues. It is then metabolized to form creatine.

guanine (gwă'nēn). $C_5H_5N_5O$. An organic compound that occurs as a natural constituent of animal and vegetable nucleic acids. It is abundant in liver, muscle, glandular tissue such as pancreas, and seeds. Uric acid is its metabolic end point.

guanosine (gwăn'ō-sĭn). The nucleoside formed from guanine and ribosone. It is a major constituent of RNA and DNA.

gubernaculum (gū"bĕr-năk'ū-lŭm) [L., helm]. A structure that guides; a cordlike structure uniting two structures.

g. dentis. A connective tissue band that connects the tooth sac of an unerupted tooth with the overlying gum.

g. testis. [NA] A fibrous cord in the fetus that extends from the caudal end of the testis through the inguinal canal to the scrotal swelling. It plays a role in the descent of the testis into the scrotum.

Gubler's line (goob'lĕrz). [Adolphe Gubler, Fr. physician, 1821–1879] The level of superficial origin of the trigeminus or fifth nerve.

Gubler's paralysis. Hemiplegia affecting parts on opposite sides of the body. SYN: *hemiplegia, alternate.*

Gubler's tumor. A fusiform swelling on the wrist in lead palsy.

Gudden's inferior commissure (gūd'ĕnz). [Bernard A. von Gudden, Ger. neurologist, 1824–1886] Fibers of optic tract.

Gudden's law. In the division of a nerve, degeneration in the proximal portion is toward the nerve cell.

guidance. The act of guiding or counseling a patient.

guide. A mechanical aid or device that assists in setting a course or directing the motion either of one's hand or of an instrument one holds.

Guillain-Barré syndrome. [G. Guillain, Fr. neurologist, 1876–1961; J. A. Barré, Fr. neurologist, b. 1880] Polyneuritis with progressive muscular weakness of extremities that may lead to paralysis. Usually occurs after recovery from an infectious disease. It has also occurred as a rare complication of immunization with influenza vaccine. Patients with this syndrome always have a high protein content in their cerebrospinal fluid. Recovery is usually complete if the acute period is uncomplicated.

This syndrome has been described by various terms: acute polyneuritis, infectious polyneuritis, acute polyneuropathy, and Landry's paralysis. All are believed to be the same syndrome.

guillotine (gĭl'ō-tēn) [Fr., instrument for beheading]. Instrument for excising tonsils and laryngeal growths.

guinea pig (gĭn'ē pĭg). 1. A small rodent used in laboratory research. 2. A colloquial term for persons being used in medical experiments.

guinea worm. Dracunculus medinensis.

gullet [L. *gula,* throat]. The esophagus.

Gull's disease. [Sir William W. Gull, Brit. physician, 1816–1890] Atrophy of the thyroid gland, which causes myxedema, q.v.

Gullstrand's slit lamp (gŭl'străndz). [Allvar Gullstrand, Swedish ophthalmologist, 1862–1920] A device for illuminating the eye so its anterior portion can be examined by use of a microscope.

gum. 1. A substance that is given out by or extracted from certain plants. It is sticky when moist but hardens upon drying. Roughly, any resinlike substance given out by plants. 2. The fleshy substance or tissue covering the alveolar processes of the jaws. SYN: *gingiva.*

DIAG: *Bleeding easily:* Indicates scurvy or inflammation as in trench mouth or pyorrhea. *Blue:* Silver poisoning. *Bluish red:* Indicates mercurial stomatitis or lead poisoning if bluish line is at edge of teeth. *Greenish line:* At edge of teeth may indicate copper poisoning. *Purplish line or color:* Scurvy. *Red line:* In youth, indicates gingivitis, pyorrhea, scurvy. *Spongy gum and ulceration:* Gingivitis; scurvy; stomatitis; leukemia; tuberculosis; and diabetes.

RS: diagnosis; gingiva; ulatrophia; ulemorrhagia; uletic; ulitis; uloglossitis; uloncus; ulorrhea.

gumboil. Abscess of the gum. SYN: *parulis.*

ETIOL: Subperiosteal infection associated with a carious tooth. May be caused by irritation or injury by a denture.

SYM: Gum is red, swollen, tender, and very painful. A fluctuating swelling may appear containing pus. It may point and break or require incision.

TREATMENT: Hot mouthwashes and applications over gum or externally. Warn patient not to swallow pus. Frequent mouthwashes after lesion is evacuated.

gumma (gŭm'mă) [L. *gummi,* gum]. A soft tumor of the tissues characteristic of the tertiary stage of syphilis. It is a granuloma varying in size from a millimeter to a centimeter or more in diameter. May be single or multiple, and tend to be encapsulated. Each consists of a central necrotic mass surrounded by an inflammatory zone and fibrosis. The necrotic portion may be firm or elastic, gelatinous or hyalinized. Infectious organisms may be present. They occur most frequently in the liver but may occur in other organs such as the brain, testis, heart, bone, and skin. SEE: *syphilis.*

SYM: Depend upon location. Bursting of a gumma leads to a gummatous ulcer that is painless but slow to heal. The base is formed by a "wash-leather" slough but surrounding tissues are healthy.

gummatous (gŭm'ă-tŭs). Having the character of a gumma.

gummose (gŭm'ōs). $C_6H_{12}O_6$. A sugar from animal gum.

gummy [L. *gummi,* gum]. Sticky, swollen, puffy.

Gunn's dots (gŭnz). [Robert M. Gunn, Brit. ophthalmologist, 1850–1909] White spots on the retina of the eye, close to the macula.

gunshot wound. Penetrating or perforating wound that may contain a foreign body, as a bullet. SEE: *wound, bullet; Wounds* in *Appendix.*

gunstock deformity. Deformity in which the long axis of the extended forearm turns outwardly from the arm, caused by fracture at the elbow.

Günther's disease. [Hans Günther, Ger. physician, 1884–1956] Congenital erythropoietic porphyria.

gurney (gĕr'nē). A litter equipped with wheels. It is used in hospitals for transporting patients.

gustation (gŭs-tā'shŭn) [L. *gustare,* to taste]. Sense of taste.

gustatory (gŭs'tă-tō-rē). Pert. to sense of taste.

gustatory sweating. Sweating and flushing over the distribution of the auriculotemporal nerve in response to chewing.

gustometry (gŭs-tŏm'ĕ-trē) [" + Gr. *metron,* measure]. Measurement of acuteness of the sense of taste.

gut [AS.]. 1. The bowel or intestine. 2. The primitive gut or embryonic digestive tube, which includes the foregut, midgut, and hindgut. 3. Short term for catgut.

gutta [L., a drop]. (pl. *guttae*) ABBR: gt. (pl. *gtt.*) A drop. The amount in a drop varies with the nature of the liquid and its temperature. It is therefore not advisable to use the number of drops per minute of a solution as anything more than a general guide to the amount of material being administered intravenously.

gutta-percha (gŭt"ă-pĕr'chă). USP. Purified dried latex of certain trees. Used in dentistry and orthopedics.

guttate [L. *gutta,* drop]. Resembling a drop, said of certain cutaneous lesions.

guttatim (gŭt-tā'tĭm) [L]. Drop by drop.

guttering (gŭt'ĕr-ĭng). Cutting a channel or groove in a bone.

guttur (gŭt'ŭr) [L. *gutter,* throat]. The throat.

guttural (gŭt'ŭ-răl). Pert. to the throat.

gutturotetany (gŭt"ŭr-ō-tĕt'ă-nē) [" + Gr. *tetanos,* tension]. Laryngeal spasm of throat with temporary stutter.

Guyon's sign (gē-yŏnz'). [Felix J. C. Guyon, Fr. surgeon, 1831–1920] Ballottement of kidney.

Gwathmey's method (gwăth'mēz). [James T. Gwathmey, U.S. surgeon, 1863–1944] Use of anesthetic consisting of ether and olive oil solution. This is placed in the rectum and colon, where it is absorbed.

gymnastics [Gr. *gymnastikos,* pert. to nakedness]. Systematic body exercise with or without special apparatus.

g., ocular. Systematic exercise of the eye muscles to improve muscular coordination and efficiency.

g., Swedish. A system of movements made by a patient against a resistance provided by the attendant.

gymnophobia (jĭm-nō-fō'bē-ă) [Gr. *gymnos,* naked, + *phobos,* fear]. Abnormal aversion to viewing a naked body.

gynander (jĭ-năn'dĕr, jī-, gī-) [Gr. *gyne,* woman, + *aner, andros,* man]. An individual possessing both male and female characteristics. SYN: *gynandromorph; pseudohermaphrodite.*

gynandrism (jĭ-năn'drĭzm). 1. Male hermaphroditism. 2. Partial female pseudohermaphroditism.

gynandroid (jĭ-năn'droyd, jī-, gī-) [" + " + *eidos,* form]. An individual having sufficient hermaphroditic sexual characteristics to be mistaken for a person of the opposite sex.

gynatresia (jĭ-nă-trē'zē-ă, jī-, gī-) [" + *a-,* not, + *tresis,* perforation]. Atresia, q.v., of the vagina.

gynecic (jĭ-nē'sĭk, jī-, gī-) [Gr. *gyne,* woman]. Pert. to women.

gyneco-, gyno- [Gr.]. Prefix meaning woman, female.

gynecogenic (jĭn"ĕ-kō-jĕn'ĭk) [" + *gennan,* to produce]. Producing female characteristics.

gynecoid (jĭn'ĕ-koyd) [" + *eidos,* form]. Resembling the female of the species.

gynecologic, gynecological (gī"nĕ-kō-lŏj'ĭk, jī"-, jĭn"ĕ-; -ĭ-kăl) [" + *logos,* study]. Pert. to gynecology or study of diseases peculiar to women.

gynecologic operative procedures. *Postoperative:* Count and chart pulse every 15 minutes for first few hours. Report immediately any change in rate or volume. Watch for shock or internal hemorrhage. Keep warm and quiet; no visitors. Fluids when tolerated, tap water being best.

Care must be taken to prevent retention of urine. Sterile, closed, continuous drainage of the bladder may be preferable to repeated catheterization. Patient catheterized every 12 hours after operation, then every 8 hours until able to void. Thrombophlebitis with embolism is a serious complication. Have the patient exercise her legs frequently. Elastic stockings up to the knees, not circular elastic bandages, should be worn continuously while the patient is bedridden.

gynecologist (gī"nĕ-kŏl'ō-jĭst, jī"-, jĭn"ĕ-). Physician who specializes in gynecology.

gynecology (gī"nĕ-kŏl'ō-jē, jī"-, jĭn"ĕ-) [" + *logos,* study]. The study of the diseases of the female reproductive organs, including the breasts.

gynecomania (jī"nĕ-kō-mā'nē-ă, gī"-, jĭn"ĕ-) [" + *mania,* madness]. Abnormal sex desire in the male. SYN: *satyriasis.*

gynecomastia (jī"nĕ-kō-măs'tē-ă, gī"-, jĭn"ĕ-) [" + *mastos,* breast]. Abnormally large mammary gland in the male; sometimes may secrete milk.

gynecopathy (jī-nĕ-kŏp'ă-thē, gī"-, jĭn"ĕ-) [" + *pathos,* disease]. Diseases peculiar to women.

gynecophonus (jī″nĕ-kŏf′ŏn-ŭs, gī″-, jĭn″ĕ-) [″ + *phone,* voice]. Having an effeminate voice.

Gyne-Lotrimin. Trade name for clotrimazole.

gynephobia (jī″nĕ-fō′bē-ă, gī″-, jĭn″ĕ-) [″ + *phobos,* fear]. Abnormal aversion to the company of women, or fear of them.

Gynergen. Trade name for ergotamine tartrate.

gynesic (gī-nē′sĭk, jī-, jĭn-ē′-) [Gr. *gyne,* woman]. Pert. to the diseases of women.

gyniatrics (jī″nē-ăt′rĭks, gī″-, jĭn″ē-) [″ + *iatrikos,* medical treatment]. Treatment of diseases of women.

gynopathic [″ + *pathos,* disease]. Pert. to diseases of women.

gynoplastics [″ + *plassein,* to form]. Reparative surgery of female genitalia.

gynoplasty. Gynoplastics.

gypsum (jĭp′sŭm) [L.; G. *gypsos,* chalk]. A natural form of hydrated calcium sulfate. When heated to 130° C., it loses its water and becomes plaster of Paris.

gyrate (jī′rāt) [Gr. *gyros,* circle]. 1. Ring-shaped, convoluted. 2. To revolve.

gyration (jī-rā′shŭn). A rotary movement.

gyre (jīr) [Gr. *gyros,* circle]. Convolution. SYN: *gyrus.*

gyrectomy (jī-rĕk′tō-mē) [″ + *ektome,* excision]. Surgical removal of a cerebral gyrus.

gyrencephalic (jī-rĕn-sĕ-făl′ĭk) [″ + *enkephale,* head]. Having a brain marked by numerous convolutions.

gyri (jī′rī). Pl. of gyrus.

gyri breves insulae. [NA] Preinsular gyri.

gyro- [Gr.]. Combining form meaning a circle, spiral, ring.

gyrochrome (jī′rō-krōm) [″ + *chroma,* color]. A nerve cell in which the stainable substance occurs in rings.

gyroma (jī-rō′mă) [″ + *oma,* tumor]. Ovarian tumor consisting of a convoluted mass.

gyrometer (jī-rŏm′ĕ-ter) [″ + *metron,* measure]. A device for measuring the cerebral gyri.

gyrose (jī′rōs). In bacteriology, marked by wavy lines or circles. Applied to bacterial colonies.

gyrospasm (jī′rō-spăzm) [″ + *spasmos,* spasm]. Spasmodic rotary head movement.

gyrous (jī′rŭs) [Gr. *gyros,* circle]. Marked by circular lines. SYN: *gyrose.*

gyrus (jī′rŭs). (pl. *gyri*) [NA] One of the convolutions of the cerebral hemispheres of the brain. The gyri are separated by shallow grooves (sulci) or deeper grooves (fissures). SEE: *convolution.*

g., angular. Gyrus of the parietal lobe that embraces the posterior end of the superior temporal sulcus.

g., annectent. Any of many short folds of gray matter that are formed as a result of short branches or twigs of sulci extending into adjacent gyri. They are not always present.

g., anterior central. Gyrus of the frontal lobe extending vertically between the precentral and central sulci.

g., Broca's. G., frontal, inferior.

g., callosal. A large gyrus on the medial surface of the cerebral hemisphere that lies directly above the corpus callosum and arches over its anterior end.

g. cerebelli. Layer of the cerebellum.

g., cingulate. Arch-shaped convolution of the cingulum, curved over the surface of the corpus callosum, from which it is separated by the callosal sulcus.

g., dentate. A gyrus marked by indentations that lie on the upper surface of the hippocampal gyrus.

g. fornicatus. Gyrus on the medial surface of the cerebrum, which includes the gyrus cinguli, the isthmus, the hippocampus, the hippocampal gyrus, and the uncus.

g., frontal, inferior. A convolution on the external suface of the frontal lobe of the cerebrum located between the sylvian fissure and the inferior frontal sulcus.

g., frontal, middle. Gyrus between the superior and inferior frontal sulci.

g., frontal, superior. Convolution of the cerebral frontal lobe situated above the superfrontal fissure.

g., fusiform. Gyrus beneath the collateral fissure joining the occipital and temporal lobes.

g., Heschl's. Transverse temporal gyrus.

g., hippocampal. Gyrus situated between the hippocampal and collateral fissures.

g., infracalcarine. G., lingual.

g., lingual. Gyrus between the calcarine and collateral fissures.

g. longus insulae. [NA] Lengthy gyrus composing the postinsula.

g., marginal. G., frontal, superior.

g., middle temporal. Gyrus located between the middle temporal sulcus and superior temporal sulcus.

g., occipital. Any of the gyri on the lateral surface of the occipital lobe. They are not always present. Classified roughly in two groups, the inferior or lateral occipital gyri and the superior occipital gyri.

g., occipitotemporal. G., fusiform.

g., orbital. One of four gyri (anterior, posterior, lateral and medial) forming the inferior surface of the frontal lobe.

g., paracentral. Area on mesial aspect of the cerebrum; the paracentral lobule. Lies above cingulate sulcus.

g., parahippocampal. Gyrus on the lower surface of each cerebral hemisphere between the hippocampal and collateral sulci.

g., paraterminal. A small area of the cerebral cortex anterior to the lamina terminalis and below the rostrum of the corpus callosum.

g., parietal. Gyrus on lateral aspect of parietal lobe. Includes posterior central gyrus, superior and inferior parietal gyri.

g., postcentral. The gyrus immediately posterior to the central sulcus of the cerebrum. It contains most of the general sensory area of the brain. SYN: *posterior central gyrus*.

g., precentral. Gyrus immediately anterior to the central sulcus of the cerebrum. It contains the pyramidal area.

g., profundi cerebri. Very deep gyri of the cerebrum.

g. rectus. [NA] Gyrus on the orbital aspect of the frontal lobe, located between the mesial margin and the olfactory sulcus.

g. Retzii. The supra- and subcallosal gyri.

g., subcallosal. A narrow band of gray matter on the medial surface of the hemisphere below the rostrum of the corpus callosum.

g., subcollateral. G., fusiform.

g., supracallosal. A rudimentary gyrus on the upper surface of the corpus callosum.

g., supracallosus. Gray matter layer covering the corpus callosum.

g., supramarginal. Gyrus in the inferior parietal lobule twisting about the upper terminus of the sylvian fissure.

g., temporal. Three gyri (superior, middle, inferior) on lateral surface of the temporal lobe.

g. transitivus. G., annectent.

g., uncinate. Anterior hooked portion of the hippocampal gyrus.

H

H. Chem. symb. for hydrogen.

H., h. *haustus,* a draft of medicine; *height; henry; hora* or *hour; horizontal; hypermetropia.*

h. Symbol for Planck's constant.

H⁺. Chem. symb. for hydrogen ion.

[H⁺]. Symbol for hydrogen ion concentration.

H¹. Chem. symb. for protium.

H². Chem. symb. for deuterium, an isotope of hydrogen.

Ha. Chem. symb. for hahnium.

Haab's reflex (hŏbz). [Otto Haab, Swiss ophthalmologist, 1850–1931] Contraction of pupils without alteration of accommodation or convergence when gazing at a bright object. May indicate a cortical lesion.

habena (hă-bē'nă) [L., rein]. (pl. *habenae*) 1. A frenum. 2. Bandage for a wound. 3. Pineal gland peduncle. SYN: *habenula* [NA].

habenal, habenar [L. *habena,* rein]. Pert. to the habena or habenula.

habenula (hă-bĕn'ū-lă) [L., little rein, strap]. 1. A frenum or any rein- or whiplike structure. 2. [NA] A peduncle or stalk attached to the pineal body of the brain. Fibers that travel posteriorly along the dorsomedial border of the thalamus to the habenular ganglia (epithalamus) resemble reins. 3. A narrow bandlike stricture.

h. urethralis. One of two whitish bands between the clitoris and meatus urethra in young females.

habenular. Pert. to the habenula, esp. the stalk of the pineal body.

habenular commissure. A band of transverse fibers connecting the two habenular areas.

habenular trigone. A depressed triangular area located on the lateral aspect of the posterior portion of the third ventricle. Each contains a medial and lateral habenular nucleus.

habilitation (hă-bĭl"ĭ-tā'shŭn). The process of education or training persons with disadvantage or disability to improve their ability to function in society.

habit [L. *habere, habitus,* to have, hold]. 1. A motor pattern executed with facility following constant or frequent repetition; an act performed in a voluntary manner but that after sufficient repetition is performed as a reflex action. Habits result from the passing of impulses through a particular set of neurons and synapses many times. 2. A particular type of dress or garb. 3. Mental or moral constitution or disposition. 4. Bodily appearance or constitution, esp. as related to a disease or predisposition to a disease, as the apoplectic habit. SYN: *habitus.* 5. Addiction to the use of drug or beverage as the drug habit or alcoholic habit.

h., chorea. H., spasm.

h., spasm. A spasmodic voluntary movement that has become involuntary. Often due to something irritating; sometimes from mimicry. SYN: *tic.*

habit training. Development by young children of specific behavior patterns concerning basic activities such as eating, dressing, using the toilet, and sleeping.

habituation. Act of becoming accustomed to anything from frequent use. In drug addiction, the mental equivalent of physical tolerance and dependence on drugs.

habitus [L., habit]. (pl. *habitus*) 1. A physical appearance that indicates a tendency to certain diseases or abnormal conditions. 2. A physical appearance that indicates a tendency for internal organs to be positioned in a specific plane.

h. apoplecticus. The supposed body build and appearance of one predisposed to develop apoplexy: short, thick-necked with flushed face and prominent temporal arteries.

h. enteroptoticus. Physical state indicating marked enteroptosis. The abdomen is long and narrow and the angle between the ribs and the long axis of the body is less than 90°.

hachement (hăsh-mŏn') [Fr., chopping]. A chopping stroke with edge of the hand in massage.

hacking cough. Recurrent, nonproductive cough. SYN: *cough, dry.*

haem. Heme.

haem-. SEE: words beginning with *hem-*.

Haemadipsa (hē"mă-dĭp'să) [Gr. *haima,* blood + *dipsa,* thirst]. A genus of terrestrial leeches found in Asia that attack man and animals.

H. ceylonica. Species of leech found in Ceylon.

Haemagogus (hē"mă-gŏg'ŭs) [" + *agogos,* leading]. A genus of mosquitoes. Includes the species H. capricorni, which serves as a vector of yellow fever.

Haemaphysalis (hĕm"ă-fĭs'ă-lĭs) [" + *physallis,* bubble]. A genus of ticks. Various species serve as vectors for diseases including tick-borne typhus and Rocky Mountain spotted fever. Some species are reservoirs for rickettsiae but do not bite man.

Haemophilus (hē-mŏf'ĭl-ŭs) [" + *philein,* to love]. Chiefly British spelling for a genus of Bacteriaceae. SEE: *Hemophilus.*

Haemosporidia (hē"mō-spō-rĭd'ē-ă). An order of sporozoa that lives in the blood cells of vertebrates and reproduces sexually in invertebrates; includes the genus Plasmodium,

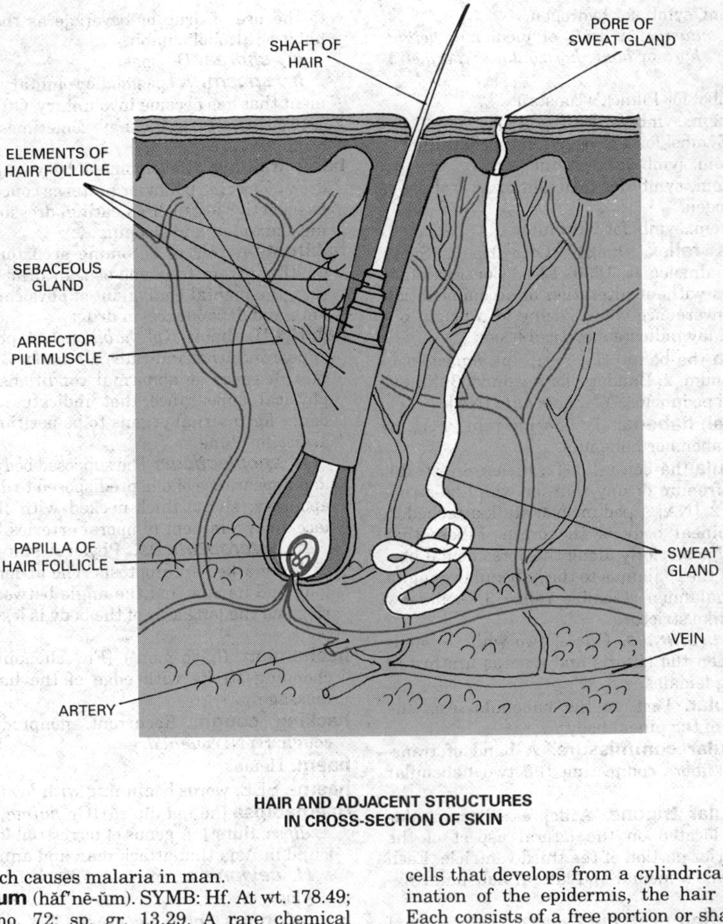

HAIR AND ADJACENT STRUCTURES IN CROSS-SECTION OF SKIN

which causes malaria in man.

hafnium (hăf'nē-ŭm). SYMB: Hf. At wt. 178.49; at no. 72; sp. gr. 13.29. A rare chemical element.

Hagedorn needle (hă'gĕ-dorn). [Werner Hagedorn, Ger. surgeon, 1831–1894] A curved surgical needle with flattened sides.

hahnium (hŏ'nē-ŭm). [Otto Hahn, Ger. physicist, 1879–1968] An element first synthesized in 1970 at the University of California, Berkeley. At. wt. 260. At. no. 105.

Hailey-Hailey disease. [W. H. Hailey, b. 1898, H. E. Hailey, b. 1909, U.S. dermatologists] Benign familial pemphigus.

hair [AS. *haer*]. 1. A keratinized, threadlike outgrowth from the skin of mammals. 2. Collectively, the threadlike outgrowths that form the fur of animals, or that grow on the human body.

A hair is a thin, flexible shaft of cornified cells that develops from a cylindrical invagination of the epidermis, the hair follicle. Each consists of a free portion or shaft (scapus pili) and a root (radix pili) embedded within the follicle. The shaft consists of three layers of cells: the cuticle or outermost layer; the cortex, forming the main horny portion of the hair; and the medulla, the central axis. SEE: illus. Hair color is due to pigment in the cortex.

Hair in each part of the body has a definite period of growth after which it is shed. In man there is a constant gradual loss and replacement of hair. Hair of the eyebrows lasts only three to five months; that of the scalp two to five years. Baldness or alopecia results when replacement fails to keep up with hair loss. It may be due to hereditary factors or pathological conditions such as infections or injury from irradiation.

h., auditory. An epithelial cell to which are attached delicate hairlike processes. These are present in the ear in the spiral organ of Corti, concerned with hearing; and the crista ampullaris, macula utriculi, and macula sacculi, concerned with equilibrium.

h., bamboo. Sparse, brittle hairs with bamboo-like nodes. These apparent nodes are actually partial fractures of the hair shaft. This is caused by an atrophic condition of the hair. SYN: *trichorrhexis nodosa.*

h., beaded. Swellings and constrictions in the hair shaft due to a developmental defect known as monilethrix, q.v.

h., burrowing. A hair that grows horizontally under the skin. This causes a foreign body reaction.

h., gustatory. One of several fine hairlike processes extending from the ends of gustatory cells in a taste bud. They project through the inner pore of a taste bud.

h., ingrown. A hair that re-enters the skin and causes a foreign body reaction.

h., kinky. Short, sparse, kinky hair that may be poorly pigmented. Associated with kinky hair disease, q.v.

h., lanugo. SEE: *lanugo.*

h., moniliform. Monilethrix, q.v.

h., pubic. Hair that appears over the pubes at the onset of sexual maturity.

h., sensory. Specialized epithelial cells with hairlike processes.

h., tactile. Hairs that are capable of receiving tactile or touching stimuli.

h., taste. Hairlike projections from the ends of the taste cells in the taste buds.

h., terminal. Long, coarse, pigmented hair of the adult.

h., twisted. Congenitally deformed hair that is short, brittle, and twisted.

hairball. A mass of hair in the stomach. SYN: *trichobezoar.*

hair bulb. The lower expanded portion of a hair root. Growth of a hair results from the proliferation of cells of the hair bulb.

hair cell. An epithelial cell possessing fine nonmotile cilia found in the maculae and the organ of Corti of the membranous labyrinth of the inner ear. They are receptors for the senses of position and hearing.

hair follicle. An invagination of the epidermis that forms a cylindrical depression, penetrating the corium into the connective tissue that holds the hair root. Sebaceous glands, which secrete an oily fluid, and tiny muscles (arrectores pili) that cause the hair to stand are attached to these follicles.

hair papilla. A projection of the corium that extends into the hair bulb at the bottom of a hair follicle. It contains capillaries through which a hair receives nourishment.

hair transplantation. A surgical procedure for placing plugs of skin containing hair follicles from one body site to another. This technique is very time consuming, but has some success in treatment of alopecia of the scalp.

hairy tongue. Tongue covered with hairlike papillae entangled with threads produced by the fungus Aspergillus niger or Candida albicans. Usually seen as the result of antibiotic therapy that inhibits growth of bacteria normally present in the mouth. This permits overgrowth of fungi. SYN: *tongue, black, hairy.*

halation (hăl-ā′shŭn) [Gr. *alos,* a halo]. Blurring of vision due to light from a wrong direction.

halazone (hăl′ă-zōn). USP. A chloramine disinfectant used in emergency sterilization of water.

halcinonide (hăl-sĭn′ō-nīd). A corticosteroid drug. Trade name is Halog.

Haldol. Trade name for haloperidol, USP.

Haldrone. Trade name for paramethasone acetate.

half-life. 1. Time required for half the nuclei of a radioactive substance to lose their activity by undergoing radioactive decay. 2. In biology and pharmacology, the time required by the body, tissue, or organ to metabolize or inactivate half the amount of a substance taken in. This is an important consideration in determining the proper amount and frequency of dose of drug to be administered. SYN: *biological half-life.* 3. Time required for radioactivity of material taken in by a living organism to be reduced to half its initial value by a combination of radioactive decay and biological elimination.

half-value layer. The amount of lead, copper, cement, or material that would dissipate the beam of radiation by 50%. The number of half-value layers required for safety in blocking the area on a patient is five, because that represents 50% of 50% and 50% of that, etc. For example, 50% + 25% + 12.5% + 6.23% + 3.12% = 96.9%. Thus the patient would be shielded from all but about 3% of the radiation. (Examples are two inches [five cm.] of lead and two feet [61 cm.] of cement.)

half-value thickness. The thickness of a substance that, when placed in the path of a given beam of rays, will lower its intensity to one half of the initial value.

halibut liver oil. An oil obtained from the liver of the halibut fish. It is rich in vitamins A and D.

halide (hăl′īd). Compound containing a halogen, i.e., bromine, chlorine, fluorine, or iodine, combined with a metal or some other radical.

halisteresis (hă-lĭs″tĕr-ē′sĭs) [Gr. *hals,* salt, + *steresis,* deprivation]. Lack of calcium (lime salt) in bone. SYN: *halosteresis*. SEE: *osteomalacia*.

halisteretic. Rel. to or affected with halisteresis.

halitosis (hăl-ĭ-tō'sĭs) [L. *halitus,* breath, + Gr. *osis,* condition]. Offensive breath.

halitus (hăl'ĭ-tŭs). 1. The breath. 2. Warm vapor.

Haller's anastomotic circle (hăl'ĕrz). [Albrecht von Haller, Swiss physiologist, 1708–1777] Circle of arteries around the intraocular portion of the optic nerve. Made up of branches of the posterior ciliary arteries.

Hallervorden-Spatz disease or syndrome. [Julius Hallervorden, 1882–1965, H. Spatz, 1888–1969, Ger. neurologists] An inherited progressive degenerative disease, beginning in childhood, of the globus pallidus, red nucleus, and reticular part of the substantia nigra of the brain. Clinically, there are progressive rigidity, athetotic movements, and mental and emotional retardation.

hallex (hăl'ĕks) [L.]. (pl. *hallices*) The great toe. SYN: *hallus; hallux.*

hallucination (hă-loo-sĭ-nā'shŭn) [L. *hallucinari,* to wander in mind]. In psychology, a false perception having no relation to reality and not accounted for by any exterior stimuli. May be visual, auditory, or olfactory. Judgement may be impaired and the patient will not be able to distinguish between the real and the imagined.

Structural disease of the sensory organ and conducting mechanism may contribute to the formation of hallucinations, e.g., the deafness of an old otitis media often is associated with tinnitus. An irritative lesion of the visual cortex may produce more directly the hallucination.

RS: acousma; delusion; hallucinosis; hypnagogic; illusion.

h., auditory. Imaginary perception of sounds, usually voices.

h., extracampine. Hallucination that arises from outside the normal sensory field or range, as people having the sensation of seeing something behind them.

h., gustatory. The sense of tasting something that is not present.

h., haptic. Hallucination pert. to touching the skin, or to sensations of temperature or pain.

h., hypnagogic. Pre-sleep phenomena having the same practical significance as a dream but experienced while consciousness persists. Includes sense of falling, sinking, or of the ceiling moving.

h., kinetic. Sensation of flying or moving the body or a part of it.

h., microptic. Hallucination in which things seem reduced in size.

h., motor. Imaginary perceptions of movement.

h., olfactory. Hallucination involving smell.

h., somatic. Sensation of pain attributed to visceral injury.

h., tactile. A false sense of touching something.

h., visual. Sensation of seeing objects that are not real.

hallucinogen (hă-loo'sĭ-nō-jĕn) [" + Gr. *gennan,* to produce]. Drug that produces hallucinations. LSD, peyote, mescaline, PCP, and sometimes ethyl alcohol are hallucinogens.

hallucinogenesis (hă-lū"sĭ-nō-jĕn'ĕ-sĭs). Production of or causing hallucinations.

hallucinosis (hă-loo"sĭn-ō'sĭs) [" + Gr. *osis,* condition]. The state of having hallucinations more or less persistently. SEE: *hallucination.*

h., acute alcoholic. Alcoholic psychosis marked by fear or anxiety and auditory hallucinations.

hallus. Hallux.

hallux (hăl'ŭks) [L.]. (pl. *halluces*) [NA] The great toe.

h. dolorosus. Pain in the metatarsophalangeal joint of the great toe due to flatfoot.

h. flexus. Hammertoe.

h. malleus. Hammertoe of the great toe.

h. rigidus. Restricted or loss of motion of the joint connecting the great toe to the metatarsal. This is painful upon walking.

h. valgus. Displacement of great toe toward other toes.

h. varus. Displacement of great toe away from other toes.

halmatogenesis (hăl"mă-tō-jĕn'ĕ-sĭs) [Gr. *halma,* jump, + *genesis,* development]. A sudden deviation of type from one generation to the other. SEE: *mutation.*

halo [Gr. *halos,* a halo]. 1. The areola, esp. of the nipple. 2. A ring surrounding the macula lutea in ophthalmoscopic images. 3. A circle of light surrounding a shining body.

h., Fick's. A colored halo around light; this is observed by some persons due to the wearing of contact lenses.

h., glaucomatous. A whitish ring surrounding the optic disk; seen in glaucoma.

h., senile peripapillary. A ring of choroidoretinal atrophy around the head of the optic nerve. This may occur in the aged.

halodermia (hăl"ō-dĕr'mē-ă). Skin eruption caused by exposure to a halogen.

Halog. Trade name for halcinonide.

halogen (hăl'ō-jĕn) [Gr. *hals,* salt, + *gennan,* to form]. A salt former; one of a group of elements (chlorine, Cl; bromine, Br; iodine, I; and fluorine, F) having very similar chemical properties. They combine with hydrogen to form acids and with metal to form salts.

haloid (hăl'oyd) [" + *eidos,* form]. Resembling

salt or a halogen.

haloid salt. A salt made up of a base and a halogen, resembling common salt.

halometer (hă-lŏm'ĕ-tĕr) [Gr. *halos,* a halo, + *metron,* measure]. 1. Device for measuring diffraction halo of a red blood cell. 2. Device for measuring the halo around the optic disk.

haloperidol (hă"lō-pĕr'ĭ-dŏl). USP. A sedative, psychotropic tranquilizer. One use is in the treatment of Gilles de la Tourette's syndrome. Trade name is Haldol.

halophilic (hăl"ō-fĭl'ĭk) [" + *philein,* to love]. Concerning or having an affinity for salt or any halogen.

halosteresis (hă-lŏs"tĕr-ē'sĭs) [Gr. *hals,* salt, + *steresis,* privation]. Deficiency of lime salts in the bones. SYN: *halisteresis.* SEE: *osteomalacia.*

halo symptom. Colored circle or circles around lights. These are seen by patients with glaucoma or with punctate lens opacities.

Halotestin. Trade name for fluoxymesterone, USP.

halothane (hăl'ō-thān). USP. A fluorinated hydrocarbon used as a general anesthetic.

Halsted's operation (hăl'stĕdz). [William Stewart Halsted, U.S. surgeon, 1852–1922] 1. Operation for inguinal hernia. 2. Radical mastectomy for cancer of the breast.

Halsted's suture. An interrupted suture for intestinal wounds.

ham [AS. *haum,* haunch]. 1. The popliteal space or region behind the knee. 2. Common name for the thigh, hip, and buttock.

hamartia (hăm-ăr'shē-ă) [Gr., defect]. Error in development due to imperfect tissue combination.

hamartoma (hăm-ăr-tō'mă) [Gr. *hamartia,* defect, + *oma,* tumor]. A tumor resulting from new growth of normal tissues. The cells grow spontaneously, reach maturity, and then do not reproduce. Thus the growth is self-limiting and benign.

h., multiple. Congenital malformations that present a slowly growing mass of abnormal tissue in multiple sites. The tissues are appropriate to the organ in which the hamartomas are located but they are not normally organized. They may appear in blood vessels as hemangiomata, and in the lung and kidney. They are not malignant but cause symptoms because of the space they occupy.

hamartomatosis (hăm"ăr-tō-mă-tō'sĭs) [" + " + *osis,* condition]. Existence of multiple hamartomas.

hamate (hăm'ăt). Hooked.

hamate bone. The medial bone in the distal row of carpal bones of the wrist.

hamatum (hă-mā'tŭm) [L. *hamatus,* hooked]. The unciform bone. SYN: *os hamatum.*

Hamman, Louis (hăm'ăn). U.S. physician, 1877–1946.

H.'s disease. Spontaneous mediastinal emphysema.

H.-Rich syndrome. [Arnold Rich, U.S. pathologist, b. 1893] A form of pulmonary disease with a rapid deterioration in clinical course due to diffuse interstitial pneumonitis or fibrosis. Symptoms vary with the degree but include dyspnea, rapid respirations, anoxia, and weight loss with subsequent weakness and fatigue. At first pulmonary symptoms are not prominent unless there is bronchial involvement with exudate. As the disease progresses, finger clubbing, cyanosis, and heart failure develop.

ETIOL: Unknown.

DIAG: Based on a characteristic chest x-ray along with exclusion of specific etiologic agent and clinical signs and symptoms.

TREATMENT: Corticosteroids are usually of considerable benefit but are not curative. Supportive therapy consists of supplemental oxygen, antibiotics, and treatment for heart failure.

hammer. 1. An instrument with a head attached crosswise to the handle for striking blows. 2. Common name for the malleus, the hammer-shaped bone of the middle ear.

h., percussion. A hammer with a rubber head used for tapping surfaces of the body in order to produce sounds for diagnostic purposes. SEE: *plexor.*

h., reflex. A hammer used for tapping parts of the body such as a muscle, tendon, or nerve in order to initiate certain reflex responses.

hammer finger. Flexion deformity of the distal joint of a finger. It is caused by avulsion of the extensor tendon. SYN: *mallet finger.*

hammertoe. A toe with dorsal flexion of 1st phalanx and plantar flexion of 2nd and 3rd phalanges. SYN: *claw toe.*

hamster. A rodent Cricetus cricetus belonging to the family Cricetidae, common in Europe and W. Asia. It is extensively used as a research animal.

hamstring [AS. *haum,* haunch]. One of the tendons that form the medial and lateral boundaries of the popliteal space.

h.'s, inner. Tendons of the semimembranosus, semitendinosus, and gracilis muscles.

h.'s, outer. The tendon of the biceps femoris.

hamstrings. Three muscles on the posterior aspect of the thigh, the semitendinosus, semimembranosus, and biceps femoris. They flex the leg and adduct and extend the thigh.

Ham test. A test for diagnosing paroxysmal nocturnal hemoglobinuria.

hamular (hăm'ū-lăr) [L. *hamulus,* a small hook]. Unciform; hook-shaped.

hamulus (hăm'ū-lŭs) [L., a small hook]. (pl. *hamuli*) 1. Any hook-shaped structure. 2.

BONES OF THE RIGHT HAND AND WRIST

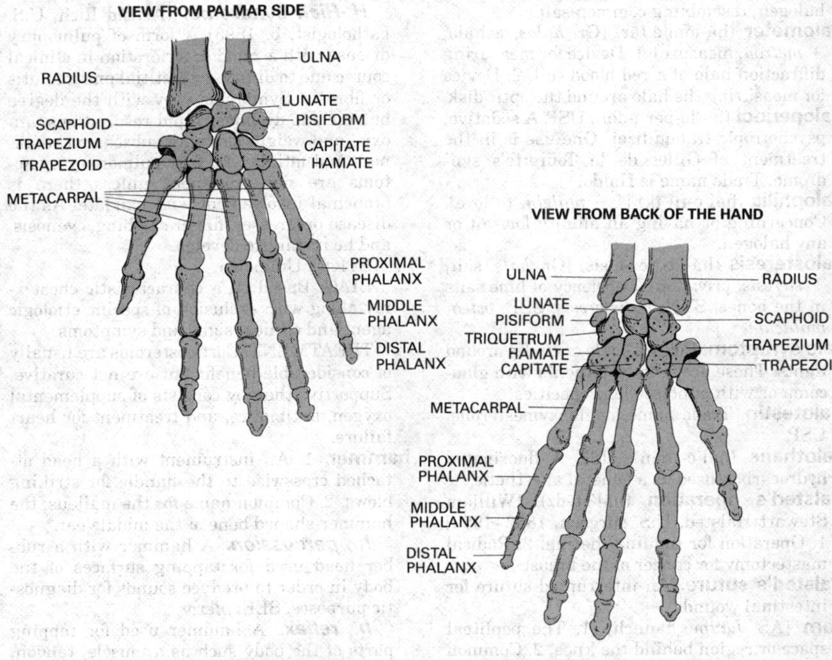

Hooklike process on the hamate bone.

h. cochleae. A hooklike process at the tip of the osseous spiral lamina of the cochlea.

h. lacrimalis. [NA] Hooklike process on the lacrimal bone.

h. pterygoideus. [NA] Hooklike process at the tip of the medial pterygoid process of the sphenoid bone.

hand [AS.]. That part of the body attached to the forearm at the wrist. It includes the wrist (carpus) with its 8 bones, the metacarpus or body of the hand (ossa metacarpalia) having 5 bones, and the phalanges (fingers) with their 14 bones. SYN: *manus* [NA]. SEE: illus.

h., ape. Deformity of the hand in which the thumb is permanently extended.

h., claw. Clawhand.

h., cleft. Deformity of the hand in which the division between the fingers, particularly between the third and fourth, extends into the carpus.

h., drop. Wrist drop.

h., functional position of. Principle used in splint fabrication whereby wrist is dorsiflexed 20–35°, there is a normal transverse arch, and the thumb is in abduction and opposition and aligned with the pads of the four fingers. Proximal interphalangeal joints are flexed 45–60°.

h., lobster-claw. Cleft hand.

h., obstetrician's. The hand in tetany with extension at the metacarpophalangeal and the interphalangeal joints, and adduction of the thumb.

h., opera-glass. Deformity of the hand caused by chronic arthritis. The phalanges appear to be telescoped into one another like an opera glass.

h., resting position of. Principle used in splint fabrication whereby the forearm is midway between pronation and supination, wrist is at 12–20° dorsiflexion, and phalanges are slightly flexed. Thumb is in partial opposition and forward.

h., writing. The tips of the thumb and first finger are touching and the other fingers are flexed as if writing. Seen in paralysis agitans.

H. and E. *hematoxylin* and *eosin,* a staining method used in histology.

handedness. The tendency to use one hand in preference to the other. Preferential use of the left hand is called sinistrality and of the right hand dextrality.

hand-foot-and-mouth disease. Painful ulcerative and vesicular lesions of the oral mucosa and tongue with vesicular lesions of the hands and feet. It is highly infectious.

Coxsackievirus Group A, type 16 predominantly, and types 4, 5, 9, and 10 cause this disease.

handicap. A mental or physical impairment that prevents or interferes with normal mental or physical activities and achievement. All living organisms have as a basic characteristic being able to adapt to handicaps. This is particularly true of human beings, some of whom are able to live useful, rewarding, and satisfying lives despite multiple handicaps. SEE: *disability.*

handpiece (hănd'pēs). Hand instrument used in dentistry. It contains a chuck for holding tools used in preparing teeth for restoration, polishing, and condensing. The tool may rotate or vibrate.

Hand-Schüller-Christian disease (hănd-shĭl'ĕr-krĭs'chăn). [Alfred Hand, Jr., U.S. pediatrician, 1868–1949; Artur Schüller, Austrian neurologist, b. 1874; Henry A. Christian, U.S. pathologist, 1876–1951] A rare disease of unknown cause in which lipids accumulate in the body and manifest as histiocytic granulomas in bone (particularly the skull), the skin, and viscera. Exophthalmos and diabetes insipidus may be present. The disease is seen in children and young adults. Adrenal cortical hormones have been of some help in treating the illness. SYN: *xanthoma disseminatum.*

handsock. A type of glove that covers the hand but, because it has no individual spaces for the fingers, makes grasping objects difficult. Use of handsocks during infancy may inhibit the rate of development of hand skills.

hanging drop culture. A method of culturing microorganisms by placing a drop of the culture medium containing organisms on a coverslip, then inverting the coverslip over a concavity of a hanging drop slide.

hangnail [AS. *hangian,* to hang, + *naegel,* nail]. Partly detached piece of skin at root or lateral edge of finger or toenail.

hangover. A nontechnical term for describing the malaise that may be present following the ingestion of a considerable amount of an alcoholic beverage or other central nervous system depressant. Usually present upon awakening after stuporous sleep. Characterized by some if not all of the following: mental depression, headache, thirst, nausea, irritability, fatigue. Symptoms and severity will vary with the individual.

The presence of congeners, q.v., in alcoholic beverages is felt to be related to the development of a hangover. Therapy of hangover is not specific. SEE: *alcoholism, acute.*

Hanot's disease (ă-nōz'). [Victor C. Hanot, Fr. physician, 1844–1896] Hypertrophic cirrhosis of liver with jaundice.

Hansen's bacillus. [Gerhard H. A. Hansen, Norwegian physician, 1841–1912] Mycobacterium leprae, the cause of leprosy, which Hansen discovered in 1871.

Hansen's disease. Leprosy.

hapalonychia (hăp"ăl-ō-nĭk'ē-ă) [Gr. *hapalos,* soft, + *onyx,* nail]. Lack of rigidity of the nails. SYN: *onychomalacia.*

haphalgesia (hăf"ăl-jē'zē-ă) [Gr. *haphe,* touch, + *algesis,* pain]. A sensation of pain upon touching the skin lightly or with an object that is not an irritant.

haphephobia (hăf"ē-fō'bē-ă) [" + *phobos,* fear]. Aversion to being touched by another person.

haplodont (hăp'lō-dŏnt) [" + *odous,* tooth]. Having teeth without ridges or tubercles on the crown.

haploid [Gr. *haploos,* simple, + *eidos,* form]. Possessing half the diploid or normal number of chromosomes found in somatic or body cells. Such is the case of the germ cells, ova or sperm, following the reduction divisions in gametogenesis, the haploid number being 23 in man. SEE: *chromosome; diploid.*

haploidy (hăp'loy-dē). The state of haploids.

haplopia (hăp-lō'pē-ă) [" + *ops,* vision]. Single vision; condition in which an object viewed by two eyes appears as a single object, in contrast to diplopia, in which it appears as two objects.

hapten(e) (hăp'tĕn, -tēn) [Gr. *haptein,* to seize]. The portion of an antigen containing the grouping on which the specificity depends.

haptic (hăp'tĭk) [Gr. *haptein,* to touch]. Pert. to touch. SYN: *tactile.*

haptics. The science of the touch sense.

haptin (hăp'tĭn). Hapten.

haptoglobin (hăp"tō-glō'bĭn). A mucoprotein to which hemoglobin released into plasma is bound. It is increased in certain inflammatory conditions and decreased in hemolytic disorders.

haptometer (hăp-tŏm'ĕ-tĕr) [" + *metron,* measure]. Device for measuring the acuteness of the sense of touch.

haptophil(e) (hăp'tō-fĭl, -fīl) [Gr. *haptein,* to touch, + *philein,* to love]. That portion of a receptor that unites with the haptophore group of a toxin.

haptophore (hăp'tō-for) [" + *pherein,* to bring]. The atom group of an antigen causing a combination with its corresponding antibody. SEE: *Ehrlich's side-chain theory.*

haptophoric, haptophorous. Pert. to the action of a haptophore.

hardening [AS. *heardian,* to harden]. 1. Rendering a pathological or histological specimen firm or compact for making thin sections for microscopic study. 2. The development of increased resistance to extremes of environmental temperature. SEE: *acclimation.*

hardness. 1. Quality of water containing certain substances, esp. soluble salts of calcium and magnesium. These react with soaps forming insoluble compounds that are precipitated out of solution, thus interfering with their cleansing action. 2. That quality of x-rays determining their penetrating power. Hardness lessens as wavelengths become longer.

h. of a gas tube. A term used to qualify the condition of a tube according to the degree of rarefaction of the residual gas. The higher the vacuum, the harder the tube and the rays emitted, the higher the voltage required to cause a discharge with a cold cathode, and hence the shorter the wavelength of the resulting roentgen rays.

harelip [AS. *hara,* hare, + *lippa,* lip]. A vertical cleft or clefts in the upper lip. It is congenital, resulting from the faulty fusion of the median nasal process and the lateral maxillary processes. Nongenetic factors may also be responsible for causing this condition. It is usually unilateral and on the left side although it may be bilateral. It may involve the lip or the upper jaw alone or both together, and often occurs with cleft palate. The incidence of harelip is from one in 600 to one in 1250 births. SYN: *cleft lip.*

harelip suture. A twisted figure-of-eight suture used in surgical correction of harelip.

harlequin fetus. A newborn infant with abnormal skin that resembles a thick horny armor. The skin is divided into areas by deep red fissures and the infants die within a few days. Also known as ichthyosis foetalis and ichthyosiform erythroderma. These were at one time regarded as separate diseases but are now known to represent different degrees of severity of the same entity.

Haroda's syndrome. [E. Haroda, contemporary Japanese physician] Uveomeningoencephalitis.

harmony (hăr'mō-nē). The condition of working or living together smoothly.

h., functional occlusal. The ideal occlusion of the teeth so that in all mandibular positions during chewing, the teeth will be functioning efficiently and without trauma to supporting tissues.

h., occlusal. Proper occlusion of the teeth in various mandibular positions.

harpoon (hăr-poon') [Gr. *harpazein,* to seize]. Device with a hook on the end for obtaining small pieces of tissue such as muscle for examination.

Harrison's groove. [Edwin Harrison, Brit. physician, 1779–1847] Depression on lower edge of the thorax caused by tug of the diaphragm; seen in rickets and any disease of infants that tends to obstruct inspiration.

Hartmann's solution. Lactated Ringer's injection. A sterile solution of 0.6 grams of sodium chloride, 0.03 grams of potassium chloride, 0.02 grams of calcium chloride, and 0.31 grams of sodium lactate diluted with water for injection to make 100 ml. Used for fluid and electrolyte treatment.

Hartnup disease. [*Hartnup,* the family name of the first reported case] A rare hereditary metabolic disease where amino acid absorption and excretion are abnormal, esp. that of tryptophan. Resorption of amino acids by the kidney is also defective. Clinical signs resemble pellagra, with a rash that is worsened by exposure to sunlight.

harvest. To obtain samples or remove bacteria or other microorganisms from a culture.

Harvey, William (hăr'vē). The British physician, 1578–1657, who described the circulation of the blood.

Hashimoto's struma. [Hakura Hashimoto, Jap. surgeon, 1881–1934] Thyroiditis, Hashimoto's, q.v.

hashish (hăsh'ĭsh) [Arabic, hemp, dried grass]. A more or less purified extract prepared from the flowers, stalks, and leaves of the hemp plant Cannabis sativa. The gummy substance is smoked or chewed for its euphoric effects. SEE: *cannabis; marijuana.*

Hasner's valve or fold. [Joseph R. Hasner, Prague ophthalmologist, 1819–1892] A fold of the mucous membrane at the opening of the nasolacrimal duct in the inferior meatus of the nasal cavity. SYN: *plica lacrimalis.*

Hassall's corpuscles. [Arthur H. Hassall, Brit. chemist and physician, 1817–1894] Spherical or oval bodies present in the medulla of the thymus. Each consists of central area of degenerated cells surrounded by concentrically arranged flattened or polygonal cells.

Hatchcock's sign. Tenderness just beyond the angle of the jaws when the finger follows on the undersurface of the mandible towards the angle. Found in mumps before any swelling can be detected.

haunch (hawnsh) [Fr. *hanche*]. The hips and buttocks.

haustra (haws'tră) [L. *haurire,* to draw, drink]. (sing. *haustrum*) The sacculated pouches of the colon.

h. coli. Sacculations of the colon resembling tucks caused by the fact that the gut is longer than the longitudinal bands or taeniae.

haustral (haw'străl). Pert. to the colonic haustra.

haustration (haws-trā'shŭn). The process of formation of a haustrum.

haustrum (haw'strŭm) [L. *haurire,* to draw, drink]. (pl. *haustra*) [NA] One of the sacculations of the colon caused by longitudinal bands that are shorter than the gut. SYN: *haustra coli.*

haustus (haws'tŭs) [L., a drink]. A swallow,

or draft, of medicine.

Haverhill fever (hā′vĕr-ĭl). [Haverhill, Mass., U.S.A., where the initial epidemic occurred] A febrile disease transmitted to man by a rat, usually by rat bite. Streptobacillus moniliformis is the etiological agent. SYN: *rat bite fever due to Streptobacillus moniliformis.*

haversian canal (hă-vĕr′shăn). [Clopton Havers, Brit. physician and anatomist, 1650–1702] Minute vascular canals found in osseous tissue.

haversian canaliculi. Delicate canals extending from the lacunae into the matrix of bone. They anastomose with canaliculi of adjacent lacunae, forming a network of fine channels that communicate with haversian and Volkmann's canals. They transmit nutrient materials.

haversian gland. Minute projections from the surface of the synovial tissue into the joint space.

haversian system. Architectural unit of bone consisting of a central tube (haversian canal) with alternate layers of intercellular material (matrix) surrounding it in concentric cylinders. Alternating layers of matrix and cells are called haversian lamellae. SEE: *bone.*

hay fever. An allergic disease of mucous membranes of nose and upper air passages induced by external irritation. SYN: *pollinosis; rhinitis, vasomotor.*

SYM: Inflammation, catarrh, watery discharges from the eyes, coryza, headache, asthmatic symptoms.

ETIOL: Air-borne pollens. Spring type is due to pollens of trees such as oak, elm, hickory, ash. The summer type is due to pollens of plants such as grasses, plantain, and sorrel. The fall type is due principally to the pollen of ragweeds. Nonseasonal hay fever may result from inhalation of irritating substances such as the danders of animals or dust such as hay, straw, or house dust or from ingestion of drugs or foods to which the subject is allergic.

TREATMENT: Either remove the patient from contact with the allergen or remove the allergen from the patient's environment. Filtration of air by masks and nasal filters may be helpful. Drug therapy in which epinephrine, antihistamines, or other drugs are given orally or used as nose drops, or nasal sprays. Prophylactic treatment consisting of desensitization by injection of pollen extracts to which the subject is sensitive may be of benefit.

Hayflick limit. [Leonard Hayflick, U.S. microbiologist, b. 1928] The limit of time cells in culture will live. Using data obtained from investigations of cell cultures, Dr. Hayflick has estimated that the limit of life of human beings could be over 100 years.

Haygarth's deformities. [John Haygarth, Brit. physician, 1740–1827] Exostoses or bony tumors on joints in rheumatoid arthritis.

Hb. *hemoglobin.*

HC Cream. Trade name for hydrocortisone cream.

HCG. *human chorionic gonadotrophin.*

HCl. *hydrochloric acid.*

H.D. *hearing distance.*

h.d. L. *hora decubitus,* the hour of going to bed.

H. disease. *Hartnup disease,* q.v.

HDL. *high-density lipoprotein.*

He. Chem. symb. for helium.

head [AS. *heafod*]. 1. Caput [NA]. That part of the animal body containing the brain and organs of sight, hearing, smell, and taste. It includes the facial bones. 2. The proximal end of a bone. 3. The larger extremity of any structure or body.

ABNORM: *Abnormal fixation* of the head may be caused by postpharyngeal abscess, arthritis deformans, swollen cervical glands, rheumatism, traumatism of the neck, sprains of cervical muscles, congenital spasmodic torticollis, caries of a molar tooth, burn scars, or eye muscle imbalance (hyperphoria). Inability to move the head may be due to caries of the cervical vertebrae and diseases of articulation between the occiput and atlas or paralysis of neck muscles.

Abnormal movements include habit spasms such as nodding. Rhythmical nodding is seen in aortic regurgitation, chorea, torticollis, q.v. A retracted head is seen in acute meningitis, cerebral abscess, tumor, thrombosis of the superior longitudinal sinus, acute encephalitis, laryngeal obstruction, tetanus, hydrophobia, epilepsy, spasmodic torticollis, strychnine poisoning, hysteria, rachitic conditions, and painful neck lesions at the back.

h., after-coming. Childbirth with the head delivered last.

h., articular. A projection on bone that articulates with another bone.

h., nerve. The optic disk.

head, words pert. to: acromegaly; caput; "ceph-" words; coryza; face; gyrospasm; macrocephalous; nutation; occipital; sinciput; skeleton; temple; vertex.

headache [AS. *heafod,* head, + *acan,* to ache]. A diffuse pain in different portions of the head and not confined to any nerve distribution area. May be acute or chronic. It may be frontal, temporal, or occipital; confined to one side of the head or to the region immediately over one eye. The character of pain may vary. It may be a dull, aching pain or an acute, almost unbearable pain. It may be an intermittent intense pain, a throbbing pain, a pressure pain when head feels as if it will burst, or a penetrating pain driving through the head. SYN: *cephalgia*. SEE: *migraine*.

ETIOL: Transient acute headaches may be due to a variety of causes including diseases of the paranasal sinuses, teeth, eye, ear, nose, or throat; acute infections; or trauma to the head. Chronic headaches may be caused by a variety of conditions including physical, emotional, psychosomatic, or psychogenic factors; fevers; metabolic conditions; or exposure to toxic chemicals. The exact cause can be determined by thorough analysis of the data obtained from history, physical examination, tests, and laboratory studies, which may include roentgenography of the skull, electroencephalography, and metabolic studies.

Toxic factors: (1) Exogenous origin: Foul air from poor ventilation; poisonous gases, including fumes from furnaces or gas fires; drugs (quinine, morphine, atropine, histamine); alcohol; tobacco; wines with high histamine content. (2) Endogenous origin: Any absorption of the toxins of bacterial infection will cause headache. Includes chronic infections (nose and sinuses, teeth, middle ear, pharynx, tonsils, appendix, gallbladder, pelvic viscera); fever; bacteremias (typhoid fever, malaria, smallpox, tuberculosis, grippe and influenza, puerperal fever).

Systemic diseases: Nephritis with uremia, biliary tract disease including acute yellow atrophy of the liver, rheumatism, diabetes, anemia, polycythemia, eclampsia, central nervous system syphilis.

Gastrointestinal disturbances: Dyspepsia, gastric hyper- and hypoacidity, intestinal stasis, and constipation. *Physicochemical disturbances:* Acidosis, alkalosis. *Cardiovascular disturbances:* Myocardial and valvular insufficiency causing congestive heart failure; constriction, dilatation, or edema of intracranial blood vessels.

Endocrine disorders: Pituitary, thyroid, adrenal, and ovarian tumors; carcinoid tumors. *Gynecological factors:* Functional disturbances of one or more of the endocrine glands; puberty, dysmenorrhea, premenstrual tension, menstruation, pregnancy, menopause. *Psychoneurological factors:* Nervous exhaustion; worry, excitement, anger, or nervous tension; migraine; hysteria; epilepsy; psychoneuroses.

Diseases of special sense organs: Iritis, glaucoma, conjunctivitis; adenoids, deviated septum; middle ear affections. *Organic disease of brain:* Causing pressure such as tumor, abscess, gumma, cyst, hydrocephaly, intracranial hemorrhage; subdural hematoma; intracranial vascular disease; arteriosclerosis; embolism, thrombosis, or aneurysm; encephalitis; various forms of meningitis; meningismus.

Miscellaneous causes: Almost any disturbance of body function may cause headache. Other causes are external pressure and constriction of head; trauma to head; sunstroke; any form of motion sickness; irritation of mucous membrane of nose and sinuses by dust, pollen; fatigue (physical or mental); insomnia; travel to an altitude sufficient to produce hypoxia. Spinal puncture or diagnostic examination involving injecting dyes or radioactive substances into cranial arteries or air into the ventricles of the brain may be followed by headache. Orgasm is a rare cause of headache.

TREATMENT: Depends entirely upon cause.

IMPORTANT: A headache that may be the symptom of a serious disease should not be treated symptomatically without attempting to find its cause.

h., cluster. A headache similar to migraine, recurring as often as two or three times a day over a period of weeks. After this cluster of headaches, the patient may be free of symptoms for weeks or months. The headaches come on abruptly and are characterized by intense throbbing pain behind the nostril and one eye. The eyes and nose water, the skin over the throbbing area becomes red, and the pupil of the eye may become constricted. An attack rarely lasts longer than two hours. Ergotamine tartrate is useful for both treatment and prophylaxis.

h., histamine. Headache resulting from ingestion of histamine (some wines contain histamine), injection of histamine, or excessive histamine in circulating blood. Due to dilatation of branches of the carotid artery. SEE: *h., cluster*.

h., post–lumbar puncture. Of patients having lumbar puncture, 10 to 40% will develop a severe headache. The headache is thought to be related to the leakage of spinal fluid through the hole that fails to close when the needle is removed from the dura. The use of a small-gauge spinal puncture needle helps to prevent this headache.

TREATMENT: Bedrest in a completely flat and prone position without use of a pillow, forced oral and intravenous fluids, and cortical steroids are useful in treating the headache. If the headache persists in spite of therapy, it is possible to stop the leakage of spinal fluid by injection of 10 ml. of the patient's blood in the epidural space at the site of the lumbar puncture. The blood may provide a patch for the hole in the dura.

h., tension. 1. Headache associated with chronic contraction of the muscles of the neck and scalp. 2. Headache associated with emotional or physical strain.

headgut. Part of the embryo that develops into the pharynx, lungs, stomach, liver, duodenum, and esophagus. SYN: *foregut.*

head injury. Injury to the head due to trauma.

head trauma. Injury to the head, esp. to the scalp and cranium. The injury may be limited to soft tissue damage or may include the cranial bones and the brain.

heal (hēl) [AS. *hael,* whole]. To cure; to make whole or healthy.

healing. The restoration to a normal mental or physical condition, but esp. of an inflammation or a wound.

Healing by first intention: This process closes the edge of a wound with little or no inflammatory reaction and in such a manner that little or no scar is left to reveal the site of the injury. New cells are formed to take the place of dead ones and the capillary walls stretch across the wound to join themselves to each other in a smooth surface. New connective tissue may form an almost imperceptible scar that proves temporary. In repairing lacerations and surgical wounds, the goal is to produce a repaired area that will heal by first intention.

Healing by second intention: This is healing by granulation or indirect union. Granulation tissue is formed to fill the gap between the edges of the wound with a thin layer of fibrinous exudate. It excludes bacteria and aids in checking bleeding by the coagulation of the blood. Connective tissue cells support the new capillaries. This form of healing is slower than that by first intention and its grayish-red surface may become pale and flabby if the healing is too long delayed. If the granulations show above the surface, they may have to be removed with caustics. If the granulations first form at the top instead of the bottom of the wound, it may have to be kept open by drainage.

Healing by third intention: Healing of an ulcer, wound, or cavity by filling with granulations. It generally results in the formation of a large scar.

COMPLICATIONS: These may result from the formation of a scar that interferes with the functioning of a part and possible deformity; the formation of a keloid, q.v., the result of overgrowth of connective tissue forming a tumor in the surface of a scar; necrosis of the skin and mucous membrane that produces a raw surface, which results in an ulcer; a sinus or fistula, which may be due to bacteria or some foreign substance remaining in the wound; proud flesh, which represents excessive growth of granulation tissue.

health (hĕlth) [AS. *haelth,* wholeness]. A condition in which all functions of the body and mind are normally active. The World Health Organization defines health as a state of complete physical, mental, or social well-being and not merely the absence of disease or infirmity.

h., bill of. Public health certificate certifying that passengers on a public conveyance or ship are free of infectious disease.

h., board of. A public body that may be appointed or elected. It is concerned with administering the laws that concern the health of the public.

h., department of. Branch of a government (city, county, or nation) for regulation and protection of the people's health.

h., industrial. The health of employees of industrial firms.

h., public. The state of health of the population of a particular community, as opposed to individual or personal health.

health certificate. An official statement signed by a physician attesting to the state of health of a particular individual.

health education. Educational process or program designed for improvement and maintenance of health. It is directed to the general public in contrast to a health education program organized for instructing persons who will become health educators.

healthful. Conducive to good health.

Health Maintenance Organization. ABBR: HMO. A prepaid health care program of group practice with comprehensive medical care being provided and with an emphasis on preventive medicine.

healthy. Being in a state of health or enjoying it.

hearing [AS. *hieran*]. The act or power of perceiving sound.

FUNCT. TESTS: Hearing acuity can be determined by the distance at which a person can hear a certain sound such as a watch tick, the use of audiometers, and bone conduction. In audiometers, electrically produced sounds are conveyed by wires to a receiver applied to the subject's ear. Intensity and pitch of sound can be altered and are indicated on the dials. Results are plotted on a graph known as an audiogram. In bone conduction tests, a device such as a tuning fork or an apparatus that converts an electrical current into mechanical vibrations is applied to the skull. This is of value in distinguishing between perceptive and conduction deafness. SEE: *audiogram; auditory evoked response; ear; Rinne's test; Weber's test.*

h., after. Perception of sound after the stimulus producing it has ceased to act.

hearing aid. An apparatus used by those with impaired hearing for amplifying sound.

hearing distance. Distance at which a given sound can be heard. On the prairies, a voice may be heard for two miles or more.

hearing hallucinations. Subjective sensations of sound such as hearing voices when none actually exists.

heart (hărt) [AS. *heorte*]. A hollow, muscular, contractile organ, the center of the circulatory system. It provides the propulsive force for circulating the blood throughout the vascular system. Its wall possesses three layers: the outer epicardium, a serous layer; the middle myocardium, composed of cardiac muscle; and the inner endocardium, a layer that lines the four chambers of the heart and covers the valves. The heart is enclosed in a fibroserous sac, the pericardium, the space between the pericardium and the epicardium forming the pericardial cavity. SEE: illus.; *circulation* for illus.

CHAMBERS: Each lower cavity, right and left, is the ventriculum or ventricle; the upper ones, the right or left atrium.

Contraction of the heart chambers is called systole; relaxation with accompanying dilation, diastole. The complete series of events that occurs in a single heartbeat is known as the cardiac cycle. In a heart beating at the rate of 72 beats per minute, each cycle lasts about 0.85 sec. The heart is divided perpendicularly from base to apex by the interatrial and interventricular septa; normally the right side has no communication with the left. The right side receives deoxygenated blood via the veins from the tissues and pumps it to the lungs; the left side receives oxygenated blood from the lungs and pumps it to the tissues via the arteries.

The atria, serving as receiving chambers and low-pressure pumps, are thin walled; the ventricles, serving as pumping chambers, are thick walled.

Accelerator impulses are conveyed over nerves and ganglia of the sympathetic division. Preganglionic neurons that lie in the thoracic portion of the spinal cord synapse with postganglionic neurons located in the cervical ganglia of sympathetic trunk whose axons pass to the heart. Impulses from these nerves increase the rate and force of heartbeats. Impulses regulating the heart arise in the cardiac center in the medulla oblongata.

Afferent fibers pass through the vagus trunks to the medulla. Some are depressor fibers originating in receptors in the base of the aorta. Impulses over these fibers reflexly slow the heart rate. Others are pressor fibers originating in receptors in the vena cavae and right atrium. These reflexly increase heartbeat. Fibers conveying pain impulses are also present.

VALVES: The atrioventricular orifice between each atrium and ventricle. The tricuspid valve is between the right atrium and ventricle. The bicuspid valve is between the left atrium and ventricle. The semilunar valve is between the right ventricle and the pulmonary artery. The aortic valve is between the left ventricle and the aorta.

NERVE SUPPLY: *Inhibitory* (Vagus): by way of the sympathetic ganglia of the autonomic system and phrenic nerve. *Afferent:* A depressor nerve running from the heart to a cardioinhibitory center in the medulla, through the sheath of the vagus nerves, causing reflex inhibition of the heart. *Efferent fibers:* Inhibitory impulses are conveyed by preganglionic fibers of the vagus nerve, which synapse with postganglionic neurons located in terminal ganglia in the wall of the heart. They are distributed to the sinoatrial node, bundles of His, and other conductile tissue of the heart.

FUNCT: At the rate of 72 times each minute, the human heart beats 104,000 times a day, 38,000,000 times during a year. At every stroke 5 cu. in. (82 ml.) of blood are forced out into the body, or 500,000 cu. in. (8,193 liters) a day. In terms of work, this is the equivalent of raising one ton (907 kg.) to a height of 41 ft. (12.5 meters) every 24 hr.

AUSCULTATION: Shows intensity, quality, and rhythm of heart sounds and detects the presence of any adventitious sounds, as murmurs. The two separate sounds heard by the use of a stethoscope over the heart have been represented by the syllables "lubb," "dupp." The first sound (systolic) results from the contraction of the ventricle, tension of the atrioventricular valves, and the impact of the heart against the chest wall, and is synchronous with the apex beat and carotid pulse. This sound is prolonged and dull; after the first sound there is a short pause, then the second sound (diastolic), which results from the closure of the aortic and pulmonary valves. This sound is short and high pitched. After the second sound a longer pause follows before the first is heard again. A very useful technique in listening to the variation in sounds from one area to another is to "inch" the stethoscope in small steps from one site to the other.

PROCEDURE: Patient should be recumbent when beginning examination; then, having elicited all the signs possible, repeat with patient sitting, standing, or leaning forward, and note any variations from change of position. First listen while patient is breathing naturally, then while holding breath in both deep inspiration and expiration, and finally have patient take three or four forced inspirations. Listen over the entire thoracic cavity and endeavor to localize the points at which heart sounds, both normal and abnor-

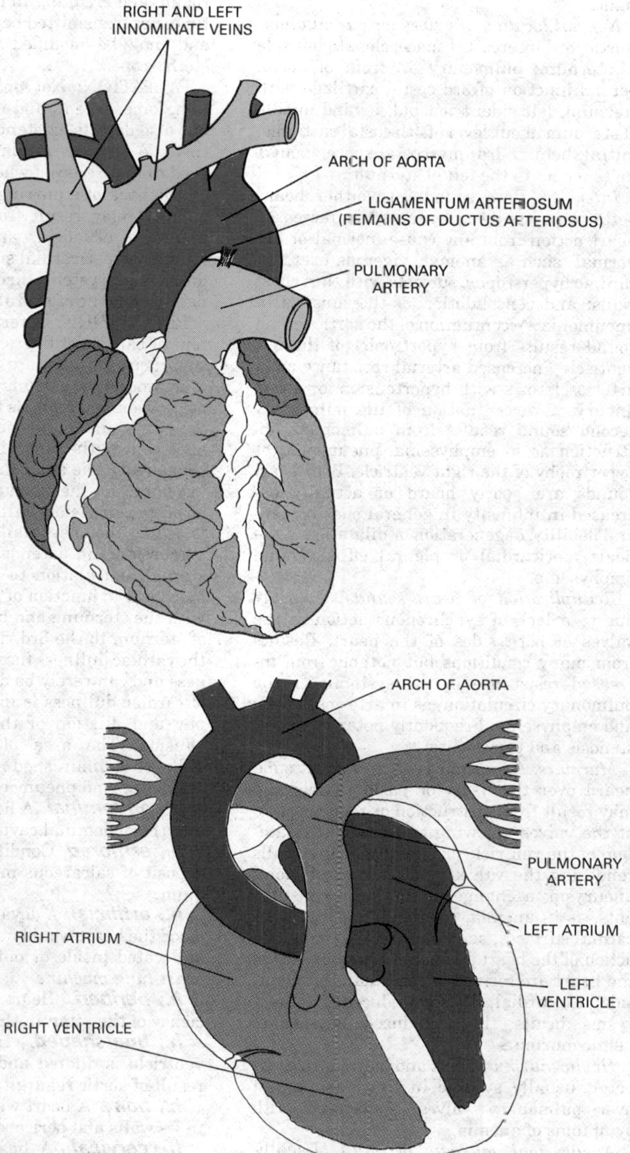

ANTERIOR VIEWS OF EXTERIOR AND INTERIOR OF HEART AND VESSELS

mal, are heard with the greatest intensity. Proceed from below upward and from left to right.

Normal location of valves for auscultation: Aortic, 3rd intercostal space, close to left side of sternum; pulmonary, in front of aorta, behind junction of 3rd costal cartilage with sternum, left side; tricuspid, behind middle of sternum about level of 4th costal cartilage; mitral, behind 3rd intercostal space about 1 in. (2.5 cm.) to the left of sternum.

Intensity: Both sounds are either heard better or actually accentuated in increased heart action from any cause, normal or abnormal, such as anemia, vigorous exercise, cardiac hypertrophy, subjects with thin chest walls, and consolidation of the lung as in pneumonia. Accentuation of the aortic second sound results from hypertrophy of the left ventricle, increased arterial resistance as in arteriosclerosis with hypertension, or aortic aneurysm. Accentuation of the pulmonary second sound results from pulmonary obstruction as in emphysema, pneumonia, or hypertrophy of the right ventricle. Both heart sounds are poorly heard or actually decreased in intensity in general obesity, general debility, degeneration or dilatation of the heart, pericardial or pleural effusion, and emphysema.

Reduplication of heart sounds: Probably due to a lack of synchronous action in the valves of both sides of the heart. Results from many conditions but notably from increased resistance in the systemic or the pulmonary circulation, as in arteriosclerosis and emphysema. Frequently noted in mitral stenosis and pericarditis.

Murmurs: A murmur is an abnormal sound heard over the heart or blood vessels and may result from obstruction or regurgitation at the valves following endocarditis; dilatation of the ventricle or relaxation of its walls rendering the valves relatively insufficient; aneurysm; a change in the blood constituents, as in anemia; roughening of the pericardial surfaces, as in pericarditis; irregular action of the heart. Murmurs produced within the heart are termed endocardial; those outside, exocardial; those produced in aneurysms, bruits; those produced by anemia, hemic murmurs.

Hemic murmurs: Soft and blowing in character, usually systolic in time, heard best over pulmonary valves. Associated with symptoms of anemia.

Aneurysmal murmur or bruit: Usually loud, booming in character, systolic in time, heard best over the aorta or base of heart, often associated with an abnormal area of dullness and pulsation, and with symptoms resulting from pressure on neighboring structures.

Pericardial friction sounds: Superficial, rough, and creaking in quality, to and fro in time, not transmitted beyond the precordium and may be modified by pressure of the stethoscope.

PALPATION: Not only determines position, force, extent, and rhythm of apex beat, but also detects existence of any fremitus or thrill. A thrill is a vibratory sensation likened to that received when the hand is placed on the back of a purring cat. Thrills at base of heart may result from valvular lesions, atheroma of aorta, aneurysm, and from roughened pericardial surfaces as in pericarditis. A presystolic thrill at apex is almost pathognomonic of mitral stenosis.

PERCUSSION: Determines shape and extent of cardiac dullness. The normal area of superficial or absolute percussion dullness (part uncovered by lung) is detected by light percussion and extends from the 4th left costosternal junction to the apex beat; from the apex beat to the juncture of the xiphoid cartilage, with the sternum, and thence up the left border of the sternum. The normal area of deep percussion dullness (the heart projected on the chest wall) is detected by firm percussion and extends from 3rd left costosternal articulation to the apex beat; from apex beat to junction of the xiphoid cartilage with the sternum; and hence up right border of sternum to the 3rd rib. The lower level of the cardiac dullness fuses with the liver dullness and can rarely be determined. The area of cardiac dullness is increased in hypertrophy and dilation of the heart; pericardial effusion. The area of detectable cardiac dullness is diminished in emphysema, pneumothorax, and pneumocardium.

h., abdominal. A heart that is displaced into the abdominal cavity.

h., armored. Condition characterized by deposit of calcareous matter in the pericardium.

h., artificial. A device that will pump the blood the heart would normally pump. It may be located inside or outside the body. SEE: *heart-lung machine*.

h., beriberi. Heart failure due to deficiency of the vitamin thiamine.

h., boatshaped. Heart in which one ventricle is dilated and hypertrophied as a result of aortic regurgitation.

h., bony. A heart with calcareous patches in its walls and pericardium.

h., cervical. A heart that is displaced into the neck region.

h., dilatation of. Enlargement of heart due to stretching of its walls. Varieties are dilatation with thickening of walls and dilatation with thinning walls.

SYM: So long as the associated hypertrophy keeps pace with the dilatation, no symptoms result. Otherwise there are dyspnea, edema, and cough, the signs of heart failure.

h., fatty degeneration of. Condition in which the myocardium has undergone fatty degeneration.

SYM: All signs of heart failure, i.e., dyspnea; cough; weak irregular pulse; edema; dyspepsia; attacks of syncope.

PROG: Unfavorable. Death may occur on slight exertion.

h., fatty infiltration of. Abnormal amount of fat deposited in and upon heart.

SYM: Shortness of breath increased by exertion; weak but regular pulse; precordial distress; tendency to pulmonary congestion with resulting bronchitis.

PROG: Depends upon cause. If due to a correctable condition, it is favorable.

h., fibroid. Chronic myocarditis in which fibrous tissue develops within the muscular tissue of the heart.

SYM: Same as fatty degeneration, condition dependent upon atheroma or sclerosis of coronary arteries.

h., hypertrophy of. Enlargement of heart due to increased size of myocardium.

h., irritable. Neurocirculatory asthenia or effort syndrome. Characterized by breathlessness, palpitation, weakness, and exhaustion.

h., left. The left atrium and ventricle. This is the portion of the heart that receives the aerated blood from the lungs and propels it into the systemic circulation.

h., palpitation of. May result from dyspepsia; mental or physical excitement; organic heart disease; hyperthyroidism; anemia; hysteria; an independent neurosis; or endocarditis, myocarditis, and pericarditis due to infection and trauma; circulatory disturbances; disorders of metabolism, nutrition, and growth.

h., right. The right atrium and ventricle. This portion of the heart receives the venous blood and propels it to the lungs.

heart attack. Myocardial infarction, q.v.

heart beat. The rhythmic contraction of the heart.

heart block. Condition in which the conductile tissue of the heart, the sinoatrial (S-A) and atrioventricular (A-V) nodes, bundle of His, Purkinje fibers, fails to conduct impulses normally from the atrium to the ventricles. This causes altered rhythm of the heartbeat. Known as arrhythmia, the condition may be present in several forms.

ETIOL: Structural changes as from tumor or damage of the myocardium due to coronary artery occlusion. Toxic effects of drugs or the toxins of infections. Nutritional or endocrine factors may also be of importance.

h. b., atrioventricular. A form in which impulses are impeded at the A-V node.

h. b., bundle branch. Condition in which impulses are blocked in one of the branches of the bundle of His, resulting in ventricles beating out of rhythm with each other so that one ventricle is stimulated to beat slightly before the other. SYN: *heart block, interventricular.*

h. b., complete or third-degree. Condition in which there is a complete dissociation between atrial and ventricular systoles. Ventricles may beat at a rate of 30 to 40/min. while atria are beating the normal 70 beats/min.

h. b., congenital. Heart block present at birth due to improper development of the impulse-conducting system.

h. b., first-degree. Heart block in which conduction time of impulses is prolonged but all atrial beats are followed by ventricular beats; usually recognized only by electrocardiograph.

h. b., interventricular. H. b., bundle branch.

h. b., partial or second-degree. Heart block in which one of two or three impulses passes from the atrium to the ventricle.

h. b., sinoatrial. Heart block in which there is interference in the passage of impulses from the sinoatrial node. May be partial or complete.

heartburn. Acid liquid raised from the stomach, causing sensation of burning in the esophagus. SYN: *brash; pyrosis.*

heart disease. Term used to describe any pathological condition of the heart.

heart failure. 1. Cessation of the beat of the heart. 2. A syndrome or clinical condition resulting from failure of the heart to maintain adequate circulation of blood. May result from failure of the right or left ventricle or both.

ETIOL: Hypertension, infections, pericardial effusion, valvular insufficiency, coronary disease, congenital malformations, arteriosclerosis, constrictive pericarditis, atherosclerosis, hyperthyroidism.

SYM: Dyspnea, cardiac asthma, stasis in systemic or portal circulation, edema, cyanosis, hypertrophy of heart. Symptoms vary depending on which side of the heart is affected.

h. f., backward. Heart failure in which venous return to the heart is reduced with resulting venous stasis and congestion. Due principally to failure of the right ventricle.

h. f., congestive. Condition characterized by weakness, breathlessness, abdominal discomfort, edema in lower portions of body resulting from venous stasis and reduced outflow of blood.

h. f., forward. Heart failure in which forward flow of blood to the tissues is inadequate due either to inability of left ventricle to pump sufficient blood or to insufficient blood arriving at the ventricle.

h. f., high output. Heart failure even though the cardiac output is high.

h. f., left. Failure of the heart to maintain left ventricular output. SYN: *left ventricular heart failure.*

h. f., left ventricular. H. f., left, q.v.

h. f., low output. Failure of the heart to maintain blood output.

h. f., right-sided. Inadequate output by the right ventricle. SYN: *right ventricular heart failure.*

h. f., right ventricular. H. f., right-sided, q.v.

heart-lung machine. Device for maintaining the functions of the heart and lungs while either, or both, is unable to continue to function adequately. The device pumps the blood and oxygenates it and removes carbon dioxide. In animal studies and in open-heart surgery, such devices take over the function of the heart and lungs while these organs are being treated or possibly replaced.

heart murmur. Sounds from the heart other than those normally present. A murmur is produced by the blood passing over a roughened valve as could be the case in rheumatic heart disease, or by flowing through a constricted opening such as a narrowed mitral valve or an interventricular septal defect.

heart pump, nuclear-powered. An artificial heart powered by nuclear energy.

heart rate. The number of beats of the heart per unit of time, usually expressed or written as number per minute.

heart reflex. Any reflex in which the stimulation of a sensory nerve brings about an increase or decrease in the heart rate. An example is the Bainbridge reflex, in which stimulation of sensory receptors in the right atrium by increased venous return results in an increase in heart rate.

heart sounds. SEE: AUSCULTATION under *heart.*

heart test. Nonspecific term for any of the various methods of clinically testing the heart.

heart transplantation. Surgical transplantation of the heart from a patient who died of trauma or some other disease that left the heart intact and capable of functioning in the recipient. This procedure became quite frequent in the 1970s and then very few were done. As techniques for matching the donor and recipient have improved, the procedure is once again being done in special centers.

heat [AS. *haetu*]. 1. Condition of being hot; warmth. Opposed to cold. 2. High temperature; generalized fever or localized heat due to an infection. Calor (fever) and dolor, rubor, and tumor (pain, redness, and swelling) represent the four classic signs of inflammation. SEE: *fever.* 3. Sexual excitement in lower animals; period of such excitement. SYN: *estrus.* 4. A form of energy that increases the temperature of surrounding tissues or objects by conduction, convection, or radiation. 5. Sensation of warmth or an increase in temperature.

Heat is constantly being produced within the body as a result of exothermic chemical processes occurring in metabolic processes. Ultimately all heat produced in the body results from oxidative processes. Body temperature (normally 98.6° F. or 37° C.) is the result of a balance between heat production (thermogenesis) and heat loss (thermolysis). SEE: table. The temperature of the body is not uniform. Oral temperatures range from 96.6° F. to 100° F. (37° to 37.8° C.). Axillary temperature is somewhat lower and rectal temperature is somewhat higher. Change in mean body temperature is not easily measured but should not be estimated to be precisely equivalent to changes in rectal or oral temperature. SEE: *core temperature.*

Reducing the temperature of the skin reflexly brings about a constriction of the blood vessels, thus reducing heat loss and conserving heat within the body. The application of

Elimination of Body Heat

The mode of elimination and the percentage of heat lost through each of the following is:

Radiation	55%
Convection and conduction	15%
Evaporation through skin and lungs	24%
Warming inspired air	2%
Elimination of CO_2 from lungs	3%
Warming ingested food and water, and loss through feces and urine	1%

Figures are approximate and vary with physiological activity of the body, type of clothing worn, relative humidity, and degree of acclimatization to a particular environment.

heat reflexly induces the dilation of blood vessels, thus increasing blood flow to the skin with consequent increase in heat loss.

The application of heat to the skin reflexly produces effects in the deeper portions of the body. It induces muscle relaxation, increases blood supply, and stimulates metabolic activity. Physiological effects resulting are hyperemia and sedation of sensory or motor activity. Application of moderate cold tends to produce the opposite effects.

Relaxation of muscular tissue results in relief of pain, which may be due to rigidity and spasm in tissues. Local hot applications may have some reflex effect on deep organs. This is the basis of treating certain conditions by means of counterirritation such as that produced by liniments or mustard plaster.

h., acclimatization to. Adjustment of an organism to heat in the environment. Exposure to high environmental temperature requires a period of adjustment in order for the body to function efficiently. The amount of time required will depend upon the temperature, humidity, and duration of exposure each day. Significant physiological adjustments will occur in five days and will be completed within two weeks to a month.

h., application of. *General:* May be dry or moist. The effect is first to produce a slight contraction of vessels in skin, thus increasing blood pressure. This makes patients feel that their head is full and bursting. However, this effect is only of very short duration, and discomfort can be avoided by application of cold compress or ice bag to head. The true effect follows immediately when the blood vessels in the skin are dilated due to the relaxation of involuntary muscle contained in their walls. The skin is reddened, increased blood supply to the sweat glands causes them to act freely, and heat loss is accelerated. During a general application of heat it is necessary to watch the patient carefully, noting any apparent discomfort, state of pulse and respiration, and color, and to be certain patient does not become dehydrated or suffer heat exhaustion, q.v.

CAUTION: Do not apply heat to extremities that have reduced blood supply as would be the case in most forms of arteriosclerosis or diabetes.

Local: May be dry or moist. Dry applications include rubber hot-water bottles; bags of hot salt previously heated in an oven; radiant heat; electric pads; and diathermy.

Moist: Considered more penetrating than dry heat but this is due more to the fact that water-soaked materials lose heat slower than dry ones. The application should be approx. 120° F. (48.9° C.). Compresses may be kept warm by keeping hot water bottles at proper temperature next to them. Do not use electric heating devices next to moist dressings. Devices that force hot water at a selected temperature through soft flexible tubing are available. These may be used to heat wet or dry compresses.

h., conductive. A term applied to heat transferred by conduction from a heat source to an object that is cold when the two materials are in contact with each other.

h., convective. Flow of heat to an object or part of the body by passage of heated particles, gas, or liquid from the heat source to the colder body.

h., conversive. Heat generated in the tissues by a current of electricity or by some form of radiant energy.

h., diathermy. Electrical energy is converted into heat by the use of diathermy and short wave.

h., dry. Heat that has no moisture. May be administered in form of hot, dry pack; hot water bottle; electric light bath; heliotherapy; hot bricks; resistance coil; electric pad or blanket; hot air bath; or therapeutic lamp.

h., initial. Muscular heat produced during contraction when tension is increasing, during maintenance of tension, and during relaxation when tension is diminishing.

h., latent. Heat that is required to convert a solid into a liquid or a liquid into a gas at a given temperature.

h., latent, of fusion. Heat that is required to convert 1 gm. of a solid into liquid at the same temperature, e.g., when 1 gm. of ice at 0° C. is converted into water at 0° C.; this process requires 80 Cal., and until it is completed there will be no rise of temperature.

h., latent, of vaporization. Heat required to change 1 gm. of a liquid at its boiling point to vapor at the same temperature. The latent heat of steam is 540 Cal.; therefore, when steam cools to liquid, each gm. gives out 540 Cal. This explains why a scald from steam is much more severe than one caused by boiling water.

h., luminous. Heat derived from light. This form may be tolerated better than other forms of radiation. Light may be converted into heat. Short infrared rays penetrate subcutaneous tissues to a greater extent than long, invisible rays.

h., mechanical equivalent of. The value of heat units in terms of work units. One Calorie (kilocalorie) is equal to 4.1855×10^4 joule.

h., moist. Heat that has moisture content. May be applied as hot bath pack, hot wet pack, hot foot bath, fomentations, poultices, or vapor bath. Watch for chill, fainting, dizziness, headache, collapse, faintness, increased pulse, weakness. Cold applications to head should be used during and after treatment. Opinion regarding therapeutic use of heat or cold differs.

h., molecular. Result of multiplying a substance's molecular weight by its specific heat.

h., prickly. Vesicles due to obstruction or acute inflammation of sweat glands. SYN: *miliaria*.

h., radiant. Heat given off from a heated body; it passes through the air in form of waves.

h., sensible. Heat producing a temperature rise when absorbed by a body.

h., specific. The heat needed to raise the temperature of 1 gm. of a substance 1° C.

heat cramps. Acute painful spasms of voluntary muscles following hard work in a hot environment without adequate fluid and salt intake.

F.A.: Remove the patient to a cool place and give a salt solution (¼ tsp. or one gram of table salt in a glass of water) by mouth. Repeat at 5- to 30-minute intervals until cramping stops.

PROPHYLAXIS: Ingestion of 1 to 2 grams (65 to 130 mg.) of salt taken three or four times a day with at least two glasses (16 ounces or ½ liter) of water with each dose.

heat exhaustion. Acute reaction to heat exposure. Not the same as heatstroke, q.v. SEE: table.

SYM: Weakness, dizziness, nausea, headache, and finally collapse. Skin is cold and clammy, pupils dilated. Body temperature is usually normal, but blood pressure may be decreased.

PROG: Favorable if properly treated.

F.A.: Remove the patient to a cool place, loosen clothing, place in a head-low position. A slow intravenous infusion of isotonic saline may be necessary if the patient is unconscious.

heat gun. Device used in splint fabrication that produces heated air to render thermoplastic splinting materials malleable for fitting.

heat labile. Thermolabile, q.v.

heatstroke. An acute and dangerous reaction to heat exposure. Characterized by high body temperature, usually above 105° F. (40.6° C.); cessation of sweating; headache; numbness; tingling and confusion prior to sudden delirium or coma; fast pulse; rapid respiratory

Comparison of Heatstroke and Heat Exhaustion

Heatstroke	Heat Exhaustion
Heatstroke. ***Definition:*** A condition or derangement of the heat-control centers due to exposure to the rays of the sun or very high temperatures. Loss of heat is inadequate or absent.	**Heat Exhaustion.** ***Definition:*** A state of very definite weakness produced by the excess loss of normal fluids and sodium chloride in the form of sweat.
History: Exposure to sun's rays or extreme heat	***History:*** Exposure to heat, usually indoors
Differential Symptoms:	***Differential Symptoms:***
Face: Red, dry, and hot	*Face:* Pale, cool, and moist
Skin: Hot, dry, and no sweating	*Skin:* Cool, clammy, with profuse diaphoresis
Temperature: High, 106° to 110° F. (41.1° to 43.3° C.)	*Temperature:* Subnormal
Pulse: Full, strong, bounding	*Pulse:* Weak, thready, and rapid
Respirations: Dyspneic and sonorous	*Respirations:* Shallow and quiet
Muscles: Tense and possible convulsions	*Muscles:* Tense and contracted
Eyes: Pupils are dilated but equal	*Eyes:* Pupils are normal, eyeballs may be soft
Treatment: Absolute rest with head elevated; cool by any means available until hospitalized, but do not use alcohol applied to skin. Take temperature every 10 minutes, and do not allow it to fall below 38.5° C. (101° F.).	***Treatment:*** Keep patient quiet; head should be lowered; keep body warm to prevent onset of shock.
Drugs: Allow no stimulants; give infusions of normal saline (to force fluids)	*Drugs:* Salty fluids and fruit juices should be given frequently in small amounts. Intravenous isotonic saline will be required if patient is unconscious.

rate; usually elevated blood pressure. The basic defect is failure of the heat-regulating mechanisms of the body. SYN: *sunstroke*. SEE: table.

TREATMENT: Effective therapy may save the patient's life. Without delay, the nude patient should be placed in a bathtub filled with cold water. This will not cause pain, shock, or cutaneous vasoconstriction. The patient's temperature will need to be monitored carefully. Remove from bath when temperature falls to 103° F. (39.4° C.). If cold water and a bathtub are not available, place wet sheets on nude body, fan vigorously, and massage the skin. Do not apply alcohol to the skin. Take temperature every 10 minutes and do not allow it to fall below 38.5° C. (101° F.) to prevent changing hyperthermia to hypothermia. The use of sedatives may be required to control convulsions. Careful observation of patient for signs of fluid imbalance and renal failure will be required for several days.

heat unit. Unit of heat produced by exposure to x-rays. It is the product of the milliamperage times the seconds of exposure times the kilovoltage peak.

heaves (hēvs). Vomiting.

heavy chain disease. Any one of several abnormalities of the plasma cells such that immunoglobulins with excessive quantities of alpha, gamma, delta, epsilon, or mu chains are produced. The immunoglobulins formed are incomplete and in some cases, this causes distinct clinical signs and symptoms including weakness, recurrent fever, susceptibility to bacterial infections, lymphadenopathy, hepatosplenomegaly, erythema, and edema of the soft palate; anemia, leukopenia, thrombocytopenia, eosinophilia, and abnormal protein electrophoretic patterns are also produced.

hebephrenia (hē″bĕ-frē′nē-ă) [Gr. *hebe,* youth, + *phren,* mind]. A chronic form of schizophrenia characterized by bizarre, illogical, and senseless thought processes and actions, delusions, and hallucinations. Wild excitement at one moment may be replaced by depression and crying. Patient may laugh often without cause and talk incoherently and excessively. Onset usually before age 20. Prognosis is poor.

hebephrenic (hē″bĕ-frĕn′ĭk). Pert. to hebephrenia.

Heberden's disease (hē′bĕr-dĕnz). [William Heberden, Brit. physician, 1710–1801] Arthritis with deformity that begins in the fingers and progresses. The concomitant deformity is caused by ankylosis, exostosis, and atrophy of soft parts. SYN: *arthritis deformans.*

Heberden's nodes. Hard nodules or enlargements of tubercles of last phalanges of fingers; seen in osteoarthritis.

hebetic (hē-bĕt′ĭk) [Gr. *hebetikos,* youthful]. Pert. to or occurring at the time of puberty.

hebetude (hĕb′ĕ-tūd) [LL. *hebetudo*]. Emotional dullness and disinterest. Patient is withdrawn and has no interest in surroundings. In late stages, indifference to personal comfort is marked. Seen in schizophrenia.

hebosteotomy (hē-bŏs″tē-ŏt′ō-mē) [Gr. *hebe,* youth, + *osteon,* bone, + *tome,* incision]. Hebotomy, q.v.

hebotomy (hē-bŏt′ō-mē). Section through the pubis to facilitate labor. SYN: *pubiotomy.*

hecateromeric, hecatomeric (hĕk″ă-tĕr″ō-mĕr′ĭk, hĕk″ă-tō-mĕr′ĭk) [Gr. *hekateros,* each of two, + *meros,* part]. Having two processes on a spinal neuron, one supplying each side of the spinal cord.

hectic (hĕk′tĭk) [Gr. *hektikos,* habitual]. 1. Habitual. 2. An afternoon rise of fever. Seen in active tuberculosis.

hecto- [Gr. *hekaton,* hundred]. In the metric system, a prefix indicating 100 times (10^2) the unit named. Thus hectoliter (10^2 liters) is 100 liters.

hectogram [″ + *gramma,* weight]. One hundred grams, or 3.527 avoirdupois ounces.

hectoliter (hĕk′tō-lē″tĕr) [″ + *litra,* a pound]. One hundred liters.

hectometer (hĕk-tŏm′ĕ-tĕr) [″ + *metron,* measure]. One hundred meters.

hedonism (hēd′ŏn-ĭzm) [Gr. *hedone,* pleasure, + *-ismos,* condition]. A theory or standard of conduct in which the principal object of life is pleasure. SEE: *pleasure principle.*

hedrocele (hĕd′rō-sēl) [Gr. *hedra,* anus, + *kele,* hernia]. Hernia or prolapse through the anus. SYN: *proctocele.*

heel [AS. *huela,* heel]. Rounded posterior portion of the foot under and behind the ankle. SYN: *calx.*

h., Thomas. [H. O. Thomas, Brit. orthopedist, 1834–1891] A corrective shoe in which the heel is approximately 12 mm. longer and 4 to 6 mm. higher on the medial edge. This produces varus of the foot and prevents depression of the head of the talus.

heel bone. Bone at back of tarsus. SYN: *calcaneus; os calcis.*

Heerfordt's disease (hār′forts). [C. F. Heerfordt, Danish ophthalmologist, b. 1871] Uveoparotid fever, a form of sarcoidosis.

Hegar's sign (hā′gărz). [Alfred Hegar, Ger. gynecologist, 1830–1914] Sign that may be present during second and third months of pregnancy. On bimanual examination, the lower part of the uterus is easily compressed between fingers placed in the vagina and those of the other hand over the pelvic area. This is due to the softening of lower segments of the uterus and to the fact that the

Height and Weight Table*

Person	Age From	Age To	Height Without Shoes Inches	Height Without Shoes Centimeters	Weight Pounds	Weight Kilograms
	Months					
Infants	0	2	22	55	9	4
	2	6	25	63	15	7
	6	12	28	72	20	9
	Years					
Children	1	2	32	81	26	12
	2	3	36	91	31	14
	3	4	39	100	35	16
	4	6	43	110	42	19
	6	8	48	121	51	23
	8	10	52	131	62	28
Male	10	12	55	140	77	35
	12	14	59	151	95	43
	14	18	67	170	130	59
	18	22	69	175	147	67
	22	35	69	175	154	70
	35	55	68	173	154	70
	55	75+	67	171	154	70
Female	10	12	56	142	77	35
	12	14	61	154	97	44
	14	16	62	157	114	52
	16	18	63	160	119	54
	18	22	64	163	128	58
	22	35	64	163	128	58
	35	55	63	160	128	58
	55	75+	62	157	128	58

* National Research Council: Recommended Dietary Allowances, ed. 7. Publication 1694, National Academy of Sciences, Washington, D.C., 1968.

fetus does not fill the uterine cavity at this stage, leaving an empty space in the lower part. The sign is not a positive one for pregnancy.

Heidenhain's demilunes (hī'dĕn-hīnz). [Rudolph P. Heidenhain, Ger. physiologist, 1834–1897] Crescent-shaped groups of serous cells at the base of, or along the sides of, the mucous alveoli of the salivary glands, esp. sublingual and submandibular. SYN: *crescents of Giannuzzi*.

height (hīt) [AS. *hiehthu*]. Vertical distance from the bottom to the top of an organ or structure. SEE: table.

Heimlich maneuver (hīm'lĭk). [H. J. Heimlich, contemporary U.S. physician] Technique for removing a foreign body from the trachea or pharynx, where it is preventing flow of air to the lungs. The obstruction usually is due to a bolus of food.

The maneuver consists of (1) wrapping your arms around the victim's waist from behind; (2) making a fist with one hand and placing it against the victim's abdomen between the navel and the rib cage; (3) clasping your fist with your free hand and pressing in with a quick forceful upward thrust. Repeat several times if necessary. If one is alone and experiences airway obstruction due to a foreign body, this technique could be self-applied.

This treatment is quite effective in dislodging the obstruction by forcing air against the mass much as pressure from a carbonated beverage will forcibly remove a cork or cap from a bottle. SEE: *choking;* illus.

Heimlich sign. [H. J. Heimlich] Grasping one's throat with the thumb and index finger to signal that the individual is choking.

Heineke-Mikulicz pyloroplasty (hī'nĕ-kĕ-mĭk'ū-lĭch). [Walter Hermann Heineke, Ger. surgeon, 1834–1901; Johann von Mikulicz-Radecki, Polish surgeon, 1850–1905] Pyloroplasty of the stomach, done to enlarge the outlet of the stomach.

Heinz bodies. [Robert Heinz, Ger. pathologist, 1865–1924] Granules in red blood cells due to damage of the hemoglobin molecules. Seen in premature infants, in certain forms of drug sensitivity, and in a certain type of hereditary hemolytic anemia. The bodies are best seen when the blood is stained with a

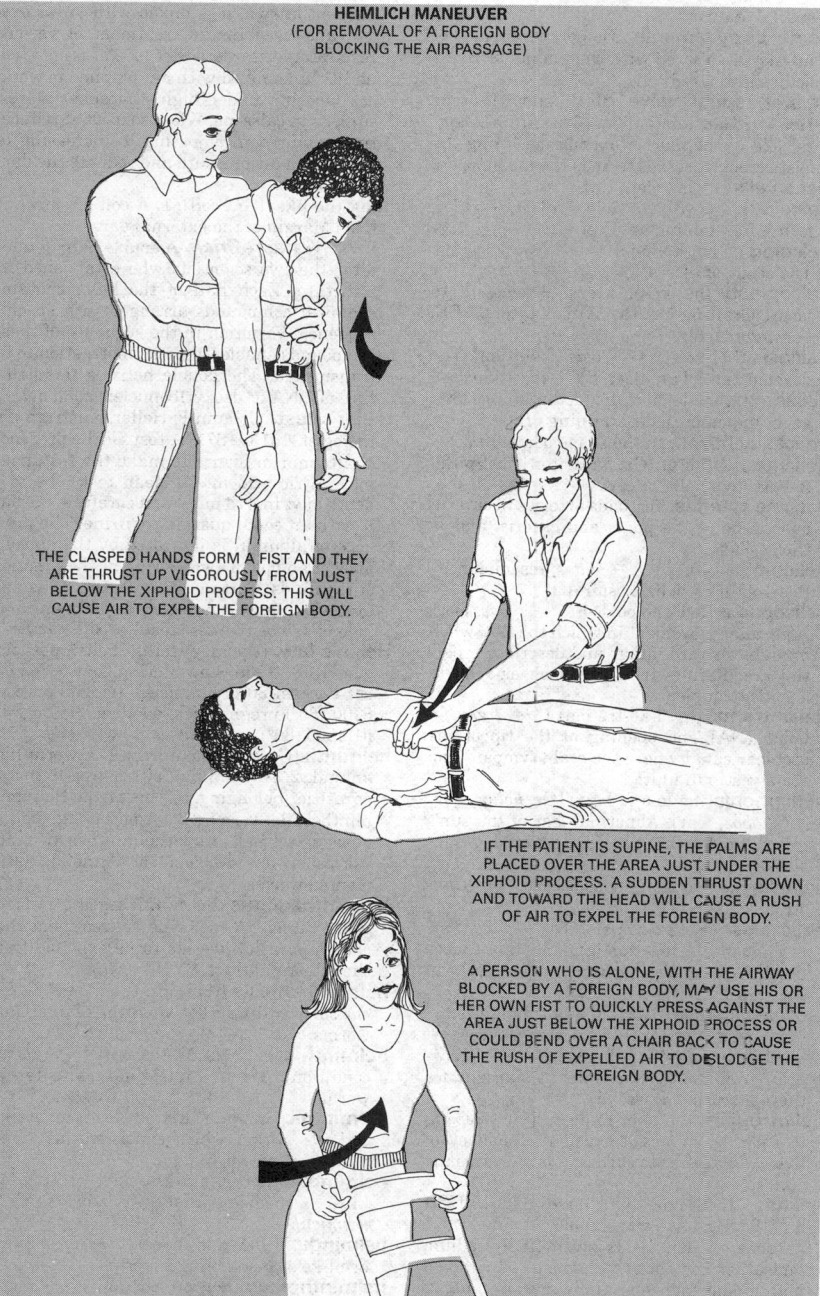

HEIMLICH MANEUVER
(FOR REMOVAL OF A FOREIGN BODY
BLOCKING THE AIR PASSAGE)

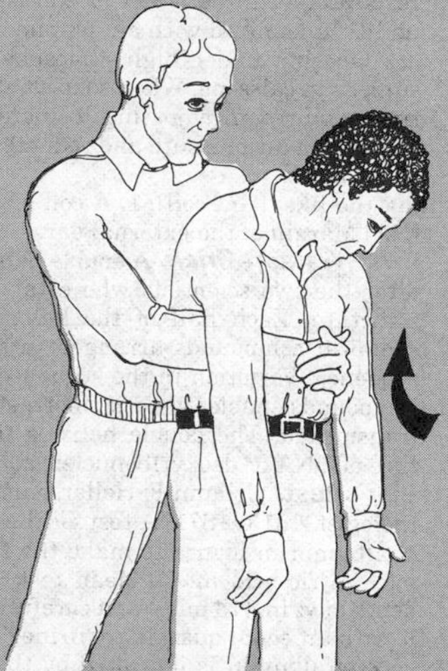

THE CLASPED HANDS FORM A FIST AND THEY ARE THRUST UP VIGOROUSLY FROM JUST BELOW THE XIPHOID PROCESS. THIS WILL CAUSE AIR TO EXPEL THE FOREIGN BODY.

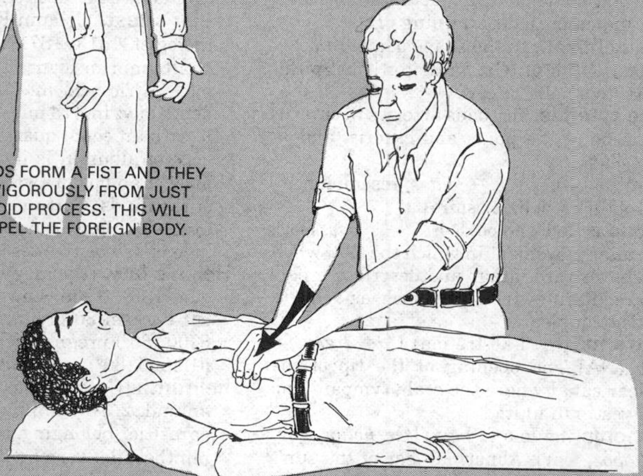

IF THE PATIENT IS SUPINE, THE PALMS ARE PLACED OVER THE AREA JUST UNDER THE XIPHOID PROCESS. A SUDDEN THRUST DOWN AND TOWARD THE HEAD WILL CAUSE A RUSH OF AIR TO EXPEL THE FOREIGN BODY.

A PERSON WHO IS ALONE, WITH THE AIRWAY BLOCKED BY A FOREIGN BODY, MAY USE HIS OR HER OWN FIST TO QUICKLY PRESS AGAINST THE AREA JUST BELOW THE XIPHOID PROCESS OR COULD BEND OVER A CHAIR BACK TO CAUSE THE RUSH OF EXPELLED AIR TO DISLODGE THE FOREIGN BODY.

special stain.

Heinz body anemia. Hemolytic anemia of infancy associated with the finding of Heinz bodies in the red cells.

Heister, spiral valve of (hī'stĕr). [Lorenz Heister, Ger. anatomist, 1683–1758] A spiral fold of the mucous membrane lining the cystic duct. It serves to keep the lumen open.

HeLa cells (hē'lă). Cell, HeLa, q.v.

helcoid (hĕl'koyd) [Gr. *helkos,* ulcer, + *eidos,* form]. Resembling an ulcer.

helcology (hĕl-kŏl'ō-jē) [" + *logos,* study]. The study of ulcers.

helcoplasty (hĕl'kō-plăs-tē) [" + *plassein,* to form]. Grafting healthy skin on ulcers. SEE: *dermatoplasty.*

helcosis (hĕl-kō'sĭs) [" + *osis,* condition]. The development of an ulcer. SYN: *ulceration.*

helianthine (hē-lē-ăn'thĭn). Methyl orange used as an indicator in determining pH.

helical (hĕl'ĭ-kăl). In the shape of a helix.

helicine (hĕl'ĭ-sĭn) [Gr. *helix,* coil]. 1. Spiral. 2. Pert. to a helix or coil.

helicine arteries. Tortuous arteries in cavernous tissue of the penis and clitoris, and in the uterus.

helicoid (hĕl'ĭ-koyd) [" + *eidos,* resemblance]. Resembling a helix or spiral.

helicopodia (hĕl"ĭ-kō-pō'dē-ă) [" + *pous,* foot]. A peculiar movement in which the foot, when brought forward, drags and describes a partial arc. Results in a gait such as seen in spastic hemiplegia.

helicotrema (hĕl"ĭ-kō-trē'mă) [" + *trema,* a hole]. [NA] The opening at the tip of the cochlear canal where the scala tympani and scala vestibuli unite.

heliophobia (hē"lē-ō-fō'bē-ă) [Gr. *helios,* sun, + *phobos,* fear]. Abnormal fear of the sun's rays, esp. by one who has suffered a sunstroke.

heliosis (hē"lē-ō'sĭs) [" + *osis,* condition]. Sunstroke.

heliotaxis (hē-lē-ō-tăk'sĭs) [" + *taxis,* arrangement]. A reaction in plants that causes them to respond negatively or positively to the sunlight.

h., negative. Turning away from the sun.

h., positive. Turning toward the sun.

heliotherapy (hē"lē-ō-thĕr'ă-pē) [" + *therapeia,* treatment]. Exposure to sunlight for therapeutic purposes.

heliotropism (hē"lē-ŏt'rō-pĭzm) [" + *trepein,* to turn, + *-ismos,* condition]. Tendency of living organisms to turn or grow towards the sun.

helium (hē'lē-ŭm) [Gr. *helios,* sun]. USP. SYMB: He. At. wt. 4.0026; at. no. 2. A gaseous element. It is given off by radium and other radioactive elements as charged helium ions known as alpha rays. Because of its low density, it being next to the lightest element known, it is mixed with air or oxygen and used in the treatment of various respiratory disorders. Because of its low solubility, it is mixed with air supplied to workers laboring under high atmospheric pressure, as in caissons. When so used, it reduces time required in adjusting to increasing or decreasing air pressure and reduces the danger of bends.

helix (hē'lĭks) [Gr., coil]. 1. A coil or spiral. 2. [NA] Margin of the external ear.

h., Watson-Crick. A double helix named after the two scientists who established its structure. Each half of the helix contains chemical compounds arranged in a specific sequence. Variation in the sequence of these compounds enables genetic information to be transmitted. The double helix is the structure of DNA or deoxyribonucleic acid, q.v.

Heller's test. [Johann F. Heller, Austrian pathologist, 1813–1871] A test for the presence of albumin in urine. To make the test, pour pure nitric acid into a clean test tube to a depth of ½ in. (13 mm.) and carefully overlay it with an equal quantity of urine. The presence of albumin is indicated by the appearance of an opaque white ring at the junction of the fluids. Certain drugs in the urine and urates in highly concentrated specimens may give false-positive test results. SEE: *urine.*

Hellin's law. [Dyonizy Hellin, Polish pathologist, 1867–1935] Law stating that twins occur once in 80 pregnancies, triplets once in 6400 (80^2) pregnancies, quadruplets once in 512,000 (80^3) pregnancies.

helminth [Gr. *helmins,* worm]. 1. A worm-like animal. 2. Any animal, either free-living or parasitic, belonging to the phyla Platyhelminthes (flatworms), Acanthocephala (spiny-headed worms), Nemathelminthes (threadworms or roundworms), or Annelida (segmented worms).

helminthagogue (hĕl-mĭnth'ă-gŏg) [" + *agogos,* leading]. A medicine or treatment that causes parasitic worms to be expelled from the intestinal tract. SYN: *vermifuge.*

helminthemesis (hĕl-mĭn-thĕm'ĕ-sĭs) [" + *emesis,* vomiting]. The vomiting of intestinal worms.

helminthiasis (hĕl-mĭn-thī'ă-sĭs) [" + *iasis,* condition]. Having intestinal parasites or worms.

helminthic (hĕl-mĭn'thĭk). 1. Pert. to worms. 2. Pert. to that which expels worms. SYN: *anthelmintic; vermifugal.*

helminthicide (hĕl-mĭn'thĭ-sīd) [" + L. *cidus,* kill]. A medicine that kills worms. SYN: *vermicide.*

helminthoid (hĕl-mĭn'thoyd) [" + *eidos,* form]. ormlike or resembling a worm.

helminthology (hĕl"mĭn-thŏl'ō-jē) [" + *logos,* study]. The study of parasitic intestinal worms.

helminthoma (hĕl″mĭn-thō′mă) [″ + *oma,* tumor]. A tumor caused by parasitic worms.

helminthophobia (hĕl-mĭn″thō-fō′bē-ă) [″ + *phobos,* fear]. Morbid dread of worms or delusion of being infested by them.

heloma (hē-lō′mă) [Gr. *helos,* nail, + *oma,* tumor]. A callosity or corn. SYN: *clavus.*

helotomy (hē-lŏt′ō-mē) [″ + *tome,* incision]. Surgical treatment of corns.

helplessness. A state that may arise when a patient has a condition in which he or she is dependent on an outside source for life support. The patients feel unable to alter their situation and experience anxiety due to inability to relieve their own discomfort. A fear of the necessary dependency on other people or even on mechanical supports may also be present. SEE: *giving-up; hopelessness.*

Helweg's bundle (hĕl′vĕgz). [Hans K. S. Helweg, Danish physician, 1847–1901] A small tract passing from the olivary body to the anterior horn cells in the cervical region. Part of the extrapyramidal motor system. SYN: *olivospinal tract.*

hema- (hē′mă, hĕm′ă) [Gr. *haima,* blood]. Combining form indicating blood.

hemachrosis (hē″mă-, hĕm″ă-krō′sĭs) [″ + *chrosis,* coloring]. Abnormal redness of blood.

hemacytometer (hē″mă-, hĕm″ă-sī-tŏm′ĭ-tĕr) [″ + *kytos,* cell, + *metron,* measure]. Apparatus used in counting blood cells.

hemacytozoon (hē″mă-, hĕm″ă-sī-tō-zō′ŏn) [″ + ″ + *zoon,* animal]. A protozoan parasite infesting red blood corpuscles.

hemad (hē′măd) [Gr. *haima,* blood, + L. *ad,* toward]. 1. Pert. to blood or blood vessels. 2. Toward the ventral or hemal aspect of the body. Opposed to neural or dorsal. SYN: *hemal.*

hemadostenosis (hē″mă-, hĕm″ă-dō-stĕn-ō′sĭs) [″ + *stenosis,* narrowing]. Contraction of blood vessels.

hemadsorption (hĕm″ăd-sorp′shŭn). Adherence of red blood cells to other cells or surfaces.

hemadynamometer (hē″mă-, hĕm″ă-dī″nă-mŏm′ĭ-ter) [″ + *dynamis,* power, + *metron,* measure]. Device for determining blood pressure.

hemafecia (hē″mă-, hĕm-ă-fē′sē-ă) [″ + L. *faeces,* refuse]. Feces containing blood.

hemagglutination (hĕm″ă-gloo-tĭn-ā′shŭn) [″ + L. *agglutinare,* to paste to]. The clumping of red blood corpuscles.

hemagglutination-inhibition. Prevention of hemagglutination by interaction or blocking of the antibody or virus that would otherwise cause hemagglutination.

hemagglutinin (hĕm″ă-gloo′tĭ-nĭn). An antibody that induces clumping of red blood corpuscles.

h., cold. Agglutination of erythrocytes (usually of sheep) at low temperatures by the serum of patients with certain diseases.

h., warm. An agglutinin effective only at body temperature, 37° C.

hemagogue (hē″mă-, hĕm′ă-gŏg) [″ + *agogos,* leading]. An agent that promotes the flow of blood, esp. menstrual flow. SEE: *emmenagogue.*

hemal (hē′măl). 1. Pert. to the blood or blood vessels. 2. Pert. to side of the body in which the heart is located. SYN: *hemad.*

hemal arch. The ribs, breastbone, and that part of the vertebrae that, together, enclose the heart and viscera.

hemal gland. A hemal or hemolymph node.

hemal node. A body resembling a lymph node in structure but associated with blood vessels instead of lymph vessels. Present in certain ungulates. SYN: *hemal gland.*

hemanalysis (hē′măn-, hĕm″ăn-ăl′ĭ-sĭs) [Gr. *haima,* blood, + *analysis,* a dissolving]. Any type of blood analysis. SEE: *blood.*

hemangiectasis (hē″măn-, hĕm″ăn-jē-ĕk′tă-sĭs) [″ + *angeion,* vessel, + *ektasis,* dilatation]. Dilatation of blood vessels.

hemangioblast (hĕ-măn′jē-ō-blăst) [″ + ″ + *blastos,* germ]. A mesodermal cell that can form either vascular endothelial cells or hemocytoblasts.

hemangioblastoma (hĕ-măn″jē-ō-blăs-tō′mă) [″ + ″ + *oma,* tumor]. A hemangioma of the brain, usually located in the cerebellum.

hemangioendothelioblastoma (hĕ-măn″jē-ō-ĕn″dō-thē″lē-ō-blăs-tō′mă) [″ + ″ + *endon,* within, + *thele,* nipple, + *blastos,* germ, + *oma,* tumor]. A neoplasm of the epithelial cells lining blood vessels.

hemangioendothelioma (hē″măn-jē-ō-ĕn″dō-thē-lē-ō′mă) [″ + ″ + ″ + ″ + *oma,* tumor]. An overgrowth of the endothelium of the minute capillary vessels. They are variable in size and are commonly seen in the capillary net of the cerebral meninges.

hemangiofibroma (hĕ-măn″jē-ō-fī-brō′mă) [″ + ″ + L. *fibra,* fiber, + Gr. *oma,* tumor]. A fibrous hemangioma.

hemangioma (hē-măn″jē-ō′mă [″ + *angeion,* vessel, + *oma,* tumor]. (pl. *hemangiomata*) A benign tumor of dilated blood vessels.

hemangiomatosis (hē-măn″jē-ō-mă-tō′sĭs) [″ + ″ + ″ + *osis,* condition]. Multiple angiomata of blood vessels.

hemangiopericytoma (hĕ-măn″jē-ō-pĕr″ĕ-sī-tō′mă). A tumor arising in capillaries. It is composed of pericytes.

hemangiosarcoma (hē-măn″jē-ō-săr-kō′mă) [″ + ″ + *sarkos,* flesh, + *oma,* tumor]. A malignant neoplasm originating from blood vessels. SYN: *angiosarcoma.*

hemaphein (hĕm′ă-fē′ĭn) [″ + *phaios,* dusky, gray]. Brown coloring material in the blood and urine.

hemapoiesis (hĕm″ă-poy-ē′sĭs) [″ + *poiesis,* formation]. Blood formation. SYN: *hematopoiesis.*

hemapoietic (hĕm-ă-poy-ĕt′ĭk) [″ + *poiein,* to form]. Pert. to hemapoiesis. SYN: *hematopoietic.*

hemapophysis (hĕm-ă-pŏf′ĭ-sĭs) [″ + *apo,* from, + *physis,* growth]. Portion of a developing vertebra that forms a rib and costal cartilage.

hemarthros, hemarthrosis (hĕm-ăr′thrŏs, hĕm-ăr-thrō′sĭs) [″ + *arthron,* joint]. Bloody effusion into cavity of a joint.

hematapostema (hĕm″ăt-ă-pŏs-tē′mă) [Gr. *haimatos,* blood, + *apostema,* abscess]. An abscess that contains blood.

hematein (hĕm″ă-tē′ĭn). A stain obtained by oxidation of hematoxylin.

hematemesis (hĕm-ăt-ĕm′ĕ-sĭs) [″ + *emesis,* vomiting]. Vomiting of blood. SEE: *hemoptysis* for table; *hemorrhage.*

SYM: Blood often clotted and mixed with food; acid in reaction. Subsequent stools may be tarry. If of gastric origin, the blood is generally dark and acid. If of pharyngeal origin, it is bright red and alkaline in reaction. If loss of blood is severe enough, shock and collapse may occur.

TREATMENT: Absolute rest, nothing by mouth. Feed intravenously if necessary. No stimulants. Have patient lie down. Surgery may be necessary.

hematencephalon (hĕm″ăt-ĕn-sĕf′ă-lŏn) [″ + *enkephalos,* brain]. Cerebral hemorrhage.

hematherapy (hĕm″ă-thĕr′ă-pē) [Gr. *haima,* blood, + *therapeia,* treatment]. Administration of fresh blood in treatment of disease.

hemathermal (hĕm″ă-, hē″mă-thĕr′măl) [″ + *therme,* heat]. Warm blooded, applied to animals whose blood remains at a fairly constant temperature. SYN: *hemathermous; hematothermal.*

hemathermous (hĕm″ă-thĕr′mŭs). Warm blooded. SYN: *hemathermal; hematothermal.*

hemathidrosis, hematidrosis (hē-măt″hĭ-drō′sĭs) [Gr. *haimatos,* blood, + *hidros,* sweat, + *osis,* condition]. Condition in which sweat contains blood.

hematic (hē-măt′ĭk). 1. Rel. to the blood. 2. A drug used in treating anemia. SYN: *hematinic.*

hematimeter (hĕm-ă-tĭm′ĕ-tĕr) [″ + *metron,* measure]. Apparatus used in counting blood corpuscles in a cu.mm. of blood. SYN: *hematometer; hemocytometer.*

hematin (hĕm′ă-tĭn). The nonprotein portion of the hemoglobin molecule wherein the iron is in the ferric (Fe^{+++}) rather than the ferrous (Fe^{++}) state. SEE: *ferritin; heme.*

hematinemia (hē-mă-, hĕm-ă-tĭn-ē′mē-ă). Heme in the circulating blood.

hematinic (hē-mă-, hĕm-ă-tĭn′ĭk) [Gr. *haima,* blood]. 1. Pert. to blood. 2. An agent that increases the amount of hemoglobin in the blood.

hematinuria (hē″mă-tĭn-ū′rē-ă). Hematin in the urine. SYN: *hemoglobinuria.*

hemato- (hē′mă-tō, hĕm′ă-tō) [Gr. *haimatos,* blood]. Prefix indicating blood.

hematobilia (hĕm″ă-tō-bĭl′ē-ă) [″ + L. *bilis,* bile]. Blood in the bile or bile ducts.

hematobium (hē″mă-, hĕm″ă-tō′bē-ŭm) [″ + *bios,* life]. A parasite that lives in the blood.

hematoblast (hē′mă-, hĕm′ă-tō-blăst) [″ + *blastos,* germ]. 1. A hemocytoblast. 2. Obsolete term for blood platelet.

hematocele (hē′mă-, hĕm′ă-tō-sēl) [″ + *kele,* hernia]. 1. A blood cyst. 2. Effusion of blood into a cavity. 3. Swelling due to effusion of blood into the tunica vaginalis testis.

h., parametric. Tumor formed by blood effusion in the cul-de-sac of Douglas walled off by adhesions.

h., pudendal. A blood-filled swollen area of the labium.

hematocelia (hĕm″ă-tō-sē′lē-ă) [″ + *koilia,* cavity]. Hemorrhage into the peritoneal cavity.

hematocephalus (hē″mă-, hĕm″ă-tō-sĕf′ă-lŭs) [″ + *kephale,* head]. Fetus born with infusion of blood in the head.

hematochezia (hĕm″ă-tō-kē′zē-ă) [″ + *chezein,* to go to stool]. Passage of stools containing red blood rather than tarry stools.

hematochromatosis (hĕm″ă-tō-krō″mă-tō′sĭs) [″ + *chroma,* color, + *osis,* condition]. A condition showing staining of tissues with blood pigment due to abnormal and excessive deposition of iron from hemoglobin or excessive ingestion of iron. SYN: *hemochromatosis.*

hematochyluria (hē″mă-, hĕm″ă-tō-kī-lū′rē-ă) [″ + *chylos,* juice, + *ouron,* urine]. Blood and chyle in the urine.

hematocolpometra (hē″mă-, hĕm″ă-tō-kŏl″pō-mē′tră) [″ + *kolpos,* vagina, + *metra,* uterus]. Retention of menstrual blood in the vagina and uterus.

hematocolpos (hē″mă-, hĕm″ă-tō-kŏl′pŏs). Retained menstrual blood in the vagina caused by an imperforate hymen.

hematocrit (hē-măt′ō-krĭt) [″ + *krinein,* to separate]. 1. Centrifuge for separating solids from plasma in the blood. 2. The volume of erythrocytes packed by centrifugation in a given volume of blood. The hematocrit is expressed as the percentage of total blood volume that consists of erythrocytes or as the volume in cubic centimeters of erythrocytes packed by centrifugation of blood. Normal values at sea level: men, average 47%, range 40–54%; women, average 42%, range 37–47%; children, varies with age from 35–

49%; newborn, 49–54%.

hematocyst (hē′mă-, hĕm′ă-tō-sĭst) [Gr. *haimatos,* blood, + *kystis,* a bladder]. 1. Hemorrhage into a cyst or the urinary bladder. 2. A blood-filled cyst.

hematocyte (hē′mă-, hĕm′ă-tō-sīt) [″ + *kytos,* cell]. 1. A red blood cell. 2. Any blood cell.

hematocytoblast (hĕm″ă-tō-sī′tō-blăst) [″ + ″ + *blastos,* germ]. Hemocytoblast, q.v.

hematocytolysis (hē″mă-, hĕm″ă-tō-sī-tŏl′ĭ-sĭs) [″ + ″ + *lysis,* dissolution]. Dissolution of blood corpuscles, thus freeing hemoglobin. SYN: *hemolysis.*

hematocytometer (hē″mă-, hĕm″ă-tō-sī-tŏm′ĕ-ter) [″ + ″ + *metron,* measure]. Device for counting number of blood cells in given quantity of blood.

hematocytozoon (hē″mă-, hĕm″ă-tō-sī-tō-zō′ŏn) [″ + ″ + *zoon,* animal]. A parasite that lives in red blood cells.

hematocyturia (hē″mă-, hĕm″ă-tō-sī-tū′rē-ă) [″ + ″ + *ouron,* urine]. Red blood cells in urine; hematuria, as differentiated from hemoglobinuria, q.v.

hematogenesis (hē″mă-, hĕm″ă-tō-jĕn′ĕ-sĭs) [″ + *genesis,* formation]. The development of blood cells. SYN: *hematopoiesis.*

hematogenic, hematogenous (hē″mă-, hĕm″ă-tō-jĕn′ĭk, -tŏj′ĕ-nŭs) [″ + *gennan,* to produce]. 1. Pert. to formation of blood. SYN: *hematopoietic.* 2. Pert. to or originating in the blood.

hematohidrosis (hē″mă-, hĕm″ă-tō-hī-drō′sĭs) [″ + *hidros,* sweat, + *osis,* condition]. Secretion of sweat containing blood. SYN: *hemathidrosis.*

hematoid (hē′mă-, hĕm′ă-toyd) [″ + *eidos,* resemblance]. Resembling blood.

hematoidin (hē″mă-, hĕm-ă-toy′dĭn). The yellow crystalline substance, biliverdin, that remains when red blood cells are destroyed in bruised tissue.

hematokolpos. Hematocolpos.

hematologist (hē″mă-, hĕm″ă-tŏl′ō-jĭst) [″ + *logos,* study]. One who specializes in the study of the blood.

hematology (hē″mă-, hĕm″ă-tŏl′ō-jē). The science concerned with blood and the blood-forming tissues.

hematolymphangioma (hē″mă-, hĕm″ă-tō-lĭmf-ăn″jē-ō′mă) [″ + L. *lympha,* lymph, + Gr. *angeion,* vessel, + *oma,* tumor]. A tumor consisting of dilated blood vessels and lymphatics.

hematolysis (hē″mă-, hĕm-ă-tŏl′ĭ-sĭs) [″ + *lysis,* dissolution]. Hemolysis.

hematolytic (hĕm-ă-tō-lĭt′ĭk). Pert. to hemolysis.

hematoma (hē″mă-, hĕm-ă-tō′mă) [Gr. *haimatos,* blood, + *oma,* tumor]. A swelling or mass of blood (usually clotted) confined to an organ, tissue, or space and caused by a break in a blood vessel.

h. auris. Hematoma beneath the perichondrium of the ear cartilage.

h., pelvic. Hematoma present in cellular tissue of the pelvis.

h., subdural. Hematoma located beneath the dura, usually the result of head injuries.

h., vulvar. Hematoma occurring on the vulva.

hematomediastinum (hē″mă-, hĕm″ă-tō-mē″dē-ă-stī′nŭm) [″ + L. *mediastinus,* in the middle]. Blood effusion into the mediastinum.

hematometer (hē-mă-tŏm′ĕ-tĕr) [″ + *metron,* measure]. Hemoglobinometer.

hematometra (hē″mă-, hĕm″ă-tō-mē′tră) [″ + *metra,* uterus]. 1. Hemorrhage in the uterus. 2. Accumulation of menstrual blood in the uterus. SEE: *hematocolpos; hydrometra; pyometra.*

hematometry (hĕm″ă-tŏm′ĕ-trē) [″ + *metron,* measure]. Determination of varieties and number of blood cells and amount of hemoglobin in the blood.

hematomphalocele (hē″mă-, hĕm″ăt-ŏm-făl′ō-sēl) [″ + *omphalos,* navel, + *kele,* hernia]. Effusion of blood into an umbilical hernia.

hematomyelia (hē″mă-, hĕm″ă-tō-mī-ē′lē-ă) [″ + *myelos,* marrow]. Hemorrhage of blood into the spinal cord.

hematomyelitis (hē″mă-, hĕm″ă-tō-mī″ĕl-ī′tĭs) [″ + ″ + *itis,* inflammation]. Inflammation of spinal cord accompanied by bloody effusion.

hematomyelopore (hē″măt-, hĕm″ăt-ō-mī′ĕl-ō-por) [″ + ″ + *poros,* opening]. Formation of cavities and channels in the spinal cord as a result of hemorrhage.

hematonephrosis (hē″mă-, hĕm″ă-tō-nĕ-frō′sĭs) [″ + *nephros,* kidney, + *osis,* condition]. Accumulation of blood in the pelvis of the kidney.

hematopathology [″ + *pathos,* disease, + *logos,* study]. The study of pathological conditions of the blood.

hematopericardium (hē″mă-, hĕm″ă-tō-pĕr″ĭ-kăr′dē-ŭm) [″ + *peri,* around, + *kardia,* heart]. Bloody effusion into the pericardial sac.

hematoperitoneum (hē″mă-, hĕm″ă-tō-pĕr″ĭ-tō-nē′ŭm) [″ + *peritonaion,* peritoneum]. Bloody effusion into the peritoneal cavity. SYN: *hemoperitoneum.*

hematopexin (hĕm″ă-tō-pĕk′sĭn) [″ + *pexis,* fixation]. Any substance that causes blood to coagulate. SYN: *hemopexin.*

hematopexis (hĕm″ă-tō-pĕk′sĭs). Coagulation of the blood. SYN: *hemopexia.*

hematophage (hĕm′ă-tō-fāj) [″ + *phagein,* to eat]. A phagocytic cell that destroys red blood cells.

hematophagia (hĕm″ă-tō-fā′jē-ă). 1. Subsistence on blood. 2. Destruction of blood cells by phagocytes.

hematophagous (hĕm-ă-tŏf′ă-gŭs). Living on blood. SEE: *hematophagia.*

hematophilia (hĕm″ă-tō-fĭl′ē-ă) [″ + *philein,* to love]. Hemophilia.

hematophobia (hē″mă-, hĕm″ă-tō-fō′bē-ă) [″ + *phobos,* fear]. Hemophobia.

hematophyte (hē′mă-, hĕm′ă-tō-fīt) [″ + *phyton,* plant]. Plant organism or bacteria in the blood.

hematoplastic [″ + *plassein,* to form]. Pert. to formation of blood. SYN: *hematopoietic.*

hematopoiesis (hē″mă-, hĕm″ă-tō-poy-ē′sĭs) [Gr. *haimatos,* blood, + *poiesis,* formation]. The production and development of blood cells, normally in the bone marrow. Tissues that produce blood cells are said to be hematopoietic.

h., extramedullary. Production of blood cells in tissues other than bone marrow. This occurs in severe anemia and other diseases affecting the blood.

hematopoietic (hē″mă-, hĕm″ă-tō-poy-ĕt′ĭk). 1. Pert. to the production and development of blood cells. 2. A substance that assists in or stimulates the production of blood cells. SYN: *hematogenic; hematoplastic.*

hematopoietic system. The blood-forming organs, esp. bone marrow and lymph nodes.

hematoporphyrin (hē″mă-, hĕm″ă-tō-por′fĭ-rĭn) [″ + *porphyra,* purple]. Iron-free heme, a decomposition product of hemoglobin present in the urine in certain conditions.

hematoporphyrinuria (hē″mă-, hĕm″ă-tō-por″fĭ-rĭn-ū′rē-ă) [″ + ″ + *ouron,* urine]. Hematoporphyrin in urine.

hematorrhachis (hĕm-ă-tor′ă-kĭs) [″ + *rhachis,* spine]. Hemorrhage into the spinal cord.

hematorrhea (hĕm″ă-tō-rē′ă) [″ + *rhoia,* flow]. Profuse hemorrhage.

hematosalpinx (hē″mă-, hĕm″ă-tō-săl′pĭnks) [″ + *salpinx,* tube]. Retained menstrual fluid in the fallopian tube.

hematoscheocele (hĕm-ă-tŏs′kē-ō-sēl) [″ + *oscheon,* scrotum, + *kele,* hernia]. Blood accumulated in the scrotum.

hematoscope (hē′mă-, hĕm′ă-tō-skōp) [″ + *skopein,* to examine]. Device for optical or spectroscopic examination of blood.

hematoscopy (hē″mă-, hĕm-ă-tŏs′kō-pē). Examination of the blood.

hematose (hē′mă-, hĕm′ă-tōs) [″ + *osis,* condition]. Full of blood.

hematosepsis (hĕm″ă-tō-sĕp′sĭs) [″ + *sepsis,* putrefaction]. Septicemia.

hematospectroscope (hĕm″ă-tō-spĕk′trō-skōp) [″ + L. *spectrum,* image, + Gr. *skopein,* to examine]. Spectroscope for examining and analyzing blood.

hematospectroscopy (hĕm″ă-tō-spĕk-trŏs′kō-pē). Examination of blood with the hematospectroscope.

hematospermatocele (hĕm″ă-tō-spĕr-măt′ō-sēl) [″ + *sperma,* seed, + *kele,* tumor]. A blood-filled spermatocele.

hematospermia (hĕm″ă-tō-spĕr′mē-ă). Semen that contains blood; hemospermia.

h. spuria. Hematospermia coming from the prostatic urethra.

h. vera. Hematospermia coming from the seminal vesicles.

hematostatic (hĕm″ă-tō-stăt′ĭk) [Gr. *haimatos,* blood, + *stasis,* standing]. 1. Retaining blood in a part. 2. Pert. to the arrest of blood flow in a hemorrhage. SYN: *hemostatic.*

hematosteon (hĕm-ă-tŏs′tē-ŏn) [″ + *osteon,* bone]. Bleeding into the medullary cavity of a bone.

hematothermal (hĕm″ă-tō-thĕr′măl) [″ + *therme,* heat]. Warm blooded. SYN: *hemathermal; hemathermous.*

hematothorax (hĕm″ă-tō-thō′răks) [″ + *thorax,* chest]. Blood in the chest. SYN: *hemothorax.*

hematotoxic (hĕm″ă-tō-tŏk′sĭk) [″ + *toxikon,* poison]. 1. Pert. to septicemia. 2. Toxic to blood cells.

hematotrachelos (hĕm″ă-tō-tră-kē′lŏs) [″ + *trachelos,* neck]. Retained menstrual blood in cervix uteri, causing distention.

hematotropic (hĕm″ă-tō-trŏp′ĭk) [″ + *tropos,* a turning]. Having special affinity for red blood cells.

hematotympanum (hĕm″ă-tō-tĭm′păn-ŭm) [″ + *tympanon,* drum]. Blood in the middle ear.

hematoxylin (hĕm″ă-tŏk′sĭ-lĭn). $C_{16}H_{14}O_6$. A colorless crystalline compound obtained by ether extraction of logwood. Upon oxidation it is converted into hematein, an oxidation product of hematoxylin, which stains certain structures a deep blue color. It is an excellent nuclear stain and widely used in histological work.

hematozoon (hē″mă-, hĕm″ă-tō-zō′ŏn) [″ + *zoon,* animal]. Any living organism in the blood.

hematozymosis (hē″mă-, hĕm″ă-tō-zī-mō′sĭs) [″ + *zymosis,* fermentation]. Blood fermentation.

hematuria (hē″mă-, hĕm″ă-tū′rē-ă) [″ + *ouron,* urine]. Blood in the urine.

NOTE: The occurrence of bright red blood in the urine and its appearance in the toilet bowl are quite frightening to the patient. The patient, the doctor, and the nurse should realize that a very small amount of blood may cause the entire toilet bowl to appear to be full of blood.

SYM: Urine may be slightly smoky, reddish, or very red.

ETIOL: Lesion of urinary tract; blood dyscrasia; contamination during menstruation or puerperium; prostatic disease; tumors; poisoning, esp. carbolic acid and cantharides; malaria; toxemias; or calculus in urinary tract.

DIAG: If blood is well mixed with urine, it probably came from the kidneys. If clotted in tubular casts of ureters, it came from the kidneys or ureters. If passed at beginning of urination, from the urethra; if at the end, from the bladder.

h., renal. Urine smoky, sometimes bright red.

h., urethral. Always bright red. Precedes urination.

h., vesical. Urine bright red, not uniform.

heme (hēm). An iron-containing nonprotein portion of the hemogloblin molecule wherein the iron is in the ferrous (Fe^{++}) state. SEE: *ferritin; hematin.*

hemeralopia (hĕm″ĕr-ăl-ō′pē-ă) [Gr. *hemera,* day, + *alaos,* blind, + *ops,* eye]. Diminished vision in bright light. Term formerly erroneously applied to night blindness or nyctalopia, q.v. Nyctalopia indicates inability to see in dim light, though otherwise vision is normal.

In hemeralopia, the sight is poor in sunlight and in good illumination; it is good at dusk, at twilight, and in poor illumination. This is noted in albinism, retinitis with central scotoma, toxic amblyopia, coloboma of the iris and choroid, opacity of the crystalline lens or cornea, and in conjunctivitis with photophobia.

hemi- (hĕm′ē) [Gr.]. Prefix meaning half.

hemiacephalus (hĕm″ē-ă-sĕf′ă-lŭs) [″ + *a-,* not, + *kephale,* head]. A malformed fetus with a markedly defective head. SEE: *anencephalus.*

hemiachromatopsia (hĕm″ē-ă-krō-mă-tŏp′sē-ă) [″ + ″ + *chroma,* color, + *opsis,* vision]. Color blindness in one half, or in corresponding halves, of the visual field.

hemiageusia (hĕm″ē-ă-gū′zē-ă) [″ + ″ + *geusis,* taste]. Loss of sense of taste on one side of the tongue.

hemialbumin (hĕm″ē-ăl-bū′mĭn) [″ + L. *albumen,* white of egg]. A product resulting from the digestion of albumin.

hemialbumose (hĕm″ē-ăl′bū-mōs). An albumoid product from the digestion of certain proteins. It is found in bone marrow.

hemialbumosuria (hĕm″ē-ăl-bū″mō-sū′rē-ă) [″ + ″ + Gr. *ouron,* urine]. Hemialbumose in the urine.

hemialgia (hĕm-ē-ăl′jē-ă) [″ + *algos,* pain]. Pain in one half of the body only.

hemiamaurosis (hĕm″ē-ăm″ŏ-rō′sĭs) [″ + *amaurosis,* darkness]. Blindness in half the visual field. SYN: *hemiamblyopia; hemianopia.*

hemiamblyopia (hĕm″ē-ăm″blē-ō′pē-ă) [″ + *amblys,* dim, + *ops,* sight]. Blindness in half the visual field. SYN: *hemiamaurosis; hemianopia.*

hemiamyosthenia (hĕm″ē-ă″mī-ŏs-thē′nē-ă) [Gr. *hemi-,* half, + *a-,* not, + *mys,* muscle, + *sthenos,* strength]. Absence of normal muscular power on one side of the body. SYN: *hemiparesis.*

hemianacusia (hĕm″ē-ăn″ă-kū′zē-ă) [″ + *an-,* not, + *akousis,* hearing]. Deafness in one ear.

hemianalgesia (hĕm″ē-ăn-ăl-jē′zē-ă) [″ + ″ + *algos,* pain]. Lack of sensibility to pain (analgesia) on one side of the body.

hemiancephaly (hĕm″ē-ăn″sĕf′ă-lē) [″ + *an-,* not, + *enkephalos,* brain]. Congenital absence of half of the brain.

hemianesthesia (hĕm″ē-ăn-ĕs-thē′zē-ă) [″ + ″ + *aisthesis,* sensation]. Anesthesia of half of the body.

hemianopia, hemianopsia (hĕm″ē-ă-nō′pē-ă, -nŏp′sē-ă) [″ + *an-,* not, + *ops,* eye]. Blindness for half the field of vision in one or both eyes. SYN: *hemiamaurosis; hemiamblyopia.*

h., altitudinal. Blindness in upper or lower half of the visual field of one or both eyes.

h., binasal. Affection of nasal half of the visual field in each eye.

h., bitemporal. Affection of temporal half of visual field in each eye.

h., complete. Blindness in half the visual field.

h., crossed. Either bitemporal or binasal hemianopsia.

h., heteronymous. H., crossed.

h., homonymous. Blindness of nasal half of the visual field of one eye and temporal half of the other or right-sided or left-sided hemianopsia of corresponding sides in both eyes.

h., incomplete. Blindness in less than half of the visual field of each eye.

h., quadrant. Blindness of symmetrical quadrant of the field of vision in each eye.

h., unilateral. Hemianopsia affecting only one eye.

hemianosmia (hĕm″ē-ăn-ŏs′mē-ă) [Gr. *hemi-,* half, + *an-,* not, + *osme,* smell]. Loss of smell in one nostril.

hemiapraxia (hĕm″ē-ă-prăks′ē-ă) [″ + *a-,* not, + *prassein,* to do]. Incapacity to exercise purposeful movements on one side of the body.

hemiarthroplasty of the hip. Replacement of the femoral head with a metal ball held in place by a stem extending into the shaft of the femur. The acetabulum is not altered. Particularly useful in patients with necrosis of the femoral head.

hemiarthrosis (hĕm″ē-ăr-thrō′sĭs) [″ + *arthron,* joint, + *osis,* condition]. A false articulation between two bones. SYN: *synchondrosis.*

hemiasynergia (hĕm″ē-ă″sĭn-ĕr′jē-ă) [″ + *a-,* not, + *syn,* with, + *ergon,* work]. Lack of coordination of parts affecting one side of the body.

hemiataxia (hĕm″ē-ă-tăks′ē-ă) [″ + *ataxia,* lack of order]. Impaired muscular coordination causing awkward movements of the affected side of the body.

hemiathetosis (hĕm″ē-ăth″ĕ-tō′sĭs) [″ + *athetos,* without fixed position, + *osis,* condition]. Athetosis of one side of the body.

hemiatrophy (hĕm-ē-ăt′rō-fē) [″ + *atrophia,* atrophy]. Impaired nutrition resulting in atrophy of one side of the face or other part; marked by white or yellow macules on affected side.

hemiballism (hĕm-ē-băl′ĭzm) [″ + *balismos,* jumping]. Jerking and twitching movements of one side of the body. SYN: *hemichorea.*

hemiblock (hĕm′ĭ-blŏk). In heart block, failure of conduction in one of the two main divisions of the left branches of the conducting bundle.

hemic (hē′mĭk, hĕm′ĭk) [Gr. *haima,* blood]. Pert. to blood. SYN: *hemal.*

hemicanities (hĕm″ē-kăn-ĭsh′ĭ-ēz) [Gr. *hemi-,* half, + L. *canities,* gray hair]. Grayness of hair on one side only.

hemicardia (hĕm-ē-kăr′dē-ă) [″ + *kardia,* heart]. Half of a four-chambered heart.

hemicellulose (hĕm-ē-sĕl′ū-lōs). One of a group of polysaccharides that differ from cellulose in that they may be hydrolyzed by dilute mineral acids, and from other polysaccharides in that they are not readily digested by amylases. Includes pentosans, galactosans (agar-agar), and pectins.

hemicentrum (hĕm-ē-sĕn′trŭm) [″ + *kentron,* center]. Either lateral half of the centrum of a vertebra.

hemicephalia (hĕm″ē-sĕ-fā′lē-ă) [″ + *kephale,* head]. Congenital absence of one half of the skull and brain.

hemicephalus (hĕm″ē-sĕf′ă-lŭs). A congenitally deformed child with only one cerebral hemisphere.

hemicerebrum (hĕm″ē-sĕr′ĕ-brŭm) [″ + L. *cerebrum,* brain]. Half of the cerebral hemisphere.

hemichorea (hĕm-ē-kō-rē′ă) [″ + *choreia,* a dancing] Convulsive movements of one side of the body. SYN: *hemiballism.*

hemichromatopsia (hĕm″ē-krō-mă-tŏp′sē-ă) [″ + *chroma,* color, + *opsis,* vision]. Blindness to color in half of the visual field. SYN: *hemiachromatopsia.*

hemicolectomy (hĕm″ē-kō-lĕk′tō-mē) [″ + *kolon,* colon, + *ektome,* excision]. Surgical removal of half or less of the colon.

hemicorporectomy (hĕm″ē-kor″pō-rĕk′tō-mē) [″ + L. *corpus,* body, + Gr. *ektome,* excision]. Surgical removal of the lower half of the body.

hemicrania (hĕm-ē-krā′nē-ă) [″ + *kranion,* skull]. 1. Unilateral head pain, usually migraine. 2. Malformed fetus having only one half of the skull development.

hemicraniectomy (hĕm″ē-krā-nē-ĕk′tō-mē) [″ + ″ + *ektome,* excision]. Surgical division of cranial vault from front backward, exposing half of the brain.

hemicraniosis (hĕm″ē-krā-nē-ō′sĭs) [″ + ″ + *osis,* condition]. Enlargement of half of cranium or face.

hemidiaphoresis (hĕm″ē-dī″ă-for-ē′sĭs) [″ + *dia,* through, + *pherein,* to carry]. Sweating on one side of the body. SYN: *hemidrosis; hemihidrosis.*

hemidiaphragm (hĕm″ē-dī′ă-frăm) [″ + ″ + *phragma,* wall]. Half of the diaphragm.

hemidrosis (hĕm″ĭ-drō′sĭs). 1. [″ + *hidrosis,* sweating] Sweating on one side of the body. SYN: *hemidiaphoresis; hemihidrosis.* 2. [Gr. *haima,* blood, + *hidrosis,* sweating] Secretion of sweat containing blood. SYN: *hemathidrosis.*

hemidysergia (hĕm″ē-dĭs-ĕr′jē-ă) [Gr. *hemi-,* half, + *dys,* bad, + *ergon,* work]. Lack of coordination of muscles on one side of the body.

hemidysesthesia (hĕm″ē-dĭs-ĕs-thē′zē-ă) [″ + ″ + *aisthesis,* sensation]. Impaired sensation of half of the body.

hemidystrophy (hĕm″ē-dĭs′trō-fē) [″ + ″ + *trophe,* nourishment]. Inequality in development of the two sides of the body.

hemiectromelia (hĕm″ē-ĕk-trō-mē′lē-ă) [″ + *ektro,* abortion, + *melos,* limb]. Deformed extremities on one side of the body.

hemiepilepsy (hĕm″ē-ĕp′ĭ-lĕp-sē) [″ + *epilepsia,* seizure]. Epilepsy with convulsions confined to lateral half of the body.

hemifacial (hĕm″ē-fā′shăl) [″ + L. *facies,* face]. Pert. to one side of the face.

hemigastrectomy (hĕm″ē-găs-trĕk′tō-mē) [″ + *gaster,* belly, + *ektome,* excision]. Excision of half of the stomach.

hemigeusia (hĕm-ē-gū′sē-ă) [″ + *geusis,* taste]. Loss of sense of taste on one side of the tongue.

hemiglossal (hĕm″ē-glŏs′săl) [″ + *glossa,* tongue]. Concerning one side of the tongue.

hemiglossectomy (hĕm″ē-glŏs-sĕk′tō-mē) [″ + ″ + ektome, excision]. Surgical removal of one half of the tongue.

hemiglossitis [″ + ″ + *itis,* inflammation]. Vesicular eruption on half of the tongue and inner surface of the cheek. Herpetic in character.

hemignathia (hĕm″ē-năth′ē-ă) [″ + *gnathos,*

jaw]. Congenital absence of one half of the lower jaw.

hemihepatectomy (hĕm″ē-hĕp″ă-tĕk′tō-mē) [″ + *hepatos,* liver, + *ektome,* excision]. Surgical removal of half the liver.

hemihidrosis (hĕm″ē-hī-drō′sĭs) [″ + *hidrosis,* perspiration]. Sweating on only one side of the body. SYN: *hemidiaphoresis; hemidrosis* (def. 1).

hemihypalgesia (hĕm″ē-hī″păl-jē′zē-ă) [″ + *hypo,* under, + *algesis,* pain]. Partial anesthesia on one side of the body.

hemihyperesthesia (hĕm″ē-hī-pĕr-ĕs-thē′zē-ă) [″ + *hyper,* over, + *aisthesis,* sensation]. Abnormal tactile and painful sensitiveness of one side of the body.

hemihyperidrosis (hĕm″ē-hī-pĕr-ĭ-drō′sĭs) [″ + ″ + *hidrosis,* sweating]. Excessive perspiration confined to one side of the body. SYN: *hemihyperhidrosis.*

hemihyperplasia (hĕm″ē-hī″pĕr-plā′zē-ă) [″ + ″ + *plassein,* to form]. Excessive development of one side or one half of the body or of an organ.

hemihypertonia (hĕm″ē-hī″pĕr-tō′nē-ă) [″ + ″ + *tonos,* tone]. Exaggerated tonicity of muscles on lateral half of the body.

hemihypertrophy (hĕm″ē-hī-pĕr′trō-fē) [″ + ″ + *trophe,* nourishment]. Hypertrophy of muscles of half of the body or face.

hemihypesthesia, hemihypoesthesia (hĕm″ē-hī″pĕs-thē′zē-ă, -pō-ĕs-thē′zē-ă) [Gr. *hemi-,* half, + *hypo,* under, + *aisthesis,* sensation]. Diminished sensibility on one side of the body.

hemihypoplasia (hĕm″ē-hī″pō-plā′zē-ă) [″ + ″ + *plassein,* to form]. Decreased development of half of the body or of an organ.

hemihypotonia (hĕm″ē-hī-pō-tō′nē-ă) [″ + ″ + *tonos,* tone]. Partial loss of tonicity of muscles on one side of the body.

hemikaryon (hĕm″ē-kăr′ē-ŏn) [″ + *karyon,* nucleus]. A cell nucleus with half the diploid number of chromosomes.

hemilaminectomy (hĕm″ē-lăm″ĭ-nĕk′tō-mē) [″ + L. *lamina,* thin plate, + Gr. *ektome,* excision]. Surgical removal of the lamina of the vertebral arch on one side.

hemilaryngectomy (hĕm″ē-lăr″ĭn-jĕk′tō-mē) [″ + *larynx,* larynx, + *ectome,* excision]. Surgical removal of the lateral half of the larynx.

hemilateral [″ + L. *latus,* side]. Rel. to one side only.

hemilesion (hĕm″ē-lē′zhŭn) [″ + L. *laesio,* a wound]. A lesion on one side of the body.

hemilingual (hĕm″ē-lĭng′gwăl) [″ + L. *lingua,* tongue]. Affecting or concerning one lateral half of the tongue.

hemimacroglossia (hĕm″ē-măk″rō-glŏs′ē-ă) [″ + *makros,* large, + *glossa,* tongue]. Enlargement of one lateral half of the tongue.

hemimandibulectomy (hĕm″ē-măn-dĭb-ū-lĕk′tō-mē) [″ + L. *mandibula,* lower jawbone, + Gr. *ektome,* excision]. Surgical removal of half of the mandible.

hemimelus (hĕm′ĭ-mē′lŭs) [″ + *melos,* limb]. A malformed fetus with defective development of the extremities, esp. the distal portion.

hemin (hē′mĭn) [Gr. *haima,* blood]. A brownish-red crystalline salt of heme formed when hemoglobin is heated with glacial acetic acid and sodium chloride. The iron is present in the ferric (Fe^{+++}) state. Used in testing for presence of blood. SEE: *heme.*

heminephrectomy (hĕm″ē-nĕ-frĕk′tō-mē) [Gr. *hemi-,* half, + *nephros,* kidney, + *ektome,* excision]. Excision or removal of a portion of a kidney.

hemineurasthenia (hĕm″ē-nū-răs-thē′nē-ă) [″ + *neuron,* nerve, + *astheneia,* weakness]. Neurasthenia affecting one side of the body only.

hemiopalgia (hĕm″ē-ŏp-ăl′jē-ă) [″ + *ops,* eye, + *algos,* pain]. Pain in one side of the head and the eye on that side.

hemiopia (hĕm-ē-ō′pē-ă) [″ + *ops,* eye]. Blindness in half of the visual field. SYN: *hemianopia.*

hemiopic (hĕm-ē-ŏp′ĭk) [″ + *ops,* eye]. Pert. to hemiopia.

hemipagus (hĕm-ĭp′ă-gŭs) [″ + *pagos,* a thing fixed]. Twins fused at the navel and thorax.

hemiparalysis [″ + *paralyein,* to loosen from the sides]. Paralysis of one side of the body only.

hemiparanesthesia (hĕm″ē-păr-ăn-ĕs-thē′zē-ă) [″ + *para,* beyond, + *an-,* not, + *aisthesis,* sensation]. Anesthesia of one lower extremity or lower half of one side.

hemiparaplegia (hĕm″ē-păr-ă-plē′jē-ă) [″ + ″ + *plege,* stroke]. Paralysis of the lower half of one side or of one leg.

hemiparesis (hĕm″ē-păr′ē-sĭs, hĕm-ē-păr-ē′sĭs) [″ + *paresis,* paralysis]. Paralysis affecting only one side of the body.

hemiparesthesia (hĕm″ē-păr-ĕs-thē′zē-ă) [″ + *para,* beyond, + *aisthesis,* sensation]. Numbness of one side of the body.

hemipelvectomy (hĕm″ē-pĕl″vĕk′tō-mē) [″ + L. *pelvis,* basin, + Gr. *ektome,* excision]. Surgical removal of one half of the pelvis, and the leg.

hemiplegia (hĕm-ē-plē′jē-ă) [″ + *plege,* a stroke]. Paralysis of only one half of the body. SEE: *Benedikt's syndrome; paralysis; thalamic syndrome.*

ETIOL: A brain lesion involving the upper motor neurons and resulting in paralysis of the opposite side of the body. May result from disturbed blood flow to a portion of the brain. This may be due to hemorrhage, cerebral thrombosis, embolism, or a tumor of the cerebrum.

F.A.: Elevate head and shoulders. See that tongue does not obstruct breathing. Avoid stimulants. Do not move patient until arrival of someone competent in emergency medical care.

NURSING IMPLICATIONS: Carefully assess the patient's neurological status. Intervene to prevent contracture formation through range of motion exercises at least once a day. Teach the patient to do quadriceps and gluteal setting exercises, and to maintain good body alignment. Frequent turning and good skin care should be done to prevent skin breakdown. Patient should cough and breathe deeply and change position every two hours to prevent hypostatic pneumonia. When able, the patient should be encouraged to assist with his or her own activities of daily living.

h., alternate. Hemiplegia affecting one side of the face and trunk and the extremities of the opposite side.

h., capsular. Hemiplegia resulting from a lesion of the internal capsule of the brain.

h., cerebral. Hemiplegia caused by brain lesion.

h., crossed. H., alternate.

h., facial. Paralysis of muscles of one side of the face.

h., spastic. Hemiplegia accompanied by spasms, usually occurring in infants.

h., spinal. Hemiplegia resulting from a lesion of the spinal cord. SEE: *Brown-Séquard's paralysis.*

hemiplegic (hĕm-ē-plē'jĭk). Pert. to hemiplegia.

Hemiptera (hĕm-ĭp'tĕr-ă) [Gr. *hemi-,* half, + *pteron,* wing]. The true bugs; an order of insects characterized by piercing and sucking mouth parts. The first pair of wings is leathery at the base and membranous at the tip; the second pair of wings is membranous. There is incomplete metamorphosis. Includes bedbugs, kissing bugs, and several other species that are pests or transmitters of pathogenic organisms.

hemipyocyanin (hĕm"ē-pī"ō-sī'ă-nĭn). Antibacterial pigment produced by Pseudomonas pyocyanea.

hemirachischisis (hĕm"ē-ră-kĭs'kĭ-sĭs) [" + *rhachis,* spine, + *schisis,* cleft]. Rachischisis in which protrusion of the spinal meninges does not occur. SYN: *spina bifida occulta.*

hemisacralization (hĕm"ē-sā"krăl-ī-zā'shŭn). Abnormal development of one half of the fifth lumbar vertebra so that it is fused with the sacrum.

hemisection (hĕm"ē-sĕk'shŭn) [" + L. *sectio,* a cutting]. In surgery or anatomy, cutting an organ or tissue in half. SYN: *bisection.*

hemisomus (hĕm"ē-sō'mŭs) [" + *soma,* body]. Fetus with lateral half of body missing or malformed.

hemispasm (hĕm'ē-spăzm) [" + *spasmos,* spasm]. Spasm of only one side of the body or face.

hemisphere (hĕm'ĭ-sfēr) [" + *sphaira,* sphere]. Either half of the cerebrum or cerebellum.

h., dominant. The cerebral hemisphere in which the higher cortical functions, esp. those rel. to speech and certain motor activities, are associated; the left one in right-handed individuals. Results in phenomenon known as cerebral dominance.

Hemispora stellata (hĕm-ĭs'pō-ră stĕl-ă'tă). A variety of fungus that causes mycosis.

hemisporosis (hĕm"ē-spō-rō'sĭs) [" + *sporos,* seed, + *osis,* condition]. Infection with a fungus, Hemispora stellata, resulting in swellings of bone and other tissue of a gummatous nature. May later ulcerate.

hemistrumectomy (hĕm"ē-stroo-mĕk'tō-mē) [" + L. *struma,* goiter, + Gr. *ektome,* excision]. Excision of approx. half of a goiter.

hemisyndrome (hĕm"ē-sĭn'drōm) [" + *syndrome,* a running with]. Syndrome indicating a unilateral lesion of the spinal cord.

hemiterata (hĕm"ē-tĕr'ă-tă) [" + *teras,* monster]. Individuals possessing congenital malformations but not to such a degree as to cause severe disability or disfigurement.

hemiteric, hemiteratic (hĕm-ē-tĕr'ĭk, -tĕr-ăt'ĭk). Congenitally deformed, but not severely so.

hemithermoanesthesia (hĕm"ē-thĕr"mō-ăn"ĕs-thē'zē-ă) [Gr. *hemi-,* half, + *therme,* heat, + *an-,* not, + *aisthesis,* sensation]. Unilateral loss of sensitivity to heat and cold.

hemithorax (hĕm"ē-thō'răks) [" + *thorax,* chest]. One half the chest.

hemithyroidectomy (hĕm"ē-thī"royd-ĕk'tō-mē) [" + *thyreos,* shield, + *eidos,* form, + *ektome,* excision]. Surgical removal of one lobe of the thyroid.

hemitomias (hĕm"ĭ-tō'mē-ăs) [Gr. *hemitomias,* half a eunuch]. A person with one testicle.

hemitremor (hĕm"ē-trĕm'or). Tremor present in one lateral half of the body.

hemivertebra (hĕm"ē-vĕr'tē-bră). Congenital absence of half of a vertebra.

hemizygosity (hĕm"ē-zī-gŏs'ĭ-tē) [" + *zygotos,* yoked]. Possessing only one of the gene pair that determines a particular genetic trait.

hemlock [AS. *hemleac*]. 1. A species of evergreen plant. 2. Volatile oil extracted from dried, unripe fruit of Conium maculatum, poison hemlock.

hemlock poisoning. SYM: Weakness, drowsiness, nausea, vomiting, difficult breathing, paralysis, and death.

TREATMENT: Empty stomach by means of a stomach pump or an emetic. Give cathartic. Treat respiratory failure with artificial respiration and oxygen.

hemo-. Prefix meaning blood. SEE: words beginning with *haemo-*, *haem-*, *hem-*, *hema-*, and *hemato-*.

hemoagglutination (hē″mō-ă-gloo″tĭ-nā′shŭn) [Gr. *haima*, blood, + L. *agglutinans*, gluing]. The clumping of red blood corpuscles.

hemoagglutinin (hē″mō-ă-gloo′tĭ-nĭn). An agglutinin that clumps the red blood corpuscles.

hemobilia (hē″mō-bĭl′ē-ă). Blood in the bile or bile ducts.

hemobilinuria (hē″mō-bĭl-ĭn-ū′rē-ă) [″ + L. *bilis*, bile, + Gr. *ouron*, urine]. Urobilin in the blood and urine.

hemoblast (hē′mō-blăst) [″ + *blastos*, germ]. The large bone marrow cell that produces red and white blood cells and platelets. SYN: *hemocytoblast*.

hemochorial (hē″mō-kor′ē-ăl) [″ + *chorion*, envelope]. Pert. to the relationship between the blood of the mother and the chorionic ectoderm. SEE: *placenta*.

hemochromatosis (hē″mō-krō″mă-tō′sĭs) [″ + *chroma*, color, + *osis*, condition]. A disease of iron metabolism in which iron accumulates in body tissues. The liver becomes enlarged; the skin is pigmented so that it has a bronze hue; and there are diabetes and frequently cardiac failure. It is a rare disease seen ten times as frequently in males as females. The majority of cases develop after the fourth decade. SYN: *diabetes, bronze*.

hemochrome (hē′mō-krōm). Hemoglobin.

hemochromogen (hē″mō-krō′mō-jĕn) [″ + *chroma*, color, + *gennan*, to produce]. General term applied to compounds of heme with nitrogen-containing substances such as a protein.

hemochromometer (hē″mō-krō-mŏm′ĕ-tĕr) [″ + ″ + *metron*, measure]. A colorimeter used for estimating the amount of hemoglobin in the blood.

hemochromoprotein (hē″mō-krō″mō-prō′tē-ĭn). Any protein combined with the blood pigment, hemochrome.

hemoclasia (hē″mō-klā′sē-ă) [″ + *klasis*, a breaking]. Hemolytic crisis.

hemoclasis (hē-mŏk′lă-sĭs). Disintegration of red blood cells. SYN: *hemolysis*.

hemoclastic (hē″mō-klăs′tĭk). Destructive of erythrocytes. SYN: *hemolytic*.

hemoconcentration. A relative increase in the number of red blood cells resulting from a decrease in the volume of plasma. SYN: *anhydremia*.

hemoconia (hē″mō-kō′nē-ă) [Gr. *haima*, blood, + *konis*, dust]. Minute colorless bodies in blood thought to be the products of disintegration of red blood cells. SYN: *blood dust; hemokonia*.

hemoconiosis (hē″mō-kō″nē-ō′sĭs) [″ + ″ + *osis*, condition]. Having an abnormal amt. of hemoconia in the blood. SYN: *hemokoniosis*.

hemocryoscopy (hē″mō-krī-ŏs′kō-pē) [″ + *kryos*, cold, + *skopein*, to view]. Determination of the freezing point of the blood.

hemocrystallin (hē″mō-krĭs′tăl-lĭn). Hemoglobin.

hemocuprein (hē″mō-kū′prē-ĭn). A blue copper-containing compound present in red blood cells.

hemocyanin (hē″mō-sī′ă-nĭn) [″ + *kyanos*, blue]. An oxygen-carrying blue pigment in the plasma of arthropods and molluscs.

hemocyte (hē′mō-sīt) [″ + *kytos*, cell]. 1. Any blood cell. 2. Red blood cell.

hemocytoblast (hē″mō-sī′tō-blăst) [″ + ″ + *blastos*, germ]. The primitive reticuloendothelial stem cell found in bone marrow from which all cells normally present in blood are thought to arise.

hemocytoblastoma (hē″mō-sī″tō-blăs-tō′mă) [″ + ″ + ″ + *oma*, tumor]. A tumor containing embryonic blood cells.

hemocytogenesis (hē″mō-sī″tō-jĕn′ĕ-sĭs) [″ + *kytos*, cell, + *genesis*, development]. The formation of blood cells. SYN: *hematopoiesis*.

hemocytology (hē″mō-sī-tŏl′ō-jē) [″ + ″ + *logos*, study]. Study of structure and function of blood cells.

hemocytolysis (hē″mō-sī-tŏl′ĭ-sĭs) [″ + ″ + *lysis*, dissolution]. Dissolution of the blood corpuscles. SYN: *hematocytolysis; hemolysis*.

hemocytometer (hē″mō-sī-tŏm′ĕ-tĕr) [″ + ″ + *metron*, measure]. Device for determining number of cells in a stated volume of blood.

hemocytopoiesis (hē″mō-sī″tō-poy-ē′sĭs) [″ + *kytos*, cell, + *poiesis*, formation]. The development of blood cells.

hemocytotripsis (hē″mō-sī″tō-trĭp′sĭs) [″ + ″ + *tribein*, to rub]. Destruction of red blood cells due to extreme pressure.

hemocytozoon (hē″mō-sī″tō-zō′ŏn) [″ + ″ + *zoon*, animal]. A protozoan parasite of the blood cells. SYN: *hematobium*.

hemodiagnosis (hē″mō-dī″ăg-nō′sĭs) [″ + *dia*, through, + *gnosis*, knowledge]. Examination of the blood for diagnostic purpose.

hemodialysis (hē″mō-, hĕm″ō-dī-ăl′ĭ-sĭs) [″ + ″ + *lysis*, dissolve]. Removal of chemical substances from the blood by passing it through tubes made of semipermeable membranes. The tubes are continually bathed by solutions that selectively remove unwanted material. Used to cleanse the blood of patients in whom one or both kidneys are defective or absent; and to remove excess accumulation of drugs or toxic chemicals in the blood.

hemodialyzer (hē″mō-dī′ă-līz″ĕr). Device used in performing hemodialysis.

hemodiastase (hē″mō-dī′ăs-tās) [″ + *dias-*

tasis, separation]. An amylolytic enzyme in the blood.

hemodilution (hē″mō-dī-lū′shŭn). An increase in the volume of blood plasma resulting in reduced relative concentration of red blood cells.

hemodynamics (hē″mō-dī-năm′ĭks) [Gr. *haima,* blood, + *dynamis,* power]. A study of the forces involved in circulating blood through the body.

hemodynamometer (hē″mō-dī″nă-mŏm′ĕ-ter) [″ + ″ + *metron,* measure]. Device for measuring blood pressure.

hemoendothelial (hē″mō-ĕn-dō-thē′lē-ăl). Pert. to the relationship between blood of the mother and the endothelium of chorionic vessels. SEE: *placenta.*

Hemofil. Trade name for antihemophilic factor (AHF), USP.

hemoflagellate (hē″mō-flăj′ĕ-lāt″) [″ + L. *flagellum,* whip]. Any flagellate protozoan of the blood. The most important genera are Trypanosoma and Leishmania.

hemofuscin (hē″mō-fū′sĭn) [″ + L. *fuscus,* brown]. Brown pigment derived from hemoglobin. In urine, it produces a reddish color.

hemogenesis (hē″mō-jĕn′ĕ-sĭs) [″ + *genesis,* formation]. Blood formation. SYN: *hemopoiesis.*

hemogenic (hē″mō-jĕn′ĭk) [″ + *gennan,* to produce]. Rel. to the production of blood.

hemoglobin (hē″mō-, hĕm″ō-glō′bĭn) [″ + L. *globus,* globe]. The iron-containing pigment of the red blood cells. Its function is to carry oxygen from the lungs to the tissues. The amount of hemoglobin in the blood averages 12–16 gm./100 ml. of blood in adult females; 14–18 in males; and somewhat less in children. One gm. of hemoglobin can combine with 1.36 cc. of oxygen, the resulting compound being oxyhemoglobin. Hemoglobin is a crystallizable, conjugated protein consisting of an iron-containing pigment called heme and a simple protein, globin. In the lungs it combines readily, by a process called oxygenation, with oxygen to form a loose, unstable compound called oxyhemoglobin. In the tissues where oxygen tension is low and carbon dioxide tension is high, oxyhemoglobin liberates its oxygen in exchange for carbon dioxide. A chemical important in these exchanges is 2,3-diphosphoglycerate, q.v. Hemoglobin liberated from disintegrating red blood cells is removed from circulation by the cells of the reticuloendothelial system, esp. those of the liver and spleen. The globin is converted to amino acids and reutilized. Iron from the iron-containing portion is stored in the liver and spleen and reutilized; the non-iron-containing pigment is converted to bilirubin, which is excreted as one of the bile pigments.

Hemoglobin combines with carbon monoxide to form the stable compound carboxyhemoglobin, which is unable to liberate oxygen for use by tissues. Oxidation of the ferrous iron of hemoglobin to the ferric state produces methemoglobin.

Many different types of hemoglobin have been discovered. Study of these has facilitated the investigation of human genetics. Hemoglobin is named according to the way the amino acid components of the globin move when studied by electrophoresis. There are more than a hundred different types of abnormal hemoglobin.

ABNORM: Abnormal forms of hemoglobin are due to mutations. Because of the size of the hemoglobin molecule, the number of possible mutant forms is enormous. Only a few of the diseases caused by these forms are described here:

Hemoglobin S: The first disease discovered to be due to a molecular abnormality of hemoglobin was sickle cell anemia. It is caused by the presence of an abnormal hemoglobin that under proper conditions alters its physical structure to cause red blood cells to assume a sickle shape. In sickle cell trait, the patient is asymptomatic because of being genetically heterozygous for hemoglobin S. In sickle cell disease, individuals are homozygous for hemoglobin S and are symptomatic. SEE: *sickle cell anemia.*

Hemoglobin C disease: This is a chronic hemolytic anemia with splenomegaly, arthralgias, and abdominal pain.

Hemoglobin E disease: This is a mild form of hemolytic anemia observed in those native to Southeast Asia.

Hemoglobin S-C disease: Present in persons who have inherited two abnormal forms of hemoglobin, S and C. Clinical symptoms may not appear until the fourth decade and even after appearing are not life threatening. Symptoms include hematuria and pain in bones, joints, abdomen, and chest.

Hemoglobin M disease: An abnormal hemoglobin associated with congenital cyanosis. The iron in the hemoglobin is present in the ferric (Fe^{+++}) state and is unable to combine with oxygen. This type of hemoglobin is called methemoglobin. There is no effective therapy; even so, the course of the disease is benign because of the presence of normal hemoglobin.

h. $\boldsymbol{A_{1c}}$. ABBR: HbA_{1c}. Hemoglobin A that contains a glucose group linked to the terminal amino acid of the beta chains of the molecule. In diabetes mellitus, when the blood glucose level is optimally and carefully regulated over a long period, five to six weeks, the HbA_{1c} level is normal. If the blood glucose level has not been controlled in the preceding five to six weeks, the HbA_{1c} blood level is increased. SYN: *glycosylated hemoglobin.*

h., fetal. Hemoglobin found in the erythrocytes of the fetus. It is capable of taking up and giving off oxygen at lower oxygen tensions than that in the erythrocytes of the adult.

h., glycosylated. Hemoglobin A_{1c}, q.v.

hemoglobinemia (hē″mō-glō-bĭn-ē′mē-ă) [Gr. *haima,* blood, + L. *globus,* globe, + Gr. *haima,* blood]. Presence of hemoglobin in the blood plasma.

hemoglobinocholia (hē″mō-glō″bĭn-ō-kō′lē-ă) [″ + ″ + Gr. *chole,* bile]. Hemoglobin in the bile.

hemoglobinolysis (hē″mō-glō-bĭn-ŏl′ĭ-sĭs) [″ + ″ + Gr. *lysis,* dissolution]. Dissolution of hemoglobin.

hemoglobinometer (hē″mō-glō-bĭn-ŏm′ĕ-ter) [″ + ″ + Gr. *metron,* measure]. Device for determining the amount of hemoglobin in the blood.

hemoglobinopathies (hē″mō-glō″bĭ-nŏp′ă-thēz). The group of diseases caused by or associated with the presence of one of several forms of abnormal hemoglobin in the blood. SEE: *hemoglobin.*

hemoglobinopepsia (hē″mō-glō″bĭn-ō-pĕp′sē-ă) [″ + L. *globus,* globe, + Gr. *pepsis,* digestion]. Destruction of hemoglobin. SYN: *hemoglobinolysis.*

hemoglobinophilic (hē″mō-glō-bĭn-ō-fĭl′ĭk) [″ + ″ + Gr. *philein,* to love]. Pert. to organisms that grow better in presence of hemoglobin.

hemoglobinous (hē″mō-glō′bĭ-nŭs). Pert. to or containing hemoglobin.

hemoglobinuria (hē″mō-glō-bĭn-ū′rē-ă) [″ + L. *globus,* globe, + Gr. *ouron,* urine]. The presence of hemoglobin in the urine, but free from red blood cells. Occurs when hemoglobin from disintegrating red blood cells or from rapid hemolysis of red cells exceeds the ability of the blood proteins to combine with the hemoglobin.

ETIOL: Hemolytic anemia; scurvy; purpura; certain chemicals such as arsenic, phosphorus; typhus fever; or septicemia.

h., cold. Hemoglobinuria following local or general exposure to cold. SYN: *h., paroxysmal.*

h., epidemic. Hemoglobinuria of the newborn characterized by jaundice, cyanosis, and fatty degeneration of heart and liver. SYN: *Winckel's disease.*

h., intermittent. Paroxysmal nocturnal hemoglobinuria.

h., malarial. Blackwater fever.

h., march. Hemoglobinuria that occurs following strenuous exercise.

h., paroxysmal. Intermittent, recurring attacks of hemoglobinuria following exposure to cold (cold hemoglobinuria) or strenuous exercise (march hemoglobinuria). Results from increased fragility of red blood cells or presence of a thermolabile autohemolysin.

h., toxic. Hemoglobinuria resulting from toxic substances such as muscarine or snake venom; toxic products of infectious diseases such as yellow fever, typhoid fever, syphilis, and certain forms of hemolytic jaundice; organisms such as Plasmodium malariae, which destroy red blood cells; foreign proteins in blood as may follow blood transfusion or serum therapy.

hemoglobinuric (hē″mō-glō′bĭ-nū′rĭk). Rel. to or marked by hemoglobinuria.

hemogram [Gr. *haima,* blood, + *gramma,* a writing]. A graph of the differential blood count. SEE: *Schilling's classification.*

hemoid (hē′moyd) [″ + *eidos,* resemblance]. Having the appearance of blood. SYN: *hematoid.*

hemokinesis (hē″mō-kī-nē′sĭs) [″ + *kinesis,* movement]. Blood flow in the body.

hemokonia (hē-mō-kō′nē-ă) [″ + *konis,* dust]. (pl. *hemokoniae*) Minute, highly refractive body in the blood, said to be a disintegrated particle of blood cell. SYN: *blood dust; hemoconia.*

hemokoniosis (hē″mō-kō-nē-ō′sĭs) [″ + ″ + *osis,* condition]. Abnormal amount of hemokoniae in the blood. SYN: *hemoconiosis.*

hemolith (hē′mō-lĭth) [″ + *lithos,* stone]. A calculus in the wall of a blood vessel.

hemolymph (hē′mō-lĭmf″) [″ + L. *lympha,* lymph]. Blood and lymph.

hemolymphangioma (hē″mō-lĭm-făn″jē-ō′mă). Hematolymphangioma, q.v.

hemolysate (hē-mŏl′ĭ-sāt). The product of hemolysis.

hemolysin (hē-mŏl′ĭ-sĭn) [″ + *lysis,* dissolution]. An agent or condition that disrupts red blood cells.

hemolysis (hē-mŏl′ĭ-sĭs) [″ + *lysis,* dissolution]. The destruction of red blood cells with the liberation of hemoglobin, which diffuses into the fluid surrounding them. May occur as a result of the effects of bacterial toxins, snake venoms, immune bodies (hemolysins), and hypotonic saline solutions. Their stroma is ruptured or dissolved and the hemoglobin is liberated into the plasma. As a result, the blood, examined grossly, appears to be more transparent and to have a richer, red color; under the microscope, the dissolution of the red corpuscles can be observed.

When hemolysis occurs within the blood vessels, the body is unable to retain the hemoglobin, which is lost through the kidneys and imparts a red color to the urine, a condition called hemoglobinuria, q.v.

Injection of a hypotonic saline solution or distilled water into the bloodstream induces hemolysis and may result in death. The red blood cells swell and become globular; their membranes rupture and hemoglobin is liberated. All solutions injected intravenously must be isotonic with the blood. Hemolysis may result from infection by certain disease organisms, e.g., certain streptococci, staphylococci and the tetanus bacillus. Hemolysis also occurs in smallpox and diphtheria and following severe burns. SYN: *hematocytolysis; hematolysis*. SEE: *fragility test*.

hemolytic (hē″mō-lĭt′ĭk). Pert. to the breaking down of red blood cells.

hemolytic anemia. Anemia resulting from hemolysis of red blood cells. Is either acquired as from the effects of toxic agents, or congenital (familial).

hemolytic disease of the newborn. Disease of the newborn characterized by anemia, jaundice, enlargement of the liver and spleen, and generalized edema (hydrops fetalis).

ETIOL: Due to transplacental transmission of maternal antibody, usually evoked by maternal and fetal blood group incompatibility. Incompatibilities of the ABO system are common but are not severe. Rh incompatibility can result in profound anemia in the fetus, causing death in utero.

Rh incompatibility develops when a Rh-negative woman carries an Rh-positive fetus. Fetal red blood cells cross the placenta and enter the maternal circulation, stimulating maternal antibody production against the Rh factor. These antibodies cross the placenta to the fetal circulation and destroy fetal red blood cells.

TREATMENT: In cases of Rh incompatibility, the condition can be controlled during pregnancy by following the anti-Rh titer of the mother's blood and the bilirubin level of the fetus by amniocentesis. These indices indicate whether the pregnancy should be allowed to go to full term or if labor should be induced earlier. The use of Rh_o(D) immune globulin (trade name: RhoGam) has been of great benefit in treating this condition. SEE: *Rh blood group*.

hemolytic jaundice. SEE: *jaundice, hemolytic*.

hemolytopoietic (hē-mŏl″ĭ-tō-poy-ĕt′ĭk) [Gr. *haima,* blood, + *lysis,* dissolution, + *poiein,* to form]. Rel. to processes of production and destruction of blood cells.

hemolyze (hē′mō-līz). To produce hemolysis.

hemomediastinum (hē″mō-mē″dē-ă-stī′nŭm) [″ + L. *mediastinus,* in the middle]. Effusion of blood into mediastinal spaces. SYN: *hematomediastinum*.

hemometra (hē″mō-mē′tră) [″ + *metra,* uterus]. Retention of blood within the uterus. SYN: *hematometra*.

hemonephrosis (hē″mō-nĕ-frō′sĭs) [″ + *nephros,* kidney, + *osis,* condition]. Blood in the pelvis of the kidney. SYN: *hematonephrosis*.

hemopathic (hē″mō-păth′ĭk) [″ + *pathos,* disease]. Rel. or due to disease of the blood.

hemopathology (hē″mō-pă-thŏl′ō-jē) [″ + ″ + *logos,* study]. The science of blood disorders.

hemopathy (hē-mŏp′ă-thē). A disease of the blood.

hemopericardium (hē″mō-pĕr″ĭ-kăr′dē-ŭm) [″ + *peri,* around, + *kardia,* heart]. Accumulation of blood in the pericardial sac.

hemoperitoneum (hē″mō-pĕr″ĭ-tō-nē′ŭm) [″ + *peritonaion,* peritoneum]. Effusion of blood into the peritoneal cavity.

hemopexin (hē″mō-pĕks′ĭn) [″ + *pexis,* fixation]. A globulin of high carbohydrate content that is capable of combining with heme.

hemophage (hē′mō-fāj) [″ + *phagein,* to eat]. A cell destroying red blood cells by phagocytosis.

hemophagocyte (hē″mō-făg′ō-sīt) [″ + ″ + *kytos,* cell]. A phagocyte that ingests red blood cells.

hemophagocytosis (hē″mō-făg″ō-sī-tō′sĭs) [″ + ″ + ″ + *osis,* condition]. Ingestion of red blood cells by phagocytes.

hemophil (hē′mŏ-fĭl) [″ + *philein,* to love]. Bacteria that grow very well on agar that contains blood.

hemophilia (hē″mō-, hĕm″ō-fĭl′ē-ă) [″ + *philein,* to love]. An hereditary blood disease characterized by greatly prolonged coagulation time. The blood fails to clot and abnormal bleeding occurs. It is a sex-linked hereditary trait, being transmitted by normal heterozygous females who carry the recessive gene. It occurs almost exclusively in males. SEE: *blood*.

The term hemophilia has been used to designate a variety of coagulation disorders of blood. This has led to confusion that can be prevented by using the word hemophilia to mean what it originally meant and to designate conditions resembling it by the name of the specific coagulation factor which is lacking.

ETIOL: The cause of true hemophilia is deficiency of a factor in plasma necessary for coagulation of blood. This factor is called by several names including factor VIII, antihemophilic globulin, and antihemophilic factor.

SYM: Abnormal tendency to bleed. May cause swelling of the joints.

PROG: The development of concentrated clotting factors VIII and IX has improved the prognosis.

NURSING IMPLICATIONS: Provide emergency care to clean the wound and stop the bleeding through application of pressure. Safety is a major concern for the patient with hemophilia, and nursing care should be done gently and carefully. Because hemarthrosis is a common complication, assess the patient for development of this condition and provide care as needed. This will include elevating the affected part, applying ice, and immobilizing the joint in a slightly flexed position. Exercise is generally not begun until at least 48 hours after a bleeding episode has subsided.

The patient and family will be anxious. In order to allay this fear, help them identify activities in which the patient may safely participate. They should also be taught ways to manage attacks of bleeding at home. It is possible for the family to administer cryoprecipitate at home to treat a bleeding episode.

TREATMENT: There is no cure for hemophilia. In an emergency, frozen factor VIII that is thawed, or lyophilized factor VIII can be administered I.V. to stop bleeding. Many hemophiliacs can self-administer lyophilized factor VIII in their homes to control bleeding episodes. Hemophiliacs should avoid trauma. In case of an accident, the individual with hemophilia should carry a card or wear a bracelet that indicates the person is a hemophiliac. Excellent pamphlets concerning home care of the hemophiliac child are available from the National Hemophilia Foundation, 25 West 39th Street, New York, N.Y. 10018.

h., vascular. SEE: *von Willebrand's disease.*

hemophilia A. Hemophilia due to a deficiency of blood coagulation factor VIII.

hemophilia B. This term refers to Christmas disease, which is a hemophilia-like disease caused by a lack of factor IX, plasma thromboplastin component. This condition can be treated with a lyophilized product that contains concentrated factor IX.

hemophiliac (hē″mō-fĭl′ē-ăk). One afflicted with hemophilia.

hemophilic (hē″mō-fĭl′ĭk). 1. Fond of blood, said of bacteria that grow well in culture media containing hemoglobin. 2. Pert. to hemophilia or hemophiliacs.

Hemophilus (hē-mŏf′ĭl-ŭs) [″ + *philein,* to love]. A genus of bacteria that require either the growth factor X or V, or both, provided by blood. The small, nonmotile, gram-negative bacilli are aerobic and do not form spores. The V factor is destroyed by enzymes present in unheated red blood cells. Thus chocolate agar is the preferred culture medium.

H. aegyptius. Koch-Weeks bacillus; the cause of one form of conjunctivitis.

H. ducreyi. The causative organism of chancroid or soft chancre.

H. influenzae. An organism found in respiratory infections and formerly thought to be the cause of influenza but now considered to be a primary and a secondary invader. It is the causative organism of influenzal meningitis, conjunctivitis, septicemia, and respiratory infections. SYN: *Pfeiffer's bacillus.*

H. pertussis. Former name for Bordetella pertussis, the causative organism of whooping cough.

H. vaginalis. Bacteria that cause vaginitis in otherwise healthy women. This organism is now called Gardnerella vaginalis.

hemophobia (hē″mō-fō′bē-ă) [Gr. *haima,* blood, + *phobos,* fear]. Aversion to seeing blood or to bleeding.

hemophoric (hē″mō-for′ĭk) [″ + *phoros,* bearing]. Conveying blood.

hemophthalmia, hemophthalmus (hē″mŏf-thăl′mē-ă, hē″mŏf-thăl′mŭs) [″ + *ophthalmos,* eye]. Effusion of blood into the eye.

hemopleura (hē″mō-ploo′ră) Blood in the pleural space. SEE: *hemothorax.*

hemopneumopericardium (hē″mō-nū″mō-pĕr″ĭ-kăr′dē-ŭm) [″ + *pneuma,* air, + *peri,* around, + *kardia,* heart]. Blood and air in the pericardial cavity.

hemopneumothorax (hē″mō-nū-mō-thō′răks) [″ + ″ + *thorax,* chest]. Blood and air in the pleural cavity.

hemopoiesis (hē″mō-poy-ē′sĭs) [″ + *poiesis,* formation]. Formation of blood cells. SYN: *hematopoiesis.*

hemoprecipitin (hē″mō-prē-sĭp′ĭ-tĭn). A precipitin in blood.

hemoprotein (hē″mō-prō′tē-ĭn). Any protein combined with the heme, blood pigment.

hemopsonin (hē″mŏp-sō′nĭn) [″ + *opsonein,* to provide]. An antibody that makes red blood cells more susceptible to phagocytosis.

hemoptysis (hē-mŏp′tĭ-sĭs) [″ + *ptyein,* to spit]. Expectoration of blood arising from the oral cavity, larynx, trachea, bronchi, or lungs. SEE: table; *bleeding; hematemesis; hemorrhage.*

SYM: Sudden attack of coughing with production of sputum containing frothy bright red blood and having a salty taste.

TREATMENT: Cold applications over the chest.

NURSING IMPLICATIONS: Keep the patient quiet and in a calm, reassuring environment. Take vital signs every 4 hours. Provide tepid fluids. Patient should be kept warm, but not hot. If you know which side the patient is bleeding from, lean the patient toward that side. Note the amount, consistency, and color of blood to assist in determining the site of bleeding. (Blood from lungs is red and frothy; blood from GI tract is dark red to black in color.) Save blood for inspection by physician.

h., endemic. Paragonimiasis.

Comparison of Hemoptysis and Hematemesis

Hemoptysis	Hematemesis
Probable previous history of tuberculosis.	Probable previous history of gastric or duodenal trouble.
Blood is coughed up.	Blood is vomited.
Blood is frothy, bright red, and alkaline in reaction.	Blood is usually (not always) dark, usually not frothy, and acid in reaction. Often clotted.
Blood may be mixed with sputum.	Blood may be mixed with food.
There is some dyspnea, pain, and a tickling sensation in the chest.	There is often nausea and pain referred to stomach.

h., parasitic. Spitting of blood resulting from infection of the lungs by Paragonimus westermani, q.v., a parasitic fluke.

hemorrhage (hĕm'ĕ-rĭj) [" + *rhegnynai*, to burst forth]. Abnormal internal or external discharge of blood. May be venous, arterial, or capillary from blood vessels into tissues, into or from the body. Venous blood is dark red; flow is continuous. Arterial blood is bright red; flows in spurts. Capillary blood is of a reddish color; exudes from tissue.

SYM: Diagnosis is obvious when hemorrhage is visible. When internal, diagnosis may be made from the general condition. Patient is in shock; pulse weak, rapid, and irregular; face pale; skin cold and moist.

NURSING IMPLICATIONS: Clean the wound and apply a sterile dressing. Hemorrhage may be decreased or stopped by elevating the body part above heart level (if possible) and by applying firm pressure over the area. A tourniquet should be applied only if bleeding can't be stopped by other methods. Extreme care must be taken to ensure that tourniquets are *never* left in place for more than 20 minutes.

h., accidental. In obstetrics and gynecology, a hemorrhage caused by premature rupture of the placenta. SEE: *ablatio placentae.*

h., antepartum. Hemorrhage appearing before the onset of labor.

h., arterial. In arterial bleeding, which is bright red, the blood ordinarily comes through in waves or spurts. However, the flow may be steady if the torn artery is deep or buried.

F.A.: It is usually necessary to make pressure along the course of the artery somewhere between the heart and bleeding point by means of fingers (digital pressure) on the pressure points and then pressure by a tourniquet above the point of injury. Tourniquet should be used only if absolutely required after other means fail to stop the bleeding. When used, apply only the pressure required to stop the bleeding. Improperly applied, a tourniquet may cause permanent damage to nerves. Elevate the part. Apply a sterile dressing and a firm bandage. Gradually release tourniquet after 12 to 15 minutes; if bleeding begins again, retighten. Do not give stimulants until bleeding is controlled. SEE: *bleeding* for table; *tourniquet.*

h., capillary. Bleeding from minute blood vessels, present in all bleeding. When large vessels are not injured, capillary bleeding may be controlled by simple elevation and pressure with a sterile dry compress.

h., carotid artery. Usually accompanied by bleeding from the jugular veins. May be fatal in a short time.

F.A.: Compression with the thumbs transversely across the neck, both above and below the wound, the fingers directed around the back of the neck to aid in compression. It may be more desirable to pack the wound with sterile gauze and compress it with the closed fist. Wounds of the jugular vein are sometimes the cause of air embolism.

h., cerebral. Escape of blood into tissues of the brain. SEE: *stroke.*

ETIOL: Hypertension, arteriosclerosis or atherosclerosis, infections.

SYM: Unconsciousness, slow pulse, stertorous breathing; hemiplegia, death. May be speech disturbance, incontinence of bladder and rectum, or constipation according to area of brain damage.

TREATMENT: Supportive therapy to maintain airway and oxygenation. Be certain patient is positioned properly to prevent nerve compression of arms. Maintain hydration and fluid and electrolyte balance.

h., concealed. Hemorrhage into an area where it is not visible. SYN: *h., internal.*

h., consecutive. Hemorrhage that occurs some time after an injury or 20 to 24 hours after an operation.

TREATMENT: Compress should be applied to main artery and wound. Elevate parts. Reopen and tie bleeding vessels.

h., contact. Hemorrhage from the cervix uteri coming on as a result of exertion or contact during coitus, douching, or instrumentation.

h., fibrinolytic. Hemorrhage due to a defect in the fibrin component in blood coagulation.

h., internal. H., concealed, q.v.

h., intracranial. Bleeding into the cranium.

h., lung. Blood bright red and frothy, frequently coughed up.

TREATMENT: Rest in cool bed, shoulders and head raised. Small pieces of ice to swallow. SEE: *hemoptysis.*

h. of knee. At the knee or below, apply pad with pressure. If behind knee, apply pad at site and bandage leg firmly. Follow same precautions as with tourniquet with respect to loosening at 12- to 15-minute intervals.

h., pancreas. Hemorrhage of dark blood in vomitus with slimy mucus, coming from pancreas, usually occurring in inflammation of pancreas. SEE: *pancreatitis, hemorrhagic.*

h., petechial. Hemorrhage in form of small rounded spots or petechiae occurring in the skin or mucous membranes.

h., postmenopausal. Bleeding from the vagina after the menopause has been established. This may be a sign of malignancy of the reproductive tract and should be carefully and thoroughly investigated.

h., postpartum. Abnormal bleeding from the uterus following childbirth.

h., primary. Hemorrhage immediately following any trauma.

h., secondary. Hemorrhage occurring some time after primary hemorrhage. It may occur after 24 hrs. or at time of separation of ligature, usually between 7th and 10th day. Usually due to sepsis.

h., stomach. Blood dark, perhaps clotted or mixed with stomach contents, usually vomited. May be from rupture of esophageal varices.

TREATMENT: Ice to swallow. Surgery may be required if bleeding continues. If hemorrhage from esophagus, compression of bleeding site with a special intraesophageal tube balloon may be helpful.

h., thigh. Upper part near groin. Insert pad of gauze into wound and apply pressure or press thumb in center of fold of groin against bone until bleeding stops below groin. Pad or tourniquet with pad under.

h., typhoid. Gross hemorrhage occurs in approx. 10% of cases of typhoid that progress to the stage of ulceration of gastrointestinal tract. Loss may be 1000 ml. It may occur singly or in succession, the latter being more serious than large hemorrhages. Hemorrhages take place at the end of the second week and during the third week of the disease.

h., unavoidable. Ceaseless, painless bleeding from placenta previa, q.v.

h., uterine. Hemorrhage into the cavity of the uterus. There are three types of uterine hemorrhage: essential uterine hemorrhage (metropathia haemorrhagica) occurs in connection with pelvic, uterine, or cervical diseases; intrapartum hemorrhage occurs during labor; and postpartum hemorrhage occurs after third stage of labor. The latter may be caused by rupture, lacerations, relaxation of the uterus, hematoma, or retained products of conception including the placenta or membrane fragments.

ETIOL: Common causes are trauma; congenital abnormalities; pathological processes such as tumors; infections, esp. of alimentary, respiratory, and genitourinary tracts; generalized vascular disorders such as various purpuras; coagulation defects; retained products of conception following criminal or therapeutic abortion.

TREATMENT: Application of an umbrella pack will apply pressure to uterine arterial supply. A retained placenta, when present and causing hemorrhage, should be removed with uterine forceps. If the uterus is flaccid, it can usually be stimulated to contract by administering oxytocin I.V. The patient may need transfusion and, in some cases, surgery will be required to prevent fatal hemorrhage. SEE: *pack, umbrella.*

h., venous. Characterized by steady, profuse bleeding of rather dark blood.

F.A.: Keep patient quiet and try to relieve anxiety; elevate the bleeding part if possible. Apply a sterile dressing and make pressure directly over the wound. Elevation and pressure will control most venous bleeding. Observe closely for signs of shock. SEE: *tourniquet.*

h., vicarious. Hemorrhage from a part due to suppression in another part. SEE: *vicarious menstruation.*

hemorrhage, words pert. to: anthemorrhagic; autotransfusion; bleeding; clotting; coagulation; hematorrhea; hemophilia; rhinorrhagia; Werlhof's disease; wound.

hemorrhagenic (hĕm″ō-ră-jĕn′ĭk) [″ + *rhegnynai,* to burst forth, + *gennan,* to form]. Producing hemorrhage.

hemorrhagic (hĕm-ō-răj′ĭk). Pert. to or marked by hemorrhage.

hemorrhagic disease of the newborn. Hemorrhaging due to inadequate supply of prothrombin received from mother or delay in establishment of bacterial flora of intestine that produces vitamin K. Administration of vitamin K corrects the condition.

hemorrhagic fevers. A group of diseases due to arthropod-borne viruses. This includes yellow fever, Omsk hemorrhagic fever, Crimean hemorrhagic fever, North and South Vietnam hemorrhagic fever, Argentinian hemorrhagic fever, Bolivian hemorrhagic fever, and Kyasanur Forest disease (India).

hemorrhagic nephrosonephritis. An acute infectious disease with abrupt onset of fever that lasts three to eight days, conjunctival injection, prostration, anorexia, and vomiting. Renal involvement may be mild or progress to acute renal failure, and this may last several weeks. The mode of transmission is unknown; the incubation period varies from 9 to 35 days; and it is apparently not transmitted from person to person. SYN: *epidemic hemorrhagic fever; Korean hemorrhagic fever.*

ETIOL: Hantan virus.

TREATMENT: Treat shock and renal failure. There is no specific therapy.

hemorrhagiparous (hĕm″ō-răj-ĭp′ă-rŭs) [″ + *rhegnynai,* to burst forth, + L. *parere,* to produce]. Producing hemorrhage. SYN: *hemorrhagenic.*

hemorrhoid (hĕm′ō-royd) [Gr. *haimorrhois*]. A mass of dilated, tortuous veins in the anorectum involving the venous plexuses of that area. There are two kinds: external, those involving veins distal to the anorectal line; internal, those involving veins proximal to the anorectal line.

TREATMENT: Depends upon the severity of the symptoms, not the extent of the hemorrhoids. In many instances, the only therapy required is improvement in anal hygiene and administration of stool softeners to prevent straining to have a bowel movement. The decision concerning the necessity of surgery or ligature with rubber bands should not be made until acute symptoms and inflammation have subsided. This allows tissues to regain their usual shape. SEE: *hemorrhoidectomy; piles.*

h., external. A dilated vein or veins at the junction of anal mucosa with the anal skin. SEE: illus.

h., internal. Dilated veins of the lower rectum at the anorectal junction. SEE: illus.

h., prolapsed. Protrusion of an internal hemorrhoid through the anus.

h., strangulated. Prolapsed hemorrhoid that is trapped by the anal sphincter, thus cutting off blood flow to the vein in the hemorrhoid.

hemorrhoidal (hĕm-ō-roy′dăl). 1. Rel. to hemorrhoids. 2. Pert. to certain anal arteries; arteria hemorrhoidalis.

hemorrhoidectomy (hĕm″ō-royd-ĕk′tō-mē) [Gr. *haimorrhois,* vein liable to bleed, + *ektome,* excision]. Removal of hemorrhoids by one of several techniques including surgery,

HEMORRHOIDS

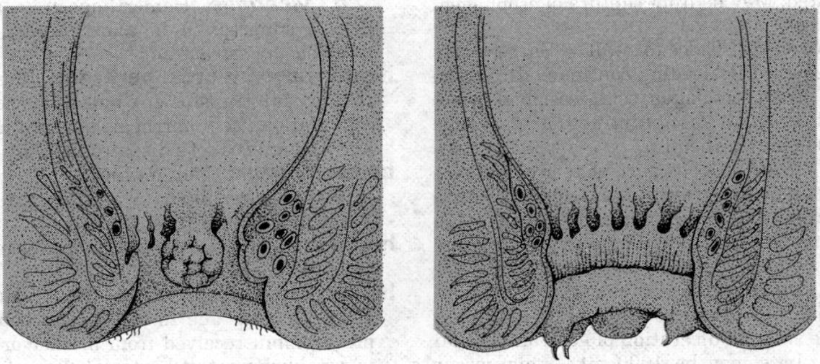

INTERNAL HEMORRHOIDS

EXTERNAL HEMORRHOIDS SHOWING SKIN TABS

cryotherapy, or ligation by use of rubber bands applied to the base of the hemorrhoid. The latter method is used mostly for external hemorrhoids.

NURSING IMPLICATIONS: *Pre-op:* Follow physician's orders for type of bowel preparation (enemas and stool softeners may be ordered, as well as a low-residue diet). Assess hemorrhoids for size, bleeding, or presence of drainage. Sitz baths should be done as ordered.

Post-op: Take vital signs every hour and check rectal area for bleeding every hour in the immediate post-op period. Keep the patient comfortable by gentle cleansing of the rectal area as often as needed, sitz baths done and ointments applied as ordered. Keep the rectal area clean and dry, and teach the patient proper perineal hygiene. Some physicians may order a rubber ring to make sitting more comfortable for the patient. Be sure that the patient uses this correctly and knows that the ring should be only partially inflated.

hemosalpinx (hē″mō-săl′pĭnks) [Gr. *haima*, blood, + *salpinx*, tube]. Blood accumulated in an oviduct. SYN: *hematosalpinx*.

hemosiderin (hē″mō-sĭd′ĕr-ĭn) [″ + *sideros*, iron]. An iron-containing pigment derived from hemoglobin from disintegration of red blood cells. It is one method whereby iron is stored until it is needed for making hemoglobin.

hemosiderosis (hē″mō-sĭd-ĕr-ō′sĭs) [″ + ″ + *osis*, condition]. Condition characterized by the deposition, esp. in liver and spleen, of hemosiderin. Occurs in diseases in which there is marked red cell destruction such as hemolytic anemias, pernicious anemia, and chronic infection.

hemospasia (hē″mō-spā′zē-ă) [″ + *spaein*, to draw]. Withdrawal of blood by cupping or leeching.

hemospermia (hē″mō-spĕr′mē-ă) [″ + *sperma*, seed]. Bloody semen. SYN: *hematospermia*.

Hemosporidia (hē-mō-spor-ĭ′dē-ă) [″ + *sporos*, seed]. An order of parasites found in the blood of various animals, including man.

hemostasis, hemostasia (hē-mŏs′tă-sĭs, hē″mō-stā′zē-ă) [″ + *stasis*, stopping]. 1. Arrest of bleeding or of circulation. 2. Stagnation of blood.

hemostat (hē′mō-stăt) [″ + *statikos*, standing]. 1. Device or medicine that arrests the flow of blood. 2. Compressor for controlling hemorrhage of the tonsils.

hemostatic (hē″mō-stăt′ĭk). 1. Checking hemorrhage. 2. Any drug, medicine, or blood component that serves to stop bleeding, such as vasopressin, gamma-aminobutyric acid, vitamin K, whole blood, or epinephrine applied locally.

hemostyptic (hē-mō-stĭp′tĭk) [″ + *styptikos*, astringent]. An astringent that stops bleeding; chemically hemostatic.

hemotherapeutics (hē″mō-thĕr″ă-pū′tĭks) [″ + *therapeutike*, medical practice]. The use of blood, by transfusion, in treatment of disease.

hemotherapy (hē″mō-thĕr′ă pē) [″ + *therapeia*, treatment]. Blood transfusion as a therapeutic measure.

hemothorax (hē″mō-thō′răks) [″ + *thorax*, chest]. Bloody fluid in the pleural cavity caused by the rupture of small blood vessels, due to inflammation of the lungs in pneumonia and pulmonary tuberculosis or to a malignant growth.

hemothymia (hē″mō-thī′mē-ă) [″ + *thymos*, anger]. An irrestible impulse to murder.

hemotoxin (hē″mō-tŏks′ĭn) [″ + *toxikon*, poison]. A toxin destructive of red blood cells. SYN: *hemolysin*.

hemotrophe (hē′mō-trŏf) [″ + *trophe*, nourishment]. Nutrients supplied to the developing embryo by the mother.

hemotrophic (hē-mō-trŏf′ĭk) [″ + *trophe*, nourishment]. Pert. to nutrient substances carried in the blood.

hemotrophic nutrition. Nutrition of the fetus by substances in the maternal blood that pass to the blood of the fetus through vessels within the villi. SEE: *histotrophic nutrition*.

hemotropic (hē-mō-trŏp′ĭk) [″ + *tropos*, turning]. Attracted to or having an affinity for blood or blood cells.

hemotympanum (hē″mō-tĭm′pă-nŭm) [″ + *tympanon*, drum]. Blood in the middle ear.

hemozoin (hē″mō-zō′ĭn). A dark pigment found within malarial organisms (plasmodia). It is derived from the disintegration of hemoglobin.

hemozoon (hē″mō-zō′ŏn). A hematozoon.

Henderson-Hasselbalch equation. In fluid and electrolyte balance, this important equation may be expressed in terms of the bicarbonate (HCO_3^-) system as: pH is equal to 6.1 + log $HCO_3^-/\alpha(PaCO_2)$ where α is equal to 0.03 mM./L./mm. Hg at 38° C. At pH of 7.4, the ratio of HCO_3^- to $\alpha(PaCO_2)$ is 20 to 1.

Henle, Friedrich G. J. (hĕn′lē). German anatomist, 1809–1885.

H.'s ampulla. A ductus deferens dilatation just above the ejaculatory duct.

H.'s fissure. Fibrous tissue between the cardiac muscle fibers.

H.'s layer. Outer layer of cells of inner root sheath of hair follicle.

H.'s ligament. The conjoint tendon of the transversus abdominis muscle.

H.'s loop. A U-shaped portion of a renal tubule lying between the proximal and distal convoluted portions. Consists of a thin descending limb and a thicker ascending limb.

H.'s membrane. Bruch's layer forming inner boundary of the choroid of the eye.

H.'s sheath. Connective tissue support of individual nerve fibers in a funiculus. SYN: *endoneurium*.

H.'s tubules. The portion of the nephron following the proximal tubule. SEE: *nephron*.

Henoch-Schönlein purpura (hĕn'ōk-shān' lĭn). [Edouard H. Henoch, Ger. pediatrician, 1820–1910; Johann L. Schönlein, Ger. physician, 1793–1864] A form of allergic purpura with erythema, urticaria, effusions of serum into subcutaneous or submucous tissue or viscera, accompanied by gastrointestinal and joint symptoms. Syndrome is seen mostly in children.

henry (hĕn'rē). [Joseph Henry, U.S. physicist, 1797–1878] Unit designating electrical inductance.

Henry's law (hĕn'rēz). [William Henry, Brit. chemist, 1774–1836] The weight of a gas dissolved by a given volume of liquid at a constant temperature is directly proportional to the pressure.

Hensen's cells (hĕn'sĕns). [Victor Hensen, Ger. anatomist and physiologist, 1835–1924] Tall columnar cells that form the outer border cells of the organ of Corti of the cochlea.

Hensen's disk. Band in center of the A disk of a sarcomere of striated muscle. During contraction it appears lighter than the remaining portion and in its center, a dark stripe, the M stripe, is seen.

Hensen's stripe. A dark band on the undersurface of the tectorial membrane of the inner ear.

hepar (hē'păr) [Gr. *hepatos,* liver]. The liver.

heparin sodium (hĕp'ă-rĭn). USP. A polysaccharide that has been isolated from the liver, lung, and other tissues. It is produced by the mast cells of the liver and by basophil leukocytes. It inhibits coagulation by preventing conversion of prothrombin to thrombin by forming an antithrombin, and by preventing liberation of thromboplastin from blood platelets. The action of heparin requires the presence of a cofactor found in serum albumin of the plasma. Trade names are Heprinar, Lipo-Hepin, Panheprin, and Liquaemin sodium.

USES: An anticoagulant in prevention and treatment of thrombosis and embolism and in treating frostbite. Sometimes employed concurrently with dicumarol, q.v. The antagonist for an overdose is protamine sulfate.

heparinize (hĕp'ĕr-ĭ-nīz). To inhibit coagulation of blood with heparin.

heparin lock flush solution. A standard solution of heparin sodium, USP, labeled to indicate it is intended for maintenance of patency of intravenous injection devices only, and is not to be used for anticoagulant therapy.

hepatalgia (hĕp"ă-tăl'jē-ă) [Gr. *hepatos,* liver, + *algos,* pain]. Pain in the liver. SYN: *hepatodynia*.

hepatalgic (hĕp"ă-tăl'jĭk). Pert. to hepatalgia.

hepatatrophia (hĕp"ăt-ă-trō'fē-ă) [" + *atrophia,* atrophy]. Atrophied condition of the liver.

hepatauxe (hĕp"ăt-awk'sē) [" + *auxe,* increase]. Enlargement or hypertrophy of the liver.

hepatectomize (hĕp"ă-tĕk'tō-mīz) [" + *ektome,* excision]. Surgical removal of the liver.

hepatectomy (hĕp"ă-tĕk'tō-mē) [" + *ektome,* excision]. Excision of part or all of the liver.

hepatic (hĕ-păt'ĭk) [Gr. *hepatikos*]. Pert. to the liver.

hepatic amebiasis. Infection of the liver by Entamoeba histolytica resulting in hepatitis and abscess formation. Usually a sequel to amebic dysentery. SEE: *amebiasis*.

hepatic coma. Impaired central nervous system function due to liver disease. The disease permits venous blood to bypass portal circulation, thus allowing an accumulation of products in the blood that are usually metabolized by the liver (e.g., ammonia). Any condition that is associated with increased ammonia production promotes hepatic coma in patients with severely impaired liver function. Causes include high-protein diet, gastrointestinal bleeding, fluid and electrolyte imbalance, infections, and drugs such as sedatives, tranquilizers, anesthetics, analgesics, diuretics, and alcohol.

SYM: Impaired consciousness, sluggish or impaired speech, drowsiness, confusion, stupor, and coma. The patient will be unable to explain the meaning of simple sayings and may have difficulty in telling the day of the week or month. Attempts to draw simple figures will be unsuccessful. A "mousy" odor of the breath (fetor hepaticus) is usually present. A distinctive type of flapping tremor of the hand called *asterixis,* q.v., will be present in severe cases. Ataxia may be present along with altered deep tendon reflexes. An electroencephalogram will be abnormal as will the blood ammonia level.

TREATMENT: Eliminate protein intake and free the intestinal tract of blood if present by enemas or mild cathartics. High-carbohydrate diet. Oral neomycin will control bacteria that favor ammonia production, and oral lactulose helps to decrease ammonia production in the intestinal tract. Exchange transfusions to remove ammonia from the blood have been used.

hepatic duct. The canal that receives bile from the liver. It unites with the cystic duct to form the common bile duct.

hepatic flexure. The right bend of the colon

under the liver. The junction of the ascending and transverse colon.

hepatic lobes. Divisions of the liver.

hepaticoduodenostomy (hĕ-păt″ĭ-kō-dū″ō-dĕ-nŏs′tō-mē) [″ + L. *duodeni,* duodenum, + Gr. *stoma,* opening]. Making an artificial opening between the hepatic duct and duodenum.

hepaticoenterostomy (hĕ-păt″ĭ-kō-ĕn-tĕr-ŏs′tō-mē) [″ + *enteron,* intestine, + *stoma,* opening]. Operation for artificial opening between the hepatic duct and intestine.

hepaticogastrostomy (hĕ-păt″ĭ-kō-găs-trŏs′tō-mē) [″ + *gaster,* stomach, + *stoma,* opening]. The operation for a passage between the hepatic duct and the stomach.

hepaticojejunostomy (hĕ-păt′ĭ-kō-jē″jū-nŏs′tō-mē) [″ + L. *jejunum,* empty, + Gr. *stoma,* opening]. Surgically joining the hepatic duct and the jejunum.

hepaticolithotomy (hĕ-păt″ĭ-kō-lĭ-thŏt′ō-mē). Surgical removal of gallstones from the hepatic duct.

hepaticolithotripsy (hĕ-păt″ĭ-kō-lĭth′ō-trĭp-sē) [″ + *lithos,* stone, + *tripsis,* a crushing]. The crushing of a biliary calculus in the hepatic duct.

hepaticostomy (hĕ-păt″ĭ-kŏs′tō-mē) [″ + *stoma,* opening]. Establishment of a permanent fistula into the hepatic duct.

hepaticotomy (hĕ-păt″ĭ-kŏt′ō-mē) [″ + *tome,* incision]. Incision into the hepatic duct.

hepatic veins. The three vessels returning blood from the liver and discharging into the inferior vena cava.

hepatic zones. Venous, arterial, and portal regions.

hepatitis (hĕp″ă-tī′tĭs) [″ + *itis,* inflammation]. Inflammation of the liver. It is usually manifest by jaundice and, in some instances, liver enlargement. Fever and other systemic disorders are usually present.

h., acute anicteric. Hepatitis marked by slight fever, gastrointestinal upset, and anorexia, but no jaundice.

h., amebic. Enlargement and tenderness of the liver occurs frequently in association with amebiasis, q.v. This is most probably due to a nonspecific inflammation of the liver and not amebic liver infection.

h., cholangiolitic. Hepatitis characterized by fatigue, jaundice, pruritus, vomiting of bile, and hepatomegaly.

h., fulminant. Hepatitis marked by sudden onset of nausea and vomiting, chills, high fever, severe and early jaundice, convulsions, shock, deep coma, and death usually within 10 days.

h., infectious. Hepatitis occurring sporadically and in epidemics. Transmitted by oral or parenteral route. Incubation period is two to six weeks. Gastrointestinal and respiratory disturbances followed by sudden onset of jaundice, enlarged and tender liver, pruritus, muscle pain, splenomegaly, loss of weight.

h., non-A, non-B. Hepatitis caused by as yet unidentified agents. It is the most common post-transfusion hepatitis in the U.S.A. Clinically and epidemiologically, the disease resembles hepatitis B.

h., post-transfusion. Hepatitis following a blood transfusion. The most common cause in the U.S.A. is whatever agent causes non-A, non-B hepatitis.

h., serum. Hepatitis in which the virus is transmitted parenterally by blood transfusion, plasma, needles, or other parenteral instruments. Incubation period varies from six weeks to six months. Marked by sudden onset of headache, fever, chills, general weakness, nausea, vomiting, abdominal pain, prostration, jaundice, pruritus, enlarged and tender liver.

h., toxic. Hepatitis caused by exposure to certain poisons (as carbon tetrachloride) or drugs (as sulfonamides), the latter causing hypersensitivity in some patients.

h., viral. Generalized inflammation of the liver caused by one of several viral agents including two known as hepatitis A virus and hepatitis B virus.

hepatitis A. Hepatitis caused by hepatitis A virus (HAV). The virus usually enters by the oral route.

hepatitis-associated antigen. An antigen present in the sera of patients with viral hepatitis, but rarely present in patients with infectious hepatitis. This antigen is also found in normal populations in the tropics and southeast Asia. It was first isolated in the serum of an Australian aborigine. SYN: *Australia antigen.*

hepatitis B. Hepatitis caused by hepatitis B virus (HBV). The virus usually enters by the parenteral route.

In 1981 in the U.S.A. a vaccine for use in preventing hepatitis B was licensed.

hepatitis B immune globulin. Standard solution consisting of globulins derived from blood plasma of human donors who have high titers of antibodies against hepatitis B surface antigen. Trade name is Hyper Hep.

hepatitis B vaccine. A vaccine prepared directly from human blood. It is used to vaccinate persons who are at high risk of coming in contact with persons who are carriers of hepatitis B, or with blood or fluids from such individuals. Included in the high-risk group are blood bank and dialysis workers, dental hygienists, drug addicts, and some homosexuals.

hepatization (hĕp″ă-tĭ-zā′shŭn). The second and third stages in consolidation in lobar pneumonia. The surface of the lung has the appearance of liver tissue.

hepato- [Gr. *hepatikos*]. Prefix indicating the liver.

hepatoblastoma (hĕp″ă-tō-blăs-tō′mă) [″ + *blastos,* germ, + *oma,* tumor]. A malignant teratoma of the liver.

hepatocarcinogen. Anything that causes cancer of the liver.

hepatocarcinoma (hĕp″ă-tō-kăr″sĭn-ō′mă) [″ + *karkinos,* crab, + *oma,* tumor]. Carcinoma of the liver.

hepatocele (hĕp′ă-tō-sēl) [+ *kele,* hernia]. Hernia of the liver.

hepatocellular (hĕp″ă-tō-sĕl′ū-lăr). Concerning the cells of the liver.

hepatocholangiocystoduodenostomy (hĕp″ă-tō-kō-lăn″jē-ō-sĭs″tō-dū″ō-dĕ-nŏs′tō-mē) [″ + *chole,* bile, + *angeion,* vessel, + *kystis,* bladder, + L. *duodenum,* duodenum, + Gr. *stoma,* opening]. Establishment of drainage of bile ducts into the duodenum through the gallbladder.

hepatocholangioduodenostomy (hĕp″ă-tō-kō-lăn″jē-ō-dū-ō-dĕ-nŏs′tō-mē) [″ + ″ + ″ + L. *duodenum,* duodenum, + Gr. *stoma,* opening]. Establishment of drainage of bile ducts into the duodenum.

hepatocholangioenterostomy (hĕp″ă-tō-kō-lăn″jē-ō-ĕn″tĕr-ŏs′tō-mē) [″ + ″ + ″ + *enteron,* intestine, + *stoma,* opening]. Establishment of a passage between the liver and intestine.

hepatocholangiogastrostomy (hĕp″ă-tō-kō-lăn″jē-ō-găs-trŏs′tō-mē) [″ + ″ + ″ + *gaster,* belly, + *stoma,* opening]. Establishment of drainage of bile ducts into the stomach.

hepatocholangiostomy (hĕp″ă-tō-kō-lăn-jē-ŏs′tō-mē) [″ + ″ + ″ + *stoma,* opening]. Establishment of free drainage by opening into the gall duct.

hepatocholangitis (hĕp″ă-tō-kō-lăn-jī′tĭs) [″ + ″ + ″ + *itis,* inflammation]. Inflammation of the cells of the liver and bile ducts.

hepatocirrhosis (hĕp″ă-tō-sĭ-rō′sĭs) [″ + *kirrhos,* tawny, + *osis,* condition]. Cirrhosis of liver.

hepatocolic (hĕp″ă-tō-kŏl′ĭk) [″ + *kolon,* colon]. Rel. to both liver and colon.

hepatocuprein (hĕp″ă-tō-koo′prĭn). A copper-containing protein in the liver.

hepatocystic (hĕp″ă-tō-sĭs′tĭk) [″ + *kystis,* bladder]. Rel. to the gallbladder or to both the liver and gallbladder.

hepatocyte (hĕp′ă-tō-sīt). A parenchymal liver cell.

hepatoduodenostomy (hĕp″ă-tō-dū″ō-dĕ-nŏs′tō-mē) [″ + L. *duodenum,* duodenum, + Gr. *stoma,* opening]. Establishment of an opening from the liver into the duodenum. SYN: *hepaticoduodenostomy.*

hepatodynia (hĕp″ă-tō-dĭn′ē-ă) [″ + *odyne,* pain]. Pain in the liver.

hepatoenteric (hĕp″ă-tō-ĕn-tĕr′ĭk) [″ + *enteron,* intestine]. Rel. to the liver and intestines.

hepatogastric (hĕp″ă-tō-găs′trĭk) [Gr. *hepatikos,* liver, + *gaster,* belly]. Rel. to the liver and stomach.

hepatogenic (hĕp″ă-tō-jĕn′ĭk) [″ + *gennan,* to produce]. Having its origin in the liver.

hepatogenous (hĕp″ă-tŏj′ĕ-nŭs). Originating in the liver.

hepatogram (hĕp′ă-tō-grăm″) [″ + *gramma,* writing]. 1. Record of the pulsations of the liver. 2. X-ray examination of the liver.

hepatography (hĕp″ă-tŏg′ră-fē) [″ + *graphein,* to write]. 1. Treatise on human liver. 2. Roentgenography of the liver.

hepatohemia (hĕp″ă-tō-hē′mē-ă) [″ + *haima,* blood]. Liver congestion.

hepatoid [″ + *eidos,* form]. Having the structural form of the liver.

hepatojugular (hĕp″ă-tō-jŭg′ū-lăr). Concerning the liver and the jugular vein.

hepatojugular reflex. Pressure on the liver causes an increase in the cervical venous pressure in persons with right-sided heart failure.

hepatolenticular (hĕp″ă-tō-lĕn-tĭk′ū-lăr) [″ + L. *lenticula,* lentil, lens]. Rel. to the lenticular nucleus of the eye and the liver.

hepatolenticular degeneration. A hereditary syndrome transmitted as an autosomal recessive trait in which a decrease of ceruloplasmin, q.v., permits accumulation of copper in various organs (brain, liver, kidney, and cornea) associated with increased intestinal absorption of copper. A pigmented ring (Kayser-Fleischer ring) at the outer margin of the cornea is pathognomonic. Syndrome is characterized by degenerative changes in the brain, cirrhosis of the liver, splenomegaly, tremor, muscular rigidity, involuntary movements, spastic contractures, psychic disturbances, dysphagia, and progressive weakness and emaciation. SYN: *Wilson's disease.*

TREATMENT: Prevention of further accumulation of copper by avoiding eating organ meats, shellfish, nuts, dried legumes, chocolate, whole cereals, and all foods and water high in copper. D-penicillamine is given orally to reduce the free plasma copper to normal levels. This therapy in carefully controlled dose will probably be required for the patient's entire lifetime.

hepatolienography (hĕp″ă-tō-lī″ĕ-nŏg′ră-fē) [″ + L. *lien,* spleen, + Gr. *graphein,* to write]. X-ray of the liver and spleen. Usually done after intravenous injection of a radiopaque material.

hepatolienomegaly (hĕp″ă-tō-lī″ĕ-nō-mĕg′ă-lē) [″ + ″ + *megas,* large]. Enlargement of the liver and the spleen.

hepatolith (hĕp'ă-tō-lĭth) [" + *lithos,* stone]. A biliary concretion of the liver.

hepatolithectomy (hĕp"ă-tō-lĭ-thĕk'tō-mē) [" + *lithos,* stone, + *ektome,* excision]. Surgical removal of a calculus from the liver.

hepatolithiasis (hĕp"ă-tō-lĭ-thī'ă-sĭs) [" + " + *-iasis,* disease condition]. Calculi or concretions in the liver.

hepatologist (hĕp"ă-tŏl'ō-jĭst) [" + *logos,* study]. A specialist in diseases of the liver.

hepatology (hĕp"ă-tŏl'ō-jē) [" + *logos,* study]. Study of the liver.

hepatolysin (hĕp"ă-tŏl'ĭ-sĭn) [" + *lysis,* dissolution]. A cytolysin specific for liver cells.

hepatolysis (hĕp"ă-tŏl'ĭ-sĭs). Liver cell destruction.

hepatolytic (hĕp"ă-tō-lĭt'ĭk). Destructive to tissues of the liver.

hepatoma (hĕp-ă-tō'mă) [" + *oma,* tumor]. A tumor of the liver.

hepatomalacia (hĕp"ă-tō-mă-lā'sē-ă) [" + *malakia,* softening]. Softening of the liver.

hepatomegaly (hĕp"ă-tō-mĕg'ă-lē) [" + *megas,* large]. Enlargement of the liver.

hepatomelanosis (hĕp"ă-tō-mĕl"ă-nō'sĭs) [" + *melas,* black, + *osis,* condition]. Pigmented deposits or melanosis in the liver.

hepatomphalocele (hĕp"ă-tŏm'fă-lō-sēl") [Gr. *hepatikos,* liver, + *omphalos,* navel, + *kele,* hernia]. Protrusion of a part of the liver through the umbilicus. The liver is covered by a membrane.

hepatonecrosis (hĕp"ă-tō-nĕ-krō'sĭs) [" + *nekrosis,* deadness]. Gangrene of the liver.

hepatonephric (hĕp"ă-tō-nĕf'rĭk) [" + *nephros,* kidney]. Concerning the liver and the kidney.

hepatonephritis (hĕp"ă-tō-nĕ-frī'tĭs) [" + " + *itis,* inflammation]. Inflammation of both liver and kidneys.

hepatonephromegaly (hĕp"ă-tō-nĕf"rō-mĕg'ă-lē) [" + " + *megas,* large]. Hypertrophy of kidneys or both liver and kidney.

h. glycogenica. Disease characterized by hypertrophy of liver and excess accumulation of glycogen resulting from failure of glycogenolysis to occur. SYN: *von Gierke's disease.*

hepatopathy (hĕp-ă-tŏp'ă-thē) [" + *pathos,* disease]. Any disease of the liver.

hepatoperitonitis (hĕp"ă-tō-pĕr"ĭ-tō-nī'tĭs) [" + *peritonaion,* peritoneum, + *itis,* inflammation]. Inflammation of the peritoneal covering of the liver. SYN: *perihepatitis.*

hepatopexy (hĕp'ă-tō-pĕks"ē) [" + *pexis,* fixation]. Fixation of a movable liver to the abdominal wall.

hepatophage (hĕp'ă-tō-fāj) [" + *phagein,* to eat]. A phagocyte that attacks liver cells.

hepatopleural (hĕp"ă-tō-ploo'răl) [" + *pleura,* side]. Concerning the liver and the pleura.

hepatopneumonic (hĕp"ă-tō-nū-mŏn'ĭk) [" + *pneumonikos,* of the lungs]. Concerning the liver and the lungs.

hepatoportogram (hĕp"ă-tō-por'tō-grăm). Roentgenography of the portal vein and its branches in the liver.

hepatoptosia, hepatoptosis (hĕp"ă-tŏp-tō'sē-ă, -tō'sĭs) [" + *ptosis,* a dropping]. Downward displacement of the liver.

hepatopulmonary (hĕp"ă-tō-pŭl'mō-năr"ē) [" + L. *pulmo,* lung]. Rel. to both liver and lungs.

hepatorenal (hĕp"ă-tō-rē'năl) [" + L. *renalis,* kidney]. Pert. to both liver and kidneys.

hepatorrhaphy (hĕp-ă-tor'ă-fē) [" + *rhaphe,* suture]. The suturing of a wound of the liver.

hepatorrhexis (hĕp"ă-tō-rĕks'ĭs) [" + *rhexis,* rupture]. Rupture of the liver.

hepatoscan (hĕp'ă-tō-skăn). A radioautograph of the liver.

hepatoscopy [" + *skopein,* to examine]. Inspection of the liver.

hepatosis (hĕp"ă-tō'sĭs) [" + *osis,* condition]. Any noninflammatory disease of the liver.

hepatosplenitis (hĕp"ă-tō-splē-nī'tĭs) [" + *splen,* spleen, + *itis,* inflammation]. Inflamed condition of both liver and spleen.

hepatosplenography (hĕp"ă-tō-splē-nŏg'ră-fē) [" + " + *graphein,* to write). X-ray examination of the liver and spleen.

hepatosplenomegaly (hĕp"ă-tō-splē"nō-mĕg'ă-lē) [" + " + *megas,* large]. Enlargement of both liver and spleen.

hepatosplenopathy (hĕp"ă-tō-splē-nŏp'ă-thē) [" + " + *pathos,* disease]. Disease that affects the liver and spleen.

hepatostomy (hĕp"ă-tŏs'tō-mē) [" + *stoma,* opening]. Surgical incision of the liver with establishment of an opening to the outside of the body.

hepatotherapy (hĕp"ă-tō-thĕr'ă-pē) [" + *therapeia,* treatment]. 1. Treatment of liver disease. 2. The use of liver or liver extract.

hepatotomy (hĕp"ă-tŏt'ō-mē) [" + *tome,* incision]. Incision into the liver.

hepatotoxemia (hĕp"ă-tō-tŏks-ē'mē-ă) [" + *toxikon,* poison, + *haima,* blood]. Autointoxication due to malfunctioning of the liver.

hepatotoxin (hĕp"ă-tō-tŏk'sĭn). A cytotoxin specific for liver cells.

Heprinar. Trade name for heparin sodium, USP.

heptachromic (hĕp"tă-krō'mĭk) [Gr. *hepta,* seven, + *chroma,* color]. Possessing normal color vision.

heptapeptide (hĕp"tă-pĕp'tīd) [" + *peptein,* to digest]. A polypeptide containing seven amino acids.

heptaploidy (hĕp'tă-ploy"dē) [" + *ploos,* fold]. Having seven sets of chromosomes.

heptose (hĕp'tōs). Any sugar containing seven

carbon atoms in its molecule.

heptosuria (hĕp″tō-sū′rē-ă) [″ + *ouron,* urine]. Heptose in the urine.

herb (ĕrb) [L. *herba,* grass]. A plant with a soft stem containing little wood, esp. one of the aromatic plants used in medicine or as seasoning.

herbivorous (hĕr-bĭv′ō-rŭs) [″ + *vorare,* to eat]. Feeding on grasses and herbs. SYN: *vegetarian.*

herd [AS. *heord*]. Any large aggregation of people or animals.

hereditary (hĕ-rĕd′ĭ-tĕr-ē) [L. *hereditarius,* an heir]. Genetic characteristic transmitted from parent to offspring. SEE: *chromosome; gene.*

heredity (hĕ-rĕd′ĭ-tē) [L. *hereditas,* heir]. The transmission of genetic characteristics from parent to offspring.

heredo- [L. *hereditas,* heir]. Prefix meaning heredity.

heredoataxia (hĕr″ĕ-dō-ă-tăks′ē-ă) [″ + Gr. *ataxia,* lack of order]. Hereditary spinal ataxia. SYN: *Friedreich's ataxia.*

heredodegeneration (hĕr″ĕ-dō-dē-jĕn″ĕr-ā′shŭn). Inherited degeneration due to defective or diseased hyaloplasm. This is seen in Marie's ataxia.

heredofamilial (hĕr″ĕ-dō-fă-mĭl′ē-ăl). Referring to any disease that occurs in families due to the inherited defect or process to develop the condition.

heredoimmunity (hĕr″ĕ-dō-ĭ-mū′nĭ-tē). Inherited immunity.

Hering, Carl Ewald K. (hĕr′ĭng). German physiologist, 1834–1918.

H.-Breuer reflex. [Josef Breuer, Ger. physician, 1842–1925] Reflex inhibition of inspiration resulting from stimulation of pressoreceptors by inflation of the lungs.

H.'s theory. A theory of color vision in which it is assumed that the retina possesses three photochemical substances that, depending on their decomposition or resynthesis, produce different color sensations by their stimulation of different nerve endings.

Hering's nerves. [Heinrich Ewald Hering, Austrian physician, 1866–1948] Afferent nerve fibers leading from the carotid sinus by way of the glossopharyngeal nerve to the brain. They are pressoreceptor nerves responding to changes in blood pressure that reflexly control heart rate. An increase in pressure diminishes heart rate.

hermaphrodism (hĕr-măf′rō-dĭzm). Hermaphroditism, q.v.

hermaphrodite (hĕr-măf′rō-dīt) [Gr. *Hermaphroditos,* son of Hermes and Aphrodite, who was man and woman combined]. One possessing genital and sexual characteristics of both sexes. The clitoris is usually enlarged, resembling the penis of the male. SYN: *androgyne.*

hermaphroditism (hĕr-măf′rō-dīt-ĭzm). Conditions in which both ovarian and testicular tissue exist in the same individual. Occurs rarely in humans. SYN: *hermaphrodism.* SEE: *intersex.*

h., bilateral. Condition in which an ovary and testicle are present on both sides.

h., complex. Having internal and external organs of both sexes.

h., dimidiate. H., lateral.

h., false. Possession of the sex glands of one sex (ovary or testis) but accompanied by secondary sexual characteristics and external genitalia of the opposite sex. SYN: *pesudohermaphroditism.*

h., lateral. Possession of a testis on one side and an ovary on the other.

h., spurious. H., false.

h., transverse. Having the outward organs of one sex and the internal organs of the other.

h., true. Hermaphroditism in which the individual possesses both ovarian and testicular gonads.

h., unilateral. Hermaphroditism in which an ovary and a testis or an ovotestis are present on one side and either an ovary or testis is present on the other side.

hermetic (hĕr-mĕt′ĭk) [L. *hermeticus*]. Airtight.

hernia (hĕr′nē-ă) [L]. The protrusion or projection of an organ or a part of an organ through the wall of the cavity that normally contains it. SYN: *rupture.* SEE: *herniotomy.*

ETIOL: Failure of certain normal openings to close during development; weakness resulting from debilitating illness, old age, or injury; prolonged distention as from tumors, pregnancy, or corpulence; increased intra-abdominal pressure resulting from lifting heavy loads or coughing.

TREATMENT: Surgery or mechanical reduction. In very large hernias, mechanical devices or trusses may be used on a temporary basis.

h., abdominal. Hernia through the abdominal wall.

h., acquired. Hernia that develops any time after birth in contrast to one present at birth (congenital hernia). Usually the result of excessive strain on the muscular wall. Frequently occurs following injuries or operations.

h., bladder. Protrusion of the bladder or a part of the bladder through a normal or abnormal orifice.

h., cerebral. Hernia of the brain through the cranial wall.

h., Cloquet's. A type of femoral hernia.

SEE: *h., femoral.*

h., complete. Hernia in which sac and its contents have passed through the aperture.

h., concealed. Hernia that is imperceptible when palpated.

h., congenital. Hernia existing from birth.

h., crural. Hernia that protrudes behind the femoral sheath.

h., cystic. H., bladder.

h., direct. H., inguinal.

h., diverticular. Protrusion of an intestinal congenital diverticulum.

h., encysted. Scrotal protrusion that, enveloped in its own sac, passes into the tunica vaginalis.

h., epigastric. Hernia of the intestine through an opening in the midline above the umbilicus.

h., fascial. Protrusion of muscular tissue through its fascial covering.

h., fatty. Protrusion of fatty tissue through the abdominal wall.

h., femoral. Descending of intestines through femoral ring.

h., funicular. Hernia into the umbilical or spermatic cord.

h., hiatus. Protrusion of the stomach upward into the mediastinal cavity through the esophageal hiatus of the diaphragm.

h., Holthouse's. H., inguinocrural.

h., incarcerated. Hernia completely obstructing the bowels.

h., incisional. Hernia through a surgical scar.

h., incomplete. Hernia that has not gone completely through the aperture.

h., indirect. H., inguinal.

h., inguinal. Protrusion of the hernial sac containing the intestine at the inguinal opening. In indirect lateral or oblique inguinal hernia, the sac protrudes through the internal inguinal ring into the inguinal canal often descending into the scrotum. In direct medial inguinal hernia, the hernial sac protrudes through the abdominal wall in the region of Hesselbach's triangle, a region bounded by the rectus abdominis muscle, inguinal ligament, and inferior epigastric vessels. Inguinal hernias account for about 80% of all hernias.

h., inguinocrural. Hernia that is both femoral and inguinal.

h., internal. Hernia that occurs within the abdominal cavity. May be intraperitoneal or retroperitoneal.

h., interstitial. Form of inguinal hernia in which the hernial sac lies between layers of the abdominal muscles.

h., irreducible. Hernia that cannot be returned to its original position out of its sac by manual methods.

h., labial. Protrusion of a loop of bowel into the labium majus.

h., lateral. H., inguinal.

h., lumbar. Hernia in lumbar regions or loins.

h., medial. H., inguinal

h., mesocolic. Hernia between the layers of the mesocolon.

h., nuckian. Hernia into canal of Nuck.

h., oblique. H., inguinal.

h., obturator. Hernia through the obturator foramen.

h. of diaphragm. There are three types: congenital, acquired or traumatic, and esophageal. In the latter, a portion of the diaphragm is pushed through the esophageal hiatus into the stomach or the hernia protrudes through the diaphragm.

h., omental. Hernia containing a portion of the omentum.

h., ovarian. Presence of an ovary in a hernial sac.

h., phrenic. Hernia projecting through the diaphragm into one of the pleural cavities.

h., posterior vaginal. Hernia of Douglas' sac downward between the rectum and posterior vaginal wall. SYN: *enterocele.*

h., properitoneal. Hernia that protrudes through the peritoneum and into the abdominal wall.

h., reducible. Hernia that can be replaced by manipulation.

h., retroperitoneal. Hernia into the peritoneal sac extending behind the peritoneum into the iliac fossa.

h., Richter's. Hernia in which only a portion of wall of intestine protrudes, the main portion of the intestine being excluded from the hernial sac and the lumen remaining open.

h., scrotal. Hernia that descends into the scrotum.

h., sliding. A form of hernia that may form and then return to normal by the viscus sliding in and out of the sac of the hernia. This may occur with hiatus hernia or in other types of abdominal hernias. In this latter type one wall of the hernia sac is the herniating viscus itself.

h., strangulated. Hernia so tightly constricted that gangrene results if surgery does not relieve it. Not reducible by ordinary means.

h., umbilical. Hernia occurring at the navel. More frequent in women than men. Treated by surgery.

h., uterine. Presence of the uterus in the hernial sac.

h., vaginal. Hernial protrusion of the vaginal wall into the surrounding area, usually the pouch of Douglas.

h., vaginolabial. Hernia of a viscus into the posterior end of the labium majus.

h., ventral. Hernia through the abdominal wall. If stretching and thinning of an abdominal scar occur, pressure from the abdomen mav cause protrusion of part of the gut. It is then protected only by a layer of thin scar tissue.

hernial (hĕr′nē-ăl) [L. *hernia,* rupture]. Pert. to a hernia.

hernial sac. The pouch of peritoneum pushed before a hernia and into which it descends.

herniated. Having a hernia.

herniated disk. Rupture or herniation of the nucleus pulposus, esp. between lumbar vertebrae. This usually causes pain in the affected side.

herniation (hĕr-nē-ā′shŭn). Development of a hernia.

h. of nucleus pulposus. Prolapse of the nucleus pulposus of the intervertebral disk into the spinal canal.

h., tonsillar. Protrusion of the cerebellar tonsils through the foramen magnum. This causes pressure on the medulla oblongata; and may be fatal.

h., transtentorial. Herniation of the uncus and adjacent structures into the incisure of the tentorium of the brain. This is caused by increased pressure in the cranium. SYN: *uncal herniation.*

hernioenterotomy (hĕr″nē-ō-ĕn″tĕr-ŏt′ō-mē) [″ + Gr. *enteron,* intestine, + *tome,* incision]. Herniotomy and enterotomy done during the same surgical procedure.

herniography (hĕr″nē-ŏg′ră-fē) [″ + Gr. *graphein,* to write]. Radiographic examination of a hernia after the introduction of a contrast medium.

hernioid (hĕr′nē-oyd) [″ + Gr. *eidos,* resemblance]. Resembling a hernia.

herniolaparotomy (hĕr″nē-ō-lăp″ă-rŏt′ō-mē) [″ + Gr. *lapara,* loin, + *tome,* incision]. Abdominal surgery for the treatment of hernia.

herniology (hĕr″nē-ŏl′ō-jē) [″ + Gr. *logos,* study]. The science of hernias.

hernioplasty (hĕr′nē-ō-plăs″tē) [″ + Gr. *plassein,* to form]. Surgical operation for hernia.

herniopuncture (hĕr″nē-ō-pŭnk′chŭr) [″ + *punctura,* puncture]. Puncture of a hernia with hollow needle for withdrawal of fluid or gas.

herniorrhaphy (hĕr-nē-or′ă-fē) [″ + Gr. *rhaphe,* a suture]. Surgical procedure for hernia.

herniotomy (hĕr-nē-ŏt′ō-mē) [″ + Gr. *tome,* incision]. Surgery for the relief of hernia; an operation for the correction of irreducible hernia, esp. strangulated hernia.

heroin (hĕr′ō-ĭn). A narcotic derived from morphine. Importation, sale, and use of this drug are illegal in the United States. SYN: *diacetylmorphine.* SEE: *drug addiction.*

heroin toxicity. Poisoning by heroin.

SYM: Acute poisoning causes euphoria, flushing, itching of the skin, miosis, drowsiness, decreased respiratory rate and depth, bradycardia, hypotension, and a decrease in body temperature. If condition is untreated, death may be the outcome.

TREATMENT: In acute toxicity, establish and maintain an airway. Remove false teeth, and clean mouth and pharynx of mucus or blood. Give mouth-to-mouth or mouth-to-nose artificial respiration if necessary. Assess and treat any abnormality of cardiac function. Use cardiac massage, defibrillator, or cardiac pacer as needed. Treat pulmonary edema with continuous positive-pressure respiration and oxygen therapy.

Intravenously administer (may have to use femoral or jugular vein) an opiate antagonist such as levallorphan tartrate or nalorphine hydrochloride according to directions in package. Also administer a respiratory stimulant such as 3 to 5 ml. of doxapram hydrochloride, USP, intravenously.

Stay with patient until he or she is fully responsive. A long-acting narcotic may continue to act after a short-acting antagonist has worn off. If patient fails to respond to treatment, look for another cause for the coma.

heroinism (hĕr′ō-ĭn-ĭzm) [*heroin* + Gr. *-ismos,* condition]. Addiction to use of heroin. SEE: *drug addiction.*

herpangina (hĕrp-ăn-jī′nă, hĕrp-ăn′jĭ-nă) [Gr. *herpes,* creeping skin disease, + L. *angina,* a choking]. A benign infectious disease of children and, less commonly, of young adults. Occurs in epidemic form throughout the world, most often in summer and early fall.

ETIOL: One of several strains of Coxsackie virus.

SYM: Sudden onset of fever, severe sore throat, nausea, vomiting, excess salivation, and malaise. The throat and posterior area of the mouth are covered with vesicles 1 to 2 mm. in diameter that rupture and form ulcers.

TREATMENT: Symptomatic and supportive. There is no specific therapy.

herpes (hĕr′pēz) [Gr. *herpes,* creeping skin disease]. A word that at one time was used to indicate a vesicular eruption caused by a virus, esp. herpes simplex, q.v., or herpes zoster, q.v., and the condition lay people call cold sore or fever blister. Its use as a single word is imprecise.

h. corneae. Inflammation of the cornea due to herpesvirus.

h. facialis. A form of herpes simplex, q.v., that occurs on the face.

h. febrilis. Herpes simplex of the lips and nasal mucosa.

h. genitalis. Infection of the genital and anorectal skin and mucosa with herpes virus type 2. It is usually spread by sexual contact and is classed as a sexually transmitted disease. This viral infection may be transmitted to the fetus during delivery and may be fatal.

SYM: Itching and soreness are usually present before a small patch of erythema develops. Then a vesicle that erodes appears. These are usually painful and heal in about 10 days. They may occur in any part of the genitalia.

TREATMENT: Acyclovir has been of considerable benefit in treating the initial infection.

CAUTION: The lesions are highly contagious and persons caring for the patient must avoid contact with the exudates.

h. labialis. A form of herpes simplex, q.v., that occurs on the lips. SYN: *cold sore; blister, fever.*

h. menstrualis. Herpetic lesions appearing at the time of the menstrual period.

h., ocular. Herpes of the eye.

h. praeputialis. Herpes simplex of the male genitals.

h. progenitalis Herpes simplex of the vulva.

h. simplex. An infectious disease caused by herpes simplex virus type 1. Characterized by thin-walled vesicles that tend to recur in the same area of the skin, usually at a site where the mucous membrane joins the skin; however, they may be limited to the gingiva, oropharynx, or conjunctiva. In newborn infants, meningoencephalitis or a panvisceral infection may occur. In adults 5 to 7% of cases of aseptic meningitis are due to herpes simplex virus.

TREATMENT: Acyclovir applied locally has been effective. Antibiotics may be helpful in treating secondary infection. Eye lesions should be treated by an ophthalmologist.

h., traumatic. Herpes at the site of a wound.

h. viruses. A group of viruses important in humans. Included are herpes simplex virus type 1; herpes simplex virus type 2; varicella-zoster; cytomegalovirus; EB-infectious mononucleosis virus (Epstein-Barr virus).

h. virus simiae encephalomyelitis. A severe, almost always fatal, encephalomyelitis due to the herpes virus simiae (also called B virus). It occurs in veterinarians, laboratory workers, and others who have come in contact with infected monkeys.

h. zoster. An acute infectious disease caused by the varicella-zoster virus. It is limited to man and is characterized by inflammation of the posterior root ganglia of only a few segments of the spinal or cranial nerves. A painful vesicular eruption occurs along the course of the nerve and is almost always unilateral. The incubation period is from 7 to 21 days. The total duration of the disease from onset to complete recovery varies from 10 days to 5 weeks. If all the vesicles appear within 24 hours, the total duration is usually short. In general, the disease lasts longer in adults than in children. The virus that causes reactivation of herpes zoster is the same as that which causes chickenpox, i.e., varicella. SYN: *shingles.*

TREATMENT: Directed toward making the patient comfortable. If the eye is affected, idoxuridine should be used and the treatment supervised by an ophthalmologist.

h. zoster ophthalmicus. Herpes zoster affecting the first division of the 5th cranial nerve. The area of the face, eye, and nose supplied by this nerve is affected. The ocular complications can be quite serious. It is important that the eye be treated early with idoxuridine and that therapy be supervised by an ophthalmologist.

herpetic (hĕr-pĕt′ĭk) [Gr. *herpes,* creeping skin disease]. Pert. to herpes.

herpetic neuralgia. Neural pain with herpes zoster.

herpetic sore throat. Herpetic tonsillitis.

herpetiform (hĕr-pĕt′ĭ-form) [″ + L. *forma,* form]. Resembling herpes.

herpetism (hĕr′pĕ-tĭzm) [″ + *-ismos,* state of]. Predisposition to herpetic eruption.

Herplex Liquifilm. Trade name for idoxuridine, USP.

Herring track. Equipment item used in rehabilitation of the upper extremity. Designed to exercise an arm in various positions and areas of motion.

hersage (ār-săzh′) [Fr., a harrowing]. Splitting of a nerve trunk into separate fibers.

Herter's disease. SEE: *glycogen storage disease, type VI.*

Herter's infantilism. [Christian A. Herter, U.S. physician, 1865–1910] A form of infantilism resulting from defective fat and calcium absorption. Resembles sprue in adults. SYN: *celiac disease.*

Hertig-Rock embryos. [Arthur T. Hertig, U.S. pathologist, b. 1904; John Rock, U.S. gynecologist, b. 1890] Very beautifully preserved and dated embryos obtained experimentally in 1952.

Hertig-Rock ovum. Fertilized human ovum 7 to 7½ days old, described in 1945.

hertz. [Heinrich R. Hertz, Ger. physicist, 1857–1894] ABBR: Hz. A unit of frequency equal to one cycle/second.

hesperidin (hĕs-pĕr′ĭ-dĭn). A chemical present

in orange and lemon peel. It increases the strength of capillaries.

Hesselbach's hernia (hĕs'ĕl-bŏks). [Franz K. Hesselbach, Ger. surgeon, 1759–1816] A lobated hernia that passes through the cribriform fascia.

Hesselbach's triangle. The triangular space bounded by Poupart's ligament below, exterior border of rectus muscle internally, and epigastric artery exteriorly.

hetacillin (hĕt"ă-sĭl'ĭn). USP. An antibiotic that in the body is rapidly hydrolyzed to ampicillin and acetone. Trade name is Versapen.

heteradelphia (hĕt"ĕr-ă-dĕl'fē-ă) [Gr. *heteros,* other, + *adelphos,* brother]. Congenitally joined fetuses in which one twin is more nearly developed than the other.

heteradenia (hĕt"ĕr-ă-dē'nē-ă) [" + *aden,* gland]. 1. Glandular substance in a part that does not normally contain glands. 2. Abnormal glandular tissue.

heteradenic (hĕt"ĕr-ă-dĕn'ĭk). Pert. to heteradenia.

heteradenoma (hĕt"ĕr-ăd-ĕ-nō'mă) [" + *aden,* gland, + *oma,* tumor]. (pl. *heteradenomata*) A glandular tumor arising from an area that does not usually contain glands.

heterecious (hĕt"ĕr-ē'shŭs) [" + *oikos,* house]. Denoting a parasite living upon different hosts at different stages of development. SYN: *metoxenous.*

heterecism (hĕt"ĕr-ē'sĭzm). Development of different cycles of existence on different hosts, said of certain parasites.

heteresthesia (hĕt"ĕr-ĕs-thē'zē-ă) [" + *aisthesis,* sensation]. Variation in degree (plus or minus) of sensory response to cutaneous stimuli.

hetero-, heter- [Gr. *heteros,* other]. Prefix indicating different, or relationship to another.

heteroagglutination (hĕt"ĕr-ō-ă-gloo"tĭ-nā'shŭn). The agglutination by one animal's serum of the red blood cells of an animal of another species.

heteroagglutinin (hĕt"ĕr-ō-ă-glū'tĭ-nĭn). 1. An agglutinin formed as the result of an injection of an antigen from an animal of a different species. 2. An agglutinin capable of agglutinating blood cells of other species of animals.

heteroalbumose (hĕt"ĕr-ō-ăl'bū-mōs) [" + L. *albumen,* white of egg]. Albumose insoluble in water but soluble in saline solutions or in acid or alkaline solutions. SYN: *hemialbumose.*

heteroantibody (hĕt"ĕr-ō-ăn"tĭ-bŏd'ē). An antibody corresponding to an antigen from another species.

heteroantigen (hĕt"ĕr-ō-ăn'tĭ-jĕn). An antigen in one species that produces a corresponding antibody in another species.

heteroautoplasty (hĕt"ĕr-ō-aw'tō-plăs-tē) [" + *autos,* self, + *plassein,* to form]. Grafting skin from one person to another.

heteroblastic (hĕt"ĕr-ō-blăs'tĭk) [" + *blastos,* germ]. Having origin in tissue of another kind. Opposed to homoblastic.

heterocellular (hĕt"ĕr-ō-sĕl'ū-lăr). Composed of different kinds of cells.

heterocephalus (hĕt"ĕr-ō-sĕf'ă-lŭs) [" + *kephale,* head]. Congenitally deformed fetus with two heads of unequal size.

heterochiral (hĕt"ĕr-ō-kī'răl) [" + *cheir,* hand]. Reversed as to right and left, but otherwise of the same form and size. Said of images in a plane mirror.

heterochromatin (hĕt"ĕr-ō-krō'mă-tĭn) [" + *chroma,* color]. A type of chromatin that stains less distinctly than the euchromatin, forming clear disks interposed between dark bands on chromosomes. In interphasic nuclei, it constitutes the chromocenters. It is thought that it controls certain metabolic activities of cells. It is genetically inert. SEE: *euchromatin.*

heterochromatosis (hĕt"ĕr-ō-krō-mă-tō'sĭs) [" + " + *osis,* condition]. 1. Pigmentation of skin from foreign substances. 2. Difference in color. SYN: *heterochromia.*

heterochromia (hĕt"ĕr-ō-krō'mē-ă). A difference in color.

h. iridis. Different color of iris or sector of iris in the two eyes. This may occur naturally or be due to previous disease in the lighter-colored eye.

heterochromosome (hĕt"ĕr-ō-krō'mō-sōm) 1. The X and Y or sex chromosomes. 2. A chromosome that contains material, heterochromatin, that stains differently from the remainder of the chromatin material.

heterochromous (hĕt"ĕr-ō-krō'mŭs) [" + *chroma,* color]. With abnormal difference in coloration.

heterochronia (hĕt"ĕr-ō-krō'nē-ă) [" + *chronos,* time]. Denoting an abnormal time for the occurrence of a phenomenon or production of a structure.

heterochronic (hĕt"ĕr-ō-krŏn'ĭk). Occurring at different or at abnormal times.

heterochthonous (hĕt"ĕr-ŏk'thō-nŭs) [Gr. *heteros,* other, + *chthon,* a particular land or country]. Having its origin in a different place from where it was found.

heterocinesia (hĕt"ĕr-ō-sĭ-nē'zē-ă) [" + *kinesis,* movement]. Movements different from those the patient is instructed to make.

heterocladic (hĕt"ĕr-ō-klăd'ĭk) [" + *klados,* branch]. Pert. to an anastomosis between branches of two different arteries. Opposed to homocladic.

heterocrisis (hĕt"ĕr-ŏk'rĭ-sĭs) [" + *krisis,* division]. Irregular crisis with abnormal symptoms.

heterocyclic (hĕt″ĕr-ō-sīk′lĭk) [″ + *kyklos,* circle]. Pert. to ring compounds that contain one or more elements other than carbon in the ring.

heterodermic (hĕt″ĕr-ō-dĕr′mĭk) [″ + *derma,* skin]. Pert. to a method of skin grafting in which grafts are taken from another person. SYN: *dermatoheteroplasty.*

heterodont (hĕt′ĕr-ō-dŏnt) [″ + *odous,* tooth]. Having teeth of various shapes.

heterodromus (hĕt″ĕr-ŏd′rō-mŭs) [″ + *dromos,* running]. Acting, arranged, or moving in the opposite direction.

heteroecious. Heterecious.

heteroecism. Heterecism.

heteroerotism (hĕt″ĕr-ō-ĕr′ō-tĭzm) [″ + *eros,* love, + *-ismos,* state of]. Sexual desire for another person. SEE: *autoerotic.*

heterogametic (hĕt″ĕr-ō-gă-mĕt′ĭk) [″ + *gamos,* marriage]. Pert. to the production of unlike gametes, applied esp. to a male that produces two types of sperm, one containing the X chromosome, the other the Y chromosome. SEE: *homogametic.*

heterogamy (hĕt″ĕr-ŏg′ă-mē). The union of gametes that are dissimilar in size and structure. Occurs in higher plants and animals. SEE: *isogamy.*

heterogeneity (hĕt″ĕr-ō-jĕ-nē′ĭ-tē). The quality of being heterogeneous.

heterogeneous (hĕt″ĕr-ō-jē′nē-ŭs) [″ + *genos,* type]. Of unlike natures; composed of unlike substances. Opposed to homogeneous.

heterogeneous vaccine. Vaccine made from some source other than patient's own tissues or cells. Opposed to autogenous vaccine.

heterogenesis (hĕt″ĕ-rō-jĕn′ĕ-sĭs) [″ + *genesis,* production]. Production of offspring that have different characteristics in alternate generations, as in the alternation of an asexual generation with a sexual one. SYN: *metagenesis.* SEE: *homogenesis.*

heterogenetic (hĕt″ĕ-rō-jĕ-nĕt′ĭk). Rel. to heterogenesis.

heterogeusia (hĕt″ĕr-ō-gū′sē-ă) [″ + *geusis,* taste]. Perception of an inappropriate quality of taste when food is present in the mouth or when it is chewed. The taste sensation is unexpected and unusual but not necessarily unpleasant.

heterograft (hĕt′ĕ-rō-grăft) [″ + L. *graphium,* grafting knife]. A graft taken from another individual or an animal of a different species from the one for whom it is intended. SEE: *autograft; graft; isograft.*

heterography (hĕt″ĕr-ŏg′ră-fē) [″ + *graphein,* to write]. Writing different words from those the writer intended.

heterohemagglutination (hĕt″ĕr-ō-hĕm″ă-gloo″tĭ-nā′shŭn). Agglutination of red blood cells by hemagglutinins from another species.

heterohemagglutinin (hĕt″ĕr-ō-hĕm″ă-gloo′tĭ-nĭn). Hemagglutinin from one species that will agglutinate red blood cells from another species.

heterohemolysin (hĕt″ĕr-ō-hē-mŏl′ĭ-sĭn). A hemolysin present in one animal that will hemolyze the red blood cells of another species.

heteroimmunity (hĕt″ĕr-ō-ĭm-mū′nĭ-tē). Having immunity to an antigen from another species.

heteroinfection (hĕt″ĕr-ō-ĭn-fĕk′shŭn) [Gr. *heteros,* other, + L. *in,* in, + *facere,* to make]. Infection by a microorganism from outside the body.

heteroinoculation (hĕt″ĕr-ō-ĭn-ŏk″ū-lā′shun) [″ + ″ + *oculus,* bud]. Inoculation with a microorganism from a source outside the body.

heterokeratoplasty (hĕt″ĕr-ō-kĕr′ă-tō-plăs″tē) [″ + *keras,* horn, + *plassein,* to form]. Plastic surgery of the cornea utilizing tissue from the cornea from another species.

heterolalia (hĕt″ĕr-ō-lā′lē-ă) [″ + *lalia,* babbling]. The use of meaningless words instead of those intended. SYN: *heterophasia; heterophemia.*

heterolateral (hĕt″ĕr-ō-lăt′ĕr-ăl) [″ + L. *latus,* side]. Situated or occurring on the other side. SEE: *ipsilateral.*

heteroliteral (hĕt″ĕr-ō-lĭt′ĕr-ăl). In speaking, pert. to an incorrect letter being substituted for the correct one.

heterologous (hĕt″ĕr-ŏl′ō-gŭs) [″ + *logos,* relation]. 1. Made up of cell tissue not normal to the part. 2. A tissue, cells, or blood obtained from a different individual or species.

heterology (hĕt″ĕr-ŏl′ō-jē). Different from the normal in structure or method of growth.

heterolysin (hĕt-ĕr-ŏl′ĭ-sĭn) [″ + *lysis,* solution]. Lysins formed from an antigen from an animal of a different species. SEE: *autolysis; hemolysis.*

heterolysis (hĕt″ĕr-ŏl′ĭ-sĭs). Hemolytic action of blood serum of an animal upon corpuscles of another species. SEE: *hemolysis; isolysis.*

heteromeric (hĕt″ĕr-ō-mĕr′ĭk) [″ + *meros,* a part]. 1. Pert. to spinal neurons with processes extending to opposite side of cord. 2. Possessing a different chemical composition.

heterometaplasia (hĕt″ĕr-ō-mĕt″ă-plā′zē-ă) [″ + *meta,* beyond, + *plassein,* to form]. Transformation of tissue to one foreign to the part where it was produced.

heterometropia (hĕt″ĕr-ō-mĕ-trō′pē-ă). The ability of one eye to refract differently as compared with the other. This produces perceived images of different size. The condition is probably prevalent in a great number of individuals who are completely unaware of it.

heteromorphosis (hĕt″ĕr-ō-mor-fō′sĭs) [″ + *morphe,* form, + *osis,* condition]. 1. The regeneration of an organ different from the one that it replaced. 2. Any disease in which malformation or deformity is characteristic. 3. Abnormal position of an organ or tissue.

heteromorphous (hĕt″ĕr-ō-mor′fŭs) [″ + *morphe,* form]. Deviating from the normal type.

heteronomous (hĕt″ĕr-ŏn′ō-mŭs) [″ + *nomos,* law]. Abnormal; differing from type.

heteronymous (hĕt″ĕr-ŏn′ĭ-mŭs) [″ + *onyma,* name]. 1. Having different names that are indicative of a correlation. 2. In opposite relation.

hetero-osteoplasty (hĕt″ĕr-ō-ŏs′tē-ō-plăs″tē) [″ + *osteon,* bone, + *plassein,* to form]. Grafting of bone, esp. with a graft from an animal.

heteropathy (hĕt″ĕr-ŏp′ă-thē) [″ + *pathos,* disease]. 1. Abnormal reaction to irritation or to stimuli. 2. Creation of a pathological condition to neutralize another disorder. SEE: *allopathy.*

heterophany (hĕt″ĕr-ŏf′ă-nē) [″ + *phainein,* to appear]. Having different expressions of the same disorder.

heterophasia (hĕt″ĕr-ō-fā′zē-ă) [″ + *phasis,* speech]. Expression of meaningless words instead of those intended. SYN: *heterolalia; heterophemia.*

heterophemia, heterophemy (hĕt″ĕr-ō-fē′mē-ă, hĕt-ĕr-ŏf′ĕ-mē) [″ + *pheme,* speech]. Expressing one thing when another is intended. SYN: *heterolalia; heterophasia.*

heterophil(e) (hĕt′ĕr-ō-fĭl, -fīl) [″ + *philein,* to love]. 1. In man, the neutrophil leukocyte. 2. Pert. to an antibody reacting with other than the specific antigen. 3. Pert. to a tissue or microorganism that takes a stain other than the ordinary one.

heterophilic (hĕt″ĕr-ō-fĭl′ĭk) [Gr. *heteros,* other, + *philein,* to love]. 1. Having affinity for something abnormal. 2. Having antibody response to an antigen other than the specific one.

heterophonia (hĕt″ĕr-ō-fō′nē-ă) [″ + *phone,* voice]. Change of voice, esp. that which occurs at puberty.

heterophoralgia (hĕt″ĕr-ō-for-ăl′jē-ă) [″ + *phoros,* bearing, + *algos,* pain]. Deviation of one eye accompanied by pain.

heterophoria (hĕt″ĕ-rō-for′ē-ă) [″ + *phoros,* bearing]. The tendency of the eyes to deviate from their normal position for visual alignment, esp. when one eye is covered; latent deviation or squint. SEE: *phoria.*

ETIOL: Imbalance or insufficiency of ocular muscles.

heterophthalmos (hĕt″ĕr-ŏf-thăl′mŏs) [″ + *ophthalmos,* eye]. Difference in appearance of the eyes due to the irides differing in color. SEE: *heterochromia.*

Heterophyes (hĕt″ĕr-ŏf′ĭ-ēz) [″ + *phye,* stature]. A genus of flukes belonging to the family Heterophyidae.

H. heterophyes. A species of intestinal fluke commonly infesting man. In heavy infestations, it may cause diarrhea, nausea, and abdominal discomfort.

heterophyiasis (hĕt″ĕr-ō-fī-ī′ă-sĭs) [″ + ″ + *-iasis,* diseased condition]. Infestation by any fluke belonging to the family Heterophyidae.

Heterophyidae. A family of Trematoda (flukes) that infests the intestines of dogs, cats, and other mammals including humans. Infestations are common in Egypt and in the Far East. Includes the genera Heterophyes, Haplorchis, Diorchitrema, and Metagonimus. Intermediate hosts are snails, the cercaria encysting in fishes, esp. mullets, or frogs.

heteroplasia (hĕt″ĕr-ō-plā′zē-ă) [″ + *plassein,* to mold]. Development of tissue at a location where that type of tissue would not normally occur. SYN: *alloplasia.*

heteroplastic (hĕt″ĕr-ō-plăs′tĭk). Rel. to heteroplasia.

heteroplasty (hĕt″ĕ-rō-plăs′tē). Grafting with tissue from another person or an animal.

heteroploid (hĕt′ĕr-ō-ployd) [″ + *ploos,* fold]. Possessing a chromosome number that is not a multiple of the haploid number common for the species.

heteroprosopus (hĕt″ĕr-ō-prō′sō-pŭs) [″ + *prosopon,* face]. A congenitally deformed fetus having one head and two faces.

heteropsia (hĕt″ĕr-ŏp′sē-ă) [″ + *opsis,* vision]. Inequality of vision in the two eyes.

heteroptics (hĕt″ĕr-ŏp′tĭks). Perversion of vision such as seeing objects that do not exist or misinterpreting what is seen.

heteropyknosis (hĕt″ĕr-ō-pĭk-nō′sĭs) [″ + *pyknos,* dense, + *osis,* condition]. The property whereby various parts of a chromosome stain with varying degrees of intensity. Thought to be due to variations in concentration of nucleic acid.

heteroscopy (hĕt″ĕr-ŏs′kō-pē) [Gr. *heteros,* other, + *skopein,* to examine]. 1. Finding range of vision in strabismus. 2. Unequal vision in the eyes.

heteroserotherapy (hĕt″ĕr-ō-sē″rō-thĕr′ă-pē) [″ + L. *serum,* whey, + Gr. *therapeia,* treatment]. Treatment by serum from another person.

heterosexual (hĕt″ĕr-ō-sĕk′shū-ăl) [″ + L. *sexus,* sex]. 1. Pertaining to the opposite sex. 2. One whose sexual orientation is to persons of the opposite sex.

heterosexuality (hĕt″ĕr-ō-sĕk″shū-ăl′ĭ-tē). Sexual attraction for one of the opposite sex.

heterosis (hĕt-ĕr-ō′sĭs) [Gr., alteration]. Greater strength, size, vigor, and growth rate seen in the first hybrid generation. SYN: *hybrid vigor.*

heterosmia (hĕt″ĕr-ŏs′mē-ă) [Gr. *heteros,* other, + *osme,* odor]. Consistent perception of an inappropriate smell when an odorant is inhaled. The smell perceived is unusual and unexpected but not unpleasant.

heterotaxia (hĕt″ĕr-ō-tăk′sē-ă) [″ + *taxis,* arrangement]. Abnormal position of organs or parts. SEE: *dextrocardia; situs inversus viscerum.*

heterotherm (hĕt′ĕr-ō-thĕrm″). An animal that is heterothermic. SEE: *heterothermy.*

heterothermy (hĕt′ĕr-ō-thĕr″mē) [″ + *therme,* heat]. Condition of animals in which the temperature varies considerably in various situations. It is *not* poikilothermic, q.v.

heterotopia (hĕt″ĕr-ō-tō′pē-ă) [″ + *topos,* place]. 1. Development of a normal tissue in an abnormal location. 2. Displacement of an organ or part from its normal location.

heterotopic (hĕt″ĕr-ō-tŏp′ĭk). Misplaced; pert. to heterotopia.

heterotopy (hĕt″ĕr-ŏt′ō-pē) [″ + *topos,* place]. Displacement of an organ or a portion of the body.

heterotoxin (hĕt″ĕr-ō-tŏk′sĭn) [″ + *toxikon,* poison]. A toxin introduced from without the patient's body.

heterotransplant (hĕt″ĕr-ō-trăns′plănt) [″ + L. *trans,* across, + *plantare,* to plant]. An organ, tissue, or structure taken from an animal and grafted into, or on, another animal of a different species. Such transplants usually atrophy.

heterotrichosis (hĕt″ĕr-ō-trĭ-kō′sĭs) [″ + *trichosis,* growth of hair]. Growth of different kinds or color of hairs on the scalp or body.

heterotroph (hĕt′ĕr-ō-trōf) [″ + *trophe,* food]. An organism such as man that requires complex organic food in order to grow and develop. In contrast to plants, which can synthesize food from inorganic materials.

heterotropia (hĕt″ĕr-ō-trō′pē-ă) [″ + *tropos,* a turning]. Manifest deviation of the eyes due to absence of binocular equilibrium. SEE: *strabismus.*

heterotypic (hĕt″ĕr-ō-tĭp′ĭk). Concerning something of a different type than that which is being discussed or examined, esp. a tissue.

heterovaccine (hĕt″ĕr-ō-văk′sēn) [″ + L. *vaccinus,* pert. to a cow]. A vaccine from a source other than that of the disease for which it is intended.

heteroxanthine (hĕt″ĕr-ō-zăn′thĭn) [″ + *xanthos,* yellow]. Methylxanthine, an alloxuric base found in the urine.

heteroxenous (hĕt″ĕr-ŏk′sē-nŭs) [″ + *xenos,* stranger]. Property of a parasite that requires two different hosts in order to complete its life cycle.

heterozygosis (hĕt″ĕr-ō-zī-gō′sĭs) [″ + *zygone,* yoke, pair, + *osis,* condition]. The state of having different alleles at a specific locus. SEE: *homozygosis.*

heterozygote (hĕt″ĕr-ō-zī′gōt). An individual with different alleles for a given characteristic. SEE: *allele.*

heterozygous (hĕt″ĕr-ō-zī′gŭs). Possessing different alleles at a given locus. SEE: *homozygous.*

hettocyrtosis (hĕt″ō-sĭr-tō′sĭs) [Gr. *hetton,* less, + *kyrtosis,* curvature]. A slight curvature.

Heubner, Johann Otto L. (hoyb′nĕr). German pediatrician, 1843–1926.

H.'s disease. Syphilitic endarteritis of the brain.

H.-Herter disease. [Christian A. Herter, U.S. pathologist, b. 1865] Nontropical sprue in infants.

heuristic (hū-rĭs′tĭk) [Gr. *heuriskein,* to find out, discover]. Helping to discover or experiment, esp. the encouragement of students to learn through their own investigation.

heurteloup (hĕr′tĕl-oop). [Charles Louis Stanislaus Baron Heurteloup, Fr. surgeon, 1793–1864] An artificial leech; a cupping apparatus.

H.E.W. U.S. Department of *H*ealth, *E*ducation, and *W*elfare. This agency is now the U.S. Department of Health and Human Services.

hex-, hexa- [Gr. *hex,* six]. Prefix indicating six.

hexabasic [Gr. *hex,* six, + *basis,* base]. An acid that contains six hydrogen atoms (H) that can be replaced by six hydroxyl (OH) radicals.

hexachlorophene (hĕks″ă-klō′rō-fēn). USP. A bactericidal and bacteriostatic compound, used in emulsions and soaps for preoperative cleansing of skin and for scrubbing the nurse's and surgeon's hands prior to surgery. Trade name is G-11.

hexachromic [″ + *chroma,* color]. Able to distinguish only six of the seven colors of the spectrum or unable to distinguish violet from indigo.

hexad (hĕk′săd). 1. Six similar things. 2. An element with a valence of six.

hexadactylism (hĕks″ă-dăk′tĭl-ĭzm) [″ + *daktylos,* finger, + *-ismos,* condition]. Possession of six fingers or six toes on one limb.

hexafluorenium bromide (hĕk″să-flūr-ĕn′ē-ŭm). USP. A neuromuscular blocking agent. Trade name is Mylaxen.

hexamethonium (hĕks″ă-mĕ-thō′nē-ŭm). A compound that acts as a ganglionic blocking agent. Used in the treatment of hypertension.

hexaploidy (hĕk′să-ploy″dē [″ + *ploos,* fold]. Condition of having six sets of chromosomes.

Hexapoda (hĕks-ăp′ō-dă) [″ + *pous,* foot]. The insects or six-legged arthropods. SYN: *Insecta.*

hexatomic (hĕks″ă-tŏm′ĭk) [″ + *atomos,* indivisible]. Pert. to a compound consisting of six atoms or a compound having six replaceable hydrogen or univalent atoms.

hexavaccine (hĕks″ă-văk′sēn) [″ + L. *vaccinus,* pert. to a cow]. A vaccine made from six different microorganisms.

hexavalent (hĕks″ă-vā′lĕnt) [″ + L. *valere,* to have power]. Having a chemical valence of six. SYN: *sexivalent.*

hexavitamin capsules or tablets. USP. A standardized vitamin preparation containing vitamins A, D, C, B, riboflavin, and niacinamide.

hexestrol (hĕk-sĕs′trŏl). A nonsteroidal estrogen.

hexobarbital (hĕk″sō-băr′bĭ-tăl). USP. A barbiturate sedative. Trade name is Sombulex.

hexocyclium methylsulfate (hĕk″sō-sī′klē-ŭm). A quaternary ammonium compound used in treating peptic ulcer. Trade name is Tral.

hexokinase (hĕks″ō-kī′nās) [″ + *kinein,* to move, + *-ase,* enzyme]. An enzyme present in muscle tissue that catalyzes the phosphorylation of glucose. It has also been isolated from yeast.

hexone (hĕk′sōn) [Gr. *hex,* six]. One of the amino acids, as histidine, arginine, and lysine, so called because they contain chains of six carbon atoms.

hexonic (hĕk-sŏn′ĭk). Rel. to hexone bases.

hexosamine (hĕk′sōs-ăm″ĭn). A sugar containing an amino group in place of a hydroxyl group. Glucosamine is one example.

hexose (hĕk′sōs). Any monosaccharide of the general formula $C_6H_{12}O_6$; the group includes particularly dextrose, q.v., and levulose, q.v.

hexosephosphate (hĕks″ōs-fŏs′fāt) [″ + *phosphoros,* phosphorus]. A phosphoric acid ester of glucose. One of several esters formed in the muscles and other tissues in the metabolism of carbohydrates.

hexuronic acid. Ascorbic acid, vitamin C.

hexylcaine hydrochloride (hĕk′sĭl-kān). USP. A local anesthetic agent. Trade name is Cyclaine.

hexylresorcinol (hĕks″ĭl-rĕ-sor′sĭ-nŏl). USP. $C_{12}H_{18}O_2$. White needle-shaped crystals used as an anthelmintic.

Hey's ligament (hāz). [William Hey, Brit. surgeon, 1736–1819] The semilunar lateral margin (falciform margin) of the fossa ovalis, which lies between the iliac and pubic portions of the fascia lata.

HF. 1. *Hageman factor,* blood coagulation factor XII. 2. *high frequency.*

Hf. Chem. symb. for hafnium.

Hg. Chem. symb. for mercury.

Hgb. *hemoglobin.*

$HgCl_2$. Chem. symb. for mercuric chloride; corrosive sublimate.

Hg_2Cl_2. Chem. symb. for mercurous chloride; calomel.

HGF. 1. *human growth factor.* 2. *hyperglycemic-glycogenolytic factor* (glucagon).

HgI_2. Chem. symb. for mercuric iodide.

HgO. Chem. symb. for mercuric oxide.

HgS. Chem. symb. for mercuric sulfide.

$HgSO_4$. Chem. symb. for mercuric sulfate.

5-HIAA. *five hydroxy indole acetic acid.*

hiatus (hī-ā′tŭs) [L., an opening]. 1. [NA] An opening, a foramen. 2. An aperture.

h. aorticus. [NA] Opening in the diaphragm through which pass the aorta and the thoracic duct.

h. canalis facialis. Hiatus of canal for greater petrosal nerve. SYN: *hiatus fallopii.*

h. esophageus. [NA] Opening in the diaphragm through which the esophagus passes.

h. fallopii. H. canalis facialis.

h. maxillaris. [NA] Opening of maxillary sinus into the nasal cavity, located on the nasal surface of the maxillary bone.

h. semilunaris. [NA] The groove in the external wall of the middle meatus of the nasal fossa into which the frontal sinus, maxillary sinus, and anterior ethmoid cells drain.

hiatus hernia. SEE: *hernia, hiatus.*

hibernation (hī″bĕr-nā′shŭn) [L. *hiberna,* winter]. Condition of spending the winter asleep and in an almost comatose condition. Some animals adapt to winter by this method.

h., artificial. State of hibernation produced therapeutically by use of drugs alone or drugs and hypothermia. The rate of metabolism is greatly reduced in this state.

hibernoma (hī″bĕr-nō′mă). A rare multilobular encapsulated tumor that contains fetal fat tissue closely resembling the fat stored in the foot pads of hibernating animals.

Hibiclens. Trade name for chlorhexidine gluconate.

Hibitane. Trade name for chlorhexidine gluconate.

hiccough, hiccup (hĭk′ŭp) [probably of imitative origin]. Spasmodic periodic closure of the glottis following spasmodic lowering of the diaphragm, causing a short, sharp, inspiratory cough. SYN: *singultus.*

ETIOL: It may be caused by indigestion, irritation of diaphragm, alcoholism, new growths of the pleura, certain cerebral lesions, or hysteria. May be due to a disturbance of the phrenic nerve. If prolonged it has serious significance.

TREATMENT: Antiemetic drugs, rebreathing in a paper bag, inhalation of carbon dioxide. Stimulation of the nasopharynx with a soft rubber tube; placement of a thin coating of dry granulated sugar in the hypopharynx. If these are not effective, anesthetization of the phrenic nerve may be helpful.

Hicks sign. [John Braxton Hicks, Brit. gynecologist, 1825–1897] Intermittent painless uterine contractions that may occur every 10 to 20 mins. These contractions may be inapparent to the individual. They appear after the third month of pregnancy. These contractions do not represent true labor pains but are often so interpreted. SYN: *Braxton Hicks sign.*

hidebound disease [AS. *hyd,* a skin, + *bindan,* to tie up]. Hardening and thickening of the skin with loss of elasticity. SYN: *scleroderma.*

hidradenitis (hī-drăd-ĕ-nī'tĭs) [Gr. *hidros,* sweat, + *aden,* gland, + *itis,* inflammation]. Inflammation of sweat glands.

hidradenoma (hī"drăd-ĕ-nō'mă) [" + " + *oma,* tumor]. Adenoma of the sweat glands.

hidrocystoma (hī"drō-sĭs-tō'mă) [" + *kystis,* cyst, + *oma,* tumor]. A cystic tumor of a sweat gland. SYN: *hydrocystoma.*

hidropoiesis (hī"drō-poy-ē'sĭs) [" + *poiesis,* formation]. The formation of sweat.

hidropoietic (hī"drō-poy-ĕt'ĭk). Pert. to hydropoiesis. SYN: *sudorific.*

hidrorrhea (hī-drō-rē'ă) [" + *rhoia,* flow]. Abnormal sweating.

hidrosadenitis (hī"drōs-ăd"ĕ-nī'tĭs) [" + *aden,* gland, + *itis,* inflammation]. Inflammation of sweat glands. SYN: *hidradenitis.*

hidroschesis (hī-drŏs'kĕ-sĭs) [" + *schesis,* a holding]. 1. Retention of perspiration. 2. Suppression of perspiration.

hidrosis (hī-drō'sĭs) [" + *osis,* condition]. 1. Formation and excretion of sweat. 2. Excessive sweating.

hidrotic (hī-drŏt'ĭk). 1. Causing the secretion and excretion of sweat. SYN: *diaphoretic; sudorific.* 2. Any drug or medicine that induces sweating.

hieralgia (hī-ĕr-ăl'jē-ă) [Gr. *hieron,* sacrum, + *algos,* pain]. Pain in the region of the sacrum.

hierolisthesis (hī"ĕr-ō-lĭs-thē'sĭs) [" + *olisthanein,* to slip]. Displacement of the sacrum.

hierophobia (hī"ĕr-ō-fō'bē-ă) [Gr. *hieros,* sacred, + *phobos,* fear]. Abnormal fear of sacred things or persons connected with religion.

high blood pressure. Blood pressure that is above the normal range. A diagnostic judgment or opinion, which must be considered with respect to the person's age, body build, previous blood pressure, and state of mental and physical health at the time the blood pressure is obtained. In general it is not advisable to declare that a person has elevated blood pressure if the opinion is based on one determination of the blood pressure.

RS: blood; blood pressure; hypertension; hypotension; pulse pressure.

high-calorie diet. Diet that includes more calories than would be normally required for that person's metabolic and energy needs. Three meals plus between-meal feedings. Fermentable and bulky foods to be avoided.

IND: Prevention of weight loss in wasting diseases; in high basal metabolism; and after long illness. In deficiency caused by anorexia, poverty, and poor dietary habits. During lactation when 1000 and 1200 extra Cal. each day are indicated.

high-cellulose diet. SEE: *high-residue diet.*

Highmore, antrum of (hī'mor). [Nathaniel Highmore, Brit. surgeon, 1613–1685] The maxillary sinus. SEE: *antrocele.*

Highmore's body. Fibrous tissue mass, a prolongation of albuginea testis, projecting forward along the posterior border of the testis. SYN: *mediastinum testis* [NA].

high-residue diet. Diet that contains considerable amounts of substances such as fiber or cellulose, which the human body is unable to metabolize and absorb. The diet is particulary useful in treating constipation. There is increasing evidence that a diet that produces high residue may be beneficial in preventing certain diseases of the gastrointestinal tract. Lay persons refer to high-residue diet as one containing a lot of roughage, q.v. SEE: *fiber.*

hila (hī'lă) [L.]. Pl. of hilum. SEE: *hilus.*

hilar (hī'lăr). Concerning or belonging to the hilus.

hilitis (hī-lī'tĭs) [L. *hilus,* a trifle, + Gr. *itis,* inflammation]. Inflammation of any hilum, esp. the hilum of the lung.

hillock (hĭl'ŏk) [ME. *hilloc*]. A small eminence or projection.

h., anal. One of two small eminences that lie lateral and posterior to the cloacal membrane and, later, the anal fissure in the embryo

h., axon. A small conical elevation on the cell body of a neuron from which the axon arises.

h., seminal. The colliculus seminalis [NA].

Hilton's law. [John Hilton, Brit. surgeon, 1804–1878] The trunk of a nerve not only sends branches to a particular muscle, but also sends branches to the joint moved by that muscle and to the skin overlying the insertion of the muscle.

Hilton's line. A white line at the junction of the skin of perineum and anal mucosa.

Hilton's muscle. The aryepiglottic muscle.

Hilton's sac. A pit along the external portion of the false vocal cords. SYN: *saccule, laryngeal.*

hilum (hī'lŭm) [L.]. (pl. *hila*) Hilus.

hilus (hī'lŭs) [L., a trifle] (pl. *hili*) [NA] 1. Depression or recess at exit or entrance of a duct into a gland or of nerves and vessels into an organ. 2. The root of the lungs at level of 4th and 5th dorsal vertebrae.

himantosis (hī″măn-tō′sĭs) [Gr. *himantosis,* a long strap]. Abnormal lengthening of the uvula.

hindbrain (hīnd′brān) [AS. *hindan,* behind, + *bragen,* brain]. The most caudal of the three divisions of the embryonic brain. It differentiates into the metencephalon, which gives rise to the cerebellum and pons, and the myelencephalon, which gives rise to the medulla oblongata. SYN: *rhombencephalon.* [NA].

hindfoot (hīnd′foot). Posterior part of the foot.

hindgut (hīnd′gŭt). The caudal portion of the entodermal tube, which develops into the alimentary canal. It gives rise to the ileum, colon, and rectum.

hind-kidney (hīnd-kĭd′nē). The most caudal of three embryonic kidneys. It persists and develops into the permanent kidney. SYN: *metanephros.*

Hines and Brown test. [Edgar H. Hines, Jr., U.S. physician, b. 1906; George Brown, U.S. physician, 1885–1935] Test designed to detect latent states of hypertension. The response of blood pressure to immersion of the patient's hand in ice water is measured; an excessive rise in pressure is thought to indicate latent hypertension.

hinge joint. An articulation that permits flexion and extension about a single axis. SYN: *ginglymus.*

Hinton's test. [William A. Hinton, U.S. bacteriologist, 1883–1959] A serological test for syphilis.

hip [AS. *hype*]. 1. Upper part of thigh, formed by the femur and innominate bones. Its three portions are the ilium, ischium, and pubis. SYN: *os coxae.* 2. The region on each side of the pelvis. SEE: *hip joint.*

h., congenital dislocation of. A congenital defect of the hip joint that is most probably due to multifactorial effects of several abnormal genes.

h., dislocation of. Dislocations of the hip are very often accompanied by a fracture and it is extremely difficult even for a well-trained surgeon to distinguish a pure dislocation from a fracture dislocation without roentgenography.

DIAG: Person has great difficulty in straightening the hip following an accident. It is always accompanied by pain. The knee on the injured side resistantly points inwardly toward the other knee, and it is difficult to straighten the leg.

SYM: Pain, rigidity, loss of function, and the dislocation may be obvious by the abnormal position in which the leg is held, or by seeing or feeling the head of the femur in an abnormal position.

F.A.: Place the patient on a large splint as in a fractured back. In addition, place a large pad, such as a pillow, under the knee of the affected side. Treat for shock if required.

h., dislocation of, backward. Dislocation of the hip onto the dorsum ilii or sciatic notch.

SYM: Inward rotation of thigh, with flexion, inversion, adduction, shortening; pain, tenderness; loss of function and immobility.

TREATMENT: Patient should be anesthetized. Dorsal position with leg flexed on thigh, and the latter upon the abdomen. Adduct thigh, rotate outward; circumduction outwardly across abdomen, back to straight position. Traction may be required.

h., dislocation of, downward. This type of hip dislocation is rare.

TREATMENT: Traction in flexed position. Outward rotation and extension.

h., dislocation of, forward. Dislocation of the hip through obturator foramen, on pubis, in perineum, or through fractured acetabulum.

SYM: Pain, tenderness, and immobility. Shortening in pubic and suprapubic forms; lengthening in obturator and perineal forms.

TREATMENT: Hyperextension and direct traction. Flexion, abduction with inward rotations, adduction.

h., snapping. A slipping around of the hip joint, sometimes producing an audible snapping sound.

h., total replacement of. Orthopedic surgical procedure involving total replacement of the head of the femur and the acetabular portion of the hip joint.

hip joint. Articulation between the femur and the innominate bone. A ball and socket (enarthrosis) formed by the head of the femur fitting into a concavity, the acetabulum.

hip-joint disease. Any disease of the hip joint, esp. tuberculosis.

Hippel's disease, von Hippel-Lindau disease (hĭp′ĕlz, vŏn hĭp′ĕl-lĭn′dow). [Eugen von Hippel, Ger. ophthalmologist, 1867–1939; Arvid Lindau, Swedish pathologist, b. 1892] Angiomatosis of the retina and various areas of the body including the central nervous system, spinal cord, and visceral organs. SYN: *angiophacomatosis.*

hippocampal (hĭp″ō-kăm′păl) [Gr. *hippokampos,* seahorse]. Pert to the hippocampus.

hippocampal commissure. A thin sheet of fibers passing transversely under posterior portion of the corpus callosum. They connect the medial margins of the crura of the fornix. SYN: *commissure of fornix.*

hippocampal fissure. Fissure above the temporal lobe on mesial surface of cerebrum.

hippocampal formation. Olfactory structures lying along the medial margin of the pallium. It includes the hippocampus, dentate gyrus, supracallosal gyrus, longitudinal striae, subcallosal gyrus, diagonal band of Broca, and hippocampal commissure.

hippocampus major. Elevation of floor of the inferior horn of the lateral ventricle of the brain, occupying nearly all of it.

h., digitations of. Three or four shallow grooves on anterior portion of hippocampus.

hippocampus minor. A small elevation on the medial wall of the lateral ventricle formed by end of the calcarine fissure. SYN: *calcar avis* [NA].

Hippocrates (hĭ-pŏk′ră-tēz). [5th and 4th centuries B.C.] Greek physician who is referred to as the Father of Medicine because he was the first healer to attempt to record medical experiences for future reference. By so doing he established the foundation for the scientific basis of medical practice. SEE: *Hippocratic oath.*

hippocratic facies. The appearance of the face at the time of impending death.

SYM: Dark brown, livid, or lead-colored skin; hollow appearances of eyes, collapse of temples, sharpness of nose, lobes of ears contracting and turning outward.

Hippocratic oath. Oath exacted of his students by Hippocrates: "I swear by Apollo the physician, and Aesculapius, and Hygeia, and Panacea, and all the gods and goddesses, that according to my ability and judgment, I will keep this oath and its stipulation—to reckon him who taught me this art equally dear to me as my parents, to share my substance with him, and to relieve his necessities if required; to look upon his offspring in the same footing as my own brothers, and to teach them this art if they shall wish to learn it, without fee or stipulation, and that by precept, lecture, and every other mode of instruction, I will impart a knowledge of the art to my own sons, and those of my teachers, and to disciples bound by a stipulation and oath according to the law of medicine, but to none other.

"I will follow that system of regimen which, according to my ability and judgment, I consider for the benefit of my patients, and abstain from whatever is deleterious and mischievous. I will give no deadly medicine to anyone if asked, nor suggest any such counsel; and in like manner I will not give to a woman a pessary to produce abortion. With purity and with holiness I will pass my life and practice my art. I will not cut persons laboring under the stone, but will leave this to be done by men who are practitioners of this work. Into whatever houses I enter, I will go into them for the benefit of the sick, and I will abstain from every voluntary act of mischief and corruption; and, further, from the seduction of females or males, of freemen and slaves. Whatever, in connection with my professional practice, or not in connection with it, I see or hear, in the life of men, which ought not to be spoken of abroad, I will not divulge, as reckoning that all such should be kept secret.

"While I continue to keep this Oath unviolated, may it be granted to me to enjoy life and the practice of this art, respected by all men, in all times. But should I trespass and violate this Oath, may the reverse be my lot."

SEE: *Declaration of Geneva; Declaration of Hawaii; Nightingale Pledge; Prayer of Maimonides.*

hippurase (hĭp′ū-rās). Hippuricase, q.v.

hippuria (hĭ-pū′rē-ă) [Gr. *hippos,* horse, + *ouron,* urine]. Large quantities of hippuric acid in the urine.

hippuric acid. An acid formed and excreted by the kidneys. It is formed in the human body from the combination of benzoic acid and glycine, the synthesis taking place in the liver and to a limited extent in the kidney.

hippuricase (hĭ-pūr′ĭ-kās). An enzyme found in the liver, kidney, and other tissues that catalyzes the synthesis of hippuric acid from benzoic acid and glycine. SYN: *hippurase.*

hippus (hĭp′ŭs) [Gr. *hippos,* horse]. Rhythmical and rapid dilatation and contraction of the pupils. Tremor of iris, spasmodic in character.

h., respiratory. Dilatation during inspiration, and contraction of pupil during expiration.

hirci (hĭr′sī) [L., goats]. (sing. *hircus*) Axillary hairs.

hircismus (hĭr-sĭs′mŭs). A malodorous condition of the axillae caused by bacterial action on the sweat.

hircus (hĭr′kŭs) [L., goat]. Sing. of hirci.

Hirschberg's reflex (hĭrsh bĕrgz). [Leonard Keene Hirschberg, U.S. neurologist, b. 1877] Adduction of foot when sole at base of great toe is irritated.

Hirschsprung's disease (hĭrsh′sprŭngz). [Harold Hirschsprung, Dan. physician, 1830–1916] Megacolon due to failure of development of the myenteric plexus of the rectosigmoid area of the large intestine. The colon above the inactive area of the sigmoid dilates and there is chronic constipation, abdominal distention, and fecal impaction.

TREATMENT: Surgical excision of affected bowel is the treatment of choice. The remaining normal colon is anastomosed to the anus. SYN: *megacolon.*

hirsute (hŭr′sūt) [L. *hirsutus,* shaggy]. Hairy.

hirsuties (hŭr-sū′shē-ēz). Hirsutism.

hirsutism (hŭr′sūt-ĭzm). Condition characterized by the excessive growth of hair or the presence of hair in unusual places, esp. in women.

hirudicide (hĭ-rū'dĭ-sīd) [L. *hirudo,* a leech, + *caedere,* to kill]. Any substance that destroys leeches.

hirudin (hĭ-rū'dĭn). A substance present in the secretion of the buccal glands of the leech that prevents coagulation of the blood by inactivating thrombin.

Hirudinea (hĭr"ū-dĭn'ē-ă). A class of Annelida. They are hermaphroditic, lack setae or appendages, and usually possess two suckers. Includes the bloodsucking leeches. A number of species, including H. medicinalis, were formerly used extensively for bloodletting.

hirudiniasis (hĭr"ū-dĭn-ī'ă-sĭs). Infestation by leeches. In external hirudiniasis, leeches attach themselves to the skin and suck blood. After the leeches drop off, bleeding may continue as a result of the action of hirudin. Bites may become infected or ulcerate.

h., internal. Results from accidental ingestion of leeches in drinking water. They may attach themselves to the wall of the pharynx, nasal cavity, or larynx.

Hirudo (hĭ-roo'dō) [L., leech]. A genus of leeches belonging to the family Gnathobdellidae.

His, Jr., Wilhelm (hĭs). German physician, 1863–1934.

H. bundle. The atrioventricular bundle (A-V bundle), a group of modified muscle fibers, Purkinje fibers, forming a part of the impulse-conducting system of the heart. It arises in the atrioventricular node and continues in the interventricular septum as a single bundle, the crus commune, which divides into two trunks that pass respectively to the right and left ventricles, fine branches passing to all parts of the ventricles. It conducts impulses from the atria to the ventricles, and this initiates ventricular contraction.

H.-Werner disease. [Heinrich Werner, Ger. physician, b. 1874] Trench fever.

histaffine (hĭs'tă-fēn) [Gr. *histos,* tissue, + L. *affinis,* having affinity for]. Having affinity for tissues.

histaminase (hĭs-tăm'ĭ-nās). An enzyme widely distributed in the body that inactivates histamine.

histamine (hĭs'tă-mĭn, -mēn). A substance normally present in the body. It exerts a pharmacologic action when released from injured cells. The red flush of a burn is due to the local production of histamine. It is produced from the amino acid histidine. If histamine is injected intradermally and if circulation is normal, it produces a triple response characterized by a small red spot that appears within a few seconds, reaches a maximum in about a minute and then becomes bluish. This is followed by a wheal surrounded by a flare, suggesting a mosquito bite. The final reaction is the development of localized edema at the site of the small red spot. This lasts about 90 seconds. Given intravenously, histamine causes gastric secretion, flushing of skin, lowered blood pressure, and headache. Blood pressure returns to normal in a short time because the circulatory system adjusts to the vascular changes and the histamine is inactivated.

Functions of histamine include increasing gastric secretion, dilatation of capillaries, and constriction of bronchial smooth muscle.

h. phosphate. USP. Water-soluble colorless crystals. Sometimes called histamine acid phosphate or histamine diphosphate. Used most frequently as a diagnostic agent in determining the acid-secreting power of the stomach.

histamine blocking agents. Drugs that block the stimulation of cells by histamine. These agents act by interfering with the action of histamine rather than by preventing its secretion. Two classes, the H_1 receptor blocking agents and the H_2 receptor blocking agents, are known and act at different receptor sites. Cimetidine is an example of an H_2 receptor blocking agent.

histamine headache. When histamine is given by injection, an intense headache may appear. The precise relationship of this to histaminic cephalalgia is not clear. Some persons will experience headache after drinking types of wine that contain histamine. This appears to be related to the histamine content of those wines.

histaminemia (hĭs-tăm"ĭ-nē'mē-ă) [*histamine* + Gr. *haima,* blood]. Histamine in the blood.

histaminia (hĭs"tă-mĭn'ē-ă). Shock induced by histamine in the body.

histase (hĭs'tās) [Gr. *histos,* tissue]. An enzyme that digests tissue.

histenzyme (hĭst-ĕn'zīm) [" + *en,* in, + *zyme,* leaven]. An enzyme in renal tissues that splits up hippuric acid into benzoic acid and glycocol. SYN: *histozyme.*

histidase. An enzyme present in the liver that acts on 1-histidine. It splits the imidazole ring with the resultant formation of glutamic and formic acids, and ammonia.

histidine (hĭs'tĭ-dĭn, -dēn). $C_6H_9N_3O_2$. An amino acid obtained by hydrolysis from tissue proteins. Necessary for tissue repair and growth.

histidinemia (hĭs"tĭ-dĭ-nē'mē-ă). A hereditary metabolic disease caused by lack of the enzyme histidase. Histidase is normally present in the urine. Clinically the symptoms are variable.

histidinuria (hĭs"tĭ-dĭ-nū'rē-ă). Presence of histidine in the urine.

histioblast (hĭs′tē-ō-blăst″). A tissue histiocyte.

histiocyte (hĭs′tē-ō-sīt″) [Gr. *histion,* little web, + *kytos,* cell]. A cell present in all loose connective tissues. It may exhibit active ameboid movement and show marked phagocytic activity. These cells easily ingest trypan blue, colloidal carbon, and other foreign substances of a particulate nature. Histiocytes belong to the reticuloendothelial system. SYN: *clasmatocyte; macrophage.*

histiocytoma (hĭs″tē-ō-sī-tō′mă) [″ + ″ + *oma,* tumor]. A tumor containing histiocytes.

histiocytosis (hĭs″tē-ō-sī-tō′sĭs) [″ + ″ + *osis,* condition]. Histocytes in the blood in unusual numbers.

h., lipid. Neimann-Pick disease.

h. X. Letterer-Siwe disease, Letterer-Christian disease.

histiogenic (hĭs-tē-ō-jĕn′ĭk) [″ + *gennan,* to form]. Formed by the tissues. SYN: *histogenous.*

histioid (hĭs′tē-oyd) [″ + *eidos,* form]. Resembling or composed of one of the body tissues. SYN: *histoid.*

histioirritative (hĭs″tē-ō-ĭr′ĭ-tā′tĭv) [″ + L. *irritare,* to excite]. Irritative to connective tissue.

histioma (hĭs″tē-ō′mă) [″ + *oma,* tumor]. A tissue tumor. SYN: *histoma.*

histionic (hĭs″tē-ŏn′ĭk). Belonging to or originating in a tissue.

histo- [Gr. *histos,* web, tissue]. Prefix indicating rel. to tissue.

histoblast (hĭs′tō-blăst) [″ + *blastos,* germ]. A tissue cell.

histochemistry (hĭs″tō-kĕm′ĭs-trē). Study of chemistry of cells and tissues. This is done by using both light and electron microscopy and by use of special chemical tests and stains.

histochromatosis (hĭs″tō-krō″mă-tō′sĭs) [″ + *chroma,* color, + *osis,* condition]. A general term for disorders of the reticuloendothelial system.

histoclastic (hĭs″tō-klăs′tĭk) [″ + *klastos,* breaking]. Decomposing tissue.

histocompatibility (hĭs″tō-kŏm-păt″ĭ-bĭl′ĭ-tē). The ability of cells to survive without immunological interference. Esp. important in blood transfusion and transplantation.

histocompatibility antigens. Antigens present on all cell types except erythrocytes and trophoblasts. These antigens, which are serologically defined in man, are controlled by genes at three loci on chromosome 6: designated HLA-A, HLA-B, and HLA-C. These loci have multiple antigens that are important in controlling transplantation reactions. The presence of specific antigens has been correlated with specific diseases; e.g., HLA-B27 with ankylosing spondylitis, Reiter's syndrome, and psoriatic arthritis; HLA-B7 with multiple sclerosis; HLA-B8 with myasthenia gravis and idiopathic Addison's disease; and insulin-dependent diabetes mellitus with HLA-B8, -Bw15, -Dw3, -DRw3, and -DRw4. SEE: *major histocompatibility complex.*

histocompatibility genes. Genes that determine the antigenicity of tissues. These genes are important in determining whether or not the recipient will reject donor tissues or a transplanted organ. SEE: *histocompatibility antigens.*

histocyte (hĭs′tō-sīt) [″ + *kytos,* cell]. A tissue cell. SYN: *histiocyte.*

histodiagnosis (hĭs″tō-dī″ăg-nō′sĭs) [″ + *dia,* through, + *gnosis,* knowledge]. Diagnosis made from examination of the tissues, esp. by use of microscopy.

histodialysis (hĭs″tō-dī-ăl′ĭ-sĭs) [″ + *dialysis,* a loosening]. Disintegration of tissue. SYN: *histolysis.*

histodifferentiation (hĭs″tō-dĭf″ĕr-ĕn″shē-ā′shŭn). The process of cellular maturation in which a primitive cell develops into specific cellular tissue types.

histogenesis (hĭs-tō-jĕn′ĕ-sĭs) [″ + *genesis,* formation]. Development into differentiated tissues of the germ layer; origin and development of tissue.

histogenetic (hĭs″tō-jĕ-nĕt′ĭk). Pert to histogenesis.

histogenous (hĭs-tŏj′ĕ-nŭs). Made by the tissues.

histogram (hĭs′tō-gram) [L. *historia,* observation, + Gr. *gramma,* a writing]. A graph showing frequency distributions.

histography [Gr. *histos,* tissue, + *graphein,* to write]. A written description of the tissues.

histohematin (hĭs″tō-hĕm′ă-tĭn) [″ + *haima,* blood]. A hemoglobin pigment in various tissues.

histohematogenous (hĭs″tō-hĕm″ă-tŏj′ĕ-nŭs) [″ + ″ + *gennan,* to form]. Arising from both the tissues and the blood.

histoid (hĭs′toyd) [″ + *eidos,* form]. 1. Resembling one of the tissues. 2. Developed from a single tissue, as fibroma.

histokinesis (hĭs-tō-kĭ-nē′sĭs) [″ + *kinesis,* movement]. Movement in the tissues of the body.

histological (hĭs″tō-lŏj′ĭ-kăl) [″ + *logos,* knowledge]. Pert. to histology.

histologist (hĭs-tŏl′ō-jĭst). An individual who specializes in the study of cells and microscopic tissues.

histology (hĭs-tŏl′ō-jē). Study of the microscopic structure of tissue.

h., normal. Study of healthy tissue.

h., pathologic. Study of diseased tissue.

histolysis (hĭs-tŏl′ĭ-sĭs) [″ + *lysis,* dissolu-

tion]. Disintegration of tissues. SYN: *histodialysis.*
histolytic (hĭs″tō-lĭt′ĭk). Pert. to histolysis.
histoma (hĭs-tō′mă) [″ + *oma,* tumor]. A tumor composed of tissue. SYN: *histioma.*
histon(e) (hĭs′tŏn, -tōn) [Gr. *histos,* web, tissue]. A class of simple proteins derived from cell nuclei that interferes with blood coagulation. They yield certain amino acids (the histone or hexone bases) as a result of hydrolysis. Histones are found in the thymus, sperm, and blood cells.
histonectomy (hĭs″tō-nĕk′tō-mē) [″ + *ektome,* excision]. Periarterial excision of parts of the sympathetic nerve.
histonomy (hĭs-tŏn′ō-mē) [″ + *nomos,* law]. The law governing development and structure of tissues.
histonuria (hĭs-tōn-ū′rē-ă) [″ + *ouros,* urine]. Excretion of histones in the urine.
histopathology (hĭs″tō-pă-thŏl′ō-jē) [″ + *pathos,* disease, + *logos,* study]. Histology of diseased tissues.
histophysiology (hĭs″tō-fĭz″ē-ŏl′ō-jē) [″ + *physis,* nature, + *logos,* study]. Study of functions of cells and tissues.
Histoplasma (hĭs″tō-plăz′mă) [″ + *plasma,* thing formed]. A genus of parasitic fungi.
H. capsulatum. The causative agent of histoplasmosis, q.v.
histoplasmin (hĭs″tō-plăz′mĭn). USP. An antigen prepared from cultures of Histoplasma capsulatum and used as a skin test for the diagnosis of histoplasmosis.
histoplasmosis (hĭs″tō-plăz-mō′sĭs) [″ + *plasma,* plasma, + *osis,* condition]. A systemic, fungal, respiratory disease due to Histoplasma capsulatum.

SYM: The signs and symptoms vary from those of a mild self-limited infection to a severe fatal disease. In the severe form there are fever, anemia, enlargement of spleen and liver, leukopenia, pulmonary involvement, adrenal necrosis, and ulcers of the gastrointestinal tract.

TREATMENT: Amphotericin B intravenously.

historetention (hĭs″tō-rē-tĕn′shŭn) [Gr. *histos,* web, tissue, + L. *re,* back, + *tenere,* to hold]. Retention of substances in the tissues.
histotherapy (hĭs″tō-thĕr′ă-pē) [″ + *therapeia,* treatment]. Administration of animal tissues in the treatment of disease. SYN: *organotherapy.*
histothrombin (hĭs″tō-thrŏm′bĭn) [″ + *thrombos,* a clot]. A thrombin derived from connective tissue.
histotome (hĭs′tō-tōm) [″ + *tome,* incision]. Instrument for cutting tissue into very thin slices for microscopic study of its minute structure. SYN: *microtome.*
histotomy (hĭs-tŏt′ō-mē) [″ + *tome,* incision]. 1. Dissection of tissue. 2. The cutting of thin sections of tissue for microscopic study. SYN: *microtomy.*
histotoxic (hĭs″tō-tŏk′sĭk) [″ + *toxikon,* poison]. Pert. to a poisonous condition within the cells.
histotribe (hĭs′tō-trīb) [″ + *tribein,* to crush]. Instrument for crushing the tissues to stop bleeding.
histotroph (hĭs′tō-trōf) [″ + *trophe,* nourishment]. Nutritive substances, other than the mother's blood, that the embryo utilizes in early development. These include endometrial tissues that have been destroyed during implantation, extravasated blood, and glandular secretions. SYN: *embryotroph.*
histotrophic (hĭs-tō-trŏf′ĭk). 1. Pert. to or favoring the formation of tissue. 2. Pert. to histotroph, q.v.
histotrophic nutrition. Nutrition of the embryo in which histotroph serves as a source of nourishment. SEE: *hemotrophic nutrition.*
histotropic (hĭs″tō-trŏp′ĭk) [″ + *trope,* a turning]. Having attraction for tissue cells, as certain parasites, stains, or chemicals.
histozoic (hĭs″tō-zō′ĭk) [″ + *zoe,* life]. Living within or on tissues, said of certain protozoan parasites.
histozyme (hĭs′tŏ-zīm) [″ + *zyme,* leaven]. A renal enzyme that converts hippuric acid into benzoic acid and glycine, causing fermentation.
histrionic (hĭs″trē-ŏn′ĭk) [L. *histrio,* an actor]. Theatrical, dramatic.
histrionic mania. Dramatic gestures, expressions, and speech in certain psychiatric states.
hives (hīvz) [of uncertain origin]. Eruption of very itchy wheals, caused by contact with or ingestion of an allergic substance or food. Sudden sharp changes in climate may produce hives in some persons who are allergic to heat or cold. SYN: *nettle rash; urticaria.*
Hl. *hectoliter; latent hyperopia.*
HLA. *human leukocyte antigen.* SEE: *histocompatibility antigens.*
Hm. *manifest hyperopia.*
HMD. *hyaline membrane disease.*
HMG. *human menopausal gonadotrophin.*
HMO. *Health Maintenance Organization.*
HMS Liquifilm Ophthalmic. Trade name for medrysone, USP.
HNO_2. Chem. symb. for nitrous acid.
HNO_3. Chem. symb. for nitric acid.
Ho. Chem. symb. for holmium.
H_2O. Chem. symb. for water.
H_2O_2. Chem. symb. for hydrogen peroxide.
hoarseness [AS. *has,* harsh]. A rough quality of the voice.

ETIOL: Simple chronic inflammations secondary to chronic nasopharyngitis, chemical irritants, tobacco, or alcohol. Specific causes of chronic laryngitis include: syphilis, tuberculosis, leprosy, neoplasms, papilloma, angioma, fibroma, singer's nodes, carcinoma, paralyses, and prolapse of ventricle of larynx. Virilization of the female usually causes hoarseness.

hobnail liver. Liver with an irregular surface. SEE: *liver, cirrhosis of, atrophic.*

ETIOL: Cirrhosis from one of a variety of causes.

Hochsinger's sign (hōk'zĭng-ĕrz). [Karl Hochsinger, Austrian pediatrician, b. 1860] Closure of fist in tetany when the inner side of the biceps muscle is pressed.

Hodara's disease (hō-dăr'ăz). [Menahem Hodara, Turkish physician, died 1926] Trichorrhexis nodosa.

Hodgkin's disease (hŏj'kĭns). [Thomas Hodgkin, Brit. physician, 1798–1866] A disease of unknown etiology producing enlargement of lymphoid tissue, spleen, and liver with invasion of other tissues. It may appear in several forms: acute, localized, latent with relapsing pyrexia, splenomegalic, and as lymphogranulomatosis.

SYM: Painless enlargement of lymph nodes beginning in the cervical region, then the axillary, inguinal, mediastinal, and mesenteric regions. There are signs due to pressure caused by lymphoid infiltration of blood vessels, bone marrow (with consequent anemia), and organs such as the liver and spleen. Other symptoms include fever, chills, night sweats, loss of appetite and weight loss. Reed-Sternberg cells, q.v., are found in the lymph nodes.

Hodgson's disease (hŏj'sŏnz). [Joseph Hodgson, Brit. physician, 1788–1869] Aneurysmal dilatation of the aorta.

hodoneuromere (hō"dō-nū'rō-mēr) [Gr. *hodos,* path, + *neuron,* nerve, + *meros,* part]. Portion of the primitive trunk including neurons and processes.

hof [Ger., court]. The hollow area of the cell cytoplasm in which the nucleus is imbedded.

Hofbauer cell (hŏf'bow-ĕr). [J. Isfred Isidore Hofbauer, U.S. gynecologist, 1879–1961] A histiocyte found in the connective tissue of chorionic villi. It is thought to be phagocytic.

Hoffman's reflex or sign. Flicking or nipping the nail of either the second, third, or fourth finger will, if the reflex is present, cause a flexion of these fingers and maybe the thumb. The test is present when tendon reflexes are hyperactive.

hol-, holo- [Gr. *holos,* entire]. Combining form indicating complete, entire, or homogenous.

holandric (hŏl-ăn'drĭk) [" + *aner,* man]. Transmitted, i.e., inherited only through the males. Thus the genes involved are located on the Y chromosome. SEE: *hologynic.*

holarthritis (hŏl"ăr-thrī'tĭs) [" + *arthron,* joint, + *itis,* inflammation]. Inflammation of all or many joints.

Holden's line (hōl'dĕnz). [Luther Holden, Brit. anatomist, 1815–1905] A wrinkle or indistinct furrow in the groin at the junction of the thigh and the abdomen.

holergastic (hŏl"ĕr-găs'tĭk). Pert. to any psychiatric disorder of major magnitude.

holism (hōl'ĭzm). The philosophy that, in nature, entities such as individuals and other complete organisms function as complete units that cannot be reduced to the sum of their parts. Originally discussed by Jan C. Smuts.

holistic (hō-lĭs'tĭk). Pert. to holism.

holistic medicine. Comprehensive and total care of a patient. In this system, the needs of the patient in all areas, such as physical, emotional, social, and economic, are considered and cared for.

Hollenhorst plaques or bodies. [R. W. Hollenhorst, U.S. ophthalmologist, b. 1913] Atheromatous plaques that have lodged in the retinal vessels after having been broken off from the lining of other vessels. They appear as shiny irregular patches in the vessels of the retina.

hollow (hŏl'ō). A depressed area, lower than the surrounding tissue.

h., Sebileau's. [Pierre Sebileau, Fr. anatomist, 1860–1953] A depression in the floor of the mouth between the tongue and the sublingual glands.

hollow-back. Anterior posterior spinal curvature. SYN: *lordosis.*

Holmgren's test (hōlm'grĕnz). [Alarik F. Holmgren, Swedish physiologist, 1831–1897] A test in which the patient matches colored skeins of yarn to test for color blindness.

holmium (hŏl'mē-ŭm). SYMB: Ho. At. wt. 164.930; at. no. 67. A rare earth metal.

holoacardius (hŏl"ō-ă-kăr'dē-ŭs) [Gr. *holos,* entire, + *a-,* not, + *kardia,* heart]. A congenitally deformed monozygotic fetus with no heart. The in utero circulation is obtained from the heart of the twin to which the deformed fetus is attached.

holoblastic ova (hŏl"ō-blăs'tĭk) [" + *blastos,* germ]. Cleavage with segmentation of the entire yolk. Complete division of the egg as opposed to partial or meroblastic cleavage.

holocrine (hŏl'ō-krĭn) [" + *krinein,* to secrete]. Pert. to a secretory gland or its secretions consisting of altered cells of the same gland. Opposite of merocrine. SEE: *apocrine.*

holodiastolic (hŏl"ō-dī"ă-stŏl'ĭk) [" + *diastellein,* to expand]. Rel. to the entire diastole, esp. a murmur that occurs during all of diastole.

holoendemic (hŏl"ō-ĕn-dĕm'ĭk) [" + *en,* in, + *demos,* people]. 1. Term used mostly by those who investigate the epidemiology of malaria. It indicates a spleen rate of 75% in children under age 10. 2. A disease that affects all of the population in the stated area.

holoenzyme (hŏl″ō-ĕn′zīm) [″ + *en,* in, + *zyme,* leaven]. A type of enzyme consisting of a protein portion (apoenzyme) and a non-amino acid part or prosthetic group. SEE: *apoenzyme; prosthetic group.*

holography (hŏl-ŏg′ră-fē) [″ + *graphein,* to write]. A method of producing pictures in which the image appears as a three-dimensional representation of the original object. The picture obtained is called a hologram, i.e., whole message.

hologynic (hŏl″ō-jĭn′ĭk) [″ + *gyne,* woman]. Inheritance through females only. SEE: *holandric.*

holomastigote (hŏl″ō-măs′tĭ-gōt) [″ + *mastix,* lash]. Having flagella over the entire surface.

holophytic (hŏl″ō-fĭt′ĭk) [″ + *phyton,* plant]. Having plant-like characteristics, esp. in reference to protozoa that resemble plants in their metabolic processes.

holoprosencephaly (hŏl″ō-prŏs″ĕn-sĕf′ă-lē) [″ + *proso,* before, + *enkephalos,* brain]. A congenital defect due to an extra chromosome, either trisomy 13-15 or trisomy 18, which causes deficiency in the forebrain.

holorachischisis (hŏl″ō-ră-kĭs′kĭ-sĭs) [″ + *rhachis,* spine, + *schisis,* fissure]. Complete spina bifida.

holosystolic (hŏl″ō-sĭs-tŏl′ĭk) [″ + *systellein,* to draw together]. Rel. to the entire systole.

holotetanus, holotonia (hŏl-ō-tĕt′ă-nŭs, hŏl″ō-tō′nē-ah) [″ + *tetanos,* tetanus; ″ + *tonos,* tension]. Muscular spasm of the entire body.

holotonic (hŏl″ō-tŏn′ĭk). Pert. to or affected by holotonia.

holotrichous (hŏl-ŏt′rĭ-kŭs) [″ + *thrix,* hair]. Covered entirely with cilia, said of certain protozoa and bacteria.

holozoic (hŏl″ō-zō′ĭk) [″ + *zoion,* animal]. Resembling an animal as to its method of nutrition in which organic materials serve as a source of energy.

Holthouse's hernia (hŏlt′howz-ĕs). [Carsten Holthouse, Brit. surgeon, 1810–1901] Inguinal hernia protruding along the folds of the groin.

homalocephalus (hŏm″ă-lō-sĕf′ă-lŭs) [Gr. *homalos,* level, + *kephale,* head]. A person with a flat skull.

Homan's sign (hō′mănz). [John Homan, U.S. surgeon, 1877–1954] Pain in the calf when the toe is passively dorsiflexed. An early sign in venous thrombosis of the deep veins of the calf.

homatropine hydrobromide (hō-măt′rō-pēn). USP. An antimuscarinic drug that acts like belladonna. Trade name is Isopto Homatropine.

homatropine methylbromide. USP. An antimuscarinic drug that acts like belladonna. Trade name is Homapin.

homaxial (hō-măk′sē-ăl) [Gr. *homos,* same, + L. *axis,* axis]. Having all axes alike, as a sphere.

homeo- [Gr. *homoios,* like, similar]. Prefix indicating likeness or resemblance.

homeomorphous (hō″mē-ō-mor′fŭs) [″ + *morphe,* form]. Of like shape but not of same composition.

homeo-osteoplasty (hō″mē-ō-ŏs′tē-ō-plăs″tē) [″ + *osteon,* bone, + *plassein,* to form]. Grafting of a piece of bone like the one upon which it is grafted.

homeopathic (hō″mē-ō-păth′ĭk) [″ + *pathos,* disease]. Pert. to homeopathy.

homeopathist (hō-mē-ŏp′ă-thĭst). One who practices homeopathy.

homeopathy (hō-mē-ŏp′ă-thē) [Gr. *homoios,* like, + *pathos,* disease]. School of medicine, founded by Dr. S. C. F. Hahnemann (1755–1843) in the late 18th century, based on the theory that large doses of drugs that produce symptoms of a disease in healthy people will cure the same symptoms when administered in small amounts. This is loosely based on the theory that "like cures like." SEE: *allopathy.*

homeoplasia (hō″mē-ō-plā′zē-ă) [″ + *plassein,* to form]. Formation of new tissue similar to that already existing in a part.

homeoplastic (hō″mē-ō-plăs′tĭk). Rel. to or resembling the structure of adjacent parts.

homeostasis (hō″mē-ō-stā′sĭs) [″ + *stasis,* a standing]. State of equilibrium of the internal environment of the body that is maintained by dynamic processes of feedback and regulation. Homeostasis is a dynamic equilibrium.

homeostatic (hō″mē-ō-stăt′ĭk). Pert. to homeostasis.

homeotherapy (hō″mē-ō-thĕr′ă-pē) [″ + *therapeia,* treatment]. Treatment or prevention of disease with a substance similar to but not identical with the active causative agent, such as jennerian vaccination.

homeothermal (hō″mē-ō-thĕr′măl) [″ + *therme,* heat]. Pert. to a homoiotherm, q.v.

homeotransplant (hō″mē-ō-trăns′plănt) [″ + L. *trans,* across, + *plantare,* to plant]. Tissue from one individual transplanted into another of the same species.

homeotransplantation (hō″mē-ō-trăns″plăn-tā′shŭn). Tissue transplantation from one to another of the same species.

homeotypical (hō″mē-ō-tĭp′ĭ-kăl) [″ + *typos,* type]. Resembling the typical or normal.

homesickness [AS. *ham,* home, + *seoc,* ill]. Sadness and depression incident to being away from home or away from loved ones.

homicide (hŏm′ĭ-sīd) [L. *homo,* man, + *caedere,* to kill]. 1. Murder. 2. A murderer.

hominid (hŏm′ĭ-nĭd) [″ + *eidos,* form]. A

primate of the Hominidae family. Man is the only surviving species.

homo- [Gr. *homos,* same]. Prefix meaning the same or a likeness.

homoblastic (hō″mō-blăs′tĭk) [″ + *blastos,* germ]. Developing from a single type of tissue. Opposite of heteroblastic.

homocentric (hō″mō-sĕn′trĭk) [″ + *kentron,* center]. Having the same center.

homochronous (hō-mŏk-rō′nŭs) [″ + *chronos,* time]. Occurring at the same time or at the same age in each generation.

homocladic (hō″mō-klăd′ĭk) [″ + *klados,* branch]. Pert. to an anastomosis between branches of the same artery. Opposite of heterocladic.

homocysteine (hō″mō-sĭs-tē′ĭn). In the catabolism of methionine, the next highest homologue.

homocystine (hō″mō-sĭs′tĭn). A homologue of cystine formed during the catabolism of methionine.

homocystinuria (hō″mō-sĭs-tĭn-ū′rē-ă). An inherited disease caused by the absence of the enzyme essential to the metabolism of homocystine. Clinically the disease is similar to Marfan's syndrome. Patients are mentally retarded, have subluxated lenses, tendency to seizures, liver disease, and failure to grow at a normal rate.

homocytotropic (hō″mō-sī″tō-trŏp′ĭk) [″ + *kytos,* cell, + *tropos,* a turning]. Having an affinity for cells of the same species.

homodromous (hō-mŏd′rō-mŭs) [″ + *dromos,* running]. Moving in the same direction or toward the same goal.

homoerotic (hō″mō-ĕ-rŏt′ĭk). Homosexuality.

homogametic (hō″mō-gă-mĕt′ĭk) [″ + *gamos,* marriage]. Pert. to the production of one kind of gamete as regards the sex chromosome. In humans, the XX female is the homogametic sex, as all ova produced contain the X chromosome. SEE: *heterogametic.*

homogenate (hō-mŏj′ĕ-nāt). The material obtained when something is homogenized.

homogeneous (hō″mō-jē′nē-ŭs) [″ + *genos,* kind]. Uniform in structure, composition, or nature. Opposite of heterogeneous.

homogenesis (hō-mō-jĕn′ĕ-sĭs) [″ + *genesis,* development]. Reproduction by the same process in succeeding generations. Opposite of heterogenesis.

homogenize (hō-mŏj′ĕ-nīz). To make homogeneous; to produce a uniform emulsion or suspension of two substances normally immiscible.

homogentisic acid. Alkaptone; an acid in the urine due to incomplete oxidation of tyrosine.

homogentisuria (hō″mō-jĕn″tĭ-sū′rē-ă). Alkaptonuria, q.v.

homoglandular (hō″mō-glăn′dū-lăr) [″ + L. *glandula,* a little acorn]. Rel. to the same gland.

homograft (hō′mō-grăft). Transplant tissue obtained from the same species. The tissues that survive best are cornea, bone, artery, and cartilage. SYN: *allograft.*

homoiopodal (hō″moy-ŏp′ō-dăl) [Gr. *homoios,* like, + *pous, pod-,* foot]. Having only one kind of process, as nerve cells.

homoiotherm (hō-moy′ō-thĕrm) [″ + *therme,* heat]. A warm-blooded organism. Opposite of poikilotherm.

homokeratoplasty (hō″mō-kĕr′ă-tō-plăs″tē). A homograft of corneal tissue.

homolateral [Gr. *homos,* same, + L. *latus,* side]. Pert. to or on the same side. Opposite of contralateral. SYN: *ipsilateral.*

homologous (hō-mŏl′ō-gŭs) [″ + *logos,* proportion]. Similar in fundamental structure and in origin but not necessarily in function.

Ex.: the arm of man, forelimb of a dog, and the wing of a bird are homologous structures.

homologous organs. Structures that are morphological equivalents, as the arm of man and forelimb of quadrupeds; penis of male and clitoris of female.

homologous series. Compounds with a similar chemical structure and properties, arranged in order of their molecular complexity, such as methane and ethane.

homologous tissues. Tissues identical in structure.

homologous vaccine. Vaccine from the microorganism infecting the patient. SYN: *vaccine, autogenous.*

homologue (hŏm′ō-lŏg). 1. An organ or part common to a number of species. 2. One that corresponds to a part or organ in another structure. 3. In chemistry, any member of a series that resembles the other members in action and general structure but will have a constant compositional difference such as a methyl, CH_3, group.

homology (hō-mŏl′ō-jē) [″ + *logos,* proportion]. Similarity in structure but not necessarily in function. Opposite of analogy.

homolysin (hō-mŏl′ĭ-sĭn) [″ + *lysis,* dissolution]. An agent in serum destructive to erythrocytes. SYN: *isolysin.*

homonomous (hō-mŏn′ō-mŭs) [″ + *nomos,* law]. Pert. to parts arranged in a series that are similar in form and structure, as metameres of a segmented animal or the fingers and toes.

homonymous (hō-mŏn′ĭ-mŭs) [″ + *onyma,* name]. Having the same name.

homonymous diplopia. Diplopia in which the image seen by the right eye is on the right side and vice versa.

homophil (hō′mō-fĭl) [″ + *philein,* to love]. Pert. to an antibody reacting only with a specific antigen.

homophile (hō-mō-fīl′). Homosexual.

homophobia. Fear or dislike of homosexuals.

homoplastic (hō″mō-plăs′tĭk) [″ + *plassein,* to form]. Having similar form and structure.

homoplasty (hō′mō-plăs″tē). Repair by tissue similar to the one replaced.

Homo sapiens (hō′mō sā′pē-ĕnz) [L. *homo,* man, + *sapiens,* wise, sapient]. The species to which modern man belongs.

homosexual (hō″mō-sĕks′ū-ăl) [Gr. *homos,* same, + L. *sexus,* sex]. 1. One sexually attracted to another of the same sex. SYN: *homophile.* 2. Pert. to attraction to another of same sex. SEE: *asexual; bisexual; heterosexual; lesbian.*

homosexuality (hō″mō-sĕks″ū-ăl′ĭ-tē). A condition in which the libido is directed toward one of the same sex. In females it is called lesbianism.

homostimulant (hō″mō-stĭm′ū-lănt) [″ + L. *stimulare,* to arouse]. Stimulating the organ from which an extract is derived.

Homo-Tet. Trade name for tetanus immune globulin.

homothallic (hŏm″ō-thăl′ĭk). In bacteriology, indicating the possibility of mating of cells of the same strain.

homotherm (hō′mō-thĕrm). An animal whose body temperature remains constant regardless of the temperature of the environment. SYN: *animal, warm-blooded.* SEE: *poikilotherm.*

homothermal (hō″mō-thĕr′măl) [″ + *therme,* heat]. Characterized by maintenance of body temperature at a fairly constant level regardless of the temperature of the environment. SYN: *homoiothermal.*

homotonic (hō″mō-tŏn′ĭk) [″ + *tonos,* tension]. Of uniform tension.

homotopic (hō″mō-tŏp′ĭk) [″ + *topos,* place]. Occurring at the same site on the body.

homotype (hō′mō-tīp) [″ + *typos,* type]. One organ or part similar in form and function to another, as one of two paired parts or organs.

homotypic (hō-mō-tĭp′ĭk). Of the same form and type.

homozygosis (hō″mō-zī-gō′sĭs) [″ + *zygon,* yoke, pair, + *osis,* condition]. Formation of a zygote by the union of gametes that have one or more identical alleles. SEE: *heterozygosis.*

homozygote (hō″mō-zī′gōt). A homozygous individual; an individual developing from gametes with similar alleles and thus possessing like pairs of genes for a given hereditary characteristic.

homozygous (hō″mō-zī′gŭs). 1. Produced by similar alleles. 2. Said of an organism when germ cells transmit nearly identical alleles resulting from inbreeding.

homunculus (hō-mŭn′kū-lŭs) [L. diminutive of *homo,* man]. A dwarf in which the parts of the body develop in their normal proportions.

honey [AS. *hunig*]. A sweet thick liquid substance produced by bees from the nectar gathered from flowers and stored by them for food. The color and flavor are determined by the flowers used. Honey has been used by man as a food since ancient times when it was early man's principal source of sugar. About 80% of honey is levulose and dextrose, the remainder mostly water.

Honey is not sterile. Its use in preparing infants' formula has caused botulism.

hook [AS. *hok,* an angle]. 1. A curved instrument. 2. Type of prehension using fingers independently of thumb and palm.

hookworm. A parasitic nematode belonging to the superfamily Strongyloidea, esp. Ancylostoma duodenale and Necator americanus, q.v.

hookworm disease. A condition brought about by the presence of the hookworm in the intestinal tract. For complete description and treatment SEE: *ancylostomiasis* and *Necator americanus.* SYN: *ancylostomiasis; uncinariasis.*

hopelessness. The reaction of feeling that a situation, condition, or illness is without solution or amelioration. This reaction can be seen in either the patient or the health care personnel or both. In certain situations such as grief reaction, q.v., or mourning, there occurs a normal period of feelings of despair, helplessness, and apathy. If this continues for an inordinately long period, then hopelessness develops. The alert medical and nursing team will be aware of the development of this reaction and take the appropriate action to prevent its continuation. When those responsible for providing medical care develop the feeling that a patient's condition is hopeless, this leads to the development of their giving up in their efforts to treat the patient effectively. SEE: *giving-up; grief reaction; helplessness.*

hordeolum (hor-dē′ō-lŭm) [L., barleycorn]. Inflammation of a sebaceous gland of the eyelid. SYN: *sty.*

h. internum. Suppuration of Zeiss or meibomian glands.

horizontal [L. *horizontalis*]. 1. Parallel to or in the plane of the horizon. 2. A transverse plane of the body that is at right angles to the vertical axis of the body.

horizontal position. A position in which the patient lies supine and parallel to the floor. Employed in palpitation and auscultation of fetal heartbeat and in operative procedures.

In the abdominal horizontal position the patient lies flat on his or her abdomen. This position is used in the examination of the back and spinal column.

hormesis (hor-mē′sĭs) [Gr. *hormesis,* rapid motion]. The stimulating effect of a small dose of a substance that is toxic in a larger dose.

hormion (hor'mē-ŏn) [Gr., little chain]. Junction of the posterior border of the vomer with the sphenoid bone.

hormonagogue (hor-mōn'ă-gŏg) [Gr. *hormon,* urging on, + *agogos,* leading]. Stimulating or increasing the production of a hormone.

hormonal (hor-mō'năl). Rel. to or acting as a hormone.

hormone (hor'mōn) [Gr. *hormon,* urging on]. 1. A substance originating in an organ, gland, or part, which is conveyed through the blood to another part of the body, stimulating it by chemical action to increased functional activity or to increase secretion of another hormone. 2. The secretion of the ductless glands, such as insulin, by the pancreas. SEE: *endocrine gland.*

h., adaptive. A hormone that is produced in response to adapting to stress or some other powerful stimulus.

h., adrenocortical. Hormone secreted by the cortex of the adrenal gland. SEE: *adrenal gland.*

h., adrenocorticotropic. ABBR: ACTH. A hormone secreted by the anterior lobe of the hypophysis (pituitary gland) that stimulates the adrenal cortex. SYN: *corticotropin.*

h., adrenomedullary. Hormones, epinephrine and norepinephrine, produced by the adrenal medulla.

h., androgenic. Hormone that regulates the development and maintenance of the male secondary sexual characteristics; an androgen, q.v. Androgens are secreted by the interstitial tissue of the testis and by the adrenal cortex of both sexes. Includes testosterone, androsterone, and dehydroandrosterone.

h., anterior pituitary. Hormones secreted by the anterior lobe of the hypophysis. Includes the growth hormone; thyrotropic (TH); gonadotropic; follicle-stimulating (FSH); interstitial cell–stimulating or luteotropic (ICSH); prolactin; melanocyte-stimulating; and adrenocorticotropic (ACTH) hormones.

h., antidiuretic. Vasopressin. A hormone formed in supraoptic and paraventricular nuclei of hypothalamus and transported to posterior lobe of hypophysis through the hypothalamo-hypophyseal tract. It has an antidiuretic and a pressor effect that elevates blood pressure.

h., calcitonin. Hormone produced in the thyroid gland. Important in regulating calcium and bone metabolism.

h., corpus luteum. Progesterone.

h., cortical. H., adrenocortical, q.v.

h., ectopic. SEE: *ectopic secretion.*

h., estrogenic. A hormone, as estrogen, that stimulates the development and maintenance of female sexual characteristics. Estrogens are secreted by the ovary, the placenta, and the adrenal cortex in both sexes. Include estradiol, estrone, and estriol.

h., follicle. Hormone secreted by the ovarian follicles; an estrogen

h., follicle-stimulating. ABBR: FSH. Hormone secreted by the anterior lobe of the hypophysis that stimulates maturation of the ovarian follicles in the female. In the male the hormone is important in maintaining spermatogenesis.

h., gastric. Gastrin.

h., gonadotropic. Anterior pituitary hormone affecting the gonads.

h., growth, human growth. ABBR: GH. Anterior pituitary hormone promoting normal growth. SYN: *somatotropin.*

h., inhibitory. Substances that inhibit the release of certain hormones from the pituitary. Somatostatin, which inhibits the release of growth hormone, is included in this group.

h., interstitial cell–stimulating. ABBR: ICSH. H., luteinizing.

h., intestinal. A hormone produced by the mucosa of the intestine. SEE: *cholecystokinin; secretin.*

h., lactogenic. Prolactin q.v.

h., luteal. Hormone produced by the corpus luteum. SYN: *progesterone.*

h., luteinizing. ABBR: LH. Hormone produced by the anterior lobe of the hypophysis that stimulates development of interstitial cells of the testes and the secretion of testosterone by those cells. In the female this hormone, working in conjunction with follicle-stimulating hormone, is responsible for maturation of the follicle of the ovary, and its rupture and transformation into the corpus luteum. SYN: *h., interstitial cell–stimulating (ICSH).*

h., luteotropic. Hormone produced by the anterior lobe of the hypophysis that stimulates the secretion of progesterone by the corpus luteum and secretion of milk by the mammary gland.

h., melanocyte-stimulating. ABBR: MSH. Hormone from the anterior pituitary. It causes pigmentation of the skin.

h., ovarian. A hormone produced by the ovary. SEE: *estradiol; estriol; estrogen; estrone; progesterone.*

h., pancreatic. Hormone produced by the islets of Langerhans of the pancreas. SEE: *insulin.*

h., parathyroid. Hormone secreted by the parathyroid glands that regulates calcium and phosphorus metabolism. Deficiency results in tetany. SEE: *parathormone.*

h., placental. Hormone secreted by the placenta. Includes chorionic gonadotropin;

hormone similar to thyroid-stimulating hormone; a type of melanocyte-stimulating hormone; a variety of ACTH.

h., posterior pituitary. Hormone secreted by the posterior lobe of the hypophysis. Includes vasopressin, which produces vasopressor and antidiuretic effects, and oxytocin, which causes contraction of smooth muscles of the uterus.

h., progestational. Progesterone, q.v. SEE: *progestational agent.*

h., progesterone. $C_{21}H_{30}O_2$, a steroid hormone obtained from the corpus luteum, adrenals, or placenta. It is responsible for changes in uterine endometrium in the second half of the menstrual cycle in preparation for implantation of the blastocyst; development of maternal placenta after implantation; and development of mammary glands.

USES: In treatment of menstrual disorders (amenorrhea, dysmenorrhea) and threatened abortion.

h., prolactin. Hormone of the anterior pituitary that is important in lactation.

h., releasing. Substances secreted by the hypothalamus that control the release of various hormones. Thyroid-stimulating hormone, follicle-stimulating hormone, and luteinizing hormone are included in this group. Growth hormone releasing factors have been discovered, but those for corticotropin, ACTH, and prolactin have not yet been isolated.

h., sex. Androgenic and estrogenic hormones.

h., somatotrophic. Growth hormone.

h., somatrophin releasing. The growth hormone releasing factor from the hypothalamus.

h., testicular. Hormone produced by the interstitial tissue of the testis, e.g., testosterone, androsterone, and dehydroandrosterone, q.v.

h., thyroid. The hormone secreted by follicles of the thyroid gland.

h., thyrotropic. Hormone produced by the anterior lobe of the hypophysis that regulates development and functioning of the thyroid gland.

hormonic (hor-mŏn'ĭk) [Gr. *hormon,* urging on]. Rel. to or acting as a hormone. SYN: *hormonal.*

hormonogenesis (hor"mō-nō-jĕn'ĕ-sĭs) [" + *genesis,* production]. Production of an internal secretion. SYN: *hormonopoiesis.*

hormonogenic (hor"mō-nō-jĕn'ĭk) [" + *gennan,* to produce]. Producing hormones. SYN: *hormonopoietic; hormopoietic.*

hormonology (hor"mō-nŏl'ō-jē) [" + *logos,* study]. The study of hormones. SYN: *clinical endocrinology.*

hormonopoiesis (hor"mō-poy-ē'sĭs) [" + *poiesis,* formation]. The production of hormones. SYN: *hormonogenesis.*

hormonopoietic (hor-mō-poy-ĕt'ĭk). Rel. to hormones and their formation.

hormonotherapy (hor"mō-nō-thĕr'ă-pē). Therapeutic use of hormones.

hormonotropic (hor"mō-nō-trŏp'ĭk). Stimulation of production of a hormone.

horn. A cutaneous outgrowth composed chiefly of keratin. A hornlike projection. SYN: *cornu.*

h., anterior, of spinal cord. The horn-shaped portion of the gray substance of anterior part of the spinal cord. SEE: *spinal cord.*

h., cicatricial. Cutaneous horn originating in scar tissue.

h., cutaneous. A hard, horny outgrowth from the skin. It is slow-growing, benign, and may be small or large, 10 to 12 cm., in diameter.

h., dorsal. Posterior projection of gray matter of the spinal cord.

h. of Ammon. Hippocampus.

h., posterior. The horn-shaped portion of the gray substance of the posterior part of the spinal cord. SEE: *spinal cord.*

h., sebaceous. A hard protrusion from a sebaceous gland.

h., ventral. Anterior projection of gray matter of the spinal cord.

h., warty. A hard outgrowth from a wart.

Horner's syndrome (hor'nĕrz). [Johann F. Horner, Swiss ophthalmologist, 1831–1886] Contraction of the pupil, partial ptosis of the eyelid, enophthalmos, and sometimes loss of sweating over the affected side of the face. Due to paralysis of the cervical sympathetic nerve trunk.

hornet sting. A general urticaria that may result from the sting of this insect.

TREATMENT: Remove the stinger; apply cold compresses. Household ammonia in 10% solution applied to the area is beneficial and subsequent soothing lotions such as calamine lotion may be used. If pain is intense, a local anesthetic may be injected. If the systemic reaction is intense, 1 ml. of epinephrine of 1:1000 concentration may be given subcutaneously to adults. An injectable antihistamine may be administered subcutaneously or intravenously if given slowly.

horny. Resembling or consisting of horn.

horopter (hō-rŏp'tĕr) [Gr. *horos,* limit, + *opter,* observer]. Sum of all points in space that have a corresponding point on the retina of the eye.

horripilation (hor"ĭ-pĭ-lā'shŭn) [L. *horrere,* to bristle, + *pilus,* hair]. Gooseflesh. SYN: *cutis anserina.*

horseshoe fistula. A fistulous tract in a semicircle in front of or behind the anus.

horseshoe kidney. A congenital abnormality in which both kidneys are united at their lower poles, thus forming a horseshoe mass generally at a lower level than normal.

hospice (hŏs'pĭs). An interdisciplinary program of palliative care and supportive services that addresses the physical, spiritual, social, and economic needs of terminally ill patients and their families. This care may be provided in the home or a hospice center.

hospital [L. *hospitalis,* pert. to a guest]. Institution for medical and surgical treatment of the sick and injured.

h., base. A hospital unit within the lines of an army for reception from the front of wounded and sick patients as well as for those within the line.

h., camp. An immobile military unit for care of sick and wounded in camp.

h., evacuation. A mobile advance hospital unit to take the place of field hospitals and to supplement base hospitals.

h., field. A portable military hospital beyond the zone of conflict and beyond the dressing stations.

hospitalism [L. *hospitalis,* pert. to a guest, + Gr. *-ismos,* condition]. 1. The air of depression and apathy that often surrounds a group of seriously ill patients, esp. if they are in the same ward and overcrowded. 2. A neurotic tendency to seek hospitalization and, once hospitalized, to resist being discharged.

hospitalization. Removal of a patient to, and confinement in, a hospital.

host [L. *hospes,* a stranger]. 1. The organism from which a parasite obtains its nourishment. 2. In embryology, the larger and relatively normal of conjoined twins. 3. In transplantation of tissue, the individual who receives the graft.

h., accidental. A host other than the usual or normal host.

h., alternate. H., intermediate.

h., definitive. 1. The final host or the host in which the parasite reaches sexual maturity. 2. The vertebrate, when the intermediate host is an invertebrate.

h., final. H., definitive.

h., intermediate. 1. Host in which a parasite passes through its larval or asexual stages of development. 2. The invertebrate host, when final host is a vertebrate.

h. of predilection. The host preferred by a parasite.

h., primary. H., final.

h., reservoir. A host other than the usual or normal one, one in which a parasite is capable of living and serving as a source of infestation.

h., secondary. H., intermediate.

h., transfer. An interim host that is not essential for the completion of the life cycle of the parasite.

hostility (hŏ-stĭl'ĭ-tē). In psychiatry, the manifestation of anger, animosity, or antagonism in a situation where such a reaction is unwarranted. Hostility may be directed toward oneself, others, or inanimate objects. It is almost always a symptom of depression.

hot [AS. *hat,* hot]. 1. Possessing a high temperature. 2. Actively conducting an electrical current. 3. Contaminated with dangerous radioactive material.

hot flashes. A symptom complex usually associated with menopause, q.v. Hot flashes, or hot flushes, may start with an aura followed by a feeling of discomfort in the abdominal area, perhaps a chill quickly followed by a feeling of heat moving toward the head. Next the face becomes red, then there is sweating followed by exhaustion. The cause of hot flashes is not completely understood and is controversial.

Hottentot apron [Hottentot, southern African population]. Excessive elongation of the labia minora seen in Hottentot women. SYN: *velamen vulvae.*

hottentotism (hŏt'ĕn-tŏt-ĭsm) [*Hottentot* + Gr. *-ismos,* condition]. Abnormal form of stuttering.

hot water bag. Rubber or plastic bag of various shapes and sizes for applying dry heat to circumscribed areas and for keeping moist applications warm.

hourglass contraction. Excessive, irregular contraction of an organ at its center, as the pregnant uterus during third stage of labor. The placenta is held in the upper part of the uterus by a tightly constricting band between the lower and upper uterine segments. SEE: *ectasia.*

hourglass stomach. Division of stomach (in form of an hourglass) by a muscular constriction; often associated with gastric ulcer.

housefly. Musca domestica, a fly belonging to the order Diptera. Serves as a transmitter of organisms of many infectious diseases.

housemaid's knee. A traumatism resulting from kneeling, which produces a swelling of the bursa anterior to the patella.

house physician. A physician, esp. an intern or resident, who is responsible for caring for patients under the direction of the medical and surgical staff.

house staff. The interns and externs of a hospital acting under direction of the general staff.

house surgeon. ABBR: H.S. The senior surgical member of the hospital staff who acts for the attending surgeon in his or her absence.

Houston's muscle (hūs'tŏns) [John Houston, Irish surgeon, 1802–1845] The anterior part of the musculus bulbocavernosus.

Houston's valves. The normal folds of mucous membrane or valves formed by them in the rectum. They are crescent-shaped. SYN:

plicae transversales recti.

Howell-Jolly bodies. [William H. Howell, U.S. physiologist, 1860–1945; Justin Jolly, Fr. histologist, 1870–1953] Spherical granules seen in erythrocytes in slides of stained blood. They are thought to be nuclear particles. The bodies are seen in cases of congenital absence of the spleen; following splenectomy; in hemolytic anemia; in pernicious anemia; in thalassemia; and in leukemia.

Howship's lacunae. [John Howship, Brit. surgeon, 1781–1841] Small pits, grooves, or depressions found where resorption of bone is occurring. They are usually occupied by osteoclasts. SEE: *osteoclast.*

Howship's symptom. Paresthesia or pain in the obturator hernia on the inner side of the thigh.

Hp. *haptoglobin.*

H.P. Acthar Gel. Trade name for corticotropin.

HPG. *human pituitary gonadotropin.*

HPL. *human placental lactogen.*

HPO_3. Metaphosphoric acid.

H_3PO_2. Hypophosphorous acid.

H_3PO_3. Phosphorous acid.

H_3PO_4. Orthophosphoric acid.

$H_4P_2O_6$. Hypophosphoric acid.

hr. *hour.*

H.S. *house surgeon.*

h.s. *hora somni,* at bedtime.

H_2S. Hydrogen sulfide.

HSA. *human serum albumin.*

H_2SO_3. Sulfurous acid.

H_2SO_4. Sulfuric acid.

H-substance. A substance similar to or identical with histamine.

5-HT. *five hydroxytryptamine,* serotonin.

Ht. *total hypermetropia.*

ht. *height.*

Hubbard tank. A tank of suitable size and shape for use in doing active or passive underwater exercises.

Huguier's canal (ē-gē-āz'). [Pierre C. Huguier, Fr. surgeon, 1804–1873] A canal through which the chorda tympani nerve exits from the cranium.

Huhner test (hoon'ĕr). [Max Huhner, U.S. urologist, 1873–1947] Test for sterility in the male that consists of aspiration of the vagina within an hour after unprotected coitus to investigate sperm motility.

hum. A soft continuous sound.

h., venous. Sound from large veins in certain anemias.

human [L. *humanus,* human]. Pert to or characterizing man or mankind.

human bite. Wound caused by human teeth.

SYM: Intense swelling, edema, and foul discharge may develop. The organisms that may be found in wounds from such bites are staphylococcus, streptococcus, anaerobic streptococcus, Vincent's bacillus, spirochete, fusiform bacillus, and gas-gangrene bacillus. The fusiform bacillus and the spirochete are believed to cause the gangrenous nature of the wounds.

TREATMENT: If lymphangitis, moderate fever, and leukocytosis occur, a wide incision may be necessary with debridement and irrigation. Bacterial examination of pustular material taken from the wound will permit appropriate antibiotic therapy. Victims of a human bite need the immediate attention of a physician.

human insulin. Insulin prepared by a synthetic process involving use of recombinant DNA technology utilizing strains of Escherichia coli. In its effect it is similar to highly purified animal insulins. Trade names are Humulin R for regular rapid-acting form; and Humulin N for intermediate-acting form.

human placental lactogen. ABBR: HPL. A hormonal substance produced by the placenta. Its actions include stimulating the metabolism of glucose and converting it to fat.

Humatin. Trade name for paromomycin sulfate.

humectant (hū-mĕk'tănt) [L. *humectus,* moist]. A moistening agent.

humeral (hū'mĕr-ăl) [L. *humerus,* upper arm]. Pert. to the humerus.

humeroradial (hū"mĕr-ō-rā'dē-ăl) [" + *radius,* wheel spoke, ray]. Pert. to the humerus and radius, esp. in comparison of their length.

humeroscapular (hū"mĕr-ō-skăp'ū-lăr) [" + *scapula,* shoulder blade]. Concerning the humerus and scapula.

humeroulnar (hū"mĕr-ō-ŭl'năr) [" + *ulna,* elbow]. Pert. to the humerus and ulna, esp. in comparison of their length.

humerus (hū'mĕr-ŭs) [L., upper arm]. Upper bone of the arm from the elbow (articulating with the ulna and radius) to the shoulder joint, where it articulates with the scapula. SEE: illus.

h., fracture of. If the fracture is of the upper end, the arm is abducted on a wire splint for about four weeks. Movements of the elbow and wrist are started early, and active movements of the shoulder are begun in about three weeks. SEE: *acromiohumeral; capitellum; cubitus; glenoid cavity.*

In a fracture of the shaft and lower end of the humerus, the limb is put in plaster in a position midway between pronation and supination with the humerus at right angles to the forearm. Movement of the shoulder, wrist, and finger is allowed at once.

humid [L. *humidus,* moist]. Moist, damp, esp. when pert. to air.

humid gangrene. Gangrene with serous exudation and rapid decomposition. SEE: *gan-*

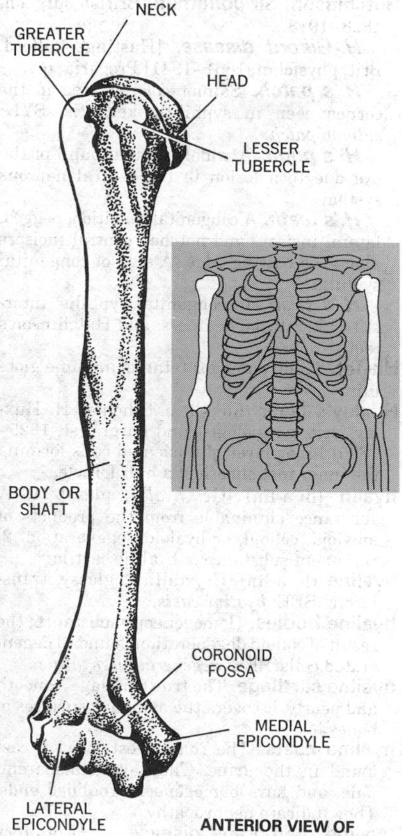

ANTERIOR VIEW OF RIGHT HUMERUS

grene.

humidifier (hū-mĭd′ĭ-fī″ĕr). Apparatus to increase moisture content of the air in a room.

humidity [L. *humiditas*]. Moisture in the atmosphere.

The moisture content of air usually is expressed as relative humidity. This indicates the amount of water vapor in the air compared to the maximum amount of moisture the air could contain at that temperature and atmospheric pressure. Air that is fully saturated with moisture has 100% relative humidity. When air that is fully saturated is cooled, the excess moisture condenses as in the case of dew or moisture on a cold glass in the summer.

Air Is Completely Saturated with Water Vapor

At:		If it Contains
F.	C.	grams
50°	10°	9.6 water/cubic meter
60°	15.5°	13.3 water/cubic meter
70°	21°	18.1 water/cubic meter
90°	32°	32.7 water/cubic meter

If air was saturated at a temperature of 70° F. (21.1° C.), water would condense on all objects if the temperature fell to 68° F. (20° C.). Air can contain at 90° F. (32.2° C.) almost twice as much water as at 70° F. (21.1° C.). SEE: table.

Moist air is less dense than completely dry air. This is another reason for humidifying oxygen or air used in inhalation therapy. Also humid air is much less irritating to the respiratory tract mucosa than dry air.

humor (hū′mor) [L. *humor*, fluid]. 1. Any fluid or semifluid substance in the body. 2. In ancient medicine, the four juices or fluids (blood, phlegm, black bile, yellow bile) of which the body was thought to be composed.

h., aqueous. The clear, watery fluid in the anterior and posterior chambers of the eye. It is produced by the ciliary processes and passes from the posterior to the anterior chamber, and then to the venous system by way of the canal of Schlemm.

h., crystalline. The fluidlike substance of the crystalline lens of the eye.

h., vitreous. The vitreous body. A semifluid, transparent substance occupying the space between the lens and retina.

humoral (hū′mor-ăl) [L. *humor*, fluid]. Pert. to body fluids or substances contained in them.

humpback (hŭmp′băk). 1. Curvature of the spine to such an extent that the back appears to have a lump or protuberance on it. 2. An individual with a humpback. SYN: *kyphosis*.

Humulin N, Humulin R. Trade names for human insulin.

hunchback (hŭnch′băk). A person with kyphosis such that there is a prominent rounded deformity of the back.

hunger [AS. *hungur*]. 1. A sensation resulting from lack of food, characterized by dull or acute pain referred to the epigastrium or lower part of chest. Usually accompanied by weakness and an overwhelming desire to eat. Hunger pains coincide with powerful contractions of the stomach. Hunger is distinguished from appetite in that the latter is a pleasant sensation based on previous experience that causes one to seek food for the purpose of tasting and enjoying it. 2. To have a strong desire.

h., air. Dyspnea; breathlessness.

hunger contractions. Contractions occurring in the normal empty stomach. They may be painful. A series of such contractions is followed by a period of rest, after which they may return with great intensity unless food is taken. Digestion may be activated under such conditions.

hunger cure. Restricted diet or fasting for cure of disease.

Hunner's ulcer (hŭn'ĕrz). [Guy LeRoy Hunner, U.S. surgeon, b. 1868] A painful, slow-to-heal ulcer of the urinary bladder.

Hunter's canal. [John Hunter, Brit. anatomist and surgeon, 1728–1793] Canalis adductorius. SEE: *canal, adductor.*

Hunter's disease. [C. H. Hunter, contemporary Canadian physician] Mucopolysaccharidosis II.

hunterian chancre. Indurated, syphilitic chancre. SEE: *chancre.*

Huntington's chorea. [G. Huntington, U.S. physician, 1850–1916] An inherited disease of the central nervous system that usually has its onset between 30 and 50 years of age. The patient has progressive dementia with bizarre involuntary movements characteristic of chorea. The posture is abnormal. The disease slowly progresses and death is usually due to an intercurrent infection. There is no effective specific therapy.

Hunt's neuralgia or syndrome. [James R. Hunt, U.S. neurologist, 1872–1937] Herpes zoster of the ganglion of the facial nerve. There is pain in the ear with a bloody serous discharge due to vesicles on the tympanic membrane. The face is paralyzed on the affected side and there is loss of sense of taste in the anterior two thirds of the tongue on the affected side.

Hurler's syndrome (hoor'lĕrz). [Gertrud Hurler, Austrian pediatrician] Congenital abnormality of bones and cartilage with deranged mucopolysaccharide metabolism, kyphosis and other skeletal deformities, possible mental deficiency, and cloudy corneae. SYN: *lipochondrodystrophy.*

Hürthle cells (hĕr'tĕl). [Karl Hürthle, Ger. histologist, b. 1860] Large eosinophil-staining cells occasionally present in the thyroid gland.

Hürthle cell tumor. A tumor of the thyroid gland composed of Hürthle cells.

Huschke's auditory teeth (hoosh'kēz). [Emil Huschke, Ger. anatomist, 1797–1858]. Tiny, toothlike protuberances at edge of cochlear labium vestibulare.

Huschke's canal. Canal formed by juncture of the annulus tympanicus tubercules. Usually present only during early childhood.

Huschke's foramen. Perforation found in arrested development near inner extremity of tympanic plate.

Huschke's valve. Plica lacrimalis.

Hutchinson, Sir Jonathan. British surgeon, 1828–1913.

H.-Gilford disease. [Hastings Gilford, Brit. physician, 1861–1941] Progeria, q.v.

H.'s patch. Salmon-colored area in the cornea seen in syphilitic keratitis. SYN: *salmon patch.*

H.'s pupil. A widely dilated pupil of the eye due to a lesion in the central nervous system.

H.'s teeth. A congenital condition; pegged, lateral incisors and notched central incisors along the cutting edge. A sign of congenital syphilis.

H.'s triad. In congenital syphilis: interstitial keratosis, deafness, and Hutchinson's teeth.

Hu-Tet. Trade name for tetanus immune globulin.

Huxley's layer (hŭks'lēz). [Thomas H. Huxley, Brit. physiologist and naturalist, 1825–1895] Inner layer of nucleated cells forming the inner root sheath of a hair follicle.

hyalin (hī'ă-lĭn) [Gr. *hyalos,* glass]. 1. A substance obtainable from the products of amyloid, colloid, or hyaloid degeneration. 2. Basement substance of hyaline cartilage.

hyaline (hī'ă-lĭn). Crystalline, glassy, translucent. SEE: *hyaline casts.*

hyaline bodies. Homogeneous substance; the result of colloid degeneration; found in degenerated cells. SEE: *degeneration, hyaline.*

hyaline cartilage. The true cartilage. Smooth and pearly, it covers the articular surfaces of bones.

hyaline casts. The commonest form of cast found in the urine. They are transparent, pale, and have homogeneous rounded ends. They indicate nephropathy.

hyaline membrane disease. A respiratory disease of the newborn infant. SEE: *respiratory distress syndrome.*

hyalinization (hī"ă-lĭn"ĭ-zā'shŭn). The development of an albuminoid mass in a cell or tissue.

hyalinosis (hī"ă-lĭn-ō'sĭs) [Gr. *hyalos,* glass, + *osis,* condition]. Waxy or hyaline degeneration.

hyalinuria (hī"ă-lĭn-ū'rē-ă) [" + *ouron,* urine]. Hyalin present in the urine.

hyalitis (hī-ă-lī'tĭs) [" + *itis,* inflammation]. Inflammation of the vitreous humor. SYN: *hyaloiditis.*

h., asteroid. Spherical or star-shaped bodies in the vitreous of the eye. Due to inflammation.

h. punctata. A form marked by minute opacities in the vitreous humor.

h. suppurativa. A purulent inflammation of the vitreous humor.

hyalo- [Gr. *hyalos,* glass]. Prefix indicating resemblance to glass.

hyaloenchondroma (hī″ă-lō-ĕn″kŏn-drō′mă) [″ + *en,* in, + *chondros,* cartilage, + *oma,* tumor]. A chondroma composed of hyaline cartilage.

hyalogen (hī-ăl′ō-jĕn) [″ + *gennan,* to produce]. A protein substance in cartilage and the vitreous humor.

hyaloid (hī′ă-loyd) [″ + *eidos,* form]. Hyaline, glassy.

hyaloid artery. A fetal artery that supplies nutrition to the lens. It disappears in later months of gestation.

hyaloid canal. Lymph channel in vitreous extending from optic disk to posterior capsule of lens; it contains the hyaloid artery in the fetus.

hyaloiditis (hī″ă-loyd-ī′tĭs) [″ + *eidos,* form, + *itis,* inflammation]. Inflammation of the hyaloid membrane of the vitreous humor. SYN: *hyalitis.*

hyaloid membrane. Membrane that envelops the vitreous humor.

hyalomere (hī′ă-lō-mēr″) [″ + *meros,* part]. Homogeneous part of a blood platelet, pale in color, as contrasted with the chromomere.

hyalomucoid (hī″ă-lō-mū′koyd) [″ + L. *mucus,* mucus, + Gr. *eidos,* form]. Mucoid in the vitreous body.

hyalonyxis (hī″ă-lō-nĭk′sĭs) [″ + *nyxis,* puncture]. The surgical procedure of puncturing the vitreous body.

hyalophagia, hyalophagy (hī″ă-lō-fā′jē-ă, hī″ă-lŏf′ă-jē) [″ + *phagein,* to eat]. The eating of glass by the demented.

hyalophobia (hī″ă-lō-fō′bē-ă) [″ + *phobos,* fear]. Fear of touching glass.

hyaloplasm (hī′ă-lō-plăzm) [″ + *plasma,* a thing formed]. The fluid portion of protoplasm. The basic ground substance; also called basic or fundamental protoplasm. SYN: *hyalotome.*

hyaloserositis (hī″ă-lō-sē″rō-sī′tĭs) [″ + L. *serum,* whey, + Gr. *itis,* inflammation]. Inflammation of a serous membrane with fibrinous exudate undergoing hyaline transformation.

h., progressive multiple. Phthisis of serous membranes.

hyalosis (hī″ă-lō′sĭs) [″ + *osis,* condition]. Pathological changes in the vitreous humor of the eye.

h., asteroid. Suspended spherical white bodies, made of calcium salts, in the vitreous of the eye.

hyalosome (hī-ăl′ō-sōm) [″ + *soma,* body]. An oval or round structure that resembles the nucleolus of a cell but stains only faintly.

hyalotome (hī-ăl′ō-tōm) [Gr. *hyalos,* glass]. Fluid portion of protoplasm. SYN: *hyaloplasm.*

hyaluronic acid. An acid mucopolysaccharide found in the ground substance of connective tissue that acts as a binding and protective agent. Also found in the synovial fluid and vitreous and aqueous humors.

hyaluronidase (hī″ă-lūr-ŏn′ĭ-dās). An enzyme found in the testes and present in semen. It depolymerizes hyaluronic acid, thereby increasing the permeability of connective tissues by dissolving the substances that hold body cells together. It acts to disperse the cells of the corona radiata about the newly ovulated ovum.

Hyazyme. Trade name for hyaluronidase.

hybrid (hī′brĭd) [L. *hybrida,* mongrel]. The offspring of parents that are different, such as different species.

hybridization (hī′brĭd-ī-zā′shŭn). The production of hybrids by crossbreeding.

hybridoma (hī″brĭ-dō′mă). The cell produced by the fusion of an antibody-producing cell and a multiple myeloma cell. This hybrid cell is capable of producing a continuous supply of antibody. SEE: *monoclonal antibody.*

hydantoin (hī-dăn′tō-ĭn). A colorless base, glycolyl urea, $C_3H_4N_2O_2$, derived from urea or allantoin.

hydatid (hī′dă-tĭd) [Gr. *hydatis,* watery vesicle]. 1. A cyst formed in the tissues, esp. liver, resulting from the development of the larval stage of the dog tapeworm, Echinococcus granulosus. The cysts develop slowly, forming a hollow bladder from the inner surface of which hollow brood capsules are formed. These are attached to the mother cyst by slender stalks or they may fall free into the fluid-filled cavity of the mother cyst. Scolices form on the inner surface of the older brood capsules. In older cysts there is a granular deposit of brood capsules and scolices called hydatid sand. Hydatids may grow for years, sometimes attaining an enormous size. There is no specific medical treatment. The cysts should be removed surgically. SYN: *echinococcosis.* 2. A small cystic remnant of an embryonic structure.

h., sessile. Morgagnian hydatid connected with a testicle.

h., stalked. Morgagnian hydatid connected with a fallopian tube.

hydatid disease. The disease produced by the cysts of the larval stage of the tapeworm Echinococcus. SYN: *echinococcosis.*

hydatid fremitus. A tremulous sensation felt on palpating a hydatid tumor

hydatidiform (hī′dă-tĭd′ĭ-form) [″ + L. *forma,* shape]. Having the form of a hyatid.

hydatid mole. Degenerative process in chorionic villi, which gives rise to multiple cysts and rapid growth of uterus with hemorrhage.

DIAG: Indicated by the hemorrhaging and expulsion of some of the cysts.

hydatidocele (hī″dă-tĭd′ō-sēl) [″ + *kele,* tumor]. Hydatid cyst of the scrotum or testicle.

hydatid of Morgagni. Cystlike remnant of the mullerian duct that is attached to the fallopian tube.

hydatidoma (hī″dă-tĭd-ō′mă) [″ + *oma,* tumor]. A tumor consisting of hydatids.

hydatidosis (hī″dă-tĭd-ō′sĭs) [Gr. *hydatis,* watery vesicle, + *osis,* condition]. Condition caused by infestation with hydatids.

hydatidostomy (hī″dă-tĭ-dŏs′tō-mē) [″ + *stoma,* opening]. Evacuation of a hydatid cyst by means of surgery.

hydatiform (hī-dăt′ĭ-form) [″ + L. *forma,* form]. Hydatidiform.

hydatism (hī′dă-tĭzm) [″ + *-ismos,* condition]. The sound produced by fluid in a cavity.

hydradenitis (hī″drăd-ĕn-ī′tĭs) [Gr. *hydros,* sweat, + *aden,* gland, + *itis,* inflammation]. Inflammation of a sweat gland.

hydradenoma (hī″drăd-ĕ-nō′mă) [″ + ″ + *oma,* tumor]. Tumor of a sweat gland.

hydraeroperitoneum (hī-dră″ĕr-ō-pĕr″ĭ-tō-nē′ŭm) [Gr. *hydor,* water, + *aer,* air, + *peritonaion,* peritoneum]. Collection of fluid and gas in the peritoneal cavity.

hydragogue (hī′dră-gŏg) [″ + *agogos,* leading]. Drug promoting watery evacuation of the bowels, such as magnesium sulfate or sodium phosphate.

hydralazine hydrochloride (hī-drăl′ă-zēn). USP. An antihypertensive drug. Trade name is Apresoline.

Hydralyn. Trade name for hydralazine hydrochloride, USP.

hydramnion, hydramnios (hī-drăm′nē-ŏn, -ŏs) [″ + *amnion,* a caul on a lamb]. An excess of liquor amnii, which leads to overdistention of the uterus and the possibility of malpresentation. The normal amount is 500 to 1,000 ml. It may increase to 2,500 ml. and not be regarded as abnormal.

Liquor amnii is secreted by the fetus, and abnormal amounts are probably due to some abnormality of the fetus. Nearly half the cases occur in twin pregnancies. Hydramnion begins about the fifth month and the pressure of the enlarged uterus gives rise to breathlessness, edema, cyanosis, and varicose veins in the mother. The uterus is large for the length of pregnancy and the fetus may be felt bobbing about in the liquor and the fetal heart is not easily heard.

hydranencephaly (hī″drăn-ĕn-sĕf′ă-lē) [″ + *an-,* not, + *enkephalos,* brain]. Internal hydrocephalus due to congenital absence of the cerebral hemispheres.

hydrargyria (hī″drăr-jĭr′ē-ă) [″ + *argyros,* silver]. Mercury poisoning.

hydrarthrosis (hī″drăr-thrō′sĭs) [″ + *arthron,* joint, + *osis,* condition]. Serous effusion in a joint cavity; white swelling.

h., intermittent. Intermittent and usually painless swelling of the same joint, a condition that lasts for three to five days. Women are affected more often than men. The period between attacks is commonly two to four weeks, during which time the joints are normal. The knee is the usual joint involved but the elbow, hip, and ankle may be affected. There is no satisfactory treatment.

hydrase (hī′drās). An enzyme that catalyzes the addition or withdrawal of water from a compound without hydrolysis occurring.

hydrate (hī′drāt). A crystalline substance formed by water combining with various compounds.

hydrated (hī′drā-tĕd) [L. *hydratus*]. Combined chemically with water, forming a hydrate.

hydration (hī-drā′shŭn). 1. The chemical combination of a substance with water. 2. Addition of water to a substance or tissue.

hydraulics (hī-draw′lĭks) [Gr. *hydor,* water, + *aulos,* pipe]. The science of fluids.

hydrazine (hī′dră-zĭn). 1. H_4N_2. A colorless gas with a peculiar odor; soluble in water. 2. One of a class derived from hydrazine.

Hydrea. Trade name for hydroxyurea, USP.

hydremia (hī-drē′mē-ă) [Gr. *hydor,* water, + *haima,* blood]. Excess of watery fluid in the blood.

hydrencephalocele (hī″drĕn-sĕf′ă-lō-sēl) [″ + *enkephalos,* brain, + *kele,* tumor]. A hernia through a cranial defect of brain substance and meninges, in which fluid occupies the space between the two. SYN: *hydroencephalocele.*

hydrencephalomeningocele (hī″drĕn-sĕf″ă-lō-mĕ-nĭng′gō-sēl) [″ + ″ + *meninx,* membrane, + *kele,* hernia]. A herniation through a defect in the skull. It contains brain substance and cerebrospinal fluid covered by meningeal tissues.

hydrencephalus (hī″drĕn-sĕf′ă-lŭs). Accumulation of fluid in the cerebral ventricles or outside of the brain. SYN: *hydrocephalus.*

hydrepigastrium (hī″drĕp-ĭ-găs′trē-ŭm) [″ + *epi,* upon, + *gaster,* belly]. Accumulation of fluid between the peritoneum and the abdominal muscles.

hydriatric (hī-drē-ăt′rĭk) [″ + *iatrikos,* healing]. Pert. to treatment of disease with water, as hydriatic procedures or hydriatric institutions.

hydriatrics (hī-drē-ăt′rĭks). Application of water in treatment of disease. SYN: *hydrotherapeutics.*

hydriatrist (hī-drī′ă-trĭst). One who practices hydrotherapy.

hydride (hī′drīd). Chemical compound containing hydrogen and an element or radical.

hydrion (hī-drī′ŏn). The hydrogen ion (H^+).

hydro- [Gr. *hydor,* water]. Prefix pert. to water

or to hydrogen.

hydroa (hĭd-rō'ă). Any bullous skin eruption.

hydroappendix (hī"drō-ă-pĕn'dĭks) [" + L. *appendere,* to hang upon]. Watery fluid distending the vermiform appendix.

hydrobilirubin (hī"drō-bĭl"ĭ-roo'bĭn) [" + L. *bilis,* bile, + *ruber,* red]. A brownish-red bile pigment, derived from bilirubin, and thought to be identical with stercobilin and urobilin.

hydrobromate (hī"drō-brō'māt) [" + *bromos,* stench]. A salt of hydrobromic acid.

hydrocalycosis (hī"drō-kăl"ĭ-kō'sĭs) [" + *kalyx,* cup, + *osis,* condition]. Cystic dilation of the renal calix due to obstruction.

hydrocarbon (hī"drō-kăr'bŏn) [" + L. *carbo,* coal]. A compound made up only of hydrogen and carbon.

h., alicyclic. Hydrocarbon that contains cyclic and straight-chain components.

h., aliphatic. A straight-chain hydrocarbon that contains no cyclic component.

h., aromatic. Hydrocarbon in which the carbon atoms are in a ring, or cyclic, configuration.

h., cyclic. Hydrocarbon in which the carbon atoms are in a ring configuration.

h., saturated. Hydrocarbon in which the carbon atoms are linked by a single electron pair and in which all valences are satisfied.

h., unsaturated. Hydrocarbon in which carbon atoms share two or three pairs of electrons.

hydrocele (hī'drō-sēl) [" + *kele,* tumor]. The accumulation of serous fluid in a saclike cavity, esp. in the tunica vaginalis testis; serous tumors of the testes or associated parts.

h., acute. Most common hydrocele. The majority of cases occur suddenly between the second and fifth years, usually the result of inflammation of the epididymis or testis.

h., cervical. Hydrocele in the neck resulting from accumulation of serous fluid in persistent cervical duct or cleft.

h., chronic. Hydrocele usually seen in men of middle age. May result from filariasis.

h., congenital. Hydrocele present at birth, resulting from failure of closure of the vaginal process.

h., encysted. Hydrocele in the vaginal process in which openings to the scrotal and peritoneal cavities are closed.

h. feminae. Hydrocele in the labium majus or canal of Nuck.

h. hernialis. Condition when hernia accompanies infantile or congenital hydrocele and there is an accumulation of peritoneal fluid in a hernial sac.

h., infantile. Peritoneal fluid in the tunica vaginalis and vaginal process with the latter closed at the abdominal ring.

h. muliebris. H. feminae

h., spermatic. Spermatic fluid in the tunica vaginalis of the testes.

h. spinalis. Spina bifida.

hydrocelectomy (hī"drō-sē-lĕk'tō-mē) [" + " + *ektome,* excision]. Surgical removal of a hydrocele.

hydrocephalic [" + *kephale,* head]. Pert. to or affected with hydrocephalus.

hydrocephalocele (hī"drō-sĕf'ă-lō-sēl) [" + " + *kele,* tumor]. Watery hernia of the brain. SYN: *hydrencephalocele.*

hydrocephaloid (hī"drō-sĕf'ă-loyd) [" + " + *eidos,* resemblance]. Resembling or pert. to hydrocephalus.

hydrocephaloid disease. Disease resembling hydrocephalus, but the fontanels of the infant are depressed due to dehydration.

hydrocephalus (hī-drō-sĕf'ă-lŭs) [" + *kephale,* head]. The increased accumulation of cerebrospinal fluid within the ventricles of the brain. Results from interference with normal circulation and with absorption of the fluid, and, esp., from destruction of the foramina of Magendie and Lushka. This may result from developmental anomalies, infection, injury, or brain tumors.

In severe cases in children, the head is usually globular or pyramidal in shape. The face is disproportionately small with eyes hidden in sockets and turned upward. Sutures are separated with bulging fontanels and thin cranial bones. In older individuals, after the skull has formed, there are headache, vomiting, choked disks, atrophy of optic nerve, and mental disturbances. SYN: *hydrencephalus.*

NURSING IMPLICATIONS: *Pre-op:* Assess for signs of increased intracranial pressure. Particularly in the infant, note bulging of the anterior fontanel and increases in head circumference. Provide adequate nutrition (the infant will need extra head support during feeding). Since the infant's head may be large, head position should be changed frequently, and the head should be assessed for signs of skin breakage. Lambs' wool may be placed under the infant's head to prevent breakdown of skin in that area.

Post-op: Take vital signs every 1–2 hours, and do systematic neurological assessment every hour in the immediate post-op period. In infants, assess the anterior fontanel for bulging or depression. Position the patient as ordered by the physician. Measure and record intake and output, and observe the patient for development of complications such as increased intracranial pressure, dehydration, intracranial infection or septicemia.

The parents will need calm reassurance and emotional support, not only concerning the surgery, but also in terms of the disease process and long-term rehabilitation of their child.

TREATMENT: If hydrocephalus progresses, the condition is treated by a surgical procedure that utilizes a shunt through which the cerebrospinal fluid flows. The shunt connects the ventricular system with a suitable cavity such as the peritoneal.

PROGNOSIS: In untreated cases of congenital hydrocephalus, the outcome is fatal in about half of the patients. The prognosis for an uncomplicated course is excellent when hydrocephalus is promptly treated by use of a surgically instituted shunt.

h., communicating. Hydrocephalus in which normal communication between the 4th ventricle and subarachnoid space is maintained.

h., congenital. Chronic type of hydrocephalus occurring in infancy.

h., external. Accumulation of fluid in subdural spaces.

h., internal. Accumulation of fluid within ventricles of the brain.

h., noncommunicating. Hydrocephalus in which a blockage at any location in the ventricular system prevents flow of cerebrospinal fluid to the subarachnoid space.

h., normal pressure. Type of hydrocephalus with enlarged ventricles of the brain with no increase in the spinal fluid pressure or no demonstrable block to the outflow of spinal fluid.

h., secondary. Hydrocephalus following injury or infections such as meningitis or syphilis.

hydrochlorate (hī″drō-klō′rāt) [Gr. *hydor,* water, + *chloros,* green]. Any salt of hydrochloric acid.

hydrochloric acid. An aqueous solution of hydrogen chloride (HCl), containing 35 to 38% HCl by weight. Crude commercial hydrochloric acid is known as muriatic acid.

This normal constituent of gastric juice is produced by the parietal (or oxyntic) cells of gastric glands. The HCl concentration in the stomach is variable, depending upon several factors, including rate of secretion of gastric juice and the type of food eaten. It serves the following functions: converts pepsinogen into pepsin and produces an acid medium favorable for the activity of pepsin; dissolves and disintegrates nucleoproteins and collagen; hydrolyzes sucrose; precipitates caseinogen; inhibits multiplication of bacteria, esp. putrefactive organisms that ferment lactic acid and certain pathogenic forms; stimulates secretion by the duodenum; inhibits the action of ptyalin and thus stops salivary digestion in the stomach.

Average amount found in the food content of stomach is small because of dilution and neutralization by alkaline contents. In pernicious anemia, hydrochloric acid is absent from the stomach (achlorhydria).

hydrochloride (hī″drō-klō′rīd). An alkaloid or other base combined with hydrochloric acid.

hydrochlorothiazide (hī″drō-klō″rō-thī′ă-zīd). USP. A diuretic. Trade names are Esidrix, HydroDIURIL, Thiuretic, and Zide.

hydrocholecystis (hī″drō-kō″lĭ-sĭs′tĭs) [″ + *chole,* bile, + *kystis,* bladder]. Dropsy of the gallbladder.

hydrocholeresis (hī″drō-kō″lĕr-ē′sĭs) [″ + ″ + *hairesis,* a taking]. Choleresis in which water content of the bile is increased, resulting in production of bile with reduced specific gravity, viscosity, and total solid content.

hydrocholeretic (hī″drō-kō″lĕ-rĕt′ĭk). Anything that increases the output of bile without increasing the solids secreted in it.

hydrocirsocele (hī″drō-sĭr′sō-sēl) [″ + *kirsos,* varix, + *kele,* tumor]. Hydrocele combined with varicose veins of spermatic cord.

hydrocodone bitartrate (hī″drō-kō′dōn). USP. An analgesic drug. Trade names are Dicodid, Didrate, and Mercodinone.

hydrocollidine (hī″drō-kŏl′ĭ-dĭn) [″ + *kolla,* glue]. A toxic substance from putrefying fish or animal flesh.

hydrocolloid (hī″drō-kŏl′loyd) [″ + *kollodes,* glutinous]. A colloidal suspension in which water is the liquid.

hydrocolpos (hī″drō-kŏl′pŏs) [″ + *kolpos,* vagina]. Retention cyst of the vagina containing watery, nonsanguineous fluid or mucus.

hydroconion (hī″drō-kō′nē-ŏn) [″ + *konis,* dust]. An atomizer that emits a fine spray.

hydrocortisone (hī″drō-kor′tĭ-sōn). The corticosteroid hormone produced by the adrenal cortex. SYN: *cortisol,* q.v.

h. acetate. Trade names are Cortef Acetate and Cortril Acetate-AF.

hydrocyanic acid. Hydrogen cyanide. SEE: *cyanide poisoning.*

hydrocyst (hī′drō-sĭst) [Gr. *hydor,* water, + *kystis,* a bladder]. A cyst containing watery fluid.

hydrocystoma [″ + ″ + *oma,* tumor]. Disease marked by small cysts that originate in the sweat gland. Sudamina on the face, esp. in women after middle age. SYN: *hidrocystoma.*

hydrodiascope (hī″drō-dī′ă-skōp) [″ + *dia,* through, + *skopein,* to examine]. Device used to treat astigmatism.

hydrodictiotomy (hī″drō-dĭk″tē-ŏt′ō-mē) [″ + *diktyon,* retina, + *tome,* incision]. A surgical procedure to correct displacement of the retina.

HydroDIURIL. Trade name for hydrochlorothiazide, USP.

hydroencephalocele (hī″drō-ĕn-sĕf′ă-lō-sēl) [″ + *enkephalos,* brain, + *kele,* tumor]. Brain substance expanded into a watery sac protruding through a cleft in the cranium. SYN: *hydrencephalocele*.

hydroflumethiazide (hī″drō-floo″mĕ-thī′ă-zīd). USP. A diuretic and antihypertensive drug. Trade names are Diucardin and Saluron.

hydrogel (hī′drō-jĕl) [″ + L. *gelare*, to congeal]. A colloid containing water that solidifies in gelatinous form.

hydrogen [″ + *gennan*, to produce]. SYMB: H. At. wt. 1.0079; at. no. 1; sp. gr. 0.069. A liter of the gas at 0° C. weighs 0.08987 gm. An element existing as a colorless, odorless, and tasteless gas, it possesses one valence electron. Three isotopes of hydrogen (protium, deuterium, and tritium) exist, having atomic weights of approx. 1, 2, and 3, respectively.

OCCURRENCE: Hydrogen is present in the sun and stars. Even though it is the most abundant element in the known universe, its concentration in the earth's atmosphere is only 0.00005%. Hydrogen occurs in its free state (in natural gases and volcanic eruptions) only in minute quantities. It occurs principally on the earth as hydrogen oxide (water, H_2O) and is a constituent of all hydrocarbons. It is present in all acids and in ionic form is responsible for the properties characteristic of acids. It is present in nearly all organic compounds and is a component of all carbohydrates, proteins, and fats.

USES: It is highly inflammable and used in the oxyhydrogen flame in welding, in hydrogenation of oils for solidifying purposes, as a reducing agent, and in many syntheses.

hydrogen acceptor. In oxidation-reduction reactions, a substance that receives hydrogen atoms from another substance, the donator. SEE: *coenzyme*.

hydrogenase (hī′drō-jĕn-ās). An enzyme that catalyzes reduction by molecular hydrogen.

hydrogenate (hī′drō-jĕn-āt″). To bring about a combination with hydrogen.

hydrogenation (hī″drō-jĕn-ā′shŭn). A process of changing an unsaturated fat to a solid saturated fat by the addition of hydrogen in the presence of a catalyst.

hydrogen cyanide. Hydrocyanic acid, q.v.

hydrogen dioxide. Hydrogen peroxide (H_2O_2).

hydrogen donator. In oxidation-reduction reactions, a substance that gives up hydrogen atoms to another substance, the acceptor.

hydrogen iodide. Acid, hydriodic, q.v.

hydrogen ion. H^+, the positively charged nucleus of a hydrogen atom.

hydrogen ion concentration. $[H^+]$, the relative proportion of hydrogen ions in a solution, the factor responsible for the acidic properties of a solution. SEE: *pH*.

hydrogen ion scale. A scale used to express the degree of acidity or alkalinity of a solution. It extends from 0.00 (total acidity) to 14 (total alkalinity), the numbers running in inverse order of H-ion concentration. The pH value is the negative logarithm of the H-ion concentration of a solution, expressed in gram ions (moles) per liter.

As the hydrogen ion concentration decreases, a change of 1 pH unit means a tenfold increase in hydrogen ion concentration or true acidity. Thus a solution with a pH of 1.0 is ten times more acid than one with a pH of 2.0 and 100 times more acid than one with a pH of 3.0. A pH of 7.0 indicates neutrality.

As the hydrogen ion concentration varies in a definite reciprocal manner with the hydroxyl ion (OH^-) concentration, a pH reading above 7.0 indicates alkalinity. The arterial blood is slightly alkaline, having a pH of 7.35. SYN: *pH scale*. SEE: *pH*

hydrogen peroxide. H_2O_2. A colorless syrupy liquid with an irritating odor and acrid taste. It decomposes readily, liberating oxygen. Light is particularly effective in activating H_2O_2; therefore it should be stored in tightly sealed glass jars in a dark place.

USES: As a commercial bleaching agent, as an oxidizing and reducing agent. In a 3% aqueous solution, as a mild antiseptic, germicide, and cleansing agent.

h. p., solution of. USP. A standardized aqueous solution of hydrogen peroxide. It has the ability to kill bacteria, and this is its most important use. However, its germicidal activity has been greatly overrated. Organic matter has a tendency to decompose it and as long as there is effervescence when the solution is applied to a wound, there is no great destruction of bacteria.

A solution of hydrogen peroxide has value as a cleansing agent for suppurating wounds and inflamed mucous membranes. It is esp. useful for this purpose because of its development of gas that tends to loosen adherent deposits and detritus, q.v., which might form a breeding place for microorganisms.

Hydrogen peroxide solution is sometimes injected into deep cavities to determine the presence of pus, which will be indicated by effervescence. Because of its lack of toxicity it is a favored disinfectant for application to various mucous membranes, esp. those of the nose and throat. Diluted with equal parts of water it is used as a gargle in pharyngitis or mouthwash in stomatitis.

hydrogen sulfide. H_2S. A poisonous, flammable, colorless compound with a characteristic odor of rotten eggs. SEE: *Poisons and Poisoning* in *Appendix*.

hydroglossa (hī″drō-glŏs′ă) [Gr. *hydor*, water, + *glossa*, tongue]. Cystic tumor beneath the tongue. SYN: *ranula*.

hydrogymnasium (hī″drō-jĭm-nā′zē-ŭm) [″ + *gymnazein,* to train naked]. Pool for underwater exercises.
hydrogymnastics (hī″drō-jĭm-năs′tĭks). Underwater exercises.
hydrohematonephrosis (hī″drō-hĕm″ă-tō-nĕf-rō′sĭs) [″ + *haima,* blood, + *nephros,* kidney, + *osis,* condition]. Bloody urine distending the pelvis of the kidney.
hydrohymenitis (hī″drō-hī″mĕn-ī′tĭs) [″ + *hymen,* membrane, + *itis,* inflammation]. Any inflammation of a serous membrane.
hydrokinetics (hī″drō-kī-nĕt′ĭks) [″ + *kinesis,* motion]. Science of fluids in motion.
hydrolabile (hī″drō-lā′bĭl). Having the tendency to lose weight because of loss of fluids, decreased intake of salt or carbohydrate, or excess loss of fluid due to gastrointestinal disease.
hydrolase (hī′drō-lās). An enzyme that causes hydrolysis.
hydrology (hī-drŏl′ō-jē) [″ + *logos,* science]. The science of water in all its aspects.
Hydrolose. Trade name for methylcellulose, USP.
hydrolysate (hī-drŏl′ĭ-sāt). That produced as a result of hydrolysis.

h., protein. The amino acids obtained from splitting proteins by hydrolysis. Used as a source of amino acids in certain diets.

hydrolysis (hī-drŏl′ĭ-sĭs) [″ + *lysis,* dissolution]. Any reaction in which water is one of the reactants, more specifically the combination of water with a salt to produce an acid and a base, one of which is more dissociated than the other. Opposed to neutralization. A chemical decomposition in which a substance is split into simpler compounds by the addition or the taking up of the elements of water.

Reactions of this kind are extremely frequent in life processes. The conversion of starch to maltose, of fat to glycerol and fatty acid, and of protein to amino acids are examples of hydrolysis, as are other reactions involved in digestion. A simple example is the reaction in which the hydrolysis of ethyl acetate yields acetic acid and ethyl alcohol: $C_2H_5C_2H_3O_2 + H_2O = CH_3COOH + C_2H_5OH$. Usually such reactions are reversible; the reversed reaction is called neutralization, esterification, or condensation. SEE: *assimilation; enzyme.*

hydrolytic (hī-drō-lĭt′ĭk). Rel. to hydrolysis.
hydrolyze (hī′drō-līz). To cause to undergo hydrolysis.
hydroma (hī-drō′mă) [Gr. *hydor,* water, + *oma,* tumor]. 1. Hygroma. 2. Any cyst containing a watery substance.
hydromeiosis (hī″drō-mī-ō′sĭs) [″ + *meiosis,* dimunition]. Swelling of the epidermis after it is exposed to water with consequent blockage of the sweat ducts. This phenomenon limits loss of fluids due to sweating, when the body is immersed in warm water.
hydromeningitis (hī″drō-mĕn″ĭn-jī′tĭs) [″ + *meninx,* membrane, + *itis,* inflammation]. 1. Inflammation of membranes of brain with serous effusion. 2. Inflammation of Descemet's membrane.
hydromeningocele (hī″drō-mĕn-ĭn′gō-sēl) [″ + ″ + *kele,* hernia]. Protrusion of meninges or spinal cord in a sac of fluid.
hydrometer (hī-drŏm′ĕ-tĕr) [″ + *metron,* measure]. An instrument that measures the density of a liquid by the depth to which a graduated scale sinks into the liquid. SYN: *areometer.*
hydrometra (hī″drō-mē′tră) [″ + *metra,* uterus]. Collection of watery fluid or mucus in the uterus.
hydrometrocolpos (hī″drō-mē″trō-kŏl′pŏs) [″ + *metra,* uterus, + *kolpos,* vagina]. Distention of the uterus by a collection of watery fluid.
hydromicrocephaly (hī″drō-mī″krō-sĕf′ă-lē) [″ + *mikros,* small, + *kephale,* head]. Condition in which there is a small head that contains an increased amount of cerebrospinal fluid.
hydromorphone hydrochloride (hī″drō-mor′fōn). USP. An analgesic drug. Trade name is Dilaudid Hydrochloride.
Hydromox. Trade name for quinethazone, USP.
hydromphalus (hī-drŏm′fă-lŭs) [″ + *omphalos,* navel]. Watery tumor at the umbilicus.
hydromyelia (hī″drō-mī-ē′lē-ă) [″ + *myelos,* marrow]. Increased fluid in the central canal of the spinal cord. SYN: *hydrorrhachis.*
hydromyelocele (hī″drō-mī-ĕl′ō-sēl) [″ + ″ + *kele,* hernia]. Protrusion of a sac with cerebrospinal fluid through a spina bifida.
hydromyelomeningocele (hī″drō-mī″ĕ-lō-mĕ-nĭng′gō-sēl) [″ + *myelos,* marrow, + *meninx,* membrane, + *kele,* hernia]. A deformity of the spine through which a fluid-filled sac containing the spinal cord tissue and membranes protrudes.
hydromyoma (hī″drō-mī-ō′mă) [″ + *mys,* muscle, + *oma,* tumor]. Cystic fibroid, usually uterine, filled with fluid.
hydronephrosis (hī″drō-nĕf-rō′sĭs) [″ + *nephros,* kidney, + *osis,* condition]. Collection of urine in the renal pelvis due to obstructed outflow, forming a cyst by production of distention and atrophy of organ. SYN: *nephrohydrosis; nephrydrosis.*

DIAG: Large, fluctuating, soft mass in region of kidney, appearing and disappearing as retained urine passes into the ureters and bladder.

TREATMENT: Aspiration, nephrectomy, or nephrotomy depending on the severity of the disease. Medical or surgical removal of the cause of the retention is indicated.

hydroparasalpinx (hī″drō-păr″ă-săl′pĭnks) [Gr. *hydor,* water, + *para,* beside, + *salpinx,* tube]. Accumulation of serous fluid in the accessory tubes of the fallopian tube.

hydroparotitis (hī″drō-păr″ō-tī′tĭs) [″ + ″ + *ous,* ear, + *itis,* inflammation]. Accumulation of fluid in the parotid gland.

hydropathic (hī″drō-păth′ĭk) [″ + *pathos,* disease]. Rel. to hydropathy.

hydropathy (hī-drŏp′ă-thē). A treatment regimen involving the use of large amounts of water internally and externally. It is falsely claimed that such treatment will cure a great variety of diseases. SEE: *hydrotherapy.*

hydropenia (hī″drō-pē′nē-ă) [″ + *penia,* poverty]. Deficiency in body water.

hydropericarditis [″ + *peri,* around, + *kardia,* heart, + *itis,* inflammation]. Serous effusion accompanying pericarditis.

hydropericardium (hī″drō-pĕr″ĭ-kăr′dē-ŭm) Pericardial dropsy. Accumulation of water in pericardial sac without inflammation.

SYM: Distress in region of heart; diminished cardiac function with signs of heart failure; dysphagia, and dyspnea.

TREATMENT: Paracentesis. Definitive therapy depends upon cause of disease.

hydroperinephrosis (hī″drō-pĕr″ĭ-nĕ-frō′sĭs) [″ + *peri,* around, + *nephros,* kidney, + *osis,* condition]. Accumulation of serum of connective tissue surrounding the kidney.

hydroperion (hī″drō-pĕr′ē-ŏn) [″ + ″ + *oon,* egg]. Fluid present between decidua capsularis and decidua parietalis; occurs early in pregnancy.

hydroperitoneum (hī″drō-pĕr″ĭ-tō-nē′ŭm) [″ + *peritonaion,* peritoneum]. Accumulation of fluid in peritoneal cavity. SYN: *ascites.*

hydropexis (hī″drō-pĕk′sĭs) [″ + *pexis,* fixation]. The retaining or fixing of water.

hydrophilia (hī-drō-fĭl′ē-ă) [″ + *philein,* to love]. Hydrophilism, q.v.

hydrophilic lyophilic colloid. Emulsoid, q.v.

hydrophilic ointment. USP. A standardized ointment preparation used topically as an emollient.

hydrophilism (hī-drŏf′ĭ-lĭzm) [″ + ″ + *-ismos,* condition]. Tendency of tissues to attract and hold water. SYN: *hydrophilia.*

hydrophilous (hī-drŏf′ĭ-lŭs). Taking up moisture. SYN: *bibulous; hygroscopic.*

hydrophobia (hī-drō-fō′bē-ă) [Gr. *hydor,* water, + *phobos,* fear]. 1. Morbid fear of water. 2. Common name for rabies, q.v., resulting from bite of a rabid animal. SYN: *lyssa.*

hydrophobophobia (hī″drō-fō″bō-fō′bē-ă) [″ + ″ + *phobos,* fear]. Morbid fear of contracting hydrophobia (rabies), sometimes resulting in a hysterical condition resembling hydrophobia.

hydrophthalmos (hī″drŏf-thăl′mŏs) [″ + *ophthalmos,* eye]. Distention of the eyeball due to accumulation of fluid within it. SYN: *glaucoma, infantile.*

hydrophysometra (hī″drō-fī″sō-mē′tră) [″ + *physa,* air, + *metra,* uterus]. Presence of water and gas in the uterus.

hydropic (hī-drŏp′ĭk) [Gr. *hydropikos*]. Dropsical or pert. to dropsy.

hydropneumatosis (hī″drō-nū″mă-tō′sĭs) [″ + *pneumatosis,* inflation]. Liquid and gas in the tissues producing combined edema and emphysema.

hydropneumogony (hī″drō-nū-mō′gō-nē) [″ + *pneuma,* air, + *gony,* knee]. Diagnosis of joint effusion by injecting air in joint. SEE: *arthrogram.*

hydropneumopericardium (hī″drō-nū″mō-pĕr-ĭ-kăr′dē-ŭm) [″ + ″ + *peri,* around, + *kardia,* heart]. Serous effusion with gas in the pericardium.

hydropneumoperitoneum (hī″drō-nū″mō-pĕr″ĭ-tō-nē′ŭm) [″ + ″ + *peritonaion,* peritoneum]. Gas and serous fluid in the peritoneal cavity.

hydropneumothorax (hī″drō-nū″mō-thō′răks) [″ + ″ + *thorax,* chest]. Gas and serous effusion in pleural cavity. SYN: *pneumohydrothorax.*

hydrops, hydropsy (hī′drŏps, hī-drŏp′sē) [Gr.]. Dropsy or edema.

h. abdominis. Edema of the abdominal cavity. SYN: *ascites.*

h., endolymphatic. H., labyrinthine.

h. fetalis. Erythroblastosis fetalis.

h. folliculi. Accumulation of fluid in the graafian follicle of the ovary.

h. gravidarum. Edema accompanying pregnancy.

h., labyrinthine. Dilatation due to an accumulation of fluid in the endolymphatic space of the ear. A characteristic of Ménière's disease, q.v.

h. tubae. Collection of fluid in a fallopian tube. SYN: *hydrosalpinx.*

h. tubae profluens. Edema of the fallopian tube in which the distention becomes so great that the tube is forced to empty itself by the pressure, the emptying taking place via the uterine cavity. SYN: *hydrosalpinx, intermittent.*

h. vesicae felleae. Fluid in the gallbladder causing distention.

hydropyonephrosis (hī″drō-pī″ō-nĕf-rō′sĭs) [Gr. *hydor,* water, + *pyon,* pus, + *nephros,* kidney, + *osis,* condition]. Dilatation of kidney pelvis with pus and urine.

hydroquinone (hī″drō-kwĭn′ōn). USP. A weak but safe depigmenting agent, used topically. Trade names are Black and white bleaching cream, Eldoquin, and Eldopaque.

hydrorheostat (hī″drō-rē′ō-stăt) [″ + *rheos,*

current, + *histanai,* to place]. A device used to control the flow of electrical current by changes in water resistance.

hydrorrhachis (hī-dror'ă-kĭs) [" + *rhachis,* spine]. Condition of increased cerebrospinal fluid between membranes and the spinal cord or its central canal or cavities. SYN: *hydromyelia.*

hydrorrhachitis (hī-dror-ă-kī'tĭs) [" + " + *itis,* inflammation]. Serous effusion from the spinal cord or its membranes with inflammation of the cord.

hydrorrhea (hī"drō-rē'ă) [" + *rhoia,* flow]. Copious watery discharge from any part, as from the nose.

h. gravidarum. Discharge of a watery fluid from the vagina during pregnancy, sometimes mistaken for amniotic fluid.

hydrosalpinx (hī"drō-săl'pĭnks) [" + *salpinx,* tube]. Distention of the fallopian tube by clear fluid.

h., intermittent. A discharge of watery fluid from the fallopian tube. SYN: *hydrops tubae profluens.*

hydrosarcocele (hī"drō-săr'kō-sēl) [" + *sarx,* flesh, + *kele,* tumor]. Hydrocele with chronic swelling of the testis.

hydroscheocele (hī-drŏs'kē-ō-sēl") [" + *oscheon,* scrotum, + *kele,* hernia]. Scrotal hernia that contains serous fluid.

hydrosis (hī-drō'sĭs). Hidrosis.

hydrosol (hī'drō-sŏl). The fluid state of a colloidal solution; a sol. State of a colloidal solution in which the colloid particles, separated by water in a continuous phase, are free to move about. SEE: *hydrogel.*

hydrosphygmograph (hī"drō-sfĭg'mō-grăf) [" + *sphygmos,* pulse, + *graphein,* to write]. A sphygmograph with indicator consisting of a column of water.

hydrostat (hī'drō-stăt) [" + *statikos,* standing]. Device that maintains the water level in a container at a predetermined level.

hydrostatic (hī"drō-stăt'ĭk) [" + *statikos,* standing]. Pert. to the pressure of liquids in equilibrium and that exerted on liquids.

hydrostatic densitometry. An underwater weighing technique for the determination of the specific gravity of an individual. The amount of water displaced by the body is corrected for the air contained in the lungs. An accurate determination of body components (e.g., the percentage of fat) can be made. SYN: *hydrostatic weighing.*

hydrostatics (hī"drō-stăt'ĭks). Science of properties of fluids in equilibrium.

hydrostatic test. Putting lungs of a dead infant in water. If they float, the infant has breathed prior to death.

hydrostatic weighing. Hydrostatic densitometry, q.v.

hydrosudotherapy (hī"drō-soo"dō-thĕr'ă-pē) [" + L. *sudor,* sweat, + Gr. *therapeia,* treatment]. Treatment of disease by sweating and hydrotherapy.

hydrosulfuric acid. Hydrogen sulfide.

hydrosyringomyelia (hī"drō-sĭr-ĭng"ō-mī-ē'lē-ă) [" + *syrinx,* tube, + *myelos,* marrow]. Distention of the central canal of the spinal cord with effusion of fluid and formation of cavities.

hydrotaxis (hī"drō-tăk'sĭs) [" + *taxis,* arrangement]. The response of an organism or cell toward or away from moisture. SEE: *hydrotropism.*

hydrotherapeutics (hī"drō-thĕr"ă-pū'tĭks) [Gr. *hydor,* water, + *therapeia,* treatment]. Treatment of disease with water. SYN: *hydrotherapy.*

hydrotherapist (hī"drō-thĕr'ă-pĭst). One who practices hydrotherapy.

hydrotherapy (hī-drō-thĕr'ă-pē) [" + *therapeia,* treatment]. Scientific application of water in treatment of disease. The therapeutic effects of hydrotherapy are as follows:

Brief hot tub and shower baths: Relieve fatigue, produce general relaxation.

Cold baths and applications: Cool the body or part and stimulate, esp. if followed by friction and percussion. They contract the small blood vessels when applied locally.

Cold and hot applications: One followed by the other stimulates the cardiovascular system both generally and locally.

Gradually elevated temperature of hot tub and vapor baths: Produces general muscular relaxation.

Hot baths: Relax tissues, including capillaries of skin, drawing blood from deeper tissues; also relieve pain.

hydrothermic (hī"drō-thĕr'mĭk). Concerning the effect of heated water.

hydrothionammonemia (hī"drō-thī"ō-năm"ō-nē'mē-ă) [" + *theion,* sulfur, + *ammoniakos,* of Amen, from near whose temple it came, + *haima,* blood]. Ammonium sulfide in the blood.

hydrothionemia (hī"drō-thī"ō-nē'mē-ă) [" + " + *haima,* blood]. Condition caused by hydrogen sulfide in the blood.

hydrothionuria (hī"drō-thī"ō-nū'rē-ă) [" + " + *ouron,* urine]. Condition caused by hydrogen sulfide in the urine.

hydrothorax (hī"drō-thō'răks) [" + *thorax,* chest]. A noninflammatory collection of fluid in the pleural cavity.

SYM: Dyspnea; absence of vesicular breath sounds; murmur; flatness over location of fluid.

hydrotis (hī-drō'tĭs) [" + *ous,* ear]. Serous effusion in the internal ear or tympanum.

hydrotomy (hī-drŏt'ō-mē) [" + *tome,* incision]. Dissection of tissue by forcible injection of water.

hydrotropism (hī″drō-trō′pĭzm) [″ + *trope*, a turning]. Response of plants toward (positive hydrotropism) or away (negative hydrotropism) from moisture.

hydrotympanum (hī″drō-tĭm′pă-nŭm) [″ + *tympanon*, drum]. Edema fluid in the middle ear.

hydroureter (hī″drō-ū-rē′tĕr) [″ + *oureter*, ureter]. Distention of ureter with fluid due to obstruction.

hydrous (hī′drŭs). Containing water. SEE: *anhydrous.*

hydrovarium (hī″drō-vā′rē-ŭm) [″ + L. *ovarium*, ovary]. Edema or cyst of the ovary.

hydroxide (hī-drŏk′sīd) [″ + *oxys*, sour]. A compound that contains the hydroxyl (—OH) group, such as NaOH (sodium hydroxide, or caustic soda).

hydroxocobalamin (hī-drŏk″sō-kō-băl′ă-mĭn). USP. A chemical that has the activity of vitamin B_{12}. Its use intramuscularly is contraindicated because it can stimulate the production of antibodies to vitamin B_{12}. Trade names are alphaRedisol, Alpha-Ruvite, and Neo-Betalin 12.

hydroxy acids (hī-drŏk′sē). Acids containing one or more hydroxyl (—OH) groups in addition to the carboxyl (C—O—O—H) group, such as lactic acid, $CH_3COHCOOH$.

hydroxyamphetamine hydrobromide (hī-drŏk″sē-ăm-fĕt′ă-mēn hī″drō-brō′mīd). USP. An amphetamine with little ability to stimulate the central nervous system. Used as a solution placed in the eye, where it has ephedrine-like action. Trade name is Paredrine.

hydroxyapatite (hī-drŏk″sē-ăp′ă-tīt). The form of calcium phosphate present in bone salts.

hydroxybenzene (hī-drŏk″sē-bĕn′zēn). Phenol.

hydroxybutyric acid. An acid present in the urine, esp. in diabetes, when fat is abnormally metabolized.

hydroxybutyric dehydrogenase. A serum enzyme that is increased in myocardial infarction.

hydroxychloroquine sulfate (hī-drŏk″sē-klō′rō-kwĭn). USP. An antimalarial drug. Trade name is Plaquenil Sulfate.

25-hydroxycholecalciferol (hī-drŏk″sē-kō″lē-kăl-sĭf′ĕ-rŏl). A vitamin A derivative.

17-hydroxycorticosterone (hī-drŏk″sē-kor″tĭ-kō-stĕr′ōn). Hydrocortisone.

hydroxydione sodium succinate (hī-drŏk″sē-dī′ōn). A steroid drug used intravenously as an anesthetic. It has no hormonal action.

hydroxyl. The univalent radical OH, that, when combined with a metallic ion or a radical that acts as a metal (e.g., NH_4), forms a hydroxide. Commonly called a base or alkali.

hydroxylase (hī-drŏk′sĭ-lās). Any enzyme that catalyzes the introduction of hydrogen into a substrate.

hydroxylysine (hī″drŏk-sĭl′ĭ-sĭn). An amino acid found in collagen.

hydroxyprogesterone caproate (hī-drŏk″sē-prō-jĕs′tĕr-ōn). USP. A progestational drug. Trade name is Delalutin.

hydroxyproline (hī-drŏk″sē-prō′lĭn). An amino acid found in collagen.

hydroxypropyl methycellulose 2910. USP. Cellulose hydroxypropyl methyl ester. A substance used to increase the viscosity of solutions. Trade names are Isopto Alkaline, Isopto Plain, Isopto Tears, and Ultra Tears.

hydroxystilbamidine isethionate (hī-drŏk″sē-stĭl-băm′ĭ-dēn). USP. An antiprotozoal drug used in treating North American blastomycosis.

5-hydroxytryptamine (hī-drŏk″sē-trĭp′tă-mēn). Serotonin.

hydroxyurea (hī-drŏk″sē-ū-rē′ă). USP. A cytotoxic drug. Trade name is Hydrea.

hydroxyzine hydrochloride (hī-drŏk′sĭ-zēn). USP. An antihistamine drug. Trade names are Atarax and Vistaril Parenteral.

hydruria (hī-droo′rē-ă) [Gr. *hydor*, water, + *ouron*, urine]. Excessive secretion and discharge of urine. As a rule the urine does not contain abnormal constituents

hygiene (hī′jēn) [Gr. *hygieinos*, healthful]. The study of health and observance of health rules. Study of the methods and means of preserving health.

h., community. That branch of hygiene that deals with the health of a large group of individuals such as city, state, or nation, and esp. with the control of communicable diseases.

h., industrial. That branch of hygiene that deals primarily with health of industrial workers, esp. study, treatment, and prevention of occupational diseases.

h., mental. Science of developing and maintaining mental health and preventing mental illness.

h., military. That branch of hygiene that deals with the health of persons in military service.

h., oral. Scientific care and prophylactic treatment of teeth and mouth.

hygienic (hī′jē-ĕn′ĭk). 1. Pert. to health or its preservation. 2. In a healthy condition.

hygienics. A system for promoting health.

hygienist (hī-jē′nĭst, hī′jē-ĕn-ĭst). A specialist in hygiene.

h., dental. An individual trained in dental prophylaxis.

hygienization (hī″jē-ĕn-ī-zā′shŭn). The establishment of sanitary conditions and rules of hygiene.

hygric (hī′grĭk) [Gr. *hygros*, moisture]. Pert. to

moisture.

hygro-. Prefix indicating relationship to moisture.

hygroblepharic (hī″grō-blĕ-făr′ĭk) [″ + *blepharon,* eyelid]. Any structure such as the lacrimal gland or agent that moistens the eye.

hygroma (hī-grō′mă) [″ + *oma,* tumor]. (pl. *hygromas* or *hygromata*) A sac or bursa containing fluid.

h., cystic. A rapidly growing hygroma of lymphatic origin. Usually located in the neck but may be in the thorax.

hygrometer (hī-grŏm′ĕ-tĕr) [″ + *metron,* measure]. An instrument for measuring the amount of moisture in the air.

hygroscopic (hī-grō-skŏp′ĭk) [″ + *skopein,* to examine]. 1. Pert. to hygroscopy. 2. Absorbing moisture readily. SYN: *bibulous; hydrophilous.*

hygroscopy (hī-grŏs′kō-pē). Estimation of the quantity of moisture in the atmosphere.

hygrostomia (hī-grō-stō′mē-ă) [″ + *stoma,* mouth]. Excess flow of saliva. SYN: *ptyalism; salivation.*

Hygroton. Trade name for chlorthalidone, USP.

hyl-, hylo- [Gr. *hyle,* matter]. Combining form indicating wood or matter.

hyla (hī′lă). A lateral extension of the aquaeductus cerebri.

hyloma (hī-lō′mă) [Gr. *hyle,* matter, + *oma,* tumor]. A tumor composed of or in the hylic tissues, such as hypohyloma and mesohyloma.

hymen (hī′mĕn) [Gr.]. [NA] A fold of mucous membrane that partially covers the entrance of the vagina. Contrary to folklore, presence or absence of the hymen cannot be used to prove or disprove virginity or history of sexual intercourse. Its rupture or absence is not evidence of loss of virginity. Conversely, pregnancy has occurred even though the hymen has not been entered.

RS: defloration; hymenorrhaphy; hymenotomy.

h., annular. Hymen with a ring-shaped opening in the center.

h. biforis. Hymen with two parallel openings with a thick septum between.

h., cribriform. Hymen with many small perforations.

h. denticulatus. Hymen with an opening with serrated edges.

h., fenestrated. H., cribriform.

h., imperforate. A hymen with no opening in it.

h., lunar. Hymen shaped like the moon.

h., ruptured. Hymen that has been torn by coitus, injury, or surgery.

h., septate. Hymen in which the opening is separated by a thin septum.

h., unruptured. H., imperforate.

hymenal (hī′mĕn-ăl). Pert. to the hymen.

hymenectomy (hī″mĕn-ĕk′tō-mē) [″ + *ektome,* excision]. 1. In surgery and gynecology, incision or removal of the hymen. 2. Excision of a membrane.

hymenitis (hī-mĕn-ī′tĭs) [″ + *itis,* inflammation]. Inflammation of the hymen or a membrane.

Hymenolepis (hī″mĕ-nŏl′ĕ-pĭs) [″ + *lepis,* rind]. A genus of tapeworm. Parasitic in birds and mammals.

H. nana. The dwarf tapeworm, a parasite in the intestine of rats and mice; also commonly found in man. It averages about 1 in. (2.5 cm.) in length and differs from other tapeworms in that it is capable of completing its life cycle within a single host. It causes severe toxic symptoms, esp. in children.

hymenology (hī′mĕn-ŏl′ō-jē) [″ + *logos,* science]. Science of the membranes and their diseases.

hymenorrhaphy (hī″mĕn-or′ă-fē) [″ + *rhaphe,* suture]. Plastic operation on the hymen to produce partial or complete closure of the vagina.

hymenotome (hī-mĕn′ō-tōm) [″ + *tome,* incision]. Knife used to divide membranes.

hymenotomy (hī″mĕn-ŏt′ō-mē) 1. Incision of the hymen. 2. Dissection of the membrane.

hyo- [Gr. *hyoeides,* U-shaped]. Prefix indicating connection with the hyoid bone.

hyobasioglossus (hī″ō-bā″sē-ō-glŏs′ŭs) [″ + *basis,* base, + *glossa,* tongue]. The part of hyoglossal muscle attached to the hyoid bone.

hyoepiglottic, hyoepiglottidean (hī″ō-ĕp″ĭ-glŏt′ĭk, hī″ō-ĕp″ĭ-glŏt-ĭd′ē-ăn) [″ + *epiglottis,* epiglottis]. Rel. to the hyoid bone and epiglottis.

hyoglossal (hī″ō-glŏs′ăl) [″ + *glossa,* tongue]. 1. Pert. to the hyoglossus. 2. Extending to the tongue from the hyoid bone.

hyoglossus (hī″ō-glŏs′ŭs). A muscle arising from the body and greater cornu of the hyoid bone and inserted into the dorsum of the tongue. It draws sides down and retracts tongue.

hyoid (hī′oyd) [Gr. *hyoeides,* U-shaped]. 1. Shaped like the Gr. letter U, *υ*. 2. Pert. to the hyoid bone, q.v.

hyoid arch. Second branchial arch.

hyoid bone. Horseshoe-shaped bone lying at the base of the tongue. SEE: illus.

hyopharyngeus (hī″ō-făr-ĭn′jē-ŭs) [″ + *pharynx,* gullet]. Middle pharyngeal constrictor.

hyoscine (hī′ō-sĭn). Scopolamine.

h. hydrobromide. Scopolamine hydrobromide.

hyoscyamus (hī″ō-sī′ă-mŭs) [Gr. *hys,* a pig, + *kyamos,* bean]. Dried leaves of the plant Hyoscyamus niger. A narcotic. SYN: *henbane.*

HYOID BONE

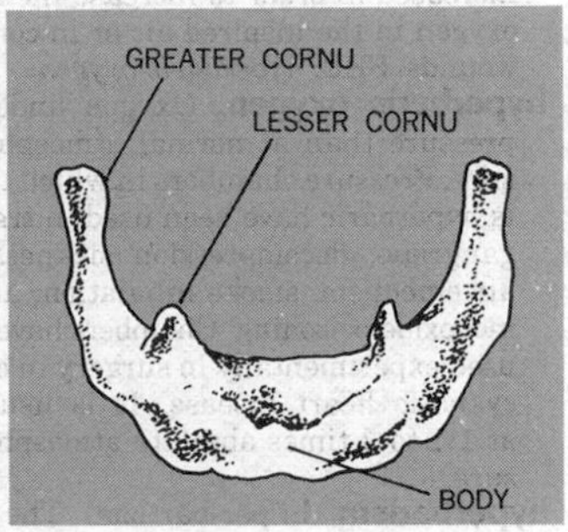

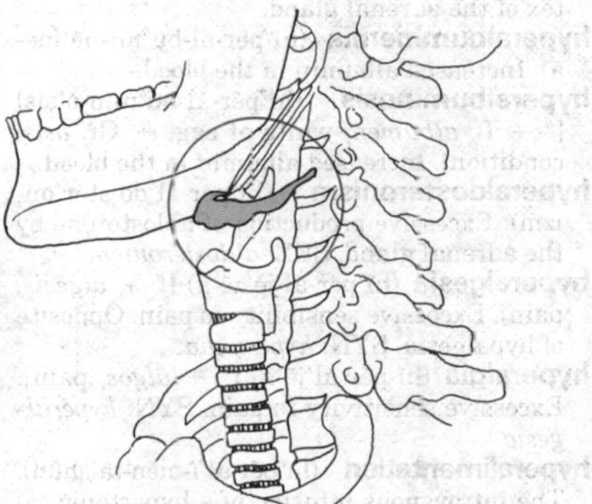

hyoscyamus poisoning. Related to atropine. SEE: *atropine* in *Poisons and Poisoning* in *Appendix.*

hypacousia, hypacusia, hypacusis (hī″pă-koo′sē-ă, -kū′sē-ă, -sĭs) [Gr. *hypo,* under, + *akousis,* hearing]. Impaired hearing. SEE: *hearing; presbyacusis.*

hypalbuminosis (hī″păl-bū-mĭn-ō′sĭs) [″ + L. *albumen,* white of egg, + Gr. *osis,* condition]. Deficiency in proportion of albumin in blood.

hypalgesia (hī-păl-jē′zē-ă) [″ + *algesis,* pain]. Lessened sensitivity to pain. Opposed to hyperalgesia.

hypalgia (hī-păl′jē-ă) [″ + *algos,* pain]. Lessened sensitivity to pain. SYN: *hypalgesia.*

hypamnios (hī-păm′nē-ŏs) [″ + *amnion,* caul of a lamb]. Deficiency in amount of amniotic fluid.

hypaphrodisia (hī-păf″rō-dĭz′ē-ă) [Gr. *hypo,* under, + *aphrodisia,* sexual pleasure]. Decreased or deficient sexual desire.

hypaxial (hī-păks′ē-ăl) [″ + *axon,* axle]. Situated beneath the body axis.

hyper- [Gr. *hyper,* above]. Prefix meaning above, excessive, or beyond.

Hyperab. Trade name for rabies immune globulin.

hyperacid (hī″pĕr-ăs′ĭd) [″ + L. *acidus,* sour]. Containing too much acid.

hyperacidaminuria (hī″pĕr-ăs″ĭd-ăm-ĭn-ū′rē-ă) [″ + ″ + *amine* + Gr. *ouron,* urine]. Presence of an excess of amino acids in the urine. SYN: *acidaminuria.*

hyperacidity (hī″pĕr-ă-sĭd′ĭ-tē) [″ + L. *acidus,* sour]. 1. An excess of acid. 2. An excess of acid in the stomach. SEE: *hyperchlorhydria.*

hyperactive child syndrome. SEE: *attention deficit disorder.*

hyperactivity 1. Increased or excessive activity that may refer to the entire organism (see below) or to a particular entity, e.g., hyperactivity of the heart or thyroid. 2. Excessive muscular activity. The term commonly refers to manifestations of disturbed behavior in children or adolescents characterized by constant overactivity, distractibility, impulsiveness, inability to concentrate, and aggressiveness. This condition is not easily defined because the claim that the child is hyperactive may be based on a low level of tolerance of the persons caring for the child. Hyperkinetic behavior usually lessens as a child grows older and usually disappears during adolescence.

ETIOL: Emotional disorders central nervous system dysfunction; mental retardation; or an exaggeration of a normal personality trait.

hyperacuity (hī″pĕr-ă-kū′ĭ-tē) [Gr *hyper,* above, + L. *acuitas,* sharpness]. Abnormal acuteness of one of the special senses such as hearing or sight.

hyperacusis (hī″pĕr-ă-kū′sĭs) [″ + *akousis,* hearing]. Abnormal sensitivity to sound. Sometimes found in hysteria. SYN: *oxyacusis.*

hyperacute (hī″pĕr-ă-kūt′). The state of any of the senses when they are very acute.

hyperadenosis (hī″pĕr-ăd″ĭ-nō′sĭs) [″ + *aden,* gland, + *osis,* condition]. Enlargement of the glands, esp. the lymph glands. SEE: *Hodgkin's disease.*

hyperadiposis, hyperadiposity (hī″pĕr-ăd″ĭ-pō′sĭs, -pŏs′ĭ-tē) [″ + L. *adeps,* fat, + Gr. *osis,* condition]. Excessive fatness.

hyperadrenalism (hī″pĕr-ă-drē′năl-ĭzm). Increased secretion from the adrenal gland.

hyperadrenocorticalism (hī″pĕr-ă-drē″nō-kor′tĭ-kăl-ĭzm). Increased secretion from the cortex of the adrenal gland.

hyperalbuminemia (hī″pĕr-ăl-bū″mĭ-nē′mē-ă). Increased albumin in the blood.

hyperalbuminosis (hī″pĕr-ăl-bū″mĭn-ō′sĭs) [″ + L. *albumen,* white of egg, + Gr. *osis,* condition]. Increased albumin in the blood.

hyperaldosteronism (hī″pĕr-ăl″dō-stĕr′ōn-ĭzm). Excessive production of aldosterone by the adrenal gland. SEE: *aldosteronism.*

hyperalgesia (hī″pĕr-ăl-jē′zē-ă) [″ + *algesis,* pain]. Excessive sensibility to pain. Opposite of hypalgesia. SYN: *hyperalgia.*

hyperalgia (hī-pĕr-ăl′jē-ă) [″ + *algos,* pain]. Excessive sensitivity to pain. SYN: *hyperalgesia.*

hyperalimentation (hī″pĕr-ăl″ĭ-mĕn-tā′shŭn). The intravenous infusion of a hypertonic solution that contains sufficient amino acids, glucose, vitamins, and electrolytes to sustain life and maintain normal growth and development. The solution is infused into the superior vena cava via a catheter threaded through the subclavian or internal jugular vein. The purpose of infusion into the superior vena cava is to have sufficient volume of blood to dilute the solution as rapidly as possible. Usually used with very sick patients, or in persons whose gastrointestinal tracts are not functioning properly.

hyperalkalinity (hī″pĕr-ăl-kă-lĭn′ĭ-tē). A condition of excess alkalinity.

hyperaminoacidemia (hī″pĕr-ăm″ĭ-nō-ăs″ĭ-dē′mē-ă). An abnormal amount of amino acids in the blood.

hyperammonemia (hī″pĕr-ăm″mō-nē′mē-ă). An excess of ammonia in the blood. SEE: *ammonia toxicity.*

h., congenital. Accumulation of an excess of ammonia in the body due to a congenital deficiency of enzymes, either carbamyl phosphate synthetase or ornithine transcarbamylase, essential to the metabolism of ammonia. Clinical signs of ammonia toxicity, q.v., are present. These include vomiting, lethargy, coma, and eventually death.

hyperamylasemia (hī″pĕr-ăm″ĭl-ās-ē′mē-ă). Increased blood amylase.

hyperanacinesia, hyperanacinesis (hī″pĕr-ăn″ă-sĭn-ē′zē-ă, -sĭs). Hyperanakinesis.

hyperanakinesis (hī″pĕr-ăn″ă-kĭ-nē′sĭs) [″ + *anakinesis,* exercise]. Excessive function or movement activity of an organ or part such as of the stomach or intestines.

hyperaphia (hī″pĕr-ā′fē-ă) [″ + *haphe,* touch]. Excessive sensitiveness to touch.

hyperaphic (hī-pĕr-ăf′ĭk). Marked by extreme sensitiveness to touch.

hyperazotemia (hī″pĕr-ăz″ō-tē′mē-ă) [″ + L. *azotum,* nitrogen, + Gr. *haima,* blood]. Increased amount of nitrogenous substances, such as urea, in the blood.

hyperazoturia (hī″pĕr-ăz″ō-tū′rē-ă) [″ + ″ + Gr. *ouron,* urine]. Excessive amount of nitrogenous matter in the urine.

hyperbaric chamber. A chamber large enough to hold a patient and a medical or surgical team. The pressure in the chamber can be increased in order to increase the amount of oxygen in the inspired air or in contact with wounds. SEE: *hyperbaric oxygen.*

hyperbaric oxygen. Oxygen under greater pressure than at normal atmospheric pressure. Pressure chambers in which the oxygen is hyperbaric have been used in treating gas gangrene, decompression sickness (bends), air embolism, smoke inhalation, and carbon monoxide poisoning. Chambers have also been used experimentally in surgery in congenital cyanotic heart disease. It is usually used at 1½ to 3 times absolute atmospheric pressure.

hyperbarism (hī″pĕr-băr′ĭzm). The condition of being exposed to or having pressure greater than atmospheric. Miners and deep sea divers are exposed to this condition. SEE: *bends; caisson disease.*

hyperbetalipoproteinemia (hī″pĕr-bā″tă-lĭp″ō-prō″tē-ĭn-ē′mē-ă). Excessive amount of β-lipoproteins in the blood. SEE: *hyperlipoproteinemia.*

hyperbilirubinemia (hī″pĕr-bĭl″ĭ-roo-bĭn-ē′mē-ă) [Gr. *hyper,* above, + L. *bilis,* bile, + *ruber,* red, + Gr. *haima,* blood]. Excessive amt. of bilirubin in the blood.

hyperbrachycephaly (hī″pĕr-brăk″ē-sĕf′ă-lē) [″ + *brachys,* short, + *kephale,* head]. Excessive degree of brachycephaly; having a cephalic index over 85.

hyperbulia (hī″pĕr-bū′lē-ă) [″ + *boule,* will]. Abnormal degree of will power.

hypercalcemia (hī″pĕr-kăl-sē′mē-ă) [″ + L. *calx,* lime, + Gr. *haima,* blood]. An excessive amount of calcium in the blood. SYN: *calcemia.*

h., idiopathic. Type of hypercalcemia seen in infants, caused by vitamin D intoxication.

hypercalciuria (hī″pĕr-kăl″sē-ū′rē-ă) [″ + ″ + Gr. *ouron,* urine]. An excessive quantity of calcium in the urine.

hypercapnia (hī″pĕr-kăp′nē-ă) [″ + *kapnos,* smoke]. Increased amount of carbon dioxide in the blood.

hypercatharsis (hī″pĕr-kă-thăr′sĭs) [″ + *katharsis,* purge]. Excessive bowel movement in response to administration of cathartics.

hypercellularity (hī″pĕr-sĕl″ū-lār′ĭ-tē). Increased number of cells in any location but esp. in the bone marrow.

hypercementosis (hī″pĕr-sē″mĕn-tō′sĭs) [″ + L. *cementum,* cement, + Gr. *osis,* condition]. Overgrowth of tooth cement (cementum).

hyperchloremia (hī″pĕr-klō-rē′mē-ă) [″ + *chloros,* green, + *haima,* blood]. Increase in chloride content of the blood.

hyperchlorhydria (hī″pĕr-klor-hī′drē-ă) [″ + ″ + *hydor,* water]. An excess of hydrochloric acid in the gastric secretion. It causes a burning sensation in the stomach in the absence of ingested foods. The amount secreted above what is needed to combine with albumoid and basic substances is known as free hydrogen chloride.

The ability of the stomach to produce hydrochloric acid can be evaluated clinically. A tube is carefully placed in the stomach and the contents aspirated prior to, and at 15-minute intervals for an hour after, stimulation of the parietal cells of the stomach. This is accomplished by giving the histamine analogue, betazole hydrochloride, USP, 2.0 mg./kg. body weight subcutaneously. If the pH of the aspirate obtained 30 minutes later is six or above, the patient has achlorhydria. The production of more than 24 millequivalents of hydrochloric acid in the four specimens obtained following the injection of betazole is considered abnormal and consistent with the presence of hyperchlorhydria. SEE: *achlorhydria; gastritis; hydrochloric acid; hypochlorhydria.*

hyperchloridation (hī″pĕr-klō″rĭ-dā′shŭn). A dosing with large amounts of sodium chloride.

hypercholesterolemia (hī″pĕr-kō-lĕs″tĕr-ŏl-ē′mē-ă) [″ + *chole,* bile, + *stereos,* solid, + *haima,* blood]. Excessive amount of cholesterol in the blood.

h., familial. A type of hyperlipoproteinemia, type IIA, in which the low-density lipoproteins are increased and the very low-density lipoproteins are normal. SEE: *hyperlipoproteinemia.*

hypercholesterolia (hī″pĕr-kō-lĕs″tĕr-ō′lē-ă) [″ + ″ + *stereos,* solid]. Excessive cholesterol in the bile.

hypercholia (hī″pĕr-kō′lē-ă) [″ + *chole,* bile]. Abnormal secretion of bile.

hyperchromasia (hī″pĕr-krō-mā′zē-ă) [Gr. *hyper,* above, + *chroma,* color]. Hyperchromatism.

hyperchromatic (hī″pĕr-krō-măt′ĭk) [″ + *chroma,* color]. Overpigmented.

hyperchromatic cell. A cell or a part of a cell that contains more than the normal number of chromosomes and hence stains more densely.

hyperchromatism (hī″pĕr-krō′mă-tĭzm) [″ + ″ + *-ismos,* state of]. 1. Excessive pigmentation. 2. Increased staining capacity of any structure. SYN: *hyperchromatosis.*

hyperchromatopsia (hī″pĕr-krō″mă-tŏp′sē-ă) [″ + ″ + *opsis,* vision]. Defect of vision in which all objects appear colored.

hyperchromatosis (hī″pĕr-krō″mă-tō′sĭs) [″ + *chroma,* color, + *osis,* condition]. 1. Excessive pigmentation, esp. of the skin. 2. Increased staining capacity. SYN: *hyperchromatism.*

hyperchromia (hī″pĕr-krō′mē-ă). Excessive pigmentation. SYN: *hyperchromatism.*

hyperchromic (hī-pĕr-krō′mĭk) 1. Pert. to excessive pigmentation. 2. Intensely colored.

hyperchylia (hī″pĕr-kī′lē-ă) [Gr. *hyper,* above, + L. *chylus,* juice]. Abnormal secretion of gastric juice.

hyperchylomicronemia (hī″pĕr-kī″lō-mī″krō-nē′mē-ă). Excess accumulation of fat particles, chylomicrons, in the blood.

hypercoagulability (hī″pĕr-kō-ăg′ū-lă-bĭl′ĭ-tē). Increased ability of anything to coagulate, but esp. the blood.

hypercorticism (hī″pĕr-kor′tĭ-sĭzm). Excessive production of adrenal cortical hormones in the body.

hypercrinism (hī″pĕr-krī′nĭzm) [″ + *krinein,* to separate, + *-ismos,* state of]. Condition due to excessive activity of any endocrine gland.

hypercryalgesia (hī″pĕr-krī″ăl-jē′zē-ă) [″ + *kryos,* cold, + *algesis,* pain]. Excessive sensitivity to cold. SYN: *hypercryesthesia.*

hypercryesthesia (hī″pĕr-krī″ĕs-thē′zē-ă) [″ + ″ + *aisthesis,* sensation]. Excessive sensitivity to cold. SYN: *hypercryalgesia.*

hypercupremia (hī″pĕr-kū-prē′mē-ă). Increased level of copper in the blood. SEE: *Wilson's disease.*

hypercyanosis (hī″pĕr-sī″ă-nō′sĭs) [″ + *kyanos,* dark blue, + *osis,* condition]. Extreme cyanosis.

hypercyanotic (hī″pĕr-sī″ă-nŏt′ĭk). Denoting extreme cyanosis.

hypercyesis (hī″pĕr-sī-ē′sĭs) [″ + *kyesis,* gestation]. Presence of more than one fetus in a uterus because of fertilization of a second ovum within a short time. SYN: *superfetation.*

hypercythemia (hī″pĕr-sī-thē′mē-ă) [″ + *kytos,* cell, + *haima,* blood]. Condition of having an excessive number of red blood corpuscles.

hypercytosis (hī″pĕr-sī-tō′sĭs) [″ + ″ + *osis,* condition]. Abnormal increase in leukocytes in the blood. SYN: *leukocytosis.*

hyperdactylia (hī″pĕr-dăk-tĭl′ē-ă) [Gr. *hyper,* above, + *daktylos,* finger]. State of having supernumerary fingers or toes.

hyperdicrotic (hī″pĕr-dī-krŏt′ĭk) [″ + *dikrotos,* beating double]. Abnormally dicrotic. SEE: *dicrotic.*

hyperdistention (hī″pĕr-dĭs-tĕn′shŭn) [″ + L. *distendere,* to stretch out]. Excessive inflation or distention.

hyperdontial (hī″pĕr-dŏn′shē-ăl). Presence of more than the normal number of teeth.

hyperdynamia (hī″pĕr-dī-nā′mē-ă) [″ + *dynamis,* force]. Muscular restlessness or extreme violence.

h. uteri. Abnormal uterine contractions in labor.

hypereccrisia, hypereccrisis (hī″pĕr-ĕk-krĭs′ē-ă, -ĕk′krĭ-sĭs) [″ + *ekkrisis,* excretion]. Abnormal amount of excretion.

hypereccritic (hī-pĕr-ĕk-krĭt′ĭk). Pert. to hypereccrisis.

hyperemesis (hī″pĕr-ĕm′ĕ-sĭs) [″ + *emesis,* vomiting]. Excessive vomiting.

h. gravidarum. Nausea and vomiting during pregnancy of such severity and duration that systemic effects such as acidosis and weight loss occur. About two out of each 1000 pregnant women have this disease with such severity as to require hospitalization. If the severe form is untreated, it can be fatal.

ETIOL: The cause is unknown.

SYM: The condition may start as a simple vomiting of early pregnancy, but with combined vomiting, first of gastric contents and later of bile, there develop a chloride depletion, acidosis, and, finally, with severe and continued vomiting, pathological changes in the liver take place.

TREATMENT: In early cases, rest in bed; small amounts of carbohydrates taken frequently; moderate restriction of fluids; mild sedation and antiemetic drugs are usually effective. In severe cases, the patient is hospitalized, with complete bedrest and no visitors until vomiting ends and eating begins. Treatment includes nothing by mouth for 48 hours; maintain nutritional and electrolyte balance by giving parenteral fluids and proteins as required. Rarely, nasogastric feeding or total parenteral nutrition will be required. The necessity for emptying the uterus should occur only rarely if the patient is seen early and the proper treatment instituted at once. When the patient improves, food taken by mouth should consist of a light solid diet given in frequent small feedings, with fruit juice or milk between feedings.

h. lactentium. Vomiting in nursing infants.

hyperemia (hī″pĕr-ē′mē-ă) [″ + *haima,* blood]. 1. Congestion. An unusual amount of blood in a part. 2. A form of macula; red areas on skin that disappear on pressure. 3. In physical therapy, increase in the quantity of blood flowing through any part of the body, shown by redness of the skin caused by the application of heat.

h., active. Hyperemia caused by increased blood inflow. SYN: *h., arterial.*

h., arterial. H., active.

h., Bier's. Passive hyperemia, q.v., produced by application of an elastic bandage and by suction. SYN: *h., constriction.*

h., constriction. H., Bier's.

h., leptomeningeal. Pia-arachnoid congestion.

h., passive. Hyperemia caused by decreased blood outflow. SYN: *h., venous.*

h., reactive. The increased presence of blood in an area after restoration of blood flow following a decreased supply.

h., venous. H., passive.

hyperemization (hī″pĕr-ē″mĭ-zā′shŭn). Hyperemia produced artificially for therapeutic purposes.

hyperemotivity (hī″pĕr-ē″mō-tĭv′ĭ-tē) [Gr. *hyper,* above, + L. *emovere,* to disturb]. Excessive emotivity or response to stimuli.

hypereosinophilia (hī″pĕr-ē″ō-sĭn-ō-fĭl′ē-ă) [″ + *eos,* dawn, + *philein,* to love]. Marked increase in number of eosinophils in the blood.

hyperepinephrinemia (hī″pĕr-ĕp″ĭ-nĕf″rĭ-nē′mē-ă) [″ + ″ + *nephros,* kidney, + *haima,* blood]. Abnormally large amount of epinephrine in the blood.

hyperequilibrium (hī″pĕr-ē″kwĭ-lĭb′rē-ŭm) [″ + L. *aequus,* equal, + *libra,* balance]. A tendency to vertigo when making even slight turning movements.

hypererethism (hī″pĕr-ĕr′ĭ-thĭzm) [″ + *erethisma,* stimulation]. Excessive irritability.

hyperergasia (hī″pĕr-ĕr-gā′sē-ă) [″ + *ergasia,* work]. Unusual functional activity.

hyperergia (hī″pĕr-ĕr′jē-ă). 1. Excessive or increased functional activity. SYN: *hyperergasia.* 2. Abnormal sensitivity to allergens.

hyperergy (hī′pĕr-ĕr″jē) [″ + *ergon,* energy]. Hypersensitivity or condition in which there is an exaggerated response. SEE: *allergy; anaphylaxis.*

hyperesophoria (hī″pĕr-ĕs″ō-fō′rē-ă) [″ + *eso,* inward, + *phorein,* to bear]. Tendency of the visual axis to deviate upward and inward due to muscular imbalance. A form of heterophoria, q.v.

hyperesthesia (hī″pĕr-ĕs-thē′zē-ă) [″ + *aisthesis,* sensation]. Increased sensitivity to sensory stimuli, such as pain or touch. SYN: *algesia; oxyesthesia.*

h., acoustic. Abnormal sensitivity to sound.

h., cerebral. Hyperesthesia caused by a cerebral lesion.

h., gustatory. Oversensitivity of taste.

h., muscular. Muscular sensitivity to pain and tiredness.

h., optic. Abnormal sensitivity to light.

h. sexualis. Abnormal increase in libido.

h., tactile. Abnormal sensitivity of touch.

hyperesthetic (hī″pĕr-ĕs-thĕt′ĭk). Pert. to hyperesthesia.

hyperexophoria (hī″pĕr-ĕks″ō-fō′rē-ă) [″ + *exo,* outward, + *phorein,* to bear]. Tendency of visual axis to deviate upward and outward due to muscular imbalance. A form of heterophoria, q.v.

hyperextension (hī″pĕr-ĕks-tĕn′shŭn) [″ +

L. *extendere*, to stretch out]. Extreme or abnormal extension.

hyperferremia (hī″pĕr-fĕr-rē′mē-ă). Excess amount of iron in the blood. SEE: *hemochromatosis*.

hyperfibrinogenemia (hī″pĕr-fī-brĭn″ō-jĕ-nē′mē-ă). Increased amount of fibrinogen in the blood.

hyperflexion (hī″pĕr-flĕk′shŭn). Increased flexion of a joint, usually due to trauma.

hyperfunction [Gr. *hyper*, above, + L. *functio*, performance]. Excessive activity.

hypergalactia (hī-pĕr-găl-ăk′shē-ă) [″ + *gala*, milk]. Excessive milk secretion.

hypergammaglobulinemia (hī″pĕr-găm″ă-glŏb″ū-lĭ-nē′mē-ă). Excess amount of gamma globulin in the blood.

hypergasia (hĭp-ĕr-gā′sē-ă). Hypoergasia, decreased sensitivity to allergens.

hypergenesis (hī″pĕr-jĕn′ĕ-sĭs) [″ + *genesis*, development]. Redundancy of organs or parts; overproduction. SYN: *hyperplasia*.

hypergenitalism (hī″pĕr-jĕn′ĭt-ăl-ĭzm) [″ + L. *genitalis*, genital]. Excessive development of the genital organs.

ETIOL: Disturbances in endocrine secretions of the adrenal gland or gonads, or hypothalamic disorders.

hypergeusesthesia, hypergeusia (hī″pĕr-gūs-ĕs-thē′sē-ă, -gū′sē-ă) [″ + *geusis*, taste, + *aisthesis*, perception]. Excessive acuteness of sense of taste.

hypergia (hī-pĕr′jē-ă). Decreased sensitivity to allergens.

hyperglandular (hī″pĕr-glăn′dū-lăr) [″ + L. *glandula*, a little acorn]. Having excessive glandular secretions.

hyperglobulinemia (hī″pĕr-glŏb″ū-lĭn-ē′mē-ă) [″ + L. *globulus*, a globule, + Gr. *haima*, blood]. Excessive globulin in the blood.

hyperglycemia (hī″pĕr-glī-sē′mē-ă) [″ + *glykys*, sweet, + *haima*, blood]. Increase of blood sugar as in diabetes. This condition increases susceptibility to infection and it often precedes diabetic coma. SEE: *hypoglycemia*.

hyperglyceridemia (hī″pĕr-glĭs″ĕr-ĭ-dē′mē-ă). Accumulation of glycerides, esp. triglycerides in the blood.

hyperglycinemia (hī″pĕr-glī″sĭ-nē′mē-ă). Accumulation of glycine in the blood. This is caused by a congenital defect in the ability to metabolize the amino acid glycine. There are at least six forms of this disease, all of which are associated with mental and growth retardation.

hyperglycogenolysis (hī″pĕr-glī″kō-jĕn-ŏl′ĭ-sĭs) [″ + ″ + *gennan*, to form, + *lysis*, dissolution]. Excessive conversion of glycogen into glucose by hydrolysis.

hyperglycoplasmia (hī″pĕr-glī″kō-plăz′mē-ă) [″ + ″ + *plasma*, matter formed]. Excessive sugar in the plasma of the blood.

hyperglycorrhachia (hī″pĕr-glī″kō-rā′kē-ă) [″ + *glykys*, sweet, + *rhachis*, spine]. Excess of sugar in the cerebrospinal fluid.

hyperglycosemia (hī″pĕr-glī-kō-sē′mē-ă) [″ + ″ + *haima*, blood]. Excessive sugar in the blood. SYN: *hyperglycemia*.

hyperglycosuria (hī″pĕr-glī″kō-sū′rē-ă) [″ + ″ + *ouron*, urine]. Excessive sugar in the urine. SEE: *glycosuria*.

hypergnosia (hī″pĕr-nō′sē-ă) [″ + *gnosis*, knowledge]. Distorted or exaggerated perception influenced by the unconscious projection of emotional subjective experiences.

hypergonadism (hī″pĕr-gō′năd-ĭzm) [″ + *gone*, seed, + *-ismos*, state of]. Excessive secretion of the sex glands.

hyperguanidinemia (hī″pĕr-gwăn″ĭ-dĭn-ē′mē-ă) [″ + Sp. *guano*, dung, + *haima*, blood]. Abnormal amt. of guanidine in blood.

hyperhedonia, hyperhedonism (hī″pĕr-hē-dŏ′nē-ă, -hē′dŏn-ĭzm) [Gr. *hyper*, above, + *hedone*, pleasure, + *-ismos*, state of]. 1. Abnormal pleasure in anything. 2. Abnormal sexual excitement.

Hyper Hep. Trade name for hepatitis B immune globulin.

hyperhidrosis (hī″pĕr-hī-drō′sĭs) [″ + *hidros*, sweat, + *osis*, condition]. Sweating greater than would be expected in the temperature of the environment.

ETIOL: Functional overactivity of sweat glands caused by debilitating disease or stimulants. Increased in rheumatic, malarial, relapsing, and septic fever. Occurs in neuralgia and migraine and follows certain drugs and hot drinks. Locally it affects hands and feet in hysteria, fright, nervous irritability, and hyperthyroidism. SEE: *sweat*.

hyperhydration (hī″pĕr-hī-drā′shŭn). Excess water in the body.

hyperimmune (hī″pĕr-ĭm-mūn′). State of immunity greater than normal.

hyperinflation (hī″pĕr-ĭn-flā′shŭn). Excess air in anything, esp. the lungs.

hyperinosemia (hī″pĕr-ī″nō-sē′mē-ă) [″ + *inos*, fiber, + *haima*, blood]. Abnormal coagulability of the blood; excess of fibrinogen in the blood.

hyperinosis (hī″pĕr-ĭ-nō′sĭs) [″ + *inos*, fiber, + *osis*, condition]. Excessive fibrinogen in the blood. SYN: *hyperinosemia*.

hyperinsulinism (hī″pĕr-ĭn′sū-lĭn-ĭzm) [″ + L. *insula*, island, + Gr. *-ismos*, state of]. An excessive amount of insulin in the blood.

ETIOL: Tumor on islets of Langerhans or excessive sensitivity of the islet tissue to an increase in blood-sugar level. May be caused by an overdose of insulin.

SYM: Those consistent with hypoglycemia, q.v. Hunger; weakness; sweating; staggering; diplopia; rarely convulsions; coma; and death. Occasionally spontaneous, in which case symptoms are similar to but last longer than those in insulin shock. SEE: *insulin; insulin shock; shock.*

hyperinvolution (hī″pĕr-ĭn″vō-lū′shŭn) [″ + L. *involvere,* to enwrap]. 1. Reduction in size of uterus below normal after childbirth. 2. Reduction in size below normal of any organ following hypertrophy. SYN: *superinvolution.*

h. uteri. Extreme atrophy of the uterus seen following prolonged lactation or severe puerperal sepsis.

hyperirritability (hī″pĕr-ĭr″ĭ-tă-bĭl′ĭ-tē). Increased response to a stimulus.

hyperisotonic [″ + *isos,* equal, + *tonos,* tension]. Said of one of two solutions that has the greater osmotic pressure. SYN: *hypertonic.*

hyperkalemia, hyperkaliemia (hī″pĕr-kă-lē′mē-ă, -kăl″ē-ē′mē-ă) [″ + L. *kalium,* potassium, + Gr. *haima,* blood]. Excessive amount of potassium in the blood.

hyperkeratinization (hī″pĕr-kĕr″ă-tĭn″ĭ-zā′shŭn) [″ + *keras,* horn]. Thickening of the horny layers of the skin, esp. of the palms and soles. May be caused by vitamin A deficiency, or chronic arsenic toxicity.

hyperkeratomycosis (hī″pĕr-kĕr″ă-tō-mī-kō′sĭs) [″ + ″ + *mykes,* fungus, + *osis,* condition]. Hypertrophy of horny layer of the epidermis due to a parasitic fungus.

hyperkeratosis [″ + ″ + *osis,* condition]. 1. Overgrowth of the cornea. 2. Overgrowth of the horny layer of the epidermis. SYN: *keratodermia; keratosis.*

h. congenitalis. Hyperkeratosis in the harlequin fetus.

h., epidermolytic. Congenital disorder characterized by hyperkeratosis, erythema, and blisters.

hyperketonemia (hī″pĕr-kē″tō-nē′mē-ă). Accumulation of an excess of ketone bodies in the blood.

hyperketonuria (hī″pĕr-kē-tō-nūr′ē-ă). Excessive quantity of ketones in urine.

hyperketosis (hī″pĕr-kē-tō′sĭs). Abnormally high ketone production in the body.

hyperkinesia, hyperkinesis (hī″pĕr-kī-nē′zē-ă, -nē′sĭs) [Gr. *hyper,* above, + *kinesis,* motion]. Increased muscular movement and physical activity. In children it may be due to minimal brain dysfunction, q.v. SEE: *hyperactivity.*

hyperlactation (hī″pĕr-lăk-tā′shŭn) [″ + L. *lactare,* to suckle]. Excessive milk secretion. SYN: *superlactation.*

hyperlipemia (hī″pĕr-lĭp-ē′mē-ă) [″ + *lipos,* fat, + *haima,* blood]. Excessive quantity of fat in the blood.

hyperlipoproteinemia (hī″pĕr-lĭp″ō-prō″tē-ĭn-ē′mē-ă). An increase in the concentration of the three fatty substances of the blood: cholesterol, phospholipid, and triglyceride. These substances do not circulate freely in the blood but are combined with the plasma proteins; they are called lipoproteins. The various forms of hyperlipoproteinemia have been classified into five major types through the use of paper electrophoresis. SEE: table.

hyperliposis (hī″pĕr-lĭ-pō′sĭs) [″ + *lipos,* fat, + *osis,* condition]. 1. Abnormal amt. of fat; adiposity. 2. Excessive fatty degeneration.

hyperlithuria (hī″pĕr-lĭth-ū′rē-ă) [″ + *lithos,* stone, + *ouron,* urine]. Excessive excretion of lithic (uric) acid in the urine.

hypermastia (hī″pĕr-măs′tē-ă) [″ + *mastos,* breast]. 1. Excessively large mammary glands. May be unilateral. SYN: *gynecomastia.* 2. Presence of abnormal number of mammary glands. SYN: *polymastia; polymazia.*

hypermature (hī″pĕr-mă-tūr′) [″ + L. *maturus,* ripe]. 1. Pert. to anything that has passed the stage of maturity. 2. Overripe, as a cataract or abscess that has gone past the optimum time for incision.

hypermegasoma (hī″pĕr-mĕg″ă-sō′mă) [″ + *megas,* large, + *soma,* body]. Excessive bodily development. SYN: *giantism.*

hypermenorrhea (hī″pĕr-mĕn″ō-rē′ă) [″ + *men,* month, + *rhoia,* flow]. Abnormal increase in the duration or amount of menstrual flow.

hypermetabolic state (hī″pĕr-mĕt″ă-bŏl′ĭk). Condition of abnormally increased rate of metabolism. Seen in fever, and in salicylate poisoning.

hypermetabolism (hī″pĕr-mĕ-tăb′ō-lĭzm). Increased rate of metabolism.

h., extrathyroidal. Increased rate of metabolism not related to thyroid disease.

hypermetaplasia (hī″pĕr-mĕt″ă-plā′sē-ă) [″ + *meta-,* after, + *plassein,* to form]. Overactivity in tissue replacement or transformation from one type of tissue to another, as cartilage to bone.

hypermetria (hī″pĕr-mē′trē-ă) [Gr. *hyper,* above, + *metron,* measure]. Unusual range of movement; state in which muscular movement overreaches the objective.

hypermetrope (hī″pĕr-mĕt′rōp) [″ + ″ + *ops,* eye]. One who is farsighted. SYN: *hyperope.*

hypermetropia (hī″pĕr-mē-trō′pē-ă). Farsightedness. Opposite of myopia. SYN: *hyperopia.*

hypermetropic (hī″pĕr-mē-trŏp′ĭk). Pert. to farsightedness.

hypermimia (hī″pĕr-mĭm′ē-ă) [″ + *mimesis,* imitation]. Use of a great number of gestures while speaking.

hypermnesia (hī″pĕrm-nē′zē-ă) [″ + *mneme,* memory]. 1. Great ability to remember names, dates, and details. 2. An exaggeration of memory involving minute details of a past experience. It occurs in manic phase of manic-depressive psychosis; in delirium and hypnoses; at the moment of shock and fright in life-threatening situations; with fever; during neurosurgical procedures where the temporal lobe is stimulated; and following some brain injuries.

hypermobility (hī″pĕr-mō-bĭl′ĭ-tē). Excess joint relaxation that permits increased mobility. It is present in certain diseases of children such as Marfan's or Ehler's-Danlos syndromes.

hypermorph (hī′pĕr-morf) [″ + *morphe,* form]. One whose length of limb and consequent standing height is high in proportion to the sitting height. SEE: *hypomorph; somatotype.*

hypermotility (hī″pĕr-mō-tĭl′ĭ-tē) [″ + L. *motio,* motion]. Unusual motility. SYN: *hyperkinesia.*

hypermyatrophy (hī″pĕr-mī-ăt′rō-fē) [″ + *mys,* muscle, + *atrophia,* atrophy]. Unusual wasting of muscle.

hypermyesthesia (hī″pĕr-mī″ĕs-thē′sē-ă) [″ + ″ + *aisthesis,* sensation]. Muscular hyperesthesia.

hypermyotonia (hī″pĕr-mī″ō-tō′nē-ă) [″ + ″ + *tonos,* tone]. Excessive muscular tonus.

hypermyotrophy (hī″pĕr-mī-ŏt′rō-fē) [″ + ″ + *trophe,* nourishment]. Abnormal muscular development.

hypernatremia (hī″pĕr-nă-trē′mē-ă) [″ + L. *natron,* sodium, + Gr. *haima,* blood]. Excess sodium in the blood.

hyperneocytosis (hī″pĕr-nē″ō-sī-tō′sĭs) [″ + *neos,* new, + *kytos,* cell, + *osis,* condition]. Abnormal increase of leukocytes in the blood (leukocytosis), including an abnormal amount of immature forms.

hypernephroma (hī″pĕr-nĕ-frō′mă) [″ + *nephros,* kidney, + *oma,* tumor]. A tumor of the kidney that to the naked eye resembles adrenal tissue.

hyperneurotization (hī″pĕr-nū-rŏt″ĭ-zā′shŭn) [″ + *neuron,* nerve]. Grafting of a motor nerve into a muscle to increase its energy.

hypernitremia (hī″pĕr-nī-trē′mē-ă) [″ + *nitron,* niter, + *haima,* blood]. Excess of nitrogen in the blood.

hypernoia (hī-pĕr-noy′ă) [″ + *nous,* mind]. Excessive mental activity or imagination.

hypernormal (hī″pĕr-nor′măl) [″ + L. *norma,* rule]. Abnormal.

hypernormocytosis (hī″pĕr-nor″mō-sī-tō′sis) [″ + ″ + Gr. *kytos,* cell, + *osis,* condition]. An increased proportion of neutrophils in the blood.

hypernutrition (hī″pĕr-nū-trĭsh′ŭn) [″ + L. *nutrire,* to nourish]. Supernutrition; overfeeding.

hyperonychia (hī″pĕr-ō-nĭk′ē-ă) [″ + *onyx,* nail]. Overgrowth (hypertrophy) of the nails.

hyperope (hī′pĕr-ōp) [″ + *ops,* eye]. One who is farsighted. SYN: *hypermetrope.*

hyperopia (hī″pĕr-ō′pē-ă) [″ + *ops,* eye]. Farsightedness. Defect in vision in which parallel rays come to a focus behind the retina due to flattening of the globe of the eye or to error in refraction. SYN: *hypermetropia.* SEE: *emmetropia* for illus.

SYM: Ocular fatigue and poor vision.

h., absolute. Hyperopia in which the eye cannot accommodate.

h., axial. Hyperopia caused by shortness of the eye's anteroposterior axis.

h., facultative. Hyperopia that can be corrected by accommodation.

h., latent. Hyperopia in which the error of refraction is overcome and disguised by ciliary muscle action.

h., manifest. Total amount of hyperopia that can be neutralized by a convex lens without interfering with clarity of vision.

h., relative. Hyperopia in which vision is clear only when excessive convergence is made.

h., total. Complete hyperopia combining both latent and manifest types; the amt. of hyperopia present when accommodation is completely suspended by paralyzing the ciliary muscle. This is done by use of a cycloplegic drug.

hyperorchidism (hī″pĕr-or kĭd-ĭzm) [Gr. *hyper,* above, + *orchis,* testicle, + *-ismos,* state of]. Abnormal activity of testicular secretion.

hyperorexia (hī″pĕr-ō-rĕks′ē-ă) [″ + *orexis,* appetite]. Abnormal hunger. Usually satisfied by frequent small meals, as in gastric diseases, diabetes, hysteria, psychosis, hyperthyroidism and brain tumors. It is found in helminthiasis, diabetes, hysteria, convalescence from acute diseases, psychosis, hyperthyroidism, brain tumors, diseases of the stomach in which hypermotility and hypersecretion are present. SYN: *bulimia.*

hyperorthocytosis (hī″pĕr-or″thō-sī-tō′sĭs) [″ + *orthos,* straight, + *kytos,* cell, + *osis,* condition]. Increased white blood cells with normal proportion of various forms and without immature forms.

hyperosmia (hī″pĕr-ŏz′mē-ă) [″ + *osme,* smell]. Abnormal sensitivity to odors.

hyperosmolar hyperglycemic nonketotic coma. ABBR: HHNC. Coma caused by increased blood osmolarity and glucose but not associated with ketoacidosis. It usually occurs in diabetes but may be present as a complication of burns, hyperalimentation, and renal dialysis. The blood glucose level may be as high as 1000 mg./dl. The metabolic disorder is treated with insulin, potassium, and sodium until the condition is corrected. The total water deficit may be as much as 10–12 liters. When adequate urine flow is established, it is essential to prevent excess

Types of Hyperlipoproteinemias

Type	Incidence	Other Name or Names	Appearance of Chilled Serum	Triglycerides	Cholesterol
I	Very rare	Exogenous hypertriglyceridemia; Familial hypertriglyceridemia; Fat-induced hyperlipidemia	Creamy layer over clear serum	May be 1000 or much more	Elevated
IIA	Common	Familial hypercholesterolemia; Hyperbetalipoproteinemia	Clear	Normal	Elevated
IIB	Common	Mixed hyperbeta- and hyperprebetalipoproteinemia; Mixed hyperlipidemia	Turbid	Elevated	Elevated
III	Relatively uncommon	Familial dysbetalipoproteinemia	Turbid	Elevated	Elevated
IV	Common	Endogenous hypertriglyceridemia; Familial hyperprebetalipoproteinemia	Turbid	Elevated	Elevated
V	Uncommon	Mixed hypertriglyceridemia; Combined exogenous and endogenous hypertriglyceridemia; Mixed hyperlipemia	Creamy layer over milky serum	Elevated	Normal or elevated

administration of potassium. This can be monitored by use of electrocardiography.

hyperosmolarity (hī″pĕr-ŏz″mō-lăr′ĭ-tē). Increased osmolarity of the blood.

hyperostosis (hī″pĕr-ŏs-tō′sĭs) [″ + *osteon,* bone, + *osis,* condition]. Abnormal growth of osseous tissue. SYN: *exostosis.*

h., frontal internal. Osteoma, usually multiple or arising from the internal area of the frontal bone.

h., infantile cortical. Increased growth of subperiosteal bone occurring most frequently in the mandible and clavicles with fever and other systemic manifestations.

h., Morgagni's. H., frontal internal.

hyperovaria [Gr. *hyper,* above, + L. *ovarium,* ovary]. Precocity of sexual development in young girls due to excessive ovarian secretion as the result of unusual and premature development of the ovaries.

hyperoxaluria (hī″pĕr-ŏk″să-lū′rē-ă). Increased oxalic acid in the urine.

h., enteric. Increased oxalic acid in the urine caused by disease of or surgical removal of the ileum.

h., primary. An inherited metabolic disease caused by a defect in glyoxalate metabolism. This causes an increased secretion of

and Their Characteristics

Clinical Features	Age of Detection	Therapy	Complications
Creamy blood; lipemia retinalis; eruptive xanthomas; hepatosplenomegaly; abdominal pain	Early childhood	Low-fat diet, 25–35 grams daily	Pancreatitis
Xanthelasma; tendon and tuberous xanthomas; juvenile corneal arcus; accelerated atherosclerosis	Early childhood in severe cases	Unstaturated fat diet; reduce cholesterol intake; cholestyramine or colestipol hydrochloride, and nicotinic acid	Coronary artery disease
Severe forms resemble IIA. Milder forms are associated with obesity or diabetes, or both	Childhood or later	Same as IIA	Coronary artery disease
Xanthoma planum; eruptive, tuberous, and tendon xanthomas; accelerated atherosclerosis of all vessels	Over age 20	Weight loss; clofibrate; nicotinic acid	Cardiovascular disease, esp peripheral atherosclerosis
Accelerated coronary artery disease; abnormal glucose tolerance; hyperuricemia	Adult	Weight loss; nicotinic acid	Cardiovascular disease; obesity
Lipemia retinalis; pancreatitis; eruptive xanthomas; hepatosplenomegaly; abdominal pain; hyperglycemia; hyperuricemia; abnormal glucose tolerance	Early adult	Weight loss; clofibrate; nicotinic acid	Obesity

oxalate in the urine, renal calculi, renal failure, and generalized deficit of oxalate crystals in tissues.

hyperoxemia (hī″pĕr-ŏk-sē′mē-ă) [″ + *oxys*, sharp, + *haima*, blood]. Extreme acidity of the blood.

hyperoxia (hī″pĕr-ŏk′sē-ă). Increased oxygen in the blood.

hyperpancreatism (hī″pĕr-păn′krē-ă-tĭzm) [″ + *pankreas*, pancreas, + *-ismos*, state of]. Abnormal amount of secretion from the pancreas.

hyperparasitism (hī″pĕr-păr′ă-sī″tĭzm). Condition in which a parasite lives in or upon another parasite.

hyperparathyroidism (hī″pĕr-păr″ă-thī′roy-dĭzm) [″ + *para*, beyond, + *thyreos*, shield, + *eidos*, form, + *-ismos*, state of]. Condition due to increased activity of the parathyroid glands. SYN: *osteitis fibrosa cystica generalisata*.

hyperpepsia (hī″pĕr-pĕp′sē-ă) [″ + *pepsis*, digestion]. Indigestion due to hyperchlorhydria.

hyperpepsinia (hī″pĕr-pĕp-sĭn′ē-ă) [″ + *pepsis*, digestion]. Excess of pepsin in the gastric secretion.

hyperperistalsis (hī″pĕr-pĕr″ĭ-stăl′sĭs) [″ +

peri, around, + *stalsis,* contraction]. Overactive peristalsis.

hyperphalangism (hī″pĕr-făl-ăn′jĭzm) [″ + *phalanx,* a line, + *-ismos,* state of]. Having an extra phalanx on a finger or toe. SYN: *polyphalangism.*

hyperphasia (hī″pĕr-fā′zē-ă) [″ + *phasis,* speech]. Abnormal desire to talk.

hyperphenylalaninemia (hī″pĕr-fĕn″ĭl-ăl″ă-nĭ-nē′mē-ă). Increased phenylalanine in the blood. SEE: *phenylketonuria.*

hyperphonia (hī″pĕr-fō′nē-ă) [″ + *phone,* voice]. 1. Stuttering or stammering due to irritability of the vocal cords. 2. Explosive speech exhibited by those who stammer.

hyperphoria (hī″pĕr-fō′rē-ă) [″ + *phorein,* to bear]. Tendency of one eye to turn upward. SYN: *anoopsia; anophoria.*

hyperphosphatasemia (hī″pĕr-fŏs″fă-tă-sē′mē-ă). Increased alkaline phosphatase in the blood.

hyperphosphatemia (hī″pĕr-fŏs″fă-tē′mē-ă) [″ + L. *phosphas,* phosphate, + Gr. *haima,* blood]. Abnormal amount of phosphorus in the blood.

hyperphosphaturia (hī″pĕr-fŏs-fă-tū′rē-ă) [″ + ″ + Gr. *ouron,* urine]. Increased amount of phosphates in the urine.

hyperphospheremia (hī″pĕr-fŏs-fĕr-ē′mē-ă) [″ + ″ + Gr. *haima,* blood]. Abnormal amount of phosphorous compounds in the blood. SYN: *hyperphosphatemia.*

hyperphrenia (hī″pĕr-frē′nē-ă) [Gr. *hyper,* above, + *phren,* mind]. 1. Excessive mental activity. Seen in the manic phase of manic-depressive psychosis. 2. Mental ability and capacity much greater than normal.

hyperpiesia, hyperpiesis (hī″pĕr-pī-ē′zē-ă, -pī′ĕ-sĭs) [″ + *piesis,* pressure]. Abnormally high blood pressure.

hyperpietic (hī″pĕr-pī-ĕt′ĭk). Rel. to extremely high blood pressure.

hyperpigmentation (hī″pĕr-pĭg″mĕn-tā′shŭn). Increased pigmentation, esp. of the skin.

hyperpituitarism (hī″pĕr-pĭ-tū′ĭ-tăr-ĭsm) [″ + L. *pituita,* mucus, + Gr. *-ismos,* state of]. Condition resulting from overactivity of the anterior lobe of the pituitary. SEE: *acromegaly; gigantism.*

hyperplasia (hī″pĕr-plā′zē-ă) [″ + *plassein,* to form]. Excessive proliferation of normal cells in the normal tissue arrangement of an organ. SYN: *hypergenesis.*

h., fibrous. Connective-tissue cell increase following any inflammation or in chronic visceral fibrosis.

h., lipoid. Increase in cells containing lipoid.

hyperplastic (hī″pĕr-plăs′tĭk). Rel. to hyperplasia.

hyperploidy (hī″pĕr-ploy′dē). Condition of having one extra chromosome and thus not balanced sets of chromosomes. SEE: *Down's syndrome; trisomy 21.*

hyperpnea (hī″pĕrp-nē′ă) [″ + *pnoia,* breath]. An increased respiratory rate or breathing that is deeper than that usually experienced during normal activity. A certain degree of hyperpnea is normal after exerise.

ETIOL: Pain, respiratory disease, febrile or cardiac disease, certain drugs, hysteria, or atmospheric conditions experienced at high altitude.

hyperporosis (hī″pĕr-por-ō′sĭs) [″ + *porosis,* callosity]. Excessive callous formation after a bone fracture.

hyperpotassemia (hī″pĕr-pŏt″ă-sē′mē-ă). Increased potassium in the blood. SYN: *hyperkalemia.*

hyperpragic (hī″pĕr-pră′jĭk) [″ + *praxis,* action]. Denoting excessive activity.

hyperpraxia (hī″pĕr-prăk′sē-ă). Excessive activity and restlessness seen in some mental disorders.

hyperprolactinemia (hī″pĕr-prō-lăk″tĭn-ē′mē-ă). Excess secretion of prolactin thought to be due to hypothalamic-pituitary dysfunction. This is usually associated with amenorrhea with or without galactorrhea.

hyperprolinemia (hī″pĕr-prō″lĭ-nē′mē-ă). An inherited metabolic disease of amino acid metabolism that results in an excess of proline in the body.

hyperproteinemia (hī″pĕr-prō″tē-ĭn-ē′mē-ă) [″ + *protos,* first, + *haima,* blood]. Excess of protein in the blood plasma.

hyperproteinuria (hī″pĕr-prō″tē-ĭn-ū′rē-ă) [″ + ″ + *ouron,* urine]. Excess of protein in the urine.

hyperpselaphesia (hī″pĕrp-sĕl″ă-fē′zē-ă) [Gr. *hyper,* above, + *pselaphesis,* touch]. Abnormal sensitivity to touch. SYN: *hyperaphia.*

hyperptyalism (hī″pĕr-tī′ăl-ĭzm) [″ + *ptyalon,* spittle]. Excessive secretion of saliva. SYN: *salivation.* SEE: *xerostomia.*

ETIOL: May be due to pregnancy, stomatitis, rabies, exophthalmic goiter, menstruation, epilepsy, hysteria, nervous conditions, and gastrointestinal disorders. May be induced by mercury, iodides, pilocarpine, and other drugs.

hyperpyretic (hī″pĕr-pī-rĕt′ĭk). Pert. to high body temperature (hyperpyrexia).

hyperpyrexia (hī″pĕr-pī-rĕks′ē-ă) [″ + *pyressein,* to be feverish]. Elevation of body temperature above 106° F. (41.1° C.). Produced by physical agents such as hot baths, diathermy, hot air, or by reaction to infection caused by microorganisms. SEE: *fever, induced.*

h., malignant. A severe form of pyrexia that occurs during the use of muscle relaxants and general inhalation anesthesia (usually succinylcholine and halothane) in those who have inherited this ability as an autosomal dominant trait. During general anesthesia the temperature rises readily and there are signs of increased muscle metabolism. This condition progresses rapidly and if it is untreated, 70% of patients die. Persons who are susceptible may be diagnosed by elevated CPK levels and histochemical studies on muscle biopsy; and history of exposure to halothane. Persons who are susceptible to this and who need anesthesia should have local anesthesia or neuroleptic anesthesia, q.v. SYN: *hyperthermia, malignant.*

hyperpyrexial (hī″pĕr-pī'rĕk'sē-ăl). Denoting high body temperature.

hyperreactive (hī″pĕr-rē-ăk'tĭv). Pert. to an increased response to stimuli.

hyperreflexia (hī″pĕr-rē-flĕk'sē-ă) [″ + L. *reflexus,* bent back]. Increased action of the reflexes.

hyperresonance (hī″pĕr-rĕz'ō-năns) [″ + L. *resonare,* to resound]. Increased resonance produced when the area is percussed.

hypersalemia (hī″pĕr-săl-ē'mē-ă). Increased salt in the blood.

hypersalivation (hī″pĕr-săl″ĭ-vā'shŭn) [″ + L. *salivatio,* salivation]. Excessive secretion of saliva.

hypersecretion (hī″pĕr-sē-krē'shŭn) [″ + L. *secretio,* separation]. Abnormal amount of secretion.

hypersensibility (hī″pĕr-sĕn″sĭ-bĭl'ĭ-tē) [″ + L. *sensibilitas,* sensibility]. Hypersensitivity of the body to a foreign protein or drug. SYN: *anaphylaxis.*

hypersensitiveness (hī″pĕr-sĕn'sĭ-tĭv-nĕs) [″ + L. *sensitivus,* sensitive]. Excessive and abnormal susceptibility to the action of a given agent, as pollen or foreign protein. SEE: *allergy; anaphylaxis; hay fever.*

hypersensitivity (hī″pĕr-sĕn″sĭ-tĭv'ĭ-tē). Abnormal sensitivity to a stimulus of any kind.

hypersensitization (hī″pĕr-sĕn″sĭ-tĭ-zā'shŭn). 1. Producing or inducing increased sensitivity to an organism or drug. 2. The condition of being sensitive to an abnormal degree to something.

hypersialosis (hī″pĕr-sī″ă-lō'sĭs). Ptyalism, q.v.

hypersomnia (hī″pĕr-sŏm'nē-ă) [″ + L. *somnus,* sleep]. Sleeping for pathological lengths of time. Occurs in certain types of encephalitis.

hypersplenism (hī″pĕr-splĕn'ĭzm). Increased activity of the spleen resulting in increased blood hemolysis, anemia, and sometimes splenomegaly.

hypersthenia (hī″pĕr-sthē'nē-ă) [Gr. *hyper,* above, + *sthenos,* strength]. Abnormal strength or excessive tension of the entire body or part of it.

hypersthenic (hī″pĕr-sthĕn'ĭk). 1. Denoting excessive strength or tension. 2. Body habitus characterized by a broad, deep thorax, short thoracic cavity, and a large abdominal cavity; a massive build.

hypersthenuria (hī″pĕr-sthĕn-ū'rē-ă) [″ + *sthenos,* strength, + *ouron,* urine]. Passage of abnormally concentrated urine. Usually due to dehydration or excess loss of fluids in sweat.

hypersusceptibility (hī″pĕr-sŭ-sĕp″tĭ-bĭl'ĭ-tē) [″ + L. *suscipere,* to take up, + *-bilis,* able]. Unusual susceptibility to a disease, pathological conditions, chemicals, or parasites. SEE: *allergy; anaphylaxis.*

hypersystole (hī″pĕr-sĭs'tō-lē) [″ + *systole,* contraction]. Unusual force or duration of the systole, q.v.

hypersystolic (hī″pĕr-sĭs-tŏl'ĭk). Pert. to hypersystole.

hypertelorism (hī″pĕr-tĕl'or-ĭzm) [″ + *telouros,* distant]. Abnormal width between two paired organs, esp. the eyes.

hypertensinogen (hī″pĕr-tĕn-sĭn'ō-jĕn). A globulin present in blood plasma that when acted upon by the enzyme renin forms angiotensin, q.v.

hypertension [″ + L. *tensio,* tension]. 1. Tension or tonus that is greater than normal. 2. A condition in which the patient has a higher blood pressure than that judged to be normal.

ETIOL: The primary factor in hypertension is an increase in peripheral resistance resulting from vasoconstriction or narrowing of peripheral blood vessels. The specific etiology for this condition can be determined in only a small number of patients with hypertension. However, it is important to attempt to define the exact etiology because, if the disease is due to certain pathological states, definitive and curative therapy can be instituted. Causes in this category include coarctation of the aorta; hyperthyroidism with thyrotoxicosis; patent ductus arteriosus; arteriovenous fistula; pheochromocytoma; psychogenic causes; certain forms of renal disease, particularly when limited to one kidney; adrenal tumors; primary aldosteronism; and polycythemia.

DIAG: There are no precise rules concerning what blood pressure reading is considered to represent hypertension. In general, if on several separate occasions the systolic pressure is above 140 mm. of mercury or the diastolic above 90 mm., the person is considered to have elevated blood pressure. Normal systolic blood pressure is not 100 plus the individual's age. Coronary artery disease and cerebral vascular disease, the great causes of death and disability, are much more frequent in those who have elevated blood pressure than those who are normotensive. On the other hand, a patient's blood pressure may register high merely because of being excited when the pressure is taken. For this reason it is advisable to take the pressure on several separate occasions to be certain that the true blood pressure is being obtained.

NURSING IMPLICATIONS: Help prevent hypertension by encouraging everyone to participate in blood pressure screening, and also by motivating people to seek and follow treatment for hypertension. Nursing interventions directed at treatment of hypertension include encouraging patients to decrease weight and to decrease sodium intake, teaching methods of stress reduction and management, and also stressing the need for periodic follow-up visits and continued medical supervision.

RS: blood pressure; diastolic pressure; hypotension; pulse; pulse pressure; systolic pressure.

h., benign. Hypertension that progresses slowly. The basic disease process may progress to the same endpoint as in malignant hypertension but at a slower rate.

h., essential. Hypertension that develops without apparent cause. SYN: *h., primary.*

h., Goldblatt. Hypertension that resembles renal hypertension produced in experimental animals by decreasing the blood flow to the kidney.

h., malignant. A form of hypertension that progresses rapidly, accompanied by severe vascular damage. It may progress to the point of death.

h., portal. Increased pressure in the portal vein caused by obstruction of flow of blood through the liver.

h., primary. H., essential, q.v.

h., renal. Hypertension accompanied by kidney disease. Hypertension produced experimentally by constriction of renal arteries. It is due to a humoral substance, renin, produced in an ischemic kidney.

hypertensive (hī″pĕr-tĕn′sĭv). Marked by a rise in blood pressure.

Hyper-Tet. Trade name for tetanus immune globulin, human.

hyperthecosis (hī″pĕr-thē-kō′sĭs). Hyperplasia of the theca interna of the ovary. Hirsutism and amenorrhea may be present.

hyperthelia (hī″pĕr-thē′lē-ă) [Gr. *hyper,* above, + *thele,* nipple]. The presence of more than two nipples.

hyperthermalgesia (hī″pĕr-thĕrm″ăl-jē′zē-ă) [″ + *therme,* heat, + *algesis,* pain]. Unusual sensitiveness to heat.

hyperthermia (hī″pĕr-thĕr′mē-ă) [″ + *therme,* heat]. 1. Unusually high fever. SYN: *hyperpyrexia.* 2. Treatment of disease by raising bodily temperature, accomplished by introduction of the malaria organism, injection of foreign proteins, or by physical means. SEE: *fever, induced.*

NURSING IMPLICATIONS: Remove excess bedclothes from the patient, and decrease the temperature of the environment. Remove all of the patient's clothes, and cover with a wet sheet. Administer antipyretics as ordered, increase oral fluid intake (unless contraindicated), provide sponging with cold water but prevent chilling by monitoring rectal temperature. The physician may order a hypothermia blanket to be utilized if other measures to decrease temperature are unsuccessful.

h., malignant. Hyperpyrexia, malignant, q.v.

hyperthermoesthesia (hī″pĕr-thĕrm″ō-ĕs-thē′zē-ă) [″ + ″ + *aisthesis,* sensation]. Unusual sensitiveness to heat. SYN: hyperthermalgesia.

hyperthrombinemia (hī″pĕr-thrŏm″bĭn-ē′mē-ă) [″ + *thrombos,* clot, + *haima,* blood]. Excess of thrombin in the blood. This tends to promote intravascular clotting.

hyperthymia (hī″pĕr-thī′mē-ă) [″ + *thymos,* mind]. 1. Pathological sensitiveness or excitability. 2. Sudden cruelty or foolhardiness.

hyperthyroidism (hī″pĕr-thī′royd-ĭzm) [″ + *thyreos,* shield, + *eidos,* form, + *-ismos,* state of]. A condition caused by excessive secretion of the thyroid glands, which increases the basal metabolic rate, causing an increased demand for food to support this metabolic activity.

SYM AND SIGNS: Exophthalmic goiter, fine tremor of the extended fingers and tongue, increased nervousness, weight loss, altered bowel activity, heat intolerance, excessive sweating, increased heart rate.

TREATMENT: Surgical, by removal of the thyroid gland following proper medical preparation. Medical, by use of antithyroid drugs (as propylthiouracil, methimazole, or carbimazole), iodide.

NURSING IMPLICATIONS: The nurse can be of great assistance in helping the patient adjust to this disease as it is being treated. Almost invariably there will be emotional and personality changes; and problems in the areas of hyperactivity, heat intolerance, and sexual dysfunction. It will be necessary to reassure the patient that these signs and symptoms will be alleviated during the course of therapy.

hyperthyrosis (hī″pĕr-thī-rō′sĭs). Hyperthyroidism.

hyperthyroxinemia (hī″pĕr-thī-rŏk″sĭ-nē′mē-ă). Excess thyroxine in the blood.

hypertonia (hī″pĕr-tō′nē-ă) [″ + *tonos,* tension]. Abnormal tension of arteries or muscles.

hypertonic (hī″pĕr-tŏn′ĭk). 1. Having a higher

osmotic pressure than a compared solution. Pert. to a solution of higher osmotic pressure than another. 2. Being in a state of greater than normal tension or of incomplete relaxation. Said of muscles. Opposite of hypotonic.

hypertonicity (hī″pĕr-tŏn-ĭ′sĭ-tē). Excess muscular tonus or intraocular pressure. SYN: *hypertonia*.

hypertonus (hī″pĕr-tō′nŭs). Increased tension, as muscular tension in spasm.

hypertoxicity (hī″pĕr-tŏk-sĭs′ĭ-tē) [″ + *toxikon*, poison]. The state of being excessively poisonous.

hypertrichiasis (hī″pĕr-trĭk-ī′ă-sĭs) [″ + *thrix*, hair, + *-iasis*, diseased condition]. Hypertrichosis.

hypertrichophobia (hī″pĕr-trĭk″ō-fō′bē-ă) [″ + ″ + *phobos*, fear]. Fear of hair on the body.

hypertrichophrydia (hī″pĕr-trĭk″ō-frĭd′ē-ă) [″ + ″ + *ophrys*, eyebrow]. Undue thickness of the eyebrows.

hypertrichosis (hī″pĕr-trĭ-kō′sĭs) [″ + ″ + *osis*, condition]. Growth of hair in excess of normal.

ETIOL: May be due to endocrine disease, esp. of the adrenal gland, and in the female, also the ovary.

hypertriglyceridemia (hī″pĕr-trī-glĭs″ĕr-ī-dē′mē-ă). Increased triglycerides in the blood.

hypertrophia (hī″pĕr-trō′fē-ă) [Gr. *hyper*, above, + *trophe*, nourishment]. Increased size of an organ, or of the body, due to growth. SYN: *hypertrophy*.

hypertrophic (hī″pĕr-trŏf′ik) [″ + *trophe*, nourishment]. Pert. to hypertrophy.

hypertrophy (hī-pĕr′trō-fē) [″ + *trophe*, nourishment]. Increase in size of an organ or structure that does not involve tumor formation. Term is generally restricted to an increase in size or bulk not resulting from an increase in number of cells or tissue elements, as in the hypertrophy of a muscle. Term sometimes used to apply to any increase in size as a result of functional activity. SYN: *hypertrophia*. SEE: *hyperplasia*.

h., adaptive. Hypertrophy in which an organ increases in size to meet increased functional demands, as hypertrophy of the heart that accompanies valvular disorders.

h., cardiac. Increase in size of the heart resulting from hypertrophy of muscle tissue but without increase in size of cavities.

h., compensatory. Hypertrophy resulting from increased function of an organ because of a defect or impaired function of the opposite of a paired organ.

h., concentric. Hypertrophy in which the walls of an organ become thickened without enlargement but with diminished capacity.

h., eccentric. Hypertrophy of an organ with dilatation.

h., false. Hypertrophy with degeneration of one constituent of an organ and its replacement by another.

h., Marie's. Chronic periostitis that causes the soft tissues surrounding the joints to enlarge.

h., numerical. Hypertrophy caused by increase in structural elements.

h., physiological. Hypertrophy due to natural rather than pathological factors.

h., pseudomuscular. A disease, usually of childhood, characterized by paralysis, depending upon degeneration of the muscles, which, however, become enlarged from a deposition of fat and connective tissue.

SYM: Weakness of muscles. Child is awkward and stumbles and seeks support in walking. As paralysis increases, the muscles, particularly those of the calf, thigh, buttocks, and back, enlarge. Upper extremities are less frequently affected. When the patient stands erect, the feet are wide apart, the abdomen protrudes and spinal column shows a marked curvature with convexity forward. Patient rises from recumbent position by grasping the knees or by resting the hands on the floor in front, extending the legs and pushing the body backwards. Gait is waddling. In course of few years paralysis becomes so marked patient is unable to leave bed This leads to muscular atrophy.

PROG: Unfavorable.

TREATMENT: Physical therapy helps to prevent contractures, but there is no effective therapy.

h., simple. Hypertrophy due to increase in size of structural parts.

h., true. Hypertrophy caused by increase in size in all the different tissues composing a part.

h., ventricular. Increased size and muscular content of the myocardium of the ventricles.

h., vicarious. Hypertrophy of an organ when another organ of allied function is disabled or destroyed.

hypertropia [Gr. *hyper*, above, + *tropos*, turning]. Vertical strabismus upward.

hyperuricemia (hī″pĕr-ū″rĭs-ē′mē-ă) [″ + *ouron*, urine, + *haima*, blood]. Abnormal amount of uric acid in the blood.

hyperuricuria (hī″pĕr-ū″rĭk-ū′rē-ă) [″ + ″ + *ouron*, urine]. Abnormal amount of uric acid in the urine.

hypervalinemia (hī″pĕr-văl″ĭn-ē′mē-ă). An inherited condition caused by a deficiency of the enzymes essential to the metabolism of valine. Clinically the child is mentally retarded, has nystagmus, vomits, and fails to thrive.

hypervascular (hī″pĕr-văs′kū-lăr) [″ + L. *vasculus*, vessel]. Excessively vascular.

hyperventilation (hī″pĕr-vĕn″tĭ-lā′shŭn) [″ + L. *ventilatio*, ventilation]. Hyperpnea as occurs in forced respiration; increased inspiration and expiration of air as a result of increase in rate or depth of respiration, or both. Results esp. in carbon dioxide depletion (acapnia) with accompanying symptoms (fall in blood pressure, vasoconstriction, and sometimes syncope). This is usually accompanied by marked anxiety. The immediate treatment involves having the patient breathe into a paper bag until the CO_2 content of the blood has an opportunity to return to normal. Just as effective is to close one nostril and be certain the patient breathes with mouth closed. In both cases the patient needs to be reassured and calmed. SEE: *Chvostek's sign.*

hyperviscosity (hī″pĕr-vĭs-kŏs′ĭ-tē) [″ + L. *viscosus*, gummy]. Excessive viscosity or exaggeration of adhesive properties. Seen in anemias and inflammatory diseases.

hypervitaminosis (hī″pĕr-vī″tă-mĭn-ō′sĭs) [″ + L. *vita*, life, + *amine* + Gr. *osis*, condition]. A condition caused by an excessive amount of vitamins in the diet, but it is most commonly due to excessive ingestion of vitamin pills.

hypervolemia (hī″per-vŏl-ē′mē-ă) [″ + L. *volumen*, volume, + Gr. *haima*, blood]. Plethora of blood; abnormal increase in the volume of circulating blood.

hypesthesia (hī″pĕs-thē′zē-ă) [Gr. *hypo*, under, + *aisthesis*, sensation]. Lessened sensibility to touch. Variant of hypoesthesia.

hypha (hī′fă) [Gr. *hyphe*, web]. (pl. *hyphae*) A filament of mold, or part of a mold mycelium.

hyphedonia (hĭp″hĕ-dō′nē-ă) [Gr. *hypo*, under, + *hedone*, pleasure]. Abnormal diminution of pleasure in acts that should normally give pleasure.

hyphema (hī-fē′mă) [Gr. *hyphaimos*, suffused with blood]. Blood in the anterior chamber of the eye, in front of the iris.

hyphidrosis (hīp-hĭd-rō′sĭs) [Gr. *hypo*, under, + *hidros*, sweat]. Diminished secretion of sweat.

Hyphomycetes (hī″fō-mī-sē′tēz) [Gr. *hyphe*, web, + *mykes*, fungus]. The Fungi Imperfecti. Filamentous fungi with branched or unbranched threads. They do not have sexual spores.

hypinosis (hīp″ĭn-ō′sĭs) [Gr. *hypo*, under, + *inos*, fiber, + *osis*, condition]. Deficiency of fibrin in the blood. SYN: *hypoinosemia.*

hypnagogic (hĭp-nă-gŏj′ĭk) [Gr. *hypnos*, sleep, + *agogos*, leading]. 1. Inducing sleep or induced by sleep. SYN: *hypnotic*. SEE: *hypnogenic zones*. 2. In psychology, pert. to hallucinations or dreams just before loss of consciousness.

hypnagogic state. A transitional state between sleeping and awaking and delusions that may result therefrom.

hypnagogue (hĭp′nă-gŏg). Concerning or causing sleep or drowsiness.

hypnalgia (hĭp-năl′jē-ă) [″ + *algos*, pain]. False sense of pain experienced in a dream.

hypnic (hĭp′nĭk) [Gr. *hypnos*, sleep]. Causing sleep. SYN: *somnifacient; somniferous.*

hypnoanalysis (hĭp″nō-ă-năl′ĭ-sĭs) [″ + *analysis*, a dissolving]. Combined psychoanalytic therapy and hypnosis.

hypnoanesthesia (hĭp″nō-ăn″ĕs-thē′zē-ă). Use of hypnosis to produce anesthesia.

hypnodontics (hĭp″nō-dŏn′tĭks). The application of controlled suggestion and hypnosis to the practice of dentistry.

hypnogenetic (hĭp″nŏ-jĕ-nĕt′ĭk) [″ + *gennan*, to produce]. Producing sleep.

hypnoidal (hĭp-noy′dăl) [Gr. *hypnos*, sleep, + *eidos*, resemblance]. Pert. to a condition between sleep and waking, resembling sleep.

hypnoidization (hĭp″noy-dī-zā′shŭn) [″ + *eidos*, form]. Induction of hypnosis.

hypnolepsy (hĭp′nŏ-lĕp″sē) [″ + *lepsis*, seizure]. Irresistible sleepiness. SYN: *narcolepsy.*

hypnology (hĭp-nŏl′ō-jē) [″ + *logos*, study]. Scientific study of sleep.

hypnonarcoanalysis (hĭp″nō-năr″kō-ă-năl′ĭ-sĭs). A psychiatric interview combining hypnosis with drug-induced sedation or narcosis.

hypnonarcosis (hĭp″nō-năr-kō′sĭs). Combination of hypnosis and narcosis.

hypnophobia (hĭp″nō-fō′bē-ă) [″ + *phobos*, fear]. Morbid fear of falling asleep.

hypnopompic (hĭp″nŏ-pŏm′pĭk) [″ + *pompe*, procession]. Pert. to dreams or visual images persisting after sleep prior to complete awakening.

hypnosis (hĭp-nō′sĭs) [″ + *osis*, condition]. A subconscious condition in which the objective manifestations of mind are more or less inactive, accompanied by abnormal sensibility to suggestions made by the hypnotist. SEE: *autohypnosis; hypnotism; sleepwalking; somnambulism.*

hypnosophy (hĭp-nŏs′ō-fē) [″ + *sophia*, wisdom]. The study of sleep.

hypnotherapy (hĭp″nō-thĕr′ă-pē) [″ + *therapeia*, treatment]. Treatment by hypnotism or by inducing prolonged sleep.

hypnotic (hĭp-nŏt′ĭk) [Gr. *hypnos*, sleep]. 1. Pert. to sleep or hypnosis. 2. An agent that induces sleep or that dulls the senses, such as chloral hydrate.

hypnotics (hĭp-nŏt′ĭks) [Gr. *hypnos*, sleep]. Drugs that cause insensibility to pain by inhibiting afferent impulses or by inhibiting the receiving of sensory impressions in the cortical centers of the brain, thus causing partial or complete unconsciousness. Hypnotics include sedatives, analgesics, anesthetics, and intoxicants. They should yield not unpleasant after effects and result in natural sleep. They are sometimes called somnifacients and soporifics when used to induce sleep.

RS: analgesic; anesthetic; intoxicant; sedative; somnifacient; soporific.

hypnotism (hĭp′nō-tĭzm) [″ + *-ismos*, state of]. An induced sleeplike state during which the patient is peculiarly susceptible to the suggestions of the hypnotist.

hypnotist (hĭp′nō-tĭst) [Gr. *hypnos*, sleep]. One who practices hypnotism.

hypnotize (hĭp′nō-tīz). To put under hypnosis.

hypnotoxin (hĭp″nō-tŏk′sĭn). Theoretically, a toxic substance that accumulates in the blood during wakefulness, the effect of which is to induce sleep.

hypo (hī′pō) [Gr. *hypo*, under]. Popular name for hypodermic syringe or injection.

hypo-, hyp- [Gr. *hypo*, under]. Prefix indicating less than, below, or under. SYN: [L.] *sub*.

hypoacidity (hī″pō-ă-sĭd′ĭ-tē) [″ + L. *acidus*, sour]. A condition of decreased acid in the stomach caused by lowered hydrochloric acid secretion. Secondary to other disorders, such as pernicious anemia.

TREATMENT: Administer dilute HCl by mouth. CAUTION: In order to protect the teeth, it is important to have the patient suck the acid solution through a straw.

hypoacusis (hī″pō-ă-kū′sĭs) [″ + *akousis*, hearing]. Decreased sensitivity to sound stimuli.

hypoadenia (hī″pō-ă-dē′nē-ă) [″ + *aden*, gland]. Defective activity of the glands.

hypoadrenalism (hī″pō-ăd-rē′năl-ĭzm) [″ + L. *ad*, to, + *renalis*, pert. to kidney, + Gr. *-ismos*, state of]. Adrenal insufficiency.

hypoadrenocorticism (hī″pō-ă-drē″nō-kor′tĭ-sĭzm). Decreased secretion or effect of the adrenal cortical hormone.

hypoaffectivity (hī″pō-ăf″fĕk-tĭv′ĭ-tē). Decreased responsiveness to emotional stimuli.

hypoalbuminemia (hīpō-ăl-bū″mĭn-ē′mē-ă). Decreased albumin in the blood.

hypoaldosteronism (hī″pō-ăl″dō-stĕr′ōn-ĭzm). Decreased aldosterone in the blood associated with hypotension and increased salt excretion.

hypoalimentation [″ + L. *alimentum*, nourishment]. Insufficient nourishment.

hypoazoturia (hī″pō-ăz-ō-tū′rē-ă) [″ + L. *azotum*, nitrogen, + Gr. *ouron*, urine]. Diminished urea in the urine.

hypobaric (hī″pō-băr′ĭk) [″ + *baros*, weight]. Decreased atmospheric pressure.

hypobaropathy (hī″pō-băr-ŏp′ă-thē) [″ + ″ + *pathos*, disease]. Symptoms produced by diminished air pressure, anoxia, mountain sickness, aviator's sickness.

hypoblast (hī′pō-blăst) [″ + *blastos*, germ]. The inner cell layer or entoderm, which develops during gastrulation. The external layer is called ectoderm.

hypoblastic (hī-pō-blăs′tĭk). Pert. to the inner layer of the blastoderm.

hypobulia (hī″pō-bū′lē-ă) [″ + *boule*, will]. Impairment of will power. SEE: *abulia*.

hypocalcemia (hī″pō-kăl-sē′mē-ă) [″ + L. *calx*, lime, + Gr. *haima*, blood]. Abnormally low blood calcium.

hypocalciuria (hī″pō-kăl″sē-ū′rē-ă). Decreased calcium in the urine.

hypocapnia (hī″pō-kăp′nē-ă) [Gr. *hypo*, under, + *kapnos*, smoke]. Decreased amount of carbon dioxide in the blood.

hypocarbia (hī″pō-kăr′bē-ă). Decreased carbon dioxide in the blood. Excess rate of respiration will cause this.

hypocellularity (hī″pō-sĕl″ū-lăr′ĭ-tē). Decreased cell content of any tissue.

hypochloremia (hī″pō-klō-rē′mē-ă) [″ + *chloros*, green, + *haima*, blood]. Deficiency of the chloride content of the blood.

hypochlorhydria (hī″pō-klor-hī′drē-ă) [″ + ″ + *hydor*, water]. Diminished secretion of hydrochloric acid. A small amount of acid may be indicative of carcinoma or anemia. It may be found in subacute and chronic gastritis and early carcinoma. SEE: *achlorhydria; hyperchlorhydria*.

hypochlorite salts. A salt of hypochlorous acid used in household bleach and as an oxidizer, deodorant, and disinfectant.

hypochlorite salts poisoning. SEE: *Poisons and Poisoning* in *Appendix*.

hypochlorization (hī″pō-klō″rī-zā′shŭn). Diminished sodium chloride in the diet. Used in treating hypertension and certain kidney diseases.

hypochlorous acid. An acid, HClO, used as a disinfectant, and as a bleaching agent. It is usually used in the form of one of its salts.

hypochloruria (hī″pō-klor-ū′rē-ă) [″ + *chloros*, green, + *ouron*, urine]. Diminution of chlorides in the urine.

hypocholesteremia (hī″pō-kō-lĕs-tĕr-ē′mē-ă) [″ + *chole*, bile, + *stereos*, solid, + *haima*, blood]. Decreased blood cholesterol.

hypochondria (hī″pō-kŏn′drē-ă) [″ + *chondros*, cartilage]. Abnormal concern about health with false belief of suffering from some disease. SYN: *hypochondriasis*.

hypochondriac (hī″pō-kŏn′drē-ăk). 1. Pert. to the region of the hypochondrium, q.v., or upper lateral region on each side of the body and below the thorax; beneath the ribs. 2. One having an abnormal and excessive interest in and fear of disease, esp. in persons who are otherwise healthy.

hypochondriac region. Part of abdomen beneath the lower ribs on both sides of the epigastrium. SYN: *hypochondrium*.

hypochondriacal (hī″pō-kŏn-drī′ă-kăl) [″ + *chondros,* cartilage]. Affected with a pathological interest in health and disease.

hypochondrial reflex (hī″pō-kŏn′drē-ăl). A sudden inspiratory act resulting from sudden pressure below the costal border.

hypochondriasis (hī″pō-kŏn-drī′ă-sĭs) [″ + *chondros,* cartilage, + *-iasis,* diseased condition]. Abnormal anxiety about one's health; a frequent symptom in depressed patients. SYN: *hypochondria.*

hypochondrium (hī″pō-kŏn′drē-ŭm). That part of the abdomen beneath the lower ribs on each side of the epigastrium.

hypochromasia (hī″pō-krō-mā′sē-ă) [″ + *chroma,* color]. Lack of hemoglobin in the red blood cells.

hypochromatism (hī″pō-krō′mă-tĭzm) [″ + *chroma,* color]. 1. Lack of or decreased color. 2. A cell, esp. its nucleus, with decreased pigment. 3. Decreased hemoglobin in the red cells.

hypochromatosis (hī″pō-krō-mă-tō′sĭs) [″ + ″ + *osis,* condition]. Disappearance of the chromatin or nucleus in a cell. SYN: *chromatolysis.*

hypochromia (hī″pŏ-krō′mē-ă). Condition of the blood in which the red blood cells have a reduced hemoglobin content.

hypochromic (hī″pō-krōm′ĭk). Pert. to hypochromia.

hypochylia (hī″pō-kī′lē-ă) [Gr. *hypo,* under, + *chylos,* juice]. Lack of normal secretion of gastric juice.

hypocinesia (hī″pō-sĭn-ē′zē-ă) [″ + *kinesis,* motion]. Diminished power of movement. SYN: *hypokinesia.*

hypocomplementemia (hī″pō-kŏm″plē-mĕn-tē′mē-ă). Concerning decreased complement in the blood.

hypocondylar (hī″pō-kŏn′dĭ-lăr) [″ + *kondylos,* condyle]. Below a condyle.

hypocone (hī′pō-kōn) [″ + *konos,* cone]. The distolingual cusp of an upper molar tooth.

hypoconid (hī″pō-kō′nĭd). The distobuccal cusp of a lower molar tooth.

hypocorticism (hī″pō-kor′tĭ-sĭzm). Decreased adrenal cortical hormone.

hypocrinism (hī″pō-krī′nĭzm) [″ + *krinein,* to separate, + *-ismos,* state of]. Deficient secretion of any gland, esp. an endocrine.

hypocupremia (hī″pō-kū-prē′mē-ă). Decreased copper in the blood.

hypocyclosis (hī″pō-sī-klō′sĭs) [″ + *kyklos,* circle]. Deficient accommodation.

h., ciliary. Weakness of ciliary muscle.

h., lenticular. Lack of elasticity in crystalline lens.

hypocystotomy (hī″pō-sĭs-tŏt′ō-mē) [″ + *kystis,* a bladder, + *tome,* incision]. Perineal opening of the bladder.

hypocythemia (hī″pō-sī-thē′mē-ă) [″ + *kytos,* cell, + *haima,* blood]. Decreased blood cells, esp. red blood cells.

hypodactylia (hī″pō-dăk-tĭl′ē-ă) [″ + *daktylos,* finger]. Having a decreased number of fingers or toes.

Hypoderma (hī″pō-dĕr′mă) [″ + *derma,* skin]. A genus of warble flies of the family Oestridae. The larvae of some species attack cattle, and rarely, man. They cause a subcutaneous channel of inflammation as they burrow under the skin. SEE: *larva migrans.*

hypodermatoclysis (hī″pō-dĕr-mă-tŏk′lĭ-sĭs). Hypodermoclysis.

hypodermatomy (hī″pō-dĕr-măt′ō-mē) [″ + *derma,* skin, + *tome,* incision]. Subcutaneous incision or section, as of a muscle or tendon.

hypodermiasis (hī″pō-dĕr-mī′ă-sĭs) [″ + ″ + *-iasis,* condition]. Infection with Hypoderma.

hypodermic (hī″pō-dĕr′mĭk) [″ + *derma,* skin]. Under or inserted under the skin, as a hypodermic injection. It may be given subcutaneously (under the skin), intracutaneously (into the skin), intramuscularly (into a muscle), intraspinally (into the spinal canal), or intravascularly (into a vein or artery). It is given to secure prompt action of a drug when the drug cannot be taken by mouth, when it may not be readily absorbed in the stomach or intestines, when it might be changed by action of the gastric secretions, or to act as an anesthetic about the site of injection.

CAUTION: When injected substance is not intended for intravascular injection, pull back on the syringe plunger after the needle is inserted to determine if the needle is in a vein or artery. If blood is obtained, the needle must be repositioned and the procedure repeated. It may be necessary to use a fresh needle and syringe. Because medicines not intended to be injected intravenously produce serious undesired effects when given intravascularly, do not inject the medicine if the needle is in a vessel.

If medicine is to be injected into an artery or vein do not administer it unless pulling back on the plunger permits blood to freely enter the syringe.

h., intracutaneous. Injection into the skin.

h., intramuscular. Injection given in gluteal or lumbar muscular region. Used when a drug is not easily absorbed, when it is irritating, or when large quantity of liquid is to be used.

h., intraspinal. Injection into the spinal canal.

h., intravenous. Injection into a vein, the usual site being the median basilic or median cephalic vein of the arm.

h., subcutaneous. Injection given just under the skin, usually in outer surface of arms and forearm.

hypodermoclysis (hī″pō-dĕr-mŏk′lĭ-sĭs) [Gr. *hypo,* under, + *derma,* skin, + *klysis,* a washing out]. The injection of fluids into the subcutaneous tissues to supply the body with liquids quickly, as after shock, hemorrhage, or diarrhea; it may be given in any condition in which it is impossible to give sufficient water by mouth, by rectum, or by vein.

When it is necessary to maintain a larger amount of water in the tissues in order to keep up proper metabolism, hypodermoclysis may be ordered. The purpose is about the same as that of intravenous infusions. Physiological salt solution (normal salt solution) is generally used because it is one of the principal constituents of the blood. There are other solutions given by this method as preferred by the attending physician. If the solution is not of the correct osmolarity, hemolysis, q.v., may occur. It is essential that the solution be the proper temperature, which should be from 108° to 115° F. (42.2° to 46.1° C.) in the flask because it cools rapidly while passing through the tubing.

Site of injection may be in the loose tissues at the base of the breasts; in the thighs or buttocks (care being taken to avoid the large blood vessels); in the axillary line (esp. for men); beneath the skin of the abdomen (halfway between the navel and the anterior superior spine); and intraperitoneally in children. The inner aspect of the thighs should be used as site of injection only with great caution because of the closeness of the femoral vessels.

hypodipsia (hī″pō-dĭp′sē-ă) [″ + *dipsa,* thirst]. Decreased intake of fluids due to lack of thirst.

hypodontia (hī″pō-dŏn′shē-ă). Diminished development, or absence of, teeth.

hypodynamia (hī″pō-dī-nā′mē-ă) [″ + *dynamis,* power]. Diminished muscular power or energy. SEE: *adynamia.*

hypoeccrisia (hī″pō-ĕk-krĭs′ē-ă) [″ + *ek,* out, + *krisis,* separation]. Diminished excretion of waste material.

hypoeccritic (hī″pō-ĕk-krĭt′ĭk). 1. Retarding normal excretion. 2. Pert. to insufficient or defective excretion.

hypoendocrinism (hī″pō-ĕn-dŏk′rĭ-nĭzm) [″ + *endon,* within, + *krinein,* to separate, + *-ismos,* state of]. Insufficiency of internal secretion in one or more glands.

hypoendocrisia (hī″pō-ĕn″dō-krĭz′ē-ă). Insufficiency of endocrine secretion. SYN: *hypoendocrinism.*

hypoeosinophilia (hī″pō-ē″ō-sĭn″ō-fĭl′ē-ă) [Gr. *hypo,* under, + *eos,* dawn, + *philein,* to love]. Diminished quantity of eosinophil leukocytes of the blood.

hypoepinephria (hī″pō-ĕp″ĭ-nĕf′rē-ă) [″ + *epi,* upon, + *nephros,* kidney]. Diminished secretion of epinephrine.

hypoergasia (hī″pō-ĕr-gā′sē-ă) [″ + *ergon,* work]. Decreased functional activity.

hypoergia (hī″pō-ĕr′jē-ă). 1. Mild allergy due to decreased response to allergic stimuli. 2. Diminished response to any stimulus.

hypoergic (hī″pō-ĕr′jĭk). 1. Concerning hypoergia 2. Pert. to decreased energy level.

hypoergy (hī″pō-ĕr′jē) [″ + *ergon,* work]. Hyposensitiveness to allergens.

hypoesophoria (hī″pō-ĕs″ō-fō′rē-ă) [″ + *eso,* inward, + *phorein,* to bear]. Downward and inward deviation of the eye.

hypoesthesia (hī″pō-ĕs-thē zē-ă) [″ + *aisthesis,* sensation]. Dulled sensitivity to touch.

hypoexophoria (hī″pō-ĕks-ō-fō′rē-ă) [″ + *exo,* outward, + *phorein,* to bear]. Downward and outward deviation of the eye.

hypoferremia (hī″pō-fĕ-rē′mē-ă). Iron deficiency as indicated by diminished iron in the blood.

hypofibrinogenemia (hī″pō-fī-brĭn″ō-jĕ-nē′mē-ă). Decreased fibrinogen in the blood.

hypofunction (hī″pō-fŭnk′shŭn). Decreased function.

hypogalactia (hī″pō-gă-lăk′shē-ă) [″ + *gala,* milk]. Deficient milk production.

hypogammaglobulinemia (hī″pō-găm″ă-glŏb″ū-lĭ-nē′mē-ă). Decreased gamma globulins in the blood. This produces a state of immunodeficiency.

h., acquired. A form of hypogammaglobulinemia that has its onset in early childhood.

h., congenital. An inherited form of hypogammaglobulinemia in which all of the immunoglobulins are decreased. This usually manifests as immunodeficiency at 6 months of age, by which time the maternal immunoglobulins have disappeared.

hypogastric (hī″pō-găs′trĭk) [″ + *gaster,* belly]. Pert. to lower middle of the abdomen or hypogastrium.

hypogastric artery. Arteria iliaca interna.

hypogastric plexus. Sympathetic nerve plexus in the pelvis.

hypogastric region. The hypogastrium. SEE: *abdominal regions.*

hypogastrium (hī″pō-găs′trē-ŭm). Region below the umbilicus or navel, between the right and left inguinal regions.

hypogenesis (hī″pō-jĕn′ĕ-sĭs) [Gr. *hypo,* under, + *genesis,* development]. ... of growth or development at ar... causing defective structure. S...

hypogenitalism (hī″pō-jĕn ĭ-t... *genitalis,* a genital, + Gr ... Condition in which the g... underdeveloped. Charact... size of genital organs, ... descend in some cases, a...

opment of secondary sex characteristics. SEE: *hypogonadism.*

hypogeusia (hī″pō-gū′sē-ă) [″ + *geusis,* taste]. Blunting of sense of taste.

h., idiopathic. A syndrome consisting of decreased taste and olfactory acuity, and with or without perverted taste (dysgeusia) and smell. Cause of the syndrome is unknown. In experimental studies, certain trace elements such as zinc added to the diet appear to correct some of the symptoms.

hypoglossal (hī″pō-glŏs′ăl) [″ + *glossa,* tongue]. Situated under the tongue.

hypoglossal alternating hemiplegia. Medulla lesion paralyzing the tongue by involving the 12th nerve fibers as they course through the uncrossed pyramid. The pathology may extend across the midline or dorsally, involving the medial fillet, causing contralateral anesthesia.

hypoglossal nerve. A mixed cranial nerve, it carries afferent proprioceptive impulses as well as efferent motor impulses. Originates in the medulla oblongata. Distribution: extrinsic and intrinsic muscles of the tongue. SYN: *twelfth cranial nerve.*

hypoglottis (hī″pō-glŏt′ĭs). Undersurface of tongue.

hypoglycemia (hī″pō-glī-sē′mē-ă) [″ + *glykys,* sweet, + *haima,* blood]. Deficiency of sugar in the blood. A condition in which the glucose in the blood is abnormally low.

ETIOL: Hyperfunction of the islets of Langerhans may cause it or injection of excessive quantity of insulin. SEE: *coma; hyperglycemia; hyperinsulinism.*

SYM: Acute fatigue, restlessness, malaise, marked irritability and weakness. In severe cases, mental disturbances, delirium, coma, and possibly death. SEE: *coma, diabetic* for table.

hypoglycemic (hī″pō-glī-sē′mĭk). Pert. to or causing hypoglycemia.

hypoglycemic agents, oral. Sulfonylurea compounds that cause a decrease in blood sugar. Acetohexamide, tolbutamide, and chlorpropamide are examples. There is no proof that their use in diabetes mellitus is beneficial in preventing the long-term complications of diabetes. Trade names for these are Dimelor, Orinase, and Diabinese, respectively.

CAUTION: The sulfonylureas should be used only in patients with diabetes of the insulin-independent type who cannot be treated with diet alone and who are unwilling or unable to take insulin if weight reduction and dietary control fail.

[hy]poglycemic shock. Production of shock, ... by induction of hypoglycemia by intra... r administration of insulin in the ... f schizophrenia.

hypoglycogenolysis (hī″pō-glī″kō-jĕn-ŏl′ĭ-sĭs) [Gr. *hypo,* under, + *glykys,* sweet, + *gennan,* to produce, + *lysis,* loosening]. Defective hydrolysis of glycogen (glycogenolysis).

hypoglycorrhachia (hī″pō-glī″kō-ră′kē-ă) [″ + ″ + *rhachis,* spine]. Decreased amount of glucose in the cerebrospinal fluid. This usually occurs in meningitis.

hypognathous (hī-pŏg′nă-thŭs) [″ + *gnathos,* jaw]. Having a lower jaw smaller than the upper jaw.

hypogonadism (hī″pō-gō′năd-ĭzm) [″ + *gone,* semen, + *-ismos,* state of]. Defective internal secretion of the gonads.

hypogonadotropic (hī″pō-gŏn″ă-dō-trŏp′ĭk). Concerning or caused by deficiency of gonadotropin.

hypohepatia (hī″pō-hĕ-pă′tē-ă) [″ + *hepar,* liver]. Deficient liver function.

hypohidrosis (hī-pō-hī-drō′sĭs) [″ + *hidros,* sweat, + *osis,* condition]. Diminished perspiration. SYN: *hyphidrosis.*

hypohyloma (hī″pō-hī-lō′mă) [″ + *hyle,* matter, + *oma,* tumor]. A tumor formed by embryonic tissue. Derived from hypoblast tissue.

hypoinsulinism [″ + L. *insula,* island, + Gr. *-ismos,* state of]. Insufficient secretion of insulin. SYN: *diabetes mellitus.*

hypoisotonic (hī″pō-ī″sō-tŏn′ĭk) [″ + *isos,* equal, + *tonos,* tension]. Hypotonic.

hypokalemia (hī″pō-kă-lē′mē-ă) [″ + Mod. L. *kalium,* potash, + Gr. *haima,* blood]. Extreme potassium depletion in the circulating blood, commonly manifested by episodes of muscular weakness or paralysis, tetany, and postural hypotension. SYN: *hypopotassemia.*

hypokalemic (hī″pō-kă-lē′mĭk). Concerning hypokalemia.

hypokinesia (hī″pō-kī-nē′zē-ă) [″ + *kinesis,* motion]. Decreased motor reaction to stimulus.

hypokinetic (hī″pō-kī-nĕt′ĭk). Pert. to hypokinesia.

hypolemmal (hī″pō-lĕm′ăl) [″ + *lemma,* sheath]. Situated below a sheath or membrane.

hypoleydigism (hī″pō-lī′dĭg-ĭzm). Decreased secretion of androgen by the interstitial (Leydig) cells of the testicles.

hypolipidemic (hī″pō-lĭp″ĭ-dē′mĭk). Decreasing the lipid concentration of the blood.

hypoliposis (hī″pō-lĭ-pō′sĭs) [″ + *lipos,* fat, + *osis,* condition]. Deficiency of fat in the tissues.

hypologia (hī-pō-lō′jē-ă) [Gr. *hypo,* under, + *logos,* word]. A cerebral symptom marked by inadequate speech.

hypolymphemia (hī″pō-lĭm-fē′mē-ă) [″ + L. *lympha,* lymph, + Gr. *haima,* blood]. Decreased lymphocytes in the blood with normal number of leukocytes.

hypomagnesemia (hī″pō-măg″nē-sē′mē-ă). Decreased magnesium in the blood. Clinically, there will be increased neuromuscular irritability.
hypomania (hī″pō-mā′nē-ă) [″ + *mania,* madness]. Mild mania and excitement with moderate change in behavior.
hypomastia (hī-pō-măs′tē-ă) [″ + *mastos,* breast]. Condition of having abnormally small breasts. SYN: *hypomazia.*
hypomazia (hī″pō-mā′zē-ă) [″ + *mazos,* breast]. Hypomastia, q.v.
hypomenorrhea (hī″pō-mĕn-ō-rē′ă) [″ + *men,* month, + *rhoia,* flow]. Deficient amount of menstrual flow, but periods are regular. SEE: *oligomenorrhea.*
hypomere (hī′pō-mēr) [″ + *meros,* part]. That portion of the mesoderm that later forms the pleuroperitoneal walls. SEE: *epimere; mesomere.*
hypometabolism (hī″pō-mĕ-tăb′ō-lĭzm) [″ + *metabole,* change, + *-ismos,* state of]. Lowered metabolism.
hypometria (hī″pō-mē′trē-ă) [″ + *metron,* measure]. Shortened range or movement.
hypometropia (hī″pō-mĕ-trōp′ē-ă) [″ + ″ + *ops,* eye]. Myopia or shortsightedness.
hypomnesia, hypomnesis (hī″pŏm-nē′zē-ă, -nē′sĭs) [″ + *mnesis,* memory]. Impaired memory.
hypomorph (hī′pō-morf) [″ + *morphe,* form]. An individual with disproportionately short legs with respect to length of trunk. Opposite of hypermorph, q.v. SEE: *somatotype.*
hypomotility (hī″pō-mō-tĭl′ĭ-tē) [″ + L. *motus,* moved]. Hypokinesia.
hypomyotonia (hī″pō-mī″ō-tō′nē-ă) [″ + *mys,* muscle, + *tonos,* tension]. Lacking in muscular tonus.
hypomyxia (hī″pō-mĭks′ē-ă) [″ + *myxa,* mucus]. Diminished secretion of mucus.
hyponanosoma (hī″pō-năn-ō-sō′mă) [″ + *nanos,* dwarf, + *soma,* body]. Extreme dwarfism.
hyponatremia (hī″pō-nă-trē′mē-ă) [″ + L. *natron,* sodium, + Gr. *haima,* blood]. Decreased concentration of sodium in the blood.
hyponeocytosis (hī″pō-nē″ō-sī-tō′sĭs) [″ + *neos,* new, + *kytos,* cell, + *osis,* condition]. Decreased number of leukocytes (leukopenia) with immature cells in the blood.
hyponoia (hī″pō-noy′ă) [″ + *nous,* mind]. Diminished or sluggish mental activity.
hyponychium (hī-pō-nĭk′ē-ŭm) [Gr. *hypo,* under, + *onyx,* nail]. [NA] The nail bed. SYN: *matrix unguis.*
hyponychon (hī-pŏn′ĭ-kŏn) [″ + *onyx,* nail]. Extravasation of blood beneath the nail.
hypo-orthocytosis (hī″pō-or″thō-sī-tō′sĭs) [″ + *orthos,* regular, + *kytos,* cell, + *osis,* condition]. Leukopenia in which the proportions of white blood cells are normal.
hypopallesthesia (hī″pō-păl″ĕs-thē′zē-ă) [″ + *pallein,* to shake, + *aisthesis,* perception]. Decreased ability to perceive vibratory sense.
hypopancreatism (hī″pō-păn′krē-ă-tĭzm) [″ + *pankreas,* pancreas, + *-ismos,* state of]. Diminished activity of the pancreas.
hypoparathyreosis (hī″pō-păr-ă-thī-rē-ō′sĭs) [″ + *para,* beside, + *thyreos,* shield, + *osis,* condition]. A condition due to lessened or absent secretion of the parathyroids. SYN: *hypoparathyroidism.*
hypoparathyroidism (hī″pō-păr-ă-thī′royd-ĭzm) [″ + ″ + ″ + *eidos,* form, + *-ismos,* state of]. Insufficient secretion of the parathyroid glands. SYN: *hypoparathyreosis.*
hypopepsia (hī″pō-pĕp′sē-ă) [″ + *pepsis,* digestion]. Impaired digestion due to lack of pepsin.
hypopepsinia (hī″pō-pĕp-sĭn ē-ă). Deficient pepsin in the gastric juice.
hypoperistalsis (hī″pō-pĕr″ĭ-stăl′sĭs). Diminished peristalsis. SEE: *paralytic ileus.*
hypophalangism (hī″pō-fă-lăn′jĭzm). Having less than the normal number of fingers or toes or both.
hypopharynx (hī″pō-făr′ĭnks) [″ + *pharynx,* pharynx]. The lowermost portion of the pharynx, which leads to the larynx and esophagus. SYN: *laryngopharynx.*
hypophonesis (hī″pō-fō-nē′sĭs) [″ + *phone,* voice]. A diminished or fainter sound in auscultation or percussion.
hypophonia (hī″pō-fō′nē-ă). Abnormally weak voice due to incoordination of speech muscles.
hypophoria (hī″pō-fō′rē-ă) [″ + *phorein,* to bear]. Tendency of one visual axis to fall below the other one.
hypophosphatasia (hī″pō-fŏs″fă-tā′zē-ă). An inherited metabolic disease in which there is a deficiency of alkaline phosphatase in the cells. Clinically there are abnormalities of the skeleton such as rickets, osteomalacia, defective tooth development, and phosphoethanolamine in the urine.
hypophosphatemia (hī″pō-fŏs″fă-tē′mē-ă) [″ + L. *phosphas,* phosphate, + Gr. *haima,* blood]. Abnormally decreased amount of phosphates circulating in the blood.
hypophosphaturia (hī″pō-fŏs″fă-tū′rē-ă) [″ + ″ + Gr. *ouron,* urine]. Decreased excretion of phosphate in the urine.
hypophrenia (hī″pō-frē′nē-ă) [″ ... *phren,* mind]. Mental deficiency.
hypophrenic (hī″pō-frĕn′ĭk) [″ + ... phragm, mind]. 1. Mental defic... low the diaphragm.
hypophyseal (hī″pō-fĭz′ē-ăl) ... growth]. Pert. to the hypophy...
hypophysectomy (hī-pŏf″ĭ-s... + *ektome,* excision]. Excisi... sis cerebri.

hypophyseoportal (hī″pō-fĭz″ē-ō-por′tăl). Concerning the portal system of the pituitary gland. SEE: *system, hypophyseoportal.*

hypophyseoprivic (hī″pō-fĭz″ē-ō-prĭv′ĭk). Deficiency of hormone secretion from the pituitary.

hypophysis (hī-pŏf′ĭ-sĭs) [Gr., an undergrowth]. (pl. *hypophyses*) 1. An undergrowth. 2. [NA] The pituitary body or gland, q.v. A gland of internal secretion lying in the sella turcica of the sphenoid bone. It consists of two portions, the adenohypophysis (anterior lobe) and the neurohypophysis (posterior lobes), which are attached to the hypothalamus of the brain by the hypophyseal stalk. SEE: *pituitary gland.*

h. cerebri. The pituitary gland.

h. sicca. Posterior pituitary.

hypophysitis (hī-pŏf″ĭ-sī′tĭs) [Gr. *hypo,* under, + *physis,* growth, + *itis,* inflammation]. Inflammation of the pituitary body.

hypopiesis (hī″pō-pī-ē′sĭs) [″ + *piesis,* pressure]. Lower than normal blood pressure.

hypopigmentation (hī″pō-pĭg″mĕn-tā′shŭn). Diminished pigment in a tissue.

hypopinealism (hī″pō-pĭn′ē-ăl-ĭzm) [″ + L. *pineus,* pert. to pine cone, + Gr. *-ismos,* state of]. Diminished secretion of the pineal gland.

hypopituitarism (hī″pō-pĭ-tū′ĭ-tă-rĭzm) [″ + L. *pituita,* mucus, + Gr. *-ismos,* state of]. A condition resulting from diminished secretion of pituitary hormones, esp. those of the anterior lobe.

hypoplasia (hī″pō-plā′zē-ă) [″ + *plasis,* formation]. Defective development of tissue. SEE: *tissue.*

hypopnea (hī″pō-nē′ă) [″ + *pnoia,* breath]. Decreased rate and depth of breathing.

hypoporosis (hī″pō-pō-rō′sĭs) [″ + *poros,* callus, + *osis,* condition]. Deficient development of a callus at site of a bone fracture.

hypoposia (hī″pō-pō′zē-ă) [″ + *posis,* drinking]. Decreased intake of fluids.

hypopotassemia (hī″pō-pō″tăs-sē′mē-ă) [″ + *potassium* + Gr. *haima,* blood]. Hypokalemia.

hypopraxia (hī″pō-prăk′sē-ă) [″ + *praxis,* action]. Decreased and inefficient activity.

hypoproteinemia (hī″pō-prō″tē-ĭn-ē′mē-ă) [″ + *protos,* first, + *haima,* blood]. Decrease in the amount of protein in the blood.

hypoproteinosis (hī″pō-prō″tē-ĭ-nō′sĭs). Condition of deficient proteins in the body or diet.

hypoprothrombinemia (hī″pō-prō-thrŏm″bĭn-ē′mē-ă) [″ + L. *pro,* for, + Gr. *thrombos,* clot, + *haima,* blood]. Deficiency of blood clotting factor II (prothrombin) in the blood.

...opselaphesia (hī″pŏp-sĕl-ă-fē′zē-ă) [″ + ...*hesis,* touch]. Blunted tactile sense.

...ism (hī″pō-tī′ăl-ĭzm) [″ + *ptyalon,* saliva, + *-ismos,* state of]. Decreased salivary secretion.

hypopyon (hī-pō′pē-ŏn) [″ + *pyon,* pus]. Pus in anterior chamber of the eye in front of iris but behind cornea, seen in corneal ulcer.

hyporeactive (hī″pō-rē-ăk′tĭv). Decreased response to stimuli.

hyporeflexia [″ + L. *reflexus,* bent back]. Diminished function of the reflexes.

hyposalemia (hī″pō-săl-ē′mē-ă) [″ + L. *sal,* salt, + Gr. *haima,* blood]. Decreased amount of sodium chloride in the blood.

hyposalivation (hī″pō-săl″ĭ-vā′shŭn). Abnormal decrease in flow of saliva.

hyposarca (hī″pō-săr′kă) [″ + *sarx,* flesh]. Extreme edema of subcutaneous connective tissue. SYN: *anasarca.*

hyposcleral (hī″pō-sklē′răl). Beneath the sclera of the eye.

hyposecretion (hī″pō-sē-krē′shŭn). Lowered amt. of secretion.

hyposensitive (hī″pō-sĕn′sĭ-tĭv) [″ + L. *sentire,* to feel]. Having reduced ability to respond to stimuli.

hyposensitization (hī″pō-sĕn″sĭ-tĭ-zā′shŭn). Production of hyposensitiveness.

hyposialadenitis (hī″pō-sī″ăl-ăd-ĕ-nī′tĭs) [Gr. *hypo,* under, + *sialon,* saliva, + *aden,* gland, + *itis,* inflammation]. Inflammation of the submandibular salivary gland.

hyposmia (hī-pŏz′mē-ă) [″ + *osme,* smell]. Defect in sense of smell.

hyposmolarity (hī-pŏz″mō-lăr′ĭ-tē). Decreased osmolar concentration, esp. of the blood or urine.

hyposomnia (hī″pō-sŏm′nē-ă). Decreased ability to sleep. SYN: *insomnia.*

hypospadia, hypospadias (hī″pō-spā′dē-ă, -ăs) [″ + *span,* to draw]. 1. An abnormal congenital opening of the male urethra upon the undersurface of the penis. 2. A urethral opening into the vagina.

hyposphresia (hī″pŏs-frē′sē-ă) [″ + *osphresis,* smell]. Hyposmia.

hypostasis (hī″pŏs′tă-sĭs) [″ + *stasis,* a standing]. 1. Diminished blood flow or circulation. 2. Deposit of sediment due to decreased flow of a body fluid such as blood or urine.

hypostatic (hī″pō-stăt′ĭk) [″ + *statikos,* standing]. 1. Of or pert. to hypostasis. 2. In genetics, hidden or suppressed, said of a gene whose effect is suppressed by the presence of another gene.

hypostatic pneumonia. SEE: *pneumonia, hypostatic.*

hyposteatolysis (hī″pō-stē-ă-tŏl′ĭ-sĭs) [″ + *stear,* fat, + *lysis,* loosening]. Diminished emulsification of fats during digestion.

hyposthenia (hī″pŏs-thē′nē-ă) [″ + *sthenos,* strength]. Subnormal strength; an enfeebled state; weakness.

hyposthenlant (hī″pŏs-thē′nē-ănt). One whose

strength and vital forces are reduced; debilitant.

hyposthenic (hī-pŏs-thĕn′ĭk). 1. Debilitant. 2. Body habitus characterized by a long, shallow thorax, a long thoracic cavity, a long, narrow abdominal cavity, and a slender build.

hyposthenuria (hī″pŏs-thĕn-ū′rē-ă) [″ + *sthenos,* strength, + *ouron,* urine]. The secretion of urine of low specific gravity, chiefly in chronic nephritis.

h., tubular. Hyposthenuria resulting from disease of the renal tubule epithelial cells.

hypostomia (hī″pō-stō′mē-ă) [″ + *stoma,* mouth]. Congenital defect in which the mouth is small.

hypostosis (hĭp″ŏs-tō′sĭs) [″ + *osteon,* bone, + *osis,* condition]. Deficient development of bone.

hypostypsis (hī″pō-stĭp′sĭs) [″ + *stypsis,* a contracting]. State of being slightly astringent.

hypostyptic (hī″pō-stĭp′tĭk). Slightly astringent.

hyposynergia (hī″pō-sĭn-ĕr′jē-ă) [″ + *syn,* together, + *ergon,* work]. Poor coordination.

hypotaxia (hī″pō-tăks′ē-ă) [Gr. *hypo,* under, + *taxis,* arrangement]. State of reduced control over voluntary actions such as occurs in early stages of hypnotism.

hypotelorism (hī″pō-tĕl′ō-rĭzm) [″ + *telouros,* distant]. Decreased distance between organs, esp. the eyes.

hypotension [″ + L. *tensio,* tension]. 1. Decrease of systolic and diastolic blood pressure below normal. 2. Deficiency in tonus or tension.

Occurs in shock, in hemorrhages, infections, fevers, cancer, anemia, neurasthenia, Addison's disease; in debilitating or wasting diseases; and approaching death.

h., orthostatic. Hypotension occurring upon suddenly arising from a recumbent position or from standing still.

hypotensive. Denoting low blood pressure.

hypothalamus (hī″pō-thăl′ă-mŭs) [″ + *thalamos,* chamber]. [NA] The portion of the diencephalon comprising the ventral wall of the third ventricle below the hypothalamic sulcus and including structures forming the ventricular floor, including the optic chiasma, tuber cinereum, infundibulum, and mammillary bodies. It lies beneath the thalamus and laterally is continuous with the subthalamic regions. It contains neurosecretions that are of importance in the control of certain metabolic activities, such as maintenance of water balance, sugar and fat metabolism, regulation of body temperature, and secretion of releasing and inhibiting hormones. It is the chief subcortical region for the integration of sympathetic and parasympathetic activities. SEE: *hormone, releasing; hormone, stimulating.*

hypothenar (hī-pŏth′ĕ-năr) [″ + *thenar,* palm]. The fleshy prominence on the inner side of the palm next to the little finger.

hypothenar eminence. Prominence on the palm below the little finger.

hypothermal (hī″pō-thĕr′măl) [″ + *therme,* heat]. 1. Tepid. 2. Subnormal temperature.

hypothermia (hī″po-thĕr′mē-ă). 1. Having a body temperature below normal. 2. A technique of lowered body temperature, usually between 78° and 90° F. (26° and 32.5° C.), to reduce oxygen need during surgery (esp. cardiovascular and neurological procedures) and in hypoxia, to reduce blood pressure, and to alleviate hyperpyrexia.

hypothermia blanket. A specially designed blanket for cooling patients with hyperthermia. The blanket has flexible tubing between the layers of cloth and cold water is pumped through the tubing.

hypothesis (hī-pŏth′ĕ-sĭs) [″ + *thesis,* a placing]. (pl. *hypotheses*) 1. An assumption not proved by experiment or observation. It is assumed for the sake of testing its soundness or to facilitate investigation of a class of phenomena. 2. A conclusion drawn before all the facts are established and tentatively accepted as a basis for further investigation.

hypothrombinemia (hī″pō-thrŏm-bĭn-ē′mē-ă) [″ + *thrombos,* clot, + *haima,* blood]. Deficiency of thrombin in the blood.

hypothymia (hī″pō-thī′mē-ă [Gr. *hypo,* under, + *thymos,* mind]. Decreased emotional response to stimuli.

hypothymism (hī″pō-thī′mĭzm) [″ + ″ + *-ismos,* state of]. Decreased activity of the thymus.

hypothyroid (hī″pō-thī′royd) [″ + *thyreos,* shield, + *eidos,* form]. Marked by insufficiency of thyroid secretion.

hypothyroidism (hī″pō-thī′royd-ĭzm). A condition due to deficiency of the thyroid secretion, resulting in a lowered basal metabolism. A lesser degree of cretinism.

SYM: May be obesity; dry skin and hair, both of which become lusterless. Low blood pressure, slow pulse, sluggishness of all functions, depressed muscular activity, goiter.

TREATMENT: Replacement therapy with natural or synthetic thyroid hormone preparations. Increase iodine in diet if iodine is deficient.

NURSING IMPLICATIONS: ...
thyroid hormone as ordered. As...
tient for symptoms of the dis...
decreased temperature, diarrh...
pation, and sensitivity to cold. ...
be protected from chilling, i...
and trauma from exposure ...
patient against (and obser...
tion during treatment with...

ment hormone.

hypotonia (hī″pō-tō′nē-ă) [″ + *tonos,* tone]. 1. Reduced tension; relaxation of arteries. 2. Loss of tonicity of the muscles or intraocular pressure.

hypotonic (hī-pō-tŏn′ĭk). 1. Pert. to defective muscular tone or tension. 2. A solution of lower osmotic pressure than another.

hypotoxicity (hī″pō-tŏks-ĭs′ĭ-tē) [″ + *toxikon,* poison]. A reduced toxic quality; only slightly poisonous.

hypotrichosis (hī″pō-trĭ-kō′sĭs) [″ + *thrix,* hair, + *osis,* condition]. Abnormal deficiency of hair.

hypotrophy (hī-pŏt′rŏ-fē) [″ + *trophe,* nourishment]. Progressive degeneration and functional loss of cells and tissues. SYN: *abiotrophy; atrophy.*

hypotropia (hī″pō-trō′pē-ă) [″ + *trope,* a turning]. Vertical strabismus downward.

hypotympanotomy (hī″pō-tĭm″pă-nŏt′ō-mē). Surgical incision of the tympanic membrane of the ear.

hypotympanum (hī″pō-tĭm′pă-nŭm). The part of the middle ear beneath the level of the tympanic membrane.

hypouricuria (hī″pō-ū-rĭ-kū′rē-ă) [″ + *ouron,* urine, + *ouron,* urine]. Deficient uric acid in the urine.

hypourocrinia (hī″po-ūr″ō-krĭn′ē-ă) [″ + ″ + *krinein,* to separate]. Deficient urinary secretion.

hypovaria (hī″pō-vā′rē-ă) [Gr. *hypo,* under, + L. *ovarium,* ovary]. Deficient internal secretion of the ovary and consequent retardation of growth and development in girls.

hypovenosity (hī″pō-vĕn-ŏs′ĭ-tē) [″ + L. *venosus,* pert. to a vein]. Incomplete development of the venous system in an area, resulting in atrophy or degeneration.

hypoventilation (hī″pō-vĕn″tĭ-lā′shŭn) [″ + L. *ventilatio,* ventilation]. Reduced rate and depth of breathing.

hypovitaminosis (hī″pō-vī″tă-mĭn-ō′sĭs) [″ + L. *vita,* life, + *amine* + Gr. *osis,* condition]. A condition due to a lack of vitamins in the diet.

hypovolemia (hī″pō-vō-lē′mē-ă) [″ + L. *volumen,* volume]. Diminished blood volume. SYN: *oligemia; oligohemia.*

hypovolia (hī″pō-vō′lē-ă). Decreased water content.

hypoxanthine (hī″pō-zăn′thĭn, -thēn) [″ + *xanthos,* yellow]. A purine derivative, $C_5H_4N_4O$, in muscles and tissues in a stage of urea and uric acid formation. It is formed during protein decomposition. It is normal in urine in small amounts.

ypoxemia (hī-pŏks-ē′mē-ă) [″ + *oxygen* + *ima,* blood]. Insufficient oxygenation of the SYN: *hypoxia.* SEE: *respiration.*

hī″pŏks′ē-ă). Deficiency of oxygen. Decreased concentration of oxygen in the inspired air. SEE: *anoxia; hypoxemia.*

HypRho-D. Trade name for $Rh_o(D)$ immune globulin, human.

hypsarrhythmia, hypsarhythmia (hĭp″săr-ĭth′mē-ă) [Gr. *hypsi,* high, + *a-,* not, + *rhythmos,* rhythm]. An abnormal electroencephalographic pattern of persistent generalized slow waves and very high voltage. Clinically it is often associated with infantile spasm and progressive mental deterioration. Etiological factors are unknown.

hypsibrachycephalic (hĭp″sē-brăk″ē-sĕ-făl′ĭk) [Gr. *hypsi,* high, + *brachys,* broad, + *kephale,* head]. Having a broad and high skull.

hypsicephalic (hĭp″sē-sĕ-făl′ĭk) [″ + *kephale,* head]. Having a skull with a cranial index above 75.1°. SYN: *hypsistenocephalic.*

hypsicephaly (hĭp-sē-sĕf′ă-lē). The condition of having a skull with a cranial index over 75.1°.

hypsiconchous (hĭp″sē-kŏng′kŭs) [″ + *konche,* shell]. Having an orbital index of about 85°.

hypsiloid (hĭp′sĭ-loyd) [Gr. *upsilon,* U or Y, + *eidos,* form]. U- or Y-shaped. SYN: *hyoid.*

hypsiloid ligament. Ligamentum iliofemorale.

hypsistaphylia (hĭp″sē-stăf-ĭl′ē-ă) [Gr. *hypsi,* high, + *staphyle,* uvula]. Having a narrow, high palatal arch.

hypsistenocephalic (hĭp″sē-stĕn″ō-sĕ-făl′ĭk) [″ + *stenos,* narrow, + *kephale,* head]. Having a cranial index over 75.1°. SYN: *hypsicephalic.*

hypsocephalous (hĭp″sō-sĕf′ă-lŭs) [Gr. *hypsos,* height, + *kephale,* head]. Having a cranial index over 75.1°. SYN: *hypsicephalic.*

hypsokinesis (hĭp″sō-kī-nē′sĭs) [″ + *kinesis,* motion]. Tendency to fall backward when standing; seen in paralysis agitans.

hypsophobia (hĭp″sō-fō′bē-ă) [″ + *phobos,* fear]. Fear of being at great heights. SYN: *acrophobia.*

hypurgia (hī-pŭr′jē-ă) [Gr. *hypourgia,* help]. Any minor factor that changes the course of a disease, esp. for the better.

hysteralgia (hĭs-tĕr-ăl′jē-ă) [Gr. *hystera,* uterus, + *algos,* pain]. Uterine pain. SYN: *hysterodynia.*

hysteratresia (hĭs″tĕr-ă-trē′zē-ă) [″ + *a-,* not, + *tresis,* perforation]. Atresia of the uterus.

hysterectomy (hĭs-tĕr-ĕk′tō-mē) [″ + *ektome,* excision]. Surgical removal of the uterus. The uterus may be removed through the abdominal wall or through the vagina. The presence of benign or malignant tumors is the most frequent reason for hysterectomy.

In preparation for abdominal hysterectomy, the patient is placed in dorsal position. The table is ready to be tipped into the Trendelenburg position. As soon as incision is made through the peritoneum, table should be put into Trendelenburg position. This procedure is the same for all abdominopelvic surgery. This position allows the intestines and abdominal organs to fall away from pelvis, so that they may be easily packed off with large pads or with a large roll of packing.

NURSING IMPLICATIONS: Postoperatively, assess the patient for bladder distention, and catheterize as needed. Administer pain medications as ordered to maintain comfort. Take the patient's vital signs and observe the patient for any bleeding or any symptoms of hemorrhage during the first few hours after surgery. Work to prevent respiratory complications by frequently (every 2 hours) turning the patient, and by having her cough and breathe deeply every 1 to 2 hours in the post-op period. Ensure that the patient wears elastic stockings, does leg exercises daily, ambulates as ordered to help prevent phlebitis. Also assess the patient for a positive Homan's sign. The patient recovering from a hysterectomy should have a high-protein diet. Explain to the patient the need for and importance of hormone replacement therapy.

h., abdominal. Removal of the uterus through an abdominal incision.

h., cesarean. Surgical removal of the uterus at the time of cesarean section.

h., Porro. Subtotal hysterectomy following cesarean section.

h., radical. Surgical removal of the uterus, tubes, ovaries, adjacent lymph nodes, and a part of the vagina. SYN: *Wertheim's hysterectomy.*

h., subtotal. Removal of the uterus, leaving the cervix uteri in place.

h., supracervical. H., subtotal.

h., supravaginal. H., subtotal.

h., total. Removal of both the body of the uterus and the cervix.

h., vaginal. Removal of the uterus through the vagina.

hysteresis (hĭs″tĕr-ē′sĭs) [Gr., a coming too late]. 1. Failure of related phenomena to keep pace with each other. 2. Failure of the manifestation of an effect to keep up with its cause. 3. A transformer loss of power due to the alternating of its magnetic field.

hystereurynter (hĭs″tĕr-ū-rĭn′tĕr) [Gr. *hystera,* uterus, + *eurynein,* to stretch]. An instrument for dilating the os uteri. SYN: *metreurynter.*

hysteria (hĭs-tē′rē-ă) [Gr. *hystera,* uterus]. A neurotic condition presenting somatic symptoms, simulating almost any type of physical disease; along with a series of mental manifestations. The condition occurs in the absence of organic disease to account for the symptoms.

The mental attitude is calm. There is a not unfriendly aloofness, but psychotic indifference is quite another matter, and not seen in hysteria. There may be easy laughing and crying episodes of emotionalism possibly without any apparent explanation, and even occurring in sleep. Episodic states known as fugues (sleepwalking is similar, occurring in sleep). In these, certain dissociated (repressed) ideas, emotions and goals develop a reality sufficient to constitute a secondary personality which now functions apart from the primary personality.

When the primary consciousness reasserts itself, there is a forgetting (amnesia) of the secondary state. The multiplication or alternation of personalities is quite distinct from schizophrenic splitting in which incongruities and confusion result from the coexistence of each phase of the personality more or less continuously.

ETIOL: Variable, as in most psychic disturbances. It occurs in both sexes before and after adolescence and at periods of emotional and physical stress.

SYM: Emotional instability, various sensory disturbances, and a marked craving for sympathy, which sometimes leads to fraud.

TREATMENT: Place patient in a quiet place devoid of spectators. Cold applications to head, face, and neck are helpful. Quiet, firm suggestions are important. Sedatives are to be used under the direction of a physician.

h., anxiety. Hysteria combined with an anxiety neurosis.

h., major. Very severe hysteria accompanied by epileptiform convulsions.

h., minor. Mild form of hysteria without loss of consciousness.

hysteriac (hĭs-tĕr′ē-ăk) [Gr. *hystera,* uterus]. A hysterical person.

hysteric, hysterical. Pert. to hysteria.

hysteric ataxia. Loss of sensation in leg muscles and skin in hysteria.

hysteric chorea. A form of hysteria with choreiform movements.

hystericoneuralgic (hĭs-tĕr″ĭk-o-nū-răl′jĭk) [″ + *neuron,* nerve, + *algos,* pain]. Pert. to pain of hysterical origin, but resembling neuralgia.

hysteritis (hĭs-tĕr-ī′tĭs) [″ + *itis,* inflammation]. Inflammation of the uterus.

hystero-, hyster- [Gr. *hystera,* wo… …fix indicating either womb or hysteri…

hysterobubonocele (hĭs″tĕr-ō-bū… + *boubon,* groin, + *kele,* herr… hernia surrounding the uterus…

hysterocatalepsy (hĭs″tĕr-ō-că… *kata,* down, + *lepsis,* seizure… with cataleptic symptoms.

hysterocele (hĭs′tĕr-ō-sēl) [

Hernia of the uterus, esp. when gravid.

hysterocleisis (hĭs″tĕr-ō-klī′sĭs) [″ + *kleisis,* closure]. Surgical closure of the os uteri.

hysterocystocleisis (hĭs″tĕr-ō-sĭs″tō-klī′sĭs) [″ + *kystis,* a bladder, + *kleisis,* a closure]. Operation fastening the cervix uteri in the wall of the bladder.

hysterodynia (hĭs″tĕr-ō-dĭn′ē-ă) [″ + *odyne,* pain]. Uterine pain. SYN: *hysteralgia.*

hysterogastrorrhaphy (hĭs″tĕr-ō-găs-tror′ă-fē) [″ + *gaster,* belly, + *rhaphe,* suture]. Fixation of uterus to the gastric wall. SYN: *hysteropexy.*

hysterogenic (hĭs″tĕr-ō-jĕn′ĭk) [″ + *gennan,* to produce]. Causing hysteria.

hysterogram (hĭs′tĕr-ō-grăm). Roentgenogram of the uterus.

hysterography (hĭs″tĕ-rŏg′ră-fē) [″ + *graphein,* to write]. Recording of the frequency and intensity of contractions of the uterus.

hysteroid (hĭs′tĕr-oyd) [″ + *eidos,* resemblance]. 1. Resembling hysteria. 2. Pert. to hysteria.

hysterolaparotomy (hĭs″tĕr-ō-lăp″ă-rŏt′ō-mē) [″ + *lapara,* flank, + *tome,* incision]. Uterine incision through abdominal wall; abdominal hysterectomy.

hysterolith (hĭs′tĕr-ō-lĭth) [″ + *lithos,* stone]. A calculus in the uterus.

hysterology (hĭs-tĕr-ŏl′ō-jē) [″ + *logos,* knowledge]. Sum of what is known about the uterus.

hysterolysis (hĭs″tĕr-ŏl′ĭ-sĭs) [″ + *lysis,* loosening]. Operation of loosening the uterus from its adhesions.

hysteromania (hĭs″tĕr-ō-mā′nē-ă) [″ + *mania,* madness]. 1. Hysterical mania. 2. Nymphomania.

hysterometer (hĭs″tĕ-rŏm′ĕ-tĕr) [″ + *metron,* measure]. Device for measuring the uterus.

hysterometry (hĭs″tĕ-rŏm′ĕ-trē). Measurement of the size of the uterus.

hysteromyoma (hĭs″tĕr-ō-mī-ō′mă) [Gr. *hystera,* womb, + *mys,* muscle, + *oma,* tumor]. Myoma or fibromyoma of the uterus.

hysteromyomectomy (hĭs″tĕr-ō-mī″ō-mĕk′tō-mē) [″ + ″ + *ektome,* excision]. Excision of a uterine fibroid.

hysteromyotomy (hĭs″tĕr-ō-mī-ŏt′ō-mē) [″ + ″ + *tome,* incision]. Uterine incision for removal of a solid tumor.

hysteroneurosis (hĭs″tĕr-ō-nū-rō′sĭs) [″ + *neuron,* nerve, + *osis,* condition]. A neurosis related to disease of the uterus.

hystero-oophorectomy (hĭs″tĕr-ō-ō″ŏ-for-ĕk′tō-mē) [″ + *oon,* egg, + *phoros,* bearing, + *ektome,* excision]. Removal of the uterus and one or both ovaries.

ysteropathy (hĭs″tĕr-ŏp′ă-thē) [″ + *pathos,* ...ease]. Any uterine disorder.

...**pexy** (hĭs′tĕr-ō-pĕk″sē) [″ + *pexis,* fix-... ...rgical fixation of the uterus. SYN: *hysterogastrorrhaphy.*

hysteropia (hĭs″tĕr-ō′pē-ă) [″ + *ops,* eye]. A hysterical visual defect.

hysteropsychosis (hĭs″tĕr-ō-sī-kō′sĭs) [″ + *psyche,* mind, + *osis,* condition]. Mental disorder due to uterine disease.

hysteroptosia, hysteroptosis (hĭs″tĕr-ŏp-tō′sē-ă, -sĭs) [″ + *ptosis,* a dropping]. Prolapse of the uterus. SYN: *procidentia.*

hysterorrhaphy (hĭs-tĕr-or′ă-fē) [″ + *rhaphe,* sewing]. Suture of the womb.

hysterorrhexis (hĭs″tĕr-ō-rĕk′sĭs) [″ + *rhexis,* rupture]. Rupture of the uterus, esp. when pregnant.

hysterosalpingectomy (hĭs″tĕr-ō-săl″pĭn-jĕk′tō-mē) [″ + *salpinx,* tube, + *ektome,* excision]. Surgical removal of the uterus and tubes.

hysterosalpingography (hĭs″tĕr-ō-săl″pĭn-gŏg′ră-fē) [″ + ″ + *graphein,* to write]. Roentgenography of the uterus and oviducts after injecting radiopaque material into those organs.

hysterosalpingo-oophorectomy (hĭs″tĕr-ō-săl-pĭng″gō-ō″ŏ-for-ĕk′tō-mē) [″ + ″ + *oon,* egg, + *phoros,* bearing, + *ektome,* excision]. Surgical removal of the uterus, oviducts, and ovaries.

hysterosalpingostomy (hĭs″tĕr-ō-săl″pĭng-ŏs′tō-mē) [″ + ″ + *stoma,* opening]. Anastomosis of the uterus with the distal end of the fallopian tube after excision of a strictured portion of the tube.

hysteroscope (hĭs′tĕr-ō-skōp) [″ + *skopein,* to examine]. Instrument for examining the uterine cavity. SYN: *metroscope.*

hysteroscopy (hĭs″tĕr-ŏs′kō-pē). Inspection of the uterus by use of a special endoscope. SEE: *hysteroscope.*

hysterospasm (hĭs′tĕr-ō-spăzm″) [Gr. *hystera,* womb, + *spasmos,* a spasm]. Uterine spasm.

hysterostomatocleisis (hĭs″tĕr-ō-stō″mă-tō-klī′sĭs) [″ + *stoma,* opening, + *kleisis,* closure]. Operation for vesicovaginal fistula. Consists of closure of the cervix uteri, making the vesical and uterine cavities into a common cavity by means of the opening between them.

hysterostomatomy (hĭs″tĕr-ō-stō-măt′ō-mē) [″ + ″ + *tome,* incision]. Surgical enlargement of the os uteri; incision of the os or cervix uteri.

hysterotome (hĭs′tĕr-ō-tōm) [″ + *tome,* incision]. Instrument for incision of the uterus.

hysterotomy (hĭs-tĕr-ŏt′ō-mē). 1. Incision of the uterus. 2. Cesarean section.

hysterotrachelectomy (hĭs″tĕr-ō-trā″kĕl-ĕk′tō-mē) [″ + *trachelos,* neck, + *ektome,* excision]. Amputation of the uterine cervix.

hysterotracheloplasty (hĭs″tĕr-ō-trā′kĕl-lō-plăs″tē) [″ + ″ + *plassein,* to form]. Plastic surgery or repair of the cervix.

hysterotrachelorrhaphy (hĭs″tĕr-ō-trā″kĕl-or′ă-fē) [″ + ″ + *rhaphe,* sewing]. Plastic surgery of a lacerated cervix by paring the edges and suturing them together.

hysterotrachelotomy (hĭs″tĕr-ō-trā″kĕl-ŏt′ō-mē) [″ + ″ + *tome,* incision]. Surgical incision of the neck of the uterus.

hysterotraumatic (hĭs″tĕr-ō-traw-măt′ĭk) [″ + *trauma,* wound]. Pert. to traumatic hysteria.

hysterotubography (hĭs″tĕr-ō-tū-bŏg′ră-fē). Hysterosalpingography, q.v.

hysterovagino-enterocele (hĭs″tĕr-ō-văj″ĭn-ō-ĕn′tĕr-ō-sēl) [″ + L. *vagina* sheath, + Gr. *enteron,* intestine, + *kele,* hernia]. Hernia surrounding the uterus, vagina, and intestines.

Hytakerol. Trade name for dihydrotachysterol, USP.

Hz. *hertz.*

HZV. *herpes zoster virus.*

I

I. Chem. symb. for iodine.

^{131}I. Radioactive iodine. At. wt. 131.

^{132}I. Radioactive iodine. At. wt. 132.

i. *optically inactive.*

-ia. Suffix indicating condition, esp. an abnormal state.

IABC. *intra-aortic balloon counterpulsation.*

IABP. *intra-aortic balloon pump.*

I and O. *intake and output.*

ianthinopsia (ī-ăn″thĭ-nŏp′sē-ă) [Gr. *ianthinos,* violet colored, + *opsis,* vision]. Abnormality of vision in which all objects appear to be violet.

-iasis [Gr.]. Suffix, same as or interchangeable with *-osis,* meaning the state or condition of, particularly a pathological condition.

iatraliptics (ī″ă-tră-lĭp′tĭks) [Gr. *iatreia,* cure, + *aleiphein,* to anoint]. Treatment by friction.

iatric (ī-ăt′rĭk) [Gr. *iatrikos,* medical]. Referring to medicine, the medical profession, or physicians.

iatro- [Gr. *iatros,* physician]. Combining form indicating relationship to medicine or a physician.

iatrochemistry (ī-ăt″rō-kĕm′ĭs-trē) [″ + *chemeia,* chemistry]. Seventeenth-century opinion that chemistry is the basis of all physiological phenomena.

iatrogenic disorder (ī″ăt-rō-jĕn′ĭk) [″ + *gennan,* to produce]. Any adverse mental or physical condition induced in a patient by effects of treatment by a physician or surgeon. Term implies that such effects could have been avoided by proper and judicious care on the part of the physician.

iatrogeny (ī″ă-trŏj′ĕ-nē). An adverse state or condition induced by a physician.

iatrology (ī″ă-trŏl′ō-jē) [″ + *logos,* science]. Medical science.

iatrotechniques (ī-ăt″rō-tĕk-nēks′) [″ + *techne,* art]. The art and technique of medicine and surgery.

I-band. Isotropic, light band (segment) of a muscle fiber.

ibuprofen. USP. A nonsteroidal anti-inflammatory agent with antipyretic and analgesic properties. Although its exact mechanism of action is unknown, it does not stimulate the pituitary-adrenal system. Used in treating chronic symptomatic rheumatoid arthritis and osteoarthritis. It may be particularly useful in patients with gastrointestinal intolerance to aspirin. Trade name in the U.S. is Motrin. This drug has antiprostaglandin activity, and is useful in treating primary dysmenorrhea.

IC. *inspiratory capacity.*

ICD. *intrauterine contraceptive device; International Classification of Diseases.*

ice (īs) [AS. *is*]. A solid form of water. Water becomes ice at a temperature of 32° F. (0° C.) Ice may be chilled lower than the freezing point. An ice bag, cap, collar, and cravat are devices for holding ice to be applied to a patient to obtain the effect of continuous cold in a circumscribed area. The part so treated should always be covered with several thicknesses of cloth to prevent cold injury to the tissues.

i., dry. Carbon dioxide cooled to the point where it is a solid. This occurs at −110° F. (−78.9° C.). Used as a commercial refrigerant and for therapeutic refrigeration in the treatment of certain skin conditions including warts. SEE: *carbon dioxide.*

ice bag. A water-tight bag with a sealable opening large enough to permit ice cubes or chipped ice to be added. Used in any localized condition requiring application of cold. In an emergency any sturdy bag made of flexible plastic can be used. That type bag can be sealed by tying a knot in the open end.

Iceland disease. Epidemic neuromyasthenia.

Iceland moss. An edible lichen containing a form of starch; a slightly tonic demulcent. SYN: *Cetraria.*

ice treatment. Use of ice applied either directly or in a suitable container to cool an injured area. It is believed that ice therapy, at least in the first 24 to 48 hours following injury, is much more beneficial than heat in treating superficial bruises, contusions, and sprains. The use of application of cold or of ice water in immediate treatment of a burn helps to reduce the extent of inflammation and pain.

ichnogram (ĭk′nō-grăm) [Gr. *ichnos,* footstep, + *gramma,* mark]. A footprint taken while standing.

ichor (ī′kor) [Gr. *ichor,* serum]. Thin, fetid discharge from an ulcer or from a wound.

ichoremia (ī″kor-ē′mē-ă) [″ + *haima,* blood]. Septicemia or blood poisoning.

ichorous (ī′kor-ŭs) [Gr. *ichor,* serum]. Resembling ichor or watery pus.

ichthammol (ĭk′thă-mŏl). USP. A reddish-brown viscous fluid obtained by the destructive distillation of certain bituminous shale. Used as a mild antiseptic and local stimulant in certain skin diseases Trad[illegible] name is Ichthyol.

ichthyism, ichthyismus (ĭk′th[illegible] ĭz′mŭs) [Gr. *ichthys,* fish, + *-is*[illegible] Poisoning from eating decom[illegible] fish. SEE: *tetrodotoxin.*

ichthyo- [Gr. *ichthys,* fish] [illegible] meaning fish.

ichthyoacanthotoxism ([illegible]

tŏk′sĭzm) [″ + *akantha*, thorn, + *toxikon*, poison, + *-ismos*, condition]. Toxin or venom present in the sting, spines, or "teeth" of certain venomous fish.

ichthyohemotoxin (ĭk″thē-ō-hē″mō-tŏk′sĭn) [″ + *haima*, blood, + *toxikon*, poison]. Toxin present in the blood of certain poisonous fish.

ichthyoid (ĭk′thē-oyd) [″ + *eidos*, form]. Fish-like.

ichthyology (ĭk″thē-ŏl′ō-jē) [″ + *logos*, study]. The study of fish.

ichthyootoxin (ĭk″thē-ō″ō-tŏk′sĭn) [″ + *oon*, egg, + *toxikon*, poison]. Toxin present in the roe of certain fish.

ichthyophagous (ĭk″thē-ŏf′ă-gŭs) [″ + *phagein*, to eat]. Subsisting on fish.

ichthyophobia (ĭk-thē-ō-fō′bē-ă) [″ + *phobos*, fear]. Aversion to fish.

ichthyosarcotoxin (ĭk″thē-ō-săr″kō-tŏk′sĭn) [″ + *sarx*, flesh, + *toxikon*, poison]. Toxin present in the flesh of certain fish.

ichthyosis (ĭk″thē-ō′sĭs) [″ + *osis*, condition]. Condition in which the skin is dry and scaly, resembling fish skin. Because ichthyosis is so easily recognized, a variety of diseases have been called by this name.

A mild nonhereditary form is called xeroderma. This is often seen on the legs of older patients, esp. during the winter months. It may be more prevalent in those who bathe frequently, thus causing excessive dryness of the skin.

TREATMENT: The application of lotions or ointments that soften and soothe the skin provide symptomatic relief for all forms of ichthyosis. Removal of dry scales can be accomplished by applying a combination of 6% salicylic acid in a gel containing propylene glycol, ethyl alcohol, hydroxy propylene cellulose, and water. This is most effective when applied to moistened skin at night, and covered with an occlusive dressing. Soaps should be used sparingly.

i. congenita. Severe form of ichthyosis present at birth. SYN: *harlequin fetus*.

i. fetalis. I. congenita.

i. hystrix. Linear nevus. The skin contains bands or lines of rough, thick, warty, hypertrophic papillary growths.

i., lamellar, of newborn. Rare form of inherited ichthyosis with lamellar desquamation.

i. vulgaris. A hereditary form of ichthyosis that includes two genetically distinct types. Dominant ichthyosis vulgaris is produced by an autosomal dominant gene. Characterized by dry, rough, scaly skin, it is not present at birth and is usually noticed between the ages of one and four. Many cases improve in later [illegible] The second type is sex-linked ichthyosis [illegible]s. It is present only in males and is [illegible]d by the female as a recessive gene. Onset of scattered large brown scales is seen in early infancy. The scalp may be involved but the face is spared except for the sides and in front of the ear. There is little tendency to improve with age.

ichthyotic (ĭk″thē-ŏt′ĭk) [Gr. *ichthys*, fish]. Rel. to ichthyosis.

ichthyotoxicology (ĭk″thē-ō-tŏk″sĭ-kŏl′ō-jē) [″ + *toxikon*, poison, + *logos*, study]. The study of poisons and toxins produced by certain fish.

ichthyotoxin (ĭk″thē-ō-tŏk′sĭn) [″ + *toxikon*, poison]. Any toxin present in fish.

icing. 1. A technique of cutaneous stimulation using ice (12 to 17° C.) to evoke or facilitate reflex muscular responses in patients with central nervous system dysfunction. 2. Application of ice to a recently traumatized area. This is done to reduce pain and swelling in the area.

ICN. *International Council of Nurses*.

iconolagny (ī-kŏn′ō-lăg′nē) [Gr. *eikon*, image, + *lagneia*, lewdness]. Sexual stimulation produced by suggestive pictures, statues, or objects.

I.C.S. *International College of Surgeons*.

ICSH. *interstitial cell–stimulating hormone*. In males, this hormone stimulates the production of testosterone from the interstitial cells of the testes. SYN: *luteinizing hormone*.

ictal (ĭk′tăl) [L. *ictus*, a blow or stroke]. Pert. to or caused by a sudden attack or stroke such as acute epilepsy. SEE: *postictal*.

icteric (ĭk-tĕr′ĭk) [Gr. *ikteros*, jaundice]. Pert. to jaundice.

icteritious (ĭk-tĕr-ĭsh′ŭs). Yellowish; resembling jaundice. SYN: *icteroid*.

icteroanemia (ĭk″tĕr-ō-ă-nē′mē-ă) [″ + *an-*, not, + *haima*, blood]. Icterus associated with anemia, hemolysis, and splenic enlargement.

icterogenic, icterogenous (ĭk″tĕr-ō-jĕn′ĭk, -ŏj′ĕn-ŭs) [″ + *gennan*, to produce]. Causing jaundice.

icterohematuric (ĭk″tĕr-ō-hĕm″ă-tū′rĭk) [″ + *haima*, blood, + *ouron*, urine]. Concerning icterus and hematuria.

icterohemoglobinuria (ĭk″tĕr-ō-hē″mō-glō″bĭ-nū′rē-ă) [″ + *haima*, blood, + L. *globus*, globe, + Gr. *ouron*, urine]. Concerning icterus and hemoglobinuria.

icterohepatitis (ĭk″tĕr-ō-hĕp-ă-tī′tĭs) [″ + *hepar*, liver, + *itis*, inflammation]. Liver inflammation with jaundice.

icteroid (ĭk′tĕr-oyd) [″ + *eidos*, form]. Resembling jaundice; yellow-hued.

icterus (ĭk′tĕr-ŭs) [Gr. *ikteros*, jaundice]. Pigmentation of the tissues, membranes, and secretions with bile pigments. SYN: *jaundice*.

i. gravis neonatorum. Hemolytic jaundice of the newborn. It is usually due to isoimmunization with the Rh factor.

i., hemolytic. Rare chronic form of icterus, frequently congenital, with periodic attacks of intense hemolysis. SYN: *icterus, nonobstructive.*

SYM: Much the same as in obstructive icterus, q.v. Sometimes found in acute yellow atrophy, the anemias, and infectious fevers. Enlarged spleen.

i. neonatorum. Hemolytic jaundice of the newborn. It is mild, self-limiting and requires no treatment.

i., nonobstructive. I., hemolytic.

i., obstructive. Jaundice caused by obstruction to the flow of bile in the common or hepatic duct.

ETIOL: Cholangitis, carcinoma, gallstones, cirrhosis of liver, cysts, parasites in ducts, pressure by tumors, hepatic abscess.

SYM: Skin, mucous membrane, sclera, and secretions stained yellow; first noticed in the conjunctivae. Stool light or clay-colored, urine dark, pulse low, temperature slightly subnormal. In extreme cases, delirium, convulsions, coma.

ictus [L., stroke]. (pl. *ictus*) Blow, sudden attack.

i. cordis. The heartbeat.

i. epilepticus. Epileptic convulsion.

i. sanguinis. Apoplexy; cerebrovascular accident.

i. solis. Sunstroke.

I.C.U. *intensive care unit.*

ID. *identification; infective dose; inside diameter; intradermal.*

ID_{50}. The infective dose of microorganisms that will produce illness in 50% of the individuals who receive that dose.

id [L. *id,* it; later translators of Freud's writings feel the word *es* should have been translated to *it* and not to id]. In psychiatry, one of the three divisions of the psyche, the others being the ego, q.v., and superego, q.v. The id is the obscure, inaccessible part of our personality that serves as a repository of instinctual drives continually striving for expression. Expression is manifest as an impulsion to obtain satisfaction for the instinctive needs in accordance with the pleasure-pain principle.

-id [Gr. *eidos,* form, shape]. Suffix indicating certain secondary skin eruptions that appear some distance from site of primary infection. If etiological agent of primary infection is known, the secondary lesion is designated by adding -id, as in tuberculid and trichophytid.

-ide. A suffix indicating a binary chemical compound, as *sodium chloride.*

idea [Gr., form]. A mental image; a concept.

i., autochthonous. A thought that comes into the mind independent of train of thoughts, in an unaccountable way.

i., compulsive. A persistent, obsessional impulse or thought.

i., dominant. An idea that controls all one's actions and thoughts.

i., fixed. An idea that completely dominates the mind despite evidence to the contrary; a delusion. SYN: *idée fixe.*

i., flight of. Rapid speech, often disconnected and incoherent, in certain mental diseases.

i. of reference. An impression that the conversation or actions of others have reference to oneself.

ideal [L. *idea,* model]. A goal or endeavor regarded as a standard of perfection.

ideation (ī-dē-ā′shŭn). The process of thinking; formation of ideas. It is slow in dementias, depressions, and other organic brain diseases, and in narcotic intoxications, but quickened in early stage of intoxications. It is unduly active in manic-depressive states.

idée fixe (ē-dā′ fēks′) [Fr.] An obsession; a fixed idea. SYN: *idea, fixed,* q.v.

identical [L. *identicus,* the same]. Exactly alike.

identification [″ + *facere,* to make]. 1. A kind of daydream, as when one identifies oneself with the hero of a book or play. 2. The process of determining the sameness of a thing or person with that described or known to exist.

identification, palm and sole system of. A system based on prints of the palmar surface of the hand and the plantar surface of the foot. SEE: *dermatoglyphics.*

identity (ī-dĕn′tĭ-tē). 1. The concept that each individual has of his or her own body in space and his or her own thought processes in relation to the social and intellectual environment. 2. The physical and mental characteristics by which an individual is known and recognized.

i., ego. The sense of self that provides a unity of personality.

i., gender. One's self-concept with respect to being male or female, or confused about one's true sexual identity.

ideo- [Gr. *idea,* form]. Prefix pert. to mental images.

ideogenous, ideogenetic (īd-ē-ŏj′ĕn-ŭs, -ō-jĕ-nĕt′ĭk) [″ + *gennan,* to produce]. Stimulated by an idea.

ideology (ī″dē-ŏl′ō-jē) [″ + *logos,* study]. 1. The science of ideas or thought. 2. A system or schema of ideas; a philosophy.

ideomotion (ī″dē-ō-mō′shŭn) [″ ... *motus,* moving]. Muscular automatic r... tivated by a dominant idea.

ideomotor (ī″dē-ō-mō′tor). Pe... tion.

ideomuscular (ī″dē-ō-mŭs′... *musculus,* muscle]. 1. Ind... activity produced in c... thought. 2. Concerning muscular activity.

ideophrenic (ĭd″ē-ō-frĕn′ĭk) [″ + *phrenitikos,* insane]. Marked by abnormal ideas of a perverted nature.

ideoplastia (ĭd-ē-ō-plăs′tē-ă) [″ + *plassein,* to form]. Condition of the mind of a hypnotized person in which the person is capable of receiving and responding to suggestions of the hypnotist.

ideovascular (ĭd″ē-ō-văs′kū-lăr). Pert. to vascular changes induced by ideas, memories, or emotions; as when a state of mental stress produces an elevation in blood pressure.

idio- [Gr. *idios,* own]. Prefix indicating individual or distinct.

idiochromosome (ĭd″ē-ō-krō′mō-sōm) [″ + *chroma,* color, + *soma,* body]. Any sex chromosome.

idiocrasy (ĭd″ē-ŏk′ră-sē) [″ + *krasis,* temperament]. Peculiarity that renders one susceptible to certain habits or drugs. SEE: *idiosyncrasy.*

idiocratic (ĭd″ē-ō-krăt′ĭk). Pert. to idiocrasy.

idiocy [Gr. *idiotes,* ignorant person]. Severe mental deficiency, usually due to an arrest in development, or defective development, as compared to the loss of mental competence. The cause, which occurs either in utero or in the first years after birth, may be genetic, traumatic, or due to severe disease. SEE: *mental retardation.*

i., complete. Idiocy in which primitive instincts are lacking, even that of self-preservation.

i., cretinoid. Endemic idiocy accompanied by goiter. SEE: *cretinism.*

i., epileptic. Idiocy accompanied by epilepsy.

i., genetous. Idiocy of congenital origin.

i., hemiplegic. Hemiplegia accompanied by idiocy in infants.

i., hydrocephalic. Idiocy accompanied by chronic hydrocephalus.

i., intrasocial. Idiocy in which the mentality permits the individual to learn an occupation.

i., microcephalic. Idiocy accompanied by microcephalia.

i., paralytic. Idiocy combined with paralysis.

i., paraplegic. Idiocy combined with paraplegia.

i., sensorial. Mental deficiency caused by loss of one of the special senses.

i., traumatic. Idiocy caused by an injury received in infancy or in early childhood.

idiogamist (ĭd″ē-ŏg′ă-mĭst) [Gr. *idios,* own, + *gamos,* marriage]. An individual who is sex- ...lly potent with only one or a few partners.

... **esis** (ĭd″ē-ō-jĕn′ĕ-sĭs) [″ + *gennan,* to ... Of self-origin or origin without ... esp. with reference to disease.

idioglossia (ĭd″ē-ō-glŏs′ē-ă) [″ + *glossa,* tongue]. Inability to articulate properly, so that the sounds emitted are like those of an unknown language.

idiogram (ĭd′ē-ō-grăm″) [″ + *gramma,* writing]. Graphic representation of the karyotype, or chromosome complement of a cell.

idioisolysin (ĭd″ē-ō-ī-sŏl′ĭ-sĭn) [″ + *isos,* equal, + *lysis,* dissolution]. A hemolysin active against the cells of an individual of the same species.

idiolalia (ĭd″ē-ō-lā′lē-ă) [″ + *lalia,* talk]. Condition in which the individual speaks in an invented language.

idiolysin (ĭd″ē-ŏl′ĭ-sĭn) [″ + *lysis,* dissolution]. A lysin normally present in blood.

idiometritis (ĭd″ē-ō-mĕ-trī′tĭs) [″ + *metra,* uterus, + *itis,* inflammation]. Inflammation of the uterine parenchyma.

idiomuscular (ĭd″ē-ō-mŭs′kū-lăr) [″ + L. *musculus,* a muscle]. Pert. to the muscles independent of nerve control.

idiomuscular contraction. Motion produced by degenerated muscles without nerve stimulus.

idioneurosis (ĭd″ē-ō-nū-rō′sĭs) [″ + *neuron,* nerve, + *osis,* condition]. Any functional neurosis arising without stimuli.

idiopathic (ĭd″ē-ō-păth′ĭk) [″ + *pathos,* disease]. Pert. to conditions without clear pathogenesis, or disease without recognizable cause, as of spontaneous origin.

idiopathy (ĭd-ē-ŏp′ă-thē). A primary disease without apparent cause.

idiophrenic (ĭd″ē-ō-frĕn′ĭk) [″ + *phren,* mind]. Pert. to or originating in the mind alone.

idiopsychologic (ĭd″ē-ō-sī″kō-lŏj′ĭk) [″ + *psyche,* mind, + *logos,* study]. Concerning ideas produced in one's own mind.

idioreflex (ĭd″ē-ō-rē′flĕks) [″ + L. *reflexus,* reflected]. A reflex resulting from a stimulus that arises within the organ in which the reflex takes place.

idiospasm (ĭd′ē-ō-spăzm) [″ + *spasmos,* convulsion]. Spasm confined to one area.

idiosyncrasy (ĭd″ē-ō-sĭn′kră-sē) [″ + *syn,* together, + *krasis,* mixture]. 1. Special characteristics by which persons differ from each other. 2. That which makes one react differently from others. A peculiar or individual reaction to an idea, an action, a drug, a food, or some other substance through unusual susceptibility.

idiosyncrasy of effect. When doses of a drug that would have a known and predictable effect cause a toxic or opposite effect, or an unusual effect, or no effect.

idiosyncrasy to a drug. An unusual response to a drug. This can manifest as an accelerated, toxic, or inappropriate response to the usual therapeutic dose of a drug.

idiosyncratic (ĭd″ē-ō-sĭn-krăt′ĭk). Pert. to an

idiosyncrasy.

idiot [Gr. *idiotes*, an ignorant person]. Former term for a person with severe mental deficiency. SEE: *idiocy; mental retardation.*

idiotic. Like an idiot; said of an idea or action.

idiotrophic (ĭd″ē-ō-trŏf′ĭk) [Gr. *idios*, own, + *trophe*, nourishment]. Capable of securing its own nourishment.

idiotropic (ĭd″ē-ō-trŏp′ĭk) [″ + *trope*, a turning]. Turning inwardly mentally and emotionally. SYN: *egocentric; introspective.*

idiotropic type. In psychology, an introvert type who is satisfied by his or her own emotions and by inner contemplation and pursuits and who is content to live apart from social contacts.

idiot-savant (ēd-jō′să-vănt) [Fr., learned idiot]. An individual who is generally mentally retarded but has the ability to do such things as recall dates or accurately and rapidly perform mathematical calculations.

idiotypic (ĭd″ē-ō-tĭp′ĭk) [Gr. *idios*, own, + *typos*, type]. Rel. to heredity.

idiovariation (ĭd″ē-ō-văr″ē-ā′shŭn) [″ + L. *variare*, to vary]. A mutation that occurs without known cause.

idioventricular (ĭd″ē-ō-vĕn-trĭk′ū-lăr) [″ + L. *ventriculus*, little belly]. Pert. to the cardiac ventricle alone when dissociated from the atrium. A heart rhythm that arises in the ventricle is an example.

idoxuridine (ī-dŏks-ūr′ĭ-dēn). 5-iodo-2′deoxyuridine. USP. ABBR: IDU. Used to treat herpesvirus infections of the eye. Trade names are Dendrid, Herplex Liquifilm, and Stoxil.

IDU. *5-iodo-2′deoxyuridine; idoxuridine.*

IgA. *immunoglobulin gamma A.*

IgD. *immunoglobulin gamma D.*

IgE. *immunoglobulin gamma E.*

IgG. *immunoglobulin gamma G.*

IgM. *immunoglobulin gamma M.*

ignatia (ĭg-nā′shē-ă) [L.]. Seeds of a climbing plant native to the Philippine Islands. The seeds contain about 3% strychnine and brucine.

igniextirpation (ĭg″nē-ĕks″tĭr-pā′shŭn) [L. *ignis*, fire, + *exstirpare*, to root out]. Cautery excision.

ignioperation (ĭg″nē-ŏp″ĕr-ā′shŭn) [″ + *operatio*, a working]. An operation by use of cautery.

ignipuncture (ĭg″nē-pŭnk′chūr) [″ + *punctura*, a piercing]. The use of heated needles in cauterization by puncture.

ignis (ĭg′nĭs) [L., fire]. Fire; cautery. SYN: *moxa.*

i. infernalis. Ergotism.

i. sacer. An inflammatory skin disease. SYN: *herpes zoster.*

i. Sancti Antonii. Acute febrile disease with localized inflammation. SYN: *erysipelas; St. Anthony's fire.*

I.H. *infectious hepatitis.*

ilea. Pl. of ileum.

ileac (ĭl′ē-ăk). 1. Pert. to the ileum. 2. Pert. to ileus.

ileal (ĭl′ē-ăl). Pert. to the ileum.

ileal bypass. Surgical procedure for decreasing absorption of nutrients from the small intestine by anastomosing one portion of the upper portion of the small intestine to another portion some distance farther along the intestine. Method is used in treating obesity.

ileal conduit. Method of diverting the urinary flow by transplanting the ureter into a prepared and isolated segment of the ileum, which is sutured closed on one end. The other end is connected to an opening in the abdominal wall. The urine is collected there in a special receptacle.

ileectomy (ĭl″ē-ĕk′tō-mē) [L. *ileum*, ileum, + Gr. *ektome*, excision]. Excision of the ileum.

ileitis (ĭl″ē-ī′tĭs) [″ + Gr. *itis*, inflammation]. Inflammation of the ileum. The membrane becomes inflamed and ulcerates, the affected portion becoming thick, rigid, and edematous, and the lumen progressively narrowed. The lymph glands enlarge and the adjacent mesentery becomes thickened. Most often found in the terminal ileum, but it may spread to other parts of the bowel and to the cecum. Adhesions may be formed. Pain is centered around the umbilicus and right lower quadrant. Abdominal distention is present. Diarrhea alternates with constipation. Vomiting may occur.

i., regional. A nonspecific chronic inflammatory granulomatous lesion involving the terminal ileum. It is nontuberculous. The disease may extend over many years with exacerbations and remissions of diarrhea, abdominal pain, anemia, loss of weight, fistula formation, and eventually obstructive intestinal symptoms. Stools are soft and grayish or brown in color with abundant fecal particles. Any part of the gastrointestinal tract may be involved, but the ileum is the principal site. The cause is unknown and the treatment is dietary and symptomatic with respect to the anemia and dehydration. Avoid raw fruits and vegetables. Antibiotics may have to be used for life. SYN: *Crohn's disease.*

ileo- (ĭl′ē-ō) [L. *ileum*]. Combining form indicating relationship to the ileum

ileocecal (ĭl″ē-ō-sē′kăl) [″ + ... d]. Rel. to the ileum and cecum.

ileocecal valve. Sphincter m... to close the ileum at the ... small intestines open i... colon. It prevents food ... entering the small intes...

ileocecostomy (ĭl″ē-ō-sē...

Gr. *stoma,* opening]. Surgical formation of an opening between the ileum and cecum.

ileocecum (ĭl″ē-ō-sē′kŭm). The ileum and cecum combined.

ileocolic (ĭl″ē-ō-kŏl′ĭk) [″ + Gr. *kolon,* colon]. Pert. to the ileum and colon.

ileocolitis (ĭl″ē-ō-kō-lī′tĭs) [″ + ″ + *itis,* inflammation]. Inflammation of mucous membrane of the ileum and colon.

ileocolostomy (ĭl″ē-ō-kō-lŏs′tō-mē) [″ + ″ + *stoma,* opening]. Anastomosis between the ileum and colon.

ileocolotomy (ĭl″ē-ō-kō-lŏt′ō-mē) [″ + ″ + *tome,* incision]. Incision of the ileum and colon.

ileocystoplasty (ĭl″ē-ō-sĭst′ō-plăs″tē) [″ + Gr. *kystis,* bladder, + *plassein,* to form]. Use of a portion of the ileum to increase the size of the bladder.

ileocystostomy (ĭl″ē-ō-sĭs-tŏs′tō-mē) [″ + ″ + *stoma,* opening]. Surgical formation of an opening between the ileum and the bladder.

ileoileostomy (ĭl″ē-ō-ĭl″ē-ŏs′tō-mē) [″ + *ileum,* small intestine, + Gr. *stoma,* opening]. Surgical formation of an opening between one part of the ileum and another part.

ileoproctostomy (ĭl″ē-ō-prŏk-tŏs′tō-mē) [″ + Gr. *proktos,* rectum, + *stoma,* opening]. Establishment of opening between ileum and rectum. SYN: *ileorectostomy.*

ileorectal (ĭl″ē-ō-rĕk′tăl) [″ + *rectum,* rectum]. Concerning the ileum and the rectum.

ileorectostomy (ĭl″ē-ō-rĕk-tŏs′tō-mē) [″ + ″ + Gr. *stoma,* opening]. Formation of a passage between the ileum and rectum. SYN: *ileoproctostomy.*

ileorrhaphy (ĭl″ē-or′ă-fē) [″ + Gr. *rhaphe,* suture]. Surgical repair of the ileum.

ileosigmoidostomy (ĭl″ē-ō-sĭg″moyd-ŏs′tō-mē) [″ + Gr. *sigma,* letter S, + *eidos,* form, + *stoma,* opening]. Surgical opening between the ileum and sigmoid flexure.

ileostomy (ĭl″ē-ŏs′tō-mē) [″ + Gr. *stoma,* opening]. Creation of a surgical passage through the abdominal wall into the ileum. The fecal material drains into a bag worn on the abdomen.

i., urinary. Surgical formation of an opening between the ileum and the urinary bladder.

ileotomy (ĭl″ē-ŏt′ō-mē) [″ + Gr. *tome,* incision]. Incision into the ileum.

ileotransversostomy (ĭl″ē-ō-trăns″vĕr-sŏs′tō-mē) [″ + *transversus,* crosswise, + Gr. *stoma,* opening]. Connection of the ileum with the transverse colon.

ileum (ĭl′ē-ŭm) [L., ileum]. (pl. *ilea*) [NA] Lower three fifths of the small intestines [illegible]rom the jejunum to the ileocecal valve. It [illegible]es in the adult male from 31 ft. 6 in. (9.6 [illegible] to 15 ft. 6 in. (4.72 meters). SEE: [illegible] *regions* and *digestive system* for illus.

i., duplex. Congenital doubling of the ileum.

ileus (ĭl′ē-ŭs) [Gr. *eileos,* a twisting]. Intestinal obstruction. Originally meant colic due to intestinal obstruction.

SYM: Acute obstruction; sudden pain, paroxysmal, then continuous; constipation; persistent fecal vomiting; abdominal distention; collapse.

i., adynamic. Ileus caused by intestinal muscle paralysis.

i., dynamic. Ileus caused by intestinal muscle contraction.

i., mechanical. Ileus produced by an obstruction.

i., meconium. Ileus of the newborn due to obstruction of the bowel with meconium.

i. paralyticus. I., adynamic.

i., postoperative. Ileus resulting from handling the bowel during surgery, anesthesia, electrolyte imbalance, or wound infection.

i., spastic. Ileus due to spasm of a segment of the intestine.

i. subparta. Ileus due to pressure of the pregnant uterus on the colon.

ilia. Pl. of ilium.

iliac [L. *iliacus,* pert. to ilium]. Rel. to the ilium.

iliac crest. The hip. Upper free margin of the ilium.

iliac fascia. Transversalis fascia over the anterior surface of the iliopsoas muscle.

iliac fossa. One of the concavities of the iliac bones of the pelvis.

iliac region. Inguinal region on either side of the hypogastrium.

iliac roll. Sausage-shaped mass in the left iliac fossa. Caused by induration of the sigmoidal walls.

iliac spine. One of four spines of the ilium, namely the anterior and posterior inferior spines and the anterior and posterior superior spines.

ilio- [L. *ilium,* flank]. Combining form indicating relationship to the ilium or flank.

iliococcygeal (ĭl″ē-ō-kŏk-sĭj′ē-ăl) [″ + Gr. *kokkyx,* coccyx]. Concerning the ilium and the coccyx.

iliocolotomy (ĭl″ē-ō-kō-lŏt′ō-mē) [″ + Gr. *kolon,* colon, + *tome,* incision]. Opening into the colon in the iliac or inguinal region.

iliocostal (ĭl″ē-ō-kŏs′tăl) [″ + *costa,* rib]. Joining or concerning the ilium and ribs.

iliofemoral (ĭl″ē-ō-fĕm′or-ăl) [″ + *femoralis,* pert. to femur]. Pert. to the ilium and femur.

ilioinguinal (ĭl″ē-ō-ĭn′gwĭ-năl) [″ + *inguinalis,* pert. to groin]. Pert. to the groin and iliac regions.

iliohypogastric (ĭl″ē-ō-hī″pō-găs′trĭk) [″ + Gr. *hypo,* under, + *gaster,* stomach]. Concerning the ilium and hypogastrium.

iliolumbar (ĭl″ē-ō-lŭm′bar) [″ + *lumbus*, loin]. Rel. to the iliac and lumbar regions.

iliopagus (ĭl″ē-ŏp′ă-gŭs) [″ + Gr. *pagos*, thing fixed]. Twins joined in the iliac region.

iliopectineal (ĭl″ē-ō-pĕk-tĭn′ē-ăl) [L. *ilium*, flank, + *pecten*, a comb]. Rel. to the ilium and the pubes.

iliopelvic (ĭl″ē-ō-pĕl′vĭk) [″ + *pelvis*, basin]. Concerning the iliac area and the pelvis.

iliopsoas (ĭl″ē-ō-sō′ăs) [″ + Gr. *psoa*, loin]. The compound iliacus and psoas magnus muscles.

iliopsoas abscess. An abscess in the psoas and iliacus muscles.

iliosacral (ĭl″ē-ō-sā′krăl) [″ + *sacralis*, pert. to sacrum]. Pert. to the sacrum and ilium.

iliosciatic (ĭl″ē-ō-sī-ăt′ĭk) [″ + *sciaticus*, pert. to the ischium]. Concerning the ilium and the ischium.

iliospinal (ĭl″ē-ō-spī′năl) [″ + *spinalis*, pert. to the spine]. Concerning the ilium and the spinal column.

iliothoracopagus (ĭl″ē-ō-thō″ră-kŏp′ă-gŭs) [″ + Gr. *thorax*, chest, + *pagos*, thing fixed]. Twins joined from the pelvis to the thorax.

iliotibial (ĭl″ē-ō-tĭb′ē-ăl) [″ + *tibialis*, pert. to tibia]. Pert. to the ilium and tibia.

iliotibial band. A thick, wide fascial layer from the iliac crest to the knee joint.

ilioxiphopagus (ĭl″ē-ō-zī-fŏp′ă-gŭs) [″ + Gr. *xiphos*, sword, + *eidos*, form, + *pagos*, thing fixed]. Twins joined from the pelvis to the xiphoid process.

ilium (ĭl′ē-ŭm) [L., groin, flank]. (pl. *ilia*) 1. One of the bones of each half of the pelvis. It is the superior and widest part and serves to support the flank. In the child, prior to fusion with adjacent pelvic bones, it is a separate bone. SYN: *os ilium* [NA]. 2. The flank. SEE: *hip bone; sacroiliac*.

ill (ĭl) [Old Norse *illr*, bad]. Sick; not healthy; diseased.

illaqueation (ĭl″ăk-wē-ā′shŭn) [L. *illaqueare*, to ensnare]. Turning an inverted eyelash by drawing a loop of thread behind it.

illegitimate. 1. Illegal; against the law. 2. Born out of wedlock.

illinition (ĭl-ĭ-nĭsh′ŭn) [L. *illinire*, to smear]. Inunction, q.v.

illness (ĭl′nĭs) [Old Norse *illr*, bad, + AS. *-ness*, state of]. 1. State of being sick. 2. Ailment.

illuminating gas. A mixture of various combustible gases, including hydrogen and carbon monoxide. Its poisonous effects are largely due to carbon monoxide, q.v. Treat by resuscitation, q.v.

illumination (ĭl-lū-mĭn-ā′shŭn) [L. *illuminare*, to light up]. 1. The lighting up of a part for examination or of an object under a microscope. 2. Amount of light thrown upon anything.

i., axial. Light transmitted along the axis of a microscope.

i., central. I., axial.

i., darkfield. Illumination of an object under a microscope in which the central or axial light rays are stopped and the object illuminated by light rays coming from the sides, the object then appearing light against a dark background. Used to observe extremely small objects such as spirochetes or colloid particles.

i., direct. Illumination of an object under a microscope by directing light rays upon its upper surface.

i., focal. The concentration of light upon an object by means of a mirror or a system of lenses.

i., oblique. Illumination of an object from one side.

i., through. SEE: *transillumination*.

i., transmitted light. Illumination in which the light is directed through the object. Light may come directly from a light source or be reflected by a mirror.

illuminism. Condition in certain psychotic states in which the patient has delusions of talking or communing with supernatural or exalted beings.

illusion [L. *illusio*]. Inaccurate perception; misinterpretation of sensory impressions, whereas a hallucination has no source in fact. Vague stimuli are conducive to the production of illusions, but essentially it is a disorder of ideation. If an illusion becomes fixed, it is said to be a delusion.

i., optical. A visual impression that is inaccurate with respect to what was available to be seen.

illusional. Pert. to, or of the nature of, an illusion.

Ilosone. Trade name for erythromycin estolate.

Ilotycin. Trade name for erythromycin, USP.

Ilozyme. Trade name for pancrelipase.

I.M. *intramuscular(ly)*.

im-. Prefix that is used in place of *in-* before words beginning with *b*, *m*, or *p*.

I.M.A. *Industrial Medical Association*.

ima (ī′mă) [L.]. Lowest.

image (ĭm′ĭj) [L. *imago*, likeness]. 1. A mental picture representing a real object. 2. A more or less accurate likeness of a thing or person. 3. The picture of an object ... h as that produced by a lens or mirror.

i., body. The concept an i... his or her physical self. M... have inappropriate self-ima... it has been shown that so... als have the body image ... person.

i., direct. Picture ...

cused.

i., double. Condition occurring in strabismus when the visual axes of the eyes are not directed toward the same object. SEE: *diplopia.*

i., false. I., double.

i., inverted. Image that is turned upside down.

i., mirror. The image of an object reflected in a mirror. Right and left are reversed in that image. The term is also used to indicate the similarity of chemical substances, or persons with quite similar personalities and looks. Identical twins are also often described as being mirror images of each other.

i., real. Image formed by convergence of rays of light from an object.

i., true. I., double.

i., virtual. I., direct.

mage intensifier. Device used in radiology to increase the brightness of an image produced in x-ray and x-ray fluoroscopy studies. The technique permits discrimination of much smaller objects in the image and greatly decreases the patient's and the examiner's exposure to the radiation.

imagery (ĭm′ĭj-rē) [L. *imago,* likeness]. Imagination; the calling up of events or mental pictures. Mental imagery may be of various types.

i., auditory. Mental image of sounds that can be recalled, as thunder or wind.

i., smell. Mental conception of odor sensations previously experienced. Often very weak.

i., tactile. Mental image of the feeling of an object.

i., taste. Mental conception of taste sensations previously experienced. Often very weak.

i., visual. Mental conception of an object seen previously. This is probably the commonest type of imagery. SEE: *afterimage.*

imagination [L. *imago,* likeness]. The power of forming mental images of things, persons, or situations that are wholly or partially different from those previously known or experienced.

imaging. The production of a picture, image, or shadow that represents the object being investigated. In diagnostic medicine the classic technique for imaging is x-ray. Newer techniques involve the use of computer-generated images produced by x-ray, ultrasound, or infrared.

imago (ĭ-mā′gō) [L., likeness]. 1. An image or shadow. 2. A memory, esp. of a loved one, ...eloped during childhood that has become ... by idealism and imagination, and ... always a correct one. 3. The adult, ...re form of an insect.

Imavate. Trade name for imipramine hydrochloride, USP.

imbalance [L. *in-,* not, + *bilanx,* two scales]. Out of balance. Without equality in power between opposing forces.

i., autonomic. An imbalance between sympathetic and parasympathetic divisions of the autonomic nervous system, esp. as pertains to vasomotor reactions.

i., sympathetic. Increased excitability of the vagus nerve. SYN: *vagotonia.*

i., vasomotor. Excessive vasoconstriction or vasodilation resulting from impulses to blood vessels.

imbecile (ĭm′bĕ-sĭl) [L. *imbecillus,* feeble]. Former term for severe mental deficiency. SEE: *mental retardation.*

imbecility. A state of severe mental deficiency.

imbed [L. *in,* in, (put) into, + AS. *bedd,* bed]. In histology, to surround with a firm substance, such as paraffin or collodium, preparatory to cutting sections. SEE: *embedding.*

imbibition (ĭm″bĭ-bĭsh′ŭn) [″ + *bibere,* to drink]. The absorption of fluid by a solid body or gel.

imbricate, imbricated (ĭm′brĭ-kāt, -ĕd) [L. *imbricare,* to tile]. Overlapping, as tiles or fish scales; overlapping aponeurotic layers.

imbrication (ĭm″brĭ-kā′shŭn) [L. *imbricare,* to tile]. 1. Overlapping, as tiles. 2. The overlapping of aponeurotic layers in abdominal surgery.

Imferon. Trade name for iron dextran.

imidazole; iminazole (ĭm″ĭd-ăz′ōl″, -ă-zōl′; ĭm″ĭn-). An organic compound, $C_3H_4N_2$, characterized structurally by the presence of the heterocyclic ring

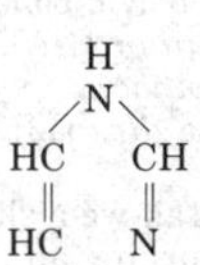

which occurs in histidine and histamine.

imide (ĭm′ĭd). A compound with the bivalent atom group (NH).

imipramine hydrochloride (ĭ-mĭp′ră-mēn). USP. An antidepressant drug of the tricyclic class. This drug is also used in treating enuresis in children over 6 years of age. Trade names are Imavate, Janimine, Presamine, SK-Pramine, and Tofranil.

immature (ĭm″mă-tūr′) [L. *in-,* not, + *maturus,* ripe]. Not fully developed or ripened.

immediate [″ + *mediare,* to be in middle]. Direct; without intervening steps.

immedicable (ĭ-mĕd′ĭ-kă-b′l) [L. *immedicabilis*]. Incurable; pert. to that which cannot be healed.

immersion (ĭm-ĕr′shŭn) [L. *in,* into, + *mergere,* to dip]. 1. Placing a body under water or other fluid. 2. In microscopy, the act of immersing the objective (then called an immersion lens) in water or oil, preventing total reflection of rays falling obliquely upon peripheral portions of the objective.

i., homogeneous. Immersion in which the stratum of air between objective and cover glass is replaced by a medium that deflects as little as possible the rays of light passing through the cover glass.

immersion foot. Damage to the entire foot due to continued exposure to water or to moisture. This can occur in a hot or cold climate in a situation wherein it is not possible to maintain proper foot hygiene. From military experience, it was found that the condition could be prevented by changing to dry socks as frequently as required. SEE: *trench foot.*

immersion lens, oil. A special lens with oil placed between the lens and the object being visualized. This produces a higher magnification than would be the case if the oil were not used.

immiscible (ĭ-mĭs′ĭ-bl) [L. *in-,* not, + *miscere,* to mix]. Pert. to that which cannot be mixed, as oil and water.

immobilization [″ + *mobilis,* movable]. The making of a part or limb immovable.

NURSING IMPLICATIONS: Assess the patient for development of any of the complications of immobilization such as: pneumonia, thrombophlebitis, fat emboli, renal calculi, urinary tract infections, decubitus ulcers, muscle atrophy, and contracture formation.

Institute nursing interventions to prevent the complications of immobilization by having the patient cough and breathe deeply every two hours, change position every two hours, wear elastic stockings, do quadriceps-setting, gluteal-setting, and range of motion exercises at least daily, ensure good body hygiene, and maintain an increased oral fluid intake. Good skin care is essential; inspect the skin daily for redness and signs of breakdown, and massage the skin; encourage good nutritional intake. If the patient has an extremity that is casted or splinted, make sure that the cast is not too tight and thereby constricting blood supply. Always assess the neurovascular status of the extremity distal to the site of the cast, splint, or traction by assessing for good color, presence of a pulse, and extremity warmth, movement, and sensation.

immune (ĭm-ūn′) [L. *immunis,* safe]. Protected from or resistant to a disease due to the development of antibodies, q.v., or cellular immunity.

immune reaction. 1. Demonstrated antigenic response to a specific antibody. 2. The specific reaction of host cells to antigenic stimulation. SEE: *immune response.*

immune response. The reaction of the body to substances that are foreign or are interpreted as being foreign.

Cell-mediated immune response: involves the production of lymphocytes by the thymus (T cells) in response to exposure to an antigen. This reaction is important in delayed hypersensitivity; rejection of tissue transplants; response to malignant growths; and in some infections. SEE: *B cells; T cells.*

Humoral immune response: involves production of plasma lymphocytes (B cells) in response to antigen exposure with subsequent antibody formation. This response can produce immunity or hypersensitivity. SEE: *B cells, T cells.*

Nonspecific immune response: does not involve antibody stimulation, but includes the inflammatory reaction, phagocytosis of microorganisms, and complement activation. SEE: *complement; phagocytosis.*

Primary immune response: The response of the immunologically competent B cells to produce a small amount of antibody in the form of immune globulin M and to differentiate into B memory cells and cells capable of becoming plasma cells. Even though the T cell response is undetectable, the T cells differentiate into T memory cells and helper or suppressor cells.

Secondary immune response (booster response): B and T cells that have undergone a primary response to an antigen will rapidly respond to a subsequent exposure to that antigen. The B cells develop into plasma cells that produce large amounts of antibody, mostly immune globulin G. The T cells change into activated lymphocytes and are responsible for inducing reactions such as delayed hypersensitivity and graft rejection.

Specific immune response: occurs in the presence of a specific antigen or disease, and involves all changes associated with antigen contact by the immune system.

immunifacient (ĭ-mū″nĭ-fā′shĕnt) [″ + *facere,* to make]. Making immune.

immunity [L. *immunitas*]. 1. State of being immune to or protected from a disease, esp. an infectious disease. Usually induced by having been exposed to the antigenic substances peculiar to the disease wh[...]fected or by having been immunized w[...] that has the capability of st[...]mul[...] tion of specific antibodies. 2. T[...] the body and its tissues t[...] antigens including red cells[...] (i.e., transplanted) tissues[...] individual's own cells (aut[...] *autoimmune disease; im*[...]

munoglobulin.

i., acquired. Immunity resulting from the development of active or passive immunity, as opposed to natural or innate immunity.

i., active. Immunity resulting from the development within the body of substances that render a person immune. This may result from antigenic stimulation produced either by having the disease or by inoculation of a vaccine or products produced by the organism. SEE: *immune response; vaccination.*

i., congenital. Immunity present at birth. It may be natural or acquired, the latter being dependent upon antibodies received from the blood of the mother.

i., herd. The level of resistance of a group or population to specific diseases.

i., local. Immunity that is limited to a given area or tissue of the body.

i., natural. A more or less permanent immunity to disease with which an individual is born, the result of natural inherent factors. It may be the heritage of an individual, a race, or a species. It may be due to the natural presence of immune bodies, but other factors such as diet, differences in metabolism or temperature, or adaptive features of infective organisms may be involved.

i., passive. Immunity acquired in utero from antibodies that pass from the mother to the fetus through the placenta, or acquired by the newborn by ingesting the mother's milk. This type of immunity can also be produced by injection of antibodies into the subject to be protected.

immunization [L. *immunitas,* immunity]. Becoming immune or the process of rendering a patient immune. SEE: *autoimmunization; immunity.*

i., deliberate. The administration, usually by injection, of immunogens as a means of protecting individuals from developing specific diseases. SEE: *immune response.*

i., natural. The development of immunity to the great number of antigens present in the bacteria to which an individual is exposed. These are the microorganisms normally present in the intestinal tract, and on the skin. SEE: *immune response.*

immunizing unit. A unit that expresses an antitoxin's strength. It varies with different antitoxins.

immunoassay (ĭm″ū-nō-ăs′sā) [L. *immunis,* safe, + O. Fr. *assai,* trial]. Measuring the protein and protein-bound molecules that are concerned with the reaction of an antigen with its specific antibody. SEE: *immunoelectrophoresis; immunofluorescence; radioim*[illegible]*noassay.*

[illegible]**biology** (ĭm″ū-nō-bī-ŏl′ō-jē) [″ + Gr. [illegible] + *logos,* study]. Study of immune phenomena in biological systems, including the immune response to infectious diseases, transplantation of organs, allergy, autoimmunity, and cancer.

immunochemistry (ĭm″ū-nō-kĕm′ĭs-trē) [″ + Gr. *chemeia,* chemistry]. The chemistry of immunization. The chemistry of antigens, antibodies, and their relation to each other.

immunochemotherapy (ĭm″ū-nō-kē′mō-thĕr″ă-pē) [″ + ″ + *therapeia,* treatment]. Alteration of the immune response or mechanisms by use of drugs. The goal of such therapy is to enhance or depress the immune response. May be used as part of the therapeutic regimen in treating certain types of malignancies.

immunocompetence (ĭm″ū-nō-kŏm′pĕ-tĕns). Being capable of developing antigenic response to stimulation by an antigen. This ability may be altered or interfered with by certain drugs used for this purpose in conditions such as organ transplantation.

immunoconglutinin (ĭm″ū-nō-kŏn-gloo′tĭ-nĭn) [″ + *conglutinare,* to glue together]. Autoantibody against certain fixed complement components of an antigen-antibody complex.

immunodeficiency (ĭm″ū-nō-dĕ-fĭsh′ĕn-sē). Decreased or compromised ability to respond to antigenic stimuli by appropriate cellular immunity reaction such as phagocytosis, or production of antibodies. SEE: *immunocompetence.*

immunodiagnosis (ĭm″ū-nō-dī″ăg-nō′sĭs). Use of specific immune responses in diagnosing medical conditions.

immunodiffusion (ĭm″ū-nō-dĭ-fū′zhŭn). A test method in which an antigen and antibody are placed in a gel where they diffuse toward each other. When they meet, a precipitate is formed.

immunoelectrophoresis (ĭ-mū″nō-ē-lĕk″trō-fō-rē′sĭs). A method of investigating the amount and character of proteins and antibodies in body fluids by using electrophoresis.

immunofluorescence (ĭm″ū-nō-floo″ō-rĕs′ĕns). The use of fluorescein-stained or fluorescein-labeled antibodies to locate antigen in tissues. The antibodies combine with the specific antigen for that antibody. Evidence of the presence of the antigen then can be determined by examining the preparation with a microscope equipped with a fluorescent light. The typical fluorescent light reaction will be present if the antigen is in the preparation.

immunofluorescent method. Detection of antibodies by using special proteins labeled with fluorescein. If the specific organism or antibody that is being searched for is present, it is observed as a fluorescent material when examined microscopically while illuminated with a fluorescent light source.

immunogen (ĭ-mū'nō-jĕn) [" + Gr. *gennan,* to produce]. A substance that stimulates the formation of an antibody.

immunogenetics (ĭm"ū-nō-jĕ-nĕt'ĭks) [" + Gr. *gennan,* to produce]. The study of genetics by use of immune responses. Included would be investigations of immunoglobulins and histocompatibility antigens.

immunogenic (ĭm"ū-nō-jĕn'ĭk). Inducing immunity.

immunogenicity (ĭm"ū-nō-jĕ-nĭs'ĭ-tē). The capacity to stimulate the formation of antibodies. Not an inherent property of the substance but a condition that exists in a particular biological system. Thus a substance may act to produce antibodies in some individuals and not others.

immunoglobulin (ĭm"ū-nō-glŏb'ū-lĭn). ABBR: Ig. One of a family of closely related though not identical proteins that are capable of acting as antibodies. Five major types of immunoglobulins are normally present in the human adult: IgG (γG), with a molecular weight of 150,000; IgA (γA), with a molecular weight of approximately 170,000; IgM (γM), with a molecular weight of 900,000; IgD (γD), with a molecular weight of 180,000; and IgE (γE), with a molecular weight of 200,000. Use of either system of naming the immunoglobulins is acceptable.

i. gamma A. ABBR: IgA. The principal immunoglobulin in exocrine secretions such as milk, respiratory and intestinal mucin, saliva, and tears. This is probably important in protecting mucosal surfaces from invasion by pathogenic bacteria and viruses.

i. gamma D. ABBR: IgD. A protein that is present in normal human serum in very small amount. The function of IgD is not known.

i. gamma E. ABBR: IgE. A gamma globulin produced by cells of the lining of the respiratory and intestinal tract. IgE is important in forming reagin, q.v., antibodies. About 50% of patients with allergic diseases have increased IgE levels.

i. gamma G. ABBR: IgG. The principal immunoglobulin in human serum. Because it moves across the placental barrier, it is important in producing immunity in the infant prior to birth. It is the major antibody for antitoxins, viruses, and bacteria.

i. gamma M. ABBR: IgM. A globulin formed in almost every immune response during the early period of the reaction.

immunohematology (ĭ-mū"nō-hēm"ă-tŏl'ō-jē) [L. *immunis,* safe, + Gr. *haima,* blood, + *logos,* study]. Study of blood diseases including certain autoimmune diseases by use of immunological techniques.

immunologic (ĭm"ū-nō-lŏj'ĭk) [" + Gr. *logos,* science]. Pert. to immunology.

immunologic diseases. Those diseases caused by the action of antibodies, as in allergic hypersensitiveness to antigens or to specific reactivity of the tissues. SEE: *anaphylaxis; serum sickness.*

immunologist (ĭm"ū-nŏl'ō-jĭst). An individual whose special training and experience is in immunology.

immunology (ĭm"ū-nŏl'ō-jē) [" + Gr. *logos,* study]. The study of immunity to diseases. SEE: *serology; serum; toxin; vaccination.*

immunopathology (ĭm"ū-nō-pă-thŏl'ō-jē). Study of tissue alterations that result from immune or allergic reactions.

immunoprecipitation (ĭm"ū-nō-prē-sĭp"ĭ-tā'shŭn). The formation of a precipitate when an antigen and antibody interact.

immunoproliferative (ĭm"ū-nō-prō-lĭf'ĕr-ă-tĭv). The proliferation of cells and tissues involved in producing antigens.

immunoprotein (ĭm"ū-nō-prō'tē-ĭn) [" + Gr. *protos,* first]. Any protein or substance that confers immunity.

immunoreaction (ĭ-mū"nō-rē-ăk'shŭn). The reaction of an antibody to an antigen.

immunoreactant (ĭ-mū"nō-rē-ăk'tănt). Any one of the substances involved in immunologic reactions. Included are immunoglobulins, complement components, and specific antigens.

immunoselection (ĭm"ū-nō-sĕ-lĕk'shŭn). Selective survival of cell lives due to their having the least amount of cell surface antigenicity. This aspect allows those cells to escape the destructive activity of either antibodies or immune lymphoid cells.

immunostimulant (ĭm"ū-nō-stĭm'ū-lănt). An agent that will cause antibody formation.

immunosuppression (ĭm"ū-nō-sū-prĕsh'ŭn). Prevention of formation of immune response.

immunosuppressive (ĭm"ū-nō-sū-prĕs'ĭv). Acting to suppress the body's natural immune response to an antigen.

immunosuppressive agent. A substance that suppresses or interferes with normal immune response. These are used in controlling autoimmune diseases and in enhancing the chances for survival of foreign tissue grafts and transplants. A wide variety of drugs and x-rays are used as immunosuppressive agents.

immunosurgery (ĭ-mū"nō-sĕr'jĕr-ē). The use of specific antigenic substances in surgical therapy.

immunosurveillance (ĭm"ū-nō-sĕr- ... ns). The immune system's recognizin... stroying newly developed abnorm... arise from mutations of cell line... occur in cancer cells that c... antigens.

immunotherapy (ĭm"ū-nō-... *therapeia,* treatment]. Th...

hancement of immunity.

immunotoxin (ĭm″ū-nō-tŏk′sĭn) [″ + Gr. *toxikon,* poison]. An antitoxin.

immunotransfusion (ĭ-mū″nō-trăns-fū′zhŭn) [″ + *trans,* across, + *fusus,* poured]. Transfusion of blood that contains known antibodies.

Immu-Tetanus. Trade name for tetanus immune globulin.

impacted [L. *impactus,* pressed on]. Pressed firmly together so as to be immovable. Term may be applied to any of the following: a fracture in which ends of bones are wedged together; a tooth so placed in the jaw bone that eruption is impossible; a fetus wedged in the birth canal; cerumen; calculi; or accumulation of feces in the rectum.

impaction (ĭm-păk′shŭn) [L. *impactio,* a pressing together]. Condition of being tightly wedged into a part; overloading of an organ, as the feces in the bowels.

impalpable (ĭm-păl′pă-bl) [L. *in-,* not, + *palpare,* to touch]. Felt with difficulty if at all; hardly perceptible to the touch.

impar (ĭm′păr) [L., unequal]. Unpaired. SYN: *azygous.*

imparidigitate (ĭm-păr″ĭ-dĭj′ĭ-tāt) [″ + *digitus,* finger]. Having an uneven number of fingers or toes.

impatent (ĭm-pă′tĕnt) [″ + *patere,* to be open]. Closed; not patent.

impedance (ĭm-pē′dăns) [L. *impedire,* to hinder]. Resistance met by alternating currents in passing through a conductor; consists of resistance, reactance, inductance, or capacitance. The resistance due to the inductive and condenser characteristics of a circuit is called reactance.

i., acoustic. The resistance to the transmission of sound waves.

imperative [L. *imperativus,* commanding]. Obligatory; not controlled by the will; involuntary.

imperception [L. *in-,* not, + *percipere,* to perceive]. Inability to form a mental picture; lack of perception.

imperforate (ĭm-pĕr′fō-rāt) [″ + *per,* through, + *forare,* to bore]. Without an opening.

imperforate hymen. A hymen without an opening. Menstruation occurs but the blood cannot escape from the vagina because of the obstruction of the hymen. The treatment is surgical incision of the hymen. SEE: *hymen.*

imperforation [L. *imperforatus,* not open]. State of being closed or occluded. SYN: *atresia.*

imperious acts. Tics and motions not under control of the will. SEE: *impulsion.*

impermeable [L. *in-,* not, + *permeare,* to pass through]. Not allowing passage, as of [illegible]; impenetrable.

[illegible]s [L. *impervius*]. Unable to be penetrated.

impetiginous (ĭm″pĕ-tĭj′ĭ-nŭs) [L. *impetiginosus*]. Rel. to impetigo.

impetigo (ĭm-pĕ-tī′gō, -tē′gō) [L.]. Inflammatory skin disease marked by isolated pustules, which become crusted and rupture. Occurs principally around the mouth and nostrils. Usually caused by either staphylococcal, streptococcal, or a combined infection.

i. contagiosa. A contagious form of impetigo. Children are esp. susceptible.

SYM: Discrete, thin-walled vesicles and bullae, which become pustular and thin-crusted, appearing in crops. They may be flat and umbilicated with no tendency to rupture, and they are filled with a straw-colored fluid. They dry up as thin yellow crusts.

ETIOL: Streptococci or staphylococci.

NURSING IMPLICATIONS: Care is given by the nurse in a hospital or by the parent at home. Note the appearance and location of the lesions. The child is placed in a single room, and isolation procedures are followed. Apply mittens or cut the fingernails short to prevent the child from injuring the area by scratching. The child is held and comforted and encouraged to play and to become involved in diversional activities. Administer medications as prescribed to relieve itching. Keep lesions clean and dry. The child will be allowed to return to school when all lesions have healed.

TREATMENT: Appropriate systemic antibiotic. Crusts can be removed by applying room-temperature aqueous soaks.

i. herpetiformis. A rare pustular eruption of unknown etiology that occurs esp. during pregnancy and in association with hypocalcemia.

implant [L. *in-,* into, + *plantare,* to plant]. 1. (ĭm-plănt′) To transfer a part, to graft, to insert. Opposite of explant. 2. (ĭm′plănt) That which is implanted, such as a piece of tissue, a tooth, a pellet of medicine, or a tube or needle containing a radioactive substance.

i., tooth. SEE: *reimplantation.*

implantation (ĭm″plăn-tā′shŭn) [″ + *plantare,* to plant]. 1. Grafting of tissue or insertion of an organ. 2. Artificial placement of a substance or material into the blood or the uterine canal. 3. Embedding of the developing blastocyst in the uterine mucosa six or seven days following fertilization.

i., hypodermic. Introduction of an implant under the skin. Usually a solid substance placed with a hypodermic needle.

i., teratic. Union of an abnormal fetus with a nearly normal fetus.

implosion. A violent collapse inward.

implosion flooding. A method of treating fear due to a phobia by exposing the person to the worst possible phobic situation. The fear is experienced at maximum intensity for up to an hour until the patient is no longer capable of experiencing further fear. The phobic situation is imagined in the first sessions and later produced in reality. SEE: *phobic desensitization.*

imponderable [L. *in-,* not, + *pondus,* weight]. Incapable of being weighed or measured.

impotence, impotency [" + *potentia,* power]. Weakness, esp. inability of the male to achieve or maintain erection.

i., anatomic. Impotence caused by a defect in the genitalia. SYN: *i., organic.*

i., atonic. Impotence resulting from paralysis of nervi erigentes, which convey impulses bringing about erection.

i., functional. Impotence not due to an organic or anatomical defect; usually of psychogenic origin.

i., organic. I., anatomic.

i., psychic. Impotence due to mental disturbance.

i., symptomatic. Impotence due to poor health, drugs, or presence of disease.

impotent (ĭm′pō-tĕnt). 1. Unable to copulate. 2. Sterile; barren.

impotentia (ĭm″pō-tĕn′shē-ă) [L.]. Impotence, q.v.

impregnate (ĭm-prĕg′nāt) [L. *impregnare,* to make pregnant]. 1. To render pregnant. To fertilize an ovum. 2. To saturate.

impregnated. 1. Rendered pregnant. 2. Saturated.

impregnated carbon. Electrode having a carbon shell with core of various metals or salts of metals for use in a carbon arc lamp.

impregnation (ĭm″prĕg-nā′shŭn) [L. *impregnare,* to make pregnant]. 1. Fertilization of an ovum. SYN: *fecundation.* 2. Saturation.

i., artificial. Artificial implantation of semen in the female reproductive tract. SYN: *artificial insemination.*

impressio (ĭm-prĕs′sē-ō) [L., impression]. [NA] A mark, as of one part upon another.

i. cardiaca. [NA] Depression on surface of the liver corresponding to the position of the heart.

i. colica. [NA] Depression on the undersurface of the right lobe of the liver where it contacts the colon.

i. digitatae. [NA] A depression on the inner cranial surface.

i. duodenalis. [NA] Depression on the undersurface of the liver beside the gallbladder indicating position of the duodenum.

i. gastrica. [NA] Hollow under the left lobe of the liver indicating position of the stomach.

i. renalis. [NA] Hollow on the undersurface of the right lobe of the liver adjacent to the right kidney.

impression [L. *impressio*]. 1. A hollow or depression in a surface. 2. Effect produced upon the mind by external stimuli. 3. The imprint of all or part of the dental arch, individual teeth, or cavity preparations, using appropriate dental materials, for the purpose of records or restorative procedures.

i., digitate. Impression on inner surface of frontal bone for convolutions of the cerebrum.

i., final. An impression that is used for making the master cast for making a dental prosthesis.

impression materials. A variety of materials appropriate for different dental procedures including special waxes, plaster of Paris modeling compounds, rubber, zinc oxide paste, reversible colloids, and alginate materials.

impression tray. A receptacle or device used to carry the impression material to the mouth and to hold it in apposition to the tissues being recorded.

imprinting. A special type of learned response that occurs in some animals at a critical period in their development.

Ex.: goslings mothered by a hen may adopt the hen as if she were their mother.

impulse (ĭm′pŭls) [L. *impulsus*]. 1. Act of driving onward with sudden force. 2. An incitement of the mind, prompting an unpremeditated act. 3. In physiology, a change transmitted through certain tissues, esp. nerve fibers and muscles, resulting in physiological activity or inhibition.

i., cardiac. 1. The heartbeat felt at the left side of the chest over the apex of the heart. This is a physical impulse. 2. Impulse transmitted over conducting pathway of the heart and responsible for the contraction of the muscular tissue of the heart. This is an electrical impulse. SEE: *heart.*

i., ectopic. A cardiac impulse arising in some part of the heart other than the sinoatrial node.

i., enteroceptive. An afferent nerve impulse arising from stimuli originating in receptors located in internal organs.

i., excitatory. An impulse that stimulates activity.

i., exteroceptive. An afferent nerve impulse arising from stimuli originating in sense organs located on the body surface.

i., inhibitory. An impulse that lessens activity.

i., nervous. A self-propagated excitatory state transmitted along a nerve fiber. It is the result of physicochemical change[illegible] ring in the membrane of the nerv[illegible] impulse on reaching the termi[illegible] fiber may induce an impulse in [illegible] cell, induce activity in a tis[illegible] muscles (contraction) or in g[illegible] or give rise to a sensati[illegible] nervous centers.

i., proprioceptive. An afferent nerve impulse arising from stimuli originating in joints, muscles, or tendons, or other sensory endings that respond to pressure or stretch.

impulsion. Idea to do something or commit some act or crime suddenly imposed upon the subject that tortures him or her until the act is accomplished. Clear consciousness of the proposed act followed by an agonizing struggle, defeat, and sense of relief following the act are characteristics of impulsions, obsessions, and of inhibitions. Impulsions may include folie du doute or doubting mania (ex.: repeatedly checking to determine whether something has been done); obsessive fears of contact or delirium of touch; agoraphobia; dipsomania; pyromania; kleptomania; homicidal or suicidal impulsion; onomatomania; arithmomania; exhibitionism.

In. Chem. symb. for indium.

in-. 1. [L. *in,* into]. Prefix indicating in, inside, within; and also intensive action. 2. [L. *in-,* not]. Negative prefix.

inaction (ĭn-ăk'shŭn) [L. *in-,* not, + *actio,* act]. Failure of or decreased response to a stimulus.

inactivate [" + *activus,* acting]. To make inactive; esp. the alteration or destruction of an enzyme system or a biologically active agent such as a microorganism or antigen.

inactivation. Rendering anything inert by using heat or other means.

inactivation of complement. Loss of activity caused by heating serum to about 55° C. (131° F.) for half an hour.

inadequacy (ĭn-ăd'ĕ-kwă-sē) [" + *adaequare,* to be equal]. Insufficiency; incompetence.

inanimate [" + *animatus,* alive]. 1. Not alive; not animate. 2. Dull, lifeless.

inanition (ĭn"ă-nĭsh'ŭn) [L. *inanis,* empty]. A debilitated condition due to lack of sufficient food material essential to the body, such as in starvation or malabsorption syndrome.

ETIOL: It may be due to causes other than the food supply, such as malabsorption, or other disease of the gastrointestinal system that prevents absorption of food.

inappetence (ĭn-ăp'ĕ-tĕns) [" + *appetere,* to long for]. Lack of craving or desire, esp. for food.

Inapsine. Trade name for droperidol.

inarticulate [" + *articulus,* joined]. 1. Not jointed; without joints. 2. Unable to pronounce distinct syllables or express oneself intelligibly. 3. Not given to expressing oneself verbally.

in articulo mortis (ĭn ăr-tĭk'ū-lō mor'tĭs) [L.]. At the very moment of death.

...similable (ĭn"ă-sĭm'ĭ-lă-bl) [" + *assimi-* ... make similar]. Not capable of being ... the body for nutrition.

inborn. 1. Innate or inherent, said of characteristics both structural and functional that are inherited or developed during intrauterine development. 2. Inherited, as in inborn error of metabolism.

inbreeding [" + AS. *bredan,* to cherish]. Mating of individuals that are closely related.

incandescent [L. *incandescere,* to glow]. Glowing with light; white hot.

incaparina. A mixture of cereal grains and oilseed meals of a given range of protein and quality fortified with vitamins and minerals. Developed at INCAP (Institute of Nutrition of Central America and Panama). Distributed in Latin America countries for feeding young children in order to prevent kwashiorkor, q.v., and other forms of malnutrition.

incarcerated [L. *incarcerare*]. Imprisoned, confined, constricted, as an irreducible hernia.

incarceration. 1. Legal confinement. 2. Imprisonment of a part; constriction as in a hernia.

incarial bone (ĭn-kā'rē-ăl). Os incae; interparietal bone.

incarnatio (ĭn"kăr-nā'shē-ō). 1. To grow in. 2. The process of being converted to flesh.

i. unguis. The ingrowing of a toenail or fingernail.

incasement. To become surrounded by a structure or wall.

incentive spirometry. Spirometry, q.v., in which visual and vocal stimuli are given to the subject in an attempt to stimulate the maximum effort in performing the test.

inception [L. *inceptio,* taking in, beginning]. 1. The beginning of anything. 2. Ingestion. 3. Intussusception.

incest (ĭn'sĕst) [L. *incestus,* unchaste, incest]. Coitus between those of near relationship. The persons are usually so closely related that a legal marriage would not be possible.

incidence [L. *incidens,* falling upon]. 1. The frequency of occurrence of any event or condition over a period of time and in relation to the population in which it occurs, as incidence of a disease. SEE: *prevalence.* 2. The falling or impinging upon, touching, or affecting in some way.

incident. 1. A happening, event, or occurrence. 2. Apt to happen, esp. in connection with some other event. 3. Falling or striking, as a ray of light.

incineration (ĭn-sĭn"ĕr-ā'shŭn) [L. *in,* into, + *cineres,* ashes]. Destruction by fire. SYN: *cremation.*

incipient (ĭn-sĭp'ē-ĕnt) [L. *incipere,* to begin]. Beginning; coming into existence.

incisal (ĭn-sī'zăl). Cutting.

incise (ĭn-sīz') [L. *incisus*]. To cut, as with a sharp instrument.

incised (ĭn-sīzd′). Cut with a knife.

incision (ĭn-sĭzh′ŭn) [L. *incisio*]. A cut made with a knife, esp. for surgical purposes.

incisive (ĭn-sī′sĭv) [L. *incisivus*]. 1. Cutting; having the power of cutting. 2. Rel. to the incisor teeth.

incisive bone. An obsolete term for the part of the maxilla that supports the incisor teeth and was derived from the median nasal process embryologically; commonly called the premaxilla.

incisor (ĭn-sī′zor) [L., a cutter]. 1. That which cuts. 2. That which applies to the incisor teeth. 3. One of the cutting teeth. The four front teeth in each jaw of the adult. SEE: *dentition.*

i., prostatic. Surgical knife for incision of an enlarged prostate.

incisura (ĭn-sī-sū′ră) [L.]. (pl. *incisurae*]. 1. An incision. 2. [NA] Incisure; notch; emargination; indentation at the edge of any structure.

incisure (ĭn-sĭz′ūr) [L. *incisura,* a cutting into]. A notch or slit.

i. of Rivinus. Tympanic incisure.

i.'s of Schmidt and Lantermann. Oblique lines on medullated nerve fiber sheaths.

inclination [L. *inclinere,* to slope]. Leaning from the normal, or from the vertical, as a tooth, or the pelvis.

inclinometer (ĭn″klĭ-nŏm′ĕ-ter) [″ + Gr. *metron,* measure]. Device for measuring ocular diameter from vertical and horizontal lines.

inclusion [L. *inclusus,* enclosed]. Being enclosed or included.

i., cell. Lifeless, temporary constituent of the protoplasm of a cell. SEE: *cell.*

i., dental. Inclusion of a tooth due to surrounding bone.

i., fetal. Malformed twins in which one, the parasite, is completely enclosed within its host, the autosite. SEE: *teratoma.*

inclusion blennorrhea. Inclusion conjunctivitis, q.v., of the newborn.

inclusion bodies. Bodies present in the nucleus of cytoplasm of certain cells in cases of infection by filtrable viruses. SEE: *Negri bodies.*

inclusion conjunctivitis. Inflammation of the conjunctiva of the eye due to the organism Chlamydia trachomatis. SYN: *swimming pool conjunctivitis.*

incoagulability (ĭn″kō-ăg″ū-lă-bĭl′ĭ-tē) [L. *in-,* not, + *coagulare,* to congeal]. Not coagulable.

incoercible (ĭn″kō-ĕr′sĭ-bl) [L. *in-,* not, + *coercere,* to restrain]. Uncontrollable; not able to be held in check.

incoherence (ĭn″kō-hēr′ĕns) [″ + *cohairens,* adhering]. Inability to express oneself coherently, or to present ideas in a related order.

incoherent (ĭn″kō-hē′rĕnt). Not coherent or understandable.

incombustible [″ + *combustus,* burned]. Incapable of being burned.

incompatibility [L. *incompatibilis*]. 1. The quality of not being suitable for mixture. Can be applied to a state that renders admixture of medicines unsuitable through chemical action or interaction, insolubility, formation of poisonous or explosive compounds, difference in solubility, or antagonistic action. The quality of not being mixed without chemical changes, or without countering the action of other ingredients in a compound. 2. Condition of not being in harmony with one's surroundings or associates, esp. a spouse or friend.

i., physiological. A condition in which one or more substances in a mixture have a physiological action antagonistic to that of one of the other compounds.

incompatible. 1. Not capable of uniting. 2. Antagonistic in action, said of some drugs. 3. Not being in harmony with one's environment, situation, or associates, esp. a spouse or friend.

incompetence, incompetency [L. *in-,* not, + *competere,* to be suitable]. Inadequate ability to perform the function or action normal to an organ or part.

i., aortic. Regurgitation of blood through the aortic valves.

i., ileocecal. Inability of ileocecal valve to stop the return of the material from the colon to the ileum.

i., mental. Mental inability to retain charge of one's self or possessions.

i., muscular. Imperfect closure of the cardiac valve due to weak action of papillary muscles.

i., pyloric. Weakness of pylorus, which permits undigested food to leave the stomach and enter the duodenum.

i., relative. Excessive dilatation of a cardiac cavity, which makes perfect closure of the cardiac valves leading in and out of the chamber impossible.

i., valvular. Leaky condition of one or more cardiac valves permitting regurgitation of blood at the time the valves should be completely closed.

incompetent. 1. One legally unable to execute a contract, such as a brain-damaged individual, or one with marked mental retardation or insanity. 2. Incapable.

incompetent palatal syndrome [...]omplete or ineffective separation b[...] palate of the nasopharynx from [...]ynx, characterized by hypernas[...] tortion of speech called rhino[...]

ETIOL: May be due to c[...]quired defects of the palat[...] disorders.

incompressible [″ + *compressus,* pressed together]. Compact; not compressible.

incontinence [″ + *continere,* to stop]. 1. Inability to retain urine, semen, or feces, through loss of sphincter control or because of cerebral or spinal lesions. 2. Absence of restraint with respect to sexual activity. SEE: *continence.*

i., active. Discharge of feces and urine in the normal way at regulated intervals but involuntarily.

i., anal. Failure of the anal sphincter to prevent involuntary expulsion of gas, liquid, or solids from the lower bowel.

i., giggle. The occurrence of involuntary uncontrollable passage of urine induced by laughter. Laughter triggers full-scale micturition that cannot be stopped, often until the bladder is empty, even if the laughter stops. It starts at about five to seven years and tends to improve or disappear with increasing age. This condition, which may be due to a central nervous system disease, is distinct from urinary stress incontinence. SEE: *i., urinary stress.*

i., intermittent. Loss of control of the bladder upon sudden pressure or movement, because of interruption of the voluntary path above the lumbar center.

i. of milk. Excessive milk flow. SYN: *galactorrhea.*

i. of urine. Inability to control urination. Sphincter muscle always relaxed. SEE: *enuresis.*

i., overflow. Incontinence characterized by small frequent voidings.

i., paralytic. Constant voiding of small amount of urine and feces due to defective nervous control of sphincters.

i., passive. Urinary incontinence of a form in which there is a full bladder that doesn't empty normally but urine drips away upon pressure.

i., urinary stress. Inability to prevent escape of urine during stress such as laughing, coughing, sneezing, lifting, or sudden movement. Occurs frequently enough in young women to be classed as normal. Nevertheless, it should be investigated to be certain it is not caused by a structural abnormality. The urine should be cultured to rule out urinary tract infection. SEE: *bladder drill; i., giggle.*

incoordinate [L. *in-,* not, + *coordinare,* to arrange]. 1. Not able to make coordinated muscular movements. 2. Unable to adjust one's work harmoniously with others.

incoordination (ĭn″kō-or″dĭ-nā′shŭn). Inability to produce harmonious, rhythmic, mus[illegible]ular action, but not due to weakness.

[illegible]OL: The condition may be sensory, due [illegible] of afferent impulses to be transmitted from muscles, bones, and joints to coordination centers, or it may be motor, due to disturbance in tone or harmony between simultaneously acting muscle groups. SYN: *asynergy.* SEE: *disdiadochokinesia.*

incorporation [L. *in,* into, + *corporare,* to form into a body]. Combining two ingredients to form a homogenous mass.

increment (ĭn′krĕ-mĕnt) [L. *incrementum*]. 1. An increase or addition in number, size, or extent; an enlargement. 2. To increase or add to. 3. Something added or gained.

incretogenous (ĭn″krē-tŏj′ĕ-nŭs) [L. *in,* into, + *secernere,* to secrete, + Gr. *gennan,* to produce]. Pert. to the internal secretions.

incrustation [L. *in,* on, + *crusta,* crust]. Formation of crusts or scabs.

incubation (ĭn″kū-bā′shŭn) [L. *incubare,* to lie on]. 1. The interval between exposure to infection and the appearance of the first symptom. SYN: *latent period* (def. 2). SEE: table. 2. In bacteriology, the period of culture development. 3. The development of an impregnated ovum. 4. The care of a premature infant in an incubator.

incubator. 1. Enclosed crib, in which the temperature and humidity may be regulated, for caring for premature babies. 2. Apparatus for providing suitable atmospheric conditions for culturing bacteria or for maintaining eggs until they hatch.

incubus (ĭn′kū-bŭs) [L. *incubare,* to lie upon]. A nightmare.

incudal (ĭng′kū-dăl) [L. *incus,* anvil]. Rel. to the incus.

incudectomy (ĭng″kū-dĕk′tō-mē) [″ + Gr. *ektome,* excision]. Surgical removal of the incus.

incudiform (ĭn-kū′dĭ-form) [″ + *forma,* shape]. Like an anvil in shape.

incudomalleal (ĭng″kū-dō-măl′ē-ăl) [″ + *malleus,* a hammer]. Pert. to the incus and malleus and articulation of the anvil and hammer in the tympanum; in the middle ear.

incudostapedial (ĭn″kū-dō-stă-pē′dē-ăl) [″ + *stapes,* a stirrup]. Pert. to the incus and stapes and the articulation between the anvil and stirrup in the tympanum; in the middle ear.

incurable [L. *in-,* not, + *curare,* to care for]. Not capable of being cured.

incurvation (ĭn″kŭr-vā′shŭn) [L. *incurvare,* to bend in]. To be bent or curved in.

incus (ĭng′kŭs) [L., anvil]. (pl. *incudes*) [NA] In the middle ear, the middle of the three ossicles in the tympanum; the anvil. SEE: *ear* for illus.

incyclophoria (ĭn-sī″klō-for′ē-ă) [L. *in-,* not, + Gr. *kyklos,* circle, + *phoros,* bearing]. Median or negative cyclophoria; the affected eye, when covered, turns inward about its

Incubation and Isolation Periods in Common Infections

	Incubation Period	Isolation of Patient
Brucellosis	Usually 5 to 21 days	None
Chickenpox	2 to 3 weeks	1 week after appearance of vesicles
Common cold	12 hours to 3 days	None
Diphtheria	Usually 2 to 5 days	Until two cultures taken at least 24 hours apart from nose and throat are negative. Cultures to be taken after cessation of antibiotic therapy.
Dysentery, amebic	5 days to 4 weeks	None
Dysentery, bacillary (shigellosis)	1 to 7 days	As long as stools remain positive
Encephalitis, mosquito-borne	7 to 14 days	None
Gonorrhea	3 to 9 days	No sexual contact until cured
Influenza	1 to 3 days	As practical
Malaria	Usually 2 weeks	Protected from mosquitoes
Measles (rubeola)	8 to 13 days	From diagnosis to 7 days after appearance of rash. Strict isolation from children under 3 years
Meningitis, meningococcal	2 to 10 days	Until 24 hours after start of chemotherapy
Mumps	12 to 26 days	Until the glands recede
Paratyphoid fevers	1 to 10 days	Until three stools are negative
Pneumonia, pneumococcal	Believed to be 1 to 3 days	Until 24 hours after administration of antibiotics
Poliomyelitis	3 to 21 days	1 week from onset
Puerperal fever, streptococcal	1 to 3 days	Transfer from maternity ward
Rabies	Usually 2 to 6 weeks	Strict for duration of illness; danger to attendants
Rubella (German measles)	14 to 21 days	None, but avoid contact with nonimmune pregnant women
Salmonellosis	6 to 72 hours, usually 12 to 36	Until stool cultures are salmonella-free on two consecutive specimens collected not less than 24 hours apart
Scarlet fever	1 to 3 days	7 days; may be terminated in 24 hours

Incubation and Isolation Periods in Common Infections *(Continued)*

	Incubation Period	Isolation of Patient
Smallpox	8 to 17 days	Strict; in screened hospital wards until all scabs have disappeared
Syphilis	2 days to 10 weeks, usually 3 weeks	In noncooperative patients, it should be enforced until surface lesions are healed
Tetanus	4 days to 3 weeks	None
Trachoma	5 to 12 days	Until lesions disappear, but usually not practical
Tuberculosis	4 to 6 weeks to primary lesion	Variable depending upon conversion of sputum to negative after specific therapy and upon ability of patient to understand and carry out personal hygiene methods
Tularemia	1 to 10 days	None
Typhoid fever	Usually 1 to 3 weeks	Until three cultures of feces and urine are negative. These should be taken not earlier than 1 month after onset
Typhus fever	7 to 14 days	None
Whooping cough	Usually a week	For 3 weeks after onset of spasmodic cough

anteroposterior axis.

incyclotropia (ĭn-sī″klō-trō′pē-ă) [″ + ″ + *tropos,* turning]. Cyclotropia in which the eye turns inward toward the nose even when both eyes are open.

in d. L. *in dies,* daily.

indagation (ĭn″dă-gā′shŭn) [L. *indagatus,* searching]. A careful, searching investigation, esp. examination of the genitalia at termination of puerperium.

indecision. Inability to make up one's mind.

indentation [L. *in,* in, + *dens,* tooth]. A depression or hollow.

independent living skills. Activities of daily living, q.v.

index (ĭn′dĕks) [L., an indicator]. (pl. *indexes* or *indices*) 1. The forefinger. 2. The ratio of the measurement of a given substance with that of a fixed standard.

i., alveolar. I., gnathic.

i., cephalic. Skull breadth multiplied by 100 and divided by its length.

i., cerebral. Ratio of greatest transverse to the greatest anteroposterior diameter of the cranium.

i., D.M.F. An index of dental health and caries experience based on the number of DMF teeth or tooth surfaces where D is the number of decayed tooth surfaces, M is missing teeth, and F is filled or restored tooth surfaces.

i., gnathic. Degree of jaw prominence expressed by a number.

i., leucopenic. In allergic individuals, a test of sensitivity to foods. The drop of more than 1000 in white blood cell count in 90 minutes following ingestion of the test food indicates the food is incompatible with that individual.

i., opsonic. The ratio of number of bacteria that are ingested by leukocytes contained in normal serum, compared with the number ingested by leukocytes in the patient's own blood serum.

i., oral hygiene. An index based on the presence and amount of debris and calculus on six preselected tooth surfaces.

i., pelvic. Ratio of pelvic conjugate and transverse diameters.

i., periodontal (Ramfjord). An extensive consideration of the periodontal status of six teeth by evaluating gingival condition, depth of gingival sulcus or pocket, plaque or calculus, attrition, tooth mobility, and extent of tooth contact.

i., phagocytic. Average of bacteria ingested per leukocyte of blood.

i., refractive. Refraction coefficient.

i., therapeutic. The maximum tolerated dose of a drug divided by the minimum curative dose.

i., thoracic. Ratio of thoracic anteroposterior diameter to transverse diameter.

i., vital. The ratio of the number of births to the number of deaths in a population over a stated period of time.

index case. The initial individual whose condition led to investigation of a hereditary disorder.

indican (ĭn′dĭ-kăn). Potassium salt of indoxylsulfate, found in sweat and urine, and formed when intestinal bacteria convert tryptophan to indole.

indicanemia (ĭn″dĭ-kăn-ē′mē-ă) [*indican* + Gr. *haima,* blood]. Indican in the blood.

indicant (ĭn′dĭ-kănt). 1. Something such as a sign or symptom that points to the presence of a disease. 2. Something such as loss of a symptom or sign that indicates the treatment of the disease is proper and effective.

indicanuria (ĭn″dĭ-kăn-ū′rē-ă) [″ + Gr. *ouron,* urine]. Excess of indoxylsulfate of potassium, a derivative of indole, in urine. It is found in small quantities in normal urine. SYN: *urocyanosis.*

indication [L. *indicare,* to point out]. A sign or circumstance that indicates the proper treatment of a disease.

i., causal. Treatment shown by a knowledge of the cause of a disease.

i., symptomatic. Treatment shown by symptoms of a disease.

indicator [L. *indicare,* to show]. In chemical analysis, a substance that can be used to determine pH. In a more general sense, any substance that can be used to determine the completeness of a chemical reaction, as in volumetric analysis. SEE: table.

USES: 1. In titration of ammonia and other weak bases. 2. Topfer's reagent, for determining free acid in gastric juice. 3. In titrating weak acids and for determining combined acid in gastric juice.

indifferent [L. *in-,* not, + *differre,* to differ]. 1. Neutral; tending in no specific direction. 2. Not responsive to normal stimuli; apathetic. 3. Pert. to cells that have not differentiated.

indigenous (ĭn-dĭj′ĕn-ŭs) [L. *indigenus,* born in]. Native to a country or region.

indigestible (ĭn″dĭ-jĕs′tĭ-bl) [L. *in-,* not, + *digerere,* to separate]. Not digestible.

indigestion [″ + *digerere,* to separate]. Incomplete or imperfect digestion, usually accompanied by one or more of the following symptoms: pain, nausea and vomiting, heartburn and acid regurgitation, accumulation of gas and belching. SYN: *dyspepsia.*

Colors of Indicators

	Color		
	Toward Acid	Toward Alkali	Range of pH
Methyl yellow	red	yellow	2.9–4.0
Congo red	blue	red	3.0–5.2
Methyl orange	red	yellow	3.1–4.4
Methyl red	red	yellow	4.2–6.2
Litmus	red	blue	4.5–8.3
Bromcresol purple	yellow	purple	5.2–6.8
Bromothymol blue	yellow	blue	6.0–7.6
Phenol red	yellow	red	6.8–8.4
Phenolphthalein	colorless	pink	8.2–10.0

indigitation (ĭn-dĭj″ĭ-tā′shŭn) [L. *in,* in, + *digitus,* finger]. Displacement of intestines by intussusception, q.v. SYN: *invagination.*

indigo. A blue dye obtained from plants or made synthetically.

Indigo Carmine. Trade name for indigotindisulfonate, USP.

indigotindisulfonate sodium (ĭn″dĭ-gō″tĭn-dī-sŭl′fō-nāt). USP. A dye used in testing renal function. Trade name is Indigo Carmine.

indigouria (ĭn″dĭ-gō-ū′rē-ă) [Gr. *indikon,* Indian dye, + *ouron,* urine]. Indigo in the urine.

indisposition [L. *in-,* not, + *dispositus,* arranged]. Disorder; any slight or temporary illness.

indium (ĭn′dē-ŭm) [L. *indicum,* indigo]. SYMB: In. At. wt. 114.82; at. no. 49; sp. gr. 7.31. A rare metallic element.

indium chlorides in 113m injection. USP. A radioactive isotope of indium, ^{113m}In, in a sterile aqueous solution suitable for intravenous administration. The half-life is 99.5 minutes.

individuation (ĭn″dĭ-vĭd′ū-ā′shŭn). During development, the emergence of specific and individual structures and functions.

Indocin. Trade name for indomethacin.

indocyanine green. USP. A dye used in testing hepatic and renal function. Trade name is Cardio Green.

indolaceturia (ĭn″dō-lăs″ē-tū′rē-ă) [*indole* + L. *acetum,* vinegar, + Gr. *ouron,* urine]. Excretion of a considerable amount of indoleacetic acid in the urine.

indole (ĭn′dōl). C_8H_7N. A solid, crystalline substance found in feces. It is the product of bacterial decomposition of tryptophan and is largely responsible for the odor of feces. In intestinal obstruction it is absorbed and eliminated in the urine in the form of indican, q.v.

indolent (ĭn'dō-lĕnt) [LL. *indolens*, painless]. 1. Indisposed to action. 2. Inactive; not developing; sluggish.

indolent ulcer. Ulcer that is slow to heal but not painful.

indologenous (ĭn"dō-lŏj'ĕn-ŭs) [*indole* + Gr. *gennan*, to produce]. Causing the production of indole.

indoluria (ĭn"dŏl-ū'rē-ă) [" + Gr. *ouron*, urine]. The presence of indole in urine.

indomethacin (ĭn"dō-mĕth'ă-sĭn). USP. Drug that has anti-inflammatory, analgesic, and antipyretic properties. Primary use is in rheumatoid arthritis, ankylosing spondylitis, and degenerative joint disease when salicylates are ineffective or can't be tolerated. Because of the high incidence and severity of side effects associated with prolonged administration, its use as a mild antipyretic or analgesic is not recommended. Has also been used in treating attacks of arthritis due to gout and as an antipyretic in Hodgkin's disease when fever fails to respond to other therapy. Trade name is Indocin.

indoxyl (ĭn-dŏk'sĭl) [Gr. *indikon*, indigo, + *oxys*, sharp]. C_8H_7NO. An oily substance sometimes found in urine of the apparently healthy, formed from the decomposition of tryptophan by intestinal bacteria.

indoxylemia (ĭn-dŏk"sĭl-ē'mē-ă) [" + " + *haima*, blood]. Indoxyl in the blood.

indoxyluria (ĭn"dŏk-sĭl-ū'rē-ă) [" + " + *ouron*, urine]. Excretion of indoxyl in urine.

induced (ĭn-dūsd') [L. *inducere*, to lead in]. Produced; caused.

inducer (ĭn-dūs'ĕr). A compound that increases the concentration of another molecule or the metabolic rate. In higher animals, these are usually hormones.

inductance. That property of an electric circuit by virtue of which a varying current induces an electromotive force in that circuit or a neighboring circuit. The unit of inductance, or self-induction, is the henry.

induction (ĭn-dŭk'shŭn) [L. *inductio*, leading in]. 1. The process of causing or producing, as induction of labor with oxytocic drugs in cases of uterine dysfunction. 2. The generation of electric current in a body by electricity in another body near it. 3. In embryology, the production of a specific morphogenic effect by a chemical substance from one part of the embryo to another. SYN: *evocation*. 4. In anesthesia, the period from the initial inhalation or injection of an anesthetic gas or drug until optimum level of anesthesia is reached.

inductor (ĭn-dŭk'tĕr). Any substance that will cause cells exposed to it to differentiate into an organized tissue.

inductorium (ĭn"dŭk-tō'rē-ŭm). Device used to produce high-voltage electrical discharges. It is used in physiological investigations.

inductotherm (ĭn-dŭk'tō-thĕrm) [L. *inducere*, to lead, + Gr. *therme*, heat]. Device for producing pyrexia by electricity.

inductothermy. Treatment of disease by artificial production of fever by electromagnetic induction.

indulin (ĭn'dū-lĭn). Any one of a group of dyes used in histology.

indulinophil(e) (ĭn"dū-lĭn'ō-fĭl, -fīl). The state of being readily stained with indulin.

indurate (ĭn'dū-rāt) [L. *in*, in, + *durus*, hard]. 1. To harden. 2. Hardened.

indurated. Hardened.

induration. 1. The act of hardening. 2. An area of hardened tissue. SEE: *sclerosis; skin*.

i., black. Anthracosis of the lung.

i., brown. Pigmentation and fibrosis of the lung due to chronic venous congestion of the lung.

i., cyanotic. An induration from long continued venous hyperemia, pressure on vessels causing transudation of blood and serum, and formation of a dark, hard mass. In the liver or spleen it leads to absorption of the parenchyma with formation of scar tissue.

i., fibrous, of the lung. A form of interstitial pneumonia in which hardened pigment forms red points on the lung.

i., granular. Fibrosis of an organ such as the liver or kidney so that small fibrotic granules are present.

i., gray. Pneumonia with fibrosis and no pigmentation.

i., red. Chronic interstitial pneumonia with severe congestion.

indurative (ĭn'dūr-ā"tĭv). Pert. to induration.

indusium (ĭn-dū'zē-ŭm) [L., tunic]. 1. A membranous covering. 2. The amnion.

i. griseum. [NA] A rudimentary gyrus located on the upper surface of the corpus callosum. SYN: *gyrus, supracallosal*.

inebriant (ĭn-ē'brē-ănt) [L. *inebrius*, drunken]. 1. Any intoxicant. 2. Making drunk.

inebriate. To make drunk or to become intoxicated.

inebriation (ĭn-ē"brē-ā'shŭn). State of intoxication. SYN: *drunkenness; intoxication*.

inelastic [L. *in-*, not, + Gr. *elastikos*, elastic]. Not elastic.

inert (ĭn-ĕrt') [L. *iners*, unskilled, idle]. 1. Not active; sluggish. 2. In chemistry, having little or no tendency or ability to react with other chemicals.

inertia (ĭn-ĕr'shē-ă) [L., inactivity]. 1. In physics, tendency of a body to remain in its state (at rest or in motion) until acted upon by an outside force. 2. Sluggishness; lack of activity.

i., uterine. Absence or weakness of uterine contractions in labor.

in extremis (ĭn ĕks-trē'mĭs) [L.]. At the point of death.

infant [L. *infans*]. A liveborn fetus from time of birth through the completion of one year of age. SEE: *neonate.*

i., development of. For three days after birth a baby loses weight; in the next four days, however, a baby should regain the loss and weigh as much as at birth.

Average weekly weight gain in the first three months is 210 gm. for boys and 195 gm. for girls; from three to six months it is 150 gm. for both girls and boys; from six to nine months, 90 gm. for boys and 105 gm. for girls; from 9 to 18 months 60 gm. for both sexes; and from 18 to 24 months 45 gm., both sexes.

The newborn is aware of shadow, movement, and voice. By the fourth week the infant lifts the head momentarily; by the 16th week, holds the head erect, coos, or laughs; walks with hands held by 52nd week; by 15th month, toddles alone and may have a vocabulary of a few words. SEE: *psychomotor and physical development of infant.*

i., post-term. Infant born after beginning of the 42nd week of gestation (longer than 288 days).

i., preterm. Infant born prior to the completion of 37 weeks (259 days) of gestation. SEE: *prematurity.*

i., respiration of. At birth, 40 to 50 per min.; first year, 20 to 40; fifth year, 20 to 25; 15th year, 15 to 20. SEE: *pulse; respiration; temperature.*

i., temperature of. Normal (rectal) temperature may have a daily variation of 1 to 1.5° C. (1.8 to 2.7° F.) It is usually highest between 5 and 8 p.m. and lowest between 3 and 6 a.m. There is therefore no specific normal temperature, but the values given should be regarded as ranging around the value of 37.6° C. (99.7° F.) when the temperature is taken rectally.

Infants have poorly developed temperature-regulating mechanisms, and need to be protected from chills and overheating.

i., term. Infant born between the beginning of the 38th week through the 41st week of gestation (260 to 287 days).

infanticide (ĭn-făn'tĭ-sīd). [LL. *infanticidium*]. The killing of an infant.

infantile (ĭn'făn-tīl) [Fr. *infantilis*]. Pert. to infancy or an infant.

infantilism (ĭn-făn'tĭl-ĭzm, ĭn"făn-tĭl-ĭzm') [" + Gr. *-ismos,* condition]. 1. A condition in which the mind and body make slow development and the individual fails to attain adult characteristics. Characterized by mental retardation, stunted growth, and sexual immaturity. 2. Childishness.

i., angioplastic. Infantilism due to defective development of vascular system.

i., Brissaud's. Cretinism.

i., cachectic. Infantilism caused by chronic infection or poisoning.

i., celiac. Infantilism caused by celiac disease. SEE: *i., Herter's.*

i., dysthyroidal. Infantilism caused by a defective thyroid.

i., hepatic. Infantilism combined with cirrhosis of the liver.

i., Herter's. Infantilism of the intestines.

i., hypophyseal. Dwarfism resulting from hyposecretion of the growth-promoting hormone and gonadotrophic hormone of the anterior lobe of the hypophysis. SYN: *i., pituitary.*

i., idiopathic. Variety of arrested physical development of unknown cause.

i., intestinal. Infantilism associated with chronic intestinal disorder, causing poor growth.

i., lymphatic. A form of infantilism associated with lymphatism.

i., myxedematous. Cretinism. SYN: *i., Brissaud's.*

i., partial. Arrest in development of a lone tissue or part.

i., pituitary. I., hypophyseal.

i., renal. Infantilism caused by a defect in renal function.

i., sex. Continuation of childish traits, esp. sex characteristics, beyond the age of puberty.

i., symptomatic. Infantilism caused by poor tissue development.

i., universal. Infantilism marked by dwarfed stature and absence of secondary sexual characteristics.

infarct [L. *infarctus*]. An area of tissue in an organ or part that undergoes necrosis following cessation of blood supply. May result from occlusion or stenosis of the supplying artery or more rarely from occlusion of the vein that drains the tissue.

i., anemic. Infarct in which blood pigment is lacking or decoloration had occurred. SYN: *i., pale; i., white.*

i., bland. Infarct in which infection is absent.

i., calcareous. Infarct in connective tissue in which calcareous salts have been deposited.

i., cicatrized. Infarct that has been replaced or encapsulated by fibrous tissue.

i., hemorrhagic. I., red.

i., infected. Infarcted tissue that has been invaded by pathogenic organisms.

i., pale. I., anemic.

i., red. An infarct that is swollen and red as a result of hemorrhage. SYN: *i., hemor-*

rhagic.

i., septic. I., infected, q.v.

i., uric acid. Infarct in kidney due to obstruction of renal tubules by uric acid crystals.

i., white. I., anemic.

infarction. 1. Formation of an infarct. 2. An infarct.

i., cardiac. Myocardial infarction.

i., cerebral. An infarct in the brain due to failure of blood supply to the area.

i., myocardial. Infarction in cardiac muscle, usually resulting from formation of a thrombus in the coronary arterial system.

The immediate therapeutic need involves assuring the patient that comprehensive care will be given; and at the same time instituting whatever needs to be done to put the patient at rest and to arrange for immediate transport to a hospital, doctor's office or any place where appropriate therapy may be provided. Because the majority of deaths occur in the first several hours following infarction, it is essential that treatment not be delayed.

i., pulmonary. Infarction in the lung usually resulting from pulmonary embolism.

Immediate therapy includes control of pain, oxygen administered continuously by mask, and treatment of the circulatory collapse (shock) if present.

infect [ME. *infecten*]. To cause pathogenic organisms to be present in or upon, as to infect a wound.

infection (ĭn-fĕk'shŭn). The state or condition in which the body or a part of it is invaded by a pathogenic agent (microorganism or virus) that, under favorable conditions, multiplies and produces effects that are injurious. Localized infection is usually accompanied by inflammation, but inflammation may occur without infection. SEE: tables.

ETIOL: The principal causes of infections are agents belonging to the following groups of microorganisms: viruses, bacteria, rickettsiae, fungi, and animal parasites.

SYM: The symptoms of infection are those of inflammation. The five classical symptoms listed by early medical writers are dolor (pain), calor (heat), rubor (redness), tumor (swelling), and functio laesa (disordered function).

Pain: This is esp. prominent when the infection is confined within closed cavities, causing pressure. The pain is in proportion to the virulence and extent of the infection. Pain associated with intra-abdominal infection often is due to contact of infected organs with peritoneum. *Redness and swelling:* Not evident when infection is within some rigid tissue or deep within some cavity; more apparent when superficial structures are involved. Discoloration would be a better term than redness, as the color is more bluish or purple in advanced infections, while tuberculosis infections have long been called white swellings. *Heat:* May not be evident on the surface, but there may be considerable elevation of body temperature even with minor infections.

Disordered function: This depends upon the part affected as well as upon the virulence. With almost all acute infections there is an increase of polymorphonuclear leukocytes either absolute or relative. The degree of prostration may be out of proportion to the extent of the injury or apparent infection. There have been many deaths from infection following pricks of needles, small splinters of bone, a trifling cut, or an infection from the bristle of a brush, in which streptococci were the inciting cause. In this type of infection, a red streak may be seen extending up the extremity from the site of injury and following the superficial lymphatics. This red line is absent in staphylococcal infections of the lymphatic vessels.

SITE: Infection may be local or general. Local infections may be at the portal of entry or remote if transferred by the blood or lymph. Microorganisms may gain entry to the tissues through the gastrointestinal tract as in typhoid fever, through the respiratory tract as in tuberculosis and common colds, through wounds as in rabies, from contaminated objects as in tetanus, or from bites of insects as in malaria and yellow fever.

Some medicines, but esp. adrenal cortical hormones and certain antibiotics, upset either the immune mechanism or the bacterial interrelations so that the growth of certain microorganisms is encouraged. The resulting superinfection may be quite difficult to control and may be so severe as to cause death. Cortisone therapy encourages the recurrence or resurgence of previous lesions of tuberculosis.

METHODS: *Airborne:* Pathogenic organisms in the respiratory tract discharged from the mouth or nose may be borne on the air and settle on food, clothing, walls, and floors. If they are of the type that resists drying for a long period, as would be the case with infections due to spore-forming organisms, they may remain virulent until transmitted to another person. Coughing, sneezing, and expectorating may be responsible for droplet infection because bacteria are expelled into the air.

Animal carriers: Some microorganisms may be carried from an animal to man by direct contact, indirect transfer, or by intermediary hosts.

Contact: This is the result of transmission from person to person as in kissing, coming

Contagious Infections

Name	Period of Incubation	Time of Eruption	Duration of Eruption	Period of Quarantine or Isolation
Scarlet Fever	1–3 days	12–24 hr. after onset	7–10 days	7 days isolation
Smallpox	8–17 days	3rd or 4th day of fever	14–21 days	21 days or until all scabs disappear
Measles (Rubeola)	8–13 days	4th day of fever	4–6 days	Isolation from diagnosis until 7 days after appearance of rash. Strict isolation from children under 3 years
Rubella	14–21 days	2nd day of fever	1–3 days	None but avoid contact with nonimmune pregnant women
Mumps	12–26 days			Until all swellings have subsided
Whooping Cough	About a week			Isolation for 3 weeks after onset of spasmodic cough
Chickenpox	14–21 days	2nd day of fever	7–21 days	7 days after onset
Diphtheria	2–5 days			7 days and until 2 successive nose and throat cultures, 24 hr apart, are negative; to be taken after cessation of antibiotic therapy
Typhus Fever	7–14 days	3rd to 8th day of fever	14 days	None
Typhoid Fever	7–21 days	4th day of fever	3–5 days for each crop of spots	Release after 3 successive negative cultures of urine and feces not less than 24 hr. apart and not earlier than one month after onset

in contact with those afflicted with communicable diseases, or with utensils handled by one with an infection.

Food-borne: Bacteria may be carried on food. Root and salad vegetables may carry bacteria from the soil or from manure used as fertilizer. Cooking safeguards by destroying microorganisms on food; but improperly prepared canned foods may contain the Clostridium botulinus toxin that causes botulism.

Human carriers: Some parasites may live in or upon the bodies of persons who themselves do not suffer from them, but the parasites may be carried by them to others. Carriers may be contact carriers or those who never show symptoms; incubationary carriers or those in whom the infection is starting but has not completed the incubation period; and convalescent carriers or those who have recovered but who still harbor the organism causing their disease.

Insect vectors: An insect may act as a physical carrier, as the housefly, which may transmit the typhoid bacillus from one point to another, or one that acts as an active

Common Protozoal Infections

Disease	Primary Site of Infection	Parasite	Mode of Transmission
Malaria:			
Benign tertian		Plasmodium vivax	
Benign quartan	Erythrocytes	P. malariae	Mosquito (Anopheles)
Malignant tertian		P. falciparum	
Sleeping sickness	Blood plasma	Trypanosoma gambiense	Tsetse fly (Glossina palpalis)
Rhodesian sleeping sickness	Blood plasma	T. rhodesiense	Tsetse fly (Glossina morsitans)
Leishmaniasis, visceral (Kala-azar)	Reticuloendothelial cells and plasma	Leishmania donovani	Sandfly (Phlebotomus argentipes)
Amebic dysentery	Wall of large intestine	Entamoeba histolytica	Fecal (cyst) contamination of food and water

intermediate host, such as the Anopheles mosquito, which transmits malaria by injecting the causative agent into the host while biting that person or animal.

Prenatal: This is the result of the fetus being infected transplacentally or from contiguity with the maternal membranes.

Soil-borne: Soil-borne, spore-forming organisms commonly enter the body through wounds, as in tetanus and gas gangrene.

Water-borne: Organisms producing typhoid, dysentery, cholera, and amebic infections may be carried through a water supply or through water in public pools used for bathing. These organisms may pass into the water from the feces of an infected person and be communicated to others.

i., acute. An infection that appears suddenly and may be of brief or prolonged duration.

i., airborne. Infectious organisms that have been transported through the air.

i., apical. Infection located at the tip of the root of a tooth.

i., chronic. Infection having a protracted course.

i., concurrent. Existence of two or more infections at the same time. SEE: *superinfection.*

i., contagious. An infectious disease communicable by contact with an infected individual.

i., cross. Transfer of an infectious organism or disease from one patient in a hospital to another.

i., droplet. Infection acquired by inhalation of a microorganism in the air, esp. one added to the air by someone's breath or cough.

i., dustborne. Airborne infection in which the infectious organism is carried by dust.

i., endogenous. Infection caused by bacteria, normally nonpathogenic and inhabiting the digestive tract.

i., exogenous. An infection caused by organisms not present in the body.

i., fungus. Infection with a fungus.

i., local. Infection caused by germs lodging and multiplying at one point in a tissue and remaining there, as a boil.

i., low-grade. Loosely used term for a subacute or chronic infection with only mild inflammation and without pus formation.

i., metastatic. Local infection caused by microorganisms circulated from a focus of infection.

i., mixed. Infection caused by two or more organisms.

i., protozoal. Infection with a protozoon, e.g., malaria.

i., pyogenic. Infection resulting from pus-forming organisms.

i., secondary. Infection caused by a different organism than the one causing the primary infection.

i., simple. Infection due to a single species of organism.

i., subacute. An infection intermediate between acute and chronic.

i., subclinical. Infection that is immunologically confirmed but does not show clinical symptoms in the individual.

i., systemic. An infection wherein the infecting agent or organisms are throughout the body rather than restricted to a local area as in an abscess.

i., terminal. Infection occurring in the late stage of a disease. Generally acute and

Fungus Infections

Disease	Causative Organisms	Structures Infected	Microscopic Appearances
Ringworm (tinea, otomycosis)	Microsporum (audouini, etc.)	Horny layer of epidermis and hairs, chiefly of scalp	Fine septate mycelium inside hairs and scales; spores in rows and mosaic plaques on hair surface
	Trichophyton (tonsurans, etc.)	Hairs of scalp, beard, and other parts; nails	Mycelium of chained cubical elements and threads in and on hairs; often pigmented
Favus (tinea favosa)	Trichophyton schönleini	Yellow disks in epidermis around a hair; all parts of body; nails	Vertical hyphae and spores in epidermis; sinuous branching mycelium and chains in hairs
Epidermophytosis (dhobie itch, etc.)	Epidermophyton (inguinale, etc.)	Inflamed patches in inguinal, axillary, and interdigital folds; hairs not affected	Long, wavy, branched and segmented hyphae and spindle-shaped cells in stratum corneum
Systemic Infections			
Thrush and other forms of candidiasis	Candida albicans	White patches on tongue, mouth, throat; also may cause lesions of vagina and skin	Yeastlike budding cells and oval thick-walled bodies in lesion
Actinomycosis	Actinomyces bovis, A. israelii	Chronic, usually in neck	Branched filaments on radiating rods, forming colonies
Nocardiosis	Nocardia asteroides	Lower extremities or lung	Closely resemble bacteria; found in pus
Blastomycosis	Blastomyces brasiliensis, B. dermatitidis	Skin and lungs	Yeastlike cells demonstrated in lesion
Coccidioidomycosis	Coccidioides immitis	Respiratory tract	Nonbudding spores containing many endospores, in sputum
Cryptococcosis	Cryptococcus neoformans	Meninges; sometimes lungs	Yeastlike fungus having gelatinous capsule; demonstrated in spinal fluid

septic, usually causing death.

i., water-borne. Infection caused by organisms present in water.

infectious (ĭn-fĕk′shŭs) [ME. *infecten*, infect]. 1. Capable of being transmitted with or without contact. 2. Pert. to a disease due to a microorganism. 3. Producing infection.

infectious disease. Any disease caused by growth of pathogenic microorganisms in the body. May or may not be contagious. SEE: *quarantine; incubation* for Incubation and Isolation Periods in Common Infections table.

infectious mononucleosis. SEE: *mononucleosis, infectious.*

infecundity (ĭn-fē-kŭn′dĭ-tē) [L. *infecunditas*, sterility]. Barrenness; sterility in women.

inferior (ĭn-fē′rē-or) [L. *inferus*, below]. 1. Beneath; lower. 2. [NA] Used medically in reference to the undersurface of an organ or indicating a structure below another structure.

inferiority complex. In psychology, a repressed state of mind in which one feels oneself inferior to others. Such a group of ideas may be manifested by the assumption of superiority, often resulting in over-compensation. Opposite of superiority complex. SEE: *complex*.

infertility. Inability or diminished ability to produce offspring; unproductivity. Condition may be present in either or both sexual partners and is usually reversible. Diagnostic investigation includes special tests of both partners as well as a complete physical examination. Some factors responsible for infertility are immature or abnormal reproductive systems, anomalies of other organs in that vicinity, infections, endocrine dysfunction, and emotional problems.

i., secondary. Infertility in which there have been one or more pregnancies prior to the present condition of infertility.

infest [L. *infestare,* to attack]. To overrun to a harmful extent. Said esp. of parasites.

infestation. The harboring of animal parasites, esp. macroscopic forms such as ectoparasites and arthropod endoparasites.

infibulation (ĭn-fĭb-ū-lā'shŭn) [L. *in,* in, + *fibula,* clasp]. The process of fastening, as in joining the lips of wounds by clasps.

infiltrate (ĭn-fĭl'trāt, ĭn'fĭl-trāt) [" + *filtrare,* to strain through]. 1. To pass into or through a substance or a space. 2. The material that has infiltrated.

infiltration (ĭn"fĭl-trā'shŭn). The process of a substance passing into and being deposited within the substance of a cell, tissue, or organ.

Ex.: infiltration of a tissue or organ with blood corpuscles, or of a cell by fatty particles. Infiltration must not be confused with degeneration; in the latter condition the foreign substances are from changes within the cell.

i., adipose. I., fatty, q.v.

i., amyloid. Infiltration of tissue or viscera with a glycoprotein.

i., anesthesia. Injection of an anesthetic solution directly into the tissue. SEE: *anesthesia*.

i., calcareous. Deposits of calcium or magnesium salts within a tissue.

i., cellular. Infiltration of cells, esp. blood cells, into tissues; invasion by cells of malignant tumors into adjacent tissue.

i., fatty. Deposit of fat in the tissues, or oil or fat globules in the cells.

i., glycogenic. Glycogen deposit in cells.

i., lymphocytic. Infiltration of tissue by lymphocytes.

i., pigmentary. Infiltration of pigments.

i., purulent. Pus cells in a tissue.

i., serous. Infiltration with diluted lymph.

i., urinous. Infiltration with urine.

i., waxy. Amyloid degeneration.

infinite distance. 1. A distance without limits. 2. In vision, light rays coming from a point of any distance beyond 20 feet (6.1 meters) are practically parallel and accommodation is unnecessary.

infinity. 1. Condition of being infinite. 2. Space, time, or quantity without limits.

infirm [L. *infirmis*]. Weak or feeble, esp. from old age or disease.

infirmary [L. *infirmarium*]. A small hospital; a place for the care of sick or infirm persons.

infirmity. 1. Weakness. 2. A sickness or illness.

Inflamase. Trade name for prednisolone sodium phosphate, USP.

inflammation [L. *inflammare,* to flame within]. Tissue reaction to injury. The succession of changes that occur in living tissue when it is injured. The inflamed area undergoes continuous change as the body repair processes start to heal and replace injured tissue. Inflammation is a conservative process modified by whatever produces the reaction, but it should not be confused with infection; the two are relatively different conditions, although one may arise from the other. SEE: *infection*.

ETIOL: The reaction of tissue to injury may be the result of blows, foreign bodies, chemicals, electricity, heat or cold (thermic causes), microorganisms, surgery (traumatic causes), or ionizing radiation.

SYM: Pain (dolor), heat (calor), redness (rubor), swelling (tumor), and impaired or disordered function. Also headache, loss of appetite, and a general feeling of discomfort.

Pathological Changes: Vascular dilatation within 30 minutes of the injury and greatly increased blood flow. This may last for hours with exudation of fluid from blood vessels into tissues with concomitant swelling, migration of leukocytes into the tissues, and gelation of fibrinogen in intercellular spaces. Depending upon the severity of the injury, some red blood cells will escape into the tissue. If the injury is not too severe, these processes reach their maximum in six to eight hours, after which reparative processes begin to take place. Blood vessels return to normal size and normal blood flow is reestablished. Leukocytes degenerate or reenter circulation, cellular disintegration or proliferation occurs, in which injured cells are replaced, and swelling disappears with resorption of tissue fluid and digestion of fibrin.

The lymphatic system plays an active and important part in the healing of inflamed tissues.

Each type of cell has a particular role to

play in the inflammatory process. The monocytes and macrophages are scavengers for all kinds of dead tissue. The neutrophils or polymorphonuclear leukocytes are active in autolysis, q.v., and the destruction of bacteria. These cells appear in inflammatory conditions in a certain order; the macrophage, for instance, antedating the polymorph by a week. SEE: *macrophage; monocyte.*

Lymphocytes both large and small are present in inflamed and healing tissues. Lymphocytes, particularly, are important in systemic immune reactions.

NOMENCLATURE: Most words denoting inflammation end with the suffix *-itis,* which in itself pertains to inflammatory conditions. The principal inflammations of the various systems follow: *Ear:* otitis externa, interna, and media; mastoiditis. *Eye:* conjunctivitis; dacryocystitis; iritis; keratitis; optic neuritis; panophthalmitis; uveitis. *Gastrointestinal tract:* appendicitis; colitis; cholangitis; cholecystitis; duodenitis; enteritis; gastritis; hepatitis; Meckel's diverticulitis; pancreatitis; peritonitis; periproctitis; periodontitis; parotitis; proctitis. *Miscellaneous organs:* arthritis; carbuncle; dermatitis; furuncle; myositis; osteitis; osteomyelitis; periostitis; cellulitis; tendovaginitis. *Nervous system:* encephalitis; leptomeningitis; myelitis; neuritis; pachymeningitis; polyneuritis. *Respiratory system:* bronchitis; empyema; laryngitis; pharyngitis; pleurisy; pleuritis; pneumoconiosis; pneumonia; rhinitis. *Urinary system:* balanitis; cystitis; cervicitis; epididymitis; endometritis; myometritis; nephritis; oophoritis; pyelitis; prostatitis; perimetritis; parametritis; pyometra; pyosalpinx; orchitis; seminal vesiculitis; salpingitis; salpingo-oophoritis; urethritis. *Vascular system:* aortitis; endarteritis; endocarditis; epicarditis; lymphangitis; lymphadenitis; myocarditis; pericarditis.

i., acute. Inflammation in which the onset is rapid and the course relatively short.

i., adhesive. Inflammation characterized by opposing tissues or sides of a cavity adhering to each other.

i., bacterial. Inflammation induced by the growth of bacteria.

i., catarrhal. Inflammation of a mucous membrane characterized by the excessive secretion of mucus.

i., chronic. Inflammation that progresses slowly, is of long duration, and usually results in the formation of scar tissue.

i., exudative. Inflammation in which there is a large accumulation of blood cells and serum with vascular congestion.

i., fibrinous. Inflammation in which the exudate is rich in fibrin.

i., granulomatous. Inflammation with considerable production of granular tissue. Seen esp. in tuberculosis, syphilis, and in some fungal infections.

i., hemorrhagic. Inflammation in which red blood cells are conspicuous in the exudate.

i., hyperplastic. Inflammation characterized by excess production of young fibrous tissue.

i., interstitial. Inflammation involving principally the noncellular or supporting elements of an organ.

i., parenchymatous. Infection in which the glandular or epithelial tissues of an organ are principally affected.

i., productive. I., hyperplastic, q.v.

i., proliferative. I., hyperplastic, q.v.

i., pseudomembranous. Inflammation in which a pseudomembrane is formed. This is due to a toxin that necrotizes the tissues. This is seen in the oral, nasal, and respiratory tract tissues in diphtheria.

i., purulent. Inflammation in which pus is formed. SYN: *i., suppurative.*

i., reactive. Inflammation around a foreign body or dead tissue.

i., serous. Inflammation in which the exudate is composed principally of serum.

i., specific. Inflammation due to a specific organism.

i., subacute. The relatively mild inflammation that may become worse and then is severe or chronic.

i., suppurative. I., purulent.

i., toxic. Inflammation due to toxin or poison.

i., traumatic. Inflammation caused by injury.

i., ulcerative. Formation of an ulcer over an area of inflammation.

inflammatory [L. *inflammare,* to flame within]. Rel. to or marked by inflammation.

inflammatory response. The tissue and cellular changes that occur with inflammation; the hemodynamic and permeability changes and migration of leukocytes to an area of tissue injury that attempt to produce a localized protective action.

inflation (ĭn-flā′shŭn) [L. *in,* into, + *flare,* to blow]. Distention of a part by air, gas, or liquid.

inflator (ĭn-flā′tor). Device for forcing air into an organ. This may be done for diagnostic or therapeutic purposes.

inflection (ĭn″flĕk′shŭn) [″ + *flectere,* to bend]. 1. An inward bending. 2. Change of tone or pitch of the voice; nuance.

influenza (ĭn″flū-ĕn′ză) [It., influence]. An acute, contagious respiratory infection characterized by sudden onset, fever, chills, headache, myalgia, and sometimes prostration. Coryza, cough, and sore throat are common.

It is usually a self-limited disease that lasts from 2 to 7 days. SYN: *flu*. SEE: *cold*.

ETIOL: The causative agent is a virus of which several genera, A, B, and C, and subtypes, such as H_0N_1 (A_0 human); H_1N_1 (A_1); H_2N_2 (A_2); H_3N_2 (A_{HK}, A_3); $H_{sw}N_1$ (swine); $H_{eq}N$ (2 equine); and $H_{av}N$ (8 avian), have been identified. The influenza virus has shown great genetic variation. This ability provides the basis for development of epidemics in populations that have previously been exposed to influenza caused by other subtypes.

EPIDEMIOLOGY: Usually more prevalent in winter and spring. Young adults, in robust health, appear to be particularly susceptible. The disease is contagious and is spread by discharges from the mouth and nose of infected persons. It may occur sporadically, epidemically, or pandemically. The incidence is highest in ages 5 to 9. The very young and the very old are most at risk of dying. Even during an epidemic, the number of people infected who remain asymptomatic is high as compared to those who are symptomatic. The influenza virus is the only organism that still causes acute nationwide epidemics.

INCUBATION: One to three days.

SYM: Begins abruptly with lassitude, malaise, chilliness, severe pain in head and back, fever from 101° to 103° F. (38.3°–39.4° C.). Prostration out of proportion to the fever. Eyes injected, sneezing, hoarseness, and hard paroxysmal cough. Coryza is moderate to severe. Less frequently, gastrointestinal symptoms including anorexia, nausea, vomiting, and diarrhea are present.

COURSE: Ordinarily lasts from four to five days, and may terminate by crisis or speedy lysis. Pulse rate is usually not increased in proportion to fever; may be 90 to 100. Blood pressure low; nosebleed not uncommon. Examination of blood demonstrates a leukopenia. Urinalysis generally demonstrates presence of albumin and casts. Even though fairly rapid recovery is the rule, some patients will experience lassitude for weeks or even months after the acute phase disappears.

The principal complications are secondary bacterial infections of the nasal sinuses, middle ear, and lungs.

DIFF. DIAG: Typhoid fever, smallpox in the prodromal stage, cerebrospinal meningitis, and rarely, pulmonary tuberculosis.

PROG: As a rule, outcome is favorable in absence of pulmonary complications. In patients with cyanosis, severe nerve disturbances, or bloody expectoration, prognosis is extremely guarded.

Death may occur but mostly in infants under one year and in those over 60 or in persons who have a chronic disease.

TREATMENT: Isolation, absolute rest, good ventilation, and selected diet as tolerated. No specific treatment; care largely symptomatic.

i., Asian. Influenza caused by a variant strain of influenza virus type A.

influenzal (ĭn″flū-ĕn′zăl) [It. *influenza*, influence]. Relating to influenza.

influenza virus vaccine. USP. A sterile aqueous suspension of suitably inactivated influenza virus types A and B either individually or combined. Trade names for influenza virus vaccine are Flu-Immune, Fluax, and Fluogen.

infolding. Process of enclosing within a fold; an operation employed in the treatment of stomach ulcer in which the walls on either side of the lesion are sutured together.

infra- [L. *infra*, beneath]. Prefix meaning below; under; beneath; inferior to; after.

infra-axillary (ĭn″fră-ăks′ĭl-ă-rē) [″ + *axilla*, little axis]. Below the axilla.

infrabulge (ĭn′fră-bŭlj). The surfaces of the tooth gingival to the height of contour.

infraclavicular (ĭn″fră-klă-vĭk′ū-lăr) [″ + *clavicula*, little key]. Below the clavicle.

infracortical (ĭn″fră-kor′tĭ-kăl) [″ + *cortex*, rind]. Beneath the cortex of any organ.

infracostal (ĭn″fră-kŏs′tăl) [″ + *costa*, rib]. Below the rib.

infracotyloid (ĭn″fră-kŏt′ĭ-loyd) [″ + Gr. *kotyloeides*, cup shaped]. Beneath the cotyloid cavity of the acetabulum of the hip.

infraction (ĭn-frăk′shŭn) [L. *infractus*, to destroy]. An incomplete fracture of a bone in which parts do not become displaced.

infradiaphragmatic (ĭn″fră-dī″ă-frăg-măt′ĭk). Below the diaphragm. SYN: *subdiaphragmatic*.

infraglenoid (ĭn″fră-glē′noyd) [L. *infra*, beneath, + Gr. *glene*, cavity, + *eidos*, form]. Beneath the glenoid fossa. SYN: *subglenoid*.

infraglottic (ĭn″fră-glŏt′ĭk) [″ + Gr. *glottis*, back of tongue]. Below the glottis.

infrahyoid (ĭn″fră-hī′oyd) [″ + Gr. *hyoeides*, U-shaped]. Below the hyoid bone.

inframammary [″ + *mamma*, breast]. Below the mammary gland.

inframandibular (ĭn″fră-măn-dĭb′ū-lăr) [″ + *mandibula*, lower jawbone]. Below the mandible.

inframarginal [″ + *margo*, a margin]. Below any edge or margin.

inframaxillary [″ + *maxilla*, little jaw]. Below the upper jaw (maxilla).

infranuclear (ĭn″fră-nū′klē-ăr) [″ + *nucleus*, kernel]. In the nervous system, peripheral to a nucleus.

infraocclusion [″ + *occlusio*, a shutting up]. Location of a tooth below the line of occlusion.

infraorbital (ĭn-fră-or′bĭ-tăl) [″ + *orbita*, track]. Beneath the orbit.

infrapatellar (ĭn″fră-pă-tĕl′ăr) [″ + *patella*, a small plate]. Below the patella.

infrapsychic (ĭn″fră-sī′kĭk) [″ + Gr. *psyche*, mind]. Below the level of consciousness; automatic.

infrapubic [″ + *pubes*, hair on genitals]. Below the pubis.

infrared rays. Invisible heat rays beyond the red end of the spectrum.

Their wavelength ranges from 7,700 Angstrom units (A.U.) to 1 mm. Long-wave infrared rays (15,000 to 150,000 A.U.) are emitted by all heated bodies and exclusively by bodies of low temperature such as hot-water bottles and electrical heating pads; short-wave infrared rays (7,200 to 15,000 A.U.) are those emitted by all incandescent heaters.

SOURCES: The sun, electric arc, incandescent globe, and so-called infrared burners.

USES: Their energy is transformed into heat in a superficial layer of the tissues. They are used therapeutically to stimulate local and general circulation and for relief of pain. The use of a device, infrared thermograph, for detecting and photographing infrared rays has been useful in studying the heat of tissues. This device has many applications such as in investigation of the rate of blood flow through a part. SEE: *radiation; ray.*

infrascapular [″ + *scapula*, shoulder blade]. Beneath the shoulder blade.

infrasonic (ĭn″fră-sŏn′ĭk) [L. *infra*, beneath, + *sonus*, sound]. Sound wave frequency lower than those normally heard.

infraspinous [″ + *spina*, a thorn]. Beneath the scapular spine.

infrasternal [″ + Gr. *sternon*, chest]. Beneath the sternum.

infratemporal (ĭn″fră-tĕm′pō-răl) [″ + *temporalis*, pert. to the temple]. Below the temporal fossa of the skull.

infratonsillar (ĭn″fră-tŏn′sĭ-lăr) [″ + *tonsilla*, almond]. In the pharynx below the tonsils.

infratrochlear (ĭn″fră-trŏk′lē-ăr) [″ + *trochlea*, pulley]. Beneath the trochlea.

infraumbilical (ĭn″fră-ŭm-bĭl′ĭ-kăl) [″ + *umbilicus*, a pit]. Below the umbilicus.

infraversion (ĭn″fră-vĕr′zhŭn) [″ + *versio*, a turning]. Downward deviation of the eye.

infriction [L. *in*, into, + *frictio*, rubbing]. Rubbing of ointments into the skin. SYN: *inunction.*

infundibulectomy (ĭn″fŭn-dĭb″ū-lĕk′tō-mē) [L. *infundibulum*, funnel, + Gr. *ektome*, excision]. Surgical excision of the infundibulum of any structure or organ, esp. the heart.

infundibuliform (ĭn″fŭn-dĭb′ū-lĭ-form) [″ + *forma*, form]. Funnel-shaped.

i. fascia. The membranous layer investing the spermatic cord.

infundibulopelvic (ĭn″fŭn-dĭb″ū-lō-pĕl′vĭk) [″ + *pelvis*, basin]. Concerning the infundibulum and pelvis of an organ, esp. the kidney.

infundibulum (ĭn″fŭn-dĭb′ū-lŭm) [L.]. 1. [NA] Funnel-shaped passage or structure. 2. Tube connecting the frontal sinus with the middle nasal meatus. 3. Stalk of the pituitary gland. 4. Any renal pelvis division. 5. Cavity formed by fallopian fimbriae. 6. Terminus of a bronchiole. 7. Terminus at upper end of cochlear canal. 8. [NA] Conelike upper anterior angle at right cardiac ventricle from which the pulmonary artery arises. SYN: *conus arteriosus.*

i., ethmoidal. The area in the middle meatus of the nose. The anterior ethmoidal air cells and the frontal nasal duct from the frontal sinus open into this area.

i. of hypothalamus. The infundibulum of the hypothalamus. It extends from the stalk of the hypothalamus to the posterior lobe of the hypothalamus.

i. of the uterine tube. The funnel-shaped opening at the lateral end of the uterine tube.

infusible. 1. [L. *in-*, not, + *fusio*, fusion] Not capable of being fused or melted. 2. [L. *in*, into, + *fundere*, to pour] Capable of being made into an infusion.

infusion (ĭn-fū′zhŭn) [L. *infusio*]. 1. A liquid substance introduced into the body via a vein for therapeutic purposes. 2 Steeping a substance in hot or cold water in order to obtain its active principle. 3. Product obtained from process described in def. 2.

i., continuous. A controlled method of prolonged drug administration that includes the ability to control the delivery rate. This system permits the drug to be available to the body at a constant level. This method of drug delivery has proved to be more effective than other regimens in the treatment of certain neoplastic diseases, including acute leukemia.

i., intravenous. Injection of a solution directly into a vein, usually the cephalic or median basilic vein of the arm. SEE: *intravenous infusion.*

i., subcutaneous. Infusion of solutions into the subcutaneous space.

infusodecoction (ĭn-fū″sō-dē-kŏk′shŭn) [″ + *de*, down, + *coquere*, to boil]. 1. Infusion followed by decoction. 2. A medicine made from a crude drug steeped in cold water and then in boiling water.

Infusoria (ĭn-fū-sō′rē-ă). Name formerly applied to a class of Protozoa, now called Ciliata, q.v.

infusum (ĭn-fū′sŭm) [L., infusion]. Product obtained from steeping a substance in hot or cold water. SYN: *infusion* (def. 3).

ingesta (ĭn-jĕs′tă) [L. *in*, into, + *gerere*, to

carry]. Food and drink received into the body through the mouth.

ingestant (ĭn-jĕs′tănt) [″ + *gerere*, to carry]. Any substance such as food and drink taken orally.

ingestion. The process of taking material (particularly food) into the gastrointestinal tract or the process by which a cell takes in foreign particles.

Ingrassia's apophyses (ĭn-gră′sē-ăs) [Giovanni Filippo Ingrassia, It. anatomist, 1510–1580] The lesser wings of the sphenoid.

ingravescent (ĭn″grăv-ĕs′ĕnt) [″ + *gravesci*, to grow heavy]. Becoming more severe.

ingredient (ĭn-grē′dē-ĕnt) [L. *ingredi*, to enter]. Any part of a compound or a mixture; a unit of a more complex substance.

ingrowing [L. *in*, into, + AS. *growan*, to grow]. Growing inward so that a portion that is normally free becomes covered.

ingrown nail. Growth of the nail edge into the soft tissue, thus causing inflammation and pain. May be due to improper paring of the nail or pressure on the nail edge from improperly fitted shoes.

inguen (ĭn′gwĕn) [L.]. (pl. *inguina*) [NA] The groin.

inguinal (ĭng′gwĭ-năl) [L. *inguinalis*, pert. to the groin]. Pert. to the region of the groin.

RS: bubo; groin; hernia; venereal bubo.

inguinal canal. The canal carrying the spermatic cord in the male and the round ligament in the female. It is 1½ in. (3.8 cm.) long. A potential source of weakness, it may be the site of a hernia or an undescended testicle.

inguinal glands. Lymph nodes of the groin.

inguinal hernia. Hernia in inguinal region. SEE: *hernia, inguinal*.

inguinal ligament. A fibrous band extending from the anterior superior iliac spine to the pubic tubercle. SYN: *Poupart's ligament*.

inguinal reflex. Reflex in females resembling cremasteric reflex, q.v., in males.

inguinal region. The iliac region on either side of the pubes. SYN: *groin*.

inguinal ring. Interior opening of the inguinal canal (abdominal inguinal ring) and the end of the inguinal canal (subcutaneous inguinal ring).

inguinocrural (ĭng″gwĭ-nō-kroo′răl) [L. *inguen*, groin, + *cruralis*, pert. to the leg]. Concerning the inguinal and thigh areas.

inguinodynia (ĭn″gwĭ-nō-dĭn′ē-ă) [″ + Gr. *odyne*, pain]. Pain in the groin or inguinal region.

inguinolabial (ĭng″gwĭ-nō-lā′bē-ăl) [″ + *labialis*, pert. to the lips]. Concerning the inguinal and the labial areas.

inguinoscrotal (ĭng″gwĭ-nō-skrō′tăl) [″+ *scrotum*, a bag]. Concerning the inguinal and scrotal areas.

INH. Abbreviation for isoniazid.

inhalant [L. *inhalare*, to inhale]. A medication or compound suitable for inhaling.

inhalation (ĭn″hă-lā′shŭn) [L. *inhalatio*]. 1. Act of drawing in of breath, vapor, or gas into the lungs; inspiration. 2. Introduction of dry or moist air or vapor into the lungs for therapeutic purposes, such as aromatic spirits of ammonia used to overcome fainting.

SUBSTANCES: Mixture of oxygen and carbon dioxide to relieve depressed breathing. Steam inhalations are given to reduce dryness of mucous membranes and to provide heat and moisture to the membranes of the lungs.

inhalation therapy. Administration of medicines, water vapors, gases (such as oxygen, carbon dioxide, or helium), or anesthetics by inhalation. The medicines usually are nebulized by using an aerosol or spray apparatus. SEE: *intermittent positive-pressure breathing*.

inhale (ĭn-hāl′) [L. *inhalare*]. To draw in the breath; to inspire.

inhaler. 1. Device for administering medicines by inhalation. 2. One who inhales.

inherent (ĭn-hē′rĕnt) [L. *inhaerens*, to inhere]. Belonging to anything naturally, not as a result of circumstances, and existing as an essential character of something. SYN: *innate; intrinsic*.

inherent cauterization. Deep cauterization.

inheritance (ĭn-hĕr′ĭ-tăns) [L. *inhereditare*, to inherit]. The sum total of all that is inherited; that which is the result of hereditary factors contained within the egg and sperm.

i., maternal. Characteristics inherited from the genes of the female, or due to uterine environment.

inherited. Received from one's parents; not acquired.

inhibin (ĭn-hĭb′ĭn). A postulated testicular hormone that acts to inhibit luteinizing hormone secretion by the anterior pituitary gland.

inhibited sexual excitement. SEE: *frigidity*.

inhibition (ĭn″hĭ-bĭsh′ŭn) [L. *inhibere*, to restrain]. 1. Repression or restraint of a function. 2. In physiology, a stopping of an action or function of an organ, as in the slowing or stopping of the heart produced by electrical stimulation of the vagus. 3. In psychiatry, restraint of one mental process almost simultaneously by another opposed mental process; an inner impediment to free activity.

i., competitive. Inhibiting the function of an active material by competing for the cell receptor site.

i., contact. Inhibition of cell division due to the close contact of similar cells.

i., noncompetitive. Inhibition of enzyme activity due only to the concentration of the inhibitor.

i., psychic. Arrest of an impulse, thought, action, or speech. The term is commonly applied to the denial of the sex instinct. SYN: *suppression.*

i., selective. I., competitive, q.v.

inhibitor. That which inhibits.

Ex.: a chemical substance that stops enzyme activity or a nerve that suppresses activity of an organ innervated by it.

inhibitory (ĭn-hĭb′ĭ-tō-rē). Restraining, preventing.

inhibitory nerve. A nerve that carries impulses that act to slow down or inhibit action in the organ or tissue supplied by its fibers.

inhibitrope (ĭn-hĭb′ĭ-trōp) [″+ Gr. *tropos,* a turning]. Person in whom certain stimuli cause partial arrest of function.

inhomogeneity (ĭn-hō″mō-jĕ-nē′ĭ-tē) [L. *in-,* not, + Gr. *homos,* same, + *genos,* kind]. Lack of uniform quality or consistency.

iniac, inial (ĭn′ē-ăk, -ăl) [Gr. *inion,* back of the head]. Pert. to the inion.

iniencephalus (ĭn″ē-ĕn-sĕf′ă-lŭs) [″ + *enkephalos,* brain]. Congenitally deformed fetus in which brain substance protrudes through a fissure in the occiput, so that the brain and spinal cord occupy a single cavity.

inion (ĭn′ē-ŏn) [Gr.]. External occipital protuberance. SEE: *antinion.*

iniopagus (ĭn″ē-ŏp′ă-gŭs) [″ + *pagos,* thing fixed]. Twins fused at the occiput.

iniops (ĭn′ē-ŏps) [″ + *ops,* eye]. A double deformity in which there is joining of the two fetuses from the posterior thorax up, so that one complete face is anterior, with the suggestion of a face posteriorly.

initial (ĭn-ĭsh′ăl) [L. *initium,* beginning]. Rel. to the beginning or commencement of a thing or process. SYN: *incipient.*

initis (ĭn-ī′tĭs) [Gr. *inos,* fiber, + *itis,* inflammation]. 1. Inflammation of fibrous tissue. SYN: *fibrositis.* 2. Inflammation of a tendon. SYN: *tendinitis.* 3. Inflamed condition of a muscle. SYN: *myositis.*

inject [L. *injicere,* to throw in]. To introduce fluid into the body or its parts artificially.

injected [L. *injectus,* thrown in]. 1. Filled by injection of fluid. 2. Congested.

injection (ĭn-jĕk′shŭn). 1. Forcing of a fluid into a vessel or cavity intramuscularly or under the skin. 2. Substance introduced in this manner. 3. State of being injected; congestion.

NURSING IMPLICATIONS: All equipment used for preparation and administration of an injection should be sterile. Wash hands before and after administration of the injection. Measure dose accurately. Carefully examine and cleanse the site for the injection. After insertion of the needle, pull back gently on the plunger to ensure that there is no blood return, which would indicate that the needle is in a small blood vessel. Administer the medication. Destroy and properly dispose of needle and syringe.

i., epidural. Injection of anesthetic solution or other medicine into the epidural space of the spinal cord.

i., hypodermic. Term originally indicating injection of a substance beneath the skin. It is preferable to state the specific route of administration, as in intramuscular.

i., intra-alveolar. An infiltration method of anesthesia where the anesthetic is introduced into the soft tissues adjacent to the tooth.

i., intracardial. Injection into the heart.

i., intracutaneous. Injection into the skin, a method employed in giving of serums and vaccines when a local reaction is desired.

i., intralingual. Injection of medicines into the tongue. Usually done as an emergency measure when a vein suitable for use is not available because of circulatory collapse.

i., intramuscular. Injection into intramuscular tissue usually in the anterior thigh, deltoid, or in one of the buttocks.

i., intraosseous. Injection of anesthetic solution directly into the cancellous bone of the alveolar process adjacent to the tooth to produce a localized effect.

i., intraperitoneal. Injection into the peritoneal cavity.

i., intravenous. Injection into a vein.

i., jet. Technique of injecting medicines and vaccines through the skin without puncturing it. This is done by the use of a nozzle that ejects a fine spray of liquid at such speed as to penetrate the skin. The skin is not harmed and the procedure is harmless. Esp. useful in immunizing a great number of persons quickly and economically. Hypospray is the trade name for a device used in this procedure.

i., rectal. Instillation, i.e., not an injection, into the rectum; an enema.

i., sclerosing. Injection into a vessel or into a tissue of a substance that will bring about obliteration of the vessel or hardening of the tissues.

i., spinal. Injection into the spinal canal.

i., subcutaneous. Injection beneath the skin.

i., vaginal. Instillation, i.e., not an injection, into the vagina. A douche.

i., Z-track. An injection technique in which after the needle is through the dermis, the point is moved laterally prior to continuing the insertion of the needle. Then insertion is continued. This makes it difficult for the injected fluid to seep back out.

injectors. Various instruments used in injection of medicinal fluids, hypodermic injections, transfusion of blood, and intravenous injection.

injury [L. *injurius,* unjust]. Trauma or damage to some part of the body. SEE: *transportation of the injured.*

SYM: These will depend on the nature, extent, and severity of the damage. If the injuries are severe, there may be signs of shock with progressive fall in blood pressure; subnormal temperature; shallow, rapid breathing; cold, clammy, pale skin.

i., egg-white. Injury resulting from biotin deficiency. It is produced in experimental animals by feeding raw egg white or its antibiotin component, avidin. SEE: *biotin.*

i., internal. SEE: *internal injury.*

i., steering wheel. An injury following an automobile accident in which the driver is thrown forward against the steering wheel. This may cause contusion of the heart and trauma to the ribcage.

ink poisoning. Many of the poisonings ascribed to ink are forms of dermatitis. Several types of materials may be responsible. Ordinary ink may cause irritation because of its composition or because of the sensitivity of particular individuals to certain ingredients. Sometimes cleaning materials used in removing ink stains have been found to be causative agents.

SYM: Redness, occasionally small pustules and cracking.

F.A.: Wash with alcohol, soap, and water. Rinse carefully and apply a bland dressing such as cold cream.

inlay (ĭn'lā) [L. *in,* in, + AS. *lecgan,* to lay]. A solid filling made to the precise shape of a cavity of a tooth and cemented into it.

inlet. Passage leading to a cavity.

i. of pelvis. The upper opening into the pelvic cavity.

I.N.N. *International Nonproprietary Names,* a list of pharmaceuticals published periodically by the World Health Organization.

innate (ĭn-nāt') [" + *natus,* born]. 1. Belonging to the essential nature of something. SYN: *inherent; intrinsic.* 2. Existing in or belonging at birth.

innervate (ĭn-nĕr'vāt, ĭn'ĕr-vāt) [" + *nervus,* nerve]. To stimulate a part, as the nerve supply of an organ.

innervation (ĭn"ĕr-vā'shŭn). 1. Stimulation of a part through the action of nerves. 2. The distribution and function of the nervous system. 3. The nerve supply of a part.

i., collateral. Development of the nerve supply in a nerve tract adjacent to the original nerve supply that has been injured or destroyed.

i., double. Innervation of an organ with both sympathetic and parasympathetic fibers.

i., reciprocal. Innervation of antagonistic muscles of a limb by which impulses of central origin that induce an action such as flexion bring about inhibition of the opposing extensors.

innidiation (ĭ-nĭd"ē-ā'shŭn) [" + *nidus,* nest]. Multiplication of cells in a part to which they have been carried by metastasis.

innocent (ĭn'ō-sĕnt) [L. *innocens*]. Harmless or benign; clinically unimportant; not malignant (a heart murmur may be called innocent in this sense). SYN: *innocuous; innoxious.*

innocuous (ĭ-nŏk'ū-ŭs) [L. *innocuus*]. Harmless or benign. SYN: *innocent; innoxious.*

innominate (ĭ-nŏm'ĭ-nāt) [L. *innominatus,* unnamed]. Nameless.

innominate artery. Right artery arising from the arch of the aorta, dividing into the right subclavian and right common carotid arteries.

innominate bone. The hip bone, composed of the ilium, ischium, and pubis. United with the sacrum and coccyx by ligaments to form the pelvis.

innominate veins. Right and left vein, each formed by union of the internal jugular with the subclavian veins.

innoxious (ĭ-nŏk'shŭs) [L. *in,* not, + *noxius,* harmful]. Not harmful. SYN: *innocent; innocuous.*

inochondritis (ĭn"ō-kŏn-drī'tĭs) [Gr. *inos,* fiber, + *chondros,* cartilage, + *itis,* inflammation]. Inflammation of a fibrocartilage.

inochondroma (ĭn"ō-kŏn-drō'mă) [" + " + *oma,* tumor]. A chondroma or tumor with much fibrous tissue. SYN: *fibrochondroma.*

inoculability (ĭn-ŏk"ū-lă-bĭl'ĭ-tē) [" + *oculus,* bud]. State of being inoculable.

inoculable. 1. Transmissible by inoculation. 2. Susceptible to a transmissible disease. 3. Capable of being inoculated.

inoculate. To inject a microorganism, serums, or toxic materials into the body. This can be accomplished by using a needle and syringe, by scarification of the skin, or by some special technique such as a very high-speed jet of air capable of a force sufficient to carry a liquid solution into the skin. SEE: *injection, jet.*

inoculation (ĭn-ŏk"ū-lā'shŭn). The process of being inoculated. SEE: *inoculate.*

i., animal. The injection of serums, microorganisms, or viral organisms into laboratory animals for the purpose of immunizing them or for the purpose of investigating the effects of the inoculated material upon the animals.

inoculum (ĭn-ŏk'ū-lŭm) [L.]. The substance introduced by inoculation.

inocyst (ĭn'ō-sĭst) [Gr. *inos,* fiber, + *kystis,* a bladder]. A fibrous capsule.

inocyte (ĭn'ō-sīt) [" + *kytos,* cell]. Fibroblast.

inogenesis (ĭn″ō-jĕn′ĕ-sĭs) [″ + *genesis*, production]. Formation of fibrous tissue.

inogenous (ĭn-ŏj′ĭ-nŭs) [″ + *gennan*, to produce]. Forming tissue or produced from it.

inoglia (ĭn-ŏg′lē-ă) [″ + *glia*, glue]. The supporting tissue of fibroblasts.

inohymenitis (ĭn″ō-hī″mĕn-ī′tĭs) [″ + *hymen*, membrane, + *itis*, inflammation]. Inflammation of any fibrous membrane or of an aponeurosis.

inolith (ĭn′ō-lĭth) [″ + *lithos*, stone]. A concretion formed from fibrous tissue.

inomyositis (ĭn″ō-mī″ō-sī′tĭs) [″ + *mys*, muscle, + *itis*, inflammation]. Chronic muscular inflammation with connective tissue hyperplasia. SYN: *fibromyositis*.

inomyxoma (ĭn″ō-mĭk-sō′mă) [″ + *myxa*, mucus, + *oma*, tumor]. A mixed myxoma and fibroma. SYN: *fibromyxoma*.

inoneuroma (ĭn″ō-nū-rō′mă) [″ + *neuron*, nerve, + *oma*, tumor]. A mixed neuroma and inoma. SYN: *fibroneuroma*.

inoperable [L. *in-*, not, + *operari*, to work]. Unsuitable for surgery. In the case of a tumor, the disease may have spread so extensively as to make surgery useless, or the patient's general condition may be so poor that surgery could cause death.

inopexia (ĭn-ō-pĕk′sē-ă) [Gr. *inos*, fiber, + *pexis*, fixation]. Tendency of blood to coagulate spontaneously in the vessels.

inorganic [L. *in-*, not, + Gr. *organon*, an organ]. 1. In chemistry, occurring in nature independently of living things. Sometimes considered to indicate chemical compounds that do not contain carbon. 2. Not pert. to living organisms.

inorganic acid. An acid composed of inorganic constituents. SYN: *mineral acid*.

inorganic chemistry. Chemistry dealing only with inorganic compounds.

inorganic compound. A compound without carbon.

inosclerosis (ĭn″ō-sklĕ-rō′sĭs) [Gr. *inos*, fiber, + *skleros*, hard]. Increased fibrous-tissue density.

inoscopy [″ + *skopein*, to examine]. Diagnosis by examining fibrinous deposits in body fluids.

inosculating [L. *in*, in, + *osculum*, little mouth]. Directly communicating. SYN: *anastomosing*.

inosculation (ĭn-ŏs″kū-lā′shŭn). Union of two vessels. SYN: *anastomosis*.

inose (ĭn′ōs). Inositol.

inosemia (ĭn-ō-sē′mē-ă) [Gr. *inos*, fiber, + *haima*, blood]. 1. An excessive amount of fibrin in the blood. 2. The presence of inositol in the blood.

inosinic acid [″ + L. *acidus*, sour]. A mononucleotide that is present in muscular tissue and also is a product of nucleic acid. Upon hydrolysis, it yields hypoxanthine and d-ribose-5-phosphoric acid.

inosite (ĭn′ō-sīt). Inositol.

inositis (ĭn″ō-sī′tĭs) [″ + *itis*, inflammation]. Inflammation of fibrous tissue.

inositol (ĭn-ŏs′ĭ-tŏl). $C_6H_6(OH)_6$. Hexahydroxycyclohexane, a sugar-like crystalline substance found in the liver, kidney, skeletal and heart muscle, and also present in the leaves and seeds of most plants. It is part of the vitamin B complex. Deficiency of inositol in experimental animals results in loss of hair, eye defects, and growth retardation. Its significance in human nutrition has not been established.

inosituria (ĭn″ō-sĭ-tū′rē-ă) [*inositol* + Gr. *ouron*, urine]. Inositol in the urine.

inosuria (ĭn-ō-sū′rē-ă). 1. [Gr. *inos*, fiber, + *ouron*, urine] Fibrinous excess in urine. 2. [*inositol* + Gr. *ouron*, urine] Inositol in the urine. SYN: *inosituria*.

inotropic (ĭn″ō-trŏp′ĭk) [Gr. *inos*, fiber, + *trepein*, to influence]. Influencing the force of muscular contractility.

inquest [L. *in*, into, + *quaerere*, to seek]. 1. In legal medicine, official examination and investigation into the cause, circumstance and manner of sudden, unexpected violent, or unexplained death. 2. The act of inquiring.

insalivation [″+ *saliva*, spittle]. The process of mixing saliva with food, as in chewing.

insalubrious (ĭn-săl-ū′brē-ŭs) [L. *in*, not, + *salus*, health]. Not healthy; not contributing to health.

insane (ĭn-sān′) [″ + *sanus*, sound]. Mentally deranged; pert. to insanity.

insanitary. Not conducive to health; unhealthful, esp. pert. to filth.

insanity [L. *insanitas*, insanity]. A severe mental disorder such as a psychosis, as distinguished from a neurosis. A general term for unsoundness of mind or any mental disorder. In legal medicine, the state or mental condition characterized by inability to distinguish between right and wrong, possession of delusions or hallucinations that prevent individuals from looking after their own affairs with ordinary prudence or that render them a menace to others, or actions resulting from impulses of such intensity that they cannot be resisted.

During lucid intervals, an insane person may enter into a legal contract, marriage, business, or buying and selling providing at the time he or she is capable of entering into such matters with an understanding of all that is implied. The mental capacity at the time determines the validity of such acts and not the condition before or after. SEE: *neurosis; psychosis*.

insatiable (ĭn-sā′shē-ă-bl) [L. *insatiabilis*]. Incapable of being satisfied or appeased.

inscriptio (ĭn-skrĭp′shē-ō) [L.]. Inscription.

i. tendinea. Tendinous band traversing a muscle.

inscription (ĭn-skrĭp′shŭn) [L. *in,* upon, + *scribere,* to write]. Body of a prescription, which gives the names of the drug(s) prescribed and dosage.

insect [L. *insectum*]. Common name for any of the class Insecta of the phylum Arthropoda. Insects of medical importance are flies, mosquitoes, lice, fleas, ticks, spiders, scorpions, bees, hornets, and wasps.

Insecta. A class of the phylum Arthropoda characterized by three distinct body divisions (head, thorax, abdomen), three pairs of jointed legs, trachea, and usually two pairs of wings. Insects are of medical significance in that some are parasitic; some serve as carriers or vectors of pathogenic organisms; and some are annoying pests causing injury by their bites or their stings. SYN: *Hexapoda.*

insect bites and stings. In some cases the venom of a stinging insect may be more toxic than that of a poisonous snake. Fortunately the insect injects a very small amount of venom into the body.

F.A.: Remove the stinger if it is present, and cool the area as quickly and efficiently as possible to prevent the venom from gaining access to the general circulation. To prevent injecting further venom, gently tease the stinger out by grasping the stinger with fingernails or forceps. If a specific therapy or antiserum is available it should be administered.

An antivenin for *black widow spiders* (Latrodectus mactans) is available. One ampule is given I.V. in 10 to 50 ml. of saline after the appropriate skin test has been done. For acute pain and muscle contraction, give 10 ml. of calcium gluconate I.V. or I.M., and repeat as necessary. SEE: *spider, black widow.*

There is no antiserum for the bite of the *brown recluse spider* (Loxosceles reclusus), but hydrocortisone in a dose of 1 to 3 mg./kg. of body weight every six hours for 4 to 8 doses is beneficial.

For *bees, wasps, and hornets* 0.2 to 0.5 ml. of epinephrine subcutaneously and an antihistamine suitable for intravenous injection should be given slowly. If shock and collapse appear to be imminent, hydrocortisone should be given. Apply an ice pack to the sting. If muscle spasms occur, intravenous infusion of calcium lactate or calcium gluconate should be given. In some cases curare (dimethyl tubocurarine chloride) will be required to relieve muscle spasms.

insecticide (ĭn-sĕk′tĭ-sīd) [L. *insectum,* insect, + *caedere,* to kill]. 1. An agent used to exterminate insects. 2. Destructive to insects.

insectifuge (ĭn-sĕk′tĭ-fūj) [″ + *fugare,* to put to flight]. Insect repellant.

Insectivora (ĭn″sĕk-tĭv′ō-ră) [″ + *vorare,* to devour]. An order of small mammals including moles and shrews.

insectivore (ĭn-sĕk′tĭ-vor). A member of the order Insectivora.

insemination (ĭn-sĕm″ĭn-ā′shŭn) [L. *in,* into, + *semen,* seed]. 1. Discharge of semen from the penis into the vagina during coitus. 2. Fertilization of an ovum.

i., artificial. ABBR: AI. Introduction of viable sperm into the vagina, cervical canal, or uterus by artificial means. SEE: *impregnation.*

i., heterologous artificial. Artificial insemination in which the semen is obtained from a donor other than the husband.

i., homologous artificial. Artificial insemination in which the semen is obtained from the husband.

insenescence (ĭn″sē-nĕs′ĕns) [″ + *senescens,* growing old]. 1. Process of growing old or the approaching of old age. 2. Old age in which infirmity and senility would normally be expected to be present but they are not.

insensible [L. *in-,* not, + *sensibilis,* appreciable]. 1. Unconscious; without feeling or consciousness. 2. Not perceptible.

insertion [L. *in,* into, + *serere,* to join]. 1. The manner or place of attachment of a muscle to the bone so that it moves. 2. A putting into or implanting.

i., velamentous. Attachment of the umbilical cord to the edge of the placenta.

insheathed (ĭn-shēthd′) [″ + AS. *sceath,* sheath]. Enclosed, as by a sheath or capsule. SYN: *encysted.*

insidious (ĭn-sĭd′ē-ŭs) [L. *insidiosus,* cunning]. Used to indicate a disease that comes on in such a manner (lacking symptoms) as to make the patient unaware of the onset of the disease.

insight. 1. Self-understanding. 2. In psychiatry, the patients' comprehension that they are ill in mind; and awareness of the character of the illness or of the unconscious factors responsible for the emotional conflict involved.

insipid (ĭn-sĭp′ĭd) [LL. *insipidus*]. Without taste; lacking in spirit or animation.

in situ (ĭn sī′tū, sĭt′ū) [L.]. In position, localized.

insolation (ĭn″sō-lā′shŭn) [L. *insolare,* to expose to the sun]. 1. Any exposure to the rays of the sun. 2. Heatstroke or sunstroke.

In the past it was felt that exposure to the sunlight was a powerful therapeutic measure. It is now known that persons who expose themselves to excess sunlight on either an acute or a chronic basis may be unwise. Acute overexposure leads to severe sunburn of the skin. People with light skin who experience chronic exposure to the sun have an increased chance of developing malignant neoplasms of the skin. SEE: *heat; heat exhaustion; hyperpyrexia.*

insoluble (ĭn-sŏl′ū-bl) [L. *insolubilis*]. Incapable of solution or of being dissolved.

insomnia (ĭn-sŏm′nē-ă) [L. *insomnis*]. Inability to sleep, or sleep prematurely ended or interrupted by periods of wakefulness. Insomnia is not a disease but may be the symptom of many diseases. It may be associated with either a trivial or serious illness; the persistence and severity of the insomnia is of little help in diagnosing the condition that causes it. The most frequent causes of insomnia are anxiety and pain.

TREATMENT: The most important advice is not to stay in bed. The insomniac should sit up and read or engage in some other type of mental or physical activity until tired. A hot foot bath, warm milk, or a mild sweet wine before retiring may be of help.

Change occupation if this is a contributing cause and if it is possible. Physical exercise during the day and a walk in fresh air at night after dinner. The several hours prior to bedtime should be as anxiety-free as possible. Peace of mind is essential to falling asleep. Those complaining about insomnia generally secure more sleep than they realize. Some people require much less sleep than others. Inability to sleep continuously through the night is not a pathological condition. If the insomnia is due to pain it is important to relieve that symptom and to attempt to cure the cause of the pain. SEE: *narcolepsy; somnambulism; vigil.*

insomniac (ĭn-sŏm′nē-ăk). One who has insomnia.

insorption (ĭn-sorp′shŭn) [L. *in*, into, + *sorbere*, to suck in]. The passage of material into the blood as is the case when substances move from the gastrointestinal tract into the bloodstream.

inspect [L. *inspectare*, to examine]. To examine visually.

inspection. Visual examination of the external surface of the body as well as of its movements and posture. SEE: *abdomen; chest; circulatory system.*

inspectionism (ĭn-spĕk′shŭn-ĭzm). Voyeurism.

inspersion (ĭn-spĕr′zhŭn) [L. *in*, upon, + *spargere*, to sprinkle]. Sprinkling with powder or a fluid.

inspiration (ĭn″spĭr-ā′shŭn) [L. *in*, in, + *spirare*, to breathe]. Inhalation; drawing air into the lungs. Opposite of expiration. The average rate is 12 to 18 respirations per minute in a normal adult at rest. SEE: *diaphragm* for illus.; *respiration.*

Inspiration may be costal or abdominal, the latter being deeper. The breaking point for breath holding is quite variable. Some professional divers and others are able to prolong this for more than two minutes.

MUSCLES: External intercostals; diaphragm; levatores costarum; pectoralis minor; scaleni; serratus posterior; and superior sternocleidomastoid.

RS: air; apnea; asphyxia breathing; chest; Cheyne-Stokes respiration; dyspnea; hyperpnea; inhalation therapy; lung; respiration; ventilation.

i., crowing. Peculiar noise in laryngismus stridulus, q.v., or spasmodic croup. SEE: *croup, spasmodic.*

i., external. Interchange of gases in the lungs.

i., forcible. Inspiration in which the muscles of inspiration are assisted by inspiration auxiliaries (i.e., muscles attached to the chest that by contraction increase the volume of the thoracic cavity directly or indirectly by furnishing fixed support whereby other muscles may act more advantageously). If movements become excessively labored, there is brought into coordinate action every muscle in the body that can either directly or indirectly increase the capacity of the thorax.

i., full. Inspiration in which lungs are filled as completely as possible (voluntarily, as in determining the amount of complemental air, or involuntarily, as in cardiac dyspnea).

i., internal. Interchange of gases in the tissues. SEE: *respiration cell.*

inspirator (ĭn′spĭ-rā″tor). A type of respirator or inhaler.

inspiratory (ĭn-spīr′ă-tor″ē). Pert. to inspiration.

inspirometer (ĭn″spĭ-rŏm′ĕ-tĕr) [″ + ″ + Gr. *metron*, measure]. Device for determining the amount of air inspired.

inspissate (ĭn-spĭs′āt) [L. *inspissatus*, thickened]. To thicken by evaporation or absorption of fluid.

inspissated (ĭn-spĭs′ā-tĕd). Thickened by absorption, evaporation, or dehydration.

inspissation (ĭn-spĭ-sā′shŭn). 1. Thickening by evaporation or absorption of fluid. 2. Diminished fluidity or increased thickness.

instep. The arched medial portion of the foot.

instillation (ĭn″stĭl-ā′shŭn) [L. *in*, into, + *stillare*, to drop]. Slowly pouring or dropping a liquid into a cavity or onto a surface.

instillator. An apparatus for introducing, drop by drop, liquids into a cavity.

instinct (ĭn′stĭngkt) [L. *instinctus*, instigation]. The inherited tendency for the members of specific species to react to certain environmental conditions and stimuli in a particular way. The nature of the reaction is that which has through many generations enabled the individuals and species involved to adapt and survive. Instincts are best understood when considered against the evolutionary background of the individuals and species being observed. Freud spoke of instinct, but present-day psychoanalytical terminology would refer to the forces Freud described as being drive instead of instinct.

i., death. In psychoanalytic theory, the unconscious will to destroy oneself. The counterinstinct for the instinct to live.

i., herd. The basic drive to be associated with a group.

instinctive. Determined by instinct.

instrument (ĭn′stroo-mĕnt) [L. *instrumentum,* tool]. 1. A mechanical device. 2. A special tool for accomplishing specific tasks. Thus a reflex hammer, a microscope, stethoscope, cystoscope, and the surgeon's scalpel are all examples of instruments. SEE: *instruments, care and sharpening of.*

instrumental. 1. Pert. to instruments. 2. An important factor in achieving a result or goal.

instrumentarium (ĭn″stroo-mĕn-tā′rē-ŭm). The instruments required for a surgical or other procedure.

instrumentation. 1. The use of instruments, and their care. 2. Accomplishment of a task by use of instruments.

Ex.: removal of a foreign body from the bronchus by means of a bronchoscope.

instruments, care and sharpening of. *Cleansing.* Following surgery, collect, count, and unlock the instruments. First rinse with warm water to remove blood, and next, wash with hot water and soap. Then place under the hot water faucet and run boiling water on and through them. Dry at once with gauze. To remove rust, use cleanser sparingly; otherwise, the surface of the instrument will be damaged in the course of time.

Reliable bacterial sterilization of instruments before an operation can always be assured by boiling in a 1% solution of sodium bicarbonate for 15 minutes. This helps to prevent rusting of the instruments. The dipping of an instrument into alcohol or even pure carbolic acid cannot be relied upon to sterilize it.

CAUTION: Boiling water does not kill the hepatitis viruses. To be certain this virus is destroyed, either autoclaving or the use of some chemical method of sterilization such as ethylene oxide gas is required.

Sharpening. Washita stone is best for sharpening dull instruments because it cuts away the metal faster. Arkansas stone is better for finishing. Glycerin is a suitable lubricant. The entire edge of the knife should be covered in one sweep. Hold knife so that the edge of the blade is at an angle of 30°. Blunt instruments should be kept highly polished. Rub with fine emery paper and polish with rouge and chamois skin or gauze. Do not use emery paper on saws. Silver instruments should not come in contact with rubber or be exposed to atmosphere. Wrap in dry gauze.

insufficiency (ĭn″sŭ-fĭsh′ĕn-sē) [L. *in-,* not, + *sufficiens,* sufficient]. The condition of being inadequate for its purpose.

i., adrenal. Decreased or abnormally low production of adrenal cortical hormone by the adrenal gland. The result is Addison's disease.

i., aortic. An imperfect closure of the aortic valve.

i., cardiac. Inability of the heart to function normally.

i., coronary. Diminished blood flow through the coronary arteries of the heart.

i., gastric. Inability of the stomach to empty itself.

i., hepatic. Inability of the liver to function properly.

i., ileocecal. Failure of the ileocecal valve to prevent the back flow of intestinal contents from the cecum to the ileum.

i., mitral. Condition in which the mitral valve closes inefficiently with rhythmic action of the heart.

i., muscular. Condition in which a muscle is unable to exert its normal force and bring about normal movement of the part to which it is attached. Term applied esp. to eye muscles.

i. of ocular muscles. Absence of dynamic equilibrium of ocular muscles.

i., pulmonary valvular. Failure of the pulmonary valve between the right atrium and right ventricle of the heart to close completely.

i., renal. Inability of the kidney to remove waste products from the blood at the normal rate.

i., respiratory. Inadequate functional capacity of the respiratory system.

i., thyroid. Hypothyroidism.

i., valvular. Imperfect cardiac valve closure, permitting leakage of blood.

i., venous. Failure of the valves of the veins to function. This interferes with venous return to the heart.

insufflate [L. *insufflare,* to blow into]. 1. To blow into, as in the lungs of a newborn infant. 2. To blow a medicated powder or medicinal vapor into a cavity.

insufflation. The act of blowing a vapor or powder into a cavity, as the lungs.

i., perirenal. Instillation of air into the perirenal space in order to visualize the adrenal gland better on x-ray.

i., tubal. Transuterine insufflation with carbon dioxide to test patency of fallopian tubes. SYN: *Rubin's test.*

insufflator (ĭn′sŭ-flā″tor). Device for blowing powders into a cavity.

insula (ĭn′sū-lă) [L.]. 1. [NA] The central lobe of the cerebral hemisphere. It is a triangular area of the cerebral cortex lying in the floor of the lateral fissure. SYN: *island of Reil.* 2. Any round cutaneous body or patch.

insular (ĭn′sū-lăr) [L. *insula,* island]. Rel. to any insula, as in pancreatic islets.

insulation [L. *insulare,* to make into an island]. 1. The protection of a body or substance with a nonconducting medium to prevent the transfer of electricity, heat, or sound. 2. The material or substance that insulates.

insulator. That which insulates. Specifically, a substance or body that interrupts the transmission of electricity to surrounding objects by conduction; anything that exerts great resistance to the passage of an electric current by conduction. The electrical resistance of an insulator is expressed in megohms, a unit representing a million ohms. SEE: *nonconductor.*

insulin [L. *insula,* island]. 1. A hormone secreted by the beta cells of the islets of Langerhans of the pancreas. It can be readily crystallized as a zinc salt, although nickel, calcium, and cobalt also are effective. It is a protein with a molecular weight of approx. 5700. Insulin is essential for the proper metabolism of blood sugar (glucose) and for maintenance of the proper blood sugar level. Inadequate secretion of insulin results in improper metabolism of carbohydrates and fats and brings on diabetes characterized by hyperglycemia and glycosuria. The secretion of insulin is primarily dependent upon the concentration of blood glucose, an increase of blood sugar bringing about an increase in the secretion of insulin.

2. USP. A protein, obtained from the pancreas of healthy bovine and porcine animals used for food by man, that affects the metabolism of glucose.

3. A preparation used in medical treatment of diabetes. Prepared from animal pancreas, usually pork or beef. First discovered and used successfully in diabetes by Sir F. G. Banting. Insulin is not a cure, and it is not necessary in every case of diabetes. Insulin when injected (it is not active orally) into an individual with diabetes produces the following effects: normal storage of glycogen in the liver and muscle tissue; reduction in blood sugar level by facilitating metabolism of glucose; disappearance of ketosis and hyperlipemia; prevention of excessive breakdown of protein; and increase in respiratory quotient.

DOSAGE: Should always be expressed in units rather than in milliliters or minims. There is no average dose of insulin for diabetics; each case must be cared for individually.

ADM: Insulin preparations are divided into three categories according to how quickly they act and their potency and duration following subcutaneous administration. The types include fast-, intermediate-, and long-acting. Examples of these are given in the subentries. SEE: table.

Syringes for use by blind patients with diabetes are available.

CAUTION: Persons taking insulin should wear an easily seen bracelet or necklace indicating they have diabetes and take insulin. This will facilitate diagnosis and treatment in case of coma due to insulin. SEE: *Medic Alert.*

STORAGE: The FDA requires that all preparations of insulin contain instructions to *keep in a cold place and to avoid freezing.* Studies have shown that Prompt Insulin Zinc Suspension, Insulin Zinc Suspension, and Extended Insulin Zinc Suspension retain their potency for 24 months when stored at a temperature of 75° F. (24° C.). Under the same conditions, Protamine Zinc Insulin Suspension and Isophane Insulin Suspension retain their potency for 36 months. However, Insulin Injection, USP, does lose potency when stored at this temperature. It is advisable to store all types of insulin in the coolest possible area if refrigeration is not available.

i., globin zinc. USP. Insulin modified by the addition of zinc chloride and globin. Its onset of effect is within one to two hours and its duration is up to 24 hours with peak activity in eight to sixteen hours.

i., human. Insulin prepared by a synthetic process involving use of recombinant DNA technology utilizing strains of Escherichia coli. In its effect it is similar to highly purified animal insulins. Trade names are Humulin R for regular rapid-acting form; and Humulin N for intermediate-acting form.

i. injection. USP. A fast-acting insulin, acting within one half to one hour of injection and lasting approx. six hours.

i., NPH. *neutral-protamine-Hagedorn.* SEE: *insulin suspension, isophane.*

i., single component or monocomponent. Highly purified insulin that contains less than 10 parts per million of proinsulin, a substance that is capable of inducing formation of anti-insulin antibodies.

i. suspension, isophane. USP. Intermediate-acting insulin with onset in a half to one hour and duration of 24 hours. SYN: *insulin, NPH.*

i. suspension, protamine zinc. USP. Long-acting insulin with onset in 6 to 8

Duration of Effect of Various Insulins When Given by Subcutaneous Injection

Type of Insulin	Synonym or Trade Name	Onset (Given in Hours)	Maximum (Given in Hours)	Duration (Given in Hours)
Insulin Injection (USP)	Insulin, Insulin Hydrochloride, Regular Insulin, Unmodified Insulin	0.5–1.0	2–3	5–7
Prompt Insulin Zinc Suspension (USP)	Semilente Insulin	0.5–0.75	3–6	12–16
Globin Zinc Insulin Injection (USP)	Globin Insulin	1–2	8–16	18–24
Isophane Insulin Suspension (USP)	Isophane Insulin, NPH Insulin	0.5–1	6–10	18–28
Insulin Zinc Suspension (USP)	Lente Insulin	1–1.5	8–12	18–24
Protamine Zinc Insulin Suspension (USP)	Protamine Zinc Insulin	6–8	14–20	30–36
Extended Insulin Zinc Suspension (USP)	Ultralente	5–8	16–18	over 36

hours and duration of 18 to 28 hours.

i., synthetic. Insulin made by the use of recombinant DNA methodology.

i. zinc suspension, extended. USP. Long-acting insulin with onset in 5 to 8 hours and duration of over 36 hours.

i. zinc suspension, prompt. USP. Fast-acting insulin with onset under 1 hour and duration of 12 to 16 hours.

insulinase (ĭn′sū-lĭn-ās). An enzyme that inactivates insulin.

insulinemia (ĭn-sū-lĭn-ē′mē-ă) [L. *insula,* island, + Gr. *haima,* blood]. An excess amount of insulin in the blood.

insulin lipodystrophy. A complication of insulin administration characterized by changes in the subcutaneous fat at the site of injection. The changes may take the form of atrophy or hypertrophy; rarely are both types present in the same patient. Atrophy develops in as many as one third of children and adult females who use insulin regularly but rarely in adult males. The subcutaneous fat appears to have melted away and leaves a saucer-like depression. Hypertrophy at the injection site occurs in the form of a spongy localized area. This complication is slightly more common in males than in females. It is usually associated with a history of prolonged use of the same injection site.

insulinogenesis (ĭn″sū-lĭn-ō-jĕn′ĕ-sĭs) [″ + Gr. *genesis,* production]. Production of insulin by the pancreas.

insulinogenic (ĭn″sū-lĭn″ō-jĕn′ĭk) [″ + Gr. *gennan,* to produce]. 1. Caused by insulin whether administered or produced by the pancreas. 2. Pert. to production of insulin.

insulinoid (ĭn′sū-lĭn-oyd) [″ + Gr. *eidos,* resemblance]. Resembling or having the properties of insulin.

insulinoma (ĭn″sū-lĭn-ō′mă) [″ + Gr. *oma,* tumor]. Insuloma, q.v.

insulin shock. A condition resulting from an overdose of insulin resulting in reduction of the blood sugar level below normal (hypoglycemia).

SYM: Rapid bounding pulse, pale moist skin, weakness, coma. Acetone odor on breath is not present.

TREATMENT: Eating sugar or candy, orange juice, glucose, other carbohydrates and injections of strong glucose solution intravenously. Epinephrine is of great but transient value.

CAUTION: Persons taking insulin should wear an easily seen bracelet or necklace indicating they have diabetes and take insulin. This will facilitate diagnosis and treatment in case of coma due to insulin. SEE: *Medic Alert.*

insulin shock therapy. Treatment of schizophrenia and other mental disorders by the administration of insulin. Sufficient insulin is injected to produce unconsciousness, the dosage being carefully regulated during the course of treatment. When a deep coma is achieved, the patient is brought out of the comatose condition by the administration of glucose followed by a meal rich in carbohydrates. Because this is a potentially dangerous procedure it should only be employed by those who are qualified, thoroughly familiar with all aspects of this method, and fully equipped to treat the side effects of hypoglycemia and convulsions. It is essential to have suitable solutions of dextrose available for intravenous use to interrupt the artificially produced hypoglycemia.

insulitis (ĭn″sū-lī′tĭs) [″ + Gr. *itis*, inflammation]. Inflammation of the islets of Langerhans of the pancreas.

insuloma (ĭn″sū-lō′mă) [″ + Gr. *oma*, tumor]. A tumor of the islets of Langerhans of the pancreas.

insulopathic (ĭn″sū-lō-păth′ĭk) [″ + Gr. *pathos*, disease]. Rel. to or caused by abnormal insulin secretion.

insultus (ĭn-sŭl′tŭs) [L.]. An attack.

insusceptibility (ĭn″sū-sĕp″tĭ-bĭl′ĭ-tē) [L. *in*, not, + *suscipere*, to take up]. Immunity or lack of susceptibility to infection or disease.

intake (ĭn-tāk′). That which is taken in, esp. food and liquids.

i. and output. ABBR: I and O. A record of the oral and parenteral intake of foods and fluids; and all of the output including urine, feces, vomitus, and if required, an estimate of loss of fluid due to perspiration.

Intal. Trade name for cromolyn sodium.

integration (ĭn″tĕ-grā′shŭn) [L. *integrare*, to make whole]. The bringing together of various parts or functions so that they function as a harmonious whole.

i., primary. Early recognition of the body and its psyche as apart from one's environment.

i., secondary. The process involved in developing the adult personality so that the individual coordinates components into unified and socialized action.

integrator (ĭn′tĕ-grā″tor). Device for measuring body surfaces.

integument (ĭn-tĕg′ū-mĕnt) [L. *integumentum*, a covering]. A covering; the skin, consisting of the corium or dermis, and epidermis.

integumentary (ĭn-tĕg-ū-mĕn′tă-rē). Rel. to the integument. SYN: *cutaneous; dermal.*

integumentary system. The skin and its appendages, including the hair and nails.

intellect [L. *intelligere*, to understand]. The mind, or understanding; conscious brain function.

intellectual. 1. Pert. to the mind. 2. Possessing intellect.

intellectualization (ĭn″tĕ-lĕk″chū-ăl-ĭ-zā′shŭn). The analysis of personal or social problems on an intellectual basis despite the individual's personal and emotional reactions to those problems.

intelligence [L. *intelligere*, to understand]. The capacity to comprehend relationships. The ability to think; to solve problems and to adjust to new situations. It is doubtful that using a single test to estimate the intelligence of persons from different social, racial, cultural, or economic backgrounds is reliable.

intelligence quotient. ABBR: IQ. An index of relative intelligence determined through the subject's answers to arbitrarily chosen questions. Intelligence quotient is merely a standard score that places an individual in reference to the scores of others within the age group. SEE: table.

intelligence test. A test designed to determine the intelligence of an individual. Tests are used as a basis for determining intelligence quotient (IQ), q.v. It is now believed that some of the standardized tests of intelligence were more nearly achievement tests.

intemperance [L. *in*, not, + *temperare*, to moderate]. Excess in the use of anything; lack of moderation.

intensifying [L. *intensus*, intense, + *facere*, to make]. Making intense; magnifying.

intensifying screen. A thin sheet of celluloid or other substance coated with a finely divided substance that fluoresces under the influence of roentgen rays and is intended to be used in close contact with the emulsion of a photographic plate or film for the purpose of reinforcing the image. SYN: *fluorescent screen.*

intensimeter (ĭn″tĕn-sĭm′ĭ-tĕr) [″ + Gr. *metron*, measure]. An instrument, often a selenium cell or ionization chamber, designed to measure the intensity of roentgen rays.

intensity (ĭn-tĕn′sĭ-tē). 1. The degree or extent of activity, strength, force, electric current, etc. 2. The state of being intense.

Classification of IQ

IQ	Classification
Above 140	Near genius or genius
120–140	Very super or intelligence
110–119	Superior intelligence
90–109	Normal or average intelligence
80–89	Dull normal
70–80	Borderline deficiency
55–69	Educable mentally retarded
40–54	Trainable
20–39	Severe mentally retarded
Below 20	Profoundly mentally retarded

intensive (ĭn-tĕn′sĭv). Rel. to or marked by intensity.

intention (ĭn-tĕn′shŭn) [″ + *tendere,* to stretch]. 1. A natural process of healing, q.v. 2. Goal or purpose.

i., first. Healing without granulation or suppuration.

i., second. Healing by adhesion of two granulated surfaces.

i., third. Healing of an ulcer, wound, or cavity by filling with granulation tissue and by cicatrization. SEE: *granulation; resolution.*

intention tremor. Tremor exhibited or intensified when attempting coordinated movements.

inter- [L.]. Prefix meaning in the midst, between.

interacinar (ĭn″tĕr-ăs′ĭ-năr) [L. *inter,* between, + *acinus,* grape]. Located between acini of a gland.

interalveolar (ĭn″tĕr-ăl-vē′ō-lăr) [″ + *alveolus,* little tub]. Between the alveoli, esp. the alveoli of the lungs.

interarticular [″ + *articulus,* joint]. 1. Between two joints. 2. Situated between two articulating surfaces.

interarytenoid (ĭn″tĕr-ăr″ē-tē′noyd) [″ + Gr. *arytaina,* ladle, + *eidos,* form]. Between the arytenoid cartilages of the larynx.

interatrial (ĭn″tĕr-ā′trē-ăl) [″ + *atrium,* hall]. Located between the atria of the heart. SYN: *interauricular* (def. 2).

interauricular (ĭn″tĕr-aw-rĭk′ū-lăr) [″ + *auricula,* little ear]. 1. Situated between the auricles or pinnae of the ears. 2. Interatrial.

interbrain [″ + AS. *braegen,* brain]. The hind original part of the forebrain including the thalamus, pineal body (epithalamus) and geniculate bodies (metathalamus). SYN: *diencephalon; thalamencephalon.*

intercadence (ĭn″tĕr-kā′dĕns) [″ + *cadere,* to fall]. A supernumerary pulse wave between two regular beats.

intercalary (ĭn-tĕr′kă-lĕr″ē) [″ + *calare,* to call]. 1. Inserted or interposed between. SYN: *extraneous; interposed.* 2. Pert. to an upstroke on a pulse tracing that comes between two pulse beats. SYN: *intercalated.*

intercalated (ĭn-tĕr′kăl-āt-ĕd). 1. Inserted between as something interposed. SYN: *extraneous.* 2. Pert. to an upstroke on a pulse tracing that comes between two pulse beats. SYN: *intercalary.*

intercalated ducts. Short, narrow ducts that lie between secretory ducts and the terminal alveoli in the parotid and submandibular glands and in the pancreas.

intercanalicular (ĭn″tĕr-kăn″ă-lĭk′ū-lăr) [″ + *canalicularis,* pert. to a canaliculus]. Between the canaliculi of a tissue.

intercapillary (ĭn″tĕr-kăp′ĭ-lăr-ē) [″ + *capillaris,* hairlike]. Between the capillaries.

intercarotic (ĭn″tĕr-kă-rŏt′ĭk) [L. *inter,* between, + Gr. *karos,* deep sleep]. Between the external and internal carotid arteries.

intercarpal (ĭn″tĕr-kăr′păl) [″ + Gr. *karpalis,* pert. to the carpus]. Between the carpal bones.

intercartilaginous (ĭn″tĕr-kăr″tĭ-lăj′ĭ-nŭs) [″ + *cartilago,* cartilage]. Connecting or between cartilages.

intercavernous (ĭn″tĕr-kăv′ĕr-nŭs) [″ + L. *caverna,* a hollow]. Between the cavernous sinuses.

intercellular (ĭn″tĕr-sĕl′ū-lăr) [″ + *cella,* compartment]. Between the cells of a structure.

intercerebral (ĭn″tĕr-sĕr′ĕ-brăl) [″ + *cerebrum,* brain]. Between the two cerebral hemispheres.

interchondral (ĭn″tĕr-kŏn′drăl) [″ + Gr. *chondros,* cartilage]. Between cartilages. SYN: *intercartilaginous.*

intercilium (ĭn″tĕr-sĭl′ē-ŭm) [″ + *cilium,* eyelash]. The space between the eyebrows. SYN: *glabella.*

interclavicular (ĭn″tĕr-klă-vĭk′ū-lăr) [″ + *clavicula,* clavicle]. Between the clavicles.

intercoccygeal (ĭn″tĕr-kŏk-sĭj′ē-ăl) [″ + Gr. *kokkyx,* coccyx]. Between the segments of the coccyx.

intercolumnar (ĭn″tĕr-kō-lŭm′năr) [″ + *columna,* column]. Between columns.

intercolumnar fascia. A membrane between pillars of the abdominal ring, enclosing the spermatic cord.

intercolumnar fibers. Intercrural fibers.

intercondylar, intercondyloid, intercondylous [″ + Gr. *kondylos,* knuckle]. Between two condyles.

intercostal [″ + *costa,* rib]. Between the ribs.

intercostal muscles, external. Outer layer of muscles between the ribs, originating on the lower margin of each rib and inserted on the upper margin of the next rib. They draw adjacent ribs together and act to increase the volume of the thorax.

intercostal muscles, internal. Muscles between the ribs, lying beneath the external intercostals. Their function is the same as the external intercostal muscles.

intercostobrachial (ĭn″tĕr-kŏs″tō-brā′kē-ăl) [″ + ″ + *brachium,* arm]. Pert. to the intercostal space and the arm, as the posterior lateral branch of the second intercostal nerve supplying the skin of the arm, or a similar branch of the third intercostal nerve. Formerly called intercostohumeralis.

intercostohumeral (ĭn″tĕr-kŏs-tō-hū′mĕr-ăl) [″ + ″ + *humerus,* upper arm]. Concerning or connecting an intercostal space and the humerus.

intercourse [L. *intercursus,* running between]. Social interaction between individuals or groups. Communication.

i., sexual. Coitus, q.v.

intercricothyrotomy (ĭn″tĕr-krī″kō-thī-rŏt′ō-mē) [L. *inter*, between, + Gr. *krikos*, ring, + *thyreos*, shield, + *eidos*, form, + *tome*, incision]. Surgical separation of the cricothyroid membrane in order to incise the larynx.

intercristal (ĭn″tĕr-krĭs′tăl) [″ + *crista*, crest]. Between two crests of a bone, organ, or process.

intercrural (ĭn″tĕr-krū′răl) [″ + *crus*, limb]. Between two crura.

intercurrent [″ + *currere*, to run]. 1. Intervening. 2. Pert. to a disease attacking a patient with another malady.

intercusping [″ + *cuspis*, point]. The natural fitting together of the surfaces of opposing teeth. SEE: *occlusion*.

interdental [″ + *dens*, tooth]. Between the teeth.

interdentium (ĭn″tĕr-dĕn′shē-ŭm). The space between any two contiguous teeth.

interdigitation [″ + *digitus*, digit]. 1. Interlocking of toothed or fingerlike processes. 2. Processes so interlocked.

interfascicular (ĭn″tĕr-făs-ĭk′ū-lăr) [″ + *fasciculus*, bundle]. Between fasciculi.

interfemoral [″ + *femoralis*, pert. to the thigh]. Between the thighs.

interference [″ + *ferire*, to strike]. Clashing or colliding.

interference of impulses. Condition in which two excitation waves, upon approaching each other and meeting in any part of the heart, are mutually extinguished.

interferometer (ĭn″tĕr-fēr-ŏm′ĕ-tĕr). Optical device that acts on the interference of two beams of light. This permits examination of the structure of spectral lines. Also used in examining prisms of lenses for faults.

interferon (ĭn-tĕr-fēr′ŏn). A protein or proteins formed when cells are exposed to viruses. Noninfected cells exposed to interferon are protected against viral infection. Interferons are specific for cells but not for viruses; thus, the same agent will induce a different interferon in different species or even in different cells in the same species. This material is extremely powerful, in that ten molecules can induce resistance of a cell to viruses. Interferons may be useful in treating a great number of diseases, including infections and neoplasms.

interfibrillar, interfibrillary (ĭn″tĕr-fĭb′rĭ-lăr, -rĭ-lăr″ē) [″ + *fibrilla*, a small fiber]. Between fibrils.

interfilamentous (ĭn″tĕr-fĭl″ă-mĕn′tŭs) [″ + *filamentum*, filament]. Between filaments.

interfilar (ĭn-tĕr-fī′lăr) [″ + *filum*, thread]. Between the fibrils of a reticulum.

interfilar mass. The fluid portion of the protoplasm.

interganglionic [″ + *ganglion*, a swelling]. Between ganglia.

intergemmal (ĭn″tĕr-jĕm′ăl) [″ + *gemma*, bud]. Between taste buds.

interglobular [″ + *globulus*, globule]. Between globules.

interglobular dentin. The dentin of the tooth that contains spaces or hypomineralized areas between mineralized globules or calcospherites.

interglobular spaces. Gaps in dentin due to failure of calcification. SYN: *Czermak's spaces*.

intergluteal (ĭn″tĕr-gloo′tē-ăl) [″ + Gr. *gloutos*, buttock]. Between the buttocks.

intergyral (ĭn″tĕr-jī′răl) [″ + Gr. *gyros*, circle]. Between the cerebral gyri.

interhemicerebral (ĭn″tĕr-hĕm″ĭ-sĕr′ĕ-brăl) [″ + Gr. *hemi*, half, + L. *cerebrum*, brain]. Intercerebral.

interictal (ĭn″tĕr-ĭk′tăl) [″ + *ictus*, a blow]. Between seizures.

interior [L. *internus*, within]. The internal portion or area of something; situated within.

interischiadic (ĭn″tĕr-ĭs″kē-ăd′ĭk) [L. *inter*, between, + Gr. *ischion*, hip]. Between the ischia of the pelvis.

interkinesis (ĭn″tĕr-kī-nē′sĭs) [″ + Gr. *kinesis*, motion]. Interval between first and second meiotic division of cells.

interlamellar (ĭn″tĕr-lă-mĕl′ăr) [″ + *lamella*, layer]. Between lamellae.

interlobar (ĭn″tĕr-lō′băr) [″ + *lobus*, lobe]. Between lobes.

interlobitis (ĭn″tĕr-lō-bī′tĭs) [″ + ″ + Gr. *itis*, inflammation]. Inflammation of the pleura separating the pulmonary lobes.

interlobular (ĭn″tĕr-lŏb′ū-lăr) [″ + *lobulus*, lobule]. Between lobules of an organ.

interlobular emphysema. Air between the lobes of the lung.

intermalleolar (ĭn″tĕr-mă-lē′ō-lăr) [″ + *malleolus*, little hammer]. Between the malleoli.

intermammary (ĭn″tĕr-măm′ă-rē) [″ + *mamma*, breast]. Between the breasts.

intermammillary (ĭn″tĕr-măm′ĭ-lăr″ē) [″ + *mammilla*, nipple]. Between the nipples of the breasts.

intermarriage [″ + *maritare*, to marry]. 1. Marriage between persons of two distinct populations. SEE: *miscegenation*. 2. Marriage between related individuals.

intermaxillary [″ + *maxilla*, jawbone]. Between two maxillae.

intermediary (ĭn″tĕr-mē′dē-ār-ē) [″ + *medius*, middle]. 1. Situated between two bodies. 2. Occurring between two periods of time.

intermediary metabolism. The series of intermediate compounds formed during digestion before the final excretion or oxidation products are formed or eliminated from the body.

intermediate (ĭn″tĕr-mē′dē-ĭt) [″ + *medius*,

middle]. Between the two extremes; after the beginning and before the end.

intermedin (ĭn″tĕr-mē′dĭn). A substance secreted by the pars intermedia of the pituitary. It is important in controlling pigment cells of the skin of some reptiles, fish, and amphibians.

intermediolateral [″ + ′ + *latus*, side]. Intermediate but not central.

intermedius (ĭn″tĕr-mē′dē-ŭs) [″ + *medius*, middle]. The middle of three structures.

intermembranous (ĭn″tĕr-mĕm′bră-nŭs) [″ + *membrana*, membrane]. Between membranes.

intermeningeal (ĭn″ter-mĕn-ĭn′jē-ăl) [″ + *meninx*, membrane]. Between the meninges.

intermenstrual (ĭn″tĕr-mĕn′stroo-ăl) [″ + Gr. *men*, month]. Between the menses or menstrual periods.

intermetacarpal (ĭn″tĕr-mĕt″ă-kăr′păl) [″ + Gr. *meta*, beyond, + *karpos*, wrist]. Between the carpal bones.

intermission [″ + *mittere*, to send]. 1. Interval between two paroxysms of a disease. 2. Temporary cessation of symptoms.

intermittence [″ + *mittere*, to send]. 1. Condition marked by intermissions in the course of a disease or of a process. 2. A loss of one or more pulse beats.

intermittent (ĭn″tĕr-mĭt′ĕnt). Suspending activity at intervals. Coming and going.

intermittent fever. Fever in which there is complete absence of symptoms between paroxysms. SEE: *malaria; undulant fever.*

intermittent positive-pressure breathing. ABBR: IPPB. Method used to assist breathing. The patient breathes through a mask connected to a device that produces intermittent positive air pressure. When the pressure is increased, the lungs are inflated, and then the pressure is released and the patient exhales.

intermittent pulse. Pulse in which a beat is dropped at intervals.

intermural (ĭn″tĕr-mū′răl) [L. *inter*, between, + *murus*, wall]. Between the walls or sides of an organ.

intermuscular [″ + *musculus*, muscle]. Between muscles.

intern (ĭn′tĕrn) [L. *internus*, within]. Physician or surgeon on a hospital staff, usually a recent graduate receiving a year of postgraduate training prior to being eligible to be licensed to practice medicine. SEE: *extern(e)*.

internal [L. *internus*, within]. Within the body. Within or on the inside; enclosed; inward. Opposite of external.

internal bleeding. Hemorrhage from an internal organ or site, esp. the gastrointestinal tract.

internal ear. The vestibule, semicircular canals, and cochlea of the ear.

internal injury. Any injury not visible from the outside, as injury to the organs occupying the thoracic, abdominal, or cranial cavities.

SYM: Vary with structures involved. Ordinarily, profound shock. Patient is pale, cold, perspiring freely, has an anxious expression, may be semicomatose. Pain usually intense at first, and may continue or gradually diminish as patient grows worse. In severe injuries, pain may not be manifested. The pulse is very feeble, fast, often irregular. Patient may be very restless, breathless, and usually has shallow respiration.

F.A.: Above all, patient should be kept very quiet and comfortably warm but not hot. Do not give anything by mouth. Do not give stimulants because they may exaggerate bleeding. Transportation must be done very cautiously. If patient is in shock, shoulders should be lowered and the lower extremities elevated at least 45°.

internalization (ĭn-tĕr″năl-ī-zā′shŭn). The unconscious mental mechanism in which the values and standards of society and one's parents are taken as one's own.

internal secretion. Secretion of the ductless glands, which, entering the bloodstream, activates other glands and organs. SYN: *hormones*. SEE: *ductless glands; endocrine; hormone; secretion*.

internarial (ĭn″tĕr-nā′rē-ăl) [L. *inter*, between, + *nares*, nostrils]. Between the nares.

internasal (ĭn″tĕr-nā′zăl) [″ + *nasus*, nose]. Between the nasal bones.

internatal (ĭn″tĕr-nā′tăl) [″ + *nates*, buttocks]. Between the buttocks.

International Classification of Diseases. A standard originated by the World Health Organization for classifying and coding diseases and medical conditions. A 5-digit code is also provided for diagnoses. This system of keeping records is encouraged to provide international standards for comparison of disease prevalence and treatment. The ninth revision (ICD-9) was adopted in January 1979. A Clinical Modification of ICD-9 has been proposed to cover health service research and the indexing of hospital records.

International Symbol of Access. A symbol used to identify buildings and facilities that are barrier-free and therefore accessible to disabled persons with restricted mobility, including wheelchair users. SEE: illus.

International System of Units. ABBR: SI. An internationally standardized system of units. The basic quantity measured and the names of the units are: meter (length), kilogram (mass), second (time), ampere (electric current), Kelvin (temperature), candela (luminous intensity), and mole (amount of a substance). All other units of measurement are derived from these seven basic units.

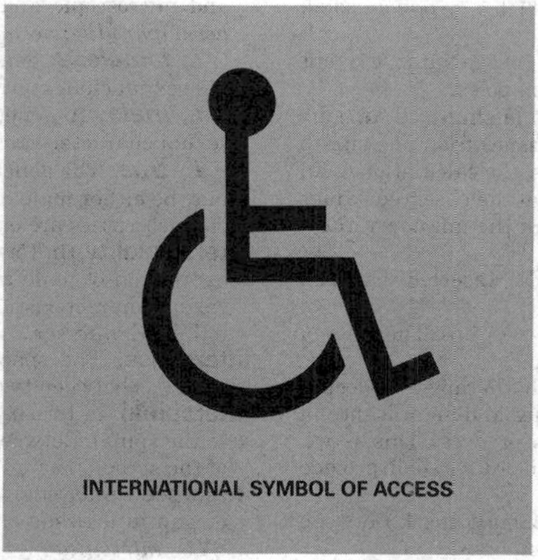

SEE: *Units of Measurement* in *Appendix*.

international unit. ABBR: I.U. An internationally accepted amount of a substance. Usually this form of expressing quantity is used for fat-soluble vitamins and some hormones, enzymes, and biologicals such as vaccines. These units are defined by the International Conference for Unification of Formulae.

interneuron (ĭn″tĕr-nū′rŏn) [L. *inter,* between, + Gr. *neuron,* nerve]. A neuron located between neurons in a chain of neurons.

internist. A physician who specializes in internal medicine.

internode [″ + *nodus,* knot]. Space between adjacent nodes.

internship (ĭn′tĕrn-shĭp). The period an intern spends in training, usually in a hospital.

internuclear (ĭn″tĕr-nū′klē-ăr) [″ + *nucleus,* a kernel]. 1. Between nuclei. 2. Between outer and inner nuclear layers of the retina.

internuncial (ĭn″tĕr-nŭn′shē-ăl) [″ + *nuncius,* messenger]. Acting as a connecting medium.

internuncial neuron. Neuron situated between two other neurons in a neural pathway.

internus (ĭn-tĕr′nŭs) [L., within]. Internal.

interocclusal (ĭn″tĕr-ŏ-kloo′zăl) [L. *inter,* between, + *occlusio,* a shutting up]. Between the occlusal surfaces of opposed teeth.

interoceptive [L. *internus,* within, + *capere,* to take]. In nerve physiology, concerned with sensations arising within the body itself, as distinguished from those arising outside the body.

interoceptor (ĭn″tĕr-ō-sĕp′tor). A receptor activated by stimuli within the body.

i., general. An end-organ carrying sensations of hunger, thirst, visceral pain, nausea, sexual and circulatory sensations.

i., special. A receptor for smell and taste.

interofective (ĭn″tĕr-ō-fĕk′tĭv) [″ + *afficere,* to influence]. Pert. to that which concerns the interior of an organism.

interoinferior (ĭn″tĕr-ō-ĭn-fē′rē-or) [″ + *inferus,* below]. Pert. to an inward and downward position.

interolivary [L. *inter,* between, + *oliva,* olive]. Between the olivary bodies.

interorbital [″ + *orbita,* orbit]. Between the orbits.

interosseous [″ + *os,* bone] (pl. *interossei*) Situated or occurring between bones, as muscles, ligaments, or vessels; specific muscles of the hands and feet.

interpalpebral (ĭn″tĕr-păl′pĕ-brăl) [″ + *palpebra,* eyelid]. Between the eyelids.

interparietal (ĭn″tĕr-pă-rī′ĕ-tăl) [″ + *paries,* wall]. 1. Between walls. 2. Between the parietal bones. 3. Between the parietal lobes of the cerebrum.

interparietal bone. Squamous portion of the occipital bone.

interparietal suture. Sagittal suture.

interparoxysmal (ĭn″tĕr-păr″ŏk-sĭz′măl) [″ + Gr. *paroxysmos,* spasm]. Between paroxysms.

interpeduncular (ĭn″tĕr-pē-dŭnk′ū-lăr) [L. *inter,* between, + *pedunculus,* peduncle]. Between peduncles.

interpersonal. Concerning the relations and interactions between persons.

interphalangeal (ĭn″tĕr-fă-lăn′jē-ăl) [″ + Gr. *phalanx,* phalanx]. In a joint between two phalanges.

interphase. 1. The resting stage of a cell between divisions. 2. The area or zone where two phases of a substance, such as a gas and a liquid, contact each other.

interpolar (ĭn″tĕr-pō′lăr) [″ + *polus*, pole]. Between two poles.

interpolar path. Path of galvanic current through tissues between poles.

interpolation (ĭn-tĕr″pō-lā′shŭn). 1. In surgery, the transfer of tissues from one site to another. 2. In statistics, the calculation of an intermediate value from the observed values larger and smaller than the unknown intermediate.

interposed (ĭn′tĕr-pōzd). Inserted between parts.

interposition (ĭn″tĕr-pō-zĭsh′ŭn). The state of being interposed.

interpretation. In psychotherapy, the deeper analysis of the meaning and significance of what the patient says or does. This is explained to the patient in order to help provide insight.

interproximal [″ + *proximus*, next]. Between two adjoining surfaces.

interproximal space. Triangular space between two adjacent teeth.

interpubic (ĭn-tĕr-pū′bĭk) [″ + *pubes*, pubes]. Between the pubic bones.

interpupillary [″ + *pupilla*, pupil]. Between the pupils.

interpupillary distance Distance between centers of the pupils of the eyes.

interradicular. Between the roots of teeth; the furcation area.

interradicular bone. The alveolar bone between the roots of multirooted teeth.

interradicular fibers. The collagen fibers of the periodontal ligament in the interradicular area, attaching the tooth to alveolar bone.

interrenal (ĭn″tĕr-rē′năl) [L. *inter*, between, + *ren*, kidney]. Between the kidneys.

interscapilium (ĭn″tĕr-skă-pĭl′ē-ŭm) [″ + *scapula*, shoulder blade]. Area between the shoulders or scapulae. SYN: *interscapular.*

interscapular. Between the scapulae.

interscapular reflex. Scapular muscular contraction following percussion or stimulus between the scapulae.

interscapulum (ĭn-tĕr-skăp′ū-lŭm). Section of back between the shoulder blades. SYN: *interscapilium.*

intersection. The site where one structure crosses another or joins a similar structure.

intersegmental (ĭn″tĕr-sĕg-mĕn′tăl) [″ + *segmentum*, a portion]. Between segments.

interseptal (ĭn″tĕr-sĕp′tăl) [″ + *saeptum*, a partition]. Between two septa.

intersex (ĭn′tĕr-sĕks). An individual having both male and female characteristics. The term has some descriptive but little or no diagnostic value. Determination of sex in individuals who appear to have both male and female characteristics is a complex task. The diagnosis should be made after careful study of the chromosomes and of the gross and microscopic anatomical findings. SEE: *hermaphrodite; hermaphroditism.*

i., female. A genetic female with external sexual characteristics of both sexes.

i., male. A genetic male with external sexual characteristics of both sexes.

i., true. The genetic sex of the individual may be either male or female and the sexual characteristics are of both sexes.

intersexuality (ĭn″tĕr-sĕks″ū-ăl′ĭ-tē). Varying expression of male and female physical and sexual characteristics in the same individual. SEE: *intersex.*

interspace. The space between two similar parts, as between two ribs.

interspinal (ĭn-tĕr-spī′năl) [″ + *spinalis*, pert. to the spine]. Between two spinous processes of the spine.

interstice (ĭn-tĕr′stĭs) [L. *interstitium*]. A space or gap in a tissue or structure of an organ. SYN: *interstitium.*

interstitial (ĭn″tĕr-stĭsh′ăl). 1. Placed or lying between. 2. Pert. to interstices or spaces within an organ or tissue.

interstitial cells of testes. Cells of Leydig located in groups between the seminiferous tubules. They produce the hormone (testosterone) of the testes.

interstitial cell–stimulating hormone. ABBR: ICSH. Luteinizing hormone. SEE: *hormone, luteinizing.*

interstitial fluid. The fluid that surrounds cells.

interstitial tissue. Intercellular connective tissue.

interstitium (ĭn″tĕr-stĭsh′ē-ŭm) [L.]. The very small space between body parts, tissues, or cells.

intersystole (ĭn″tĕr-sĭs′tō-lē) [L. *inter*, between, + Gr. *systole*, contraction]. The period between the end of the atrial systole and the commencement of the ventricular systole.

intertarsal (ĭn″tĕr-tăr′săl) [″ + Gr. *tarsos*, a broad, flat surface]. Between the tarsal bones of the foot.

intertransverse (ĭn″tĕr-trăns-vĕrs′) [″ + *transversus*, turned across]. Between vertebrae or joining the transverse processes of a vertebra.

intertriginous (ĭn″tĕr-trĭj′ĭ-nŭs). Having the character of intertrigo or having intertrigo.

intertrigo (ĭn″tĕr-trī′gō) [″ + *terere*, to rub]. A superificial dermatitis in the folds of the skin. SEE: *erythema intertrigo.*

intertrochanteric (ĭn″tĕr-trō″kăn-tĕr′ĭk) [″ + Gr. *trochanter*, trochanter]. Situated between the greater and lesser trochanters of the femur.

intertrochanteric line. The ridge between the greater and lesser trochanters of the femur on the posterior aspect of the bone.

intertubular (ĭn″tĕr-tū′bū-lăr) [″ + *tubulus*,

tubule]. Between or among tubules.

interureteral, interureteric (ĭn″tĕr-ū-rē′tĕr-ăl, ĭn″tĕr-ū″rē-tĕr′ĭk) [″ + Gr. *oureter,* ureter]. Between the two ureters.

intervaginal (ĭn″tĕr-văj′ĭ-năl) [″ + *vagina,* sheath]. Between sheaths.

interval [″ + *vallum,* a breastwork]. 1. The space or time between two objects or periods. 2. Break in the course of disease or between paroxysms.

i., atriocarotid. In a venous pulse tracing, the interval between onset of the presystolic wave (a) and the systolic (c) wave. It indicates the time required for impulses to travel from the S-A node to the ventricle, normally about 0.2 sec.

i., A-V. Interval between the beginning of atrial systole and ventricular systole, measured in man from an electrocardiogram.

i., cardioarterial. The time between the apex beat and radial pulsation.

i., focal. Distance between the anterior and posterior focal points of the eyes.

i., isometric. Distance between onset of ventricular systole and opening of the semilunar valves. SYN: *i., presphygmic.*

i., lucid. Brief remission of symptoms in a psychosis.

i., passive. The rest period of the heart.

i., postsphygmic. Interval between closure of the semilunar valves and opening of semilunar valves and opening of atrioventricular valves.

i., P-R. In the electrocardiogram, period between the onset of the P wave and the beginning of the QRS complex.

i., presphygmic. Brief period between the ventricular systole and opening of the semilunar valves. SYN: *i., isometric.*

i., Q-R. In the electrocardiogram, period between the onset of the QRS complex and the peak of the R wave.

i., QRST. The ventricular complex of the electrocardiogram. SEE: *electrocardiogram* for illus.

intervalvular (ĭn″tĕr-văl′vū-lăr) [L. *inter,* between, + *valva,* a fold]. Between valves, esp. the heart valves.

intervascular [″ + *vasculum,* a vessel]. Situated between blood vessels.

intervention (ĭn″tĕr-vĕn′shŭn). Taking actions so as to modify an effect.

i., crisis. In psychiatry, the immediate institution of all appropriate forms of therapy for an individual experiencing a personal crisis.

i., nursing. The activities of a nurse in caring for patients. This may include activities at all levels from the usual patient-care tasks to noting changes in the patient's condition that require immediate nursing staff action or notification of the attending physician or both.

interventricular [″ + *ventriculum,* a small cavity]. Between the ventricles.

intervertebral [″ + *vertebra,* joint]. Situated between two adjacent vertebrae.

intervertebral disk. Broad and flattened disk of fibrocartilage between the bodies of vertebrae. SEE: *herniated disk.*

intervillous (ĭn″tĕr-vĭl′ŭs) [″ + *villus,* tuft]. Between villi.

intestinal [L. *intestinum,* intestine]. Pert. to the intestines. SEE: *digestion; intestine.*

intestinal bypass surgery. Production of controlled intestinal malabsorption by surgically short-circuiting the small intestine. This is done by anastomosing the jejunum to the ileum and removing the small intestine between the anastomotic sites. This surgical procedure is used in treatment of massive obesity.

intestinal flora. The bacteria present in the intestines. The chemical nature of the contents of the intestines varies considerably with respect to the portion of the tract being considered. There are no bacteria in the intestines at birth but they are present very shortly thereafter. Favorable bacteria may protect the body from invasion by unfavorable ones, which cannot thrive in an acid condition. Also, certain medicines, particularly antibiotics, may cause drastic alterations in the number and kinds of bacteria present.

intestinal gases. Gaseous compounds, such as carbon dioxide, hydrogen, methane, methylmercaptan, and hydrogen sulfide, present in the intestinal tract. These are produced by digestive processes. SEE: *digestion.*

intestinal juice. An imprecise term used to denote the liquid substances secreted into the intestine, esp. the small intestine. It contains a number of enzymes, peptidases, lipase, maltase, and sucrase. Each is important in digesting food.

intestinal obstruction. Blockage of the lumen of the intestine.

Acute: Small intestine usually involved. Due to intussusception, strangulation, volvulus (twists), foreign bodies, adhesions, tumors, stricture, and gallstones in intestines. Auscultation of the abdomen may reveal a high-pitched tinkle or no sound at all.

SYM: Pain localized and intense. Temperature subnormal or normal; vomiting, constipation, and distention of abdomen.

TREATMENT: Relief of intestinal and gastric distention by use of gastric and intestinal suction tubes. Fluid balance must be maintained. Surgical exploration may be necessary to determine the cause. Parenteral antibodies are indicated for peritonitis.

Chronic: Involves large intestine. Due to

stricture, inflammation, abscesses, tumors, fecal matter or chronic peritonitis; gallstones may obstruct feces. Gradual constipation, pain becoming more severe in a few days followed by acute symptoms.

intestinal perforation. Abdominal crisis due to escape of contents of perforated intestines into the peritoneal cavity. SEE: *perforation of stomach or intestine*.

Test: Administration of 50 to 60 ml. of diatrizoate by mouth. If there is an intestinal perforation, the substance will enter the peritoneal cavity and be absorbed and excreted in the urine. If the gastrointestinal tract is intact, diatrizoate will not be absorbed. The test is negative if the intestinal perforation is sealed off prior to administration of the dye.

Diatrizoate is detected by precipitating it in the urine and adding concentrated hydrochloric acid one drop at a time. Some antibiotics, particularly penicillin, will also cause a precipitation in the urine when hydrochloric acid is added. However diatrizoate in the urine causes a greater increase in specific gravity than penicillin.

intestinal putrefaction. The chemical changes by bacteria in the intestine, forming the following: indole, skatole, paracresol, phenol, phenylpropionic acid, phenylacetic acid, paraoxyphenylacetic acid, hydroparacumaric acid, fatty acids, carbon dioxide, hydrogen, methane, methylmercaptan, and sulfurated hydrogen.

intestinal reflex. Intestinal contraction and relaxation above a portion of bowel that is stimulated.

intestinal tubes. Flexible tubes, usually made of plastic or rubber, placed in the intestinal tract for the purpose of sucking gas, fluid, or solids from the stomach or intestines; or for administering fluids, electrolytes, or nutrients to the patient. The tubes may be passed through the nose, mouth, or anus, or through a colostomy opening.

NURSING IMPLICATIONS: When an intestinal tube is inserted, the nurse must aid its movement into the intestinal tract. The patient is usually placed on the right side for a half hour, then the left side for a half hour, and then on the back. These position changes, as well as ambulation, will facilitate movement of the tube into the intestinal tract.

Because the tube may drain feces, the drainage should be kept from the patient's view. Frequent oral hygiene is needed to prevent oral ulceration because the patient will not be taking fluids by mouth. When the tube is removed, the patient's emotional reaction must be considered. Immediate oral hygiene is done, particularly since drainage from the tube can easily cause the patient to become nauseated.

While the tube is in, teach the patient not to mouth breathe or to swallow air. These enhance the entry of air into the gastrointestinal tract and work counter to the principle of intestinal tubes and drainage.

intestine (ĭn-tĕs'tĭn) [L. *intestinum*]. The alimentary canal extending from the pylorus to the anus. It is divided into the small intestine and large intestine or colon. The length of the intestine given is based on measurements made at autopsy. During life the small intestine is approx. 7 meters (23 feet) long. The total surface of the inside of the small intestine is estimated to be 800 square meters (8,611 square feet or 956.8 square yards).

PALPATION: Fecal accumulations feel similar to tumors but are hard and resistant; however, if one finger is pressed steadily upon them for one or two minutes, they will indent. They most frequently collect in descending colon.

PERCUSSION: In normal conditions, the large intestine furnishes a more amphoric percussion sound than the stomach. When filled with liquid or solid accumulations, the situation of these accumulations can be marked out on the surface by dullness on percussion. Because these accumulations most frequently occur in the descending colon, the percussion sound over this portion is usually less resonant than over the ascending or transverse colon.

i., large. The large intestine extends from the ileum to the anus and consists of the cecum with vermiform appendix, colon, and rectum. The mucous coat resembles that of small intestine, although glands are smaller. The large intestine resorbs fluid from the intestinal contents. If the bowel is hyperactive, diarrhea is likely to occur.

The beginning of the large intestine is the cecum, a pouch situated on the right side, adjoining the ascending colon. Attached to the cecum is the vermiform appendix, about 7.5 to 10.4 cm. (3 to 4 in.) long. The colon is approx. 1.5 meters (5 ft.) in length. The first portion of ascending colon extends from the cecum to the undersurface of the liver, where it turns to the left as the transverse colon. Its bend is the right colic or hepatic flexure. The transverse colon passes horizontally to the left to the region of the spleen, where it turns downward as the descending colon. This turn is the splenic flexure. The descending colon continues downward on the left side of the abdomen until it reaches the pelvic brim and curves like the letter S and is placed in front of the sacrum to become the rectum. This S-shaped section is known as the sigmoid colon. The rectum, about 10.2 to 12.7 cm. (4 to 5 in.) long, passes downward to terminate in the lower opening of the tract, the anus or anal opening.

i., small. The small intestine begins with the duodenum, approx. 20.3 cm. to 25.4 cm. (8 to 10 in.) long, which receives the food mass from the stomach through the pylorus, the bile from the liver and gallbladder, and the pancreatic juice from the pancreas. It connects with the jejunum, about 2.8 meters (9 feet) long. The jejunum, in turn, joins the ileum or twisted intestine, about 4.2 meters (13.7 ft.) long, which is attached to the large intestine by the ileocecal or colic valve, which controls passage of food into the large intestine.

In the wall of the small intestine are the Brunner's glands, intestinal glands (crypts of Lieberkühn), blood and lymph vessels (lacteals), and lymphatic tissue in the form of solitary nodules or aggregated nodules (Peyer's patches). The inner surface is thrown into folds (circular folds). Lining the entire surface are minute fingerlike villi through which the products of digestion (simple sugars, amino acids, and fatty acids and carbohydrates) are absorbed. The villi are from 0.5 to 1.5 mm. long and there are from 10 to 40 per sq. mm. of intestinal mucosa. SEE: *digestive system* for illus.

intestinum (ĭn″tĕs-tī′nŭm) [L.]. (pl. *intestina*) Intestine.

i. crassum. [NA] The large intestine.

i. rectum. The rectum.

i. tenue. [NA] The small intestine.

intima (ĭn′tĭ-mă) [L.]. [NA] Innermost coat of a structure, as a blood vessel. SYN: *tunica intima.*

intimal (ĭn′tĭ-măl). Pert. to the inner coat of a blood vessel, the intima.

intimitis (ĭn″tĭ-mī′tĭs) [L. *intima*, innermost, + Gr. *itis*, inflammation]. Inflammation of an intima.

intolerance [L. *in-*, not, + *tolerare*, to bear]. Inability to endure or incapacity for bearing pain or the effects of a drug or other substance.

intorsion (ĭn-tor′shŭn) [L. *in*, toward, + *torsio*, twisting]. Rotation of the eye inward toward the nose on the anterior-posterior axis of the eye. In this condition, twelve o'clock on the corneal margin would be closer to the nose than normal.

intoxicant (ĭn-tŏks′ĭ-kănt). An agent that produces intoxication.

intoxication [L. *in*, in, + Gr. *toxikon*, poison]. 1. State of being intoxicated, esp. of being poisoned by a drug or toxic substance. 2. Intoxicated from overindulgence in alcoholic beverages.

The determination of alcohol content of the blood (i.e., ethyl alcohol, the alcohol present in commercial beverages such as beer, wine, and whiskey) is frequently of value in the diagnosis of intoxication from alcohol, esp. in differentiating other disorders. Normally the alcohol content of body tissues and fluids is negligible. Upon ingestion, alcoholic fluids are absorbed slowly or quickly depending upon the amount swallowed, presence of food in the stomach, and rate of gastric emptying. The amount of alcohol found in each ml. of blood will also depend upon body size. Thus if 70 kg. (154 lb.) and 90 kg. (198 lb.) individuals drink the same amount of alcohol in the same time and under similar conditions, the concentration of alcohol in each ml. of blood will be least in the person who weighs the most.

The amount of alcohol present in expired air will also provide an estimate of the alcohol content of the blood. The amount of alcohol present in the blood does not provide completely valid information about the degree of intoxication because of the ability of the central nervous system to adapt to alcohol. SEE: *alcoholism; breathalyzer.*

i., water. Intoxication resulting from excessive intake or undue retention of water.

intra- [L.]. Prefix meaning within.

intra-abdominal [L. *intra*, within, + *abdomen*, belly]. Within the abdomen.

intra-acinous (ĭn-tră-ăs′ĭ-nŭs) [″ + *acinus*, grape]. Within an acinus.

intra-aortic balloon counterpulsation. ABBR: IABC. The use of a balloon attached to a catheter inserted through the femoral artery into the descending thoracic aorta for producing alternating inflation and deflation during diastole and systole respectively. This permits lowering resistance to aortic blood flow during systole and increasing resistance during diastole. The result is to decrease the work of the heart and to increase flow of blood to the coronary arteries. The inflation of the balloon is accomplished by using helium. This method is useful in treating shock.

intra-arterial [″ + Gr. *arteria*, artery]. Within the artery(ies).

intra-articular (ĭn″tră-ăr-tĭk′ū-lăr) [″ + *articulus*, little joint]. Within a joint.

intra-atrial (ĭn″tră-ā′trē-ăl [″ + Gr. *atrion*, hall]. Within the atrium or atria of the heart.

intrabronchial (ĭn″tră-brŏng′kē-ăl) [″ + Gr. *bronchos*, windpipe]. Within a bronchus.

intrabuccal (ĭn″tră-bŭk′ăl) [″ + *bucca*, cheek]. Within the tissue of the cheek or within the mouth.

intracanalicular (ĭn″tră-kăn″ă-lĭk′ū-lăr) [″ + *canalicularis*, pert. to a canaliculus]. Within a canaliculus.

intracapsular [″ + *capsula*, little box]. Within a capsule.

intracapsular fracture. A fracture occurring within the capsule of a joint.

intracardiac. Within the heart.
intracarpal (ĭn″tră-kăr′păl) [″ + Gr. *karpalis,* pert. to the carpus]. Within the wrist.
intracartilaginous (ĭn″tră-kăr″tĭ-lăj′ĭn-ŭs) [″ + *cartilago,* gristle]. Within a cartilage or cartilaginous tissue.
intracellular (ĭn″tră-sĕl′ū-lăr) [″ + *cellula,* cell]. Within cells.
intracerebellar (ĭn″tră-sĕr″ĕ-bĕl′ăr) [″ + *cerebellum,* little brain]. Within the cerebellum of the brain.
intracerebral (ĭn″tră-sĕr′ĕ-brăl) [″ + *cerebrum,* brain]. Within the main portion of the brain.
intracervical (ĭn″tră-sĕr′vĭ-kăl) [″ + *cervicalis,* pert. to the neck]. In the cervical canal of the uterus.
intracisternal (ĭn″tră-sĭs-tĕr′năl) [″ + *cisterna,* cavity]. Within a cistern of the brain.
intracostal (ĭn″tră-kŏs′tăl) [″ + *costa,* rib]. On the inner surface of a rib.
intracranial [″ + Gr. *kranion,* skull]. Within the cranium or skull.
intractable (ĭn-trăk′tă-b′l) Incurable or resistant to therapy.
intracutaneous [″ + *cutis,* skin]. Within the substance of the skin. SYN: *intradermal.*
intracutaneous injection. Hypodermic injection into the skin.
intracutaneous reaction. Reaction following injection of a substance into the skin. SYN: *intradermoreaction.*
intracystic [″ + Gr. *kystis,* bladder]. Inside a bladder or cyst.
intrad (ĭn′trăd). Inwardly; toward the inner part.
intradermal [″ + Gr. *derma,* skin]. ABBR: ID. Within the substance of the skin. SYN: *intracutaneous.*
intradermoreaction (ĭn′tră-dĕr″mō-rē-ăk′shŭn) [″ + ″ + L. *re,* back, + *agere,* to do]. Reaction resulting from the injection of a reagent into substance of the skin. SYN: *intracutaneous reaction.*
intraduct (ĭn′tră-dŭkt) [″ + *ductus,* a canal]. Inside a duct.
intraduodenal (ĭn″tră-dū″ō-dē′năl) [″ + *duodeni,* twelve]. Within the duodenum.
intradural (ĭn-tră-dū′răl) [″ + *durus,* hard]. Within or enclosed by the dura mater.
intraepidermal (ĭn″tră-ĕp″ĭ-dĕr′măl) [L. *intra,* within, + Gr. *epi,* upon, + *derma,* skin]. Within the epidermis.
intraepithelial (ĭn″tră-ĕp″ĭ-thē′lē-ăl) [″ + ″ + *thele,* nipple]. Within the epithelium or located between its cells.
intrafebrile [″ + *febris,* fever]. During the febrile stage. SYN: *intrapyretic.*
intrafilar (ĭn-tră-fī′lăr) [″ + *filum,* thread]. Within a network or reticulum.
intragastric [″ + Gr. *gaster,* belly]. Within the stomach.
intragemmal (ĭn″tră-jĕm′ăl) [″ + *gemma,* bud]. Within a bud or the expanded ending of a nerve, as a taste bud.
intraglandular [″ + *glans,* acorn]. Within a gland.
intragyral (ĭn″tră-jī′răl) [″ + Gr. *gyros,* circle]. Within a gyrus of the brain.
intrahepatic (ĭn″tră-hĕ-păt′ĭk) [″ + Gr. *hepatikos,* pert. to the liver]. Within the liver.
intraintestinal [″ + *intestinum,* intestine]. Within the intestine.
intralaryngeal (ĭn″tră-lă-rĭn′jē-ăl) [″ + Gr. *larynx,* larynx]. Within the larynx.
intralesional (ĭn″tră-lē′zhŭn-ăl) [″ + *laesio,* a wound]. Within a lesion.
intraligamentary [″ + *ligamentum,* a binding]. Within the leaves of a ligament. Usually used in referring to fibroid tumors or cysts of the ovary that have grown within the broad ligament.
intraligamentous. Within a ligament.
intralobar (ĭn″tră-lō′băr) [″ + *lobus,* a lobe]. Within a lobe.
intralobular (ĭn″tră-lŏb′ū-lăr) [″ + *lobulus,* a lobule]. Within a lobule.
intralocular (ĭn″tră-lŏk′ū-lăr) [″ + *loculus,* a cavity]. Within the cavity of any structure.
intralumbar [″ + *lumbus,* loin]. Within the lumbar region or portion of the spinal cord.
intraluminal (ĭn″tră-lū′mĭ-năl) [″ + *lumen,* light]. Within any tubular structure. SYN: *intratubal.*
intramastoiditis (ĭn″tră-măs″tŏyd-ī′tĭs) [″ + Gr. *mastos,* breast, + *eidos,* form, + *itis,* inflammation]. Inflammation of the antrum and mastoid process. SYN: *endomastoiditis.*
intramedullary (ĭn″tră-mĕd′ū-lăr″ē) [″ + *medullaris,* marrow]. 1. Within the medulla oblongata of the brain. 2. Within the spinal cord. 3. Within the marrow cavity of a bone.
intramural [″ + *murus,* a wall]. Within the walls of a hollow organ or cavity.
intramuscular [″ + *musculus,* a muscle]. ABBR: I.M. Within a muscle.
intramuscular injection. Injection of drugs into a muscle.
intranasal [″ + *nasus,* nose]. Within the nasal cavity.
intraocular [″ + *oculus,* eye]. Within the eyeball.
intraoperative (ĭn″tră-ŏp′ĕr-ă″tĭv) [L. *intra,* within, + *operativus,* working]. Occurring during surgery.
intraoral [″ + *oralis,* pert. to the mouth]. Within the mouth.
intraorbital [″ + *orbita,* mark of a wheel]. Within the orbit.
intraosseous (ĭn″tră-ŏs′ē-ŭs) [″ + *os,* bone]. Within the bone substance.
intraovarian (ĭn″tră-ō-vā′rē-ăn) [″ + *ovarium,* ovary]. Within the ovary.
intraparietal (ĭn″tră-pă-rī′ĕ-tăl) [″ + *paries,*

wall]. 1. Within the parietal lobe of the cerebrum. 2. Intramural.

intrapartum (ĭn″tră-păr′tŭm) [″ + *partus,* birth]. Happening during childbirth.

intrapelvic (ĭn″tră-pĕl′vĭk) [″ + *pelvis,* basin]. Within the pelvis.

intraperitoneal [″ + Gr. *peritonaion,* peritoneum]. Within the peritoneal cavity.

intraplacental (ĭn″tră-plă-sĕn′tăl) [″ + *placenta,* a flat cake]. Within the placenta.

intrapleural [″ + Gr. *pleura,* rib]. Within the pleural cavity.

intrapontine (ĭn″tră-pŏn′tĭn) [″ + *pons,* bridge]. Within the pons varolii.

intrapsychic, intrapsychical (ĭn″tră-sī′kĭk, -kĭ-kăl) [″ + Gr. *psyche,* mind]. Having a mental origin or basis, such as conflicts and complexes.

intrapulmonary [″ + *pulmo,* lung]. Within the lung substance.

intrapyretic (ĭn″tră-pī-rĕt′ĭk) [″ + Gr. *pyretos,* fever]. During the period of fever. SYN: *intrafebrile.*

intrarectal (ĭn″tră-rĕk′tăl) [″ + *rectum,* straight]. Within the rectum.

intrarenal (ĭn″tră-rē′năl) [″ + *renalis,* pert. to the kidney]. Within the kidney.

intraretinal (ĭn″tră-rĕt′ĭ-năl) [″ + *retina,* retina]. Within the retina of the eye.

intrascrotal (ĭn″tră-skrō′tăl) [″ + *scrotum,* a bag]. Within the scrotum.

intraspinal [L. *intra,* within, + *spina,* spine]. 1. Ensheathed, within a sheath. 2. Within the spinal canal.

intrathecal (ĭn″tră-thē′kăl) [″ + Gr. *theke,* sheath]. 1. Within the spinal canal. 2. Within a sheath.

intrathoracic (ĭn″tră-thō-răs′ĭk) [″ + Gr. *thorax,* chest]. Within the thorax.

intratracheal (ĭn″tră-trăk′ē-ăl) [″ + Gr. *tracheia,* trachea]. Introduced into, or inside, the trachea.

intratracheal anesthesia. Anesthesia administered through a catheter passed down the trachea.

intratubal [″ + *tubus,* hollow tube]. Within a tube, esp. the fallopian tube. SYN: *intraluminal.*

intratympanic (ĭn″tră-tĭm-păn′ĭk) [″ + Gr. *tympanon,* drum]. Within the tympanic cavity.

intrauterine (ĭn″tră-ū′tĕr-ĭn) [″ + *uterus,* womb]. Within the uterus.

intrauterine contraceptive device. ABBR: I.U.C.D. or I.U.D. Device made in a variety of shapes and from several different materials, including plastic and copper, and placed in the uterus for a prolonged period of time to prevent conception.

intravasation (ĭn-trăv″ă-zā′shŭn) [″ + *vas,* vessel]. Passage into the blood vessels of matter formed outside of them through traumatic or pathological lesions

intravascular. Within blood vessels.

intravenous (ĭn-tră-vē′nŭs) [′ + *vena,* vein]. ABBR: I.V. Within or into a vein.

intravenous feeding. Providing total nutritional requirements intravenously; essential in treating some diseases. This is accomplished by carefully controlling the composition of fluid given with respect to total calories derived from protein hydrolysate and dextrose, and the electrolytes, minerals, and vitamins. Patients have been maintained for months on nothing but the nutrients and fluids given intravenously, usually through a major vein, such as the subclavian or the jugular. SEE: *parenteral hyperalimentation.*

intravenous infusion. Injection into a vein of a solution to secure an immediate result as in hemorrhage, shock, or collapse. SEE: illus.

SOLUTIONS: Many liquid preparations are given by intravenous infusion. Those commonly used include isotonic saline, Ringer's solution, 1/6 molar sodium lactate, dextrose

INTRAVENOUS INFUSION TECHNIQUE

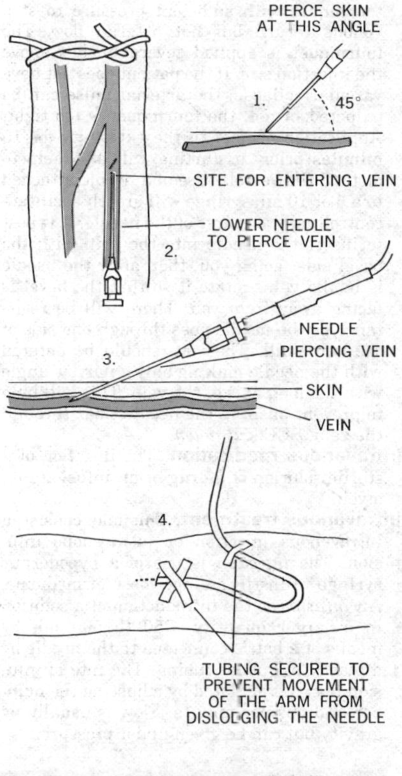

5% in water, potassium chloride 0.2% in 5% dextrose. The quantity depends on the needs of the patient. May be given continuously at the rate of from 1 to 2 or more liters per day. In severe shock up to 4 liters may be necessary.

SITE: Usually, in the arm, the median basilic or median cephalic vein but veins at various areas may be used. Preparation is the same as for intravenous injection but a needle or cannula is used. The vein must be exposed if cannula is used. Introduction of solution should be at the rate required to deliver the amount of fluid and contained electrolytes, medicines, or nutrients in a prescribed time.

intravenous infusion pump. A special pump designed to provide constant but adjustable rate of flow of solutions given intravenously. The pump may work by applying intermittent pressure on the tubing carrying the solution so that the fluid is not actually in contact with the pump itself.

intravenous injection. Inserting the needle requires a degree of skill that is easily obtained if the proper instruction is available. The vein may be distended by applying a tourniquet with sufficient pressure to stop venous return but not arterial flow. The tourniquet is applied several inches above the injection site. If the patient does not have vascular collapse, the arterial pulse can be palpated; if not, the tourniquet is too tight. Application of heat to the extremity for 15 minutes prior to starting will also help to distend the vessels. Use of a needle attached to a 5 or 10 ml. syringe will greatly facilitate controlling the course of the needle. It is best to insert the needle into the vein with the bevel side facing you, then after the needle is in the vein, rotate it so that the bevel is facing away from you. There will be resistance as the needle goes through one side of the vein wall. The vein should be entered with the needle making only a narrow angle with the long axis of the vein. This will help to prevent pushing the needle clear through the vein. SEE: *cut-down.*

intravenous medication. The injection of a sterile solution of a drug or an infusion into a vein.

intravenous treatment. This may consist of intravenous injection or intravenous infusion. The *injection* is use of a hypodermic syringe to instill a single dose of medicine. An *infusion* is the introduction of a solution in a larger quantity—250 to 500 ml. by means of a bottle connected to the needle by a plastic or rubber tubing. The rate of infusion may be regulated by adjusting the number of drops per minute. Flow is usually by gravity but can be given under pressure.

CAUTION: I.V. infusions should be discontinued or infusion fluid replenished when the bottle being administered is depleted. If this is not done it is possible for air to be introduced into the bloodstream. Clotting of blood in needle occurs when infusion is not continuous.

NURSING IMPLICATIONS: Nurses' responsibilities include: ensuring that the correct fluid is infusing; observing the I.V. infusion site every half hour for symptoms of infiltration; calculating and maintaining the correct flow rate; ensuring that the needle is properly secured and the patient restrained as needed to maintain the I.V. Change the dressing on the infusion site daily, according to hospital policy. Also assess the patient for development of the complications of I.V. therapy such as circulatory or electrolyte overload, thrombophlebitis, and air embolism.

intraventricular [L. *intra,* within, + *ventriculus,* ventricle]. Within a ventricle.

intravesical (ĭn″tră-vĕs′ĭ-kăl) [″ + *vesica,* a bladder]. Within the urinary bladder.

intravital [″ + *vita,* life]. During period of life.

intravital stain. One that when introduced into a living organism is taken up by living cells.

intra vitam (ĭn′tră vī′tăm) [L.]. During life.

intravitelline (ĭn″tră-vī-tĕl′ĭn) [″ + *vitellus,* yoke]. Within the vitelline or yolk.

intravitreous (ĭn″tră-vĭt′rē-ŭs) [″ + *vitreus,* glassy]. Within the vitreous of the eye.

intrinsic [L. *intrinsicus,* on the inside]. 1. Belonging to the essential nature of a thing. It is both essential and natural, not merely apparent or accidental. SYN: *inherent; innate.* 2. In anatomy, structures belonging solely to a certain body part, as intrinsic nerves or muscles. 3. Due to causes or elements within the body, an organ, or a part.

intrinsic factor. A substance normally present in the gastric juice of humans. Its presence makes absorption of vitamin B_{12} possible. Absence of this factor leads to vitamin B_{12} deficiency and pernicious anemia.

intrinsic muscles. Muscles that have their origin and insertion entirely within a structure, as the intrinsic muscles of the tongue, larynx, or eye.

intro- [L.]. Prefix meaning in or into.

introducer [L. *intro,* into, + *ducere,* to lead]. Device for controlling, directing, and placing an intubation tube within the trachea, a blood vessel, or the heart (as in Swan-Ganz catheter placement). SYN: *intubator.*

introflexion (ĭn″trō-flĕk′shŭn) [″ + *flexus,* bent]. A bending inward.

introitus (ĭn-trō′ĭ-tŭs) [L.]. [NA] An opening or entrance into a canal or cavity, as the vagina.

i. canalis sacralis. Terminal opening of

the spinal canal at the end of the sacrum.

i. laryngis. Upper opening of larynx.

i. vaginae. Exterior orifice of vagina.

introjection [" + *jacere,* to throw]. In psychoanalysis, identification of the self with another or with some object, the victim assuming the supposed feelings of the other personality.

intromission (ĭn″trō-mĭsh′ŭn) [" + *mittere,* to send]. An insertion or placing of one part into another, esp. insertion of the penis into the vagina.

intromittent (ĭn-trō-mĭt′ĕnt). Conveying or injecting into a cavity or body.

Intropin. Trade name for dopamine hydrochloride.

introspection [" + *spicere,* to look]. Looking within, esp. examination of one's own mind.

introsusception (ĭn″trō-sŭ-sĕp′shŭn) [" + *suscipere,* to receive]. Intussusception.

introversion (ĭn″trō-vĕr′shŭn) [" + *versio,* a turning]. 1. Turning inside out of a part or organ. 2. Condition of an introvert, q.v. Preoccupation with one's self.

introvert. 1. A personality-reaction type characterized by withdrawal from reality; fantasy formation, and stress on the subjective side of life adjustments, seen pathologically in extreme form in schizophrenia. 2. To turn one's psychic energy inward upon oneself.

intubate (ĭn′tū-bāt) [L. *in,* into, + *tuba,* a tube]. To insert a tube in a part, esp. the larynx. SEE: *catheterization.*

intubation (ĭn″tū-bā′shŭn). Insertion of a tube into any hollow organ, as into the larynx or trachea through the glottis for entrance of air, or to dilate a stricture.

POSITION: Patient, who is usually anesthetized, so held that body, neck, and head are kept in a straight line. Neck hyperextension may aid in endotracheal intubation.

intubator. Device used in inserting a tube into the larynx. SYN: *introducer.*

intumesce (ĭn-tū-mĕs′) [L. *intumescere*]. To enlarge or swell.

intumescence. 1. A swelling. 2. The process of enlarging. SYN: *tumefaction.*

intumescent (ĭn-tū-mĕs′ĕnt). Swelling or becoming enlarged.

intussusception (ĭn″tŭ-sŭ-sĕp′shŭn) [L. *intus,* within, + *suscipere,* to receive]. Invagination. The slipping of one part of an intestine into another part just below it. Noted chiefly in children, usually in the ileocecal region. SYN: *indigitation; introsusception; invagination.*

PROG: Good if surgery is performed immediately. High mortality if untreated within 24 hours. SEE: *ileus.*

intussusceptum (ĭn″tŭ-sŭ-sĕp′tŭm) [L.]. The inner segment of intestine that has been pushed into another segment.

intussuscipiens (ĭn″tŭ-su-sĭp′ē-ĕns). [L.]. That portion of intestine that receives the intussusceptum.

Inuit [Eskimo people]. People native to Arctic America.

inulase (ĭn′ū-lās). An enzyme that converts inulin into levulose.

inulin. A polysaccharide found in plants. Yields levulose when hydrolyzed. It is used to study renal function.

inunction (ĭn-ŭngk′shŭn) [L. *in,* into, + *unguere,* to anoint]. Ointment or medicated substance rubbed into the skin to secure a local or a more general systemic effect. SYN: *enepidermic.*

inustion (ĭn-ŭs′chŭn) [" + *urere,* to burn]. 1. To apply cautery. 2. Deep cauterization.

in utero (ĭn ū′tĕr-ō) [L.]. Within the uterus.

in vacuo (ĭn văk′ū-ō) [L.]. Within a cavity or a space from which air has been exhausted.

invaginate (ĭn-văj′ĭn-āt) [L. *invaginatio*]. 1. To ensheath. 2. To insert one part of a structure within a part of the same structure. SYN: *intussusception.* 3. In embryology, to grow in or from an ingrowth or inpocketing, esp. the ingrowth of the wall of the blastula, which results in the formation of the gastrula.

invaginated. Enclosed in a sheath; ensheathed.

invagination. The process of becoming ensheathed. SYN: *intussusception.* SEE: *evagination.*

invalid [L. *in-,* not, + *validus,* strong]. 1. Not well; weak. 2. A sickly person, particularly one who is confined to a bed or wheelchair.

invasion [L. *in,* into, + *vadere,* to go]. 1. That period of a disease following entrance of infective organisms and preceding the appearance of symptoms. 2. The entrance of bacteria or other infectious organisms into the body and their distribution to the tissues.

invasive. Tending to spread, esp. the tendency of a malignant process or growth to spread into healthy tissue.

invermination [" + *vermis,* worm]. Infestation by intestinal worms.

inverse-square law. Law stating that the intensity of radiation or light at any distance is inversely proportional to the square of the distance between the irradiated surface and a point source. Thus a light with a certain intensity at a 4-foot distance will have only one fourth that intensity at 8 feet and would be four times as intense at a 2-foot distance.

Inversine. Trade name for mecamylamine hydrochloride.

inversion (ĭn-vĕr′zhŭn) [L. *inversio,* to turn inward]. 1. Reversal of normal relationship. 2. Turning inside out of an organ, e.g., the uterus. 3. In chemistry, the process of converting sucrose (which rotates the plane of polarized light to the right) into a mixture of dextrose and levulose, which mixture rotates the plane to the left. The resulting mixture is called invert sugar, and the enzyme that catalyzes this conversion is called invertase. SEE: *enzyme*.

i., uterine. A condition in which the uterus is turned inside out so that the internal surface protrudes into the vagina or beyond it.

invert (ĭn-vĕrt'). To turn inside out or upside down.

invertase (ĭn-vĕr'tās). A sugar-splitting enzyme found in the intestinal juice. It causes the inversion of sugar. SYN: *invertin*.

invertebrate [L. *in-*, not, + *vertebratus*, vertebrate]. Without a backbone; species of animals that do not have a backbone.

invertin (ĭn-vĕr'tĭn). An intestinal ferment that converts cane sugar into invert sugar. SYN: *invertase; zymose*.

invertor (ĭn-vĕr'tor). Muscle that rotates a part inward.

invert sugar. A term usually applied to a mixture of levulose and dextrose, formed by inversion of sucrose by the enzyme invertase. SEE: *carbohydrates; inversion; sugar*.

investing [L. *in*, into, + *vestire*, to clothe]. Ensheathing, encircling with a sheath or coating, as tissue; surrounding.

investment. A covering or sheath.

inveterate [" + *vetus*, old]. Chronic; firmly seated, as a disease or a habit.

inviscation (ĭn"vĭs-kā'shŭn) [L. *in*, among, + *viscum*, slime]. The mixing of saliva with food during chewing.

in vitro (ĭn vē'trō) [L., in glass]. In glass, as in a test tube. An in vitro test is one done in the laboratory, usually involving isolated tissue, organ, or cell preparations. SEE: *in vivo*.

in vivo (ĭn vē'vō) [L., in the living body]. In the living body or organism. A test performed on a living organism. SEE: *in vitro*.

involucre, involucrum (ĭn'vō-lū"kĕr, ĭn"vō-lū'krŭm) [" + *volvere*, to wrap]. 1. A sheath or covering. 2. The covering of newly formed bone enveloping the sequestrum in infection of the bone.

involuntary [L. *in-*, not, + *voluntas*, will]. Independent of or even contrary to volition.

involution (ĭn"vō-lū'shŭn) [" + *volvere*, to roll]. 1. A turning or rolling inward. 2. The reduction in size of the uterus following delivery. 3. The retrogressive change in vital processes after their functions have been fulfilled, such as the change that follows the menopause. 4. A backward change. 5. Diminishing of an organ in vital power or in size. 6. In bacteriology, digression from the usual morphological type such as occurs in certain bacteria, esp. when grown under unfavorable conditions; degeneration.

i. of uterus. Return of uterus to normal size after childbirth.

i., senile. Atrophy of an organ or part from old age.

i., sexual. Cessation of menstrual function. SYN: *climacteric; menopause*.

involutional (ĭn-vō-lū'shŭn-ăl). Concerning involution or a turning inward.

involutional melancholia. Depressive psychosis that occurs during the involutional period (40 to 55 years of age in women; 50 to 65 in men). There is usually no previous history of mental illness. Characteristic symptoms include depression; delusions of sin, guilt, or poverty; an obsession with death; imagined gastrointestinal tract disease; and sometimes delusions of being persecuted. The patient manifests agitation and dejection. The condition may be successfully treated with antidepressant drugs or electroconvulsive therapy.

Io. Chem. symb. for ionium.

iocetamic acid. USP. A radiopaque agent used in certain x-ray studies. Trade name is Cholebrine.

Iodamoeba (ī"ō-dă-mē'bă). A genus of amebas found in the intestinal tract. Their cysts are peculiar in that they are irregular in shape, the nucleus usually is single, and they possess a vacuole filled with glycogen that stains brown in iodine.

I. bütschlii. A small, sluggish ameba found in the large intestine of man. Also found in monkeys and pigs. It is usually nonpathogenic. Also: *I. williamsi*.

iodide (ī'ō-dīd). A compound of iodine containing another radical or element, as potassium iodide.

iodide I 125 solution, sodium. USP. A standardized solution of radioactive iodide, ^{125}I.

iodinate (ī-ō'dĭ-nāt). To combine with iodine.

iodinated I 131 albumin injection. USP. A standardized preparation of albumin iodinated with the use of radioactive iodine, ^{131}I.

iodine (ī'ō-dīn, ī'ō-dēn) [Gr. *ioeides*, violet colored]. USP. SYMB: I. At. wt. 126.904; at. no. 53.; sp. gr. (solid, 20° C.) 4.93. A nonmetallic element belonging to the halogen group. It is a black crystalline substance having a melting point of 113.5° C.; it boils at 184.4° C., giving off a characteristic violet vapor.

FUNCTIONS: Iodine aids in the development and functioning of the thyroid gland, formation of thyroxine and prevention of goiter. The amount of iodine in the entire body averages 50 mg., of which one-third to one-fifth (10 to 15 mg.) is found in the thyroid. Adult daily requirement for iodine is from 100 to 150 μg. A growing child or a pregnant woman needs more than this amount. Those under emotional strain and adolescents likewise need more iodine.

DEFICIENCY SYM: Iodine deficiency in diet may lead to simple goiter characterized by thyroid enlargement and hypothyroidism. This may result in retardation of physical, sexual, and mental development in the young, a condition called cretinism.

SOURCES: In vegetables, esp. those growing near the seacoast, in iodized salt, and in seafoods, esp. in liver of halibut and cod, or the fish liver oils.

USES: Tincture of iodine contains 2% iodine and 2.4% sodium iodide diluted in 50% ethyl alcohol. It is used as a disinfectant for the skin, and as a germicide. It may be used to make contaminated water safe for drinking. Adding three drops of tincture of iodine to a quart of water will kill amebae and bacteria within 30 minutes, and the water will still be palatable. If water to be treated by this method is cloudy or turbid, it should be allowed to settle. Then decant the clear portion and treat it with iodine.

i., protein-bound. Iodine that is attached to serum protein.

i., radioactive. ^{131}I, an isotope of iodine with an at. wt. of 131. Used in diagnosis of thyroid disorders and in the treatment of toxic goiter and thyroid carcinoma.

i., tincture of. A 2% solution of iodine and sodium iodide in dilute alcohol.

iodine poisoning. Iodism. SEE: *Poisons and Poisoning* in *Appendix*.

SYM: Brown stains on lips and mouth; burning pain in mouth, throat, and stomach; vomiting (blue vomitus if stomach contained starches, otherwise yellow vomitus); bloody diarrhea.

F.A.: Give immediately by mouth a cornstarch or flour solution, 15 gm. in 500 ml. (2 cups) of water. Lavage with starch solution or 2% sodium-thiosulfate solution. Morphine for pain; and mild stimulants as indicated. Following this therapy, promote catharsis with 30 gm. of sodium sulfate and 15 gm. of starch in 250 ml. (one cup) of water.

INCOMPAT: Alkaloids.

iodine tincture. USP. A standardized preparation of iodine in alcohol and water.

iodinophilous (ī″ō-dĭn-ŏf′ĭ-lŭs) [Gr. *ioeides,* violet colored, + *philos,* love]. Easily stained with iodine.

iodipamide meglumine injection. USP. A combination of iodipamide and meglumine used to aid in x-ray examination of the gallbladder. Trade name is Cholografin Meglumine.

iodipamide sodium I 131. USP. Radioactive chemical used in examining body organs and cavities. Trade name is Radio-Cholografin.

iodism (ī′ō-dĭzm). Condition induced by prolonged and excessive use of iodine or its compounds. SEE: *iodine poisoning.*

iodize. To administer or impregnate with iodine.

iodized. Impregnated with iodine.

iodized salt. In the U.S.A., salt containing about 100 μg. of sodium or potassium iodide in each gram of salt. SEE: *salt.*

5-iodo-2′-deoxyuridine. ABBR: IDU. A substance used to treat herpesvirus infections of the eye. SEE: *mace.* SYN: *idoxuridine.*

iododerma (ī-ō″dō-dĕr′mă) [″ + *derma,* skin]. Dermatitis due to iodine.

iodoform (ī-ō′dō-form) [Gr. *ioeides,* violet colored, + L. *forma,* form]. CHI_3. Yellow crystals having a disagreeable odor. Produced by the action of iodine on acetone in the presence of an alkali. Used topically it has mild antibacterial action.

iodoformism (ī′ō-dō-form″ĭzm) [″ + ″ + Gr. *-ismos,* state of]. Poisoning caused by iodoform.

iodoglobulin (ī″ō-dō-glŏb′ū-lĭn) [″ + L. *globus,* globe]. A globulin protein that contains iodine.

iodohippurate sodium I 131 injection (ī-ō″dō-hĭp′ū-rāt). USP. A radioactive dye used in testing renal function. Trade names are Hippuran-131 and Hippuran I 131.

iodophilia (ī″ō-dō-fĭl′ē-ă) [″ + *philein,* to love]. Condition in which certain cells, when stained, esp. polymorphonuclear leukocytes, show a pronounced affinity for iodine, the cells acquiring a brownish-red color. Seen in pathologic conditions such as acute infections and anemia.

i., intracellular. Iodophilia in which color changes occur within the cells.

i., extracellular. Iodophilia in which substances in the plasma outside the cells are colored.

iodophor (ī-ō′dō-for). A combination of iodine and a solubilizing agent or carrier that liberates free iodine in solution. Some forms are used as general antiseptics; they are less irritating than elemental forms of iodine. SEE: *povidone-iodine.*

iodopyracet (ī″ō′dō-pī′ră-sĕt). A radiopaque medium used in intravenous pyelography and urography. Proprietary name is Diodrast.

iodoquinol (ī-ō″dō-kwĭn′ŏl). USP. $C_9H_5I_2NO$. An antiamebic agent used in the treatment of amebiasis and Trichomonas hominis infection of intestines. Previously used name was diiodohydroxyquin. Trade name is Yodoxin. Outside the U.S.A. this drug is sold under a great number of names.

CAUTION: Use of this drug has been associated with production of a severe disease of the central nervous system called subacute myelo-optic neuropathy, q.v.

iodotherapy [Gr. *ioeides,* violet colored, + *therapeia,* treatment]. Use of iodine medica-

tion.

iodum (ī-ō′dŭm) [L.]. Iodine.

I.O.M.L. *infraorbitomeatal line;* line through the infraorbital margin and the external auditory meatus.

ion [Gr. *ion,* going]. A particle carrying an electric charge, consisting of an atom or group of atoms into which the molecules of an electrolyte are divided or one of the electrified particles into which the molecules of a gas are divided by ultraviolet rays, gamma rays, or x-rays, or by other ionizing agents.

Ions occur in gases, esp. at low pressures, under the influence of strong electrical discharges, x-rays, and radium; in solutions of acids, bases, and salts. Such moving particles render the gas or solution capable of conducting the electric current and, on reaching the electrodes, they are discharged.

Ions that carry positive charges and that consequently discharge at the negative electrode (cathode) are called cations.

Ex.: hydrogen in aqueous solutions of acids and sodium in aqueous solutions of sodium chloride.

Ions that carry negative charges will appear at the positive electrode (anode) and are, therefore, called anions.

Ex.: chlorine in aqueous solutions of hydrochloric acid or of sodium chloride. Thus the reaction in ionization of hydrogen chloride (hydrochloric acid) when dissolved in water is represented as

$$HCl \rightarrow H^+ + Cl^-$$

It means that when the electric current is passed through the solution, hydrogen gas will appear as bubbles at the cathode while chlorine will appear at the anode.

i., dipolar. An ion that contains both positive and negative charges.

i., hydrogen. A hydrogen atom that has lost an electron. It has a positive charge, and its symbol is H^+.

i., hydroxyl. The negatively charged ion of hydrogen and oxygen. The symbol for it is OH^-.

Ionamin. Trade name for phentermine.

ion-exchange resins. Synthetic organic substances of high molecular weight. They replace certain negative or positive ions that they encounter in solutions.

ionic [Gr. *ion,* going]. Pert. to ions.

ionic medication. The therapeutic introduction of ionized substances into the superficial tissues by means of a carefully controlled direct electric current. The basic rules are: substances of like electric charge repel each other; unlike forms attract each other. Bases, metallic radicals, and alkaloids are electropositive and should be placed at the positive pole. Acids and acid radicals are electronegative and should be placed at the negative pole. SYN: *iontophoresis* (def. 2).

Ex.: potassium iodide for the introduction of free iodine should be placed at the negative pole; cocaine hydrochloride for local anesthesia at the positive pole.

ionium (ī-ō′nē-ŭm). A natural radioactive isotope of thorium. It has a mass number of 230.

ionization. The dissociation of compounds (acids, bases, salts) into their constituent ions.

ionization chamber. Device for determining the number of ions produced by a radioactive source.

ionize. To separate into ions; ionization.

ionogen (ī-ŏn′ō-jĕn) [Gr. *ion,* going, + *gennan,* to produce]. Anything that can be ionized.

ionometer [″ + *metron,* measure]. An instrument consisting of an ionization chamber, an electroscope, and an electric charging current designed to measure the amount of radiation used by roentgen rays or radium and to measure the intensity of the rays themselves. SYN: *iontoquantimeter; iontoradiometer.*

ionophose (ī′ō-nō-fōz) [″ + *phos,* light]. Production of a violet color.

ionotherapy (ī″ŏn-ō-thĕr′ă-pē) [″ + *therapeia,* treatment]. Introduction of ions into the body. SYN: *iontophoresis.*

iontophoresis (ī-ŏn″tō-fō-rē′sĭs) [″ + *phorein,* to carry]. 1. Process of electrical current traveling through salt solution causing migration of metal (positive) ion to negative pole and radical (negative) ion to positive pole. 2. Introduction of various ions into tissues through the skin by means of electricity. SYN: *ionic medication.*

iontoquantimeter (ī-ŏn″tō-kwŏn-tĭm′ĕ-ter) [″ + L. *quantus,* how much, + Gr. *metron,* measure]. Instrument used to measure the amount of radiation used by, and the intensity of, roentgen rays. SYN: *ionometer; iontoradiometer.*

iontoradiometer (ī-ŏn″tō-rā″dē-ŏm′ĭ-tĕr) [″ + L. *radius,* ray, + Gr. *metron,* measure]. Instrument for measuring the amount and intensity of roentgen rays. SYN: *ionometer; iontoquantimeter.*

iontotherapy (ī-ŏn″tō-thĕr′ă-pē) [″ + *therapeia,* treatment]. Treatment by introducing ions into the body electrically.

IOP. *intraocular pressure.*

iopanoic acid. USP. A radiopaque dye used in x-ray studies of the gallbladder. Trade name is Telepaque.

iophendylate (ī″ō-fĕn′dĭ-lāt). USP. A radiopaque material used in myelography.

iophobia (ī″ō-fō′bē-ă) [Gr. *ios,* poison, + *pho-*

bos, fear]. 1. Fear of being poisoned. SYN: *toxicophobia.* 2. Fear of touching any rusty object.

iotacism (ī-ō'tă-sĭzm) [Gr. *iota,* letter i]. Defective utterance marked by constant substitution of an ē sound (Greek iota) for other vowels.

iothalamate meglumine injection (ī-ō-thăl'ă-māt). USP. A radiopaque material used in investigation of arteries of the brain as well as in the rest of the body, and in studying kidney function. Trade names are Conray, Cysto-Conray.

I.P. intraperitoneal; isoelectric point.

ipecac (ĭp'ĕ-kăk). USP. Dried root of the plant ipecacuanha grown in Brazil. It is the source of emetine, q.v. SEE: *Poisons and Poisoning* in *Appendix.*

ACTION AND USES: Emetic.

I.P.L. *interpupillary line;* line between the center of both pupils.

ipodate calcium (ī'pō-dāt). USP. A radiopaque material used in x-ray studies of the gallbladder. Trade name is Oragrafin Calcium.

ipodate sodium. USP. A radiopaque material used in x-ray studies of the gallbladder. Trade name is Oragrafin Sodium.

IPPB. *intermittent positive-pressure breathing.*

IPPV. *intermittent positive-pressure ventilation.*

iproniazid (ī"prō-nī'ă-zĭd). An antitubercular drug.

ipsation (ĭp-sā'shŭn) [L. *ipse,* same]. Masturbation.

ipsi- [L. *ipse,* same]. Combining form indicating the same.

ipsilateral (ĭp"sĭ-lăt'ĕr-ăl) [" + *latus,* side]. On the same side; affecting the same side of the body. Thus, when the right patellar tendon is tapped, a knee-jerk is observed on the same side. Said of findings (paralysis) appearing on same side of body as brain or spinal cord lesion producing them. Opposite of crossed, contralateral. SYN: *homolateral.*

IPSP. *inhibitory postsynaptic potential.*

IQ. *intelligence quotient.*

IR. *infrared.*

I.R. *internal resistance.*

Ir. Chem. symb. for iridium.

iralgia (ĭr-ăl'jē-ă) [Gr. *iris,* colored circle, + *algos,* pain]. Pain felt in the iris. SYN: *iridalgia.*

irascible (ĭ-răs'ĭ-bl) [LL. *irascibilis*]. Marked by outbursts of temper or irritability. Easily angered.

irid- [Gr. *iridos,* colored circle]. Combining form indicating relationship to the iris of the eye.

iridadenosis (ĭr"ĭd-ăd-ĭn-ō'sĭs) [L. *iris,* colored circle, + Gr. *aden,* gland, + *osis,* condition]. A glandular affection of the iris.

iridal (ī'rĭd-ăl). Rel. to the iris. SYN: *iridic; iritic.*

iridalgia (ī"rĭd-ăl'jē-ă) [" + *algos,* pain]. Pain felt in the iris. SYN: *iralgia.*

iridauxesis (ĭr"ĭd-ŏk-sē'sĭs) [" + *auxesis,* increase]. Increase in thickness of the iris.

iridectome (ĭr"ĭ-dĕk'tōm) [" + *tome,* incision]. Instrument for cutting the iris in iridectomy.

iridectomesodialysis (ĭr"ĭ-dĕk"tō-mĕs"ō-dī-ăl'ĭ-sĭs) [" + *ektome,* excision, + *mesos,* middle, + *dialysis,* loosening]. Formation of an artificial pupil, by separating adhesions on inner margin of iris.

iridectomize (ĭr"ĭd-ĕk'tō-mīz) [" + *ektome,* excision]. To excise a portion of the iris.

iridectomy. Surgical removal of a portion of the iris.

i., optical. Iridectomy done for purpose of making an artificial pupil

iridectropium (ĭr-ĭ-dĕk-trō'pē-ŭm) [" + *ektrope,* a turning aside]. Partial eversion of the iris.

iridemia (ĭr-ĭ-dē'mē-ă) [" + *haima,* blood]. Bleeding from the iris.

iridencleisis (ĭr"ĭ-dĕn-klī'sĭs) [" + *enklein,* to lock in]. An operation for relieving increased intraocular pressure, as in glaucoma, in which the iris and a portion of the limbus are excised to allow increased volume of the aqueous humor under the conjunctiva.

iridentropium (ĭr"ĭ-dĕn-trō'pē-ŭm) [" + *en,* in, + *tropein,* to turn]. Partial inversion of the iris.

irideremia (ĭr"ĭd-ĕr-ē'mē-ă) [" + *eremia,* lack]. Partial or total congenital absence of the iris. SYN: *aniridia.*

irides (ĭr'ĭ-dēz) [Gr.]. Plural of iris.

iridescence (ĭr"ĭ-dĕs'ĕns) [L. *iridescere,* to gleam like a rainbow]. Having the capability to disperse light into the colors of the spectrum.

iridesis (ī-rĭd'ĕ-sĭs) [" + *desis,* a binding]. Formation of an iris artificially, by ligation. SYN: *iridodesis.*

iridic (ī-rĭd'ĭk) [Gr. *iris,* colored circle]. Rel. to the iris. SYN: *iridal; iritic.*

iridis, rubeosis. SEE: *rubeosis iridis.*

iridium (ī-rĭd'ē-ŭm) [Gr. *iris,* colored circle]. SYMB: Ir. At. wt. 192.2; at. no. 77. A white, hard metallic element.

irido- [Gr. *iridos,* colored circle]. Combining form pert. to the iris.

iridoavulsion (ĭr"ĭ-dō-ă-vŭl'shŭn) [" + L. *avulsio,* a pulling away from]. Tearing away (avulsion) of the iris.

iridocapsulitis (ĭr"ĭd-ō-kăp-sū-lī'tĭs) [" + L. *capsula,* little box, + Gr. *itis,* inflammation]. Iritis with inflammation of the capsule of the lens.

iridocele (ī-rĭd'ō-sēl) [" + *kele,* hernia]. Protrusion of a portion of the iris through a defect in the cornea.

iridochorioiditis, iridochoroiditis (ĭr"ĭ-dō-kō"

rē-oy-dī'tĭs, ĭr"ĭ-dō-kō-roy-dī'tĭs) [" + *chorioeides,* skinlike, + *itis,* inflammation]. Inflamed condition of both iris and choroid.

iridocoloboma (ĭr"ĭd-ō-kŏl"ō-bō'mă) [" + *koloboma,* mutilation]. Congenital defect or fissure of the iris.

iridoconstrictor (ĭr"ĭ-dō-kŏn-strĭk'tor). A muscle or drug that acts to constrict the pupil of the eye.

iridocyclectomy (ĭr"ĭ-dō-sī-klĕk'tō-mē) [" + *kyklos,* circle, + *ektome,* excision]. Surgical removal of iris and ciliary body.

iridocyclitis (ĭr"ĭd-ō-sī-klī'tĭs) [" + " + *itis,* inflammation]. Inflammation of iris and ciliary body.

i., heterochromic. Inflammation of the iris of the eye with depigmentation of the iris.

iridocyclochoroiditis (ĭr"ĭ-dō-sī"klō-kō"roy-dī'tĭs) [" + " + *chorioeides,* skinlike, + *itis,* inflammation]. Inflammation of the iris, ciliary body, and choroid of the eye.

iridocystectomy (ĭr"ĭ-dō-sĭs-tĕk'tō-mē) [" + *kystis,* bladder, + *ektome,* excision]. An operation for removal of a cyst from the iris.

iridodesis (ĭr-ĭ-dŏd'ĕ-sĭs) [" + *desis,* a binding]. Ligature of part of the iris to form an artificial one. SYN: *iridesis.*

iridodiagnosis [" + *dia,* through, + *gnosis,* knowledge]. Diagnosis of disease by examination of the iris.

iridodialysis (ĭr"ĭd-ō-dī-ăl'ĭ-sĭs) [" + *dialysis,* loosening]. The separation of the outer margin of the iris from its ciliary attachment.

iridodilator [" + L. *dilatare,* to dilate]. Substance causing dilatation of the pupil.

iridodonesis (ĭr"ĭd-ō-dō-nē'sĭs) [" + *donesis,* tremor]. Tremulousness of iris, seen in an aphakic eye or one with subluxated lens. SYN: *hippus.*

iridokeratitis (ĭr"ĭ-dō-kĕr"ă-tī'tĭs) [" + *keras,* horn, + *itis,* inflammation]. Inflammation of the iris and the cornea.

iridokinesis (ĭr"ĭd-ō-kĭn-ē'sĭs) [Gr. *iridos,* colored circle, + *kinesis,* motion]. The contracting and expanding movements of the iris.

iridoleptynsis (ĭr"ĭ-dō-lĕp-tĭn'sĭs) [" + *leptynsis,* attenuation]. Thinning or atrophy of the iris.

iridology (ĭr"ĭ-dŏl'ō-jē) [" + *logos,* study]. The study of changes in the iris during the course of a disease.

iridomalacia (ĭr"ĭd-ō-mă-lā'shē-ă) [" + *malakia,* softness]. Softening of the iris.

iridomedialysis (ĭr"ĭd-ō-mē-dē-ăl'ĭ-sĭs) [" + L. *medius,* in middle, + Gr. *dialysis,* loosening]. Separation of inner marginal adhesions of the iris. SYN: *iridomesodialysis.*

iridomesodialysis (ĭr"ĭd-ō-mĕs"ō-dī-ăl'ĭ-sĭs) [" + *mesos,* middle, + *dialysis,* loosening]. Separation of adhesions around the inner border of iris. SYN: *iridomedialysis.*

iridomotor [" + L. *motor,* that which moves]. Rel. to movements of the iris.

iridoncus (ĭr-ĭ-dong'kŭs) [" + *onkos,* bulk]. Tumefaction of the iris or development of a tumor.

iridoparalysis [" + *paralysis,* a loosening]. Paralysis of the iris. SYN: *iridoplegia.*

iridoparelkysis (ĭr"ĭ-dō-păr-ĕl'kĭ-sĭs) [" + *parelkysis,* protraction]. Surgically induced prolapse of the iris in order to displace the pupil artificially.

iridopathy (ĭr"ĭ-dŏp'ă-thē) [" + *pathos,* disease]. Disease of the iris of the eye.

iridoperiphacitis, iridoperiphakitis (ĭr"ĭ-dō-pĕr"ĭ-fă-sī'tĭs, -pĕr"ĭ-fă-kī'tĭs) [" + *peri,* around, + *phakos,* lens, + *itis,* inflammation]. Inflammation of the iris and anterior portion of the capsule of the lens.

iridoplegia (ĭr"ĭd-ō-plē'jē-ă) [" + *plege,* stroke]. Paralysis of the sphincter of the iris. SYN: *iridoparalysis.*

i., accommodative. Inability of iris to contract when stimulated by accommodation.

i., complete. Iridoplegia in which the iris fails to respond to any stimulation. Seen in Adie's pupil, q.v.

i., reflex. Absence of light reflex with retention of accommodation reflex (Argyll Robertson pupil).

iridoptosis (ĭr"ĭ-dŏp-tō'sĭs) [" + *ptosis,* a falling]. Prolapse of the iris.

iridopupillary (ĭr"ĭ-dō-pū'pĭ-lĕr"ē) [" + L. *pupilla,* pupil]. Concerning the iris and the pupil of the eye.

iridorrhexis (ĭr"ĭd-ō-rĕk'sĭs) [" + *rhexis,* rupture]. Rupture of or a tearing of the iris away from its attachment.

iridoschisis (ĭr"ĭ-dŏs'kĭ-sĭs) [" + *schistos,* split]. Separation of the stroma of the iris into two layers with disintegration of the anterior layer.

iridosclerotomy (ĭr"ĭd-ō-sklē-rŏt'ō-mē) [" + *skleros,* hard, + *tome,* incision]. Piercing of the sclera and the border of the iris.

iridosteresis (ĭr"ĭ-dō-stē-rē'sĭs) [" + *steresis,* loss]. Removal of the iris or a portion of it.

iridotasis (ĭr-ĭ-dŏt'ă-sĭs) [" + *tasis,* a stretching]. Stretching the iris in treatment of glaucoma.

iridotomy (ĭr-ĭ-dŏt'ō-mē) [" + *tome,* incision]. Incision of the iris without excising a portion, done for the purpose of making a new aperture in the iris when the pupil is closed. Indicated in eyes that had been operated on for cataract but that have lost their sight through subsequent iridocyclitis. SYN: *iritomy; irotomy.*

iris [Gr.]. (pl. *irides*) The colored contractile membrane suspended between the lens and the cornea in the aqueous humor of the eye, separating the anterior and posterior chambers of the eyeball and perforated in the center by the pupil. By contraction and dilatation it regulates the entrance of light.

ANAT: The free inner edge rests on the lens when the pupil is contracted or partially dilated. The iris contains two muscles, the sphincter pupillae (circular fibers), about one millimeter wide, and the dilator pupillae (meridionally arranged fibers), extending from the sphincter pupillae to the root of the iris. The former is supplied through the oculomotor nerve with parasympathetic fibers derived from the ciliary ganglion; the latter by sympathetic fibers from the superior cervical ganglion. The color of the iris depends on the pigment in the stroma cells and in the cells of the retinal layers. SEE: *aniridia; choroidoiritis; heterochromia iridis; rubeosis iridis; "irid-" words.*

i. bombé. Condition seen in annular posterior synechia. The iris is bulged forward by the pressure of the aqueous humor, which cannot reach the anterior chamber.

i., chromatic asymmetry of. Difference in color of the two irides (heterochromia). One may be blue or gray and the other brown. May occur in early iritis or cyclitis, or may be present without an associated pathological process.

i., piebald. Dark discoloration in irregularly shaped area. May be in one or both eyes.

Irish moss. A genus of seaweeds, Chondrus crispus; source of a demulcent used in pharmacologic preparations. SYN: *carrageen.*

irisopsia (ī″rĭs-ŏp′sē-ă) [Gr. *iris,* colored circle, + *opsis,* vision]. Visual defect in which colored circles are seen around lights.

iritic (ī-rĭt′ĭk) [Gr. *iris,* colored circle]. Rel. to the iris. SYN: *iridal; iridic.*

iritis [″ + *itis,* inflammation]. Inflammation of the iris.

SYM: Pain, photophobia, lacrimation, diminution of vision. The iris appears swollen, dull, and muddy, and the pupil is contracted, irregular, and sluggish in reaction.

TREATMENT: One percent atropine is used, as an ointment or in drop form, frequently enough to keep the pupil dilated. Cortisone or hydrocortisone is used systemically as well as topically. If the primary disease causing the iritis is known it should be treated. However, the etiological factor is usually not known.

i., plastic. Iritis in which the fibrinous exudate forms new tissue.

i., primary. Condition in which the process develops in the iris itself. Seen in general diseases as syphilis, tuberculosis; metastatic in infectious diseases, gonorrhea, and focal infections; also occurs in trauma and sympathetic ophthalmia.

i., purulent. Iritis with a purulent exudate.

i., secondary. Iritis in which the inflammation has spread from neighboring parts as diseases of cornea and sclera.

i., serous. Serum forming the exudate.

iritoectomy (ī″rĭ-tō-ĕk′tō-mē) [″ + *ektome,* excision]. In cataract treatment, excision of the part of the iris that is inflamed and occluding the pupil.

iritomy (ī-rĭt′ō-mē) [″ + *tome,* incision]. Formation of an artifical pupil, or incision into the iris. SYN: *iridotomy; irotomy.*

iron (ī′ĕrn) [AS. *iren;* L. *ferrum*]. SYMB: Fe. At. wt. 55.847; at. no. 26. A metallic element widely distributed in nature. Compounds (oxides, hydroxides, salts) exist in two forms: ferrous, in which iron has a valence of two (Fe^{++}), and ferric, in which it has a valence of three (Fe^{+++}). It is widely used in the treatment of certain forms of anemia. Iron is essential for the formation of chlorophyll in plants, although it is not a constituent of chlorophyll. It is part of the hemoglobin and myoglobin molecules. SEE: *ferritin.*

FUNCT: Because it is essential to hemoglobin formation, it is essential to life. Iron is also present in enzymes that permit cellular respiration to occur. It plays a role in the nutrition of epithelial tissues. There are approximately 4 to 5 gm. of iron in the adult body, distributed as follows: 60–70% in hemoglobin, 15% in the iron-protein compound ferritin, and the remainder is present in enzymes and myoglobin. Iron is stored in the tissues principally as ferritin. Iron is absorbed from the food in the small intestine; it passes, in the blood, to the bone marrow; here it is used in making hemoglobin, which is incorporated into the red corpuscles. A corpuscle, after circulating in the blood for approx. 120 days, is destroyed, and its iron is used over again. The adult male requires from 0.5 to 1.0 mg. of iron a day. A female of menstrual age will require about double this amount. During pregnancy and lactation from 2 to 4 mg. of iron per day will be required. Prior to puberty and after menopause the female requires no more iron than the male.

Because only a fraction of the iron present in food is absorbed, it is necessary to provide from 15 to 30 mg. of iron in the diet to be certain that 1.0 to 4.0 mg. will be absorbed.

Copper in the food is necessary for the utilization of iron. It is stored in the body and reused repeatedly.

In the first few months of life, the infant will use up most of its iron stores, and the typical diet or formula may not have sufficient iron to replenish those stores. It is therefore important to add iron-containing foods to the diet of an infant by age six months.

Manganese and cobalt, in addition to copper, are necessary for proper utilization of iron.

Iron, as a component of hemoglobin, is essential in the transportation of oxygen. It is needed for tissue respiration and the development of blood cells.

DEFICIENCY SYM: Anemia, lowered vitality, pale complexion, conjunctival pallor, retarded development, decreased amount of hemoglobin in each red cell.

NOTE: Sometimes a disturbance in iron metabolism occurs in which an iron-containing pigment, hemosiderin, and hemofuscin are deposited in the tissues. This gives rise to hemochromatosis. Excessive deposition of hemosiderin in the tissues, such as may occur as a result of excessive breakdown of red cells, is called hemosiderosis.

SOURCES: Almonds; asparagus; bran; beans; cauliflower; celery; chard; dandelions; Boston brown bread; graham bread; egg yolk; kidney; lettuce; liver; oatmeal; oysters; soy beans; whole wheat. Other good sources are apricots; greens; beets; beef; cabbage; cucumbers; currants; dates; duck; goose; lamb; molasses; oranges; parsnips; peppers; peas; potatoes; prunes; radishes; raisins; rhubarb; pineapple; tomatoes; peanuts; turnips; cornmeal; mushrooms. Only 50% of the iron in spinach and similar vegetables is assimilable by the body.

iron dextran injection. USP. A preparation of iron suitable for parenteral use. Trade names are Feostat, Ferrospan, and Imferon.

CAUTION: At time of intravenous use, one or two drops are administered over a period of five minutes to determine whether any signs of anaphylaxis appear.

iron lung. Device for automatically providing artificial respiration for patients whose respiratory muscles are paralyzed.

iron poisoning. Acute poisoning usually caused by the accidental ingestion by infants or small children of iron-containing medications intended for the use of adults.

SYM: Vomiting, usually within an hour of taking the iron. Vomiting of blood and melena may occur. If untreated, restlessness, hypotension, rapid respirations, and cyanosis may be followed within a few hours by coma and death.

F.A.: Prompt emptying of the stomach. By digital stimulation of the pharynx if done in the home or by gastric lavage if done in the emergency room. Administration of warm solution of baking soda may help to induce vomiting and the bicarbonate helps to prevent absorption of the iron. Gastric lavage with a solution containing 4 gm. of sodium bicarbonate per 100 ml. is done and then either 60 ml. of the bicarbonate solution or 5 to 10 gm. of deferoxamine, q.v., in solution is left in the stomach. The deferoxamine may be administered intramuscularly in an initial dose of 1 gm. This dose may be repeated intramuscularly in four to eight hours and then at 12-hour intervals if needed. If the patient is in shock, treat by the usual methods.

iron sorbitex injection. USP. A preparation of iron suitable for parenteral use.

iron storage disease. Hemochromatosis, q.v.

Irospan. Trade name for ferrous sulfate.

irotomy (ī-rŏt'ō-mē) [Gr. *iris*, colored circle, + *tome*, incision]. Formation of an artificial pupil. SYN: *iridotomy; iritomy.*

irradiate (ĭ-rā'dē-āt) [L. *in*, into, + *radiare*, to emit rays]. 1. To expose to radiation. 2. To treat with roentgen rays or other forms of radiation. SEE: *irradiation.*

irradiating. Diverging or spreading out from a common center.

irradiation. 1. Therapeutic application of roentgen rays, radium rays, ultraviolet rays or other radiation to a patient. 2. Application of form of radiation to an object or substance to give it therapeutic value, or increase that which it already has. 3. Phenomenon in which a bright object on a dark background appears larger than a dark object of the same size on a bright background. 4. The spreading in all directions from a common center, as nerve impulses, the sensation of pain.

RS: heliotherapy; lamp; light therapy; radiotherapy; radiothermy; radium therapy; radium; radon; ray, roentgen; roentgenotherapy; ultraviolet.

i., interstitial. Therapeutic irradiation by the insertion into the tissues of capillary tubes containing radon.

i. of reflexes. The spread of a reflex to an increasing number of motor units upon increasing the strength of the stimulus.

irreducible (ĭr"rē-dū'sĭ-bl) [L. *in-*, not, + *re*, back, + *ducere*, to lead]. Not capable of being reduced or made smaller, as a fracture or dislocation.

irrelevance [" + *relevans*, raising]. Inappropriate to or unrelated to that which was asked or being discussed.

irrespirable (ĭr"rĕ-spī'ră-bl) [" + *respirare*, to breathe again]. Unfit for breathing, as a gas, or incapable of being breathed.

irreversible. Not being possible to reverse.

irrigate [L. *in*, into, + *rigare*, to carry water]. To wash out with a fluid.

irrigation. The cleansing of a canal by flushing with water or other fluids; the washing of a wound. SYN: *lavage.* SEE: *lavage, gastric.*

Solutions should be sterile and have an approx. temperature slightly warmer than body temperature (100° to 115° F. or 37.8° to

46.1° C.).

i., bladder. Washing out of the bladder for treatment of inflammation. Can be accomplished by forcing oral fluids.

NURSING IMPLICATIONS: Assemble necessary equipment and the ordered irrigation solution. Follow hospital procedure for catheterization. Insert catheter. Instill irrigation solution in the specified amount using a bulb syringe, and then clamp the catheter and allow the solution to remain in the bladder for the specified amount of time. Unclamp the catheter and allow the irrigation solution to flow into a basin. Repeat the irrigation as often as ordered. Carefully observe the return from the irrigation and particularly note the presence of any drainage. The catheter should be removed when the irrigations have been completed. Record treatment done, amount and type of solution used, return from irrigation, and response of patient to procedure.

i., colonic. The flushing of the colon with water. This procedure is done to wash out material in the colon and to cleanse the bowel as high as possible.

irrigator. Device with hose attachment used for purpose of flushing or washing a part or cavity with fluids.

irritability [L. *irritabilis,* irritable]. 1. Excitability. 2. The ability to respond in a specific way to a change in environment, a property of all living tissue. 3. Condition in which a person, organ, or a part responds excessively to a stimulus. 4. Quick response to annoyance; impatience.

i., muscular. Normal response of muscle to a stimulus.

i., nervous. Response of nerve to stimulus.

irritable. 1. Capable of reacting to a stimulus. 2. Sensitive to stimuli.

irritant. An agent that, when used locally, produces more or less local inflammatory reaction. Anything that induces or gives rise to irritation, such as iodine.

irritant poisons. These include a large number of poisons of great variety, not including the corrosive acids or alkalies. They cause pain in the mouth, esophagus, and stomach; nausea; vomiting; great thirst; abdominal cramping; bloody diarrhea; diminished urine.

TREATMENT: SEE: individual poisons in *Poisons and Poisoning* in *Appendix.*

irritation [L. *irritatio*]. 1. Reaction to that which is irritating. 2. Extreme reaction to pain or pathological conditions. 3. Normal response to stimulus of a nerve or muscle.

i., spinal. A neurasthenic condition characterized by tenderness along the spinal column, numbness and tingling in the limbs, and susceptibility to fatigue.

i., sympathetic. The response of an organ to irritation in another organ.

irritative. Pert. to that which causes irritation.

I.S. *intercostal space.*

ischemia (ĭs-kē′mē-ă) [Gr. *ischein,* to hold back, + *haima,* blood]. Local and temporary deficiency of blood supply due to obstruction of the circulation to a part.

i., myocardial. Insufficient blood supply to the heart muscle.

ischesis (ĭs-kē′sĭs). Suppression of a discharge, esp. a normal one.

ischia (ĭs′kē-ă) [L.]. Pl. of ischium.

ischiac, ischiadic (ĭs′kē-ăk ĭs-kē-ăd′ĭk). Ischiatic; sciatic.

ischial (ĭs′kē-ăl) [Gr. *ischion,* hip]. Pert. to the ischium.

ischialgia (ĭs″kē-ăl′jē-ă) [″ + *algos,* pain]. Neuralgic pain in the hip. SYN: *sciatica.*

ischiatic (ĭs″kē-ăt′ĭk) [Gr. *ischion,* hip]. Pert. to ischium or hip bone. SYN: *ischiac; ischiadic; sciatic.*

ischiatitis (ĭs″kē-ă-tī′tĭs) [″ + *itis,* inflammation]. Sciatic nerve inflammation.

ischidrosis (ĭs″kĭ-drō′sĭs) [Gr. *ischein,* to hold back, + *hidrosis,* sweat]. Suppression of perspiration.

ischio- [Gr. *ischion,* hip]. Prefix pert. to the ischium.

ischioanal (ĭs″kē-ō-ā′năl) [″ + L. *anus,* anus]. Concerning the ischium and the anus.

ischiobulbar (ĭs″kē-ō-bŭl′băr) [″ + L. *bulbus,* bulb]. Rel. to the ischium and urethral bulb.

ischiocapsular (ĭs″kē-ō-kăp′sū-lăr) [″ + L. *capsula,* capsule]. Concerning the ischium and the capsule of the hip.

ischiocavernosus (ĭs″kē-ō-kă″vĕr-nō′sŭs) [″ + L. *cavernosus,* cavernous]. A muscle extending from the ischium to the penis or clitoris and assisting in their erection.

ischiocele (ĭs′kē-ō-sēl) [″ + *kele,* hernia]. Hernia through the sciatic notch.

ischiococcygeus (ĭs″kē-ō-kŏk-sĭj′ē-ŭs) [″ + *kokkyx,* coccyx]. 1. Coccygeus muscle. 2. Posterior portion of the levator ani.

ischiodynia (ĭs″kē-ō-dĭn′ē-ă) [″ + *odyne,* pain]. Pain in the ischium.

ischiofemoral (ĭs″kē-ō-fĕm′or-ăl) [″ + L. *femur,* thigh]. Rel. to the ischium and femur.

ischiofibular (ĭs″kē-ō-fĭb′ū-lăr) [″ + L. *fibula,* buckle]. Rel. to the ischium and fibula.

ischiohebotomy (ĭs″kē-ō-hē-bŏt′ō-mē) [″ + *hebe,* pubes, + *tome,* incision]. Surgical division of the ascending ramus of the pubes and the ischiopubic ramus. SYN: *ischiopubiotomy.*

ischioneuralgia (ĭs″kē-ō-nū-răl′jē-ă) [″ + *neuron,* nerve, + *algos,* pain]. Neuralgic pain in the hip. SYN: *sciatica.*

ischionitis (ĭs″kē-ō-nī′tĭs) [″ + *itis,* inflammation]. Inflammation of the tuberosity of the ischium.

ischiopubic (ĭs″kē-ō-pū′bĭk) [″ + L. *pubes*, the pubes]. Rel. to the ischium and pubes.

ischiopubiotomy (ĭs″kē-ō-pū″bē-ŏt′ō-mē). Ischiohebotomy.

ischiorectal (ĭs″kē-ō-rĕk tăl) [″ + L. *rectus*, straight]. Pert. to the ischium and rectum.

ischiorectal abscess. Collection of pus in fatty tissue on either side of the rectum.

ischiosacral (ĭs″kē-ō-sā′krăl) [″ + L. *sacralis*, pert. to the sacrum]. Concerning the ischium and the sacrum.

ischiovaginal (ĭs″kē-ō-văj′ĭ-năl) [″ + L. *vagina*, sheath]. Concerning the ischium and the vagina.

ischium (ĭs′kē-ŭm) [Gr. *ischion*, hip]. (pl. *ischia*) Lower portion of the innominate or hip bone.

ischo- (ĭs′kō) [Gr. *ischein*, to hold back]. Prefix meaning to suppress or restrain.

ischogalactic (ĭs″kō-gă-lăk′tĭk) [″ + *gala*, milk]. 1. Causing suppression of breast milk. 2. Agent that checks milk secretion. SYN: *antigalactic.*

ischuretic (ĭs″kū-rĕt′ĭk) [″ + *ouron*, urine]. 1. Relieving or pert. to ischuria. 2. That which relieves urinary retention or suppression.

ischuria (ĭs-kū′rē-ă) [″ + *ouron*, urine]. Suppression or retention of the urine.

I.S.C.L.T. *International Society of Clinical Laboratory Technologists.*

iseikonia (ĭs″ī-kō′nē-ă) [Gr. *isos*, equal, + *eikon*, image]. Condition in which the image in both eyes is the same. SYN: *isoiconia.*

isinglass (ī′sĭn-glăs). A transparent gelatin prepared from the bladder of certain fish.

island [AS. *igland*, island]. A structure detached from surrounding tissues or characterized by difference in structure; an islet.

i., blood. A small area of blood accumulation present in the yolk sac of the early embryo.

i.'s of Calleja. Groups of densely packed, small cells in the cortex of the gyrus hippocampi.

i.'s of Langerhans. Clusters of cells in the pancreas. The cells are of three types: alpha, beta, and delta cells. The beta cells are found in greatest abundance and produce insulin. Destruction or impairment of function of the islands of Langerhans may result in diabetes or hypoglycemia.

i. of Reil. The insula, a lobe of the cerebral cortex comprising a triangular area lying in the floor of the lateral or sylvian fissure. It is overlapped and hidden by the gyri of the fissure, which constitute the operculum of the insula.

i., pancreatic. I.'s of Langerhans.

islet (ī′lĕt). A tiny isolated mass of one kind of tissue within another type.

i.'s of Calleja. Islands of Calleja.

i.'s of Langerhans. Islands of Langerhans.

i.'s, Walthard's. [Max Walthard, Swiss gynecologist, b. 1867] Embryological nests of epithelial-like cells in the superficial part of the ovaries, tubes, and uterine ligaments. They may also appear as minute cysts. Brenner's tumor is thought to arise from these islets.

-ism [Gr. *-ismos*]. Suffix meaning condition or theory of; principle or method.

Ismelin. Trade name for guanethidine sulfate, USP.

I.S.O. *International Standards Organization.*

iso- [Gr. *isos*, equal]. Combining form meaning equal.

isoagglutination (ī″sō-ă-gloo″tĭ-nā′shŭn) [″ + L. *agglutinare*, to glue to]. Agglutination of red blood cells by agglutinins from the blood of another member of the same species.

isoagglutinin (ī″sō-ă-glū′tĭn-ĭn) [″ + L. *agglutinare*, to glue to]. Antibody in a serum that agglutinates the blood cells of those of the same species from which it is derived. SEE: *agglutinin; blood groups; isohemagglutinin.*

isoagglutinogen (ī″sō-ă-ğlū-tĭn′ō-jĕn). One of two substances designated A and B that may be present on the surface of red blood cells. Cells containing these substances become agglutinated when mixed with serum containing corresponding isoagglutinins (anti-A or anti-B). SEE: *blood groups.*

isoamyl nitrite (ī″sō-ăm′ĭl nī′trīt). Amyl nitrite.

isoanaphylaxis (ī″sō-ăn″ă-fĭ-lăk′sĭs) [″ + *ana*, against, + *phylaxis*, protection]. Anaphylaxis produced by serum from another member of the same species.

isoantibody (ī″sō-ăn″tĭ-bŏd′ē). An antibody produced by an isoantigen, q.v.

isoantigen (ī″sō-ăn′tĭ-jĕn) [″ + L. *anti*, against, + *gennan*, to produce]. A substance present in certain individuals that stimulates production of antibodies in other members of the same species but not in the donor. SYN: *alloantigen.*

Ex.: blood group isoantigens that are harmless to the donor but may produce severe antibody response in a recipient of a different blood group or type.

isobar (ī′sō-băr) [″ + *baros*, weight]. In chemistry, one of two or more chemical bodies having same atomic weight, but with different atomic numbers.

isobaric (ī″sō-băr′ĭk). Specific gravity equal to that with which it is being compared. Thus an anesthetic solution used in spinal anesthesia, if isobaric, would be of the same specific gravity as the spinal fluid.

isobucaine hydrochloride (ī″sō-bū′kān). USP. A local anesthetic agent.

isocaloric (ī″sō-kă-lō′rĭk) [″ + L. *calor*, heat].

Containing the same number of calories as the food or diet with which it is being compared.

isocarboxazid (ī″sō-kăr-bŏk′să-zĭd). USP. An antidepressant drug. Trade name is Marplan.

isocellular [″ + L. *cellula,* cell]. Composed of equal and similar cells.

isochromatic (ī″sō-krō-măt′ĭk) [″ + *chroma,* color]. 1. Having the same color. 2. Of uniform color. SYN: *isochroous.*

isochromatophil(e) (ī″sō-krō-măt′ō-fĭl, -fīl) [″ + ″ + *philein,* to love]. Having the same affinity for a dye.

isochromosome (ī″sō-krō′mō-sōm) [″ + ″ + *soma,* body]. A chromosome with arms that are morphologically identical and contain the same genetic loci. This is the result of the transverse rather than the longitudinal splitting of a chromosome.

isochronal (ī-sŏk′rō-năl) [″ + *chronos,* time]. Acting in uniform time, or taking place at regular intervals. SYN: *isochronous.*

isochronia (īs-sō-krō′nē-ă) [Gr. *isos,* equal, + *chronos,* time]. The correspondence of events with respect to time, rate, or frequency.

isochronous (ī-sŏk′rō-nŭs). Isochronal, q.v.

isochroous (ī-sŏk′rō-ŭs) [″ + *chroa,* color]. Of uniform color. SYN: *isochromatic.*

isocitrate dehydrogenase (ī″sō-cĭt′rāt dē″hī-drŏj′ĕn-ās) An enzyme present in tissues. It catalyzes the conversion of isocitric acid to α-ketoglutaric acid.

isocolloid (ī-sō-kŏl′oyd) [″ + *kollodes,* glutinous]. A colloid having the same composition in every transformation.

isocomplement [″ + L. *complere,* to complete]. Complement from an individual of the same species.

isocoria (ī″sō-kō′rē-ă) [″ + *kore,* pupil]. Equality of size of both pupils. SEE: *anisocoria.*

isocortex (ī″sō-kor′tĕks) [″ + L. *cortex,* bark]. The neopallium or non-olfactory portion of the cerebral cortex. It is composed of six layers of fibrous and cellular tissue having a similar distribution pattern. SYN: *neocortex; neopallium.*

isocytosis (ī″sō-sī-tō′sĭs) [″ + *kytos,* cell, + *osis,* condition]. Cells of equal size.

isocytotoxin (ī″sō-sī″tō-tŏk′sĭn) [″ + ″ + *toxikon,* poison]. A cytotoxin destructive to homologous cells of the same species.

isodactylism (ī-sō-dăk′tĭl-ĭzm) [″ + *daktylos,* finger]. Condition of having fingers or toes of equal length.

isodiametric (ī″sō-dī-ă-mĕt′rĭk) [″ + *dia,* across, + *metron,* measure]. Having equal diameters.

isodontic (ī″sō-dŏn′tĭk) [″ + *odous,* tooth]. Having teeth of equal size.

isodose (ī′sō-dōs). In radiology, to have equal doses of radiation to different areas.

isodynamic (ī″sō-dī-năm′ĭk) [″ + *dynamis,* power]. Having equal power.

isoelectric (ī″sō-ē-lĕk′trĭk) [″ + *elektron,* amber]. Having equal electric potentials.

isoelectric period. In an occurrence that normally produces an electric force, such as a muscle contraction, the time or point when no electric energy is produced. In an electrocardiogram, the period when the electrical tracing is at zero and is neither positive or negative.

isoenergetic [Gr. *isos,* equal + *energeia,* energy]. Showing equal force or activity.

isoenzyme (ī″sō-ĕn′zīm) [″ + *en,* in, + *zyme,* leaven]. One of several forms in which an enzyme may exist in various tissues. Although the isoenzymes are similar in catalytic qualities, they may be separated from each other by special chemical tests. SYN: *isozyme.* SEE: *lactic dehydrogenase.*

isoetharine hydrochloride (ī-sō-ĕth′ă-rēn). USP. A sympathomimetic drug used as a bronchodilator. Trade name for 1% solution is Bronkosol.

Isofedrol. Trade name for ephedrine sulfate, USP.

isoflurophate (ī-sō-floo′rō-fāt). USP. An anticholinesterase drug used in treating glaucoma as well as atony of the smooth muscle of the intestinal tract and urinary bladder. Trade name is Floropryl.

isogamete (ī″sō-găm′ēt) [″ + *gamete,* wife, *gametes,* husband]. 1. A cell that, through conjugation or fusion with a similar cell, reproduces. 2. A gamete of the same size as the one with which it fuses or unites.

isogamy (ī-sŏg′ă-mē) [″ + *gamos,* marriage]. Reproduction resulting from conjugation of isogametes or identical cells.

isogeneic (ī″sō-jĕn-ē′ĭk). Syngeneic, q.v.

isogeneric (ī″sō-jĕ-nĕr′ĭk) [″ + L. *genus,* kind]. Of the same kind; concerning or obtained from members of the same genus.

isogenesis (ī″sō-jĕn′ĕ-sĭs) [″ + *genesis,* production]. Similarity in morphological development.

isogenic (ī″sō-jĕn′ĭk). Isologous, q.v.

isograft [″ + L. *graphium,* grafting shoot]. A graft taken from another individual or animal of the same genotype as the recipient. SEE: *cutograft.*

isohemagglutination (ī″sō-hĕm″ă-gloo″tĭ-nā′shŭn) [″ + *haima,* blood, + L. *agglutinare,* to glue to]. Isoagglutination, q.v.

isohemagglutinin (ī″sō-hĕm″ă-glū′tĭn-ĭn) [″ + *haima,* blood, + L. *agglutinare,* to glue to]. Substance normally present in most human blood serum; responsible for the clumping of corpuscles observed when incompatible bloods are mixed. The clumping is ascribed to the interaction of an agglutinogen in the corpuscles with a specific agglutinin in the foreign serum. In transfusions, the corpuscles of the donor are exposed to an overwhelming quantity of the recipient's plasma; therefore the agglutinogen content of the donor's corpuscles and the agglutinin content of the recipient's serum are the factors that determine compatibility.

Assuming that there are but two possible agglutinogens, red corpuscles from a given donor may contain both, either, or neither. If the agglutinin, alpha, can react only with agglutinogen A, one can construct a table to illustrate which blood types will be compatible or incompatible with other types. SEE: *agglutinin; agglutinogen.*

isohemolysin (ī″sō-hē-mŏl′ĭ-sĭn) [″ + ″ + *lysis,* dissolution]. Substance that destroys red blood corpuscles of animals of the same species from which it is obtained. SYN: *isolysin.* SEE: *hemolysin.*

isohemolysis (ī″sō-hē-mŏl′ĭ-sĭs). Action of an isohemolysin. SYN: *isolysis.* SEE: *hemolysis.*

isohypercytosis (ī″sō-hī″pĕr-sī-tō′sĭs) [″ + *hyper,* above, + *kytos,* cell, + *osis,* condition]. Condition in which the total number of white blood cells is increased but the proportions of the polymorphonuclear leukocytes remain stable.

isohypocytosis (ī″sō-hī″pō-sī-tō′sĭs) [″ + *hypo,* under, + *kytos,* cell, + *osis,* condition]. Condition in which the total number of white blood cells is decreased but the proportions of polymorphonuclear leukocytes remain stable.

isoiconia (ī″sō-ī-kō′nē-ă) [Gr. *isos,* equal, + *eikon,* image]. Equality of both retinal images.

isoiconic (ī″sō-ī-kŏn′ĭk). Having equal retinal images.

isoimmunization [″ + L. *immunis,* safe]. Immunization of an individual against the blood of an individual of the same species, esp. the development of Rh-negative agglutinins in an Rh-negative mother in response to agglutinogens present in transfused Rh-positive blood or developed in an Rh-positive fetus.

isokinetic exercise. Contraction of a muscle during which the force exerted while the muscle shortens is maximal. SEE: *isometric exercise.*

isolate [It. *isolato,* isolated]. 1. To separate or detach from other persons, as during an infectious disease. 2. In chemistry, to obtain a substance in pure form from the mixture or solution that contains it.

isolation. Limitation of movement and social contacts of patient suffering from, or a known carrier of, communicable disease, in contradistinction to quarantine, which limits the movements of exposed or contact persons. SEE: *incubation* for table; *quarantine.*

NURSING IMPLICATIONS: A patient is placed in isolation to prevent the spread of the disease-causing agents. The rules to be followed are based on the mode of transmission of the organism, e.g., if the organism is spread by droplet, then all items that come in contact with the upper respiratory tract of the patient are isolated and destroyed or disinfected. Most institutions use readily disposed of paper plates, cups, and plastic utensils for patients who are isolated. The hands of the personnel caring for the patient, the doctor, nurse, allied health personnel, and family are the commonest means of transmitting infection. Handwashing and keeping the hands away from the face, esp. the nose and mouth, is the best method of control of spread of disease. Upon leaving the patient, gowns, masks, and caps used in the sickroom should be removed and placed in an appropriate container. Follow hospital procedure for the specific type of isolation that is in effect. The purpose for isolation precautions should be explained to the patient and family to decrease their fears and increase compliance.

isolation ward. Hospital ward where patients suffering from communicable disease may be kept apart from the rest of the patients.

isoleucine (ī″sō-lū′sēn). USP. An amino acid formed during hydrolysis of fibrin and other proteins. It is essential in the diet.

isologous (ī-sŏl′ō-gŭs). Genetically identical. In transplantations, being isologous (or isogenic) indicates the absence of any tissue incompatibility between the recipient of tissue and the tissue or organ itself. SYN: *isogenic; syngeneic.*

isolophobia (ī″sō-lō-fō′bē-ă) [It. *isolato,* isolated, + Gr. *phobos,* fear]. Fear of being alone. SEE: *agoraphobia.*

isolysin (ī-sŏl′ĭ-sĭn) [Gr. *isos,* equal, + *lysis,* dissolution]. Substance that dissolves red corpuscles of animals of the same species from which it is obtained. SYN: *isohemolysin.*

isolysis (ī-sŏl′ĭ-sĭs). Destruction of red blood corpuscles produced by an isolysin. SYN: *isohemolysis.* SEE: *hemolysis.*

isolytic (ī-sō-lĭt′ĭk). Rel. to isolysis.

isomer (ī′sō-mĕr) [Gr. *isos,* equal, + *meros,* part]. One of two or more chemical substances that have the same molecular formula but different chemical and physical properties due to different arrangement of the atoms in the molecule. Dextrose is an isomer of levulose. SEE: *polymer.*

isomerase (ī-sŏm′ĕr-ās). Any enzyme that catalyzes the isomerization of its substrate. For example, phosphoglucose isomerase interconverts glucose and fructose-6-phosphate. SEE: *isomerism.*

isomeric (ī″sō-mĕr′ĭk). Pert. to isomerism.

isomerism (ī-sŏm′ĕr-ĭzm). State of being composed of compounds of the same number of atoms but having different atomic arrangement in the molecule. SEE: *metamerism; polymerism.*

isomerization (ī-sŏm″ĕr-ī-zā′shŭn). The conversion of one chemical substance to an isomer. SEE: *isomer; isomerism.*

isometric [″ + *metron,* measure]. Having equal dimensions. SEE: *isotonic.*

isometric contraction. Contraction of a muscle in which shortening or lengthening is prevented. Tension is developed but no mechanical work performed, all energy being liberated as heat.

isometric contraction phase. The first phase in contraction of the ventricle of the heart in which ventricular pressure increases but there is no decrease in volume of contents because semilunar valves are closed.

isometric exercise. Contraction of a muscle that is not accompanied by movement of the joints that would normally be moved by that muscle's action. The muscle length is not changed by this type of exercise. SEE: *isotonic exercise.*

isometric muscle. Contraction in which a muscle increases its tension without shortening.

isometropia (ī″sō-mĕ-trō′pē-ă) [″ + ″ + *ops,* eye]. Same refraction of the two eyes.

isomorphism (ī-sō-mor′fĭzm) [″ + *morphe,* form, + *-ismos,* state of]. Condition marked by possession of the same form.

isomorphous (ī″sō-mor′fŭs). Possessing the same shape.

isoniazid (ī″sō-nī′ă-zĭd). USP. ABBR: INH. $C_6H_7N_3O$. An odorless compound occurring as colorless or white crystals or as a white crystalline powder. An antibacterial, used principally in treating tuberculosis. Trade names are Cotinazin, Dinacrin, and Nydrazid.

isonicotinoylhydrazine (ī″sō-nĭk″ō-tĭn″ō-ĭl-hī′dră-zēn). Isoniazid.

isonormocytosis (ī″sō-nor″mō-sī-tō′sĭs) [″ + L. *norma,* rule, + Gr. *kytos,* cell, + *osis,* condition]. State of having leukocytes of the blood normal in number and proportion of varieties.

isopathy (ī-sŏp′ă-thē) [Gr. *isos,* equal, + *pathos,* disease]. Therapeutic administration of the causative agent of the disease or its products. SYN: *isotherapy.*

isophoria (ī″sō-fō′rē-ă) [″ + *phorein,* to carry]. Equal tension of vertical muscles of each eye with visual lines in the same horizontal plane. Absence of hyperphoria, q.v., and hypophoria, q.v.

isopia (ī-sō′pē-ă) [″ + *ops,* vision]. Equal vision in the eyes.

isoplastic (ī″sō-plăs′tĭk) [″ + *plastos,* formed]. Term applied to a graft taken from one individual and transplanted to another of the same species. SEE: *isograft.*

isoprecipitin (ī″sō-prē-sĭp′ĭ-tĭn) [″ + L. *praecipitare,* to cast down]. A precipitin that reacts with antigens from other members of the same species, but they are genetically dissimilar.

isopropamide iodide (ī″sō-prō′pă-mīd). USP. A synthetic antimuscarinic drug that acts similarly to belladonna. Trade name is Darbid.

isopropanol (ī″sō-prō′pă-nŏl). Isopropyl alcohol.

isopropyl alcohol. C_3H_8O. A clear flammable liquid similar to ethyl alcohol and propyl alcohol. Used in medical preparations for external use, antifreeze, cosmetics, and as a solvent.

CAUTION: Toxic when taken internally. SEE: *Poisons and Poisoning* in *Appendix.*

isoproterenol hydrochloride (ī″sō-prō″tē-rē′nŏl). USP. A sympathomimetic amine used to relieve bronchoconstriction in asthma. It is also used as a cardiac stimulant in heart block. Trade names are Isuprel Hydrochloride, Norisodrine Hydrochloride, and Vapo-Iso.

CAUTION: Overdosage administered by inhalation can be fatal.

isopters (ī-sŏp′tĕrz) [″ + *opter,* observer]. Lines on a chart of the field of vision that connect points of equal visual acuity.

Isopto Atropine. Trade name for atropine sulfate.

Isopto Carbachol. Trade name for carbachol.

Isopto Carpine. Trade name for pilocarpine hydrochloride, USP.

Isopto Cetamide. Trade name for sulfacetamide sodium, USP.

Isopto Eserine. Trade name for physostigmine salicylate, USP.

Isopto Frin. Trade name for phenylephrine hydrochloride, USP.

Isopto Homatropine. Trade name for homatropine hydrobromide.

Isopto Hyoscine. Trade name for scopolamine hydrobromide.

isopyknosis (ī″sō-pĭk-nō′sĭs) [″ + *pyknosis,* condensation]. Having uniform density, esp. being in a state of equal condensation as in comparing different chromosomes.

Isordil. Trade name for isosorbide dinitrate.

isoserotherapy (ī″sō-sē″rō-thĕr′ă-pē) [″ + L. *serum,* whey, + Gr. *therapeia,* therapy]. Treatment with serum from one having had the same disease as the patient.

isoserum (ī″sō-sē′rŭm). A serum from one having had the disease for which a patient is to receive treatment.

isosexual (ī″sō-sĕks′ū-ăl). Concerning or characteristic of the same sex.

isosmotic (ī″sŏs-mŏt′ĭk) [″ + *osmos,* impulsion]. Having the same total concentration of osmotically active molecules or ions in solution as the solution or body fluid to which it is being compared. SEE: *isotonic*.

isosorbide dinitrate tablets (ī″sō-sor′bīd). USP. An antiaginal drug used sublingually. Trade names are Isordil, Sorbitrate, and Sorquad.

Isospora (ī-sŏs′pō-ră) [″ + *sporos*, spore]. A genus of Sporozoa belonging to the order Coccidia.

I. hominis. A parasitic protozoon inhabiting the small intestine of man. It is nonpathogenic.

isospore (ī′sō-spor) [Gr. *isos*, equal, + *sporos*, spore]. A nonsexual spore from plants with only one kind of spore. It grows to maturity without conjugating.

isosthenuria (ī″sŏs-thĕn-ū′rē-ă) [″ + *sthenos*, strength, + *ouron*, urine]. Condition of the urine being of a uniform specific gravity and osmolarity despite variations in fluid intake. A sign of marked impairment of renal function.

isostimulation [″ + L. *stimulare*, to goad]. Stimulation of an animal by the use of antigenic material derived from another animal of the same species.

isotherapy (ī″sō-thĕr′ă-pē) [″ + *therapeia*, treatment]. Treatment of disease by active causative agent of the same disease. SYN: *isopathy*.

isothermal [″ + *therme*, heat]. Having equal temperature.

isothermognosis (ī″sō-thĕrm″ŏg-nō′sĭs) [″ + ″ + *gnosis*, knowledge]. Abnormal perception in which stimulation by pain, heat, and cold are all felt as heat.

isotherms (ī′sō-thĕrmz). Lines on a chart or map connecting points that have the same temperature.

isotones (ī′sō-tōnz). Nuclides with the same number of neutrons but a different number of protons in their nuclei.

isotonia (ī″sō-tō′nē-ă) [″ + *tonos*, tone]. The state of equal osmotic pressure of two or more solutions or substances.

isotonic (ī″sō-tŏn′ĭk). 1. Having the same tension or tone. An isotonic muscle contraction occurs when equal tension on the muscle is maintained while the length of the muscle is decreased during the performance of work or exercise. SEE: *isometric*. 2. Having the same osmotic pressure.

isotonic exercise. Contraction of a muscle during which the force of resistance to the movement remains constant throughout the range of motion.

isotonicity (ī″sō-tō-nĭs′ĭ-tē). The state or condition of being isotonic.

isotonic solution. A solution that has a concentration of electrolytes, nonelectrolytes, or a combination of the two that will exert equivalent osmotic pressure as that solution with which it is being compared.

Ex.: Either 0.16 molar sodium chloride solution (approx. 0.95% salt in water) or 0.3 molar nonelectrolyte solution is approx. isotonic with human red blood cells.

isotope (ī′sō-tōp) [″ + *topos*, place]. One of a series of chemical elements that have nearly identical chemical properties but that differ in their atomic weights and electric charge. Many isotopes are radioactive.

i., radioactive. Radioisotope. An isotope in which the nuclear composition is unstable.

isotope cisternography. Use of a radioactive tracer to investigate the circulation of cerebrospinal fluid. A tracer such as ^{131}I serum albumin is injected in the lumbar subarachnoid space. Flow of the tracer toward the head and into areas of the brain can be recorded by means of serial scintillation scanning. This technique is useful in studying hydrocephalus.

isotropic (ī″sō-trŏp′ĭk) [″ + *tropos*, a turning]. 1. Possessing similar qualities in every direction. 2. Having equal refraction.

isotropy (ī-sŏt′rō-pē). State of being isotropic, q.v.

isotypical (ī-sō-tĭp′ĭ-kăl) [″ + *typos*, mark]. Belonging to the same variety or classification.

isovaleric acidemia (ī″sō-vă-lĕr′ĭk ăs″ĭ-dē′mē-ă). An inherited metabolic disease in which leucine metabolism is affected. Isovaleric acid accumulates in the blood during periods of increased amino acid metabolism, i.e., during infections or following ingestion of proteins. Coma and death may occur.

isoxsuprine hydrochloride (ī-sŏk′sū-prēn). USP. A vasodilator drug. Its therapeutic usefulness has not been established. Trade name is Vasodilan.

isozyme (ī′sō-zīm). Isoenzyme, q.v.

issue (ĭsh′ū) [ME.]. 1. Offspring. 2. A suppurating sore maintained by a foreign body in the tissue to act as a counterirritant. 3. A discharge of pus or blood.

isthmectomy (ĭs-mĕk′tō-mē) [Gr. *isthmos*, isthmus, + *ektome*, incision]. Excision of an enlarged isthmus, esp. of the thyroid gland.

isthmian (ĭs′mē-ăn). Rel. to an isthmus.

isthmitis (ĭs-mī′tĭs) [″ + *itis*, inflammation]. Inflammation of the throat or fauces.

isthmoparalysis (ĭs″mō-pă-răl′ĭ-sĭs) [″ + *para*, beyond, + *lyein*, to loosen]. Paralysis of the muscles of the fauces. SYN: *isthmoplegia*.

isthmoplegia (ĭs″mō-plē′jē-ă) [″ + *plege*, a stroke]. Faucial paralysis. SYN: *isthmoparalysis*.

isthmospasm (ĭs′mō-spăzm″) [″ + *spasmos*, spasm]. Isthmian spasm, as of the fauces or of the fallopian tubes.

isthmus (ĭs′mŭs) [L.; Gr. *isthmos,* isthmus]. (pl. *isthmuses* or *isthmi*) 1. A narrow passage connecting two cavities. 2. A narrow structure connecting two larger parts. 3. A constriction between two larger parts of an organ, or anatomical structure.

i., aortic. Constriction in the fetal aorta between the ductus arteriosus and left subclavian artery. Sometimes persists in adults.

i. faucium. [NA] A constriction connecting the posterior mouth cavity proper with the pharynx.

i. glandulae thyreoideae. [NA] A narrow portion of the thyroid gland connecting the left and right lobes. SYN: *i. of thyroid.*

i. of eustachian tube. I. tubae auditivae.

i. of thyroid. I. glandulae thyreoideae.

i. of uterine tube. I. tubae uterinae.

i. of uterus. I. uteri.

i., pharyngeal. I. pharyngonasalis.

i. pharyngonasalis. [NA] The opening between the naso- and oral pharynx. SYN: *i., pharyngeal.*

i. tubae auditivae. [NA] Narrowest portion of the eustachian tube. SYN: *i. of eustachian tube.*

i. tubae uterinae. [NA] The constricted portion (the medial third) of the uterine (fallopian) tube nearest the uterus. SYN: *i. of uterine tube.*

i. uteri. [NA] A slight constriction on the surface of the uterus midway between the uterine body and the cervix. SYN: *i. of uterus.*

Isuprel Hydrochloride. Trade name for isoproterenol hydrochloride, USP.

isuria (ī-sū′rē-ă) [Gr. *isos,* equal, + *ouron,* urine]. Excretion of urine at a uniform rate.

itch [ME. *icchen*]. 1. Irritation of skin, inducing desire to scratch. SYN: *pruritus.* 2. Scabies.

i., baker's. Rash that occurs on the hands and forearms of bakers. It may be due to mechanical or chemical factors.

i., barber's. A fungus infection of the bearded portion of the face and neck. SYN: *tinea barbae.*

i., dhobie. A fungus infection of the groin and perineum. SYN: *jock itch; tinea cruris.*

i., grain. Dermatitis caused by mites.

i., grocer's. Dermatitis caused by mites in grain or cheese; dermatitis caused by sugar.

i., ground. Local irritation produced by penetration of the skin of the foot by hookworm larvae, especially Necator americanus.

i., jock. A fungus infection of the groin and perineum. SYN: *dhobie itch; tinea cruris.*

i., seven-year. Scabies.

i., swimmer's. Dermatitis that develops after swimming in water containing the larval form of schistosomes.

i., winter. Dermatitis that occurs in the winter. SYN: *pruritus hiemalis.*

itching. Pruritus; irritation of the skin, causing desire to rub or scratch the part.

itch mite. Sarcoptes scabiei. SEE: *scabies.*

-ite [Gr.]. 1. Suffix meaning of the nature of. 2. In chemistry, a salt of an acid having the termination *-ous.*

iter (ī′tĕr) [L.]. Passageway between two anatomical parts.

iteral (ī′tĕr-ăl). Pert. to an iter.

iteroparity (ĭt″ĕr-ō-păr′ĭ-tē) [L. *iterare,* to repeat, + *parere,* to bear]. Condition of reproducing more than once in a lifetime.

ithycyphosis, ithyokyphosis (ĭth″ĭ-sī-fō′sĭs, ĭth″ē-ō-kī-fō′sĭs) [Gr. *ithys,* straight, + *kyphos,* humped]. Kyphosis with backward projection of the spine.

ithylordosis (ĭth″ĭ-lor-dō′sĭs) [″ + *lordosis,* a bending forward]. Lordosis without lateral curvature of the spine.

-itis (ī′tĭs) [Gr.]. Suffix meaning inflammation of.

ITP. *idiopathic thrombocytopenic purpura.*

I.U. *immunizing unit; international unit.*

I.U.C.D. *intrauterine contraceptive device.*

I.U.D. *intrauterine device.*

I.V. *intravenous(ly).*

Ivadantin. Trade name for nitrofurantoin sodium, USP.

I.V.P. *intravenous pyelography;* radiographic examination of the kidneys, ureters, and bladder after introduction of a contrast medium.

I.V. push. Administration of medicine intravenously by quick and forcible injection.

I.V.T. *intravenous transfusion.*

I.V.U. *intravenous urography.*

Ivy method (ī′vē). [Andrew C. Ivy, Chicago physiologist, b. 1893] SEE: *bleeding time.*

ivy poisoning. Dermatitis caused by contact with poison ivy. SEE: *poison ivy dermatitis.*

Ixodes (ĭks-ō′dēz) [Gr. *ixodes,* like birdlime]. A genus of ticks of the family Ixodidae, q.v., many of which are parasitic on man and animals.

ixodiasis (ĭks″ō-dī′ă-sĭs). 1. Lesions of the skin caused by tick bites. 2. Any disease caused by ticks, as Rocky Mountain fever.

ixodic (ĭks-ŏd′ĭk). Pert. to or caused by ticks.

Ixodidae (ĭks-ŏd′ĭ-dē). A family of ticks belonging to the order Acarina, class Arachnida. Comprises the hard-bodied ticks including the genera Amblyomma, Boophilus, Dermacentor, Haemaphysalis, Hyalomma, Ixodes, and Rhipicephalus. All are parasitic and of importance as pests or in the transmission of disease in domestic animals and man. Among diseases transmitted are Rocky Mountain spotted fever, relapsing fever, and tularemia.

Ixodides (ĭks-ŏd′ĭ-dēz). Ticks.

Ixodoidea (ĭks″ō-doy′dē-ă). A superfamily of

Acarina, the ticks, in which the adults have a thick cuticle.

ixomyelitis (ĭks″ō-mī-ĕ-lī′tĭs) [Gr. *ixodes,* like birdlime, + *myelos,* marrow, + *itis,* inflammation]. Inflammation of the spinal cord in the lumbar region.

J. Symb. for joule.

Jaboulay's amputation (zhă″boo-lāz′). [Mathieu Jaboulay, Fr. surgeon, 1860–1913] Amputation of the thigh and removal of the hip bone.

Jaboulay's button. Two cylinders that may be screwed together for lateral intestinal anastomosis without the use of sutures.

jacket [O. Fr. *jacquet,* jacket]. A bandage that is usually applied to the trunk to immobilize the spine or to correct deformities.

j., Sayre's. Plaster-of-Paris jacket used as a support for deformity of the spinal column.

j., strait. Device for restraining a patient or criminal who is violent. It has sleeves that extend beyond the hands. The ends of these may be secured, thereby preventing movement of the arms and trunk. SYN: *camisole.*

jack-knife position. Position in which the patient lies on the back with shoulders elevated, lower legs flexed on thighs and the thighs are at right angles to the trunk. Employed when passing a urethral sound. SYN: *position, reclining.*

jackscrew. A threaded screw used for expanding the dental arch or for positioning bone fragments after a fracture.

jacksonian epilepsy. [John Hughlings Jackson, Brit. neurologist, 1835–1911] A localized form of epilepsy with spasms confined to one part or one group of muscles. SEE: *epilepsy.*

Jacob, Arthur. Irish ophthalmologist, 1790–1874.

J.'s membrane. Retinal layer of rods and cones.

J.'s ulcer. Epithelioma, usually of the face, that slowly destroys soft tissue and bones. SYN: *rodent ulcer.*

Jacobson, Ludwig. Danish anatomist, 1783–1843.

J.'s cartilage. One of two narrow longitudinal cartilages lying along the anterior inferior border of the nasal septum. They are rudimentary in man.

J.'s nerve. Tympanic nerve.

J.'s organ. Rudimentary sac in nasal septum. SYN: *vomeronasal organ.* SEE: *organ of Jacobson.*

J.'s sulcus. Portion of the middle ear containing branches of the tympanic plexus.

Jacquemier's sign (zhăk-mē-āz′). [Jean Jacquemier, Fr. obstetrician, 1806–1879] Blue or purplish color of the vaginal mucosa. A presumptive sign of pregnancy.

jactatio (jăk-tā′shē-ō) [L.]. Restless tossing of the head and body. Seen in acute illness.

jactitation (jăk″tĭ-tā′shŭn) [L. *jactitatio,* tossing]. In acute disease, the restless to-and-fro movement of the body.

Jadelot's lines (zhăd-lōz′). [François N. Jadelot, Fr. physician, 1791–1830] Lines on the face, said to indicate disease in children.

Ocular line: Down from corner of mouth; seen in respiratory diseases.

Nasal line: From lower border of ala nasi about outer side of orbicularis oris muscle; seen in abdominal disorders.

Labial line: From inner canthus toward glenoid fossa; observed in cerebral disease.

Jaeger's test types (yā′gĕrz). [Edward Jaeger von Jastthal, Austrian ophthalmologist, 1818–1884] Lines of type of various sizes, printed on a card for testing near vision. The smallest type read at the closest distance is recorded.

jalap (jăl′ăp) [Jalapa, a city in Mexico]. The dried tuberous root of Exogonium purga. Formerly used as a cathartic. Now considered to be unapproved for this use.

jamais vu (zhăm′ā voo) [Fr., never seen]. Subjective mental reaction of being in a completely strange environment when in familiar surroundings. May be associated with temporal lobe lesions. SEE: *déjà vu.*

James fibers. Pathway for conduction of cardiac impulses so they bypass the atrioventricular node. This alternate fiber pathway permits preexcitation of the ventricle with resultant tachycardia.

Janeway lesions. [E. G. Janeway, U.S. physician, 1841–1911] Small, painless red-blue macular lesions a few mm. in diameter found on the palms and soles in acute bacterial endocarditis. SEE: *Roth's spots.*

janiceps (jăn′ĭ-sĕps) [L. *Janus,* a two-faced god, + *caput,* head]. Deformed embryo with a face on the anterior and posterior aspects of the single head.

Janimine. Trade name for imipramine hydrochloride.

Jansky-Bielschowsky syndrome (jăn′skē-bē-ăl-show′skē). [Jan Jansky, Czech physician, 1873–1921; Max Bielschowsky, Ger. neuropathologist, 1869–1940] Early juvenile cerebral sphingolipidosis, q.v.

jar. 1. A container that is made of glass, plastic, or other sturdy or impervious materials. It is usually taller than it is wide and may be cylindrical, square, or in other shapes. 2. A sudden movement, as a jolt or shock.

j., bell. A glass vessel with an opening at only one end.

j., heel. The production of pain by having the patient stand on tiptoes and suddenly bring the heels to the floor. This may be diagnostic of tuberculosis of the spine or of renal calculus.

jargon (jăr′gŭn) [O. Fr., a chattering]. 1. Unintelligible speech. SYN: *paraphasia.* 2. Speech or writing that includes unfamiliar terms or abbreviations peculiar to persons in a special field or of science.

Jarvis' snare. [William C. Jarvis, U.S. laryngologist, 1855–1895] A snare for removing growths in the nasal cavities.

jaundice (jawn′dĭs) [Fr. *jaune,* yellow]. A condition characterized by yellowness of skin and whites of eyes, mucous membranes, and body fluids due to deposition of bile pigment resulting from excess bilirubin in the blood (hyperbilirubinemia). It may be caused by obstruction of bile passageways, excess destruction of red blood cells (hemolysis), or disturbances in functioning of liver cells.

Jaundice is a symptom that may be the indicator of a benign and curable disease, such as a gallstone blocking the common duct. It may be due to carcinoma of the head of the pancreas involving the opening of the bile duct into the duodenum. It is therefore important to make the correct diagnosis. Sometimes diagnosis can be made only after exploratory surgical procedures. SYN: *icterus.*

j., acholuric. Jaundice without bile pigment in the urine.

j., cholestatic. Jaundice due to failure of bile to reach the duodenum, whether due to blockage of the flow of bile or to liver cell changes.

j., congenital. Jaundice occurring at or shortly after birth due to maldevelopment of biliary apparatus.

j., hematogenous. J., hemolytic.

j., hemolytic. A rare chronic form that causes jaundice as a result of increased destruction of red blood cells. The serum bilirubin may be only slightly elevated even though bile pigment production may be increased as much as six times normal. The bilirubin, which is mostly unconjugated and therefore insoluble in water, does not appear in the urine. The spleen usually is enlarged. SYN: *icterus, hemolytic.*

j., hemorrhagic. Jaundice present with leptospirosis.

j., hepatocanalicular. Jaundice resulting from changes in the bile canaliculi, the liver cells remaining relatively normal.

j., hepatocellular. Jaundice resulting from disease of liver cells.

j., hepatogenous. Jaundice due to disease of the liver.

j., infectious. Infectious hepatitis.

j., leptospiral. Jaundice present with leptospirosis.

j., malignant. Acute yellow atrophy of the liver.

j., nonhemolytic. Jaundice due to abnormal metabolism of bilirubin. By implication, the jaundice is not due to excessive destruction of red blood cells.

j., obstructive. Jaundice due to a mechanical impediment in the flow of bile from the liver to the duodenum. SYN: *icterus, obstructive.*

j. of newborn. Jaundice affecting newborn infants. SYN: *icterus neonatorum.*

j., parenchymatous. J., hepatocellular.

j., physiologic. Simple jaundice in infants. It lasts only a few days, and does not require therapy.

j., posthepatic. Jaundice resulting from obstruction of flow of bile ducts. May be incomplete or complete.

j., regurgitation. Jaundice due to bile entering lymph channels of the liver and thence being conveyed to the blood. May result from biliary obstruction or lesions involving bile capillaries.

j., retention. Jaundice resulting from inability of liver cells to remove bile pigment from circulation.

j., spirochetal. An acute infectious disease due to a spirochete, Leptospira icterohemorrhagica. SYN: *Weil's disease.*

j., toxic. Jaundice resulting from bacterial toxins or poisons such as phosphorus, arsphenamine, carbon tetrachloride.

Javelle water (zhŭ-vĕl′) [Javel, a city now part of Paris]. An aqueous solution of potassium or sodium hypochlorite used as a bleach and disinfectant.

jaw [ME. *iawe*]. Either or both of the maxillary and mandibular bones, bearing the teeth and forming the mouth framework. SEE: illus.

j., dislocation of. Jaw dislocations are uncomfortable and extremely embarrassing to the patient. They may occur on either side, in which instance the tip of the jaw is pointed away from the dislocation. On the normal side, just in front of the ear, may be felt a little hollow or depression that is often tender. If both sides of the jaw are dislocated, the jaw is pushed downward and forward. In either event, there is pain and difficulty in speech and the condition is often accompanied by shock. Backward dislocation of jaw is rare.

CAUSES: Most often caused by a blow to the face or a fall on the chin, but occasionally caused by chewing large chunks of food, by yawning, or by hearty laughing.

REDUCTION: These dislocations are reduced by placing well-padded thumbs inside of the mouth on the lower molar (back) teeth with the fingers running along the jawbone as a lever. The thumbs should be pressed downward toward the patient's lips and the fingers upward toward the patient's nose.

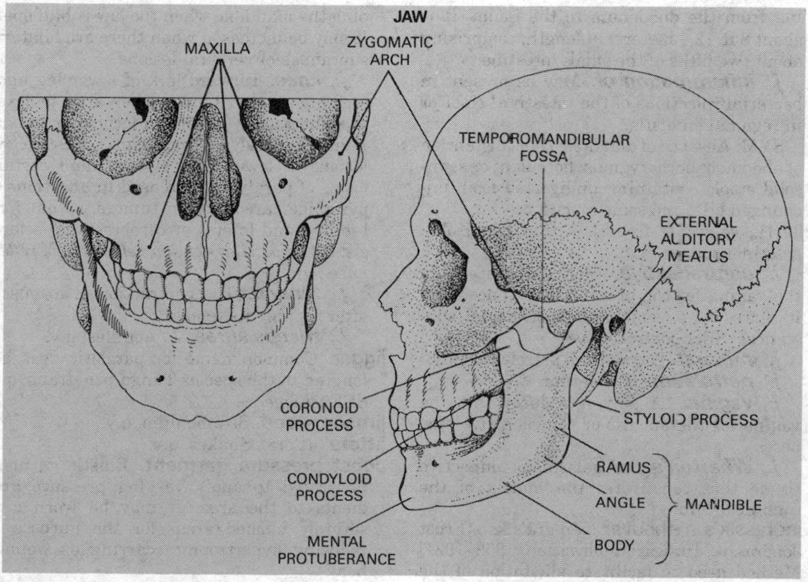

Give a twisting motion to the jaw and at the same time with the wrist and elbows press backward toward the neck. The jaw gliding over the ridge of bone may be felt and just as this occurs the jaw usually snaps into place. When this motion is noted, move the thumbs laterally toward the cheeks to avoid the thumbs being crushed between the molars.

This snapping into place is due to an involuntary spasm of the muscles pulling the jaw as though an overstretched rubber band were attached to it. Following the reduction, an immobilizing bandage or double cravat should be applied.

j., lumpy. Fungus disease affecting the jaw, brain, lungs, and gastrointestinal tract. Common in cattle and sometimes affecting humans. SYN: *actinomycosis.*

j., swelling of. *Lower:* May be due to alveolar abscess, a cyst, gumma, sarcoma, or actinomycosis. *Upper:* Occurs in alveolar abscess, parotid tumor, parotitis, carcinoma, sarcoma, necrosis of bone, or disease of antrum.

jaw, words pert. to: agnathia; alveolar; alveolate; alveolus; epulis; genyplasty; "gnath-" words; hypognathous; mandible; maxilla; prognathism; ramus; submaxillary; temporomandibular syndrome; tetanus; trismus.

jaw winking. Congenital disorder in which ptosis of the eyelid is momentarily improved by movement of the jaw.

jejunal (jē-jū'năl) [L. *jejunum,* empty]. Rel. to the jejunum.

jejunectomy (jē″jū-nĕk'tō-mē) [″ + Gr. *ektome,* excision]. Excision of part or all of the jejunum.

jejunitis (jē″jū-nī'tĭs) [″ + Gr. *itis,* inflammation]. Inflammation of the jejunum.

jejuno- [L.]. Combining form referring to the jejunum.

jejunocecostomy (jĕ-joo″nō-sē-kŏs'tō-mē) [″ + *caecum,* blindness, + Gr. *stoma,* mouth]. Surgical joining of the cecum and jejunum.

jejunocolostomy (jē-jū″nō-kōl-ŏs'tō-mē) [″ + Gr. *kolon,* colon, + *stoma,* mouth]. Formation of an artificial passage between the jejunum and colon.

jejunoileal (jĕ-joo″nō-ĭl'ē-ăl) [″ + *ileum,* small intestine]. Concerning the jejunum and ileum.

jejunoileitis (jē-jū″nō-ĭl″ē-ī'tĭs) [″ + ″ + Gr. *itis,* inflammation]. Inflamed condition of the jejunum and ileum.

jejunoileostomy (jē-jū″nō-ĭl″ē-ŏs'tō-mē) [″ + ″ + Gr. *stoma,* mouth]. Formation of a passage between the jejunum and ileum.

jejunojejunostomy (jē-jū″nō-jē″jū-nŏs'tō-mē) [″ + *jejunum,* empty, + Gr. *stoma,* mouth]. Formation of a passage between two parts of the jejunum.

jejunorrhaphy (jĕ″joo-nor'ă-fē) [″ + Gr. *rhaphe,* suture]. Surgical repair of the jejunum.

jejunostomy (jē″jū-nŏs'tō-mē) [″ + Gr. *stoma,* mouth]. Surgical creation of a permanent opening into the jejunum.

jejunotomy (jē″jū-nŏt'ō-mē) [″ + Gr. *tome,* incision]. Surgical incision into the jejunum.

jejunum (jē-jū'nŭm) [L., empty]. [NA] The second portion of the small intestine extending from the duodenum to the ileum. It is about 8 ft. (2.4 meters) in length, comprising about two fifths of the small intestine.

j., inflammation of. May be present in bacterial infections of the intestinal tract or in regional enteritis.

SYM: Absence of diarrhea; colic, distention of abdomen, borborygmus; flocculent or semisolid stools containing undigested food, unchanged bile, and some mucus.

jelly [L. *gelare,* to freeze]. A thick semisolid, gelatinous mass.

j., contraceptive. A jelly introduced into the vagina for the prevention of conception. It serves as a vehicle for spermicidal substances. SEE: *contraceptive.*

j., mineral. Petrolatum, petroleum jelly.

j., petroleum. Petrolatum.

j., vaginal. A jelly introduced into the vagina for therapeutic or contraceptive purposes.

j., Wharton's. Soft gelatinous connective tissue that constitutes the matrix of the umbilical cord.

Jendrassik's maneuver (yĕn-dră'sĭks). [Ernst Jendrassik, Hungarian physician, 1858–1921] Method used to facilitate elicitation of the deep tendon reflexes of the lower extremities. The patient hooks together the fingers of the hands and attempts to pull them apart. While this pressure is maintained the patellar or Achilles' tendon reflex is tested.

Jenner, Edward. A British physician, 1749–1823, who invented the vaccination for smallpox. Prior to Jenner's work, it was known that individuals exposed to a mild case of the disease for the first time would suffer a mild case and then be immune to smallpox. Jenner observed that individuals exposed to cowpox, such as those who milked cows, would develop a minor lesion and then be immune to smallpox. From this observation Jenner developed a vaccine from cowpox lesions, now known to be the vaccinia virus, that gives immunity to smallpox.

Jenner's stain. [Louis Jenner, Brit. physician, 1866–1904] Eosin methylene blue stain.

jerk (jĕrk). 1. A sudden muscular movement. 2. Certain reflex actions resulting from striking or tapping a muscle or tendon. SEE: *reflex.*

j., Achilles; j., ankle. Contraction of the calf muscles produced by tapping the stretched Achilles tendon.

j., biceps. Reflex contraction produced by tapping over the lower end of the radius. The elbow will flex due to contraction of the biceps and supinator muscles.

j., elbow. Involuntary extension of forearm produced by external stimulation of the stretched triceps tendon.

j., jaw. Movement that is a result of tapping the mandible when the jaw is half open. It may be increased when there are bilateral supranuclear cerebral lesions.

j., knee. Forward jerk of lower leg upon striking patellar tendon when knee is flexed at right angles. Absent in locomotor ataxia, infantile paralysis, meningitis, destructive lesions of lower part of cord, and certain forms of paralysis. Increased in affections of pyramidal areas, brain tumors, spinal irritability, and lateral or cerebrospinal sclerosis. SYN: *patellar-tendon reflex.* SEE: *reflex, knee-jerk.*

j., tendon. The contraction of a muscle after tapping its tendon.

j., triceps surae. J., Achilles, q.v.

jigger. Common name for parasitic fleas belonging to the species Tunga penetrans, q.v. SEE: *chiggers.*

jimson weed. Stramonium, q.v.

jitters (jĭt'ĕrz). Shakes, q.v.

Jobst pressure garment. Elastic garment fabricated to apply varying pressure gradients to the area. It may be worn over severely burned areas for the purpose of reducing hypertrophic scarring as wounds heal.

Jocasta complex (jō-kăs'tă) [Jocasta, mother in the Oedipus complex, who was the wife and mother of Oedipus]. A term implying psychological or emotional fixation of a mother to her son. SEE: *Oedipus complex.*

Joffroy's reflex (zhŏf-rwhăz'). [Alexis Joffroy, Fr. physician, 1844–1908] Twitching of gluteal muscles when pressure is made against buttocks.

Joffroy's sign. 1. Absence of facial muscle contraction when eyes turn upward in exophthalmic goiter. 2. Inability to do simple sums in arithmetic. An early sign of general paralysis of the insane caused by central nervous system syphilis.

jogger's heel. Irritation of the fibrous and fatty tissue covering the heel. Due to the type of running characteristic of jogging wherein the heel strikes the surface first, rather than the toes as in sprinting. Persons prone to develop this may diminish the risk by wearing pads on their heels and by running on surfaces softer than wood, concrete, or asphalt.

jogging. Running for enjoyment or to maintain physical fitness. In contrast to running, jogging is not a competitive exercise.

joint [L. *junctio,* a joining]. An articulation. The point of juncture between two bones. A joint is usually formed of fibrous connective tissue and cartilage. It is classified as being immovable (synarthrosis), slightly movable (amphiarthrosis), and freely movable (diarthrosis). *Synarthrosis* is a joint in which the two bones are separated only by an interven-

TYPICAL SYNOVIAL JOINT

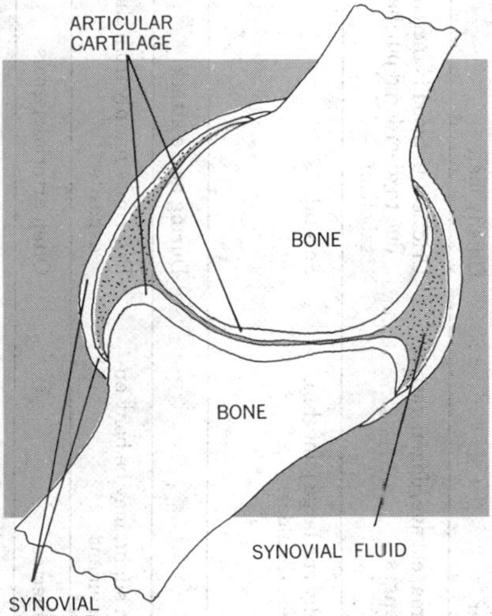

ing membrane, as the cranial sutures. *Amphiarthrosis* is a joint having a fibrocartilaginous disk between the bony surfaces (symphysis), such as the symphysis pubis, or a joint with a ligament uniting the two bones (syndesmosis), such as the tibiofibular articulation. *Diarthrosis* is a joint in which the adjoining bone ends are covered with a thin cartilaginous sheet and joined by ligament lined by a synovial membrane, which secretes a lubricant. SEE: illus.

Joints are grouped according to motion: ball and socket (enarthrosis); hinge (ginglymus); condyloid, pivot (trochoid); gliding (arthrodia); and saddle joint.

Joints can move in four ways: *gliding,* in which one bony surface glides on another without angular or rotatory movement; *angular,* occurring only between long bones, increasing or decreasing the angle between the bones; *circumduction,* occurring in joints composed of the head of a bone and an articular cavity, the long bone describing a series of circles, the whole forming a cone; and *rotation,* in which a bone moves about a central axis without moving from this axis. In angular movement, if it occurs forward or backward, it is called flexion or extension respectively; away from the body, abduction; and toward the median plane of the body, adduction.

Joints, because of their location and constant use, are prone to stress, injuries, and inflammation. The main diseases affecting the joints are rheumatic fever, rheumatoid arthritis, osteoarthritis, and gout. Injuries are contusions, sprains, dislocations, and penetrating wounds. SEE: table.

j., amphidiarthrodial. Joint that is both ginglymoid and arthrodial.

j., arthrodial. Diarthrosis permitting a gliding motion. SYN: *j., gliding.*

j., ball-and-socket. Joint in which the round end of one bone fits into the cavity of another bone. SYN: *enarthrosis; j., multiaxial; j., polyaxial.*

j., biaxial. Joint possessing two chief movement axes at right angles to each other.

j., bilocular. Joint separated into two sections by interarticular cartilage.

j., bleeders'. Joint hemorrhage in hemophiliacs.

j., Brodie's. Arthrodial neuralgia due to hysteria.

j., Budin's. Congenital cartilaginous band between squamous and condylar parts of the occipital bone.

j., cartilaginous. A joint in which there is cartilage connecting the bones.

j., Charcot's. A disease in tabes dorsalis or syringomyelia. Joint enlargement owing to wasting away of muscles below the joint.

j., Chopart's. Union of remainder of tarsal bones with os calcis and astragalus.

j., cochlear. Hinge joint permitting lateral motion. SYN: *j., spiral.*

j., compound. Joint made up of several bones.

Comparison of Joint Diseases*

	Rheumatic Fever	Rheumatoid Arthritis	Osteoarthritis	Gout
Age	Children and young adults	25 and over	Middle and old age	Middle and old age
Sex	Either	Chiefly women	Either	Chiefly men
Cause	Unknown. Autoimmune reaction to streptococci	Unknown. Autoimmune (collagen) disease	Trauma, old age, degenerative changes	Uric acid in blood is increased due to disordered purine metabolism
Joints	Usually large joints, subsiding in one and commencing in another	Multiple, including small joints of hands and feet, usually not axial joints	Usually one large joint (hip, knee, shoulder)	Several
Pyrexia	At onset	In acute stages	None	During acute attack
Permanent deformity	None	Spindle-shaped joints; often gross deformity	Often slight; may be bony enlargement	Deformity mainly from chalky deposits
Heart	Often affected	Infrequently affected	Not affected	Often arteriosclerosis
Treatment	Salicylates; rest in bed. Adrenal cortical hormones may be required in acute state.	Local heat; physiotherapy; gold; nonsteroidal anti-inflammatory agents; phenylbutazone; indomethacin; analgesics	Analgesics, physiotherapy plus orthopedic measures	Colchicine; probenecid; phenylbutazone; allopurinol; diet

*Adapted from Sears, W. G., and Winwood, R. S.: Medicine for Nurses, ed. 11. Edward Arnold Publishers Ltd., London, 1970.

j., condyloid. Joint permitting all forms of angular movements except axial rotation.

j.'s, craniomandibular. The encapsulated, double, synovial joints between the heads of the mandible and the temporal bones of the cranium. SYN: *j.'s, temporomandibular.*

j., diarthrodial. A joint characterized by the presence of a cavity within the capsule separating the bony elements, thus permitting considerable freedom of movement.

j., dry. Arthritis of chronic villous type.

j., ellipsoid. Joint having two axes of motion through the same bone.

j., enarthrodial. J., ball-and-socket. SYN: *j., multiaxial.*

j., false. False joint formation subsequent to a fracture.

j.'s, fibrous. Joints connected by fibrous tissue.

j., flail. Joint that is extremely relaxed, the distal portion of the limb being almost beyond the control of the will.

j., ginglymoid. A synovial joint having only forward and backward motion, as a hinge. SYN: *ginglymus; j., hinge.*

j., gliding. Diarthrosis permitting a gliding motion. SYN: *j., arthrodial.*

j., hemophiliac. J., bleeders'.

j., hinge. Joint having only a forward and backward motion, as a hinge. SYN: *j., ginglymoid.*

j., hip. A stable ball-and-socket type of joint in which the head of the femur fits into the acetabulum of the hip bone.

j., immovable. Joint in which a cavity is lacking between the bones. SYN: *synarthrosis.*

j.'s, intercarpal. Articulations that the carpal bones form in relation to one another.

j., irritable. Inflamed spasmodic condition of joint of unknown cause.

j., knee. The joint between the femur, patella, and tibia.

j., midcarpal. Joint separating the navicular, lunate, and triangular bones from the distal row of carpal bones.

j., mixed. Joint with surfaces joined by fibrocartilaginous disks.

j., movable. Slightly movable or freely movable joint, amphiarthrosis and diarthrosis, respectively.

j., multiaxial. J., ball-and-socket. SYN: *j., enarthrodial; j., polyaxial.*

j., pivot. A joint that permits rotation of a bone, the joint being formed by a pivotlike process that turns within a ring, or by a ringlike structure that turns on a pivot. SYN: *j., rotary; j., trochoid.*

j., plane. Synovial joint between bone surfaces. Only gliding movements are possible.

j., polyaxial. J., ball-and-socket. SYN: *j., enarthrodial; j., polyaxial.*

j., receptive. J., saddle.

j., rotary. J., pivot. SYN: *j., trochoid.*

j., saddle. A joint in which the opposing surfaces are reciprocally concavoconvex. SYN: *j., receptive.*

j., simple. Joint composed of two bones.

j., spheroid. Multiaxial joint with spheroid surfaces.

j., spiral. J., cochlear.

j., synarthrodial. J., immovable.

j., synovial. Joint separated by space containing synovial fluid.

j.'s, tarsometatarsal. Joint made up of three arthrodial joints, the bones of which articulate with the bases of the metatarsal bones.

j.'s, temporomandibular. J.'s, craniomandibular, q.v.

j., trochoid. J., pivot. SYN: *j., rotary.*

j., uniaxial. Joint moving on a single axis.

j., unilocular. Joint with a single cavity.

joint approximation. A rehabilitation technique used to inhibit spastic musculature. Also: *joint compression.*

joint capsule. The saclike structure that encloses the ends of bones in a diarthrodial joint. Consists of an outer fibrous layer and an inner synovial layer and contains synovial fluid.

joint cavity. The articular cavity or space enclosed by the synovial membrane and articular cartilages. It contains synovial fluid.

joint mice. Free bits of cartilage or bone present in the joint space, esp. the knee joint. These are usually the result of previous trauma. They may or may not be symptomatic. SYN: *loose bodies.*

joint protection. Techniques for minimizing stress on joints, including proper body mechanics and the avoidance of continuous weight-bearing or deforming postures. Also: *joint preservation.*

joule (jūl). [James P. Joule, Brit. physicist, 1818–1899] Work done in one second by current of one ampere against a resistance of one ohm. One kilogram calorie (kcal. or Calorie) is equal to 4185.5 joules. One calorie (small calorie) is equal to 4.1855 joules.

jugal [L. *jugalis*]. 1. Connected or united as by a yoke. 2. Pert. to the malar or zygomatic bone.

jugal bone. Malar or zygomatic bone.

jugale (jū-gā′lē). The point at the margin of the zygomatic process.

jugal process. Temporal bone process forming the zygomatic arch. SYN: *zygomatic process.*

jugate (jū′gāt) [L. *jugatus*, joined]. 1. Coupled, yoked. 2. Having ridges.

jugomaxillary (joo″gō-măk′sĭ-lār″ē). Concerning the maxilla and the zygomatic bone.

jugular (jŭg'ū-lăr). [L. *jugularis*]. Pert. to the throat.

jugular foramen. Opening formed by jugular notches of the occipital and temporal bones.

jugular fossa. Depression in the petrosal portion of the temporal bone for the jugular vein.

jugular ganglion. Nodes of vagus root and glossopharyngeal nerve in jugular foramen.

jugular process. Projection from occipital bone toward the temporal bone.

jugular veins. *External,* receives the blood from the exterior of the cranium and the deep parts of the face. It lies superficial to the sternocleidomastoid muscle as it passes down the neck to join the subclavican vein. *Internal,* receives blood from the brain and superficial parts of the face and neck. It is directly continuous with the transverse sinus, accompanying the internal carotid as it passes down the neck, and joins with the subclavian vein to form the innominate vein. They are more prominent during expiration than during inspiration, and also during cardiac decompensation.

The height of the jugular veins and their pulsations when the patient is sitting or in a semirecumbent position can provide an accurate estimation of central venous pressure and give important information about cardiac compensation.

jugulate (jŭg'ū-lāt) [L. *jugulare,* to cut the throat]. To arrest quickly a process or disease by therapeutic measures.

jugulation (jŭg"ū-lā'shŭn). Sudden arrest of a disease by therapeutic means.

jugulum (jŭg'ū-lŭm) [L.]. Neck or throat.

jugum (jū'gŭm) [L., a yoke]. (pl. *juga*) 1. [NA] Ridge or furrow connecting two points. 2. A type of forceps.

j. penis. Forceps for temporarily compressing the penis.

j. petrosum. Eminence on petrous section of the temporal bone showing the position of the superior semicircular canal. SYN: *arcuate eminence.*

juice [L. *jus,* broth]. Liquid that is excreted, secreted, or is expressed from any part of an organism.

j., alimentary. The digestive juices.

j., gastric. Secretions of the stomach, consisting of water, salts, pepsin, and free hydrochloric acid.

j., intestinal. A clear, yellowish, viscid fluid; alkaline in reaction, secreted by Lieberkühn's crypts. SYN: *succus entericus.*

j., pancreatic. A clear, viscid, alkaline digestive juice of the pancreas poured into the duodenum. It contains the enzymes trypsin, amylase, and lipase or steapsin.

jujitsu, jiujitsu (jū-jĭt'sū) [Jap.]. A system of physical training for developing the art of self-defense without weapons. The opponent's weight and strength are used to his or her disadvantage.

jumentous (jū-mĕn'tŭs) [L. *jumentum,* beast of burden]. Like that of a horse, said of odor of urine in certain diseased conditions.

Jumping Frenchmen of Maine. A condition, prevalent in persons of almost any nationality and geographic location, characterized by a sudden, single, sometimes violent, movement or cry that occurs in response to a sharp unexpected sound or touch. The individual may also blurt out whatever was being thought of at the time of the stimulus. The condition may begin in childhood and last forever. It has been most frequently described in persons of French descent living in Maine. The cause is unknown and there is no effective therapy. SEE: *Gilles de la Tourette disease; miryachit.*

junction (jŭnk'shŭn) [L. *junctio,* a joining]. The place of union or coming together of two parts.

j., mucocutaneous. A junction between the skin and a mucous membrane.

j., myoneural. Meeting point of a nerve with the muscle to which it is distributed. SYN: *motor endplate.*

j., sclerocorneal. Meeting point between the sclera and the cornea marked on the external surface of the eyeball by the outer scleral sulcus.

junctura (jŭnk-tū'ră) [L., a joining]. (pl. *juncturae*) Suture of bones; articulation.

juniper tar (joo'nĭ-pĕr). USP. A volatile oil obtained from the wood of Juniperus oxycedrus. It is used in shampoos and bath emulsions.

junket [L. *juncus*]. 1. Curds and whey; a type of cream cheese. 2. Commonly, a flavored and sweetened custard set by rennet.

jurisprudence, medical (joor"ĭs-proo'dĕns) [L. *juris prudentia,* knowledge of law]. The interrelation of law and its application to the practice of medicine or dentistry.

jurymast (jūr'ē-măst) [L. *jurare,* to be right, + AS. *masc,* a stick]. Apparatus for support of head in disease of the spine.

jusculum (jŭs'kū-lŭm) [L.]. Broth or soup.

Juster's reflex. Finger extension instead of flexion when palm of hand is irritated.

justo major (jŭs'tō mā'jor) [L.]. Bigger than normal, as a pelvis.

justo minor (jŭs'tō mī'nor) [L.]. Smaller than normal, as a pelvis.

jute (jūt) [Sanskrit *juta,* matted hair]. Fiber obtained from tropical shrubs. Once used in making dressings.

juvenile (jū'vĕ-nīl") [L. *juvenis,* young]. 1. Pert. to youth or childhood. 2. Young; immature.

juvenile cell. The early developmental form of white blood cells.

juvenile rheumatoid arthritis. SEE: *arthritis, juvenile rheumatoid.*

juxta- [L., near]. Prefix indicating close proximity.

juxta-articular (jŭks″tă-ăr-tĭk′ū-lăr) [″ + *articulus,* joint]. Situated close to a joint.

juxtaglomerular (jŭks″tă-glō-mĕr′ū-lăr) [″ + *glomus,* ball]. Near or adjacent to a glomerulus.

juxtaglomerular apparatus. A structure consisting of myoepithelioid cells forming a cuff surrounding the arteriole leading to a glomerulus of the kidney. It is concerned with the production of renin, and it is involved in sodium metabolism.

juxtaglomerular cells. Myoepithelioid cells resembling those of the carotid body present in the juxtaglomerular apparatus. Function unknown.

juxtangina (jŭks″tăn-jī′nă) [″ + *angina,* a choking]. Inflamed condition of pharyngeal muscles.

juxtaposition (jŭks″tă-pō-zĭ′shŭn) [″ + *positio,* place]. Position that is adjacent or side by side. SYN: *apposition; contiguity.*

juxtapyloric (jŭks″tă-pī-lor′ĭk) [″ + Gr. *pyloros,* pylorus]. Near the pylorus or pyloric orifice.

juxtaspinal (jŭks″tă-spī′năl) [″ + *spina,* thorn]. Near the spinal column.

K

K, k. 1. Chem. symb. for potassium. 2. Symb. for Gr. letter *kappa.* 3. Used in some formulae in chemistry and physics to indicate a constant or value that does not change. 4. Kelvin temperature scale.

Ka. *cathode;* also Ca.

Kabikinase. Trade name for streptokinase.

Kader's operation (kă'dĕrs). [Bronislaw Kader, Polish surgeon, 1863–1937] Surgical formation of a gastric fistula with the feeding tube inserted through a valvelike flap.

Kaes' feltwork (kīz). [Theodor Kaes, Ger. neurologist, 1852–1913] Nerve fiber network in the cerebral cortex.

Kafocin. Trade name for cephaloglycin dihydrate.

Kahler's disease (kă'lĕrz). [Otto Kahler, Viennese physician, 1849–1893] Multiple myeloma.

kaif (kīf) [Arabic, quiescence]. A dreamy, tranquil state induced by drugs.

kainophobia (kī-nō-fō'bē-ă) [Gr. *kainos,* new, + *phobos,* fear]. Abnormal aversion to new situations and things. SYN: *neophobia.*

kaiserling (kī'zĕr-lĭng). [Karl Kaiserling, Ger. pathologist, 1869–1942] Liquid used in preserving pathological specimens.

kakidrosis (kăk-ĭ-drō'sĭs) [Gr. *kakos,* bad, + *hidrosis,* sweat]. Unpleasant odor of the sweat. SYN: *bromidrosis.*

kakke (kŏk'kā) [Jap.]. Endemic form of polyneuritis. SYN: *beriberi.*

kakosmia (kăk-ŏz'mē-ă) [Gr. *kakos,* bad, + *osme,* smell]. Perception of bad odors that do not exist. SYN: *cacosmia.* SEE: *parosmia.*

kakotrophy (kăk-ŏt'rō-fē) [" + *trophe,* nourishment]. Malnutrition. SYN: *cacotrophy.*

kala-azar (kă'lă ă-zăr') [Hindi, black fever]. An infectious disease, common in the rural parts of tropical and subtropical areas of the world. There are several types, which differ as to preference for children or adults, incidence in domestic animals, and transmitting agent. The disease is characterized by lesions of the reticuloendothelial system, esp. the liver and spleen. It is often fatal. SYN: *leishmaniasis, visceral.*

ETIOL: Leishmania donovani, a flagellated protozoon. The organism is transmitted by the bite of infected sandflies of the genus Phlebotomus.

TREATMENT: Sodium antimony gluconate, available in the U.S.A. only from the Centers for Disease Control, Atlanta, Georgia (telephone: 404-329-3670); or meglumine antimoniate.

PROPHYLAXIS: Control of the sandflies that transmit the organisms can be accomplished by use of insecticides that have residual action. In addition elimination of breeding grounds of the flies is helpful as is avoidance of animals that are known reservoirs. If exposure to flies is inevitable, then protective clothing should be worn.

kaliemia (kā-lē-ē'mē-ă) [L. *kali,* potash, + Gr. *haima,* blood]. Potassium in the blood.

kaligenous (kā-lĭj'ĕ-nŭs) [" + Gr. *gennan,* to produce]. Forming potash.

kalimeter (kă-lĭm'ĕ-ter) [" + Gr. *metron,* measure]. Device for determining degree of alkalinity of a substance. SYN: *alkalimeter.*

kaliopenia (kă"lē-ō-pē'nē-ă) [L. *kalium,* potassium, + Gr. *penia,* poverty]. Hypokalemia, i.e., decreased potassium in the blood.

kalium (kā'lē-ŭm) [L.]. SYMB: K. A mineral element necessary to the growth of cells, esp. those of the muscles and blood. SYN: *potassium.*

kaliuresis (kă"lē-ū-rē'sĭs) [" + Gr. *ouresis,* urination]. Excretion of potassium in the urine.

kallidin (kăl'ĭ-dĭn). A plasma kinin. SEE: *kinin.*

kallikrein (kăl-ĭ-krē'ĭn) [Gr. *kallikreas,* pancreas]. An enzyme normally present in blood plasma, urine, and body tissue in an inactive state. When activated, kallikrein is one of the most potent vasodilators. It forms kinin, q.v.

kallikreinogen (kăl"ĭ-krī'nō-jĕn) [" + *gennan,* to produce]. The precursor of kallikrein, q.v., in blood plasma.

kanamycin sulfate (kăn"ă-mī'sĭn). USP. An antibiotic. Trade names are Kantrex, Kantrim, and Klebcil.

Kanner syndrome. [Leo Kanner, Austrian psychiatrist in the U.S., b. 1894] Infantile autism. SEE: *autism; autistic child.*

Kantrex. Trade name for kanamycin sulfate, USP.

Kaochlor. Trade name for potassium chloride, USP.

kaolin (kā'ō-lĭn) [Fr., from Mandarin Chinese *kao,* high, + *ling,* mountain]. A yellowish-white or gray clay powder, occurring in a natural state as a form of hydrated aluminum silicate. Used internally as an absorbent; externally as a protective by absorbing moisture. SYN: *China clay.*

kaolinosis (kā"ō-lĭn-ō'sĭs). Pneumoconiosis caused by inhaling kaolin particles.

Kaon. Trade name for potassium gluconate.

Kaon-Cl. Trade name for potassium chloride, USP.

Kaopectate. Trade name for a combination product containing kaolin, USP.

Kaposi, Moritz K. (kăp'ō-sē"). Austrian dermatologist, 1837–1902.

K.'s disease. Xeroderma pigmentosum,

q.v. SYN: *xanthelasmoidea.*

K.'s sarcoma. Malignant neoplasm of the skin. For an unexplained reason, homosexual men are especially prone to develop this disease. SEE: *acquired immune deficiency syndrome.*

K.'s varicelliform eruption. Skin disease that results from infection with herpes simplex or vaccinia virus in the presence of another skin disease such as eczema.

Kappadione. Trade name for menadiol sodium diphosphate.

karaya gum (kăr'ā-ă). Dried gum from Sterculia plants. It becomes gelatinous when moist. Used as an adhesive and as a bulk laxative.

Karman catheter. [Harvey Karman, contemporary U.S. psychologist] Catheter used in performing suction curettage of the uterus.

Kartagener's syndrome (kăr'tă-gā"nĕrz). [Manes Kartagener, Swiss physician, b. 1897] Hereditary syndrome consisting of bronchiectasis, maldevelopment of the sinuses, and transposition of the viscera.

karyo- [Gr. *karyon,* nucleus]. Prefix referring to a cell's nucleus.

karyochromatophil (kăr"ē-ō-krō-măt'ō-fĭl) [" + *chroma,* color, + *philein,* to love]. Having a nucleus that stains.

karyochrome (kăr'ē-ō-krōm"). The cell of a nerve with an easily staining nucleus.

karyoclasis (kăr-ē-ŏk'lă-sĭs) [Gr. *karyon,* nucleus, + *klasis,* a breaking]. The fragmentation of a cell nucleus. SYN: *karyorrhexis.*

karyocyte (kăr'ē-ō-sīt) [" + *kytos,* cell]. Normoblast, the nucleated red blood cell.

karyogamy (kăr-ē-ŏg'ă-mē) [" + *gamos,* marriage]. Union of nuclei in cell conjugation.

karyogenesis (kăr"ē-ō-jĕn'ĕ-sĭs) [" + *genesis,* production]. Formation and development of a cell nucleus.

karyogram (kăr'ē-ō-grăm) [" + *gramma,* mark]. A picture of the interphase of mitosis in somatic chromosomes.

karyokinesis (kăr"ē-ō-kĭn-ē'sĭs) [" + *kinesis,* movement]. The equal division of nuclear material that occurs in cell division. SEE: *cytokinesis; mitosis.*

karyokinetic (kăr"ē-ō-kĭ-nĕt'ĭk). 1. Pert. to karyokinesis. 2. Ameboid.

karyoklasis (kăr"ē-ŏk'lă-sĭs) [" + *klasis,* a breaking]. Disintegration of the cell nucleus.

karyolobism (kăr"ē-ō-lō'bĭzm) [Gr. *karyon,* nucleus, + L. *lobus,* lobe, + Gr. *-ismos,* state of]. Condition in which the nucleus of a cell is lobed as in polymorphonuclear leukocytes.

karyolymph [" + L. *lympha,* lymph]. Fluid in meshes of the nucleus. This fluid is now known to contain active submicroscopic components of the nucleoplasm. Thus the terms karyolymph and nuclear sap do not describe clearly definable entities and should not be used. SEE: *cell; organelle.*

karyolysis (kăr-ē-ŏl'ĭ-sĭs) [" + *lysis,* dissolution]. The destruction of a nucleus or loss of affinity for basic dyes. SYN: *chromatolysis.*

karyolytic (kăr-ē-ō-lĭt'ĭk). Producing or rel. to karyolysis.

karyomegaly (kăr"ē-ō-mĕg'ă-lē) [" + *megas,* large]. Abnormal enlargement of the cell nucleus.

karyomere (kăr'ē-ō-mēr") [" + *meros,* part]. 1. Chromomere (def. 1), q.v. 2. A vesicle containing only a small portion of the nucleus.

karyomicrosome (kăr"ē-ō-mī'krō-sōm) [" + *mikros,* small, + *soma,* body]. 1. Any one of the small particles in the karyoplasm. 2. Any one of the small tangible bodies or segments of chromatin fiber.

karyomitome (kăr-ē-ŏm'ĭ-tōm) [" + *mitos,* thread]. The nuclear network.

karyomitosis (kăr"ē-ō-mī-tō'sĭs) [" + *mitos,* thread, + *osis,* condition]. Nuclear changes in mitosis or cell division. SYN: *karyokinesis.*

karyomorphism (kăr-ē-ō-mor'fĭzm) [" + *morphe,* form, + *-ismos,* state of]. The form of a cell nucleus.

karyon (kăr'ē-ŏn) [Gr.]. The nucleus of a cell.

karyophage (kăr'ē-ō-fāj) [" + *phagein,* to eat]. An intracellular protozoan parasite that destroys the nucleus of a cell.

karyopyknosis (kăr"ē-ō-pĭk-nō'sĭs) [" + *pyknos,* thick, + *osis,* condition]. Shrinkage of the nucleus of the cell with condensation of the chromatin.

karyorrhexis (kăr"ē-ō-rĕk'sĭs) [" + *rhexis,* rupture]. Fragmentation of the chromatin in nuclear disintegration. SYN: *karyoclasis.*

karyosome (kăr'ē-ō-sōm) [" + *soma,* body]. Irregular clumps of chromatin material seen in the nuclei of cells that are not dividing. SYN: *chromocenter; prochromosome.*

karyostasis (kăr"ē-ŏs'tă-sĭs) [" + *stasis,* standing]. Stage of resting of a cell nucleus.

karyotheca (kăr"ē-ō-thē'kă) [" + *theke,* sheath]. The enveloping membrane of a cell nucleus.

karyotype (kăr'ē-ō-tīp) [" + *typos,* mark]. A photomicrograph of a single cell in the metaphase, q.v., stage of division that is arranged to show the chromosomes in descending order of size. SEE: *chromosome* for illus.

karyozoic (kăr"ē-ō-zō'ĭk) [" + *zoon,* animal]. Living in the cell nucleus as would occur with a protozoal parasite.

Kasabach-Merritt syndrome. [Haig H. Kasabach, contemporary U.S. pediatrician; K. K. Merritt, U.S. physician, b. 1886] Capillary hemangioma associated with thrombocytopenic purpura. SYN: *hemangioma-thrombocytopenia syndrome.*

Kashin-Beck disease. [N. I. Kashin, Russian physician, 1825–1872; E. V. (Bek) Beck] Endemic polyarthritis limited to certain areas of Asia including the Urov River. It is believed to be a form of mycotoxicosis caused by eating grain contaminated with the fungus Fusarium sporotrichiella.

kata- [Gr. *kata,* down]. Prefix meaning down, reversing process, wrongly, back, against. SEE: words beginning with *cata-*.

katabolism (kă-tăb'ō-lĭsm) [" + *ballein,* to throw, + *-ismos,* state of]. Catabolism.

kataplasia (kăt-ă-plā'sē-ă). Cataplasia.

katathermometer (kăt"ă-thĕr-mŏm'ĕ-ter) [" + *therme,* heat, + *metron,* measure]. Two thermometers, one a dry bulb and the other a wet bulb. Both are heated to 110° F. (43.3° C.) and the time required for each thermometer to fall from 100° to 90° F. (37.8° to 32.2° C.) is noted. The dry kata gives the cooling power by radiation and convection. The wet kata gives the cooling power by radiation, convection, and evaporation.

katatonia (kăt-ă-tō'nē-ă) [" + *tonos,* tension]. Catatonia.

kathisophobia (kăth"ĭ-sō-fō'bē-ă) [Gr. *kathizein,* to sit down, + *phobos,* fear]. Fear of sitting down, and subsequent inability to sit still.

kation (kăt'ē-ŏn) [Gr., descending]. Cation.

katophoria (kăt"ō-fō'rē-ă). Katotropia, q.v.

katotropia (kăt"ō-trō'pē-ă) [Gr. *kato,* below, + *tropos,* a turning]. Tendency of the eyeball to drop too far downward. SYN: *katophoria.*

katzenjammer (kăts'ĕn-yăm'ĕr) [Ger.]. Symptoms of a "hangover" following excess intake of alcohol. Nausea, cerebral edema, and neurological signs may be present.

kava [Tongan, bitter]. 1. Root of Piper methysticum, a tropical shrub. 2. A Polynesian beverage made from the root of Piper methysticum. Its acute effect is to cause excitement and loss of use of legs. If used habitually, it causes debility and a scaly skin disease. SEE: *arevareva.*

Kawasaki disease [Tomsaku Kawasaki, contemporary Japanese pediatrician]. Mucocutaneous lymph node syndrome, q.v.

Kay Ciel. Trade name for potassium chloride, USP.

Kayser-Fleischer ring (kī'zĕr-flī'shĕr). [Bernard Kayser, b. 1869, Bruno Fleischer, 1848–1904, Ger. physicians] SEE: *Wilson's disease.*

KBr. Potassium bromide.

kc. *kilocycle.*

$KC_2H_3O_2$. Potassium acetate.

KCl. Potassium chloride.

KClO. Potassium hypochlorite.

$KClO_3$. Potassium chlorate.

K_2CO_3. Potassium carbonate.

k.c.p.s. *kilocycles per second.*

kefir, kefyr (kĕf'ĕr) [Caucasus region of Russia]. A preparation of curdled milk made originally in the Caucasus by adding kefir grains to milk.

Keflex. Trade name for cephalexin, USP.

Keflin. Trade name for cephalothin sodium, USP.

Kegel exercises. [A. H. Kegel, contemporary U.S. physician] Exercises for strengthening the perineal muscles of the female, esp. the pubococcygeus and the levator ani. This aids in the childbirth process and in sexual enjoyment. The exercises involve resisting increased abdominal pressure during forced expiration or resisting the passage of urine.

Keith's bundle, node (kēths). [Sir Arthur Keith, London anatomist, 1866–1955] Sinoatrial node of the heart.

Keith-Flack node. [Sir Arthur Keith; Martin William Flack, physiologist in London, 1882–1931] Sinoatrial node of the heart.

Keith-Wagener-Barker classification. Classification of the fundoscopic findings in hypertensive patients. Grades one to four indicate progressive pathological changes. Grade 1 is moderate narrowing of the retinal arterioles; Grade 2 has retinal hemorrhages in addition to arteriolar narrowing; Grade 3 has cotton-wool exudates; Grade 4 has papilledema.

kelis (kē'lĭs) [Gr., blemish]. Keloid.

Kell blood group. One of the human blood groups. It is composed of antigens present on the surface of the red blood cells with three alternate forms. SEE: *blood groups.*

Kelly's pad. [Howard A. Kelly, U.S. surgeon, 1858–1943] A drainage pad for the operating table or bed made by wrapping one end of a rubber sheet over a rolled small blanket, forming a bolster. The bolster is twisted round like a horseshoe to form the pad, the free part of the sheet forming the apron. A commercial inflatable rubber pad of horseshoe shape may be used in same way.

keloid (kē'lŏyd) [Gr. *kele,* tumor, + *eidos,* form]. Scar formation in the skin following trauma or surgical incision. The tissue response is out of proportion to the amount of scar tissue required for normal repair and healing. The result is a raised, firm, thickened red scar that may grow for a prolonged period of time. Blacks are esp. prone to developing keloids.

k., acne. Keloid that develops at site of acne pustule.

keloidosis (kē"loy-dō'sĭs) [" + " + *osis,* condition]. The formation of keloids.

kelotomy (kē-lŏt'ō-mē) [" – *tome,* incision]. Operation for strangulated hernia through tissues of the constricting neck.

kelp. 1. Any member of the brown seaweeds of the order Laminariales. 2 The ash of seaweed from which potassium and iodine salts are prepared.

Kelvin scale. [William Thompson Kelvin, Brit.

physicist, 1824–1907] ABBR: K. Temperature scale in which absolute zero is equal to minus 273° on the Celsius scale. On the Kelvin scale the freezing point of water is 273° K; and the boiling point of water is 373° K.

Kemadrin. Trade name for procyclidine hydrochloride.

Kempner rice-fruit diet (kĕmp'nĕr). [Walter Kempner, U.S. physician, b. 1903] Rigid salt restriction diet used in treating hypertension. It consists of rice, fruit, and sugar for no more than 2000 Calories per day and 7 mEq. of sodium per day.

Kenacort. Trade name for triamcinolone.

Kenalog. Trade name for triamcinolone acetonide.

Kenny treatment. [Sister Elizabeth Kenny, Australian nurse, 1886–1952] A specified form of physical therapy used in treating poliomyelitis. Consists of application of hot, moist packs to affected muscles and early reeducation of muscles, first through passive exercise and then by active movements as soon as possible. Rigid fixation of paralyzed limbs is disparaged.

kenophobia (kĕn″ō-fō'bē-ă) [Gr. *kenos,* empty, + *phobos,* fear]. Fear of empty spaces.

kenotoxin (kē'nō-tŏk-sĭn) [″ + *toxikon,* poison]. A postulated toxin associated with muscular fatigue.

Kent's bundles. [A. F. S. Kent, Brit. physiologist, 1863–1958] Accessory conduction fiber bundles in the heart. They rapidly convey atrial impulses across the atrioventricular tissue. They are usually present in the Wolff-Parkinson-White syndrome, q.v.

kerasin (kĕr'ă-sĭn). A cerebroside isolated from brain tissue.

keratalgia (kĕr″ă-tăl'jē-ă) [Gr. *keras,* horn, + *algos,* pain]. Neuralgia of the cornea.

keratectasia (kĕr″ă-tĕk-tā'sē-ă) [″ + *ektasis,* extension]. Conical protrusion of the cornea.

keratectomy (kĕr-ă-tĕk'tō-mē) [″ + *ektome,* excision]. Excision of a portion of the cornea.

keratiasis (kĕr-ă-tī'ă-sĭs) [″ + *-iasis,* condition]. Horny wart formations on the skin.

keratic (kĕr-ăt'ĭk). 1. Rel. to keratin. SYN: *horny.* 2. Rel. to the cornea.

keratin (kĕr'ă-tĭn). An extremely tough protein substance in hair, nails, and horny tissue, insoluble in water, weak acids, or alkalis, and unaffected by most proteolytic enzymes.

keratinase (kĕr'ă-tĭ-nās). Enzyme that hydrolyzes the protein keratin.

keratinize (kĕr'ă-tĭn-īz) [Gr. *keras,* horn]. To become hard or horny. Usually said of tissue.

keratinocyte (kĕ-răt'ĭ-nō-sīt) [″ + *kytos,* cell]. Any one of the cells in the skin that synthesize keratin.

keratinous (kĕr-ăt'ĭ-nŭs). Pert. to or composed of keratin.

keratitic precipitates. Inflammatory cells of the anterior chamber of the eye that adhere to the endothelial surface of the cornea. These may be large, heavy, fat precipitates, or small and punctate.

keratitis (kĕr-ă-tī'tĭs) [″ + *itis,* inflammation]. Inflammation of the cornea.

k., band-shaped. Whitish or grayish band extending across the cornea.

k. bullosa. The formation of large, quite resistant blebs with increased tension in the cornea of blind trachomatous eyes.

k., deep. K., interstitial.

k., dendritic. Superficial branching corneal ulcers.

k. disciformis. Gray disk-shaped opacity in the middle of the cornea.

k., fascicular. Corneal ulcer resulting from phlyctenules that spread from limbus to center of cornea accompanied by fascicle of blood vessels.

k., herpetic. Vesicular keratitis in herpes zoster.

k., hypopyon. Serpent-like ulcer with pus in the anterior chamber of the eye.

k., interstitial. Deep form of nonsuppurative keratitis with vascularization, occurring usually in syphilis and rarely in tuberculosis. Commonly found between fifth and fifteenth years. SYN: *k., deep; k., parenchymatous.*

SYM: Pain, photophobia, lacrimation, and loss in vision.

k., lagophthalmic. Drying due to air exposure of cornea due to defective closure of lids.

k., mycotic. Keratitis produced by fungi.

k., neuroparalytic. Dull and slightly cloudy insensitive cornea seen in lesions of the fifth nerve.

k., parenchymatous. K., interstitial, q.v.

k., phlyctenular. Circumscribed inflammation of conjunctiva and cornea accompanied by formation of small projections called phlyctenules, which consist of accumulations of lymphoid cells. The phlyctenules soften at the apices, forming ulcers.

k., punctate. Cellular deposits on the posterior surface of the cornea seen in diseases of uveal tract.

k., purulent. Keratitis with formation of pus.

k., sclerosing. Triangular opacity in deeper layers of cornea, associated with scleritis.

k., superficial punctate. Small gray spots in superficial layers of cornea beneath Bowman's membrane. Occurs in young persons.

k., trachomatous. Keratitis with abnormal membrane on cornea. SYN: *pannus.*

k., traumatic. Keratitis caused by a wound of the cornea.

k., xerotic. Softening, desiccation, and ulceration of cornea due to dryness of the conjunctiva.

kerato-, kerat- [Gr. *keras,* horn]. Combining form indicating relation to horny substances or to the cornea.

keratoacanthoma (kĕr″ă-tō-ăk″ăn-thō′mă) [″ + *akantha,* thorn, + *oma,* tumor]. A papular lesion filled with a keratin plug that can resemble squamous cell carcinoma. It is benign and usually subsides spontaneously within 6 months.

keratocele (kĕr-ăt′ō-sēl) [″ + *kele,* hernia]. Protrusion or herniation of Descemet's membrane through a weakened or absent corneal stroma as a result of injury or ulcer.

keratoconjunctivitis (kĕr″ă-tō-kŏn-jŭnk″tĭ-vī′tĭs). Inflammation of the cornea and the conjunctiva.

k., epidemic. An acute, self-limited keratoconjunctivitis due to a highly infectious virus. SYN: *k., virus.*

k., flash. Painful keratoconjunctivitis resulting from exposure of the eyes to intense ultraviolet irradiation. Arc welders whose eyes are not properly protected will develop this acute condition.

k., phlyctenular. Acute inflammation of the conjunctiva due to decreased lacrimal function. The corneal epithelium may be thickened and visual acuity may be impaired.

k. sicca. Dryness with hyperemia of the conjunctiva due to decreased lacrimal function. The corneal epithelium may be thickened and visual acuity may be impaired.

k., virus. K., epidemic.

keratoconus (kĕr-ă-tō-kō′nŭs) [″ + *konos,* cone]. Conical protrusion of the center of the cornea without inflammation. Occurs most often in pubescent females.

keratoderma (kĕr″ă-tō-dĕr′mă) [″ + *derma,* skin]. A localized or disseminated disease of the horny layer of the skin.

k. climactericum. Hyperkeratosis of the palms and soles of women. This may occur during menopause.

k. blennorrhagica. Prominent cone-shaped pustular lesions. As new lesions develop they tend to merge and produce a relief map appearance.

ETIOL: Not clear; probably due to a virus. May be associated with nonspecific urethritis or gonorrhea but is not considered to be caused by bacteria. SEE: *Reiter's syndrome.*

keratodermatitis (kĕr″ă-tō-dĕr″mă-tī′tĭs) [″ + ″ + *itis,* inflammation]. Inflammation of the horny layer of the skin with proliferation.

keratodermia. Hypertrophy of the stratum corneum or horny layer of the epidermis, esp. on the palms of hands and soles of feet, producing a horny condition of the skin.

keratogenous (kĕr-ă-tŏj′ĕ-nŭs) [″ + *gennan,* to produce]. Causing horny tissue development.

keratoglobus (kĕr″ă-tō-glō′bŭs) [″ + L. *globus,* circle]. Globular protrusion and enlargement of cornea seen in congenital glaucoma.

keratohelcosis (kĕr″ă-tō-hĕl-kō′sĭs) [″ + *helkosis,* ulceration]. Corneal ulceration.

keratohemia (kĕr″ă-tō-hē′mē-ă) [″ + *haima,* blood]. Presence of blood in the cornea of the eye.

keratohyalin. A substance present in the form of granules in the cytoplasm of cells in the stratum granulosum of keratinized mucosa or epidermis of the skin.

keratoid (kĕr′ă-toyd) [″ + *eidos,* form]. Horny; resembling corneal tissue.

keratoiditis (kĕr″ă-toyd-ī′tĭs) [″ + ″ + *itis,* inflammation]. Inflammation of the cornea.

keratoiritis (kĕr″ă-tō-ī-rī′tĭs) [″ + *iris,* iris, + *itis,* inflammation]. Inflammation of the cornea and iris.

keratoleptynsis (kĕr″ă-tō-lĕp-tĭn′sĭs) [″ + *leptynein,* to make thin]. A cosmetic operation performed on a sightless eye. The procedure involves removal of the corneal surface, and covering the area with bulbar conjunctiva.

keratoleukoma (kĕr″ă-tō-lū-kō′mă) [″ + *leukos,* white, + *oma,* tumor]. White corneal opacity.

keratolysis (kĕr-ă-tŏl′ĭ-sĭs) [″ + *lysis,* loosening]. 1. Loosening of horny layer of the skin. 2. Shedding of the skin at regular intervals.

k., pitted; k. plantare sulcatum. Hyperkeratotic areas of the soles and palms with erosion and pitting. Etiology is unknown but may be due to infection with Corynebacterium or Streptomyces. It occurs mostly in barefooted adults in the tropics.

keratolytic (kĕr″ă-tō-lĭt′ĭk). 1. Rel. to or causing keratolysis. SYN: *desquamative.* 2. An agent that causes or promotes keratolysis.

keratoma (kĕr″ă-tō′mă) [″ + *oma,* tumor]. 1. A callosity. 2. A horny growth. SYN: *keratosis.*

keratomalacia (kĕr″ă-tō-mă-lā′shē-ă) [″ + *malakia,* softness]. Softening of the cornea seen in early childhood due to deficiencies of vitamin A. SYN: *xerotic keratitis.*

keratome (kĕr′ă-tōm) [″ + *tome,* incision]. Knife for incising the cornea.

keratometer (kĕr-ă-tŏm′ĕ-ter) [″ + *metron,* a measure]. An instrument for measuring the curves of the cornea.

keratometry (kĕr″ă-tŏm′ĕ-trē) [″ + *metron,* measure]. Measurement of the cornea.

keratomileusis (kĕr″ă-tō-mī-loo′sĭs). Plastic surgery of the cornea in which a portion is removed, frozen, its curvature reshaped, and then reattached to the cornea.

keratomycosis (kĕr″ă-tō-mī-kō′sĭs) [″ + *mykes*, fungus, + *osis*, condition]. Fungus growth on the cornea.

keratonosis (kĕr″ă-tō-nō′sĭs) [″ + *nosos*, disease]. Any noninflammatory disease or deformity of the horny layer of the skin.

keratonyxis (kĕr″ă-tō-nĭks′ĭs) [″ + *nyssein*, to puncture]. Corneal puncture, esp. surgical puncture.

keratopathy, band (kĕr″ă-tŏp′ă-thē) [″ + *pathos*, disease]. Calcium deposits in the superficial layer of the cornea and Bowman's membrane. Occurs with chronic intraocular inflammation; and with systemic diseases in which there is hypercalcemia.

keratoplasty (kĕr′ă-tō-plăs″tē) [″ + *plassein*, to form]. Plastic operation on the cornea.

k., optic. Removal of a corneal scar and replacing it with corneal tissue.

k., tectonic. Use of corneal tissue to replace that lost due to trauma or disease.

keratoprotein (kĕr″ă-tō-prō′tē-ĭn) [″ + *protos*, first]. The protein of the hair, nails, and epidermis.

keratorrhexis (kĕr″ă-tō-rĕks′ĭs) [″ + *rhexis*, rupture]. Corneal rupture.

keratoscleritis (kĕr″ă-tō-sklĕr-ī′tĭs) [″ + *skleros*, hard, + *itis*, inflammation]. Inflammation of both cornea and sclera.

keratoscope (kĕr′ăt-ō-skōp) [″ + *skopein*, to examine]. An instrument for examination of the cornea.

keratoscopy. Examination of the cornea and its reflection of light.

keratose (kĕr′ă-tōs) [Gr. *keras*, horn]. Horny.

keratosis (kĕr-ă-tō′sĭs) [″ + *osis*, condition]. (pl. *keratoses*) 1. Horny growth. 2. Any condition of the skin characterized by the formation of horny growths or excessive development of the horny growth.

k., actinic. A horny, keratotic, premalignant lesion of the skin caused by excess exposure to sunlight.

k. climatericum. A skin disease occurring in women during the menopause, characterized by a circumscribed hyperkeratosis of the palms and soles.

k. follicularis. A rare hereditary condition characterized by verrucous papular growths that coalesce into plaques of various sizes on the scalp, face, neck, trunk, and axillae. SYN: *Darier's disease.*

k. nigricans. Acanthosis nigricans.

k., oral. Keratinization of the mucosa of the mouth to an unusual extent or in locations that are normally nonkeratinized.

k. palmaris et plantaris. Congenital abnormality of the palms and soles, characterized by dense thickening of the keratin layer of the palms and soles.

k. pharyngea. Horny projections from the pharyngeal tonsils and adjacent lymphoid tissue.

k. pilaris. Chronic inflammatory disorder of area surrounding the hair follicles. Etiology is unknown.

SYM: Accumulation of horny material at follicular orifices of persons with rough, dry skin. Most pronounced in winter on lateral aspects of thighs and upper arms with possible extension to legs, forearms, and scalp.

TREATMENT: There is no specific therapy. Keratolytic lotions may be of some value.

k. punctata. Discrete horny projections from the sweat pores of the palms and soles.

k., seborrheic. A benign skin tumor that may be pigmented. Quite common in the elderly. It is composed of immature epithelial cells. SYN: *wart, seborrheic.*

ETIOL: Unknown.

SYM: Keratoid, nevoid, acanthoid, or verrucose types occurring in elderly and in those with long-standing dry seborrhea, on face, scalp, interscapular or sternal regions, and backs of hands. Yellowish, grayish, brownish sharply circumscribed lesions covered with a firmly adherent scale, greasy or velvety on trunk or scalp but harsh, rough, and dry on face or hands. The tendency as time passes is for the lesions to increase in number. It is doubtful that they ever become malignant.

TREATMENT: Thorough curettage is quite effective. This leaves a flat surface that becomes covered with normal skin within about a week. Pedunculated lesions can be removed surgically. Cautery may produce scarring; therefore it should not be used.

k. senilis. Dry, harsh skin of the aged.

keratotome (kĕr-ăt′ō-tōm) [″ + *tome*, incision]. A knife for incising the cornea. SYN: *keratome.*

keratotomy (kĕr-ă-tŏt′ō-mē). Incision of cornea.

keraunoneurosis (kē-raw″nō-nū-rō′sĭs) [Gr. *keraunos*, lightning, + *neuron*, nerve, + *osis*, condition]. A neurosis caused by fear of a thunderstorm or stroke of lightning.

keraunophobia (kē-raw″nō-fō′bē-ă) [″ + *phobos*, fear]. Dread of thunder and lightning.

Kerckring's folds (kĕrk′rĭngz). [Theodorus Kerckring, Dutch anatomist, 1640–1693] Transverse folds of the mucous membrane of the small intestine. SYN: *plicae circulares; valvulae conniventes.*

kerectomy (kē-rĕk′tō-mē) [Gr. *keras*, horn, + *ektome*, excision]. Excision of a portion of the cornea.

kerion (kē′rē-ŏn) [Gr., honeycomb]. A form of tinea capitis due to Trichophyton tonsurans. A lesion secondary to tinea capitis.

keritherapy [Gr. *keros*, wax, + *therapeia*, treatment]. Treatment of burns and denuded surfaces with liquid paraffin.

Kerley lines. [P. J. Kerley, Brit. radiologist, b. 1900] Thickening of the interlobular septa, seen in chest roentgenography. May be due to cellular infiltration or edema associated with pulmonary vein hypertension.

kernicterus (kĕr-nĭk'tĕr-ŭs) [Ger.]. A form of icterus neonatorum occurring in infants. The basal ganglia and other areas of the brain and spinal cord are infiltrated with bilirubin, a yellow pigmented substance produced by the breakdown of hemoglobin. Develops during the second to eighth day of life. Prognosis is quite poor if untreated. For prevention and treatment, SEE: *erythroblastosis fetalis.*

Kernig's sign (kĕr'nĭgz). [Vladimir Kernig, Russ. physician, 1840–1917] A symptom of meningitis evidenced by reflex contraction and pain in the hamstring muscles when attempting to extend the leg after flexing the thigh upon the body.

kerosene (kĕr'ō-sēn). An inflammable liquid fuel distilled from petroleum. It is used as a solvent as well as a fuel source.

Ketaject. Trade name for ketamine hydrochloride, USP.

Ketalar. Trade name for ketamine hydrochloride, USP.

ketamine hydrochloride. USP. A nonbarbiturate substance, $C_{13}H_{16}ClNO$, that is used intravenously or intramuscularly to produce anesthesia. The patient becomes cataleptic and may appear to be awake, but is unaware of the environment and unresponsive to pain. Laryngeal reflexes are depressed, and for this reason an endotracheal tube should be used to prevent aspiration. Most frequently used for diagnostic procedures and minor operations where muscle relaxation is not required. Trade names are Ketaject, Ketaset, and Ketalar. SEE: *anesthesia, dissociative.*

ketoacid (kē"tō-ăs'ĭd). Any chemical compound containing the ketone, CO, and carboxyl, COOH, groups.

ketoacidosis (kē"tō-ă"sĭ-dō'sĭs) [*ketone* + L. *acidus,* sour, + Gr. *osis,* condition]. Acidosis due to an excess of ketone bodies.

ketoaciduria (kē"tō-ăs"ĭ-dū'rē-ă) [" + " + Gr. *ouron,* urine]. Presence of ketoacids in the urine.

ketogenesis (kē-tō-jĕn'ĕ-sĭs) [" + Gr. *genesis,* production]. Production of ketones or acetone substances.

ketogenic diet (kē-tō-jĕn'ĭk) [" + Gr. *gennan,* to produce]. Diet that produces acetone or ketone bodies, or mild acidosis.

ketohexose (kē"tō-hĕks'ōs). A nonsaccharide consisting of a six-carbon chain and containing a ketone group in addition to alcohol groups. Fructose is an example.

ketolysis (kē-tŏl'ĭ-sĭs) [*ketone* + Gr. *lysis,* dissolution]. The dissolution of acetone or ketone bodies.

ketolytic. Pert. to ketolysis.

ketone (kē'tōn). A substance containing the carbonyl group (C = O). Oxidation product of a secondary alcohol. Organic chemical substance of the general formula:

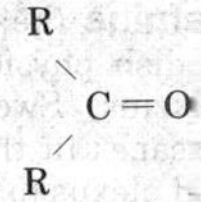

Acetone is an example of a simple ketone. The ketone acids in the body are the end products of fat metabolism.

ketone bodies. A group of compounds produced during the oxidation of fatty acids, including acetoacetic acid, β-hydroxybutyric acid, and acetone. SEE: *acetone; ketosis.*

ketonemia (kē"tō-nē'mē-ă) [*ketone* + Gr. *haima,* blood]. Acetone bodies in the blood. Their presence causes the characteristic fruity breath odor in ketoacidosis. SYN: *acidosis.*

ketone threshold. Level of ketone in the blood above which ketone bodies appear in the urine.

ketonuria (kē-tō-nū'rē-ă) [" + Gr. *ouron,* urine]. Acetone bodies in the urine.

ketoplasia (kē-tō-plā'sē-ă) [" + Gr. *plassein,* to form]. The formation or excretion of ketones.

ketoplastic [" + Gr. *plastikos,* formed]. Pert. to ketoplasia or formation of ketones.

ketose. A carbohydrate containing the ketones.

ketosis (kē-tō'sĭs) [*ketone* + Gr. *osis,* condition]. The accumulation in the body of the ketone bodies: acetone, beta-hydroxybutyric acid, and acetoacetic acid. It is frequently associated with acidosis and is often miscalled acidosis. Ketosis results from the incomplete metabolism of fatty acids, generally from carbohydrate deficiency or inadequate utilization, and is commonly observed in starvation, high-fat diet, pregnancy, following ether anesthesia, and most significantly in diabetes mellitus. Large quantities of these ketone bodies may be eliminated in the urine (ketonuria). The presence of ketosis is easily determined by testing for the presence of acetone or diacetic acid in the urine. Ketonuria is an early sign of acidosis in patients with diabetes mellitus.

17-ketosteroid. One of a group of neutral steroids having a ketone group in carbon position 17. They are produced by the adrenal cortex and gonads and appear normally in the urine. Among them are androsterone, dehydroisoandrosterone, corticosterone, compound E, and 11-hydroxyisoandrosterone. A greater than normal or less than normal excretion in the urine is indicative of certain endocrine disorders. SEE: *perhydrocyclopentanophenanthrene.*

ketosuria (kē″tō-sū′rē-ă). Presence of ketone bodies in the urine. SEE: *ketosis.*

ketotic. Pertaining to ketosis.

KEV. *kilo electron volts.*

Key-Retzius foramina (kē′rĕt′zē-ŭs). [Ernst A. H. Key, Swedish physician, 1832–1901; Magnus G. Retzius, Swedish histologist, 1842–1919] Passages in the pia mater carrying the choroid plexus to the fourth ventricle. SYN: *Luschka's foramen.*

kg. *kilogram.*

kg.-m. *kilogram-meter.*

$KHCO_3$. Potassium bicarbonate.

$KHSO_4$. Potassium bisulfate.

kHz. *kilohertz.*

KI. Potassium iodide.

kibe (kīb) [Welsh *cibi,* chilblain]. Inflamed patch on hands or feet caused by exposure to cold. SYN: *chilblain.*

kidney [ME. *kidenei*]. Paired organs, purplish-brown in color, situated at the back (retroperitoneal area) of the abdominal cavity, one on each side of the spinal column. Their function is to excrete urine and to help regulate the water, electrolyte, and acid-base content of the blood.

The upper level of the kidneys is opposite the 12th thoracic (dorsal) vertebra, the lower level is opposite the 3rd lumbar vertebra. The right kidney is slightly lower than the left one.

Weight: 113 to 170 gm. (4 to 6 oz.). Size: about 11.4 cm. (4½ in.) long, 5 to 7.5 cm. (2 to 3 in.) broad, and 2.5 cm. (1 in.) thick. The kidneys in the newborn are about three times as large in proportion to body weight as in the adult.

ANAT: Each kidney is surrounded by fatty tissue and by the renal fascia, a sheath of fibrous tissue, which helps to hold the kidney in place. The concave border of the kidney faces the median line, the center of the concave border opening into a fissure called the hilum or hilus.

The ureter enters the kidney through the hilum into the pelvis of the kidney. The outer portion of the kidney is the cortex, a mass of cortical substance; the inner portion (medullary substance) is the medulla. Within the cortical substance are found the arteries, veins, convoluted tubules, and glomerular capsules, while the medulla contains the renal pyramids, conical masses with papillae projecting into the cuplike cavities (calyces) of the pelvis. Each kidney contains 8 to 18 pyramids made up of collecting tubules, lymphatics, and blood vessels, the pyramids being penetrated by the cortical substance and supporting them. These extensions are known as the renal columns, or columns of Bertini.

The cortical and medullary substance is composed of renal tubules, connective tissue, blood vessels, nerves, and lymphatics. The renal tubule or nephron constitutes the structural and functional unit of the kidney. Each consists of a capsule, proximal convoluted portion, loop of Henle, and distal convoluted portion, which leads to a collecting duct. The capsule, called the glomerular or Bowman's capsule, encloses a globular mass of capillaries, the glomerulus. The capsule and the enclosed glomerulus comprise the malpighian or renal corpuscle. The renal corpuscles are located principally in the cortex. SEE: illus.

FORMATION OF URINE: Urine consists of water (95%) and solids (5%), the latter being in solution. The solids include organic constituents (urea, hippuric acid, uric acid, creatinine) and inorganic constituents, principally salts of sodium and potassium. The kidneys remove these substances from the blood, thus acting to maintain homeostasis of the blood and body fluids. Urine is formed by the processes of filtration and reabsorption. As blood passes through the glomerulus, water and dissolved substances are filtered through the capillary walls and the inner or visceral layer of Bowman's capsule, resulting in formation of the glomerular filtrate. Blood cells and colloidal substances such as proteins are retained within the capillaries. The glomerular filtrate passes through the renal tubules to the collecting ducts, during the course of which all of the sugar and some of the salts and other substances are selectively reabsorbed into the capillaries surrounding the tubule. Substances such as uric acid and hydrogen ions may be added to the urine by the cells of the tubules through the process of secretion. The final product now known as urine passes through straight collecting ducts into larger collecting ducts (papillary ducts) that open on the tips of the renal papillae. There urine is discharged into the minor calyces of the renal pelvis, and then is conveyed by the ureters to the bladder. Periodically the bladder is voluntarily emptied and discharges its contents to the outside through the urethra. This is called micturition, urination, or voiding. If a normally hydrated individual ingests a large volume of aqueous fluids, in about 42 min. a sufficient quantity will have been excreted into the bladder to cause the urge to urinate.

Substances that are entirely or almost entirely reabsorbed during passage through the tubule are known as high-threshold substances. These include glucose and chlorides of sodium, potassium, calcium, and magne-

KIDNEY

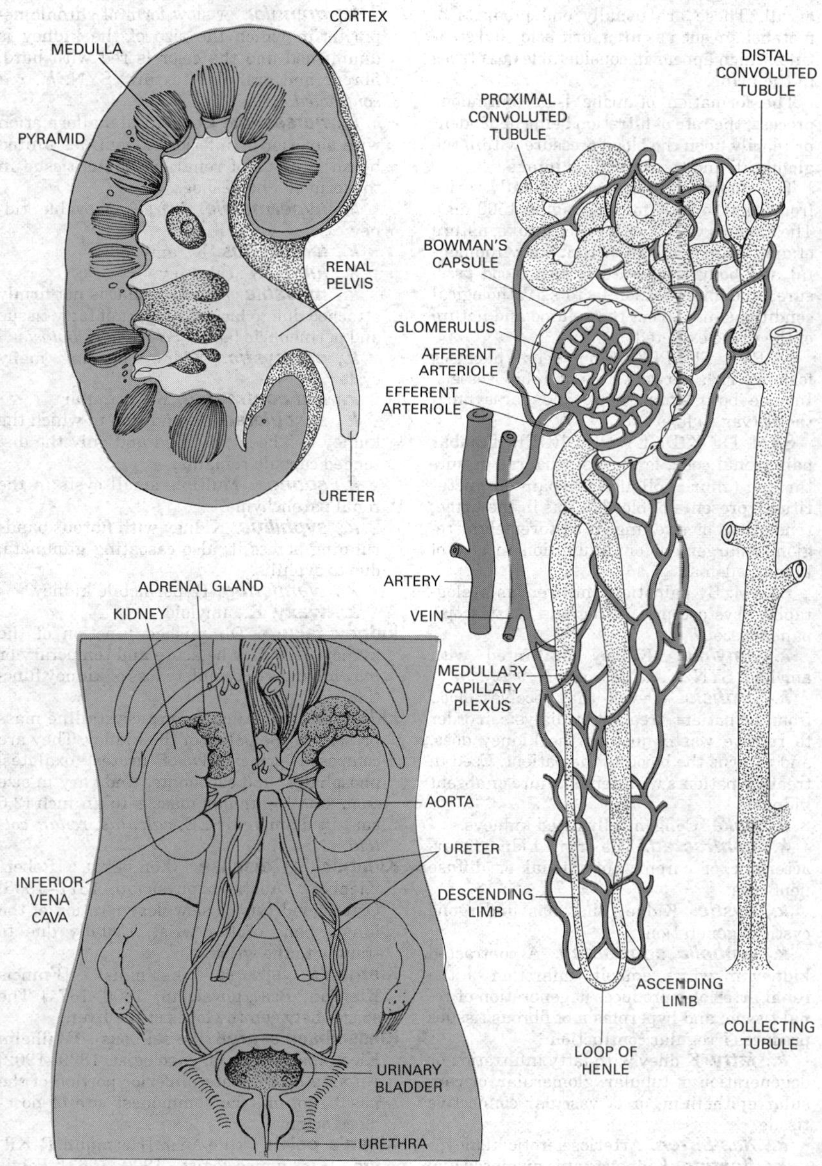
CORTEX
MEDULLA
PYRAMID
RENAL PELVIS
URETER
PROXIMAL CONVOLUTED TUBULE
DISTAL CONVOLUTED TUBULE
BOWMAN'S CAPSULE
GLOMERULUS
AFFERENT ARTERIOLE
EFFERENT ARTERIOLE
ARTERY
VEIN
MEDULLARY CAPILLARY PLEXUS
DESCENDING LIMB
ASCENDING LIMB
LOOP OF HENLE
COLLECTING TUBULE
ADRENAL GLAND
KIDNEY
AORTA
URETER
INFERIOR VENA CAVA
URINARY BLADDER
URETHRA

sium. These are important blood constituents and excreted only when their concentrations in the blood are above normal. Low or nonthreshold substances are those that are reabsorbed only in limited quantities or not at all. These are usually end products of metabolism such as urea, uric acid, and creatine, which appear in considerable quantities in the urine.

The formation of urine is a continuous process, the rate of filtration being dependent primarily upon the blood pressure within the glomeruli and the daily fluid intake.

The volume of urine excreted daily varies from 1000 to 2000 ml. (averaging 1500 ml.). The amount varies with water intake, nature of diet, degree of body activity, environmental and body temperature, age, blood pressure, and many other factors. Pathological conditions may affect the volume and nature of the urine excreted.

NERVE SUPPLY: From renal plexuses forming rich networks about renal vessels. Include both sympathetic and parasympathetic (vagal) fibers.

SYM. OF KIDNEY DISORDER: Lumbar pain, renal colic, fever, disturbances in micturition (anuria, oliguria, or pain on micturition), presence of blood or pus in the urine, tenderness or swelling in costovertebral region, enlargement or diminution in size of kidney, edema.

EXAM: By palpation, intravenous pyelography, cystoscopy, retrograde cystoscopy, panendoscopy.

k., amyloid. Kidney infiltrated with amyloid. SYN: *k., lardaceous; k., waxy.*

k., artificial. Device that receives blood from the patient, treats it by dialysis in order to remove wastes just as the kidney does, and returns the blood to the patient. Used in treating patients with renal failure or absent kidneys.

k., cake. Congenitally fused kidneys.

k., contracted. The small kidney characteristic of chronic interstitial or diffuse nephritis.

k., cystic. Kidney that has undergone cystic degeneration.

k., embolic contracted. A contracted kidney in which embolic infarction of the renal arterioles produces degeneration of renal tissue, and hyperplasia of fibrous tissues produces irregular contraction.

k., fatty. Kidney with fatty infiltration or degeneration of tubular, glomerular, or capsular epithelium, or of vascular connective tissue.

k., flea-bitten. Arteriosclerotic kidney.

k., floating. Kidney that is displaced and movable.

k., fused. The two kidneys are fused.

k., Goldblatt. Kidney with impaired blood supply and resulting hypertension. Named after the U.S. physician Harry Goldblatt, who produced the same type of kidney experimentally in animals.

k., granular. A slow form of chronic nephritis in which the size of the kidney is diminished and the color is red with hard, fibrous and granular texture. SYN: *k., red contracted.*

k., horseshoe. Congenital malformation with superior or inferior extremities united by an isthmus of renal or fibrous tissue in the form of a horseshoe.

k., hypermobile. A freely movable kidney.

k., lardaceous. K., amyloid.

k., lump. K., cake, q.v.

k., movable. A kidney that is not firmly attached due to lack of support of fatty tissue and perinephric fascia. SYN: *nephroptosis.*

k., polycystic. Kidney bearing many cysts.

k., red contracted. K., granular.

k., sacculated. A condition in which the kidney has been absorbed and only the distended capsule remains.

k., sponge. Multiple small cysts in the renal parenchyma.

k., syphilitic. Kidney with fibrous bands running across it, also caseating gummata, due to syphilis.

k., wandering. Hypermobile kidney.

k., waxy. K., amyloid.

kidney failure. Diminished function of the kidney. This may be acute and temporary or may progress to complete loss of kidney function.

kidney stone. Calculus or a crystalline mass present in the pelvis of the kidney. They are composed principally of urates, oxalates, phosphates, and carbonates and vary in size from small granular masses to an inch (2.5 cm.) in diameter. SEE: *calculus, renal; colloid.*

Kienböck's disease (kēn'běks). [Robert Kienböck, Austrian physician, 1871–1953] Osteochondrosis or slow degeneration of the lunate bone of the wrist. Usually due to trauma to the wrist.

Kiernan's spaces (kēr'nănz). [Francis Kiernan, Brit. physician, 1800–1874] The spaces between the lobes of the liver.

Kiesselbach's area (kē'sěl-bŏks). [Wilhelm Kiesselbach, Ger. laryngologist, 1839–1902] An area on the anteroinferior portion of the nasal septum, the commonest site of nosebleed origin.

Kilian's pelvis (kĭl'ē-ănz). [Hermann F. Kilian, Ger. gynecologist, 1800–1863] Pelvis affected with osteomalacia. SYN: *pelvis spinosa.*

kilo- [Fr.]. Combining form indicating 1,000.
kilocalorie. ABBR: C.; kcal. A unit of measure for heat. In nutrition, a kilocalorie is known as a large Calorie and is always written with a capital C. SEE: *calorie*.
kilocycle (kĭl'ō-sī"k'l). ABBR: kc. A thousand cycles.
kilogram [Fr. *kilo*, a thousand, + *gramme*, a weight]. ABBR: kg. One thousand gm. or 2.2 lb. avoirdupois.
kilogram-meter. ABBR: kg.-m. The work required to raise one kilogram one meter.
kilohertz. In electricity, a unit of a thousand cycles. Formerly called kilocycle.
kilojoule. One thousand joules.
kiloliter (kĭl'ō-lē"tĕr) [Fr. *kilolitre*]. ABBR: kl. One thousand liters.
kilomegacycles. 10^9 cycles per second, i.e., 1000 megacycles per second.
kilometer [Fr. *kilometre*]. ABBR: km. One thousand meters, or 3281 feet (roughly 0.6 of a mile).
kilounit (kĭl"ō-ū'nĭt). One thousand units.
kilovolt [Fr. *kilo*, a thousand, + *volt*]. ABBR: kv. One thousand volt unit.
kilovoltage peak. The highest voltage occurring during an electrical cycle.
kilowatt. ABBR: kw. A unit of electrical energy equal to one thousand watts.
Kimmelstiel-Wilson syndrome. A syndrome that may develop in patients in whom diabetes mellitus has been present for several years. Hypertension, glomerulonephrosis, edema, and retinal lesions are present and arteriosclerosis of the renal artery is a common complication. SEE: *diabetes*.
kinanesthesia (kĭn-ăn-ĕs-thē'zē-ă) [Gr. *kinesis*, movement, + *an-*, not, + *aisthesis*, sensation]. Inability to perceive extent of movement or direction, resulting in ataxia.
kinase (kĭn'ās). An enzyme that catalyzes the transfer of phosphate from ATP to an acceptor.
kinematics [Gr. *kinematos*, movement]. Science of motion.
kinematograph (kin"ĕ-măt'o-grăf). A device for viewing photographs of objects in motion; used in diagnosis.
kineplastic (kĭn"ĭ-plăs'tĭk) [Gr. *kinein*, to move, + *plastikos*, formed]. Pert. to kineplasty.
kineplasty. A form of amputation so that the muscles of the stump can be used to impart motion to an artificial limb. SEE: *Boston arm; cineplastics*.
kinergety (kĭn'ĕr-jĕt-ē) [Gr. *kinein*, to move, + *ergon*, energy]. The potential capacity for kinetic energy.
kinesalgia (kĭn"ĕ-săl'jē-ă) [Gr. *kinesis*, movement, + *algos*, pain]. Pain associated with muscular movement. SYN: *kinesialgia*.
kinescope (kĭn'ĕ-skōp) [" + *skopein*, to examine]. A device for testing the refraction of the eye. A slit of variable width moves as the patient observes a fixed object.
kinesia (kī-nē'sē-ă). Sickness caused by motion, as seasickness, car sickness.
kinesialgia (kĭ-nē"sē-ăl'jē-ă) [" + *algos*, pain]. Pain caused by muscular movements. SYN: *kinesalgia*.
kinesiatrics (kĭ-nē"sē-ăt'rĭks) [" + *iatrikos*, curative]. Treatment involving active and passive movements. SYN: *kinesitherapy*.
kinesics (kī-nē'sĭks). Systematic study of the body and the use of its static and dynamic position as a means of communication. SEE: *body language*.
kinesimeter (kĭn"ĕ-sĭm'ĕ-tĕr) [" + *metron*, measure]. An apparatus for determining the extent of movement of a part.
kinesiodic (kĭ-nē"sē-ŏd'ĭk) [" + *hodos*, path]. Pert. to paths through which motor impulses pass.
kinesiology (kĭ-nē"sē-ŏl'ō-jē) [" + *logos*, study]. The study of muscles and muscular movement. SEE: *biomechanics*.
kinesioneurosis (kĭ-nē"sē-ō-nū-rō'sĭs) [" + *neuron*, nerve, + *osis*, condition]. Functional disorder marked by tics and spasms.
  k., external. Kinesioneurosis affecting external muscles.
  k., vascular. Kinesioneurosis of the vasomotor system.
  k., visceral. Kinesioneurosis affecting muscles of internal organs
kinesiotherapy (kĭ-nē"sē-ō-thĕr'ă-pē) [" + *therapeia*, therapy]. Therapeutic exercises. SYN: *kinesitherapy; kinetotherapy*.
kinesis (kĭn-ē'sĭs) [Gr.]. Motion.
kinesitherapy [" + *therapeia*, therapy]. Treatment by movements or exercises. SYN: *kinesiotherapy; kinetotherapy*. SEE: *physical therapy*.
kinesodic (kĭn"ē-sŏd'ĭk) [" + *hodos*, path]. Rel. to the conveyance of motor impulses.
kinesthesia (kĭn"ĕs-thē'zē-ă) [" + *aisthesis*, sensation]. Ability to perceive extent, direction, or weight of movement.
kinesthesiometer (kĭn"ĕs-thē-zē-ŏm'ĕ-tĕr) [" + " + *metron*, measure]. Instrument for testing ability to determine the position of the muscles.
kinesthetic. Rel. to kinesthesia.
kinetic (kĭ-nĕt'ĭk) [Gr. *kinesis*, motion]. Pert. to or consisting of motion.
kinetocardiography. Record of precordial vibrations of such low frequency that they are inaudible.
kinetosis (kĭn"ĕ-tō'sĭs) [" + *osis*, condition]. Any disorder caused by motion, such as seasickness, car sickness. SYN: *kinesia*.
kinetotherapy (kĭ-nĕt"ō-thĕr'ă-pē) [" + *therapeia*, treatment]. Treatment that employs active and passive movements. SYN: *kinesiotherapy; kinesitherapy*.

kingdom [AS. *cyningdom*]. In classifying living entities, the broadest category is kingdom. Thus there are the animal and plant kingdoms. SEE: *taxonomy*.

kinin (kī'nĭn) [Gr. *kinesis*, movement]. A general term for a group of polypeptides that have considerable biological activity. They are capable of influencing smooth muscle contraction; inducing hypotension; increasing the blood flow and permeability of small blood capillaries, and inciting pain.

kininases, plasma. Plasma carboxypeptidases that inactivate plasma kinins.

kininogen. A substance that produces a kinin when acted upon by certain enzymes.

kink [Low Ger. *kinke*, a twist in rope]. Unnatural angle or bend in a duct or tube such as the intestine, umbilical cord, or ureter.

kinky hair disease. Congenital syndrome due to an autosomal recessive gene, consisting of short, sparse, kinky hair that frequently is poorly pigmented. Both physical and mental development are retarded. The disease is due to a metabolic defect that causes an abnormality in the fatty acid composition of the grey matter of the brain. Death follows progressive severe degenerative changes in the central nervous system.

kino- (kī'nō) [Gr. *kinein*, to move]. Combining form indicating movement.

kinocilium (kī"nō-sĭl'ē-ŭm) [" + L. *cilium*, eyelash]. Protoplasmic filament on the cell surface.

kinomometer (kī"nō-mŏm'ĕ-tĕr) [" + *metron*, measure]. Device that measures degree of motion in a joint.

kinship (kĭn'shĭp). The descendants from a common ancestor.

kiotome (kī'ō-tōm) [Gr. *kion*, column, + *tome*, incision]. Instrument for amputating the uvula.

kiotomy (kī-ŏt'ō-mē) Use of the kiotome in amputating the uvula.

Kirschner's wire (kĕrsh'nĕrz). [Martin Kirschner, Ger. surgeon, 1879–1942] SEE: *wire, Kirschner's*.

Kisch's reflex (kĭsh'ĕs). [Bruno Kisch, Ger. physiologist, 1890–1966] Closure of an eye resulting from stimulation of heat or some tactile irritant on the auditory meatus. SYN: *auriculopalpebral reflex*.

kitasamycin (kĭt"ă-să-mī'sĭn). An antibiotic substance produced by Streptomyces kitasatoensis. Also: *leucomycin*.

Kite apparatus. [Joseph H. Kite, U.S. orthopedic surgeon, b. 1891] Apparatus for reeducation of weak muscles and for assistance in overcoming contractures of forearm, wrist, and fingers.

KJ. *knee jerk*.

KK. *knee kick* (knee jerk).

kl. *kiloliter*.

Klebcil. Trade name for kanamycin sulfate, USP.

Klebsiella (klĕb"sē-ĕl'ă). [T. A. Edwin Klebs, Ger. bacteriologist, 1834–1913] A genus of bacteria of the family Enterobacteriaceae. They are short, plump, gram-negative bacilli that form capsules but not spores. Frequently associated with respiratory infections and may cause urinary tract infections.

K. ozaenae. Species found in ozena.

K. pneumoniae. A species that can cause pneumonia. Also found as a secondary invader in other respiratory infections such as bronchitis or sinusitis. SYN: *Friedländer's bacillus; pneumobacillus*.

K. rhinoscleromatis. Species that can cause rhinoscleroma, a destructive granuloma of the nose and pharnyx.

Klebs-Loeffler bacillus (klĕbs-lĕf'lĕr). [T. A. E. Klebs; Friedrich Loeffler, Ger. bacteriologist, 1852–1915] The bacillus of diphtheria. SYN: *Corynebacterium diphtheriae*.

klepto- (klĕp'tō) [Gr. *kleptein*, to steal]. Combining form meaning to steal.

kleptolagnia (klĕp"tō-lăg'nē-ă) [" + *lagneia*, lust]. Sexual gratification derived from stealing.

kleptomania (klĕp-tō-mā'nē-ă) [" + *mania*, madness]. Impulsive stealing, the motive not being in the intrinsic value of the article to the patient. In almost all cases, the individual has enough money to pay for the stolen goods. The stealing is done without prior planning and without the assistance of others. There is increased tension prior to the theft and a sense of gratification while committing the act.

kleptomaniac. 1. Pert. to kleptomania. 2. A psychopathic personality suffering from impulsive stealing.

kleptophobia (klĕp-tō-fō'bē-ă) [" + *phobos*, fear]. Morbid fear of stealing.

Klieg eye (klēg). Conjunctivitis, lacrimation, and photophobia from exposure to the intense lights used in making motion pictures or television films.

Klinefelter's syndrome (klĭn'fĕl-tĕrs). [Harry F. Klinefelter, Jr., U.S. physician, b. 1912] Congenital endocrine condition of primary testicular failure that usually is not evident prior to puberty. The classical form is associated with the presence of an extra X chromosome. The testes are small and firm, and gynecomastia, abnormally long legs, and subnormal intelligence usually are present. In variant forms the chromosomal abnormalities vary and the severity and number of abnormal findings are diversified. The syndrome is estimated to occur in one of 700 live male births. Diagnosis may by confirmed by chromosomal analysis of tissue culture.

Klippel's disease (klĭ-pĕlz'). [Maurice Klippel, Fr. neurologist, 1858–1942] Weakness or pseudoparalysis due to generalized arthritis.

Klippel-Feil syndrome. [Maurice Klippel; André Feil, Fr. physician, b. 1884] Congenital anomaly characterized by a short and wide neck, low hairline, reduction in the number of cervical vertebrae, and fusion of the cervical spine. The hairline on the back of the neck is quite low. The central nervous system may also be affected.

K-Lor. Trade name for potassium chloride, USP.

Klumpke's paralysis (kloomp'kĕz). [Madame A. Dejerine Klumpke, Fr. neurologist, 1859–1927] Atrophic paralysis of forearm.

K-Lyte. Trade name for potassium bicarbonate.

K-Lyte/Cl. Trade name for potassium chloride, USP.

km. *kilometer.*

kMc. *kilomegacycle.*

$KMnO_4$. Potassium permanganate.

Knapp's forceps (năps). [Herman J. Knapp, U.S. ophthalmologist, 1832–1911] A forceps with blades like rollers for expressing trachomatous granulations on the palpebral conjunctiva.

kneading (nēd'ĭng) [AS. *cnedan*]. A form of massage consisting of grasping, wringing, lifting, rolling, or pressing part of a muscle or group of muscles. SYN: *pétrissage.*

knee [AS. *cneo*]. 1. The anterior aspect of the leg at the articulation of the femur and tibia and the articulation itself, covered anteriorly with the patella or kneecap. Formed by the femur, tibia, and patella. SEE: illus. 2. Any structure shaped like a semiflexed knee. SYN: *geniculum.*

RS: geniculate; geniculum; "genu-" words; "gon-" words; patella; popliteal.

k., Brodie's. A chronic fungoid synovitis of the knee joint in which the affected parts become soft and pulpy.

k., dislocation of. Displacement of the knee. Dislocations in themselves are unusual. The so-called dislocation of the knee is usually due to various injuries of the joint and of the complicating structures of the knee, such as the tearing of the crushed tendons or ligaments or the slipping of cartilages. They should be treated either by a straight splint, as in a fracture of the kneecap, or by two splints, one on either side of the knee, as in a fracture involving the knee joint. The patient should be transported to a

ANATOMY OF THE SUPPORTING STRUCTURES OF THE KNEE

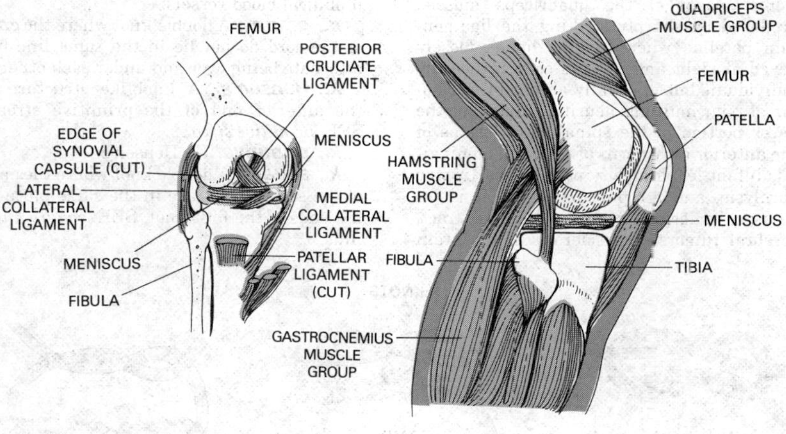

hospital as quickly as possible.

k., game. A lay term for internal derangement of the knee joint.

PATH: Usually a torn internal cartilage, a fracture of the tibial spine, or an injury to the collateral or cruciate ligaments.

SYM: Pain or instability, locking, and weakness.

F.A.: Immobilize with a posterior splint. Surgical exploratory arthrotomy may be necessary.

k., housemaid's. Inflamed condition of the bursa anterior to the patella with accumulation of fluid therein. May be seen in those who have to kneel frequently or continually while working.

k., knock. The condition in which the knees come together while the ankles are far apart, caused by an outward distortion of the leg that throws the knee inside the normal line. SYN: *genu valgum*. SEE: *bowleg; genu varum*.

k., locked. Condition in which the leg cannot be extended. Usually due to displacement of semilunar cartilage.

kneecap. The patella.

knee-chest position. Position in which the patient is on knees with thighs upright, head and upper part of chest resting on table, and arms crossed above the head. Employed in displacement of prolapsed fundus, dislodgement of impacted head of fetus, management of transverse presentation, replacement of retroverted uterus or displaced ovary, or endoscopic examination of the rectum and colon. SYN: *genupectoral position*. SEE: *position* for illus.

knee-jerk reflex. The reflex contraction or clonic spasm of the quadriceps muscle, produced by sharply striking the ligamentum patellae when the leg hangs loosely flexed at right angles. It is seen in healthy individuals but is usually absent in locomotor ataxia, multiple neuritis, lesions of the lower portion of the spinal cord, lesions of the anterior gray horns of the cord, meningitis, infantile paralysis, pseudohypertrophic paralysis, and atrophic paralysis. It is increased in lesions of the pyramidal tract, cerebral tumors, and sclerosis of the brain and cord. SYN: *patellar reflex*. SEE: *Jendrassik's maneuver; jerk*.

knee-joint. The articulation of the femur and tibia.

knee of internal capsule. The curve at the meeting place of the anterior and posterior limbs of the internal capsule of the brain.

Kneipp cure (nīp). [Rev. Father Sebastian Kneipp, Ger. priest, 1821–1897] Application of water in various forms and degrees of temperature in the cure of disease, esp. wading in cold, dewy grass. SEE: *hydrotherapy*.

kneippism (nīp′ĭzm). Walking barefoot in dewy grass, or bathing in cold water as a form of hydrotherapy.

knife (nīf) [AS. *cnif*]. A cutting instrument.

k., electric. A knife that functions by use of a high-frequency cutting current.

knismogenic (nĭs″mō-jĕn′ĭk) [Gr. *knismos*, tickling, + *gennan*, to produce]. Producing a tickling sensation.

knitting [AS. *cnyttan*, to make knots]. The process of healing by union of pieces of a fractured bone.

KNO_3. Potassium nitrate, niter, q.v., saltpeter.

knob (nŏb) [ME. *knobbe*]. A protuberance on a surface or extremity; a mass, q.v., or nodule, q.v.

knock-knee. Knee, knock, q.v.

knot [AS. *cnotta*]. 1. An intertwining of a cord or cordlike structure to form a lump or knob. 2. In surgery, the intertwining of the ends of a suture, ligature, bandage, or sling so that the ends will not slip or become separated. SEE: *square knot;* illus. 3. In anatomy, an enlargement forming a knoblike structure.

k., false. An external bulging of the umbilical cord resulting from the coiling of the umbilical blood vessels.

k., granny. A double knot where the ends of the cord do not lie in the same line but alternate being over and under each other.

k., Hensen's. A knoblike structure at the anterior end of the primitive streak. SEE: *primitive streak*.

k., primitive. K., Hensen's.

k., square. A double knot where the ends of the second knot are in the same place as the ends of the first knot. SEE: *square knot;* illus.

KNOTS

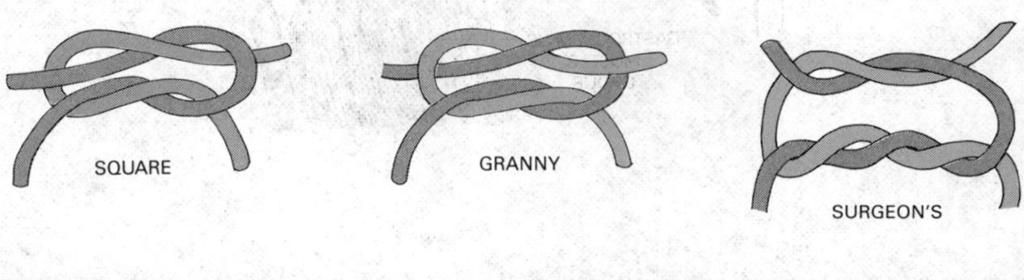

k., surgical. A double knot in which the cord is passed through the first loop twice.

k., syncytial. A protuberance formed by many nuclei of the syntrophoblast and found on the surface of a chorionic villus.

k., true. A knot formed by the fetus slipping through a loop of the umbilical cord.

knuckle (nŭk'ĕl) [Middle Low Ger. *knokel*]. Prominence of the dorsal aspect of any of the phalangeal joints, esp. of the distal heads of the metacarpals when the fist is clenched.

knuckle pads. Discrete fibromatous pads appearing over the fingerjoints. Usually appear between ages of 15 and 30. Etiol. is unknown but trauma is not a significant factor.

K.O.C. *cathodal opening contraction.* SYN: *COC.*

Koch, Robert (kōk). German bacteriologist, 1843–1910.

K.'s bacillus. The bacillus causing tuberculosis in mammals. SYN: *Mycobacterium tuberculosis.*

K.'s law. Criterion used in proving an organism is the cause of a disease or lesion: the microorganism in question is regularly found in the lesions of the disease; pure cultures can be obtained from it; pure cultures when inoculated into susceptible animals can reproduce the disease or pathological condition; and the organism can be obtained again in pure culture from the inoculated animal.

K.'s phenomenon. Local inflammatory reaction resulting from injection of tuberculin into the skin of a person who has been previously exposed to the tubercle bacillus.

K.'s postulates. K.'s law, q.v.

Koch, Walter (kōk). German surgeon, b. 1880.

K.'s node. The atrioventricular node.

kocherization (kōk"ĕr-ī-zā'shŭn). Operative technique in opening the duodenum to expose the ampulla of the common bile duct.

Kocher's reflex (kō'kĕrz). [Theodor Kocher, Swiss surgeon, 1841–1917] Contraction of abdominal muscles following moderate compression of the testicle.

Koebner phenomenon. Linear papules in a line on the skin that has been scratched.

KOH. Potassium hydroxide.

Köhler's disease (kā'lĕrz). [Alban Köhler, Ger. physician, 1874–1947] 1. Aseptic necrosis of the navicular bone of the wrist. 2. Osteochondrosis of the head of the second metatarsal bone of the foot.

Kohlrausch's fold (kōl'rowsh-ĕs). [Otto L. B. Kohlrausch, Ger. physician, 1811–1854] The rectal valve; horizontal folds of the mucosa of the rectum. SYN: *Houston's valves; plica transversales recti* [NA].

Kohnstamm's phenomenon (kōn'stămz). [Oscar Kohnstamm, Ger. physician, 1871–1917] Persistent and spontaneous contraction of a muscle after a strong contraction against resistance has ceased. This is easily demonstrated by standing and forcibly pushing the arm against a wall while standing with the frontal plane perpendicular to the wall. When this is stopped and you have moved away from the wall, the arm will involuntarily adduct and be elevated. SYN: *aftermovement.*

koilocytotic atypia (koy"lō-sī-tŏt'ĭk ā-tĭp'ē-ă) [Gr. *koilos,* hollow, + *kytos,* cell, + *osis,* condition, + *a-,* not, + *typicalis,* typical]. Abnormality of the top layers of the epithelium of the uterine cervix wherein the cells undergo vacuolization and enlargement.

koilonychia (koy-lō-nĭk'ē-ă) [" + *onyx,* nail]. Dystrophy of the fingernails in which they are thin and concave with raised edges. Sometimes associated with iron-deficiency anemia.

koilorrhachic (koy"lō-răk'ĭk) [" + *rhachis,* spine]. Pert. to a spinal column that has an excessive anterior curve.

koilosternia (koy"lō-stĕr'nē-ă) [" + Gr. *sternon,* sternum]. Condition where the chest has a funnel-like depression in the middle of the thoracic wall.

kolp- [Gr. *kolpos,* vagina]. Prefix indicating vagina. SEE: words beginning with *colp-.*

kolpitis (kŏl-pī'tĭs) [" + *itis,* inflammation]. Inflammation of vaginal mucous membrane. SYN: *colpitis.*

kolypeptic (kō"lē-pĕp'tĭk) [Gr. *kolyein,* to hinder, + *pepsis,* digestion]. Retarding digestion.

Konakion. Trade name for phytonadione, USP.

Kondoleon's operation (kŏn-dō'lē-ŏnz). [Emmanuel Kondoleon, Gr. surgeon, 1879–1939] Surgical removal of layers of subcutaneous tissue to relieve elephantiasis.

Kondremul. Trade name for mineral oil.

koniocortex (kō"nē-ō-kor'tĕks) [Gr. *konis,* dust, + L. *cortex,* rind]. The cortex of the sensory areas, so named because of its granular appearance.

koniology [" + *logos,* study]. Science of dust and its effects. SYN: *coniology.*

koniometer (kō-nē-ŏm'ĕ-tĕr) [" + *metron,* measure]. Device for estimating amount of dust in the air.

koniosis (kō-nē-ō'sĭs) [" + *osis,* condition]. Any disease condition caused by dust. SYN: *coniosis.* SEE: *pneumoconiosis.*

Konyne. Trade name for factor IX complex.

kopf-tetanus [Ger. *Kopf,* head, + *tetanos,* tetanus]. Tetanus developing subsequent to a head wound.

kophemia (kō-fē'mē-ă). Word deafness.

Koplik's spots. [Henry Koplik, U.S. pediatrician, 1858–1927] Small red spots with bluish-white centers on the oral mucosa, particularly in the region opposite the molars. A diagnostic sign in measles before the rash appears. Not infrequently, the spots disappear as the eruption develops.

kopophobia (kŏp″ō-fō′bē-ă) [Gr. *kopos,* fatigue, + *phobos,* fear] Abnormal fear of fatigue or exhaustion.

Korányi's sign (kō-răn′yēz). Increased resonance on percussion of the dorsal spine, a sign of pleural effusion.

koro (kō′rō). In China and Southeast Asia, a hysterical phobia that the penis will retract into the abdomen.

koronion (kō-rō′nē-ŏn) [Gr. *korone,* crest]. Apex of coronoid process of the mandible.

Korotkoff's sounds (kō-rŏt′kŏfs). [Nicolai S. Korotkoff, Russ. physician, b. 1874] Sounds heard in auscultation of blood pressure. SEE: *blood pressure.*

Korsakoff's syndrome (kor′să-kŏfs). [Sergei S. Korsakoff, Russ. neurologist, 1854–1900] Personality characterized by a psychosis with polyneuritis, disorientation, muttering delirium, insomnia, illusions, and hallucinations. Painful extremities, rarely a bilateral wrist drop, more frequently bilateral foot drop with pain or pressure over the long nerves. May occur as a sequel to chronic alcoholism. SYN: *polyneuritic psychosis.*

kosam (kō′săm). A shrub, Brucea sumatrana, of Southeast Asia and Australia, the seeds of which are used medicinally to treat diarrhea and uterine hemorrhage.

kosher (kō′shĕr) [Hebrew *kasher,* proper]. Food prepared and served according to Jewish dietary laws.

koumiss (koo′mĭs) [Tartar *kumyz*]. Fermented cow's milk or substance used for fermenting cow's milk. Also spelled kumiss and kumyss.

Kr. Chem. symb. for krypton.

Krabbe's disease (krăb′ēz) [Knud H. Krabbe, Danish neurologist, 1885–1961] Leukodystrophy due to the accumulation of a sphingolipid in the tissues. This is the result of a deficiency of β-galactosidase. Clinically, the infant develops seizures, blindness, paralysis, and marked mental deficiency.

Kraepelin's classification (krā′pă-lĭnz). [Emil Kraepelin, Ger. psychiatrist, 1856–1926] A classification of mental disease into two groups: the manic-depressive and the schizophrenic.

krait (krāt). Small venomous snake of the genus Bungarus indigenous to India.

kraurosis (krŏ-rō′sĭs) [Gr. *krauros,* dry]. Atrophy and dryness of skin and any mucous membrane, esp. of the vulva. The subcutaneous fat of the mons pubis and labia disappears, clitoris and prepuce atrophy, and stenosis of the vaginal orifice is common. Fissures may develop.

ETIOL: Probably hypoestrinism.

k. penis. Kraurosis in which the glans penis atrophies and becomes shriveled.

k. vulvae. Atrophic disease affecting the female external genitalia seen most often in older women. Characterized by severe itching and a white marble-like appearance of the skin, frequently with excoriations. If untreated, the skin may undergo malignant degeneration. SYN: *Breisky's disease; leukoplakia vulvae.*

Krause, Karl (krowz). German anatomist, 1797–1868.

K.'s glands. Small mucous acinous glands located beneath the fornix conjunctiva. They are accessory lacrimal glands that open into the fornix.

K.'s valve. Fold of mucous membrane of the lacrimal sac at the junction of the lacrimal duct. SYN: *Beraud's valve.*

Krause, Wilhelm (krowz). German anatomist, 1833–1910.

K.'s bulbs; K.'s end bulbs. Widely distributed encapsulated nerve endings present superficially in the skin and cornea and in organs such as the testicles.

K.'s membrane. A thin, dark disk that transversely crosses through and bisects the clear zone of a striated muscle and bisects the clear zone (isotropic disk) of a striated muscle fiber. The portion between two disks constitutes a sarcomere. SYN: *Z disk.*

Krebs cycle. [Sir Hans Krebs, Ger. biochemist, 1900–1981, who was co-winner of a Nobel prize in 1953. He lived and worked in Britain.] A complicated series of reactions in the body involving the oxidative metabolism of pryuvic acid and liberation of energy. It is the main pathway of terminal oxidation in the process of which not only carbohydrates but proteins and fats are utilized. SYN: *citric acid cycle; tricarboxylic acid cycle.* SEE: illus.

Krönig's area (krā′nĭgz). [Georg Krönig, Ger. physician, 1856–1911] Resonant region in the thorax over the apices of the lungs.

Krukenberg's tumor (kroo′kĕn-bĕrgz). [Frederick Krukenberg, Ger. pathologist, 1871–1946] A malignant tumor of the ovary, usually bilateral and frequently secondary to malignancy of the gastrointestinal tract. Histologically, these tumors consist of myxomatous connective tissue and cells having a signet ring arrangement of their nuclei. The epithelial tissue resembles malignancy of the original site.

krypton (krĭp′tŏn) [Gr. *kryptos,* hidden]. SYMB: Kr. At. wt. 83.80; at. no. 36. A gaseous element found in small amounts in the atmosphere.

K_2SO_4. Potassium sulfate.

KUB. *kidney, ureter, bladder.* Used in reference to x-ray study of the abdomen.

kubisagari (koo-bĭs″ă-gă′rē) [Japanese, hanghead]. A form of paralytic vertigo endemic in Japan.

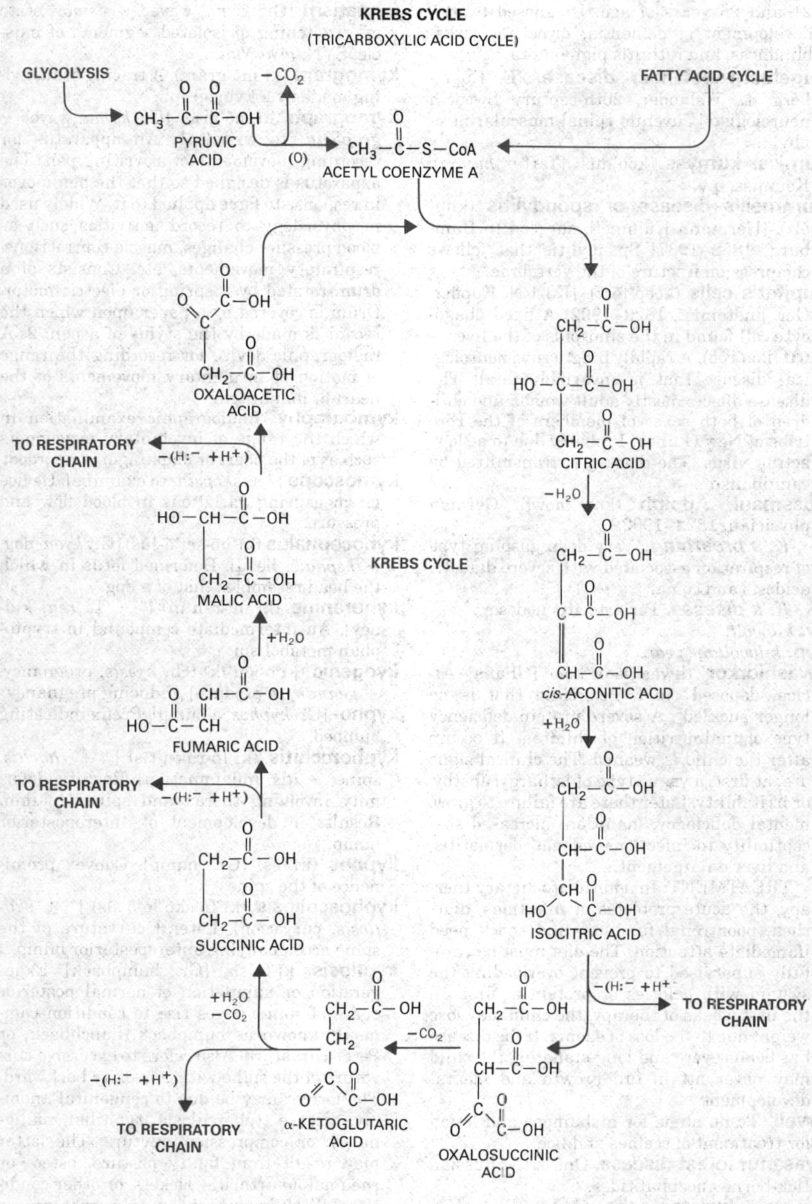
KREBS CYCLE
(TRICARBOXYLIC ACID CYCLE)
GLYCOLYSIS
FATTY ACID CYCLE
PYRUVIC ACID
ACETYL COENZYME A
OXALOACETIC ACID
CITRIC ACID
TO RESPIRATORY CHAIN
KREBS CYCLE
MALIC ACID
cis-ACONITIC ACID
FUMARIC ACID
TO RESPIRATORY CHAIN
SUCCINIC ACID
ISOCITRIC ACID
TO RESPIRATORY CHAIN
α-KETOGLUTARIC ACID
OXALOSUCCINIC ACID
TO RESPIRATORY CHAIN

Kufs' disease. [H. Kufs, Ger. psychiatrist, 1871–1955] Adult form of cerebral sphingolipidosis, q.v. Onset of symptoms is between 21 and 26 years of age. Diagnosed by the development of dementia, myoclonic jerks, blindness, and retinitis pigmentosa.

Kugelberg-Welander disease. [E. Kugelberg, L. Welander, 20th-century Swedish neurologists] Juvenile spinal muscular atrophy.

kumiss, kumyss (koo'mĭs) [Tartar *kumyz*]. Koumiss, q.v.

Kümmell's disease or spondylitis (kĭm'ĕlz). [Hermann Kümmell, surgeon in Hamburg, 1852–1937] Spondylitis that follows compression fracture of the vertebrae.

Kupffer's cells (koop'fĕrz). [Karl N. Kupffer, Ger. anatomist, 1829–1902] A fixed phagocyte cell found in the sinusoids of the liver.

kuru (koo'roo). A rapidly progressive neurological disease that is invariably fatal. The disease affects mostly adult women and children of both sexes of members of the Fore tribe of New Guinea. Probably due to a slow-acting virus. The disease is transmitted by cannibalism.

Kussmaul, Adolph (koos'mowl). German physician, 1822–1902.

K.'s breathing. Very deep gasping type of respiration associated with severe diabetic acidosis and coma.

K.'s disease. Periarteritis nodosa.

kv. *kilovolt.*

kvp. *kilovoltage peak.*

kwashiorkor (kwăsh-ē-or'kor) [Ghana, Africa, deposed child, i.e., child that is no longer suckled]. A severe protein-deficiency type of malnutrition of children. It occurs after the child is weaned. The clinical signs are, at first, a vague type of lethargy, apathy, or irritability. Later there are failure to grow, mental deficiency, inanition, increased susceptibility to infections, edema, dermatitis, and liver enlargement.

TREATMENT: In addition to dietary therapy, the acute problems of infections, diarrhea, poor renal function, and shock need immediate attention. The diet must be carefully supervised to prevent overloading the system with calories or protein at first. In the first weeks of therapy, the child may lose weight due to the loss of edema. If the disease has been severe and long-standing, the child may never attain full growth and mental development.

Kwell. Trade name for a shampoo and lotion for treatment of scabies and lice.

kyasanur forest disease. One of the Russian tick-borne encephalitides.

kyestein, kyesthein (kī-ĕs'tē-ĭn, -thē-ĭn) [Gr. *kyesis*, pregnancy]. A scum or film on stale urine; formerly thought to be a sign of pregnancy.

kyllosis (kĭl-lō'sĭs) [Gr., crippling]. Clubfoot. SEE: *talipes.*

kymatism [Gr. *kyma*, wave, + *-ismos*, state of]. Twitching of isolated segments of muscle. SYN: *myokymia.*

kymogram (kī'mō-grăm). A tracing or recording made by a kymograph.

kymograph (kī'mō-grăf) [Gr. *kyma*, wave, + *graphein*, to write]. 1. An apparatus for recording movements of a writing pen. The apparatus is designed so that the pen moves in response to force applied to it. Widely used in physiology to record activities such as blood pressure changes, muscle contractions, respiratory movements, etc. Consists of a drum rotated by a spring or electric motor. Drum is covered by a paper upon which the record is made by the stylus of a pen. 2. A radiographic device for recording the range of motion of involuntary movements of the heart or diaphragm.

kymography. Radiographic examination in which the range of involuntary movements such as of the heart or diaphragm is recorded.

kymoscope [" + *skopein*, to examine]. Device for measuring variations in blood flow and pressure.

kynocephalus (kī"nō-sĕf'ă-lŭs) [Gr. *kyon*, dog, + *kephale*, head]. Deformed fetus in which the head resembles that of a dog.

kynurenine (kī"nū-rĕn'ĭn) [" + L. *ren*, kidney]. An intermediate compound in tryptophan metabolism.

kyogenic (kī"ō-jĕn'ĭk) [Gr. *kyesis*, pregnancy, + *gennan*, to produce]. Inducing pregnancy.

kypho- [Gr. *kyphos*, a hump]. Prefix indicating humped.

kyphorachitis (kī"fō-răk-ī'tĭs) [" + *rhachis*, spine, + *itis*, inflammation]. Rachitic deformity involving thorax and spinal column. Results in development of anteroposterior hump.

kyphos (kī'fŏs) [Gr., hump]. Convex prominence of the spine.

kyphoscoliosis (kī"fō-skō"lē-ō'sĭs) [" + *skoliosis*, curvation]. Lateral curvature of the spine accompanying anteroposterior hump.

kyphosis (kī-fō'sĭs) [Gr., humpback]. Exaggeration or angulation of normal posterior curve of spine. Gives rise to condition commonly known as humpback, hunchback, or Pott's curvature. Also refers to excessive curvature of the spine with convexity backward. The former may be due to congenital anomaly, disease (tuberculosis, syphilis), malignancy, or compression fracture. The latter may result from faulty posture, osteo- or rheumatoid arthritis, rickets, or other conditions. SYN: *humpback; spinal curvature.*

kyphotic (kī-fŏt'ĭk). Affected by or pert. to kyphosis.

kyrtorrhachic (kĭr″tō-răk′ĭk) [Gr. *kyrtos,* curved, + *rhachis,* spine]. Spinal curvature with posterior concavity.

kysthitis (kĭs-thī′tĭs) [Gr. *kysthos,* vagina, + *itis,* inflammation]. Inflammation of the vagina. SYN: *colpitis; vaginitis.*

kysthoptosis (kĭs-thŏp-tō′sĭs) [″ + *ptosis,* a falling]. Prolapse of the vagina.

kyto- [Gr. *kytos,* cell]. Prefix denoting a cell. SEE: words beginning with *cyto-*.

L

Λ, λ. In the Greek alphabet, symbol for lambda.

L., l. *Lactobacillus; Latin; left; left eye; length; lethal; light sense; liter.*

L_+. Symb. for limes tod.

L_0. Symb. for limes nul.

L-. In chemistry, a symbol used as a prefix. Written as a small capital letter to indicate the structure of certain organic compounds with asymmetric carbon atoms. If the asymmetric carbon atom is represented as

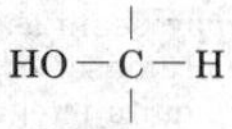

the name of the compound is preceded by L-. If it is represented as

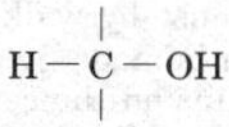

its name would be preceded by D-.

If an L-form compound that has an asymmetric carbon is also capable of rotating light and does so levorotatory, its name is preceded by L(−) and if dextrorotatory preceded by L(+). If the asymmetric carbon is of the D-form and it rotates light dextrorotatory, its name is preceded by D(+) and if levorotatory preceded by D(−).

In chemical nomenclature, a small letter *l*- or *d*- indicates the direction of rotation of polarized light shown through a solution of the compound. When the plane of the light is rotated to the left (levorotatory), the compound's name is preceded by *l*-. If the light is rotated to the right (dextrorotatory), the name is preceded by *d*-.

La. Chem. symb. for lanthanum.

lab. 1. German for the enzyme rennin. 2. Colloquial for laboratory.

Labbé's vein (lăb-āz′). [Léon Labbé, Fr. surgeon, 1832–1916] Vein that connects the superficial middle cerebral vein and the transverse sinus of the brain. SYN: *inferior anastomotic vein.*

la belle indifference [Fr., beautiful indifference]. An unrealistic degree of indifference to, or complacency about, startling and gross symptoms of hysterical anesthesia or paralysis. Seen in conversion reaction.

labia (lā′bē-ă) [L.]. Plural of labium.

l. majora. The two folds of cellular adipose tissue lying on either side of the vaginal opening and forming the lateral borders of the vulva. Their medial surfaces unite anteriorly above the clitoris to form the anterior commissure; posteriorly they are connected by a poorly defined posterior commissure. They are separated by a cleft, the rima pudendi, into which the urethra and vagina open. In young girls, their medial surfaces are in contact with each other, concealing the labia minora and vestibule. In older women, the labia minora may protrude between them.

l. minora. Two thin folds of integument that lie just inside the vestibule of the vagina and between the labia majora and the hymen. They enclose the vestibule. Anteriorly each divides into two smaller folds that unite with similar folds from the other side and enclose the clitoris, the more anterior one forming the prepuce (preputium clitoridis) of the clitoris, the posterior one forming the frenulum clitoridis. In younger children, they are entirely hidden by the labia majora.

RS: clitoris; Hottentot apron; mons veneris; nympha; nymphoncus; nymphotomy; smegma; vagina.

labial (lā′bē-ăl) [L. *labialis*]. Pert. to the lips.

labial glands. Many racemose glands between the labial mucosa and orbicularis muscle opening on the lip's inner surface.

labialism (lā′bē-ăl-ĭzm) [″ + Gr. *-ismos,* state of]. Defective speech in which labial sounds are stressed.

LaBID. Trade name for theophylline, USP.

labile (lā′bīl) [L. *labi,* to glide]. Not fixed; unsteady; easily disarranged.

l., heat. Easily altered or decomposed by heat. SYN: *thermolabile.*

lability (lă-bĭl′ĭ-tē). State of being unstable or changeable.

labioalveolar (lā″bē-ō-ăl-vē′ō-lăr) [L. *labium,* lip, + *alveolus,* little hollow]. Pert. to lips and tooth sockets.

labiocervical (lā″bē-ō-sĕr′vĭ-kl) [″ + *cervix,* neck]. Pert. to the buccal surface of the lips and the neck of a tooth.

labiochorea (lā″bē-ō-kō-rē′ă) [″ + Gr. *choreia,* dance]. Spasm of the lips in chorea. This causes stammering.

labioclination (lā″bē-ō-klī-nā′shŭn) [″ + Gr. *klinein,* to slope]. In dentistry, deviation of a tooth from the normal vertical toward the labial side.

labiodental (lā″bē-ō-dĕn′tăl) [″ + *dens,* tooth]. 1. Concerning the lips and the teeth, esp. the labial surface of a tooth. 2. Referring to the pronunciation of certain letters that require interaction of the teeth and the lips.

labiogingival (lā″bē-ō-jĭn′jĭ-văl) [″ + *gingiva,* gum]. Concerning the lips and the gums or referring to the labial and gingival surfaces of a tooth.

labioglossolaryngeal (lā″bē-ō-glŏs″ō-lăr-ĭn′jē-ăl) [″ + Gr. *glossa,* tongue, + *larynx,* larnyx]. Pert. to lips, tongue, and larynx.

labioglossopharyngeal (lā″bē-ō-glŏs″ō-făr-ĭn′jē-ăl) [″ + ″ + *pharynx,* throat]. Pert. to the lips, tongue, and pharynx.

labiograph (lā′bē-ō-grăf) [″ + Gr. *graphein,* to write]. Device for registering lip movements in speaking.

labiomental (lā″bē-ō-mĕn′tăl) [″ + *mentum,* chin]. Pert. to the lower lip and chin.

labiomycosis (lā″bē-ō-mī-kō′sĭs) [″ + Gr. *mykes,* fungus, + *osis,* condition]. Any disease of the lips due to presence of a fungus.

labionasal (lā″bē-ō-nā′zăl) [″ + *nasus,* nose]. Concerning the nose and the lips.

labiopalatine (lā″bē-ō-păl′ă-tīn) [″ + *palatum,* palate]. Rel. to the lips and palate.

labioplasty (lā′bē-ō-plăs″tē) [″ + Gr. *plassein,* to form]. Plastic surgery of the lips. SYN: *cheiloplasty.*

labiotenaculum (lā″bē-ō-tĕn-ăk′ū-lŭm) [″ + *tenaculum,* a hook]. Instrument for holding lips during an operation.

labioversion (lā″bē-ō-vĕr′zhŭn) [″ + *versio,* a turning]. State of being twisted in a labial direction, esp. a tooth.

labium (lā′bē-ŭm) [L.]. (pl. *labia*) [NA] A lip or a structure like one; an edge or fleshy border.

l. cerebri. Margin of the cerebral hemispheres overlapping the corpus callosum.

l. inferius oris. [NA] Lower lip.

l. majus. SEE: *labia majora.*

l. minus. SEE: *labia minora.*

l. minus pudendi. Nympha, q.v.

l. oris. [NA] The skin and muscular tissue surrounding the mouth; lips of the mouth.

l. superius oris. [NA] The upper lip.

l. tympanicum. Outer edge of organ of Corti.

l. urethrae. Lateral margin of meatus urinarius externus.

l. uteri. Thickened margin of the cervix uteri.

l. vestibulare. Vestibular or inner edge of organ of Corti.

labor [L., work]. The physiological process by which the fetus is expelled from the uterus into the vagina and then to the outside of the body. SYN: *childbirth; parturition.* SEE: illus.

Approx. 95% of normal full-term babies are born 265 to 300 days from the first day of the last menstrual period. Average duration of normal pregnancy is 282 days.

Traditionally labor is divided into three stages, but *lightening* most often occurs a few days up to four weeks prior to onset of labor in primigravidous women. It may occur during labor in a woman who has borne a previous child or children. The shape of the abdomen changes, with the lower portion becoming more pendulous and the costal area looking flatter. This change is due to the presenting part having descended into the pelvis to the level of the ischial spines.

FIRST STAGE (stage of dilatation): Period from the onset of regular contractions of the uterus until the cervix is fully dilated and effaced. Averages 12 hours in primigravidas and eight in multiparas.

Identification of this stage is particularly important to the woman who is having her first baby. Diagnosis is complicated by the fact that many persons experience *false labor pains.* These may begin as early as three to four weeks before onset of true labor. False labor pains are quite irregular, usually confined to the lower part of the abdomen and groin, and do not extend from the back around the abdomen as in true labor. False labor pains do not increase with time and are not made more intense by walking. The conclusive distinction is made by determining the effect of the pains on the cervix. False labor pains do not cause effacement and dilatation of the cervix as do true labor pains. SEE: *Braxton Hicks sign.*

A reliable sign of impending labor is *show.* The appearance of a slight amount of vaginal blood-tinged mucus is a good indication that labor will begin within the next 24 hours. Loss of more than a few milliliters of blood at this time must be regarded as being due to a pathological process. SEE: *placenta previa.*

SECOND STAGE (stage of expulsion): Period from complete dilatation of the cervix through the birth of the fetus. Averages 50 minutes' duration in primigravidas and 20 minutes in multigravidas. Labor pains are severe, occur at two- or three-minute intervals, and last from a little less than one minute to a little more than a minute and a half.

Rupture of the membranes (bag of waters) usually occurs during the early part of this stage, accompanied by a gush of amniotic fluid from the vagina. The muscles of the abdomen contract involuntarily during this portion of labor. The patient directs all her strength to *bearing down* during the pains. She may be quite flushed during the pains and perspire. As labor continues the perineum bulges and, in a head presentation, the scalp of the fetus appears through the vulvar opening. With cessation of each pain the fetus recedes from its position and then advances a little more when the pains return. This continues until more of the head is visible and the vulvar ring encircles the head. This is called *crowning.*

At this time the decision is made concerning an incision in the perineum, i.e., episiotomy, to facilitate delivery. If done, it is most

SEQUENCE OF LABOR AND CHILDBIRTH

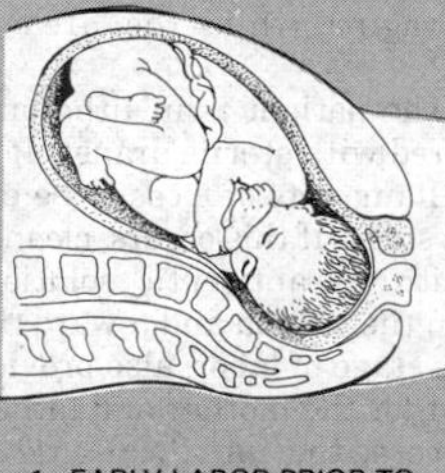

1. EARLY LABOR PRIOR TO BREAKING OF BAG OF WATERS (RUPTURE OF MEMBRANES)

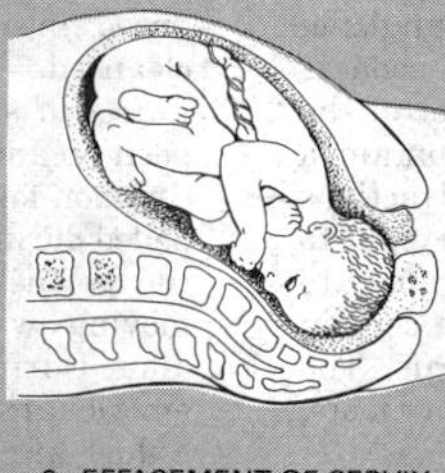

2. EFFACEMENT OF CERVIX

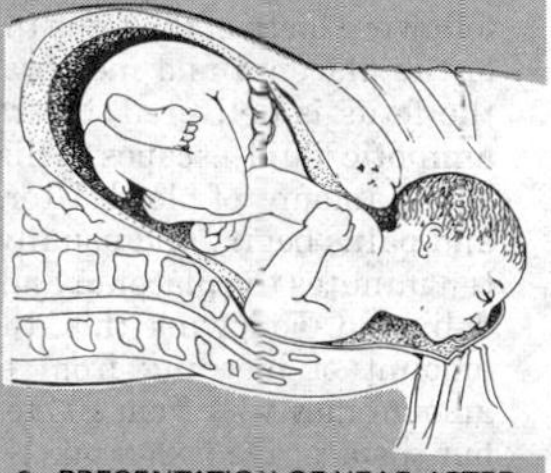

3. PRESENTATION OF HEAD AFTER RUPTURE OF MEMBRANES

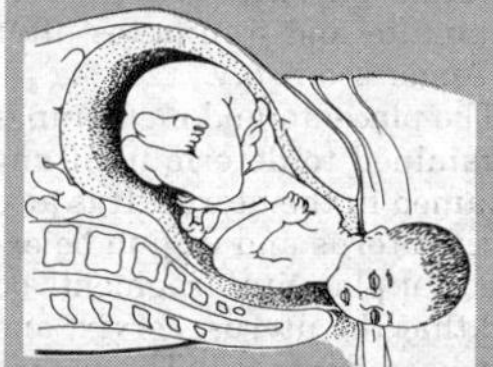

4. BEGINNING OF DELIVERY OF THE HEAD

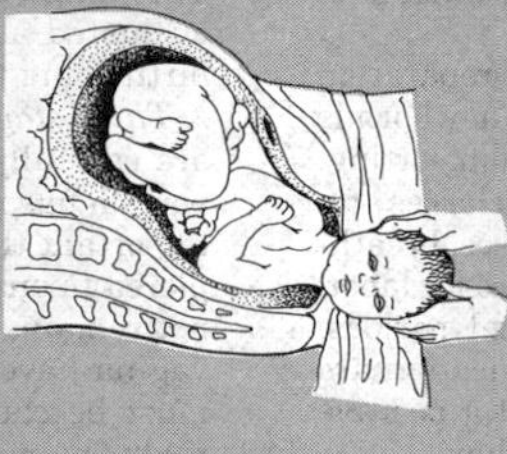

5. ROTATION AND DELIVERY OF HEAD

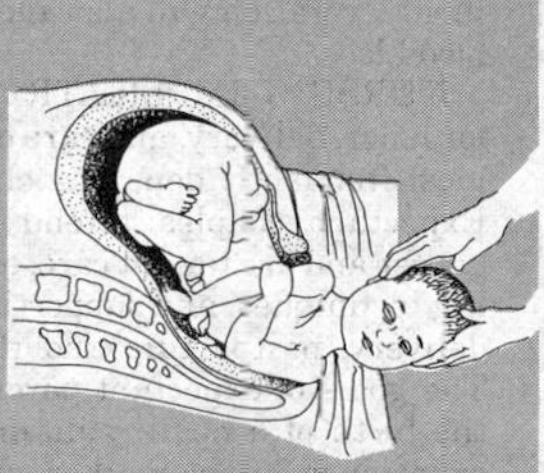

6. DELIVERY OF SHOULDER

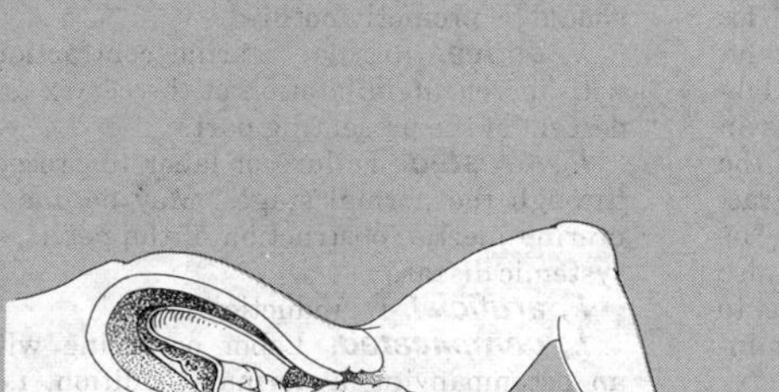

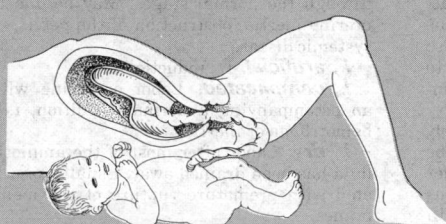

7. INFANT HAS BEEN DELIVERED AND UTERUS BEGINS TO CONTRACT FOR DELIVERY OF PLACENTA

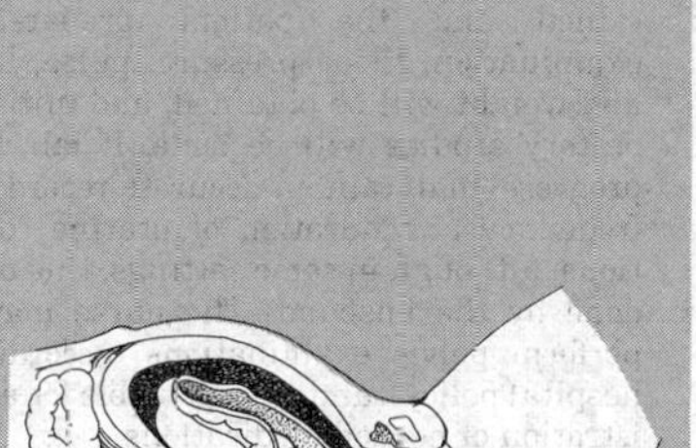

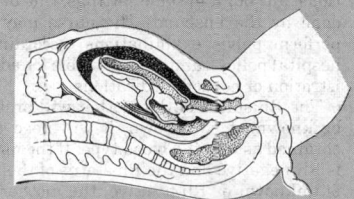

8. UMBILICAL CORD HAS BEEN CUT, PLACENTA IS SEPARATING FROM UTERUS AND WILL ALSO BE DELIVERED

commonly a midline posterior episiotomy. When the head is completely removed from the vagina it falls posteriorly; later the head rotates as the shoulders turn to come through the pelvis. There is a gush of amniotic fluid as the shoulders are delivered.

THIRD STAGE (placental stage): Period following birth of the fetus through expulsion of the placenta and membranes. As soon as the fetus is delivered, the remainder of the amniotic fluid escapes. This will contain a small amount of blood. Uterine contractions and pains begin, and usually within eight to ten minutes the placenta and membranes are delivered. Following this, there is a certain amount of bleeding from the uterus. The amount may vary from 100 to 500 ml. or more, but the average is 200 ml.

Amount of blood loss will vary directly with the size of the fetus. The probability that blood loss will exceed 500 ml. is less than 5% if the fetus weighs 5 pounds (2268 gm.) or less. The chances that blood loss will exceed 500 ml. is 25% if the fetus weighs more than 9 lb. (4082 gm.) Other factors such as episiotomy or perineal laceration will also affect the amount of blood loss.

NURSING IMPLICATIONS: Preparation for labor, delivery, and care of the newborn is most frequently done in a classroom setting. Expectant couples attend the classes together and are taught care, exercises, breathing techniques, and supportive care for labor, delivery, postpartum and neonatal periods. The goals of expectant parent education are the birth of a healthy infant and a positive experience for the mother and father.

Upon the patient's admission to the hospital, or at home, the medical, surgical, obstetrical, and gynecologic history will be obtained and the patient prepared for examination. Blood pressure, pulse, height, and weight will be obtained, and initial laboratory studies will be done. If labor is in progress, maintain an accurate record of the frequency and duration of uterine contractions, although in some settings, this may be done by the husband. The nurse may also perform pelvic examinations (according to hospital policy), and is responsible for administration of needed medications.

The Rh status of the mother will probably be known; if not known, it will need to be obtained as will the blood type. If the mother is Rh-negative and the Rh status of the fetus is unknown or Rh-positive, the mother will be given Rh immune globulin. This should be done within 72 hours after delivery.

First stage: In the past, it has been customary to shave the perineum, thighs, and lower abdominal area in preparation for delivery. This may or may not be done, in accordance with hospital and physician practice. The patient should be asked to urinate and have a bowel movement. If she is unable to void, and if the bladder is distended, catheterization is indicated. When labor begins, the perineal area is thoroughly cleansed. The introitus is covered to prevent water from being introduced into the vagina while the area is cleansed.

Second stage: The patient is in lithotomy position and covered with sterile drapes. It is common for small amounts of feces to be expelled during this stage. If this occurs, cleanse the perineum with an antiseptic solution, moving away from the vagina and toward the anus. During this stage of labor, also provide emotional support for the mother and father.

Just after delivery, the umbilical cord is clamped using a disposable clamp, and the cord is cut. The cord clamp may be left in place for two or three days or it may be left on to drop off with the cord stump.

The infant's nose and oropharynx are aspirated. Prophylaxis for gonococcal eye infections using Credé's method should be done. The infant's overall physical condition is evaluated at 1 minute and 5 minutes after birth using the Apgar score, q.v.

Third stage: The placenta and membranes are carefully examined to determine if any portion has remained in the uterus. It is also important that the uterus and vagina be explored to ensure that placental fragments do not remain, and that the uterus, cervix, and vagina have not been damaged. The uterus must be carefully assessed during this period. The nurse uses palpation to assess the fundus, and should massage the fundus as needed to maintain contractions. If the uterus fails to contract, the physician in charge should be promptly notified.

l., active. Regular uterine contractions with increasing dilatation of the cervix and descent of the presenting part.

l., arrested. Failure of labor to proceed through the normal stages. May be due to uterine inertia, obstruction of the pelvis, or systemic disease.

l., artificial. L., induction of.

l., complicated. Labor occurring with an accompanying abnormal condition, i.e., hemorrhage or inertia.

l., dry. Labor after most of the amniotic fluid has been drained away. Usually associated with premature rupture of the membranes.

l., false. Uterine contractions occurring before the onset of actual labor. These contractions eventually subside.

l., induction of. Use of oxytocics or other methods to stimulate uterine contractions prior to the time they normally would occur.

l., instrumental. Labor completed by mechanical means, such as the use of forceps.

l., missed. 1. Labor, false, q.v. 2. True labor pains begin but subside. This may be a sign of a dead fetus or extrauterine pregnancy.

l., normal. Progressive dilatation and effacement of the cervix with descent of the presenting part.

l., precipitate. Labor that lasts less than 2 to 3 hours from onset to delivery.

l., premature. Labor that begins prior to the completion of 37 weeks' gestation. SEE: *gestation*.

l., spontaneous. Labor that is completed without mechanical or operative interference.

l., trial of. Permitting labor to continue long enough to determine if normal birth appears to be possible.

labor, words pert. to: abortion; "amni-" words; afterbirth; afterpains; ante partum; axis traction; bag of waters; ballottement; bipara; biparous; bradytocia; breech presentation; bruit, placental; caput succedaneum; caul; cephalhematoma; cephalic version; cephalotomy; cesarean section; cesarotomy; cleidotomy; conception; conjugate; Credé's method; cross birth; delivery; disengagement; dystocia; ecbolic; eclampsia; embryectomy; embryo; embryoctony; embryotocia; eutocia; fetus; gestation; Hegar's sign; herpes; hourglass contraction; hydramnion; impetigo herpetiformis; Lamaze technique or method; Leboyer method; maneuver; midwife; multipara; nullipara; nurse-midwife; obstetrician; obstetrics; ophthalmia neonatorum; oxytocic principle; oxytocin; parturient; parturifacient; partus; placenta; placenta previa; postpartum; presentation, brow; primipara; puerpera; puerperal; puerperium; quintuplet; restitution; Rh; show; twins; uterus.

laboratory (lăb′ră-tor″ē) [L. *laboratorium*]. A room or building equipped for scientific experimentation, research, testing, or clinical studies of materials, fluids, or tissues obtained from patients.

Laborde's method (lă-bordz′). [Jean B. V. Laborde, Fr. physician, 1830–1903] Stimulation of the respiratory center in asphyxiation by a series of rhythmical traction movements upon the tongue.

labret (lā′brĕt) [L. *labrum,* lip]. A distinctive plug of ivory, bone, stone, or bottle top worn by some primitive people in a hole artificially produced in the lips of adolescent boys.

labrocyte (lăb′rō-sīt) [Gr. *labros,* greedy, + *kytos,* cell]. A mast cell.

labrum (lā′brŭm) [L., lip]. (pl. *labra*) 1. Lip or liplike structure. 2. The upper lip of an insect.

LABYRINTH OF INNER EAR

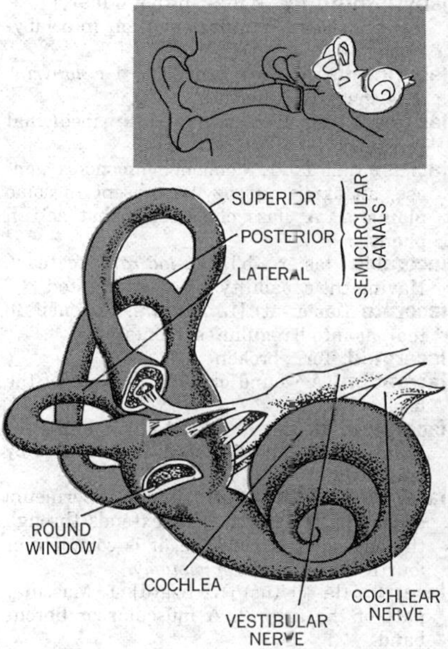

labyrinth (lăb′ĭ-rĭnth) [Gr. *labyrinthos,* maze]. 1. Intricate communicating passages. 2. The internal ear consisting of osseous and membranous labyrinths. These structures are essential to maintaining physical equilibrium of the body. SEE: illus.

l., bony. L., osseous.

l., ethmoidal. The lateral mass of the ethmoid bone. Includes the superior and middle conchae and encloses the ethmoidal air cells. SYN: *l., olfactory.*

l., membranous. Structure in osseous labyrinth consisting of utricle and saccule of vestibule, three semicircular ducts, and the cochlear duct. All are filled with endolymph.

l., olfactory. L., ethmoidal.

l., osseous. Consists of vestibule, three semicircular canals, and cochlea. Channeled out of the petrous portion of the temporal bone. SYN: *l., bony.*

labyrinthectomy (lăb-ĭ-rĭn-thĕk′tō-mē) [″ + *ektome,* excision]. Excision of the labyrinth.

labyrinthine (lăb-ĭ-rĭn′thĭn) 1. Pert. to a labyrinth. 2. Intricate or involved, as a labyrinth.

labyrinthitis (lăb″ĭ-rĭn-thī′tĭs) [″ + *itis,* inflammation]. Inflammation (acute or chronic) of labyrinth; otitis externa. SEE: *Ménière's disease.*

ETIOL: Primary infection; complication of influenza, otitis media, or meningitis.

SYM: Vertigo, vomiting, nystagmus.

labyrinthotomy (lăb″ĭ-rĭn-thŏt′ō-mē) [″ + *tome,* incision]. Surgical incision into labyrinth.

labyrinthus (lăb″ĭ-rĭn′thŭs) [L., Gr. *labyrinthos,* maze]. A labyrinth.

lac (lăk) [L.]. 1. Milk. 2. Milky medicinal substance.

laccase (lăk′ās). 1. Monophenol mono-oxygenase, an oxidizing enzyme present in some plants. 2. A class of oxidases that act on phenols.

lacerable (lăs′ĕr-ă-b′l) [L. *lacerare,* to tear]. Having the capability of being lacerated.

lacerate (lăs′ĕr-āt) [L. *lacerare,* to tear]. To tear, as into irregular segments.

lacerated. Torn; broken.

laceration. A wound or irregular tear of the flesh.

laceration of cervix. Bilateral, stellate, or unilateral tear of the cervix uteri caused by childbirth.

laceration of perineum. Injury of perineum caused by childbirth. If it extends through the sphincter ani muscle, it is complete or fourth degree. SEE: *episiotomy.*

lacertus (lă-sĕr′tŭs) [L., lizard]. 1. Muscular part of the arm. 2. A muscular or fibrous band.

l. cordis. A muscular tissue band on the inner cardiac surface. SYN: *trabeculae carneae cordis* [NA].

l. fibrosus. Aponeurotic band from the biceps tendon to the bicipital or semilunar fascia of forearm.

laciniate (lă-sĭn′ē-āt) [L. *lacinia,* fringe]. Being jagged or fringed.

lacrima (lăk′rĭ-mă) [L.]. Tear.

lacrimal (lăk′rĭm-ăl) [L. *lacrima,* tear]. Pert. to the tears.

lacrimal apparatus. Structures concerned with secretion and conduction of tears. Includes lacrimal gland and its excretory ducts, lacrimal canaliculi, lacrimal sac, and nasolacrimal duct, which empties into the nasal cavity. SEE: illus.

The patency of the lacrimal duct may be tested by placing a dilute solution of sugar in the conjunctival sac; if the duct is patent, the individual will report the sensation of sweetness in the mouth; if not, the sugar will not be perceived.

lacrimal bone. Bone at inner side of the orbital cavity.

lacrimal duct. One of two ducts (superior and inferior) that conveys tears from the lacrimal lake to the lacrimal sac.

lacrimal gland. Gland that secretes tears. A tubuloalveolar gland located in orbit, superior and lateral to the eyeball. Consists of a large superior portion (pars orbitalis) and a smaller inferior portion (pars palpebralis).

LACRIMAL APPARATUS

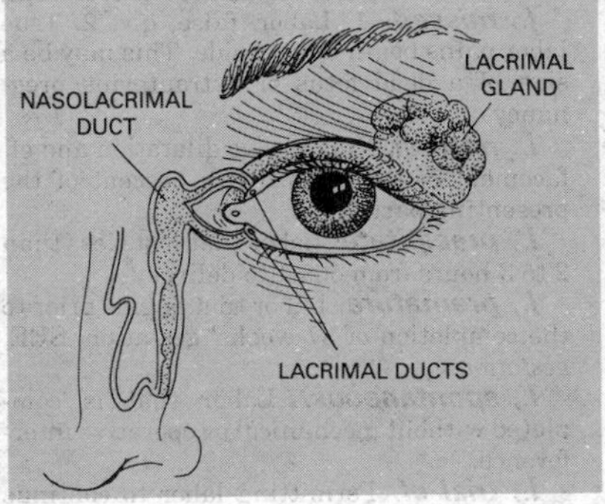

lacrimal reflex. Secretion of fluid resulting from irritation of corneal conjunctiva.

lacrimal sac. Upper dilated portion of nasolacrimal duct situated in groove of lacrimal bone. The upper part is behind the internal tarsal ligament. Measures 12 to 15 mm. in length.

lacrimation [L. *lacrima,* tear]. Secretion and discharge of tears.

lacrimator. A substance that increases the flow of tears.

lacrimatory (lăk′rĭ-mă-tō″rē). Causing the production of tears.

lacrimonasal (lăk″rĭ-mō-nā′zăl) [″ + *nasus,* nose]. Concerning the nose and lacrimal apparatus.

lacrimotome (lăk′rĭ-mō-tōm) [″ + Gr. *tome,* incision]. A cutting instrument used for incising the lacrimal sac or duct.

lacrimotomy (lăk″rĭm-ŏt′ō-mē) [″ + Gr. *tome,* incision]. Incision of lacrimal duct.

lactacid. Lactic acid.

lactacidase (lăk-tăs′ĭ-dās) [L. *lac,* milk, + *acidus,* sour, + *-ase,* enzyme]. Enzyme in lactic acid bacteria that causes fermentation of lactic acid.

lactacidemia (lăk-tăs″ĭ-dē′mē-ă) [″ + ″ + Gr. *haima,* blood]. Accumulation of an excess of lactic acid in the blood. This occurs normally following strenuous and prolonged exercise.

lactaciduria (lăkt-ă-sĭd-ū′rē-ă) [″ + ″ + Gr. *ouron,* urine]. Lactic acid excreted in the urine.

lactagogue (lăk′tă-gŏg) [″ + Gr. *agogos,* leading]. Agent that induces secretion of milk. SYN: *galactagogue.*

lactalbumin [″ + *albumen,* coagulated white of egg]. The albumin of milk and cheese; a soluble simple protein. Lactalbumin is present in higher concentration in human milk than in cow's milk. When milk is heated, the lactalbumin coagulates and appears as a film on the surface of the milk.

lactam (lăk'tăm). An organic chemical that contains the —NH—CO group in a ring form. It is formed by the removal of a molecule of water from certain amino acids.

β-lactamase (bā"tă-lăk'tă-mās). One of two enzymes, β-lactamase I, which is penicillinase, or β-lactamase II, which is cephalosporinase.

β-lactamase-resistant antibiotics. Antibiotics that are resistant to the action of β-lactamase. This property makes them effective against microbial organisms that produce β-lactamase.

lactase [" + *-ase,* enzyme]. An intestinal sugar-splitting enzyme converting lactose into dextrose and galactose; found in intestinal juice. SEE: *enzyme; maltase; sucrase; sugar.*

lactate (lăk'tāt). 1. Any salt derived from lactic acid. 2. To secrete milk.

lactate dehydrogenase. Lactic dehydrogenase, q.v.

lactation (lăk-tā'shŭn) [L. *lactatio,* a sucking]. 1. The period of suckling in mammals. 2. The function of secreting milk.

DIET: During this period the mother needs additional calcium to offset her loss of milk; and adequate intake of fluids and protein. Fruits, vegetables, and whole-grain cereal should also be included.

lacteal (lăk'tē-ăl) [L. *lacteus,* of milk]. 1. Pert. to milk. 2. An intestinal lymphatic that takes up chyle and passes it to the lymph circulation and, by way of the thoracic duct, to the blood vascular system. SEE: *lymph.*

lactenin (lăk'tĕn-ĭn). An antistreptococcal factor present in milk.

lactescence (lăk-tĕs'ĕns) [L. *lactescere,* to become milky]. Condition of becoming or resembling milk.

lactic (lăk'tĭk) [L. *lac,* milk]. Pert. to milk.

lactic acid. USP. A mixture of lactic acid, $C_3H_6O_3$, and lactic acid lactate, $C_6H_{10}O_5$, equivalent to a total of not less than 85% and not more than 90%, by weight, of $C_3H_6O_3$. A colorless syrupy liquid formed in milk, sauerkraut, and in certain types of pickles by the fermentation of the sugars by microorganisms. It is also formed during muscular activity by the breakdown of glycogen (glycolysis).

lactic acid fermentation. The production of lactic acid from carbohydrates by the action of various bacteria. Occurs commonly in milk and milk products.

lactic dehydrogenase. ABBR: LDH. An enzyme present in various tissues and serum that is important in catalyzing the oxidation of lactate. In man, LDH is present in several molecular forms called isoenzymes. Some LDH isoenzymes are present in certain tissues to a greater extent than in others. When one of these particular tissues is damaged, an isoenzyme of LDH is released into the blood. In that case, determination of the pattern of LDH isoenzymes in serum may help to identify which tissue has been damaged. SYN: *lactate dehydrogenase.*

lacticemia (lăk-tĭ-sē'mē-ă) [" + Gr. *haima,* blood]. Lactic acid in the blood. SYN: *lactacidemia.*

lactiferous (lăk-tĭf'ĕr-ŭs) [" + *ferre,* to bear]. Secreting and conveying milk.

lactiferous ducts. Ducts of the mammary gland.

lactiferous glands. 1. The mammary glands. 2. Montgomery's glands, consisting of 20 to 24 glands in the areola of the nipples.

lactification (lăk"tĭ-fĭ-kā'shŭn) [" + *facere,* to make]. Lactic acid production.

lactifuge (lăk'tĭ-fūj) [" + *fugare,* to expel]. 1. Stopping milk secretion. 2. Agent stopping milk secretion.

lactigenous (lăk-tĭj'ĕn-ŭs) [" + Gr. *gennan,* to produce]. Producing milk.

lactigerous (lăk-tĭj'ĕr-ŭs) [" + *gerere,* to carry]. Secreting or conveying milk.

lactin [L. *lac,* milk]. Lactose, milk sugar.

lactinated (lăk'tĭ-nāt"ĕd). Containing or prepared with milk sugar.

lactivorous (lăk-tĭv'or-ŭs) [" + *vorare,* to devour]. Living upon milk.

Lactobacillus (lăk-tō-bă-sĭl'ŭs) [" + *bacillus,* little rod]. A genus of bacteria belonging to the family Lactobacillaceae. They are gram-positive, nonmotile, rod-shaped organisms that do not produce spores and are acid resistant. They produce lactic acid from carbohydrates. They are responsible for the souring of milk.

L. acidophilus. An organism that produces lactic acid by fermenting the sugars in milk. Found in milk, feces of infants fed by bottle, and adults. Also present in carious teeth, saliva, and the vagina.

L. bulgaricus. The bacillus found in fermented milk. Milk fermented with this organism is known as Bulgarian milk.

L. casei. A bacillus found in milk and cheese.

L. helveticus. A bacillus found in Swiss cheese.

L. panis. A bacillus occurring in sour dough.

lactobutyrometer (lăk"tō-bū-tĭ-rŏm'ĕ-tĕr) [" + Gr. *boutyron,* butter, + *metron,* measure]. Instrument for estimating the cream content of milk

lactocele (lăk'tō-sēl) [" + Gr. *kele,* hernia]. Cystic tumor of the breast due to occlusion of a milk duct. SYN: *galactocele.*

lactochrome (lăk'tō-krōm) [" + Gr. *chroma,* color]. Riboflavin, q.v.

lactocrit (lăk'tō-krĭt) [" + Gr. *krites,* judge]. Device for determining the fat content of milk.

lactodensimeter (lăk"tō-dĕn-sĭm'ĕ-tĕr) [" + *densus,* thick, + Gr. *metron,* meter]. Lactocrit, q.v.

lactoflavin (lăk'tō-flā"vĭn) [" + *flavus,* yellow]. Riboflavin.

lactogen (lăk'tō-jĕn) [L. *lac,* milk, + Gr. *gennan,* to produce]. Any substance that stimulates the production of milk. SEE: *prolactin.*

lactogenic [" + Gr. *gennan,* to produce]. Inducing the secretion of milk.

lactogenic hormone. Prolactin.

lactoglobulin (lăk"tō-glŏb'ū-lĭn) [" + *globulus,* globule]. A protein found in milk.

l.'s, immune. Antibodies present in the colostrum.

lactolase (lăk'tō-lās) [" + *-ase,* enzyme]. An enzyme forming lactic acid. SYN: *lactacidase.*

lactometer (lăk-tŏm'ĕ-tĕr) [" + Gr. *metron,* measure]. Device for determining the specific gravity of milk.

lactone (lăk'tōn). An organic anhydride formed by the elimination of a molecule of water from an oxyacid.

lacto-ovovegetarian (lăk"tō-ō"vō-vĕj"ĕ-tā'rē-ăn). A person who is a vegetarian but also utilizes eggs and dairy products in his or her diet.

lactophosphate (lăk"tō-fŏs'fāt) [" + *phosphas,* phosphate]. A salt derived jointly from lactic and phosphoric acid.

lactoprotein (lăk"tō-prō'tē-ĭn) [" + Gr. *protos,* first]. Any protein present in milk.

lactorrhea (lăk-tō-rē'ă) [" + Gr. *rhoia,* flow]. Discharge of milk between nursings and after weaning of offspring. SYN: *galactorrhea.*

lactoscope (lăk'tō-skōp) [" + Gr. *skopein,* to examine]. Device for determining amount of cream in milk.

lactose. USP. $C_{12}H_{22}O_{11}$ + H_2O. 1. A disaccharide that on hydrolysis yields glucose and galactose. Bacteria can convert it into lactic and butyric acids, as in the souring of milk. The milk of mammals contains 4 to 7% lactose. Its presence in the urine may be indicative of obstruction to flow of milk after cessation of nursing. Commercially, a fine powdered, white substance that will not dissolve in cold water. 2. USP. A sugar, $C_{11}H_{22}O_{11}$, obtained from evaporation of cow's milk. Used, in manufacturing tablets, as a diluent, and in making capsules.

lactose intolerance. Intolerance to milk characterized by gastrointestinal symptoms.

ETIOL: Deficiency of the enzyme lactase, which is essential to the absorption of lactose from the intestinal tract. The deficiency may be present in the newborn or it may be acquired as an adult.

TREATMENT: Avoid foods that contain lactose.

lactoserum (lăk-tō-sēr'ŭm) [" + *serum,* whey]. Blood serum of an animal inoculated with milk; used to precipitate specific caseins from milk.

lactosuria (lăk-tō-sū'rē-ă) [" + Gr. *ouron,* urine]. Occurrence of milk sugar (lactose) in the urine. Frequent during pregnancy and lactation.

lactotherapy (lăk-tō-thĕr'ă-pē) [" + Gr. *therapeia,* therapy]. 1. Treatment with milk diet. 2. Medicinal treatment of nursing infant with drugs given to mother to be excreted in milk. SYN: *galactotherapy.*

lactotoxin (lăk"tō-tŏks'ĭn) [" + Gr. *toxikon,* poison]. Any toxic substance occurring in milk that has decomposed.

lactotrophin (lăk"tō-trō'fĭn) [" + Gr. *trephein,* to nourish]. Prolactin, q.v.

lactovegetarian. 1. Pert. to milk and vegetables. 2. One who lives on a diet of milk and dairy products and vegetables.

lactulose. A synthetic disaccharide, β-1, 4-galactosido-fructose, that is not hydrolyzed or absorbed in man. It is metabolized by bacteria in the colon with the production of organic acids. Used in treating the encephalopathy that develops in patients with advanced cirrhosis of the liver. The unabsorbed sugar produces diarrhea and the acid pH helps to contain ammonia in the feces. Trade names are Cephulac and Chronulac.

lacuna (lă-kū'nă) [L., a pit]. (pl. *lacunae*) [NA] 1. A small hollow space, such as that found in bones, in which lie the osteoblasts. 2. A gap or hiatus found in cartilage or bone in which lie cartilage or bone cells.

l., absorption. L., Howship's.

l., blood. L., trophoblastic.

l., bone. One of the isolated ovoid spaces between osseous lamellae, connected by canaliculi, containing a protoplasmic body or bone cell.

l., Howship's. A pit or groove in bone where resorption or dissolution of bone is occurring. Usually containing osteoclasts. SYN: *l., absorption.*

l., intervillous. A space in the placenta occupied by maternal blood and into which fetal placenta villi project.

l. laterales. Irregular diverticula on either side of the superior sagittal sinus of the brain into which the arachnoidal granulations project.

l. magna. The largest pitlike recess in the fossa navicularis of the distal end of the male urethra.

l. of the urethra. One of several recesses in the mucous membrane of the urethra, esp.

along the floor and in the bulb. They compose the openings of the urethral glands.

l. pharyngis. Pit at pharyngeal end of the eustachian tube.

l., trophoblastic. Irregular cavities in the syntrophoblast that develop into intervillous spaces or lacunae. SYN: *l., blood.* SEE: *l., intervillous.*

l. vasorum. [NA] Space for passage of femoral vessels to the thigh.

l., venous. Endothelial lined spaces in the dura mater that communicate with the meningeal veins and blood sinuses, esp. the superior sagittal sinus.

lacunae (lă-kū'nē) [L.]. Pl. of lacuna.

lacunar (lă-kū'năr) [L. *lacuna,* pit]. Pert. to lacunae.

lacunes (lă-kūnz'). Small, irregularly jagged cavities in the brain ranging in size from 0.5 to 15 mm. in diameter. They are believed to be small, deep, cerebral infarcts. Principal locations are the lenticular nucleus, pons, thalamus, caudate nucleus, internal capsule, and corona radiata. They are absent from the cerebral and cerebellar cortex. Although they are important in explaining cerebral pathology, they are not completely understood.

lacunula (lă-kū'nū-lă) [L., little pit]. Small or minute lacuna.

lacunule (lă-kū'nūl) [L. *lacunula*]. A small lacuna.

lacus (lā'kŭs) [L., lake]. Collection of fluid in small hollow or cavity.

l. lacrimalis. [NA] Space at the inner canthus of the eye where tears collect.

Laënnec's cirrhosis (lā"ĕ-nĕks'). [René T. H. Laënnec, Fr. physician and the inventor of the stethoscope, 1781–1826] Cirrhosis of the liver associated with chronic excessive alcohol ingestion. SYN: *hobnail liver.* SEE: *liver, cirrhosis of.*

Laënnec's pearls. Round gelatinous masses seen in asthmatic sputum.

Laënnec's thrombus. Globular thrombus in the heart.

Laetrile. In the U.S., amygdalin. Amygdalin is a glycoside derived from pits or other seed parts of plants, including apricots and almonds. Amygdalin contains sufficient cyanide to be fatal when taken in large doses. Laetrile, also known as vitamin B-17, has no known therapeutic or nutritional value. SYN: *amygdalin.*

There is no evidence that Laetrile is effective in treating cancer.

CAUTION: Those who administer Laetrile should be prepared to treat acute cyanide poisoning. Signs of chronic cyanide poisoning (weakness of arms and legs and disorders of the central nervous system) should also be kept in mind.

Lafora, Gonzalo R. (lă-fō'ră). Spanish physician, born in 1887.

L.'s bodies. Cytoplasmic inclusion bodies, made of acid mucopolysaccharides, present in neuronal tissue of the brain in familial myoclonus epilepsy.

L.'s disease. Familial progressive epilepsy.

lag. 1. Period of time between application of stimulus and resulting reaction. 2. Early period following bacterial inoculation into culture medium. Growth is slow during this time. SYN: *lag phase; latent period.*

lageniform (lă-jĕn'ĭ-form) [L. *lagena,* flask, + *forma,* shape]. Flask-shaped.

lagophthalmos, lagophthalmus (lăg"ŏf-thăl'mŏs, -mŭs) [Gr. *lagos,* hare, + *ophthalmos,* eye]. Incomplete closure of palpebral fissure when an attempt is made to shut the eyelids. This results in exposure and injury to bulbar conjunctiva and cornea.

ETIOL: Contraction of a scar of the eyelid, facial nerve injury, atony of orbicularis palpebrarum, exophthalmos. Incomplete closure of the lids during sleep is seen in hysteria, in exhausted adults, and often in healthy children.

lag phase. Latent period (def. 2), q.v.; lag (def. 2), q.v.

la grippe (lă grĭp') [Fr.]. Influenza.

laity (lā'ĭ-tē) [Gr. *laos,* the people]. 1. The collective of individuals not in the clergy. 2. Individuals who are not members of a particular profession such as law, medicine, or the ministry.

lake [L. *lacus*]. A small cavity of fluid. SEE: *lacus.*

laked. Said of the blood in hemolysis, q.v., or disintegration of the red blood corpuscles, freeing the hemoglobin into the blood plasma.

laking. Freeing of hemoglobin from red blood corpuscles.

La Leche League. An organization whose purpose is to promote breast feeding. The address is Franklin Park, Illinois 60131, U.S.A.

laliatry (lăl-ī'ă-trē) [Gr. *lalia,* talk, + *iatria,* therapy]. Study and treatment of speech disorders and defects.

lallation (lă-lā'shŭn) [L. *lallatio*]. A babbling form of stammering. Infantile form of speech.

lalognosis (lăl-ŏg-nō'sĭs) [Gr. *lalia,* talk, + *gnosis,* understanding]. Science of understanding speech, particularly lallation.

lalopathology (lăl"ō-pă-thŏl'ō-jē) [" + *pathos,* disease, + *logos,* study]. The medical area that is concerned with speech pathology.

lalopathy (lă-lŏp'ă-thē) [" + *pathos,* disease]. Any disorder of the speech.

lalophobia (lăl"ō-fō'bē-ă) [" + *phobos,* fear]. Morbid reluctance to speak due to fear of stammering or committing errors.

laloplegia (lăl-ō-plē'jē-ă) [" + *plege,* a stroke].

A paralysis of speech muscles without affecting action of tongue.

lalorrhea (lăl″ō-rē′ă) [″ + *rhoia,* flow]. Abnormal flow of speech.

Lamarck's theory (lă-mărks′). [Jean Baptiste P. A. Lamarck, Fr. naturalist, 1744–1829] Theory, popular in the 19th century, that evolutionary changes are the result of environmental changes, and that acquired characters are inherited and passed on to descendants. This theory has been rejected. SEE: *natural selection.*

Lamaze technique or method (lă-măz′). [Fernand Lamaze, contemporary Fr. obstetrician] A method of psychoprophylaxis for childbirth in which the mother is instructed in breathing techniques that permit her to facilitate delivery by relaxing at the proper time with respect to the involuntary contractions of abdominal and uterine musculature. Those who are able to use the method require little if any anesthesia during delivery.

lambda (lăm′dă) [Gr.]. 1. Letter in Gr. alphabet (Λ, λ). Also signified by letter L or l. 2. Point or angle of junction of lambdoid and sagittal sutures.

lambdacism (lăm′dă-sĭzm) [Gr. *lambdakismos*]. 1. Stammering of "l" sound. 2. Inability to pronounce "l" sound properly. 3. Substitution of "l" for "r" in speaking.

lambdoid, lambdoidal (lăm′doyd, lăm-doyd′ ăl) [Gr. *lambda,* L, + *eidos,* form]. Shaped like Gr. letter Λ.

lambdoid suture. Suture between the occipital and two parietal bones.

lambert. [Johann H. Lambert, Ger. physicist, 1728–1777] A unit of brightness equal to that seen when a perfectly diffusing surface radiates or reflects one lumen of light per square centimeter. SEE: *lumen* (def. 2).

Lamblia intestinalis (lăm′blē-ă). [Wilhelm D. Lambl, Bohemian physician, 1824–1895] Flagellate protozoan parasite found in intestine. SYN: *Giardia lamblia,* q.v.

lambliasis (lăm-blī′ă-sĭs). Infection with Giardia lamblia. SYN: *giardiasis.*

lame [AS. *lama*]. Disabled in one or more limbs, esp. in a leg or foot, so that ability for normal locomotion is impaired. Also applied to a weak or painful condition as a lame back.

lamella (lă-mĕl′ă) [L., a little plate]. (pl. *lamellae*) 1. A thin plate or scale. 2. A medicated disk of gelatin inserted under lower eyelid and against the eyeball; used as a local application to eye.

l., bone. Thin layer of ground substance of osseous tissue.

l., circumferential. A layer of bone that underlies the periosteum.

l., concentric. Plate of bone surrounding a haversian canal.

l., ground. L., interstitial, q.v.

l., haversian. L., concentric, q.v.

l., interstitial. Bone lamella filling irregular spaces between the haversian system.

l., medullary. The osseous lamella surrounding and forming the wall of the medullary cavity of tubular bones.

l., periosteal. Bone lamella next to and parallel with the periosteum, forming the external portion of bone.

l., triangular. Small fibrous lamina between the choroid plexuses of the third ventricle of the brain.

l., vitreous. Innermost layer of the choroid next to the retina. SYN: *Bruch's membrane; lamina basalis of choroid.*

lamellar (lă-mĕl′ăr). 1. Arranged in thin plates or scales. 2. Pert. to lamella.

lameness. Limping, abnormal gait, or hobbling resulting from partial loss of function in a leg. May be due to maldevelopment, injury, or disease.

lamina (lăm′ĭ-nă) [L.]. (pl. *laminae*) [NA] 1. A thin flat layer or membrane. 2. The flattened part of either side of the arch of a vertebra.

l., alar. Alar plate of the spinal cord in the human embryo; later becomes the sensory portion.

l., anterior elastic. Thin, tough membrane just below the corneal epithelium. SYN: *Bowman's membrane; l., Bowman's.*

l., basal. Basal plate of spinal cord in the human embryo; later becomes the motor portion.

l. basalis of choroid. The membrane covering the inner surface of the choroid. SYN: *Bruch's membrane.*

l. basilaris ductus cochlearis. The membranous portion of the spiral lamina of the cochlea of the inner ear.

l., Bowman's. Basement membrane beneath the epithelium of the cornea. SYN: *l., anterior elastic; Bowman's membrane.*

l. cartilaginis cricoideae. [NA] The posterior portion of the cricoid cartilage.

l. choriocapillaris. [NA] Middle layer of the choroid, containing close mesh of capillaries.

l. cribrosa. [NA] Cribriform plate of the ethmoid bone.

l. cribrosa sclerae. Portion of sclera forming a sievelike plate through which pass fibers of the optic nerve to the retina.

l., dental. An epithelial plate that grows gumward from the labial lamina. From it arise the enamel organs of the future teeth.

l. dura. A radiographic term describing the compact bone (alveolar bone proper) that surrounds the roots of teeth; in a state of health, it appears on a radiograph as a dense radiopaque line.

l., epithelial. The epithelial layer covering the choroid plexus of the eye.

l. fusca sclerae. Layer of thin pigmented connective tissue on the inner surface of the sclera of the eye.

l. ganglionaris. Ganglionic layer of the isocortex, which is the nonolfactory cerebral cortex.

l. granularis externa. External granular layer of the isocortex.

l. granularis interna. The internal granular layer of the isocortex.

l., interpubic fibrocartilaginous. Part of the articulation of the pubic bones; it connects the opposing surfaces of these bones.

l., labial. A thickened band of epithelium that grows from the ectodermal covering of the primitive jaw. The ectodermal plate splits and separates lip from gum.

l., medullary, internal. A layer of white substance that divides the gray substance of the thalamus into three parts: anterior, medial, and lateral.

l. multiformis. Polymorphic layer of the isocortex of the cerebral cortex.

l. of vertebral arch. Laminae of the vertebral arch. They extend from the pedicles of the vertebral arches and fuse together to form the dorsal portion of the arch. The spinous process extends from the center of these laminae.

l. papyracea. A thin, smooth plate of bone on the lateral surface of the ethmoid bone; it forms part of the orbital plate.

l., perpendicular. Thin sheet of bone forming the perpendicular plate of the ethmoid bone. Supports the upper portion of the nasal septum.

l. propria mucosae. A thin layer of fibrous connective tissue that lies immediately beneath the surface epithelium of mucous membranes. SYN: *tunica propria.*

l. pyramidalis. The pyramidal cell layer of the isocortex of the cerebral cortex.

l., rostral. Continuation of the rostrum of the corpus callosum and the lamina terminalis of the third ventricle.

l. spiralis. Lamina that divides the interior of the spiral canal of the cochlea into two scalae and divides into lamina spiralis ossea and lamina spiralis membrana.

l. suprachoroidea. [NA] Outermost layer of the choroid.

l., terminal. Thin sheet of tissue forming the anterior border of the third ventricle.

l. vitrea. L. basalis of choroid.

l. zonalis. The outer or plexiform layer of the isocortex.

laminae (lăm'ĭ-nē). Pl. of lamina.

laminagram (lăm'ĭ-nă-grăm) [L. *lamina,* thin plate, + Gr. *gramma,* writing]. A roentgenogram taken of a section of the body so that the area being investigated appears as if only a slice through the tissue is depicted. SEE: *tomogram.*

laminagraph (lăm'ĭ-nă-grăf) [" + Gr. *graphein,* to write]. An x-ray technique for producing a laminagram, q.v.

laminagraphy (lăm"ĭ-năg'ră-fē) [" + Gr. *graphein,* to write]. Study of body tissues by use of laminagrams. SEE: *tomography.*

laminar air flow. Filtered air moving along separate parallel flow planes to surgical theaters, nurseries, bacteriology work areas, or food preparation areas. This method of air flow helps to prevent bacterial contamination and collection of hazardous chemical fumes in areas where they would pollute the work environment.

Laminaria digitata (lăm-ĭ-năr ē-ă dĭj-ĭ-tā'tă). Genus of kelp or seaweed that when dried has the ability to absorb water and expand with considerable force. Has been used to dilate the uterine cervical canal in induced abortion.

laminarin (lăm"ĭ-nā'rĭn). A polysaccharide obtained from Laminaria species of seaweed. It consists principally of glucose residues.

laminated (lăm'ĭn-āt"ĕd) [L. *lamina,* thin plate]. Arranged in layers or laminae.

lamination (lăm"ĭn-ā'shŭn). 1. Layerlike arrangement. 2. In embryotomy the slicing of the skull.

laminectomy (lăm"ĭ-nĕk'tō-mē) [" + Gr. *ektome,* excision]. The excision of a vertebral posterior arch.

laminitis (lăm-ĭn-ī'tĭs) [" + Gr. *itis,* inflammation]. Inflammation of a lamina.

laminotomy (lăm"ĭ-nŏt'ō-mē) [" + Gr. *tome,* incision]. Division of one of the vertebral laminae.

lamp [Gr. *lampein,* to shine]. Device for producing and applying light, heat, radiation, and various forms of radiant energy for the treatment of disease.

l., Gullstrand's. L., slit, q.v.

l., infrared. Heat lamp; a lamp that develops a high temperature, emitting infrared rays. Rays penetrate only a short distance (5 to 10 mm.) into the skin. Principal effect is to cause heating of the skin.

l., slit. Lamp constructed so that an intense light is emitted through a slit; used for examination of the eye.

l., sun. A light that produces ultraviolet light.

l., ultraviolet. L., sun, q.v.

lamprophonia (lăm"prō-fō'nē-ă) [Gr. *lampros,* clear, + *phone,* voice]. Marked distinctness or clearness of voice.

lamprophonic (lăm"prō-fŏn'ĭk). Possessing a clear voice.

lana (lăn'ă) [L.]. Wool.

lanatoside C (lăn-ăt'ō-sīd). Glycoside of Digitalis lanata; an agent used for digitalization.

Trade name is Cedilanid.

lance (lăns) [L. *lancea*]. 1. Two-edged surgical knife. 2. To incise with a lancet.

Lancefield classification (lăns′fēld). [Rebecca Lancefield, U.S. bacteriologist, b. 1895] A classification of hemolytic streptococci into various groups by antigenic structure.

lancet (lăn′sĕt) [L. *lancea,* lance]. Pointed surgical knife with two edges.

lancinating (lăn′sĭ-nāt″ĭng) [L. *lancinare,* to tear]. Sharp or cutting, as pain.

L and A. The reaction of the pupils of the eye to *light* and *accommodation.*

Landouzy-Dejerine atrophy (lăn-dū-zē′ dĕ″zhĕ-rēn′). [Louis T. J. Landouzy, Fr. physician, 1845–1917; Joseph Jules Dejerine, Fr. neurologist, 1849–1917] Atrophy of muscles of face and scapulohumeral group.

Landry's paralysis (lăn-drēz′). [Jean Baptiste O. Landry, Fr. neurologist, 1826–1865] Acute febrile polyneuritis. A disease of unknown etiology but thought to have an autoimmune basis. Onset is usually preceded by a history of nonspecific febrile illness. From one to three weeks later, signs and symptoms of multiple nerve involvement develop. Characterized by pain; and weakness that is symmetrical and begins in the extremities and ascends to involve the entire limb and may involve the trunk and abdominal and thoracic muscles. The muscles of the head and face may be paralyzed bilaterally. Almost all of the patients have some sensory nerve symptoms but these are usually mild. Recovery after a period varying from several weeks or months is the usual outcome. There is no specific therapy. Usually the spinal fluid contains an increased amount of protein but only rarely will the cells in the fluid be increased.

This disease has been described by various terms: acute polyneuritis with facial diplegia, acute infectious polyneuritis, Guillain-Barré syndrome, and neuritis with albuminocytologic dissociation. All are believed to be the same disease.

NURSING IMPLICATIONS: Assess patient for extent of involvement and paralysis. Note and document swallowing difficulty and signs of respiratory distress. Take appropriate measures if either or both occur. Administer analgesic in accordance with medication orders. Place emergency tracheostomy tray at bedside. Provide passive range of motion exercises three to four times a day to prevent formation of contractures. Maintain fluid and electrolyte balance if swallowing reflex is impaired.

Landsteiner's classification (lănd′stī-nĕrz). [Karl Landsteiner, Austrian-born U.S. biologist, 1868–1943; Nobel prize winner in medicine in 1930] A classification of blood types designating O, A, B, and AB based on the presence of antigens on the erythrocytes.

Lane's kinks. [Sir W. Arbuthnot Lane, Brit. surgeon, 1856–1943] Bending or twisting of the last few centimeters of the ileum with external adhesions between the folded loops of intestines. This may cause intestinal obstruction.

Langerhans' islands (lăng′ĕr-hănz). [Paul Langerhans, Ger. pathologist, 1847–1888] Clusters of cells in the pancreas. They are made up of three types: alpha, beta, and delta cells. The beta cells, which produce insulin, are the predominant type. Destruction or impairment of function of the islands may result in diabetes or hypoglycemia.

Langer's lines (lăng′ĕrz). [Carl Ritter von Langer, Austrian anatomist, 1819–1887] The structural orientation of the fibrous tissue of the skin. They form the natural cleavage lines that, though present in all body areas, are visible only in certain sites such as the creases of the palm. These lines are of particular importance in surgery. Incisions made parallel to them make a much smaller scar upon healing than those made at right angles to the lines. SEE: illus.

Langer's muscle. Muscular fibers from insertion of pectoralis major muscle, over the bicipital groove to the insertion of the latissimus dorsi.

Lange's test (lăng′ĕz). [Carl Lange, Ger. physician, b. 1883] Diagnosis of cerebrospinal syphilis by degree of gold precipitation in varying concentrations of colloidal gold solution and spinal fluid.

Langhans' layer (lăng′hăns). [Theodor Langhans, Ger. pathologist, 1839–1915] A cellular layer present in chorionic villi of the placenta. SYN: *cytotrophoblast.*

languor (lăng′gĕr) [L. *languere,* to languish]. Feeling of weariness or exhaustion as from illness; lack of vigor or animation; lassitude.

laniary (lăn′ē-ā″rē) [L. *laniare,* to tear to pieces]. Adapted or designed for tearing, as are the canine teeth.

lanolin (lăn′ō-lĭn) [L. *lana,* wool]. USP. The purified, fatlike substance obtained from the wool of sheep. Used as an ointment base.

l., anhydrous. USP. Wool fat containing not more than 0.25% water. Used as an ointment base that has the ability to absorb water.

Lanoxin. Trade name for digoxin, USP.

lanthanum (lăn′thă-nŭm). SYMB: La. At. wt. 138.906; at. no. 57. A metallic element. One of a group of elements called lanthanides.

lanuginous (lă-nū′jĭn-ŭs). Covered with lanugo.

lanugo (lă-nū′gō) [L. *lana,* wool]. 1. Downy hair covering the body. 2. Fine downy hairs that cover the body of the fetus, esp. when

LANGER'S LINES

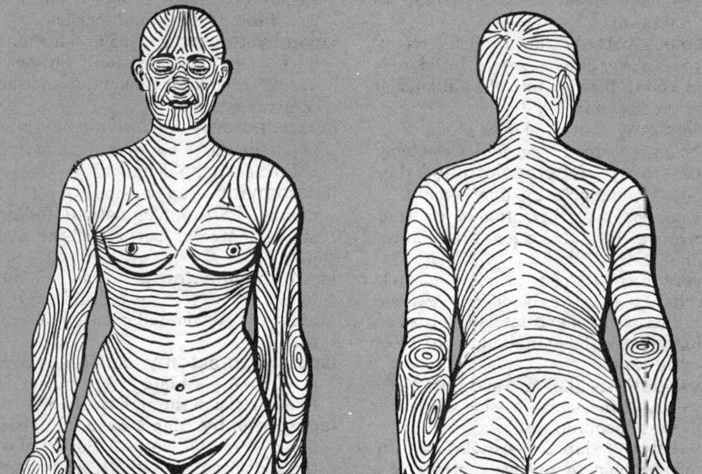

Reproduced with permission from May, *Plastic and Reconstructive Surgery,* third edition. F. A. Davis, Philadelphia, 1971.

premature.

laparectomy (lăp″ă-rĕk′tō-mē) [Gr. *lapara,* loin, + *ektome,* excision]. Excision of strips or gores in abdominal wall to relieve extreme weakness of abdominal muscles.

laparo- [Gr. *lapara,* flank]. Combining form pert. to the flank and to operations through the abdominal wall.

laparocele (lăp′ă-rō-sēl) [″ + *kele,* hernia]. An abdominal hernia.

laparocholecystotomy (lăp″ăr-ō-kōl″ē-sĭs-tŏt′ō-mē) [″ + *chole,* bile, + *kystis,* bladder, + *tome,* incision]. Incision into the gallbladder through the abdominal wall.

laparocolectomy (lăp″ă-rō-kō-lĕk′tō-mē) [″ + *kolon,* colon, + *ektome,* excision]. Colectomy.

laparocolostomy, laparocolotomy (lăp″ăr-ō-kō-lŏs′tō-mē, lăp″ăr-ō-kō-lŏt′ō-mē) [″ + ″ + *stoma,* opening]. Formation of a permanent opening into the colon through the abdominal wall.

laparocystectomy (lă″pă-rō-sĭs-tĕk′tō-mē) [Gr. *lapara,* flank, + *kystis,* bladder, + *ektome,* excision]. Removal of extrauterine fetus or a cyst through an abdominal incision. SYN: *laparocystotomy.*

laparocystidotomy (lăp″ăr-ō-sĭst-ĭ-dŏt′ō-mē) [″ + ″ + *tome,* incision]. Incision of bladder through the abdominal wall.

laparocystotomy (lăp″ăr-ō-sĭs-tŏt′ō-mē). Incision of abdomen to remove contents of a cyst or an extrauterine fetus. SYN: *laparocystectomy.*

laparoenterostomy (lăp″ă-rō-ĕn″tĕr-ŏs′tō-mē) [″ + *enteron,* intestine, + *stoma,* opening]. Formation of an artificial opening into the intestine through the abdominal wall.

laparoenterotomy (lăp″ăr-ō-ĕn″tĕr-ŏt′ō-mē) [″ + ″ + *tome,* incision]. Opening into the intestinal cavity by incision through the loins.

laparogastroscopy (lăp″ă-rō-găs-trŏs′kō-pē) [″ + *gaster,* belly, + *skopein,* to examine]. Inspection of the inside of the stomach after gastrotomy.

laparogastrostomy (lăp″ăr-ō-găs-trŏs′tō-mē) [″ + ″ + *stoma,* opening]. Formation of a permanent gastric fistula through the abdominal wall. SYN: *celiogastrostomy.*

laparogastrotomy (lăp″ă-rō-găs-trŏt′ō-mē) [″ + ″ + *tome,* incision]. Abdominal incision into the stomach.

laparohepatotomy (lăp″ăr-ō-hĕp″ă-tŏt′ō-mē) [″ + *hepar,* liver, + *tome,* incision]. Incision of the liver through the abdominal wall.

laparohysterectomy (lăp″ăr-ō-hĭs″tĕr-ĕk′tō-mē) [″ + *hystera,* uterus, + *ektome,* excision]. Removal of the uterus through an incision in the abdominal wall.

laparohystero-oophorectomy (lăp″ăr-ō-hĭs″tĕr-ō-ō″ō-for-ĕk′tō-mē) [″ + ″ + *oon,* ovum, + *phoros,* bearer, + *ektome,* excision]. Removal of uterus and ovaries through an abdominal incision.

laparohysteropexy (lăp″ăr-ō-hĭs′tĕr-ō-pĕks-ē) [″ + ″ + *pexis,* fixation]. Abdominal fixation of the uterus.

laparohysterosalpingo-oophorectomy (lăp″ăr-ō-hĭs″tĕr-ō-săl-pĭn″gō-ō″ō-fō-rĕk′tō-mē) [″ + *hystera,* uterus, + *salpinx,* tube, + *oon,* ovum, + *phoros,* bearer, + *ektome,* excision]. Removal of uterus, fallopian tubes, and ovaries through abdominal incision.

laparohysterotomy (lăp″ăr-ō-hĭs″tĕr-ŏt′ō-mē) [″ + ″ + *tome,* incision]. Surgery of the uterus through an abdominal incision. SEE: *cesarean section.*

laparoileotomy (lăp″ăr-ō-ĭl-ē-ŏt′ō-mē) [″ + L. *ileum,* ileum, + Gr. *tome,* incision]. Abdominal incision into ileum.

laparomyitis (lăp″ăr-ō-mī-ī′tĭs) [″ + *mys,* muscle, + *itis,* inflammation]. Inflammation of the muscular portion of the abdominal wall.

laparomyomectomy (lăp″ăr-ō-mī″ō-mĕk′tō-mē) [″ + ″ + *oma,* tumor, + *ektome,* excision]. Abdominal excision of a muscular tumor.

laparonephrectomy (lăp″ăr-ō-nē-frĕk′tō-mē) [″ + *nephros,* kidney, + *ektome,* excision]. Renal excision through the loin.

laparorrhaphy (lăp-ă-ror′ă-fē) [Gr. *lapara,* flank, + *rhaphe,* suture]. Suture of wound in the abdominal wall. SYN: *celiorrhaphy.*

laparosalpingectomy (lăp″ăr-ō-săl-pĭn-jĕk′tō-mē) [″ + *salpinx,* tube, + *ektome,* excision]. Excision of a fallopian tube through an abdominal incision.

laparosalpingo-oophorectomy (lăp″ăr-ō-săl-pĭn″gō-ō″ŏf-ō-rĕk′tō-mē) [″ + ″ + *oon,* ovum, + *phoros,* bearer, + *ektome,* excision]. Removal of fallopian tubes and ovaries through an abdominal incision.

laparosalpingotomy (lăp″ăr-ō-săl-pĭn-gŏt′ō-mē) [″ + ″ + *tome,* incision]. Incision of a fallopian tube through an abdominal incision. SYN: *celiosalpingotomy.*

laparoscope (lăp′ă-rō-skōp″) [″ + *skopein,* to examine]. An endoscope designed to permit visual examination of the peritoneal cavity.

laparoscopy (lăp-ăr-ŏs′kō-pē) [″ + *skopein,* to examine]. Abdominal exploration employing a type of endoscope called a laparoscope.

laparosplenectomy (lăp″ăr-ō-splēn-ĕk′tō-mē) [″ + *splen,* spleen, + *ektome,* excision]. Abdominal excision of the spleen.

laparosplenotomy (lăp″ăr-ō-splēn-ŏt′ō-mē) [″ + ″ + *tome,* incision]. Incision of the spleen through the abdominal wall.

laparotomy (lăp-ăr-ŏt′ō-mē) [″ + *tome,* incision]. The surgical opening of the abdomen; an abdominal operation.

PREOPERATIVE PREPARATION: Follow the physician's orders regarding diet, shaving of abdomen and pubic area, enemas, douches, and collecting of urine specimens.

NURSING IMPLICATIONS: Perform and document preoperative teaching. Prepare the patient in accordance with prescribed routine. Apply antiembolic hose as prescribed. Precribe postoperative nursing care plan including diet, maintenance of fluid and electrolyte balance, respiratory toiletry, oral hygiene, positioning and ambulation, care of the incision, pain relief, drainage monitoring, and establish discharge plans.

laparotrachelotomy (lăp″ăr-ō-trā-kĕl-ŏt′ō-mē) [″ + *trachelos,* neck, + *tome,* incision]. Cesarean section with the incision through the lower segment of the uterus.

laparotyphlotomy (lăp″ăr-ō-tĭ-flŏt′ō-mē) [″ + *typhlon,* cecum, + *tome,* incision]. Incision of cecum through lateral abdominal incision.

lapinization (lăp″ĭn-ī-zā′shŭn) [Fr. *lapin,* rabbit]. In virology, serial passage of a virus through rabbits in order to modify the virus.

lapis (lă′pĭs) [L.]. Stone.

lard [L. *lardum,* fat]. Purified fat from the hog. The sole nutrient is fat; a 100-gm. portion contains 902 Cal.

l., benzoinated. Lard containing 1% benzoin. It is used as a vehicle for certain types of topically applied medicines.

lardaceous (lăr-dā′shŭs) [L. *lardum,* fat]. Resembling lard; waxy, fatty.

Largon. Trade name for propiomazine hydrochloride.

Larodopa. Trade name for levodopa, USP.

larva [L., mask]. (pl. *larvae*) General term applied to the developing form of an insect after it has emerged from the egg and before it transforms into a pupa, from which it emerges as an adult.

l. currens. A type of larva migrans. The organism, Strongyloides stercoralis, travels subcutaneously at the rate of about 10 cm. an hour rather than at the slow rate of larva migrans.

l. migrans, cutaneous. A skin lesion characterized by a tortuous elevated red line that progresses at one end while fading out at the other. It is caused by the subcutaneous migration of the larvae of certain nematodes, esp. Ancylostoma braziliense and A. canis, that occur as accidental invaders of man.

l. migrans, visceral. Infestation of viscera by larvae of animal nematodes such as Toxocara canis. These migrate and cause eosinophilia, hepatomegaly, fever and hyperglobulinemia. Occurs mostly in children who play in soil or sand contaminated with dog and cat feces. SEE: *toxocariasis.*

CAUTION: The ocular symptoms may lead to the erroneous clinical diagnosis of retinoblastoma. There is no specific therapy but cortisone may be useful in controlling hypersensitivity reaction.

larval (lăr′văl) [L. *larva,* mask]. Concerning larva.

larvate [L. *larva,* mask]. Hidden, concealed. Term applied to an atypical or hidden symptom.

larvicide [″ + *caedere,* to kill]. An agent that destroys insect larvae.

larviphagic (lăr″vĭ-fă′jĭk) [″ + Gr. *phagein,* to eat]. Consuming larva, as is done by certain fish.

laryngalgia (lăr-ĭn-găl′jē-ă) [Gr. *larynx,* larynx, + *algos,* pain]. Neuralgia of the larynx.

laryngeal (lăr-ĭn′jē-ăl) [Gr. *larynx,* larynx]. Pert. to the larynx.

laryngeal reflex. Cough as result of irritation of larynx or fauces.

laryngectomee (lăr″ĭn-jĕk′tō-mē) [″ + *ektome,* excision]. An individual whose larynx has been removed.

laryngectomy (lăr″ĭn-jĕk′tō-mē) [″ + *ektome,* excision]. Excision of larynx.

NURSING IMPLICATIONS: The patient must be prepared for the changes that will occur both to the voice and to the airway following surgery. Diagrams should be used to explain the altered airway. In addition, it is essential that the patient be fully prepared for communicating in the immediate post-surgical period. A magic slate is quite helpful as are flash cards in facilitating communication. All of this is reviewed and practiced prior to surgery. Inform the patient what to expect concerning post-op procedure, including use of oxygen and nothing per os for seven days post-op.

laryngemphraxis (lăr″ĭn-jĕm-frăk′sĭs) [″ + *emphraxis,* an obstruction]. Obstruction of the larynx.

laryngismal (lăr″ĭn-jĭs′măl) [″ + *-ismos,* condition of]. Concerning or resembling affection with laryngeal spasm.

laryngismus (lăr″ĭn-jĭs′mŭs) [″ + *-ismos,* condition of]. Spasm of the larynx.

laryngitic (lăr-ĭn-jĭt′ĭk) [Gr. *larynx,* larynx]. 1. Resulting from laryngitis. 2. Rel. to laryngitis.

laryngitis (lăr-ĭn-jī′tĭs) [″ + *itis,* inflammation]. Inflammation of larynx. SEE: *croup.*

l., acute catarrhal. Acute congestive laryngitis; catarrhal inflammation of laryngeal mucosa and the vocal cords.

SYM: Hoarseness and aphonia and occasionally pain on phonation and deglutition.

ETIOL: Improper use or over-use of voice; exposure to cold and wet; extension from infections in nose and throat; inhalation of irritating vapors and dust; associated with systemic diseases as whooping cough or measles.

TREATMENT: Complete rest of voice; promotion of diaphoresis; liquid or soft diet; medicated steam inhalations such as compound tincture of benzoin; codeine or nonnarcotic cough suppressants for cough and pain.

l., atrophic. Laryngitis leading to diminished secretion and atrophy of the mucous membrane.

SYM: Tickling sensation in throat, hoarseness, cough, dyspnea when crusts are thick and accumulate on vocal cords so as to narrow the breathing aperture.

TREATMENT: Inhalants and medicated sprays to loosen the crusts; strict attention to associated nose and throat pathology.

l., chronic. A type of laryngitis due to a recurrent irritation, or following the acute form. Often secondary to sinus or nasal pathology, improper use of voice, excessive smoking, drinking, or neoplasms.

SYM: Tickling in throat, huskiness of voice, dysphonia.

TREATMENT: Correction of preexisting nose and throat pathology, discontinuance of alcohol and tobacco, avoidance of excessive use of voice and proper vocal placement.

l., croupous. Laryngitis occurring mainly in infants and young children and characterized by a barky cough, hoarseness, and stridor.

l., croupous hypertrophic. Hypertrophy of tissues accompanying chronic laryngitis.

l., diphtheritic. Invasion of larynx by diphtheria bacilli, usually with formation of membrane.

l., membranous. Laryngitis characterized by inflammation of larynx with the formation of a false membrane of nondiphtheritic origin.

l., phlegmonous. Inflamed larynx with edema and submucous suppuration.

l., syphilitic. A chronic form of laryngitis due to syphilis.

SYM: Hoarseness, cough, simple catarrh, formation of broad condylomata, follicular hyperplasia, syphiloma, syphilitic perichondritis.

Secondary stage in form of mucous patches or tertiary in form of gumma. Secondary syphilis is a diffuse infection and one sees luetic patches spread over large areas of larynx. In tertiary syphilis, the gummatous lesion can occur in any part of larynx. There is marked redness over the infiltrated area as well as in the surrounding mucous membrane. When there is breakdown, the resultant ulceration is deep with sharp edges. Pain is usually absent and fixation of the cord is late. Cicatrization and deformity follow healing of gumma.

TREATMENT: Appropriate antibiotic therapy for syphilis.

l., tuberculous. Laryngitis secondary to pulmonary tuberculosis.

SYM: Hoarseness, aphonia, pain in swallowing, cough. Lesion located in interarytenoid area, vocal cords, epiglottis, or false cords. Lesions are relatively pale; ulceration occurs early.

laryngo- [Gr. *larynx,* larynx]. Prefix pert. to the larynx.

laryngocele (lăr-ĭn′gō-sēl) [″ + *kele,* hernia]. A congenital air sac connected to the larynx. Its presence is normal in some animals but abnormal in man.

laryngocentesis (lăr-ĭn″gō-sĕn-tē′sĭs) [″ + *kentesis,* puncture]. Incision or puncture of the larynx.

laryngofissure (lăr-ĭng″gō-fĭsh′ūr) [″ + L. *fissura,* a cleft]. The operation of opening the larynx by a median line incision through the thyroid cartilage.

laryngogram (lă-rĭng′gō-grăm) [″ + *gramma,* writing]. Roentgenogram of the larynx.

laryngograph (lăr-ĭng′ō-grăf) [″ + *graphein,* to write]. Device for making a record of laryngeal movements.

laryngography (lăr″ĭn-gŏg′ră-fē). 1. Description of the larynx. 2. Roentgenography of the larynx after application of a radiopaque dye.

laryngologist (lăr″ĭn-gŏl′ō-jĭst) [″ + *logos,* study]. Specialist in laryngology.

laryngology. The area of medicine dealing with the pharynx, throat, larynx, nasopharynx, and tracheobronchial tree.

laryngomalacia (lăr-ĭng″gō-mă-lā′shē-ă) [″ + *malakia,* softness]. Softening of the tissues of the larynx.

laryngometry (lăr″ĭn-gŏm′ĕ-trē) [″ + *metron,* measure]. Systematic measurement of the larynx.

laryngoparalysis (lăr-ĭn″gō-păr-ăl′ĭ-sĭs) [″ + *paralyein,* to disable at one side]. Paralysis of muscles of the larynx.

laryngopathy (lăr″ĭn-gŏp′ă-thē) [″ + *pathos,* disease]. Any disease of the larynx.

laryngophantom (lăr″ĭn-gō-făn′tŏm) [″ + *phantasma,* image]. Plastic model of the larynx.

laryngopharyngeal (lăr-ĭn″gō-făr-ĭn′jē-ăl) [″ + *pharynx,* pharynx]. Rel. jointly to larynx and pharynx.

laryngopharyngectomy (lăr-ĭn″gō-făr-ĭn-jĕk′tō-mē) [″ + ″ + *ektome,* excision]. Removal of the larynx and pharynx.

laryngopharyngeus (lă-rĭng″gō-fă-rĭn′jē-ŭs). The muscle that constricts the inferior pharynx.

laryngopharyngitis (lăr-ĭn″gō-făr-ĭn-jī′tĭs) [″ + ″ + *itis,* inflammation]. Inflammation of the larynx and pharynx. SYN: *pharyngolaryngitis.*

laryngopharyngography (lă-rĭng″gō-fă-rĭn-jŏg′ră-fē) [″ + ″ + *graphein,* to write]. Radiographic examination of the larynx and pharynx when filled with air.

laryngopharynx (lăr-ĭn″gō-făr′ĭnks) [Gr. *larynx*, larynx, + *pharynx*, pharynx]. Lower portion of the pharynx that extends from the cornua of the hyoid bone or vestibule of the larynx to the lower border of the cricoid cartilage.

laryngophony (lăr″ĭn-gŏf′ō-nē) [″ + *phone*, voice]. Voice sounds heard in auscultating the pharynx.

laryngophthisis (lăr″ĭng-gŏf′thĭ-sĭs) [″ + *phthisis*, a wasting]. Tuberculosis of the larynx.

laryngoplasty (lăr-ĭn′gō-plăs″tē) [″ + *plassein*, to form]. Plastic reparative surgery of the larynx.

laryngoplegia (lă-rĭng″gō-plē′jē-ă) [″ + *plege*, stroke]. Paralysis of laryngeal muscles.

laryngoptosis (lă-rĭng″gō-tō′sĭs) [″ + *ptosis*, a dropping]. Condition in which the larynx is positioned, at birth, somewhat lower than usual. This may also occur in old age.

laryngorhinology (lăr-ĭn″gō-rīn-ŏl′ō-jē) [″ + *rhis*, nose, + *logos*, study]. The branch of medical science concerned with diseases of the larynx and nose.

laryngorrhagia (lăr″ĭn-gō-rā′jē-ă) [″ + *rhegnynai*, to flow forth]. Laryngeal hemorrhage.

laryngorrhea (lăr″ĭn-gō-rē′ă) [″ + *rhoia*, flow]. Excessive discharge of laryngeal mucus.

laryngoscleroma (lăr-ĭn″gō-sklē-rō′mă) [″ + *skleros*, hard, + *oma* tumor]. Scleroma affecting the larynx.

laryngoscope (lăr-ĭn′gō-skōp) [″ + *skopein*, to examine]. Instrument for examining the larynx.

laryngoscopic (lăr″ĭn-gō-skŏp′ĭk) [″ + *skopein*, to examine]. Pert. to observation of the interior of the larynx with the aid of a small long-handled mirror. SEE: *laryngoscopy*.

laryngoscopist (lăr″ĭng-gŏs′kō-pĭst) [″ + *skopein*, to examine]. An individual trained in laryngoscopy.

laryngoscopy (lăr″ĭn-gŏs′kō-pē). Examination of the interior of the larynx.

NURSING IMPLICATIONS: Explain procedure to patient. Assist physician as necessary. Reassure patient during the procedure. After procedure, place patient in semi-Fowler's position until swallow reflex is reestablished. Omit oral intake until swallowing reflex returns. Monitor patient for any adverse effects. Instruct patient not to smoke for at least 24 hours to prevent irritation.

l., direct. Laryngoscopy with laryngeal speculum or laryngoscope.

l., indirect. Laryngoscopy with a mirror.

laryngospasm (lăr-ĭn′gō-spăzm) [″ + *spasmos*, spasm]. Spasm of laryngeal muscles.

laryngostenosis (lăr-ĭng″gō-stē-nō′sĭs) [″ + *stenosis*, a narrowing]. Stricture of the larynx.

l., compression. Stricture of the larynx due to outside causes such as abscess, tumor, or goiter.

l., occlusion. Stricture of the larynx due to congenital bands or membranes, foreign bodies, tumors, cicatricial contraction following ulceration as in diphtheria and tertiary syphilis, penetrating wounds, or corrosive fluid.

SYM: Dyspnea, esp. on inspiration and exertion. Loud breathing that becomes a stridulous choking respiration; pulse small and frequent; face anxious and cyanotic.

PROG: Grave.

TREATMENT: Depends on cause. Tracheotomy is often necessary.

laryngostomy (lăr-ĭn-gŏs′tō-mē) [″ + *stoma*, opening]. Establishing a permanent opening through the neck into the larynx.

laryngostroboscope (lăr″ĭn-gō-strō′bō-skōp) [″ + *strobos*, whirl, + *skopein*, to view]. Instrument for inspection of vibration of vocal cords.

laryngotomy (lăr-ĭn-gŏt′ō-mē) [″ + *tome*, incision]. Incision of larynx.

l., inferior. Surgical incision of the larynx through the cricoid cartilage.

l., median. Surgical incision of the larynx through the thyroid cartilage.

l., subhyoid or superior. Surgical incision of the larynx through the thyroid membrane.

laryngotracheal (lă-rĭng″gō-trā′kē-ăl) [″ + *tracheia*, trachea]. Concerning the larynx and trachea.

laryngotracheitis (lăr-ĭn″gō-trā-kē-ī′tĭs) [″ + ″ + *itis*, inflammation]. Inflamed condition of the larynx and trachea.

laryngotracheobronchitis (lă-rĭng″gō-trā″kē-ō-brŏng-kī′tĭs) [″ + ″ + *bronchos*, windpipe, + *itis*, inflammation]. Inflammation of the larynx, trachea, and bronchi.

laryngotracheotomy (lăr-ĭn″gō-trā-kē-ŏt′ō-mē) [″ + ″ + *tome*, incision]. Incision of the larynx with section of upper tracheal rings.

laryngoxerosis (lăr-ĭn″gō-zēr-ō′sĭs) [″ + *xeros*, dry, + *osis*, condition]. Abnormal dryness of the larynx.

larynx (lăr′ĭnks) [Gr.]. (pl. *larynges*) The enlarged upper end of the trachea below the root of the tongue; a musculocartilaginous structure lined with mucous membrane; the organ of voice. SEE: illus.

STRUCTURE: Consists of nine cartilages bound together by an elastic membrane and moved by muscles. Cartilages include three single (cricoid, thyroid, and epiglottic) and three paired (arytenoid, corniculate, and cuneiform). The extrinsic muscles include the omohyoid, sternohyoid, sternothyroid, and several others; intrinsic muscles include the cricothyroid, external and internal thyroar-

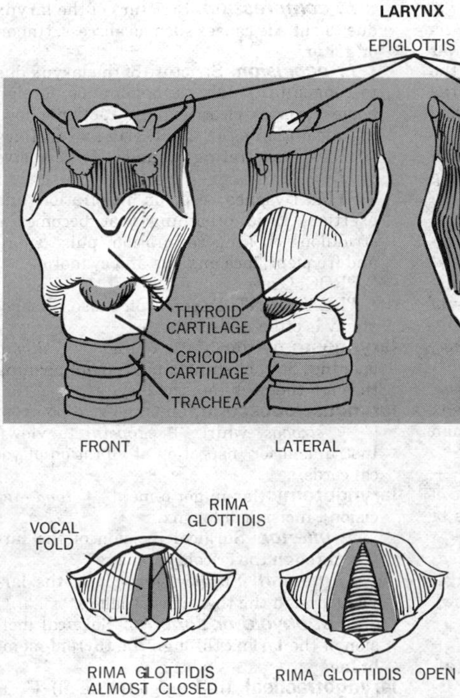

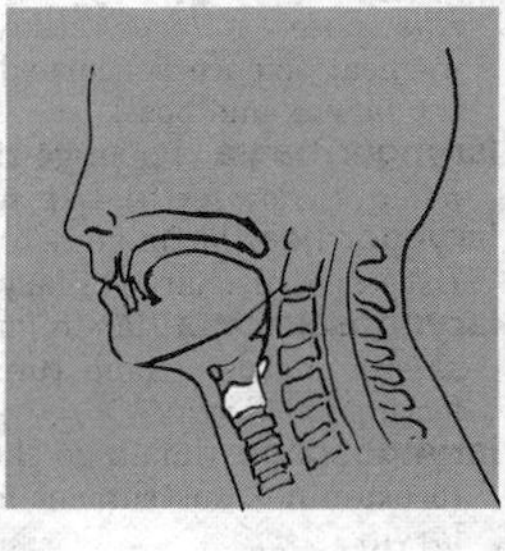

ytenoid, transverse and oblique arytenoid, and external and internal thyroarytenoid. The cavity of the larynx contains two pairs of folds, the ventricular folds (false vocal cords) and vocal folds (true vocal cords), and is divided into three regions (vestibule, ventricle, and inferior entrance to the glottis). An opening between the true vocal folds forms a narrow slit, the rima glottidis or glottis.

NERVES: From interior and external branches of superior laryngeal.

BLOOD SUPPLY: Inferior thyroid, branch of thyroid axis and superior thyroid, branch of external carotid.

RS: cricoarytenoid; epiglottis; glottis; "laryng-" words; prominentia laryngea; vestibule; vocal cord.

l., foreign bodies in. SYM: Violent spasmodic cough and dyspnea; fixed pain at particular spot; loss of voice.

NURSING IMPLICATIONS: American Heart Association recommendations for aspiration of foreign body include recognition of foreign body obstruction. If patient is able to speak or cough, do not interfere with patient's attempts to expel the object. If patient is unable to speak, cough, or breathe, follow Heimlich maneuver, q.v. If unconscious, patient should be rolled onto side. Deliver four sharp back blows between the shoulder blades. Roll patient onto back and apply four manual abdominal thrusts between the xiphoid and umbilicus. Continue until you can successfully ventilate. Tracheostomy may be required.

Lasan. Trade name for anthralin, USP.

lascivia (lă-sĭv′ē-ă) [L. *lascivire,* to be wanton]. Abnormal sexual desire. SEE: *nymphomania; satyriasis.*

Lasègue's sign (lă-sĕgz′). [Ernest C. Lasègue, Fr. physician, 1816–1883] Pain and discomfort in the back when the fully extended leg of the supine patient is gently raised.

laser (lā′zĕr). Acronym for *l*ight *a*mplification by *s*timulated *e*mission of *r*adiation. A device that emits intense heat and power at close range, a tool used in surgery and in diagnosis. The instrument converts various frequencies of light into one small and extremely intense unified beam of one

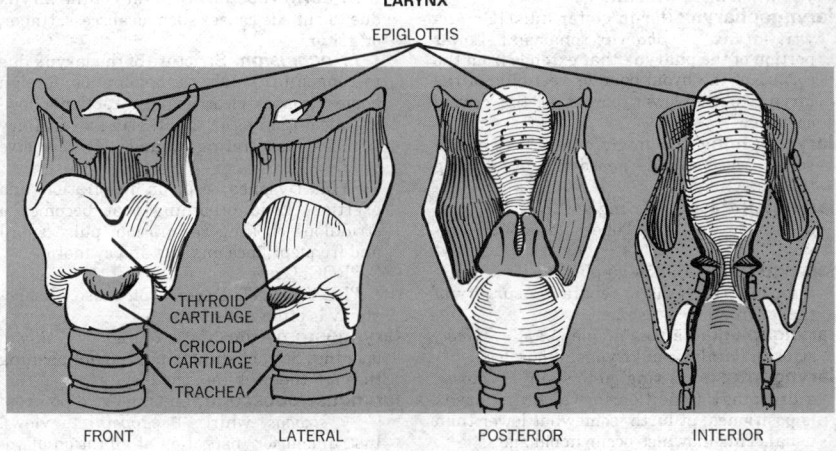

wavelength radiation.

laser cane. An experimental cane that helps a blind person detect objects ahead of, above, and below his or her path.

Lasix. Trade name for furosemide, USP.

Lassa fever. [Lassa, city in Africa] A disease caused by the Lassa virus, first reported in Nigeria in 1969.

SYM AND SIGNS: Abrupt onset of high fever that is continuous or intermittent spiking with generalized myalgia, chest and abdominal pain, headache, sore throat, cough, dizziness with flushing of the face, conjunctival injection, and nausea, diarrhea, and vomiting. Hemorrhagic areas of the skin and mucous membranes may appear on the fourth day. Mortality may be over 50%.

TREATMENT: No specific therapy is known. Transfusion of blood or plasma from individuals who have recovered from the disease is indicated. Patients are isolated in special isolation units that filter the air leaving the room and in which negative pressure may be maintained. All sputum, blood, excreta, and objects that the patient has contacted are disinfected.

Lassa virus. An arenavirus that causes Lassa fever. Its reservoir may be a species of rat, Mastomys natalensis.

lassitude (lăs'ĭ-tūd) [L. *lassitudo,* weariness]. Weariness; exhaustion.

last sacraments. A religious rite performed by a clergyman to the individual just prior to death.

latah (lă'tă). A type of mental disorder that occurs in people of Southeast Asia, esp. in women. It is characterized by imitative behavior, coprolalia, echolalia, and automatic obedience. It may be provoked by startling, tickling, or frightening the patient. SEE: *jumping Frenchmen of Maine; miryachit.*

latency (lā'tĕn-sē) [L. *latens,* lying hidden]. State of being concealed, hidden, inactive, or inapparent. SYN: *latent period.*

latency period. The time between the initiation of a stimulus, or contracting of a disease, and the response or clinical manifestation of the disease, respectively.

latent. 1. Lying hidden. 2. Quiet; not active.

latent content. In psychology, that part of a dream or unconscious mental content that cannot be brought into the objective consciousness through any effort of will to remember.

latent heat. Caloric or heat energy absorbed by matter changing from solid to liquid or liquid to vapor without a change in temperature.

latent image. Invisible image formed on the radiographic film because of exposure to x-rays, made visible by the development process.

latent period. 1. Time between a stimulus and its response. SYN: *lag phase.* 2. Time during which a disease is supposed to be existent without manifesting itself; period of incubation.

laterad (lăt'ĕr-ăd) [L. *latus,* side, + *ad,* toward]. Toward a side or lateral aspect.

lateral (lăt'ĕr-ăl) [L. *lateralis*]. Pert. to the side.

lateralis (lăt"ĕr-ā'lĭs) [L.]. Indicating that the structure is located away from the mid-plane of the body.

laterality (lăt"ĕr-ăl'ĭ-tē). Condition of being on one side or toward the side. Term is used to specify which side of the body or brain is dominant.

l., crossed. Mixed dominance of certain body parts so that the left arm and right leg would be dominant.

l., dominant. Preferential dominance and use of the parts of one side of the body such as the eye, arm, leg, or hand.

lateral sinus. Transverse and sigmoid portion of two cranial venous sinuses. Extends from occipital protuberance to jugular bulb.

latericeous, lateritious (lăt"ĕr-ĭsh'ŭs) [L. *later,* brick]. Resembling brick dust.

lateroabdominal (lăt"ĕr-ō-ăb-dŏm'ĭ-năl) [L. *lateralis,* pert. to side, + *abdomen,* belly]. Concerning the side of the body and the abdominal area.

laterodeviation (lăt"ĕr-ō-dē"vē-ā'shŭn) [" + *deviare,* to turn aside]. To push or displace to one side.

lateroduction (lăt"ĕr-ō-dŭk'shŭn) [" + *ducere,* to lead]. To draw to one side, esp. the eye.

lateroflexion (lăt"ĕr-ō-flĕk'shŭn) [" + *flexis,* bending]. Bending or curvature toward a side.

lateroposition (lăt"ĕr-ō-pō-zĭsh'ŭn) [" + *positio,* position]. To be displaced to one side.

lateroprone position (lăt"ĕr-ō-prōn'). Position where patient is on left side leaning forward on chest, right knee and thigh drawn up, left arm along back of patient. SYN: *Sims' position.*

lateropulsion (lăt"ĕr-ō-pŭl'shŭn) [L. *lateralis,* pert. to side, + *pulsus,* driving]. Involuntary tendency in cerebellar and labyrinthine disease to fall to one side.

laterotorsion (lăt"ĕr-ō-tor'shŭn) [" + *torsio,* a twisting]. To be twisted to one side.

lateroversion (lăt"ĕr-ō-vĕr'shŭn) [" + *versio,* a turning]. Tendency or a turning toward one side.

latex (lā'tĕks) [L., fluid]. The fluid or sap produced by some plants. Natural rubber is produced from the latex of certain tropical trees.

lathyrism (lăth'ĭr-ĭzm) [Gr. *lathyros,* vetch]. Disease presumably caused by eating certain plants of the genus Lathyrus. Characterized by muscular weakness and paraplegia that are irreversible.

lathyrogen (lăth'ĭ-rō-jĕn) [" + *gennan,* to produce]. Something that produces lathyrism.

latissimus (lă-tĭs'ĭ-mŭs) [L., widest]. Denoting a broad anatomical structure such as a muscle.

latitude. In radiology, a range of exposure that would result in a diagnostic radiograph.

latrine (lă-trēn') [L. *latrina*]. A toilet, particularly one in a military camp.

latrodectism (lăt"rō-dĕk'tĭzm) [*Latrodectus* + Gr. *-ismos,* condition]. The toxic reaction to the bite of the Latrodectus genus of spiders. SEE: *spider, black widow.*

Latrodectus (lăt"rō-dĕk'tŭs) [L. *latro,* robber, + Gr. *daknein,* biting]. A genus of small black spiders belonging to the family Theriidae.

L. mactans. The black widow or hourglass spider, a species widely distributed in the United States. The bite of the female produces serious symptoms and may result in death. SEE: *spider, black widow.*

LATS. *long-acting thyroid stimulator.*

lattice (lăt'ĭs). 1. A network or framework formed by structures intertwined usually at right angles with each other. 2. In physics, the arrangement of atoms in a crystal.

latus (lā'tŭs) [L., broad]. (pl. *latera*) [NA] The side; the flank.

latus, lata, latum (lā'tŭs, lā'tă, lāt'ŭm) [L., broad]. Broad, as the uterine broad ligament.

laudable [L. *laudabilis,* praiseworthy]. Commendable; healthy; normal; formerly said erroneously of pus.

laudanum (lăw'dăn-ŭm). Tincture of opium. SEE: *morphine.*

laugh (lăf) [ME. *laughen,* to laugh]. 1. Sound produced by laughing. SYN: *risus.* 2. To express emotion, usually happiness or mirth, by a series of inarticulate sounds. Typically the mouth is open and a wide smile is present.

l., sardonic. Spasm of facial muscles producing a grinning effect that is inappropriate to the situation. SYN: *risus sardonicus.*

laughing gas (lăf'ĭng). Nitrous oxide gas.

laughter, compulsive. Laughter without cause, occurring in certain psychoses, esp. schizophrenia.

laughter reflex (lăf'tĕr). Uncontrollable laughter resulting from tickling or pretense of tickling.

Laurence-Moon-Biedl syndrome (law'rĕns-moon'bē'dĕl). [John L. Laurence, Brit. ophthalmologist, 1830–1874; Robert C. Moon, U.S. ophthalmologist, 1844–1914; Arthur Biedl, Prague endocrinologist, 1869–1933] The combination of girdle-type obesity, sexual underdevelopment, mental retardation, retinal degeneration, polydactyly, and deformity of the skull. The condition is inherited as an autosomal recessive trait.

lavage (lă-văzh') [Fr., from L. *lavare,* to wash]. Washing out of a cavity. SYN: *irrigation.*

l., gastric. Washing out of the stomach. A stomach tube or catheter is used with a solution of sterile water, normal saline, or 1 to 5% sodium bicarbonate.

Quantity of solution: Not more than 10 oz. at a time repeated until fluid runs clear.

Temperature and time: 105° F. (40.6° C.). Preferably before breakfast.

Position: Semirecumbent or low enough to prevent inhalation of returning fluid. In poisoning, save siphoned fluid for examination. If patient is unconscious, use a mouth gag.

Purpose: To remove irritants or poisons, to cleanse the stomach preoperatively or postoperatively. SEE: *colonic irrigation; irrigation, bladder.*

law [AS. *laga,* law]. Scientifically, a statement that is found to hold true uniformly for a whole class of natural occurrences.

l., all-or-none. The weakest stimulus capable of producing a response produces the maximum response contraction in cardiac and skeletal muscles and nerves.

l., Avogadro's. If temperature and external pressure are the same, all gases contain the same number of molecules in equal volumes.

l., Bell's. Anterior spinal nerve roots are motor, and posterior spinal nerve roots are sensory. SYN: *l. of Magendie.*

l., biogenetic. Ontogeny recapitulates phylogeny, i.e., an individual in its development recapitulates stages in its evolutionary development. SYN: *l., Haeckel's.*

l., Boyle's. The volume occupied by a fixed quantity of every gas is inversely proportional, and density directly proportional, to pressure applied to the gas. SYN: *l., Mariotte's.*

l., Charles'. When pressure is constant, volume of a gas varies as the absolute temperature.

l., Courvoisier's. When the common bile duct is obstructed by a calculus, dilatation of the gallbladder is rare; when otherwise obstructed, dilatation is common.

l., Fechner's. The intensity of sensation is proportional to the logarithm of the strength of the stimulus.

l., Gay-Lussac's. L., Charles', q.v.

l., Graham's. The rate at which a gas diffuses through a porous membrane is inversely proportional to the square root of the density of the gas.

l., Haeckel's. L., biogenetic.

l., Hilton's. A nerve trunk supplying any joint supplies the muscles that move the joint and skin over insertion of such muscles.

l., Hooke's. The stress used to stretch or compress a body is proportional to the strain as long as the elasticity of the body is within normal limits.

l., Koch's. To prove an organism to be the cause of a given disease or lesion: the microorganism in question is regularly found in the lesions of the disease; pure cultures can be obtained from it; pure cultures when introduced into susceptible animals reproduce the disease or pathological condition; the organism can be obtained again in pure culture from the inoculated animal. SYN: *Koch's postulate*.

l., Marey's. Heart rate varies inversely to arterial blood pressure; that is, a rise or fall in arterial blood pressure brings about, respectively, a slowing or speeding up of heart rate.

l., Mariotte's. L., Boyle's.

l.'s, Mendel's. A number of principles of heredity established by Mendel (1822–1884) that laid the foundation for the modern science of genetics. Includes the principles of unit characters, dominance, segregation, and independent assortment. SEE: *Mendel's laws*.

l., Murphy's. If something can go wrong, it will.

l., Nysten's. Rigor mortis travels progressively from muscles of mastication, through the face, neck, trunk, and arms, reaching the legs and feet last.

l. of definite proportions. Two or more elements when united to form a new substance do so in a constant and fixed proportion by weight.

l. of the heart. Other things being equal, the stroke volume of the heart varies as the extent of diastolic filling or the energy of contraction is a function of the initial length of the muscle fibers.

l. of the intestine. Moderate distention of the intestine at a point causes relaxation below (aborally to the point) and contraction above.

l. of Magendie. L., Bell's.

l. of mass action. In chemical reactions, the amount of change taking place is proportional to the action mass of the reacting substance.

l. of multiple proportions. When two substances unite to form a series of chemical compounds, the proportions in which they unite are simple multiples of one another or of one common proportion.

l. of reciprocal proportions. In chemistry, the proportions in which two elementary bodies unite with a third one are simple multiples or simple fractions of the proportions in which these two bodies unite with each other.

l. of specificity of nervous energy. — Law that states excitation of a receptor always gives rise to the same sensation regardless of the nature of the stimulus.

l., periodic. The physical and chemical properties of chemical elements are periodic functions of their atomic weight. A natural classification of elements is according to their atomic weight. When arranged in order of their atomic weight or atomic number, elements show regular variations in most of their physical and chemical properties.

l.'s, Rubner's. 1. Law of constant energy consumption: Rapidity of growth is proportional to intensity of the metabolic process. 2. Law of constant growth quotient: The same proportional part, or growth quotient, of total energy is utilized for growth.

l., Sutton's. SEE: *Sutton's law*.

l., Waller's, of degeneration. If a spinal nerve is completely divided, the distal portion undergoes fatty degeneration.

l., Weber's. The increase in stimulus necessary to produce the smallest perceptible increase in sensation bears a constant ratio to the strength of the stimulus already acting.

l., Wolff's. Changes in form and function of bones result in definite changes in their internal structure.

lawrencium (lă-rĕn'sē-ŭm) [Ernest O. Lawrence, U.S. physicist, 1901–1958] SYMB: Lr. At. wt. 256.0986; at no. 103. A synthetic transuranic chemical element.

lax (lăks) [L. *laxus*, slack]. 1. Without tension. 2. Loose and not easily controlled. Said of bowel movements.

laxation (lăk-sā'shŭn) [L. *laxare*, to loosen]. Bowel movement.

laxative (lăk'să-tĭv) [L. *laxare*, to loosen]. A food or chemical substance that acts to loosen the bowels (i.e., facilitate passage of bowel contents at time of defecation), and, therefore, to prevent or treat constipation. Laxatives may act by increasing peristalsis by irritating the intestinal mucosa, lubricating the intestinal walls, softening the bowel contents by increasing the amount of water in the intestines, and increasing the bulk of the bowel contents. Many feel it is essential to have one or more bowel movements a day. These individuals may develop the habit of taking some form of laxative daily. They should be instructed that missing a bowel movement is not harmful and bowel movements do not necessarily occur at regular intervals. SYN: *aperient; cathartic; purgative*. SEE: *constipation*.

CAUTION: A sudden change in bowel habits may be the first sign of a malignancy of the intestinal tract. When this happens, the individual should consult a physician without delay.

laxative regimen. The diet may be modified to avoid chronic constipation by maintaining adequate volume of food; eating high-bulk foods that contain high fiber content; eating foods that tend to stimulate bowel activity such as stewed fruits and vegetables; maintaining adequate fluid intake; and participating in regular exercise. In addition, avoid foods that the individual has found cause constipation. Some persons are esp. liable to be constipated by certain cheeses.

laxator (lăk-sā'tor) [L. *laxare*, to loosen]. That which has a relaxing effect.

l. tympani. One of two muscles or ligaments of the malleus of the inner ear.

Laxinate 100. Trade name for docusate sodium.

layer (lā'ĕr) [ME. *leyer*]. A stratum; a thin sheetlike structure of more or less uniform thickness.

l., ameloblastic. Enamel layer of the tooth.

l., bacillary. Rod and cone layer of the retina of the eye.

l., basal. The outermost layer of the uterine endometrium lying next to the myometrium.

l., blastodermic. L., germ, q.v.

l., choriocapillary. Lamina choriocapillaris.

l., claustral. Layer of gray matter between the external capsule and insula.

l., clear. Stratum lucidum of the skin.

l., columnar. 1. Stratum basale epidermidis of the skin. 2. The rod and cone layer of the retina of the eye.

l., compact. The compact surface layer of the uterine endometrium.

l., cuticular, of epithelium. A striated layer secreted by and covering the free surface of an epithelial sheet, esp. that on the surface of columnar epithelium of the intestine.

l., enamel. L., ameloblastic, q.v.

l., ependymal. Inner layer of cells of the embryonic neural tube.

l., ganglionic. 1. Fifth layer of cerebral cortex. 2. An inner layer of ganglion cells in the retina whose axons form the fibers of the optic nerve.

l., germ. One of the three primary layers of the developing embryo from which the various organ systems develop. SEE: *ectoderm; endoderm; mesoderm.*

l., germinative. The innermost layer of the epidermis, consisting of a basal layer of cells and a layer of prickle cells (stratum spinosum). SYN: *malpighian layer; stratum germinativum.*

l., granular exterior. Second layer of cerebellar cortex, lying within the molecular layer and separated from it by a single row of Purkinje cells. Consists principally of granule cells.

l., granular interior. The fourth layer of the cerebral cortex, consisting principally of closely packed stellate cells.

l., half-value. In radiology, the thickness of an absorber that will reduce the intensity of a beam of radiation by one half.

l., Henle's. A layer of clear cells forming the outermost layer of the inner epithelial root sheath of a hair.

l., horny. Outermost layer of the skin, consisting of clear, dead, scalelike cells, those of the surface layer being constantly desquamated. SYN: *stratum corneum.*

l., Huxley's. The middle layer of the inner epithelial root sheath of a hair.

l., Langhans'. Cytotrophoblast of a chorionic villus of the placenta.

l., malpighian. L., germinative.

l., mantle. The middle layer of the neural tube of the developing embryo.

l., molecular. 1. Outermost layer of the cerebral or cerebellar cortex. 2. Inner or outer plexiform layer of the retina.

l., nervous. The nerve-containing portion of the retina of the eye.

l., odontoblastic. Layer of connective tissue cells at the outer edge of the pulp of a tooth.

l. of pyramidal cells. The exterior pyramidal layer; the third layer of the cerebral cortex.

l. of rods and cones. The layer of the retina of the eye next to the pigment layer. It contains the rods and cones.

l., osteogenic; l., Ollier's. Innermost or bone-forming layer of the periosteum.

l., outer-nuclear. A layer of the retina containing the nuclei of the visual cells (rods and cones).

l., papillary. Superficial layer of the corium lying immediately under the epidermis into which it extends, forming dermal papillae.

l., pigment. Outermost layer of the retina. Cells contain a pigment called fuscin.

l., prickle cell. Stratum spinosum epidermidis; the layer between the granular and basal layers of the skin. Prickle cells are present in this layer.

l., Purkinje. A single row of large flask-shaped cells (Purkinje cells, q.v.) lying between molecular and granular layers of the cerebellar cortex.

l., reticular. The inner layer of the corium lying beneath the papillary layer.

l., somatic. In the embryo, a layer of extra-embryonic mesoderm that forms a part of the somatopleure, the outer wall of the coelom.

l., spinous. L., prickle cell, q.v.

l., splanchnic. A layer of extra-embryonic mesoderm that with the endoderm forms the splanchnopleure.

l., spongy. The middle layer of the uterine endometrium. Contains dilated portions of uterine glands. SYN: *stratum spongiosum.*

l., subendocardial. Layer of loose connective tissue immediately under the endocardium that binds it to the myocardium. Contains fibers of the conducting system of the heart.

l., subendothelial. Layer of fine fibers and fibroblasts lying immediately under the endothelium of the tunica intima of larger arteries and veins.

l., zonal, of hypothalamus. Layer of myelinated fibers covering the thalamus of the brain.

lazaretto (lăz"ă-rĕt'ō) [It. *lazzaro,* a leper]. 1. A quarantine station. 2. Hospital for treatment of contagious diseases.

lb. *pound.*

LD. *lethal dose.*

LD_{50}. *median lethal dose* of a substance, which will kill 50% of the animals receiving that dose. Dose is usually calculated on amount of material given per gram or kilogram of body weight or amount per unit of body surface area.

LDH. *lactic dehydrogenase.*

LDL. *low-density lipoprotein.*

L-dopa. L-3,4-dihydroxyphenylalanine. A drug used in the treatment of Parkinson's disease. SYN: *levodopa.*

L.E. *lupus erythematosus.*

leaching (lēch'ĭng) [AS. *leccan,* to wet]. Extraction of a substance from a mixture by washing the mixture with a solvent in which only the desired substance is soluble. SYN: *lixiviation.*

lead (lēd) [AS. *laedan,* to guide]. A conductor attached to an electrocardiograph. The three common leads are: lead I, right arm to left arm; lead II, right arm to left leg; lead III, left arm to left leg. These are known as standard leads, bipolar limb leads, or indirect leads. SEE: *electrocardiogram* for illus.

l., bipolar. In electrocardiography, any lead that consists of an electrode at one site and another at a different body site. A standard limb lead, I, II, or III, is a bipolar lead.

l., esophageal. One lead is placed in the esophagus.

l., limb. Any lead, unipolar or bipolar, in which a limb is the location of one of the electrodes.

l., precordial. Record taken when one electrode is placed over the precordium, the other over an indifferent region.

l., unipolar. Record made when one electrode is placed on chest wall overlying the heart, where potential changes are of considerable magnitude and the other (distant or indifferent electrode) placed where potential changes are of small magnitude.

lead (lĕd). Latin *plumbum.* SYMB: Pb. At. wt. 207.2; at. no. 82; sp. gr. 11.35. A metallic element. Its compounds are poisonous. Accumulation and toxicity occur if more than 0.5 mg. per day is absorbed.

Most cases of lead poisoning occur in children who live in homes where lead was used in the paint. Children eat the paint and thus develop signs of lead toxicity. SEE: *lead poisoning, acute; lead poisoning, chronic; pica.*

l. acetate. A lead compound that is used in solution as an astringent.

l. monoxide. A reddish-brown compound used to prepare lead subacetate.

lead apron. An apron that contains lead but is sufficiently pliable to allow it to be worn as protection from ionizing radiation. Used by fluoroscopists and dental technicians as well as patients to protect the gonads during x-ray studies of other parts of the body.

lead colic. Colic due to lead poisoning.

lead encephalopathy. A syndrome seen mostly in children that follows rapid absorption of a large amount of lead. Initially there is clumsiness, vertigo, ataxia, falling, headache, insomnia, restlessness, and irritability. With progression of the syndrome, there will be forceful vomiting, excitement, confusion, convulsions, and coma. There is also a sudden and marked increase in intracranial pressure. About 25% of those poisoned will die, and about half of the survivors show evidence of permanent damage to the central nervous system, including mental retardation, EEG abnormalities, cerebral palsy, and optic atrophy.

TREATMENT: Corticosteroids and intravenous urea will relieve increased intracranial pressure. Lead can be removed from the body by giving calcium disodium edetate, USP, followed by prolonged oral administration of penicillamine, USP.

CAUTION: Penicillamine is contraindicated in individuals with a history of sensitivity to penicillin.

lead line. Bluish line on gums in lead poisoning.

lead pipe contraction. Cataleptic condition during which limbs remain in any position in which placed.

lead poisoning, acute. Ingestion or inhalation of a large amount of lead causes anorexia, vomiting, diarrhea, headache, stupor, convulsions, and coma.

TREATMENT: Establish adequate urine flow; control convulsions with diazepam. Calcium disodium edetate and dimercaprol are administered to promote removal of lead from the body. After acute therapy is completed, penicillamine is given orally for three to six months for children and up to two months for adults.

CAUTION: Patients on penicillamine therapy must be monitored weekly for adverse reactions including diffuse erythematous rashes, angioneurotic edema, proteinuria, and neutropenia.

lead poisoning, chronic. Chronic ingestion or inhalation of lead causes damage to the central and peripheral nervous systems, the blood-forming organs, and the gastrointestinal tract.

TREATMENT: Remove patient from exposure and do not allow return to that environment or condition. Provide adequate diet with added vitamins. If hematologic disorders are present, give penicillamine as if poisoning were acute.

NURSING IMPLICATIONS: Identify causative factors and remove. Administer antiemetic as prescribed for nausea and vomiting, hemopoietic for anemia, antispasmodic for abdominal cramps, and analgesic and muscle relaxant for muscle and joint pain.

Provide tissues and disposal containers for salivation. Establish an active or passive range of motion exercise schedule to prevent muscle atrophy.

leaf (lēf) [AS.]. A plant organ usually shooting out from the side of a stem or branch; somewhat flattened and oval in shape, and green in color. SEE: *belladonna; digitalis; hyoscyamus.*

lean (lēn) [AS. *hlaene,* without flesh]. Without flesh, emaciated.

lean body mass. The weight of the body minus the fat content.

learning, latent. Learning that is inapparent, to the individual, at the time it occurs but becomes evident at a later time when the learning is facilitated beyond what would be expected in the area of the original learning.

learning disability. Inability or defect in ability to learn. Occurs in children and is manifested by difficulty in learning basic skills such as writing, reading, and mathematics.

Leber's disease (lā'bĕrz). [Theodor Leber, Ger. ophthalmologist, 1840–1917] Hereditary form of atrophy of the optic nerve that usually affects young males.

Leber's plexus. Plexus of venules in the eye between Schlemm's canal and Fontana's spaces.

Leboyer method (lĕ-boy-yā'). [Frederick Leboyer, contemporary French obstetrician] A procedure for childbirth that emphasizes the provision of a gentle and peaceful environment for the birth process. Basic to this is the physical contact between the mother and the child immediately after delivery. Caressing and massaging the infant begins immediately and is continued daily for several months. The method is believed to facilitate mental and physical development of the child.

Lecat's gulf (lā-kăz'). [Claude N. Lecat, Fr. surgeon, 1700–1768] The hollow of the bulbous portion of the urethra.

L.E. cell. Abbrev. for *lupus erythematosus,* q.v., cell. A mature neutrophilic polymorphonuclear leukocyte characteristic in lupus erythematosus.

A distinctive cell that may form when the blood of patients with systemic lupus erythematosus is incubated and further processed according to a specified method. The plasma of some patients contains an antibody to the nucleoprotein of leukocyte nuclei. These altered nuclei, which are swollen, pink, and homogenous, are ingested by phagocytes. These are the L.E. cells. The ingested material, when stained properly, is lavender in color and displaces the nucleus of the phagocyte to the edge of the cell wall. The L.E. cell phenomenon can be demonstrated in most patients with systemic lupus erythematosus but it is not essential for the diagnosis. SEE: *lupus erythematosus, systemic.*

lechery (lĕtch'ĕr-ē) [Fr. *lecher,* to lick]. Lewdness; sensualism.

lecithal (lĕs'ĭ-thăl) [Gr. *lekithos,* egg yolk]. Concerning the yolk of an egg.

lecithin (lĕs'ĭth-ĭn) [Gr. *lekithos,* egg yolk]. A fatty substance, of the group called phospholipids, found in blood, bile, brain, egg yolk, nerves, and other animal tissues, and yielding stearic acid, glycerol, phosphoric acid, and choline on hydrolysis.

lecithin/sphingomyelin ratio. ABBR: L/S ratio. The ratio of lecithin to sphingomyelin in the amniotic fluid. This is used to assess maturity of the fetal lung. Until about the 34th week of gestation the lungs produce less lecithin than sphingomyelin. As the fetal lung begins to mature, more lecithin than sphingomyelin is produced. Delivery prior to the reversal of the ratio is associated with an increased risk of hyaline membrane disease in the infant. Use of the test enables the obstetrician to determine the optimum time for elective termination of pregnancy.

NURSING IMPLICATIONS: Assist in the performance of the test. Support obstetrician's decision for pregnancy termination and provide support to mother.

lecithinase (lĕs'ĭ-thĭn-ās). An enzyme that catalyzes the decomposition of lecithin.

l., cobra. An enzyme present in certain snake venoms.

lecithoblast (lĕs'ĭ-thō-blăst") [" + *blastos,* germ]. One of the cells that proliferates to form the yolk-sac.

lecithoprotein (lĕs"ĭ-thō-prō'tē-ĭn) [" + *protos,* first]. A protein in which lecithin is part of the conjugate.

lectin (lĕk′tĭn) [L. *legere,* to pick and choose]. One of several plant proteins that stimulate lymphocytes to proliferate. Phytohemagglutinin, q.v. and concanavilin A, q.v., are lectins.

lectual (lĕkt′ū-ăl) [L. *lectus,* bed]. Pert. to a bed or couch.

LED. *light-emitting diode.*

leech (lētch) [AS. *laece*]. A bloodsucking water worm, belonging to the phylum Annelida, class Hirudinea. It is parasitic on man and other animals, producing a condition known as hirudiniasis, q.v. Leeches were at one time used as a means of blood-letting, a practice common up to the middle of the 19th century but that now has been almost completely abandoned. They are a source of hirudin, an anticoagulating principle secreted by their buccal glands.

l., artificial. Cup and suction pump or syringe for drawing blood.

lees. The sediment obtained by allowing a solution to settle, esp. the dregs at the bottom of a wine bottle.

Lee's ganglion (lēz). Cervical uterine ganglion formed from 3rd and 4th sacral nerves and hypogastric and ovarian plexuses.

Leeuwenhoek's disease (lū′ĕn-hōks). [Antonj van Leeuwenhoek, Dutch microscopist, 1632–1723] Repetitive involuntary contractions of the diaphragm and accessory muscles of respiration. The patient complains of shortness of breath and epigastric pulsations. SYN: *respiratory myoclonus.*

ETIOL: Abnormality of the respiratory control system of the brain stem.

TREATMENT: Diphenylhydantoin may be effective. If not, section of the phrenic nerve may be necessary.

left. The opposite of right. SYN: *sinistral.*

left-handedness. Condition of being more adept in use of left hand. SYN: *sinistrality.*

left lateral recumbent position. Position where patient is on left side with right knee and thigh drawn up. Used in rectal operations and sometimes used in obstetrics.

leg (lĕg) [ME.]. One of the two lower extremities, including the femur, tibia, fibula, and patella; specifically the part between the knee and ankle. SEE: illus.

RS: Buerger's disease; calf; crural; crus; saphena; saphenous; sura; systremma; thrombophlebitis; tibia.

l., Anglesey. A form of jointed artificial leg.

l., badger. Inequality in the length of the legs.

l., baker. Genu valgum; knock-knee.

l., bandy. L., bow-.

l., Barbadoes. Elephantiasis of the legs.

l., bayonet. Uncorrected backward displacement of the knee bones, followed by ankylosis at the joint.

l., bird. Reduction in size of the leg as a result of atrophy of the muscles.

l., boomerang. A disease of the leg bones occurring among Australian natives, causing a curvature of the leg resembling a boomerang.

l., bow-. An outward curving of the legs at the knees. SYN: *bandy leg; genu varum.*

l., milk. Phlebitis of the femoral vein occasionally following parturition and typhoid fever. It is characterized by swelling of the leg, usually without redness. SYN: *phlegmasia alba dolens; white leg.*

l., restless. A sense of uneasiness and uncomfortableness of the legs that comes on at bedtime. Moving the legs tends to relieve the condition. This syndrome is sometimes present at the onset of renal colic due to renal calculi.

l., scissor. Crossed-leg deformity, a result of double hip disease, in which the patient walks with the legs swinging across the midline with each step.

l., white. L., milk. SEE: *phlegmasia alba dolens.*

Legg-Calvé-Perthes' disease (lĕg′kăl-vā′pĕr′tĕz). [Arthur T. Legg, Boston surgeon, 1874–1939; Jacques Calvé, Fr. orthopedist, 1875–1954; Georg C. Perthes, Ger. surgeon, 1869–1927] Legg's disease, q.v.

Legg's disease (lĕgz). [Arthur T. Legg] Osteochondritis of the upper femoral epiphysis. SYN: *Legg-Calvé-Perthes' disease.*

leggings (lĕg′gĭngs) [ME. *leg,* leg]. Sterile leg coverings used on patient while in operating room.

Legionnaires disease. [after individuals stricken while attending an American Legion convention in Philadelphia, PA, in 1976] A severe, often fatal disease characterized by pneumonia, dry cough, myalgia, and sometimes gastrointestinal symptoms. As the disease progresses, there is evidence of dysfunction of other major organs, and in fatal cases, there is eventual cardiovascular collapse. SYN: *legionellosis.*

ETIOL: A gram-negative bacillus not previously recognized as an agent of human disease. The organism has been termed Legionella pneumophila.

TREATMENT: Erythromycin given early in the course of the disease and for a prolonged period is the drug of choice.

legitimacy (lĕ-jĭt′ĭ-mă-sē) [L. *legitimus,* lawful]. 1. Condition of being legal. 2. Condition of being born in wedlock.

legume (lĕ′gūm) [L. *legumen,* pulse, bean]. Fruit or pod of beans, peas, or lentils.

COMP: Nitrogen: almost equal to that in meat. Legumin, a globulin, is present.

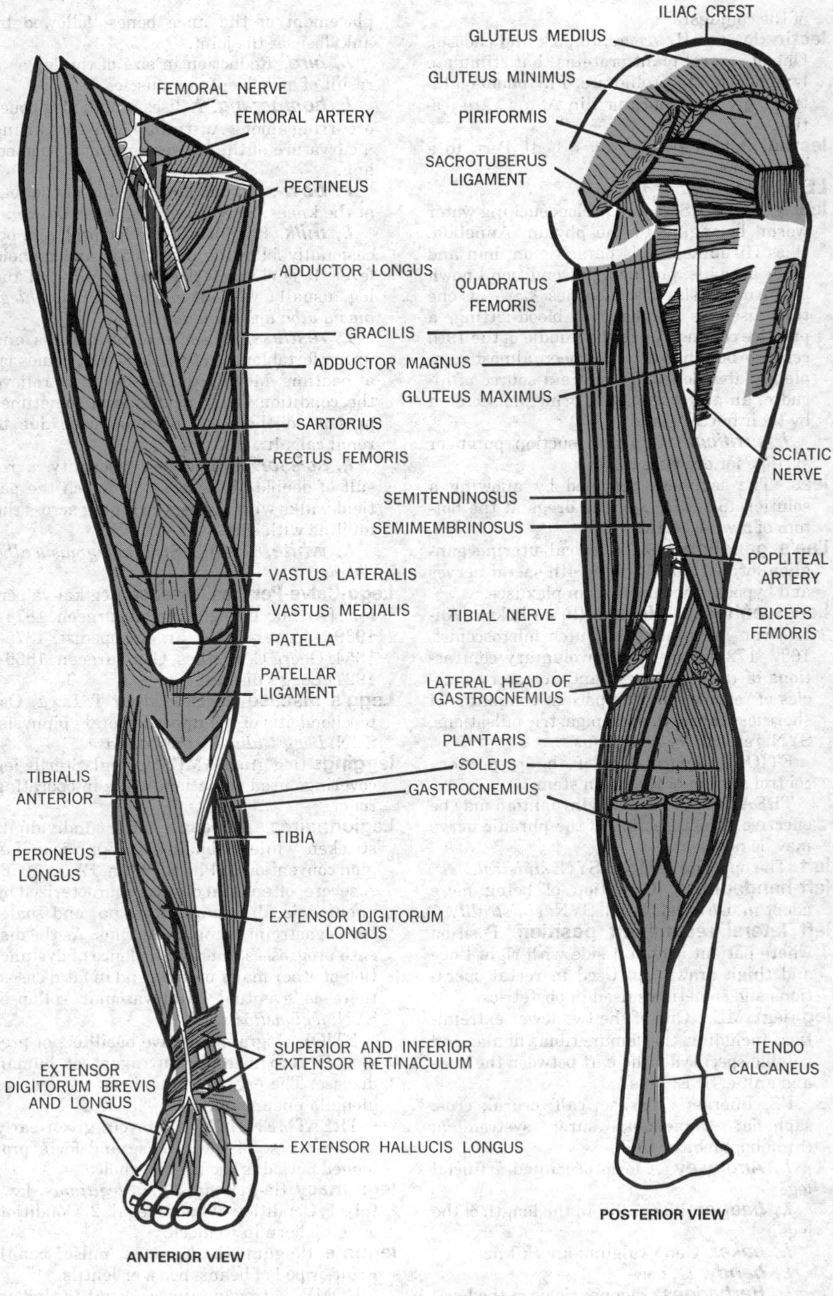
ILIAC CREST
GLUTEUS MEDIUS
GLUTEUS MINIMUS
PIRIFORMIS
SACROTUBERUS LIGAMENT
QUADRATUS FEMORIS
GLUTEUS MAXIMUS
SCIATIC NERVE
SEMITENDINOSUS
SEMIMEMBRINOSUS
POPLITEAL ARTERY
TIBIAL NERVE
BICEPS FEMORIS
LATERAL HEAD OF GASTROCNEMIUS
PLANTARIS
SOLEUS
GASTROCNEMIUS
TENDO CALCANEUS
POSTERIOR VIEW
FEMORAL NERVE
FEMORAL ARTERY
PECTINEUS
ADDUCTOR LONGUS
GRACILIS
ADDUCTOR MAGNUS
SARTORIUS
RECTUS FEMORIS
VASTUS LATERALIS
VASTUS MEDIALIS
PATELLA
PATELLAR LIGAMENT
TIBIALIS ANTERIOR
TIBIA
PERONEUS LONGUS
EXTENSOR DIGITORUM LONGUS
SUPERIOR AND INFERIOR EXTENSOR RETINACULUM
EXTENSOR DIGITORUM BREVIS AND LONGUS
EXTENSOR HALLUCIS LONGUS
ANTERIOR VIEW

MUSCLES OF LEG

VITAMINS: (sprouted beans): A good source of vitamin B complex. Vitamin A and ascorbic acid are present in small amounts.

CARBOHYDRATES: Generally in the form of starch in about the same proportion as the cereals but with more cellulose.

legumelin (lĕg-ū'mĕl-ĭn) [L. *legumen*, pulse, bean]. An albumin present in many leguminous seeds, as in peas. SEE: *legume; legumin*.

legumin (lĕ-gū'mĭn). A globulin present in legumes such as peas and beans.

Leiner's disease (lī'nĕrz). [Karl Leiner, Austrian pediatrician, 1871–1930] Exfoliative dermatitis.

leiodermia (lī"ō-dĕr'mē-ă) [Gr. *leios*, smooth, + *derma*, skin]. Dermatitis characterized by abnormal glossiness and smoothness of the skin.

leiomyofibroma (lī"ō-mī"ō-fī-brō'mă) [" + *mys*, muscle, + L. *fibra*, fiber, + Gr. *oma*, tumor]. A benign tumor composed principally of smooth muscle and fibrous connective tissue.

leiomyoma (lī"ō-mī-ō'mă) [" + " + *oma*, tumor]. Myoma consisting principally of smooth muscle tissue.

l., epitheloid. Smooth muscle tumor, usually of the stomach.

l. uteri. Fibroma, uterine, q.v.

leiomyosarcoma (lī"ō-mī"ō-săr-kō'mă) [" + " + *sarx*, flesh, + *oma*, tumor]. Combined leiomyoma and sarcoma.

leiotrichous (lī-ŏt'rĭ-kŭs) [" + *thrix*, hair]. Possessing smooth or straight hair.

Leishman-Donovan bodies. SEE: *body, Leishman-Donovan*.

Leishmania (lēsh-mā'nē-ă). [Sir William B. Leishman, Brit. medical officer, 1865–1926] A genus of parasitic flagellate protozoa that occur as typical leishmanian forms in vertebrate hosts but as leptomonad forms in invertebrate hosts or in cultures. They are transmitted by the bite of the female phlebotomines (sandflies).

L. braziliensis. Causative agent of American leishmaniasis.

L. donovani. Causative agent of kala-azar (visceral leishmaniasis).

L. tropica. Causative agent of Oriental sore (cutaneous leishmaniasis).

leishmaniasis (lēsh"mă-nī'ă-sĭs). Infection with a species of Leishmania, affecting the skin, nasal cavities, and pharynx. One form causes Oriental sore and another kala-azar.

l., American. Leishmaniasis caused by L. braziliensis, involving principally nasopharyngeal and mucocutaneous membranes. Common in Central and South America.

l., cutaneous. Leishmaniasis due to infection with L. tropica. SYN: *aleppo boil; Oriental sore*.

l., mucocutaneous. A form of cutaneous leishmaniasis found in parts of Central and South America. The causative organism is Leishmania braziliensis transmitted by sandflies usually of the genus Lutzomyia. SYN: *American leishmaniasis*.

l., visceral. Leishmaniasis caused by L. donovani. SYN: *kala-azar*.

lema (lē'mă) [Gr. *leme*]. The dried secretion of the tarsal glands that collects in the inner canthus of the eye. SYN: *sebum palpebrale*.

lemic (lē'mĭk) [Gr. *loimos*, plague]. Concerning an epidemic disease.

lemmocyte (lĕm'ō-sīt) [Gr. *lemma*, husk, + *kytos*, cell]. A cell that becomes a neurilemma cell. SEE: *nerve fiber*.

lemniscus (lĕm-nĭs'kŭs) [Gr. *lemniskos*, a ribbon]. (pl. *lemnisci*) [NA] A bundle of sensory fibers (lateral or exterior and median or interior) in the medulla and pons.

lemon [Persian *limun*, lemon]. Fruit of the tree Citrus limonia, containing citrus acid. Lemons contain enough ascorbic acid to prevent or treat scurvy.

May be used in place of vinegar, spices, and aromatic substances by those who cannot use the latter. Diabetics may use.

CAUTION: Food faddists who drink large quantities of lemon juice by sucking directly from the raw fruit may develop erosion of the enamel of their teeth.

lemoparalysis (lē"mō-pă-răl'ĭ-sĭs) [Gr. *laimos*, gullet, + *para*, beside, + *lyein*, to loosen]. Paralysis of the esophagus.

lemostenosis [" + *stenosis*, a narrowing]. Stricture of the esophagus.

length. Measurement of the distance between two points.

l., basialveolar. Distance from the basion of the foramen magnum of the skull to the intermaxillary suture of the jaw.

l., basinasal. Distance from the basion of the foramen magnum of the skull to the center of the suture between the frontal and nasal bones.

l., crown-heel. In the embryo, fetus, or newborn, the distance from the crown of the head to the heel.

l., crown-rump. In the embryo, fetus, or newborn, the distance from the crown of the head to the apex of the buttocks.

l., focal. In optics, the distance from the lens to the point of focus of light rays passing through the lens.

l., wave. In the line of progression of a wave, the distance from one point on the wave to the same point on the next wave. The length of a wave determines whether or not the wave is visible light, x-ray, gamma, or radio waves.

lenitive (lĕn'ĭ-tĭv) [L. *lenire*, to soothe]. 1. Demulcent, soothing, slightly laxative. 2. A palliative.

lens (lĕnz) [L. *lens,* lentil]. 1. A transparent refracting medium; usually made of glass. 2. [NA] The crystalline lens of the eye.

RS: capsulociliary; circle of diffusion; vitreous chamber.

l., achromatic. Lens that corrects chromatic aberration.

l., aplanatic. Lens that corrects spherical aberrations.

l., apochromatic. Lens that corrects both spherical and chromatic aberrations.

l., biconcave. A lens that has a concave surface on each side. SEE: *biconcave* for illus.

l., biconvex. A lens that has a convex surface on each side. SEE: *biconvex* for illus.

l., bifocal. Corrective lens containing in either its upper or lower segment a lens of different power. The main lens is for distant vision; the secondary lens is for near vision.

l., concave spherical. Lens formed of prisms with their apices together and, therefore, thin at the center and thick at the edge. Used in myopia.

l., contact. A custom-fitted curved lens of glass or synthetic material that is applied to the eye for correction of refractive errors.

l., convexconcave. A lens that has a convex surface on one side and a concave surface on the opposite side.

l., convex spherical. Lens formed of prisms with their bases together and, therefore, thick at the center and thin at the edge. Used in hyperopia.

l., corneal contact. A type of contact lens that adheres to and covers only the cornea.

l., crystalline. Transparent colorless structure in the eye, biconvex in shape, enclosed in a capsule, and held in place just behind the pupil by the suspensory ligament. Consists principally of lens fibers that at the periphery are soft, forming the cortex lentis, and in the center of harder consistency, forming the nucleus lentis. Beneath the capsule on the anterior surface is a thin layer of cells, the lens epithelium. Function is to focus rays so they form a perfect image on the retina.

l., cylindrical. Segment of a cylinder parallel to its axis, used in correcting astigmatism.

l., implanted. An artificial lens implanted at the time a cataract is removed. This procedure may also be used in correcting other lens defects.

l., omnifocal. A lens used in making eyeglasses. Its power to alter light rays varies from the top to the bottom of the lens. This permits a smooth transition from one power lens to the other as one moves the eyes. This is in contrast to an eyeglass lens that has the usual two component bifocal lenses.

l., orthoscopic. A lens that produces no distortion of the periphery of the image.

l., soft contact. Contact lens for correcting refractive errors. They are of soft plastic material and cause less discomfort than conventional contact lenses.

l., spherical. A lens in which all surfaces are spherical.

l., trial. Any lens used in testing the vision.

l., trifocal. Corrective lens containing three segments: one for near, intermediate, and distant vision.

lentectomy (lĕn-tĕk'tō-mē) [L. *lens,* lentil, + Gr. *ektome,* excision]. Surgical removal of the lens of the eye.

lenticonus (lĕn"tĭ-kō'nŭs) [" + *conus,* cone]. Conical protrusion of the anterior or posterior surface of the lens.

lenticular [L. *lenticularis,* pert. to a lens]. 1. Lens shaped. SYN: *lentiform.* 2. Pert. to a lens.

lenticular fossa. Depression in the anterior surface of the vitreous for reception of the crystalline lens.

lenticular glands. Small masses of lymphatic tissue in the lamina propria of the pyloric region of the stomach.

lenticular nucleus. Mass of gray matter forming part of the corpus striatum. Consists of the putamen and globus pallidus.

lenticulostriate (lĕn-tĭk"ū-lō-strī'āt) [" + *striatus,* streaked]. Rel. to the lenticular nucleus and corpus striatum.

lenticulothalamic. Pert. to the lenticular nucleus and the thalamus.

lentiform (lĕnt'ĭ-form) [L. *lens,* lentil, + *forma,* shape]. Lentil or lens shaped. SYN: *lenticular.*

lentiginosis (lĕn-tĭj"ĭ-nō'sĭs) [L. *lentigo,* freckle, + Gr. *osis,* condition]. Presence of multiple lentigines.

lentiginous (lĕn-tĭj'ĭn-ŭs) [L. *lentigo,* freckle]. 1. Affected by lentigo. 2. Covered with very small dots.

lentiglobus (lĕn"tĭ-glō'bŭs) [L. *lens,* lentil, + *globus,* sphere]. A lens of the eye that has extreme anterior spherical bulging.

lentigo (lĕn-tī'gō) [L., freckle]. (pl. *lentigines*) Small brown macules or yellow-brown pigmented areas on skin sometimes caused by exposure to sun and weather. SYN: *ephelis; freckle.*

l. maligna. A noninvasive malignant melanotic freckle. SYN: *freckle, Hutchinson's.*

lentitis (lĕn-tī'tĭs) [L. *lens,* lentil, + Gr. *itis,* inflammation]. Inflammation of the crystalline lens. SYN: *phakitis.*

leontiasis (lē"ŏn-tī'ă-sĭs) [Gr. *leon,* lion, + *-iasis,* condition]. Lionlike appearance of the face, accompanying certain diseases, esp.

lepromatous leprosy.

l. ossea. Enlargement and distortion of facial bones, giving one the appearance of a lion. The condition is rare and not fatal.

leotropic (lē-ō-trŏp'ĭk) [Gr. *laios,* left, + *tropos,* a turning]. Wound in a spiral form going from right to left.

leper (lĕp'ĕr) [Gr. *lepros,* scaly]. Person afflicted with leprosy.

lepidic (lĕ-pĭd'ĭk) [Gr. *lepis,* scale]. Concerning scales, or a scaly covering.

lepido- [Gr. *lepis,* scale]. Combining form referring to flakes or scales.

Lepidoptera (lĕp"ĭ-dŏp'tĕr-ă) [" + *pteron,* feather, wing]. An order of the class Insecta that includes the butterflies, moths, and skippers. Characterized by scaly wings, sucking mouth parts, and complete metamorphosis.

lepidosis (lĕp"ĭ-dō'sĭs) [" + *osis,* condition]. Any scaly or desquamating eruption such as pityriasis.

lepothrix (lĕp'ō-thrĭks) [" + *thrix,* hair]. Condition in which the shaft of the hair is encased in hardened, scaly, sebaceous matter.

lepra (lĕp'ră) [Gr. *lepra,* leprosy]. A term formerly used for leprosy. Now used to indicate a reaction that occurs in leprosy patients consisting of aggravation of lesions accompanied by fever and malaise. This can occur in any form of leprosy and may be prolonged.

l. alba. Skin is anesthetic and white, and different forms of paralysis follow.

l. anesthetica. Leprosy with anesthetic areas on body.

l. Arabum. True or nodular leprosy.

l. maculosa. Form of lepra with pigmented cutaneous areas.

l. mutilans. Final stage of true leprosy.

l. nervorum. Maculo-anesthetic leprosy.

leprechaunism (lĕp'rĕ-kŏn"ĭzm). Hereditary disease in which the elfin features of the face are accompanied by retardation of physical and mental development, a variety of endocrine disorders, emaciation, and susceptibility to infections. SYN: *Donohue's syndrome.*

leprid (lĕp'rĭd) [Gr. *lepra,* leprosy, + *eidos,* form]. Leprous cutaneous lesion.

leprology (lĕp-rŏl'ō-jē) [" + *logos,* study]. The study of leprosy and methods of treating it.

leproma (lĕp-rō'mă) [" + *oma,* tumor]. A cutaneous nodule or tubercle characteristic of leprosy.

lepromatous (lĕp-rō'mă-tŭs). Concerning lepromas. SEE: *leprosy.*

lepromin (lĕp'rō-mĭn). A substance prepared from lepromatous nodules of leprosy.

lepromin skin test. Test in which lepromin is introduced intradermally to attempt to diagnose leprosy. The test is positive in individuals with tuberculoid leprosy and is negative in individuals with the lepromatous form.

leprosarium. An institution for the care of lepers.

leprostatic (lĕp"rō-stăt'ĭk) [" + *statikos,* standing]. Either inhibiting the growth of Mycobacterium leprae, or an agent that inhibits that organism's growth.

leprosy (lĕp'rō-sē) [Gr. *lepros,* scaly]. A chronic communicable disease caused by the acid-fast Mycobacterium leprae. It may occur in various clinical forms. The two principal forms are lepromatous and tuberculoid. SYN: *Hansen's disease.*

The *lepromatous* form is characterized by skin lesions and symmetrical involvement of peripheral nerves with anesthesia, muscle weakness, and paralysis. In this form, the lesions are limited to the cooler portions of the body such as skin, upper respiratory tract, and testes. In *tuberculoid* leprosy, which is usually benign, the nerve lesions are asymmetrical and skin anesthesia is an early occurrence. Visceral involvement is not seen. Because of the anesthesia, rats have been able to remove digits while the patient sleeps. For some time this loss of digits was thought, erroneously, to be due only to spontaneous amputation as a part of the disease process.

Lepromatous leprosy is much more contagious than the tuberculoid form. In the latter, Mycobacterium leprae are found only rarely except during reactions.

Between the two major forms are *borderline* and *indeterminate* leprosy. In the borderline group, the clinical and bacteriological features represent a combination of the two principal types. In the indeterminate group, there are fewer skin lesions and bacteria are much less abundant in the lesions. In many respects, this infection resembles tuberculosis and for many years was regarded as incurable, a conclusion no longer considered true.

ETIOL: Caused by Mycobacterium leprae. May occur at practically any age.

INCUBATION: From 1 to 30 years.

SYM: Onset very gradual. The first signs of infection are usually skin changes, but they may be so nonspecific and so slow to progress as to go unrecognized for years.

DIAG: Biopsy of a suspected skin lesion. The bacilli may not be present in tuberculoid lesions. In vitro tests of the immunologic response can be accomplished by the lymphocyte transformation test and the leukocyte migration inhibition test. SEE: *lepromin skin test.*

COMPLICATIONS: Bacterial infections of skin, ulcers, traumatic amputation of fingers due to anesthesia. Tuberculosis is a much more common complication in untreated cases of lepromatous leprosy than in the tuberculoid form. Amyloidosis may be the cause of death in advanced cases.

PROG: With proper therapy, the outlook for recovery is good.

TREATMENT: Dapsone (4,4′-diaminodiphenyl sulfone, DDS) is the form of sulfone most commonly used. If dapsone is not tolerated, sulfoxone may be substituted. Rifampin, clofazimine, and thalidomide (not to be used in those at risk of becoming pregnant) are experimentally used in patients with sulfone-resistant bacilli.

Treatment may be complicated by an acute reversal reaction in tuberculoid or indeterminate forms of leprosy in which the lesions become erythematous and edematous and may become necrotic and ulcerated. Also, the erythema nodosum leprosum (ENL) reaction may develop. This occurs most commonly during the end of the first year of therapy. In this reaction, multiple painful red nodules develop and then may become ulcerated and necrotic; they may last a short time, but new lesions appear. The ENL reaction may be of short or long duration.

The management of patients with leprosy is complex and may require expert consultation. Such assistance may be obtained by contacting physicians at the U.S. Public Health Service Hospital, Carville, Louisiana 70721.

Segregation of patients in colonies or hospitals until bacterial tests have been negative for six months is not the preferred or effective method of isolating patients. Ambulatory treatment of patients at general clinics has been found to be much more effective. Because they are more susceptible to this disease than adults, children should be removed from contact with leprosy patients.

leprotic (lěp-rŏt′ĭk) [Gr. *lepra,* leprosy]. 1. Rel. to leprosy. 2. Affected with leprosy. SYN: *leprous.*

leprous (lěp′rŭs). 1. Pert. to leprosy. 2. Affected by leprosy. SYN: *leprotic.*

leptocephalia (lěp″tō-sĕ-fā′lē-ă) [Gr. *leptos,* slender, + *kephale,* head]. Having an abnormally vertically elongated, narrow skull.

leptocephalus. An individual possessing an abnormally vertically elongated, narrow skull.

leptochromatic (lěp″tō-krō-măt′ĭk) [″ + *chromatin*]. Having a fine chromatin network.

leptocyte (lěp′tō-sīt) [″ + *kytos,* cell]. Target cell, q.v.

leptocytosis (lěp″tō-sī-tō′sĭs) [″ + ″ + *osis,* condition]. Presence of leptocytes in the blood. SEE: *target cell.*

leptodactyly (lěp″tō-dăk′tĭ-lē) [″ + *daktylos,* finger]. Abnormally slim fingers.

leptomeninges (lěp″tō-mĕn-ĭn′jēs) [″ + *meninx,* membrane]. (sing. *leptomeninx*) The pia mater and arachnoid as distinct from the dura mater, because of their thinner and more delicate structure.

leptomeningitis (lěp″tō-mĕn-ĭn-jī′tĭs) [″ + ″ + *itis,* inflammation]. Inflammation of the pia and arachnoid membranes. SYN: *piarachnitis.* SEE: *meningitis.*

ETIOL: Tubercle bacillus, spirochete of syphilis, and other organisms.

SYM: Acute headache, pain in back, rigidity of spine, irritability, drowsiness ending in coma. Clinically, it cannot be distinguished from pachymeningitis, q.v.

leptomeningopathy (lěp″tō-mĕn″ĭn-gŏp′ă-thē) [″ + ″ + *pathos,* disease]. Disease of the leptomeninges of the brain.

leptomeninx. Sing. of leptomeninges.

leptonema (lěp″tō-nē′mă) [″ + *nema,* thread]. Early stage of prophase in meiosis. At this stage the chromatin contracts into long, thin filaments. SEE: *cell division.*

leptopellic (lěp″tō-pĕl′ĭk) [″ + *pellis,* basin]. Having an abnormally narrow pelvis.

leptophonia (lěp″tō-fō′nē-ă) [″ + *phone,* voice]. Weakness or feebleness of voice.

leptoprosopia (lěp″tō-prō-sō′pē-ă) [″ + *prosopon,* face]. Narrowness of the face.

leptorhine, leptorrhine (lěp′tor-rīn) [″ + *rhis,* nose]. Having a very thin or slender nose.

leptoscope (lěp′tō-skōp) [″ + *skopein,* to examine]. Optical device for measuring the thickness of cell membranes.

leptosome (lěp′tō-sōm) [″ + *soma,* body]. Person of thin, slight stature.

Leptospira (lěp-tō-spī′ră) [″ + *speira,* coil]. Genus of thin, spiral, and hook-ended spirochetes.

L. autumnalis. A species of spirochetes first isolated in Japan. Causes a nonicteric infection in man called pretibial or Fort Bragg fever.

L. hebdomadis. Species causing seven-day fever in Japan.

L. icterohaemorrhagiae. Species causing infectious, hemorrhagic, spirochetal jaundice (Weil's disease, q.v.).

leptospire (lěp′tō-spīr). Any organism belonging to the genus Leptospira.

leptospirosis (lěp″tō-spī-rō′sĭs) [″ + ″ + *osis,* condition]. Condition resulting from Leptospira infection.

leptospiruria (lěp″tō-spīr-ū′rē-ă) [″ + ″ + *ouron,* urine]. Presence of Leptospira organisms in the urine.

leptotene (lěp′tō-tēn) [″ + *tainia,* ribbon]. The initial stage of the prophase of cell division. The chromosomes become visible as separate entities but are not yet paired.

leptothricosis (lěp″tō-thrī-kō′sĭs) [″ + *thrix,* hair]. Disease from Leptothrix infection.

Leptus autumnalis. Parasitic mite larvae causing itch and sometimes wheals. SEE:

chiggers.

leresis (lĕ-rē'sĭs) [Gr.]. Loquacity in old age; garrulousness.

Leriche's syndrome (lĕ-rēsh'ēz). [René Leriche, Fr. surgeon, 1879–1955] Occlusion of the abdominal aorta by a thrombus at its bifurcation. This causes intermittent ischemic pain, i.e., claudication, in the lower extremities and buttocks, impotence, and absent or diminished femoral pulses.

Leri's pleonosteosis (lā'rēz). [André Leri, Fr. physician, 1875–1930] A form of hereditary physical malformation characterized by upward slanting palpebral fissures, broad thumbs, short stature, and flexion contractures of the fingers.

lesbian (lĕs'bē-ăn) [Gr. *lesbios,* pert. to island of Lesbos]. 1. Pert. to lesbianism, q.v., or sexual desire in women for those of their own sex. SEE: *homosexual; bisexual.* 2. One who practices lesbianism.

lesbianism. Sexual desire of women for one of their own sex. SYN: *sapphism.*

Named from the Island of Lesbos wherein the practice of lesbianism was reputed to have been general in ancient days.

Lesch-Nyhan disease. [M. Lesch, b. 1939, W. L. Nyhan, b. 1926, U.S. pediatricians] An inherited metabolic disease that affects only males. Clinically there is mental retardation, aggressive behavior, self-mutilation, and renal failure. Biochemically there is excess uric acid production due to a virtual absence of an enzyme essential for purine metabolism.

lesion (lē'zhŭn) [L. *laesio,* a wound]. 1. A circumscribed area of pathologically altered tissue. 2. An injury or wound. 3. Single infected patch in a skin disease.

Primary or initial lesions include macules, vesicles, blebs or bullae, chancres, pustules, papules, tubercles, wheals, and tumors, q.v. Secondary lesions are the result of primary lesions. They may be crusts, excoriations, fissures, pigmentations, scales, scars, and ulcers, q.v.

RS: abscess; boil; cancer; carbuncle; cerebropsychosis; chancre; chancroid; felon; gumma; mole; neoplasm; pimple; pus; rash; sebaceous cyst; tumefaction; verruca; wound.

l., degenerative. Lesion caused by or showing degeneration.

l., diffuse. Lesion spreading over a large area.

l., discharging. 1. Brain lesion that discharges nervous impulses. 2. Lesion that discharges an exudate.

l., focal. Lesion of a small definite area.

l., indiscriminate. Lesion affecting separate systems of the body.

l., initial, of syphilis. Hard chancre. SEE: *chancre; syphilis.*

l., irritative. Lesion that stimulates or excites activity in the part of the body where it is situated.

l., local. Lesion of nervous system origin giving rise to local symptoms.

l., peripheral. Lesion of the nerve endings.

l., primary. First lesion of a disease, esp. used in referring to chancre of syphilis, q.v.

l., structural. A lesion that causes change in tissue.

l., systemic. Lesion confined to organs of common function.

l., toxic. Lesion resulting from poisons or toxins from microorganisms.

l., vascular. Lesion of a blood vessel.

L.E.T. *linear energy transfer.* A measure of the rate of energy transfer from ionizing radiation to soft tissue.

lethal [Gr. *lethe,* oblivion]. Pert. to or that which causes death.

lethargic (lĕ-thăr'jĭk) [Gr. *lethargos,* drowsiness]. 1. Affected with lethargy. 2. Rel. to lethargy. 3. Sluggish.

lethargy (lĕth'ăr-jē) [Gr. *lethargos,* drowsiness]. A condition of functional torpor or sluggishness; stupor.

l., African. Sleeping sickness. SEE: *encephalitis lethargica.*

l., hysteric. The sleep of hypnotic lethargy, the state in which many cases of apparent death and resurrection are found.

l., induced. Hypnotic trance.

l., lucid. Retention of intellect but loss of will power with a consequent total lack of muscular response. The subject knows what is going on, resents it perhaps, but is unable to exercise sufficient will to bring about muscular defense.

lethe (lē'thē) [Gr., oblivion]. Amnesia.

lethologica (lĕth-ō-lŏj'ĭ-kă) [Gr. *lethe,* forgetfulness, + *logos,* word]. Temporary inability to remember a word or name, or an intended action.

Letterer-Siwe disease (lĕt'ĕr-ĕr-sī'wē). [Erich Letterer, Ger. physician, b 1895; S. August Siwe, Ger. physician, b. 1897] A histiocytosis syndrome characterized by proliferation of histiocytes in the viscera and bones. The spleen and liver are enlarged, and there is widespread pulmonary infiltration. There is bone marrow failure accompanied by fever and severe infections. The skin is involved and a variety of lesions are present, including papulovesicular eruption and inflamed pruritic lesions around the anal and vaginal areas. The cause is unknown and there is no specific treatment. If the visceral lesions progress, death is the usual outcome. It is felt that this disease, eosinophilic granuloma of bone, Hand-Schüller-Christian syndrome, histiocytosis X, and reticuloendotheliosis share a common pattern of the development of granulomatous lesions with histiocytic proliferation.

Leu. *leucine.*

leuc-. SEE: words beginning with *leuk-*.

leucine (loo'sĭn) [Gr. *leukos,* white]. $C_6H_{13}NO_2$. Alpha-amino-isobutyl acetic acid, an amino acid found among the products of digestion of proteins. It is present in body tissues and is essential for normal growth and metabolism.

leucine aminopeptidase. ABBR: LAP. A proteolytic enzyme present in the pancreas, liver, and small intestine. Its serum level is elevated in disease of the pancreas, esp. acute pancreatitis, and in obstruction of the common bile duct.

leucinosis (loo"sĭn-ō'sĭs) [" + *osis,* condition]. Excess of leucine in the body, thus producing leucine in the urine.

leucinuria (loo"sĭn-ū'rē-ă) [" + *ouron,* urine]. Presence of leucine in urine.

leucism (loo'sĭzm) [" + *-ismos,* condition]. A form of incomplete albinism.

leucismus (loo-sĭz'mŭs) [" + *-ismos,* condition]. Condition of being white.

leucitis (loo-sī'tĭs) [" + *itis,* inflammation]. Inflammation of the sclera. SYN: *scleritis.*

leucovorin calcium (loo"kō-vō'rĭn). USP. The calcium salt of folic acid. It is used in the treatment of megaloblastic anemias. It is also used to antagonize the effect of methotrexate on normal cells when methotrexate is being used to treat malignancies. When so used, large doses of leucovorin are required and the optimum timing and dosage are difficult to establish. This use is called leucovorin "rescue."

leukapheresis (loo"kă-fĕ-rē'sĭs) [" + *aphairesis,* removal]. Separation of leukocytes from blood that is then transfused back into the patient.

leukemia (loo-kē'mē-ă) [Gr. *leukos,* white, + *haima,* blood]. A chronic or acute disease of unknown etiological factors characterized by unrestrained growth of leukocytes and their precursors in the tissues. Leukemia is classified according to the dominant cell type and severity of the disease.

l., acute granulocytic. L., acute myeloblastic, q.v.

l., acute lymphatic. Progressive type of leukemia that causes death in untreated patients within four to six months of onset. Certain types of acute leukemia are described below but the symptoms of various forms are similar.

SYM AND SIGNS: Most of the clinical abnormalities are due to failure of the bone marrow to function adequately. Thus the patient develops anemia, infections, bleeding as a result of thrombocytopenia, and fatigue. Other abnormalities are due to interference by infiltrating leukocytes with the function of organs such as the spleen and liver and function of the lymph nodes and nervous system. Patients are pale and have purpura, bone pain, esp. children, and usually hepatosplenomegaly with splenomegaly being more frequent. The white cell count is usually between 10,000 and 50,000/cu. mm. (normally 5,000 to 10,000), but may be leukopenic.

NURSING IMPLICATIONS: Monitor hematology results and establish infectious precautions for patients experiencing leukopenia. Administer chemotherapeutic agents as prescribed and document. Teach the patient and family about the chemotherapeutic agents being administered and the importance of compliance to the regimen. Provide support and reassurance during periods of exacerbation. Reassure patient that adverse side effects from chemotherapy will subside shortly after the drug is discontinued.

TREATMENT: A variety of chemotherapeutic agents are used in treating those with acute leukemia, and new drugs and combinations of old and new drugs are being developed and tried. These include: cytarabine, mercaptopurine, vincristine, prednisone, cyclophosphamide, and daunorubicin. Therapy of acute granulocytic leukemia is less effective than that of acute lymphocytic leukemia. Even though the agents used are effective in interfering with the proliferation of leukemic cells, they also destroy normal cells.

PROG: About 90% of patients treated while under age 20 will experience a remission that will last one to three years. Apparent cure may be achieved in one third of patients treated for 30 months.

l., acute monoblastic. A form of acute leukemia in which the basic abnormality is a generalized progressive proliferation of reticuloendothelial elements with invasion of the blood, bone marrow, and other tissues by abnormal monocytes.

l., acute myeloblastic. Leukemia that usually occurs in adults. There are six different types, classified according to the type of myelocyte involved, i.e., myeloblastic cell without maturation; myeloblastic cell with maturation; promyelocyte; myelomonocyte; monocytic; and erythroleukemia. The clinical signs and symptoms are similar to those of acute lymphatic leukemia.

TREATMENT: Combinations of daunomycin, cytarabine, and thioguanine are used. Allopurinol is used to prevent uric acid uropathy. Marrow transplant has been used in young patients who are in complete remission and who have a histocompatible sibling.

PROG: Fifty percent of treated patients will have a remission that will last about one year. Survival may be for as long as several years.

l., aleukemic. Any type of leukemia in which the total white blood count is normal or subnormal.

l., basophilic. A rare form of leukemia in which the predominant cell in the peripheral blood is the basophil.

l., chronic lymphatic. A generalized and progressive leukemia in which there is abnormal proliferation of lymphoid tissues affecting esp. the small lymphocytes.

ETIOL: Unknown, but it has been observed that this type of leukemia appears in families with the disease with much greater frequency than in control groups. Chronic lymphatic leukemia is rare under age 30 and is quite rare in Orientals.

SYM AND SIGNS: The accumulation of abnormal lymphocytes varies considerably from patient to patient and thus the progress of the disease varies from almost acute to benign. Fatigue with diminished exercise tolerance is an early clinical manifestation. Lymph nodes are superficial and the spleen may be enlarged.

l., chronic myelocytic. A neoplastic disease associated with a unique chromosome abnormality (Philadelphia chromosome). The clinical manifestations relate to the excessive overgrowth of granulocytes in the bone marrow.

ETIOL: About 90% of the patients have an abnormality of the chromosome that has been named the Philadelphia chromosome (Ph^1). This abnormality is thought to be acquired or induced rather than being present from birth. Ionizing radiations have been proven to have the ability to induce chronic lymphocytic leukemia but not over 1 in 15 to 20 of individuals who develop the disease have a history of exposure to radiation.

SYM AND SIGNS: Fatigue, malaise, pallor, anemia, aching of bones, bleeding tendency with retinal hemorrhages, ecchymoses, and hematuria. Hepatosplenomegaly, fever, warm moist skin, and sternal tenderness are usually present.

TREATMENT: A variety of chemotherapeutic agents that have the ability to control cell proliferation.

l., eosinophilic. A rare form of leukemia in which the predominant cell in the peripheral blood is the eosinophil.

l., lymphosarcoma cell. A term used to describe a type of lymphocytic leukemia in which the circulating lymphocytes are large, reticulated, and immature.

l., mast cell. A rare form of leukemia caused by proliferation of mast cells.

l., myelocytic; l., myelogenous; l., myeloid. L., acute myeloblastic, q.v.

l., plasma cell. Leukemia in which the predominant cell in the peripheral blood is the plasma cell.

l., promyelocytic. A form of acute granulocytic leukemia.

l., stem cell. A form of leukemia in which the predominant cell type is a cell too immature to classify.

l., subleukemic. L., aleukemic, q.v.

leukemic (loo-kēm′ĭk) [″ + *haima,* blood]. 1. Rel. to leukemia. 2. Affected with leukemia.

leukemid (loo-kē′mĭd). Any nonspecific skin lesion associated with leukemia. The lesions may or may not contain leukemia cells.

leukemogenesis (loo-kē″mō-jĕn′ĕ-sĭs) [″ + ″ + *genesis,* production]. The induction of leukemia.

leukemoid (loo-kē′moyd) [″ + ″ + *eidos,* form]. Having symptoms of leukemia that are actually due to other conditions.

Leukeran. Trade name for chlorambucil, USP.

leukin (loo′kĭn). A thermostable bactericidal substance present in leukocytes.

leuko-, leuk- [Gr. *leukos,* white]. Combining forms signifying white, colorless, or rel. to leukocyte.

leukoagglutinin (loo″kō-ă-gloo′tĭ-nĭn) [″ + L. *agglutinans,* gluing]. An antibody that agglutinates white blood cells.

leukoblast (loo′kō-blăst) [″ + *blastos,* germ]. General term applied to a cell that is an immature leukocyte.

leukoblastosis (loo″kō-blăs-tō′sĭs) [″ + ″ + *osis,* condition]. Proliferation of excessive numbers of immature leukocytes.

leukocidin (loo-kō-sī′dĭn) [″ + L. *caedere,* to kill]. A bacterial toxin that destroys leukocytes.

leukocytal (loo″kō-sī′tăl) [″ + *kytos,* cell]. Rel. to leukocytes.

leukocyte (loo′kō-sīt) [″ + *kytos,* cell]. White blood corpuscle. There are two types: granulocytes (those possessing granules in their cytoplasm) and agranulocytes (those lacking granules). Granulocytes include juvenile neutrophils (3 to 5%), segmented neutrophils (54 to 62%), basophils (0 to 0.75%), and eosinophils (1 to 3%). Agranulocytes include lymphocytes, large and small (25 to 33%), and monocytes (3 to 7%).

Not all leukocytes are formed in the same place nor in the same manner. Granulocytes are formed in the bone marrow, arising from large cells called megakaryocytes. Lymphocytes are formed in the lymph nodes and probably in bone marrow. Monocytes are formed from the cells lining the capillaries in various organs, perhaps principally in the spleen and bone marrow. SEE: *B cells; T cells.*

FUNCT: Leukocytes act as scavengers, helping to combat infection. They travel by ameboid movement and are able to penetrate tissue and then return to the bloodstream. The direction of movement is probably due to the stimuli from injured cells, called chemotaxis. When invading bacteria destroy them, the dead leukocytes collect in the form of pus, causing an abscess if a ready outlet is not available.

Leukocytes, esp. the granular forms, are markedly phagocytic, i.e., have the power to ingest particulate substances. Neutrophils ingest bacteria and small particles; other cells such as the monocytes and histiocytes in the tissues ingest larger particles. They are important in both defensive and reparative functions of the body. Basophils most probably function by delivering anticoagulants to facilitate blood clot absorption or to prevent blood coagulation. Eosinophils increase in number in certain conditions such as asthma and infestations of animal parasites. Lymphocytes are not phagocytic. B-cell lymphocytes produce antibodies and T-cell lymphocytes are important in producing cellular immunity.

A greatly diminished number of erythrocytes is found in the anemias, and a greatly increased number of leukocytes (leukocytosis) is usually indicative of bacterial infection. A leukocyte count is usually taken preoperatively if infection is suspected, such as in appendicitis. A count may also be taken following surgery to be sure that an occult wound infection has not developed.

How to recognize: White blood cells are round with edges occasionally broken, nucleated, granular, of grayish color, sometimes clumped, and can be stained as polynuclears.

Microscopic examination: Leukocytes are usually found in mucus and can be stained by ordinary blood stains. Normally 1 cu. mm. of blood contains 5,000 to 10,000 leukocytes.

Two determinations are usually made regarding the leukocytes: their total number (total count) and the percentage of each type (differential count). A decrease in total number below the normal (5000) is called leukopenia; an increase in total number above normal (10,000) is called leukocytosis. Relative increase or decrease of any particular type is denoted by adding the suffix "-philia" (denoting increase) or "-penia" (denoting decrease). Ex.: neutrophilia, granulocytopenia, neutropenia, eosinophilia.

Sometimes immature white cells (myelocytes, myeloblasts, or lymphoblasts) are discharged into the bloodstream and may be observed in blood smears.

In a smear of blood, the white cells vary in size, shape, appearance, and the color they assume when stained. Some of the cells contain minute granules and these cells are called granulocytes. The granules in some cells stain bright red and these cells are called eosinophils. Others stain deep blue and these are called basophils. In most of the cells, however, the granules take a neutral purplish color and these are called neutrophils.

l., acidophil. L., eosinophil.

l., agranular. L., nongranular, q.v.

l., basophil. Leukocyte with cytoplasmic granules that stain with basic dyes. Stain a deep purple with Wright's stain. Comprise 0 to 0.75% of white cell count.

l., eosinophil. A granular leukocyte with cytoplasmic granules that stain with acid dyes. Appear reddish when stained with Wright's stain. Comprise 1 to 3% of white cell count. SYN: *l., acidophil.*

l., granular. Leukocyte containing granules in cytoplasm.

l., heterophilic. Neutrophil leukocyte of certain animals whose granules stain with an acid stain.

l., lymphoid. L., nongranular, q.v.

l., neutrophil. Leukocyte with fine cytoplasmic granules that do not stain with acid or basic stains but have an affinity for neutral stains.

l., nongranular. An agranulocyte; a lymphocyte or monocyte.

l., polymorphonuclear. Leukocyte with a nucleus consisting of several lobes. One of the granulocytes (neutrophil, eosinophil, basophil).

leukocythemia (loo"kō-sī-thē'mē-ă) [Gr. *leukos,* white, + *kytos,* cell, + *haima,* blood]. Leukemia, q.v.

leukocytic (loo"kō-sĭt'ĭk) [" + *kytos,* cell]. Pert. to leukocytes.

leukocytoblast (loo"kō-sī'tō-blast) [" + " + *blastos,* germ]. Cell from which leukocytes arise.

leukocytogenesis (loo"kō-sī"tō-jĕn'ĕ-sĭs) [" + *kytos,* cell, + *genesis,* formation]. Leukocyte formation. SYN: *leukopoiesis.*

leukocytoid (loo'kō-sī"toyd) [" + " + *eidos,* form]. Resembling a leukocyte.

leukocytolysin. A lysin that destroys leukocytes. SEE: *leukocidin.*

leukocytolysis (loo"kō-sī-tŏl'ĭ-sĭs) [" + *kytos,* cell, + *lysis,* dissolution]. Destruction of leukocytes.

leukocytoma (loo"kō-sī-tō'mă) [" + " + *oma,* tumor]. 1. Tumor composed of cells resembling leukocytes. 2. Tumorlike mass of leukocytes.

leukocytopenia (loo"kō-sī"tō-pē'nē-ă) [" + " + *penia,* want]. An abnormal decrease in leukocytes, usually below 5000 per cu. mm. SYN: *leukopenia.*

leukocytoplania (loo"kō-sī"tō-plā'nē-ă) [" + " + *plane,* wandering]. The passage of leukocytes from blood vessels into the tissues, or through membranes.

leukocytopoiesis (loo″kō-sī″tō-poy-ē′sĭs) [″ + ″ + *poiein,* to make]. Formation of white blood cells.

leukocytosis (loo″kō-sī-tō′sĭs) [″ + *kytos,* cell, + *osis,* condition]. Increase in number of leukocytes (above 10,000 per cu. mm.) in the blood, generally caused by presence of infection and is usually transient. It also may accompany or occur after the following conditions: hemorrhage, extensive operations, coronary occlusion, malignant growth, pregnancy, certain intoxications, and toxemias. Eosinophilic leukocytosis occurs in some allergies, animal parasite infestation, and Hodgkin's disease.

Leukemias, however, are associated with production of immature leukocytes due to abnormal condition of blood-forming organs. Leukocytosis is present in most infections but not usually in those due to a virus.

In leukocytosis the numbers of white cells may vary from a 50% increase to many times more than normal. In leukemia there may be as many as one million white cells per cu. mm. Leukocytosis is early and marked in severe infections when the patient's resistance is good; if infection and resistance are less marked it appears later to a lesser degree and disappears more quickly. Leukocytosis may occur in unusually virulent infections, such as diphtheria, pneumonia, and sepsis. SEE: *leukopenia.*

l., basophilic. An increase in the basophils in the blood.

l., mononuclear. An increase in the monocytes in the blood.

l., pathologic. Leukocytosis due to a disease such as an infection.

leukocytotaxis (loo″kō-sī″tō-tăk′sĭs) [Gr. *leukos,* white, + *kytos,* cell, + *taxis,* arrangement]. The movement of leukocytes either toward or away from an area such as a traumatized or infected site.

leukocytotoxin (loo″kō-sī″tō-tŏk′sĭn) [″ + ″ + *toxikon,* poison]. A toxin that destroys leukocytes.

leukocyturia (loo″kō-sī-tū′rē-ă) [″ + ″ + *ouron,* urine]. Leukocytes in the urine.

leukoderma (loo-kō-dĕr′mă) [″ + *derma,* skin]. Deficiency of pigmentation of the skin, esp. in patches. SEE: *vitiligo.*

l., syphilitic. Macular depigmentation esp. of the skin of the neck and shoulders. Seen in late syphilis.

leukodiagnosis (loo″kō-dī″ăg-nō′sĭs) [″ + *dia,* through, + *gnosis,* knowledge]. Diagnosis by observance of number, variety, or reaction of leukocytes.

leukodystrophy (lu″kō-dĭs′trō-fē). Sclerosis of the white matter of the brain.

l., metachromatic. A type of hereditary leukodystrophy caused by a deficiency of the enzyme aryl sulfatase, an enzyme that is essential for the degradation of sulfatide. Deficiency of the enzyme allows excess deposition of sulfatide in nerve tissues. Clinical signs of this disease usually appear at about one year of age. They include gait disturbance, inability to learn to walk, spasticity of limbs, hyperreflexia, dementia, and eventually death. There is no specific therapy.

leukoedema (loo″kō-ē-dē′mă) [″ + *oidema,* swelling]. A benign leukoplakia-like abnormality of the mucosa of the mouth or tongue. The affected areas are opalescent or white, and wrinkled.

leukoencephalitis (loo″kō-ĕn-sĕf-ă-lī′tĭs) [″ + *enkephalos,* brain + *itis,* inflammation]. Inflammation of the white matter of the brain.

leukoerythroblastosis (loo″kō-ĕ-rĭth″rō-blăs-tō′sĭs) [″ + *erythros,* red, + *blastos,* germ + *osis,* condition]. Anemia due to any condition that causes the bone marrow to be infiltrated and thus inactivated.

leukokeratosis (loo″kō-kĕr-ă-tō′sĭs) [″ + *keras,* horn, + *osis,* condition]. White patch formation on the surface of the mucosa of the tongue, cheek, and gums. SYN: *leukoplakia.*

leukokoria (loo″kō-kō′rē-ă) [″ + *kore,* pupil]. A white reflection from the pupil due to the presence of a mass in the pupillary area of the eye.

leukokraurosis (loo″kō-kraw-rō′sĭs) [″ + *kraurcs,* dry, + *osis,* condition]. Kraurosis vulvae, q.v.

leukolymphosarcoma (loo″kō-lĭm″fō-săr-kō′mă) [″ + L. *lympha,* lymph, + Gr. *sarx,* flesh, + *oma,* tumor]. Leukemia, lymphosarcoma cell, q.v.

leukolysis (loo-kŏl′ĭ-sĭs) [″ + *lysis,* dissolution]. Destruction of leukocytes. SYN: *leukocytolysis.*

leukoma (loo-kō′mă) [″ + *oma,* tumor]. A white, opaque corneal opacity.

l. adherens. Corneal scar with incarcerated iris tissue.

leukomaine (loo′kō-mān) [Gr. *leukoma,* whiteness]. A group of substances that are normally present in living tissues. They resemble alkaloids, some are toxic, and some are physiologically active

leukomainemia (loo″kō-mā-nē′mē-ă) [″ + *haima,* blood]. Excess of leukomaines in the blood.

leukomatous (loo-kō′mă-tŭs) [Gr. *leukos,* white, + *oma,* tumor]. 1. Pert. to leukoma. 2. Suffering from leukoma.

leukomyelitis (loo″kō-mī-ĕ-lī′tĭs) [″ + *myelos,* marrow, + *itis,* inflammation]. Inflammation of the white matter of the spinal cord.

leukomyelopathy (loo″kō-mī-ĕl-ŏp′ă-thē) [″ + ″ + *pathos,* disease]. Disease involving the white matter of the spinal cord or myelon.

leukonecrosis (loo″kō-nĕ-krō′sĭs) [″ + *nekrosis,* deadness]. Dry, light-colored, or white gangrene.

leukonychia (loo″kō-nĭk′ē-ă) [″ + *onyx,* nail]. White spots or streaks on the nails. SYN: *canities unguium.*

leukopathia (loo″kō-păth′ē-ă) [″ + *pathos,* disease]. 1. Absence of pigment in the skin. SEE: *leukoderma.* 2. Disease involving leukocytes.

l. unguium. Leukonychia, q.v.

leukopedesis (loo″kō-pĕ-dē′sĭs) [″ + *pedan,* to leap]. Passage of leukocytes through walls of blood vessels.

leukopenia (loo″kō-pē′nē-ă) [″ + *penia,* lack]. Abnormal decrease of white blood corpuscles usually below 5000 per cu. mm. A great number of drugs may cause leukopenia, as can failure of the bone marrow. SYN: *granulocytopenia; leukocytopenia.*

leukoplakia (loo″kō-plā′kē-ă) [″ + *plax,* plate]. Formation of white spots or patches on the mucous membrane of the tongue or cheek. The spots are smooth, irregular in size and shape, hard, and occasionally fissured. The lesions may become malignant.

l. buccalis. Leukoplakia of the mucosa of the cheek.

l. lingualis. Leukoplakia of the tongue.

l. vulvae. Atrophic disease affecting the female external genitalia seen most often in older women. Characterized by severe itching and a white marble-like appearance of the skin, frequently with excoriations. Without medical intervention, the skin may undergo malignant degeneration. SYN: *Breisky's disease; kraurosis vulvae.*

leukoplasia (loo-kō-plā′zē-ă). White patch formation on buccal mucosa. SYN: *leukoplakia.*

leukopoiesis (loo″kō-poy-ē′sĭs) [″ + *poiesis,* formation]. Leukocyte production. SYN: *leukocytogenesis.*

leukopoietic (loo″kō-poy-ĕt′ĭk) [″ + *poiein,* to make]. Forming leukocytes.

leukoprotease (loo-kō-prō′tē-ās) [″ + *protos,* first, + *-ase,* enzyme]. An enzyme in polynuclear leukocytes that splits protein.

leukopsin. A substance formed in the rods of the retina from rhodopsin under the influence of light.

leukorrhagia (loo″kō-rā′jē-ă) [″ + *rhegnynai,* to burst forth]. Profuse white vaginal discharge. SYN: *leukorrhea.*

leukorrhea (loo″kō-rē′ă) [″ + *rhoia,* flow]. Usually white or yellowish mucous discharge from the cervical canal or the vagina. There is frequently a so-called physiological leukorrhea that may be constantly present but somewhat increased preceding and following menstruation, and during sexual excitement. It may be of considerable concern to the young girl at the time of menarche because she has not been told this white fluid would tend to collect on the vulvae. Leukorrhea may be abnormal if it is increased in amount; has a change in color; is malodorous; or contains blood.

ETIOL: Pathological states of the endocervix and vagina. Infection by Trichomonas vaginalis, Candida albicans, and other pathogens.

SYM: Usually indications of acute inflammation—pain, heat, redness of parts involved. Pain in groin, hypogastrium, sacral regions, and small of back. Urethra often implicated, causing painful micturition. Symptoms that may occur in connection with chronic leukorrhea are innumerable. Discharge may be of any consistency: thin and watery or viscid and tenacious; and it may or may not have a foul odor.

TREATMENT: If due to a specific microorganism, treat with appropriate antibiotic. In general douches are ineffective in curing the cause of this symptom. If due to senile changes in the vagina, estrogen-containing cream or ointment applied locally is quite effective.

leukosarcoma (loo″kō-săr-kō′mă) [Gr. *leukos,* white, + *sarx,* flesh, + *oma,* tumor]. A variation of malignant lymphoma where the blood cells become leukemic.

leukosis (loo-kō′sĭs) [″ + *osis,* condition]. Abnormal proliferation of leukocyte-forming tissues.

leukotactic (loo″kō-tăk′tĭk) [″ + *taxis,* arrangement]. Possessing the power of attracting leukocytes.

leukotaxine (loo″kō-tăk′sĭn). A noncellular nitrogenous substance present in injured tissue.

leukotaxis (loo″kō-tăks′ĭs). Possessing the power of attracting (positive leukotaxis) or repelling (negative leukotaxis) leukocytes.

leukotomy (loo-kŏt′ō-mē) [″ + *tome,* incision]. Lobotomy, q.v.

leukotoxic (loo″kō-tŏks′ĭk) [″ + *toxikon,* poison]. Destructive to leukocytes.

leukotoxin (loo″kō-tŏk′sĭn) [″ + *toxikon,* poison]. Leukocytotoxin, q.v.

leukotrichia (loo″kō-trĭk′ē-ă) [″ + *thrix,* hair]. Whiteness of the hair. SYN: *canities.*

leukous (loo′kŭs) [Gr. *leukos,* white]. White, esp. rel. to the skin.

levallorphan tartrate. (lĕv″ăl-lor′făn). USP. A narcotic antagonist used to counteract morphine or opioid-induced respiratory depression. Trade name is Lorfan.

lavarterenol bitartrate (lĕv″ăr-tē-rē′nŏl bī-tăr′trāt). The preferred term is norepinephrine bitartrate, q.v. A sympathomimetic agent that, due to its vasopressor effect, may be useful in treating hypotension that accompanies shock. It is usually administered intravenously because it is rapidly inactivated. Trade name is Levophed. SYN: *noradrenalin; norepinephrine.*

levator (lē-vā′tor) [L., lifter]. (pl. *levatores*) 1. [NA] A muscle that raises or elevates a part. Opposite of depressor. 2. An instrument that lifts depressed portions.

l. ani. A broad muscle that helps to form the floor of the pelvis.

l. palpebrae superioris. A muscle that elevates the upper eyelid.

level of activities. In the nervous system, connector neurons are grouped into levels corresponding to different stages of development: spinal cord level; medullary level; midbrain level; basal ganglial level; cortical level. Each level is responsible for certain activities but controlled by the one above it.

lever (lĕv′ĕr, lē′vĕr) [L. *levare,* to raise]. Rigid bar used to modify direction, force, and motion. A type of simple machine that provides the user with a mechanical advantage. Levers are used to facilitate in moving and lifting of objects too heavy or awkward to move unassisted. SEE: illus.

levigation (lĕv″ĭ-gā′shŭn) [L. *levigare,* to render smooth]. The grinding of a substance into a fine state, usually in water, and then letting the material settle in order to separate the coarser particles from the fine.

Levin's tube (lĕ-vĭnz′). [Abraham L. Levin, New Orleans physician, 1880–1940] A catheter, usually introduced through the nose, that extends through the stomach into the duodenum. It is used to help prevent accumulation of intestinal liquids and gas during and following intestinal surgery.

levitation [L. *levitas,* lightness]. The subjective sensation of rising in the air or moving through the air unsupported. Occurs in dreams, altered states of consciousness, and certain mental disorders.

levocardia (lē″vō-kăr′dē-ă) [L. *laevus,* left, + Gr. *kardia,* heart]. Term describing the normal position of the heart when other viscera are inverted. SEE: *dextrocardia.*

levoclination (lē″vō-klī-nā′shŭn) [″ + *clinatus,* leaning]. Torsion or twisting of the upper meridians of the eyes to the left.

levocycloduction (lē″vō-sī″klō-dŭk′shŭn) [″ + Gr. *kyklos,* circle, + L. *ducere,* to lead]. Levoduction, q.v.

levodopa. USP. L-3,4-dihydroxyphenylala-

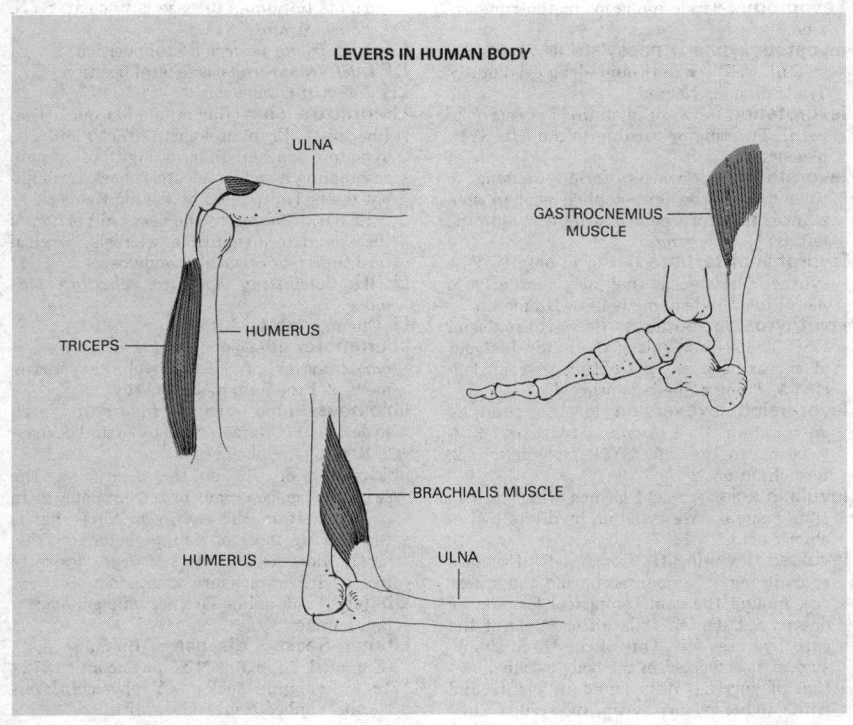

LEVERS IN HUMAN BODY

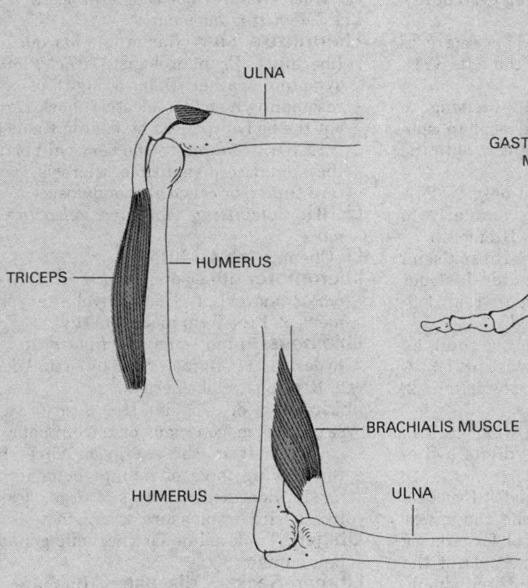

nine. Drug used in the treatment of Parkinson's disease. Trade names are Bendopa, Dopar, and Larodopa. SYN: *L-dopa.*

Levo-Dromoran. Trade name for levorphanol tartrate, USP.

levoduction (lē″vō-dŭk′shŭn) [L. *laevus,* left, + *ducere,* to lead]. Movement or drawing toward the left, esp. of an eye.

levography (lē-vŏg′ră-fē) [″ + Gr. *graphein,* to write]. Radiographic examination of the left side of the heart after introduction of a contrast medium.

levogyration (lē″vō-jī-rā′shŭn) [″ + *gyrare,* to turn]. Levorotatory, q.v.

levogyrous (lē″vō-jī′rŭs) [″ + *gyrare,* to turn]. Causing to turn toward the left, applied esp. to substances that turn polarized light rays to the left. SYN: *levorotatory.*

levonordefrin (lē″vō-nor′dĕ-frĭn). USP. A vasoconstrictor drug used to prolong the action of local anesthetic agents. Trade name is Neo-Cobefrin.

Levopa. Trade name for levodopa, USP.

Levophed. Trade name for norepinephrine bitartrate.

levophobia (lĕv″ō-fō′bē-ă) [″ + Gr. *phobos,* fear]. Morbid dread of objects on the left side of the body.

Levoprome. Trade name for methotrimeprazine.

levopropoxyphene napsylate (lē″vō-prō-pŏk′sĕ-fēn). USP. An anticough drug used orally. Trade name is Novrad.

levorotation (lē″vō-rō-tā′shŭn) [″ + *rotare,* to turn]. Twisting or turning to the left. SYN: *levotorsion.*

levorotatory (lē″vō-rō′tă-tor-ē). Causing to turn toward the left, applied esp. to substances that turn polarized light rays to the left. SYN: *levogyrous.*

levorphanol tartrate (lēv-or′fă-nŏl). USP. A synthetic analgesic that acts similarly to morphine. Trade name is Levo-Dromoran.

levothyroxine sodium (lē″vō-thī-rŏk′sēn). USP. The sodium salt of the natural isomer of thyroxine used in treating thyroid deficiency. Trade name is Synthroid.

levotorsion, levoversion (lē″vō-tor′shŭn, lē″vō-vĕr′shŭn) [″ + *torsio,* a twisting]. 1. A twisting to the left. SYN: *levorotation.* 2. Levoclination, q.v.

levulinic acid. An acid formed when certain simple sugars are acted on by dilute hydrochloric acid.

levulose (lĕv′ū-lōs) [L. *laevus,* left]. Fructose or fruit sugar, a monosaccharide and a hexose, having the same empirical formula as dextrose, $C_6H_{12}O_6$. It is an example of the carbohydrates, q.v. One of the three simple sugars, it is formed in the body by the digestion of sucrose. It is found in plants and fruits, in honey, corn syrup, and syrup resulting from the inversion of sucrose.

levulosemia (lĕv″ū-lō-sē′mē-ă) [″ + Gr. *haima,* blood]. Presence of fructose in the blood.

levulosuria (lĕv″ū-lō-sū′rē-ă) [″ + Gr. *ouron,* urine]. Presence of fructose in the urine.

levurid (lĕv′ū-rĭd). A sterile usually vesicular lesion of the skin due to the spread through the blood of substances from Candida albicans. SYN: *candidid.*

lewisite (lū′ĭ-sīt). [W. L. Lewis, U.S. chemist, 1879–1943] A toxic gas similar in action to mustard gas used in warfare to disable and kill. It acts as a vesicant in the lungs.

TREATMENT: dimercaprol, USP, q.v.

Leyden jar (lī′dĕn). [Ernst V. von Leyden, Ger. physician, 1832–1910] A glass jar coated partially inside and out with metal; it is used as a capacitor or collector of electricity.

Leydig cells (lī′dĭg). [Franz von Leydig, Ger. anatomist, 1821–1908] Interstitial tissue cells in the testicles, believed to be responsible for internal secretion of the testicles, testosterone.

L.F.A. *left fronto-anterior* fetal position.

L-forms [named for *Lister* institute]. Spontaneous variants of bacteria that replicate as pleomorphic, filterable elements with defective or absent cell walls. The relation of these variants to human disease is unclear. SYN: *L-phase variants.*

L.F.P. *left fronto-posterior* fetal position.

L.F.T. *left fronto-transverse* fetal position.

LH. *luteinizing hormone.*

Lhermitte's sign (lār′mĭts). [Jacques Jean Lhermitte, Fr. neurologist, 1877–1959] The symptom (rather than a sign) of a pain resembling a sudden electric shock throughout the body produced by flexing the neck.

ETIOL: Trauma to the cervical portion of the spinal cord, multiple sclerosis, cervical cord tumor, or cervical spondylosis.

LHRH. *luteinizing hormone releasing hormone.*

Li. Chem. symb. for lithium.

liberomotor (lĭb″ĕr-ō-mō′tor) [L. *liber,* free, + *motor,* mover]. 1. Pert. to voluntary movement. 2. Free from motor energy.

libidinous (lĭ-bĭd′ĭ-nŭs) [L. *libidinosus,* pert. to desire]. 1. Characterized by sexual desires. 2. Rel. to psychic energy.

libido (lĭ-bī′dō, -bē′dō) [L., desire]. 1. The sexual drive, conscious or unconscious. 2. In psychoanalysis, the energy or force that is the driving force of human behavior. Variously identified as the sex urge, desire to live, desire for pleasure or satisfaction.

Libigen. Trade name for chorionic gonadotropin, human.

Libman-Sacks disease (lĭb′măn-săks′). [Emanuel Libman, N.Y. physician, 1872–1946; Benjamin Sacks, N.Y. physician] Verrucous, nonbacterial endocarditis.

Libritabs. Trade name for chlordiazepoxide.

Librium. Trade name for chlordiazepoxide hydrochloride, USP.

lice. Pl. of louse.

licensure. In the health care profession, the granting of official or legal, or both, permission to perform medical actions that are legally forbidden to be done by persons who are not so licensed. Whether or not one is qualified for such a license is usually determined by some official body representing the federal or state government.

l., individual. In the health care profession, licensure of an individual to perform certain medical actions.

l., institutional. In the health care business, the licensing of institutions such as hospitals, clinics, or corporations to perform certain medical care functions.

licentiate (lī-sĕn′shē-ăt). 1. An individual who practices a profession by the authority granted by a license. 2. In some countries, a medical practitioner who does not have a medical degree.

lichen (lī′kĕn) [Gr. *leichen,* lichen]. 1. Any form of papular skin disease; usually noting lichen planus. 2. In botany, any one of numerous plants consisting of a fungus growing symbiotically with certain algae. They form characteristic scaly or branching growths on rocks or barks of trees.

l., myxedematous. Generalized eruption of asymptomatic nodules due to mucinous deposits in the upper layers of the skin and in vessels and organs.

l. nitidus. A rare skin condition characterized by small, chronic, asymptomatic papules that are usually pink and are usually located only on the male genitalia, abdomen, and flexor surfaces of the elbows and palms.

l. pilaris. L. spinulosus, q.v.

l. planopilaris. A form of lichen planus in which white shiny follicular papules are present along with the usual plane papules.

l. planus. Inflammatory skin disease of many varieties. Usually occurs in otherwise healthy persons who are emotionally tense.

SYM: Begins with pinhead size papules, reddish or violaceous, glistening, then coalescing, forming rough, scaly patches; acute, subacute, or chronic itching situated on extremities. According to type of lesion the disease may be lichen planus atrophicus, erythematosus, hypertrophicus, linearis or ruber moniliformis.

ETIOL: Unknown.

PROG: Prolonged but favorable.

TREATMENT: Therapy for the anxiety. Locally, soothing antipruritic ointment. There is no specific therapy. The disease is self-limiting but may last years, or recur.

l. ruber moniliformis. Large verrucous lesions of lichen planus arranged as the beads in a necklace.

l. ruber planus. L. planus, q.v.

l. sclerosus et atrophicus. Chronic skin eruption consisting of discrete or confluent flat-topped ivory-white papules, each of which contains a black keratotic plug. The lesions may be associated with intractable itching, esp. when they are in the anal and genital areas. Kraurosis vulvae, q.v., is frequently associated with this disease.

l. scrofulosus. An eruption of tiny punctate reddish-brown papules arranged in circles or groups in young persons with tuberculosis. The lesions are caused by the spread of the tubercle bacilli through the blood to the skin.

l. simplex chronicus. An itching papular eruption that is circumscribed and located on skin that has become thickened and pigmented due to the rubbing of it. SYN: *Vidal's disease.*

l. spinulosus. Form of lichen with a spine developing in each follicle. SYN: *keratosis pilaris.*

l. striatus. A papular eruption usually seen on one extremity of a child. It is arranged in linear groups and consists of pink papules. The disease, though self-limiting, may last for a year or longer.

l. tropicus. Form of lichen with redness and inflammatory reaction of the skin. SYN: *miliaria rubra; prickly heat.*

l. urticatus. Urticaria papulosa, q.v.

lichenification (lī-kĕn″ĭ-fĭ-kā′shŭn) [Gr. *leichen,* lichen, + L. *facere,* to make]. 1. Cutaneous thickening and hardening from continued irritation. 2. Changing of an eruption into one resembling a lichen.

lichenin (lī′kĕ-nĭn). A starch obtained from Icelandic moss. SYN: *moss starch.*

lichenoid (lī′kĕn-oyd) [″ + *eidos,* form]. Resembling lichen.

Lichtheim's syndrome (lĭkt′hīmz). [Ludwig Lichtheim, Ger. physician, 1845–1928] Subacute combined degeneration of the spinal cord associated with pernicious anemia.

licorice (lĭk′ĕr-ĭs, -ĕr-ĭsh [ME.]. A dried root of Glycyrrhiza glabra used as a flavoring agent, demulcent, and mild expectorant. Glycyrrhiza is prepared from licorice. Ingestion of large amounts of licorice can cause salt retention, excess potassium loss in the urine, and elevated blood pressure. SYN: *glycyrrhiza.*

lid [ME.]. An eyelid.

Lida-Mantle. Trade name for lidocaine hydrochloride, USP.

lidocaine (lī′dō-kān). USP. A local anesthetic drug. Trade name is Xylocaine.

l. hydrochloride. USP. A local anesthetic that is also used intravenously to treat certain cardiac arrhythmias. Trade names are Dolicaine, Lida-Mantle, and Xylocaine.

lid reflex. Closure of eyelids resulting from direct corneal stimulation. SYN: *corneal reflex.*

lie, transverse. A position of the fetus in utero in which the long axis of the fetus is across the long axis of the mother. SEE: *presentations of fetus* for illus.

Lieberkühn crypts (lē'bĕr-kēn). [Johann N. Lieberkühn, Ger. anatomist, 1711–1756] Simple tubular glands present in the intestinal mucosa. In their epithelium are found goblet cells, cells of Paneth, and argentaffine cells. The glands form minute invaginations opening between the bases of the villi. They lie in the lamina propria, their blind ends extending to the muscularis mucosa. In the large intestine they are longer, contain few if any Paneth cells and more goblet cells. They are arranged vertically with much regularity. SYN: *glands, Lieberkühn's.*

lie detector. A polygraph; an instrument for determining minor physiological changes assumed to occur under the stress of lying (or any other emotion). Variations in respiratory rhythm, pulse rate, blood pressure, and sweating of the hands are among the functions that are monitored. Increased perspiration lessens resistance to passage of electrical current. The test has popular appeal among law enforcement departments but results obtained are presumptive and not absolute.

lien (lī'ĕn) [L.]. [NA] The spleen.

l. accessorius. [NA] Accessory spleen.

l. mobilis. Floating spleen.

lienal (lī-ē'năl) [L. *lien,* spleen]. Rel. to the spleen. SYN: *splenic.*

lienitis (lī"ĕ-nī'tĭs) [" + Gr. *itis,* inflammation]. Inflammation of the spleen. SYN: *splenitis.*

lienocele (lī-ē'nō-sēl) [" + Gr. *kele,* hernia]. Splenic hernia. SYN: *splenocele.*

lienography (lī"ē-nŏg'ră-fē) [" + Gr. *graphein,* to write]. Radiographic examination of the spleen after introduction of a contrast medium.

lienomalacia (lī-ē"nō-mă-lā'shē-ă) [" + Gr. *malakia,* softening]. Softening of the spleen. SYN: *splenomalacia.*

lienomedullary (lī-ē"nō-mĕd'ū-lăr-ē) [" + *medulla,* marrow]. Rel. to both spleen and bone marrow.

lienomyelogenous (lī-ē"nō-mī-ĕl-ŏj'ĕ-nŭs) [" + Gr. *myelos,* marrow, + *gennan,* to produce]. Derived from both the spleen and bone marrow.

lienomyelomalacia (lī-ē"nō-mī"ĕl-ō-mă-lā'shē-ă) [" + " + *malakia,* softening]. Softening of the spleen and bone marrow.

lienopancreatic (lī-ē"nō-păn"krē-ăt'ĭk) [" + Gr. *pankreas,* pancreas]. Rel. to the spleen and pancreas.

lienorenal (lī-ē"nō-rē'năl) [" + *renalis,* pert. to kidney]. Rel. to the spleen and kidney.

lienotoxin (lī-ē"nō-tŏk'sĭn) [" + Gr. *toxikon,* poison]. Splenotoxin, q.v.

lientery (lī'ĕn-tĕr"ē) [Gr. *leios,* smooth, + *enteron,* intestine]. Diarrhea in which the stool contains undigested food.

lienunculus (lī"ĕn-ŭng'kū-lŭs). Accessory spleen.

life (līf) [AS.]. 1. State of being alive; quality manifested by metabolism, growth, reproduction, and adaptation to environment; state in which the organs of an animal or plant are capable of performing all or any of their functions. 2. Time between birth or inception and death of an organism. Biologically, unitary life begins at the moment of conception and ends at death. However, for legal and other reasons the definition of when life begins has been subject to a variety of interpretations. 3. The sum total of those properties that distinguish living things (animals or plants) from nonliving inorganic chemical matter or dead organic matter.

RS: antibiotic; "bio-" words; death; vital; vitality.

life expectancy. The number of years that an average person of a given age may be expected to live as determined by mortality tables.

ligament (lĭg'ă-mĕnt) [L. *ligamentum,* a band]. 1. A band or sheet of strong fibrous connective tissue connecting the articular ends of bones serving to bind them together and to facilitate or limit motion. 2. A thickened portion or fold of peritoneum or mesentery that supports a visceral organ or connects it to another viscus. 3. A band of fibrous connective tissue connecting bones, cartilages, and other structures and serving for support or for attachment of fascia or muscles. 4. A cordlike structure representing the vestigial remains of a fetal blood vessel.

l., accessory. A ligament that supplements another, esp. one on the lateral surface of a joint. One outside of and independent of the capsule of a joint.

l., acromioclavicular. Ligament extending from the clavicle to the acromial process of the scapula.

l., alar. Ligament connecting the odontoid process of the atlas to the occipital bone. SYN: *l., apical.*

l., annular. A circular ligament, esp. one enclosing a head or radius or one holding the footplate of the stapes in the fenestra vestibuli.

l., apical. A single median ligament extending from the odontoid process to the occipital bone. SYN: *l., alar.*

l.'s, arcuate. The lateral, medial, and exterior ligaments that extend from the 12th rib to the transverse process of the 1st lumbar vertebra to which the diaphragm is attached.

l., arterial. A fibrous cord extending from the pulmonary artery to the arch of the aorta, the remains of the ductus arteriosus of the fetus.

l.'s, auricular. The anterior, posterior, and superior auricular ligaments uniting the external ear to the temporal bone.

l., broad, of liver. A wide, sickle-shaped fold of peritoneum, attached to the lower surface of the diaphragm, the internal surface of the right rectus abdominis muscle, and the convex surface of the liver.

l., broad, of uterus. Folds of peritoneum attached to lateral borders of the uterus from insertion of the fallopian tube above to the pelvic wall. It consists of two leaves between which are found the remnants of the wolffian ducts, cellular tissues, and the major blood vessels of the pelvis.

l.'s, capsular. Heavy fibrous structures, lined with synovial membrane and surrounding articulations.

l.'s, carpal. Ligaments uniting the carpal bones.

l., caudal. Bundles of fibrous tissue uniting dorsal surfaces of the two lower coccygeal vertebrae and superjacent skin.

l., check. Ligament that restrains motion of a joint, esp. the lateral odontoid ligaments.

l., conoid. Posterior portion of the coracoclavicular ligament.

l., coracoacromial. Broad triangular ligament attached to the outer edge of the coracoid process of the scapula and the tip of the acromion.

l., coracoclavicular. Ligament uniting the clavicle and coracoid process of the scapula.

l., coracohumeral. Broad ligament connecting the coracoid process of the scapula to the greater tubercle of the humerus.

l., coronary, of liver. A fold of peritoneum extending from the posterior edge of the liver to diaphragm.

l., costocolic. Ligament attaching the splenic flexure of the colon to the diaphragm.

l., costocoracoid. Ligament joining the first rib and coracoid process of the scapula.

l.'s, costotransverse. Ligaments uniting ribs with transverse processes of vertebrae.

l., costotransverse, middle. Ligament consisting of parallel fibers extending between a vertebra and its adjacent rib.

l.'s, costovertebral. Ligaments uniting the ribs and vertebrae.

l., cricopharyngeal. A ligamentous bundle between the upper and posterior border of the cricoid cartilage and the anterior wall of the pharynx.

l.'s, cricothyroid. Ligaments uniting cricoid and thyroid cartilages.

l., cricotracheal. The ligamentous structure uniting the upper ring of the trachea and the cricoid cartilage.

l., cruciate. 1. Ligament of the ankle passing transversely across the dorsum of the foot that holds tendons of the anterior muscle group in place. 2. A cross-shaped ligament of the atlas consisting of the transverse ligament and superior and inferior bands, the former passing upwards and attaching to the margin of the foramen magnum, the latter passing downwards and attaching to the body of the atlas. 3. Two ligaments of the knee, the anterior passing from tibia to medial aspect of the lateral condyle of the femur, the posterior passing from the tibia to the lateral aspect of the medial condyle.

l., cruciform. A structure consisting of one ligament crossing another.

l., crural. L., inguinal.

l., deltoid. Interior lateral ligament of the ankle.

l., dentate. A fibrous band of pia mater extending the length of the spinal cord on each side between the spinal nerves. It has a scalloped appearance as it pierces the arachnoid to attach to the dura mater at regular intervals.

l., falciform, of liver. A wide, sickle-shaped fold of peritoneum attached to the lower surface of the diaphragm, internal surface of the right rectus abdominis muscle, and convex surface of the liver.

l., fundiform, of penis. Ligament extending from lower portion of the linea alba and Scarpa's fascia to dorsum of the penis.

l., gastrophrenic. A fold of peritoneum between the esophageal end of the stomach and the diaphragm.

l., Gimbernat's. Triangular flat expansion of aponeurosis of abdominal external oblique muscle. Forming medial boundary of femoral ring. SYN: *l., lacunar.*

l., glenohumeral. Fibers of the coracohumeral ligament passing into the joint and inserted into the inner and upper part of the bicipital groove.

l., glenoid. Ligament that extends between palmar surfaces of phalanges and corresponding metacarpal bone.

l., Henle's. The lateral extension of the tendinous insertion of the rectus abdominus muscle. It is posterior to the falx inguinalis.

l., hepaticoduodenal. A fold of peritoneum from transverse fissure of liver to vicinity of the duodenum and right flexure of colon, forming anterior boundary of foramen of Winslow.

l., ileopectineal. A portion of the pelvic fascia attached to the ileopectineal line and to the capsular ligament of the hip joint.

l., iliofemoral. Bundle of fibers forming the upper and anterior portion of the capsular ligament of the hip joint. Ligament that extends from ilium to intertrochanteric line. SYN: *Y ligament.*

l., iliolumbar. Ligament extending from 4th and 5th lumbar vertebrae to iliac crest.

l., infundibulopelvic. The upper free edge of the broad ligament in which the ovarian artery is found. SYN: *l., suspensory of ovary.*

l., inguinal. Ligament extending from anterior superior iliac spine to pubic tubercle. Forms lower margin of aponeurosis of exterior oblique muscle. SYN: *l., crural; l., Poupart's.*

l., interclavicular. Bundle of fibers between sternal ends of the clavicles, attached to interclavicular notch of sternum.

l., interspinal. Ligament extending from the superior margin of a spinous process of one vertebra to lower margin of one above.

l., ischiocapsular. Ligament extending from ischium to ischial border of acetabulum.

l., lacunar. L., Gimbernat's, q.v.

l.'s, lateral, of liver. Folds of peritoneum extending from lower surface of diaphragm to adjacent borders of right and left lobes of the liver. SYN: *triangular ligaments.*

l., lateral occipitoatlantal. A ligament on each side between transverse processes of atlas and jugular process of the occipital bone.

l.'s, lateral odontoid. Strong ligaments extending between sides of odontoid process of the axis and inner sides of condyles of the occipital bone.

l.'s, Lisfranc's. Cuneometatarsal interosseous ligaments. Ligaments that join the cuneiform bone to the metatarsal bone.

l., Lockwood's. Suspensory ligament of the eye.

l., medial. A broad ligament that connects the medial malleolus of the tibia to the tarsal bones.

l.'s, meniscofemoral. Two small ligaments of the knee, one anterior and one posterior. The anterior one attaches to the posterior area of the lateral meniscus and the anterior cruciate ligament. The posterior one attaches to the posterior area of the lateral meniscus and the medial condyle of the femur.

l.'s, nephrocolic. Fibrous strands that connect the kidneys with the ascending and descending colon.

l., nuchal. The upward continuation of the supraspinous ligament, extending from the 7th cervical vertebra to the occipital bone.

l., palpebral. Two ligaments, medial and lateral, extending from tarsal plates of the eyelids to the frontal process of maxilla and the zygomatic bone respectively.

l., patellar. A strong, flat band securing the patella to the tibia. It is a continuation of the tendon of the quadriceps femoris muscle.

l., pectineal. A triangular-shaped ligament that extends from the medial end of the inguinal ligament and the pectineal line of the pubis.

l., periodontal. The connective tissue that surrounds the roots of teeth and holds them in the sockets of the teeth.

l., Petit's. A thickened portion of the pelvic fascia between the cervix and vagina. It passes posteriorly in the rectouterine fold to attach to the anterior surface of the sacrum.

l., phrenocolic. A fold of peritoneum joining the left colic flexure of the colon to the adjacent costal portion of the diaphragm.

l., popliteal, arcuate. Ligament on the posterolateral side of the knee, extending from the head of the fibula to the joint capsule.

l., Poupart's. L., inguinal.

l., pterygomandibular. Band of fiber extending between apex of internal pterygoid plate of sphenoid bone and the posterior extremity of internal oblique line of mandible.

l.'s, pubic. Those connecting the pubic bones at the symphysis pubis. Include anterior and superior pubic ligaments and the arcuate (inferior) ligament.

l., pulmonary. A fold of pleura that extends from the hilus of the lung to the base of the medial surface of the lung.

l., rhomboid. A strong structure extending from the tuberosity of the clavicle to outer surface of the cartilage of the first rib.

l., round, of femur. A ligament of the head of the femur that is attached to the anterior superior part of the fovea of the head of the femur and to the sides of the acetabular notch.

l., round, of liver. Fibrous cord extending upward from the umbilicus and enclosed in lower margin of the falciform ligament. Represents obliterated left umbilical vein of the fetus.

l., round, of uterus. Ligament attached to uterus immediately below and in front of the entrance of the fallopian tube. Each extends laterally in the broad ligament to the pelvic wall, where it passes through inguinal ring, terminating in the labium majus.

l.'s, sacroiliac. Two ligaments, the anterior and posterior, that connect sacrum and ilium.

l., sacrospinous. Ligament extending from the spine of the ischium to sacrum and coccyx in front of the sacrotuberous ligament.

l., sacrotuberous. Ligament extending from tuberosity of the ischium to posterior superior and inferior iliac spines and to lower part of sacrum and coccyx.

l., sphenomandibular. Ligament attached superiorly to spine of sphenoid and inferiorly to lingula of mandible.

l., spiral. The thickened periosteum of the peripheral wall of the osseous cochlear canal. The basilar membrane is attached to its inner surface.

l., stylohyoid. A thin fibroelastic cord between lesser cornu of hyoid bone and apex of styloid process of the temporal bone.

l., stylomandibular. A thin fibrous band of tissue extending between styloid process of temporal bone and lower part of posterior border of ramus of the mandible. SYN: *stylomaxillary ligament*.

l., suprascapular. A thin fibrous band of tissue extending from base of coracoid process of scapula to inner margin of suprascapular notch.

l., supraspinal. Ligament uniting apices of spinous processes of vertebrae.

l., suspensory. Ligament suspending an organ.

l., suspensory, of axilla. The continuation of the clavipectoral fascia down to attach to the axillary fascia.

l., suspensory, of lens. The zonula ciliaris (ciliary zonule); the fibers holding the crystalline lens in position.

l., suspensory, of ovary. Ligament extending from tubal end of ovary laterally to pelvic wall. It lies in layers of the broad ligament. SYN: *l., infundibulopelvic*.

l., suspensory, of penis. A triangular bundle of fibrous tissue extending from anterior surface of the symphysis pubis and adjacent structures to the dorsum of the root of the penis.

l.'s, suspensory, of uterus. The broad ligaments, the round ligaments, and the rectouterine folds of the uterus.

l.'s, sutural. Thin, fibrous layers interposed between articulating surfaces of bones united by suture.

l., temporomandibular. The thickened portion of the joint capsule that passes from the articular tubercle at the root of the zygomatic arch to attach to the subcondylar neck of the mandible.

l., tendinotrochanteric. A ligament that forms a part of the capsule of the hip joint.

l., transverse, of atlas. A strong ligament passing over the odontoid process of the axis.

l., transverse, of hip joint. A ligamentous band extending across cotyloid notch of the acetabulum.

l., transverse, of knee joint. A fibrous band extending from anterior margin of external semilunar fibrocartilage of knee to extremity of the internal semilunar fibrocartilage.

l., transverse crural. Ligament lying on anterior surface of leg just above ankle.

l., transverse humeral. A fibrous band that bridges the bicipital groove of the humerus in connecting the lesser and greater tuberosities.

l., trapezoid. Anterior exterior portion of the coracoclavicular ligament.

l.'s, triangular, of liver. Two ligaments, right and left, that connect posterior aspects of right and left lobes with corresponding portions of the diaphragm.

l., umbilical, lateral. Fibrous cord extending from bladder to umbilicus. Represents obliterated interior iliac artery of fetus.

l., umbilical, median. Fibrous cord extending from apex of bladder to umbilicus. Represents the remains of the urachus of fetus.

l., uterorectosacral. Ligament that arises from the sides of the cervix and passes upwards and backwards, passing around the rectum, to the second sacral vertebra. They are enclosed within the rectouterine folds, which demarcate borders of the rectouterine pouch.

l., uterosacral. L., Petit's, q.v.

l., venous. A solid fibrous cord representing obliterated ductus venosus of the fetus. It lies between the caudate and left lobes of the liver and connects the left branch of the portal vein to the interior vena cava.

l., ventricular, of larynx. The lateral free margin of the quadrangular membrane. It is enclosed within and supports the ventricular fold.

l., vesicouterine. Ligament that attaches the anterior aspect of the uterus to the bladder.

l., vestibular. A thin fibrous band attached anteriorly to the lamina of the thyroid cartilage and posteriorly to the anterior portion of the arytenoid cartilage.

l., vocal, of larynx. The thickened free edges of the elastic cone extending from thyroid angle to vocal processes of arytenoid cartilages. They support the vocal folds, q.v.

l., Weitbrecht's. The oblique band connecting the ulna and radius.

l., yellow. One of a series of ligaments connecting laminae of adjacent vertebrae.

ligamenta. Pl. of ligamentum.

ligamentopexis (lĭg″ă-mĕn″tō-pĕks′ĭs) [L. *ligamentum,* band, + Gr. *pexis,* fixation]. Suspension of uterus on the round ligament.

ligamentous (lĭg″ă-mĕn′tŭs) [L. *ligamentum,* band]. 1. Rel. to a ligament. 2. Like a ligament.

ligamentum (lĭg″ă-mĕn′tŭm) [L., a band]. (pl. *ligamenta*) [NA] Ligament.

ligand (lī′gănd, lĭg′ănd) [L. *ligare,* to bind]. 1. In chemistry, an organic molecule attached to a central metal ion by multiple bonds. 2. In immunology, a small molecule bound to a protein by non-covalent forces. The term may be used to include haptens and antigens.

ligase (lī′gās, lĭg′ās). General term for a class of enzymes that catalyze the joining of the ends of two chains of DNA.

ligate (lī′gāt). To apply a ligature.

ligation (lī-gā′shŭn). The application of a ligature.

ligature (lĭg′ă-chūr) [L. *ligatura,* a binding]. 1. Process of binding or tying. 2. A band or bandage. 3. A thread or wire for tying a blood vessel or other structure in order to constrict it. Cord or material used may be catgut, q.v., synthetic suture materials such as nylon or Dacron, kangaroo gut, polyglycollic acid, and natural fibers such as silk or cotton. Sometimes strips of fascia obtained from the patient are used as a ligature.

light (līt) [AS. *leohte,* not heavy]. 1. Not heavy. 2. Pale.

light (līt) [AS. *lihtan,* to shine]. The sensation produced by electromagnetic radiation that falls on the retina. Radiant energy producing a sensation of luminosity on the retina is limited to a wavelength of from about 390 to 770 nanometers. SEE: *laser; ray.*

l., axial. Light with rays parallel to each other and to optic axis.

l., cold. Any form of light that is not perceptibly warm. The heat of ordinary light rays is dissipated when they are passed through some medium such as quartz.

l., diffused. Rays broken by refraction.

l., idioretinal; l., intrinsic. The sensation of light when there are no retinal stimuli to produce that sensation.

l., oblique. Light that strikes a surface obliquely.

l., polarized. Light in which waves vibrate in one direction only.

l., reflected. Light rays that are thrown back by an illuminated object such as a mirror.

l., refracted. Rays bent from original course.

l., transmitted. Light that passes through an object.

l., white. Light that contains all of the visible wavelengths of light.

l., Wood's. Ultraviolet light of approximately 365 nanometers wavelength, used in diagnosing fungus infections of the scalp and in detecting materials that fluoresce.

light, words pert. to: "actin-" words; Fraunhofer's lines; heliotherapy; lambert; lumen; lux; "phot-" words; "radi-" words; ray; reflection; reflector; refraction; spectrum.

light adaptation. Changes that occur in a dark-adapted eye in order for vision to occur in moderate or bright light. Principal changes are contraction of pupil and bleaching of visual purple in the rods.

light diet. Diet consisting of all foods allowed in soft diet, q.v., plus whole-grained cereals, easily digested raw fruits and vegetables. Foods not pureed or ground. Used as an intermediate regimen for patients who do not require a soft diet but are not yet able to resume a full diet.

light difference. The difference with respect to sensitiveness to intensity of light between the two eyes.

lightening [AS. *leohte,* not heavy]. Descent of presenting part of fetus into the pelvis. This often occurs two to three weeks prior to the beginning of the first stage of labor. It may not occur in multiparas until active labor begins. SEE: *labor.* SYN: *engagement.*

light reflex. Constriction of the pupil when light is flashed into the eye.

light therapy. The use of light rays in the treatment of disease. Includes use of ultraviolet and infrared radiations. SYN: *phototherapy.*

light unit. A foot candle. This is the amount of light measured one foot from a standard candle. The ideal amount of light required for work varies with the specific type of work being done. The term foot candle took the place of candle power, but light intensity is best described by the word lumen, q.v.

Lignac-Fanconi disease. Fanconi's syndrome, q.v.

lignin (lĭg′nĭn). A polysaccharide present in plants that combines with cellulose to form the cell walls.

lignocaine (lĭg′nō-kān). A local anesthetic. SEE: *lidocaine hydrochloride.*

lignoceric acid. A saturated fatty acid present in one type of sphingomyelin.

limb (lĭm) [AS. *lim*]. 1. An arm or leg. 2. An extremity. 3. A limblike extension of a structure.

RS: anisomelia; appendicular; extremity; member.

l., anacrotic. The ascending portion of the pulse wave.

l., anterior, of internal capsule. The lenticulocaudate portion that lies between lenticular and caudate nuclei.

l., ascending, of renal tubule. Portion of tubule between the bend in Henle's loop and the distal convoluted section.

l., catacrotic. The descending portion of the pulse wave.

l., descending, of renal tubule. Portion of tubule between proximal convoluted section and the bend in Henle's loop.

l., pectoral. The arm.

l., pelvic. The lower extremity.

l., phantom. The perception and sensation that an amputated limb is still present. It may be associated with painful paresthesias, pain, and itching.

l., thoracic. The upper extremity.

limbic (lĭm'bĭk) [L. *limbus,* border]. Pert. to a limbus or border. SYN: *marginal.*

limbic system. A group of brain structures including the hippocampus, amygdala, dentate gyrus, cingulate gyrus, gyrus fornicatus, the archicortex, and their interconnections and connections with the hypothalamus, septal area, and a medial area of the mesencephalic tegmentum. The system is activated by motivated behavior and arousal, and it influences the endocrine and autonomic motor systems.

limbus (lĭm'bŭs) [L., border]. [NA] The edge or border of a part.

l. alveolaris. 1. The upper free edge of the alveolar process of the mandible. 2. The lower free edge of the alveolar process of the maxilla. SYN: *arcus alveolaris maxillae.*

l. conjunctivae. The edge of the conjunctiva overlapping the cornea.

l. corneae. [NA] The edge of the cornea where it unites with the sclera.

l., corneoscleral. In the eye, a transitional dome 1 to 2 mm. wide where the cornea joins the sclera and conjunctiva.

l. fossa ovalis. [NA] The thickened margin of the fossa ovalis, esp. the rim of the septum secundum bounding the fossa.

l. lamina spiralis. Thickening of the periosteum of the osseus spiral lamina of the cochlea to which the tectorial membrane is attached.

l. palpebralis, anterior. The anterior margin of the free edge of the eyelid from which the cilia or eyelashes grow.

l. palpebralis, posterior. The posterior margin of the free edge of the eyelid; the region of transition of skin to conjunctival mucous membrane.

l. sphenoidalis. Ridge on anterior portion of upper surface of sphenoid bone.

lime (līm) [AS. *lim,* glue]. USP. Calcium oxide, CaO. A substance obtained from limestone. Calcium oxide is prepared from limestone, $CaCO_3$, by heating it sufficiently to drive off the carbon dioxide. When lime is mixed with water, heat is produced. Lime is an ingredient of cement and mortar.

CAUTION: Avoid contact with eyes when working with lime. SYN: *calcium oxide; quicklime.* SEE: *calcium.*

l., chlorinated. Substance resulting from chlorinization of slaked lime, consisting chiefly of calcium chloride and calcium hypochlorite. Used principally as a disinfectant and in aqueous solution as a bleaching agent.

l., slaked. The substance produced when lime is allowed free access to water and carbon dioxide from the atmosphere. It is a mixture of calcium hydroxide, $Ca(OH)_2$, and calcium carbonate, $CaCO_3$.

l., soda. A combination of calcium oxide and sodium hydroxide.

l., sulfurated. USP. Solution of lime, sublimated sulfur, and water. Used as a topical solution in treating skin disease.

l. water. Alkaline solution of calcium hydroxide, $Ca(OH)_2$, in water; a weak base used as an antacid.

lime [Fr.]. Fruit of Citrus aurantifolia. Its juice is antiscorbutic.

limen (lī'mĕn) [L.]. (pl. *limina*) [NA] Entrance, threshold.

l. nasi. The boundary line between the bony and cartilaginous portion of the nasal cavity. It is also at this point that the nasal cavity proper and the vestibule of the nose meet.

l. of insula. The portion of the cortex of the brain that provides a threshold to the insula. The middle cerebral artery passes over this threshold to extend to the insula.

limes tod. The least amount of toxin that when mixed with one unit of antitoxin and injected into a guinea pig weighing 250 gm. will kill it within 96 hours. SYMB: L_+.

limes nul. The greatest amount of toxin that when mixed with one unit of antitoxin and injected into a guinea pig weighing 250 gm. will cause no local reaction. SYMB: L_0.

liminal (lĭm'ĭ-năl) [L. *limen,* threshold]. Hardly perceptible; rel. to a threshold as of consciousness or vision.

limit (lĭm'ĭt). 1. A boundary. 2. A point or line beyond which something cannot or may not progress.

l., assimilation. The amount of carbohydrate that can be absorbed or ingested without causing glycosuria.

l., audibility. The limits of sound frequencies at both the low and high ends of the sound scale beyond which sound cannot be heard. The lower limit is approximately 8–16 Hz and the upper limit between 12,000 and 20,000 Hz, depending upon various factors, including age. In general, the upper limit of audible sound decreases with age.

l., elastic. The extent to which something may be stretched or bent and still have the ability to return to its original shape.

l., Hayflick's. The number of cell divisions that will take place in human cell cultures prior to dying out. This is estimated to be about 50 cell divisions.

l. of flocculation. The amount of a toxin or toxoid that causes the most rapid flocculation when combined with its antitoxin.

l. of perception. The smallest object that can be detected by the eye. Such an object usually subtends a visual image of one minute. This produces a retinal image slightly larger than the diameter of a retinal cone, i.e., about 0.004 mm. SYN: *normal limit of visual acuity.*

l., quantum. The minimum wavelength present in the spectrum produced by x-rays.

limitans (lĭm′ĭ-tăns) [L. *limitare,* to limit]. 1. Used in conjunction with other words to denote limiting. 2. Used synonymously to indicate membrane limitans.

limitation (lĭm″ĭ-tā′shŭn). Condition of being limited.

limitation of motion. The restriction of movement or range of motion of a part or joint. Esp. that imposed by disease or trauma to joints and soft tissues.

limosis (lī-mō′sĭs) [Gr. *limos,* hunger]. Abnormal hunger; perverted appetite.

limotherapy (lī″mō-thĕr′ă-pē) [″ + *therapeia,* treatment]. Treatment of obesity by restriction of diet or by fasting.

limulus amebocyte lysate test. ABBR: LAL test. Limulus amebocyte lysate is formed from the lysed circulating amebocytes of the horseshoe crab (Limulus polyphemus). The lysate is used to detect minute quantities of bacterial endotoxins, and has been used to test for pyrogens in various materials. It is also used to detect septicemia due to gram-negative bacteria.

Lincocin. Trade name for lincomycin.

Lincocin Hydrochloride. Trade name for lincomycin hydrochloride, USP.

lincomycin hydrochloride (lĭn″kō-mī′sĭn). USP. An antibiotic obtained from Streptomyces lincolnensis. Trade name is Lincocin Hydrochloride.

lincture, linctus (lĭnk′tūr, -tŭs) [L. *linctus,* a licking]. A thick, sweet, syrupy medicinal preparation given for its effect on the throat. Usually taken in sips or may be licked or sucked as with a throat lozenge.

lindane (lĭn′dān). USP. A miticide used in treating scabies. The trade name products Gamene and Kwell include this chemical in their formulation.

Lindau's disease (lĭn′dowz). [Arvid Lindau, Swedish pathologist, b. 1892] Lindau-von Hippel disease, q.v.

Lindau-von Hippel disease (lĭn′dow-vŏn-hĭp′ĕl). [Arvid Lindau; Eugen von Hippel, Ger. ophthalmologist, 1867–1939] Angiomata of the retina and cysts and angiomata of the brain and certain visceral organs.

line (līn) [L. *linea*]. 1. Any long, relatively narrow mark. 2. A boundary or an outline. 3. A wrinkle.

l., abdominal. Line indicating abdominal muscle boundaries.

l., absorption. A black line in the continuous spectrum of light passing through an absorbing medium.

l., alveolobasilar. Line from basion to alveolar point.

l., alveolonasal. Line from alveolar point to nasion.

l., auriculobregmatic. Line from auricular point to bregma.

l.'s, axillary. Anterior, posterior, and midaxillary lines that extend downward from the axilla.

l., base. Line from the infraorbital ridge through the middle of the external auditory meatus to midline of occiput.

l., basiobregmatic. Line from basion to bregma.

l., Baudelocque's. Exterior conjugate diameter of pelvis.

l.'s, Beau's. Transverse lines on the fingernails formed at the base of the nail, usually in response to local trauma, malnutrition, or systemic disease. They become visible as the nail grows. Their distance from the base of the nail can provide a rough estimate of the time of occurrence of the cause.

l., biauricular. Line from one auditory meatus over vertex to the other.

l., blue. Line seen on gums in chronic lead poisoning.

l., cervical. 1. Line of junction of cementum and enamel of a tooth. 2. Line on neck of tooth where gum is attached.

l., cement. The refractile boundary of an osteon of the haversian system of a bone.

l.'s, cleavage. Langer's lines, q.v.

l., costoarticular. Line from sternoclavicular joint to point on 11th rib.

l., costoclavicular. Line midway between nipple and sternum border.

l., Douglas'. A crescent-shaped line at the lower limit of the posterior sheath of the rectus abdominis muscle. It is sometimes indistinct.

l., epiphyseal. The line at the junction of the epiphysis and diaphysis of a long bone. It is at this junction that bone growth occurs.

l., gingival. A line determined by the extent of coverage of the tooth by gingiva; the shape of the gingival lines is similar to the curvature of the cervical line but they rarely coincide. Also: *free gingival margin.*

l.'s, gluteal. Three lines, anterior, posterior, and inferior, on exterior surface of ilium.

l., gum. The line formed by the gingival

margin of the neck of the tooth.

l., iliopectineal. Bony ridge marking the brim of the pelvis.

l., incremental. One of the lines seen in a microscopic section of the enamel of a tooth. They resemble growth lines in a tree.

l., incremental, of Retzius. Periodic dark lines seen in the enamel of a tooth that represent occasional metabolic disturbances of mineralization.

l., incremental, of von Ebner. Very light lines in the dentin of a tooth that represent the boundary between the layers of dentin produced daily.

l., interauricular. Line joining the two auricular points.

l., intercondylar. Transverse ridge joining condyles of femur above the intercondyloid fossa.

l., intertrochanteric. Ridge upon posterior surface of femur exterior between the greater and lesser trochanters.

l., intertuberal. Line joining inner borders of the ischial tuberosities below the small sciatic notch.

l., Kerley's. Lines present on roentgenograms of the chest of patients with any disease that causes thickening or infiltration of the interlobular septa. Those in the costophrenic angle area are called Kerley B lines and those extending peripherally from the hilum are termed Kerley A lines.

l., lead. An irregular dark line in the gingival margin. The line is present in chronic lead poisoning and is caused by the deposition of lead in that portion of the gum.

l., lip. The highest or lowest point the lips reach on the teeth or gums during a broad smile.

l., mammary. Horizontal line from one nipple to the other.

l., mammillary. Vertical line through the center of the nipple.

l., median. Line joining any two points in the periphery of the median plane of the body or one of its parts.

l., milk. The mammary ridge, an ectodermal thickening in the embryo exterior between bases of limb buds.

l., mylohyoid. A ridge on the inner surface of the mandible. It extends from a point beneath the mental spine upward and back to the ramus past the last molar. The mylohyoid and superior constrictor muscle of the pharynx attach to this ridge.

l., nasobasilar. Line through basion and nasion.

l., nuchal, superior and inferior. Two curved ridges on occipital bone extending laterally from exterior occipital crest.

l., oblique, of fibula. The medial crest of posteromedial border; a line extending from the medial side of the head and terminating distally at the interosseous crest.

l., oblique, of radius. Faint ridge on anterior surface passing downward and laterally from radial tuberosity.

l. of demarcation. Line of division between healthy and diseased tissue.

l. of femur, internal supracondylar. Inner of two ridges into which linea aspera of femur divides.

l. of fibula, oblique. Prominent ridge on the interior surface of the shaft of the fibula.

l. of fixation. Imaginary line drawn from subject viewed to the fovea centralis.

l. of ilium, intermediate. Ridge upon crest of ilium between inner and outer lip.

l. of mandible, internal oblique. Ridge on interior surface of lower jaw.

l.'s of Owen. [Sir Richard Owen, Brit. anatomist, 1804–1982] Occasional prominent growth lines or bands in the dentin of a tooth. They provide a record of the growth of the coronal or radicular dentin. SYN: *contour lines.*

l., parasternal. Line midway between nipple and border of sternum.

l., pectineal. Line on posterior surface of femur extending downward from lesser trochanter. That portion of the iliopectineal line formed by the os pubis.

l., popliteal. Line of posterior surface of tibia, extending obliquely downward from the fibular facet on lateral condyle to the medial border of bone.

l., scapular. Line extending downward from the lower angle of the scapula.

l., semilunar. The curved groove in the external abdominal wall. This is over the lateral border of the sheath of the rectus abdominis muscle. SYN: *spigelian line.*

l., Shenton's. In a roentgenogram of the hip joint, a curved line formed by the obturator foramen.

l., sight. Line from center of pupil to viewed object.

l., sternal. Medial line of the sternum.

l., sternomastoid. Line from between heads of sternomastoid muscle to mastoid process.

l., supracondylar, medial and lateral. Two ridges on posterior surface of distal end of femur, formed by diverging lips of the linea aspera.

l., supraorbital. Line across forehead above root of exterior angular process of frontal bone.

l., temporal, superior and inferior. Two curved lines on lateral surface of skull, passing upwards and backwards from zygomatic process of frontal bone and terminating posteriorly at supramastoid crest.

l., umbilicopubic. That portion of median line extending from umbilicus to symphysis pubis.

l., visual. Line that extends from object to macula lutea passing through the nodal point. SYN: *visual axis.*

l.'s, Zollner's. Parallel lines, usually three long ones, with a series of short lines drawn at regular intervals across one of the lines at approximately 60°. Similar lines are drawn across the second line at the angle of approximately 120°. Short lines are drawn across the third line at the same angle as on the first lines. These lines produce the optical illusion that the long lines are converging or diverging. SEE: illus.

linea (lĭn'ē-ă) [L., line]. (pl. *lineae*) [NA] An anatomical line.

l. alba. [NA] The white line of connective tissue in middle of abdomen from sternum to pubis.

l. albicans. Lines seen on the abdomen, buttocks, and breasts. Frequently due to pregnancy, obesity or prolonged adrenal cortical hormone therapy but may occur as the result of abdominal distention due to any cause. SYN: *stria atrophica.*

l. aspera. [NA] A longitudinal ridge on posterior surface of middle third of the femur.

l. atrophicae. The lines, or striae, of atrophic skin. Seen esp. in Cushing's syndrome.

l. costoarticularis. A line between the sternoclavicular articulation and point of the 11th rib.

l. nigra. Black line or discoloration of the abdomen that may be seen in pregnant women during latter part of term. It runs from above the umbilicus to the pubes.

l. semilunaris. Spigelian line, q.v.

l. splendens. A thickening of the pia mater extending along the anterior median surface of the spinal cord. It ensheaths the anterior spinal artery.

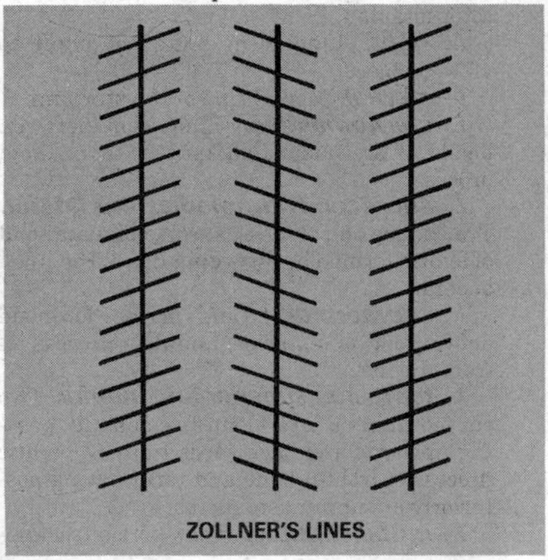

ZOLLNER'S LINES

l. sternalis. Median line of the sternum.

l. terminalis. [NA] Bony ridge on inner surface of ilium continued on to pubis that divides true and false pelvis.

l. transversae ossis sacralis. Ridges formed by lines of union of the 5th sacral vertebrae.

linear (lĭn'ē-ăr) [L. *linea,* line]. Pert. to or resembling a line.

linear energy transfer. A measure of the rate of energy transfer from ionizing radiation to soft tissue.

liner (līn'ĕr). Anything applied to the inside of a hollow body or structure.

lingua (lĭng'gwă) [L.]. (pl. *linguae*) [NA] Tongue or tonguelike structure.

l. fraenata. A tongue with a very short frenum, resulting in tongue-tie. SYN: *ankyloglossia.*

l. geographica. Geographic tongue.

l. nigra. Condition in which tongue has a brown furlike area on its dorsum. The area is composed of hypertrophied filiform papillae pigment and possibly microorganisms. Sometimes results from excessive use of oxygen-liberating mouthwashes or antibiotic therapy. SYN: *tongue, black hairy.*

l. plicata. A fissured tongue.

lingual (lĭng'gwăl) [L. *lingua,* tongue]. 1. Pert. to the tongue. 2. Tongue-shaped.

linguiform (lĭng'gwĭ-form) [" + *forma,* shape]. Tongue-shaped.

lingula (lĭng'gū-lă) [L., little tongue]. [NA] Tongue-shaped process, esp. lingula cerebelli.

l. cerebelli. [NA] Tongue of cerebellum prolonged forward on upper surface of superior medullary velum.

l. of lung. Projection of lung that separates cardiac notch from inferior margin of left lung.

l. of mandible. Projection of bone that forms the medial boundary of the mandibular foramen.

l. of sphenoid. Ridge between the body and ala magna of the sphenoid.

l. Wrisbergi. Connecting fibers of motor and sensory roots of the trigeminal nerve.

lingulectomy (lĭng"gū-lĕk'tō-mē) [L. *lingula,* little tongue, + Gr. *ektome,* excision]. Surgical removal of the lingula of the upper lobe of the left lung.

linguoclasia (lĭng"gwō-klā'zē-ă) [" + Gr. *klasis,* destruction]. Displacement of a tooth toward the tongue.

linguoclination (lĭng"gwō-klī-nā'shŭn) [L. *lingua,* tongue, + *clinatus,* leaning]. Angulation of a tooth in its vertical axis toward the tongue.

linguodistal (lĭng"gwō-dĭs'tăl) [" + *distare,* to be distant]. Concerning the distal part of a tooth and the tongue.

linguogingival (lĭng″gwō-jĭn′jĭ-văl) [″ + *gingiva,* gum]. Concerning the tongue and the gingiva.

linguo-occlusal (lĭng″gwō-ŏ-kloo′zăl) [″ + *occludere,* to shut up]. Concerning or bounded by the lingual and occlusal surfaces of a tooth.

linguopapillitis (lĭng″gwō-păp″ĭ-lī′tĭs) [″ + *papilla,* nipple, + Gr. *itis,* inflammation]. Small ulcers of the papillae of the edge of the tongue.

linguoversion (lĭng″gwō-vĕr′zhŭn) [″ + *versio,* a turning]. Displacement of a tooth toward the tongue.

liniment [L. *linimentum,* smearing substance]. A liquid containing a medicament and oil, alcohol, or water for use externally. Applied by friction method or on a bandage.

l., camphor. A preparation of camphor and a suitable vehicle, such as an oil, that is used topically as an irritant.

l., medicinal soft soap. Tincture of green soap.

linimentum (lĭn-ĭ-mĕn′tŭm) [L.]. Liquid preparation for external use and usually applied by rubbing. SYN: *liniment.*

linitis (lĭn-ī′tĭs) [Gr. *linon,* flax, + *itis,* inflammation]. Inflammation of the lining of the stomach.

l. plastica. Linitis with thickening of the wall of the stomach usually due to neoplastic tissue. SYN: *stomach, leather-bottle.*

linkage. In genetics, the association between distinct genes that occupy closely situated loci on the same chromosome. This results in an association in the inheritance of these genes.

l., sex. A genetic characteristic that is located on the X or Y chromosome.

linseed [AS. *linsaed*]. Seeds of the common flax, Linum usitatissimum. It is the source of linseed oil. Linseed is used as a demulcent and emollient. SYN: *flaxseed.*

lint (lĭnt) [L. *linteum,* made of linen]. 1. Linen scraped until soft and wooly for dressing wounds. 2. Cotton fiber. 3. Household dust.

lintin (lĭn′tĭn). Prepared absorbent cotton; fabric used in dressings.

liothyronine sodium (lī″ō-thī′rō-nēn). USP. Sodium salt of triiodothyronine. Used in treating hypothyroidism. Trade name is Cytomel. SEE: *thyroid function tests.*

liotrix tablets (lī′ō-trĭks). USP. A combination of levothyroxine sodium and liothyronine sodium. Used in treating thyroid deficiency. Trade names are Euthroid and Thyrolar.

lip [AS. *lippa*]. 1. Soft external structure that forms the boundary of the mouth or opening to the oral cavity. SYN: *labium* or *labia oris.* 2. One of the lips of the pudendum (labium majus or minus). 3. A liplike structure forming the border of an opening or groove.

PATH: *Chancre:* It is not unusual to have the initial lesion of syphilis appear upon the lip of the mouth as an indurated base with a thin secretion and accompanied by enlargement of the submaxillary glands. *Condyloma latum:* This appears as a mucous patch, flattened, coated with gray exudate, with strictly delimited area, usually at the angle of the mouth. *Eczema:* Dry fissures, often covered with a crust, bleeding easily, and occurring on both lips. *Epithelioma:* May be confused with chancre. Seldom appears before the age of 40, but there are exceptions. It may appear as a common cold sore, a painless fissure, or other break of the lower lip. A crust or scab covers the lesion, leaving a raw surface if removed. Pain does not appear until the lesion is well advanced. Much more common on lower lip than upper. *Herpes:* Appears on the lips in pneumonia, typhoid, common cold, other febrile diseases, and idiopathically. *Tuberculous ulcer:* At inner portion of lip close to angle of mouth. Pathological examination necessary for verification.

DIAG: Examination is considered to be incomplete unless lips are everted to expose buccal surfaces. *Bluish or purplish:* May appear in the aged, in those exposed to great cold, and in carbon monoxide poisoning. *Dry:* May be seen in fevers or be caused by drugs such as atropine, by thirst, or by mouth breathing. *Fissured:* May occur after exposure to cold, in avitaminosis, and in children with congenital syphilis. The dribbling of saliva and a toothless condition may cause fissures in the corners of the mouth. *Pale:* May be seen in anemia and wasting diseases, in prolonged fever, and after a hemorrhage. *Rashes:* May be manifestations of typhoid fever, meningitis, or pneumonia. Mucous patches may appear in secondary syphilis, chancre, cancer, and epithelioma.

RS: buccal; cheilitis; cheilosis; "chil-" words; labia; labium; labrum.

l., cleft. Harelip.

l., double. A redundant fold of mucous membrane in the mouth on either side of the midline of the lip.

l., glenoid. Thickened fibrocartilaginous structure surmounting margin of acetabulum.

l., Hapsburg. A thick, overdeveloped lower lip.

l.'s, oral. Upper and lower lips that surround mouth opening and form anterior wall of buccal cavity.

l., tympanic. Lower border of the sulcus spiralis internus of the cochlea.

l., vestibule. Upper border of the sulcus spiralis internus of the cochlea.

lipacidemia (lĭp″ăs-ĭ-dē′mē-ă) [Gr. *lipos,* fat, + L. *acidus,* acid, + Gr. *haima,* blood]. Excess fatty acids in the blood.

lipaciduria (lĭp″ăs-ĭ-dū′rē-ă) [″ + ″ + Gr. *ouron,* urine]. Fatty acids in the urine.

liparocele (lĭp′ă-rō-sēl) [″ + *kele,* hernia]. 1. Scrotal hernia containing fat. 2. A fatty tumor.

liparous (lĭp′ă-rŭs) [Gr. *lipos,* fat]. Obese; fat.

lipase (lī′pās, lĭ′pās) [″ + *-ase,* enzyme]. A lipolytic or fat-splitting enzyme found in the blood, pancreatic secretion, and tissues. Emulsified fats of cream and egg yolk are changed in the stomach to fatty acids and glycerol by gastric lipase. SEE: *digestion; enzyme.*

l., pancreatic. Steapsin, q.v.

lipasuria (lĭp″ăs-ū′rē-ă) [″ + ″ + Gr. *ouron,* urine]. Lipase in the urine.

lipectomy (lĭ-pĕk′tō-mē) [″ + *ektome,* excision]. Excision of fatty tissues.

lipedema (lĭp″ĕ-dē′mă) [″ + *oidema,* swelling]. Swelling of the skin, esp. of the lower extremity, due to accumulation of fat and fluid subcutaneously.

lipemia (lĭ-pē′mē-ă) [″ + *haima,* blood]. Abnormal amount of fat in the blood.

l., alimentary. Accumulation of fat in the blood after eating.

l. retinalis. Condition in which retinal vessels appear reddish white or white. Found in cases of hyperlipidemia. SEE: *hyperlipoproteinemia.*

lipid(e) (lĭp′ĭd, -īd) [Gr. *lipos,* fat]. Any one of a group of fats or fatlike substances, characterized by their insolubility in water and solubility in fat solvents such as alcohol, ether, and chloroform. The term is descriptive rather than a chemical name such as protein or carbohydrate. Includes true fats (esters of fatty acids and glycerol); lipoids (phospholipids, cerebrosides, waxes); and sterols (cholesterol, ergosterol). SEE: *fat; lipoprotein.*

lipid histiocytosis. Niemann-Pick disease.

lipidosis. Any disorder of fat metabolism. SYN: *lipoidosis.*

lipiduria (lĭp″ĭ-dū′rē-ă) [″ + Gr. *ouron,* urine]. Lipids in the urine.

lipin (lĭp′ĭn) [Gr. *lipos,* fat]. SEE: *lipid.*

Lipiodol (lĭp-ī′ō-dŏl) [″ + L. *oleum,* oil]. Proprietary name for an iodized oil obtained by fixation of iodine in poppyseed oil. It contains 40% of pure iodine by weight. Being opaque to x-rays, it is used for radiological studies. It is introduced into cavities by a catheter, into the trachea for outlining the bronchial tree by x-ray, and into the spinal canal to locate tumors. It is eliminated completely and does not cause iodism.

lipo-, lip- [Gr. *lipos,* fat]. Combining forms pert. to fat.

lipoarthritis (lĭp″ō-ărth-rī′tĭs) [″ + *arthron,* joint, + *itis,* inflammation]. Inflammation of fatty tissues of joints.

lipoatrophia, lipoatrophy (lī″pō-ă-trō′fē-ă, lī″pō-ăt′rō-fē) [″ + *a-,* not, + *trophe,* nourishment]. Atrophy of fat tissue. May occur at the site of insulin injection. SEE: *lipodystrophy.*

lipoblast (lĭp′ō-blăst) [″ + *blastos,* germ]. An immature fat cell.

lipoblastoma (lĭp″ō-blăs-tō′mă) [″ + ″ + *oma,* tumor]. A benign tumor of fatty tissue. SYN: *adipoma; lipoma.*

lipocardiac (lĭp″ō-kăr′dē-ăk) [″ + *kardia,* heart]. 1. Pert. to fatty heart degeneration. 2. Sufferer from fatty degeneration of heart.

lipocatabolic (lĭp″ō-kăt″ă-bŏl′ĭk) [″ + *katabole,* a casting down]. Concerning the breaking down of fat tissue during metabolism.

lipocele (lĭp′ō-sēl) [″ + *kele,* hernia]. Presence of fatty tissue in a hernia sac. SYN: *adipocele; liparocele.*

lipoceratous (lĭp″ō-sĕr′ă-tŭs) [″ + L. *cera,* wax]. Concerning the waxy substance formed when a body decomposes in a moist area, as when buried in wet soil. SYN: *adipoceratous.*

lipocere (lĭp′ō-sēr) [″ + L. *cera,* wax]. Waxy substance resulting from exposure of fleshy tissue to moisture with the exclusion of air. SYN: *adipocere.*

lipochondrodystrophy (lĭp″ō-kŏn″drō-dĭs′trō-fē) [″ + *chondros,* cartilage, + *dys,* bad, + *trephein,* to nourish]. Congenital abnormality in the skeletal bones and cartilage with deranged mucopolysaccharide metabolism, kyphosis and other deformity, possible mental deficiency, and cloudy corneae. SYN: *Hurler's syndrome; mucopolysaccharidosis I.*

lipochondroma (lĭp″ō-kŏn-drō′mă) [″ + ″ + *oma,* tumor]. Tumor that is both fatty and cartilaginous.

lipochrome (lĭp′ō-krōm) [″ + *chroma,* color]. A group of fat-soluble pigments. SEE: *carotene.*

Ex.: carotene, the fat-soluble yellow pigment found in carrots, sweet potatoes, egg yolk, butter, body fat and corpus luteum.

lipoclasis (lĭp-ŏk′lă-sĭs) [″ + *klasis,* breaking]. Splitting up of fat. SYN: *lipolysis.*

lipoclastic (lĭp-ō-klăs′tĭk) Rel. to or causing lipoclasis. SYN: *lipolytic.*

lipocyte (lĭp′ō-sīt) [″ + *kytos,* cell]. Fat cell.

lipodieresis (lĭp″ō-dī-ĕr′ē-sĭs) [″ + *diairesis,* a taking]. Splitting or destructive to fat.

lipodystrophy (lĭp″ō-dĭs′trō-fē) [″ + *dys,* bad, + *trophe,* nourishment]. Disturbance or defectiveness of fat metabolism.

l., insulin. A complication of insulin administration characterized by changes in the subcutaneous fat at the site of injection. The changes may take the form of atrophy or hypertrophy; rarely are both types present in the same patient. Atrophy develops in as many as one third of children and adult females who use insulin regularly but rarely in adult males. The subcutaneous fat appears to have melted away and leaves a saucer-like depression. Hypertrophy at the injection site occurs in the form of a spongy localized area. This type of complication of insulin administration is slightly more common in males than females. It is usually associated with a history of prolonged use of the same injection site.

l., intestinal. Disease characterized principally by fat deposits in intestinal and mesenteric lymphatic tissue, fatty diarrhea, loss of weight and strength, and arthritis.

l., progressive. A pathological condition in which there is progressive, symmetrical loss of subcutaneous fat from the upper part of the trunk, face, neck, and arms.

lipoferous (lĭp-ŏf′ĕr-ŭs) [″ + L. *ferre,* to carry]. Causing or carrying fat.

lipofibroma (lĭp″ō-fī-brō′mă) [″ + L. *fibra,* fiber, + Gr. *oma,* tumor]. A lipoma having much fibrous tissue. SYN: *fibrolipoma.*

lipofuscin (lĭp″ō-fŭs′sĭn). One of a class of partly insoluble lipid pigments present in cardiac and smooth muscle cells.

lipofuscinosis (lĭp″ō-fū″sĭn-ō′sĭs) [*lipofuscin* + Gr. *osis,* condition]. Abnormal deposition of lipofuscin in tissues.

Lipo Gantrisin. Trade name for sulfisoxazole acetyl, USP.

lipogenesis (lĭp″ō-jĕn′ĕ-sĭs) [Gr. *lipos,* fat, + *genesis,* formation]. Fat formation.

lipogenetic, lipogenic (lĭp″ō-jĕ-nĕt′ĭk, lĭp″ō-jĕn′ik). Fat producing. SYN: *lipogenous.*

lipogenous (lĭp-ŏj′ĕ-nŭs). Producing fat. SYN: *lipogenetic.*

lipogranuloma (lĭp″ō-grăn-ū-lō′mă) [″ + L. *granulum,* granule, + Gr. *oma,* tumor]. Inflammation of fatty tissue with granulation and development of oily cysts.

lipogranulomatosis (lĭp″ō-grăn″ū-lō-mă-tō′sĭs) [″ + ″ + ″ + *osis,* condition]. A disorder of fat metabolism in which a nodule of fat undergoes central necrosis and the surrounding tissue becomes granulomatous.

Lipo-Hepin. Trade name for heparin sodium, USP.

lipoid (lĭp′oyd) [″ + *eidos,* form]. 1. Similar to fat. 2. Substance resembling fats in appearance and solubility, but containing other groups than the glycerol and fatty acids that make up the true fats. SYN: *lipid.*

Ex.: cholesterol; kephalin; lecithin.

lipoidemia (lĭp″oy-dē′mē-ă) [″ + ″ + *haima,* blood]. Excess of lipoids in the blood.

lipoidosis (lĭp-oy-dō′sĭs) [″ + ″ + *osis,* condition]. Condition in which lipids accumulate in excessive quantities in body tissue. SYN: *lipidosis.* SEE: *xanthomatosis.*

l., arterial. Arteriosclerosis.

l., cerebral infantile. A hereditary disorder due to a defect in lipid metabolism in which sphingolipids accumulate in the brain.

l., cerebroside. A familial disease characterized by deposition of kerasin, a cerebroside, in cells of the reticuloendothelial system. SYN: *Gaucher's disease.*

l., primary. Lipoidosis of unknown etiology in which serum lipids are abnormal in quantity or in quality, or else serum lipids are normal but lipids accumulate intracellularly.

lipoiduria (lĭp″oy-dū′rē-ă) [″ + ″ + *ouron,* urine]. Lipoids in the urine.

lipolipoidosis (lĭp″ō-lĭp″oy-dō′sĭs) [″ + *lipos,* fat, + *eidos,* form, + *osis,* condition]. Infiltration of fats and lipoids into a tissue.

lipolysis (lĭp-ŏl′ĭ-sĭs) [″ + *lysis,* dissolution]. The decomposition of fat. SYN: *lipoclasis.*

lipolytic (lĭp-ō-lĭt′ĭk). Rel. to lipolysis.

lipolytic digestion. The conversion of neutral fats by hydrolysis into fatty acids and glycerol; fat splitting.

lipolytic enzyme. Fat-splitting ferment. SYN: *lipase.* SEE: *enzyme.*

lipoma (lĭ-pō′mă) [Gr. *lipos,* fat, + *oma,* tumor]. A fatty tumor. They are frequently multiple but not metastatic. SYN: *adipoma.* SEE: *chondrolipoma.*

l. arborescens. An abnormal treelike accumulation of fatty tissue in a joint.

l., cystic. Lipoma containing cysts.

l., diffuse. Lipoma not definitely circumscribed.

l. diffusum renis. Condition in which fat displaces parenchyma of the kidney.

l. durum. Lipoma in which there is marked hypertrophy of the fibrous stroma and capsule.

l., hernial. Lipocele.

l., nasal. A fibrous growth of the subcutaneous tissue of the nostrils.

l., osseous. Lipoma in which the connective tissue has undergone calcareous degeneration.

l. telangiectodes. A rare form of lipoma containing a large number of blood vessels.

lipomatoid (lĭ-pō′mă-toyd) [″ + ″ + *eidos,* form] Similar to a lipoma.

lipomatosis (lĭp″ō-mă-tō′sĭs) [″ + *oma,* tumor + *osis,* condition]. Condition marked by excessive deposit of fat in a localized area. SYN: *liposis; obesity.*

l. renis. Fatty infiltration of renal parenchyma. SYN: *lipoma diffusum renis.*

lipomatous (lĭp-ō′mă-tŭs). 1. Of the nature of lipoma. 2. Affected with lipoma.

lipomeningocele (lĭp″ō-mĕ-nĭng′gō-sēl) [″ + *meninx,* membrane, + *kele,* hernia]. A meningocele associated with lobules of fat tissue.

lipomeria (lī″pō-mē′rē-ă) [Gr. *leipein,* to leave, + *meros,* a part]. In a deformed fetus, congenital absence of a limb.
lipometabolic (lĭp″ō-mĕt″ă-bŏl′ĭk) [″ + *metabole,* change]. Rel. to metabolism of fat.
lipometabolism (lĭp-ō-mĕ-tăb′ŏl-ĭzm) [″ + ″ + *-ismos,* state of]. Fat metabolism.
lipomyoma (lĭp″ō-mī-ō′mă) [″ + *mys,* muscle, + *oma,* tumor]. A myoma containing fatty tissue.
lipomyxoma (lĭp″ō-mĭks-ō′mă) [″ + *myxa,* mucus, + *oma,* tumor]. A mixed lipoma and myxoma. SYN: *myxolipoma.*
lipopectic (lĭp-ō-pĕk′tĭk) [″ + *pexis,* fixation]. Characterized by lipopexia.
lipopenia (lĭp″ō-pē′nē-ă) [″ + *penia,* poverty]. Deficiency of lipids.
lipopenic (lĭp″ō-pē′nĭk). Concerning lipopenia.
lipopeptid, lipopeptide (lĭp″ō-pĕp′tĭd, -tīd). A complex of lipids and amino acids.
lipopexia (lĭp″ō-pĕk′sē-ă). Accumulation of fat in the body.
lipophage (lĭp′ō-fāj) [″ + *phagein,* to eat]. Fat-absorbing cell.
lipophagia, granulomatous (lĭp″ō-fā′jē-ă). Lipodystrophy, intestinal, q.v.
lipophagic (lĭp-ō-fā′jĭk). Consuming, destroying, or absorbing fat.
lipophagy (lĭ-pŏf′ă-jē). The absorption of fat.
lipophanerosis (lĭp″ō-făn″ĕ-rō′sĭs) [″ + *phaneros,* visible, + *osis,* condition]. The alteration of fat in a cell so that it becomes visible as droplets.
lipophil (lĭp′ō-fĭl) [″ + *philein,* to love]. 1. Having an affinity for fat. 2. Absorbing fat.
lipophilia (lĭp″ō-fĭl′ē-ă) [″ + *philos,* love]. Affinity for fat.
lipopolysaccharide (lĭp″ō-pŏl″ē-săk′ă-rīd). The linkage of molecules of lipids with polysaccharides.
lipoproteins. Conjugated proteins consisting of simple proteins combined with lipid components: cholesterol, phospholipid, and triglyceride. Most plasma lipids do not circulate in an unbound state, but are chemically linked with proteins. These large molecules are categorized with respect to their chemical properties and densities as determined by ultracentrifugation. Analysis of their concentrations and proportions in the blood can provide important clues as to their role in certain diseases, particularly cardiovascular abnormalities, hypertension, atherosclerosis, and coronary artery disease. Lipoproteins are classified as very low density (VLDL), low-density (LDL), and high-density (HDL). It is thought that individuals with high blood levels of HDL are less predisposed to coronary heart disease as compared to those with high blood levels of VLDL or LDL. SEE: *hyperlipoproteinemia.*

l., high-density. ABBR: HDL. Plasma lipids bound to albumin, consisting of lipoproteins. They contain more protein than either very low-density lipoproteins or low-density lipoproteins.

l., low-density. ABBR: LDL. Plasma lipids bound to albumin, consisting of lipoproteins that contain more protein than the very low density lipoproteins.

l., very low density. ABBR: VLDL. Plasma lipids bound to albumin consisting of chylomicrons and pre-lipoproteins. This class of plasma lipoproteins contains a greater ratio of lipid than the low-density lipoproteins and is the least dense.

liposarcoma (lĭp″ō-săr-kō′mă) [Gr. *lipos,* fat, + *sarx,* flesh, + oma, tumor]. A malignant tumor derived from embryonal lipoblastic cells.
liposis (lĭ-pō′sĭs) [″ + *osis,* condition]. Abnormal accumulation of fat in the body. SYN: *adiposis.*
liposoluble (lĭp″ō-sŏl′ū-b′l) [″ + L. *solubilis,* soluble]. Soluble in fats.
liposome (lĭp′ō-sōm) [″ + *soma,* body]. A particle of lipoidal substances held in suspension in tissues.
lipostomy (lī-pŏs′tō-mē) [Gr. *leipein,* to fail, + *stoma,* mouth]. Congenital absence or extreme smallness of the mouth.
lipothymia (lī″pō-thī′mē-ă) [″ + *thymos,* mind]. Faintness; syncope.
lipotrophy (lĭ-pŏt′rō-fē) [Gr. *lipos,* fat, + *trophe,* nourishment]. Increase in body fat.
lipotropic (lĭp-ō-trŏp′ĭk) [″ + *trope,* a turning]. Having an affinity for lipids.

Ex.: certain dyes such as Sudan III, which stains fat readily.

lipotropic factors. Compounds that promote the transportation and utilization of fats and help to prevent accumulation of fat in the liver.
lipotropism, lipotropy (lĭ-pŏt′rō-pĭzm, -pē) [″ + *trope,* a turn, + *-ismos,* condition]. 1. To have the action of removing fat deposits in the liver. 2. An agent that acts to remove fat from the liver.
lipovaccine (lĭp″ō-văk′sēn). A vaccine suspended in vegetable oil.
lipoxeny (lĭ-pŏks′ĕ-nē) [Gr. *leipein,* to fail, + *xenos,* host]. Desertion of host by parasitic organism after completion of its development.
lipoxidase (lĭ-pŏk′sĭ-dās). An enzyme that catalyzes the oxidation of the double bonds of an unsaturated fatty acid.
lipoxygenase (lĭ-pŏks′ĭ-jĕ-nās). Lipoxidase, q.v.
Lippes loop (lĭ′pēz). A type of intrauterine contraceptive device.
lipping (lĭp′ĭng). A growth of bony tissue beyond the joint margin in degenerative joint disease.

lippitude (lĭp′ĭ-tūd) [L. *lippitudo,* fr. *lippus,* blear-eyed]. Ulcerations of the margins of the eyelids.

lip reading. Interpreting what is being said by watching the speaker's lip movements. This method is used very effectively by deaf people.

lip reflex. Reflex movement of lips when angle of mouth is suddenly and lightly tapped during sleep.

lipsis (lĭp′sĭs) [Gr. *leipein,* to fail]. Ending or cessation.

l. animi. Fainting.

lipuria (lĭ-pū′rē-ă) [Gr. *lipos,* fat, + *ouron,* urine]. Fat in the urine.

Liquaemin Sodium. Trade name for heparin sodium, USP.

Liquamar. Trade name for phenprocoumon.

liquefacient (lĭk″wĕ-fā′shĕnt) [L. *liquere,* to flow, + *facere,* to make]. 1. Agent that converts a solid substance into liquid. 2. Converting a solid into liquid.

liquefaction (lĭk″wĕ-făk′shŭn) 1. The conversion of a solid into a liquid. 2. Conversion of solid tissues to a fluid or semifluid state.

liquescent (lĭk-wĕs′sĕnt) [L. *liquescere,* to become liquid]. Becoming liquid. SYN: *deliquescent.*

liqueur (lĭ-kĕr′) [Fr.]. Alcoholic beverage, aromatically flavored, often colored, and sweetened. A cordial.

Liqui-Cee. Trade name for sodium ascorbate, USP.

liquid (lĭk′wĭd) [L. *liquere,* to flow]. 1. Flowing easily. 2. State of matter where a substance flows without being melted. SEE: *emulsion; liquefacient; liquefaction.*

liquid air therapy. Therapeutic application of air that is so cold as to be liquefied. SEE: *CO_2 therapy; cryotherapy; hypothermia.*

liquid crystals. Substances that alter their color or change from opaque to transparent when subjected to changes in temperature, electric current, pressure, electromagnetic waves, or when impurities are present. They have been used to detect temperature fluctuation in infants. Liquid crystals are of two general classes: cholestric, which change color, and nematic, which can change back and forth from transparent to opaque.

liquid diet. Coffee with hot milk; tea; water; milk in all forms; milk and cream mixtures; cocoa; strained cream soups; fruit juices; meat juices; beef tea; clear broths; gruels; strained meat soups; eggnogs. SEE: *fluid diet.*

liquid measure. Measure of liquid capacity.

liquor (lĭk′ĕr) [L.]. 1. Any liquid or fluid. 2. An alcoholic beverage. 3. Solution of medicinal substance in water.

l. amnii. The amniotic fluid, a clear watery fluid that surrounds the fetus in the amniotic sac. SEE: *hydramnion.*

l. folliculi. The fluid contained in the graafian follicle.

l. puris. Liquid portion of pus.

l. sanguinis. Blood serum or plasma.

liquor solutions. Aqueous solutions of nonvolatile substances presenting the greatest variety in strength, character and method of preparation. They are usually very active medicinal preparations.

Lisfranc's ligament (lĭs-frănks′). [Jacques Lisfranc, Fr. surgeon, 1790–1847] The ligament joining the first cuneiform bone of the ankle to the second metatarsal.

lisping (lĭsp′ĭng) [AS. *wlisp,* lisping]. Substitution of sounds due to defect in speech, as of "th" sound for "s" and "z."

lissencephalous (lĭs″sĕn-sĕf′ă-lŭs) [Gr. *lissos,* smooth, + *enkephalos* brain]. Pert. to condition in which the brain is smooth owing to failure of development of cerebral gyri.

lissotrichy (lĭs-sŏt′rĭ-kē) [″ + *thrix,* hair]. Condition of having straight hair.

Lister, Baron Joseph (lĭs′tĕr). British surgeon, 1827–1912, who developed the technique of antiseptic surgery. Without this, modern surgery would not be possible.

listeriosis, listerosis (lĭs-tĕr″ē-ō′sĭs, lĭs″tĕr-ō′sĭs). A disease affecting many domestic animals, wild animals, and man. Caused by Listeria monocytogenes, a soil saprophyte that becomes pathogenic for animals or man under favorable circumstances. The most common manifestation in the adult is meningitis. It may be transmitted transplacentally to the fetus, in which case it may cause abortion. In newborns, the disease is much more serious than in the adult. The mortality may be 100% when it occurs in the first four days. Although man has a high degree of resistance to the bacteria hygienic precautions should be taken when handling infected animals.

TREATMENT: penicillin or ampicillin.

liter (lē′tĕr) [Fr. *litre,* liter]. Metric fluid measure; equivalent to 1000 milliliters (ml.), 270 fl. drams, 61 cu. in., 33.8 fl. oz., or 1.0567 qt. The volume occupied by 1 kg. of water at 4° C. and 760 mm. of mercury pressure. SEE: *metric system.*

NOTE: It is common to define a liter as 1000 cubic centimeters (cc.). This is almost but not quite correct because 1 ml. is equal to 1.000028 cc. Thus liquid volume should be expressed in ml. rather than cc.

lithagogue (lĭth′ă-gŏg) [Gr. *lithos,* stone, + *agogos,* leading]. 1. Agent that expels calculi. 2. Expelling calculi.

Lithane. Trade name for lithium carbonate, USP.

lithecbole (lĭ-thĕk′bō-lē) [″ + *ekbole,* expulsion]. Ejection or passage of a calculus.

lithectasy (lĭth-ĕk′tă-sē) [″ + *ektasis,* dilatation]. Removal of a calculus from the bladder through the dilated urethra.

lithectomy (lĭ-thĕk'tō-mē) [" + *ektome,* excision]. Surgical removal of a calculus.

lithemia (lĭth-ē'mē-ă) [" + *haima,* blood]. Excess of lithic or uric acid in the blood due to imperfect metabolism of the nitrogenous substances.

lithiasis (lĭth-ī'ă-sĭs). 1. Formation of calculi and concretions. 2. Uric acid diathesis.

l. biliaris. Gallstones.

l. nephritica. Stone formation in the kidneys. SYN: *nephrolithiasis.* SEE: *calculus, renal.*

l. renalis. Kidney stones. SEE: *calculus, renal.*

lithic acid (lĭth'ĭk). Uric acid.

lithicosis (lĭth"ĭ-kō'sĭs) [Gr. *lithikos,* made of stone]. Stone cutters' silicosis; pneumoconiosis.

lithium (lĭth'ē-ŭm) [Gr. *lithos,* stone]. SYMB: Li. At. wt. 6.941; at. no. 3. A metallic element.

l. carbonate. USP. A drug that is particularly useful in treating the manic phase of manic-depressive illness. Trade names are Eskalith, Lithane, Lithonate, and Lithotabs. Given orally it is readily absorbed and eliminated at a fast rate for 5 to 6 hrs. and then eliminated at a much slower rate over the next 24 hrs. It is essential to monitor the blood level of the drug in patients on this therapy; samples should be taken 8 to 10 hrs. after the last dose and at intervals after medication.

A dose of 1200 mg. each day is initially given and adjusted as needed to produce a plasma level of 0.8 mEq. per liter. When the dose has been found to produce the optimal plasma concentration, blood analysis is done every three months. Plasma levels of two or more mEq. per liter cause serious toxic effects including stupor or coma, muscular rigidity, marked tremor, and in some cases epileptic seizure.

Side effects including fatigue, weakness, fine tremor of the hands, nausea and vomiting, thirst, and polyuria may be noticed in the first week of therapy. If these are mild, most will disappear, but the thirst, polyuria and tremor tend to persist.

CAUTION: Decreased dietary sodium intake lowers the excretion rate of lithium. It should not be administered to patients on a salt-free diet.

litho-, lith- [Gr. *lithos,* stone]. Prefixes pert. to stone or calculus.

lithocenosis (lĭth"ō-sĕn-ō'sĭs) [" + *kenosis,* evacuation]. Removal of crushed fragments of calculi from the bladder.

lithoclast (lĭth'ō-klăst) [" + *klastos,* broken]. Forceps for breaking up large calculi.

lithoclasty (lĭth'ō-klăs"tē). The crushing of a stone into fragments that may pass through natural channels.

lithoclysmia (lĭth-ō-klĭz'mē-ă) [" + *klysma,* a clyster]. Injection into urinary bladder of substances that have the ability to dissolve calculi.

NOTE: There are no such substances that are both effective and safe to use.

lithocystotomy (lĭth"ō-sĭs-tŏt'ō-mē) [" + *kystis,* bladder, + *tome,* incision]. Incision of the bladder to remove a calculus.

lithodialysis (lĭth"ō-dī-ăl'ĭ-sĭs) [" + *dialyein,* to dissolve]. Fragmentation or dissolution of calculi by injection of a solvent. SYN: *litholysis.*

lithogenesis (lĭth"ō-jĕn'ĕ-sĭs) [" + *gennan,* to produce]. Formation of calculi.

lithokelyphopedion (lĭth"ō-kĕl"ĭ-fō-pē'dē-ŏn) [" + *kelyphos,* sheath, + *paidion,* child]. Calcification of both the fetus and the membranes of a lithopedion.

lithokelyphos (lĭth"ō-kĕl'ĭ-fŏs) [" + *kelyphos,* sheath]. A type of lithopedion in which only the membranes are calcified.

lithokonion (lĭth"ō-kō'nē-ŏn) [" + *konios,* dusty]. Instrument for pulverizing vesical calculi. SYN: *lithomyl.*

litholabe (lĭth'ō-lāb) [" + *lambanein,* to hold]. Device for holding a calculus during its removal.

litholapaxy (lĭth-ŏl'ă-păks"ē) [Gr. *lithos,* stone, + *lapaxis,* evacuation]. The operation of crushing a stone in the bladder followed by immediate washing out of the crushed fragments through a catheter.

lithology (lĭth-ŏl'ō-jē) [" + *logos,* science]. The science dealing with calculi.

litholysis (lĭth-ŏl'ĭ-sĭs) [" + *lysis,* dissolution]. Dissolving of calculi. SYN: *lithodialysis.*

lithometer (lĭth-ŏm'ĕ-tĕr) [" + *metron,* measure]. Instrument for estimating the size of calculi.

lithometra (lĭth-ō-mē'tră) [" + *metra,* uterus]. Uterine tissue ossification.

lithomyl (lĭth'ō-mĭl) [" + *myle,* mill]. Instrument for crushing a vesical stone. SYN: *lithokonion.*

Lithonate. Trade name for lithium carbonate, USP.

lithonephritis (lĭth"ō-nē-frī'tĭs) [" + *nephros,* kidney, + *itis,* inflammation]. Inflammation of the kidney due to a calculus.

lithonephrotomy (lĭth"ō-nē-frŏt'ō-mē) [" + *nephros,* kidney, + *tome,* incision]. Incision of kidney for removal of renal calculus.

lithontriptic (lĭth-ŏn-trĭp'tĭk) [" + *tribein,* to rub]. An agent that tends to dissolve calculi. There are no drugs, medicines, or chemicals that will do this without harming the patient. SYN: *lithotriptic.*

lithopedion (lĭth"ō-pē'dē-ŏn) [" + *paidion,*

child]. A uterine or extrauterine fetus that has died and become calcified. SYN: *ostembryon; osteopedion.*

lithophone (lĭth'ō-fōn) [" + *phone,* sound]. Instrument for determining the presence of calculi in the bladder by sound.

lithoscope (lĭth'ō-skōp) [" + *skopein,* to examine]. Instrument for examining calculi in the bladder.

Lithotabs. Trade name for lithium carbonate, USP.

lithotome (lĭth'ō-tōm) [" + *tome,* incision]. Instrument for performing lithotomy.

lithotomy (lĭth-ŏt'ō-mē) [" + *tome,* incision]. Incision of a duct or organ, esp. of the bladder, for removal of a calculus.

NURSING IMPLICATIONS: Perform catheter care every shift according to hospital procedure. Observe catheter for drainage and document description. Monitor intake and output, and incision site.

l., bilateral. Lithotomy performed with the incision across the perineum.

l., high. Lithotomy performed through a suprapubic incision.

l., lateral. Lithotomy performed with incision from front of the rectum to one side of the raphe.

l., median. Lithotomy performed with incision in median line in front of the anus.

l., rectal. Lithotomy performed through the rectum.

l., vaginal. Lithotomy performed through the vaginal wall.

lithotomy position. Position in which the patient lies upon her back with thighs flexed upon abdomen and legs upon thighs, which are abducted. SYN: *dorsosacral position.* SEE: *position* for illus.

lithotony (lĭth-ŏt'ō-nē) [Gr. *lithos,* stone, + *teinein,* to stretch]. Removal of a calculus through a small incision that is instrumentally dilated.

lithotresis (lĭth"ō-trē'sĭs) [" + *tresis,* boring]. Drilling or boring of holes in a calculus to facilitate crushing.

lithotripsy (lĭth'ō-trĭp"sē) [" + *tribein,* to rub]. Crushing of a calculus in the bladder or urethra.

lithotriptic (lĭth-ō-trĭp'tĭk). 1. Pert. to lithotripsy. SYN: *lithontriptic.* 2. An agent that dissolves calculi.

NOTE: There are no substances that have this capability and are harmless to the patient.

lithotriptor (lĭth'ō-trĭp"tor) [" + *tripsis,* a crushing]. Device for crushing a calculus in the bladder.

lithotriptoscopy (lĭth"ō-trĭp-tŏs'kō-pē) [" + " + *skopein,* to examine]. Crushing of a renal calculus under direct vision by using a lithotriptoscope.

lithotrite (lĭth'ō-trīt) [" + *tribein,* to rub]. Instrument for crushing bladder stones. SEE: *lithotrity.*

lithotrity (lĭth-ŏt'rĭ-tē). Crushing of a stone to small fragments in the bladder.

lithous (lĭth'ŭs) [Gr. *lithos,* stone]. Rel. to a calculus or stone. SYN: *calculous.*

lithoxiduria (lĭth"ŏks-ĭ-dū'rē-ă) [" + L. *oxidum,* oxide, + Gr. *ouron,* urine]. Presence of xanthic oxide in the urine.

lithuresis (lĭth"ū-rē'sĭs) [" + *ouresis,* urination]. Passage of calculus through the urethra during urination.

lithureteria (lĭth"ū-rē-tē'rē-ă) [" + *oureter,* ureter]. Disease of the ureter due to presence of calculi.

lithuria (lĭth-ū'rē-ă) [" + *ouron,* urine]. Excess of uric acid or of urates in the urine.

litmus (lĭt'mŭs). A blue dyestuff made by treating coarsely powdered lichens, such as those of the family Rocella species, with ammonia.

litmus paper. Chemically prepared blue paper that is turned red by acids and remains blue in alkali solutions; pH range is 4.5 to 8.5. SEE: *indicator.*

litter (lĭt'tĕr) [O. Fr. *litiere,* offspring at birth, bed]. 1. A stretcher for carrying the wounded or the sick. 2. The young produced at one birth by a multiparous mammal.

Little's disease. [William John Little, Brit. physician, 1810–1894] Congenital spastic paralysis on both sides (diplegia), although it may be paraplegic or hemiplegic in form. SYN: *paralysis, cerebral spastic infantile.*

ETIOL: Possible birth injury.

SYM: Child has urinary incontinence and is mentally deficient. Stiff, awkward movements, legs crossed and pressed together, arm adducted, forearm flexed, hand pronated, scissors gait.

Littre's glands (lē'trz). [Alexis Littre, Fr. surgeon, 1658–1725] Urethral glands.

littritis (lĭt-trī'tĭs). Inflammation of the urethral glands.

Litzmann's obliquity. Posterior parietal presentation of the fetal head during labor. SYN: *asynclitism, posterior.*

live birth. A term used for statistical purposes indicating an infant born with signs of life such as heartbeat, respiration, or movement of voluntary muscle. In some countries a live birth is considered not to have occurred if the infant dies in the 24 hours following delivery. Obviously, which of these two definitions is used has considerable effect on various vital statistics concerned with the viability of the fetus at time of delivery.

livedo (lĭv-ē'dō) [L. *livedo,* lividness]. Patchy or general bluish discoloration of the skin, as a bruise. SYN: *lividity.*

l. reticularis. Semipermanent bluish

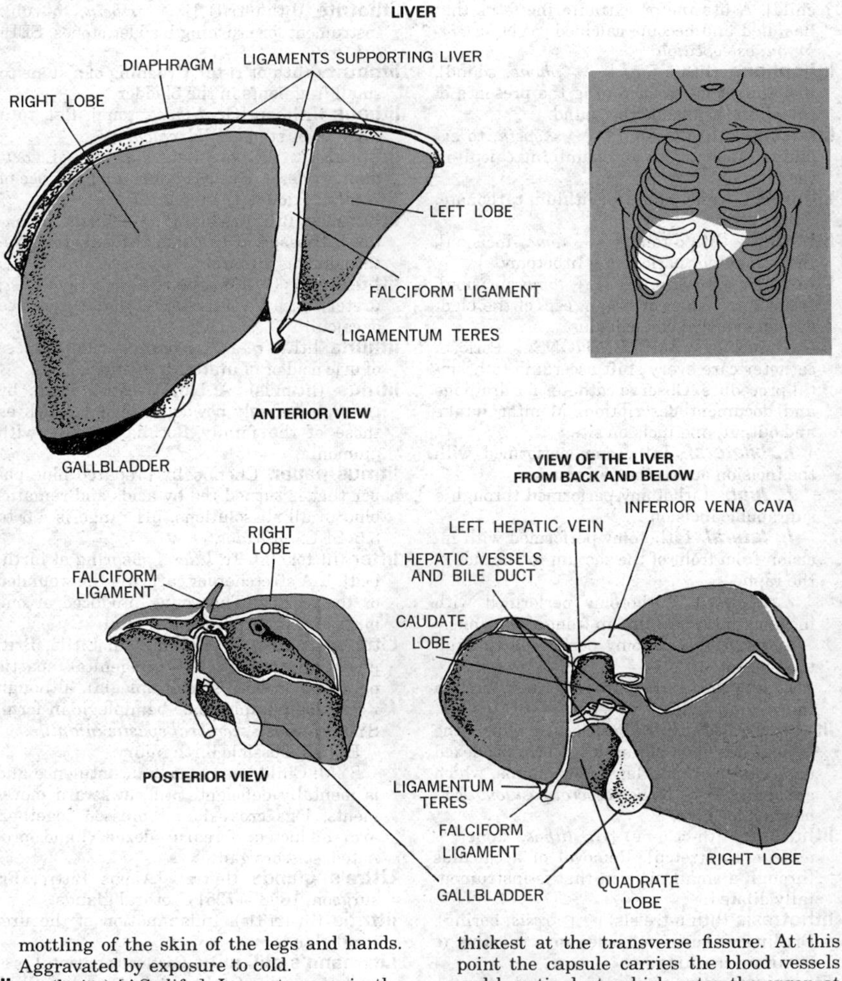

mottling of the skin of the legs and hands. Aggravated by exposure to cold.

liver (lĭv′ĕr) [AS. *lifer*]. Largest organ in the body, approx. 21 to 22.5 cm. in its greatest transverse diameter, 15 to 17.5 cm. in its greatest vertical height, and 10 to 12.5 cm. in its anteroposterior depth, weighing 1200 to 1600 gm., situated on right side beneath the diaphragm; occupies the right hypochondrium, epigastrium, and part of left hypochrondrium; level with bottom of sternum; undersurface concave; covers stomach, duodenum, hepatic flexure of colon, right kidney, and suprarenal capsule; secretes bile and is the site of a great many metabolic functions. SEE: illus.

ANAT: Completely covered by a tough fibrous sheath, Glisson's capsule, which is thickest at the transverse fissure. At this point the capsule carries the blood vessels and hepatic duct, which enter the organ at the hilus. Strands of connective tissue originating from the capsule enter the liver parenchyma and form the supporting network of the organ and separate the functional units of the liver, the hepatic lobules.

The many intrahepatic bile passages converge and anastomose, finally leading into the hepatic duct, the excretory channel of the liver. This structure receives the cystic duct, on the end of which is situated the gallbladder. The union of the cystic and the hepatic ducts forms the common bile duct or the ductus choledochus, which enters the duodenum at the papilla of Vater. A ring of smooth muscle at the terminal portion of the choledochus, the sphincter of Oddi, permits the passage of bile into the duodenum by relaxing. The bile leaving the liver enters the gallbladder, where it undergoes concentration principally through loss of fluids absorbed by the gallbladder mucosa. When bile is needed in the small intestine for digestive purposes, the gallbladder contracts and the sphincter relaxes, thus permitting escape of the viscid gallbladder bile. Ordinarily, the sphincter of Oddi is contracted, shutting off the duodenal entrance and forcing the bile to enter the gallbladder after leaving the liver.

Within the sinusoids of the liver and attached to their walls are found the cells of Kupffer, which are highly phagocytic. They remove cellular detritus, bacteria, and other foreign particulate substances from the bloodstream.

The liver has four lobes, five ligaments, five fissures, derives its blood supply from the hepatic artery and portal vein, and secretes 800 to 1000 ml. of bile in 24 hours. The rate of bile secretion is greatly increased during digestion.

BLOOD SUPPLY: From the hepatic artery, a branch of the celiac artery and the hepatic portal vein, which drains the intestine.

NERVE SUPPLY: Parasympathetic fibers from the vagi and sympathetic fibers from celiac plexus via hepatic artery.

FUNCT: The liver receives blood from the portal vein and thus is the first organ to receive blood from the intestines, where the blood has absorbed the final products of digestion and decomposition products. From this blood the liver removes glucose, from which it synthesizes glycogen, which it stores. Glucose not stored as glycogen or used to form amino acids is converted to fatty acids, carbon dioxide, and water. It deaminizes amino acids with the resultant formation of ammonia, which is converted into urea. Hippuric acid and uric acid are synthesized in the liver. The liver incorporates amino acids into proteins. The liver probably makes such proteins as albumin, prothrombin component, fibrinogen, transferrin, and glycoprotein. The liver is important in the biotransformation (i.e., so-called detoxification) of such substances as indole and skatole, which may be absorbed into the blood from the intestine.

The liver excretes bile pigments bilirubin and biliverdin, formed in the cells of the reticuloendothelial system in various parts of the body from hemoglobin derived from effete (exhausted and no longer functioning) red corpuscles. The liver synthesizes fibrinogen and prothrombin, blood constituents essential for clotting. It is the source of heparin, an anticoagulant. It is the source of red blood cells in the fetus and is the main site for the production of plasma proteins. Reticuloendothelial cells (Kupffer cells), present in the linings of the sinusoids, act to filter out and destroy bacteria present in the bloodstream.

The liver also performs the following functions. It is a storage place for vitamin B_{12} (the anti–pernicious anemia factor) and the fat-soluble vitamins A, D, E, and K. It plays a role in the regulation of blood volume and is one of the main sources of body heat. It is important in lipid metabolism. Cholesterol, which is found in most body cells and is a major constituent of bile, is manufactured mainly in the liver.

l., abscess of. ETIOL: Pathogenic bacteria, esp. pyogenic organisms such as Streptococcus, Staphylococcus, and Pneumococcus; trauma; infection by Entamoeba histolytica.

SYM: Temperature elevated in evening, low in morning; sweats and chills; liver enlarged, painful, tender, may be bulging and fluctuating. Pus may be detected by aspiration.

PROG: Embolic (multiple) abscesses are generally fatal. Traumatic abscesses, or those due to an amebic dysentery, may terminate favorably after spontaneous or induced evacuation.

l., acute yellow atrophy of. A rare and grave disease, characterized anatomically by a rapid destruction of the liver tissues, and manifested by jaundice and hemorrhages, a reduction in size of liver and marked cerebral phenomena. Usually due to viral hepatitis B infection or toxic reaction to a drug. SYN: *hepatitis, fulminant.* SEE: *asterixis; hepatic coma.*

SYM: Malaise, slight fever, nausea, vomiting, jaundice, severe headache, tremor, delirium, convulsions, and coma. Urine is scanty, contains albumin, blood, and casts; renal failure may occur. Hemorrhages are common, the skin may be covered with ecchymoses, and bleeding from the mucous membranes may occur. Hepatic dullness diminished; splenic increased.

PROG: Generally fatal.

TREATMENT: Constitutional and palliative.

l., amyloid. An enlargement of liver due to the deposition of an albuminoid substance.

SYM: Failure of general health with anemia. Liver is enlarged, smooth, firm, and painless. Spleen and kidneys share in the degeneration, so the spleen is enlarged and the urine albuminous.

PROG: Unfavorable.

TREATMENT: Therapy must be directed to the causal disease, usually prolonged suppuration, syphilis, tuberculosis, or chronic malaria.

l., biliary cirrhotic. Cirrhosis of liver due to fibrous tissue formed as a result of infection or obstruction of the bile ducts.

l., cancer of. Male sex and heredity are predisposing factors. Malignancy in the liver as a result of spread from a primary source is many times more frequent than primary tumor of the liver. The liver is the most usual site of metastatic spread of tumors that disseminate through the bloodstream.

SYM: Severe pain and tenderness; cachexia, i.e., loss of weight; pressure symptoms; jaundice common; liver enlarged, surface is nodular and a central depression or umbilications can often be detected; symptoms of the primary growth. Fever generally absent, but secondary perihepatitis or suppuration of cancerous nodules may produce it.

PROG: Fatal; duration from few months to year.

TREATMENT: Palliative, constitutional in first stage.

l., cirrhosis of. Generalized pathology of the liver with disturbed normal architecture of the lobes due to infiltration of fibrous tissue and nodule formation. These changes are accompanied by impaired liver function. The disease can progress to the stage of complete liver failure. SEE: *asterixis; hepatic coma.*

ETIOL: In the U.S.A., the most frequent cause is chronic alcoholism. About 20% of those who drink alcohol heavily for a 5- to 10-yr. period develop cirrhosis. Cirrhosis may occur in individuals with no history of alcoholism. It can develop due to contact with toxic substances such as methotrexate, methanol, halothane, or oxyphenisatin. Other causes include infectious hepatitis; metabolic disorders, including glycogen storage diseases, tyrosinosis, thalassemia, and hemochromatosis; heart disease with chronic passive congestion of the liver; biliary obstruction; and as a complication of intestinal bypass surgery.

SYM: Abdominal swelling due to ascites, jaundice, weakness, weight loss, anorexia, nausea, fetor hepaticus, and mild continuous fever. As cirrhosis progresses, portal blood finds new channels, and the superficial abdominal veins enlarge, notably about the umbilicus, forming the so-called caput medusae; hemorrhoids and esophageal varices result from the same cause. In the final stages, hepatic encephalopathy develops. This is due in part to substances including ammonia absorbed from the intestines that have not been metabolized by the liver. These reach the brain and produce encephalopathy. Clinically the patient is mentally dulled, may have hallucinations and a peculiar type of flapping tremor. SEE: *asterixis.*

PROG: Unfavorable except in first stages.

TREATMENT: Depends on the etiology. Major complications that occur regardless of etiology include portal hypertension, upper gastrointestinal tract bleeding, ascites, and hepatic coma.

l., cysts of. May be simple cysts, usually small and single, hydatid cysts, or cysts associated with cystic disease of the liver, a rare condition usually associated with congenital cystic kidneys. SEE: *Echinococcus granulosus; hydatid.*

l., fatty. Degenerative changes in liver cells due to fat deposits in the cells.

l., floating. An easily displaced liver.

l., foamy. Presence of gas bubbles in the liver as a result of infection with anaerobic bacteria. This produces a honeycomb appearance in the liver tissue.

l., hobnail. Degeneration of the liver characterized by fatty changes, fibrous scarring, nodular degeneration, and atrophy of the liver with the surface covered with brown or yellow nodules. Seen in chronic alcoholism and malnutrition.

l., inflammation of. The usual cause of inflammation is the same as that causing viral hepatitis. The clinical picture may be so mild as to be almost unnoticed or may be so severe that the jaundice is followed rapidly by hepatic encephalopathy and death. SYN: *hepatitis.*

TREATMENT: Treated as if the condition were going to progress to the severe form; bedrest; diet as requested by patient but should be high caloric; cortisone should not be given routinely. There is no specific treatment and in general the disease is self-limiting.

l., lardaceous. L., amyloid, q.v.

l., nutmeg. Chronic passive congestion of the liver, which produces a reddened central portal area and a yellowish periportal zone.

l., wandering. L., floating, q.v.

l., waxy. L., albuminoid, q.v.

liver, words pert. to: anhepatia; anhepatic; bile; -acids; -calculi; -colic; -pigments; "bili-" words; capsule, Glisson's; cardiohepatic; choleresis; cirrhosis; facies hepatica; flexure; "glyco-" words; "hepa-" words; jaundice; perihepatitis.

liver extract. A dry brown powder obtained from mammalian livers that contains the hematinic factor (antianemic factor), which stimulates erythropoiesis. Was important in treatment of pernicious anemia until vitamin B_{12} was discovered.

liver failure. Inability of the liver to function because of a disease process within the liver or because of demands beyond its capability.

liver flap. A characteristic flapping type of tremor seen in patients with severe impairment of liver function. SYN: *asterixis*.

liver fluke, human. Clonorchis sinensis common in Far East. Adults infest biliary and pancreatic ducts. Eggs pass from the body with feces and continue development in snails of the sub-family Buliminae (family Hydrobiidae). Cercaria emerge and infest numerous species of freshwater fishes in which they encyst. Infestation results from eating raw fish containing encysted metacercaria.

liver spots. Yellowish-brown spots on skin. SYN: *chloasma hepaticum*.

livid (lĭv'ĭd) [L. *lividus*, lead-colored]. 1. Ashen, cyanotic. 2. Discolored, black and blue.

lividity (lĭv-ĭd'ĭ-tē). 1. Skin discoloration, as from a bruise or venous congestion. 2. State of being livid.

living will. A statement prepared at a time when the individual was well. It attests to the wish that heroic measures such as use of life-support devices not be used to prolong life when it is obvious that such actions will not permit recovery from the condition.

livor (lī'vor) [L., a black-and-blue spot]. Lividity.

l. mortis. Cutaneous dark spot on dependent portion of a cadaver due to gravitational pooling of blood.

lixiviation (lĭks"ĭv-ē-ā'shŭn) [L. *lixivia*, lye]. Separation of soluble from insoluble substances by washing and filtration. SYN: *leaching*.

L.L.E. *left lower extremity*.

LLQ. *left lower quadrant* (of abdomen).

L.M.A. *left mentoanterior* fetal position.

L.M.P. *left mentoposterior* fetal position.

L.M.T. *left mentotransverse* fetal position.

L.O.A. *left occipitoanterior* fetal position.

Loa loa (lō'ă) [W. African]. The African eyeworm, a species of filarial worm that infests the subcutaneous tissues and conjunctiva of man. Its migration causes itching and a creeping sensation. Sometimes causes itchy edematous areas known as calabar swellings. It is transmitted by flies of the genus Chrysops.

load. 1. The weight supported or force imposed. 2. A substance given to test body function, esp. metabolic function. SEE: *loading test*.

loading, carbohydrate. SEE: *carbohydrate loading*.

loading test. The administration of a substance in order to determine the individual's ability to metabolize or excrete it. Thus a glucose tolerance test is one form of this test.

loaiasis. Loiasis, q.v.

lobar (lō'băr) [Gr. *lobos*, lobe]. Pert. to a lobe.

lobar pneumonia. Inflammation of one or more lobes of the lungs.

lobate (lō'bāt) [L. *lobatus*, lobed]. 1. Pert. to a lobe. 2. Having a deeply undulated border. 3. Producing lobes.

lobe (lōb) [Gr. *lobos*, lobe]. A fairly well defined part of an organ separated by boundaries.

l., anterior, of hypophysis. Anterior portion of the hypophysis or pituitary gland, consisting of the pars distalis and pars tuberalis.

l., azygos. An anomalous lobe at the apex of the right lobe of the lung.

l., caudate. A lobe on the posterior surface of the liver. SYN: *l., spigelian*.

l., central. Island of Reil, which forms the floor of the lateral cerebral fossa.

l., flocculonodular. A lobe of the cerebellum consisting of the flocculi, nodulus, and their connecting peduncles.

l., frontal. That part of a cerebral hemisphere in front of the central and sylvian fissures.

l., hepatic. Lobe of the liver.

l., insular. L., central.

l.'s, lateral, of prostate. The portions on each side of the urethra.

l.'s, lateral, of thyroid gland. The two main portions, one on each side of the trachea, united below by the thyroid isthmus.

l., limbic. Marginal section of the cerebral hemisphere on the medial aspect. SYN: *gyrus fornicatus*.

l., occipital. Caudal region of either hemicerebrum.

l.'s of cerebrum. Frontal, parietal, occipital, and temporal lobes and the insula or island of Reil (central lobe.)

l. of ear. Lower portion of the auricle having no cartilage.

l.'s of lungs. Large divisions of the lungs: superior and inferior lobes of the left lung; superior, middle, and inferior lobes of the right lung.

l. of mamma. One of the 15 to 20 divisions of the glandular tissue of the breast separated by connective tissue and each possessing a duct (lobar duct) opening via the nipple.

l.'s of pancreas. Roundish aggregations of glandular tissue separated by connective tissue.

l. of parotid, accessory. A small lobe, variable in size, on the anterior surface of the parotid gland superior to the exit of the parotid duct.

l.'s of prostate. The lateral lobes and the middle lobe of the prostate gland.

l., olfactory. A series of convolutions below the horizontal portion of the intraparietal fissure of the cerebrum, containing the olfactory bulb. SYN: *rhinencephalon*.

l.'s, orbital. The convolutions above the

orbit.

l., parietal. Upper and lateral portion of the hemisphere of the cerebrum.

l., posterior, of hypophysis. The posterior portion of the pituitary gland, consisting of the pars intermedia and the processus infundibuli (pars nervosa).

l., prefrontal. The frontal portion of the frontal lobe of the brain.

l., pyramidal, of thyroid. A portion of the thyroid gland extending upward from the isthmus. It is extremely variable in size.

l., quadrate, of liver. An oblong elevation on the lower surface of the liver.

l., Riedel's. An anomalous tongue-like extension from the right lobe of the liver to the gallbladder.

l., spigelian. Irregular quadrangular portion of liver behind fissure for portal vein and between fissures for vena cava and ductus venosus. SYN: *l., caudate.*

l., temporal. The portion of the cerebral hemisphere lying below the lateral fissure of Sylvius. It is continuous posteriorly with the occipital lobe.

lobectomy (lō-běk'tō-mē) [Gr. *lobos,* lobe, + *ektome,* excision]. Surgical removal of a lobe of any organ or gland.

lobelia (lō-bē'lē-ă). Substance obtained from the dried leaves and tops of the herb, Lobelia inflata. The chief constituent, lobeline, has the same action as nicotine but is less potent. SYN: *Indian tobacco.*

lobeline (lŏb'ē-lĭn). The chief constituent of lobelia, q.v.

lobi. Pl. of lobus.

lobitis (lō-bī'tĭs) [" + *itis,* inflammation]. Inflammation of a lobe.

Loboa loboi. Fungus that causes keloidal blastomycosis (Lobo's disease). It has been identified in tissues but has not been cultured.

Lobo's disease. Keloidal blastomycosis. SEE: *blastomycosis, keloidal.*

lobotomy (lō-bŏt'ō-mē) [Gr. *lobos,* lobe, + *tome,* incision]. Incision of a lobe. An operation that is performed for relief of some forms of mental disturbances. Accomplished by a small bilateral trephination in the plane of the coronal suture through which the white matter of the brain is sectioned, disconnecting the diencephalon, esp. the hypothalamic area, from the prefrontal cortex by section of the white fiber connecting pathways subcortically in a plane that passes adjacent to the anterior tip of the lateral ventricle and the posterior margin of the sphenoid wing.

Lobstein's disease (lōb'stīnz). [Johann F. G. C. M. Lobstein, Strasbourg surgeon, 1777–1835] Osteogenesis imperfecta, q.v.

lobular (lŏb'ū-lăr) [L. *lobulus,* small lobe]. Composed of small lobes; pert. to a lobule. SYN: *lobulate.*

lobulate, lobulated (lŏb'ū-lāt, -lāt-ĕd). 1. Consisting of lobes or lobules. 2. Pert. to lobes or lobules. 3. Resembling lobes. SYN: *lobular.*

lobule (lŏb'ūl) [L. *lobulus,* small lobe]. A small lobe.

l., central, of cerebellum. A small lobe at anterior part of the superior vermiform process.

l. of epididymis. Conelike divisions of the head of the epididymis formed by the much coiled distal ends of the efferent ducts of the testis.

l. of kidney. Subdivision of the renal cortex consisting of a medullary ray and surrounding glandular tissue.

l. of liver. Structural unit consisting of hepatic cells arranged in irregular, branching, and interconnected groups and anastomosing blood channels (sinusoids) surrounding a central vein. Polyhedral in shape with branches of portal vein, hepatic artery, and interlobular bile ducts at its periphery.

l. of lung. Physiological unit of the lung consisting of a respiratory bronchiole and its branches (alveolar ducts, alveolar sacs, and alveoli).

l. of testis. One of the pyramidal divisions separated from each other by incomplete partitions called septulae. Each consists of one to three coiled seminiferous tubules.

l. of thymus. Subdivisions of a lobe, each consisting of a cortex and medulla.

l., paracentral. Superior convolution of ascending frontal and parietal convolutions of the brain, forming a union of both.

l., parietal. One of two subdivisions of the parietal lobe of the brain. The superior parietal lobule comprises the posterior part of the upper portion, and the inferior parietal lobule comprises a lateral area continuous with temporal and occipital lobes.

l., primary pulmonary. The functional unit of the lung. Included are the respiratory bronchiole, alveolar ducts, sacs, and alveoli. SYN: *respiratory lobe.*

lobuli. Pl. of lobulus.

lobulus (lŏb'ū-lŭs) [L.]. (pl. *lobuli*) [NA] A lobule or small division of a lobe.

lobus (lō'bŭs) [L.]. (pl. *lobi*) [NA] Lobe.

local (lō'kăl) [L. *locus,* place]. Limited to one place or part.

localization (lō-kăl-ĭ-zā'shŭn). 1. Limitation to a definite area. 2. Determination of the seat of an infection. 3. Relation of a sensation to its point of origin.

l., cerebral. Determination of centers of various faculties and functions in particular parts of the brain.

localized (lō'kăl-īzd). Restricted to a limited

region.

localizer. Apparatus used for locating solid opaque bodies in the eye or other areas by roentgenographic examination.

locator (lō'kā-tĕr). Device for locating or discovering an object such as a foreign body.

lochia (lō'kē-ă) [Gr. *lochia*]. The discharge from the uterus of blood, mucus, and tissue during the puerperal period. The first six days it is distinctly blood-tinged and is known as lochia rubra or cruenta; the following three or four days the discharge becomes brownish and is known as lochia serosa; after this it becomes yellowish, turning to white, and is known as lochia alba. It is diminished or suppressed in high fever. If the odor is offensive it is the result of contamination with saprophytic organisms. Position the patient to favor drainage.

l. alba. The whitish postpartum vaginal discharge that is no longer blood-tinged.

l. cruenta. The bloody postpartum vaginal discharge.

l. purulenta L. alba, q.v.

l. rubra. L. cruenta, q.v.

l. serosa. A thin, watery postpartum vaginal discharge.

lochial (lō'kē-ăl). Pert. to the lochia.

lochiocolpos (lō"kē-ō-kŏl'pŏs) [Gr. *lochia,* discharge following childbirth, + *kolpos,* vagina]. Distention of the vagina due to retention of lochia.

lochiometra (lō"kē-ō-mē'tră) [" + *metra,* uterus]. Retention of lochia in the uterus.

lochiometritis (lō"kē-ō-mē-trī'tĭs) [" + " + *itis,* inflammation]. Puerperal inflammation of the uterus.

lochiorrhagia (lō"kē-ō-rā'jē-ă) [" + *rhegnynai,* to break forth]. Excessive flow of lochia.

lochiorrhea (lō"kē-ō-rē'ă) [" + *rhoia,* flow]. Abnormal flow of lochia.

lochioschesis (lō"kē-ŏs'kĕ-sĭs) [" + *schesis,* retention]. Retention or suppression of the lochia.

lochometritis (lō"kō-mē-trī'tĭs) [" + *metra,* uterus, + *itis,* inflammation]. Puerperal inflammation of uterus.

loci [L.]. Pl. of locus.

Locke's solution, Locke-Ringer's solution. [Frank S. Locke, Brit. physician, 1871–1949; Sydney Ringer, Brit. physiologist, 1835–1910] A solution used in experiments in physiology. It contains sodium, potassium, calcium, and magnesium chlorides; sodium bicarbonate, dextrose, and water.

lockjaw. Tonic spasm of muscles of jaw. SEE: *tetanus.*

Lockwood's ligament. [Charles B. Lockwood, Brit. surgeon, 1856–1914] The suspensory ligament of the eyeball.

loco (lō'kō) [Sp., cracked brain]. 1. Locoweed disease, a nervous disorder that affects cattle that eat the locoweed. 2. Slang for insane.

locomotion (lō"kō-mō'shŭn) [L. *locus,* place, + *movere,* to move]. Movement or power of movement from one place to another.

locomotor (lō"kō-mō'tor). Pert. to locomotion.

locomotor ataxia. A sclerosis affecting the posterior columns of the spinal cord. SEE: *ataxia, locomotor; Charcot's joint.*

locomotorium (lō"kō-mō-tō'rē-ŭm). The locomotor apparatus of the body.

locular (lŏk'ū-lăr) [L. *loculus,* a small space]. Divided into small cavities.

loculated (lŏk'ū-lāt-ĕd). Containing or divided into loculi. SYN: *locular.*

loculi (lŏk'ū-lī). Pl. of loculus.

loculus (lŏk'ū-lŭs) [L.]. (pl. *loculi*) A small space or cavity.

locum tenens (lō'kŭm tĕn'ĕns) [L. *locus,* place, + *tenere,* to hold]. A substitute. Physician who temporarily substitutes for another.

locus (lō'kŭs) [L. *locus,* a place]. (pl. *loci*) 1. A spot or place. 2. In genetics, the site of a gene on a chromosome.

l. ceruleus. [NA] A dark-colored depression in floor of 4th ventricle of the brain at its upper part.

l. niger. Gray matter separating the crusta and tegmentum of the crura cerebri of the brain. SYN: *substantia nigra* [NA].

Loeffler's bacillus (lĕf'lĕrz). [Friedrich A. J. Loeffler, Ger. bacteriologist, 1852–1915] The bacillus of diphtheria, Corynebacterium diphtheriae. SYN: *Klebs-Loeffler bacillus.* SEE: *diphtheria.*

Loeffler's endocarditis (lĕf'lĕrz). [Wilhelm Loeffler, Swiss physician] Endocarditis associated with eosinophilia and fibroplastic thickening of the endocardium. The cause is unknown.

logadectomy (lŏg"ă-dĕk'tō-mē) [Gr. *logades,* the whites of the eyes, + *ektome,* excision]. Excision of a portion of the conjunctiva.

logaditis (lŏg"ă-dī'tĭs) [" + *itis,* inflammation]. Inflammation of the sclerotic coat of the eye. SYN: *scleritis.*

logagnosia (lŏg"ăg-nō'sē-ă) [Gr. *logos,* word, + *a-,* not, + *gnosis,* knowledge]. A type of aphasia in which words are seen but not identified with respect to their meaning. SEE: *aphasia.*

logagraphia (lŏg-ă-grăf'ē-ă) [" + " + *graphein,* to write]. Loss of ability to express ideas in writing. SYN: *agraphia.*

logamnesia (lŏg-ăm-nē'zē-ă) [" + *amnesia,* forgetfulness]. Aphasia of a sensory character. Inability to recognize spoken or written words.

logaphasia (lŏg"ă-fā'zē-ă) [" + *a-,* not, + *phasis,* speaking]. Motor aphasia. It is usually due to a cerebral lesion.

logasthenia (lŏg"ăs-thē'nē-ă) [" + " + *sthenos,*

strength]. Mental impairment characterized by defective ability to understand the spoken word.

logoklony (lŏg′ō-klŏn-ē) [″ + *klonein,* to agitate]. Intermittent repetition of the last syllable of a word.

logokophosis (lŏg″ō-kō-fō′sĭs) [″ + *kophosis,* deafness]. Inability to understand spoken language; word deafness.

logomania (lŏg-ō-mā′nē-ă) [″ + *mania,* madness]. Repetitious, continuous, and excessive flow of speech seen in monomania.

logoneurosis (lŏg″ō-nū-rō′sĭs) [″ + *neuron,* nerve, + *osis,* condition]. Any neurosis marked by speech disorders.

logopathia (lŏg-ō-păth′ē-ă) [″ + *pathos,* disorder]. Any disorder of speech arising from derangement of the central nervous system.

logopedia (lŏg″ō-pē′dē-ă) [″ + *pais,* child]. Science dealing with speech defects and their correction.

logoplegia (lŏg-ō-plē′jē-ă) [″ + *plege,* stroke]. Paralysis of the speech organs.

logorrhea (lŏg″ō-rē′ă) [″ + *rhoia,* flow]. Unusual loquacity seen in insanity. SYN: *logomania.*

logospasm (lŏg′ō-spăzm) [″ + *spasmos,* spasm]. Spasmodic word enunciation.

-logy [Gr. *logos,* word]. Suffix meaning discourse, science or study of.

loiasis (lō-ī′sĭs). Infestation with Loa loa, q.v.

loin (loyn) [O. Fr. *loigne,* long part]. Lower part of back and sides between the ribs and pelvis. SYN: *lumbus* [NA].

lolism. Poisoning by the seeds of Lolium temulentum, darnel ryegrass.

lomustine (lō-mŭs′tēn). A chemotherapeutic agent used in treating certain neoplastic conditions. Also called *CCNU.* Trade name is CeeNU.

Long, Crawford Williamson. U.S. physician, 1815–1878, who in 1842 first administered an anesthetic during surgery.

long-acting thyroid stimulator. ABBR: LATS. A serum globulin that causes hyperfunction of the thyroid. There are probably other similar substances involved in affecting the thyroid gland in thyrotoxicosis.

longevity (lŏn-jĕv′ĭ-tē) [L. *longaevus,* aged]. Long duration of life. Age was reckoned by the Romans in six stages: *pueritia,* childhood, to 5 years; *adolescentia,* youth, to 18 years; *juventus,* young man, to 25 years; *majores,* man, to 50 years; *senectus,* old man, to 60 years; *crepita aetas,* decrepit, 60 years to death.

longing. A persistent desire or craving for something, usually that which is remote or unattainable.

longissimus (lŏn-jĭs′ĭ-mŭs) [L.]. Anatomical term indicating a long structure.

longitudinal (lŏn″jĭ-tū′dĭ-năl) [L. *longitudo,* length]. Parallel to the long axis of the body or part.

longsightedness. Farsightedness. SYN: *hyperopia.*

longus (lŏng′gŭs) [L.]. Anatomical term indicating a long structure.

loop [ME. *loupe*]. A curve or bend in a cord or cordlike structure, forming roughly an oval.

l., capillary. Minute blood vessels in the papillae of the skin.

l., closed. A biological system in which a substance produced affects the output of the substance by a feedback mechanism.

l., Henle's. The descending and ascending loops of the renal tubule.

l., Lippes. Lippes loop, q.v.

loosening of associations. Thinking characterized by speech in which ideas shift from one subject to another that is completely unrelated or only obliquely related. The speaker is apparently unaware that the subjects are unrelated. This may be seen in schizophrenia and in manic episodes.

L.O.P. *left occipitoposterior* fetal position.

lophotrichea (lŏf-ō-trĭk′ē-ă) [Gr. *lophos,* tuft, + *thrix,* hair]. Microorganisms possessing flagella in tufts.

lophotrichous (lŏf-ŏt′rĭ-kŭs). Having bunches of flagella at one end.

lordoma (lor-dō′mă) [Gr.]. Lordosis.

lordoscoliosis (lor″dō-skō″lē-ō′sĭs) [Gr. *lordosis,* bending, + *skoliosis,* curvation]. Forward curvation of the spine complicated by lateral curvature.

lordosis (lor-dō′sĭs) [Gr.]. Abnormal anterior convexity of the spine.

Lorfan. Trade name for levallorphan tartrate, USP.

Loridine. Trade name for cephaloridine.

L.O.T. *left occipitotransverse* fetal position.

lotio (lō′shē-ō) [L.]. Lotion.

l. alba. Lotion, white, q.v.

lotion (lō′shŭn) [L. *lotio*]. Liquid medicinal preparation for local application to, or bathing of, a part.

l., calamine. SEE: *calamine.*

l., hydrocortisone. USP. A lotion containing hydrocortisone. Used in treating certain skin diseases.

l., white. A combination of 4% zinc sulfate with 4% sulfurated potash.

Lotrimin. Trade name for clotrimazole.

Lotusate. Trade name for talbutal.

Louis-Bar syndrome (loo-wē′băr). [Denise Louis-Bar] A degenerative brain disease characterized by a specific immunologic dysfunction and progressive cerebellar degeneration, telangiectasis of the bulbar conjunctiva, and increased tendency to experience malignancy. It is transmitted as an autosomal recessive. Death usually occurs in adolescence or early adulthood. Parents should be informed that subsequent children have a 25% risk of having this condition. SYN: *ataxia-telangiectasia.*

loupe (loop) [Fr.]. A magnifying lens used in the form of a monocular or binocular lens. Surgeons, dentists, jewelers, and watchmakers frequently use this device.

louse [AS. *lus*]. (pl. *lice*) A small wingless insect that lives as an ectoparasite on birds and mammals. Sucking lice belong to the order Anoplura; biting or chewing lice belong to the order Mallophaga. Human lice are the primary transmitters of epidemic typhus, trench fever, and relapsing fever. They may also be the mechanical transmitters of other diseases such as plague. SYN: *pediculus.* SEE: illus.; *Pediculus.*

l., body. Pediculus humanus corporis; lives principally in or on clothing.

l., crab. Phthirus pubis; lives principally in hair in pubic region but also found in beard, eyebrows, and eyelashes.

l., head. Pediculus humanus capitis; lives in hair of the head.

lousiness. State of being infested with lice. SYN: *pediculosis.*

love [ME.]. 1. Concern and affection for another person. This may be to such a degree as to cause individuals to risk losing their lives in their concern for the safety, care, and well-being of another. 2. In psychiatry, love is equated to pleasure, particularly as it applies to the gratifying sexual experiences between individuals.

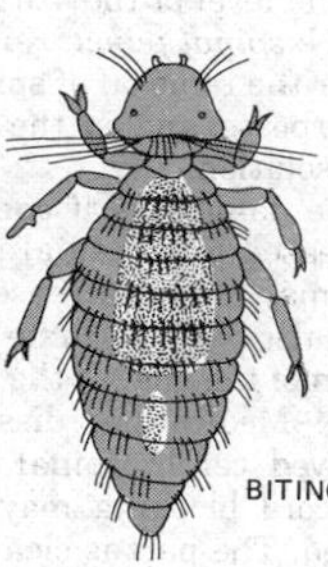

BITING LOUSE

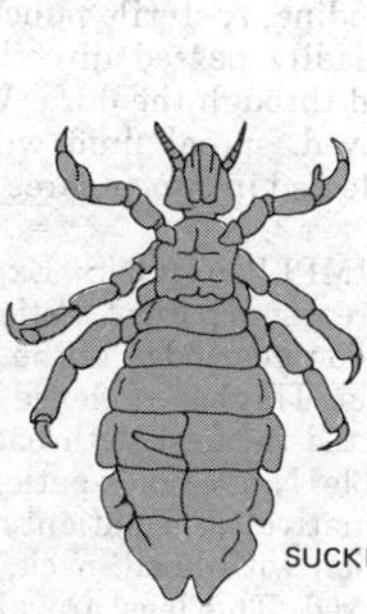

SUCKING LOUSE

LOUSE

Loven's reflex (lō-vānz'). [Otto K. Loven, Swed. physician, 1835–1904] Vasodilation with corresponding increase in size of organ resulting from stimulation of afferent nerve or organ.

lower motor neuron lesion. Injury occurring in the anterior horn cells, nerve roots, or peripheral nervous system that results in diminished reflexes, flaccid paralysis, and atrophy.

Lowe's syndrome (lōz). [Charles U. Lowe, U.S. pediatrician, b. 1921] Oculocerebrorenal dystrophy characterized by hypotonia, loss of reflexes, mental deterioration, glaucoma, cataracts, and renal tubular dysfunction. Transmitted as a sex-linked recessive.

Lowman balance board. [Charles LeRoy Lowman, U.S. orthopedist, b. 1879] Tilted board for walking with feet inverted to restore proper muscle balance and to correct static faults.

low-protein diet. Diet that contains limited amount of protein. The principal sources of food energy are fats and carbohydrates. Used in treating hepatic coma.

low-salt diet. Diet in which no salt is allowed on patient's tray and no salty foods are served. Used in treating hypertension as well as congestive heart failure.

lox. *liquid oxygen.*

loxapine succinate (lŏks'ă-pēn). An antipsychotic agent of the tricyclic class.

loxarthron (lŏks-ăr'thrŏn) [Gr. *loxos,* slanting, + *arthron,* joint]. Oblique deformity of a joint without dislocation.

loxia (lŏks'ē-ă) [Gr., slanting]. Stiff neck caused by spasmodic contraction of the neck muscles drawing the head to one side with the chin pointing to the other side. SYN: *torticollis; wryneck.*

Loxosceles (lŏks-ŏs'sĕ-lēz). A genus of spiders.

loxoscelism (lŏk-sŏs'sĕ-lĭzm). The disease produced by the bite of the brown spider, Loxosceles laeta, or L. reclusa. Symptoms include a painful red vesicle that eventually becomes gangrenous and sloughs.

loxotic (lŏks-ŏt'ĭk) [Gr. *loxos,* slanting]. Distorted in an awry manner.

loxotomy (lŏks-ŏt'ō-mē) [" + *tome,* incision]. Amputation by oblique section.

lozenge (lŏz'ĕnj) [Fr.]. Small, dry, medicinal solid to be held in mouth until it dissolves. SYN: *troche.*

L-phase variants. L-forms q.v.

L.P.N. *licensed practical nurse.*

Lr. Chem. symb. for lawrencium.

L.R.C.P. *licentiate of the Royal College of Physicians.*
L.R.C.S. *licentiate of the Royal College of Surgeons.*
LRF. *luteinizing hormone releasing factor.*
L.S.A. *left sacroanterior* fetal position.
L.Sc.A. *left scapuloanterior* fetal position.
L.Sc.P. *left scapuloposterior* fetal position.
LSD. *lysergic acid diethylamide,* a derivative of an alkaloid in ergot. LSD is used legally only for experimental purposes. It is used illegally for its hallucinogenic effects.
L.S.P. *left sacroposterior* fetal position.
L/S ratio. *lecithin/sphingomyelin ratio,* q.v.
L.S.T. *left sacrotransverse* fetal position.
LTH. *luteotropic hormone.*
Lu. Chem. symb. for lutetium.
lubb-dupp (lŭb-dŭp′). The two sounds heard in auscultation marking a complete cycle of the heart. Pause following the cycle is slightly longer than that between the two sounds. SEE: *heart, auscultation of.*
lubricant (loo′brĭ-kănt) [L. *lubricans*]. Agent, usually a liquid oil, that reduces friction between parts that brush against each other as they move. Joints are lubricated by synovial fluid.
lubricating enema. Enema given to soften feces and lubricate anal canal after hemorrhoidectomy, or to soften fecal impaction. SEE: *enema, lubricating.*
Lucas-Championnière′s disease (lū-kă′ shaw″pē-ŏn-ē-ayrz′). [J. M. M. Lucas-Championnière, Fr. surgeon, 1843–1913] Pseudomembranous bronchitis.
lucid (lū′sĭd) [L. *lucidus,* clear]. Clear, esp. applied to clarity of the mind.
lucid interval. Period of normal mental functioning between attacks of mental illness.
lucidity (lū-sĭd′ĭ-tē). Quality of clearness or brightness, esp. with regard to mental conditions.
luciferase (loo-sĭf′ĕr-ās). An enzyme that acts on luciferins to oxidize them and cause bioluminescence. It is present in certain organisms such as the firefly, or insects, that emit light either continuously or intermittently.
luciferin (loo-sĭf′ĕr-ĭn). General term for substances present in some organisms. It becomes luminescent when acted upon by luciferase.
lucifugal (loo-sĭf′ū-găl) [L. *lux,* light, + *fugere,* to flee from]. Being repelled by bright light.
lucipetal (loo-sĭp′ĭ-tăl) [″ + *peter,* to seek]. Being attracted by bright light.
lucotherapy (lū″kō-thĕr′ă-pē) [″ + Gr. *therapeia,* treatment]. Therapeutic use of light rays. SYN: *phototherapy.*
Ludwig′s angina (lūd′vĭgz). [Wilhelm F. von Ludwig, Ger. surgeon, 1790–1865] A suppurative inflammation of subcutaneous connective tissue adjacent to a submaxillary gland.
L.U.E. *left upper extremity.*
Luer-Lok syringe (lū′ĕr-lŏk′). A glass syringe made to permit rapid and firm attachment of the needle.
lues (lū′ēz) [L.]. Syphilis.
luetic (lū-ĕt′ĭk). 1. Pert. to syphilis. 2. Affected with syphilis. SYN: *syphilitic.*
Lugol′s solution (lū′gŏlz). [Jean G. A. Lugol, Fr. physician, 1786–1851] Strong iodine solution used in iodine therapy. Iodine 5 gm., potassium iodide 10 gm., and water to make 100 ml.
lumbago (lŭm-bā′gō) [L. *lumbus,* loin]. A general nonspecific term for dull, aching pain in the lumbar region of the back.
lumbar (lŭm′băr) [L. *lumbus,* loin]. Pert. to the loins; the part of the back between the thorax and pelvis.
lumbarization (lŭm″băr-ĭ-zā′shŭn). Fusion of the 1st sacral vertebra with the last lumbar vertebra.
lumbar nerves. Five pairs of nerves, corresponding with the lumbar vertebrae.
lumbar plexus. A nerve plexus formed by the ventral branches of the second to fifth lumbar nerves.
lumbar puncture. Puncture made by placing an aspiration needle into the subarachnoid space of the spinal cord. Usually done in the lumbar area at the level of the 4th intervertebral space. SYN: *spinal puncture.*

PURPOSE: For the removal of spinal fluid for diagnostic purposes, and for the injection of an anesthetic solution.

NOTE: May be dangerous if done in the presence of increased intracranial pressure. The brain stem may, upon decrease of pressure in the spinal canal, herniate into the foramen magnum of the base of the skull.

PROCEDURE: Medication, dissolved in previously removed cerebrospinal fluid, or anesthetics for cord blocking may be cautiously introduced. The part is cleansed and painted with iodine. A sterile puncture needle is then readily passed directly in the midline, to and through the dura. When the stylet is removed, spinal fluid will escape and can be collected in two or three tubes for examination.

NURSING IMPLICATIONS: Explain the procedure and reassure patient. Patient should be turned on side near edge of the bed with back to operator. Thighs are flexed on trunk and head lowered to chest with back bowed as far as possible. Nurse holds patient in this position. Alternatively, the patient may be in a sitting position with head, neck, and thoracic spine flexed. The legs are allowed to dangle over the side of the bed or table. The nurse stands in front of the patient to support him or her in this position.

After the procedure, assess the vital signs and neurological status, looking particularly for signs of paralysis, weakness, and loss of sensation in the legs or trunk. In order to decrease the chance of the development of a headache, instruct the patient to remain flat in bed. The head may be moved from side to side but not elevated.

ARTICLES NECESSARY: Sterilized lumbar puncture needles, gloves for physician, alcohol, sterilized gauze and sponge, sterile towel, 5 ml. of 0.5% solution of procaine hydrochloride, two sterile test tubes. If spinal fluid pressure is to be determined, sterile manometer tubes and a 3-way stop-cock adaptor for connecting the manometer to the spinal puncture needle will be required.

The use of a small-gauge needle will lessen the chance that spinal fluid will continue to seep from the spinal canal after the needle is removed, and thus the possibility of development of post–spinal tap headache will be diminished. SEE: *cerebrospinal fluid; cisternal puncture; headache; Queckenstedt's sign; spinal puncture.*

lumbar reflex. Irritation of the skin over the erector spinae muscles causing contraction of muscles of the back.

lumbar region. Each side of umbilical region above the iliac, below the hypochondriac.

lumbar vertebrae. Five bones of the spinal column between the sacrum and thoracic vertebrae. SEE: *spinal column* for illus.

lumbo- [L. *lumbus,* loin]. Combining form pert. to the loins.

lumboabdominal (lŭm″bō-ăb-dŏm′ĭ-năl) [″ + *abdomen,* belly]. Concerning the lateral and frontal areas of the abdomen.

lumbocolostomy (lŭm″bō-kō-lŏs′tō-mē) [″ + Gr. *kolon,* colon, + *stoma,* opening]. Colostomy by lumbar incision.

lumbocolotomy (lŭm″bō-kō-lŏt′ō-mē) [″ + ″ + *tome,* incision]. Incision into the colon through the lumbar region.

lumbocostal (lŭm″bō-kŏs′tăl) [″ + *costa,* rib]. Rel. to the loins and ribs.

lumbodynia (lŭm″bō-dĭn′ē-ă) [″ + Gr. *odyne,* pain]. Pain and rigidity in the loins. SYN: *lumbago.*

lumboiliac (lŭm″bō-ĭl′ē-ăk) [″ + *iliacus,* pert. to ilium]. Concerning the lumbar and inguinal areas.

lumboinguinal (lŭm″bō-ĭng′gwĭ-năl) [″ + *inguinalis,* pert. to the groin]. Lumboiliac, q.v.

lumbosacral. Pert. to the lumbar vertebrae and the sacrum.

lumbosacral plexus. Nerve plexus formed by union of lumbar, sacral, and coccygeal nerves.

lumbrical (lŭm′brĭ-kăl) [L. *lumbricus,* earthworm]. Like a worm. SYN: *vermiform.*

lumbricalis. One of the muscles of the hand or foot that are wormlike in shape.

lumbricide (lŭm′brĭ-sīd) [″ + *caedere,* to kill]. An agent that kills lumbricoid worms, i.e., ascarides or intestinal worms.

lumbricoid (lŭm′brĭ-koyd) [″ + Gr. *eidos,* form]. Resembling a roundworm.

lumbricosis (lŭm″brĭ-kō′sĭs) [″ + Gr. *osis,* condition]. State of being infested with lumbricoid worms.

Lumbricus (lŭm-brĭ′kŭs). A genus of worms that includes earthworms.

lumbricus (lŭm-brī′kŭs). Ascaris lumbricoides.

lumbus [L.]. [NA] The loin; part of back between thorax and pelvis.

lumen (lū′mĕn) [L., light]. (pl. *lumina*) 1. The space within an artery, vein, intestine, or tube. 2. Unit of light, the amount of light emitted in a unit solid angle by a uniform point source of one international candle. SEE: *light unit; candela.*

Luminal. Trade name for phenobarbital, USP.

luminal (lū′mĭ-năl). Rel. to lumen of tubular structure, such as a blood vessel.

Luminal Sodium. Trade name for phenobarbital sodium, USP.

luminescence (loo″mĭ-nĕs′ĕns). Production of a light without production of heat. SEE: *bioluminescence.*

luminiferous (loo″mĭ-nĭf′ĕr-ŭs) [L. *lumen,* light, + *ferre,* to bear]. Producing or conveying light.

luminophore (loo′mĭ-nō-for″) [″ + Gr. *phoros,* bearing]. A chemical present in organic compounds that permits luminescence of those compounds.

luminous (loo′mĭ-nŭs). Emitting light.

lumirhodopsin (loo″mĭ-rō-dŏp′sĭn). In the retina of the eye, the intermediate between rhodopsin and all-*trans*-retinal, plus opsin during bleaching of rhodopsin by light.

lumpectomy (lŭm-pĕk′tō-mē) [*lump* + Gr. *ektome,* excision]. Surgical removal of a tumor from the breast, esp. to remove only the tumor and no other tissue or lymph nodes.

lunacy (lū′nă-sē) [L. *luna,* moon]. Obsolete term for insanity. Insanity was formerly thought to be affected by the moon.

lunar. Pert. to the moon, a month, or silver.

lunar caustic. Silver nitrate.

lunate. 1. Moon-shaped or crescent. 2. A bone in the proximal row of the carpus. SYN: *semilunar bone.*

lunatic (lū′nă-tĭk) [L. *luna,* moon]. Obsolete term for an insane person. SEE: *lunacy.*

lunatomalacia (loo-nā″tō-mă-lā′shē-ă). Kienböck's disease, q.v.

lung (lŭng) [AS. *lungen*]. One of two cone-shaped spongy organs of respiration contained within the pleural cavity of the thorax. SEE: illus.; *alveolus of lung* for illus.

ANAT: Connected with the pharynx through the trachea and larynx. The base

LUNGS

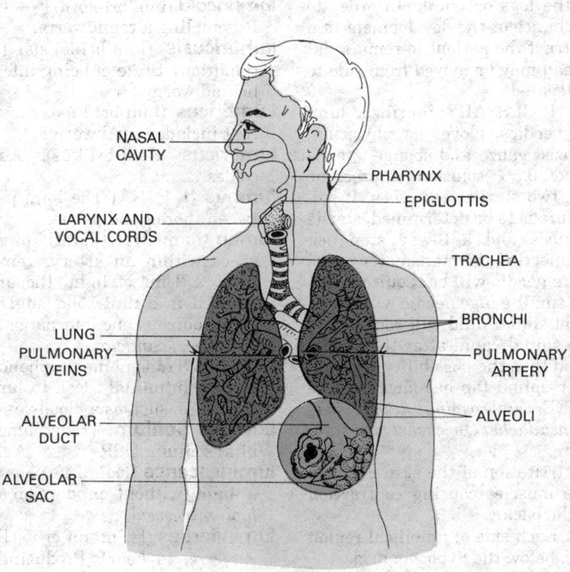

rests on the diaphragm and the apex rises from 2.5 to 5 cm. above the sternal end of the first rib, the collarbone, supported by its attachment to the hilum or root structures. The lungs include the lobes, lobules, bronchi, bronchioles, infundibula, and alveoli or air cells.

The right lung has three lobes and the left two. Approx. weight in the adult male: right lung 625 gm., left 570 gm. The lungs contain 300,000,000 alveoli and the respiratory surface is about 70 square meters. Averages 18 respirations per minute in adult. The total capacity of the lung varies from 3.6 to 9.4 liters in adult men and 2.5 to 6.9 in adult women.

The left lung has an indentation for the normal placement of the heart, which is called the cardiac depression. Behind this is the hilum, through which the blood vessels, lymphatics, and bronchi enter and leave the lung.

Air travels from the mouth and nasal passage to the pharynx and the trachea. Two main bronchi, one on each side, extend from the trachea. The main bronchi divide into smaller bronchi, one for each of five lobes. These further divide into a great number of smaller bronchioles. The pattern distribution of these into the segments of each lobe is important in pulmonary and thoracic surgery. There are 10 bronchopulmonary segments in the right lung and eight in the left, but the number is variable. There are 50 to 80 terminal bronchioles in each lobe. Each of these divides into two respiratory bronchioles, which in turn divide to form 2 to 11 alveolar ducts. The alveolar sacs and alveoli arise from these ducts. The spaces between the alveolar sacs and alveoli are called atria.

The alveolus is the point at which the blood and inspired air are separated only by a very thin wall or membrane that allows O_2 and nitrogen to diffuse into the blood and CO_2 and other gases to pass from the blood into the alveoli. This wall is so thin (0.07 to 2.0 microns) that it is best seen by using an electron microscope. The alveoli contain small pores that serve to connect adjacent alveoli to each other.

NERVE SUPPLY: Parasympathetic fibers via vagus nerve and sympathetic fibers from anterior and posterior pulmonary plexuses.

BLOOD VESSELS: Bronchial and pulmonary arteries and pulmonary veins. Blood passing through lungs gives off carbon dioxide and receives oxygen.

FUNCT: The primary purpose of the lung

is to bring air and blood into intimate contact so that oxygen can be added to the blood and carbon dioxide can be removed. This is achieved by two pumping systems, one moving a gas and the other a liquid. The blood and air are brought together so closely that approximately one micrometer (10^{-6} meter) of tissue separates them. The volume of the pulmonary capillary circulation is 150 ml., but this is spread out over a surface area of approx. 750 sq. feet (69.68 sq. meters). This capillary surface area surrounds 300 million air sacs called alveoli. The blood that is poor in oxygen but high in CO_2 is in contact with the air that is high in oxygen and low in CO_2 for less than one second.

l.'s, compliance of. A measure of the distensibility of the lungs. It is expressed as the change in volume of the lungs in liters when the transpulmonary pressure is changed by 1 cm. of water pressure. Normally it is between 0.08 and 0.33 liters/cm. H_2O. It is reduced by anything that obstructs the normal flow of air in and out of the lung, whether due to changes in the airway or the mechanical forces that move the ribs and diaphragm.

l., edema of. Effusion of serous fluid into air vesicles and into interstitial tissue of lungs. SYN: *pulmonary edema.*

SYM: Extreme dyspnea; rapid, labored breathing; cough with frothy bloodstained expectoration; cyanosis; cold extremities.

PROG: Grave. Often a final symptom of some pulmonary disease.

TREATMENT: Directed toward altering the condition that caused the difficulty. Usually this includes vigorous treatment of the heart condition, oxygen, and morphine; in extreme cases phlebotomy may be required. But prior to this, tourniquets are applied to the limbs in an attempt to have the excess tissue fluid collect in the extremities rather than the lungs.

NOTE: Tourniquets should be applied to only one limb at a time for 15 minutes and with pressure sufficient to block venous return but not enough to interfere with arterial blood flow to the limb.

l., iron. Drinker respirator, q.v.

lung, words pert. to: air; air vesicle; alveobronchiolitis; alveolar; alveolus; alveolus pulmoneus; anthracosis; anthrax; artificial pneumothorax; asbestosis; atelectasis; auscultation; "bronch-" words; byssinosis; cardiopulmonary; chest; embolism; emphysema; hilum; pectoriloquy; "pleur-" words; "pneum-" words; pulmonary; rales; siderosis; silicosis; tuberculosis.

lung abscess. Circumscribed suppuration of lung.

SYM: High and irregular fever, rigors, sweats, and pallor. Dyspnea, cough, and purulent expectoration. May be bubbling rales and later cavernous breathing and pectoriloquy.

PROG: Fair, except in embolic abscesses.

TREATMENT: Nutritious food. Remedies called for by general condition. Abscess should be opened and drained.

lung cancer. Cancer that may appear in trachea, air sacs, and other lung tubes. It may appear as an ulcer in the windpipe, as a nodule or small flattened lump, or on the surface blocking air tubes. It may invade surface of tubes extending to lymphatics into blood vessels.

lung collapse. Condition resulting from a lowering of intrapulmonic pressure or an increase in intrathoracic pressure. It may be focal, involving only a few lobules, or massive, in which an entire lobe or the complete lung is involved. It may result from obstruction of the bronchial tubes (obstructive atelectasis) or pressure upon the lung by air or fluid in the pleural cavity, an intrathoracic tumor, or a greatly enlarged heart (compressive atelectasis). Air may be introduced artificially into the pleural cavity (artificial pneumothorax) or it may be derived from emphysematous lesions. Collapse may occur in the newborn as a result of blockage of bronchioles by mucus or from failure of the lung to distend because of weak inspiratory movements. SYN: *atelectasis.*

SYM: In a sudden collapse, there is pronounced dyspnea and circulatory collapse. When collapse occurs gradually, symptoms are less pronounced or may not occur at all.

PROG: Depends upon extent of collapse and gravity of preexisting disease.

TREATMENT: In the newborn, aspirate the excess mucus from the bronchus and gently inflate lung with a catheter. In acquired varieties, direct remedies to the original disease. SEE: *auscultation; chest; emphysema; tuberculosis.*

l.c., hypostatic. Congestion of dependent portions of the lungs occurring in asthenic diseases that necessitate a protracted recumbent position.

SYM: Dyspnea, cough, scanty expectoration. Slight dullness, subcrepitant rales, and feeble bronchial breathing.

TREATMENT: Development of congestion should be prevented by frequent change in position and timely use of cardiac stimulants.

l.c., passive. Results from obstruction to the flow of blood from the lungs to the heart.

SYM: Dyspnea, hard cough, mucous expectoration containing pigmented cells and rales. Slight dullness, feeble breathing.

lung fluke. Paragonimus westermani.

lung hemorrhage. Hemoptysis.

lung inflammation. Pneumonia.

lung motor. An apparatus designed for forcing air or a mixture of air and oxygen into the lungs.

lung surfactant. A substance in the lung that acts to regulate the amount of surface tension of the fluid lining the alveoli.

lungworm (lŭng'wĕrm). Nematodes that infest the lungs of man and animals.

lunula (lū'nū-lă) [L., little moon]. (pl. *lunulae*) [NA] A crescent-shaped area.

l. of valves of heart. One of two narrow portions on the free edges of the semilunar valves on each side of the nodulus.

lupiform (lū'pĭ-form) [L. *lupus,* wolf, + *forma,* shape]. Resembling lupus.

lupoid (loo'poyd) [" + Gr. *eidos,* form]. 1. Resembling lupus. 2. Boeck's sarcoid.

lupous (lū'pŭs) 1. Pert. to lupus. 2. Affected with lupus.

lupus (lū'pŭs) [L., wolf]. Originally any chronic, progressive, usually ulcerating, skin disease. In current usage when the word is used alone, it has no precise meaning.

l. erythematosus, cutaneous. A chronic disease of unknown etiology that causes skin lesions of the face, neck, and upper extremities. Macules, papules, plaques, scales, follicular plugging and atrophic areas are present. There is usually a history of exposure to sunlight prior to onset. The typical lesion progresses from the center as the central area atrophies. About 10% of patients will develop systemic lupus erythematosus. SEE: *collagen diseases.*

TREATMENT: Topical application of corticosteroids and then systemic antimalarials if the lesion fails to respond to topical therapy. The possibility of retinal damage from the antimalarials must be considered, and the medication discontinued if this develops. The antimalarial quinacrine does not cause retinal damage.

l. erythematosus, systemic. A chronic inflammatory disease of connective tissue, of unknown etiology, that affects the skin, joints, kidneys, nervous system, and mucous membranes. A characteristic butterfly rash or erythema may be present on the malar areas and across the nose. The disease may begin acutely with fever, joint pain and malaise or smolder over a period of years with intermittent fever and malaise. Symptoms from any organ system may be present. The disease occurs most frequently in young women. Antinuclear antibodies and the L.E. cell factor, q.v., are usually present but are not required for a positive diagnosis. SEE: *collagen diseases.*

DIAGNOSIS: Diagnosis can be made if four or more of the following are present either at one time or sequentially: butterfly rash; characteristic discoid skin lesion; Raynaud's phenomenon; alopecia; photosensitivity; oral or nasopharyngeal ulceration; arthritis without deformity; L.E. cells; chronic pleuritis or pericarditis; chronic false-positive serological test for syphilis; over 35 grams of protein in the urine in 24 hrs.; cellular casts in the urine; psychosis or convulsions; hemolytic anemia, less than 4000 white blood cells/cu. mm., thrombocytopenia of less than 100,000/cu. mm.

TREATMENT: In mild cases, salicylates or indomethacin if fever and joint pain are present. For severe cases, antimalarial therapy such as hydroxychloroquine, chloroquine or quinacrine is indicated as are corticosteroids. It is preferable to give corticosteroids on alternate days if this will control symptoms. Dosage is determined by the patient's response. Immunosuppressive agents are useful when life-threatening or severe crippling disease is present, or when there is failure to respond to conventional therapy, or when intolerable side effects have developed. When antimalarials are used, the patient must be closely observed for retinal damage. In general patients should not be exposed to the sun, and intercurrent infections should be treated early and vigorously.

l. pernio. Sarcoidosis; Boeck's sarcoid.

l. vulgaris. Tuberculosis of the skin. Characterized by patches that break down and ulcerate, leaving scars on healing.

LUQ. *left upper quadrant* of abdomen.

Lust's reflex (lŭsts). Dorsal flexion and abduction of foot resulting from percussion of external branch of sciatic nerve.

lusus naturae (loo'sŭs nă-chū'rē). A congenital anomaly.

luteal [L. *luteus,* yellow]. Pert. to the corpus luteum, its cells, or its hormone.

luteal hormone. Progesterone, q.v. Secreted by the corpus luteum. SEE: *corpus luteum; endocrine; estrogen; hormone; ovary.*

lutein (lū'tē-ĭn). Yellow pigment derived from corpus luteum, egg yolk, and fat cells or lipochromes.

lutein cells. Ovarian cells that contain a yellow pigment and are involved in the formation of the corpus luteum. They are of two types: granulosa-lutein cells of follicular origin and theca-lutein cells from the theca interna.

luteinic (loo"tē-ĭn'ĭk). Concerning the corpus luteum of the ovary.

luteinization (lū"tē-ĭn-ĭ-zā'shŭn). Process of development of the corpus within a ruptured graafian follicle.

luteinizing hormone. ABBR: LH. Hormone secreted by anterior lobe of the hypophysis that stimulates development of the corpus luteum.

luteinizing hormone releasing hormone. ABBR: LHRH. A hormone that is produced in the hypothalamus and controls the release and synthesis of luteinizing hormone.

Lutembacher's syndrome (loo'tĕm-băk"ĕrz). [René Lutembacher, Fr. physician, b. 1884] Atrial septal defect of the heart with mitral stenosis.

luteohormone (loo"tē-ō-hor'mōn). Progesterone.

luteoma (lū"tē-ō'mă) [L. *luteus,* yellow, + Gr. *oma,* tumor]. An ovarian tumor containing lutein cells.

luteotropin (loo"tē-ō-trō'pĭn). The luteotropic hormone of the anterior pituitary.

lutetium (lū-tē'shē-ŭm). SYMB: Lu. At. wt. 174.97; at. no. 71. A rare element.

luteum (lū'tē-ŭm) [L.]. Yellow.

l., corpus. Yellow cellular mass in the ovary that forms after the graafian follicle has erupted. It persists and enlarges if pregnancy occurs. SEE: *ovary* for illus.

lutin (lū'tĭn). Hormone of corpus luteum that aids in preparation of endometrium for fertilized ovum. SYN: *progesterone.*

Lutz-Splendore-Almeida disease. [Alfredo Lutz, contemporary Brazilian physician; A. Splendore, contemporary Italian physician; Floriano P. de Almeida, contemporary Brazilian physician] Brazilian or South American blastomycosis, paracoccidioidosis, q.v.

lux (lŭks) [L., light]. A unit of light intensity equivalent to one lumen per square meter.

luxation (lŭks-ā'shŭn) [L. *luxatio,* dislocation]. Displacement of organs or articular surfaces; dislocation of a joint.

luxus (lŭks'ŭs) [L.]. Excess of anything.

Luys' body (lū-ēz'). [Jules B. Luys, Fr. physician, 1828–1898] Small mass of gray matter lying on the dorsal surface of the peduncle dorsolateral to the substantia nigra of the brain. Luys' nucleus is located in the posterior portion of the thalamus.

lyase (lī'ās). The class name for enzymes that remove chemical groups other than by hydrolysis. Ex.: decarboxylase, aldolase, and synthases.

lycanthropy (lī-kăn'thrō-pē) [Gr. *lykos,* wolf, + *anthropos,* man]. Mania in which one believes oneself a wild beast, esp. a wolf.

lycopene (lī'kō-pēn). The red pigment, a carotene, of tomatoes. It is also present in other red fruits and berries.

lycopenemia (lī"kō-pē-nē'mē-ă) [*lycopene* + Gr. *haima,* blood]. A type of carotenemia, q.v., caused by eating excessive amount of foods that contain lycopene, q.v.

lycoperdonosis (lī"kō-pĕr"dŏn-ō'sĭs) [Gr. *lykos,* wolf, + *perdesthai,* to break wind, + *osis,* condition]. Respiratory disease caused by inhaling large quantities of spores from the mature mushroom commonly called puffball. Lycoperdon is the genus of fungi to which most puffballs belong.

lycopodium (lī-kō-pō'dē-ŭm). A yellow powder formed from spores of Lycopodium clavatum, a club moss. Used as a dusting powder and as a desiccant and absorbent.

lycorexia (lī-kō-rĕk'sē-ă) [Gr. *lykos,* wolf + *orexis,* appetite]. Bulimia; voracious, insatiable appetite.

lye (lī) [AS. *leag*]. 1. Liquid from leaching of wood ashes. 2. Any strong alkaline solution, esp. sodium or potassium hydroxide. SEE: *alkali; potassium hydroxide; sodium hydroxide.*

lye poisoning. SEE: *Poisons and Poisoning* in *Appendix.*

lying-in. 1. The puerperal state. 2. Being hospitalized for the purpose of childbearing.

Lyme disease, Lyme arthritis. [Lyme, Connecticut, U.S.A., where the disease was originally described] A recurrent inflammatory disorder accompanied by distinctive skin lesions, erythema chronicum migrans (ECM); polyarthritis, and involvement of the heart and nervous system. The onset, usually in the summer, consists of a red macule or papule that expands to a large annular lesion (ECM). There may be several of these lesions. They are associated with fever, fatigue, malaise, headache, and a stiff neck that lasts several weeks. Within the next few days or as late as two years later, polyarthritis without joint swelling develops. This develops into chronic arthritis within weeks or months after the skin lesion. Neurological symptoms of neuritis of cranial and somatic nerves appear. These may last months. The cardiac abnormalities including myopericarditis and cardiomegaly develop within weeks of the initial skin lesion. There is good evidence that the disease is caused by a spirochete called Ixodes dammini after the tick-host of the organism.

TREATMENT: Salicylates for the arthritis. Penicillin causes the ECM to disappear but does not prevent the other aspects of the disease.

lymph (lĭmf) [L. *lympha*]. An alkaline fluid found in the lymphatic vessels and the cisterna chyli. It is usually a clear, transparent, colorless fluid; however, in vessels draining the intestines it may appear milky owing to presence of absorbed fats. It differs from blood in that red blood corpuscles are absent and the protein content is lower. Osmotic pressure is slightly higher than in blood plasma; viscosity, slightly less. Sp. gr. 1.016–1.023.

Lymph may vary considerably in composition in different parts of the body. In peripheral vessels, it is similar to blood plasma except that the protein content is usually much lower. Lymph contains proteins (serum albumin, serum globulin, serum fibrinogen), salts, organic substances (urea, creatinine, neutral fats, glucose), and water. Cells present are principally lymphocytes, formed in lymph nodes and other lymphatic organs. Lymph from the intestine (called chyle) contains fats and other substances absorbed from the intestine.

The lymph is formed in tissue spaces all over the body and is gathered into small vessels that carry it centrally. All lymph eventually enters into either the thoracic duct or right lymph duct, each terminating at the junction of the internal jugular and subclavian veins, where the lymph reenters the bloodstream. The thoracic duct commences in the abdomen as a dilated sac, the cisterna (receptaculum) chyli, which receives lymph vessels from the lower limbs and pelvis and from the intestines and digestive organs. It continues upward through the thorax receiving intercostal lymph vessels, and near its termination, it receives the left subclavian trunk, draining left upper extremity, and the left jugular trunk, draining left side of head and neck. The right lymph duct drains the right sides of the thorax, head, and neck. SEE: *lymphatic system* for illus.

Lymph, in passing from any region of the body to the main lymph ducts, must pass through lymph vessels that lead to regional lymph nodes. These filter the lymph, freeing it of foreign particulate matter, esp. bacteria.

The absorption of fatty matter chiefly takes place through the epithelial cells of the intestines, and those of the villi. These cells carry it to the lacteals, the lymph vessels of the small intestine.

Absorption is most active in the alimentary canal, the digested material passing into the bloodstream through the vessels of the portal circulation and into the lacteals.

l., animal. Lymph or vaccine from an animal.

l., inflammatory. Exudate due to inflammation.

l., intercellular. Tissue fluid.

lymphadenectasis (lĭm-făd″ĕ-nĕk′tă-sĭs) [L. *lympha,* lymph, + Gr. *aden,* gland, + *ektasis,* dilatation]. Dilatation or distention of a lymph node.

lymphadenectomy (lĭm-făd″ĕ-nĕk′tō-mē) [″ + ″ + *ektome,* excision]. Surgical removal of a lymph node.

lymphadenia (lĭm″fă-dē′nē-ă). Hyperplasia affecting lymph nodes.

l. ossea. Bone marrow hyperplasia accompanied by Bence Jones protein in urine.

SYM: Neuralgic pains followed by painful swellings on ribs and skull and possible occurrence of spontaneous fractures. SYN: *myeloma, multiple.*

lymphadenitis (lĭm-făd″ĕn-ī′tĭs) [″ + ″ + *itis,* inflammation]. Inflammation of the lymph nodes. SYN: *adenolymphitis.*

ETIOL: Drainage of bacteria or toxic substances into lymph nodes. May be specific, as by the organisms of typhoid, syphilis, or tuberculosis, or nonspecific, in which causative organism is not identified.

SYM: Marked increase of tissue; possible suppuration. Swelling, pain, tenderness. Usually accompanies lymphangitis.

TREATMENT: Hot, moist dressings; incision and drainage if abscesses occur. Antibiotics as indicated.

l., tuberculous. Tuberculosis of lymph nodes.

ETIOL: Mycobacterium tuberculosis.

SYM: Possible loss of weight and strength; gradual onset and enlargement of lymph nodes; may become adherent, necrotic, and discharge pus through skin.

TREATMENT: Antituberculosis drugs.

lymphadenocele (lĭm-făd′ĕ-nō-sēl″) [″ + ″ + *kele,* hernia]. Cyst of a lymph node.

lymphadenogram (lĭm-făd′ĕ-nō-grăm″) [″ + ″ + *gramma,* writing]. Roentgenogram of a lymph gland.

lymphadenography (lĭm-făd″ĕ-nŏg′ră-fē) [″ + ″ + *graphein,* to write]. X-raying of lymph glands after a radiopaque material has been injected.

lymphadenoid (lĭm-făd′ĕ-noyd) [″ + ″ + *eidos,* form]. Resembling a lymph node or lymph tissue.

lymphadenopathy (lĭm-făd″ĕ-nŏp′ă-thē) [″ + ″ + *pathos,* disease]. Disease of the lymph nodes.

l., dermatopathic. Widespread lymphadenopathy secondary to various skin disorders.

lymphadenosis benigna cutis (lĭm-făd″ĕ-nō′sĭs) [″ + ″ + *osis,* condition]. A benign collection of lymphocytes in the skin.

lymphadenotomy (lĭm-făd″ĕ-nŏt′ō-mē) [″ + ″ + *tome,* incision]. Surgical incision of a lymph node.

lymphadenovarix (lĭm-făd″ĕ-nō-vā′rĭks) [″ + ″ + L. *varix,* a twisted vein]. Enlargement of lymph nodes due to increased pressure in the lymph vessels.

lymphagogue (lĭmf′ă-gŏg) [L. *lympha,* lymph, + Gr. *agogos,* leading]. An agent that stimulates the production or flow of lymph.

lymphangial (lĭm-făn′jē-ăl) [″ + Gr. *angeion,* vessel]. Concerning lymph vessels.

lymphangiectasis (lĭm-făn″jē-ĕk′tă-sĭs) [″ + ″ + *ektasis,* dilatation]. Dilatation of lymphatic vessels. SYN: *lymphectasia.*

lymphagiectomy (lĭm-făn″jē-ĕk′tō-mē) [″ + ″ + *ektome,* excision]. Surgical removal of lymph vessels.

lymphangiitis (lĭm-făn″jē-ī′tĭs) [″ + ″ + *itis,* inflammation]. Inflammation of lymph vessels.

lymphangioendothelioma (lĭm-făn″jē-ō-ĕn″dō-thē-lē-ō′mă) [″ + ″ + *endon,* within, + *thele,* nipple, + *oma,* tumor]. Endothelioma originating from lymph vessels. SYN: *lymphendothelioma.*

lymphangiofibroma (lĭm-făn″jē-ō-fī-brō′mă) [″ + Gr. *angeion,* vessel, + L. *fiber,* fiber, + Gr. *oma,* tumor]. Fibroma and lymphangioma combined.

lymphangiogram (lĭm-făn′jē-ō-grăm) [″ + ″ + *gramma,* writing]. Roentgenogram of the lymph vessels.

lymphangiography (lĭm-făn″jē-ŏg′ră-fē) [″ + ″ + *graphein,* to write]. Roentgenography of the lymph vessels after a radiopaque substance has been injected into the vessels.

lymphangiology (lĭm-făn″jē-ŏl′ō-jē) [″ + ″ + *logos,* study]. The branch of medical science concerned with the lymphatic system.

lymphangioma (lĭm-făn″jē-ō′mă) [″ + ″ + *oma,* tumor]. Tumor composed of lymphatic vessels.

l., cavernous. Dilated lymph vessels filled with lymph.

l., cystic. Multilocular cysts filled with lymph. The condition is usually congenital.

lymphangiophlebitis (lĭm-făn″jē-ō-flĕ-bī′tĭs) [″ + ″ + *phleps,* vein, + *itis,* inflammation]. Inflammation of lymphatic vessels and veins.

lymphangioplasty (lĭm-făn′jē-ō-plăs″tē) [″ + Gr. *angeion,* vessel, + *plassein,* to form]. Formation of artificial lymphatics.

lymphangiosarcoma (lĭm-făn″jē-ō-săr-kō′mă) [″ + ″ + *sarx,* flesh, + *oma,* tumor]. A malignant neoplasm that develops from the endothelial lining of lymphatics.

lymphangiotomy (lĭm-făn″jē-ŏt′ō-mē) [″ + ″ + *tome,* incision]. 1. Dissection of the lymphatics. 2. Anatomy of the lymphatics. SYN: *lymphotomy.*

lymphangitis (lĭm″făn-jī′tĭs) [″ + Gr. *angeion,* vessel, + *itis,* inflammation]. Inflammation of lymphatic channels or vessels.

ETIOL: May be due to a variety of organisms but is frequently due to streptococci.

SYM: Onset of chill and high fever, moderate swelling and pain. Deep general flush with raised border on affected area if infection is in deep layers of skin. The red inflamed area is commonly called blood poisoning by lay persons.

NURSING IMPLICATIONS: Elevate affected area. If affected area is an extremity, elevate above the level of the heart. Apply warm moist dressings as ordered. Administer antibiotics as prescribed. Force fluids. Dispose of dressings in an appropriate waste container.

lymphatic (lĭm-făt′ĭk) [L. *lymphaticus*]. 1. Of or pert. to lymph. 2. A lymph vessel.

ANAT: A lymph vessel conveys toward the heart; contains valves like the veins. The intestinal parts of the lymphatics that take up some of the products of digestion are called lacteals. After the chyle enters the lacteals, it is known as lymph. The lymphatics, or lacteals, carry the food material in the form of lymph, which has not hitherto been taken directly into the blood vessels of the alimentary canal, into the bloodstream.

Fluids exuded from the blood vessels into the tissues are collected and returned to the blood via the lymphatics. They appear like small veins with thin walls, and they are provided with valves. They commence as lymph capillaries, microscopic in size, and empty into two trunks that open into the large veins near the heart.

Unlike blood, the fluid contained in the lymphatics flows only in one direction from the small capillaries to the main trunk (the thoracic duct and a smaller duct on the right side) and then to the large veins. When the lymph enters the blood it becomes part of its constituents.

RS: angiolymphitis; angiolymphoma; bubo; chylangioma; varix; "vas-" words.

l., afferent. Any of the small vessels carrying lymph to a lymph node.

l., efferent. Any one of the small vessels carrying lymph from a lymph node.

lymphatic blockade. Local defense mechanism in which minute bits of material, such as fibrinous exudate from injured tissue, enter local lymphatic vessels, tending to obstruct them and thus prevent foreign substances, esp. bacteria, from passing to other parts of the body.

lymphatic capillary. The smallest lymph vessel. A minute tube consisting of a single layer of endothelium ending blindly in a swollen or rounded end. Tissue fluid enters the lymphatic system through the lymph capillaries. In intestinal villi they are called lacteals.

lymphatic organ. A structure composed principally of lymphatic tissue. Includes lymph nodes, spleen, tonsil, and thymus.

lymphaticostomy (lĭm-făt′ĭ-kŏs′tō-mē) [L. *lymphaticus,* lymphatic, + Gr. *stoma,* opening]. Making of a permanent aperture into a lymphatic duct.

lymphatic system. That system including all structures involved in the conveyance of lymph from the tissues to the bloodstream. It includes the lymph capillaries, lacteals, lymph nodes, lymph vessels, and main lymph ducts (thoracic and right lymphatic duct). SEE: *lymph;* illus.

lymphatic vessels. Thin-walled vessels conveying lymph from the tissues. They resem-

LYMPHATIC DRAINAGE OF ABDOMINAL AND THORACIC AREA

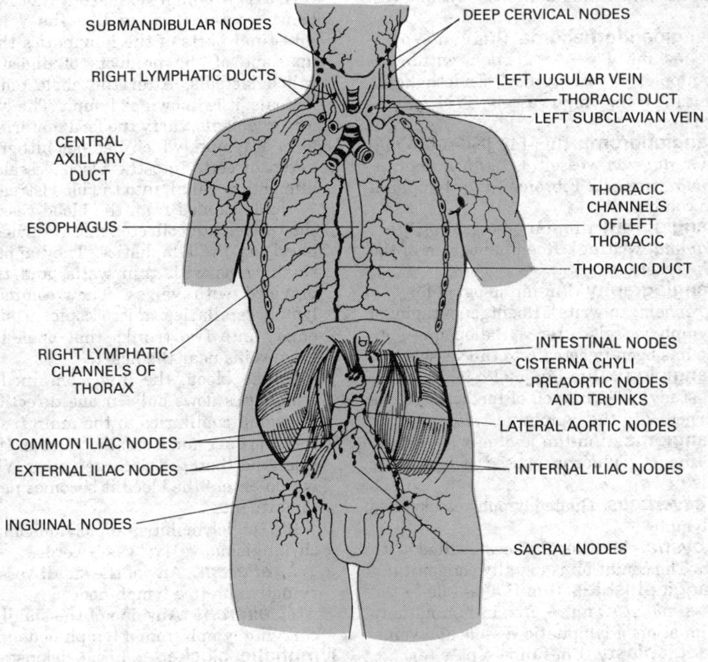

ble veins in structure, possessing three layers: the intima, media, and adventitia. They possess paired valves.

lymphatism (lĭm′fă-tĭzm) [″ + Gr. *-ismos,* condition]. Condition of an excess of lymphatic or tonsillar tissue.

lymphatitis (lĭm″fă-tī′tĭs) [″ + Gr. *itis,* inflammation]. Inflammation of the lymphatic system.

lymphatology (lĭm″fă-tŏl′ō-jē) [″ + Gr. *logos,* study]. Study of the lymphatic system.

lymphatolysis (lĭm″fă-tŏl′ĭ-sĭs) [″ + Gr. *lysis,* dissolution]. Destruction of lymphatic vessels or tissue.

lymphatolytic (lĭm″fă-tō-lĭt′ĭk). Destructive to lymphatics.

lymph cell. Lymphocyte.

lymph channel. Lymph sinus.

lymphectasia (lĭmf″ĕk-tā′zē-ă) [L. *lympha,* lymph, + Gr. *ektasis,* dilatation]. Dilatation of the lymphatics. SYN: *lymphangiectasis.*

lymphedema (lĭmf-ĕ-dē′mă) [″ + Gr. *oidema,* swelling]. Edema due to obstruction of lymphatics. SEE: *phlegmasia alba dolens.*

l., congenital. Chronic pitting edema of the lower extremities. SYN: *Meige-Milroy's disease.*

lymphemia (lĭm-fē′mē-ă) [″ + Gr. *haima,* blood]. An increased number of lymphocytes in the blood.

lymphendothelioma (lĭmf″ĕn-dō-thē-lē-ō′mă) [″ + Gr. *endon,* within, + *thele,* nipple, + *oma,* tumor]. Tumor from proliferation and dilatation of lymphatics with overgrowth of myxomatous tissue.

lymphenteritis (lĭmf″ĕn-tĕr-ī′tĭs) [″ + Gr. *enteron,* intestine, + *itis,* inflammation]. Serous infiltration accompanying inflammation of bowels.

lymph follicle. An irregular and inconstant aggregation of lymphocytes, usually seen in the lamina propria of a mucosal layer; an old term for lymph node.

lymphization (lĭm″fĭ-zā′shŭn). Production of lymph.

lymph node. A rounded body consisting of accumulations of lymphatic tissue found at intervals in the course of lymphatic vessels. Lymph nodes vary in size from a pinhead to an olive and may occur singly or in groups. One side bears an indentation, the hilum, from which blood vessels enter and leave and efferent lymph vessels leave. Afferent vessels enter on the side opposite from the hilum.

The node is enclosed in a capsule, from which trabeculae project inwardly, dividing the node into compartments called ampullae or alveoli. An outer compact region comprises the cortex; the inner diffuse portion is the medulla. The cortex is tightly packed with lymph nodules, which are separated from the capsule by the cortical sinus. The lymphatic tissue of the medulla is arranged in the form of medullary cords. Irregular tortuous spaces, called lymph sinuses, are present throughout the node. The nodes are aggregated in regions, the principal ones of which are in the neck (cervical), the armpit (axillary), and the groin (inguinal). Lymph nodes as well as vessels are divided into superficial and deep groups. Among the deep groups are those draining lymph from the visceral organs of the thorax and abdomen.

FUNCT: Lymph nodes produce lymphocytes and monocytes. They act as filters keeping particulate matter, esp. bacteria, from gaining entrance to the bloodstream. They may stop cancer cells, but in turn may become a metastatic site.

lymphnoditis (lĭmf″nō-dī′tĭs) [″ + *nodus,* knot, + Gr. *itis,* inflammation]. Inflamed condition of a lymph node.

lymph nodule. A small, compact, densely staining mass of cells each containing a lighter-staining central area in which lymphocytes are formed. They comprise the structural unit of lymphatic tissue. May occur singly, in groups as in Peyer's patches, or in encapsulated organs as lymph nodes.

lymphoblast (lĭm′fō-blăst) [″ + Gr. *blastos,* germ]. A cell that gives rise to a lymphocyte.

lymphoblastic (lĭm″fō-blăs′tĭk) [″ + Gr. *blastos,* germ]. Concerning a lymphoblast.

lymphoblastoma (lĭm″fō-blăst-ō′mă) [″ + ″ + *oma,* tumor]. Tumor composed of lymphocytes. SYN: *lymphosarcoma.*

lymphoblastomatosis (lĭm″fō-blăs″tō-mă-tō′sĭs) [″ + ″ + *oma,* tumor, + *osis,* condition]. Condition produced by lymphoblastomas.

lymphoblastosis (lĭm″fō-blăs-tō′sĭs) [″ + ″ + *osis,* condition]. Excessive number of lymphoblasts in the blood.

lymphocyte (lĭm′fō-sīt) [L. *lympha,* lymph, + Gr. *kytos,* cell]. Lymph cell or white blood corpuscle without cytoplasmic granules. They normally number from 20 to 50% of total white cells. May increase to 90% in lymphatic leukemia.

Lymphocytes average 10 to 12 micrometers in diameter but may be as large as 20 micrometers. Characterized by deeply staining, compact nucleus taking a dark blue. The nucleus occupies all or most of the cell, either in the center or at one side. The cytoplasm is usually clear but in some cells bright red-dish-violet granules are seen. SEE: *blood cells* for illus.

l., B-. A type of lymphocyte that arises in the bone marrow. They are present in the blood, lymph, and connective tissue. When stimulated by certain antigens, the small B-cell lymphocytes transform into large lymphocytes and some of these further differentiate into plasma cells, which are important in producing circulating antibodies. In lower animals, the bursa of Fabricus is important in the development of B cells The structure in mammals that corresponds to the bursa of Fabricus has not been identified. SYN: *B cells.*

l., T-. Lymphocytes migrate to the thymus, where they develop into T cells and begin to mature. From the thymus they go to a particular area of the peripheral lymphoid tissues and from there they circulate between blood and lymph. Three subpopulations of T cells are known: helper or cooperator cells, which enhance the production of antibody-forming cells from B-lymphocytes; cytotoxic or killer T cells, which are formed after mature T cells interact with some antigens present on foreign cells—these cells cause graft rejection and kill foreign cells in vitro; suppressor T cells, which suppress production of antibody-forming cells from B-lymphocytes.

lymphocythemia (lĭm″fō-sī-thē′mē-ă) [″ + Gr. *kytos,* cell, + *haima,* blood]. Excess of lymph cells in the blood. SYN: *lymphocytosis.*

lymphocytoblast (lĭm″fō-sī′tō-blăst″) [″ + ″ + *blastos,* germ]. Lymphoblast.

lymphocytoma (lĭm″fō-sī-tō′mă) [″ + ″ + *oma,* tumor]. A malignant mass of lymphocytes.

lymphocytopenia (lĭm″fō-sīt″ō-pē′nē-ă) [″ + ″ + *penia,* lack]. Less than normal number of lymphocytes in the blood.

lymphocytopoiesis (lĭm″fō-sīt″ō-poy-ē′sĭs) [″ + ″ + *poiesis,* production]. Lymphocyte production.

lymphocytosis (lĭm″fō-sī-tō′sĭs) [″ + ″ + *osis,* condition]. Excess of lymph cells. SYN: *lymphocythemia.*

lymphocytotoxin (lĭm″fō-sīt″ō-tŏks′ĭn) [″ + ″ + *toxikon,* poison]. A toxin destructive to lymphocytes.

lymphoduct (lĭm′fō-dŭkt) [″ + *ducere,* to lead]. A lymph vessel.

lymphoepithelioma (lĭm″fō-ĕp″ĭ-thē-lē-ō′mă) [″ + Gr. *epi,* at, + *thele,* nipple, + *oma,* tumor]. A poorly differentiated squamous cell carcinoma that involves the lymphoid tissue of the tonsils and nasopharynx.

lymphogenesis (lĭm″fō-jĕn′ĕ-sĭs) [″ + Gr. *genesis,* production]. Production of lymph.

lymphogenous (lĭm-fŏj′ĕn-ŭs) [″ + Gr. *gennan,* to produce]. 1. Forming lymph. 2. Derived from lymph.

lymphoglandula (lĭm″fō-glăn′dū-lă) [″ + *glandula,* little gland]. Lymph gland.

lymphogonia (lĭm″fō-gō′nē-ă) [″ + Gr. *gonos,*

offspring]. Large lymphocytes with large nuclei appearing in lymphatic leukemia.

lymphogram (lĭm′fō-grăm) [″ + Gr. *gramma*, writing]. Roentgenogram of a lymph vessel and nodes.

lymphogranuloma inguinale. Previous term for lymphogranuloma venereum.

lymphogranulomatosis (lĭm″fō-grăn-ū-lō″mă-tō′sĭs) [″ + *granulum*, granule, + Gr. *oma*, tumor, + *osis*, condition]. 1. Infectious granuloma of the lymphatics. 2. Hodgkin's disease.

lymphogranuloma venereum (lĭm″fō-grăn″ū-lō′mă) [″ + ″ + Gr. *oma*, tumor]. ABBR: LGV. An infectious venereal disease. SYN: *lymphogranuloma inguinale; lymphopathia venereum.*

ETIOL: Group A Chlamydiae (C. trachomatis) and rarely group B (C. psittaci).

SYM: From 7 to 12 days after exposure, a vesicle similar to that caused by herpes will appear usually on the genitals. This ruptures and heals painlessly. Then from one to eight weeks later, the regional lymph nodes enlarge, become tender, and may suppurate. These enlarged glands are called buboes. They heal and leave scars that may obstruct lymph channels. The perirectal lymph nodes in women may scar and cause rectal obstruction.

DIAG: Usually by clinical findings, but a skin reaction to injected killed organisms may help to confirm the clinical evidence.

TREATMENT: Tetracyclines cure the acute clinical signs but do not affect the previous scarring.

lymphogranuloma venereum antigen. USP. An antigen used in a skin test for lymphogranuloma venereum. SEE: *Frei test.*

lymphography (lĭm-fŏg′ră-fē) [L. *lympha*, lymph, + Gr. *graphein*, to write]. X-raying of a lymph vessel and nodes after a radiopaque substance has been injected in the lymphatic system.

lymphoid (lĭm′foyd) [″ + Gr. *eidos*, form]. Resembling lymph or lymph tissue.

lymphoid cells. Lymphocytes.

lymphoidectomy (lĭm″foyd-ĕk′tō-mē) [″ + ″ + *ektome*, excision]. Surgical removal of lymphoid tissue.

lymphoidocyte (lĭm-foyd′ō-sīt) [″ + ″ + *kytos*, cell]. A hemocytoblast.

lymphokines (lĭm′fō-kīnz). Substances released by sensitized lymphocytes when they contact specific antigens. They help to produce cellular immunity by stimulating macrophages and monocytes.

lymphokinesis (lĭm″fō-kī-nē′sĭs) [″ + Gr. *kinesis*, motion]. 1. Circulation of lymph in the lymphatic system. 2. Movement of lymph in the semicircular canals of the inner ear.

lymphology (lĭm-fŏl′ō-jē) [″ + Gr. *logos*, study]. Science of the lymphatics.

lymphoma (lĭm-fō′mă) [″ + Gr. *oma*, tumor]. (pl. *lymphoma* or *-mata*) A general term for growth of new tissue in the lymphatic system. Included in this general group are Hodgkin's disease, lymphatic leukemia, and reticuloses.

l., African. L., Burkitt's, q.v.

l., Burkitt's. A malignant lymphoma that causes bone-destroying lesions of the jaw. The Epstein-Barr virus is believed to be the causative agent. Initially reported from central Africa.

l., clasmocytic. L., malignant, histiocytic, q.v.

l., giant follicular. A well-differentiated lymphocytic malignant lymphoma.

l. granulomatosum. Small, white lymphatic nodule in the liver in Hodgkin's disease.

l., lymphoblastic. Poorly differentiated lymphocytic malignant lymphoma.

l., lymphocytic. L., malignant, well-differentiated, q.v.

l., malignant, histiocytic. A lymphoma composed mostly of neoplastic histiocytes. SYN: *reticulum cell sarcoma.*

l., malignant, mixed cell. A lymphoma that contains both histiocytes and monocytes.

l., malignant, poorly differentiated diffuse lymphocytic. Lymphoma in which the predominant cell is similar to the lymphoblast. The cells contain one or more nuclei.

l., malignant, undifferentiated. Lymphoma in which the predominant cell is a large stem cell with pale cytoplasm and indistinct cell borders.

l., malignant, well-differentiated diffuse lymphocytic. Lymphoma in which the predominant cells are mature lymphocytes.

lymphomatoid (lĭm-fō′mă-toyd) [L. *lympha*, lymph, + Gr. *oma*, tumor, + *eidos*, form]. Resembling lymphoma.

lymphomatosis (lĭm″fō-mă-tō′sĭs) [″ + ″ + *osis*, condition]. General lymphatic engorgement; deposition of lymphomata throughout the body.

lymphomatous (lĭm-fō′mă-tŭs). 1. Pert. to a lymphoma. 2. Affected with lymphomata.

lymphomyxoma (lĭm″fō-mĭk-sō′mă) [″ + Gr. *mys*, muscle, + *oma*, tumor]. A soft, nonmalignant tumor that contains lymphoid tissue.

lymphonodus (lĭm″fō-nō′dŭs) [″ + *nodus*, knot]. Lymphatic node.

lymphopathia venereum. Venereal disease marked by ulceration and enlargement of lymph nodes in inguinal area. SYN: *lymphogranuloma venereum.*

lymphopathy (lĭm-fŏp′ă-thē) [″ + Gr. *pathos*,

disease]. Any disease of the lymphatic system.

lymphopenia (lĭm-fō-pē′nē-ă) [″ + Gr. *penia,* a lack]. Deficiency of lymphocytes in the blood.

lymphoplasty (lĭm′fō-plăs″tē) [″ + Gr. *plassein,* to form]. Lymphoangioplasty, q.v.

lymphopoiesis (lĭm″fō-poy-ē′sĭs) [″ + Gr. *poiesis,* production]. Formation of lymphocytes or of lymphoid tissue.

lymphopoietic (lĭm″fō-poy-ĕt′ĭk) [″ + Gr. *poiein,* to produce]. Forming lymphocytes.

lymphoproliferative (lĭm″fō-prō-lĭf′ĕr-ă-tĭv). Concerning proliferation of lymphoid tissue.

lymphoprotease. Protein-splitting enzyme secured from a suspension of lymphatic tissue.

lymphoreticular (lĭm″fō-rĕ-tĭk′ū-lăr) [″ + *reticula,* net]. Pert. to reticuloendothelial cells of the lymph node.

lymphoreticular disorders. A great variety of poorly understood and inadequately classified diseases of the lymphoreticular system. Included are self-limited proliferation of lymph glands, lymphocytes, and monocytes; infectious mononucleosis; benign abnormalities of immunoglobulin synthesis; leukemias; lymphomas such as Hodgkin's disease, lymphosarcoma, reticulum cell sarcoma, and mycosis fungoides; malignant proliferative response or abnormal immunoglobulin synthesis such as plasma cell myeloma, macroglobulinemia, and amyloidosis; histiocytosis and lipid storage disease.

lymphoreticular system. In general the lymphatic tissue and the reticuloendothelial system. Specifically the system includes fixed and mobile cellular tissue involved in body defense by macrophage activity and immunologic mechanisms but does not include the granulocytic cells of the blood, i.e., neutrophils, eosinophils, and basophils.

lymphoreticulosis, benign, of inoculation (lĭm″fō-rē-tĭk″ū-lō′sĭs) [″ + ″ + Gr. *osis,* condition]. A benign self-limited granulomatous lymphadenitis transmitted by cat scratches. A pustular lesion appears about 10 days after the cat scratch. Then regional lymph nodes enlarge and may progress to suppuration. The causative organism is unknown; and there is no specific treatment. SYN: *cat-scratch disease.*

lymphorrhagia (lĭm″fō-rā′jē-ă) [″ + Gr. *rhegnynai,* to burst forth]. Flow of lymph from ruptured lymph vessels. SYN: *lymphorrhea.*

lymphorrhea (lĭm″fō-rē′ă) [″ + Gr. *rhoia,* flow]. Internal or external discharge of lymph through a wound. SYN: *lymphorrhagia.*

lymphorrhoid (lĭm′fō-royd). Dilated lymph channels that resemble hemorrhoids.

lymphosarcoma (lĭm″fō-săr-kō′mă) [″ + Gr. *sarx,* flesh, + *oma,* tumor]. A malignant disease of lymphatic tissue. Clinically may be quite similar to Hodgkin's disease. Diagnosis is made by biopsy rather than by clinical examination.

lymphosarcomatosis (lĭm″fō-săr″kō-mă-tō′sĭs) [″ + ″ + ″ + *osis,* condition]. Condition characterized by the development of lymphosarcoma.

lymphostasis (lĭm″fŏs′tă-sĭs) [L. *lympha,* lymph, + Gr. *stasis,* a stoppage]. Stoppage of flow of lymph.

lymphotaxis (lĭm″fō-tăk′sĭs) [″ + Gr. *taxis,* arrangement]. The effect of attracting or repelling lymphocytes.

lymphotome (lĭm′fō-tōm) [″ + Gr. *tome,* incision]. Instrument for removing glandular growths from tonsils and adenoids.

lymphotomy (lĭm-fŏt′ō-mē) [″ + Gr. *tome,* incision]. Lymphangiotomy, q.v.

lymphotoxin (lĭm″fō-tŏk′sĭn) [″ + Gr. *toxikon,* poison]. A lymphokine, q.v., that is produced by activated lymphocytes. The toxin affects a variety of cells.

lymphotrophy (lĭm-fŏt′rō-fē) [″ + Gr. *trophe,* nourishment]. Lymph nourishment of cells in regions devoid of blood vessels.

lymph sinus. One of several irregular tortuous vessels found in lymphatic organs. Lined with cells belonging to the reticuloendothelial system. SYN: *lymph channel.*

lymph spaces. Spaces in connective tissue filled with lymph.

lymphuria (lĭm-fū′rē-ă) [″ + Gr. *ouron,* urine]. Lymph in the urine.

lymphvascular (lĭmf-văs′kū-lăr) [″ + *vasculus,* a little vessel]. Rel. to the lymphatic vessels.

lynestrenol (lĭn-ĕs′trĕ-nōl). A progestational agent.

Lyon hypothesis (lī′ŏn). [Mary Lyon, Brit. geneticist, b. 1925] The idea that one of the X chromosomes of the female is inactivated during embryogenesis and becomes hyperpyknotic. This chromosome forms, in the cell nucleus, the sex chromatin mass, or Barr body, q.v. This X chromosome remains in this state throughout the cell's progeny so that in the adult only one X chromosome is active in each cell.

lyo- [Gr. *lyein,* to dissolve]. Combining form meaning dissolved or loose

lyochrome (lī′ō-krōm) [″ + *chroma,* color]. Flavin.

lyoenzyme (lī″ō-ĕn′zīm) [″ + *en,* in, + *zyme,* leaven]. An extracellular enzyme.

lyogel (lī′ō-jĕl). A gel containing much water.

lyophil(e) (lī′ō-fĭl, -fīl). Lyophilic, q.v.

lyophilic (lī″ō-fĭl′ĭk) [Gr. *lyein,* + *to dissolve,* + *philos,* love]. Concerning a colloid that forms a stable colloidal solution. It is not easily precipitated, but once precipitated, the action is readily reversed.

lyophilization (lī-ŏf″ĭ-lī-zā′shŭn). Process of rapidly freezing a substance at an extremely low temperature and then dehydrating in a high vacuum. SYN: *freeze-drying.*

lyophobe, lyophobic (lī′ō-fōb, lī″ō-fō′bĭk) [Gr. *lyein,* to dissolve, + *phobos,* fear]. Tending not to go into solution; applied to colloidal systems in which there is no strong affinity between dispersed phase and dispersion medium.

Lyophrin. Trade name for epinephrine bitartrate, USP.

lyosorption (lī″ō-sorp′shŭn) [″ + *sorbere,* to suck in]. The absorption, in a colloid, of a substance on the surface of the particles in the dispersed phase.

lyotrope (lī′ō-trōp) [″ + *tropos,* a turning]. A substance that goes into solution readily. Opposite of lyophobe.

lyotropic (lī″ō-trŏp′ĭk) [″ + *tropikos,* turning]. Lyophilic, q.v.

lypressin (lī-prĕs′ĭn). USP. A posterior pituitary hormone obtained from the pituitary gland of healthy pigs. Used as an antidiuretic. It is also used in treating von Willebrand's disease. Trade name is Diapid. SEE: *vasopressin.*

lyra (lī′ră) [L., Gr., *lyre*]. One of several anatomical structures so called because of their resemblance to the shape of a lyre.

lysate (lī′sāt). 1. The products of hydrolysis. 2. That which is produced when cells are lysed by the actions of agents such as chemicals, enzymes, or physical agents.

lyse (līz) [Gr. *lysis,* dissolution]. To cause lysis.

lysemia (lī-sē′mē-ă) [″ + *haima,* blood]. Lysis of red blood cells with release of hemoglobin into the plasma.

lysergic acid diethylamide. *LSD.*

lysimeter (lī-sĭm′ĕ-tĕr) [Gr. *lysis,* dissolution, + *metron,* measure]. Apparatus for determining solubilities of various substances.

lysin (lī′sĭn). A specific antibody acting destructively upon cells and tissues. SEE: *immune bodies.*

lysine (lī′sēn). An amino acid that is a hydrolytic cleavage product of digested protein. It is essential for growth and repair of tissues.

lysinogen (lī-sĭn′ō-jĕn) [Gr. *lysis,* dissolution, + *gennan,* to produce] An antibody that forms lysins.

lysis (lī′sĭs) [Gr., dissolution]. 1. The gradual decline of a fever or disease. Opposite of crisis. 2. Destruction of blood cells by a lysin, as when rabbit's red corpuscles are dissolved by dog's serum.

-lysis. 1. Combining form meaning dissolution or decomposition of. 2. Combining form indicating, in medicine, reduction or relief of.

lysocephalin (lī″sō-sĕf′ă-lĭn). Partial hydrolysis of a cephalin. This can be caused by the action of cobra venom.

Lysodren. Trade name for mitotane, USP.

lysogen (lī′sō-jĕn) [″ + *gennan,* to produce]. Something capable of producing a lysin.

lysogenesis (lī″sō-jĕn′ĕ-sĭs) [″ + *genesis,* production]. The production of cell-dissolving substances known as lysin.

lysogenic (lī-sō-jĕn′ĭk) [″ + Gr. *gennan,* to produce]. Producing lysins.

lysogeny (lī-sŏj′ĕ-nē). A special type of virus-bacterial cell interaction maintained by a complex cellular regulatory mechanism. Bacterial strains freshly isolated from their natural environment may contain a low concentration of bacteriophage. This phage will lyse other related bacteria. Cultures that contain these substances are said to be lysogenic.

Lysol (lī′sŏl). A proprietary preparation of a mixture of cresols. Because of its potential for causing toxicity, its use should be confined to disinfecting inanimate objects, feces, and urine.

Lysol poisoning. When swallowed, Lysol causes corrosion, edema of the lungs, immobility of pupils, and collapse. Vomiting may occur; death sometimes occurs after symptoms have abated.

TREATMENT: Prompt emptying of the stomach by emesis and lavage if the esophagus is not injured. Treat shock and convulsions symptomatically. Correct acidosis and maintain airway. Do tracheotomy if indicated.

lysolecithin (lī″sō-lĕs′ĭ-thĭn). A substance obtained from lecithin through the action of an enzyme present in cobra venom. Exerts a powerful hemolytic action.

lysosome (lī′sō-sōm). Part of an intracellular digestive system that exists as separate particles in the cell. Inside their limiting membrane, they contain a number of hydrolytic enzymes capable of breaking down proteins and certain carbohydrates. Even though their importance in health and disease is certain, all of the precise ways lysosomes effect changes are not understood.

lysozyme (lī′sō-zīm) [Gr. *lysis,* dissolution, + *zyme,* leaven]. An enzyme that is now called muramidase.

lyssa (lĭs′să) [Gr., frenzy]. An acute infectious disease, transferable by inoculation, attacking the nervous system in particular. SYN: *hydrophobia; rabies.*

lyssa virus. The genus of the family Rhabdoviridae. The previous term was rabies virus.

lyssoid (lĭs′oyd) [Gr. *lyssa,* frenzy, + *eidos,* resemblance]. Resembling lyssa or rabies.

lyssophobia (lĭs-ō-fō′bē-ă) [″ + *phobos,* fear]. 1. Hysteria resembling rabies. 2. Fear of rabies.

lyterian (lī-tĕr′ē-ăn) [Gr. *lyein,* to dissolve]. Indicative of the lessening of a disease process.

lytic (lĭt′ĭk). Rel. to lysis or a lysin.

lyze (līz) [Gr. *lysis,* dissolution]. To bring about lysis.

M

μ [*mu,* the twelfth letter of the Greek alphabet]. Symbol for micro-, a prefix indicating one one-millionth (10^{-6}) of the quantity, e.g., microgram or 0.000001 gram.

M. *master* or *medicine* in professional titles; *mille,* a thousand; *misce,* mix; *molar.*

m. *meter* and *minim;* in chemistry, for *meta-,* and for *mol* or *mole.*

MA. *mental age.*

M.A. *Master of Arts.*

ma. *milliampere.*

Maalox. Trade name for magnesia and alumina tablets.

M.A.C. *maximum allowable concentration.*

Mace. A proprietary substance for which the name is an acronym for *me*thylchloroform chloro-*ace*tophenone, a chemical compound used at one time in riot control because of its ability to irritate the eyes. Now it is considered to be too toxic for that purpose. SEE: *IDU.*

TREATMENT: Instillation of 0.1% aqueous solution of idoxuridine (IDU) into the eye. Contact lenses must be removed immediately.

mace (mās) [L. *macis*]. A spice from the outer covering of the nutmeg; employed as a condiment.

macerate (măs′ĕr-āt). To soften by steeping or soaking in water. Usually pertains to the skin.

maceration (măs-ĕr-ā′shŭn) [L. *macerare,* to make soft]. Process of softening a solid by steeping in a fluid.

Mache unit (mă′kē). [Heinrich Mache, Austrian physicist, b. 1876] ABBR: M.u., or German, M.E. The unit of measurement of concentration of radium emanation.

macies (mā′shē-ēz) [L., wasting]. Atrophy, wasting, emaciation.

machine. Any mechanical device or apparatus.

macrencephalia, macrencephaly (măk-rĕn″sĕ-fā′lē-ă, -sĕf′ă-lē) [Gr. *makros,* large, + *enkephalos,* brain]. Abnormally large size of the brain.

macro-, macr- [Gr. *makros,* large]. Combining forms meaning large or long.

macroamylase (măk″rō-ăm′ĭ-lās). A form of amylase that has a molecular weight much greater than ordinary amylase. The macroamylase molecule is too large to be excreted by the glomerulus of the kidney. Clinically important because routine blood-amylase study of an individual with macroamylase in the blood would indicate amylase to be elevated. This could lead the physician to believe the patient needs surgical exploration of the abdomen. In such a patient the urinary amylase would be within normal limits, which would not be true if the elevation of blood amylase were due to an actual increase in amylase present.

macroamylasemia (măk″rō-ăm″ĭl-ā-sē′mē-ă). Macroamylase in the serum. The presence of increased amounts of macroamylase in the blood has not been correlated with a specific single disease state.

macrobiosis (măk″rō-bī-ō′sĭs) [Gr. *makros,* large, + *biosis,* life]. Longevity.

macrobiota (măk″rō-bī-ō′tă). The macroscopic living organisms, flora and fauna, of an area.

macroblepharia (măk″rō-blĕ-fā′rē-ă) [Gr. *makros,* large, + *blepharon,* eyelid]. Abnormal largeness of eyelid.

macrobrachia (măk″rō-brā′kē-ă) [″ + *brachion,* arm]. Abnormal size or length of the arm.

macrocardius (măk″rō-kăr′dē-ŭs) [″ + *kardia,* heart]. Deformed individual with an abnormally large heart.

macrocephalia (măk″rō-sĕ-fā′lē-ă) [″ + *kephale,* head]. Abnormal largeness of head. SYN: *macrocephaly.*

ETIOL: Found in acromegaly, hydrocephalus, rickets, osteitis deformans, leontiasis ossea, myxedema, leprosy, and pituitary disturbances.

macrocephalic. Megalocephalic, q.v.

macrocephalous (măk″rō-sĕf′ă-lŭs). Pert. to or having an excessively large head.

macrocephaly (măk-rō-sĕf′ă-lē). Abnormal largeness of the head. SYN: *macrocephalia.*

macrocheilia (măk″rō-kī′lē-ă) [″ + *cheilos,* lip]. Abnormal size of lip characterized by swelling of glands of lip. It is a congenital condition. SYN: *macrolabia.*

macrocheiria (măk-rō-kī′rē-ă) [″ + *cheir,* hand]. Excessive size of the hands.

macrochemistry. Use of chemical tests that produce changes that are detectable by the unaided eye.

macrocnemia (măk″rŏk-nē′mē-ă) [″ + *kneme,* shin]. A condition in which the legs below the knees are excessively large.

macrocolon (măk″rō-kō′lŏn) [″ + *kolon,* colon]. Megacolon.

macroconidium (măk″rō-kō-nĭd′ē-ŭm). A large conidium or exospore.

macrocornea (măk-rō-kor′nē-ă) [″ + L. *cornu,* horn]. Abnormal size of the cornea. SYN: *megalocornea.*

macrocyst (măk′rō-sĭst) [″ + *kystis,* bladder]. A large cyst.

macrocyte [″ + *kytos,* cell]. Erythrocyte that is abnormally large, exceeding 10 microns in diameter.

macrocythemia, macrocytosis (măk″rō-sī-thē′mē-ă, măk″rō-sī-tō′sĭs) [″ + ″ + *haima,* blood]. A condition in which erythrocytes are larger than normal.

macrodactylia (măk″rō-dăk-tĭl′ē-ă) [″ + *daktylos,* finger]. Excessive size of one or more of the digits.

Macrodantin. Trade name for nitrofurantoin.

Macrodex. Trade name for dextran 70.

macrodontia (măk″rō-dŏn′shē-ă) [″ + *odous,* tooth]. An abnormal increase in size of the teeth.

macroesthesia (măk″rō-ĕs-thē′zē-ă) [Gr. *makros,* large, + *aisthesis,* sensation]. A state in which objects seen or felt appear to be greatly magnified.

macrofauna (măk″rō-faw′nă). In a particular location or area, the animal life visible to the naked eye.

macroflora (măk″rō-flō′ră). In a particular area or location, the plant life visible to the naked eye.

macrogamete (măk″rō-găm′ĕt) [″ + *gamete,* wife]. A large immobile reproductive cell formed in certain protozoa and simple plants. Corresponds to the ovum in higher forms.

macrogametocyte (măk″rō-gă-mē′tō-sīt). A large nonmotile reproductive cell developing from the merozoite of certain protozoans. Red blood cell infected with female form of the malarial parasite. SEE: *Plasmodium.*

macrogenitosomia praecox (măk″rō-jĕn″ĭ-tō-sō′mē-ă prē′kŏks) [″ + L. *genitalis,* genital, + Gr. *soma,* body, + L. *praecox,* early]. Abnormal size of genitalia due to excess androgens (male hormones) from the fetal adrenal. In the female this causes pseudohermaphroditism and in the male enlarged external genitalia.

macrogingivae (măk″rō-jĭn-jī′vē) [″ + L. *gingiva,* gum]. Hypertrophy of the gums.

macroglia (măk-rŏg′lē-ă) [″ + *glia,* glue]. Astrocyte.

macroglobulin (măk″rō-glŏb′ū-lĭn). A globulin of high molecular weight, about 1,000,000, normally present in the blood but increased in disease states such as multiple myeloma, collagen disorders, cirrhosis of the liver, and amyloidosis.

macroglobulinemia (măk-rō-glŏb″ū-lĭn-ē′mē-ă). Presence of globulins of high molecular weight in serum.

m., Waldenström's. Excessive growth of plasma cells, which are responsible for synthesis of IgM globulins. This causes excess production of IgM globulins. The patients are usually middle aged or elderly and the frequency is slightly higher in men than in women. Anemia due to infiltration of the bone marrow with lymphocytes and plasma cells, generalized lymphadenopathy, chronic lymphocytic leukemia, and hyperviscosity of the blood are present. The last causes lassitude, confusion, and bleeding tendency.

TREATMENT: Reduce tumor mass by use of cytotoxic agents; symptomatic therapy for complications.

macroglossia [Gr. *makros,* large, + *glossa,* tongue]. Hypertrophied condition of the tongue; a congenital disorder.

macrognathia (măk-rō-nā′thē-ă) [″ + *gnathos,* jaw]. Abnormal size of the jaw.

macrography (măk-rŏg′ră-fē) [″ + *graphein,* to write]. Writing with large letters.

macrogyria [″ + *gyros,* circle]. Excessively large size of convolutions (gyri) of cerebral hemispheres.

macrolabia (măk-rō-lā′bē-ă) [″ + L. *labium,* lip]. Abnormal size of lip. SYN: *macrocheilia.*

macroleukoblast (măk″rō-lū′kō-blăst) [″ + *leukos,* white, + *blastos,* germ]. A large leukoblast.

macrolymphocyte (măk″rō-lĭmf′ō-sīt) [″ + L. *lympha,* lymph, + Gr. *kytos,* cell]. A large lymphocyte.

macromania (măk″rō-mā′nē-ă) [″ + *mania,* madness]. 1. Megalomania, q.v. 2. The delusion that the affected individual or his or her parts or surroundings are extremely large.

macromastia (măk-rō-măs′tē-ă) [″ + *mastos,* breast]. Abnormally large breasts.

macromelia [″ + *melos,* limb]. Excessive size of an organ or a part, esp. an extremity.

macromelus (măk-rŏm′ē-lŭs) [″ + *melos,* limb]. An individual with abnormally large extremities.

macromere (măk′rō-mēr) [″ + *meros,* a part]. Blastomere of large size.

macromethod (măk′rō-mĕth″ŏd). Chemical examinations or analysis wherein ordinary quantities of the material being studied are used.

macromolecule (măk″rō-mŏl′ĕ-kūl). A large molecule such as a protein, polymer, or polysaccharide.

macromonocyte (măk″rō-mŏn′ō-sīt). A large monocyte.

macromyeloblast (măk″rō-mī′ĕ-lō-blăst) [″ + *myelos,* marrow, + *blastos,* germ]. A large myeloblast.

macronormoblast (măk″rō-nor′mō-blăst) [″ + L. *norma,* rule, + Gr. *blastos,* germ]. Large nucleated red blood corpuscle.

macronucleus (măk″rō-nū′klē-ŭs). A nucleus that occupies most of the cell.

macronychia (măk″rō-nĭk′ē-ă) [″ + *onyx,* nail]. Abnormal length of the fingernails.

macropathology (măk″rō-pă-thŏl′ō-jē). The pathological changes in the gross anatomical structures.

macrophage, macrophagus (măk′rō-fāj, măk-rŏf′ă-gŭs) [″ + *phagein,* to eat]. Cells of the reticuloendothelial system having the ability to phagocytose particulate substances and to store vital dyes and other colloidal substances. They are found in loose connective tissues and various organs of the body. They include Kupffer cells of the liver, splenocytes of the spleen, dust cells of the lung, microglia of spinal cord and brain, and histiocytes of loose connective tissue.

m., fixed. A nonmotile macrophage. SYN: *histiocyte.*

m., free. A wandering or ameboid macrophage. Found esp. in areas where inflammatory processes are in progress. SYN: *polyblast.*

macrophage activating factor. A substance that stimulates macrophages to change in appearance and metabolic activities and to become more effective killers of certain microbial cells.

macrophage migration inhibiting factor. A substance that blocks the migration of macrophages in culture.

macrophagocyte (măk″rō-făg′ō-sīt). A large phagocyte.

macrophallus (măk″rō-făl′ŭs) [Gr. *makros,* large, + *phallos,* penis]. Abnormally large penis.

macrophthalmia (măk″rŏf-thăl′mē-ă) [″ + *ophthalmos,* eye]. Abnormally large eyeball.

macroplasia (măk″rō-plā′zē-ă) [″ + *plasis,* forming]. Abnormally large size of a part or specific tissue.

macropodia (măk-rō-pō′dē-ă) [″ + *pous,* foot]. Abnormally large feet.

macropolycyte (măk″rō-pŏl′ē-sīt) [″ + *polys,* many, + *kytos,* cell]. A large polymorphonuclear leukocyte with a multisegmented nucleus.

macropromyelocyte (măk″rō-prō-mī′ĕ-lō-sīt). A large promyelocyte.

macroprosopia (măk″rō-prō-sō′pē-ă) [″ + *prosopon,* face]. Large facial features.

macropsia (măk-rŏp′sē-ă) [″ + *opsis,* vision]. Condition in which objects look larger than they really are.

macrorhinia (măk-rō-rĭn′ē-ă) [″ + *rhis,* nose]. Excessive size of the nose, either congenital or pathological.

macroscelia (măk-rō-sē′lē-ă) [″ + *skelos,* leg]. Abnormally large legs.

macroscopic (măk-rō-skŏp′ĭk) [″ + *skopein,* to examine]. Large enough to be seen by the naked eye. Opposite of microscopic.

macroscopy (măk-rŏs′kō-pē). Examination of an object with the naked eye.

macrosigmoid (măk″rō-sĭg′moyd). Abnormally large sigmoid colon.

macrosis (mă-krō′sĭs) [″ + *osis,* condition]. Increase in size.

macrosmatic (măk″rŏs-măt′ĭk) [″ + *osmasthai,* to smell]. Indicating an abnormally keen sense of smell.

macrosomatia, macrosomia (măk″rō-sō-mā′shē-ă, măk-rō-sō′mē-ă) [Gr. *makros,* large, + *soma,* body]. Abnormally large body.

macrospore (măk′rō-spor). In certain fungi and protozoa with two spores, the larger of the two.

macrostereognosis (măk″rō-stē″rē-ō-nō′sĭs) [″ + *stereos,* solid, + *gnosis,* knowledge]. A misperception that objects appear to be larger than they are.

macrostomia (măk-rō-stō′mē-ă) [″ + *stoma,* mouth]. Excessively wide mouth.

macrostructure (măk′rō-strŭk′tūr). The gross structure of an entity.

macrotia (măk-rō′shē-ă) [″ + *ous,* ear]. Abnormally large ears.

macrotome (măk′rō-tōm) [″ + *tome,* incision]. Device for cutting large anatomical sections. SEE: *microtome.*

macrotooth. Abnormally enlarged tooth.

macula (măk′ū-lă) [L., spot]. (pl. *maculae*) 1. [NA] A small spot or colored area. SEE: *roseola.* 2. A macule.

m. acusticae. Thickened oval areas in the saccule and utricle in which fibers of the vestibular branch of the acoustic nerve terminate. They are sensory receptors containing hair cells that respond to movement of the endolymph. They include macula sacculi and macula utriculi.

m. albida. White mark found on the visceral layer of the peritoneum or epicardium in some contagious diseases.

m. atrophica. Glistening white spot on skin due to atrophy.

m. caerulea. Steel-gray or blue stain of epidermis without elevation. It does not disappear on pressure and occurs esp. with pediculosis pubis or bites from fleas.

m., cerebral. Reddened line that becomes deeper and persists for some time when the fingernail is drawn across the skin, esp. in tuberculous meningitis. SYN: *tache cérébrale.*

m. cornea. Opaque spot in cornea.

m. cribrosa. [NA] One of the tiny foramina in the wall of the vestibule of the bony labyrinth of the ear through which pass filaments of the acoustic nerve.

m. densa. Closely packed cells in the distal tubular epithelium of each nephron. These cells are close to the juxtaglomerular apparatus and may function as chemoreceptors.

m. flava laryngis. A small yellow spot at the ventral end of each vocal cord formed by a small mass of elastic tissue or, sometimes, cartilage.

m. folliculi. The point on the ovarian follicle where it ruptures.

m. germinativa. The germinal area in eggs with large yolks.

m. gonorrhoeica. Red spot at orifice of

Bartholin's gland. Seen in gonorrheal vulvitis.

m. lutea retinae. A yellow spot in the center of the retina approx. 2 mm. lateral to the optic nerve's exit. Contains a pit, fovea centralis, where the retina is reduced to a layer of closely packed cones, which functions as the area of most acute vision (central vision).

m. sacculi. [NA] Thickened area in the saccule where vestibular impulses are received and transmitted.

m. utriculi. [NA] Thickened area in the utricle where vestibular impulses are received and transmitted.

macular (măk'ū-lăr) [L. *macula,* spot]. 1. Rel. to macules. 2. Having macules.

maculate(d) (măk'ū-lāt, -lāt-ĕd). Spotted, as with macules.

maculation (măk-ū-lā'shŭn) [L. *macula,* spot]. Process of becoming maculate; development of macules.

macule (măk'ūl) [L. *macula,* spot]. Discolored spot or patch on the skin, neither elevated nor depressed, of various colors, sizes, and shapes. Macules include hyperemia, roseola, erythema, telangiectasis, nevi vasculosi, areola, achromia, chloasma, purpura, petechiae, ecchymosis, vibices, albinism, vitiligo, lentigines, nevi pigmentosi, nevi spili, and discolorations.

Macules occur in pellagra, pityriasis rosea, pediculosis corporis, rubella, scurvy, serum sickness, peliosis, anemia, leukemia, cancer, infectious diseases, erysipelas, acne rosacea, nevus pigmentosus, vitiligo, leprosy, morphea, and facial hemiatrophy. SYN: *macula.*

maculocerebral (măk"ū-lō-sĕr'ē-brăl) [" + *cerebrum,* brain]. Concerning the macula of the retina and the brain.

maculopapular (măk"ū-lō-păp'ū-lăr). Consisting of or pert. to macules and papules. An eruption consisting of both macules and papules.

maculopathy (măk"ū-lŏp'ă-thē) [L. *macula,* spot, + Gr. *pathos,* disease]. Retinal pathology involving the macula of the eye.

mad. 1. Not rational. SYN: *insane.* 2. Angry. 3. Rash, foolish, frantic. 4. Suffering from infection with rabies. SYN: *rabid.*

madarosis (măd-ă-rō'sĭs) [Gr. *madaros,* bald]. Loss of eyelashes or eyebrows.

madder (măd'ĕr). Root of the plant Rubia tinctoria, a source of the red dye alizarin.

Madelung's deformity. [Otto W. Madelung, Strasbourg surgeon, 1846–1926] Displacement of the hand to the radial side due to relative overgrowth of the ulna.

Madelung's disease. Generalized symmetrical deposits of fatty tissue, lipomata, on the upper back, shoulders, and neck. SYN: *Madelung's neck.*

madescent (măd-ĕs'ĕnt) [L. *madescere,* to become moist]. Slightly moist or becoming so.

madidans (măd'ĭ-dăns) [L. *madidus,* wet]. Exuding moisture as in some skin lesions.

Madura foot. Fungus disease of the foot. SYN: *maduromycosis; mycetoma.*

maduromycosis (măd-ū"rō-mī-kō'sĭs). Chronic infection of the foot or hand characterized by marked swelling and development of nodules, vesicles, abscesses, and sinuses. A type of mycetoma, q.v.

ETIOL: Various fungi.

mafenide acetate (măf'ĕn-īd). USP. An antibacterial drug of the sulfonamide class. It is used topically in cream form for treating burns.

magaldrate (măg'ăl-drāt). USP. A complex of magnesium oxide and aluminum oxide used as a gastric antacid. Trade name is Riopan.

Magendie's foramen (mă-jĕn'dēz). [François Magendie, Fr. physiologist, 1783–1855] The median of three openings in the roof of the 4th ventricle. It is in front of the cerebellum and behind the pons varolii, connecting the ventricle with the subarachnoid space.

magenstrasse (măg"ĕn-străs'ĕ) [Ger. *magen,* stomach, + *strasse,* street]. A groove along the lesser curvature of the stomach from cardia to pylorus.

magenta (mă-jĕn'tă). The dye, basic fuchsin.

maggot. Larva of an insect, esp. the soft-bodied footless larva of flies (order Diptera). Many are parasitic, giving rise to myiasis, q.v.

maggot treatment. An obsolete method of treating septic wounds. Meat maggots, introduced into a sloughing septic wound, ingested the necrotic material, leaving the wound with a clean granulating surface. The maggots were then removed and destroyed.

magic thinking. A person feeling that his or her thoughts or actions have the ability to cause actions or effects that would defy the normal laws of cause and effect.

magistery (măj'ĭs-tĕr"ē) [L. *magister,* master]. 1. Specially compounded remedy. 2. A precipitate.

magistral (măj'ĭs-trăl). Concerning medicines prescribed by a physician for a particular case. SEE: *officinal.*

magma (măg'mă) [Gr.]. 1. Mass left after extraction of principal. 2. Salve or paste. 3. A suspension of finely divided material in a small amount of water.

magnesia (măg-nē'zē-ă) [magnetic stone found in Magnesia, region of ancient Thessaly]. Magnesium oxide. MgO.

m., milk of. Aperient composed of magnesium hydroxide and water.

magnesia and alumina (tablets). An antacid preparation comprised of aluminum hydroxide and magnesium hydroxide. Trade name is Maalox.

magnesium [L.]. SYMB: Mg. At. wt. 24.312; at. no. 12; sp. gr. 1.738. A white mineral element found in soft tissue, muscles, bones, and to some extent in the body fluids. It is a naturally occurring element on earth, being extracted from well and sea water. The human body contains approx. 25 gm. of magnesium, most of which is in the bones. Muscles contain less of it than they do of calcium. Concentration of magnesium in the blood serum is between 1.5 and 2.5 mEq./liter.

Magnesium is widely distributed in foods; therefore deficiency rarely occurs. It is obtained in sufficient quantities in whole grains, fruits, and vegetables so that it is unnecessary to make special dietary plans. A typical diet contains 200 to 400 mg. but very little of this is absorbed. Deficiency may be present in patients with chronic diarrhea or diseases that interfere with absorption.

FUNCT: Magnesium activates enzymes that catalyze reactions between phosphate ions and adenosine triphosphate (ATP). It is also associated with regulation of body temperature, neuromuscular contraction, and synthesis of protein.

DEFICIENCY SYM: Tetany quite similar to that produced by hypocalcemia, weakness, and mental depression.

m. carbonate. USP. $MgCO_3 \cdot 3H_2O$. A bulky, white, odorless powder. Taken by mouth to neutralize acid in stomach.

m. chloride. USP. $MgCl_2 \cdot 6H_2$. It is used in treating electrolyte disturbances and in dialysis solutions.

m. citrate oral solution. USP. A solution containing an amount of magnesium citrate corresponding to approx. 1.6% magnesium oxide. Used as a purgative. Trade name is Eval-Q-Mag.

m. gluconate. USP. A medicine used to replace magnesium in the body.

m. hydroxide. $Mg(OH)_2$. USP. A bulky white powder that, in aqueous suspension, is milk of magnesia. Used as a laxative and antacid.

m. oxide. USP. MgO. Calcined magnesia. Light magnesia. A white, very bulky powder. In Great Britain called light magnesium oxide. Used as an antacid and laxative.

m. phosphate. USP. A white, odorless powder. Used as an antacid and laxative.

m. salicylate. USP. An antipyretic and analgesic drug. Trade name is Magan.

m. stearate. USP. Compound of magnesium and palmitic and stearic acids. Used in manufacture of pharmaceutical tablets.

m. sulfate. USP. $MgSO_4 \cdot 7H_2O$. Small colorless crystals with a bitter saline taste. SYN: *Epsom salt.* Used as a cathartic, anticonvulsant and topically as an anti-inflammatory agent.

INCOMPAT: Ammonium chloride, soapsuds enema, quinine, ferric chloride, sulfanilamide.

m. trisilicate. USP. Magnesium oxide, silicon dioxide, and water. Used as an antacid. Trade names are Azolid-A and Trimax.

magnet [Gr. *magnes,* magnet]. Any body that has the property of attracting iron. This may be a natural iron oxide or a mass of iron or steel that has this property given to it artificially. A piece of iron may be magnetized by passage of an electric current through an insulated wire wound around it.

m., horseshoe. Magnet in shape of a horseshoe.

magnetic. Pert. to a magnet or having magnetism.

magnetic field. The space permeated by the magnetic lines of force surrounding a permanent magnet or coil of wire carrying electric current.

magnetic lines of force. The lines indicating the direction of the magnetic force in the space surrounding a magnet or constituting a magnetic field.

magnetism (măg′nĕ-tĭzm) [Gr *magnes,* magnet, + *-ismos,* condition]. The property of repulsion and attraction of certain substances that have magnetic properties. SEE: *magnet.*

magnetoelectricity (măg-nē″tō-ē″lĕk-trĭs′ĭ-tē) [″ + *elektron,* amber]. Electricity generated by use of magnets.

magnetometer (măg″nĕ-tŏm′ĕ-tĕr) [″ + *metron,* measure]. Device for measuring magnetic fields.

magneton (măg′nĕ-tŏn). The unit of nuclear magnetic force.

magnetotherapy (măg-nē″tō-thĕr′ă-pē) [″ + *therapeia,* treatment]. Application of magnets or magnetism in treating diseases.

magnetropism (măg-nĕt′rō-pĭzm) [″ + *trope,* a turn]. The change in direction of growth of a plant or organism in response to the action of a magnetic field.

magnification (măg-nĭ-fĭ-kā′shŭn) [L. *magnus,* great, + *facere,* to make]. Process of increasing apparent size of an object, esp. under microscope.

magnum [L.]. 1. Large or great. 2. Old term for capitate bone (os magnum), the largest of the carpals.

Mahaim fibers. [I. Mahaim, contemporary Fr. physician] Fibers for conducting cardiac impulses. They connect the proximal main atrioventricular bundle to the septal myocardium and permit ventricular preexcitation with resultant tachycardia.

maidenhead. Lay term for the thin crescentic fold surrounding vaginal opening. At one time considered to be a sign of virginity.

However, it may be present in those who have had sexual intercourse and may be absent in those who have never experienced sexual intercourse. SYN: *hymen.*

maim (mām) [ME. *maymen,* to cripple]. 1. To injure seriously; to disable. 2. To deprive of the use of a part, such as an arm or leg.

main (măn) [Fr.]. Hand.

m. en griffe. Flexion and atrophy of the hand in a claw shape. SYN: *clawhand.*

m. succulente. Edema of a hand.

Majocchi's disease (mă-yŏk'ēz). [Domenico Majocchi, It. physician, 1849–1929] Ring-shaped purplish eruption of lower limbs. SYN: *purpura annularis telangiectodes.*

Majocchi's granuloma. Allergic granulomata of the skin due to fungal infections.

major histocompatibility complex. ABBR: MHC. The chromosomal region that controls for strong transplantation antigens. In humans, antibodies to MHC-controlled antigens have been found in sera from women with multiple pregnancies and from persons who have received multiple blood transfusions. Investigation of these antigens led to the work indicating that these antigens are controlled by genes at three loci on chromosome 6. These loci have been designated HLA-A, HLA-B, and HLA-C. HLA indicates human leukocyte antigen. SEE: *histocompatibility antigens.*

makro- [Gr.]. SEE: words beginning with *macro-.*

mal-. Combining form meaning ill, bad, poor.

mal (măl) [Fr., from L. *malum,* an evil]. A sickness, or a disorder.

m. de Cayenne. Elephantiasis.

m. de mer. Seasickness.

m. perforant. A perforating ulcer of the foot.

m. perforant palatin. A perforating ulcer of the palate.

mala (mā'lă) [L.]. 1. [NA] The cheek. 2. The cheekbone.

malabsorption syndrome. Disordered or inadequate absorption of nutrients from the intestinal tract, esp. the small intestine. May be associated with or due to a number of diseases, including those that affect the intestinal mucosa, as infections, tropical sprue, gluten enteropathy, pancreatic insufficiency, or surgery such as gastric resection and ileal bypass, or may be due to antibiotic therapy such as neomycin.

malacia (mă-lā'shē-ă) [Gr. *malakia,* softening]. Abnormal softening of tissues of an organ or of tissues themselves.

malacoma (măl-ă-kō'mă). Softening of an organ or part of the body. SYN: *malacia; malacosis.*

malacoplakia (măl"ă-kō-plā'kē-ă) [Gr. *malakos,* soft, + *plax,* plaque]. Existence of soft patches in mucous membrane of a hollow organ.

m. vesicae. Soft, fungus-like patches on mucosa of the bladder and ureters.

malacosarcosis (măl"ă-kō-săr-kō'sĭs) [" + *sarx,* flesh, + *osis,* condition]. Softness of tissue, esp. muscular.

malacosis (măl-ă-kō'sĭs) [" + *osis,* condition]. Abnormal softening of an organ or tissue. SYN: *malacia; malacoma.*

malacosteon (măl-ă-kŏs'tē-ŏn) [" + *osteon,* bone]. Softening of the bones. SYN: *mollities ossium; osteomalacia.*

malacotic (măl-ă-kŏt'ĭk). 1. Soft. 2. Affected with malacia. 3. Rel. to malacia.

malacotomy (măl-ă-kŏt'ō-mē) [Gr. *malakos,* soft, + *tome,* incision]. Incision of soft areas of the body, esp. of the abdominal wall.

malactic (mă-lăk'tĭk) [Gr. *malakos,* soft]. Emollient.

maladie de Roger (măl"ă-dē'). Congenital interventricular septal defect.

maladjusted. Poorly adjusted; unhappy or unsuccessful because of inability or failure to adjust to life stresses. Marked by depression, anxiety, and irritability.

malady (măl'ă-dē) [Fr. *maladie,* illness, from L. *malum,* an evil]. A disease or disorder. SYN: *disease.*

malaise (mă-lāz') [Fr.]. Discomfort, uneasiness, or indisposition, often indicative of infection.

malalignment (măl"ă-līn'mĕnt). Improper alignment of structures such as teeth, or portions of a fractured bone.

malar (mā'lăr) [L. *mala,* cheek]. Pert. to the cheek or cheekbones.

malar bone. A four-pointed bone on each side of the face, uniting the frontal and superior maxillary bones with the zygomatic process of the maxilla. SYN: *cheekbone; mala; zygoma; zygomatic bone.*

malaria (mă-lā'rē-ă) [It. *malaria,* bad air]. An acute and sometimes chronic infectious disease due to the presence of protozoan parasites within red blood cells.

The parasites undergo an asexual cycle in man and a sexual cycle in the mosquito. Sporozoites injected by the bite of a mosquito or by blood transfusion go through an exoerythrocytic cycle in tissue cells, such as liver cells where they undergo schizogony. After an interval of 7 to 10 days, they invade erythrocytes in which they undergo several divisions (schizogony), forming many merozoites. These break free and invade other corpuscles. The destruction of corpuscles with liberation of pigment and waste products brings on the characteristic paroxysms of chills and fever. This occurs at 48-hour intervals in tertian malaria and 72-hour intervals in quartan malaria.

After several generations of schizonts, some merozoites develop into micro- and macrogametocytes, which, when sucked up by a mosquito, feeding on the patient, undergo further development. The microgametocytes produce several flagellated bodies that unite with a macrogamete to form a zygote. This elongates, forming a vermicule or ookinete, which penetrates the stomach wall of the mosquito, forming an oocyst in which sporozoites develop. The oocyst bursts when mature, liberating sporozoites into the body cavity through which the sporozoites then make their way to salivary glands. They are discharged through salivary ducts when the mosquito bites a person.

ETIOL: Four species of a sporozoan, Plasmodium (P. vivax, P. falciparum, P. malariae, P. ovale). The causative organism is transmitted through bites of infected female mosquitoes of the genus Anopheles; may be transmitted by blood transfusion.

INCUBATION: Average 12 days for P. falciparum; 14 days for P. vivax and P. ovale; and 30 days for P. malariae.

SYM: Various derangements of the digestive and nervous systems. Characterized by periodicity, chills, fever, and sweats in the order mentioned, having pathological manifestations of progressive anemia, splenic enlargement, and deposition in various organs of a melanin, resulting from biological activity of the Plasmodia.

TREATMENT: Chloroquine phosphate is indicated in all types of malaria except that due to drug-resistant P. falciparum. In drug-resistant P. falciparum, treatment with combinations of quinine, pyrimethamine, and a sulfonamide is indicated. Malaria due to other species should be treated with both chloroquine and primaquine in a dose of 15 mg. of the base each day for 14 days. This may be given at the same time as the chloroquine. Persons with glucose-6-phosphate-dehydrogenase deficiency may develop hemolysis of red blood cells, but this is a rare complication.

PROPHYLAXIS: When traveling to areas where falciparum malaria is endemic, one should take 500 mg. of chloroquine phosphate daily for one week, and upon arrival 500 mg. should be taken twice weekly. The medication should be continued for 6 weeks after leaving the area. In areas where chloroquine-resistant falciparum malaria occurs, primaquine and sulfadoxine are given. These should be continued for 6 weeks after leaving the area.

Prevention of other forms of malaria requires the addition of primaquine phosphate to the chloroquine regimen.

m., cephalgic. Malaria with unusually severe headache, nausea, and vomiting. Meningitis and intracranial lesions are characteristic.

m., cerebral. Falciparum malaria in which brain is affected due to tendency of parasites to agglutinate, resulting in clogging of capillaries, which, in the brain, leads to coma or sometimes sudden death.

m., estivoautumnal. Previous name for falciparum malaria.

m., falciparum. Malaria caused by Plasmodium falciparum. More prevalent in tropics. Symptoms more severe than in other types but runs a shorter course without relapses.

m., latent. Malaria in which parasites exist within the bloodstream but give rise to no recognizable symptoms. An individual having this form is a reservoir for the disease.

m., quartan. Malaria with short and less severe paroxysms. Sporulation occurs each 72 hours, causing seizures every 4 days. Caused by Plasmodium malariae.

m., quotidian. Malaria in which paroxysms occur with daily periodicity due to 24-hour sporulation of two groups of P. vivax. Abrupt rise and fall of temperature.

m., tertian. Malaria in which sporulation occurs each 48 hours. Symptoms more common during the day. Paroxysms divided into chill, fever, and sweating stages. Cold stage usually is 10 to 15 minutes but may last an hour or more. Febrile stage varies from 4 to 6 hours. Benign tertian malaria is caused by Plasmodium vivax, malignant tertian by Plasmodium falciparum.

m., vivax. Malaria caused by Plasmodium vivax. It is the most common form of malaria. Marked by frequent recurrence.

malariacidal (mă-lā″rē-ă-sī′dăl) [It. *malaria,* bad air, + L. *caedere,* to kill]. Having the property of killing malaria parasites.

malarial (mă-lăr′ē-ăl) [It. *malaria,* bad air]. 1. Affected with malaria. 2. Causing malaria. 3. Resembling malaria. 4. Pert. to malaria. SYN: *malarious.*

malariology (mă-lăr-ē-ŏl′ō-jē) The scientific study of malaria.

malariotherapy (mă-lăr-ē-ō-thĕr′ă-pē). A now obsolete method of treating syphilis of the central nervous system by injecting malarial organisms into the body. The organisms produce hyperthermia, which is then terminated by administering an antimalarial.

malarious (mă-lăr′ē-ŭs). Of the nature of, or afflicted with malaria. SYN: *malarial.*

Malassezia (măl″ă-sē′zē-ă). [Louis C. Malassez, Fr. physiologist, 1842–1910] A genus of fungi.

malassimilation (măl″ă-sĭm-ĭ-lā′shŭn) [L. *malus,* ill, + *assimilatio,* making like]. Defective, incomplete, or faulty assimilation, esp. of nutritive material. SEE: *malabsorption syndrome.*

malate (mā′lāt). A salt or ester of malic acid.

malathion (măl″ă-thī′ŏn). An effective pesticide.

malaxate (măl′ăk-sāt) [L. *malaxare,* to soften]. To knead, as in massaging a part.

malaxation (măl-ăks-ā′shŭn) [L. *malaxare,* to soften]. Kneading movement used in massage.

maldigestion (măl″dī-jĕs′chŭn). Disordered digestion.

male [O. Fr.]. 1. Masculine. 2. The sex that has organs for producing sperm for fertilization of ova.

RS: female; organ; penis; sperm; testicle; virile; virilescence; virilism; virility.

malemission (măl″ē-mĭsh′ŭn) [L. *malus,* evil, + *e,* out, + *mittere,* to send]. Failure of semen to be ejaculated from the urinary meatus during coitus.

maleruption (măl-ē-rŭp′shŭn). Incorrect eruption of teeth.

malformation (măl-for-mā′shŭn) [″ + *formatio,* a shaping]. Deformity; abnormal shape or structure, esp. congenital.

malfunction (măl-fŭnk′shŭn). Defective function.

malic (mā′lĭk, măl′ĭk) [L. *malum,* apple]. Pert. to apples.

malic acid. An acid found in some fruits, such as apples. SEE: *acid, malic.*

malign (mă-līn′) [ME. *maligne*]. Tending to injure or harm; malignant.

malignancy (mă-lĭg′năn-sē) [L. *malignus,* of bad kind]. 1. State of being malignant. 2. A neoplasm or tumor that is cancerous as opposed to benign. SYN: *virulence.*

malignant (mă-lĭg′nănt). Growing worse; resisting treatment, said of cancerous growths. Tending or threatening to produce death; harmful. SYN: *virulent.*

malinger (mă-lĭng′ĕr) [Fr. *malingre,* weak, sickly]. To feign illness, usually to arouse sympathy, to escape work, or to continue to receive compensation. SEE: *factitious disorder; Münchhausen syndrome.*

malingerer (mă-lĭng′gĕr-ĕr). 1. One who pretends to be ill or to be suffering from a nonexistent disorder to arouse sympathy. 2. One who pretends slow recuperation from a disease once suffered in order to continue to receive benefits of medical insurance.

malinterdigitation (măl″ĭn-tĕr-dĭj″ĭ-tā′shŭn). Abnormal intercuspal relation of the upper and lower teeth.

malleable (măl′ē-ă-b′l) [L. *mallere,* to hammer]. Having the property of being shaped by pressure.

malleation (măl-lē-ā′shŭn) [L. *mallere,* to hammer]. Spasmodic action of the hands in which they seem drawn to strike any near object, as spasmodic rapping against thighs or furniture. SEE: *tic.*

malleoincudal (măl″ē-ō-ĭng′kū-dăl) [L. *malleus,* hammer, + *incus,* anvil]. Concerning or pert. to the malleus and incus.

malleolar (măl-ē′ō-lăr) [L. *malleolus,* little hammer]. Concerning the malleolus.

malleolus (măl-ē′ŏ-lŭs) [L.]. (pl. *malleoli*) The protuberance on both sides of the ankle joint, the lower extremity of the fibula being known as the lateral malleolus and lower end of the tibia as the medial malleolus.

m., external. Process on outer edge of fibula at lower end.

m., internal. Round process on inner edge of tibia at lower end.

malleotomy (măl″ē-ŏt′ō-mē) [″ + Gr. *tome,* incision]. 1. Division of the malleus of the inner ear. 2. Severing the ligaments attached to the malleoli of the ankle.

mallet finger. Flexion deformity of the distal joint of a finger. It is caused by avulsion of the extensor tendon. SYN: *hammer finger.*

mallet toe. Abnormal flexion or loss of power of extension of a toe. SYN: *hammertoe.*

malleus (măl′ē-ŭs) [L., hammer]. (pl. *mallei*) 1. [NA] The largest of the three auditory ossicles in the middle ear, attached to the eardrum, and articulating with the incus. SEE: *ear.* 2. Glanders, an acute febrile disease with suppuration and necrosis of cartilage and bone.

Mallophaga (măl-ŏf′ă-gă) [Gr. *mallos,* wool, + *phagein,* to eat]. An order of insects that includes biting lice.

Mallory-Weiss syndrome. [G. Kenneth Mallory, U.S. pathologist, b. 1900; Soma Weiss, U.S. internist, 1898–1942] Hemorrhage from the upper gastrointestinal tract due to a tear in the mucosa of the esophagus or gastroesophageal junction. The syndrome is associated with chronic alcoholism and is usually preceded by severe vomiting.

malnutrition (măl″nū-trĭ′shŭn). Lack of necessary or proper food substances in the body or improper absorption and distribution of them. Any disorder of nutrition; may be due to a deficient diet or deficient breakdown, assimilation, or utilization of food. SEE: table.

malocclusion. Malposition and imperfect contact of the mandibular and maxillary teeth.

m., classification of. The designation by angle of the types of malocclusion based on the relative positions of the first molar in the two arches when in occlusion: *Class I*—normal anteroposterior relationship but with crowding and rotated teeth. *Class II*—the lower arch is distal to the upper arch on one or both sides; the lower first molar is distal to the upper first molar. *Class III*—the lower

Physical Signs of Malnutrition and Deficiency State*

Infants and Children	Adolescents and Adults
Lack of subcutaneous fat	Red swollen lingual papillae
Wrinkling of skin on light stroking	Glossitis
Poor muscle tone	Papillary atrophy of tongue
Pallor	Stomatitis
Rough skin (toad skin)	Spongy, bleeding gums
Hemorrhage of newborn, vitamin K deficiency	Muscle tenderness in extremities
Bad posture	Poor muscle tone
Nasal area is red and greasy	Loss of vibratory sensation
Sores—at angles of mouth, cheilosis	Increase or decrease of tendon reflexes
Rapid heartbeat	Hyperesthesia of skin
Red tongue	Bilateral symmetrical dermatitis
Square head, wrists enlarged, rib beading	Purpura
Vincent's angina, thrush	Dermatitis: facial butterfly, perineal, scrotal, vulval
Serious dental abnormalities	Thickening and pigmentation of skin over bony prominences
Corneal and conjunctival changes	Nonspecific vaginitis
	Follicular hyperkeratosis of extensor surfaces of extremities
Adolescents and Adults	Rachitic chest deformity
Nasolabial sebaceous plugs	Anemia not responding to iron
Sores at corners of mouth, cheilosis	Fatigue of visual accommodation
Vincent's angina	Vascularization of cornea
Minimal changes in tongue color or texture	Conjunctival changes

* Committee on Medical Nutrition, National Research Council.

arch is anterior to the upper arch on one or both sides; the lower first molar is anterior to the upper first molar.

malonylurea (măl″ō-nĭl-ū′rē-ă). Barbituric acid. SEE: *acid, barbituric.*

malpighian body (măl-pĭg′ē-ăn). [Marcello Malpighi, It. anatomist, founder of histology, 1628–1694] 1. A malpighian capsule, q.v. 2. A splenic nodule; a spherical, ovoid body found in the white pulp of the spleen. Similar in structure to a lymphatic nodule.

malpighian capsule. A spherical body found in cortex of kidney consisting of a glomerulus and Bowman's capsule.

malpighian layer. The innermost layer of the epidermis. SYN: *stratum germinativum.*

malpighian pyramid. A renal pyramid.

malposition (măl-pō-zĭ′shŭn) [L. *malus,* evil, + *positio,* placement]. Faulty or abnormal position or placement, esp. of the body or one of its parts.

malpractice [″ + Gr. *praxis,* an action]. Incorrect or negligent treatment of a patient by persons responsible for health care, such as physicians and nurses. SEE: *iatrogeny.*

malpresentation [″ + *praesentatio,* a presenting]. Abnormal position of fetus rendering natural delivery difficult or impossible.

malrotation (măl″rō-tā′shŭn). During embryogenesis, failure of normal rotation of the viscera or a portion of them.

malt [AS. *mealt*]. Germinated grain, usually

barley, used in manufacture of ale and beer. Contains carbohydrates (dextrin, maltose), a diastase, and proteins. Used as a food, esp. in wasting diseases.

Malta fever. Brucellosis, q.v.

maltase (mawl'tās) [AS. *mealt,* grain]. A salivary and pancreatic enzyme that acts on maltose, converting it by hydrolysis to glucose. SEE: *digestion; enzyme.*

malt extract. A viscous, light brown fluid obtained from malt steeped in water.

maltose (mawl'tōs). $C_{12}H_{22}O_{11}$. A disaccharide present in malt, malt products, and sprouting seeds. It is formed by the hydrolysis of starch and is converted into glucose by the enzyme maltase. SYN: *malt sugar.* SEE: *carbohydrates; disaccharose.*

maltosuria (mawl"tō-sūr'ē-ă) [" + Gr. *ouron,* urine]. Presence of maltose in urine.

malt sugar. Maltose.

malturned. Abnormally turned, said of a tooth turned on its long axis.

malum (mă'lŭm) [L., an evil]. A disease.

m. articulorum senilis. Arthritis in the aged.

m. coxae senilis. Hip disease in the aged, esp. osteoarthritis.

m. perforans pedis. Perforating ulcer of the foot. Begins with thickening epidermis.

m. venereum. Syphilis.

malunion [L. *malus,* evil, + *unio,* oneness]. Growth of the fragments of a fractured bone in a faulty position, forming an imperfect union.

mamanpian (mă-măn"pē-ăn') [Fr. *maman,* mother, + *pian,* yaw]. A mother yaw.

mamelon (măm'ĕ-lŏn) [Fr., nipple]. One of the three cusps present on the cutting edge of an incisor tooth when it erupts. These are worn away by use.

mamill-. SEE: words beginning with *mammill-.*

mamma (măm'ă) [L., breast]. (pl. *mammae*) [NA] Cutaneous glandular structure in the female that secretes milk. In the human female, there are two, situated over the anterolateral area between the 3rd and 6th ribs. SYN: *breast; mammary gland.*

mammal (măm'ăl). An animal of the class Mammalia. Characterized by having breasts from which milk is available for the nourishment of the newborn.

mammalgia (măm-ăl'jē-ă) [L. *mamma,* breast, + Gr. *algos,* pain]. Pain in the breast. SYN: *mastalgia; mastodynia.*

mammaplasty (măm'ă-plăs"tē) [" + Gr. *plassein,* to form]. Plastic surgery of the breast.

mammary (măm'ă-rē) [L. *mamma,* breast]. Pert. to the breast.

mammary glands. Two compound glands of the female breast that secrete milk. They are made up of lobes and lobules bound together by areolar tissue. The main ducts are 15 to 20 in number and are known as lactiferous ducts, each one discharging through a separate orifice upon the surface of the nipple. The dilatations of the ducts form reservoirs for the milk during lactation, q.v, The pink, or dark-colored, skin around the nipple is called the areola, q.v. SYN: *mammae.*

RS: breast; caked breast; galactagogue; gynecomastia; mammectomy; mastectomy; mastopathy; nipple.

mammectomy (măm-mĕk'tō-mē) [" + Gr. *ektome,* excision]. Removal of the breast. SYN: *mastectomy.*

mammilla (mă-mĭl'lă) [L., nipple]. 1. Nipple. 2. Any structure resembling a nipple.

mammillary (măm'ĭl-lăr-ē) [L. *mammilla,* nipple]. Shaped like or concerning a nipple.

mammillated (măm'mĭl-lā-tĕd). Having protuberances like a nipple.

mammillation (măm-ĭl-lā'shŭn). 1. Condition of having a granulated appearance or nipplelike projections. 2. A nipplelike protuberance.

mammilliform (măm-mĭl'ĭ-form) [" + *forma,* shape]. Shaped like a nipple.

mammilliplasty (măm-mĭl'ĭ-plăs"tē) [" + Gr. *plassein,* to form]. Plastic operation on a nipple. SYN: *theleplasty.*

mammillitis (măm"mĭl-ī'tĭs) [" + Gr. *itis,* inflammation]. Inflammation of a nipple. SYN: *acromastitis; thelitis.*

mammitis (măm-ī'tĭs) [L. *mamma,* breast, + Gr. *itis,* inflammation]. Inflamed condition of the breast. SYN: *mastitis.*

mammogen (măm'ō-jĕn) [" + Gr. *gennan,* to produce]. Prolactin, q.v.

mammogram (măm'ō-grăm) [" + Gr. *gramma,* writing]. X-ray of the breast.

mammography (măm-ŏg'ră-fē) [" + Gr. *graphein,* to write]. Roentgenographic study of the breast. Used in the diagnosis of cancer.

mammoplasty (măm'ō-plăs"tē) [" + Gr. *plassein,* to form]. Surgical reconstruction of the breasts; sometimes augmented by substances such as fat tissue or silicone to alter the size and shape.

m., augmentation. Plastic surgery of the breast involving increasing the size of the breast.

m., reduction. Plastic surgery of the breast involving decreasing the amount of breast tissue.

mammose (măm'ōs) [L. *mammosus*]. 1. Having unusually large breasts. 2. Shaped like a breast.

mammotomy (măm-ŏt'ō-mē) [L. *mamma,* breast, + Gr. *tome,* incision]. Surgery of a breast. SYN: *mastotomy.*

mammotrophic (măm"ō-trŏf'ĭk) [" + Gr. *trophe,* nourishment]. To have the effect of stimulating size or function of the breast.

man [AS. *mann*]. 1. Member of the human species; Homo sapiens. 2. Male member of the species as distinguished from female. 3. The human race, collectively; mankind. SEE: words beginning with *anthro-*.

manchette (măn-chĕt′) [Fr., a cuff]. A circular band consisting of microtubules around the caudal pole of the developing sperm.

manchineel (măn″kĭ-nēl′) [Sp. *manzanilla*, small apple]. A tropical tree native to America, Hippomane mancinella, that contains a milky, poisonous sap. Contact with the sap causes blistering of the skin. The fruit is poisonous also.

mancinism (măn′sĭn-ĭzm) [L. *mancus*, crippled]. State of being left-handed.

Mandelamine. Trade name for methenamine mandelate, USP.

mandelic acid. $C_8H_8O_3$. A colorless hydroxy acid, q.v. Its salt is used in urinary tract infections.

mandible (măn′dĭ-bl) [L. *mandibula*, lower jawbone]. The horseshoe-shaped bone forming the lower jaw. SEE: illus. SYN: *mandibula* [NA].

mandibula (măn-dĭb′ū-lă) [L.]. (pl. *mandibulae*) [NA] The bone of the lower jaw, having a horseshoe shape.

mandibular (măn-dĭb′ū-lăr). Rel. to the lower jaw.

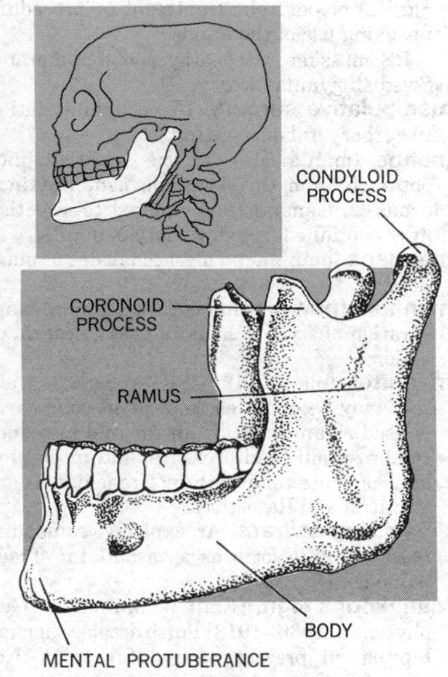

MANDIBLE—LEFT LATERAL VIEW

mandibular reflex. Clonic movement resulting from percussing or stroking lower jaw.

mandibulopharyngeal (măn-dĭb″ū-lō-fă-rĭn′jē-ăl) [″ + Gr. *pharynx*, pharynx]. Concerning the mandible and pharynx.

mandrel, mandril (măn′drĕl). The handle that holds a dental tool so that the tool may be rotated. A variety of tools for grinding, polishing, and buffing may be attached to the handle.

mandrin (măn′drĭn) [Fr.]. A guide or stylet for a flexible catheter.

maneuver [Fr. *manoeuvre*, from L. *manu operari*, to work by hand]. 1. Any dextrous or skillful procedure. 2. In obstetrics, manipulation of the fetus to aid in delivery. SEE: *labor*.

m., Crede's. Method of expressing the placenta in which the hand is placed on the fundus of the uterus with the thumb on the anterior wall and the fingers on the posterior wall, the placenta being pushed out by pressure in the direction of the birth canal.

m., Heimlich. Technique for removing a foreign body from the trachea or pharynx, where it is preventing flow of air to the lungs. The obstruction is usually a bolus of food. The maneuver consists of (1) wrapping your arms around the victim's waist from behind, and allowing victim's upper torso to hang forward; (2) making a fist with one hand and placing it against the victim's abdomen between navel and rib cage; (3) clasping your fist with your free hand and pressing in with a quick, forceful upward thrust. Repeat several times if necessary. The sudden expulsion of air should dislodge the obstruction.

If the victim is sitting, stand behind victim and perform the maneuver the same way. If victim is unconscious, place in a supine position, kneel astride the torso, place both hands on the abdomen as described above, and push forcefully with an upward thrust. SEE: *Heimlich maneuver* for illus.

m., Leopold's. Method of abdominal palpation for the diagnosis of presentation and position of the fetus in utero.

m., Mauriceau-Smellie-Veit. Method employed to deliver the aftercoming head in breech presentation. Straddling the baby over the right arm, one introduces the index finger of that hand into the mouth of the child and applies it over the maxilla; two fingers of the other hand are then hooked over the neck, grasping the shoulders. Downward traction is made until the occiput appears under the symphysis pubis. The body of the child is now raised up toward the mother's abdomen and the mouth nose, brow, and occiput are successively brought over the perineum.

m., Muller's. Inspiratory effort with a

closed glottis at the end of expiration. This produces negative intrathoracic pressure and may cause engorgement of blood vessels and thus allow those structures to be better visualized during x-ray studies. Esp. useful in demonstrating esophageal varices.

m., Munro Kerr. A method for determining the presence of disproportion between the fetal head and the maternal pelvis. The fetal head is pushed into the pelvis with the right hand on the abdomen while, with two fingers of the left hand in the vagina, one notes the possibilities of engagement of the head. At the same time the thumb of the left hand feels over the brim of the pelvis to determine the degrees of overlapping.

m., Pinard's. A method used in breech presentation. Fingers are placed behind the fetal knee, pushing it toward and past the fetal body, causing flexion of the knee. The foot is then grasped and brought down.

m., Prague. A method for the delivery of the aftercoming head in a breech delivery when the occiput is posterior.

m., Scanzoni. Double application of forceps in posterior position of the occiput.

m., Valsalva's. Forcible expiration against the closed glottis with both mouth and nose closed. This produces increased intrathoracic pressure and also increases the pressure in the eustachian tube. If the tubes are patent, air will be forced into the middle ear. A useful maneuver in "clearing" ears that have become blocked during a descent from altitude.

manganese (măn′gă-nēz) [L. *manganesium*]. SYMB: Mn. At. wt. 54.938; at. no. 25; sp. gr. 7.21. A metal element found in many foods, in some plants, and in the tissues of the higher animals. An essential element needed for normal bone metabolism and many enzyme reactions. Deficiency in humans has not been demonstrated.

SOURCES: Bananas, bran, beans, beets, blueberries, chard, chocolate, peas, leafy vegetables, and whole grains.

manganese poisoning. A rather uncommon cause of toxicity in workers exposed to manganese on a regular basis.

SYM: Muscular weakness, peculiar gait, tremors, central nervous system disturbances, salivation.

mange (mānj). A cutaneous communicable disease of domestic animals, including dogs and cats. A number of mites, such as Chorioptes, Demodex, Psoroptes, and Sarcoptes are causative agents. In man, this condition is known as scabies, q.v.

mania (mā′nē-ă) [Gr., madness]. 1. Mental disorder characterized by excessive excitement. 2. A form of psychosis characterized by exalted feelings, delusions of grandeur, elevation of mood, psychomotor overactivity, and overproduction of ideas. SEE: *psychosis, manic-depressive*. 3. Used as combining form to signify obsessive preoccupation.

m., puerperal. A form of mental derangement that occurs occasionally following childbirth.

m., religious. Mania resulting from excessive religious fervor.

m., transitory. Attacks of severe frenzy, of short duration.

m., unproductive. Behavior characteristic of mania with lack of spontaneity in speech or muteness, sometimes seen in manic-depressive psychosis. SEE: *alcoholism*.

maniac (mā′nē-ăk). Person afflicted by mania.

maniacal (mă-nī′ă-kl). 1. Rel. to or characterized by mania. 2. Afflicted with mania.

manic (măn′ĭk). Maniacal, q.v.

manic-depressive psychosis. Cyclic affective psychosis in which there are alternating moods of depression and mania. SEE: *psychosis, manic-depressive*.

manifest squint. Tropia, q.v.

manikin [D. *manneken*, little man]. A model of the human body or its parts, used esp. in teaching anatomy and nursing procedures.

maniphalanx (măn″ĭ-fā′lănks) [L. *manus*, hand, + Gr. *phalanx*, closely knit row]. A phalanx, or finger, of the hand. SEE: *pediphalanx*.

manipulation [L. *manipulare*, to handle]. Skillful or dextrous treatment or procedure involving use of the hands.

RS: massage; osteopathy; spondylotherapy; Swedish gymnastics.

manipulative surgery. Use of manipulation in surgery or bone-setting.

manna (măn′ă) [L.]. 1. The sweetish juice obtained from the flowering ash, Fraxinus ornus. 2. General term applied to sweetish juices obtained from a variety of plants.

mannans (măn′ănz). Polysaccharides of mannose.

mannerism. A peculiar modification or exaggeration of style or habit of dress, speech, or action.

mannitol (măn′ĭ-tŏl). USP. A carbohydrate that may be obtained from plant sources. It is used as an osmotic diuretic and to reduce cerebrospinal fluid pressure, and in prophylaxis of acute renal failure. Trade names are Osmitrol and Resectisol.

m. hexanitrate. An explosive compound used in dilute form as a vasodilator. Trade name is SDM No. 5.

Mannkopf's sign. [Emil W. Mannkopf, Ger. physician, 1836–1918] Pulse acceleration exhibited on pressing a painful point. Not present in feigned pain.

mannose (măn′ōs). A polysaccharide present in certain plants. It is an aldohexose.

mannoside (măn′ō-sīd). A glycoside of mannose.

mannosidosis (măn″ōs-ĭ-dō′sĭs). An inborn error of metabolism in which the deficiency of α-mannosidase is associated with mental deficiency, kyphosis, enlarged tongue, abnormal lymphocytes, and accumulation of mannose in tissues.

manometer (măn-ŏm′ĕt-ĕr) [Gr. *manos,* thin, + *metron,* measure]. Device for determining liquid or gaseous pressure such as blood, spinal fluid, or atmospheric. The measurement is expressed in millimeters of either mercury or water; or in torr.

m., saline. Manometer that utilizes a special hollow tube shaped like a U and with both ends open. This tube, called a U tube, is partially filled with saline. The pressure is determined by connecting one end of the U tube to the system in which pressure is to be measured. The pressure, in millimeters of saline, is the measured distance between the fluid level in one side of the U tube and that in the other side.

Mansonella (măn″sō-nĕl′ă). A genus of filarial nematodes.

M. ozzardi. A filaria that occurs in Central and South America and the Caribbean. They are unsheathed, and usually harmless, but they may cause hydrocele or lymphadenopathy.

mansonelliasis (măn″sō-nĕl-ī′ă-sĭs) [*Mansonella* + Gr. *-iasis,* condition]. Infection in man with Mansonella ozzardi.

Mansonia (măn-sō′nē-ă). A genus of mosquitoes in tropical countries; transmits microfilaria to man.

mantle [AS. *mentel,* a garment]. A covering structure or layer.

Mantoux reaction (măn-tū′). [Charles Mantoux, Fr. physician, 1877–1947] Intracutaneous injection of Old Tuberculin. Within 24 to 72 hours the area becomes hard (indurated) and red if either an active or inactive tuberculous infection is present.

manual (măn′ū-ăl) [L. *manus,* hand]. 1. Pert. to the hands. 2. Performed by or with the hands.

manubrium (mă-nū′brē-ŭm) [L., handle]. (pl. *manubria*) Any handle-shaped structure.

m. sterni. [NA] The upper segment of the sternum articulating with the clavicle and first pair of costal cartilages.

manudynamometer (măn″ū-dī″nă-mŏm′ĕ-tĕr) [L. *manus,* hand, + Gr. *dynamis,* force, + *metron,* measure]. A device for measuring the force of a thrust.

manus (mā′nŭs) [L.]. (pl. *manus*) [NA] The hand.

MAO. *monoamine oxidase.*

map. A graphic presentation in two dimensions of the location of items.

m., genetic. Map of chromosomes indicating the location of genes on a chromosome.

m., linkage. Map of chromosomes indicating the relationship of genes to each other on the chromosome.

maple bark disease. A pneumonitis caused by inhalation of spores from the mold, Cryptostroma corticale, present in the bark of maple trees.

maple syrup urine disease. An inherited metabolic disease involving defective amino acid metabolism so named because of the characteristic odor of the urine and sweat. The amino acids involved are leucine, isoleucine, valine, and alloisoleucine. Clinically, in the first few months of life, there is rapid deterioration of the nervous system and then death at an early age.

TREATMENT: Controlling the intake of these amino acids; exchange transfusion; and peritoneal dialysis.

mapping. Location of the genes on a chromosome.

marantic (mă-răn′tĭk) [Gr. *marantikos,* wasting away]. 1. Pert. to marasmus. 2. Wasting away. SYN: *marasmic.*

marantology (mă″răn-tŏl′ō-jē) [Gr. *marasmos,* a dying away, + *logos,* study]. Study, care, and treatment of debilitated, elderly, and chronically ill patients whose outlook for recovery is poor.

marasmic (mă-răz′mĭk) [Gr. *marasmos,* a dying away]. Affected with marasmus; wasting away. SYN: *marantic.*

marasmoid (mă-răz′moyd) [″ + *eidos,* form]. Similar to marasmus.

marasmus (măr-ăz′mŭs) Emaciation and wasting due to malnutrition in an infant. Caused by caloric deficiency secondary to acute diseases, esp. diarrheal diseases of infancy. May also be due to deficiency in nutritional composition, inadequate food intake, malabsorption, child abuse, failure to thrive syndrome, deficiency of vitamin D, or scurvy. Most common in children over two years.

SYM: Extreme wasting is seen. Failure to gain weight is followed by a loss of weight. Brain and skeletal growth continue, resulting in a long body and a large head in proportion to weight. Subcutaneous fat is minimal, the eyes are sunken, and tissue turgor is lost. The skin appears loose and sags. The infant is not active, muscles are flabby and relaxed, and the cry is weak and shrill.

PROG: Death will occur in 40% of the children.

TREATMENT: Initial feedings should be small and low in calories because digestive capacity is poor. Diluted formula or breast milk is best. The amount of calories and protein, carbohydrates, and fat should be gradually increased. The goal for protein intake is 5 gm./kg. body weight per day. If diarrhea due to disaccharidase deficiency is present, a low-lactose diet will be of benefit. Parenteral fluid therapy is indicated if shock or fluid and electrolyte imbalance exists.

marble bones. Abnormally calcified bones with spotted appearance in a roentgenogram. SEE: *Albers-Schönberg disease; osteopetrosis.*

Marburg virus disease. [Marburg, Germany] Febrile illness characterized by acute onset of prostration, headache, myalgia, nausea, and vomiting, followed two days later by diarrhea, drowsiness, and mental disturbances. Most patients develop an erythematous rash on the fifth to seventh day of the illness. About a fourth of the patients will die between the eighth and sixteenth day of the illness.

ETIOL: Ebola-Marburg virus, which is contracted by laboratory workers handling tissues and cell cultures from African green monkeys.

TREATMENT: No specific therapy but convalescent serum may be helpful.

marc (mărk) [Fr.]. The remaining substance after a drug has been percolated.

Marchiafava-Micheli syndrome (măr"kē-ă-fă'vă-mē-kā'lē). [Ettore Marchiafava, It. pathologist, 1847–1935; F. Micheli, It. clinician] A rare hemolytic anemia associated with paroxysmal nocturnal hemoglobinuria.

marcid (măr'sĭd) [L. *marcere,* to waste away]. 1. Wasted or emaciated. 2. Exhausted.

Marezine Hydrochloride. Trade name for cyclizine hydrochloride, USP.

Marfan's syndrome. [Bernard-Jean Antonin Marfan, Fr. physician, 1858–1942] A hereditary condition of connective tissue, bones, muscles, ligaments, and skeletal structures.

SYM: Irregular and unsteady gait, a tall lean body type with long extremities including fingers and toes. There is abnormal joint flexibility, flat feet, stooped shoulders and dislocation of the optic lens. The aorta will usually be dilated and may become sufficiently weakened to allow an aneurysm to develop. SEE: *arachnodactyly.*

margarine. Artificial butter substitute made from refined vegetable oils or a combination of vegetable oils and animal fats. Coloring material and vitamin A are added. Contains 7.2 Cal. per gram. SYN: *oleomargarine.*

margin [L. *marginalis,* border]. 1. A boundary, such as the edge of a structure of the anatomy. SYN: *margo.* 2. In dentistry, the apical extent or boundary of enamel adjacent to cementum of the tooth root; the junction of a restoration with the cavosurface angle of a prepared cavity in enamel.

marginal (măr'jĭn-ăl). Concerning a margin or border. SYN: *limbic.*

margination (măr"jĭ-nā'shŭn). Adhesion of leukocytes to walls of blood vessel in first stages of inflammation.

marginoplasty (mar-jĭn'ō-plăs"tē) [L. *marginalis,* border, + Gr. *plassein,* to mold]. Plastic surgery of a border, as of an eyelid.

margo (măr'gō) [L.]. (pl. *margines*) [NA] A border or edge.

m. acutus. A sharp margin of the heart extending from the apex to the right.

m. obtusus. Portion of a line extending from apex to root of the pulmonary artery that lies along the rounded left side of the left ventricle.

Marie's ataxia (mă-rēz'). [Pierre Marie, Fr. physician, 1853–1940] Hereditary cerebellar ataxia caused by bilateral cortical atrophy of the cerebellum.

Marie's disease. Chronic condition with enlargement of bones and soft tissues of hands, feet, and face. SYN: *acromegaly,* q.v.

Marie's sign. Hand tremor seen in exophthalmic goiter.

marijuana, marihuana (măr"ĭ-wă'nă). The dried flowering tops of the Cannabis sativa (hemp) plant.

There is controversy over the effects of marijuana. This substance has dose-related effects on mood, perception, and psychomotor coordination. Driving and other machine-operating skills may therefore be seriously affected. The users have impairment of short-term memory and its use slows learning. Depending on the dose of the drug and the underlying psychological conditions of the user, marijuana may cause transient episodes of confusion, anxiety, or even frank toxic delirium. Use may exacerbate pre-existing mental illness, esp. schizophrenia. Long-term, relatively heavy use may be associated with behavioral disorders, and a kind of ennui called the "amotivational syndrome," but it is not known whether use of the drug is a cause or a result of this condition. Transient symptoms occur on withdrawal, indicating that the drug can lead to physical dependence. Research has demonstrated a significant correlation between heavy marijuana use by pregnant women and impaired fetal growth and development.

Because marijuana smoke contains many of the components of tobacco smoke, it is felt that prolonged heavy smoking of marijuana would probably lead to impaired pulmonary function and could cause cancer of the lung.

Marijuana, its constituents or its derivatives, may be useful in the acute treatment of glaucoma, and in the control of the severe nausea and vomiting caused by cancer chemotherapy.

One of the most important constituents of marijuana is delta-9-tetrahydrocannabinol. SYN: *cannabis*. SEE: *hashish*.

mark [AS. *mearc*]. Any nevus, bruise, cut, or spot on the surface of a body.

m., birth-. Blemish on the skin at birth. SYN: *nevus*.

m., port-wine. A congenital hemangioma or nevus vascularis.

m., strawberry. Nevus vascularis.

marker. 1. A device or substance used to indicate or mark something. 2. An identifying characteristic or trait that allows apparently similar materials or disease conditions to be differentiated.

m., fecal. A substance, such as carmine, ingested to mark the beginning and end of fecal collection periods.

Marmo's method (măr'mōz). [Serafino Marmo, contemporary It. obstetrician] A manner of performing artificial respiration on asphyxiated infants. The physician places his or her hands in the infant's axillae and thereby raises the subject up in the air and suddenly releases the child. A sudden drop of a foot or two will cause inspiration to occur; expiration is effected by pressure of the physician's hands against the chest wall.

Marplan. Trade name for isocarboxazid.

marrow [AS. *mearh*]. The soft tissue occupying the medullary cavities of long bones, some haversian canals, and spaces between trabeculae of cancellous or spongy bone. Marrow is of two types: red and yellow. The yellow marrow is found esp. in medullary cavity of long bones, and the red in spongy bones.

m., gelatinous. Yellow marrow of old or emaciated persons, almost devoid of fat and having a gelatinous consistency.

m., red. Marrow found in cancellous tissue of bone. Concerned with the production of blood cells and hemoglobin, i.e., hematopoiesis.

m., spinal. The spinal cord.

m., yellow. Marrow found in the medullary canal of long bones. Consists principally of fat cells and connective tissue. It does not participate in hematopoiesis.

marrow aspiration. Procedure using a special aspirating needle to obtain a specimen of bone marrow for examination. The material is usually obtained from the upper portion of the sternum or the iliac crest. Examination of the stained marrow is helpful in diagnosing a great number of blood disorders, infections, and malignant diseases.

marrow transplantation. SEE: *bone marrow transplantation*.

marsh fever. Malaria.

marsh gas. Methane.

Marsh's test. [James Marsh, Brit. chemist, 1789–1846] A test to detect the presence of arsenic.

marsupialization (măr-sū"pē-ăl-ĭ-zā'shŭn) [L. *marsupium*, pouch]. Process of raising the borders of an evacuated tumor sac to the edges of the abdominal wound and stitching them there to form a pouch. The interior of the sac suppurates and gradually closes by granulation.

marsupium (măr-sū'pē-ŭm) [L., pouch]. 1. Scrotum. 2. A sac or pouch that serves to hold the young of a marsupial.

M.A.S. In radiology, the *milliamperage* times the *seconds*, or time of exposure.

maschaladenitis (măs"kăl-ăd"ĕ-nī'tĭs) [Gr. *maschale*, armpit, + *aden*, gland, + *itis*, inflammation]. Inflammation of axillary glands.

maschaliatry (măs-kăl-ī-ă'trē) [" + *iatreia*, healing]. Medication by axillary inunctions.

maschaloncus (măs"kăl-ŏng'kŭs) [" + *onkos*, tumor]. A new growth in the axilla.

masculation (măs-kū-lā'shŭn) [L. *masculus*, a male]. Development of male secondary sexual characteristics.

masculine (măs'kū-lĭn). 1. Pert. to the male sex. 2. Having male characteristics. SYN: *virile*.

masculinization. 1. The normal development of secondary male sex characteristics that occur at puberty. 2. The abnormal development of masculine characteristics in the female. This may be caused by certain testosterone-producing tumors or medication that contains testosterone or anabolic steroids. SYN: *virilization*.

masculinovoblastoma (măs"kū-lĭn-ō"vō-blăs-tō'mă). A benign ovarian tumor that resembles, microscopically, adrenal cortical tissue. Usually results in masculinization.

maser. Acronym for *m*icrowave *a*mplification by *s*timulation *e*mission of *r*adiation. A device that produces a small, nondiverging radiation beam.

mask [Fr. *masque*]. 1. A covering for the face, as the gauze mask of a surgeon or nurse. 2. The countenance or appearance of the face such as appears in certain pathological conditions. 3. To conceal or prevent detection.

m., BLB. A mask for administering oxygen to aviators or to patients during anesthesia. Invented by Boothby Lovelace, and Bulbulian, working at the Mayo Clinic.

m., death. A plaster cast of the face molded soon after death.

m., ecchymotic. Cyanotic facies accompanying traumatic asphyxia.

m., Hutchinson's. A feeling of compression over face as though one is wearing a mask.

m., luetic. Blotchy brown pigmentation

of cheeks, forehead, and temples, seen in tertiary syphilis.

m. of pregnancy. Pigmented areas seen on the face of some pregnant women. SYN: *chloasma gravidarum*.

m., Parkinson's. Immobile facial appearance as a result of paralysis agitans (Parkinson's disease). The face is devoid of expression.

masked. Concealed, esp. as in masked infection.

Ex.: women exposed to rubella during the first trimester of pregnancy may be given immune globulin. This may prevent clinical symptoms of rubella in the mother, yet the fetus may be adversely affected and may be born with congenital defects.

masochism (măs'ō-kĭzm). [Leopold von Sacher-Masoch, Austrian novelist, 1835–1895] A general orientation to life that suffering relieves guilt and leads to a reward. Opposite of sadism. SEE: *algolagnia; flagellation*.

m., sexual. Sexual excitement produced in an individual by his or her own suffering. The individual with this condition usually prefers to be bound, beaten, or made to suffer or be humiliated.

masochist (măs'ō-kĭst). A person addicted to masochism.

mass [L. *massa*]. 1. A quantity of material, such as cells that unite or adhere to each other. 2. Soft solid preparation for internal use and of such consistency that it may be molded into pills. It is frequently prescribed alone or with other agents and may be given in pill form or put into capsules. 3. The characteristic of matter that gives it inertia.

m., cell. An aggregation of cells that serves as the primordium (anlage) of a future organ or part.

m., epithelial. Inner portion of a developing gonad enclosed within the germinal epithelium.

m., inner cell. Mass of cells within the blastocyst, q.v., from which the embryo, yolk sac, and amnion develop.

m., intermediate cell. A plate of nonsegmented mesoderm lying lateral to the segments (somites) and connecting them to the nonsegmented lateral mesoderm. SYN: *nephrotome*.

massa [L.]. (pl. *massae*) [NA] Mass.

m. intermedia. The middle commissure of the brain, an inconstant mass of gray matter extending across the third ventricle and connecting adjacent surfaces of the thalami.

massage [Gr. *massein*, to knead]. Manipulation, methodical pressure, friction, and kneading of the body.

RS: anatripsis; effleurage; flagellation; friction; frolement; fustigation; kneading; malaxation; masseur; petrissage; Swedish gymnastics; tapotement; vibration.

m., auditory. Massage of the eardrum.

m., cardiac. Manual compression of the heart to restore heartbeat after heart has stopped. Accomplished either through an incision in the chest wall or over the sternum. This forces blood out of the heart and, when pressure is removed, allows the heart to fill as if the heart were beating.

m., electrovibratory. Massage by means of an electric vibrator.

m., general. Consists of centripetal stroking in connection with some muscular kneading from the toes upward. Principally used for nervousness, being an important part of the well-known rest cure. Useful in connection with certain baths, duration 30 to 40 minutes. As soon as a part is massaged, it should be given a few passive rotary movements and afterwards covered up.

m., introductory. Massage consisting of centripetal strokings around the affected part.

Ex.: an affection of the knee joint, where introductory massage should be used on lower part of thigh and somewhat below the knee. Very useful in cases where it is impossible for operator to apply treatment directly to diseased parts.

m., local. Massage confined to particular parts.

m., tremolo. A type of mechanical massage.

m., vapor. Treatment of a cavity by a medicated and nebulized vapor under interrupted pressure.

m., vibratory. Massage by rapidly repeated tapping of the affected surface by means of a vibrating hammer or sound.

masseter (măs-sē'tĕr) [Gr. *maseter*, chewer]. The muscle that closes the mouth and is the principal muscle in mastication.

masseur (mă-soor') [Fr.]. 1. A man who gives massages. 2. An instrument for massaging.

masseuse (mă-sooz') [Fr.]. A woman who gives massages.

massive (măs'sĭv) [Fr. *massif*]. Bulky; consisting of a large mass; huge.

massive collapse of the lung. Dyspnea, cyanosis, shock, and pain in chest, esp. in patients who have suffered severe shock and collapse after abdominal operation or thyroidectomy. Collapse is due to obstruction of a main bronchus by a mucous plug or foreign body or a tension pneumothorax. SEE: *lung*.

TREATMENT: If caused by mucus—CO_2 inhalation and breathing exercises, antibiotics, and oxygen. If due to foreign body—remove the foreign body.

mass number. Total number of neutrons and protons in the nucleus of an atom.

massotherapy (măs-ō-thĕr'ă-pē) [Gr. *mas-*

sein, to knead, + *therapeia,* treatment]. Use of massage in treatment of disease.

mastadenitis (măst-ăd-ĕ-nī′tĭs) [Gr. *mastos,* breast, + *aden,* gland, + *itis,* inflammation]. A mammary gland inflammation.

mastadenoma (măst″ă-dĕ-nō′mă) [″ + ″ + *oma,* tumor]. A tumor of the breast.

mastalgia (măst-ăl′jē-ă) [″ + *algos,* pain]. Pain in the breast. SYN: *mammalgia; mastodynia.*

mastatrophia, mastatrophy (măst-ă-trō′fē-ă, măst-ăt′rō-fē) [″ + *atrophia,* want of nourishment]. Atrophy of breasts.

mastauxe (măs-tawk′sē) [″ + *auxe,* increase]. Enlargement of the breast.

mast cells [Gr. *masten,* to feed]. Connective tissue cells that contain heparin and histamine in their granules. Important in cellular defense mechanisms including blood coagulation needed during injury or infection.

mastectomy (măs-tĕk′tō-mē) [Gr. *mastos,* breast, + *ektome,* excision]. Excision of the breast.

NURSING IMPLICATIONS: Preoperative care includes helping the patient express feelings, and preparation of the breast and the donor site if skin graft is to be done. Explain the postoperative course, the need for exercise, and the availability of various types of prostheses. Postoperative care includes frequent inspection of the operative site and donor site (if graft was done), elevating the arm, frequent checking of arm and hand for signs of impaired circulation, providing food and fluids, ambulating early, exercising the arm, and supporting the expression of such reactions as crying, withdrawal, and anger.

Master two-step test. [A. M. Master, U.S. physician, 1895–1973] A standardized exercise test used to assess cardiac function. The patient participates in a standardized exercise of repeatedly walking up and down on a step. The electrocardiogram is monitored during the study and the exercise is stopped if abnormal changes appear. SEE: *exercise tolerance test.*

masthelcosis (măs″thĕl-kō′sĭs) [Gr. *mastos,* breast, + *helkosis,* ulceration]. Ulcerated condition of the breast.

mastic (măs′tĭk). A resin obtained from the tree, Pistacia lentincus. It has been used in industry and in coating tablets.

mastication (măs-tĭ-kā′shŭn) [L. *masticare,* to chew]. Chewing. The comminution and insalivation of the food in the mouth is the first stage of digestion. Certain muscles close the mouth, raise and lower the mandible, tense the cheeks, and accomplish the highly coordinated movements of the tongue. The smell and taste of food stimulate sensory nerves, which reflexly elicit both motor and secretory activity in various digestive organs. Thus the salivary glands begin to secrete at once, and both the glands and the musculature of the stomach gradually become active. The saliva dissolves some substances, dilutes materials too concentrated for the stomach, hydrolyzes (due to the salivary enzyme ptyalin) some of the starch to maltose, and lubricates material to be swallowed.

RS: absorption; amasesis; enzyme; digestion.

masticatory (măs′tĭk-ă-tō″rē) [L. *masticare,* to chew]. 1. Pert. to mastication. 2. Any substance chewed to stimulate secretion of saliva.

Mastigophora (măs″tĭ-gŏf′ō-ră). A subphylum of protozoa characterized by the possession of one or more flagella. Includes both free-living and parasitic forms.

mastigote (măs′tĭ-gōt). A member of the protozoon class Mastigophora.

mastitis (măs-tī′tĭs) [Gr. *mastos,* breast, + *itis,* inflammation]. Inflammation of the breast. Most common in women during lactation but it may occur at any age.

ETIOL: May be due to entry of disease-producing germs through the nipple. In most cases there is a crack or abrasion of the nipple. Infection begins in one lobule but may extend to other areas.

SYM: The earliest sign is a triangular flush generally underneath the breast. There may be a high temperature and pulse rate.

m., cystic. Mastitis resulting in formation of cysts that give the breast a nodular feeling upon palpation.

m., interstitial. Inflammation of connective tissue of the breast.

m., parenchymatous. Inflammation of the secreting tissue of the breast.

m., puerperal. Mastitis in later portion of puerperium and often accompanied by suppuration. Breast may become indurated owing to retention of milk.

m., stagnation. Painful distention of breast occurring during early lactation. SYN: *caked breast.*

mastocarcinoma (măst″ō-kăr-sĭn-ō′mă) [″ + *karkinos,* crab, + *oma,* tumor]. Carcinoma of the breast.

mastochondroma (măst′ō-kŏn-drō′mă) [″ + *chondros,* cartilage, + *oma,* tumor]. Cartilaginous breast tumor.

mastocyte (măs′tō-sīt) [Gr. *masten,* to feed, + *kytos,* cell]. Mast cell.

mastocytoma (măs″tō-sī-tō′mă) [″ + ″ + *oma,* tumor]. An accumulation of mast cells that resembles a neoplasm.

mastocytosis (măs″tō-sī-tō′sĭs) [″ + ″ + *osis,* condition]. Neoplastic mast cells that manifest as urticaria pigmentosa. In some cases bone and spleen are involved.

mastodynia (măst-ō-dĭn'ē-ă) [Gr. *mastos,* breast, + *odyne,* pain]. Pain in the breast. SYN: *mammalgia; mastalgia.*

mastography [" + *graphein,* to write]. Roentgenography of the breasts.

mastoid (măs'toyd) [" + *eidos,* form]. 1. Formed like a breast. 2. Pert. to mastoid process of the temporal bone. 3. The mastoid process of temporal bone.

mastoidal (măs-toy'dăl). Rel. to mastoid process.

mastoidale (măs-toy-dā'lē). The lowest point of the mastoid process.

mastoidalgia (măs-toyd-ăl'jē-ă) [Gr. *mastos,* breast, + *eidos,* form, + *algos,* pain]. Pain in the mastoid.

mastoid antrum. Small chamber through which the mastoid cells communicate with the tympanic cavity.

mastoid cells. Air spaces in the mastoid process of the temporal bone.

mastoidectomy [" + " + *ektome,* excision]. Excision of mastoid cells. Rarely indicated since advent of antibiotics. May be simple, involving exenteration of the air cells of the mastoid process alone, or radical involving the middle ear.

NURSING IMPLICATIONS: Inspect dressing at frequent intervals, reinforcing as necessary. Utilize aseptic technique during dressing changes. Observe for bright red drainage, neck stiffness, vomiting, dizziness, disorientation, headache, and facial paralysis. If any of above symptoms occur, notify physician immediately.

mastoideocentesis (măs-toyd"ē-ō-sĕn-tē'sĭs) [Gr. *mastos,* breast, + *eidos,* form, + *kentesis,* puncture]. Surgical puncture of the mastoid process and subsequent paracentesis of mastoid cells.

mastoiditis (măs-toyd-ī'tĭs) [" + " + *itis,* inflammation]. Inflammation of the air cells of the mastoid process.

COMPLICATIONS: Perisinus abscess, periphlebitis, lateral sinus thrombosis. Involvement is metastatic through blood vessels without erosion of sinus plate or extension of suppuration directly through sinus plate into the sinus.

SYM: Fever, chills, tenderness over emissary vein, leukocytosis, sepsis.

TREATMENT: Surgical. Myringotomy and antibiotics, mastoidectomy.

m., Bezold's. Abscess underneath insertion of sternocleidomastoid muscle due to pus breaking through the tip cell.

m. externa. Inflammation of the periosteum of the mastoid process.

m., sclerosing. Mastoiditis in which there is thickening and hardening of trabeculae between mastoid cells.

mastoidotomy (măs-toyd-ŏt'ō-mē) [" + " + *tome,* incision]. Incision into the mastoid process.

mastoid portion of temporal bone. Portion of the temporal bone lying behind the external opening of the ear and below the temporal line. Contains mastoid cells and antrum, and its inner surface bears a deep, curved, sigmoid groove that contains a part of the transverse sinus. The opening of the mastoid foramen is visible in it.

mastoid process. Nipple-shaped process of mastoid portion of temporal bone extending downward and forward behind the external auditory meatus. Serves for attachment of sternocleidomastoid, splenius capitis, and longissimus capitis muscles.

mastology (măs-tŏl'ō-jē) [" + *logos,* study]. The branch of medicine concerned with study of the breast.

mastomenia (măs-tō-mē'nē-ă) [Gr. *mastos,* breast, + *menes,* menses]. Vicarious menstruation from the breast.

mastoncus (măst-ŏng'kŭs) [" + *onkos,* bulk]. Any tumor of the breast.

masto-occipital (măs"tō-ŏk-sĭp'ĭ-tăl). Rel. to the mastoid process and occipital bone.

mastoparietal (măs"tō-pă-rī'ĕ-tăl). Concerning the mastoid process and the parietal bone.

mastopathy (măs-tŏp'ă-thē) [Gr. *mastos,* breast, + *pathos,* disease]. Any disease of the mammary glands.

mastopexy (măs'tō-pĕks-ē) [" + *pexis,* fixation]. Correction of a pendulous breast by surgical fixation and plastic surgery. SYN: *mazopexy.*

mastoplasia (măst-ō-plā'zē-ă) [" + *plassein,* to form]. Hyperplasia of mammary gland tissue. SYN: *mazoplasia.*

mastoplasty (măs'tō-plăs"tē) [" + *plassein,* to form]. Plastic surgery of the breast.

mastoptosis (măs"tō-tō'sĭs) [" + *ptosis,* fall]. Pendulous breasts.

mastorrhagia (măs-tor-ā'jē-ă) [" + *rhegnynai,* to burst forth]. Hemorrhage from the breast.

mastoscirrhus (măs-tō-skĭr'ŭs) [" + *skirros,* hardness]. A hardening of the breast.

mastosquamous (măs-tō-skwā'mŭs). Relating to the mastoid process and the squamous portion of the temporal bone.

mastostomy (măs-tŏs'tō-mē) [" + *stoma,* opening]. Incision into the breast in order to drain a cyst or to obtain tissue for microscopic study.

mastotomy (măs-tŏt'ō-mē). Surgical incision of a breast. SYN: *mammotomy.*

masturbate (măs'tĕr-bāt) [L. *masturbari,* to pollute one's self]. 1. To induce sexual self-excitement through manipulation of the genital organs or other erogenous areas. 2. To perform masturbation on another.

masturbation (măs″tĕr-bā′shŭn). Stimulation of genitals or other erogenous areas, usually to orgasm, by some means other than sexual intercourse.

match [ME. *macche,* lamp wick]. A narrow strip of wood tipped with a compound that ignites by friction. Lucifer matches usually are made of phosphorus, q.v., and potassium chlorate. Safety matches contain antimony, sulfide, and potassium chlorate and must be lit by striking a rough surface.

matching. 1. Comparison in order to select objects with similar characteristics. 2. Being identical, equal, or exactly alike.

m., cross. Technique of determining the compatibility of the patient's blood with that of blood being considered for use in transfusion. SEE: *blood groups.*

m. of blood. Technique and procedure for determining the immunologic and genetic characteristics of the patient's blood so that appropriate blood may be used for transfusion. SEE: *blood groups.*

match poisoning. SYM: Gastrointestinal irritation with blood changes.

F.A.: Wash out stomach with water or very dilute potassium permanganate. Repeated catharsis.

maté (mă-tā′) [Sp., vessel for preparing leaves]. Tea made from the leaves of Ilex paraguayensis. Contains caffeine and tannin.

USES: Diaphoretic and diuretic when taken in large quantities.

materia alba (mă-tē′rē-ă ăl′bă) [L., white matter]. White cheeselike deposit along gum line about the necks of teeth, consisting of mucus, epithelial cells, food particles, leukocytes, and microorganisms.

material. The substance from which something may be made, constructed, or created.

m., base. The basic ingredient in a denture. It may be a polymer, shellac, or metal.

m., impression. Any material used to make an impression of teeth.

materia medica (mă-tē′rē-ă mĕd′ĭ-kă) [L., medical matter]. 1. That branch of science dealing with all drugs used in treatment of diseases, their source, preparation, dosage, and use. SYN: *pharmacology.* 2. A substance used to prepare a medicine.

materies morbi (mă-tē′rē-ēz mor′bē) [L., substance of disease]. Any substance that is the direct cause of death.

maternal [L. *maternus*]. 1. Rel. to the mother. 2. From a mother.

maternal deprivation syndrome. Emotional, physical, and nutritional neglect of an infant or young child. Children suffering from this are emotionally disturbed, withdrawn, apathetic, and retarded in growth and development. The lack of expected growth and development is due to a combination of nutritional and emotional neglect.

maternity (mă-tĕr′nĭ-tē). 1. The condition of motherhood. 2. The obstetrical department of a hospital.

mating [ME. *mate,* companion]. Pairing of male and female, esp. for reproduction.

m., assortative. Pairing of male and female that is not random.

m., random. Pairing of male to female when each individual has the same chance of mating with those of other genetic make-up.

matrilineal (mā″trĭ-lĭn′ē-ăl) [L. *mater,* mother, + *linea,* line]. Concerning descent through the female line.

matrix (mā′trĭks) [L.]. (pl. *matrices*) 1. The womb. 2. The basic substance from which a thing is made or develops. 3. The intercellular material of a tissue. 4. Mold for casting amalgams in dental restoration.

m. unguis. [NA] Nailbed.

matrixitis (mā-trĭks-ī′tĭs). Inflammation of the nailbed. SYN: *onychia.* SEE: *paronychia.*

matter. 1. Anything that occupies space. May be gaseous, liquid, or solid. 2. Pus.

m., gray. The gray substance of the spinal cord and brain, consisting principally of nerve-cell bodies, dendrites, and portions of axons. Also found in peripheral ganglia and retina of eye. SYN: *substantia grisea.*

m., white. The white substance of spinal cord and brain, consisting principally of nerve fibers (myelinated and unmyelinated). SYN: *substantia alba.*

Matulane. Trade name for procarbazine hydrochloride, USP.

maturate (măt′ū-rāt) [L. *maturus,* ripe]. 1. To ripen; to mature. 2. To suppurate.

maturation (măt″ū-rā′shŭn). 1. Maturing; ripening, as a graafian follicle. 2. Suppuration. 3. The process in the development of germ cells (spermatozoa and ova) occurring in spermatogenesis or oogenesis in which the number of chromosomes is reduced from the diploid number to the haploid number (one half of diploid). Includes two cell divisions. SEE: *oogenesis; spermatogenesis.* 4. The completion of the mineralization pattern or crystalline structure of calcified tissues.

m., enamel. The process of changing from approximately 30% inorganic mineral in enamel matrix to the 96% inorganic content in mature enamel; maturation is accomplished by the ameloblast cells over a long period of time, with a decrease in water and organic content, and an increase in mineral content and size or density of hydroxyapatite crystals.

mature (mă-tūr′). 1. Fully developed or ripened. 2. To become fully developed.

maturity. State of completed growth; fully developed; time when an individual becomes capable of reproducing.

matutinal (mă-tū'tĭ-năl) [L. *matutinalis,* morning]. Pert. to or occurring early in the day, as morning sickness.

matzoon (măt-zūn') [Armenian]. Milk with a ferment containing lactic acid, bacilli, and other organisms. Similar to yogurt.

Maurer's dots (mow'ĕrz) [Georg Maurer, Ger. physician in Sumatra] In malaria due to Plasmodium falciparum, coarse stippling of the red cells.

Maxidex. Trade name for dexamethasone, USP.

maxilla [L., jawbone]. (pl *maxillae*) [NA] The upper jawbone. SEE: *skeleton.*

maxillary (măk'sĭ-lĕr"ē). Pert. to the upper jaw.

maxillary sinus. The antrum of Highmore, air cavity in maxilla opening into middle meatus of nose.

maxillitis (măks"ĭl-ī'tĭs) [L. *maxilla,* jawbone, + Gr. *itis,* inflammation]. Inflammation of maxilla.

maxillodental (măk-sĭl"ō-dĕn'tăl) [" + *dens,* tooth]. Concerning the maxilla and the teeth it contains.

maxillofacial (măks-ĭl"ō-fā'shăl). Pert. to the maxilla and face.

maxillojugal (măk-sĭl"ō-jū'găl). Concerning the maxilla and the zygomatic bone.

maxillomandibular (măk-sĭl"ō-măn-dĭb'ū-lăr) [" + *mandibula,* lower jawbone]. Concerning the maxilla and the mandible.

maxillopalatine (măk-sĭl"ō-păl'ă-tĭn). Concerning the maxilla and the palatine bone.

maxillotomy (măk"sĭ-lŏt'ō-mē) [" + Gr. *tome,* incision]. Surgical incision of the maxilla.

maxima (măk'sĭ-mă) [L.]. Pl. of maximum.

maximal (măks'ĭ-măl) [L. *maximus,* greatest]. Greatest possible; highest. Opposite of minimal.

maximum (măks'ĭ-mŭm) [L.]. (pl. *maxima*) 1. The greatest quantity or effect. 2. Height of a disease.

maximum allowable concentration. ABBR: MAC. The upper limit of concentration of certain atmospheric contaminants allowed in the workplace. SEE: *threshold limit value.*

maximum breathing capacity. The greatest amount of air that can be breathed in a specified period of time, usually 30 seconds. It is expressed in liters of air/minute.

maximum permissible dose. ABBR: M.P.D. Maximum dose of radiation allowed a person occupationally exposed over a stated length of time.

Mayo-Robson's point. [Arthur Mayo-Robson, Brit. surgeon, 1853–1933] A point just above and to right of the umbilicus where pressure causes tenderness in pancreatic disease.

maze. A labyrinth of communicating paths.

mazindol. USP. An anorexic drug. Trade name is Sanorex.

mazopexy (mā'zō-pĕk"sē) [Gr. *mazos,* breast, + *pexis,* fixation]. Correction of a pendulous breast by surgical fixation and plastic surgery. SYN: *mastopexy.*

mazoplasia (mā"zō-plā'zē-ă) [" + *plassein,* to form]. Degenerative hyperplasia of mammary gland tissue. SYN: *mastoplasia.*

M.B. *Bachelor of Medicine.*

m.b. Prescription sign meaning L. *misce bene,* mix well.

MBC. *maximum breathing capacity.*

M.B.D. *minimal brain dysfunction.*

μc. *microcurie.*

M.C. 1. *Master of Surgery.* 2. *Medical Corps.*

Mc. *megacurie.*

mc. *millicurie.*

McArdle's disease. [B. McArdle, contemporary Brit. pediatrician] One of the glycogen storage diseases (type V) in which there is an abnormal accumulation of glycogen in muscle tissue due to deficiency of myophosphorylase B.

SYM: Pain, fatiguability, and muscle stiffness after prolonged exertion.

McBurney's incision. [Charles McBurney, U.S. surgeon, 1845–1914] Abdominal incision employed in appendectomy. An incision is made parallel to path of external oblique muscle, 1 to 2 in. (2.5–5.1 cm.) away from the anterosuperior spine of the right ilium, incision through the external oblique to the internal oblique and transversalis, separating their fibers.

McBurney's point. Point of tenderness in acute appendicitis, situated on a line between the umbilicus and the right anterosuperior iliac spine, about 1 or 2 in. (2.5–5.1 cm.) above the latter.

McBurney's sign. Tenderness and rigidity at McBurney's point, may be indicative of appendicitis.

McCarthy's reflex. [Daniel J. McCarthy, U.S. neurologist, 1874–1958] Contraction of orbicularis palpebrarum with closure of lids resulting from percussion above the supraorbital nerve.

McCormac's reflex. Adduction of one leg resulting from percussion of the patellar tendon of the opposite leg.

mcg. *microgram.*

MCH. *mean corpuscular hemoglobin.*

mc.h. *millicurie hour.*

MCHC. *mean corpuscular hemoglobin concentration,* average hemoglobin concentration in each red blood cell, expressed as a percentage value.

μCi. *microcurie.*

mCi. *millicurie.*

McMurray's sign. [Thomas P. McMurray, Brit. orthopedic surgeon, b. 1887] Manipulation of the tibia, with the leg flexed, produces a pronounced click if the meniscus has been injured.

M.C.P. *metacarpophalangeal joint.*

MCV. *mean corpuscular volume.* Expressed as the average volume of individual cells in cubic microns.

M.D. [L. *Medicinae,* Doctor]. *Doctor of Medicine.* Often shortened to Doctor, but this usage leads to confusion. Doctor may mean dentist, veterinarian, or other persons possessing a doctoral degree (e.g., Ph.D., Doctor of Philosophy). Thus, the word physician is preferred over doctor when doctor of medicine is intended.

Md. Chem. symb. for mendelevium.

meal (mēl) [AS. *mael,* measure, meal]. 1. Portion of food eaten at a particular time to satisfy the appetite. 2. The edible portion of any cereal grain that has been coarsely ground, as in corn meal.

mean [L. *medius,* middle]. The average or central tendency of a set of values. In statistics, a number derived from a series of other numbers by a prescribed method of computation. SEE: *median.* Thus the arithmetic mean is obtained by adding all the numbers or values and dividing the sum by the number of values.

Ex.: 100, 100, 98, 96, 97, 97, 85, 85, 85 = 843
843 divided by 9 = 93.6
93.6 is the mean.

mean corpuscular hemoglobin. ABBR: MCH. A measure of hemoglobin content of red corpuscles. The formula for determining this is

$$\text{MCH} = \frac{\text{hemoglobin in grams/1000 ml. of blood}}{\text{red cell count in millions/cubic micrometers}}$$

Ex.: if the hemoglobin is 13.6 gm. per 100 ml. and the red cell count is 3,600,000, then

$$\text{MCH} = \frac{13.6 \times 10}{3.6} = 37.8$$

This is the amount of hemoglobin in each red cell.

mean corpuscular hemoglobin concentration. ABBR: MCHC. A measure of concentration of hemoglobin in the average red cell. The formula used is

$$\frac{\text{hemoglobin, gm./100 ml.} \times 100}{\text{vol. of packed red cells, ml./100 ml.}}$$

Ex.: if the hemoglobin is 13.6 gm. and the volume of packed red cells (hematocrit) is 39.2 ml. per 100 ml., then

$$\text{MCHC} = \frac{13.6 \times 100}{39.2} = 35\%$$

mean corpuscular volume. ABBR: MCV. A measure of the volume of red corpuscles expressed in cubic micrometers. The formula for determining this is

$$\frac{\text{vol. of packed red cells/1000 ml. of blood}}{\text{red cell count in millions/cubic millimeter}}$$

Ex.: if the volume of packed red cells (hematocrit) is 39.2 per 100 ml. and the red cell count is 3,600,000, then

$$\text{MCV} = \frac{39.2 \times 10}{3.6} = 108.9 \text{ cubic millimeters}$$

measles (mē'zls) [Dutch *maselen*]. A highly communicable disease characterized by fever, general malaise, sneezing, nasal congestion, brassy cough, conjunctivitis, spots on the buccal mucosa (Koplik's spots), and a maculopapular eruption over the entire body caused by the rubeola virus. It is most common in school-age children with outbreaks occurring in the winter and spring. The occurrence of measles before the age of six months is relatively uncommon, because of passively acquired maternal antibodies from the immune mother.

An attack of measles almost invariably confers permanent immunity. Active immunization can be produced by administration of measles vaccine, preferably that containing the live attenuated virus, although measles vaccine containing the inactivated virus is available for individuals in whom the live attenuated type is contraindicated. Passive immunization is afforded by administration of gamma globulin. SYN: *rubeola.*

INCUBATION: From 10 to 21 days.

SYM: Onset gradual; coryza, rhinitis, drowsiness, loss of appetite, gradual elevation of temperature for first two days, when fever may rise to 101° to 103° F. (38.3° to 39.4° C.). Koplik's spots appear on the buccal mucosa opposite the molars on the second or third day. Photophobia and cough soon develop, although some recession in the temperature may occur. About the fourth day, fever usually reaches a higher elevation than previously, at times as high as 104° to 106° F. (40° to 41.1° C.). With this recurrence the rash appears.

Eruption first appears on face, being seen early as small maculopapular lesions that increase rapidly in size and coalesce in places, often causing a swollen, mottled appearance. The rash extends to the body and extremities and in some areas may resemble the rash of scarlet fever.

A cough, present at this time, is due to bronchitis produced by the inflammatory condition of the mucous membranes which undoubtedly corresponds to the rash seen on the skin. Ordinarily, the rash lasts from 4 to 5 days and as it subsides the temperature declines. Consequently, by the end of 5 days from appearance of rash, temperature should be normal, or approx. normal in uncomplicated cases. Early in the disease leukopenia, esp. of polymorphonuclear cells, may be present.

COMPLICATIONS: Encephalitis is a grave complication. Of those who develop encephalitis about one in eight will die, approx. half will have permanent central nervous system injury, and the remainder will recover completely. Bronchopneumonia is a serious complication of measles. Otitis media, followed by mastoiditis, brain abscess, or even meningitis, is not rare. Cervical adenitis with marked cellulitis sometimes leads to fatal consequences. Tracheitis and laryngeal stenosis, due to edema of glottis, are sometimes seen in the course of measles. Eye complications are not common in measles, although a marked conjunctivitis usually occurs.

DIFF. DIAG: Scarlet fever, German measles, the prodromal rash of smallpox, or even cases of confluent smallpox may have to be considered. If the measles patient is observed prior to appearance of rash, or sometimes even after rash has developed, a definite decision may be based on the presence of Koplik's spots, q.v.

Hemorrhagic spots are also seen on the hard palate and mucous membrane many times before rash is evident on the skin. These spots probably correspond to the typical maculopapular eruption of the disease.

PROG: While usually favorable in the well-nourished child, the seriousness of the possible complications of measles should not be minimized.

NURSING IMPLICATIONS: Maintain bedrest and provide quiet activities for child. If photophobia occurs, keep room dimly lit. Remove eye secretions with warm saline or water. Encourage child not to rub eyes. Promote adequate hydration. Administer antipyretics and tepid sponge baths as ordered. Use cool mist vaporizer to relieve cough and coryza. Apply antipruritic medication as ordered to prevent itching.

PREVENTION: All children who have not had measles or who have not been vaccinated previously should be immunized with live attenuated measles vaccine at 12 months of age. Inactivated vaccine is not recommended because of the short-lived protection it produces.

Live attenuated vaccine is contraindicated in pregnancy, leukemia, lymphomas, and other generalized neoplasms; when agents that depress resistance such as steroids and antimetabolites are being given; during severe illness; in active tuberculosis that is not being treated; in individuals with neomycin, duck, or egg sensitivity; and after blood transfusion or injection of immune serum globulin. In these latter two cases wait 12 weeks before administering vaccine.

Measles immune serum globulin is effective in preventing measles if it is given not later than 5 days after exposure.

m., black. A severe form of measles in which the eruption is dark in color due to an effusion of blood into the skin. SYN: *m., hemorrhagic.*

m., German. Rubella.

m., hemorrhagic. M., black.

measles and mumps virus vaccine, live. A standardized vaccine containing live measles and mumps viruses.

measles and rubella virus vaccine, live. A standardized vaccine containing live measles and rubella viruses.

measles, mumps, and rubella virus vaccine, live. A standardized vaccine containing live measles, mumps, and rubella viruses. Trade name is M-M-R-II.

measles virus vaccine, live. USP. A standardized live virus vaccine for use in immunizing against measles. Trade name is Attenuvax.

measly (mē′zlē). Description of pork that is infected with the cysticerci of Taenia solium or saginata.

measure (mĕ′zhūr) [L. *mensura,* a measuring]. 1. The dimensions, capacity, or quantity of anything that can be so evaluated. Length, area, volume, and mass are basic properties of matter and materials that can be measured. 2. To determine the extent of length, area, mass, or volume of a substance or object. 3. A device used in measuring, for ex., a marked tape or a graduated beaker. SEE: In *Appendix: Metric System; Weights and Measures;* and *Household Measures and Weights.*

Measurin. Trade name for aspirin.

meat [AS. *mete,* food]. 1. The edible portion of anything. 2. The flesh of animals, including poultry, that is used for food.

Meat from animals is a source of vitamins, esp. those of the B complex (thiamine, riboflavin, niacin). Pork is especially rich in thiamine. Liver has an unusually high vitamin content, esp. of vitamin A. The glandular organs such as liver and kidney contain a considerably higher percentage of certain mineral elements and vitamins than are found in other forms of meat.

Most meats have the same nutritive value but differ greatly in flavor and tenderness. Muscle contains about 20% protein, 20% fat, and 60% water. Lean meat is rich in phosphorus, potassium, and iron; it has a good percentage of other minerals but is deficient in calcium. In all meats the acid-forming elements are decidedly in excess of the base-forming.

Many myths about meat have been repudiated. For instance, one kind of meat is as easily digested as another and tough meat is just as nutritious as tender meat.

meatal (mē-ā'tăl) [L. *meatus,* passage]. Pert. to a meatus or passage.

meatometer (mē-ă-tŏm'ĕt-ĕr) [" + Gr. *metron,* measure]. Device for measuring the size of a passage or opening.

meatorrhaphy (mē"ă-tor'ăf-ē) [" + Gr. *rhaphe,* a sewing]. Suture of the severed end of the urethra to the glans penis following surgical procedure to enlarge the meatus.

meatoscope (mē-ăt'ō-skōp) [" + Gr. *skopein,* to examine]. A speculum for examining a meatus.

meatoscopy (mē-ă-tŏs'kō-pē) [" + Gr. *skopein,* to examine]. Instrumental examination of a meatus, esp. the meatus of the urethra.

meatotome (mē-ăt'ō-tōm) [" + Gr. *tome,* incision]. Knife with probe or guarded point for enlarging meatus by direct incision.

meatotomy (mē"ă-tŏt'ō-mē). Incision of urinary meatus to enlarge the opening.

meatus (mē-ā'tŭs) [L.]. (pl. *meattus*) [NA] A passage or opening.

m. acusticus externus. [NA] External auditory canal from the eardrum to the external ear.

m. acusticus internus. [NA] Canal in the petrous portion of temporal bone, containing facial and auditory nerves and vessels.

m. nasi communis. Common nasal cavity on either side of septum, into which three meattus open.

m. nasi inferior. [NA] Space beneath inferior turbinate of the nose.

m. nasi medius. [NA] Space beneath middle turbinate or concha of the nose.

m. nasi superior. [NA] Space beneath superior turbinate or concha of the nose.

m. nasopharyngeus. [NA] Posterior portion of nasal cavity, which communicates with the nasopharynx.

m. urinarius. External opening of the urethra.

Mebaral. Trade name for mephobarbital, USP.

mebendazole (mĕ-bĕn'dă-zōl). A broad-spectrum antihelmintic drug. It is used in treating tapeworm infections and is the drug of choice in treating Ascaris lumbricoides, Trichuris trichuria, hookworm, and Strongyloides stercoralis. Trade name is Vermox.

CAUTION: This drug should not be used during pregnancy.

mebutamate (mĕ-bū'tă-māt). A sedative-hypnotic drug that also has antihypertensive action.

mecamylamine hydrochloride (mĕk"ă-mĭl'ă-mĭn). USP. An antihypertensive drug of the ganglionic blocking agent type. Trade name is Inversine.

mechanical rectifier. A device that, by changing contacts at the proper moment in a cycle, changes alternating current into pulsating direct current.

mechanics [Gr. *mechane,* machine]. Science of force and matter.

mechanism. 1. Involuntary and consistent response to a stimulus. 2. A habit or response pattern to achieve a result. 3. A machine or machine-like structure.

m., countercurrent. The mechanism used by the kidneys in making it possible to excrete excess solutes in the urine with little loss of water from the body.

m., defense. The means utilized in coping with stress. Included are denial, rationalization, repression, sublimation, and conversion.

m., Duncan's. Delivery of the placenta from the uterus with the rough side presenting first.

mechanocyte (mĕk'ă-nō-sīt") [" + *kytos,* cell]. In in-vitro tissue cell culture, a fibroblast.

mechanoreceptor (mĕk"ă-nō-rē-sĕp'tor). A receptor that receives mechanical stimuli such as pressure from sound or touch.

mechanotherapy (mĕk"ăn-ō-thĕr'ă-pē) [Gr. *mechane,* machine, + *therapeia,* treatment]. Use of various types of mechanical apparatus to perform passive movements and to exercise various parts of the body.

mechlorethamine (mĕk"lor-ĕth'ă-mēn). USP. A cytotoxic drug of the nitrogen mustard type. Trade name is Mustargen.

mecism (mē'sĭzm) [Gr. *mekos,* length]. Abnormal lengthening of the body.

Meckel, Johann Friedrich [the elder] (mĕk'ĕl). German anatomist, 1724–1774.

M.'s ganglion. Ganglion located in the sphenomaxillary fossa giving off nerves to eyes, nose, and palate. SYN: *sphenopalatine ganglion.*

M.'s space. Area in dura holding the gasserian ganglion.

Meckel, Johann Friedrich [the younger] (mĕk'ĕl). German anatomist, 1781–1833, grandson of J. F. Meckel, the elder.

M.'s cartilage. A cartilaginous bar about which the mandible develops.

M.'s diverticulum. A congenital sac or blind pouch sometimes found in lower portion of the ileum. It represents the persistent proximal end of the yolk stalk. Sometimes it is continued to the umbilicus as a cord or as a tube forming a fistulous opening at the umbilicus. Strangulation may cause intestinal obstruction. SEE: *diverticulitis; diverticulum.*

meckelectomy (mĕk-ĕl-ĕk′tō-mē). Excision of Meckel's ganglion.

meclizine hydrochloride (mĕk′lĭ-zēn). USP. Antiemetic esp. effective for control of nausea and vomiting of motion sickness. Trade names are Antivert and Bonine.

meclocycline sulfosalicylate. USP. An antibacterial drug used topically. Trade name is Meclan cream.

meconium (mĕ-kō′nē-ŭm) [Gr. *mekonion,* poppy juice]. 1. Opium; poppy juice. 2. First feces of a newborn infant, made up of salts, liquor amnii, mucus, bile and epithelial cells. Greenish black to light brown, almost odorless and of a tarry consistency. The first meconium stool should appear during the first 24 hrs. and persist for about 3 days.

meconium ileus. Ileus due to impacted meconium in the intestines. This is usually associated with newborn children with cystic fibrosis.

mecystasis (mē-sĭs′tă-sĭs). Process in which a muscle maintains its original degree of tension although its length is increased.

M.E.D. *minimal effective dose.*

medi- [L.]. Prefix indicating middle.

media (mē′dē-ă) [L.]. 1. Pl. of medium. 2. Middle or muscular coat of an artery. SYN: *tunica media.*

mediad (mē′dē-ăd) [L. *medium,* middle, + *ad,* toward]. Toward the median line or plane of the body.

medial [L. *medialis*]. 1. Pert. to middle. 2. Nearer the medial plane.

medialis (mē″dē-ā′lĭs) [L.]. Term indicating something is close to the midline of the body.

median (mē′dē-ăn) [L. *medianus*]. 1. Middle; central. 2. In statistics, a number obtained by arranging the given series in order of size and taking the middle number; one then has an equal number of values above and below that number. Thus, in the series 5, 7, 8, 9, 10, the median is 8. SYN: *mesial.* SEE: *mean.*

median line. An imaginary line extending longitudinally on the anterior or posterior surface of the body marking the edges of the median plane.

median nerve. A combined motor and sensory nerve having its origin in the brachial plexus.

median plane. A vertical plane through the trunk and head dividing the body into right and left halves. SYN: *midsagittal plane.* SEE: *plane* for illus.

mediastinal (mē″dē-ăs-tī′năl) [L. *mediastinalis*]. Rel. to the mediastinum.

mediastinitis (mē″dē-ăs″tĭ-nī′tĭs) [″ + Gr. *itis,* inflammation]. Inflammation of tissue of the mediastinum.

mediastinography (mē″dē-ăs″tĭ-nŏg′ră-fē) [″ + Gr. *graphein,* to write]. X-raying of the mediastinum.

mediastinopericarditis (mē-dē-ăs″tĭ-nō-pĕr″ĭ-kăr-dī′tĭs) [″ + Gr. *peri,* around, + *kardia,* heart, + *itis,* inflammation]. Inflammatory condition of the mediastinum and pericardium.

mediastinoscopy (mē″dē-ăs″tĭ-nŏs′kō-pē) [″ + *skopein,* to examine]. Endoscopic examination of the mediastinum.

mediastinotomy (mē″dē-ăs″tĭ-nŏt′ō-mē) [″ + *tome,* incision]. Surgical incision of the mediastinum.

mediastinum (mē″dē-ăs-tī′nŭm) [L., in the middle]. (pl. *mediastina*) 1. A septum or cavity between two principal portions of an organ. 2. The mass of organs and tissues separating the lungs. It contains the heart and its large vessels, trachea, esophagus, thymus, lymph nodes, and connective tissue.

m. testis. [NA] The thickened portion of the tunica albuginea on posterior surface of the testis. SYN: *corpus highmorianum.*

mediate (mē′dē-āt). 1. Accomplished by indirect means. 2. Between two parts or sides.

mediation (mē″dē-ā′shŭn). The action of an intermediary, i.e., mediating, substance.

mediator (mē′dē-ā″tor). That which acts to mediate. The mediator may be a person, a nerve, a chemical substance, or a cellular substance.

medic. A member of the medical team in the U.S. Armed Forces. SYN: *medical corpsman.*

medicable (mĕd′ĭ-kă-bl) [L. *medicari,* to heal]. Possibly responsive to therapy; curable.

Medicaid. In the U.S.A., a government program for providing medical care for the poor. The program is jointly funded by the Federal and state governments.

medical (mĕd′ĭ-kăl). 1. Pert. to medicine or the study of the art and science of caring for those who are ill. 2. Requiring therapy with medicines as distinct from surgical treatment.

medical assistant. An individual who assists a qualified physician in an office or other clinical setting, performing administrative (secretary, receptionist, bookkeeper) and technical (vital signs, height, weight, laboratory tests) duties as delegated and in accordance with state laws governing medical practice.

medical audit. Professional evaluation of a sample of the medical records of hospitals and practices in order to evaluate the quality of medical care and compare it with accepted standards and criteria.

medical corpsman. An enlisted man in the U.S. Armed Forces who works as a member of the medical team. SYN: *corpsman; medic.*

Medic Alert. A nonprofit organization that provides a bracelet or pendant with an emblem on which is contained information and a warning in case of emergency. They also keep a file of the medical information and a toll-free number for emergency consultation. The purpose is the prevention of a serious or fatal mistake in rendering aid or medical care to an injured or unconscious person who may have an additional condition or allergy, e.g., diabetes, penicillin allergy. Applications may be obtained from Medic Alert, P.O. Box 1009, Turlock, CA 95381. Persons wishing to donate organs may also acquire an emblem from the Medic Alert company stating that fact. SEE: illus.

medical examiner. A physician who is trained and qualified for the task of investigating the cause of death and the circumstances surrounding it. Training usually includes study of pathology and forensic medicine. The examiner is empowered by governmental agencies to represent them, and is expected to make a comprehensive report of findings to judicial or police authorities. The skill of a medical examiner is especially important in investigating deaths wherein malpractice, homicide, suicide or other criminal actions are suspected of being a contributing factor.

medical history. That portion of a patient's life history, including ancestry, social, occupational, and medical, that is important in diagnosing and caring for the medical or surgical condition or conditions present. This information, which is recorded in the patient's permanent record, may be obtained from all available sources if for some reason the patient isn't able or willing to provide full details. The importance of an accurate and complete medical history for proper care of the patient cannot be overestimated. SEE: *nursing history form.*

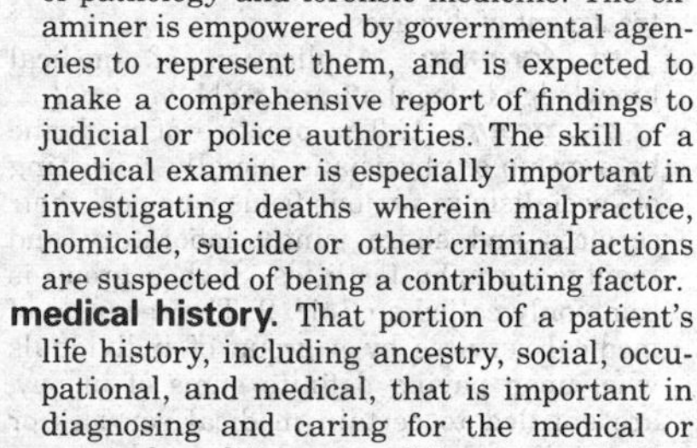

MEDIC ALERT SYMBOL

medical jurisprudence. Principles of medicine in their application to questions of law.

medical preparations. SOLID SUBSTANCES: Capsule or capsula, confection, extract, lozenge, lamella, ointment, plaster, powder or pulvis, pill or pilula, paper, suppository or suppositorium, tablet or tabella.

FLUIDS: Fluidextract, tincture infusion, decoction, wine, oleoresin.

SUSPENSIONS: Mixture emulsion.

SOLUTIONS: Water, mucilage, solution or liquor, elixir, syrup, spirit, glycerite, vinegar.

MISC: Liniment or linimentum, oleate or oleatum

RS: active principle; alkaloid; antidote; dosage; drug action; drug administration; names of individual drugs; names of individual poisons; poison; poisoning; prescription writing.

medical record. Transcript of information obtained from a patient, guardian, or professionals and presented in tabular, outline, or written form. It may contain history, diagnoses, treatment, prognosis, etc. Utilized by the school, place of employment, personal physician, hospital, etc.

medical record, problem-oriented. A technique of clinical record keeping described by Lawrence Weed, a contemporary U.S. physician. The patient's record is organized in a logical and efficient manner including a list of problems and flow charts determining diagnostic and therapeutic plans and indicating what has been done.

medical records librarian. An individual who is trained and experienced in maintaining, storing, and retrieving all of the medical records collected for the patients treated at a medical care facility.

medicament [L. *medicamentum*]. A medicine or remedy.

medicamentosus (mĕd″ĭ-kă-mĕn-tō′sŭs). Concerning drugs.

Medicare. Federal medical and hospital care program for the elderly.

medicate (mĕd′ĭ-kāt) [L. *medicatus*]. 1. To treat a disease with drugs. 2. To permeate with medicinal substances.

medication (mĕd-ĭ-kā′shŭn). 1. Treatment with remedies. 2. Impregnation with medicine.

m., hypodermic. Treatment by injection of medicine into the body through the skin, using a syringe and needle.

m., ionic. Introduction of ions of drugs into the body by cataphoresis, q.v.

m., sublingual. Treatment with an agent, usually in tablet form, placed under the tongue.

m., substitutive. Medical therapy to cause a nonspecific inflammation to counteract a specific one.

medication route. The way that a drug is introduced into the body. The route of administration is chosen according to the speed of absorption desired, and the site of action of the medication. Some medications are formulated for a specific route only and must be given in that manner. Various routes of administration used are as follows:

Oral and *enteral* administration require that the medication not be destroyed by the environment of the stomach and digestive enzymes. It is too slow if rapid absorption is required, and cannot be used if the patient is vomiting. Rectal administration in the form of liquids or suppositories circumvents this problem in enteral administration.

Mucosal routes of administration other than the above include absorption through the nasal mucosa, the buccal mucosa, or the bronchioles, the latter usually achieved through inhalation of an aerosol. Vaginal administration is also a mucosal route of medication.

Percutaneous administration is used for iontophoresis or by direct absorption through the skin.

Parenteral administration is used when a drug can not be given by mouth. The speed of absorption varies greatly with the specific route used. These include: subcutaneous, intravenous, intramuscular, intra-arterial, intraperitoneal, intrathecal, intracardiac, and intrasternal.

medicinal (mĕ-dĭ'sĭn-ăl) [L. *medicina*, medicine]. Pert. to medicine.

medicinal enema. An enema to which some drug or medication has been added, for retention or absorption, particularly in cases where medication cannot be administered by mouth. SEE: *enema, medicinal; medication route.*

medicine. 1. A drug or remedy. 2. The act of maintenance of health, and prevention and treatment of disease and illness. 3. Treatment of disease medically as distinguished from surgical treatment.

m., aerospace. Branch of medicine concerned with the selection of individuals for duty as pilots or crew members for flight and space missions. Includes study of the pathology and physiology of persons and animals who travel in airplanes and spacecraft in the Earth's atmosphere and in outer space.

m., clinical. Observation and treatment at the bedside; the practice of medicine in the clinical setting as distinguished from laboratory science.

m., community. Medical care directed toward service of the entire population of the community, with emphasis on preventive medicine.

m., disaster. Large-scale application of emergency medical services in a community following a natural or man-made catastrophe. The aim is to save lives and restore every survivor to maximum health as promptly as possible. Its success depends upon prompt sorting of patients according to their immediate needs and prognosis. SEE: *triage.*

m., emergency. The medical specialty concerned with those who are acutely ill or suddenly injured and thus require immediate care.

m., environmental. Branch of medicine concerned with the effects of the environment (temperature, population size, pollution, radiation) on man.

m., experimental. The scientific study of disease or pathological conditions through experimentation upon laboratory animals or through clinical research.

m., family. The area of medical specialization concerned with providing or supervising the medical care of all members of the family.

m., folk. The use of home remedies for treatment of diseases.

m., forensic. Application of medical knowledge to legal affairs. SYN: *m., legal.*

m., group. 1. The practice of medicine by a group of physicians, usually consisting of specialists in various fields who pool their services and share jointly laboratory and roentgenography facilities. Such a group is commonly called a clinic. 2. The securing of medical services by a group of individuals who, upon paying definite sums of money, are entitled to certain medical services or hospitalization in accordance with prearranged rules and regulations.

m., industrial. M., occupational, q.v.

m., internal. 1. That branch of medicine that treats diseases of the internal organs by other than surgical means. 2. Treatment of diseases nonsurgical in nature.

m., legal. M., forensic.

m., nuclear. The branch of medicine involved with the use of radioactive substances for diagnosis, therapy, and research.

m., occupational. The branch of medicine concerned with the problems peculiar to the workplace, and with the prevention and treatment of diseases and injuries that are especially liable to occur at work.

m., patent. A medicine for which a patent has been granted. May be purchased without a doctor's prescription. SEE: *patent medicine.*

m., physical. Treatment of disease by physical agents such as heat, cold, light, electricity, manipulation, or the use of mechanical devices. SYN: *physical therapy; physiotherapy.*

m., preclinical. 1. Preventive medicine,

q.v. 2. Term used to indicate the first two years of medical school training, during which there is little or no exposure to patients for teaching purposes.

m., preventive. The study and practice of preventing disease.

m., proprietary. Medicine in which exclusive interests have been secured by patent, copyright of labels, or secrecy of composition. SEE: *proprietary medicine.*

m., psychosomatic. A branch of medicine that recognizes the importance of mind-body interrelationship in all illnesses and in which therapy and management are based on this fact.

m., socialized. Practice of medicine under control and direction of agency of the government. The cost of medical care under this plan usually is financed by levying taxes or through a national medical insurance program.

m., sports. Field of medicine concerned with all aspects of physiology, pathology, and psychology as they apply to persons who participate in sports whether at the recreational, amateur, or professional level. An important facet of sports medicine is the application of medical knowledge to the prevention of injuries in those who participate in sports.

m., tropical. Branch of medical science that deals principally with diseases common in tropical or subtropical regions, esp. of parasitic origin.

m., veterinary. Branch of medical science that deals with diagnosis and treatment of diseases of animals.

medicine man. Shaman, q.v.

medicinerea (mĕd″ĭ-sĭn-ē′rē-a) [L. *medius,* middle, + *cinerea,* ashen]. Internal gray matter of the claustrum and lenticula of the brain.

medicochirurgical (mĕd″ĭ-kō-kī-rŭr′jĭ-kăl) [L. *medicus,* medical, + Gr. *cheir,* hand, + *ergon,* work]. Concerning both medicine and surgery.

medicolegal (mĕd″ĭ-kō-lē′găl) [″ + *legalis,* legal]. Rel. to medical jurisprudence or forensic medicine.

medicomechanical (mĕd″ĭ-kō-mĕ-kăn′ĭ-kăl). Concerning both medical and mechanical aspects of treating patients.

medicopsychology (mĕd″ĭ-kō-sī-kŏl′ō-jē). The relationship of medicine with the mind or with mental illness.

medicopter. Helicopter equipped for emergency care of sick or injured while they are being evacuated to a hospital.

medicornu (mĕd″ĭ-kor′nū) [L. *medius,* middle, + *cornu,* horn]. The inferior horn of the lateral ventricle of the brain.

Medihaler-Epi. Trade name for epinephrine bitartrate, USP.

Medina worm. Dracunculus medinensis.

medio- [L. *medius,* middle]. Prefix meaning middle.

mediocarpal (mē″dē-ō-kăr′păl). Concerning the middle part of the carpal bone.

mediolateral (mē″dē-ō-lăt′ĕr-ăl). Concerning the middle and side of a structure.

medionecrosis (mē″dē-ō-nē-krō′sĭs) [″ + *nekrosis,* deadness]. Necrosis of the tunica media of a blood vessel.

mediopontine (mē″dē-ō-pŏn′tīn) [″ + *pons,* bridge]. Rel. to center of the pons varolii.

mediotarsal (mē″dē-ō-tăr′săl). Rel. to the middle of the tarsus.

medisect (mē′dĭ-sĕkt) [″ + *secare,* to cut]. To cut on the median line of the body or structure.

Mediterranean anemia. A hereditary anemia due to an abnormality in the synthesis of hemoglobin. Usually occurs in Mediterranean populations. There is no specific therapy. SYN: *Cooley's anemia; thalassemia.*

Mediterranean fever, familial. A disease, esp. one originally common in people of the Middle East, but now seen in various parts of the world. This familial disease is characterized by short attacks of fever, signs of peritonitis, pleuritis, and arthritis. The most frequent cause of death is amyloidosis, which occurs as the disease progresses. There is no specific diagnostic test.

TREATMENT: Symptomatic. SYN: *polyserositis, recurrent.*

medium (mē′dē-ŭm). (pl. *media*) 1. An agent through which an effect is obtained. 2. Substance used for the cultivation of microorganisms or cellular tissue. SYN: *culture medium.* 3. Substance through which impulses are transmitted.

medium-chain triglycerides. Triglycerides with 8 to 10 carbon atoms. They are digested and absorbed differently than the usual dietary fats and, for that reason, have been useful in treating malabsorption.

medius (mē′dē-ŭs) [L.]. Middle. Indicating the middle one of three similar structures.

MEDLARS [*Med*ical *L*iterature *A*nalysis and *R*etrieval *S*ystem]. Acronym indicating the U.S. National Library of Medicine's system of computerized bibliography. Index Medicus is produced by this system. A MEDLARS search is use of this system to retrieve medical references of specific interest.

MEDLINE [*MED*LARS on *line*]. The system where telephone lines may be linked to the MEDLARS system so bibliographic data may be transmitted from the National Library of Medicine to a great number of locations.

medrogestone (mĕd-rō-jĕs′tōn). A progestin.

Medrol. Trade name for methylprednisolone.

medroxyprogesterone acetate (mĕd-rŏk″sē-prō-jĕs′tĕr-ōn). USP. A progestational agent. It is used intramuscularly in appropriate dose. It is effective for as long as 90 days. Trade names are Depo-Provera and Provera.

medrysone (mĕd′rĭ-sōn). USP. An adrenal corticosteroid drug. Trade name is HMS Liquifilm.

medulla (mĕ-dŭl′lă) [L.]. (pl. *medullae*) [NA] 1. The marrow. 2. Inner or central portion of an organ in contrast to the outer portion or cortex. 3. Medulla oblongata.

m., adrenal. Inner portion of the adrenal gland composed of chromaffin tissue. Secretes epinephrine. SEE: *adrenal gland.*

m. nephrica. Pyramids of kidneys.

m. oblongata. [NA] Enlarged portion of spinal cord in cranium after it enters the foramen magnum of the occipital bone; the lower portion of the brain stem.

m. of hair. Central axis of a hair.

m. of kidneys. Renal pyramids. SEE: *pyramid, renal.*

m. of ovary. Central portion of the ovary composed of loose connective tissue, blood vessels, lymphatics, and nerves.

m. ossium. [NA] Marrow in bone.

m. spinalis. [NA] Spinal cord.

medullary (mĕd′ū-lār-ē) [L. *medularis*]. Concerning marrow or medulla.

medullated (mĕd′ū-lāt″ĕd). Covered by or containing marrow or medulla; myelinated.

medullated nerve fiber. A nerve fiber possessing a myelin or medullary sheath; a myelinated nerve fiber.

medullation. Acquiring a myelin sheath.

medullectomy (mĕd″ū-lĕk′tō-mē) [L. *medulla,* marrow, + Gr. *ektome,* excision]. Surgical excision of a part of the medulla of the brain.

medullitis (mĕd-ū-lī′tĭs) [″ + Gr. *itis,* inflammation]. Inflammation of marrow. SYN: *myelitis.*

medullization (mĕd″ū-lī-zā′shŭn). Abnormal conversion to marrow.

medulloadrenal (mē-dŭl″ō-ă-drē′năl) [″+ *ad,* to, + *ren,* kidney]. Concerning the medulla of the adrenal gland.

medulloarthritis (mĕ-dŭl″ō-ăr-thrī′tĭs) [L. *medulla,* marrow, + Gr. *arthron,* joint, + *itis,* inflammation]. Inflammation of marrow elements of bone ends.

medulloblast (mĕ-dŭl′ō-blăst) [″ + Gr. *blastos,* germ]. An immature cell of the neural tube that may develop into either a nerve or neuroglial cell.

medulloblastoma (mĕ-dŭl″ō-blās-tō′mă) [″ + Gr. *blastos,* germ, + *oma,* tumor]. A soft infiltrating malignant tumor of the roof of the 4th ventricle and cerebellum. Often invades the meninges.

medulloepithelioma (mĕ-dŭl″ō-ĕp″ĭ-thēl-ē-ō′mă) [″ + Gr. *epi,* upon, + *thele,* nipple, + *oma,* tumor]. Tumor composed of retina epithelium and of neuroepithelium. SYN: *glioma; neuroepithelioma.*

Mees line. A transverse white line that appears above the lunula of the fingernails about 5 weeks after exposure to arsenic.

mefenamic acid. An analgesic and antipyretic drug that also has anti-inflammatory action. Trade name is Ponstel.

mega- [Gr. *megas,* large]. 1. Combining form that means great or large. 2. Indicates one million (10^6) when used in combination with terms indicating units of measure; thus megaton is one million tons. SEE: words beginning with *megalo-.*

megabladder (mĕg″ă-blăd′ĕr) [″ + AS. *blaedre,* bladder]. Permanent abnormal distention of the urinary bladder. SYN: *megalocystis.*

megabuck (mĕg′ă-bŭk). A million dollars, possession of which may contribute to either health or disease. Colloquially used to refer to large amounts of money.

megacardia (mĕg″ă-kăr′dē-ă). Enlargement of the heart. SYN: *cardiomegaly.*

Megace. Trade name for megestrol acetate.

megacephalic (mĕg-ă-sĕf-ăl′ĭk). Having an abnormally large head. SYN: *macrocephalous.*

megacolon (mĕg-ă-kō′lŏn) [″ + *kolon,* colon]. Extremely dilated colon. Usually congenital but occurs also in infancy or childhood. SEE: *Hirschsprung's disease.*

m., toxic. Acute dilatation of the colon that may progress to rupture. Seen in acute attacks of ulcerative colitis.

megacurie (mĕg″ă-kū′rē) [″ + *curie*]. ABBR: Mc. A radioactivity unit, 10^6 curies.

megadontia (mĕg″ă-dŏn′shē-ă) [″ + *odous, odont-,* tooth]. Possessing very large teeth.

megadyne (mĕg′ă-dīn). A unit equal to one million dynes. SEE: *dyne.*

megaesophagus (mĕg″ă-ē-sŏf′ă-gŭs) [″ + *oisophagos,* esophagus]. A grossly dilated esophagus, usually associated with achalasia.

megahertz (mĕg′ă-hĕrtz). ABBR: MHz. One million, 10^6, cycles per second (i.e., hertz).

megakaryoblast (mĕg″ă-kăr′ē-ō-blăst). An immature megakaryocyte.

megakaryocyte (mĕg″ă-kăr′ē-ō-sīt″) [″ + *karyon,* nucleus, + *kytos,* cell]. Large bone marrow cell with large or multiple nuclei. SYN: *giant cell; myeloplax.*

megakaryocytosis (mĕg″ă-kăr″ē-ō-sī-tō′sĭs) [″ + ″ + ″ + *osis,* condition]. An increased number of megakaryocytes in the bone marrow; presence of megakaryocytes in the blood.

megalecithal (mĕg″ă-lĕs′ĭ-thăl) [″ + *lekithos,* egg yolk]. An egg that has a large amount of yolk.

megalencephaly (mĕg″ăl-ĕn-sĕf′ă-lē) [″ + *enkephalos,* brain]. Abnormally large size of the brain, usually accompanied by mental deficiency.

megalgia (mĕg-ăl'jē-ă) [" + *algos*, pain]. Very severe pain.

megalo- [Gr. *megas*, large]. Combining form meaning of great size.

megaloblast (mĕg'ă-lō-blăst) [" + *blastos*, germ]. A large-size nucleated abnormal red blood corpuscle, from 11 to 20 microns in diameter, oval and slightly irregular. Found in the blood in cases of pernicious anemia.

megalocardia (mĕg"ă-lō-kăr'dē-ă) [" + *kardia*, heart]. Cardiac hypertrophy. SYN: *cardiomegaly.*

megalocephalic (mĕg-ă-lō-sĕf-ăl'ĭk) [" + *kephale*, head]. Having an abnormally large skull. SYN: *megacephalic; macrocephalic.*

megalocephaly (mĕg"ă-lō-sĕf'ă-lē) [" + *kephale*, head]. 1. Abnormal size of the head. SYN: *macrocephaly.* 2. A rare disease characterized by hyperostosis of bones of the skull. SYN: *leontiasis ossea.*

megalocheiria (mĕg"ă-lō-kī'rē-ă) [" + *cheir*, hand]. Abnormally large hands.

megalocornea (mĕg"ă-lō-kor'nē-ă) [" + L. *cornu*, horn]. An enlarged cornea due to a developmental anomaly. SYN: *macrocornea.*

megalocystis (mĕg"ă-lō-sĭs'tĭs) [" + *kystis*, bladder]. Abnormal permanent enlargement of the bladder. SYN: *megabladder.*

megalocyte (mĕg'ă-lō-sīt) [" + *kytos*, cell]. A larger than average red blood corpuscle.

megalodactylous (mĕg"ă-lō-dăk'tĭl-ŭs) [" + *daktylos*, finger]. Having very large fingers or toes.

megalodontia (mĕg"ă-lō-dŏn'shē-ă) [" + *odous*, tooth]. Abnormally large teeth.

megaloesophagus (mĕg"ă-lō-ē-sŏf'ă-gŭs) [" + *oisophagos*, esophagus]. Megaesophagus, q.v.

megalogastria (mĕg"ă-lō-găs'trē-ă) [" + *gaster*, belly]. Excessive size of stomach. SYN: *gastromegaly.*

megaloglossia (mĕg"ă-lō-glŏs'sē-ă) [" + *glossa*, tongue]. Enlargement of the tongue. SYN: *macroglossia.*

megalographia (mĕg"ă-lō-gră'fē-ă) [" + *graphein*, to write]. Macrography, q.v.

megalohepatia (mĕg"ă-lō-hĕ-păt'ē-ă) [" + *hepar*, liver]. Abnormal enlargement of the liver. SYN: *hepatomegaly.*

megalokaryocyte (mĕg"ă-lō-kăr'ē-ō-sīt) [" + *karyon*, nucleus, + *kytos*, cell]. A large bone marrow cell with multiple nuclei. SYN: *megakaryocyte.*

megalomania (mĕg"ă-lō-mā'nē-ă) [" + *mania*, madness]. A psychosis characterized by ideas of personal exaltation and delusions of grandeur.

megalomelia (mĕg"ă-lō-mĕl'ē-ă) [" + *melos*, limb]. Abnormally large size of the limbs. SYN: *macromelia.*

megalonychosis (mĕg"ă-lō'nĭ-kō'sĭs) [" + *onyx*, nail]. Hypertrophy of the nails.

megalopenis (mĕg"ă-lō-pē'nĭs) [" + L. *penis*, penis]. Abnormally large penis. SYN: *macrophallus.*

megalophthalmus (mĕg"ă-lŏf-thăl'mŭs) [" + *ophthalmos*, eye]. Abnormally large eyes.

megalopodia (mĕg"ă-lō-pō'dē-ă) [" + *pous*, foot]. Abnormally large feet.

megalopsia (mĕg"ă-lŏp'sē-ă) [" + *opsis*, vision]. An affection of the eyes in which objects appear enlarged. SYN *macropsia.*

megaloscope (mĕg'ă-lō-skōp") [" + *skopein*, to examine]. A large magnifying lens; a speculum fitted with a magnifying lens.

megalosplenia (mĕg"ă-lō-splēn'ē-ă) [" + *splen*, spleen]. Hypertrophy of the spleen. SYN: *splenomegaly.*

megalospore (mĕg'ă-lō-spor"). Macrospore q.v.

megalosyndactyly (mĕg"ă-lō-sĭn-dăk'tĭl-ē) [" + *syn*, with, + *daktylos*, finger]. A condition of large and webbed digits.

megaloureter (mĕg"ă-lō-ū-rē'tĕr, -ūr'ĕ-tĕr) [" + *oureter*, ureter]. Increase in diameter of the ureter.

megaprosopous (mĕg"ă-prŏs'ō-pŭs) [" + *prosopon*, face]. Possessing a large face.

megarectum (mĕg-ă-rĕk'tŭm) [" + L. *rectum*, straight]. Excessive dilatation of the rectum.

megaseme (mĕg'ă-sēm) [" + *sema*, sign]. Having an orbital aperture with an index exceeding 89, said of a skull.

megavitamin (mĕg"ă-vī'tă-mĭn). A dose of one or more vitamins that is in huge excess of the normal daily requirements.

megavolt (mĕg'ă-vōlt). A million, 10^6, volts.

megestrol acetate (mĕ-jĕs'trōl). A synthetic progestin that is also used in treating certain neoplasms. Trade name is Megace.

meglumine (mĕg'lū-mēn). USP. A radiopaque compound used in x-ray studies.

m. antimonate. A drug used in treating leishmaniasis.

megohm (mĕg'ōm). A million, 10^6, ohms.

megophthalmos (mĕg-ŏf-thăl'mŏs) [" + *ophthalmos*, eye]. Abnormally large eyes. SYN: *megalophthalmus.*

megrim (mē'grĭm). Migraine.

meibomian cyst (mī-bō'mē-ăn). [Heinrich Meibom, Ger. anatomist, 1638–1700] Small tumor on eyelid, the result of inflammation of a meibomian gland. SYN: *chalazion.*

meibomian gland. One of the sebaceous glands between the tarsi and conjunctiva of eyelids. SYN: *tarsal gland.*

meibomitis (mī-bō"mī'tĭs). Inflammation of the meibomian glands.

meio- [Gr. *meioun*, diminution]. Combining form indicating decrease in size or number. SEE: words beginning with *mio-*.

meiogenic (mī"ō-jĕn'ĭk) [Gr. *meiosis*, diminution, + *gennan,* to produce]. Causing meiosis.

meiosis (mī-ō'sĭs) [Gr., diminution]. A type of cell division of germ cells (sperm or ova) in which two successive divisions of the nucleus produce cells that contain half the number of chromosomes present in somatic cells. When fertilization occurs, the nuclei of the sperm and ovum fuse and produce a zygote with the full chromosome complement. SEE: *chromosome; mitosis.*

Meissner's corpuscles (mīs'nĕrz). [Georg Meissner, Ger. histologist, 1829–1905] An encapsulated end-organ of touch found in dermal papillae close to epidermis. Each is an ovoid body containing endings of myelinated and unmyelinated nerve fibers. Most numerous in hairless portion of skin, esp. volar surface of hands, fingers, feet, and toes; also present in lips, eyelids, tip of tongue, and nipple.

Meissner's plexus. Small aggregations of ganglion cells located in submucosa of intestine.

mel [L.]. Honey.

melagra (mĕl-ă'gră) [Gr. *melos,* limb, + *agra,* seizure]. Muscular pain in the limbs.

melalgia (mĕl-ăl'jē-ă) [" + *algos,* pain]. Pain of neural origin in the limbs.

melancholia (mĕl-ăn-kō'lē-ă) [Gr. *melankholia,* sadness]. A mental disorder characterized by marked depression, physical and mental apathy, brooding, mournful and doleful notions, and inhibition of activity.

m., affective. Melancholia observed in depressed phase of manic-depressive psychoses. SEE: *psychosis, manic-depressive.*

m. agitata. Agitated depression.

m., climacteric. Melancholia occurring at the time of menopause.

m., involutional. Despondency, suicidal tendencies, feelings of unworthiness and mental agitation occurring in late middle age.

m., panphobic. Melancholia characterized by dread of everything.

m., sexual. Melancholia associated with fear of impotence, venereal disease, unsatisfied sexual desires.

m. simplex. A mild form without delusions or great excitement.

m. stuporosa. Melancholia in which patient lies silent and motionless, indifferent to surroundings.

m., suicidal. Impulse to commit suicide combined with melancholia.

melanedema (mĕl-ăn-ē-dē'mă) [Gr. *melas,* black, + *oidema,* swelling]. Black deposit in the lungs; melanosis of the lungs. SYN: *anthracosis.*

melanemia (mĕl-ăn-ē'mē-ă) [" + *haima,* blood]. Unnaturally dark color of blood, due to presence of free dark pigment. Seen mainly in pernicious anemia.

melanephidrosis, melanidrosis (mĕl"ăn-ĕf"ĭ-drō'sĭs, mĕl"ăn-ĭd-rō'sĭs) [" + *ephidrosis,* sweating]. A form of chromhidrosis in which the sweat is black.

melaniferous (mĕl"ăn-ĭf'ĕr-ŭs) [" + L. *ferre,* to carry]. Containing melanin or some other black pigment.

melanin [Gr. *melas,* black]. The pigment that gives color to hair, skin, the substantia nigra of the brain, and the choroid of the eye. Exposure to sunlight stimulates melanin production. It can be prepared chemically. It is present in some cancers such as melanoma.

melanism (mĕl'ăn-ĭzm) [" + *-ismos,* state of]. Abnormal black pigmentation of the organs and tissues. SYN: *melanosis.*

melano- [Gr. *melas,* black]. Prefix meaning black or darkness.

melanoameloblastoma (mĕl"ă-nō-ă-mĕl"ō-blăs-tō'mă) [" + O. Fr. *amel,* enamel, + Gr. *blastos,* germ, + *oma,* tumor]. Melanotic neuroectodermal tumor.

melanoblast (mĕl'ăn-ō-blăst", mĕl-ăn'ō-blăst) [" + *blastos,* germ]. A cell originating from the neural crest that differentiates into a melanocyte.

melanoblastoma (mĕl"ă-nō-blăs-tō'mă) [" + " + *oma,* tumor]. A tumor containing melanin.

melanocarcinoma (mĕl"ă-nō-kăr-sĭn-ō'mă) [" + *karkinos,* cancer, + *oma,* tumor]. Malignant melanoma.

melanocyte (mĕl'ăn-ō-sīt, mĕl-ăn'ō-sīt) [" + *kytos,* cell]. Melanin-forming cell.

melanocyte-stimulating hormone. ABBR: MSH. Hormone that regulates skin pigmentation in man.

melanocytoma (mĕl"ă-nō-sī-tō'mă) [" + *kytos,* cell, + *oma,* tumor]. A rare pigmented benign tumor of the optic disk.

melanoderm (mĕl'ăn-ō-dĕrm) [Gr. *melas,* black, + *derma,* skin]. A person belonging to one of the black races.

melanoderma (mĕl"ăn-ō-dĕr'mă). A patchy or generalized skin discoloration caused by either an increase in the production of melanin by the normal number of melanocytes or an increase in the number of melanocytes. SYN: *melanopathy.*

melanodermatitis (mĕl"ă-nō-dĕr"mă-tī'tĭs) [" + " + *itis,* inflammation]. Dermatitis in which an excess of melanin is deposited in the involved area.

melanoepithelioma (mĕl"ăn-ō-ĕp"ĭ-thē-lē-ō'mă) [" + *epi,* upon, + *thele,* nipple, + *oma,* tumor]. A malignant epithelioma containing melanin.

melanogen (mĕ-lăn'ō-jĕn) [" + *gennan,* to produce]. A colorless substance that may be converted into melanin.

melanogenesis (mĕl″ăn-ō-jĕn′ĕ-sĭs) [″ + *genesis*, production]. Formation of melanin.
melanoglossia (mĕl″ăn-ō-glŏs′ē-ă) [″ + *glossa*, tongue]. Black tongue. SYN: *glossophytia*.
melanoid (mĕl′ă-noyd) [″ + *eidos*, form]. 1. Concerning or resembling melanin. 2. Artificial melanin that is chemically prepared.
melanoleukoderma (mĕl″ăn-ō-lū″kō-dĕr′mă) [″ + *leukos*, white, + *derma*, skin]. Mottled skin.

m. colli. Mottled skin of the neck sometimes seen in syphilis. SYN: *collar of Venus; venereal collar*.

melanoma (mĕl″ă-nō′mă) [″ + *oma*, tumor]. A pigmented mole or tumor that may or may not be malignant. SEE: *nevus pigmentosus*.
melanomatosis (mĕl″ă-nō″mă-tō′sĭs) [″ + ″ + *osis*, condition]. Formation of numerous melanomas on or beneath the skin.
melanonychia (mĕl″ă-nō-nĭk′ē-ă) [″ + *onyx*, nail]. Black pigmentation of the nails.
melanopathy (mĕl″ă-nŏp′ă-thē) [″ + *pathos*, disease]. 1. Dark pigmentation of skin. 2. Any disease with dark pigmentation of the skin. SYN: *melanoderma*.
melanophage (mĕl′ă-nō-fāj″) [″ + *phagein*, to eat]. A phagocytic cell that contains ingested melanin.
melanophore (mĕl′ăn-ō-for) [″ + *phoros*, bearing]. Cell containing dark pigment.
melanoplakia (mĕl″ăn-ō-plā′kē-ă) [″ + *plax*, a flat plain]. Condition marked by pigmented patches on the tongue and buccal mucosa.
melanorrhagia, melanorrhea (mĕl″ăn-ō-rā′jē-ă, mĕl″ăn-ō-rē′ă) [″ + *rhegnynai*, to burst forth]. Black feces. SYN: *melena*.
melanosarcoma (mĕl″ă-nō-săr-kō′mă) [″ + *sarx*, flesh, + *oma*, tumor]. Sarcoma containing melanin.
melanoscirrhus (mĕl″ă-nō-skĭr′ŭs) [Gr. *melas*, black, + *skirros*, hardness]. Black-pigmented cancer; an unusual form of melanoma. SYN: *melanocarcinoma*.
melanosis (mĕl-ăn-ō′sĭs) [″ + *osis*, condition]. 1. Unusual deposit of black pigments in different parts of body. 2. Disorder of pigment metabolism.

m. lenticularis. Rare skin disease beginning in early youth and characterized by scattered pigment discolorations, ulcers, and atrophy. SYN: *Kaposi's disease; xeroderma pigmentosum*.

melanosome (mĕl′ă-nō-sōm″) [″ + *soma*, body]. The pigment granule produced by melanocytes.
melanotic. 1. Black in color. 2. Pert. to melanosis.
melanotrichia linguae (mĕl″ăn-ō-trĭk′ē-ă lĭng′gwē) [″ + *thrix*, hair, + L. *linguae*, tongue]. Black, hairy tongue.
melanotroph (mĕl′ă-nō-trōf″) [″ + *trophe*, nutrition]. A cell of the pituitary that produces melanocyte-stimulating hormone.
melanuria (mĕl-ăn-ū′rē-ă) [″ + *ouron*, urine]. Dark pigments in urine.
melasma (mĕl-ăz′mă) [Gr., a black spot]. Any discoloration of the skin.

m. gravidarum. Discoloration of the skin during pregnancy.

melatonin (mel″ă-tō′nĭn). Hormone produced by the pineal gland in mammals. Its function in humans is not known.
melena (mĕl′ē-nă, mĕl-ē′nă) [Gr. *melaina*, black]. 1. Black tarry feces due to action of intestinal secretions on free blood. Common in the newborn. SYN: *melanorrhagia*. 2. Black vomitus.

m. neonatorum. Melena in the newborn.

melicera, meliceris (mĕl-ĭ-sēr′ă, -ĭs) [Gr. *meli*, honey, + *keros*, wax]. 1. Cyst containing matter of honeylike consistency. 2. Viscid, syrupy.
melioidosis (mē″lē-oy-dō′sĭs) [Gr. *melis*, a distemper of asses, + *eidos*, resemblance, + *osis*, condition]. An acute or chronic disease due to Pseudomonas pseudomallei (formerly called Malleomyces pseudomallei). Acute form causes pneumonia, multiple abscesses, septicemia, and possibly death.
melissophobia (mĕ-lĭs″ō-fō′bē-ă) [Gr. *melissa*, bee, + *phobia*, fear]. Abnormal fear of bee or wasp stings.
melitagra. Eczema with honeycomb crusting.
melitemia (mĕl-ĭ-tē′mē-ă) [Gr. *meli*, honey, + *haima*, blood]. Abnormal amount of sugar in the blood.
melitensis (mĕl-ĭ-tĕn′sĭs). Undulant fever; brucellosis.
melitis (mĕl-ī′tĭs) [Gr. *melon*, cheek, + *itis*, inflammation]. Inflammation of the cheek.
melitoptyalism (mĕl″ĭ-tō-tī′ă-lĭzm) [″ + *ptyalon*, saliva]. Saliva containing glucose. SYN: *glycoptyalism*.
melituria (mĕl-ĭ-tū′rē-ă) [″ + *ouron*, urine]. Presence of sugar in the urine.
Mellaril. Trade name for thioridazine hydrochloride, USP.
mellitum (mĕ-lī′tŭm) [L.]. A pharmaceutical preparation with honey as the vehicle or excipient
melo-, mel-. 1. [Gr. *melon*, cheek]. Combining form meaning cheek. 2. [Gr. *melos*, limb]. Combining form meaning extremity.
melomelus (mē-lŏm′ē-lŭs) [Gr. *melos*, limb, + *melos*, limb]. A malformed fetus with rudimentary limb attached to normal limb.
meloncus (mĕl-ŏn′kŭs) [Gr. *melon*, cheek, + *onkos*, bulk]. Tumor of the cheek.
melonoplasty (mĕl′ŏn-ō-plăs′tē) [″ + *plassein*, to form]. Plastic surgery of the cheek.
meloplasty (mĕl′ō-plăs-tē) 1. [″ + *plassein*, to form]. Plastic surgery of the face. 2. [Gr. *melos*, limb, + *plassein*, to form]. Reparative

surgery of the extremities.

melorheostosis (mĕl″ō-rē″ŏs-tō′sĭs) [Gr. *melos,* limb, + *rhein,* to flow, + *osteon,* bone, + *osis,* condition]. A rare disease of long bones in which new bone is formed so that the bone looks like candle wax had dripped down the sides.

melosalgia (mĕl″ō-săl′jē-ă) [″ + *algos,* pain]. Pain in the lower limbs.

meloschisis (mĕ-lŏs′kĭ-sĭs) [Gr. *melon,* cheek, + *schistos,* split]. A congenitally cleft cheek.

melotia (mĕ-lō′shē-ă) [″ + *ous,* ear]. Congenital displacement of the ear on the cheek.

melphalan (mĕl′fă-lăn). USP. A cytotoxic drug of the nitrogen mustard class. Trade name is Akeran.

melting point. Temperature at which conversion of a solid to a liquid begins.

member [L. *membrum*]. An organ or part of the body, esp. a limb.

membrane (mĕm′brān) [L. *membrana*]. A thin, soft, pliable layer of tissue that lines a tube or cavity, covers an organ or structure, or separates one part from another.

m., alveolocapillary. Very thin tissue that separates the air inside the pulmonary alveolus from blood in the surrounding capillaries.

m., alveodental. Periodontium, q.v.

m., arachnoid. Middle layer of membranes covering brain and spinal cord.

m., atlanto-occipital. A single midline ligamentous structure that extends from the arch of the atlas to borders of the foramen magnum.

m., basement. A delicate, noncellular membrane underlying a layer of epithelial cells and serving for their support and attachment. SYN: *basement lamina.*

m., basilar. Membrane extending from the tympanic lip of the osseous spiral lamina to the crest of the spiral ligament in the cochlea of the ear. It separates the scala tympani from the cochlear duct and forms supporting structure for the organ of Corti.

m., Bowman's. Thin homogeneous membrane separating corneal epithelium from proper substance of the cornea.

m., Bruch's. Inner layer of the choroid of the eye. SYN: *lamina basalis of choroid.*

m., buccopharyngeal. In the embryo, the membrane that separates the oral cavity from the foregut until the fourth week of development. SYN. *m., oral; m., pharyngeal.*

m., cell. Surface layer of the cytoplasm of a cell. SYN: *m., plasma.*

m., choroid. The choroid, the portion of the vascular tunic or uvea of the eye that extends posteriorly from the ora serrata.

m., costocoracoid. Dense fascia between the pectoralis minor and subclavius muscles.

m., cricothyroid. Membrane connecting thyroid and cricoid cartilages of the larynx.

m., croupous. False yellowish-white membrane in the larynx during croup.

m., decidual. One of the membranes formed in the endometrium of a pregnant uterus. Includes the decidua basalis, decidua capsularis, and decidua parietalis.

m., Descemet's. Elastic membrane forming the lining surface of the cornea. SYN: *m., vitreous.*

m., diphtheritic. Fibrinous false membrane on mucous surfaces in diphtheria.

m., drum. Tympanic membrane.

m., egg. One of the protective membranes or envelopes enclosing an ovum. May be primary (formed by egg itself, e.g., vitelline membrane); secondary (formed by follicle cells, e.g., zona pellucida); or tertiary (formed by oviduct or uterus, e.g., albumin and shell of hen's egg).

m., elastic. One of several membranes formed of elastic connective tissue fibers.

m., enamel. 1. Cuticula dentis. 2. Thin calcified internal layer of cells of the enamel organ.

m., false. Fibrinous exudate on a mucous surface of a membrane, as in diphtheria.

m., fenestrated. A layer of elastic connective tissue possessing minute round or oval openings. Found in tunica intima and tunica media of medium-sized and large arteries. SYN: *m., Henle's elastic.*

m., fetal. One of the membranous structures that serve to protect and support the embryo. The structures are yolk sac, allantois, amnion, chorion, decidua, and placenta.

m., fibrous. Membrane composed entirely of connective tissue. Examples include the fasciae, aponeuroses, perichondrium, periosteum, dura mater, and capsules of some organs.

m., glassy. 1. Transparent capsule that separates membrana granulosa from the theca of the graafian follicle. 2. Internal layer of a hair follicle separating the epithelial and connective tissues.

m., glial. Extremely delicate membrane, formed of foot plates of astrocytes, that surrounds all blood vessels in the brain, spinal cord, and in lining of pia mater separating these vessels from nervous tissue proper. Thought to be one of the components of the blood-brain barrier, q.v.

m., Henle's elastic. M., fenestrated.

m., homogeneous. A fine membrane covering villi of the placenta.

m., Huxley's. SEE: *layer, Huxley's.*

m., hyaline. 1. Basement lamina. 2. Membrane between outer root sheath of a hair follicle and inner fibrous layer.

m., hyaloid. Membrane investing the

vitreous humor of the eye, seen on longitudinal section.

m., hyoglossal. A transverse fibrous lamella uniting tongue to hyoid bone.

m., interosseous. 1. A fibrous membrane in the arm connecting ulna to radius. 2. A fibrous membrane in the leg connecting tibia to fibula.

m., Krause's. Dark membranous band limiting the sarcomere in striated muscle. SYN: *myofibril; Z disk.*

m., limiting, external. 1. Outer layer of cells of the embryonic neural tube. 2. Membrane in retina of eye separating rods and cones from their cell bodies.

m., limiting, internal. 1. Inner layer of ependymal cells lining embryonic neural tube. 2. Glial membrane forming innermost layer of the retina and of the iris.

m., medullary. Endosteum.

m., mucous. Membrane lining cavities and canals communicating with the air and kept moist by secretion of mucus.

m., Nasmyth's. A thin cuticle that consists of the cellular remnants of the enamel organ and the mucopolysaccharide basement membrane that attaches them to the enamel surface. This covering is very friable and usually lost after eruption of the tooth into the oral cavity but may persist in protected areas, such as the labial surface of maxillary incisors. SYN: *m., enamel.*

m., nictitating. A third eyelid present in lower vertebrates and represented in man by a fold of the conjunctiva, the plica semilunaris.

m., nuclear. A two-layered membrane surrounding the nucleus, q.v. Prior to electron microscopy, the nucleus was thought to be surrounded by a single thin membrane.

m., obturator. Fibrous membrane closing the obturator foramen.

m., olfactory. The olfactory portion of the membrane lining the nasal fossa.

m., oral. The buccopharyngeal membrane. SYN: *m., pharyngeal.*

m., oronasal. A double epithelial layer separating the nasal pits from the embryonic oral cavity.

m., otolithic. A layer of gelatinous substance containing otoconia or otoliths, found on the surface of maculae in the inner ear.

m., peridental. Connective tissue between the root of a tooth and the alveolar bone.

m., permeable. A membrane that permits the passage of water and certain substances in solution. SEE: *m., selectively permeable; m., semipermeable.*

m., pharyngeal. The buccopharyngeal membrane. SYN: *m., oral.*

m., placental. The membrane of the placenta that separates the maternal blood from fetal blood.

m., plasma. M., cell.

m., pseudoserous. Membrane resembling a serous membrane but differing in structure as the endothelium.

m., pupillary. Transparent membrane closing the fetal pupil. If it persists after birth it is known as persistent pupillary membrane.

m., pyogenic. Granular lining of an abscess or fistula.

m., quadrangular. Upper portion of the elastic membrane of the larynx.

m., Reissner's. Delicate membrane separating cochlear canal from scala vestibuli.

m., Ruysch's. Middle layer of the choroid membrane of the eye, composed of a close capillary network. SYN: *lamina choriocapillaris* [NA].

m., Scarpa's. The membrane that covers the opening to the fenestra cochleae of the inner ear.

m., schneiderian. Mucosa of the nasal fossae.

m., selectively permeable. A membrane that allows a substance such as water to pass through more readily than another, such as salt or sugar.

m., semipermeable. Membrane that allows passage of water but not substances in solution.

m., serous. Membrane consisting of mesothelium lying on thin layer of connective tissue that lines the closed cavities (peritoneal, pleural, and pericardial) of the body. Surface is moistened by a thin fluid similar to lymph.

m., Shrapnell's. That portion of the tympanic membrane filling the notch of Rivinus.

m., synovial. Membrane lining a joint and secreting synovia.

m., tectorial. Thin, jellylike membrane projecting from vestibular lip of osseous spiral lamina and overlying the spiral organ of Corti of the ear.

m., thyrohyoid. Membrane joining the hyoid bone and the thyroid cartilage.

m., tympanic. Membrane separating the tympanic cavity from the external auditory canal. SYN: *m., drum.*

m., unit. A thin intracellular plasma membrane that has three layers. It can only be visualized by use of electron microscopy.

m., virginal. The hymen.

m., vitelline. Membrane that forms the surface layer of an ovum.

m., vitreous. Descemet's membrane.

m., yolk. A membrane surrounding the ovum. SYN: *vitelline membrane; zona pellucida.*

membranectomy (mĕm″bră-nĕk′tō-mē) [L. *membrana,* membrane, + Gr. *ektome,* excision]. Surgical removal of a membrane.

membranella (mĕm″bră-nĕl′ă). A thin membrane composed of fused cilia.

membrane potential. The electrical potential difference across the membrane of a cell.

membraniform (mĕm-brā′nĭ-form). Resembling or of the nature of a membrane. SYN: *membranoid; membranous.*

membranocartilaginous (mĕm″brăn-ō-kăr-tĭ-lăj′ĭ-nŭs). 1. Pert. to both membrane and cartilage. 2. Derived from both membrane and cartilage.

membranoid (mĕm′bră-noyd) [L. *membrana,* membrane, + Gr. *eidos,* form]. Resembling a membrane. SYN: *membraniform; membranous.*

membranous. Rel. to or resembling a membrane. SYN: *membraniform, membranoid.*

membrum muliebre (mĕm′brŭm mū-lē-ĕ′brē) [L., female member]. The clitoris.

membrum virile (mĕm′brŭm vĭr-ĭl′ē) [L., male member]. The penis.

memory [L. *memoria*]. The mental registration, retention, and recall of past experience, knowledge, ideas, sensations, and thoughts. Registration of experience is favored by clear comprehension during intense consciousness. Retention of memory differs greatly with individuals. Memory recall, esp. its intentional recall, means the reproduction of a memory in consciousness. Clear comprehension greatly favors retention. Recall may fail because the memory has been obliterated or because the stream of ideas is that which one does not wish to remember. Various memory defects occur in many diseases.

Memory is confused or obliterated in maniacal states, lively in paranoia, abolished in senile psychosis and organic brain disease, but undisturbed in depressions. In dementia from senile causes there is accurate memory for remote events but little or none for recent occurrences.

RS: amnesia; anamnesis; association; consciousness; mnemic; mnemonics; recall; retention; retention defect; subconscious.

m., anterograde. Ability to remember events occurring in the remote past but lacking ability to remember recent events. SYN: *amnesia, anterograde.*

m., retrograde. Ability to recall events of recent occurrence but lacking ability to recall knowledge with which patient had previously been familiar. SYN: *amnesia, retrograde.*

menacme (mĕn-ăk′mē) [Gr. *men,* month, + *akme,* top]. The height of the menstrual activity of a woman.

menadiol sodium diphosphate. USP. A synthetic water-soluble vitamin, having same activity as natural vitamin K. Used as an antihemorrhagic agent in hypoprothrombinemia or hemorrhagic disorders due to hypoprothrombinemia. Trade names are Kappadione and Synkayvite.

menadione (mĕn″ă-dī′ōn). USP. A synthetic drug that acts like vitamin K. It is used parenterally in oil, or orally in tablet form.

CAUTION: Menadione powder is irritating to the respiratory tract and skin. In alcoholic solution, it is a vesicant.

m. sodium bisulfite. USP. Synthetic vitamin K. Trade name is Hykinone.

menarchal, menarcheal, menarchial. Pert. to menarche.

menarche (mĕn-ăr′kē) [Gr. *men,* month, + *arche,* beginning]. The initial menstrual period. Occurs normally between the 9th and 17th year. The average age of menarche in the U.S.A. is 12.8 years. SEE: *puberty; adrenarche.*

mendelevium (mĕn-dĕ-lē′vē-ŭm). SYMB: Md. At. wt. 257.0956; at no. 101. A transuranium element.

mendelism (mĕn′dĕl-ĭzm). The principles of heredity expressed in Mendel's laws.

Mendel's laws. [Gregor Johann Mendel, Austrian monk, 1822–1884] Mendel carefully studied the heredity characteristics of garden peas, and was able to explain the transmission of certain traits from one generation to the next.

Some inherited characteristics are controlled by the combination of two units, genes, from the reproductive cells of each parent. Each of these cells, gametes, has a pair of chromosomes that contain the genes for a specific trait at paired locations. Alternate forms of the gene for a specific trait are called alleles. During meiosis, q.v., the cells of each parent divide and contribute half their chromosome complement to the offspring. SEE: *allele; chromosome; gamete; gene.*

Mendel's law of segregation states that as the gametes are formed, the gene pairs separate and do not influence each other.

Mendel's law of dominance resulted from his observation that crossing a tall strain of peas with a short strain resulted in the expression of the dominant trait, in this case tallness. Thus, some alleles will dominate others in physical expression.

Mendel's law of independent assortment states that traits controlled by different gene pairs (such as height and color) pass to the offspring independently of each other.

Mendel's reflex. [Kurt Mendel, Ger. neurologist, 1874–1946] Dorsal flexion of second to fifth toes upon percussion of the dorsum of the foot.

Ménétrier's disease (mān″ă-trē-ārz′). [Pierre Ménétrier, Fr. physician, 1859–1935] Diffuse giant hypertrophic gastritis of unknown etiology.

menhidrosis, menidrosis (mĕn-hī-drō'sĭs, mĕn"ĭ-drō'sĭs) [Gr. *men,* month, + *hidros,* sweat]. Vicarious menstruation through the sweat glands.

Ménière's disease (mān"ē-ārz'). [Prosper Ménière, Fr. physician, 1799–1862] A recurrent and usually progressive group of symptoms including progressive deafness, ringing in the ears, dizziness, and a sensation of fullness or pressure in the ears. SYN: *vertigo, labyrinthine.*

ETIOL: Unknown, but edema of the membranous labyrinth has been found in autopsy studies.

TREATMENT: In acute attacks, bedrest is the most effective treatment. Also antihistamines; discontinuation of smoking; rarely, surgical treatment.

meningeal (mĕn-ĭn'jē-ăl). Rel. to the meninges.

meningeocortical (mĕ-nĭn"jē-ō-kor'tĭ-kăl) [Gr. *meninx,* membrane, + L. *corticalis,* pert. to cortex]. Concerning the meninges and cortex of the brain.

meningeorrhaphy (mĕ-nĭn"jē-or'ă-fē) [" + *rhaphe,* suture]. Suture of membranes, esp. those of the brain and spinal cord.

meninges (mĕn-ĭn'jēz) [Gr.]. (sing. *meninx*) 1. Membranes. 2. [NA] The three membranes investing the spinal cord and brain: the dura mater (external), the arachnoid (middle), and pia mater (internal).

meningioma (mĕn-ĭn"jē-ō'mă) [Gr. *meninx,* membrane, + *oma,* tumor]. A slow-growing tumor that originates in the arachnoidal tissue.

meningiomatosis (mĕ-nĭn"jē-ō-mă-tō'sĭs) [" + " + *osis,* condition]. Multiple meningiomas.

meningism (mĕn-ĭn'jĭzm) [" + *-ismos,* state of]. Irritation of the brain and spinal cord with symptoms simulating meningitis, but without actual inflammation.

meningismus. Meningism.

meningitic (mĕn-ĭn-jĭt'ĭk) [Gr. *meninx,* membrane]. Pert. to meningitis.

meningitis (mĕn-ĭn-jī'tĭs) [" + *itis,* inflammation]. (pl. *meningitides*) Inflammation of the membranes of the spinal cord or brain.

SEE: *choriomeningitis; Kernig's sign; leptomeningitis; pachymeningitis.*

m., acute. SYM: Moderate, irregular fever; loss of appetite; constipation; intense headache; intolerance to light and sound; contracted pupils; delirium; retraction of head; convulsions; and coma.

ETIOL: Caused by bacteria, viruses, or other organisms that reach the meninges from other foci in the body via blood or lymph, through trauma, or from adjacent bony structures (sinuses, mastoid cells).

PROG: Favorable with prompt diagnosis and appropriate therapy.

TREATMENT: Antibiotics such as ampicillin, penicillin G, chloramphenicol, kanamycin, and gentamicin are the drugs of choice if the organism is susceptible. Supportive symptomatic therapy is also indicated

NURSING IMPLICATIONS: Isolate patient for at least 24 hours following initiation of antibiotic therapy. If causative organism is meningococcus, follow strict isolation techniques. Force fluids; provide high-protein diet. Administer antipyretics and tepid sponge baths as ordered. Dispose of drainage and soiled bandages in an appropriate waste container. Assess neurological status at frequent intervals to determine presence of increased intracranial pressure. Provide personal hygiene. Change position frequently and protect bony prominences from injury. Provide dark, quiet atmosphere. Place padded tongue blade at bedside. Pad siderails. Administer analgesics and apply cool compresses to forehead to relieve headache. Administer intravenous fluids or tube feedings as ordered and monitor intake and output. Assess for complications that may include shock, respiratory distress, and intravascular coagulation.

DIET: A fluid diet is necessary during the acute stage, but later as much nourishment should be given as possible. Milk, eggs, beef tea, water, and fruit juices may be given freely. A more solid diet may be given during convalescence. Tube feeding is necessary with stuporous patients; and children and some adults may have to be fed with a spoon or a medicine dropper.

m., acute aseptic. A nonpurulent form of meningitis usually running a short, benign course with recovery. Usually due to viral infection.

m., basilar. Inflammation of the meninges at base of brain, usually due to tuberculosis.

m., cerebral. Acute or chronic meningitis of the brain.

m., cerebrospinal. Meningitis of brain and spinal cord.

m., listeria. Listeriosis.

m., pneumococcal. Meningitis that is caused by the pneumococcus. Common in young children.

m., serosa circumscripta. Meningitis accompanied by the formation of cystic accumulations of fluid that simulate tumors.

m., serous. Meningitis with serous exudation into the cerebral ventricles.

m., spinal. Meningitis of spinal cord membranes.

m., sterile. Meningitis in which infectious organisms are absent. Usually caused by injection of contrast media.

m., traumatic. Meningitis resulting from traumatism or injury.

m., tuberculous. An acute inflammation of the cerebral meninges caused by the tubercle bacillus. Occurs in children.

SYM: Loss of weight, gradual wasting of strength, evening rise of temperature, restlessness, irritability, and sleeplessness may exist for some time before acute symptoms come on. These are severe headache, occasional convulsions, delirium, vomiting, fever, optic neuritis.

meningitophobia (mĕn″ĭn-jĭt″ō-fō′bē-ă) [Gr. *meninx,* membrane, + *phobos,* phobia]. A condition that simulates meningitis and is caused by fear of meningitis.

meningo- (mĕn-ĭn′gō) [Gr. *meninx,* membrane]. A combining form that denotes relationship to the membranes covering the spinal cord or brain.

meningoarteritis (mĕn-ĭn″gō-ăr″tĕr-īt′ĭs) [″ + *arteria,* artery, + *itis,* inflammation]. Inflammatory condition of the meningeal arteries.

meningocele (mĕn-ĭn′gō-sēl) [″ + *kele,* hernia]. Congenital hernia in which the meninges protrude through an opening of the skull or spinal column.

meningococcal polysaccharide vaccine group A. A vaccine used to immunize against meningococci group A during epidemics or to immunize persons traveling to epidemic areas.

meningococcal polysaccharide vaccine group C. A vaccine used to immunize against meningococci group C during epidemics or to immunize persons traveling to epidemic areas. This vaccine is much less effective in children younger than two years of age than it is in older children and adults.

meningococcemia (mĕn-ĭn″gō-kŏk-sē′mē-ă) [″ + *kokkyx,* coccyx, + *haima,* blood]. Meningococci in the circulating blood.

meningococci (mĕn-ĭn″gō-kŏk′sī) Pl. of meningococcus.

meningococcidal (mĕ-nĭng″gō-kŏk-sī′dăl) [″ + ″ + L. *caedere,* to kill]. Lethal to meningococci.

meningococcus (mĕn-ĭn″gō-kŏk′ŭs). (pl. *meningococci*). A microorganism of Neisseria meningitidis, the causative agent of epidemic cerebral meningitis (cerebrospinal fever, spotted fever).

meningocortical (mĕn-ĭn″gō-kor′tĭ-kăl). Pert. to the meninges and the cortex of the brain.

meningocyte (mĕ-nĭng′gō-sīt) [″ + *kytos,* cell]. A macrophage of the meninges of the brain.

meningoencephalitis (mĕn-ĭn″gō-ĕn-sĕf″ă-lī′tĭs) [Gr. *meninx,* membrane, + *enkephalos,* brain, + *itis,* inflammation]. Inflammation of the brain and its meninges. The usual cause is a bacterial infection; but the free-living amebae, such as the Naegleria and Acanthamoeba species, have also caused this condition.

meningoencephalocele (mĕn-ĭn″gō-ĕn-sĕf′ăl-ō-sēl) [″ + ″ + *kele,* hernia]. Hernial protrusion of brain and meninges through a defect in the skull.

meningoencephalomyelitis (mĕn-ĭn″gō-ĕn-sĕf″ăl-ō-mī-ĕl-ī′tĭs) [″ + ″ + *myelos,* marrow, + *itis,* inflammation]. Inflammation of the brain, spinal cord, and their meninges.

meningoencephalopathy (mĕ-nĭng″gō-ĕn-sĕf″ă-lŏp′ă-thē) [″ + ″ + *pathos,* disease]. Disease of the meninges and the brain.

meningomalacia (mĕn-ĭn″gō-mă-lā′shē-ă) [″ + *malakia,* softening]. Softening of any membrane.

meningomyelitis (mĕn-ĭn″gō-mī″ĕl-ī′tĭs) [″ + *myelos,* marrow, + *itis,* inflammation]. Inflammation of spinal cord and its enveloping arachnoid and pia mater, and, less commonly, of the dura mater.

meningomyelocele (mĕn-ĭn″gō-mī-ĕl′ō-sēl) [″ + ″ + *kele,* hernia]. Hernia of the spinal cord and membranes through a defect in the vertebral column.

meningomyeloradiculitis (mĕ-nĭng″gō-mī″ĕ-lō-ră-dĭk″ū-lī′tĭs) [″ + ″ + L. *radicula,* radicle, + Gr. *itis,* inflammation]. Inflammation of the meninges, spinal cord, and the brain.

meningo-osteophlebitis (mĕ-nĭng″gō-ŏs″tē-ō-flē-bī′tĭs) [″ + *osteon,* bone, + *phleps,* vein, + *itis,* inflammation]. Parosteitis and inflammation of the veins of the bone.

meningopathy (mĕn-ĭn-gŏp′ă-thē) [″ + *pathos,* disease]. Any pathological condition of the meninges.

meningoradicular (mĕ-nĭng″gō-ră-dĭk′ū-lăr) [″ + L. *radicula,* radicle]. Concerning the meninges, and the spinal and cerebral nerve roots.

meningoradiculitis (mĕ-nĭng″gō-ră-dĭk″ū-lī′tĭs) [″ + ″ + Gr. *itis,* inflammation]. Inflammation of the meninges and roots of the spinal nerves.

meningorrhachidian (mĕn-ĭn″gō-ră-kĭd′ē-ăn) [″ + *rhachis,* spine]. Concerning the spinal cord and meninges.

meningorrhagia (mĕn-ĭn″gō-rā′jē-ă) [″ + *rhegnynai,* to burst forth]. Hemorrhage of the cerebral or spinal membrane.

meningorrhea (mĕn-ĭn″gō-rē′ă) [″ + *rhoia,* flow]. Effusion of blood on or between the meninges.

meningosis (mĕn″ĭn-gō′sĭs) [″ + *osis,* condition]. The fibrous tissue union of some bones.

meningotyphoid (mĕn-ĭn″gō-tī′foyd). Typhoid fever with symptoms of meningitis.

meningovascular (mĕn-ĭn″gō-văs′kū-lăr). Pert. to blood vessels of the meninges.

meninguria (mĕn″ĭn-gū′rē-ă) [Gr. *meninx,* membrane, + *ouron,* urine]. Presence of membraniform shreds in urine.

meninx (mē'nĭnks) [Gr., membrane]. (pl. *meninges*) [NA] Any membrane, but esp. one of the coverings of the brain or spinal cord.

meniscectomy (mĕn"ĭ-sĕk'tō-mē) [" + *ektome,* excision]. Removal of meniscus cartilage of the knee.

menisci (mĕn-ĭs'ē). Pl. of meniscus.

meniscitis (mĕn"ĭ-sī'tĭs) [Gr. *meniskos,* crescent, + *itis,* inflammation]. Inflamed condition of an interarticular cartilage, esp. the semilunar cartilage of the knee joint.

meniscocyte (mĕn-ĭs'kō-sīt) [" + *kytos,* cell]. A crescent-shaped red blood cell. SYN: *sickle cell.*

meniscocytosis (mĕn-ĭs"kō-sī-tō'sĭs) [" + " + *osis,* intensive]. Sickle cell anemia.

meniscus (mĕn-ĭs'kŭs) [Gr. *meniskos,* crescent]. (pl. *menisci*) 1. Concavoconvex lens. 2. Interarticular fibrocartilage of crescent shape, found in certain joints, esp. the lateral and medial menisci (semilunar cartilages) of the knee joint. 3. The curved upper surface of a liquid in a container. The surface is convex if the liquid does not wet the container and concave if it does.

m. articularis. [NA] Crescent-shaped interarticular fibrocartilage found in certain synovial joints.

menometrorrhagia (mĕn"ō-mĕt-rō-rā'jē-ă) [Gr. *men,* month, + *metra,* womb, + *rhegnynai,* to burst forth]. Irregular or excessive menstrual bleeding. SEE: *menorrhagia; metrorrhagia.*

menopause (mĕn'ō-pawz) [" + *pausis,* cessation]. That period which marks the permanent cessation of menstrual activity. Usually occurs between 35 and 58 years of life. The menses may stop suddenly, there may be a decreased flow each month until there is a final cessation, or the interval between periods may be lengthened until complete cessation is accomplished.

Natural menopause will occur in 25% of women by age 47, in 50% by age 50, 75% by age 52, and in 95% by age 55. Menopause due to surgical removal of the ovaries occurs in almost 30% of U.S. women past age 50. SYN: *change of life; climacteric.*

SYM: The symptoms that may be associated with menopause begin soon following the cessation of ovarian function. This is true whether menopause occurs naturally, or is due to surgical removal of the ovaries, or due to failure of the pituitary gland to function. Symptoms that may last from a few months to years vary from being hardly noticeable to severe. Included are symptoms of vasomotor instability, nervousness, hot flashes, chills, excitability, fatigue, apathy, mental depression, crying following circumstances that would not normally cause that reaction, insomnia, palpitation, vertigo, headache, numbness, tingling, myalgia, urinary disturbances such as frequency and incontinence, and various disorders of the gastrointestinal system.

Hot flashes, or hot flushes, may start with an aura followed by a feeling of discomfort in the abdominal area, perhaps a chill quickly followed by a feeling of heat moving toward the head. Next the face becomes red, and sweating is followed by exhaustion. The cause, or causes, of hot flashes is not completely understood and is controversial.

TREATMENT: Hormone replacement as required. However, the use of estrogen as a cure-all in treating the symptoms of menopause has been seriously questioned due to the possibility of undesired side effects. Yearly pelvic examination to include Papanicolaou test for cancer of the cervix.

m., artificial. Menopause occurring subsequent to surgical castration, x-ray irradiation, or radium implantation into the uterus.

m., premature. Natural or artificial menopause occurring before age 35.

m., surgical. A form of artificial menopause that follows surgical removal of the ovaries.

menophania (mĕn-ō-fā'nē-ă) [Gr. *men,* month, + *phainesthai,* to appear]. First appearance of the menses at puberty.

menoplania (mĕn-ō"plā'nē-ă) [" + *plane,* deviation]. Menstruation through other than the normal outlet, as through the nose. SYN: *vicarious menstruation.*

menorrhagia (mĕn"ō-rā'jē-ă) [" + *rhegnynai,* to burst forth]. Excessive bleeding at the time of a menstrual period, either in number of days or amount of blood or both. SEE: *hemorrhage, uterine.*

ETIOL: Endocrine disturbances: pituitary gland, thyroid, and ovary. General systemic diseases: hypertension, diabetes mellitus, blood dyscrasias, chronic nephritis. Malpositions of the uterus: retroversion and retroflexion. New growths of the uterus: particularly fibroids of the intramural and submucous types, adenomyosis of the uterus, fibrosis of the uterus with hyperplastic changes of the endometrium. Conditions of the cervix uteri: erosions or polypi. Inflammations in the pelvis: acute salpingitis, acute metritis, acute endometritis, chronic metritis, and endometritis.

menorrhalgia (mĕn-ō-răl'jē-ă) [" + *rhoia,* flow, + *algia,* pain]. Painful menstruation or pelvic pain accompanying menstruation, sometimes a symptom of endometriosis. SYN: *dysmenorrhea.*

menorrhea (mĕn"ō-rē'ă). 1. Normal menstruation. 2. Free or profuse menstruation. SYN: *menorrhagia.*

menostasis (mĕn-ŏs′tă-sĭs) [″ + *stasis*, halt]. Suppression of the menses.

menostaxis (mĕn″ō-stăk′sĭs) [″ + *staxis*, dripping]. Prolonged menstruation.

menotropins (mĕn″ō-trō′pĭns). USP. Combination of follicle-stimulating and luteinizing hormones (FSH and LH) used to promote growth and maturation of the follicle of the ovary. Menotropins is obtained from the urine of postmenopausal women and a standard extract is used with human chorionic gonadotropin (HCG) to induce ovulation. Trade names are Humegon and Pregova.

menoxenia (mĕn-ŏk-sē′nē-ă) [″ + *xenos*, strange]. Abnormal menstruation.

menses (mĕn′sēz) [L., month]. Monthly flow of bloody fluid from the uterine mucous membrane.

menstrual (mĕn′stroo-ăl) [L. *menstrualis*]. Pert. to menstruation. SYN: *catamenial*.

menstrual cycle. The periodically recurrent series of changes occurring in the uterus and associated sex organs (ovaries, cervix, and vagina) associated with menstruation and the intermenstrual period. The human cycle averages 28 days in length, measured from the beginning of menstruation. The menstrual cycle is, however, quite variable in length even in the same person from month to month. Variations in the length of the cycle are due principally to variation in the length of the proliferative phase.

The menstrual cycle is divided into four phases characterized by histological changes that take place in the uterine endometrium. They are:

Proliferative Phase: Uterine epithelium is restored to normal; endometrium becomes thicker and more vascular; glands elongate. During this period the ovarian follicle is maturing and secreting estrogens. Period is terminated by rupture of follicle and liberation of ovum at about 14 days before next menstrual period begins.

Luteal or Secretory Phase: Endometrium increases in thickness; glands become more tortuous and produce an abundant secretion containing glycogen. Coiled arteries make their appearance; endometrium becomes edematous; stroma becomes compact. During this period the corpus luteum in an ovary is developing and secreting progesterone. Lasts 10 to 14 days.

Premenstrual or Ischemic Phase: A day or two before menstruation, coiled arteries constrict and endometrium becomes anemic and shrinks. Corpus luteum of ovary begins involution. Phase lasts about two days and is terminated by opening up of constricted arteries, the breaking off of small patches of necrotic endometrium, and the beginning of menstruation with the flow of menstrual fluid.

Menstruation: Period of uterine bleeding accompanied by shedding of the endometrium. Averages 4 to 5 days in length.

menstrual extraction. Vacuum or suction curettage of the uterus done just prior to the date of the next menstrual period. The procedure, which is done by using carefully controlled suction and a soft flexible catheter, is used to be certain the menstrual period is induced even though in a sexually active individual the uterus may contain a fertilized ovum.

menstrual regulation. Vacuum or suction curettage of the uterus done within the first two weeks following the expected date of the onset of menstruation. If the amenorrhea was due to pregnancy, the procedure is classed as a form of fertility control.

menstruant (mĕn′stroo-ănt) [L. *menstruare*, to discharge the menses]. 1. In the condition of menstruating. 2. One who menstruates.

menstruate (mĕn′stroo-āt). To discharge menses.

menstruation (mĕn-stroo-ā′shŭn) [L. *menstruare*, to discharge the menses]. The periodic discharge of a bloody fluid from the uterus occurring at more or less regular intervals during the life of a woman from age of puberty to menopause. The discharge contains altered blood with normal, hemolyzed, and sometimes agglutinated, red blood cells; disintegrated endometrial and stroma cells; and secretions of glands. In general, menstrual blood does not coagulate, but the passage of occasional clots is not unusual. Menstruation is brought on by the reduction in production of ovarian hormones, esp. progesterone, that results from involution of the corpus luteum following failure of the ovum to become fertilized. SEE: *menstrual cycle; ovary* for illus.

Menstruation has its onset at puberty (9 to 17 years of age). Length of flow varies from 3 to 7 days (av. 4 to 5 days). It occurs on an average every 27 to 28 days, although time may vary from 18 to 40 days. Menstruation ceases during pregnancy; may or may not cease during lactation; and ceases permanently with the completion of menopause. Its failure to occur may result from congenital abnormalities, physical disorders (disease, obesity, malnutrition), emotional or hormonal disturbances, esp. diseases involving the ovaries, hypophysis, thyroid, or adrenal glands.

Menstrual irregularities: Absence of flow when normally expected is called *amenorrhea;* scanty flow is known as *oligomenorrhea;* painful menstruation is *dysmenorrhea.* Excessive loss of blood is termed *menorrhagia;* loss of blood during intermenstrual periods is known as spotting or *metrorrhagia.*

m., anovulatory. Menstruation occurring without discharge of ovum, i.e., ovulation, from ovary.

m., retrograde. Backflow of menstrual fluid through fallopian tubes into peritoneal cavity.

m., suppressed. Failure of menstruation to occur when normally expected.

m., vicarious. Menstruation from site other than the uterus when menstrual flow is expected.

menstruous (mĕn'stroo-ŭs). Rel. to menstruation.

menstruum (mĕn'stroo-ŭm) [L. *menstruus,* menstrual fluid; once it was believed that this fluid had solvent qualities]. A solvent; a medium. SEE: *vehicle.*

mensual (mĕn'sū-ăl) [L. *mensis,* month]. Monthly.

mensuration (mĕn-sū-rā'shŭn) [L. *mensuratio*]. The process of measuring.

Menta-Bal. Trade name for mephobarbital, USP.

mentagrophyton (mĕn"tă-grŏf'ĭ-tŏn) [L. *mentagra,* sycosis, + Gr. *phyton,* plant]. Former name for the fungus that causes infection in the hair of the scalp and beard and in the skin and nails. SEE: *Trichophyton.*

mental. 1. [L. *mens,* mind] Rel. to the mind. 2. [L. *mentum,* chin]. Rel. to the chin.

mental age. ABBR: MA. Age of a person with respect to the intellectual development as contrasted with the chronological age.

mental deficiency. Mental retardation.

mental disorder. An imprecise and quite general term, but it may be described briefly as a clinically significant behavioral or psychological syndrome or pattern that is typically associated with either a distressing symptom or impairment of function. It is important to bear in mind that individuals described as having the same mental disorder are not alike in the way they react to their illness and how they will need to be treated.

mental fog. Clouding of consciousness, usually with some loss of memory.

mental hygiene. Science of maintaining healthy mental and emotional responses and preventing development of psychoses.

mental illness. Any disorder that affects the mind or behavior.

mental retardation. Below normal intellectual function that has its cause or onset during the developmental period and usually in the first years after birth. There is impaired learning, social adjustment, and maturation. The causes may be but do not have to be genetic. Rubella in the first trimester of pregnancy may be associated with mental retardation. Intrauterine trauma or infection may also cause this condition. The degree of intellectual impairment is classed on the basis of the Wechsler I.Q. scale as follows: 1. Mild, I.Q. 69–55. These children are educable. 2. Moderate, I.Q. 54–40. These children are trainable. 3. Severe, I.Q. 39–25. 4. Profound, I.Q. below 25.

mentality. Mental power or activity.

mentation (mĕn-tā'shŭn). Mental activity. During sleep it is possible to determine the level of mental activity by studying eye movements observed through the closed eyelids and by monitoring the electrical activity of the brain by use of electroencephalography. SEE: *R.E.M.*

Mentha [L.]. Mint; a genus of labiate plants.

M. piperita. Peppermint.

M. pulegium. Pennyroyal.

M. viridis. Spearmint.

menthol. USP. $C_{10}H_{20}O$. An alcohol obtained from oil of peppermint or other mint oils. May be prepared synthetically. Occurs in crystalline form. It is an antipruritic.

menton (mĕn'tŏn) [L. *mentum,* chin]. Gnathion, q.v.

mentulagra (mĕn"tū-lăg'ră) [L. *mentula,* penis, + Gr. *agra,* seizure]. Painful involuntary erection of the penis, sometimes curved. SYN: *priapism.* SEE: *chordee.*

mentulate (mĕn'tū-lāt) [L. *mentula,* penis]. Possessing a large penis.

mentulomania (mĕn"tū-lō-mā'nē-ă) [" + Gr. *mania,* madness]. Mental state characterized by addiction to masturbation.

mentum [L.]. [NA] The chin. SYN: *genion.*

mepacrine hydrochloride (mĕp'ă-krĭn). Quinacrine hydrochloride, USP. An antimalarial drug. Trade name is Atabrine.

mepazine (mĕp'ă-zēn). An antipsychotic drug.

mepenzolate bromide (mĕ-pĕn'zō-lāt). USP. An anticholinergic drug used as an antispasmodic in treating peptic ulcer. Its action mimics belladonna. Trade name is Cantil.

meperidine hydrochloride (mĕ-pĕr'ĭ-dēn). USP. A narcotic analgesic sold under the trade names of Demerol and Pethadol.

mephenesin (mĕ-fĕn'ĕ-sĭn). Chemical formerly used as a skeletal muscle relaxant.

mephentermine sulfate (mĕ-fĕn'tĕr-mēn). USP. A drug used for its pressor effect in treating hypotension. Trade name for mephentermine sulfate is Wyamine Sulfate.

mephenytoin (mĕ-fĕn'ĭ-tō-ĭn). USP. An anticonvulsive drug that is used in the lowest concentration possible in combination with other drugs. This is done because of its toxicity. Trade name is Mesantoin.

mephitic [L. *mephiticus, mephitis,* foul exhalation]. Noxious, foul, as a poisonous odor.

mephobarbital (mĕf"ō-băr'bĭ-tăl). USP. A

hypnotic and sedative drug of the barbiturate class. Trade names are Mebaral and Menta-Bal.

Mephyton. Trade name for phytonadione, USP.

mepivacaine hydrochloride (mĕ-pĭv′ă-kān). USP. A local anesthetic drug. Trade name is Carbocaine.

meprednisone (mĕ-prĕd′nĭ-sōn). USP. An adrenocorticosteroid drug. Trade name is Betapar.

meprobamate (mĕ-prō′bă-māt). USP. A tranquilizing agent, used for relief of anxiety and mental tension. Trade names are Equanil, Miltown, and Meprospan. SEE: *Poisons and Poisoning* in *Appendix*.

Meprospan. Trade name for meprobamate, USP.

meprylcaine hydrochloride (mĕp′rĭl-kān). USP. A local anesthetic drug.

mEq. *milliequivalent.*

meralgia (mĕr-ăl′jē-ă) [Gr. *meros,* thigh, + *algos,* pain]. Pain in the thigh.

m. paresthetica. Paresthesia and disturbed sensation of the lateral area of the thigh; due to injury to the external cutaneous femoral nerve.

merbromin (mĕr-brō′mĭn). An organic mercury compound used as a topical antiseptic. Its effectiveness is doubtful. Trade name is Mercurochrome.

mercaptan (mĕr-kăp′tăn). Any organic chemical that contains the ⁻SH radical. They are formed when the oxygen of an alcohol is replaced by sulfur.

mercaptomerin sodium injection (mĕr-kăp″tō-mĕr′ĭn). USP. A diuretic of the organomercurial type. Trade name is Thiomerin.

mercaptopurine (mĕr-kăp″tō-pū′rēn). USP. An antineoplastic and immunosuppressive agent used in treating acute leukemia. Trade name is Purinethol.

Mercier's bar (mĕr-sē-āz′). [Louis A. Mercier, Fr. urologist, 1811–1882] A curved fold at neck of bladder forming posterior margin of trigonum vesicae.

mercurial (mĕr-kū′rē-ăl) [L. *mercurialis*]. 1. Pert. to mercury. 2. A substance containing mercury.

mercurial diuretics. A class of organic mercurial compounds that produce diuresis.

mercurialism (mĕr-kū′rē-ăl-ĭzm) [L. *mercurius,* mercury, + Gr. *-ismos,* state of]. Chronic poisoning by mercury. Seen as a result of continuous administration of mercury or occurs in workmen who work with the metal or inhale its vapors.

SYM: Soreness of gums and loosening of teeth; increased salivation; fetor of breath; griping, and diarrhea.

mercurialized (mĕr-kū′rē-ăl-īzd). 1. Impregnated with mercury. 2. Influenced by or treated with mercury.

mercurial palsy. Paralysis induced by mercury poisoning.

mercurial rash. Rash caused by local application of mercurial preparations.

mercuric (mĕr-kū′rĭk). Rel. to bivalent mercury.

m. chloride. $HgCl_2$. A common compound of mercury used in the past as a topical antiseptic.

m. oxide, yellow. HgO. A powder, usually yellow in color. Previously used in ointments as an antibacterial agent.

mercuric chloride poisoning. SEE: *Poisons and Poisoning* in *Appendix.*

SYM: *Acute:* Those of any severe gastrointestinal irritation with pain, cramping, constriction of the throat, vomiting, and a metallic taste in the mouth. Stronger solution causes a white coating due to coagulation. Abdominal pain may be so severe as to cause fainting, bloody diarrhea, bloody vomitus, scanty urine, prostration, convulsions, and unconsciousness. Death is the usual outcome unless treatment is begun immediately.

Chronic: Bad breath, loosening of teeth, fever, urinary difficulties, nausea, diarrhea, sore tongue, paralysis, weakness, and death.

F.A.: Evacuate stomach, wash out with milk or with a baking soda solution made by dissolving a teaspoonful of sodium bicarbonate in 6 oz. (177 ml.) of water. Treatment with BAL (British anti-lewisite) should begin as soon as possible after poisoning has occurred. Maintain fluid and electrolyte balance.

Mercurochrome. Trade name for merbromin.

mercurous (mĕr-kū′rŭs, mĕr′kū-rŭs). Rel. to monovalent mercury.

m. chloride. HgCl. A heavy white powder used in small doses in medicine as a laxative. It is used in powder form as an application in ulcers and skin rashes.

mercurous chloride poisoning. SEE: *mercuric chloride* in *Poisons and Poisoning* in *Appendix*. SYM: Salivation, abdominal discomfort, and diarrhea.

mercury (mĕr′kū-rē) [L. *mercurius*]. A metallic element. SYMB: Hg. At. wt. 200.59; at. no. 80. Insoluble in ordinary solvents but soluble in hydrochloric acid upon boiling. It is a silvery liquid at ordinary temperatures. Forms two series of salts: mercurous, in which it has a valence of one (univalent), and mercuric, in which it has a valence of two (bivalent). SYN: *hydrargyrum; quicksilver.*

NOTE: Metallic mercury swallowed in small quantities, as from a broken thermometer, is not harmful.

m., ammoniated. USP. A topical antiseptic used in treating certain skin diseases.

CAUTION: Chronic use can cause mercury poisoning.

m. bichloride. $HgCl_2$. Corrosive sublimate that is no longer used in medicine.

m. chloride, mild. Mercurous chloride. SYN: *calomel.*

mercury poisoning. SYM: In large doses, increased salivation, abdominal cramps, and interference with kidney function. SEE: *mercuric chloride; mercuric chloride* in *Poisons and Poisoning* in *Appendix.*

meridian (mĕ-rĭd'ē-ăn). An imaginary line encircling a globular body at right angles to its equator and passing through the poles, or a half of such a line.

m. of eye. A circle passing through anterior and posterior poles of the eyeball.

merinthophobia (mĕr-ĭn"thō-fō'bē-ă) [Gr. *merinthos,* a cord, + *phobia,* fear]. Morbid fear of being tied.

merispore (mĕr'ĭ-spor) [Gr. *meros,* a part, + *sporos,* seed]. A secondary spore resulting from the division of another spore.

meristic (mĕr-ĭs'tĭk) [Gr. *meristikos,* fit for dividing]. Bilaterally symmetrical.

mero- [Gr. *meros*]. Combining form meaning a part.

meroacrania (mĕr"ō-ă-krā'nē-ă) [" + *a-,* not, + *kranion,* skull]. Congenital absence of a part of the cranium.

meroblastic (mĕr-ō-blăst'ĭk) [" + *blastos,* germ]. Pert. to a type of ovum containing considerable yolk or a type of cleavage in which cleavage divisions are restricted to the protoplasmic region of the animal pole. SEE: *holoblastic ova.*

merocele (mĕr'ō-sēl) [" + *kele,* hernia]. Femoral hernia.

merocoxalgia (mĕr"ō-kŏk-săl'jē-ă) [" + L. *coxa,* hip, + Gr. *algos,* pain]. Painful condition of the thigh and hip.

merocrine (mĕr'ō-krĭn) [" + *krinein,* to separate]. Pert. to a type of secretion in which the glandular cell remains intact during the process of elaborating and discharging its product. SEE: *apocrine; eccrine; holocrine.*

merodiastolic (mĕr"ō-dī-ă-stŏl'ĭk). Concerning a part of diastole of the cardiac cycle.

meroergasia (mĕr"ō-ĕr-gā'zē-ă) [Gr. *meros,* a part, + *ergasia,* work]. Partial mental disorder with symptoms of emotional instability. SEE: *holergasia.*

merogenesis (mĕr"ō-jĕn'ĕ-sĭs) [" + *genesis,* production]. Multiplication or reproduction by segmentation.

merogony (mĕ-rŏg'ō-nē) [" + *gonos,* procreation]. Incomplete development of fragments of an ovum.

meromelia (mĕr"ō-mē'lē-ă) [" + *melos,* limb]. Partial absence of a limb.

meromicrosomia (mĕr"ō-mī"krō-sō'mē-ă) [" + *mikros,* small, + *soma,* body]. Abnormal smallness of some part or structure of the body.

meromyosin (mĕr"ō-mī'ō-sĭn). That produced by tryptic digestion of myosin.

meronecrosis (mĕr"ō-nĕk-rō'sĭs) [" + *nekrosis,* deadness]. Death of cells.

meropia (mĕr-ō'pē-ă) [" + *ops,* vision]. Partial blindness.

merorrhachischisis (mĕ"rō-rā-kĭs'kĭ-sĭs) [" + *rhachis,* spine, + *schisis,* fissure]. Fissure of a portion of the spinal cord.

merosmia (mĕr-ŏs'mē-ă) [" + *osme,* odor]. Inability to detect certain odors.

merosystolic (mĕr"ō-sĭs-tŏl'ĭk) [" + *systole,* a contraction]. Rel. to a portion of the systole.

merotomy (mĕr-ŏt'ō-mē) [" + *tome,* incision]. Division into sections or segments.

merozoite (mĕr"ō-zō'īt) [" + *zoon,* animal]. A body formed by segmentation or breaking up of schizont in asexual reproduction of certain sporozoans such as Plasmodium. Merozoites when formed are liberated and invade other corpuscles, where they repeat the process of schizogony, or develop into gametocytes.

merozygote (mĕr"ō-zī'gōt) [" + *zygotos,* yoked together]. A bacterial mechanism of gene transfer in which part of the genome, or chromosome complement, is transferred into an intact recipient cell.

Merthiolate. Trade name for thimerosal.

Meruvax. Trade name for rubella virus vaccine, live.

mesad (mē'săd) [Gr. *mesos,* middle, + L. *ad,* toward]. Toward a median point, line, or plane.

mesal (mē'săl). In a middle line or plane.

mesangium (mĕs-ăn'jē-ŭm). The suspensory structure of the renal glomerulus.

Mesantoin. Trade name for mephenytoin, USP.

mesaortitis (mĕs"ā-or-tī'tĭs) [" + *aorte,* aorta + *itis,* inflammation]. Inflammation of the middle aortic coat.

mesaraic, mesareic (mĕs-ă-rā'ĭk, -rī'ĭk) [Gr. *mesaraion,* the mesentery]. Rel. to the mesentery. SYN: *mesenteric.*

mesarteritis (mĕs-ăr-tĕr-ī'tĭs). Inflammation of the tunica media or middle coat of an artery.

mesaticephalic (mĕs-ăt"ĭ-sĕf-ăl'ĭk) [Gr. *mesatos,* medium, + *kephale,* brain]. Having a skull with a cephalic index of 75 to 79.9 degrees.

mesatipellic, mesatipelvic (mĕs-ăt"ĭ-pĕl'lĭk, -pĕl'vĭk) [" + *pella,* bowl]. Having a pelvis with an index between 90 and 95 degrees.

mescaline (mĕs'kă-lēn). A poisonous alkaloid, the active ingredient of the mescal cactus, that causes hallucinations, esp. those involving color and music.

mescalism (mĕs'kă-lĭzm). Intoxication produced by ingesting mescal.

mesectic (mĕs-ĕk'tĭk) [Gr. *mesos,* middle, + *echein,* to hold]. Using an average amount of oxygen. SEE: *mionectic.*

mesectoderm (mĕs-ĕk′tō-derm). Migratory cells derived from ectoderm, esp. from the neural crest of the cephalic area in young embryos; they become pigment cells.

mesencephalitis (mĕs″ĕn-sĕf″ă-lī′tĭs) [″ + *enkephalos,* brain, + *itis,* inflammation]. Inflammation of the mesencephalon.

mesencephalon (mĕs-ĕn-sĕf′ă-lŏn) [″ + *enkephalos,* brain]. [NA] The midbrain, one of three primitive cerebral vesicles from which develop the corpora quadrigemina, the crura cerebri, and the aqueduct of Sylvius.

mesencephalotomy (mĕs″ĕn-sĕf″ă-lŏt′ō-mē) [″ + ″ + *tome,* incision]. Surgical incision of the midbrain. Usually done to relieve intractable pain.

mesenchyme (mĕs′ĕn-kīm) [″ + *enchyma,* infusion]. A diffuse network of cells forming the embryonic mesoderm and giving rise to connective tissues, blood and blood vessels, the lymphatic system, and cells of the reticuloendothelial system.

mesenchymoma (mĕs″ĕn-kī-mō′mă). A neoplasm containing a mixture of mesenchymal and fibrous tissue.

mesenterectomy (mĕs″ĕn-tĕ-rĕk′tō-mē) [″ + *enteron,* intestine, + *ektome,* excision]. Surgical removal of the mesentery.

mesenteric (mĕs″ĕn-tĕr′ĭk) [Gr. *mesenterikos*]. Pert. to the mesentery. SYN: *mesaraic.*

mesenteriolum (mĕs-ĕn″tĕr-ī′ō-lŭm) [L.]. A small mesentery, as that of a diverticulum of the intestine.

mesenteriopexy (mĕs″ĕn-tĕr′ē-ō-pĕk″sē) [″ + *enteron,* intestine, + *pexis,* fixation]. Operation for attaching a torn mesentery.

mesenteriorrhaphy (mĕs″ĕn-tĕr-ē-or′ă-fē) [″ + ″ + *rhaphe,* suture]. Suturing of the mesentery. SYN: *mesorrhaphy.*

mesenteriplication (mĕs″ĕn-tĕr″ĭ-plĭ-kā′shŭn) [″ + ″ + L. *plicare,* to fold]. Shortening the mesentery by taking tucks in it surgically.

mesenteritis (mĕs″ĕn-tĕr-ī′tĭs) [″ + ″ + *itis,* inflammation]. Inflamed condition of the mesentery.

mesenterium (mĕs″ĕn-tē′rē-ŭm). Mesentery.

mesenteron (mĕs-ĕn′tĕr-ŏn). Middle portion of the embryonic digestive tract.

mesentery (mĕs′ĕn-tĕr″ē) [″ + *enteron,* intestine]. A peritoneal fold encircling the greater part of the small intestines and connecting the intestine to the posterior abdominal wall.

MESH. *Me*dical *S*ubject *H*eadings. A list of the medical words used in storing and retrieving medical references by the U.S. National Library of Medicine. SEE: *MEDLARS.*

mesiad (mē′zē-ăd) [″ + L. *ad,* toward]. Toward the median plane of a body or part. SYN: *mesad.*

mesial (mē′zē-ăl). Located near the median plane of the body. SYN: *median.*

mesio- [Gr. *mesos,* middle]. In dentistry, combining form meaning pert. to or facing the median plane of the mouth.

mesiobuccal (mē″zē-ō-bŭk′kăl). Concerning the mesial and buccal surfaces of a tooth or the surfaces involved in a cavity in the tooth.

mesiobucco-occlusal (mē″zē-ō-bŭk″kō-ŏ-kloo′zăl). Concerning the mesial, buccal, and occlusal surfaces of a tooth.

mesiobuccopulpal (mē″zē-ō-bŭk″kō-pŭl′păl). Concerning the mesial, buccal, and pulpal sides of a tooth cavity.

mesiocervical (mē″zē-ō-sĕr′vĭ-kăl). Concerning the mesial surface of the neck of a tooth.

mesioclusion (mē″zē-ō-kloo′zhŭn). Malocclusion of the lower teeth. They are in a position in front of the position they are normally in with respect to the upper teeth.

mesiodens (mē′zē-ō-dĕnz). A supernumerary tooth between the maxillary and central incisors and on the palatal side of the maxilla.

mesiodistal (mē″zē-ō-dĭs′tăl). Concerning the mesial and distal surfaces of a tooth.

mesiogingival (mē″zē-ō-jĭn′jĭ-văl). Concerning the mesial and gingival walls of a tooth cavity.

mesiolabial (mē″zē-ō-lā′bē-ăl). Concerning the mesial and labial surfaces of a tooth or cavity.

mesiolingual (mē″zē-ō-lĭng′gwăl). Concerning the mesial and lingual surfaces of a tooth or cavity.

mesiolinguo-occlusal (mē″zē-ō-lĭng″gwō-ŏ-kloo′zăl). Concerning the mesial, lingual, and occlusal surfaces of a tooth.

mesiolinguopulpal (mē″zē-ō-lĭng″gwō-pŭl′păl). Concerning the mesial, lingual, and pulpal sides of a tooth cavity.

mesion (mē′sē-ŏn) [Gr. *mesos,* middle]. The imaginary plane dividing the body into right and left symmetric halves. SYN: *meson* (def. 2).

mesiopulpal (mē″zē-ō-pŭl′păl). Concerning the mesial and pulpal sides of a tooth cavity.

mesioversion (mē″zē-ō-vĕr′zhŭn). Displacement of a tooth posteriorly in the dental arch.

mesiris (mĕs-ī′rĭs). Middle portion of the iris.

mesmeric (mĕs-mĕr′ĭk). [Franz Anton Mesmer, Austrian physician, 1734–1815] Rel. to or induced by hypnotism.

mesmerism (mĕs′mĕr-ĭzm). Originally Mesmer's theory of animal magnetism, it now means therapeutics employing hypnotism or hypnotic suggestion.

meso- [Gr. *mesos,* middle]. Combining form meaning (1) middle; (2) in anatomy, pert. to a mesentery; (3) in medicine, secondary or partial.

mesoappendicitis. Inflamed condition of the mesoappendix.

mesoappendix (mĕs″ō-ă-pĕn′dĭks) [Gr. *mesos,* middle + L. *appendix,* an appendage]. [NA] Mesentery of the vermiform appendix.
mesoarium (mĕs″ō-ā′rē-ŭm). Mesovarium, q.v.
mesoblast (mĕs′ō-blăst) [″ + *blastos,* germ]. Mesoderm.
mesobronchitis (mĕs″ō-brŏng-kī′tĭs). Inflammation of the middle layer of the bronchi.
mesocardia (mĕs″ō-kăr′dē-ă) [″ + *kardia,* heart]. Location of the heart in the middle line of the thorax, being a normal position in fetal stage but a malposition after birth.
mesocardium (mĕs-ō-kăr′dē-ŭm). An embryonic mesentery supporting the heart. The dorsal mesocardium connects the heart to the foregut and the ventral mesocardium connects the heart to the central body wall.
mesocarpal (mĕs″ō-kăr′păl). Mediocarpal.
mesocecum (mĕs″ō-sē′kŭm) [″ + L. *caecum,* blindness]. Part of the mesentery that connects the cecum to the right iliac fossa.
mesocele (mĕs′ō-sēl) [″ + *koilia,* hollow]. Sylvian aqueduct in the brain.
mesocephalic (mĕs″ō-sĕ-făl′ĭk) [″ + *kephale,* head]. 1. Pert. to the midbrain. 2. Having a medium-sized head, with a cranial index of 76.0 to 80.9.
mesocephalon (mĕs″ō-sĕf′ă-lŏn). The mesencephalon, q.v.
mesocolic (mĕs″ō-kŏl′ĭk). Concerning the mesocolon.
mesocolon (mĕs″ō-kō′lŏn) [″ + *kolon,* colon]. [NA] Mesentery connecting the colon with the posterior abdominal wall.
mesocolopexy (mĕs″ō-kō′lō-pĕk″sē) [″ + ″ + *pexis,* fixation]. The taking of tucks in the mesocolon and then suturing it to make it shorter in order to correct unneeded mobility and ptosis.
mesocoloplication (mĕs″ō-kō″lō-plī-kā′shŭn) [″ + ″ + L. *plicare,* to fold]. Plication of the mesocolon in order to stabilize it.
mesocord. A portion of umbilical cord attached to the placenta by means of an amniotic fold.
mesocuneiform (mĕs″ō-kū′nē-ĭ-form). The intermediate cuneiform bone of the ankle.
mesoderm (mĕs′ō-dĕrm) [″ + *derma,* skin]. A primary germ layer of the embryo lying between ectoderm and entoderm. From it arise all connective tissues; muscular, skeletal, circulatory, lymphatic, and urogenital systems; and the linings of the body cavities. SEE: *ectoderm; entoderm.*

m., axial. That portion of the mesoderm that gives rise to the notochord and prechordal plate.

m., extraembryonic. Mesoderm lying outside the embryo proper. It is involved in formation of amnion, chorion, yolk sac, and body stalk.

m., intermediate. Mesoderm lying between somite and lateral mesoderm. Gives rise to embryonic and definitive kidneys and their ducts. SYN: *mesomere, nephrotome.*

m., lateral. Unsegmented mesoderm lying lateral to the intermediate mesoderm. In it develops a cavity, the coelom, separating it into layers, the somatic and splanchnic mesoderm. SYN: *hypomere.*

m., paraxial. Mesoderm lying immediately lateral to the neural tube and notochord.

m., somatic. Outer layer of lateral mesoderm. Becomes intimately associated with ectoderm, forming the somatopleure, from which ventral and lateral walls of the embryo develop.

m., splanchnic. Inner layer of lateral mesoderm. Becomes intimately associated with entoderm, forming the splanchnopleure, from which the gut and lungs and their coverings arise.

mesodiastolic (mĕs″ō-dī″ă-stŏl′ĭk). In mid-diastole of the heart beat sequence.
mesodont (mĕs′ō-dŏnt). To have teeth of medium size; a dental index of 42 to 43.9.
mesoduodenum (mĕs″ō-dū″ō-dē′nŭm). Mesentery connecting the duodenum to the abdominal wall.
mesoepididymis (mĕs″ō-ĕp″ĭ-dĭd′ĭ-mĭs). A fold of the tunica vaginalis that is not always present. It binds the epididymis to the testicle.
mesogastric (mĕs″ō-găs′trĭk). 1. Pert. to umbilical region. 2. Pert. to the mesogastrium.
mesogastrium (mĕs″ō-găs′trē-ŭm) [″ + *gaster,* belly]. 1. [NA] The umbilical region. 2. The part of the mesentery of the embryo attached to the primitive stomach.
mesoglia (mĕ-sŏg′lē-ă). Phagocytes present in the neuroglia. They probably arise in the mesoderm.
mesogluteal (mĕs″ō-gloo′tē-ăl). Concerning the gluteus medius muscle.
mesogluteus (mĕs″ō-gloo′tē-ŭs). The gluteus medius muscle.
mesognathic (mĕs″ŏg-nă′thĭk) [″ + *gnathos,* jaw]. Having a gnathic index between 98 and 103.
mesognathion (mĕs-ŏg-nā′thē-ŏn). The intermaxillary or premaxillary bone.
mesohyloma (mĕs″ō-hī-lō′mă) [Gr. *mesos,* middle, + *hyle,* matter, + *oma,* tumor]. Tumor derived from the mesothelium.
meso-ileum (mĕs″ō-ĭl′ē-ŭm). Mesentery of the ileum.
mesojejunum (mĕs″ō-jē-jū′nŭm). Mesentery of the jejunum.
mesolymphocyte (mĕs″ō-lĭm′fō-sīt). A moderate-sized lymphocyte.
mesomere (mĕs′ō-mēr) [″ + *meros,* part]. 1. Portion of mesoderm between epimere and hypomere. SYN: *nephrotome; mesoderm, in-*

termediate. 2. A blastomere that is intermediate in size between a micromere and a macromere.

mesometritis (mĕs-ō-mē-trī'tĭs) [" + *metra,* uterus, + *itis,* inflammation]. Inflammation of the uterine musculature. SYN: *myometritis.*

mesometrium (mĕs"ō-mē'trē-ŭm). 1. The uterine musculature. 2. [NA] The broad ligament below the mesovarium.

mesomorph (mĕs'ō-morf). Body build characterized by predominance of tissues derived from the mesoderm; a well-proportioned individual. SEE: *ectomorph; endomorph; somatotype.*

meson (mĕs'ŏn, mē'sŏn) [Gr. *mesos,* middle]. 1. Particle of mass intermediate between that of the electron and proton. Mesons of more than one variety and of both positive and negative charge occur. SYN: *mesotron.* 2. Mesion.

mesonasal (mĕs"ō-nā'zăl). In the middle of the nose.

mesonephric (mĕs"ō-nĕf'rĭk) [" + *nephros,* kidney]. Pert. to the mesonephros.

mesonephric duct. Embryonic duct that gives rise in the male to reproductive ducts (ductus epididymidis, ductus deferens, seminal vesicle, and ejaculatory duct). In the female, it gives rise to Gartner's duct of the epoophoron, a rudimentary structure. SYN: *wolffian duct.*

mesonephric tubules. Embryonic tubules consisting of two groups, cranial and caudal. The cranial group gives rise in the male to the efferent ductules of the testes and appendix epididymis; in the female, it gives rise to the epoophoron and vesicular appendices. The caudal group gives rise in the male to the paradidymis and aberrant ductules; in the female, it gives rise to the paroophoron. All structures except the efferent ductules of the testes are vestigial. SYN: *wolffian tubules.*

mesonephroma (mĕs"ō-nē-frō'mă) [" + *nephros,* kidney, + *oma,* tumor]. A relatively rare tumor derived from mesonephric cells developing in reproductive organs, esp. ovary or genital tract.

mesonephros (mĕs"ō-nĕf'rŏs). (pl. *mesonephroi*) [NA] A type of kidney that develops in all vertebrate embryos of classes above the Cyclostomes. It is the permanent kidney of fishes and amphibians but is replaced by the metanephros in reptiles and mammals. SYN: *wolffian body.*

mesoneuritis (mĕs-ō-nū-rī'tĭs) [" + *neuron,* nerve, + *itis,* inflammation]. Inflammation of the substance of a nerve or of its lymphatics.

meso-ontomorph (mĕs"ō-ŏn'tō-morf). A broad, husky body type.

mesopexy (mĕs'ō-pĕks"ē) [" + *pexis,* fixation]. Surgery to attach a torn mesentery.

mesophilic (mĕs-ō-fĭl'ĭk) [" + *philein,* to love]. Preferring moderate temperature, as some bacteria, which develop best at temperatures between 15° and 43° C.

mesophlebitis (mĕs"ō-flē-bī'tĭs). Inflammation of the medial layer of the wall of a vein.

mesophragma (mĕs"ō-frăg'mă) [" + *phragmos,* a fencing in]. A band in the center of the A-band in the myofibrils of a striated muscle.

mesophryon (mĕs-ŏf'rē-ŏn) [" + *ophrys,* eyebrow]. Midpoint in smooth space between the eyebrows. SEE: *glabella.*

mesopic (mĕs-ŏp'ĭk). Pert. to vision at low levels of light, e.g., at twilight.

mesopneumon (mĕs"ō-nū'mŏn) [" + *pneumon,* lung]. Meeting point of two pleural layers at hilus of the lung.

mesoporphyrin. $C_{34}H_{38}O_4N_4$. An iron-free derivative of hemin.

mesoprosopic (mĕs"ō-prō-sŏp'ĭk) [" + *prosopon,* face]. Pert. to a face of moderate width; a facial index of 90.

mesopulmonum (mĕs"ō-pŭl-mō'nŭm). The mesentery of the lung.

mesorchium (mĕs-or'kē-ŭm) [" + *orchis,* testicle]. [NA] Peritoneal fold that holds fetal testes in place.

mesorectum (mĕs"ō-rĕk'tŭm). Mesentery of the rectum.

mesoridazine besylate (mĕs"ō-rĭd'ă-zēn). USP. A drug used in treating psychoses.

mesoropter (mĕs-ō-rŏp'tĕr) [" + *horos,* boundary, + *opter,* observer]. Normal eye position with muscles at rest.

mesorrhachischisis (mĕs"ō-ră-kĭs'kĭ-sĭs) [" + *rhachis,* spine, + *schisis,* cleft]. Fissure of a portion of the spinal cord. SYN: *merorrhachischisis.*

mesorrhaphy (mĕs-or'ă-fē) [" + *rhaphe,* suture]. Suture of the mesentery. SYN: *mesenteriorrhaphy.*

mesorrhine (mĕs'ō-rīn) [" + *rhis,* nose]. With a nasal index variously quoted to range anywhere between 48 and 53.

mesosalpinx (mĕs"ō-săl'pĭnks) [" + *salpinx,* tube]. [NA] The free margin of the upper division of the broad ligament within which lies the oviduct.

mesoseme (mĕs'ō-sēm) [" + *sema,* sign]. Possessing an orbital index between 83 and 89.

mesosigmoid (mĕs-ō-sĭg'moyd). Mesentery of the sigmoid flexure.

mesosigmoiditis (mĕs"ō-sĭg"moy-dī'tĭs). Inflammation of the sigmoid colon.

mesosigmoidopexy (mĕs"ō-sĭg-moy'dō-pĕk"sē). Surgical fixation of the sigmoid colon.

mesoskelic (mĕs-ō-skĕl'ĭk) [" + *skelos,* leg]. Legs of normal length.

mesosome (mĕs′ō-sōm) [″ + *soma,* body]. In some bacteria, one or more large irregular convoluted invaginations of the cytoplasmic membrane. Mesosomes are larger in gram-positive than in gram-negative bacteria. Their function in the cell is not well understood.

mesosternum (mĕs″ō-stĕr′nŭm) [″ + *sternon,* chest]. The middle or second section of the sternum. SYN: *gladiolus.*

mesosystolic (mĕs″ō-sĭs-tŏl′ĭk). Midsystolic portion of the cardiac cycle.

mesotarsal (mĕs″ō-tăr′săl). Mediotarsal, q.v.

mesotendineum (mĕs″ō-tĕn-dĭn′ē-ŭm). The part of the synovial sheath of a tendon that connects the lining of the tendon sheath to the fibrous sheath covering the tendon.

mesotendon. Tissue lining a fibrous sheath attaching the sheath to the tendon.

mesothelial (mĕs″ō-thē′lē-ăl). Concerning the mesothelium.

mesothelioma (mĕs″ō-thē-lē-ō′mă). A rare malignant tumor of the mesothelium of the pleura, pericardium, or peritoneum.

mesothelium (mĕs″ō-thē′lē-ŭm) [″ + *epi,* at, + *thele,* nipple]. [NA] The layer of cells derived from the mesoderm lining the primitive body cavity. In the adult it becomes the epithelium covering the serous membranes.

mesothenar (mĕs″ō-thē′năr) [″ + *thenar,* palm]. The adductor pollicis muscle.

mesothorium (mĕs″ō-thō′rē-ŭm). The first two disintegration products of thorium.

mesotron. A subatomic particle of weight intermediate between light particles (electrons) and heavy particles (protons). SYN: *meson* (def. 1).

mesouranic (mĕs″ō-ū-răn′ĭk). Having a palatal index between 110 and 114.9.

mesovarium (mĕs″ō-vā′rē-ŭm). [NA] The portion of the peritoneal fold that connects the anterior border of the ovary to the posterior layer of the broad ligament.

Mestinon. Trade name for pyridostigmine bromide, USP.

mestranol (mĕs′tră-nōl). USP. A estrogen used in combination with progestational drugs in some birth control pill formulations.

MET. *metabolic equivalent.*

meta- (mĕt′ă) [Gr. *meta,* after, beyond, over]. 1. Prefix denoting change, transformation, or following something in a series. 2. In chemistry, prefix indicating the 1,3 position of benzene derivatives.

metabiosis (mĕt″ă-bī-ō′sĭs) [″ + *biosis,* way of life]. Dependence of an organism for its existence upon another. SYN: *commensalism.* SEE: *symbiosis.*

metabolic (mĕt″ă-bŏl′ĭk) [Gr. *metaballein,* to turn about, alter]. Pert. to metabolism.

metabolic balance. Comparison of the intake and excretion of a specific nutrient. The balance may be negative when an excess of the nutrient is excreted or positive when more is taken in than excreted.

metabolic body size. Body weight in kilograms to the three-fourths power ($kg.^{0.75}$), representative of the active tissue mass or metabolic mass of an individual.

metabolic equivalent. ABBR: MET. Unit used to estimate the metabolic cost of physical activity. One MET = uptake of 3.5 ml. of oxygen per kilogram of body weight per minute.

metabolic failure. Rapid failure of physical and mental functions ending in death.

metabolic gradient. A gradient in metabolic activity that exists in certain structures such as the small intestine from duodenum to ileum or in embryos from animal to vegetal poles in which metabolic activity is highest in one region and becomes progressively lower away from this region.

metabolic rate. The rate of utilization of energy. This is usually measured at a time when the subject is completely at rest and in a fasting state. Energy used is calculated from the amount of oxygen used during the test. The clinical usefulness of this test is doubtful. SEE: *basal metabolic rate; metabolism, basal.*

metabolimeter (mĕt″ă-bō-lĭm′ĕ-tĕr) [″ + *metron,* measure]. Device for measuring the metabolic rate.

metabolism [″ + *-ismos,* state of]. The sum of all physical and chemical changes that take place within an organism; all energy and material transformations that occur within living cells. It includes material changes, i.e., changes undergone by substances during all periods of life (growth, maturity, senescence) and energy changes, i.e., all transformations of chemical energy of foodstuffs to mechanical energy or heat. It involves two fundamental processes: anabolism (assimilation or building-up processes) and catabolism (disintegration or tearing-down processes). Anabolism is the conversion of ingested substances into the constituents of protoplasm; catabolism is the breakdown of substances into simpler substances, the end products usually being excreted.

Inborn errors of metabolism are a group of inherited metabolic diseases caused by the absence or deficiency of specific enzymes essential to the metabolism of basic substances such as amino acids, carbohydrates, vitamins, or essential trace elements. Examples include phenylketonuria, and hereditary fructose intolerance.

m., basal. Lowest level of energy expenditure. This is determined when the body is at complete rest. For an average person, this is, in terms of Cal., approx. 1500 to 1800 per day; in terms of body weight, 1 Cal. per kilogram per hour; in terms of body surface, 40 Cal. per sq. meter per hour.

m., carbohydrate. All carbohydrates are digested to monosaccharides and absorbed as such principally in the form of hexoses, of which glucose is the principal one. In the liver and muscles, glucose is converted to glycogen or it may be oxidized to carbon dioxide and water, the ultimate fate of all carbohydrates. These reactions require the presence of insulin and other hormones. In the process, many intermediate compounds are formed, among them lactic acid. The basic reaction is

$$C_6H_{12}O_6 + 6O_2 \rightarrow 6CO_2 + 6H_2O$$

which is the basis for the determination of the respiratory quotient (R.Q.). SEE: *quotient, respiratory.*

m., constructive. The building-up processes by which complex substances are synthesized. SYN: *anabolism; assimilation.*

m., destructive. The breakdown or decomposition of substances into their simple constituents. SYN: *catabolism.*

m., fat. Fats are digested to fatty acids and glycerol. Following absorption they may be reconverted to neutral fats and stored as adipose tissue or oxidized to CO_2 and H_2O. Fats may be formed from carbohydrates or proteins. In the utilization of fats, the liver plays an important role in the desaturation of fatty acids. Fat metabolism also involves the formation and utilization of substances related to fats, such as sterols and phospholipids.

m., general. Includes all processes involved in utilization of substances entering the body.

m., protein. Proteins are digested to amino acids and absorbed as such. In the body these are synthesized into body proteins, which form an integral part of protoplasm; hence they are essential for normal growth and the repair of tissues. Those not utilized thus are deaminized, i.e., the amino, NH, group is removed. This results in the production of urea, which is excreted; the remainder, a fatty acid residue (COOH), may be oxidized or converted to glucose, which may be stored as glycogen or converted to fat.

m., purine. Metabolism involving nucleic acids, present in nuclei of cells, in which they are combined with proteins to form nucleoproteins. In the breakdown of nucleic acid, uric acid, one of the end products, is formed.

m., special. Applies to all changes involved in utilization of particular substances such as carbohydrates, proteins, fats, minerals, or water. Referred to as carbohydrate metabolism, protein metabolism, etc.

metabolite (mĕ-tăb'ō-līt). Any product of metabolism.

metabolize (mĕ-tăb'ō-līz) [Gr. *metaballein,* to turn about, alter]. To alter the character of a food substance by metabolic reactions.

metacarpal [Gr. *meta,* beyond, + *karpos,* wrist]. Pert. to the bones of the metacarpus or bones of the hand. SEE: *skeleton.*

metacarpectomy (mĕt"ă-kăr-pĕk'tō-mē) [" + " + *ektome,* excision]. Surgical excision or resection of one or more wrist bones.

metacarpophalangeal (mĕt"ă-kăr"pō-fă-lăn'jē-ăl). Concerning the metacarpus and the phalanges.

metacarpus (mĕt"ă-kăr'pŭs) [" + *karpos,* wrist]. [NA] The five metacarpal bones of the palm of the hand. SEE: *carpometacarpal.*

metacentric (mĕt"ă-sĕn'trĭk). Term indicating a chromosome with the centromere in the median position. Thus the arms of the chromosome are of equal length.

metacercaria (mĕt"ă-sĕr-kā'rē-ă). The encysted stage in the life history of a trematode. This stage occurs in an intermediate host prior to transfer to the definitive host.

metachromasia, metachromatism (mĕt-ă-krō-mā'zē-ă, -krōm'ă-tĭzm) [Gr. *meta,* change, + *chroma,* color]. Condition in which different components of the same tissue assume different colors or shades of color. The colors are different from those of the dye used.

metachromatic (mĕt"ă-krō-măt'ĭk). Pert. to metachromatism.

metachromatic granules. Granules that stain a different color from that of the dye used.

metachromatic leukodystrophy. A fatal disease of infancy, caused by a deficiency of the enzyme aryl sulfatase A. Metachromatic material is deposited in the brain, peripheral nerves, liver, kidney, and frequently the urine. This material, sulfated lipids, would normally be degraded to cerebrosides. There is no specific therapy.

metachromophil (mĕt-ă-krōm'ō-fĭl) [" + *chroma,* color, + *philein,* to love]. Not reacting normally to staining.

metachrosis (mĕt-ă-krō'sĭs). Change of color in animal life, e.g., chameleon.

metacone [Gr. *meta,* beyond, + *konos,* cone]. The distobuccal cusp of an upper molar tooth.

metaconid (mĕt-ă-kŏn'ĭd). The mesiolingual cusp of a lower molar tooth.

metaconule (mĕt-ă-kŏn'ūl). The distal intermediate cusp of an upper molar tooth.

metacyesis (mĕt-ă-sī-ē'sĭs) [" + *kyesis,* pregnancy]. Extrauterine gestation.

metagenesis [" + *genesis,* formation]. Alternation of generations, esp. involving regular alternation of sexual with asexual reproduction. Seen in some fungi.

metagglutinin (mĕt″ă-gloo′tĭn-ĭn) [″ + L. *agglutinare,* glue]. A partial agglutinin; an agglutinin present in immune serum that acts on organisms closely related to the one acting as the specific antigen.

Metagonimus (mĕt″ă-gŏn′ĭ-mŭs) [″ + *gonimos,* productive]. A genus of flukes belonging to the family Heterophyidae.

M. yokogawai. A species of intestinal flukes common in the Middle and Far East. Normally infests the intestines of dogs, cats, and other animals, but commonly found in man also. Intermediate hosts: snails and fish, esp. a series of trout, Plecoglossus altivelis.

Metahydrin. Trade name for trichlormethiazide.

metaicteric (mĕt″ă-ĭk-tĕr′ĭk) [″ + *ikteros,* jaundice]. Occurring as a result of jaundice.

metainfective (mĕt″ă-ĭn-fĕk′tĭv). Occurring subsequent to an infection.

metakinesis (mĕt″ă-kī-nē′sĭs). Moving apart, esp. the moving of the two chromatids of each chromosome away from each other as they move to opposite poles in the anaphase of mitosis.

metalbumin (mĕt-ăl-bū′mĭn). The mucin present in ovarian cysts. SYN: *pseudomucin.*

metal fume fever. A syndrome resembling influenza produced by inhalation of excessive concentrations of metallic oxide fumes such as zinc oxide or antimony, arsenic, cadmium, cobalt, copper, iron, lead, magnesium, manganese, mercury, nickel, or tin. Occurs in persons whose occupations lead to exposure to these metals.

SYM: Onset of symptoms is usually delayed. Chills, weakness, lassitude, profound thirst, followed after some hours by sweating and anorexia; occasionally there is mild inflammation of the eyes and respiratory tract. The symptoms are more acute at the beginning of the work week than at the end. This is felt to be due to the individual adapting to the fumes as exposure continues.

F.A.: Fresh air and symptomatic treatment.

metallesthesia (mĕt″ăl-ĕs-thē′sē-ă) [Gr. *metallon,* metal, + *aisthesis,* perception]. Recognition of metals by touching them.

metallic. 1. Pert. to metal. 2. Composed of or resembling a metal.

metallic tinkling. A peculiar ringing or bell-like auscultatory sound in pneumothorax over large pulmonary cavities.

metalloenzyme (mĕ-tăl″ō-ĕn′zīm). An enzyme that contains a metal ion in its structure.

metalloid (mĕt′ăl-loyd) [″ + *eidos,* resemblance]. Resembling a metal.

metallophilia (mĕ-tăl″ō-fĭl′ē-ă) [″ + *philein,* to love]. The property of some tissues of binding certain metal salts.

metallophobia (mĕ″tăl-ō-fō′bē-ă) [″ + *phobos,* fear]. Abnormal fear of metals and metallic objects and of touching them.

metalloporphyrin (mĕ-tăl″ō-por′fĭ-rĭn). Porphyrin combined with a metal. Ex.: iron with heme to form hemoglobin; magnesium in chlorophyll.

metalloprotein (mĕ-tăl″ō-prō′tē-ĭn). A protein bound with metal ions.

metalloscopy (mĕt-ăl-ŏs′kō-pē) [″ + *skopein,* to examine]. Determination of the effects of applying metals to the body and the body's sensitivity to them.

metallotherapy (mĕt″ăl-ō-thĕr′ă-pē) [″ + *therapeuein,* to heal]. Treatment of disease by applying metals to the affected part.

metallurgy (mĕt″ăl-ŭr′jē) [″ + *ergon,* work]. Science of obtaining metals from their ores, refining them, and making them into various shapes and forms.

metamer (mĕt′ă-mĕr). Something similar to but different from something else. Ex.: isomers of chemical compounds.

metamere (mĕt′ă-mēr) [Gr. *meta,* beyond, + *meros,* part]. One of a series of similar segments arranged in a linear series and making up the body of an animal such as an earthworm.

metameric (mĕt-ă-mĕr′ĭk). Rel. to metamerism. SYN: *isomeric.*

metamerism (mĕ-tăm′ĕr-ĭzm). 1. Isomerism, q.v. 2. Isomerism consisting of segments or metameres.

metamorphopsia (mĕt″ă-mor-fŏp′sē-ă) [Gr. *meta,* change, + *morphe,* form, + *opsis,* vision]. In ophthalmology, visual distortion of objects; found in refractive errors, esp. astigmatism, retinal disease, choroiditis, detachment of retina, and tumors of retina and choroid.

metamorphosis (mĕt″ă-mor′fō-sĭs) [″ + *morphosis,* bringing into shape]. 1. A change in form or structure, esp. the transition from one form to another as in complete metamorphosis of an insect (egg, larva, pupa, adult). 2. In pathology, a degenerative change.

m., fatty. Transformation of fat by infiltration or degeneration.

m., platelet. The fusion of platelets during blood coagulation.

m., retrograde. Degeneration.

m., structural. M., platelet, q.v.

m., viscous. M., platelet, q.v.

Metamucil. Trade name for psyllium.

metamyelocyte (mĕt″ă-mī-ĕl′ō-sīt). A transitional cell intermediate in development between a myelocyte and a mature granular leukocyte. SYN: *juvenile cell.*

Metandren. Trade name for methyltestosterone.

metanephrine (mĕt″ă-nĕf′rĭn). An inactive

metabolite of epinephrine.

metanephrogenic (mĕt″ă-nĕf′rō-jĕn′ĭk) [″ + *nephros,* kidney, + *gennan,* to produce]. The part of the caudal mesoderm of the embryo that forms metanephric tubules of the kidney.

metanephros (mĕt″ă-nĕf′rōs) [″ + *nephros,* kidney]. (pl. *metanephroi*) The permanent kidney of amniotes (reptiles, birds, and mammals). A portion of it develops from the caudal portion of the intermediate cell mass or nephrotome; the remaining portion is derived from a bud of the mesonephric duct.

metaneutrophil (mĕt-ă-nū′trō-fĭl) [″ + L. *neuter,* neither, + Gr. *philein,* to love]. Not reacting normally with neutral dyes.

metaphase (mĕt′ă-fāz) [″ + *phasis,* to appear]. Stage in mitosis in which the chromosomes are arranged in an equatorial plane prior to separation. Follows the prophase and precedes the anaphase in which longitudinal halves of chromosomes diverge. SEE: *mitosis.*

metaphrenia (mĕt″ă-frē′nē-ă) [″ + *phren,* mind]. The mental status of turning away from family interests toward personal goals such as business.

metaphysis (mĕ-tăf′ĭ-sĭs) [Gr. *meta,* beyond, + *phyein,* to grow]. (pl. *metaphyses*) Portion of a developing long bone between the diaphysis or shaft and epiphysis; the growing portion of a bone.

metaphysitis (mĕt″ă-fĭs-ī′tĭs) [″ + ″ + *itis,* inflammation]. Inflammation of the metaphysis of a bone.

metaplasia (mĕt″ă-plā′zē-ă) [″ + *plassein,* to form]. Conversion of one kind of tissue into a form that is not normal for that tissue.

m., myeloid. The development of marrow tissue at sites in which it would not normally occur.

metaplasm (mĕt′ă-plăzm). Reserve material present in protoplasm of a cell, esp. stored nutritive substance.

metaplastic (mĕt-ă-plăs′tĭk) [″ + *plastikos,* formed]. Pert. to or formed by metaplasia.

metapneumonic (mĕt″ă-nū-mŏn′ĭk). Succeeding or as a consequence of pneumonia.

metapophysis (mĕt″ă-pŏf′ĭ-sĭs) [″ + *apophysis,* a process]. Mammillary process on the superior articular processes of a vertebra.

Metaprel. Trade name for metaproterenol sulfate.

metaprotein. Derived protein resulting from the action of acids or alkalies, in which the molecule is changed to form protein insoluble in neutral solvents but soluble in alkalies and weak acids. SEE: *protein.*

metaproterenol sulfate (mĕt″ă-prō-tĕr′ĕ-nōl). An adrenergic stimulant used to treat bronchospasm and bronchial asthma. It is effective when given by inhalation. Trade name is Metaprel.

metapsychology (mĕt″ă-sī-kŏl′ō-jē). Any concept of mental processes that is unverifiable by factual evidence and that cannot be discredited by reasoning.

metaraminol bitartrate (mĕt″ă-răm′ĭ-nōl). USP. A drug used for its pressor effect in treating hypotension. Trade names are Aramine and Pressonex Bitartrate.

metarteriole (mĕt″ăr-tē′rē-ōl). A small vessel connecting an arteriole to a venule from which true capillaries are given off. SYN: *precapillary.*

metarubricyte (mĕt″ă-roo′brĭ-sīt). A normally staining normoblast.

metastable [″ + L. *stabilis,* stable]. Marked by a slight margin of stability. Will change into another phase when conditions change. Term used in chemistry and physics.

metastasis (mĕ-tăs′tă-sis) [″ + *stasis,* stand]. (pl. *metastases*) 1. Movement of bacteria or body cells (esp. cancer cells) from one part of the body to another. 2. Change in location of a disease or of its manifestations or transfer from one organ or part to another not directly connected.

The usual application is to the manifestation of a malignancy as a secondary growth arising from the primary growth in a new location. Spread is by the lymphatics or bloodstream.

metastasize (mĕ-tăs′tă-sīz). To invade by metastasis.

metastatic (mĕt″ă-stăt′ĭk). Pert. to metastasis.

metasternum (mĕt″ă-stĕr′nŭm). Xiphoid process of the sternum.

metatarsal (mĕt″ă-tăr′săl). Concerning the metatarsal arch of the foot.

metatarsalgia (mĕt″ă-tăr-săl′jē-ă) [Gr. *meta,* beyond, + *tarsos,* a flat surface, + *algos,* pain]. Severe pain or cramp in anterior portion of metatarsus. SEE: *Morton's disease, syndrome.*

metatarsectomy (mĕt″ă-tăr-sĕk′tō-mē). [″ + ″ + *ektome,* excision]. Removal of the metatarsus or a metatarsal bone.

metatarsophalangeal (mĕt″ă-tăr″sō-fă-lăn′jē-ăl) [″ + ″ + *phalanx,* closely knit row]. Concerning the metatarsus and phalanges of the toes.

metatarsus (mĕt″ă-tăr′sŭs) [″ + *tarsos,* tarsus]. [NA] The region of the foot between the tarsus and phalanges. Includes the five metatarsal bones.

metatarsus primus varus. Inturning of the first metatarsal bone of the foot.

metatarsus varus. Congenital deformity of the feet in which the inner border is off the ground and the sole turned inward, so the child walks on the outer border of the foot.

metathalamus (mĕt″ă-thăl′ă-mŭs) [″ + *thalamos,* a chamber]. [NA] The posterior part of the thalamus including the two geniculate bodies.

metathesis (mĕ-tăth'ĕ-sĭs) [" + *thesis,* placement]. 1. A changing of places. 2. Forcible transference of a disease process from one part to another where it will be more accessible for treatment or where it causes less inconvenience. 3. Double decomposition of two chemical compounds.

metatrophia (mĕt-ă-trō'fē-ă) [" + *trophe,* nourishment]. 1. A wasting due to malnutrition. 2. A change in diet.

metatrophic. 1. Pert. to metatrophia. 2. Requiring lifeless organic matter for food.

metatypical (mĕt"ă-tĭp'ĭ-kăl). Tissue elements similar to those other tissues at that site, but the components are not in a normal pattern.

metaxalone (mĕ-tăks'ă-lōn). A centrally acting muscle relaxant. Trade name is Skelaxin.

Metazoa [" + *zoon,* animal]. Division of the animal kingdom that includes all multicellular forms, in contrast to unicellular forms or Protozoa.

Metchnikoff's theory (mĕch'nĭ-kŏfs). [Elie Metchnikoff, Russian zoologist in France, 1845–1916] The theory that the body is protected against infection by cells such as leukocytes and phagocytes that attack and destroy invading microorganisms. SEE: *phagocytosis.*

metencephalon (mĕt"ĕn-sĕf'ă-lŏn) [Gr. *meta,* after, + *enkephalos,* brain]. [NA] The anterior portion of the embryonic rhombencephalon, from which the cerebellum and pons arise. SYN: *hindbrain.*

meteorism (mē'tē-or-ĭzm) [Gr. *meteorizein,* to raise up]. Distention by gas in the abdomen or intestines. SYN: *tympanites.*

meteoropathy (mē"tē-ĕ-rŏp'ă-thē) [" + *pathos,* disease]. Illness due to climatic conditions.

meteorotropic (mē"tē-ĕ-rō-trŏp'ĭk) [" + *trope,* a turn]. Pert. to diseases that are affected in their occurrence rate by weather.

meteorotropism (mē"tē-ĕ-rŏt'rō-pĭzm). The influence of meteorological events on biological conditions and events such as death rate, disease incidence, and birth rate.

meter [Gr. *metron,* measure]. A linear standard of measurement in the SI measurement system that is equal to 39.37 inches.

metergasis (mĕt"ĕr-gā'sĭs) [Gr. *meta,* change, + *ergon,* work]. Change or alteration in function.

metestrus (mĕ-tĕs'trŭs) [" + L. *oistros,* mad desire]. Period following estrus and preceding diestrus. SEE: *estrus.*

methacholine chloride (mĕth"ă-kō'lēn). USP. A cholinergic drug that is rarely used because of the unpredictability of the intensity of response.

methacycline hydrochloride. USP. An antibacterial drug. Trade name is Rondomycin.

methadone hydrochloride. USP. A synthetic analgesic drug with potency equal to that of morphine, but the narcotic action is weaker than that of morphine. Methadone is a habit-forming agent and its use should be carefully supervised. Used experimentally in treatment of drug dependence due to use of opium derivatives. Trade names are Dolophine and Methadone.

methallenestril (mĕth"ăl-ĕ-nĕs'trĭl). A nonsteroidal estrogenic substance.

methamphetamine hydrochloride (mĕth"ăm-fĕt'ă-mēn). A sympathomimetic agent that is now used principally as a drug of abuse.

methane. CH_4. A colorless, odorless, inflammable gas. It is produced as a result of putrefaction and fermentation of organic matter. SYN: *marsh gas.*

methandriol (mĕth-ăn'drē-ōl). An anabolic steroid drug. Trade name is Cytobolin.

methandrostenolone (mĕth-ăn"drō-stĕn'ō-lōn). USP. An anabolic steroid used as replacement therapy in treating deficient endocrine function of the testes. Trade name is Dianabol.

methanol. CH_3OH. A poisonous volatile, inflammable alcohol that may be mistaken for ethyl alcohol. If ingested, can cause blindness and death. SYN: *methyl alcohol; wood alcohol.* SEE: *Poisons and Poisoning* in *Appendix.*

methantheline bromide (mĕ-thăn'thĕ-lēn). USP. An anticholinergic drug that acts similarly to belladonna. Trade name is Banthine.

methapyrilene fumarate hydrochloride (mĕth"ă-pĭr'ĭ-lēn). USP. An antihistamine drug.

methaqualone hydrochloride (mĕ-thă'kwă-lōn). USP. A hypnotic and sedative drug that has become a drug of abuse. Because of the illegal and abused use of this drug, it is no longer distributed in the United States. Trade name is Quaalude.

metharbital (mĕ-thăr'bĭ-tăl). USP. An anticonvulsant drug of the barbiturate class. Trade name is Gemonil.

methazolamide (mĕth"ă-zō'lă-mīd). USP. A carbonic acid inhibitor used in treating glaucoma. Trade name is Neptazane.

methdilazine (mĕth-dĭ'lă-zēn). USP. An antihistamine drug. Trade name is Tacaryl Hydrochloride.

methemalbumin (mĕt"hēm-ăl-bū'mĭn). The abnormal combination of heme with albumin instead of globulin. This is present in blackwater fever and paroxysmal nocturnal hemoglobinuria.

methemoglobin (mĕt-hē"mō-glō'bĭn) [Gr. *meta,* across, + *haima,* blood, + L. *globus,* globe]. A form of hemoglobin wherein the ferrous iron in it has been oxidized to ferric iron. This may be due to toxic substances such as aniline dyes, potassium chlorate, or nitrate-contaminated water. Methemoglobin is also present when there is a hereditary deficiency of NADH-diaphorase, q.v.

m. reductase. Nicotinamide adenine dinucleotide-diaphorase. SYN: *NADH-diaphorase,* q.v.

methemoglobinemia (mĕt″hē-mō-glōb″ĭ-nē′mē-ă) [″ + ″ + ″ + *haima,* blood]. The clinical condition in which more than 1% of hemoglobin in blood has been oxidized to the ferric (Fe^{+++}) form. The principal sign is cyanosis because the oxidized hemoglobin is incapable of transporting oxygen.

m., congenital. Condition due to a hereditary deficiency of NADH-diaphorase.

methemoglobinuria (mĕt″hē-mō-glōb″ĭ-nū′rē-ă) [″ + ″ + ″ + *ouron,* urine]. Presence of methemoglobin in the urine.

methenamine (mĕth-ĕn′ă-mēn). USP. A urinary antiseptic drug. Previously used name was hexamethylenamine.

m. mandelate. USP. A urinary antiseptic that derives its activity from the release of formaldehyde. Trade names are Mandelamine and Manese.

USES: In the treatment of urinary infection, esp. pyelitis and cystitis. It is necessary that the acidity of the urine be controlled; thus an acidifying agent, such as ammonium chloride, usually is required to maintain a urine pH of 5.5. This drug should not be used as the sole therapeutic agent in acute urinary tract infections.

methene. Methylene, q.v.

Methergine. Trade name for methylergonovine maleate, USP.

methicillin sodium (mĕth″ĭ-sĭl′ĭn). USP. A semisynthetic penicillinase-resistant penicillin. Trade names are Azapen, Celbenin, and Staphcillin.

methimazole (mĕth-ĭm′ă-zōl). USP. An antithyroid drug. Trade name is Tapazole.

methiodal sodium (mĕth-ī′ō-dăl). USP. A radiopaque compound used in x-ray examination of the urinary tract. Trade name is Skiodan Sodium.

methionine (mĕth-ī′ō-nĭn). USP. $C_5H_{11}NO_2S$. A sulfur-bearing compound; an essential amino acid.

methisazone (mĕ-thĭs′ă-zōn). An antiviral agent. Trade name is Marboran.

methixene hydrochloride (mĕ-thĭks′ēn). A smooth muscle relaxant drug. Trade name is Trest.

methocarbamol (mĕth″ō-kăr′bă-mŏl). USP. A centrally acting muscle relaxant drug. Trade name is Robaxin.

method [Gr. *methodos*]. The systematic manner, procedure, or technique in performing details of an operation, tests, treatment, or any act. SEE: *maneuver; stain; test; treatment.*

methodology (mĕth″ō-dŏl′ō-jē) [″ + *logos,* study]. The system of principles and procedures used in scientific endeavors.

methohexital sodium (mĕth″ō-hĕk′sĭ-tăl). USP. An ultrashort-acting barbiturate. Used in anesthesia. Trade name is Brevital Sodium.

methomania (mĕth″ō-mā′nē-ă) [Gr. *methe,* drunkenness, + *mania,* madness]. Pathological craving for intoxicating drinks or other intoxicants.

methotrexate (mĕth″ō-trĕk′sāt). USP. An antimetabolite that acts as a folic acid antagonist. It is used in treating acute lymphoblastic leukemia in children, and in treating choriocarcinoma and psoriasis. Previously used name was amethopterin. Trade name is Mexate.

methotrimeprazine (mĕth″ō-trī-mĕp′ră-zēn). USP. A tranquilizer and analgesic drug. Trade name is Levoprome.

methoxamine hydrochloride (mĕ-thŏk′să-mēn). USP. An adrenergic drug used to maintain blood pressure in hypotensive states by causing vasoconstriction. It is also used to end attacks of paroxysmal atrial tachycardia. Trade name is Vasoxyl.

methoxsalen (mĕ-thŏk′să-lĕn). USP. A psoralen used in treating vitiligo, eczema, mycosis fungoides, and psoriasis. Trade name is Oxsoralen. SEE: *psoralen; PUVA therapy; trioxsalen.*

methoxyflurane (mĕ-thŏk″sē-floo′rān). USP. A general anesthetic administered by inhalation. Its renal toxicity prevents its being used for prolonged anesthesia. Trade name is Penthrane.

methoxyphenamine hydrochloride (mĕ-thŏk″sē-fĕn′ă-mēn). USP. A sympathomimetic drug used in treating bronchospasm. Trade name is Orthoxine Hydrochloride.

methscopolamine bromide (mĕth″skō-pŏl′ă-mēn). USP. An anticholinergic drug that is used in treating gastric hyperacidity and hypermotility. Trade name is Pamine Bromide.

methsuximide (mĕth-sŭk′sĭ-mīd). USP. An anticonvulsant drug used in treating epilepsy. Trade name is Celontin.

methyclothiazide (mĕth″ĭ-klō-thī′ă-zīd). USP. An antihypertensive and diuretic drug. Trade names are Aquatensen and Enduron.

methyl (mĕth′ĭl) [Gr. *methy,* wine, + *hyle,* wood]. In organic chemistry, the radical CH_3, seen, for instance, in the formula for methyl alcohol, CH_3OH.

m. alcohol. A colorless liquid with an alcoholic odor largely used as a solvent for paints or varnishes.

m. ether. An anesthetic gas without color.

m. orange. A dye used as a pH indicator.

m. purine. An oxidation product of purine. Includes caffeine, theophylline and theobromine. SEE: *aminopurine; oxypurine.*

m. salicylate. Oil of wintergreen, oil of gaultheria. Produced from distillation of leaves of sweet birch; it has a characteristic odor.

ACTION AND USES: Commonly used in preparations in the form of liniment or ointment for topical use as an analgesic balm and counterirritant.

m. violet. Stain employed in histology and bacteriology.

methyl alcohol poisoning. Symptoms are different from those of ordinary alcoholism. Depression, weakness, nausea, headache, abdominal cramping, difficult breathing, cold sweats, coma, and convulsions. May be confused with cerebrovascular accident. Blindness, which often follows, may appear in several hours or not for several days; it may be permanent.

TREATMENT: Gastric lavage, q.v., or induce vomiting. Intravenous alkali solution (5% sodium bicarbonate) in large amounts, supportive therapy. To prevent formation of formic acid, 10 ml. of ethyl alcohol per hour will help to prevent metabolism of methyl alcohol. Hemodialysis may be necessary.

methylate (mĕth′ĭ-lāt). 1. To introduce the methyl group, CH_3, into a chemical compound. 2. To mix with methyl alcohol. 3. A compound of methyl alcohol and a base.

methylation (mĕth″ĭ-lā′shŭn). The addition of methyl groups to a compound.

methylatropine nitrate (mĕth″ĭl-ăt′rō-pēn). A quaternary ammonium derivative of atropine, with action similar to that drug. Trade name is Eumydrin.

methylbenzethonium chloride (mĕth″ĭl-bĕn″zĕ-thō′nē-ŭm). USP. A deodorant used topically. It acts by reducing the number of resident bacteria on the skin. Trade name is Diaparene.

methylcellulose. USP. A tasteless powder that becomes swollen and gummy when wet. Used as a bulk substance in foods and laxatives, also as an adhesive or emulsifier. Trade names are Cologel and Methocel A.

methylcytosine (mĕth″ĭl-sī′tō-sĭn). A derivative of pyrimidine present in some nucleic acids.

methyldopa (mĕth″ĭl-dō′pă). USP. An antihypertensive drug used in treating essential hypertension. Previously used name was alpha-methyldopa. Trade name is Aldomet.

methyldopate hydrochloride (mĕth″ĭl-dō′pāt). USP. An antihypertensive drug used in treating essential hypertension. Trade name is Aldomet Ester Hydrochloride.

methylene (mĕth′ĭ-lēn). The chemical radical $-CH_2-$. SYN: *methene.*

methylene blue (mĕth′ĭ-lēn). A dark green crystalline powder, producing a distinct blue stain.

USES: As an antidote for carbon monoxide and cyanide poisoning. It is also valuable in the treatment of drug-induced methemoglobinemia (1 mg. of dye per kilogram of body weight).

methylenophil (mĕth″ĭ-lĕn′ō-fĭl). Something that stains easily with methylene blue.

methylergonovine maleate (mĕth″ĭl-ĕr″gō-nō′vēn). USP. A drug of the ergot alkaloid type. It is used to stimulate uterine contractions and in the treatment of migraine. Trade name is Methergine.

methylglucamine (mĕth″ĭl-gloo′kă-mĭn). Meglumine, USP, q.v.

methylmalonic acidemia. An inherited metabolic disease caused by inability to convert methylmalonic acid to succinic acid. Clinically there are failure to grow, mental retardation, and severe metabolic acidosis. This disease has been treated in utero.

methylparaben (mĕth″ĭl-păr′ă-bĕn). An antifungal agent used as a preservative in pharmaceuticals.

methylphenidate hydrochloride (mĕth″ĭl-fĕn′ĭ-dāt). USP. A drug that is chemically related to amphetamine. It is used in treating narcolepsy. Trade name is Ritalin Hydrochloride.

methylprednisolone (mĕth″ĭl-prĕd′nĭ-sō-lōn). USP. An adrenal corticosteroid drug. Trade name is Medrol.

methylrosaniline chloride (mĕth″ĭl-rō-zăn′ĭ-lĭn). Previously used name for gentian violet, q.v.

methyltestosterone (mĕth″ĭl-tĕs-tŏs′tĕr-ōn). USP. An androgenic steroid hormone. Trade names are Metandren, Oreton-Methyl, and Testred.

methylthiouracil (mĕth″ĭl-thī″ō-ū′ră-sĭl). USP. An antithyroid drug used in treating hyperthyroidism.

methyltransferase (mĕth″ĭl-trăns′fĕr-ās). An enzyme that catalyzes the transfer of a methyl group from one compound to another.

methyprylon (mĕth″ĭ-prī′lŏn). USP. A sedative and hypnotic drug. Trade name is Noludar.

methysergide maleate (mĕth″ĭ-sĕr′jīd). USP. A vasoconstrictor drug used in treating migraine. Trade name is Sansert. SEE: *carcinoid syndrome; serotonin.*

Meticorten. Trade name for prednisone, USP.

Meti-Derm. Trade name for prednisolone, USP.

metmyoglobin (mĕt-mī″ō-glō′bĭn). Myoglobin with the ferrous ion in the heme oxidized to the ferric ion.

metocurine iodide (mĕt″ō-kū′rēn). USP. A drug that relaxes skeletal muscle. It is used as an adjuvant in surgical anesthesia. Previously used name was dimethyl tubocurarine iodide. Trade name is Metubine Iodine.

CAUTION: An overdose may be lethal due to prolonged apnea and cardiac collapse. This drug should be used only by those familiar with its pharmacology and where facilities and staff for respiratory and cardiovascular resuscitation are immediately available.

metonymy (mĕ-tŏn'ĭ-mē) [Gr. *meta,* beyond, + *onyma,* name]. Mental confusion exhibited by the patient's use of a word that is not the precise term but of similar meaning.

Ex.: rifle in place of war; apple in place of ball.

metopagus (mĕ-tŏp'ă-gŭs) [Gr. *metopon,* forehead, + *pagos,* thing fixed]. Conjoined twins united at the forehead.

metopic (mē-tŏp'ĭk) [Gr. *metopon,* forehead]. Rel. to the forehead.

metopion (mē-tō'pē-ŏn). Craniometric point in forehead midway between frontal eminences. SYN: *glabella.*

metopism (mĕt'ō-pĭzm). Persistence of the metopic suture in an adult.

metopodynia (mĕt"ō-pō-dĭn'ē-ă) [" + *odyne,* pain]. Frontal headache.

metoprolol tartrate. USP. An antiadrenergic drug. Trade name is Lopressor.

metoxenous (mĕt"ŏk-sē'nŭs) [Gr. *meta,* change, + *xenos,* host]. Denoting a parasite that spends each of its two cycles on a different host. SYN: *heterecious.*

metoxeny (mĕt-ŏk'sĕ-nē). Condition of being metoxenous.

metra (mē'tră) [Gr.]. Combining form meaning the uterus. SEE: *metro-.*

metralgia (mē-trăl'jē-ă) [Gr. *metra,* uterus, + *algos,* pain]. Pain in the uterus. SYN: *metrodynia.*

metratome (mē'tră-tōm) [" + *tome,* incision]. Instrument for incising the uterus.

metratomy (mē-trăt'ō-mē). Surgical incision of the uterus. SYN: *hysterotomy; metrotomy.*

metratonia (mē"tră-tō'nē-ă). Uterine atony occurring after childbirth.

metratrophia (mē"tră-trō'fē-ă). Atrophy of the uterus.

Metrazol (mĕt'ră-zōl). Trade name for a preparation of pentylenetetrazole. A white powder, chemically neutral substance.

USES: A diagnostic aid in epilepsy. It is injected intravenously as the EEG is being recorded. This may activate epileptic foci with production of characteristic EEG changes.

metre (mē'tĕr) [Gr. *metron,* measure]. Meter.

metrechoscopy (mĕt"rē-kŏs'kō-pē) [" + *echo,* sound, + *skopein,* to examine]. Combined mensuration, auscultation, and inspection.

metrectasia (mē"trĕk-tā'zē-ă) [Gr. *metra,* uterus, + *ektasis,* extension]. Dilatation of nonpregnant uterus.

metrectopia (mē"trĕk-tō'pē-ă) [" + *ektopos,* displaced]. Displacement of the uterus.

metreurynter (mē-troo-rĭn'tĕr) [Gr. *metra,* uterus, + *eurynein,* to stretch]. An inflatable bag that is inserted in the os uteri and distended to dilate the cervix.

metreurysis (mē-troo'rĭ-sĭs). Dilatation of the cervix uteri with the metreurynter.

metria (mē'trē-ă). Inflammation of the uterus during pregnancy.

metric system. A system of weights and measures based upon the meter (39.37 in.) as the unit of measurement; the gram (15.432 gr.) as the unit of weight; the liter (1.057 qt. liquid, or 0.908 qt. dry measure) as the unit of volume.

CONVERSION RULES: (Approximate) To change gm. to gr. multiply by 15 or divide by 0.064. To change gr. to gm. divide by 15 or multiply by 0.064. To change gm. to avoirdupois oz., divide by 28.35. To change fluid oz. to ml. multiply by 30. SEE: *avoirdupois; SI units; Troy weight; Weights and Measures* in *Appendix.*

metriocephalic (mĕt"rē-ō-sĕ-făl'ĭk) [Gr. *metrios,* moderate, + *kephale,* head]. A skull with a vertical index of 72 to 76.9.

metritis (mĕ-trī'tĭs) [Gr. *metra,* uterus, + *itis,* inflammation]. Inflammation of the uterus. Designated endometritis if the endometrium is involved and myometritis if the musculature (myometrium) is involved.

m., chronic. Condition in which there are an increase in fibrous tissue and infiltration of lymphocytes.

metro- [Gr. *metra,* uterus]. Combining form meaning rel. to the uterus.

metrocarcinoma (mē"trō-kăr-sĭ-nō'mă) [" + *karkinos,* cancer, + *oma,* tumor]. Uterine carcinoma.

metrocele (mē'trō-sēl) [" + *kele,* hernia]. Uterine hernia.

metrocolpocele (mē"trō-kŏl'pō-sēl) [" + *kolpos,* vagina, + *kele,* hernia]. Protrusion of the uterus into the vagina, which pushes the vaginal wall downward.

metrocystosis (mē"trō-sĭs-tō'sĭs) [" + *kystis,* cyst, + *osis,* intensive]. Formation of uterine cysts.

metrodynia (mē"trō-dĭn'ē-ă) [" + *odyne,* pain]. Uterine pain. SYN: *metralgia.*

metrofibroma (mē-trō-fī-brō'mă) [" + L. *fibra,* fiber, + *oma,* tumor]. Uterine fibroma.

metromalacia (mē"trō-măl-ā'shē-ă) [" + *malakia,* softness]. Softening of the uterus.

metromalacosis (mē"trō-măl-ă-kō'sĭs) [" + " + *osis,* condition]. Malacia or softening of uterine tissues.

metronidazole. USP. Medicine used in treating infections due to Trichomonas vaginalis or Giardia lamblia, and in treating amebiasis. Trade name is Flagyl.

CAUTION: This drug may depress the level of white blood cells. Drinking alcohol while taking it may cause abdominal pain, nausea, or vomiting; and central nervous system symptoms such as vertigo, dizziness, and ataxia.

metronome (mĕt'rō-nōm) [Gr. *metron,* measure, + *nomos,* law]. Apparatus for recording intervals or periods of time.

metronoscope (mĕ-trŏn'ō-skōp). A device for exposing written material to the eye at timed intervals in order to facilitate development of reading skills and speed.

metroparalysis (mē"trō-pă-răl'ĭ-sĭs) [Gr. *metra,* uterus, + *paralyein,* to disable]. Uterine paralysis during or immediately following childbirth.

metropathia hemorrhagica (mē"trō-păth'ē-ă hĕm"ō-răj'ĭk-ă) [" + *pathos,* disease, + *haima,* blood, + *rhegnynai,* to burst forth]. Condition of the uterus characterized by hemorrhage, usually accompanied by hypertrophy of the uterine mucous membranes and ovarian cystic disease.

metropathic (mē"trō-păth'ĭk). Pert. to or caused by uterine disease.

metropathy (mē-trŏp'ă-thē). Any uterine disease.

metroperitoneal (mē"trō-pĕr"ĭ-tō-nē'ăl) [" + *peritonaion,* peritoneum]. Concerning the uterus and the peritoneum.

metroperitonitis (mē"trō-pĕr"ĭ-tō-nī'tĭs) [" + " + *itis,* inflammation]. Inflamed condition of uterus and peritoneum.

metrophlebitis (mē"trō-flē-bī'tĭs) [" + *phleps,* vein, + *itis,* inflammation]. Inflamed condition of the uterine veins.

metroplasty (mē"trō-plăs'tē) [" + *plastikos,* formed]. Any plastic operation on the uterus.

metroptosis (mē-trō-tō'sĭs) [" + *ptosis,* falling]. Downward displacement or prolapse of the uterus.

metrorrhagia (mĕt"rō-rā'jē-ă) [" + *rhegnynai,* to burst forth]. Bleeding from the uterus, esp. at any time other than during the menstrual period. May be caused by lesions of the cervix uteri. Its occurrence should lead one to suspect and search for a malignancy in the genital tract, specifically cancer of the cervix. SEE: *menorrhagia.*

metrorrhea (mē"trō-rē'ă) [" + *rhoia,* flow]. Abnormal uterine discharge.

metrorrhexis (mē"trō-rĕk'sĭs) [" + *rhexis,* rupture]. Rupture of the uterus.

metrorthosis (mē"tror-thō'sĭs) [" + *orthosis,* a straightening]. Correction of uterine displacement.

metrosalpingitis (mē"trō-săl"pĭn-jī'tĭs) [" + *salpinx,* tube, + *itis,* inflammation]. Inflamed condition of uterus and oviducts.

metrosalpingography (mē"trō-săl"pĭng-gŏg'ră-fē) [" + " + *graphein,* to write]. X-raying of the uterus and the fallopian tubes after the injection of air or an opaque medium into them.

metroscope (mē'trō-skōp) [" + *skopein,* to examine]. Instrument for examining the uterus. SYN: *hysteroscope.*

metrostaxis (mē"trō-stăk'sĭs) [" + *staxis,* a dripping]. Persistent but slight hemorrhage from the uterus.

metrostenosis (mē"trō-stĕn-ō'sĭs) [" + *stenosis,* contraction]. Contraction or narrowing of the uterine cavity.

metrotherapy [Gr. *metron,* measure, + *therapeia,* treatment]. Treatment of a condition by measurement.

Ex.: in restoration of joint function following injury, measurement of the angle of joint motion and recording the progress has a psychological effect on the patient.

metrotome (mē'trō-tōm) [Gr. *metra,* uterus, + *tome,* incision]. Instrument used in incising the uterus.

metrotomy (mē-trŏt'ō-mē). Incision of the uterus. SYN: *hysterotomy; metratomy.*

metrourethrotome (mĕt"rō-ū-rē'thrō-tōm) [Gr. *metron,* measure, + *ourethra,* urethra, + *tome,* incision]. Device for incising the urethra and measuring depth to be incised.

-metry [Gr. *metrein,* to measure]. Suffix meaning to measure.

metyrapone (mĕ-tĕr'ă-pōn). USP. A drug that reduces adrenocortical secretion from the adrenal gland. It is used to treat excessive adrenocortical hormone secretion and to test the function of the adrenal gland. Trade name is Metopirone.

mev. *million electron volts.*

Mexate. Trade name for methotrexate sodium.

Meynert's commissure (mī'nĕrts) [Theodor H. Meynert, Austrian neurologist, 1833–1892] Fibrous tract extending from subthalamic body to base of 3rd ventricle.

Meynet's nodosities (mā-năz'). [Paul C. H. Meynet, Fr. physician, 1831–1892] In rheumatic disease, nodules attached to the tendon sheaths and joints.

M.F.D. *minimum fatal dose.*

μg. *microgram.*

Mg. Chem. symb. for magnesium.

mg. *milligram.*

mgh. *milligram hour.* Dosage of radiation obtained by application of 1.0 mg. radium for 1 hr.

MHC. *major histocompatibility complex.*

mho (mō). Siemens.

miasm, miasma (mī'ăzm, mī-ăz'mă) [Gr. *miasma,* stain]. A foul emanation or odor from the earth. Formerly thought to cause disease endemic to certain regions, esp. fevers such as malaria.

miasmatic (mī"ăz-măt'ĭk). Pert. to miasm.

mica (mī'kă) [L.]. 1. A crumb. 2. A mineral

composed of various silicates of metals. It occurs in thin, laminated scales.

mication (mī-kā'shŭn). A sudden movement such as eye blinking.

micella, micelle (mī-sĕl'ă, mī-sĕl'). One of the ultramicroscopic units of protoplasm.

miconazole nitrate (mĭ-kŏn'ă-zōl). An antifungal used as a vaginal cream. Trade names are Monistat-Derm and Monistat Cream.

micra. Pl. of micron.

micracusia (mī"kră-kū'zē-ă) [Gr. *mikros,* small, + *akousis,* hearing]. An auditory illusion in which sounds appear to be remote. May occur at the onset of an epileptic seizure. SEE: *macracusia.*

micrencephalon (mī"krĕn-sĕf'ă-lon) [Gr. *mikros,* small, + *enkephalos,* brain]. 1. Cerebellum. 2. Smallness of the brain; cretinism, q.v.

micrencephalous (mī"krĕn-sĕf'ă-lŭs). Possessing a small brain.

micrencephaly (mī"krĕn-sĕf'ă-lē). Abnormal smallness of the brain.

micro-, micr- [Gr. *mikros,* small]. Combining forms denoting small size or extent. Indicates one millionth of a unit; thus microgram is one millionth of a gram. SYMB: μ.

microabscess (mī"krō-ăb'sĕs) [" + L. *abscessus,* a going away]. A very small abscess.

microaerophilic (mī"krō-ā'ĕr-ō-fĭl"ĭk) [" + *aer,* air, + *philein,* to love]. Growing at low amounts of oxygen; said of certain bacteria.

microanalysis. Analytical examination of tiny granules.

microanatomy. Microscopic anatomy; histology.

microaneurysm (mī"krō-ăn'ū-rĭzm) [" + *aneurysma,* a widening]. A microscopic aneurysm.

microangiitis (mī"krō-ăn"jē-ī'tĭs). Inflammation of very small blood vessels.

microangiopathy (mī"krō-ăn"jē-ŏp'ă-thē) [" + *angeion,* vessel, + *pathos,* disease]. Pathology of small blood vessels.

m., thrombotic. Formation of thrombi in small blood vessels.

microangioscopy (mī"krō-ăn"jē-ŏs'kō-pē) [" + " + *skopein,* to examine]. Use of microscopy to diagnose pathological changes in capillaries.

microbalance (mī'krō-băl"ăns). A scale or balance for measuring very small weight changes.

microbe (mī'krōb) [" + *bios,* life]. 1. A minute one-celled form of life not distinguishable as to its vegetable or animal nature. 2. Bacteria, germs producing fermentation, putrefaction, and disease. SYN: *microorganism.*

microbial (mī-krō'bē-ăl). Rel. to microbes. SYN: *microbian; microbic.*

microbian (mī-krō'bē-ăn). Rel. to microbe. SYN: *microbial; microbic.*

microbic (mī-krōb'ĭk). Concerning microbes. SYN: *microbial; microbian.*

microbicidal (mī-krō"bĭ-sī'dăl) [" + *bios,* life, + L. *cidus,* kill]. Lethal to microbes.

microbicide (mī-krō'bĭ-sīd). An agent that kills microbes.

microbiology (mī"krō-bī-ŏl'ō-jē) [" + *bios,* life, + *logos,* study]. Scientific study of microorganisms.

microbiophobia (mī"krō-bī"ō-fō'bē-ă) [" + " + *phobia,* fear]. An abnormal fear of germs. SYN: *microphobia* (def. 1).

microbiota (mī"krō-bī-ō'tă). Microscopic organisms of an area. SEE: *macrobiota.*

microbiotic (mī"krō-bī-ŏt'ĭk). Pertinent to microbial forms of life.

microbism (mī'krōb-ĭzm) [" + *bios,* life, + *ismos,* state of]. Infection with microbes.

microblast (mī'krō-blăst) [" + *blastos,* germ]. Minute red blood corpuscle.

microblepharism, microblephary (mī"krō-blĕf'ăr-ĭzm, -ăr-ē) [" + *blepharon,* eyelid]. Condition of having abnormally small eyelids.

microbodies. Small, spherical, cytoplasmic bodies approx. 0.5 μ in diameter. They have been found in the cells of the liver and kidney tubule.

microbrachia (mī"krō-brā'kē-ă) [" + *brachion,* arm]. Abnormally small arms.

microbrachius (mī"krō-brā'kē-ŭs) [" + *brachion,* arm]. A fetus with very small arms.

microcalorie (mī"krō-kăl'ō-rē) [Gr. *mikros,* small, + L. *calor,* heat]. A unit of heat, the amount required to raise the temperature of 1 ml. of distilled water from 0° to 1° C. One thousand microcalories equal one Calorie.

NOTE: A microcalorie is also called calorie (spelled with a small "c"). A thousand calories equal one kilocalorie (kcal.). This is also called a Calorie (with a capital "C").

The energy value of food is expressed in Calories, i.e., kilocalories.

microcardia (mī"krō-kăr'dē-ă) [" + *kardia,* heart]. Unusually small heart.

microcaulia (mī"krō-kaw'lē-ă) [" + *kaulos,* penis]. Unusually small size of penis. SYN: *microphallus.*

microcentrum (mī"krō-sĕn'trŭm) [" + *kentron,* center]. 1. Centrosome. 2. Motor or dynamic center of a cell.

microcephalia (mī"krō-sĕf-ā'lē-ă) [" + *kephale,* head]. Abnormal smallness of the head. SYN: *microcephalism; microcephaly.*

microcephalic (mī"krō-sĕf-ăl'ĭk). Having or pert. to a small head; one below 1350 cc. capacity.

microcephalous (mī"krō-sĕf'ă-lŭs). Having an abnormally small head. SYN: *microcephalic.*

microcephalus (mī"krō-sĕf'ă-lŭs). Individual with an exceptionally small head.

microcephaly (mī″krō-sĕf′ă-lē). Abnormal smallness of head often seen in mental retardation; it is congenital.
microcheilia (mī″krō-kī′lē-ă) [Gr. *mikros,* small, + *cheilos,* lip]. Abnormal smallness of lips.
microchemistry (mī″krō-kĕm′ĭs-trē) [″ + *chemeia,* chemistry]. Chemical work in which minute quantities and small instruments are utilized.
microchiria, microcheiria (mī″krō-kī′rē-ă) [″ + *cheir,* hand]. Abnormal smallness of the hand.
microcinematography (mī″krō-sĭn″ĕ-mă-tŏg′ră-fē) [″ + *kinema,* motion, + *graphein,* to write]. Motion pictures of microscopic objects.
microcirculation (mī″krō-sĭr″kū-lā′shŭn). Blood or lymph flow in the very small vessels.
Micrococcaceae (mī″krō-kŏk-ā′sē-ē). A family of bacteria belonging to the order Eubacteriales. Contains the genera Micrococcus, Sarcina, and Staphylococcus.
Micrococcus (mī″krō-kŏk′ŭs) [Gr. *mikros,* small, + *kokkos,* berry]. A genus of spherical gram-positive bacteria belonging to the family Micrococcaceae. Cells occur singly or in irregular groups.

M. albus. Staphylococcus albus, the current name of which is Staphylococcus epidermidis.

M. melitensis. Brucella melitensis. Cause of undulant fever.

micrococcus (mī″krō-kŏk′ŭs). 1. An organism of the genus Micrococcus. 2. A very small spherical microorganism.
microcolon. Abnormally small colon.
microcoria (mī″krō-kō′rē-ă) [″ + *kore,* pupil]. Smallness of the pupil of the eye.
microcornea. Abnormally small cornea.
microcoulomb (mī″krō-koo′lŏm). A microunit of quantity of current electricity; one millionth part (10^{-6}) of a coulomb, q.v.
microcrystalline (mī″krō-krĭs′tăl-ĭn, -ēn). Composed of microscopic crystals.
microcurie. Measure of radiation. One-millionth of a curie.
microcurie-hour. The radiation produced by radioactive decay at the rate of 3.7×10^4 atoms per second.
microcyst (mī′krō-sĭst). A very small cyst.
microcytase (mī″krō-sī′tās) [″ + *kytos,* cell, + *-ase,* enzyme]. Enzyme in leukocytes that is capable of destroying microorganisms.
microcyte. A small erythrocyte or red blood corpuscle; one less than 5 microns in diameter.
microcythemia (mī″krō-sī-thē′mē-ă) [″ + ″ + *haima,* blood]. Smallness of the red blood cells.
microcytosis. Condition characterized by presence of abnormal numbers of microcytes in the blood.
microdactylia (mī″krō-dăk-tĭl′ē-ă) [″ + *daktylos,* digit]. Abnormal smallness of the digits.
microdetermination. The chemical examination of extremely minute quantities of a substance.
microdissection (mī″krō-dī-sĕk′shŭn) [″ + L. *dissectio,* a cutting apart]. Dissection with the aid of a microscope, esp. by utilization of a micromanipulator.
microdont (mī′krō-dŏnt) [″ + *odous,* tooth]. Possessing very small teeth.
microdontia (mī″krō-dŏn′shē-ă) [″ + *odous,* tooth]. Abnormal smallness of the teeth or a single tooth.
microdontism (mī″krō-dŏn′tĭzm) [″ + ″ + *-ismos,* state of]. Unusual smallness of the teeth.
microdose. Minute dose.
microdrepanocytic (mī″krō-drĕp′ă-nō-sĭt′ĭk). Containing the genes of sickle cell and thalassemia. This produces a chronic hemolytic anemia.
microdrepanocytosis (mī″krō-drĕp″ă-nō-sī-tō′sĭs). Condition combining sickle cell disease and thalassemia.
microelectrophoresis. Electrophoresis of minute quantities of a solution.
microembolus (mī″krō-ĕm′ɔō-lŭs) [″ + *embolos,* plug]. A very small embolus.
microencephaly (mī″krō-ĕn-sĕf′ă-lē) [″ + *enkephalos,* brain]. Having a very small head.
microenvironment. The environment at the microscopic or cellular level.
microerythrocyte (mī″krō-ĕ-rĭth′rō-sīt) [″ + *erythros,* red, + *kytos,* cell]. Microcyte, q.v.
microfarad (mī-krō-făr′ăd). A microunit of electrical capacity; one-millionth of a farad, q.v.
microfauna (mī″krō-faw′nă). In a specific location, the animal life that is microscopic in size.
microfibril (mī″krō-fī′brĭl). A very small fibril.
microfiche (mī′krō-fēsh″) [Gr. *mikros,* small, + Fr. *fiche,* index card]. A sheet of microfilm that enables a large number of library data and medical records to be stored in a small space.
microfilament (mī″krō-fĭl′ă-mĕnt). Submicroscopic elements of the cell.
microfilaremia (mī″krō-fĭl″ă-rē′mē-ă). Microfilaria in the blood.
microfilaria (mī″krō-fī-lā′rē-ă). The embryos of filarial worms. They are present in the blood and tissues and are of importance in the diagnosis of filarial infections.
microfilm. A film containing the photograph of something greatly reduced in size.
microflora (mī″krō-flō′ră). In a specific area, the plant life that is visible by use of a microscope.

microgamete (mī-krō-găm′ēt) [″ + *gametes,* spouse]. Male element in conjugation of protozoa.
microgametocyte (mī″krō-gă-mē′tō-sīt) [″ + ″ + *kytos,* cell]. Mother cell of the microgamete.
microgamy (mī-krŏg′ă-mē). Union of male and female cells in certain lower forms.
microgastria (mī″krō-găs′trē-ă) [″ + *gaster,* stomach]. Unusual smallness of the stomach.
microgenia (mī″krō-jĕn′ē-ă) [″ + *geneion,* chin]. Abnormal smallness of the chin.
microgenitalism (mī″krō-jĕn′ĭ-tăl-ĭzm) [″ + L. *genitalia,* genitals, + Gr. *-ismos,* state of]. Abnormal smallness of the external genitals.
microglia (mī-krŏg′lē-ă) [″ + *glia,* glue]. Neuroglia tissue probably derived from the mesoderm, forming a portion of the adventitial structure of the central nervous system.
microgliacyte (mī″krŏg′lē-ă-sīt) [″ + ″ + *kytos,* cell]. An embryonic cell of the microglia.
microglioma (mī″krō-glī-ō′mă) [″ + ″ + *oma,* tumor]. A tumor composed of microglial cells.
microglossia (mī-krō-glŏs′ē-ă) [″ + *glossa,* tongue]. Abnormally small tongue.
micrognathia (mī-krō-nā′thē-ă) [″ + *gnathos,* jaw]. Abnormal smallness of jaws, esp. the lower jaw.
microgonioscope (mī″krō-gō′nē-ō-skōp) [″ + *gonia,* angle, + *skopein,* to examine]. Device for measuring the angles of the anterior chamber of the eye. Used in studying glaucoma.
microgram. ABBR: μg. or mcg. One-millionth part of a gram. One-thousandth of a milligram.
micrograph (mī′krō-grăf) [Gr. *mikros,* small, + *graphein,* to write]. 1. Apparatus for magnifying and recording minute movements. 2. Photograph of an object through a microscope. SYN: *photomicrograph.*
micrography (mī-krŏg′ră-fē). 1. Study of physical appearance and characteristics of microscopic objects. 2. Very minute writing, engraving, etc. 3. Study of an object by use of a microscope.
microgyria (mī-krō-jĭr′ē-ă) [″ + *gyros,* circle]. Smallness of cerebral convolutions.
microgyrus (mī″krō-jī′rŭs) [″ + *gyros,* circle]. A small, malformed gyrus of the brain.
microhematocrit (mī″krō-hē-măt′ō-krĭt). Packed red cell volume of blood determined by using very small amount of blood collected in a capillary tube and placed in high-speed centrifuge.
microhepatia (mī″krō-hē-păt′ē-ă) [″ + *hepar,* liver]. Abnormally small size of the liver.
microhm (mī′krōm). A microunit of electrical resistance; one-millionth of an ohm.
microincineration. Determination of presence and distribution of inorganic matter in tissues by subjecting a microscopic section of tissue to a high temperature, which destroys organic matter and leaves mineral matter as ash.
microinjection. Injection of substances into cells or minute vessels by means of a micropipette.
microinvasion (mī″krō-ĭn-vā′zhŭn). Invasion of the cellular tissue adjacent to a carcinoma in situ.
microlentia (mī″krō-lĕn′shē-ă). Possessing a very small crystalline lens.
microleukoblast [″ + *leukos,* white, + *blastos,* germ]. A small leukoblast. SYN: *myeloblast.*
microlesion (mī″krō-lē′zhŭn). A very small lesion.
microliter (mī′krō-lē″tĕr). One-millionth part of a liter.
microlith (mī′krō-lĭth) [″ + *lithos,* stone]. A very tiny calculus.
microlithiasis (mī″krō-lĭ-thī′ă-sĭs) [″ + ″ + *-iasis,* process]. The development of very minute calculi.

m., pulmonary alveolar. Deposition of microscopic granules of bone throughout the lungs.

micrology (mī-krŏl′ō-jē) [″ + *logos,* study]. Science of microscopic investigations.
micromanipulator. Apparatus by which extremely minute pipettes or needles can be manipulated under a microscope for microinjection or microsurgery.
micromastia (mī-krō-măs′tē-ă). Micromazia.
micromazia (mī-krō-mā′zē-ă) [Gr. *mikros,* small, + *mazos,* breast]. Abnormally small size of the breasts.
micromelia (mī″krō-mē′lē-ă) [″ + *melos,* limb]. Abnormally small or short limbs.
micromelus (mī-krŏm′ē-lŭs) [″ + *melos,* limb]. One who has micromelia.
micromere (mī′krō-mēr) [″ + *meros,* part]. A small blastomere.
micrometer. 1. (mī′krō-mē-ter) ABBR: μm. A millionth part of a meter (10^{-6}); one-thousandth part of a millimeter (0.001 mm.). SEE: *micron.* 2. (mī-krŏm′ĕ-tĕr) Device for measuring small distances.
micromethod (mī″krō-mĕth′ŏd). Any chemical or physical method involving small amounts of material or very small tissues, respectively.
micrometry (mī-krŏm′ĕ-trē) [″ + *metron,* measure]. Use of device, esp. a micrometer, to measure small objects or thickness.
micromicrogram (mī″krō-mī′krō-grăm). ABBR: μμg. One millionth of a microgram. Now called a picogram, or 10^{-12} gram.
micromicron (mī″krō-mī′krŏn). ABBR: μμ. Former name for picometer or 10^{-12} meter.
micromillimeter (mī-krō-mĭl′ĭ-mē-tĕr). ABBR: μmm. One-millionth part of a millimeter. SYN: *millimicron.*

micromole (mī′krō-mōl). One millionth, 10^{-6}, of a mole. SEE: *mole* (def. 2).

micromolecular (mī″krō-mō-lĕk′ū-lăr). Composed of small molecules.

Micromonospora (mī″krō-mō-nŏs′por-ă). A genus of fungi belonging to the family Streptomycetaceae.

micromyces (mī-krŏm′ĭ-sēs) [Gr. *mikros,* small, + *mykes,* fungus]. (pl. *micromycetes*) Minute fungus.

micromyelia (mī″krō-mī-ē′lē-ă) [″ + *myelos,* marrow]. Abnormally small size of spinal cord.

micromyeloblast (mī-krō-mī′ĕl-ō-blăst) [″ + *myelos,* marrow, + *blastos,* germ]. A small, immature myelocyte; often the predominating cell in myeloblastic leukemia.

micromyelolymphocyte (mī″krō-mī″ē-lō-lĭm′fō-sīt) [″ + ″ + L. *lympha,* lymph, + Gr. *kytos,* cell]. Micromyeloblast, q.v.

micron. (pl. *micra, microns*) Unit of linear measure; equal to .001 millimeter (10^{-3} mm.). In the International System (SI) of units, micron has been designated micrometer. The abbr. for micrometer is μm.

microne (mī′krōn). A colloid particle that is distinguishable with the microscope.

microneedle. Extremely minute needle used in a micromanipulator for microdissection.

micronize. To pulverize a substance into particles only a few micra in size.

micronodular (mī″krō-nŏd′ū-lăr). Having small nodules.

micronucleus (mī-krō-nū′klē-ŭs) [″ + L. *nucleus,* kernel]. (pl. *micronuclei*) 1. A small nucleus. 2. The smaller of the two nuclei of Infusoria considered as containing the inheritable germ substance.

micronutrient (mī″krō-nū′trē-ĕnt). Essential nutrient required only in small amounts.

micronychia (mī″krō-nĭk′ē-ă) [″ + *onyx,* nail]. Possessing abnormally small nails.

microorganism (mī-krō-or′găn-ĭzm) [″ + *organon,* organ, + *-ismos,* condition]. Minute living body not perceptible to the naked eye, esp. a bacterium or protozoon.

Microorganisms may be carried from one host to another as follows:

Animal sources: Some organisms are pathogenic for animals as well as man and may be communicated to man through direct, indirect, or intermediary hosts.

By air: Pathogenic microorganisms in the respiratory tract may be discharged from the mouth or nose and settle on food, dishes or clothing. They may carry infection if they resist drying.

Contact infections: These are the result of direct transmission of bacteria from one to another, as in venereal diseases.

Food-borne: Food and water may contain pathogenic organisms acquired from infected persons handling the food or through fecal or insect contamination.

Fomites: Inanimate objects such as linens, books, cooking utensils, or clothing that will harbor microorganisms and could serve to transport them from one location to another.

Human carriers: Persons who have recovered from an infectious disease remain carriers of the organism causing the infection and may transfer the organism to another host.

Insects: They may be physical carriers, such as the housefly, or act as intermediate hosts, such as the Anopheles mosquito.

Soil-borne: Spore-forming organisms in the soil may enter the body through a cut or wound. Vegetables and fruits, esp. roots, need thorough cleansing before being eaten raw.

m., pathologic. Any disease-causing microorganism. Includes rickettsias, bacteria, spirochetes, yeasts, molds, protozoons, and some helminths.

microparasite (mī″krō-păr′ă-sīt). A parasitic microorganism.

micropathology (mī″krō-păth-ŏl′ō-jē) [Gr. *mikros,* small, + *pathos,* disease, + *logos,* study]. Study of microorganismal diseases and resulting cell and tissue changes.

micropenis (mī″krō-pē′nĭs). A very small penis.

microphage, microphagus (mī′krō-fāj, mī-krŏf′ă-gŭs) [″ + *phagein,* to eat]. A small phagocyte.

RS: bacteria; bacteriolysin; leukocyte; opsonic index; opsonin.

microphagocyte (mī″krō-făg′ō-sīt) [″ + ″ + *kytos,* cell]. Microphage.

microphakia (mī″krō-fā′kē-ă) [″ + *phakos,* lens]. Abnormally small crystalline lens.

microphallus (mī-krō-făl′ŭs) [″ + *phallos,* penis]. Abnormally small size of penis. SYN: *microcaulia.*

microphobia (mī-krō-fō′bē-ă) [″ + *phobos,* fear]. 1. Psychopathic fear of microbes. 2. Morbid dread of small objects. SYN: *microbiophobia.*

microphone (mī′krō-fōn) [″ + *phone,* voice]. Device for detecting and transmitting sound.

microphonia (mī-krō-fō′nē-ă). Weakness of the voice.

microphonoscope (mī″krō-fō′nō-skōp) [Gr. *mikros,* small, + *phone,* voice, + *skopein,* to examine]. Form of binaural stethoscope for magnifying sound.

microphotograph (mī″krō-fō′tō-grăf) [″ + *phos,* light, + *graphein,* to write]. 1. A photograph of extremely small size. 2. A photograph on microfilm. 3. A photomicrograph.

microphthalmia (mī-krŏf-thăl′mē-ă) [″ + *ophthalmos,* eye]. Abnormally small size of one or both eyes.

microphthalmus (mī-krŏf-thăl′mŭs). 1. Person with unusually small eyes. 2. Condition characterized by abnormally small eyes.

microphysics (mī-krō-fĭz'ĭks). The branch of science dealing with the forces controlling the ultimate structure of matter.

microphyte (mī'krō-fīt) [" + *phyton,* plant]. Any microscopic plant, esp. if parasitic.

micropia (mī-krō'pē-ă) [" + *opsis,* vision]. A condition in which objects seem diminished in size. SYN: *micropsia.*

micropipette. An extremely small pipette used for measuring small amounts of fluid substances.

microplasia (mī"krō-plā'zē-ă) [" + *plassein,* to form]. Dwarfism.

microplethysmography (mī"krō-plĕth"ĭs-mŏg'ră-fē) [" + *plethysmos,* increase, + *graphein,* to write]. Detection of small changes in the volume of a part due to alteration in blood flow.

micropodia (mī-krō-pō'dē-ă) [" + *pous,* feet]. Unusually small size of the feet.

micropolariscope (mī"krō-pōl-ăr'ĭ-skōp). A microscope with a polarizer.

microprobe (mī'krō-prōb). A very small probe, suitable for use in microsurgery.

microprojection. Projection of images of microscopic objects upon a screen.

microprosopia (mī"krō-prō-sō'pē-ă) [" + *prosopon,* face]. Abnormal smallness of the face.

micropsia (mī-krŏp'sē-ă) [" + *opsis,* vision]. Condition in which objects seem smaller than they usually are. Seen in paralysis of accommodation, retinitis, and choroiditis. SYN: *micropia.*

micropuncture (mī"krō-pŭnk'chŭr). A very small incision or puncture of a structure such as a single cell.

micropus (mī-krō'pŭs) [" + *pous,* feet]. One with unusually small feet.

micropyle (mī'krō-pīl) [" + *pyle,* gate]. The opening in the ovum for entrance of the spermatozoon. Seen in ovum of some animals.

microradiography (mī"krō-rā"dē-ŏg'ră-fē). Technique of x-raying microscopic objects. The pictures are usually enlarged.

microrefractometer (mī"krō-rē"frăk-tŏm'ĕ-tĕr). Refractometer used to study cells, esp. red blood cells.

microrespirometer (mī"krō-rĕs"pĭ-rŏm'ĕ-tĕr). Device for measuring oxygen consumption of very small bits of tissue.

microrhinia (mī"krō-rĭn'ē-ă) [" + *rhis,* nose]. Abnormal smallness of the nose.

microscelous (mī-krŏs'kĕ-lŭs) [" + *skelos,* leg]. Possessing short legs.

microscope (mī'krō-skōp) [" + *skopein,* to examine]. Optical instrument that greatly magnifies very minute objects.

m., binocular. Microscope possessing two eyepieces or oculars.

m., compound. Microscope with two or more lenses or lens systems for use in observing the minutest bodies.

m., darkfield. Microscope using darkfield illumination. SYN: *ultramicroscope.* SEE: *illumination, darkfield.*

m., electron. A microscope that utilizes streams of electrons deflected from their course by an electrostatic or electromagnetic field for the magnification of objects. The final image is viewed on a fluorescent screen or recorded on a photographic plate. Because of greater resolving power, images may be magnified up to 400,000 diameters. SEE: *m., scanning electron.*

m., light. A microscope that uses visible light to allow viewing of the object.

m., operating. A microscope designed for use during surgery involving small tissues such as vessels, the inner ear, or fallopian tubes.

m., phase. A compound microscope to which two elements have been added, namely, a diffraction or phase plate and a specialized condenser diaphragm. This makes it possible to view details of objects characterized by differences in refractive index and thus delineates a change of phase such as brightness or color.

m., polarization. Microscope for examining specimens that polarize light or have double refraction.

m., scanning electron. ABBR: SEM. An electron microscope that scans the image point-by-point and displays the image on a photographic film or television screen. The SEM, unlike other types of microscopes, allows a three-dimensional view of the tissue and tissues do not need to be extensively handled and prepared in order to be visualized. The magnification ranges from 20 to 100,000 times.

m., simple. One with a simple or single lens; magnifying glass.

m., slit lamp. A microscope with slit illumination for examining the eye, esp. the cornea.

m., stereoscopic. A binocular microscope with an objective lens for each eyepiece. This permits the object to be viewed stereoscopically.

m., ultraviolet. Microscope utilizing ultraviolet radiations as a light source and having an optical system for transmitting them. Used in observing a specimen that fluoresces such as tissues stained with a fluorescent dye.

m., x-ray. Microscope for utilizing x-rays to reveal structure of objects through which light cannot pass. The image is usually reproduced on film.

microscopic, microscopical (mī-krō-skŏp'ĭk,

-ĭ-kăl). 1. Pert. to the microscope. 2. Visible only by using the microscope.

microscopy (mī-krŏs'kōp-ē). Inspection with the microscope.

microsecond (mī'krō-sĕk"ŭnd). One millionth of a second; 10^{-6} second.

microseme (mī'krō-sēm) [Gr. *mikros,* small, + *sema,* sign]. Possessing an orbital index of less than 83.

microsmatic (mī"krŏs-măt'ĭk) [" + *osmasthai,* to smell]. Having a poorly developed sense of smell.

microsoma (mī"krō-sō'mă) [" + *soma,* body]. Unusually small stature.

microsome (mī'krō-sōm). Particles derived from the endoplasmic reticulum of cell nuclei. Obtained when cells are broken up by centrifuging with a force 100,000 times that of gravity. They can be seen only by use of electron microscopy.

microsomia (mī-krō-sō'mē-ă). Abnormally small size of body.

microspectrophotometry (mī"krō-spĕk"trō-fō-tŏm'ĕ-trē). Method for the histochemical study of substances present in cells, such as nucleic acid, based on absorption in the ultraviolet spectrum. Permits quantitative and qualitative studies of certain cellular components with a high degree of sensitivity.

microspectroscope [" + L. *spectrum,* image, + Gr. *skopein,* to examine]. A combined spectroscope and microscope.

microspherocyte (mī"krō-sfē'rō-sīt) [" + *sphaira,* globe, + *kytos,* cell]. Red blood cells, small and shaped like spheres. Seen in certain kinds of anemia.

microspherocytosis (mī"krō-sfē"rō-sī-tō'sĭs) [" + " + *osis,* condition]. Spherocytosis.

microsphygmia (mī-krō-sfĭg'mē-ă) [" + *sphygmos,* pulse]. A pulse difficult to palpate.

microsplanchnic (mī"krō-splănk'nĭk). Having an abdominal cavity relatively small compared to the rest of the body.

microsplenia (mī-krō-splē'nē-ă) [" + *splen,* spleen]. Abnormal smallness of the spleen.

microsporid (mī-krŏs'pō-rĭd). A skin eruption distant from the site of infection with Microsporum, and due to hypersensitivity to the organism.

Microsporon (mī"krŏs'por-rŏn) [" + *sporos,* seed]. Former name of Microsporum.

microsporosis (mī"krō-spō-rō'sĭs). Ringworm infection due to fungi of the genus Microsporum.

Microsporum (mī"krŏs'por-ŭm). A genus of ringworm fungi that causes disease of the skin, hair, and nails.

M. audouini. Causative agent of tinea capitis (ringworm of scalp), q.v.

M. canis. Cause of ringworm of cats and dogs. May be transmitted to children.

microstomia (mī-krō-stō'mē-ă) [" + *stoma,* mouth]. Unusual smallness of the mouth.

microstrabismus (mī"krō-stră-bĭs'mŭs) [" + *strabismos,* a squinting]. Movement of the eyes in divergent directions or at different speeds. These movements are too small and too quick to be seen, but they have been detected by analyzing high-speed motion pictures.

microsurgery. Dissection of tissues under the microscope, usually involving the use of a micromanipulator.

microsyringe. A special syringe for injecting very small quantities of solutions.

microthelia (mī"krō-thē'lē-ă) [" + *thele,* nipple]. Very small nipples.

microtia (mī-krō'shē-ă) [" + *ous,* ear]. Unusually small size of the auricle or external ear.

microtome (mī'krō-tōm) [" + *tome,* incision]. Instrument for preparing thin sections of tissue for microscopic study.

m., freezing. Microtome equipped to cut frozen tissues.

m., sliding. Microtome in which the tissue being sectioned slides along a track.

microtomy (mī-krŏt'ō-mē). The process of incision thin sections of tissues.

microtonometer (mī"krō-tō-nŏm'ĕ-tĕr). Device for determining oxygen and carbon dioxide concentration in blood.

microtrauma (mī"krō-traw'mă). A very small lesion.

microtropia (mī"krō-trō'pē-ă) [" + *trope,* a turning]. Strabismus with very small deviation, usually less than 4°.

microtubule (mī"krō-tū'būl) An elongated (200 to 300 Ångstrom), hollow or tubular structure present in the cell. Microtubules are important in helping certain cells maintain their rigidity and in converting chemical energy into work. They increase in number during mitosis.

microtus (mī-krō'tŭs) [" + *ous,* ear]. Individual with very small ears.

microvascular (mī"krō-văs'kū-lăr). Pert. to the very fine blood vessels of the body.

microvilli (mī"krō-vĭl'ī) [L., tufts of hair]. (sing. *microvillus*) Microscopic projections from the free surface of cell membranes. They greatly increase the exposed surface area of the cell. SEE: *border, brush.*

microvolt. One-millionth part of a volt.

microwave (mī'krō-wāv). That portion of the radio wave spectrum between a wavelength of 1 mm. and 30 cm.

microxycyte (mī-krŏk'sĭ-sīt) [Gr. *mikros,* small, + *oxys,* sharp, + *kytos,* cell]. Any fine granular cell.

microxyphil (mī-krŏk'sĭ-fĭl) [" + " + *philein,* to love]. Microxycyte.

microzoon (mī"krō-zō'ŏn) [" + *zoon,* animal]. Microscopic animal.

micrurgy (mī'krŭr-jē) [Gr. *mikros,* small, +

ergos, work]. Microsurgery, q.v.

miction (mĭk′shŭn). Urination.

micturate (mĭk′tū-rāt) [L. *micturire*]. To pass the urine. SYN: *urinate*.

micturition (mĭk-tū-rĭ′shŭn). The voiding of urine. SYN: *urination*

M.I.D. *minimum infective dose*.

midbody (mĭd′bŏd-ē). Microtubules that appear as a granule between daughter cells during telophase of mitosis.

midbrain [AS. *mid*, middle, + *braegen*, brain]. The corpora quadrigemina, the crura cerebri, and aqueduct of Sylvius, which connect the pons and cerebellum with the hemispheres of the cerebrum. SYN: *mesencephalon*.

midcarpal (mĭd-kăr′păl). 1. Between the two rows of carpal bones. 2. Mediocarpal.

middle lobe syndrome. Atelectasis, bronchiectasis, or chronic pneumonitis of the right middle lobe of the lung. May be due to calcified lymph nodes compressing the right middle lobe bronchus.

midget. A very small person; an adult who is perfectly formed but has not attained and will not attain full growth.

midgut [AS. *mid*, middle, + *gut*, intestine]. The midportion of the embryonic gut that opens ventrally into the yolk stalk.

midline (mĭd′līn). Any line that bisects a structure that is bilaterally symmetrical.

midoccipital (mĭd″ŏk-sĭp′ĭ-tăl). In the middle of the occiput.

midpain (mĭd′pān). Intermenstrual pain.

midplane (mĭd′plān). 1. The plane bisecting a symmetrical structure. 2. In obstetrics, the plane of least dimensions in the pelvic outlet.

midriff (mĭd′rĭf) [″ + *hrif*, belly]. The diaphragm; the middle region of the torso.

midsection (mĭd-sĕk′shŭn) [″ + L. *secare*, to cut]. A section through the middle of a structure.

midsternum (mĭd-stĕr′nŭm). The largest and middle portion of the sternum.

midstream specimen. A urine specimen collected during the passage of the urine after the flow has begun and prior to the end. This is done to obtain a specimen with little urethral contamination.

midtarsal (mĭd-tăr′săl). Between the two rows of bones that comprise the tarsus of the foot.

midwife [″ + *wif*, wife]. A female who practices the art of aiding in the delivery of children.

m., nurse-. A nurse who has received special training in obstetrics and is qualified to deliver infants.

midwifery (mĭd-wĭf′ĕr-ē) The art of assisting at childbirth. SYN: *obstetrics*.

migraine (mī′grān) [Fr. from Gr. *hemikrania*, half skull]. Paroxysmal attacks of headache, frequently unilateral, usually accompanied by disordered vision and gastrointestinal disturbances. Thought to be the result of vasodilation of extracerebral cranial arteries.

ETIOL: Unknown but a family history of migraine will be found in over half of the patients. It may be precipitated by allergic hypersensitivity or emotional disturbances.

SYM: Headaches associated with the sensation of seeing zigzags of light, called scintillating scotomata, vomiting, and at times diplopia, unilateral sweating, and focal symptoms. Sharp stabbing pains frequently in temporofrontal region.

DIAG: It must be distinguished from other types of headache, but the history, the course of the disorder, and the peculiar combination of symptoms rarely permit much uncertainty. The frequency may vary from several times a week to several times a year.

TREATMENT: Rest in quiet, darkened room during attack. Ergotamine tartrate proves efficacious in most cases but should be taken at the onset of the attack.

migration (mī-grā′shŭn) [L. *migrare*, to move from place to place]. Passage of cells from one position to another.

Ex.: migration of an ovum from the ovary into the fallopian tube; movement of leukocytes through the wall of a blood vessel into surrounding tissues.

m., internal, of ovum. Passage of the ovum through the uterine (fallopian) tube to the uterus.

m. of leukocytes. Passage of white blood corpuscles through walls of capillaries. SYN: *diapedesis*.

m. of testicle. Descent of testicle into the scrotum. SYN: *descensus testis*.

migratory. 1. Pert. to migration. 2. Changing or capable of changing positions.

mikro-. SEE: words beginning with *micro-*.

Mikulicz's drain (mĭk′ū-lĭch″ĕs). [Johann von Mikulicz-Radecki, Polish surgeon, 1850–1905] Drain formed by pushing a single layer of gauze into a cavity or wound, then packing with several layers of gauze as the original layer is pushed farther and farther into the defect.

Mikulicz's mask. Gauze-covered frame worn over nose and mouth during performance of operation.

Mikulicz's pad. Folded gauze pad for packing off the viscera in abdominal operations and used as a sponge in general.

Mikulicz's syndrome. Chronic infiltration with lymphocytes and painless enlargement of lacrimal and salivary glands.

mildew [AS. *mildeaw*]. Lay term for a discoloration or superficial coating on various materials caused by the growth of fungi. Occurs in damp conditions.

milia (mĭl′ē-ă). Pl. of milium.

miliaria (mĭl-ē-ā′rē-ă) [L. *milium*, millet]. Vesicles caused by obstruction of ducts of sweat glands. Acute inflammation of the sweat glands will result if the obstruction persists. The three forms of miliaria (sudamina, rubra, and profunda) represent different levels of obstruction of the sweat ducts. Occurs most commonly in infants, the obese, and in those exposed to excessive heat for prolonged periods. Excessive clothing and hyperhidrosis are contributing factors. SYN: *prickly heat.*

ETIOL: Exposure to excessive heat, skin irritants, and tendency to hyperhidrosis.

SYM: Sudden appearance of red patches of small papules. Vesicles are discrete and accompanied by red areolae. They usually appear on the trunk and are accompanied by itching, burning, and fever of short duration. They occur in hot weather, in tropical countries, and in individuals sweating profusely. Papules may become eczematous if irritated.

TREATMENT: The only effective treatment and prevention is avoidance of further sweating. Calamine lotion helps to relieve symptoms.

m. crystallina. Sweat escaped into or just below the stratum corneum. SYN: *sudamen.*

m. profunda. Nearly always follows attacks of miliaria rubra. Seen almost exclusively in the tropics. Area is covered with pale, firm papules 1 to 3 mm. across. These are painless and do not cause itching.

m. rubra. An eruption of papulovesicles at the mouth of sweat follicles and accompanied by inflammation, resulting from obstruction to the ducts of the sweat glands. Sweat escapes into the epidermis. Symptoms oscillate with the heat load of the individual. SYN: *prickly heat.*

miliary (mĭl′ē-ă-rē) [L. *miliaris,* like a millet seed]. Characterized by presence of small nodules or lesions resembling millet seed.

miliary fever. Sudden onset of fever with drenching sweats, followed by miliary vesicles and erythema. May be related to influenza.

miliary tubercles. Small gray nodules in first stage of tuberculosis.

miliary tuberculosis. Acute, generalized tuberculosis with minute tubercles in the affected part or organ.

milieu (mē-lyŭ′) [Fr.]. Environment.

m. interieur. Internal environment of extracellular fluids of the body.

milieu therapy. A method of psychotherapy that controls the environment of the patient to provide interpersonal contacts that will develop trust, assurance, and personal autonomy.

milium (mĭl′ē-ŭm) [L., millet seed]. (pl. *milia*) White pinhead-size papules occurring on face, and sometimes the trunk of a newborn, and that usually disappear in several weeks; keratin-filled cysts.

TREATMENT: Mechanical keratolytics (pumice stone, soap), salicylic acid and sulfur ointment, or incision and expression of contents.

m., colloid. Tiny papule formed beneath the epidermis due to colloid degeneration.

milk [AS. *meolc*]. A secretion of the mammary glands for feeding the young. Sp. gr. about 1.032.

COMP: Milk consists of water, organic substances, and mineral salts. SEE: table. *Organic substances:* Proteins: The principal proteins are caseinogen, lactoalbumin, and lactoglobulin; in the presence of calcium ions, soluble caseinogen is converted into insoluble casein by the action of acids, rennet, or pepsin. This brings about the curdling of milk. Lactoglobulin is identical with serum globulin of blood and hence contains maternal antibodies. Carbohydrates: Lactose or milk sugar is the principal sugar, although small quantities of other sugars are present. Fats: The principal fats are glycerides of oleic, palmitic, and myristic acids. Smaller quantities of stearic acid and short-chain fatty acids with carbon chains of C_4 to C_{24} are present. Sterols and phosphatides (lecithin and cephalin) are also present. Churning causes the fat globules to unite into a solid mass and separate from the whey to form butter. *Mineral salts:* The principal cations are calcium, potassium, and sodium; the principal anions are phosphate and chloride. Citrates and lactates are present in

Composition of Milk in Percent

	Human Milk	Cow's Milk
Water	87–88	85–88
Minerals	0.2	0.7
Protein	1.0–1.5	3.5–4.0
Fat	3.5–4.0	3.5–4.0
Sugar (lactose, carbohydrate)	6.5–7.0	4.5
Reaction	Alkaline	Acid

small quantities. Milk is low in iron and magnesium.

Vitamins: Vitamins A and those of the B complex (thiamine, riboflavin, and pantothenic acid) are present in adequate quantities to meet the needs of a growing child. Milk is low in vitamins C and D.

On standing at room temperature milk sours as a result of the action of lactic acid bacilli on lactose converting it into lactic acid. When the pH reaches 5.34, coagulation occurs, resulting in production of a curd. The remaining watery portion is called whey.

Milk contains antibodies that are present in the mother's blood. Milk also contains a number of enzymes (catalase, oxidase, reductase, phosphatase).

m., acidophilus. Milk inoculated with Lactobacillus acidophilus, a bacterium that grows best in an acid medium. Used to modify the bacterial flora of the digestive tract.

m., butter-. That portion of milk left after removal of butter following churning.

m., casein. Milk prepared with a large quantity of casein and fat but little sugar and salts.

m., certified. Milk certified by a milk commission as pure.

m., condensed. Partly evaporated and sweetened milk.

m., cows'. Fluid, whole, 1 cup (244 gm.): Cal. 165; protein 9 gm.; carbohydrate 12 gm.; calcium 285 mg.; vitamin A 390 I.U. Minimum standards for fat content vary from state to state. National average is 3.7% fat.

m., evaporated. Cows' milk that has been concentrated by evaporating some of the water. It can be canned after pasteurization, q.v., and stored for long periods of time. SEE: *milk, lactic acid evaporated.*

m., filled. A product made by combining fats or oils other than milk fat with milk solids. The product resembles milk.

m., fortified. Milk enriched by the addition of cream, albumin, or vitamins.

m., homogenized. Milk that has been processed so that fats are combined with the body of the milk; thus the cream does not separate.

m., instant dry nonfat. Dried skimmed milk. It may be stored at room temperature until needed. Reconstituted by adding water to the granules.

m., lactic acid evaporated. Evaporated milk to which sugar and lactic acid have been added. To prepare this milk, add 17 oz. (503 ml.) of water to 13 oz. (384 ml.) of evaporated milk, 2 level tbsp. (1 oz. or 28 gm.) of granulated sugar and 3 tbsp. (45 ml.) of vinegar. This mixture contains 77 Cal. per 100 ml.

May be used for normal infants from birth to 12 months. For older children omit the sugar. This reduces the Cal. to about 67 per 100 ml. (20 per oz.).

m., modified. Milk altered so that its composition more closely approximates that of human milk.

m., mother's. Milk from the mammary glands of a woman.

m., nonfat. M., skimmed.

m. of bismuth. USP. A suspension of bismuth hydroxide and bismuth subcarbonate in water. It is an antacid. Previously used name was bismuth magma.

m., pasteurized. Milk heated to a specified temperature for a precise length of time and then cooled rapidly. This kills pathogenic bacteria without appreciably altering the taste of the milk. SEE: *pasteurization.*

m., protein. Milk with high protein and low carbohydrate and fat content.

m., red. Milk contaminated by blood, chromogenic bacteria, or plant pigments.

m., ropy. Milk that has become viscid due to formation of vegetable gums from carbohydrates or mucinlike substances from proteins as a result of bacterial action.

m., skimmed. Milk that has the cream portion removed. SYN: *m., nonfat.*

m., sour. Milk with lactic acid caused by lactic acid bacteria.

m., sterilized. Milk that has been boiled to kill bacteria.

m., uterine. Whitish fluid found between villi in placenta of pregnant uterus.

m., uviol. Milk sterilized by ultraviolet rays.

m., vegetable. 1. The latex of plants. 2. A synthetic milk prepared from juices of various plants, such as soybean.

m., vitamin D. Milk in which vitamin D content has been increased by addition of concentrates, ultraviolet irradiation, or by feeding irradiated yeast to milk-producing animals.

m., witch's. Milk secreted in the breast of the newborn.

milk-alkali syndrome. Elevated blood calcium without an increase in calcium or phosphate in the urine, renal insufficiency, and alkalosis due to prolonged intake of excessive amounts of milk and soluble alkali. This condition is usually found as an undesired side effect in conjunction with treating a peptic ulcer. SYN: *Burnett's syndrome.*

milker's nodules. Painless smooth or warty lesions on the hands and arms, produced by the virus that causes paravaccinia, a viral disease that affects the udders of cows and may be transmitted to man. SEE: *paravaccinia.*

milk fever. Fever during the puerperium due to infection.

milking. Removal of the contents of a tubular structure by compressing the tube with the fingers and moving them along the course of the tube. This maneuver forces material out of the tube which might not otherwise be seen or available for study.

Ex.: milking to express purulent material from the urethra. SEE: *strip.*

milk leg. Thrombosis of the iliac or femoral vein followed by swelling of the leg. So named because it is often a complication of puerperium. SYN: *phlegmasia alba dolens.*

Milkman's syndrome (mĭlk'mănz). [Louis A. Milkman, U.S. roentgenologist, 1895–1951] Failure of reabsorption of phosphate by the renal tubules. This causes a special type of demineralization of bones that produces a transverse striped area of multiple pseudofractures in roentgenograms of the bones.

milk of magnesia. USP. Magnesium hydroxide in suspension, used as an antacid and a cathartic. Previously used name was magnesia magma. Trade name is Mint-O-mag.

milk teeth. The first or deciduous teeth.

milk tumor. Retention of milk in the mammary gland.

Miller-Abbott tube. [T. Grier Miller, U.S. physician, b. 1886; W. Osler Abbott, U.S. physician, 1902–1943] A double-channel intestinal tube used to relieve intestinal distention. Inserted through a nostril, the tube is passed through the stomach into the small intestine.

milli- [L. *milli,* thousand]. Prefix used in metric system to denote one-thousandth (10^{-3}).

milliammeter. Ammeter registering in milliamperes. SEE: *ammeter.*

milliampere (mĭl″ē-ăm'pēr). ABBR: ma. One-thousandth of an ampere.

milliampere minute. An electrical unit of quantity, equivalent to that delivered by 1 milliampere in 1 minute.

milliampere-seconds. Product of the time of radiation exposure times the milliamperage used.

millibar (mĭl'ĭ-băr). One thousandth of a bar, which is 100 newtons per square meter. The normal atmospheric pressure of 14.7 pounds per square inch is equal to 1013 millibars.

millicoulomb (mĭl″ĭ-koo'lŏm). A unit of electric current, one one-thousandth, 10^{-3}, of a coulomb.

millicurie (mĭl″ĭ-kū'rē). ABBR: mc. One-thousandth of a curie.

millicurie hour. A practical unit of dosage for radon: 1 mc. of radon applied for one hour. The biological effect depends on time, filtration, and distance.

milliequivalent. ABBR: mEq. The concentration of electrolytes in a certain volume of solution. Usually expressed as milliequivalent per liter (mEq./L.). It is calculated by multiplying the milligrams per liter by the valence of the chemical and dividing by the molecular weight of the substance:

$$\text{mEq./L.} = \frac{(\text{mg./L.}) \times \text{Valence}}{\text{molecular weight}}$$

milligram (mĭl'ĭ-grăm). ABBR: mg. One-thousandth of a gram.

millilambert (mĭl″ĭ-lăm'bĕrt). A unit of light intensity, one one-thousandth of a lambert. About one foot-candle, but more accurately, it is 0.929 lumens per square foot.

milliliter. ABBR: ml. One-thousandth of a liter. For practical purposes it is equivalent to one cubic centimeter. The term milliliter is used when refering to *liquid* volume; cubic centimeter is used when referring to the volume of a gas.

millimeter. ABBR: mm. One-thousandth of a meter.

millimicrocurie (mĭl″ĭ-mī″krō-kū'rē). A nanocurie or 10^{-9} curie.

millimicrogram (mĭl″ĭ-mī'krō-grăm). A nanogram or 10^{-9} gram.

millimicron (mĭl-ĭ-mī'krŏn). ABBR: mμ or mmm. One-thousandth of a micron; one-millionth of a millimeter.

millimole (mĭl'ĭ-mōl). ABBR: mM. One-thousandth of a mole.

milling-in. A method of adjusting the occlusion of teeth by moving the teeth against each other while an abrasive substance is between them.

millinormal (mĭl″ĭ-nor'măl). Strength of a solution equal to one one-thousandth normal.

milliosmole (mĭl″ē-ŏs'mōl). The osmotic pressure equal to one one-thousandth of the molecular weight of a substance divided by the number of ions that the substance forms in a liter of solution.

millipede (mĭl'ĭ-pēd). A wingless, worm-like insect with a pair of legs on each body segment. Some produce an irritating venom.

millisecond (mĭl″ĭ-sĕk'ŏnd). One one-thousandth of a second.

millivolt (mĭl'ĭ-vōlt). One one-thousandth of a volt.

Milontin. Trade name for phensuximide.

milphae (mĭl'fē) [Gr. *milphai*]. Loss of eyebrow hair.

milphosis (mĭl-fō'sĭs) [Gr.]. Loss of eyebrows or eyelashes.

Milroy's disease (mĭl'roys). [William F. Milroy, U.S. physician, 1853–1942] Chronic hereditary edema of the legs.

Miltown. Trade name for meprobamate, USP.

Milwaukee brace. A steel and leather brace extending from a chin cup with neck pad to the pelvis, used to correct minimal curve scoliosis.

mimesis [Gr.]. Imitation, mimicry. Term applied to a disease that exhibits symptoms of another disease or to conditions in hysteria that simulate organic disease.

mimetic, mimic (mī-mĕt'ĭk, mĭm'ĭk) [Gr. *mimetikos*]. Imitative.

mimmation (mī-mā'shŭn). A form of stuttering in which the "m" sound is inappropriately used.

mimosis (mī-mō'sĭs). Mimesis, q.v.

min. *minim; minute.*

Minamata disease (mĭn"ă-maw'tă). Neurological disease due to ingestion of alkyl mercury, an organic mercury compound used in industrial processes. Present in fish taken from Minamata Bay, Japan. SYN: *yushi.*

SYM: Paresthesias, loss of peripheral vision, dysarthria, ataxia, tremors, excessive salivation, sweating, and mental disturbances.

PROG: Poor. Death may occur.

mind [AS. *gemynd*]. Integration of functions of the brain resulting in the ability to perceive surroundings, to have emotions, imagination, memory, and will, and to process information in an intelligent manner.

mineral [L. *minerale*]. 1. An inorganic element or compound occurring in nature, esp. one that is solid. 2. Inorganic; not of animal or plant origin. 3. Impregnated with minerals, as mineral water. 4. Pert. to minerals.

mineral acid. An acid containing no carbon atoms. SYN: *inorganic acid.*

mineral compounds. Compounds of mineral elements, excepting carbon, constitute the mineral constituents of the body. SEE: *acid-base balance; names of elements; buffer.*

FUNCT: Minerals are essential constituents of all cells; they form the greater portion of the hard parts of the body (bone, teeth, nails); they are essential components of respiratory pigments, enzymes, and enzyme systems; they regulate the permeability of cell membranes and capillaries; they regulate the excitability of muscular and nervous tissue; they are essential for regulation of osmotic pressure equilibria; they are necessary for maintenance of proper acid-base balance; they are essential constituents of secretions of glands; they play an important role in water metabolism and regulation of blood volume.

Mineral salts and water are excreted daily from the body. These must be replaced through food intake. Daily requirements for principal minerals for a normal adult are as follows: calcium and phosphorus, 0.8–1.4 gm.; sodium, 10–18 mg.; copper, 1–2 mg.; iodine, 50–75 μg (micrograms); magnesium, 100 mg.; sodium, about 1 gm. of sodium chloride per kg. of water intake. Requirements are greater for growing children and pregnant women and in certain pathological conditions.

mineralization (mĭn"ĕr-ăl-ī-zā'shŭn). Normal or abnormal deposition of minerals in tissues.

mineralocorticoid (mĭn"ĕr-ăl-ō-kor'tĭ-koyd). A biologically active principle of the adrenal cortex predominantly involved in the regulation of fluid and electrolytes by its effects on ion transport and on the renal tubules.

mineral oil. USP. Liquid petrolatum.

mineral spring. A spring in which water contains mineral salts thought to have a therapeutic value in certain diseases, but usually the principal action is as a cathartic. SYN: *spa.*

mineral water. Water that contains sufficient inorganic salts to cause it to have characteristic properties.

minim (mĭn'ĭm) [L. *minimum,* least]. ABBR: m., min. One-sixtieth part of a fluidram or 0.06 milliliter.

minimal (mĭn'ĭ-măl). Least; the smallest possible.

minimal brain damage. SEE: *attention deficit disorder.*

minimal brain dysfunction. ABBR: MBD. A poorly defined concept rather than a specific diagnosis. SEE: *attention deficit disorder.*

minimal cerebral dysfunction. SEE: *attention deficit disorder.*

minimal dose. Smallest dose producing an effect.

minimum (mĭn'ĭ-mŭm). (pl. *minima*) Least quantity or lowest limit. SEE: *threshold.*

minimum daily requirements. ABBR: MDR. The daily requirements of vitamins and minerals needed to prevent symptoms of deficiency. SEE: *Dietary Allowances* in *Appendix.*

minimum lethal dose. Smallest quantity of a substance capable of producing death.

minin light (mĭn'ĭn). A special light that produces violet or ultraviolet light.

Minipress. Trade name for prazosin hydrochloride.

Minocin. Trade name for minocycline hydrochloride, USP.

minocycline hydrochloride (mī-nō-sī'klēn). USP. An antibiotic of the tetracycline class. Trade names are Minocin and Vectrin.

minor. Person not of legal age and thus requiring consent for medical, surgical, or dental care. Legal age in the U.S.A. is variable from state to state.

m., emancipated. A person not of legal age who is either in the armed services, married or mother of a child whether married or not, or has left home and is self-sufficient. Some state legislatures do not require such an individual to have parental consent in order to receive medical or surgical care.

Minot-Murphy diet (mī'nŏt). [George R.

Minot, U.S. physician, 1885–1950; William P. Murphy, U.S. physician, b. 1892] Diet for pernicious anemia containing large quantities of liver.

Mintezol. Trade name for thiabendazole, USP.

Mint-O-mag. Trade name for milk of magnesia, USP.

minute volume. The volume of air breathed in a minute.

mio- (mī'ō) [Gr. *meion,* less]. Combining form meaning less, smaller.

miocardia (mī-ō-kăr'dē-ă) [" + *kardia,* heart]. Lessening of heart's volume during systolic contraction. SYN: *systole.*

Miochol. Trade name for acetylcholine chloride.

miodidymus (mī"ō-dĭd'ĭ-mŭs) [" + *didymos,* twin]. A fetus with two heads joined at the occiput.

miolecithal (mī"ō-lĕs'ĭ-thăl) [" + *lekithos,* egg yolk]. Pert. to an egg with a small amount of yolk.

mionectic (mī-ō-nĕk'tĭk) [Gr. *meionektikos,* disposed to taking too little]. Pert. to or having or using a subnormal amount of oxygen, esp. blood. SEE: *mesectic.*

mioplasmia. Abnormal lessening of the amount of blood plasma.

miopragia (mī-ō-prā'jē-ă) [Gr. *meion,* less, + *prassein,* to perform]. Decrease of functional activity.

miopus (mī'ō-pŭs) [" + *ops,* face]. Conjoined twins with one having a rudimentary face.

miosis (mī-ō'sĭs) [Gr. *meiosis,* a lessening]. 1. Abnormal contraction of the pupils.

ETIOL: May be due to irritation of the oculomotor system, or paralysis of dilators. Occurs in certain fevers, congestion of iris, in typhus, in early stages of meningitis, and in some forms of drug poisoning. Also seen in brain lesions and sunstroke.

2. The stage of disease during which intensity of signs and symptoms diminishes.

Miostat. Trade name for carbachol (intraocular).

miotic. 1. An agent that causes the pupil to contract, such as eserine or pilocarpine. 2. Pert. to or causing contraction of the pupil. 3. Diminishing. SYN: *myotic.*

miracidium (mī"ră-sĭd'ē-ŭm) [Gr. *meirakidion,* lad]. (pl. *miracidia*) A ciliated free-swimming larva of a digenetic fluke. On emerging from an ovum, it penetrates a snail of a particular species and metamorphoses into a sporocyst. SEE: *fluke.*

mire (mēr) [L. *mirari,* to look at]. A test object on the ophthalmometer, the images of which denote the amount of astigmatism.

mirror [Fr. *miroir*]. A polished surface that reflects rays of light and thus reproduces visible images of objects in front of it.

m., dental. A dental instrument commonly used for viewing occlusal and distal surfaces of teeth and for retracting soft tissues from the field of operation. SYN: *mouth mirror.*

miryachit (mĭr-ē'ă-chĭt) [Russian]. A type of "jumping disorder" seen in Siberia. It is similar to the Jumping Frenchmen of Maine, q.v. SYN: *saltatory spasm.*

mis- [AS. *mis,* wrong]. Prefix implying bad, wrong, improper or negative.

misanthropia (mĭs"ăn-thrō'pē-ă) [" + Gr. *anthropos,* man]. Hatred of mankind.

miscarriage [" + L. *carrus,* cart]. Lay term for termination of pregnancy at any time before the fetus has attained extrauterine viability. Usually refers specifically to expulsion of fetus in period between fourth month and viability. SYN: *abortion.*

misce (mĭs'ē) [L., mix]. ABBR: M. A direction given on prescriptions, instructing the pharmacist to mix the ingredients.

miscegenation (mĭs"ĕ-jē-nā'shŭn) [L. *miscere,* to mix, + *genus,* race]. Sexual relations or marriage bet. those of different races.

miscible (mĭs'ĭ-bl). Capable of being mixed.

misocainia (mĭs-ō-kī'nē-ă) [Gr. *miseio,* to hate, + *kainos,* new]. An aversion to new ideas. SYN: *misoneism.*

misogamy (mĭ-sŏg'ă-mē) [" + *gamos,* marriage]. Aversion to marriage.

misogynist (mĭs-ŏj'ĭ-nĭst) [" + *gyne,* woman]. One who hates women.

misogyny (mĭs-ŏj'ĭn-ē). Abnormal hatred of women.

misologia (mĭs-ō-lō'jē-ă) [Gr. *miseio,* to hate, + *logos,* study]. Aversion to mental activity.

misoneism (mĭ-sō-nē'ĭzm) [" + *neos,* new]. Aversion to new things or new ideas; conservatism. SYN: *misocainia.*

misopedia (mĭ-sō-pē'dē-ă) [" + Gr. *pais,* child]. Abnormal dislike for children or the young.

Mist., mist. *mistura.*

mistura (mĭs-tū'ră) [L.]. Mixture. Preparation intended for internal use and containing suspended insoluble substances that do not unite chemically. Should always be shaken before using.

Mitchell's disease (mĭch'ĕlz). [Silas W. Mitchell, Philadelphia neurologist, 1829–1914] Erythromelalgia, q.v.

mite (mīt) [AS.]. A minute arachnid, a member of the order Acarina. Some are parasitic and are the cause of conditions such as mange and scabies. Some serve as vectors of disease organisms and as intermediate hosts for certain Cestodes.

m., follicle. Mite that lives in hair follicles and sebaceous glands. SYN: *Demodex folliculorum.*

m., itch. Sarcoptes scabiei. SEE: *scabies.*

m., mange. Mites belonging to the families Sarcoptidae and Psoroptidae. The cause of mange and scabies in many species of animals. SEE: *mange; scabies.*

m., red. Redbugs or chiggers, members of the family Thrombiculidae. SEE: *chiggers.*

mitella (mī-tĕl′ă) [L.]. A sling for the arm.

Mithracin. Trade name for mithramycin, USP.

mithramycin (mĭth″ră-mī′sĭn). USP. An antibiotic with antineoplastic action. It is also used experimentally in treating Paget's disease of bone. Trade name is Mithracin.

mithridatism (mĭth′rĭ-dāt″ĭzm). [Mithridates, king of Pontus, 132–63 B.C., supposed to have acquired immunity in this fashion] Immunity to a poison acquired by taking it in doses of gradually increasing size.

miticide (mī′tĭ-sīd) [AS. *mite,* mite, + L. *caedere,* to kill]. A substance that kills mites.

mitigated (mĭt′ĭ-gāt-ĕd) [L. *mitigare,* to soften.]. Diminished in severity. SYN: *allayed; moderated.*

mitis (mī′tĭs) [L.]. Mild.

mitochondria (mīt″ō-kŏn′drē-ă) [Gr. *mitos,* thread, + *chondros,* cartilage]. (sing. *mitochondrion*) Slender microscopic filaments or rods 0.5 micrometer in diameter that can be seen in cells by using phase-contrast microscopy or electron microscopy. They are the source of energy in the cell and are involved in protein synthesis and lipid metabolism. SEE: *cell; organelle* for illus.

mitogen (mī′tō-jĕn). Something that induces cell mitosis.

mitogenesis (mī″tō-jĕn′ĕ-sĭs) [″ + *osis,* condition, + *genesis,* production]. To cause cell mitosis.

mitoma, mitome [Gr. *mitos,* thread]. A fine network support or framework of protoplasm in a cell.

mitomycin (mī″tō-mī′sĭn). USP. An antibiotic with antineoplastic action. Trade name is Mutamycin.

mitoplasm (mī′tō-plăzm) [″ + *plassein,* to form]. The chromatic substance in a cell nucleus.

mitosis (mī-tō′sĭs) [″ + *osis,* condition]. (pl. *mitoses*) Type of cell division of somatic cells where each daughter cell contains the same number of chromosomes as the parent cell. It is the process by which the body grows, and by which somatic cells are replaced. SEE: *cell division* for illus.; *meiosis.*

Mitosis is a continuous process divided into four phases:

Prophase: the chromatin granules of the nucleus stain more densely and become organized into chromosomes that first appear as long, delicate, spiral structures, each consisting of two spiral filaments called chromatids. Each chromosome possesses a clear region (centromere) usually in the midregion. As the prophase progresses, the chromosomes become shorter, more compact, and stain densely; the nuclear membrane and the nucleoli disappear. At the same time, the centriole divides and the two daughter centrioles, each surrounded by a centrosphere, move to opposite poles of the cell. They are connected by fine protoplasmic fibrils that form the achromatic spindle.

Metaphase: the chromosomes (paired chromatids) arrange themselves in an equatorial plane midway between the two centrioles forming the equatorial plate.

Anaphase: the chromatids (now called daughter chromosomes) diverge and move toward their respective centrosomes. The end of their migration marks the beginning of the next phase.

Telophase: the chromosomes at each pole of the spindle undergo changes the reverse of those in the prophase, each becoming a long, loosely spiraled thread. The nuclear membrane reforms and nucleoli reappear. Outlines of chromosomes disappear and chromatin appears as granules scattered throughout nucleus and connected by a lightly staining net. The cytoplasm becomes separated into two parts, resulting in two complete cells. This is accomplished in animal cells by constriction in the equatorial region; in plant cells, a cell plate that gives rise to the cell membrane forms in a similar position. The period between two successive divisions is called interphase.

Mitosis is of particular significance in that genes are distributed equally to each daughter cell and a fixed number of chromosomes is maintained in all somatic cells of an organism.

m., heterotypic. The first or reduction division in the maturation of germ cells.

m., homeotypic. The second or equational division in the maturation of germ cells.

mitosome (mī′tō-sōm) [Gr. *mitos,* thread, + *soma,* body]. 1. A body giving rise to the middle piece of the spermatozoon. 2. Chromatin mass in a cellular nucleus.

mitotane (mī′tō-tān). USP. A drug that selectively acts against the cells of the adrenal cortex. It is used in treating inoperable adrenal cortical carcinoma. Previously used name was o, p′-DDD. Trade name is Lysodren.

mitotic (mī-tŏt′ĭk). Pert. to mitosis.

mitral (mī′trăl). Pert. to the bicuspid or mitral valve. SEE: *facies mitralis.*

mitral commissurotomy. Surgical procedure for treating stenosis of the mitral valve of the heart.

mitral disease. Disease of the mitral valve. SEE: *heart.*

mitralization (mī″trăl-ī-zā′shŭn). In the roentgenogram of the heart, straightening of the left border, as seen in the anterior-posterior view, due to mitral valve disease.

mitral murmur. Murmur produced at the mitral valve.

mitral orifice. Left atrioventricular aperture.

mitral regurgitation. Backflow of blood from the left ventricle into the left atrium due to failure of the valve to close completely.

mitral stenosis. Narrowing orifice of the mitral valve obstructing free flow from atrium to ventricle.

mitral valve. Bicuspid valve, q.v.; valvula bicuspidalis.

mitral valve prolapse. A common and occasionally serious condition in which the cusp or cusps of the mitral valve prolapse into the left atrium during systole. There may be no symptoms, but in some patients, non-anginal chest pain, palpitations, dyspnea, and fatigue may be present.

TREATMENT: Prophylaxis against subacute bacterial endocarditis.

mittelschmerz (mĭt′ĕl-shmărts) [Ger.]. Abdominal pain midway between menstrual periods, occurring at time of ovulation and from the ovulation site.

Mittendorf's dot. A grayish dot on the posterior lens capsule. It is the remnant of the fetal hyaloid artery of the eye.

mittor [L. *mittere,* to send]. A neuron terminal that transmits impulses to ceptors of the adjoining neuron.

mixed [L. *mixtus*]. Consisting of two or more intermingling substances.

mixoscopia [Gr. *mixis,* intercourse, + *skopein,* to examine]. Sexual perversion in which sexual gratification is obtained through observation of others in coition.

mixture (mĭks′tūr) [L. *mistura*]. A combination of two or more substances without chemical union. SEE: *mistura.*

MKS, mks. *meter-kilogram-second.* Indicates measurements used with meter for length, kilogram for weight, and second for time.

ml. *milliliter.*

M.L.A. *left mento-anterior* fetal position.

M.L.D., m.l.d. *minimum lethal dose.*

mM. *millimole.*

mm. *millimeter.*

mmm. *millimicron.*

Mn. Chem. symb. for manganese.

mnemasthenia (nē″măs-thē′nē-ă) [Gr. *mneme,* memory, + *a-,* not, + *sthenos,* strength]. Poor memory not resulting from organic disease.

mnemic (nē′mĭk). Rel. to memory.

mnemonics (nē-mŏn′ĭks) [Gr. *mnemonikos,* pert. to memory]. The art of improving or assisting memory. A device to help recall a series of related data, names, or anatomical terms.

M.O. *Medical Officer.*

Mo. Chem. symb. for molybdenum.

mo. *month.*

mobile [L. *mobilis*]. Movable.

mobile arm support. A device for support of the forearm, usually mounted on a wheelchair, that assists weak shoulder and elbow muscles in positioning the hand, as in feeding. Also: *ball bearing feeder; ball bearing forearm orthosis.*

mobile spasm. Tonic spasm with irregular, slow movements of limbs following hemiplegia. SYN: *athetosis.*

mobility [L. *mobilitas*]. State or quality of being mobile; facility of movement.

mobilization (mō″bĭl-ĭ-zā′shŭn). 1. The making of a fixed or ankylosed part movable. 2. Restoration of motion to a joint. 3. Freeing an organ or making it movable. 4. The freeing, or making available, of substances held in reserve as glycogen or fat.

m., stapes. Surgical treatment to restore mobility to the stapes. Used in treatment of deafness.

mobilize (mō′bĭl-īz). 1. To incite to physiological action. 2. To render movable; to put in movement.

Möbius' disease (mē′bē-ŭs). [Paul J. Möbius, Ger. neurologist, 1853–1907] Migraine accompanied by paralysis of the oculomotor nerves.

Möbius' sign. A symptom in Graves' disease in which one eye converges and the other diverges when looking at the tip of one's nose.

modal (mōd′l) [L. *modus,* mode]. Pert. to, or characteristic of, a mode. Thus pert. to the most frequent, common or typical.

modality. 1. Quality of being modal. 2. A method of application or the employment of any therapeutic agent; limited usually to physical agents. 3. Any specific sensory stimulus such as taste, touch, vision, pressure, or hearing.

Modane. Trade name for danthron.

Modane Soft. Trade name for docusate sodium.

mode (mōd). In statistics, the value or item of the class occurring most frequently in a series of variables.

model. 1. The pattern or form to be used in duplicating or constructing something. In dentistry, the cast or impression of teeth or a single tooth or cavity. 2. The ideal that would be used as a guide for action or imitation, e.g., model conduct or behavior.

m., animal. The study of anatomy, physiology, or pathology in an animal with respect to the possibility of applying the information obtained to human function and disease.

moderated. Mitigated, q.v.

modification (mŏd″ĭ-fĭ-kā′shŭn). The result of

having changed something such as the shape or character of an object or structure.

modiolus (mō-dī′ō-lŭs) [L., hub]. [NA] Central pillar or axial part of cochlea extending from the base to the apex.

modulation (mŏd″ū-lā′shŭn). The alteration in function or status of something in response to a stimulus or altered chemical or physical environment.

modulus (mŏj′ŭ-lŭs) [L., a small measure]. In physics, a constant or coefficient that indicates to what extent a substance possesses some property.

modus [L.]. A method or a mode.

modus operandi. Method of performing an act.

mogilalia (mŏj-ĭ-lā′lē-ă) [Gr. *mogis,* with difficulty, + *lalia,* chatter]. Any speech defect, as stuttering.

mogiphonia (mōj-ĭ-fō′nē-ă) [″ + *phone,* voice]. Difficulty in emitting vocal sounds.

Mohrenheim's space (mor′ĕn-hīmz). [Baron J. J. Freiherr von Mohrenheim, Austrian surgeon, died 1799] Space between the pectoralis major and deltoid muscles just beneath the clavicle.

Mohs' chemosurgery technique. [F. E. Mohs, U.S. surgeon, 1910–1979] A method of excising tumors of the skin. The tumor tissue is fixed in place and a layer is removed. That portion is then examined microscopically. This procedure is repeated until the entire tumor is removed. Use of this technique ensures complete removal. It is esp. useful in treating basal cell epitheliomas.

moiety (moy′ĕ-tē) [Fr. *moitié,* fr. L. *medietas,* middle]. A part of something that can be divided.

moist (moyst). Damp, wet.

mol. Mole, def. 2, q.v.

molal (mō′lăl). One mole of solute per kilogram of solvent. SEE: *molar.*

molality (mō-lăl′ĭ-tē). The number of moles of a solute per kilogram of solvent.

molar. 1. [L. *molaris,* grinding] A grinding or back tooth, one of three on each side of the jaws. The first permanent molar erupts at the 6th year; the second one about the 12th year. The third molars (wisdom teeth) are extremely variable, usually erupting between 17th and 25th years. However, they may erupt later or not at all. SEE: *dentition; teeth.* 2. [L. *moles,* a mass] Pert. to a mass; not molecular. 3. Pert. to a mole (def. 2). 4. Gram-molecule. SYN: *mole* (def. 2).

molariform (mŏl-ăr′ĭ-form). Resembling a molar tooth.

molarity. The number of gram molecular weights (moles) of a substance per liter of solution. Thus 1/M (also expressed as 1 M) means one mole of a substance per liter. 0.1/M indicates 0.1 mole per liter.

molar solution. One in which there is one mole of the solute dissolved in each liter of the solution.

mold. 1. A fuzzy coating due to growth of a fungus on the surface of decaying vegetable matter or on nonorganic objects. 2. Any one of a group of parasitic or saprophytic fungi that causes mold, such as black molds (Mucorales) and blue and green molds (Aspergillales). The latter include Penicillium, the source of the antibiotic, penicillin. 3. To shape a mass, as a pill. 4. To shape the fetal head, adapting it to the pelvic inlet.

molding. 1. Shaping of the fetal head, adapting itself to the pelvic inlet. 2. A protective border, used in plastic surgery. 3. Casting of a reproduction.

mole (mōl). 1. [AS. *mael*] A congenital discolored spot elevated above the surface of the skin.

ETIOL: Not clear. May arise from local or static condition of circulation in a small area. Harmless unless irritated.

TREATMENT: Protect against irritation.

CAUTION: Do not tie a thread about a mole in an attempt to remove it. Consult a physician. SYN: *nevus.* SEE: *racemose; melanoma.*

2. [Ger. *Mol,* abbr. for *Molekulargewicht,* molecular weight] A quantity of a chemical compound whose weight in grams equals its molecular weight. Thus 18.016 gm. of water would be one mole. 3. [L. *moles,* a shapeless mass] A uterine mass arising from a poorly developed or degenerating ovum.

m., blood. A mass made up of blood clots, membranes, and placenta, retained following abortion.

m., Breus'. Malformation of the ovum, a decidual tuberous subchorional hematoma.

m., carneous. Blood mole that assumes a fleshlike appearance when retained in uterus for some time. SYN: *m., fleshy.*

m., false. Mole formed from a uterine tumor or polypus.

m., fleshy. M., carneous.

m., hydatid. A polycystic mass in which the chorionic villi have undergone cystic degeneration.

m., pigmented. Nevus pigmentosus.

m., stone. A fleshy mole that has undergone calcareous degeneration in the uterus.

m., true. Mole representing the degenerated embryo or fetus.

m., vascular. A hemangioma.

m., vesicular. M., hydatid.

molecular (mō-lĕk′ū-lăr) [L. *molecula,* little mass]. Pert. to a molecule.

molecular biology. Branch of biology dealing with analysis of the structure and development of biological systems with respect to the chemistry and physics of their molecular constituents.

molecular disease. Disease due to a defect in a single molecule. The abnormal hemoglobin molecule found in persons with sickle cell anemia causes the abnormally shaped red cells characteristic of this disease.

molecular layer. 1. Cortical layer of cerebellar or cerebral substance. 2. (Inner). Inner retinal plexiform layer. 3. (Outer). Outer retinal plexiform layer.

molecular lesion. Defect or absence of a basic organic molecule that is of sufficient importance to cause disease. Sickle cell anemia is an example of this type of lesion.

molecular weight. ABBR: mol. wt. Weight of a molecule attained by totalling the atomic weight of its constituent atoms. SEE: *atomic weight.*

molecule (mŏl'ĕ-kūl) [L. *molecula,* little mass]. 1. The smallest quantity into which a substance may be divided without loss of its characteristics. 2. Any small portions of a substance. 3. A chemical combination of two or more atoms that form a specific chemical compound; the chemical elements are formed by the combination of atoms.

Combinations of dissimilar atoms form chemical compounds. In normal molecules the positive and negative electrical charges exactly balance. Excess or deficiency of either positive or negative charge by the loss or acquisition of electrons results in the formation of an ion.

The molecule is designated by the number of atoms it contains, as monatomic (one atom); diatomic (two); triatomic (three); tetratomic (four); pentatomic (five); or hexatomic (six). SEE: *cleavage.*

molimen (mō-lī'mĕn) [L., effort]. (pl. *molimina*) Effort to establish any normal function, esp. that necessary to establish the menstrual flow.

Mol-Iron. Trade name for ferrous sulfate, USP.

Moll's glands. [Jacob A. Moll, Dutch oculist, 1832–1914] Modified sweat glands at border of eyelids. SYN: *ciliary glands.*

mollities (mōl-ĭsh'ē-ēz) [L.]. Abnormal softening of a part.

m. ossium. Softening of the bones. SYN: *malacosteon; osteomalacia.*

mollusc, mollusk. Any member of the phylum Mollusca.

Mollusca. A phylum of animals that includes the bivalves (mussels, oysters, clams), slugs, and snails. Snails serve as intermediate hosts of many parasitic flukes. Oysters and clams may transmit the virus of infectious hepatitis, esp. if improperly cooked.

molluscous (mŏ-lŭs'kŭs). Concerning molluscum.

molluscum (mŏ-lŭs'kŭm) [L., soft]. A mildly infective skin disease characterized by tumor formations on the skin.

m. contagiosum. The usual mildly contagious form of molluscum that affects mainly children and young adults.

SYM: Characterized by small waxy globular epithelial tumors that are umbilicated containing semifluid caseous matter or solid masses, healing without scarring though they may suppurate and break down, commonly on face, eyelids, breasts, genitalia, and inner surface of thigh. These may only be a few millimeters in diameter, but are sometimes 2 or 3 cm. wide. On pressure a substance resembling sebum is expressed.

ETIOL: A large virus of the pox group.

TREATMENT: Incision, expression of contents, followed by application of tincture of iodine.

m. fibrosum. A form of molluscum showing masses of fibrocellular tissue.

molt. To shed a covering such as feathers or skin that is replaced by new growth.

mol. wt. *molecular weight.*

molybdenum (mō-lĭb'dĕ-nŭm). SYMB: Mo. At. wt. 95.94; at. no. 42. A hard, heavy, metallic element.

molysmophobia (mō-lĭz"mō-fō'bē-ă) [Gr. *molysma,* stain, + *phobia,* fear]. Morbid fear of contamination or infection. SYN: *mysophobia.*

momentum (mō-mĕn'tŭm) [L.]. 1. In physics, the description of a quantity obtained by multiplying the mass of a body by its linear velocity. 2. Force of motion acquired by a moving object as a result of continuance of its motion; impetus.

monad [Gr. *monas,* a unit]. 1. A univalent element. 2. A unicellular organism. 3. One of the four components of a tetrad.

monamide (mŏn-ăm'ĭd). An amide with one amide group.

monamine (mŏn-ăm'ĭn). An amine with one amine group.

monarthric (mŏn-ăr'thrĭk) [Gr. *monos,* single, + *arthron,* joint]. Concerning a single joint.

monarthritis (mŏn"ăr-thrī'tĭs) [" + " + *itis,* inflammation]. Arthritis affecting a single joint.

monarticular (mŏn-ăr-tĭk'ŭ-lăr). Concerning or affecting one joint.

monaster (mŏn-ăs'tĕr) [" + *aster,* star]. Single starlike figure formed in mitosis.

monathetosis (mŏn"ăth-ē-tō'sĭs) [" + *athetos,* not fixed, + *osis,* condition]. Athetosis affecting a single part of the body.

monatomic (mŏn"ă-tŏm'ĭk) [" + *atomos,* indivisible]. 1. Concerning a single atom. 2. Univalent.

monaural (mŏn-aw'răl). Concerning an ear.

monaxonic (mŏn"ăk-sŏn'ĭk) [" + Gr. *axon,* axis]. A neuron with one axon.

Mondonesi's reflex (mŏn-dō-nā'zēz). [Filippo Mondonesi, It. physician] In coma, contraction of facial muscles following pressure on eyeball. SYN: *bulbomimic reflex; facial reflex.*

Mondor's disease (mŏn'dorz). [Henri Mondor, Fr. physician, 1885–1962] Thrombosis and sclerosis of a subcutaneous vein or veins in the breast area of either sex. May occur after trauma or appear without apparent cause. The long firm tender cord or stringlike structure extends from the breast up into the axilla or down toward the epigastrium. It is a benign self-limiting disease that is important because its appearance may be confused with cancer of the breast.

monecious (mŏn-ē'shŭs). Monoecious, q.v.

monesthetic (mŏn"ĕs-thĕt'ĭk) [Gr. *monos,* single, + *aisthesis,* sensation]. Affecting only one of the senses.

monestrous (mŏn-ĕs'trŭs). Having a single estrous cycle in a single sexual season.

mongolian spots (mŏn-gō'lē-ăn). Blue-grey areas of discoloration of the skin of the lower back, thighs, and sometimes the shoulders of the newborn. They gradually fade. Eighty percent of nonwhite and 10% of white infants have these benign spots.

mongolism. Previous term for Down's syndrome or trisomy 21. A severe form of mental deficiency due to deletion of a chromosome or the triplication of a chromosome. Children have a characteristic appearance: small head, slanting eyes with inner epicanthal fold (thus the name mongol), and a fissured tongue that usually is large and protruding. About one in eight of all mentally defective infants are afflicted with this syndrome. About 70% of children with this syndrome are born to women over 30. The risk of a mother who has had one Down's syndrome child having another one is increased four times.

mongoloid (mŏn'gō-loyd). 1. Concerning Mongols. 2. Characterized by mongolism, i.e., Down's syndrome.

monilethrix (mŏn-ĭl'ĕ-thrĭks) [L. *monile,* necklace, + Gr. *thrix,* hair]. A genetic defect of the hair shaft in which the hair becomes beaded and brittle. The defect usually appears by the second month of life. No effective treatment.

Monilia [L. *monile,* necklace]. Former name for the genus of fungi now called Candida, q.v.

monilial (mō-nĭl'ē-ăl). Concerning Monilia.

moniliasis (mō"nĭ-lī'ă-sĭs). Infection of the skin or mucous membranes by yeastlike fungi. Usually localized in skin, nails, mouth, vagina, bronchi, or lungs, but may invade bloodstream. SYN: *candidiasis.*

ETIOL: Various species of Candida but chiefly C. albicans.

moniliform (mŏn-ĭl'ĭ-form) [L. *monile,* necklace, + *forma,* shape]. Resembling a necklace or string of beads.

moniliid (mō-nĭl'ē-ĭd). A skin eruption due to hypersensitivity to a Monilia infection in another part of the body.

moniliosis (mō-nĭl-ē-ō'sĭs). Moniliasis.

monitor (mŏn'ĭ-tor) [L., one who warns]. 1. One who observes an operation, procedure, or apparatus, esp. one who is responsible for detecting and preventing malfunction. 2. A device that provides a warning if that which is being observed fails or malfunctions. 3. To check by using an electronic device.

m., blood pressure. Monitor that provides a record of systolic and diastolic blood pressure.

m., cardiac. Monitor of heart function, providing visual and audible record of heartbeat.

m., fetal. 1. Monitor that detects and displays fetal heartbeat. 2. Assessment of fetus in utero with respect to its heart rate by use of electrocardiogram or by chemical analysis of the amniotic fluid or fetal blood.

m., personal radiation. Small device carried by an individual to measure the accumulated radiation dosage over a period of time. SEE: *dosimeter.*

m., temperature. Monitor for measuring and recording temperature of the body or some particular portion of the body.

mono-, mon- [Gr. *monos,* single]. Prefix designating one, single.

monoacidic (mŏn"ō-ă-sĭd'ĭk). Having one replaceable hydroxyl (OH) group.

monoamide. Monamide.

monoamine. Containing one amine radical.

monoamine oxidase inhibitors. ABBR: MAO inhibitors. A group of drugs that are effective in treating depression. Their mode of action in addition to inhibiting monoamine oxidase is not clearly understood. Because of their toxic potential, they should be used with caution. Hypertensive crises have been observed in persons who eat certain kinds of cheese while taking MAO inhibitors. SEE: *tyramine.*

monoanesthesia (mŏn"ō-ăn-ĕs-thē'sē-ă). Anesthesia of a single member or organ.

monobacillary (mŏn"ō-băs'ĭ-lă"rē). Concerning a single species of bacilli.

monobacterial (mŏn"ō-băk-tē'rē-ăl). Concerning a single species of bacteria.

monobasic (mŏn-ō-bā'sĭk) [Gr. *monos,* single, + *basis,* a base]. Having one hydrogen atom replaceable by a metal or positive radical.

monobenzone (mŏn"ō-bĕn'zōn). USP. A drug used in treating hyperpigmentation conditions. Trade name is Benoquin.

monoblast (mŏn'ō-blăst) [" + *blastos,* germ]. A cell that gives rise to a monocyte.

monoblastoma (mŏn″ō-blăs-tō′mă) [″ + ″ + *oma,* tumor]. A neoplasm that contains both monoblasts and monocytes.

monoblepsia (mŏn-ō-blĕp′sē-ă) [″ + *blepsis,* sight]. 1. Condition in which vision is more distinct when only one eye is used, hence tendency to close one eye to see clearly. 2. A type of colorblindness in which only one color can be seen.

monobrachius (mŏn″ō-brā′kē-ŭs) [″ + *brachion,* arm]. 1. State of having only one arm. 2. Fetus with only one arm.

monobromated (mŏn″ō-brō′māt-ĕd). Pert. to chemical compound with only one atom of bromine in each molecule.

monocalcic (mŏn-ō-kăl′sĭk). Pert. to a chemical compound containing only one atom of calcium in the molecule.

monocardian (mŏn-ō-kăr′dē-ăn) [″ + *kardia,* heart]. Individual possessing a heart with only one atrium and one ventricle.

monocelled (mŏn′ō-sĕld). Composed of a single cell.

monocephalus (mŏn″ō-sĕf′ă-lŭs) [″ + *kephale,* head]. A congenitally deformed fetus with duplicated parts except for the head. SYN: *syncephalus.*

monochord (mŏn′ō-kord) [″ + *chorde,* cord]. An instrument for testing upper tone audition by means of friction.

monochorea (mŏn″ō-kō-rē′ă) [″ + *choreia,* dance]. Chorea that affects but a single part or extremity.

monochorionic (mŏn-ō-kor″ē-ŏn′ĭk). Possessing a single chorion, as in the case of identical twins.

monochromasy (mŏn″ō-krō-mā′sē) [″ + *chroma,* color]. Colorblindness in which all colors are perceived as shades of gray.

monochromatic (mŏn″ō-krō-măt′ĭk). 1. Having but one color. 2. A colorblind person to whom all colors appear to be of one hue.

monochromatism (mŏn″ō-krō′mă-tĭzm) [Gr. *monos,* single, + *chroma,* color, + *-ismos,* condition]. Complete color blindness.

monochromatophil (mŏn″ō-krō-măt′ō-fĭl) [″ + ″ + *philein,* to love]. A cell or tissue that accepts only one stain.

monochromator (mŏn-ō-krō′mā-tor). Instrument for selective transmission of homogeneous radiant energy.

monoclinic (mŏn″ō-klĭn′ĭk) [″ + *klinein,* to incline]. Pert. to crystals in which the vertical axis is inclined to one lateral axis but at right angles to the other.

monoclonal (mŏn″ō-klōn′ăl). Arising from a single cell.

monoclonal antibodies. Antibodies derived from hybridoma cells, q.v. Such antibodies are of exceptional purity and specificity; they are being used to identify antigens on a number of viruses, and bacteria; in addition, they are used in tissue and blood typing, in identifying hormones such as human chorionic gonadotropin, in diagnosis of infectious diseases, and in identifying tumor antigens. These antibodies are being extensively studied for their potential for treating cancer.

monococcus (mŏn-ō-kŏk′ŭs) [″ + *kokkos,* berry]. A form of coccus existing singly instead of as part of the usual group or chain.

monocontaminated (mŏn″ō-kŏn-tăm′ĭ-nāt″ ĕd). Infected with a single species of organism.

monocrotic (mŏn″ō-krŏt′ĭk) [″ + *krotos,* beat]. Indicating a single pulse wave with no notches in it.

monocular (mŏn-ŏk′ū-lar) [″ + L. *oculus,* eye]. 1. Concerning or affecting but one eye. 2. Possessing a single eyepiece as in a monocular microscope.

monoculus (mŏn-ŏk′ū-lŭs). 1. A bandage for shielding one eye. 2. A fetus with only one eye. SYN: *cyclops.*

monocyclic (mŏn″ō-sī′klĭk). Concerning one cycle.

monocyesis (mŏn″ō-sī-ē′sĭs) [″ + *kyesis,* pregnancy]. Pregnancy with a single fetus.

monocyte (mŏn′ō-sīt) [″ + *kytos,* cell]. A large mononuclear leukocyte having more protoplasm than a lymphocyte. SEE: *blood cell* for illus.

monocytic (mŏn-ō-sĭt′ĭk). Concerning or resembling monocytes.

monocytopenia (mŏn″ō-sī″tō-pē′nē-ă) [″ + *kytos,* cell, + *penia,* lack]. Diminished number of monocytes in the blood.

monocytosis (mŏn″ō-sī-tō′sĭs) [″ + ″ + *osis,* condition]. Excessive number of monocytes in the blood.

monodactylism (mŏn-ō-dăk′tĭl-ĭzm) [″ + *daktylos,* digit]. Condition, usually congenital, of having only one digit on a hand or foot.

monodal (mŏn-ō′dăl) [″ + *hodos,* road]. Connected with one terminal of a resonator so that the patient acts as a capacitor for entrance and exit of high-frequency currents.

monodermoma (mŏn″ō-dĕr-mō′mă) [″ + *derma,* skin, + *oma,* tumor]. A neoplasm originating in one germinal layer.

monodiplopia (mŏn″ō-dĭ-plō′pē-ă) [″ + *diploos,* double, + *ops,* eye]. Double vision in one eye only.

monodromia. Condition of muscles or nerves in which conduction occurs in one direction only.

monoecious (mŏn-ē′shŭs) [″ + *oikos,* house]. Pert. to the presence of functioning male and female sex organs in the same individual.

monogamy (mō-nŏg′ă-mē) [″ + *gamos,* marriage]. The practice of being married to only one person at a time.

monogenesis (mŏn″ō-jĕn′ĕ-sĭs) [Gr. *monos,* single, + *genesis,* production]. 1. Production of offspring of only one sex. 2. The theory that all organisms arise from a single cell. 3. Asexual reproduction.

monogerminal (mŏn″ō-jĕr′mĭ-năl). Produced from a single ovum.

monogony (mō-nŏg′ō-nē) [″ + *gone,* seed]. Asexual reproduction.

monograph (mŏn′ō-grăf) [″ + *graphein,* to write]. A treatise dealing with a single subject.

monohybrid [″ + L. *hybrida,* mongrel]. Offspring of a cross between parents differing in a single character.

monohydrated (mŏn-ō-hī′drāt-ĕd) [″ + *hydor,* water]. United with only one molecule of water.

monohydric (mŏn″ō-hī′drĭk). Having a single replaceable hydrogen atom.

monoideaism, monoideism (mŏn″ō-ī-dē′ă-ĭzm, -dē′ĭzm) [″ + *idea,* idea]. Preoccupation with only one idea; a slight degree of monomania.

monoinfection (mŏn″ō-ĭn-fĕk′shŭn). Infection with a single species of organism.

monoiodotyrosine (mŏn″ō-ī-ō″dō-tī′rō-sēn). An amino acid intermediate in the synthesis of thyroxine and triiodothyronine.

monolayer (mŏn″ō-lā′ĕr). Having a single layer, esp of cells growing in culture.

monolocular (mŏn″ō-lŏk′ū-lar) [″ + L. *loculus,* a small chamber]. Having only one cell or cavity. SYN: *unilocular.*

monomania (mŏn-ō-mā′nē-ă) [″ + *mania,* madness]. Mental illness characterized by distortion of thought processes concerning a single subject or idea.

monomaniac. One afflicted with monomania.

monomastigote (mŏn-ō-măs′tĭ-gōt) [″ + *mastix,* whip]. Possessing only one flagellum.

monomelic (mŏn-ō-mĕl′ĭk) [″ + *melos,* limb]. Affecting a single limb.

monomer (mŏn′ō-mĕr). Any molecule that can be bound to similar molecules to form a polymer.

monomeric (mŏn-ō-mĕr′ĭk) [″ + *meros,* part]. Consisting of, or affecting, a single piece or segment of a body.

monometallic (mŏn″ō-mĕ-tăl′ĭk). Containing a single atom of a metal in the formula.

monomicrobic (mŏn″ō-mī-krō′bĭk). Concerning organisms of a single species.

monomolecular (mŏn″ō-mō-lĕk′ū-lăr). Concerning one molecule.

monomorphic (mŏn-ō-mor′fĭk) [″ + *morphe,* form]. Unchangeable in form; keeping the same form throughout every stage of development.

monomyoplegia (mŏn″ō-mī″ō-plē′jē-ă) [″ + *mys,* muscle, + *plege,* stroke]. Paralysis of only one muscle.

monomyositis (mŏn″ō-mī-ō-sī′tĭs) [″ + ″ + *itis,* inflammation]. Inflamed condition of only one muscle.

mononeural (mŏn-ō-nū′răl) [″ + *neuron,* nerve]. Supplied by or concerning a single nerve.

mononeuritis (mŏn″ō-nū-rī′tĭs) [″ + ″ + *itis,* inflammation]. Inflamed condition of a single nerve.

m. multiplex. Inflammation of nerves in separate body areas.

mononeuropathy (mŏn″ō-nū-rŏp′ă-thē) [″ + ″ + *pathos,* disease]. Disease of a single nerve.

mononoea (mŏn″ō-nē′ă) [″ + *nous,* mind]. Mental fixation on a single subject.

mononuclear (mŏn-ō-nū′klē-ăr) [″ + L. *nucleus,* kernel]. Having one nucleus, particularly a blood cell such as a monocyte or lymphocyte. SYN: *uninuclear.*

mononucleosis (mŏn-ō-nū″klē-ō′sĭs) [″ + *nucleus,* kernel, + *osis,* condition]. Presence of an abnormally high number of mononuclear leukocytes in the blood.

m., infectious. An acute infectious disease that affects lymphoid tissue primarily. Characterized by enlarged, often tender, lymph nodes and enlarged spleen with great increase of atypical or abnormal mononuclear leukocytes in the blood. Abnormal liver function test will be found in about 90% of cases. The disease is associated with the Epstein-Barr virus. Incubation period may be as long as 4 to 7 weeks.

SYM: Constitutional symptoms, fever, sore throat, and generalized lymphadenopathy; hyperplasia of lymphatic tissue. Blood contains heterophile antibodies.

TREATMENT: There is no specific therapy but, for serious complications (for example, hemolytic anemia, pharyngeal swelling interfering with swallowing), cortisone is indicated.

mononucleotide (mŏn″ō-nū′klē-ō-tīd″). A product resulting from hydrolysis of nucleic acid. Contains phosphoric acid combined with a glucoside or pentoside. SYN: *nucleotide.*

monoparesis (mŏn-ō-păr-ē′sĭs) [Gr. *monos,* single, + *paresis,* weakness]. Paralysis of a single part of the body.

monoparesthesia (mŏn″ō-păr-ĕs-thē′sē-ă) [″ + *para,* beside, + *aisthesis,* sensation]. Paresthesia of only one region or limb.

monopathy (mō-nŏp′ă-thē) [″ + *pathos,* disease]. A disease attacking only one part of the body.

monophagia (mŏn-ō-fā′jē-ă) [″ + *phagein,* to eat]. 1. Appetite for only one kind of food. Said especially of insects. 2. The habit of eating only one meal a day.

monophasia (mŏn-ō-fā′zē-ă) [″ + *phasis,* speech]. Inability to utter anything but one word or phrase repeatedly.

monophobia (mŏn-ō-fō′bē-ă) [″ + *phobos,* fear]. Abnormal fear of being alone.

monophthalmus (mŏn″ŏf-thăl′mŭs) [″ + *ophthalmos,* eye]. A cyclops, q.v.

monophyletic (mŏn″ō-fīl-ĕt′ĭk) [″ + *phyle,* tribe]. Originating from a single source. Opposite of polyphyletic.

monophyletism (mŏn″ō-fī′lĕ-tĭzm). Concerning the concept that all blood cells are derived from a single stem cell.

monophyodont (mŏn″ō-fī′ō-dŏnt) [″ + *phyein,* to grow, + *odous,* tooth]. Having a single set of teeth, which are permanent.

monoplasmatic (mŏn″ō-plăz-măt′ĭk) [″ + *plasma,* plasm]. Made up of a single substance or tissue.

monoplast (mŏn′ō-plăst) [″ + *plastos,* formed]. A single-cell type of organism that does not change during its life cycle.

monoplegia (mŏn-ō-plē′jē-ă) [″ + *plege,* stroke]. Paralysis of a single limb or a single group of muscles.

monopodia (mŏn″ō-pō′dē-ă) [″ + *pous,* foot]. The condition of having only one foot; usually the two feet are fused.

monopolar (mŏn-ō-pōl′ăr) [″ + L. *polus,* pole]. Using one terminal only, the ground acting as the second terminal. SYN: *monoterminal.*

monops (mŏn′ŏps) [″ + *ops,* eye]. Cyclops, q.v.

monopsychosis (mŏn″ō-sī-kō′sĭs) [Gr. *monos,* single, + *psyche,* mind, + *osis,* condition]. Monomania, q.v.

monopus (mŏn′ō-pŭs) [″ + *pous,* foot]. Individual exhibiting monopodia, q.v.

monorchia (mŏn-or′kē-ă). Monorchism.

monorchid (mŏn-or′kĭd) [″ + *orchis,* testicle]. Person having only one testicle or ovary.

monorchidism, monorchism (mŏn-or′kĭd-ĭzm, mŏn′or-kĭzm). Condition in which there is only one descended testicle.

monorhinic (mŏn″ō-rĭn′ĭk) [″ + *rhis,* nose]. 1. Having a single nose as conjoined twins. 2. Having a single fused nasal cavity.

monosaccharide (mŏn-ō-săk′ă-rīd) [″ + Sanskrit *sarkara,* sugar]. A simple sugar that cannot be decomposed by hydrolysis, such as fructose, galactose, or glucose.

monosodium glutamate. ABBR: MSG. Sodium salt of glutamic acid, $C_5H_8O_4NaN$. A white crystalline substance that has a meatlike taste. Used to flavor foods, esp. in the Orient. When ingested in large amounts causes chest pain, facial pressure, headaches, burning sensation, and excessive sweating. This has been termed the Chinese restaurant syndrome, q.v. Suitability of its general use as a food additive is being investigated. Its use to enhance the flavor of foods prepared for infants is especially questionable. Manufactured and sold under various names as Ajinomoto, Accent, Vetsin.

monosome (mŏn′ō-sōm) [″ + *soma,* body]. An accessory chromosome that, without dividing, goes into only one of the daughter cells. The unpaired sex chromosome.

monosomy (mŏn′ō-sō″mē). Condition of having one member of a chromosome pair missing.

monospasm (mŏn′ō-spăzm) [″ + *spasmos,* convulsion]. Spasm of a single limb or part.

monospermy (mŏn′ō-spĕr″mē) [″ + *sperma,* seed]. Fertilization by a single spermatozoon entering an ovum.

monostotic (mŏn″ŏs-tŏt′ĭk) [″ + *osteon,* bone]. Concerning a single bone.

monostratal (mŏn″ō-strā′tăl). Consisting of a single layer.

monosubstituted (mŏn″ō-sŭb′stĭ-tūt″ĕd). Having only a single molecule replaced.

monosymptomatic (mŏn″ō-sĭmp-tō-măt′ĭk) [″ + *symptomatikos,* pert. to symptom]. Having only one dominant symptom.

monosynaptic (mŏn″ō-sī-năp′tĭk). Transmitted through only a single synapse.

monosyphilide (mŏn-ō-sĭf′ĭl-īd) [″ + Fr. *syphilide,* syphilitic lesion]. Characterized by a single syphilitic lesion.

monoterminal [″ + *terma,* a limit]. Using one terminal only in the giving of treatments, the ground acting as the second terminal for the completion of the electrical circuit. SYN: *monopolar.*

monothermia (mōn-ō-thĕrm′ē-ă) [″ + *therme,* heat]. Condition in which body temperature is stable; absence of rise in evening temperature.

monotocous (mō-nŏt′ō-kŭs) [Gr. *monos,* single, + *tokos,* birth]. Production of a single offspring at birth.

Monotricha (mō-nŏt′rĭ-kă) [″ + *thrix,* hair]. Bacteria having a single flagellum at one pole.

monotrichous (mŏn-ŏt′rĭ-kŭs). Pert. to or having a single flagellum.

monovalent (mŏn-ō-vā′lĕnt) [″ + L. *valere,* to have power]. Having the combining power of a single hydrogen atom. SYN: *univalent.*

monoxenous (mō-nŏks′ĕn-ŭs) [″ + *xenos,* stranger]. Said of a parasite that requires only one species as a host.

monoxide (mŏn-ŏk′sīd). An oxide having only one atom of oxygen.

monozygotic (mŏn″ō-zī-gŏt′ĭk) [″ + *zygotos,* yoked]. Originating from a single fertilized ovum, said of identical twins

monozygotic twins. Two offspring developed from a single fertilized ovum. At an early stage the ovum separates into independent cells that develop into offspring of the same sex with identical genetic characteristics. SEE: *twins.*

Monro's foramen (mŏn-rōz′). [Alexander Monro, Scot. anatomist, 1737–1817] Point of communication between 3rd and lateral ventricles of the brain.

Monro's sulcus. Sulcus on lateral wall of 3rd ventricle from the foramen interventriculare to the aditus ad aquaeductum cerebri.

mons (mŏns) [L., mountain]. (pl. *montes*) An anatomical eminence above the surface of the body.

m. pubis. [NA] Pubic eminence. SYN: *mons veneris.*

m. veneris. A pad of fatty tissue and coarse skin overlying the symphysis pubis. After puberty it is covered with hair. SYN: *mons pubis.*

monster [L. *monstrum*]. A grossly deformed fetus or infant, usually due to faulty development; is usually nonviable. The term should never be used when discussing such a patient with those who are emotionally attached to him or her. Terms such as handicapped, congenitally deformed, or abnormal are more appropriate.

monstriparity (mŏn″strĭ-păr′ĭ-tē) [″ + *parere,* to give birth to]. To give birth to an abnormally formed infant.

monstrosity [L. *monstrositas*]. A congenitally deformed child or infant.

Monteggia's fracture (mŏn-tĕj′ăz). [Giovanni B. Monteggia, It. surgeon, 1762–1815] Fracture of the upper portion of the ulna with dislocation of the radial head.

Montgomery's glands. [William F. Montgomery, Ir. obstetrician, 1797–1859] Small prominences around the nipple of the breast that enlarge during pregnancy and lactation. SEE: *areola; mamma.*

Montgomery's straps. Adhesive straps affixed to the skin arranged opposite to each other; and with the middle ends turned back on each other so that gauze straps can be placed between holes of each end of the middle of the paired tapes. This provides a method of securing a bandage and subsequently changing it without having to replace the tape each time. SEE: illus.

monticulus (mŏn-tĭk′ū-lŭs) [L., little mountain]. (pl. *monticuli*) A protuberance.

m. cerebelli. In the cerebellum, protuberance of the superior vermis, the anterior portion of which is called the culmen and the posterior portion, the declive.

mood [AS. *mod,* mind, feeling]. A pervasive and sustained emotion that may have a major influence on a person's perception of the world. Examples of mood include depression, joy, elation, anger, and anxiety.

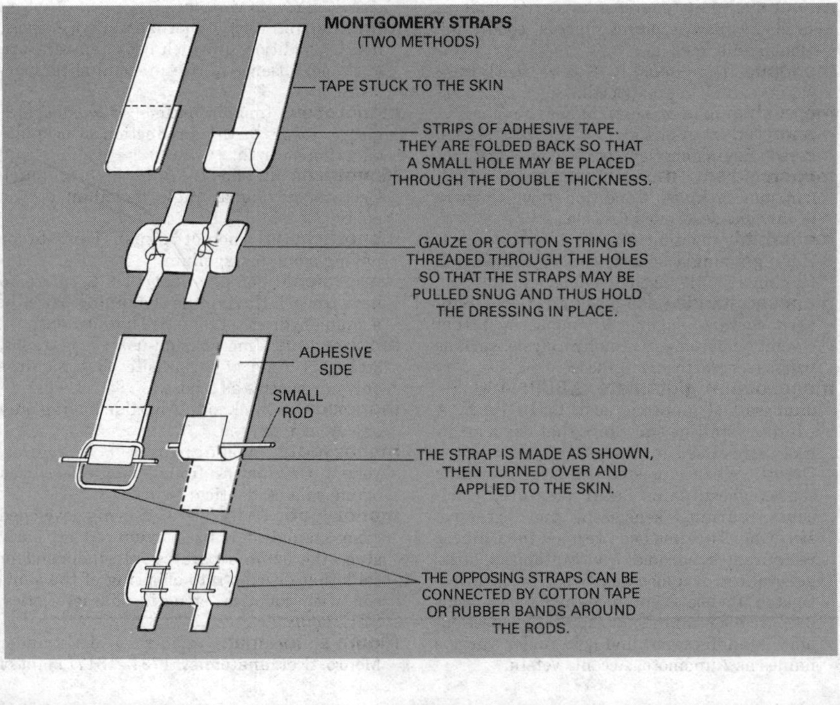
MONTGOMERY STRAPS
(TWO METHODS)
TAPE STUCK TO THE SKIN
STRIPS OF ADHESIVE TAPE. THEY ARE FOLDED BACK SO THAT A SMALL HOLE MAY BE PLACED THROUGH THE DOUBLE THICKNESS.
GAUZE OR COTTON STRING IS THREADED THROUGH THE HOLES SO THAT THE STRAPS MAY BE PULLED SNUG AND THUS HOLD THE DRESSING IN PLACE.
ADHESIVE SIDE
SMALL ROD
THE STRAP IS MADE AS SHOWN, THEN TURNED OVER AND APPLIED TO THE SKIN.
THE OPPOSING STRAPS CAN BE CONNECTED BY COTTON TAPE OR RUBBER BANDS AROUND THE RODS.

moon-face. The development of a round full face in response to excess secretion of adrenal cortical hormone or prolonged therapy with this hormone.

Moraxella (mor-ăx-ĕl'ă). Genus of bacteria sometimes confused with Neisseria. Morax-Axenfeld species is associated with conjunctivitis.

morbid (mor'bĭd) [L. *morbidus,* sick]. 1. Diseased. 2. Pert. to disease. 3. Preoccupied with unwholesome ideas and circumstances.

morbidity [L. *morbidus,* sick]. 1. State of being diseased. 2. The number of sick persons or cases of disease in relationship to a specific population. SEE: *incidence.*

morbidity rate. Number of cases of a specific disease in a specified period of time (usually a year) per unit of population (usually 1,000, 10,000 or 100,000) alive.

morbific (mor-bĭf'ĭk) [" + *facere,* to make]. Causing or producing disease.

morbilli (mor-bĭl'ī) [L. *morbillus,* little disease]. Measles.

morbilliform [" + *forma,* shape]. Like measles or its rash.

morbillous (mor-bĭl'ŭs). Concerning measles.

morbus [L.]. Disease.

m. caeruleus. Cyanosis that is congenital.

m. miseriae. Any condition due to neglect and want.

morcellation, morcellement (mor-sĕl-ā'shŭn, -ā-mŏn') [Fr. *morceller,* to subdivide]. Method of removing a fetus, tumor, or organ by pieces.

mordant (mor'dănt) [L. *mordere,* to bite]. A substance that fixes a stain or dye, as alum and phenol.

mores (mō'rāz) [L.]. Habits and customs of society. Usually those that come to be regarded as being essential to the survival and well-being of the society.

Morgagni (mor-găn'yē). [Giovanni B. Morgagni, It. pathological anatomist, 1682–1771].

M.'s caruncle. The middle prostatic lobe.

M.'s cataract. Cataract that is hypermature with a softened cortex and a hard nucleus. SEE: *cataract.*

M.'s hydatid. Cystlike remains of müllerian duct attached to testicle or oviduct.

M.'s hyperostosis. Hyperostosis of the frontal bones of the head. Associated with obesity, headache, amenorrhea, diabetes, multiple endocrine abnormalities, and various neuropsychiatric disturbances.

M.'s ventricle. Ventriculus laryngis. SEE: *ventricle of the larynx.*

morgagnian (mor-găn'yē-ăn). Pert. to or described by Morgagni, q.v.

morgagnian cyst. Cystlike remnant of the müllerian duct that is attached to the fallopian tube.

morgue (morg) [Fr.]. A public mortuary; a place for holding dead bodies for identification and burial. SYN: *mortuary.*

moria (mō'rē-ă) [Gr. *moria,* folly]. 1. Simple dementia. 2. Foolishness. SEE: *witzelsucht.*

moribund (mor'ĭ-bŭnd) [L. *moribundus*]. In a dying condition; dying.

morioplasty (mō'rē-ō-plăs-tē) [Gr. *morion,* piece, + *plassein,* to form]. Plastic surgery to restore portions of the body that have been lost through accident or disease.

morning care. The care provided for the patient which includes taking temperature, pulse, and respiration, oral hygiene, bath, change of linen on bed, and breakfast.

morning sickness. The nausea and vomiting that affect some women during first few months of pregnancy, particularly in the morning. Headache, dizziness, and exhaustion also may be experienced. It may clear up after the 3rd month. SEE: *hyperemesis gravidarum.*

Occurs usually about the 5th or 6th week and symptoms vary from simple morning sickness to pernicious vomiting of pregnancy. Usually clears up without treatment in 1 to 3 weeks. Occurs in about 50% of pregnancies.

TREATMENT: Dietary management will help in most cases. Frequent small feedings of bland foods such as crackers, broths, and clear soups will be beneficial. If the sickness persists, an antinausea medicine suitable for use during pregnancy is usually effective.

CAUTION: The use of any drug during pregnancy should be carefully monitored due to possible damage to the fetus.

morning stiffness. Generalized joint and muscle stiffness that is present upon awakening. This tends to subside as activity is increased during the day. The stiffness is associated with various types of inflammatory arthritis.

moron [Gr. *moros,* stupid]. A feebleminded person, not beyond the intellectual development level of age 12, having the mentality ordinarily attained between 7 and 12, or an I.Q. of 50 to 70. The term implies no moral defect. SEE: *mental retardation.*

Moro reflex. [Ernst Moro, Ger. pediatrist, 1874–1951] A defensive reflex consisting of the infant's drawing of its arms across its chest in an embracing manner in response to stimuli produced by striking the surface on which the infant rests. SYN: *embrace reflex.*

morphea (mor-fē'ă) [Gr. *morphe,* form]. A rare skin disease of unknown etiology, characterized by widespread sclerosis of the skin which may be localized or widespread. There is no specific treatment but physiotherapy or infiltration with cortisone solution may help to prevent contractures.

morpheme (mor'fēm). The smallest meaningful unit in phonetics. SEE: *phoneme.*

morphia. Morphine.

morphine (mor'fēn) [L. *morphina,* from *Morpheus,* god of sleep]. Main alkaloid found in opium, occurring in bitter colorless crystals. Widely used as an analgesic and sedative.

m. sulfate. USP. The sulfate of an alkaloid obtained from opium and occurring as feathery white crystals, incompatible with alkalies, tannic acid, and iodides. Loses water of crystallization when exposed to air. Trade name is Epimorph.

ACTION AND USES: Hypnotic and analgesic.

CAUTION: Morphine sulfate is used by drug addicts due to its action on the central nervous system. For this reason, its security in the hospital and pharmacy must be strictly maintained.

morphine poisoning. Brief mental exhilaration; languor; followed by weariness, sleepiness, pinpoint pupils; rapid forcible pulse that becomes slow and feeble. Respiration slow and shallow. Unconsciousness from which patient may be aroused with difficulty. Muscles become relaxed, reflexes diminished, and temperature low. The skin is pale, cold, and moist, and the pupils dilated. If dose is large enough, coma and death follow.

TREATMENT: Establish airway and provide ventilation. Give a narcotic antagonist such as naloxone, which is the treatment of choice, in small doses and repeat if necessary at 30-minute intervals. Pulmonary edema may occur; treat with positive-pressure respiration.

morphinism (mor'fĭn-ĭzm) [L. *morphina,* morphine, + *-ismos,* condition]. Morbid condition due to habitual or excessive use of morphine. Morphine habit. SEE: *morphine poisoning.*

morphinomania, morphiomania (mor″fĭn-ō-mā'nē-ă, -fē-ō-mā'nē-ă) [″ + *mania,* madness]. 1. Morbid craving for morphine. 2. Insanity resulting from use of morphine.

morphogenesis (mor″fō-jĕn'ĕ-sĭs) [Gr. *morphe,* form, + *genesis,* production]. The various processes occurring during development by which the form of the body and its organs is established.

morphogenetic (mor″fō-jĕn-ĕt'ĭk). Stimulating growth and development of form.

morphogenetic processes. Processes by which morphogenesis is accomplished. Include cell migration, cell aggregation, localized growth, splitting including delamination and cavitation, folding including invagination and evagination.

morphogenetic substance. Chemical substances present in eggs or early embryos that induce morphologic differentiation. SEE: *induction.*

morphography (mor-fŏg'ră-fē) [″ + *graphein,* to write]. The classification of organisms by describing their form and structure.

morphology (mor-fŏl'ō-jē) [Gr. *morphe,* form, + *logos,* study]. Science of structure and form without regard to function.

morphometry (mor-fŏm'ĕ-trē) [″+ *metron,* measure]. The measurement of forms of organisms.

morphon (mor'fŏn) [Gr., forming]. Any individual structure making up part of an organism.

morphosis (mor-fō'sĭs) [Gr., a shaping]. The formation of a structure.

morpio, morpion (mor'pē-ō, -pē-ŏn) [L.]. (pl. *morpiones*) The crab louse, Phthirus pubis, that infests the pubic area. SEE: *lice.*

Morquio's syndrome (mor-kē'ōz). [Louis Morquio, Uruguayan physician, 1867–1935] Mucopolysaccharidosis IV.

morrhuate sodium injection (mor'ū-āt). USP. A sclerosing agent used to obliterate varicose veins.

mors [L.]. Death.

m. putativa. Apparent death.

m. subita. Sudden death.

morsal (mor'săl) [L. *morsus,* bite]. Involved in biting and chewing as the occlusal surfaces of teeth.

morsulus (mor'sū-lŭs) [L. dim. of *morsus,* bite]. Troche, q.v.

mortal [L. *mortalis*]. 1. Causing death. 2. Subject to death. 3. Human.

mortality. 1. State of being mortal. 2. The death rate; ratio of number of deaths to a given population.

mortar [L. *mortarium*]. Vessel with a smooth interior in which crude drugs are crushed or ground by using a pestle.

mortician [L. *mors,* death]. Undertaker; person trained to attend to the dead.

mortification (mor″tĭ-fĭ-kā'shŭn) [″ + *facere,* to make]. Death or failure of a tissue, organ, or part. SYN: *gangrene; necrosis.*

mortinatality (mor″tĭ-nā-tăl'ĭ-tē) [″ + *natus,* birth]. Ratio of stillbirths to general birth rate. SYN: *natimortality.*

mortise joint. Ankle joint.

Morton's disease, syndrome (mor'tŭnz). [Thomas G. Morton, U.S. surgeon, 1835–1903] The condition of having a short hypertrophied second metatarsal bone with tenderness over the head of that bone, callosities under the second and third metatarsals, and pain and tenderness of the metatarsal area.

Morton's foot syndrome. SEE: *Morton's disease, syndrome.*

Morton's neuralgia. Pain in the metatarsal area due to a fallen transverse arch with pressure on the lateral plantar nerve. SYN: *Morton's metatarsalgia.*

Morton's neuroma. A neuroma-like mass of the neurovascular bundle of the intermetatarsal spaces.

mortuary (mor'chū-ā-rē) [L. *mortuarium,* a tomb]. 1. Temporary place for keeping dead bodies before burial. SYN: *morgue.* 2. Rel. to the dead or to death.

morula (mor'ū-lă) [L. *morus,* mulberry]. Solid mass of cells, resembling a mulberry, resulting from cleavage of an ovum. SEE: *fertilization* for illus.

morulation (mor"ū-lā'shŭn). The formation of morula.

moruloid (mor'ū-loyd) [" + Gr. *eidos,* form]. 1. A bacterial colony made up of a mass resembling a mulberry. 2. Resembling a mulberry.

Morvan's disease (mor'vănz). [Augustin M. Morvan, Fr. physician, 1819–1897] A form of syringomyelia, q.v., in which there are trophic changes in the extremities with formation of slowly healing lesions.

mosaic. 1. A picture or design made of many small colored pieces interspersed in some other material. 2. An individual whose tissues are of different genetic kinds even though they were derived from the same cell. Caused by a genetic mutation. 3. Spotted condition in plants as in tobacco mosaic, a disease caused by a virus.

mosaic bone. Bone appearing as small pieces fitted together, characteristic of Paget's disease.

mosaic development. Type of development exhibited by ova that undergo determinate cleavage in which each blastomere has a characteristic position and unalterable fate.

mosaicism (mō-zā'ĭ-sĭzm). Presence of cells of two different genetic materials in the same individual.

mosquito [Sp., little fly]. (pl. *mosquitoes)* A blood-sucking insect belonging to the order Diptera, family Culicidae, q.v. Important genera are Anopheles, Culex, Aedes, Haemagogus, Mansonia, and Psorophora. They serve as transmitting agents of many diseases, including malaria, filariasis, yellow fever, dengue, viral encephalitis, and dermatobiasis.

mosquitocide [" + L. *caedere,* to kill]. An agent that is lethal to mosquitoes or their larvae.

mosquito forceps. A very small, delicately pointed hemostat. SYN: *Halsted's forceps.*

moss. 1. Any low-growing green plant of the class Musci. 2. In general, any one of a number of lichens and seaweeds.

m., sphagnum. Peat moss. It has been used as a surgical bandage and by some primitive people for menstrual protection.

mossy cell. A protoplasmic astrocyte, a neuroglia cell with many branching processes. SEE: *neuroglia.*

mossy fibers. Afferent fibers to the cerebellar cortex. They give off many collaterals, each ending in a glomerulus.

mother [AS. *modor*]. 1. Female parent. 2. A structure that gives rise to others.

mother cell. A cell that, by fission or budding, gives rise to similar cells.

mother cyst. An echinococcus cyst enveloping smaller ones.

mother liquor. Portion left after removal of crystals from a solution.

mother's mark. A birthmark. SEE: *mark.*

motile (mō'tĭl) [L. *motilis,* moving]. Able to move spontaneously.

motility (mō-tĭl'ĭ-tē). Power to move spontaneously.

motion (mō'shŭn) [L. *motio,* movement]. 1. A change of place or position; movement. 2. Evacuation of the bowels. 3. Matter evacuated from bowels. SEE: words beginning with *cine-* and *kine-.*

m., active. Movement caused by the patient's own intention.

m., passive. Movement as the result of the attendant's causing the part to be moved.

motion sickness. Nausea, vomiting, and vertigo induced by irregular or rhythmic movements.

Ex.: seasickness, airsickness, car sickness, swing sickness.

motivation (mō"tĭ-vā'shŭn). The internal drive or externally arising stimulus to action or thought.

motive (mō'tĭv). The mental condition or state that affects, alters, or stimulates behavior.

motofacient (mō"tō-fā'shĕnt). Producing motion.

motoneuron (mō"tō-nū'rŏn). A motor neuron.

m.'s, lower. Peripheral motor neurons that originate in the ventral gray columns of the spinal cord and terminate in skeletal muscles.

m.'s, peripheral. Motor neurons that transmit stimuli to skeletal muscles.

m.'s, upper. Neurons of the cerebral cortex that conduct stimuli from the motor cortex of the brain to motor nuclei of cerebral nerves or the ventral gray columns of the spinal cord.

motor [L. *motus,* moving]. 1. Causing motion. 2. A part or center that induces movements, as nerves or muscles.

motor aphasia. A condition in which patients understand but cannot express themselves in words or cannot read aloud.

motor area. Posterior part of frontal lobe anterior to the central sulcus, from which impulses for volitional movement arise.

motor endplate. Flat expansion ending a

motor nerve fiber where it connects with a muscle fiber.

motor fibers. Axons of motor neurons that innervate skeletal muscles.

motorial (mō-tor'ē-ăl) [L. *motus,* moving]. Concerning motion or a motor center.

motoricity (mō-tor-ĭs'ĭ-tē). Capability of movement.

motorium (mō-tor'ē-ŭm) [L., power of motion]. Motor center of a body or organism.

motorius (mō-tor'ē-ŭs). Any motor nerve.

motor nerve. A nerve composed entirely of motor fibers.

motor neuron. 1. A neuron that innervates muscle tissue. 2. A neuron that carries impulses initiating muscle contraction.

motor neuron disease. One of several types of disease of the motor neurons: progressive muscle atrophy, progressive bulbar palsy, and amyotrophic lateral sclerosis. These diseases are characterized by degeneration of anterior horn cells of the spinal cord, the motor cranial nerve nuclei, and the pyramidal tracts. They occur principally in males. In the U.S.A., amyotrophic lateral sclerosis is known to the laity as Lou Gehrig's disease. He was a well-known athlete whose baseball career and life were prematurely ended as a result of this disease.

motorpathy (mō-tor'păth-ē) [L. *motus,* moving, + Gr. *pathos,* disease]. Treatment of a condition by prescribed movements. SYN: *kinesitherapy; kinetotherapy.*

motor points. Points where the motor nerve enters the muscle and where visible contraction can be elicited with a minimal amount of stimulation.

motor sense. The kinesthetic sense.

motor speech area. Area in the hemisphere of the brain that controls movements of tongue, lips, and vocal cords. In right-handed people, this area is in the left hemisphere; and in left-handed persons, in the right hemisphere. Loss of speech may follow hemorrhage into this area. SYN: *Broca's area.*

motor unit. A single motor neuron and the muscle fibers its branches innervate.

Motrin. Trade name for ibuprofen.

mottled enamel. Condition in which the enamel of the teeth becomes discolored. Often associated with excessive fluorine or fluoride in drinking water. SEE: *fluorosis.*

mottling (mŏt'lĭng) [ME. *motteley,* many colored]. A condition that is marked by discolored areas.

moulage (moo-lăzh') [Fr.]. 1. A wax model or reproduction of the configuration of some part of the anatomy such as the face or nose, or of a pathological skin lesion. 2. Molding of a wax model.

mounding [origin uncertain]. The rising of a lump, as the mounding of a wasting muscle when struck a quick, firm blow. SYN: *myoedema.*

mountain fever. Condition occurring in individuals ascending to high altitudes (over 10,000 ft. or 3,048 meters) or to those subjected to rarefied atmospheres. Due to anoxia resulting from reduced oxygen tension. SYN: *hypobaropathy.* SEE: *bends.*

SYM: euphoria, tachycardia, headache, nausea, increased respiratory rate, fatigue, and cerebral disorders (loss of memory, errors of judgment).

mounting (mownt'ĭng) [ME. *mounten,* to mount]. 1. The arrangement of specimens on slides, frames, chart boards, display boards, or any background for study. 2. In dentistry, attaching a cast of the mandible or maxilla to an articulator.

mourning [AS. *murnan*]. Normal grief usually produced by the death of a loved one. Not synonymous with depression or melancholia.

mouse (mows). 1. A small rodent of the genus Mus. Used extensively in research. 2. A small piece of tissue that has become free or unattached, esp. in a body cavity or joint.

m., joint. Pieces of synovial membrane or cartilage that because of trauma or osteoarthritis are free in the joint space.

m., NZB. SEE: *NZB mouse.*

mouse unit. The smallest amount of estrogen that will produce cornified cells in the vaginal epithelium of a spayed mouse. SYN: *Allen-Doisy unit.*

mouth [AS. *muth*]. 1. The opening of any cavity. SYN: *buccal cavity; cavity, oral.* 2. The cavity within the cheeks, containing the tongue and teeth and communicating with the pharynx. SEE: illus.

ABNORM: *Tongue:* dry, coated, smooth, strawberry, large, pigmented, geographic, deviated, tremulous, sore. *Gums and teeth:* gingivitis, sordes, lead line, pyorrhea, atrophy, hypertrophy, dental caries, alveolar abscesses. *Mucous membrane and other parts of mouth:* eruptions accompanying exanthematous diseases, stomatitis, canker sores, herpes simplex, thrush, trench mouth, cysts, tumors, carcinoma, lesions of syphilis such as chancre, mucous patches, gumma, lesions of tuberculosis, abscesses.

Disorders of the mouth cavity may be indications of purely local disease or they may be symptoms of systemic disturbances such as dehydration, pernicious anemia, nutritional deficiencies, esp. avitaminoses.

Rashes of the mouth may indicate stomatitis, measles, or scarlet fever. Rashes on lips may indicate typhoid fever, meningitis, or pneumonia. In secondary syphilis, chancre, cancer, and epithelioma, mucous patches appear.

EXAM: In addition to visual examination,

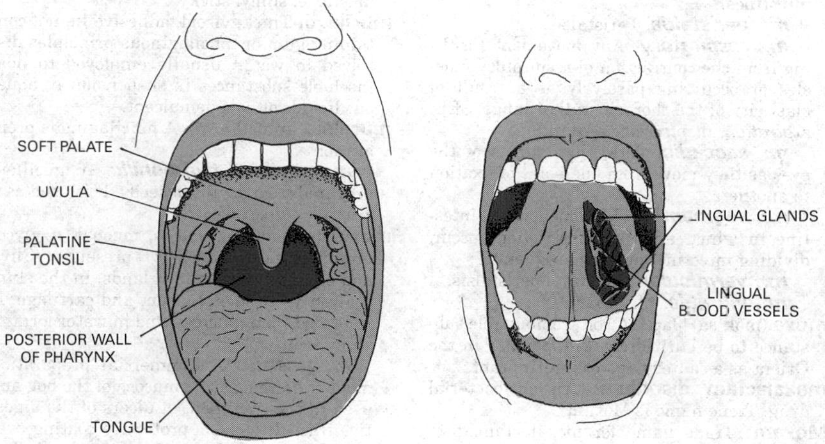

MOUTH, TONGUE, AND PHARYNX

careful digital examination should be made because it reveals areas of tenderness and alterations of texture characteristic of leukoplakia, cancer, cystic swellings, and lymphadenopathy.

Excessive moisture of the mouth is seen in stomatitis, irritation of the vagus nerve, ingestion of irritating drugs or foods, nervous disorders, teething, seeing appetizing foods, and smelling pleasant odors.

RS: antitrismus; bucca; cancrum oris; canker; catarrh; chalinoplasty; Escherich's reflex, mandible; maxilla; oral; orifice; palate; palatine stoma; stomatitis; tongue; xerostomia.

m., trench. SEE: *trench mouth.*

mouthstick. Adapted device consisting of a stick attached to a molded dental mouthpiece that permits page-turning and other tasks through head movement.

movement [L. *movere,* to move]. 1. Act of passing from place to place or changing position of body or its parts. 2. Evacuation of feces.

m., active. Voluntary movement accomplished without external assistance.

m., ameboid. Movement resembling that of an ameba in which the protoplasm of a cell flows into a projection of the cell membrane forming a pseudopodium. Characteristic of leukocytes and certain protozoa.

m., associated. Involuntary movement of a part occurring coincident with and subsequent to the movement of another part, as in the eyes.

m., autonomic. A spontaneous, involuntary movement independent of external stimulation.

m., brownian. The peculiar jiggling or dancing movement of minute particles suspended in liquids or gases when observed under the microscope due to bombardment of the particles by molecules of their surrounding medium.

m., ciliary. Rhythmic movement of the cilia of a ciliated cell or epithelium. SYN: *m., vibratile.*

m., circus. A phenomenon after injury to a corpus striatum, optic thalamus, or crus cerebri, causing an odd circular gait.

m., disorders of. May be due to injury or disease of muscle, nerve ending, motor nerve, spinal cord, or the brain. Types are hemiplegia, ataxia, monoplegia, tremors, rigors, chorea, athetosis, convulsions, spasm (clonic or tonic), reflex (hysterical, habit spasm, tics), and spastic paralysis.

m.'s, fetal. Muscular movements performed by the fetus in utero.

m., molecular. The movement of molecules of a substance, the basis of the kinetic theory of matter. SEE: *m., brownian.*

m. of restitution. A partial rotation of the fetal head in cases of head presentation.

m., passive. Movement of the body or a part due to outside forces.

m., pendular. Swaying movements of the intestines caused by rhythmic contractions of the longitudinal muscles of the walls of the intestines.

m., peristaltic. Peristalsis.

m., respiratory. Any movement resulting from the contraction of respiratory muscles or occurring passively as a result of elasticity of the thoracic wall or lungs. SEE: *expiration; inspiration; respiration.*

m., saccadic. Jerky movements of the eyes as they move from one point of fixation to another.

m., segmenting. Movement of the intestine in which annular constrictions occur, dividing intestine into ovoid segments.

m., vermicular. Intestinal peristalsis.

m., vibratile. M., ciliary.

moxa (mŏk'sa) [Jap.]. A soft, combustible substance to be burned on skin, popular in the Orient as a cautery and counterirritant.

moxalactam disodium. An antibacterial drug. Trade name is Moxam.

Moxam. Trade name for moxalactam disodium.

moxibustion (mŏks-ĭ-bŭs'chŭn) [" + L. *combustus,* burned]. Cauterization by means of a cylinder or cone of cotton wool, called a moxa, placed on the skin and fired at the top. Used to produce counterirritation.

M.P.D. *maximum permissible dose.*

M.P.H. *Master of Public Health.*

M.P.N. *most probable number* (of bacteria present in a quantity of solution, esp. water).

mR. *milliroentgen.*

M.R.L. *medical record librarian.*

mRNA. *messenger RNA.*

MS. *multiple sclerosis.*

M.S. *Master of Surgery; Master of Science.*

msec. *millisecond.*

MSH. *melanocyte-stimulating hormone.*

M.T. *medical technologist*

M.u. *Maché unit.*

m.u. *mouse unit.*

mu (mū) [Gr. μ, letter m]. SYMB: μ; u. Symb. used for the prefix *micro-* which stands for multiplication by 10^{-6}. Thus, μm. would stand for 10^{-6} meter.

mucedin (mū'sĕ-dĭn) [L. *mucedo,* mucus]. A substance obtained from gluten.

muciferous (mū-sĭf'ĕr-ŭs) [" + *ferre,* to carry]. Secreting or producing mucus. SYN: *mucigenous; muciparous.*

muciform (mū'sĭ-form) [" + *forma,* shape]. Appearing similar to mucus.

mucigen (mŭ'sĭ-jĕn) [" + Gr. *gennan,* to produce]. A substance present in mucous cells that, upon being extruded from the cell, is converted into mucin.

mucigenous (mū-sĭj'ĕn-ŭs). Producing mucus. SYN: *muciferous; muciparous.*

mucilage (mū'sĭ-lĭj) [L. *mucilago,* moldy juice]. Vegetable preparation used in pharmaceuticals. SEE: *mucilago.*

mucilaginous (mū-sĭl-ăj'ĭn-ŭs). Resembling mucilage; slimy; sticky.

mucilago. Thick, viscid, adhesive liquid, containing gum or mucilaginous principles dissolved in water, usually employed to hold insoluble substances in suspension in aqueous liquids or as a demulcent.

mucilloid (mū'sĭl-loyd). A mucilaginous preparation.

m., psyllium hydrophilic. A mucilloid prepared from psyllium seeds. It is used as a bulk-type laxative.

mucin (mū'sĭn) [L. *mucus,* mucus]. A glycoprotein found in mucus. It is present in saliva and bile and in salivary glands, in the skin, connective tissues, tendon, and cartilage. It is formed from mucigen and in water forms a slimy solution.

m., gastric. A commercial preparation made from the gastric mucosa of the hog and used in the treatment of ulcers of the digestive tract. It forms a protective coating over the ulcer or erosion, which prevents irritation from the passing of bile and acid secretions in the duodenum and from acid conditions irritating peptic ulcer of the stomach.

mucinase (mū'sĭ-nās). Any enzyme that acts on mucin.

mucinemia (mū"sĭn-ē'mē-ă) [" + Gr. *haima,* blood]. Mucin in the blood. SYN: *myxemia.*

mucinogen (mū-sĭn'ō-jĕn) [" + Gr. *gennan,* to produce]. A glycoprotein that forms mucin.

mucinoid (mū'sĭn-oyd) [" + Gr. *eidos,* resemblance]. Appearing similar to mucin.

mucinolytic (mū"sĭ-nō-lĭt'ĭk) [" + Gr. *lysis,* dissolution]. Hydrolyzing or dissolving mucin.

mucinuria (mū-sĭn-ū'rē-ă) [" + Gr. *ouron,* urine]. Presence of mucin in the urine.

muciparous (mū-sĭp'ăr-ŭs) [" + *parere,* to bring forth]. Producing or secreting mucus. SYN: *muciferous; mucigenous.*

muco- [L. *mucus,* mucus]. Combining form indicating rel. to mucus.

mucocele (mū'kō-sēl) [" + Gr. *kele,* tumor]. 1. Enlargement of the lacrimal sac. 2. A mucous cyst. 3. A mucous polypus. 4. Cystic disease of the air cavities of the cranial bones causing erosion of the bone.

mucocolpos (mū"kō-kŏl'pŏs) [" + Gr. *kolpos,* vagina]. Accumulation of mucus in the vagina.

mucocutaneous (mū"kō-kū-tā'nē-ŭs) [" + *cutis,* skin]. Concerning mucous membrane and the skin. SYN: *mucodermal.*

mucocutaneous lymph node syndrome. An acute febrile disease of children that resembles scarlet fever. The fever is present on the first day of the illness and may last from one to three weeks. The child is irritable, lethargic, and has bilateral congestion of the conjunctivae. The oral mucosa is deep red and strawberry tongue is prominent. Lips are dry, cracked and red. On the third to fifth day the palms and soles are distinctly red and edema of the hands and feet is present. The skin on the tips of the fingers and toes peels in layers. A macular erythematous rash free of crusts and vesicles spreads from the extremities to the trunk. Cervical lymphadenopathy is present in the first three days and lasts over three weeks. The disease is rarely fatal in the acute phase but children may die suddenly from coronary artery disease some years later. SYN: *Kawasaki disease.* SEE: *toxic shock syndrome.*

ETIOL: Unknown.

TREATMENT: There is no specific therapy.

mucodermal (mū-kō-dĕr′măl) [″ + Gr. *derma,* skin]. Pert. to mucous membrane and the skin. SYN: *mucocutaneous.*

mucoenteritis (mū″kō-ĕn-tĕr-ī′tĭs) [″ + Gr. *enteron,* intestine, + *itis,* inflammation]. Inflammation of intestinal mucosa.

mucoglobulin (mū″kō-glŏb′ū-lĭn) [″ + *globulus,* globule]. A type of glycoprotein, q.v.

mucoid (mū′koyd) [″ + Gr. *eidos,* resemblance]. 1. Glycoprotein similar to mucin. 2. Muciform similar to mucus.

mucomembranous (mū″kō-mĕm′bră-nŭs) [″ + *membrana,* membrane]. Concerning mucous membrane.

mucoperiosteum (mū″kō-pĕr″ē-ŏs′tē-ŭm). Periosteum that has a mucous surface; or mucous and periosteal surfaces combined to form a membrane.

mucopolysaccharidase (mū″kō-pŏl″ē-săk′ă-rī-dās). An enzyme that catalyzes the hydrolysis of polysaccharides.

mucopolysaccharide (mū″kō-pŏl″ĭ-săk′ă-rīd). Polysaccharides that form chemical bonds with water. They contain hexosamine and sometimes proteins. Thick gelatinous material that is found many places in the body; it forms intercellular ground substance and basement membranes of cells; it is in mucous secretions and synovial fluid. SYN: *glycosaminoglycans.*

mucopolysaccharidosis. ABBR: MPS. One of a group of inherited diseases wherein mucopolysaccharide metabolism is defective and these substances accumulate in the tissues. Clinically there are severe skeletal deformities and usually mental retardation.

m. I. An inherited metabolic disease characterized by dwarfism, mental retardation, skeletal deformities including lumbar gibbus and clawhand, heart disease, and liver enlargement. Death usually occurs in the first decade. SYN: *Hurler's syndrome.*

m. II. A milder form of mucopolysaccharidosis I with a different inheritance pattern in that only males are affected. Patients may survive to age 60. SYN: *Hunter's disease.*

m. III. An inherited metabolic disease wherein the skeletal deformities are milder than in mucopolysaccharidosis I. Mental retardation is severe. SYN: *Sanfilippo's disease.*

m. IV. An inherited metabolic disease with severe skeletal deformities, corneal disease with clouding, and flat vertebrae. As the child starts to grow, cardiorespiratory symptoms develop. Most patients die in the second decade.

m. V. An inherited metabolic disease that becomes clinically apparent at about ten years of age. At that time stiff joints of the hands and feet, corneal clouding, generalized hypertrichosis, and valvular heart disease develop. The mouth is abnormally broad. Intellect is impaired little if at all. Patients may survive until the fifth decade of life.

mucopolysachariduria (mū″kō-pŏl″ē-săk″ă-rĭ-dū′rē-ă). Mucopolysaccharides in the urine.

mucoprotein (mū″kō-prō′tē-ĭn). A complex of protein and mucopolysaccharide. Usually the polysaccharide contains hexosamine.

mucopurulent (mū-kō-pūr′ū-lĕnt) [L. *mucus,* mucus, + *purulentus,* made up of pus]. Consisting of mucus and pus.

mucopus (mū′kō-pŭs). Mucus combined with or resembling pus.

Mucor (mū′kor) [L.]. A genus of mold fungi seen on dead and decaying matter. Sometimes responsible for infections of external ear, skin, and respiratory passageways.

mucoriferous (mū″kor-ĭf′ĕr-ŭs) [L. *mucor,* mold, + *ferre,* to carry]. Covered with mold or a moldlike substance.

mucorin (mū′kor-ĭn). An albuminoid substance derived from molds.

mucormycosis (mū″kor-mī-kō′sĭs) [″ + Gr. *mykes,* fungus, + *osis,* condition]. Zygomycosis, q.v.

mucorrhea [″ + *rhoia,* to flow]. Increased cervical discharge at ovulation. Usually covers a 3- to 4-day span and has character and appearance of raw egg white. SEE: *spinnbarkheit.*

mucosa (mū-kō′să) [L., mucous]. (pl. *mucosae*) Mucous membrane.

mucosal (mū-kō′săl). Concerning any mucous membrane.

mucosanguineous (mū″kō-săn-gwĭn′ē-ŭs) [″ + *sanguineus,* bloody]. Containing mucus and blood.

mucosedative (mū″kō-sĕd′ă-tĭv) [″ + *sedativus,* allaying]. Soothing to mucosae of the body. SYN: *demulcent.*

mucoserous (mū″kō-sĕr′ŭs). Composed of mucus and serum.

mucosin (mū′kō-sĭn). Mucin found in thick sticky mucus.

mucositis (mū″kō-sī′tĭs) [″ + Gr. *itis,* inflammation]. Inflammation of a mucous membrane.

mucosocutaneous (mū-kō"sō-kū-tā'nē-ŭs). Concerning mucous membrane and skin.

mucostatic (mū"kō-stăt'ĭk) [" + *statikos,* standing]. Stopping the secretion of mucus.

mucous (mū'kŭs). 1. Having the nature of or resembling mucus. 2. Secreting mucus. 3. Depending on presence of mucus.

mucous colitis. Inflammation of the mucosa of the colon. SEE: *colitis; irritable bowel syndrome.*

mucous membrane. Membrane lining passages and cavities communicating with the air. Consists of a surface layer of epithelium, a basement membrane, and an underlying layer of connective tissue, the lamina propria. Mucus-secreting cells or glands usually are present in the epithelium but may be absent. Examination should reveal degree of moisture, cyanosis, pallor, hyperemia, pigmentation, lesions or their absence, and hemorrhage. Pallor is seen in all anemias. If temporary, may indicate shock, vasomotor spasm, or may occur in severe hemorrhages. Blanching and flushing alternately accompanies aortic regurgitation.

Hyperemia or excessive redness of the mucous membranes is indicative of certain pathologies.

Buccal mucous membrane: Due to decayed teeth, traumatism, stomatitis. SEE: *mouth.*

Nasal mucosa: Ulceration of nose, rhinitis, inflammation. SEE: *nose.*

Eyes (local irritation): Foreign body, ulcer, inflammation. SEE: *jaundice.*

Dryness is seen in fevers, chronic gastritis, some liver disturbances, excitement, shock, prostration, fatigue, thirst, and certain drugs.

mucous polypus. Small growth from mucous lining of the cervix or uterus.

mucoviscidosis (mū"kō-vĭs"ĭ-dō'sĭs). Cystic fibrosis, q.v.

mucro (mū'krō) [L., a sharp point]. The pointed end of a structure.

mucus (mū'kŭs) [L.]. A viscid fluid secreted by mucous membranes and glands, consisting of mucin, leukocytes, inorganic salts, water, and epithelial cells. A good example is the almost ropy secretion from the sublingual and submandibular glands.

RS: amyxorrhea, expectorant; expectoration; glairy; goblet cell; "blenn-" and "muc-" words.

mulatto (mū-lăt'tō) [Sp. *mulato,* of mixed breed]. A person with one black parent and one white parent; popularly, anyone of mixed white and black ancestry.

muliebria (mū"lē-ĕb'rē-ă) [L.]. The female genitalia.

muliebrity (mū"lē-ĕb'rĭ-tē) [L. *muliebritas*]. 1. Femininity; womanliness. The assumption of womanly qualities at puberty. 2. The assumption of female characteristics by a male.

mull (mŭl). 1. To grind or pulverize. 2. A type of soft muslin.

Müller, Heinrich (mĭl'ĕr). German anatomist, 1820–1864.

M.'s fibers. Fine fibers of neuroglia cells that form supporting elements of the retina.

M.'s muscle. 1. Circular fibers of ciliary muscle. 2. The superior tarsal muscle of the eyelid. 3. Smooth muscle covering over the sphenomaxillary fissure.

M.'s trigone. Portion of tuber cinereum folding over the optic chiasm.

Müller, Johannes B. (mĭl'ĕr). German physician, 1801–1858.

M.'s ducts. Embryonic tubes from which the oviducts, uterus, and vagina develop in the female; in the male, they atrophy.

M.'s ring. Muscular ring at the junction of the cervical canal and the gravid uterus.

M.'s tubercle. Projection on the dorsal wall of the cloaca at which Müller's ducts terminate.

müllerian duct. SEE: *appendix testis.*

mult-, multi- [L. *multus*]. Prefixes indicating many or much.

multangular. Having many angles.

multangular bone, greater. The first or outermost of the distal row of carpal bones. SYN: *trapezium.*

multangular bone, lesser. The second in distal row of carpal bones. SYN: *trapezoid bone.*

multiallelic (mŭl"tē-ă-lĕl'ĭk). Concerning a large number of genes affecting hereditary characteristics.

multiarticular (mŭl"tē-ăr-tĭk'ū-lăr) [L. *multus,* many, + *articulus,* joint]. Concerning, having, or affecting many joints. SYN: *polyarticular.*

multicapsular (mŭl"tĭ-kăp'sū-lăr) [" + *capsula,* a little box]. Composed of many capsules.

multicellular (mŭl"tĭ-sĕl'ū-lăr) [" + *cellula,* small chamber]. Consisting of many cells.

Multiceps. A genus of tapeworms.

multicuspid, multicuspidate (mŭl"tĭ-kŭs'pĭd, -pĭ-dāt) [" + *cuspis,* point]. Having several cusps.

multifactorial. The result of many factors, as in a disease resulting from the combined action of several factors.

multifamilial (mŭl"tĭ-fă-mĭl'ē-ăl). Concerning a familial disease that affects children in several generations.

multifid (mŭl'tĭ-fĭd) [" + *fidus,* from *findere,* to split]. Divided into many sections.

multifocal (mŭl"tĭ-fō'kăl). Concerning many foci.

multiform (mŭl'tĭ-form) [" + *forma,* shape]. Having many forms or shapes. SYN: *poly-*

morphic; polymorphous.

multiglandular (mŭl″tĭ-glănd′ū-lar) [″ + *glandula,* a little acorn]. Concerning several glands.

multigravida (mŭl″tĭ-grăv′ĭ-dă) [″ + *gravida,* pregnant]. A woman who has been pregnant two or more times. May be written as gravida II or III, etc., according to the number of pregnancies. SEE: *multipara.*

multi-infection (mŭl″tĭ-ĭn-fĕk′shŭn) [L. *multus,* many, + *infectio,* an infection]. A mixed infection with several organisms developing at the same time.

multilobular (mŭl″tĭ-lŏb′ū-lar) [″ + *lobulus,* a small lobe]. Formed of or possessing many lobules.

multilocular (mŭl″tĭ-lŏk′ū-lar) [″ + *loculus,* a cell]. Having many cells or compartments. SYN: *multicellular.*

multimammae (mŭl″tĭ-măm′mē) [″ + *mamma,* breast]. Condition of possessing more than the normal number of breasts. SYN: *polymastia.*

multinodal (mŭl-tĭ-nō′dăl). Having many nodes or knots.

multinodular (mŭl-tĭ-nŏd′ū-lar) [″ + *nodulus,* little knot]. Possessing many nodules or small knots.

multinuclear, multinucleate (mŭl-tĭ-nū′klē-ăr, -āt). Possessing several nuclei. SYN: *polynuclear.*

multipara (mŭl-tĭp′ă-ră) [″ + *parere,* to bear]. A woman who has borne more than one viable fetus, whether or not the offspring were alive at birth. May be written para II or III, etc., according to the number of pregnancies. SEE: *multigravida.*

m., grand. A woman who has given birth seven or more times.

multiparity (mŭl-tĭ-păr′ĭ-tē). 1. Condition of having borne more than one child. 2. Production of more than one child at one birth.

multiparous (mŭl-tĭp′ăr-ŭs). 1. Having borne more than one child. 2. Producing more than one child at birth.

multipartial (mŭl″tĭ-păr′shăl). Concerning a polyvalent antiserum.

multiphasic screening. Attempting to determine an individual's health through a variety of methods and techniques. Usually consists of one or more of the following: self-completed medical history, variety of laboratory examinations of urine and blood, chest x-ray, serological test for syphilis, Papanicolaou smear, tonometry, pulmonary vital capacity, electrocardiogram, breast examination, height, weight, vision test, blood pressure. The cost-effectiveness of this approach in screening the apparently well has not been demonstrated.

multiple (mŭl′tĭ-pl) [L. *multiplex,* many folded]. 1. Consisting of or containing more than one; manifold. 2. Occurring simultaneously in various parts of the body.

multiple myeloma. SEE: *myeloma, multiple.*

multiple personality. Condition in which the subject may develop two or more personalities. SEE: *dissociation of personality; dual personality.*

multiple sclerosis. A chronic, slowly progressive disease of the central nervous system characterized by development of disseminated demyelinated glial patches called plaques. Symptoms and signs are numerous, but in later stages those of Charcot's triad (nystagmus, scanning speech, and intention tremor) are common. Occurs in the form of many clinical syndromes, the most common being the cerebral, brain stem–cerebellar, and spinal. A history of remissions and exacerbations is diagnostic. Etiology is unknown and there is no specific therapy.

multipolar (mŭl-tĭ-pōl′ăr) [L. *multus,* many, + *polus,* a pole]. 1. Possessing more than two poles. 2. Possessing more than two processes, said of neurons.

multisynaptic (mŭl″tē-sĭ-năp′tĭk). Polysynaptic.

multiterminal [″ + Gr. *terma,* a limit]. Providing several sets of terminals, making possible the use of several electrodes.

multivalent (mŭl-tĭ-vā′lĕnt) [″ + *valere,* to have power]. 1. Having ability to combine with more than two atoms of a univalent element or radical. 2. Active against several strains of an organism.

mummification (mŭm″mĭ-fĭ-kā′shŭn) [Arabian *mumiyaa,* mummy, + L. *facere,* to make]. 1. Mortification producing a hard, dry mass. SYN: *gangrene, dry.* 2. Drying and shriveling of a body, as a dead fetus.

mumps (mŭmps). An acute contagious, febrile disease characterized by inflammation of the parotid glands and other salivary glands. SYN: *parotitis.*

ETIOL: Mumps virus.

SYM: Onset gradual. There may be chilliness, malaise, headache, pain below ears, moderate fever of 101–102° F. (38.3–38.9° C.) or higher followed by swelling of one or both parotid glands. Usually swelling in one gland is subsiding as other swells. Swelling is below and in front of the ear. The lobe of the ear is sometimes pushed forward, surrounding tissues are edematous, and the features may be greatly distorted. Movements of the jaw are painful and restricted. Saliva may be increased or diminished. In a third of cases only one parotid is involved. Occasionally the parotid glands seem to escape, and swelling is confined to the submaxillary gland. Swelling usually lasts from 5 to 7 days.

COMPLICATIONS: Complications usually develop about the time the swelling in the parotids subsides. The most common complication in the postpubertal male is orchitis, which occurs in about 20 to 30% of cases; in the female, oöphoritis and mastitis. In rare cases permanent impairment of hearing follows an attack of mumps. Meningoencephalitis has been estimated to occur in 10% of patients.

DIFF. DIAGNOSIS: Cases of symptomatic parotitis may be excluded. Instances of trauma, infections about teeth and mouth, or a blocking of Stensen's duct may be suggestive of mumps.

PROG: Favorable, although the possibility of sexual sterility may occur in rare instances of bilateral orchitis.

TREATMENT: Rest in bed, a soft diet, and analgesics for headache and general malaise. Cold local applications may control swelling of testicles in orchitis.

mumps skin test antigen. USP. A standardized suspension of sterile formaldehyde–inactivated mumps virus. It is used in diagnosing mumps.

Mumpsvax. Trade name for mumps virus vaccine, live, USP.

mumps virus vaccine, live. USP. A sterile preparation of live mumps virus used to immunize against mumps. Trade name is Mumpsvax.

mumps virus vaccine, live attenuated. A vaccine made from the Jeryl Lynn strain of mumps virus for active immunization against mumps. Should not be given to pregnant women or to those who are sensitive to eggs, chicken, chicken feathers, or neomycin.

Münchhausen syndrome (mĕn-chow'zĕn). [Baron Karl F. H. von Münchhausen, known for his tall tales] A type of malingering or factitious disorder in which the patient may practice self-multilation and deception in order to feign illness. When detected, such patients leave one hospital and appear in the emergency room of another. Patients of this type are seldom recognized in time to receive psychiatric diagnoses and therapy, which they need.

mural (mū'răl) [L. *murus*, a wall]. Pert. to a wall of an organ or part.

muramidase. An enzyme found in blood cells of the granulocytic and monocytic series. Its serum and urine level is increased in patients with acute or chronic leukemia. It is also normally present in saliva, sweat, and tears. Formerly called lysozyme.

Murchison-Pel-Ebstein fever (mŭr'chĭ-sŏn-pĕl-ĕb'stīn). [Charles Murchison, Brit. physician, 1830–1879; Pieter K. Pel, Dutch physician, 1852–1919; Wilhelm Ebstein, Ger. physician, 1836–1912] SEE: *Pel-Ebstein fever*.

muriate (mūr'ē-āt) [L. *muria*, brine]. Former term for chloride.

muriatic acid (mū"rē-ăt'ĭk). Commercial hydrochloric acid.

murine (mū'rīn) [L. *mus*, mouse]. Concerning rodents, esp. rats and mice.

murmur [L.]. A soft blowing or rasping sound heard on auscultation. An adventitious sound heard on auscultation of the heart. It results from vibrations produced by movement of the blood within the heart and adjacent large blood vessels. May be heard during systole, diastole, or both. Two of the valves give forth a "lubb" sound and the other two a "dupp" sound, known as the first and second heart sounds. A blowing sound is heard if the valve does not close tightly, indicating an incompetent valve. A great vessel irregularity, such as an aortic aneurysm, or the flow of blood through a narrowed orifice, as in aortic or mitral stenosis, may produce a murmur.

A murmur does not necessarily indicate organic pathology, and heart disease may not result in any murmur; this may also be true in angina pectoris and coronary disorders. Air in the lungs may simulate sounds similar to heart murmurs.

RS: auscultation; bruit; circulation of blood; heart; hum, venous.

m., aneurysmal. Whizzing systolic sound heard over an aneurysm.

m., aortic obstructive. Harsh systolic murmur heard with and after the first heart sound. Loudest at the base.

m., aortic regurgitant. Blowing and hissing following second heart sound.

m., apex. Inorganic murmur over apex of heart.

m., arterial. Soft flowing murmur, synchronous with pulse.

m., Austin Flint. A presystolic or late diastolic heart murmur best heard at the apex of the heart. It is present in some cases of aortic insufficiency and is thought to be due to the vibration of the mitral valve caused by the backward-flowing blood from the aorta meeting the blood flowing in from the left atrium.

m., bronchial. Murmur heard over large bronchi, resembling respiratory laryngeal murmur.

m., cardiac. A sound arising due to blood flow through the heart.

m., cardiopulmonary. Murmur caused by movement of heart against lungs.

m., continuous. A continuous murmur that extends through systole and diastole.

m., crescendo. A murmur that builds up in intensity and subsides.

m., Cruveilhier-Baumgarten. A murmur, heard on the abdominal wall, from the collateral veins connecting the caval and portal veins.

m., diastolic. Murmur during dilation of

heart.

m., Duroziez's. A diastolic and systolic murmur heard over peripheral arteries of patients with aortic insufficiency.

m., ejection. A systolic murmur that is most intense at the time of maximum flow of blood from the heart; associated with pulmonary and aortic stenosis.

m., endocardial. Abnormal sound produced by any cause and arising within the heart.

m., exocardial. A cardiac murmur produced outside the cavities of the heart.

m., Flint's. M., Austin Flint, q.v.

m., friction. Murmur caused by rubbing of two inflamed mucous surfaces.

m., functional. Murmur occurring in the absence of any pathological change in structure of heart valves or orifices. It does not indicate organic disease of the heart. It may disappear upon a return to health. It must not be mistaken for true pathological murmurs.

m., Gibson. A continuous, machinery-like murmur heard in patent ductus arteriosus.

m., Graham Steell's. An early systolic murmur associated with pulmonic insufficiency caused by pulmonary hypertension.

m., heart. Cardiac murmur.

m., hemic. Sound heard on auscultation of anemic persons without a valvular lesion. Result of an abnormal, usually anemic, blood condition.

m., machinery. A continuous rough murmur heard in patients with a patent ductus arteriosus.

m., mitral. Murmur produced at orifice of mitral or bicuspid valve.

m., musical. A cardiac murmur that occurs when the sounds have an intermittent harmonic pattern.

m., organic. Murmur due to structural changes.

m., pansystolic. A heart murmur heard throughout systole.

m., pericardial. A friction sound produced within the pericardium.

m., physiologic. M., functional.

m., prediastolic. Systolic murmur.

m., presystolic. Murmur occurring just before systole, due to mitral or tricuspid obstruction.

m., pulmonary. Murmur produced at the orifice of the pulmonary artery.

m., regurgitant. Murmur due to leakage or backward flow of blood current through a dilated valvular orifice.

m., seagull. A murmur that mimics the cry of a seagull.

m., Still's. A benign, functional midsystolic murmur heard in children. The maximum sound is heard over the left lower sternal border.

m., systolic. Murmur heard during contraction of heart due to obstruction of flow of blood at one or several of the heart valves or in the aorta.

m., to-and-fro. Pericardial murmur heard during both systole and diastole.

m., tricuspid. Murmur produced at orifice of tricuspid valve, caused by disease.

m., vascular. Murmur occurring within a blood vessel.

m., vesicular. Normal breathing sounds.

Murphy's button. [John B. Murphy, U.S. surgeon, 1857–1916] Mechanical device used for intestinal anastomosis. Consists of two buttonlike hollow cylinders, each one sutured to an open end of the intestine and fitted together. After firm union of intestines, cylinders are passed in stools.

Murphy's sign. When the inflamed gallbladder is palpated by pressing the fingers under the rib cage, deep inspiration causes pain because the gallbladder is forced down to touch the fingers.

Mus (mŭs) [L., mouse]. A genus of rodents including mice and rats.

M. musculus. The common house mouse.

Musca (mŭs'kă) [L., fly]. A genus of flies belonging to the order Diptera, family Muscidae.

M. domestica. The common house fly, the transmitting agent for causative organisms of typhoid fever, bacillary and amebic dysentery, cholera, trachoma, and many other diseases.

muscae volitantes (mŭs'sē vŏl-ĭ-tăn'tēz) [L., flitting flies]. Black specks seen floating in the vitreous humor of the eye. They are sometimes apparent to the individual. This benign phenomenon is present in most individuals.

muscarine (mŭs'kă-rĭn) [L. *muscarius,* pert. to flies]. A highly toxic organic compound present in Amanita muscaria, a form of mushroom. SEE: *muscaria mushroom* in *Poisons and Poisoning* in *Appendix; mushroom and toadstool poisoning; Poison Control Centers* in *Appendix.*

muscegenetic (mŭs″ē-jĕ-nĕt'ĭk) [L. *musca,* fly, + Gr. *genesis,* production]. Causing muscae volitantes, q.v.

muscicide (mŭs'ĭ-sīd) [″ + *cidus,* killing]. Lethal to flies.

muscle (mŭs'ĕl) [L. *musculus*]. A type of tissue composed of contractile cells or fibers that effects movement of an organ or part of the body. The outstanding characteristic of muscular tisue is its ability to shorten or contract. It also possesses the properties of irritability, conductivity, and elasticity. Muscle tissue possesses little intercellular material, hence its cells or fibers lie close together. SYN: *musculus* [NA]. SEE for illus.: *arm; cells; face; leg; muscle.*

TYPES: Three types of muscle differentiated on basis of histologic structure occur in the body, namely, smooth, striated, and cardiac. SEE: table.

Smooth, Nonstriated: Cells are fusiform or spindle-shaped, each containing a central nucleus. Cells usually arranged in sheets or layers but may occur as isolated units in connective tissue. Called involuntary because they are not under conscious control. Found principally in the internal organs, esp. digestive tract, respiratory passages, urinary and genital ducts, urinary bladder and gallbladder, and walls of blood vessels. Smooth muscle lacks the cross striations characteristic of other types of muscle.

Striated, Skeletal: The cytoplasm (sarcoplasm) contains numerous myofibrillae. The cytoplasmic cell membrane is called the sarcolemma. Muscle fibers are grouped into bundles called fasciculi, each of which is surrounded by a sheath or connective tissue called perimysium. The fibers within a fasciculus are surrounded by and held together by delicate reticular fibrils forming the endomysium. Striated muscle is found in all skeletal muscles and movement is under conscious control. It also occurs in the tongue, pharynx, and upper portion of esophagus.

Cardiac: Fibers branch and anastomose, forming a continuous network or syncytium.

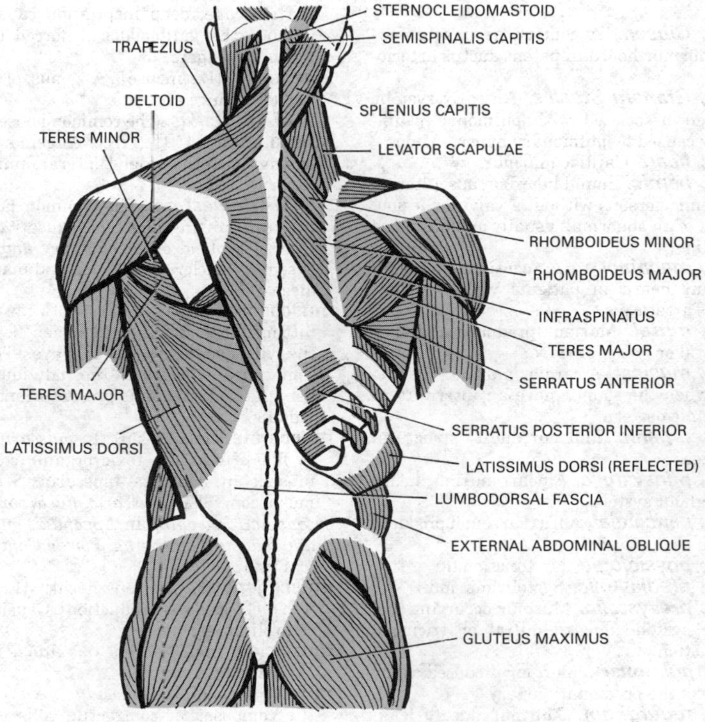

MUSCLES OF BACK

Comparison of Properties of Three Types of Muscle

	Smooth	Cardiac	Striped
Synonyms	Involuntary Nonstriated Visceral Plain	Myocardium	Voluntary Skeletal Striated
Fibers:			
Length (in micrometers)	50–200		25,000
Thickness (in micrometers)	4–8		75
Shape	Spindles		Cylinders
Marking	No striation	Striation	Marked striation
Nuclei	Single	Single	Multiple
Speed of contraction	Very slow	Moderate	Very quick
Effects of cutting related nerve	Slight	Slight	Complete paralysis

At intervals, prominent bands or intercalated disks cross the fibers. Certain fibers, called Purkinje fibers, form the impulse-conducting system of the heart.

ANAT: A contractile organ consisting of muscle tissue, which effects movements of parts of the body, esp. a structure composed of striated muscle and attached to a part of the skeleton. A typical muscle consists of a central fleshy portion or belly and its attachments. One end called the head is attached to a fixed structure termed the origin; the other end is attached to a movable part called the insertion. Some muscles are spindle-shaped; others form flat sheets or bands. Muscles may be attached directly to the periosteum of bones or they may be attached by means of tough cords of connective tissue (tendons) or broad flat sheets (aponeuroses). The connective tissue enclosing a muscle is called epimysium; it is continuous with the deep fascia.

BLOOD SUPPLY: Obtained from small blood vessels that enter the muscular tissue and subdivide into capillaries that permeate throughout.

NERVE SUPPLY: *Voluntary:* From branches of the peripheral cerebrospinal nervous system. It is because of this that the skeletal muscles are under conscious control. *Involuntary:* Smooth and cardiac receive their nerve supply from autonomic nervous system and function involuntarily without conscious control.

m., abductor. Muscle that draws away from the midline.

m., adductor. Muscle that draws toward the midline.

m., antagonistic. Muscle that counteracts the action of another muscle.

m.'s, antigravity. Muscles that pull against the constant force of gravity to maintain posture.

m., appendicular. One of the skeletal muscles of the limbs.

m., arrector pili. SEE: *arrectores pilorum.*

m., articular. Muscle attached to capsule of a joint.

m., axial. A skeletal muscle of the head or trunk.

m., bipennate. Muscle in which the fibers converge toward a central tendon on both sides.

m., constrictor, of pharynx. A muscle that constricts the pharynx.

m., digastric. Muscle that lowers the jaw.

m., extensor. Muscle that extends a part.

m., extrinsic. Muscle whose origin lies outside the part moved.

m., fixation. A muscle that acts to steady a part in order that more precise movements in a related structure may be accomplished.

m., flexor. Muscle that bends a part.

m., fusiform. A muscle resembling a spindle.

m., intrinsic. A muscle that has both its origin and insertion within a structure, as intrinsic muscles of the tongue, eye, or limb.

m., involuntary. Muscle not under conscious control; mainly smooth muscle.

m.'s, mastication. The four pairs of muscles that move the mandible and provide the primary forces of mastication; the masseter, temporalis, medial pterygoid, and lateral pterygoid muscles.

m.'s, mimetic. Superficial muscles of the facial region that by skin movements produce the facial expressions. Also: *muscles of facial expression.*

m., multipennate. Muscle with several tendons of origin and several tendons of insertion in which fibers pass obliquely from a tendon of origin to a tendon of insertion on each side.

m., nonstriated. M., smooth.

m., papillary. Muscle on inner surface of ventricle of heart to which chordae tendineae are attached.

m., pectinate. Muscle on inner surface of right atrium giving it a ridged appearance.

m., postaxial. Muscle on the posterior or dorsal aspect of a limb.

m., preaxial. Muscle on the anterior or ventral aspect of a limb.

m., skeletal. Muscle that is connected with a bone; mainly striated.

m., smooth. Muscle tissue that lacks cross striations on its fibers; involuntary in action and found principally in visceral organs. SYN: *m., nonstriated.*

m., somatic. Muscle derived from mesodermal somites. Includes most skeletal muscle.

m., sphincter. Muscle that encircles a duct, tube, or orifice, thus controlling its opening.

m., striated. Muscle fibers that possess alternate light and dark bands or striations; mainly voluntary and comprise skeletal muscles.

m.'s, synergistic. Muscles aiding one another in function.

m., unipennate. Muscle whose fibers converge on only one side of a tendon.

m., unstriated. Muscle without markings; mainly involuntary. SYN: *m., smooth.*

m., voluntary. Muscle whose action is controlled by will. Except for the cardiac muscle, all striated muscles are voluntary.

muscular [L. *muscularis*]. 1. Pert. to muscles. 2. Possessing well-developed muscles.

muscular contractions, graduated. Accomplished by use of electrical current of varying strength and duration. Used in muscles with an intact nerve supply when muscles are atonic, wasted away, or when voluntary exercise is not feasible; and in denervated muscles as in cases following nerve injury or poliomyelitis.

muscular dystrophy. Wasting away and atrophy of muscles. SEE: *dystrophy, progressive muscular.*

muscularis (mŭs-kū-lā'rĭs) [L.]. Muscular layer of an organ or tubule.

m. mucosae. Unstriated muscular tissue layer of mucous membrane.

muscularity. State or quality of being muscular.

muscularize (mŭs'kū-lăr-īz). To change into muscle tissue.

musculature [L. *musculus,* muscle]. The arrangement of muscles in the body or its parts.

musculin. A globulin in muscle.

musculo- [L. *musculus,* muscle]. Combining form pert. to a muscle.

musculoaponeurotic (mŭs-kū-lō-ăp"ō-nū-rŏt'ĭk). Composed of muscle and an aponeurosis of fibrous connective tissue.

musculocutaneous (mŭs"kū-lō-kū-tān'ē-ŭs) [" + *cutis,* skin]. 1. Pert. to the muscles and skin. 2. Supplying or affecting the muscles and skin. 3. The specific nerve from the brachial plexus that innervates the coracobrachialis, biceps branchii, and brachialis muscles and provides cutaneous sensory distribution to the forearm.

musculofascial (mŭs"kū-lō-făsh'ē-ăl). Composed of muscle and fascia.

musculomembranous (mŭs"kū-lō-mĕm'brān-ŭs). Pert. to or consisting of muscle and membrane.

musculophrenic (mŭs"kū-lō-frĕn'ĭk). Pert. to muscles of the diaphragm.

musculoskeletal (mŭs"kū-lō-skĕl'ĕ-tăl). Pert. to the muscles and the skeleton.

musculospiral (mŭs"kū-lō-spī'răl) [" + *spira,* coil]. Concerning the musculospiral nerve.

musculotendinous. Composed of both muscle and tendon.

musculotropic (mŭs"kū-lō-trŏp'ĭk) [" + Gr. *tropikos,* turning]. Affecting, acting on, or having an affinity for muscular tissue.

musculus [L.]. (pl. *musculi*) [NA] Muscle.

mushbite (mŭsh'bīt). Making a dental impression by having the patient bite into a soft wax or plastic material. The technique is little used.

mushroom [Fr. *mousseron*]. Umbrella-shaped fungus, belonging to the Basidiomycetes, that grows on decaying vegetable matter; common in woods and damp places. Some of the poisonous varieties are commonly called toadstools. SEE: *muscaria mushrooms* in *Poisons and Poisoning* in *Appendix; toadstool.*

COMP: Low in carbohydrates and fats; high in protein. Their relationship and similarity to poisonous fungi are so close that only those who are thoroughly capable of distinguishing the poisonous varieties from the edible ones should attempt to gather and eat them.

mushroom and toadstool poisoning. Poisoning resulting from ingestion of mushrooms such as Amanita muscaria, which contains muscarine, or other species that contain phalloidine, a component of the amanita toxin. SEE: *muscaria mushrooms* in *Poisons and Poisoning* in *Appendix.*

musicogenic (mū″zĭ-kō-jĕn′ĭk) [L. *musica,* music, + *gennan,* to produce]. Caused by music, esp. epileptic convulsions.

musicomania [″ + Gr. *mania,* madness]. Insane love of music.

musicotherapy [″ + *therapeia,* treatment]. Treatment of disease with music.

musk (mŭsk) [Sanskrit *muska,* testicle]. An oily secretion obtained from the musk bag, a gland beneath the abdominal skin of the male musk deer. Has a very strong odor. Used in manufacturing perfume.

mussel. A freshwater bivalve mollusc belonging to the class Pelecypoda.

mussel poisoning. Poisoning common on the Pacific coast of the United States resulting from eating mussels or clams that have ingested a poisonous dinoflagellate. Occurs from June to October. The poison is not destroyed by cooking.

Musset's sign (mū-sāz′). [Louis C. A. de Musset, Fr. poet, 1810–1857] Repetitive jerking movements of the head and neck in synchrony with ventricular contractions of the heart. Seen in advanced aortic incompetence, or aortic aneurysm.

mussitation (mŭs-sĭ-tā′shŭn) [L. *mussitare,* to mutter]. The muttering of delirium or the moving of the lips without sound.

mustard [Fr. *moustarde*]. Yellow powder of mustard seed used as a counterirritant, rubefacient, emetic, stimulant, and condiment SEE: *plaster.*

m., nitrogen. SEE: *nitrogen mustards.*

mustard gas. Dichlorodiethyl sulfide, a war gas that causes burns and destruction on tissue internally and externally.

Mustargen. Trade name for mechlorethamine hydrochloride, USP.

mutacism (mū′tă-sĭzm). A form of speech impediment in which the "m" sound is often substituted for other sounds.

mutagen (mū′tă-jĕn) [L. *mutare,* to change, + Gr. *gennan,* to produce]. Any agent that causes genetic mutations. Many medicines, chemicals, and physical agents such as ionizing radiations and ultraviolet light have this ability.

mutagenesis (mū″tă-jĕn′ĕ-sĭs). The induction of genetic mutation. SEE: *mutation* (defs. 2 and 3); *teratogenesis.*

mutagenicity (mū″tă-jĕ-nĭs′ĭ-tē). Property of causing genetic mutation.

mutant (mū′tănt) [L. *mutare,* to change]. A variation of genetic structure that breeds true.

mutase (mū′tās) [″ + *ase,* enzyme]. 1. Enzyme that accelerates oxidation-reduction reactions through activation of oxygen and hydrogen. 2. A food preparation made from leguminous plants high in protein content.

mutation (mū-tā′shŭn). 1. Change; transformation; instance of such change. 2. Permanent variation in genetic structure with offspring differing from parents in a characteristic. Differentiated from gradual variation through many generations. 3. A change in a gene potentially capable of being transmitted to offspring.

m., induced. Mutation resulting from exposure to x-rays, radioactive substances, and certain drugs and chemicals.

m., natural. Mutation occurring without artificial external intervention; thought to be a primary factor in evolutionary change.

m., somatic. Mutation occurring in somatic cells.

mute (mūt) [L. *mutus,* dumb]. 1. One who is unable to speak. 2. Dumb, without ability to speak.

m., deaf. Individual who is unable to hear or to speak.

mutilate [L. *mutilatus,* to maim]. To deprive of a limb or a part; to maim or disfigure.

mutilation (mū″tĭ-lā′shŭn). Maiming; the act of removing or destroying a conspicuous or essential part or organ.

mutism (mū′tĭzm) [L. *mutus,* dumb]. 1. Condition of being unable to speak. 2. Persistent inhibition to speech; seen in some severe forms of mental disorder.

m., akinetic. Syndrome consisting of mutism, loss of physical movement, and apparent loss of feeling.

m., hysterical. Inability to speak due to hysteria.

mutualism (mū′tū-ăl-ĭzm) [L. *mutuus,* exchanged]. A form of symbiosis in which organisms of two different species live in close association to the mutual benefit of each.

mutualist (mū′tū-ăl-ĭst). Organism associated with another organism to the mutual benefit of each.

M.V. *Medicus Veterinarius.* Latin for veterinary physician.

Mv. Chem. symb. for mendelevium.

mv. *millivolt.*

M.W.I.A. *Medical Women's International Association.*

my-, myo- [Gr. *mys,* muscle]. Prefix denoting rel. to muscle.

myalgia (mī-ăl′jē-ă) [″ + *algos,* pain]. Tenderness or pain in the muscles; muscular rheumatism. SYN: *myodynia.*

Myambutrol. Trade name for ethambutol hydrochloride.

myasis (mī-ā'sĭs) [Gr. *myia,* a fly]. Condition that arises from infestation with larvae of flies or maggots in the body or upon mucous membranes. SYN: *myiasis.*

myasthenia (mī-ăs-thē'nē-ă) [Gr. *mys,* muscle, + *astheneia,* weakness]. Muscular weakness.

m., angiosclerotic. Vascular changes producing excessive muscular fatigue.

m. cordis. Weakness of the heart muscle. SYN: *amyocardia.*

m. gastrica. Loss of muscular tone in coats of the stomach.

m. gravis. A disease characterized by great muscular weakness (without atrophy) and progressive fatigability. It is due to a functional abnormality, lack of acetylcholine or excess of cholinesterase at the myoneural junction, in which nerve impulses fail to induce normal muscle contractions. SEE: *edrophonium test.*

ETIOL: Unknown. More common in females. Occurs most frequently between ages of 20 and 50.

SYM: Abnormal fatigability and weakness of muscles. Muscles of the face and neck primarily involved, those of the trunk and extremities secondarily. Onset gradual; symptoms worse in the evening. Patient complains of difficulty in chewing, swallowing, and talking. Expressionless facies and ptosis usually present.

PROG: Some cases mild; others rapidly fatal, death resulting from respiratory failure. Course is variable. Prolonged remissions may occur.

TREATMENT: Restricted activity; complete rest in severe cases. Soft or liquid diet; tube feedings sometimes essential. Physostigmine and neostigmine given intramuscularly or orally are effective. Potassium chloride, ephedrine, and guanidine are also used as adjuvants of pyridostigmine bromide (Mestinon), the drug of choice.

myasthenic. Marked by muscular weakness.

myatonia (mī-ă-tō'nē-ă). Deficiency or loss of muscular tone.

m. congenita. A noninherited but sometimes familial disease characterized by absence of muscular development, with the lower extremities being the first involved. It is seen shortly after birth. SYN: *amyotonia congenita; Oppenheim's disease.*

myatrophy (mī-ăt'rō-fē). Muscular wasting.

My-B-Den. Trade name for adenosine.

myc-, myco- [Gr. *mykes,* fungus]. Combining form meaning fungus.

mycelioid (mī-sē'lē-oyd) [" + *eidos,* form]. Moldlike; resembling mold colonies in which filaments radiate from a center, said of bacterial colonies.

mycelium (mī-sē'lē-ŭm) [Gr. *mykes,* fungus, + *helos,* nail]. The mass of filaments (hyphae) that constitutes the vegetative body of fungi such as molds.

mycetes (mī-sē'tēz). The fungi.

mycethemia (mī-sĕ-thē'mē-ă) [" + *haima,* blood]. Fungi in the blood. SYN: *mycohemia.*

mycetism, mycetismus (mī'sĕ-tĭzm, mī-sĕ-tĭz'mŭs) [" + *-ismos,* condition]. Poisoning from eating fungi, esp. poisonous mushrooms.

mycetogenetic (mī-sē"tō-jĕn-ĕt'ĭk) [" + *gennan,* to produce]. Induced by fungi.

mycetoma (mī-sĕ-tō'mă) [" + *oma,* tumor]. A syndrome caused by a variety of aerobic actinomycetes and fungi. It is characterized by swelling and suppuraton of subcutaneous tissues; and formation of sinus tracts, with granules present in the pus draining from the sinus tracts. These tracts usually appear on the lower body.

TREATMENT: Sulfones, trimethoprim-sulfamethoxazole, or sulfonamides may benefit lesions caused by actinomycetes. If lesions are due to fungi, there is no specific therapy.

Mycifradin Sulfate. Trade name for neomycin sulfate, USP.

mycobacteriosis (mī"kō-băk-tē"rē-ō'sĭs). A tuberculosis-like disease not caused by Mycobacterium tuberculosis.

Mycobacterium [" + *bakterion,* little rod]. A genus of acid-fast organisms belonging to the Mycobacteriaceae that includes the causative organisms of tuberculosis and leprosy. They are slender, nonmotile, gram-positive rods and do not produce spores or capsules.

M., atypical. Species of mycobacteria that are classified with respect to their growth characteristics, ability to produce pigment, and on the basis of chemical and agglutination tests. Some cause disease in lower animals, some cause a mild form of tuberculosis in man; and some are nonpathogenic. Species include: M. avium intracellulare, M. chelonei, M. fortuitum, M. gastri, M. gordonae, M. kansasii, M. marinum, M. scrofulaceum, M. terrae, M. triviale, and M. xenopi.

M. balnei. The organism that causes a chronic skin lesion called swimming pool granuloma.

M. bovis. The organism that causes tuberculosis in cows.

M. kansasii. A cause of tuberculosis-like pulmonary disease in humans.

M. leprae. The causative agent of leprosy.

M. marinum. An atypical mycobacterium that produces skin infection resembling sporotrichosis. The organism has been cultured from tropical fish aquariums.

M. tuberculosis. Causative agent of tuberculosis in mammals.

mycocidin (mī″kō-sī′dĭn). An antibiotic derived from molds of the family Aspergillaceae.

mycoderma [Gr. *mykos,* mucus, + *derma,* skin]. Mucous membrane.

mycodermatitis (mī″kō-dĕr″mă-tī′tĭs). A nonspecific term for any skin disease caused by fungi, yeasts, or molds.

mycodermomycosis (mī″kō-dĕr″mō-mī-kō′sĭs). Candidiasis.

mycohemia (mī″kō-hē′mē-ă) [Gr. *mykes,* fungus, + *haima,* blood]. Mycethemia, q.v.

mycoid (mī′koyd) [″ + *eidos,* form]. Funguslike.

mycology (mī-kŏl′ō-jē) [″ + *logos,* study]. Science of fungi.

mycomyringitis (mī″kō-mĭr-ĭn-jī′tĭs) [″ + L. *myringa,* drum membrane, + *itis,* inflammation]. Fungus inflammation of the tympanic membrane SYN: *myringomycosis; otomycosis.*

mycophthalmia (mī-kŏf-thăl′mē-ă). Ophthalmia resulting from fungus infection.

mycoplasmas. Several bacteria of the Mycoplasma genus that are found in the human. Includes M. hominis types 1 and 2, M. salivarium, M. orale, M. fermentans, and M. pneumoniae. Most forms have no cell wall. Mycoplasma that were called pleuropneumonia-like organisms (PPLO) have been proven to be the cause of primary atypical pneumonia (called viral pneumonia at one time). Their relationship to other diseases such as Reiter's syndrome, q.v., has not been proven. T (for *tiny*) strains, so called because they produce small colonies on agar, inhabit the urogenital tract.

mycoprecipitin (mī″kō-prē-sĭp′ĭ-tĭn). A precipitin for extracts of yeast and fungi.

mycosis (mī-kō′sĭs) [″ + *osis,* condition]. Any disease induced by a fungus.

m. fungoides. A rare, poorly understood, malignant disease that originates in the reticuloendothelial cells of the skin. The lymph nodes and internal organs become involved.

SYM: Urticarial, erythematous, or eczematous patches of irregular shape and size, with well-defined margins usually upon scalp and skin of trunk. Itching intense; frequently the patches become hypertrophic and firm. Hard nodules varying from size of pea to apple, either sessile or pedunculated, develop on them. These eventually break down and form ulcers that contain sensitive, fungating granulation tissue, and discharge thin pus and serum. Death results from progressive cachexia.

TREATMENT: General supportive measures. Electron beam radiation and cytotoxic agents have been used.

m., superficial. A dermatomycosis; a fungus infection of the skin. Includes erythrasma; tinea barbae, tinea capitis, tinea corporis, tinea cruris, tinea favosa, tinea pedis, tinea unguium; trichomycosis axillaris.

m., systemic. A deep mycosis; a fungus infection involving various bodily systems or regions. Includes aspergillosis, blastomycosis, chromoblastomycosis, coccidioidomycosis, conidiosporosis, cryptococcosis, geotrichosis, histoplasmosis, maduromycosis, moniliasis, mucormycosis, nocardiosis, paraactinomycosis, penicilliosis, rhinosporidiosis, sporotrichosis.

mycostasis (mī-kŏs′tă-sĭs) [Gr. *mykes,* fungus, + *stasis,* standing]. Stopping the growth of fungi.

mycostat (mī′kō-stăt) [″ + *statikos,* standing]. Anything that stops the growth of fungi.

Mycostatin. Trade name for nystatin, USP.

mycotic (mī-kŏt′ĭk). Caused by or affected with microorganisms; concerning mycosis.

mycotoxicosis (mī″kō-tŏk″sĭ-kō′sĭs) [″ + *toxikon,* poisoning, + *osis,* condition]. Disease either caused by toxins on or produced by molds.

mycotoxinization (mī″kō-tŏk″sĭn-ī-zā′shŭn). Inoculation with a fungal toxin.

mycotoxins. Substances, produced by mold growing in food or animal feed, that cause illness or death when ingested by man or animals. SEE: *ergotism.*

mycterophonia (mĭk″tĕr-ō-fō′nē-ă) [Gr. *mykter,* nostril, + *phone,* voice]. Phonation in which the voice possesses a nasal quality.

mydaleine (mĭd-ā′lē-ēn) [Gr. *mydaleos,* moldy]. A poisonous ptomaine from putrefied visceral organs, acting mainly on the heart.

Mydfrin. Trade name for phenylephrine hydrochloride, USP.

Mydriacyl. Trade name for tropicamide, USP.

mydriasis (mĭd-rī′ă-sĭs) [Gr.]. Pronounced or abnormal dilation of the pupil.

ETIOL: Fright, sudden emotion, first and third stages of anesthesia, drugs, coma, hysteria, botulism, or irritation of cervical sympathetic nerve.

m., alternating. Mydriasis that affects one eye, then the other.

m., paralytic. Mydriasis resulting from paralysis of oculomotor nerve.

m., spastic. Mydriasis resulting from overactivity of dilator muscle of iris or of sympathetic nerves supplying that muscle.

m., spinal. Mydriasis resulting from a lesion of, or irritation of, ciliospinal center of spinal cord.

mydriatic (mĭd-rē-ăt′ĭk). 1. Causing pupillary dilatation. 2. Any drug that dilates the pupil. In certain eye diseases it is essential that the pupil be dilated during the course of treatment to prevent adhesions of the pupils.

Ex.: atropine, cocaine, ephedrine, euphthalmine, homatropine.

myectomy (mī-ĕk'tō-mē) [Gr. *mys,* muscle, + *ektome,* excision]. Excision of a portion of a muscle.

myectopia (mī-ĕk-tō'pē-ă) [" + *ek,* out, + *topos,* place]. Muscle dislocation.

myelalgia (mī-ĕl-ăl'jē-ă) [Gr. *myelos,* marrow, + *algos,* pain]. Pain of the spinal cord or its membranes.

myelanalosis (mī"ĕl-ăn"ăl-ō'sĭs) [" + *analosis,* wasting]. Gradual wasting of the spinal cord.

myelapoplexy (mī"ĕl-ăp'ō-plĕks-ē) [" + *apoplexia,* stroke]. Hemorrhagic effusion into the spinal cord.

myelasthenia (mī"ĕl-ăs-thē'nē-ă) [Gr. *myelos,* marrow, + *astheneia,* weakness]. Spinal exhaustion; neurasthenia arising from disease of the spinal cord.

myelatelia (mī"ĕl-ă-tē'lē-ă) [" + *ateleia,* imperfection]. Defective development of spinal cord.

myelatrophy (mī-ĕl-ăt'rō-fē) [" + *atrophia,* atrophy]. Wasting of the spinal cord.

myelauxe (mī-ĕl-awks'ē) [" + *auxe,* increase]. Abnormal enlargement of spinal cord.

myelemia (mī-ĕl-ē'mē-ă) [" + *haima,* blood]. Abnormal number of marrow cells in the blood. SYN: *myelocytosis.*

myelencephalon (mī"ĕl-ĕn-sĕf'ă-lŏn) [Gr. *myelos,* marrow, + *enkephalos,* brain]. [NA] The most posterior portion of the embryonic hindbrain (rhombencephalon), which gives rise to the medulla oblongata.

myelic. Pert. to the spinal cord.

myelin. 1. A fatlike substance forming a sheath around the axons of certain nerves. Composed of lipids and protein. 2. A complex lipoid substance present in the brain in small quantities.

myelination (mī"ĕl-ĭn-ā'shŭn) [Gr. *myelos,* marrow]. Process of acquiring a myelin sheath. SYN: *myelinization.*

myelinic (mī-ĕl-ĭn'ĭk). Concerning or composed of myelin.

myelinization (mī"ĕl-ĭn-ĭ-zā'shŭn). Acquisition of myelin sheath for nerve fibers. SYN: *myelination.*

myelinoclasis (mī"ĕ-lĭn-ŏk'lă-sĭs) [" + *klasis,* breaking]. Destruction of myelin.

myelinogenesis (mī"ĕ-lĭn"ō-jĕn'ĕ-sĭs) [" + *genesis,* production]. Myelinization.

myelinogenetic (mī"ĕl-ĭn-ō-jĕn-ĕt'ĭk) [" + *gennan,* to produce]. Producing myelin or a myelin sheath.

myelinolysis (mī"ĕ-lĭn-ŏl'ĭ-sĭs) [" + *lysis,* dissolution]. Destructive of the myelin sheaths of nerves.

myelinosis (mī"ĕl-ĭn-ō'sĭs) [" + *osis,* condition]. Fatty degeneration during which myelin is produced.

myelitic (mī-ĕl-ĭt'ĭk). Concerning myelitis.

myelitis (mī-ĕ-lī'tĭs) [" + *itis,* inflammation]. 1. Inflammation of bone marrow. 2. Inflammation of the spinal cord.

SYM: Moderate fever (101°–103° F. or 38.3°–39.4° C.), loss of appetite and constipation, followed by pain in back radiating into the limbs. Various forms of paresthesia, such as numbness, tingling, or burning, may be present. Frequently a sense of painful constriction, girdle pain, also develops. Paralysis soon develops and may become more or less complete. At first there may be retention of feces, later incontinence. Bedsores are likely to develop if care is not taken to prevent them. Death may result in a few days from upward extension and involvement of respiratory muscles. In rare cases, a spontaneous arrest of inflammation and slow recovery follow, attended with partial paralysis. SEE: *axophage; osteomyelitis; poliomyelitis.*

m., acute. Simple acute form of myelitis that develops following injury.

m., ascending, acute. Myelitis that moves progressively upward in the spinal cord.

m., bulbar. Myelitis involving the medulla oblongata.

m., central. 1. Inflammation of the spinal cord. 2. Inflammation of the bone marrow.

m., compression. Myelitis caused by pressure on the spinal cord, as by a hemorrhage or tumor.

m., descending. Myelitis affecting successively lower areas of the spinal cord.

m., disseminated. Inflammation of several separate areas of the spinal cord.

m., focal. Myelopathy, q.v., of small areas of the spinal cord.

m., hemorrhagic. Myelitis with hemorrhage.

m., sclerosing. Myelopathy wherein there is hardening of the spinal column.

m., transverse. Myelitis involving the whole thickness of the spinal cord, but limited longitudinally.

m., transverse, acute. Acute form of myelitis involving entire thickness of spinal cord, developing subsequent to injury to spinal cord.

m., traumatic. Myelitis due to spinal cord injury.

myelo- [Gr. *myelos,* marrow]. Prefix denoting the spinal cord or bone marrow.

myeloblast (mī'ĕl-ō-blăst) [" + *blastos,* germ]. Immature bone marrow cell that develops into a myelocyte. It matures to develop into a promyelocyte, and eventually the granular leukocyte. SYN: *microleukoblast.*

myeloblastemia (mī"ĕl-ō-blăst-ē'mē-ă) [" + " + *haima,* blood]. Occurrence of myeloblasts in the blood.

myeloblastoma (mī″ĕl-ō-blăst-ō′mă) [″ + ″ + *oma,* tumor]. Tumor containing myeloblasts, seen in the myelogenic form of leukemia.

myeloblastosis (mī″ĕ-lō-blăs-tō′sĭs) [″ + ″ + *osis,* condition]. Excess production of myeloblasts and their presence in circulating blood.

myelocele (mī′ĕ-lō-sēl). [″ + *kele,* hernia]. A form of spina bifida with spinal cord protrusion.

myelocyst (mī′ĕl-ō-sĭst) [″ + *kystis,* bladder]. Cyst arising from the rudimentary medullary canal of the spinal cord.

myelocystocele (mī″ĕl-ō-sĭst′ō-sēl) [″ + ″ + *kele,* hernia]. Cystic tumor of spinal cord substance through a defect in the canal.

myelocystomeningocele (mī″ĕl-ō-sĭst″ō-mĕn-ĭn′gō-sēl) [″ + *kystis,* bladder, + *meninx,* membrane, + *kele,* hernia]. Combined myelocystocele and meningocele.

myelocyte (mī′ĕl-ō-sīt) [″ + *kytos,* cell]. A large cell in red bone marrow from which leukocytes are derived.

myelocythemia (mī″ĕl-ō-sī-thē′mē-ă) [″ + ″ + *haima,* blood]. Presence of an excess number of myelocytes in the blood. SYN: *myelemia; myelocytosis.*

myelocytic (mī″ĕl-ō-sĭt′ĭk). Characterized by presence of, or pert. to, myelocytes.

myelocytoma (mī″ĕl-ō-sī-tō′mă) [″ + *kytos,* cell, + *oma,* tumor]. Leukemia with leukocytes arising from both myeloid and lymphoid substance.

myelocytosis (mī″ĕl-ō-sī-tō′sĭs) [″ + ″ + *osis,* condition]. Myelocytes in large quantities in the blood. SYN: *myelemia; myelocythemia.*

myelodiastasis (mī″ĕl-ō-dī-ăs′tă-sĭs) [Gr. *myelos,* marrow, + *diastasis,* separation]. Destruction and disintegration of spinal cord.

myelodysplasia (mī″ĕl-ō-dĭs-plā′zē-ă) [″ + *dys,* bad, + *plassein,* to form]. Defective formation of the spinal cord.

myeloencephalic (mī″ĕl-ō-ĕn-sĕf-ăl′ĭk) [″ + *enkephalos,* brain]. Concerning the spinal cord and brain.

myeloencephalitis (mī″ĕl-ō-ĕn-sĕf″ă-lī′tĭs) [″ + ″ + *itis,* inflammation]. Inflamed condition of spinal cord and brain.

myelofibrosis (mī″ĕ-lō-fī-brō′sĭs). Replacement of bone marrow by fibrous tissue.

myelogenesis (mī″ĕl-ō-jĕn′ĕ-sĭs) [″ + *genesis,* development]. 1. The development of brain and spinal cord. 2. Development of the myelin sheath of nerve fiber.

myelogenic, myelogenous (mī-ĕ-lō-jĕn′ĭk, -lŏj′ĕn-ŭs) [″ + *gennan,* to produce]. Producing or originating in marrow.

myelogeny (mī″ĕ-lŏj′ĕ-nē). Maturation of the myelin sheaths during the development of the central nervous system.

myelogram (mī′ĕ-lō-grăm) [″ + *gramma,* writing]. 1. Roentgenogram of the spinal canal after injection of a radiopaque dye. 2. Differential count of bone marrow cells.

myelography (mī-ĕ-lŏg′ră-fē) [″ + *graphein,* to write]. Roentgenographic inspection of the spinal cord by use of a radiopaque medium injected into the intrathecal space.

m., air. Myelography in which oxygen or air is used instead of radiopaque dye.

myeloid (mī′ĕ-loyd) [″ + *eidos,* form]. 1. Medullary; like marrow. 2. Resembling a myelocyte, but not necessarily originating from bone marrow.

myeloidosis (mī″ĕ-loy-dō′sĭs) [″ + ″ + *osis,* condition]. Development of myeloid tissue.

myelolymphangioma (mī″ĕ-lō-lĭm-făn″jē-ō′mă). Elephantiasis.

myelolymphocyte (mī″ĕ-lō-lĭmf′ō-sīt) [″ + L. *lympha,* lymph, + Gr. *kytos,* cell]. Tiny lymphocyte formed abnormally in bone marrow.

myelolysis (mī″ĕ-lŏl′ĭ-sĭs) [″ + *lysis,* dissolution]. Dissolution of myelin.

myeloma (mī-ĕ-lō′mă) [″ + *oma,* tumor]. A tumor originating in cells of the hematopoietic portion of bone marrow.

m., multiple. A neoplastic disease characterized by the infiltration of bone and bone marrow by myeloma cells forming multiple tumor masses. Usually progressive and generally fatal. Accompanied by anemia, renal lesions, and high globulin levels in blood. Common in sixth decade of life. More frequent in males by ratio of 2:1. SYN: *myelomatosis.*

myelomalacia (mī″ĕ-lō-mă-lā′sē-ă) [Gr. *myelos,* marrow, + *malakia,* softening]. Abnormal softening of spinal cord.

myelomatosis (mī″ĕl-ō-mă-tō′sĭs) [″ + *oma,* tumor, + *osis,* intensive]. Myeloma, multiple.

myelomenia (mī-ĕ-lō-mē′nē-ă) [″ + *men,* month]. A form of vicarious menstruation with periodic hemorrhage into the spinal cord.

myelomeningitis (mī″ĕ-lō-mĕn-ĭn-jī′tĭs) [″ + *meninx,* membrane, + *itis* inflammation]. Inflammation of the spinal cord and its membranes; spinal meningitis.

myelomeningocele (mī″ĕ-lō-mĕn-ĭn′gō-sēl) [″ + ″ + *kele,* hernia]. Spina bifida with portion of cord and membranes protruding.

myelomere (mī′ĕ-lō-mēr) [″ + *meros,* part]. A segment of the developing spinal cord.

myelomyces (mī″ĕ-lō-mī′sēs) [″ + *mykes,* fungus]. Malignant growth resembling brain substance. SYN: *encephaloma.*

myeloneuritis (mī″ĕ-lō-nū-rī′tĭs) [″ + *neuron,* nerve, + *itis,* inflammation]. Multiple neuritis and myelitis combined.

myelopathy (mī-ĕ-lŏp′ă-thē) [″ + *pathos,* disease]. Any pathological condition of the spinal cord.

m., ascending. Myelopathy that ascends along the spinal cord toward the head.

m., descending. Myelopathy that descends along the spinal cord toward the feet.

m., focal. Myelopathy of small areas.

m., sclerosing. Myelopathy in which there is hardening of the spinal cord.

m., transverse. Myelopathy extending across the spinal cord.

m., traumatic. Myelopathy due to trauma to the spinal cord.

myelopetal (mī-ĕ-lŏp′ĕt-ăl) [″ + L. *petere,* to seek for]. Proceeding toward the spinal cord, said of certain nerve impulses.

myelophage (mī′ĕ-lō-fāj) [″ + *phagein,* to eat]. A myelin-ingested macrophage.

myelophthisis (mī-ĕ-lŏf′thĭ-sĭs) [″ + *phthisis,* a wasting]. 1. Atrophy of the spinal cord. SYN: *myelanalosis.* 2. Replacement of the bone marrow by a disease process such as a neoplasm.

myeloplast (mī′ĕ-lō-plăst) [″ + *plastos,* formed]. A leukocyte cell of the bone marrow.

myeloplax [Gr. *myelos,* marrow, + *plax,* plate]. Large multinuclear bone-marrow cell. SYN: *megakaryocyte; megaloblast.*

myeloplaxoma (mī″ĕ-lō-plăk-sō′mă) [″ + ″ + *oma,* tumor]. Tumor composed of myeloplaxes.

myeloplegia (mī″ĕl-ō-plē′jē-ă) [″ + *plege,* stroke]. Paralysis of spinal origin.

myelopoiesis (mī″ĕl-ō-poy-ē′sĭs) [″ + *poiein,* to form]. The development of bone marrow or formation of cells derived from bone marrow.

m., ectopic. M., extramedullary.

m., extramedullary. Development of myeloid elements (erythrocytes and granular leukocytes) in regions other than bone marrow. SYN: *m., ectopic.*

myelopore. An opening in the spinal cord.

myeloproliferative (mī″ĕ-lō-prō-lĭf″ĕr-ā′tĭv). Concerning proliferation of bone marrow either in the bone marrow or extramedullary.

myeloradiculitis (mī″ĕ-lō-rā-dĭk″ū-lī′tĭs) [″ + L. *radiculus,* rootlet, + Gr. *itis,* inflammation]. Inflammation of spinal cord and dorsal roots of spinal nerves.

myeloradiculodysplasia (mī″ĕ-lō-rā-dĭk″ū-lō-dĭs-plā′sē-ă) [″ + ″ + Gr. *dys,* bad, + *plassein,* to form]. Congenital abnormality of spinal cord and spinal nerve roots.

myeloradiculopathy (mī″ĕ-lō-ră-dĭk″ū-lŏp′ă-thē) [″ + ″ + Gr. *pathos,* disease]. Disease of the spinal cord and spinal nerves.

myelorrhagia (mī-ĕ-lō-rā′jē-ă) [″ + *rhegnynai,* to burst forth]. Hemorrhage into the spinal cord.

myelorrhaphy (mī-ĕl-or′ă-fē) [″ + *rhaphe,* suture]. Suture of a cut or wound of the spinal cord.

myelosarcoma (mī″ĕl-ō-săr-kō′mă) [″ + *sarx,* flesh, + *oma,* tumor]. Sarcoma composed of bone marrow cells and tissue. SYN: *osteosarcoma.*

myelosarcomatosis (mī″ĕ-lō-săr-kō″mă-tō′sĭs) [″ + ″ + ″ + *osis,* condition]. Disseminated myelosarcomas.

myeloschisis (mī″ĕ-lŏs′kĭ-sĭs) [″ + *schisis,* cleft]. Cleft spinal cord resulting from failure of neural tube to close. SEE: *rachischisis; spina bifida.*

myelosclerosis (mī″ĕ-lō-sklĕr-ō′sĭs) [″ + *sklerosis,* hardening]. Sclerosis of the spinal cord.

myelosis (mī-ĕ-lō′sĭs) [″ + *osis,* condition]. Formation of a myeloma or medullary tumor.

m., erythremic. A malignancy involving the erythropoietic tissue. Symptoms and signs include anemia, fever, hepatosplenomegaly, bleeding tendency, and abnormal cells in the circulating blood.

myelospongium (mī″ĕ-lō-spŏn′jē-ŭm) [Gr. *myelos,* marrow, + *spongos,* sponge]. Embryonic network from which the neuroglia arises.

myelosuppressive (mī″ĕ-lō-sū-prĕs′ĭv). Concerning inhibition of bone marrow function.

myelosyphilis (mī″ĕ-lō-sĭf′ĭ-lĭs). Syphilis of the spinal cord.

myelosyringosis (mī″ĕ-lō-sĭr″ĭng-gō′sĭs) [″ + *syrinx,* pipe, + *osis,* condition]. Syringomyelia.

myelotome (mī-ĕl′ō-tōm) [″ + *tome,* incision]. Instrument used to dissect the spinal cord.

myelotomy (mī-ĕl-ŏt′ō-mē). Surgical severance of nerve fibers of the spinal cord.

myelotoxic (mī-ĕl-ō-tŏk′sĭk) [″ + *toxikon,* poison]. 1. Destroying bone marrow. 2. Pert. to or arising from diseased bone marrow.

myelotoxin (mī″ĕl-ō-tŏk′sĭn). Toxin that destroys marrow cells.

myenteric (mī″ĕn-tĕr′ĭk) [Gr. *mys,* muscle, + *enteron,* intestine]. Concerning the myenteron.

myenteric reflex. Intestinal contraction above and relaxation below the point of stimulation.

myenteron (mī-ĕn′tĕr-ŏn). Muscular coat of the intestine.

Myerson's sign. In Parkinson's disease, inability to stop blinking in response to tapping the forehead, nasal bridge, or maxilla.

myesthesia (mī″ĕs-thē′zē-ă) [″ + *aisthesis,* sensation]. Muscle sense; consciousness of muscle contraction.

myiasis (mī′ă-sĭs) [Gr. *myia,* fly, + *-iasis,* condition]. Condition resulting from infestation by the larvae (maggots) of flies. Infestation may be cutaneous, intestinal, atrial (within a cavity such as mouth, nose, eye, sinus, vagina, urethra), via a wound, or external.

myiocephalon (mī″yō-sĕf′ă-lŏn) [″ + *kephale,* head]. Extrusion of a part of the iris through a tear in the cornea.

myiodesopsia (mī″ē-ō-dĕs-ŏp′sē-ă) [Gr. *myiodes*, flylike, + *opsis*, vision]. Condition in which spots are seen before the eyes. SEE: *muscae volitantes*.

myiosis (mī-yō′sĭs) [″ + *osis*, condition]. Myiasis.

myitis (mī-ī′tĭs) [Gr. *mys*, muscle, + *itis*, inflammation]. Inflamed condition of a muscle. SYN: *myositis*.

Mylaxen. Trade name for hexafluorenium bromide.

Myleran. Trade name for busulfan, USP.

Mylicon. Trade name for simethicone.

mylodus. A molar tooth.

mylohyoid (mī″lō-hī′oyd) [Gr. *myle*, mill, + *hyoid*, U-shaped]. 1. Pert. to the hyoid bone and the molar teeth. 2. The paired muscles attached to the mandible that fuse in the midline and form the floor of the mouth.

myo- [Gr. *mys*, muscle]. Combining form pert. to muscle.

myoalbumin (mī″ō-ăl-bū′mĭn) [″ + L. *albus*, white]. Albumin found in muscular tissue.

myoalbumose (mī″ō-ăl′bū-mōs). A protein derived from muscle.

myoarchitectonic (mī″ō-ăr″kĭ-tĕk-tŏn′ĭk) [Gr. *mys*, muscle, + *architekton*, master workman]. Pert. to or resembling structural arrangement of muscle or of fibers.

myoatrophy (mī-ō-ăt′rō-fē). Muscular wasting.

myoblast (mī′ō-blăst) [″ + *blastos*, germ]. An embryonic cell that develops into muscle fiber cell.

myoblastoma (mī″ō-blăs-tō′mă) [″ + ″ + *oma*, tumor]. A tumor consisting of cells resembling myoblasts.

myobradia (mī″ō-brā′dē-ă) [″ + *bradys*, slow]. Slow muscular reaction to stimulation.

myocardial, myocardiac (mī-ō-kăr′dē-ăl, -ăk) [″ + *kardia*, heart]. Concerning the myocardium.

myocardial infarction. Condition caused by occlusion of one or more of the coronary arteries. The symptoms include prolonged heavy pressure or squeezing pain in the center of the chest behind the sternum. Typically the patient will describe this by clenching a fist and holding it over the heart to demonstrate the character of the pain. The pain may spread to the shoulder, neck, arm, and fourth and fifth fingers of the left hand; to the back, to the teeth, or to the jaw. These symptoms may be accompanied by nausea and vomiting, sweating, and shortness of breath. They may come and go.

It is imperative that medical care be obtained without delay. About half of myocardial infarction patients die prior to reaching the hospital. Delaying the institution of specific therapy may cause loss of life. SYN: *heart attack*. SEE: *angina; artificial respiration; cardiopulmonary resuscitation*.

myocardial insufficiency. Inability of the heart to perform its usual function. Eventually this results in cardiac failure.

myocardiograph (mī″ō-kăr′dē-ō-grăf) [″ + ″ + *graphein*, to write]. Instrument for recording heart movements.

myocardiopathy (mī″ō-kăr″dē-ŏp′ă-thē) [″ + ″ + *pathos*, disease]. Any disease of the myocardium.

myocardiosis (mī″ō-kăr-dē-ō′sĭs) [″ + ″ + *osis*, condition]. Noninflammatory cardiac disorder.

myocarditis (mī″ō-kăr-dī′tĭs) [″ + *kardia*, heart, + *itis*, inflammation]. Inflammation of the myocardium.

ETIOL: Associated with a number of conditions including many types of infections, nephritis, carbon monoxide poisoning, heat stroke, and burns. Occurs commonly after rheumatic fever and diphtheria and rarely after viral infections, or it may be idiopathic.

PHYS. SIGNS: Apex beat is extremely weak and rapid; pulse is irregular and weak; tenderness over precordium, percussion is negative, auscultation reveals first sound of heart resembling second heart sound, being high pitched and wanting in muscular quality.

NURSING IMPLICATIONS: Initially establish complete bedrest until symptoms have resolved. Provide for adequate rest periods and sleep. Provide light diet, stress-free environment, and proper elimination regimen. Assess cardiac status at frequent intervals for signs of increased cardiac workload and fatigue. If these occur, provide more rest periods. Increase activity gradually after acute phase. In period of recuperation, avoid travel to high altitudes, frequent stair climbing, and mental stress.

m., acute primary. Acute interstitial inflammation of the myocardium.

m., acute secondary. Acute inflammation of the heart muscle.

ETIOL: Secondary to acute inflammation of pericardium or endocardium, or may occur during some infectious disease.

SYM: Marked by primary disease; great weakness; cardiac palpitation with irregularity; small, feeble pulse, and dyspnea; precordial pain and distress.

m., acute septic. Localized, suppurative inflammation of the heart muscle.

ETIOL: Distant infection, suppurating pericardium or endocardium.

m., chronic. Myocarditis characterized by round cell infiltration of interstitial tissue, followed by parenchymatous changes of muscle fibers.

ETIOL: Nephritis, syphilis, grave anemias, diabetes, rheumatic fever, malaria, toxic substance, or excessive use of alcohol and tobacco. Certain wasting diseases, disease of coronary arteries, joint affections, or extension from endocardium and pericardium.

SYM: Cardiac insufficiency. Rapid heart rate that does not immediately recover following exercise. On first exertion the heart and blood pressure rise quickly but become slower with prolonged exertion.

PHYS. SIGNS: Face appears cyanosed, esp. about the lips and ears; also about the fingertips. Apex beat of heart not displaced unless the heart was previously hypertrophied, in which case apex beat will be displaced downward and to the left, or downward if dilatation exists. Pulse is weak, blood pressure is either low or high. Auscultation reveals a short, feeble first sound with reduplication. It is lacking in muscular quality. Second sound, esp. the aortic, is accentuated. Systolic murmur is present at apex over a small area if dilatation exists.

m., fragmentation. Fragmentation of the myocardium.

m., indurative. Chronic myocarditis causing hardening of muscular walls of the heart.

myocardium (mī-ō-kăr′dē-ŭm) [″ + *kardia,* heart]. [NA] The middle layer of the walls of the heart, composed of cardiac muscle.

myocardosis (mī″ō-kăr-dō′sĭs) [″ + ″ + *osis,* condition]. 1. A noninflammatory disorder of the myocardium. 2. Any degenerative condition (except myofibrosis) of the heart muscle.

myocele (mī′ō-sēl) [″ + *kele,* hernia]. 1. Muscular protrusion through a muscle sheath. 2. Cavity within a somite of an embryo.

myocelialgia (mī″ō-sē-lē-ăl′jē-ă) [″ + *koilia,* belly, + *algos,* pain]. Abdominal muscle pain.

myocelitis (mī″ō-sē-lī′tĭs) [″ + ″ + *itis,* inflammation]. Inflamed condition of abdominal muscles.

myocellulitis (mī″ō-sĕl-ū-lī′tĭs) [″ + L. *cellula,* little chamber, + Gr. *itis,* inflammation]. Myositis combined with cellulitis.

myoceptor (mī′ō-sĕp″tor) [″ + L. *capere,* to take]. The endplates of a nerve supplying a muscle.

myocerosis (mī″ō-sē-rō′sĭs) [″ + *keros,* wax]. Waxy degeneration of a muscle.

myochorditis (mī″ō-kor-dī′tĭs) [″ + *chorde,* cord, + *itis,* inflammation]. Inflammation of the muscles of the vocal cord.

myochrome (mī′ō-krōm) [″ + *chroma,* color]. 1. Any muscle pigment. 2. Cytochrome C.

myochronoscope (mī″ō-krō′nō-skōp) [″ + *chronos,* time, + *skopein,* to examine]. Device for determining time for producing a muscular contraction.

myocinesimeter (mī″ō-sĭn″ĕ-sĭm′ĕ-tĕr). Device for measuring muscle activity.

myoclonia (mī-ō-klō′nē-ă) [″ + *klonos,* tumult]. Condition of intermittent clonic spasm or twitching of a muscle or muscles.

myoclonus (mī-ŏk′lō-nŭs). Twitching or clonic spasm of a muscle or group of muscles.

m. multiplex. Condition marked by persistent and continuous muscular spasms in unrelated muscles. SYN: *paramyoclonus multiplex.*

m., palatal. Rapid clonus of one or both sides of the palate.

myocoele (mī′ō-sēl) [″ + *koila,* hollow]. Cavity within a somite of an embryo.

myocolpitis (mī″ō-kŏl-pī′tĭs) [″ + *kolpos,* vagina, + *itis,* inflammation]. Inflammation of vaginal muscular tissue.

myocomma (mī-ō-kŏm′mă) [″ + *komma,* cut]. (pl. *myocommata*) Septum dividing the myotomes.

myocrismus (mī-ō-krĭs′mŭs) [″ + *krizein,* to creak]. A peculiar crackling sound sometimes heard in auscultation resulting from contraction of a muscle.

myocyte (mī′ō-sīt) [″ + *kytos,* cell]. A muscular tissue cell.

myocytoma (mī″ō-sī-tō′mă) [″ + ″ + *oma,* tumor]. Tumor containing muscle cells.

myodemia (mī-ō-dē′mē-ă) [″ + *demos,* fat]. Fatty degeneration of muscular tissue. Muscular fiber cells become filled with fat granules and are ultimately destroyed.

myodesopsia (mī″ō-dĕs-ŏp′sē-ă) [Gr. *myiodes,* flylike, + *opsis,* vision]. The presence of muscae volitantes.

myodiastasis (mī″ō-dī-ăs′tă-sĭs) [Gr. *mys,* muscle, + *diastasis,* separation]. Division or rupture of a muscle.

myodiopter (mī″ō-dī-ŏp′tĕr). The force of the ciliary muscle to increase the refraction of the eye one diopter more than when the eye is at rest.

myodynamia (mī″ō-dī-năm′ē-ă) [″ + *dynamis,* force]. Muscular force or strength.

myodynamometer (mī″ō-dī″nă-mŏm′ĕt-ĕr) [″ + ″ + *metron,* measure]. Device for measurement of muscular strength.

myodynia (mī″ō-dĭn′ē-ă) [″ + *odyne,* pain]. Muscle pain. SYN: *myalgia.*

myodystonia (mī″ō-dĭs-tō′nē-ă) [″ + *dys,* bad, + *tonos,* tension]. Disorder of muscle tone.

myodystrophy (mī″ō-dĭs′trō-fē) [″ + ″ + *trophe,* nutrition]. Muscular dystrophy.

myoedema (mī″ō-ĕ-dē′mă) [″ + *oidema,* swelling]. 1. Lumping in a wasting muscle when struck. May also be seen in normal muscle. SYN: *mounding.* 2. Edema of a muscle.

myoelastic. Pert. to muscle and elastic tissue.

myoelectric. Pert. to electrical properties of muscles.

myoelectric prosthesis. An advanced prosthetic device operated by battery-powered electric motors that are activated through electrodes by the myoelectric potentials provided by muscles.

myoendocarditis (mī″ō-ĕn″dō-kăr-dī′tĭs) [″ + *endon,* within, + *kardia,* heart, + *itis,* inflammation]. Inflammation of the cardiac muscular wall and membranous lining.

myoepithelial (mī″ō-ĕp″ĭ-thē′lē-ăl). Pert. to contractile epithelial cells.

myoepithelial cells. Spindle-shaped or branched contractile epithelial cells found between glandular cells and basement membrane of sweat, mammary, and salivary glands.

myoepithelioma (mī″ō-ĕp″ĭ-thē″lē-ō′mă) [″ + *epi,* upon, + *thele,* nipple, + *oma,* tumor]. A slow-growing tumor of the sweat gland.

myoepithelium (mī″ō-ĕp″ĭ-thē′lē-ŭm) [″ + ″ + *thele,* nipple]. Tissue containing contractile epithelial cells.

myofascitis (mī″ō-făs-ī′tĭs) [″ + L. *fascia,* band, + Gr. *itis,* inflammation]. Inflamed condition of a muscle and its fascia.

myofibril, myofibrilla (mī-ō-fī′brĭl, -fī-brĭl′lă) [″ + L. *fibrilla,* a small fiber]. (pl. *myofibrillae*) A tiny fibril found in muscular tissue, running parallel to the cellular long axis, from one cell to another. May be the contractile element.

myofibroma (mī″ō-fī-brō′mă) [″ + L. *fibra,* fiber, + Gr. *oma,* tumor]. Tumor containing muscular and fibrous tissue.

myofibrosis (mī″ō-fī-brō′sĭs) [″ + ″ + Gr. *osis,* condition]. Increase of connective or fibrous tissue with degeneration of muscular tissue.

myofibrositis (mī″ō-fī″brō-sī′tĭs) [Gr. *mys,* muscle, + L. *fibra,* fiber, + Gr. *itis,* inflammation]. Inflammation of the perimysium, the fibrous tissue that encloses muscle tissue.

myofilament (mī″ō-fĭl′ă-mĕnt). Filament in the fine structure of muscles. Thick ones contain myosin and thin ones actin. These are seen by use of electron microscopy.

myofunctional (mī″ō-fŭnk′shŭn-ăl). Concerning muscle function.

myogelosis (mī″ō-jē-lō′sĭs) [″ + L. *gelare,* to congeal]. Hardening of a portion of muscle.

myogen (mī′ō-jĕn) [″ + *gennan,* to produce]. Cold water–extractable proteins in muscle. These consist mainly of enzymes concerned with glycolysis. SYN: *myosinogen.*

myogenesis (mī-ō-jĕn′ĕ-sĭs) [″ + *genesis,* development]. Formation of muscular tissue, esp. in embryos.

myogenetic, myogenic (mī″ō-jĕn-ĕt′ĭk, mī″ō-jen′ĭk) [″ + *gennan,* to produce]. Having origin in muscle.

myoglia (mī-ŏg′lē-ă) [″ + *glia,* glue]. A fibrous network in muscular tissue resembling neuroglia in appearance.

myoglobin. Myohemoglobin.

myoglobulin (mī″ō-glŏb′ū-lĭn) [″ + L. *globulus,* globule]. A coagulable globulin present in muscular tissue.

myoglobinuria (mī″ō-glō″bĭn-ū′rē-ă). Myoglobin in the urine. It may occur following muscular activity, trauma, or as a result of a deficiency of muscle phosphorylase.

myognathus (mī-ŏg′nă-thŭs) [″ + *gnathos,* jaw]. Deformed individual with a rudimentary conjoined twin.

myogram [″ + *gramma,* a marking]. A tracing made by the myograph of muscular contractions.

myograph (mī′ō-grăf) [″ + *graphein,* to write]. Instrument for tracing movements caused by muscular contractions.

myographic (mī-ō-grăf′ĭk). Pert. to a myograph, or the tracings made by it.

myographic tracing. A myogram or muscular tracing.

myography (mī-ŏg′ră-fē). 1. Recording of muscular contractions by a myograph. 2. Description of the muscles and their action.

myohematin (mī″ō-hĕm′ă-tĭn). Cytochrome C.

myohemoglobin (mī″ō-hē″mō-glō′bĭn). ABBR: MHb. A respiratory pigment in muscle tissue that serves as an oxygen carrier. SYN: *myoglobin.*

myohysterectomy (mī″ō-hĭs-tĕr-ĕk′tō-mē) [Gr. *mys,* muscle, + *hystera,* uterus, + *ektome,* excision]. Excision of the body of the uterus leaving the cervix in place. SYN: *hysterectomy, subtotal.*

myoid (mī′oyd) [″ + *eidos,* resemblance]. Resembling muscle.

myoidema (mī-oy-dē′mă) [″ + *oidema,* swelling]. Myoedema.

myoischemia (mī″ō-ĭs-kē′mē-ă) [″ + *ischein,* to hold back, + *haima,* blood]. Localized deficiency of blood supply in muscle tissue.

myokerosis (mī″ō-kē-rō′sĭs) [″ + *keros,* wax, + *osis,* intensive]. Waxy degeneration of muscle or muscular tissue.

myokinase (mī″ō-kĭn′ās). An enzyme present in muscle that catalyzes the synthesis of adenosine triphosphate.

myokinesimeter (mī″ō-kĭn″ĕ-sĭm′ĕ-tĕr) [″ + *kinesis,* motion, + *metron,* measure]. Myocinesimeter, q.v.

myokinesis (mī″ō-kĭn-ē′sĭs) [″ + *kinesis,* motion]. 1. Muscular activity. 2. Surgical displacement of muscular fibers.

myokymia (mī-ō-kĭm′ē-ă) [″ + *kyma,* wave]. Twitching of fibers of a muscle. It may be functional and is also seen in organic affections and general paresis. SYN: *kymatism.*

myolemma (mī″ō-lĕm′ă) [″ + *lemma,* sheath]. Sarcolemma, q.v.

myolipoma (mī″ō-lī-pō′mă) [″ + *lipos,* fat, + *oma,* tumor]. Muscle tissue tumor containing fatty elements.

myology (mī-ŏl′ō-jē) [″ + *logos,* study]. The

science or study of the muscles and their parts.

myolysis (mī-ŏl′ĭ-sĭs) [″ + *lysis,* destruction]. Fatty degeneration and infiltration with destruction of muscular tissue accompanied by separation and disappearance of muscle cells.

myoma (mī-ō′mă) [″ + *oma,* tumor]. (pl. *myomas* or *myomata*) A tumor containing muscle tissue. SEE: *chondromyoma.*

m., nonstriated. A tumor of unmarked muscle tissue. SYN: *leiomyoma.*

m. striocellulare. Fibroma with striated muscular fibers. SYN: *rhabdomyoma.*

m. telangiectodes. Coiled blood vessel tumor in muscular fibers. SYN: *angiomyoma.*

m. uteri. Fibroid tumor of the uterus.

myomalacia (mī″ō-mă-lā′sē-ă) [Gr. *mys,* muscle, + *malakia,* softening]. Softening of muscular tissue.

m. cordis. Softening of the heart muscle.

myomatosis (mī″ō-mă-tō′sĭs) [″ + *oma,* tumor, + *osis,* condition]. The development of multiple myomata.

myomatous (mī-ō′mă-tŭs). Pert. to or resembling a myoma.

myomectomy (mī″ō-mĕk′tō-mē) [″ + *oma,* tumor, + *ektome,* excision]. 1. Removal of a portion of muscle or muscular tissue. 2. Removal of a myomatous tumor, generally uterine, usually by abdominal section, leaving the uterus in place. SYN: *myomotomy.*

myomelanosis (mī″ō-mĕl-ă-nō′sĭs) [″ + *melanosis,* blackening]. Abnormal darkening of muscle tissue.

myomere (mī′ō-mēr) [″ + *meros,* part]. Myotome.

myometer (mī-ŏm′ĕt-ĕr) [″ + *metron,* measure]. Device for measurement of muscular contractions.

myometritis (mī″ō-mē-trī′tĭs) [″ + *metra,* uterus, + *itis,* inflammation]. Inflamed condition of the muscular wall of the uterus. SYN: *mesometritis.*

myometrium (mī″ō-mē′trē-ŭm). [NA] Muscular wall of the uterus forming the main mass of the uterus.

myomohysterectomy (mī-ō″mō-hĭs-tĕr-ĕk′tō-mē) [″ + *oma,* tumor, + *hystera,* uterus, + *ektome,* excision]. Hysterectomy performed to remove a myomatous uterus.

myomotomy (mī″ō-mŏt′ō-mē) [″ + ″ + *tome,* excision]. Excision of a myoma, usually uterine. SYN: *myomectomy* (def. 2).

myon [Gr. *mys,* muscle]. A single muscle unit.

myonarcosis (mī″ō-năr-kō′sĭs) [″ + *narkosis,* a numbing]. Muscular numbness.

myonecrosis (mī″ō-nĕ-krō′sĭs) [″ + *nekrosis,* deadness]. Necrosis of muscle tissue.

myonephropexy (mī″ō-nĕf′rō-pĕk″sē) [″ + *nephros,* kidney, + *pexis,* fixation]. Fixation of a movable kidney by attaching it to a portion of muscular tissue with sutures.

myoneural. Pert. to muscle and nerve, esp. nerve terminations in muscles.

myoneuralgia (mī″ō-nū-răl′jē-ă) [″ + *neuron,* nerve, + *algos,* pain]. Muscle pain.

myoneural junction. Ending of a nerve in a muscle. SEE: *motor endplate.*

myoneurasthenia (mī″ō-nūr″ăs-thē′nē-ă) [″ + ″ + *astheneia,* weakness]. Relaxed condition of muscular system associated with neurasthenia.

myoneuroma (mī″ō-nū-rō′mă) [″ + ″ + *oma,* tumor]. A neuroma partially composed of muscular elements.

myonosus (mī-ŏn′ō-sŭs) [″ + *nosos,* disease]. A disease of muscular tissue. SYN: *myopathy.*

myonymy (mī-ŏn′ĭ-mē) [″ + *onoma,* name]. Nomenclature of muscles.

myopachynsis (mī″ō-păk-ĭn′sĭs) [″ + *pachynsis,* thickening]. Abnormal thickening of muscle tissue.

myopalmus (mī-ō-păl′mŭs) [″ + *palmos,* a twitching]. Twitching of muscles.

myoparalysis (mī″ō-pă-răl′ĭ-sĭs). Paralysis of a muscle.

myoparesis (mī″ō-păr′ē-sĭs). Weakness or incomplete paralysis of a muscle.

myopathic (mī-ō-păth′ĭk) [″ + *pathos,* disease]. 1. Pert. to muscular disease. 2. One suffering from a muscular disease.

myopathic facies. Facial expression caused by relaxation of facial muscles.

myopathy (mī-ŏp′ă-thē). Any disease or abnormal condition of striated muscle. SYN: *myonosus.*

m., centronuclear. Myopathy in which the muscle fibers resemble those seen in fetal development. The nuclei of the cells are surrounded by a halo. SYN: *m., myotubular.*

m., cortisone. Myopathy, esp. of the limbs, following high dosage of corticosteroid preparations for an extensive period of time. Recovery takes place upon lowering the dose or discontinuing administration of the drug.

m., distal. Myopathy of the hands.

m., facial. Atrophy of facial muscles.

SYM: Lips pouted, smile twisted. Sometimes ptosis of upper eyelids; inability to whistle or to blow out the cheeks, depending upon the muscles affected.

m., metabolic. Myopathy resulting from enzymatic defects in the muscle walls.

m., myotubular. M., centronuclear, q.v.

m., nemaline. Congenital nonprogressive weakness, esp. of the proximal muscles. The muscles contain threadlike rods.

m., ocular. Hereditary dystrophy of the extraocular muscles. This may progress to complete paralysis of these muscles.

m., thyrotoxic. A chronic disease characterized by progressive muscular weakness and atrophy and hyperthyroidism.

myope (mī'ōp) [Gr. *myein,* to shut, + *ops,* eye]. One afflicted with myopia or nearsightedness.

myopericarditis (mī"ō-pĕr-ĭ-kar-dī'tĭs) [Gr. *mys,* muscle, + *peri,* around, + *kardia,* heart, + *itis,* inflammation]. Inflammation of the pericardium and cardiac muscular wall.

myophage (mī'ō-fāj) [" + *phagein,* to eat]. A macrophage that destroys muscular tissue.

myophone (mī'ō-fōn) [" + *phone,* voice]. Device for conveying sound of muscular contractions.

myopia [Gr. *myein,* to shut, + *ops,* eye]. Defect in vision in which parallel rays come to a focus in front of the retina; objects can only be seen distinctly when very close to the eyes. SYN: *nearsightedness.* SEE: *emmetropia* for illus.

m., axial. Myopia due to elongation of the axis of the eye.

m., chromic. Colorblindness only when viewing distant objects.

m, curvature. Myopia due to curvature of the eye's refracting surfaces.

m., index. Myopia resulting from abnormal refractivity of the media.

m., malignant. Progressive myopia leading to retinal detachment and blindness. SYN: *m., pernicious.*

m., pernicious. M., malignant.

m., prodromal. Myopia in which reading without glasses becomes possible; seen in incipient cataract.

m., progressive. Myopia that increases steadily during adult life.

m., stationary. Myopia that comes to a stop after adult growth is attained.

m., transient. Myopia seen in spasm of accommodation, as in acute iritis or iridocyclitis.

myopic (mī-ŏp'ĭk). Pert. to or affected with myopia.

myopic crescent. Posterior crescentic protrusion seen in myopia.

myoplasm (mī'ō-plăzm) [Gr. *mys,* muscle, + *plasma,* a thing formed]. The contractile part of the muscle cell, as differentiated from the sarcoplasm.

myoplastic (mī-ō-plăs'tĭk) [" + *plassein,* to form]. Pert. to plastic use of muscle tissue or plastic surgery on muscles.

myoplasty (mī'ō-plăs"tē). Plastic surgery of muscle tissue.

myopolar (mī"ō-pō'lăr). The muscle tissue between electrodes.

myoporthosis (mī"ŏp-or-thō'sĭs). Correction of myopia or nearsightedness.

myoprotein (mī"ō-prō'tēn). A protein found in muscle tissue.

myopsis (mī-ŏp'sĭs). Myodesopsia, q.v.

myopsychopathy (mī"ō-sī-kŏp'ă-thē) [" + *psyche,* mind, + *pathos,* disease]. Any muscle dysfunction associated with mental disorder.

myoreceptor (mī"ō-rē-sĕp'tor). A proprioceptor in the muscle.

myorrhaphy (mī-or'ă-fē) [Gr. *mys,* muscle, + *rhaphe,* a sewing]. Suture of a muscle wound.

myorrhexis (mī-or-ĕk'sĭs) [" + *rhexis,* a rupture]. Rupture of a muscle.

myosalgia (mī-ō-săl'jē-ă) [" + *algos,* pain]. Pain in a muscle. SYN: *myalgia.*

myosalpingitis (mī"ō-săl-pĭn-jī'tĭs) [" + *salpinx,* tube, + *itis,* inflammation]. Inflamed condition of muscular tissue of a fallopian tube.

myosarcoma (mī"ō-sar-kō'mă) [" + *sarx,* flesh, + *oma,* tumor]. A malignant tumor derived from myogenic cells.

myosclerosis (mī"ō-sklĕr-ō'sĭs) [" + *skleros,* hardening]. Hardening of muscle.

myoseism (mī'ō-sīzm) [" + *seismos,* shake, + *-ismos,* condition]. Nonrhythmic spasmodic muscle contractions.

myosin [Gr. *mys,* muscle]. A protein present in muscle fibrils and comprising about 65% of total muscle protein. It consists of long chains of polypeptides joined to each other by side chains. The molecular structure of myosin is thought to be responsible for the properties of muscle tissue, namely, birefringence, double refraction, contractility, and elasticity. Myosin combines with another muscle protein, actin, to form actomyosin.

myosinase (mī"ō-sĭn-ās'). An enzyme that catalyzes the conversion of myosinogen to myosin.

myosinogen (mī"ō-sĭn'ō-jĕn) [Gr. *mys,* muscle, + *gennan,* to produce]. A protein present in the muscle tissue, the precursor of myosin. SYN: *myogen.*

myosinose (mī-ōs'ĭn-ōs). A proteose resulting from the hydrolysis of myosin.

myosinuria (mī"ō-sĭn-ū'rē-ă). The occurrence of myosin in the urine. SYN: *myosuria.*

myositis (mī-ō-sī'tĭs) [" + *itis,* inflammation]. Inflammation of muscle tissue, esp. voluntary muscles. SYN: *myitis.* SEE: *fibrositis.*

ETIOL: Infection, trauma, diathetic states, or infestation by parasites.

m., epidemic. Epidemic pleurodynia.

m. fibrosa. Myositis accompanied by infiltration of fibrous tissue.

m., interstitial. Myositis with hyperplasia of connective tissue.

m., multiple. Polymyositis.

m. ossificans. Myositis marked by ossification of muscles.

m., parenchymatous. Myositis of substance of a muscle.

m. purulenta. Suppurative myositis with abscesses; caused by bacterial infection.

m., traumatic. May be simple with pain

and swelling or may be suppurative.

m. trichinosa. Myositis due to infestation with trichinae. SYN: *trichinous myositis.*

myospasm (mī'ō-spăzm) [" + *spasmos,* spasm]. Spasmodic contraction of a muscle.

myosteoma (mī-ŏs"tē-ō'mă) [" + *osteon,* bone, + *oma,* tumor]. A bony growth found in muscle tissue.

myosthenometer (mī"ō-sthĕn-ŏm'ĕ-tĕr) [" + *sthenos,* strength, + *metron,* measure]. Device for measuring muscle power.

myostroma (mī"ō-strō'mă) [" + *stroma,* mattress]. The framework of muscle tissue.

myosuria (mī-ō-sū'rē-ă) [" + *ouron,* urine]. Presence of myosin in the urine. SYN: *myosinuria.*

myosuture (mī"ō-sū'chūr) [" + L. *sutura,* sewing]. Stitching of a muscle.

myosynizesis (mī"ō-sĭn"ĭ-zē'sĭs) [Gr. *mys,* muscle, + *synizesis,* sitting together]. Adhesion of muscular layers of tissue.

myotactic (mī"ō-tăk'tĭk) [" + L. *tactus,* touch]. Pert. to muscle or kinesthetic sense.

myotasis (mī-ŏt'ă-sĭs) [" + *tasis,* stretching]. Stretching of a muscle.

myotatic. Pert. to the stretching of muscles.

myotatic reflex. Stretch reflex.

myotenontoplasty (mī'ō-tĕn-ŏn'tō-plăst"ē) [" + *tenon,* tendon, + *plassein,* to form]. Plastic operation involving muscles and tendons. SYN: *tenomyoplasty; tenontomyoplasty.*

myotenositis (mī"ō-tĕn-ō-sī'tĭs) [" + " + *itis,* inflammation]. Inflamed condition of a muscle and its tendon.

myotenotomy (mī"ō-tĕn-ŏt'ō-mē) [" + " + *tome, incision*]. Division of the tendon of a muscle.

myothermic (mī"ō-thĕrm'ĭk) [" + *therme,* heat]. Pert. to rise in muscle temperature due to its activity.

myotic (mī-ŏt'ĭk). Miotic. q.v.

myotility (mī-ō-tĭl'ĭ-tē) [Gr. *mys,* muscle]. Contractility of a muscle.

myotome (mī'ō-tōm) [" + *tome,* incision]. 1. Knife for cutting muscles. 2. That portion of an embryonic somite that gives rise to somatic (striated) muscles. SYN: *myomere.*

myotomy (mī-ŏt'ō-mē). Division or anatomical dissection of muscles.

myotonia (mī"ō-tō'nē-ă) [" + *tonos,* tension]. Tonic spasm of a muscle or temporary rigidity after muscular contraction.

m. atrophica. M. dystrophica.

m. congenita. A benign disease characterized by tonic spasms of the muscles induced by voluntary movements; usually congenital and transmitted from one generation to another. SYN: *Thomsen's disease.*

SYM: Disease appears in early childhood, is manifested by a tonic spasm of the muscles every time they are put in use. In a few minutes, rigidity wears away and the movements become free from repeated contractions, the muscles becoming firm and extremely well developed.

PROG: Incurable but may improve with age.

TREATMENT: Quinine or procainamide for relief of myotonia. Avoid obesity. Neostigmine is contraindicated.

m. dystrophica. A hereditary disease characterized by muscular wasting, myotonia, and cataract. SYN: *myotonia atrophica; Steinert's disease.*

myotonic. Pert. to tonic muscular spasm, as differentiated from myokinetic spasm.

myotonoid (mī-ŏt'ō-noyd). Similar to myotonia.

myotonometer (mī"ō-tō-nŏm'ĕt-ĕr) [" + *tonos,* tension, + *metron,* measure]. Instrument used to measure muscular tonus.

myotonus (mī-ŏt'ō-nŭs). A tonic muscle spasm with temporary rigidity.

myotony (mī-ŏt'ō-nē). Myotonia.

myotrophy (mī-ŏt'rō-fē) [" + *trophe,* nourishment]. Nutrition of muscle tissues.

myotropic (mī"ō-trŏp'ĭk) [" + *trope,* a turn]. Attracted to muscle tissue.

myotube (mī'ō-tūb). The developing stage of skeletal muscle. The central nucleus occupies most of the cell.

myovascular (mī"ō-văs'kū-lăr). Concerning muscles and blood supply to them.

myriachit (mĭr-ē'ă-chĭt) [Russian]. SEE: *miryachit.*

Myriapoda (mĭr-ē-ăp'ō-dă) [Gr. *myrios,* numberless, + *pous,* foot]. Group of arthropods including millipedes and centipedes.

myriapodiasis (mĭr"ē-ăp-ō-dī'ă-sĭs). Infestation with one of the Myriapoda.

myricin (mĭr'ĭ-sĭn). The principal ingredient in beeswax.

myringa (mĭr-ĭn'gă) [L.]. The tympanic membrane.

myringectomy (mĭr-ĭn-jĕk'tō-mē) [" + Gr. *ektome,* excision]. Myringodectomy.

myringitis (mĭr-ĭn-jī'tĭs) [L. *myringa,* drum membrane, + Gr. *itis,* inflammation]. Inflammation of the tympanum or eardrum.

m. bullosa. Myringitis with serous or hemorrhagic blebs or vesicular inflammation of the eardrum and adjacent wall.

myringodectomy (mĭr-ĭn"gō-dĕk'tō-mē) [" + Gr. *ektome,* excision]. Excision of a part or the entire tympanic membrane. SYN: *myringectomy.*

myringomycosis (mĭr-ĭn"gō-mī-kō'sĭs) [" + Gr. *mykes,* fungus, + *osis,* condition]. Inflammation of the tympanic membrane resulting from infection by parasitic fungi. SYN: *mycomyringitis; otomycosis.*

myringoplasty (mĭr-ĭn'gō-plăst"ē) [" + Gr. *plassein,* to form]. Plastic operation of the tympanic membrane.

myringoscope (mĭr-ĭn′gō-skōp) [″ + Gr. *skopein,* to examine]. Instrument used for examination of the eardrum.

myringotome (mĭ-rĭn′gō-tōm) [″ + Gr. *tome,* incision]. Knife for incising the tympanic membrane.

myringotomy (mĭr-ĭn-gŏt′ō-mē). Incision of the tympanic membrane.

myrmecia (mŭr-mē′shē-ă) [Gr. *myrmex,* ant]. A dome-shaped wart.

myrrh (mŭr) [Gr. *myrra*]. A gum resinous substance used by man for many centuries. In antiquity, cherished as a constituent of incense and perfume; most important use today is as an aromatic astringent mouthwash. Tincture of myrrh provides symptomatic relief when applied to canker sores.

mysophilia (mī″sō-fĭl′ē-ă). Erotic interest in body excretions.

mysophobia (mī″sō-fō′bē-ă) [Gr. *mysos,* filth, + *phobos,* fear]. Abnormal aversion to dirt or contamination. SYN: *molysmophobia.*

mytacism (mī′tă-sĭzm) [Gr. *mytakismos* from Gr. letter μ]. Excessive or incorrect use of the letter *m* or the *m* sound, in writing or speaking.

mythomania (mĭth″ō-mā′nē-ă) [Gr. *mythos,* myth, + *mania,* madness]. Abnormal tendency to lie and exaggerate.

mythophobia (mĭth″ō-fō′bē-ă) [″ + *phobos,* fear]. Abnormal dread of making a false or incorrect statement.

mytilotoxin (mĭt″ĭ-lō-tŏk′sĭn). A neurotoxin present in certain mussels.

myxadenitis (mĭks″ăd-ĕn-ī′tĭs) [Gr. *myxa,* mucus, + *aden,* gland, + *itis,* inflammation]. Inflammation of mucous gland or glands.

m. labialis. Painless inflammation of the mucous glands of the lips. SYN: *cheilitis glandularis.*

myxadenoma (mĭks″ăd-ē-nō′mă) [″ + ″ + *oma,* tumor]. 1. A tumor with the structure of a mucous gland. SYN: *myxoadenoma.* 2. A tumor of glandular structure containing mucous elements.

myxangitis (mĭks″ăn-jī′tĭs) [″ + *angeion,* vessel, + *itis,* inflammation]. Inflammation of mucous gland ducts.

myxasthenia (mĭks″ăs-thē′nē-ă) [″ + *astheneia,* weakness]. Imperfect or insufficient secretion of mucus.

myxedema (mĭks-ĕ-dē′mă) [Gr. *myxa,* mucus, + *oidema,* swelling]. Condition resulting from hypofunction of the thyroid gland. Occurs in older children and adults.

ETIOL: Iodine deficiency in diet; surgical excision or atrophy of thyroid gland; excessive use of antithyroid drugs. May occur secondary to hypofunction of anterior pituitary and is complicated by adrenal and gonadal deficiencies.

SYM: Decreased metabolic rate, low radioactive iodine uptake by thyroid, decreased protein-bound iodine, anemia, myxedematous facies, large tongue, slow speech, puffiness of hands and face, coarse and thickened edematous skin, loss and dryness of hair, mental apathy, drowsiness, and sensitivity to cold.

TREATMENT: Thyroid hormone replacement.

m., childhood. Myxedema occurring before puberty.

m., operative. Myxedema following removal of thyroid gland. SYN: *cachexia strumipriva.*

m., pituitary. Myxedema occurring secondary to anterior pituitary hypofunction.

myxedematoid (mĭks-ĕ-dĕm′ă-toyd) [Gr. *myxa,* mucus, + *oidema,* swelling, + *eidos,* resemblance.]. Resembling myxedema.

myxedematous (mĭks-ĕ-dĕm′ă-tŭs). Marked by or concerning myxedema.

myxemia (mĭks-ē′mē-ă) [″ + *haima,* blood]. Accumulation of mucin in the blood. SYN: *mucinemia.*

myxiosis (mĭks-ē-ō′sĭs) [″ + *osis,* condition]. A mucous discharge or secretion.

myxo-, myx- [Gr. *myxa*]. Combining form designating rel. to mucus.

myxoadenoma (mĭks″ō-ăd-ē-nō′mă) [″ + *aden,* gland, + *oma,* tumor]. Myxadenoma.

Myxobacterales (mĭks″ō-băk-tē-rā′lēz). An order of bacteria found in soil and dung. Characterized by a slimy spreading colony.

myxochondrofibrosarcoma (mĭks″ō-kŏn″drō-fī″brō-săr-kō′mă). A malignant tumor composed of myxomatous, chondromatous, fibrous, and sarcomatous elements.

myxochondroma (mĭks″ō-kŏn-drō′mă). A benign tumor composed of myxomatous and chondromatous elements.

myxocystoma (mĭks″ō-sĭs-tō′mă) [Gr. *myxa,* mucus, + *kystis,* cyst, + *oma,* tumor]. A benign cystic tumor containing mucus.

myxocyte (mĭk′sō-sīt) [″ + *kytos,* cell]. A characteristic cell of mucous tissue.

myxoedema (mĭks″ĕ-dē′mă) [″ + *oidema,* swelling]. Myxedema.

myxoenchondroma (mĭks″ō-ĕn-kŏn-drō′mă) [″ + *en,* in, + *chondros,* cartilage, + *oma,* tumor]. A cartilaginous tissue tumor that has undergone partial mucous degeneration.

myxofibroma (mĭks″ō-fī-brō′mă) [″ + L. *fibra,* fiber, + Gr. *oma,* tumor]. Tumor composed of mucous and fibrous elements. SYN: *myxoinoma.*

myxofibrosarcoma (mĭk″sō-fī″brō-săr-kō′mă) [″ + ″ + Gr. *sarx,* flesh, + *oma,* tumor]. Fibrosarcoma that contains primitive mesenchymal tissue.

myxoglioma (mĭk″sō-glī-ō′mă) [Gr. *myxa,* mucus, + *glia,* glue, + *oma,* tumor]. Tumor composed of myxomatous and gliomatous elements.

myxoid (mĭk'soyd) [" + *eidos,* resemblance]. Similar to or resembling mucus.

myxoinoma (mĭk"sō-ĭn-ō'mă) A myxofibroma.

myxolipoma (mĭk"sō-lĭ-pō'mă) [" + *lipos,* fat, + *oma,* tumor]. Mucous tumor with fatty tissue elements in it. SYN: *lipomyxoma.*

myxoma (mĭk-sō'mă) [" + *oma,* tumor]. (pl. *myxomas* or *myxomata)* A tumor composed of mucous connective tissue similar to that present in the embryo or umbilical cord. Cells are stellate or spindle-shaped and separated by mucoid tissue. The tumors are usually soft, gray, lobulated, and translucent and are not completely encapsulated. May be pure or of mixed types involving other types of tissue.

m., cartilaginous. Chondromyxoma.

m., cystic. Tumor with parts fluid enough to resemble cysts.

m., enchondromatous. Tumor with nodules of hyaline cartilage.

m., erectile. Myxoma containing an excess of vessels, resembling an angioma.

m., fibrous. Fibromyxoma.

m., intracanalicular, of mamma. Myxoma that develops in the interstitial connective tissue of the mamma.

m., odontogenic. A tumor of the jaw that appears to arise from mesenchymal tissue.

m., telangiectatic, vascular. Myxoma of highly vascular structure.

myxomatosis (mĭk"sō-mă-tō'sĭs) [" + " + *osis,* condition]. 1. Formation of multiple myxomas. 2. Myxomatous degeneration.

myxomycetes (mĭk"sō-mī-sē'tēz) [Gr. *myxa,* mucus, + *mykes,* fungus]. A group of organisms of uncertain classification, but thought to be fungus-like. Includes slime molds. SEE: *Myxobacterales.*

myxomyoma (mĭks-ō-mī-ō'mă) [" + *mys,* muscle, + *oma,* tumor]. Muscle tissue tumor that has undergone mucous degeneration.

myxoneuroma (mĭks"ō-nū-rō'mă) [" + *neuron,* nerve, + *oma,* tumor]. Tumor composed of mucous and nerve tissue elements.

myxopapilloma (mĭk"sō-păp"ĭl-ō'mă) [" + L. *papilla,* nipple, + Gr. *oma,* tumor]. Combination of myxomatous and papillomatous tumor or tumors.

myxopoiesis (mĭk"sō-poy-ē'sĭs) [" + *poiesis,* creation]. Formation of mucus.

myxorrhea (mĭk-sō-rē'ă) [" + *rhoia,* flow]. Free discharge from mucous surfaces. SYN: *blennorrhea.*

m. gastrica. Excessive mucous secretion in the stomach.

m. intestinalis. Secretion of mucus from the bowel in neurotic persons in times of mental stress.

myxosarcoma (mĭk"sō-săr-kō'mă) [" + *sarx,* flesh, + *oma,* tumor]. Mixed tumor, partly myxomatous and partly sarcomatous, having undergone partial degeneration.

myxosarcomatous (mĭk"sō-săr-kō'mă-tŭs). Pert. to or of the nature of myxosarcoma.

myxospore (mĭks'ō-spor) [" + *sporos,* seed]. Spore embedded in a gelatinous mass, seen in some fungi and protozoa.

Myxosporidia (mĭks-ō-spor-ĭd'ē-ă). Parasitic sporozoans, most commonly found in epithelial cells of lower vertebrates.

myxoviruses. Family of viruses including those that cause influenza. SEE: *paramyxoviruses.*

myzesis (mī-zē'sĭs) [Gr. *myzan,* to suck]. Sucking.

Myzomyia (mī"zō-mī'ă) [" + *myia,* fly]. Subgenus of anopheline mosquitoes. Some species transmit malarial parasites.

Myzorhynchus (mī"zō-rĭng'kŭs) [" + *rhynchos,* snout]. Subgenus of anopheline mosquitoes. Some species transmit malarial parasites.

N

N. 1. Chem. symb. for nitrogen. 2. *normal,* esp. with reference to solutions.

n. 1. Symb. for *index of refraction.* 2. *nasal; number.*

n_1, n_2, n_3 . . . n_n. In statistical terminology, the notations used for subjects, i.e., n_1 is subject number one, n_2 subject number two, and the last subject n_n, where the subscript $_n$ would be the last subject in the series.

^{15}N. Symb. for radioactive isotope of nitrogen.

NA. *nicotinic acid; Nomina Anatomica; numerical aperture; nurse's aide.*

N.A.A.C.O.G. *Nurses Association of the American College of Obstetricians and Gynecologists.*

Na. Chem. symb. for sodium.

nabothian cysts (nă-bō'thē-ăn). Retention cysts formed by the nabothian glands at the neck of the uterus.

ETIOL: Due to closing of mouths of glands by new epithelium of a healed ectropion. They always denote an ectropion has been present.

NaBr. Sodium bromide.

NaCl. Sodium chloride.

NaClO. Sodium hypochlorite.

Na_2CO_3. Sodium carbonate.

nacreous (nă'krē-ŭs) [L. *nacer,* mother of pearl]. Having an iridescent pearl-like luster, as bacterial colonies.

NAD. *nicotinamide adenine dinucleotide.*

NAD^+. Oxidized form of NAD. This enzyme is important in accepting electrons in the course of metabolic reactions. When NAD^+ gives up its electron, it is converted to the reduced form, NADH.

N.A.D. *no appreciable disease.*

NADH. The reduced form of NAD^+. SYN: *TPN; coenzyme.*

NADH-diaphorase. The reduced form of the enzyme nicotinamide adenine dinucleotide-diaphorase. It is important in reducing the ferric iron (Fe^{+++}) to its ferrous (Fe^{++}) form; thus it is one of the enzymes that converts methemoglobin (which is unable to transport oxygen) to hemoglobin (which can transport oxygen). Deficiency of NADH-diaphorase causes congenital methemoglobinemia. SYN: *methemoglobin reductase.*

NADP. *nicotinamide adenine dinucleotide phosphate,* reduced form of $NADP^+$, an enzyme important in accepting electrons in the course of metabolic reactions.

$NADP^+$. Oxidized form of NADP.

Naegele's obliquity (nā'gĕ-lēz). [Franz Carl Naegele, Ger. obstetrician, 1777–1851] Anterior parietal presentation of the fetal head in labor. SYN: *asynclitism, anterior.*

Naegele's pelvis. An obliquely contracted pelvis, caused by disease in infancy.

Naegele's rule. A system to estimate the day in the year labor will begin: count back exactly 90 days from the day the last menstrual period began and add seven days to that date.

NaF. Sodium fluoride.

Nafcil. Trade name for nafcillin sodium, USP.

nafcillin sodium (năf-sĭl'ĭn). USP. A semisynthetic penicillin that is penicillinase-resistant. Trade names are Nafcil and Unipen.

$NaHCO_3$. Sodium bicarbonate.

$NaHSO_3$. Sodium bisulfite.

nail [AS. *naegel*]. 1. A rod made of metal, bone, or solid material used to attach the ends or pieces of broken bones. 2. A horny cell structure of the epidermis forming flat plates upon the dorsal surface of the terminal phalanges. Called toenail and fingernail on the toes and fingers respectively. SYN: *unguis* (def. 1) (L.); *onyx* (def. 1) (Gr.).

A nail consists of a body, composed of keratin, the exposed portion, and a root, the proximal portion hidden by the nail fold, both of which rest on the nailbed or matrix. The latter consists of epithelium and corium continuous with the epidermis and dermis of the skin of the nail fold. The crescent-shaped white area near the root is the lunula. The epidermis extending from the margin of the nail fold over the root is called eponychium; that underlying the free border of the distal portion is called hyponychium.

A nail grows in length and thickness through activity of cells in the stratum germinativum of the root. Average rate of growth in fingernails is about 1 mm. per week. It is slower in toenails and slower in summer than in winter. Nail growth varies with age and is affected by disease and certain hormone deficiencies.

DIFF. DIAG: Changes in the nails, such as *ridges,* may occur in defective nutrition or after a serious illness. In achlorhydria and hypochromic anemia, excessive spoon-shaped nails, which are depressed in the center, may occur. In chronic pulmonary conditions and congenital heart disease, excessive curving of the nails may be associated with clubbed fingers.

Atrophy may occur as a result of hereditary or congenital tendencies. Permanent atrophy may follow injuries, scars from disease, frostbite, nerve injuries, and hyperthyroidism. Nail shedding is due to the same causes.

Nails that are *fragile* or *split* often may occur as a congenital condition, due to prolonged contact with chemicals, or too frequent manicuring.

Dry, malformed nails may be due to trophic changes resulting from injury to nerve or finger, neuritis, Raynaud's disease, pulmonary osteoarthropathy, syphilis, onychia, scleroderma, acrodermatitis, and granuloma fungoides of the fingers.

Longitudinal striations are often found in those past middle life; frequently they are associated with onychorrhexis, splitting at the free margins. Also noted in association with a focus of infection in the bowel or at root of a tooth. Vitamin deficiency may be a cause. Microscopic examination of nail clippings should be made for ringworm.

Transverse lines (Beau's lines) may result from previous interference of nail matrix growth. May be caused by local or systemic conditions. Approximate date of lesion may be determined, because it takes 4 to 6 months for the fingernail to replace itself.

Chancre may be suspected if a small indolent ulcer appears near the nail, esp. if indurated and associated with enlarged lymph glands above the inner condyle.

Quincke's capillary pulsation, indicated by a rhythmic flushing and blanching under the nails, is seen most frequently in aortic regurgitation and often in anemia.

Discolorations: Black: In diabetes and other forms of gangrene. *Blue-black:* Common condition, usually due to hemorrhage, bleeding diseases such as hemophilia, and trauma. May be painful and can be relieved by drilling a small hole in the nail at the site of hemorrhage. This may be done by using a dental drill or the heated tip of a paper clip or similar rigid wire of small diameter. *Brown:* May be due to arsenical poisoning. *Brownish-black:* This discoloration often indicates chronic mercurial poisoning due to formation of sulfide of mercury in the tissues. *Cyanosis:* Usually indicates anemia, poor circulation, or venous stasis. *Slate:* This is an early manifestation of argyria, and administration of silver should be stopped at once. *White spots:* Striate lesions may be due to trauma and are more frequent in women. Transverse white bands in all nails may be a sign of acute or chronic arsenical poisoning or, rarely, of thallium acetate poisoning. SEE: *Mees line.*

n., eggshell. A condition in which the nail plate is soft and semitransparent, bends easily, and splits at the end. Associated with arthritis, peripheral neuritis, leprosy, and hemiplegia. May be the only visible sign of late syphilis.

n., hang. Broken epidermis at edge of the nail.

n., ingrown. Growth of the nail edge into the soft tissue, thus causing inflammation and sometimes an abscess. May be due to improper paring of the nail or pressure on the nail edge from improperly fitted shoes.

n., reedy. Nail marked by longitudinal fissures.

n., Smith-Peterson. A three-flanged nail employed to fix fractures of the neck of the femur.

n., spoon. A nail with central portion depressed and lateral edges elevated.

nailbed. The portion of a finger or toe covered by the nail. SYN: *nail matrix.*

nail biting. A nervous affliction or neurosis in which the free edges of the nails are bitten down. SYN: *onychophagy.*

nail fold. Groove in the cutaneous tissue surrounding the margins and proximal edges of the nail.

nail groove. The space between the nail wall and the nailbed.

nail matrix. Nailbed.

nail-patella syndrome. Onycho-osteodysplasia, q.v.

nail root. Proximal portion of nail covered by nail fold.

nail wall. Epidermis covering edges of the nail. SYN: *vallum unguis.*

Naja-naja. The Indian cobra, a poisonous snake.

naked (nā'kĕd) [AS. *naced,* nude]. Uncovered, exposed to view, nude, bare, devoid of clothing.

Nalfon. Trade name for fenoprofen calcium.

nalidixic acid. USP. An antibiotic used in treating certain urinary tract infections. Trade names are NegGram, Wintomylon, and Cybis.

Nalline. Trade name for nalorphine hydrochloride, USP.

nalorphine hydrochloride (năl-or'fēn). USP. A narcotic antagonist. Used in treatment of certain kinds of narcotic overdose, esp. with morphine.

naloxone hydrochloride (năl-ŏks'ōn). USP. A drug that prevents or reverses the action of morphine and other opioid drugs. Trade name is Narcan.

nandrolone decanoate (năn'drō-lōn). USP. An anabolic androgenic steroid. Trade name is Deca-Durabolin.

nandrolone phenpropionate. USP. An anabolic androgenic steroid. Trade name is Durabolin.

nanism (nā'nĭzm) [L. *nanus,* dwarf, + Gr. *-ismos,* condition]. Condition of being dwarflike in build. SYN: *nanosomia.*

n., symptomatic. Nanism with deficient dentition, sexual development, and ossification.

nano- (nā'nō) [L. *nanus,* dwarf]. Prefix indicating one-billionth (10^{-9}) of the unit following. Thus a nanogram is one-billionth (10^{-9})

of a gram.
nanocephalism (nā-nō-sĕf′ăl-ĭzm) [″ + Gr. *kephale,* head, + *-ismos,* condition]. Condition of having an abnormally small head.
nanocephalous (nā-nō-sĕf′ă-lŭs). Having an abnormally small head.
nanocormia (nā″nō-kor′mē-ă) [L. *nanus,* dwarf, + Gr. *kormos,* trunk]. Abnormally dwarfed thorax or body.
nanocurie (nā″nō-kū′rē). A unit of radioactivity equal to 10^{-9} curie.
nanogram. One-billionth (10^{-9}) of a gram. SEE: *picogram.*
nanoid (nā′noyd) [″ + Gr. *eidos,* like]. Dwarflike.
nanomelus (nā-nŏm′ĕ-lŭs) [″ + Gr. *melos,* limb]. Fetus with congenital deformity characterized by undersized extremities.
nanometer (nā″nō-mē′tĕr). A unit of length equal to 10^{-9} meter.
nanophthalmos (năn″ŏf-thăl′mŭs) [″ + *ophthalmos,* eye]. Abnormal smallness of one or both eyes. SYN: *microphthalmia.*
nanosecond (nā″nō-sĕk′ŏnd). A unit of time measurement equal to 10^{-9} second.
nanosoma, nanosomia (nā″nō-sō′mă, nā-nō-sō′mē-ă) [L. *nanus,* dwarf, + Gr. *soma,* body]. State of being a dwarf. SYN: *nanism.*
nanosomus (nā-nō-sō′mŭs). A person of stunted size; a dwarf.
nanous (nā′nŭs) [L. *nanus,* dwarf]. Dwarfed or stunted.
nanukayami (nă″nū-kă-yă′mē). A form of leptospirosis present in Japan.
nanus (nā′nŭs) [L.]. 1. A dwarf. 2. Stunted; dwarflike.
NaOH. Sodium hydroxide.
nap (năp) [AS. *hnappian,* nap]. 1. To slumber. 2. A short sleep; a doze.
napalm (nā′pălm) [from *na*phthene + *palmi*tate]. Gasoline made thick or jellylike for use in incendiary bombs and flame throwers.
napalm burn. Burn due to use of napalm, usually during war.
nape (nāp, năp) [origin uncertain]. Back of neck. SYN: *nucha; scruff.*
napex (nā′pĕks) [origin uncertain]. Scalp beneath the occipital protuberance.
naphazoline hydrochloride (năf-ăz′ō-lēn). USP. A vasoconstrictor drug used topically esp. on nasal mucosa. Trade names are Privine Hydrochloride, Albalon Liquifilm, Naphcon Forte, and Vasocon.
Naphcon Forte. Trade name for naphazoline hydrochloride, USP.
naphtha (năf′thă). 1. A volatile inflammable liquid distilled from carbonaceous substances. 2. Petroleum, esp. more volatile varieties.
naphthalene (năf′thă-lēn). $C_{10}H_8$. A hydrocarbon, one of principal constituents of coal tar. SEE: *Poisons and Poisoning* in *Appendix.*
USES: As a disinfectant, in moth balls, and in manufacture of dyes and explosives.
naphthol (năf′thōl). $C_{10}H_7OH$. Coal tar substance used as an antiseptic and in certain dyes. It is prepared from naphthalene.
napiform (nā′pĭ-form) [L. *napus,* turnip, + *forma,* shape]. In bacteriology, formed like a turnip, as gelatin liquefaction in a culture.
N.A.P.N.A.P. *National Association of Pediatric Nurse Associates and Practitioners.*
N.A.P.N.E.S. *National Association for Practical Nurse Education and Service.*
naprapathy (nă-prăp′ăth-ē) [Bohemian *napravit,* correction, + Gr. *pathos,* disease]. Method of therapeutic manipulation based upon the assumption that all disease is caused by faulty functioning of ligaments.
Naprosyn. Trade name for naproxen, USP.
N.A.P.T. *National Association of Physical Therapists.*
Naqua. Trade name for trichlormethiazide.
Narcan. Trade name for naloxone hydrochloride, USP.
narcissism (năr-sĭs′ĭzm). [Narcissus, a Gr. mythical character who fell in love with his own reflection] 1. Self-love or self-admiration. 2. Sexual pleasure derived from observing one's own naked body.
narcissistic (năr-sĭs-sĭst′ĭk). Pert. to narcissism.
narcissistic object choice. Selection of another like one's own self as the object of love, friendship, or liking.
narco- [Gr. *narke,* numbness]. Combining form meaning numbness, stupor.
narcoanalysis (năr″kō-ă-năl′ĭ-sĭs) [″ + *analysis,* a dissolving]. A form of psychotherapy in which light anesthesia is produced by use of I.V. barbiturates. Patients are encouraged to talk about their experiences and may discuss events that would ordinarily be suppressed.
narcoanesthesia (nar″kō-ăn-ĕs-thē′zē-ă). Anesthesia produced by a narcotic, as scopolamine and morphine.
narcohypnia (năr″kō-hĭp′nē-ă) [Gr. *narke,* numbness, + *hypnos,* sleep]. Numbness following sleep.
narcohypnosis (năr″kō-hĭp-nō′sĭs). Stupor or deep sleep produced by hypnosis.
narcolepsy (năr′kō-lĕp″sē) [Gr. *narke,* numbness, + *lepsis,* seizure]. A chronic ailment consisting of recurrent attacks of drowsiness and sleep. The patient is unable to control these spells of sleep but is easily awakened. Except for frequent sleep patterns, the electroencephalogram is normal. SEE: *epilepsy.*
TREATMENT: Symptomatic with drugs such as ephedrine or amphetamine.
narcoleptic (năr-kō-lĕp′tĭk) [″ + *lepsis,* seizure]. Pert. to or marked by an overwhelming

desire to sleep.

narcomatous (năr-kō'mă-tŭs) [Gr. *narke,* numbness, + *koma,* coma]. Pert. to a state of stupor from use of narcotics.

narcosis [Gr. *narkosis,* a benumbing]. Unconscious state due to narcotics. SYN: *narcotism.*

n., basal. Initial narcosis produced by sedatives used prior to administration of a general anesthetic.

n., medullary. General anesthesia induced by a local anesthetic injected in the sheath of the spinal cord in lumbar region. SYN: *spinal anesthesia.*

narcosynthesis (năr"kō-sĭn'thĕ-sĭs) [" + *synthesis,* synthesis]. Narcoanalysis.

narcotic [Gr. *narkotikos,* benumbing]. 1. Producing stupor or sleep. 2. A drug that in moderate doses depresses the central nervous system, thus relieving pain and producing sleep, but that in excessive doses produces unconsciousness, stupor, coma, and possibly death.

Ex.: opium, morphine, codeine, papaverine, heroin, and many synthetics. Most are habit-forming. 3. Anything that soothes, relieves, or lulls. 4. One addicted to the use of narcotics.

RS: drug action; drug addiction; drug dependence; drug reaction; drugs and their administration; narcotism.

narcotic addict. One who has become physiologically or psychologically dependent upon narcotics. SEE: *drug addiction.*

narcotic poisoning. Caused by narcotic or sleep-producing poisons such as opium and its derivatives, chloral combinations, barbital and its myriad subvarieties.

SYM. AND SIGNS: Depression, slowing of heart rate and respiration, sleep, followed by coma.

F.A.: Remove poison by gastric lavage. Administer nalorphine if poisoning is due to a derivative of opium such as morphine.

narcotism (năr'kō-tĭzm) [Gr. *narke,* stupor, + *-ismos,* condition]. 1. State of stupor induced by a narcotic. SYN: *narcosis.* 2. An addiction to the use of narcotics. Addiction may be said to exist when discontinuance causes abstinence symptoms that are speedily relieved by a dose of the drug.

TREATMENT: Ordinarily successful only during hospitalization. Relapses are frequent, and the adoption of an alternate philosophy of life is of prime importance.

narcotize [Gr. *narkotikos,* benumbing]. To place under the influence of a narcotic.

Nardil. Trade name for phenelzine sulfate.

naris (nā'rĭs) [L.]. (pl. *nares*) [NA] The nostril. SEE: *nose.*

n., anterior. External nostril.

n., posterior. The opening between the nasal cavity and the nasopharynx.

RS: anosmia; epistaxis; hyperosmia; nasal; parosmia; septum; smell.

NASA. *National Aeronautics and Space Administration.*

nasal (nā'zl) [L. *nasus,* nose]. 1. Pert. to the nose. 2. Uttered through the nose. 3. A nasal bone.

nasal bleeding. SEE: *epistaxis.*

nasal bones. The two small bones forming the arch of the nose.

nasal cartilages. Cartilages forming the principal portion of the framework of the external nose.

nasal cavity. Cavity between floor of cranium and roof of mouth.

nasal concha. (pl. *nasal conchae*). SEE: *concha, nasal.*

nasal douche. Injection of fluid into nostril with fluid escaping by way of the nasopharynx out of the mouth. Patient should keep mouth open and glottis closed to prevent fluid from entering the throat and bronchus. Force must not be great. Atomized spray is faster. Container should not be suspended more than 6 in. (9.2 cm.) above patient, who should not blow the nose during treatment.

nasal feeding. Nasal gavage.

nasal fossa. One of the two halves of the nasal cavity.

nasal gavage. Feeding through a tube in the nasal passage leading to the stomach. This is resorted to when it is the only route available or when the patient refuses to eat.

nasal height. Distance between lower border of nasal aperture and the nasion.

nasal index. The greatest width of the nasal aperture in relation to a line from the lower edge of the nasal aperture to the nasion.

nasal line. Line from lower edge of the ala nasi curving to outer side of the orbicularis oris muscle. SEE: *Jadelot's line.*

nasal meatus. SEE: *meatus.*

nasal obstruction. Commonest causes: irregular septum; enlarged turbinates; nasal polypi; in children foreign bodies such as food, buttons, or pins. Complications such as infections, sinusitis, and otitis may develop.

TREATMENT: Nasal douches, inhalations, and operative care: resection of septum; turbinectomy; removal of polypi; opening and draining sinuses; removal of foreign body.

nasal reflex. Sneezing resulting from irritation of nasal mucosa.

nasal septum. The wall or septum between the two nasal cavities. SEE: illus.

nasal sinuses, accessory. The paranasal sinuses, q.v. SEE: *sinuses, accessory nasal.*

nasal width. Maximum width of nasal aperture.

nascent (năs'ĕnt; nā'sĕnt) [L. *nascens,* born].

TWO VIEWS OF NASAL CAVITY

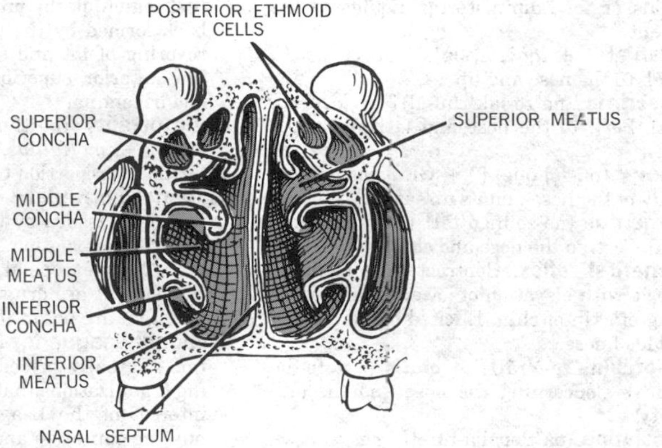

FRONTAL SECTION THROUGH NASAL CAVITIES

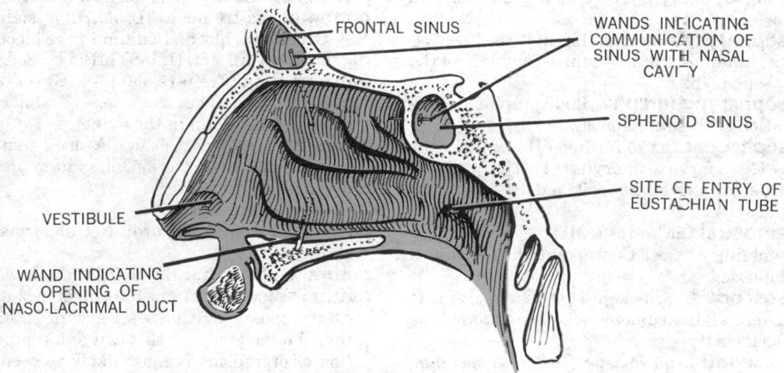

VIEW TOWARD NASAL SEPTUM FROM LATERAL AREA OF THE NOSE

1. Just born; incipient or beginning. 2. Pert. to a substance being set free from a compound.

nasioiniac (nā″zē-ō-ĭn′ē-ăk) [L. *nasus,* nose, + Gr. *inion,* back of the head]. Concerning the nasion and the inion.

nasion (nā′zē-ōn) [L. *nasus,* nose]. The point at which the nasofrontal suture is cut across by the median anteroposterior plane.

nasitis (nā-zī′tĭs) [″ + Gr. *itis,* inflammation]. Inflammation of the nose. SEE: *rhinitis.*

Nasmyth's membrane (năz′mĭths). [Alexander Nasmyth, Scottish dental surgeon, died 1847] Epithelial membrane that envelops the enamel of a tooth for a short period after birth.

naso- [L. *nasus,* nose]. Combining form indicating rel. to the nose.

nasoantral (nā″zō-ăn′trăl) [″ + Gr. *antrum,* cavity]. Concerning the nose and the maxillary antrum, or sinus.

nasoantritis (nā″zō-ăn-trī′tĭs) [″ + ″ + *itis,* inflammation]. Inflammation of nose and antrum of Highmore.

nasociliary (nā″zō-sĭl′ē-ār-ē) Pert. to nose, eyebrow, and eyes. Applied esp. to nerve supplying these structures.

nasofrontal [″ + *frontalis,* forehead]. Pert. to nasal and frontal bones.

nasogastric tube (nā″zō-găs′trĭk) [″ + Gr.

gaster, belly]. A tube inserted through the nose that extends into the stomach. It may be used for emptying the stomach of gas and liquids or for administering liquids to the patient.

nasolabial [" + *labium,* lip]. Connected with or rel. to the nose and lip.

nasolacrimal (nā"zō-lăk'rĭm-ăl) [" + *lacrima,* tear]. Pert. to the nose and lacrimal apparatus.

nasology (nā-zŏl'ō-jē) [" + Gr. *logos,* study]. Study of the nose and its diseases.

nasomental (nā"zō-mĕn'tăl) [" + *mentum,* chin]. Pert. to the nose and chin.

nasomental reflex. Contraction of mentalis muscle with elevation of lower lip and wrinkling of skin of chin. Elicited by percussion of side of nose.

naso-oral (nā"zō-ō'răl) [" + *oralis,* pert. to the mouth]. Concerning the nose and the oral cavity.

nasopalatine (nā"zō-păl'ă-tĭn) [L. *nasus,* nose, + *palatum,* palate]. Pert. to both nose and palate.

nasopharyngeal (nā"zō-făr-ĭn'jē-ăl) [" + Gr. *pharynx,* pharynx]. Pert. to the pharynx and nose.

nasopharyngitis (nā"zō-făr-ĭn-jī'tĭs) [" + " + *itis,* inflammation]. Inflamed condition of the nasopharynx.

nasopharyngography. Radiographic examination of the nasopharynx.

nasopharynx (nā"zō-făr'ĭnks) [L. *nasus,* nose, + Gr. *pharynx,* pharynx]. Part of pharynx situated above the soft palate (postnasal space).

nasorostral (nā"zō-rŏs'trăl) [" + *rostralis,* resembling a beak]. Concerning the rostrum of the nose.

nasoscope (nā'zō-skōp) [" + Gr. *skopein,* to examine]. Instrument for examination of the nasal cavity.

nasoseptitis (nā"zō-sĕp-tī'tĭs) [" + *saeptum,* partition, + Gr. *itis,* inflammation]. Inflamed condition of the nasal septum.

nasosinusitis (nā"zō-sī"nū-sī'tĭs) [" + *sinus,* cavity]. Inflammation of the nasal accessory sinuses and cavities.

nasospinale (nā"zō-spīn'ăl-ē). Point at which median sagittal plane intersects line joining lowest points on nasal margins.

nasus (nā'sŭs) [L.]. [NA] The nose, organ for respiration and sense of smell. SEE: *nose.*

Natacyn. Trade name for natamycin, USP.

natal (nā'tăl). 1. [L. *natus,* birth]. Pert. to birth or the day of birth. 2. [L. *nates,* buttocks]. Pert. to the buttocks.

natality [L. *natalis,* birth]. The birth rate; ratio of births to population of a given community.

natamycin (năt"ă-mī'sĭn). USP. An antibiotic agent used topically. Trade name is Natacyn.

natant (nā'tănt) [L. *natare,* to swim]. Floating; swimming.

nates (nā'tēz) [L.]. (sing. *natis*) 1. [NA] Gluteal region; fleshy prominences on the lower back formed by the gluteal muscles with a covering of fat and skin. SYN: *buttocks.* 2. The anterior, superior, or upper two corpora quadrigemina.

natimortality (nā"tĭ-mor-tăl'ĭ-tē) [L. *natus,* birth, + *mortalitas,* death]. Rate of stillbirths in proportion to birth rate.

National Formulary. ABBR: NF. Formulary originally issued by the American Pharmaceutical Association. Now published by the U.S. Pharmacopeial Convention, Inc. Included in it are drugs of established usefulness that are not in the U.S. Pharmacopeia.

National League for Nursing. An organization originally formed from three other nursing organizations that merged. The principal interest of the League is in the areas of nursing education and service.

native (nā'tĭv) [L. *nativus*]. 1. Born with; inherent. 2. Natural, normal. SYN: *indigenous.* 3. Belonging to, as place of one's birth.

Native American. An American Indian.

natremia (nă-trē'mē-ă) [L. *natrium,* sodium, + Gr. *haima,* blood]. Sodium in the blood.

natrium (nā'trē-ŭm) [L.]. SYMB: Na. Sodium.

natriuresis (nā"trē-ū-rē'sĭs) [" + Gr. *ouresis,* make water]. The excretion of abnormal amounts of sodium in the urine.

natriuretic (nā"trē-ūr-ĕt'ĭk). A drug that increases rate of excretion of sodium in the urine. SEE: *diuretic.*

natron. Sodium carbonate.

natural [L. *natura,* nature]. Not abnormal or artificial.

natural childbirth. SEE: *childbirth, natural.*

natural selection. A mechanism of evolution, q.v., proposed by Charles Darwin. It states that the tendency for survival and reproduction of organisms is most likely to occur in those who are best adapted to their environment.

Naturetin. Trade name for bendroflumethiazide, USP.

naturopath (nā'tūr-ō-păth) [" + Gr. *pathos,* suffering]. One who practices naturopathy.

naturopathy (nā"tūr-ŏp'ă-thē). A therapeutic system that does not use drugs or therapy but employs natural forces such as light, heat, air, water, and massage.

nausea (naw'sē-ă) [Gr. *nausia,* seasickness]. Unpleasant sensation usually preceding vomiting. It is present in seasickness, early pregnancy, diseases of the central nervous system, neurasthenia, or hysteria. It may be due to the sight or odor of obnoxious matter or conditions or to mental images of same. It may be present, without vomiting, in certain gallbladder disturbances, in carsickness, and in other types of motion sickness.

NURSING IMPLICATIONS: Remove any materials or environmental factors that precipitate the nausea. Note frequency, time, amount, and characteristics of emesis. Test vomitus for blood when indicated. Record and report any pertinent factors to physician. SEE: *vomitus*.

n. gravidarum. Morning sickness of pregnancy.

n. navalis. Seasickness. SYN: *mal de mer.*

nauseant (naw'shē-ănt, naw'sē-ănt). 1. Provoking nausea. 2. That which causes nausea.

nauseate (naw'shē-āt, naw'sē-āt). To cause nausea.

nauseous (naw'shŭs, naw'shē-ŭs). 1. Producing nausea, disgust, or loathing. 2. To be nauseated.

Navane. Trade name for thiothixene hydrochloride.

navel (nā'vĕl) [AS. *nafela*]. The depression or scar in the center of the abdomen where the umbilical cord was attached to the fetus. SYN: *umbilicus*.

navicula (nă-vĭk'ū-lă) [L. *navicula,* boat]. Fossa navicularis, q.v.

navicular (nă-vĭk'ū-lăr). 1. Shaped like a boat. 2. Scaphoid bones in the carpus (wrist) and in the tarsus (ankle). SEE: *skeleton*.

navicular fossa. Fossa navicularis.

Nb. Chem. symb. for niobium (columbium).

nc. *nanocurie*.

N.C.A.P. *National Coalition for Action in Politics*.

N.C.I. *National Cancer Institute*.

N.C.S.N.N.E. *National Commission for the Study of Nursing and Nursing Education*.

Nd. Chem. symb. for neodymium.

N.D.A. *National Dental Association*.

Ne. Chem. symb. for neon.

near point. ABBR: n.p. Closest point of distinct vision with maximum accommodation. It recedes with age, varying from about 3 in. (7.62 cm.) at 2 yr. to 40 in. (101.60 cm.) at 60 yr. SYN: *punctum proximum*.

nearsight. Ability to see clearly only those objects held close to the eye. SYN: *myopia.* SEE: *nearsighted*.

nearsighted. Able to see clearly only those objects held close to the eye. Caused by error in refraction in which rays are focused in front of the retina. A negative (concave) lens will correct this condition. SYN: *myopic*.

RS: eye; eyeball; farsightedness; hypermetropia; hyperopia; lens; presbyopia.

nearsightedness. Error in refraction in which rays are focused in front of the retina, thus the person is able to see distinctly for only a short distance. A negative (concave) lens will correct this condition. SYN: *myopia*.

nearthrosis (nē"ăr-thrō'sĭs) [Gr. *neos,* new, + *arthron,* joint, + *osis,* condition]. A false joint or abnormal articulation. SYN: *neoarthrosis.*

Nebcin. Trade name for tobramycin sulfate.

nebula (nĕb'ū-lă) [L., mist, cloud]. (pl. *nebulae*) 1. Slight haziness on the cornea. 2. Cloudiness in urine. 3. Aqueous or oily substance for use in an atomizer.

nebulization. Production of particles such as a spray or mist from liquid. The size of particles produced depends upon the method used. SEE: *nebulizer*.

nebulizer (nĕb'ū-lī"zĕr) [L. *nebula,* mist]. An apparatus for producing a fine spray or mist. This may be done by rapidly passing air through a liquid or by vibrating a liquid at a high frequency so the particles produced are extremely small. SEE: *aerosol, atomizer; vaporizer*.

Necator (nē-kā'tor) [L., murderer]. A genus of nematode hookworms belonging to the family Ancylostomidae.

N. americanus. A species of hookworm widely distributed in tropical regions and common in the southern United States. Adults live in the small intestine of man attached to mucosa by their mouths. Adults lay eggs, which pass out with feces and under proper conditions of warmth and moisture hatch within 24 hours into rhabditiform larvae. After two molts, the larvae become strongyliform. After two more molts occurring within five days, they become infective larvae. They enter the body through the skin, enter the venous system, and are carried to the lungs. Here they burrow into air spaces from which they pass via bronchial tubes and trachea to the pharynx from which they are expectorated or swallowed. If swallowed, they reach the intestine, bury themselves among the villi, molt again, acquire a mouth part, and attach themselves to the mucosa. Worms may live 5 years. Disease is contracted by walking barefoot or otherwise exposing the skin to soil that has been contaminated by feces of persons who are infected with the worm.

SYM: Anemia, weakness, failure to grow.

DIAG: Microscopic examination of preparation of feces reveals eggs of the worm.

TREATMENT: Mebendazole (trade name Vermox) is the drug of choice. Pyrantel pamoate is also effective.

RS: Ancylostoma; ancylostomiasis; hookworm.

necatoriasis (nē-kā"tō-rī'ă-sĭs). Infestation by Necator americanus. SEE: *ancylostomiasis*.

neck [AS. *hnecca,* nape]. 1. Part of body between the head and shoulders. SEE: illus.; *muscle* for illus. 2. The constricted portion of an organ, or that resembling a neck. 3. Region between crown and root of a tooth.

n., anatomical, of humerus. Constriction just below the head of the humerus.

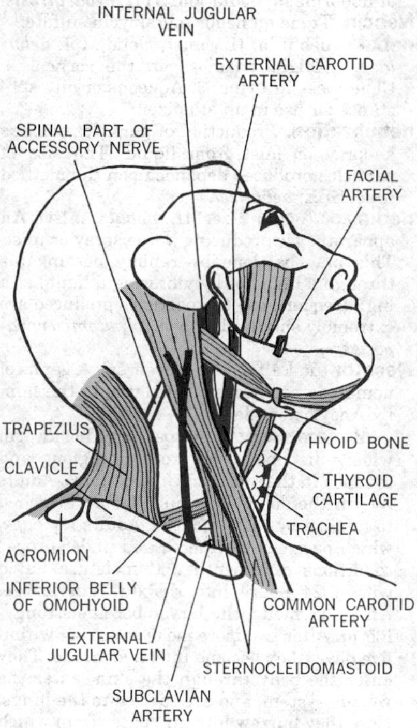

LATERAL ASPECT OF NECK

n., Madelung's. Diffuse lipoma of the neck.

n. of femur. The heavy column of bone that connects the head of the femur to the shaft.

n. of tooth. The constricted area that connects the crown of a tooth to the root of a tooth.

n. of uterus. The cervix uteri.

n., surgical, of humerus. Narrow part of humerus below the tuberosity. Fracture here is common.

n., webbed. A broad neck as seen anteriorly or posteriorly. The breadth is due to a fold of skin that extends from the clavicle to the head. This is present in Turner's syndrome.

n., wry. Torsion of the neck caused by contracted muscles. SYN: *torticollis*.

neck conformer. Splint, usually fabricated of thermoplastic material, that positions the neck to prevent flexion contractures due to burns of the anterior neck.

necklace, Casal's. In pellagra, a ring of pigmented, reddened skin around the neck.

neck-righting reflex. SEE: *reflex, neck-righting*.

necrectomy (nĕ-krĕk'tō-mē) [Gr. *nekros,* dead, + *ektome,* excision]. Surgical removal of necrotic tissue.

necro- [Gr. *nekros,* dead]. Combining form meaning pert. to death, dead cells or tissue.

necrobiosis (nĕk-rō-bī-ō'sĭs) [" + *biosis,* life]. Gradual degeneration and swelling of collagen bundles in the dermis. SEE: *necrosis*.

n. lipoidica diabeticorum. A skin disease common in diabetics characterized by necrobiosis of connective and elastic tissue and discoloration of skin.

necrobiotic (nĕ"krō-bī-ŏt'ĭk). Pert. to or affected by necrobiosis.

necrocytosis (nĕ"krō-sī-tō'sĭs) [" + *kytos,* cell, + *osis,* condition]. Cellular death or decomposition.

necrocytotoxin (nĕk"rō-sī"tō-tŏks'ĭn). A toxin that causes death of cells.

necrogenic, necrogenous (nĕ-krō-jĕn'ĭk, -krŏj'ĕn-ŭs) [" + *gennan,* to produce]. Caused by, pert. to, or originating in dead matter.

necrologist (nĕk-rŏl'ō-jĭst) [" + *logos,* study]. A student of mortality statistics.

necrology (nĕk-rŏl'ō-jē). The study of mortality statistics.

necrolysis (nĕ-krŏl'ĭ-sĭs) [" + *lysis,* dissolution]. Necrosis and dissolution of tissue.

necromania (nĕk-rō-mā'nē-ă) [" + *mania,* madness]. 1. Abnormal interest in dead bodies or in death. 2. Mania with desire for death.

necrometer (nĕk-rŏm'ĕt-ĕr) [" + *metron,* measure]. Device for measurement of organs from dead bodies.

necromimesis (nĕk"rō-mī-mē'sĭs) [" + *mimesis,* imitation]. A delusion in which one believes oneself to be dead or acts as though one were dead.

necronectomy (nĕk-rō-nĕk'tō-mē) [" + *ektome,* excision]. Excision of a necrotic part, esp. of necrotic ossicles.

necroparasite (nĕk"rō-păr'ă-sīt) [" + *parasitos,* fellow guest]. Saprophyte.

necrophagous (nĕ-krŏf'ă-gŭs) [" + *phagein,* to eat]. Feeding or existing on dead bodies or matter.

necrophile (nĕk'rō-fĭl) [" + *philein,* to love]. One who has a morbid interest in dead bodies or who has intercourse with corpses.

necrophilia (nĕk"rō-fĭl'ē-ă) [" + *philein,* to love]. 1. Abnormal concern with corpses. 2. Sexual intercourse with a dead body.

necrophilic (nĕk"rō-fĭl'ĭk) [" + *philein,* to love]. 1. Concerning necrophilism. 2. Descriptive of bacteria that prefer dead tissue.

necrophilism (nĕk-rŏf'ĭl-ĭzm). Sexual perversion in which there is insane love for, or intercourse with the dead.

necrophilous (nĕk-rŏf'ĭl-ŭs). 1. Having a

morbid fondness for, or feeding on, dead tissue. 2. Pert. to or affected with necrophilism.

necrophobia (nĕk-rō-fō'bē-ă) [" + *phobos,* fear]. 1. Abnormal aversion to dead bodies. 2. Insane dread of death. SYN: *thanatophobia.*

necropneumonia (nĕk"rō-nū-mō'nē-ă) [" + *pneumon,* lung]. Pulmonary gangrene.

necropsy (nĕk'rŏp-sē) [" + *opsis,* view]. Examination of a dead body to determine cause of death or pathological conditions. SYN: *autopsy; necroscopy; postmortem examination.*

necrosadism (nĕk"rō-sā'dĭzm) [" + *sadism*]. Sexual gratification derived from the mutilation of dead bodies.

necroscopy (nĕ-krŏs'kō-pē) [" + *skopein,* to examine]. Examination of a dead body to find cause of death or pathological condition. SYN: *autopsy; necropsy; postmortem examination.*

necrose (nĕk-rōs') [Gr. *nekros,* dead]. To cause or to undergo necrosis.

necrosin. A substance obtained from inflamed tissues. It induces inflammatory changes in normal tissue.

necrosis (nĕ-krō'sĭs) [Gr. *nekrosis,* a killing]. (pl. *necroses*) Death of areas of tissue or bone surrounded by healthy parts; death in mass as distinguished from necrobiosis, which is a gradual degeneration. The dead part in bone is called a sequestrum; in soft tissue it is called a slough or sphacelus. Term is usually applied to bone destruction or small areas of tissue, while gangrene is generally applied to destruction of specific parts or larger areas. SYN: *gangrene; mortification.*

ETIOL: Insufficient blood supply; physical agents such as trauma, radiant energy (electricity, infrared, ultraviolet, roentgen, and radium rays); chemical agents acting locally, acting internally following absorption, or placed into the wrong tissue. For example, some medicines cause necrosis if injected into the tissues rather than the vein, and iron dextran causes necrosis if injected into areas other than deep muscle or vein.

n., anemic. Necrosis caused by disturbed circulation in a part.

n., aseptic. Necrosis occurring without infection.

n., Balser's fatty. Pancreatitis with gangrenous areas in the fatty tissues.

n., caseous. N., cheesy.

n., central. Necrosis that affects only the center of a part.

n., cheesy. Necrosis with soft, dry, cheeselike formation. Usually seen in tuberculosis or syphilis. SYN: *n., caseous.*

n., coagulation. Necrosis occurring esp. in infarcts in which coagulation occurs in necrotic area, converting it into a homogenous mass and depriving the organ or tissue of blood. SYN: *n., fibrinous.*

n., colliquative. Necrosis caused by liquefaction of tissue due to autolysis or bacterial putrefaction. SYN: *n., liquefactive.*

n., dry. Necrosis with dryness of the sequestrum.

n., embolic. Necrosis resulting from an embolus, which causes anemic necrosis.

n., fat. Necrosis in small scattered areas in the fatty tissue.

n., fibrinous. N., coagulative.

n., focal. Necrosis in small scattered areas, often seen in infection.

n., gummatous. Necrosis resulting from syphilis forming a dry rubbery mass.

n., ischemic. N., coagulation.

n., liquefactive. N., colliquative.

n., medial. Necrosis of cells in tunica media of arteries.

n., moist. Necrosis with softening and moist condition of the dead tissue.

n., postpartum pituitary. The cause of Sheehan's syndrome, q.v.

n., putrefactive. Necrosis caused by bacterial decomposition.

n., subcutaneous fat, of newborn. An inflammatory disorder of fat tissue that may occur in the newborn at the site of application of forceps during delivery, and occasionally in premature infants. The cause is unknown.

n., superficial. Necrosis affecting only the outer layers of bone or any tissue.

n., thrombotic. Necrosis due to thrombus formation.

n., total. Necrosis affecting an entire organ or part.

n. ustilaginea. Dry necrosis due to ergot poisoning.

n., Zenker's. SEE: *Zenker's degeneration.*

necrospermia (nĕk-rō-spĕr'mē-ă) [Gr. *nekros,* death, + *sperma,* seed]. Condition in which spermatozoa in the ejaculate are immobile or lifeless.

necrotic [Gr. *nekrosis,* a killing]. Rel. to death of a portion of tissue.

necrotizing (nĕk'rō-tīz"ĭng). Causing necrosis.

necrotomy (nĕ-krŏt'ō-mē) [" + *tome,* incision]. 1. Dissection of a cadaver. 2. Excision of a sequestrum or other necrotic tissue.

necrotoxin (nĕk"rō-tŏk'sĭn) [" + *toxikon,* poison]. A general term for any toxin that causes necrosis.

need. Something required or wanted, a requisite. Essential for the physical and mental health of humans are certain needs. Included in physical needs are oxygen, water, food, shelter, freedom from fear and physical harm, usually some form of acceptable human (loving) relationship, and stress in its positive sense. Not an absolute need, but highly desirable, is that each individual have some goal no matter how trivial or grandiose, and the feeling that the goal is being attained. Most human beings seem to need some form of physical exercise over and above that required for ordinary daily living.

needle [AS. *naedl*]. A pointed instrument for stitching, ligaturing, or puncturing. It may be straight, half curved, full curved, semicircular, double curved (sometimes called "S" or sigmoid-shaped), or double ended. There are two classifications: cutting edge and round point. Cutting edge type is used in skin and dense tissue, while round point needles are used for more delicate operations. All curved needles are used with a holder and the straight needles usually without a holder.

n., aneurysm. A blunt, curved needle with an eye in tip; used for passing a suture around a vessel.

n., aspirating. A hollow needle, usually fitted to a syringe, for withdrawing fluids from a cavity.

n., cataract. Needle used in removing a cataract.

n., discission. A special cataract needle for making multiple cuts into the lens capsule.

n., Hagedorn. A curved, flattened needle with a cutting edge near the end.

n., hypodermic. A hollow needle for administration of hypodermic solutions.

n., knife. A narrow needle-pointed knife.

n., ligature. N., aneurysm, q.v.

n., Reverdin's. A needle used to carry a suture. It has an eye at the tip that can be opened and closed by use of a lever.

n., stop. A needle with an eye at its tip and a flange or shelf extending out from its shank end. This prevents the needle being inserted any farther than the shelf.

N.E.F. *Nurses' Educational Funds, Inc.*

NEFA. *nonesterified fatty acids.*

negation (nē-gā'shŭn) [L. *negare,* to deny]. Denial.

negative (nĕg'ă-tĭv) [L. *negare,* to deny]. 1. Possessing a numerical value that is less than zero. 2. Lacking results or indicating an absence, as in a test result. 3. Marked by resistance or retreat.

negative culture. A culture that does not reveal the suspected organism.

negative electrode. The pole by which electric current leaves the generating source.

negative glow. The luminous glow that is adjacent to the cathode in a vacuum tube through which an electrical discharge is passing.

negative sign. Minus sign (−) used in subtraction and to indicate a lack.

negativism. Behavior peculiarity marked by not performing suggested actions (passive negativism) or in doing the opposite (active negativism), as seen in dementia praecox. A patient may refuse to respond to suggestions because of sluggish mental reflexes or from fear. Retardation may be slow, or sudden and intense, as in manic-depressive insanity. Opposition caused by fear must be considered apart from dementia praecox, in which the patient performs acts directly contrary to those suggested.

negatron (nĕg'ă-trŏn). Negative electron.

NegGram. Trade name for nalidixic acid, USP.

Negri bodies (nā'grē). [Adelchi Negri, It. physician, 1876–1912] Very minute bodies formed in nerve cells of the brain of one affected by rabies.

Neisseria (nī-sē'rē-ă). [Albert Neisser, Ger. physician, 1855–1916] A genus of bacteria belonging to the family Neisseriaceae. They are gram-negative and usually occur in pairs with flattened sides but may occur singly or in irregular groups. The two species most often associated with disease in man are Neisseria meningitis and Neisseria gonorrhoeae, which cause meningitis and gonorrhea respectively.

N. catarrhalis. Species of Neisseria found in catarrhal inflammations of the upper respiratory tract. They may be confused with meningococci.

N. gonorrhoeae. Species causing gonorrhea. SYN: *gonococcus.* SEE: *gonorrhea.*

N. meningitidis. Species causing epidemic cerebrospinal meningitis, usually called meningococcal meningitis.

N. sicca. Species found in mucous membrane of respiratory tract. Occasionally may cause bacterial endocarditis.

Neisseriaceae (nīs-sē"rē-ā'sē-ē). A family of bacteria that are spherical, gram-negative, and nonmotile. The two genera are Neisseria and Veillonella.

Nelaton's line (nā-lă-tŏnz'). [Auguste Nelaton, Fr. surgeon, 1807–1873] Line from the anterior superior spine of the ilium to tuberosity of the ischium.

nemathelminth (nĕm"ă-thĕl'mĭnth) [Gr. *nema,* thread, + *helmins,* worm]. A roundworm belonging to the phylum Nemathelminthes.

Nemathelminthes (nĕm"ă-thĕl-mĭn'thēz). The phylum of the roundworm.

nematocide (nĕm'ă-tō-sīd") [Gr. *nema,* thread, + L. *caedere,* to kill]. An agent that kills nematode worms.

nematocyst (nĕm'ă-tō-sĭst) [" + *kystis,* bladder]. A small stinger present in the cnidoblasts of some coelenterates including jellyfish and Portuguese man-of-war. The stinger can penetrate the skin upon contact.

Nematoda (nĕm"ă-tō'dă) [" + *eidos,* form]. A

class of the phylum Nemathelminthes that includes the true roundworms or threadworms, many species of which are parasitic. They are cylindrical or spindle-shaped worms possessing a resistant cuticle, have a complete alimentary canal, and lack a true coelom. The sexes usually separate, and development usually is direct and simple.

nematode (nĕm′ă-tōd) [Gr. *nema,* thread, + *eidos,* like]. A member of the class Nematoda.

nematodiasis (nĕm″ă-tō-dī′ă-sĭs) [″ + ″ + *iasis,* infection]. Infestation by a parasite belonging to the class Nematoda.

nematoid (nĕm′ă-toyd). Threadlike, like a nematode.

nematology (nĕm″ă-tŏl′ō-jē). The division of parasitology that deals with worms belonging to the class Nematoda.

nematospermia (nĕm″ă-tō-spĕr′mē-ă) [″ + *sperma,* seed]. Spermatozoa with long tails.

Nembutal (nĕm′bū-tăl). Trade name for pentobarbital. It is a short-acting drug used as a preanesthetic, sedative, and hypnotic.

neo- [Gr. *neos*]. Combining form meaning new or recent.

neoantigen (nē″ō-ăn′tĭ-jĕn) [″ + *anti,* against, + *gennan,* to produce]. A nonspecific term for various tumor antigens.

neoarthrosis (nē″ō-ăr-thrō′sĭs) [″ + *arthron,* joint, + *osis,* condition]. A false joint. SYN: *nearthrosis.*

Neo-Betalin 12. Trade name for hydroxocobalamin (vitamin B_{12}), USP.

neobiogenesis (nē″ō-bī″ō-jĕn′ĕ-sĭs) [″ + *bios,* life, + *genesis,* origin]. The theory that life can arise from inorganic compounds.

Neobiotic. Trade name for neomycin sulfate, USP.

neoblastic [″ + *blastos,* germ]. Pert. to, or constituting, a new growth of tissue.

neocerebellum (nē″ō-sĕr-ĕ-bĕl′ŭm) [Gr. *neos,* new, + L. *cerebellum,* little brain]. The portion of the corpus cerebelli of the cerebellum that lies between the primary and prepyramidal fissures. Consists principally of the ansiform lobules. Phylogenetically, it develops last, in conjunction with cerebral cortex, and is concerned with the integration of voluntary movements. It is the posterior lobe of the cerebellum.

neocinetic (nē″ō-sī-nĕt′ĭk) [″ + *kinetikos,* pert. to movement]. Concerning the portion of the nervous system that regulates voluntary muscular control. SYN: *neokinetic.*

neocortex (nē″ō-kor′tĕks). Neopallium.

Neo-Cultol. Trade name for mineral oil.

neodymium (nē″ō-dĭm′ē-ŭm). SYMB: Nd. At. wt. 144.24; at. no. 60. A shiny, silvery, rare-earth chemical element.

neofetus (nē-ō-fē′tŭs) [″ + L. *foetus,* offspring]. Embryo during eighth or ninth week of intrauterine life.

neoformation (nē″ō-for-mā′shŭn) [″ + L. *formatio,* a shaping]. 1. Regeneration. 2. A neoplasm or new growth.

neogala (nē-ŏg′ă-lă) [″ + *gala,* milk]. The first milk following childbirth. SEE: *colostrum.*

neogenesis (nē-ō-jĕn′ĕ-sĭs) [″ + *genesis,* formation]. Regeneration or reformation, as of tissue.

neogenetic (nē″ō-jĕn-ĕt′ĭk). Newly formed; rel. to new formations.

neohymen (nē-ō-hī′mĕn) [Gr. *neos,* new, + *hymen,* membrane]. A false or new membrane. SYN: *pseudomembrane.*

neolalism (nē″ō-lăl′ĭzm) [″ + *laleo,* to chatter]. Use of neologisms in speech. This may be associated with schizophrenia.

neologism (nē-ŏl′ō-jĭzm) [″ + *logos,* study, + *-ismos,* state]. 1. A new word or phrase, or a new meaning attached to an old word or phrase. 2. A mental condition in which the patient coins new words that are meaningless or words to which he or she gives special significance without being aware of their normal significance.

Neoloid. Trade name for castor oil.

neomembrane (nē-ō-mĕm′brān) [″ + L. *membrana,* membrane]. A false or a new membrane. SYN: *pseudomembrane.*

neomorph (nē′ō-morf) [″ + *morphe,* form]. A new formation or development that is not inherited from a similar structure in an ancestor.

neomycin sulfate (nē″ō-mī′sĭn) [″ + *mykes,* fungus]. USP. An antibiotic from a species of Streptomyces, isolated from soil. Active against gram-positive and gram-negative bacteria, as well as streptomycin-resistant strains of Mycobacterium tuberculosis. It is toxic to kidneys and to the eighth nerve. The ototoxicity may cause hearing difficulties. Trade names are Neobiotic and Mycifradin Sulfate.

neon (nē′ŏn) [Gr. *neos,* new]. SYMB: Ne. At. wt. 20.183; at. no. 10. A rare, inert, gaseous element in the air. Only 18 parts per million parts of air are neon.

neonatal (nē″ō-nā′tăl) [″ + L. *natus,* born]. Concerning the first six weeks after birth.

neonate (nē′ō-nāt). A newborn infant up to six weeks of age.

neonatologist (nē″ō-nā-tŏl′ō-jĭst) [″ + ″ + Gr. *logos,* study]. A physician who specializes in the study of and care and treatment of neonates.

neonatology (nē″ō-nā-tŏl′ō-jē). The study of and care and treatment of neonates.

neon gas. Colorless gas that makes a reddish-orange glow when an electric charge strikes it.

neopallium (nē″ō-păl′ē-ŭm) [Gr. *neos,* new, +

L. *pallium,* cloak]. That portion of cerebral hemisphere not belonging to the rhinencephalon or corpus striatum, comprising most of the convoluted cortex and its associated white fibers. Phylogenetically, it is the new part of the pallium. SYN: *isocortex; neocortex.*

neopathy (nē-ŏp'ă-thē) [" + *pathos,* disease]. 1. A newly found disease. 2. A new complication or new condition of a disease.

Neopavrin. Trade name for ethaverine hydrochloride.

neophilism (nē-ŏf'ĭl-ĭzm) [" + *philein,* to love, + *-ismos,* state]. Morbid love of novelty and new persons and scenes.

neophobia (nē"ō-fō'bē-ă) [" + *phobos,* fear]. Fear of new scenes or novelties; aversion to all that is unknown or not understood.

neophrenia (nē"ō-frē'nē-ă) [" + *phren,* mind]. Mental deterioration in early youth.

neoplasia (nē"ō-plā'zē-ă) [" + *plassein,* to form]. The development of neoplasms.

neoplasm (nē'ō-plăzm) [" + *plasma,* a thing formed]. A new and abnormal formation of tissue, as a tumor or growth. It serves no useful function, but grows at the expense of the healthy organism.

n., benign. A growth not spreading by metastases or infiltration of tissue.

n., histoid. A neoplasm in which structure resembles the tissues and elements that surround it.

n., malignant. A growth that infiltrates tissue, metastasizes, and often recurs after attempts at surgical removal. SYN: *cancer.*

n., mixed. A neoplasm composed of tissues from two of the germinal layers.

n., multicentric. A growth arising from a number of distinct groups of cells.

n., organoid. A neoplasm in which the structure is similar to some organ of the body.

n., unicentric. A growth having origin in one group of cells.

neoplastic (nē"ō-plăs'tĭk) [Gr. *neos,* new, + *plastikos,* formed]. Pert. to, or of the nature of, new, abnormal tissue formation.

neoplasty (nē'ō-plăs-tē) [" + *plassein,* to form]. Surgical formation or restoration of parts.

neostigmine (nē-ō-stĭg'mĭn). A cholinergic drug used clinically in the form of a bromide or methylsulfate.

n. bromide. USP. A preparation of neostigmine used for oral administration in the treatment of myasthenia gravis. Ophthalmic solution used for glaucoma. Trade name is Prostigmin.

n. methylsulfate. USP. A preparation of neostigmine used for parenteral administration in treatment of myasthenia gravis. Trade name is Prostigmin.

neostomy (nē-ŏs'tō-mē) [" + *stoma,* opening]. Surgical formation of artificial opening into an organ or between two organs.

neostriatum (nē"ō-strī-ā'tŭm) [" + L. *striatum,* grooved]. The caudate nucleus and the putamen considered together.

Neo-synephrine Hydrochloride (nē"ō-sĭn-ĕf'rĭn). Trade name for phenylephrine hydrochloride, USP.

neoteny (nē-ŏt'ĕ-nē) [" + *teinein,* to extend]. In zoology, maturation while remaining in the larval stage.

neothalamus (nē"ō-thăl'ă-mŭs) [" + L. *thalamus,* thalamus]. The lateral and dorsomedial nuclei of the thalamus.

nephelometer (nĕf"ĕl-ŏm'ĕ-ter) [Gr. *nephele,* mist, + *metron,* measure]. Apparatus for measuring the turbidity of a fluid. This apparatus also may be used in estimating the degree of contamination of air by particulate matter.

nephelometry (nĕf"ĕl-ŏm'ĕ-trē). The employment of the nephelometer.

nephelopia (nĕf"ĕ-lō'pē-ă) [Gr. *nephele,* mist, + *ops,* eye]. Dim or cloudy vision from lessened transparency of the ocular media.

nephradenoma (nĕf"răd-ē-nō'mă) [Gr. *nephros,* kidney, + *aden,* gland, + *oma,* tumor]. Renal adenoma.

nephralgia (nĕ-frăl'jē-ă) [" + *algos,* pain]. Renal pain. In absence of other symptoms, may alone be symptomatic of an obstructive renal process, but commonly presents a problem in differential diagnosis.

nephralgic (nĕ-frăl'jĭk). Pert. to renal pain.

nephrapostasis (nĕf"ră-pŏs'tă-sĭs) [" + *apostasis,* suppuration]. Renal abscess or purulent inflammation of the kidney.

nephratony (nē-frăt'ō-nē) [" + *a,* not, + *tonos,* tension]. Lack of normal renal tone. SYN: *nephratonia.*

nephrauxe (nĕf-rawks'ē) [" + *auxe,* increase]. Renal enlargement.

nephrectasia, nephrectasis, nephrectasy (nĕf-rĕk-tā'zē-ă, -rĕk'tă-sĭs, -tă-sē) [Gr. *nephros,* kidney, + *ektasis,* distention]. Distention of the kidney.

nephrectomize (nĕ-frĕk'tō-mīz) [" + *ektome,* excision]. Surgical removal of one or both kidneys.

nephrectomy (nĕ-frĕk'tō-mē) [" + *ektome,* excision]. Removal of a kidney.

NURSING IMPLICATIONS: Provide adequate pre- and post-operative instruction. Physically prepare the patient according to prescribed protocol such as skin preparation, laboratory studies, and preoperative medications. Provide activities that are interesting but not tiring. Prevent or control complications of fluid or electrolyte imbalance and weigh daily.

Post-op: Administer analgesics and other prescribed medications. Report and record any excessive bleeding. Turn patient so you can view entire dressing area. Assist with cough and deep breathing exercises at frequent intervals. Turn and position frequently, observing operative site and dressing, changing as necessary. Institute range of motion exercises. Check drainage tubes at frequent intervals to be certain they are functioning. Monitor and record intake and output. Change position frequently to prevent complications (operative side may be most comfortable). Provide frequent mouth care while the patient is not taking anything by mouth. Then encourage progressive diet. Establish discharge teaching plan including diet, activities, incision care, and medications. Instruct patient concerning engaging in activities that could injure the remaining kidney.

COMPLICATIONS: Spontaneous pneumothorax and secondary hemorrhage.

n., abdominal. Nephrectomy through an incision in the abdominal wall.

n., paraperitoneal. Removal of a kidney through an extraperitoneal incision.

nephrelcosis (něf-rěl-kō'sĭs) [Gr. *nephros,* kidney, + *helkosis,* ulceration]. Ulceration of the mucosa of the kidney.

nephrelcus (něf-rěl'kŭs). Renal ulcer.

nephremia (něf-rē'mē-ă) [" + *haima,* blood]. Congested state of kidney.

nephremphraxis (něf"rěm-frăks'ĭs) [" + *emphraxis,* obstruction]. Obstruction in the renal vessels.

nephric (něf'rĭk) [Gr. *nephros,* kidney]. Pert. to the kidney or kidneys. SYN: *renal.*

nephridium (ně-frĭd'ē-ŭm) [Gr. *nephridios,* pert. to the kidney]. A segmented excretory tubule present in many invertebrates.

nephritic (nē-frĭt'ĭk). 1. Rel. to the kidney. 2. Pert. to nephritis. 3. An agent used in nephritis.

nephritic syndrome. A clinical classification that includes almost all forms of glomerular disease that are severe enough to cause loss of blood from the glomerulus and red blood cell casts. SEE: *glomerular disease; nephritis; nephrotic syndrome.*

nephritis (něf-rī'tĭs) [" + *itis,* inflammation]. (pl. *nephritides*) Inflammation of the kidney. The glomeruli, tubules, and interstitial tissue may be affected. It may be either acute or chronic.

ETIOL: Bacteria or their toxins; streptococcal infections; diphtheria; septicemia; or toxic drugs such as mercury; arsenic, alcohol.

NURSING IMPLICATIONS: Maintain bedrest if indicated for elevated blood pressure. Observe, record, and report any hematuria. Monitor blood pressure using same arm, same cuff, same position each time. Observe or question concerning headache, restlessness, lethargy, convulsions, tachycardia, cardiac gallop. Administer antihypertensive as prescribed. Maintain adequate hydration and prescribed dietary restrictions. Carefully monitor prescribed I.V. fluids. Anticipate and attempt to avoid complications of hypertension.

RS: arteriosclerosis; glomerulonephritis; kidney; nephritic syndrome; nephrosclerosis; nephrotic syndrome.

n., acute. An inflammatory form of nephritis involving the glomeruli, the tubules, or the entire kidney. It is of various types depending on the portion of the kidney involved: degenerative, diffuse, suppurative, hemorrhagic, interstitial, and parenchymatous.

n., chronic. Progressive form of nephritis in which entire structure of kidney may be affected or affection may be confined to the glomerular or tubular processes. One variety of nephritis may merge with another, causing a diffuse nephritis. Symptoms depend upon the tissues involved.

n., glomerular. Glomerulonephritis.

n., interstitial. Nephritis associated with pathological changes in the renal interstitial tissue that in turn may be primary or due to a toxic agent such as drugs, or chemicals. The end result is that the nephrons are destroyed and renal function is seriously impaired.

n., salt-losing. A rare disease of the renal tubules that causes abnormal salt loss even though salt intake is normal. This progresses to cause azotemia, renal failure, shock, and death. The cause is unknown. SYN: *Thorn's syndrome.*

n., scarlatinal. Acute glomerulonephritis complicating scarlet fever.

n., suppurative. Nephritis associated with abscesses in the kidney.

n., transfusion. Renal failure and tubular disease caused by transfusion of incompatible blood.

nephritogenic (ně-frĭt"ō-jěn'ĭk) [" + *gennan,* to produce]. Causing nephritis.

nephro-, nephr- [Gr. *nephros,* kidney]. Combining form pert. to the kidney.

nephroabdominal (něf"rō-ăb-dŏm'ĭ-năl) [" + L. *abdominalis,* abdomen]. Concerning the kidney and abdomen.

nephroblastoma (něf"rō-blăs-tō'mă) [" + *blastos,* germ, + *oma,* tumor]. Wilms' tumor, q.v.

nephrocalcinosis (něf-rō"kăl"sĭn-ō'sĭs) [" + L. *calx,* lime, + Gr. *osis,* condition]. Calcinosis of the kidney characterized by deposits of calcium phosphate in renal tubules.

nephrocapsectomy (něf"rō-kăp-sěk'tō-mē) [" + L. *capsula,* capsule, + Gr. *ektome,* excision]. Renal decapsulation.

nephrocardiac (něf"rō-kăr'dē-ăk) [" + *kardia,* heart]. Concerning the heart and kidney.

nephrocele (nĕf′rō-sēl) [″ + *kele,* hernia]. Renal hernia.

nephrocolic (nĕf″rō-kŏl′ĭk) [Gr. *nephros,* kidney, + *kolikos,* colic]. 1. Severe colicky pain in ureter due to passage of stone. 2. Concerning the colon and kidney.

nephrocolopexy (nĕf″rō-kŏl′ō-pĕks″ē) [″ + Gr. *kolon,* colon, + *pexis,* fixation]. Surgical suspension of the kidney and colon using the nephrocolic ligament.

nephrocoloptosis (nĕf″rō-kō″lŏp-tō′sĭs) [″ + ″ + *ptosis,* a dropping]. Condition in which the kidney and colon are displaced downward.

nephrocystanastomosis (nĕf″rō-sĭst-ă-năs″tō-mō′sĭs) [″ + *kystis,* bladder, + *anastomosis,* outlet]. Surgical formation of an artificial connection between kidney and bladder in permanent ureteral obstruction.

nephrocystitis (nĕf″rō-sĭs-tī′tĭs) [″ + ″ + *itis,* inflammation]. Inflamed condition of the kidneys and bladder.

nephrocystosis (nĕf″rō-sĭs-tō′sĭs) [″ + ″ + *osis,* condition]. Formation of renal cysts.

nephroerysipelas (nĕf″rō-ĕr″ĭ-sĭp′ĕ-lăs) [″ + *erythros,* red, + *pella,* skin]. Acute nephritis occurring as a complication of erysipelas.

nephrogenetic (nĕf″rō-jĕn-ĕt′ĭk) [″ + *gennan,* to produce]. Arising in or from the renal organs; capable of giving rise to kidney tissue. SYN: *nephrogenic; nephrogenous.*

nephrogenic. Nephrogenetic, q.v.

nephrogenous (nĕ-frŏj′ĕ-nŭs). Arising from the kidney.

nephrogram. A roentgenogram of the kidney.

nephrography (nĕ-frŏg′ră-fē) [″ + *graphein,* to write]. Roentgenography of the kidney.

nephrohydrosis (nĕf″rō-hī-drō′sĭs) [″ + *hydor,* water, + *osis,* condition]. Accumulation of urine in renal pelvis and calyces due to obstruction. SYN: *hydronephrosis; nephrydrosis.*

nephrohypertrophy (nĕf″rō-hī-pĕr′trō-fē) [″ + *hyper,* over, + *trophe,* nourishment]. Increased size of kidneys.

nephroid (nĕf′royd) [″ + *eidos,* form]. Resembling a kidney; kidney-shaped. SYN: *reniform.*

nephrolith (nĕf′rō-lĭth) [″ + *lithos,* stone]. Stone in the kidney.

nephrolithiasis (nĕf″rō-lĭth-ī′ă-sĭs). The presence of calculi in the kidney. SEE: *calculus, renal.*

nephrolithotomy (nĕf″rō-lĭth-ŏt′ō-mē) [″ + *lithos,* stone, + *tome,* incision]. Renal incision for removal of calculus.

nephrology (nē-frŏl′ō-jē) [″ + *logos,* study]. Science of the structure and function of the kidney.

nephrolysine (nĕ-frŏl′ĭ-sĭn) [″ + *lysis,* dissolution]. A toxic substance, esp. an antigen, that can destroy renal tissue.

nephrolysis (nē-frŏl′ĭ-sĭs) [″ + *lysis,* loosening]. 1. Surgical detachment of an inflamed kidney from paranephric adhesions. 2. Destruction of kidney tissue by action of a nephrotoxin.

nephroma (nĕ-frō′mă) [″ + *oma,* tumor]. Renal tumor.

nephromalacia (nĕf″rō-mă-lā′sē-ă) [″ + *malakia,* softening]. Abnormal renal softness or softening.

nephromegaly (nĕf″rō-mĕg′ă-lē) [″ + *megas,* great]. Extreme enlargement of one or both kidneys.

nephromere (nĕf′rō-mēr) [″ + *meros,* part]. Segment in embryo from which kidney develops. The intermediate mesoderm in an embryo from which the kidney develops. SYN: *nephrotome.*

nephron (nĕf′rŏn) [Gr. *nephros,* kidney]. The structural and functional unit of the kidney, consisting of a renal (malpighian) corpuscle (a glomerulus enclosed within Bowman's capsule), and its attached tubule, consisting of the proximal convoluted portion, loop of Henle, and distal convoluted portion. These connect by arched collecting tubules with straight collecting tubules. Urine is formed by filtration in renal corpuscles, and selective reabsorption and secretion by cells of the renal tubule. There are approximately one million nephrons in each kidney. SYN: *renal tubule.* SEE: *kidney* for illus.; *malpighian corpuscle; urine.*

nephroncus (nĕf-rŏn′kŭs) [″ + *onkos,* tumor]. A renal tumor.

nephroparalysis (nĕf″rō-păr-ăl′ĭ-sĭs) [″ + *paralyein,* to disable]. Paralyzed renal function.

nephropathy (nē-frŏp′ă-thē) [″ + *pathos,* disease]. Disease of the kidney. This term includes inflammatory (nephritis), degenerative (nephrosis), and sclerotic (arteriosclerotic) lesions of the kidney.

n., analgesic. Renal impairment resulting from ingestion of a large amount of specific analgesics such as phenacetin or salicylate over an extended period of time.

n., hypercalcemic. Renal damage due to hypercalcemia. This is usually caused by hyperparathyroidism, sarcoidosis, excess vitamin D intake, excess ingestion of milk and alkali, multiple myeloma, malignant disease, and occasionally immobilization or Paget's disease. If the underlying cause is allowed to persist, the damage to the renal tubules may be permanent.

TREATMENT: Correction of the primary disease.

n., hypokalemic. Renal damage due to abnormal depletion of potassium regardless of the basic cause of the electrolyte abnormality. Characteristically, there are multiple vacuoles in microscopic sections of the renal tubular epithelium. Clinically, the patient is unable to concentrate urine.

TREATMENT: Therapy for the primary cause of the hypokalemia may allow the kidney lesions to become completely reversed.

n., membranous. A glomerular disease of unknown etiology that produces the nephrotic syndrome, q.v. It may be distinguished from lipoid nephrosis by the use of immunofluorescence and electron microscopy. SEE: *glomerular disease; nephrotic syndrome.*

TREATMENT: High-protein diet and diuretics. Adrenocortical hormones may be of benefit in young patients.

nephropexy (nĕf'rō-pĕks-ē) [" + *pexis,* fixation]. Surgical attachment of a floating kidney.

nephrophthisis (nĕ-frŏ'thĭ-sĭs) [" + *phthisis,* a wasting]. 1. Tuberculosis of the kidney with caseous degeneration. 2. Suppurative nephritis with wasting of the kidney substance.

nephroptosis (nĕf"rŏp-tō'sĭs) [" + *ptosis,* a dropping]. Prolapse or downward displacement of the kidney.

nephropyelitis (nĕf"rō-pī-ĕl-ī'tĭs) [" + *pyelos,* pelvis, + *itis,* inflammation]. Inflammation of the renal pelvis and parenchyma of kidney. SYN: *pyelonephritis.*

nephropyelography (nĕf"rō-pī"ĕ-lŏg'ră-fē) [" + *pyelos,* pelvis, + *graphein,* to write]. Roentgenogram of the kidney and the renal pelvis.

nephropyeloplasty (nĕf"rō-pī'ĕ-lō-plăs"tē) [" + " + *plassein,* to form]. Plastic surgery on the kidney and renal pelvis.

nephropyosis (nĕf"rō-pī-ō'sĭs) [" + *pyosis,* suppuration]. Purulence of a kidney.

nephrorrhagia (nĕf-ror-ā'jē-ă) [" + *rhegnynai,* to burst forth]. Renal hemorrhage into pelvis and tubules.

nephrorrhaphy (nĕf-ror'ă-fē) [" + *rhaphe,* suture]. Surgical procedure of suturing the kidney.

nephros (nĕf'rŏs) [Gr.]. The kidney.

nephrosclerosis (nĕf"rō-sklĕ-rō'sĭs) [" + *sklerosis,* a hardening]. Renal sclerosis or hardening.

n., arterial. Arteriosclerosis of kidney arteries. Results in ischemia, atrophy of parenchyma, and fibrosis of kidney.

n., arteriolar. Sclerosis of the smaller renal arterioles, esp. the afferent glomerular arterioles with resulting fibrosis, ischemic necrosis, and glomerular degeneration and failure. Occurs in most cases of essential hypertension.

n., malignant. Nephrosclerosis that develops rapidly in patients with severe hypertension. SEE: *hypertension, malignant.*

nephrosis (nĕf-rō'sĭs) Gr. *nephros,* kidney, + *osis,* condition]. (pl. *nephroses*) 1. Condition in which there are degenerative changes in the kidneys, esp. the renal tubules, without the occurrence of inflammation. 2. Clinical classification of kidney disease wherein protein loss is so extensive that edema and hypoproteinemia are produced. SEE: *nephrotic syndrome.*

n., acute. Nephrosis accompanying acute infectious disease or resulting from poisoning or metabolic disturbances such as toxemias of pregnancy or obstructive jaundice. Marked by decreased secretion of urine.

n., amyloid. Nephrosis due to deposition of amyloid within the walls of the renal blood vessels and at the base of the cells of the tubules. Marked degeneration of kidney tissue results.

n., lipoid. A chronic disease of unknown etiology in which large amounts of albumin are lost in urine, resulting in depletion of the plasma protein and development of edema. The cause is unknown.

SYM: Gradual development of severe edema. Oliguria, albumin, casts of hyaline and granular type, and lipids in urine. Blood serum proteins markedly reduced, but nitrogenous constituents remain normal. Blood cholesterol and globulin elevated. Hypertension absent. Anemia occurs.

PROG: Guarded.

TREATMENT: High-protein and low-sodium diet. Adrenocortical hormones are useful in most cases but are not curative. SEE: *nephropathy, membranous.*

n., lower nephron. Nephrosis due to pathological changes in the cells of the lower nephron. This causes uremia and renal failure.

nephrosonephritis (nĕ-frō"sō-nĕ-frī'tĭs) [" + *osis,* condition, + *nephros,* kidney, + *itis,* inflammation]. Renal disease with characteristics of nephritis and nephrosis.

nephrospasis (nĕf"rō-spăs'ĭs) [" + Gr. *span,* to draw]. A kidney with poor supporting tissue. This allows the kidney to be suspended by its pedicle.

nephrostoma (nĕ-frŏs'tō-mă) [" + *stoma,* mouth]. The internal orifice of a wolffian tubule, connected with the coelom in the human embryo.

nephrostomy (nĕ-frŏs'tō-mē). Formation of an artificial fistula into the renal pelvis.

nephrotic (nĕ-frŏt'ĭk) [Gr. *nephros,* kidney]. Rel. to, or caused by, nephrosis.

nephrotic syndrome. Disease of the basement membrane of the glomerulus that causes hyponatruria, severe proteinuria, hypoalbuminemia, generalized edema, lipiduria, and hyperlipemia. Blood pressure is normal.

NURSING IMPLICATIONS: Monitor and record blood pressure. Plan care to provide adequate rest periods. Monitor and record intake and output, as well as daily weights. Prevent abrasions and injury to skin. Prevent friction in skin folds by applying talcum powder or cornstarch. Give attractive, small, frequent feedings of preferred high-protein foods. Carefully monitor I.V. protein infusions. Promote activity as tolerated. Provide pulmonary toilet for inactive child. Reassure child that physical changes are temporary. Prevent contact with persons who show signs of infection.

nephrotome (nĕf′rō-tōm) [″ + *tome,* a section]. Embryonic bridge of cells connecting primitive segments along neural tube to the somatic and splanchnic mesoderm from which arises the urogenital system. SYN: *mesomere; nephromere.*

nephrotomogram (nĕf″rō-tō′mō-grăm). A tomogram of the kidney.

nephrotomography (nĕf″rō-tō-mŏg′ră-fē) [″ + ″ + *graphein,* to write]. Tomograph, q.v., of the kidney after the intravenous injection of a radiopaque dye that is excreted by the kidney.

nephrotomy (nĕ-frŏt′ō-mē) [″ + *tome,* incision]. Surgical incision of the kidney.

nephrotoxin (nĕf″rō-tŏk′sĭn) [″ + *toxikon,* poison]. A toxic substance that damages kidney tissues.

nephrotresis (nĕf-rō-trē′sĭs) [″ + *tresis,* piercing]. Formation of a permanent excretory opening in the kidney through the loin.

nephrotropic (nĕf″rō-trŏp′ĭk) [″ + *tropos,* turning]. 1. Affecting the kidneys. 2. An agent or drug that exerts its effect principally on the kidney or renal function.

nephrotuberculosis (nĕf″rō-tū-bĕr″kū-lō′sĭs) [″ + *tuberculum,* a little swelling, + *osis,* condition]. Infection of the kidney due to Mycobacterium tuberculosis.

nephrotyphoid (nĕf″rō-tī′foyd) [″ + *typhos,* stupor, + *eidos,* form]. Renal disease complicating typhoid fever.

nephroureterectomy (nĕf″rō-ū-rē″tĕr-ĕk′tō-mē) [″ + *oureter,* ureter, + *ektome,* excision]. Surgical excision of the kidney with the ureter or part of it.

nephrourography. Radiographic examination of the nephron phase during urography.

nephrydrosis (nĕf″rĭ-drō′sĭs) [″ + *hydor,* water, + *osis,* condition]. Distention and dilatation of renal pelvis resulting from obstruction. SYN: *hydronephrosis; nephrohydrosis.*

Neptazane. Trade name for methazolamide, USP.

neptunium [planet Neptune]. SYMB: Np. At. wt. 237; at. no. 93. An element obtained by bombarding uranium with neutrons.

nerve [L. *nervus,* sinew; Gr. *neuron,* sinew]. A bundle or a group of bundles of nerve fibers outside the central nervous system that connect the brain and spinal cord with various parts of the body. Nerves conduct afferent impulses centrally from receptor organs and efferent impulses peripherally to effector tissues and organs. The fibers of peripheral nerves are the processes of neurons whose cell bodies are located within the brain, spinal cord, or in ganglia. A bundle of nerve fibers is called a fasciculus, q.v. The fibers within a fasciculus are surrounded and held together by delicate connective tissue fibers forming the endoneurium. Each fasciculus is surrounded by a sheath of connective tissue, the perineurium. The entire nerve is enclosed in a thick sheath of connective tissue, the epineurium, which may contain numerous fat cells. Small nerves may lack an epineurium. SYN: *nervus* [NA]. SEE: *cell* and *nerve cell* for illus.; *Nerves* in *Appendix.*

Test for loss of function: It is important to know the extent of peripheral nerve damage and to follow the course of healing. This may be done for injury of nerves of the hand by observing the wrinkling of the hand when it is soaked in warm water for 30 minutes. If the nerve supply is intact, skin of the fingers show characteristic wrinkling; however, the fingers remain unwrinkled over the area in which the nerve supply is absent.

n.'s, accelerator. Nerves to the heart that carry sympathetic fibers that convey impulses. These impulses, when stimulated, accelerate the heartbeat.

n., acoustic. Eighth cranial nerve. SEE: *vestibulocochlear nerve* for illus.

n., adrenergic. A sympathetic nerve that liberates norepinephrine at a synapse when it transmits a stimulus.

n., afferent. Any nerve that transmits impulses from the periphery to the central nervous system.

n., autonomic. A nerve of the autonomic nervous system, q.v.

n., cerebrospinal. A nerve originating from the brain or spinal cord.

n., cholinergic. A parasympathetic nerve that liberates acetylcholine when it transmits a stimulus.

n., cranial. One of the 12 pairs of nerves arising from the brain. They exit through foramina of the cranium. SEE: *cranial nerves; Cranial Nerves* in *Appendix.*

n., depressor. Any afferent nerve that, when stimulated, depresses the activity of an organ or nerve center.

n., efferent. A nerve that transmits impulses from a nerve center to the periphery. SYN: *n., motor.*

n., excitatory. Nerve that transmits impulses that stimulate function.

n., excitoreflex. A visceral nerve that, when stimulated, causes reflex action.

n., facial. Seventh cranial nerve. SEE: *facial nerve* for illus.

n., gangliated. Any sympathetic nervous system nerve.

n., glossopharyngeal. Ninth cranial nerve. SEE: *glossopharyngeal nerve* for illus.

n., inhibitory. A nerve that, upon stimulation, lessens activity in a part.

n., mixed. Nerve containing both afferent (sensory) and efferent (motor) fibers.

n., motor. Nerve containing motor fibers and conveying motor impulses. SYN: *efferent nerve.*

n.'s, olfactory. First pair of cranial nerves. SEE: *olfactory nerve* for illus.

n., optic. Second cranial nerve.

n., parasympathetic. A nerve of the parasympathetic division of the autonomic nervous system. SEE: *parasympathetic nervous system.*

n., peripheral. Any nerve that connects the brain or spinal cord with peripheral receptors or effectors.

n., pilomotor. A nerve that innervates the arrectores pilorum muscles of hair follicles.

n., pressor. An afferent nerve that, when stimulated, excites the vasoconstrictor center and thus increases blood pressure.

n., secretory. Nerve whose stimulation excites secretion in a gland or a tissue.

n., sensory. A nerve that conducts afferent impulses from sensory receptors to the brain or spinal cord.

n., somatic. A nerve that innervates somatic structures, i.e., those comprising the body wall and extremities.

n., spinal. One of 31 pairs of peripheral nerves that connect with the spinal cord. Includes 8 cervical, 12 thoracic, 5 lumbar, 5 sacral, 1 coccygeal. SEE: *cranial nerves.*

n., splanchnic. Nerves that supply the visceral organs.

n., sudomotor. Nerves that supply sweat glands.

n., sympathetic. Nerve of the sympathetic division of the autonomic nervous system. SEE: *autonomic nervous system.*

n., trophic. Any nerve involved in regulating nutrition of tissues.

n., vagus. Tenth cranial nerve. SEE: *vagus nerve* for illus.

n., vasoconstrictor. A nerve that conducts impulses that bring about constriction of a blood vessel.

n., vasodilator. A nerve that conducts impulses that bring about dilation of a blood vessel.

n., vasomotor. Nerve that controls the caliber of a blood vessel. A vasoconstrictor or vasodilator nerve, q.v.

n., vasosensory. Any nerve providing sensory fibers for a vessel.

nerve block. The induction of regional anesthesia by preventing sensory nerve impulses from reaching centers of consciousness. This is usually done on a temporary basis, by using chemical or electrical means. In the former case, it is accomplished by injecting an anesthetic solution, such as procaine, around the nerve but some distance from the region, or by anesthetizing nerve endings in the region itself (infiltration).

nerve cell. A neuron, q.v.; consists of a cell body and its processes, an axon and one or more dendrites. SEE: illus.

nerve ending. The termination of a nerve fiber (axon or dendrite) in a peripheral structure. May be sensory (receptor) or motor (effector). Sensory endings can be nonencapsulated, such as free nerve endings, peritrichal endings, or tactile corpuscles of Merkel, or they can be encapsulated as in the end-bulbs of Krause, Meissner's corpuscles, Vater-Pacini corpuscles, or neuromuscular and neurotendinous spindles.

nerve fiber. An elongated process of a nerve cell or neuron, usually the axon, concerned primarily with the condition of impulses. Nerve fibers form the major portion of the white matter of the brain and spinal cord and all nerves. Most fibers in peripheral nerves are myelinated (also called medullated, which means they are covered by a noncellular sheath of myelin, a fatty substance). The myelin sheath is interrupted at intervals by the nodes of Ranvier. Outside the myelin sheath and closely investing it is another sheath, the neurilemma or sheath of Schwann. Between the two sheaths are Schwann cells, thin cells having flat, oval-shaped nuclei. One Schwann cell occurs at each internode length. Fibers lacking a myelin sheath are called nonmedullated (unmyelinated). The neurilemma is lacking in all fibers of the central nervous system.

n.f., adrenergic. Nerve fiber that liberates norepinephrine at its synapse when an impulse is transmitted. Includes most postganglionic fibers of the sympathetic division.

n.f., arcuate. Arch-shaped nerve fiber in the medulla. They comprise three groups, the external dorsal, external ventral, and internal.

n.f., association. Nerve fiber that connects one region of the cerebral cortex with another region in the same hemisphere.

n.f., cholinergic. Nerve fiber that liberates acetylcholine at its synapse when an impulse is transmitted. Includes preganglionic fibers ending in sympathetic ganglia,

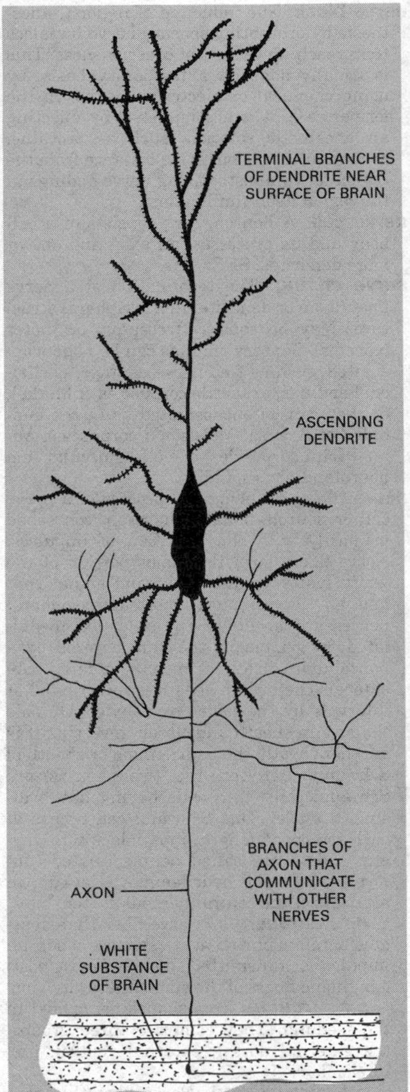

NERVE CELL FROM CEREBRAL CORTEX

postganglionic parasympathetic fibers, and efferent somatic fibers ending in skeletal muscle.

n.f.'s, climbing, of cerebellum. 1. Afferent nerve fibers entering the cortex and synapsing with dendrites of Purkinje cells. SYN: *mossy fibers*. 2. Collateral branches of Purkinje cell axons that return to molecular layer terminating about Purkinje of basket cell dendrites.

n.f., collateral. A small branch of nerve fibers extending at a right angle from an axon.

n.f., commissural. Nerve fiber that passes from one cerebral hemisphere to the other.

n.f., myelinated. A nerve fiber possessing a myelin sheath.

n.f., nonmedullated. Nerve fiber containing only an axis cylinder and a neurilemma.

n.f., postganglionic. Nerve fiber of the autonomic nervous system that terminates in smooth or cardiac muscle or a gland. Its cell body lies in an autonomic ganglion.

n.f., preganglionic. Nerve fiber of the autonomic nervous system that terminates and synapses in one of the autonomic ganglia. Its cell body lies in the brain or spinal cord.

n.f., projection. 1. Nerve fiber arising in the diencephalon and passing to the cerebral cortex. 2. Nerve fiber arising in the cerebral cortex and terminating in lower portions of the brain or in the spinal cord.

nerve fibril. A fine fiber in the cytoplasm and cell processes of a neuron. SYN: *neurofibrilla*.

nerve impulse. The excitatory process that travels along a nerve fiber when stimulated. SEE: *impulse, nervous*.

nerve plexus. A network of nerves.

nerve trunk. The main stem of a peripheral nerve.

nervi. Pl. of nervus.

n. terminales. [NA] Terminal nerves, accompanying the olfactory nerve to the brain. Consist principally of sensory fibers from mucosa of nasal septum.

nervimotility (nĕr″vĭ-mō-tĭl′ĭ-tē) [L. *nervus*, nerve, + *motilis*, moving]. Capability for motion or movement in response to nervous stimulation.

nervimotor (nĕr″vĭ-mō′tor) [″ + *motus*, moving]. Concerning a motor nerve.

nervo- [L. *nervus*, nerve]. Combining form pert. to a nerve.

nervomuscular [″ + *musculus*, a muscle]. Rel. to nerve supply of muscles.

nervone. A cerebroside present in brain tissue; contains nervonic acid.

nervous [L. *nervosus*]. 1. Anxious. 2. Characterized by excitability. 3. Pert. to the nerves.

nervous breakdown. A lay term for any mental condition or illness, esp. one with acute onset, that interferes with normal function, thought, or action.

nervous debility. Nervous fatigue with resultant physical exhaustion. SYN: *neurasthenia.*

nervous impulse. The excitatory process set up in nerve fibers by stimuli. It is probably in the nature of a wave of electrochemical disturbance traveling at the comparatively slow rate (even in fastest conducting mammalian nerves) of 50 to 80 meters per second. The velocity varies in different fibers according to the diameter. SEE: *impulse, nervous.*

nervousness. State of being nervous.

nervous prostration. Neurasthenia, q.v.

nervous system. A system of extremely delicate nerve cells, elaborately interlaced with each other. Made up collectively of the brain, cranial nerves, spinal cord, spinal nerves, autonomic ganglia, ganglionated trunks and nerves, maintaining the vital function of reception and response to stimuli. The nervous system regulates and coordinates body activities and brings about responses by which the body adjusts to changes of environment, either external or internal. These changes constitute stimuli that initiate impulses in receptors or sense organs. The principal organs of this group are the eye, ear, the organs of taste and smell, and sensory receptors located in the skin, joints, muscles, and various parts of the body.

The nervous system is divided into two divisions: the central nervous system, which includes the brain and spinal cord; and the peripheral nervous system, which includes all the other neural elements. SEE: *autonomic nervous system; central nervous system; parasympathetic nervous system; sympathetic nervous system.*

nervous tissue. The tissue that comprises the nervous system. Includes the nervous elements proper (neurons) and the interstitial tissue (neuroglia, neurilemma cells, and satellite cells).

nervus [L.]. (pl. *nervi*) [NA] Nerve. SEE: *Nerves* in *Appendix.*

n. erigens. [NA] A scattered bundle of craniosacral autonomic fibers originating from the 2nd to 4th sacral nerves and passing to terminal ganglia from which postganglionic fibers pass to the pelvic organs (bladder, colon, rectum, prostate gland, seminal vesicles, external genitalia).

n. intermedius. [NA] A branch of the facial nerve consisting principally of sensory fibers.

n. nervorum. Nerve fibers that innervate sheaths of nerves.

n. vasorum. Nerve fibers that innervate the walls of blood vessels.

Nesacaine. Trade name for chloroprocaine hydrochloride, USP.

nesidiectomy (nē-sĭd″ē-ĕk′tō-mē) [Gr. *nesidion,* islet, + *ektome,* excision]. Surgical excision of islet cell tissue of the pancreas.

nesidioblastoma (nē-sĭd″ē-ō-blăs-tō′mă) [″ + *blastos,* germ, + *oma,* tumor]. Islet-cell tumor of the pancreas.

nesslerize (nĕs′lĕr-īz). To test with Nessler's reagent.

Nessler's reagent (nĕs′lĕrz). [A. Nessler, Ger. chemist, 1827–1905] A solution used to test for ammonia. It contains potassium iodide, mercuric chloride, and potassium hydroxide.

nest. A small mass of cells, resembling a bird nest, and that is alien to the surrounding tissue.

n., cancer. A mass of cells extending from a common center; seen in cancerous growths.

n., cell. A small mass of epithelial cells set apart from surrounding cells by connective tissue.

nesteostomy (nĕs″tē-ŏs′tō-mē) [Gr. *nestis,* jejunum, + *stoma,* mouth]. Jejunostomy, q.v.

nestiatria (nĕs″tē-ā′trē-ă) [Gr. *nestis,* fasting, + *iatreia,* medical treatment]. Fasting therapy.

n. et m. *nocte et mane,* night and morning.

net reproductive rate. ABBR: NRR. A measure of whether a population is reproducing at a greater or lesser rate than needed for its replacement. It is determined by calculating the average number of surviving daughters born to the women in that population during their reproductive years. An NRR of 1 indicates that each woman in the population has one surviving daughter during her lifetime.

ne tr. s. num. *ne tradas sine nummo,* do not deliver unless paid.

nettle. Plants of the genus Urtica. Their saw-toothed leaves contain hairs that secrete a fluid that irritates the skin.

nettle rash [AS. *netel*]. Skin rash with intense itching, resembling condition produced by stinging with nettles. SYN: *hives; urticaria.*

network [AS. *net,* net, + *wyrcan,* to work]. Fiber arrangement in a structure resembling a net. SYN: *rete; reticulum.*

Neumann's disease (noy′mănz). [Isidor Neumann, Austrian dermatologist, 1832–1906] Pemphigus vegetans.

neuragmia (nū-răg′mē-ă) [Gr. *neuron,* sinew, + *agmos,* break]. The tearing or rupturing of a nerve trunk.

neurad (nū′răd) [Gr. *neuron,* sinew, + L. *-ad,* toward]. Toward a nerve or its axis.

neural (nū′răl) [L. *neuralis*]. Pert. to nerves or connected with the nervous system.

neural crest. A band of cells extending longitudinally along the neural tube of an embryo from which cells forming cranial, spinal, and autonomic ganglia arise. They also give rise to cells (ectomesenchyme) that migrate into the forming facial region and become odontoblasts, which form the dentin of the tooth.

neural fold. One of two longitudinal elevations of the neural plate of an embryo that unite to form the neural tube.

neuralgia (nū-răl′jē-ă) [Gr. *neuron,* sinew, + *algos,* pain]. Severe sharp pain along the course of a nerve. SYN: *neurodynia.* SEE: *sciatica.*

ETIOL: Pressure on nerve trunks, faulty nerve nutrition, toxins, neuritis. Usually no morphologic changes can be detected.

n., cardiac. Angina pectoris.

n., degenerative. Neuralgia caused by degenerative changes in the nerves or nerve cells; occurs in the elderly.

n., facial. N., trigeminal, q.v.

n., facialis vera. N., geniculate, q.v.

n., Fothergill's. N., trigeminal, q.v.

n., geniculate. Neuralgia characterized by pain over all or any part supplied by sensory fibers of facial nerve. Pain may be deep in facial muscles, within the ear, or in pharynx. SYN: *n., Hunt's.*

n., glossopharyngeal. Neuralgia along the course of the glossopharyngeal nerve characterized by severe pain in back of throat, tonsils, and middle ear.

n., hallucinatory. Impression of local pain without an actual stimulus to cause the pain.

n., Hunt's. N., geniculate.

n., idiopathic. Neuralgia without structural lesion or pressure from a lesion.

n., intercostal. Neuralgia where pain follows course of intercostal nerves; frequently associated with eruption of herpes zoster. Spots of tenderness near vertebral column, in middle of nerve, and near sternum. May be dependent upon spinal caries or thoracic aneurysm. SYN: *pleuralgia.*

n., mammary. Neuralgia of the breast. SYN: *mastodynia.*

n., Morton's. Neuralgia of joint of third and fourth toes. SYN: *metatarsalgia.*

n., nasociliary. Neuralgia of eyes, brows, and root of nose.

n., occipital. Neuralgia involving upper cervical nerves. A spot of tenderness found between mastoid process and upper cervical vertebrae. May be due to spinal caries.

n., otic. N., geniculate.

n., reminiscent. Continued mental perception of pain after neuralgia has ceased.

n., sphenopalatine. Neuralgia of the sphenopalatine ganglion, causing pain in the area of the upper jawbone and radiating into the neck and shoulders.

SYM: Pain on one side of face radiating to eyeballs, ear, occipital and mastoid areas of skull; sometimes to nose, upper teeth, and shoulder of same side.

PROG: Good.

n., stump. Neuralgia due to pressure on nerves at site of amputation.

n., symptomatic. Neuralgia not primarily involving the nerve structure but occurring as a symptom of local or systemic disease.

n., trifacial. Old term for trigeminal neuralgia.

n., trigeminal. Neuralgia involving the gasserian ganglion or one or more branches of the trigeminal nerve. SYN: *n., facial; n., Fothergill's; tic douloureux.*

ETIOL: Unknown. Attacks often precipitated by initiation of pain by obvious stimuli on certain hypersensitive areas called trigger zones of face, lips, or tongue.

SYM: Tender points correspond to supraorbital, infraorbital, and mental foramina. Often violent spasm of muscles. In long-standing cases, hair on affected side sometimes becomes coarse and bleached.

TREATMENT: Use of drugs such as phenytoin or dibenzazepine has been useful in suppressing or shortening attacks. Their use for temporary relief may permit spontaneous remission. If, however, the syndrome persists, then the nerve is injected with alcohol or phenol, or it is surgically sectioned.

neuralgic (nū-răl′jĭk) [Gr. *neuron,* sinew, + *algos,* pain]. Of, or concerning, neuralgia.

neuralgiform (nū-răl′jĭ-form) [″ + ″ + L. *forma,* form]. Similar to neuralgia.

neural plate. A thickened band of ectoderm along the dorsal surface of an embryo. The nervous system develops from this tissue.

neural spine. Spinous vertebral process.

neural tube. Tube formed from fusion of the neural folds from which the brain and spinal cord arise.

neuramebimeter (nū″răm-ē-bĭm′ĕt-ĕr) [″ + *amoibe,* response, + *metron,* a measure]. Device for determining time of response of a nerve to a stimulus.

neuraminidase (nūr-ăm′ĭn-ĭ-dās″). An enzyme present on the surface of influenza virus particles. Activity of this enzyme enables the virus particle to separate itself from cells. Persons with increased levels of antibodies against neuraminidase in their serum may have increased resistance to influenza infection.

neuranagenesis (nū″răn-ă-jĕn′ĕ-sĭs) [″ + *anagennan,* to regenerate]. Regeneration of a nerve.

neurapophysis (nū″ră-pŏf′ĭ-sĭs) [″ + *apo,* from, + *physis,* growth]. Either of the two sides of a vertebra that unite to form the neural arch.

neurapraxia (nū″ră-prăks′ē-ă) [″ + *apraxia,*

nonactive]. Cessation in function of a peripheral nerve without degenerative changes occurring. Recovery is the usual outcome.

neurarchy (nū'răr-kē) [" + *arche,* rule]. The domination of the nervous system over the body.

neurarthropathy (nū"răr-thrŏp'ă-thē) [" + *arthron,* joint, + *pathos,* disease]. Neuroarthropathy, q.v.

neurasthenia (nū"răs-thē'nē-ă) [" + *astheneia,* weakness]. A term previously used for persons with unexplained chronic fatigue and lassitude. Accompanying these symptoms were usually nervousness, irritability, anxiety, depression, headache, insomnia, and sexual disorders. Those individuals are now diagnosed according to their total condition, such as some form of psychiatric illness, esp. anxiety neurosis or tension state.

neurasthenic (nū-răs-thē'nĭk). 1. Individual suffering from neurasthenia. 2. Suffering from or concerning neurasthenia.

neuratrophia, neuratrophy (nū-ră-trō'fē-ă, -răt'rō-fē) [" + *atrophia,* a wasting]. Atrophy of the nervous tissue or deficient nutrition of the nervous system.

neuraxis (nū-răk'sĭs) [" + L. *axon,* axis]. The cerebrospinal axis.

neuraxitis (nū-răks-ī'tĭs) [" + " + *itis,* inflammation]. Encephalitis.

n., epidemic. Epidemic encephalitis.

neuraxon(e) (nū-răks'ŏn). The axis cylinder process of a nerve cell. SYN: *axon.* SEE: *nerve fiber.*

neurectasia, neurectasis, neurectasy (nū"rĕk-tā'sē-ă, -rĕk'tă-sĭs, -rĕk'tă-sē) [" + *ektasis,* a stretching]. Surgical nerve stretching. SYN: *neurotension.*

neurectomy (nū-rĕk'tō-mē) [" + *ektome,* excision]. Partial or total excision or resection of a nerve.

neurectopia, neurectopy (nū-rĕk-tō'pē-ă, nūr-ĕk'tō-pē) [" + *ek,* out, + *topos,* place]. Displacement or abnormal position of a nerve.

neurenteric (nū-rĕn-tĕr'ĭk) [" + *enteron,* intestine]. Rel. to the neural canal and intestinal tube of the embryo.

neurenteric canal. Temporary canal of the embryo, between the neural and intestinal tubes. In human development, the temporary communication between cavities of the yolk sac and the amnion.

neurepithelium (nūr"ĕp-ĭ-thē'lē-ŭm) [" + *epi,* upon, + *thele,* nipple]. 1. Epithelial structures forming the terminations of nerves of special sense. 2. Embryonic layer from which arises the cerebrospinal axis. SYN: *neuroepithelium.*

neurergic (nū-rĕr'jĭk) [" + *ergon,* work]. Concerning the activity of a nerve.

neurexeresis (nūr"ĕks-ĕr'ĕ-sĭs) [" + *exairein,* to draw out]. Ripping or tearing out of a nerve to relieve neuralgia.

neuriatry (nū-rī'ă-trē) [" + *iatreia,* medication]. Neurology, q.v.

neurilemma (nū'rĭ-lĕm"mă) [" + *lemma,* husk]. A thin membranous sheath enveloping a nerve fiber. SYN: *neurolemma; sheath of Schwann.* SEE: *nerve fiber.*

neurilemmitis (nū"rĭ-lĕm-mī'tĭs) [" + " + *itis,* inflammation]. Inflamed condition of a neurilemma.

neurilemoma, neurilemmoma (nū"rĭ-lĕm-ō'mă) [" + *eilema,* tight sheath, + *oma,* tumor]. A firm, encapsulated fibrillar tumor of peripheral nerves. SYN: *neurinoma; neurofibroma; peripheral glioma; schwannoma.*

neurilemosarcoma (nū"rĭ-lĕm"ō-săr-kō'mă). A malignant neurilemoma.

neurimotility (nū"rĭ-mō-tĭl'ĭ-tē) [" + *motilus,* moving]. Nervimotility, q.v.

neurimotor [" + L. *motor,* a mover]. Concerning a motor nerve.

neurinoma (nū-rĭ-nō'mă) [" + *oma,* tumor]. A peripheral glioma. A tumor of a peripheral nerve arising from endoneurium or sheath of Schwann. SYN: *neurilemmoma; neurofibroma; schwannoma.*

neurinomatosis (nū"rĭ-nō-mă-tō'sĭs) [" + " + *osis,* condition]. Condition of having multiple neurinomas on nerve fibers. SYN: *neurofibromatosis.*

neurite (nū'rīt) [Gr. *neuron,* sinew]. The axis cylinder process of a neuron. Both axites and dendrites are neurites. SYN: *neuraxon.*

neuritis (nū-rī'tĭs) [" + *itis,* inflammation]. Inflammation of a nerve or nerves, usually associated with a degenerative process. SEE: *Guillain-Barré syndrome; polyneuritis.*

ETIOL: Mechanical factors: compression, contusion, trauma. Infections: localized involving direct infection of nerves or may accompany diseases such as leprosy, tetanus, tuberculosis, malaria, or measles. Toxins: esp. poisoning by heavy metals (arsenic, lead, mercury), alcohol, or carbon tetrachloride. Metabolic factors: as in thiamine deficiency, gastrointestinal dysfunction, diabetes, or toxemias of pregnancy. Vascular: as in neuritis accompanying peripheral vascular disease.

SYM: Neuralgia in part affected; hyperesthesia, paresthesia, dysesthesia, hypesthesia, or anesthesia; muscular atrophy of part supplied by affected nerve; paralysis; lack of reflexes.

NURSING IMPLICATIONS: Maintain bedrest. Provide passive range of motion exercises to all joints. Apply wrist splints and footboard as indicated. Administer analgesics prescribed for hyperesthesias. Assess, record, and report any neurological dysfunction. Remove causative factors. Promote dietary therapy for metabolic disorders. Avoid application of temperature extremes to affected areas. Provide daily skin care and massage.

n., adventitial. Inflammation of nerve sheath.

n., ascending. Neuritis moving upward along a nerve trunk away from periphery.

n., axial. Inflammation of inner portion of a nerve.

n., degenerative. Neuritis with rapid degeneration of nerve.

n., descending. Neuritis that leads away from the central nervous system.

n., dietetic. Beriberi.

n., diphtheritic. Neuritis following diphtheria.

n., disseminated. Neuritis involving a large group of nerves.

n., endemic. Beriberi.

n., interstitial. Neuritis involving connective tissue of a nerve.

n., intraocular. Neuritis of retinal fibers of optic nerve.

SYM: Disturbed vision, contracted field, enlarged blind spot, fundus findings such as exudates, hemorrhages, and abnormal condition of blood vessels.

TREATMENT: Depends on etiology such as brain tumors, meningitis, syphilis, nephritis, diabetes.

n. migrans. Neuritis that passes along a nerve trunk, affecting one area and then another. May be ascending or descending, q.v.

n., multiple. Simultaneous impairment of a number of peripheral nerves. SYN: *polyneuritis.*

SYM: Related to suddenness of onset and severity; usually lower limbs are affected first with weakness that may progress until the entire body is affected. Muscle strength, deep tendon reflexes, sensory nerves, and autonomic nerves become involved.

ETIOL: Infectious diseases such as diphtheria; metabolic disorders including alcoholism, diabetes, pellagra, beriberi, and sprue; various poisons, including lead. In some instances the disease arises without apparent cause.

TREATMENT: Remove causative factors if possible. Skilled nursing with particular care taken to prevent bedsores. Dietary therapy depending upon the etiology.

n. nodosa. Neuritis with formation of nodes on nerves.

n., optic. Neuritis of optic nerve.

n., parenchymatous. Neuritis of nerve fiber substance.

n., peripheral. Neuritis of terminal nerves or end-organs.

n., retrobulbar. Neuritis of optic nerve behind the eyeball.

SYM: Acute loss of vision in one or both eyes. Pain may be absent or unbearable and may last for days or only a brief period.

ETIOL: May be caused by a variety of illnesses but is most frequently caused by multiple sclerosis, pernicious anemia, diabetes, alcohol ingestion, or excessive use of tobacco.

n., rheumatic. Neuritis with symptoms of rheumatism.

n., sciatic. Inflammation of the sciatic nerve. SEE: *sciatica.*

n., segmental. Neuritis affecting segments of a nerve interspersed with healthy segments.

n., senile. Neuritis in the elderly, usually affecting the extremities.

n., sympathetic. Neuritis of the opposite nerve without attacking nerve center.

n., tabetic. Neuritis in locomotor ataxia. Caused by syphilis.

n., toxic. Neuritis resulting from poisons. Metallic poisons such as arsenic, mercury, and thallium or nonmetallic poisons such as various hydrocarbons and organic solvents can cause this.

n., traumatic. Neuritis following an injury.

neuro- [Gr. *neuron,* sinew, nerve]. Combining form indicating rel. to a nerve, nervous tissue, or nervous system.

neuroallergy (nū″rō-ăl′ĕr-jē) [″ + *allos,* other, + *ergon,* work]. Allergy in nervous tissue.

neuroanastomosis (nū″rō-ă-năs″tō-mō′sĭs) [″ + *anastomosis,* opening]. Surgical attachment of one end of a severed nerve to the other end.

neuroanatomy (nū″rō-ăn-ăt′ō-mē). Study of anatomy of the nervous system.

neuroarthritism (nū″rō-ăr′thrĭ-tĭzm) [″ + *arthron,* joint, + *-ismos,* condition]. Tendency toward contraction of nervous and gouty disorders.

neuroarthropathy (nū″rō-ăr-thrŏp′ăth-ē) [″ + ″ + *pathos,* disease]. Disease of a joint combined with disease of the central nervous system.

neuroastrocytoma (nū″rō-ăs″trō-sī-tō′mă) [″ + *kytos,* cell, + *oma,* tumor]. A tumor of the central nervous system composed of neurons and glial cells.

neurobiology (nū″rō-bī-ŏl′ō-jē) [″ + *bios,* life, + *logos,* study]. Biology of the nervous system.

neurobiotaxis (nū″rō-bī-ō-tăk′sĭs) [″ + *bios,* life, + *taxis,* order]. The phenomenon involving growth of dendrites and migration of nerve-cell bodies during development toward the region from which their dominant impulses are initiated.

neuroblast (nū′rō-blăst) [″ + *blastos,* germ]. An embryonic cell derived from neural tube or neural crest, giving rise to a neuron.

neuroblastoma (nū″rō-blăs-tō′mă) [″ + ″ + *oma,* tumor]. A malignant hemorrhagic tumor composed principally of cells resembling neuroblasts that give rise to cells of the sympathetic system, esp. adrenal medulla. Occurs chiefly in infants and children. Primary sites are in the mediastinal and retroperitoneal regions.

neurocanal (nū″rō-kă-năl′) [″ + L. *canalis,* passage]. The central canal of the spinal cord.

neurocardiac (nū″rō-kăr′dē-ăk) [″ + *kardia,* heart]. 1. Pert. to the nerves supplying the heart or nervous system and the heart. 2. Concerning a cardiac neurosis.

neurocele (nū′rō-sēl) [″ + *koilia,* cavity]. Ventricles and cavities in the cerebrospinal axis.

neurocentral (nū″rō-sĕn′trăl) [″ + *kentron,* center]. Pert. to the centrum of a vertebra and the neural arch.

neurocentrum (nū″rō-sĕn′trŭm). The body of a vertebra.

neurochemistry (nū″rō-kĕm′ĭs-trē). Physiological chemistry dealing with nervous tissue.

neurochitin (nū″rō-kī′tĭn). Neurokeratin, q.v.

neurochorioretinitis (nū″rō-kō″rē-ō-rĕ″tĭn-ī′tĭs) [Gr. *neuron,* sinew, + *chorion,* skin, + L. *retina,* retina, + Gr. *itis,* inflammation]. Inflammation of choroid and retina combined with optic neuritis.

neurochoroiditis (nū″rō-kō-roy-dī′tĭs) [″ + ″ + *eidos,* resemblance, + *itis,* inflammation]. Inflamed condition of the choroid coat and optic nerve.

neurocirculatory (nū″rō-sŭr′kū-lă-tō″rē) [″ + L. *circulatio,* circulation]. Pert. to circulation and the nervous system.

neurocirculatory asthenia. A combination of functional nervous and circulatory disturbances with fatigue and precordial pain.

neurocladism (nū-rŏk′lă-dĭzm) [″ + Gr. *klados,* a young branch]. Phenomenon occurring after a nerve is severed, where an outgrowth of fibrils closes the gap and begins the process of nerve repair. SYN: *odogenesis.*

neuroclonic (nū″rō-klŏn′ĭk) [″ + *klonos,* spasm]. Marked by spasms of nervous origin.

neurocoele (nū′rō-sēl) [″ + *koilia,* cavity]. System of cavities in cerebrospinal axis. SYN: *neurocele.*

neurocranium (nū″rō-krā′nē-ŭm) [″ + *kranion,* skull]. The part of the skull enclosing the brain.

neurocrine (nū′rō-krĭn) [″ + *krinein,* to secrete]. 1. Indicating an endocrine influence on nerves or the influence of nerves on endocrine tissue. 2. A chemical transmitter.

neurocutaneous (nū″rō-kū-tā′nē-ŭs) [″ + L. *cutis,* skin]. Pert. to the nervous system and skin.

neurocyte (nū′rō-sīt) [″ + *kytos,* cell]. A nerve cell. SYN: *neuron.*

neurocytoma (nū″rō-sī-tō′mă) [″ + ″ + *oma,* tumor]. A tumor formed of cells, usually ganglionic, of nervous origin. SEE: *neuroma.*

neurodealgia (nū-rō″dē-ăl′jē-ă) [Gr. *neurodes,* retina, + *algos,* pain]. Pain in the retina.

neurodendrite, neurodendron (nū″rō-dĕn′drīt, -drŏn) [Gr. *neuron,* sinew, + *dendron,* tree]. Protoplasmic branched process of a nerve cell. SYN: *dendrite; dendron.* SEE: *dendrite* and *nerve cell* for illus.

neurodermatitis (nū″rō-dĕr-mă-tī′tĭs) [″ + *derma,* skin, + *itis,* inflammation]. Cutaneous inflammation with itching that is associated with, but not entirely due to, emotional disturbance. Circumscribed neurodermatitis is used as a synonym for lichen simplex.

n., disseminated. Chronic superficial inflammation of skin characterized by thickening, excoriation, and lichenification, beginning usually in infancy. Common in families with high familial incidence of allergic diseases. SYN: *dermatitis, atopic.*

neurodermatosis (nū″rō-dĕr-mă-tō′sĭs) [″ + ″ + *osis,* condition]. Any skin disease of neural origin. Includes neurofibromatosis (von Recklinghausen's disease), von Hippel-Lindau disease, Sturge-Weber syndrome, and tuberous sclerosis. SYN: *phacomatosis.*

neurodermatrophia (nū″rō-dĕrm″ă-trōf′ē-ă). Atrophy of the skin from nervous disease.

neurodiagnosis (nū″rō-dī-ăg-nō′sĭs). Diagnosis of nervous disorders.

neurodynamic (nū″rō-dī-năm′ĭk). Concerning nervous force or energy.

neurodynia (nū″rō-dĭn′ē-ă) [Gr. *neuron,* nerve, + *odyne,* pain]. Pain in a nerve or nerves. SYN: *neuralgia.*

neuroectoderm (nū″rō-ĕk′tō-dĕrm) [″ + *ektos,* outside, + *derma,* skin]. The embryonic tissue that gives rise to nerve tissue.

neuroencephalomyelopathy (nū″rō-ĕn-sĕf″ă-lō-mī″ĕ-lŏp′ă-thē) [″ + *enkephalos,* brain, + *myelos,* marrow, + *pathos,* disease]. Disease of the brain, spinal cord, and nerves.

neuroendocrine (nū″rō-ĕn′dō-krĭn). Pert. to the nervous and endocrine systems as an integrated functioning mechanism.

neuroendocrinology (nū″rō-ĕn″dō-krĭ-nŏl′ō-jē) [″ + *endon,* within, + *krinein,* to secrete, + *logos,* study]. Study of the relationship between the nervous and endocrine systems.

neuroenteric (nū″rō-ĕn-tĕr′ĭk). Concerning the nervous system and intestines.

neuroepidermal (nū″rō-ĕp-ĭ-dĕr′măl) [″ + *epi,* upon, + *derma,* skin]. Pert. to or giving rise to the nervous system and epidermis.

neuroepithelioma (nū″rō-ĕp″ĭ-thē-lē-ō′mă) [″ + ″ + *thele,* nipple, + *oma,* tumor]. A relatively rare tumor of neuroepithelium in a nerve of special sense.

neuroepithelium (nū″rō-ĕp″ĭ-thē′lē-ŭm). 1. A specialized epithelial structure forming the termination of a nerve of special sense. Includes gustatory cells, olfactory cells, hair cells of inner ear, and rods and cones of retina. 2. Embryonic layer of the epiblast from which the cerebrospinal axis is developed. SYN: *neurepithelium.*

neurofibril, neurofibrilla (nū-rō-fī′brĭl, -fī-brĭl′ă) [″ + L. *fibrilla,* a small fiber]. (pl. *neurofibrils, neurofibrillae*) Many tiny fibrils that extend in every direction in the cytoplasm of the nerve cell body. They extend into the axon and dendrites of the cell. SEE: *neuron.*

neurofibroma (nū″rō-fī-brō′mă) [Gr. *neuron,* nerve, + L. *fibra,* fiber, + Gr. *oma,* tumor]. (pl. *neurofibromata* or *-mas*) A tumor of connective tissue of a nerve including medullated layer of a nerve fiber. May occur in mouth, pleura, or stomach. SYN: *pseudoneuroma.*

neurofibromatosis (nū″rō-fī-brō″mă-tō′sĭs) [″ + ″ + ″ + *osis,* condition]. Condition in which there are tumors of various sizes on peripheral nerves. They may be neuromas or fibromas. SYN: *neurinomatosis.* SEE: *neuroma, multiple; von Recklinghausen's disease.*

neurofibrosarcoma (nū″rō-fī″brō-săr-kō′mă) [″ + ″ + Gr. *sarx,* flesh, + *oma,* tumor]. A malignant neurofibroma. SYN: *neurogenic sarcoma.*

neurofibrositis (nū″rō-fī″brō-sī′tĭs) [″ + ″ + Gr. *itis,* inflammation]. Inflammation of nerve fibers and sensory nerve fibers in muscular tissue.

neurogangliitis (nū″rō-găn-glē-ī′tĭs) [″ + *ganglion,* knot, + *itis,* inflammation]. Inflamed condition of a neuroganglion.

neuroganglion (nū″rō-găn′glē-ŏn). A mass of nervous tissue.

neurogastric (nū″rō-găs′trĭk) [″ + *gaster,* belly]. Concerning the nerves of the stomach.

neurogenesis (nū″rō-jĕn′ĕ-sĭs) [″ + *genesis,* production]. 1. Growth or development of nerves. 2. Development from nervous tissue.

neurogenetic (nūr″ō-jĕn-ĕt′ĭk). 1. Pert. to nerve formation. 2. Pert. to origin in nerves.

neurogenic, neurogenous (nū-rō-jĕn′ĭk, -rŏj′ĕn-ŭs). 1. Originating from nervous tissue. 2. Due to or resulting from nervous impulses.

neuroglia (nū-rŏg′lē-ă) [″ + *glia,* glue]. The tissue that forms the interstitial or supporting elements—cells and fibers—of the nervous system. Neuroglia, also called glia, includes astrocytes, oligodendroglias, microglia (mesoglia), ependyma, neurilemma sheath cells or nerve fibers (cells of Schwann), and satellite (capsule) cells surrounding cranial and spinal ganglia. All except the microglia are of ectodermal origin. Neuroglia acts as connective or supporting tissue and also plays an important role in the reaction of the nervous system to injury or infection.

neurogliacyte (nū-rŏg′lē-ă-sīt) [″ + ″ + *kytos,* cell]. Any one of the cells found in neuroglial tissue. SYN: *glia cell.*

neuroglial (nū-rŏg′lē-ăl). Pert. to the neuroglia.

neuroglioma (nū″rō-glī-ō′mă) [Gr. *neuron,* nerve, + *glia,* glue, + *oma,* tumor]. Tumor of neuroglial tissue. SYN: *glioma.*

n., ganglionar. Glioma with ganglion cells.

neurogliomatosis (nū″rō-glī″ō-mă-tō′sĭs) [″ + ″ + ″ + *osis,* condition]. Multiple glioma formation in the nervous system.

neurogliosis (nū-rŏg″lē-ō′sĭs) [″ + ″ + *osis,* condition]. Development of numerous neurogliomas.

neurogram (nū′rō-grăm). Engram, q.v.

neurography (nū-rŏg′ră-fē) [″ + *graphein,* to write]. A study or description of the nervous system.

neurohematology (nū″rō-hĕm″ă-tŏl′ō-jē) [″ + *haima,* blood, + *logos,* study]. The study of blood changes in neural diseases.

neurohistology (nū″rō-hĭs-tŏl′ō-jē) [″ + *histos,* tissue, + *logos,* study]. Study of the microscopic anatomy of nervous tissue.

neurohormone (nū′rō-hor″mōn) [″ + *hormon,* urging on]. 1. A hormone that affects nervous system function. 2. A hormone released due to nervous stimuli.

neurohumor (nū-rō-hū′mor). A chemical substance liberated at a nerve ending that excites or activates an adjacent structure (neuron or muscle fiber). Ex.: acetylcholine, epinephrine, norepinephrine. These substances are essential for transmission of impulses across synapses or myoneural junctions.

neurohypophysis (nū″rō-hī-pŏf′ĭs-ĭs) [″ + *hypo,* under, + *physis,* growth]. Posterior portion or pars nervosa of the pituitary gland.

neuroid (nū′royd) [″ + *eidos,* form]. Similar to a nerve.

neuroinduction (nū″rō-ĭn-dŭk′shŭn) [″ + L. *inductus,* leading]. Mental suggestion.

neurokeratin (nū″rō-kĕr′ă-tĭn) [″ + *keras,* horn]. The type of keratin found in myelinated nerve fibers.

neurokyme (nū′rō-kīm) [″ + *kyma,* wave]. A nerve process or action.

neurolemma. Neurilemma.

neurolemmitis (nū″rō-lĕ-mī′tĭs) [″ + *lemma,* husk]. Neurilemmitis, q.v.

neurolemmoma (nū″rō-lĕ-mō′mă) [″ + ″ + *oma,* tumor]. Neurilemoma, q.v.

neuroleptanesthesia (nū″rō-lĕp″tăn-ĕs-thē′zē-ă) [″ + *leptos,* slender, + *-an,* not, + *ais-*

thesis, sensation]. General anesthesia involving intravenous administration of a neuroleptic drug, and an analgesic.

neuroleptic (nū"rō-lĕp'tĭk) [" + *lepsis,* a taking hold]. 1. An agent or drug that modifies psychotic behavior. 2. Indicating a condition produced by a neuroleptic agent.

neuroleptic anesthesia. SEE: *anesthesia, neuroleptic.*

neuroleptic drugs. Medicines that produce symptoms resembling those of diseases of the nervous system.

neurologic, neurological (nū-rō-lŏj'ĭk, -ĭ-kăl) [" + *logos,* study]. Pert. to the study of nervous diseases.

neurologist (nū-rŏl'ō-jĭst). A specialist in diseases of the nervous system.

neurology (nū-rŏl'ō-jē) [" + *logos,* study]. The branch of medicine that deals with the nervous system and its diseases. SEE: *psychiatry and neurology, words pert. to.*

n., clinical. The branch of medicine that is concerned with study and treatment of diseases of the nervous system.

neurolymphomatosis (nū"rō-lĭm"fō-mă-tō'sĭs) [" + L. *lympha,* lymph, + Gr. *oma,* tumor, + *osis,* condition]. Malignant lymphoma involving the nervous system.

neurolysin (nū-rŏl'ĭs-ĭn) [" + *lysis,* destruction]. A substance that destroys nerve cells.

neurolysis (nū-rŏl'ĭs-ĭs). 1. Stretching of a nerve to relieve tension. 2. Loosening of adhesions surrounding a nerve. 3. Disintegration or destruction of nerve tissue.

neurolytic (nū-rō-lĭt'ĭk). Concerning neurolysis.

neuroma (nū-rō'mă) [" + *oma,* tumor]. Former term for any type of tumor composed of nerve cells. New growth of nerves is now categorized with respect to the specific portion of the nerve involved. SEE: *ganglioneuroma; neurilemoma.*

n., acoustic. A benign tumor of the eighth cranial nerve. The symptoms may include hearing loss, balance disturbances, pain, headache, and tinnitus.

n., amputation. Neuroma occurring on a stump after amputation.

n., amyelinic. Neuroma composed principally of unmyelinated nerve fibers.

n., appendiceal. Neuroma found in mucosa and submucosa of the appendix.

n. cutis. Neuroma in the skin.

n., cystic. Neuroma with cystic formations.

n., false. Tumor arising from connective tissue of nerves, including the myelin sheath. SYN: *neurofibroma; pseudoneuroma.*

n., ganglionated. Neuroma composed of true nerve cells.

n., multiple. Neurofibromatosis.

n., myelinic. Neuroma composed of medullated nerve fibers.

n., plexiform. Neuroma of nerve trunks that appear to be twisted.

n. telangiectodes. Neuroma with an abundance of blood vessels contained within it.

n., traumatic. Unorganized mass of nerve fibers occurring in wounds or on an amputation stump; result of accidental or intentional incision of the nerve.

neuromalacia (nū"rō-măl-ā'sē-ă) [" + *malakia,* softening]. Pathological softening of neural tissue.

neuromatosis (nū-rō"mă-tō'sĭs) [" + *oma,* tumor, + *osis,* condition]. Multiple neuromas occurring in the body.

neuromatous (nū-rō'mă-tŭs). Rel. to a neuroma.

neuromechanism (nū"rō-mĕk'ăn-ĭzm). The neural structure controlling organic and systemic function.

neuromere (nū'rō-mēr) [" + *meros,* part]. One of a series of segmental elevations on the ventrolateral surface of the rhombencephalon.

neuromimesis (nū"rō-mĭ-mē'sĭs) [" + *mimesis,* imitation]. Hysterical or neurotic simulation of organic disease.

neuromuscular (nū"rō-mŭs'kū-lăr) [" + L. *musculus,* a muscle]. Concerning both nerves and muscles.

neuromyasthenia (nū"rō-mī"ăs-thē'nē-ă) [" + *mys,* muscle, + *astheneia,* weakness]. Muscular weakness usually due to an emotional disorder.

neuromyelitis (nū"rō-mī-ĕl-ī'tĭs) [" + *myelos,* marrow, + *itis,* inflammation]. Inflammation of nerves and the spinal cord.

n. optica. A syndrome resulting from demyelinization occurring in the spinal cord, optic nerves, and chiasma. Etiology is unknown. May be a variant form of multiple sclerosis.

neuromyopathic (nū"rō-mī"ō-păth'ĭk) [" + *mys,* muscle, + *pathos,* disease]. Pert. to pathological conditions involving both muscles and nerves.

neuromyositis (nū"rō-mī"ō-sī'tĭs) [" + " + *itis,* inflammation]. Neuritis complicated by inflammation of muscles that come in contact with affected nerves.

neuron (nū'rŏn) [Gr. *neuron,* nerve, sinew]. A nerve cell, the structural and functional unit of the nervous system. A neuron consists of a cell body or perikaryon and its processes, an axon, and one or more dendrites. Neurons function in initiation and conduction of impulses. SEE: *nerve; nervous impulse; nervous system.*

n., afferent. Neuron that conducts impulses toward brain or spinal cord.

n., associative. Neuron that mediates

impulses between a sensory and a motor neuron.

n., bipolar. Neuron that bears two processes.

n., central. Neuron confined entirely to central nervous system.

n., commissural. Neuron whose axon crosses to opposite side of brain or spinal cord.

n., efferent. Neuron that conducts impulses away from the brain or spinal cord.

n., motor. Neuron that conveys impulses initiating muscle contraction. SEE: illus.

n., motor, lower. Neuron whose cell body lies in anterior gray column of spinal cord. Its axon innervates striated muscle fibers.

n., motor, upper Neuron whose cell body lies in motor area of cerebral cortex. Its axon passes down spinal cord and synapses with lower motor neurons.

n., multipolar. Neuron with one axon and many dendrites.

n., peripheral. Neuron whose process constitutes a part of the peripheral nervous system (cranial, spinal, or sympathetic nerves).

n., postganglionic. Neuron whose body lies in an autonomic ganglion and whose axon terminates in an effector organ (smooth or cardiac muscle or glands).

n., preganglionic. Neuron of autonomic nervous system whose cell body lies in central nervous system and axon terminates in peripheral ganglia.

n., sensory. An afferent neuron that conveys impulses that give rise to sensations.

n., unipolar. Neuron whose cell body bears one process.

MOTOR NEURON

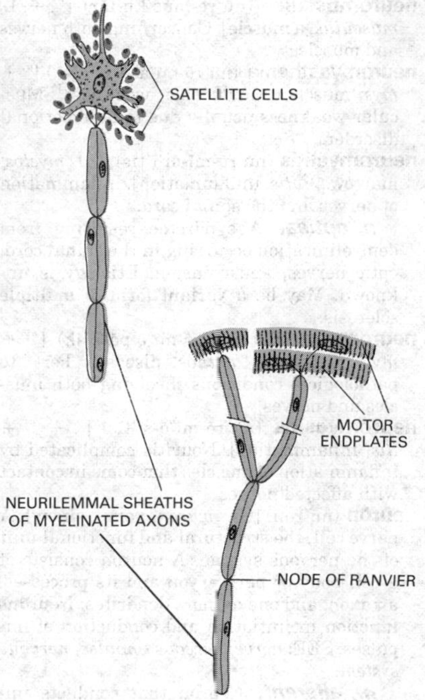

neuronal (nū'rō-năl). Pert. to one or more neurons.

neurone (nū'rōn). Neuron.

neuronephric (nū"rō-nĕf'rĭk) [" + *nephros,* kidney]. Concerning the nervous and renal systems.

neuronevus (nū"rō-nē'vŭs). Intradermal nevus.

neuronitis (nū-rō-nī'tĭs) [Gr. *neuron,* nerve, + *itis,* inflammation]. Inflammation or degenerative inflammation of nerve cells.

neuronophage (nū-rŏn'ō-fāj) [" + *phagein,* to eat]. A phagocyte that destroys tissue in the nervous system.

neuronophagia, neuronophagy (nū-rŏn"ō-fā'jē-ă, -ŏf'ă-jē). Destruction of nerve cells by phagocytes.

neuro-ophthalmology (nū"rō-ŏf"thăl-mŏl'ō-jē) [" + *ophthalmos,* eye, + *logos,* study]. The branch of ophthalmology concerned with the neurology of the visual system.

neuropacemaker. An implantable device for electrical stimulation of the dorsal column of the spinal tract. The electrical energy is provided in pulses at an appropriate rate in order to inhibit perception of pain.

neuropapillitis (nū"rō-păp"ĭ-lī'tĭs) [" + L. *papilla,* nipple, + Gr. *itis,* inflammation]. Optic neuritis.

neuroparalysis (nū"rō-pă-răl'ĭ-sĭs) [" + *paralyein,* to disable]. Paralysis due to disease of the nervous system.

neuropathic (nū-rō-păth'ĭk) [" + *pathos,* disease]. Rel. to neuropathy.

neuropathogenesis (nū"rō-păth"ō-jĕn'ĕ-sĭs) [" + " + *genesis,* production]. The origin and development of a neural disease.

neuropathogenicity (nū"rō-păth"ō-jĕ-nĭs'ĭ-tē) [" + *pathos,* disease, + *gennan,* to produce]. The ability to cause pathological changes in nerves.

neuropathology (nū"rō-pă-thŏl'ō-jē) [" + " + *logos,* study]. The study of diseases of the nervous system and structural and functional changes occurring in them. The diseases are divided into (1) congenital defects in development, those in which a degeneration reveals itself only after a period of time, and (2) those in which destructive influences act upon a brain that was normal initially. The latter are mainly inflammatory, toxic, traumatic, mechanical, or neoplastic in type. Circulatory impairment as well as failure to use elements of the nervous system will cause impaired function.

neuropathy (nū-rŏp′ă-thē). Any disease of the nerves.

n., ascending. Pathological condition of the nervous system that ascends from the lower body to the upper.

n., descending. Pathological condition of the nervous system that descends from the upper part of the body to the lower.

n., entrapment. Pathological changes in a nerve due to its inflammation in a confined space, such as the median nerve in the carpal tunnel.

n., hypertrophic interstitial. A slowly progressive neuritis that appears in late infancy or early childhood. There is gait disturbance with foot drop and ataxia due to loss of position sense. Pes cavus and scoliosis may be present. These patients have a normal life span.

neuropharmacology (nū″rō-făr″mă-kŏl′ō-jē) [″ + *pharmakon,* drug, + *logos,* study]. The branch of pharmacology concerned with the effects of drugs on the nervous system.

neurophilic (nū″rō-fĭl′ĭk) [″ + *philos,* fond]. Having an affinity for nervous tissue.

neurophonia (nū″rō-fō′nē-ă) [Gr. *neuron,* nerve, + *phone,* voice]. A tic or spasm of muscles of speech resulting in an involuntary cry or sound.

neurophthalmology (nū″rŏf-thăl-mŏl′ō-jē) [″ + *ophthalmos,* eye, + *logos,* study]. Neuro-ophthalmology, q.v.

neurophthisis (nū-rŏf′thĭ-sĭs) [″ + *phthisis,* wasting]. Wasting of nervous tissue.

neurophysin (nū″rō-fī′zĭn). Neurosecretory material in the hypothalamus. They are proteins and are involved in the transport of oxytocin and vasopressin.

neurophysiological treatment approach. In occupational and physical therapy, various techniques used in sensorimotor rehabilitation that rely on voluntary and involuntary activation, facilitation, and inhibition of muscle action through the reflex arc.

neurophysiology (nū″rō-fĭz-ē-ŏl′ō-jē) [″ + *physis,* growth, + *logos,* study]. Physiology of the nervous structure of the body.

neuropil (nū′rō-pĭl) [″ + *pilos,* felt]. Network of unmyelinated fibrils into which nerve processes of central nervous system divide.

neuroplasm (nū′rō-plăzm) [″ + *plasmos,* a thing formed]. The undifferentiated cytoplasmic substance of a neuron that surrounds and separates the neurofibrils.

neuroplasmic (nū″rō-plăz′mĭk). Concerning the protoplasm of a neuron.

neuroplasty (nū′rō-plăs″tē) [″ + *plassein,* to form]. Reparative surgery of the nerves.

neuropodia (nū″rō-pō′dē-ă) [″ + *podion,* little feet]. (pl. of *neuropodium*) Small bulblike expansions of axon terminals at a synaptic junction.

neuropore (nū′rō-pōr″) [″ + *poros,* an opening]. Embryonic opening from neural canal to exterior.

neuropotential (nū″rō-pō-tĕn shăl) [″ + L. *potentia,* power]. Nerve energy.

neuropraxia [″ + Gr. *praxis,* action]. The condition in which, due to trauma, a nerve no longer conducts even though the anatomic continuity of nerve is not interrupted.

neuropsychiatrist (nū″rō-sī-kī′ă-trĭst) [″ + *psyche,* mind, + *iatreia,* healing]. A specialist in neuropsychiatry.

neuropsychiatry (nū″rō-sī-kī′ă-trē). The branch of medicine pert. to study and treatment of nervous and mental diseases.

neuropsychopathy (nū″rō-sī-kŏp′ăth-ē) [″ + ″ + *pathos,* disease]. Disease of the nerves combined with mental disorder.

neuropsychopharmacology nū″rō-sī″kō-făr″mă-kŏl′ō-jē) [″ + ″ + *pharmakon,* drug, + *logos,* study]. The study of the effects of drugs on mental illness.

neuroradiography (nū″rō-rā″dē-ŏg′ră-fē) [″ + L. *radius,* ray, + Gr. *graphein,* to write]. Radiography of the structures of the nervous system.

neuroradiology (nū″rō-rā″dē-ŏl′ō-jē) [″ + ″ + Gr. *logos,* study]. X-ray study of the nervous system.

neurorelapse (nū″rō-rē-lăps′ [Gr. *neuron,* sinew, + L. *relapsus,* fallen back]. Reappearance of neurological symptoms in syphilis subsequent to institution of therapy.

neuroretinitis (nū″rō-rĕt″ĭn-ī′tĭs) [″ + L. *retina,* retina, + Gr. *itis,* inflammation]. Inflamed condition of optic nerve and retina.

neuroretinopathy (nū″rō-rĕt″ĭ-nŏp′ă-thē) [″ + ″ + Gr. *pathos,* disease]. Pathology of the retina and optic nerve.

neurorentgenography (nū″rō-rĕnt″gĕn-ŏg′ră-fē) [″ + *roentgen* + Gr. *graphein,* to write]. Neuroradiology, q.v.

neurorrhaphy (nū-ror′ă-fē) [″ + *rhaphe,* a sewing]. Suturing of ends of a severed nerve. SYN: *neurosuture.*

neurosarcokleisis (nū″rō-săr″kō-klī′sĭs) [″ + *sarx,* flesh, + *kleisis,* closure]. Operation for relief of neuralgia by resection of a wall of the osseous canal carrying a nerve and by transplanting the nerve to soft tissues.

neurosarcoma (nū″rō-săr-kō′mă) [″ + ″ + *oma,* tumor]. A sarcoma containing neuromatous components.

neuroscience (nū″rō-sī′ĕns). Any one of the various branches of science such as embryology, anatomy, histopathology, biochemistry, and pharmacology concerned with growth, development, and function of the nervous system.

neurosclerosis (nū″rō-sklĕ-rō′sĭs) [″ + *sklerosis,* a hardening]. Hardening of nervous tissue.

neurosecretion (nū″rō-sē-krē′shŭn) [″ + L. *secretio,* separation]. The elaboration and discharge of a chemical substance by a neuron.

Ex.: secretion of hormones by cells of the hypothalamus.

neurosensory (nū″rō-sĕn′sō-rē) [″ + L. *sensorius,* pert. to a sensation]. Concerning a sensory nerve.

neurosis (nū-rō′sĭs) [″ + *osis,* condition]. (pl. *neuroses)* The definition of this term is controversial. Some feel its use should be limited to describe an unpleasant mental symptom in an individual with intact reality testing; others would have it apply to the etiological process, i.e., unconscious conflict that arouses anxiety and leads to maladaptive use of defensive mechanisms that result in symptom formation. The various types of neuroses listed below are of both the descriptive and etiological types. SYN: *psychoneurosis.* SEE: *neurotic disorder.*

TREATMENT: Psychotherapy, tranquilizers, and sedatives. It must be remembered that in general a symptom due to a neurotic reaction to a situation is just as real to the patient as if it were due to organic disease. Usually such a symptom is much more difficult to treat than it would be if due to organic disease.

n., accident. A nervous disorder caused by injury or an accident. SYN: *n., traumatic.*

n., anxiety. Neurosis in which vague anxiety or apprehension is the essential symptom to the point where it interferes with daily living.

n., association. Neurosis in which association of ideas causes mental repetition of an experience.

n., cardiac. Asthenia, neurocirculatory, q.v.

n., compensation. Neurosis that develops after an accident in people who think they can obtain compensation by being ill. SYN: *n., pension.*

n., compulsion. Neurosis marked by overpowering impulse to perform acts against the will.

n., craft. N., occupational.

n., expectation. Condition in which anticipation of an occurrence produces nervous symptoms.

n., fatigue. Neurasthenia.

n., obsessional. Neurosis in which uncontrollable obsessions dominate the victim's behavior.

n., occupational. Neurosis due to the occupation or profession of a patient. SYN: *n., craft.*

n., pension. N., compensation.

n., sexual. Neurosis involving sexual function.

n., traumatic. N., accident.

n., war. Neurosis brought on by conditions of war, seen in soldiers.

neuroskeletal (nū″rō-skĕl′ĕ-tăl) [Gr. *neuron,* nerve, + *skeleton,* skeleton]. Concerning the skeletal and nervous system.

neuroskeleton (nū″rō-skĕl′ĕ-tŏn) [″ + *skeleton,* skeleton]. That portion of the skeleton that surrounds and protects the nervous system, i.e., the cranium, and spinal column.

neurosome (nū′rō-sōm) [″ + *soma,* body]. 1. The body of a neuron. 2. Minute granules in the protoplasm of nerve cells.

neurospasm (nū′rō-spăzm) [″ + *spasmos,* spasm]. Spasmodic muscular twitching due to a nervous disorder.

neurosplanchnic (nū″rō-splăngk′nĭk) [″ + *splanchnikos,* pert. to the viscera]. Concerning the sympathetic and cerebrospinal nervous system.

neurospongioma (nū″rō-spŏn″jē-ō′mă) [″ + *spongos,* sponge, + *oma,* tumor]. Spongioblastoma.

Neurospora (nū-rŏs′pō-ră). Genus of fungi belonging to the Ascomycetes class. Includes certain bread molds.

neurosurgeon (nū″rō-sŭr′jŭn). A physician specializing in surgery of the nervous system.

neurosurgery [Gr. *neuron,* sinew, + L. *chirurgia,* hand, + *ergon,* work]. Surgery of the nervous system.

neurosuture (nū″rō-soo′chūr) [″ + L. *sutura,* a stitch]. Stitching of ends of a cut nerve. SYN: *neurorrhaphy.*

neurosyphilis (nū″rō-sĭf′ĭ-lĭs). Syphilis affecting the nervous structures. SEE: *dementia paralytica.*

n., asymptomatic. Neurosyphilis preceding symptomatic neurosyphilis but showing no symptoms. Diagnosed by changes in spinal fluid.

n., meningovascular. A form of neurosyphilis involving the meninges and vascular structures in the brain or spinal cord or both.

n., paretic. Dementia paralytica.

n., tabetic. Tabes dorsalis.

neurotendinous (nū″rō-tĕn′dĭ-nŭs) [″ + L. *tendinosus,* tendinous]. Concerning a nerve and tendon.

neurotension (nū″rō-tĕn′shŭn) [″ + L. *tensio,* a stretching]. Operative stretching of a nerve. SYN: *neurectasis.*

neurothecitis (nū″rō-thē-sī′tĭs) [″ + *theke,* sheath, + *itis,* inflammation]. Inflamed condition of a nerve sheath.

neurothele (nū″rō-thē′lē) [″ + *thele,* nipple]. A nerve papilla.

neurotherapeutics (nū″rō-thĕr-ă-pū′tĭks) [″ + *therapeutike,* treatment]. Treatment of disorders of the nervous system. SYN: *neurotherapy.*

neurotherapy (nū″rō-thĕr′ă-pē) [″ + *therapeia,* treatment]. Treatment of nervous disorders. SYN: *neurotherapeutics.*

neurotic (nū-rŏt′ĭk) [Gr. *neuron,* sinew, nerve]. 1. One suffering from a neurosis. 2. Pert. to neurosis. 3. Nervous.

neurotic disorder. A mental disorder in which the predominant disturbance is a symptom or group of symptoms that is distressing the individual and is recognized by that person as being unacceptable, undesirable, and alien (ego-dystonic). Reality testing is grossly intact and behavior is socially acceptable. This disorder is chronic unless treated. This term does not imply that there is a special etiological process. SEE: *neurosis.*

neuroticism (nū-rŏt′ĭ-sĭzm) [″ + *-ismos,* state of]. A condition or trait of neurosis.

neurotization (nū″rŏt-ĭ-zā′shŭn) [Gr. *neuron,* sinew]. 1. Regeneration of a nerve after division. 2. Surgical introduction of a nerve into a paralyzed muscle.

neurotmesis (nū″rŏt-mē′sĭs) [″ + *tmesis,* cutting]. Nerve injury with complete loss of function of the nerve even though there is little apparent damage anatomically.

neurotology (nū″rō-tŏl′ō-jē) [″ + *ous,* ear, + *logos,* study]. The division of otology that deals with the inner ear, esp. its nerve supply, nerve connections with the brain, and auditory and labyrinthine pathways and centers within the brain. SYN: *otoneurology.*

neurotome (nū′rō-tōm). Fine knife used in the division of a nerve.

neurotomy (nū-rŏt′ō-mē) [″ + *tome,* an incision]. Division or dissection of a nerve.

neurotonic (nū″rō-tŏn′ĭk) [″ + *tonos,* tension]. 1. Concerning neural stretching. 2. Having a stimulating effect upon nerves or the nervous system.

neurotony (nū-rŏt′ō-nē). Nerve stretching, usually to ease pain.

neurotoxic (nū″rō-tŏks′ĭk) [″ + *toxikon,* poison]. Poisonous to the nerve cells.

neurotoxicity (nū″rō-tŏk-sĭs′ĭ-tē) [″ + *toxikon,* poison]. To have the capability of harming nerve tissue.

neurotoxin (nū″rō-tŏks′ĭn). A toxin that attacks nerve cells. SYN: *neurolysin.*

neurotransmitter (nū″rō-trăns′mĭt-ĕr). Substance such as norepinephrine, acetylcholine, and dopamine that is released when the axon terminal of a presynaptic neuron is excited. The substance then travels across the synapse to act on the target cell to either inhibit or excite it.

neurotrauma (nū-rō-traw′mă) [″ + *trauma,* wound]. Injury of a nerve.

neurotripsy (nū″rō-trĭp′sē) [″ + *tripsis,* a rubbing]. Surgical crushing of a nerve.

neurotrophasthenia (nū″rō-trŏf-ăs-thē′nē-ă) [″ + *trophe,* nourishment, + *astheneia,* weakness]. Malnutrition of the nervous system.

neurotrophic. Pert. to the influence of nervous impulses upon the nutrition and function of an organ or structure.

neurotrophy (nū-rŏt′rō-fē). Nutrition and maintenance of nervous tissue.

neurotropism (nū-rŏt′rō-pĭzm) [Gr. *neuron,* nerve, + *trope,* a turning, + *-ismos,* condition]. Attraction that materials including nutritive elements, basic dyes, and microorganisms have for nervous tissue.

neurotropy (nū-rŏt′rō-pē). Neurotropism.

neurotrosis (nū″rō-trō′sĭs) [″ + *trosis,* a wound]. Injury of a nerve.

neurotubule (nū″rō-too′būl) [″ + L. *tubulus,* a tubule]. A microtubule seen by use of electron microscopy in nerve cells, dendrites, and axons.

neurovaccine (nū″rō-văk′sĭn). A standardized vaccine virus of specific strength. Usually prepared by cultivation in a rabbit's brain.

neurovaricosis (nū″rō-văr″ĭ-kō′sĭs) [″ + L. *varicosus,* pert. to a swollen vein, + *osis,* condition]. Multiple swellings along the pathway of a nerve.

neurovascular (nū″rō-văs′kū-lar) [″ + L. *vasculus,* a small vessel]. Concerning both the nervous and vascular systems.

neurovegetative (nū″rō-vĕj′ĕ-tā″tĭv). Concerning the autonomic nervous system.

neurovirus (nū″rō-vī′rŭs). Virus that has been modified by its growing in nervous tissue. Used in preparing a vaccine.

neurovisceral (nū″rō-vĭs′ĕr-ăl) [″ + L. *viscera,* body organs]. Neurosplanchnic, q.v.

neurula (nū′roo-lă). Stage in development of an embryo, esp. amphibian embryos, during which the neural plate develops and axial embryonic nervous structures are elaborated.

neurulation (nū″roo-lā′shŭn). Formation of the neural plate in the embryo and development and closure of the neural tube.

neutral (nū′trăl) [L. *neutralis,* neither]. 1. Neither alkaline nor acid. 2. Indifferent; having no positive qualities or opinions.

neutral fat. One of the lipids commonly found in the tissues; an ester of fatty acids with glycerol. Ex.: tristearin; triolein; tripalmitin.

neutralization (nū″trăl-ĭ-zā′shŭn). 1. The opposing of one force or condition with an opposite force or condition to such degree as to cause counteraction that permits neither to dominate. 2. In chemistry, the process of destroying the peculiar properties or effect of a substance, i.e., the neutralization of an acid with a base or vice versa. 3. In medicine, the process of checking or counteracting the effects of any agent that produces a morbid effect.

neutralize (nū'trăl-īz). 1. To counteract and make ineffective. 2. In chemistry, to destroy peculiar properties or effect; to make inert.

neutral point. A point on the pH scale (pH 7.0) that represents neutrality, i.e., the solution is neither acid or alkaline in reaction.

neutral red. A dye used as an indicator and as a vital stain.

neutrino (nū-trē'nō). In physics, subatomic particle with no mass, at rest, and no electric charge. These particles are constantly flowing through the universe, including the Earth. They are not known to affect the matter through which they pass.

neutroclusion (nū"trŏ-kloo'zhŭn) [L. *neuter,* neither, + *occludo,* to close]. State in which the anteroposterior occlusal positions of the teeth or the mesiodistal positions are normal, but malocclusion of the other positions exists.

neutrocyte (nū'trō-sīt) [" + Gr. *kytos,* cell]. A neutrophil leukocyte.

neutrocytopenia (nū"trō-sī"tō-pē'nē-ă) [" + " + *penia,* poverty]. Neutropenia.

neutrocytosis (nū"trō-sī-tō'sĭs) [" + " + *osis,* condition]. Neutrophilia.

neutron (nū'trŏn) [L. *neuter,* neither]. Subatomic particle equal in mass to a proton but without an electric charge. A constituent of the atomic nucleus, it has a mass 1,839 times that of an electron. As a free particle, it has an average life of little less than 17 minutes.

neutron capture analysis. Use of the ability of a neutron to be absorbed (i.e., captured) by an atomic nucleus to detect the presence of various substances.

neutropenia (nū-trō-pē'nē-ă) [" + Gr. *penia,* lack]. Abnormally small number of neutrophil cells in the blood.

n., malignant. Agranulocytosis.

neutrophil(e) (nū'trō-fĭl, -fīl) [" + Gr. *philein,* to love]. 1. Staining easily with neutral dyes. 2. A leukocyte that stains easily with neutral dyes. SEE: *blood cell* for illus.; *leukocyte.*

neutrophilia (nū"trō-fĭl'ē-ă). Increase in the number of neutrophil leukocytes in the blood.

neutrophilic, neutrophilous (nū-trō-fĭl'ĭk, -trŏf'ĭ-lŭs) [" + Gr. *philein,* to love]. Staining readily with neutral dyes.

neutrotaxis (nū"trō-tăk'sĭs) [*neutrophil* + Gr. *taxis,* arrangement]. The phenomenon in which neutrophils are repelled from or attracted to something.

nevocarcinoma (nē"vō-kăr"sĭ-nō'mă) [L. *naevus,* birthmark, + Gr. *karkinos,* crab, + *oma,* tumor]. Malignant melanoma.

nevoid (nē'voyd) [" + Gr. *eidos,* form]. Resembling a nevus.

nevolipoma (nē"vō-lĭ-pō'mă) [" + Gr. *lipos,* fat, + *oma,* tumor]. Rare lipoma containing numerous blood vessels and fatty tissue, probably a degenerated nevus. SYN: *nevus lipomatodes.*

nevose (nē'vōs) [L. *naevus,* birthmark]. Spotted or marked with nevi. SEE: *nevus.*

nevoxanthoendothelioma (nē"vō-zăn"thō-ĕn"dō-thē"lē-ō'mă) [" + *xanthos,* yellow, + *endon,* within, + *thele,* nipple, + *oma,* tumor]. Juvenile xanthogranuloma. SEE: *xanthogranuloma, juvenile.*

nevus (nē'vŭs) [L. *naevus,* birthmark]. (pl. *nevi)* 1. A congenital discoloration of a circumscribed area of the skin due to pigmentation. SYN: *birthmark; mole.* 2. Circumscribed vascular tumor of the skin, usually congenital, due to hyperplasia of the blood vessels. SEE: *angioma.*

n. angiectodes. N. vascularis.

n. angiomatodes. Extensive diffuse angiomatous condition of the subcutaneous tissues.

n. araneus. Acquired or congenital dilatation of the capillaries, marked by red lines radiating from a central red dot. SYN: *n., spider.*

n., blue. A dark blue nevus covered by smooth skin. It is composed of melanin-pigmented spindle cells in the mid-dermis.

n., blue rubber bleb. A rubbery blue cavernous hemangiomatous nodule that is erectile and easily compressed. Present in the skin and gastrointestinal tract.

n., capillary. Nevus of dilated capillary vessels, elevated above the skin. Usually treated by ligature and excision.

n. comedonicus. A horny nevus that contains a hard plug of keratin. Caused by failure of the pilosebaceous follicles to develop normally.

n., connective tissue. A nevus composed of collagenous tissue.

n., cutaneous. Nevus formation on the skin.

n., epidermal. Raised lesions present at birth; they may be hyperkeratotic and widely distributed.

n. flammeus. Reddish discoloration of the face or neck, usually not elevated above the skin. A serious deformity due to its large size and color. SYN: *port-wine stain.*

n., hairy. A nevus, usually pigmented, from which hair grows.

n., halo. A nevus surrounded by a depigmented area. SYN: *leukoderma acquisitum centrifugum.*

n., intradermal. Nevus in which the melanocytes are found in nests in the dermis and have no connection with the deeper layers from which they were formed.

n., Ito's. A mongolian spot, q.v., innervated by lateral branches of the supraclavicular nerve and the lateral cutaneous nerve of the arm.

n., junction. A nevus in the basal cell zone at the junction of the epidermis and dermis. They are slightly raised, do not contain hair, and are pigmented. These may become malignant.

n. lipomatodes. Fatty connective tissue tumor, probably a degenerated nevus containing numerous blood vessels. SYN: *nevolipoma.*

n. maternus. A birthmark; congenital angioma.

n., melanocytic. Any nevus that contains melanocytes.

n., nevocytic. A common mole. They may appear at any age. They are classified according to their stage of growth and as to whether or not they are still growing.

n., Ota's. A mongolian spot, q.v., occurring in the skin surrounding the eye.

n. pigmentosus. Congenital pigment spot varying in color from light yellow to black. Intradermal, or common moles, are benign. Other types are or may become malignant.

TREATMENT: Malignant or suspicious lesions should be treated by wide surgical excision. Benign lesions do not require treatment except when located at sites of friction causing bleeding or ulceration. Some are removed for cosmetic reasons.

n. pilosus. A nevus covered with hair.

n., sebaceous. A nevus composed of sebaceous-gland tissue.

n., spider. N. araneus.

n. spilus. Pigmented nevus with smooth surface.

n. spongiosus albus mucosae. A white, spongy nevus that may occur in the mouth, labia, vagina, or rectum.

n., strawberry. N. vascularis.

n., telangiectatic. Nevus containing dilated capillaries.

n. unius lateralis. Congenital nevus that occurs in streaks or linear bands on one side of the body. They usually occur between the neurotomes of the lumbar or sacral area.

n. vascularis. Nevus in which superficial blood vessels are enlarged. Nevi are usually congenital and of variable size and shape; slightly elevated; reddish or purplish; on face, head, neck, and arms though no region is exempt. Usually disappear spontaneously but wrinkling, pigmentation, and scarring are sometimes seen. SYN: *nevus angiectodes; strawberry mark.*

n. venosus. Nevus formed of dilated venules.

n. verrucosus. Nevus with a raised wartlike surface.

n., white sponge. N. spongiosus albus mucosae, q.v.

newborn. Born recently. Term applied to human infants less than a month old. SYN: *neonate.*

Newcastle disease (nū′kăs-ĕl). An acute viral disease of birds, particularly chickens. It occasionally produces accidental infections in man, usually a mild conjunctivitis.

new growth. Any new growth of tissue. Usually considered to be abnormal but not always so; the normal fetus is in fact a new growth. SYN: *neoplasm.*

newton. SYMB: N. In SI units, the unit of force is *newton,* which is equal to 1 kilogram times 1 meter per second squared, or 1N = 1 kg./s^2.

newton meter. SYMB: Nm. In SI units, one newton per square meter. This is called one pascal (Pa). Thus 1 Pa = 1N/M^2.

nexus (nĕk′sŭs) [L., bond]. (pl. *nexus*) A connection or link; a binding together. Used to designate a bond between components of a group.

NF. *National Formulary.*

N.F.L.P.N. *National Federation for Licensed Practical Nurses.*

ng. nanogram.

NH_3. Ammonia.

NH_4^+. The univalent ammonium radical.

NH_4Br. Ammonium bromide.

NH_4Cl. Ammonium chloride.

N.H.I. *National Heart Institute.*

N.H.L.I. *National Heart and Lung Institute.*

NH_4NO_3. Ammonium nitrate.

NH_4OH. Ammonium hydroxide. SYN: *ammonia water; aqua ammonia.*

Ni. Chem. symb. for nickel.

niacin (nī′ă-sĭn). USP. Nicotinic acid. A vitamin used in preventing and treating pellagra. Trade names are Nicobid, Nicocap, and Nicolar.

niacinamide (nī″ă-sĭn-ăm′ĭd). USP. A niacin derivative used in the prophylaxis and treatment of pellagra. SYN: *nicotinamide.*

N.I.A.I.D. *National Institute of Allergy and Infectious Diseases.*

N.I.A.M.D. *National Institute of Arthritis and Metabolic Diseases.*

niche (nĭch) [Fr.]. A depression or recess on a smooth surface, esp. an erosion in the wall of a hollow organ, detected by roentgenography.

n., enamel. One of two depressions that develop between the dental lamina and the enamel organ.

N.I.C.H.H.D. *National Institute of Child Health and Human Disease.*

nickel [L. *niccolum*]. SYMB: Ni. At. wt. 58.70, at. no. 28. Metallic element.

n. carbonyl. An industrial chemical, $Ni(CO)_4$, used in plating metals. It is toxic when inhaled, causing pulmonary edema.

nicking. 1. Compression of the retinal vessels of the eye at the point where a vein and an artery cross. Seen in hypertensive cardiovascular disease. 2. To notch a tissue.

niclosamide (nī-klō′să-mīd). A teniacide esp. effective against the cestodes that infect man. Trade names are Niclocide and Yomesan.

Nicobid. Trade name for niacin, USP.

Nicocap. Trade name for niacin, USP.

Nicolar. Trade name for niacin, USP.

Nicolas-Favre disease (nē″kō-lă-făv′r). [Josef Nicolas and M. Favre, Fr. physicians] Venereal disease marked by involvement of inguinal lymph glands with an exuding lesion. SYN: *lymphogranuloma venereum.*

nicotinamide (nĭk″ō-tĭn′ă-mīd). Member of vitamin B complex, used in management or prevention of pellagra. The peripheral flush that often accompanies therapy with nicotinic acid, q.v., is avoided with nicotinamide. SYN: *niacinamide.*

n. adenine dinucleotide. SEE: NAD^+.

n. adenine dinucleotide-dehydrogenase. SYN: *nicotinamide adenine dinucleotide diaphorase; methemoglobin reductase.* SEE: *NADH-diaphorase.*

n. adenine dinucleotide-diaphorase. SEE: *NADH-diaphorase.*

n. adenine dinucleotide phosphate. A coenzyme that contains adenine, nicotinamide, D-ribose, and phosphoric acid. It serves as an electron carrier in catabolic and anabolic reactions.

n. adenine diphosphate. SEE: *NADP.*

nicotine (nĭk′ō-tēn, -tĭn) [L. *nicotiana,* tobacco]. A poisonous alkaloid found in all parts of the tobacco plant, but esp. in the leaves. When pure, it is a colorless oily fluid with little odor but a sharp burning taste. On exposure to air or in crude materials, it becomes deep brown with the characteristic tobacco-like smell. Nicotine is one of the most toxic and addicting of all poisons. Cigarette tobacco contains varying amounts of nicotine per cigarette. SEE: *nicotine poisoning, acute.*

nicotine poisoning, acute. Nicotine is an extremely toxic substance that acts as swiftly as cyanide. The fatal dose for an adult is estimated to be less than 5 mg./kg. body weight.

SYM: Nausea, salivation, abdominal pain, vomiting, diarrhea, sweating, dizziness, and mental confusion. If dose is sufficient, the patient will collapse, develop shock, convulse, and die of respiratory failure due to paralysis of respiratory muscles. For treatment, SEE: *Poisons and Poisoning* in *Appendix.*

TREATMENT: If patient is conscious, oral administration of universal antidote, q.v., tannic acid, activated charcoal, or strong tea, followed by gastric lavage or an emetic. If patient is unconscious, use gastric lavage. Keep patient warm with external heat and maintain the airway. Artificial or mechanical respiration and oxygen therapy if necessary. If convulsions are severe or persist, intravenous barbiturates in small doses are indicated.

nicotinic acid (nĭk″ō-tĭn′ĭk). The antipellagra principle of vitamin B complex. Occurs naturally in liver, yeast, milk, cheese, and cereals. Used orally or parenterally for treatment of pellagra. SYN: *niacin.*

nicotinism (nĭk′ō-tĭn-ĭzm). Poisoning from excessive use of tobacco or nicotine.

nictation [L. *nictitare,* to wink]. Involuntary winking. SYN: *nictitation.*

nictitate (nĭk′tĭ-tāt). To wink.

nictitating (nĭk′tĭ-tāt-ĭng). Winking.

nictitating membrane. SEE: *membrane, nictitating.*

nictitating spasm. Clonic spasm of eyelid with continuous winking.

nictitation [L. *nictitare,* to wink]. Involuntary winking. SYN: *nictation.*

nidal (nī′dăl) [L. *nidus,* nest]. Pert. to a nidus.

nidation (nī-dā′shŭn). Implantation of the fertilized ovum in the lining of the uterus (endometrium).

N.I.D.R. *National Institute of Dental Research.*

nidus (nī′dŭs) [L., nest]. (pl. *nidi*) 1. A cluster; nestlike structure. 2. Focus of infection. 3. A nucleus or origin of a nerve.

n. avis cerebelli. A deep sulcus on each side of the inferior vermis separating it from adjacent lobes of hemispheres.

n. hirundis. Swallow's nest, q.v.

Niemann-Pick disease (nē′măn-pĭk). [Albert Niemann, Ger. pediatrician, 1880–1921; Ludwig Pick, Ger. physician, 1868–1935] A disturbance of sphingolipid metabolism characterized by enlargement of liver and spleen (hepatosplenomegaly), anemia, lymphadenopathy, and progressive mental and physical deterioration. A hereditary disease, its onset is in early infancy. Death usually occurs before the third year. Typical cell, having a foamy appearance and filled with a lipoid believed to be sphingomyelin, can be found in bone marrow, spleen, or lymph nodes and aids in establishing the diagnosis.

night blindness. Absence of, or defective vision in the dark. Due to lack of visual purple in the rods or to its slowness in regenerating after exposure to light. May result from vitamin A deficiency or hereditary factors. SYN: *nyctalopia.* SEE: *night vision.*

Nightingale, Florence (nīt′ĭn-găl). British

philanthropist, 1820–1910, who was founder of modern nursing and reformer of hospital conditions. Served as a nurse in Crimean War. Founded a training school for nurses.

Nightingale Pledge. An oath used universally by nurses upon capping or graduation as a pledge of ethical standards of their profession. The pledge was formulated by a committee of the Farrand School of Nursing, Harper Hospital, Detroit, Michigan.

"I solemnly pledge myself before God and in the presence of this assembly to pass my life in purity and to practice my profession faithfully. I will abstain from whatever is deleterious and mischievous, and will not take or knowingly administer any harmful drug. I will do all in my power to maintain and elevate the standard of my profession, and will hold in confidence all personal matters committed to my keeping and all family affairs coming to my knowledge in the practice of my calling. With loyalty will I endeavor to aid the physician in his work, and devote myself to the welfare of those committed to my care." SEE: *Declaration of Hawaii; Declaration of Geneva; Hippocratic Oath; Prayer of Maimonides.*

nightmare (nīt'mār) [AS. *nyht,* night, + *mara,* a demon]. A bad dream accompanied by great fear. SYN: *incubus; oneirodynia.* SEE: *paralysis, sleep.*

nightshade (nīt'shād) [AS. *nihtscada*]. Any of several of the plants of the genus Solanum. SEE: *belladonna.*

n., deadly. Belladonna, q.v.

night sweat [AS. *nyht,* night, + *swat,* sweat]. Profuse sweating during sleep at night. Often it is an early sign of disease, esp. with intermittent temperature. In children, it occurs in rickets and in debilitated states. Patient should be rubbed down, sponged, and changed into dry clothing.

night terrors [" + L. *terror,* state of fear]. Form of nightmare in children causing them to awaken in terror, screaming. Fear continues for a period after the return to consciousness. SYN: *pavor nocturnus.*

night vision. The ability to see at night or in light of low intensity. Results from dark adaptation in which pupil dilates, visual purple increases, and intensity threshold of the retina is lowered. Any decrease in oxygen content of the blood is accompanied by some loss of night vision. Thus smoking cigarettes or being in an atmosphere with decreased oxygen content decreases night vision. SYN: *scotopic vision.*

nightwalking. State in which individual habitually walks about while sleeping. SYN: *somnambulism.*

N.I.G.M.S. *National Institute of General Medical Sciences.* A division of the National Institutes of Health of the U.S. Department of Health and Human Services.

nigra (nī'gră) [L., black]. Mass of gray matter between the dorsal and pedal parts of the crus cerebri. SYN: *substantia nigra.*

nigri-, nigro- [L. *nigra,* black]. Combining forms pert. to blackness.

nigricans (nī'grĭ-kăns). Blackened.

nigrities (nī-grĭsh'ĭ-ēz). Blackness; black pigmentation.

n. linguae. A black pigmentation of the tongue.

nigrosin (nī'grō-sĭn). An aniline dye used in staining nervous tissue and certain bacteria, and to discriminate between live and dead cells.

nigrostriatal (nī"grō-strī-ā'tăl). Concerning a bundle of nerve fibers that connect the substantia nigra of the brain to the corpus striatum.

NIH. *National Institutes of Health* (of the U.S. Department of Health and Human Services).

nihilism (nī'ĭ-lĭzm) [L. *nihil,* nothing, + Gr. *-ismos,* state of]. 1. Disbelief in efficacy of medical therapy. 2. A delusion in which everything is unreal or does not exist.

nikethamide (nĭ-kĕth'ă-mīd). A drug that is supposed to selectively stimulate central respiratory centers. Use for this purpose in treating respiratory depression due to poisoning from sedative-hypnotic drugs is ineffective. Trade name is Coramine.

Nikolsky's sign (nĭ-kŏl'skēz) [Pyotr Nikolsky, Russ. dermatologist, 1855–1940] Condition of the external layer of the skin in which it can be rubbed off by slight friction or injury. Seen in pemphigus.

Nilstat. Trade name for nystatin, USP.

N.I.M.H. *National Institute of Mental Health.* A division of the National Institutes of Health of the U.S. Department of Health and Human Services.

N.I.N.D.B. *National Institute of Neurological Diseases and Blindness.* A division of the National Institutes of Health of the U.S. Department of Health and Human Services.

ninth cranial nerve. Glossopharyngeal nerve. SEE: *glossopharyngeal nerve* for illus.; *Cranial Nerves* in *Appendix.*

niobium (nī-ō'bē-um). [Legendary Gr. woman, Niobe, who was turned into stone] SYMB: Nb. At. wt. 92.906; at. no. 41. A chemical element formerly called columbium.

niphablepsia (nĭf"ă-blĕp'sē-ă) [Gr. *nipha,* snow, + *ablepsia,* blindness]. Blindness caused by light glare on snow. SYN: *niphotyphlosis.*

niphotyphlosis (nĭf"ō-tĭf-lō'sĭs) [" + *typhlosis,* blindness]. Snow blindness. SYN: *niphablepsia.*

nipple (nĭp'l) [AS. *neble,* a little protuberance]. 1. The conical protuberance in each breast from which the lactiferous ducts discharge in the female. SYN: *mammilla; papilla mamma* [NA]; *teat.* 2. Artificial substitute for female nipple to be used on a nursing bottle.

The nipple contains erectile tissue and is surrounded by a pigmented area called the areola. The areola may be darker in those who have borne children. It is supplied with a row of small sebaceous glands around its base called areolar glands that secrete an oily substance to keep it supple. SEE: *breast* for illus.

NURSING IMPLICATIONS: *Postpartum:* Wash with warm water and pat dry. Apply emollient for dry, cracked nipples. Instruct mother to position infant's mouth properly or apply nipple shield to prevent trauma.

RS: acromastitis; areola; breast; halo; mamma; mammary glands; mammillation; Paget's disease of nipple; "thel-" words.

n., crater. N., retracted.

n., retracted. Nipple whose tip lies below the level of the surrounding skin. Caused by deficiency of muscle tissue or flattening of erectile tissue.

nipple shield. A device consisting of an artificial nipple used by some nursing mothers to protect the natural nipple.

Nipride. Trade name for sodium nitroprusside, USP.

Nisentil. Trade name for alphaprodine hydrochloride.

Nissl bodies (nĭs'l). [Franz Nissl, Ger. neurologist, 1860–1919] Chromophil substance in the form of granules found in the cell bodies and dendrites of neurons but lacking in the most peripheral region of the nerve cell cytoplasm and the area where the axis cylinder (axon hillock) originates and from the axon cylinder. They are stained selectively by toluidine and other basic aniline dyes. They consist principally of the ribose type of nucleic acid and nucleoprotein.

They are concerned with protein synthesis and metabolism; their condition varies with physiological and pathological conditions. In fatigue and certain pathological states, they may dissolve and disappear, a phenomenon called chromatolysis. SYN: *tigroid bodies.*

nisus (nī'sŭs) [L.]. Effort, exertion, or a strong force.

nit (nĭt) [AS. *hnitu*]. The egg of a louse or any other parasitic insect. SEE: *pediculosis; Pediculus.*

niter (nī'ter) [Gr. *nitron,* salt]. Sodium nitrate or potassium nitrate (saltpeter).

niton (nī'tŏn). Radon.

nitrate (nī'trāt) [L. *nitratum*]. A salt of nitric acid.

nitrated. Combined with nitric acid or a nitrate.

nitration. Combination with nitric acid or a nitrate.

nitre (nī'tĕr) [Fr.]. British spelling of niter, q.v.

nitremia (nī-trē'mē-ă). Azotemia.

nitric acid. HNO_3. A colorless, corrosive, poisonous liquid in concentrated form, employed as a caustic. It is widely used in industry and in chemical laboratories.

n.a., fuming. Concentrated nitric acid, which emits toxic fumes that cause choking if inhaled. SEE: *fumes; nitrous fumes* in *Poisons and Poisoning* in *Appendix.*

nitric acid poisoning. Symptoms are essentially same as those produced by sulfuric acid poisoning, q.v. Pain, burning, vomiting, thirst, and shock.

TREATMENT: Dilute with large volumes of water. Neutralize with weak alkalies; give magnesium oxide, milk of magnesia, milk, or egg white in large amounts. Avoid emetics and stomach tubes because they may cause rupture of the esophagus or stomach.

nitridation (nī-trĭ-dā'shŭn). Combination with nitrogen to form a nitride.

nitride (nī'trīd). A binary compound formed by direct combination of nitrogen with another element, e.g., lithium nitride (Li_3N), formed from nitrogen and lithium.

nitrification (nī"trĭ-fĭ-kā'shŭn). The process by which the nitrogen of ammonia or other compounds is oxidized to nitric or nitrous acid or their salts (nitrates, nitrites). Takes place continually in the soil through the action of nitrifying bacteria.

nitrifying (nī'trĭ-fī"ĭng). The process of nitrification.

nitrifying bacteria. Bacteria that induce nitrification. Include the nitrite bacteria Nitrosomonas, which convert ammonia to nitrites, and nitrate bacteria Nitrobacter, which convert nitrites to nitrates.

nitrile (nī'trĭl). An organic compound in which trivalent nitrogen is attached to a carbon atom.

nitrite (nī'trīt) [Gr. *nitron,* salt]. A salt of nitrous acid. Nitrites dilate blood vessels, reduce blood pressure, depress motor centers of the spinal cord, and act as antispasmodics. Principal nitrites used in medicine are amyl, ethyl, potassium, and sodium nitrite, q.v.

nitritoid (nī'trĭ-toyd) [" + *eidos,* resemblance]. Resembling a nitrite.

n. crisis. A syndrome resembling symptoms produced by the use of a nitrite, usually occurring after arsphenamine injection.

nitrituria (nī-trĭ-tū'rē-ă) [" + *ouron,* urine]. Nitrites present in the urine.

nitro-, nitr- [Gr. *nitron,* salt]. Combining form denoting combination with nitrogen or presence of the group NO_2.

nitrobenzene (nī"trō-bĕn'zēn). A toxic derivative of benzene. It is used in making aniline.

nitroblue tetrazolium test. A test of the ability of leukocytes to transform nitroblue tetrazolium from a colorless state to deep blue. Failure to cause this reaction indicates that the leukocytes do not have the capability of reacting in a normal manner to the ingestion of the particular bacteria used in the test.

nitrocellulose (nī"trō-sěl'ū-lōs). Pyroxylin, q.v.

nitrofurantoin (nī"trō-fū-răn'tō-ĭn). USP. An antibacterial drug used in treating certain urinary tract infections. Trade names are Dantafur, Furadantin, and Macrodantin.

nitrofurazone (nī"trō-fū'ră-zōn). USP. An antibacterial agent used topically. Trade names are Amifur and Furacin.

nitrogen (nī'trō-jěn) [Fr. *nitrogene*]. SYMB: N. At. wt. 14.0067; at. no. 7. A colorless, odorless, tasteless gaseous element occurring free in the atmosphere, forming approx. 80% of its volume.

A component of all proteins, nitrogen is essential to plant and animal life for tissue building. Generally it is found in organic nature only in the form of compounds such as ammonia, nitrites, and nitrates. These are transformed by plants into proteins and, being consumed by animals, are converted into animal proteins of the blood and tissues. SYN: *azote*.

n. monoxide. N_2O. Laughing gas; nitrous oxide.

n. mustards. 1. A term embracing certain therapeutic mustard compounds that act as alkylating agents and therefore have the ability to disturb cell growth during a cell's growth phase. Used because they destroy lymphoid tissue in Hodgkin's disease. They are also used in treating lymphosarcoma, giant follicular lymphoblastoma, chronic lymphoid myeloid leukemia, rheumatoid arthritis, and nephritis. Nitrogen mustards include mechlorethamine, cyclophosphamide, uracil mustard, melphalan, and chlorambucil. 2. Gases used in chemical warfare. SEE: *gas, mustard; gas, vesicant*.

n., nonprotein. That nitrogen that appears in food, blood, or other substance but is not present as a protein.

nitrogenase (nī'trō-jěn-ās) [*nitrogen* + *-ase*, enzyme]. An enzyme that catalyzes the reduction of nitrogen to ammonia.

nitrogen balance. The difference between the amount of nitrogen ingested and that excreted each day. If intake is greater, a positive balance exists; if less, there is a negative balance. SEE: *nitrogen equilibrium*.

nitrogen cycle. A natural cycle in which nitrogen is discharged from animal life into the soil; it is then taken up from soil into plants for their nourishment; and in turn nitrogen returns to animal life through plants eaten.

nitrogen equilibrium. Condition during which nitrogen excreted in the urine, feces, and sweat equals amount taken in by the body in food.

nitrogen fixation. Conversion of atmospheric nitrogen into nitrates through the action of bacteria in the soil.

nitrogen lag. Extent of time required after a given protein is ingested before an amount of nitrogen equal to that in protein has been excreted.

nitrogen narcosis. Condition of euphoria, impaired judgment, and decreased coordination and motor ability seen in persons exposed to high air pressure such as divers and submariners. The effects, caused by the increased concentration of nitrogen gas in body tissues, including the brain are similar to those produced by alcoholic intoxication.

nitrogenous (nī-trŏj'ěn-ŭs). Pert. to or containing nitrogen. Foods that contain nitrogen are the proteins; those that do not contain nitrogen are the fats and carbohydrates. The retention of nitrogenous products in the blood is marked in kidney diseases.

nitroglycerin (nī"trō-glĭs'ěr-ĭn) [Gr. *nitron*, salt, + *glycerin*]. Any nitrate of glycerol. Specifically the trinitrate—a heavy oily, explosive, colorless liquid obtained by treating glycerol with nitric and sulfuric acids. Even though it is the explosive constituent of dynamite, it is not used medically in an explosive form. In medicine it has the action of nitrites and is a vasodilator. Used esp. in angina pectoris.

Persons who use nitroglycerin regularly should be told that the tablets must be stored in a tightly sealed dark-tinted glass (not plastic) container without a cotton plug. Nitroglycerin ointment is available for treatment of angina. It is especially helpful when used in the prophylactic treatment of angina. It is used in a 2% ointment rubbed into the chest wall. A long-term transdermal delivery system is also available for nitroglycerin.

nitroglycerin tablets. USP. A standardized preparation of nitroglycerin, q.v. Trade names are Klavikordal, Nitrospan, Nitrostat, and Nitrong. Previously used name was glyceryl trinitrate.

nitromersol (nī"trō-měr'sŏl). USP. An organic mercurial antiseptic used topically. It penetrates poorly and the mercury is fixed by tissues so that its bacteriostatic action is prevented.

nitrometer (nī-trŏm'ĕ-těr) [*nitrogen* + Gr. *metron*, measure]. Device for measuring the amount of nitrogen produced in a chemical reaction.

nitromuriatic acid (nī"trō-mū-rē-ăt'ĭk) [" + L. *muriaticus*, briny]. A mixture of one part nitric acid and three parts hydrochloric acid used in commercial industries because it dissolves all the metals including platinum and gold. SYN: *aqua regia*.

Nitrong. Trade name for nitroglycerin, USP.

Nitropress. Trade name for sodium nitroprusside, USP.

Nitrosomonas. A genus of gram-negative, aerobic bacteria that oxidize ammonia to nitrate.

nitrous (nī'trŭs) [Gr. *nitron*, salt]. Containing nitrogen in its lowest valency.

nitrous acid. A chemical reagent, HNO_2, used in biological laboratories.

nitrous oxide. USP. N_2O. Colorless sweet-tasting gas with pleasing smell causing temporary general anesthesia when inhaled in proper concentration. It is given in various amounts with oxygen; and is used as an adjuvant with other anesthetic agents. It should not be used as the sole anesthetic agent because the concentration required to produce anesthesia is close to the concentration that would also lead to hypoxia. Its action as an anesthetic can be potentiated by other classes of drugs—barbiturates, narcotics, and tranquilizers. Nitrous oxide is not flammable but it will support combustion when it is present in proper concentration with a flammable anesthetic. SYN: *laughing gas*.

Nitrous oxide has little or no effect on body temperature, blood pressure, volume or composition of blood, metabolism, or the genitourinary system. Diaphoresis, increased muscle tone, or both may occur with induction of anesthesia with nitrous oxide.

Asphyxiation may occur if it is not administered properly. Prolonged administration of nitrous oxide will cause depression of bone marrow.

SYM: Signs of deep nitrous oxide anesthesia are a slight increase in respirations, some dyspnea. Cyanosis becomes deeper; eyeballs are fixed either upward or downward. There is muscular rigidity; cyanosis increases to a grayish pallor; pupils become fixed in a dilated form; and respirations cease.

TREATMENT: The patient who suffers from an overdose should be resuscitated and given oxygen under pressure.

N.J.P.C. *National Joint Practice Commission.*

N.L.N. *National League for Nursing.*

NMRI. *Naval Medical Research Institute* (U.S. Navy).

N.M.S.S. *National Multiple Sclerosis Society.*

N.N.D. *New and Nonofficial Drugs*, a former publication of the American Medical Association, which described new drugs that had not been admitted to the U.S. Pharmacopeia.

NO. *nitrous oxide.*

No. 1. L. *numero*, to the number of. 2. Chem. symb. for nobelium.

N_2O. Nitrous oxide.

N_2O_3. Nitrogen trioxide.

N_2O_5. Nitrogen pentoxide.

nobelium (nō-bē'lē-ŭm). [Named for Nobel Institute, where it was first isolated] SYMB: No. At. wt. of the most stable isotope is 254 (other isotopes vary in weight from 252 through 256); at. no. 102. Element obtained from bombardment of curium.

Nobel prize. [Alfred B. Nobel, Swedish chemist and philanthropist, 1833–1896, whose will provided funds for awarding the annual prizes] Awards consisting of a medal and monetary prize of over $100,000 usually given annually to those selected for excellence in the fields of chemistry, literature, medicine, physics, and physiology. The first prizes were awarded in 1901. A prize in economics has also been established.

Nocardia. [Edmund I. E. Nocard, Fr. veterinary pathologist, 1850–1903] A genus of gram-positive aerobic bacteria. Some species are acid-fast and thus may when stained be confused with the causative organism for tuberculosis. Species pathogenic for man cause the disease nocardiosis.

N. asteroides. Species of Nocardia pathogenic for man. The invasion site may be the lungs or skin. Abscesses called mycetomas arise in the skin.

N. brasiliensis. Species of Nocardia pathogenic for man. Chronic subcutaneous abscesses are formed.

nocardial (nō-kăr'dē-ăl). Concerning Nocardia.

nocardiosis. Pathological condition resulting from infection by any species of Nocardia. May occur as a pulmonary infection that spreads, resulting in abscesses in the skin, brain, or other areas. May also give rise to tumors that occur most frequently in lower extremities, esp. the foot, in which case it is called maduromycosis or Madura foot. Nocardiosis is distinguishable from actinomycosis by identification of organism.

TREATMENT: Sulfadiazine daily for several months.

noci- (nō'sē) [L. *nocere*, to injure]. A combining form indicating pain or injury.

nociassociation (nō"sē-ă-sō"sē-ā'shŭn) [" + *ad*, to, + *socius*, companion]. The involuntary release of nervous energy during surgical shock or following trauma.

nociceptive (nō"sĭ-sĕp'tĭv) [" + *ceptus*, receiving]. Pert. to stimuli to the brain.

nociceptive impulses. Impulses giving rise to sensations of pain.

nociceptive reflex. A reflex initiated by painful stimuli.

nociceptor (nō"sē-sĕp'tor) [" + L. *receptor*, receiver]. A nerve for receiving and transmitting painful stimuli.

noci-influence (nō″sē-ĭn′floo-ĕns) [″ + *influence*]. Injurious or harmful influence.

nociperception (nō″sĭ-pĕr-sĕp′shŭn) [″ + *perceptio,* apprehension]. The perception by the nerve centers of injurious influences or painful stimuli.

Noct. L. *nocte,* night.

noctalbuminuria (nŏk″tăl-bū-mĭn-ū′rē-ă) [L. *nocte,* at night, + *albumen,* white of egg, + Gr. *ouron,* urine]. Excess of albumin voided in urine at night. SYN: *nyctalbuminuria.*

noctambulation (nŏk″tăm-bū-lā′shŭn) [″ + *ambulare,* to move about]. Sleepwalking.

noctambulism (nŏk-tăm′bū-lĭzm) [″ + ″ + Gr. *-ismos,* state of]. Sleepwalking. SYN: *somnambulism.*

Noctec. Trade name for chloral hydrate, USP.

noctiphobia (nŏk″tĭ-fō′bē-ă) [″ + Gr. *phobos,* fear]. Fear of the night and darkness. SYN: *nyctophobia; scotophobia.*

nocturia (nŏk-tū′rē-ă) [″ + Gr. *ouron,* urine]. Urination, esp. excessive, during the night. SYN: *nycturia.* SEE: *enuresis.*

nocturnal [L. *nocturnus,* at night]. Pert. to or occurring in the night. Opposed to diurnal. SEE: words beginning with *nyct-.*

nocturnal emission. Harmless involuntary discharge of semen during sleep. Usually occurs in conjunction with an erotic dream. SYN: *wet dream.*

nocturnal enuresis. Urinary incontinence during sleep at night. SYN: *bedwetting.* SEE: *enuresis.*

nocuous (nŏk′ū-ŭs) [L. *nocuus*]. Noxious, injurious, harmful, poisonous.

nodal (nō′dăl) [L. *nodus,* knot]. Pert. to a protuberance.

nodal points. A pair of points situated on the axis of an optical system so that any incident ray sent through one will produce a parallel emergent ray sent through the other.

nodal rhythm. Cardiac rhythm with origin at atrioventricular node.

nodding (nŏd′ĭng). Involuntary allowing of head to fall downward as when momentarily dozing. SYN: *nutation.*

nodding spasm. Nodding of the head due to spasm of the sternomastoid muscles. SYN: *salaam convulsion.*

node (nōd) [L. *nodus,* knot]. 1. A knot, knob, protuberance, or swelling. 2. A constricted region. 3. A small rounded organ or structure.

n., Aschoff's. Atrioventricular node of the heart.

n., atrioventricular. A tangled mass of Purkinje fibers located in the lower part of the interatrial septum from which the atrioventricular bundle (bundle of His) arises. SEE: *bundle, atrioventricular.*

n., A-V. Atrioventricular node.

n., Bouchard's. In osteoarthritis, bony enlargement of the proximal interphalangeal joints. SEE: *n., Heberden's.*

n., Flack's. The sinoatrial node of the heart.

n.'s, Haygarth's. Joint swelling in arthritis deformans.

n.'s, Heberden's. Node on fingers seen in osteoarthritis, usually on the terminal phalangeal joints.

n., hemal. A lymphoid structure in which blood sinuses are present instead of lymph sinuses. These occur in animals but most probaby not in man.

n., Hensen's. A mass of rapidly proliferating cells at the anterior end of the primitive streak of the embryo.

n., lymph. Mass of lymphoid tissue along the course of lymphatic vessels.

n.'s, Meynet's. Nodes in capsules of joints and in tendons in rheumatism, esp. in children.

n.'s of Ranvier. Constrictions of the myelin sheath of a myelinated nerve fiber.

n., Osler's. Tender cutaneous nodes, usually in fingers and toes, that may be seen with subacute bacterial endocarditis.

n.'s, Parrot's. Osteophytes around anterior fontanel seen in hereditary syphilis.

n., piedric. Node on the hair shaft seen in piedra, q.v.

n., Schmorl's. A node seen in roentgenograms of the spine. They are caused by prolapse of the nucleus pulposus into the end plate of the vertebra.

n., sentinel. N., signal.

n., signal. Enlargement of one of the supraclavicular lymph nodes. Usually indicative of primary carcinoma of thoracic or abdominal organs.

n., singer's. Small white node that develops on vocal cords caused by overuse or improper use of the voice. SEE: *chorditis nodosa.*

n., sinoatrial. Node in wall of right atrium near entrance of superior vena cava, consisting of dense network of Purkinje fibers. Source of impulses initiating heartbeat. SYN: *pacemaker* (def. 2); *n., sinoauricular; n., sinus.*

n., sinoauricular. N., sinoatrial.

n., sinus. N., sinoatrial.

n., syphilitic. Circumscribed swelling at end of long bones due to congenital syphilis. Sensitive and painful during inflammation, esp. at night. SEE: *n., Parrot's.*

n., teacher's. N., singer's, q.v.

n., Troisier's. An enlarged node above the clavicle. It is caused by metastasis usually from an intrathoracic neoplasm.

n., Virchow. N., signal, q.v.

nodi (nō′dī). Plural of nodus.

nodose (nō′dōs) [L. *nodosus,* knotted]. Swollen or knotlike at intervals; marked by nodes or projections.

nodosity (nō-dŏs′ĭ-tē) [L. *nodositas,* a knot]. 1. A protuberance or knot. 2. Condition of having nodes.

nodular (nŏd′ū-lăr). Containing or resembling nodules.

nodulation (nŏd″ū-lā′shŭn). Formation of nodules.

nodule (nŏd′ūl) [L. *nodulus,* little knot]. 1. A small node. 2. A small aggregation of cells.

n.′s, aggregate. A group of solitary lymph nodules, such as Peyer's patches of the small intestine.

n., Albini's. Nodules sometimes seen on free edges of atrioventricular valves of the heart in infants.

n., apple jelly. The jelly-like lesion of lupus vulgaris.

n.′s, Arantius′. Central fibrous tubercles in segments of semilunar valves. SYN: *corpora Arantii; n.'s, Morgagni.*

n., Aschoff's. Nodule found in myocardium, a characteristic lesion of rheumatic carditis.

n.′s, cortical. Lymph nodules located in cortex of a lymph node.

n.′s, Gamna. Yellowish-brown nodules in the spleen in certain enlargements.

n., lymph. A mass of densely packed lymphocytes forming the structural unit of lymphatic tissue. Each contains a germinal center where new lymphocytes are formed.

n., lymphatic. N., lymph.

n., milker's. A nodule due to poxvirus that is transmitted from the udder of infected cows to the hands of milkers.

n.′s, Morgagni. N.'s, Arantius'.

n. of semilunar valve. N.'s, Arantius'.

n., rheumatic. Subcutaneous nodes of fibrous tissue that may be present in patients with rheumatic fever.

n., Schmorl's. A node seen in roentgenograms of the spine. They are caused by prolapse of the nucleus pulposus into the end plate of the vertebra.

n.′s, siderotic. Small brown nodules, seen in spleen and other organs, consisting of necrotic tissue encrusted by iron salts.

n., solitary. An isolated nodule of lymphatic tissue such as occurs in mucous membranes.

n., subcutaneous. Small, non-tender swellings resembling Aschoff bodies and found over bony prominences on hands and feet, occurring in persons with rheumatic fever.

n., surfer's. Surfer's knots, q.v.

n.′s, typhoid. Nodules characteristic of typhoid fever and found in the liver.

n., typhus. Small nodules of the skin seen in typhus. They are composed of mononuclear cell infiltration around vessels.

no diagnosis. The condition when a patient is studied extensively but no evidence of mental or physical disease can be established.

nodulus (nŏd′ū-lŭs) [L.]. (pl. *noduli*) [NA] 1. Nodule. 2. Anterior portion of vermis of the cerebellum.

nodus (nō′dŭs) [L.]. (pl. *nodi*) [NA] Node; anatomically, a small circumscribed mass of undifferentiated tissue.

noematachograph (nō-ē″mă-tăk′ō-grăf) [Gr. *noema,* thought, + *tachys,* swift, + *graphein,* to write]. Device for recording time taken in mental activity.

noematachometer (nō-ē″mă-tăk-ŏm′ĕ-tĕr) [″ + ″ + *metron,* measure]. Device for measurement of the time taken in a simple perception.

noematic (nō″ē-măt′ĭk) [Gr. *noema,* thought]. Concerning the mental process of thinking.

noesis (nō-ē′sĭs) [Gr. *noesis,* thought]. The act of thinking, cognition.

Noguchia (nō-goo′chē-ă). [Hideyo Noguchi] A genus of microorganisms of the family Brucellaceae. They are slim, gram-negative, flagellated rods. They are present in the conjunctiva of man and animals with follicular conjunctivitis.

noise [O. Fr. *noise,* strife, brawl]. 1. Sound of any sort. Loud, harsh, confused, or senseless. 2. In electronics or physics, any electronic disturbance that interferes with the signal that is being recorded or monitored. In electrocardiography, the 60-cycle alternating current used to power the machine may be inadvertently recorded. This obscures the signal from the electrical activity of the heart.

noli-me-tangere (nō″lĭ-mē-tăn′jĕ-rē) [L., touch me not]. Cancerous ulcer, generally of the face, which eats away bone and soft tissue; rodent ulcer.

Noludar. Trade name for methyprylon, USP.

Nolvadex. Trade name for tamoxifen citrate.

noma (nō′mă) [Gr. *nome,* a spreading]. A gangrenous progressive condition, generally found in undernourished children, spreading rapidly from the mucous membrane of the cheek or gum to the cutaneous surface. SYN: *cancrum oris; stomatitis, gangrenous.*

n. pudendi. An ulcerative condition affecting the labia majora, esp. in young children.

nomadism [Gr. *nomas,* roaming about]. Impulse to wander about aimlessly; restlessness.

nomenclature (nō′mĕn-klā″chūr) [L. *nomen,* name, + *calare,* to call]. Classified system of technical or scientific names. SYN: *terminology.*

n., binomial. The system of classifying plants and animals by the use of two Latin-derived words to indicate the genus and species.

Nomina Anatomica (nō′mĭ-nă ăn-ă-tŏm′ĭ-kă) [″ + Gr. *anatome,* dissection]. ABBR: NA. Anatomical terminology adopted as official by the International Congress of Anatomists at various meetings since 1950. The Tenth International Congress was held in Tokyo, Japan, in 1975. The 1977 publication *Nomina Anatomica,* containing the nomenclature, is published by Excerpta Medica Foundation, New York, London, Paris, Amsterdam, Tokyo, and Buenos Aires.

nomogram (nŏm′ō-gram) [Gr. *nomos,* law, + *gramma,* mark]. Representation by graphs, diagrams, or charts of the relationship between numerical variables.

nomography (nō-mŏg′ră-fē) [″ + *graphein,* to write]. A graphic representation of the relationship between numerical variables.

nomotopic (nō-mō-tŏp′ĭk) [″ + *topos,* place]. Occurring at the normal site.

non- [L.]. Prefix denoting negation or absence.

nona-, non- [L. *nonus,* ninth]. Prefix meaning ninth.

nona (nō′nă) [L. *nonus,* ninth]. Old term for acute or chronic infectious disease of central nervous system. SYN: *encephalitis lethargica; sleeping sickness.*

nonan (nō′năn). Having increased symptoms or reappearing every ninth day, as the paroxysms of malaria.

non compos mentis (nŏn kŏm′pŏs mĕn′tĭs) [L.]. Not of sound mind; mentally incompetent to handle one's affairs.

nonconductor [L. *non,* not, + *con,* with, + *ductor,* a leader]. Any substance that does not transmit heat, sound, or electricity or that conducts it with difficulty. Strictly speaking, there is no perfect nonconductor. On the application of a sufficiently high voltage, current may be caused to flow through materials usually spoken of as nonconductors. SYN: *insulator.*

nondisjunction. Failure of a pair of chromosomes to separate at meiosis. This allows one daughter cell to have two chromosomes and the other to have none.

nonelectrolyte [″ + *electron,* amber + *lytos,* dissolved]. A solution that will not conduct electricity because its chemical constituents are not sufficiently dissociated into ions.

nonigravida (nō″nĭ-gră′vĭ-dă) [L. *nonus,* ninth, + *gravida,* pregnant]. A woman pregnant for the ninth time. Written gravida IX. SEE: *nonipara.*

noninvasive. 1. Not tending to spread as certain tumors. 2. Devices or procedures that do not require entering the body or puncturing the skin.

noninvasive neoplasm. A tumor that has not spread or does not spread.

nonipara (nō-nĭp′ăr-ă) [″ + *parere,* to bring forth]. A woman who has given birth nine times. Written para IX.

nonlaxative diet. Low-residue diet with boiled milk and toasted crackers. No strained oatmeal, vegetable juice, or fruit juice given. Fats and concentrated sweets are restricted.

nonmedullated (nŏn-mĕd′ū-lāt″ĕd) [L. *non,* not, + *medulla,* marrow]. Containing no myelin.

nonmyelinated (nŏn-mī′ĕ-lĭ-nāt″ĕd) [″ + *myelos,* marrow]. Containing no myelin.

non-nucleated (nŏn-nū′klē-āt″ĕd) [″ + *nucleatus,* having a kernel]. Containing no nucleus.

nonocclusion (nŏn″ō-kloo′zhŭn) [″ + *occlusio,* occlusion]. A type of malocclusion in which the teeth fail to make contact.

nonopaque (nŏn″ō-pāk′). Not opaque, esp. to x-rays.

nonose (nŏn′ōs) [L. *nonus,* ninth]. A nine-carbon carbohydrate.

nonoxynol (nō-nŏks′ĭ-nōl). A general class of surface-active agents with the basic formula of $C_{15}H_{24}O(C_2H_4O)_n$; they are named with respect to the value of *n.* Thus nonoxynol 10 is $C_{15}H_{24}O(C_2H_4O)_{10}$.

n. 9. A spermicide.

nonparous (nŏn-păr′ŭs) [L. *non,* not, + *parere,* to bear]. Nulliparous.

nonpolar [″ + *polus,* a pole]. Not having separate poles; sharing electrons.

nonpolar compound. Compound formed by the sharing of electrons.

nonproprietary name. The name of a drug other than its proprietary or trademarked name. The nonproprietary name for new drugs is usually the same as that selected by United States Adopted Name (USAN) Council. The official name for older drugs may be different from the nonproprietary name. In some but not all cases, the generic name is the same as the nonproprietary name. Drugs also have chemical names; and in most cases that name is too long and complex to permit its use. Thus the use of a USAN-selected name simplifies and standardizes drug nomenclature. SEE: *proprietary medicine.*

nonprotein [L. *non,* not, + Gr. *protos,* first]. Any substance not a protein.

nonprotein nitrogen. 1. A nitrogenous constituent of blood that is not a protein. 2. Sum of all nonprotein nitrogen in the blood. SEE: *nitrogen.*

non repetat [L.]. Do not repeat.

nonrestraint (nŏn″rē-strānt′) [L. *non,* not, + *re,* back, + *stringere,* to bind back]. Treatment of the insane without using mechanical repression.

nonrotation (nŏn″rō-tā′shŭn) [″ + *rotare,* to turn]. Failure of a part or organ to rotate, esp. during embryological development.

n. of intestine. In embryonic development, the intestines fail to rotate so the descending colon is on the left side of the abdominal cavity instead of the right.

nonsecretor (nŏn″sē-krē′tor) [″ + *secretio,* separation]. An individual whose saliva does not contain the ABO blood antigens.

nonseptate (nŏn-sĕp′tāt) [″ + *septum,* a partition]. Having no dividing walls.

nonsexual (nŏn-sĕk′shū-ăl). Without sex. SYN: *asexual.*

nonspecific. Term used in reference to the cause of a disease when the exact organism or agent has not been identified.

nonspecific urethritis. Urethritis not due to a provable specific virus or bacteria.

nontoxic (nŏn-tŏk′sĭk) [Gr. *non,* not, + Gr. *toxikon,* poison]. Not poisonous or productive of poison.

nontoxic substances. For those involved in patient care, it is important to know that some of the common materials that children and adults can accidentally ingest are not toxic. A list of substances considered to be generally nontoxic is provided in the Appendix. SEE: *Generally Nontoxic Substances* in *Appendix.*

nonunion (nŏn-ūn′yŭn) [″ + *unio,* oneness]. Failure of fragments of a fractured bone to knit together.

nonus [L.]. 1. Ninth. 2. Hypoglossal nerve, formerly regarded as ninth cranial nerve.

nonvalent (nŏn-vā′lĕnt) [L. *non,* not, + *valens,* powerful]. Having no chemical valency.

nonviable (nŏn-vī′ă-bl) [″ + *via,* life]. Incapable of life or of living; frequently used to indicate a fetus that has died in utero, born prior to 20th week of gestation.

nonyl. A univalent radical, $CH_3(CH_2)_8$, that contains 9 carbon atoms.

nookleptia (nō-ō-klĕp′tē-ă) [Gr. *nous,* mind, + *kleptein,* to steal]. An obsession that one's thoughts are being stolen by others.

Noonan's syndrome. A syndrome quite similar to Turner's. There are low-set ears, webbing of the neck, pulmonary valve stenosis, and in some cases severe mental retardation.

noopsyche (nō′ō-sī″kē) [Gr. *nous,* mind, + *psyche,* soul]. Mental processes.

noradrenalin bitartrate (nor″ă-drĕn′ă-lĭn) Norepinephrine bitartate, USP.

nordefrin hydrochloride (nor-dĕf′rĭn). A vasoconstrictor drug. Trade name is Cobefrin.

norepinephrine (nor-ĕp″ĭ-nĕf′rĭn). A hormone produced by the adrenal medulla, similar in chemical and pharmacological properties to epinephrine, but it is chiefly a vasoconstrictor and has little effect on cardiac output.

n. bitartrate. USP. A standardized preparation of norepinephrine, q.v. Trade name is Levophed. Previously used name was levarterenol bitartrate.

norethandrolone (nor″ĕth-ăn′drō-lōn). An anabolic steroid.

norethindrone (nor-ĕth′ĭn-drōn). USP. A steroid hormone similar in action to progesterone. Used in progestational agents for birth control. Trade names are Micronor, Nor-Q.D., and Norlutin.

norethynodrel (nor″ĕ-thī′nō-drĕl). USP. A progestational agent used in certain birth control pils.

Norflex. Trade name for orphenadrine citrate, USP.

norflurane (nor-floor′ān). An inhalation anesthetic.

norgestrel (nor-jĕs′trĕl). USP. A progestational agent used in certain birth control pills. Trade names are Microlut and Ovrette.

Norisodrine Hydrochloride. Trade name for isoproterenol hydrochloride, USP.

Norisodrine Sulfate. Trade name for isoproterenol sulfate, USP.

Norlutate. Trade name for norethindrone acetate, USP.

Norlutin. Trade name for norethindrone, USP.

norm [L. *norma,* rule]. 1. A standard or ideal for a specific group. 2. Normal.

norma [L., rule]. A view or aspect, esp. with reference to the skull.

n., anterior. N. frontalis.

n. basilaris. N. ventralis.

n. facialis. N. frontalis.

n. frontalis. Outline of the skull viewed from the front. SYN: *n. anterior; n. facialis.*

n., inferior. N. ventralis.

n. lateralis. View as seen from the side; a profile view.

n. occipitalis. View of the skull as seen from behind.

n. sagittalis. View as seen in sagittal section.

n., superior. N. verticalis.

n. ventralis. View of inferior surface of skull. SYN: *n., inferior; n. basilaris.*

n. verticalis. View of skull as seen from above. SYN: *n., superior.*

normal (nor′măl) [L. *normalis,* according to pattern]. 1. Standard; performing proper functions; natural; regular. 2. In biology, not affected by experimental treatment; occurring naturally and not because of disease or experimentation. 3. In psychology, free from mental disorder; or of average development or intelligence. 4. In chemistry, a term used to describe a solution so made that 1 liter contains 1 gram equivalent of the solute.

normalization (nor″măl-ī-zā′shŭn) [L. *normalis,* according to pattern]. Modification or reduction to the normal standard.

normal salt. An ionic compound containing no replaceable hydrogen or hydroxyl ions.

normal solution. 1. SEE: *normal* (def. 4). 2. A solution that neutralizes an equal volume of a normal solution of any base or acid.

normergic (nor-mĕr′jĭk). Reacting, or pert. to that which reacts, in a normal manner.

normetanephrine (nor-mĕt″ă-nĕf′rĭn). A metabolite of epinephrine.

normo- [L. *norma,* rule]. A combining form indicating normal or usual.

normoblast (nor′mō-blăst) [″ + Gr. *blastos,* germ]. A nucleated red blood corpuscle similar in size to an ordinary erythrocyte.

normoblastosis (nor″mō-blăs-tō′sĭs) [″ + ″ + *osis,* condition]. Increased production of normoblasts.

normocalcemia (nor″mō-kăl-sē′mē-ă). Normal level of blood calcium.

normocapnia (nor″mō-kăp′nē-ă). Presence of carbon dioxide in the blood and serum in normal concentration.

normocapnic (nor″mō-kăp′nĭk). Having the normal amount of carbon dioxide in the blood.

normocholesterolemia (nor″mō-kō-lĕs″tĕr-ō-lē′mē-ă). Presence of cholesterol in the blood in normal concentration.

normochromasia (nor″mō-krō-mā′zē-ă) [″ + Gr. *chroma,* color]. Average staining capacity in a cell or tissue.

normochromia (nor″mō-krō′mē-ă). Blood possessing normal color and hemoglobin content.

normocyte (nor′mō-sīt) [″ + Gr. *kytos,* cell]. An average-sized red blood corpuscle. SYN: *erythrocyte; normoerythrocyte.*

normocytosis (nor″mō-sī-tō′sĭs) [″ + ″ + *osis,* condition]. A normal state of the corpuscular elements of the blood.

normoerythrocyte (nor″mō-ĕ-rĭth′rō-sīt) [″ + Gr. *erythros,* red, + *kytos,* cell]. Normocyte.

normoglycemia (nor″mō-glī-sē′mē-ă) [″ + Gr. *glykys,* sweet, + *haima,* blood]. Normal state of sugar content of the blood.

normoglycemic (nŏr″mō-glī-sē′mĭk). Having a normal amount of sugar in the blood.

normokalemia (nor″mō-kă-lē′mē-ă). Normal level of blood potassium.

normoorthocytosis (nor″mō-or″thō-sī-tō′sĭs) [L. *norma,* rule, + Gr. *orthos,* correct, + *kytos,* cell, + *osis,* condition]. Increase of the number of leukocytes in the blood but with normal proportion of the different varieties.

normoskeocytosis (nor″mō-skē″ō-sī-tō′sĭs) [″ + *skaios,* left, + *kytos,* cell, + *osis,* condition]. Normal number of the leukocytes of the blood with shift to the left, i.e., with immature forms present.

normospermic (nor″mō-spĕr′mĭk) [″ + *sperma,* seed]. The production of normal spermatozoa.

normosthenuria (nor″mō-sthĕn-ū′rē-ă) [″ + Gr. *sthenos,* strength, + *ouron,* urine]. Urination of normal amount and specific gravity.

normotensive (nor″mō-tĕn′sĭv). 1. Normal blood pressure. 2. A person with normal blood pressure.

normothermia (nor″mō-thĕr′mē-ă) [″ + Gr. *therme,* heat]. Normal body temperature.

normotonic (nor″mō-tŏn′ĭk) [″ + Gr. *tonos,* tension]. 1. Having normal muscular tonus. 2. One who has normal muscle tonus.

normotopia (nor″mō-tō′pē-ă) [″ + Gr. *topos,* place]. Situation in the regular place.

normotopic (nor″mō-tŏp′ĭk). In the right location; pert. to the normal situation.

normovolemia (nor″mō-vō-lē′mē-ă) [″ + *volumen,* volume, + Gr. *haima,* blood]. Normal state of blood volume.

Norpace. Trade name for disopyramide phosphate, USP.

Norpramin. Trade name for desipramine hydrochloride, USP.

Norrie's disease. [G. Norrie, contemporary Danish ophthalmologist] A rare form of sex-linked hereditary blindness. Also present are peripheral vascular pathology, retinal malformation, vitreous opacities, microphthalmia, and sometimes mental retardation and loss of hearing.

nortriptyline hydrochloride (nor-trĭp′tĭ-lēn). USP. An antidepressant drug of the tricyclic class. Trade names are Aventyl Hydrochloride and Pamelor.

Norwalk agent [virus first identified in Norwalk, Ohio, U.S.A.]. The viral agent that causes epidemic acute nonbacterial gastroenteritis, q.v.

Norwegian itch. Severe form of scabies marked by pustules and crusts.

noscapine (nŏs′kă-pēn). A naturally occurring opium alkaloid that is used as an antitussive in cough preparations.

nose [AS. *nosw*]. Projection in center of face; the organ of olfaction and the entrance that warms, moistens, and filters the air as it passes through en route to the respiratory tract. SYN: *nasus* [NA]; *organum olfactus.*

ANAT: The external portion of the nose is a triangle of cartilage and bone covered with skin and lined with mucous membrane. Internally, a septum divides the nose into two chambers. Each chamber contains three meattus, which are found underneath the corresponding turbinates. Orifices of frontal, anterior, ethmoid, and maxillary sinuses are in middle meatus. Orifices of posterior ethmoids and sphenoids are in superior meatus.

Communicating sinuses: Ethmoidal, frontal, maxillary, and sphenoidal. *Nerves:* Facial, olfactory, ophthalmic, and maxillary. *Blood supply:* External and internal maxillary arteries from the external carotid and ethmoidal artery from the internal carotid.

EXAM: Note shape, size, color, state of the alae nasi, discharge, interference with respiration, evidences of injury, deflected or perforated septum, enlarged turbinates, and tenderness over frontal and maxillary sinuses.

DIAG: *Chronic red nose:* dilated capillaries as a result of alcoholism, lupus erythematosus, acne rosacea, pustules, and boils. *Superficial ulceration:* tuberculous ulcer, epithelioma, syphilis. *Broad and coarse:* cretinism, myxedema, acromegaly. *Sunken:* syphilis or injury. *Pinched with small nares:* hypertrophied adenoid tissue or chronic obstructions; tumors. *Inoffensive watery discharge:* present in nasal catarrh, early stages of measles, hay fever, acute irritation of lining membranes. *Offensive discharge:* nasopharyngeal diphtheria, lupus, local infection, impacted foreign bodies, caries, rhinitis, glanders, syphilitic infection.

n., bridge of. Superior portion of external nose formed by union of the two nasal bones.

n., foreign body in. Irritation of nose resulting in coughing or watery or purulent discharge. Occasionally pain and obstruction of nose. If not recognized immediately, it often causes a foul discharge on the affected side of the nose. There may be obstruction to breathing in one nostril. If the foreign body is very small, symptoms may be absent.

TREATMENT: Take the patient to a physician. Vigorous blowing of the nose is dangerous because it may spread infection to the various cavities and sinuses about the nose or to the middle ear. Attempts to dislodge it may cause it to slip further into the nose or down the throat and into the windpipe.

n., hammer. Rhinophyma.

n., saddle. Nose with depressed bridge seen in tertiary syphilis due to gummatous destruction of septal supporting structure, and following operations that are complicated by suppuration and destruction of supporting framework.

nose, words pert. to: ala nasi; alinasal; anosmia; bulb, olfactory; choana; columella nasi; epistaxis; hyperosmia; Kiesselbach's area; naris; nasal; nostril; parosmia; rhinalgia; septum, nasal; sinuses, accessory nasal; sinusitis; smell; vestibule of nose; vibrissae; vomer; and "nas-" and "rhino-" words.

nosebleed. Hemorrhage from nose. SYN: *epistaxis.* SEE: *Kiesselbach's area.*

Nosema (nō-sē′mă). A genus of parasites of the Microsporidia order.

nosepiece (nōz′pēs). The portion of a microscope to which the objective lenses attach.

nosetiology (nŏs″ē-tē-ŏl′ō-jē) [Gr. *nosos,* disease, + *aitia,* cause, + *logos,* study]. Study of the cause of disease.

nosh. 1. Between-meal snacks. 2. To eat or nibble between meals.

noso- [Gr. *nosos,* disease]. Combining form pert. to disease.

nosochthonography (nŏs″ŏk-thō-nŏg′ră-fē) [″ + *chthon,* earth, + *graphein,* to write]. Study of geographical distribution of diseases; medical geography. SYN: *nosogeography.*

nosocomial (nŏs″ō-kō′mē-ăl) [″ + *komeion,* to care for]. Pert. to a hospital or infirmary.

nosocomial infection. Infection acquired in a hospital.

nosogenesis, nosogeny (nŏs″ō-jĕn′ĕ-sĭs, nō-sŏj′ĕn-ē) [Gr. *nosos,* disease, + *gennan,* to produce]. The development and progress of a disease.

nosogeography (nŏs″ō-jē-ŏg′ră-fē) [″ + *ge,* earth, + *graphein,* to write]. Study of medical geography. SYN: *nosochthonography.*

nosography (nō-sŏg′ră-fē) [″ + *graphein,* to write]. The written description of a disease.

nosohemia (nŏs-ō-hē′mē-ă) [″ + *haima,* blood]. Disease of the blood.

nosology (nō-sŏl′ō-jē) [″ + *logos,* study]. The science of description or classification of diseases.

nosomania (nŏs″ō-mā′nē-ă) [″ + *mania,* madness]. The delusion that one is diseased.

nosomycosis (nŏs″ō-mī-kō′sĭs) [″ + *mykes,* fungus, + *osis,* condition]. Any disease caused by a parasitic fungus or Schizomycete.

nosonomy (nō-sŏn′ō-mē) [″ + *nomos,* law]. The science of disease classification.

nosophilia (nŏs″ō-fĭl′ē-ă) [″ + *philein,* to love]. An abnormal desire to be ill.

nosophobia (nō″sō-fō′bē-ă) [″ + *phobos,* fear]. Abnormal aversion to illness or to a particular affection.

nosophyte (nŏs′ō-fīt) [″ + *phyton,* plant]. A disease-causing plant microorganism.

nosopoietic (nŏs″ō-poy-ĕt′ĭk) [″ + *poiein,* to form]. Producing or causing disease.

Nosopsyllus (nŏs″ŏ-sĭl′ŭs) [″ + *psylla,* flea]. A genus of fleas belonging to the order Siphonaptera.

N. fasciatus. A species of rat fleas responsible for transmission of murine typhus and perhaps of plague.

nosotaxy (nŏs′ō-tăk″sē) [″ + *taxis,* arrangement]. Classification of disease.

nosotherapy (nŏs″ō-thĕr′ă-pē) [″ + *therapeia,* treatment]. Treatment of one disease by voluntarily introducing another microorganism into the body.

Ex.: In the past, the use of malaria parasites to cause fever in treatment of central nervous system syphilis.

nosotoxic (nŏs″ō-tŏk′sĭk) [″ + *toxikon,* poison]. Anything that produces a disease-causing toxin.

nosotoxicosis (nŏs″ō-tŏk″sī-kō′sĭs) [″ + ″ + *osis,* condition]. Any disease caused by poisoning.

nosotrophy (nō-sŏt′rō-fē) [″ + *trophe,* nourishment]. Nursing care and feeding of the sick.

nosotropic (nō″sō-trŏp′ĭk) [″ + *tropos,* turning]. Directed against the symptoms or effects of a disease. Opposite of etiotropic.

nostalgia (nŏs-tăl′jē-ă) [Gr. *nostos,* a return home, + *algos,* pain]. Homesickness; longing to return home.

nostomania (nŏs″tō-mā′nē-ă) [″ + *mania,* madness]. Nostalgia verging on insanity.

nostril [AS. *nosu,* nose, + *thyrel,* a hole]. One of the external apertures of the nose. SYN: *naris.* SEE: *nose.*

nostril reflex. Reduction of opening of naris on affected side in lung disease in proportion to lessened alveolar air capacity on affected side.

nostrum (nŏs′trŭm) [L., our]. A patent, secret, or quack remedy.

notal (nō′tăl) [Gr. *noton,* back]. Concerning the back. SYN: *dorsal.*

notalgia (nō-tăl′jē-ă) [″ + *algos,* pain]. Painful condition of the back. SYN: *dorsalgia.*

notancephalia (nō″tăn-sĕ-fā′lē-ă) [″ + *-an,* not, + *kephale,* head]. Congenital absence of the back of the skull.

notanencephalia (nō″tăn-ĕn-sĕ-fā′lē-ă) [″ + ″ + *enkephalos,* brain]. Absence of the cerebellum.

notch (nŏch). A rather deep indentation or narrow gap in the edge of a structure. SYN: *incisura* [NA].

n., acetabular. Notch in inferior border of acetabulum. SYN: *n., cotyloid.*

n., aortic. Notch in sphygmogram from rebound at aortic valve closure.

n., cardiac. Concavity on anterior border of left lung into which the heart projects.

n., cerebellar, anterior and posterior. Deep notches separating the hemispheres of the cerebellum.

n., clavicular. Notch at the upper angle of the sternum with which the clavicle articulates.

n., costal. One of seven pairs of indentations on lateral surfaces of the sternum, for articulation with costal cartilages.

n., cotyloid. N., acetabular.

n., ethmoidal. Notch separating the two orbital portions of frontal bone.

n., frontal. Notch on supraorbital arch that transmits frontal artery and nerve.

n., interclavicular. A rounded notch at the top of the manubrium of the sternum, between surfaces articulating with the clavicles.

n., jugular (of occipital bone). Notch that forms the posterior and middle portions of jugular foramen.

n., jugular (of sternum). Notch on upper surface of manubrium between the two clavicular notches.

n., mandibular. Notch on superior border of ramus of mandible separating coronoid and condyloid processes.

n., nasal. 1. Deep notch on anterior surface of maxilla and forming lateral border of piriform aperture. 2. Notch between internal angular processes of frontal bone.

n. of Rivinus. N., tympanic, q.v.

n., pancreatic. Notch on lateral surface of head of pancreas for superior mesenteric artery and vein. It separates uncinate process of head from remaining portion.

n., parotid. The space between the ramus of the mandible and the mastoid process of the temporal bone.

n., radial. Notch on lateral surface of coronoid process of ulna for receiving circumference of head of radius.

n., scapular. A deep notch on superior border of scapula. Transmits suprascapular nerve.

n., sciatic, greater. Large notch on the posterior border of the hip bone between the posterior inferior iliac spine and the spine of ischium.

n., sciatic, lesser. Notch immediately below the spine of the ischium on the posterior border of the hip bone. Converted into a foramen by the sacrotuberous ligament.

n., semilunar. Notch on anterior aspect of proximal end of ulna for articulation with trochlea of humerus.

n., sphenopalatine. Notch between orbital and sphenoidal processes of palatine bone.

n., tentorial. Notch in free border of tentorium cerebelli through which brain stem passes.

n., thyroid. Deep notch on superior border of thyroid cartilage of larynx separating the two laminae.

n., tympanic. Notch in superior portion of the tympanic ring. SYN: *n of Rivinus.*

n., ulnar. Notch on distal end of radius for receiving head of ulna.

n., umbilical. Notch on anterior border of liver where it is crossed by falciform ligament.

n., vertebral. Concavity on inferior surface of root of vertebral arch. When two vertebrae are in position, the notches form the intervertebral foramina.

note [L. *nota,* a mark]. 1. A sound of definite pitch. 2. A brief comment or condensed report.

note blindness. Inability to recognize musical notes; due to a central lesion.

notencephalocele (nō″tĕn-sĕf′ăl-ō-sēl) [Gr. *noton,* back, + *enkephalos,* brain, + *kele,* hernia]. Protrusion of brain substance at the back of the head.

notencephalus (nō″tĕn-sĕf′ă-lŭs) [″ + *enkephalos,* brain]. A deformed fetus with notencephalocele.

nothing by mouth. An instruction used in patient care to indicate the patient is to take or receive no food, liquid, or medicine, i.e., *nothing,* by mouth. Usually abbreviated NPO.

notifiable diseases. The laws of the various states require that certain diseases when existing shall be reported to the local health authorities, such as a Board of Health. A fine may be levied for not doing so. Among the diseases that may be required to be reported are all communicable or contagious diseases such as smallpox, scarlet fever, diphtheria; enteric fevers such as typhoid fever; cholera; typhus; meningococcal meningitis; acute anterior poliomyelitis; polioencephalitis; encephalitis lethargica; tuberculosis; epidemic of acute diarrheal disease; rubella; chickenpox; gonorrhea; syphilis. SEE: *quarantine; reportable diseases.*

noto- [Gr. *noton,* back]. Combining form indicating a relationship to the back.

notochord (nō'tō-kord) [" + *chorde,* cord]. A rod of cells lying dorsal to the intestine and extending from anterior to posterior end. It forms axial skeleton in embryos of all chordates. In vertebrates it is replaced partially or completely by the bodies of vertebrae. A remnant persists in man as a portion of nucleus pulposus of intervertebral disk.

notogenesis (nō"tō-jĕn'ĕ-sĭs) [" + *genesis,* production]. Development of the notochord.

notomelus (nō-tŏm'ĕ-lŭs) [" + *melos,* limb]. A deformed fetus with one or more accessory limbs attached to the back.

noumenal (nū'mē-năl) [Gr. *nooumenon,* a thing perceived]. Pert. to noumenon, q.v. Pert. to that which arises because of intellectual intuition rather than sensory perception.

noumenon (nū'mē-nŏn) [Gr. *nooumenon*]. That which one knows or perceives by intellectual intuition alone, as distinguished from something perceived through sensory perception.

nourishment [L. *nutrire,* to nurse]. 1. Act of nourishing or of being nourished. 2. Sustenance; nutriment. SEE: *center, trophic; trophic.*

Novafed. Trade name for pseudoephedrine hydrochloride, USP.

Novocain. Trade name for procaine hydrochloride, USP.

Novrad. Trade name for levopropoxyphene napsylate, USP.

noxa (nŏk'să) [L., injury]. (pl. *noxae*) Anything harmful to health.

noxious (nŏk'shŭs) [L. *noxius,* injurious]. Harmful; not wholesome.

NP. *nucleoprotein; nurse practitioner; nursing practice; nursing procedure; neuropsychiatrist; neuropsychiatry.*

Np. Chem. symb. for neptunium.

NPH insulin. *neutral protamine Hagedorn insulin.*

NPN. *nonprotein nitrogen.*

n.p.t. *normal pressure and temperature.*

N.R.E.M. sleep. Non–rapid eye movement sleep. SEE: *sleep, N.R.E.M.*

N.R.M.S. *National Registry of Medical Secretaries.*

ns. 1. *nanosecond.* 2. *nonsignificant.*

NSA. *Neurosurgical Society of America.*

NSCC. *National Society for Crippled Children.*

NSD. *nominal standard dose* in ret. Ret indicates *r*adiation *e*quivalent *t*herapy, which is analogous to the rem (*r*oentgen *e*quivalent *m*an) used in radiation protection.

nsec. *nanosecond.*

N.S.N.A. *National Student Nurse Association.*

NSPB. *National Society for the Prevention of Blindness.*

Nt. Chem. symb. for niton.

nth (ĕnth). Used in medical statistics to indicate the continuation of data or subjects to large numbers in that progression or series. Thus, one would indicate patients numbered beginning P1, P2, P3, and so forth through P nth. P nth would be the last patient indicated.

Nubain. Trade name for nalbuphine hydrochloride.

nubecula (nū-bĕk'ū-lă) [L., little cloud]. Cloudiness of the cornea or the urine.

nubile (nū'bĭl) [L. *nubere,* to marry]. Pert. to a girl who has attained puberty.

nubility (nū-bĭl'ĭ-tē). Marriageableness, said of the female.

nucha (nū'kă) [L.]. [NA] Nape of neck.

nuchal (nū'kăl) [L. *nucha,* back of neck]. Pert. to the neck or nucha.

Nuck's canal (nŭks). [Anton Nuck, Dutch anatomist, 1650–1692] An anomalous peritoneal pouch extending for a variable distance into the labium of the external female genitalia. Homologous to processus vaginalis of the male.

nuclear (nū'klē-ăr) [L. *nucleus,* a kernel]. Resembling or concerning a nucleus.

nuclear arc. Spiral patterns on the surface of the lens due to concentric pattern of fiber growth.

nuclear envelope. Consists of two parallel membranes enclosing a narrow perinuclear space, enveloping the nucleus. Prior to electron microscopy, the nucleus of a cell was thought to be surrounded by a single, thin membrane.

nuclear family. The basic family unit consisting of parents and their children.

nuclear magnetic resonance imaging. ABBR: NMR. A technique by which the quantitative analysis of a biological structure of tissue sample may be determined. This technique provides a means of evaluating the chemical and biological state of tissues.

nuclear medicine. That branch of medicine concerned with the diagnostic, therapeutic, and investigative use of radionuclides, q.v.

nuclease (nū'klē-ās) [L. *nucleus,* kernel, + *-ase,* enzyme]. Any enzyme in animals and plants that facilitates hydrolysis of nuclein and nucleic acids.

nucleate (nū'klē-āt) [L. *nucleatus,* having a kernel]. 1. Having a nucleus. 2. To form a nucleus. 3. A salt or ester of nucleic acid.

nucleic acid. A group of high–molecular weight substances found in cells of all living things. They have a complex chemical structure being formed of sugars (pentoses), phosphoric acid, and nitrogen bases (purines and pyrimidines). Most important are deoxyribonucleic acid, q.v., and ribonucleic acid, q.v.

nucleiform (nū'klē-ĭ-form) [L. *nucleus,* kernel, + *forma,* shape]. Shaped like a nucleus.

nuclein (nū'klē-ĭn) [L. *nucleus,* a kernel]. A normal chemical constituent of a cell nucleus; a colorless, shapeless substance obtained by hydrolysis of nucleoproteins to form nucleic acid and proteins.

nuclein bases. Bases formed from decomposition of nuclein.

Ex.: adenine, guanine, xanthine, hypoxanthine.

nucleinase. Nuclease.

nucleo- [L. *nucleus*]. Pert. to a nucleus.

nucleocapsid (nū"klē-ō-kăp'sĭd). In a virus, the protein coat and the viral nucleic acid.

nucleochylema (nū"klē-ō-kī-lē'mă) [" + Gr. *chylos,* juice]. Karyolymph or nuclear sap.

nucleochyme (nū'klē-ō-kīm) [" + Gr. *chymos,* juice]. Karyolymph.

nucleofugal (nū-klē-ŏf'ū-găl) [" + *fugere,* to flee]. Directed or moving away from a nucleus in the cell.

nucleohistone (nū"klē-ō-hĭs'tŏn, -tōn) [" + *histos,* tissue]. A substance composed of nuclein and histone, found in sperm of various animals.

nucleoid (nū'klē-oyd) [" + Gr. *eidos,* resemblance]. Resembling a nucleus.

nucleolar (nū-klē'ō-lăr) [L. *nucleolus,* a little kernel]. Pert. to a nucleolus.

nucleoli (nū-klē'ō-lī). Pl. of nucleolus.

nucleoliform (nū-klē-ō'lĭ-form) [" + *forma,* shape]. Like a nucleolus.

nucleoloid (nū'klē-ō-loyd). Similar to a nucleus.

nucleolonema (nū"klē-ō"lō-nē'mă) [" + Gr. *nema,* thread]. A fine network in the nucleolus of a cell.

nucleolus (nū-klē'ō-lŭs) [L., little kernel]. (pl. *nucleoli*) A spherical body within the cell nucleus.

nucleomicrosome (nū"klē-ō-mī'krō-sōm) [L. *nucleus,* kernel, + Gr. *mikros,* tiny, + *soma,* body]. Any one of the minute granules that make up the fibers of nuclear fibers.

nucleons (nū'klē-ŏnz). Collective name of the particles that make up the nucleus of an atom.

nucleopetal (nū-klē-ŏp'ĕ-tăl) [L. *nucleus,* kernel, + *petere,* to seek]. Seeking or moving toward the nucleus.

nucleophilic (nū"klē-ō-fĭl'ĭk) [" + *philein,* to love]. Having an attraction to nuclei.

nucleoplasm (nū'klē-ō-plăzm") [" + Gr. *plasma,* a thing formed]. The protoplasm of a cell nucleus.

nucleoplasmic. Pert. to nucleoplasm.

nucleoplasmic index. The ratio of nuclear volume to cytoplasmic volume, expressed thus:

$$NP = \frac{\text{vol. of nucleus}}{\text{vol. of cell} - \text{vol. of nucleus}}$$

nucleoprotein (nū"klē-ō-prō'tē-ĭn) [" + Gr. *protos,* first]. The combination of one of the proteins with nucleic acid to form a conjugated protein found in cell nuclei.

nucleoreticulum (nū"klē-ō-rē-tĭk'ū-lŭm) [" + *reticulum,* network]. Any mesh framework in a nucleus.

nucleosidase (nū"klē-ō-sī'dās). An enzyme that catalyzes the hydrolysis of nucleosides.

nucleoside. A glycoside formed by the union of a purine or pyrimidine base with a sugar (pentose).

nucleospindle (nū"klē-ō-spĭn'dl). Spindle-shaped body occurring in karyokinesis, q.v.

nucleotidase (nū"klē-ŏt'ĭ-dās). An enzyme (nucleophosphatase) that splits phosphoric acid from nucleotides leaving a nucleoside.

5-nucleotidase. An enzyme present in serum. Its serum level is increased in carcinoma of the pancreas when there is common bile duct obstruction or metastasis to the liver.

nucleotide (nū'klē-ō-tīd) [L. *nucleus,* kernel]. A compound formed of phosphoric acid, a sugar, and a base (purine or pyrimidine), all of which constitute the structural unit of nucleic acid. SYN: *mononucleotide.*

nucleotidyl (nū"klē-ō-tīd'ĭl). The residue of a nucleotide.

nucleotidyltransferase (nū"klē-ō-tīd'ĭl-trăns'fĕr-ās). Enzyme that transfers nucleotidyls from nucleosides into dimer or polymer forms.

nucleotoxin [" + Gr. *toxikon,* poison]. A toxin acting upon or produced by cell nuclei.

nucleus (nū'klē-ŭs) [L., kernel]. (pl. *nuclei*) 1. A central point about which matter is gathered, as in a calculus. 2. The vital body in the protoplasm of a cell; the essential agent in growth, metabolism, reproduction, and transmission of characteristics of a cell. SEE: *cell.* 3. [NA] Group of nerve cells or mass of gray matter in the central nervous system, esp. the brain. 4. In chemistry, a heavy central atomic particle in which most of the mass and total positive electric charge are concentrated.

n., abducent. A gray nucleus, the origin of the abducens nerve, on the floor of the 4th ventricle, behind the trigeminal nucleus.

n., ambiguous. Nucleus of the glossopharyngeal and vagus nerves in medulla oblongata. Lies in lateral half of reticular formation.

n., amygdaloid. Nucleus projecting into inferior cornua of lateral ventricle. Constitutes part of basal ganglia.

n., angular. The superior vestibular nucleus. SYN: *n., Bechterew's*. SEE: *n., vestibular.*

n., anterior, of thalamus. Nucleus located in rostral part of thalamus. Receives fibers of mammillothalamic tract.

n., arcuate. 1. Nucleus located on basal aspect of pyramid of medulla. 2. The posteromedial ventral nucleus of the thalamus.

n., atomic. The central part of atoms, which contains protons and electrons.

n., auditory. Nest of nerve cells where auditory nerves arise.

n., Bechterew's, Bekhterev's. N., angular.

n., caudate. A comma-shaped mass of gray matter forming part of the corpus striatum. Constitutes part of the basal ganglia. SYN: *n., intraventricular.*

n., central, of thalamus. A group of nuclei in middle part of thalamus. SYN: *n., centromedian.*

n., centromedian. N., central, of thalamus.

n., cerebellar. One of the nuclei of the cerebellum.

n., cochlear, dorsal. Nucleus in medulla oblongata lying dorsal to restiform body. Receives fibers of cochlear nerve.

n., cochlear, ventral. Nucleus in medulla oblongata lying anterior and lateral to restiform body. Receives fibers from cochlear nerve.

n., cornucommissural, posterior. A column of cells that extends the entire length of the spinal cord and lies along the medial border of the posterior column near the posterior gray commissure.

n., cuneate. Nucleus in inferior portion of medulla oblongata in which fibers of the fasciculus cuneatus terminate. SYN: *n. of Burdach.*

n., Deiter's. Lateral vestibular nucleus. SEE: *n., vestibular.*

n., dentate. Large convoluted mass of gray matter in lateral portion of cerebellum. It is folded so as to enclose some of the central white matter. Gives rise to fibers of the superior cerebellar peduncle.

n., diploid. A nucleus that contains the normal double complement of chromosomes.

n., dorsal, of spinal cord. A column of gray matter lying at base of dorsal horn of the gray matter and extending from 7th cervical to 3rd lumbar segments. Cells give rise to fibers of the dorsal spinocerebellar tract. SYN: *Clarke's column.*

n., dorsal motor, of vagus. A column of cells in medulla oblongata lying lateral to hypoglossal nucleus. Its cells give rise to most of the efferent fibers of vagus nerve.

n., dorsal sensory, of vagus. Nucleus lying lateral to dorsal motor nucleus of vagus. Receives fibers of solitary tract.

n., ectoblastic. Nucleus in cells of the epiblast.

n., Edinger-Westphal. Nucleus of midbrain located dorsomedially to oculomotor nucleus. Gives rise to visceral efferent fibers terminating in ciliary ganglion, axons from which innervate ciliary muscle and sphincter iridis.

n., emboliform. Nucleus of cerebellum lying between dentate and globose nuclei. Receives axons of Purkinje cells and sends efferent fibers into branchium conjunctivum.

n., facial motor. Nucleus in medulla oblongata in floor of 4th ventricle giving rise to efferent fibers of facial nerve.

n., fastigial. Nucleus in medullary portion of cerebellum. Receives afferent fibers from vestibular nerve and superior vestibular nucleus. Afferent fibers form fasciculus uncinatus and fastigiobulbar tract.

n., fertilization. The nucleus produced by the joining of the male and female nuclei in fertilization of the ovum.

n., free. A nucleus that is no longer surrounded by the other cellular elements.

n. funiculi gracilis. Elongated mass of gray matter in dorsal pyramid of medulla oblongata.

n., germinal. Nucleus resulting from union of male and female pronuclei.

n., globose. Nucleus of the cerebellum located medial to the emboliform nucleus.

n., gonad. Micronucleus (def. 1).

n. gracilis. [NA] Nucleus in medulla oblongata in which fibers of the fasciculus gracilis terminate.

n., habenular. Nucleus of the diencephalon located in the habenular trigone. Functions as an olfactory correlation center.

n., haploid. Cell nucleus with half the normal number of chromosomes. This is true for germ cells, i.e., ova or sperm, following the normal reduction divisions in gametogenesis.

n., hypoglossal. An elongated mass of gray matter in the medulla oblongata in floor of 4th ventricle. Gives rise to motor fibers of hypoglossal nerve.

n., hypothalamic. One of the nuclei occurring in four groups found in hypothalamus. Includes the following nuclei: dorsomedial, intercalatus, lateral, mammillary (lateral and medial), paraventricular, posterior, supraoptic, tuberal, ventromedial. Cells of these nuclei, esp. the supraoptic and paraventricular, in addition to serving a neural function, are secretory and produce the vasopressor oxytocin as well as antidiuretic principles of the hypophysis. These hormones pass through efferent fibers of the infundibular stalk to the pars nervosa (posterior lobe) of the hypophysis, where they are stored and liberated.

n., interpeduncular. Nucleus of the midbrain near superior border of pons. Receives fibers of the habenulopeduncular tract.

n., interstitial, of Cajal. Nucleus in superior portion of midbrain. Receives fibers from vestibular nuclei, basal ganglia, and occipital regions of cerebral cortex. Efferent fibers pass to ipsi- and contralateral fasciculi and interstitiospinal tracts.

n., intraventricular. N., caudate.

n., lenticular. One of the nuclei forming part of the basal ganglia of the cerebrum. Consists of globus pallidus and putamen. With the caudate nucleus, it forms the corpus striatum.

n. lentis. [NA] The core or inner dense section of the crystalline lens.

n., mother. Nucleus that divides into two or more parts to form daughter nuclei.

n., motor. Nucleus giving rise to motor fibers of a nerve.

n., motor, of trigeminal nerve. Nucleus in medulla oblongata near first margin of superior part of 4th ventricle. Gives rise to motor fibers of trigeminal nerve.

n., oculomotor. Nucleus in central gray matter of midbrain lying below rostral end of cerebral aqueduct.

n. of Burdach. N., cuneate, q.v.

n. of origin. Any collection of nerve cells giving rise to fibers of a nerve or nerve tract.

n. of termination. Clusters of cells in the brain and medulla in which fibers of a nerve or nerve tract terminate.

n., olivary, inferior. A large convoluted mass of cells lying in ventral part of medulla oblongata and forming part of the reticular system. Gives rise to fibers of the olivocerebellar tract.

n., olivary, superior. A small nucleus located in mid-lateral tegmental region of pons. Receives fibers from ventral cochlear nucleus.

n., paraventricular. Nucleus of hypothalamus lying in supraoptic portion. Its axons with those of supraoptic nucleus form supraopticohypophyseal tract. SEE: *n., hypothalamic.*

n., pontine. One of several groups of nerve cells located in the pons. Receives afferent fibers from cerebral cortex; efferent fibers pass through brachium pontis to cerebellum.

n. pulposus. [NA] The center cushioning gelatinous mass lying within an intervertebral disk; remains of the notochord.

n., pyramidal. Band of gray matter near olivary nucleus in the medulla.

n., red. Large oval pigmented mass in upper portion of midbrain and extending upward into subthalamus. Receives fibers from cerebral cortex and cerebellum; efferent fibers give rise to rubrospinal tracts.

n., reproductive. Micronucleus (def. 2).

n., reticular. A column of neurons in spinal cord, brain stem, and thalamus affecting local reflex activity, muscle tone, and wakefulness.

n. ruber. [NA] Mass of red-colored gray matter in crus cerebri located in the anterior portion of the tegmentum and extending into the posterior portion of the subthalamic region.

n., salivatory, inferior. Nucleus located in pons near level of dorsal motor nucleus of the vagus. Gives rise to preganglionic parasympathetic fibers that pass to otic ganglion via hypoglossal nerve. Impulses regulate secretion of parotid gland.

n., salivatory, superior An ill-defined nucleus in pons lying dorsomedial to facial nucleus. Gives rise to preganglionic parasympathetic fibers passing through chorda tympani and lingual nerve to submaxillary ganglion. Impulses regulate secretion of submaxillary and sublingual glands.

n., segmentation. Nucleus of zygote formed by fusion of male and female pronuclei.

n., sensory. A nucleus of termination, q.v., of afferent fibers of a peripheral nerve.

n., sensory, of trigeminal nerve. A group of nuclei in pons and medulla oblongata consisting of the spinal nucleus, which extends inferiorly into the spinal cord; the main nucleus, which lies dorsal and lateral to the motor nucleus; and the mesencephalic nucleus, which lies in the lateral wall of the 4th ventricle.

n., sperm. The head of the sperm.

n., subthalamic. N., hypothalamic.

n., supraoptic. Nucleus of the hypothalamus lying above rostral ends of the optic tracts and lateral to the optic chiasma. SEE: *n., hypothalamic.*

n., thalamic. Any of the nuclei of the thalamus. Include a large number belonging to the following groups: anterior, intralaminar, lateral, and medial thalamic nuclei.

n., thoracic. A column of large neurons in the posterior gray column of the spinal cord. These cells give rise to the dorsal spinocerebellar tract on the same side.

n., vesicular. Nucleus having deeply staining membrane and a pale center.

n., vestibular. One of four nuclei in medulla oblongata in which fibers of the vestibular nerve terminate. Include medial (Schwalbe's), superior (Bechterew's), lateral (Deiter's), and inferior.

n., vitelline. Nucleus formed by union of male and female pronuclei within the vitellus. SYN: *n., yolk.*

n., white. Central white substance of corpus dentatum of olive.

n., yolk. A part of the cytoplasm of an ovum in which the initial process of accumulation of food supplies probably is located. SYN: *n., vitelline.*

nuclide (nū'klīd). Any atomic nucleus identified by its atomic number, mass, and energy state.

nude [L. *nudus,* naked]. 1. Bare; naked; unclothed. 2. An unclothed body.

nude mice. Mice that are devoid of hair. They are T-lymphocyte deficient. They are used in immunological investigations.

nudism. 1. In psychiatry, morbid desire to remove clothing. 2. The cult or practice of living in a nude condition.

nudo- [L. *nudus*]. Combining form denoting uncovered, naked.

nudomania (nū"dō-mā'nē-ă) [" + Gr. *mania,* madness]. Abnormal desire to be nude.

nudophobia (nū"dō-fō'bē-ă) [" + Gr. *phobos,* fear]. Abnormal fear of being unclothed. SEE: *gymnophobia.*

Nuel's space (nū'ĕlz). [Jean P. Nuel, Bel. oculist, 1847–1920] Space in organ of Corti between outer pillar and outer phalangeal cells (Dieter's cells).

Nuhn's glands (noonz). [Anton Nuhn, Ger. anatomist, 1814–1889] Anterior lingual glands on each side of frenum of the tongue. SYN: *Blandin's glands.*

null hypothesis. The assumption or hypothesis that the observed difference between two groups of patients studied is accidental or due to chance and is not due to one of the groups having received a specific treatment.

nulligravida. A woman who never conceived a child.

nullipara (nŭl-ĭp'ă-ră) [L. *nullus,* none, + *parere,* to bear]. A woman who has never produced a viable offspring.

nulliparity (nŭl"ĭ-păr'ĭ-tē). Condition of not having given birth to a child.

nulliparous (nŭl-lĭp'ăr-ŭs). Never having borne a child.

nullisomatic (nŭl"ĭ-sō-măt'ĭk) [" + Gr. *soma,* body]. Lacking one pair of chromosomes.

numb (nŭm). 1. Insensible; lacking in feeling as from cold. 2. Deadened or lacking in power to move as numb with cold.

number [L. *numerus,* number]. 1. A total of units. 2. A symbol graphically representing an arithmetical sum.

RS: mean; median; modality; mode; numeral.

n., atomic. The numeral indicating the number of negatively charged electrons in an uncharged atom, or the number of protons in the nucleus. This number determines the position of elements in the periodic table of elements.

n., Avogadro's. Number of molecules, 6.0225×10^{23}, in one gram-molecular weight of a compound.

n., mass. The mass of the atom of a specific isotope relative to the mass of hydrogen. In general, this number is equal to the total of the protons and electrons in the atomic nucleus of that specific isotope.

numbness. Lack of sensation in a part, esp. from cold. SEE: *narcohypnia; obdormition.*

numeral (nū'mĕr-ăl) [L. *numerus,* number]. 1. Denoting or pert. to a number. 2. A conventional symbol expressing a number.

nummiform (nŭm'mĭ-form) [L. *nummus,* a coin, + *forma,* shape]. 1. Coin-shaped, said of some mucous sputum. 2. Arranged like a stack of coins.

nummular (nŭm'ū-lăr) [L. *nummus,* coin]. 1. Coin-shaped. 2. Stacked like coins, as in rouleau of red blood cells.

nummulation (nŭm-ū-lā'shŭn) The formation of a coin-shaped mass.

Numorphan. Trade name for oxymorphone hydrochloride, USP.

nunnation (nŭn-ā'shŭn) [Heb. *nun,* letter N]. Frequent and abnormal use of the n sound.

Nupercainal. Trade name for dibucaine, USP.

Nupercaine Hydrochloride (nū'pĕr-kān). Trade name for dibucaine hydrochloride, USP, a white powder or crystals manufactured from cinchoninic acid. Used as a local anesthetic when prolonged anesthesia is required.

nurse [L. *nutrix,* nurse]. 1. An individual who provides health care. The extent of participation varies from simple patient-care tasks to the most expert professional techniques necessary in acute life-threatening situations. The ability of a nurse to function in making self-directed judgments and to act independently will depend on his or her professional background, motivation, and opportunity for professional development. The health care team includes the technical nurse, who is technique-oriented and deals with the commonly recurring nursing problems and knows standardized procedures and medically delegated techniques. Also included in the team is the professional nurse, who is prepared to assume responsibility for the care of individuals and groups through a colleague relationship with a physician. The roles of nurses constantly change in response to the growth of biomedical knowledge, changes in patterns of demand for health services, and the evolution of professional relationships among nurses, physicians, and other health care professionals. 2. To feed an infant at the breast. 3. To perform the duties of caring for an invalid. 4. To care for a young child.

n., charge. SEE: *n., head.*

n., clinical (nurse) specialist. A nurse with particular competence in certain areas such as intensive care, cardiology, oncology, obstetrics, or psychiatry. A clinical nurse specialist holds a master's degree in nursing, preferably with emphasis in clinical nursing.

n., community health. A nurse who combines principles and practices of nursing and public health to provide care to people in a community rather than an institution.

n., flight. Nurse who cares for patients being transported in an aircraft.

n., general duty. Nurse not specializing in a particular field of nursing but available for any duty.

n., graduate. Nurse who is a graduate of an accredited school of nursing.

n., head. A nurse in charge of a group of patients, usually a unit within an institution, and the nursing staff required to care for the patients.

n., health. A community or visiting nurse whose duty is to give information on hygiene and prevention of disease. SEE: *n., community health.*

n., licensed practical. A nurse who has graduated from a school of practical nursing and has passed the practical nursing state board examination.

n., practical. Nurse who is licensed to administer care, usually working under direction of a licensed physician or a registered nurse. May be a graduate of an accredited school for practical nursing.

n., private duty. A nurse who on a fee-for-service basis cares for one or two patients, usually in an institution. The nurse is not a staff member of the institution.

n.'s, probationer. Student nurses who are on probation until the instructors have had sufficient time to determine their suitability for the nursing profession.

n., public health. SEE: *n., community health.*

n., registered. A nurse who has graduated from a state-approved school of nursing, and has passed the professional nursing state board examination, and has been granted a license to practice within a given state.

n., school. A nurse who is responsible for the health of children, adolescents, and young adults in school.

n., scrub. The nurse who assists at surgery primarily by passing instruments and supplies to the surgeon(s).

n., special. N., private duty.

n., specialist. Clinical nurse specialist.

n., student. An individual who is enrolled in a school of nursing.

n., trained. N., graduate.

n., visiting. N., community health.

n., wet. A woman who breast feeds a child that is not her own.

nurse anesthetist. A registered nurse who administers anesthesia to patients in the operating room and delivery room. The knowledge and skill required to provide this service are attained through an organized program of study recognized by the American Association of Nurse Anesthetists.

nurse clinician. A registered nurse with preparation in a specialized educational program. The nurse clinician is capable of working independently in solving patient-care problems and is able to teach and work successfully with others on the medical care team. Term was first used by Frances Reiter, R.N., M.A., Dean, Graduate School of Nursing, New York Medical College.

nurse-midwife. A registered nurse who manages the care of mothers and babies throughout the maternity cycle including the postpartum period. The knowledge and skill required to provide this service are attained through an organized program of study recognized by the American College of Nurse-Midwives.

nurse practitioner. A nurse who has skills in the assessment of physical and psychosocial status of individuals and families and can manage some of the common illnesses of people in a colleague relationship with a physician. This nurse includes medical skills in his or her practice of nursing.

nursery. Department of a hospital where the newborn are cared for.

n., day. A nursery in which children, usually of preschool age, are cared for during the day.

nurse's aide. An individual who assists nurses by doing the patient-care procedures that do not require special technical training, such as feeding and bathing patients, and by taking temperature, pulse, and respiration.

nursing. 1. Scientific care of the sick by a graduate, registered nurse. 2. Loosely applied to any care of the sick. 3. Breast feeding. 4. Lactation.

nursing audit. A procedure to evaluate the quality of nursing care provided for a patient.

Established criteria for care is the yardstick for the evaluation of the care.

nursing diagnosis. Nurses, esp. those involved in patient care, are in virtually constant need to make decisions and diagnoses based on their clinical experience and judgment. In many instances, that process dictates a course of nurse-action that is of vital importance to the patient. As the nursing profession evolves and develops, nursing diagnosis will be defined and indeed specified in accordance with the specialized training and experience of nurses, particularly for nurse practitioners and clinical nurse specialists.

nursing histories. The assessment stage of the nursing process that leads to development of a nursing care plan. Valuable information can be obtained from this history and reactions to previous hospitalization can be recorded and utilized in managing the patient's care during the current stay. SEE: *Nursing History Form* illus.

nursing intervention. The activities of a nurse in caring for patients. This may include activities at all levels from the usual patient-care tasks to noting changes in the patient's condition that require immediate nursing staff action or notification of the attending physician or both.

nursing process. The systematic method used to provide nursing care. The method includes assessment of the client, formation of a nursing diagnosis, a plan of care, implementation of the plan, and evaluation.

nutation (nū-tā′shŭn) [L. *nutatio*]. Nodding, as of the head. SEE: *nodding*.

nutgall (nŭt′gawl). A growth on certain oak trees. It is produced by insect eggs and larvae in the twigs of the tree. Gallic and tannic acid are obtained from these growths.

Nutracort. Trade name for hydrocortisone, USP.

nutrient (nū′trē-ĕnt) [L. *nutriens*]. 1. Food or any substance that supplies the body with elements necessary for metabolism. 2. Nourishing; supplying nutriment.

Certain nutrients (carbohydrates, fats, proteins, and alcohol) provide energy; other nutrients (water, electrolytes, minerals, and vitamins) are essential to the metabolic process. Those containing carbon are organic food nutrients. Organic food nutrients may or may not contain nitrogen.

RS: calorie; carbohydrate; fat; food; mineral; nitrogen; protein; vitamin.

nutrilite (nū′trĭ-līt). Any essential nutrient, esp. ones that are required in only trace quantities.

nutriment (nū′trĭ-mĕnt) [L. *nutrimentum*,

Nursing History Form*†

Admission date ______ History taken by ______ Date ______
Diagnosis ______ Date of injury/illness ______
Special circumstances of present illness ______
Previous hospitalization ______
List nursing activities or omissions which were helpful or deleterious to the patient during previous hospitalization______
Is patient transient?______
Family background
married ____ single ____ widowed ____ divorced ____ estranged ____ common law ____
Religion ______
Does patient wish visitors excluded? ______ If so, give reason ______
Daily living habits:
Food and fluid likes and dislikes ______
Sleeping habits: preferred time of retiring and arising ______
dreams______ nightmares______ insomnia______
Television, radio, and phone preference ______
Bowel and urinary habits ______
Medicines taken regularly ______ Known allergies ______
Menstrual-age female patients: Is a personal supply of pads or tampons available? ______
Interests, hobbies, pastimes ______
List wounds or special medical care ______
Cultural factors, vocabulary, native language, education ______
Questions patient asked ______
Additional observations ______

*Adapted from Shaw, J. S., McLaughlin, M.: Nursing Histories in a Naval Hospital, U.S. Navy Medical News Letter. 54:43–46, 1969.

(addressograph plate) Date ______
Time ______

Understanding of illness or reason for hospitalization: ______

Expectations regarding hospitalization: ______

Brief social and cultural history: ______

DATA ABOUT USUAL:

1. Activities: ______
2. Recreation: ______
3. Eating and drinking: ______
4. Elimination: ______
5. Hygiene: ______
6. Breathing: ______
7. Sleeping: ______
8. Interpersonal relationships: ______
9. Temperament or moods: ______
10. Independent and dependent behaviors: ______
11. Medications used: ______

DATA ABOUT

1. Hearing: ______
2. Eyesight: ______
3. Handedness: ______
4. Smelling: ______
5. Tasting: ______

ADDITIONAL PERTINENT DATA: ______

PROBLEMS:

Subjective: ______

Objective: ______

Assessment: ______

Plan for nursing care: ______

†Adapted from Saperstein, A. and Frazier, M.: *Introduction to Nursing Practice.* F.A. Davis Co., Philadelphia, 1980.

nourishment]. That which nourishes; nutritious substance.

nutrition (nū-trĭ'shŭn) [L. *nutritio,* nourish]. The sum total of the processes involved in the taking in and utilization of food substances by which growth, repair, and maintenance of activities in the body as a whole or in any of its parts are accomplished. Includes ingestion, digestion, absorption, and metabolism (assimilation). Some but not all nutrients are capable of being stored by the body in various forms and drawn upon when the food intake is not sufficient. An example of a nutrient that is not stored is vitamin C.

nutritional (nū-trĭsh'ŭn-ăl). Rel. to nutrition.

nutritional adequacy. The relationship between intake of nutrients and individual requirements.

nutritious (nū-trĭsh'ŭs) [L. *nutritius*]. Affording nutriment. SYN: *nutritive.*

nutritive (nū'trĭ-tĭv). Pert. to the process of assimilating food; having the property of nourishing.

nutritive enema. Enema containing predigested foods to give sustenance to a patient unable to take nourishment in the usual way.

nutriture (nū'trĭ-tūr). The state of body nutrition.

nux vomica (nŭks vŏm'ĭ-kă). A poisonous seed from an East Indian tree, containing several alkaloids, the principal ones being brucine and strychnine, q.v.

nyctalbuminuria (nĭk"tăl-bū"mĭn-ū'rē-ă) [Gr. *nyx,* night, + L. *albus,* white, + Gr. *ouron,* urine]. A cyclic albuminuria occurring at night. SYN: *noctalbuminuria.*

nyctalgia (nĭk-tăl'jē-ă) [" + *algos,* pain]. Pain during the night.

nyctalopia (nĭk-tă-lō'pē-ă) [" + *alaos,* blind, + *ops,* eye]. 1. A condition in which the individual cannot see well in a faint light or at night. Occurs in retinitis pigmentosa and choroidoretinitis. Also may be due to vitamin A deficiency. Smoking tobacco impairs ability to see at night. SYN: *night blindness.* 2. Incorrectly used to indicate the condition of having better sight at night or in semidarkness than by day; night vision. SEE: *hemeralopia.*

nyctamblyopia (nĭk"tăm-blē-ō'pē-ă) [Gr. *nyx,* night, + *amblyopia,* poor sight]. Poor vision at night without visible eye changes.

nyctaphonia (nĭk-tă-fō'nē-ă) [" + *a,* not, + *phone,* voice]. Hysterical loss of voice during the night.

nycterine (nĭk'tĕr-īn) [Gr. *nykterinos,* by night]. 1. Taking place at night. 2. Obscure.

nycthemerus (nĭk-thĕm'ĕ-rŭs) [Gr. *nychthemeros*]. 1. Space of a day and a night. 2. Pert. to a night and day.

nycto- (nĭk'tō) [Gr. *nyx,* night]. Combining form indicating night or darkness.

nyctohemeral (nĭk"tō-hĕm'ĕr-ăl). Rel. to both day and night.

nyctophilia (nĭk"tō-fĭl'ē-ă) [Gr. *nyx,* night, + *philein,* to love]. Abnormal preference for darkness or night. SYN: *scotophilia.*

nyctophobia (nĭk"tō-fō'bē-ă) [" + *phobos,* fear]. Abnormal dread of the night or of darkness. SYN: *scotophobia.*

nyctophonia (nĭk"tō-fō'nē-ă) [" + *phone,* voice]. Hysterical loss of voice only during the day.

nyctotyphlosis (nĭk"tō-tĭf-lō'sĭs) [" + *typhlosis,* blindness]. Poor vision at night. SYN: *night blindness; nyctalopia.*

nycturia (nĭk-tū'rē-ă) [" + *ouron,* urine]. Urination, esp. excessive, during the night. SYN: *nocturia.* SEE: *enuresis.*

Nydrazid. Trade name for isoniazid, USP.

nylidrin hydrochloride (nĭl'ĭ-drĭn). USP. A drug used to produce peripheral vasodilation. Trade name is Arlidin.

nymph (nĭmf) [Gr. *nymphe,* a maiden]. The immature stage of insect development in which wings and genitalia have not fully developed.

nympha [Gr. *nymphe,* a maiden]. (pl. *nymphae*) One of the labia minora, q.v., the small folds of mucous membrane forming the inner lips of the vulva. So called from the nymphs or goddesses of the fountain. SYN: *labium minus pudendi.*

nymphectomy (nĭm-fĕk'tō-mē) [" + *ektome,* excision]. Excision of hypertrophied nymphae.

nymphitis (nĭm-fī'tĭs) [" + *itis,* inflammation]. Inflamed condition of the nymphae.

nympho- (nĭm'fō) [Gr. *nymphe,* a maiden]. A combining form indicating relationship to the labia minora.

nymphocaruncular sulcus (nĭm"fō-kăr-ŭn'kū-lăr sŭl'kŭs) [" + L. *caruncula,* little mass of flesh, + *sulcus,* a groove]. The depression between the caruncula of the hymen and the labium minus.

nymphohymenal sulcus (nĭm"fō-hī'mĕn-ăl sŭl'kŭs) [" + *hymen,* membrane, + *sulcus,* a groove]. Trench between the labium minus and the hymen on either side.

nympholepsy (nĭm'fō-lĕp"sē) [" + *lepsis,* a seizure]. 1. Frenzied ecstasy, usually erotic in nature. 2. Obsession for something that is unattainable.

nymphomania (nĭm"fō-mā'nē-ă) [" + *mania,* madness]. Abnormally excessive sexual desire in a female. SYN: *furor femininus.* SEE: *satyriasis.*

nymphomaniac (nĭm"fō-mā'nē-ăk) [" + *mania,* madness]. 1. Woman who is afflicted with excessive sexual desire. 2. Affected by excessive sexual desire.

nymphoncus (nĭm-fŏn'kŭs) [" + *onkos,* a swelling]. Swelling or tumor of the nymphae.

nymphotomy (nĭm-fŏt'ō-mē) [" + *tome,* incision]. 1. Removal of the nymphae. SYN: *nymphectomy.* 2. Incision into a nympha or clitoris.

nystagmic (nĭs-tăg′mĭk) [Gr. *nystagmos,* to nod]. Rel. to or suffering from condition of involuntary eyeball movements.

nystagmiform (nĭs-tăg′mĭ-form) [″ + L. *forma,* shape]. Like or resembling nystagmus. SYN: *nystagmoid.*

nystagmograph (nĭs-tăg′mō-grăf) [″ + *graphein,* to write]. Apparatus for recording the oscillations of the eyeball in nystagmus.

nystagmoid (nĭs-tăg′moyd) [″ + *eidos,* resemblance]. Similar to or resembling nystagmus.

nystagmus (nĭs-tăg′mŭs) [Gr. *nystagmos,* to nod]. Constant, involuntary, cyclical movement of the eyeball. Movement may be in any direction.

ETIOL: May be congenital and inapparent to the patient; seen in bilateral amblyopia; occupational, as in miners and train dispatchers; labyrinthine irritability; neurologic diseases.

n., aural. Nystagmus due to disorder in the labyrinth of the ear. Eye movement is spasmodic.

n., Cheyne's. Rhythmic nystagmus that resembles the rhythm of Cheyne-Stokes breathing, q.v.

n., convergence. Slow abduction of eyes followed by rapid adduction. Usually accompanies other types of nystagmus.

n., dissociated. Nystagmus in one eye that is not synchronized with that in the other eye.

n., end-position. Nystagmus that occurs when eyes are turned to extreme positions. May occur normally in debilitation or fatigue. May be due to pathology of the subcortical centers for conjugate gaze.

n., fixation. Nystagmus that occurs only when the eyes gaze at an object.

n., jerk. N., rhythmic.

n., labyrinthine. Nystagmus due to disease of the labyrinthine vestibular apparatus.

n., latent. Nystagmus that occurs only when one eye is covered.

n., lateral. Horizontal movement of eyes from side to side.

n., miner's. Nystagmus occurring in those who work in comparative darkness for long periods.

n., opticokinetic. A rhythmic jerk nystagmus occurring while looking at constantly moving objects, such as telephone poles from a moving car or train.

n., pendular. Nystagmus characterized by movement that is approximately equal in both directions. Usually seen in those who have congenital absence of central vision or who lost it prior to the age of two.

n., retraction. Nystagmus associated with drawing of the eye backward into the orbit.

n., rhythmic. Nystagmus in which the eyes move slowly in one direction and then are jerked back rapidly. SYN: *n., jerk.*

n., rotatory. Nystagmus in which eyes rotate about the visual axis.

n., vertical. Up and down ocular movements.

n., vestibular. Nystagmus due to ear disturbances.

n., voluntary. A rare type of pendular nystagmus in persons who have learned to oscillate their eyes rapidly, usually by extreme convergence. It is an acquired art that has no clinical significance.

nystatin (nĭs′tă-tĭn). USP. An antifungal agent. Trade names are Mycostatin and O-V Statin.

nystaxis (nĭs-tăk′sĭs) [Gr.]. Nystagmus.

Nysten's law (nē-stănz′). [Pierre Hubert Nysten, Fr. pediatrician, 1774–1817] Law stating that rigor mortis begins with muscles of mastication and progresses from the head down the body, affecting legs and feet last. SEE: *rigor mortis.*

nyxis (nĭk′sĭs) [Gr.]. Puncture or piercing. SYN: *paracentesis.*

NZB mouse [New Zealand Black mouse]. A mouse bred for the genetic trait of spontaneously developing autoimmune hemolytic anemia.

O

O. 1. Chem. symb. for oxygen. 2. *octarius,* pint; *oculus,* eye. 3. Symb. for a particular blood type.

o-. *ortho-,* prefix commonly used in chemical terminology.

O_2. Symb. for the molecular formula of oxygen.

O_3. Chem. symb. for ozone.

O.A. *occiput anterior.*

oakum (ō'kŭm) [AS. *acumba,* tow]. Loose fiber obtained from old hemp ropes, formerly used as a surgical dressing.

oarialgia (ō"ăr-ē-ăl'jē-ă) [Gr. *oarion,* little egg, + *algos,* pain]. Ovarian pain. SYN: *oophoralgia; ovaralgia.*

oario-, oari- [Gr. *oarion,* little egg]. Prefix pert. to the ovary. SEE: words beginning with *ovario-* or *oophor-*.

oasis (ō-ā'sĭs) [Gr., a fertile area in an arid region]. (pl. *oases*) Area of healthy tissue surrounded by a diseased portion.

oasthouse urine disease. Methionine malabsorption syndrome, which is associated with mental retardation, diarrhea, convulsions, phenylketonuria, and a peculiar odor. The latter is due to the absorption from the intestinal tract of fermentation products of methionine. SYN: *Smith-Strang disease.*

oat [AS. *ate,* oat]. Grain or seed of a cereal grass used as food.

oath [AS. *ooth*]. A solemn attestation or affirmation. SEE: *Hippocratic oath; Nightingale pledge.*

oatmeal [AS. *ate,* oat, + *mele,* meal]. A meal made from oats. Usually cooked to make porridge. Oatmeal is sometimes used in a tepid bath to soothe inflamed or irritated skin. It is rich in fats and lecithins.

O.B. *obstetrics.*

ob- [L.]. Combining form meaning toward, against, in the way of.

obcecation (ŏb"sē-kā'shŭn). Partial blindness.

obdormition (ŏb-dor-mĭsh'ŭn) [L. *ob,* towards, + *dormire,* to sleep]. Numbness followed by tingling in an extremity produced by pressure of the nerve trunk supplying it. Limb is commonly referred to as being asleep.

obduction (ŏb-dŭk'shŭn) [" + *ducere,* to lead]. Inspection of a dead body to learn pathological conditions and cause of death. SYN: *autopsy; necropsy; postmortem examination.*

obelion (ō-bē'lē-ōn) [Gr. *obelos,* a spit]. A craniometric point on the sagittal suture between the two parietal foramina.

obese (ō-bēs') [L. *obesus*]. Extremely fat. SYN: *corpulent.*

obesity (ō-bē'sĭ-tē) [L. *obesitas,* corpulence]. Abnormal amount of fat on the body. The term is usually not employed unless the individual is from 20 to 30% over average weight for his or her age, sex, and height. SYN: *adiposity; corpulence.*

ETIOL: Obesity is the result of an imbalance between food eaten and energy expended, but the underlying cause usually is quite complex and difficult to diagnose and treat.

TREATMENT: Prophylaxis in children of families with a tendency to obesity in the form of establishing moderate eating and exercise habits; dieting.

DIET: Caloric intake should be less than maintenance requirements, but all other essential nutrients must be included. Maintenance requirements are based on what the average or desired weight should be. A slow reduction regimen is 1200 to 1600 Cal. per day; 1000 to 1200 Cal. will provide a more rapid loss of weight.

The average basic reducing diet is about 9 Cal. per pound of ideal body weight per day. Thus a 160-pound person whose ideal wt. is 135 should eat a diet of about 1200 Cal. a day. These calories should be obtained from foods that would provide adequate protein, carbohydrates, fats, minerals, and vitamins, and not from a fad diet. Adherence to this diet should cause the person to lose the excess weight. After that the diet is adjusted so that caloric intake is just equal to total energy required. Obviously this is different for each individual.

Losing weight by fasting is effective but is not recommended unless done under strict medical and nursing supervision.

RS: anorexia nervosa; caloric excess; carbohydrate; diet; dietetics; emaciation; fat; mineral compounds; protein; starch; starvation; sugar; vegan; vitamin; weight.

o., endogenous. Obesity caused by some metabolic abnormality within the body.

o., exogenous. Obesity due to excessive intake of food.

o., hypothalamic. Obesity resulting from dysfunction of hypothalamus, esp. the appetite-regulating center.

o., morbid. Obesity of such degree as to interfere with normal activities, including respiration. SEE: *pickwickian syndrome.*

obex (ō'bĕks) [L., a band]. [NA] A thin, crescent-shaped band of tissue covering the calamus scriptorius, q.v., at the point of convergence of nervous tissue at the caudal end of the fourth ventricle.

obfuscation (ŏb-fŭs-kā'shŭn) [L. *obfuscare,* to darken]. 1. The act of making obscure or confusing. 2. Mental confusion.

object [L. *objectus*]. That which is visible or

tangible to the senses.

object blindness. Affection in which brain fails to recognize things seen correctly by eyes. SEE: *apraxia.*

objective (ŏb-jĕk′tĭv). 1. Perceptible to other persons, said of symptoms. Opposite of subjective. 2. Directed toward external things. 3. The lens of a microscope that is closest to the object.

o., achromatic. A microscope objective in which chromatic aberration is corrected for red and blue light.

o., apochromatic. A microscope objective in which chromatic aberration is corrected for red, blue, and green light.

o., immersion. A microscope objective designed so that the space between the objective lens and the specimen is filled with oil or water.

objective sign. In physical diagnosis, a sign that can be seen, heard, measured, or felt by the diagnostician. Finding of such a sign(s) can be used to confirm or deny the diagnostician's impressions of the disease suspected of being present.

objective symptoms. Symptoms apparent to physical means of diagnosis.

object relations. Emotional attachment for other persons or objects.

obligate (ŏb′lĭ-gāt) [L. *obligatus*]. To make necessary or require; without alternative. SEE: *anaerobe, obligatory.*

oblique (ō-blēk′, ō-blīk′) [L. *obliquus*]. Slanting, diagonal.

obliquimeter (ŏb″lĭ-kwĭm′ĕt-ĕr) [″ + Gr. *metron,* measure]. Apparatus for indicating the angle of the pelvic brim with the upright body.

obliquity (ŏb-lĭk′wĭ-tē) [L. *obliquus,* slanting]. The state of being oblique or slanting.

o., Litzmann's. Inclining of the fetal head until the posterior parietal bone presents to the uterine canal.

o., Naegele's. Presentation of the fetal head with anterior parietal bone toward the uterine canal with oblique biparietal diameter in relation to the pelvic brim.

o. of pelvis. Inclination of pelvis.

o., Roederer's. Presentation of fetal head with occiput at pelvic brim.

obliquus (ŏb-lĭk′wŭs). Oblique.

obliquus reflex. Contraction of the entire external obliquus muscle on application of stimulus to skin of thigh below Poupart's ligament.

obliteration (ŏb-lĭt″ĕr-ā′shŭn) [L. *obliterare,* to remove]. Extinction or complete occlusion of a part by degeneration, disease, or surgery.

oblongata (ŏb″lŏng-gă′tă) [L. *oblongus,* long]. Oblong. Sometimes used to designate the cylindrical extension of the spinal cord as it enters the brain, about an inch long, reaching to the pons, and forming part of the base of the fourth ventricle. SYN: *medulla oblongata.*

obmutescence (ŏb″mū-tĕs′ĕns) [L. *obmutescere,* to become dumb]. Loss of vocal power. SYN: *aphonia.*

obscure (ŏb-skūr′) [L. *obscurus,* hide]. 1. Hidden, indistinct, as the cause of a condition. 2. To make less distinct or to hide.

observerscope (ŏb-zĕr′vĕr-skōp). Type of endoscope designed so that two persons can view the site simultaneously.

obsession [L. *obsessus,* besiege]. The neurotic mental state of having an uncontrollable desire to dwell on an idea or an emotion. The patient is usually aware of the abnormality and resists these thoughts. SEE: *compulsion.*

o., impulsive. An obsession accompanied by action.

o., inhibitory. An obsession accompanied by impediments to action.

obsessional neurosis. A psychoneurosis marked by obsessions controlling the behavior of the individual. SYN: *compulsion neurosis.*

obsessive-compulsive. Marked by an inclination to perform certain rituals repetitiously in order to relieve anxiety.

obsolescence [L. *obsolescere,* to grow old]. The condition of becoming useless, or out of date.

obstetric (ŏb-stĕt′rĭk) [L. *obstetrix,* midwife]. Pert. to obstetrics or midwifery.

obstetrician (ŏb-stĕ-trĭsh′ăn). A physician who treats women during pregnancy and parturition and delivers infants.

obstetrics (ŏb-stĕt′rĭks) [L. *obstetrix,* midwife]. Branch of medicine that concerns management of women during pregnancy, childbirth, and the puerperium.

RS: ballottement; breech presentation; brow presentation; cesarean section; childbirth; childbirth, psychological preparation for; delivery; fetus; gestation; labor; maneuver; midwife; nurse-midwife; parturition; position; postpartum hemorrhage; pregnancy; puerpera; puerperal.

obstipation (ŏb″stĭ-pā′shŭn) [L. *obstipatio*]. Obstinate or extreme constipation.

obstruction (ŏb-strŭk′shŭn). 1. Blocking of a structure that prevents it from functioning normally. 2. A thing that impedes; an obstacle.

o., aortic. Blocking of the aorta, thereby preventing the flow of blood.

o., intestinal. Blockage of the lumen of the intestine.

obstructive lung disease, chronic. ABBR: COLD. Increased resistance to the passage of air in and out of the lung due to narrowing of the bronchial tree. It is diagnosed by determining that the amount of air forcibly expired from the lung in one second is less than normal. The disease process may be caused by a number of irritants or diseases that damage the bronchial tree, including pulmonary tuberculosis, cigarette smoking, and silicosis.

obstruent (ŏb′stroo-ĕnt) [L. *obstruens*]. 1. Blocking up. 2. That which closes a normal passage in the body. 3. Any agent or agency causing obstruction.

obtund (ŏb-tŭnd′) [L. *obtundere,* to beat against]. To dull or blunt, as sensitivity or pain. SEE: *consciousness, levels of.*

obtundent (ŏb-tŭn′dĕnt) [L. *obtundens*]. 1. Having the capacity to deaden sensibility of a part or reduce irritability. 2. A soothing remedy.

obturation (ŏb-tūr-ā′shŭn) [L. *obturare,* to stop up]. Closure of a passage or opening, as in intestinal obstruction.

obturator (ŏb′tū-rā″tor). 1. Anything that obstructs or closes a cavity or opening. 2. Rel. to the obturator membrane. 3. Bridge for spanning the gap in the cleft palate.

obturator foramen. Obturator in the anterior part of the os innominatum between the pubis and ischium.

obturator membrane. Strong obturator occluding the obturator foramen.

obturator muscles. Two muscles on each side of the pelvic region that rotate the thighs outward. SEE: *Muscles* in *Appendix.*

obturator sign. Obturator test of inward rotation of the hip so that the obturator internus muscle is stretched. This test result may be positive in acute appendicitis.

obtuse (ŏb-tūs′) [L. *obtusus*]. 1. Not pointed or acute; dull or blunt. 2. Dull mentality.

obtusion (ŏb-tū′zhŭn). Blunting or weakening of normal sensation, as in certain diseases.

O.C. *oral contraceptive.*

Occam's razor (ŏck′hăms). [William of Occam, or Ockham, Brit. Franciscan and philosopher, c. 1285–1350] The concept that entities do not have to be proven beyond the point of proof; or "what can be done with fewer (assumptions) is done in vain with more."

occipital (ŏk-sĭp′ĭ-tăl) [L. *occipitalis*]. Concerning the back part of the head.

occipital bone. Bone in lower back part of skull between the parietal and temporal bones.

occipitalis (ŏk-sĭp″ĭ-tā′lĭs) [L.]. The posterior portion of the occipitofrontalis muscle at the back of the head.

occipitalization (ŏk-sĭp″ĭ-tăl-ĭ-zā′shŭn). Fusion of the atlas and occipital bones.

occipital lobe. Posterior lobe of the cerebral hemisphere that is shaped like a three-sided pyramid.

occipito- [L. *occiput*]. Combining form showing relationship between the occiput and another part.

occipitoatloid (ŏk-sĭp″ĭ-tō-ăt′loyd). Concerning the occipital and atlas bones.

occipitoaxoid (ŏk-sĭp″ĭ-tō-ăk′soyd). Concerning the occipital and axis bones.

occipitobregmatic (ŏk-sĭp′ĭ-tō-brĕg-măt′ĭk). Concerning the occiput and the bregma.

occipitocervical (ŏk-sĭp″ĭ-tō-sĕr′vĭ-kăl). Concerning the occiput and the neck.

occipitofacial (ŏk-sĭp″ĭ-tō-fā′shăl). Concerning the occiput and the face.

occipitofrontal (ŏk-sĭp″ĭ-tō-frŏn′tăl). Concerning the occiput and the forehead.

occipitomastoid (ŏk-sĭp″ĭ-tō-măs′toyd). Concerning the occiput and the mastoid process.

occipitomental (ŏk-sĭp″ĭ-tō-mĕn′tăl). Concerning the occiput and the chin.

occipitoparietal (ŏk-sĭp″ĭ-tō-pă-rī′ĕ-tăl). Concerning the occiput and the parietal bones or lobes of the brain.

occipitotemporal (ŏk-sĭp″ĭ-tō-tĕm′pō-răl). Concerning the occiput and the temporal bones.

occipitothalamic (ŏk-sĭp″ĭ-tō-thă-lăm′ĭk). Concerning the occiput and the thalamus.

occiput (ŏk′sĭ-pŭt) [L.]. [NA] The back part of the skull.

occlude (ŏ-klūd′) [L. *occludere,* to shut up]. To close up, obstruct, or join together, as bringing the biting surfaces of opposing teeth together.

occlusal (ŏ-kloo′zăl). Pert. to the closure of an opening.

occlusal plane. The imaginary surface extending from the tip of the mandibular incisors back along the cusp tips of the mandibular molar teeth to contact the cranium; more precise points are used for some dental records but generally it is considered a curve of the occlusal surface rather than a true plane.

occlusal surface. The masticating surface of the premolar and molar teeth.

occlusal wear. The attritional loss of substance on opposing occlusal surfaces in natural or artificial teeth; the modification of tooth cusps, ridges, and grooves by functional use.

occlusion (ŏ-kloo′zhŭn) [L. *occlusio*]. 1. The closure, or state of being closed, of a passage. May be acquired or congenital. SYN: *imperforation.* 2. Adsorption of gas by a substance that does not thereby lose its characteristic property. 3. The alignment of the mandibular and maxillary teeth when the jaw is closed or in functional contact.

o., abnormal. Malocclusion of the teeth.

o., centric. The maximum occlusal contact of the teeth. This occurs when the mandible is in centric relationship with the maxilla.

o., coronary. Obstruction of a coronary vessel by thrombosis or as a result of spasm. SYN: *coronary thrombosis.*

o., eccentric. Any occlusion other than centric.

occlusive (ŏ-kloo'sĭv). Concerning occlusion.

occlusive dressing. SEE: *dressing, occlusive.*

occlusometer (ŏk″loo-sŏm'ĕ-tĕr). Device for measuring the force exerted during forcible occlusion of the teeth. SYN: *gnathodynamometer.*

occult (ŭ-kŭlt') [L. *occultus*]. Obscure; concealed, as a hemorrhage.

occult blood. Blood in such minute quantity that it can be recognized only by microscopic examination or by chemical means.

occult blood test. A chemical test or microscopic examination for blood, esp. in feces, that is not apparent on visual inspection.

occupational therapist. One who evaluates the self-care, work, play, and leisure time task performance skills of well and disabled clients of all ages; plans and implements programs, social and interpersonal activities designed to restore, develop, and maintain the client's ability to accomplish satisfactorily those daily tasks required of his or her specific age and necessary to his or her particular role adjustment.

occupational therapist assistant. One who works under the supervision of the occupational therapist in evaluating clients, planning and implementing programs designed to restore or develop a client's self-care, work, play, or leisure time task performance skills. Although requiring supervision in conducting a remedial program, the assistant can function independently when conducting a maintenance program.

occupational therapy. The use of work-related skills to treat or train the physically or emotionally ill, to prevent disability, to evaluate behavior, and to restore disabled persons to health, social, or economic independence.

occupational therapy aide. An individual who has had on-the-job training or experience in occupational therapy who performs routine tasks under the direction of an occupational therapist.

occupation neurosis. A functional disorder caused by certain occupations.

ochlesis (ŏk-lē'sĭs) [Gr., crowding]. Any disease caused by conditions of overcrowding.

ochlophobia (ŏk″lō-fō'bē-ă) [Gr. *ochlos,* crowd, + *phobos,* fear]. Abnormal dread of crowds or populated places.

ochrometer (ō-krŏm'ĕt-ĕr) [″ + *metron,* measure]. Device for estimating the capillary blood pressure by recording the pressure required to compress a finger until the skin becomes blanched.

ochronosis (ō-krō-nō'sĭs) [″ + *nosos,* disease]. A rare condition marked by dark pigmentation of the ligaments, cartilage, fibrous tissues, skin, and urine. May be caused by an inborn error of metabolism, alkaptonuria. This allows formation of homogentisic acid, part of which is excreted in the urine and part of which is stored in the tissues. The condition also may be caused by chronic phenol poisoning.

octa-, octo- [Gr. *okto,* L. *octo*]. Combining forms meaning eight.

octahedron (ŏk-tă-hē'drŏn). An eight-sided solid figure.

octamethyl pyrophosphoramide (ŏk″tă-mĕth'ĭl pĭr″ō-fŏs-for'ă-mīd). An insecticide that acts by inhibiting cholinesterase.

octan (ŏk'tăn) [L. *octo,* eight]. Reappearing on every eighth day, as a fever.

octane (ŏk'tān). C_8H_{18}. A hydrocarbon of the paraffin series.

octapeptide (ŏk″tă-pĕp'tīd). A peptide that contains eight amino acids.

octaploid (ŏk'tă-ployd). 1. Concerning octaploidy. 2. Having eight pairs of chromosomes.

octaploidy (ŏk'tă-ploy″dē). The condition of having eight sets or pairs of chromosomes.

octarius (ŏk-tā'rē-ŭs) [L.]. ABBR: O. Pint.

octavalent (ŏk″tă-vā'lĕnt) [L. *octo,* eight, + *valeo,* to have power]. Having a valency of eight.

octigravida (ŏk″tĭ-grăv'ĭ-dă) [″ + *gravida,* pregnant]. One who has been pregnant eight times.

octipara (ŏk-tĭp'ă-ră) [″ + L. *parere,* to bear]. A woman who has given birth to eight children.

octogenarian (ŏk″tō-jĕn-ĕr'ē-ĕn) [L. *octogenarius,* containing eighty]. A person who is in his or her eighties.

ocular (ŏk'ū-lăr) [L. *oculus,* eye]. 1. Concerning the eye or vision. 2. Eyepiece of a microscope.

oculi (ŏk'ū-lī). Pl. of oculus.

oculist (ŏk'ū-lĭst). Former term for ophthalmologist, a physician who is a specialist in diseases of the eye.

oculo- (ŏk'ū-lō) [L. *oculus,* eye]. Combining form indicating relationship to the eye.

oculocardiac reflex. Slowing of the pulse following pressure applied to the eyeball or carotid sinus. SYN: *Aschner's phenomenon.*

oculocephalogyric reflex (ŏk″ū-lō-sĕf″ă-lō-jī'rĭk). Associated movements of eye, head, and body in focalizing vision upon an object.

oculocerebrorenal syndrome. A sex-linked condition characterized by hydrophthalmia, cataracts, mental retardation, aminoaciduria, impaired renal ammonia production, and rickets that resists vitamin D therapy.

oculocutaneous (ŏk″ū-lō-kū-tā'nē-ŭs). Concerning the eye and the skin.

oculofacial (ŏk″ū-lō-fā′shē-ăl). Concerning the eye and the face.

oculogyration (ŏk″ū-lō-jī-rā′shŭn) [″ + Gr. *gyros,* circle]. Circular motion of the eyeball around its anterior-posterior axis.

oculogyria (ŏk″ū-lō-jī′rē-ă). The limits of rotation of the eyeballs.

oculogyric (ŏk″ū-lō-jī′rĭk). Producing or concerning movements of the eye. SYN: *oculomotor; ophthalmogyric.*

oculogyric crisis. Attack of involuntary deviation and fixation of the eyeballs, usually upward. The crisis may last for several minutes or hours. May be seen with postencephalitic parkinsonism or encephalitis lethargica.

oculomotor (ŏk″ū-lō-mō′tor) [″ + *motor,* mover]. Rel. to eye movements. SYN: *oculogyric.*

oculomotorius (ŏk″ū-lō-mō-tō′rē-ŭs) [L.]. Oculomotor nerve.

oculomotor nerve. Nerve that originates in the medial surface of the cerebral peduncle of the midbrain and consists of general somatic efferent, general visceral efferent, and general somatic afferent fibers. It is distributed through all extrinsic muscles of the eye except the exterior rectus and superior oblique, through the levator palpebrae superioris of the eyelid, through the ciliary muscle, and through the sphincter muscle of the iris. It has primarily a motor function, but it also contains proprioceptive fibers. SYN: *third cranial nerve. SEE: Cranial Nerves* in *Appendix.*

oculomycosis (ŏk″ū-lō-mī-kō′sĭs) [″ + Gr. *mykes,* fungus, + *osis,* condition]. Any disease of the eye or its parts caused by fungus.

oculonasal (ŏk″ū-lō-nā′săl) [″ + *nasus,* nose]. Concerning both eye and nose.

oculopathy (ŏk″ū-lŏp′ă-thē) [″ + Gr. *pathos,* disease]. Ophthalmopathy, q.v.

oculopupillary (ŏk″ū-lō-pū′pĭ-lăr-ē). Concerning the pupil of the eye.

oculoreaction (ŏk″ū-lō-rē-ăk′shŭn) [L. *oculus,* eye, + *re,* back, + *actus,* acting]. A reaction observed in the conjunctiva of the eye when toxins of tuberculosis and typhoid are instilled into the conjunctival space. Of diagnostic value. SYN: *ophthalmic reaction; ophthalmoreaction.*

oculozygomatic (ŏk″ū-lō-zī″gō-măt′ĭk) [″ + Gr. *zygon,* yoke]. Pert. to the eye and zygoma.

oculozygomatic line. Line appearing between the inner canthus of eye and cheek, supposedly indicative of neural disorders.

oculus (ŏk′ū-lŭs) [L.]. (pl. *oculi*) [NA] Eye; the organ of vision made up of the eyeball and optic nerve.

o. dexter. ABBR. O.D. The right eye.

o. sinister. ABBR: O.S. The left eye.

o. uterque. ABBR. O.U. Each eye.

Ocusert. Trade name for pilocarpine, USP.

O.D. *oculus dexter,* right eye; *Doctor of Optometry; overdose.*

OD′d. Street term for a person who died due to a drug overdose, esp. a drug of abuse.

odaxesmus (ō″dăk-sĕz′mŭs) [Gr. *odaxesmos,* an irritation]. The biting of the tongue, lip, or cheek during an epileptic attack.

odaxetic (ō″dăk-sĕt′ĭk). Producing a stinging or itching sensation.

Oddi′s sphincter (ŏd′ēz). [Ruggero Oddi, 19th-century It. physician] A sphincter at the opening of the common bile duct into the duodenum at the papilla of Vater.

odditis (ŏd-dī′tĭs) [*Oddi* + Gr. *itis,* inflammation]. Inflammation of the sphincter of Oddi.

odogenesis (ō″dō-jĕn′ĕ-sĭs) [Gr. *hodos,* pathway, + *genesis,* formation]. The branching and growth of axons from the proximal end of a severed nerve. This allows the space between the nerves to be bridged and thus repaired.

odontagra (ō-dŏn-tă′gră) [Gr. *odous,* tooth, + *agra,* seizure]. Toothache, esp. when originating from gout.

odontalgia (ō-dŏn-tăl′jē-ă) [″ + *algos,* pain]. Toothache. SYN: *odontia; odontodynia.*

o., phantom. Pain felt in the area from which a tooth has been pulled.

odontatrophy (ō″dŏn-tăt′rō-fē) [″ + *atrophia,* atrophy]. Imperfect development of the teeth.

odontectomy (ō-dŏn-tĕk′tō-mē) [″ + *ektome,* excision]. Surgical removal of a tooth.

odonterism (ō-dŏn′tĕr-ĭzm) [″ + *erismos,* quarrel]. Chattering of the teeth.

odontia (ō-dŏn′shē-ă) [Gr. *odous,* tooth]. 1. Pain in a tooth. SYN: *odontalgia; odontodynia.* 2. Condition or abnormality of the teeth.

odontic (ō-dŏn′tĭk) [Gr. *odous,* tooth]. Concerning the teeth.

odontitis (ō″dŏn-tī′tĭs) [″ + *itis,* inflammation]. Inflammation of a tooth.

odonto-, odont- [Gr. *odous,* tooth]. Combining form rel. to the tooth or teeth.

odontoblast (ō-dŏn′tō-blăst) [″ + *blastos,* germ]. One of the cells forming the surface layer of the dental papilla that is responsible for the formation of the dentin of a tooth. After a tooth is formed, the odontoblasts line the pulp cavity and continue to produce dentin for years after the tooth has erupted.

odontoblastoma [″ + ″ + *oma,* tumor]. A tumor composed principally of odontoblasts.

odontobothrion (ō-dŏn″tō-bŏth′rē-ŏn) [″ + *bothrion,* pit]. Socket of a tooth.

odontobothritis [″ + ″ + *itis,* inflammation]. Inflammation of alveolar process of the tooth.

odontocele (ō-dŏn′tō-sēl) [″ + *kele,* hernia]. An alveolodental cyst.

odontochirurgical (ō-dŏn″tō-kī-rŭr′jĭ-kăl) [″ + *chirurgia,* surgery]. Pert. to dental surgery.

odontoclasis (ō″dŏn-tŏk′lă-sĭs) [″ + *klasis,* fracture]. The breaking or fracture of a tooth.

odontoclast. A cell that brings about the absorption of the roots of deciduous teeth.

odontodynia (ō-dŏn″tō-dĭn′ē-ă) [″ + *odyne,* pain]. Toothache. SYN: *odontalgia; odontia.*

odontogenesis, odontogeny (ō-dŏn″tō-jĕn′ĕ-sĭs, -tŏj′ĕn-ē) [″ + *genesis,* production]. The origin and formation of the teeth.

o. imperfecta. A congenital anomaly of the developing teeth in which there is deficient production of enamel and dentin in affected teeth. There is decreased density of the teeth and enlarged pulp chambers.

odontograph (ō-dŏn′tō-grăf) [″ + *graphein,* to write]. Device for determining the degree of uneven surface of tooth enamel.

odontography (ō-dŏn-tŏg′ră-fē). Descriptive anatomy of the teeth.

odontoid (ō-dŏn′toyd) [″ + *eidos,* resemblance]. Toothlike.

odontoid process. The toothlike projection from upper surface of the body of the second cervical vertebra.

odontolith (ō-dŏn′tō-lĭth) [″ + *lithos,* stone]. The accretion of a calcareous substance on the teeth; tartar.

odontologist (ō″dŏn-tŏl′ō-jĭst). A dentist or dental surgeon.

odontology (ō″dŏn-tŏl′ō-jē) [″ + *logos,* study]. The art and science of dentistry, q.v.

odontolysis (ō-dŏn-tŏl′ĭ-sĭs) [Gr. *odous,* tooth, + *lysis,* dissolution]. Loss of calcium from a tooth.

odontoma (ō″dŏn-tō′mă) [″ + *oma,* tumor]. Tumor of a tooth or tumor originating in the dental tissue.

o., ameloblastic. A neoplasm that contains enamel, dentin, and odontogenic tissue that does not develop to form enamel.

o., composite. An odontoma in which the epithelial and mesenchymal cells are completely differentiated. This causes enamel and dentin to be formed in an abnormal manner.

o., coronary. Bony tumor at the crown of a tooth.

o., follicular. Bony shell in gums below the tooth margin, usually after the second dentition. SYN: *cyst, dentigerous.*

ETIOL: Excessive number of dental follicles.

SYM: Crepitating to pressure. Tumor often involves one or more teeth.

o., radicular. Odontoma close to or on the root of a tooth.

odontonecrosis (ō-dŏn″tō-nē-krō′sĭs) [″ + *nekros,* dead, + *osis,* condition]. Extensive decay of a tooth.

odontonomy (ō″dŏn-tŏn′ō-mē) [″ + *onoma,* name]. Dental nomenclature.

odontopathy (ō-dŏn-tŏp′ă-thē) [″ + *pathos,* disease]. Any disease of the teeth.

odontophobia (ō-dŏn″tō-fō′bē-ă) [″ + *phobos,* fear]. 1. Abnormal aversion to the sight of teeth. 2. Abnormal fear of dental surgery.

odontoprisis (ō-dŏn″tō-prī′sĭs) [″ + *prisis,* sawing]. Grinding of the teeth. SYN: *bruxism.*

odontorrhagia (ō-dŏn″tō-rā′jē-ă) [″ + *rhegnynai,* to burst forth]. Hemorrhage from a tooth socket following extraction.

odontoschism (ō-dŏn′tō-skĭzm) [″ + *schisma,* cleft]. Fissure of a tooth.

odontoscopy (ō″dŏn-tŏs′kō-pē) [″ + *skopein,* to view]. 1. Examination of the teeth and oral cavity by use of an odontoscope. 2. An impression made of the biting marks made by teeth. These are used as a means of identification.

odontosis (ō-dŏn-tō′sĭs) [″ + *osis,* condition]. 1. Development of teeth. 2. Eruption of teeth.

odontotherapy (ō-dŏn″tō-thĕr′ă-pē) [″ + *therapeia,* treatment]. Care of diseased teeth.

odontotripsis (ō-dŏn″tō-trĭp′sĭs) [″ + *tripsis,* a rubbing]. Natural abrasion or wearing away of the teeth.

odor (ō′dĕr) [L.]. 1. That quality of a substance that renders it perceptible to sense of smell. 2. Any smell. 3. Any sensation of sense of smell.

Each odoriferous substance causes its own sensations, the description of which is complex and subjective. Odors have been classed as (1) pure odors, (2) those mixed with sensations from the mucous membrane, and (3) those mixed with the sensation of taste. A suggested classification of odors includes aromatic, burning, fragrant, fetid, nauseating, and repulsive. Another classification is spicy, flowery, fruity, resinous, foul, and scorched. Although classification attempts are useful, it is important to realize that most complex substances do not produce a single odor.

RS: "brom-" words; deodorant; effluvium; nose; olfactology; olfactory; osmolagnia; "osmo-" words; osphresiolagnia; osphresiometer; pungent; smell; taste.

odorant (ō′dor-ănt). Something that stimulates the sense of smell.

odoriferous (ō″dor-ĭf′ĕ-rŭs) [L. *odor,* smell, + *ferre,* to bear]. Bearing scent, having an odor; fragrant; perfumed.

odorimetry. The measurement of the ability of a substance to induce olfactory sensations.

odoriphore (ō-dor′ĭ-for) [″ + Gr. *phoros,* bearing]. The portion of a molecule that imparts odor to the substance.

odorography (ō″dor-ŏg′ră-fē) [″ + Gr. *graphein,* to write]. Description of odors.

odorous [L. *odor,* smell]. Having an odor, scent, or fragrance.

odynacusis (ō″dĭn-ă-kū′sĭs) [Gr. *odyne,* pain, + *akousis,* hearing]. A condition in which noises cause pain in the ear.

-odynia (ō-dĭn′ē-ă) [Gr. *odyne,* pain]. Combining form meaning pain.

odynometer (ō″dĭn-om′ĕt-ĕr) [″ + *metron,* measure]. Device for measuring pain.

odynophagia (ŏd″ĭn-ō-fā′jē-ă) [″ + *phagein,* to eat]. Pain upon swallowing.

odynophobia (ŏd″ĭn-ō-fō′bē-ă) [″ + *phobos,* fear]. Abnormal dread of pain.

Oedipus complex (ĕd′ĭ-pŭs). [Oedipus, a character in Gr. tragedy who unwittingly fell in love with his mother, Jocasta, killed his father in jealousy, and married his mother] Abnormally intense love of the child for parent of the opposite sex retained in adulthood. Usually involves jealous dislike of the other parent. Most commonly love of a son for his mother. SEE: *Electra complex; Jocasta complex.*

oenology (ē-nŏl′ō-jē) [Gr. *oinos,* wine, + *logos,* study]. The science of production and evaluation of wine.

oersted (ĕr′stĕd). [Hans Christian Oersted, Danish physicist, 1777–1851] A unit of magnetic field intensity. An oersted is the magnetism that exerts a force of one dyne on a unit magnetic pole.

oesophagostomiasis (ē-sŏf″ă-gō-stō-mī′ă-sĭs) [Gr. *oisophagos,* esophagus, + *stoma,* mouth, + *-iasis,* state]. Infection with the nematode of the genus Oesophagostomum.

Oesophagostomum (ē-sŏf″ă-gŏs′tō-mŭm) [Gr. *oisophagos,* esophagus, + *stoma,* mouth]. A genus of nematodes belonging to the suborder Strongylata; parasitic in the intestinal walls of animals and men.

O. apiostomum. The nodular nematode worm parasitic to monkeys. Occasionally infests man.

oestrus. Estrus.

Oestrus ovis. A botfly that may cause ocular myiasis in man.

O.F.D. *object film distance.* Distance from the radiographic film to the object being radiographed.

official. Said of medicines authorized as standard in the U.S. Pharmacopeia and in the National Formulary.

officinal (ŏf-ĭs′ĭn-ăl) [L. *officina,* shop]. Regularly kept in a druggist's stock. SEE: *magistral.*

Ogen. Trade name for estropipiate, USP.

Oguchi's disease (ō-goot′chēz). [Chuta Oguchi, Jap. ophthalmologist, 1875–1945] Hereditary night blindness with onset in infancy. Commonly found in Japan; rare in the United States.

OH^-. Chemical symbol for the hydroxyl ion.

ohm (ōm). Unit of electrical resistance equal to that of a conductor in which a current of one ampere is produced by a potential of one volt across the terminals. SEE: *electromotive force.*

ohmammeter (ōm′ăm-mē″tĕr). Combined ohmmeter and ammeter.

Ohm's law. [George S. Ohm, Ger. physicist, 1787–1854] The strength of an electric current, expressed in amperes, is equal to the electromotive force, expressed in volts, divided by the resistance, expressed in ohms. SEE: *electricity.*

ohmmeter (ōm′mē-tĕr). Device for determining the electrical resistance of a conductor.

-oid [Gr. *eidos,* form]. Suffix indicating resemblance to the item designated in the first part of the word.

oikofugic (oy″kō-fū′jĭk) [Gr. *oikos,* house, + L. *fugere,* to flee]. Having a compulsion to leave home.

oikomania (oy″kō-mā′nē-ă) [″ + *mania,* madness]. Nervous disorder induced by unhappy home surroundings.

oikophobia (oy″kō-fō′bē-ă). Morbid dislike of the home.

oil (oyl) [L. *oleum*]. A greasy liquid not miscible with water, usually obtained from and classified as mineral, vegetable, or animal. According to character, oils are subdivided principally as fixed or fatty and volatile or essential.

Ex.: *Fixed:* castor oil, olive oil, cod liver oil. *Volatile:* oils of mustard, peppermint, rose.

RS: oleaginous; oleate; oleic, olein; "oleo-" words; oleum; unctuous.

o., essential. Volatile oils, esp. those that have an odor and produce taste sensations, obtained from certain plants by steam distillation. These oils are used in flavors, perfumes, and medicines. They are usually complex chemicals that are difficult to purify.

o., ethereal. O., volatile.

o., fixed. Oils present in plants and animals that are glyceryl esters of fatty acids. These oils serve as food reserves in animals. They are non-volatile and contain no acid.

ointment (oynt′mĕnt) [Fr. *oignement*]. A medicated, fatty, soft substance for external application to the body, having antiseptic, cosmetic, or healing properties. Usually its base is petroleum jelly, lard, or lanolin to which the medicament is added. These forms are not water soluble. However, some ointments are composed of ingredients that are water soluble. SYN: *salve; unguent.*

o., hydrophilic. USP. A standardized ointment preparation used topically as an emollient.

o., white. USP. An ointment containing white wax and white petrolatum.

o., yellow. USP. An ointment containing yellow wax and petrolatum.

O.L. *oculus laevus,* left eye.

ol. L. *oleum,* oil.

-ol. Suffix indicating a substance is an alcohol or phenol.

O.L.A. L. *occipito laevo anterior,* fetal presentation with the occiput toward the maternal left acetabulum. SYN: *L.O.A.* SEE: *position.*

olea (ō′lē-ă) [L.]. 1. Olive. 2. Pl. of oleum.

oleaginous (ō-lē-ăj′ĭ-nŭs) [L. *oleaginus*]. Greasy; oily; unctuous.

oleander (ō″lē-ăn′dĕr). An ornamental evergreen shrub, Nerium oleander. It is toxic.

oleate (ō′lē-āt) [L. *oleatum*]. 1. Any salt of oleic acid. 2. Salt of oleic acid dissolved in an excess of the acid. Used as an ointment.

oleatum (ō-lē-ā′tŭm) [L.]. Preparation made by dissolving metallic salts or alkaloids in oleic acid. SYN: *oleate.*

olecranal (ō-lĕk′răn-ăl) [Gr. *olekranon,* elbow]. Concerning the elbow.

olecranarthritis (ō-lĕk″răn-ăr-thrī′tĭs) [″ + *arthron,* joint, + *itis,* inflammation]. Inflamed condition of the elbow joint.

olecranarthrocace (ō-lĕk″răn-ăr-thrŏk′ă-sē) [″ + ″ + *kake,* badness]. Tuberculous ulceration of the elbow joint.

olecranarthropathy (ō-lĕk″răn-ăr-thrŏp′ă-thē) [″ + ″ + *pathos,* disease]. Any disease of the elbow joint.

olecranoid (ō-lĕk′ră-noyd) [″ + *eidos,* resemblance]. Similar to the olecranon.

olecranon (ō-lĕk′răn-ŏn) [Gr., elbow]. [NA] A large process of the ulna projecting behind the elbow joint and forming the bony prominence of the elbow. SEE: *elbow; skeleton; ulna.*

o., fracture of. In treating this type of injury, prevent spasm of triceps muscle to avoid separation of fragments. The latter may have to be wired.

TREATMENT: Prevent spasm of the triceps by either placing the arm in a sling or bandaging the arm to the side.

oleic (ō-lē′ĭk) [L. *oleum,* oil]. Derived from or pert. to oil.

oleic acid. $C_8H_{34}O_2$. A colorless oily liquid prepared from tallow and other fats, the salts of which are oleates.

olein (ō′lē-ĭn) [L. *oleum,* oil]. An oleate of glyceryl found in nearly all fixed oils and fats; an important part of oils. SYN: *triolein.*

oleo- [L. *oleum,* oil]. Combining form meaning oil.

oleoarthrosis (ō″lē-ō-ăr-thrō′sĭs) [″ + Gr. *arthron,* joint, + *osis,* condition]. Therapeutic introduction of oil into a joint.

oleogranuloma (ō″lē-ō-grăn″ū-lō′mă) [″ + L. *granulum,* little grain, + Gr. *oma,* tumor]. A granuloma caused by continuous contact with oil, or at sites of subcutaneous injection of oily substances.

oleoinfusion (ō″lē-ō-ĭn-fū′zhŭn) [″ + *in,* into, + *fusus,* poured]. A formulation of a drug in oil.

oleoma (ō″lē-ō′mă) [″ + Gr. *oma,* tumor]. Oleogranuloma.

oleomargarine (ō″lē-ō-măr′jă-rĭn) [″ + *margarine*]. Butter substitute that may be salted or plain. It is made from refined vegetable and animal fats. These may be saturated or polyunsaturated. Vitamins, preservatives, and coloring agents usually are included. Caloric content is 7.2 Calories per gram. SYN: *margarine.*

oleometer (ō″lē-ŏm′ĕ-tĕr). Device for testing the purity of oil.

oleoresin (ō″lē-ō-rĕz′ĭn) [″ + *resina,* resin]. Extract of plant containing resinous substance and oil, prepared by dissolving the crude drug in ether, acetone, or alcohol.

oleosaccharum (ō-lē-ō-săk′ă-rŭm) [″ + *saccharum,* sugar]. A substance compounded of sugar and volatile oil.

oleostearate (ō″lē-ō-stē′ăr-āt). A combination of a base with oleic and stearic acids.

oleosus (ō″lē-ō′sŭs) [L.]. Greasy.

oleotherapy (ō″lē-ō-thĕr′ă-pē) [L. *oleum,* oil, + Gr. *therapeia,* treatment]. Therapeutic injection of oil. SYN: *eleotherapy.*

oleothorax (ō-lē-ō-thō′răks) [″ + Gr. *thorax,* chest]. Therapeutic injection of oil into the pleural cavity, as in pulmonary tuberculosis.

oleovitamin (ō″lē-ō-vī′tă-mĭn). A vitamin preparation in an edible oil.

o. A and D. A standardized preparation of vitamins A and D in fish liver oil or in an edible vegetable oil.

oleum (ō′lē-ŭm) [L.]. (pl. *olea*) Oil.

o. morrhuae. Cod liver oil.

o. olivea. Olive oil.

o. percomorphum. Mixture of oils from livers of various members of order Percomorphi. More potent in vitamins A and D than cod liver oil.

o. ricini. Castor oil.

olfactie (ŏl-făk′tē) [L. *olfacere,* to smell]. Unit of smell; the threshold of olfactory stimulation.

olfaction (ŏl-făk′shŭn) [L. *olfacere,* to smell]. 1. The sense of smell. 2. The act of smelling.

olfactive (ŏl-făk′tĭv) [L. *olfacere,* to smell]. Pert. to the sense of smell. SYN: *olfactory.*

olfactology (ŏl-făk-tŏl′ō-jē) [″ + Gr. *logos,* study]. Scientific investigation of sense of smell.

olfactometer (ŏl″făk-tŏm′ĕt-ĕr) [″ + Gr. *metron,* measure]. Apparatus for testing the power of the sense of smell.

olfactory (ŏl-făk′tō-rē). Pert. to smell.

olfactory area. Area in the hippocampal convolution, the anterior portion of the callosal gyrus and the uncus of the brain. Includes the olfactory bulb, tract, and trigone and is perforated by many blood vessels.

olfactory bulb. Enlarged anterior extremity of the olfactory tract.

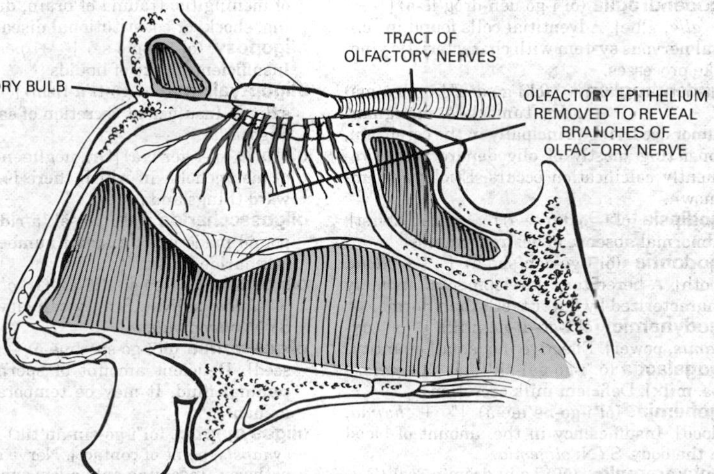

RIGHT OLFACTORY NERVE
(1st CRANIAL)

olfactory cortex. Portion of the cerebral cortex concerned with the olfactory sense. Includes the pyriform lobe and the hippocampal formation.

olfactory esthesioneuroma. Slowly growing malignant tumor of the nasal fossa, developing from epithelial and neural tissues of the olfactory mucosa.

olfactory lobe. A cranial lobe projecting from the anterior lower part of each cerebral hemisphere.

olfactory membrane. Membrane in the upper part of the nasal cavity that contains olfactory receptors.

olfactory nasal sulcus. An anterior-posterior groove in the wall of the nasal cavity. It passes from the anterior area to the lamina cribrosa.

olfactory nerves. The nerves supplying the nasal olfactory mucosa. Consist of delicate bundles of unmyelinated fibers, the fila olfactoria, that pass through cribriform plate and terminate in olfactory glomeruli of olfactory bulb. The fila are central processes of bipolar receptor neurons of olfactory mucous membrane. SEE: illus.; *cranial nerves*.

olfactory organ. The nose.

olfactory striae. Three bands of fibers (lateral, intermediate, and medial) that form the roots of the olfactory tract.

olfactory tract. Band of fibers that extends posteriorly from the olfactory bulb to the anterior perforated substance. Here it enlarges and divides into the olfactory striae.

olfactory trigone. Small triangular area between lateral and medial olfactory striae.

olfactory tubercle. An elevation at rostral end of anterior perforated substance. Well developed in lower mammals but rudimentary in man.

oligemia (ŏl-ĭg-ē′mē-ă) [Gr. *oligos*, little, + *haima*, blood]. Deficient volume of blood in the body. SYN: *oligohemic*.

oligergasia (ŏl-ĭ-gĕr-gā′sē-ă). Mental disorder based on intellectual inadequacy or feeblemindedness.

oligo-, olig- [Gr. *oligos*, little]. Combining form meaning small or few.

oligoamnios (ŏl″ĭ-gō-ăm′nē-ŏs) [″ + *amnion*, lamb]. Oligohydramnios, q.v.

oligocholia (ŏl″ĭ-gō-kō′lē-ă) [″ + *chole*, bile]. Lack or deficiency of bile.

oligochromemia (ŏl″ĭg-ō-krō-mē′mē-ă) [″ + *chroma*, color, + *haima*, blood]. Reduction of total amount of hemoglobin in the blood.

oligochylia (ŏl″ĭ-gō-kī′lē-ă) [″ + *chylos*, juice]. Deficiency of gastric juice

oligochymia (ŏl″ĭg-ō-kī′mē-ă) [″ + *chymos*, juice]. Deficiency of chyme.

oligocystic (ŏl-ĭ-gō-sĭs′tĭk) [″ + *kystis*, a bladder]. Having just a few cysts.

oligodactylia (ŏl-ĭ-gō-dăk-tĭl′ē-ă) [″ + *daktylos*, digit]. Subnormal number of fingers or toes.

oligodendroblast (ŏl″ĭ-gō-dĕn′drō-blăst) [″ + Gr. *dendron*, tree, + *blastos*, germ]. A primitive precursor cell of the oligodendrocyte.

oligodendroblastoma (ŏl″ĭ-gō-dĕn″drō-blăs-tō′mă) [″ + ″ + ″ + *oma*, tumor]. A neoplasm derived from oligodendroblasts.

oligodendrocyte [″ + ″ + *kytos*, cell]. Neuroglial cells having few and delicate processes.

oligodendroglia (ŏl″ĭ-gō-dĕn-drŏg′lē-ă) [″ + ″ + *glia*, glue]. Adventitial cells found in central nervous system with characteristic vine-like processes.

oligodendroglioma (ŏl″ĭ-gō-dĕn″drō-glī-ō′mă) [″ + ″ + ″ + *oma*, tumor]. A malignant tumor occurring principally in the cerebrum, consisting mostly of oligodendrocytes. Frequently calcification occurs. Etiology is unknown.

oligodipsia (ŏl″ĭ-gō-dĭp′sē-ă) [″ + *dipsa*, thirst]. Abnormal absence of desire for fluids.

oligodontia (ŏl″ĭ-gō-dŏn′shē-ă) [″ + *odont*, tooth]. A hereditary developmental anomaly characterized by fewer teeth than normal.

oligodynamic (ŏl″ĭ-gō-dī-năm′ĭk) [″ + *dynamis*, power]. Effective in a small quantity.

oligogalactia (ŏl″ĭ-gō-găl-ăk′tē-ă) [″ + *galaktos*, milk]. Deficient milk secretion.

oligohemia (ŏl″ĭ-gō-hē′mē-ă) [″ + *haima*, blood]. Insufficiency in the amount of blood in the body. SYN: *oligemia*.

oligohydramnios (ŏl″ĭg-ō-hī-drăm′nē-ōs) [″ + *hydor*, water, + *amnion*, amnion]. Abnormally small amount of amniotic fluid.

oligolecithal (ŏl″ĭg-gō-lĕs′ĭ-thăl) [″ + *lethikos*, yolk]. An egg with a small yolk.

oligoleukocythemia (ŏl″ĭ-gō-lū″kō-sī-thē′mē-ă) [Gr. *oligos*, little, + *leukos*, white, + *kytos*, cell, + *haima*, blood]. Reduction in leukocytic content of blood. SYN: *leukopenia*.

oligomastigate (ŏl″ĭ-gō-măs′tĭ-gāt) [″ + *mastix*, whip]. Characterized by two flagella.

oligomenorrhea (ŏl″ĭ-gō-mĕn″ō-rē′ă) [″ + *men*, month, + *rhoia*, flow]. Scanty or infrequent menstrual flow.

oligomorphic (ŏl″ĭ-gō-mor′fĭk) [″ + *morphe*, form]. Indicating organisms, esp. microorganisms, that go through only a few changes in form during development.

oligonucleotide (ŏl″ĭ-gō-nū′klē-ō-tīd) [″ + *nucleotide*]. A compound made up of a small number of nucleotide units.

oligophosphaturia (ŏl″ĭ-gō-fŏs-fă-tū′rē-ă) [″ + *phosphas*, phosphate, + *ouron*, urine]. Scanty amount of phosphates in the urine.

oligophrenia (ŏl″ĭg-ō-frē′nē-ă) [″ + *phren*, mind]. Mental retardation due to faulty development. SYN: *mental retardation*.

o., phenylpyruvic. Phenylpyruvic acid oligophrenia, q.v.

oligoplastic (ŏl″ĭ-gō-plăs′tĭk) [″ + Gr. *plassein*, to form]. Deficient repair of tissue.

oligopnea (ŏl-ĭ-gŏp′nē-ă) [″ + *pnoia*, breath]. Infrequent respiration. Respiration shallow or abnormally deep; rate as slow as 6 to 10 per minute. Usually accompanied by slow pulse, although high in some conditions.

ETIOL: Increased intracranial pressure, meningeal or pontine hemorrhage, cerebral or cerebellar tumors, abscess, gumma of meninges, osteoma of cranium, some forms of meningitis, trauma of brain, drug poisoning, shock, or constitutional diseases.

oligoposy (ŏl-ĭ-gŏp′ō-sē) [″ + *posis*, drink]. Insufficient intake of liquids.

oligoptyalism (ŏl-ĭ-gō-tī′ă-lĭzm) [″ + *ptyalon*, saliva]. Insufficient secretion of saliva. SYN: *oligosialia*.

oligoria (ŏl-ĭ-gor′ē-ă) [Gr., negligence]. A form of melancholia in which there is apathy toward things and people.

oligosaccharide (ŏl″ĭ-gō-săk′ă-rīd). A compound made up of a small number of monosaccharide units.

oligosialia (ŏl″ĭ-gō-sī-ā′lē-ă) [Gr. *oligos*, little, + *sialon*, saliva]. Scanty salivary secretion. SYN: *oligoptyalism*.

oligospermia (ŏl″ĭ-gō-spĕr′mē-ă) [″ + *sperma*, seed]. Deficient amount of spermatozoa in seminal fluid. It may be temporary or permanent.

oligosynaptic (ŏl″ĭ-gō-sĭn-ăp′tĭk) [″ + Gr. *synapsis*, point of contact]. Nerve conducting pathways involving only a few synapses.

oligotrichia (ŏl″ĭ-gō-trĭk′ē-ă) [″ + *thrix*, hair]. Congenital scantiness of hair.

oligotrophy (ŏl-ĭ-gŏt′rō-fē) [″ + *trophe*, nourishment]. Inadequate nutrition.

oligozoospermatism, oligozoospermia (ŏl″ĭ-gō-zō″ō-spĕr′mă-tĭzm, -spĕr′mē-ă) [″ + ″ + *ismos*, condition]. Oligospermia, q.v.

oliguresis (ŏl-ĭg-ū-rē′sĭs) [″ + *ouresis*, urination]. Scantiness of urine or infrequent urination.

oliguria (ŏl-ĭg-ū′rē-ă) [″ + *ouron*, urine]. Diminished amount of urine formation.

ETIOL: Seen after profuse perspiration, bleeding, diarrhea, and renal failure due to any disease. Also in retention of urine due to disease of the central nervous system, shock, drug poisoning, deep coma, or hypertrophy of the prostate.

oliva (ō-lī′vă) [L., olive]. (pl. *olivae*) [NA] An olive-shaped gray body behind the anterior pyramid of the medulla oblongata. SYN: *olivary body*.

olivary [L. *oliva*, olive]. Shaped like an olive; oval.

olivary body. A rounded mass located in the anterolateral portion of the medulla oblongata. Consists of a convoluted sheet of gray matter enclosing white matter. SYN: *oliva*.

olive (ŏl′ĭv) [L. *oliva*, olive]. Oliva.

o., accessory. One of two masses of gray matter lying adjacent to the inferior olive of the brain.

o., inferior. Olivary body.

o., superior. The superior olivary nucleus. SEE: *nucleus, olivary, superior*.

olive oil. Oil obtained by pressing the ripe fruit of olives (olea europaea). Used as an emollient in treating skin diseases and as a nutrient.

olivifugal (ŏl″ĭ-vĭf′ū-găl) [″ + *fugerea,* to flee]. In a direction away from the olivary nucleus of the brain.

olivipetal (ŏl″ĭ-vĭp′ĕ-tăl) [″ + *peter,* to seek]. In a direction toward the olivary nucleus of the brain.

olivopontocerebellar (ŏl″ĭ-vō-pŏn″tō-sĕr″ĕ-bĕl′ăr). Concerning the olivary nucleus, the pons, and the cerebellum of the brain.

Ollier, Léopold L. X. E. (ŏl″ē-ā′). French surgeon, 1830–1900.

O.'s disease. Chondrodysplasia, q.v.

O. layer. The deepest layer of the periosteum closest to the bone. The osteoblasts are in this layer.

O.-Thiersch graft. [Karl Thiersch, Ger. surgeon, 1822–1895] A split-thickness skin graft that is quite thin.

-ology [Gr. *logos,* study]. Suffix pert. to study of, knowledge, or science of.

olophonia (ŏl-ō-fōn′ē-ă) [Gr. *oloos,* destroyed, + *phone,* voice]. Malformation of vocal organs with resultant unnatural speech.

O.L.P. L. *occipito laeva posterior,* fetal presentation with its occiput toward the left posterior quadrant of the pelvis. SYN: *L.O.P.* SEE: *position.*

o.m. L. *omni mane,* every morning.

-oma [Gr.]. Suffix denoting a tumor.

omagra (ō-mă′gră) [Gr. *omos,* shoulder, + *agra,* seizure]. Attack of gout in the shoulder.

omalgia (ō-măl′jē-ă) [″ + *algos,* pain]. Neuralgia of the shoulder.

omarthritis (ō″măr-thrī′tĭs) [″ + *arthron,* joint, + *itis,* inflammation]. Inflamed condition of the shoulder joint.

omasitis (ō-mă-sī′tĭs). Inflammation of the omasum, q.v.

omasum (ō-mā′sŭm) [L.]. The third division of a ruminant's stomach.

ombrophobia (ŏm-brō-fō′bē-ă) [Gr. *ombros,* rain, + *phobos,* fear]. Fear and anxiety induced by storms, threatening clouds, or rain.

omenta (ō-mĕn′tă) [L.]. Pl. of omentum.

omental (ō-mĕn′tăl) [L. *omentum,* covering]. Pert. to the omentum, the peritoneal fold supporting the viscera.

omental bursa. A cavity within the layers of peritoneum forming the great omentum. Its opening into the main peritoneal cavity is the epiploic foramen (foramen of Winslow).

omentectomy (ō-mĕn-tĕk′tō-mē) [″ + Gr. *ektome,* excision]. Surgical removal of a portion of the omentum.

omentitis (ō-mĕn-tī′tĭs) [″ + Gr. *itis,* inflammation]. Inflamed condition of omentum.

omentofixation (ō-mĕn″tō-fĭk-sā′shŭn). Omentopexy, q.v.

omentopexy (ō-mĕn′tō-pĕks″ē) [″ + Gr. *pexis,* fixation]. Fixation of the omentum to the abdominal wall or adjacent organ.

omentoplasty (ō-mĕn′tō-plăs″tē) [L. *omentum,* a covering, + Gr. *plassein,* to form]. Use of tissue from the greater omentum as a graft in rejoining tissues.

omentorrhaphy (ō-mĕn-tor′ră-fē) [″ + Gr. *rhaphe,* suture]. Suturing of the omentum.

omentosplenopexy (ō-mĕn″tō-splē′nō-pĕks-ē) [″ + Gr. *splen,* spleen, + *pexis,* fixation]. Fixation of the spleen and omentum. Combined omentopexy and splenopexy.

omentotomy (ō-mĕn-tŏt′ō-mē) [″ + Gr. *tome,* incision]. Incision of the omentum.

omentovolvulus (ō-mĕn″tō-vŏl′vū-lŭs) [″ + *volvere,* to roll]. Volvulus, i.e., twisting, of the omentum.

omentum (ō-mĕn′tŭm) [L. a covering]. (pl. *omenta*) A double fold of peritoneum attached to the stomach and connecting it with certain of the abdominal viscera. It contains a cavity, the omental bursa (lesser peritoneal cavity). The omenta are the greater or gastrocolic omentum; and the lesser or gastrohepatic omentum. SEE: illus.

PALPATION: Infiltration of the omentum by malignant cells or tubercular enlargements is distinguished by the fact that they extend across the abdomen, cannot be traced backward, do not ascend behind the ribs, and are rough, hard, and uneven.

RS: abdomen; caul; epiploon; kidney; ovary; spleen.

o., gastrocolic. O., greater, q.v.

o., gastrohepatic. O., lesser, q.v.

o., greater. Portion of the omentum that is suspended from the greater curvature of the stomach and covers the intestines like an apron. It dips in among the folds of the intestines and is attached to the transverse colon and mesocolon. It contains fat, aids in keeping the intestines warm, prevents friction, and aids in localizing infections.

o., lesser. Portion of the omentum that passes from the lesser curvature of the stomach to the transverse fissure of the liver.

omentumectomy (ō-mĕn″tŭm-ĕk′tō-mē) [″ + Gr. *ektome,* excision]. Omentectomy, q.v.

omitis (ō-mī′tĭs) [Gr. *omos,* shoulder, + *itis,* inflammation]. Inflamed condition of the shoulder.

OML. *orbitomeatal line.*

omn. bih. L. *omni bihora,* every two hours.

omn. hor. L. *omni hora,* every hour.

omni- (ŏm′nĭ) [L. *omnis*]. Prefix designating all.

Omnipen. Trade name for ampicillin, USP.

Omnipen-N. Trade name for ampicillin sodium, USP.

omnipotence of thought. In psychiatry, infantile concept of reality whereby one expects all one's wishes to be instantly accomplished.

RELATIONSHIP OF GREATER OMENTUM TO ABDOMINAL ORGANS

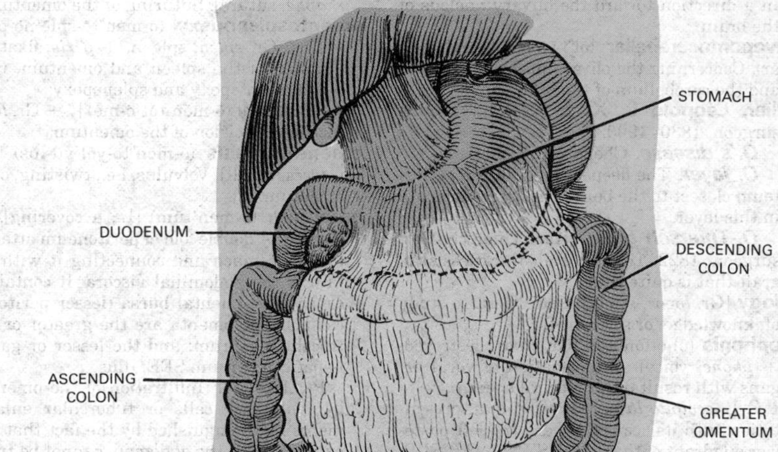

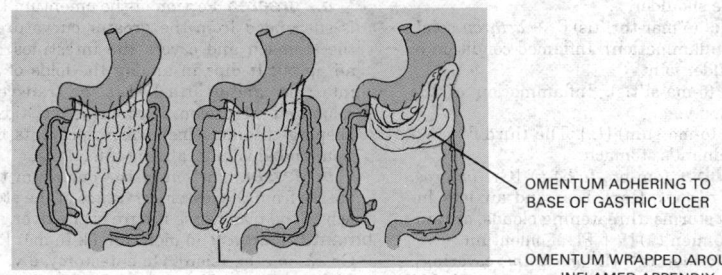

OMENTUM

Ex.: Children who gain their objectives through crying come to believe in their own omnipotence because of a parent's surrender to their demands.

omnivorous (ŏm-nĭv′ō-rŭs) [L. *omnis*, all, + *vorare*, to eat]. Eating both vegetable and animal foods.

omn. noct. L. *omni nocte*, every night.

omn. quad. hor. L. *omni quadrante hora*, every quarter of an hour.

omo- [Gr. *omos*, shoulder]. Combining form pert. to the shoulder.

omoclavicular (ō″mō-klă-vĭk′ū-lăr). Concerning the shoulder and the clavicle.

omodynia (ō-mō-dĭn′ē-ă) [Gr. *omos*, shoulder, + *odyne*, pain]. Pain of the shoulder.

omohyoid (ō-mō-hī′oyd). 1. Concerning the scapula and the hyoid bone. 2. Muscle attached to the hyoid bone and the scapula. SEE: *Muscles* in *Appendix*.

omophagia (ō-mō-fā′jē-ă) [Gr. *omos*, raw, + *phagein*, to eat]. The custom of eating raw foods, esp. flesh.

OMPA. *octamethyl pyrophosphoramide;* used as cholinesterase inhibitor.

omphal-, omphalo- [Gr. *omphalos,* the navel]. Combining form designating relationship to the navel.

omphalectomy (ŏm-făl-ĕk'tō-mē) [" + *ektome,* excision]. Surgical removal of the umbilicus.

omphalelcosis (ŏm"făl-ĕl-kō'sĭs) [" + *helkosis,* ulceration]. Ulceration of the umbilicus.

omphalic (ŏm-făl'ĭk) [Gr. *omphalikos*]. Concerning the umbilicus.

omphalitis (ŏm-făl-ī'tĭs) [" + *itis,* inflammation]. Inflamed condition of the navel.

omphaloangiopagus (ŏm"fă-lō-ăn"jē-ŏp'ă-gŭs) [" + *angeion,* vessel, + *pagos,* thing fixed]. Conjoined twins united by vessels of the umbilical cord.

omphalocele (ŏm-făl'ō-sēl) [" + *kele,* hernia]. Congenital hernia of the navel. SEE: *hernia.*

omphalochorion (ŏm"fă-lō-kō'rē-ŏn). A chorion supplied with blood by the omphalomesenteric blood vessels of the yolk sac.

omphalomesenteric (ŏm"făl-ō-mĕs-ĕn-tĕr'ĭk) [" + *mesenterion,* mesentery]. Concerning the umbilicus and mesentery.

omphaloncus (ŏm"făl-ŏn'kŭs) [" + *onkos,* tumor]. Umbilical tumor or swelling.

omphalopagus (ŏm"fă-lŏp'ă-gŭs) [" + *pagos,* thing fixed]. Conjoined twins joined at the abdomen.

omphalophlebitis (ŏm"făl-ō-flē-bī'tĭs) [" + *phleps,* vein, + *itis,* inflammation]. Inflamed condition of umbilical veins.

omphalorrhagia (ŏm"făl-ō-rā'jē-ă) [" + *rhegnynai,* to burst forth]. Umbilical hemorrhage.

omphalorrhea (ŏm"făl-ō-rē'ă) [" + *rhoia,* flow]. Discharge of lymph at the navel.

omphalorrhexis (ŏm"făl-ō-rĕk'sĭs) [" + *rhexis,* rupture]. Rupture of the navel.

omphalos (ŏm'făl-ŏs) [Gr.]. Umbilicus. SYN: *navel.*

omphalosite (ŏm'fă-lō-sīt") [" + *sitos,* food]. The underdeveloped twin of the omphaloangiopagus twins.

omphalosotor (ŏm"făl-ō-sō'tor) [" + *soter,* preserver]. Device used in replacing the prolapsed umbilical cord at childbirth.

omphalospinous (ŏm"făl-ō-spī'nŭs) [" + L. *spina,* thorn]. Concerning the navel and the anterior superior spine of the ilium.

omphalotomy (ŏm-făl-ŏt'ō-mē) [" + *tome,* incision]. Division of umbilical cord at birth.

omphalotripsy (ŏm"făl-ō-trĭp'sē) [" + *tripsis,* a rubbing]. Severing of the umbilical cord by a crushing method.

omphalus (ŏm'fă-lŭs) [Gr. *omphalos*]. The umbilicus.

ON. *orthopedic nurse.*

o.n. L. *omni nocte,* every night.

onanism (ō'năn-ĭzm). [So named because it was practiced by the Biblical character Onan, son of Judah] Coitus interruptus; withdrawal before ejaculation. Term was previously used erroneously to designate masturbation, q.v.

onanist (ō'nă-nĭst). One who practices coitus interruptus. Erroneously used to indicate one who masturbates.

Onanoff's reflex (ŏn-ă-nŏfs'). [Jacques Onanoff, Fr. physician, b. 1859] Contraction of bulbocavernous muscle resulting from compression of glans penis.

Onchocerca (ŏng"kō-sĕr'kă) [Gr. *onkos,* hook, + *kerkos,* tail]. A genus of filarial worms. They live in subcutaneous and connective tissues and usually are enclosed in fibrous cysts or nodules.

O. volvulus. A species of Onchocerca that infests man, frequently invading the tissues of the eye. Transmitted by species of the blackfly Simulium and Eusimulium.

onchocerciasis (ŏng"kō-sĕr-kī'ă-sĭs) [" + " + *iasis,* infestation]. Condition produced by infestation with one of the worms of Onchocerca. It is characterized by a nodular swelling over the coiled parasite. SYN: *oncocercosis.*

onco- [Gr. *onkos,* mass, bulk]. Combining form indicating rel. to a tumor, swelling, or mass.

Oncocerca. Onchocerca.

oncocercosis. Onchocerciasis.

oncocyte (ŏn'kō-sīt) [" + *kytos,* cell]. A large columnar cell with granular, acidophilic cytoplasm and a large number of mitochondria. They may become neoplastic.

oncocytoma (ŏng"kō-sī-tō'mă) [" + " + *oma,* tumor]. An adenoma composed of eosinophilic epithelial cells, esp. one of the salivary or parathyroid glands. These are benign tumors.

oncofetal (ŏng"kō-fē'tăl). Concerning tumors in the fetus.

oncogenesis (ŏng"kō-jĕn'ĕ-sĭs) [" + *genesis,* production]. Tumor formation and development.

oncogenic (ŏng"kō-jĕn'ĭk). Giving rise to tumors, esp. malignant tumors.

oncogenic virus. Virus that produces tumors. Although there is a relationship between viruses and human cancer, their exact role is not fully understood.

oncograph (ŏng'kō-grăf) [Gr. *onkos,* mass, + *graphein,* to write]. Device attached to oncometer for making record of the size and configuration of internal organs.

oncoides (ŏng-koy'dēz) [" + *eidos,* form]. Turgescence.

oncology (ŏng-kŏl'ō-jē) [" + *logos,* study]. The branch of medicine dealing with tumors.

oncolysis (ŏng-kŏl'ĭ-sĭs) [" + *lysis,* dissolution]. The absorption or dissolution of tumor cells.

oncolytic (ŏng"kō-lĭt'ĭk). Destructive to tumor

cells.

oncometer (ŏng-kŏm′ĕt-ĕr) [″ + *metron,* measure]. Apparatus for measurement of variations in size of internal organs. SEE: *plethysmograph.*

oncometric (ŏng″kō-mĕt′rĭk). Pert. to oncometry.

oncometry. The measurement of variations in size of internal organs.

oncosis (ŏng-kō′sĭs) [″ + *osis,* condition]. 1. A condition characterized by the development of tumors. 2. A swelling or tumor.

oncosphere (ŏng′kō-sfēr) [″ + *sphaira,* sphere]. Embryonic stage of a tapeworm in which it has hooks.

oncotherapy (ŏng″kō-thĕr′ă-pē) [″ + *therapeia,* treatment]. Treatment of tumors.

oncothlipsis (ŏng″kō-thlĭp′sĭs) [″ + *thlipsis,* pressure]. Pressure caused by presence of a tumor.

oncotic (ŏng-kŏt′ĭk) [Gr. *onkos,* tumor]. Concerning, caused, or marked by swelling.

oncotic pressure, colloidal. The total influence of the protein on the osmotic activity of plasma water.

oncotomy (ŏng-kŏt′ō-mē) [″ + *tome,* incision]. The incision of a tumor, abscess, or boil.

oncotropic (ŏng″kō-trŏp′ĭk) [″ + *tropos,* a turning]. Possessing special attraction for tumor cells.

Oncovin. Trade name for vincristine sulfate, USP.

oncovirus (ŏn′kō-vī″rŭs) [″ + *virus*]. Any virus that causes malignant neoplasms.

Ondine's curse. [Fr. Undine, mythical water nymph whose human lover was cursed to continuous sleep] 1. Primary alveolar hypoventilation due to reduced responsiveness of the respiratory center to carbon dioxide. 2. Loss of automatic respiratory function due to a lesion in the cervical portion of the spinal cord.

oneir(o)- (ō-nī′rō) [Gr. *oneiros,* dream]. Combining form indicating or concerning dreams.

oneiric (ō-nī′rĭk) [Gr. *oneiros,* dream]. Resembling, rel. to, or accompanied by dreams.

oneirism (ō-nī′rĭzm) [″ + *-ismos,* state of]. Dreamlike hallucination in a waking state.

oneirodynia (ō-nī″rō-dĭn′ē-ă) [″ + *odyne,* pain]. Painful dreaming; nightmare.

oneirogmus (ō″nī-rŏg′mŭs) [Gr. *oneirogmos,* an effusion during sleep]. Emission of semen during an erotic dream. SYN: *wet dream.*

oneirology (ō″nī-rŏl′ō-jē) [Gr. *oneiros,* dream, + *logos,* study of]. The scientific study of dreams.

oneiroscopy (ō″nī-rŏs′kō-pē) [″ + *skopein,* to examine]. Analysis of dreams in order to diagnose the individual's emotional state.

oniomania (ō″nē-ō-mā′nē-ă) [Gr. *onios,* for sale, + *mania,* madness]. A psychoneurotic urge to spend money.

onion (ŭn′yŭn) [AS. *oignon*]. The edible bulb of the onion plant, cultivated as a vegetable. Latin name for the common onion is alium cepa. The characteristic odor of onions is due to several volatile chemicals, some of which contain sulfur. The ability of onions to cause persons who peel them to shed tears probably is caused by a derivative of cysteine containing sulfur and oxygen.

onkinocele (ŏng-kĭn′ō-sēl) [Gr. *onkos,* mass, + *inos,* fiber, + *kele,* swelling]. Inflammation with swelling of a tendon sheath.

onlay. A graft applied to the surface of a tissue, esp. a bone graft applied to bone.

onomatology (ŏn″ō-mă-tŏl′ō-jē) [Gr. *onoma,* name, + *logos,* study]. Science of names. SYN: *nomenclature; terminology.*

onomatomania (ŏn″ō-mă″tō-mā′nē-ă) [″ + *mania,* madness]. A mental derangement characterized by an abnormal impulse to dwell upon or repeat certain words by attaching significance to their imagined hidden meanings or by trying frantically to recall a particular word.

onomatophobia (ŏn″ō-mă″tō-fō′bē-ă) [″ + *phobos,* fear]. Abnormal fear of hearing a certain name or word because of an imaginary dreadful meaning attached to it.

onomatopoiesis (ŏn″ō-mă″tō-poy-ē′sĭs) [Gr. *onoma,* name, + *poiein,* to make]. In psychiatry, created, usually meaningless, imitative words and sounds formed by the psychotic.

ontogenesis (ŏn″tō-jĕn′ĕ-sĭs). Ontogeny.

ontogenetic (ŏn″tō-jĕ-nĕt′ĭk). Concerning ontogeny.

ontogeny (ŏn-tŏj′ĕn-ē) [Gr. *on,* being, + *gennan,* to produce]. The history of the development of an individual. SYN: *ontogenesis.*

onych(o)- [Gr. *onyx,* nail]. Combining form indicating a relationship to finger- or toenails.

onychalgia (ŏn″ĭ-kăl′jē-ă) [Gr. *onyx,* nail, + *algos,* pain]. Pain in the nails.

o. nervosa. Extreme sensitivity of nails.

onychatrophia (ō″nĭk-ă-trō′fē-ă) [″ + *trophe,* nourishment]. Atrophy of the nails.

onychauxis (ŏn″ĭ-kawk′sĭs) [″ + *auxein,* to increase]. Overgrowth of the nails.

onychectomy (ŏn″ĭ-kĕk′tō-mē) [″ + *ektome,* to cut]. Surgical removal of the nail of a finger or toe.

onychia (ō-nĭk′ē-ă) [Gr. *onyx,* nail]. Inflammation of the nailbed with suppuration and frequently loss of the nail. SYN: *matrixitis; onychitis; onyxitis.* SEE: *paronychia.*

o. craquele. Fragility of nails.

o. lateralis. Suppuration of tissues in the area lateral to the fingernail. SYN: *paronychia.*

o. maligna. Type of onychia in debilitated persons in which there is fetid ulceration and loss of the nail.

o. parasitica. Any parasitic disease of the nails. SYN: *onychomycosis*.

o., piannic. Hyperkeratotic plaques that occur in the periungual region and cause deformities of the nail fold. ETIOL: Yaws.

o. punctata. Condition in which a nail possesses small punctiform depressions.

onychitis (ŏn″ĭ-kī′tĭs) [″ + *itis*, inflammation]. Inflammation of the nail bed. SYN: *onychia*.

onychocryptosis (ŏn″ĭ-kō-krĭp-tō′sĭs) [″ + *kryptein*, to conceal]. Ingrowing of the toenail.

onychodystrophy (ŏn″ĭ-kō-dĭs′trō-fē) [″ + *dys*, bad, + *trophe*, nutrition]. Any maldevelopment of a nail.

onychogenic (ŏn″ĭ-kō-jĕn′ĭk) [″ + *gennan*, to produce]. Concerning nail formation.

onychograph (ŏn-ĭk′ō-grăf) [″ + *graphein*, to write]. Device for making record of capillary blood pressure under the fingernails.

onychogryposis (ŏn″ĭ-kō-grĭ-pō′sĭs) [″ + *gryposis*, a curving]. Abnormal overgrowth of the nails with inward curvature.

onychoheterotopia (ŏn″ĭ-kō-hĕt″ĕr-ō-tō′pē-ă) [″ + *heteros*, other, + *topos*, place]. Abnormally located nails.

onychoid (ŏn′ĭ-koyd) [″ + *eidos*, resemblance]. Similar to a nail, esp. a fingernail.

onycholysis (ŏn″ĭ-kŏl′ĭ-sĭs) [″ + *lysis*, destruction]. Loosening or detachment of the nail from the nailbed.

onychoma (ŏn-ĭ-kō′mă) [″ + *oma*, tumor]. Tumor of the nail or nailbed.

onychomadesis (ŏn″ĭ-kō-mă-dē′sĭs) [Gr. *onyx*, nail, + *madesis*, loss of hair]. Complete loss of nails.

onychomalacia (ŏn″ĭ-kō-mă-lā′sē-ă) [″ + *malakia*, softening]. Abnormal softening of the nails. SYN: *hapalonychia*.

onychomycosis (ŏn″ĭ-kō-mī-kō′sĭs) [″ + *mykes*, fungus, + *osis*, condition]. Disease of the nails due to a parasitic fungus.

onycho-osteodysplasia (ŏn″ĭ-kō-ŏs″tē-ō-dĭs-plā′zē-ă). A genetic disease involving ectodermal and mesodermal tissues. The nails and patellae may be absent and other bones and joints are affected. SYN: *nail-patella syndrome*.

onychopathology (ŏn″ĭ-kō-pă-thŏl′ō-jē) [″ + *pathos*, disease, + *logos*, study]. Study of diseases of the nails.

onychopathy (ŏn-ĭ-kŏp′ăth-ē) [″ + *pathos*, disease]. Any disease of the nails. SYN: *onychosis*.

onychophagy (ŏn-ĭ-kŏf′ă-jē) [″ + *phagein*, to eat]. The practice of nail biting.

onychophosis (ŏn″ĭk-ō-fō′sĭs). Accumulation of horny layers of epidermis under the toenail.

onychophyma (ŏn″ĭ-kō-fī′mă) [″ + *phyma*, a growth]. Painful degeneration of the nail with hypertrophy.

onychoptosis (ŏn″ĭk-ŏp-tō′sĭs) [″ + *ptosis*, a falling]. Dropping off of the nails.

onychorrhexis (ŏn″ĭ-kō-rĕk′sĭs) [″ + *rhexis*, a rupture]. Abnormal brittleness and nail splitting. SYN: *fragilitas unguium*.

onychoschizia (ŏn″ĭ-kō-skĭz′ē-ă) [″ + *schizein*, to divide]. Loosening and eventual separation of the nail from its bed.

onychosis (ŏn-ĭ-kō′sĭs) [″ + *osis*, disease]. Any diseased condition of the nails. SYN: *onychopathy*.

onychotillomania (ŏn″ĭ-kō-tĭl″ō-mā′nē-ă) [″ + *tillein*, to pluck, + *mania*, insanity]. A neurotic tendency to pick the nails.

onychotomy (ŏn″ĭ-kŏt′ō-mē) [″ + *tome*, incision]. Surgical incision of a fingernail or toenail.

onychotrophy (ŏn-ĭ-kŏt′rō-fē) [″ + *trophe*, nourishment]. Nourishment of the nails.

onyx (ŏn′ĭks) [Gr., nail]. 1. A fingernail or toenail. 2. Pus collection between the corneal layers of the eye. SYN: *hypopyon*.

onyxis (ō-nĭk′sĭs). Ingrowing of the nails.

onyxitis (ŏn-ĭk-sī′tĭs) [″ + *itis*, inflammation]. Onychia.

oo- (ō-ō) [Gr. *oon*, egg]. Combining form denoting an egg or the primordial cell that develops into an ovule. SEE: words beginning with *ovo-*.

ooblast (ō′ō-blăst) [″ + *blastos*, germ]. The primitive cell from which the ovum is developed.

oocyesis (ō″ō-sī-ē′sĭs) [″ + *kyesis*, pregnancy]. Ectopic pregnancy in the ovary.

oocyst (ō′ō-sĭst) [Gr. *oon*, egg, + *kystis*, bladder]. The encysted form of a fertilized gamete (zygote) occurring in certain Sporozoa. SEE: *ookinete*.

oocytase (ō″ō-sī′tās) [″ + *kytos*, cell, + *-ase*, enzyme]. An enzyme destructive of ovarian cells.

oocyte (ō′ō-sīt) [″ + *kytos*, cell]. The early or primitive ovum before it has developed completely.

o., primary. The oocyte at end of growth period of oogonium and before first maturation division has occurred.

o., secondary. The larger of two oocytes resulting from first maturation division. SEE: *body, polar*.

oocytin (ō″ō-sī′tĭn). A substance that causes the formation of fertilization membranes in ova.

oogenesis (ō″ō-jĕn′ĕ-sĭs) [″ + *genesis*, formation]. Formation and development of the ovum. SYN: *ovigenesis*.

oogenetic (ō″ō-jĕ-nĕt′ĭk). Concerning oogenesis.

oogonium (ō″ō-gō′nē-ŭm) [″ + *gone*, seed]. (pl. *oogonia*) 1. The primordial cell from which an oocyte originates. 2. Descendant of the primordial cell from which the oocyte arises.

ookinesis (ō″ō-kĭn-ē′sĭs) [″ + *kinesis,* movement]. Mitotic phenomena taking place within an ovum during maturation and fertilization.

ookinete (ō″ō-kī-nēt′) [″ + *kinetos,* motile]. An elongated motile zygote occurring in the life cycle of certain sporozoan parasites, esp. Plasmodium. It penetrates the stomach wall of a mosquito and gives rise to an oocyst.

oolemma (ō″ō-lĕm′ă) [″ + *lemma,* sheath]. The plasma membrane of the oocyte.

oophagy (ō-ŏf′ă-jē) [″ + *phagein,* to eat]. Eating of eggs.

oophor- [Gr. *oophoros,* bearing eggs]. Combining form indicating rel. to the ovary.

oophoralgia (ō″ŏf-ō-răl′jē-ă) [″ + *algos,* pain]. Pain in an ovary. SYN: *oarialgia; ovarialgia.*

oophorauxe (ō″ŏf-ō-rawks′ē) [″ + *auxein,* to increase]. Ovarian enlargement.

oophorectomy (ō″ŏf-ō-rĕk′tō-mē) [″ + *ektome,* excision]. Excision of an ovary. SYN: *ovariectomy.*

oophoritis (ō″ŏf-ō-rī′tĭs) [″ + *itis,* inflammation]. Inflamed condition of the ovary. SYN: *ovaritis.*

o., follicular. Inflammation of the graafian follicles.

oophorocystectomy (ō-ŏf″ō-rō-sĭs-tĕk′tō-mē) [″ + *kystis,* cyst, + *ektome,* excision]. Surgical removal of an ovarian cyst.

oophorocystosis (ō-ŏf″ō-rō-sĭs-tō′sĭs) [Gr. *oophoros,* bearing eggs, + *kystis,* cyst, + *osis,* condition]. Development of an ovarian cyst.

oophorohysterectomy (ō-ŏf″ō-rō-hĭs″tĕr-ĕk′tō-mē) [″ + *hystera,* uterus, + *ektome,* excision]. Surgical removal of the uterus and ovaries. SYN: *oothecohysterectomy; ovariohysterectomy.*

oophoroma (ō-ŏf″ō-rō′mă) [″ + *oma,* tumor]. Malignant ovarian tumor.

oophoron (ō-ŏf′ō-rŏn) [Gr. *oophoros,* bearing eggs]. An ovary. SYN: *ootheca.*

oophoropathy (ō-ŏf″or-ŏp′ă-thē) [″ + *pathos,* disease]. Any pathological condition of the ovary.

oophoropeliopexy (ō-ŏf″ō-rō-pē′lē-ō-pĕk″sē) [″ + *pellis,* pelvis, + *pexis,* fixation]. Suture of a displaced ovary to the pelvic wall.

oophoropexy (ō-ŏf″ō-rō-pĕk′sē) [″ + *pexis,* fixation]. Fixation of a displaced ovary. SYN: *oophoropeliopexy.*

oophoroplasty (ō-ŏf′ō-rō-plăs″tē) [″ + *plassein,* to form]. Plastic surgery on the ovary.

oophorosalpingectomy (ō-ŏf″ō-rō-săl-pĭn-jĕk′tō-mē) [″ + *salpinx,* tube, + *ektome,* excision]. Excision of an oviduct and ovary. SYN: *ovariosalpingectomy.*

oophorosalpingitis (ō-ŏf″or-ō-săl″pĭn-jī′tĭs) [″ + ″ + *itis,* inflammation]. Inflammation of the ovary and oviduct.

oophorostomy (ō-ŏf″ō-rŏs′tō-mē) [″ + *stoma,* opening]. Creation of an artificial opening into the ovarian cyst for drainage.

oophorotomy (ō-ŏf″ō-rŏt′ō-mē) [″ + *tome,* excision]. Surgical incision of the ovary.

oophorrhagia (ō″ŏf-ō-rā′jē-ă) [″ + *rhegnynai,* to burst forth]. Hemorrhage from an ovulatory site severe enough to cause clinical symptoms or signs.

oophorrhaphy (ō-ŏf-or′ă-fē) [″ + *rhaphe,* suture]. Suture of a displaced ovary to the pelvic wall.

ooplasm (ō′ō-plăzm) [Gr. *oon,* egg, + *plasma,* a thing formed]. The cytoplasm of an ovum.

oosperm (ō′ō-spĕrm) [″ + *sperma,* seed]. The cell formed by union of the spermatozoon with the ovum; the fertilized ovum.

oosporangium (ō″ō-spō-răn′jē-ŭm). The female portion in the sexual formation of oospores.

oospore (ō′ō-spor) [″ + *sporos,* seed]. A spore formed by the union of opposite sexual elements.

ootheca (ō-ō-thē′kă) [Gr. *ootheke,* ovary]. An ovary. SYN: *oophoron.*

oothecohysterectomy (ō-ō-thē″kō-hĭs″tĕr-ĕk′tō-mē) [Gr. *ootheke,* ovary, + *hystera,* uterus, + *ektome,* excision]. Excision of the uterus and ovaries. SYN: *oophorohysterectomy; ovariohysterectomy.*

ootid (ō′ō-tĭd). The ripe ovum after first maturation has been completed and the second has begun.

OP. *operative procedure; outpatient.*

O.P. *occiput position.*

opacification (ō-păs″ĭ-fĭ-kā′shŭn) [L. *opacitas,* shadiness, + *facere,* to make]. 1. The process of making something opaque. 2. Formation of opacities.

opacity (ō-păs′ĭ-tē) [L. *opacitas,* shadiness]. 1. State of being opaque. 2. An opaque area or spot.

opalescent (ō″păl-ĕs′ĕnt). Similar to an opal with respect to colors produced.

opaque (ō-pāk′) [L. *opacus,* dark]. 1. Impenetrable by visible light rays or by other forms of radiant energy such as x-rays. 2. Not transparent. 3. Dense or slow to learn.

OPC. *outpatient clinic.*

OPD. *outpatient department.*

open [AS.]. 1. Not shut. 2. Uncovered, exposed, as a wound to air. 3. To puncture, as to open a boil. 4. Interrupted, said of an electric circuit, when current cannot pass because a switch is open.

opening. 1. A hole, or aperture, or the entrance to a hole. 2. An open space that serves as an entrance to a tissue or organ. 3. The act of becoming open.

o., aortic. The opening in the diaphragm through which the aorta passes.

o., cardiac. The opening of the esophagus into the cardiac end of the stomach.

o., pyloric. The opening between the stomach and duodenum.

open reduction. In orthopedics, realigning the fractured segments after incising the skin and tissues in order to expose the fractured bone. SEE: *reduction, closed.*

operable (ŏp'ĕr-ă-bl) [L. *operor,* to work]. 1. Practicable. 2. Admitting of treatment by surgery with reasonable expectation of cure.

operant conditioning. Conditioning or influencing behavior by rewarding an individual for certain forms of behavior. This reward, also called reinforcement, induces the person to act in such a way as to receive the award.

operate (ŏp'ĕr-āt) [L. *operatus,* worked]. 1. To perform an excision or incision or to make a suture on the body or any of its organs or parts to restore health. 2. To produce an effect, as a drug.

operation (ŏp-ĕr-ā'shŭn) [L. *operatio,* a working]. 1. The act of operating. 2. A surgical procedure. 3. The effect or method of action of any type of therapy. SEE: *surgery.*

Even though many surgeons feel that preoperative shaving of the skin over the surgical site is unnecessary insofar as bacterial considerations are concerned, it is still utilized in order to facilitate access to the operative site.

o., ablative. Operation in which a part is removed.

o., cosmetic. An operation for the purpose of improving the appearance of some part of the body.

o., exploratory. Operation performed for diagnostic purposes.

o., flap. Surgical procedure in which a flap of tissue or periosteum is raised. An amputation flap is a tissue flap produced to cover the amputation stump.

o., major. Operation involving a considerable hazard to the patient.

o., minor. Operation not serious or risking life.

o., plastic. Operation for reconstruction and repair of surface and other structures.

o., radical. Operation performed to remove a large amount of damaged or neoplastic tissue.

o., reconstructive. Operation to repair a loss or defect.

o., subtotal. Operation in which only a portion of the organ is removed, as subtotal removal of the thyroid gland.

operative (ŏp'ĕr-ă-tĭv) [L. *operativus,* working]. 1. Effective, active. 2. Pert. to or brought about by an operation.

operative dentistry. The area of dentistry concerned with operations to restore or replace the hard dental tissues; such operations necessitated by caries, trauma, or malocclusions that may be restored by silver amalgam, gold, porcelain, or a variety of plastic dental materials. SYN: *restorative dentistry.*

operator (ŏp'ĕr-ā-tor). A person who performs surgical operations.

opercular (ō-pĕr'kū-lăr) [L. *operculum,* a cover]. Concerning a covering structure.

operculitis (ō-pĕr"kū-lī'tĭs) [" + Gr. *itis,* inflammation]. Inflammation of the gingiva over a partially erupted tooth.

operculum (ō-pĕr'kū-lŭm) [L., a covering]. (pl. *opercula*) 1. Any covering. 2. Plug of mucus that fills up the opening of the cervix upon impregnation. 3. [NA] Convolutions of the cerebrum, the margins of which are separated by the lateral cerebral (Sylvian) fissure. The opercula cover the insula.

o., dental. The soft tissue overlying the crown of a partially erupted tooth.

o., trophoblastic. The plug of fibrin that covers the opening in the endometrium made by the implanting ovum.

operon (ŏp'ĕr-ŏn). In genetics, a group of linked genes and regulatory elements that functions as a unit of transcription.

ophiasis (ō-fī'ă-sĭs) [Gr. *ophis,* snake]. Baldness occurring in winding streaks across the head.

ophidiasis (ō-fĭ-dī'ă-sĭs). Ophidism, q.v.

ophidiophobia (ō-fĭd"ē-ō-fō'bē-ă) [Gr. *ophidion,* snake, + *phobos,* fear] Abnormal fear of snakes.

ophidism (ō'fĭd-ĭzm) [" + *-ismos,* condition]. Poisoning from snake bite.

ophiotoxemia (ō"fē-ō-tŏk-sē'mē-ă) [" + *toxikon,* poison, + *haima,* blood]. Poisoning due to venom injected by a snake

ophritis, ophryitis (ŏf-rī'tĭs, -rē-ī'tĭs) [Gr. *ophrys,* eyebrow, + *itis,* inflammation]. Inflammation of the eyebrow.

ophryon (ŏf'rē-ŏn). Meeting point of the facial median line with a transverse line across the forehead's narrowest portion.

ophryosis (ŏf'rē-ō'sĭs) [" + *osis,* condition]. Eyebrow spasm.

Ophthaine. Trade name for proparacaine hydrochloride, USP.

Ophthalgan. Trade name for glycerin, USP.

ophthalmagra (ŏf"thăl-măg'ră) [Gr. *ophthalmos,* eye, + *agra,* seizure]. Sudden development of eye pain.

ophthalmalgia (ŏf"thăl-măl'jē-ă) [" + *algos,* pain]. Pain in the eye. SYN: *ophthalmodynia.*

ophthalmatrophy (ŏf-thăl-măt'rō-fē) [" + *atrophia,* a wasting]. Atrophy of eyeball.

ophthalmectomy (ŏf-thăl-mek'tō-mē) [Gr. *ophthalmos,* eye, + *ektome,* excision]. Surgical excision of an eye.

ophthalmencephalon (ŏf"thăl-mĕn-sĕf'ă-lŏn) [" + *enkephalos,* brain]. The vision apparatus from the retina, to the optic nerves, optic chiasm, optic tract, and the visual centers of the brain.

ophthalmia (ŏf-thăl′mē-ă) [Gr. *ophthalmos,* eye]. Severe inflammation of the eye, usually including the conjunctiva.

o., catarrhal. Conjunctivitis of a severe, frequently purulent, form.

o., Egyptian. Granular conjunctivitis. SYN: *trachoma.*

o., electric. Ophthalmia marked by pain in the eye, intolerance to light, and tearing (lacrimation). Occurs following exposure, usually prolonged, to intense light as that in arc welding.

o., gonorrheal. Severe purulent form due to infection with gonococcus.

o., granular. Severe purulent conjunctivitis with formation of granules on the eyelids. SYN: *trachoma.*

o., metastatic. Sympathetic inflammation of the choroid due to pyemia or metastasis.

o. neonatorum. Severe purulent conjunctivitis in the newborn.

ETIOL: Infection of the birth canal at the time of delivery. Gonococcus is responsible for a great majority of cases. Symptoms present 12 to 48 hrs. after birth when due to gonorrhea.

PROPHYLAXIS: Introduction of two drops of a 1% silver nitrate solution into each eye of newborn at birth.

o., neuroparalytic. Ophthalmia resulting from injury or disease involving semilunar ganglion or branches of the trigeminal nerve supplying eyeball.

o., phlyctenular. Vesicular formations on epithelium of conjunctiva or cornea. SYN: *o., scrofulous.*

o., purulent. Purulent inflammation of eye, usually due to gonococcus.

o., scrofulous. O., phlyctenular.

o., spring. Conjunctivitis in the spring of the year, usually an allergic reaction to tree pollen. SYN: *conjunctivitis, vernal.*

o., sympathetic. Rare bilateral granulomatous inflammation of the entire uveal tract of both eyes. Occurs in the untraumatized eye following perforation of the globe of the other eye.

SYM: Photophobia, lacrimation, pain, blurring of vision, eyeball tenderness, deposits on posterior surface of cornea. Exudate appears in pupillary area with posterior synechia, seclusio pupillae, secondary atrophy with blindness.

TREATMENT: Mydriatics, analgesics, steroids, other anti-inflammatory therapy. Sympathetic ophthalmia does not occur immediately following injury; thus it is not necessary to remove the injured eye as an emergency procedure.

o., varicose. Ophthalmia seen in varicose veins of the conjunctiva.

ophthalmiatrics (ŏf″thăl-mē-ăt′rĭks) [″ + *iatreia,* treatment]. The treatment of eye diseases.

ophthalmic (ŏf-thăl′mĭk) Pert. to the eye.

ophthalmic nerve. A branch of the trigeminal (5th cranial) nerve. It is sensory and its branches are the lacrimal, frontal, and nasociliary.

ophthalmic reaction. Reaction of the eye following instillation into the eye of toxins of typhoid or tuberculosis. SYN: *Calmette's reaction; oculoreaction; ophthalmoreaction.*

ophthalmitis (ŏf″thăl-mī′tĭs) [″ + *itis,* inflammation]. Inflamed condition of the eye.

ophthalmo- [Gr. *ophthalmos,* eye]. Combining form pert. to the eye.

ophthalmoblennorrhea (ŏf-thăl″mō-blĕn″ō-rē′ă) [″ + *blenna,* mucus, + *rhoia,* flow]. Purulent inflammation of the eye or conjunctiva, usually due to the gonococcus.

ophthalmocele (ŏf-thăl′mō-sēl) [″ + *kele,* swelling]. Abnormal protrusion of the eyeballs. SYN: *exophthalmos.*

ophthalmocopia (ŏf-thăl″mō-kō′pē-ă) [″ + *kopos,* fatigue]. Ocular fatigue; eyestrain. SYN: *asthenopia.*

ophthalmodesmitis (ŏf-thăl″mō-dĕs-mī′tĭs) [″ + *desmos,* ligament, + *itis,* inflammation]. Inflammation of tendons of the eye.

ophthalmodiagnosis (ŏf-thăl″mō-dī″ăg-nō′sĭs) [″ + *dia,* through, + *gnosis,* knowledge]. Diagnosis of eye conditions by means of the ophthalmoreaction, q.v.

ophthalmodiaphanoscope (ŏf-thăl″mō-dī-ă-făn′ō-skōp) [″ + ″ + *phainein,* to appear, + *skopein,* to examine]. A device for examining the retina by transillumination, the source of which may be a light in the oral cavity.

ophthalmodonesis (ŏf-thăl″mō-dō-nē′sĭs) [″ + *donesis,* trembling]. A tremor or oscillatory movement of the eye.

ophthalmodynamometer (ŏf-thăl″mō-dī″nă-mŏm′ĕ-tĕr) [″ + *dynamis,* power, + *metron,* measure]. Instrument for determining pressure in ophthalmic arteries. Device is placed against conjunctiva of eye. If pressure is higher on one side than the other, appropriate studies to attempt to define the cause are indicated.

ophthalmodynamometry (ŏf-thăl″mō-dī″nă-mŏm′ĕ-trē). Determination of pressure in the ophthalmic artery by use of an instrument that produces pressure on the eyeball until pulsations in the ophthalmic artery are seen through the ophthalmoscope. That pressure is diastolic. As the pressure is increased, the vessel collapses; this is systolic pressure.

ophthalmodynia (ŏf-thăl″mō-dĭn′ē-ă) [″ +

odyne, pain]. Pain in the eye. SYN: *ophthalmalgia.*

ophthalmoeikonometer (ŏf-thăl″mō-ī″kō-nŏm′ĕ-tĕr) [″ + *eikon,* image, + *metron,* measure]. Device for measuring the relative size of ocular images in the eyes.

ophthalmofundoscope (ŏf-thăl″mō-fŭn′dō-skōp) [″ + L. *fundus,* base, + Gr. *skopein,* to examine]. Apparatus used in examining the fundus of the eye.

ophthalmography (ŏf″thăl-mŏg′răf-ē) [″ + *graphein,* to write]. Description of the eye.

ophthalmogyric (ŏf-thăl″mō-jī′rĭk) [″ + *gyros,* circle]. Causing or concerning concentric ocular movements. SYN: *oculogyric; oculomotor.*

ophthalmolith (ŏf-thăl′mō-lĭth) [″ + *lithos,* stone]. A calculus of the lacrimal duct.

ophthalmologist (ŏf-thăl-mŏl′ō-jĭst) [″ + *logos,* study]. A physician who specializes in the treatment of disorders of the eye; an oculist.

NOTE: The preferred term for a physician who treats and studies diseases of the eye is ophthalmologist. An optometrist is not a physician, but one who is skilled in testing visual acuity and prescribing corrective lenses. An optician sells or makes optical materials.

ophthalmology (ŏf-thăl-mŏl′ō-jē) [″ + *logos,* study]. The science dealing with the eye and its diseases.

ophthalmomalacia (ŏf-thăl″mō-măl-ā′sē-ă) [″ + *malakia,* softening]. Abnormal shrinkage or softening of the eye. SYN: *ophthalmophthisis.*

ophthalmometer (ŏf-thăl-mŏm′ĕt-ĕr) [″ + *metron,* measure]. 1. Instrument for measuring error of refraction. 2. Instrument for measuring the volume of various chambers of the eye. 3. Instrument for measuring the anterior curvatures of the eye. 4. Device for measuring the size of the eye.

ophthalmometry (ŏf-thăl-mŏm′ĕt-rē). Measurement of the ocular defects and refractive powers.

ophthalmomyiasis (ŏf-thăl″mō-mī′yă-sĭs) [Gr. *ophthalmos,* eye, + *myia,* a fly, + *-iasis,* condition]. Eye infestation by larvae of the fly Oestrus ovis.

ophthalmomycosis (ŏf-thăl″mō-mī-kō′sĭs) [″ + *mykes,* fungus, + *osis,* condition]. Any fungus disease of the eye.

ophthalmomyitis (ŏf-thăl″mō-mī-ī′tĭs) [″ + *mys,* muscle, + *itis,* inflammation]. Inflammation of the ocular muscles.

ophthalmomyositis (ŏf-thăl″mō-mī″ō-sī′tĭs). Ophthalmomyitis.

ophthalmomyotomy (ŏf-thăl″mō-mī-ŏt′ō-mē) [″ + *mys,* muscle, + *tome,* incision]. Surgical section of the muscles of the eyes.

ophthalmoneuritis (ŏf-thăl″mō-nū-rī′tĭs) [″ + *neuron,* sinew, + *itis,* inflammation]. Inflamed condition of the optic nerve.

ophthalmopathy (ŏf″thăl-mŏp′ă-thē) [″ + *pathos,* disease]. Any eye disease.

ophthalmophlebotomy (ŏf-thăl″mō-flē-bŏt′ō-mē) [″ + *phleps,* vein, + *tome,* incision]. Incision of the eye to overcome congestion of conjunctival veins.

ophthalmophthisis (ŏf″thăl-mŏf′thĭ-sĭs) [″ + *phthisis,* wasting]. Ophthalmomalacia.

ophthalmoplasty (ŏf-thăl′mō-plăs″tē) [″ + *plassein,* to form]. Ocular plastic surgery.

ophthalmoplegia (ŏf-thăl″mō-plē′jē-ă) [″ + *plege,* stroke]. Paralysis of ocular muscles.

o. externa. Paralysis of extraocular muscles.

o. interna. Paralysis of iris and ciliary muscle.

o., nuclear. Ophthalmoplegia due to lesion of nuclei of origin of the ocular motor nerves.

o., Parinaud's. Paralysis of conjugate movement of the eyes upward. Convergence is not affected. The pathological lesion is in the midbrain.

o. partialis. Incomplete paralysis, involving only one or two of the ocular muscles.

o. progressiva. Form of ophthalmoplegia in which all muscles become involved slowly, caused by deterioration of the motor nerve nuclei.

o. totalis. Paralysis that affects both internal and external ocular muscles.

ophthalmoptosis (ŏf-thăl″mŏp-tō′sĭs) [″ + *ptosis,* fall]. Protrusion of the eyeball. SYN: *exophthalmos.*

ophthalmoreaction (ŏf-thăl″mō-rē-ăk′shŭn) [″ + L. *re,* back, + *actus,* acted]. Reaction of the conjunctiva following instillation of a drop of tuberculin or typhoid fever toxin into the eye of persons suffering from tuberculosis or typhoid diseases. Of diagnostic value. SYN: *oculoreaction; ophthalmic reaction.*

ophthalmorrhagia (ŏf-thăl″mō-rā′jē-ă) [″ + *rhegnynai,* to burst forth]. Ocular hemorrhage.

ophthalmorrhea (ŏf-thăl″mō-rē′ă) [″ + *rhoia,* flow]. Discharge from the eye.

ophthalmorrhexis (ŏf-thăl″mō-rĕk′sĭs) [″ + *rhexis,* rupture]. Rupture of an eyeball.

ophthalmoscope (ŏf-thăl′mō-skōp) [″ + *skopein,* to examine]. Instrument for examining interior of the eye, esp. the retina.

ophthalmoscopy (ŏf-thăl-mŏs′kō-pē). Examination of the interior of the eye.

o., medical. Use of ophthalmoscopy to diagnose systemic disease.

o., metric. 1. Use of the ophthalmoscope to determine the refractive error of the lens of the eye. 2. Use of ophthalmoscopy to measure the height of the head of the optic nerve in cases of papilledema.

ophthalmospasm (ŏf-thăl'mō-spăsm). Spasm of ocular muscles.
ophthalmostasis (ŏf'thăl-mŏs'tă-sĭs) [Gr. *ophthalmos,* eye, + *stasis,* standing]. Fixation of the eyeball during surgery on it.
ophthalmostat (ŏf-thăl'mō-stăt) [" + *statos,* made to stand]. Instrument used to hold the eye still during an operation.
ophthalmostatometer (ŏf-thăl"mō-stăt-ŏm'ĕt-ĕr) [" + " + *metron,* measure]. Instrument for ascertaining position of eyes.
ophthalmosynchysis (ŏf-thăl"mō-sĭn'kĭ-sĭs) [" + *synchisis,* a mixing]. Effusion into one of the cavities of the eye.
ophthalmothermometer (ŏf-thăl"mō-thĕr-mŏm'ĕt-ĕr) [" + *therme,* heat, + *metron,* measure]. Instrument for determining local temperature in eye diseases.
ophthalmotomy (ŏf"thăl-mŏt'ō-mē) [" + *tome,* incision]. Surgical incision of the eyeball.
ophthalmotonometer (ŏf-thăl"mō-tō-nŏm'ĕt-ĕr) [" + *tonos,* tension, + *metron,* measure]. Instrument for determining tension within the eye.
ophthalmotoxin (ŏf-thăl"mō-tŏk'sĭn) [" + *toxikon,* poison]. Cytotoxin derived on injection of emulsions of the ciliary body.
ophthalmotrope (ŏf-thăl'mō-trōp) [" + *trope,* a turning]. Instrument or model of the eye used to demonstrate the movements of the extraocular muscles.
ophthalmotropometer (ŏf-thăl"mō-trō-pŏm'ĕt-ĕr) [" + " + *metron,* measure]. Instrument for measuring the eye movements.
ophthalmovascular (ŏf-thăl"mō-văs'kū-lăr) [" + L. *vasculum,* a small vessel]. Pert. to blood vessels of the eye.
ophthalmoxerosis (ŏf-thăl"mō-zē-rō'sĭs) [" + *xeros,* dry, + *osis,* condition]. Xerophthalmia, q.v.
ophthalmoxyster (ŏf-thăl"mŏks-ĭs'tĕr) [" + *xyster,* scraper]. Instrument used to scrape the conjunctiva.
Ophthetic. Trade name for proparacaine hydrochloride, USP.
opiate (ō'pē-ăt). Any drug containing or derived from opium.
opiate abstinence syndrome. Withdrawal symptoms range from restlessness, depression, and mild disturbances in function of the autonomic nervous system, to chills, nausea, vomiting, and diarrhea. The severity of the symptoms correlates with the dosage of the drug. Emotional reactions may be pronounced.
opiate poisoning. SYM: Acute poisoning causes euphoria, flushing, itching of the skin, miosis, drowsiness, decreased respiratory rate and depth, bradycardia, hypotension, and a decrease in body temperature. If condition is untreated, death may be the outcome.
opiate receptor. Specific sites on cell surfaces that interact in a highly selective fashion with opiate drugs. These receptors mediate the major known pharmacological actions of opiates and the physiologic functions of the endogenous opiate-like substance, endorphins, and enkephalins, q.v.
opioid (ō'pē-oyd) [L. *opium,* opium, + Gr. *eidos,* form]. 1. Non-opium-derived synthetic narcotics. 2. Indicating substances such as enkephalins or endorphins occurring naturally in the body that act on the brain to decrease the sensation of pain.
opiomania (ō"pē-ō-mā'nē-ă) [" + Gr. *mania,* madness]. Insane craving for opium or its derivatives.
opiophagism (ō"pē-ŏf'ă-jĭzm) [" + Gr. *phagein,* to eat]. Addiction to the use of opium, esp. the eating of it.
opisthenar (ō-pĭs'thē-năr) [Gr. *opisthen,* behind, + *thenar,* palm]. Back of the hand.
opisthiobasial (ō-pĭs"thē-ō-bā'sē-ăl). Concerning the opisthion and basion of the skull.
opisthion (ō-pĭs'thē-ŏn) [Gr., rear]. Craniometric point at middle of lower border of the foramen magnum.
opisthionasial (ō-pĭs"thē-ō-nā'zē-ăl). Concerning the opisthion and nasion of the skull.
opistho-, opisth- [Gr. *opisthen*]. Combining form meaning backward or indicating rel. to the back.
opisthognathism (ō"pĭs-thō'nă-thĭzm) [" + *gnathos,* jaw, + *ismos,* state of]. Skull abnormality marked by a receding lower jaw.
opisthoporeia (ō-pĭs"thō-pō-rē'ă) [" + *poreia,* walk]. Involuntary walking backward due to loss of motor control.
opisthorchiasis (ō"pĭs-thor-kī'ă-sĭs). Infestation of the liver by flukes of the genus Opisthorchis.
Opisthorchis (ō"pĭs-thor'kĭs) [Gr. *opisthen,* behind, + *orchis,* testicle]. A genus of parasitic flukes characterized by having testicles near the posterior end of the tapered body.
O. felineus. A species of liver flukes in dogs, cats, foxes. Occasionally infest man through raw or partially cooked fish.
O. sinensis. A common liver fluke in man, esp. in the Far East. It develops in those who eat inadequately cooked fish that are infected with the larval form.
opisthotic (ō"pĭs-thŏt'ĭk) [Gr. *opisthen,* behind, + *ous,* ear]. Located behind the ear or in the interior ear.
opisthotonoid (ō"pĭs-thŏt'ō-noyd) [" + *tonos,* tension, + *eidos,* form]. Resembling opisthotonos.
opisthotonos (ō"pĭs-thŏt'ō-nŏs) [" + *tonos,* tension]. Form of spasm in which head and heels are bent backward and body bowed forward. Caused by a tetanic spasm. Seen in strychnine poisoning, tetanus, hysteria, epilepsy, the convulsions of rabies, and in severe

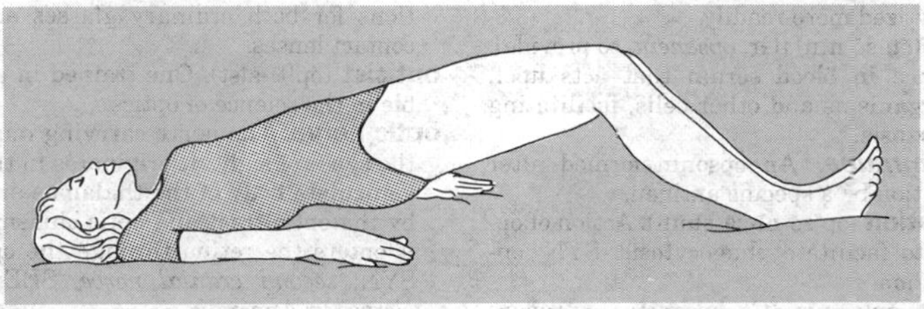

OPISTHOTONOS

cases of meningitis. In the latter case, the patient's neck is rigid and the head retracted, seeming to press into the pillow. SEE: illus.; *emprosthotonos; pleurothotonos.*

opium (ō'pē-ŭm) [L.]. 1. The substance obtained by air-drying of the juice from the unripe capsule of the poppy, Papaver somniferum. It contains a number of important alkaloids such as morphine, codeine, heroin, and papaverine. Opium is not permitted to be used in the United States. The growing and transportation of the poppy as well as the manufacture of drugs from the juice are controlled by national and international laws. 2. USP. A standardized preparation of the air-dried milky exudate from unripe capsules of the poppy, Papaver somniferum, or its variety album DeCandolle. It contains not less than 9.5% anhydrous morphine.

opium poisoning. SEE: *morphine* in *Poisons and Poisoning* in *Appendix*.

opiumism (ō'pē-ŭm-ĭzm). 1. Opium habit; addiction to use of opium. 2. Physical condition resulting from overuse of opium.

opo- [Gr. *opos,* juice]. Prefix meaning derived from juice; used in trade names of some organic extracts.

opocephalus (ō"pō-sĕf'ă-lŭs) [Gr. *ops,* face, + *kephale,* head]. A congenitally deformed fetus without nose or mouth, fused at the ears. There is either a single orbit or two very close together.

opodidymus (ō"pō-dĭd'ĭ-mŭs) [" + *didymos,* twin]. Congenitally deformed twins in which there is a single body, two fused heads, and partial fusion of the sense organs.

Oppenheim's disease (ŏp'ĕn-hīmz). [Hermann Oppenheim, Ger. neurologist, 1858–1919] A noninherited but sometimes familial disease, characterized by absence of muscular development with the lower extremities being the first involved. It is first seen at, or shortly after, birth. SYN: *amyotonia congenita; myatonia congenita.*

Oppenheim's gait. Gait wherein there is a wide swinging motion of the head, body, and extremities. This is a variation of the gait seen in multiple sclerosis.

oppilation (ŏp"ĭ-lā'shŭn) [L. *oppilatio,* an obstruction]. 1. An obstruction. 2. Act or state of being obstructed. 3. Constipation.

opponens (ō-pō'nĕns) [L.]. Opposing, a term applied to muscles of hand or foot by which one of the lateral digits may be opposed to one of the other digits. SEE: *Muscles* in *Appendix.*

opponens splint. A splint designed to maintain the thumb in a position to oppose the other fingers.

opportunistic infections. Infections with any organism, but esp. fungi and bacteria, that occur due to the opportunity afforded by the altered physiological state of the host. Thus when certain antibiotics or adrenal cortical steroids are given for long periods, certain microorganisms that would otherwise be nonpathogenic become pathogenic due to the suppression of the more prevalent microorganism.

opposition. The ability to move the thumb into contact with the other fingers.

opsialgia (ŏp"sē-ăl'jē-ă) [Gr. *ops,* face, + *algos,* pain]. Neuralgic pain of the face.

opsin (ŏp'sĭn). The protein portion of the rhodopsin molecule.

opsinogen (ŏp-sĭn'ō-jĕn). An antigen that causes the production of opsonins.

opsinogenous (ŏp"sĭn-ŏj'ĕn-ŭs). Capable of forming opsonins.

opsiometer (ŏp"sē-ŏm'ĕ-tĕr). Optometer, q.v.

opsiuria (ŏp-sē-ū'rē-ă) [Gr. *opse,* late, + *ouron,* urine]. Condition in which excretion of urine is more rapid during fasting than after a meal.

opsoclonus. Irregular and nonrhythmical jerking movements of the eyes. Seen in comatose patients with lesions of the brain stem.

opsogen (ŏp'sō-jĕn). An opsinogen, q.v.

opsomania (ŏp"sō-mā'nē-ă) [Gr. *opson,* food, + *mania,* madness]. Craving for some special article of food.

opsonic (ŏp-sŏn'ĭk) [Gr. *opsonein,* to prepare food for]. Pert. to opsonins or their use in therapy.

opsonification (ŏp-sŏn"ĭ-fĭ-kā'shŭn). Effect of

opsonins in rendering cells or bacteria phagocytized more readily.

opsonin (ŏp-sō'nĭn) [Gr. *opsonein,* to provide]. Substance in blood serum that acts upon microorganisms and other cells, facilitating phagocytosis.

o., immune. An opsonin formed after stimulation by a specific antigen.

opsonization (ŏp"sō-nī-zā'shŭn). Action of opsonins to facilitate phagocytosis. SYN: *opsonification.*

opsonize (ŏp'sō-nīz) [Gr. *opsonein,* to prepare food for]. To facilitate phagocytosis.

opsonocytophagic (ŏp"sŏn-ō-sī"tō-fā'jĭk) [" + *kytos,* cell, + *phagein,* to eat]. Pert. to phagocytic action of blood when serum opsonins are present.

opsonometry (ŏp-sō-nŏm'ĕt-rē) [" + *metron,* measure]. Estimation of amount of opsonins in the blood serum. SEE: *opsonic index.*

opsonophilia (ŏp"sō-nō-fĭl'ē-ă) [" + *philein,* to love]. Attraction for opsonins.

opsonophilic. Having attraction to opsonins.

opsonotherapy (ŏp"sō-nō-thĕr'ă-pē). Treatment by stimulation of a specific opsonin with bacterial vaccines. SEE: *vaccine.*

Optacon. Acronym for *Op*tical to *Ta*ctile *Con*verter, a proprietary name of a portable electronic reading assistance device for use by the blind. It translates printed material to patterns of raised pins under the user's fingers. Manufactured by Telesensory Systems Inc., Palo Alto, CA, (415) 413-2626.

optesthesia (ŏp"tĕs-thē'zē-ă) [Gr. *optikos,* optical, + *aisthesis,* sensation]. Visual sensibility; perception of visual stimuli.

optic (ŏp'tĭk) [Gr. *optikos*]. Pert. to the eye or the sight.

optical (ŏp'tĭ-kăl) [L. *opticus;* Gr. *optikos*]. Pert. to vision, the eye, or optics.

optical activity. In chemistry, the property of rotating the plane of polarized light. Measurement of this property is called polarimetry, and is useful in the determination of optically active substances such as dextrose. Sugars are classified according to this criterion. Optical activity of a substance in solution can be detected by placing it between polarizing and analyzing prisms.

optic chiasm. An x-shaped crossing of the optic nerve fibers in the brain. Past this point, the fibers travel in optic tracts. Fibers that originated in the outer half of the retina end up on the same side of the brain; those from the inner half cross over.

optic disk. Area in retina for entrance of optic nerve; the blind spot, q.v. SYN: *optic papilla.*

optic foramen. Groove for optic nerve and ophthalmic artery at the orbit's apex.

optician (ŏp-tĭsh'ăn). One who is a specialist in the making of optical apparatus.

opticianry (ŏp-tĭsh'ăn-rē). The science and art of optics applied to filling optical prescriptions for both ordinary glasses as well as contact lenses.

opticist (ŏp'tĭ-sĭst). One trained in and capable in the science of optics.

optic nerve. The nerve carrying impulses for the sense of sight. It originates in the lateral geniculate body of the thalamus and travels by the optic tract and optic chiasma, where it enters the retina through the optic disk. SYN: *second cranial nerve.* SEE: *Cranial Nerves* in *Appendix.*

optico- [Gr. *optikos*]. Combining form indicating rel. to the eye or vision.

opticociliary (ŏp"tĭ-kō-sĭl'ē-ăr-ē). Concerning the optic and ciliary nerves.

opticokinetic (ŏp"tĭ-kō-kī-nĕt'ĭk) [" + *kinesis,* movement]. Concerning the movement of the eye.

opticonasion (ŏp"tĭ-kō-nā'sē-ŏn). Length of an imaginary line drawn from the posterior edge of the optic foramen to the nasion.

opticopupillary (ŏp"tĭ-kō-pū'pĭl-ĕr"ē). Concerning the optic nerve and the pupil.

optic papilla. Optic disk.

optics (ŏp'tĭks) [Gr. *optikos,* pert. to vision]. The science dealing with light and its relationship to vision.

optic tract. Fibers of the optic nerve that continue beyond the optic chiasma, most of which terminate in the lateral geniculate body of the thalamus. Some continue to the superior colliculus of the midbrain, others enter the hypothalamus and terminate in the supraoptic and medial nuclei.

Optimine. Trade name for azatadine maleate, USP.

optimum (ŏp'tĭ-mŭm) [L. *optimus,* best]. (pl. *optima*) The condition that is most conducive to a function or functions such as growth and development.

optimum temperature. That temperature that is most suitable for a procedure or operation, esp. the development of bacterial cultures.

opto- [Gr. *optos,* seen]. Combining form meaning vision or eye.

optogram (ŏp'tō-grăm) [Gr. *optos,* seen, + *gramma,* mark]. Image of external object fixed on the retina by photochemical bleaching action of light on the visual purple.

optokinetic (ŏp"tō-kī-nĕt'ĭk) [" + *kinesis,* movement]. Concerning the appearance of twitching of the eye, as in nystagmus when the eyes gaze at moving objects.

optomeninx (ŏp"tō-mē'nĭngks) [" + *meninx,* membrane]. The retina of the eye.

optometer (ŏp-tŏm'ĕt-ĕr) [" + *metron,* measure]. Instrument for measurement of the eye's refractive power. SYN: *opsiometer.*

optometrist (ŏp-tŏm'ĕ-trĭst). A person specifically trained and licensed to examine the eyes in order to test visual acuity and to prescribe and adapt lenses to preserve or restore maximum efficiency of vision. The optometrist's professional degree is Doctor of Optometry (O.D.).

optometry (ŏp-tŏm'ĕt-rē). Measurement of the visual refractive power; correction of visual defects with eyeglasses or optical aids excluding drugs.

optomyometer (ŏp"tō-mī-ŏm'ĕt-ĕr) [" + *mys,* muscle, + *metron,* a measure]. Instrument for determining strength of the muscles of the eye.

optophone (ŏp'tō-fōn) [" + *phone,* voice]. Instrument converting light energy into sound waves. Used by the blind.

optostriate (ŏp-tō-strī'āt) [" + L. *striatus,* grooved]. Concerning the optic thalamus and the corpus striatum.

optotype (ŏp'tō-tīp). The test type used in determining visual acuity.

OR. *operating room.*

ora (ō'ră) [L.]. 1. Pl. of os. 2. (pl. *orae*) A border or margin.

o. serrata retinae. [NA] Notched anterior edge of sensory portion of retina.

orad (ō'răd) [L. *oris,* mouth, + *ad,* toward]. Toward the mouth or oral region.

oral (or'ăl) [L. *oralis*]. Concerning the mouth.

oral contraceptive. SEE: *contraceptive.*

oral diagnosis. The procedure or special area of dentistry devoted to the compilation and study of the patient's dental history, and a detailed clinical examination of the oral tissues and radiographs to assess the level of oral health, with the object of developing a treatment plan to restore tooth structure and proper occlusion, and to promote healing and better oral health.

orale (ō-rā'lē). Point on hard palate in the midsagittal plane where lines drawn tangent to the lingual margins of the alveoli of the medial incisor teeth intersect.

orality (ō-răl'ĭ-tē). The oral stage of psychosexual development such as sucking, or chewing on objects other than food.

oralogy (ō-răl'ō-jē) [" + Gr. *logos,* study of]. 1. The science of dental hygiene. 2. Study of diseases of the mouth. SYN: *stomatology.*

orange, methyl. A chemical used as an indicator in acid-base titrations.

Orasone. Trade name for prednisone, USP.

Oratestryl. Trade name for fluoxymesterone, USP.

Oratrol. Trade name for dichlorphenamide, USP.

orb [L. *orbis,* circle, disk]. A spherical body, esp. the eyeball.

orbicular (or-bĭk'ū-lăr) [L. *orbiculus,* a small circle]. Circular.

orbicular bone. The ossicle in the middle ear that frequently becomes attached to the incus. SYN: *orbiculare.*

orbicular muscle. Muscle encircling an opening.

orbicular process. End of long process of the incus. SYN: *process, lenticular.*

orbiculare (or-bĭk"ū-lā'rē). The middle ear ossicle that frequently becomes attached to the incus at the end of its long process. SYN: *orbicular bone.*

orbiculus (or-bĭk'ū-lŭs) [L., little circle]. (pl. *orbiculi*) Muscle surrounding an orifice; a sphincter muscle.

o. ciliaris. The ciliary muscles of the eye. SYN: *ring, ciliary.*

o. oculi. Measure encircling the opening of orbit of the eye.

o. oris. Circular muscle surrounding the mouth.

orbit (or'bĭt) [L. *orbita,* track]. The bony pyramid-shaped cavity of the skull that contains and protects the eyeball. It is pierced posteriorly by the optic foramen, which transmits the optic nerve and ophthalmic artery, the superior and inferior orbital fissures, and several foramina. It is formed by the frontal, malar, ethmoid, maxillary, lacrimal, sphenoid, and palatine bones.

orbita (or'bĭ-tă) [L.]. (pl. *orbitae*) [NA] Orbit.

orbital (or'bĭ-tăl) [L. *orbitalis*]. Concerning the orbit.

orbitomeatal line. Imaginary line through the mid-orbit and external auditory meatus.

orbitonasal (or"bĭ-tō-nā'zăl). Concerning the orbit and the nasal cavity of the skull.

orbitonometer (or"bĭ-tō-nŏm'ĕ-tĕr). Device for measuring the resistance of the eye to being pushed back into the orbit.

orbitonometry (or"bĭ-tō-nŏm'ĕ-trē). Determining the displacement of the eye into the orbit when pressure is placed on the eye.

orbitopagus (or"bĭ-tŏp'ă-gŭs) [L. *orbita,* track, + Gr. *pagos,* thing fixed]. A congenitally deformed fetus in which the small fetus is attached to the orbit of the more nearly normal twin.

orbitotomy (or-bĭ-tŏt'ō-mē) [' + Gr. *tome,* incision]. Surgical incision into the orbit.

orcein (or-sī'ĭn). A chemical used as a histological stain.

orchectomy (or-kĕk'tō-mē) [Gr. *orchis,* testicle, + *ektome,* excision]. Surgical removal of a testicle. SYN: *orchidectomy; orchiectomy.*

orcheoplasty (or'kē-ō-plăs"tē) [" + *plassein,* to form]. Plastic repair work of the testicle.

orchialgia (or-kē-ăl'jē-ă) [" + *algos,* pain]. Pain in the testes. SYN: *orchidalgia; orchiodynia; orchioneuralgia.*

orchi(o)-. A combining form indicating relationship to the testicles.

orchichorea (or"kĭ-kō-rē'ă) [" + *choreia,* a dance]. Involuntary jerking movements of the testicles.

orchidalgia (or-kĭ-dăl′jē-ă) [″ + *algos*, pain]. Neuralgia in the testicles. SYN: *orchialgia; orchioneuralgia.*

orchidectomy (or″kĭ-dĕk′tō-mē) [″ + *ektome*, excision]. Surgical removal of a testicle. SYN: *orchectomy; orchiectomy.*

orchidic (or-kĭd′ĭk). Concerning or rel. to the testes.

orchiditis (or″kĭ-dī′tĭs) [″ + *itis*, inflammation]. Orchitis, q.v.

orchido- [Gr. *orchidion*]. Combining form indicating relationship to the testicle. SEE: words beginning with *orchio-*.

orchidoncus (or-kĭ-dŏng′kŭs) [″ + *onkos*, mass]. A neoplasm of the testicle. SYN: *orchioncus.*

orchidopexy (or′kĭd-ō-pĕk″sē) [″ + *pexis*, fixation]. Surgical transfer of an imperfectly descended testicle into the scrotum and suturing it there. SYN: *orchiopexy; orchiorrhaphy.*

orchidoplasty (or′kĭd-ō-plăs″tē) [″ + *plassein*, to form]. Operative transfer of an undescended testicle to the scrotum.

orchidoptosis (or″kĭd-ŏp-tō′sĭs) [″ + *ptosis*, a falling]. Downward displacement of the testes.

orchidorrhaphy (or″kĭ-dor′ă-fē) [″ + *rhaphe*, suture]. Orchiopexy, q.v.

orchidotomy (or-kĭd-ŏt′ō-mē) [″ + *tome*, incision]. Incision into the testes.

orchiectomy (or″kē-ĕk′tō-mē) [″ + *ektome*, excision]. Surgical excision of a testicle. SYN: *orchectomy; orchidectomy.* SEE: *castration.*

orchiepididymitis (or″kē-ĕp″ĭ-dĭd″ĭ-mī′tĭs) [″ + *epi*, upon, + *didymos*, testis, + *itis*, inflammation]. Inflamed condition of a testicle and epididymis.

orchilytic (or″kĭ-lĭt′ĭk) [″ + *lysis*, dissolution]. Destructive to testicular tissue.

orchiocele (or′kē-ō-sēl) [″ + *kele*, hernia]. 1. Scrotal hernia. SYN: *orchidocele.* 2. A tumor of the testicle.

orchiodynia (or″kē-ō-dĭn′ē-ă) [″ + *odyne*, pain]. Testicular pain. SYN: *orchialgia; orchidalgia; orchioneuralgia.*

orchioncus (or″kē-ŏng′kŭs) [″ + *onkos*, tumor]. Neoplasm of the testicle. SYN: *orchidoncus.*

orchioneuralgia (or″kē-ō-nū-răl′jē-ă) [″ + *neuron*, sinew, + *algos*, pain]. Neuralgia of the testicles. SYN: *orchialgia; orchidalgia.*

orchiopathy (or″kē-ŏp′ăth-ē) [″ + *pathos*, disease]. Any diseased condition of the testes.

orchiopexy (or″kē-ō-pĕk′sē) [″ + *pexis*, fixation]. The suturing of an undescended testicle in the scrotum. SYN: *orchidopexy; orchiorrhaphy.*

orchioplasty (or′kē-ō-plăs″tē) [″ + *plassein*, to form]. Plastic repair of the testicle.

orchiorrhaphy (or″kē-or′ră-fē) [″ + *rhaphe*, suture]. The suturing of an undescended testicle to surrounding tissue in the scrotum. SYN: *orchidopexy; orchiopexy.*

orchioscheocele (or″kē-ŏs′kē-ō-sēl) [″ + *oscheon*, scrotum, + *kele*, hernia]. Scrotal hernia with enlargement or tumor of testicle.

orchioscirrhus (or″kē-ō-skĭr′rŭs) [″ + *skirros*, hard]. Testicular hardening due to tumor formation.

orchiotomy (or″kē-ŏt′ō-mē) [″ + *tome*, incision]. Surgical incision of a testicle.

orchis (or′kĭs) [Gr.]. A testicle.

orchitic (or-kĭt′ĭk). Concerning or caused by orchitis.

orchitis (or-kī′tĭs) [″ + *itis*, inflammation]. Inflammation of a testis due to trauma, metastasis, mumps, or infection elsewhere in the body.

SYM: Swelling, severe pain, possibly gangrene, chills, fever, vomiting, hiccough, delirium. May end in atrophy of organ.

TREATMENT: Confine patient to bed first eight days, immobilize organ, and use ice bag.

o., gonorrheal. Orchitis due to gonococcus.

o., metastatic. Orchitis due to infection from organisms in blood stream.

o., syphilitic. Orchitis due to syphilis.

SYM: Usually begins painlessly in body of gland but apt to be bilateral. Causes dense, irregular, knotty induration but little enlargement in size.

o., tuberculous. Form of orchitis generally arising in the epididymis. It may be accompanied by formation of chronic sinuses, and destruction of tissues.

SYM: Little or no pain. Begins as hard, irregular enlargement at lower and posterior aspect of gland, gradually increases, and sometimes extends along vas deferens. Later whole gland undergoes caseous degeneration.

orchitolytic (or″kĭt-ō-lĭt′ĭk) [″ + *lysis*, destruction]. Destructive to testicular tissue.

orchotomy (or-kŏt′ō-mē) [″ + *tome*, incision]. Incision, but not excision, of a testicle.

orcin, orcinol (or′sĭn, -ŏl). A white, crystalline substance derived from lichens and used as a reagent.

order [L. *ordo*, a row, series]. 1. An arrangement or sequence of events; rules; regulations; procedures. 2. In biological classification, the main division under class and superior to family.

orderly (or′dĕr-lē). An attendant in a hospital who does general work to assist nurses. Responsible for lifting patients, transporting patients, and preparing patients for surgery (shaving, catheterizing, or administering enemas).

ordinate (or′dĭ-năt). In a graph wherein horizontal and perpendicular lines are crossed in order to provide a frame of reference, the ordinate is the horizontal line or x-axis. The abscissa, q.v., is the vertical line or y-axis. SEE: *abscissa* for illus.

ordure (or′dūr). Feces or other excrement.

Oretic. Trade name for hydrochlorothiazide, USP.

Oreton. Trade name for testosterone, USP.

Oreton-Methyl. Trade name for methyltestosterone, USP.

Oreton Propionate. Trade name for testosterone propionate, USP.

orexia (ō-rĕk′sē-ă) [Gr. *orexis*]. Appetite.

orexigenic (ō-rĕk″sĭ-jĕn′ĭk) [Gr. *orexis*, appetite, + *gennan*, to produce]. Stimulating the appetite.

oreximania (ō-rĕk″sĭ-mā′nē-ă) [″ + *mania*, madness]. Abnormal desire for food because of fear of becoming thin.

orf. A contagious pustular dermatitis mainly affecting lambs and occurring in the spring. The disease rarely occurs in humans. When it does, it usually is confined to a single pustular lesion on a finger, which encrusts and finally heals.

ETIOL: Orf virus, which is related to the vaccinia-variola subgroup of poxviruses.

organ (or′găn) [Gr. *organon;* L. *organum*]. A part of the body having a special function. Many organs are in pairs. In such pairs, one organ may be extirpated and the remaining one can perform all necessary functions peculiar to it. From one third to two fifths of some organs may be removed without loss of function necessary to support life. SEE: Size, Weight, and Capacity of Various Organs and Parts of the Body table.

o., accessory. An organ that has a subordinate function.

o., acoustic. Organ of Corti.

o., enamel. A knoblike thickening that develops on dental lamina, giving rise to a double-walled cup-shaped organ that encloses the dental papilla. It functions in the shaping of the tooth and the formation of enamel.

o., end. The specialized termination of a sensory nerve fiber that serves as a receptor. May be nonencapsulated or encapsulated.

o., excretory. An organ that is concerned with the excretion of waste products from the body. SEE: *excretion.*

o., Golgi's. A spindle-shaped structure at junction of a muscle and tendon. Functions as a receptor for proprioceptive sense. SYN: *Golgi's corpuscle.*

o., gustatory. The organ that controls the sense of taste; a taste bud. SYN: *organum gustus* [NA].

o. of Corti. Terminal acoustic apparatus in the cochlea. SYN: *organum spirale.* SEE: *Claudius' cells; ear.*

o. of Giraldès. A small body on the spermatic cord above the epididymis. SYN: *paradidymis.*

o. of Jacobson. A blind tubular sac that develops in the medial wall of the nasal cavity. Becomes a functional olfactory organ in lower animals but degenerates or remains rudimentary in man. SYN: *o., vomeronasal.*

o. of Ruffini. Sensory receptor of warmth located principally at tips of fingers. SYN: *Ruffini's corpuscles.*

o.'s of Zuckerkandl. A pair of organs containing chromaffin tissue present in the embryo and persisting until shortly after birth. Located adjacent to the anterior surface of the abdominal aorta. The cells secrete epinephrine. SYN: *corpora paraaortica.*

o., reproductive. Any organ concerned with the production of offspring. Includes the primary organs (testes and ovaries) and accessory structures (penis and spermatic cord in the male and fallopian tubes, uterus, and vagina in the female). SYN: *o., sex.*

o., sense. A sensory receptor; a structure consisting of specialized sensory nerve endings that are capable of reacting to a stimulus (an environmental change) by giving rise to nerve impulses that pass through afferent nerves to the central nervous system. These impulses may give rise to sensations or reflexly bring about responses in the body.

o., sex. O., reproductive

o.'s, special sense. The organs of smell, taste, sight, and hearing.

o., spiral. The spiral organ of the inner ear, which contains the special sensory apparatus for hearing.

o., target. The organ upon which a chemical or hormone acts.

o., vestigial. An organ that is immature or underdeveloped in humans but is fully functional in some animals.

o., vomeronasal. O. of Jacobson.

o., Weber's. Residual prostatic pouch in the male, the remains of the müllerian ducts.

organelle (or″găn-ĕl′). A specialized part of a cell that performs a definite function. Ex.: mitochondria; Golgi apparatus; endoplasmic reticulum; lysosomes; and cell centriole. SEE: illus.

organic (or-găn′ĭk) [Gr. *organikos*]. 1. Pert. to an organ or organs. 2. Structural. 3. Pert. to or derived from animal or vegetable forms of life. 4. Denoting chemical substances containing carbon.

organic acid. Any acid containing one or more —COOH or carboxyl groups. Acetic, formic, lactic, and all fatty acids are organic.

organic brain syndromes. A large group of acute and chronic mental disorders associated with brain damage or impaired cerebral function.

SYM: The clinical characteristics vary not

Size, Weight, and Capacity of Various Organs and Parts of the Body ♂ male ♀ female*

Description	Size	Weight	Capacity
Adrenal gland	3 to 5 cm. long, 4 to 6 cm. thick	3.5–5.0 gm.	
Bladder	12 cm. in diameter		500 ml. (when moderately full)
Blood volume			♂ 4200 ml. ♀ 5000 ml.
Brain		♂ 1430 gm. ♀ 1294 gm.	
Esophagus	23 to 25 cm.		
Fallopian tube	10 cm.		
Gallbladder	7 to 10 cm. long 2.5 cm. wide		30 to 35 ml.
Heart	12 × 8 to 9 × 6.0 cm.	♂ 280–340 gm. ♀ 230–280 gm.	
Intestines—small	Quite variable 472 to 970 cm. long		
Intestines—large	150 cm. long		
Intestines—vermiform appendix	2 to 20 cm. long Average 8.3 cm.		
Intestines—rectum	12 cm. long		
Kidney	11.25 cm. long, 5 to 7.5 cm. broad, 2.5 cm. thick	♂ 125–170 gm. ♀ 115–155 gm.	
Liver		♂ 1400–1600 gm. ♀ 1200–1400 gm.	6500 cc.
Lung		Rt. 625 gm. Lt. 567 gm.	
Ovaries	4 × 2 × 0.8 cm.	2–3.5 gm.	

*Adapted from *Gray's Anatomy,* ed. 27. Lea & Febiger, Philadelphia, 1959; Growth, Federation of American Societies for Experimental Biology, Washington, D.C., 1962.

Size, Weight, and Capacity of Various Organs and Parts of the Body ♂ male ♀ female* (*Continued*)

Description	Size	Weight	Capacity
Pancreas	12.5 to 15 cm. long	♂ 74–106 gm. ♀ 70–100 gm.	
Pharynx	12.5 cm. long		
Prostate	2 × 4 × 3 cm.	20 gm.	
Skeleton		Average adult male, 4957 gm.	
Skull		Average (without teeth), 642 gm.	
Spinal cord	42 to 45 cm. long	30 gm.	
Spleen	12 × 7 × 3 to 4 cm.	100–250 gm. Decreases with age	
Stomach	Quite variable 25 cm. long, 10 cm. wide		Quite variable 1000 ml.
Testes	4 to 5 × 2.5 × 3.0 cm.	10.5–14 gm.	
Thoracic duct	38 to 45 cm. long		
Thymus		Newborn, 10.9 gm. 10–15 yrs., 29.5 gm. 20–25 yrs., 18.6 gm.	
Thyroid	Each lobe 5 × 3 × 2 cm.	30 gm. total	
Trachea	11 cm. long, 2 to 2.5 cm. in diameter		
Ureter	28 to 34 cm. long		
Urethra	♂ 17.5 to 20 cm. long ♀ 4 cm. long		
Uterus	7.5 × 5.0 × 2.5 cm.	30–40 gm. (nonpregnant)	

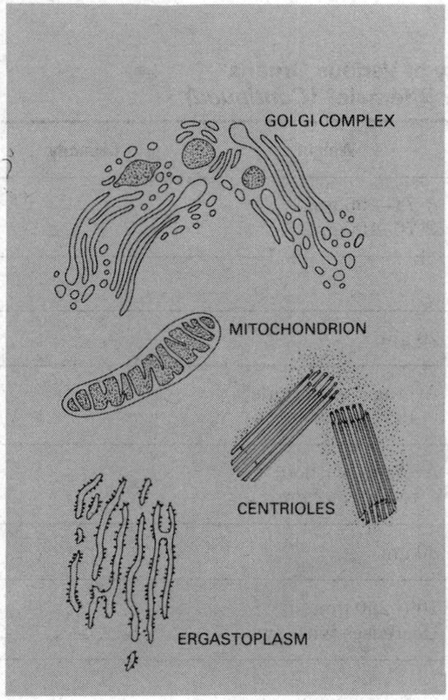

ORGANELLE

only with the nature and severity of the underlying organic disorder but also from time to time in each individual. The following functions may be impaired: consciousness, orientation, memory, intellect, judgment and insight, and thought content such as hallucinations, illusions, and mood.

ETIOL: Any acute or chronic disease or injury that interferes with cerebral function such as infection, intoxication, trauma, circulatory disturbance, epilepsy, metabolic and endocrine diseases, or intracranial neoplasms.

DIAG: May be difficult because of the possibility of attributing all of the signs and symptoms to a psychiatric disorder and ignoring the organic disease or vice versa.

TREATMENT: Treat basic organic disease and provide psychiatric care.

organic chemistry. Branch of chemistry dealing with substances containing carbon compounds.

organic disease. A disease associated with observable or detectable changes in the organs or tissues of the body.

organicism (or-găn'ĭ-sĭzm). The theory that all diseases are due to organic disease.

organicist (or-găn'ĭ-sĭst). One who believes in organicism.

organic psychoses. A general term applied to those psychoses induced by structural brain changes. In general, a character change is manifested in behavior and disposition. The patient is less stable than before. Emotional instability, irritability, and angry outbursts become frequent. Attention fluctuates widely; gradually the patient deteriorates. At any time in the course of the disease, memory, comprehension, ideation, and orientation may become defective.

ETIOL: Alcohol, narcotics, trauma, syphilis, drugs, poisons, chronic infections, encephalitis, and brain tumors among many others.

Organidin. Trade name for glycerol, iodinated.

organism (or'găn-ĭzm) [Gr. *organon,* organ, + *-ismos,* condition]. Any living thing, plant, or animal. May be unicellular (bacteria, yeasts, protozoa) or multicellular (all complex organisms including man).

organization (or"găn-ĭ-zā'shŭn). 1. Process of becoming organized. 2. Systematic arrangement. 3. That which is organized; an organism.

organization center. 1. An embryonic group of cells, which induces the development of another structure. 2. A region in an ovum that is responsible for the mode of development of the fertilized ovum.

organize (or'găn-īz). To develop from an amorphous state to that having structure and form.

organo- (or'gă-nō). A combining form indicating a relationship to an organ.

organoferric (or"gă-nō-fĕr'ĭk). Concerning iron and an organic molecule.

organogel (or-găn'ō-jĕl). A gel in which the continuous phase is an organic liquid instead of water.

organogenesis (or"găn-ō-jĕn'ĕ-sĭs) [" + *genesis,* production]. The formation and development of body organs from embryonic tissues.

It is important that the fetus not be exposed to harmful chemicals. This is particularly important during organogenesis. The first critical period for the effects of teratogenic drugs on the human fetus is between the 13th and 56th day of gestation. The second period of high risk is during the last trimester when metabolic enzyme systems are beginning to be defined. The third period is during labor when the physiologic changes required for transition of the fetus to life outside the womb are taking place.

SYN: *organogeny.*

organogeny (or"gă-nŏj'ĕ-nē). Organogenesis, q.v.

organography (or-găn-ŏg'ră-fē) [" + *graphein,* to write]. 1. The description of the body organs. 2. Roentgenographic visualization of the organs of the body.

organoid [" + *eidos,* form]. 1. Resembling an

organ. 2. An organelle.

organoleptic (or″găn-ō-lĕp′tĭk) [″ + *lepsis,* a seizure]. 1. Affecting an organ, esp. the organs of special sense. 2. Susceptible to sensory impressions.

organology (or-gă-nŏl′ō-jē) [″ + *logos,* study]. The science dealing with the body organs.

organoma (or-gă-nō′mă) [″ + *oma,* tumor]. A neoplasm that contains cellular elements that can be definitely identified as being specific or certain tissues and organs.

organomegaly (or″gă-nō-mĕg′ă-lē) [″ + *megas,* large]. Enlargement of visceral organs.

organomercurial (or″gă-nō-mĕr-kū′rē-ăl). Any organic mercurial compound.

organometallic (or-gă-nō-mĕ-tăl′ĭk). A compound containing a metal combined with an organic molecule.

organon (or′gă-nŏn) [Gr.]. (pl. *organa)* Organum, q.v.

organonomy (or″gă-nŏn′ō-mē) [″ + *nomos,* law]. The laws regulating the biological processes of living organisms.

organopathy (or″gă-nŏp′ă-thē) [″ + *pathos,* disease]. Any disease affecting an organ of the body.

organopexy (or′găn-ō-pĕk″sē) [″ + *pexis,* fixation]. Surgical fixation of an organ that is detached from its proper position.

organophilic (or″gă-nō-fĭl′ĭk) [″ + *philos,* to love]. The attraction of organic molecules for particular organs.

organoscopy (or-gă-nŏs′kō-pē) [″ + *skopein,* to examine]. Examination of abdominal organs of the body by means of an endoscope.

organotherapy (or″găn-ō-thĕr′ă-pē) [″ + *therapeia,* treatment]. The treatment of disease by preparations of the endocrine glands of animals or by extracts made from the same.

organotrope, organotropic (or-găn′ō-trōp, -găn-ō-trŏp′ĭk) [″ + *tropos,* turning]. Having affinity for tissues or certain organs.

organotrophic (or″gă-nō-trŏf′ĭk) [″ + *trophe,* nutrition]. Concerning the nutrition of organs.

organotropism (or″gă-nŏt′rō-pĭzm) [″ + *trope,* a turn, + *-ismos,* condition]. Organophilic, q.v.

organ perfusion system. A mechanical device equipped to supply metabolic, oxygen, and electrolyte needs in order to keep viable for transplantation an organ obtained from a cadaver or donor. The organ and the perfusion solution pumped through it can be kept at the ideal temperature for organ survival. Together they can be transported by any means required to deliver the organ to the patient.

organ-specific (or′găn-spĕ-sĭf′ĭk). Originating in a single organ or affecting only one specific organ.

organum [L.]. (pl. *organa)* [NA] An organ.

o. auditus. O. vestibulocochleare.

o. gustus. [NA] Organ of taste.

o. olfactus. [NA] Organ of smell; olfactory region in the nasal cavity.

o. spirale. [NA] Spiral organ in the cochlea. SYN: *organ of Corti.*

o. vestibulocochleare. [NA] Organ of hearing. SYN: *organum auditus.* SEE: *ear.*

o. visus. [NA] The organ of sight; the eye and its adnexa.

o. vomeronasale. [NA] Canal opening into the nasal septum. SYN: *organ of Jacobson.*

orgasm (or′găzm) [Gr. *orgasmos,* swelling]. A state of physical and emotional excitement, esp. that which occurs at the climax of sexual intercourse. In the male it is accompanied by the ejaculation of semen. SYN: *climax.*

Oriental sore. An ulcerating, chronic, nodular skin lesion prevalent in the Orient and tropics and due to infection with Leishmania tropica. SYN: *Aleppo boil; leishmaniasis, cutaneous.*

orientation (or″ē-ĕn-tā′shŭn) [L. *oriens,* to arise]. Ability to comprehend and to adjust one's self in an environment with regard to time, location, and identity of persons. Partially or completely absent in some psychoses.

orifice (or′ĭ-fĭs) [L. *orificium*]. Mouth, entrance, or outlet to any aperture.

o., anal. The anus.

o., atrioventricular. The opening between the atrium and the ventricle on each side of the heart.

o., cardiac. Opening of esophagus into the stomach.

o., mitral. Opening between the atrium and ventricle.

o., pyloric. Opening from the stomach into the duodenum. SEE: *pylorus.*

o., ureteric. Opening of ureter into the bladder.

o., urethral, external. Exterior opening of the urethra. In male, located at tip of glans penis; in female, located anterior and cephalad to vaginal opening.

o., urethral, internal. Opening from which urethra makes its exit from bladder.

orificial (or″ĭ-fĭ′shăl) [L. *orificium,* outlet]. Pert. to or forming an orifice.

orificium (or″ĭ-fĭsh′ē-ŭm) [L.] An opening or orifice.

origin (or′ĭ-jĭn) [L. *origo,* beginning]. 1. The source of anything; a starting point. 2. The beginning of a nerve. 3. The more fixed attachment of a muscle.

o., deep. The region within the brain where the fibers that comprise a cranial nerve terminate.

o., superficial. Point where a cranial

nerve exits from the brain.

Orimune. Trade name for poliovirus vaccine, live oral, USP.

Orinase. Trade name for tolbutamide sodium, USP.

Ormond's disease. Retroperitoneal fibrosis causing ureteral obstruction.

ornithine (or'nĭ-thĭn). An amino acid formed when arginase hydrolyzes arginine. It is not present in proteins.

Ornithodoros (or"nĭ-thŏd'ō-rōs). A genus of ticks belonging to the family Argasidae, which infest mammals including man. Several species serve as transmitters of the causative agents of disease, including spotted fever, tick fever, Q fever, tularemia, Russian encephalitis, and relapsing fever.

ornithosis (or"nĭ-thō'sĭs) [Gr. *ornithos,* bird, + *osis,* condition]. An acute generalized infectious disease of birds and domesticated fowls, communicated to man. SYN: *parrot fever; psittacosis.*

SYM: Headache, chills and fever, anorexia, myalgia, sore throat, nausea, and vomiting.

ETIOL: Chlamydia psittaci.

TREATMENT: Tetracyclines continued for 10–14 days after temperature returns to normal.

oro-. Combining form denoting the mouth.

orodiagnosis (or"ō-dī-ăg-nō'sĭs) [Gr. *oros,* serum, + *dia,* through, + *gnosis,* knowledge]. Diagnosis by using serums or serum reactions.

orofaciodigital syndrome. The condition of mental retardation and deformities of the mouth, tongue, fingers, and sometimes the face.

orolingual (or"ō-lĭng'gwăl) [L. *oris,* mouth, + *lingua,* tongue]. Concerning the mouth and tongue.

oromeningitis (or"ō-mĕn"ĭn-jī'tĭs) [" + Gr. *meninx,* membrane, + *itis,* inflammation]. Orrhomeningitis, q.v.

oronasal (or"ō-nā'zăl) [" + *nasus,* nose]. Concerning the mouth and nose.

oropharynx (or"ō-făr'ĭnks) [" + Gr. *pharynx,* pharynx]. Central portion of the pharynx lying between the soft palate and upper portion of the epiglottis.

orosomucoid (or"ŏ-sō-mū'koyd). An alpha 1-globulin in plasma.

orotherapy (or"ō-thĕr'ă-pē) [" + Gr. *therapeia,* treatment]. Treatment of disease with injection of blood serum from immune persons or animals. SYN: *serotherapy.*

orotic acid. Uracil-6-carboxylic acid. It is a precursor in the formation of pyrimidine nucleotides.

orotic aciduria. An inherited disorder of pyrimidine metabolism wherein orotic acid accumulates in the body. Clinically, children fail to grow and have megaloblastic anemia and leukopenia. The disease responds to administration of uridine or cytidine.

Oroya fever [Oroya, a region of Peru]. An acute infectious disease endemic in Peru and other S.A. countries. The first clinical stage of bartonellosis. SYN: *bartonellosis; Carrion's disease.*

SYM: Intermittent fever; lymphadenopathy; severe anemia; and pains in joints and long bones.

TREATMENT: SEE: *bartonellosis.*

orphenadrine citrate (or-fĕn'ă-drēn). USP. An antiparkinsonism drug. Trade names are Banflex and Norflex.

orrhology (or-ŏl'ō-jē) [Gr. *orrhos,* blood serum, + *logos,* study]. The study of serums and their reactions. SYM: *serology.*

orrhomeningitis (or"ō-mĕn"ĭn-jī'tĭs) [" + *meninx,* membrane, + *itis,* inflammation]. Inflammation of a serous membrane.

orrhoreaction (or"ō-rē-ăk'shŭn) [" + *re,* back, + *actus,* acted]. A reaction from injection of serum. SYN: *seroreaction; serum sickness.*

orrhorrhea (or"ō-rē'ă) [" + *rhoia,* flow]. Any watery, thin, colorless discharge from a body structure. Usually it is the result of inflammation.

orrhotherapy (or"rō-thĕr'ă-pē) [" + *therapeia,* treatment]. Therapeutic use of serums. SYN: *serotherapy.*

orris root (or'ĭs). The powder made from the root of certain varieties of iris. It is used in making some types of cosmetics. It is a sensitizer either by contact or inhalation.

O.R.T. *operating room technician.*

orthergasia (or"thĕr-gā'zē-ă) [Gr. *orthos,* straight, + *ergon,* work]. The state of normal mental condition.

orthesis (or-thē'sĭs). Orthosis, q.v.

orthetics (or-thĕt'ĭks). Orthotics, q.v.

orthetist (or'thĕ-tĭst). Orthotist, q.v.

ortho- [Gr. *orthos,* straight]. Combining form meaning straight, correct, normal, in proper order.

orthoacid (or"thō-ăs'ĭd). An acid with as many hydroxyl groups as the number of valences of the acid-forming portion of the molecule.

orthobiosis (or"thō-bī-ō'sĭs) [" + *bios,* life]. Right living. A term used by Metchnikoff to encompass all the factors that may affect longevity and well-being.

orthocephalic (or"thō-sē-făl'ĭk) [" + *kephale,* head]. Having a well-proportioned head; a head with a height-length index between 70 and 75.

orthochorea (or"thō-kō-rē'ă) [" + *choreia,* dance]. A type of chorea in which attacks appear mainly when the person is in an erect position.

orthochromatic (or"thō-krō-măt'ĭk) [" + *chroma,* color]. Having normal color or staining normally.

orthochromophil (or″thō-krō′mō-fĭl) [″ + ″ + *philein,* to love]. Staining normally with neutral dyes.

orthocytosis (or″thō-sī-tō′sĭs) [″ + *kytos,* cell, + *osis,* condition]. Condition in which only mature cells are present in the blood.

orthodentin (or″thō-dĕn′tĭn). Tubular dentin as in human teeth.

orthodiagraph (or″thō-dī′ă-grăf) [″ + *dia,* through, + *graphein,* to write]. An instrument for accurate recording of the outlines and positions of organs or foreign bodies as seen by radiographic apparatus.

orthodigita (or″thō-dĭj′ĭ-tă) [″ + L. *digitus,* finger or toe]. The division of podiatry that deals with the correction of deviated toes; the prevention and correction of deformities of the fingers or toes.

orthodontia (or″thō-dŏn′shē-ă) [″ + *odous,* tooth]. Division of dentistry dealing with prevention and correction of abnormally positioned or aligned teeth. SYN: *orthodontics.*

orthodontics (or″thō-dŏn′tĭks). The branch of dentistry that deals with the prevention and correction of irregularities of the teeth. SYN: *orthodontia.*

orthodontist. A dentist who is an expert in orthodontia.

orthodromic (or″thō-drŏm′ĭk) [Gr. *orthodromein,* to run straight forward]. The transmission of nerve impulses in the normal direction.

orthogenesis (or″thō-jĕn′ĕ-sĭs) [Gr. *ortho,* straight, + *genesis,* development]. A biological principle that evolution of an animal species is in a given direction, governed by intrinsic factors, and independent of external factors.

orthogenic. Pert. to, or related to, the correction, treatment, or rehabilitation of children with mental or emotional difficulties.

orthogenics (or″thō-jĕn′ĭks). Eugenics, q.v.

orthognathous (or-thŏg′nă-thŭs) [″ + *gnathos,* jaw]. Having straight jaws with a gnathic index of 97.9 or less.

orthograde (or′thō-grād) [″ + L. *gradi,* to walk]. Walking with the body vertical or upright; pert. to bipeds, esp. man. Opposite of pronograde.

orthokinetic cuff. An elastic device fitted around a muscle and employing the principle that tactile stimulation over a muscle belly will facilitate contraction in the muscle or inhibit contraction in its antagonist.

orthokinetics. Various tactile stimulation techniques to stimulate the proprioceptors of muscles and tendons and thereby enhance motor performance in rehabilitation.

orthomelic (or″thō-mē′lĭk) [″ + *melos,* limb]. Correcting deformed arms and legs.

orthometer (or-thŏm′ĕ-tĕr) [″ + *metron,* measure]. Device for determining the degree of protrusion or retraction of the eyeballs.

orthomolecular (or″thō-mō-lĕk′ū-lăr). Indicating the normal chemical constituents of the body; or restoring those constituents to normal.

orthomyxoviruses (or″thō-mĭk″sō-vī′rŭs-ĕs). Influenza viruses.

Ortho-Novum. Trade name for estrogen combined with progestogen.

orthopedia (or″thō-pē′dē-ă [Gr. *orthos,* straight, + *pais,* child]. Orthopedics.

orthopedic (or″thō-pē′dĭk). Concerning orthopedics; prevention or correction of deformities.

orthopedics (or″thō-pē′dĭks) [″ + *pais,* child]. Branch of medical science that deals with prevention or correction of disorders involving locomotor structures of the body, esp. the skeleton, joints, muscles, fascia and other supporting structures such as ligaments and cartilage.

orthopedic surgery. Surgical prevention and correction of deformities.

orthopedist (or″thō-pē′dĭst). A specialist in orthopedics.

orthopercussion (or″thō-pĕr-kŭsh′ŭn) [″ + L. *percussio,* a striking through]. Percussion with the distal phalanx of the percussing finger held perpendicularly to the surface percussed.

orthophoria (or″thō-fō′rē-ă) [″ + *pherein,* to bear]. Parallelism of visual axes, the normal muscle balance.

orthophrenia (or″thō-frē′nē-ă) [″ + *phren,* mind]. The normal mental state in social relations.

orthopnea (or″thŏp-nē′ă) [″ + *pnoia,* breath]. Respiratory condition in which there is discomfort in breathing in any but erect sitting or standing position.

ETIOL: Seen in heart failure, bronchial and cardiac asthma, pulmonary edema, severe emphysema, pneumonia, angina pectoris, spasmodic cough.

SYM: Respiratory rate, slow or rapid; sitting or standing posture necessary; muscles of respiration forcibly used; patients feel necessity of bracing themselves in order to breathe. Anxious expression, face cyanosed. Struggle to inhale and exhale.

RS: dyspnea; hyperpnea; oligopnea; posture; respiration.

orthopneic position (or″thŏp-nē′ĭk). The upright or nearly upright position of the upper trunk of the patient in bed or a chair. This facilitates breathing in those with congestive heart failure and some forms of pulmonary disease.

orthopraxis (or″thō-prăk′sĭs) [″ + *prassein,* to make]. Mechanical or surgical correction of deformities.

orthopsychiatry (or″thō-sī-kī′ă-trē) [″ + *psy-*

che, soul, + *iatreia,* treatment]. Branch of psychiatry dealing with mental and emotional development; it encompasses child psychiatry and mental hygiene.

orthoptic (or-thŏp′tĭk) [″ + *optikos,* pert. to vision]. Pert. to or producing normal binocular vision.

orthoptics. 1. The science of correcting defects in binocular vision resulting from defects in optic musculature. 2. The technique of eye exercises for correcting faulty eye coordination affecting binocular vision.

orthoptic training. Eye muscle exercises for the purpose of correcting squint. SYN: *orthoptics.*

orthoroentgenography (or″thō-rĕnt-gĕn-ŏg′ră-fē). Accurate measurement of size and position of internal organs, using radiographic apparatus. A radiographic procedure used for the accurate measurement of long bones. SEE: *orthodiagraph.*

orthoscopic (or″thō-skŏp′ĭk). 1. Having correct and undistorted vision. 2. Made to correct optical distortion.

orthoscopy (or-thŏs′kō-pē). Ocular examination with an orthoscope.

orthosis [Gr., making straight]. The straightening or correction of a deformity or disability.

orthostatic (or″thō-stăt′ĭk) [Gr. *orthos,* straight, + *statikos,* causing to stand]. Concerning an erect position. SYN: *orthotic.*

orthostatic hypotension. Postural hypotension, q.v.

orthostatism (or′thō-stăt″ĭzm) [″ + ″ + *-ismos,* condition]. An upright standing position of the body.

orthotast (or′thō-tăst) [″ + *tassein,* to arrange]. Instrument for straightening bone curvatures.

orthotic [Gr. *orthosis,* making straight]. 1. Rel. to orthosis. 2. Orthostatic.

orthotics (or-thŏt′ĭks). 1. The science pert. to mechanical appliances for orthopedic use. 2. The use of orthopedic appliances.

orthotist (or′thō-tĭst) [Gr. *orthosis,* making straight]. One skilled in orthosis.

orthotonos, orthotonus (or-thŏt′ō-nŏs, -nŭs) [″ + *tonos,* tension]. Tetanic spasm marked by rigidity of the body in a straight line. SEE: illus.

orthotopic (or″thō-tŏp′ĭk). In the correct place.

orthovoltage (or″thō-vŏl′tĭj). Median voltage used in x-ray therapy. Approx. 250 kilovolts.

Orthoxine Hydrochloride. Trade name for methoxyphenamine hydrochloride, USP.

orthropsia (or-thrŏp′sē-ă) [Gr. *orthros,* time near dawn, + *opsis,* sight]. Characteristic of human vision by which sight is better at dawn or dusk than in bright sunlight.

orthuria (orth-ū′rē-ă) [Gr. *orthos,* normal, + *ouron,* urine]. Normal frequency of urination.

O.S., o.s. L. *oculus sinister,* left eye.

Os. Chem. symb. for osmium.

os (ōs) [L.]. (pl. *ora*) [NA] Mouth, opening.

o. uteri. Mouth of the uterus.

o. uteri externum. The opening of the cervical canal of the uterus into the vagina.

o. uteri internum. The internal opening of the cervical canal into the uterus.

o. ventriculi. The cardia of the stomach.

os (ŏs) [L.]. (pl. *ossa*) [NA] Bone.

o. calcis. [NA] Heel bone. SYN: *calcaneus* [NA].

o. coxae. [NA] Hip bone.

o. hamatum. [NA] Hooked bone in second row of carpus (wrist). SYN: *unciform bone.*

o. hyoideum. [NA] U-shaped bone at the base of the tongue. SYN: *hyoid bone.*

o. ilium. [NA] The ilium.

o. innominatum. Hip bone.

o. magnum. A carpal bone, the third in the second distal row. SYN: *capitatum.*

o. orbiculare. Tiny bone in the ear that becomes attached to the incus, forming the lenticular process.

o. peroneum. Bone occasionally found in the tendon of peroneus longus muscle.

o. planum. 1. [NA] Flat bone; any bone that has a slight thickness only. 2. Orbital plate of ethmoid bone.

o. pubis. [NA] The pubic bone; anteroinferior part of the hip bone. In the adult, it

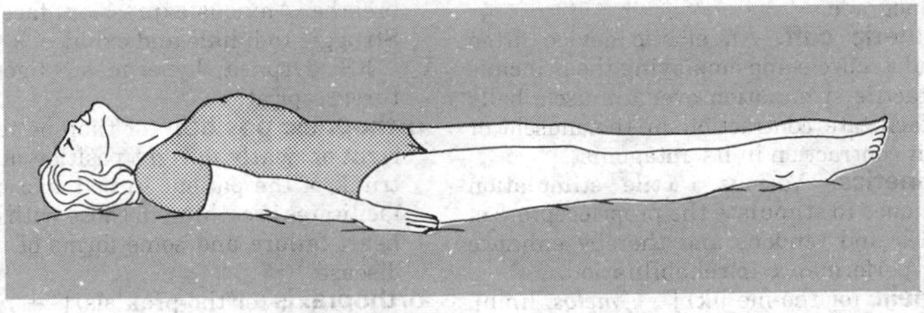

ORTHOTONOS

unites the innominate bone with the ilium and ischium to form the pelvis. It is irregular in shape, divided into a horizontal, ascending, and descending ramus. The outer extremity constitutes approx. one fifth of the acetabulum. The inner ramus forms the symphysis pubis.

o. scaphoideum. Scaphoid, q.v.

o. temporale. Temporal bone, q.v.

o. trigonum. [NA] Bone of foot that develops from an extra center of ossification along posterior surface of the talus.

o. unguis. Lacrimal bone.

o. vesalianum. Bone that develops from ossification of the posterior tubercle of the fifth metatarsal.

osazone (ō'sā-zōn). Any of a series of compounds resulting from heating sugars with acetic acid and phenylhydrazine.

oscedo (ŏs-sē'dō) [L.]. 1. Yawning. 2. White spots on the mucosa of the mouth. SYN: *aphtha.*

oscheal (ŏs'kē-ăl) [Gr. *oscheon,* scrotum]. Concerning the scrotum.

oscheitis (ŏs-kē-ī'tĭs) [" + *itis,* inflammation]. Inflamed condition of the scrotum. SYN: *oschitis.*

oschelephantiasis (ŏsk"ĕl-ĕ-făn-tī'ă-sĭs). Elephantiasis of the scrotum.

oscheo- [Gr. *oscheon*]. Combining form meaning the scrotum.

oscheocele (ŏs'kē-ō-sēl) [" + *kele,* swelling]. A scrotal swelling or tumor. SYN: *oscheoma.*

oscheohydrocele (ŏs"kē-ō-hī'drō-sēl) [" + *hydor,* water, + *kele,* hernia]. Scrotal hydrocele; collection of fluid in the sac of a scrotal hernia.

oscheolith (ŏs'kē-ō-lĭth) [" + *lithos,* stone]. A concretion in the scrotal sebaceous glands.

oscheoma (ŏs-kē-ō'mă) [" + *oma,* tumor]. Scrotal tumor. SYN: *oscheoncus.*

oscheoncus (ŏs"kē-ŏng'kŭs) [" + *onkos,* tumor]. A tumor of the scrotum. SYN: *oscheoma.*

oscheoplasty (ŏs'kē-ō-plăs"tē) [" + *plassein,* to form]. Plastic surgical repair of the scrotum.

oschitis (ŏs-kī'tĭs). Oscheitis.

oscillation (ŏs"sĭl-ā'shŭn) [L. *oscillare,* to swing]. A swinging, pendulum-like movement; a vibration; fluctuation.

oscillator (ŏs'ĭ-lā"tor). 1 Device for producing oscillations. 2. An electronic circuit that will produce an oscillating current of a certain frequency.

oscillogram (ŏs'ĭl-ō-grăm) [" + Gr. *gramma,* a mark]. Graphic record made by the oscillograph.

oscillograph (ŏs'ĭl-ō-grăf) [" + Gr. *graphein,* to write]. An electronic device for detecting and recording variations in electrical phenomena. In medicine, it is used for recording electrical activity of the heart and other muscular tissues. Electrocardiographs and electroencephalographs are examples of the application of this technique. SEE: *oscilloscope.*

oscillometer (ŏs-ĭl-ŏm'ĕt-ĕr) [" + Gr. *metron,* measure]. Machine to measure oscillations, esp. those of the blood stream.

oscillometry (ŏs-ĭl-ŏm'ĕ-trē). The measurement of oscillations with a machine.

oscillopsia. Sensation of oscillation or swinging of the visual field. It is illusory and may be associated with a severe form of labyrinthine nystagmus.

oscilloscope (ŏ-sĭl'ō-skōp) [L. *oscillare,* to swing, + Gr. *skopein,* to examine]. An instrument for making visible the presence, nature, and form of oscillations or irregularities of an electric current. SEE: *oscillograph.*

Oscinidae. The eye flies. A family of small hairless flies that includes the genera Hippelates, Siphunculina, and Oscinis. They are serious pests and transmit a number of infectious diseases.

oscitation (ŏs-ĭ-tā'shŭn) [L. *oscitatio*]. Yawning, gaping.

osculation [L. *osculum,* little mouth, kiss]. 1. The union of two vessels or structures by their mouths. 2. Kissing.

osculum (ŏs'kū-lŭm) [L.]. (pl. *oscula*) Any tiny aperture or pore.

-ose. 1. Chemical suffix indicating that the substance is a carbohydrate as glucose. 2. Suffix indicating a primary alteration product of a protein, as proteose.

Osgood-Schlatter disease (ŏz-good-shlăt'ĕr). [Robert B. Osgood, U.S. orthopedist, b. 1873; Carl Schlatter, Zurich surgeon, 1864–1934] Osteochondritis of the epiphysis of the tibial tuberosity.

OSHA. *Occupational Safety and Health Administration.* A U.S. governmental regulatory agency that is concerned with the health and safety of workers.

-osis [Gr.]. Suffix added to words of Greek origin. Indicates the condition, status, or process. Usually denotes an increase in the condition. SEE: *-sis.*

Osler, Sir William (ŏs'lĕr). Canadian-born physician, 1849–1919. In his career he was associated with McGill, Johns Hopkins, and Oxford Universities. During that time, he prepared a number of editions of his monumental *The Principles and Practice of Medicine.*

O.'s disease. Disease of the blood in which the red cells are increased in number, the spleen becomes enlarged, and the face is a deep red rather than truly cyanotic. SYN: *erythremia; polycythemia vera; Vaquez's disease.*

O.'s nodes. A small, raised, red, tender area present in the pads of the fingers and toes in bacterial endocarditis. The areas are due to infected emboli from the heart.

O.-Vaquez disease. Polycythemia vera.

O.-Weber-Rendu disease. [Frederick P. Weber, Brit. physician, 1863–1962; Henri J. L. M. Rendu, Fr. physician, 1844–1902] A hereditary disease of capillaries. SEE: *telangiectasia, hereditary hemorrhagic.*

osmate. A salt of osmic acid.

osmatic (ŏz-măt'ĭk) [Gr. *osmasthai,* to smell]. Pert. to, or having, a keen sense of smell.

osmesis (ŏz-mē'sĭs) [Gr. *osmesis,* smelling]. 1. The sense of smell. 2. The act of smelling. SYN: *olfaction.*

osmesthesia (ŏz"mĕs-thē'zē-ă) [Gr. *osme,* odor, + *aisthesis,* sensation]. Olfactory sensibility; power of perceiving and distinguishing odors.

osmic acid (ŏz'mĭk). OsO_4. Volatile colorless compound formed by heating osmium in air. Used as a caustic, stain for fats, tissue fixative for electron microscopy. SYN: *osmium tetroxide.*

CAUTION: Vapors are extremely toxic to eyes, skin, and respiratory tract. Container must not be opened without safeguarding eyes from vapors released both from uncapping and possible spilling.

osmicate (ŏz'mĭ-kāt). To impregnate or stain with osmic acid.

osmics (ŏz'mĭks) [Gr. *osme,* odor]. The science of odors.

osmidrosis (ŏz-mĭ-drō'sĭs) [" + *hidros,* perspiration]. Condition in which perspiration has a very strong odor. SYN: *bromidrosis.*

osmiophilic (ŏz"mē-ō-fĭl'ĭk). Having an affinity for the staining material osmium tetroxide.

osmiophobic (ŏz"mē-ō-fō'bĭk). Having resistance to the staining material osmium tetroxide.

Osmitrol. Trade name for mannitol, USP.

osmium (ŏz'mē-ŭm) [Gr. *osme,* smell]. SYMB: Os. At. wt. 190.2; at. no. 76. A metallic element.

o. tetroxide. OsO_4 Osmic acid.

osmo-. 1. [Gr. *osme,* odor]. Combining form indicating relationship to odor or smell. 2. [Gr. *osmos,* impulse]. Combining form indicating a thrusting forth. 3. [Gr. *osmos,* impulse]. Pert. to osmosis.

osmodysphoria (ŏz-mō-dĭs-fō'rē-ă) [Gr. *osme,* odor, + *dys,* bad, + *pherein,* to bear]. Deep-seated and abnormal dislike of certain odors.

osmolagnia (ŏz"mō-lăg'nē-ă) [" + *lagneia,* lust]. Erotic satisfaction derived from odors, usually of the body. SYN: *osphresiolagnia.*

osmolality (ŏs"mō-lăl'ĭ-tē). Osmotic concentration, the characteristic of a solution determined by the ionic concentration of the dissolved substances per unit of solvent.

o., serum. The osmotic concentration of the serum.

o., urine. The osmotic concentration of the urine.

osmolar (ŏz-mō'lăr). Concerning the osmotic concentration of a solution.

osmolarity (os"mō-lăr'ĭ-tē). Concentration of osmotically active particles in solution.

osmology (ŏz-mŏl'ō-jē). 1. [Gr. *osme,* odor, + *logos,* study]. The study of odors. SYN: *osphresiology.* 2. [Gr. *osmos,* impulse, + *logos,* study]. Study of osmosis.

osmometer (ŏz-mŏm'ĕt-ĕr). 1. [Gr. *osme,* odor, + *metron,* measure]. Device for measuring acuity of sense of smell. 2. [Gr. *osmos,* impulse, + *metron,* measure]. A device for measuring osmotic pressure.

osmonosology (ŏz"mō-nō-sŏl'ō-jē) [Gr. *osme,* odor, + *nosos,* disease, + *logos,* study]. Branch of medicine dealing with diseases and disorders of the organs of smell.

osmophilic (ŏz"mō-fĭl'ĭk) [Gr. *osmos,* impulse, + *philos,* to love]. The character that promotes osmosis.

osmophobia [Gr. *osme,* odor, + *phobia,* fear]. Morbid fear of odors.

osmophore (ŏz'mō-for) [" + *phoros,* bearing]. The portion of a chemical that is responsible for the odor of the compound.

osmoreceptor (ŏz"mō-rē-sĕp'tor). 1. A receptor in the hypothalamus that is sensitive to the osmotic pressure of the serum. 2. A receptor in the brain that is sensitive to olfactory stimuli.

osmoregulation (ŏz"mō-rĕg"ū-lā'shŭn). The regulation of osmotic pressure.

osmose (ŏz'mōs) [Gr. *osmos,* impulse]. 1. To subject to osmosis. 2. To undergo osmosis.

osmosis (ŏz-mō'sĭs) [Gr. *osmos,* impulse, + *osis,* condition]. The passage of solvent through a semipermeable membrane separating solutions of different concentrations. The solvent, usually water, passes through the membrane from the region of lower concentration of solute to that of a higher concentration of solute, thus tending to equalize the concentrations of the two solutions. The rate of osmosis is dependent primarily upon the difference in osmotic pressures of the solutions on the two sides of a membrane, the permeability of the membrane, and the electric potential across the membrane and charge upon walls of the pores in it. SEE: illus.

RS: absorption; dialysis; diffusion; hypotonic; isotonic solution.

osmotherapy (ŏz"mō-thĕr'ă-pē) [" + *therapeia,* treatment]. Intravenous administration of hypertonic solutions in order to increase the osmolar concentration of the serum. This is used in treating cerebral edema.

osmotic (ŏz-mŏt'ĭk) [Gr. *osmos,* impulse]. Pert. to osmosis.

OSMOSIS

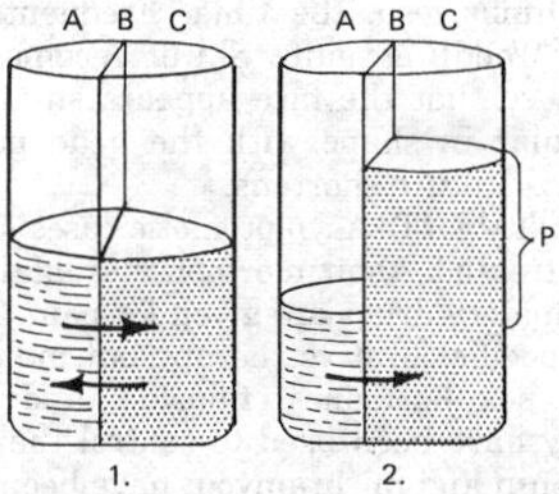

A. CHAMBER CONTAINING WATER
B. MEMBRANOUS PARTITION BETWEEN CHAMBERS
C. CHAMBER CONTAINING A SOLUTION OF SALT IN WATER
1. B IS PERMEABLE TO ALL SUBSTANCES
2. B IS SEMIPERMEABLE. IMPERMEABLE TO SALT PARTICLES BUT PERMEABLE TO WATER PARTICLES.
P OSMOTIC PRESSURE THAT CAUSES THE DIFFERENCE IN LEVELS BETWEEN CHAMBERS A AND C WHEN SEPARATED BY A SEMIPERMEABLE MEMBRANE.

OSMOSIS IN WHOLE BLOOD AND IN SALT SOLUTIONS THAT HAVE INCREASED OR DECREASED SALT CONCENTRATION

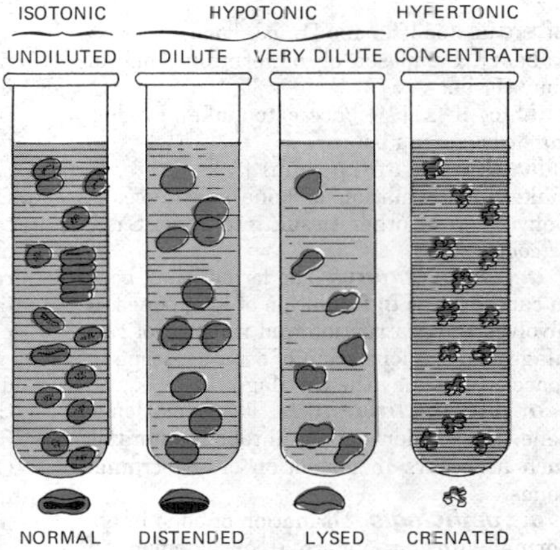

THE ERYTHROCYTES SWELL IN HYPOTONIC AND CONTRACT (BECOME CRENATED) IN HYPERTONIC SALT SOLUTIONS.

osmotic pressure. 1. The pressure that develops when two solutions of different concentrations are separated by a semipermeable membrane. 2. The pressure that would develop if a solution were enclosed in a membrane impermeable to all solutes present and surrounded by pure solvent. Osmotic pressure varies with concentration of the solution and with temperature increase. Animal cells have an osmotic pressure approximately equal to that of the circulating fluid, the blood. Solutions exerting this osmotic pressure are said to be isotonic or isosmotic; stronger solutions that cause cells to shrink are hypertonic; weaker solutions that cause cells to swell are hypotonic.

osphresiolagnia (ŏs-frē″zē-ō-lăg′nē-ă) [Gr. *osphresis,* smell, + *lagneia,* lust]. Excitement of an erotic nature produced by odors. SYN: *osmolagnia.*

osphresiology (ŏs″frē-zē-ŏl′ō-jē) [″ + *logos,* study]. Science of odors and the sense of smell. SYN: *osmology.*

osphresiometer (ŏs″frē-zē-ŏm′ĕt-ĕr) [″ + *metron,* measure]. Apparatus for measuring the acuteness of the sense of smell. SYN: *osmometer.*

osphresis (ŏs-frē′sĭs) [Gr.]. The sense of smell. SYN: *olfaction.*

osphretic (ŏs-frĕt′ĭk). Concerning the sense of smell. SYN: *olfactory.*

osphus (ŏs′fŭs) [Gr. *osphys*]. Loin.

osphyalgia (ŏs-fē-ăl′jē-ă) [″ − *algos,* pain]. Pain in the loins or hips. SEE: *lumbago; sciatica.*

osphyitis (ŏs-fē-ī′tĭs) [″ + *itis,* inflammation]. Inflammation of the lumbar region.

osphyomyelitis (ŏs″fē-ō-mī″ĕl-ī′tĭs) [″ + *myelos,* marrow, + *itis,* inflammation]. Inflamed condition of the lumbar region of the spinal cord.

ossa (ŏs′ă) [L., bones]. Pl. of os.

ossein (ŏs′ē-ĭn) [L. *ossa,* bones]. The collagen of bone. It forms the framework of bone.

osseocartilaginous (ŏs″ē-ō-kăr″tĭ-lăj′ĭ-nŭs). Concerning bone and cartilage.

osseofibrous (ŏs″ē-ō-fī′brŭs) [″ + *fibra,* fiber]. Composed of bone and fibrous tissue.

osseomucin (ŏs″ē-ō-mū′sĭn). Ground substance of bone.

osseous (ŏs′ē-ŭs) [L. *osseus,* bony]. Bonelike; concerning bones. SYN: *bony.*

ossicle (ŏs′ĭ-kl) [L. *ossiculum,* little bone]. Any small bone, esp. one of the three bones of the ear.

o.'s, auditory. The three bones of the inner ear: incus, malleus, and stapes. SEE: *ear* for illus.

ossicula (ō-sĭk′ū-lă) [L.]. (sing. *ossiculum*) Little bones.

ossiculectomy (ŏs″ĭk-ū-lĕk′tō-mē) [L. *ossiculum,* little bone, + Gr. *ektome,* excision]. Excision of an ossicle, esp. one of the ear.

ossiculotomy (ŏ″sĭk-ū-lŏt′ō-mē) [″ + Gr. *tome,* incision]. Surgical incision of one or more of the ossicles of the ear.

ossiculum (ŏ-sĭk′ū-lŭm) [L.]. (pl. *ossicula*) Tiny bone, esp. one of the three in the middle ear.

ossiferous (ŏs-ĭf′ĕr-ŭs) [L. *os,* bone, + *ferre,* to bear]. Composed of, or forming, bone or bony tissue.

ossific (ŏs-ĭf′ĭk) [″ + *facere,* to make]. Producing or becoming bone.

ossification (ŏs″ĭ-fĭ-kā′shŭn) [″ + *facere,* to make]. 1. Formation of bone substance. 2. Conversion of other tissue into bone. SYN: *osteogenesis.*

o., endochondral. The formation of bone in cartilage, as in formation of long bones. It involves the destruction and removal of cartilage and the formation of osseous tissue in space occupied by the cartilage.

o., intramembranous. The formation of bone in or underneath a fibrous membrane, such as occurs in formation of the cranial bones.

o., pathologic. Formation of bone in abnormal sites or abnormal development of bone.

ossifluence (ŏ-sĭf′lū-ĕns). Osteolysis or softening of bone.

ossiform (ŏs′ĭ-form). Resembling bone. SYN: *osteoid.*

ossify (ŏs′ĭ-fī) [″ + *facere,* to make]. To turn into bone.

ostalgia (ŏs-tăl′jē-ă) [Gr. *osteon,* bone, + *algos,* pain]. Pain in a bone. SYN: *osteodynia.*

osteal (ŏs′tē-ăl). Pert. to bone.

ostealgia (ŏs″tē-ăl′jē-ă) [″+ *algos,* pain]. Bone pain.

osteanagenesis (ŏs″tē-ăn-ă-jĕn′ĕ-sĭs) [″ + *anagenesis,* reproduction]. Regeneration or re-formation of bone.

ostearthrotomy (ŏs″tē-ăr-thrŏt′ō-mē) [″ + *arthron,* joint, + *tome,* incision]. Surgical excision of the articular end of a bone. SYN: *osteoarthrotomy.*

ostectomy, osteectomy (ŏs-tĕk′tō-mē, -tē-ĕk′tō-mē) [″+ *ektome,* excision]. Surgical excision of a bone or a portion of one.

osteectopia (ŏs″tē-ĕk-tō′pē-ă) [″ + *ektopos,* out of place]. Displacement of a bone.

osteitis (ŏs-tē-ī′tĭs) [″ + *itis,* inflammation]. Inflammation of a bone.

o., condensing. Osteitis in which the marrow cavity becomes filled with osseous tissue. Bone becomes denser and heavier. SYN: *o., sclerosing.*

o. deformans. Skeletal disease of older people. Chronic form of osteitis with thickening and hypertrophy of the long bones and deformity of the flat bones. SYN: *Paget's disease.*

ETIOL: Unknown.

SYM: Slow and insidious in onset. Pain in lower limbs, esp. the tibia. Frequent fractures. Waddling gait. Skull becomes enlarged, so that the face appears small and triangular in shape with the head pushed forward. Stature shortens.

TREATMENT: Asymptomatic cases should not be treated. Aspirin or non-steroidal anti-inflammatory drugs are given for pain. There is no specific curative therapy but male and female sex hormones, fluoride, and x-ray therapy have been used to control the pain. Calcitonin and mithramycin have been used to control the resorption of bone and thus are of assistance in alleviating bone pain. Etidronate sodium has reduced bone resorption in most patients and produced clinical improvement in some.

o. fibrosa cystica generalisata. A condition resulting from overactivity of the parathyroid glands with resulting disturbances in calcium and phosphorus metabolism. Characterized by decalcification and softening of bone, nephrolithiasis, and elevation of blood calcium and lowering of blood phosphorus. Cysts form and tumors may develop. SYN: *hyperparathyroidism.*

o. fragilitans. Osteogenesis imperfecta, q.v.

o., gummatous. Chronic osteitis associated with syphilis and characterized by the formation of gummas.

o., rarefying. Form of osteitis in which inorganic matter is lessened and bone tissue becomes lattice-like in structure. SYN: *osteoporosis.*

o., sclerosing. O., condensing.

ostembryon (ŏs-tĕm′brē-ŏn) [Gr. *osteon,* bone, + *embryon,* fetus]. A fetus that has become ossified. SYN: *lithopedion; osteopedion.*

ostemia (ŏs-tē′mē-ă) [″ + *haima,* blood]. Congestion of blood in a bone.

ostempyesis (ŏs″tĕm-pī-ē′sĭs) [″ + *empyesis,* suppuration]. Purulent inflammation within a bone.

osteo- [Gr. *osteon,* bone]. Combining form indicating relationship to a bone.

osteoanagenesis (ŏs″tē-ō-ăn″ă-jĕn′ĕ-sĭs) [″ + *anagenesis,* reproduction]. Regeneration of bone.

osteoanesthesia (ŏs″tē-ō-ăn″ĕs-thē′zē-ă) [″ + *an-,* not, + *aisthesis,* sensation]. The condition of the bone being insensitive, esp. to stimuli that would normally produce pain.

osteoaneurysm (ŏs″tē-ō-ăn′ū-rĭzm) [″ + *aneurysma,* a widening]. Aneurysm, or dilatation of a blood vessel filled with clotted blood, occurring within a bone.

osteoarthritis (ŏs″tē-ō-ăr-thrī′tĭs) [″ + *ar-*

thron, joint, + *itis,* inflammation]. A chronic disease involving the joints, esp. those bearing weight. Characterized by destruction of articular cartilage, overgrowth of bone with lipping and spur formation, and impaired function. SYN: *arthritis, degenerative.*

osteoarthropathy (ŏs″tē-ō-ăr-thrŏp′ă-thē) [″ + ″ + *pathos,* disease]. Any disease involving the joints and bones, accompanied by severe pain.

o., hypertrophic pulmonary. An affection characterized by enlargement of distal phalanges of fingers and toes and a thickening of their distal ends, accompanied by a peculiar longitudinal curving of nails. Wrist and interphalangeal joints may become enlarged as well as distal ends of tibia and fibula and the jaw.

ETIOL: Found in pulmonary tuberculosis, chronic bronchitis, bronchiectasis, and congenital heart disease.

osteoarthrosis (ŏs″tē-ō-ăr-thrō′sĭs) [″ + ″ + *osis,* condition]. Osteoarthritis.

osteoarthrotomy (ŏs″tē-ō-ăr-thrŏt′ō-mē) [″ + ″ + *tome,* incision]. Excision of joint end of a bone. SYN: *ostearthrotomy.*

osteoblast (ŏs′tē-ō-blăst) [Gr. *osteon,* bone, + *blastos,* germ]. A cell of mesodermal origin that is concerned with the formation of bone.

osteoblastoma (ŏs″tē-ō-blăs-tō′mă) [″ + ″ + *oma,* tumor]. A large benign tumor of osteoblasts in a patchy osteoid matrix. It occurs mostly in the vertebral column of young people.

osteocampsia (ŏs″tē-ō-kămp′sē-ă) [″ + *kamptein,* to bend]. Curvature of a bone, as in osteomalacia.

osteocarcinoma (ŏs″tē-ō-kăr-sĭn-ō′mă) [″ + *karkinos,* cancer, + *oma,* tumor]. 1. Combined osteoma and carcinoma. 2. Carcinoma of a bone.

osteocartilaginous (ŏs″tē-ō-kăr″tĭ-lăj′ĭ-nŭs). Concerning bone and cartilage.

osteocele (ŏs′tē-ō-sēl) [″ + *kele,* hernia]. 1. A testicular or scrotal tumor that contains bony tissue. 2. A bone-containing hernia.

osteocephaloma (ŏs″tē-ō-sĕf″ă-lō′mă) [″ + *kephale,* head, + *oma,* tumor]. Encephaloma, a malignant neoplasm of brainlike texture in a bone.

osteochondral (ŏs″tē-ō-kŏn′drăl). Concerning bone and cartilage.

osteochondritis (ŏs″tē-ō-kŏn-drī′tĭs) [″ + *chondros,* cartilage, + *itis,* inflammation]. Inflammation of bone and cartilage.

o. deformans juvenilis. Chronic inflammation of the head of the femur in children. Results in atrophy and shortening of the neck of femur with a wide flat head. SYN: *Waldenström's disease.*

o. dissecans. Condition affecting a joint in which a fragment of cartilage and its underlying bone become detached from articular surface. Occurs commonly in the knee joint.

osteochondrodystrophy (ŏs″tē-ō-kŏn″drō-dĭs′trō-fē) [″ + ″ + *dys,* bad, + *trephein,* to nourish]. A disorder of skeletal growth resulting from bone and cartilage malformation. Produces a form of dwarfism. SYN: *Morquio's syndrome.*

o., familial. Morquio syndrome. SEE: *mucopolysaccharidosis IV.*

osteochondrolysis (ŏs″tē-ō-kŏn-drŏl′ĭ-sĭs) [″ + ″ + *lysis,* dissolution]. Osteochondritis dissecans.

osteochondroma (ŏs″tē-ō-kŏn-drō′mă) [″ + ″ + *oma,* tumor]. Tumor composed of both cartilaginous and bony substance.

osteochondromatosis (ŏs″tē-ō-kŏn″drō-mă-tō′sĭs) [″ + ″ + ″ + *osis,* condition]. A disease in which there are multiple osteochondromata.

osteochondrosarcoma (ŏs″tē-ō-kŏn″drō-săr-kō′mă) [″ + ″ + *sarx,* flesh, − *oma,* tumor]. Chondrosarcoma occurring in bone.

osteochondrosis (ŏs″tē-ō-kŏn-drō′sĭs) [″ + ″ + *osis,* condition]. Degenerative changes in the ossification centers of the epiphyses of bones, particularly during periods of rapid growth in children. The process continues to the stage of avascular and aseptic necrosis and then there is slow healing and repair.

o. deformans tibiae. Degeneration or aseptic necrosis of the medial condyle of the tibia.

osteochondrous (ŏs″tē-ō-kŏn′drŭs). Containing bone and cartilage.

osteoclasia, osteoclasis (ŏs″tē-ō-klā′zē-ă, -ŏk′lă-sĭs) [″ + *klasis,* a breaking]. 1. Surgical fracture of a bone in order to remedy a deformity. 2. Bony tissue absorption and destruction.

osteoclast (ŏs′tē-ō-klăst) [″ + *klan,* to break]. 1. Device for fracturing bones for therapeutic purposes. 2. Giant multinuclear cell formed in bone marrow of growing bones. Found in depressions (called Howship's lacunae) on the surface of the bone. Concerned with absorption and removal of unwanted tissue.

osteoclast activating factor. Factor produced in certain conditions associated with resorption of bone. Periodontal disease and lymphoid proliferative diseases such as multiple myeloma and malignant lymphoma are included.

osteoclastic (ŏs″tē-ō-klăs′tĭk). Concerning osteoclasts.

osteoclastoma (ŏs″tē-ō-klăs-tō′mă) [″ + ″ + *oma,* tumor]. Giant cell tumor of bone.

osteoclasty (ŏs′tē-ō-klăs″tē). Osteoclasis.

osteocope (ŏs′tē-ō-kōp) [″ + *kopos,* pain]. Extreme pain in the bones, esp. in syphilitic bone disease.

osteocopic (ŏs″tē-ō-kŏp′ĭk). Concerning severe pain in the bone.

osteocranium (ŏs″tē-ō-krā′nē-ŭm) [″ + *kranion,* skull]. The portion of the cranium formed of membrane bones in contrast to that formed of cartilage (chondrocranium).

osteocystoma (ŏs″tē-ō-sĭs-tō′mă) [″ + *kystis,* sac, bladder, + *oma,* tumor]. Cystic tumor of a bone.

osteocyte (ŏs′tē-ō-sīt″) [″ + *kytos,* cell]. A mesodermal bone-forming cell that has become entrapped within the bone matrix; it lies within a lacuna with processes extending outward through canaliculi, and by its metabolic activity helps to maintain bone as a living tissue.

osteodensitometer. Device for determining the density of bones. Usually x-ray technique is used.

osteodermia (ŏs″tē-ō-dĕr′mē-ă) [″ + *derma,* skin]. The formation of bony deposits in the skin.

osteodesmosis (ŏs″tē-ō-dĕs-mō′sĭs) [″ + *desmos,* tendon, + *osis,* condition]. Transformation of tendon into bone.

osteodiastasis (ŏs″tē-ō-dī-ăs′tă-sĭs) [″ + *diastasis,* separation]. Separation of two adjacent bones.

osteodynia (ŏs″tē-ō-dĭn′ē-ă) [″ + *odyne,* pain]. Persistent pain in a bone. SYN: *ostealgia.*

osteodystrophia (ŏs″tē-ō-dĭs-trō′fē-ă) [″ + *dys,* ill, + *trophe,* nourishment]. Defective bone development. SYN: *osteodystrophy.*

osteodystrophy (ŏs″tē-ō-dĭs′trō-fē). Defective bone development.

o., renal. Generalized pathological changes in bone with resemblance to osteitis fibrosa cystica, osteomalacia, and osteoporosis. These changes are associated with renal failure. The serum phosphorus is elevated, calcium is low or normal, and there is increased parathyroid gland activity.

osteoectomy (ŏs″tē-ō-ĕk′tō-mē) [″ + *ektome,* excision]. Ostectomy, q.v.

osteoepiphysis (ŏs″tē-ō-ē-pĭf′ĭs-ĭs) [″ + *epi,* upon, + *physis,* growth]. A small piece of bone that is separated in childhood from the larger bone by cartilage; during later growth, the two bones join.

osteofibroma (ŏs″tē-ō-fī-brō′mă) [″ + L. *fibra,* fiber, + Gr. *oma,* tumor]. Tumor of bony and fibrous tissues. SYN: *fibro-osteoma.*

osteogen (ŏs′tē-ō-jĕn) [″ + *gennan,* to produce]. Substance of the inner periosteal layer from which bone is formed.

osteogenesis, osteogeny (ŏs″tē-ō-jĕn′ĕ-sĭs, -ŏj′ĕ-nē). Formation and development of bone taking place in connective tissue or in cartilage. SYN: *ossification.*

o. imperfecta. An inherited disorder of connective tissue characterized by defective bone matrix with calcification occurring normally on whatever matrix is present. Clinical findings are multiple fractures with minimal trauma, blue sclerae, early deafness, opalescent teeth, tendency to capillary bleeding, translucent skin, and joint instability. Although the disease is heterogeneous, two different classifications of osteogenesis imperfecta are still used for clinical distinction: osteogenesis imperfecta congenita with early fractures occurring even in utero; and osteogenesis imperfecta tarda with delayed onset of fracturing and much milder manifestations. Healing of bone fractures progresses normally. Later in life, the tendency to fracture decreases and often disappears. The vast majority of cases are inherited as an autosomal dominant trait, although a small percentage of congenital cases are transmitted as an autosomal recessive. There is no known cure for osteogenesis imperfecta; therefore, treatment is still supportive and palliative. Definition provided by the American Brittle Bone Society, Inc.

osteogenic. Pert. to osteogenesis.

osteography (ŏs″tē-ŏg′răf-ē) [Gr. *osteon,* bone, + *graphein,* to write]. Descriptive treatise on the bones.

osteohalisteresis (ŏs″tē-ō-hăl-ĭs″tĕr-ē′sĭs) [″ + *hals,* salt, + *sterein,* to deprive]. Softening of the bones, caused by deficiency of mineral constituents of the bone.

osteoid (ŏs′tē-oyd) [″ + *eidos,* resemblance]. Resembling bone; ossiform.

osteolipochondroma (ŏs″tē-ō-lĭ-pō″kŏn-drō′mă) [″ + *lipos,* fat, + *chondros,* cartilage, + *oma,* tumor]. A chondroma containing fatty and bony tissue.

osteologist (ŏs″tē-ŏl′ō-jĭst) [″ + *logos,* study]. A specialist in the study of bone.

osteology (ŏs-tē-ŏl′ō-jē) [″ + *logos,* study]. The science of structure and function of bones.

osteolysis (ŏs″tē-ŏl′ĭ-sĭs) [″ + *lysis,* dissolution]. Softening and destruction of bone, as in caries.

osteolytic (ŏs″tē-ō-lĭt′ĭk). Causing osteolysis.

osteoma (ŏs-tē-ō′mă) [″ + *oma,* tumor]. (pl. *osteomata, osteomas*) A benign bony tumor; a bonelike structure that develops on a bone or, occasionally, at other sites. SYN: *exostosis; osteoncus.*

o., cancellous. A tumor that is soft and spongy. Its thin and delicate trabeculae enclose large medullary spaces similar to cancellous bone.

o., cavalryman's. Bony outgrowth of femur at the insertion of the adductor femoris longus.

o. cutis. Benign formation of bone nodules in the skin.

o., dental. A bony outgrowth or exostosis of the root of a tooth.

o. durum, eburneum. A very hard osteoma in which the bone is ivory-like.

o. medullare. An osteoma containing medullary spaces.

o., osteoid. A rare benign tumor of bone composed of sheets of osteoid tissue partially calcified and ossified. Occurs esp. in extremities of young.

o. spongiosum. Spongy tumor in the bone. SYN: *osteospongioma.*

osteomalacia (ŏs″tē-ō-măl-ā′shē-ă) [Gr. *osteon,* bone, + *malakia,* softening]. Softening of the bones. A disease marked by increasing softness of the bones, so that they become flexible and brittle, thus causing deformities. Osteomalacia is the adult form of rickets, q.v.

SYM: Rheumatic pains in the limbs, spine, thorax, and esp. the pelvis; anemia and signs of deficiency disease; progressive weakness.

ETIOL: Deficiency or loss of calcium salts due to vitamin D deficiency.

TREATMENT: If the diet contains an adequate amount of calcium and phosphorus, a daily dose of 1600 IU of vitamin D for about a month will cause great improvement. The dose can then be gradually decreased to the normal daily requirement for vitamin D.

osteomalacic (ŏs″tē-ō-măl-ā′sĭk) [″ + *malakia,* softening]. Concerning or characterized by softening of the bone.

osteomatoid (ŏs-tē-ō′mă-toyd) [″ + *oma,* tumor, + *eidos,* resemblance]. Resembling a bonelike tumor.

osteomatosis (ŏs″tē-ō″mă-tō′sĭs) [″ + ″ + *osis,* condition]. Formation of multiple osteomas.

osteomere (ŏs′tē-ō-mēr) [″ + *meros,* part]. One in a series of similar bony segments, as the vertebrae.

osteometry (ŏs-tē-ŏm′ĕt-rē) [″ + *metron,* measure]. The study of the measurement of parts of the skeletal system.

osteomyelitis (ŏs″tē-ō-mī″ĕl-ī′tĭs) [″ + *myelos,* marrow, + *itis,* inflammation]. Inflammation of bone, esp. the marrow, caused by a pathogenic organism.

SYM: Pain in the affected part, fever, sweats, leukocytosis, overlying muscles usually rigid, skin inflamed, pain on pressure over affected part. Suppuration may occur.

TREATMENT: Prompt and adequate doses of antibiotics; sedation for pain and anxiety; aspiration of abscess; immobilization of affected extremity; surgery if abscess persists.

osteomyelodysplasia (ŏs″tē-ō-mī″ĕ-lō-dĭs-plā′sē-ă) [″ + ″ + *dys,* bad, + *plassein,* to form]. Condition in which the marrow space of the bones is increased, the bony tissue becomes thin, and there are leukopenia and fever.

osteon (ŏs′tē-ŏn) [Gr., bone]. The microscopic bone unit of compact bone, consisting of the haversian canals and the surrounding lamellae.

osteoncus (ŏs-tē-ŏng′kŭs) [″ + *onkos,* tumor]. A bone tumor. SYN: *exostosis; osteoma.*

osteonecrosis (ŏs″tē-ō-nē-krō′sĭs) [″ + *nekrosis,* death]. Generalized death of bone tissue rather than isolated areas of necrosis.

osteoneuralgia (ŏs″tē-ō-nū-răl′jē-ă) [″ + *neuron,* nerve, + *algos,* pain]. Pain of a bone.

osteopath (ŏs′tē-ō-păth) [″ + *pathos,* disease]. A practitioner of osteopathy.

osteopathic (ŏs″tē-ō-păth′ĭk). Concerning osteopathy.

osteopathology (ŏs″tē-ō-păth-ŏl′ō-jē) [″ + *pathos,* disease, + *logos,* study]. 1. Any bone disease. SYN: *osteopathy* (def. 1.) 2. Study of bone diseases.

osteopathy (ŏs-tē-ŏp′ă-thē) [″ + *pathos,* disease]. 1. Any bone disease. 2. A system of medicine based upon the theory that the normal body is a vital mechanical organism in which structural and functional states are of equal importance and that the body is able to rectify itself against toxic conditions when it has favorable environmental circumstances and satisfactory nourishment. Therefore it is the osteopathic physician's responsibility to remove any internal or external peculiarities to the system. Although using manipulation for the most part to restore structural and functional balance, osteopaths also rely upon physical, medicinal, and surgical methods. Osteopathy, which was founded by Doctor Andrew Taylor Still (1828–1917), is recognized as a standard method or system of medical and surgical care.

osteopecilia (ŏs″tē-ō-pē-sĭl′ē-ă) [″ + *poikilia,* spottedness]. Osteosclerosis fragilis generalisata.

osteopedion (ŏs″tē-ō-pē′dē-ŏn) [″ + *paidion,* child]. A calcified or hardened fetus. SYN: *lithopedion; ostembryon.*

osteopenia (ŏs″tē-ō-pē′nē-ă) [″ + *penia,* lack]. 1. Condition of diminished amount of bone tissue, without respect to cause. 2. Decreased bone density caused by failure of rate of osteoid tissue synthesis to keep up with the normal rate of bone lysis. SEE: *osteoporosis.*

osteoperiosteal (ŏs″tē-ō-pĕr″ē-ŏs′tē-ăl) [″ + *peri,* around, + *osteon,* bone]. Concerning bone and its periosteum, the protective connective tissue covering bone.

osteoperiostitis (ŏs″tē-ō-pĕr″ē-ŏs-tī′tĭs) [″ + ″ + ″ + *itis,* inflammation]. Inflammation of a bone and its protective membrane, the periosteum.

osteopetrosis (ŏs″tē-ō-pĕ-trō′sĭs) [″ + *petra,* stone, + *osis,* condition]. Hereditary condition marked by excessive calcification of bones causing spontaneous fractures and marble-like appearance. SYN: *Albers-Schönberg disease.* SEE: *marble bones.*

osteophage (ŏs′tē-ō-făj) [″ + *phagein,* to eat]. Large multinuclear cell that causes absorption of bone. SEE: *osteoclast.*

osteophagia (ŏs″tē-ō-fā′jē-ă). Craving to eat bones, caused by a calcium or phosphorus deficiency.

osteophlebitis (ŏs″tē-ō-flē-bī′tĭs) [″ + *phleps, phleb-,* vein, + *itis,* inflammation]. Inflammation of veins of a bone.

osteophone (ŏs′tē-ō-fōn″) [Gr. *osteon,* bone, + *phone,* voice]. Device used by the deaf for conducting sound through facial bones.

osteophony (ŏs″tē-ŏf′ō-nē). Bone conduction of sound.

osteophore (ŏs′tē-ō-for) [″ + *pherein,* to carry]. A forceps for crushing bone.

osteophyma (ŏs″tē-ō-fī′mă) [″ + *phyma,* growth]. A swelling or growth of bone.

osteophyte (ŏs′tē-ō-fīt) [″ + *phyton,* plant]. A bony excrescence or outgrowth, usually branched in shape.

osteoplaque (ŏs′tē-ō-plăk). A layer of bone.

osteoplast (ŏs′tē-ō-plăst) [″ + *plastos,* formed]. Osteoblast.

osteoplastic (ŏs″tē-ō-plăs′tĭk) [″ + *plastikos,* formed]. 1. Pert. to bone repair by plastic surgery or grafting. 2. Concerning bone formation.

osteoplasty (ŏs′tē-ō-plăs″tē) [″ + *plassein,* to form]. Plastic repair of the bones.

osteopoikilosis (ŏs″tē-ō-poy″kĭ-lō′sĭs) [″ + *poikilos,* spotted]. Hereditary disease of bones marked by excessive calcification in spots less than 1 cm. in diameter. It is a benign disease.

osteoporosis (ŏs″tē-ō-por-ō′sĭs) [″ + *poros,* a passage, + *osis,* condition]. Increased porosity of bone seen most often in the elderly. SEE: *osteomalacia.*

SYM: Softening of bone, widening of haversian canals, absorption of calcareous matter.

o. circumscripta cranii. Localized osteoporosis of the skull associated with Paget's disease of bone.

o. of disuse. Osteoporosis due to lack of stress to the bones. This may occur while in bed for a prolonged period or while flying in outer space in a weightless condition.

o., posttraumatic. Loss of bone tissue following trauma, esp. when there is damage to a nerve supplying the injured area. The condition may also be caused by disuse.

osteoporotic (ŏs″tē-ō-por-ŏt′ĭk). Concerning a porous condition of the bones.

osteoradionecrosis (ŏs″tē-ō-rā″dē-ō-nē-krō′sĭs) [Gr. *osteon,* bone, + L. *radiatio,* radiation, + Gr. *nekrosis,* a killing]. Death of bone following irradiation.

osteorrhagia (ŏs″tē-ō-rā′jē-ă) [″ + *rhegnynai,* to burst forth]. Hemorrhagic flow of blood from a bone.

osteorrhaphy (ŏs-tē-or′ă-fē) [″ + *rhaphe,* a sewing]. Suture of bone or the wiring of bone fragments. SYN: *osteosuture.*

osteosarcoma (ŏs″tē-ō-săr-kō′mă) [″ + *sarx,* flesh, + *oma,* tumor]. A malignant sarcoma of the bone. SYN: *myelosarcoma.*

osteosarcomatous (ŏs″tē-ō-săr-kō′măt-ŭs). Concerning or like an osteosarcoma.

osteosclerosis (ŏs″tē-ō-sklē-rō′sĭs) [″ + *skleros,* hard, + *osis,* condition]. Hardening of bone with increased heaviness.

o. congenita. Achondroplasia, q.v.

osteoscope (ŏs′tē-ō-skōp) [″ + *skopein,* to examine]. Appliance used to test x-ray machines by observing certain bones of the forearm that are considered as a standard.

osteoseptum (ŏs″tē-ō-sĕp′tŭm) [″ + L. *septum,* a partition]. The bony area of the nasal septum.

osteosis (ŏs″tē-ō′sĭs) [″ + *osis,* condition]. Presence of bone-containing nodules in the skin.

o. cutis. Diffuse thickening of skin and subcutaneous tissue.

osteospongioma (ŏs″tē-ō-spŏn″jē-ō′mă) [″ + *spongos,* sponge, + *oma,* tumor]. A spongy neoplasm of bone. SYN: *osteoma spongiosum.*

osteosteatoma (ŏs″tē-ō-stē″ă-tō′mă) [″ + *stear,* fat, + *oma,* tumor]. A benign fatty tumor with bony elements.

osteostixis (ŏs″tē-ō-stĭk′sĭs) [″ + *stixis,* a puncture]. Therapeutic diagnostic puncture of a bone.

osteosuture (ŏs″tē-ō-sū′chūr) [″ + L. *sutura,* a stitch]. Suture or wiring of bone fragments. SYN: *osteorrhaphy.*

osteosynovitis (ŏs″tē-ō-sĭn″ō-vī′tĭs) [″ + *syn,* with, + *oon,* egg, + *itis,* inflammation]. Inflammation of a synovial membrane and the surrounding bones.

osteosynthesis (ŏs″tē-ō-sĭn′thē-sĭs) [″ + *synthesis,* a joining]. Surgical fastening of the ends of a fractured bone by mechanical means.

osteotabes (ŏs″tē-ō-tā′bēz) [″ + L. *tabes,* wasting]. Atrophy of the bone in infants, beginning with wasting of the marrow and gradually including the rest of the bone.

osteotelangiectasia (ŏs″tē-ō-tĕl-ăn″jē-ĕk-tā′zē-ă) [″ + *telos,* end, + *angeion,* vessel, + *ektasis,* a stretching]. Sarcomatous tumor of the bone containing dilated blood vessels.

osteothrombosis (ŏs″tē-ō-thrŏm-bō′sĭs) [″ + *thrombosis,* a clotting]. Clot formation in the veins of a bone.

osteotome (ŏs′tē-ō-tōm) [″ + *tome,* incision]. A chisel bevelled on both sides for cutting through bones.

osteotomoclasis (ŏs″tē-ō-tō-mŏk′lă-sĭs) [Gr. *osteon,* bone, + *tomos,* section, + *klasis,* breaking]. Correction of a pathologically curved bone by bending it after a wedge has been chiseled out of it by use of an osteotome.

osteotomy (ŏs-tē-ŏt'ō-mē) [" + *tome,* incision]. The operation for cutting through a bone.

o., cuneiform. The excision of a wedge of bone.

o., linear. Lengthwise division of a bone.

o., Macewen's. Supracondylar section of the femur for correction of knock-knee.

o., subtrochanteric. Division of shaft of femur below lesser trochanter to correct ankylosis of hip joint.

o., transtrochanteric. Section of the femur through the lesser trochanter for deformity about the hip joint.

osteotribe (ŏs'tē-ō-trīb") [" + *tribein,* to rub]. A bone rasp.

osteotrite (ŏs'tē-ō-trīt) [" + *tribein,* to grind or rub]. Instrument used to scrape away diseased bone.

osteotrophy (ŏs-tē-ŏt'rō-fē) [" + *trophe,* nutrition]. Bone nutrition.

osteotylus (ŏs"tē-ŏt'ī-lŭs) [" + *tylos,* callus]. The callus around the ends of bones that have been fractured.

osteotympanic (ŏs"tē-ō-tĭm-păn'ĭk). Craniotympanic, q.v.

ostial (ŏs'tē-ăl) [L. *ostium,* a little opening]. Concerning an orifice.

ostitis (ŏs-tī'tĭs) [" + *itis,* inflammation]. Inflammation of a bone. SYN: *osteitis.*

ostium (ŏs'tē-ŭm) [L.]. (pl. *ostia*) [NA] Small opening, esp. one into a tubular organ.

o. abdominale tubae uterinae. [NA] Fimbriated end of fallopian tube.

o. arteriosum. [NA] Arterial orifice of ventricle of the heart into the aorta or pulmonary artery.

o. internum. Uterine end of a fallopian tube.

o. pharyngeum. Pharyngeal opening of the auditory (eustachian) tube.

o. primum. The primary opening in the lower part of the septum of the atria of the embryonic heart. This closes shortly after birth.

o. primum defect. Atrial septal defect located low in septum.

o. secundum. An opening in the higher part of the septum of the atria of the embryonic heart. This closes shortly after birth.

o. secundum defect. Atrial septal defect located high in septal wall.

o. tympanicum. Tympanic opening of the auditory (eustachian) tube.

o. urethrae externum. [NA] External opening of the urethra.

o. uteri. The opening from the uterus to the vagina. SYN: *cervical os.*

o. uterinum tubae. The opening of the uterine tube into the uterus.

o. vaginae. [NA] External opening of the vagina.

ostomate (ŏs'tō-māt) [L. *ostium,* little opening]. One who has a surgically formed fistula connecting the bowel or intestine to the outside, usually through the abdominal wall. Thus an artificial anus exists at the ostomy site. SEE: *colostomy; ileostomy.*

ostomy (ŏs'tō-mē). The surgically formed artificial opening that serves as the exit site for connections that the surgeon has made from the bowel or intestine to the outside. SEE: *colostomy; ileostomy.*

OSTOMY CARE: Whether the ostomy is temporary or permanent, assure the patient that it will be possible to carry on normal activities with a minimum of inconvenience. Prior to being discharged from the hospital, the patient should be provided full explanation and demonstration of ostomy care. It is esp. important to have the patient and family become involved in ostomy care as soon as possible. This will promote confidence that a normal life will be possible. Consultation with another patient who has become competent in ostomy care will be esp. helpful. Those individuals may be contacted through ostomy clubs that have been organized in various cities. The patient should be provided with precise directions concerning places that sell ostomy care equipment. Detailed instructions for care and use of ostomy devices are included in the package.

Specific care involves the stoma (enterostomal care) and irrigation of the bowel leading from the stoma. In caring for a double-barrel colostomy, it is important to irrigate only the proximal stoma.

STOMA CARE: Character of material excreted through the stoma will depend on the portion of the bowel to which it is attached; excretions from the ileum will be fluid and quite irritating to skin; those from the upper right colon will be semi-fluid; those from the upper left colon are mushy; and those from the sigmoid colon will tend to be solid. Care of the stoma whether for ileostomy or colostomy is directed toward maintaining the peristomal skin and mucosa of the stoma in a healthy condition. This is more difficult to achieve with an ileostomy than with a lower colon colostomy. The skin surrounding the stoma can be protected by use of commercially available discs, or washers, made of karaya gum or hypoallergenic skin shields. The collecting bag or pouch can be attached to the karaya gum washer or skin shield so that a water-tight seal is made. The karaya gum washers can be used on weeping skin, but the skin shields cannot. New skin will grow beneath the karaya gum. The stoma may require only a gauze pad covering in the case of a sigmoid colostomy that is being irrigated daily or every other day. If a plastic bag is used for collecting drainage, it will need to be emptied periodically and changed as directed. At each change of the bag, meticulous but gentle skin care will be given. The stoma should not be manually dilated except by those experienced in enterostomal care.

IRRIGATION OF COLOSTOMY: Many individuals will be able to regulate the character of their diet so that the feces may be removed from the colon at planned intervals. The stoma is attached to a plastic bag held in place with a self-adhering collar or a belt. The irrigating fluid, tap water, or saline (1 teaspoonful salt, 4 grams, to one pint, 500 ml., of water) solution at 40°C (104°F) is introduced slowly through a soft rubber catheter. Catheter is inserted about 10 to 15 cm. and container for irrigating fluid is hung at height that will allow fluid to flow slowly. The return from the irrigation may be collected in a closed or open-ended bag. The latter will allow the return to empty into a basin or toilet. The return of fluid and feces should be completed in less than one half hour after irrigating fluid has entered bowel.

At the completion, clean the skin and stoma carefully and replace the dressing or the pouch. Then clean equipment thoroughly and store in a dry, well-ventilated space. When irrigation of ostomy is provided for a hospitalized patient, chart amount and kind of fluid instilled, amount and character or return, care provided for stoma and condition of stoma. If pouch or bag is attached, note whether or not it was replaced.

MISCELLANEOUS CONSIDERATIONS: *Odor* may be controlled by avoiding foods that the individual finds to cause undesirable odors. *Gas* may be controlled by avoiding foods known to produce gas, which will vary from patient to patient. *Diet* should be planned to provide stool consistency that will be neither hard and constipating nor loose and watery. The patient may learn this by trial and error and by consulting with nutritionists and ostomy club members. *Daily activities* including physical activity, sexual relations, and swimming are all possible. *References for Patient:* ET Journal—Official Publication of the International Association of Enterostomal Therapy, P.O. Box 67, Des Plaines, Illinois 60016; Journal of the Colostomy/Ileostomy Rehabilitation Association, P.O. Box 121, Philadelphia, Pennsylvania 19105.

ostosis (ŏs-tō'sĭs). Osteogenesis.

ostraceous (ŏs-trā'shŭs). Shaped like an oyster shell.

ostraco-, ostrac- [Gr. *ostrakon,* shell]. Combining form meaning hard shell.

ostreotoxismus (ŏs"trē-ō-tŏks-ĭz'mŭs) [Gr. *ostreon,* oyster, + *toxikon,* poison]. Poisoning from eating contaminated oysters.

O.T. *occupational therapy.*

otacoustic (ō"tă-koo'stĭk) [Gr. *otakousteo,* to listen]. 1. Aiding or concerning the hearing. 2. Device to aid hearing; an ear trumpet.

otalgia (ō-tăl'jē-ă) [Gr.]. Pain in the ear. SYN: *earache; otodynia; otoneuralgia.*

TREATMENT: *Local:* Heat in the form of compresses, hot water bottle, or warm glycerin dropped in ear. *General:* Nasal astringents to help maintain patency of the eustachian tube; relieve pain; use appropriate systemic antibiotic if there is an infection.

otantritis (ō"tăn-trī'tĭs) [Gr. *otos,* ear, + L. *antrum,* sinus, + Gr. *itis,* inflammation]. Inflammation of the mastoid antrum.

O.T.C. *over the counter.* Refers to drugs and devices available without a prescription.

OTD. *organ tolerance dose,* limitation of radiation tolerated by particular tissues.

otectomy (ō-tĕk'tō-mē) [Gr. *otos,* ear, + *ektome,* excision]. Surgical excision of the contents of the middle ear.

othelcosis (ō-thĕl-kō'sĭs) [" + *helkosis,* ulceration]. Ulceration or suppuration of the ear.

othematoma (ōt"hē-mă-tō'mă) [" + *haima,* blood, + *oma,* tumor]. Effusion of blood, causing a hard swelling between perichondrium and cartilage of pinna. Common in fighters and wrestlers. SYN: *hematoma auris.* SEE: *cauliflower ear.*

othemorrhea (ōt-hĕm"ō-rē'ă) [" + " + *rhoia,* flow]. Bleeding from the ear.

othygroma (ōt-hī-grō'mă) [" + *hygros,* moist, + *oma,* tumor]. Edema of ear lobe.

otic (ō'tĭk) [Gr. *otikos*]. Concerning the ear.

oticodinia (ō"tĭ-kō-dĭn'ē-ă) [Gr. *otikos,* aural, + *dine,* whirl]. Vertigo due to ear disease. SEE: *Ménière's disease; vertigo.*

otitic (ō-tĭt'ĭk). Concerning inflammation of the ear.

otitis (ō-tī'tĭs) [Gr. *otos,* ear, + *itis,* inflammation]. Inflamed condition of the ear. It is differentiated as externa, media, and interna, depending upon the portion of the ear which is inflamed.

o., aero-. Otitis resulting from pressure changes when auditory tubes are obstructed. Occurs commonly in aviators or divers.

o., aviation. Barotitis, q.v.

o. externa. Inflammation of the external auditory canal.

o., furuncular. Furuncle formation in the external meatus of the ear.

o. interna, labyrinthica. Labyrinthitis, q.v.

o. labyrinthica. Inflammation of the labyrinth of the ear.

o. mastoidea. Inflamed condition of the middle ear that involves the mastoid spaces.

o. media. Inflammation of the middle

ear.

o. mycotica. Inflammation of the ear caused by a fungal infection.

o. parasitica. Inflammation of the ear caused by a parasite.

o. sclerotica. Inflammation of inner ear accompanied by hardening of the aural structures.

oto-, ot- [Gr. *otos,* ear]. Combining form rel. to the ear.

otoantritis (ō″tō-ăn-trī′tĭs) [″ + *antron,* cavity, + *itis,* inflammation]. Inflamed condition of mastoid antrum and the tympanic attic.

otoblennorrhea (ō″tō-blĕn″ō-rē′ă) [″ + *blenna,* mucus, + *rhoia,* flow]. Mucous discharge from the ear.

otocatarrh (ō″tō-kă-tăr′) [″ + *katarrhein,* to flow down]. Catarrhal discharge of the ear.

otocephalus (ō″tō-sĕf′ă-lŭs). One with otocephaly.

otocephaly (ō″tō-sĕf′ă-lē) [″ + *kephale,* head]. Congenital absence of the lower jaw and fusion or near fusion of the ears on the front of the neck.

otocleisis (ō-tō-klī′sĭs) [″ + *kleisis,* closure]. Occlusion of any auditory passages.

otoconium (ō″tō-kō′nē-ŭm) [″ + *konis,* dust]. (pl. *otoconia*) Minute particles, composed chiefly of calcium carbonate, found in otolithic membrane on surface of maculae of inner ear. SYN: *ear dust; otolith.*

otocyst (ō′tō-sĭst) [″ + *kystis,* sac, bladder]. Primordial chamber from which arises the membranous labyrinth.

otodynia (ō″tō-dĭn′ē-ă) [″ + *odyne,* pain]. Pain in the ear; earache. SYN: *otalgia; otoneuralgia.*

otoganglion (ō″tō-găng′glē-ŏn) [″ + *ganglion,* ganglion]. The otic ganglion.

otogenic, otogenous (ō″tō-jĕn′ĭk, ō-tŏj′ĕn-ŭs) [″ + *gennan,* to produce]. Having its origin in the ear.

otography (ō-tŏg′ră-fē) [″ + *graphein,* to write]. A description of the ear.

otolaryngologist (ō″tō-lar″ĭn-gŏl′ō-jĭst) [″ + *larynx,* larynx, + *logos,* study]. A specialist in otolaryngology.

otolaryngology (ō″tō-lar″ĭn-gŏl′ō-jē). The division of medical science that includes otology, rhinology, and laryngology.

otolith (ō′tō-lĭth) [″ + *lithos,* stone]. Otoconium.

otological (ō″tō-lŏj′ĭ-kăl) [″ + *logos,* study]. Rel. to study of diseases of the ear.

otologist (ō-tŏl′ō-jĭst). One knowledgeable in the anatomy, physiology, and pathology of the ear. A specialist in diseases of the ear.

otology (ō-tŏl′ō-jē) [Gr. *otos,* ear, + *logos,* study]. The science dealing with the ear, its function, and its diseases.

otomassage [″ + *massein,* to knead]. Massage of the tympanic membrane and bones of the middle ear by means such as sound waves, puffs of air in the ear canal, or by vibratory percussion of the tympanic membrane.

otomucormycosis (ō″tō-mū″kor-mī-kō′sĭs) [″ + L. *mucor,* mold, + Gr. *mykes,* fungus, + *osis,* condition]. Mucormycosis, q.v., of the ear.

otomyasthenia (ō″tō-mī″ăs-thē′nē-ă) [″ + *mys,* muscle, + *astheneia,* weakness]. 1. Weakened condition of the ear muscles. 2. Defective hearing caused by paresis of the tensor tympani and stapedius muscles.

otomyces (ō″tō-mī′sēz) [″ + *mykes,* fungus]. Any fungus infection of the ear.

otomycosis (ō″tō-mī-kō′sĭs) [″ + ″ + *osis,* condition]. An infection of the external auditory meatus of the ear caused by a fungus infestation. SYN: *mycomyringitis; myringomycosis; otitis mycotica.*

otoncus (ō-tŏng′kŭs) [″ + *onkos,* tumor]. Tumor of the ear.

otonecrectomy, otonecronectomy (ō″tō-nē-krĕk′tō-mē, ō″tō-nē″krō-nĕk′tō-mē) [″ + *nekros,* dead, + *ektome,* excision]. Excision of necrosed areas from the ear.

otoneuralgia (ō″tō-nū-răl′jē-ă) [″ + *neuron,* sinew, + *algos,* pain]. Pain in the ear. SYN: *otalgia; otodynia.*

otoneurasthenia (ō″tō-nū″răs-thē′nē-ă) [″ + ″ + *astheneia,* weakness]. Neurasthenia caused by ear disease.

otoneurology (ō″tō-nū-rŏl′ō-jē) [″ + ″ + *logos,* study]. The division of otology that deals with the inner ear, esp. its nerve supply, nerve connections with the brain, and auditory and labyrinthine pathways and centers within the brain. SYN: *neurotology.*

otopathy (ō-tŏp′ă-thē) [″ + *pathos,* disease]. Any diseased condition of the ear.

otopharyngeal (ō″tō-făr-ĭn′jē-ăl) [″ + *pharynx,* pharynx]. Concerning the ear and pharynx.

otopharyngeal tube. Passage between the tympanic cavity and the pharynx. SEE: *eustachian tube.*

otoplasty (ō′tō-plăs″tē) [″ + *plassein,* to form]. Plastic surgery of the ear to correct defects and deformities.

otopolypus (ō″tō-pŏl′ĭ-pŭs) [″ + *polypous,* a morbid excrescence]. Smooth growth occurring in the ear.

otopyorrhea (ō″tō-pī″ō-rē′ă) [″ + *pyon,* pus, + *rhein,* to flow]. Purulent discharge from the ear.

otopyosis (ō″tō-pī-ō′sĭs) [″ + ″ + *osis,* infection]. Ear disease marked by discharge of pus.

otorhinolaryngology (ō″tō-rī″nō-lăr″ĭn-gŏl′ō-jē) [″ + *rhis,* nose, + *larynx,* larynx, + *logos,* study]. The science of ear, nose, and larynx and their functions and diseases.

otorhinology (ō″tō-rī-nŏl′ō-jē) [″ + ″ + *logos,* study]. Branch of medicine dealing with the ear and nose and their diseases.

otorrhagia (ō-tō-rā′jē-ă) [Gr. *otos,* ear, + *rhegnynai,* to burst forth]. Discharge of blood from the ear.

otorrhea (ō″tō-rē′ă) [″ + *rhoia,* flow]. Inflammation of ear with purulent discharge. SEE: *otitis.*

otosalpinx (ō″tō-săl′pĭnks) [″ + *salpinx,* trumpet]. Passage connecting pharynx and tympanic cavity. SYN: *eustachian tube; otopharyngeal tube.*

otoscleronectomy (ō″tō-sklē″rō-nĕk′tō-mē) [″ + *skleros,* hard, + *ektome,* excision]. Surgical excision of sclerosed and ankylosed ear ossicles.

otosclerosis (ō″tō-sklē-rō′sĭs) [″ + *sklerosis,* hardening]. Condition characterized by chronic progressive deafness, esp. for low tones. Caused by formation of spongy bone, esp. around the oval window with resulting ankylosis of stapes. In late stages, atrophy of the organ of Corti may occur. More common in females. May be made worse by pregnancy.

ETIOL: Unknown. In some cases, condition is familial.

TREATMENT: Various surgical procedures have been used with considerable improvement in hearing.

otoscope (ō′tō-skōp) [″ + *skopein,* to examine]. Device for examination of the ear.

otoscopy (ō-tŏs′kō-pē). Use of the otoscope in examining the ear.

otosis (ō-tō′sĭs) [″ + *osis,* condition]. Mishearing or misunderstanding of spoken sounds.

otosteal (ō-tŏs′tē-ăl) [″ + *osteon,* bone]. Concerning the bones or ossicles of the ear.

ototomy (ō-tŏt′ō-mē) [″ + *tome,* incision]. Incision into or dissection of the ear.

ototoxic (ō″tō-tŏk′sĭk) [″ + *toxikon,* poison]. Having a detrimental effect on the eighth nerve or the organs of hearing.

ototoxicity (ō″tō-tŏks-ĭs′ĭ-tē). The quality of being ototoxic.

O.T.R. *occupational therapist, registered.*

Otrivin Hydrochloride. Trade name for xylometazoline hydrochloride, USP.

Otto pelvis (ŏt′ō). [Adolph W. Otto, Ger. surgeon, 1786–1845] Protrusion of the acetabulum into the pelvic cavity. This may occur in association with severe osteoarthritis of the hip.

O.U., o.u. L. *oculus uterque,* for each eye.

ouabain (wă-bā′ĭn). USP. A glycoside prepared from Strophanthus gratus. Its action is similar to digitalis.

oulitis (oo-lī′tĭs) [Gr. *oulon,* gum, + *itis,* inflammation]. Ulitis.

oulorrhagia (oo-lō-rā′jē-ă) [″ + *rhegnynai,* to burst forth]. Hemorrhage from the gums. SYN: *ulorrhagia.*

ounce (owns) [L. *uncia,* a twelfth]. ABBR: oz. A measure of weight and liquid volume used in the apothecaries' system. When used in the avoirdupois system, ounce indicates only a unit of weight.

Apothecary or *troy* weight: SYMB: ℥. Equivalent to 1/12 pound, 480 grains, 31.103 grams. When used in U.S. Pharmacopeia, 1 oz. contains 8 drams.

Avoirdupois measure: Equivalent to 1/16 pound, 437.5 grains, 28.349 grams.

o., fluid. Apothecaries' measure for liquid medicines, 8 fluid drams (1/16 pint, 29.6 milliliters).

outflow. In neurology, the passage of impulses outwardly from the central nervous system.

o., craniosacral. Impulses passing through parasympathetic nerves.

o., thoracolumbar. Impulses passing through sympathetic nerves.

outlet. A vent or opening for something to escape.

o., pelvic. SEE: *pelvic outlet.*

outpatient. One who receives treatment at a hospital, clinic, or dispensary but is not hospitalized.

outpocketing. Evagination, q.v.

output (owt′poot). That which is produced, ejected, or expelled.

o., cardiac. Volume of blood pumped into the arterial system per unit of time. The stroke volume multiplied by the heart rate per minute gives the cardiac output.

o., energy. The work expended per unit of time by the body.

o., stroke. The amount of blood pumped in a single heartbeat.

o., urinary. The amount of urine produced by the kidneys.

ova (ō′vă) [L. *ovum,* egg]. Pl. of ovum.

oval (ō′văl) [L. *ovalis,* egg shaped]. 1. Concerning an ovum, the reproductive cell of the female. 2. Having an elliptical shape like an egg.

ovalbumin (ō″văl-bū′mĭn) [″ + *albumen,* albumin]. Albumin occurring in egg white.

ovalocyte (ō′văl-ō-sīt″) [″ + Gr. *kytos,* cell]. Elliptical red blood corpuscle.

ovalocytosis (ō-văl″ō-sī-tō′sĭs) [″ + ″ + *osis,* condition]. Abnormally large amount of elliptical red blood corpuscles in the blood.

oval window. Oval-shaped aperture in the middle ear into which fits the base of the stapes.

ovaralgia, ovarialgia (ō″văr-ăl′jē-ă, -ē-ăl′jē-ă) [L. *ovarium,* ovary, + Gr. *algos,* pain]. Ovarian pain. SYN: *oarialgia, oophoralgia.*

ovarian (ō-vā′rē-ăn) [L. *ovarium,* ovary]. Concerning or resembling the ovary.

ovarian cyst. A sac that develops in the ovary proper. It consists of one or more chambers containing fluid. These loculi, or chambers, may contain an enormous amount of fluid. Although nonmalignant, the cyst may have to be surgically removed because of twisting of the pedicle, which causes gangrene, or because of pressure. SEE: *polycystic ovaries.*

ovariectomy (ō″vā-rē-ĕk′tō-mē) [″ + Gr. *ektome,* excision]. Excision of an ovary or a portion of it. SYN: *oophorectomy.*

ovario- [Gr. *ovarium,* ovary]. Combining form indicating relationship to the ovary.

ovariocele (ō-vā′rē-ō-sēl) [″ + Gr. *kele,* mass]. Ovarian tumor or hernia.

ovariocentesis (ō-vā″rē-ō-sĕn-tē′sĭs) [″ + Gr. *kentesis,* puncture]. Surgical puncture and drainage of an ovarian cyst.

ovariocyesis (ō-vā″rē-ō-sī-ē′sĭs) [″ + Gr. *kyesis,* pregnancy]. Pregnancy in the ovary. SEE: *ectopic gestation.*

ovariodysneuria (ō-vā″rē-ō-dĭs-nū′rē-ă) [″ + Gr. *dys,* ill, + *neuron,* sinew]. Neuralgia in an ovary.

ovariogenic (ō-vā″rē-ō-jĕn′ĭk) [″ + *gennan,* to produce]. Originating in the ovary.

ovariohysterectomy (ō-vā″rē-ō-hĭs″tĕr-ĕk′tō-mē) [″ + Gr. *hystera,* uterus, + *ektome,* excision]. Excision of the ovaries and uterus. SYN: *oophorohysterectomy; oothecohysterectomy.*

ovariopathy (ō-vā″rē-ŏp′ă-thē) [″ + *pathos,* disease]. Disease of the ovary.

ovariopexy (ō-vā″rē-ō-pĕk′sē) [″ + *pexis,* fixation]. Surgical fixation of the ovary to the abdominal wall.

ovariorrhexis (ō-vā″rē-ō-rĕk′sĭs) [″ + Gr. *rhexis,* a rupture]. Rupture of an ovary.

ovariosalpingectomy (ō-vā″rē-ō-săl″pĭn-jĕk′tō-mē) [″ + Gr. *salpinx,* tube, + *ektome,* excision]. Removal of an ovary and oviduct. SYN: *oophorosalpingectomy.*

ovariosteresis (ō-vā″rē-ō-stĕr-ē′sĭs) [″ + Gr. *steresis,* loss]. Removal of an ovary.

ovariostomy (ō-vā″rē-ŏs′tō-mē) [″ + Gr. *stoma,* opening]. Creation of an opening in an ovarian cyst for drainage purpose.

ovariotexy. Surgical procedure for encompassing the ovaries in a Silastic bag in order to prevent contact of the ovum with sperm.

ovariotomy (ō-vā″rē-ŏt′ō-mē) [L. *ovarium,* ovary, + Gr. *tome,* incision]. 1. Incision into, or removal of, an ovary. 2. Removal of a tumor of the ovary.

ovariotubal (ō-vā″rē-ō-tū′băl) [″ + *tuba,* a narrow duct]. Concerning the ovary and the oviducts.

ovariprival (ō-vā″rĭ-prī′văl) [″ + *privare,* to remove]. Resulting from loss of the ovaries.

ovaritis (ō″vă-rī′tĭs) [″ + Gr. *itis,* inflammation]. Inflamed condition of an ovary. Usually involved secondarily in inflammation of the oviducts or pelvic peritoneum. May involve the substance of the organ (oophoritis) or its surface (perioophoritis), and may be acute or chronic.

ovarium (ō-vā′rē-ŭm) [L.]. (pl. *ovaria*) [NA] The ovary.

ovary (ō′vă-rē) [L. *ovarium,* ovary]. One of two glands in the female that produce the reproductive cell, the ovum, and two known hormones. The ovaries are almond-shaped bodies lying in the fossa ovarica on either side of the pelvic cavity, attached to the uterus by the utero-ovarian ligament and lying close to the fimbria ovarica of the fallopian tube. About 4 cm. long, 2 cm. wide, and 8 mm. thick. Each ovary is attached to the broad ligament by the mesovarium and to the side of the pelvis by the suspensory ligament. The surface of the ovary in early life is smooth and in later life is markedly pitted as an end result of the atrophy of corpora lutea.

STRUCTURE: Each ovary consists of two parts, an outer portion or cortex, which encloses a central medulla. The medulla consists of a stroma of connective tissue containing nerves, blood, and lymphatic vessels, and some smooth muscle tissue at region of hilus. The cortex consists principally of follicles in various stages of development (primary, growing, and mature or graafian). Its surface is covered by a single layer of cells, the germinal epithelium, beneath which is a layer of dense connective tissue, the tunica albuginea. Other structures (corpus luteum, corpus albicans, q.v.) may be present. SEE: illus.

BLOOD SUPPLY: Mainly derived from the ovarian artery, which reaches the ovary through the infundibulopelvic ligament.

FUNCT: 1. The production of ova. 2. The production of hormones, among which are estrogen, secreted by the follicles, and progesterone, secreted by the corpus luteum. These hormones are responsible for development and maintenance of secondary sexual characteristics, preparation of uterus for pregnancy, and development of the mammary gland.

Functional activity of the ovary is controlled primarily by gonadotrophins of the hypophysis, esp. the follicle-stimulating hormone (FSH) and luteinizing hormone (LH) or interstitial cell hormone (ICH).

ovary, words pert. to: adnexitis; albuginea; castrate; cell, interstitial; conception; corpus albicans; facies ovarina; fertilization; fimbria ovarica; folliculoma; graafian follicle; hyperovaria; Krukenberg's tumor; menstrual cycle; menstruation; mesosalpinx; mesovarium; oarialgia; polycystic ovaries; pyoovarium; spay; spermatozoon; teratoma; tunica albuginea; and words beginning with "oophor-" and "ov-".

overbite. The vertical extension of the incisal

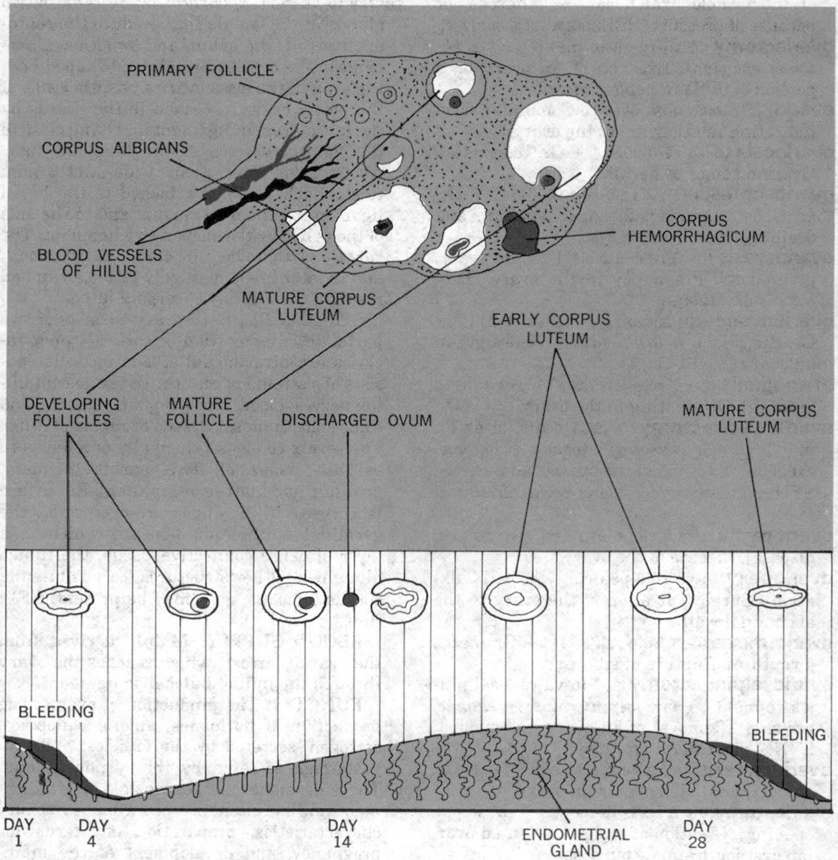

ENDOMETRIAL CYCLE
CORRELATED WITH FOLLICLE,
AND CORPUS LUTEUM DEVELOPMENT

ridges of the upper teeth over the incisal ridges of the lower anterior teeth when the jaws are in occlusion.

Ovcon. Trade name for estrogen combined with progestogen.

overclosure. A form of defective bite in which the mandible closes too far before the teeth make contact.

overcompensation. The process by which a person substitutes an opposite trait or exerts effort in excess of that needed to compensate for, or conceal, a psychological feeling of guilt, inadequacy, or inferiority. May lead to maladjustment.

overcorrection. The use of too powerful a lens to correct the defect in refractive power of the eye.

overdenture. A denture supported by the soft tissue and whatever natural teeth remain. These have been altered so the denture will fit over them.

overdetermination. The idea in psychoanalysis that every symptom and dream may have several meanings, being determined by more than a single association.

overdose. ABBR: O.D. A dose of a drug, esp.

a drug of abuse, sufficient to cause an acute reaction such as coma, mania, hysteria, or even death.

overeruption. Condition in which the occluding surface of a tooth projects beyond the line of occlusion.

overexertion. Physical exertion to a state of abnormal exhaustion.

overextension. 1. Extension beyond that which usually occurs. SYN: *hyperextension.* 2. In dentistry, the assessment of the vertical extent of a root canal filling, denoting an extrusion beyond the apical foramen.

overflow. The continuous escape of fluid from a vessel or viscus, as of urine or tears.

overgrowth. 1. Excessive growth. SYN: *hyperplasia; hypertrophy.* 2. In bacteriology, the growth of one type of microorganism on a culture plate so that it covers and obscures the growth of other types.

overhang. The extension beyond the margins of a cavity of the excess filling material used. This is not the desired outcome.

overhydration. An excess of fluids in the body.

overjet. Horizontal overlap of the teeth.

overlap. Something that covers the tissue or object but also extends past the border.

overlay. 1. An addition superimposed upon an already existing state. 2. In dentistry, a cast restoration that restores the occlusal surface of one or more cusps of a tooth but not a three-quarter- or full-cast crown.

o., psychogenic. The emotional component of a symptom or illness that has an organic basis.

overproduction. Excessive output of an organic element during the reparative process, as excessive callous development after a bone fracture.

overresponse. An abnormally intense reaction to a stimulus; inappropriate degree of response.

overriding. The slipping of one end of a fractured bone past the other part.

overtoe. Hallux varus of the great toe to the extent that it rests over the other toes.

overtone. In music and acoustics, a harmonic.

overvalued idea. An unreasonable and strongly held belief or idea that is maintained with less than delusional intensity. Such a belief is beyond the norm of beliefs held or accepted by other members of the person's culture or subculture.

overventilation. Hyperventilation, q.v.

ovi- [L. *ovum,* egg]. Combining form meaning egg.

ovi albumen (ō″vē-ăl-bū′mĭn) [L.]. White of egg. SYN: *ovalbumin.*

ovicide (ō′vĭ-sīd) [L. *ovum,* egg, + *caedere,* to kill]. Destructive to ova.

oviduct (ō′vĭ-dŭkt) [″ + *ductus,* a path]. One of two tubes extending laterally from superior angles of the uterus; serves to convey the ovum from the ovary to the uterus. Each oviduct consists of the infundibulum, expanded portion surrounding the ostium or opening through which the ovum enters, bearing many fingerlike processes called fimbria; the ampulla, the tube itself; and the isthmus, a straight narrow portion that connects with the uterus.

Each oviduct is a muscular tube consisting of three layers: mucosa, muscular layer, and serosa. The mucosa consists of columnar epithelial cells, some ciliated, others glandular. In addition to conveying the ovum, the oviduct provides a passageway through which sperm travel from the uterus toward the ovary. It is the usual site of fertilization of the ovum. SYN: *fallopian tube; uterine tube.*

oviferous (ō-vĭf′ĕr-ŭs) [″ + *ferre,* to bear]. Containing or producing ova.

oviform (ō′vĭ-form) [″ + *forma,* shape]. 1. Having the shape of an egg. SYN: *ovoid.* 2. Resembling an ovum.

ovigenesis [″ + Gr. *gennan,* to produce]. Oogenesis.

ovigerm (ō′vĭ-jĕrm) [″ + *germen,* a bud]. The cell that produces or develops into an ovum.

ovination (ō″vĭ-nā′shŭn) [L. *ovinus,* of a sheep]. Inoculation with the virus of sheep-pox.

ovine (ō′vīn) [L. *ovinus,* of a sheep]. Concerning sheep

ovinia (ō-vĭn′ē-ă) [L. *ovinus,* of a sheep]. Sheep-pox.

oviparity (ō″vĭ-păr′ĭ-tē). Quality of being oviparous.

oviparous (ō-vĭp′ăr-ŭs) [L. *ovum,* egg, + *parere,* to produce]. Producing eggs that are hatched outside the body; egg laying. Opposite of ovoviviparous.

oviposition [″ + *ponere,* to place]. The laying of eggs as in oviparous reproduction.

ovipositor (ō″vĭ-pŏs′ĭ-tor). A specialized tubular structure found in many female insects, through which they lay their eggs in plants or soil.

ovisac (ō′vĭ-săk). The graafian follicle.

ovo- [L. *ovum,* egg]. Combining form indicating rel. to an egg.

ovocenter. The centrosome of a fertilized ovum.

ovocyte (ō′vō-sīt) [″ + *kytos,* cell]. Oocyte.

ovoflavin (ō″vō-flā′vĭn) [″ + *flavus,* yellow]. A flavin derived from eggs; identical to riboflavin.

ovogenesis (ō″vō-jĕn′ĕ-sĭs) [″ + Gr. *genesis,* production]. Production of ova. SYN: *oogenesis.*

ovoglobulin (ō″vō-glŏb′ū-lĭn) [″ + *globulus,* globule]. The globulin found in egg white. SEE: *albumin; protein, simple.*

ovogonium (ō″vō-gō′nē-ŭm). Oogonium.

ovoid (ō′voyd) [L. *ovum,* egg, + Gr. *eidos,*

form]. Egg shaped. SYN: *oviform.*

ovomucin (ō″vō-mū′sĭn). A glycoprotein in the white of an egg.

ovomucoid (ō″vō-mū′koyd) [″ + *mucus,* mucus, + Gr. *eidos,* form]. A glycoprotein principle derived from egg white.

ovoplasm (ō′vō-plăzm) [″ + Gr. *plasma,* anything formed]. Protoplasm of an unfertilized egg. SEE: *ooplasm.*

ovotestis (ō″vō-tĕs′tĭs). A gonad that contains both testicular and ovarian tissue.

ovovitellin (ō″vō-vī-tĕl′ĭn) [″ + *vitellus,* yolk]. Protein found in an egg yolk.

ovoviviparous (ō″vō-vī-vĭp′ă-rŭs) [″ + *vivus,* alive, + *parere,* to bear]. Reproducing by eggs that have a well-developed membrane and that hatch inside the maternal organism. Opposite of oviparous.

Ovral. Trade name for estrogen combined with progestogen.

Ovrette. Trade name for norgestrel, USP.

ovula (ŏv′ū-lă) [L.]. Pl. of ovulum.

ovular (ō′vū-lăr) [L. *ovulum,* little egg]. Concerning an ovule or ovum.

ovulation (ŏv″ū-lā′shŭn) [L. *ovulum,* little egg]. The periodic ripening and rupture of the mature graafian follicle and the discharge of the ovum from the cortex of the ovary. Ovulation occurs approximately 14 days before the next menstrual period. It is virtually impossible to determine when ovulation will occur by counting from the first day of the preceding menstrual period. Following ovulation, a corpus luteum develops within the collapsed follicle. The ovum, being liberated from the follicle, enters the fallopian tube and is transported slowly toward the uterus. If sperm are present, it may become fertilized; if not, the ovum degenerates within the oviduct and is passed out of the body with the menstrual flow.

RS: anovular; conception; corpus luteum; fertilization; follicle; menstruation; ovary; ovum; spermatozoon.

ovulatory (ŏv′ū-lă-tō″rē). Concerning ovulation.

ovule (ō′vūl) [L. *ovulum*]. 1. The ovum in the graafian follicle. 2. A small egg.

Ovulen. Trade name for estrogen combined with progestogen.

ovulogenous (ō-vū-lŏj′ĕn-ŭs). 1. Giving rise to ovules or ova. 2. Originating from an ovule or ovum.

ovulum (ŏv′ū-lŭm) [L. *ovulum,* little egg]. (pl. *ovula*) A small egglike structure; the ovum.

ovum (ō′vŭm) [L., egg]. (pl. *ova*) [NA] The female reproductive or germ cell; a cell that is capable of developing into a new organism of the same species. Usually fertilization by a spermatozoon is necessary, although in some lower animals ova develop without fertilization (parthenogenesis).

The various parts of the ovum have been named as follows: The protoplasm is known as the vitellus or yolk; the outer layer is referred to as the ectoplasm; zona pellucida, or zona radiata; the inner layer, the cell membrane, is the vitelline membrane; the nucleus is called the germinal vesicle; and the nucleolus, the germinal spot.

The cellular layers proliferate, becoming cuboid in shape, and in the center a clear albuminous fluid, the liquor folliculi, forms. The follicular cells surrounding the fluid-filled cavity are known as the membrana granulosa. The layer surrounding the egg cell, or oocyte, is known as the discus proligerus or cumulus oophorus.

As the follicular layer enlarges to form the graafian follicle, the term for the developed ovum before it leaves the ovary, there is a slight protrusion of the ovarian surface. Rupture through the ovarian surface frees the ovum, which then proceeds through the fallopian tube and into the uterus. This process is known as ovulation, q.v. It usually takes the ovum from 5 to 7 days to go from the ovary to the uterus. Normally, only one graafian follicle matures each month, not necessarily in alternate ovaries. SEE: illus.;

HUMAN OVUM

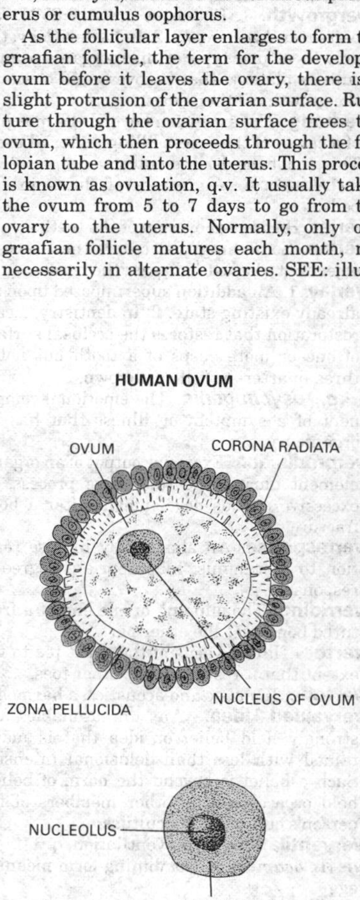

conception; fertilization; menstrual cycle; menstruation.

o., alecithal. Ovum with a small yolk portion that is distributed throughout the protoplasm.

o., centrolecithal. Ovum having a large central food yolk, as in a bird's egg.

o., holoblastic. Ovum that undergoes complete cleavage.

o., human. The female reproductive cell that develops within the graafian follicle of the ovary. It develops from an oogonium that undergoes a process of maturation (oogenesis) during which primary and secondary oocytes are produced, finally giving rise to the mature ovum. During this process, the number of chromosomes is reduced from 46 to 23 and the egg is prepared for fertilization.

A mature ovum is approximately 0.130 to 0.140 mm. (.0051 to .0055 in.) in diameter. Each contains a spherical nucleus, bounded by a nuclear membrane, enclosing chromatin material and one or more nucleoli. The cytoplasm is granular and contains yolk granules or deuteroplasm and other characteristic organoids of cells. Its surface layer is the vitelline membrane. When liberated from the ovary as a primary oocyte, it is surrounded by a clear layer, zona pellucida, and several layers of adhering follicular cells, the latter constituting the corona radiata.

The length of time a human ovum retains its ability to be fertilized and develop is not known precisely but it is probably at least 48 hours. If fertilized, it undergoes development. If not fertilized, it degenerates. SEE: *cleavage; conception; embryo, development of; fertilization; follicle; menstruation; ovulation; spermatozoon.*

o., isolecithal. O., alecithal.

o., meroblastic. Ovum in which only the protoplasmic region undergoes cleavage; characteristic in ova containing a large amount of yolk.

o., permanent. An ovum that is ready for fertilization.

o., primordial. Germ cells that arise very early in development of the embryo, usually in the yolk sac endoderm, migrate into the urogenital ridge, and possibly serve as progenitors of functional sex cells.

o., telolecithal. Ovum in which yolk is fairly abundant and tends to concentrate in one hemisphere.

Owren's disease. Parahemophilia.

ox-. Combining form indicating presence of oxygen.

oxa-. Combining form indicating presence of oxygen in place of carbon.

oxacillin (ŏks″ă-sĭl′ĭn). A semisynthetic penicillin.

o. sodium. USP. An antibiotic drug. Trade names are Prostaphlin and Bactocill.

oxal-, oxalo-. Combining forms indicating derivation from oxalic acid.

oxalacetic acid (ŏks″ăl-ă-sē′tĭk). A product of carbohydrate metabolism HOOC·CH_2·CO·COOH resulting from oxidation of malic acid. May be derived from other sources.

oxalate (ŏk′să-lāt) [Gr. *oxalis,* sorrel]. A salt of oxalic acid.

o., potassium. The potassium salt of oxalic acid.

oxalemia (ŏk″să-lē′mē-ă) [″ + *haima,* blood]. Excess oxalates in the blood.

oxalic acid (ŏks-ăl′ĭk). A white crystalline powder often used about the home as a stain remover or bleach, resembling Epsom salts in appearance. SYN: *ethanedioic acid.*

SOURCES: Cranberries, chard, rhubarb, gooseberries, spinach, beet leaves. When these are eaten they should be accompanied by liberal portions of calcium foods, such as eggs, beans, and milk.

oxalic acid poisoning. Acute poisoning occurs when oxalic acid is accidentally ingested; or by eating large quantities of foods rich in oxalic acid. Ingestion of 5 grams may be fatal. Chronic poisoning may result from inhalation of vapors. SEE: *Poisons and Poisoning* in *Appendix.*

SYM: Corrosive action on mucosa of mouth, esophagus, and stomach; sour taste; burning in mouth, throat, and stomach; great thirst; bloody vomitus; collapse; sometimes convulsions and coma.

TREATMENT: Prompt treatment with any soluble calcium salt such as powdered chalk in water or milk, lime, water, or calcium lactate. This procedure inactivates the acid by precipitating it as an insoluble calcium salt. Careful gastric lavage with dilute lime water. Do not induce vomiting. Intravenous calcium gluconate or calcium chloride to treat tetany. Morphine may be required for pain.

Oxalid. Trade name for oxyphenbutazone, USP.

oxalism (ŏks′ăl-ĭzm) [Gr. *oxalis,* sorrel, + *-ismos,* state of]. Poisoning from oxalic acid or an oxalate.

oxalosis. An autosomal recessive hereditary disease due to faulty metabolism of glyoxylic acid. Oxalic acid is elevated in the urine due to increased production of oxalic acid. Calcium oxalate is deposited in body tissues but especially in the kidneys.

oxaluria (ŏk-să-lū′rē-ă) [″ + *ouron,* urine]. Excess excretion of oxalates in the urine, esp. calcium oxalate.

oxalylurea (ŏk″săl-ĭl-ū-rē′ă). An oxidation product of uric acid.

oxandrolone (ŏk-săn′drō-lōn). USP. An anabolic steroid. Trade name is Anavar.

oxazepam (ŏks-ăz′ĕ-păm). USP. A tranquilizer drug. Trade name is Serax.

oxidant (ŏk′sĭ-dănt). In oxidation-reduction reactions, the acceptor of an electron.

oxidase (ŏk′sĭ-dās) [Gr. *oxys,* sharp]. A class of enzymes present in animal and vegetable life. It catalyzes an oxidation reaction; a respiratory enzyme.

o., cytochrome. Enzyme, present in most cells, that oxidizes reduced cytochrome back to cytochrome.

oxidation (ŏk′sĭ-dā′shŭn) [Gr. *oxys,* sharp]. 1. The process of a substance combining with oxygen. 2. The loss of electrons in an atom with an accompanying increase in positive valence. SEE: *reduce* (def. 2).

oxidation-reduction reaction. Chemical interaction wherein one substance is oxidized and loses electrons and, thus, is increased in positive valence, while another substance gains an equal number of electrons by being reduced. This is called a redox system or reaction.

oxide (ŏk′sīd). Any chemical compound in which oxygen is the negative radical.

oxidize (ŏk′sĭ-dīz). 1. To combine with oxygen. 2. To increase the positive valence, or to decrease the negative valence, by bringing about a loss of electrons. SYN: *oxygenize.* SEE: *oxidation-reduction reaction.*

oxidoreductase (ŏk″sĭ-dō-rē-dŭk′tās). An enzyme that catalyzes oxidation-reduction reactions.

oxim, oxime (ŏk′sĭm). Any compound produced by the action of hydroxylamine on an aldehyde or ketone. When an aldehyde is involved, the general formula RCH=NOH is produced. When a ketone is acted upon, $R_2CH{=}NOH$ is produced.

oximeter (ŏk-sĭm′ĕ-ter) [Gr. *oxys,* sharp, + *metron,* measure]. Photoelectric apparatus for determining the amount of oxygen in the blood. Usually done by measuring the amount of light transmitted through a translucent part of the skin.

o., ear. Oximeter that attaches to the pinna of the ear to determine the degree of oxygen saturation of blood flowing through the ear.

Oxlopar. Trade name for oxytetracycline hydrochloride, USP.

oxonemia (ŏk″sō-nē′mē-ă) [L. *oxone,* acetone, + Gr. *haima,* blood]. Excess of acetone bodies found in the blood. SYN: *acetonemia.*

oxophenarsine hydrochloride. An antitrypanosomal compound containing 30% arsenic.

oxprenolol hydrochloride (ŏks-prĕn′ō-lōl). A beta-adrenergic blocking agent. It is used as a coronary vasodilator.

oxtriphylline (ŏks-trĭf′ĭ-lēn). USP. A drug that resembles theophylline in its actions. Trade name is Choledyl.

oxy- [Gr. *oxys*]. Combining form indicating (1) sharp, keen, acute, acid, pungent; (2) presence of oxygen in a compound; (3) presence of a hydroxyl group.

oxyacoia (ŏk″sē-ă-koy′ă). Oxyecoia, q.v.

oxyacusis (ŏk″sē-ă-kū′sĭs) [Gr. *oxys,* sharp, + *akousis,* hearing]. Abnormally acute hearing. SYN: *hyperacusis.*

oxybenzene (ŏk″sē-bĕn′zēn). Phenol.

oxybenzone (ŏk″sē-bĕn′zōn). USP. A sunscreen agent used topically. Trade names are Spectra-Sorb UV9 and Uvinul M-40.

oxyblepsia (ŏk″sē-blĕp′sē-ă) [Gr. *oxys,* sharp, + *blepsis,* vision]. Extraordinary acuteness of vision.

oxybutyria (ŏk″sē-bū-tĭr′ē-ă). Oxybutyric acid in the urine.

oxycalcium (ŏk″sē-kăl′sē-ŭm). Of or pert. to oxygen and calcium.

Oxycel. Trade name for cellulose, oxidized, USP.

oxycephalia, oxycephaly (ŏk″sē-sĕf-ā′lē-ă, -sĕf′ă-lē) [Gr. *oxys,* sharp, + *kephale,* head]. State of having a high and pointed skull.

oxycephalous (ŏk-sē-sĕf′ă-lŭs). Denoting a head that is pointed and conelike.

oxychloride (ŏk″sē-klō′rīd) [Gr. *oxys,* sharp, + *chloros,* green]. A compound consisting of an element or radical combined with oxygen and chlorine or the hydroxyl radical (OH) and chlorine.

oxychromatic (ŏk″sē-krō-măt′ĭk) [″ + *chroma,* color]. Staining readily with acid dyes.

oxychromatin (ŏk″sē-krō′mă-tĭn). That part of chromatin that stains readily with acid dyes.

oxycinesia (ŏk″sē-sĭ-nē′zē-ă) [″ + *kinesis,* movement]. The experiencing of pain when movement occurs.

oxyecoia (ŏk″sē-ē-koy′ă) [″ + *akoe,* hearing]. Abnormal sensitivity to noises.

oxyesthesia (ŏk″sē-ĕs-thē′zē-ă) [″ + *aisthesis,* sensation]. Abnormal acuteness of sensation. SYN: *algesia; hyperesthesia.*

oxygen (ŏk′sĭ-jĕn) [Gr. *oxys,* sharp, + *gennan,* to produce]. USP. 1. A standardized preparation of oxygen used as a medicinal gas. 2. SYMB: O. At. wt. 15.9994; at. no. 8. A nonmetallic element occurring free in the atmosphere as a colorless, odorless, tasteless gas. It is a constituent of animal, vegetable, and mineral substances. Oxygen is essential to respiration of most forms of animal and plant life and is the most important and abundant element. At sea level, it represents 10 to 16% of venous and 17 to 21% of arterial blood.

It is the only element that enters the animal organism in a free state. It is absorbed by plants in the form of water and carbon dioxide, converted by them into organic substances that are used as food by man, and returned to the atmosphere by man in form of waste products of water and carbon dioxide. Thus the balance of oxygen and carbon dioxide in the atmosphere is maintained.

When oxygen combines with another substance, the process is called oxidation. When combination takes place rapidly enough to produce light and heat, the process is called burning or combustion. Oxygen combines readily with other elements to form oxides.

USES: In conditions in which there is insufficient oxygen carried by the blood to the tissues. Therefore oxygen is used in cases of severe anemia, shock or circulatory collapse, pulmonary edema, pneumonia; or by mountain climbers, astronauts, or aviators when at heights where the amount of oxygen present in the atmosphere is insufficient to support life.

Frequently oxygen is employed with ether or other agents used for the induction of general anesthesia. Following extensive surgery, it reduces reactions to the anesthetic. Also employed in septicemia, gas gangrene, peritonitis, and intestinal obstruction.

Oxygen is used in pressure chambers for cardiac surgery; in treating aerobic infections such as gas gangrene; vascular disorders; bends, q.v.; carbon monoxide poisoning; and in connection with radiation therapy for tumors. When oxygen is administered in this manner it is called hyperbaric oxygenation.

ADM: Oxygen is administered by mask, nasal tube, tent, or by placing the patient in an airtight chamber in which pressure may be increased. No matter how much oxygen is given, it is important to have it adequately humidified. It is desirable to administer oxygen at whatever rate is necessary to increase the oxygen content of inspired air to 50%.

CAUTION: Inhalation of high concentrations of oxygen, esp. at pressures of more than one atmosphere, may produce deleterious effects such as irritation of respiratory tract, reduced vital capacity, and sometimes neurological symptoms. Serious eye defects may result if premature infants are exposed as part of their therapy to a high concentration of oxygen. SEE: *retrolental fibroplasia*.

Because oxygen provides perfect support of combustion, it should not be used in the presence of oil, lighted cigarettes or open flames or where there is the possibility of electrical or spark hazards.

oxygenase (ŏk′sĭ-jĕn-ās″) [Gr. *oxys*, sharp, + *gennan*, to produce, + *-ase*, enzyme]. An enzyme that enables an organism to use atmospheric oxygen in respiration.

oxygenate (ŏk′sĭ-jĕn-āt). To combine or supply with oxygen.

oxygenation (ŏk″sĭ-jĕn-ā′shŭn). Saturation or combination with oxygen, as the aeration of the blood in the lungs.

o., hyperbaric. Administration of oxygen under increased pressure while the patient is in an airtight chamber. Used for certain surgical procedures, treatment of aerobic infections such as gas gangrene, and in conjunction with radiation therapy of tumors.

oxygenator (ŏk″sĭ-jĕ-nā′tor). A device for mechanically oxygenating anything but esp. blood. When used to oxygenate blood, it is usually used during thoracic surgery or open-heart surgery.

o., bubble. Device for bubbling oxygen through the blood during extracorporeal circulation.

o., rotating disk. Device for oxygenating blood during extracorporeal circulation. A thin film of blood attaches to a disk as it dips into the blood flow. The portion of the disk not in the blood is rotating in an atmosphere of oxygen

o., screen. During extracorporeal circulation, the blood passes over a series of screens that are in an oxygen atmosphere. Oxygen is exchanged in the thin film of blood on the screens.

oxygen capacity. The maximum amount of oxygen expressed in volume percent (cc. per 100 ml.) that a given amount of blood will absorb. For normal blood it is about 20 cc.

oxygen content. The amount of oxygen in volume percent that is present in the blood at any one moment.

oxygen debt or deficit. After strenuous, i.e., anaerobic, physical activity, the oxygen required, in addition to that required while resting, in the recovery period to oxidize the excess lactic acid produced; and to replenish the depleted stores of adenosine triphosphate and phosphocreatinase.

oxygen dissociation curve. A curve that shows relationship between partial pressure of oxygen and the percentage saturation of hemoglobin with oxygen, i.e., the proportion of oxyhemoglobin to reduced hemoglobin. Factors that favor shift of curve to the right, accelerating the decomposition of hemoglobin, are a rise in temperature and an increase of H ions that results from liberation of CO_2 and formation of lactic acid.

oxygenic (ŏk″sĭ-jĕn′ĭk) [″ − *gennan*, to produce]. Concerning, resembling, containing, or consisting of oxygen.

oxygenize. Oxidize.

oxygen saturation. Oxygen content of blood divided by oxygen capacity and expressed in volume percent.

oxygen tent. An airtight enclosure for a patient's head and shoulders in which the oxygen content of the air can be raised above normal.

oxygen therapy. The administration of oxygen for the treatment of conditions resulting from oxygen deficiency. It is used to combat acute arterial anoxia that may result from pneumonia, pulmonary edema, or obstruction to breathing. It is also employed in congestive heart failure, coronary thrombosis, and following surgery. It may be administered by nasal catheter, mask (nasal or oronasal), funnel or cone, oxygen tent, or special oxygen chamber, and usually in a concentration of 70 to 100%.

oxygen toxicity. Progressive failure of ventilation of the lungs that develops when pure oxygen is breathed for a prolonged period. Failure of ventilation leads to decreased oxygen tension in the blood.

oxygeusia (ŏk"sē-gū'sē-ă) [Gr. *oxys,* sharp, + *geusis,* taste]. Abnormally keen sense of taste.

oxyhematin (ŏk"sē-hĕm'ă-tĭn). An iron compound that constitutes the coloring matter in oxyhemoglobin. When oxidized it yields hematinic acid; when reduced, hematoporphyrin.

oxyhematoporphyrin (ŏk"sē-hĕm"ă-tō-por'fĭ-rĭn). A derivative of hematoporphyrin. It is sometimes present in urine.

oxyhemoglobin (ŏk"sē-hē"mō-glō'bĭn) [" + *haima,* blood, + L. *globus,* a sphere]. The combined form of hemoglobin and oxygen. Hemoglobin with oxygen is found in arterial blood and is the oxygen carrier to the body tissues.

oxyhemoglobinometer (ŏk"sē-hē"mō-glō"bĭn-ŏm'ĕt-ĕr) [" + " + " + Gr. *metron,* a measure]. Apparatus for measurement of amount of oxygen in the blood.

oxyhydrocephalus (ŏk"sē-hī-drō-sĕf'ăl-ŭs) [" + *hydor,* water, + *kephale,* brain]. Type of hydrocephalus in which the head has a pointed shape.

oxyiodide (ŏk"sē-ī'ō-dīd) [" + *ioeides,* violet colored]. Compound of iodine and oxygen with an element or radical.

oxylalia (ŏk"sē-lā'lē-ă) [" + *lalein,* to speak]. Abnormal rapidity of speech.

Oxylone. Trade name for fluorometholone, USP.

oxymetazoline hydrochloride (ŏk"sē-mĕt-ăz'ō-lēn). USP. A vasoconstrictor drug used topically for nasal decongestion. Trade names are Afrin and Duration.

oxymetholone (ŏk"sē-mĕth'ō-lōn). USP. An anabolic steroid. Trade names are Androyd and Anadrol.

oxymorphone hydrochloride (ŏk"sē-mor'fōn). USP. A semisynthetic analgesic narcotic similar in action to morphine. Trade name is Numorphan.

oxymyoglobin (ŏk"sē-mī"ō-glō'bĭn). The compound formed when myoglobin is exposed to air.

oxyntic (ŏk-sĭn'tĭk) [Gr. *oxynein,* to make acid]. Producing or secreting acid.

oxyopia (ŏk"sē-ō'pē-ă) [Gr. *oxys,* sharp, + *ops,* sight]. Unusual acuteness of vision.

oxyopter (ŏk"sē-ŏp'tĕr). A unit of measuring visual acuity; the reciprocal of the visual angle expressed in degrees.

oxyosmia (ŏk"sē-ŏz'mē-ă) [" + *osme,* odor]. Unusual acuity of sense of smell.

oxyosphresia (ŏk"sē-ŏs-frē'zē-ă) [" + *osphresis,* smell]. Abnormal acuity of the sense of smell.

oxypathia, oxypathy (ŏk"sē-păth'ē-ă, -sĭp'ăth-ē) [" + *pathos,* feeling]. 1. Unusual acuity of sensation. 2. An acute condition. 3. Condition in which the body is unable to eliminate unoxidizable acids, which combine with fixed alkalies of the tissues and harm the organism.

oxyperitoneum (ŏk"sĭ-pĕr-ĭ-tō-nē'ŭm) [" + *peritonaion,* peritoneum]. Introduction of oxygen into the peritoneal cavity.

oxyphenbutazone (ŏk"sē-fĕn-bū'tă-zōn). USP. An anti-inflammatory and antipyretic drug similar in action to phenylbutazone. Trade names are Oxalid and Tandearil.

oxyphencyclimine hydrochloride (ŏk"sē-fĕn-sī'klĭ-mēn). USP. A belladonna-like drug. Trade name is Daricon.

oxyphil(e) (ŏk'sē-fĭl, -fīl) [" + *philein,* to love]. 1. Staining readily with acid dyes. 2. A cell that stains readily with acid dyes.

oxyphilous (ŏk-sĭf'ĭl-ŭs). Having an affinity for acid dyes. SYN: *oxyphil.*

oxyphonia (ŏk"sē-fō'nē-ă). An abnormally sharp or shrill pitch to the voice.

oxypurine (ŏk"sē-pū'rēn) [" + L. *purus,* pure, + *urina,* urine]. An oxidation product of purine. Includes hypoxanthine, xanthine, and uric acid. SEE: *aminopurine; methyl purine.*

oxyrhine (ŏk'sē-rīn) [" + *rhis,* nose]. 1. Having a sharp-pointed nose. 2. Possessing an acute sense of smell.

oxytalan (ŏks-ĭt'ă-lăn). A type of connective tissue fiber present in periodontal tissues.

oxytetracycline (ŏks"ē-tĕt"ră-sī'klēn). USP. One of a group of broad-spectrum antibiotic substances called tetracyclines. Originally obtained from a strain of Streptomyces, it is now prepared synthetically. Trade name is Terramycin.

oxytocia (ŏk"sē-tō'sē-ă) [" + *tokos,* childbirth]. Unusual rapidity of childbirth.

oxytocic (ŏk"sē-tō'sĭk). 1. Agent that stimulates uterine contractions. 2. Accelerating childbirth.

oxytocic principle. A hormone stored in the posterior lobe of the hypophysis that acts specifically on the smooth musculature of the uterus, therefore increasing tone of, and inducing, uterine contractions. SYN: *oxytocin.*

oxytocin (ŏk"sē-tō'sĭn). USP. A pituitary hormone that stimulates the uterus to contract, thus inducing parturition. It also acts on the mammary gland to stimulate the release of milk. Trade names are Syntocinon and Pitocin.

oxytocin challenge test. Test usually done in late pregnancy to judge the fetal response to induced uterine contractions. Labor is simulated by giving a dilute concentration of I.V. oxytocin and simultaneously monitoring uterine contractions and fetal heart rate. The character of the response is assessed by the physician in order to determine whether or not the fetus can withstand the stress of labor.

NURSING IMPLICATIONS: Assist patient during study. Monitor and record fetal heart rate and uterine contractions (force and duration).

oxyuriasis (ŏk"sē-ū-rī'ăs-ĭs) [Gr. *oxys,* sharp, + *oura,* tall, + *iasis,* infection]. Infestation with Enterobius vermicularis (pinworm), q.v. SYN: *enterobiasis.*

oxyuricide (ŏk"sē-ū'rĭ-sīd) [" + " + L. *caedere,* to kill]. Destructive to pinworms, such as an agent that destroys them.

oxyurid (ŏk"sē-ūr'ĭd). Pinworm or seatworm. SEE: *Enterobius vermicularis.*

Oxyuris [" + *oura,* tail]. Former name for genus of nematode intestinal worms that includes the pinworms or seatworms. SEE: *Enterobius.*

O. vermicularis. Enterobius vermicularis.

Oxyuroidea (ŏk"sē-ū"roy-dē'ă). A superfamily of nematodes that includes the pinworm Enterobius vermicularis.

oyster [AS. *oistre*]. Shellfish eaten raw or cooked. When eaten raw or partially cooked, it may be source of infectious hepatitis virus.

oz. *ounce.*

oz. ap. *ounce apothecary's* (pharmaceutical term).

oz. av. *ounce avoirdupois.*

ozena (ō-zē'nă) [Gr. *oze,* stench]. Disease of the nose characterized by atrophy of the turbinates and mucous membrane accompanied by considerable crusting, discharge, and a very offensive odor. It is present in various forms of rhinitis.

ozochrotia (ō"zō-krō'shē-ă) [" + *chros,* skin]. Strong odor given off by the skin. SYN: *bromidrosis.*

ozonator (ō'zō-nā"tor). Device for generating ozone.

ozone (ō'zōn) [G. *ozein,* to smell]. A form of oxygen in which three atoms of the element combine to form the molecule O_3. In even very low concentration in inhaled air, ozone is toxic.

ozonization (ō"zō-nĭ-zā'shŭn). The act of converting to, or impregnating with, ozone.

ozonize (ō'zō-nīz) [Gr. *ozein,* to smell]. 1. To convert oxygen to ozone, q.v. 2. To impregnate the air of a substance with ozone.

ozonometer (ō"zō-nŏm'ĕt-ĕr) [Gr. *oze,* stench, + *metron,* a measure]. An apparatus for estimating the quantity of ozone in the atmosphere.

ozonoscope (ō-zō'nō-skōp) [" + *skopein,* to examine]. A device for showing the presence or amount of ozone.

ozostomia (ō"zō-stō'mē-ă) [Gr. *oze,* stench, + *stoma,* mouth]. Fetid breath, halitosis.

P

P. 1. *position; posterior; postpartum; pressure; pulse; pupil.* 2. Chem. symb. for phosphorus.
p. *page; probability* (in statistics); *pupil.*
p-. *para-* in chemical formulas.
P_1. *first parental generation* (in genetics); *first pulmonic heart sound.*
P_2. *pulmonic second sound.*
P^{32}, ^{32}P. Chem. symb. for radioactive isotope of phosphorus.
P.A. *physician's assistant.*
Pa. Chem. symb. for protactinium.
P-A, p-a. *posteroanterior.*
P & A. *percussion and auscultation.*
PABA. Trade name for para-aminobenzoic acid, previously used name for aminobenzoic acid.
Pabanol. Trade name for para-aminobenzoic acid, previously used name for aminobenzoic acid.
Pablum (păb′lŭm). Trade name for a cereal food for infants.
pabular (păb′ū-lăr) [L. *pabulum,* food]. Pert. to nourishment.
pabulum (păb′ū-lŭm) [L.]. Food; nourishment.
PAC. *phenacetin, aspirin,* and *caffeine.* (Also: *APC.*)
pacchionian bodies (păk″ē-ō′nē-ăn). [Antonio Pacchioni, It. anatomist, 1665–1726] Enlarged villi, small pedunculated or rounded growths of fibrous tissue along longitudinal fissure of the cerebrum growing on arachnoid membrane.
pacchionian depressions. Small pits produced on inner surface of skull by protuberance of the pacchionian bodies.
pacemaker (pās′māk-ĕr) [L. *passus,* a step, + AS. *macian,* to make]. 1. Anything that influences the rate and rhythm of occurrence of some activity or process. 2. In cardiology, a cell or group of cells that automatically generate impulses that may spread to other regions of the heart. The normal cardiac pacemaker is the sinoatrial node, a group of cells in the atrium near the entrance of the superior vena cava into the right atrium.

p., cardiac, artificial. An electrical device that can substitute for a defective natural pacemaker and control the beating of the heart by a series of rhythmic electrical discharges. If the electrodes that deliver the discharges to the heart are placed on the outside of the chest, the device is called an external pacemaker. If the electrodes are placed within the chest wall, it is called an internal pacemaker.

p., demand. An implanted pacemaker that is designed to permit its electrical output to be inhibited by the heart's electrical impulses. This decreases the chances for the pacemaker to induce ventricular fibrillation.

p., ectopic. Any endogenous cardiac pacemaker other than the sinoatrial node.

p., external. An artificial cardiac pacemaker that is located outside the body. The electrodes for delivering the stimulus are located on the chest wall or may be introduced through an intravenous catheter.

p., fixed rate. An artificial pacemaker that stimulates the heart at a fixed rate.

p., wandering. A cardiac arrhythmia in which the site of origin of the pacemaker stimulus shifts from one site to another, usually from the A-V node to some other part of the atrium.

pacer. Pacemaker.
pachismus (păk-ĭz′mŭs) [Gr. *pachys,* thick, + *-ismos,* condition]. Condensation or thickening of an organ or part.
pachy-, pach- [Gr. *pachys,* thick]. Combining form meaning thick, large, heavy, massive.
pachyacria, pachyakria (păk″ē-ā′krē-ă) [Gr. *pachys,* thick, + *akron,* end]. Hypertrophy of soft portions of the extremities.
pachyblepharon (păk″ē-blĕf′ă-rŏn) [″ + *blepharon,* eyelid]. A thickening of the border of the eyelid.
pachyblepharosis (păk′ē-blĕf″ă-rō′sĭs). Chronic thickening of the eyelid.
pachycephalic (păk″ē-sĕ-făl′ĭk) [″ + *kephale,* brain]. Possessing an abnormally thick skull. SYN: *pachycephalous.*
pachycephalous (păk″ē-sĕf′ă-lŭs). Thick skulled. SYN: *pachycephalic.*
pachycephaly (păk″ē-sĕf′ă-lē). Unusual thickness of the walls of the skull.
pachycheilia (păk″ē-kī′lē-ă) [″ + *cheilos,* lip]. Unusual thickness of the lips
pachycholia (păk″ē-kō′lē-ă) [″ + *chole,* bile]. Thickening or inspissation of the bile.
pachychromatic (păk″ē-krō-măt′ĭk) [″ + *chroma,* color]. Possessing a coarse chromatin network.
pachycolpismus (păk″ē-kŏl-pĭz′mŭs) [″ + *kolpos,* vagina, + *-ismos,* condition]. Chronic inflammation of the vagina with thickened vaginal walls. SYN: *pachyvaginitis.*
pachydactylia, pachydactyly (păk″ē-dăk-tĭl′ē-ă, -dăk′tĭ-lē) [″ + *daktylos,* digit]. Condition marked by unusually large fingers and toes.
pachyderma (păk-ē-dĕr′mă) [″ + *derma,* skin]. Unusual thickness of the skin. SYN: *pachydermatosis.* SEE: *elephantiasis.*

p. circumscripta. P. laryngis, q.v.

p. laryngis. Irregular thickening and hypertrophy of mucous membrane in the larynx seen in chronic laryngitis.

p. lymphangiectatica. A diffuse form of skin thickening due to blocked or defective lymph drainage.

p., occipital. A disease in which the skin of the scalp, esp. in the occipital region, falls into thickened folds.

p. vesicae. Condition in which there is a thickened mucous membrane in the urinary bladder.

pachydermatocele (păk″ē-děr-măt′ō-sēl) [″ + ″ + *kele,* swelling]. 1. A pendulous state of the skin with thickening. SYN: *cutis laxa; dermatolysis.* 2. Huge neurofibroma.

pachydermatosis (păk″ē-děr″mă-tō′sĭs) [″ + ″ + *osis,* condition]. Unusual thickness of the skin. SYN: *pachyderma; pachydermia.*

pachydermatous (păk-ē-děr′mă-tŭs) [″ + *derma,* skin]. Possessing a thick skin.

pachydermoperiostosis (păk″ē-děr″mō-pěr″ē-ŏs-tō′sĭs). Hereditary form of osteoarthropathy with marked thickening of the skin over the face and extremities. It is self-limiting with an active progressive phase during adolescence.

pachyemia (păk-ē-ē′mē-ă) [Gr. *pachys,* thick, + *haima,* blood]. Thickness of the blood.

pachyglossia (păk″ē-glŏs′sē-ă) [″ + *glossa,* tongue]. Unusual thickness of the tongue.

pachygnathous (pă-kĭg′năth-ŭs) [″ + *gnathos,* jaw]. Having a thick or large jaw.

pachygyria (păk-ē-jī′rē-ă) [″ + *gyros,* a circle]. Flat, broad formation of the cerebral convolutions.

pachyhematous (păk-ē-hěm′ă-tŭs) [″ + *haima,* blood]. Having, or pert. to, thickened blood.

pachyhemia (păk-ē-hē′mē-ă). A thickened state of the blood.

pachyleptomeningitis (păk-ē-lěp″tō-měn″ĭn-jī′tĭs) [″ + *leptos,* thin, + *meninx,* membrane, + *itis,* inflammation]. Inflammation of pia and dura of the brain and spinal cord.

pachylosis (păk-ē-lō′sĭs) [″ + *osis,* condition]. A chronic condition of rough, dry, thickened skin. SYN: *xerosis.*

pachymenia (păk-ē-mē′nē-ă) [″ + *hymen,* membrane]. Thickening of the skin or membranes.

pachymeningitis (păk-ē-měn″ĭn-jī′tĭs) [″ + *meninx,* membrane, + *itis,* inflammation]. Inflamed condition of the dura mater. Inflammation of either the pia, dura, or the arachnoid membranes is sure to extend to one or both of the others, and the consequence in any form is suppuration, abscess, effusion into the ventricles, and softening of cerebral tissue if brain is involved. SYN: *perimeningitis.*

p., external. Inflammation of outer layer of dura mater.

p., hemorrhagic. Circumscribed effusion of blood on inner surface of dura with inflammation.

SYM: Intermittent headache, choked disks, hemiparesis, dilated pupil, unconsciousness in varying degrees.

ETIOL: Usually the result of trauma, such as a blow, resulting in a venous tear. Blood oozes into subdural space and a blood clot is formed, becomes encysted, and gives rise to a hematoma.

p., internal. Inflammation of inner layer of dura mater.

p., spinal. Inflammation of the dura of the spinal cord.

pachymeningopathy (păk″ē-měn″ĭn-gŏp′ă-thē) [″ + ″ + *pathos,* disease]. Any noninflammatory disease of the dura mater.

pachymeninx (păk-ē-mē′nĭnks) [″ + *meninx,* membrane]. The dura mater.

pachynema (păk″ē-nē′mă) [″ + *nema,* thread]. Pachytene, q.v.

pachynsis (pă-kĭn′sĭs) [Gr.]. Thickening, esp. pathological thickening.

pachyonychia (păk″ē-ō-nĭk′ē-ă) [Gr. *pachys,* thick, + *onyx,* nail]. Abnormal thickening of fingernails or toenails.

p. congenita. A congenital condition characterized by thickening of the nails, thickening of the skin on palms of hands and soles of feet, follicular keratosis at knees and elbows, and corneal dyskeratosis.

pachyostosis (păk″ē-ŏs-tō′sĭs) [″ + *osteon,* bone, + *osis,* condition]. A benign condition of thickening of the bones.

pachyotia (păk-ē-ō′shē-ă) [″ + *ous,* ear]. Abnormal thickness of the ears.

pachypelviperitonitis (păk″ē-pěl″vĭ-pěr″ĭ-tō-nī′tĭs) [″ + L. *pelvis,* basin, + Gr. *peritonaion,* peritoneum, + *itis,* inflammation]. Inflammation of the pelvic and peritoneal membranes with hypertrophy and thickening of their surfaces.

pachyperiostitis (păk″ē-pěr″ē-ŏs-tī′tĭs) [″ + *periosteon,* periosteum, + *itis,* inflammation]. Thickening of the periosteum due to inflammation.

pachyperitonitis (păk″ē-pěr″ĭ-tō-nī′tĭs) [″ + *peritonaion,* peritoneum, + *itis,* inflammation]. Inflammation of the peritoneum with thickening of the membrane.

pachypleuritis (păk-ē-plū-rī′tĭs) [″ + *pleura,* side, + *itis,* inflammation]. Inflamed condition of the pleura with thickening.

pachypodous (pă-kĭp′ō-dŭs) [″ + *pous,* foot]. Having abnormally thick feet.

pachyrhinic (păk″ē-rī′nĭk) [″ + *rhis,* nose]. Having a thick, flat nose.

pachysalpingitis (păk″ē-săl″pĭn-jī′tĭs) [″ + *salpinx,* tube, + *itis,* inflammation]. Chronic inflammation of an oviduct with thickening of the walls.

pachysalpingoovaritis (păk″ē-săl-pĭng″gō-ō″văr-ī′tĭs) [″ + ″ + L. *ovarium,* ovary, + Gr. *itis,* inflammation]. Chronic inflamed condition of an ovary and oviduct with thickening of the membranes.

pachysomia (păk-ē-sō′mē-ă) [Gr. *pachys,* thick, + *soma,* body]. Pathological thickening of the soft parts of the body.

pachytene (păk′ē-tēn) [″ + *tainia,* band]. The stage in meiosis, or cell division, in which the paired homologous chromosomes contract due to their becoming intertwined in a spiral fashion and then become much thicker than in the preceding leptotene and zygotene stages.

pachyvaginalitis (păk″ē-văj″ĭn-ă-lī′tĭs) [″ + L. *vagina,* sheath, + Gr. *itis,* inflammation]. Inflamed condition of the tunica vaginalis of the testes.

pachyvaginitis (păk″ē-văj″ĭn-ī′tĭs). Chronic inflammation of the vagina with thickening of the vaginal walls. SYN: *pachycolpismus.*

pacing (pās′ĭng) [L. *passus,* a step]. Setting the rate or pace of an event, esp. the heartbeat. SEE: *pacemaker.*

pacinian corpuscles (pă-sĭn′ē-ăn). [Filippo Pacini, It. anatomist, 1812–1883] Encapsulated sensory nerve endings found in subcutaneous tissue and many other parts of the body (pancreas, penis, clitoris, nipple). These corpuscles are sensitive to deep or heavy pressure. SYN: *Vater's corpuscles.*

pack (păk) [AS. *pak*]. 1. A dry or moist, hot or cold blanket or sheet wrapped around a patient and used for treatment. 2. The procedure in which one enwraps a person. 3. To fill up a cavity with cotton, gauze, or a similar substance.

p., cold. A physiological sedative and hypnotic employed for relief of restlessness and insomnia; used extensively in psychiatric conditions. Patient is wrapped in two or more sheets that have been placed in cold water and wrung out before application. The patient's body is then wrapped in heavy blankets to prevent loss of cooling and evaporation of moisture.

p., dry. Procedure used in combination with hot bath to induce perspiration. When leaving the hot bath the patient is placed in a dry warm sheet and wrapped in several warm blankets.

p., full. Any pack that enwraps the entire body.

p., half. Wet-sheet pack extending from the axillae to below the knees.

p., hot. The envelopment of a patient in a hot dry blanket or a moist blanket wrung from very hot water (150° to 160° F. or 65.6° to 71.1° C.). Given to relax contracted muscles, relieve convulsions, or induce profuse perspiration.

p., ice. A substitute for an ice bag; a local cold application made by folding a soft towel so it will fit the area and filling it with crushed ice.

p., one-sheet. A wet-sheet pack in which only one large sheet, 84 × 96 in. (213.4 × 243.8 cm.), is used.

p., partial. A wet pack that covers a portion of the body.

p., three-quarter. Pack that uses same temperatures as the wet-sheet pack, but the body is enveloped upward as far as the armpits.

p., umbrella. A pack inserted through the abdominal incision following hysterectomy to stop arterial bleeding. The pack itself consists of a piece of absorbent cloth about 24 in. (61 cm.) square into the middle of which is placed about 60 ft. (18.28 meters) of 2 in. (5 cm.) gauze. The tails of the pack are pulled through the vagina from below and the corners of the cloth are brought together to form the tail of the pack. After placement, the tail is pulled firmly, and the bolus of gauze in the cloth exerts enough pressure against the blood vessels to stop arterial bleeding. In Greece this is known as the Logothetopulos tampon, named after the physician who developed it in 1926.

p., wet-sheet. The envelopment of a patient in one, two, or three linen or soft cotton sheets that have been wrung out of water. These are held against the body by large woolen blankets. Temperature of the water used for the sheets varies depending upon the purpose.

package insert. An informational leaflet placed inside the container or package of prescription drugs. The Food and Drug Administration requires that the drug's generic name, indications, contraindications, adverse effects, dosage, and route of administration be described in the leaflet.

packed cells. Red blood cells that have been separated from the plasma. Used in treating conditions that require red blood cells but not the liquid components of whole blood. This prevents excess hydration of the vascular system.

packer (păk′ĕr). Device for packing a cavity or a wound.

packing (păk′ĭng). 1. The process of filling a cavity or wound with gauze sponges or gauze strips. 2. Material used to fill a cavity or wound.

$PaCO_2$. Partial pressure of CO_2 in the arterial blood. Arterial carbon dioxide concentration, or tension. Usually expressed in mm. Hg.

pad (păd). 1. Cushion of soft material used to apply pressure, relieve pressure, or support an organ or part. Usually cotton or rayon. 2. A fleshlike or fatty mass.

p., abdominal. Dressing for absorbing discharges from surgical wounds of the abdomen.

p., dinner. Pad placed on stomach prior

to application of a plaster cast. Pad is then removed, leaving space for abdominal distention after meals.

p., fat. 1. The sucking pad in the infant's cheek. 2. A pad of fat behind and below the patella.

p., kidney. Air or water pad fixed on abdominal belt for compression over a movable kidney.

p.'s, knuckle. Congenital condition in which small nodules appear on dorsal side of fingers.

p., Malgaigne's. Mass of fat in knee joint on either side of the patella's upper end.

p., Mikulicz's. Pad of folded gauze used in surgery.

p., perineal. Pad covering the perineum. Used to cover a wound or to absorb the menstrual flow.

p., sucking. A pad of fat seen inside the cheeks of infants.

p., surgical. Soft rubber pad with apron and inflatable rim for drainage of escaping fluids. Used in surgery and obstetrics.

p. ae. Abbr. in prescription writing for L. *partes aequales,* in equal parts.

paed-, paedo-. SEE: words beginning with *ped-, pedia-, pedo-.*

Paget, Sir James (păj'ĕt). British surgeon, 1814–1899.

P.'s disease. Skeletal disease of the elderly with chronic inflammation of bones, resulting in thickening and softening of bones, and bowing of long bones. SYN: *osteitis deformans.*

TREATMENT: Asymptomatic cases should not be treated. There is no specific curative therapy but vitamin D three times a week and anabolic hormones may be of help in treating osteoporosis. Calcitonin, etidronate disodium, and mithramycin have been used to control resorption of bone and thus are of assistance in alleviating bone pain.

P.'s disease, extramammary. A plaque with a definite margin found in the anogenital area and in the axilla. It is a rare malignant disease.

TREATMENT: Surgical excision.

P.'s disease, mammary. Carcinoma of the mammary ducts.

pagetoid (păj'ĕ-toyd) [*Paget* + Gr. *eidos,* form]. Similar to Paget's disease.

Pagitane Hydrochloride. Trade name for cycrimine hydrochloride.

pagophagia [Gr. *pagos,* frost, + *phagein,* to eat]. A form of pica, q.v., characterized by the deliberate eating of large quantities of ice.

-pagus [Gr. *pagos,* thing fixed]. A terminal combining form indicating twins joined together at the site indicated in the initial part of the word. SEE: *craniopagus.*

PAH. *PAHA, para-aminohippuric acid.*

pain (pān) [L. *poena,* a fine, a penalty]. A sensation in which a person experiences discomfort, distress, or suffering due to irritation of or stimulation of sensory nerves, esp. pain sensors.

Pain is one of the cardinal symptoms of inflammation. It may vary in intensity from mild discomfort to intolerable agony. In most cases, pain stimuli are harmful to the body and tend to bring about reactions by which the body protects itself. Adaptation to pain stimuli does not readily occur.

p., abdominal. Pain in the abdomen that usually increases with respiration. Experienced in a great variety of conditions including appendicitis; broken ribs; intercostal neuralgia; wounds; herpes zoster; pleurisy; pleurodynia; myalgia; periostitis; acute peritonitis; colic; hepatic, gastric, or renal ulcer; gallbladder disorders; carcinoma in late stages; and gummata of this region.

p., aching. Generalized aching that may accompany infectious disease such as influenza, smallpox, or rheumatic fever. It is also found in myalgia and various headaches.

p., acute. A short, sharp, cutting pain. Usually associated with acute inflammation or inflammation of serous membranes as in pleurisy and pericarditis; also posterior spinal-root pains. SYN: *p., lancinating.*

p.'s, after-. Pains following labor, caused by contraction of uterine muscles during their involution.

p., agonizing. Intense, torturing pain of mind or body. May be due to coronary thrombosis, angina pectoris, aortic aneurysm, mediastinitis. May occur in milder form in asthma, tracheobronchitis, or it may be due to referred pain from gallbladder, intestinal obstruction, diaphragmatic hernia, pancreatitis, or a perforated ulcer.

p., angina pectoris. Severe paroxysmal pain due to decreased blood supply to the myocardium, radiating through the shoulder down arm, or rarely from the heart to the abdomen, ear, or back. At the same time the patient may experience a feeling that the chest is being crushed or compressed. Lasts from a few seconds to several minutes. SEE: *angina pectoris.*

p., appendicitis. If the attack is acute, there is abdominal pain, usually severe, generally throughout the abdomen, followed by localization of pain in lower right quadrant of abdomen with tenderness over right rectus muscle with rigidity. Rebound pain at McBurney's point is a classic symptom.

p.'s, bearing-down. Pain and pressure of the second stage of labor that causes the female to strain or bear down as one does to defecate.

p., boring. Pain deep in tissues that gives the sensation of being produced by a boring instrument.

p., Brodie's. Pain caused near a joint affected with neuralgia when the skin is folded near it.

p., burning. Pain experienced in heat burns, superficial skin lesions, herpes zoster, and in circumscribed neuralgias.

p., cardiac. Angina pectoris.

p., causalgic. A spontaneous pain, esp. burning in character, when associated with anesthesia or hyperesthesia in a given nerve. SYN: *causalgia.*

p., central. Pain due to a lesion in the central nervous system.

p., cephalgic. P., head.

p., chest. Severe pain in chest from exercise may be due to heart disease. If due to pleurisy, it comes with a deep breath. If pain accompanies stiff shoulder or neck, it may be due to arthritis or fibrositis. If it comes when patient is bending over after a meal, it may be due to diaphragmatic or hiatal hernia.

p., chronic. Pain that is constantly present.

p., cramplike. Muscular spasm such as epigastric pain. Significance depends upon location of pain. Menstrual pain is often cramplike.

p., dental. Pain in the oral area in general may be of two origins; soft tissue pain may be acute or chronic, and a burning pain is due to surface lesions, and usually can be discretely localized; pulpal pain or tooth pain will vary whether acute or chronic but often is difficult to localize.

p.'s, dilating. Rhythmic pains occurring during the first stage of labor accompanying dilatation of the cervix.

p., dull. Continuous mild throbbing.

p., ear. May indicate inflammation of the external auditory canal, except in young children. Also may indicate a furuncle in the meatus; or middle ear disease. SYN: *earache; otalgia; otodynia.*

p., eccentric. Pain occurring in peripheral structures due to a lesion involving posterior roots of spinal nerves.

p., epigastric. Severe pain occurring in paroxysms in gastric disorders. In general, may accompany any gastric or intestinal disorder or pleural and some cardiac affections. SYN: *p., gastralgic.* SEE: *cardialgia.*

p.'s, expulsive. Pains of the second and third stages of labor.

p., false. Pain mistaken for a true labor pain; an ineffective pain of labor. Braxton-Hicks, q.v., contractions are often confused with labor particularly by the female experiencing her first pregnancy.

p., fulgurant. P., lightning, q.v.

p., gallbladder. Pain in upper right abdominal quadrant, dull pain just below the last rib in infection, or sharp pain in same area radiating to the back and up under the right shoulder, esp. if calculi are present.

p., gas. Pain in the intestines due to accumulation of gas therein.

p., gastralgic. Severe pain occurring in paroxysms in gastric disorders. SYN: *p., epigastric.*

p., girdle. Pain resembling sensation of a constricting cord around the waist, occurring in spinal cord disease.

p.'s, growing. Pain felt in the joints or limbs of growing children; may be rheumatic. An imprecise term indicating ill-defined pain in the muscular system of young persons. There is no evidence that the pain is related to rapid growth.

p., head. An ache or pain located in the head, esp. one experienced in region of cranial vault. Headache may be a symptom of acute systemic infections; intracranial tumors; infections; vascular lesions; hypertension; acute and chronic infections of the nose, sinuses, pharynx, eye, and ear; and toxic states such as alcoholism or uremia. Headache may occur after the injection of histamine, following a lumbar puncture, in infections of the meninges, and in subarachnoid hemorrhages. Headache occurs in many febrile diseases, in anemia, hypoxia, and following head injuries (post-traumatic). Migraine, q.v., is a common cause of headache. SYN: *cephalalgia; headache.*

p., heterotopic. P., referred.

p., homotopic. Pain felt at the point of injury.

p., hunger. Pain due to need for food; coincides with powerful contractions of the stomach. May be indicative of gastric disorder. SEE: *hunger.*

p., hypogastric. Pain in the hypogastrium.

p., imperative. A persistent sensation of pain occurring in psychasthenia.

p., inflammatory. Pain in presence of inflammation that is increased by pressure.

p., intermenstrual. Pelvic pain arising during the cycle between the menses; may accompany ovulation. SYN: *mittelschmerz.*

p., intractable. Pain that cannot be easily relieved, as that occurring from certain neoplastic invasions.

p.'s, labor. Rhythmical uterine contractions at childbirth; increasing in frequency and severity, climaxing in vaginal delivery.

p., lancinating. A short, sharp, cutting pain. SYN: *p., acute.*

p., lightning. A sudden brief pain that may be repetitive. It is usually in the legs but may be at any location. These pains are associated with tabes dorsalis.

p., lingual. Pain in tongue that may be due to local lesions, glossitis, fissures, or pernicious anemia.

p., lung. Sharp pain in the region of the lungs. SYN: *p., pulmonary.*

p., menstrual. Pain, usually cramping, occurring just prior to onset or during the menstrual period. SYN: *dysmenorrhea.*

p., mental. Pain of psychic origin such as mental distress or grief. If persistent, it may cause true physical pain.

p., middle. Pain between menstrual periods. SYN: *p., intermenstrual; mittelschmerz.*

p., migraine. Headache accompanied by nausea and vomiting. It may arise from a number of causes, esp. those of neurological origin. SEE: *migraine.*

p., mind. Pain of mental origin or pain occurring subsequent to mental effort, noted esp. in melancholia.

p., mobile. Pain that moves from one area to another.

p., movement. Kinesalgia, q.v.

p., neuralgic. Pain, frequently paroxysmal, occurring along the branches of a nerve. Temporarily relieved by heat or pressure. May be rheumatic in origin.

p., night. Pain in hip or knee during muscular relaxation in sleep.

p., noise. Pain of ear caused by noise. SYN: *odynacusis.*

p., objective. Pain induced by some external or internal irritant, by inflammation, or by injury to nerves, organs, or other tissues that interfere with the function, nutrition, or circulation of the affected part. Usually traceable to a definite pathological process.

p., organic. Pain due to organic causes. SYN: *somatalgia.*

p., osteocopic. Pain in bones. SEE: *osteocope.*

p., parenchymatous. Pain felt at the peripheral end of a nerve.

p., paresthesic. Stinging or tingling sensation manifested in central and peripheral nerve lesions. SEE: *paresthesia.*

p., phantom limb. Pain that seems to be in a certain limb following amputation of that limb. SEE: *phantom limb.*

p., postprandial. Abdominal pain after eating.

p., premonitory. Ineffective contractions of the uterus prior to the beginning of true labor.

p., pseudomyelic. False sensation of movement in a paralyzed limb or of no movement in a moving limb. Not a true pain.

p., psychic. Mental suffering such as that resulting from a sense of unworthiness or from feelings of guilt.

p., psychogenic. Pain having mental origin as opposed to organic origin.

p., psychosomatic. Pain in which some part of etiology is due to mental or emotional disorders.

p., pulmonary. Sharp pain in the region of the lungs.

p., rectal, constant. Pain in rectal area. Usually aggravated by defecation. May be due to ischiorectal abscess, anal abscess, inflamed or strangulated hemorrhoids, carcinoma, periproctitis, prostatic abscess, seminal vesiculitis, fecal impaction, acute salpingitis, tabes dorsalis, irritation from diarrhea, foreign bodies, fissures, rectal polyps, or adenoma. Pain during defecation may result from anal fissure, ulcer, hemorrhoids, anal abscess, stenosis, stricture, dysentery, impaction, foreign body, or any inflammation. SEE: *proctalgia fugax.*

p., referred. Pain seeming to arise in an area other than its origin, as pain from appendicitis, which often seems to occur in areas other than that of the appendix. SYN: *p., heterotopic; p., sympathetic; synalgia.*

p., remittent. Pain with temporary abatements in severity. Characteristic of neuralgia and colic.

p., rest. Pain due to ischemia that comes on when sitting or lying.

p., root. Cutaneous pain caused by disease of sensory nerve roots.

p., shifting. Pain that seems to arise from different sites from time to time. Present in rheumatism, hysteria, and locomotor ataxia.

p.'s, spot. Pains that seem to be located in patches of the skin.

p.'s, starting. Pains accompanied by muscular spasm during early stages of sleep.

p., subdiaphragmatic. A sharp stitch-like pain occurring during breathing. When the breath is held, the pain ceases. Pressure against the lower rib cage eases the pain.

p., subjective. Pain that has no apparent physical basis for its existence. It may be found among the highly imaginative neurotics in whom mild sensations are perceived as pain.

p., sympathetic. P., referred.

p., tenesmic. Pain accompanying urination or defecation. SEE: *tenesmus.*

p., terebrant. A boring or piercing type of pain.

p., thermalgesic. Pain caused by heat.

p., thoracic. A sharp pain over the sternum, primarily in the chest or thoracic region, often running down the arm to the elbow. May be indicative of angina pectoris, although it must not be confused with pain from gastric pressure in the region of the heart, caused by an accumulation of gas. It is increased with respiration. It is experienced in broken ribs; intercostal neuralgia; wounds; herpes zoster; pleurisy; pleurodynia; myalgia; periostitis; acute peritonitis; colic; hepatic, gastric, or renal ulcer; gallbladder disorders; carcinoma in late stages; and gumma of this region.

p., throbbing. Pain found in dental caries, headache, and localized inflammation.

p., tongue. P., lingual.

p., tracheal. Trachealgia.

p., wandering. Pain that changes its location repeatedly.

paint (pānt). 1. A solution of medication for application to skin. 2. To apply a medicated liquid to the skin.

p., Castellani's. A germicide consisting of phenol, resorcinol, boric acid, acetone, and basic fuchsin.

painters' colic. Colic accompanying lead poisoning. SEE: *lead* in *Poisons and Poisoning* in *Appendix*.

pair. Two of anything similar in shape, size, and conformation.

p., base. A pair of nucleotides, one a purine and the other a pyrimidine, joined by hydrogen bonds. These pairs make up DNA, q.v.

PAL. *posterior axillary line.*

palatable (păl'ăt-ă-bl) [L. *palatum,* palate]. Pleasing to the palate or taste, as food.

palatal (păl'ă-tăl). Pert. to the roof of the mouth, the palate.

palatal reflex. Swallowing induced by stimulation of the soft palate.

palate (păl'ăt) [L. *palatum,* palate]. The horizontal structure separating the mouth and the nasal cavity; the roof of the mouth. SEE: *mouth* for illus.

DIFF. DIAG: *Koplik's spots:* A rash frequently seen upon the palate in measles. *Secondary syphilis:* Indicated by mucous patches on the palate. *Herpes of the throat:* Shown by vesicles in circles upon the pharyngeal walls and soft palate. *Swelling of uvula:* Noted in inflammations of pharynx and tonsil, in nephritis, severe anemia, angioneurotic edema, and general debility. In diphtheria and Vincent's angina, a membranous exudate appears. In purpura hemorrhagica and some hemorrhagic diatheses, bloody extravasation appears. *Paralysis:* May result from diphtheria, bulbar paralysis, neuritis, basal meningitis, tumor at base of brain. *Anesthesia:* Seen in pathological conditions of second division of the 5th nerve.

RS: Avellis' paralysis syndrome; Bednar's aphthae; cheilognathopalatoschisis; cleft; "palat-," "staphyl-," "uran-," "uvul-" words.

p., artificial. Prosthetic device molded to fill a cleft in the palate.

p., bony. P., hard, q.v.

p., cleft. Palate with a congenital opening.

p., falling. Abnormally long uvula.

p., gothic. An excessively high palatal arch.

p., hard. Anterior part of the palate supported by the maxillary and palatine bones.

p., pendulous. Uvula.

p., primary. In the embryo, the partition between the nasal cavities and the mouth.

p., secondary. In the embryo, the palate formed from the maxillary arches and the frontonasal process.

p., soft. Posterior musculomembranous fold partly separating the mouth and pharynx. SYN: *velum palatinum* [NA].

palate bones. Bones forming the posterior part of the hard palate and lateral nasal wall between the interior pterygoid plate of the sphenoid bone and maxilla.

palatiform (pă-lăt'ĭ-form) [L. *palatum,* palate, + *forma,* form]. Resembling the palate.

palatine (păl'ă-tīn) [L. *palatinus*]. 1. Concerning the palate. 2. The palate bones.

palatine arches. Two archlike folds of mucous membrane (glossopalatine and pharyngopalatine arches) that form the lateral margins of faucial and pharyngeal isthmuses. They are continuous above with the soft palate.

palatine artery, greater. A branch of the maxillary artery that supplies the palate, upper pharynx, and pharyngotympanic tube.

palatine bone. Palate bones.

palatitis (păl-ăt-ī'tĭs) [L. *palatum,* palate, + Gr. *itis,* inflammation]. Inflamed condition of the palate.

palatoglossal (păl"ă-tō-glŏs'ăl). Concerning the palate and the tongue.

palatoglossus (păl"ă-tō-glŏs ŭs) [" + Gr. *glossa,* tongue]. Muscle arising from sides and undersurface of tongue. Fibers pass upward through glossopalatine arch and are inserted in palatine aponeurosis. It constricts faucial isthmus by raising root of tongue and drawing sides of soft palate downward. SYN: *glossopalatinus.*

palatognathous (păl"ă-tŏg'nă-thŭs) [" + Gr. *gnathos,* jaw]. Having a congenital cleft in the palate.

palatograph (păl'ă-tō-grăf). A device that records the movements of the palate during speech.

palatography (păl"ă-tŏg'ră-fē) [" + Gr. *graphein,* to write]. 1. The recording of the movements of the palate in speech. 2. Radiographic examination of the soft palate after injection of a contrast medium.

palatomaxillary (păl"ă-tō-măk'sĭ-lĕr"ē). Concerning the palate and the maxilla.

palatomyograph (păl"ă-tō-mī'ō-grăf) [" + Gr.

mys, muscle, + *graphein,* to write]. Palatograph, q.v.

palatonasal (păl″ă-tō-nā′zăl). Concerning the palate and the nasal cavity.

palatopharyngeal (păl″ă-tō-fă-rĭn′jē-ăl). Concerning the palate and the pharynx.

palatopharyngeus (păl″ăt-ō-făr″ĭn-jē′ŭs) [″ + Gr. *pharynx,* pharynx]. Muscle arising from thyroid cartilage and pharyngeal wall, extending upward in posterior pillar, and inserting into aponeurosis of soft palate. Constricts pharyngeal isthmus, raises larynx, and depresses soft palate.

palatoplasty (păl′ăt-ō-plăs″tē) [″ + Gr. *plassein,* to form]. Plastic surgery of the palate, usually to correct a cleft. SYN: *staphylorrhaphy; uranoplasty.*

palatoplegia (păl″ă-tō-plē′jē-ă) [″ + Gr. *plege,* stroke]. Paralysis of muscles of the soft palate. SEE: *palate.*

palatorrhaphy (păl-ă-tor′ă-fē) [″ + Gr. *rhaphe,* a sewing]. Operation for uniting of a cleft palate. SYN: *staphylorrhaphy.*

palatosalpingeus (păl″ă-tō-săl-pĭn′jē-ŭs) [″ + Gr. *salpinx,* tube]. The tensor palati muscle.

palatoschisis (păl-ă-tŏs′kĭ-sĭs) [″ + *schisis,* fissure]. Palate with cleft in it.

palatum (păl-ă′tŭm) [L.]. (pl. *palata*) [NA] The palate.

paleencephalon, paleoencephalon (pā″lē-ĕn-sĕf′ă-lŏn, -ō-ĕn-sĕf′ă-lŏn) [Gr. *palaios,* old, + *enkephalos,* brain]. Phylogenetically older portion of the brain; includes all of it except the cerebral cortex and its allied structures.

paleo- [Gr. *palaios,* old, ancient]. Combining form meaning old or ancient.

paleocerebellum (păl″ē-ō-sĕr″ĕ-bĕl′ŭm) [Gr. *palaios,* old, + L. *cerebellum,* little brain]. Phylogenetically, the older portion of the cerebellum including the flocculi, certain parts of the vermis (lingula, nodulus, uvula), and the lobulus centralis (culmen, pyramis, uvula, and simple lobule). These parts are concerned primarily with equilibrium and movements of locomotion.

paleogenesis (pā″lē-ō-jĕn′ĕ-sĭs) [″ + *genesis,* production]. Reproduction of ancestral characteristics, esp. abnormalities, without change in a later generation. SYN: *atavism; palingenesis.*

paleogenetic (pā″lē-ō-jĕn-ĕt′ĭk) [″ + *gennan,* to produce]. Having origin in a previous generation.

paleokinetic (pā″lē-ō-kĭ-nĕt′ĭk) [″ + Gr. *kinetikos,* concerning movement]. Noting a peripheral motor nervous system controlling automatic associated movements. It is older phylogenetically than the system controlling voluntary movement.

paleontology (pā″lē-ŏn-tŏl′ō-jē) [Gr. *palaios,* old, + *onta,* existing things, + *logos,* study]. Branch of biology dealing with ancient plant and animal life of the earth.

paleopathology (pā″lē-ō-pă-thŏl′ō-jē) [″ + *pathos,* disease, + *logos,* study]. The study of diseases in remains of bodies and fossils of ancient times.

paleostriatal (pā″lē-ō-strī-ā′tăl) [″ + L. *striatus,* ridged]. Concerning the primitive portion of the corpus striatum.

paleostriatum (pā″lē-ō-strī-ā′tŭm). Primitive portion of corpus striatum, the globus pallidus. SEE: *neostriatum.*

paleothalamus (pā″lē-ō-thăl′ă-mŭs) [″ + *thalamos,* chamber]. Medial portion of thalamus (the medullary or noncortical part), which is older phylogenetically. SEE: *thalamus.*

pali-, palin- [Gr. *palin,* backward, again]. Prefix meaning recurrence or repetition.

palikinesia (păl″ĭ-kĭn-ē′zē-ă) [″ + *kinesis,* motion]. Continued, involuntary, repetitious movements.

palilalia (păl-ĭ-lā′lē-ă) [″ + *lalein,* to speak]. Pathological repetitious use of words and phrases with increasing rapidity. SYN: *paliphrasia.*

palinal (păl′ĭn-ăl) [Gr. *palin,* backward]. Moved or moving backward.

palindromia (păl-ĭn-drō′mē-ă) [″ + *dromos,* a running]. The recurrence of a disease or a relapse.

palindromic (păl-ĭn-drŏm′ĭk). Recurring, as the symptoms of a disease. SYN: *relapsing.*

palindromic rheumatism. A disease of unknown etiology characterized by intermittent joint pain with tenderness, heat, and swelling that lasts from a few hours to as long as a week. The knees or fingers are most often involved but the disease does not necessarily return to the same joint(s). Between attacks there is no evidence of the disease. Symptomatic treatment is usually sufficient.

palinesthesia (păl″ĭn-ĕs-thē′zē-ă) [Gr. *palin,* again, + *aisthesis,* sensation]. Return of power of sensation, as after recovery from anesthesia or coma.

palingenesis (păl″ĭn-jĕn′ĕ-sĭs) [″ + *genesis,* formation]. 1. Regeneration or restoration of an organism or part of one. 2. Reappearance of ancestral characteristics, esp. abnormal ones, in successive generations. SYN: *atavism; paleogenesis.*

palingraphia (păl″ĭn-grăf′ē-ă) [″ + *graphein,* to write]. Pathological repetition of words or phrases in writing.

palinopsia [″ + *opsis,* vision]. Persistence or recurrence of visual images after the stimulus of the image has been removed. Occurs in visual field defects, in acute mental and visual defects, and in association with auditory or somatic hallucinations. SEE: *afterimage.*

paliphrasia (păl-ĭ-frā'zē-ă) [" + *phrasis,* speech]. Pathological condition in which there is coherent speech but certain words or phrases frequently are repeated. SYN: *palilalia.*

palladium (pă-lā'dē-ŭm) [L.]. SYMB: Pd. At. wt. 106.4; at. no. 46. Metallic element used in dentistry and surgical instruments.

pallanesthesia (păl"ăn-ĕs-thē'zē-ă) [Gr. *pallein,* to shake, + *anaisthesia,* anesthesia]. Loss of ability to sense vibrations. SYN: *apallesthesia.* SEE: *pallesthesia.*

pallescence (păl-lĕs'ĕns) [L. *pallescere,* to grow pale]. Diminution of body color; a pale appearance. SYN: *pallor.*

pallesthesia (păl-ĕs-thē'zē-ă) [Gr. *pallein,* to shake, + *aisthesis,* sensation]. The sensation of vibration felt in skin or bones, as that produced by a tuning fork when held against the body.

palliate (păl'ē-āt) [L. *palliatus,* cloaked]. To ease or reduce effect or intensity, esp. of a disease; to allay temporarily, as pain, without curing.

palliative (păl'ē-ā"tĭv). 1. Serving to relieve or alleviate, without curing. 2. An agent that alleviates or eases.

pallid (păl'ĭd) [L. *pallidus,* pale]. Lacking color; pale, wan.

pallidal (păl'ĭ-dăl). Concerning the pallidum of the brain.

pallidectomy (păl"ĭ-dĕk'tō-mē) [L. *pallidum,* pallidum, + Gr. *ektome,* excision]. Surgical, chemical, or cryogenic removal or inactivation of the globus pallidus of the brain.

pallidoansotomy (păl"ĭ-dō-ăn-sŏt'ō-mē) [" + *ansa,* a handle, + Gr. *tome,* incision]. Production of lesions in the globus pallidus and ansa lenticularis of the brain.

pallidotomy (păl"ĭ-dŏt'ō-mē) [" + Gr. *tome,* incision]. Surgical destruction of the globus pallidus done to treat involuntary movements or muscular rigidity.

pallidum (păl'ĭ-dŭm) [L.]. The globus pallidus of the lenticular nucleus in the corpus striatum.

pallium (păl'ē-ŭm) [L., cloak]. [NA] The cerebral cortex with its adjacent white substance, considered as a cover for the rest of the brain.

pallor (păl'or) [L.]. Lack of color; paleness. SEE: *skin.*

palm [L. *palma,* hand]. Anterior or flexor surface of the hand from wrist to fingers. SYN: *vola manus.* SEE: *antithenar; thenar.*

palma (păl'mă) [L.]. The palm of the hand.

palmar (păl'măr). Concerning the palm of the hand.

palmar grasp reflex. SEE: *reflex, palmar grasp.*

palmaris (păl-mā'rĭs). [NA] One of two muscles, palmaris brevis and palmaris longus. SEE: *Muscles* in *Appendix.*

palmar reflex. A grasping reflex in infants, more highly developed in some than in others. It gradually disappears and is absent after 4 or 5 months.

palmature (păl'mă-tūr) [L. *palma,* hand]. The pathological condition in which the fingers are joined or united.

palm-chin reflex. When the thenar eminence is scratched with a sharp object, contraction of the superficial muscles of the eye and chin is produced on the same side as the palmar area that was stimulated.

palmic (păl'mĭk) [Gr. *palmikos*]. 1. Concerning palpitation or pulse. 2. Concerning palmus.

palmitic acid (păl-mĭt'ĭk). $CH_3(CH_2)_{14}COOH$. A fatty acid found in palm oil, solid fats, some waxes, and many fatty oils.

palmitin (păl'mĭ-tĭn). An ester of glycerol and palmitic acid, derived from fat of both animal and vegetable origin.

palmomental reflex. Palm-chin reflex, q.v.

palmoplantar (păl"mō-plăn'tăr). Pert. to the palms of the hands and soles of the feet.

palmus (păl'mŭs) [Gr. *palmos,* pulsation, quivering]. 1. Palpitation; a throb. 2. Jerking; a disease with convulsive nervous twitching of the leg muscles, similar to jumping. 3. Heartbeat.

palpable (păl'pă-bl) [L. *palpabilis,* stroke, touch]. Perceptible, esp. by touch.

palpate (păl'pāt) [L. *palpare,* to touch]. To examine by touch; to feel.

palpation (păl-pā'shŭn) [L. *palpatio*]. Process of examining by application of the hands or fingers to the external surface of the body to detect evidence of disease or abnormalities in the various organs.

p., light-touch. Determining the outline of abdominal organs by lightly palpating the abdominal wall with the fingers.

palpatopercussion (păl"pă-tō-pĕr-kŭsh'ŭn). Palpation combined with percussion.

palpebra (păl'pĕ-bră) [L.]. (pl *palpebrae*) An eyelid.

p. inferior. [NA] The lower eyelid.

p. superior. [NA] The upper eyelid.

palpebral (păl'pē-brăl). Concerning an eyelid.

palpebral cartilages. Thin plates of condensed tissue resembling cartilage that form the framework of the eyelid. SYN: *tarsal cartilages.*

palpebral commissure. The union of the eyelids at each end of the palpebral fissure.

palpebral fissure. The opening between the eyelids.

palpebral ligament. One of two ligamentous structures (medial and lateral) that fix the two ends of the tarsi to the orbital wall.

palpebral muscles. 1. Palpebral portion of muscularis orbicularis oculi. 2. Levator palpebra muscle.

palpebrate (păl′pĕ-brāt). 1. [L. *palpebrare*]. To wink. 2. [L. *palpebra,* eyelid]. Possessing eyelids.

palpebritis (păl″pĕ-brī′tĭs) [L. *palpebra,* eyelid, + Gr. *itis,* inflammation]. Blepharitis, q.v.

palpitant (păl′pĭ-tănt) [L. *palpitare,* to quiver]. Throbbing; trembling.

palpitate (păl′pĭ-tāt) [L. *palpitatus,* throbbing]. 1. To cause to throb. 2. To throb or beat intensely or rapidly, usually said of the heart.

palpitation (păl-pĭ-tā′shŭn). Rapid, violent, or throbbing pulsation, as an abnormally rapid throbbing or fluttering of the heart. The palpitation is perceptible to the patient. SEE: *heart.*

p., arterial. Palpitation felt in course of an artery.

palsy (pawl′zē) [ME. *palesie,* from L. *paralysis*]. Temporary or permanent loss of sensation or loss of ability to move or to control movement. SYN: *paralysis.*

p., Bell's. Paralysis of the facial nerve in its peripheral distribution. Muscles of unaffected side of face pull the face into a distorted position.

p., birth. Palsy arising from an injury received at birth.

p., bulbar. Palsy caused by degeneration of the nuclear cells of the lower cranial nerves. This causes progressive muscular paralysis.

p., cerebral. Bilateral, symmetrical, nonprogressive paralysis resulting from developmental defects in brain or trauma at birth. SYN: *paralysis, cerebral spastic infantile; Little's disease.*

p., crutch. Palsy resulting from pressure on nerves in the axilla from use of a crutch.

p., diver's. Paralysis caused by decompression illness, q.v. SEE: *bends; caisson disease.*

p., Erb's. A paralysis of the deltoid, biceps, long supinator, and brachialis anticus muscles due to a lesion of the brachial plexus or of the fifth and sixth cervical nerves.

p., facial. P., Bell's, q.v.

p., lead. Paralysis of extremities in lead poisoning.

p., night. Form of paresthesia in which numbness is a symptom, esp. at night.

p., progressive supranuclear. Chronic progressive degenerative disease of the central nervous system that has its onset in middle age. There are conjugate ocular palsies, dystonia of the neck, and widespread rigidity.

p., Saturday night. Paralysis, musculospiral, q.v.

p., scrivener's. Writer's cramp.

p., shaking. Progressive muscular weakness and tremor with impaired voluntary motion. SYN: *paralysis agitans; Parkinson's disease.*

p., wasting. Chronic condition in which there is atrophy and paralysis of muscles; grows progressively worse. SYN: *progressive muscular atrophy.*

paludal (păl′ū-dăl) [L. *palus,* a marsh]. Concerning, or originating in, marshes. SYN: *malarial.*

paludism (păl′ū-dĭzm) [″ + Gr. *-ismos,* condition]. Swamp fever. SYN: *malaria.*

palynology [Gr. *palumein,* to sprinkle, + *logos,* study]. Study of pollens, spores or microscopic segments of organisms present in sediments.

Pamelor. Trade name for nortriptyline hydrochloride.

Pamine Bromide. Trade name for methscopolamine bromide.

pampiniform (păm-pĭn′ĭ-form) [L. *pampinus,* tendril, + *forma,* shape]. Convoluted like a tendril.

pampiniform plexus. 1. A mesh of spermatic or ovarian veins. 2. Network of nerves supplying the testicles.

pampinocele (păm-pĭn′ō-sēl) [″ + Gr. *kele,* swelling]. A swollen, painful condition of the veins of the spermatic cord. SYN: *varicocele.*

pan- [Gr.]. Combining form indicating all.

panacea (păn-ă-sē′ă) [Gr. *panakeia,* universal remedy]. A remedy for all ills; cure-all.

panagglutinable (păn″ă-gloo′tĭ-nă-b′l) [Gr. *pan,* all, + L. *agglutinare,* to glue to]. Blood cells that are agglutinable by every blood group serum of the species.

panagglutinin (păn″ă-glū′tĭn-ĭn) [Gr. *pan,* all, + L. *agglutinare,* to glue to]. Substance capable of agglutinizing corpuscles of every blood group.

panangiitis (păn″ăn-jē-ī′tĭs) [″ + *angeion,* vessel, + *itis,* inflammation]. Inflammation of all of the coats of a blood vessel.

panaris (păn′ă-rĭs) [L. *panaricium,* disease of the fingernail]. Inflammation of the skin fold surrounding the nail. SYN: *paronychia.*

panarteritis (păn″ăr-tĕ-rī′tĭs) [″ + *arteria,* artery, + *itis,* inflammation]. Inflammation of all of the coats of an artery.

panarthritis (păn-ăr-thrī′tĭs) [″ + *arthron,* joint, + *itis,* inflammation]. 1. Inflammation of all parts of a joint. 2. Inflamed condition of all the joints of the body.

panasthenia (păn″ăs-thē′nē-ă) [″ + *astheneia,* weakness]. Generalized weakness or exhaustion without evidence of organic disease. SYN: *neurasthenia.*

panatrophy (păn-ăt′rō-fē) [″ + *a-,* not, + *trophe,* nourishment]. Wasting away of an entire structure; generalized wasting away of the body.

panblastic (păn-blăs′tĭk) [″ + *blastos,* germ]. Concerning all of the layers of the blastoderm.

pancarditis (păn-kăr-dī′tĭs) [″ + *kardia,* heart, + *itis,* inflammation]. Inflamed condition involving all the structures of the heart.

panchreston (păn-krē′stŏn) [″ + *chrestos,* useful]. A remedy for every disease. SYN: *panacea.*

panchromia (păn-krō′mē-ă) [″ + *chroma,* color]. Power of staining with numerous dyes.

Pancoast syndrome. [H. K. Pancoast, U.S. physician, 1875–1939] Production of Horner's syndrome, q.v., by a malignant neoplasm of the cervical area with involvement of the brachial plexus and cervical sympathetic nerves. The neoplasm is called Pancoast's tumor.

pancolectomy (păn″kō-lĕk′tō-mē) [Gr. *pan,* all, + *kolon,* colon, + *ektome,* excision]. Surgical excision of the entire colon.

pancreas (păn′krē-ăs) [″ + *kreas,* flesh]. (pl. *pancreata*) [NA] A compound tubuloacinar or racemose gland situated behind the stomach in front of the 1st and 2nd lumbar vertebrae in a horizontal position, its head attached to the duodenum and its tail reaching to the spleen. The portion between the head and the tail constitutes the body.

The gland is composed of lobules that form lobes connected by strands of tissue with ducts that lead from the lobules into a main one, the pancreatic duct or duct of Wirsung. This duct is connected with the duodenum. Scattered throughout the substance are differentiated masses of cells that are the islets of Langerhans. An accessory pancreatic duct or duct of Santorini frequently is present. It is smaller than the main duct and opens into the duodenum cephalad to the main duct with which it communicates SEE: illus.

FUNCT: The pancreas produces both an external and an internal secretion. The external secretion, called pancreatic juice, q.v., is produced by the cells of the acini. It passes through the pancreatic ducts into the duodenum, where it plays an important role in the digestion of all classes of foods. The internal secretion, which is elaborated by the islets of Langerhans, includes the hormones insulin and glucagon (hyperglycemic-glycogenolytic factor). These hormones in conjunction with hormones from other endocrine glands (adrenal cortex, medulla, anterior hypophysis), play a primary role in the regulation of carbohydrate metabolism.

Diminished secretion of insulin by the islets of Langerhans results in a clinical entity called diabetes mellitus, q.v. In this disease there are disturbances in the metabolism of carbohydrates and fats resulting in the elevation of blood glucose, cholesterol, and ketone bodies. Urinary output is greatly increased and the urine usually contains glucose and ketone bodies.

Excessive secretion of insulin, called hyperinsulinism, q.v., may sometimes occur. This results in the lowering of blood sugar (hypoglycemia, q.v.).

p., accessory. Small mass of pancreatic

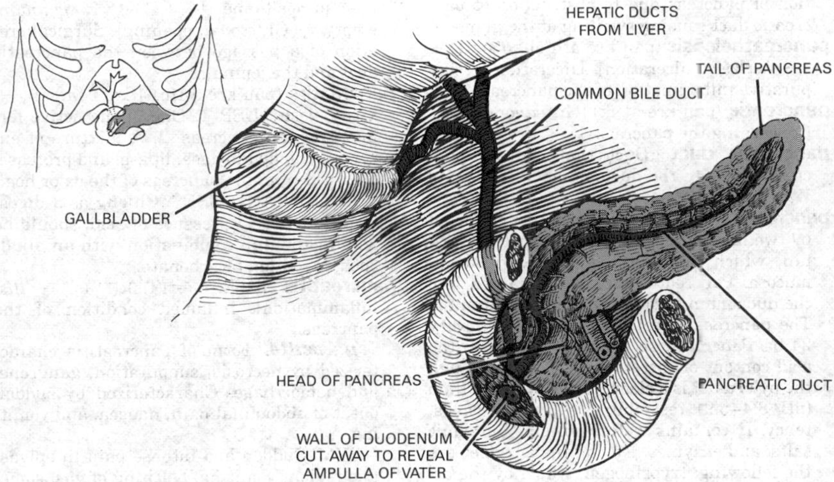

PANCREAS AND ITS RELATIONSHIP TO THE DUODENUM

tissue close to the pancreas but detached from it.

p., annular. An anomalous condition in which a portion of the pancreas encircles the duodenum.

p. divisum. A congenital anomaly wherein the two portions of the embryonic pancreas fail to unite.

p., dorsal. A dorsal outpocketing of the embryonic gut that gives rise to the body and tail of the adult pancreas.

p., lesser. Semi-detached lobular part of the posterior surface of the head of the pancreas, sometimes having a separate duct opening into the principal one. SYN: *p., Willis'*.

p., ventral. An outgrowth at the angle of the hepatic diverticulum and the embryonic gut that migrates and fuses with the dorsal pancreas. It forms the head of the definitive organ.

p., Willis'. P., lesser.

pancreatalgia (păn″krē-ă-tăl′jē-ă) [″ + *kreas,* flesh, + *algos,* pain]. Pain in the pancreas.

pancreatectomy (păn″krē-ăt-ĕk′tō-mē) [″ + ″ + *ektome,* excision]. Operation for removal of part or all of the pancreas. Total pancreatectomy will produce diabetes because of a complete lack of insulin. Following a subtotal (or partial) pancreatectomy, diabetes will develop some time later because the remaining islets will be unable to take care of the excessive demands placed upon them. SEE: *diabetes.*

pancreatemphraxis (păn″krē-ăt-ĕm-frăk′sĭs) [″ + ″ + *emphraxis,* stoppage]. Congestion of pancreas due to obstruction of pancreatic duct causing swelling of the gland.

pancreathelcosis (păn″krē-ăth″ĕl-kō′sĭs) [″ + ″ + *helkosis,* ulceration]. Ulceration or suppurative inflammation of the pancreas.

pancreatic (păn″krē-ăt′ĭk) [Gr. *pancreaticus*]. Concerning the pancreas.

pancreatic duct. Duct that conveys pancreatic juice to the duodenum. SYN: *duct of Wirsung.*

pancreatic juice. Its secretion is brought about by two hormones, secretin and cholecystokinin, which are secreted by the duodenal mucosa. Pancreatic juice is discharged into the duodenum through the duct of Wirsung. The pancreas secretes 500 to 800 ml. every 24 hr. Pancreatic secretion begins when the acid content of the stomach passes through the pylorus. It is a clear, viscid, alkaline fluid (pH 8.4–8.9) resembling saliva in consistency. It contains water, protein, inorganic salts, and enzymes. Among the enzymes are the following: trypsinogen, which by the action of intestinal enterokinase is converted into trypsin, a proteolytic enzyme; chymotrypsinogen, which is converted by trypsin into chymotrypsin, a milkcurdling enzyme; amylopsin, a maltase that acts on carbohydrates; and steapsin, a lipase that acts on fats. Amylopsin hydrolyzes starch to maltose; steapsin hydrolyzes fats to fatty acids and glycerol; trypsinogen, by the action of enterokinase in the duodenum, is converted into the active form trypsin which hydrolyzes proteins to amino acids. The alkaline secretion from the pancreas neutralizes the acidity of the chyme entering the duodenum from the stomach. SEE: *enzyme; pancreas; secretion.*

pancreaticocholecystostomy (păn″krē-ăt″ĭ-kō-kō″lē-sĭs-tŏs′tō-mē) [Gr. *pan,* all, + *kreas,* flesh, + *chole,* bile, + *kystis,* bladder, + *stoma,* opening]. Surgical creation of passage between the gallbladder and pancreas.

pancreaticoduodenal (păn″krē-ăt″ĭ-kō-dū-ō-dē′năl) [″ + ″ + L. *duodeni,* twelve]. Concerning the duodenum and pancreas.

pancreaticoduodenostomy (păn″krē-ăt″ĭ-kō-dū″ō-dē-nŏs′tō-mē) [″ + ″ + ″ + Gr. *stoma,* opening]. Surgical creation of an artificial passage between the pancreas and duodenum.

pancreaticoenterostomy (păn″krē-ăt″ĭ-kō-ĕn″tĕr-ŏs′tō-mē) [″ + ″ + *enteron,* intestine, + *stoma,* opening]. Surgical creation of a passage between the pancreatic duct and the intestine.

pancreaticogastrostomy (păn″krē-ăt′ĭ-kō-găs-trŏs′tō-mē) [″ + ″ + *gaster,* belly, + *stoma,* opening]. Surgical creation of a passage between the pancreas and stomach.

pancreaticojejunostomy (păn″krē-ăt″ĭ-kō-jĕ″jū-nŏs′tō-mē) [″ + ″ + L. *jejunum,* empty, + Gr. *stoma,* opening]. Surgical creation of a passage between the pancreatic duct and the jejunum.

pancreatin (păn′krē-ă-tĭn) [Gr. *pan,* all, + *kreas,* flesh]. USP. 1. One of the active ferments of the pancreas. 2. A mixture of enzymes, chiefly amylase, lipase, and protease, obtained from the pancreas of the ox or hog.

ACTION AND USES: Chiefly as a digestant. Inactive in presence of acid, should be administered in combination with an alkali such as sodium bicarbonate.

pancreatitis (păn″krē-ă-tī′tĭs) [″ + ″ + *itis,* inflammation]. Inflamed condition of the pancreas.

p., acute. Form of pancreatitis characterized by necrosis, suppuration, gangrene, and hemorrhage. Characterized by sudden onset of abdominal pain, nausea, and vomiting.

SYM: Sudden and intense pain in epigastric region, vomiting, belching of gas, sometimes hiccough, collapse. Rigidity and tenderness over umbilicus. Constipation, slow pulse, possible jaundice.

p., acute hemorrhagic. Form of pancreatitis with hemorrhage into pancreatic tissue.

SYM: Paroxysms of deep-seated pain in epigastrium, nausea, retching, constipation. Slight rise in temperature, blood and mucus in vomitus, delirium, tympanites, jaundice, hiccough, cyanosis, collapse.

p., calcareous. Pancreatitis accompanied by calculi formation.

p., centrilobar. Pancreatitis located around divisions of the pancreatic duct.

p., chronic. Form of pancreatitis marked by formation of scar tissue associated with malfunction.

SYM: Pain, mild or severe. Pain has tendency to radiate to the back. Jaundice, weakness, emaciation, diarrhea.

p., interstitial. Pancreatitis with overgrowth of inter- and intra-acinar connective tissue.

p., perilobar. Fibrosis of the pancreas between acinous groups.

p., purulent. Pancreatitis with suppuration.

p., suppurative. Form of pancreatitis marked by development of many small abscesses. Symptoms may be those of acute or chronic form.

pancreatoduodenectomy (păn″krē-ă-tō-dū″ō-dē-nĕk′tō-mē) [Gr. *pan,* all, + *kreas,* flesh, + L. *duodeni,* twelve, + Gr. *ektome,* excision]. Excision of the head of the pancreas and the adjacent portion of the duodenum.

pancreatoduodenostomy (păn″krē-ă-tō-dū″ō-dĕ-nŏs′tō-mē) [″ + ″ + ″ + *stoma,* opening]. Surgical anastomosis of the pancreatic duct, or a pancreatic fistula, to the duodenum.

pancreatogenic, pancreatogenous (păn″krē-ă-tō-jĕn′ĭk, -tŏj′ĕ-nŭs) [″ + ″ + *gennan,* to produce]. Produced in or by the pancreas; having origin in the pancreas.

pancreatography (păn″krē-ă-tŏg′ră-fē) [″ + ″ + *graphein,* to write]. Combined surgical and radiographic procedure in which a roentgenogram of the pancreas is taken after iodinated contrast medium is injected into the duct of Wirsung.

pancreatolith (păn″krē-ăt′ō-lĭth) [″ + *kreas,* flesh, + *lithos,* stone]. A calculus of the pancreas.

pancreatolithectomy (păn″krē-ăt-ō-lĭth-ĕk′tō-mē) [″ + ″ + ″ + *ektome,* excision]. Removal of a calculus from the pancreas. SYN: *pancreatolithotomy; pancreolithotomy.*

pancreatolithiasis (păn″krē-ă-tō-lĭ-thī′ă-sĭs) [″ + ″ + ″ + *-iasis,* condition]. Calculi in the duct system of the pancreas.

pancreatolithotomy (păn″krē-ăt-ō-lĭth-ŏt′ō-mē) [″ + ″ + ″ + *tome,* an incision]. Removal of a calculus from the pancreas. SYN: *pancreatolithectomy; pancreolithotomy.*

pancreatolysis (păn″krē-ă-tŏl′ĭ-sĭs) [″ + *kreas,* flesh, + *lysis,* dissolution]. Destruction of the pancreatic substance by pancreatic enzymes.

pancreatolytic (păn″krē-ăt-ō-lĭt′ĭk). Destructive to the pancreatic tissues. SYN: *pancreolytic.*

pancreatomy (păn-krē-ăt′ō-mē) [″ + *kreas,* flesh, + *tome,* incision]. Pancreatotomy, q.v.

pancreatoncus (păn-krē-ăt-ŏng′kŭs) [″ + ″ + *onkos,* tumor]. A pancreatic tumor.

pancreatopathy (păn″krē-ă-tŏp′ă-thē) [″ + ″ + *pathos,* disease]. Any pathological state of the pancreas. SYN: *pancreopathy.*

pancreatotomy (păn″krē-ă-tŏt′ō-mē) [″ + ″ + *tome,* incision]. Surgical incision into the pancreas. SYN: *pancreatomy.*

pancreatotropic (păn-krē″ă-tō-trŏp′ĭk) [″ + ″ + *tropikos,* turning]. Having an affinity for or action on the pancreas.

pancreectomy (păn″krē-ĕk′tō-mē) [″ + ″ + *ektome,* excision]. Partial or total excision of the pancreas.

pancrelipase (păn″krē-lī′pās). USP. A standardized preparation of enzymes, principally lipase, with amylase and protease, obtained from the pancreas of the hog. Used in treating conditions associated with deficient secretion from the pancreas. Trade names are Cotazym, Ilozyme, and Accelerase.

pancreolithotomy (păn″krē-ō-lĭth-ŏt′ō-mē) [″ + *kreas,* flesh, + *lithos,* stone, + *tome,* incision]. Surgical removal of a pancreatic concretion. SYN: *pancreatolithectomy; pancreatolithotomy.*

pancreolysis (păn″krē-ŏl′ĭ-sĭs) [″ + ″ + *lysis* dissolution]. Enzymatic destruction of the pancreas.

pancreolytic (păn″krē-ō-lĭt′ĭk) [″ + ″ + *lysis,* dissolution]. Destructive to the pancreas. SYN: *pancreatolytic.*

pancreopathy (păn″krē-ŏp′ă-thē) [″ + ″ + *pathos,* disease]. Any diseased condition of the pancreas. SYN: *pancreatopathy.*

pancreoprivic (păn″krē-ō-prĭv′ĭk). Having no pancreas.

pancreozymin-cholecystokinin. A polypeptide that has various effects on the gastrointestinal tract including stimulation of the pancreas to produce insulin and pancreatic enzymes. This substance has also been found in the brain.

pancuronium bromide (păn″kū-rō′nē-ŭm). A neuromuscular blocking agent. Trade name is Pavulon.

pancytopenia (păn″sī-tō-pē′nē-ă) [″ + *kytos,* cell, + *penia,* poverty]. A reduction in all cellular elements of the blood. SEE: *anemia, aplastic.*

pandemia (păn-dē′mē-ă) [″ + *demos,* the people]. Epidemic affecting the major portion of the population of a district.

pandemic (păn-dĕm'ĭk). A disease affecting the majority of the population of a large region, or a disease that is epidemic at the same time in many different parts of the world.

pandiculation (păn"dĭk-ū-lā'shŭn) [L. *pandiculari*, to stretch one's self]. Stretching of the limbs and yawning, as on awakening from normal sleep.

panencephalitis (păn"ĕn-sĕf"ă-lī'tĭs) [Gr. *pan*, all, + *enkephalos*, brain, + *itis*, inflammation]. A cerebral degenerative disease thought to be secondary to entrance of the measles virus into the brain. The first signs are due to a progressive decrease in higher cerebral functions, usually manifested as failure to progress in school. There are personality changes, emotional instability, and generalized myoclonic jerks. In late stages, dementia and generalized rigidity occur. There is no treatment and most patients die of the disease. SYN: *subacute sclerosing panencephalitis.*

panendoscope (păn-ĕn'dō-skōp) [" + *endon*, within, + *skopein*, to view]. A cystoscope that gives a wide view of the bladder.

panesthesia (păn"ĕs-thē'zē-ă) [" + *aisthesis*, perception]. The sum of all of the stimuli and sensations coming from the body at one time.

Paneth, cells of (pă'nāt). [Josef Paneth, Ger. physician, 1857–1890] Large secretory cells, containing coarse granules, found at the blind end of the crypts of Lieberkühn (the intestinal glands).

pang. 1. A paroxysm of extreme agony. 2. A sudden attack of any emotion.

pangamic acid. A substance of disputed composition with no known therapeutic or nutritional properties. SYN: *"vitamin B-15."*

pangenesis (păn-jĕn'ĕ-sĭs) [" + *genesis*, production]. The discredited hypothesis that each cell of the parent is represented by a particle in the reproductive cell, and thus each part of the organism reproduces itself in the progeny.

panglossia (păn-glŏs'sē-ă) [Gr.]. Excessive talkativeness, esp. in psychotic persons.

Panheprin. Trade name for heparin sodium, USP.

panhidrosis (păn"hĭd-rō'sĭs) [Gr. *pan*, all, + *hidros*, perspiration]. Perspiration over the entire surface of the body.

panhyperemia (păn"hī-pĕr-ē'mē-ă) [" + *hyper*, over, + *haima*, blood]. Widespread or complete hyperemia.

panhypopituitarism (păn-hī"pō-pĭ-tū'ĭ-tăr-ĭzm) [" + *hypo*, under, + L. *pituita*, mucus, + Gr. *-ismos*, condition]. Defective or absent function of the entire pituitary gland. SEE: *Simmonds' disease.*

panhysterectomy (păn"hĭs-tĕr-ĕk'tō-mē) [" + *hystera*, uterus, + *ektome*, excision]. Excision of entire uterus including the cervix uteri. SEE: *hysterectomy.*

panhysterocolpectomy (păn-hĭs"tĕr-ō-kŏl-pĕk'tō-mē) [" + " + *kolpos*, vagina, + *ektome*, excision]. Total excision of the uterus and vagina.

panhystero-oophorectomy (păn-hĭs"tĕr-ō-ō"ŏf-ō-rĕk'tō-mē) [" + " + *oophoros*, bearing eggs, + *ektome*, excision]. Excision of uterus, cervix uteri, and one or both ovaries.

panhysterosalpingectomy (păn-hĭs"tĕr-ō-săl"pĭn-jĕk'tō-mē) [" + " + *salpinx*, tube, + *ektome*, excision]. Surgical removal of the uterus, cervix, and fallopian tubes.

panhysterosalpingo-oophorectomy (păn-hĭs"tĕr-ō-săl"pĭng-gō-ō"ŏf-ō-rĕk'tō-mē) [" + " + " + *oophoros*, bearing eggs, + *ektome*, excision]. Excision of entire uterus, including the cervix, ovaries, and uterine tubes.

panic (păn'ĭk). Acute anxiety, terror or fright, usually of sudden onset, that may be uncontrollable and require sedation. Because it is difficult to know the cause of this reaction, it is quite difficult to evaluate the response. If hyperventilation and tetany are present, the patient should breathe with the mouth closed and one nostril held closed. This will alleviate the symptoms in a short time.

p., homosexual. An acute anxiety syndrome due to unconscious homosexual conflicts. Symptoms include fear, paranoid ideas, and excitement, and sometimes hallucinations and combative behavior are present.

panimmunity (păn"ĭ-mū'nĭ-tē) [" + L. *immunitas*, immunity]. General immunity to a large number of bacterial diseases.

panis (păn'ĭs) [L.]. Bread.

Panmycin Hydrochloride. Trade name for tetracycline hydrochloride, USP.

panmyeloid (păn-mī'ĕ-loyd) [" + *myelos*, marrow, + *eidos*, form]. Concerning all of the elements of the bone marrow.

panmyelophthisis (păn"mī-ĕl-ŏf'thĭ-sĭs) [Gr. *pan*, all, + *myelos*, marrow, + *phthisis*, a wasting]. 1. General wasting away of the bone marrow. 2. Aplastic anemia.

panmyelosis (păn"mī-ĕl-ō'sĭs) [" + " + *osis*, condition]. Increase in all the elements of the bone marrow.

panneuritis (păn"ū-rī'tĭs) [" + *neuron*, sinew, + *itis*, inflammation]. Generalized neuritis.

p. endemica. Deficiency disease in which there is lack of vitamin B_1. SYN: *beriberi.*

panniculitis (păn-ĭk"ū-lī'tĭs) [L. *panniculus*, a small piece of cloth, + *itis*, inflammation]. Inflamed condition of a layer of fatty connective tissue in the anterior wall of the abdomen.

SYM: Pain and tenderness and hypertrophy of tissue in parts where fat is the thickest.

p., nodular nonsuppurative. A rare disease of unknown etiology characterized by intermittent fever and groups of tender nodules in the subcutaneous fat tissue. SYN: *Weber-Christian disease.*

p., relapsing febrile nodular nonsuppurative. P., nodular nonsuppurative, q.v.

panniculus (păn-ĭk'ū-lŭs) [L., a small piece of cloth]. Any clothlike sheet or layer of tissue.

p. adiposus. [NA] The subcutaneous layer of fat, esp. where fat is abundant; the superficial fascia that is heavily laden with fat cells.

p. carnosus. Thin layer of muscular tissue in the superficial fascia. SEE: *platysma myoides.*

pannus (păn'nŭs) [L., cloth]. Newly formed superficial vascular tissue over the cornea. The area is cloudy and its surface is uneven because it is covered with a film of new capillary blood vessels. May cover the entire cornea. May be seen in trachoma, acne rosacea, eczema, and as a result of irritation in granular conjunctivitis.

p. carateus. Pinta.

p. carnosus. P. crassus.

p. crassus. Pannus that is highly vascularized, thick, and opaque. SYN: *p. carnosus.*

p. degenerativus. P. siccus.

p., phlyctenular. Pannus that occurs in conjunction with phlyctenular conjunctivitis.

p. siccus. Pannus accompanying xerophthalmia; composed principally of connective tissue; poorly vascularized and dry. SYN: *p. degenerativus.*

p. tenuis. Pannus that is thin, poorly vascularized, and with slight opacity.

panodic (pă-nŏd'ĭk). Radiating in all directions, esp. a nerve impulse.

panography (pă-nŏg'ră-fē). Radiographic procedure that provides a panoramic view of an entire dental arch on one film.

panophobia (păn-ō-fō'bē-ă) [Gr. *pan,* all, + *phobos,* fear]. Morbid fear of some unknown evil or of everything in general; general apprehension. SYN: *pantophobia.*

panophthalmia, panophthalmitis (păn-ŏf-thăl'mē-ă, -thăl-mī'tĭs) [" + *ophthalmos,* eye, + *itis,* inflammation]. Inflammation of entire eye.

panoptic (păn-ŏp'tĭk) [" + *optikos,* vision]. Making every part visible.

panoptic stain. Stain that causes every part of the tissue to be differentiated.

panoptosis (păn-ŏp-tō'sĭs) [" + *ptosis,* falling]. General prolapse of the abdominal organs.

pan-oral radiography. Radiographic procedure that provides a panoramic view of an entire dental arch on one film.

panosteitis (păn"ŏs-tē-ī'tĭs) [Gr. *pan,* all, + *osteon,* bone, + *itis,* inflammation]. Inflammation of every structure of a bone.

panotitis (păn-ō-tī'tĭs) [" + *ous,* ear, + *itis,* inflammation]. Inflammation involving all the parts of the ear.

Panoxyl. Trade name for benzoyl peroxide, USP.

panphobia (păn-fō'bē-ă) [" + *phobos,* fear]. Groundless fear of everything. SYN: *pantophobia.*

panplegia (păn-plē'jē-ă) [" + *plege,* stroke]. Total paralysis.

pansclerosis (păn"sklē-rō'sĭs) [" + *sklerosis,* hardening]. Hardening of all of an organ.

pansinusitis (păn"sī-nŭs-ī'tĭs) [" + *sinus,* cavity, + *itis,* inflammation]. Inflammation of all of the paranasal sinuses.

pansphygmograph (păn-sfĭg'mō-grăf) [" + *sphygmos,* pulse, + *graphein,* to write]. Apparatus for registering cardiac movements, the pulse wave, and chest movements at the same time.

Panstrongylus (păn-strŏn'jĭ-lŭs). A genus of insects belonging to the order Hemiptera, family Reduviidae.

P. megistus. Species that serves as vector for Trypanosoma cruzi, the causative agent of Chagas' disease.

pant [ME. *panten*]. 1. To gasp for breath. 2. A short and shallow breath.

ETIOL: Produced by physical overexertion, as in running, or from fear.

pant-, panto- [Gr. *pantos,* all]. Combining form indicating all or the whole of something.

pantachromatic (păn"tă-krō-măt'ĭk) [" + *achromatos,* colorless]. Entirely colorless.

pantalgia (păn-tăl'jē-ă) [" + *algos,* pain]. Pain felt over the entire body.

pantamorphia (păn"tă-mor'fē-ă) [" + *a-,* not, + *morphe,* form]. Generalized malformation.

pantanencephaly (păn"tăn-ĕn-sĕf'ă-lē) [" + *an-,* not, + *enkephalos,* brain]. Complete absence of the brain in the fetus.

pantankyloblepharon (păn-tăng"kĭ-lō-blĕf'ă-rŏn) [" + *ankyle,* noose, + *blepharon,* lid]. Generalized adhesion of the eyelids to the eyeball.

pantatrophia, pantatrophy (păn-tă-trō'fē-ă, -tăt'rō-fē) [" + *atrophia,* atrophy]. General wasting and atrophy.

Panteric. Trade name for pancreatin.

pantetheine (păn-tē-thē'ĭn). The naturally occurring amide of pantothenic acid. It is a growth factor for Lactobacillus bulgaricus.

panthodic (păn-thŏd'ĭk) [" + *hodos,* way]. Radiating to all parts of the body, esp. applied to nervous impulses.

panting (pănt'ĭng) [ME. *panten*]. Short, shallow, rapid respirations.

pantograph (păn'tō-grăf) [Gr. *pantos,* all, + *graphein,* to write]. A device that will reproduce, through a system of levers connected to a stylus, a duplicate of whatever figure or drawing is being copied by the device.

pantomography (păn″tō-mŏg′ră-fē). Tomography of curved surfaces.

pantomorphia (păn″tō-mor′fē-ă) [″ + *morphe*, form]. 1. State of being symmetrical. 2. Being able to assume any shape.

pantophobia (păn-tō-fō bē-ă) [″ + *phobos*, fear]. Morbid, groundless fear of everything in general. SYN: *panophobia*.

pantoscopic (păn″tō-skŏp′ĭk) [″ + *skopein*, to examine]. Adjusted to view both close and distant objects.

pantoscopic glasses. Glasses with two segments of different focal lengths for near and far objects. SYN: *lenses, bifocal*.

pantothenate (păn-tō′thĕn-āt). A salt of pantothenic acid.

pantothenic acid (păn-tō-thĕn′ĭk). $C_9H_{17}NO_5$. A vitamin of the B-complex group widely distributed in nature, occurring naturally in yeast, liver, heart, salmon, eggs, and various grains. It was synthesized in 1940.

pantothermia (păn″tō-thĕr′mē-ă) [″ + *therme*, heat]. Condition in which there is a variation in bodily temperature without any apparent reason.

pantropic (păn-trō′pĭk, -trŏp′ĭk) [″ + *tropos*, turning]. Showing affinity to many organs, as pantropic viruses. SYN: *polycytotropic*.

panturbinate (păn-tŭr′bĭ-nāt) [″ + L. *turbinatus*, shaped like a top]. All of the turbinate structure of the nose; the nasal concha.

Panwarfin. Trade name for warfarin sodium, USP.

panzootic (păn″zō-ŏt′ĭk) [″ + *zoon*, animal]. Any animal disease that is widespread.

PaO_2. The partial pressure of oxygen in arterial blood. Arterial oxygen concentration, or tension. Usually expressed in mm. Hg.

pap (păp) [L. *pappa*, infant's sound for food]. Any soft, semiliquid food.

papain (pă-pā′ĭn). USP. Proteolytic enzyme obtained from the fruit of the papaya, Carica papaya. Used to tenderize meat. Trade name is Caroid.

Papanicolaou test. [George Papanicolaou, U.S. scientist, 1883–1962] A study for early detection of cancer cells. It involves collecting material from areas of the body that shed cells or in which shed cells collect, esp. the cervix and vagina. This material is then prepared for microscopic study by special staining. Analysis of the cells is extremely helpful in diagnosing cancer.

ABBR: Pap smear; Pap test.

papaverine hydrochloride (pă-păv′ĕr-ēn) [L., poppy]. USP. The salt of an alkaloid obtained from opium. Used as an a smooth muscle relaxant, esp. in gastric and intestinal distress, and recommended in bronchial spasm. Trade names are Tutag, Cerespan, Pavabid, and Therapav.

papaya (pă-pă′yă) [Sp. AmerInd.]. 1. A tropical tree, Carica papaya. 2. Large, oblong, edible fruit from that tree. Source of papain, q.v.

paper [L. *papyrus*, paper]. 1. Cellulose pulp prepared in thin sheets from fibers of wood, rags, and other substances. 2. A piece of paper prepared with a medicinal solution. SYN: *charta*. 3. Thin sheet of cellulosic material impregnated with specific chemicals that react in a definite manner when exposed to certain solutions. This permits use of these papers for testing purposes.

p., articulating. Paper coated on both sides with a pigment that marks the teeth when their occlusal surfaces contact the paper. This allows the contact points of the teeth to be demonstrated.

p., bibulous. Paper that absorbs water readily.

p., blistering. A paper saturated with a substance, such as cantharides, that causes vesiculation when applied to the skin.

p., filter. A porous, unglazed paper used for filtration.

p., indicator. Paper saturated with an indicator solution of known strength and then dried. Used for testing the pH (acidity or alkalinity) of a solution.

p., litmus. An indicator paper impregnated with litmus, which in alkalies turns blue and in acids turns red.

p., occluding. P., articulating, q.v.

p., test. Paper impregnated with a substance that will change color when exposed to solutions of a certain pH, or to specific chemicals.

papilla (pă-pĭl′ă) [L.]. (pl. *papillae*) [NA] A small, nipplelike protuberance or elevation.

p., acoustic. The spiral organ of the ear.

p., Bergmeister's. A veil in front of the retina of the eye. It is made of a conical mass of glial elements that are the developmental tissue of the eye that has not been reabsorbed.

p., circumvallate. One of the large papillae near the base on the dorsal aspect of the tongue, arranged in a V-shape. The taste buds are located in the epithelium of the trench surrounding the papilla.

p., clavate. P., fungiform, q.v.

p., conical. 1. Papillae on the dorsum of the tongue. 2. Papillae in the ridge-like projections in the corium of the surface of the skin.

p., dental. A mass of connective tissue that becomes enclosed by the developing enamel organ. It gives rise to dentin and dental pulp.

p., dermal. Small elevations of the corium that indent the inner surface of the epidermis.

p., duodenal. Papilla of Vater.

p., filiform. One of the very slender papillae at the tip of the tongue.

p., foliate. Folds, which are rudimentary papillae, in the sides of the tongue.

p., fungiform. One of the broad flat papillae resembling a fungus, chiefly found on the dorsal central area of the tongue.

p., gingival. The gingiva that fills the proximal space between adjacent teeth.

p., gustatory. Taste papilla of tongue; one of those possessing a taste bud.

p., incisive. Projection on the anterior portion of the raphe of the palate.

p., interdental. The triangular shaped part of the gingivae that fits between adjacent teeth, including both free gingiva and attached gingiva.

p., interproximal. The gingival papillae between adjacent teeth. These include the projections seen from the lingual, buccal, or labial sides.

p., lacrimal. An elevation in medial edge of each eyelid, in the center of which is the opening of the lacrimal duct.

p., lenticular. A small rounded elevation underlying lymphatic nodules in mucosa of the root of the tongue.

p., lingual. Any one of the tiny eminences covering the anterior two thirds of the tongue, including circumvallate, filiform, fungiform, and conical papillae.

p. mammae. [NA] The nipple of the mammary gland.

p., optic. Point at which optic nerve fibers leave the eyeball. SYN: *blind spot; optic disk.*

p. of corium. P., conical (def. 2).

p. of hair. A conical process of the corium that projects into undersurface of a hair bulb. It contains capillaries through which a hair receives its nourishment.

p. of Vater. The duodenal end of the drainage systems of the pancreatic and common bile ducts. Commonly, but inaccurately, called ampulla of Vater. SYN: *p., duodenal.*

p., palatine. P., incisive, q.v.

p., parotid. The projections around the opening of the parotid duct into the mouth.

p. pili. Papilla of hair, q.v.

p., renal. Apex of a malpighian pyramid in the kidney.

p., tactile. A dermal papilla that contains a sensory end-organ for touch.

p., taste. P., gustatory.

p., urethral. The small projection in the vestibule of the vagina at the entrance of the urethra.

p., vallate. P., circumvallate, q.v.

papillary (păp'ĭ-lăr-ē) [L. *papilla,* nipple]. 1. Concerning a nipple or papilla. 2. Resembling or composed of papillae.

papillary ducts of Bellini. Short ducts that open on tip of renal papilla. They are formed by union of the straight collecting tubules.

papillary layer. The layer of the corium that adjoins the epidermis. SYN: *stratum papillare.*

papillary muscles. Muscular eminences in ventricles of the heart.

papillary tumor. Neoplasm composed of or resembling enlarged papillae. SEE: *papilloma.*

papillate (păp'ĭ-lāt) [L. *papilla,* nipple]. Having nipplelike growths on the surface, as a culture in bacteriology.

papillectomy (păp"ĭ-lĕk'tō-mē) [" + Gr. *ektome,* excision]. Excision of any papilla or papillae.

papilledema (păp"ĭl-ĕ-dē'mă) [" + Gr. *oidema,* swelling]. Edema and inflammation of the optic nerve at its point of entrance into the eyeball. SYN: *choked disk.*

ETIOL: Intracranial pressure, often caused by tumor of the brain pressing on optic nerve.

PROG: Blindness may result very rapidly unless relieved.

papilliferous (păp"ĭ-lĭf'ĕr-ŭs) [" + *ferre,* to carry]. Having or containing papillae.

papilliform (pă-pĭl'ĭ-form) [" + *forma,* shape]. Having the characteristics or appearance of papillae.

papillitis (păp-ĭ-lī'tĭs) [" + Gr. *itis,* inflammation]. Inflammation of the optic disk, usually accompanied by swelling. SYN: *choked disk.*

papilloadenocystoma (păp"ĭl-ō-ăd"ĕ-nō-sĭs-tō'mă) [" + Gr. *aden,* gland, + *kystis,* a cyst, + *oma,* tumor]. A tumor composed of elements of papilloma, adenoma, and cystoma.

papillocarcinoma (păp"ĭl-ō-kăr-sĭ-nō'mă) [" + Gr. *karkinos,* crab, + *oma,* tumor]. 1. A malignant tumor of hypertrophied papillae. 2. Carcinoma with papillary growths.

papilloma (păp-ĭ-lō'mă) [" + Gr. *oma,* tumor]. 1. Any benign epithelial tumor. 2. Epithelial tumor of skin or mucous membrane consisting of hypertrophied papillae covered by a layer of epithelium. Included in this group are warts, condylomas, and polyps. SEE: *acanthoma; papillomaviruses.*

p. durum. A hardened papilloma, as a wart or corn.

p., fibroepithelial. A skin tag containing fibrous tissue.

p., hard. Papilloma that develops from squamous epithelium.

p., Hopman. A papillomatous overgrowth of the nasal mucosa. SYN: *Hopman's polyp.*

p., intracystic. Papilloma within a cystic adenoma.

p. molle. A papilloma with only a thin, horny layer covering it. SYN: *condyloma.*

p., soft. Papilloma formed from columnar epithelium; applies to any small, soft growth.

p., villous. Papilloma with thin, long excresences present in the urinary bladder, breast, intestinal tract, or choroid plexus of the cerebral ventricles.

papillomatosis (păp″ĭ-lō-mă-tō′sĭs) [″ + Gr. *oma*, tumor, + *osis*, condition]. 1. Widespread formation of papillomas. 2. Condition of being afflicted with many papillomas.

papillomaviruses. Viruses that cause papillomas or warts in man and animals. They belong to the papovaviruses family or group.

papilloretinitis (păp″ĭ-lō-rĕt-ĭn-ī′tĭs) [″ + *rete*, net, + Gr. *itis*, inflammation]. Inflamed condition of the papilla and retina extending to the optic disk.

papovaviruses (păp″ō-vă-vī′rŭs-ĕs) [*pa*pilloma + *po*lyoma + *va*cuolating agent + *virus*]. A group of viruses important in investigating viral carcinogenesis. Included are polyoma virus, simian virus 40 (SV40), and papilloma viruses.

pappataci fever. Sandfly fever.

pappose (păp′pōs) [L. *pappus*, down]. Covered with fine, downy hair.

pappus [L.]. The first growth of beard hair appearing on the cheeks and chin as fine, downy hair.

paprika (păp′rĭ-kă, păp-rē′kă) [Gr. *peperi*, pepper]. A mild, powdered seasoning made from sweet red peppers. Also used to color food.

Pap smear; Pap test. Papanicolaou test.

papula (păp′ū-lă) [L.]. A small, inflammatory, congested spot on the skin; a pimple. SYN: *papule*.

papular (păp′ū-lĕr). Concerning an eruption of the nature of papules.

papular fever. Mild fever with maculopapular eruptions and rheumatoid pains.

papulation (păp-ū-lā′shŭn). 1. The development of papules. 2. The stage of pimple formation in a disease.

papule (păp′ūl) [L. *papula*, pimple]. Red elevated area on the skin, solid and circumscribed. Papules often precede vesicular or pustular formation and may appear in erythema multiforme, eczema papulosum, prurigo, syphilis, measles, and smallpox, and they may develop after use of bromides, iodides, or coal tar preparations.

DIFF. DIAG: In *measles* they are small and run together. In *smallpox* they are hard and feel like pellets, terminating in umbilicated vesicles that itch. In *prurigo* they are small, pale, deep seated, and accompanied by intense itching. In *syphilis* they are dark colored and widely distributed, esp. on the trunk and surfaces of the extremities; they do not cause itching. In *eczema* they are small, often associated with pustules and vesicles, and are closely aggregated; there is intense itching and the skin is thickened. In *erythema multiforme* they are found with macules and tubercles and are bright red or purple and flat, appearing esp. on the extremities; they do not suppurate or cause itching.

p., dry. Hard papule that is primary lesion of syphilis, occurring at site of infection. SYN: *chancre*.

p., moist. A syphilitic eruption of papules with flat tops. SYN: *condyloma latum; p., mucous*.

p., mucous. P., moist.

p., split. Fissures at the corners of the mouth. Seen in some cases of secondary syphilis.

papuliferous (păp″ū-lĭf′ĕr-ŭs) [L. *papula*, pimple, + *ferre*, to bear]. Having papules or pimples.

papulo- [L. *papula*, pimple]. Combining form indicating a pimple or a papule.

papuloerythematous (păp″ū-lō-ĕr″ĕ-thĕm′ă-tŭs) [″ + Gr. *erythema*, redness]. Occurrence of papules on an erythematous surface.

papulopustular (păp″ū-lō-pŭs′tū-lăr) [″ + *pustula*, blister]. The presence of both pustules and papules.

papulosis (păp-ū-lō′sĭs) [″ + Gr. *osis*, condition]. Presence of numerous and generalized papules.

papulosquamous (păp″ū-lō-skwā′mŭs) [″ + *squamosus*, scalelike]. Presence of both papules and scales.

papulovesicular (păp″ū-lō-vē-sĭk′ū-lăr) [″ + *vesicula*, tiny bladder]. Presence of both papules and vesicles.

papyraceous (păp-ĭ-rā′shŭs) [L.]. Parchmentlike. In obstetrics it denotes a fetus retained in the uterus beyond natural term, thus assuming a mummified appearance.

par [L., equal]. A pair, esp. a pair of cranial nerves.

para [L. *parere*, to bring forth, to bear]. A woman who has produced a viable infant (weighing 500 grams or more or over 20 weeks gestation) regardless of whether the infant is alive at birth. Multiple births are considered to be a single parous experience. The term is used with numerals to designate the number of pregnancies. SEE: *gravida*.

Ex.: para 0 (nullipara)
para 1 (primipara)
para 2 (secundipara)
para 3 (tertipara)

para-, par- [Gr. *para*, beyond; L. *par*, equal, pair]. ABBR: p- when used in chemistry to indicate *para-*. Combining forms meaning near, beside, past, beyond, the opposite, abnormal, irregular, or two like parts.

para-actinomycosis. Pseudoactinomycosis.

para-aminobenzoic acid (păr″ă-ăm″ĭ-nō-bĕn-zō'ĭk). ABBR: PABA. Previously used name for aminobenzoic acid, $C_7H_7NO_2$. A crystalline substance which is part of the folic acid molecule. Used as a dietary supplement and a reagent. It is effective in treating rickettsial diseases but is not the drug of choice. Inhibits bacteriostatic action of sulfonamides; hence contraindicated during sulfonamide therapy.

para-aminohippuric acid. ABBR: PAHA. A derivative of aminobenzoic acid. The salt, para-aminohippurate, is used to test the excretory capacity of the renal tubules.

para-aminosalicylic acid (păr"ă-ăm"ĭ-nō-săl"ĭ-sĭl'ĭk). USP. ABBR: PAS. $C_7H_7NO_3$. A white or nearly white and practically odorless powder that darkens when exposed to air or light. It is an antituberculosis drug, but its effectiveness is greatly enhanced when used in combination with streptomycin and isoniazid; it is believed to delay development of bacterial resistance. SYN: *aminosalicylic acid*.

para-anesthesia (păr"ă-ăn-ĕs-thē'zē-ă) [" + *an-*, negative, + *aisthesis*, sensation]. Anesthesia of two corresponding sides, esp. of lower half of body.

para-aortic bodies. Small masses of chromaffin tissue along the abdominal aorta. They secrete epinephrine.

para-appendicitis (păr"ă-ă-pĕn"dĭ-sī'tĭs) [" + L. *appendix*, appendix, + Gr. *itis*, inflammation]. Inflammation involving the connective tissue adjacent to the appendix.

parabionts (păr-ăb'ē-ŏnts) [" + *bioun*, to live]. Two individuals living in the condition of parabiosis, q.v.

parabiosis (păr"ă-bī-ō'sĭs) [" + *biosis*, living]. 1. Joining together of two individuals. This may occur congenitally as with Siamese twins or may be produced surgically for experimentation in animals. 2. Temporary suppression of excitability of a nerve.

parabiotic (păr"ă-bī-ŏt'ĭk). Concerning parabiosis.

parablepsia, parablepsis (păr"ă-blĕp'sē-ă, -sĭs) [Gr. *para*, beside, + *blepsis*, vision]. Abnormality of the vision.

parabulia (păr"ă-bū'lē-ă) [" + *boule*, will]. Perversion or abnormality of will power.

paracanthoma (păr"ă-kăn-thō'mă) [Gr. *para*, beside, + *akantha*, thorn, + *oma*, tumor]. A tumor involving the prickle-cell layer of the epidermis.

paracasein (păr-ă-kā'sē-ĭn). A substance formed when rennin or pepsin acts on the casein of milk. In the presence of calcium ions, an insoluble protein is formed, resulting in the curdling of milk.

Paracelsus (păr-ă-sĕl'sŭs). [Philippus Aureolus Theophrastus Bombastus von Hohenheim, 1493–1541] Swiss alchemist and physician who introduced several chemicals (lead, sulfur, iron, and arsenic) into pharmaceutical chemistry. Remembered because of his independent spirit, observant mind, and his fearlessness in breaking with traditional practice.

paracenesthesia (pă"ă-sē"nĕs-thē'zē-ă) [Gr. *para*, beside, + *koinos*, common, + *aisthesis*, feeling]. Decrease in the sense of well-being.

paracentesis (păr"ă-sĕn-tē'sĭs) [Gr. *para*, beside, + *kentesis*, a puncture]. Puncture of a cavity with removal of fluid, as in pleural effusion or ascites.

NURSING IMPLICATIONS: Explain procedure to patient and have patient void prior to treatment. Position patient as directed by physician. Assist physician during procedure. Monitor vital signs and observe for signs of shock (such as cold and clammy skin). Measure and record amount of fluid removed and describe its appearance, specific gravity, and whether or not it clots upon standing. Observe and redress puncture site as necessary. Send specimens to laboratories as directed. Document procedure and patient's response.

p., abdominal. Paracentesis of the abdominal cavity.

p. capitis. Paracentesis of the cranium.

p. cordis. Surgical puncture of the heart.

p. pericardii. Puncture of the pericardial sac.

p. pulmonis. Removal of fluid from a lung.

p. thoracis. Drainage of fluid from the cavity of the chest. SEE: *aspiration*.

p. tunicae vaginalis. Puncture of the tunica vaginalis.

p. tympani. Drainage or irrigation through incision of the tympanic membrane.

p. vesicae. Puncture of the wall of the urinary bladder.

paracentetic (păr"ă-sĕn-tĕt'ĭk). Concerning paracentesis.

paracentral (păr"ă-sĕn'trăl) [" + L. *centralis*, center]. Located near the center.

paracentral lobule. Cerebral convolution on mesial surface joining the upper terminations of the ascending parietal and frontal convolutions.

paracephalus (păr"ă-sĕf'ă-lŭs) [" + *kephale*, head]. A parasitic placental twin with a small rudimentary head.

parachlorophenol (păr"ă-klō"rō-fē'nŏl). USP. A drug that has the same actions and uses as phenol, q.v.

p., camphorated. USP. A mixture of parachlorophenol, q.v., and camphor. Its activity as a topical antiseptic in root canal therapy is markedly decreased by blood and necrotic tissue.

paracholera (păr"ă-kŏl'ĕr-ă) [" + L. *cholera*,

cholera]. A disease resembling cholera, but it is caused by vibrio other than true Vibrio cholerae.

paracholia (păr″ă-kō′lē-ă) [″ + *chole,* bile]. Condition of disturbed bile secretion.

parachordal (păr-ă-kor′dăl) [Gr. *para,* beside, + *chorde,* cord]. Lying alongside the anterior portion of the notochord in the embryo.

parachordal cartilage. One of a pair of cartilages in the cephalic portion of the notochord of the embryo that unite in man to form a single basal plate that is the forerunner of the occipital bone.

parachromatism (păr″ă-krō′mă-tĭzm) [″ + *chroma,* color, + *-ismos,* condition]. Incorrect perception of colors but not true color blindness.

parachromatopsia (păr″ă-krō-mă-tŏp′sē-ă) [″ + ″ + *opsis,* vision]. Colorblindness.

parachute reflex (reaction). SEE: *reflex, parachute.*

paracinesia, paracinesis (păr″ă-sĭ-nē′zē-ă, -sĭs) [″ + *kinesis,* motion]. Condition in which there is perversion of motor powers; motor abnormality. SYN: *parakinesia.*

paracme (păr-ăk′mē) [″ + *akme,* point]. Denoting the stage at which symptoms or a fever begins to decline.

Paracoccidioides (păr″ă-kŏk-sĭd″ē-oy′dēz). A genus of yeastlike fungi.

P. brasiliensis. The causative agent of paracoccidioidomycosis. SYN: *Blastomyces brasiliensis.*

paracoccidioidomycosis (păr″ă-kŏk-sĭd″ē-ŏy″dō-mī-kō′sĭs). A chronic granulomatous disease of the skin caused by Paracoccidioides brasiliensis. SYN: *South American blastomycosis.*

paracolitis (păr″ă-kō-lī′tĭs). Inflammation of the tissue surrounding the colon.

paracolon bacilli. Colonlike bacilli that ferment lactose. They can cause urinary tract infections, and occasionally gastroenteritis.

paracolpitis (păr″ă-kŏl-pī′tĭs) [″ + *kolpos,* vagina, + *itis,* inflammation]. Inflammation of tissues surrounding the vagina.

paracolpium (păr″ă-kŏl′pē-ŭm). The connective tissue adjacent to the vagina.

paracone (păr′ă-kōn) [″ + *konos,* cone]. The mesiobuccal cusp of an upper molar tooth.

paraconid (păr″ă-kō′nĭd). The mesiobuccal cusp of a lower molar tooth.

paracousis (păr″ă-koo′sĭs). Paracusis, q.v.

paracrisis (păr-ăk′rĭ-sĭs, păr″ă-krī′sĭs) [″ + *krinein,* to secrete]. Any abnormality of body secretions.

paracusia (păr″ă-kū′sē-ă) [″ + *akousis,* hearing]. Any abnormality or disorder of the sense of hearing.

p. acris. Excessively acute hearing.

p. duplicata. The hearing of one sound as two. SYN: *diplacusis.*

p. loci. Difficulty in locating the direction of sound.

p. willisiana. An apparent ability to hear better in a noisy place, found in deafness due to stapes fixation and adhesive processes. SYN: *paracusis of Willis.*

paracusis (păr″ă-kū′sĭs). Paracusia.

p. of Willis. Paracusia willisiana.

paracystic (păr″ă-sĭs′tĭk) [Gr. *para,* beside, + *kystis,* bladder]. Located close to a bladder, esp. the urinary bladder.

paracystitis (păr″ă-sĭs-tī′tĭs) [″ + ″ + *itis,* inflammation]. Inflamed condition of connective tissues and other structures around the urinary bladder.

paracystium (păr-ă-sĭs′tē-ŭm). The connective tissue surrounding the urinary bladder.

paracytic (păr″ă-sĭt′ĭk) [″ + *kytos,* cell]. Concerning cells other than those normally present in a specific location.

paradenitis (păr″ăd-ĕn-ī′tĭs) [″ + *aden,* gland + *itis,* inflammation]. Inflammation of tissues around a gland.

paradental (păr″ă-dĕn′tăl) [″ + L. *dens,* tooth]. 1. Concerning the practice of dentistry. 2. Periodontal, q.v.

paradentium (păr″ă-dĕn′shē-ŭm). Periodontium, q.v.

paradidymal (păr″ă-dĭd′ĭ-măl) [″ + *didymos,* testicle]. 1. Concerning the paradidymus. 2. Adjacent to the testis.

paradidymis (păr-ă-dĭd′ĭ-mĭs) [″ + *didymos,* testicle]. [NA] The atrophic remnants of the tubules of the wolffian body, situated on the spermatic cord above the epididymis. SYN: *organ of Giraldès.*

Paradione. Trade name for paramethadione, USP.

paradipsia (păr″ă-dĭp′sē-ă) [″ + *dipsa,* thirst]. Perverted desire for fluids irrespective of the need for liquids.

paradox, Weber's. A muscle loaded beyond its ability to contract may elongate.

paradoxic, paradoxical (păr″ă-dŏk′sĭk, -sĭ-kăl) [Gr. *paradoxos,* conflicting with expectation]. Seemingly contradictory, but demonstrably true.

paradoxical respiration. 1. Respiration occurring in open pneumothorax in which lung fills on expiration and is deflated on inspiration. 2. Condition seen in paralysis of diaphragm in which diaphragm ascends during inspiration.

paraequilibrium (păr″ă-ē″kwĭ-lĭb′rē-ŭm). Vertigo caused by disease or malfunction of the vestibular apparatus of the ear. Sometimes this is accompanied by nystagmus and nausea.

paraffin (păr′ă-fĭn) [L. *parum,* little, + *affinis,* neighboring]. 1. A waxy, white, tasteless, odorless mixture of solid hydrocarbons obtained from petroleum. Used as ointment base or wound dressing. SEE: *petrolatum*. 2. One of a series of saturated aliphatic hydrocarbons having the formula C_nH_{2n+2}. Paraffins constitute the methane or paraffin series.

p., hard. Solid paraffin with a melting point between 45° C. and 60° C.

p., liquid. Liquid hydrocarbon. Mineral oil.

p., soft. A semisolid paraffin. Petrolatum.

p., white soft. White petrolatum. SEE: *petrolatum*.

p., yellow soft. Petrolatum, q.v.

paraffinoma (păr″ă-fĭn-ō′mă) [″ + ″ + Gr. *oma,* tumor]. A tumor that arises at site of injection of paraffin.

paraffinum (păr-ă-fē′nŭm) [L.]. Paraffin.

Paraflex. Trade name for chlorzoxazone.

paraformaldehyde (păr″ă-for-măl′dĕ-hīd). A white, powdered antiseptic and disinfectant, a polymer of formaldehyde.

paragammacism (păr″ă-găm′mă-sĭzm) [″ + *gamma,* Gr. letter G, + *-ismos,* condition]. Inability to pronounce "g," "k," and "ch" sounds, with substitution of other consonants such as "d" or "t."

paraganglia (păr″ă-găng′lē-ă) [″ + *ganglion,* knot]. (sing. *paraganglion*) [NA] Groups of chromaffin cells, similar in staining reaction to cells of the adrenal medulla, associated anatomically and embryologically with the sympathetic system. They are located in various organs and parts of the body.

paraganglioma (păr″ă-găng-lē-ō′mă) [″ + ″ + *oma,* tumor]. A tumor derived from chromaffin cells. Includes tumors of the adrenal medulla and the paraganglia. SYN: *pheochromocytoma*.

paraganglion (păr″ă-gang′lē-ŏn) [″ + *ganglion,* knot]. Sing. of paraganglia.

parageusia, parageusis (păr-ă-gū′sē-ă, -sĭs) [″ + *geusis,* taste]. Disorder or abnormality of the sense of taste.

paraglobulin (păr″ă-glŏb′ū-lĭn) [″ + L. *globulus,* a small sphere]. A globulin found in blood plasma, lymph, and other body fluids; associated with coagulation. SYN: *fibroplastin*.

paraglobulinuria (păr″ă-glŏb″ū-lĭn-ū′rē-ă) [″ + ″ + Gr. *ouron,* urine]. Excessive excretion of paraglobulin in the urine.

paraglossa (păr-ă-glŏs′să) [″ + *glossa,* tongue]. 1. Enlargement of the tongue. 2. Congenital hypertrophy of the tongue.

paraglossia (păr″ă-glŏs′sē-ă). Inflammation of the tissues underlying the tongue.

paragnathus (păr-ăg′nă-thŭs) [″ + *gnathos,* jaw]. 1. A congenital deformity in which there is an accessory jaw. 2. A parasitic fetus attached to the outer part of the jaw of the autosite.

paragonimiasis (păr″ă-gŏn″ĭ-mī′ă-sĭs) [*Paragonimus* + *-iasis,* condition]. Infection with worms of genus Paragonimus. The clinical signs depend on the path the worm takes in migrating through the body, after the larvae contained in partially cooked freshwater crabs or crayfish are eaten. The larvae migrate from the duodenum to various organs, including the lungs, intestinal wall, lymph nodes, brain, subcutaneous tissues, and genitourinary tract. When the lungs are involved, the symptoms are cough and hemoptysis. In peritoneal infections, there may be an abdominal mass, pain and dysentery. When the larvae invade the brain, paralysis, epilepsy, homonymous hemianopsia, optic atrophy, and papilledema are common. In some cases, the infected person may appear to be well.

TREATMENT: Biothionol available from the Centers for Disease Control (CDC) in Atlanta, Georgia.

Paragonimus (păr″ă-gŏn′ĭ-mŭs). Genus of trematode worms.

P. westermani. The lung fluke, a common parasite of certain mammals including man, dog, cat, pig, and mink. Human infestation occurs through eating partially cooked crabs or crayfish, the second intermediate host. Infestation endemic in certain parts of the Orient.

paragrammatism. A speech defect characterized by improper use of words and inability to arrange them grammatically.

paragranuloma (păr″ă-grăn″ū-lō′mă) [Gr. *para,* beside, + L. *granulum,* little grain, + Gr. *oma,* tumor]. A benign form of Hodgkin's disease usually limited to lymph nodes.

paragraphia (păr-ă-grăf′ē-ă) [″ + *graphein,* to write]. The writing of letters or words other than those intended.

parahemophilia (păr-ă-hē″mō-fĭl′ē-ă) [″ + *haima,* blood, + *philein,* to love]. A rare, congenital, idiopathic disorder due to deficiency of coagulation factor V, characterized by prolonged prothrombin and coagulation times.

parahepatic (păr″ă-hē-păt′ĭk) [″ + *hepar,* liver]. Adjacent to the liver.

parahepatitis (păr″ă-hĕp″ă-tī′tĭs) [″ + ″ + *itis,* inflammation]. Inflamed condition of parts immediately adjacent to the liver.

parahormone [″ + *hormaein,* to set in motion]. A substance that is conveyed through the circulatory system and exerts a stimulating effect like hormones, yet not originating in endocrine tissue. Carbon dioxide is an example.

parahypnosis [Gr. *para,* beside, + *hypnos,* sleep]. Abnormal or disordered sleep.

parahypophysis (păr″ă-hī-pŏf′ĭ-sĭs) [″ + *hypophysis,* an undergrowth]. Accessory to the pituitary tissue.

parainfection [" + L. *in*, into, + *facere*, to make]. The symptomatology of an infectious disease without evidence of the presence of the microorganisms causing the disease.

parainfluenza viruses. A group of viruses that cause acute respiratory infections in man, esp. in children. Virtually all children in the U.S.A. have been infected by age six.

parakeratosis (păr"ă-kĕr"ă-tō'sĭs) [" + *keras*, horn, + *osis*, condition]. The persistence of nuclei within the keratinocytes of the stratum corneum of epidermis or mucosal layers that indicates a partial keratinization process; a general term applied to disorders of the keratinized layer of the skin.

p. ostracea. Parakeratosis scutularis, q.v.

p. psoriasiformis. Scab formation resembling that of psoriasis.

p. scutularis. Scalp disease with hairs encircled by epidermic crust formation.

parakinesia. Paracinesia.

Paral. Trade name for paraldehyde, USP.

paralalia (păr"ă-lā'lē-ă) [" + *lalein*, to babble]. Any speech defect characterized by sound distortion.

p. literalis. Stammering.

paralambdacism (păr"ă-lăm'dă-sĭzm) [" + *lambda*, Gr. letter L, + *-ismos*, condition]. Inability to sound the letter "l" correctly, substituting some other letter for it.

paralbumin (păr"ăl-bū'mĭn) [" + L. *albumen*, white of egg]. An albumin found in fluid content in ovarian cysts and in ascites.

paraldehyde (păr-ăl'dĕ-hīd). USP. $C_6H_{12}O_3$. A liquid polymer of acetaldehyde that is colorless. It has an unpleasant taste and a characteristic odor. Made by action of hydrochloric acid on acetic aldehyde. Trade name is Paral.

ACTION AND USES: Hypnotic, having low toxicity and prompt action as a sedative. Useful in treating acute alcoholism and delirium tremens. Sometimes used as an analgesic in obstetrics, esp. in combination with rectal ether.

CAUTION: Do not dispense paraldehyde from a bottle that has been open longer than 24 hours. In partially filled containers, oxidation occurs, forming acetic acid.

paraldehyde poisoning. Symptoms resemble those of chloral hydrate: cardiac and respiratory depression, dizziness, collapse with partial or complete anesthesia. Odor on the breath is a constant distinct sign.

F.A.: Maintain airway and physiological responses by use of tracheostomy, artificial ventilation, and oxygen. If poisoning is mild, induce vomiting. Because of the danger of asphyxiation, gastric lavage is dangerous unless the airway is protected.

paraldehydism (păr-ăl'dĕ-hīd"ĭzm). Poisoning from an overdose of paraldehyde, q.v.

paralepsy (păr'ă-lĕp"sē) [" + *lepsis*, seizure]. Temporary attack of mental inertia and hopelessness, or sudden alteration in mood or mental tension. SYN: *psycholepsy.*

paralexia (păr"ă-lĕk'sē-ă) [" + *lexis*, speech]. Inability to comprehend printed words or sentences with substitution of meaningless combinations of words.

paralgesia (păr"ăl-jē'zē-ă) [" + *algesis*, sense of pain]. Any unusual sensation that is painful. SYN: *paralgia.*

paralgia (păr-ăl'jē-ă) [" + *algos*, pain]. An abnormal sensation that is painful.

parallactic. Concerning parallax.

parallagma (păr"ăl-ăg'mă) [Gr., alternation]. Overlapping or displacement of the fragments of a fractured bone.

parallax (păr'ă-lăks) [Gr. *parallaxis*, change of position]. The apparent movement or displacement of objects caused by change in the observer's position or by movement of the head or eyes.

p., binocular. The basis of stereoscopic vision. The difference in the angles formed by the lines of sight to two objects at different distances from the eyes. This is important in depth perception.

p., heteronymous. When one eye is closed, the object viewed appears to move closer to the closed eye.

p., homonymous. When one eye is covered, the object viewed appears to move closer to the uncovered eye.

parallelism (păr'ă-lĕl"ĭzm). The condition of being parallel.

parallelometer (păr"ă-lĕl-ŏm'ĕ-tĕr). A device used in dentistry to determine whether or not lines and tooth surfaces are parallel to each other.

parallergic (păr"ă-lĕr'jĭk). Concerning parallergy.

parallergy (păr-ăl'ĕr-jē). The condition of being allergic to nonspecific stimuli after having been sensitized with a specific allergen.

paralogia (păr"ă-lō'jē-ă) [Gr. *para*, beside, + *logos*, understanding]. A disorder of the reasoning.

p., benign. Disordered thinking and communication of thought. Delusions, bizarre thoughts, hallucinations, and regressive behavior are absent. The patient is not severely incapacitated and should not be considered to have schizophrenia.

paralogy (pă-răl'ō-jē). Paralogia, q.v.

paralysis (pă-răl'ĭ-sĭs) [Gr. *paralyein*, to disable]. (pl. *paralyses*) Temporary suspension or permanent loss of function, esp. loss of sensation or voluntary motion.

Any voluntary movement depends on the integrity of two motor neurons: one, the upper motor neuron, arising in the motor cortex, coursing across the brain stem, and ending in the anterior gray horn of the spinal cord; and the lower neurons, arising in the anterior horn cell and passing to the muscle. If the latter are destroyed, the muscle loses tone, atrophies (withers away), and shows reaction of degeneration (R.D.).

The flaccidity and absent muscular reflexes reveal the loss of tonus. If the upper neuron is paralyzed, the patient is equally unable to move the affected part, but the intact lower neuron may permit other motor centers to act on the muscle. In addition, tone is increased, there is no R.D., and no atrophy except that of disuse. So-called pathological reflexes may appear in addition to the increase of normal deep reflexes.

Paralyses are divided into two groups: *spastic* when due to lesion of upper motor neuron and *flaccid* when due to lesion of lower motor neuron. Psychic inhibition of motor function occurs most characteristically in hysteria, but the evidence of organic disease is always lacking in these hysterical paralyses.

p., acoustic. Deafness.

p., acute ascending spinal. An acute type of paralysis that may be caused by a number of diseases. The flaccid paralysis starts in the lower part of the body and progresses to the trunk, arms, and muscles of respiration.

p., acute atrophic. P., infantile.

p., acute infectious. P., infantile.

p. agitans. A disease of middle and late life producing a picture of rigid tremulousness, progressive in its course and marked by weakness, delay of voluntary motion, a peculiar festinating gait, and muscular contraction, causing peculiar and characteristic positions of the limbs and head. While movement is slow, there is no true paralysis. The face appears expressionless, there is general flexion attitude, the balance tends to be lost (in a forward direction). Sometimes occurs following encephalitis lethargica; others are due to an unknown cause. SYN: *palsy, shaking; Parkinson's disease.*

p., alcoholic. Paralysis due to habitual drunkenness.

p., anesthesia. Paralysis that develops following administration of anesthesia.

p., anterior spinal. P., infantile.

p., arsenical. Paralysis following poisoning from arsenic.

p., ascending. Paralysis beginning with the lower limbs and progressing upward.

p., association. P., bulbar.

p., asthenic bulbar. Myasthenia gravis, q.v.

p., atrophic spinal. Paralysis caused by acute poliomyelitis.

p., Bell's. Facial paralysis.

ETIOL: Lesion of the facial nerve or of its nucleus; a neuritis of this nerve. Pressure on the nerve as it reaches the face through its bony canal near the ear.

SYM: One side of entire face may be affected, corner of mouth may drop, or eyelid may droop or be unable to close. Patient may be unable to close lips or to speak, or may lose ability to close the eye

p., Bernhardt's. Pain and hyperesthesia on the outer femoral surface from lesion or disease of the external cutaneous nerve of the thigh. SEE: *meralgia paresthetica.*

p., birth. Paralysis caused by injury received at birth.

p., brachial. Paralysis of one or both arms.

p., brachiofacial. Paralysis of the face and an arm.

p., Brown-Sequard's. 1. Paralysis due to cutting through of the spinal cord. On the side of the lesion there is paralysis with loss of position and vibration sense. On the opposite side there is loss of sensation of pain and temperature. 2. Reflex flaccid paraplegia occurring during some urinary tract disorders.

p., bulbar. Paralysis caused by changes in the motor centers of the brain stem.

p., central. Any paralysis from a lesion of the brain or spinal cord.

p., cerebral spastic, infantile. Nonprogressive paralysis resulting from developmental defects in brain or from trauma at birth. SYN: *Little's disease.*

p., complete. Paralysis in which there is total loss of function and sensation.

p., compression. Paralysis due to prolonged pressure on a nerve, as by a crutch or during sleep.

p., conjugate. Paralysis of the conjugate movement of the eyes in all directions even though the fixation axis remains parallel.

p., crossed. Paralysis affecting one side of the face and limbs of the opposite side of the body.

p., crutch. Paralysis due to pressure on nerves in the axilla caused by a crutch.

p., decubitus. Paralysis due to pressure on a nerve from lying in one position for a long time, as in sleep.

p., diphtheritic. Paralysis of the muscles of the palate, eyes, limbs, diaphragm, and intercostal muscles that occurs as a complication of diphtheria. It is caused by a toxin produced by the diphtheria bacillus.

p., diver's. Paralysis due to decrease in pressure after a deep-sea diver has been exposed to pressure greater than atmospheric pressure. SYN: *beads; caisson disease.*

p., Duchenne's. P., bulbar, q.v.

p., Duchenne-Erb. Paralysis of the muscles of the upper arm due to injury of the upper nerves, fifth and sixth cervical roots, of the brachial plexus. The hand muscles are unaffected.

p., exhaustion. Paralysis due to prolonged voluntary movements involving exhaustion of the nerve centers.

p., facial. P., Bell's.

p., familial periodic. A rare familial disease in which attacks of flaccid paralysis, often at time of awakening, occur. This condition is usually associated with hypokalemia, but is sometimes present even though the blood potassium level is normal or elevated. The condition may, in affected individuals, be precipitated by administration of glucose.

p., flaccid. Paralysis in which there is loss of muscle tone, loss of or reduction of tendon reflexes, atrophy and degeneration of muscles, and reaction of degeneration. Due to lesions of lower motor neurons of spinal cord.

p., general. Progressive loss of power and mental faculties resulting eventually in dementia and death. SYN: *paresis.*

p., ginger. P., Jamaica ginger, q.v.

p., glossolabial. Paralysis of the tongue and lips. Occurs in bulbar paralysis.

p., Gubler's. A form of alternate hemiplegia in which a brain stem lesion causes paralysis of the cranial nerves on one side and the body on the opposite side.

p., histrionic. Paralysis of certain facial muscles, producing a fixed facial expression of a certain emotion.

p., hyperkalemic periodic. P., familial periodic, q.v.

p., hypokalemic periodic. P., familial periodic, q.v.

p., hysteric. Apparent loss of movement that may simulate any form of paralysis with no adequate causative lesion.

p., immunological. Inability to form antibodies after exposure to large doses of the antigen.

p., incomplete. Partial paralysis of the body or a part.

p., infantile. Motor paralysis in children with atrophy of a group of muscles, following an acute infectious disease that is transmitted by a filtrable virus. SYN: *paralysis, acute atrophic; paralysis, acute infectious; paralysis, anterior spinal; poliomyelitis, acute anterior.*

p., infantile cerebral ataxic. Palsy, cerebral, q.v.

p., infantile spinal. Paralysis due to acute poliomyelitis.

p., infectious bulbar. Pseudorabies, q.v.

p., ischemic. Paralysis resulting from impaired blood supply. SYN: *Volkmann's contracture.*

p., jake. P., Jamaica ginger, q.v.

p., Jamaica ginger. Paralysis due to polyneuropathy that affects the muscles of the distal portions of the limbs. It is caused by drinking an alcoholic beverage called Jamaica ginger that contains the toxic substance triorthocresylphosphate.

p., Klumpke's. Wasting paralysis of the arms and hands; often resulting from birth injury.

p., Kussmaul's. P., Landry's.

p., labial. Progressive bulbar paralysis affecting the lips, tongue, and larynx.

p., Landry's. Flaccid paralysis that begins in the lower extremities and rapidly ascends to the trunk. SYN: *p., Kussmaul's.*

p., lead. Paralysis following poisoning by lead.

p., local. Paralysis of a single muscle or one group of muscles.

p., mimetic. Paralysis of the facial muscles.

p., mixed. Paralysis of motor and sensory nerves.

p., muscular. Loss of the capacity of muscles to contract. May be due to a structural or functional disorder in the muscle at the myoneural junction, in efferent nerve fibers, in cell bodies of nuclei of origin of brain or gray matter of spinal cord, in conducting pathways of brain or spinal cord, or in motor centers of the brain.

p., musculospiral. Paralysis due to prolonged ischemia of the musculospiral nerve incident to compressing the arm against a hard edge. This occurs if the patient has been comatose or in a stupor or has fallen asleep with the arm hanging over the edge of a bed or chair. Sometimes called Saturday night paralysis because in some cultures individuals traditionally become intoxicated on Saturday night; while stuporous, they may remain in a position that allows the nerve to be compressed.

p., normokalemic periodic. P., familial periodic, q.v.

p., nuclear. Paralysis caused by lesion of a nerve nucleus in the central nervous system.

p., obstetrical. P., birth.

p., ocular. Paralysis of the extraocular and intraocular muscles.

p. of accommodation. Inability of the eye to adjust itself to various distances due to paralysis of ciliary muscles.

p., periodic. Paralysis that recurs and abates temporarily.

p., phonetic. Paralysis of vocal cords.

p., postdiphtheritic. P., diphtheritic, q.v.

p. posticus. Paralysis of the posterior

cricothyroid muscles.

p., Pott's. Paralysis of the lower part of the body due to tuberculosis of the spine (Pott's disease).

p., progressive bulbar. P., bulbar.

p., pseudobulbar. Paralysis caused by cerebral center lesions, simulating the bulbar types of paralysis.

p., pseudohypertrophic muscular. Dystrophy, pseudohypertrophic muscular, q.v.

p., radial. Paralysis, musculospiral, q.v.

p., Saturday night. P., musculospiral.

p., sensory. Loss of sensation. May be due to a structural or functional disorder of the sensory end-organs, sensory nerves, conducting pathways of spinal cord or brain, or sensory centers in the brain.

p., sleep. Condition of being unable to speak or move even though fully aware of external events. Most commonly occurs upon awakening but may appear just prior to falling asleep. The attack usually is of short duration but to the patient the elapsed time may seem like hours. The exact cause or explanation of this condition is unknown.

p., spastic. Paralysis usually involving groups of muscles. Characterized by excessive tone and spasticity of muscles, exaggeration of tendon reflexes but loss of superficial reflexes, positive Babinski response, no atrophy or wasting except from prolonged disuse, and absence of reaction of degeneration. Due to lesions of upper motor neurons or cerebrum.

p., spinal. Paralysis due to injury or disease of the spinal cord.

p., supranuclear. Paralysis resulting from disorders in pathways or centers above nuclei of origin.

p., tick-bite. Paralysis resulting from bites of certain species of ticks, esp. of the genera Ixodes and Dermacentor, presumably due to a toxin present in saliva of tick. Affects domestic animals and humans, esp. children. Causes a progressive ascending, flaccid, motor paralysis. Recovery usually occurs after removal of ticks.

p., Todd's. A transitory paralysis following an epileptic seizure.

p., tourniquet. Paralysis, esp. of the arm, resulting from a tourniquet being applied for too long a time.

p., vasomotor. Paralysis of vasomotor centers resulting in lack of tone and dilation of blood vessels.

p., Volkmann's. Volkmann's contracture.

p., wasting. Progressive wasting away of the muscles. SYN: *atrophy, progressive muscular.*

paralytic (păr"ă-lĭt'ĭk) [Gr. *paralyein,* to disable]. 1. Concerning paralysis. 2. One afflicted with paralysis.

paralytic dementia. Progressive paralysis with mental deterioration. SYN *paresis.*

paralytic ileus. Paralysis of intestines with distention and symptoms of acute obstruction and prostration. May occur after any abdominal surgery.

paralyzant (păr'ă-līz"ănt) [Fr. *paralyser,* paralyze]. 1. Causing paralysis. 2. A drug or other agent that induces paralysis.

paralyze (păr'ă-līz) [Fr. *paralyse*]. 1. To cause temporary or permanent loss of muscular power or sensation. 2. To render ineffective.

paralyzer (păr'ă-līz"ĕr). 1. That which causes paralysis. 2. A substance that inhibits a chemical reaction.

paramagnetic (păr"ă-măg-nĕt'ĭk). Anything that is attracted by the poles of a magnet, and becomes parallel to the lines of magnetic force.

paramania (păr"ă-mā'nē-ă) [Gr. *para,* beside, + *mania,* madness]. A type of emotional disturbance in which the individual derives pleasure from complaining.

paramastigote (păr"ă-măs'tĭ-gōt) [" + *mastix,* lash]. Having a small supernumerary flagellum next to a larger one.

paramastitis (păr"ă-măs-tī'tĭs) [" + *mastos,* breast, + *itis,* inflammation]. Inflammation around the breast.

paramastoid (păr"ă-măs'toyd) [" + " + *eidos,* form]. Next to the mastoid.

paramedian (păr"ă-mē'dē-ăn) [" + L. *medianus,* median]. Close to the midline.

paramedian incision. A surgical incision, esp. of the abdominal wall, close to the midline.

paramedic (păr"ă-mĕd'ĭk) [Gr. *para,* beside, + L. *medicus,* doctor]. A trained medical assistant who participates in rescue operations or assists a physician.

paramedical. Supplementing the work of medical personnel in related fields: social work; physical, occupational, and speech therapy.

paramedical personnel. Those health manpower who are not physicians, such as medical technicians, emergency technicians, or physician's assistants.

paramenia (păr"ă-mē'nē-ă) [" + *meniaia,* menses]. Irregular, abnormal, or difficult menstruation.

paramesial (păr"ă-mē'sē-ăl) [" + *mesos,* middle]. Paramedian, q.v.

parameter (păr-ăm'ĕ-tĕr) [" + *metron,* measure]. In mathematics, an arbitrary constant, each value of which determines the specific form of the equation in which it appears. Often misused by biologists to indicate a variable.

paramethadione (păr"ă-mĕth"ă-dī'ōn). USP. Anticonvulsive drug used in treating absence seizures. Trade name is Paradione.

paramethasone acetate (păr″ă-mĕth′ă-sōn). USP. A glucocorticosteroid drug. Trade names are Haldrone, Monocortin, and Stemex.

parametric (păr″ă-mĕt′rĭk) [Gr. *para,* beside, + *metra,* uterus]. 1. Concerning the area near the uterus. 2. Rel. to the parametrium, the tissue surrounding the uterus. 3. [Gr. *para,* beside, + *metron,* measure] Adjectival form of parameter, q.v.

parametritic (păr″ă-mē-trĭt′ĭk). Concerning parametritis, q.v.

parametritis (păr″ă-mē-trī′tĭs) [″ + *metra,* uterus, + *itis,* inflammation]. Inflamed condition of parametrium, the cellular tissue adjacent to the uterus. SYN: *cellulitis, pelvic.*

parametrium (păr-ă-mē′trē-ŭm) [″ + *metra,* uterus]. [NA] Loose connective tissue around the uterus.

paramimia (păr″ă-mĭm′ē-ă) [″ + *mimeisthai,* to imitate]. Use of gestures that are inappropriate to the spoken words that they accompany.

paramnesia (păr″ăm-nē′zē-ă) [″ + *amnesia,* loss of memory]. 1. The use of words without meaning. 2. The distortion of memory in which there is inability to distinguish imaginary or suggested experiences from those that have actually occurred. 3. Seeming recall of events that never have occurred.

paramolar (păr″ă-mō′lăr). A supernumerary tooth close to a molar.

paramorphia (păr″ă-mor′fē-ă) [″ + *morphe,* form]. Abnormality of shape or structure.

paramucin (păr″ă-mū′sĭn). A glycoprotein found in ovarian and some other cysts.

paramusia (păr″ă-mū′zē-ă) [″ + *mousa,* music]. A form of aphasia in which the ability to render music correctly is lost.

paramyloidosis (păr-ăm″ĭ-loy-dō′sĭs) [″ + L. *amylum,* starch, + Gr. *eidos,* form, + *osis,* condition]. The presence and build-up of atypical amyloid in tissues.

paramyoclonus multiplex (păr-ă-mī-ŏk′lō-nŭs mŭl′tĭ-plĕks) [″ + *mys,* muscle, + *klonos,* tumult]. Sudden and frequent shock-like contractions usually affecting muscles of both legs, and trunk muscles particularly. The contractions, which disappear during sleep and motion, may occur 10 to 50 times each minute. Usually the condition develops spontaneously but has been known to follow fright, trauma, infectious diseases, and poliomyelitis.

paramyosinogen (păr″ă-mī″ō-sĭn′ō-jĕn) [Gr. *para,* beside, + *myosin,* protein globin of muscle, + *gennan,* to produce]. Protein derived from muscle plasma.

paramyotonia (păr″ă-mī″ō-tō′nē-ă) [″ + *mys,* muscle, + *tonos,* tone]. A disorder marked by muscular spasms and abnormal muscular tonicity.

p. ataxia. Tonic muscular spasm with slight ataxia or paresis when making any attempt at movement.

p. congenita. Congenital condition of tonic muscular spasms when body is exposed to cold. SYN: *Eulenburg's disease.*

p., symptomatic. Temporary muscular rigidity when first trying to walk, as in paralysis agitans.

paramyotonus (păr″ă-mī-ŏt′ō-nŭs) [″ + ″ + *tonos,* tone]. A condition in which there is tonic muscular spasm.

paramyxoviruses. A subgroup of the myxoviruses that are similar in physical, chemical, and biological characteristics. However, they are quite different pathogenetically. Includes parainfluenza, measles, mumps, Newcastle disease, and respiratory syncytial viruses.

paranalgesia (păr″ăn-ăl-jē′sē-ă) [″ + *an-,* not, + *algos,* pain]. Analgesia of the lower half of the body.

paranasal (păr″ă-nā′săl) [″ + L. *nasalis,* pert. to nose]. Situated near or alongside the nasal cavities.

paranasal sinuses. Accessory nasal sinuses that open into the nasal cavities. They are the frontal, ethmoidal, sphenoidal, and maxillary. All are lined with a ciliated mucous membrane continuous with that of the nasal cavities.

paraneoplastic syndromes. Term used to describe indirect effects of neoplasms that may be so severe as to be the actual cause of death rather than the tumor itself. These include endocrine effects of neoplasms of the lungs or kidneys, and various neoplasms of the endocrine glands.

paranephric (păr″ă-nĕf′rĭk) [″ + *nephros,* kidney]. 1. Close to the kidney. 2. Concerning the adrenal glands.

paranephritis (păr″ă-nē-frī′tĭs) [″ + ″ + *itis,* inflammation]. 1. Inflamed condition of the suprarenal capsules. 2. Inflammation of connective tissue about kidney. SYN: *perinephritis.*

paranephros (păr-ă-nĕf′rŏs). A suprarenal or adrenal capsule.

paranesthesia (păr″ăn-ĕs-thē′zē-ă) [″ + *an-,* not, + *aisthesis,* sensation]. Para-anesthesia, q.v.

paraneural (păr″ă-nū′răl) [″ + *neuron,* nerve] Adjacent to a nerve.

paranoia (păr″ă-noy′ă) [Gr. *para,* beside, + *nous,* mind]. The diagnostic criteria for this illness are: persistent persecutory delusions or delusional jealousy; emotion and behavior appropriate to the content of the delusional system; the disorder has been present at least one week; symptoms of schizophrenia such as bizarre delusions or incoherence are present; no prominent hallucinations; a full depressive or manic syndrome is either not present or is of brief duration; the illness is not due to organic disease of the brain.

This disorder, which usually occurs in middle or late adult life and may be chronic, often includes resentment and anger that may lead to violence. These patients rarely seek medical attention. They are brought for care by associates or relatives.

p., litigious. Paranoia in which the patient institutes or threatens to institute legal action because of the imagined persecution.

paranoiac (păr-ă-noy'ăk). 1. Concerning or afflicted with paranoia. 2. One suffering from paranoia.

paranoid (păr'ă-noyd) [" + *nous,* mind, + *eidos,* resemblance]. 1. Resembling paranoia. 2. A person afflicted with paranoia.

paranoid reaction type. Individual who has fixed systematized delusions, is suspicious, has a persecution complex, is resentful and bitter, and is a megalomaniac. Many states approach true paranoia and resemble it but lack one or more of its distinguishing features. Some of these are transitory paranoid states due to toxic conditions, a paranoid type of schizophrenia, and paranoid states due to alcoholism.

paranomia (păr"ă-nō'mē-ă) [" + *onoma,* name]. Form of aphasia in which there is inability to remember correct name of objects shortly after seeing or using them.

paranormal. 1. Pert. to experiences that are not within the range of normal experiences or are not scientifically explainable. SEE: *extrasensory perception.* 2. Moderately abnormal.

paranuclear (păr"ă-nū'klē-ăr). Adjacent to the nucleus of a cell.

paranucleate (păr"ă-nū'klē-ăt). Concerning or having a paranucleus.

paranucleolus (păr"ă-nū-klē'ō-lŭs). A small basophil body in the sac enclosing the nucleus.

paranucleus (păr"ă-nū'klē-ŭs) [Gr. *para,* beside, + L. *nucleus,* a kernel]. A small body lying close to a cell nucleus.

paraomphalic (păr"ă-ŏm-făl'ĭk) [" + *omphalos,* navel]. Adjacent to the navel. SYN: *paraumbilical.*

paraoperative (păr"ă-ŏp'ĕr-ă-tĭv) [" + L. *operari,* to work]. Concerning all the details and accessories of surgery and preparation of the patient.

paraosteoarthropathy (păr"ă-ŏs"tē-ō-ăr-thrŏp'ăth-ē) [" + *osteon,* bone, + *arthron,* joint, + *pathos,* disease]. Paralysis of lower portion of the body in addition to bone and joint disease.

parapancreatic (păr"ă-păn"krē-ăt'ĭk) [" + *pan,* all, + *kreas,* flesh]. Located close to the pancreas.

paraparesis (păr"ă-păr-ē'sĭs, -păr'ĕ-sĭs) [" + *paresis,* paralysis]. Partial paralysis affecting the lower limbs.

parapedesis (păr"ă-pĕd-ē'sĭs) [" + *pedesis,* leaping]. Secretion or excretion through other than normal channels.

parapeptone (păr"ă-pĕp'tōn) [" + *peptein,* to digest]. Intermediate digestion product of albumin. SEE: *peptone.*

paraperitoneal (păr"ă-pĕr"ĭ-tō-nē'ăl) [" + *peritonaion,* peritoneum]. Near the peritoneum.

parapestis (păr"ă-pĕs'tĭs) [" + L. *pestis,* plague]. Ambulatory plague.

paraphasia (păr-ă-fā'zē-ă) [" + *aphasis,* speech loss]. The misuse of spoken words or word combinations; a form of aphasia. SEE: *paraphrasia.*

paraphemia (păr"ă-fē'mē-ă) [" + *pheme,* speech]. A disorder marked by consistent use of the wrong words, or mispronunciation of words.

paraphia (păr-ā'fē-ă) [" + *haphe,* touch]. Abnormality of the sense of touch. SYN: *parapsia.*

paraphilia [" + *philein,* to love]. A psychosexual disorder in which unusual or bizarre imagery or acts are necessary for realization of sexual excitement. Included in this disorder are fetishism, transvestism, zoophilia, pedophilia, exhibitionism, voyeurism, sexual masochism, and sexual sadism.

paraphimosis (păr"ă-fī-mō'sĭs) [" + *phimoun,* to muzzle, + *osis,* condition]. Strangulation of glans penis due to retraction of narrowed or inflamed foreskin.

paraphimosis oculi. Retraction of the eyelid behind a protruding eyeball.

paraphobia (păr"ă-fō'bē-ă) [" + *phobos,* fear]. A mild form of phobia.

paraphonia (păr"ă-fō'nē-ă) [" + *phone,* voice]. Partial loss, weakness, or abnormal change of the voice.

p. puberum. A deep voice that develops in boys during puberty.

paraphora (păr-ăf'ō-ră) [Gr., a wandering]. A mental disorder of minor degree.

paraphrasia (păr-ă-frā'zē-ă) [Gr. *para,* beside, + *phrasis,* speech]. A condition characterized by loss of the ability to use words correctly and coherently. The words spoken are so jumbled and misused as to make speech unintelligible. SEE: *paraphasia.*

paraphrenitis (păr"ă-frē-nī'tĭs) [" + *phren,* diaphragm, + *itis,* inflammation]. Inflammation of the tissues around the diaphragm.

paraphronia (păr"ă-frō'nē-ă). A mental disorder in which character and disposition are altered.

paraphyseal (păr"ă-fĭz'ē-ăl) Concerning the paraphysis.

paraphysis (pă-răf'ĭ-sĭs) [Gr., offshoot]. The

vestigial structure that originates from the roof plate of the telencephalon. Presumably the colloid cyst of the third ventricle arises from it. A midline organ that develops from the roof plate of the diencephalon of some lower vertebrates.

paraplasm (păr'ă-plăzm) [" + *plasma*, a thing formed]. 1. Any abnormal new formation or malformation. 2. The fluid portion of protoplasm. SYN: *hyaloplasm*.

paraplastic (păr"ă-plăs'tĭk) [" + *plastikos*, formed]. 1. Misshapen; deformed. 2. Pert. to fluid portion of protoplasm.

paraplectic (păr"ă-plĕk'tĭk) [Gr. *paraplektikos*, striking at the side]. Afflicted with paralysis of lower extremities. SYN: *paraplegic*.

paraplegia (păr-ă-plē'jē-ă) [Gr. *paraplegia*, stroke on one side]. Paralysis of lower portion of the body and of both legs.

ETIOL: A lesion involving the spinal cord that may be due to the following: maldevelopment, epidural abscess, hematomyelia, acute transverse myelitis, spinal neoplasms, multiple sclerosis, syringomyelia, or trauma.

p., alcoholic. Paraplegia of spinal origin due to excessive use of alcohol.

p., ataxic. Lateral and posterior sclerosis of the spinal cord characterized by slowly progressing ataxia and paresis.

p., cerebral. Paraplegia from a bilateral cerebral lesion.

p., congenital spastic. P., infantile spastic, q.v.

p. dolorosa. Paraplegia due to pressure of a neoplasm on the posterior spinal cord and nerve roots. Extremely painful despite paralysis.

p., infantile spastic. Spastic paraplegia that occurs in infants. It is usually due to birth injury. SEE: *p., spastic*.

p., peripheral. Paraplegia due to pressure on, injury to, or disease of peripheral nerves.

p., Potts. Paraplegia associated with tuberculosis of the spine.

p., senile. Paraplegia resulting from sclerosis of arteries supplying spinal cord.

p., spastic. Paraplegia characterized by increased muscular tone and accentuated tendon reflexes. Seen in multiple sclerosis and other conditions involving the pyramidal tracts. SYN: *p., tetanoid*.

p., spastic, primary. Paraplegia from degeneration in pyramidal tracts.

p., superior. Paralysis of both arms.

p., tetanoid. P., spastic.

paraplegic (păr-ă-plē'jĭk) [Gr. *paraplegia*, stroke on one side]. Pert. to, or affected with, paraplegia. SYN: *paraplectic*.

paraplegiform (păr"ă-plĕj'ĭ-form) [" + L. *forma*, form]. Similar to paraplegia.

parapleuritis (păr"ă-plū-rī'tĭs) [Gr. *para*, beside, + *pleura*, a side, + *itis*, inflammation]. 1. Inflammation in the thoracic wall. 2. Mild inflammation of the pleura. 3. Pain in the pleura. SYN: *pleurodynia*.

parapoplexy (păr-ăp'ō-plĕk"sē) [" + *apoplexia*, apoplexy]. A mild or slight apoplexy with partial stupor; a stupor resembling apoplexy. SYN: *pseudoapoplexy*.

parapraxia (păr-ă-prăk'sē-ă) [" + *praxis*, doing]. Disturbed mental processes producing inaccuracy, forgetfulness, and tendency to misplace things and make slips of speech or pen. SYN: *parapraxis*.

paraproctitis (păr"ă-prŏk-tī'tĭs) [Gr. *para*, beside, + *proktos*, anus, + *itis*, inflammation]. Inflamed condition of tissues near the rectum.

paraproctium (păr"ă-prŏk'shē-ŭm) [" + *proktos*, anus]. The connective tissue around the anus and rectum.

paraprostatitis (păr"ă-prŏs"tă-tī'tĭs) [" + *prostates*, prostate, + *itis*, inflammation]. Inflammation of the tissues around the prostate.

paraprotein (păr"ă-prō'tē-ĭn). An abnormal plasma protein, such as a macroglobulin, cryoglobulin, or the protein present in myeloma.

paraproteinemia. A general term for abnormalities of the immunoglobulins, associated with one of several disease states. SEE: *Bence Jones protein*.

parapsia, parapsis (păr-ăp'sē-ă, -sĭs) [" + *hapsis*, touch]. Any disorder of touch. SYN: *paraphia*.

parapsoriasis (păr"ă-sō-rī'ă-sĭs) [" + *psoriasis* itching]. A chronic disorder of the skin marked by scaly red lesions.

p. en plaque. A form of parapsoriasis that is often the precursor of mycosis fungoides.

p. lichenoides chronica. A form of parapsoriasis that forms a widespread network over the extremities and trunk. It is red to bluish in color and sometimes resembles psoriasis and at other times lichen planus.

parapsychology (păr"ă-sī-kŏl'ō-jē). The division of psychology that deals with extrasensory perception, telepathy, psychokinesis, clairvoyance, and associated phenomena.

paraquat (păr'ă-kwăt). A toxic chemical used in agriculture to kill certain weeds. It damages the skin on contact and if ingested may cause liver, renal, and pulmonary disease. This chemical is sometimes present as a contaminant in marijuana.

TREATMENT: Remove from stomach and gastrointestinal tract by emesis, gastric lavage, and cartharsis. Clay and charcoal should be administered to absorb the poison. Cortisone I.V. and hemodialysis are helpful.

pararectal (păr"ă-rĕk'tăl) [" + L. *rectum*,

straight]. Close to the rectum.

parareflexia (păr″ă-rē-flĕk′sē-ă). An abnormal condition of the reflexes.

pararenal (păr″ă-rē′năl) [″ + L. *ren,* kidney]. Near the kidneys.

pararhotacism (păr″ă-rō′tă-sĭzm) [″ + *rho,* Gr. letter R, + *-ismos,* condition]. Constant erroneous use of letter "r" or the placing of undue emphasis on letter "r."

pararrhythmia (păr″ă-rĭth′mē-ă) [″ + *a-,* not, + *rhythmos,* rhythm]. A cardiac rhythm caused by action of two pacemakers. It is not caused by a disturbance of the normal conducting pathways.

pararthria (păr-ăr′thrē-ă) [″ + *arthron,* articulation]. A speech disorder characterized by difficulty in uttering sounds.

parasacral (păr″ă-sā′krăl) [″ + L. *sacrum,* sacred]. Close to the sacrum.

parasalpingitis (păr″ă-săl-pĭn-jī′tĭs) [″ + *salpinx,* tube, + *itis,* inflammation]. Inflamed condition of tissues around an oviduct or a eustachian tube.

parasecretion (păr″ă-sē-krē′shŭn) [″ + L. *secretio,* secretion]. 1. An abnormality in secretion. 2. A substance abnormally secreted.

parasexuality (păr″ă-sĕks″ū-ăl′ĭ-tē) [″ + L. *sexus,* sex]. Any sexually deviant act.

parasigmatism (păr″ă-sĭg′mă-tĭzm) [″ + *sigma,* Gr. letter S, + *-ismos,* condition]. Imperfect pronunciation of the letter "s" and "z." SYN: *lisping.*

parasinoidal (păr″ă-sĭ-noy′dăl) [″ + L. *sinus,* a curve]. Close to a sinus.

parasite (păr′ă-sīt) [Gr. *parasitos,* fellow guest]. 1. An organism that lives within, upon, or at expense of another organism, known as the host, without contributing to survival of the host. 2. The smaller or incomplete element of conjoined twins that is attached to and dependent upon the more nearly normal twin, called the autosite.

p., accidental. Parasite infesting a host that is not its normal host. SYN: *p., incidental.*

p., external. Parasite that lives on the outer surface of its hosts, such as fleas, lice, mites, or ticks. SYN: *ectoparasite.*

p., facultative. Parasite capable of living independently of its host at times. Opposite of obligate parasite.

p., incidental. P., accidental.

p., intermittent. Parasite that visits its host at intervals for nourishment. SYN: *p., occasional.*

p., internal. Parasite such as protozoa or worms that lives within the body of the host, occupying the digestive tract or body cavities, or living within body organs, blood, tissues, or even cells.

p., malarial. Any one of the four species of Plasmodium that can cause malaria when transmitted by anopheline mosquitoes.

p., obligate. Parasite completely dependent on its host. Opposite of facultative parasite.

p., occasional. Parasite that seeks its host at intervals to obtain nourishment. SYN: *p., intermittent.*

p., periodic. Parasite that lives upon the host for short periods of time.

p., permanent. Parasite that lives upon its host until maturity or spends its entire life upon its host such as flukes or itch mites.

p., specific. Parasite that requires a specific host in order to complete its life cycle.

p., temporary. Parasite that is free-living during a part of its life cycle.

parasitemia (păr″ă-sī-tē′mē-ă) [Gr. *parasitos,* fellow guest, + *haima,* blood]. Presence of parasites in the blood.

parasitic (păr″ă-sĭt′ĭk) [Gr. *parasitikos*]. Like, caused by, or concerning, a parasite.

parasitic disease drug service. The Centers for Disease Control (CDC), Public Health Service, U.S. Department of Health and Human Services, maintains a supply of antiparasitic agents which otherwise are difficult to obtain. These drugs are available to licensed physicians by writing the Centers for Disease Control, Atlanta, GA, 30333, U.S.A. SEE: table (Antiparasitic Drugs).

parasiticide (păr″ă-sĭt′ĭ-sīd) [Gr. *parasitos,* fellow guest, + L. *caedere,* to kill]. 1. Destructive to parasites. 2. An agent that will kill parasites.

parasitism (păr′ă-sīt″ĭzm) [″ + *-ismos,* condition]. 1. The state or condition of being infected or infested with parasites. 2. The behavior of a parasite.

parasitize (păr′ă-sĭt-īz″, -sīt-īz″). To infest or infect with a parasite.

parasitogenic (păr″ă-sī″tō-jĕn′ĭk) [″ + *gennan,* to produce]. 1. Caused by parasites. 2. Favoring parasitic development.

parasitologist (păr″ă-sī-tŏl′ō-jĭst) [″ + *logos,* study]. One who specializes in the science of parasitology.

parasitology (păr″ă-sī-tŏl′ō-jē) [″ + *logos,* study]. The study of parasites and parasitism.

parasitophobia (păr″ă-sī″tō-fō′bē-ă) [″ + *phobos,* fear]. Unusual fear of parasites.

parasitosis (păr″ă-sī-tō′sĭs) [″ + *osis,* condition]. A disease or condition resulting from parasitism.

parasitotropic (păr″ă-sī″tō-trŏp′ĭk) [″ + *tropos,* turning]. Having attraction for parasites, esp. certain drugs that act chiefly upon parasites in the body.

parasitotropism (păr″ă-sī-tŏt′rō-pĭzm) [″ + ″ + *-ismos,* condition]. The special affinity of

Antiparasitic Drugs Available from the Centers for Disease Control

Infection	Drug
Onchocerciasis	Suramin
Dracunculiasis	Niridazole
Leishmaniasis	Pentostam
Central nervous system trypanosomiasis	Melarsoprol (Mel B)
Early infection with Trypanosoma rhodesiense	Suramin
Early infection with T. gambiense	Pentamidine
Chagas' disease	Nifurtimox
Amebiasis	Dehydroemetine, furamide
Malaria	Parenteral quinine

From Most, H: Treatment of parasitic infections of travelers and immigrants. N Engl J Med 310:299, 1984, with permission.

drugs or other agents for parasites.

parasitotropy (păr″ă-sī-tŏt′rō-pē). Parasitotropism, q.v.

paraspadia (păr-ă-spā′dē-ă) [Gr. *paraspadein,* to draw aside]. Condition in which the urethra has an opening through one side of the penis.

paraspasm (păr′ă-spăzm) [L. *paraspasmus*]. 1. Muscular spasm of the lower extremities. 2. Spastic paralysis of the lower extremities.

parasteatosis (păr″ă-stē″ă-tō′sĭs) [Gr. *para,* beside, + *steatos,* fat, + *osis,* condition]. Any disordered condition of the sebaceous secretions.

parasternal (păr-ă-stĕrn′ăl) [″ + *sternon,* chest]. Beside the sternum.

parasternal line. Imaginary vertical line running midway between sternal margin and line passing through the nipple.

parasternal region. Area between sternal margin and parasternal line.

parasthenia (păr″ăs-thē nē-ă) [″ + *sthenos,* strength]. Condition characterized by abnormal functioning of organic tissue at odd intervals.

parastruma (păr″ă-stroo′mă) [″ + L. *struma,* goiter]. Goiterlike tumor due to hypertrophy of a parathyroid gland.

parasympathetic (păr″ă-sĭm″pă-thĕt′ĭk) [″ + *sympathetikos,* sympathetic nerve]. Of or pert. to the craniosacral division of the autonomic nervous system.

parasympathetic nervous system. The craniosacral division of the autonomic nervous system. Preganglionic fibers originate from nuclei in the midbrain, medulla, and sacral portion of the spinal cord. They pass through the 3rd, 7th, 9th, and 10th cranial nerves and the 2nd, 3rd, and 4th sacral nerves, and synapse with postganglionic neurons located in autonomic (terminal) ganglia that lie in the walls of or near the organ innervated.

Some effects of parasympathetic stimulation are constriction of pupil, contraction of smooth muscle of alimentary canal, constriction of bronchioles, slowing of heart rate, and increased secretion by glands, except sweat glands. Parasympathetic effects are specific rather than general. SEE: *autonomic nervous system; sympathetic nervous system.*

parasympathicotonia (păr″ă-sĭm-păth″ĭk-ō-tō′nē-ă) [″ + *sympathetikos,* sympathetic nerve, + *tonos,* tension]. Condition in which there is an imbalance in functioning of the autonomic nervous system, the parasympathetic division dominating over the sympathetic. SYN: *vagotonia.*

parasympatholytic (păr″ă-sĭm″pă-thō-lĭt′ĭk) [″ + ″ + *lytikos,* dissolving]. Having a destructive effect on or blocking parasympathetic nerve fibers.

parasympathomimetic (păr″ă-sĭm″pă-thō-mĭm-ĕt′ĭk) [″ + ″ + *mimetikos,* imitative]. Producing effects similar to those resulting from stimulation of parasympathetic nervous system.

parasynapsis (păr″ă-sĭ-năp′sĭs) [″ + *synapsis,* conjunction]. The side-to-side union of chromosomes in the process of reduction division of meiosis.

parasynovitis (păr″ă-sĭn″ō-vī′tĭs) [″ + *syn,* with, + *oon,* egg, + *itis,* inflammation]. Inflamed condition of tissues around a synovial sac.

parasystole (păr-ă-sĭs′tō-lē) [″ + *systole,* contraction]. An ectopically originating cardiac rhythm independent of the normal sinus rhythm.

paratarsium (păr-ă-tăr′sē-ŭm) [″ + *tarsos,* tarsus]. The covering and connective tissues of the tarsus of the feet.

paratenon (păr″ă-tĕn′ŏn) [″ + *tenon,* tendon]. Fatty and areolar tissue that surrounds the tendon and fills the spaces around the tendon.

paratereseomania (păr″ă-tĕr-ē″sē-ō-mā′nē-ă) [Gr. *parateresis,* observation, + *mania,* madness]. Insane desire to investigate new scenes and subjects.

parathion (păr″ă-thī′ŏn). An agricultural insecticide, highly poisonous to humans and animals.

parathion poisoning. Contracted by accidental inhalation or ingestion while working with the pesticide or by inadvertent contamination of food products. SEE: *Poisons and Poisoning* in *Appendix.*

SYM: Shortly after exposure, headache, sweating, salivation, lacrimation, vomiting, diarrhea, muscular twitching, convulsions, dyspnea, and blurred vision occur.

parathormone (păr″ă-thor′mōn) [Gr. *para,* beside, + *thyreos,* shield, + *eidos,* form, + *hormaein,* to excite]. Hormone secreted by the parathyroid glands that regulates calcium and phosphorus metabolism. Deficiency results in tetany, carpopedal spasm, wheezing, muscle cramps, urinary frequency, mood changes, and lassitude. An extract from fresh or frozen parathyroid glands of domestic animals that contains the active principle or principles of these glands is used therapeutically. SEE: *parathyroid.* SYN: *hormone, parathyroid.*

parathymia (păr″ă-thī′mē-ă) [″ + *thymos,* mind, spirit]. Disordered or inappropriate mood.

parathyroid (păr-ă-thī′royd) [″ + *thyreos,* shield, + *eidos,* form]. 1. Located close to the thyroid gland. 2. One of four small endocrine glands about 6 mm. long by 3 to 4 mm. broad on the back of, and at lower edge of, the thyroid gland, or embedded within its substance. These glands secrete a hormone, parathyroid hormone (parathormone), that regulates calcium and phosphorus metabolism.

ABNORM: Hypoparathyroidism or hyposecretion results in neuromuscular hyperexcitability manifested by convulsions and tetany, carpopedal spasm, wheezing, muscle cramps, urinary frequency, mood changes and lassitude. Blood calcium falls and blood phosphorus rises. Other symptoms include blurring of vision due to cataracts, teeth may be poorly formed if onset was in childhood, maldevelopment of hair and nails, and dry and scaly skin. Hyperparathyroidism or hypersecretion results in a rise in blood calcium and fall in phosphorus. Calcium is removed from bones, resulting in increased fragility. Muscular weakness, reduced muscular tone, and general neuromuscular hypoexcitability occur. Generalized osteitis fibrosa or osteitis fibrosa cystica (von Recklinghausen's disease) is a clinical entity associated with hyperplasia and resulting hypersecretion of the parathyroids. Parathormone, q.v., secreted by these glands contains the active principle or principles.

parathyroidectomy (păr″ă-thī-royd-ĕk′tō-mē) [″ + ″ + ″ + *ektome,* excision]. Excision of one or more of the parathyroid glands.

parathyroid injection. USP. A standard preparation of the water-soluble hormone obtained from the parathyroid glands of mammals used for food by man. It acts to increase the calcium content of the blood.

parathyroprivia (păr″ă-thī″rō-prī′vē-ă) [″ + ″ + L. *privus,* deprived of]. Condition that results when the parathyroids are removed or cease functioning.

parathyroprivic (păr″ă-thī″rō-prĭv′ĭk). Resulting from loss of function of, or removal of, parathyroid glands.

parathyrotropic (păr″ă-thī-rō-trŏp′ĭk) [″ + ″ + ″ + *tropikos,* turning]. Having an affinity for the parathyroid gland.

paratonsillar (păr″ă-tŏn′sĭl-ăr) [″ + L. *tonsillaris,* pert. to tonsil]. Near or about the tonsil.

paratope (păr′ă-tōp) [″ + *topos,* a place]. The site on an antibody to which an antigen attaches. SEE: *epitope.*

paratrichosis (păr″ă-trĭ-kō′sĭs) [″ + *trichosis,* being hairy]. Abnormality of hair or its location.

paratripsis (păr″ă-trĭp′sĭs) [″ + *tribein,* to rub]. Rubbing, chafing.

paratrophic (păr″ă-trō′fĭk) [″ + *trophe,* nourishment]. 1. Requiring living substances for food; parasitic. 2. Pert. to abnormal nutrition.

paratrophy (păr-ăt′rō-fē) [″ + *trophe,* nourishment]. 1. The obtaining of nutrition from the host by a parasite. 2. Atrophy due to a nutritional defect.

paratyphlitis (păr″ă-tĭf-lī′tĭs) [″ + *typhlos,* blind, + *itis,* inflammation]. Inflammation of the connective tissue close to the cecum.

paratyphoid (păr-ă-tī′foyd) [″ + *typhos,* fever, + *eidos,* like]. Similar to typhoid.

paratyphoid fever. An infectious fever resembling typhoid.

ETIOL: Bacteria of the genus Salmonella, esp. the species S. paratyphi (A and B strains) and S. schottmulleri. However, any Salmonella pathogenic to man may cause a similar disease.

SYM: Fever with gastroenteritis. Incubation period may be less than in typhoid. Usually patient's condition is less severe than that found in typhoid fever, but symptoms vary from a mild transient diarrhea to those quite similar to typhoid fever, q.v.

paratypic (păr″ă-tĭp′ĭk) [″ + *typos,* type]. Diverging from a type.

paraumbilical (păr″ă-ŭm-bĭl′ĭk-ăl) [″ + L. *umbilicus,* navel]. Close to the navel.

paraurethral (păr″ă-ū-rē′thrăl) [″ + *ourethra,* urethra]. Located close to the urethra.

parauterine (păr″ă-ū′tĕr-ĭn) [″ + L. *uterus*, womb]. Located close to or around the uterus.
paravaccinia (păr″ă-văk-sĭn′ē-ă). A viral disease that affects the udders of cows and may be transmitted to man. In man, the virus produces painless, smooth or warty lesions, called "milker's nodules," on the hands and arms. SEE: *milker's nodules*.
paravaginal (păr″ă-văj′ĭn-ăl) [″ + *vagina*, sheath]. Located close to or around the vagina.
paravaginitis (păr″ă-văj-ĭn-ī′tĭs) [″ + ″ + Gr. *itis*, inflammation]. Inflammation of the tissue surrounding the vagina.
paravenous (păr″ă-vē′nŭs) [″ + L. *vena*, vein]. Close to a vein.
paravertebral (păr″ă-vĕr′tē-brăl) [″ + L. *vertebralis*, pert. to vertebrae]. Alongside or near the vertebral column.
paravertebral anesthesia. Injection of a local anesthetic at roots of spinal nerves.
paravesical (păr″ă-vĕs-ĭk′ăl) [″ + L. *vesica*, bladder]. Near the urinary bladder.
paravitaminosis (păr″ă-vī″tă-mĭ-nō′sĭs). 1. Any disease indirectly associated with a vitamin deficiency. 2. A disease that mimics avitaminosis but is not due to a vitamin deficiency.
paraxial (păr-ăk′sē-ăl) [″ + L. *axis*, axis]. On either side of the axis of the body, or one of its parts.
paraxon (păr-ăk′sŏn) [″ + *axon*, axis]. A collateral branch of an axon.
parazoon (păr″ă-zō′ŏn) [″ + Gr. *zoon*, animal]. An animal that lives as a parasite upon another animal.
parched [ME. *parchen*]. Extremely dry.
Paré, Ambroise (păr-ā′). French surgeon, 1510–1590, who instituted certain refined techniques into surgery and obstetrics.
parectasia (păr″ĕk-tā′sē-ă) [″ + *ektasis*, stretching]. Excessive dilatation or stretching of a structure.
parectasis (păr-ĕk′tă-sĭs). Parectasia.
parectropia (păr″ĕk-trō′pē-ă) [″ + Gr. *ek*, out, + *trope*, a turn]. Apraxia, q.v.
paregoric (păr-ĕ-gor′ĭk) [L. *paregoricus*, soothing]. 1. USP. Camphorated tincture of opium, a narcotic-containing drug that in large doses is poisonous. Used in the symptomatic treatment of diarrhea. 2. Soothing.
paregoric poisoning. SEE: *morphine*.
parelectronomic (păr″ē-lĕk″trō-nŏm′ĭk) [Gr. *para*, beside, + *elektron*, amber, + *nomos*, law]. Not stimulated by an electric stimulus.
parencephalia (păr″ĕn-sĕ-fā′lē-ă) [″ + *enkephalos*, brain]. Congenital defect of the brain.
parencephalocele (păr″ĕn-sĕf′ă-lō-sēl) [″ + ″ + *kele*, hernia]. Herniation of the cerebellum through a defect in the cranium.
parencephalous (păr″ĕn-sĕf′ă-lŭs) [″ + *enkephalos*, brain]. A fetus with imperfect development of the cranium.
parenchyma (păr-ĕn′kĭ-mă) [Gr. *parenkheim*, to pour in beside]. [NA] The essential parts of an organ that are concerned with its function in contradistinction to its framework.

p. testis. [NA] The functional portion of the testis, including the seminiferous tubules within the lobules.

parenchymatitis (păr″ĕn-kĭm″ă-tī′tĭs) [″ + *itis*, inflammation]. Inflamed condition of parenchyma or substance of a gland.
parenchymatous (păr″ĕn-kĭm′ă-tŭs). Concerning the essential substances of an organ.
parent [L. *parens*]. A father or a mother; one who begets offspring.
parenteral (păr-ĕn′tĕr-ăl) [Gr. *para*, beside + *enteron*, intestine]. Denoting any route other than the alimentary canal, such as intravenous, subcutaneous, intramuscular or mucosal. SEE: *medication routes*.
parenteral digestion. Digestion of foreign substances by body cells as opposed to enteral digestion, which occurs in the alimentary canal.
parenteral hyperalimentation. Providing the total caloric needs by intravenous route for a patient who is unable to take food orally. Although this is extremely difficult, patients have been maintained in a healthy state for prolonged periods by providing nutrients through a catheter extending through the subclavian vein to the superior vena cava.

The daily feeding of 2500–3000 kcal. for an adult includes 2500–3000 ml. of water; 100–130 gm. protein hydrolysate (amino acids); 12–18 gm. nitrogen; 525–625 gm. dextrose; 125–150 mEq sodium; 75–120 mEq potassium; 4–8 mEq magnesium; vitamins A, D, E, C, thiamine, riboflavin, niacin, and pantothenic acid. Calcium, phosphorus, and iron given as required; vitamin B_{12}, folic acid, and vitamin K given intramuscularly as needed. Trace elements required after one month of continuous feeding.

NURSING IMPLICATIONS: Explain procedure to patient. Obtain a nutritional assessment of the patient. Monitor and record intake and output. Assist with the catheter insertion. Observe for adverse affects. Document procedure and initial fluid administration. Monitor fluid flow with mechanical device and frequent nursing observations. Inspect and redress catheter site every 24 to 48 hours using strict aseptic technique. Document condition of site and position of catheter. Evaluate for catheter leakage and if present, report to physician immediately. Monitor electrolytes. Administer (I.M.) weekly vitamin supplements as prescribed. Observe for presence of edema or dehydration. If diarrhea or nausea occurs, slow the infusion rate.

Observe for aphasia. Perform urine sugar and acetone every six hours. Monitor blood sugar levels as ordered. Weigh patient daily. Never discontinue solution abruptly; always taper off with hypertonic solutions. In the event of catheter blockage or removal, notify physician immediately. Provide discharge teaching for patient and those in the household who will be caring for the patient.

parenting. 1. Caring for and raising a child or children. 2. Producing offspring.

parepididymus (păr″ĕp-ĭ-dĭd′ĭ-mĭs). Paradidymus, q.v.

parepithymia (păr″ĕp-ĭ-thī′mē-ă) [″ + *epithymia*, desire]. Abnormal desire or craving.

paresis (păr′ē-sĭs, pă-rē′sĭs) [Gr. *parienai*, to let fall]. 1. Partial or incomplete paralysis. 2. An organic mental disease with somatic, irritative, and paralytic focal symptoms and signs running a slow, chronic, progressive course and tending to a fatal termination. SYN: *dementia paralytica.*

ETIOL: Diffuse and focal involvement of brain and spinal cord due to syphilis, usually occurring 5–15 years after primary infection.

PATH: A diffuse meningoencephalitis with degenerative changes dependent upon vascular and toxic factors.

SYM: May simulate any psychoneurosis or psychosis. Pupillary changes, facial tremors, tremors of the lips and tongue, speech disturbances. Usually Argyll-Robertson pupil, impaired vision, headache, speech slurred with letters and syllables often omitted. Epileptic convulsions. Unequal exaggeration of the reflexes. Always a positive serologic test for syphilis in the spinal fluid with increase of protein and lymphocytes. Colloidal gold curve is abnormal in more than half the cases. Memory defective, expansive delusions, depression, dementia.

TREATMENT: Penicillin.

p., juvenile. General paresis due to congenital syphilis; seen in children.

Parest. Trade name for methaqualone hydrochloride.

paresthesia (păr″ĕs-thē′zē-ă) [″ + *aisthesis*, sensation]. Sensation of numbness, prickling, or tingling; heightened sensitivity. Experienced in central and peripheral nerve lesions and in locomotor ataxia.

p., Berger's. Paresthesia of the legs that occurs in young people.

paretic (pă-rĕt′ĭk, pă-rē′tĭk) [Gr. *parienai*, to let fall]. Affected with or concerning paresis.

Parfuran. Trade name for nitrofurantoin, USP.

pargyline hydrochloride (păr′gĭ-lēn). USP. An antihypertensive drug. Trade name is Eutonyl.

paridrosis (păr″ĭ-drō′sĭs) [″ + *hidrosis*, perspiration]. Any disordered secretion of perspiration.

paries (pā′rē-ēs) [L., a wall]. (pl. *parietes*) [NA] The enveloping wall of any structure; applied esp. to hollow organs.

parietal (pă-rī′ĕ-tăl) [L. *parietalis*]. 1. Pert. to, or forming, the wall of a cavity. 2. Pert. to the parietal bone.

parietal bone. One of two bones that together form the roof and sides of the skull.

parietal cells. Large cells on margin of the peptic glands of the stomach. SYN: *cell, oxyntic.*

parietal lobe. The division of each side of the brain lying beneath each parietal bone.

parietes (pă-rī′ĕ-tēs) [L.]. Pl. of paries; walls of an organ or hollow part.

parietofrontal (pă-rī″ĕ-tō-frŏn′tăl). Concerning the parietal or frontal bones or lobes.

parietography (pă-rī″ĕ-tŏg′ră-fē) [″ + Gr. *graphein*, to write]. X-ray study of the walls of an organ.

parieto-occipital (pă-rī″ĕ-tō-ŏk-sĭp′ĭ-tăl). Concerning the parietal and occipital bones or lobes.

parietosplanchnic (pă-rī″ĕ-tō-splănk′nĭk). Parietovisceral, q.v.

parietosquamosal (pă-rī″ĕ-tō-skwă-mō′săl). Concerning the parietal bone and the squamous part of the temporal bone.

parietotemporal (pă-rī″ĕ-tō-tĕm′pō-răl). Concerning the parietal and temporal bones or lobes.

parietovisceral (pă-rī″ĕ-tō-vĭs′ĕr-ăl). Concerning the wall of a body cavity and the viscera within.

Parinaud, Henri (pă-rĭ-nō′). French ophthalmologist, 1844–1905.

P.'s oculoglandular syndrome. Conjunctivitis with palpable preauricular lymph nodes.

P.'s ophthalmoplegia syndrome. Palsy of vertical gaze that may or may not be associated with pupillary or oculomotor nerve paresis. It is caused by a lesion at the level of the anterior corpora quadrigemina of the brain.

pari passu (păr′ē păs′ū) [L., with equal speed]. Occurring at the same time or at the same rate; side by side.

parity (păr′ĭ-tē). 1. [L. *par*, equal]. Equality, similarity. 2. [L. *parere*, to bear]. The ability of a woman to carry a pregnancy to a point of viability (500 g. birth weight or 20 weeks gestation) regardless of the outcome. SEE: *multiparity; nulliparity; primiparity; secundiparity.*

Parkinson, James. British physician, 1755–1824.

P.'s disease. A chronic nervous disease characterized by a fine, slowly spreading tremor, muscular weakness and rigidity, and a peculiar gait. SYN: *paralysis agitans;*

shaking palsy.

SYM: Onset may be abrupt; generally insidious. First symptom is a fine tremor beginning in hand or foot that may spread until it involves all the members. At first paroxysmal but becomes almost continuous. Face becomes expressionless. Speech slow and measured, later muscular rigidity. Head bowed, body bent forward, arms flexed, thumbs turned into palms, knees slightly bent. Gait characteristic by this time; steps grow faster and faster, body inclines more and more forward until patient falls, seeks some support; this is termed festination. Occasionally a tendency to fall backwards, retropulsion, replaces festination. Numbness, tingling, and sensation of heat may be present.

PROG: Recovery rarely if ever occurs. Duration indefinite.

TREATMENT: General supportive measures plus medicines to combat muscle rigidity and lethargy. Drugs used include levodopa, levodopa and carbidopa, amantadine hydrochloride, and anticholinergics.

P.'s facies. The immobile, masklike facies characteristic of parkinsonism.

P.'s mask. Expressionless appearance of the face. Eyebrows are raised, wrinkles are smoothed out, and there is immobility of the facial muscles. A typical symptom seen in Parkinson's disease and in post-encephalitic states.

parkinsonian (păr″kĭn-sŏn′ē-ăn). Concerning parkinsonism.

parkinsonism (păr′kĭn-sŏn-ĭzm″). Parkinson's disease.

Parlodel. Trade name for bromocriptine mesylate.

Parnate. Trade name for tranylcypromine sulfate.

paroccipital (păr-ŏk-sĭp′ĭt-ăl) [Gr. *para,* beside, + L. *occiput,* occiput]. 1. Close to the occipital bone. 2. The paramastoid process.

parodontitis (păr″ō-dŏn-tī′tĭs) [″ + *odous,* tooth, + *itis,* inflammation]. Inflamed condition of tissues around a tooth.

parodontium (păr″ō-dŏn′shē-ŭm). Periodontium.

parodynia (păr-ō-dĭn′ē-ă) [L. *parere,* to bear, + Gr. *odyne,* pain]. 1. Labor pains. 2. Difficult or abnormal labor or birth. SYN: *dystocia.*

p. perversa. Presentation with fetus lying transversely across the uterus.

Paroidin. Trade name for parathyroid hormone.

parolivary (păr-ŏl′ĭ-vă″rē) [Gr. *para,* beside, + L. *oliva,* olive]. Situated close to the olivary body.

parolivary bodies. Nuclei in medulla oblongata, lying close to the olivary bodies.

paromomycin sulfate (păr′ō-mō-mī″sĭn). USP. An aminoglycoside antibiotic used in treating intestinal amebiasis and various tapeworms. It is not effective against extraintestinal infections with amebae. Trade name is Humatin.

paromphalocele (păr″ŏm-făl′ō-sēl″) [″ + *omphalos,* navel, + *kele,* hernia]. Hernia or tumor close to the umbilicus.

paroniria (păr-ō-nī′rē-ă) [″ + *oneiros,* dream]. Abnormal or terrifying dreams.

p. ambulans. Sleepwalking.

p. salax. Restlessness in sleep with lascivious dreams and nocturnal emissions.

paronychia (păr-ō-nĭk′ē-ă) [″ + *onyx,* nail]. Acute or chronic infection of marginal structures about the nail. SYN: *felon; panaris; runaround; whitlow.*

ETIOL: Trauma, infection. SYM: Redness, swelling, and suppuration around nail edge.

TREATMENT: Heat to area unless there is inadequate blood supply; surgery in severe cases.

p. tendinosa. Inflammation of sheath of a digital tendon due to sepsis.

paronychomycosis (păr″ō-nĭk″ō-mī-kō′sĭs) [″ + ″ + *mykes,* fungus, + *osis,* condition]. Fungus infection about the nails.

paronychosis (păr-ō-nī-kō′sĭs). Growth of a nail in an abnormal position.

paroophoritis (păr″ō-ŏf-ō-rī′tĭs) [″ + *oophoros,* bearing eggs, + *itis,* inflammation]. Inflammation of the tissues around the ovary.

paroophoron (păr-ō-ŏf′ō-rŏn) [″ + *oophoros,* bearing eggs]. A group of minute tubules located in the mesosalpinx between the uterus and ovary. It is a vestigial structure consisting of the remains of the caudal group of mesonephric tubules and is a homologue of the paradidymis of the male.

parophthalmia (păr-ŏf-thăl′mē-ă) [″ + *ophthalmos,* eye]. Inflamed condition of tissue around the eye.

parophthalmoncus (păr″ŏf-thăl-mŏn′kŭs) [″ + ″ + *onkos,* mass]. A tumor located near the eye.

paropsis (păr-ŏp′sĭs) [″ + *opsis,* vision]. Any disorder of sense of sight.

parorchidium (păr-or-kĭd′ē-ŭm) [″ + *orchis,* testicle]. Abnormal position, or nondescent, of a testicle. SYN: *ectopia testis.*

parorchis (păr-or′kĭs) [″ + *orchis,* testicle]. The epididymis.

parorexia (păr-ō-rĕk′sē-ă) [″ + *orexis,* appetite]. An abnormal or perverted craving for special or strange foods. SEE: *appetite, perverted; taste.*

parosmia (păr-ŏz′mē-ă) [″ + *osme,* odor]. Any disorder or perversion of the sense of smell; a false sense of odors or perception of those that do not exist. Agreeable ones are considered offensive and disagreeable odors are accepted as pleasant. SYN: *parosphresia.* SEE:

cacosmia; kakosmia.

parosphresia, parosphresis (păr″ŏs-frē′zē-ă, -sĭs) [″ + *osphresis,* smell]. Disordered sense of smell. SYN: *parosmia.*

parosteal (păr-ŏs′tē-ăl). Concerning the outermost layer of the periosteum.

parosteitis, parostitis (păr-ŏs-tē-ī′tĭs, -tī′tĭs) [Gr. *para,* beside, + *osteon,* bone, + *itis,* inflammation]. Inflammation of tissues next to the bone.

parosteosis, parostosis (păr″ŏs-tē-ō′sĭs, -tō′sĭs) [″ + *osteon,* bone, + *osis,* condition]. 1. Bone formation outside of the periosteum. 2. Bone development in an unusual location.

parotic (pă-rŏt′ĭk) [″ + *ous,* ear]. Near the ear.

parotid (pă-rŏt′ĭd). Located near the ear; esp. the parotid gland.

parotid duct. Approx. 2 in. (5.08 cm.) long. Extends from anterior border of the parotid gland crossing the masseter muscle and piercing the buccinator muscle, and then runs between the buccinator and the mucous membrane. It opens into the mouth opposite the 2nd upper molar. The transverse facial artery is above the duct and the buccal branch of the 7th cranial nerve below. The duct transports secretions from the parotid gland to the oral cavity. Stenosis of the duct causes pain and swelling in the parotid gland. SYN: *Stensen's duct.* SEE: *saliva.*

parotidectomy (pă-rŏt″ĭ-dĕk′tō-mē) [″ + *ous,* ear, + *ektome,* excision]. Excision of the parotid gland.

parotid gland. A nearly pure serous gland, its secreting tubules and acini being long and branched. It is enclosed in a sheath, the parotid fascia. The parotid gland is one of the salivary glands of the mouth. Its secretion helps to lubricate food and makes it easier to chew and swallow.

parotiditis (pă-rŏt″ĭ-dī′tĭs) [″ + ″ + *itis,* inflammation]. Parotitis.

parotidoscirrhus (pă-rŏt″ĭd-ō-skĭr′ŭs) [″ + ″ + *skirrhos,* hardness]. 1. Hardening of the parotid gland. 2. A scirrhous cancer of the parotid area.

parotitis (pă″rō-tī′tĭs) [″ + *ous,* ear, + *itis,* inflammation]. Inflammation of the parotid gland, either simple or epidemic. SYN: *mumps.*

parous (pā′rŭs) [L. *pario,* to bear]. Parturient; fruitful; having borne at least one child.

parovarian (păr-ō-vā′rē-ăn) [″ + L. *ovarium,* ovary]. 1. Situated near or beside the ovary. 2. Pert. to the parovarium, a residual structure in the broad ligament.

parovariotomy (păr″ō-vā″rē-ŏt′ō-mē) [″ + ″ + Gr. *tome,* incision]. Removal of a parovarian cyst.

parovaritis (păr″ō-vă-rī′tĭs) [″ + L. *ovarium,* ovary, + Gr. *itis,* inflammation]. Inflammation of the epoophoron.

parovarium (păr″ō-vā′rē-ŭm). Lateral portion of the vestigial remains of the mesonephric tubules. Located in the mesosalpinx between the ovary and the fallopian tube. SYN: *epoophoron* [NA].

paroxysm (păr′ŏk-sĭzm) [Gr. *paroxysmos,* irritation]. 1. A sudden, periodic attack or recurrence of symptoms of a disease; an exacerbation of the symptoms of a disease. 2. A sudden spasm or convulsion of any kind. 3. Sudden emotional state, as of fear, grief, or joy.

paroxysmal (păr″ŏk-sĭz′măl). 1. Occurring in or concerning paroxysms. 2. Of the nature of a paroxysm.

paroxysmal cold hemoglobinuria. A rare form of an autoimmune hemolytic syndrome that occurs idiopathically, in association with syphilis, or following viral or presumed viral diseases such as measles, mumps, chicken pox, infectious mononucleosis, and influenza.

SYM: Acute onset of back and extremity pain and abdominal cramps following chilling. Hemoglobinuria if sufficient numbers of red blood cells have been destroyed. Fever may be as high as 40° C. (104° F.).

TREATMENT: Therapy of primary disease if caused by an unknown virus; otherwise protection from the cold is the only practical therapy in the idiopathic form.

parricide (păr′ĭ-sīd) [L. *parricida*]. The murdering of one's own parent or a close relative. SYN: *patricide.*

Parrot, Jules Marie (păr-ō′). French physician, 1839–1883.

P.'s disease. 1. Osteochondritis that occurs in infants with congenital syphilis. 2. A form of dwarfism that is transmitted as an autosomal dominant.

P.'s nodes. Bony nodules on the skull of infants with congenital syphilis. SYN: *P.'s sign.*

P.'s pseudoparalysis. Pseudoparalysis caused by syphilitic osteochondritis.

P.'s sign. P.'s nodes.

P.'s ulcer. Lesions seen in thrush or stomatitis.

parrot fever. Psittacosis.

Parry's disease (păr′ēz). [Caleb H. Parry, Brit. physician, 1755–1822] Hyperthyroidism.

pars (părz) [L.]. (pl. *partes*) [NA] A part; portion of a larger structure.

p. anterior hypophyseos. The anterior lobe of the hypophysis.

p. basilaris ossis occipitalis. [NA] Basilar process of the occipital bone.

p. buccalis hypophyseos. Developmental protrusion in primitive buccal cavity of anterior lobe of hypophysis.

p. caeca oculi. The optic disk.

p. caeca retinae. The parts of the retina not sensitive to light (pars ciliaris retinae and pars iridica retinae).

p. cavernosa urethra. Cavernous portion of the male urethra.

p. cephalica nervi sympathici. Plexus, ganglia, and nerves derived from sympathetic nerve.

p. ciliaris retinae. [NA] Portion of the retina situated in front of the ora serrata and covering the ciliary body.

p. distalis. That part of the hypophysis forming the major portion of the anterior lobe.

p. flaccida. A portion of the membrane of the eardrum that fills the notch of Rivinus. SYN: *Shrapnell's membrane.*

p. intermedia. The intermediate lobe of the hypophysis cerebri.

p. iridica retinae. [NA] Portion of the retina on the posterior surface of the iris.

p. mastoidea ossis temporalis. The mastoid portion of the temporal bone.

p. membranacea urethrae. The membranous portion of the urethra.

p. nervosa hypophyseos. Posterior lobe of the pituitary gland.

p. optica hypothalami. The optic chiasma.

p. optica retinae. [NA] The sensory portion of the retina extending from the optic disk to the ora serrata.

p. petrosa ossis temporalis. The petrous portion of the temporal bone.

p. plana corporis ciliaris. Ciliary ring of the eye.

p. radiata. Ray, medullary, q.v.

p. squamosa ossis temporalis. The flat portion of the temporal bone that forms part of the lateral wall of the skull.

p. tensa. The larger portion of the tympanic membrane, a tightly stretched membrane lying inferior to the malleolar folds.

p. tuberalis. The portion of the anterior lobe of the hypophysis cerebri that invests the infundibular stalk.

p. tympanica ossis temporalis. The tympanic portion of the temporal bone.

pars planitis (păr̆s plā-nī'tĭs). Inflammation of the peripheral retina characterized by aggregations of inflammatory cells on the anterior inferior retina. These are called "snowbanks." This chronic condition, which occurs mostly in the young, is of unknown etiology. It may cause loss of vision.

TREATMENT: Systemic corticosteroids or by injection behind the eye.

part. aeq. *partes aequales,* equal parts.

partes (păr'tēs). Pl. of pars.

parthenogenesis (păr"thĕn-ō-jĕn'ĕ-sĭs) [Gr. *parthenos,* virgin, + *genesis,* origin]. Reproduction arising from a female egg that has not been fertilized by the male; unisexual reproduction.

parthenophobia (păr"thĕ-nō-fō'bē-ā) [" + *phobos,* fear]. Fear of virgins or girls.

particle [L. *particula*]. 1. A very small piece or part of matter; a tiny fragment or trace. 2. One of several subatomic components of the nucleus of radioactive elements such as alpha and beta particles. 3. Attraction particle or centriole, q.v., of the nucleus of a cell. 4. Viral particle or virion, q.v.

p., alpha. A charged particle emitted from the nucleus of a radioactive atom. The particle is weakly penetrating.

p., beta. An electron of positive or negative charge emitted during the decay of a radioactive substance.

p., Dane. A very small round particle present in the serum of some patients with viral hepatitis.

p., elementary. The subatomic parts of the atomic nucleus.

p., elementary, of the mitochondria. A surface particle on the mitochondrial cristae.

particulate (păr-tĭk'ū-lāt). Made up of particles.

parts per million. ABBR: PPM; ppm. Phrase used with a number to indicate the concentration of one substance with respect to another. For example, a chemical substance may be said to be present in air at a level of 50 parts per million (parts of air). The units also may be expressed as weight of one substance to the weight of another. This is called weight-to-weight comparison, or the concentration may be expressed as volume-to-volume.

parturient (păr-tū'rē-ĕnt) [L. *parturiens,* in labor]. Concerning childbirth or parturition; giving birth.

parturifacient (păr-tū-rĭ-fā'shĕnt) [" + *facere,* to make]. 1. Inducing or accelerating labor. 2. Drug used to cause or hasten delivery of the fetus.

parturiometer (păr"tū-rē-ŏm'ĕ-tĕr) [" + Gr. *metron,* measure]. A device for determining the force of uterine contractions during childbirth.

parturiphobia [" + Gr. *phobos,* fear]. Fear of childbirth.

parturition (păr-tū-rĭsh'ŭn) [L. *parturitio*]. Act of giving birth to young. SYN: *childbirth; delivery.*

parturition, words pert. to: accouchement; accoucheur; accoucheuse; afterbirth; afterpains; amniocentesis; ante partum; axis traction; bag of waters; ballottement; bipara; bradytocia; breech presentation; cephalic version; cephalotomy; cesarean section; childbirth; dystocia; hourglass contraction; labor; maneuver; multipara; nullipara; obstetrics; oxytocia; parturient; parturifacient; partus; placenta; placenta previa; postpartum; puerperium; Rh; uterus.

part. vic. *partibus vicibus*, in divided doses.

parulis (păr-ū'lĭs) [Gr. *para*, beside, + *oulon*, gum]. Abscess of a gum. SYN: *gumboil*.

parumbilical (păr"ŭm-bĭl'ĭ-kăl) [" + L. *umbilicus*, navel]. Close to the navel.

paruria (păr-ū'rē-ă) [Gr. *para*, beside, + *ouron*, urine]. Any abnormality in discharge of urine.

parvicellular (păr-vĭ-sĕl'ū-lăr) [L. *parvus*, small, + *cellula*, little box]. Concerning, or composed of, tiny cells.

parvoline (păr'vō-lĭn). A ptomaine formed in decaying fish.

parvovirus (păr"vō-vī'rŭs) [" + *virus*, poison]. A group of viruses similar to adeno-associated viruses. They are pathogenic in animals but not in man.

parvule (păr'vūl) [L. *parvulus*, very small]. A small pill, pellet, or granule.

PAS, PASA. *para-aminosalicylic acid*.

pascal. A unit of pressure equal to the force of one newton acting uniformly over one square meter. SEE: *newton*.

Paschen bodies (pă'shĕn). [Enrique Paschen, Ger. pathologist, 1860–1936] Particles thought to be the pathogenic virus of vaccinia and variola found in great numbers in skin exanthemas.

passage (păs'ăj) [ME., to pass]. 1. A channel between cavities and body structures or with the external surface of an organ. 2. Act of passing. 3. An evacuation of the bowels. 4. Introduction of a probe or catheter. 5. Incubation of a pathogenic organism, esp. a virus in one or a series of tissue cultures or living organisms.

passion (păsh'ŭn) [L. *passio*, suffering]. 1. Suffering. 2. Great emotion or zeal; frequently associated with sexual excitement.

passional (păsh'ŭn-ăl). Concerning any passion. SEE: *emotional*.

passive (păs'ĭv) [L. *passivus*, capable of suffering]. Submissive; acted upon; not active.

passive congestion. Congestion due to obstruction in venous return or, if general, due to myocardial insufficiency.

passive exercise. Muscular exercise without any effort on part of patient; accomplished by use of a machine or an assistant. SYN: *passive motion; passive movement*.

passive hyperemia. Increased blood in an area or part due to decreased outflow.

passive motion. Passive exercise.

passive movement. Passive exercise.

passive smoking. Breathing the smoke produced by persons smoking in one's immediate environment.

passivism (păs'ĭ-vĭzm) [" + Gr. *-ismos*, condition]. 1. Passive behavior or character. 2. Sexual perversion with subjugation of the will to another.

passivity (păs-sĭv'ĭ-tē) [L. *passivus*, capable of suffering]. In psychiatry, the condition of being dependent on others and a reluctance to be assertive or to be responsible.

paste. A semisolid gelatinous substance usually intended for external application. It may contain specific active ingredients or simple materials such as oils, waxes, and starch.

Pasteur, Louis (pă-stĕr'). French chemist and bacteriologist, 1822–1895, who founded the science of microbiology. His greatest accomplishments were in the field of bacteriology and immunology. He developed the technique of immunization and produced vaccines.

P. effect. Inhibition of fermentation by bacteria when oxygen is abundant.

P. treatment. Used for the prevention of rabies. Daily injection of increasingly virulent suspensions prepared from the brain or spinal cord of rabbits that have died of rabies. The treatment is continued for 21 days. Suspension is treated so as to kill or inactivate the virus. This treatment is no longer used, but is presented here for historical purposes. SEE: *rabies*.

Pasteurella (pās-tĕr-ĕl'ă). [Louis Pasteur] A genus of bacteria that at one time included the species P. pestis, P. tularensis, P. multocida, and P. pseudotuberculosis. P. pestis, the organism that causes plague, is now classed as Yersinia pestis. P. tularensis, the causative organism of tularemia, is now classed as Francisella tularensis. P. pseudotuberculosis, which can cause acute mesenteric lymphadenitis or enterocolitis, is now classed as Yersinia pseudotuberculosis.

P. multocida. A small nonmotile gram-negative coccobacillus that frequently causes disease in animals and birds. In man the organism may cause soft tissue infection or even osteomyelitis following an animal bite or may cause a systemic infection, such as bacteremia or meningitis, or a respiratory tract infection.

pasteurellosis (păs"tĕr-ĕ-lō'sĭs). Disease caused by infection with bacteria of the Pasteurella species.

pasteurization (păs"tūr-ī-zā'shŭn). [Louis Pasteur] The process of heating a fluid at a moderate temperature for a definite period of time in order to destroy undesirable bacteria without changing to any extent its chemical composition.

In pasteurization of milk, pathogenic bacteria are destroyed by heating at 62° C. for 30 minutes, or by "flash" heating to higher temperatures for less than a minute. The pasteurization process, reducing total bacterial count of the milk by 97 to 99%, is effective because the common milk-borne pathogens (tubercle bacillus, Salmonella,

Streptococcus, and Brucella) do not form spores and are quite sensitive to heat. However, pasteurization should not be considered as a substitute for cleanliness in milk production. SEE: *milk*.

pastille (păs-tēl′, -tĭl′) [L. *pastillus*, a little roll]. 1. A medicated disk used for local action on the mucosa of the throat and mouth. SYN: *lozenge; troche*. 2. A small cone used to fumigate or scent the air of a room.

past-pointing. Term used to describe the inability to place finger or some other part of the body accurately on a selected point. Seen in certain neurologic disorders.

patagia (pă-tā′jē-ă) [L.]. Pl. of patagium.

patagium (pă-tā′jē-ŭm) [L.]. (pl. *patagia*) A weblike membrane. SEE: *pterygium*.

patch (păch) [ME. *pacche*]. A small circumscribed area distinct from surrounding surface in character and appearance.

p., cotton wool. The appearance of exudative areas in the retina. Usually seen in connection with hypertensive retinopathy.

p., herald. Solitary oval patch of efflorescence showing before the general eruption of pityriasis rosea, often several days before.

p., Hutchinson's. Salmon-yellow area seen on cornea in syphilitic keratitis.

p., mucous. A syphilitic eruption having an eroded, moist surface; generally on mucous membrane of mouth or external genitals, or on surface subject to moisture and heat.

p., opaline. Whitish patch in mouth sometimes present in syphilis.

p.'s, Peyer's. Masses of lymphoid follicles found on mucous membrane of small intestine. SEE: *typhoid fever*.

p., salmon. Salmon-colored area of cornea seen in interstitial keratitis due to syphilis.

p., smoker's. Leukoplakia of the oral mucosa.

p., soldier's. SEE: *spot, milk*.

patch test. SEE: *test, patch*.

patefaction (păt″ĕ-făk′shŭn) [L. *patefacere*, to lay open]. A laying open.

patella (pă-tĕl′ă) [L., a small pan]. (pl. *patellae*) [NA] A lens-shaped sesamoid bone situated in front of the knee in the tendon of the quadriceps femoris muscle. SEE: *osteochondritis dissecans*. SYN: *kneecap*.

p., bipartite. Bipartite patella, q.v.

p., floating. A patella that rides up from the condyles due to a large effusion in the knee.

p., fracture of. TREATMENT: Suture of bone fragments. A plaster cast is applied from the toes to the groin, remaining on for 6 to 8 weeks. Following removal of cast, gradual exercise and weight upon the leg for a few weeks, after which the patient may walk.

p., rider's painful. Tenderness and pain in patella from horseback riding.

p., slipping. An easily dislocated patella.

patellapexy (pă-tĕl′ă-pĕk″sē) [L. *patella*, small pan, kneecap, + Gr. *pexis*, fixation]. Fixation of the patella to the lower end of the femur to stabilize the joint.

patellar (pă-tĕl′ăr). Concerning the patella.

patellar ligament. The ligamentous continuation of the tendon of the quadriceps femora to extend beyond the distal portion of the patella to attach to the tuberosity of the tibia.

patellar reflex. Involuntary jerk of leg due to sudden spasm of quadriceps following percussion of patellar ligament. SYN: *knee-jerk reflex*. SEE: *Jendrassik's maneuver*.

patellectomy (păt″ĕ-lĕk′tō-mē) [″ + Gr. *ektome*, excision]. Surgical removal of the patella.

patelliform (pă-tĕl′ĭ-form) [″ + *forma*, shape]. Shaped like the patella.

patellofemoral (pă-tĕl″ō-fĕm′ō-răl). Concerning the patella and the femur.

patellometer (păt″ĕ-lŏm′ĕ-tĕr) [″ + Gr. *metron*, measure]. Device for measuring the patellar reflex.

patency (pā′tĕn-sē) [L. *patens*, open]. The state of being freely open.

patent (păt′ĕnt, pā′tĕnt). Wide open; evident; accessible.

patent ductus arteriosus. SEE: *ductus arteriosus, patent*.

patent medicine. A drug or medical preparation that is protected by patent and sold without a physician's prescription. The law requires that it be labeled with names of active ingredients, the quantity or proportion of the contents, and directions for its use, and that it may not have misleading statements as to curative effects on the label. This term is rarely used. SEE: *nonproprietary name; prescription; proprietary medicine*.

paternal (pă-tĕr′năl) [L. *paternis*, fatherly]. Of, pert. to, or inherited from the father.

paternity test. Test to determine whether it would be possible for an individual to have fathered a specific child. The results can be used only to exclude the possibility of paternity; they cannot be used to prove paternity. Test results are analyzed with respect to the blood type of the child and that of the suspected father. Thus paternity may be excluded if the child had a blood type it could not have inherited from the mother and the alleged father.

path. SEE: *pathway*.

path-, patho- [Gr. *pathema*, disease]. Prefix indicating disease.

pathema (pă-thē′mă) [Gr.]. (pl. *pathemas;*

pathemata) Disease.

pathergasia (păth″ĕr-gā′zē-ă) [Gr. *pathos,* disease, + *ergasia,* work]. Adolf Meyer's term for personality maladjustment associated with organic, functional, or structural changes.

pathergia (pă-thĕr′jē-ă). Pathergy.

pathergy (păth′ĕr-jē). 1. Any lesion caused by an altered immune state of body tissues. 2. Allergic response to a great number of antigens.

pathetic (pă-thĕt′ĭk) [L. *patheticus*]. 1. Pert. to, or arousing, the emotions of pity, sympathy, or tenderness. 2. Pert. to trochlear nerve.

pathetism (păth′ĕ-tĭzm) [Gr. *pathein,* to suffer, + *-ismos,* condition]. State of overcoming another's will by suggestion. SYN: *hypnotism; mesmerism.*

pathfinder [AS. *paeth,* road, + *findan,* to locate]. 1. Instrument for locating stricture of the urethra. 2. Dental instrument for tracing the course of root canals.

-pathic (pă′thĭk) [Gr. *pathos,* disease]. Suffix indicating (1) a feeling that is affected in a specific way, as in telepathic; (2) a diseased condition, as in cardiopathic; (3) a form of therapy or system of medicine, as allopathic, homeopathic, or osteopathic.

Pathilon. Trade name for tridihexethyl chloride.

patho- (păth′ō) [Gr. *pathos,* disease]. Combining form indicating disease or suffering.

pathoamine (păth″ō-ăm′ĭn). A toxic ptomaine.

pathoanatomy (păth″ō-ă-năt′ō-mē). Anatomical pathology.

pathobiology (păth″ō-bī-ŏl′ō-jē). Pathology.

Pathocil. Trade name for dicloxacillin sodium, USP.

pathoclisis (păth″ō-klĭs′ĭs). A specific tendency to be sensitive to certain toxins.

pathocrine (păth′ō-krīn, -krēn, -krĭn) [Gr. *pathos,* suffering, + *krinein,* to secrete]. Concerning an endocrine disorder.

pathodixia [″ + Gr. *deiknunia,* to show]. An unusual desire to exhibit one's illness or injury. SEE: *anosognosia.*

pathodontia (păth″ō-dŏn′shē-ă) [″ + *odous,* tooth]. The science of dental pathology.

pathoformic (păth″ō-for′mĭk) [″ + L. *forma,* form]. Concerning the earliest signs of a disease, esp. mental disorder.

pathogen (păth′ō-jĕn) [″ + *gennan,* to produce]. A microorganism or substance capable of producing a disease.

pathogenesis (păth″ō-jĕn′ĕ-sĭs). Origination and development of a disease.

pathogenetic, pathogenic (păth″ō-jĕn-ĕt′ĭk, -jĕn′ĭk). Productive of disease. SYN: *morbific.*

pathogenicity (păth″ō-jĕ-nĭs′ĭ-tē) [″ + *gennan,* to produce]. The state of producing or being able to produce pathological changes and disease.

pathogeny (păth-ŏj′ĕn-ē). The origin and development of a disease. SYN: *pathogenesis.*

pathognomonic (păth″ŏg-nō-mŏn′ĭk) [Gr. *pathognomonikos,* skilled in diagnosing]. Indicative of a disease, esp. its characteristic symptoms.

pathognomy (păth-ŏg′nō-mē) [Gr. *pathos,* disease, + *gnome,* a means of knowing]. To diagnose the cause of an illness by carefully studying the signs and symptoms of a disease.

pathognostic (păth″ŏg-nŏs′tĭk) [″ + *gnosis,* knowledge]. Pathognomonic, q.v.

pathologic, pathological (păth-ō-lŏj′ĭk, -ĭ-kăl) [Gr. *pathos,* disease, + *logos,* study]. 1. Concerning pathology. 2. Diseased; due to a disease. SYN: *morbid.*

pathological reaction to alcohol. An exceedingly severe reaction to ingestion of alcohol, esp. to small amounts. Manifested by irrational violent behavior followed by exhaustion, sleep, and loss of recall of the event. Patient may not be intoxicated. SEE: *alcoholism.*

ETIOL: Unknown but is associated with hypoglycemia, exhaustion, and stress,

pathologist (pă-thŏl′ō-jĭst) [″ + *logos,* study]. A specialist in diagnosing the abnormal changes in tissues removed at operations and postmortem examinations.

pathology (pă-thŏl′ō-jē). 1. Study of the nature and cause of disease, which involves changes in structure and function. 2. Condition produced by disease.

p., anatomic. Field of pathology that deals with structural changes in disease.

p., cellular. Pathology that is based upon microscopic changes in body cells during disease.

p., chemical. The study of chemical changes that occur in disease.

p., clinical. Pathology as it is used to aid in the diagnosis of disease and care for patients.

p., comparative. The observation of pathological condition, spontaneous or artificial, in the lower animals or in vegetable organisms as compared to those of the human body.

p., dental. The science of diseases of the mouth.

p., experimental. Study of diseases induced artificially and intentionally, esp. in animals.

p., functional. The study of alterations of functions that occur in disease processes without associated structural changes.

p., geographical. Pathology in its relationship to climate and geography.

p., humoral. Pathology of the fluids of the body.

p., medical. The pathology of disorders that are not accessible for surgical procedures.

p., molecular. Study of the pathological effects of specific molecules.

p., oral. P., dental, q.v.

p., special. The pathology of particular diseases or organs.

p., surgical. Application of pathologic procedures and techniques for investigating tissues removed surgically.

pathomimesis (păth″ō-mĭm-ē′sĭs) [Gr. *pathos,* disease, + *mimesis,* imitation]. Intentional (conscious or unconscious) imitation of a disease. SYN: *malingering; pathomimicry.*

pathomimicry (păth″ō-mĭm′ĭ-krē). Pathomimesis.

pathomorphism (păth″ō-mor′fĭzm) [″ + *morphe,* form, + *-ismos,* condition]. Study of abnormal form and structure of organisms.

pathonomia (păth-ō-nō′mē-ă) [″ + *nomos,* law]. Study of the laws of disease processes.

pathophilia (păth″ō-fĭl′ē-ă) [″ + *philein,* to love]. Adjustment of habits to conditions made mandatory by some chronic disease.

pathophobia (păth-ō-fō′bē-ă) [″ + *phobos,* fear]. Morbid fear of disease.

pathophoric (păth″ō-for′ĭk) [″ + *phoros,* carrying]. Carrying or transmitting disease, as certain insects.

pathophysiology (păth″ō-fĭz″ē-ŏl′ō-jē) [″ + *physis,* nature, + *logos,* study]. The study of how normal physiological processes are altered by disease.

pathopoiesis (păth″ō-poy-ē′sĭs) [″ + *poiesis,* production]. 1. The generation of disease. 2. Tendency to become diseased.

pathopsychology (păth″ō-sī-kŏl′ō-jē) [″ + *psyche,* soul, + *logos,* study]. The branch of psychology dealing with mental processes during disease.

pathosis. A diseased state or condition.

pathotropism (pă-thŏt′rō-pĭzm) [″ + *trope,* a turn, + *-ismos,* condition]. The attraction of drugs to diseased tissues.

pathway. 1. A path or a course; more specifically a pathway formed by neurons (cell bodies and their processes) over which impulses pass from their point of origin to their destination. 2. A chemical or metabolic pathway; the various chemical reactions that occur in metabolism as specific substances are absorbed, metabolized, and altered as they are biotransformed in the body.

p., afferent. Pathway leading from a receptor to the spinal cord and/or brain.

p., biosynthetic. The chemical and metabolic events that lead to the formation of substances in the body.

p., central. Pathway within the brain or spinal cord.

p., conduction. A group of fibers in a nerve, spinal cord, or brain over which impulses are conducted.

p., efferent. Pathway from the central nervous system to an effector.

p., Embden-Myerhof. The anaerobic series of enzymatic reactions involved in the metabolism of glucose to form lactic acid, and to produce adenosine triphosphate, which releases energy for muscular and other cellular activity.

p., metabolic. The sequence of chemical reactions that occur as a substance is metabolized.

p., motor. Pathway over which motor impulses are conveyed from a motor center to muscles.

p., pentose phosphate. A pathway of glucose metabolism in tissues during which five-carbon sugars are formed. SYN: *hexose monophosphate shunt.*

p., sensory. Pathway over which sensory impulses are conveyed from sense organs or receptors to sensory or reflex centers of the spinal cord or brain.

patient (pā′shĕnt) [L. *patiens*]. 1. One who is sick with, or being treated for, an illness or injury. 2. An individual receiving medical care. This includes persons with no demonstrable illness who are being investigated for signs of insidious pathology such as altered blood chemical values or physical changes such as asymptomatic cardiovascular abnormalities.

patient day. The basic unit for calculating the cost of keeping a patient in a hospital for one day.

patient mix. The numbers and types of patients served by a hospital or other health program.

patricide (păt′rĭ-sīd) [L. *patricida*]. Parricide.

Patrick's test (păt′rĭks). [Hugh T. Patrick, U.S. neurologist, 1860–1938] A test for arthritis of the hip. The thigh and knee of the supine patient are flexed and the external malleolus of the ankle is placed over the patella of the opposite leg. The test is positive if depression of the knee produces pain.

patrilineal (păt-rĭ-lĭn′ē-ăl) [L. *pater,* father, + *linea,* line]. Tracing descent through the father.

patten (păt′ĕn) [Fr. *patin,* wooden shoe]. Support applied under one shoe as part of the treatment for hip disease or unequal length of the legs.

pattern. 1. A design, figure, model, or example. 2. In psychology, a set or arrangement of ideas or behavior reactions.

patterning. Physical therapy method used in treating children and adults with brain damage. The patient is guided through movements such as creeping or crawling, based on the theory that undamaged sections of the brain will develop the ability to perform these functions.

patulous (păt'ū-lŭs) [L. *patulus*]. Open, distended, spread apart. SYN: *patent.*

paucisynaptic (paw"sĭ-sĭn-ăp'tĭk) [L. *paucus,* few, + Gr. *synapsis,* point of contact]. A neural pathway made up of relatively few synapses.

Paul-Bunnell test. [John R. Paul, U.S. physician, b. 1893; Walls W. Bunnell, U.S. physician, b. 1902] Test for heterophil antibodies in the serum of patients thought to have infectious mononucleosis.

pause [ME.]. An interruption; a temporary cessation of activity.

p., compensatory. The long interval following an extrasystole, so-called because its duration is such that the next beat occurs at the exact time of the succeeding normal beat.

Pavabid. Trade name for papaverine hydrochloride.

pavementing. Condition occurring during inflammation in which leukocytes adhere to the lining of capillaries.

Paveril Phosphate. Trade name for dioxyline phosphate.

Pavlik harness. A device used to stabilize the hip in neonates with congenital hip dislocation.

Pavlov, Ivan Patrovich (păv'lŏv). Russian physiologist, 1849–1936; winner of Nobel prize in medicine in 1904. He is remembered particularly for his work on conditioned response. SEE: *reflex, conditioned.*

pavor (pā'vor) [L.]. Anxiety, dread.

p. diurnus. Attacks of terror or fright during the day, esp. in children.

p. nocturnus. Night terror during sleep in children and the aged.

Pavulon. Trade name for pancuronium bromide.

P.B. *Pharmacopoeia Britannica,* British pharmacopeia.

Pb. Chem. symb. for plumbum, lead.

PBI. *protein-bound iodine.*

P.B.W. *posterior bite wing* in dentistry.

PBZ. *pyribenzamine.*

p.c. L. *post cibum,* after meals.

PCG. *phonocardiogram.*

pCO_2. Symb. for *carbon dioxide pressure* or *tension.*

PCV. *packed cell volume.*

P.D. *Doctor of Pharmacy.*

Pd. Chem. symb. for palladium.

p.d. *prism diopter; pupilla diameter; pupillary distance.*

PDR. *Physician's Desk Reference.*

peanut oil. A refined oil obtained from the seed kernels of one or more of the cultivated varieties of Arachis hypogaea. Used as a solvent for medicines that are injected intramuscularly.

pearl [ME. *perle*]. 1. Small, tough mass in sputum in asthma. 2. Small capsule containing a medicinal fluid for inhalation. Capsule is crushed in handkerchief and inhaled. 3. Small mass of cells.

p.'s, enamel. Small rounded globules of highly mineralized material seen near or attached to the enamel margin or furcation of the tooth roots.

p., epithelial. Concentric squamous epithelial cells in carcinoma.

p., gouty. Sodium urate concretion on cartilage of the ear seen in people with gout.

p., Laënnec's. A mucous cast of the bronchus or bronchiole sometimes present in the sputum of asthmatic patients.

peau d'orange (pō"dō-rănj') [Fr., orange skin]. Dimpled skin condition that resembles an orange. Seen in lymphatic edema, and may be present over the area of carcinoma of the breast.

peccant (pĕk'ănt) [L. *peccans* sinning]. Corrupt; producing disease. SYN: *morbid; pathogenic; unhealthy.*

peccatiphobia (pĕk"ăt-ĭ-fō'bē-ă) [L. *peccata,* sins, + Gr. *phobos,* fear]. Abnormal dread of sinning.

pecilo-. SEE: words beginning with *poikilo-.*

pectase (pĕk'tās) [Gr. *pektos* congealed, + *-ase,* enzyme]. Enzyme facilitating the conversion of pectin to pectic acid and methanol.

pecten (pĕk'tĕn) [L., comb] (pl. *pectines*) 1. A comblike organ. 2. The pubic bone. 3. Middle portion of the anal canal.

p. ossis pubis. [NA] A sharp ridge on the superior ramus of the pubis that forms the pubic portion of the terminal (iliopectineal) line.

pectenosis (pĕk"tē-nō'sĭs) [" + Gr. *osis,* condition]. Narrowing of the anal canal.

pectic acid (pĕk'tĭk) [Gr. *pektos,* congealed]. An acid, derived from pectin by hydrolyzing the methyl ester group, which is found in many fruits.

pectin (pĕk'tĭn) [Gr. *pektos,* congealed]. USP. Purified carbohydrate obtained from peel of citrus fruits, or from apple pulp. When pectin is cooked with sugar at the proper pH a gel forms. SEE: *pectose.*

pectinase (pĕk'tĭ-nās). An enzyme that catalyzes the formation of sugars and galacturonic acid from pectin.

pectinate (pĕk'tĭ-nāt) [L. *pecten,* comb]. Having teeth like a comb. SYN: *pectiniform.*

pectineal (pĕk-tĭn'ē-ăl). Rel. to the os pubis or the pectineus muscle.

pectineal line. The line or ridge on the os pubis separating the true from the false pelvis.

pectineus (pĕk-tĭn-ē'ŭs) [L. *pecten,* comb]. A flat quadrangular muscle at the upper and inner part of the thigh, arising from the superior ramus of pubis and inserted between the lesser trochanter and linea aspera of the femur, which flexes and adducts the thigh. SEE: *Muscles* in *Appendix*.

pectiniform (pěk-tĭn′ĭ-form) [″ + *forma,* shape]. Toothed like a comb. SYN: *pectinate*.

pectization (pěk-tĭ-zā′shŭn) [Gr. *pektos,* congealed]. In colloidal chemistry, the conversion of a substance from sol to gel state.

pectora (pěk′tor-ă) [L.]. Pl. of pectus.

pectoral (pěk′tō-răl) [L. *pectoralis*]. 1. Concerning the chest. 2. Efficacious in relieving chest conditions, as a cough.

pectoralgia (pěk″tō-răl′jē-ă) [″ + Gr. *algos,* pain]. Neuralgic pain in the chest.

pectoralis (pěk″tō-rā′lĭs) [L.] 1. Pert. to the breast or chest. 2. One of four muscles of the anterior upper portion of the chest.

p. major. A large triangular muscle that extends to the humerus, drawing the arm forward and downward and aiding in chest expansion.

p. minor. A muscle beneath the pectoralis major, extending to the scapula, that lowers the scapula and depresses the shoulder point.

pectoriloquy (pěk″tō-rĭl′ō-kwē) [L. *pectoralis,* chest, + *loqui,* to speak]. The distinct transmission of vocal sounds to the ear through the chest wall in auscultation, q.v. The words seem to emanate from the spot that is ausculted. Heard over cavities that communicate with a bronchus and areas of consolidation near a large bronchus, over pneumothorax when the opening in the lung is patulous, and over some pleural effusions. SYN: *pectorophony*. SEE: *chest*.

p., aphonic. In auscultation, whispered sound heard over a lung with a cavity or pleural effusion.

p., whispering. Sound over a lung with a cavity of limited extent when patient whispers, in auscultation of the chest.

pectorophony (pěk″tō-rŏf′ō-nē) [″ + Gr. *phone,* voice]. Exaggeration of vocal sounds heard on auscultation of the chest. SYN: *pectoriloquy*.

pectose (pěk′tōs) [Gr. *pektos,* congealed]. A substance found in some fruits and vegetables. It yields pectin when boiled.

pectunculus (pěk-tŭn′kū-lŭs) [L., little comb]. One of the tiny longitudinal ridges on the sylvian aqueduct of the brain.

pectus (pěk′tŭs) [L.]. (pl. *pectora*) [NA] The chest, breast, or thorax.

p. carinatum. Abnormal prominence of the sternum. SYN: *chicken breast; pigeon breast*.

p. excavatum. Congenital condition in which sternum is abnormally depressed. SYN: *funnel breast*.

p. recurvatum. P. excavatum, q.v.

ped- [L.]. Combining form denoting foot.

pedal (pěd′l) [L. *pedalis*]. Concerning the foot.

pedarthrocace (pē″dăr-thrŏk′ă-sē) [Gr. *paidos,* child, + *arthron,* joint, + *kakos,* bad]. Carious condition of joints of children.

pedatrophia. Pedatrophy.

pedatrophy (pē-dăt′rō-fē) [Gr. *paidos,* child, + *atrophia,* want of nourishment]. 1. Marasmus. 2. Any wasting disease in children. 3. Tabes mesenterica.

pederast (pĕd′ĕr-ăst) [Gr. *paiderastes,* a lover of boys]. A male who indulges in anal intercourse with young boys.

pederasty (pĕd′ĕr-ăs″tē). Anal intercourse between a man and a young boy.

pedes (pē′dēz). Pl. of pes.

pedesis (pē-dē′sĭs) [Gr., leaping]. The incessant dancing or to-and-fro movements of particles in a colloidal system or minute particles of any substance in a liquid or gaseous medium. SYN: *brownian movement*. SEE: *diapedesis*.

pedi- (pĕd′ĭ) [L. *pedalis*]. Combing form denoting foot.

pedia- [Gr. *paidos,* child]. Combining form denoting relationship to a child.

Pediaflor. Trade name for sodium fluoride, USP.

pedialgia (pĕd-ē-ăl′jē-ă, pē-dē-) [Gr. *pedion,* foot, + *algos,* pain]. Pain of the foot.

Pediamycin. Trade name for erythromycin ethylsuccinate, USP.

pediatric (pē-dē-ăt′rĭk) [Gr. *paidos,* child, + *iatreia,* treatment]. Concerning the treatment of children.

Pediatric Nurse Practitioner. A registered nurse who provides primary health care to children. Special preparation is required. Abbreviation is P.N.P. and is used after one's name, e.g.: Jane Grey, R.N., P.N.P.

pediatrician (pē-dē-ă-trĭsh′ăn) [″ + *iatrikos,* healing]. A specialist in treatment of children's diseases. SYN: *pediatrist*.

pediatrics (pē-dē-ăt′rĭks) [″ + *iatreia,* treatment]. Medical science relating to care of children and treatment of their diseases. SYN: *pediatry*.

pediatrist (pē″dē-ăt′rĭst) [″ + *iatrikos,* healing]. Physician who specializes in treatment of children's diseases. SYN: *pediatrician*.

pediatry (pĕd″ē-ăt′rē, pē′dē-ăt″rē). The treatment of children's diseases. SYN: *pediatrics*.

pedicel (pĕd′ĭ-sĕl). 1. Foot process or footplate. 2. A secondary process of a pedocyte that in conjunction with other pedocytes helps form the visceral capsule of a renal corpuscle.

pedicellation (pĕd″ĭ-sĕl-ā′shŭn) [L. *pediculus,* a little foot; stalk]. Formation and development of a pedicle.

pedicle (pĕd′ĭ-kl). 1. The stem that attaches a new growth. 2. The bony process that projects backward from the body of a vertebra connecting with the lamina on each side. Forms the root of the vertebral arch. SYN: *peduncle.*

pedicle flap. In plastic surgery, a type of flap that is attached by a pedicle to its source of blood supply. The other end may be attached to a site from which a new blood supply will develop. This permits the eventual severance of the original pedicle, so the flap may be moved step-by-step to where it is needed in the plastic surgical procedure.

pedicterus (pē-dĭk'tĕr-ŭs) [Gr. *paidos,* child, + *ikteros,* jaundice]. Jaundice of the newborn. SYN: *icterus neonatorum.*

pedicular (pē-dĭk'ū-lar). 1. [L. *pediculus,* a louse] Infested with or concerning lice. 2. [L. *pediculus,* a little foot] Concerning a stalk or stem.

pediculate (pē-dĭk'ū-lāt) [L. *pediculus,* a little foot]. Having a pedicle or stem. SYN: *pedunculate.*

pediculation (pē-dĭk"ū-lā'shŭn) [L. *pediculatio*]. 1. Infestation with lice. 2. Development of a pedicle.

pediculicide (pē-dĭk'ū-lĭ-sīd) [L. *pediculus,* a louse, + *caedere,* to kill]. Destroying or that which destroys lice.

Pediculidae. A family of lice belonging to the order Anoplura. Includes the species parasitic on primates including man. SEE: *Pediculus.*

pediculophobia (pē-dĭk"ū-lō-fō'bē-ă) [" + Gr. *phobein,* to fear]. Abnormal dread of lice. SYN: *phthiriophobia.*

pediculosis (pē-dĭk"ū-lō'sĭs) [" + Gr. *osis,* condition]. Lousiness; infestation with lice. SEE: *Pediculus.*

p. capitis. Pediculosis due to infestation with the head louse, Pediculus humanus capitis. Transmission is by personal contact or common use of brushes, combs, or headgear.

SYM: Itching and eczematous dermatitis. In long-standing, neglected cases, scratching may result in marked inflammation and secondary infection by bacteria may occur with formation of pustules, crusts, and suppuration. Hair may become matted and give rise to an unpleasant odor.

TREATMENT: Apply 1% gamma benzene hexachloride to the scalp or affected areas once each day for two days. Repeat this in 10 days to destroy nits that may have survived. All possible sources of infection should be examined and treated if necessary. Headgear, combs, and brushes should be disinfected by heat or use of disinfection solutions. If lice have infested the eyelashes and eyelids, the lice will have to be removed with forceps.

p. corporis. Pediculosis due to infestation with body louse, Pediculus humanus corporis, q.v. Transmitted by direct contact or use of infested wearing apparel. Occurs as a result of crowding or unhygienic conditions.

SYM: Intense itching. In heavy infestations there is generalized red skin eruption, mild fever, tiredness, irritability, and in severe cases weakness and debility.

TREATMENT: As for pediculosis capitis, q.v. In addition, clothing and bedding should be sterilized by dry heat (140° F. or 60° C. for 5 min.), hot water (150° F. or 65.6° C. for 5 min.), or by dry cleaning.

p. palpebrarum. Infestation by lice of the eyebrows and eyelashes.

p. pubis. Pediculosis due to infestation with the crab louse, Phthirus pubis, q.v. Generally confined to hairs of genital region but hair of the axilla, eyebrows, eyelashes, beard, and in hairy individuals body surface may be involved. Lice may be acquired through personal contact, by wearing contaminated clothing, from toilet seats, or from bed clothes. For treatment, SEE: *pediculosis capitis.*

SYM: Itching and irritation of the external genital area (not introital), esp. the mons. The pubic louse bite produces in light-skinned individuals bluish or slate-colored macules that do not blanch when pressure is applied.

p. vestimenti. Infestation by lice of the clothing.

pediculous (pē-dĭk'ū-lŭs). Infested with lice.

Pediculus (pē-dĭk'ū-lŭs). A genus of parasitic insects commonly called lice that infests humans and other primates. Lice are sucking insects belonging to the family Pediculidae, order Anoplura. They are of medical importance in that they are the transmitters of the causative organisms of epidemic typhus, trench fever, and relapsing fever. They may serve as mechanical transmitters of bubonic plague and possibly other diseases.

P. humanus capitis. The head louse that lives in fine hair of the head, although beard and eyebrows may be infested Its eggs, commonly called nits, are glued to hairs and frequently form nests in the vicinity of the ears. Cause of pediculosis capitis, q.v.

P. humanus corporis. The body louse that inhabits the seams of clothing worn next to the body and feeds on regions of the body covered by that clothing. Eggs are attached to fibers of the clothing. The cause of pediculosis corporis, q.v.

pediculus (pē-dĭk'ū-lŭs) [L.]. (pl. *pediculi*) 1. A footlike part. SYN: *pedicle.* 2. Louse. SEE: *Pediculus.*

pedicure (pĕd'ĭ-kūr) [L. *pes,* foot, + *cura,* care]. 1. Care of the feet. 2. Cosmetic care of the feet and toenails. 3. A podiatrist.

pediform (pĕd'ĭ-form) [" + *forma,* shape]. Having the shape of a foot.

pedigree. A chart, diagram, or table of an individual's ancestors used in human genetics in the analysis of mendelian inheritance.

pediluvium (pĕd-ĭ-lū'vē-ŭm) [" + *luere,* to wash]. A foot bath.

pedionalgia (pē"dē-ō-năl'jē-ă) [Gr. *pedion,* metatarsus, + *algos,* pain]. Neuralgic pain in the sole of the foot.

pediphalanx (pĕd"ĭ-fā'lănks) [L. *pes,* foot, + Gr. *phalanx,* closely knit row]. Phalanx of the foot. SEE: *maniphalanx.*

pediophobia (pē"dē-ō-fō'bē-ă) [Gr. *paidos,* child, + *phobos,* fear]. Unnatural dread of young children or of dolls.

pedobaromacrometer (pē"dō-băr"ō-mă-krŏm'ĕt-ĕr) [" + *baros,* weight, + *makros,* long, + *metron,* measure]. Apparatus for determining measurement and weight of infants.

pedodontia, pedodontics (pē"dō-dŏn'shē-ă, -tĭks) [Gr. *paidos,* child, + *odous,* tooth]. Phase of dentistry dealing with care of children's teeth.

pedodontist (pē"dō-dŏn'tĭst). Dentist who specializes in care of children's teeth.

pedodynamometer (pĕd"ō-dī-nă-mŏm'ĕ-tĕr) [L. *pes,* foot, + Gr. *dynamis,* power, + *metron,* measure]. Device for measuring the strength of the leg muscles.

pedograph (pĕd'ō-grăf) [L. *pes,* foot, + Gr. *graphein,* to write]. Imprint of the foot on paper.

pedologist (pē-dŏl'ō-jĭst) [Gr. *paidos,* child, + *logos,* study]. One who has made a study of children and their development.

pedology (pē-dŏl'ō-jē). The study of children and their development.

pedometer. 1. (pē-dŏm'ĕt-ĕr) [Gr. *pais, paidos,* child, + *metron,* measure] Device for measurement of infants. 2. (pĕd-ŏm'ĕt-ĕr) [L. *pes,* foot, + Gr. *metron,* measurement] An instrument that indicates number of steps taken while walking.

pedomorphism (pē"dō-mor'fĭzm) [Gr. *paidos,* child, + *morphe,* form, + *-ismos,* condition]. Retention of juvenile characteristics in the adult.

pedophilia (pē"dō-fĭl'ē-ă) [" + *philein,* to love]. 1. Fondness for children. 2. In psychology, an unnatural desire for sexual relations with children.

peduncle (pē-dŭn'kl) [L. *pedunculus,* a little foot]. 1. A stem or stalk. SYN: *pedicle.* 2. A brachium of the brain; a band connecting parts of the brain. SYN: *pedunculus.* SEE: *cimbia; crus; sessile.*

p., cerebellar, inferior. A band of fibers running along the lateral border of the 4th ventricle, connecting spinal cord and medulla with the cerebellum. SYN: *restiform body.*

p., cerebellar, middle. A band of fibers connecting cerebellum with basilar portion of the pons. SYN: *brachium pontis.*

p., cerebellar, superior. A band of fibers connecting cerebellum with midbrain. SYN: *brachium conjunctivum.*

p., cerebral. A pair of white bundles from upper part of the pons to the cerebrum. It constitutes the ventral portion of the midbrain. SYN: *crus cerebri.*

p., mammillary. A band of fibers extending from tegmentum of midbrain to mammillary body.

p. of flocculus. A band of fibers connecting flocculus of cerebellum with vermis.

p. of superior olive. A slender band of fibers extending from the superior olivary nucleus in the medulla to the nucleus of the abducens nerve.

p., olfactory. The long stalk of the olfactory bulb.

p., pineal. A band from either side of the pineal gland to the anterior pillars of the fornix.

p., thalamic. One of four groups of fibers known as thalamic radiations that connect thalamus with the cerebral cortex. SEE: *radiation, thalamic.*

peduncular (pē-dŭn'kū-lăr) [L. *pedunculus,* a little foot]. Concerning a peduncle.

pedunculate, pedunculated (pē-dŭn'kū-lāt, -ĕd). Possessing a stalk or peduncle. SYN: *pediculate.*

pedunculotomy (pē-dŭng"kū-lŏt'ō-mē) [" + Gr. *tome,* incision]. Surgical section of a cerebral peduncle. This is done in treating involuntary movement disorders.

pedunculus (pē-dŭng'kū-lŭs) [L.]. Peduncle.

peeling [ME. *pelen,* to peel]. Shedding of surface layer of skin. SYN: *desquamation.*

peenash (pē'năsh) [Indian]. Rhinitis due to insect larvae in the nose.

PEEP. *positive end-expiratory pressure.*

peer (pēr). 1. [ME.] One who has an equal standing with another in age, class, or rank. 2. To observe closely.

peer review. The evaluation by practicing physicians or other health professionals of the effectiveness and efficiency of the services ordered or performed by physicians or other health professionals.

peg, rete. The downward extension of thickened epidermis between the dermal papillae.

Peganone. Trade name for ethotoin.

pejorative (pĭ-jor'ă-tĭv, pē"jă-rā'tĭv) [L. *pejor,* worse]. Tending to become or make worse.

PEL. *permissible exposure limits.*

pelade (pĕl-ăd') [Fr., to remove hair]. Loss of body hair in patchy areas. SYN: *alopecia areata.*

pelage (pĕl'ĭj) [Fr.]. The collective hair of the body.

Pel-Ebstein fever. [Pieter K. Pel, Dutch physician, 1852–1919; Wilhelm Ebstein, Ger. physician, 1836–1912] Cyclic fever occurring in Hodgkin's disease in which periods of fever lasting from 3 to 10 days are separated by an afebrile period of about the same length.

Pelger-Huët anomaly (pĕl″jĕr hū′ĕt). [Karel Pelger, Dutch physician, 1885–1931; G. J. Huet, Dutch physician, b. 1879] Granulocytes of the blood with rodlike, dumb-bell, peanut-shaped, and spectacle-like nuclei. The chromatin of the nuclei is unusually coarse. The condition is inherited as a non-sex-linked dominant. The cells function in a normal manner and carriers have no demonstrably lowered resistance to infection.

pelioma (pē-lē-ō′mă) [Gr.]. A livid cutaneous patch. SYN: *ecchymosis.*

peliosis (pē-lē-ō′sĭs) [Gr.]. A disease marked by purple patches on the mucous membranes and skin. SYN: *purpura.*

SYM: Sore throat, urticaria, moderate fever, and purpuric spots over extremities or trunk. Tenderness, swelling, and pain in joints.

pellagra (pĕl-ă′gră, pĕ-lăg′ră) [L. *pellis,* skin, + Gr. *agra,* rough]. A deficiency disease or syndrome endemic in certain parts of the world, characterized by cutaneous, gastrointestinal, mucosal, neurologic, and mental symptoms.

ETIOL: Due to deficiency in diet or failure of body to absorb niacin (nicotinic acid) or its amide (niacinamide, nicotinamide). Usually associated with a deficiency of tryptophan-containing proteins, such as occurs in a high-corn diet. Pellagra may occur secondary to gastrointestinal diseases, and alcoholism.

SYM: In advanced cases, scarlet stomatitis and glossitis, diarrhea, dermatitis, and central nervous system involvement. Cutaneous lesions include erythema followed by vesiculation, crusting, and desquamation. Skin may become dry, scaly, and atrophic. The mucous membranes of mouth, esophagus, and vagina may undergo atrophy; ulcers and cysts may develop. Anemia is common. Nausea, vomiting, and diarrhea occur, the latter being characteristic. Involvement of the central nervous system is first manifested by neurasthenia, followed by organic psychosis characterized by disorientation, impairment of memory, and confusion. Later delirium and clouding of consciousness may occur.

TREATMENT: A diet adequate in all vitamins, minerals, and amino acids supplemented by 500 to 1000 mg. of niacinamide given orally three times daily. If there is any doubt about the ability of the intestinal tract to absorb vitamins, the vitamins should be given parenterally.

p. sine pellagra. Pellagra in which the characteristic erythematous rash is absent.

pellagrazein (pĕl-ă-grā′zē-ĭn). Poisonous substance in decomposed cornmeal. At one time was regarded erroneously as the cause of pellagra.

pellagrin (pĕ-lā′grĭn, -lăg′rĭn). A person afflicted with pellagra.

pellagroid (pĕ-lăg′royd, -lăg′royd) [L. *pellis,* skin, + Gr. *agra,* rough, + *eidos,* form]. Resembling pellagra.

pellagrous (pĕ-lā′grŭs, -lăg′rŭs). Concerning or affected with pellagra.

pellant (pĕl′ănt) [L. *pellere,* to drive]. Cleansing and tending to purify.

Pellegrini's disease, Pellegrini-Stieda disease (pĕl″ā-grē′nē-stē′dă). [Augusto Pellegrini, It. surgeon; Alfred Stieda, Ger. surgeon, 1869–1945] Following trauma, ossification of the superior portion of the medial collateral ligament of the knee.

pellet (pĕl′ĕt) [Fr. *pelote,* a ball]. A tiny pill or small ball of medicine or food.

pellicle (pĕl′ĭ-kl) [L. *pellicula,* a little skin]. 1. A thin piece of cuticle or skin. 2. Film or surface on a liquid. 3. A thin nonliving sheath forming the surface layer of certain one-celled animals. SYN: *scum.*

p., salivary. The thin layer of salivary proteins and glycoproteins that quickly adhere to the tooth surface after the tooth has been cleaned; this amorphous, bacteria-free layer may serve as an attachment medium for bacteria, which in turn form plaque. SYN: *acquired pedicle.*

pellotine (pĕl′ō-tēn). A white, crystalline alkaloid used as a hypnotic.

pellucid (pĕl-lū′sĭd) [L. *pellucidus*]. Translucent; transparent.

pellucid zone. Clear layer covering the oocyte. SYN *zona pellucida.*

pelotherapy (pĕ″lō-thĕr′ă-pē) [Gr. *pelos,* mud, + *therapeia,* treatment]. Therapeutic use of mud, peat, moss, or clay applied to all or part of the body.

pelvic (pĕl′vĭk) [L. *pelvis,* basin]. Pert. to a pelvis, usually the bony pelvis.

pelvic bone. Os coxae, which is the hip bone. This includes the ilium, ischium, and pubis.

pelvic diameter. Any one of several diameters of the pelvis. SEE: *diameter of the pelvis.*

pelvicephalography (pĕl″vē-sĕf″ă-lŏg′ră-fē) [″ + Gr. *kephale,* head, + *graphein,* to write]. X-ray and measurement of the fetal head and the pelvic outlet.

pelvicephalometry (pĕl″vē-sĕf″ă-lŏm′ĕ-trē) [″ + ″ + *metron,* measure]. Measurement of the diameters of the fetal head and comparing these with the diameters of the maternal pelvis.

pelvic girdle. Arch made by the innominate bones.

pelvic inflammatory disease. ABBR: PID. Ascending infection from the vagina or cervix to the uterus, fallopian tubes, and broad ligaments.

SYM: A mucopurulent vaginal discharge caused by cervicitis; there may be associated dysuria, due to urethritis; anorectal pain and bleeding due to proctitis are sometimes present; the abdominal pain may be in the midline or bilateral in the lower abdominal area; when salpingitis is present, the pain and tenderness are severe and usually accompanied by nausea and vomiting.

ETIOL: Almost any bacterium may cause PID, but the most frequent agents are Neisseria gonorrhoeae and Chlamydia trachomatis.

DIAG: History of previous PID or of sexual intercourse with a man with urethritis; insertion of an IUD, abortion, or childbirth; fever and increased white blood count; severe pain during pelvic examination when the cervix is moved or the adnexa are moved; and lower genital tract infection as evidenced by the preponderance of white blood cells in the vaginal fluid. Laparoscopy and ultrasonography may also be useful in making the diagnosis. PID must be distinguished from ectopic pregnancy and other pelvic disease, esp. surgical emergencies such as acute appendicitis.

TREATMENT: Early therapy with appropriate antibiotics is important if subsequent infertility due to occlusion of the fallopian tubes by adhesions is to be prevented. Pelvic and tubal abscesses may need to be drained but may subside with conservative therapy. All sexual partners should be examined for evidence of sexually transmitted diseases and, if positive, treated with the appropriate antibiotic. PID patients should be followed for several days after discontinuation of therapy to be certain they are cured as judged by culture of the cervix and vagina.

pelvic inlet. Upper pelvic entrance, the brim of the pelvis forming its boundary.

pelvic outlet. Lower pelvic opening.

pelvifixation (pěl″vē-fĭk-sā′shŭn) [″ + *fixatio*, fixation]. Surgical stabilization of loose pelvic organs.

pelvilithotomy (pěl″vĭ-lĭ-thŏt′ō-mē) [″ + Gr. *lithos*, stone, + *tome*, incision]. Surgical removal of a stone from the renal pelvis. SYN: *nephrolithotomy; pelviolithotomy; pyelolithotomy.*

pelvimeter (pěl-vĭm′ĕ-tĕr) [″ + Gr. *metron*, measure]. Device for measuring the pelvis.

pelvimetry (pěl-vĭm′ĕt-rē). Measurement of the pelvic dimensions or proportions. Helps determine whether or not it will be possible to deliver a fetus through the normal route. Done by manual or x-ray methods or both. SEE: *pelvis*.

pelviolithotomy (pěl″vē-ō-lĭ-thŏt′ō-mē) [L. *pelvis*, basin, + Gr. *lithos*, stone, + *tome*, incision]. Incision of the renal pelvis to remove a calculus.

pelvioplasty (pěl′vē-ō-plăs″tē) [″ + Gr. *plassein*, to form]. 1. Enlargement of the pelvic outlet to facilitate childbirth. SYN: *pelviotomy* (def. 1); *pubiotomy; symphysiotomy.* 2. Plastic surgical procedure on the pelvis of the kidney.

pelvioscopy (pěl″vē-ŏs′kō-pē) [L. *pelvis*, basin, + Gr. *skopein*, to examine]. Inspection of the pelvis.

pelviotomy (pěl-vē-ŏt′ō-mē) [″ + Gr. *tome*, incision]. 1. Enlargement of the pelvic outlet to facilitate childbirth. 2. Incision of the renal pelvis. Usually done in order to remove a calculus.

pelviperitonitis (pěl″vĭ-pěr-ĭ-tō-nī′tĭs) [″ + Gr. *peritonaion*, peritoneum, + *itis*, inflammation]. Inflammation of the peritoneum lining the pelvic cavity.

pelvirectal (pěl″vē-rěk′tăl) [″ + *rectum*, straight]. Concerning the pelvis and the rectum.

pelvis (pěl′vĭs) [L., basin]. (pl. *pelves*). 1. [NA] Any basin-shaped structure or cavity. 2. The bony structure formed by the innominate bones, the sacrum, the coccyx, and the ligaments uniting them. The structure serves as a support for the vertebral column and for articulation with the lower limbs. SEE: illus. 3. The cavity included within these bones.

ANAT: The pelvis is separated into a false or superior pelvis and a true or inferior pelvis by the iliopectineal line and the upper margin of the symphysis pubis. The circumference of this area constitutes the inlet of the true pelvis. The lower border of the true pelvis, termed the outlet, is formed by the coccyx, the protuberances of the ischia, the ascending rami of the ischia, and the descending rami of the ossa pubis and the sacrosciatic ligaments. The floor of the pelvis is formed by the perineal fascia, levator ani, and the coccygeus muscles. All diameters normally are larger in the female than in the male.

EXTERNAL DIAMETERS: *Interspinous:* Distance between outer edges of the anterosuperior iliac spines, diameter normally measuring 26 cm. (10¼ in.). *Intercristal:* Distance between outer edges of the most prominent portion of the iliac crests, diameter normally being 28 cm. (11 in.). *Intertrochanteric:* Distance between most prominent points of the femoral trochanters 32 cm. (12½ in.). *Oblique* (right and left): Distance from one posterosuperior iliac spine to the opposite anterosuperior iliac spine, 22 cm. (8½ in.), right being slightly greater than the left. *External conjugate:* Distance from the undersurface of the spinous process of last lumbar vertebra to the upper margin of anterior surface of the symphysis pubis, 20 cm.

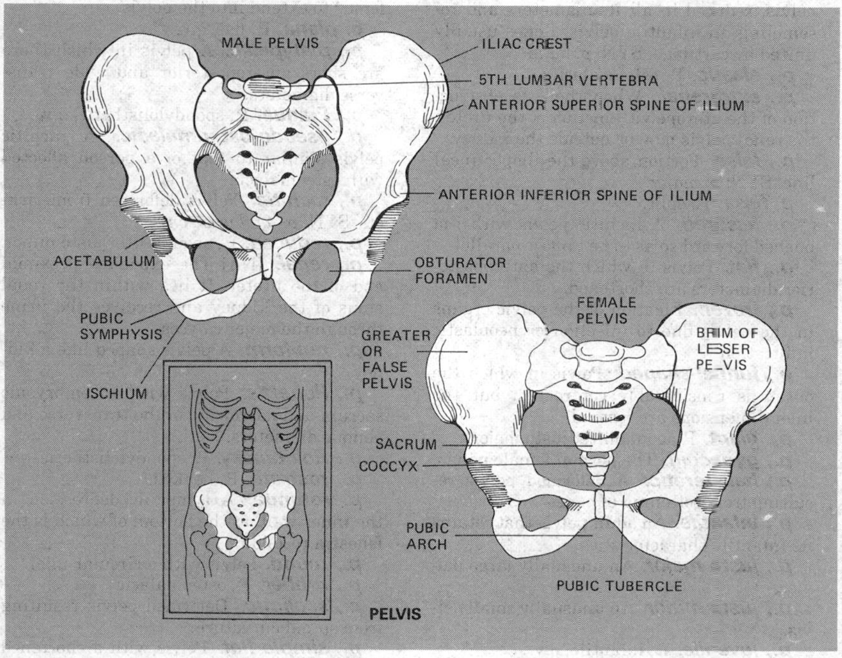

PELVIS

(7⅞ in.). SYN: *Baudelocque's diameter.*

INTERNAL DIAMETERS: *True conjugate:* Anteroposterior diameter of the pelvic inlet, 11 cm. (4¼ in.), the most important single diameter of the pelvis. *Diagonal conjugate:* Distance between the promontory of the sacrum to undersurface of symphysis pubis, 13 cm. (5⅛ in.). Two cm. (¾ in.) is deducted for the height and inclination of symphysis pubis to obtain diameter of conjugate. *Transverse:* Distance between ischial tuberosities, 11 cm. (4¼ in.). *Anteroposterior* (of outlet): Distance between the lower border of symphysis pubis and tip of sacrum, 11 cm. (4¼ in.). *Anterior sagittal:* Distance from undersurface of symphysis pubis to center of line between the ischial tuberosities, 7 cm. (2¾ in.). *Posterior sagittal:* Distance from the center of line between ischial tuberosities to the tip of the sacrum, 10 cm. (4 in.).

RS: acanthopelvis; brim; cavity, pelvic; Claudius' fossa; conjugate diameter of pelvis; endopelvic fasciae; pelvic; "pelvi-" words; sacrum; symphysis pubis.

p. aequabiliter justo major. A pelvis that is symmetrically larger than the standard in all its dimensions. SYN: *pelvis, giant.*

p. aequabiliter justo minor. A pelvis with all its dimensions uniformly smaller than the standard. SYN: *p., reduced.*

p., android. A female pelvis that resembles that of a male. SYN: *p., masculine.*

p., anthropoid. A female pelvis that is long and narrow.

p., assimilation. Abnormal pelvis in which the transverse processes of the last lumbar vertebra are fused with the sacrum; or the last sacral vertebra is fused with the coccyx.

p., beaked. Pelvis with the pelvic bones laterally compressed and pushed forward so that the outlet is narrow and long. SYN: *p., rostrate; p., triradiate.*

p., brachypellic. An oval pelvis in which the transverse diameter is at least one cm. but no more than three cm. longer than the anterior-posterior diameter of the pelvis.

p., brim of. Inlet of pelvis. SEE: *brim* (def. 2).

p., contracted. Pelvis in which one or more of the principal diameters is reduced to a degree that parturition is impeded.

p., cordate. A pelvis possessing a heart-shaped inlet.

p., coxalgic. A pelvis deformed subsequent to hip joint disease.

p., dolichopellic. An abnormal pelvis in which the anterior-posterior diameter is greater than the transverse diameter.

p., dwarf. An aequabiliter justo minor

pelvis, reduced in all its diameters and resembling an infantile pelvis. Bones usually united by cartilage. SYN: *p. nana.*

p., elastic. P., osteomalacic.

p., extrarenal. When there is obstruction of the uteropelvic junction of the ureter, the renal pelvis may be outside the kidney.

p., false. Portion above the iliopectineal line. SYN: *p. major.*

p. fissa. P., split.

p., fissured. A rachitic pelvis with ilia pushed forward so as to be almost parallel.

p., flat. Pelvis in which the anteroposterior diameters are shortened.

p., frozen. Fixation of the pelvic organs in the pelvis due to infection or neoplastic infiltration.

p., funnel-shaped. Pelvis in which the outlet is considerably contracted, but the inlet dimensions are normal.

p., giant. P. aequabiliter justo major.

p., gynecoid. The normal female pelvis.

p., halisteretic. A deformed pelvis resulting from softening of bones.

p., infantile. An adult pelvis that retains its infantile characteristics.

p., justo major. An unusually large pelvis.

p., justo minor. An unusually small pelvis.

p., juvenile. P., infantile, q.v.

p., Kilian's. P., osteomalacic.

p., kyphoscoliotic. A deformed pelvis due to rickets.

p., kyphotic. Deformed pelvis characterized by increase of the conjugate diameter at the brim with reduction of the transverse diameter at the outlet.

p., large. P., justo major, q.v.

p., lordotic. Deformed pelvis in which the spinal column has an anterior curvature in the lumbar region.

p. major. [NA] P., false.

p., malacosteon. P., rachitic.

p., masculine. A female pelvis that resembles a male pelvis, esp. in that it is narrower, more conical, heavier boned, and with heart-shaped inlet. SYN: *p., android.*

p., mesatipellic. P., round, q.v.

p., minor. P., justo minor, q.v.

p., Naegele. An obliquely contracted pelvis in which the conjugate diameter assumes an oblique direction.

p. nana. P., dwarf.

p. obtecta. A deformed pelvis in which the vertebral column extends across the pelvic inlet.

p., osteomalacic. A pelvis distorted as a consequence of osteomalacia. SYN: *p., elastic; p., rubber.*

p., Otto. A pelvis in which the acetabulum is depressed. This allows the head of the femur to extend into the pelvis.

p. plana. P., flat, q.v.

p., platypellic. A pelvis in which there are short anteroposterior and wide transverse diameters.

p., Prague. P., spondylolisthetic, q.v.

p., pseudo-osteomalacic. A rachitic pelvis similar to that of a person affected with osteomalacia.

p., rachitic. Pelvis deformed from rickets. SYN: *p., malacosteon.*

p., reduced. P., aequabiliter justo minor.

p., renal. [NA] The expanded proximal end of the ureter. It lies within the renal sinus of the kidney and receives the urine through the major calyces.

p., reniform. A pelvis shaped like a kidney.

p., Robert's. Pelvis with an embryonic sacrum and narrowing of the transverse and oblique diameters.

p., Rokitansky. P., spondylolisthetic, q.v.

p., rostrate. P., beaked.

p. rotunda. A tympanic depression in the inner wall, at the bottom of which is the fenestra rotunda.

p., round. Pelvis with a circular inlet.

p., rubber. P., osteomalacic.

p., scoliotic. Deformed pelvis resulting from spinal curvature.

p., simple flat. Pelvis with a shortened anteroposterior diameter.

p., small. P., justo minor, q.v.

p. spinosa. A rachitic pelvis with a pointed pubic crest.

p., split. Pelvis with a congenital division at the symphysis pubis.

p., spondylolisthetic. A pelvis in which the last lumbar vertebra is dislocated in front of the sacrum causing occlusion of the brim.

p. spuria. P., justo major, q.v.

p., triangular. Pelvis whose inlet is triangular.

p., triradiate. P., beaked.

p., true. The part of the pelvis below the iliopectineal line.

pelvitherm (pĕl′vĭ-thĕrm) [L. *pelvis,* basin + Gr. *therme,* heat]. Device for applying heat to the pelvis through the vagina.

pelvoscopy (pĕl-vŏs′kō-pē) [″ + Gr. *skopein,* to examine]. Inspection of pelvis.

pelvospondylitis (pĕl″ vō-spŏn″dĭ-lī′tĭs) [′ + Gr. *spondylos,* vertebra, + *itis,* inflammation]. Inflammation of the pelvic portion of the spine.

p. ossificans. Rheumatoid spondylitis.

pemoline (pĕm′ō-lēn). A central nervous system stimulating drug that is used in treating children with hyperkinesis and minimal brain damage. Trade name is Cylert.

pemphigoid (pĕm′fĭ-goyd) [Gr. *pemphigodes,*

breaking out in blisters]. A skin condition similar to pemphigus.

p., benign mucosal. A chronic bullous skin disease that produces scarring of the conjunctiva and oral mucosa.

p., bullous. A chronic bullous eruption over many sites. It is rarely fatal.

p., cicatricial. P., benign mucosal, q. v.

pemphigus (pĕm'fĭ-gŭs) [Gr. *pemphix,* a blister]. An acute or chronic disease of adults characterized by occurrence of successive crops of bullae that appear suddenly on apparently normal skin and disappear, leaving pigmented spots. It may be attended by itching and burning and constitutional disturbance. The disease if untreated is usually fatal. A characteristic finding is a positive Nikolsky sign: when pressure is applied tangential to the surface of affected skin, the outer layer of epidermis will detach from the lower layers.

ETIOL: Unknown but is probably due to an autoimmune phenomenon.

TREATMENT: Care of general health. In severe and extensive cases, the patient should be kept on air or water mattress and given meticulous care of the skin. Large doses of corticosteroids, and certain cytotoxic agents will control the disease. But the latter have serious undesired side effects.

p. acutus. A form of pemphigus in which constitutional symptoms are severe and the outcome is often fatal. Bullae, 1 to 10 cm. in diameter, often contain blood and serum. If coalescing, denuded areas are formed.

p., benign familial. A hereditary bullous and vesicular skin disease that recurs persistently. It affects the axillae, groin, and neck principally.

p. circinatus. Pemphigus with circular eruptions.

p., erythematous. Scaling, erythematous macules and blebs of the scalp, face, and trunk. The disease resembles both lupus erythematosus and pemphigus vulgaris.

p. foliaceus. Rare type of pemphigus with a chronic course. Large flaccid bullae that develop rapidly, rupture soon, and leave a moist, raw surface covered with seropurulent fluid. Bullous contents are purulent from beginning with sickening odor.

p. neonatorum. Impetigo bullosa.

p., ocular. Benign pemphigoid lesions affecting the conjunctivae.

p. vegetans, Hallopeau type. A form of pemphigus vulgaris characterized by pustules instead of bullae. Pustules are followed by warty vegetations. Prognosis, even prior to corticosteroids, was good.

p. vegetans, Neumann type. Variant of pemphigus vulgaris. Initial stage similar, but the lesions persist instead of drying up, resulting in papillary excrescences with no tendency to heal, secreting foul-smelling seropurulent fluid and sodden decomposing masses of epidermis. Prior to the use of corticosteroids most patients with this form of pemphigus died.

p. vulgaris. Uncomplicated form of pemphigus in which replacement of epidermis follows. Lesions develop suddenly and are round or oval, thin walled, tense and translucent with contents bilateral in distribution. The lesions have little tendency to heal and bleed easily when they burst. Prior to the use of corticosteroids, the outcome was fatal. With the use of corticosteroids, the mortality is 40%.

Pen A/N. Trade name for ampicillin sodium, USP.

Penapar VK. Trade name for penicillin V potassium, USP.

Penbritin. Trade name for ampicillin, USP.

Penbritin-S. Trade name for ampicillin sodium, USP.

pendular (pĕn'dū-lĕr) [L. *pendulus*]. Hanging so as to swing by an attached part; oscillating like a pendulum.

pendulous (pĕn'dū-lŭs). Swinging freely like a pendulum; hanging.

penetrance. 1. The frequency of manifestation of the hereditary condition in individuals who have the dominant or double recessive gene. Failure of manifestation of the condition in those individuals is due to interaction with other genes and nongenetic factors. 2. The extent to which something enters an object.

penetrate (pĕn'ĕ-trāt) [L. *penetrare*]. To enter or force into the interior; pierce.

penetrating (pĕn'ĕ-trāt-ĭng). Entering beyond the exterior.

penetrating power. Penetrating capacity of a lens.

penetrating wound. Wound entering the interior of an organ or cavity.

penetration (pĕn"ĕ-trā'shŭn) [L. *penetrare,* to go within]. 1. Process of entering within a part. 2. Capacity to enter within a part. 3. Power of a lens to give a clear focus at varying depths. 4. Ability of radiation to pass through a substance.

penetrometer (pĕn"ĕ-trŏm'ĕ-tĕr) [" + Gr. *metron,* measure]. An instrument that compares roughly the comparative absorption of roentgen rays in various metals, esp. silver, lead, and aluminum; hence, it gives a rough estimation of the ability of x-rays to penetrate tissues. SYN: *qualimeter.*

penicillamine (pĕn"ĭ-sĭl'ă-mēn). USP. A hydrolytic degradation product of penicillin. It is used to treat copper, mercury, zinc, or lead poisoning. It promotes the urinary excretion of those metals.

penicillic acid. An antibiotic, $C_8H_{10}O_4$, produced by some species of penicillium.

penicillin (pĕn-ĭ-sĭl′ĭn). One of a group of antibiotics biosynthesized by several species of molds, esp. Penicillium notatum and P. chrysogenum. Penicillin is bacteriostatic, inhibiting the growth of most gram-positive bacteria and certain gram-negative forms. It is effective also against certain molds, spirochetes, and rickettsias. There are many different penicillins, including synthetic ones, and their effectiveness varies for different organisms.

p., beta-lactamase resistant. Synthetic penicillins that resist the action of the enzyme beta-lactamase, produced by some organisms. Bacteria that produce the enzyme are not susceptible to the action of non-beta-lactamase resistant penicillins.

p. G benzathine. USP. An antibiotic of the penicillin class. It is available in a variety of dosage forms. It is used orally and parenterally. Trade names are Bicillin L-A and Permapen.

p. V. USP. An antibiotic of the penicillin class. It is relatively stable in an acid medium and is therefore not inactivated by gastric acid when taken orally. Trade names are Compocillin-V, Ledercillin VK, Pfizerpen VK, Robincillin-VK, SK-Penicillin VK, Uticillin VK, V-Cillin Drops, and V-Pen.

penicillinase (pĕn-ĭ-sĭl′ĭ-nās). A bacterial enzyme that inactivates most but not all penicillins.

penicillinase-producing Neisseria gonococcus. ABBR: PPNG. Penicillin-resistant strains of Neisseria gonococcus.

penicilliosis (pĕn″ĭ-sĭl″ē-ō′sĭs) [L. *penicillum,* brush, + *osis,* condition]. Infection with the fungi of the genus Penicillium.

Penicillium (pĕn″ĭ-sĭl′ē-ŭm) [L. *penicillum,* brush]. A genus of molds belonging to the Ascomycetes (sac fungi). They form the blue molds that grow on fruits, bread, and cheese. A number of species (P. chrysogenum, P. notatum) are the source of penicillin. Occasionally in man they produce infections of the external ear, skin, or respiratory passageways. They are common allergens.

penicilloyl-polylysine (pĕn″ĭ-sĭl′oyl-pŏl″ē-lī′sēn). A substance used to determine sensitivity to some forms of penicillin. When it is injected intradermally into a sensitive individual, a wheal appears within 20 minutes.

penicillus (pĕn″ĭ-sĭl′ŭs) [L., paint brush]. (pl. *penicilli*) [NA] A group of the branches of arteries in the spleen that are arranged like the bristles of a brush. Each consists of successive portions: the pulp arteries, sheathed arteries, and terminal arteries.

penile (pē′nĭl, -nīl) [L. *penis,* penis]. Pert. to the penis.

penile reflex. 1. Sudden downward movement of penis when the prepuce or gland of a completely relaxed penis is pulled upward 2. Contraction of bulbocavernous muscle on percussing dorsum of penis. 3. Contraction of bulbocavernous muscle resulting from compression of glans penis.

penis (pē′nĭs) [L.]. (pl. *penises* or *penes*) [NA] The male organ of copulation and, in mammals, urination. It is a cylindrical pendulous organ suspended from the front and sides of the pubic arch. Contrary to popular myths, the size of the penis has no physical bearing on the male's or female's enjoyment of sexual intercourse.

ANAT: The penis is composed mainly of erectile tissue arranged in three columns, the whole being covered with skin. The two lateral columns are the corpora cavernosa penis. The third or median column, known as the corpus spongiosum, contains the urethra. The body is attached to the descending portion of the pubic bone by the crura of the penis. The cone-shaped head of the penis, the glans penis, contains the urethral orifice. It is covered with a movable hood known as the foreskin or prepuce, under which is secreted the substance called smegma. SEE: illus.

Hyperemia of the genitals fills the corpora cavernosa with blood as the result of sexual excitement or stimulation, thus causing an erection. The hyperemia subsides following orgasm and ejaculation of the seminal fluid. The organ then returns to its flaccid condition. The size of the flaccid penis does not necessarily correlate with that of the erect penis.

p. captivus. Condition in which the penis is erroneously thought to be held within the vagina and unable to be withdrawn during copulation as a result of vaginismus and contraction of the perineal muscles. There is no evidence that this can happen in the human.

p., clubbed. A condition in which the penis is curved during erection.

p., double. A congenital deformity in which the penis in the embryo is completely divided by the urethral groove.

p. lunatus. Painful curved erection in gonorrhea. SYN: *chordee.*

p. palmatus. Penis enclosed by the scrotum.

p., webbed. P. palmatus.

penis, words pert. to: balanitis; cavernitis; cavernosum; chordee, circumcision; condyloma; cord, spermatic; corpus cavernosum; Cowper's glands; ductus deferens; epispadias; erection; foreskin; frenulum preputii; genitalia, male; gonorrhea; hypospadia; nervus erigens; penis captivus; Peyronie's disease; prepuce; priapism; prostate; scrotum;

PENIS, INCLUDING TESTICLES AND SCROTUM

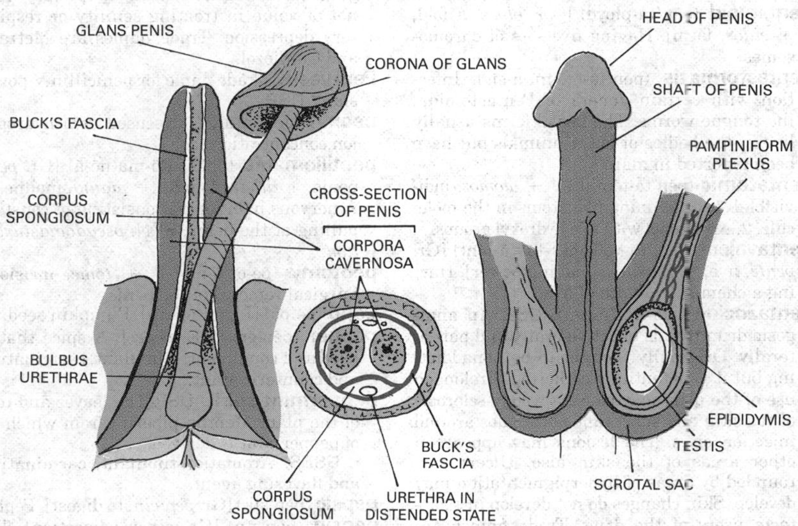

seminal vesicle; smegma; testes; Tyson's glands; urethra; vas deferens; "balano-" and "phall-" words.

penischisis (pĕ-nĭs′kĭ-sĭs) [L. *penis*, penis, + Gr. *schisis*, splitting]. Epispadias, hypospadias, paraspadias, or any fissured condition of the penis.

penitis (pĕ-nī′tĭs) [″ + Gr. *itis*, inflammation]. Inflammation of the penis.

pennate (pĕn′āt) [L. *penna*, feather]. An object in which parts extend at an angle from a central portion, as the barbs do from a feather.

penniform (pĕn′ĭ-form) [″ + *forma*, shape]. Feather-shaped.

pennyroyal (pĕn″ĭ-roy′ăl). Name for various plants, esp. Hedeoma and Mentha, that yield commercial oil used as a carminative and stimulant.

pennyweight. Troy weight containing 24 grains or 1/20 of a troy ounce. Equal to 1.555 grams.

penoscrotal (pē″nō-skrō′tăl). Concerning the penis and the scrotum.

pension neurosis. A form of malingering that develops subsequent to an injury in the belief that financial or other forms of compensation can be obtained or will be continued by being ill. SEE: *neurosis, compensation.*

pent-, penta- [Gr. *pente*, five]. Combining form meaning five.

pentabasic (pĕn″tă-bā′sĭk). 1. A compound that contains five replaceable hydrogen atoms. 2. An alcohol that contains five hydroxyl groups.

pentad (pĕn′tăd) [Gr. *pente*, five]. 1. A radical or element with a valence of five. 2. Group of five.

pentadactyl (pĕn″tă-dăk′tĭl) [″ + *dakytlos*, finger]. Having five digits on each hand and foot.

pentaerythritol tetranitrate (pĕn″tă-ē-rĭth′rĭ-tōl). USP. An organic nitrate drug used in treating angina pectoris. Trade names are Pentritol, Pentryate 80, Peritrate, and SDM N.35.

pentagastrin (pĕn″tă-găs′trĭn). A synthetic gastrin that is used to determine the capacity of the stomach to secrete hydrochloric acid.

pentalogy (pĕn-tăl′ō-je). The occurrence of five factors in combination, e.g., symptoms or signs of a disease.

pentamethylenediamine (pĕn″tă-mĕth″ĭl-ĕn-dī′ă-mĕn). A ptomaine occurring in tissue decomposed by certain bacteria.

pentamidine (pĕn-tăm′ĭ-dĕn). A drug used in treating leishmaniasis, early cases of Gambian and Rhodesian trypanosomiasis, and pneumonia due to Pneumocystis carinii. This drug is available in the U.S.A. only from the Parasitic Drug Service of the Centers for Disease Control, Atlanta, Georgia, phone: (404) 452-4174.

pentane (pĕn′tān). C_5H_{12}. One of the hydrocarbons of the methane series. A product of petroleum distillation.

pentapeptide (pĕn″tă-pĕp′tīd). A polypeptide with five amino acid groups.

pentaploid (pĕn′tă-ployd) [″ + *ploos,* a fold, + *eidos,* form]. Having five sets of chromosomes.

pentastomiasis (pĕn″tă-stō-mī′ă-sĭs). Infection with certain genera of Pentastomida, the tongue worms. The larval forms usually live in the bodies of lower animals but have been reported in man.

pentatomic (pĕn″tă-tŏm′ĭk) [″ + *atomos,* indivisible]. 1. Containing five atoms in the molecule. 2. An alcohol with five hydroxyl groups.

pentavalent (pĕn″tă-vā′lĕnt, -tăv′ă-lĕnt) [Gr. *pente,* five, + L. *valens,* having power]. Having a chemical valence of five.

pentazocine (pĕn-tăz′ō-sēn). USP. An analgesic drug that is effective orally and parenterally. Originally thought to be nonaddicting but it is potentially addicting. Prolonged use of the drug may cause a woody sclerosis of the skin and subcutaneous tissues around injection sites. The lesions may appear on other areas of the skin also. Ulcers surrounded by areas of hyperpigmentation may develop. Skin changes do not develop in short-term users of the drug. Trade names are Talwin and Fortral.

Pentids. Trade name for penicillin G potassium, USP.

pentobarbital (pĕn″tō-băr′bĭ-tăl). USP. A hypnotic sedative drug of the barbiturate class.

p. sodium. A barbituric acid derivative used as an oral or intravenous hypnotic agent in preanesthetic medication. Used in labor with or without scopolamine. Trade name is Nembutal Sodium.

pentosazon (pĕn″tō-sā′zŏn). Crystalline compound formed when a pentose is treated with phenylhydrazine. It is not normally present in urine.

pentose (pĕn′tōs) [Gr. *pente,* five].$C_5H_{10}O_5$. A simple sugar with five atoms of carbon in the molecule.

pentosemia (pĕn″tō-sē′mē-ă). Pentose in the blood.

pentoside (pĕn′tō-sīd). Pentose combined with some other substance. Pentoses combined with purine or pyrimidine bases are present in nucleic acid.

pentostam. A drug used in leishmaniasis available in U.S.A. only from the Parasitic Disease Drug Service of the Centers for Disease Control, Atlanta, Georgia 30333, (404) 452-4154.

pentosuria (pĕn″tō-sū′rē-ă). A condition in which pentose is found in the urine.

Pentothal Sodium. Trade name for thiopental sodium, USP.

pentoxide (pĕn-tŏk′sīd). A chemical molecule containing five atoms of oxygen.

pentylenetetrazol (pĕn″tĭ-lēn-tĕt′ră-zōl). A drug used to activate the electroencephalogram as a diagnostic acid in epilepsy. It is not of value in treating senility or respiratory depression. Trade names are Metrazol and Cardiozol.

Pen-Vee-K. Trade name for penicillin V potassium, USP.

peonin (pē′ō-nĭn). A dye used as a hydrogen ion concentration test.

peotillomania (pē″ō-tĭl″ō-mā′nē-ă) [Gr. *peos,* penis, + *tillein,* to pull, + *mania,* madness]. A nervous habit or tic consisting of constant pulling at the penis. SYN: *pseudomasturbation.*

peotomy (pē-ŏt′ō-mē) [″ + *tome,* incision]. Surgical removal of the penis.

pepo (pē′pō) [L., pumpkin]. Pumpkin seed.

pepper (pĕp′ĕr) [ME. *peper*]. A spice that is used as a condiment, stimulant, carminative, and counterirritant.

peppermint spirit. USP. The leaves and tops of the plant Mentha piperita from which oil of peppermint is derived.

USES: Aromatic stimulant, carminative, and flavoring agent.

pepsic (pĕp′sĭk) [Gr. *peptein,* to digest]. Peptic.

pepsin (pĕp′sĭn) [Gr. *pepsis,* digestion]. The chief enzyme of gastric juice, which converts proteins into proteoses and peptones. It is formed by the chief cells of gastric glands and produces its maximum activity at a pH of 1.5 to 2. It is obtainable in granular form. In the presence of HCl, it will digest proteins in vitro.

pepsinogen (pĕp-sĭn′ō-jĕn) [″ + *gennan,* to produce]. The antecedent of pepsin existing in the form of granules in the chief cells of gastric glands.

pepsinuria (pĕp″sĭ-nū′rē-ă) [″ + *ouron,* urine]. Excretion of pepsin in the urine.

peptic (pĕp′tĭk) [Gr. *peptikos*]. 1. Concerning digestion. 2. Concerning pepsin.

peptic ulcer. An ulcer occurring in the lower end of the esophagus; in the stomach usually along the lesser curvature; in the duodenum; or on the jejunal side of a gastrojejunostomy.

SYM: Pain is the most characteristic symptom, tending to be of uniform quality and usually described as "gnawing." It is localized in the epigastrium and exhibits a rhythmicity and periodicity usually appearing one to three hours after a meal. It is absent before breakfast but may occur during the night. It is relieved by foods and alkalies; it is aggravated by alcohol and condiments. Often periods of remission occur in which pain is absent.

Other symptoms include dyspepsia, heartburn, acid eructations, nausea, vomiting, and anorexia. Diarrhea with loss of weight may occur. In some cases, physical signs may be absent, the first indication of the condition being hemorrhage or perforation.

PROG: Guardedly favorable. Hemorrhage or perforation may occur without warning.

NURSING IMPLICATIONS: Reduce emotional stress during hospitalization, and at home and work. Provide physical rest. Control gastric acidity with prescribed medication and diet.

In the acute state, test vomitus and stools for blood. Observe for complications such as perforation or hemorrhage. Prevent injuries that may occur due to drowsiness associated with use of sedatives and tranquilizers.

Develop coping mechanism to relieve anxiety. Advise that all activities should be done in moderation. Establish teaching plan including prescribed medications; drugs to avoid because of gastric irritation; diet; discontinuation of or decreased smoking; and significance of follow-up care.

TREATMENT: Symptoms may disappear and the ulcers heal without benefit of any medical therapy, and symptoms may subside without evidence of healing by x-ray evaluation. Therapy includes combinations of the following.

General: Bedrest is indicated if pain is severe, or if patient has lost considerable blood or is heavily sedated. Otherwise it is optional according to the physician's instructions. Sedatives probably will be helpful if the patient is under severe and chronic emotional stress.

Diet: The Sippy diet, q.v., is used in the acute phase of the disease. In general, however, diet has probably been overemphasized as a means of treating peptic ulcer. Frequent small feedings are usually more effective in relieving pain than three widely spaced meals. Alcoholic beverages usually are not allowed, but some patients will be greatly relaxed by their use. If alcohol is allowed, be certain it is consumed well diluted and not taken on an empty stomach. This will help to counteract its ability to stimulate gastric acid secretion. Patients may be aware of specific foods that aggravate their symptoms. These should, of course, be avoided. Spices except for black pepper are not harmful. Smoking, being generally detrimental to health, should be discontinued.

Antacids: Excess gastric acid secretion is an important factor in the cause of peptic ulcer; therefore, antacids usually provide prompt relief of pain. Antacids leave the stomach quite rapidly if taken on an empty stomach. They should therefore be taken hourly while awake. Alternatively the antacids can be taken 1 hour and 3 hours after each meal and at bedtime. Antacids commonly used include calcium carbonate, aluminum hydroxide, aluminum carbonate, magnesium carbonate, magnesium trisilicate, and sodium bicarbonate. The latter should not be used because of its several disadvantages, including gastric distention and the potential for causing edema in those who retain sodium.

Histamine H_2 receptor antagonists: The use of histamine H_2 receptor blocking agents has added a new approach to the control of gastric secretions. An example of this type of drug is cimetidine.

Anticholinergics: Used to reduce secretion of acid following food intake. These act synergistically with antacids by causing gastric retention and thus allowing greater time for the antacids to be effective. They are also useful when given at night to help prevent excess acid secretion during sleep. Anticholinergics are increased in dose until blurring of vision and dryness of mouth occur.

CAUTION: Anticholinergics should not be used in patients who have glaucoma, gastric retention, pyloric obstruction, prostatic hypertrophy, or other conditions that cause retention of urine. Also the use of adrenal corticosteroids, phenylbutazone, aspirin, and other drugs that have the ability to irritate the gastric mucosa should be discontinued in patients with peptic ulcer.

Psychotherapy: Some patients will need extensive psychotherapy in order to change lifestyles or situations from those that are stressful to those more compatible with this condition.

peptidase. An enzyme that converts peptides to amino acids.

peptide (pĕp'tīd) [Gr. *peptein,* to digest]. Compound formed by hydrolytic cleavage of peptones and containing two or more amino acids. A class of substances prepared by synthesis from amino acids and intermediate in molecular weight and chemical properties between the amino acids, which may be made artificially, and the proteins, which may not.

RS: dipeptide; polypeptide; tripeptide.

peptidolytic (pĕp"tĭ-dō-lĭt'ĭk) [" + *lytikos,* dissolving]. Causing the splitting up or digestion of peptides.

peptinotoxin (pĕp"tĭn-ō-tŏk'sĭn) [" + *toxikon,* poison]. Poisonous ptomaine found in the body as a result of disordered or defective digestion.

peptization (pĕp'tĭ-zā'shŭn) [Gr. *peptein,* to digest]. In the chemistry of colloids, the process of making a colloidal solution more stable; conversion of a gel to a sol.

Pepto-Bismol. Trade name for bismuth subsalicylate

Peptococcus (pĕp"tō-kŏk'ŭs). Strictly anaerobic gram-positive cocci that are normally present in the oral cavity, on the skin, and in the intestinal and urinary tracts. They are usually associated with infections, when they act synergistically with other organisms.

peptogenic, peptogenous (pĕp-tō-jĕn′ĭk, -tŏj′ĕn-ŭs) [″ + *gennan,* to produce]. 1. Producing peptones and pepsin. 2. Promoting digestion.

peptoid (pĕp′toyd) [″ + *eidos,* resemblance]. A product of protein digestion that does not give the biuret reaction.

peptolysis (pĕp-tŏl′ĭ-sĭs) [Gr. *peptein,* to digest, + *lysis,* dissolution]. The splitting up or hydrolysis of peptones. SYN: *peptonolysis.*

peptolytic (pĕp-tō-lĭt′ĭk). Pert. to the splitting up of peptone.

peptone (pĕp′tōn) [Gr. *pepton,* digesting]. A secondary protein formed by the action of proteolytic enzymes, acids, or alkalies on certain proteins. Peptones are nitrogenous compounds soluble in water; they are not coagulated by boiling.

peptonemia (pĕp″tō-nē′mē-ă) [″ + *haima,* blood]. Peptones in the blood.

peptonization (pĕp″tō-nĭ-zā′shŭn) [Gr. *pepton,* digesting]. Process of changing protein substance into peptones by action of proteolytic enzymes.

peptonize. To convert into peptones; to predigest with pepsin.

peptonolysis (pĕp″tō-nŏl′ĭ-sĭs) [Gr. *pepton,* digesting, + *lysis,* dissolution]. The breakdown of peptones into simpler products (peptides or amino acids). SYN: *peptolysis.*

peptonuria (pĕp″tō-nū′rē-ă) [″ + *ouron,* urine]. Excretion of peptones in the urine.

Peptostreptococcus (pĕp″tō-strĕp″tō-kŏk′ŭs). Strictly anaerobic gram-positive cocci that are normally present in the oral cavity, on the skin, and in the intestinal and urinary tracts. They are usually associated with infections, when they act synergistically with other organisms.

peptotoxin (pĕp″tō-tŏk′sĭn) [″ + *toxikon,* poison]. Any toxin produced from a peptone.

per, per- [L. *per,* through]. 1. A word used as a prefix or by itself meaning through, by, or by means of. 2. In chemistry, the highest valence of an element.

peracephalus (pĕr″ă-sĕf′ă-lŭs) [″ + Gr. *a-,* not, + *kephale,* head]. A parasitic twin of the placenta. It does not contain a head or arms, and the thorax is malformed.

peracid (pĕr-ăs′ĭd). 1. An acid that contains the highest valence possible. 2. An acid containing the peroxide group, O — OH.

peracidity (pĕr″ă-sĭd′ĭt-ē) [L. *per,* through, + *acidus,* sour]. Abnormal acidity.

peracute (pĕr″ă-kūt′) [″ + *acutus,* keen]. Very acute or violent.

per anum (pĕr ā′nŭm) [L.]. Through or by way of the anus.

perarticulation (pĕr″ăr-tĭk″ū-lā′shŭn) [L. *per,* through, + *articulatio,* joint]. Diarthrosis, q.v.

peratodynia (pĕr″ăt-ō-dĭn′ē-ă) [Gr. *peran,* to pierce, + *odyne,* pain]. Heartburn; pain in region of cardia of stomach.

percent. Per hundred. For or out of each hundred. Its symbol, %, is used to indicate that the preceding number is a percentage.

percentile (pĕr-sĕn′tīl). One of 100 equal divisions of a series of items or data. Thus if a value, such as a test score, is higher than 92% of all the other test scores, that result is above the 92nd percentile of the range of scores.

percept (pĕr′sĕpt). The mental image of an object seen.

perception (pĕr-sĕp′shŭn) [L. *percepitio,* perceive]. 1. Process of being aware of objects; consciousness. 2. The process of receiving sensory impressions. 3. The elaboration of a sensory impression; the ideational association modifying, defining, and usually completing the primary impression or stimulus. Vague or inadequate association occurs in confused and depressed states.

p., depth. Term used in evaluating visual function. The ability to recognize that an object has depth as well as height and width. It is generally believed that it is essential that both eyes be functioning normally for a person to have normal ability to perceive depth. Sometimes this is true, but most persons with the use of only one eye learn to judge depth quite accurately.

p., extrasensory. ABBR: ESP. Perception not through the recognized senses.

p., stereognostic. Recognition of objects by touch.

perceptivity (pĕr-sĕp-tĭv′ĭ-tē). Power to receive sense impressions.

percolate (pĕr′kō-lāt) [L. *percolare,* to strain through]. 1. To allow a liquid to seep through a powdered substance. 2. Any fluid that has been filtered or percolated. 3. To strain a fluid through powdered substances in order to impregnate it with soluble principles of such substances.

percolation (pĕr″kō-lā′shŭn) [L. *percolatio*]. 1. Filtration. 2. Process of extracting soluble portions of a drug of powdered composition by filtering a liquid solvent through it.

percolator (pĕr′kō-lā″tor). Apparatus used for extraction of a drug with a liquid solvent.

per contiguum (pĕr kŏn-tĭg′ū-ŭm) [L.]. Touching, as in the spread of an inflammation from one part to an adjacent structure.

per continuum (pĕr kŏn-tĭn′ū-ŭm) [L.]. Continuous, as the spread of an inflammation from part to part.

Percorten Acetate. Trade name for desoxycorticosterone aceate, USP.

Percorten Pivalate. Trade name for desoxycorticosterone pivalate.

perculsion. Inability to perform movement.

percuss (pĕr-kŭs′) [L. *percutere*]. To tap parts of the body to aid diagnosis by sound emitted.

percussible (pĕr-kŭs′ĭ-b′l). Able to be detected by percussion.

percussion (pĕr-kŭsh′ŭn) [L. *percussio,* a striking]. Use of the fingertips to tap the body lightly but sharply to determine position, size, and consistency of an underlying structure and the presence of fluid or pus in a cavity. These conditions are established by alterations felt and heard in resonance and pitch of the sound emitted, vibration elicited, or resistance encountered.

RS: abdomen; bladder; box-note; chest; heart; intestines; kidney; liver; ovary; palpation; spleen; uterus.

p., auscultatory. Percussion combined with auscultation.

p., bimanual. P., mediate, q.v.

p., deep. Forceful percussion used to elicit a note from a deeply seated tissue or organ.

p., direct. P., immediate.

p., finger. Striking of the finger resting upon the body with a finger of the other hand.

p., immediate. Percussion performed by striking the surface directly with the fingers. SYN: *p., direct.*

p., indirect. P., mediate.

p., mediate. Percussion performed by using fingers of one hand as a plexor and those of the opposite hand as a pleximeter. SYN: *p., indirect.*

p., palpation. Percussion in which the fingers perceive the tactile impression rather than the examiner relying on the sounds produced.

p., threshold. Percussing lightly with the fingers on a glass-rod pleximeter, the far end of which is covered with a rubber cap. The cap is usually placed on an intercostal space. This technique is used to confine the percussion to a very small area. SYN: *Goldscheider's percussion.*

percussor (pĕr-kŭs′or) [L., striker]. Device used for diagnosis by percussion, consisting of a hammer with a rubber or metal head.

percutaneous (pĕr″kū-tā′nē-ŭs) [L. *per,* through, + *cutis,* skin]. Effected through the skin. Applying a medicated ointment by friction, or removal or injection by needle.

percutaneous ultrasonic lithotripter. A device that employs ultrasound to break up kidney stones. The sound waves are applied to the outside of the body.

percutaneous transluminal angioplasty. A method of treating localized arterial narrowing due to atherosclerosis. A special double-lumen catheter is designed so that a cylindrical balloon surrounds a portion of it. Inflation of the balloon with pressure of up to 90 p.s.i. dilates the narrowed vessel. This technique may be used on various arteries including those of the coronary circulation of the heart.

per diem cost. Hospital or other inpatient institutional cost per day.

perencephaly (pĕr″ĕn-sĕf′ă-lē) [Gr. *pera,* pouch, + *enkephalos,* brain]. Porencephaly, q.v.

perfectionism (pĕr-fĕk′shŭn-ĭzm). A type of neurosis in which the individual attempts to achieve goals of behavior or performance that are unrealistic or unnecessary.

perflation (pĕr-flā′shŭn) [L. *perflatio*]. The process of blowing air into a cavity to expand its walls or to force out secretions or other matter.

perforans (pĕr′fō-răns) [L.]. Perforating or penetrating, as a nerve or muscle.

perforate (pĕr′fō-rāt) [L. *perforatus,* pierced with holes]. 1. To puncture or to make holes. 2. Pierced with holes.

perforation (pĕr″fō-rā′shŭn). 1. The act or process of making a hole, such as that caused by ulceration. 2. The hole made through a substance or part.

p., Bezold's. Perforation on the inner surface of the mastoid bone.

perforation of stomach or intestine. Abdominal crisis due to escape of contents of the perforated viscus into the peritoneal cavity. Peritonitis is certain to develop unless there is immediate surgical intervention. SEE: *intestinal perforation; peritonitis.*

SYM: Onset is accompanied by acute pain, which begins over perforated area and spreads all over the abdomen, which has become rigid. Face is anxious with beads of perspiration on it. Nausea and vomiting will occur. Pulse rapid and feeble and respiration rapid and shallow. Temperature drops, but rises as peritonitis sets in, and pulse becomes stronger.

TREATMENT: Surgical. Pending operation give no fluids. Complete rest.

perforator (pĕr′fō-rā-tor) [L., a piercing device]. Instrument for piercing the skull and other bones.

p., tympanum. Instrument for perforating the tympanum.

perforatorium (pĕr″fō-ră-tō′rē-ŭm). The pointed tip of the acrosome of the spermatozoa.

perfrication (pĕr-frĭ-kā′shŭn) [L. *perfricare,* to rub]. Thorough rubbing with an ointment. SYN: *inunction.*

perfrigeration (pĕr-frĭj″ĕr-ā′shŭn) [L. *per,* through, + *frigere,* to be cold]. Frostbite.

perfusate (pĕr-fū′zāt). The fluid used to perfuse a tissue or organ.

perfusion (pĕr-fū′zhŭn) [L. *perfundere,* to pour through]. 1. Passing of a fluid through spaces. 2. The pouring of a fluid. 3. Supplying an organ or tissue with nutrients and oxygen by injecting blood or a suitable fluid into an artery.

Pergonal. Trade name for menotropins.

perhydrocyclopentanophenanthrene (pĕr-hī″drō-sī″klō-pĕn-tăn″ō-phĕn-ăn′thrēn). Name of the ring structure of the chemical nucleus of the steroids. SEE: *steroid hormone* for illus.

peri- [Gr.]. Prefix meaning around or about.

periacinal, periacinous (pĕr″ē-ăs′ĭ-năl, -nŭs) [Gr. *peri,* around + L. *acinus,* grape]. Placed around a saclike dilation.

Periactin. Trade name for cyproheptadine hydrochloride.

periadenitis (pĕr″ē-ă″dē-nī′tĭs) [″ + *aden,* gland, + *itis,* inflammation]. Inflamed condition of tissues surrounding a gland.

p. mucosae necrotica recurrens. Recurring necrotic or ulcerative lesions on the buccal and pharyngeal mucosa. These start as small hard nodules that ulcerate and leave a deep crater. These may be associated with Behçet's syndrome.

perialienitis (pĕr″ē-ā″lē-ĕn-ī′tĭs) [″ + L. *alienus,* foreign, + Gr. *itis,* inflammation]. Noninfectious inflammation around a foreign body. SYN: *perixenitis.*

periamygdalitis (pĕr″ē-ăm-ĭg″dăl-ī′tĭs) [″ + *amygdale,* tonsil, + *itis,* inflammation]. Inflammation of connective tissue around the tonsil. SYN: *peritonsillitis.*

perianal (pĕr″ē-ā′năl) [″ + L. *anus,* anus]. Around or close to the anus.

periangiitis (pĕr″ē-ăn″jē-ī′tĭs) [″ + *angeion,* vessel, + *itis,* inflammation]. Inflamed condition of tissue around a blood or lymphatic vessel.

periangiocholitis (pĕr″ē-ăn″jē-ō-kō-lī′tĭs) [″ + ″ + *chole,* bile, + *itis,* inflammtion]. Inflamed condition of tissues around the bile ducts. SYN: *pericholangitis.*

periaortic (pĕr″ē-ā-or′tĭk) [″ + *aorte,* aorta]. Around the aorta.

periaortitis (pĕr″ē-ā-or-tī′tĭs) [″ + *aorte,* aorta, + *itis,* inflammation]. Inflamed condition of adventitia and tissues around the aorta.

periapex (pĕr″ē-ā′pĕks) [″ + L. *apex,* tip]. Area around the apex of a tooth.

periapical (pĕr″ē-ăp′ĭ-kăl) [″ + L. *apex,* tip]. Around the apex of the root of a tooth.

periappendicitis (pĕr″ē-ă-pĕn″dĭ-sī′tĭs) [″ + L. *appendix,* appendage, + Gr. *itis,* inflammation]. Inflamed condition of the appendix and its surrounding tissues.

p. decidualis. Condition in which there are decidual cells in the peritoneum of the appendix vermiformis in cases of tubal pregnancy due to adhesions between fallopian tubes and the appendix.

periappendicular (pĕr″ē-ăp″ĕn-dĭk′ū-lăr) [″ + L. *appendix,* appendage]. Surrounding an appendix.

periarterial (pĕr″ē-ăr-tē′rē-ăl) [″ + *arteria,* artery]. Placed around an artery.

periarteritis (pĕr″ē-ăr-tĕr-ī′tĭs) [″ + ″ + *itis,* inflammation]. Inflammation of the external coat of an artery.

p. gummosa. Gummas in the blood vessels in syphilis.

p. nodosa. Polyarteritis nodosa, q.v.

periarthric (pĕr″ē-ăr′thrĭk) [″ + *arthron,* joint]. Surrounding a joint. SYN: *circumarticular; periarticular.*

periarthritis (pĕr″ē-ăr-thrī′tĭs) [″ + ″ + *itis,* inflammation]. Inflammation of area around a joint.

periarticular (pĕr″ē-ăr-tĭk′ū-lăr) [Gr. *peri,* around, + L. *articulus,* a joint]. Surrounding a joint. SYN: *circumarticular; periarthric.*

periatrial (pĕr″ē-ā′trē-ăl) [″ + L. *atrium,* corridor]. Around the atria, or auricles, of the heart.

periaxial (pĕr-ē-ăk′sē-ăl) [″ + *axon,* axis]. Located around an axis.

periaxillary (pĕr″ē-ăk′sĭl-ĕ″rē) [″ + L. *axilla,* armpit]. Occurring around the axilla.

periaxonal (pĕr″ē-ăk′sō-năl) [″ + *axon,* axis]. Around an axon.

periblast (pĕr′ĭ-blăst) [″ + *blastos,* germ]. That portion of the yolk surface adjacent to the blastoderm in telolecithal eggs.

peribronchial (pĕr″ĭ-brŏng′kē-ăl) [″ + *bronchos,* windpipe]. Surrounding a bronchus.

peribronchiolar (pĕr″ĭ-brŏng-kī′ō-lăr) [″ + L. *bronchiolus,* bronchiole]. Surrounding a bronchiole.

peribronchiolitis (pĕr″ĭ-brŏng″kē-ō-lī′tĭs) [″ + ″ + *itis,* inflammation]. Inflammation of area around the bronchioles.

peribronchitis (pĕr″ĭ-brŏng-kī′tĭs) [″ + *bronchos,* windpipe, + *itis,* inflammation]. Inflammation of all tissues surrounding the bronchi or bronchial tubes.

peribulbar (pĕr″ĭ-bŭl′băr) [″ + L. *bulbus,* bulbous root]. Surrounding a bulb, esp. the bulb of the eye.

peribursal (pĕr″ĭ-bĕr′săl) [″ + *bursa,* leather sack]. Around a bursa.

pericanalicular (pĕr″ĭ-kăn″ă-lĭk′ū-lăr) [″ + L. *canaliculus,* small canal]. Around a canaliculus.

pericardiac, pericardial (pĕr-ĭ-kăr′dē-ăk, -ăl) [″ + *kardia,* heart]. Concerning the pericardium.

pericardial rub. A friction sound heard when the inflamed or roughened pericardial surfaces rub against each other.

pericardicentesis (pĕr″ĭ-kăr″dĭ-sĕn-tē′sĭs) [″ + ″ + *kentesis,* puncture]. Surgical perforation of the pericardium. SYN: *pericardiocentesis.*

pericardiectomy (pĕr″ĭ-kăr-dē-ĕk′tō-mē) [″ + ″ + *ektome,* excision]. Excision of part or all of the pericardium.

pericardiocentesis (pĕr′ĭ-kăr″dē-ō-sĕn-tē′sĭs) [Gr. *peri,* around, + *kardia,* heart, + *ken-*

tesis, puncture]. Surgical perforation of the pericardium. SYN: *pericardicentesis.*

pericardiolysis (pĕr″ĭ-kăr″dē-ŏl′ĭ-sĭs) [″ + ″ + *lysis*, dissolution]. Separation of adhesions between the visceral and parietal pericardium.

pericardiomediastinitis (pĕr″ĭ-kăr″dē-ō-mē-dē-ăs″tĭ-nī′tĭs) [″ + ″ + L. *mediastinum*, + Gr. *itis*, inflammation]. Inflamed condition of the pericardium and mediastinum.

pericardiopexy [″ + ″ + *pexis*, fixation]. Surgical procedure designed to increase the blood supply to the heart by joining the pericardium to an adjacent tissue.

pericardiophrenic (pĕr-ĭ-kăr″dē-ō-frĕn′ĭk) [″ + *kardia*, heart, + *phren*, diaphragm]. Concerning the pericardium and diaphragm.

pericardiopleural (pĕr″ĭ-kăr″dē-ō-ploo′răl) [″ + ″ + *pleura*, rib]. Concerning the pericardium and pleura.

pericardiorrhaphy (pĕr″ĭ-kăr″dē-or′ă-fē) [″ + ″ + *rhaphe*, a sewing]. Suture of a wound in the pericardium.

pericardiostomy (pĕr″ĭ-kăr″dē-ŏs′tō-mē) [″ + *kardia*, heart, + *stoma*, opening]. Formation of an opening into the pericardium for drainage.

pericardiosymphysis (pĕr″ĭ-kăr″dē-ō-sĭm′fĭ-sĭs) [″ + ″ + *symphysis*, a joining]. Adhesion between the layers of the pericardium.

pericardiotomy (pĕr″ĭ-kăr-dē-ŏt′ō-mē) [″ + ″ + *tome*, incision]. Incision of the pericardial sac around the heart.

pericarditic (pĕr″ĭ-kăr-dĭt′ĭk). Concerning the pericardium.

pericarditis (pĕr-ĭ-kăr-dī′tĭs) [″ + *kardia*, heart, + *itis*, inflammation]. Inflammation of the pericardium.

ETIOL: Tuberculosis, mycoses, infection by pyogenic organisms, collagen disease, uremia, myocardial infarction, neoplasms, trauma.

SYM: Moderate fever, precordial pain and tenderness, dry cough, dyspnea, and palpitation. Pulse, first rapid, forcible, then weak and irregular.

First stage: Auscultation reveals to and fro friction sound heard over 4th left intercostal space near sternum. Inspection and palpation sometimes reveal a diffuse apex beat. Friction rub may sometimes be palpated.

Second stage: Serofibrinous effusion. Bulging of precordium. Increased area of dullness, triangular in shape, base down. Heart sounds muffled, distant, feeble. Purulent effusion yields similar signs, but in addition high, irregular fever; sweats; chills, and progressive pallor; sometimes edema over the precordium. In doubtful cases the aspirating needle reveals pus.

PROG: Fair in early stages but extremely grave in purulent and fibrinous stages.

TREATMENT: *General:* Absolute bedrest, light diet. For relief of pain apply ice bag over precordium or administer pain-relieving drugs, depending on its intensity. *Specific:* Appropriate antibiotic for specific organisms involved. If purulent effusion occurs, aspiration or surgical drainage. If gallop rhythm or signs of heart failure occur, restrict fluids and salt. For chronic constrictive pericarditis, resection of pericardium.

p., acute fibrinous. Pericarditis characterized by fibrinous exudation.

p., acute nonspecific. A disease of unknown etiology usually following respiratory infections. SYN: *p., idiopathic.*

p., adhesive. Form of pericarditis in which the layers of pericardium adhere.

p., constrictive. Pericarditis in which adhesions form between visceral and parietal layers of the peritoneum.

p., external. Inflammation of exterior surface of the pericardium.

p., fibrinous. Pericarditis in which the membrane is covered with butterlike exudate that organizes and unites the pericardial surfaces.

SYM: Precordial bulging, a weak apex beat with loud sounds, a systolic retraction at apex and over a large part of the precordium, peculiar diastolic collapse of jugular veins, feeble apex beat with a forcible impulse over body of the heart. Signs of heart failure, as dyspnea, generalized edema, cyanosis.

p., hemorrhagic. Pericarditis in which the exudate contains blood.

p., idiopathic. P., acute nonspecific.

p., ischemic. Pericarditis resulting from myocardial infarction.

p., neoplastic. Pericarditis due to invasion of the pericardium by malignant tumors of adjoining structures.

p. obliterans. Pericardial inflammation causing adhesions and obliteration of the pericardial cavity.

p., serofibrinous. Pericarditis in which there is a considerable quantity of serous exudate but little fibrin.

p., uremic. Pericarditis resulting from uremia.

pericardium (pĕr″ĭ-kăr′dē-ŭm) [Gr. *peri*, around, + *kardia*, heart]. [NA] The double membranous fibroserous sac enclosing the heart and the origins of the great blood vessels. It is composed of an inner serous layer (visceral pericardium or epicardium) and an outer fibrous layer (parietal pericardium). The space between the two constitutes the pericardial cavity, which is normally filled with a small amount of serous fluid. Its base is attached to the diaphragm, its apex extending upward as far as the first subdivision of the great blood vessels. It is attached in front to the sternum, laterally to the mediastinal pleura, and posteriorly to the esophagus, trachea, and principal bronchi. Normally, the pericardium contains a thin serous fluid.

p., adherent. Condition in which fibrous bands form between the two layers of the pericardium, obliterating the pericardial cavity. SEE: *pericarditis, constrictive.*

p., bread and butter. Condition seen in fibrinous pericarditis in which the pericardium has a peculiar appearance due to fibrinous deposits on the two opposing surfaces.

p. externum. The outer fibrous layer of the pericardium. SYN: *p., parietal.*

p., fibrous. The strong fibrous tissue on the outer surface of the pericardial sac.

p. internum. Serous inner layer of the pericardium.

p., parietal. The outer fibrous layer of the pericardium. SYN: *p. externum.*

p., serous. The smooth lining of the pericardial sac.

p., shaggy. Condition occurring in fibrinous pericarditis in which loose shaggy deposits of fibrin are seen on the surfaces of the pericardium.

p., visceral. Serous inner layer of the pericardium.

pericardotomy (pĕr″ĭ-kăr-dŏt′ō-mē) [Gr. *peri,* around, + *kardia,* heart, + *tome,* incision]. Incision of the pericardium.

pericecal (pĕr″ĭ-sē′kăl) [″ + L. *caecum,* blind]. Situated around the cecum.

pericecitis (pĕr″ĭ-sē-sī′tĭs) [″ + ″ + Gr. *itis,* inflammation]. Inflamed condition of area around the cecum.

pericellular (pĕr″ĭ-sĕl′ū-lăr) [″ + L. *cellula,* cell]. Around a cell.

pericemental (pĕr″ĭ-sē-mĕn′tăl) [″ + L. *caementum,* cement]. Concerning the pericementum, i.e., the periodontal ligament.

pericementitis (pĕr″ĭ-sē-mĕn-tī′tĭs) [″ + ″ + Gr. *itis,* inflammation]. Progressive necrosis of the alveoli of the teeth. SYN: *periodontitis.*

p., apical. Apical abscess of the tooth.

pericementoclasia (pĕr″ĭ-sē-mĕn″tō-klā′zē-ă) [″ + ″ + Gr. *klasis,* a breaking]. Dissolution of the pericementum with alveolar absorption. SYN: *pyorrhea alveolaris.*

pericementum (pĕr″ĭ-sē-mĕn′tŭm). Fibrous tissue covering the root of a tooth.

pericentral (pĕr″ĭ-sĕn′trăl) [″ + *kentron,* center]. Around the center.

perichareia (pĕr″ĭ-kă-rī′ă) [Gr.]. Excessive or abnormal rejoicing, seen in certain psychoses.

pericholangitis (pĕr″ĭ-kō-lăn-jī′tĭs) [Gr. *peri,* around, + *chole,* bile, + *angeion,* vessel, + *itis,* inflammation]. Inflammation of tissues surrounding a bile duct. SYN: *periangiocholitis.*

pericholecystitis (pĕr″ĭ-kō-lē-sĭs-tī′tĭs) [″ + ″ + *kystis,* a sac, + *itis,* inflammation]. Inflammation of tissues situated around the gallbladder.

perichondral, perichondrial (pĕr-ĭ-kŏn′drăl, -drē-ăl) [″ + *chondros,* cartilage]. Concerning the membrane that covers cartilage.

perichondritis (pĕr-ĭ-kŏn-drī′tĭs) [″ + ″ + *itis,* inflammation]. Inflamed condition of the perichondrium.

perichondrium (pĕr-ĭ-kŏn′drē-ŭm) [″ + *chondros,* cartilage]. [NA] Membrane of fibrous connective tissue around the surface of cartilage.

perichondroma (pĕr″ĭ-kŏn-drō′mă) [″ + ″ + *oma,* tumor]. A tumor arising from fibrous tissue that covers cartilage.

perichord (pĕr′ĭ-kord) [″ + *chorde,* cord]. The sheath of the notochord.

perichordal (pĕr-ĭ-kor′dăl) [″ + *chorde,* cord]. Placed around the notochord.

perichorioidal, perichoroidal (pĕr″ĭ-kō-rē-oy′dăl, -roy′dăl) [″ + *chorioeides,* skinlike]. Situated around the choroid coat.

perichrome (pĕr′ĭ-krōm) [″ + *chroma,* color]. A nerve cell in which the Nissl body is arranged in rows throughout the protoplasm.

pericolic (pĕr-ĭ-kō′lĭk) [″ + *kolon,* colon]. Around or encircling the colon.

pericolitis (pĕr″ĭ-kō-lī′tĭs) [″ + ″ + *itis,* inflammation]. Inflammation of area around the colon.

pericolonitis (pĕr″ĭ-kō-lŏn-ī′tĭs). Inflamed condition of region around the colon.

pericolpitis (pĕr″ĭ-kŏl-pī′tĭs) [Gr. *peri,* around, + *kolpos,* vagina, + *itis,* inflammation]. Inflammation of connective tissues surrounding the vagina.

periconchal (pĕr-ĭ-kŏng′kăl) [″ + *konche,* concha]. Around the concha of the ear.

pericorneal (pĕr″ĭ-kor′nē-ăl) [″ + L. *cornu,* horn]. Placed around the cornea.

pericoronal (pĕr″ĭ-kor′ō-năl) [″ + *korone,* crown]. Around the crown of a tooth.

pericoronitis (pĕr″ĭ-kor″ō-nī′tĭs) [″ + ″ + *itis,* inflammation]. Inflammation around the crown of a tooth.

pericranial (pĕr″ĭ-krā′nē-ăl) [″ + *kranion,* skull]. Pert. to the periosteum of the skull.

pericranitis (pĕr″ĭ-krā-nī′tĭs) [″ + ″ + *itis,* inflammation]. Inflamed condition of pericranium.

pericranium (pĕr″ĭ-krā′nē-ŭm). [NA] Fibrous membrane surrounding the cranium; periosteum of the skull.

p. internum. Lining surface of the cranium. SYN: *endocranium.*

pericystic (pĕr″ĭ-sĭs′tĭk) [″ + *kystis,* bladder]. Surrounding a cyst.

pericystitis (pĕr″ĭ-sĭs-tī′tĭs) [″ + ″ + *itis,* inflammation]. Inflamed condition of tissues about the bladder.

pericystium (pĕr″ĭ-sĭs′tē-ŭm) [″ + *kystis,* bladder]. 1. The vascular wall surrounding a cyst. 2. Tissues around the urinary bladder or the gallbladder.

pericyte (pĕr′ĭ-sīt) [″ + *kytos,* cell]. A flat, undifferentiated connective tissue cell around the capillary walls. It may become a macrophage, fibroblast, or smooth muscle cell.

pericytial (pĕr-ĭ-sĭsh′ăl) [″ + *kytos,* cell]. Placed around a cell.

peridectomy (pĕr″ĭ-dĕk′tō-mē) [″ + *ektome,* excision]. Peritectomy, q.v.

peridendritic (pĕr″ĭ-dĕn-drĭt′ĭk) [″ + *dendron,* a tree]. Surrounding a dendrite of a nerve cell.

peridens (pĕr′ĭ-dĕns) [Gr. *peri,* around, + L. *dens,* tooth]. A supernumerary tooth not situated in the dental arch.

peridental (pĕr″ĭ-dĕn′tăl) [″ + L. *dens,* tooth]. Surrounding a tooth or part of one. SYN: *periodontal.*

peridentitis [″ + ″ + *itis,* inflammation]. Inflammation of tissues surrounding a tooth. SYN: *periodontoclasia.*

peridentium (pĕr″ĭ-dĕn′shē-ŭm) [″ + L. *dens,* tooth]. Periodontium, q.v.

periderm [″ + *derma,* skin]. Thin layer of flattened cells forming a transient layer of embryonic epidermis. SYN: *epitrichial layer; epitrichium.*

peridesmitis (pĕr″ĭ-dĕz-mī′tĭs) [″ + *desmion,* band, + *itis,* inflammation]. Inflammation of the areolar tissue around a ligament.

peridesmium (pĕr″ĭ-dĕz′mē-ŭm). The connective tissue membrane sheathing a ligament.

perididymis (pĕr″ĭ-dĭd′ĭ-mĭs) [″ + *didymos,* testicle]. The tunica vaginalis of the testicle.

perididymitis (pĕr″ĭ-dĭd″ĭ-mī′tĭs) [″ + ″ + *itis,* inflammation]. Inflammation of the perididymis.

peridiverticulitis (pĕr″ĭ-dī″vĕr-tĭk″ū-lī′tĭs) [″ + L. *diverticulare,* to turn aside, + Gr. *itis,* inflammation]. Inflammation of tissues situated around an intestinal diverticulum.

periductal (pĕr-ĭ-dŭk′tăl) [″ + L. *ductus,* a passage]. Situated around a duct.

periduodenitis (pĕr″ĭ-dū″ō-dē-nī′tĭs) [″ + L. *duodeni,* twelve, + Gr. *itis,* inflammation]. Inflammation around the duodenum often causing adhesions attaching it to the peritoneum.

peridural (pĕr″ĭ-dū′răl) [″ + L. *durus,* hard]. Outside the dura mater of the spinal cord.

periencephalitis (pĕr″ē-ĕn-sĕf″ă-lī′tĭs) [″ + *enkephalos,* brain, + *itis,* inflammation]. Inflamed condition of the surface of the brain.

periencephalomeningitis (pĕr″ē-ĕn-sĕf″ă-lō-mĕn″ĭn-jī′tĭs) [″ + ″ + *meninx,* membrane, + *itis,* inflammation]. Inflamed condition of cerebral cortex and the meninges.

periendothelioma (pĕr″ē-ĕn″dō-thē″lē-ō′mă) [″ + *endon,* within, + *thele,* nipple, + *oma,* tumor]. A tumor arising from the endothelium of the lymphatics and the perithelium of blood vessels.

perienteric (pĕr″ē-ĕn-tĕr′ĭk) [Gr. *peri,* around, + *enteron,* intestine]. Around the intestines.

perienteritis (pĕr″ē-ĕn″tĕr-ī′tĭs) [″ + ″ + *itis,* inflammation]. Inflammation of the intestinal peritoneum.

perienteron (pĕr″ē-ĕn′tĕr-ŏn) [″ + *enteron,* intestine]. The peritoneal cavity of the embryo.

periependymal (pĕr″ē-ĕp-ĕn′dĭ-măl) [″ + *ependyma,* an upper garment]. Around the ependyma.

periesophagitis (pĕr″ē-ē-sŏf″ă-jī′tĭs) [″ + *oisophagos,* esophagus, + *itis,* inflammation]. Inflamed condition of tissues around the esophagus.

perifistular (pĕr-ĭ-fĭs′tū-lĕr) [″ + L. *fistula,* pipe]. Located around a fistula.

perifocal (pĕr″ĭ-fō′kăl) [″ + L. *focus,* hearth]. Around a focus, esp. around an infected focus.

perifollicular (pĕr″ĭ-fŏl-lĭk′ū-lăr) [″ + L. *folliculus,* a little sac]. Around a follicle.

perifolliculitis (pĕr″ĭ-fō-lĭk″ū-lī′tĭs) [″ + ″ + Gr. *itis,* inflammation]. Inflamed condition of area around the hair follicles.

perigangliitis (pĕr″ĭ-găng″lē-ī′tĭs) [″ + *ganglion,* knot, + *itis,* inflammation]. Inflamed condition of region around a ganglion.

periganglionic (pĕr″ĭ-găng″glē-ŏn′ĭk) [″ + *ganglion,* knot]. Around a ganglion.

perigastric (pĕr″ĭ-găs′trĭk) [″ + *gaster,* belly]. Around the stomach.

perigastritis (pĕr″ĭ-găs-trī′tĭs) [″ + ″ + *itis,* inflammation]. Inflammation of peritoneal covering of the stomach.

perigemmal (pĕr″ĭ-jĕm′ăl) [″ + L. *gemma,* bud]. Around any bud, esp. a taste bud.

periglandulitis (pĕr″ĭ-glăn″dū-lī′tĭs) [″ + L. *glandula,* small gland, + Gr. *itis,* inflammation]. Inflammation of tissues around a gland.

periglottic (pĕr″ĭ-glŏt′ĭk) [″ + *glotta,* tongue]. Around the base of the tongue and epiglottis.

perihepatic (pĕr″ĭ-hē-păt′ĭk) [Gr. *peri,* around, + *hepar,* liver]. Around the liver.

perihepatitis (pĕr″ĭ-hĕp-ă-tī′tĭs) [″ + ″ + *itis,* inflammation]. Inflammation of peritoneal covering of the liver, usually occurring in circumscribed areas.

perihernial (pĕr″ĭ-hĕr′nē-ăl) [″ + L. *hernia,* rupture]. Around a hernia.

perijejunitis (pĕr″ĭ-jē-jū-nī′tĭs) [″ + L. *jejunum,* empty, + Gr. *itis,* inflammation]. Inflamed condition of tissues around the jejunum.

perikaryon (pĕr″ĭ-kăr′ē-ŏn) [″ + *karyon,* nucleus]. The cell body of a neuron.

perikeratic (pĕr″ĭ-kĕr-ă′tĭk) [″ + *keras,* horn].

About the cornea. SYN: *pericorneal.*

perikymata (pěr″ĭ-kī′mă-tă) [″ + *kyma,* wave]. The transverse wave-like grooves most apparent in surface enamel of newly erupted anterior teeth; they are more pronounced at eruption and are reduced in depth with wear in advancing age.

perilabyrinthitis (pěr″ĭ-lăb″ĭr-ĭn-thī′tĭs) [″ + *labyrinthos,* a maze of canals, + *itis,* inflammation]. Inflammation of tissues around the labyrinth.

perilaryngeal (pěr″ĭ-lă-rĭn′jē-ăl) [″ + *larynx,* larynx]. Around the larynx.

perilaryngitis (pěr″ĭ-lăr″ĭn-jī′tĭs) [″ + ″ + *itis,* inflammation]. Inflamed condition of tissues around the larynx.

perilenticular (pěr″ĭ-lĕn-tĭk′ū-lăr) [″ + L. *lenticularis,* pert. to a lens]. Around the lens of the eye.

periligamentous (pěr″ĭ-lĭg″ă-mĕn′tŭs) [″ + L. *ligamentum,* a band]. Around a ligament.

perilymph (pěr′ĭ-lĭmf) [″ + L. *lympha,* serum]. The pale limpid fluid contained in the space between the membranous and bony labyrinth of the internal ear.

perilympha (pěr″ĭ-lĭm′fă). Perilymph, q.v.

perilymphangeal (pěr″ĭ-lĭm-făn′jē-ăl) [″ + ″ + Gr. *angeion,* vessel]. Around a lymphatic vessel.

perilymphangitis (pěr″ĭ-lĭmf-ăn-jī′tĭs) [″ + ″ + *angeion,* vessel, + *itis,* inflammation]. Inflammation of tissues around a lymphatic vessel.

perimastitis (pěr″ĭ-măs-tī′tĭs) [Gr. *peri,* around, + *mastos,* breast, + *itis,* inflammation]. Inflammation of the fibrous tissue around a breast.

perimeningitis (pěr″ĭ-mĕn″ĭn-jī′tĭs) [″ + *meninx,* membrane, + *itis,* inflammation]. Inflamed condition of the dura mater. SYN: *pachymeningitis.*

perimeter (pěr-ĭm′ĕt-ĕr) [″ + *metron,* measure]. 1. The outer edge or periphery of a body or measure of the same. 2. Device for determining the extent of the field of vision.

perimetric (pěr″ĭ-mĕt′rĭk). 1. [″ + *metron,* measure] Concerning perimetry, q.v. 2. [″ + *metra,* uterus] Around the uterus.

perimetritic (pěr″ĭ-mē-trĭt′ĭk) [″ + *metra,* uterus, + *itis,* inflammation]. Concerning perimetritis.

perimetritis (pěr″ĭ-mē-trī′tĭs) [″ + ″ + *itis,* inflammation]. Inflammation of the peritoneal covering of the uterus. May be associated with parametritis.

perimetrium (pěr-ĭ-mē′trē-ŭm). [NA] Serous coat of the uterus.

perimetry (pěr-ĭm′ĕ-trē) [″ + *metron,* measure]. 1. Circumference, edge, border of a body. 2. Measurement of the scope of the field of vision with a perimeter.

perimyelis (pěr″ĭ-mī′ĕ-lĭs) [″ + *myelos,* marrow]. Endosteum.

perimyelitis (pěr″ĭ-mī″ĕ-lī′tĭs) [″ + ″ + *itis,* inflammation]. 1. Inflammation of the pia mater and arachnoid of the brain or spinal cord. SYN: *leptomeningitis.* 2. Inflammation of the endosteum or membrane around medullary cavity of a bone.

perimyelography (pěr″ĭ-mī″ĕ-lŏg′ră-fē) [″ + ″ + *graphein,* to write]. X-ray examination of the area around the spinal cord.

perimyoendocarditis (pěr″ĭ-mī″ō-ĕn″dō-kăr-dī′tĭs) [″ + *mys,* muscle, + *endon,* within, + *kardia,* heart, + *itis,* inflammation]. Inflammation of the muscular wall of the heart, its endothelial lining, and the pericardium.

perimyositis (pěr″ĭ-mī″ō-sī′tĭs) [″ + ″ + *itis,* inflammation]. Inflammation of the connective tissue around a muscle.

perimysia (pěr″ĭ-mĭs′ē-ă). Pl. of perimysium.

perimysial (pěr-ĭ-mĭs′ē-ăl). Concerning, or of the nature of, the fibrous sheath of a muscle.

perimysiitis (pěr″ĭ-mĭs″ē-ī′tĭs) [″ + *mys,* muscle, + *itis,* inflammation]. Inflamed condition of the perimysium, the sheath surrounding a muscle.

perimysium (pěr″ĭ-mĭs′ē-ŭm). (pl. *perimysia*) [NA] Connective tissue sheath that envelops each primary bundle of muscle fibers. Sometimes called perimysium internum.

p. externum. The epimysium.

perinatal (pěr″ĭ-nā′tăl) [″ + L. *natalis,* birth]. Concerning the period beginning after the 28th week of pregnancy through 28 days following birth.

perinatology. Study of the fetus and infant during the perinatal period. SEE: *perinatal.*

perineal (pěr″ĭ-nē′ăl) [Gr. *perinaion,* perineum]. Concerning, or situated on, the perineum.

perineal body. Mass of tissue composed of skin, muscle, and fascia between the vagina and rectum in the female and the penis and rectum in the male.

perineal fascia. Three layers of tissue between the muscles of the perineum.

perineal hernia. Hernia perforating the perineum. SYN: *perineocele.*

perineal section. Surgical incision through the perineum. SYN: *perineotomy.*

perineo- [Gr. *perinaion*]. Combining form pert. to the perineum.

perineocele (pěr″ĭ-nē′ō-sēl) [Gr. *perinaion,* perineum, + *kele,* hernia]. Hernia in the region of the perineum, between the rectum and vagina or between the rectum and prostate.

perineocolporectomyomectomy (pěr″ĭ-nē-ō-kŏl″pō-rĕk″tō-mī″ō-mĕk′tō-mē) [″ + *kolpos,* vagina, + L. *rectus,* straight, + Gr. *mys,* muscle, + *oma,* tumor, + *ektome,* excision]. Excision of a myoma by incising the perineum, vagina, and rectum.

perineometer (pĕr″ĭ-nē-ŏm′ĕ-ter) [Gr. *perinaion,* perineum, + *metron,* measure]. Apparatus for measuring pressure or force that is produced in the vagina when pubococcygeus and levator ani muscles are contracted voluntarily. SEE: *Kegel exercises.*

perineoplasty (pĕr″ĭ-nē′ō-plăs″tē) [″ + *plassein,* to form]. Reparative surgery on the perineum.

perineorrhaphy (pĕr″ĭ-nē-or′ă-fē) [″ + *rhaphe,* a sewing]. Suture of the perineum to repair a laceration made during the delivery of the fetus.

NURSING IMPLICATIONS: Prevent infection by thorough washing of the perineum after each elimination. Be certain washing solutions drain down toward the anal area. Keep sutures dry and clean. Assess perineum daily for signs of infection. Utilize a heat lamp or sitz baths or both several times a day to promote pain relief and healing. Encourage ambulation. Check for daily bowel movement and adjust diet and fluid intake to prevent constipation.

p., anterior. Surgical repair of anterior perineum and vaginal wall to correct a cystocele.

p., colpo-. Removal of part of posterior vaginal wall and suturing of torn perineal body.

p., posterior. Removal and repair of rectocele.

perineoscrotal (pĕr″ĭ-nē-ō-skrō′tăl) [″ + L. *scrotum,* a bag]. Concerning the perineum and scrotum.

perineotomy (pĕr″ĭ-nē-ŏt′ō-mē) [″ + *tome,* incision]. Surgical incision into the perineum. SYN: *perineal section.*

perineovaginal (pĕr″ĭ-nē″ō-văj′ĭn-ăl) [″ + L. *vagina,* sheath]. Concerning the perineum and vagina.

perinephrial (pĕr″ĭ-nĕf′rē-ăl). Concerning the perinephrium.

perinephric (pĕr″ĭ-nĕf′rĭk) [Gr. *peri,* around, + *nephros,* kidney]. Located or occurring around the kidney.

perinephric abscess. Abscess formation in the peritoneal membrane surrounding the kidney.

perinephritis (pĕr″ĭ-nē-frī′tĭs) [″ + ″ + *itis,* inflammation]. Inflammation of peritoneal tissues around the kidney. SYN: *paranephritis.*

perinephrium (pĕr″ĭ-nĕf′rē-ŭm). The connective and fatty tissue surrounding the kidney.

perineum (pĕr″ĭ-nē′ŭm) [Gr. *perinaion*]. 1. [NA] The structures occupying the pelvic outlet and comprising the pelvic floor. 2. The external region between the vulva and anus in a female or between the scrotum and anus in a male. It is made up of skin, muscle, and fasciae. The muscles of the perineum are the anterior portion of the intact levator ani muscle, the transverse perineal muscle, and the pubococcygeus muscle. SEE: illus.; *body, perineal; "perine-" words.*

perineum, tears of the. There are four degrees of severity caused by overstretching of the vagina and perineum in delivery. Fetal malposition increases the chance of tears occurring.

A first-degree tear involves superficial tissues of the perineum and vaginal mucosa but does not injure muscular tissue. A second-degree tear involves those tissues included in a first-degree tear and the muscles of the perineum but not the muscles of the anal sphincter. A third-degree tear involves all of the tissues of the second-degree tear and the muscles of the anal sphincter. A fourth-degree tear extends completely through the perineal skin, vaginal mucosa, perineal body, anal sphincter muscles, and the rectal mucosa.

COMPLICATIONS: Hemorrhage, infection, cystocele, rectocele, descent of uterus, perhaps loss of bowel control.

TREATMENT: Surgery.

perineural (pĕr″ĭ-nū′răl) [Gr. *peri,* around, + *neuron,* nerve]. Around a nerve.

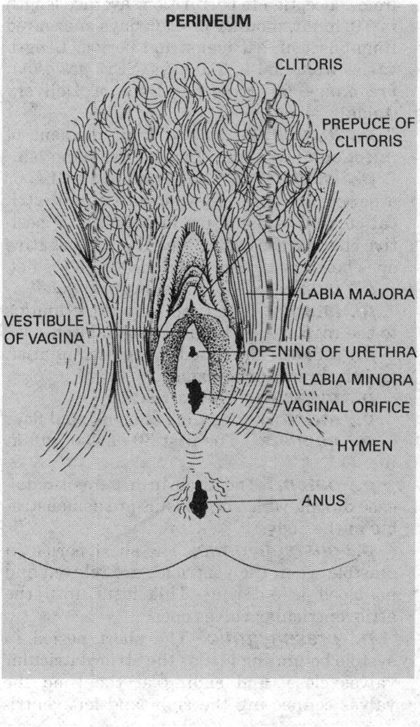

perineurial (pĕr″ĭ-nū′rē-ăl) [″ + *neuron,* sinew]. Concerning the perineurium, the sheath around a bundle of nerve fibers.

perineuritis (pĕr″ĭ-nū-rī′tĭs) [″ + ″ + *itis,* inflammation]. Inflammation of the sheath enveloping nerve fibers.

perineurium (pĕr″ĭ-nū′rē-ŭm) [″ + *neuron,* sinew]. A connective tissue sheath investing a fasciculus or bundle of nerve fibers.

perinuclear (pĕr″ĭ-nū′klē-ăr) [″ + L. *nucleus,* a kernel]. Around a nucleus.

periocular (pĕr″ē-ŏk′ū-lăr) [″ + L. *oculus,* eye]. Located around the eye. SYN: *circumocular.*

period [L. *periodus*]. 1. The interval of time between two successive occurrences of any regularly recurring phenomenon or event; a cycle. 2. The menses. 3. Time occupied by a disease in running its course, or by a stage of a disease, such as an incubation period.

p., absolute refractory. Following contraction of a muscle, the period in which a stimulus, no matter how strong, will not elicit a response.

p., childbearing. The period in the female during which she is capable of procreation; puberty to the menopause.

p., ejection. P., sphygmic, q.v.

p., gestation. Period of pregnancy; time from conception to parturition. Average length is 10 lunar months or 280 days measured from onset of last menstrual period. Length varies from 250 to 310 days. SEE: *gestation; pregnancy* for Expected Date of Delivery (table).

p., incubation. Time from moment of infection until appearance of first symptom.

p., isoelectric. The period in an EKG or other electrical record when either no electrical current is being produced or those positive charges are exactly equal to the negative ones being produced. Thus the tracing is flat.

p., isometric. P., postsphygmic, q.v.

p., latency. The time from the stimulus to the response of the tissue stimulated.

p., latent. The time between stimulation and the resulting response.

p., menstrual. Menstruation.

p., monthly. The time of menstrual flow.

p., neonatal. The first 30 days of infant life.

p., patent. The time in a parasitic disease during which organisms are demonstrable in the body.

p., postsphygmic. The short period in diastole when the ventricles are relaxed and no blood is entering. This lasts until the atrioventricular valves open.

p., presphygmic. The short period in systole beginning just as the atrioventricular valves close, and ending at the time the valves connecting the right and left ventricles to the pulmonary artery and aorta, respectively, open.

p., puerperal. Interval of time from birth of a child to approximately six weeks later, at which time complete involution of the uterus has occurred.

p., relative refractory. The period after activation of a nerve or muscle, during recovery, when it can be excited only by a stronger than normal stimulus.

p., safe. The time during the menstrual cycle when conception is allegedly not possible. Because of the great variability of the menstrual cycle, it is extremely difficult to predict the portion of the cycle in which intercourse may take place and be "safe" from conception.

p., silent. 1. The time in the course of a disease in which the signs and symptoms are so mild as to be difficult to detect. 2. A pause in normally continuous electrical events such as an EKG or EEG.

p., sphygmic. The period in the cardiac cycle when the blood is being ejected into the arterial system.

p., Wenckebach. The time when a systolic beat of the heart is skipped. This follows a series of ever-lengthening P-R intervals.

periodic (pēr-ē-ŏd′ĭk) [Gr. *periodikos*]. Recurring after definite intervals.

periodic law. Law stating that the chemical and physical properties of the chemical elements are periodic functions of their atomic numbers.

periodic table. A chart with the chemical elements arranged by their atomic numbers according to the periodic law, q.v.

periodicity (pēr″ē-ō-dĭs′ĭ-tē). 1. State of being regularly recurrent. 2. The rate of rise and fall or interruption of a unidirectional current in physical therapy.

periodontal (pĕr″ē-ō-dŏn′tăl) [Gr. *peri,* around, + *odous,* tooth]. Located around a tooth. SYN: *peridental.*

periodontal abscess. A localized area of acute or chronic inflammation with pus formation found in the gingiva, periodontal pockets, or periodontal ligament.

periodontal disease. Any abnormality, inflammatory or degenerative, of the tissue around the tooth.

periodontal ligament. The structural unit of oriented collagen fiber bundles that attaches the tooth to the surrounding alveolar bone proper and gingiva; may be subdivided into gingival ligament, alveolodental ligament, and interdental ligament according to the attachment of its fibers.

periodontal pocket. A gingival sulcus enlarged beyond normal limits as a result of poor oral hygiene; the space bordered on one side by the tooth and the other side by ulcerated sulcular epithelium; it will be several millimeters deep when probed and limited at its apex by attachment epithelium.

periodontia (pĕr″ē-ō-dŏn′shē-ă) [Gr. *peri,* around, + *odous,* tooth]. 1. Plural of periodontium. 2. The study and treatment of diseases of the periodontal tissues.

periodontics (pĕr″ē-ō-dŏn′tĭks) [″ + *odous,* tooth]. The branch of dentistry concerned with study and treatment of the periodontal tissues.

periodontitis (pĕr″ē-ō-dŏn-tī′tĭs) [″ + ″ + *itis,* inflammation]. Inflammation or degeneration, or both, of the dental periosteum, alveolar bone, cementum, and adjacent gingiva. Suppuration usually occurs, supporting bone is resorbed, teeth become loose, and recession of gingivae occurs. Usually follows chronic gingivitis, Vincent's infection, or poor dental hygiene. Systemic factors may predispose. SYN: *pyorrhea alveolaris; Riggs' disease.*

p., apical. Periodontitis of periapical region usually leading to formation of periapical abscess.

periodontium (pĕr-ē-ō-dŏn′shē-ŭm). [NA] The supporting apparatus for the tooth, including the gingiva, periodontal ligament, and alveolar bone proper.

periodontoclasia (pĕr″ē-ō-dŏn″tō-klā′zē-ă) [″ + *odous,* tooth, + *klasis,* breaking]. Condition characterized by inflammation accompanied by degenerative and retrogressive changes in the periodontium. SYN: *peridentitis.*

periodontology (pĕr″ē-ō-dŏn-tŏl′ō-jē) [″ + ″ + *logos,* study of]. Branch of dentistry dealing with treatment of diseases of the tissues around the teeth.

periodontosis (pĕr″ē-ō-dŏn-tō′sĭs) [″ + ″ + *osis,* condition]. Any degenerative disease of the periodontal tissues.

periodoscope (pĕr″ē-ŏd′ō-skōp) [LL. *periodus,* interval of time, + *skopein,* to examine]. Table or dial for calculation of expected date of delivery. SEE: *pregnancy* for Expected Date of Delivery (table).

periomphalic (pĕr″ē-ŏm-făl′ĭk) [Gr. *peri,* around, + *omphalos,* navel]. Located around or near the umbilicus.

periontogenic [″ + *on,* existing, + *gennan,* to produce]. Diseases caused by the environment.

perionychia (pĕr″ē-ō-nĭk′ē-ă) [″ + *onyx,* nail]. Inflammation around a nail.

perionychium (pĕr″ē-ō-nĭk′ē-ŭm). The epidermis surrounding a nail.

perionyx (pĕr″ē-ō′nĭks) [″ + *onyx,* nail]. The remnant of the eponychium that persists as a band across the root of the nail.

perionyxis (pĕr″ē-ō-nĭk′sĭs). Inflammation of epidermis surrounding a nail.

perioophoritis (pĕr″ē-ō-ŏf″ō-rī′tĭs) [″ + *oophoron,* ovary, + *itis,* inflammation]. Inflammation of the surface membrane of the ovary. SYN: *perioothecitis.*

perioophorosalpingitis (pĕr″ē-ō-ŏf″ō-rō-săl″pĭn-jī′tĭs) [″ + ″ + *salpinx,* tube, + *itis,* inflammation]. Inflamed condition of tissues around an ovary and oviduct. SYN: *perioothecosalpingitis; perisalpingoovaritis.*

perioothecitis (pĕr″ē-ō″ō-thē-sī′tĭs) [″ + *oon,* egg, + *theke,* box, + *itis,* inflammation]. Inflammation of the tissues around the ovary. SYN: *perioophoritis.*

perioothecosalpingitis (pĕr″ē-ō″ō-thē″kō-săl-pĭn-jī′tĭs) [″ + ″ + ″ + *salpinx,* tube, + *itis,* inflammation]. Inflammation of peritoneal membrane around the ovary and oviduct. SYN: *perioophorosalpingitis; perisalpingoovaritis.*

periophthalmic (pĕr″ē-ŏf-thăl′mĭk) [″ + *ophthalmos,* eye]. Around the eye.

perioptometry (pĕr″ē-ŏp-tŏm′ĕ-trē) [″ + *optos,* visible, + *metron,* a measure]. Measurement of the visual field. SYN: *perimetry.*

perioral (pĕr″ē-ō′răl) [″ + L. *oralis,* mouth]. Surrounding the mouth. SYN: *circumoral.*

periorbita (pĕr″ē-or′bĭ-tă) [″ + L. *orbita,* orbit]. [NA] Connective tissue covering the socket of the eye.

periorbital (pĕr″ē-or′bĭ-tăl). Surrounding the socket of the eye. SYN: *circumorbital.*

periorbititis (pĕr″ē-or″bĭ-tī′tĭs) [″ + L. *orbita,* orbit, + Gr. *itis,* inflammation]. Inflamed condition of the periorbita.

periorchitis (pĕr″ē-or-kī′tĭs) [″ + *orchis,* testicle, + *itis,* inflammation]. Inflamed condition of the tissues investing a testicle.

p. hemorrhagica. Chronic hematocele of the tunica vaginalis coat of the testis.

periosteal (pĕr-ē-ŏs′tē-ăl) [″ + *osteon,* bone]. Concerning the periosteum. SYN: *periosteous.*

periosteitis (pĕr″ē-ŏs″tē-ī′tĭs) [″ + ″ + *itis,* inflammation]. Inflammation of membrane investing a bone, the periosteum. SYN: *periostitis.*

periosteoedema (pĕr″ē-ŏs″tē-ō-ē-dē′mă) [Gr. *peri,* around, + *osteon,* bone. + *oidema,* swelling]. Edema of the periosteum, the membrane surrounding a bone.

periosteoma (pĕr″ē-ŏs-tē-ō′mă) [″ + ″ + *oma,* tumor] 1. An abnormal growth surrounding a bone. 2. Tumor of the periosteum, the tissue surrounding a bone.

periosteomyelitis (pĕr″ē-ŏs″tē-ō-mī″ĕ-lī′tĭs) [″ + ″ + *myelos,* marrow, + *itis,* inflammation]. Inflammation of bone, including the periosteum and marrow.

periosteophyte (pĕr″ē-ŏs′tē-ō-fīt) [″ + *osteon,* bone + *phyton,* growth]. Abnormal bony growth on periosteum, or arising from it.

periosteorrhaphy (pĕr″ē-ŏs″tē-or′ă-fē) [″ + ″ + *rhaphe,* a sewing]. Joining by suture the margins of a severed periosteum.

periosteosis (pĕr″ē-ŏs″tē-ō′sĭs) [″ + ″ + *osis,* condition]. Periostosis, q.v.

periosteotome (pĕr″ē-ŏs′tē-ō-tōm) [″ + *osteon,* bone, + *tome,* incision]. Instrument for cutting the periosteum or removing it from the bone.

periosteotomy (pĕr″ē-ŏs-tē-ŏt′ō-mē). Incision into the periosteum.

periosteous (pĕr″ē-ŏs′tē-ŭs) [″ + *osteon,* bone]. Concerning, or of the nature of, periosteum. SYN: *periosteal.*

periosteum (pĕr-ē-ŏs′tē-ŭm) [Gr. *periosteon*]. [NA] The fibrous membrane that forms the investing covering of bones except at their articular surfaces. Consists of a dense external layer containing numerous blood vessels and an inner layer of connective tissue cells that, when the bone is injured, function as osteoblasts and participate in new bone formation. Periosteum serves as a supporting structure for blood vessels nourishing bone and for attachment of muscles, tendons, and ligaments. It extends over the whole surface except at the cartilaginous articulations.

p., alveolar. The periodontal ligament.

p. externum. Periosteum covering external surfaces of bones.

p. internum. Interior periosteum lining the medullary canal of a bone.

periostitis (pĕr″ē-ŏs-tī′tĭs) [″ + *itis,* inflammation]. Inflamed condition of periosteum, the membrane investing a bone.

ETIOL: Infectious diseases, esp. syphilis; also trauma.

SYM: Pain over part, esp. under pressure, fever, sweats, leukocytosis, skin inflamed, rigidity of overlying muscles.

p., albuminous. Periostitis with albuminous serous fluid exudate beneath the membrane affected.

p., alveolar. Inflammation of the peridental membrane. SYN: *periodontitis.*

p., dental. Periostitis of a tooth sheath.

p., diffuse. Periostitis of the long bones.

p., hemorrhagic. Periostitis with extravasation of blood under the periosteum.

periostoma (pĕr″ē-ŏs-tō′mă) [″ + *osteon,* bone, + *oma,* tumor]. A bony neoplasm around a bone or arising from its membranous sheath.

periostomedullitis (pĕr″ē-ŏs″tō-mĕd-ū-lī′tĭs) [″ + ″ + L. *medulla,* marrow, + Gr. *itis,* inflammation]. Inflammation of the marrow or sheath of a bone. SYN: *periosteomyelitis.*

periostosis (pĕr″ē-ŏs-tō′sĭs) [″ + ″ + *osis,* condition]. A bony neoplasm around a bone or arising from it.

periostosteitis (pĕr″ē-ŏs-tŏs″tē-ī′tĭs) [″ + ″ + *osteon,* bone, + *itis,* inflammation]. Osteoperiosteitis, q.v.

periostotome (pĕr″ē-ŏs′tō-tōm) [″ + ″ + *tome,* incision]. A device for cutting the periosteum. SYN: *periosteotome.*

periostotomy (pĕ″ē-ŏs-tŏt′ō-mē) [″ + ″ + *tome,* incision]. Incision of the periosteum, the sheath covering a bone. SYN: *periosteotomy.*

periotic (pĕr-ē-ō′tĭk) [Gr. *peri,* around, + *ous,* ear]. Situated around the ear, esp. the internal ear.

periotic bone. The mastoid and petrous portions of the temporal bone.

periovaritis (pĕr″ē-ō″vă-rī′tĭs) [″ + L. *ovarium,* ovary, + Gr. *itis,* inflammation]. Periooophoritis, q.v.

periovular (pĕr″ē-ō′vū-lăr) [″ + L. *ovulum,* little egg]. Around an ovum.

peripachymeningitis (pĕr″ĭ-pak″ē-mĕn″ĭn-jī′tĭs) [″ + *pachys,* thick, + *meninx,* membrane, + *itis,* inflammation]. Inflamed condition of connective tissue between the dura mater and the bone that encloses the central nervous system.

peripapillary (pĕr″ĭ-păp′ĭ-lĕr″ē) [″ + L. *papilla,* nipple]. Around a papilla.

peripancreatitis (pĕr″ĭ-păn″krē-ă-tī′tĭs) [″ + *pankreas,* pancreas, + *itis,* inflammation]. Inflammation of tissues about or around the pancreas.

peripatetic (pĕr″ĭ-pă-tĕt′ĭk) [L. *peripateticus,* to walk about while teaching]. Moving from place to place.

peripenial (pĕr″ĭ-pē′nē-ăl) [″ + L. *penis,* penis]. Around the penis.

periphacitis (pĕr-ĭ-fă-sī′tĭs) [″ + *phakos,* lens, + *itis,* inflammation]. Inflamed condition of the capsule of the crystalline lens of the eye.

periphakus (pĕr″ĭ-fā′kŭs). The elastic capsule surrounding the crystalline lens.

peripharyngeal (pĕr″ĭ-fă-rĭn′jē-ăl) [″ + *pharynx,* pharynx]. Around the pharynx.

peripherad (pĕr-ĭf′ĕr-ăd) [″ + *pherein,* to bear, + L. *ad,* to]. In the direction of the periphery.

peripheral (pĕr-ĭf′ĕr-ăl). Located at, or pert to, the periphery; occurring away from the center.

peripheral nervous system. That portion of the nervous system outside the central nervous system. Included are the 12 pairs of cranial nerves, 31 pairs of spinal nerves, and their branches to the entire body. Also included are all sensory nerves, the sympathetic and parasympathetic nerves.

peripheral vascular disease. An imprecise term indicating diseases of the arteries and veins of the extremities, esp. those conditions that interfere with adequate flow of blood to or from the extremities, such as atherosclerosis with narrowing of the arterial lumen.

peripheraphose (pĕr-ĭf′ĕr-ă-fōs). Subjective sensation of darkness or shadow that originates in peripheral optic structures (optic nerve or eyeball).

peripherocentral (pĕ-rĭf″ĕr-ō-sĕn′trăl) [″ + *pherein,* to bear, + *kentron,* center]. Concerning both the periphery and central part of an organ.

peripherophose (per-ĭf′ĕr-ō-fōs). A subjective sensation of light or color that originates in peripheral optic structures (optic nerve or eyeball).

periphery (pĕr-ĭf′ĕ-rē) [Gr. *periphereia*]. Outer part or surface of a body; the part away from the center.

periphlebitis (pĕr″ĭ-flĕ-bī′tĭs) [Gr. *peri,* around, + *phleps,* vein, + *itis,* inflammation]. Inflamed condition of external coat of a vein or tissues around it.

periphoria (pĕr-ĭ-fō′rē-ă) [″ + *phoros,* bearing]. Tendency of the axis of the eye to deviate from the normal due to weakness of oblique muscles. SYN: *cyclophoria.*

periphrastic (pĕr″ĭ-frăs′tĭk) [Gr. *periphrastikos*]. Rel. to the use of superfluous words in expressing a thought. Appears in the writings and speech of some schizophrenics.

periphrenitis (pĕr″ĭ-frē-nī′tĭs) [Gr. *peri,* around + *phren,* diaphragm, + *itis,* inflammation]. Inflamed condition of the structures around the diaphragm.

Periplaneta (pĕr″ĭ-plă-nē′tă). A genus of cockroaches belonging to the order Orthoptera. Roaches contaminate food by mechanically transporting disease-producing bacteria, ova, and protozoa to the food.

P. americana. The American cockroach.

P. australasiae. The Australian cockroach.

periplasmic vesicles. A specialized apparatus in bacteria for excreting certain substances such as penicillinase.

periplast (pĕr′ĭ-plăst) [″ + *plassein,* to form]. Peripheral protoplasm of a cell exclusive of the nucleus.

peripleural (pĕr″ĭ-plū′răl) [″ + *pleura,* rib]. Encircling the pleura.

peripleuritis (pĕr-ĭ-plū-rī′tĭs) [″ + ″ + *itis,* inflammation]. Inflamed condition of the connective tissues between the pleura and wall of the chest.

peripolar (pĕr″ĭ-pō′lăr) [″ + L. *polus,* pole]. Around a pole.

peripolesis (pĕr″ĭ-pō-lē′sĭs) [Gr., a going about]. In tissue culture, the collecting of lymphocytes around macrophages.

periporitis (pĕr″ĭ-por-ī′tĭs) [Gr. *peri,* around, + L. *porus,* pore, + Gr. *itis*]. Multiple abscesses around sweat glands, esp. as a complication of malaria in children.

periportal (pĕr″ĭ-por′tăl) [″ + L. *porta,* gate]. Around the portal vein and its branches.

periproctic (pĕr″ĭ-prŏk′tĭk) [″ + *proktos,* anus]. Around the anus.

periproctitis (pĕr″ĭ-prŏk-tī′tĭs) [″ + ″ + *itis,* inflammation]. Inflammation of areolar tissues in region of the rectum and anus. SYN: *perirectitis.*

periprostatic (pĕr″ĭ-prŏs-tăt′ĭk) [″ + *prostates,* prostate]. Surrounding or occurring about the prostate.

periprostatitis (pĕr″ĭ-prŏs-tă-tī′tĭs) [″ + ″ + *itis,* inflammation]. Inflamed condition of tissues surrounding the prostate.

peripylephlebitis (pĕr″ĭ-pī″lē-flē-bī′tĭs) [″ + *pyle,* gate, + *phleps,* vein, + *itis,* inflammation]. Inflamed condition of tissues about the portal vein.

peripyloric (pĕr″ĭ-pī-lor′ĭk) [″ + *pyloros,* pylorus]. Extending around the pylorus.

perirectal (pĕr″ĭ-rĕk′tăl) [″ + L. *rectus,* straight]. Extending around the rectum.

perirectitis (pĕr″ĭ-rĕk-tī′tĭs) [″ + ″ + Gr. *itis,* inflammation]. Inflamed condition of tissues about rectum and anus. SYN: *periproctitis.*

perirenal (pĕr″ĭ-rē′năl) [Gr. *peri,* around, + L. *ren,* kidney]. Extending around the kidney. SYN: *circumrenal; perinephric.*

perirhinal (pĕr″ĭ-rī′năl) [″ + *rhis,* nose]. Located about the nose or nasal fossae.

perirhizoclasia (pĕr″ĭ-rī″zō-klā zē-ă) [″ + *rhiza,* root, + *klasis,* destruction]. Inflammation and destruction of tissues extending around the roots of a tooth.

perisalpingitis (pĕr″ĭ-săl″pĭn-jī′tĭs) [″ + *salpinx,* tube, + *itis,* inflammation]. Inflamed condition of peritoneal coat about the oviduct. SYN: *perioophorosalpingitis; perioothecosalpingitis.*

perisalpingoovaritis (pĕr″ĭ-săl-pĭn″gō-ō″văr-ī′tĭs) [″ + ″ + L. *ovarium,* ovary, + Gr. *itis,* inflammation]. Inflammation of peritoneal tissues surrounding the fallopian tubes and ovaries. SYN: *perioophorosalpingitis; perioothecosalpingitis.*

perisalpinx (pĕr″ĭ-săl′pĭnks) [″ + *salpinx,* tube]. The peritoneum covering the upper borders of the uterine tubes.

perisclerium (pĕr″ĭ-sklē′rē-ŭm) [″ + *skleros,* hard]. Fibrous tissue encircling ossifying cartilage.

periscopic (pĕr″ĭ-skŏp′ĭk) [″ + *skopein,* to examine]. Viewing on all sides; providing a wide range of vision.

perish (pĕr′ĭsh) [ME. *perisshen*]. To disintegrate or die, esp. by other than natural causes.

perisigmoiditis (pĕr″ĭ-sĭg″moy-dī′tĭs) [″ + *sigma,* Gr. letter S, + *eidos,* like, + *itis,* inflammation]. Inflamed condition of peritoneal tissues around the sigmoid flexure of the colon.

perisinusitis (pĕr″ĭ-sī″nū-sī′tĭs) [″ + L. *sinus,* cavity, + Gr. *itis,* inflammation]. Inflammation of membranes about a sinus, esp. a venous sinus of the dura mater.

perispermatitis (pĕr″ĭ-spĕr″mă-tī′tĭs) [″ +

sperma, seed, + *itis,* inflammation]. Inflamed condition of tissues about the spermatic cord.

p. serosa. Hydrocele of spermatic cord.

perisplanchnic (pĕr″ĭ-splăngk′nĭk) [″ + *splanchnon,* viscus]. Extending around a viscus or the viscera.

perisplanchnitis (pĕr″ĭ-splăngk-nī′tĭs) [″ + ″ + *itis,* inflammation]. Inflamed condition of the tissues around the viscera. SYN: *perivisceritis.*

perisplenic (pĕr″ĭ-splĕn′ĭk) [″ + *splen,* spleen]. Near or around the spleen.

perisplenitis (pĕr″ĭ-splē-nī′tĭs) [″ + ″ + *itis,* inflammation]. Inflammation of peritoneal coat of the spleen, the splenic capsule.

p. cartilaginea. Inflammation of capsule of the spleen resulting in thickening and hardening.

perispondylic (pĕr″ĭ-spŏn-dĭl′ĭk) [Gr. *peri,* around, + *spondylos,* vertebra]. Around a vertebra.

perispondylitis (pĕr″ĭ-spŏn-dĭl-ī′tĭs) [″ + ″ + *itis,* inflammation]. Inflamed condition of the parts around a vertebra.

perissodactylous (pĕr-ĭs″sō-dăk′tĭ-lŭs) [Gr. *perissos,* odd, + *daktylos,* digit]. Having an odd number of digits on a hand or foot. SYN: *imparidigitate.*

peristalsis (pĕr-ĭ-stăl′sĭs) [Gr. *peri,* around, + *stalsis,* contraction]. A progressive wavelike movement that occurs involuntarily in hollow tubes of the body, esp. the alimentary canal. It is characteristic of tubes possessing longitudinal and circular layers of smooth muscle fibers.

Peristalsis is induced reflexly by distention of the walls of the tube. The wave consists of contraction of the circular muscle above the distention with relaxation of the region immediately distal to the distended portion. The simultaneous contraction and relaxation progresses slowly for a short distance as a wave that causes the contents of the tube to be forced onward.

p., mass. Forced peristaltic movements of short duration, moving contents from one section of the colon to another, occurring three or four times daily.

p., reverse. Peristalsis in a direction opposite to the normal direction. SYN: *antiperistalsis.*

peristaltic (pĕr″ĭ-stăl′tĭk). Concerning, or of the nature of, peristalsis.

peristaphyline (pĕr″ĭ-stăf′ĭ-lĭn) [″ + *staphyle,* uvula]. About the uvula.

peristasis (pĕr-rĭs′tă-sĭs) [″ + *stasis,* standing]. 1. In the early stage of inflammation, the decrease in blood flow in the affected area. 2. Environment.

peristomatous (pĕr″ĭ-stŏm′ă-tŭs) [″ + *stoma,* mouth]. Around the mouth.

peristome (pĕr′ĭ-stōm) [″ + *stoma,* mouth]. Channel leading to the cytosome or mouth in certain types of protozoa.

peristrumitis (pĕr″ĭ-stroo-mī′tĭs) [″ + L. *struma,* goiter, + *itis,* inflammation]. Inflamed condition of tissues around a goiter. SYN: *perithyroiditis.*

peristrumous (pĕr″ĭ-stroo′mŭs) [″ + *struma,* goiter]. Around a goiter.

perisynovial (pĕr″ĭ-sĭ-nō′vē-ăl) [Gr. *peri,* around, + L. *synovia,* joint fluid]. Extending around a synovial structure.

perisystole (pĕr″ĭ-sĭs′tō-lē) [″ + *systole,* contraction]. The period preceding the systole in the cardiac rhythm. SYN: *presystole.*

peritectomy (pĕr″ĭ-tĕk′tō-mē) [″ + *ektome,* excision]. Surgical removal of a ring of conjunctiva around the cornea.

peritendineum (pĕr″ĭ-tĕn-dĭn′ē-ŭm) [″ + L. *tendo,* tendon]. [NA] A sheath of fibrous connective tissue investing a fiber bundle of a tendon.

peritendinitis (pĕr″ĭ-tĕn″dĭ-nī′tĭs) [″ + ″ + Gr. *itis,* inflammation]. Inflamed condition of the sheath of a tendon. SYN: *peritenonitis; tenosynovitis.*

p. calcarea. The deposition of calcareous material in tendons and associated regions, characterized by pain, tenderness, and limitation of motion.

p. serosa. Peritendinitis with effusion into the sheath.

peritenon (pĕr″ĭ-tē′nŏn) [″ + *tenon,* tendon]. 1. The sheath of a tendon. 2. Peritendineum.

peritenonitis (pĕr″ĭ-tĕn″ō-nī′tĭs). Inflammation of sheath investing a tendon. SYN: *peritendinitis.*

perithelioma (pĕr″ĭ-thē-lē-ō′mă) [″ + *thele,* nipple, + *oma,* tumor]. A tumor derived from the perithelial layer of the blood vessels.

perithelium (pĕr″ĭ-thē′lē-ŭm). Fibrous outer layer of the smaller blood vessels and capillaries.

p., Eberth's. An incomplete layer of cells covering capillaries.

perithoracic (pĕr″ĭ-thō-răs′ĭk) [″ + *thorax,* chest]. Around the thorax.

perithyroiditis (pĕr″ĭ-thī-roy-dī′tĭs) [″ + *thyreos,* shield, + *eidos,* form, + *itis,* inflammation]. Inflammation of capsule or tissues sheathing the thyroid gland. SYN: *peristrumitis.*

peritomist (pĕ-rĭt′ō-mĭst) [″ + *tome,* incision]. One who performs circumcision, i.e., peritomy.

peritomize (pĕ-rĭt′ō-mīz) [″ + *tome,* incision]. To perform peritomy.

peritomy (pĕr-ĭt′ō-mē) [″ + *tome,* incision]. 1. Excision of narrow strip of conjunctiva around the cornea in treatment of pannus. SYN: *syndectomy.* 2. Circumcision.

peritoneal (pĕr″ĭ-tō-nē′ăl) [Gr. *peritonaion,*

peritoneum]. Concerning the peritoneum.

peritoneal cavity. A potential space between layers of the parietal and visceral peritoneum. A small amount of fluid is contained in the space. Thus friction is minimized as the viscera glide on each other, or against the wall of the abdominal cavity.

peritoneal dialysis. Removal of toxic substances from the body by perfusing specific warm sterile chemical solutions through the peritoneal cavity. Used in treating renal failure or in certain poisonings. Some of the drugs and chemicals that may be so removed are salicylates, barbiturates, meprobamate, amphetamines, bromide, methanol, boric acid, sulfonamide, and various antibiotics.

CAUTION: Peritoneal dialysis may be dangerous and may cause death if not done with adequate supervision of body fluid and electrolyte balance.

p.d., continuous ambulatory. SEE: *continuous ambulatory peritoneal dialysis.*

peritoneal fluid. The clear straw-colored serous fluid secreted by the cells of the peritoneum. The few milliliters present in the peritoneal cavity moisten the surfaces of the viscera and allow them to glide over each other as the intestinal tract changes shape during the process of digestion and absorption. In certain disease states the amount of peritoneal fluid is increased. If this is not due to inflammation, the fluid is called ascitic fluid. SEE: illus.; *ascites.*

peritonealgia (pĕr″ĭ-tō″nē-ăl′jē-ă) [″ + *algos,* pain]. Pain of the peritoneum.

peritonealize. During abdominal surgery, to cover a tissue with peritoneum.

peritoneocentesis (pĕr″ĭ-tō″nē-ō-sĕn-tē′sĭs) [Gr. *peritonaion,* peritoneum, + *kentesis,* puncture]. Piercing of the peritoneal cavity to obtain fluid. SEE: *paracentesis.*

peritoneoclysis (pĕr″ĭ-tō″nē-ō-klī′sĭs) [″ + *klysis,* a washing out]. Introduction of fluid into the peritoneal cavity.

peritoneopathy (pĕr″ĭ-tō-nē-ŏp′ăth-ē) [″ + *pathos,* disease]. Any disordered condition of the peritoneum.

peritoneopericardial (pĕr″ĭ-tō-nē′ō-pĕr″ĭ-kăr′dē-ăl) [″ + *peri,* around, + *kardia,* heart]. Concerning the peritoneum and pericardium.

peritoneopexy (pĕr″ĭ-tō′nē-ō-pĕks″ē) [Gr. *peritonaion,* peritoneum, + *pexis,* fixation]. Fixation of the uterus by way of the vagina.

peritoneoplasty (pĕr″ĭ-tō′nē-ō-plăs″tē) [″ + *plassein,* to form]. Reparative surgery to prevent reformation of loosened adhesions.

peritoneoscope (pĕr″ĭ-tō′nē-ō-skōp″) [Gr. *peritonaion,* peritoneum, + *skopein,* to examine]. Long, slender periscope or telescope device with a light at one end and an eyepiece at the other. Used to inspect the peritoneal and abdominal cavities through a small incision in the abdominal wall.

peritoneoscopy (pĕr″ĭ-tō″nē-ŏs′kō-pē). Examination of peritoneal cavity with the peritoneoscope.

peritoneotomy (pĕr″ĭ-tō″nē-ŏt′ō-mē). Process of incising the peritoneum.

peritoneum (pĕr″ĭ-tō-nē′ŭm) [LL., Gr. *peritonaion*]. [NA] The serous membrane reflected over the viscera and lining the abdominal cavity.

PALPATION: If palmar surface of hand is applied to side of abdomen at level of the liquid in ascites and light percussion is performed on the opposite side, a sense of fluctuation will be communicated to the hand.

p., parietal. Peritoneum lining abdominal and pelvic walls and undersurface of diaphragm.

p., visceral. The peritoneum that invests the abdominal organs. The peritoneum holds the viscera in position by its folds.

PERITONEAL FLUID

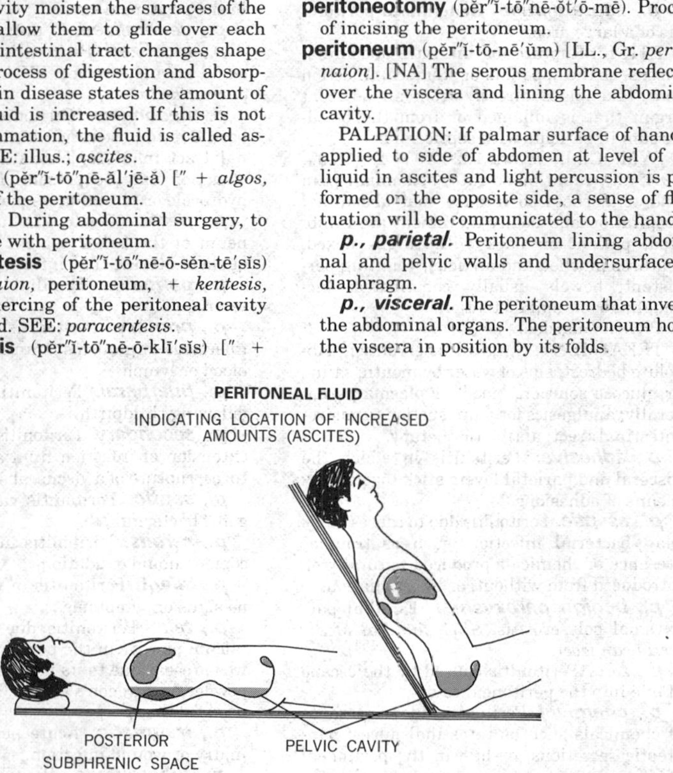

peritonism (pĕr'ĭ-tō-nĭzm) [Gr. *peritonaion,* peritoneum, + *-ismos,* condition]. 1. The clinical signs of shock and peritonitis but without inflammation of the peritoneum. 2. A neurosis in which the patient's complaints are consistent with peritonitis.

peritonitic (pĕr"ĭ-tō-nĭt'ĭk) [" + *itis,* inflammation]. Affected with or concerning peritonitis.

peritonitis (pĕr"ĭ-tō-nī'tĭs) [Gr. *peritonaion,* peritoneum, + *itis,* inflammation]. Inflammation of the peritoneum, the membranous coat lining the abdominal cavity and investing the viscera.

ETIOL: Infectious organisms that gain access by way of rupture or perforation of viscus or associated structures, via the female genital tract, piercing of abdominal wall, bloodstream or lymphatic vessels, surgical incisions, and failure to practice aseptic techniques during surgery. Prophylactic measures to prevent development of peritonitis are of utmost importance in the care of all patients.

TREATMENT: Antibiotic therapy.

p., acute diffuse. Generalized peritonitis of a large area.

ETIOL: Rupture of an intra-abdominal viscus, as the appendix or stomach. Infection may take place directly from an adjacent organ that is inflamed or from the bloodstream in patients with septicemia.

SYM: Chill; fever, 102°–103° F. (38.9°–39.4° C.); rapid pulse rate; abdominal pain and tenderness so intense that abdominal respiration and bodily movement are inhibited; patient on back with thighs flexed; features pinched and anxious; vomiting persistent; bowels usually constipated; hiccough; abdominal distention.

PROG: Guarded.

TREATMENT: Surgical intervention. Absolute bedrest; sips of water by mouth; saline or glucose solution, blood, or plasma parenterally; analgesics for pain; suction to gastrointestinal tract; antibiotic therapy.

p., adhesive. Peritonitis in which the visceral and parietal layers stick together by means of adhesions.

p., aseptic. Peritonitis due to causes other than bacterial infection, such as trauma, presence of chemicals produced naturally or introduced from without, or by irradiation.

p., benign paroxysmal. Familial paroxysmal polyserositis. *SEE: familial Mediterranean fever.*

p., bile. Peritonitis caused by the escape of bile into the peritoneal cavity.

p., chemical. Peritonitis due to presence of chemicals such as intestinal juices, pancreatic secretions, or bile in the peritoneal cavity.

p., chronic. Peritonitis that is usually due to tuberculosis or cancer.

SYM: Fever slight or absent. Pain not severe; paroxysms; usually diffuse tenderness; anemia and emaciation may be marked.

PROG: Guarded.

TREATMENT: Rest; light diet; paracentesis. Laparotomy.

p., circumscribed. P., localized.

p. deformans. Chronic peritonitis with thickened membrane and adhesions contracting and causing retraction of the intestines.

p., diaphragmatic. Peritonitis in which the peritoneal surface of the diaphragm is mainly affected.

p., diffuse. Peritonitis that is widespread, involving most of the peritoneum. SYN: *p., generalized.*

p. encapsulans. A localized abscess in the peritoneal cavity. This may occur after generalized peritonitis has subsided.

p., fibrocaseous. Peritonitis with fibrosis and caseation. Usually due to tuberculosis.

p., gas. Peritonitis in which gas is present in the peritoneal cavity.

p., generalized. P., diffuse.

p., localized. Peritonitis in which only a small area is involved. SYN: *peritonitis, circumscribed.*

p. meconium. Peritonitis in the newborn due to perforation of the gastrointestinal tract in utero. Neonatal intestinal obstruction may be present. In males a soft hydrocele or scrotal mass may be found.

p., pelvic. Peritonitis involving peritoneum of the pelvic region, usually the sequela of uterine tube infection in female.

p., periodic. Familial Mediterranean fever, q.v.

p., primary. Peritonitis resulting from infectious organisms transmitted through blood or lymph.

p., puerperal. Peritonitis that develops following childbirth.

p., secondary. Peritonitis resulting from extension of infection from adjoining structures, rupture of a viscus, abscess, or trauma.

p., septic. Peritonitis caused by a pyogenic bacterium.

p., serous. Peritonitis in which there is copious liquid exudation.

p., silent. Peritonitis in which there are no signs or symptoms.

p., talc. Peritonitis due to particles of talcum powder in the peritoneal cavity. Talc was present due to its having been used as a powder on surgeon's gloves. Talc is no longer used for that purpose.

p., traumatic. Acute peritonitis due to injury or wound infection.

p., tuberculous. Peritonitis caused by

numerous tubercle bacilli on the peritoneum.

peritonize (pěr'ĭ-tō-nīz) [Gr. *peritonaion,* peritoneum]. Peritonealize, q.v.

peritonsillar (pěr"ĭ-tŏn'sĭ-lăr) [Gr. *peri,* around, + L. *tonsilla,* tonsil]. Extending around a tonsil.

peritonsillitis (pěr"ĭ-tŏn"sĭ-lī'tĭs) [" + " + Gr. *itis,* inflammation]. Inflamed condition of tissues around the tonsils. SYN: *periamygdalitis.*

peritracheal (pěr"ĭ-trā'kē-ăl) [" + *tracheia,* trachea]. Around the trachea.

Peritrate. Trade name for pentaerythritol tetranitrate.

Peritricha (pěr-ĭt'rĭ-kă) [Gr. *peri,* around, + *thrix,* hair]. A group of protozoa having flagella over the entire surface.

peritrichal, peritrichic (pĕ-rĭt'rĭ-kăl, pěr"ē-trĭk'ĭk) [" + *thrix,* hair]. Uniform distribution of flagellae over a cell, usually a bacterial cell. SYN: *peritrichous.*

peritrichous (pĕ-rĭt'rĭk-ŭs) [" + *thrix,* hair]. Indicating microorganisms that have cilia or flagella covering the entire surface.

peritrochanteric (pěr"ĭ-trō"kăn-tĕr'ĭk) [" + *trokhanter,* runner]. Around a trochanter.

perityphlic (pěr"ĭ-tĭf'lĭk) [" + *typhlon,* cecum]. Around the cecum.

perityphlitis (pěr"ĭ-tĭf'lī-tĭs) [" + " + *itis,* inflammation]. Inflamed condition of tissues around the cecum and appendix. SYN: *appendicitis.*

periumbilical (pěr"ē-ŭm-bĭl'ĭ-kăl) [" + L. *umbilicus,* a pit]. Around the navel, i.e., umbilicus.

periungual (pěr"ē-ŭng'gwăl) [" + L. *unguis,* nail]. Around a nail.

periureteral (pěr"ē-ū-rē'tĕr-ăl) [" + *oureter,* ureter]. Around the ureter.

periureteritis (pěr"ē-ū-rē"tĕr-ī'tĭs) [" + " + *itis,* inflammation]. Inflamed condition of parts about the ureter.

periurethral (pěr"ē-ū-rē'thrăl) [" + *ourethra,* urethra]. Located about the urethra.

periurethritis (pěr"ē-ū"rē-thrī'tĭs) [" + " + *itis,* inflammation]. Inflammation of the tissues around the urethra.

periuterine (pěr"ē-ū'tĕr-ĭn) [" + L. *uterus,* womb]. Located about the uterus. SYN: *perimetric.*

periuvular (pěr"ē-ū'vū-lăr) [" + L. *uvula,* little grape]. Around the uvula.

perivaginal (pěr"ĭ-văj'ĭ-năl) [" + L. *vagina,* sheath]. Around the vagina.

perivaginitis (pěr"ĭ-văj"ĭ-nī'tĭs) [" + " + Gr. *itis,* inflammation]. Inflammation of region around the vagina. SYN: *pericolpitis.*

perivascular (pěr"ĭ-văs'kū-lăr) [" + L. *vasculus,* a little vessel]. Located around a vessel, esp. a blood vessel.

perivasculitis (pěr"ĭ-văs"kū-lī'tĭs) [" + " + Gr. *itis,* inflammation]. Inflamed condition of tissues surrounding a blood vessel. SYN: *periangiitis.*

perivenous (pěr"ĭ-vē'nŭs) [" + L. *vena,* vein]. Surrounding or occurring around a vein.

perivertebral (pěr"ĭ-vĕr'tĕ-brăl) [" + L. *vertebra,* vertebra]. Around a vertebra.

perivesical (pěr"ĭ-vĕs'ĭ-kăl) [" + L. *vesicula,* little bladder]. Around the urinary bladder.

perivesiculitis (pěr"ĭ-vĕ-sĭk"ū-lī'tĭs) [" + " + Gr. *itis,* inflammation]. Inflammation of tissues around a seminal vesicle.

perivisceral (pěr"ĭ-vĭs'ĕr-ăl) [" + L. *viscera,* internal organs]. Around the viscera or a seminal vesicle.

perivisceritis (pěr"ĭ-vĭs"ĕr-ī'tĭs) [" + " + Gr. *itis,* inflammation]. Inflamed condition of the tissues surrounding the viscera.

perivitelline (pěr"ĭ-vī-tĕl'ĕn) [" + L. *vitellus,* yolk]. Around a vitellus or yolk.

perixenitis (pěr"ĭ-zĕ-nī'tĭs) [" + *xenos,* strange, + *itis,* inflammation]. Inflammation occurring around a foreign body in a tissue or organ. SYN: *perialienitis.*

perle (pěrl) [Fr., pearl]. A soft capsule containing medicine.

perlèche (pěr-lĕsh') [Fr.]. Disorder marked by fissures and epithelial desquamation at corners of the mouth, esp. seen in children. May be due to oral candidiasis or may be a symptom of dietary deficiency, esp. riboflavin deficiency.

perlingual (pěr-lĭng'gwăl) [L. *per,* through, + *lingua,* tongue]. By way of the tongue; method of administering medicines.

permanent (pěr'mă-nĕnt) [" + *manere,* to remain]. Enduring; without change.

permanent teeth. Teeth developing at the second dentition. SEE: *dens permanens; teeth, permanent* for illus.

permanganate (pěr-măn'gă-nāt). Any one of the salts of permanganic acid.

Permapen. Trade name for penicillin G benzathine, USP.

permeability (pěr"mē-ă-bĭl'ĭ-tē) [LL. *permeabilis*]. The quality of being permeable; that which may be traversed.

p., capillary. The condition of the capillary wall that enables substances in the blood to diffuse into tissue spaces or into cells, or vice versa.

permeable (pěr'mē-ă-bl). Capable of allowing the passage of fluids or substances in solution.

permeation (pěr"mē-ā'shŭn) [L. *permeare,* permeate]. Penetration of, and spreading throughout, an organ, tissue, or space.

permissible exposure limits. The limits, usually expressed as a combination of time and concentration, to which humans may be safely exposed to physical agents, ionizing radiations, or chemical substances in the environment in general and in work areas specifically. SEE: *maximum allowable concentration; threshold limit values.*

Permitil. Trade name for fluphenazine hydrochloride, USP.

permutation (pĕr″mū-tā′shŭn) [L. *per,* completely, + *mutare,* to change]. Transformation; complete change; act of altering objects in a group.

perniciosiform (pĕr-nĭsh″ē-ō′sĭ-form) [L. *perniciosus,* destructive, + *forma,* form]. Pert. to a condition that is apparently but not actually pernicious.

pernicious (pĕr-nĭsh′ŭs) [L. *perniciosus,* destructive]. Destructive; fatal; harmful.

pernicious anemia. Severe form of blood disease marked by progressive decrease in red blood corpuscles, muscular weakness, and gastrointestinal and neural disturbances. May be fatal if not treated with vitamin B_{12}, iron, and diet. SEE: *anemia, pernicious.*

pernicious trend. A psychological term indicating an abnormal departure from conventional ideas and social interests.

pernio (pĕr′nē-ō) [L.]. Chilblain. Congestion and swelling of the skin due to cold.

SYM: Attended with severe burning or itching; ulceration may result from vesicles and bullae that sometimes form.

pero- [Gr. *peros,* maimed]. Combining form meaning deformed.

perobrachius (pē″rō-brā′kē-ŭs) [″ + *brachion,* arm]. Condition in which forearms and hands are deformed.

perocephalus (pē″rō-sĕf′ă-lŭs) [″ + *kephale,* head]. An individual with a congenitally defective head.

perochirus (pē″rō-kī′rŭs) [″ + *cheir,* hand]. An individual with congenitally deformed hands.

perocormus (pē″rō-kor′mŭs) [″ + *kormos,* trunk]. An individual with a congenitally deformed trunk.

perodactylia (pē″rō-dăk-tĭl′ē-ă) [″ + *daktylos,* finger]. Condition in which one or more fingers or toes are deformed.

perodactylus (pē″rō-dăk′tĭ-lŭs) [″ + *daktylos,* finger]. An individual with congenitally deformed fingers or toes.

peromelia (pē″rō-mē′lē-ă) [″ + *melos,* limb]. Congenital absence or deformity of the terminal part of a limb or limbs.

peromelus (pē-rŏm′ĕ-lŭs) [″ + *melos,* limb]. An individual with malformation of extremities, including absence of hand or foot.

perone (pĕr-ō′nē) [Gr. *perone,* pin]. The fibula.

peroneal (pĕr″ō-nē′ăl) [Gr. *perone,* pin]. Concerning the fibula.

peroneal sign. In patients with tetany, tapping on the fibular side over the peroneal nerve causes eversion and dorsiflexion of the foot.

peroneo- [Gr. *perone,* pin]. Combining form pert. to the fibula.

peroneotibial (pĕr″ō-nē″ō-tĭb′ē-ăl) [″ + L. *tibia,* shinbone]. Concerning the fibula and tibia.

peroneus (pĕr″ō-nē′ŭs) [Gr. *perone,* pin]. One of several muscles of the leg that act to move the foot.

peronia (pē-rō′nē-ă) [Gr. *peros,* maimed]. Malformation.

peropus (pē′rō-pŭs) [″ + *pous,* foot]. An individual with congenitally deformed feet.

peroral (pĕr-or′ăl) [L. *per,* through, + *oris,* mouth]. Administered through the mouth.

per os [L.]. By mouth.

perosomus (pē″rō-sō′mŭs) [Gr. *peros,* maimed, + *soma,* body]. An individual with a congenitally defective body.

perosplanchnia (pē″rō-splănk′nē-ă) [″ + *splanchnon,* viscus]. Congenital malformation of the viscera.

perosseous (pĕr-ŏs′ē-ŭs) [L. *per,* through, + *os,* bone]. Through bone.

peroxidase (pĕr-ŏk′sĭ-dās) [″ + *oxys,* acid, + *-ase,* enzyme]. An enzyme that hastens the transfer of oxygen from peroxide to a tissue that requires oxygen. This process is essential to intracellular respiration.

peroxide (pĕr-ŏk′sīd). In chemistry, a compound containing more oxygen than the other oxides of the element in question.

Ex.: peroxides of hydrogen, H_2O_2; sodium, Na_2O_2; magnesium, MgO_2; and nitrogen, NO_2.

peroxisome (pĕ-rŏks′ĭ-sōm). A microbody present in vertebrate animal cells. They contain a great number and variety of enzymes important in cell metabolism.

perphenazine (pĕr-fĕn′ă-zēn). USP. An antipsychotic drug that is also used as an antiemetic. Trade name is Trilafon.

perplication (pĕr-plĭ-kā′shŭn) [″ + *plicare,* to fold]. Inserting the cut end of an artery through an incision in its own wall to arrest bleeding.

per primam, per primam intentionem (pĕr prī′măm ĭn-tĕn-shē-ō′nĕm) [L.]. By first intention. SEE: *healing.*

per rectum (pĕr rĕk′tŭm) [L.]. By the rectum; through the rectum.

PERRLA. *pupils equal, regular, react to light, and accommodation.*

Persadox. Trade name for benzoyl peroxide, USP.

persalt (pĕr′sawlt). In chemistry, a salt containing the largest possible amount of an acid radical.

Persantine. Trade name for dipyridamole.

per secundam intentionem (pĕr sē-kŭn′dăm) [L.]. By second intention. SEE: *healing.*

perseveration (pĕr-sĕv″ĕr-ā′shŭn) [L. *perseverare,* to persist]. Continued repetition of a meaningless word or phrase, or repetition of answers that are not related to successive questions asked.

person. A human being.

persona (pĕr-sō′nă) [L., mask]. The outer attitude or appearance a person presents to others.

personal [L. *personalis*]. Characteristic of an individual.

personality [LL. *personalitas*]. The unique organization of traits, characteristics, and modes of behavior of an individual, setting the individual apart from others and at the same time determining how others react to the individual. Personality refers to the mental aspects of an individual, in contrast to physique.

RS: consciousness; dissociation; somnambulism; vigilambulism.

p., alternating. SEE: *p., multiple.*

p., antisocial. A type of personality disorder characterized by disregard of the rights of others. It usually begins prior to age 15. In early childhood there are lying, stealing, fighting, truancy, and disregard of authority. In adolescence there are usually aggressive sexual behavior, excessive use of alcohol, and use of drugs of abuse. In adulthood these behavior patterns continue with the addition of poor work performance, inability to function responsibly as a parent, and inability to accept normal restrictions imposed by laws. This type of personality disorder is not due to mental retardation, schizophrenia, or manic episodes. It is much more common in males than females.

p., compulsive. A type of personality disorder in which there is inability to express warm and tender emotions. The individual's perfectionism, q.v., interferes with ability to consider the entire situation but is instead preoccupied with trivial details, rules, orderliness, organization, schedules, and lists. These individuals resist the authority of others but insist that others conform to their wishes. The desire for work and productivity precludes enjoying a vacation or warm interpersonal relations. Because of fear of making a mistake, decision-making is difficult. This disorder may be incapacitating with respect to success in an occupation.

p., double. P., dual.

p., dual. Mental dissociation in which one individual shows in alternation two very different personalities. SEE: *dual personality.*

p., extroverted. Personality in which activities or libido are directed to other individuals or the environment.

p., histrionic. A disorder in which the individuals are active and dramatic, draw attention to themselves, are prone to exaggerate, and are subject to emotional excitability such as irrational, angry outbursts or tantrums. They are bored with normal routines and crave novelty and excitement. Even though these individuals are usually attractive and productive, their behavior in interpersonal relationships is perceived to be shallow, vain, demanding, dependent, and constantly seeking reassurance.

p., inadequate. Personality in which the individual is ineffective, and is physically and emotionally unstable to the extent of being unable to cope with the normal stress of living.

p., introverted. Personality in which activities or libido are directed to the individual him- or herself.

p., multiple. State in which three or more personalities alternate in the same individual, usually with each personality unaware of the others.

p., neurotic. Personality characterized by behavior intermediate between normal and that of a neurotic individual.

p., obsessive-compulsive. SEE: *p., compulsive.*

p., paranoid. A disorder characterized by a continuing and unwarranted suspiciousness, mistrust of people, and hypersensitivity. It is not a psychosis but those affected have great difficulty with interpersonal relations. They are quite critical of others but virtually unable to accept criticism.

p., passive-aggressive. Personality in which individuals resist demands for adequate performance in work and social situations. The resistance is indirectly expressed. This is done by misplacing work assignments, or being late to appointments or forgetting them. Persons with this type of personality are ineffective at work and socially.

p., psychopathic. An obsolete term. SEE: *p., antisocial.*

p., schizoid. Personality characterized by shyness, oversensitivity, seclusiveness, dissociation from close interpersonal or competitive relationships, eccentricity, daydreaming, and inability to express hostility and aggression in situations that would call for such reactions.

persons in need of supervision. ABBR: PINS. A legal term for children who because of behavioral problems require supervision, usually in an institution.

perspiration (pĕr″spĭr-ā′shŭn) [L. *perspirare*, breathe through]. Salty fluid secreted through the sweat glands of the skin; sweat. Essentially it is a weak solution of sodium chloride, but it also contains potassium, lactate, and urea. Perspiration is a means of removing heat from the body. This is best accomplished by sweat evaporating from the skin rather than dripping off. Evaporation of a liter of sweat removes 580 Cal. of heat from the body.

Sweat loss will vary from 100 to 1000 ml. per hour but may be more than that in a hot climate.

Perspiration is increased by temperature and humidity of the atmosphere, exercises, pain, nausea, nervousness, mental excitement, dyspnea, diaphoretics, and shock. Perspiration is decreased by cold, diarrhea, voiding large quantities of urine, and using certain drugs.

p., insensible. Evaporation of water vapor from the body without appearing as moisture on the skin.

p., sensible. Perspiration that forms moisture on the skin.

perspiration, words pert. to: adiaphoresis; anhidrosis; apocrine gland; bromohyperhidrosis; bromidrosis; chromidrosis; diaphoresis; eccrine gland; polyhidrosis; secretion; sudor; sweat; sweating; transpiration.

perspire (pĕr-spīr′) [L. *perspirare,* breathe through]. To excrete fluid through the pores of the skin. SYN: *sweat.*

persuasion (pĕr-swā′zhŭn). In psychiatry, the attempt to influence behavior by authority, reason, or argument.

persulfate (pĕr-sŭl′fāt). One of a series of sulfates containing more sulfuric acid than the others in the same series.

per tertiam intentionem (pĕr tĕr′shē-ăm ĭn-tĕn-shē-ō′nĕm) [L.]. By third intention. SEE: *healing.*

Perthes' disease (pĕr′tēz). [Georg C. Perthes, Ger. surgeon, 1869–1927] Disease in which changes take place in bone at the head of the femur with deformity resulting. SYN: *osteochondritis deformans juvenilis.*

SYM: Similar to tuberculous hip joint disease.

Pertofrane. Trade name for desipramine hydrochloride.

per tubam (pĕr tū′băm) [L.]. Through a tube.

perturbation (pĕr″tĕr-bā′shŭn) [L. *perturbare,* thoroughly disordered]. State of being greatly disturbed or agitated; uneasiness of mind.

pertussis (pĕr-tŭs′ĭs) [L. *per,* through, + *tussis,* cough]. An acute, infectious disease characterized by a catarrhal stage, followed by a peculiar paroxysmal cough, ending in a whooping inspiration. Pertussis may be prevented by immunization of infants beginning at three months of age. SYN: *whooping cough.*

ETIOL: Due to a small, nonmotile, gram-negative bacillus, Bordetella pertussis.

INCUBATION: Seven to 10 days.

SYM: Elevated white blood count with marked lymphocytosis. May be in excess of 30,000 per cubic millimeter.

Often divided into the following three stages: *Catarrhal:* At this time the symptoms are chiefly suggestive of the common cold—slight elevation of fever, sneezing, rhinitis, and dry cough; irritability and loss of appetite.

Paroxysmal: Sets in after approx. 2 weeks. The cough is more violent and consists of a series of several short coughs, followed by long drawn inspiration during which the typical whoop is heard, this being occasioned by the spasmodic contraction of the glottis. Often with the beginning of each paroxysm, the patient assumes a worried expression, sometimes even one of terror. The face becomes cyanosed, eyes injected, veins distended. With conclusion of the paroxysm, vomiting is common. Also at this time there may be epistaxis, subconjunctival hemorrhages, or hemorrhages in other portions of body. Number of paroxysms in 24 hours may vary from 3 to 4 up to 40 to 50. Cough is precipitated by eating, drinking, or by pressing on the trachea. It is associated often with vomiting.

Decline: Begins after an indefinite period of several weeks. Paroxysms grow less frequent and less violent. Nutrition of child improves, and after a period that may be prolonged for several months, the cough finally ceases.

pertussis immune human globulin. USP. A sterile solution of globulins derived from the blood of adults who have been immunized with pertussis vaccine. Used to produce passive immunity to pertussis.

pertussis vaccine. USP. Sterile bacterial fraction of killed pertussis bacilli. Used for active immunization against pertussis.

pertussoid (pĕr-tŭs′oyd) [L. *per,* through, + *tussis,* cough, + Gr. *eidos,* resemblance]. 1. Of the nature of whooping cough. 2. A cough generally similar to that of whooping cough.

per vaginam (pĕr vă-jī′năm) [L.]. Through the vagina.

perversion (pĕr-vĕr′zhŭn) [L. *perversus,* perverted]. Deviation from the normal path, whether it be in the area of one's intellect, emotions, actions, or reactions. SEE: *paraphilia.*

p., sexual. Maladjustment of sexual life in which satisfaction is sought in ways deviating from the accepted norm. In judging the sexual actions of individuals, it is important to remember that what is normal behavior in one society may be regarded as grossly abnormal or perverted in another.

pervert [L. *pervetere,* to turn the wrong way]. 1. (pĕr-vĕrt′) To turn from the normal; to misuse. 2. (pĕr′vĕrt) One who has turned from the normal or socially acceptable path, esp. sexually.

per vias naturales (pĕr vē′ăs năt″ū-rā′lēz) [L.]. Through natural ways.

pervigilium (pĕr″vĭ-jĭl′ē-ŭm) [L.]. Inability to sleep. SYN: *insomnia; wakefulness.*

pervious (pĕr'vē-ŭs) [L. *pervius*]. 1. Capable of being penetrated. SYN: *permeable*. 2. Penetrating.

pes (pĕs) [L.]. (pl. *pedes*) [NA] The foot or a footlike structure.

p. abductus. Talipes valgus, q.v.

p. adductus. Talipes varus, q.v.

p. anserinus. 1. Three primary branches of the facial nerve after leaving the stylomastoid foramen. 2. The tendinous expansions of the sartorius, gracilis, and semitendinosus muscles at the medial border of the tibia's tuberosity.

p. cavus. Abnormal hollowness or concavity of the sole of the foot.

p. contortus. Clubfoot. SYN: *talipes*.

p. equinovalgus. Talipes equinovalgus. The heel is elevated and turned laterally.

p. equinovarus. Talipes equinovarus. The heel is turned inward and the foot is plantar flexed.

p. equinus. Deformity marked by walking without touching the heel to the ground. SYN: *talipes equinus*.

p. gigas. An abnormally large foot. SYN: *macropodia*.

p. hippocampi. [NA] Lower portion of the hippocampus major.

p., infraorbital. Terminal radiating branches of the infraorbital nerve after exit from the infraorbital canal.

p. planus. Flatfoot.

p. valgus. Clubfoot in which sole turns outward. SYN: *talipes valgus*.

p. varus. Clubfoot in which sole turns inward. SYN: *talipes varus*.

pessary (pĕs'ă-rē) [L. *pessarium*]. A device inserted into the vagina to function as a supportive structure for the uterus.

p., cup. Pessary that has a cup-shaped hollow that fits over the os uteri.

p., diaphragm. Cup-shaped rubber pessary used as a contraceptive device.

p., Gariel's. Inflatable hollow rubber pessary.

p., Hodge's. Pessary used to correct retrodeviations of the uterus.

p., lever. Pessary design according to the principles of a lever.

p., Menge's. A ring pessary with a fixed cross bar to which a detachable stem may be affixed.

p., ring. Round pessary.

p., stem. Pessary with stem that fits into the uterine canal.

pessimism [L. *pessimus*, worst]. Morbid state of mind in which outlook toward life is gloomy or the worst interpretation is applied to events occurring; lacking in hope. Opposed to optimism.

p., therapeutic. Tendency not to believe in the effectiveness of therapeutic measures, esp. of drugs.

pest (pĕst) [L. *pestis*, plague]. 1. Fatal epidemic disease, esp. plague. 2. A noxious, destructive insect.

pesticemia (pĕs"tĭ-sē'mē-ă) [" + Gr. *haima*, blood]. Presence of plague organisms in the blood.

pesticide (pĕs'tĭ-sīd) [" + *cida*, killer]. Any chemical used to kill pests, esp. rodents and insects.

pesticide residue. The amount of any pesticide remaining on or in food or beverages intended for human consumption.

pestiferous (pĕs-tĭf'ĕr-ŭs) [L *pestiferus*]. Producing a pestilence; carrying infection. SYN: *pestilential*.

pestilence (pĕs'tĭl-ĕns) [L. *pestilentia*]. 1. An epidemic contagious disease. 2. An epidemic caused by such a disease.

pestilential (pĕs-tĭ-lĕn'shăl). Concerning or causing a pestilence. SYN: *pestiferous*.

pestis (pĕs'tĭs) [L.]. Plague.

p. ambulans. Ambulatory plague.

p. fulminans. The most severe form of plague.

p. major. P. fulminans, q.v.

p. minor. P. ambulans, q.v.

p. siderans. Septicemic plague.

p. variolosa. Smallpox.

pestle (pĕs'l) [L. *pistillum*]. Device for macerating drugs in a mortar.

petechiae (pē-tē'kē-ē) [It. *petecchia*, skin spot]. (sing. *petechia*) 1. Small, purplish, hemorrhagic spots on the skin that appear in certain severe fevers and are indicative of great prostration, as in typhus. May be due to abnormality of blood-clotting mechanism. Also applied to similar spots occurring on mucous membranes or serous surfaces. 2. Red spots from bite of a flea.

petechial (pē-tē'kē-ăl). Marked by presence of petechiae.

pethidine hydrochloride (pĕth'ĭ-dĭn). The international nonproprietary name for meperidine hydrochloride, USP, q.v.

petiole (pĕt'ē-ōl) [LL. *petiolus*]. A slender stalk or stem, as petiole of the epiglottic cartilage.

petiolus (pĕ-tī'ō-lŭs) [LL.]. The stalk or stem of a fruit. A pedicle.

p. epiglottidis. The pedicle of the cartilage of the epiglottis. It is attached to the superior notch of the thyroid cartilage.

Petit, François Pourfour du (pĕt-ē'). French anatomist and surgeon, 1664–1741.

P.'s canal. A space or cleft encircling lens between points of attachment of fibers of suspensory ligament. SYN: *zonular spaces*.

P.'s sinuses. Hollows in aortic and pulmonary arteries behind semilunar valves.

Petit, Jean Louis (pĕt-ē'). French surgeon, 1674–1750.

P.'s ligament. The uterosacral ligament.

P.'s triangle. Area on lateral abdominal wall bounded by crest of ilium, posterior margin of exterior oblique, and lateral margin of latissimus dorsi. SYN: *trigonum lumbale.*

petit mal (pĕt-ē′ măl′) [Fr., little illness]. Mild form of epileptic attack. Consciousness may be lost, but there is an absence of convulsions. SEE: *epilepsy; pyknolepsy.*

Petri dish (pā′trē). [Julius Petri, Ger. bacteriologist, 1852–1921] A shallow dish made of plastic or glass with a cover. Used to hold solid media for culturing bacteria.

petrifaction (pĕt-rĭ-făk′shŭn) [L. *petra,* stone, + *facere,* to make]. Process of changing into stone or hard substance.

petrified (pĕt′rĭ-fīd). Changed into stone; rigid.

petrify (pĕt′rĭ-fī). Convert into stone; make rigid.

pétrissage (pā″trē-săzh′) [Fr.]. A kneading movement in massage. Performed generally by the tips of the thumbs, with index finger and thumb, or with palm of hand. It is used principally on the extremities. The operator picks up a special muscle or tendon and, placing one finger on each side of the part, proceeds in centripetal motion with a firm pressure. SYN: *kneading.*

petro- [L. *petra,* stone]. Combining form meaning stone. Pert. to the petrous portion of the temporal bone.

Petrogalar. Trade name for mineral oil, USP.

petrolatoma (pĕt″rō-lă-tō′mă) [L. *petrolatum,* petroleum]. Tumor or swelling caused by introduction of liquid petrolatum under the skin.

petrolatum (pĕt″rō-lā′tŭm) [L.]. USP. A purified semisolid mixture of hydrocarbons obtained from petroleum. SYN: *paraffin, soft.*

ACTION AND USES: As a base for ointments. It is not suitable for use as a vaginal lubricant because it is not miscible in body secretion.

p., liquid. A mixture of liquid hydrocarbons obtained from petroleum.

ACTION AND USES: A vehicle for medicinal substances for local applications. Light petrolatum is employed as a spray while heavy petrolatum is given internally in treatment of constipation.

p., white. USP. Purified mixture of semisolid hydrocarbons obtained from petroleum. It is decolorized and may contain a suitable stabilizer. Trade name is Moroline.

petroleum (pĕ-trō′lē-ŭm) [L. *petra,* stone, + *oleum,* oil]. An oily inflammable liquid found in the upper strata of the earth; a hydrocarbon mixture.

petromastoid (pĕt″rō-măs′toyd). Pert. to the petrous and mastoid portions of the temporal and occipital bones.

petro-occipital (pĕt″rō-ŏk-sĭp′ĭ-tăl) [″ + *occipitalis,* occipital]. Concerning the petrous portion of the temporal bone and the occipital bone.

petropharyngeus (pĕt″rō-făr-rĭn′jē-ŭs) [″ + Gr. *pharynx,* pharynx]. A small muscle joining the lower surface of the petrous portion of the temporal bone and the pharynx. It helps to constrict the pharynx.

petrosa (pĕ-trō′să) [L., stony]. The petrous part of the temporal bone.

petrosal (pĕt-rō′săl) [L. *petrosus,* stony]. Of, pert. to, or situated near the petrous portion of the temporal bone.

petrosalpingostaphylinus (pĕt″rō-săl-pĭng″gō-stăf″ĭ-lī′nŭs) [L. *petra,* stone, + Gr. *salpinx,* tube, + *staphyle,* uvula]. Musculus levator veli palatini.

petrositis (pĕt″rō-sī′tĭs) [″ + Gr. *itis,* inflammation]. Inflamed condition of the petrous region of the temporal bone.

petrosomastoid (pĕ-trō″sō-măs′toyd) [″ + Gr. *mastos,* breast, + *eidos,* form]. Concerning the petrous portion of the temporal bone and its mastoid process.

petrosphenoid (pĕt″rō-sfē′noyd) [″ + Gr. *sphen,* wedge, + *eidos,* form]. Pert. to the petrous portion on the temporal and sphenoid bones.

petrosquamous (pĕt″rō-skwā′mŭs) [″ – *squamosus,* scaly]. Pert. to the petrous and squamous portions of the temporal bones.

petrostaphylinus (pĕt″rō-stăf″ĭ-lī′nŭs) [″ – Gr. *staphyle,* uvula]. Musculus levator veli palatini.

petrous (pĕt′rŭs) [L. *petrosus*]. 1. Resembling stone. 2. Rel. to the petrous portion of the temporal bone. SYN: *petrosal.*

petrous ganglion. Inferior ganglion of the glossopharyngeal nerve.

Peutz-Jeghers syndrome (pūtz-jā′kĕrs). [J. L. A. Peutz, 20th-cent. physician; H. Jeghers, U.S. physician, b. 1904] Polyps of the small intestine and melanin pigmentation of the lips, mucosa, fingers, and toes. Anemia due to bleeding from the intestinal polyps is a common finding. It is an inherited disorder.

pexin (pĕk′sĭn). Rennet.

-pexy [Gr. *pexis,* fixation]. A combining form meaning fixation.

Peyer's patch (pī′ĕrz). [Johann Conrad Peyer, Swiss anatomist, 1653–1712] An aggregation of solitary nodules or groups of lymph nodules found chiefly in the ileum near its junction with the colon. They are circular or oval, about 1 cm. wide and 2 to 3 cm. long. They lie in the mucosa and submucosa and always occur on side of intestine opposite to attachment of mesentery. In typhoid fever, they undergo hyperplasia and often become ulcerated. SYN: *aggregated follicles.*

peyote (pā-ō′tē). 1. The cactus plant, Lophophora williamsii, from which the hallucinogen mescaline is obtained. 2. The drug from the flowering heads, buttons, of L. williamsii, used by some Indians of the North American continent to produce altered states of consciousness. In certain tribes the buttons are used in religious ceremonies and for that reason members of that tribe are permitted to use this substance even though the drug is classed as a narcotic and its use otherwise restricted to research.

Peyronie's disease (pā-rō-nēz'). [François de la Peyronie, Fr. surgeon, 1678–1747] Hardening of the corpora cavernosa of the penis. This causes distortion or deflection of the penis, esp. when erect.

TREATMENT: The disease is self-limiting in many instances. Persistence or progression of the penile deformity requires therapy but of the several medical, surgical and radiological approaches none seem to be completely effective. There are devices that will assist the individual with the disease to participate in sexual intercourse.

Pfeiffer, Emil (fī'fĕr). German physician, 1846–1921.

P.'s disease. Infectious mononucleosis, q.v.

Pfeiffer, Richard F. (fī'fĕr). German bacteriologist, 1858–1945.

P.'s bacillus. Hemophilus influenzae.

P.'s phenomenon. A discovery announced in 1894 stating that serum of guinea pigs immunized with cholera vibrios destroyed cholera organisms in peritoneal cavity of immune and nonimmune guinea pigs and that the same reaction occurred in vitro. Also that same lytic reaction occurred with typhoid and colon bacteria.

PG. Abbr. for *prostaglandin.*

pg. *picogram.*

PGA. *pteroylglutamic acid.*

Ph. 1. *Pharmacopoeia.* SEE: *pharmacopeia.* 2. Chem. symb. for phenyl.

pH [potential of Hydrogen]. In chemistry, the degrees of acidity or alkalinity of a substance are expressed in pH values. The neutral point, where a solution would be neither acid or alkaline, is pH 7. Increasing acidity is expressed as a number less than 7 and increasing alkalinity as a number greater than 7. Maximum acidity is pH 0 and maximum alkalinity is pH 14. Because each unit on the scale represents a logarithm, there is a tenfold difference between each unit.

Ex.: pH 5 is 10 times as acid as pH 6 and pH 4 is 100 times as acid as pH 6. Expressed mathematically, pH is logarithm of the hydrogen ion concentration divided into one, i.e.,

$$\text{Log}\ \frac{1}{H^+}$$

The pH of a solution may be determined electrically by a pH meter or colorimetrically by the use of indicators. A list of indicators and the pH range registered by each is given under indicator, q.v. SEE: table.

phacitis (fă-sī'tĭs) [Gr. *phakos,* lens, + *itis,* inflammation]. Inflamed condition of the crystalline lens. SYN: *phakitis; lentitis.*

phaco- [Gr. *phakos*]. Prefix pert. to lens of the eye.

phacoanaphylaxis (făk"ō-ăn"ă-fī-lăk'sĭs) [" + *ana,* excessive, + *phylaxis,* protection]. Hypersensitivity to protein of the crystalline lens.

phacocele (făk'ō-sēl) [" + *kele,* hernia]. Displacement of the crystalline lens into the interior chamber of the eye. SYN: *phacometachoresis.*

phacocyst (făk'ō-sĭst) [Gr. *phakos,* lens, + *kystis,* a sac]. Capsule of the crystalline lens.

phacocystectomy (făk"ō-sĭs-tĕk'tō-mē) [" + " + *ektome,* excision]. Surgical excision of part of crystalline lens capsule for treatment of cataract.

phacocystitis (făk"ō-sĭs-tī'tĭs) [" + " + *itis,* inflammation]. Inflamed condition of the capsule of the crystalline lens.

phacoemulsification (făk"ō-ē-mŭl'sĭ-fĭ-kā"shŭn). A method of treating cataracts of the crystalline lens of the eye. An ultrasonic device is used to disintegrate the cataract, which is then aspirated and removed.

phacoerysis (făk"ō-ĕr-ē'sĭs) [" + *eresis,* removal]. Removal of the lens of the eye by attaching a suction device, an erysiphake, to it. SEE: *erysiphake.*

phacoglaucoma (făk"ō-glaw-kō'mă) [" + *glaukos,* green, + *oma,* tumor]. Glaucoma and the changes it induces in the crystalline lens. SEE: *glaucoma.*

phacohymenitis (făk"ō-hī"mĕn-ī'tĭs) [" + *hymen,* membrane, + *itis,* inflammation]. Inflamed condition of the capsule of the crystalline lens.

phacoid (făk'oyd) [" + *eidos,* form]. Lentil- or lens-shaped.

phacoiditis (făk"oy-dī'tĭs) [" + " + *itis,* inflammation]. Phakitis, q.v.

pH of Some Fluids

Material	pH
Decinormal HCl	1.0
Gastric juice	1.0 to 5.0
Thousandth-normal HCl	3.0
Pure water (neutral) at 25° C	7.0
Blood plasma	7.35 to 7.45
Pancreatic juice	8.4 to 8.9
Thousandth-normal NaOH	11.0
Decinormal NaOH	13.0

phacoidoscope (fă-koyd′ō-skōp) [″ + ″ + *skopein,* to examine]. Instrument for observing accommodative changes of the lens. SYN: *phacoscope.*

phacolysis (făk-ŏl′ĭ-sĭs) [″ + *lysis,* dissolution]. 1. Dissection and removal of the lens of the eye in treatment of cataract. 2. Any dissolution or disintegration of the crystalline lens.

phacoma (fă-kō′mă) [″ + *oma,* tumor]. Phakoma, q.v.

phacomalacia (făk″ō-mă-lā′shē-ă) [″ + *malakia,* softening]. A softening of the lens usually due to a soft cataract.

phacomatosis (fă″kō-mă-tō′sĭs) [″ + *oma,* tumor, + *osis,* condition]. One of a group of diseases that are congenital and probably hereditary in origin, manifested by cutaneous and neurological syndromes. They include the following: neurofibromatosis (von Recklinghausen's disease); von Hippel-Lindau disease; Sturge-Weber syndrome; and tuberous sclerosis. SYN: *neurodermatosis.*

phacometachoresis (făk″ō-mĕt″ă-kō-rē′sĭs) [″ + *metachoresis,* displacement]. Dislocation of the crystalline lens. SYN: *phacocele.*

phacometer (făk-ŏm′ĕ-tĕr) [Gr. *phakos,* lens, + *metron,* measure]. Device for ascertaining refractive power of a lens.

phacoplanesis (făk″ō-plăn-ē′sĭs) [″ + *planesis,* wandering]. Abnormal mobility of the crystalline lens.

phacosclerosis (făk″ō-sklĕr-ō′sĭs) [″ + *sklerosis,* a hardening]. Hardening of crystalline lens of the eye.

phacoscope (făk′ō-skōp) [″ + *skopein,* to examine]. Instrument for observing change of curvature of crystalline lens during accommodation.

phacoscotasmus (făk″ō-skō-tăs′mŭs) [″ + *skotasmos,* clouding]. Clouding of crystalline lens of the eye.

phacotoxic (făk″ō-tŏk′sĭk) [″ + *toxikon,* poison]. Concerning the toxicity of material in the lens of the eye.

Phaedra complex. [Wife of King Theseus of Athens] The love and attraction between a stepparent and a stepchild. So named because of Phaedra's tragic love for the son (Hippolytus) of her husband by a previous marriage.

phag-, phago- [Gr. *phagein,* to eat]. Combining form meaning an eater, or pert. to ingestion, or engulfing.

phage (fāj) [Gr. *phagein,* to eat]. A virus with a specific affinity for inducing lysis of certain bacterial cells. Phages are widely distributed in nature, and have been isolated in feces, sewage, and polluted surface waters. They are regarded as bacterial viruses, the phage particle consisting of a head composed of RNA or DNA and a tail by which it attaches to host cells. SYN: *bacteriophage.*

phagedena (făj-ē-dē′nă) [Gr. *phagedaina*]. A sloughing ulcer that spreads rapidly.

p., sloughing. Hospital gangrene; bedsores.

phagedenic (făj-ē-dĕn′ĭk). Concerning, or of the nature of, phagedena.

phage typing. A method of identifying particular strains of bacteria that are lysed only by strain-specific bacteriophages.

phagocyte (făg′ō-sīt) [Gr. *phagein,* to eat, + *kytos,* cell]. A cell that has the ability to ingest and destroy particulate substances such as bacteria, protozoa, cells and cell debris, dust particles, and colloids by ingesting them.

Ex.: Cells of the reticuloendothelial system (macrophages or histiocytes, reticular cells of lymph nodes, Kupffer's cells of liver, dust cells of lung) and leukocytes. SEE: *histiocyte; macrophage; reticuloendothelial system.*

phagocytic (făg″ō-sĭt′ĭk). Concerning phagocytes or phagocytosis.

phagocytic index. The average number of bacteria ingested by each leukocyte after incubation of the bacteria in a mixture of serum and bacterial culture. SEE: *opsonic index.*

phagocytize (făg′ō-sīt″īz). The ingestion of bacteria and foreign particles by phagocytes.

phagocytoblast (făg″ō-sī′tō-blăst) [″ + ″ + *blastos,* germ]. A cell that develops into a phagocyte.

phagocytolysis (făg″ō-sī-tŏl′ĭ-sĭs) [″ + *kytos,* cell, + *lysis,* dissolution]. Destruction or disintegration of phagocytes. SYN: *phagolysis.*

phagocytolytic (făg″ō-sī″tō-lĭt′ĭk). Destroying phagocytes.

phagocytose (făg″ō-sī′tōs) [″ + *kytos,* cell]. Phagocytize, q.v.

phagocytosis (făg″ō-sī-tō′sĭs) [″ + ″ + *osis,* condition]. Ingestion and digestion of bacteria and particles by phagocytes. SEE: illus.

p., induced. Phagocytosis that is aided or stimulated by the effect of serum opsonins or bacteria.

p., spontaneous. Phagocytosis occurring in an indifferent medium such as physiologic salt solution.

phagodynamometer (făg″ō-dī″nă-mŏm′ĕ-tĕr) [″ + *dynamis,* power, + *metron,* measure]. Device that measures energy expended in chewing food.

phagokaryosis (făg″ō-kăr″ē-ō′sĭs) [″ + *karyon,* nucleus, + *osis,* condition]. Phagocytic action that is performed by a cell nucleus.

phagolysis (făg-ŏl′ĭ-sĭs) [″ + *lysis,* dissolution]. Disintegration of phagocytes. SYN: *phagocytolysis.*

phagomania (făg″ō-mā′nē-ă) [″ + *mania,* madness]. Abnormal craving for food.

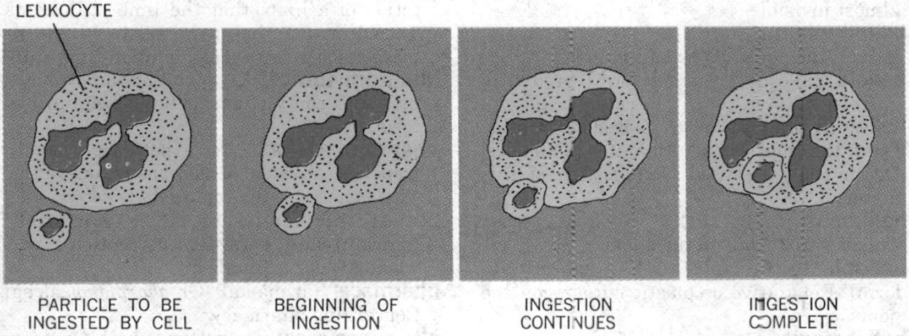

PHAGOCYTOSIS

phagophobia (făg″ō-fō′bē-ă) [″ + *phobos,* fear]. Dread of being eaten.

phagopyrism (făg″ō-pī′rĭzm) [″ + *pyr,* fever, + *-ismos,* condition]. Hypersensitiveness to certain foods that induce symptoms of poisoning upon ingestion.

phagotherapy (făg″ō-thĕr′ă-pē) [″ + *therapeia,* treatment]. Treatment by feeding or overfeeding.

phagotype (făg′ō-tīp) [″ + *typos,* mark]. The classification of bacteria by their sensitivity to phage types. SEE: *phage typing.*

phakitis (făk-ī′tĭs) [Gr. *phakos,* lens, + *itis,* inflammation]. Inflamed condition of the crystalline lens of the eye. SYN: *phacitis; lentitis.*

phakolysis (făk-ŏl′ĭ-sĭs) [″ + *lysis,* dissolution]. Disintegration or removal of the crystalline lens of the eye. SYN: *phacolysis.*

phakoma (fă-kō′mă) [″ + *oma,* tumor]. 1. Microscopic gray white tumor present in the retina in tuberous sclerosis. 2. Area of myelinated nerve fibers rarely seen in the retina in association with neurofibromatosis.

phalacrosis (făl-ă-krō′sĭs) [Gr. *phalakrosis*]. Baldness. SYN: *alopecia.*

phalacrotic (făl-ă-krŏt′ĭk). Bald; bald-headed.

phalacrous (făl-ăk′rŭs). Bald. SYN: *phalacrotic.*

phalangeal (fă-lăn′jē-ăl) [Gr. *phalanx,* closely knit row]. Concerning a phalanx.

phalangeal cells, inner. A row of cells along surface of inner pillar cells in the organ of Corti.

phalangeal cells, outer. Cells arranged in rows that support the outer hair cells in the organ of Corti. SYN: *Deiters' cells.*

phalangectomy (făl-ăn-jĕk′tō-mē) [″ + *ektome,* excision]. Excision of one or more phalanges.

phalanges (fă-lăn′jēz). (sing. *phalanx*) [NA] Bones of a finger or toe. SEE: *skeleton.*

phalangette (făl″ăn-jĕt′). The distal phalanx of a digit.

p., drop. Falling of the distal phalanx of a digit with loss of power to extend it when the hand is prone. This is due to trauma or overstretching of the extensor tendon.

phalangitis (făl″ăn-jī′tĭs) [Gr *phalanx,* closely knit row, + *itis,* inflammation]. Inflamed condition of one or more phalanges.

phalanx (făl′ănks) [Gr., closely knit row]. (pl. *phalanges*) 1. [NA] Any one of the bones of the fingers or toes. 2. One of a set of plates formed of phalangeal cells (inner and outer) forming the reticular membrane of the organ of Corti.

p., distal. The phalanx most remote from the metacarpus or metatarsus. SYN: *p., terminal; p., ungual; p., ungucular.*

p., metacarpal. Any phalanx that articulates with a metacarpal bone. SYN: *p., proximal.*

p., metatarsal. Any phalanx that articulates with a metatarsal bone. SYN: *p., proximal.*

p., middle. The phalanx (where there are three) intermediate between distal and proximal phalanges.

p., proximal. Any phalanx that articulates with a metacarpal or metatarsal bone.

p., terminal. P., distal.

p., ungual. P., distal. SYN: *p., terminal.*

phallalgia (făl-ăl′jē-ă) [Gr. *phallos,* penis, + *algos,* pain]. Pain in the penis.

phallectomy (făl-ĕk′tō-mē) [″ + *ektome,* excision]. Surgical removal of the penis.

phallic (făl′ĭk). Concerning the penis.

phalliform (făl′ĭ-form) [″ + L. *forma,* form]. Shaped like a penis.

phallitis (făl-ī′tĭs) [″ + *itis,* inflammation]. Inflamed condition of the penis.

phallocampsis (făl-ō-kămp′sĭs) [″ + *kampsis,* a bending]. Painful downward curvature of the penis when erect.

phallocrypsis (făl″ō-krĭp′sĭs [″ + *krypsis,*

hiding]. Contraction of the penis so that it is almost invisible.

phallodynia (făl-ō-dĭn'ē-ă) [" + *odyne*, pain]. Pain in the penis. SYN: *phallalgia*.

phalloid (făl'oyd) [" + *eidos*, form]. Similar to a penis.

phalloidin (fă-loyd'ĭn). A poisonous peptide from the mushroom Amanita phalloides. Death can be caused by ingestion of this material.

phalloncus (făl-ŏn'kŭs) [" + *onkos*, mass]. Tumor or swelling on the penis.

phalloplasty (făl'ō-plăs"tē) [" + *plassein*, to form]. Reparative or plastic surgery on the penis.

phallorrhagia (făl-ō-rā'jē-ă) [" + *rhegnynai*, to burst forth]. Hemorrhage from the penis.

phallus (făl'ŭs) [Gr. *phallos*, penis]. 1. The penis. 2. An artificial penis, used as a symbol. 3. Embryonic structure developing at tip of the genital tubercle that, in the male, develops into the penis and, in the female, the clitoris.

phanero-, phaner- [Gr. *phaneros*, visible]. Combining forms meaning evident, visible.

phanerogenic (făn"ĕr-ō-jĕn'ĭk) [" + *gennan*, to produce]. Indicating a disease with a known cause.

phaneromania (făn"ĕr-ō-mā'nē-ă) [" + *mania*, madness]. Abnormal tendency to bite the nails or pick, scratch, or pull a pimple, wart, hair, beard, or mustache.

phanerosis (făn"ĕr-ō'sĭs) [Gr.]. The process of becoming visible.

phanic (făn'ĭk) [Gr. *phainein*, to show]. Manifest; apparent.

phantasia (făn-tā'zē-ă) [Gr.]. An appearance that is imaginary.

phantasm (făn'tăzm) [Gr. *phantasma*]. An optical illusion; an apparition, or illusion of something that does not exist.

phantasmatomoria (făn-tăz"măt-ō-mō'rē-ă) [" + *moria*, folly]. Dementia with silly fancies; childishness in the demented.

phantasmology (făn"tăz-mŏl'ō-jē) [" + *logos*, study]. The study of dreams, phantoms, and spiritually derived apparitions.

phantasy (făn'tă-sē) [Gr. *phantasia*, imagination]. A daydream. Phantasy-thinking is a form of wish fulfillment, a disregard for reality, from which one would escape through revelling in imaginative possibilities.

RS: delirium; delusion; hallucination; hysteria; illusion; phobia.

phantogeusia (făn-tō-gū'sē-ă) [" + *geusis*, taste]. An intermittent or persistent taste sensation in the mouth not produced by an external stimulus.

phantom (făn'tŭm) [Gr. *phantasma*, an appearance.]. 1. An apparition. 2. A model of the body or of one of its parts.

phantom corpuscle. A colorless erythrocyte.

phantom limb. An illusion, following amputation of a limb, that the limb still exists. The sensation that pain exists in the removed part is known as phantom-limb pain.

phantom tumor. An apparent tumor due to muscular contractions or flatus seen in hysteria.

phantom vision. An experience, usually transient, of visual sensations in an eye that has been surgically removed.

phantosmia (făn-tŏs'mē-ă) [" + *osme*, smell]. Intermittent or persistent perception of odor when no odor is inhaled.

pharmacal (făr'mă-kăl) [Gr. *pharmakon*, drug]. Concerning pharmacy.

pharmaceutical (făr-mă-sū'tĭ-kăl) [Gr. *pharmakeutikos*]. Concerning drugs or pharmacy.

pharmaceutical chemistry. The chemistry of medicines, their composition, synthesis, analysis, storage, and actions.

pharmaceutics (făr-mă-sū'tĭks). Science of dispensing medicines. SYN: *pharmacy*.

pharmacist (făr'mă-sĭst) [Gr. *pharmakon*, drug]. A druggist; one licensed to prepare and dispense drugs. SYN: *apothecary*.

pharmaco- [Gr. *pharmakon*, drug]. Combining form meaning drug, medicine, poison.

pharmacochemistry (făr"mă-kō-kĕm'ĭs-trē) [" + *chemeia*, chemistry]. Pharmaceutical chemistry, q.v.

pharmacodiagnosis (făr"mă-kō-dī"ăg-nō'sĭs) [" + *dia*, through, + *gnosis*, knowledge]. Use of drugs in making a diagnosis.

pharmacodynamics (făr"mă-kō-dī-nam'ĭks) [" + *dynamis*, power]. Study of drugs and their actions on living organisms.

pharmacoendocrinology (făr"mă-kō-ĕn"dō-krĭ-nŏl'ō-jē) [" + *endon*, within, + *krinein*, to secrete, + *logos*, study]. The pharmacology of the function of endocrine glands.

pharmacogenetics (făr"mă-kō-jĕn-ĕt'ĭks) [" + *genesis*, production]. Study of the influence of hereditary factors on response of individual organisms to drugs.

pharmacognosy (făr"mă-kŏg'nō-sē) [" + *gnosis*, knowledge]. The science of natural drugs and their physical, botanical, and chemical properties.

pharmacography (făr"mă-kŏg'ră-fē) [" + *graphein*, to write]. Treatise on the properties of drugs.

pharmacokinetics (făr"mă-kō-kī-nĕt'ĭks). Study of the metabolism and action of drugs with particular emphasis on the time required for absorption, duration of action, distribution in the body, and method of excretion.

pharmacologist (făr"mă-kŏl'ō-jĭst). An individual who by training and experience is a specialist in pharmacology.

pharmacology (făr"mă-kŏl'ō-jē) [" + *logos*, a study]. The study of drugs and their origin, nature, properties, and effects upon living organisms.

pharmacomania (făr″mă-kō-mā′nē-ă) [″ + *mania,* madness]. Abnormal desire for giving or taking medicines.

pharmacopedia (făr″mă-kō-pē′dē-ă) [″ + *paideia,* education]. Information concerning drugs and their preparation.

pharmacopeia (far″mă-kō-pē′ă) [Gr. *pharmakopoeia,* preparation of drugs]. Authorized treatise on drugs and their preparation, esp. a book containing formulas and information that provide a standard for preparation and dispensation of drugs.

Pharmacopeia, United States. ABBR: USP. A pharmacopeia issued every five years, prepared under supervision of a national committee of pharmacists, pharmacologists, physicians, chemists, biologists, and other scientific and allied personnel. The United States Pharmacopeia was adopted as standard in 1906. Beginning with the U.S. Pharmacopeia XIX, 1975, the National Formulary has been included in that publication.

pharmacophilia (făr″mă-kō-fĭl′ē-ă) [Gr. *pharmakon,* drug, + *philos,* love]. Pathological fondness for drugs and medicines.

pharmacophobia (făr″mă-kō-fō′bē-ă) [″ + *phobos,* fear]. Abnormal fear of taking medicines.

pharmacophore (făr′mă-kō-for) [″ + *phoros,* bearing]. The particular group or arrangement of atoms in a molecule that gives the material its medicinal activity.

pharmacopsychosis (făr″mă-kō-sī-kō′sĭs) [″ + *psyche,* soul, + *osis,* condition]. Mental disorder associated with addiction to drugs or alcohol.

pharmacotherapy (făr″mă-kō-thĕr′ă-pē) [″ + *therapeia,* treatment]. Use of medicine in treatment of disease.

pharmacy (făr′mă-sē) [Gr. *pharmakon,* drug]. 1. The practice of compounding and dispensing medicinal preparations. 2. A drugstore.

Pharm.D. *Doctor of Pharmacy.*

pharyngalgia (făr″ĭn-găl′jē-ă) [Gr. *pharynx,* pharynx, + *algos,* pain]. Pain in the pharynx. SYN: *pharyngodynia.*

pharyngeal (făr-ĭn′jē-ăl) [L. *pharyngeus*]. Concerning the pharynx.

pharyngeal bursa. A small blind sac often present in lower portion of pharyngeal tonsil.

pharyngeal hypophysis. A small structure anterior to pharyngeal bursa. It is derived from the lower portion of Rathke's pouch and occasionally gives rise to a cyst or tumor.

pharyngeal reflex. Attempt to swallow following any application of stimulus to pharynx.

pharyngeal tonsil. Lymphoid tissue on posterior superior wall of the pharynx. When hypertrophied, it is called adenoids, q.v.

pharyngectomy (făr-ĭn-jĕk′tō-mē) [″ + *ektome,* excision]. Partial excision of the pharynx to remove growths or abscesses.

pharyngemphraxis (făr″ĭn-jĕm-frăk′sĭs) [″ + *emphraxis,* stoppage]. Pharyngeal obstruction.

pharyngismus (făr″ĭn-jĭz′mŭs) [″ + *-ismos,* condition]. Spasm of the muscles in the pharynx. SYN: *pharyngospasm.*

pharyngitis (făr″ĭn-jī′tĭs) [″ + *itis,* inflammation]. Inflammation of pharynx.

p., acute. Inflammation of the pharynx with pain in the throat.

SYM: Malaise, fever, dysphagia, pain in throat, postnasal secretion.

TREATMENT: *Local:* Gargles, lozenges, topical application to oral pharynx. *General:* Bedrest, adequate fluids, analgesics. Appropriate antibiotic after material has been taken for bacterial study, esp. for beta-hemolytic streptococci.

p., atrophic. Chronic form of pharyngitis with some atrophy of mucous glands and abnormal secretion. SYN: *p sicca.*

p., chronic. Pharyngitis associated with pathology in nose and sinuses, mouth breathing, excessive smoking, and chronic tonsillitis.

SYM: Dryness and irritation of throat; cough.

TREATMENT: Intranasal medication and removal of pathological factors in sinuses; tonsillectomy.

p., croupous. Pharyngitis with the false membrane of croup.

p., diphtheritic. Sore throat with general symptoms of diphtheria and formation of a true membrane.

p., follicular. P., granular.

p., gangrenous. Gangrenous inflammation of mucous membrane of the pharynx. SYN: *angina maligna.*

p., granular. Chronic pharyngitis with granulations seen on the pharynx. SYN: *p., follicular.*

p. herpetica. Pharyngitis characterized by formation of vesicles and ulcers.

p., hypertrophic. A chronic form with thickened red mucous membrane on each side with a glazed central portion.

p., membranous. Pharyngitis in which there is a membranous exudate that forms a false membrane.

p. sicca. P., atrophic.

p. ulcerosa. Pharyngitis with fever, pain, and the formation of ulcerations.

pharyngo- [Gr. *pharynx,* pharynx]. Combining form pert. to the pharynx.

pharyngoamygdalitis (fă-rĭn″gō-ă-mĭg″dăl-ī′tĭs) [″ + *amygdale,* tonsil, + *itis,* inflammation]. Inflamed condition of the pharynx and tonsil.

pharyngocele (făr-ĭn′gō-sēl) [″ + *kele,* hernia]. Hernia through pharyngeal wall.

pharyngoceratosis (fă-rĭng″gō-sĕr″ă-tō′sĭs) [″ + *keras,* horn, + *osis,* condition]. Pharyngokeratosis, q.v.

pharyngoconjunctival fever, acute. ABBR: APC. A form of acute disease consisting of fever, pharyngitis, and conjunctivitis. ETIOL: Adenovirus Type 3. It is particularly predisposed to occur in children in summer camp, and may temporarily disable more than half of the campers in a few weeks. Treatment is symptomatic.

pharyngodynia (făr-ĭn″gō-dĭn′ē-ă) [″ + *odyne,* pain]. Pain in the pharynx. SYN: *pharyngalgia.*

pharyngoepiglottic, pharyngoepiglottidean (fă-rĭng″gō-ĕp″ĭ-glŏt′ĭk, -glŏ-tĭd′ē-ăn) [″ + *epi,* upon, + *glottis,* glottis]. Concerning the pharynx and the glottis.

pharyngoesophageal (fă-rĭng″gō-ē-sŏf′ă-jē″ăl) [″ + *oisophagos,* esophagus]. Concerning the pharynx and the esophagus.

pharyngoglossal (fă-rĭng″gō-glŏs′ăl) [″ + *glossa,* tongue]. Concerning the pharynx and the tongue.

pharyngography. Radiographic examination of the pharynx after ingestion of a contrast medium.

pharyngokeratosis (făr-ĭn″gō-kĕr″ă-tō′sĭs) [″ + *keras,* horn, + *osis,* condition]. Thickening and hardening of mucous lining of the pharynx.

pharyngolaryngeal (fă-rĭng″gō-lă-rĭn′jē-ăl) [″ + *larynx,* larynx]. Concerning the pharynx and the larynx.

pharyngolaryngitis (făr-ĭn″gō-lăr-ĭn-jī′tĭs) [″ + ″ + *itis,* inflammation]. Inflamed condition of the pharynx and larynx. SYN: *laryngopharyngitis.*

pharyngolith (făr-ĭn′gō-lĭth) [″ + *lithos,* stone] Concretion in pharyngeal walls.

pharyngology (făr″ĭn-gŏl′ō-jē) [″ + *logos,* a study]. Branch of medicine dealing with the pharynx.

pharyngolysis (făr″ĭn-gŏl′ĭ-sĭs) [″ + *lysis,* dissolution]. Paralysis of the pharynx.

pharyngomaxillary (fă-rĭng″gō-măk′sĭ-lĕr″ē) [Gr. *pharynx,* pharynx, + L. *maxilla,* jawbone]. Concerning the pharynx and the maxillae.

pharyngomycosis (făr-ĭn″gō-mī-kō′sĭs) [″ + *mykes,* fungus, + *osis,* condition]. Disease of the pharynx due to fungi.

pharyngonasal (fă-rĭng″gō-nā′săl) [″ + L. *nasus,* nose]. Concerning the pharynx and the nose.

pharyngo-oral (fă-rĭng″gō-ō′răl) [″ + L. *os,* mouth]. Concerning the pharynx and the mouth.

pharyngopalatine (fă-rĭng″gō-păl′ă-tīn) [″ + L. *palatum,* palate]. Concerning the pharynx and the palate.

pharyngoparalysis (făr-ĭn″gō-păr-ăl′ĭ-sĭs) [″ + *paralysis,* a loosening at the side]. Paralysis of the muscles of the pharynx. SYN: *pharyngoplegia.*

pharyngopathy (făr″ĭn-gŏp′ă-thē) [″ + *pathos,* disease]. Any disorder of the pharynx.

pharyngoperistole (făr-ĭn″gō-pĕr-ĭs′tō-lē) [″ + *peristole,* contracture]. Narrowing or stricture of the lumen of the pharynx.

pharyngoplasty (făr-ĭn′gō-plăs″tē) [″ + *plassein,* to form]. Reparative surgery of the pharynx.

pharyngoplegia (făr-ĭn″gō-plē′jē-ă) [″ + *plege,* a stroke]. Paralysis of muscles of the pharynx. SYN: *pharyngoparalysis.*

pharyngorhinitis (făr-ĭn″gō-rī-nī′tĭs) [″ + *rhis,* nose, + *itis,* inflammation]. Inflamed condition of the nasopharynx.

pharyngorhinoscopy (făr-ĭn″gō-rī-nŏs′ko-pē) [″ + ″ + *skopein,* to examine]. Inspection of the nasopharynx and posterior nares.

pharyngorrhea (făr″ĭn-gō-rē′ă) [″ + *rhoia,* flow]. Discharge of mucus from the pharynx.

pharyngoscleroma (făr-rĭng″gō-sklē-rō′mă) [″ + *skleroma,* induration]. An indurated patch, or scleroma, in the pharynx.

pharyngoscope (făr-ĭn′gō-skōp) [Gr. *pharynx,* pharynx, + *skopein,* to examine]. Instrument for visual examination of the pharynx.

pharyngoscopy (făr″ĭn-gŏs′kō-pē). Visual examination of the pharynx.

pharyngospasm (făr-ĭn′gō-spăzm) [″ + *spasmos,* a spasm]. Spasmodic contraction of muscles of the pharynx. SYN: *pharyngismus.*

pharyngostenosis (fă-rĭng″gō-stē-nō′sĭs) [″ + *stenosis,* narrowing]. Narrowing or stricture of the pharynx.

pharyngotherapy (făr-ĭn″gō-thĕr′ă-pē) [″ + *therapeia,* treatment]. Treatment of pharyngeal disturbances or diseases.

pharyngotome (făr-ĭn′gō-tōm) [″ + *tome,* incision]. Instrument for incision of the pharynx.

pharyngotomy (făr-ĭn-gŏt′ō-mē). Incision of the pharynx.

pharyngotonsillitis (fă-rĭng″gō-tŏn″sĭ-lī′tĭs) [″ + L. *tonsilla,* almond, + Gr. *itis,* inflammation]. Inflammation of the pharynx and the tonsils.

pharyngoxerosis (fă-rĭng″gō-zē-rō′sĭs) [″ + *xerosis,* dryness]. Dryness of the pharynx.

pharynx (făr′ĭnks) [Gr.]. (pl. *pharynges*) [NA] Passageway for air from nasal cavity to larynx and food from mouth to esophagus. Also acts as a resonating cavity. A musculomembranous tube extending from base of skull to level of the 6th vertebra, where it becomes continuous with the esophagus. Upper portion is lined with pseudostratified ciliated epithelium, middle portion with stratified columnar epithelium, and lower portion with stratified squamous epithelium.

Communicates with the posterior nares, eustachian tube, mouth, esophagus, and larynx. The nasopharynx is the section above the palate; the oropharynx lies between the palate and hyoid bone; and the laryngopharynx is below the hyoid bone.

The nerves are autonomic, vagus, and glossopharyngeal. Blood vessels branch from the exterior carotid artery. Veins form an extensive pharyngeal plexus and drain into the interior jugular vein. SEE: *mouth* for illus.

phase (fāz) [Gr. *phasis,* an appearance]. 1. A stage of development. 2. A transitory appearance. 3. The state of a component of a heterogeneous system, as when oil is mixed with water, which is homogeneous throughout itself and bounded by an interface with other phases of the system.

p., continuous. State of substance in a heterogeneous system in which particles are continuous.

Ex.: The water particles in which oil has been dispersed.

p., disperse. State of a substance in a heterogeneous system in which particles are separated from each other.

Ex.: Oil particles in water.

phase-shift balloon pumping. A device for aiding circulation of blood. A balloon attached to a catheter is inserted through the femoral artery in the aorta. As the heart rests in diastole, the balloon is quickly filled with helium so that blood is forced on its way peripherally as well as into the coronary arteries. The balloon, which is 15 cm. long, deflates just before systole. This inflation-deflation cycle is timed and activated by the electrical activity of the patient's heart. This complicated device requires a team of physicians and nurses to work it. It is used as an emergency procedure in patients with shock due to myocardial infarction.

phasic (fā'sĭk). Of, or pert. to, a phase.

phatnorrhagia (făt"nō-rā'jē-ă) [" + *rhegnynai,* to burst forth]. Hemorrhage from the socket of a tooth.

Ph.D. *Doctor of Philosophy.*

Phe. *phenylalanine.*

phenacaine hydrochloride (fĕn'ă-kān). USP. A local anesthetic drug used in ophthalmology.

phenacemide (fĕ-năs'ĕ-mīd). USP. An anticonvulsive drug. Serious adverse side effects limit its usefulness. Trade name is Phenurone.

phenacetin (fĕ-năs'ĕ-tĭn). USP. An analgesic and antipyretic drug.

phenakistoscope (fē"nă-kĭs'tō-skōp) [Gr. *phenakistos,* deceiver, + *skopein,* to view]. A device that produces a stroboscopic-like view of the figures seen through slits that revolve in the same direction. The figures are seen in a mirror, and they appear to move.

phenanthrene (fē-năn'thrēn). A coal tar derivative, $C_{14}H_{10}$, that is carcinogenic.

Phenaphen. Trade name for acetaminophen, USP.

phenate (fē'nāt). A salt of phenic acid (phenol).

phenazopyridine hydrochloride (fĕn"ă-zō-pēr'ĭ-dēn). USP. A drug with analgesic action on the urinary tract. It causes a red or orange color of the urine. Trade name is Pyridium.

phencyclidine hydrochloride. An anesthetic used in veterinary medicine. It is also used illegally as a hallucinogen, referred to as PCP or angel dust. Moderate doses cause elevated blood pressure, rapid pulse, increased skeletal muscle tone and sometimes, myoclonic jerks. Large doses can cause seizures, ataxia, nystagmus, respiratory depression and death. Pupils are usually of normal size or small.

TREATMENT: For agitation caused by acute intoxication, diazepam is indicated. After initial therapy the patient should be observed in a quiet room. Efforts to "talk down" the patient are contraindicated.

phenelzine sulfate (fĕn'ĕl-zēn). USP. An antidepressant drug. Trade name is Nardil.

Phenergan. Trade name for promethazine hydrochloride, USP.

phenethicillin potassium (fĕ-nĕth"ĭ-sĭl'ĭn). USP. A penicillin that may be used orally because its activity is not appreciably affected by gastric acid. Trade names are Syncillin and Maxipen.

phenformin hydrochloride (fĕn-for'mĭn). An oral hypoglycemic agent that is no longer marketed in the U.S.A. because of its tendency to cause lactic acidosis.

phengophobia (fĕn"gō-fō'bē-ă) [Gr. *phengos,* light, + *phobos,* fear]. Abnormal dread of light. SYN: *photophobia.*

phenic acid (fē'nĭk). Phenol.

phenindione (fĕn"ĭn-dī'ōn). USP. An anticoagulant drug. Trade name is Hedulin.

pheniramine maleate (fĕn-ĭr'ă-mēn). An antihistamine drug. Trade name is Inhiston.

phenmetrazine hydrochloride (fĕn-mĕt'ră-zēn). A sympathomimetic drug. Its effectiveness in treating obesity is unpredictable. Trade name is Preludin.

phenobarbital (fē"nō-băr'bĭ-tăl). USP. Phenylethylbarbituric acid, a white crystalline substance soluble in alcohol. Trade names are Eskabarb, Luminal, SK-phenobarbital, Sulfoton, and Talpheno.

ACTION AND USES: A hypnotic, long-acting sedative, and anticonvulsant. Used, often in combination with diphenylhydantoin sodium, in treatment of epilepsy because it has a depressive effect on motor areas of the cerebral cortex.

p., sodium. USP. Soluble phenobarbital. More rapidly absorbed than phenobarbital but has the same uses. Trade name is Luminal sodium.

phenocopy (fē'nō-kŏp″ē) [Gr. *phainein,* to show, + *copy*]. An individual with a biochemical or physical characteristic that resembles that produced by a genetic mutation, but is instead due to an environmental condition.

phenol (fē'nōl). USP. C_6H_5OH. 1. A crystalline, colorless or light pink solid, melting at 43° C., obtained from the distillation of coal tar. It has a characteristic odor, and is dangerous because of its rapid corrosive action on tissues. When used carefully and properly diluted, it is effective as a bacteriostatic agent. SYN: *carbolic acid; phenic acid.* 2. Any of the aromatic derivatives of benzene with one or more hydroxyl groups attached.

p. red. An indicator used in determining hydrogen ion concentration.

Phenolax. Trade name for phenolphthalein.

phenolemia (fē″nō-lē'mē-ă) [*phenol* + Gr. *haima,* blood]. Presence of phenol in the blood.

phenology (fē-nŏl'ō-jē) [Gr. *phainesthai,* to appear, + *logos,* study]. Study of the effects of climate on living things.

phenolphthalein (fē″nŏl-thăl'ē-ĭn, fē″nōl-thăl'ēn). USP. A white or yellowish crystallized powder, produced by the interaction of phenol and phthalic anhydride. Trade names are Phenolax and Evac-Q-Tabs.

ACTION AND USES: Laxative.

phenol poisoning. Phenol is rapidly corrosive on tissues.

SYM: Strong solutions cause burning pain and, later, anesthesia. The skin and mucous membrane first become pale, then grayish-white, opalescent, and finally brown to black. Even a 1% solution may cause local gangrene. It is absorbed from intact skin wounds and mucous membrane to cause general effects, including collapse and coma. When taken by mouth, it causes whitish discoloration of mucous membranes, intense burning, nausea and rarely vomiting, followed shortly by faintness, weakness, and collapse. Pulse slow and weak and hypothermia with respiratory arrest may be present. Perspiration is increased and there is renal damage. Profound coma may occur within 30 minutes of exposure of skin to phenol.

NURSING IMPLICATIONS: Remove poison from stomach as soon as possible. While waiting to do this, administer 5 to 6 tsp. (25 to 30 ml.) of activated charcoal in water. Turn the patient from side to side to ensure all portions of the stomach come in contact with the charcoal.

A well-lubricated gastric tube should be used with caution. Give extensive lavage with charcoal. If this isn't available, use olive oil, leaving some in the stomach. If olive oil is not available, use cottonseed oil or water. Do not use ethyl alcohol as lavage fluid because it speeds absorption of phenol. Demulcents such as egg whites or milk may be left in the stomach when lavage is finished.

Remove contaminated clothing instantly and wash external burns with large amounts of water or with olive oil. Use external heat, oxygen therapy, and morphine as required. Intravenous sodium bicarbonate may provide symptomatic relief, but its mechanism of action is not understood.

PROG: A guarded prognosis should always be given because, although the patient may improve at first, damage to the mucous membrane and absorption of phenol may lead to serious complications later.

phenolsulfonphthalein (fē″nŏl-sŭl″fōn-thăl'ē-ĭn). USP. A dye that is given parenterally. It is used to test renal function.

phenoluria (fē″nŏl-ū'rē-ă). Elimination of phenols in the urine.

phenomenology (fē-nŏm″ē-nŏl'ō-jē) [Gr. *phainomenon,* appearing + *logos,* study]. The study and classification of phenomena.

phenomenon (fē-nŏm'ē-nŏn) [Gr. *phainomenon,* appearing]. (pl. *phenomena*) A change, perceivable by the senses, that occurs in an organ or vital function; an objective symptom.

p., Bell's. Rolling of the eyeball upward and outward when an attempt is made to close the eye on the side of the face affected in peripheral facial paralysis.

phenothiazine (fē″nō-thī'ă-zēn). An organic compound used in manufacturing a certain class of tranquilizers and in the production of insecticides, anthelmintics for livestock, and dyes.

CAUTION: Overdose may cause severe postural hypotension, drowsiness, tachycardia, nausea, drying of the mouth, ataxia, fever, tremor, blurring of vision, and occasionally paralytic ileus.

TREATMENT: Symptomatic therapy; remove drug from stomach by gastric lavage. SEE: *chlorpromazine* in *Poisons and Poisoning* in *Appendix.*

phenotype (fē'nō-tīp) [Gr. *phainein,* to show, + *typos,* type]. 1. The physical appearance or makeup of an individual. Some phenotypes, such as the blood groups, are completely determined by heredity, while others, such as stature, are readily altered by environmental agents. 2. A group of individuals who resemble each other in appearance. SEE:

genotype.

phenoxybenzamine hydrochloride (fē-nŏk″sē-bĕn′ză-mēn). USP. An α-adrenergic blocking agent used to produce peripheral vasodilation. Trade name is Dibenzyline.

phenozygous (fē-nŏz′ĭ-gŭs) [″ + *zygon,* yoke]. Possessing a cranium much narrower than the face.

phenprocoumon (fĕn-prō′koo-mŏn). USP. An anticoagulant drug. Trade name is Liquamar.

phensuximide (fĕn-sŭk′sĭ-mīd). USP. An anticonvulsant drug used in treating absence seizures. Trade name is Milontin.

phentermine (fĕn′tĕr-mēn). A sympathomimetic drug used as an anorexic.

phentolamine hydrochloride (fĕn-tŏl′ă-mēn). USP. An α-adrenergic blocking agent used in diagnosing pheochromocytoma. Trade name is Regitine hydrochloride.

Phenurone. Trade name for phenacemide.

phenyl (fĕn′ĭl, fē′nĭl). The univalent radical of phenol, C_6H_5.

phenylalanine (fĕn″ĭl-ăl′ă-nīn). An essential amino acid formed from protein.

phenylamine. $C_6H_5NH_2$. The simplest aromatic amine, an oily liquid derived from benzene. Used in manufacture of dyes for medical and industrial purposes. SYN: *aminobenzene.*

phenylbutazone (fĕn″ĭl-bū′tă-zōn). USP. An antiarthritic and anti-inflammatory drug originally developed for use in various forms of arthritis. Because of the possibility of serious side effects the drug is used only when it is possible to supervise the patient carefully. Its long-term unsupervised use is contraindicated. Trade names are Azolid and Butazolidin.

phenylephrine hydrochloride. USP. Adrenergic compound used in a suitably weak concentration to produce nasal decongestion. May also be used in ophthalmic solutions.

phenylethyl alcohol. USP. An antibacterial agent that has been used as a preservative in ophthalmic solutions.

phenylhydrazine (fĕn″ĭl-hī′dră-zēn). Oily nitrogenous base used as a test for presence of sugar in the urine.

phenylketonuria (fĕn″ĭl-kē″tō-nū′rē-ă). ABBR: PKU. 1. Phenylpyruvic acid in the urine. 2. A recessive hereditary disease caused by the body's failure to oxidize an amino acid (phenylalanine) to tyrosine, because of a defective enzyme. If the disease is not treated early, brain damage may occur, causing severe mental retardation. Test for phenylketonuria should be made at birth; some states require it. The disease is seen equally in the sexes and in the U.S. the incidence is approximately 1:40,000 births. The incidence in England is 1:25,000 births.

SYM: Tremor, spasticity, convulsions, hyperactivity, mental deficiency, eczema, unusual hand posturing, and offensive odor of urine and sweat.

TREATMENT: Low-phenylalanine diet.

PROG: Excellent if treatment is started early postnatal. If started after three years, no improvement will occur because of brain damage.

phenylmercuric acetate (fĕn″ĭl-mĕr-kū′rĭk). A bacteriostatic agent that also acts as a fungicide and herbicide.

phenylmercuric nitrate. A bacteriostatic agent that has been used in treating wounds and as a preservative for intravenous solutions.

phenylpropanolamine hydrochloride (fĕn″ĭl-prō″pă-nŏl′ă-mēn). USP. A sympathomimetic drug used to produce bronchodilation. Trade name is Propadrine.

phenylpyruvic acid (fĕn″ĭl-pī-roo′vĭk). A metabolic derivative of phenylalanine.

phenylpyruvic acid oligophrenia. A form of inherited mental deficiency resulting from phenylketonuria.

phenylthiocarbamide (fĕn″ĭl-thī″ō-kăr′bă-mīd). ABBR: PTC. A chemical used in studying medical genetics to detect the presence of a marker gene. About 70% of the population inherit the ability to note the taste of phenylthiocarbamide to be extremely bitter. To the remainder of the population, it is tasteless. The inheritance of this trait is due to a single dominant gene pair.

phenylthiourea (fĕn″ĭl-thī″ō-ū-rē′ă). Phenylthiocarbamide, q.v.

phenytoin (fĕn′ĭ-tō-ĭn). USP. An anticonvulsant drug. Trade name is Dilantin. SYN: *diphenylhydantoin.*

pheochrome (fē′ō-krōm) [Gr. *phaios,* dusky, + *chroma,* color]. Staining darkly with chrome salts.

pheochromoblast (fē″ō-krō′mō-blăst) [″ + *blastos,* germ]. Embryonic cells that develop into pheochromocytes.

pheochromoblastoma (fē″ō-krō″mō-blăs-tō′mă) [″ + ″ + *oma,* tumor]. Pheochromocytoma, q.v.

pheochromocyte (fē″ō-krō′mō-sīt) [″ + ″ + *kytos,* cell]. A chromaffin cell, such as those in the adrenal medulla, that gives a positive chromaffin reaction, i.e., it gives a yellowish reaction with chrome salts.

pheochromocytoma (fē-ō-krō″mō-sī-tō′mă) [″ + ″ + ″ + *oma,* tumor]. A chromaffin cell tumor of the sympatho-adrenal system that produces catecholamines, i.e., norepinephrine and epinephrine. Although the tumor usually is benign, it produces hypertension that may be paroxysmal in about half the patients. The patient will complain of attacks of pounding headaches, sweating, palpitation, apprehension, flushing of the face, nausea and vomiting, and tingling of the extremities. SYN: *paraganglioma.*

TREATMENT: Surgical removal of the tumor.

pheromone (fĕr'ō-mōn). A substance that provides chemical means of communication between animals and between certain insects, of the same species. It is probably detected by smell. May affect development, reproduction, or behavior of other individuals.

Ph.G. *Graduate in Pharmacy; German Pharmacopeia.*

phial (fī'ăl) [Gr. *phiale,* a bowl]. A small vessel for medicine; a vial.

Philadelphia chromosome. An abnormal chromosome 21 that has lost part of its long arm. Found in leukocyte cultures of many patients with chronic myeloctyic leukemia.

-philia (fĭl'ē-ă) [Gr. *philein,* to love]. Combining form meaning love for, tendency towards, craving for.

philiater (fĭ-lī'ă-tĕr) [" + *iatreia,* healing]. A student of medicine.

philoneism (fĭ-lō'nē-ĭzm) [Gr. *philein,* to love, + *neos,* new, + *-ismos,* condition]. Excessive love or fondness for newness or change. Opposed to misoneism.

philoprogenitive (fĭ"lō-prō-jĕn'ĭ-tĭv) [" + *pro,* for, + *gennan,* to produce]. Producing a large number of offspring. SYN: *prolific.*

philter, philtre [Gr. *philtron*]. A potion or drug that is supposed to induce love or promote sexual activity.

philtrum. [NA] The median groove on the external surface of the upper lip.

phimosis (fī-mō'sĭs) [Gr., a muzzling]. Stenosis or narrowness of preputial orifice so that the foreskin cannot be pushed back over the glans penis.

TREATMENT: Circumcision.

p. vaginalis. Narrowness or closure of the vaginal orifice.

pHisoHex (fī'sō-hĕks). Trade name for an antibacterial skin cleanser containing hexachlorophene as the main ingredient.

pHisoScrub. Trade name for a combination product that contains hexachlorophene and entsulfon sodium.

phlebalgia (flĕ-băl'jē-ă) [Gr. *phleps,* vein, + *algos,* pain]. Pain arising from a vein.

phlebangioma (flĕb"ăn-jē-ō'mă) [" + *angeion,* vessel, + *oma,* tumor]. An aneurysm occurring in a vein.

phlebarteriectasia (flĕb"ăr-tē"rē-ĕk-tā'zē-ă) [" + *arteria,* artery, + *ektasis,* dilatation]. Dilatation of blood vessels.

phlebarteriodialysis (flĕb"ar-tē"rē-ō-dī-ăl'ĭ-sĭs) [" + " + *dialysis,* separation]. Arteriovenous aneurysm.

phlebectasia, phlebectasis (flĕb-ĕk-tā'zē-ă, -ĕk'tă-sĭs) [" + *ektasis,* dilatation]. Venous dilatation. SYN: *varicosity.*

phlebectomy (flĕb-ĕk'tō-mē) [" + *ektome,* excision]. Surgical removal of a vein or part of a vein.

phlebectopia (flĕb"ĕk-tō'pē-ă) [" + *ek,* out, + *topos,* place]. Abnormal position of a vein.

phlebemphraxis (flĕb"ĕm-frăk'sĭs) [" + *emphraxis,* stoppage]. Artificial obstruction of a vein.

phlebismus (flĕb-ĭz'mŭs) [" + *-ismos,* condition]. Venous congestion and dilatation.

phlebitis (flĕ-bī'tĭs) [" + *itis,* inflammation]. Inflammation of a vein. SYN: *milk leg; phlegmasia alba dolens; thrombophlebitis.*

ETIOL: Unknown. May occur in acute or chronic infections or following operations or childbirth.

SYM: Pain and tenderness along course of vein; discoloration of skin; inflammatory swelling and acute edema below obstruction; rapid pulse; mild elevation of temperature; pain in joints.

p., adhesive. Phlebitis in which vein tends to become obliterated. SYN: *p., plastic, p., proliferative.*

p., migrating. A transitory phlebitis that appears in a portion of a vein, then clears up only to reappear later in another location.

p. nodularis necrotisans. Circumscribed inflammation of cutaneous veins resulting in nodules that ulcerate.

p., obliterative. Phlebitis in which the lumen of a vein becomes permanently closed

p., plastic. P., adhesive.

p., proliferative. P., adhesive.

p., puerperal. Venous inflammation following childbirth.

p., sclerosing. Phlebitis in which the veins become obstructed and hardened.

p., sinus. Inflammation of a sinus of the cerebrum.

p., suppurative. Phlebitis characterized by the formation of pus.

phlebo- [Gr. *phleps, phlebos*]. Combining form meaning vein.

phleboclysis (flĕb-ŏk'lĭ-sĭs) [" + *klysis,* injection]. The introduction of medicinal substances intravenously.

p., drip. Intravenous injection instilled slowly drop by drop.

phlebogram (flĕb'ō-grăm) [Gr. *phlebos,* vein, + *gramma,* mark]. A tracing of the venous pulse.

phlebograph (flĕb'ō-grăf) A device for recording the venous pulse.

phlebography (flĕ-bŏg'ră-fē) [" + *graphein,* to write]. A study of the structure and function of the veins.

phleboid (flĕb'oyd) [" + *eidos,* form]. Pert. to, resembling, or of the nature of a vein; venous.

phlebolith, phlebolite (flĕb'ō-lĭth, -līt) [" + *lithos,* a stone]. A calcareous concretion in a vein.

phlebolithiasis (flĕb"ō-lĭ-thī'ă-sĭs) [" + *lithiasis,* forming stones]. The formation of phleboliths in veins.

phlebology (flĕb-ŏl'ō-jē) [Gr. *phlebos,* vein, + *logos,* study]. The science of veins and their diseases.

phlebomanometer (flĕb"ō-mă-nŏm'ĕ-tĕr) [" + *manos,* thin, + *metron,* measure]. A device for direct measurement of venous pressure.

phlebometritis (flĕb"ō-mē-trī'tĭs) [" + *metra,* uterus, + *itis,* inflammation]. Inflammation of uterine veins.

phlebomyomatosis (flĕb"ō-mī"ō-mă-tō'sĭs) [" + *mys,* muscle, + *oma,* tumor, + *osis,* condition]. Thickening of the tissue of a vein from overgrowth of muscular fibers.

phlebopexy (flĕb'ō-pĕk"sē) [Gr. *phlebos,* vein, + *peksis,* fixation]. Extraserous transplantation of the testes for varicocele, with preservation of venous network.

phlebophlebostomy (flĕb"ō-flĕ-bŏs'tō-mē) [" + *phlebos,* vein, + *stoma,* opening]. Surgical anastomosis of veins.

phleboplasty (flĕb'ō-plăs"tē) [" + *plassein,* to form]. Plastic repair of an injured vein.

phleborrhagia (flĕb"ō-rā'jē-ă) [" + *rhegnynai,* to burst forth]. Bleeding from a vein.

phleborrhaphy (flĕb-or'ă-fē) [" + *rhaphe,* a sewing]. Suturing of a vein.

phleborrhexis (flĕb"ō-rĕk'sĭs) [" + *rhexis,* rupture]. Rupture of a vein.

phlebosclerosis (flĕb"ō-sklē-rō'sĭs) [" + *sklerosis,* hardening]. Fibrous hardening of a vein's walls.

phlebostasia, phlebostasis (flĕb-ō-stā'zē-ă, -ŏs'tă-sĭs) [" + *stasis,* stoppage]. Compression of veins temporarily to restrict an amount of blood from the general circulation. SYN: *phlebotomy, bloodless.*

phlebostenosis (flĕb"ō-stē-nō'sĭs) [" + *stenosis,* narrowing]. Constriction of a vein.

phlebothrombosis (flĕb"ō-thrŏm-bō'sĭs) [" + *thrombos,* a clot]. Clotting in a vein; phlebitis with secondary thrombosis.

phlebotome (flĕb'ō-tōm) [" + *tome,* incision]. Lancet used in incising a vein.

phlebotomist (flĕ-bŏt'ō-mĭst) [" + *tome,* incision]. One who practices venesection, i.e., draws blood by use of a syringe and needle.

phlebotomize (flĕ-bŏt'ō-mīz). To take blood from a person.

Phlebotomus (flĕ-bŏt'ō-mŭs) [" + *tome,* incision]. A genus of insects, the sandflies, belonging to the family Psychodidae, order Diptera. The bloodsucking insects are annoying and transmit various forms of leishmaniasis, sandfly (pappataci) fever, and Oroya fever.

P. argentipes. In India, the transmitter of Leishmania donovani, causative agent of kala-azar.

P. chinensis. Transmitter of kala-azar in China.

P. papatasii. Transmitter of the causative agent of sandfly fever. The virus is capable of being transmitted through the offspring of flies.

P. sergenti. Transmitter of kala-azar in Middle East and India.

P. verrucarum. The transmitter of Bartonella bacilliformis, causative agent of Oroya fever (Carrion's disease), in S. America.

phlebotomus fever (flĕ-bŏt'ō-mŭs). Sandfly fever, q.v.

phlebotomy (flĕ-bŏt'ō-mē) [" + *tome,* incision]. Surgical opening of a vein to withdraw blood. SYN: *venesection.*

p., bloodless. Compression of veins of the extremities, restricting some of the blood from the general circulation. SYN: *phlebostasia.*

phlegm (flĕm) [Gr. *phlegma*] 1. Thick mucus, esp. that from the respiratory passages. 2. One of the four "humors" of early physiology.

phlegmasia (flĕg-mā'zē-ă) [Gr. *phlegmasia*]. Inflammation.

p. alba dolens. Acute edema, esp. of the leg, from venous obstruction, usually a thrombosis. SYN: *milk leg; white leg.*

SYM: Usually begins, esp. in women who have recently given birth, with slight fever. Pain in lower part of abdomen follows, extends to hips and back, passes under Poupart's ligament, and thence down the thigh into the calf of the leg. Sometimes proceeds from calf upwards. Whole extremity becomes excessively swollen, hot, and painful, but not red, hence the name.

Tenderness on pressure most marked along course of the femoral vein, and veins of the affected region together with associated lymphatics may be felt to be hard and cordlike. Sometimes marked by faint red line. Progress is rapid, frequently doubling size of limb in 24 hours or less. Often there is difficulty in evacuating the bladder and rectum; glands in the groin sometimes swell and suppurate; and abscesses may form in different parts of the limb.

TREATMENT: Elevate limb, protect with a cradle, and apply heat. Anticoagulants to prevent clot formation. Vasodilator drugs and paracervical block may be used to combat vasospasm. Ligation of main venous channel proximal to thrombus may be done to prevent embolus.

NURSING IMPLICATIONS: Maintain strict bedrest. Utilize leg and foot cradle. Immobilize the limb. Apply anti-emboli stockings as ordered by the physician. Administer anticoagulants and other medications as ordered. Apply warm compresses as ordered by the physician. Instruct patient concerning the importance of bedrest and immobilization to prevent thrombi from becoming emboli.

p., cellulitic. Septic inflammation of connective tissue of the leg following childbirth.

p. malabarica. Inflammation with hypertrophy and induration of the skin. SYN: *elephantiasis.*

phlegmatic (flĕg-măt'ĭk) [Gr. *phlegmatikos*]. Of sluggish or dull temperament; apathetic.

phlegmon (flĕg'mŏn) [Gr. *phlegmone,* inflammation]. Acute suppurative inflammation of subcutaneous connective tissue, esp. a pyogenic inflammation that spreads along fascial planes or other natural barriers.

p., bronze. Gaseous phlegmon following renal surgery, causing bronze spots near the incision.

p., diffuse. Diffuse inflammation of subcutaneous tissues with sepsis.

p., gas. Gas gangrene.

p., Holz. A chronic cellulitis of the deep tissues of the floor of the mouth.

phlegmonous (flĕg'mŏn-ŭs). Pert. to inflammation of subcutaneous tissues.

phlogistic (flō-jĭs'tĭk) [Gr. *phlogistos*]. Pert. to, or inducing, inflammation.

phlogogenic, phlogogenous (flō-gō-jĕn'ĭk, -gŏj'ĕn-ŭs) [Gr. *phlogosis,* inflammation, + *gennan,* to produce]. Producing or exciting inflammation.

phlorhizin (flō-rī'zĭn). A glycoside present in the bark of some fruit trees. It is a powerful inhibitor of sugar transport in some animals.

phlyctena (flĭk-tē'nă) [Gr. *phlyktaina*]. (pl. *phlyctenae*) A vesicle, esp. one of many after a first-degree burn.

phlyctenar (flĭk'tē-năr). Concerning a vesicle.

phlyctenoid (flĭk'tĕ-noyd) [" + *eidos,* resemblance]. Resembling a blister or pustule.

phlyctenosis (flĭk"tĕ-nō'sĭs) [" + *osis,* condition]. Appearance of blisters or pustules.

phlyctenula (flĭk-tĕn'ū-lă) [L.]. (pl. *phlyctenulae*) A tiny vesicle or pustule, esp. that seen on the cornea.

phlyctenular (flĭk-tĕn'ū-lăr). Resembling or pert. to vesicles or pustules.

phlyctenule (flĭk'tĕn-ūl) [Gr. *phlyktaina,* a blister; L. *phlyctenula*]. A small vesicle or blister, as on cornea or conjunctiva.

phlyctenulosis (flĭk-tĕn-ū-lō'sĭs) [" + *osis,* condition]. The formation of many phlyctenules.

phobia (fō'bē-ă) [Gr. *phobos,* fear]. Any persistent and irrational fear of a specific object, activity, or situation that results in a compelling desire to avoid the feared or phobic stimulus. Phobias are classified into three types: agoraphobia, social phobia, and simple phobias. SEE: *Phobias* in *Appendix.*

-phobia [Gr.]. Suffix indicating abnormal fear of, or aversion to, a subject.

phobic (fō'bĭk) [Gr. *phobos,* fear]. Concerning a phobia.

phobic desensitization. Method of treating phobias in which the patient is taught to relax while slowly re-entering the phobic situation, first in imagination and then in real life. Anxiety and fear are kept to a minimum at all times. SEE: *implosion flooding.*

phobophobia (fō"bō-fō'bē-ă) [" + *phobos,* fear]. Morbid fear of acquiring a phobia.

phocomelia (fō"kō-mē'lē-ă) [Gr. *phoke,* seal, + *melos,* limb]. A congenital malformation wherein the proximal portion of the extremities is poorly developed or absent. Thus the hands and feet are attached to the trunk directly or by means of a poorly formed bone. In some cases this was due to the administration of thalidomide, a sleeping pill, during early pregnancy. That drug is no longer approved for such use.

phocomelus (fō-kŏm'ĕ-lŭs). A person with phocomelia, q.v.

phon-. SEE: *phono-.*

phonacoscope (fō-năk'ō-skōp) [Gr. *phone,* voice, + *skopein,* to examine]. A device for increasing the percussion note or voice sounds.

phonacoscopy (fō-nă-kŏs'kō-pē). Inspection of the chest with the phonacoscope.

phonal (fō'năl) [Gr. *phone,* voice]. Concerning the voice.

phonasthenia (fōn-ăs-thē'nē-ă) [" + *asthenia,* weakness]. Vocal weakness or hoarseness due to straining the voice.

phonation (fō-nā'shŭn). Process of uttering vocal sounds.

phonatory (fō'nă-tō"rē) [Gr. *phone,* voice]. Concerning utterance of vocal sounds.

phonautograph (fōn-aw'tō-grăf) [" + *autos,* self, + *graphein,* to write]. Device for registering the voice's vibrations.

phone (fōn) [Gr. *phone,* voice]. An element of speech; a single speech sound.

-phone [Gr. *phone,* voice]. Combining form indicating sound or voice.

phoneme (fō'nēm) [Gr. *phonema,* an utterance]. In linguistics, the smallest unit of speech that distinguishes one sound from another.

phonendoscope (fō-nĕn'dō-skōp) [Gr. *phone,* voice, + *endon,* within, + *skopein,* to examine]. A stethoscope that intensifies sounds.

phonendoskiascope (fō-nĕn"dō-skī'ă-skōp) [" + " + *skia,* shadow, + *skopein,* to examine]. Device for observing the cardiac movements and for hearing heart sounds.

phonetics (fō-nĕt'ĭks) [Gr. *phonetikos,* spoken]. Science of speech and pronunciation. SYN: *phonology.*

phoniatrics (fō″nē-ăt′rĭks) [Gr. *phone,* voice, + *iatrikos,* treatment]. The study of the voice and treatment of its disorders.

phonic (fō′nĭk). Concerning the voice or sound.

phonism (fō′nĭzm) [″ + *-ismos,* condition]. An auditory sensation occurring when another sense is stimulated. SEE: *synesthesia.*

phono- [Gr. *phone,* voice]. Combining form indicating sound, voice.

phonocardiogram (fō″nō-kăr′dē-ō-grăm) [″ + *kardia,* heart, + *gramma,* mark]. Graphic recording of the heart sounds.

phonocardiography (fō″nō-kăr″dē-ŏg′ră-fē) [″ + ″ + *graphein,* to write]. Mechanical or electronic registration of heart sounds.

phonocatheter (fō″nō-kăth′ĕ-tĕr) [″ + *katheter,* something inserted]. A catheter with a microphone at its end.

phonogram (fō′nō-grăm) [″ + *gramma,* a mark]. A graphic curve indicating intensity and duration of a sound.

phonograph (fō′nō-grăf) [″ + *graphein,* to write]. Instrument used for reproduction of sounds.

phonology (fō-nŏl′ō-jē) [″ + *logos,* a study]. Science of vocal sounds. SYN: *phonetics.*

phonomania (fŏn″ō-mā′nē-ă) [Gr. *phone,* murder, + *mania,* madness]. Insanity characterized by tendency to commit murder.

phonomassage (fō″nō-mă-sahzh′) [Gr. *phone,* voice, + *massein,* to knead]. Exciting movements of the ossicles of the ear by means of noise or alternating suction and pressure directed through the external auditory meatus.

phonometer (fō-nŏm′ĕ-tĕr) [″ + *metron,* measure]. Device for determining intensity of vocal sounds.

phonomyoclonus (fō″nō-mī-ŏk′lō-nŭs) [″ + *mys,* muscle, + *klonos,* a contraction]. Invisible fibrillary muscular contractions revealed by auscultation.

phonomyogram (fō″nō-mī′ō-grăm) [″ + ″ + *gramma,* mark]. A recording of sound produced by action of a muscle.

phonomyography (fō″nō-mī-ŏg′ră-fē) [″ + ″ + *graphein,* to write]. The recording of sounds made by contracting muscular tissue.

phonopathy (fō-nŏp′ă-thē) [″ + *pathos,* disease]. Any disease of organs affecting speech.

phonophobia (fō″nō-fō′bē-ă) [″ + *phobos,* fear]. 1. Morbid fear of sound or noise. 2. Fear of speaking or hearing one's own voice.

phonophotography. Photography of the vibrations produced by speech.

phonopsia (fō-nŏp′sē-ă) [″ + *opsis,* vision]. The subjective perception of sensations upon hearing certain sounds.

phonoreceptor. A receptor for sound waves.

phonorenogram (fō″nō-rē′nō-grăm) [″ + L. *ren,* kidney, + Gr. *gramma,* mark]. A recording of the pulse in the renal artery.

phonoscope (fō′nō-skōp) [″ + *skopein,* to examine]. Device for recording heart sounds.

phonoscopy (fō-nŏs′kō-pē). A recording made by use of a phonoscope.

-phoresis (fō-rē′sĭs) [Gr. *phoresis,* being borne]. A word termination denoting the migration of ions through a membrane by the action of an electric current. The direction of movement is distinguished by the use of prefixes, as in cataphoresis and anaphoresis for migrations toward cathode and anode, respectively.

-phoria [Gr. *phoresis,* being borne]. In ophthalmology, a combining form meaning a turning with reference to the visual axis, such as cyclophoria, q.v.

Phormia (for′mē-ă). A genus of blowflies belonging to the family Calliphoridae. Their larvae normally live in decaying flesh of dead animals, but they may infest neglected wounds or sores giving rise to myiasis.

phorology (fō-rŏl′ō-jē) [Gr. *phoros,* carrying, + *logos,* study]. Science dealing with disease carriers.

phorotone (fō′rō-tōn) [Gr. *phora,* motion, + *tonos,* tension]. Device for exercising eye muscles.

phorozoon (fō″rō-zō′ŏn) [Gr. *phoros,* fruitful, + *zoon,* animal]. The nonsexual stage of an animal that in its life cycle passes through several stages.

phose (fōz) [Gr. *phos,* light]. A subjective sensation of light or color. SEE: *centraphose; centrophose; chromophose; erythrophose.*

phosgene (fŏs′jēn) [″ + *genes,* born]. Carbonyl chloride ($COCl_2$), a poisonous gas causing nausea and suffocation when inhaled. Used in chemical warfare, esp. during World War I. Now used in industry in preparation of pharmaceutical and chemical products. SEE: *nitrous fumes* in *Poisons and Poisoning* in *Appendix.*

phosphagen (fŏs′fă-jĕn). Several chemicals including phosphocreatine that release energy when split. They are high-energy phosphate compounds.

Phosphalgel. Trade name for aluminum phosphate.

phosphatase (fŏs′fă-tās). One of a group of enzymes that catalyzes the hydrolysis of phosphoric acid esters. They are of importance in absorption and metabolism of carbohydrates, nucleotides, and phospholipids and are essential in the calcification of bone.

p., acid. Phosphatase whose optimum pH is between 4.0 and 5.4. Present in kidney, semen, serum, and prostate gland.

p., alkaline. Phosphatase whose optimum pH is about 9.0. Present in teeth, developing bone, plasma, kidney, and intestine. It is excreted by the liver, hence increases in blood in obstructive jaundice. It is also elevated in diseases of the pancreas, lung, bone, some malignancies without metastases, and in pregnancy; in the first month of life, it may be as high as 6 times the normal level in adults. The level gradually decreases during childhood and puberty. Alkaline phosphatase can by use of special techniques be separated into bone, intestinal, and placental fractions.

phosphate (fŏs′fāt) [Gr. *phosphas*]. A salt of phosphoric acid. Phosphates are important in maintenance of acid-base balance of the blood, the principal ones being monosodium and disodium phosphate. The former is acid, the latter alkaline. In the blood, because of their low concentration, they exert a minor buffering action. In the formation of urine, by altering the proportions of acid and alkaline phosphates, an acid urine is formed and the body's fixed base, chiefly Na but also K, Mg, and Ca, is conserved.

Decreased phosphate excretion in urine occurs when alkaline reserve is high; in nephritis, tetany (hypoparathyroidism), adrenal cortical deficiency, and certain bone diseases.

Increased phosphate excretion in urine occurs when alkali reserve is low; in starvation, hyperparathyroidism, high-protein diet, and extreme muscular exercise.

p., acid. Phosphate in which only one or two of hydrogen atoms of phosphoric acid have been replaced by a metal.

p., calcium. Any one of three salts of calcium and phosphate. Used as an antacid and as a dietary supplement.

p., creatine. Phosphocreatine, q.v.

p., normal. Phosphate in which all three hydrogen atoms of phosphoric acid have been replaced by metals.

p., triple. Calcium, ammonium, and magnesium phosphate.

phosphate-bond energy. Energy derived from phosphorylated compounds such as adenosine triphosphate (ATP) and creatine phosphate.

phosphatemia (fŏs″fă-tē′mē-ă) [Gr. *phosphas,* phosphate, + *haima,* blood]. Phosphates in the blood.

phosphatide (fŏs′fă-tīd). A phospholipid.

phosphatoptosis (fŏs″fă-tŏp-tō′sĭs) [″ + *ptosis,* a dropping]. Spontaneous precipitation of phosphates in urine.

phosphaturia (fŏs″fă-tū′rē-ă) [″ + *ouron,* urine]. Excessive amount of phosphates in the urine. Often causes renal calculi. SYN: *phosphoruria; phosphuria.*

SYM: Cloudy urine, opaque and pale. Reaction alkaline. Pearly or pinkish-white deposits of phosphates in standing urine.

phosphene (fŏs′fēn) [Gr. *phos,* light, + *phainein,* to show]. A subjective sensation of light caused by pressure upon the eyeball.

p., accommodation. Phosphene resulting from contraction of ciliary muscles in accommodation. Seen esp. in the dark.

phosphide (fŏs′fīd) [″ + *phorein,* to carry]. Binary compound of phosphorus with an element or radical.

phosphite (fŏs′fīt). A salt of phosphoric acid.

phosphoamidase (fŏs″fō-ăm′ĭ-dās). An enzyme that catalyzes the conversion of phosphocreatine to creatine and orthophosphate.

phosphocreatine (fŏs″fō-krē′ă-tĭn). A compound found in muscle. It is important in muscle metabolism, yielding inorganic phosphate and creatine in this process.

phosphofructokinase (fŏs″fō-frŭk″tō-kī′nās). A glycolytic enzyme that catalyzes phosphorylation of fructose-6-phosphate by adenosine triphosphate.

Phospholine Iodide. Trade name for echothiophate iodide, USP.

phospholipase (fŏs″fō-lĭp′ās). An enzyme that catalyzes hydrolysis of a phospholipid.

phospholipid (fŏs″fō-lĭp′ĭd) [Gr. *phos,* light, + *phorein,* to carry, + *lipos,* fat]. A lipoid substance containing phosphorus, fatty acids, and nitrogenous base, as lecithin. SYN: *phosphatide; phospholipin.*

phospholipin (fŏs″fō-lĭp′ĭn). A lipoid compound containing phosphorus. SYN: *phosphatide; phospholipid.*

phosphonecrosis (fŏs″fō-nē-krō′sĭs) [″ + *phorein,* to carry, + *nekros,* dead, + *osis,* condition]. Necrosis of the alveolar process in persons working with phosphorus.

phosphonuclease (fŏs″fō-nū′klē-ās). An enzyme that catalyzes the hydrolysis of nucleotides to nucleosides and phosphoric acid.

phosphopenia (fŏs″fō-pē′nē-ă) [″ + *phorein,* to carry, + *penia,* lack]. Deficiency of phosphorus in the body.

phosphoprotein (fŏs″fō-prō′tē-ĭn) [″ + ″ + *protos,* first]. One of a group of proteins in which the protein is combined with a phosphorus-containing compound. Caseinogen and vitellin are examples. Formerly called nucleoalbumin.

phosphorated (fŏs′fō-rā″tĕd) [″ + *phorein,* to carry]. Impregnated with phosphorus.

phosphorescence (fŏs-fō-rĕs′ĕns). The induced luminescence that persists after cessation of the irradiation that caused it. The emission of light without appreciable heat.

phosphorhidrosis (fŏs″for-hĭd-rō′sĭs) [″ + *phorein,* to carry, + *hidrosis,* sweating]. Secretion of luminous perspiration. SYN: *phosphoridrosis.*

phosphoribosyltransferase (fŏs″fō-rī″bō-sĭl-trăns′fĕr-ās). An enzyme that catalyzes reconversion to the ribonucleotide stage of the purine bases, hypoxanthine and guanine. A deficiency of the enzyme causes gout. The deficiency is inherited as an X chromosome–linked trait.

phosphoric acid (fŏs-for′ĭk). Orthophosphoric acid, H_3PO_4, a tribasic acid.

phosphoridrosis (fŏs″for-ĭd-rō′sĭs) [″ + *phorein,* to carry, + *hidrosis,* perspiration]. Secretion of perspiration that is luminous. SYN: *phosphorhidrosis.*

phosphorism (fŏs′for-ĭzm) [″ + ″ + *-ismos,* condition]. Chronic poisoning from phosphorus.

phosphorolysis (fŏs″fō-rŏl′ĭ-sĭs). The chemical reaction of incorporating phosphoric acid into a molecule.

phosphorous acid (fŏs-fō′rŭs, fŏs′for-ŭs) [″ + *phoros,* carrying]. H_3PO_3. Crystalline acid formed when phosphorus is oxidized in moist air.

phosphoruria (fŏs″for-ū′rē-ă) [″ + *phorein,* to carry, + *ouron,* urine]. Phosphorus in the urine in excess of normal. SYN: *phosphaturia; phosphuria.*

phosphorus (fŏs′fō-rŭs) [Gr. *phos,* light, + *phoros,* carrying]. SYMB: P. At. wt. 30.9738; at. no. 15. A nonmetallic element not found in a free state but in combination with alkalies.

The adult body contains from 600 to 900 gm. of phosphorus in various forms: 70–80% in bones and teeth, principally combined with calcium; 10% in muscle; and 1% in nerve tissue. Minimum daily requirement is approx. 800 mg. Amount should be increased during pregnancy and lactation. Vitamin D is important in the absorption and metabolism of phosphorus. Excesses of phosphorus are excreted by kidney and intestine, about 60% being excreted in urine principally as phosphates.

Phosphorus compounds (adenosine triphosphate and phosphocreatine) are the principal sources of energy in muscle contraction, and phosphorus is essential in the conversion of glycogen to glucose.

OCCURRENCE: Phosphorus is found in many foods. Excellent sources are: almonds, beans, barley, bran, cheese, cocoa, chocolate, eggs, lentils, liver, milk, oatmeal, peanuts, peas, walnuts, whole wheat, and rye. Good sources are: asparagus, beef, cabbage, carrots, celery, cauliflower, chard, chicken, clams, corn, cream, cucumbers, eggplant, fish, figs, meat, prunes, pineapples, pumpkin, raisins, and string beans.

DEFICIENCY SYM: Perverted appetite, retarded growth, loss of weight, weakness, rickets, imperfect bone and teeth development.

phosphorus poisoning. Prior to the introduction of safety matches (which contain no yellow phosphorus), phosphorus poisoning was quite common. However, acute phosphorus poisoning still is seen following ingestion of rat and roach poisons, which contain yellow phosphorus.

SYM: Acute irritation of gastrointestinal tract followed by symptoms resembling acute yellow atrophy of liver and marked blood changes. Bloody vomitus, garlic odor of breath, cramps, headache, liver and kidney damage. Profound weakness, hemorrhage, heart failure. Occasionally nervous symptoms predominate.

NURSING IMPLICATIONS: Prolonged gastric lavage, part of which should contain 100 ml. of mineral oil and cupric sulfate (250 mg. in 250 ml. of water, or 0.2%), or potassium permanganate, which may aid in oxidizing the phosphorus. This should, of course, be washed out. Protect patient and attendants from vomitus, gastric washings, and feces because the phosphorus in them can burn the skin and eyes. Oils, creams, and fats should be avoided because these promote absorption of phosphorus. Intravenous transfusion with fresh blood. Otherwise treat symptomatically. SEE: *Poisons and Poisoning* in *Appendix.*

phosphoryl (fŏs′for-ĭl). The radical [PO]≡.

phosphorylase (fŏs-for′ĭ-lās). An enzyme that catalyzes the formation of glucose-1-phosphate from glycogen.

phosphorylation (fŏs″for-ĭ-lā′shŭn). The combining of a phosphate with an organic compound.

phosphuria (fŏs-fū′rē-ă) [Gr. *phos,* light, + *phoros,* a bearer, + *ouron,* urine]. Excess of phosphorus in the urine. SYN: *phosphaturia; phosphoruria.*

phot (fōt) [Gr. *photos,* light] ABBR: ph. The unit of photochemical energy equal to 1 lumen per square centimeter or about 929 foot candles.

phot-. SEE: words beginning with *photo-.*

photalgia (fō-tăl′jē-ă) [Gr. *photos,* light, + *algos,* pain]. Pain produced by light. SYN: *photodynia.*

photaugiaphobia (fō-taw″jē-ă-fō′bē-ă) [Gr. *photaugeia,* glare, + *phobos,* fear]. Intolerance of bright light.

photechy (fō′tĕk-ē) [Gr. *photos,* light, + *echo,* echo]. The acquisition of radioactivity by having been exposed to a radioactive source.

photesthesis (fō″tĕs-thē′sĭs) [″ + *aisthesis,* sensation]. Sensitivity to light.

photic (fō′tĭk). 1. Concerning light. 2. In biology, pert. to the production of light by certain organisms.

photic driving. In neurology, altering the electroencephalogram by intermittently flashing light into the eyes.

photic sneezing. Sneezing initiated or hastened in its onset by light stimulus. Sometimes due to light causing tears that, upon draining into the nasal area, cause sneezing.

photism (fō′tĭzm) [″ + *-ismos,* condition]. A subjective sensation of color or light produced by a stimulus of another sense, such as smell, hearing, taste, or touch. SEE: *synesthesia.*

photo- [Gr. *photos*]. Combining form indicating light.

photoactinic (fō″tō-ăk-tĭn ĭk). Emitting both luminous and actinic rays.

photoallergic contact dermatitis. Inflammation of the skin due to substances made allergenic by the effect of ultraviolet or light in the visible spectrum. SEE: *photoallergy.*

photoallergy (fō″tō-ăl′ĕr-jē) [″ + *allos,* other, + *ergon,* work]. An immunological reaction produced by interaction of light rays and certain chemicals. It is a form of contact allergic reaction wherein light is necessary to cause the sensitivity reaction. Some of the photocontact allergens are phenothiazine, sulfonamides, hexachlorophene, sunscreen agents, optical bleaches, and topical antihistamines. SEE: *photosensitivity; phototoxic.*

photobacterium (fō″tō-băk-tē′rē-ŭm). A bacterium that produces light.

photobiology (fō″tō-bī-ŏl′ō-jē) [″ + *bios,* life, + *logos,* study]. Study of the effect of light on living things.

photobiotic (fō″tō-bī-ŏt′ĭk) [″ + *bios,* life]. Capable of living only in the light.

photocatalysis (fō″tō-kă-tăl′ĭ-sĭs) [″ + *katalysis,* dissolution]. Catalysis of a chemical reaction by light.

photoceptor (fō″tō-sĕp′tor) [″ + L. *ceptor,* a receiver]. A nerve ceptor receiving light ray sensations.

photochemistry (fō″tō-kĕm′ĭs-trē) [Gr. *photos,* light, + *chemeia,* chemistry]. Branch of chemistry concerned with the effects of light rays. SYN: *actinochemistry.*

photochromogen [″ + *chroma,* color, + *gennan,* to produce]. Certain microorganisms in which a pigment develops when it is grown in the presence of light, such as Mycobacterium kansasii.

photocoagulation. Alteration of proteins in tissue by the use of light energy in the form of ordinary light rays or a laser beam. Used esp. in treating retinal detachments or bleeding from the retina.

photodermatitis (fō″tō-dĕr-mă-tī′tĭs) [″ + *dermatos,* skin, + *itis,* inflammation]. Sensitivity of the epithelium to light. May be due to photoallergy, q.v., or to phototoxic, q.v., reaction.

photodromy (fō-tŏd′rō-mē) [″ + *dromos,* running]. The condition of particles in suspension wherein they move toward (positive photodromy) or away from (negative photodromy) light.

photodynamic (fō″tō-dī-năm′ĭk) [″ + *dynamis,* force]. Pert. to the energy or force effected by light on organisms.

photodynamic action. Action exerted by certain dyes, such as methylene blue and eosin, on certain biological systems when subjected to light.

photodynia (fō″tō-dĭn′ē-ă) [″ + *odyne,* pain]. Pain produced by rays of light. SYN: *photalgia.*

photodysphoria (fō″tō-dĭs-for′ē-ă) [″ + *dysphoria,* distress]. Extreme intolerance of light. SYN: *phengophobia; photophobia.*

photoelectricity (fō″tō-ē-lĕk-trĭ′sĭ-tē) [″ + *elektron,* amber]. Electricity formed by action of light.

photoelectron (fō″tō-ē-lĕk′trŏn) [″ + *elektron,* amber]. An electron set free by the action of light.

photoerythema (fō″tō-ĕr″ĭ-thē′mă) [″ + *erythema,* redness]. Erythema of the skin caused by light.

photofluorography (fō″tō-flū″ĕr-ŏg′ră-fē). Photographing the images seen during fluoroscopic examination.

photogastroscope (fō″tō-găs′trō-skōp) [″ + *gaster,* belly, + *skopein,* to view]. A device for viewing and taking photographs of the interior of the stomach.

photogene (fō′tō-jēn) [″ + *gennan,* to produce]. Prolonged retinal image. SYN: *afterimage.*

photogenic, photogenous (fō″tō-jĕn′ĭk, -tŏj′ĕn-ŭs). Induced by, or inducing, light.

photogenic epilepsy. Epileptic seizures induced by the intermittent flashing of light into the eyes.

photographic radiometer. An instrument containing a half-tone color index for strips of photographic paper after exposure to roentgen rays and, after development, used to estimate the quantity of roentgen rays.

photohemotachometer (fō″tō-hĕm″ō-tăk-ŏm′ĕ-tĕr) [″ + *haima,* blood, + *tachys,* swift, + *metron,* measure]. Device for photographing rate of blood flow.

photokinetic (fō″tō-kĭn-ĕt′ĭk) [″ + *kinetikos,* motion]. Reacting with motion to stimulus of light.

photokymograph (fō″tō-kī′mō-grăf) [″ + *kyma,* wave, + *graphein,* to write]. A device for making continuous photographs of a physiologic event.

photoluminescence (fō″tō-lū-mĭ-nĕs′ĕns) [″ + L. *lumen,* light]. The power of an object to become luminescent when acted on by light.

photolysis (fō-tŏl′ĭ-sĭs) [″ + *lysis,* dissolution]. Dissolution or disintegration under stimulus of light rays.

photolyte (fō′tō-līt). A substance decomposed by light.

photolytic (fō″tō-lĭt′ĭk). Dissolved by stimulus of light rays.

photomania (fō″tō-mā′nē-ă) [″ + *mania,* madness]. 1. A psychosis produced by prolonged exposure to intense light. 2. A psychotic desire for light.

photometer (fō-tŏm′ĕt-ĕr) [″ + *metron,* measure]. A device for measuring the intensity of light.

photometry (fō-tŏm′ĕ-trē). Measurement of light rays.

photomicrograph (fō″tō-mī′krō-grăf) [″ + *mikros,* small, + *graphein,* to write]. Photograph of an object under the microscope.

photomotor. Pert. to muscular contraction induced by light.

photon (fō′tŏn) [Gr. *photos,* light]. A light quantum or unit of energy of a light ray or other form of radiant energy. Generally considered to be a discrete particle with zero mass, no electric charge, and of indefinitely long life.

photoncia (fō-tŏn′sē-ă) [″ + *onkos,* tumor]. Swelling produced by light.

photonosus (fō-tŏn′ō-sŭs) [″ + *nosos,* disease]. Disease due to prolonged exposure to intense light.

photo-ophthalmia (fō″tō-ŏf-thăl′mē-ă) [″ + *ophthalmos,* eye]. Keratoconjunctivitis produced by excess exposure to intense light rays.

photopathy (fō-tŏp′ă-thē) [″ + *pathos,* disease]. Pathologic effect produced by light.

photoperceptive (fō″tō-pĕr-sĕp′tĭv) [″ + *percipere,* to receive]. Capable of perceiving light.

photoperiod (fō″tō-pēr′ē-ŏd) [″ + LL. *periodus,* period]. The daily duration of exposure to light of a living thing.

photoperiodism (fō″tō-pēr′ē-ō-dĭzm) [″ + ″ + Gr. *-ismos,* condition]. The periodic occurrence of biological phenomena in relationship to the presence or absence of light. In most animals, the sleep-wakefulness cycle is a form of periodism.

photophilic (fō-tō-fĭl′ĭk) [″ + *philein,* to love]. Seeking, or fond of, light.

photophobia (fō″tō-fō′bē-ă) [″ + *phobos,* fear]. Unusual intolerance of light. Occurs in measles and rubella, meningitis, and inflammation of the eyes.

photophone (fō′tō-fōn) [″ + *phone,* voice]. Device for production of sound by action of light.

photophthalmia (fō″tŏf-thăl′mē-ă) [″ + *ophthalmos,* eye]. Photo-ophthalmia, q.v.

photopia. Adjustment of the eye for vision in bright light. Opposite of scotopia.

photopic (fō-tŏp′ĭk). Pert. to bright light.

photopsia, photopsy (fō-tŏp′sē-ă, fō-tŏp′sē) [Gr. *photos,* light, + *opsis,* vision]. Subjective sensation of sparks or flashes of light in retinal, optic, or brain diseases.

photopsin (fō-tŏp′sĭn). The protein portion or opsin of the pigment in the cover of the retina of the eye.

photoptarmosis (fō″tō-tăr-mō′sĭs) [″ + *ptarmosis,* sneezing]. Sneezing caused by the effect of light. SYN: *photic sneezing.*

photoptometer (fō-tŏp-tŏm′ĕ-tĕr) [″ + *opsis,* vision, + *metron,* measure]. Device for determining the smallest amount of light that will make an object visible.

photoptometry (fō″tŏp-tŏm′ĕ-trē). Measurement of light perception.

photoradiometer (fō″tō-rā″dē-ŏm′ĕ-tĕr) [″ + L. *radius,* ray, + Gr. *metron,* measure]. Device for determining the ability of ionizing radiation to penetrate substances.

photoreaction (fō″tō-rē-ăk′shŭn) [″ + LL. *reactus,* reacted]. A chemical reaction produced or influenced by light.

photoreactivation (fō″tō-rē-ăk″tĭ-vā′shŭn). Enzymatic repair of lesions such as can be produced in DNA by ultraviolet light.

photoreception (fō″tō-rē-sĕp′shŭn) [″ + L. *recipere,* to receive]. The perception of light rays in the visible light spectrum.

photoreceptive (fō″tō-rē-sĕp′tĭv) [″ + *receptor,* a receiver]. Capable of perceiving light rays.

photoreceptor (fō″tō-rē-sĕp′tor). Sensory nerve endings or cells that are capable of being stimulated by light. In man, rods and cones of the retina.

photoretinitis (fō″tō-rĕt″ĭ-nī′tĭs) [Gr. *photos,* light, + L. *retina,* retina, + Gr. *itis,* inflammation]. Damage to the macula of the eye due to exposure to intense light. SEE: *blindness, eclipse.*

photoscan. A representation of the concentration of a radioisotope outlining an organ in the body. The map is printed on photographic paper. SEE: *scintiscan.*

photoscope (fō′tō-skōp) [″ + *skopein,* to examine]. A variety of fluoroscope used to observe light.

photoscopy (fō-tŏs′kō-pē). Examination with a fluorescent screen. SYN: *fluoroscopy.*

photosensitivity [″ + L. *sensitivus,* feeling]. Sensitive to light. SEE: *photoallergy.*

photosensitization (fō″tō-sĕn″sĭ-tĭ-zā′shŭn). Condition in which the skin reacts abnormally to light, esp. ultraviolet rays or sunlight; due to the presence of drugs, hormones, or heavy metals in the system. SEE: *photoallergy.*

photosensitizer (fō″tō-sĕn′sĭ-tĭ′zĕr). Substance that, in combination with light, will cause a sensitivity reaction in the substance or organism.

photostable (fō′tō-stā″b′l) [″ + L. *stabilis,* stable]. Uninfluenced by exposure to light.

photosynthesis (fō″tō-sĭn′thĕ-sĭs) [″ + *synthesis,* placing together]. The process by which plants are able to manufacture carbohydrates by combining carbon dioxide from the air and water from the soil, utilizing light energy in the presence of chlorophyll.

The basic chemical reaction is as follows:

$$6CO_2 + 6H_2O + \text{light energy} \rightarrow C_6H_{12}O_6 + 6O_2$$

Only plants containing chlorophyll are capable of thus producing sugars. The red and blue waves of the spectrum are absorbed by the chlorophyll, but all other rays are reflected. CO_2 and H_2O are also necessary factors.

When simple sugar is formed, the plant utilizes the light energy plus water and CO_2 to form carbohydrate. The sources of energy for this synthesis are the blue and red rays that are absorbed by the plant. To make 1 gm. of natural sugar the plant uses 750 cu. ft. (21.24 cubic meters) of CO_2.

phototaxis (fō″tō-tăk′sĭs) [Gr. *photos,* light, + *taxis,* arrangement]. The reaction and movement of cells and microorganisms under the stimulus of light.

phototherapy (fō″tō-thĕr′ă-pē) [″ + *therapeia,* treatment]. 1. Exposure to sunlight or artificial light for therapeutic purposes. 2. Reduction of serum bilirubin concentration in the newborn infant by exposure to sunlight or artificial blue light. Infant's eyes must be protected from the light used.

photothermal (fō″tō-thĕr′măl) [″ + *therme,* heat]. Concerning heat produced by light.

photothermal radiation. Radiation of heat by a source of light, as that from an electric bulb.

phototimer. A device that automatically terminates a radiographic exposure after a preset amount of radiation has reached it.

phototonus (fō-tŏt′ō-nŭs) [″ + *tonos,* tension]. Sensitivity in an organism produced by exposure to light.

phototopia (fō″tō-tō′pē-ă). A subjective sensation of light.

phototoxic (fō″tō-tŏk′sĭk) [″ + *toxikon,* poison]. Pert. to the harmful reaction produced by light energy, esp. that produced in the skin. Simple sunburn of the skin is an example of phototoxicity.

phototoxis (fō″tō-tŏk′sĭs). Disorder produced by effects of overexposure to light or radiation.

phototrophic (fō″tō-trŏf′ĭk) [″ + *trophe,* nutrition]. Concerning the ability to use light in metabolism.

phototropism (fō-tŏt′rō-pĭzm) [″ + *tropos,* turning, + *-ismos,* condition]. A tendency exhibited by green plants and some microorganisms to turn toward or grow toward light.

photuria (fō-tū′rē-ă) [″ + *ouron,* urine]. Excretion of phosphorescent urine.

phren (frēn) [Gr.]. 1. The mind. 2. The diaphragm.

phrenalgia (frē-năl′jē-ă). 1. [Gr. *phren,* mind, + *algos,* pain] Pain of hysterical origin. SYN: *psychalgia.* 2. [Gr. *phren,* diaphragm, + *algos,* pain] Pain in the diaphragm.

phrenectomy (frĕ-nĕk′tō-mē) [Gr. *phren,* diaphragm, + *ektome,* excision]. 1. Surgical excision of all or part of the diaphragm. 2. Surgical resection of part of the phrenic nerve.

phrenemphraxis (frĕn″ĕm-frăk′sĭs) [″ + *emphraxis,* stoppage]. Crushing of the phrenic nerve in order to induce temporary paralysis of the diaphragm; a therapeutic measure that was previously employed in treatment of pulmonary tuberculosis.

phrenetic (frĕn-ĕt′ĭk) [Gr. *phren,* mind]. 1. Maniacal; frenzied. 2. A maniac.

-phrenia. Combining form indicating mental disorder.

phrenic (frĕn′ĭk). 1. [Gr. *phren,* diaphragm] Concerning the diaphragm, as the phrenic nerve. 2. [Gr. *phren,* mind] Concerning the mind.

phrenic avulsion. Elevation of a side of the diaphragm and semi-collapse of the corresponding lung by means of excision of part of the phrenic nerve.

phrenicectomy (frĕn-ĭ-sĕk′tō-mē) [″ + *ektome,* excision]. Resection of a part of the phrenic nerve. Used to collapse the lung on one side by paralyzing the diaphragm.

phreniclasia (frĕn″ĭ-klā′zē-ă) [″ + *klasis,* destruction]. Phrenemphraxis, q.v.

phrenic nerve. Nerve arising in the cervical plexus, entering the thorax, and passing to the diaphragm. A motor nerve to the diaphragm with sensory fibers to the pericardium.

phrenicoexeresis (frĕn″ĭ-kō-ĕk-sĕr′ĕ-sĭs) [″ + *exairesis,* taking out]. Excision of part of the phrenic nerve.

phreniconeurectomy (frĕn″ĭ-kō-nū-rĕk′tō-mē) [″ + *neuron,* nerve, + *ektome,* excision]. Excision of part of the phrenic nerve.

phrenicotomy (frĕn″ĭ-kŏt′ō-mē) [″ + *tome,* incision]. Cutting of the phrenic nerve to produce immobilization of a lung by inducing paralysis of one side. This causes the diaphragm to rise; it compresses the lung and diminishes respiratory movement, thus resting the lung on that side.

phrenicotripsy (frĕn″ĭ-kō-trĭp′sē) [″ + *tripsis,* a crushing]. Crushing of the phrenic nerve.

phrenitis (frē-nī′tĭs) [″ + *itis,* inflammation]. 1. Acute delirium or frenzy. 2. Inflammation of the brain. SYN: *encephalitis.* 3. [Gr. *phren,* diaphragm, + *itis,* inflammation] Inflammation of the diaphragm.

phreno- [Gr. *phren,* mind; L. *phrenicus,* diaphragm]. Combining form meaning mind or diaphragm.

phrenocardia (frē″nō-kăr′dē-ă) [Gr. *phren,* mind, + *kardia,* heart]. Cardiovascular neurasthenia.

SYM: Cardiac arrhythmia, dyspnea with psychic disturbances, and submammary pain.

phrenocolic (frĕn″ō-kŏl′ĭk) [Gr. *phren,* diaphragm, + *kolon,* colon]. Concerning the diaphragm and the colon.

phrenocolopexy (frĕn″ō-kō′lō-pĕk″sē) [″ + *kolon*, colon, + *pexis*, fixation]. Suture of the transverse colon to the diaphragm.

phrenodynia (frĕn″ō-dĭn′ē-ă) [″ + *odyne*, pain]. Pain in the diaphragm.

phrenogastric (frĕn″ō-găs′trĭk) [″ + *gaster*, belly]. Concerning the diaphragm and the stomach.

phrenoglottic (frĕn″ō-glŏt′ĭk) [″ + *glottis*, back of tongue]. Concerning the diaphragm and the glottis.

phrenograph (frĕn′ō-grăf) [″ + *graphein*, to write]. Device for registering movements of the diaphragm.

phrenohepatic (frĕn″ō-hĕ-păt′ĭk) [″ + *hepar*, liver]. Concerning the diaphragm and the liver.

phrenologist (frĕ-nŏl′ō-jĭst) [Gr. *phren*, mind, + *logos*, study]. A person who claims to use the shape of the head to diagnose and predict mental capabilities. There is no evidence that such efforts can be scientifically validated.

phrenology (frĕ-nŏl′ō-jē) [″ + *logos*, study]. The imagined ability to predict mental capabilities by studying the shape of the head.

phrenopericarditis (frē″nō-pĕr″ĭ-kar-dī′tĭs) [Gr. *phren*, diaphragm, + *peri*, around, + *kardia*, heart, + *itis*, inflammation]. Attachment of the heart by adhesions to the diaphragm.

phrenoplegia (frĕn-ō-plē′jē-ă) 1. [Gr. *phren*, mind, + *plege*, stroke]. A sudden attack of mental illness. 2. [Gr. *phren*, diaphragm, + Gr. *plege*, stroke] Paralysis of the diaphragm.

phrenoptosis (frĕn″ŏp-tō′sĭs) [Gr. *phren*, diaphragm, + *ptosis*, falling]. Downward displacement of the diaphragm.

phrenosin (frĕn′ō-sĭn). A cerebroside isolated from brain tissue.

phrenospasm (frĕn′ō-spăzm) [″ + *spasmos*, convulsion]. Spasm of the diaphragm.

phrenosplenic (frĕn″ō-splĕn′ĭk) [″ + *splen*, spleen]. Concerning the diaphragm and the spleen.

phrenotropic (frĕn″ō-trŏp′ĭk) [Gr. *phren*, mind, + *tropikos*, turning]. Affecting the brain.

phrictopathic (frĭk-tō-păth′ĭk) [Gr. *phriktos*, shuddering, + *pathos*, disease]. Pert. to or having a shuddering sensation; applied to a shuddering sensation due to irritating a hysterical anesthetic area.

phronesis (frō-nē′sĭs) [Gr.]. Soundness of mind.

phrynoderma (frĭn-ō-dĕr′mă) [Gr. *phryne*, toad, + *derma*, skin]. A form of follicular keratosis of unknown etiology but thought to be related to one of several vitamin deficiencies.

phthalylsulfathiazole (thăl″ĭl-sŭl″fă-thī′ă-zōl). USP. A poorly absorbed sulfonamide that has no therapeutic usefulness.

phthiriasis (thĭr-ī′ă-sĭs) [Gr. *phtheiriasis*]. Condition of being infested with lice. SYN: *pediculosis*.

phthiriophobia (thĭr″ē-ō-fō′bē-ă) [Gr. *phtheir*, louse, + *phobos*, fear]. Abnormal dread of lice. SYN: *pediculophobia*.

Phthirus (thĭr′ŭs) [Gr. *phtheir*, louse]. A genus of sucking lice belonging to the order Anoplura.

P. pubis. The crab louse. Infests primarily the pubic region but is also found in armpits, beard, eyebrows, and eyelashes. SEE: *pediculosis pubis*.

phthisic (tĭz′ĭk) [Gr. *phthisikos*]. 1. Affected with pulmonary tuberculosis. 2. One afflicted with phthisis.

phthisical (tĭz′ĭ-kăl). Concerning, or afflicted with, phthisis.

phthisis (tī′sĭs) [Gr., a wasting]. 1. Pulmonary tuberculosis. 2. Any wasting or atrophic disease.

p., abdominal. Intestinal tuberculosis.

p., black. Lung disease from inhaled coal dust. SYN: *anthracosis; black lung; p., miner's*.

p. bulbi. Atrophy of the eyeball following intraocular inflammation.

p., fibroid. 1. Interstitial pneumonia. 2. Pulmonary tuberculosis with dense layers of fibrous tissues surrounding a cavity.

p., grinders'. The combination of tuberculosis and pneumoconiosis in knife grinders who inhale the dust from the grinding wheel.

p., miner's. P., black.

p., pulmonary. Tuberculosis of the lungs.

p., stonecutter's. A wasting form of bronchopneumonia due to inhalation of silica-containing dust with consequent irritation.

phycobilin (fī″kō-bĭl′ĭn). A chemical that acts as light absorbers in algae.

phycochrome (fī′kō-krōm) [Gr. *phykos*, seaweed, + *chroma*, color]. A blue-green pigment present in algae.

phycocyanin (fī″kō-sī′ăn-ĭn). A blue pigment present in blue-green algae.

phycoerythrin (fī″kō-ĕr′ĭ-thrĭn). A red pigment present in the chloroplasts of some red algae.

phycology (fī-kŏl′ō-jē) [Gr. *phykos*, seaweed, + *logos*, study]. Study of algae.

Phycomycetes (fī″kō-mī-sē′tēz) [″ + *mykes*, fungus]. A class of fungi several genera of which occasionally cause disease in humans.

phycomycosis (fī″kō-mī-kō′sĭs) [″ + ″ + *osis*, condition]. A disease caused by the phycomycetes fungi. The Rhizopus species is the most common cause of disease in man, but the genera Absidia, Mortierella, and Basidobolus may also cause infection.

Infection is contracted through inhalation of the spores, but may also enter the body through breaks in the skin or mucous membranes. Patients with poorly controlled diabetes can contract severe infection of the central nervous system with Phycomycetes. Visceral infections can occur secondary to severe malnutrition, uremia, liver failure, or in those on corticosteroid or broad-spectrum antibiotic therapy. Infection spreads to adjacent areas by direct contact.

TREATMENT: Therapy for the primary condition; and administration of amphotericin B.

phylactic (fĭ-lăk'tĭk) [Gr. *phylaktikos,* preservative]. Concerning or producing phylaxis.

phylaxis (fĭ-lăk'sĭs) [Gr., protection]. The active defense of the body against infection.

phyletic (fĭ-lĕt'ĭk) [Gr. *phyletikos*]. Pert. to a phylum or race. SYN: *phylogenetic.*

phyllo- [Gr. *phyllon,* leaf]. Combining form meaning leaf.

phylloquinone (fĭl"ō-kwĭn'ōn). Phytonadione, q.v.

phylogenesis (fĭ"lō-jĕn'ĕ-sĭs) [Gr. *phyle,* tribe, + *genesis,* generation]. The evolutionary development of a group, race, or species. SEE: *phylogeny.*

phylogenetic (fĭ"lō-jĕ-nĕt'ĭk). Concerning the development of a race or group.

phylogeny (fĭ-lŏj'ĕ-nē). Development and growth of a race or group of animals. SEE: *ontogeny.*

phylum (fĭ'lŭm) [Gr. *phylon,* tribe]. (pl. *phyla*) One of the primary divisions of the animal or plant kingdom, next higher than a class.

phyma (fĭ'mă) [Gr., a growth]. (pl. *phymata*) A small, rounded skin tumor.

phymatoid (fĭ'mă-toyd) [" + *eidos,* resemblance]. Like a tumor.

phymatorrhysin (fĭ"mă-tō-rĭ'sĭn). A pigment present in hair and melanotic tumors.

phymatosis (fĭ-mă-tō'sĭs) [Gr. *phyma,* a growth, + *osis,* condition]. A disease marked by the presence of phymata or small nodules in the skin.

physaliform, physalliform (fĭ-săl'ĭ-form) [Gr. *physallis,* bubble, + L. *forma,* shape]. Resembling a bleb or bubble.

physaliphore (fĭ-săl'ĭ-for) [" + *phorein,* to carry]. Physaliphorous cell.

physaliphorous (fĭs"ă-lĭf'ō-rŭs). Pert. to a highly vacuolated cell present in a chordoma.

physalis (fĭs'ă-lĭs) [Gr. *physallis,* bubble]. A large vacuole present in the cell of certain malignancies such as a chondroma.

Physaloptera (fĭs"ă-lŏp'tĕr-ă) [" + *pteron,* wing]. A genus of nematode worms belonging to the suborder Spiruata.

P. caucasica. Species that occurs in and damages the upper gastrointestinal tract.

physiatrics (fĭz"ē-ăt'rĭks) [Gr. *physis,* nature, + *iatrikos,* treatment]. The curing of disease by natural methods, esp. physical therapy.

physiatrist (fĭz"ē-ăt'rĭst). A physician who specializes in physical medicine.

physic (fĭz'ĭk) [Gr. *physikos,* natural]. 1. The art of medicine and healing. 2. A medicine, esp. a cathartic.

physical (fĭz'ĭ-kăl). 1. Of or pert. to nature or material things. 2. Concerning or pert. to the body; bodily.

physical examination. Examination of the body by auscultation, palpation, percussion, inspection, and smelling.

physical fitness. The ability to carry out daily tasks with vigor and alertness, without undue fatigue, and with ample energy to enjoy leisure-time pursuits and meet unforeseen emergencies. It is the ability to withstand stress and persevere under difficult circumstances where an unfit person would quit. Implied in this is more than lack of illness; it is a positive quality that everyone has to some degree. Physical fitness is minimal in the severely ill and maximum in the highly trained athlete.

physical signs. Disease symptoms revealed by physical examination.

physical therapist. An individual who is legally responsible for planning, conducting and evaluating a physical therapy program for patients referred by physicians.

physical therapist aide. An individual with on-the-job training and experience who performs routine tasks under direction of the physical therapist.

physical therapist assistant. An individual who works within a physical therapy service carrying out a planned program under the direction of a physical therapist.

physical therapy. Rehabilitation concerned with restoration of function and prevention of disability following disease, injury, or loss of body part. The therapeutic properties of exercise, heat, cold, electricity, ultraviolet, and massage are used to improve circulation, strengthen muscles, encourage return of motion, and train or retrain an individual to perform the activities of daily living.

physician (fĭ-zĭsh'ŭn) [O. Fr. *physicien*]. A person who has successfully completed the prescribed course of studies in medicine in a medical school officially recognized by the country in which it is located and who has acquired the requisite qualifications for licensure in the practice of medicine.

p., attending. Physician who is on the staff of a hospital and regularly cares for patients therein.

p., family. SEE: *p., primary care.*

p., primary care. The physician to whom a family or individual goes initially when ill or for a periodic health check. This physician assumes medical coordination of care with other physicians for the patient with multiple health concerns.

p., resident. A physician who works full or part time in a hospital to continue training after internship. Commonly called resident.

physician's assistant. ABBR: P.A. A specially trained and (when necessary) licensed individual who performs tasks usually done by physicians under the direction of a supervising physician. Physician's assistants are usually salaried rather than reimbursed on a fee-for-service basis although the supervising physician may receive fee-for-service for their services.

Physician's Desk Reference. ABBR: PDR. An annual compendium of information concerning drugs, primarily prescription and diagnostic products. The information is largely that included in the labeling or package insert as required by the Food and Drug Administration: indication for use, effects, dosages, administration, warnings, hazards, contraindications, side effects, and precautions.

physician shortage area. An area with an inadequate supply of physicians, usually with a physician to population ratio less than 1 to 4,000.

physicist (fĭz'ĭ-sĭst) [L. *physics,* natural sciences]. A specialist in the science of physics.

physico- [Gr. *physikos*]. Combining form indicating physical or natural.

physicochemical (fĭz"ĭ-kō-kĕm'ĭ-kăl) [" + *chemeia,* chemistry]. Concerning the application of the laws of physics to chemical reactions.

physics (fĭz'ĭks) [Gr. *physis,* nature]. The study of the laws of matter and their interactions with energy. Included are the fields of acoustics, optics, mechanics, electricity, and thermodynamics, and the study of ionizing radiation.

physio- [Gr. *physis*]. Combining form indicating relationship to nature.

physiochemical (fĭz"ē-ō-kĕm'ĭ-kăl) [Gr. *physis,* nature, + *chemeia,* chemistry]. Concerning clinical chemistry.

physiocogenic (fĭz"ē-ō-kō-jĕn'ĭk) [" + *gennan,* to produce.]. Originating from physical causes.

physiocopyrexia (fĭz"ē-ō-kō"pī-rĕk'sē-ă) [" + *pyressein,* feverish]. Fever produced artificially by physical means.

physiognomy (fĭz"ē-ŏg'nō-mē) [Gr. *physis,* nature, + *gnomon,* a judge]. 1. The countenance. 2. Assumed ability to judge the mental or moral character and qualities by the face.

physiognosis (fĭz"ē-ŏg-nō'sĭs) [" + *gnosis,* knowledge]. Diagnosis determined from one's facial expression and appearance of the eyes.

physiological (fĭz"ē-ō-lŏj'ĭ-kăl) [Gr. *physis,* nature, + *logos,* study]. Concerning body function.

physiological salt solution. ABBR: P.S.S. A sterile solution consisting of 0.85% sodium chloride in distilled water It is isotonic to body fluids. A teaspoonful of table salt in a pint of water approximates a physiological salt solution. Used in irrigating mucous membranes and raw surfaces, in replenishing of body water in dehydration, and in shock or hemorrhage to restore circulating blood volume. SEE: *saline solution.*

physiologicoanatomical (fĭz"ē-ō-lŏj"ĭ-kō-ăn"ă-tŏm'ĭ-kăl) [" + " + *anatome,* dissection]. Concerning physiology and anatomy.

physiologist (fĭz"ē-ŏl'ō-jĭst). A person trained in and capable in the field of physiology.

physiology (fĭz"ē-ŏl'ō-jē) [Gr. *physis,* nature, + *logos,* study]. The science of the functions of the living organism and its components and the chemical and physical processes involved.

p., cell. The physiology of cells.

p., comparative. Study and comparison of the physiology of different species.

p., general. The broad scientific basis of physiology.

p., pathologic. The physiological explanation of pathological events.

p., special. Physiology of special organs or systems.

physiomedical (fĭz"ē-ō-mĕd'ĭ-kăl) [" + L. *medicina,* medicine]. Practice of medicine utilizing only bland plant-derived medicines.

physiopathologic (fĭz"ē-ō-păth"ō-lŏj'ĭk) [" + *pathos,* disease, + *logos,* study]. 1. Concerning physiology and pathology. 2. Pertaining to a pathological alteration in a normal function.

physiotherapy (fĭz"ē-ō-thĕr'ă-pē) [" + *therapeia,* treatment]. Treatment with physical and mechanical means, as massage or electricity. SYN: *physical therapy.*

physique (fĭ-zēk') [Fr.]. Body build; the structure and organization of the body.

physis (fī'sĭs) [Gr. *phyein,* to generate]. The portion of a long bone involved with the linear growth of a bone.

physo- [Gr. *physa,* air]. Combining form indicating air or gas.

physocele (fī'sō-sēl) [Gr. *physa,* air, + *kele,* tumor]. 1. A tumor filled with gas or circumscribed swelling due to gas. 2. A gas-distended hernial sac.

physocephaly (fī"sō-sĕf'ă-lē [" + *kephale,* head]. Swelling of the head due to the abnormal presence of air under the skin of the scalp.

physohematometra (fī"sō-hĕm"ă-tō-mē'tră) [" + *haima,* blood, + *metra,* uterus]. Gas and blood distending the uterus.

physohydrometra (fī"sō-hī"drō-mē'tră) [" + *hydor,* water, + *metra,* uterus]. Air or gas and serum in the uterus.

physometra (fī″sō-mē′tră) [″ + *metra,* uterus]. Air or gas in the uterine cavity.

physopyosalpinx (fī″sō-pī″ō-săl′pĭnks) [″ + *pyon,* pus, + *salpinx,* tube]. Pus and gas in the fallopian tube.

physostigmine salicylate (fī″sō-stĭg′mĭn săl-ĭs′ĭl-āt). USP. The salicylate of an alkaloid usually obtained from the dried ripe seed of Physostigma venenosum. Trade names are Antilirium and Isopto Eserine.

ACTION AND USES: Cholinergic. It inactivates cholinesterase, thus prolonging and intensifying the action of acetylcholine. It improves the tone and action of skeletal muscle; it increases intestinal peristalsis through its effects on the parasympathetic nervous system; and it acts as a miotic in the eye. It is used in tetanus and strychnine poisoning and in the treatment of myasthenia gravis.

phytalbumose (fī-tăl′bū-mōs) [Gr. *phyton,* plant, + L. *albumen,* white protein]. An albumose found in plants and vegetables.

phytase (fī′tās) [″ + *ase,* enzyme]. An enzyme found in grains and present in the kidneys; important in splitting phytin or phytic acid into inositol and phosphoric acid.

phytin (fī′tĭn). A calcium or magnesium salt of inositol and hexaphosphoric acid, present in cereals. SEE: *inositol.*

phyto-, phyt- [Gr. *phyton*]. Combining forms indicating a plant or that which grows.

phytoagglutinin (fī″tō-ă-gloo′tĭ-nĭn) [Gr. *phyton,* plant, + L. *agglutinans,* gluing]. A lectin that agglutinates red blood cells and leukocytes.

phytoalexins. Substances produced by plants. These counteract plant infections.

phytobezoar (fī″tō-bē′zor) [″ + Arabic *bazahr,* protecting against poison]. A mass composed of vegetable matter found in the stomach. SYN: *food ball.* SEE: *bezoar.*

phytochemistry (fī″tō-kĕm′ĭs-trē) [″ + *chemeia,* chemistry]. Study of plant chemistry.

phytocholesterol (fī″tō-kō-lĕs′tĕr-ŏl) [″ + *chole,* bile, + *stereos,* solid]. Phytosterol, q.v.

phytogenesis (fī″tō-jĕn′ĕ-sĭs) [″ + *genesis,* generation]. The origin and development of plants. SYN: *phytogeny.*

phytogenous (fī-tŏj′ĕ-nŭs) [″ + *gennan,* to produce]. Arising in or caused by plants.

phytohemagglutinin (fī″tō-hĕm-ă-glū′tĭ-nĭn) [″ + *haima,* blood, + L. *agglutinare,* to glue to]. ABBR: PHA. A specific substance, called a lectin, derived from plants. It agglutinates red blood cells.

phytoid (fī′toyd) [″ + *eidos,* like]. 1. Plantlike. 2. Any disease of vegetable parasitic origin. 3. The production of a disease by plant parasites. 4. The presence of plant parasites in an organism.

phytomenadione (fī″tō-mĕn″ă-dī′ōn). Phytonadione, q.v.

phytonadione (fī″tō-nă-dī′ōn). 1. USP. Synthetic vitamin K_1. Used as a prothrombogenic agent. 2. USP. An anticoagulant drug that is little used because of its toxicity. Trade names are Aqua Mephyton, Konakion, and Mephyton.

phytoparasite (fī″tō-păr′ă-sīt) [Gr. *phyton,* plant, + *parasitos,* fellow guest]. A vegetable parasite.

phytopathogenic (fī″tō-păth″ō-jĕn′ĭk) [″ + *pathos,* disease, + *gennan,* to produce]. Causing disease in plants.

phytopathology (fī″tō-pă-thŏl′ō-jē) [″ + ″ + *logos,* study]. Study of plant diseases.

phytophagous (fī-tŏf′ă-gŭs) [″ + *phagein,* to eat]. 1. Plant eating. 2. Vegetarian.

phytopharmacology (fī″tō-făr″mă-kŏl′ō-jē) [″ + *pharmakon,* drug, + *logos,* study]. The study of the effects of drugs and chemicals on plants.

phytophotodermatitis (fī″tō-fō″tō-dĕr″mă-tī′tĭs) [″ + *photos,* light, + *derma,* skin, + *itis,* inflammation]. A dermatitis produced by exposure to certain plants and then sunlight.

phytoplankton (fī″tō-plănk′tŏn) [″ + *planktos,* wandering]. Plankton that are classed as vegetable life rather than animal.

phytoplasm (fī′tō-plăzm) [″ + *plasma,* thing formed]. Vegetable protoplasm.

phytoprecipitin (fī″tō-prē-sĭp′ĭ-tĭn). A precipitin produced by immunization with a plant protein.

phytosis (fī-tō′sĭs) [″ + *osis,* condition]. 1. A disease caused by a vegetable parasite. 2. Presence of vegetable parasites.

phytosterol (fī″tō-stē′rŏl). Any sterol present in vegetable oil or fat.

phytotoxic (fī″tō-tŏk′sĭk). 1. Concerning a substance poisonous to plants. 2. Concerning a phytotoxin.

phytotoxin (fī″tō-tŏk′sĭn) [Gr. *phyton,* plant + *toxikon,* a poison]. A toxin produced by or derived from a plant. SEE: *ricin.*

pI. The pH of the isoelectric point of a substance in solution.

pia (pī′ă, pē′ă) [L.]. Tender, soft.

pia-arachnitis (pī″ă-, pē″ă-ăr″ăk-nī′tĭs). Piarachnitis.

pia-arachnoid. Piarachnoid.

pial (pī′ăl). Concerning the pia mater.

pia mater (pī′ă mā′tĕr, pē′ă mă′tĕr) [L. *pia,* soft, + *mater,* mother]. A thin vascular membrane closely investing the brain and spinal cord and proximal portions of the nerves. Innermost of the three meninges. The other portions of the covering are dura mater and the arachnoid. SEE: *meninges.*

pian (pē-ăn′) [Fr.]. Contagious skin disease of the tropics. SYN: *yaws.*

pianists' cramp. Spasm, or occupational neurosis, of muscles of fingers and forearms from piano playing.

piarachnitis (pī″ăr-ăk-nī′tĭs) [L. *pia,* tender, + Gr. *arachne,* spider, + *itis,* inflammation]. Inflammation of the arachnoid and pia mater. SYN: *leptomeningitis.*

piarachnoid (pī″ăr-ăk′noyd) [″ + ″ + *eidos,* like]. The pia mater and arachnoid membranes when regarded as one structure. SYN: *leptomeninges.*

pica (pī′kă) [L., magpie]. A perversion of appetite with ingestion of material not fit for food, as starch, clay, ashes, or plaster. Condition seen in pregnancy, chlorosis, hysteria, helminthiasis, and in certain psychoses. SEE: *appetite; taste.*

piceous (pĭ′sē-ŭs) [L. *piceus,* pitch]. Like pitch.

Pick, Arnold. Czechoslovakian physician, 1851–1924.

P.'s disease. A form of presenile dementia due to atrophy of the frontal and temporal lobes. Usually occurs between the ages of 40 and 60, more often in women than men. Involves progressive, irreversible loss of memory, deterioration of intellectual functions, disordered emotions, apathy, speech disturbances, and disorientation. Course may take from a few months to 4 or 5 years to progress to complete loss of intellectual function. SEE: *Alzheimer's disease.*

Pick, Friedel. Czechoslovakian physician, 1867–1926.

P.'s disease. Nonrheumatic chronic pericarditis of unknown etiology.

Pick, Ludwig. German physician, 1868–1935.

P.'s cells. A foamy, lipid-filled cell present in the spleen and bone marrow in Niemann-Pick's disease. SYN: *cell, Niemann-Pick.*

P.'s disease. Niemann-Pick disease.

pick 1. A sharp, pointed, curved dental instrument used to explore tooth surfaces and restorations for defects. 2. To remove bits of food from teeth.

pickling. 1. A method of preserving and flavoring food in which the food is soaked in a solution of salt and vinegar. 2. Use of a chemical solution to remove scales and oxides from metals prior to plating them.

pickwickian syndrome. [Inspired by Joe, an obese character in Pickwick Papers by Charles Dickens] Obesity, decreased pulmonary function, and polycythemia.

pico- [It. *pico,* small]. Combining form used to indicate a unit of measurement that is one trillionth of the basic unit. This is 10^{-12} of the basic unit. Thus a picogram is:

$$\frac{1}{10^{12}} \text{ or } 0.000000000001 \text{ gram}$$

picogram. ABBR: pg. 1×10^{-12} gram or one trillionth of a gram.

picornaviruses (pī-kor″nă-vī′rŭ-sĕs) [″ + *RNA,* ribonucleic acid, + L. *virus,* virus]. Very small viruses that are insoluble in a lipid solvent such as ether. Those that affect humans have been classified as Coxsackievirus A (23 species), Coxsackievirus B (6 species), ECHO virus (31 species), poliovirus (3 species), and rhinovirus (approx. 89 species).

picrate (pĭk′răt). A salt of picric acid.

picric acid. SEE: *acid, picric.*

picro-, picr- [Gr. *pikros,* bitter]. Combining forms meaning bitter.

picrocarmine (pĭk″rō-kăr′mĭn). A stain used in microscopy.

picroformal (pĭk″rō-for′măl). Solution of picric acid, formaldehyde, and water used as a fixing agent.

picrol (pĭk′rōl). Antiseptic powder used as a dressing for wounds.

picrotoxin (pĭk″rō-tŏk′sĭn) [″ + *toxikon,* poison]. A powerful stimulant to the central nervous system, obtained from the seed of Anamirta cocculus, a shrub. It is used as a respiratory stimulant.

pictograph (pĭk′tō-grăf). A set of test pictures used for testing vision in children and illiterate adults.

P.I.D. *pelvic inflammatory disease,* q.v.

piebald skin (pī′băld) [ME. *pie,* magpie, + *ballede,* bald]. Skin with spots of pigmentation, or patches with loss of pigment. SEE: *leukoderma; vitiligo.*

piedra (pē-ā′dră) [Sp., stone]. A fungus disease, affecting only the hair, in which hard nodules form on the hair shafts. Black piedra is caused by the fungus Piedraia hortae and white piedra by Trichosporon beigelii. Either form of the disease is cured by shaving the hair. SYN: *tinea nodosa.*

Pierre Robin syndrome. [Pierre Robin, French pediatrician, 1867–1950] Unusual smallness of the jaw combined with cleft palate, downward displacement of the tongue, and an absent gag reflex.

piesesthesia (pī-ē″zĕs-thē′zē-ă) [Gr. *piesis,* pressure, + *aisthesis,* sensation]. Sensitivity to pressure.

piesimeter, piesometer (pī″ĕ-sĭm′ĕ-tĕr, -sŏm′ĕ-tĕr) [″ + *metron,* measure]. Device for measurement of skin's sensitiveness to pressure.

-piesis. A combining form used at the end of a word to indicate pressure.

piezochemistry (pī-ē′zō-kĕm″ĭs-trē) [Gr. *piezo,* to squeeze, + *chemeia,* chemistry]. The study of the effect of high pressure on chemical reactions.

piezoelectricity [″ + *elektron,* amber]. Production of an electric current by application of pressure to certain crystals such as mica, quartz, or Rochelle salt.

piezogenic pedal papules (pī-ē'zō-jĕn"ĭk) [" + *gennan,* to produce]. Soft painful skin-colored papules present on the non-weight-bearing portion of the heel. They disappear when weight is taken off the foot and heel. Caused by herniation of fat through connective tissue defects.

piezometer (pī"ē-zŏm'ĕ-tĕr) [" + *metron,* measure]. Piesimeter, q.v.

PIF. *proliferation inhibiting factor.* SEE: *factor, proliferation inhibiting.*

pigeon breast. Deformity in which the sternum projects anteriorly. Caused by rickets or obstructed respiration in childhood. SYN: *chicken breast.*

pigeon-breeder's disease. Attacks of chills, fever, and cough with shortness of breath in persons who are closely associated with birds such as pigeons and parakeets. In some patients the onset is slow rather than acute. The symptoms are due to antigenic substances in the bird's excreta. Symptoms usually subside when exposure to the birds ceases.

pigeon-toed. Walking with feet turned inward. SYN: *pes varus.*

pigment (pĭg'mĕnt) [L. *pigmentum,* paint]. Any organic coloring matter in the body. SEE: *albino;* words beginning with *chrom-.*

p.'s, bile. Complex, highly colored substances found in bile derived from the red pigment (hemoglobin) of the blood and imparting brown color to intestinal contents and feces. Included are bilirubin, biliverdin and their derivatives (urobilinogen, urobilin, bilicyanin, and bilifuscin).

p., blood. Pigment in blood (hemoglobin) or a derivative of it (hematin, hemin, methemoglobin, hemosiderin).

p., endogenous. Pigment produced within the body, as melanin.

p., exogenous. Pigment produced outside the human body.

p., hematogenous. Pigment from hemoglobin of the erythrocytes.

p., hepatogenous. Pigment from hemoglobin destruction in the liver. SYN: *bile pigment.*

p., respiratory. Any pigment such as hemoglobin, myoglobin, cytochrome, or flavine that has a part in oxidative processes of the body.

p., skin. Melanin, melanoid, and carotene.

p., urinary. Urochrome and sometimes urobilin.

p., uveal. Pigment found in cells on the inner or posterior surface of the iris, choroid, and ciliary processes.

pigmentary (pĭg'mĕn-tĕr"ē) [L. *pigmentum,* paint]. Concerning, or like, a pigment.

pigmentation (pĭg"mĕn-tā'shŭn). Coloration due to deposition of pigments. SEE: *albinism; carotenemia; "chrom-" words.*

p., hematogenous. Pigmentation produced by the collection of hemoglobin, or pigment carried to a site through the blood.

pigmented (pĭg'mĕnt-ĕd). Colored by a pigment.

pigmentolysin (pĭg"mĕn-tŏl'ĭ-sĭn) [" + Gr. *lysis,* dissolution]. A substance that destroys a pigment.

pigmentophage (pĭg-mĕn'tō-fāj) [" + Gr. *phagein,* to eat]. Any cell that ingests a pigment.

pigmentophore (pĭg-mĕn'tō-for) [" + Gr. *phorein,* to carry]. A cell that carries pigment.

pigmentum nigrum (pĭg-mĕn'tŭm nī'grŭm) [L., black paint]. The black pigment of the lamina vitrea of the choroid of the eye.

piitis (pī-ī'tĭs) [L. *pia,* tender, + Gr. *itis,* inflammation]. Inflamed condition of the pia mater.

Pil. L. *pilula,* pill, or *pilulae,* pills.

pila (pī'lă) [L., pillar]. (pl. *pilae*) A pillarlike structure in spongy bone.

pilar, pilary (pī'lăr, pĭl'ă-rē) [L. *pilaris*]. Concerning, or covered with, hair.

pilaster (pī-lăs'tĕr) [L. *pilastrum,* small pillar]. A prominent ridge sometimes seen on the femur.

pile [L. *pila,* a ball, a pillar]. 1. A single hemorrhoid. SEE: *piles.* 2. The hair. 3. A battery for production of electricity. 4. An apparatus for producing and regulating a nuclear chain-reaction fission process.

p., sentinel. A localized thickening of the mucous membrane at the distal end of an anal fissure.

pileous (pī'lē-ŭs) [L. *pilus,* hair]. Hairy; hirsute.

piles (pīls) [L. *pila,* a mass]. Dilated blood vessels in the rectal mucosa forming a vascular tumor. SYN: *hemorrhoid.*

pileum (pī'lē-ŭm) [L., a cap]. 1. A membrane or portion of the amnion sometimes covering a baby's head at birth. SYN: *caul; pileus* (def. 2). 2. Great omentum.

pileus (pī'lē-ŭs) [L., a cap]. 1. A hemisphere of the cerebellum. 2. Membrane that sometimes covers the head of an infant at birth. SYN: *caul; pileum* (def. 1).

pili (pī'lē). (sing. *pilus*) Hairs.

p. annulata. Condition in which hairs have a ringed appearance; monilethrix.

p. incarnati. Condition of ingrowing hair, esp. in the beard area.

p. tactiles. Sensitive or tactile hairs.

p. torti. Condition in which hairs are broken and twisted.

piliation (pī-lē-ā'shŭn) [L. *pilus,* hair]. Formation and development of hair.

piliform (pī'lĭ-form) [" + *forma,* shape]. Hairlike.

pilimiction (pī″lĭ-mĭk′shŭn) [″ + *mictio,* micturition]. Passing of urine containing hairlike or filamentous substances.

pill (pĭl) [L. *pilula,* small mass]. Medicine in the form of a tiny solid mass or pellet to be swallowed or chewed. May be coated.

pillar (pĭl′ĕr) [L. *pila,* a column]. An upright support, column, or structure resembling a column.

p.'s, anterior, of fornix. Two diverging columns extending downward from anterior extremity of body of the fornix of cerebrum.

p.'s of Corti. Two layers resting on membrana basilaris in the ear. SYN: *rods of Corti.*

p.'s of diaphragm. Crura of diaphragm, two bundles of muscle fibers extending from lumbar vertebrae to the central tendon and forming sides of hiatus aorticus.

p.'s of fauces. Folds of mucous membrane, one on each side of the fauces, q.v., and between which is situated the tonsil. SYN: *arches, glossopalatine; arches, pharyngopalatine.*

pillar cells. Two groups of cells (inner and outer) resting on basement membrane of organ of Corti in which elongated bodies (pillars) develop. These enclose the inner tunnel (Corti's tunnel).

pillet (pĭl′ĕt). A small pill.

pillion (pĭl′yŭn) [L. *pellis,* skin]. Temporary form of artificial leg, esp. a peg-leg type of stump.

pilo- [L. *pilus*]. Combining form indicating hair.

pilobezoar (pī″lō-bē′zor) [″ + Arabic *bazahr,* protecting against poison]. Trichobezoar, q.v.

pilocarpine hydrochloride (pī″lō-kăr′pīn). USP. $C_{11}H_{16}N_2O_2$•HCl. Hydrochloride of an alkaloid obtained from leaflets of Pilocarpus jaborandi and P. microphyllus. Trade names are Almocarpine, Pilomiotin, and Isopto Carpine.

ACTION AND USES: Cholinergic. Causes contraction of the pupil. Used topically as a miotic, esp. in glaucoma.

pilocarpine nitrate. USP. Nitrate of the alkaloid obtained from leaves of the jaborandi tree. Trade name is P.V. Carpine liquifilm.

ACTION AND USES: Same as pilocarpine hydrochloride.

pilocystic (pī″lō-sĭs′tĭk) [L. *pilus,* hair, + Gr, *kystis,* bladder]. Encysted and containing hair, said of a dermoid cyst.

piloerection. Hair erection or apparent stiffening due to stimulation and contraction of the arrector pili muscles. SYN: *goose flesh.*

pilojection [″ + *jacere,* to throw]. Introduction of hairs, by use of a pneumatic gun, into an aneurysm to induce clotting in the aneurysmal sac. Has been used in treating intracranial aneurysms.

pilomatrixoma. Benign calcifying tumor of the skin. It is small and firm with normal skin over it.

Pilomiotin. Trade name for pilocarpine hydrochloride, USP.

pilomotor (pī″lō-mō′tor) [″ + *motor,* mover]. Causing movements of hairs, as the arrectores pilorum, q.v.

pilomotor nerve. A nerve that stimulates an arrector pili muscle. SEE: *arrectores pilorum.*

pilomotor reflex. Goose flesh formation when skin is cooled or as a result of emotional reaction.

pilonidal (pī″lō-nī′dăl) [″ + *nidus,* nest]. Containing hairs in a dermoid cyst in nest formation.

pilonidal cyst. A cyst in the sacrococcygeal region, usually at the upper end of the intergluteal cleft. The cyst is due to a developmental defect that permits epithelial tissue to be trapped below the skin. May become symptomatic in early adulthood when an infected draining sinus forms.

pilonidal fistula. Fistula beneath the skin at the lower end of the spinal column resulting from a pilonidal cyst.

pilonidal sinus. SEE: *pilonidal cyst.*

pilose (pī′lōs) [L. *pilosus*]. Hairy, downy.

pilosebaceous (pī″lō-sē-bā′shŭs) [″ + *sebaceus,* fatty]. Concerning the hair and sebaceous glands.

pilosis (pī-lō′sĭs) [L. *pilosus,* hairy, + Gr. *osis,* condition]. Excessive formation of hair.

pilosity (pī-lŏs′ĭ-tē). Hairiness.

pilous (pī′lŭs) [L. *pilus,* hair]. Covered with hair; hirsute.

Piltz's reflex (pĭlts′ĕz). [Jan Piltz, Polish neurologist, 1870–1931] Change in size of pupil on sudden fixation of attention. SYN: *pupillary reflex.*

pilula (pĭl′ū-lă) [L., pill]. (pl. *pilulae*) A small amount of medicine intended to be swallowed whole and to produce medicinal action.

pilular (pĭl′ū-lar). Pert. to, or of the nature of, pills.

pilule (pĭl′ūl) [L. *pilula*]. A small pill.

pilus (pī′lŭs) [L.]. (pl. *pili*) [NA] A hair.

p. cuniculatus. A hair that burrows into the skin.

p. incarnatus. An ingrown hair.

p. tortus. A twisted hair.

pimel- [Gr. *pimele,* fat]. Combining form or prefix indicating an association with fat.

pimelitis (pĭm-ĕl-ī′tĭs) [Gr. *pimele,* fat, + *itis,* inflammation]. Inflammation of adipose tissue and of connective tissue in general.

pimeloma (pĭm″ĕ-lō′mă) [″ + *oma,* tumor]. A fatty tumor. SYN: *lipoma.*

pimelopterygium (pĭm″ĕ-lō-tĕ-rĭj′ē-ŭm) [″ + *pterygion,* wing]. A fatty outgrowth of the conjunctiva.

pimelorrhea (pĭm″ĕl-or-ē′ă) [″ + *rhoia,* flow].

Discharge of fat in loose stools.

pimelorthopnea (pĭm″ĕl-or″thŏp′nē-ă) [″ + *orthos,* straight, + *pnoia,* breath]. Difficulty in breathing when lying down, resulting from obesity.

pimelosis (pĭm″ĕ-lō′sĭs) [″ + *osis,* condition]. 1. Conversion into fat. 2. Fatty degeneration of any tissue. 3. Corpulence; obesity.

pimeluria (pĭm″ĕl-ū′rē-ă) [″ + *ouron,* urine]. Excretion of fat or oil in urine. SYN: *lipuria.*

pimple (pĭm′pl) [ME. *pinple*]. A papule or pustule of the skin, sometimes going on to suppuration. Often seen in clusters on skin of the adolescent with acne. Patients should be warned not to pick at pimples because infection may result.

pin. A short, slim piece of wire, plastic, or metal. It may or may not have one end blunt and the other sharp.

p., Steinmann. A metal rod used for internal fixation of the adjacent sections of a fractured bone.

pincement (păns-mŏn′) [Fr.]. Pinching or nipping of the flesh in massage.

pinch. A type of hand prehension. The pinch of the human hand is achieved principally through holding objects between the thumb and index finger or the index and long fingers.

Hand pinch is classified according to the anatomical parts involved, as follows:

Pinch, finger tip—pinch using the tips of strongly arched digits, primarily the thumb and index finger. Used to pick up very small objects such as pins and needles.

Pinch, palmar tripod or three jaw chuck—pinch using the palmar pads of the thumb and index and long fingers.

Pinch, lateral—pinch accomplished by clamping the palmar surface of the distal portion of the thumb against the side of the index finger.

pinch meter. A device for objectively measuring the strength of hand pinch in grams or pounds.

pindolol (pĭn′dō-lōl). A β-adrenergic blocking agent.

pineal (pĭn′ē-ăl) [Fr., pine cone]. 1. Shaped like a pine cone. 2. Pert. to the pineal body.

pineal body. A glandlike structure in the brain, shaped like a pine cone, and located in a pocket near the splenium of the corpus collosum. It appears to be the major site of melatonin biosynthesis in most mammals and in man, but the effect of melatonin on the body and the exact function of the pineal body remain unknown.

pinealectomy (pĭn″ē-ăl-ĕk′tō-mē) [L. *pineus,* pineal body, + Gr. *ektome,* excision]. Removal of the pineal body.

pineal gland. SEE: *pineal body.*

pinealism (pĭn′ē-ăl-ĭzm) [″ + Gr. *-ismos,* condition]. Disorder caused by abnormal secretion of the pineal body.

pinealoblastoma (pĭn″ē-ă-lō-blăs-tō′mă) [″ + Gr. *blastos,* germ, + *oma,* tumor]. Pineoblastoma, q.v.

pinealocyte (pĭn′ē-ă-lō-sīt″) [″ + Gr. *kytos,* cell]. The principal cell of the pineal body. It contains pale-staining cytoplasm and has long processes that terminate in bulbous expansions.

pinealoma (pĭn″ē-ă-lō′mă) [″ + Gr. *oma,* tumor]. A tumor of the pineal body, usually encapsulated. Often associated with precocious puberty.

pinealopathy (pĭn″ē-ă-lŏp′ă-thē) [″ + Gr. *pathos,* disease]. Any disorder of the pineal gland.

Pinel, Philippe (pē-nĕl′). French psychologist, 1745–1826, who developed a method or system of treating the mentally ill without the use of restraint, at a time when use of restraint was the accepted form of therapy.

pineoblastoma (pĭn″ē-ō-blăs-tō′mă) [L. *pineus,* pineal body, + Gr. *blastos,* germ, + *oma,* tumor]. A blastoma of the pineal body.

pine tar. USP. A product obtained from the distillation of pine wood. Used as an expectorant, and in certain skin preparations.

pinguecula (pĭn-gwĕk′ū-lă) [L. *pinguiculus,* fatty]. Yellowish thickening of bulbar conjunctiva, triangular in shape, on inner and outer margins of the cornea. The base of the triangle is toward the limbus. Yellowish color is due to increase in elastic fibers.

pinhole (pĭn′hōl) [AS. *pinn,* pin, + *hol,* hole]. Small perforation made by, or size of that made by, a pin.

pinhole os. A very small opening to the uterus from the vagina. This may be present in very young women.

pinhole pupil. Extreme contraction of the iris. The condition is seen in locomotor ataxia, after use of miotics, in some brain diseases, and in opium poisoning.

piniform (pĭn′ĭ-form) [L. *pineas,* pine cone, + *forma,* shape]. Conical; shaped like a pine cone.

pink disease. A disease of infancy characterized by lesions of the skin on the hands and feet, swelling of the extremities, digestive disturbances, and itching of hands and feet, which, along with the cheeks and tip of nose, are intensely pink. It is frequently followed by arthritis involving multiple joints; and muscle weakness. Caused by hypersensitivity to mercury. SYN: *acrodynia.*

pinkeye [D. *pinck oog*]. Epidemic form of acute conjunctivitis caused by various organisms. Sporadic noninfectious cases may result from irritation by various agents such as intense light, or they may accompany exanthematous disease such as measles.

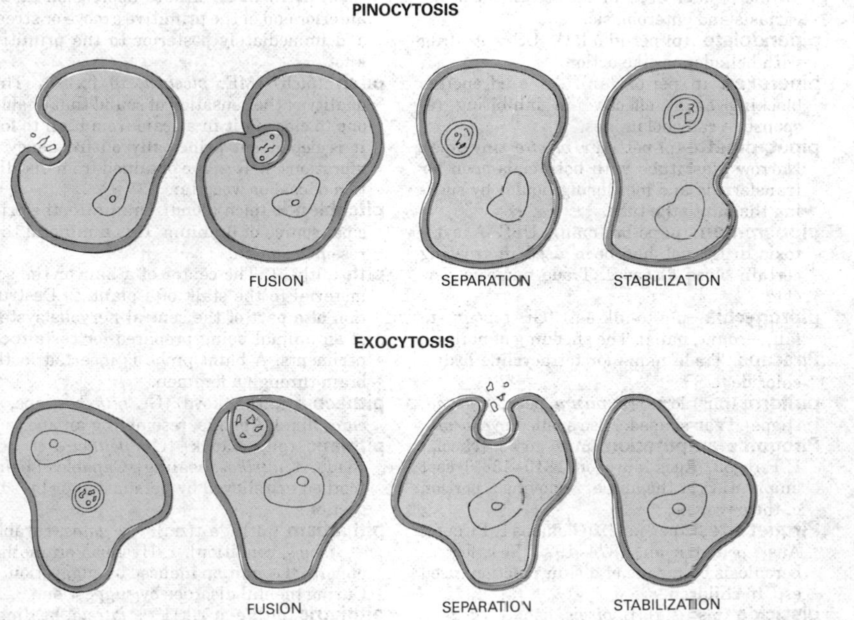

pinna (pĭn′ă) [L., feather]. (pl. *pinnae*) 1. The auricle or projected part of the exterior ear. It collects and directs sound waves into the external acoustic meatus and thence to the tympanic membrane. 2. A feather, fin, wing, or similar appendage.

p. nasi. Protruding cartilaginous extension on each nostril. SYN: *ala nasi* [NA].

pinnal (pĭn′ăl). Concerning pinna.

pinocyte (pī′nō-sīt) [Gr. *pinein,* to drink, + *kytos,* cell]. A cell that exhibits pinocytosis.

pinocytosis (pī″nō-sī-tō′sĭs) [″ + ″ + *osis,* condition]. Process by which cells absorb or ingest nutrients and fluid. A hollowed-out portion of the cell membrane is filled with liquid and the area closes to form a small sac or vacuole. The nutrient, now inside, is available for use in the cell's metabolism. SEE: illus.

pinosome (pī′nō-, pĭn′ō-sōm) [″ + *soma,* body]. The fluid-filled vacuole formed during pinocytosis, q.v.

PINS. *persons in need of supervision,* q.v.

Pins' sign. [Emil Pins, Aust. physician, 1845–1913] In pericarditis, the disappearance of symptoms of pleurisy when patient assumes knee-chest position.

pint (pīnt) [ME. *pinte*]. ABBR: pt. In the U.S.A. a measure of capacity equal to ½ qt.; 16 fl. oz.; 473.2 ml. SEE: *Weights and Measures* in *Appendix.*

pinta (pēn′tă) [Sp., paint]. A nonvenereal disease caused by the spirochete Treponema carateum. This infection is spread by body contact. Manifested by depigmented spots or patches.

TREATMENT: penicillin.

pintid (pĭn′tĭd). A flat red skin lesion present in the second stage of pinta, q.v.

pinus (pī′nŭs) [L.]. The pineal gland.

pinworm. A parasitic nematode Enterobius vermicularis, q.v., causing enterobiasis, infection of intestines and rectum.

pioepithelium (pī″ō-ĕp″ĭ-thē′lē-ŭm) [Gr. *pion,* fat, + *epi,* upon, + *thele,* nipple]. Epithelium that contains fat globules.

pionemia (pī″ō-nē′mē-ă) [″ + *haima,* blood]. An abnormally large amount of fat in the blood. SYN: *lipemia.*

pion therapy. Experimental use of the subatomic particle, the pion, in treating cancer.

piorthopnea (pī″or-thŏp-nē′ă) [″ + *orthos,* straight, + *pnoia,* breath]. Pimelorthopnea, q.v.

Piper (pī′pĕr) [L.]. Genus of plants that produce pepper.

piperacetazine (pĭp″ĕr-ă-sĕt′ă-zēn). USP. An antipsychotic drug. Trade name is Quide.

piperazine (pī-pĕr′ă-zēn). USP. A white crystalline powder used in the treatment of ascariasis and enterobiasis.

piperidolate (pī″pĕr-ĭd′ō-lāt). USP. A drug with belladonna-like action.

piperoxan (pī″pĕr-ŏks′ăn). An α-adrenergic blocking agent effective in inhibiting response to catecholamines.

pipet, pipette (pī-pĕt′) [Fr. *pipette,* tiny pipe]. Narrow glass tube with both ends open for transferring and measuring liquids by sucking them into the tube.

pipobroman (pī″pō-brō′măn). USP. A cytotoxic drug that has been used in treating certain blood diseases. Trade name is Vercyte.

piptonychia (pĭp″tō-nĭk′ē-ă) [Gr. *piptein,* to fall, + *onyx,* nails]. The shedding of nails.

Piracaps. Trade name for tetracycline hydrochloride, USP.

piriform (pĭr′ĭ-form) [L. *pirum,* pear, + *forma,* shape]. Pear-shaped. Also spelled *pyriform.*

Pirogoff's amputation (pĭr″ō-gŏfs′). [Nicolai I. Pirogoff, Russ. surgeon 1810–1881] Foot amputation at the ankle, removing a portion of the os calcis.

Pirquet's test (pĕr-kāz′). [Clemens P. Pirquet, Aust. pediatrician, 1874–1929] Test for tuberculosis by means of a skin reaction, used esp. in children.

piscicide (pĭs′ĭ-sīd) [L. *piscis,* fish, + *caedere,* to kill]. An agent that kills fish.

pisiform (pī′sĭ-form) [L. *pisum,* pea, + *forma,* shape]. 1. Pea shaped. 2. The smallest carpal bone, located in the proximal row on the ulnar side.

pit (pĭt) [ME. *pitt,* hole]. 1. A tiny hollow or pocket. SYN: *depression; fossa.* 2. To be or become marked with a shallow depression; to cause a depression on pressure in edema.

p., anal. The proctodeum, q.v.

p., auditory. A pit that develops in auditory placode.

p., costal. The inferior facet on the body of a vertebra. It articulates with the head of a rib. SYN: *inferior costal facet; fovea costalis inferior.*

p., gastric. One of many minute depressions (foveolae) in gastric mucosa into which the gastric glands open.

p., lens. The depression on the skin of the embryonic head where the lens will develop.

p., nasal. One of two horseshoe-shaped depressions on the ventrolateral surface of the head bounded by lateral and median nasal processes. It gives rise to nostrils and a portion of the nasal fossa.

p. of stomach. 1. Depression at end of the ensiform process. 2. The center of the abdominal region above the navel. SYN: *scrobiculus cordis.*

p., olfactory. P., nasal.

p., primitive. Minute depression at the anterior end of the primitive groove or streak and immediately posterior to the primitive knot.

pitch (pĭch) [ME. *picchen,* to fix]. 1. That quality of the sensation of sound that enables one to classify it in a scale from high to low. It is dependent principally on frequency of vibrations. 2. Residue obtained from distillation of coal or wood tar.

pitchblende (pĭch′blĕnd). Uraninite, the principal source of uranium. It is a mineral that resembles pitch.

pith (pĭth). 1. The center of a hair or the soft material in the stalk of a plant. 2. Destruction of a part of the central nervous system of an animal being prepared for certain experiments. A blunt probe is inserted in the brain through a foramen.

pithecoid (pĭth′ĕ-koyd) [Gr. *pithekos,* ape, + *eidos,* like]. Apelike; resembling an ape.

pithiatic (pĭth-ē-ăt′ĭk) [Gr. *peithein,* to persuade, + *iatrikos,* healing]. Capable of being soothed or relieved by persuasion or by suggestion.

pithiatism (pĭth-ī′ă-tĭzm) [″ + *iatos,* curable, + *-ismos,* condition]. 1. Hysteria or another abnormal condition induced by suggestion. 2. Curing mental disorder by suggestion.

pithiatric (pĭth″ē-ăt′rĭk) [″ + *iatreia,* healing]. Curable by persuasion or suggestion.

pithiatry (pĭth-ī′ă-trē) [″ + *iatreia,* healing]. Treatment of disease by persuasion or suggestion.

pithing (pĭth′ĭng) [ME. *pithe*]. Destruction of the central nervous system by the piercing of brain or spinal cord, as in vivisection. Done on experimental animals to render them insensible to pain and to inhibit controlling effects of the central nervous system during research and experimentation. SEE: *decerebration.*

pithode (pī′thōd) [Gr. *pithose,* wine cask, + *eidos,* form]. The barrel-shaped spindle formed during karyokinesis.

Pitocin. Trade name for oxytocin.

Pitres' sections (pē-trēs′). [Jean A. Pitres, Fr. physician, 1848–1927] Series of six coronal vertical sections of the brain for study. The sections are prefrontal, pediculofrontal, frontal, parietal, pediculoparietal, and occipital.

Pitressin (pĭt-rĕs′ĭn). Trade name for vasopressin, a product obtained from the posterior lobe of the pituitary gland. It contains pressor and antidiuretic principles. SEE: *principle, antidiuretic; vasopressin.*

USES: Increasing blood pressure, increasing the muscular contraction of the intestinal tract, and diminishing urinary output in diabetes insipidus.

Pitressin Tannate (synthetic). Trade name for

argipressin tannate.

pitting (pĭt′ĭng) [ME. *pitt*, hole]. 1. The formation of pits, depressions, or scars, as in smallpox. 2. In the spleen, removal of the remains of red blood cells that have completed their lifespan or have been injured. Nucleated red blood cells are also removed in this pitting function. 3. In dentistry, the formation of depressions in the materials used in restoring teeth.

pitting edema. Edema, usually of the skin of the extremities, that when pressed firmly with a finger will maintain the depression produced by the finger.

pituicyte (pĭ-tū′ĭ-sīt) [L. *pituita*, phlegm, + Gr. *kytos*, cell]. A modified branched neuroglia cell characteristic of pars nervosa of the posterior lobe of the pituitary gland. Also present in the infundibular stalk.

pituita (pĭ-tū′ĭ-tă) [L., phlegm]. Glue-like mucus.

pituitarism (pĭt-ū′ĭ-tă-rĭzm) [″ + Gr. *-ismos*, condition]. Any disorder of the pituitary gland and its function.

pituitarium (pĭ-tū″ĭ-tār′ē-ŭm) [L.]. Pituitary.

pituitary (pĭ-tū′ĭ-tār″ē) [L. *pituitarius*, phlegm]. 1. Concerning phlegm. 2. The pituitary body or gland, q.v. SYN: *hypophysis*. SEE: *hormone, releasing; hormone, inhibiting*.

p., anterior. Preparation consisting of dried, defatted, powdered anterior lobe of the pituitary gland of domestic animals.

p., posterior. Dried, powdered posterior lobe of the pituitary gland of animals used as food by man.

p., whole. Dried, defatted, powdered entire pituitary gland of domestic animals.

pituitary gland. A small, gray, rounded body attached to the base of the brain by the infundibular stalk, a downward extension of the floor of the third ventricle. It averages 1.3 × 1.0 × 0.5 cm. in size and 0.55 to 0.6 gm. in weight. SYN: *hypophysis cerebri*. SEE: illus.

FUNCT: The pituitary is an endocrine gland secreting a number of hormones that regulate many bodily processes including growth, reproduction, and various metabolic activities. It is often referred to as the master gland of the body. Evidence indicates that the hormones are secreted by neurosecretory cells of the hypothalamus and pass through fibers of the supraopticohypophyseal tracts in the infundibular stalk to the neurohypophysis, where they are stored.

Hormones are secreted in the following lobes: *Intermediate lobe:* In cold-blooded animals, intermedin is secreted, influencing the activity of pigment cells (chromatophores) of fishes, amphibians, and reptiles. In warm-blooded animals, no effects are known.

Anterior lobe: somatotrophic, or growth, hormone (STH), which regulates growth; adrenocorticotrophic hormone (ACTH), which regulates functional activity of the adrenal cortex; thyrotrophic hormone (TTH), which regulates functional activity of the thyroid gland; gonadotrophic hormones, which include follicle-stimulating hormone (FSH), which stimulates development of ovarian follicles and spermatogenesis in the testis, luteinizing hormone (LH), also called interstitial cell–stimulating hormone (ICSH), which in conjunction with FSH induces secretion of estrogens, ovulation, and development of corpus luteum, and luteotrophic hormone (LTH), which maintains mature corpora lutea and induces secretion of progesterone. It also induces secretion of milk in a fully developed mammary gland. Because of this action, it is sometimes called the lactogenic hormone.

Posterior lobe: oxytocin, which acts specifically on smooth muscle of the uterus, increasing tone and contractility; vasopressin, which induces contraction of smooth muscles of the blood vessels. The latter is associated with an antidiuretic principle, which prevents excessive loss of water through the kidneys.

DISORDERS OF: *Hypersecretion of anterior lobe:* gigantism, acromegaly, pituitary basophilism (Cushing's disease). *Hyposecretion of anterior lobe:* dwarfism, pituitary cachexia (Simmond's disease), Sheehan's syndrome, acromicria, eunuchoidism or hypogonadism. *Posterior lobe deficiency or hypothalamic lesion:* diabetes insipidus. *Anterior and posterior lobe deficiency and hypothalamic lesion:* Frohlich's syndrome (adiposogenital dystrophy), pituitary obesity.

pituitary (injection), posterior. USP. Antidiuretic hormone.

pituitous (pĭ-tū′ĭ-tŭs). Concerning mucus.

Pituitrin (pĭ-tū′ĭ-trĭn). Trade name for posterior pituitary extract.

ACTION AND USES: Used to stimulate contraction of blood vessels, peristalsis in intestines, and uterine contractions in labor.

pityriasis (pĭt″ĭ-rī′ă-sĭs) [Gr. *pityron*, bran, + *-iasis*, disease]. A skin disease characterized by branny scales.

p. alba. Patches of round or oval, macular skin lesions with fine adherent scales. These are usually and commonly seen in children. The lesions are virtually painless, and usually require no therapy. They disappear spontaneously. The etiology is unknown but the disease is regarded as a mild form of eczema.

p. amiantacea. Sticky scaling of the scalp following infection or trauma. SYN: *tinea amiantacea*.

p. capitis. Dandruff.

p. lichenoides, acute. A skin disorder characterized by development of an edema-

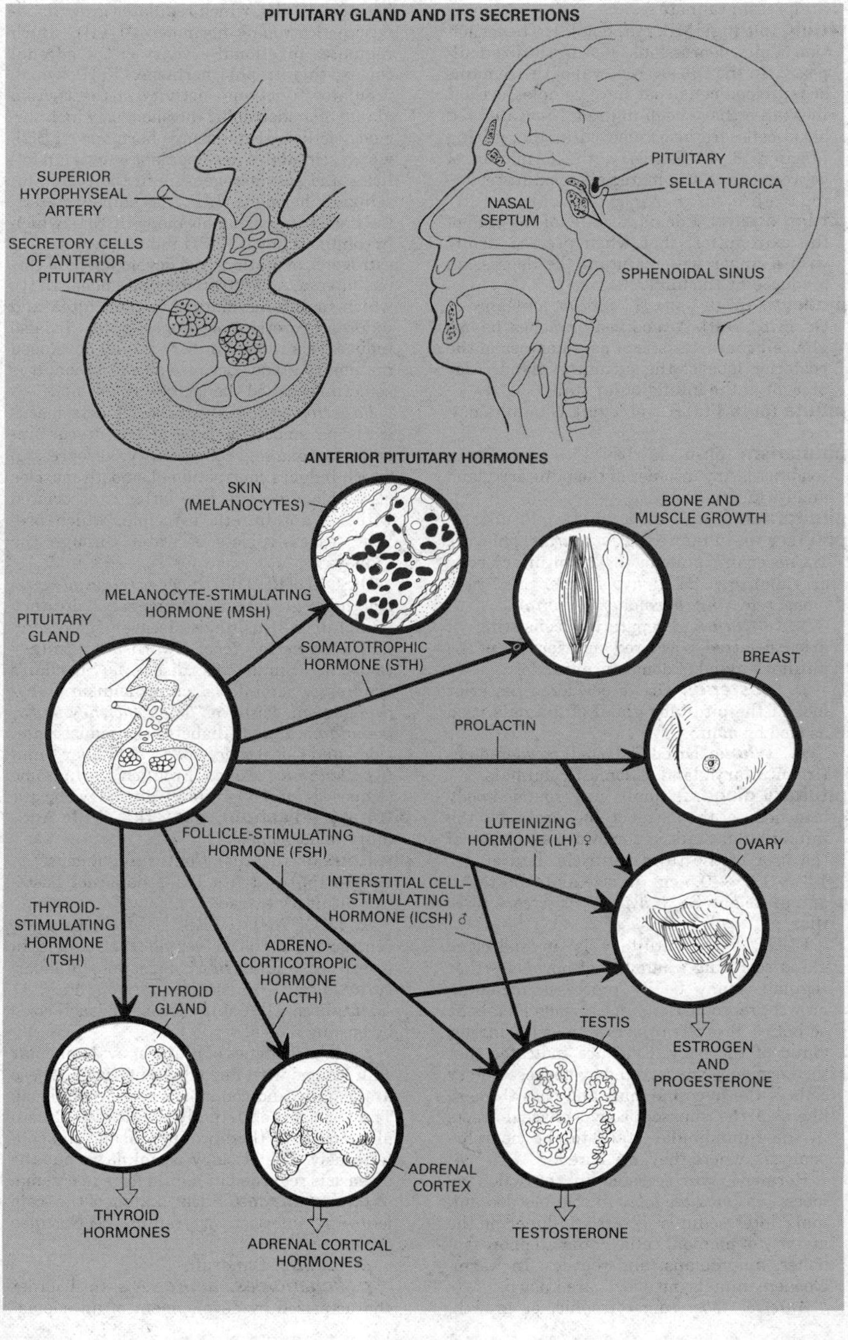
PITUITARY GLAND AND ITS SECRETIONS
SUPERIOR HYPOPHYSEAL ARTERY
SECRETORY CELLS OF ANTERIOR PITUITARY
PITUITARY
SELLA TURCICA
NASAL SEPTUM
SPHENOIDAL SINUS
ANTERIOR PITUITARY HORMONES
SKIN (MELANOCYTES)
BONE AND MUSCLE GROWTH
MELANOCYTE-STIMULATING HORMONE (MSH)
PITUITARY GLAND
SOMATOTROPHIC HORMONE (STH)
BREAST
PROLACTIN
LUTEINIZING HORMONE (LH) ♀
FOLLICLE-STIMULATING HORMONE (FSH)
OVARY
INTERSTITIAL CELL–STIMULATING HORMONE (ICSH) ♂
THYROID-STIMULATING HORMONE (TSH)
ADRENO-CORTICOTROPIC HORMONE (ACTH)
THYROID GLAND
TESTIS
ESTROGEN AND PROGESTERONE
ADRENAL CORTEX
THYROID HORMONES
TESTOSTERONE
ADRENAL CORTICAL HORMONES

tous pink papule that undergoes central vesiculation and hemorrhagic necrosis. This may progress to a depressed scar or ulcer.

p. linguae. Transitory benign plaques of the tongue.

p. nigra. Tinea nigra.

p. rosea. Acute inflammatory skin disease marked by a macular eruption on the trunk, obliquely to the ribs, and the upper extremities. Rose red and somewhat scaly with a clearing in the center, or reddish ring-shaped patches symmetrically distributed over the limbs.

ETIOL: Unknown.

SYM: Macular or circinate lesions; yellowish, salmon, or red; rounded, oval, or irregular; thinly covered with fine branny scales, increasing in size. When centers clear up, giving rise to slightly elevated reddish rings with fawn-colored centers, coalescence of rings results in segmental or gyrate lesions of various sizes. Spontaneous disappearance within three to four weeks but may last several months.

TREATMENT: Locally: antipruritics.

p. rubra pilaris. Persistent general exfoliative dermatitis of unknown etiology.

p. versicolor. A mild, chronic, symptomless fungus infection of the superficial layer of the skin. Characterized by scaly discolored areas. Due to a fungus Malassezia furfur. Treatment is necessary only for cosmetic purposes. SYN: *tinea versicolor*.

pityroid (pĭt'ĭ-royd) [Gr. *pituron*, bran, + *eidos*, like]. Branny; resembling bran.

pivot (pĭv'ŭt). In dentistry, a part used for attaching an artificial crown to the base of a natural tooth.

pix (pĭks) [L.]. Pitch or tar.

PK. *psychokinesis.*

pK. Abbr. for the negative logarithm of the ionization constant, called K, of an acid. The closer the pK to the pH, the greater the buffering power of the system.

PKU. *phenylketonuria.*

placebo (plă-sē'bō) [L., I shall please]. Inactive substance given to satisfy patient's demand for medicine. Also used in controlled studies of drugs. The placebo is given to a group of patients and the drug being tested is given to a similar group; then the results obtained in the two groups are compared.

placenta (plă-sĕn'tă) [L., a flat cake]. (pl. *placentae, placentas*) [NA] The oval or discoid spongy structure in the uterus of eutherian mammals through which the fetus derives its nourishment. SEE: illus.

ANAT: The placenta consists of a fetal

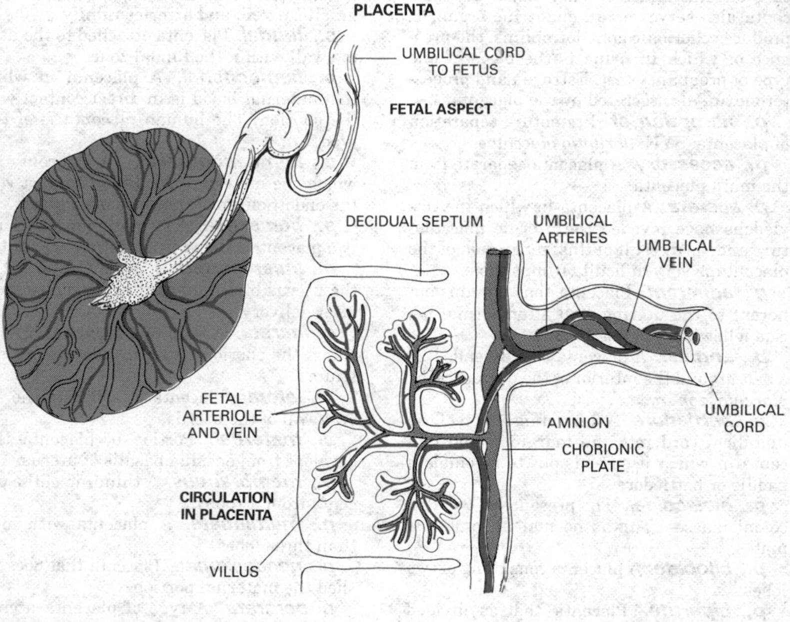

portion, the chorion frondosum, bearing many chorionic villi that interlock with the decidua basalis of the uterus which constitutes the maternal portion. The chorionic villi lie in spaces in the uterine endometrium where they are bathed in maternal blood and lymph. Groups of villi are separated by placental septa forming about twenty distinct lobules called cotyledons.

Attached to the margin of the placenta is a membrane that encloses the embryo. It is a composite of several structures (decidua parietalis, decidua capsularis, chorion laeve, and amnion). At the center of the concave side is attached the umbilical cord through which the umbilical vessels (two arteries and one vein) pass to the fetus. The cord is approx. 50 cm. long at full term.

The mature placenta is 15 to 18 cm. (6 to 7 in.) in diameter and weighs about 450 gm. (approx. 1 lb.). When expelled following parturition, it is known as the afterbirth.

Maternal blood enters the intervillous spaces of the placenta through spiral arteries, branches of the uterine arteries. It bathes the chorionic villi and flows peripherally to the marginal sinus, which leads to uterine veins. Food substances, oxygen, and antibodies pass into fetal blood of the villi; metabolic waste products pass from fetal blood into the mother's blood. In general, there is no admixture of fetal and maternal blood. The placenta also serves as an endocrine organ. It produces chorionic gonadotrophins, the presence of which in urine is the basis of one type of pregnancy test. Estrogen and progesterone are also secreted by the placenta.

p., abruption of. Premature separation of placenta. SYN: *abruptio placentae.*

p., accessory. A placenta separate from the main placenta.

p. accreta. A placenta in which the cotyledons have invaded the uterine musculature and, as a result of this, separation of the placenta is very difficult or impossible.

p., adherent. Placenta that remains adherent to the uterine wall after normal period following childbirth.

p., annular. A placenta that extends like a belt around the interior of the uterus. SYN: *placenta, zonary.*

p., battledore. A form of insertion of the umbilical cord into the margin of the placenta in which it spreads out to resemble a paddle or battledore.

p., bidiscoidal. The presence of two discoidal masses. This is normal in some primates.

p., bilobate. A placenta consisting of two lobes.

p., bipartite. Placenta that is divided into two separate parts. SYN: *placenta, duplex.*

p., chorioallantoic. A placenta in which the allantoic mesoderm and vessels fuse with the inner face of the serosa to form the chorion.

p., circinate. Placenta that is cup-shaped.

p. circumvallata. A cup-shaped placenta with raised edges.

p., cirsoid. Placenta with appearance of varicose veins.

p., cordiform. Placenta having a marginal indentation giving it a heart shape.

p., deciduate. A placenta of which the maternal part escapes with delivery.

p., dimidiate. P., bilobate, q.v.

p., discoid. Placenta that constitutes practically one mass, circumscribed and circular in form.

p., double. A placental mass of the two placentae of a twin gestation.

p., duplex. P., bipartite.

p., endotheliochorial. A placenta in which the syncytial trophoblasts of the chorion penetrate to the blood vessels of the uterus.

p., epitheliochorial. A placenta in which the chorion is next to the lining of the uterus but does not invade or erode the lining.

p. fenestrata. Placenta in which there is thinning or absence of placental tissue.

p., fetal. That part of the placenta formed by aggregation of chorionic villi in which the umbilical vein and arteries ramify.

p., fundal. Placenta attached to the uterine wall within the fundal zone.

p., hemochorial. A placenta in which the maternal blood is in direct contact with the chorion. The human placenta is of this type.

p., hemoendothelial. A placenta in which the maternal blood is in contact with the endothelium of the chorionic vessels.

p., horseshoe. A formation in which the two placentae of a twin gestation are united.

p., incarcerated. Placenta retained in the uterus by irregular uterine contractions after delivery.

p. increta. A form of placenta accreta in which the chorionic villi invade the myometrium.

p., lateral. Placenta attached to the lateral wall of the uterus.

p., maternal. Portion of placenta that develops from decidua basalis of uterus.

p., membranous. A thinning of the placenta from atrophy.

p., multilobate. A placenta with more than three lobes.

p., nondeciduate. Placenta that does not shed the maternal portion.

p. percreta. A type of placenta accreta in which the myometrium is invaded to the serosa of the peritoneum covering the uterus. This may cause rupture of the uterus.

p. previa. Placenta that is implanted in the lower uterine segment. There are three types: centralis, lateralis, and marginalis. *Placenta previa centralis* is the condition in which the placenta has been implanted in the lower uterine segment and has grown to completely cover the internal cervical os. *Placenta previa lateralis* is the condition in which the placenta lies just within the lower uterine segment. *Placenta previa marginalis* is the condition in which the placenta partially covers the internal cervical os.

SYM: Slight hemorrhage, recurrent with greater severity, appears 7th or 8th month; gradual anemia, pallor, rapid weak pulse, air hunger, low blood pressure.

DIAG: Painless bleeding during last three months; placenta in lower portion of uterus.

PROG: Depends upon control of hemorrhage and asepsis.

TREATMENT: Conserve blood supply during delivery and before; prevent and control postpartum hemorrhage; combat anemia before and after labor; prevent sepsis.

p. previa partialis. A placenta that only partially covers the internal os of the uterus.

p. reflexa. An abnormal placenta in which the margin is thickened and appears to turn back on itself.

p., reniform. A kidney-shaped placenta.

p., retained. Placenta not expelled for two hours after second stage of labor.

p. spuria. An outlying portion of the placenta that has not maintained its vascular connection with the decidua vera.

p., succenturiate. An accessory placenta that has a vascular connection.

p., trilobate. A placenta with three lobes.

p., tripartite. A three-lobed placenta with a single fetus.

p., triple. A placental mass of three lobes in a triple gestation.

p. uterina. The uterine part of the placenta.

p., velamentous. A placenta with the umbilical cord attached to the membrane a short distance from the placenta, the vessels entering the placenta at its margin.

p., villous. A placenta in which the chorion forms villi.

p., zonary. P., annular.

placental (plă-sĕn′tăl) [L. *placenta*, a flat cake]. Rel. to the placenta.

placental souffle. Sound heard in auscultation over the placenta in pregnancy; due to circulation of the blood.

placentation (plă″sĕn-tā′shŭn). The process of formation and attachment of the placenta.

placentitis (plă″sĕn-tī′tĭs) [″ + Gr. *itis*, inflammation]. Inflamed condition of the placenta.

placentography (plă″sĕn-tŏg′ră-fē) [″ + Gr. *graphein*, to write]. Examination of the placenta by roentgenography.

p., indirect. Measurement of the space between the placenta and the head of the fetus by means of x-ray. This is done to diagnose placenta previa.

placentoid (plă-sĕn′toyd) [″ + Gr. *eidos*, like]. Like the placenta.

placentolysin (plă″sĕn-tŏl′ĭ-sĭn) [″ + Gr. *lysis*, dissolution]. A lysin obtained by injecting placental tissue into an animal, the serum thus obtained being destructive to placental cells of the species of animal from which the placenta was originally taken.

placentoma (plă″sĕn-tō′mă) [″ + Gr. *oma*, tumor]. A neoplasm derived from retained placental tissue.

placentotherapy (plă-sĕn″tō-thĕr′ă-pē) [″ + Gr. *therapeia*, treatment]. Therapeutic use of placental extract.

Placido's disk (plă-sē′dōz). [Antonio Placido, Portuguese ophthalmologist, 1848–1916] A disk marked with black and white circles used in determining the amount and character of corneal astigmatism.

Placidyl. Trade name for ethchlorvynol.

placing reflex. SEE: *reflex, placing*.

placode (plăk′ōd) [Gr. *plax*, plate, + *eidos*, form]. In embryology, a platelike thickening of epithelium, usually ectoderm, that serves as the anlage of an organ or structure.

p., auditory. A dorsolateral placode located alongside the hindbrain that gives rise to the otocyst, which in turn develops into the internal ear.

p., lens. Placode developing in the ectoderm directly overlying the optic vesicle. Forms the lens vesicle, which becomes enclosed in the optic cup and eventually becomes the lens of the eye.

p., olfactory. Placode that gives rise to the olfactory pit and finally the major portion of the nasal cavity.

placoid (plăk′oyd) [″ + *eidos*, form]. Platelike.

pladaroma (plăd-ă-rō′mă) [Gr. *pladaros*, damp, + *oma*, tumor]. A soft growth like a wart on the eyelid.

pladarosis (plăd-ă-rō′sĭs) [″ + *osis*, condition]. Pladaroma.

plagiocephalic (plā-jē″ō-sē-făl′ĭk) [Gr. *plagios*, oblique, + *kephale*, head]. Marked by or rel. to plagiocephaly.

plagiocephalism (plā″jē-ō-sĕf′ă-lĭzm). Plagiocephaly.

plagiocephaly (plā″jē-ō-sĕf′ă-lē). Malformation of the skull producing the appearance of a twisted and lopsided head. Due to irregular closure of the cranial sutures.

plague (plāg) [ME., calamity]. A word once

used to describe any widespread contagious disease associated with a high death rate. Now applied specifically to the highly fatal disease caused by Yersinia pestis (previously classed as Pasteurella pestis) infection.

SYM: High fever, restlessness, staggering gait, mental confusion, prostration, delirium, shock, and coma. Exists in several forms: bubonic with acutely inflamed lymph nodes (buboes); septicemic with absence of buboes; primary pneumonic characterized by pulmonary symptoms. The pneumonic form may be spread from man to man by droplets.

TREATMENT: Streptomycin, tetracyclines, and chloramphenicol are effective in treating plague.

p., ambulatory. Mild but often fatal form of bubonic plague.

p., black. SEE: *black death.*

p., bubonic. The more common form of plague marked by formation of buboes.

p., glandular. P., bubonic, q.v.

p., hemorrhagic. A severe form of bubonic plague in which there is hemorrhage into the skin.

p., larval. P., ambulatory, q.v.

p., murine. Plague infecting rats.

p., pneumonic. A highly virulent form of plague with extensive involvement of the lungs. Occurs as sequela of bubonic plague or as a primary infection.

p., septicemic. Plague characterized by massive infection of the bloodstream before the formation of buboes.

p., sylvatic. Plague infecting various species of rodents.

p., white. Tuberculosis.

plague vaccine. USP. A standard preparation of specific plague bacilli that have been killed by the addition of formaldehyde.

plan. The conscious design of desired future states, the goals, objectives and activities required.

p., medical care. The goals and objectives of the physician's care and the treatment instituted to accomplish the goal.

p., nursing care. The statement of the goals and objectives of the nursing care provided for the client and the activities or tasks required to accomplish the plan, including the criteria that will be utilized to evaluate the effectiveness and appropriateness of the plan.

planaria (plă-năr′ē-ă). Free-living flatworms of the Turbellaria class. They are used extensively in studying regeneration.

planchet (plăn′chĕt). A small flat container or dish upon which a radioactive sample is placed.

plane (plān) [L. *planus*]. 1. A flat or relatively smooth surface. SYN: *planum.* 2. A flat surface formed by making a cut, imaginary or real, through the body or a part of it. Planes are used as points of reference by which positions of parts of the body are indicated. In the human subject, all planes are based on the body being in an upright anatomic position. SEE: illus.; *position, anatomic.* 3. A certain stage, as in levels of anesthesia. 4. To rub away.

p.'s, Addison's. Planes used as landmarks in thoracoabdominal topography.

p., Aeby's. Plane perpendicular to the median plane of the cranium through the basion and nasion.

p., alveolocondylar. Plane tangent to the alveolar point with most prominent points on lower aspects of condyles of the occipital bone.

p., axiolabiolingual. A plane that passes through an incisor or canine tooth parallel to the long axis of the tooth and in a labiolingual direction.

p., axiomesiodistal. A plane that passes through a tooth parallel to the axis and in a mesiodistal direction.

p., Baer's. Plane through upper border of the zygomatic arches.

p., bite. The plane formed by the biting surfaces of the teeth.

p., coccygeal. The fourth parallel plane of the pelvis.

p., coronal. Vertical plane at right angles to a sagittal plane dividing the body into anterior and posterior portions. SYN: *p., frontal.*

p., datum. An assumed horizontal plane from which craniometric measurements are taken.

p., Daubenton's. Plane passing through the opisthion and inferior bones of the orbits.

p.'s, focal. Two planes through the anterior and posterior principal foci of a dioptric system and perpendicular to the line connecting the two.

p., Frankfort horizontal. A cephalometric plane joining porion and orbitale, the upper part of the ear openings and the lowest margin of the orbit, to establish a reproducible position of the head for radiographic and cephalometric studies.

p., frontal. P., coronal.

p., Hodge's. Plane running parallel to the pelvic inlet and passing through the 2nd sacral vertebra and upper border of the os pubis.

p., horizontal. A transverse plane at right angles to the vertical axis of the body. SYN: *p., transverse.*

p.'s, inclined, of pelvis. Anterior and posterior inclined planes of the pelvic cavity, two unequal sections divided by the sciatic spines. In the larger, anterior section, the lateral walls slope toward the symphysis and

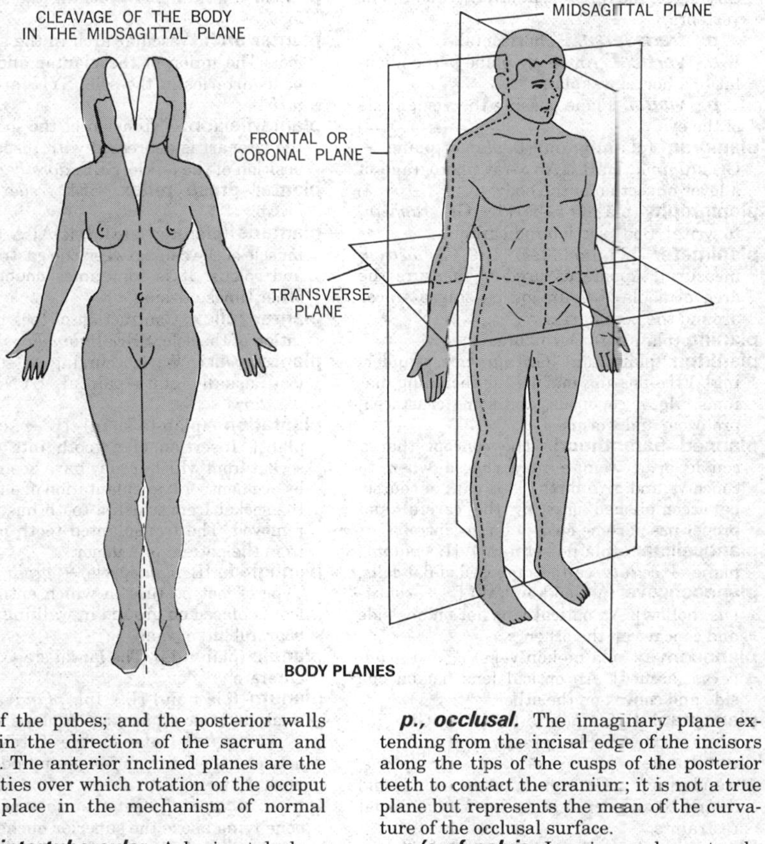

BODY PLANES

arch of the pubes; and the posterior walls slope in the direction of the sacrum and coccyx. The anterior inclined planes are the declivities over which rotation of the occiput takes place in the mechanism of normal labor.

p., intertubercular. A horizontal plane passing through the tubercles of the crests of the ilia. Lies approx. at level of the 5th lumbar vertebra.

p., Listing's. A transverse vertical plane lying perpendicular to the anteroposterior axis of the eye and containing the center of motion of the eyes. In it also lie the transverse and vertical axes of voluntary ocular rotation.

p., Meckel's. Plane through the auricular and alveolar points.

p., median. Anteroposterior plane dividing a body or organ into two equal and symmetrical parts. The median plane of the body is known as the mesion.

p., midsagittal. Vertical plane dividing the body into symmetrical right and left halves.

p., Morton's. Plane passing through the most projecting points of the parietal and occipital protuberances.

p., occlusal. The imaginary plane extending from the incisal edge of the incisors along the tips of the cusps of the posterior teeth to contact the cranium; it is not a true plane but represents the mean of the curvature of the occlusal surface.

p.'s of pelvis. Imaginary planes touching the same parts of the pelvic canal on both sides.

p. of refraction. Plane passing through a refracted ray of light and drawn perpendicular to the surface at which refraction takes place.

p. of regard. Plane through the fovea of the eye and fixation point.

p.'s, parallel, of pelvis. Planes intersecting the axis of the pelvic canal at right angles. The first plane is that of the superior strait. The second plane is that extending from the middle of the sacral vertebra to the level of the subpubic ligament. The third plane is at the level of the spines of the ischia and the fourth plane is at the outlet.

p., sagittal. Vertical plane parallel to the midsagittal plane. One that divides the body into right and left portions.

p., subcostal. Horizontal plane passing through the lowest points of the 10th costal cartilages. Lies approx. at level of 3rd lumbar vertebra.

p., transverse. P., horizontal.

p., vertical. Any body plane perpendicular to a horizontal plane.

p., visual. Plane passing the visual axis of the eye.

planigram (plā'nĭ-grăm) [L. *planus,* plane, + Gr. *gramma,* mark]. An x-ray photograph of a layer or section of the body.

planigraphy (plă-nĭg'ră-fē) [" + Gr. *graphein,* to write]. Body section radiography.

planimeter (plā-nĭm'ĕ-tĕr) [" + Gr. *metron,* measure]. Apparatus used to measure the area of a plane figure by passing a tracer around the boundaries.

planing (plā'nĭng). Dermabrasion, q.v.

plankton (plănk'tŏn) [Gr. *planktos,* wandering]. Free-floating marine life including diatoms, algae, copepods, and some crustacea, protozoa, and worms.

planned parenthood. The concept that a couple or a woman may choose when to conceive and give birth. This can, of course, be accomplished only by the careful and proper use of some form of birth control.

planocellular (plā"nō-sĕl'ū-lăr) [L. *planus,* plane, + *cellula,* cell]. Composed of flat cells.

planoconcave (plā"nō-kŏn'kāv) [" + *concavus,* hollow]. An optical lens flat on one side and concave on the other.

planoconvex (plā"nō-kŏn'vĕks) [" + L. *convexus,* arched]. An optical lens flat on one side and convex on the other.

planography (plă-nŏg'ră-fē) [" + Gr. *graphein,* to write]. Planigraphy, q.v.

planomania (plā"nō-mā'nē-ă) [Gr. *plane,* wandering, + Gr. *mania,* madness]. Morbid desire to wander and to be free of social restraints.

Planorbis (plăn-or'bĭs). A genus of freshwater snails serving as intermediate hosts for certain species of blood flukes (Schistosoma).

planotopokinesia (plā"nō-tŏp"ō-kī-nē'zē-ă) [" + *topos,* place, + *kinesis,* movement]. Loss of orientation in space.

plant (plănt) [L. *planta,* a sprout]. An organism that contains chlorophyll and manufactures carbohydrates from carbon dioxide and water or, if lacking these characteristics, is similar in structure and life history to those organisms that do possess chlorophyll and manufacture food. SEE: *chlorophyll.*

planta (plăn'tă) [L.]. (pl. *plantae*) [NA] The sole of the foot.

p. pedis. Sole of the foot.

plantago seed (plăn-tā'gō). USP. The cleaned, dried, ripe seed of Plantago psyllium or indica. It is used as a cathartic, but usually in a powdered form rather than the whole seeds.

plantalgia (plăn-tăl'jē-ă) [L. *planta,* sole, + Gr. *algos,* pain]. Pain in the sole of the foot.

plantar (plăn'tăr). Concerning the sole of the foot.

plantar arch. Vascular arch in the sole of the foot. The union of the plantar and dorsalis pedis arteries in the sole. SYN: *arcus plantaris.*

plantarflexion. Extension of the foot so that the forepart is depressed with respect to the position of the ankle. SEE: *dorsiflexion.*

plantar grasp reflex. SEE: *reflex, plantar grasp.*

plantaris (plăn-tăr'ĭs) [L.]. [NA] A long slim muscle of the calf between the gastrocnemius and soleus. It is sometimes double and at other times missing.

plantar reflex. Contraction of toes upon irritation of the sole. SEE: *Babinski's reflex.*

plantar wart. Wart occurring on sole of the foot; usually quite painful. SYN: *verruca plantaris.*

plantation (plăn-tā'shŭn) [L. *plantare,* to plant]. Insertion of a tooth into the bony socket from which it may have been removed by accident; or transplantation of a tooth into the socket from which a tooth has just been removed. The transplanted tooth may come from the patient or a donor.

plantigrade [L. *planta,* sole, + *gradi,* to walk]. Type of foot posture in which entire sole of foot is placed on ground in walking as in the bear, rabbit, or man.

planula (plăn'ū-lă). The larval stage of a coelenterate.

planum (plā'nŭm) [L.]. (pl. *plana*) A flat or relatively smooth surface. A plane.

p., nuchal. Outer surface of occipital bone between the foramen magnum and superior nuchal line.

p., occipital. Outer surface of occipital bone lying above the superior nuchal line.

p., orbital. Portion of maxilla that forms greater part of floor of orbit.

p., popliteal. Smooth triangular area on posterior surface of distal end of femur. Bordered by medial and lateral supracondylar lines and forms floor of popliteal fossa.

p., sternal. Anterior or ventral surface of sternum.

p., temporal. Depressed area on side of skull below inferior temporal line. Underlies the temporal fossa.

planuria (plā-nū'rē-ă) [Gr. *plane,* wandering, + *ouron,* urine]. The voiding of urine from an abnormal passage of the body.

plaque (plăk) [Fr., a plate]. 1. A patch on the skin or on a mucous surface. 2. A blood platelet.

p., atheromatous. A yellow swollen area of the lining of an artery. This is formed by deposition of lipid in the area.

p., bacterial. P., dental, q.v.

p., dental. A gummy mass of microorganisms that grows on the crowns and spreads along the roots of teeth. It usually is too small to be seen and is both colorless and transparent. Dental plaques are the forerunners of dental caries and periodontal disease. They may be prevented by proper daily self-care of the teeth. SEE: *caries; periodontitis; pyorrhea alveolaris.*

p., Hollenhorst. Orange-yellow emboli in the retinal vessels.

p., mucous. Condyloma latum, q.v.

Plaquenil Sulfate. Trade name for hydroxychloroquine sulfate, USP.

plasm (plăzm) [Gr. *plasma,* a thing formed]. Plasma.

plasma (plăz′mă) [Gr. *plasma,* a thing formed]. 1. The liquid part of the lymph and of the blood. 2. Protoplasm, cell substance outside the nucleus. 3. An ointment base of glycerol and starch.

In the blood, corpuscles and platelets float in plasma. It consists of serum, q.v., and protein substances in solution. Blood plasma consists of water in which numerous chemical compounds, both solids and gases, are dissolved. Included are water, electrolytes, sugar, glucose, proteins, nonprotein nitrogenous compounds, fats, bile pigment or bilirubin, and gases.

In general, plasma is a medium for circulation of blood cells, it carries nutritive substances to various structures, and it removes waste products of metabolism from those structures. Plasma makes possible chemical communication between different portions of the body, carrying minerals, hormones, vitamins, and antibodies.

Different constituents of plasma have specific functions within the blood. Proteins, bicarbonates, carbon dioxide, chlorides, phosphates, and ammonia serve to keep the acid-base equilibrium of the blood constant when acid or base substances are added to it. Proteins, esp. albumin, by virtue of their osmotic pressure, tend to prevent undue leakage of fluids out of the capillaries and to maintain a proper exchange of fluid between capillaries and tissues.

Normal plasma is thin and colorless when free from corpuscles, or it has a faint yellow tinge when seen in thick layers.

After clotting of the blood, the liquid squeezed out by the clot is called blood serum. If whole blood is prevented from clotting either by chilling it or by adding anticoagulants, such as sodium citrate, it can be centrifuged. The clear fluid that then occupies the upper half of the centrifuge tube is called plasma. SEE: *blood; coagulation; serum.*

p., antihemophilic human. Human plasma in which the antihemophilic globulin has been preserved. It is used to correct temporarily the bleeding tendency in some forms of hemophilia.

p., blood. Fluid in which cellular elements of the blood are suspended.

p., lymph. Lymph without its corpuscles.

p., normal human. Pooled plasma from eight or more human donors. The plasma is sterile and the donors are free from diseases that could be transmitted by transfusion.

plasmablast (plăz′mă-blăst) [Gr. *plasma,* a thing formed, + *blastos,* germ]. The primitive cell that is the precursor of the plasma cell.

plasmacyte (plăz′mă-sīt) [" + *kytos,* cell]. A plasma cell, one of those found in connective tissue, with an eccentrically placed round nucleus and filled with a chromatin mass that stains deeply.

plasmacytoma (plăz″mă-sī-tō′mă) [" + " + *oma,* tumor]. A plasma cell myeloma occurring in bone marrow. SEE: *myeloma, multiple.*

plasmacytosis (plăz″mă-sī-tō′sĭs) [" + " + *osis,* condition]. An excess of plasma cells in the blood.

plasmagel (plăz′mă-jĕl″) [" + L. *gelare,* to congeal]. The peripheral portion of the endoplasm of a cell such as in an ameba. It is immobile and of the nature of a gel.

plasmagene (plăz′mă-jēn″) [" + *gennan,* to produce]. A cytoplasmic hereditary determiner.

plasmalemma (plăz″mă-lĕm′ă) [" + *lemma,* husk]. Plasma, or cell, membrane.

Plasmanate. Trade name for plasma protein fraction, USP.

plasmapheresis (plăz″mă-fĕr-ē′sĭs) [" + *aphairesis,* removal]. The removal of blood from the body and centrifuging it in order to separate the cellular elements from the plasma. The packed red cells then are suspended in a physiological solution. They may be reinjected into the donor or injected into a patient who requires red cells rather than whole blood.

plasma protein fraction. USP. A standard sterile preparation of serum albumin and globulin obtained by fractionating blood, serum, or plasma from healthy human donors and testing for absence of hepatitis B surface antigen. Trade names are Plasmanate, Plasma-Plex, Plasmatein, and Protenate.

plasmasome (plăz′mă-sōm) [" + *soma,* body]. A leukocyte granule; nucleolar substance (nonchromatin-staining) in the cytoplasm.

plasmatherapy (plăz″mă-thĕr′ă-pē) [" + *therapeia,* service]. The use of blood plasma for therapeutic purposes, as injection in treatment of shock.

plasmatic (plăz-măt′ĭk). 1. Rel. to plasma. 2. Formative or plastic.

plasmatogamy (plăz″mă-tŏg′ă-mē) [″ + *gamos,* marriage]. The union of the cytoplasm of two or more cells without joining of the nuclei.

Plasmatein. Trade name for plasma protein fraction, USP.

plasmatorrhexis (plăz″mă-tō-rĕk′sĭs) [″ + *rhexis,* rupture]. Rupture of a cell with loss of its plasma, caused by internal pressure due to swelling.

plasma volume expander. A nontoxic substance composed of high–molecular weight compounds in a solution suitable for intravenous use. The materials such as dextran or certain proteins are used in treating shock due to loss of blood volume.

plasmic (plăz′mĭk) [Gr. *plasma,* a thing formed]. Concerning protoplasm.

plasmid. Any inclusion in a cell that has a genetic function but is not located in the nucleus. Found in bacteria. Plasmids are divided into two classes: the large plasmids include certain bacteriocinogens; the small plasmids include those from 1.5 to 15 μm. in length.

plasmin (plăz′mĭn). Fibrinolytic enzyme derived from its precursor plasminogen.

plasminogen (plăz-mĭn′ō-jĕn). A protein found in many tissues and body fluids. It is important in preventing fibrin clot formation.

plasmocyte (plăz′mō-sīt) [″ + *kytos,* cell]. Cells found in bone marrow, connective tissue, and sometimes in blood plasma. Considered by some to be abnormal leukocytes. They are numerous in plasma cell myeloma.

plasmocytoma (plăz″mō-sī-tō′mă) [″ + ″ + *oma,* tumor]. Plasmacytoma, q.v.

plasmodesma (plăz″mō-dĕz′mă). Singular of plasmodesmata.

plasmodesmata (plăz″mō-dĕz′mă-tă) [″ + *desmos,* bond]. Tunnels in plant cells. These facilitate communication between cells.

plasmodial (plăz-mō′dē-ăl). Concerning Plasmodia.

plasmodicidal (plăz″mō-dĭ-sī′dăl) [″ + *eidos,* form, + L. *caedere,* to kill]. Lethal to Plasmodia.

Plasmodium (plăz-mō′dē-ŭm). (pl. *Plasmodia)* A genus of protozoa belonging to subphylum Sporozoa, class Telosporidea. Includes causative agents of malaria in man and lower animals. SEE: *malaria; mosquito.*

P. falciparum. Causative agent for malignant tertian (estivoautumnal) malaria.

P. malariae. Causative agent for quartan malaria.

P. ovale. Causative agent for benign tertian or ovale malaria.

P. vivax. Causative agent for benign tertian or vivax malaria.

plasmodium (plăz-mō′dē-ŭm) [Gr. *plasma,* a thing formed, + *eidos,* form]. (pl. *plasmodia)* 1. A multinucleate mass of naked protoplasm, occurring commonly among slime molds. 2. An organism in the genus Plasmodium.

plasmogamy (plăs-mŏg′ă-mē) [″ + *gamos,* marriage]. The fusion of cells.

plasmogen (plăz′mō-jĕn) [″ + *gennan,* to produce]. Essential part of protoplasm.

plasmology (plăz-mŏl′ō-jē) [″ + *logos,* a study]. The study of the cells and plasma. SYN: *histology.*

plasmolysis (plăz-mŏl′ĭ-sĭs) [″ + *lysis,* dissolution]. Shrinking of cytoplasm in a living cell due to loss of water by osmosis.

plasmolyzable (plăz″mō-līz′ă-b′l). Capable of being plasmolyzed.

plasmolyze (plăz′mō-līz). To bring about loss of water by osmosis.

plasmoma (plăz-mō′mă) [″ + *oma,* tumor]. 1. A collection of plasma cells. 2. Plasmacytoma.

plasmon (plăz′mŏn). The genetic portion of the cell cytoplasm.

plasmoptysis (plăz-mŏp′tĭ-sĭs) [″ + *ptyein,* to spit]. Escape of cytoplasm from a cell.

plasmorrhexis (plăz″mō-rĕk′sĭs) [″ + *rhexis,* rupture]. Rupture of a cell with loss of plasma. SYN: *erythrocytorrhexis; erythrorrhexis; plasmatorrhexis.*

plasmoschisis (plăz-mŏs′kĭ-sĭs) [″ + *schisis,* a splitting]. The splitting of a cell.

plasmotomy (plăz-mŏt′ō-mē) [″ + *tome,* incision]. Mitosis in which the cytoplasm divides into two or more masses.

plasmotropism (plăz-mŏt′rō-pĭzm) [″ + *tropein,* to turn, + *-ismos,* condition]. The action of spleen, liver, and bone marrow, causing the destruction of red blood cells.

plasson (plăs′sŏn) [Gr. *plasson,* forming]. Primitive protoplasm in cytode or nonnucleated cell stage.

plastein (plăs′tē-ĭn). Proteins or polypeptides synthesized by proteolytic enzymes following the peptic digestion of proteins.

plaster [Gr. *emplastron*]. 1. Material, usually plaster of Paris, that is applied to a part and allowed to harden in order to immobilize the part or to make an impression. 2. External medicinal preparation in which the constituents are formed into a tenacious mass of substance harder than an ointment and spread upon muslin, linen, skin, or paper. Mustard or belladonna may be applied to check secretions, allay pain, or act as a counterirritant.

p., adhesive. Plaster made of a strong cloth coated on one side with an adhesive substance. Used to immobilize a part, to relieve pressure upon sutures, to protect wounds, to secure traction in fractures, to exert pressure, or to hold dressings in place. Hair on the area should be removed before applying any plaster. Plaster should never be applied to abraded or raw surfaces. In reapplying, dead skin should be removed. Surface should be dry and clean. Removal should be made by stripping from both ends up to the wound, first moistening with benzine or ether.

p., blistering. Plaster made of cantharides.

p., mustard. Plaster made of powdered mustard paste spread on cloth; used as a rubefacient. SYN: *sinapism.*

p. of Paris. Gypsum cement, hemihydrated calcium sulfate ($CaSo_4 \cdot \frac{1}{2}H_2O$), mixed with water to form a paste that sets rapidly; used to make casts and stiff bandages.

p., porous. Plaster spread on a cloth perforated with holes.

p., resin. Plaster containing resin, wax, and lead plaster; used as a soothing agent, esp. for children.

p., salicylic acid. A uniform mixture of salicylic acid spread on an appropriate base such as paper, cotton, or fabric. It is applied topically for use as a keratolytic agent.

p., warming. Plaster of cantharides and pitch employed as a counterirritant.

plaster cast. Rigid dressing made of gauze impregnated with plaster of Paris, used to immobilize an injured part, esp. in bone fractures.

NURSING IMPLICATIONS: Prevent complications after application. Allow cast to dry (approximately 48 hours). Do not cover until completely dry. Prevent cast dents by not allowing the cast to rest on hard or sharp surfaces. Keep affected limb elevated above the level of the heart. Encourage range of motion exercise in the digits of the casted extremity.

Observe for swelling, which may indicate circulatory constriction. Color of skin distal to cast should be pink, and temperature should be warm to touch if there is no circulatory impairment. Perform blanch test at frequent intervals to test circulatory status (blue tinge indicates venous obstruction and white tinge indicates arterial obstruction). Immediately report unrelieved pain, swelling, blanching, discoloration, tingling, numbness, immobility of the fingers or toes, and any temperature changes. Immediate attention to these signs and symptoms will help to prevent paralysis and necrosis.

Inspect skin surfaces around cast edges for irritation. Bathe skin surfaces; and massage with an emollient. Smooth bedclothes next to the weight-bearing part of the body. Pad edge of the cast with moleskin if indicated. Provide a padded back scratcher to the patient in a body cast. Protect the perineal area of a cast by placing a towel over the perineum and spraying the cast with polyethylene spray (once the cast is dry).

On a daily basis, remove plaster crumbs from inside the cast. When normal activity is permitted, establish a prescribed exercise schedule. Do not cover the cast with plastic or rubber boots. (These promote cast softening.) Avoid getting the cast wet. Report cast breaks or deterioration immediately to the physician Cleanse soiled areas of the cast with a damp cloth. Avoid skin breakdown by not allowing sharp objects to be used to scratch beneath the cast.

If patient is unable to turn unassisted, turn frequently to prevent respiratory complications and skin breakdown. Use a mirror to inspect the skin under the cast (skin taut—flash light into the space between the skin and the cast) and teach the patient the method of self-examination. Place supportive pillows along entire length of casted area. Never use cast braces when turning the patient. Provide adequate fluids and nutrition to promote tissue repair and elimination.

plastic (plăs′tĭk) [Gr. *plastikos,* fit for molding]. 1. Capable of being molded. 2. Contributing to building tissues.

plastic bronchitis. Bronchitis with fibrin exudate adhering in the form of a cast to the bronchial tubes.

plastic surgery. Surgery for the restoration, repair, or reconstruction of body structures.

plasticity (plăs-tĭs′ĭ-tē). The ability to be molded.

plastid (plăs′tĭd) [Gr. *plastos,* formed]. A cytoplasmic organoid found in plant cells. Includes chloroplasts (which contain chlorophyll), leukoplasts (colorless), chromoplasts (which contain pigment), and amyloplasts (which store starch). Plastids are centers of chemical activity involved in cell metabolism.

plastogamy (plăs-tŏg′ă-mē) [″ + *gamos,* marriage]. Plasmatogamy, q.v.

plastron [Fr., breastplate]. The sternum and attached cartilages.

-plasty [Gr. *plastos,* formed]. A word ending meaning molding or surgically forming.

plate (plāt) [Gr. *plate,* flat]. 1. A thin flattened part or portion, such as a flattened process of a bone. SYN: *lamella; lamina.* 2. An incorrect reference to a full denture. 3. A shallow covered dish for culturing microorganisms. 4. To inoculate and culture microorganisms in a culture plate.

p., approximation. A disk of decalcified bone used in intestinal surgery.

p., auditory. Bony roof of the external auditory meatus.

p., axial. The primitive streak of the embryo.

p., bite. In dentistry a plate made of some suitable plastic material into which the patient bites in order to have a record of the relationship between the upper and lower jaw. The device may be reinforced with wire and used as a splint in the mouth or to treat temporomandibular joint difficulties.

p., blood. Platelet.

p., bone. Flat, round or oval, decalcified bone or metal disk, employed in pairs, used in approximation.

p., cortical. The compact layers of bone forming the surfaces of the alveolar processes of the mandible and maxilla.

p., deck. The roof plate of the embryonic neural tube.

p., dental. An old term for the denture base of metal or acrylic material that rests on the oral mucosa and to which artificial teeth are attached, by extension *incorrectly* used to mean the complete denture.

p., dorsal. One of two prominences of the notochord in the embryo.

p., end. The terminal mass of a nerve fiber ending on a muscle cell.

p., epiphyseal. The thin layer of cartilage between the epiphysis and the shaft of a bone. Growth in length of the bone occurs at this layer.

p., equatorial. The plate-like mass of chromosomes at the equator of the spindle in cell division.

p., floor. The floor of the embryonic neural tube.

p., foot. [NA] Flat portion of stapes.

p., medullary. Central portion of the ectoderm in the embryo developing into the neural canal. SYN: *p., neural.*

p., muscle. In the somite, the myotome from which the striated muscles are formed.

p., neural. P., medullary.

p., palate. Part of the palate bone forming the lateral half of roof of the mouth.

p., polar. In some cells, the flattened plate-like bodies seen at the end of the spindle during mitosis.

p., roof. P., deck, q.v.

p., tarsal. A plate of dense fibrous tissue inside of and supporting each eyelid.

p., tympanic. Bony plate between the anterior wall of the external auditory meatus and the tympanum.

p., ventral. P., floor, q.v.

plateau. An elevated and usually flat area. Thus a steady and consistent fever appears as a plateau on the patient's chart of vital signs.

p., ventricular. The flat portion of the record of intraventricular pressure during the end of the ejection phase of ventricular systole.

platelet (plāt′lĕt) [Gr. *plate,* flat]. A round or oval disk, 2 to 4 micra (micrometers) in diameter, found in the blood of vertebrates. Platelets number 200,000 to 300,000/cu. mm. They contain no hemoglobin. SYN: *thrombocyte.* SEE: *blood.*

FUNCT: Platelets play an important role in blood coagulation, hemostasis, and blood thrombus formation. When a small vessel is injured, platelets adhere to each other and the edges of the injury and form a plug that covers the area. The plug or blood clot formed soon retracts and stops the loss of blood.

DISORDERS OF: Thrombocytopenia (reduced platelet count) occurs in acute infections, anaphylactic shock, and certain hemorrhagic diseases and anemias. Thrombocytosis (increased platelet count) occurs after operations, esp. splenectomy, and following violent exercise and also following tissue injury.

platelet concentrate. USP. Platelets prepared from a single unit of whole blood or plasma and suspended in a specific volume of the original plasma. This blood fraction must be used prior to the indicated expiration date on its label. Platelets are stored at either room temperature (22° C.) in plasma or in a concentrated form as platelet-rich plasma.

plateletpheresis. The process of treatment of donor blood to remove platelets and then returning the remaining blood to the donor.

plating. In bacteriology, inoculation of liquefiable, solid media (gelatin or agar) with microorganisms and pouring of medium into a shallow flat dish.

platinic (plă-tĭn′ĭk). Pert. to a compound containing quadrivalent platinum.

Platinol. Trade name for cisplatin.

platinosis. Cutaneous and respiratory allergic reactions to exposure to complex salts of platinum.

platinous (plăt′ĭ-nŭs). A compound containing divalent platinum.

platinum (plăt′ĭ-nŭm) [Sp. *platina*]. SYMB: Pt. At. wt. 195.09; at. no. 78.; sp. gr. 21.45. Heavy silver-white metal.

platy- [Gr. *platys,* broad]. Combining form meaning broad.

platybasia (plăt″ē-bā′sē-ă). A developmental defect of the skull in which the floor of the posterior fossa of the skull around the foramen magnum protrudes upward.

platycelous (plăt-ē-sē′lŭs) [Gr. *platys,* broad, + *koilos,* hollow]. Concave ventrally and convex dorsally, said of vertebrae.

platycephalic (plăt″ē-sē-făl′ĭk) [″ + *kephale,* head]. Having a wide skull with vertical index less than 70.

platycephalous (plăt″ē-sĕf′ă-lŭs). Platycephalic.

platycephaly (plăt″ē-sĕf′ă-lē). Flattening of the skull.

platycnemia (plăt-ĭk-nē′mē-ă) [″ + *kneme,*

leg]. 1. Condition of having an unusually broad tibia. 2. Broadlegged condition.

platycnemic (plăt″ĭk-nē′mĭk). Having an unusually broad tibia.

platycnemism (plăt″ĭk′nē-mĭzm). Platycnemia.

platycoria (plăt″ē-kor-ē′ă) [″ + *kore,* pupil]. Dilatation of the pupil. SYN: *mydriasis.*

platycoriasis (plăt″ē-kor-ī′ă-sĭs). Platycoria.

platycrania (plăt″ē-krā′nē-ă) [″ + *kranion,* skull]. Platycephaly, q.v.

platyglossal (plăt″ē-glŏs′ăl) [Gr. *platys,* broad, + *glossa,* tongue]. Having a broad, flat tongue.

platyhelminth (plăt″ē-hĕl′mĭnth). Common name for any flatworm.

Platyhelminthes (plăt″ē-hĕl-mĭn′thēz) [″ + *helmins,* worm]. A phylum of flatworms including the classes Turbellaria, Trematoda (flukes), and Cestoidea (tapeworms). The last two are parasitic and include many species of medical importance. SEE: *Cestoda; Cestoidea; fluke; tapeworm; trematode.*

platyhieric (plăt″ē-hī-ĕr′ĭk) [″ + *hieron,* sacrum]. Having a broad sacrum with a sacral index over 100.

platymeric (plăt″ē-mē′rĭk) [″ + *meros,* thigh]. Having an unusually broad femur.

platymorphia (plăt″ē-mor′fē-ă) [″ + *morphe,* form]. Having an eye with a shortened anteroposterior diameter. Results in hyperopia, q.v.

platyopia (plăt″ē-ō′pē-ă) [″ + *ops,* face]. Having a very broad face, the nasomalar index being less than 107.5.

platyopic (plăt″ē-ŏp′ĭk). Having a broad, flattened face.

platypellic, platypelvic (plăt″ē-pĕl′ĭk, -vĭk) [″ + *pella,* a basin]. Having a broad pelvis.

platypodia (plăt″ē-pō′dē-ă) [″ + *pous,* foot]. Condition of being flatfooted.

platyrrhine (plăt′ĭr-īn) [″ + *rhis,* nose]. 1. Having a very wide nose in proportion to length. 2. Pert. to a skull with a nasal index between 51.1 and 58.

platysmal reflex (plă-tĭz′măl rē′flĕks). Dilation of pupil resulting from sharp pinching of platysma myoides.

platysma myoides (plă-tĭz′mă mī-oy′dēz) [Gr. *platysma,* plate, + *mys,* muscle, + *eidos,* form]. Broad, thin, platelike layer of muscle that extends from the fascia of both sides of the neck to jaw and muscles around the mouth. Acts to wrinkle the skin of the neck and to depress the jaw.

platyspondylia (plăt″ē-spŏn-dĭl′ē-ă). Platyspondylisis, q.v.

platyspondylisis (plăt″ĭ-spŏn-dĭl′ĭ-sĭs) [Gr. *platys,* flat, + *spondylos,* vertebra]. Flatness of the vertebral bodies.

platystencephaly (plăt″ĭ-stĕn-sĕf′ă-lē) [″ + *kephale,* head]. Having a skull wide at the occiput.

pleasure principle. In psychology, the avoidance of pain and the seeking of pleasure, indicative of the early stages of man's development. SYN: *hedonism.*

pledget (plĕj′ĕt) [origin uncertain]. Small, flat compress, usually of gauze or absorbent cotton, used to apply or absorb fluid, to protect, or to exclude air.

plegaphonia (plĕg″ă-fō′nē-ă) [Gr. *plege,* stroke, + *a-,* not, + *phone,* voice]. A sound produced in percussion of the larynx when the glottis is open during auscultation of the chest.

-plegia (plē′jē-ă) [Gr. *plege,* stroke]. Suffix meaning paralysis or stroke.

Plegine. Trade name for phendimetrazine tartrate.

pleio-, pleo-, plio- [Gr. *pleion, pleon,* more]. Combining forms meaning more.

pleiotropia (plī″ō-trō′pē-ă) [Gr. *pleion,* more, + *trope,* turn]. The ability of a gene to have many effects.

pleiotropism (plī-ŏt′rō-pĭzm) [″ + ″ + *-ismos,* condition]. Pleiotropia, q.v.

pleochroic (plē″ō-krō′ĭk) [Gr. *pleon,* more, + *chroia,* color]. Pleochromatic

pleochroism (plē-ŏk′rō-ĭzm) [″ + ″ + *-ismos,* condition]. The property of a crystal that produces different colors when light passes through it at different angles.

pleochromatic (plē″ō-krō-măt′ĭk) [″ + *chroma,* color]. Pert. to the property of crystals and some other bodies in which they show different colors when seen from different axes. SYN: *pleochroic.*

pleocytosis (plē″ō-sī-tō′sĭs) [″ + *kytos,* cell, + *osis,* condition]. Increased number of lymphocytes in the cerebrospinal fluid.

pleomastia, pleomazia (plē″ō-măs′tē-ă, -mā′zē-ă) [Gr. *pleon,* more, + *mastos, mazos,* breast]. The state of having more than two mammae. SYN: *polymastia.*

pleomorphic (plē-ō-mor′fĭk) [″ + *morphe,* form]. Having many shapes.

pleomorphism (plē-ō-mor′fĭzm) [″ + ″ + *-ismos,* condition]. 1. Property of crystallizing into two or more different forms. 2. Occurrence of more than one form in a life cycle. SYN: *polymorphism.*

pleomorphous (plē-ō-mor′fŭs). Having many shapes or crystallizing into several forms.

pleonasm (plē′ō-năzm) [Gr. *pleonasmos,* exaggeration]. 1. State of having more than normal number of organs or parts. 2. The use of more words than necessary to express an idea.

pleonexia (plē″ō-nĕk′sē-ă) [Gr.]. Having morbid desire for possession of material things; greediness.

pleonosteosis (plē″ŏn-ŏs″tē-ō′sĭs) [Gr. *pleon,* more, + *osteon,* bone, + *osis,* condition]. Premature and excessive ossification of bones.

p., Leri's. A hereditary syndrome manifesting as pleonosteosis of the long bones, esp. of the digits, with short stature, and mongolian facies. It is apparent during the first year of age and is inherited as an autosomal dominant trait.

pleoptics (plē-ŏp'tĭks) [" + *optikos,* sight]. A method of eye exercises created to stimulate and train an amblyopic eye.

plerocercoid. The solid worm-like larva of certain tapeworms. Plerocercoids develop in secondary hosts.

plerosis (plē-rō'sĭs) [Gr. *plerosis,* filling up]. Restoration of lost tissue by the normal recuperative ability of the body.

plesiomorphism (plē"sē-ō-mor'fĭzm) [Gr. *plesios,* close, + *morphe,* form, + *-ismos,* condition]. Similarity of form.

plesiomorphous (plē"sē-ō-mor'fŭs) [" + *morphe,* form]. Of, like, or nearly the same in form.

plesiopia (plē"sē-ō'pē-ă) [+ *ops,* eye]. Increase in convexity of lens of eye.

plessesthesia (plĕs"ĕs-thē'zē-ă) [Gr. *plessein,* to strike, + *aisthesis,* sensation]. Palpatory percussion with left middle finger pressed against body and the index finger of right hand percussing in contact with the left finger.

plessimeter (plĕs-sĭm'ĕ-tĕr) [" + *metron,* a measure]. A disk that is struck in mediate percussion while being held over the surface of the body. SYN: *pleximeter.*

plessor (plĕs'or) [Gr. *plessein,* to strike]. A hammer for performing percussion. SYN: *plexor.*

plethora (plĕth'ō-ră) [Gr. *plethore,* fullness]. 1. Overfullness of blood vessels or of the total quantity of any fluid in the body. SEE: *sanguine.* 2. Congestion causing distention of blood vessels.

plethoric (plĕ-thor'ĭk, plĕth'ō-rĭk). Pert. to, or characterized by, plethora; overfull.

plethysmograph (plē-thĭz'mō-grăf) [Gr. *plethysmos,* to increase, + *graphein,* to write]. Device for finding variations in size of a part due to variations in amount of blood passing through or contained in the part.

plethysmography (plĕth"ĭz-mŏg'ră-fē). Use of a plethysmograph to record the changes in volume of an organ or extremity.

pleur-, pleuro- [Gr. *pleura,* rib, side]. Prefix indicating rel. to the pleura, the side, or a rib.

pleura (ploo'ră) [Gr., side]. (pl. *pleurae*) [NA] Serous membrane that enfolds both lungs and is reflected upon the walls of the thorax and diaphragm. The pleurae are moistened with a serous secretion that reduces friction during respiratory movements of the lungs. SEE: *mediastinum; thorax.*

p., costal. P., parietal.

p. diaphragmatica. [NA] Part of the pleura covering the upper surface of the diaphragm. SYN: *p. phrenica.*

p., mediastinal. That portion of the parietal pleura that extends to cover the mediastinum.

p., parietal. The portion of the pleura that extends from the roots of the lungs and covers the sides of the pericardium to chest wall and backward to the spine. The visceral and costal pleural layers are separated only by a lubricating secretion. These layers may become adherent or separated by fluid or air in diseased conditions. SYN: *pleura, costal.*

p. pericardiaca. Portion of the pleura covering the pericardium.

p. phrenica. P. diaphragmatica [NA].

p. pulmonalis. [NA] The pleura investing the lungs and fissures between the lobes.

p., visceral. Pleura that invests the lungs and enters into and lines the interlobar fissures. It is loose at the base and at sternal and vertebral borders to allow for lung expansion.

pleuracentesis (ploor"ă-sĕn-tē'sĭs) [Gr. *pleura,* side, + *kentesis,* puncture]. Thoracentesis.

pleuracotomy (ploor"ă-kŏt'ō-mē) [" + *tome,* incision]. Incision into the pleura through the chest wall.

pleural (ploo'răl) [Gr. *pleura,* a side]. Concerning the pleura.

pleural cavity. Space between the parietal and visceral layers of the pleura.

pleural fibrosis. Condition occurring in pulmonary tuberculosis in which the pleura becomes thickened and the pleural cavity often is obliterated.

pleuralgia (ploo-răl'jē-ă) [" + *algos,* pain]. Pain in the pleura, or in the side. SYN: *neuralgia, intercostal.*

pleurapophysis (ploo-ră-pŏf'ĭ-sĭs) [" + *apo,* from, + *physis,* a growth]. A rib or a vertebral lateral process.

pleurectomy (ploo-rĕk'tō-mē) [Gr. *pleura,* a side, + *ektome,* excision]. Excision of part of the pleura.

pleurisy (ploo'rĭs-ē) [Gr. *pleuritis*]. Inflammation of the pleura. It may be primary or secondary; unilateral, bilateral, or local; acute or chronic; fibrinous, serofibrinous, or purulent.

NURSING IMPLICATIONS: Administer analgesics as prescribed. Splint the chest when the patient coughs and teach the patient to assist. Apply warm or cool compresses to the pain area to decrease inflammation and relieve pain. Assess vital signs at regular intervals. Provide chest physiotherapy. Provide adequate rest periods. Reduce risk factors. Assist physician with local nerve block. Provide adequate fluids to liquefy secretions. Instruct patient to lie on affected side to prevent transfer of pathogenic organisms to unaffected side. Encourage cessation of use of tobacco.

p., acute. Chilliness, stabbing pain or stitch in affected side, intensified by coughing or deep breathing. Fever of 101° to 103° F. (38.3° to 39.4° C.); a short, dry, partially suppressed cough; pale, anxious face; patient usually lies on affected side. An effusion of fluid, which remains unabsorbed, in the pleural space characterizes chronic pleurisy.

p., adhesive. Pleurisy in which the exudate causes the parietal pleura to adhere to the visceral. If this is extensive, the pleural space is obliterated.

p., diaphragmatic. Inflammation of the diaphragmatic pleura.

SYM: Intense pain under margin of the ribs, sometimes referred into abdomen, with tenderness on pressure; thoracic breathing; tenderness over the phrenic nerve referred to the supraclavicular region in the neck or same side; hiccough; extreme dyspnea.

p., dry. Condition in which the pleural membrane is covered with a fibrinous exudate. It clings together, causing pain during respiration. There is slight pain when apical pleura is inflamed, but there is acute stabbing pain in costal or diaphragmatic pleural inflammation.

p., encysted. Pleurisy with effusion limited by adhesions.

p., fibrinous. Pleurisy with severe and continuous pain. Aspiration gives negative results, later much retraction of affected side.

p., hemorrhagic. Pleurisy with hemorrhage.

p., interlobar. Pleurisy in interlobar spaces.

p., plastic. P., dry.

p., pulmonary. Inflammation of the pleura covering the lung.

p., purulent. Pleurisy with high, irregular fever; sweats; chills; anemia; sometimes pitting from edema of surface; purulent effusion found on aspiration. SYN: *empyema; p., suppurative.*

p., sacculated. Pleurisy in which there are inflammatory areas, sealed off and filled with fluid.

p., serofibrinous. Pleurisy with fibrinous exudate and serous effusion.

p., serous. Pleurisy with a serous effusion.

p., suppurative. P., purulent.

p., tuberculous. Inflammation of the pleura as a result of tuberculosis. The effusion may be bloody.

p., typhoid. Pleurisy with symptoms of typhoid.

p., visceral. P., pulmonary.

p., wet. P., serous, q.v.

p. with effusion. P., serous, q.v.

pleuritic (ploo-rĭt'ĭk) [Gr. *pleuritis,* pleurisy]. Rel. to, or like, pleurisy.

pleuritis (ploo-rī'tĭs) [Gr.]. Inflammation of the pleura. SYN: *pleurisy.*

pleuritogenous (ploor"ĭ-tŏj'ĕ-nŭs) [" + *gennan,* to produce]. Causing pleurisy.

pleurocele (ploo'rō-sēl) [Gr. *pleura,* a side, + *kele,* a swelling]. 1. Hernia of the lungs or pleura. 2. A serous pleural effusion.

pleurocentesis (ploo"rō-sĕn-tē'sĭs) [" + *kentesis,* a piercing]. Surgical puncture of the pleural cavity. SYN: *thoracentesis; thoracocentesis.*

pleurocentrum (ploo"rō-sĕn'trŭm) [" + *kentron,* center]. (pl. *pleurocentra*) The lateral half of the centrum of a vertebra.

pleurocholecystitis (ploo"rō-kō"lē-sĭst-ī'tĭs) [" + *chole,* bile, + *kystis,* bladder, + *itis,* inflammation]. Inflamed condition of the pleura and gallbladder.

pleuroclysis (ploo-rŏk'lĭ-sĭs) [" + *klysis,* a washing]. Injection of fluid into the pleural cavity and washing out the cavity.

pleurodesis (ploo"rō-dē'sĭs) [" + *desis,* binding]. Production of adhesions between the parietal and visceral pleura. Usually done surgically. Method is useful in treating recurrent pneumothorax.

pleurodynia (ploo"rō-dĭn'ē-ă) [" + *odyne,* pain]. Pain of sharp intensity in the intercostal muscles due to chronic inflammatory changes in the chest fasciae; pain of the pleural nerves.

p., epidemic. An epidemic disease caused by coxsackie B virus. Characterized by sudden onset of pain in the chest and fever. SYN: *Bornholm disease.*

pleurogenic (ploo"rō-jĕn'ĭk) [" + *gennan,* to produce]. Arising in the pleura. SYN: *pleurogenous.*

pleurogenous (ploo-rŏj'ĕn-ŭs). Having origin in the pleura. SYN: *pleurogenic.*

pleurography (ploo-rŏg'ră-fē) [" + *graphein,* to write]. X-ray examination of the lungs and pleura.

pleurohepatitis (ploo"rō-hĕp"ă-tī'tĭs) [" + *hepatos,* liver, + *itis,* inflammation]. Inflammation of pleura and the liver.

pleurolith (ploo'rō-lĭth) [" + *lithos,* stone]. A calculus in the pleura.

pleurolysis (ploo-rŏl'ĭ-sĭs) [" + *lysis,* a loosening]. Loosening of parietal pleura from intrathoracic fascia to facilitate contraction of the lung or artificial pneumothorax.

pleuromelus (ploor"ō-mē'lŭs) [Gr. *pleura,* a side, + *melos,* limb]. A congenital anomaly in which an accessory limb arises from the thorax or flank.

pleuroparietopexy (ploo"rō-păr-ī'ĕt-ō-pĕk"sē) [" + L. *parietalis,* wall, + Gr. *pexis,* fixation]. Fastening of the lung to the wall of the chest by binding the visceral pleura to the wall of its cavity.

pleuropericardial (ploor″ō-pĕr-ĭ-kăr′dē-ăl) [″ + *peri,* around, + *kardia,* heart]. Concerning the pleura and pericardium.

pleuropericarditis (ploo″rō-pĕr″ĭ-kăr-dī′tĭs) [″ + ″ + *itis,* inflammation]. Pleuritis accompanied by pericarditis.

pleuroperitoneal (ploo′rō-pĕr″ĭ-tō-nē′ăl) [″ + *peritonaion,* peritoneum]. Rel. to the pleura and peritoneum.

pleuroperitoneal cavity. The body cavity. SYN: *celom.*

pleuropneumonia (ploo″rō-nū-mō′nē-ă) [″ + *pneumon,* lung]. Pleurisy accompanied by pneumonia.

pleuropneumonia-like organisms. ABBR: PPLO. The name once given organisms that are now called mycoplasmas, q.v.

pleuropneumonolysis (ploo″rō-nū″mōn-ŏl′ĭ-sĭs) [Gr. *pleura,* a side, + *pneumon,* lung, + *lysis,* a loosening]. Resection of one or more ribs from one side to collapse the lung in unilateral pulmonary tuberculosis. This procedure is rarely necessary.

pleuropulmonary (ploor″ō-pŭl′mō-nĕr″ē) [″ + L. *pulmo,* lung]. Concerning the pleura and the lung.

pleurorrhea (ploor″ō-rē′ă) [″ + *rhoia,* flow]. Effusion of fluid into the pleura.

pleuroscopy (ploo-rŏs′kō-pē) [″ + *skopein,* to examine]. Inspection of the pleural cavity through an incision into the thorax.

pleurosoma (ploor″ō-sō mă) [″ + *soma,* body]. A fetus with a cleft in the abdominal wall and thorax with protrusion of the contents of the thoracic and abdominal cavities.

pleurothotonos (ploo″rō-thŏt′ō-nŏs) [Gr. *pleurothen,* from the side, + *tonos,* tension]. Tetanic spasm in which the body position is arched to one side.

RS: emprosthotonos; opisthotonos; orthotonos; position; posture.

pleurotomy (ploo-rŏt′ō-mē) [Gr. *pleura,* a side, + *tome,* incision]. Incision of the pleura.

pleurotyphoid (ploo″rō-tī′foyd) [″ + *typhos,* fever, + *eidos,* form]. Typhoid fever with pleural involvement.

pleurovisceral (ploo″rō-vĭs′ĕr-ăl) [″ + L. *viscera,* viscera]. Concerning the pleura and the viscera.

plexal (plĕk′săl) [L. *plexus,* a braid]. Pert. to, or of the nature of, a plexus.

plexectomy (plĕk-sĕk′tō-mē) [″ + Gr. *ektome,* excision]. Surgical removal of a plexus.

plexiform (plĕk′sĭ-form) [″ + *forma,* shape]. Resembling a network or plexus.

pleximeter (plĕks-ĭm′ĕ-tĕr) [Gr. *plexis,* stroke, + *metron,* measure]. Device for receiving the blow of the percussion hammer. SYN: *plessimeter.*

plexitis (plĕk-sī′tĭs) [L. *plexus,* a braid, + Gr. *itis,* inflammation]. Inflammation of a nerve plexus.

plexometer (plĕk-sŏm′ĕ-tĕr). Pleximeter, q.v.

plexor (plĕks′or). Hammer or other device for striking upon the pleximeter in percussion. SYN: *plessor.*

plexus (plĕks′ŭs) [L., a braid]. (pl. *plexus* or *plexuses*) [NA] A network of nerves or of blood or lymphatic vessels. SEE: *rete; Nerve Plexuses* in *Appendix.*

p., cavernous. A plexus of a cavernous part of the body. The following are included. *Of the nose:* a venous plexus in the mucosa covering the superior and middle conchae. *Of the penis:* nerve plexus at the base of the penis giving rise to large and small cavernous nerves. *Of the clitoris:* nerve plexus at the base of the clitoris, formed of fibers from the uterovaginal plexus. *Of the cavernous sinus:* a sympathetic plexus that supplies fibers to the internal carotid artery and its branches within the cranium.

p., enteric. One of two plexuses of nerve fibers and ganglion cells that lie in the wall of the alimentary canal. Include myenteric (Auerbach's) and submucosal (Meissner's) plexuses.

p., myenteric. One of the two plexuses in the wall of the alimentary canal. SYN: *Auerbach's plexus.*

p., nerve. A plexus made of nerve fibers. SEE: *Nerve Plexuses* in *Appendix.*

p., pampiniform. In the male, a complicated network of veins lying in the spermatic cord and draining the testis. In the female, a network of veins lying in the mesovarium and draining the ovary.

p., prevertebral. One of three plexuses of autonomic nerve division that lie in body cavities. Includes cardiac, celiac, and hypogastric (pelvic) plexuses. SEE: *Nerve Plexuses* in *Appendix.*

pliability (plī″ă-bĭl′ĭ-tē) [O. Fr. *pliant,* bend, + L. *abilis,* able]. Capacity of being bent or twisted easily.

plica (plī′kă) [L.]. (pl. *plicae*) [NA] A fold. SEE: *fold.*

p., circular. One of the transverse folds in the small intestine. SYN: *Kerckring's folds.*

p., epiglottic. One of three folds of mucosa between the tongue and the epiglottis.

p., lacrimal. Mucosal fold at the lower orifice of the nasolacrimal duct.

p., palmate. Radiating fold in the uterine mucosa on the anterior and posterior walls of the cervical canal.

p. polonica. Tangled matted hair in which crusts and vermin are embedded.

p., semilunar, of colon. Transverse fold of mucosa of the large intestine lying between sacculations.

p., semilunar, of conjunctiva. Mucosal fold at the inner canthus of the eye.

p., synovial. A fold of synovial membrane that projects into a joint cavity.

p., transverse, of rectum. One of the mucosal folds in the rectum.

plicate (plī'kāt) [L. *plicatus*]. Braided or folded.

plication (plī-kā'shŭn) [L. *plicare,* to fold]. The stitching of folds or tucks in an organ's walls to reduce its size.

p. of stomach. Surgical creation of tucks in the wall of the stomach. This technique has been used experimentally in treating obesity.

plicotomy (plī-kŏt'ō-mē) [" + Gr. *tome,* incision]. Section of the posterior fold of the tympanic membrane.

plinth [Gr. *plinthos,* tile]. A table, seat, or apparatus that a patient lies or sits on while doing remedial exercise.

ploidy (ploy'dē) [Gr. *ploos,* a fold, + *eidos,* form]. The number of chromosome sets in a cell, e.g., haploidy, diploidy, and triploidy for one, two, and three sets, respectively, of chromosomes.

plombage (plŏm-băzh') [Fr. *plomber,* to plug]. A method of collapsing the apex of the lung by stripping the parietal pleura from the chest wall at the site of desired collapse and packing the space between the lung and chest wall with an inert substance such as small balls made of certain plastic materials.

plototoxin (plō"tō-tŏk'sĭn). A toxic substance present in the catfish, Plotosus lineatus.

plug (plŭg) [MD. *plugge*]. A mass obstructing a hole or intended for closing a hole.

p., Dittrich's. A mass of foul-smelling bacteria, and fatty acid crystals, in the sputum in bronchiectasis or gangrenous bronchitis.

p., epithelial. A mass of epithelial cells temporarily plugging an orifice in the embryo, esp. the nasal openings.

p., mucous. A mass of cells and mucus that closes the cervical canal of the uterus during pregnancy and between menstrual periods.

p., Traube's. P., Dittrich's, q.v.

p., vaginal. Closed tube for maintaining patency of the vagina following operation for fistula.

plugger. A hand- or machine-operated device for condensing amalgam, or gold foil, in the cavity of a tooth.

p., automatic. A plugger that is run by a machine rather than by hand.

p., back action. A plugger with a bent shank so that the pressure applied is back toward the operator.

p., foot. A plugger having a broad, foot-shaped tip.

plumbic (plŭm'bĭk) [L. *plumbicus,* leaden]. Pert. to, or containing, lead.

plumbism (plŭm'bĭzm) [L. *plumbum,* lead, + Gr. *-ismos,* condition]. Poisoning from lead.

plumbum (plŭm'bŭm) [L.]. Lead; a bluish-white metal. SEE: *lead.*

Plummer-Vinson syndrome (plŭm'ĕr-vĭn'sŏn). [Henry S. Plummer, U.S. physician, 1874–1937; Porter P. Vinson, U.S. surgeon, b. 1890]. Iron-deficiency anemia, dysphagia, gastric achlorhydria, splenomegaly, spooning of the nails due to an esophageal web. This occurs most commonly in premenopausal women. Treatment consists of disrupting the web. SEE: *esophageal web.*

plumose (plū'mōs) [L. *plumosus*]. Having a delicate, feathery growth.

plumper (plŭm'pĕr) [Middle Low Ger. *plump,* to fill]. Pad for filling out sunken cheeks, sometimes in form of a flange or extension from artificial dentures.

pluri- [L. *plus,* more]. Prefix meaning several or more.

pluriceptor (ploo"rĭ-sĕp'tor) [L. *plus,* more, + *ceptor,* a receiver]. A receptor that has more than two groups uniting with the complement.

pluridyscrinia (ploo"rĭ-dĭs-krĭn'ē-ă) [" + Gr. *dys,* bad, + *krinein,* to secrete]. Disorder of several endocrine organs at the same time.

pluriglandular (ploo"rĭ-glănd ū-lăr) [" + *glandula,* gland]. Pert. to several glands. SYN: *polyglandular.*

plurigravida (ploo"rĭ-grăv'ĭ-dă) [L. *plus,* more, + *gravida,* pregnant]. A pregnant woman who has had three or more pregnancies.

plurilocular (ploo"rĭ-lŏk'ū-lăr) [" + *loculus,* a cell]. Composed of several compartments or cavities. SYN: *multilocular.*

plurinuclear (ploor"ĭ-nū'klē-ăr) [" + *nucleus,* kernel]. Having a number of nuclei.

pluripara (ploo-rĭp'ă-ră) [" + *parere,* to bring forth]. A woman who has given birth three or more times.

pluriparity (ploo"rĭ-păr'ĭ-tē). Condition of having three or more pregnancies that have reached a point of viability regardless of the outcome.

pluripotent, pluripotential (ploo-rĭp'ō-tĕnt, ploor"ĭ-pō-tĕn'shăl) [" + *potentia,* power]. 1. Concerning an embryonic cell that can form different kinds of cells. 2. Having a number of different actions.

pluripotentiality (ploor"ĭ-pō-tĕn"shē-ăl'ĭ-tē). Having the potential for developing in several ways or acting in different ways.

pluriresistant (ploor"ĭ-rē-zĭs'tănt) [" + *resistens,* standing back]. Resistant to several drugs, esp. antibiotics.

plutomania (ploo"tō-mā'nē-ă) [Gr. *ploutos,* wealth, + *mania,* madness]. Delusion that one is very rich.

plutonium (ploo-tō'nē-ŭm). [Named after the planet *Pluto*] SYMB: Pu. At. wt. of the most stable isotope is 244; at. no. 94. A chemical element obtained from neptunium, which in turn is obtained from uranium.

Pm. Chem. symb. for promethium.

PMS. *premenstrual syndrome,* q.v.

PMSG. *pregnant mare serum gonadotrophin.* SEE: *gonadotrophin, chorionic.*

PMT. *premenstrual tension.*

pneo- (nē'ō) [Gr. *pnein,* to breathe]. Combining form meaning pert. to breath or breathing. SEE: words beginning with *pneum-.*

pneocardiac reflex (nē"ō-kăr'dē-ăk) [Gr. *pnein,* to breathe, + *kardia,* heart]. Change in rate and rhythm of heart and blood pressure when an irritant vapor is inhaled.

pneodynamics (nē"ō-dī-năm'ĭks) [" + *dynamis,* force]. The mechanism of breathing. SYN: *pneumodynamics.*

pneogram (nē'ō-grăm) [" + *gramma,* mark]. Spirogram, q.v.

pneograph (nē'ō-grăf) [" + *graphein,* to write]. Apparatus for recording the frequency and intensity of respiratory movements.

pneometer (nē-ŏm'ĕ-tĕr) [Gr. *pnein,* to breathe, + *metron,* a measure]. Instrument for measuring the volume of air moved in and out of the lungs during respiration. SYN: *spirometer.*

pneopneic reflex (nē-ŏp-nē'ĭk) [" + *pnein,* to breathe]. Change in respiratory depth and rate, coughing, suffocation, and pulmonary edema when an irritant vapor is inhaled.

pneoscope (nē'ō-skōp) [" + *skopein,* to examine]. Device for measuring movements of respiration.

pneum-, pneuma-, pneumato- [Gr. *pneuma, pneumatos,* air, breath]. Combining form meaning pert. to air or gas, or respiration.

pneumarthrogram (nū-măr'thrō-grăm) [Gr. *pneuma,* air, + *arthron,* joint, + *gramma,* mark]. Roentgenogram of a joint into which air has been injected.

pneumarthrography (nū"măr-thrŏg'ră-fē) [" + " + *graphein,* to write]. X-ray study of a joint into which air has been injected.

pneumarthrosis (nū-măr-thrō'sĭs) [" + " + *osis,* condition]. Accumulation of gas or air in a joint.

pneumascope (nū'mă-skōp) [" + *skopein,* to examine]. Pneumatoscope.

pneumatic (nū-măt'ĭk) [Gr. *pneumatikos,* pert. to air]. 1. Concerning gas or air. 2. Rel. to respiration. 3. Rel. to rarefied or compressed air.

pneumatics (nū-măt'ĭks). The branch of physics that is concerned with the physical and mechanical properties of gases and air.

pneumatinuria (nū"măt-ĭn-ū'rē-ă) [" + *ouron,* urine]. Excretion of urine containing free gas. SYN: *pneumaturia.*

pneumatization (nū"mă-tī-zā'shŭn). The formation of air-filled cells or cavities, esp. of the mastoid areas.

pneumatized (nū'mă-tīzd). Filled with air.

pneumatocardia (nū"măt-ō-kăr'dē-ă) [" + *kardia,* heart]. Air or gas in the heart chambers.

pneumatocele (nū-măt'ō-sēl) [" + *kele,* hernia]. 1. Hernia protuberance of lung tissue. 2. A swelling containing gas or air, esp. a swelling of the scrotum. SYN: *pneumocele; pneumonocele.*

p., extracranial. A collection of gas under the scalp, caused by a fracture of the skull that communicates with a paranasal sinus.

p., intracranial. A collection of gas within the skull.

pneumatodyspnea (nū"măt-ō-dĭsp'nē-ă) [" + *dys,* bad, + *pneia,* breath]. Dyspnea caused by pulmonary emphysema.

pneumatogram (nū-măt'ō-grăm) [" + *gramma,* a mark]. A tracing or record made by a pneumatograph.

pneumatograph (nū-măt'ō-grăf) [" + *graphein,* to write]. Device for registering respiratory movements. SYN: *pneograph.*

pneumatology (nū"mă-tŏl'ō-jē) [" + *logos,* a study]. Science of gases and air and their chemical properties and use in treatment.

pneumatometer (nū"măt-ŏm'ĕ-tĕr) [" + *metron,* a measure]. Device for measuring quantity of air involved in inspiration and expiration. SYN: *spirometer.*

pneumatometry (nū"măt-ŏm'ĕ-trē). Measurement of respiratory force as a means of diagnosis.

pneumatorrhachis (nū"măt-or'ă-kĭs) [" + *rhachis,* spine]. Air in the spinal canal.

pneumatoscope (nū-măt'ō-skōp) [" + *skopein,* to inspect]. 1. Apparatus used to measure the gas in expired air. 2. Instrument used to measure the respiratory movements. SYN: *pneumascope.*

pneumatosis (nū"mă-tō'sĭs) [Gr. *pneumatosis*]. Presence of air or gas in an abnormal location in the body.

p. abdominis. Air in the peritoneal cavity. SYN: *pneumoperitoneum.*

p. cystoides intestinalis. Presence of thin-walled gas-filled cysts in the intestines. The cause is unknown. The cysts usually disappear but will occasionally rupture and cause pneumoperitoneum.

pneumatotherapy (nū"măt-ō-thĕr'ă-pē) [Gr. *pneumatos,* air, + *therapeia,* treatment]. 1. Treatment of diseases by use of rarefied or condensed air. 2. Treatment of diseases of the lungs. SYN: *pneumotherapy.*

pneumatothorax (nū"măt-ō-thō'răks) [" + *thorax,* chest]. Air or gas accumulation in the pleural cavities. SYN: *pneumothorax.*

pneumaturia (nū"măt-ū'rē-ă) [" + *ouron,* urine]. Excretion of urine containing free gas. SYN: *pnematinuria.*

pneumatype (nū'mă-tīp) [" + *typos,* type]. Deposit of moisture on glass from the breath exhaled through the nostrils with the mouth closed for purpose of comparing the airflow through the nostrils.

pneumectomy (nū-mĕk'tō-mē) [Gr. *pneumon,* lung, + *ektome,* excision]. Excision of all or part of a lung.

pneumo-, pneumono- [Gr. *pneumon,* lung]. Combining forms meaning air; lung.

pneumoangiography (nū"mō-ăn"jē-ŏg'ră-fē) [" + *angeion,* vessel, + *graphein,* to write]. X-ray study of the vessels of the lungs. This is usually done by using a contrast medium.

pneumoarthrography (nū"mō-ăr-thrŏg'ră-fē) [" + *arthron,* joint, + *graphein,* to write]. Pneumarthrography, q.v.

pneumobulbar (nū"mō-bŭl'băr) [" + L. *bulbus,* bulbous root]. Concerning the lungs and the respiratory center in the medulla oblongata of the brain.

pneumocardial (nū"mō-kăr'dē-ăl) [" + *kardia,* heart]. Concerning the lungs and the heart.

pneumocele (nū'mō-sēl). Pneumatocele.

pneumocentesis (nū"mō-sĕn-tē'sĭs) [" + *kentesis,* a piercing]. Paracentesis, q.v., or surgical puncture of a lung to evacuate a cavity.

pneumocephalus (nū"mō-sĕf'ă-lŭs) [" + *kephale,* head]. Gas or air in the cavity of the cranium.

pneumocholecystitis (nū"mō-kō"lē-sĭs-tī'tĭs) [" + *chole,* bile, + *kystis,* bladder, + *itis,* inflammation]. Cholecystitis with gas in the gallbladder.

pneumococcal (nū"mō-kŏk'ăl) [" + *kokkos,* berry]. Concerning or caused by pneumococci.

pneumococcal vaccine, polyvalent. A vaccine that contains 14 of the known 83 pneumococcal capsular polysaccharides. The vaccine induces immunity for 3 to 5 years. This vaccine is estimated to protect against 80% of the pneumococcal types that produce serious disease in patients over 2 years of age. Children at high risk can be vaccinated at 6 months of age and reinoculated at 2 years. The vaccine is particularly indicated in high-risk groups such as persons with sickle cell diseases, the elderly, and persons with chronic debilitating disease or with immunologic defects.

pneumococcemia (nū"mō-kŏk-sē'mē-ă). Presence of pneumococci in the blood.

pneumococci (nū"mō-kŏk'sī). Pl. of pneumococcus.

pneumococcidal (nū"mō-kŏk-sī'dăl) [" + " + L. *cidus,* killing]. Killing pneumococci.

pneumococcolysis (nū"mō-kŏk-ŏl'ĭ-sĭs) [" + *kokkos,* berry, + *lysis,* destruction]. Destruction or lysis of pneumococci.

pneumococcus (nū"mō-kŏk'ŭs) [" + *kokkos,* berry]. (pl. *pneumococci*) An oval-shaped, encapsulated, non-spore-forming, gram-positive organism occurring usually in pairs (diplococcus) having lancet-shaped ends. There are more than 75 serological types of pneumococci. In addition to causing pneumonia, pneumococci are also found to be the cause of infections such as otitis media, mastoiditis, meningitis, bronchitis, bloodstream infections, keratitis, and conjunctivitis. Pneumococcal infections are effectively treated with penicillin. Erythromycin may be used if the patient is allergic to penicillin. SEE: *pneumonia.*

pneumocolon (nū"mō-kō'lŏn) [" + *kolon,* colon]. Air in the colon. This may be introduced as an aid in X-ray diagnosis

pneumoconiosis (nū"mō-kō"nē-ō'sĭs) [" + *konis,* dust, + *osis,* condition]. A condition of the respiratory tract due to inhalation of dust particles. An occupational disorder such as that caused by mining or stonecutting. SEE: *bituminosis.*

RS: anthracosis; chalicosis; coal worker's pneumoconiosis; pneumomelanosis; siderosis; silicosis.

pneumocranium (nū"mō-krā'nē-ŭm) [" + *kranion,* skull]. Pneumocephalus, q.v.

Pneumocystis carinii (nū"mō-sĭs'tĭs). The causative organism of pneumocystis pneumonia, q.v.

pneumocystis pneumonia. An acute interstitial plasma cell pneumonia characterized by slight if any fever, nonproductive cough, tachypnea, and dyspnea. It is caused by Pneumocystis carinii, an organism thought to be a protozoon. This disease is seen in marasmic and other debilitated children, and in immunodeficient adults. SYN: *pneumonia, interstitial plasma cell.*

DIAG: Made by finding the organism in tissue obtained by lung biopsy.

TREATMENT: Sulfamethoxazole-trimethoprim. If the pneumonia is untreated, mortality is quite high.

pneumocystography (nū"mō-sĭs-tŏg'ră-fē) [Gr. *pneumon,* lung, + *kystis,* bladder, + *graphein,* to write]. Cystogram done after air has been introduced into the urinary bladder.

pneumocystosis (nū"mō-sĭs-tō'sĭs). SEE: *pneumocystis pneumonia.*

pneumoderma (nū"mō-dĕr'mă) [" + *derma,* skin]. Emphysema under the skin.

pneumodynamics (nū"mō-dī-năm'ĭks) [" + *dynamis,* force]. Branch of science dealing with force employed in respiration.

pneumoempyema (nū"mō-ĕm-pī-ē'mă) [" + *en,* in + *pyon,* pus]. Empyema accompanied by an accumulation of gas.

pneumoencephalitis (nū"mō-ĕn-sĕf"ă-lī'tĭs)

[" + *enkephalos,* brain, + *itis,* inflammation]. Newcastle disease, q.v.

pneumoencephalogram (nū"mō-ĕn-sĕf'ă-lō-grăm) [" + " + *gramma,* mark]. Roentgenogram of the brain during pneumoencephalography, q.v.

pneumoencephalography (nū"mō-ĕn-sĕf"ă-lŏg'ră-fē) [" + " + *graphein,* to write]. Roentgenographic examination of ventricles and subarachnoid spaces of the brain following withdrawal of cerebrospinal fluid and injection of air or gas via lumbar puncture.

pneumoenteritis (nū"mō-ĕn"tĕr-ī'tĭs) [" + *enteron,* intestine, + *itis,* inflammation]. Pneumonia and enteritis combined.

pneumofasciogram (nū"mō-făs'ē-ō-grăm) [" + L. *fascia,* band, + Gr. *gramma,* mark]. Roentgenogram of fascial tissues and spaces after air has been injected in the fascia.

pneumogalactocele (nū"mō-găl-ăk'tō-sēl) [" + *gala,* milk, + *kele,* hernia]. A breast tumor containing milk and gas.

pneumogastric (nū"mō-găs'trĭk) [" + *gaster,* stomach]. Pert. to the lungs and stomach.

pneumogastric nerve. Term formerly used for the vagus nerve.

pneumogastrography (nū"mō-găs-trŏg'ră-fē) [" + " + *graphein,* to write]. X-ray study of the stomach after air has been introduced into it.

pneumogram (nū'mō-grăm) [" + *gramma,* a mark]. 1. A record of respiratory movements. 2. A roentgenogram following injection of air. SYN: *pneumatogram.*

pneumograph (nū'mō-grăf) [" + *graphein,* to write]. A device for recording frequency and intensity of respiration.

pneumography (nū-mŏg'ră-fē) [" + *graphein,* to write]. 1. Anatomical description or illustration of the lung. 2. Recording of respiratory movements on a graph. 3. Roentgenography of a part or organ after air is injected.

p., pelvic. Roentgenography of the pelvis after CO_2 has been injected into the peritoneal cavity.

pneumohemia (nū"mō-hē'mē-ă) [" + *haima,* blood]. Presence of air or gas in blood vessels.

pneumohemopericardium (nū"mō-hēm"ō-pĕr-ĭ-kăr'dē-ŭm) [Gr. *pneumon,* lung, + *haima,* blood, + *peri,* around, + *kardia,* heart]. The accumulation of air and blood in the pericardium.

pneumohemorrhagica (nū"mō-hēm-ō-rā'jĭ-kă) [" + " + *rhegnynai,* to burst forth]. Hemorrhage into pulmonary air cells; apoplexy of the lungs.

pneumohemothorax (nū"mō-hēm"ō-thō'răks) [" + " + *thorax,* chest]. Gas or air and blood collected in the pleural cavity.

pneumohydrometra (nū"mō-hī"drō-mē'tră) [" + *hydor,* water, + *metra,* uterus]. The accumulation of gas and fluid in the uterus.

pneumohydropericardium (nū"mō-hī"drō-pĕr-ĭ-kăr'dē-ŭm) [" + *hydor,* water, + *peri,* around, + *kardia,* heart]. Air and fluid accumulated in the pericardium.

pneumohydrothorax (nū"mō-hī"drō-thō'răks) [" + " + *thorax,* chest]. Gas or air and fluid in the pleural cavity.

pneumohypoderma (nū"mō-hī"pō-der'mă) [" + *hypo,* under, + *derma,* skin]. Air in the tissues under the skin.

pneumokidney (nū"mō-kĭd'nē) [" + ME. *kydney,* kidney]. Air in the pelvis of the kidney.

pneumolith (nū'mō-lĭth) [" + *lithos,* stone]. A pulmonary calculus.

pneumolithiasis (nū"mō-lĭth-ī'ăs-ĭs) [" + " + *-iasis,* condition]. Formation of concretions in the lungs.

pneumology (nū-mŏl'ō-jē) [" + *logos,* a study]. The scientific study of diseases of the lungs and air passages.

pneumolysin (nū-mŏl'ĭ-sĭn). A hemolytic toxin produced by pneumococci.

pneumolysis (nū-mŏl'ĭs-ĭs) [" + *lysis,* a loosening]. Separation of an adherent lung from costal pleura. SYN: *pneumonolysis.*

pneumomalacia (nū"mō-mă-lā'shē-ă) [Gr. *pneumon,* lung, + *malakia,* a softening]. Abnormal softening of the lung.

pneumomassage (nū"mō-mă-săzh') [" + *massein,* to knead]. Massage of the tympanum with air to cause movement of the ossicles of the inner ear.

pneumomediastinum (nū"mō-mē"dē-ăs-tī'nŭm) [" + L. *mediastinum,* in the middle]. Presence of air or gas in the mediastinal tissues. This may be present due to disease or following injection of air into the area for diagnostic purposes.

pneumomelanosis (nū"mō-mĕl-ăn-ō'sĭs) [" + *melano,* black, + *osis,* condition]. Pigmentation of the lung seen in pneumoconiosis, q.v.

pneumometer (nū-mŏm'ĕt-ĕr) [" + *metron,* measure]. Instrument for measuring the amount of air inspired and expired in respiration. SYN: *spirometer.*

pneumomycosis (nū"mō-mī-kō'sĭs) [" + *mykes,* fungus, + *osis,* condition]. A fungal pulmonary disease. SYN: *pneumonomycosis.*

pneumomyelography (nū"mō-mī-ĕl-ŏg'ră-fē) [" + *myelos,* marrow, + *graphein,* to write]. X-ray inspection of the spinal canal following injection of air or gas.

pneumonectasia, pneumonectasis (nū"mŏn-ĕk-tā'zē-ă, -ĕk'tă-sĭs) [" + *ektasis,* dilatation]. Distention of lungs with air.

pneumonectomy (nū"mŏn-ĕk'tō-mē) [" + *ektome,* excision]. Removal of a lung. SYN: *pneumectomy; pulmonectomy.*

pneumonia (nū-mō'nē-ă) [Gr.]. Inflammation of the lungs caused primarily by bacteria, viruses, and chemical irritants. There are more than 50 causes; the most common ones are listed in the accompanying table.

SYM: Pneumonia caused by pneumococci, staphylococci, streptococci, or bacilli often begins suddenly. Chills, high fever, pain in the chest, cough, purulent and often bloody sputum. Mortality is high unless treated with an appropriate antibiotic.

NURSING IMPLICATIONS: Follow implications under pleurisy. Obtain sputum specimens. Administer antimicrobial agents as prescribed. Evaluate for shock. Assess level of orientation at regular intervals. Anticipate and recognize complications. Administer cough medications as prescribed. Administer oxygen as needed. Maintain bedrest but passive range of motion exercises are indicated. Provide oral hygiene at frequent intervals. Keep patient warm and dry. Maintain well-balanced diet. Teach the patient the importance of follow-up therapy and prevention, e.g., pneumococcal vaccine.

p., abortive. Mild pneumonia with a brief course.

p., acute lobar. Pneumonia caused by pneumococci. SYN: *p., croupous*.

p. alba. A fatal pneumonia of the newborn caused by congenital syphilis.

p., anthrax. Anthrax that affects the

Pneumonias

Specific Microbial Causes	Diseases That May Be Accompanied by Pneumonia	Pneumonia Not Caused by Infections
Viruses	Tularemia	Oil aspiration
Adenoviruses	Brucellosis	Radiation
influenza	Rheumatic fever	Chemicals
Rhinoviruses	Syphilis	Vegetable dusts
respirosyncytial	Typhus	Silo-filler's disease
Coxsackie	Typhoid	
Coronaviruses	Rocky Mountain fever	
	Q fever	
	Acute viral respiratory disease	
Mycoplasmas	Infectious mononucleosis	
Mycoplasma pneumoniae		
	Trichiniasis	
Cocci	Acquired immune deficiency syndrome	
Pneumococcus		
Staphylococcus	Psittacosis	
Hemolytic streptococcus	Plague	
	Legionnaire's disease	
Protozoon (probable)	Rickettsial diseases	
Pneumocystis carinii		
Bacilli		
Hemophilus influenzae		
Mycobacterium tuberculosis		
Klebsiella pneumoniae (Friedländer's bacillus)		
Gram-negative bacilli		
Chlamydiae		
C. trachomatis		
C. psittaci		
Fungi		
Histoplasma capsulatum		
Coccidioides immitis		
Rickettsiae		
Rickettsia rickettsii		
Rickettsia burnetii		

lungs.

p., apex, apical. Pneumonia limited to the apices of the lungs; a form of lobar pneumonia.

p., aspiration. Pneumonia after inhaling foreign matter into the lungs.

p., atypical. P., primary atypical.

p., bronchial. A general classification of pneumonias that defines pneumonia due to mixed bacterial infections usually associated with a complication of surgery, aspiration, anesthesia, chronic illnesses, or chronic pulmonary diseases such as bronchiectasis or emphysema. SYN: *bronchopneumonia.*

p., caseous. Pneumonia associated with tuberculosis; and in which the lung has undergone necrosis and appears to be cheese-like.

p., catarrhal. P., bronchial, q.v.

p., central. P., lobar, q.v.

p., chronic interstitial. Chronic disease of the lung with overgrowth of fibrous tissue.

SYM: Moderate dyspnea and chronic cough, expectoration, which is slight or profuse and fetid from being retained in the bronchiectatic cavities. No fever.

PROG: The patient may live for years.

p., congenital aspiration. Pneumonia that existed prior to birth or is due to aspiration during the birth process.

p., contusion. P., traumatic, q.v.

p., croupous. P., acute lobar.

p., deglutition. P., aspiration, q.v.

p., desquamative interstitial. Pneumonia accompanied by cellular infiltration or fibrosis in the pulmonary interstitium. The cause is unknown.

SYM: Progressive dyspnea and nonproductive cough. Clubbing of the fingers is a common finding. Diffusion of oxygen and carbon dioxide is abnormal. Diagnosis is made by lung biopsy.

TREATMENT: Corticosteroids.

p., double. Pneumonia that involves both lungs.

p., Eaton agent. Pneumonia caused by Mycoplasma pneumoniae.

p., embolic. Pneumonia following embolization of a pulmonary blood vessel.

p., eosinophilic. Inflammation of the lung characterized by transient or prolonged pulmonary changes. The principal causes are parasites such as roundworms or filariae; fungus infection; drugs or chemicals such as nickel, penicillin, aminosalicylic acid, nitrofurantoin, and sulfonamides. In most cases, however, the cause is unknown.

p., fibrinous. Acute lobar pneumonia.

p., fibrous. Pneumonia followed by formation of scar tissue.

p., Friedlander's. A form of lobar pneumonia caused by the specific organism Klebsiella pneumoniae.

p., gangrenous. Pulmonary gangrene.

p., giant cell. An interstitial pneumonitis of infancy and childhood. The lung tissue contains multinucleated giant cells. The disease often occurs in connection with measles. SYN: *Hecht pneumonia.*

p., hypostatic. Pneumonia occurring in the elderly or debilitated patient who constantly remains in the same position. Gravity causes blood to become congested in one part of the lung. Infection aids development of true pneumonia.

NURSING IMPLICATIONS: SEE: *Nursing Implications* under *pneumonia.* Prevention is the most important factor, especially in the elderly and those who are immobile.

p., influenzal. 1. Pneumonia that occurs in association with influenza. The disease may be fatal. 2. Pneumonia caused by Hemophilus influenzae.

p., interstitial. Pneumonia with inflammation of the tissues surrounding the air passages rather than the bronchi, bronchioles, and alveoli themselves.

p., interstitial plasma cell. Pneumocystis pneumonia, q.v.

p., intrauterine. Pneumonia contracted prior to birth.

p., Legionella. An acute lobar pneumonia caused by Legionella pneumophila. SEE: *Legionnaires' disease.*

p., lipid. Pneumonia after aspiration of oily substances such as oily nose drops or mineral or other bland oil.

p., lobar. Pneumonia infecting one or more lobes of the lung. It is usually caused by Streptococcus pneumoniae. The pathological changes are, in order, first congested; then red and firm due to exudate and red blood cells in the alveoli; and gray hepatization as the exudate degenerates and is absorbed.

p., migratory. Pneumonia in which infected area shifts from one part of the lung to another part.

p., pneumocystis. SEE: *pneumocystis pneumonia.*

p., primary atypical. A relatively mild pneumonia characterized by cough, fever, pharyngitis, and x-ray evidence of lung infiltration out of proportion to the minimal findings upon examining the lungs. Caused by Mycoplasma pneumoniae.

TREATMENT: Tetracyclines and erythromycin are effective.

p., secondary. Pneumonia that occurs in connection with a specific systemic disease such as typhoid, diphtheria, or plague.

p., staphylococcal. Pneumonia due to infection with staphylococci.

p., streptococcal. Pneumonia due to infection with Streptococcus pneumoniae.

p., terminal. Lethal pneumonia that occurs secondary to another disease.

p., traumatic. Pneumonia that occurs after trauma to the lung or the thoracic cage. SYN: *p., contusion.*

p., tuberculous. Pneumonia caused by the tubercle bacilli. May result in rapid and widespread inflammatory exudation. If untreated, it may run a malignant course, ending fatally, or may subside and become chronic.

p., tularemic. Pneumonia caused by Francisella tularensis. May be primary or associated with tularemia, q.v.

p., typhoid. Pneumonia complicating typhoid fever.

p. varicella. Pneumonia complicating chickenpox.

p., viral. An acute systemic disease caused by a variety of viruses, including childhood exanthems. Symptoms may vary from those of the common cold to those of progressive respiratory insufficiency. Prognosis is influenced by the type of viral agent, age of the patient, extent of pulmonary involvement, and underlying systemic disease. SEE: *influenza.*

p., woolsorter's. Pulmonary anthrax.

pneumonic (nū-mŏn′ĭk) [Gr. *pneumon,* lung]. Concerning the lungs or pneumonia.

pneumonitis (nū″mō-nī′tĭs) [″ + *itis,* inflammation]. Inflammation of the lung. SYN: *pneumonia.*

p., hypersensitivity. A diffuse granulomatous lung disease caused by hypersensitivity to inhalation of organic dusts. Usually occurs in those with a hobby or occupation that involves heavy exposure to dust. SYN: *allergic alveolitis.* SEE: *bagassosis; farmer's lung.*

pneumono- [Gr. *pneumon,* lung]. Combining form pert. to the lung.

pneumonocele (nū-mŏn′ō-sēl) [″ + *kele,* hernia]. A pulmonary hernia. SYN: *pneumatocele; pneumocele.*

pneumonocentesis (nū-mō″nō-sĕn-tē′sĭs) [″ + *kentesis,* puncture]. Pneumocentesis, q.v.

pneumonoconiosis (nū-mō″nō-kō″nē-ō′sĭs) [″ + *konis,* dust, + *osis,* condition]. Fibrous inflammation or chronic induration of the lungs resulting from inhalation of dust. SYN: *pneumoconiosis.*

pneumonograph (nū-mŏn′ō-grăf) [″ + *graphein,* to write]. A roentgenogram of the lungs.

pneumonography (nū″mŏn-ŏg′ră-fē). Roentgenography of the lungs.

pneumonolysis (nū″mŏn-ŏl′ĭs-ĭs) [″ + *lysis,* loosening]. Loosening of an adherent lung from the chest wall to induce collapse of the lung. SYN: *pneumolysis.*

p., extrapleural. Separation of parietal pleura from the chest wall. SEE: *apicolysis.*

p., intrapleural. Separation of adhering visceral and parietal layers of pleura.

pneumonomelanosis (nū″mō-nō-mĕl″ăn-ō′sĭs) [″ + *melano,* black, + *osis,* condition]. Darkening of the lung tissue as a result of inhalation of black dust particles such as coal dust. SYN: *pneumomelanosis.*

pneumonomycosis (nū-mōn″ō-mī-kō′sĭs) [″ + *mykes,* fungus, + *osis,* condition]. Disease of the lungs caused by fungi. SYN: *pneumomycosis.*

pneumonopathy (nū″mō-nŏp′ăth-ē) [″ + *pathos,* disease]. Any diseased condition of the lung.

pneumonoperitonitis (nū″mō-nō-pĕr″ĭ-tō-nī′tĭs) [″ + *peritonaion,* peritoneum, + *itis,* inflammation]. Peritonitis with gas in the peritoneal cavity.

pneumonopexy (nū-mō″nō-pĕk′sē) [″ + *pexis,* fixation]. Surgical attachment of the lung to the chest wall. SYN: *pneumopexy.*

pneumonopleuritis (nū-mō″nō-ploo-rī′tĭs) [Gr. *pneumon,* lung, + *pleura,* a side, + *itis,* inflammation]. Pneumopleuritis, q.v.

pneumonorrhaphy (nū″mō-nor′ă-fē) [″ + *rhaphe,* a sewing]. Suture of a lung.

pneumonosis (nū-mō-nō′sĭs) [″ + *osis,* condition]. Any noninfective disease or disorder of the lungs, esp. those resulting from degenerative processes.

pneumonotherapy. Pneumotherapy.

pneumonotomy (nū-mō-nŏt′ō-mē) [″ + *tome,* incision]. Incision into the lung. SYN: *pneumotomy.*

pneumopathy (nū-mŏp′ă-thē) [″ + *pathos,* disease]. Any disease of the lungs.

pneumopericardium (nū″mō-pĕr-ĭ-kăr′dē-ŭm) [″ + *peri,* around, + *kardia,* heart]. Air or gas in the pericardial sac.

ETIOL: Traumatism or communication between the esophagus, stomach, or lungs and the pericardium.

SYM: Unusual metallic heart sounds, tympany over precordial area.

pneumoperitoneography. Radiographic examination of the peritoneum and internal organs after introduction of sterile air into the peritoneal cavity.

pneumoperitoneum (nū″mō-pĕr-ĭ-tō-nē′ŭm) [″ + *peritonaion,* peritoneum]. Condition in which air or gas is collected in the peritoneal cavity. May be artificially induced to treat tuberculous peritonitis. SYN: *pneumatosis abdominis.*

pneumoperitonitis (nū″mō-pĕr-ĭ-tō-nī′tĭs) [″ + *peritonaion,* peritoneum + *itis,* inflammation]. Peritonitis with gas accumulation.

pneumopexy (nū′mō-pĕks″ē) [″ + *pexis,* fixation]. Surgical attachment of a lung to the thoracic wall. SYN: *pneumonopexy.*

pneumopleuritis (nū″mō-ploo-rī′tĭs) [″ + *pleura,* a side, + *itis,* inflammation]. Inflamed condition of lungs and pleura.

pneumopleuroparietopexy (nū″mō-ploo″rō-pă-rī′ĕt-ō-pĕk″sē) [″ + ″ + L. *paries*, wall, + Gr. *pexis*, fixation]. The operation of attaching the lung with its parietal pleura to the border of a thoracic wound.

pneumopyelography (nŭ″mō-pī-ĕ-lŏg′ră-fē) [″ + *pyelos*, pelvis, + *graphein*, to write]. X-ray examination of the renal pelvis and ureters after they are injected with oxygen.

pneumopyopericardium (nū″mō-pī″ō-pĕr-ĭ-kar′dē-ŭm) [″ + *pyon*, pus, + *peri*, around, + *kardia*, heart]. Air, gas, and pus collected in the pericardial sac.

pneumopyothorax (nū″mō-pī″ō-thō′răks) [″ + ″ + *thorax*, chest]. Air and pus collected in the pleural cavity.

pneumoradiography (nū″mō-rā-dē-ŏg′ră-fē) [″ + L. *radius*, ray, + Gr. *graphein*, to write]. Injection of air into a part for the purpose of taking an x-ray picture.

pneumoretroperitoneum (nū″mō-rē″trō-pĕr″ĭ-tō-nē′ŭm) [″ + L. *retro*, backwards, + Gr. *peritonaion*, peritoneum]. Air or gas in the retroperitoneal space.

pneumorrhachis (nū″mō-rā′kĭs) [Gr. *pneumon*, lung, + *rhachis*, spine]. Gas accumulation in the spinal canal.

pneumorrhagia (nū″mō-rā′jē-ă) [″ + *rhegnynai*, to burst forth]. Pulmonary hemorrhage. SYN: *hemoptysis*.

pneumoserothorax (nū″mō-sē-rō-thō′răks) [″ + L. *serum*, whey, + Gr. *thorax*, chest]. Air or gas and serum collected in the pleural cavity.

pneumosilicosis (nū″mō-sĭl″ĭ-kō′sĭs) [″ + L. *silex*, flint, + Gr. *osis*, condition]. Silicosis, q.v.

pneumotachograph (nū″mō-tăk′ō-grăf) [Gr. *pneuma*, air, + *tachys*, swift, + *graphein*, to write]. Device for registering velocity of inspiration and expiration of air.

pneumotachometer (nū″mō-tăk-ŏm′ĕ-tĕr) [″ + *tachos*, speed, + *metron*, measure]. Device for measuring expired air flow.

pneumotaxic (nū″mō-tăk′sĭk) [″ + *taxis*, arrangement]. Concerning the regulation of breathing.

pneumotherapy (nū-mō-thĕr′ă-pē) [Gr. *pneumon*, lung, + *therapeia*, treatment]. 1. Treatment of diseases of the lungs. 2. Treatment of diseases by the use of rarefied or condensed gases. SYN: *pneumonotherapy*.

pneumothermomassage (nū″mō-thĕr″mō-măs-ăzh′) [Gr. *pneuma*, air, + *therme*, heat, + *massein*, to knead]. Application to the body of air of varying temperature and pressure.

pneumothorax (nū-mō-thō′răks) [″ + *thorax*, chest]. A collection of air or gas in the pleural cavity. The gas enters as the result of a perforation through the chest wall or the pleura covering the lung (visceral pleura). This perforation may be the result of an injury or the rupture of an emphysematous bleb or superficial lung abscess. The most common cause of the latter condition is a tuberculous abscess in the presence of pulmonary tuberculosis. SEE: illus. SYN: *aeropleura; aerothorax; pneumatothorax*.

SYM: The onset is sudden, usually with a severe sticking pain in the side and marked dyspnea. Fluid very frequently is found, developing within 48 hours (hydropneumothorax). The physical signs are those of a distended unilateral chest, tympanitic resonance, absence of breath sounds, and if fluid is present, a splash or succussion on shaking the patient.

p., artificial. Pneumothorax induced intentionally by artificial means, employed in the treatment of pulmonary tuberculosis or pneumonia. Pneumothorax gives the diseased lung temporary rest. The lung collapses when the air enters the pleural space.

Scattered adhesions may afford only a partial collapse. Effusion may occur in about one third of the cases. Hazards are minimal.

NURSING IMPLICATIONS: Explain the procedure for chest tube insertion to the patient and assist as necessary. Assess vital signs, breath sounds, chest expansion, chest tube site, drainage, and blood gas analysis. Administer oxygen as prescribed. Implement coughing and deep breathing and chest physiotherapy. Place patient in semi-Fowler's position to promote drainage, comfort, and ease of breathing. Provide adequate rest periods. Establish range of motion exercises and activity as tolerated. Administer medications as prescribed (analgesics, antibiotics, expectorants). Monitor intake and output. Maintain adequate nutrition and fluid intake to promote tissue healing and repair and to promote secretion liquefication. Observe catheter site daily and redress daily or as necessary. Have patient avoid excessive exercises and avoid smoking. Stress the importance of follow-up. Perform patient teaching as to the care of the insertion site after discharge.

p., extrapleural. Formation of a pneumothorax by introducing air into the space between the pleura and the inside of the rib cage.

p., open. Pneumothorax in which the pleural cavity is exposed to the atmosphere through an open wound in the chest wall.

p., spontaneous. Spontaneous entrance of air into the pleural cavity. The pressure may collapse the lung and displace the heart.

SYM: Sudden sharp pain, dyspnea, and cough. Pain may be referred to the shoulder. Majority of cases are mild and require only rest. Rarely shock and collapse occur.

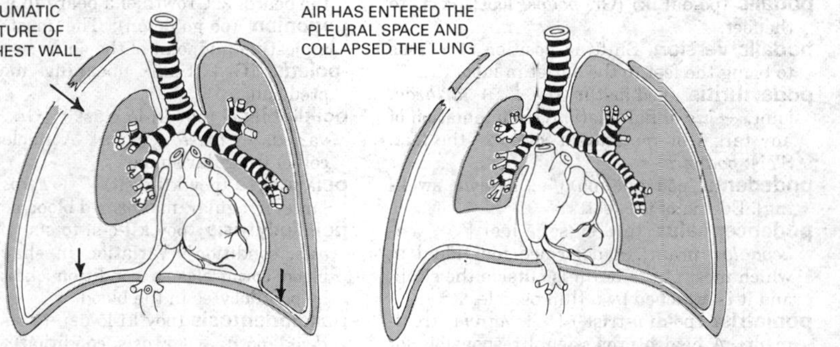
PNEUMOTHORAX
(OPEN—THE CHEST WALL INJURY PERMITS AIR TO FLOW IN AND OUT OF THE PLEURAL SPACE ON THE AFFECTED SIDE)
TRAUMATIC RUPTURE OF THE CHEST WALL
AIR HAS ENTERED THE PLEURAL SPACE AND COLLAPSED THE LUNG
INHALATION: AIR ENTERS THE INJURED SIDE, CAUSING COLLAPSE OF THE LUNG AND SHIFT OF THE MEDIASTINUM AND HEART TOWARD THE UNAFFECTED SIDE
EXHALATION: THE AIR IS PARTIALLY FORCED FROM THE AFFECTED SIDE PLEURAL SPACE AND THE MEDIASTINUM SHIFTS TOWARD THE AFFECTED SIDE

p., tension. A type of pneumothorax in which the air can enter the pleural space but cannot escape via the route of entry. This leads to an increase of pressure in the pleural space with collapse of the lung.

p., therapeutic. P., artificial, q.v.

p., valvular. Pneumothorax characterized by an opening through the pleura, which has a slit with a valvelike action, allowing the air to pass in but not out. SYN: *tension pneumothorax.*

pneumotomy (nū-mŏt′ō-mē) [Gr. *pneumon,* lung, + *tome,* incision]. Incision of the lung.

pneumotoxin (nū″mō-tŏks′ĭn) [″ + *toxikon,* poison]. A toxin produced by pneumococcus.

pneumotyphus (nū″mō-tī′fŭs) [″ + *typhos,* fever]. 1. Typhoid fever with pneumonia at onset. 2. Development of pneumonia during typhoid fever.

pneumouria (nū″mō-ū′rē-ă) [Gr. *pneuma,* air, + *ouron,* urine]. Excretion of urine with free gas. SYN: *pneumaturia.*

pneumoventricle (nū″mō-vĕn′trĭ-kl) [″ + L. *ventriculus,* little belly]. Air accumulation in the cerebral ventricles.

pneumoventriculography (nū″mō-vĕn-trĭk″ū-lŏg′ră-fē) [″ + ″ + Gr. *graphein,* to write]. Radiography of the lateral ventricles of the brain after removal of fluid content and injection with air. SYN: *ventriculography.*

pneusis (nū′sĭs) [Gr. *pnein,* to breathe]. 1. Respiration. 2. Panting. SYN: *anhelation.*

pnigophobia (nī″gō-fō′bē-ă) [Gr. *pnigos,* choking, + *phobos,* fear]. Morbid fear of choking; sometimes experienced in angina pectoris.

P.O. *per os,* i.e., by mouth.

Po. Chem. symb. for polonium.

Po_2. Abbr. for *partial pressure of oxygen.*

pock (pŏk) [AS. *poc,* pustule]. A pustule of an eruptive fever, esp. of smallpox.

pocket (pŏk′ĕt) [ME. *poket,* pouch]. A saclike cavity.

p., gingival. A gingival sulcus of abnormal depth. SYN: *periodontal pocket.*

p., pseudo-. A pocket that results from gingival inflammation with edema that produces an apparent abnormal depth of the gingival sulcus without apical movement of the bottom of the sulcus; a false pocket.

pocketing. Method of treating the pedicle in ovariotomy by enclosing it within the edges of the wound.

pockmarked. Pitted or marked with cicatrices from healed pustules, esp. those due to smallpox.

poculum Diogenis (pŏk′ū-lŭm dī-ŏj′ĕ-nĭs) [L. *poculum,* cup, + Diogenes, Gr. philosopher, 412–323 B.C.]. The concavity formed by contracting the muscles of the hand so the palm becomes cupped instead of flat.

podagra (pō-dăg′ră) [Gr. *podos,* foot, + *agra,* seizure]. Gout, esp. of the joints of the foot or of the great toe.

podalgia (pō-dăl′jē-ă) [″ + *algos,* pain]. Pain in the feet.

podalic (pō-dăl′ĭk) [Gr. *podos,* foot]. Pert. to the feet.

podalic version. Shifting position of a fetus to bring the feet to the outlet in labor.

podarthritis (pŏd″ăr-thrī′tĭs) [″ + *arthron,* joint, + *itis,* inflammation]. Inflammation of any tarsal or metatarsal joints of the feet. SYN: *podagra.*

podedema (pŏd″ē-dē′mă) [″ + *oidema,* swelling]. Edema of the feet.

podencephalus (pŏd″ĕn-sĕf′ă-lŭs) [″ + *enkephalos,* brain]. A deformed individual in which most of the brain is outside the skull, and it is attached by a thin pedicle.

podiatrist (pō-dī′ă-trĭst″) [″ + *iatreia,* treatment]. A health professional responsible for the examination, diagnosis, prevention, treatment, and care of conditions and functions of the human foot. A podiatrist performs surgical procedures, prescribes corrective devices and drugs and physical therapy as legally authorized in the state in which he or she is practicing. SYN: *chiropodist.*

podiatry (pō-dī′ă-trē). The diagnosis, treatment, and prevention of conditions of human feet. SYN: *chiropody.*

podium (pō′dē-ŭm) [Gr. *podos,* foot]. A footlike projection.

podo-, pod- [Gr. *pous, podos,* foot]. Combining forms indicating rel. to the foot.

podobromidrosis (pŏd″ō-brō″mĭ-drō′sĭs) [″ + *bromos,* stench, + *hidros,* perspiration]. Offensive perspiration of the feet.

podocyte (pŏd′ō-sīt) [″ + *kytos,* cell]. A special epithelial cell that forms an incomplete covering for the glomerulus of the kidney.

pododynamometer (pŏd″ō-dī″nă-mŏm′ĕ-ter) [″ + *dynamis,* force, + *metron,* measure]. A device for testing strength of the leg and foot muscles.

pododynia (pŏd″ō-dĭn′ē-ă) [″ + *odyne,* pain]. Pain in the feet, esp. a neuralgic pain in the heel with swelling and redness.

podogram (pŏd′ō-grăm) [″ + *gramma,* a mark]. An imprint or outline of the sole of the foot.

podograph (pŏd′ō-grăf) [″ + *graphein,* to write]. A device for taking an imprint of the sole of the foot.

podology (pŏd-ŏl′ō-jē) [″ + *logos,* a study]. The study of the anatomy and physiology of the foot.

podophyllum (pŏd-ō-fĭl′ŭm) [″ + *phyllon,* leaf]. USP. The dried rhizome and roots of Podophyllum peltatum. Used for treating, by direct application, certain papillomas such as verruca acuminata. SEE: *verruca acuminata.*

podophyllum resin (pŏd″ō-fĭl′ŭm). USP. The resinous extract from podophyllum, q.v.

pogoniasis (pō″gō-nī′ă-sĭs) [Gr. *pogon,* beard, + *-iasis,* disorder]. 1. Excessive growth of the beard. 2. Growth of a beard in a woman.

pogonion (pō-gō′nē-ŏn). The most anterior projecting midpoint of the chin.

-poietic [Gr.]. Suffix meaning making or producing.

poikiloblast (poy′kĭ-lō-blăst″) [Gr. *poikilos,* varied, + *blastos,* germ]. A nucleated red cell of irregular shape.

poikilocyte (poy′kĭl-ō-sīt) [″ + *kytos,* cell]. A large, irregular, malformed blood corpuscle.

poikilocytosis (poy″kĭl-ō-sī-tō′sĭs) [″ + ″ + *osis,* condition]. Variation in shape of red blood corpuscles, a condition characterized by poikilocytes in the blood.

poikilodentosis (poy″kĭ-lō-dĕn-tō′sĭs) [″ + L. *dens,* tooth, + Gr. *osis,* condition]. Mottling of the teeth usually due to an excess of fluoride in the drinking water.

poikiloderma (poy-kĭl-ō-dĕr′mă) [″ + *derma,* skin]. A skin disorder characterized by pigmentation, telangiectasia, purpura, pruritus, and atrophy.

p. atrophicus vasculare. A generalized dermatitis of unknown cause. It is symmetrical and occurs almost exclusively in adults. There is widespread telangiectasia, pigmentation, and atrophy of the skin.

p. of Civatte. Reticulated pigmentation and telangiectasia of the sides of the face and neck. Seen quite commonly in middle-aged women.

poikilonymy (poy″kĭ-lŏn′ĭ-mē) [″ + *onoma,* name]. The use of terms from several nomenclature systems.

poikilotherm (poy-kĭl′ō-thĕrm) [″ + *therme,* heat]. An animal whose body temperature varies according to the temperature of the environment. SYN: *allotherm.* SEE: *homotherm.*

poikilothermal, poikilothermic (poy″kĭ-lō-thĕr′măl, -mĭk). Concerning poikilothermy.

poikilothermy (poy″kĭ-lō-thĕr′mē). The condition of having the temperature of the organism or animal assume the same temperature as the environment. Reptiles have this property. SEE: *homoiotherm.*

poikilothrombocyte (poy-kĭl″ō-thrŏm′bō-sīt) [″ + *thrombos,* clot, + *kytos,* cell]. A blood platelet of abnormal shape.

point (poynt) [O. Fr., a prick, a dot]. 1. The sharp end of any object. 2. Stage at which the surface of an abscess is about to rupture.

3. A minute spot. 4. Position in space, time, or degree.

p., absorbent. A cone of paper used in drying or in keeping liquid medicines in a root canal of a tooth.

p., auricular. Center of the external orifice of the auditory canal. SYN: *p., Broca's.*

p., Boas'. A tender spot left of the 12th thoracic vertebra in patients with gastric ulcer.

p., boiling. The temperature at which a liquid will boil.

p., Broca's. P., auricular.

p.'s, Capuron's. Four fixed points in the pelvic inlet, the two iliopectineal eminences and the two sacroiliac joints. SYN: *p.'s, cardinal* (def. 2).

p.'s, cardinal. 1. Six points determining the direction of light rays emerging from and entering the eye. SEE: *p.'s, nodal; p.'s, principal.* 2. P.'s, Capuron's.

p., cold rigor. The temperature at which cell activity ceases.

p., contact. The point on a tooth that touches an opposed tooth.

p., convergence. 1. The point to which rays of light converge. 2. The closest point to the patient on which the eyes can converge as the object is moved closer and closer.

p.'s, corresponding. Point in the retina of each eye that, when stimulated simultaneously, results in a single visual sensation.

p., craniometric. One of the fixed points of the skull used in craniometry.

p., critical, of gases. Temperature at or above which a gas can no longer be liquefied by pressure.

p., critical, of liquids. Temperature above which no pressure may retain a substance in a liquid form.

p.'s, deaf, of ear. Several points or areas close to the external auditory meatus where a vibrating tuning fork will not be heard.

p., dew. The temperature at which moisture begins to be condensed and deposited as dew.

p.'s, disparate. Points on the retinae unequally paired.

p., Erb's. The point on the side of the neck, 2–3 cm. above the clavicle and in front of the transverse process of the sixth cervical vertebra. Electrical stimulation over this area causes various arm muscles to contract.

p., external orbital. The prominent point at outer edge of orbit above the frontomalar suture.

p., far. The point (20 ft. [6.1 meters] or more) at which distinct vision is possible without aid of the muscles of accommodation. It may be nearer than 20 ft. (6.1 meters) according to degree of myopia. There is no far point in the hypermetropic eye.

p., fixation. Point at which the two visual axes converge.

p., flash. The lowest temperature at which a volatile liquid will ignite.

p., focal. The point at which a group of light rays converge.

p., freezing. Temperature at which liquids become solid.

p., fusion. Melting point.

p., Guéneau de Mussy's. Pressure on this point causes pain in cases of diaphragmatic pleurisy. The point is located at the junction of a line extending down from the left border of the sternum with a horizontal line at the level of the bony part of the anterior portion of the tenth rib.

p., gutta-percha. Cone made of gutta-percha combined with other material that is used in filling root canals of teeth.

p., Halle's. A point at the intersection of a horizontal line drawn from the anterior superior iliac spines and an angled line extending up from the public spine. At that point, the ureter is palpable as it crosses the pelvic brim.

p., hot. A spot on the skin that perceives hot but not cold stimuli.

p.'s, hysterogenic. Circumscribed areas of the body that produce symptoms of a hysterical aura, and eventually a hysterical attack when rubbed or pressed.

p., ice. The temperature at which there is equilibrium between ice and air-saturated water at one atmosphere of pressure.

p.'s, identical retinal. Points in the two retinae upon which the images are seen as one.

p., isionic. The pH at which a solution of ionized material has as many negative as positive ions.

p., isoelectric. The particular pH of a solution of an amphoteric electrolyte such as an amino acid or protein in which the charged molecules do not migrate to either electrode. Proteins are least soluble at this point. Thus at the appropriate pH, proteins may be precipitated.

p., jugal. Posterior border of frontal process of the malar bone where cut by a line tangent to upper border of zygoma.

p., lacrimal. Outlet of lacrimal canaliculus. SYN: *punctum lacrimale* [NA].

p., Lanz's. Point on the line between the two anterior superior iliac spines, one third of the distance from the right spine, indicating origin of the vermiform appendix.

p., Lian's. Point at junction of outer and middle thirds of a line from the umbilicus to the anterior superior spine of ilium where a trocar may be introduced safely for paracentesis.

p., malar. The most prominent point on

the external tubercle of the malar bone.

p., maximum occipital. The point on the occipital bone farthest from the glabella.

p., McBurney's. Point 1½ to 2 in. (4.1 to 5.1 cm.) above the anterosuperior spine of the ilium on a line between the ilium and umbilicus where pressure produces tenderness in acute appendicitis.

p., median mandibular. Point on the anterior-posterior center of the mandibular ridge in the median sagittal plane.

p., melting. The temperature at which a solid becomes a liquid. This is a constant for each material.

p., mental. The most anterior point of the midline of the chin. SYN: *pogonion*.

p., metopic. Glabella, q.v.

p., motor. A point usually about the middle of a muscle where a motor nerve enters the muscle at which a minimal electrical stimulus to the overlying skin will elicit a visible contraction.

p., Munro's. Point halfway between the left anterior iliac spine and the umbilicus.

p., nasal. Nasion, q.v.

p., near. Nearest point at which the eye can accommodate for distinct vision.

p.'s, nodal. An anterior and posterior cardinal point on the surface of lens of the eye so related that every ray directed toward the anterior point is represented after refraction by a ray emanating from the posterior point.

p., occipital. The most posterior point on the occipital bone.

p. of maximal impulse. ABBR: P.M.I. The point on the chest wall over the heart at which the contraction of the heart is best seen or felt.

p. of regard. The point at which the eye is looking.

p.'s, painful. Points over which a neuralgic nerve is tender on pressure. SYN: *p.'s, Valleix's*.

p., preauricular. The point immediately in front of the auricular point.

p.'s, pressure. 1. Points on the skin that, when stimulated, give rise to sensation of pressure. 2. Points where arteries come near the surface and at which pressure may be applied to stop arterial bleeding.

p.'s, principal. Two points so situated that the optical axis is cut by the two principal planes.

p., spinal. P., subnasal, q.v.

p., subnasal. Center of the root of the anterior nasal spine.

p., supra-auricular. A point on the skull on the posterior root of the zygomatic process of the temporal bone, directly above the auricular point.

p., supraorbital. 1. A point on the skull in the midline of the forehead, just above the glabella. SYN: *ophryon*. 2. A neuralgic point just above the supraorbital notch.

p., supranasal. P., supraorbital, q.v.

p., thermal death. The temperature required to kill all of the organisms in a culture in a specified time.

p., trigger. A spot at which the application of pressure will cause pain. The pain is not necessarily in the area of the pressure.

p.'s, Trousseau's apophysiary. Sensitive points over the dorsal and lumbar vertebrae in neuralgia.

p., triple. The temperature and pressure at which a substance that can exist in three phases, liquid, solid, and gas, is at equilibrium.

p.'s, Valleix's. Tender spots upon pressure over the course of a nerve in neuralgia. SYN: *p.'s, painful*.

p., vital. The point in the medulla oblongata close to the floor of the fourth ventricle, puncture of which causes instant death due to destruction of the respiratory center.

p., Voillemier's. Point on the linea alba of the abdominal wall about 6 to 7 cm. below a line connecting the anterior superior iliac spines. Suprapubic puncture of the bladder may be made at this point in obese or edematous individuals.

pointillage (pwăn″tĭ-yăzh′) [Fr.]. Massage with finger tips.

pointing. Reaching a point.

poise (poyz). [J. M. Poiseuille] The unit of viscosity. The tangential shearing force required to be applied to an area of one square cm. between two parallel planes of one square cm. in area and one cm. apart in order to produce a velocity of flow of the liquid of one cm. per second.

Poiseuille's law (pwă-zŭ′yĕz). [Jean Marie Poiseuille, Fr. physiologist, 1799–1869] A law that states that the rapidity of the capillary current is in direct proportion to the fourth power of the radius of the capillary tube, the pressure on the fluid, and indirectly to the viscosity of the liquid and length of the tube. The formula is:

$$\text{rate of flow} = \frac{\pi p r^4}{8 l n}$$

where p = pressure; r = radius of tube; l = length of tube; and n = coefficient of viscosity of the liquid.

Poiseuille's space. The inert capillary current in which leukocytes close to the wall of the vessel move slowly; the erythrocytes travel more rapidly in the middle current.

poison (poy′zn) [L. *potio*, a poisonous draft]. Any substance taken into the body by ingestion, inhalation, injection, or absorption that interferes with normal physiological functions. Virtually any substance can be poisonous if consumed in sufficient quantity; therefore the term poison more often implies an excessive degree of dosage rather than a specific group of substances. Aspirin is not usually thought of as a poison, but overdoses of this drug kill more children accidentally each year than any of the traditional poisons. Since the list of poisonous substances is infinite, it defies classification in any simple way. For a list of commonly encountered hazardous substances in the home, SEE: *Poisons and Poisoning* in *Appendix*.

p., pesticidal. Chemicals whose toxic properties are commercially exploited in agriculture, industry, or commerce to increase quantity, improve quality, or generally to promote consumer acceptability of a variety of products. Common types include insecticides, rodenticides, herbicides, defoliants, fungicides, insect repellants, molluscicides, and some kinds of food additives. The wide variety of poisons commonly found in and around the home constitutes an important group in accidental poisonings. SEE: *Poisons and Poisoning* in *Appendix*.

poison control center. A facility meeting the staffing and equipment standards of the American Association of Poison Control Centers and recognized to be able to give information on, or treatment to patients suffering from, poisoning. A poison information center consists only of a reference library and does not have treatment facilities. Over 400 poison centers of these two types are scattered throughout the U.S. Staffed largely by volunteer personnel, they offer 24-hour service. By virtue of their function, they are commonly associated with or are part of large hospitals or medical schools. A government agency—the Bureau of Drugs Division of the Poison Control Branch of the Food and Drug Administration, U.S. Department of Health and Human Services—is also active in poison control programs and in coordinating the efforts of individual centers. For address and telephone number of state or province control center, SEE: *Poison Control Centers* in *Appendix*.

poisoning [L. *potio,* a poisonous draft]. 1. The state produced by introduction of a poison into the body. 2. Administration of a poison. Symptoms of poisoning vary widely with the agent. SEE: *Poisons and Poisoning* in *Appendix*.

NURSING IMPLICATIONS: Identify the poison and contact the local poison control center for directions. In certain types of poisons, a physical, mechanical, or physiological antidote will help to decrease absorption, protect body tissues, or reverse the effects of the poison.

Establish and maintain the airway; administer oxygen as ordered. If indicated and safe to do so, induce vomiting by tickling the back of the throat or administering large quantities of water, saline, milk, soap suds, or ipecac syrup.

Support the patient physically and psychologically. Hospitalize for treatment and close observation. Treat for shock. Keep the patient warm. Provide appropriate nursing measures to the convulsing patient to prevent injury. Monitor intake and output. Monitor fluid and electrolyte balance. Reduce elevated temperature by use of cool or alcohol sponge bath and use of antipyretics. Assist with medical procedures such as dialysis.

Teach patient and family methods to avoid food contamination, to place toxic substances in a safe place out of children's reach, and to place the poison control center's phone number with the list of emergency numbers. Instruct the family to have ipecac syrup in the household.

NOTE: Do not be hasty in concluding that a patient has been poisoned. Many disease states mimic the symptoms of poisoning. Cerebral hemorrhage, epilepsy, overdose of insulin, diabetic coma, meningitis, thrombosis, and uremia may simulate poisoning. Acute indigestion, appendicitis, gastritis, renal colic, or peptic ulcer may mimic poisoning by corrosive substances.

p., arsenic. In acute poisoning, symptoms may appear in a few minutes. When arsenic is ingested with solid food, symptoms may not appear for many hours. Symptoms are: metallic taste and odor of garlic on breath, burning pain throughout gastrointestinal tract, vomiting and purging, dehydration, shock syndrome, coma, convulsions, paralysis, and death.

F.A.: Lavage stomach with copious amounts of water. If this cannot be done, induce vomiting. Administer dimercaprol (British antilewisite).

TREATMENT: After first aid, maintain fluid and electrolyte balance. Morphine for pain. Treat for shock and pulmonary edema. Blood transfusion may be required.

p., blood. Presence of pathogenic bacteria in the blood. If allowed to progress, the organisms may multiply and cause an overwhelming infection and death. Symptoms and signs usually include chills and fever, petechiae, purpuric pustules, and abscesses. SYN: *septicemia.*

p., convulsive. Common convulsive poisons are strychnine and infrequently used drugs such as picrotoxin. For symptoms and treatment, SEE: *convulsant poisons.*

p., corrosive. Poisoning by strong acids, alkalies, strong antiseptics including bichloride of mercury, carbolic acid (phenol), Lysol, cresol compounds, tincture of iodine, and arsenic compounds. These are destructive and cause tissue damage similar to that caused by burns. If the substances have been swallowed, any part of the alimentary canal may be affected. Tissues involved are easily perforated. Death comes very shortly from shock or swelling of throat and pharynx, which causes choking, or by closure of esophagus, causing slow starvation. For symptoms and treatment, SEE: *corrosive poisoning*.

p., fish. A form of food poisoning caused by eating fish that are inherently poisonous; poisonous through decomposition, infection, or because the fish had been feeding on other poisonous life forms. For symptoms and treatment, SEE: *fish poisoning*.

p., food. Illness resulting from ingestion of foods containing poisonous substances. This includes mushrooms, shellfish, foods contaminated with pesticides, lead, or mercury, milk sickness (milk from cows that have fed on poisonous plants), or foods that have putrefied or decomposed due to bacterial action.

p., lead. Symptoms of acute poisoning include a metallic taste in mouth, burns in throat and pharynx, and later abdominal cramps and prostration. Chronic lead poisoning is characterized by anorexia, nausea, vomiting, excess salivation, anemia, a lead line on the gums, abdominal pains, muscle cramps, and pains in the joints.

F.A.: In acute poisoning, wash out stomach. Administration of magnesium sulfate (Epsom salts) or sodium sulfate, which precipitates the lead, and helps to remove it by purging. Give 10% dextrose in water intravenously to increase urine flow.

TREATMENT: If children have signs of lead encephalopathy, administer dimercaprol 4 mg./kg. I.M. every four hours for 30 doses. Four hours after the last of that series of doses give calcium disodium edetate, 12.5 mg./kg. I.M. every four hours in a 20% solution with 0.5% procaine added for a total of 30 doses. Adults with signs of acute encephalopathy should be given the same therapy. Treatment for chronic poisoning depends on the severity of the symptoms.

p., mercury. Mercury per se, i.e., mass of mercury, is not poisonous, but its bivalent salt, mercuric chloride ($HgCl_2$), is highly poisonous. Symptoms of acute poisoning include: severe gastrointestinal irritation with pain, cramping, constriction of the throat, vomiting, and a metallic taste in the mouth. A stronger solution causes a white coating due to coagulation. Abdominal pain is very severe, bloody diarrhea and vomitus appear, urine flow is scanty. Prostration, convulsions, unconsciousness, and death occur. Chronic poisoning is characterized by bad breath, loosening of teeth, fever, urinary difficulties, nausea, diarrhea, sore tongue, paralysis, weakness, and death.

F.A.: Evacuate stomach, wash out with milk or with a solution of a teaspoon of sodium bicarbonate dissolved in 6 oz. (177 ml.) of water. Treatment with dimercaprol (British antilewisite) should be instituted immediately. Maintain fluid and electrolyte balance.

p., mushroom. Ingestion of mushrooms such as Amanita muscaria, which contains muscarine, or species that contain phalloidine, a component of the amanita toxin, cause poisoning. The nearest Poison Control Center should be called for emergency treatment.

p., potato. Poisoning due to ingestion of potatoes that contain excess amounts of solanine, q.v. This toxic substance is present in the potato peel and in the green sprouts. Potatoes usually contain about 7 mg. of solanine per 100 grams; the toxic dose of solanine is about 20–25 grams. Boiling but not baking removes most of the solanine from the potato. Symptoms of poisoning include headache, vomiting, abdominal pain, diarrhea, and fever. Neurological disturbances include apathy, restlessness, drowsiness, confusion, stupor, hallucinations, and visual disturbances.

TREATMENT: There is no specific therapy.

PROGNOSIS: With appropriate supportive and symptomatic therapy, prognosis is good.

p., unknown substances. Cases where there is no information concerning the nature of the poison taken, and the signs and symptoms are not recognized as being due to any particular substance. Specific antidotes cannot be given in this situation. There are, however, certain agents that act in a general manner and may be efficacious.

One of these is activated charcoal, which is available from many sources. Although a slurry of this in water is messy and offensive to the patient, it is a highly effective adsorbent for certain kinds of poisons. Another substance is referred to as the universal antidote. It consists of a mixture of 2 parts activated charcoal, 1 part magnesium oxide, and 1 part tannic acid. The universal antidote has been used empirically for a number of years and prepackaged units now are available commercially. It is doubtful if this mixture offers any real advantage over activated charcoal, which has a proven effectiveness against many substances. Both these materials may be given as a slurry made from several heaping teaspoonsful in a glass of water. Since the ingredients are essentially harmless and since the efficiency is increased by increasing the amount of adsorbent relative to the amount of poison, the dose may be repeated several times.

poison ivy. A climbing vine, Rhus toxicodendron, which on contact produces a severe form of dermatitis. Rhus species contain urushiol, an extremely irritating oily resin. Urushiol may also be a potent sensitizer since in many cases subsequent contacts produce increasingly severe reactions. SEE: illus.

poison ivy dermatitis. Dermatitis resulting from irritation or sensitization of the skin by the resin of the poison ivy plant. There is no absolute immunity although susceptibility varies greatly even in the same individual. SYN: *ivy poisoning.*

SYM: An interval of time between skin contact of poison and first appearance of symptoms, varying from a few hours to several days and depending on sensitivity of the patient and possibly condition of the skin. Moderate itching or burning sensation soon followed by small blisters; later manifestations vary. Blisters usually rupture and are followed by oozing of serum and subsequent crusting.

NURSING IMPLICATIONS: Instruct the patient concerning recognition of the plant, avoiding contact with it, and to wear long-sleeved shirts and long pants in wooded areas. If contact occurs, wash with soap and water immediately to remove the toxic oil. Apply antipruritic lotion (e.g., calamine) or a cool wet dressing of aluminum acetate (Burow's) solution or epsom salts. Cover this with plastic wrap to retain moisture. Topical or systemic steroids or both may be prescribed in severe cases. Antihistamines are of little value.

TREATMENT: In mild dermatitis, a lotion to relieve itching is usually sufficient. In severe dermatitis, cool, wet dressings or compresses, potassium permanganate baths, and perhaps a course of intramuscular or oral corticosteroid therapy will be required. Sedation is also necessary in some cases.

Tepid water is used to provide symptomatic relief from itching and burning. The affected area is massaged with water as hot as can be tolerated for 1 or 2 minutes. The relief from itching is dramatic and may last several hours.

poison oak. A climbing vine, Rhus radicans or R. diversiloba, closely related to poison ivy and containing the same active principle. The symptoms and treatment are identical with those for poison ivy dermatitis, q.v. SEE: illus.

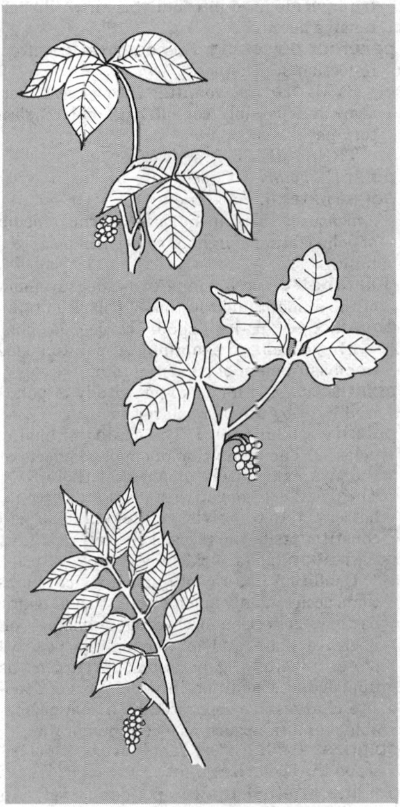

POISON IVY - POISON OAK
POISON SUMAC
(FROM TOP TO BOTTOM)

poisonous (poy'zŏn-ŭs) [L. *potio,* a poisonous draft]. Having the properties or qualities of a poison. SYN: *toxic; venomous.*

poisonous plants. *Do not eat:* castor bean, chinaberry, European bittersweet, wild or black cherry, horse chestnuts, poison hemlock, laurel, death cup, black nightshade or deadly nightshade, jimsonweed. *Do not touch:* poison ivy, poison oak, poison sumac.

poison sumac. A shrublike plant, Rhus vernix, widely distributed in the U.S., as are all Rhus species. Since it contains the same active principle as poison ivy, the symptoms and treatment are the same as for poison ivy dermatitis, q.v. SEE: illus.

poker back. Stiffness of the spine. May result from spondylitis, q.v., or rheumatoid arthritis. SEE: *arthritis, rheumatoid.*

pokeroot (pōk'root). The dried root of Veratrum viride used internally as an antihypertensive agent.

pokeroot poisoning. Poisoning resulting from ingestion of pokeroot.

SYM: Nausea, vomiting, drowsiness, vertigo, and possibly convulsions and respiratory paralysis.

TREATMENT: Emetic or lavage.

polar [L. *polaris*]. Concerning a pole.

polarimeter (pō″lăr-ĭm′ĕ-tĕr) [″ + Gr. *metron*, a measure]. Instrument for measuring amount of polarization of light or rotation of polarized light.

polarimetry (pō″lăr-ĭm′ĕ-trē). Measurement of the amount and rotation of polarized light.

polariscope (pō-lăr′ĭ-skōp) [L. *polaris*, pole, + Gr. *skopein*, to examine]. Apparatus used in measurement of polarized light.

polariscopy (pō″lăr-ĭs′kō-pē). Study of polarized light by use of a polariscope.

polarity (pō-lăr′ĭ-tē). 1. The quality of having poles. 2. The exhibition of opposite effects at the two extremities in physical therapy. 3. The positive or negative state of an electrical battery. 4. In cell division, the relation of cell constituents to the poles of the cell.

polarization (pō″lăr-ī-zā′shŭn) [L. *polaris*, pole]. 1. Condition in a ray of light in which vibrations occur in only one plane. 2. In a galvanic battery, collection of hydrogen bubbles on negative plate and oxygen on the positive plate, whereby generation of current is impeded. 3. Condition in which ions of opposite charges are separated by a semipermeable membrane such as a cell membrane.

polarizer (pō′lă-rīz″ĕr). The part of a polariscope that polarizes light.

poldine methylsulfate (pŏl′dēn). USP. An anticholinergic drug with action similar to belladonna.

pole (pōl) [L. *polus*]. 1. The extremity of any axis about which forces acting on it are symmetrically disposed. SYN: *polus*. 2. One of two points in a magnet, cell, or battery having opposite physical qualities.

p., animal. Pole opposite the yolk in an ovum. At this point, polar bodies are formed and pinched off and protoplasm is concentrated and has its greatest activity.

p., frontal. Most projecting part of the anterior extremity of both cerebral hemispheres.

p., germinal. The pole of an ovum at which the development begins.

p., occipital. The posterior extremity of the occipital lobe.

p.'s of eye. The anterior and posterior extremities of the optic axis.

p.'s of kidney. The kidney's upper and lower extremities.

p.'s of testicle. The upper and lower extremities of a testicle.

p., pelvic. Breech of a fetus.

p., placental, of chorion. Spot at which the domelike placenta is situated.

p., temporal. The anterior extremity of the temporal lobe.

p., vegetal. Part of the egg containing the food yolk.

policlinic (pŏl″ĭ-klĭn′ĭk) [Gr. *polis*, city, + *kline*, bed]. Polyclinic, q.v.

polio. *poliomyelitis, acute anterior.*

polio- [Gr. *polios*, gray]. Combining form indicating rel. to the gray matter of the nervous system.

polioclastic (pŏl″ē-ō-klăs′tĭk) [″ + *klastos*, breaking]. Destructive to gray matter of the nervous system.

polioencephalitis (pŏl″ē-ō-ĕn-sĕf″ă-lī′tĭs) [″ + *enkephalos*, brain, + *itis*, inflammation]. Condition characterized by inflammatory lesions of the gray matter of the brain.

p., anterior superior. A disease involving necrotic changes in gray matter about the 3rd ventricle, anterior portion of the 4th ventricle, and aqueduct of Sylvius. Characterized by ocular abnormalities, mental disturbances, and ataxia. Of nutritional origin, probably thiamine (vitamin B_1) deficiency. SYN: *Wernicke's syndrome.*

p. hemorrhagica. Polioencephalitis accompanied by hemorrhagic lesions.

p., posterior. Polioencephalitis involving gray matter about the 4th ventricle.

polioencephalomeningomyelitis (pŏl″ē-ō-ĕn-sĕf″ăl-ō-mĕn-ĭn″gō-mī-ĕl-ī′tĭs) [″ + ″ + *meninx*, membrane, + *myelos*, marrow, + *itis* inflammation]. Inflammation of the gray matter of the brain and spinal cord and their meninges.

polioencephalomyelitis (pŏl″ē-ō-ĕn-sĕf″ăl-ō-mī″ĕl-ī′tĭs). Inflamed condition of the gray matter of the brain and spinal cord.

polioencephalopathy (pŏl″ē-ō-ĕn-sĕf″ăl-ŏp′ă-thē) [Gr. *polios*, gray, + *enkephalos*, brain, + *pathos*, disease]. Diseased condition of the gray matter of the brain.

poliomyelencephalitis (pŏl″ē-ō-mī″ĕl-ĕn-sĕf″ăl-ī′tĭs) [″ + *myelos*, marrow, + *enkephalos* brain, + *itis*, inflammation]. Poliomyelitis with polioencephalitis.

poliomyelitis (pŏl″ē-ō-mī″ĕl-ī′tĭs) [″ + ″ + *itis*, inflammation]. Inflammation of the gray matter of the spinal cord. An acute viral disease characterized by fever, sore throat, headache, vomiting, and often stiffness of the neck and back. There may also be subsequent atrophy of groups of muscles ending in contraction and permanent deformity.

p., abortive. Poliomyelitis in which illness is mild with no involvement of central nervous system.

p., acute anterior. An acute infectious inflammation of the anterior horns of the gray matter of the spinal cord. This is an acute, systemic, infectious disease in which paralysis may or may not occur. In the majority of patients, the disease is mild, being limited to respiratory and gastrointestinal symptoms, such constituting the minor illness or the abortive type, which lasts only a few days. In the major illness, paralysis or weakness of muscles occurs with loss of superficial and deep reflexes. In such cases characteristic lesions are found in the gray matter of the spinal cord, medulla, motor area of cerebral cortex, and cerebellum. SYN: *paralysis, infantile polio.*

ETIOL: Causative agent is a virus consisting of particles from 270 to 300 Ångstrom units in diameter. The virus that is excreted in the feces is resistant and stable, remaining viable for months outside the body. Three immunologic types exist.

SYM: Onset often is abrupt, although the ordinary manifestations of a severe cold or some gastrointestinal disturbances may come on gradually, accompanied by slight elevation of temperature, frequently enduring for not more than three days. At the end of this period, paralysis may or may not develop. The extent of any paralysis necessarily depends upon degree of nerve involvement. Consequently, paralysis may be confined to one small group of muscles or affect one or all extremities. In some instances, the respiratory muscles also are involved and it is in these cases that death is so likely to ensue. In the average paralytic case it is the extensor muscles in particular that are affected.

COMPLICATIONS: Paralysis, atrophy of muscles, and ultimate deformities. Aside from bronchopneumonia, which may develop in very severe cases, other complications are surprisingly few.

DIFF. DIAG: Among the diseases confused with this infection are the various types of meningitis, postinfection encephalomyelitis, and hysteria.

INCIDENCE: Poliomyelitis is endemic throughout the world but occurs in epidemics in certain countries, including the U.S. However, the disease in the U.S. has been brought under almost complete control by vaccination. Epidemics are seasonal, occurring in summer and fall. Children are more susceptible than adults. Infection is spread by direct contact, the virus probably entering the body via the mouth. It reaches the central nervous system through the blood.

INCUBATION: Ranges from 5 to 35 days, but usually 7 to 12 days.

PROG: Ordinarily the outcome as to life is good. It is only the bulbar and respiratory types in which death is likely to occur. These two types constitute nearly all of the fatal cases. Even when paralysis develops, 50% of the cases make a full recovery and about 25% have mild permanent paralysis. In the more severe types, however, some paralysis may remain.

PROPHYLAXIS: Active immunization with either Live poliovirus vaccine or Inactivated poliovirus vaccine has greatly reduced the incidence of paralytic poliomyelitis. The oral vaccine containing all three types of the virus should be given to young infants beginning at 6 to 12 weeks with a second dose about 2 months later and then a third dose 8 to 12 months later. Older children who have not been previously immunized with trivalent oral poliovirus vaccine should be given two doses at 8-week intervals and a third dose 6 months to 1 year later. SEE: *poliovirus vaccine, inactivated.*

PREDISPOSING: Tonsillectomy and other nose and throat operations, routine immunizations, excessive physical strain, and fatigue. Pregnant women are especially susceptible during epidemics.

NURSING IMPLICATIONS: Encourage immunization at an early age to prevent disease. Enforce isolation with concurrent disinfection of throat discharge and feces to prevent transmission of polio virus. Maintain a calm, reassuring manner. Maintain a patent airway and observe closely for respiratory distress; administer oxygen as needed; and keep a tracheostomy tray at the bedside.

Maintain strict bedrest during the acute phase. Alleviate muscle pain by gentle, passive range of motion exercises and application of hot moist packs at 20-minute intervals or tub baths for children. Maintain proper body alignment and turn frequently to prevent deformity and decubiti. Administer mild sedative or analgesic to decrease pain and anxiety and to promote rest. Observe for distended bladder due to transitory paralysis. Promote personal hygiene, and provide oral hygiene. Provide appetizing food because anorexia is common. Administer antipyretic to reduce fever. Closely monitor fluid and electrolyte balance and elimination. Apply a footboard to prevent foot drop. Provide emotional support to the patient who is coping with loss of body function and paralysis.

p., anterior. Inflamed state of the anterior horns of the spinal cord

p., ascending. Poliomyelitis in which paralysis begins in the lower extremities and progresses up the legs, thighs, trunk, and finally involves respiratory muscles.

p., bulbar. Poliomyelitis in which gray matter of the medulla oblongata is involved, resulting in paralysis and usually respiratory failure. SEE: *poliomyelitis, acute anterior.*

p., chronic anterior. Progressive wasting of the muscles. Myelopathic progressive muscular atrophy.

p., nonparalytic. Pain and stiffness in the muscles of the axial skeleton, esp. of the neck and back; mild fever; increased proteins and leukocytes in the cerebrospinal fluid. Diagnosis depends on the isolation of the virus and serological reactions.

p., paralytic. Poliomyelitis with a variable combination of signs of damage of the central nervous system. These include weakness, incoordination, muscle tenderness and spasms, flaccid paralysis, and disturbance of consciousness.

poliomyelopathy (pŏl″ē-ō-mī″ĕl-ŏp′ă-thē) [Gr. *polios,* gray, + *myelos,* marrow, + *pathos,* disease]. Any diseased condition of the gray matter of the spinal cord.

polioplasm (pōl′ē-ō-plăzm) [″ + *plasma,* a thing formed]. Granular protoplasm.

poliosis (pŏl″ē-ō′sĭs) [″ + *osis,* condition]. Whiteness of the hair, esp. when due to a hereditary condition or as a result of infection. SYN: *canities.*

poliovirus (pō″lē-ō-vī′rŭs). Etiological agent of poliomyelitis, q.v., separable into three serotypes based on the specificity of the neutralizing antibody. The three serotypes are type I, II, and III. A virus found worldwide, it spreads directly or indirectly from infected persons or convalescent carriers. Epidemics of poliomyelitis that were characteristic of infections with this virus have been virtually eliminated by poliovirus vaccine. SEE: *poliovirus vaccine, inactivated.*

poliovirus vaccine, inactivated. ABBR: IPV. USP. A poliovirus vaccine recommended for prevention of paralytic poliomyelitis. The vaccine contains inactivated types I, II, and III polioviruses. It is suitable for parenteral administration to all infants and children.

Infants should be given three doses, the first at 2 months of age, followed by two more doses at 8-week intervals. A fourth dose should be given at 18 months unless poliomyelitis is endemic in the area, in which case the fourth dose is given at 6 to 12 months after the third. Additional doses are recommended prior to school entry and then every 5 years until age 18.

poliovirus vaccine, live oral. USP. ABBR: OPV. A standard preparation of one or a combination of the three types of live, attenuated polioviruses. It is suitable for immunizing children and adults against all three types of poliovirus; but the inactivated poliovirus vaccine is preferred for adults because of the slightly high risk of vaccine-associated paralysis. The schedule for infants is first dose at 6–12 weeks, the second about 2 months later, a third 8–12 months after the second. No additional "boosters" are recommended. For children and adolescents not previously immunized prior to age 18, 2 doses are given 8 weeks apart and a third dose 6 to 12 months later. Trade name is Orimune.

polishing (pŏl′ĭsh-ĭng). Producing a smooth, glossy finish on a denture or a dental restoration.

politzerization (pŏl″ĭt-sĕr-ĭ-zā′shŭn). The inflation of the middle ear by means of a Politzer bag, q.v.

Politzer bag (pŏl′ĭt-zĕr). [Adam Politzer, Hungarian otologist, 1835–1920] Soft rubber bag with rubber tip for inflating the middle ear by increasing the pressure in the nasopharynx.

pollakiuria (pŏl″ă-kē-ū′rē-ă) [Gr. *pollakis,* often, + *ouron,* urine]. Abnormally frequent passage of urine.

pollen (pŏl′ĕn) [L., dust]. The microspores of a seed plant that develop in the anther at the tip of the stamen. Each pollen grain develops a pollen tube and constitutes the male gametophyte. Within it develops a tube nucleus and two sperm nuclei, the latter constituting the male reproductive elements. Many airborne pollens are allergens, q.v. SEE: *hay fever.*

pollenogenic (pŏl″ĕn-ō-jĕn′ĭk) [″ + Gr. *gennan,* to produce]. Caused by the pollen of plants, or producing plant pollen.

pollenosis (pŏl″ĕn-ō′sĭs) [″ + Gr. *osis,* condition]. Pollinosis.

pollex (pŏl′ĕks) [L.]. (pl. *pollices*) [NA] The thumb.

p. extensus. Backward deviation of the thumb.

p. flexus. Permanent flexion of the thumb.

p. valgus. Abnormal deviation of the thumb toward the ulnar side.

p. varus. Abnormal deviation of the thumb toward the radial side.

pollicization (pŏl″ĭs-ĭ-zā′shŭn) [L. *pollex,* thumb]. The plastic surgical procedure of constructing a thumb from adjacent tissues.

pollinosis (pŏl-ĭn-ō′sĭs) [L. *pollen,* dust, + Gr. *osis,* disease]. Nasal congestion of mucous membranes due to contact with pollen. SYN: *hay fever.*

pollodic (pŏl-lō′dĭk) [Gr. *polloi,* many, + *hodos,* way]. Concerning nerve stimuli that originate from one center.

pollution (pŭ-loo′shŭn) [ME. *polluten*]. State of making impure or defiling.

polocyte (pō′lō-sīt) [Gr. *polos,* pole, + *kytos,* cell]. Body, polar, q.v.

polonium (pō-lō′nē-ŭm). [L. *Polonia,* Poland, native country of its discoverers, the Curies]. SYMB: Po. At. wt. 210; at. no. 84. Radioactive element isolated from pitchblende.

poltophagy (pŏl-tŏf′ă-jē) [Gr. *poltos,* porridge,

+ *phagein,* to eat]. Thorough chewing of food so that it is reduced to a finely divided mass. SEE: *fletcherism.*

polus (pō'lŭs) [L.]. (pl. *poli*) [NA] The extremity of an organ. SYN: *pole.*

poly (pŏl'ē). *polymorphonuclear leukocyte.*

poly- [Gr. *polys,* many]. Prefix indicating many or much.

polyacid (pŏl"ē-ăs'ĭd). An alcohol or a base with two or more hydroxyl groups that will combine with an acid.

polyadenitis (pŏl"ē-ăd"ĕ-nī'tĭs) [" + Gr. *aden,* gland, + *itis,* inflammation]. Condition of inflamed lymph nodes, esp. the cervical lymph nodes.

polyadenomatosis (pŏl"ē-ăd"ĕ-nō-mă-tō'sĭs) [" + " + *oma,* tumor, + *osis,* condition]. Adenomas in many glands.

polyadenopathy (pŏl"ē-ăd"ĕ-nŏp'ă-thē) [" + " + *pathos,* disease]. Any disease in which many glands are involved.

polyadenous (pŏl"ē-ăd'ĕ-nŭs). Involving or rel. to many glands.

polyalgesia (pŏl"ē-ăl-jē'zē-ă) [" + *algesis,* sensation]. A single stimulus of a part, producing sensation in many parts.

polyandry (pŏl"ē-ăn'drē) [Gr. *polyandria*]. The practice of having more than one husband at the same time. SEE: *polygamy.*

polyangiitis (pŏl"ē-ăn"jē-ī'tĭs) [Gr. *polys,* many, + *angeion,* vessel, + *itis,* inflammation]. Inflammation of a number of blood vessels.

polyarteritis (nodosa) (pŏl"ē-ăr"tĕr-ī'tĭs) [" + *arteria,* artery, + *itis,* inflammation]. A disease of medium and small arteries, particularly at the point of bifurcation and branching. Segmental inflammation, infiltration with fibrinoid, and necrosis of the vessel lining and walls lead to a diminished flow of blood to the areas normally supplied by these arteries. Signs and symptoms depend on the location of the affected vessels and may affect any organ or body system. SYN: *periarteritis nodosa.* SEE: *collagen disease.*

ETIOL: Unknown, but associated with hypersensitivity. Drug therapy, vaccines, bacterial and viral infections have been associated with the onset of polyarteritis.

PROG: Without therapy, only one person in 8 will live 5 years. Death is due to failure of a function of a vital organ such as the heart or kidney; hemorrhage from the gastrointestinal tract; or a ruptured aneurysm.

TREATMENT: Corticosteroids in large doses initially and tapered off may be of benefit. General supportive therapy. The value of immunosuppressive therapy is questionable.

polyarthric (pŏl"ē-ăr'thrĭk) [" + *arthron,* joint]. Affecting or pert. to several joints.

polyarthritis (pŏl-ē-ăr-thrī'tĭs) [" + " + *itis,* inflammation]. Inflammation of more than one joint. SYN: *amarthritis*

p., chronic villous. Chronic inflammation of the synovial membrane of several joints.

p. rheumatica, acute. Acute rheumatic fever.

polyarticular (pŏl"ē-ăr-tĭk'ū-lăr) [" + L. *articulus,* a joint]. Affecting many joints. SYN: *multiarticular.*

polyatomic (pŏl"ē-ă-tŏm'ĭk) [" + *atomon,* atom]. 1. Having several atoms. 2. Having more than two replaceable hydrogen atoms.

polyavitaminosis (pŏl"ē-ă-vī"tă-mĭn-ō'sĭs) [" + *a-,* not, + L. *vita,* life, + *amine* + Gr. *osis,* condition]. A deficiency of more than one vitamin.

polybasic (pŏl"ē-bā'sĭk) [Gr. *polys,* many, + *basis,* base]. Pert. to an acid with two or more hydrogen ions that will combine with a base.

polyblast (pŏl'ē-blăst) [" + *blastos,* a germ]. Large mononuclear phagocyte, derived from an embryonic wandering cell, that is present in inflammation.

polyblennia (pŏl"ē-blĕ'nē-ă) [" + *blennos,* mucus]. Secretion of an abnormal amount of mucus.

polycarbophil (pŏl"ē-kăr'bō-fĭl). USP. A hydrophilic substance that is used as a bulk-forming laxative. Trade name is Mitrolan.

polycentric (pŏl"ē-sĕn'trĭk) [" + *kentron,* center]. Condition of having many centers.

polycheiria (pŏl"ē-kī'rē-ă) [" + *cheir,* hand]. Having more than two hands.

polychemotherapy (pŏl"ē-kē"mō-thĕr'ă-pē) [" + *chemeia,* chemistry, + *therapeia,* treatment]. Treatment with several chemotherapeutic agents at once.

polycholia (pŏl"ē-kō'lē-ă) [" + *chole,* bile]. Abnormal secretion of bile.

polychondritis (pŏl"ē-kŏn-drī'tĭs) [" + *chondros,* cartilage, + *itis,* inflammation]. Inflammation of several cartilages of the body.

p., chronic atrophic relapsing. A degenerative disease of cartilage associated with polyarthritis, involvement of the cartilage of the nose, ears, joints, bronchi, and trachea. The cause is unknown and there is no specific therapy. Because of the collapse of the bronchial walls, repeated infections of the lungs will occur and death may result from these infections.

polychrest (pŏl'ē-krĕst) [" + *chrestos,* useful]. A medicine useful in many diseases.

polychromasia (pŏl"ē-krō-mā'zē-ă) [" + *chroma,* color]. Quality of having many colors.

polychromatic (pŏl"ē-krō-măt'ĭk). Multicolored

polychromatocyte (pŏl"ē-krō-măt'ō-sīt) [" + " + *kytos,* cell]. Polychromatophilia (def. 2), q.v.

polychromatophil(e) (pŏl"ē-krō-măt'ō-fĭl) [Gr.

polys, many, + *chroma*, color, + *philein*, to love]. A cell, esp. an erythrocyte, that is stainable with more than one kind of stain.

polychromatophilia (pŏl″ē-krō-măt″ō-fĭl′ē-ă). 1. The quality of being stainable with more than one stain. 2. Excess of polychromatophil cells in the blood.

polychromophilia (pŏl″ē-krō-mō-fĭl′ē-ă) [″ + ″ + *philos*, to love]. Polychromatophilia, q.v.

polychylia (pŏl″ē-kī′lē-ă) [″ + L. *chylus*, juice]. Excessive secretion of chyle.

Polycillin-N. Trade name for ampicillin sodium, USP.

polyclinic (pŏl″ē-klĭn′ĭk) [″ + *kline*, bed]. Hospital or clinic treating all kinds of diseases; a general hospital.

polyclonal (pŏl″ē-klōn′ăl). Arising from different cell lines.

polyclonia (pŏl″ē-klō′nē-ă) [″ + *klonos*, tumult]. A disease characterized by many clonic spasms, but distinct from chorea or tic.

polycoria (pŏl″ē-kō′rē-ă) [″ + *kore*, pupil]. The state of having more than one pupil in one eye.

polycrotic (pŏl″ē-krŏt′ĭk) [″ + *krotos*, beat]. Having several pulse waves for each heartbeat.

polycrotism (pŏl-ĭk′rō-tĭzm) [″ + ″ + *-ismos*, condition]. Condition of having several pulse waves for each heartbeat.

polycyesis (pŏl″ē-sī-ē′sĭs) [″ + *kyesis*, pregnancy]. Multiple pregnancy.

polycystic (pŏl″ē-sĭs′tĭk) [″ + *kystis*, cyst]. Composed of many cysts.

polycystic ovary syndrome. An endocrine disturbance that causes primary anovulation and polycystic ovaries due to the continued stimulation of the ovary by pituitary luteinizing hormone. SYN: *Stein-Leventhal syndrome.*

TREATMENT: Clomiphene, gonadotropins, or wedge resection of the ovary.

polycythemia (pŏl″ē-sī-thē′mē-ă) [″ + *kytos*, cell, + *haima*, blood]. An excess of red blood cells. SYN: *erythrocytosis; polyemia; polyhemia.*

p., compensatory. P., secondary, q.v.

p., myelopathic. P. vera.

p., primary. P. vera.

p., relative. Relative increase in number of erythrocytes that occurs in hemoconcentration.

p. rubra; p. rubra vera. P. vera, q.v.

p., secondary. Polycythemia resulting from some physiological condition, such as lowered oxygen tension in blood, that stimulates erythropoiesis. SYN: *erythrocytosis.*

p., splenomegalic. P. vera.

p. vera. A chronic life-shortening myeloproliferative disorder involving all bone marrow elements. Characterized by an increase in red blood cell mass and hemoglobin concentration. SYN: *erythremia.*

SYM AND SIGNS: Weakness, fatigue, vertigo, tinnitus, irritability, enlarged spleen, flushing of face, redness and pain of extremities, black-and-blue spots. Bone marrow shows increased cellularity.

ETIOL: Unknown.

TREATMENT: Permanent cure cannot be achieved today, but remissions of many years can be produced. Phlebotomy and radioactive phosphorus (^{32}P) are effective. Phlebotomy followed by chemotherapy with either chlorambucil or cyclophosphamide has been used, but requires much closer follow-up than phlebotomy and use of ^{32}P.

polycytotropic. Pantropic, q.v.

polydactylism (pŏl″ē-dăk′tĭ-lĭzm) [Gr. *polys*, many, + *daktylos*, digit, + *-ismos*, condition]. State of having supernumerary fingers or toes.

polydactyly (pŏl″ē-dăk′tĭ-lē) [″ + *daktylos*, finger]. Condition of having more than the normal number of fingers and toes.

polydentia (pŏl″ē-dĕn′shē-ă) [″ + L. *dens*, tooth]. Polyodontia, q.v.

polydipsia (pŏl″ē-dĭp′sē-ă) [″ + *dipsa*, thirst]. Excessive thirst.

polydysplasia (pŏl″ē-dĭs-plā′zē-ă) [″ + *dys*, bad, + *plassein*, to form]. Condition of having multiple developmental abnormalities.

polydystrophic (pŏl″ē-dĭs-trō′fĭk). Concerning or having polydystrophy.

polydystrophy (pŏl″ē-dĭs′trō-fē) [″ + ″ + *trophe*, nourishment]. Condition of having multiple congenital anomalies of the connective tissues.

polyemia (pŏl″ē-ē′mē-ă) [″ + *haima*, blood]. Abnormal amount of blood in the system. SYN: *polycythemia; polyhemia.*

polyendocrine (pŏl″ē-ĕn′dō-krĭn) [″ + *endon*, within, + *krinein*, to secrete]. Concerning several endocrine glands.

polyene (pŏl-ē′ēn). An organic compound containing alternating, or conjugate, double bonds. An example is butadiene, $CH_2{=}CHCH{=}CH_2$.

polyergic (pŏl″ē-ĕr′jĭk) [″ + *ergon*, work]. Having the ability to act in several different ways.

polyesthesia (pŏl″ē-ĕs-thē′zē-ă) [″ + *aisthesis*, sensation]. Abnormal sensation of touch in which a single stimulus is felt at two or more places.

polyesthetic (pŏl″ē-ĕs-thĕt′ĭk). 1. Pert. to polyesthesia. 2. Pert. to several senses or sensations.

polyestrous (pŏl″ē-ĕs′trŭs) [″ + *oistros*, mad desire]. Having two or more estrous cycles in each mating season.

polyethylene (pŏl″ē-ĕth′ĭ-lēn). A polymerized resin of ethylene. Used to make a wide variety of products, including tubing used in intravenous sets.

p. glycol 400. A polymer of ethylene oxide and water. The formula is $H(OCH_2CH_2)_nOH$, in which the value of n is from 8.2 to 9.1. Used as a water-soluble ointment base.

p. glycol 4000. A polymer of ethylene oxide and water. The formula is $H(OCH_2CH_2)_nOH$, in which the value of n is from 68 to 84. Used as a water-soluble ointment base.

polygalactia (pŏl″ē-gă-lăk′shē-ă) [Gr. *polys,* many, + *gala,* milk]. Excessive secretion or flow of milk.

polygalacturonase (pŏl″ē-gă-lăk-tū′rō-nās). An enzyme present in plant tissues that hydrolyses pectins to cause them to form gels.

polygamy (pō-lĭg′ă-mē) [″ + *gamos,* marriage]. Practice of having several wives, husbands, or mates at the same time. SEE: *polyandry.*

polyganglionic (pŏl″ē-găng″glē-ŏn′ĭk) [″ + *ganglion,* ganglion]. 1. Concerning many ganglia. 2. Affecting many glands.

polygastria (pŏl″ē-găs′trē-ă) [″ + *gaster,* stomach]. Excessive secretion or flow of gastric juice.

polygen (pŏl′ĕ-jĕn). 1. An element with more than one valency and that can form more than one series of compounds. 2. An antigen that will cause the formation of two or more specific antibodies.

polygenic (pŏl″ē-jĕn′ĭk) [″ + *gennan,* to produce]. Pert. to or caused by several genes.

polyglandular (pŏl″ē-glăn′dū-lar) [″ + L. *glandula,* a little kernel]. Pert. to or affecting many glands. SYN: *pluriglandular.*

polyglycolic acid. A polymer of glycolic acid anhydride units. It is used in surgical sutures.

polygnathus (pō-lĭg′nă-thŭs) [″ + *gnathos,* jaw]. Conjoined twins of unequal size in which the smaller is attached to the jaw of the larger.

polygram (pŏl′ē-grăm) [″ + *gramma,* mark]. A tracing or record made by a polygraph.

polygraph (pŏl′ē-grăf) [″ + *graphein,* to write]. A device that records simultaneously tracings of several different pulsations, as arterial and venous pulse waves, and the apex beat of the heart. Has been used as a so-called lie detector. The scientific basis for the validity of this test is disputed. SYN: *sphygmograph.*

polygyria (pŏl″ē-jī′rē-ă) [″ + *gyros,* circle]. Excess of the normal number of convolutions in the brain.

polyhedral (pŏl″ē-hē′drăl) [Gr. *polys,* many, + *hedra,* base]. Having many surfaces.

polyhemia (pŏl″ē-hē′mē-ă) [″ + *haima,* blood]. Abnormal increase in amount of the blood. SYN: *polycythemia; polyemia.*

polyhidrosis (pŏl″ē-hī-drō′sĭs) [″ + *hidrosis,* perspiration]. Excessive perspiration.

polyhistor (pŏl″ē-hĭs′tŭr) [″ + *histor,* learned]. A scholar or physician who has great and varied abilities and knowledge. SYN: *polymath.*

Ex.: Hippocrates, Galen, Paracelsus, Leonardo da Vinci, Boerhaave, Richard Mead, and Thomas Jefferson.

polyhybrid (pŏl″ē-hī′brĭd) [″ + L. *hybrida,* mongrel]. The offspring of parents that are different with respect to three or more characteristics.

polyhydramnios (pŏl″ē-hī-drăm′nē-ŏs) [″ + *hydor,* water, + *amnion,* amnion]. An excess of amniotic fluid in the bag of waters in pregnancy. SEE: *amnion.*

polyhydric (pŏl″ē-hī′drĭk). Containing more than two hydroxyl groups.

polyhydruria (pŏl″ē-hī-droo′rē-ă) [″ + ″ + *ouron,* urine]. Excessive amount of water in the urine.

polyhypermenorrhea (pŏl″ē-hī″pĕr-mĕn″ō-rē′ă) [″ + *hyper,* over, + *men,* month, + *rhoia,* flow]. Frequent menstruation with excessive discharge.

polyhypomenorrhea (pŏl″ē-hī″pō-mĕn″ō-rē′ă) [″ + *hypo,* under, + *men,* month, + *rhoia,* flow]. Frequent menstruation with scanty discharge.

Poly I:C. A complex of synthetic polyriboinosinic and polyribocytidylic acids. They are a form of double-stranded ribonucleic acids that may help to induce resistance to virus infection. Poly I:C stimulates production of interferon, q.v.

polyidrosis (pŏl″ē-ĭd-rō′sĭs) [″ + *hidrosis,* perspiration]. Hyperhydrosis, q.v.

polyinfection (pŏl″ē-ĭn-fĕk′shŭn) [″ + ME. *infecten,* infect]. Infection with two or more microorganisms. SYN: *multi-infection.*

polykaryocyte (pŏl″ē-kăr′ē-ō-sīt) [″ + *karyon,* nucleus, + *kytos,* cell]. A cell possessing several nuclei.

polyleptic (pŏl″ē-lĕp′tĭk) [″ + *lepsis,* a seizure]. Characterized by numerous remissions and exacerbations, as malaria.

polylysine (pŏl″ē-lī′sĭn). A polypeptide in which two lysine molecules are joined by a peptide linkage.

polymastia (pŏl″ē-măs′tē-ă) [Gr. *polys,* many, + *mastos,* breast]. Condition of having more than two breasts. SYN: *multimammae; polymazia.*

polymastigote (pŏl″ē-măs′tĭ-gōt) [″ + *mastix,* whip]. Possessing several flagella.

polymath. Polyhistor, q.v.

polymazia [″ + *mazos,* breast]. Condition of having more than two breasts. SYN: *multimammae; polymastia.*

polymelia (pŏl″ē-mē′lē-ă) [″ + *melos,* limb]. A

congenital abnormality in which there are supernumerary limbs.

polymelus (pō-lĭm′ĕ-lŭs) [″ + *melos,* limb]. One having polymelia.

polymenia (pŏl″ē-mē′nē-ă) [″ + *men,* month]. Polymenorrhea.

polymenorrhea (pŏl″ē-mĕn-ō-rē′ă) [″ + ″ + *rhoia,* a flow]. Menstrual periods occurring with abnormal frequency. SYN: *polymenia.*

polymer (pŏl′ĭ-mĕr) [″ + *meros,* a part]. A natural or synthetic substance formed by a combination of two or more molecules (and up to millions) of the same substance.

Ex.: paraformaldehyde $(HCHO)_3$ formed from three molecules of formaldehyde, HCHO.

polymerase (pŏl-ĭm′ĕr-ās). An enzyme that catalyzes polymerization of nucleosides to form DNA.

polymer fume fever. Condition resulting from breathing fumes produced by certain polymers when they are heated to 300° to 700° C. or higher. SEE: *metal fume fever.*

SYM: Tight gripping sensation of the chest associated with shivering, sore throat, fever, and weakness.

TREATMENT: Discontinue exposure to fumes.

polymeria (pŏl-ĭ-mē′rē-ă). Condition of having supernumerary parts of the body. SYN: *polymerism.*

polymeric (pŏl″ĭ-mĕr′ĭk). 1. Having the characteristics of a polymer. 2. Muscles derived from more than one myotome.

polymerid (pō-lĭm′ĕr-ĭd). A polymer.

polymerism (pŏl′ĭ-mĕr″ĭzm, pō-lĭm′ĕr-ĭzm) [″ + *meros,* part, + *-ismos,* condition]. Condition of having more than normal number of parts. SYN: *polymeria.*

polymerization (pŏl″ĭ-mĕr″ĭ-zā′shŭn). Process of changing a simple chemical substance or substances into another compound having the same elements usually in the same proportions but with a higher molecular weight.

polymerize (pŏl′ĭ-mĕr-īz). To cause polymerization.

polymicrobial (pŏl″ē-mī-krō′bē-ăl) [Gr. *polys,* many, + *mikros,* small, + *bios,* life]. Concerning a number of species of microorganisms.

polymicrobic infections. Bacterial infections caused by two or more different microorganisms.

polymicrogyria (pŏl″ē-mī″krō-jī′rē-ă) [″ + ″ + *gyros,* convolution]. A malformed brain in which multiple small convolutions have developed.

polymitus (pō-lĭm′ĭ-tŭs) [″ + *mitos,* thread]. Stage in reproduction of microorganisms in which threads of protoplasm, now being detached, constitute the microgamete.

polymorph (pŏl′ē-morf) [″ + *morphe,* form]. A polymorphonuclear leukocyte.

polymorphic. Occurring in more than one form. SYN: *multiform; polymorphous.*

polymorphism [″ + *morphe,* form, + *-ismos,* condition]. 1. Capacity for appearing in many forms. 2. Existence of several types in the same group or species. SYN: *pleomorphism.*

polymorphocellular (pŏl″ē-mor″fō-sĕl′ū-lăr) [″ + ″ + L. *cellula,* a small chamber]. Composed of cells of many forms.

polymorphonuclear (pŏl″ē-mor″fō-nū′klē-ăr) [″ + ″ + L. *nucleus,* a kernel]. Possessing a nucleus consisting of several parts or lobes connected by fine strands.

polymorphonuclear leukocyte. A white blood cell that possesses a nucleus composed of two or more lobes or parts; a granulocyte (neutrophil, eosinophil, basophil).

polymorphous (pŏl″ē-mor′fŭs). Appearing in many forms. SYN: *multiform; polymorphic.*

Polymox. Trade name for amoxicillin.

polymyalgia arteritica (pŏl″ē-mī-ăl′jē-ă) [″ + *mys,* muscle, + *algos,* pain]. Polymyalgia rheumatica, q.v.

polymyalgia rheumatica. A poorly understood condition almost always found in patients over 50 years of age and four times more frequently in women. It is characterized by the following: pain in the muscles of the shoulder and pelvic girdle; marked elevation of erythrocyte sedimentation rate; absence of evidence of inflammatory arthritis of any kind; absence of signs of muscle disease such as atrophy, weakness, or fibrillation; and prompt and dramatic response to low doses of corticosteroid therapy.

Corticosteroids relieve symptoms and the sedimentation rate approaches normal. Temporal and cranial arteritis may be associated with this disease.

polymyoclonus (pŏl″ē-mī-ŏk′lō-nŭs) [″ + ″ + *klonos,* tumult]. A shocklike muscular contraction, occurring in various parts at the same time. SYN: *myoclonus multiplex; paramyoclonus multiplex.*

polymyopathy (pŏl″ē-mī-ŏp′ă-thē) [″ + ″ + *pathos,* disease]. Disease that affects several muscles.

polymyositis (pŏl″ē-mī″ō-sī′tĭs) [″ + ″ + *itis,* inflammation]. A disease of the connective tissue characterized by edema, inflammation and degeneration of the muscles, and dermatitis. Etiology is unknown. SYN: *dermatomyositis.*

polymyxin (pŏl″ē-mĭks′ĭn). One of several closely related antibiotics isolated from various strains of Bacillus polymyxa and designated polymyxins A, B, C, D, and E. Most polymyxins cause renal toxicity.

p. B. Least toxic of the antibiotic fractions of polymyxin, and the only one used therapeutically for treating infection.

p. B sulfate. USP. An antibiotic substance produced by Bacillus polymyxa. Trade name is Aerosporin.

polynesic (pŏl″ē-nē′sĭk) [″ + *nesos,* island]. Appearing in many separate locations or foci.

polyneural (pŏl″ē-nū′răl) [″ + *neuron,* sinew]. Pert. to, innervated, or supplied by many nerves.

polyneuralgia (pŏl″ē-nū-răl′jē-ă) [″ + ″ + *algos,* pain]. Neuralgia in several nerves.

polyneuritic (pŏl″ē-nū-rĭt′ĭk) [″ + ″ + *itis,* inflammation]. Inflammation of several nerves at once.

polyneuritic psychosis. Psychosis seen in chronic alcoholism with disturbed orientation, polyneuritis, hallucinations, and falsification of memory. SYN: *Korsakoff's syndrome.*

polyneuritis (pŏl″ē-nū-rī′tĭs) [″ + ″ + *itis,* inflammation]. A neuritis involving two or more nerves, usually a large number. SYN: *neuritis, multiple.*

p., acute idiopathic. Landry's paralysis.

p., Jamaica ginger. Polyneuritis, esp. of the nerves of the extremities following ingestion of Jamaica ginger beverage. SYN: *ginger paralysis.*

p., metabolic. Polyneuritis resulting from metabolic disorders such as nutritional deficiency, esp. the lack of thiamine; gastrointestinal disorders; or pathological conditions such as diabetes, pernicious anemia, and toxemias of pregnancy.

p., toxic. Polyneuritis resulting from poisons such as heavy metals, alcohol, carbon monoxide, or various organic compounds.

polyneuromyositis (pŏl″ē-nū″rō-mī″ō-sī′tĭs) [″ + ″ + *mys,* muscle, + *itis,* inflammation]. Disease in which there are polyneuritis and polymyositis together.

polyneuropathy (pŏl″ē-nū-rŏp′ă-thē) [Gr. *polys,* many, + *neuron,* sinew, + *pathos,* disease]. Term applied to any disorder or affection of peripheral nerves, but preferably restricted to those of a noninflammatory nature. SYN: *neuritis, multiple; polyneuritis.*

p., amyloid. Polyneuropathy characterized by deposition of amyloid in nerves.

p., buckthorn. A symmetrical progressive polyneuropathy that starts in the lower limbs and ascends until there is respiratory paralysis when the brain stem becomes affected. If the patient survives, improvement is slow but may progress to almost complete functional recovery. There is no specific therapy.

Disease is due to ingestion of the fruit of the poisonous shrub of the buckthorn (Rhamnus) family. This plant grows in central and northern Mexico and in Texas and New Mexico.

p., erythredema. A condition of unknown etiological factors, occurring in children, and characterized by degenerative changes in peripheral nerves, skin disorders, and motor and sensory disturbances. SYN: *acrodynia.*

p., porphyric. Polyneuropathy resulting from acute porphyria, characterized by pains and paresthesias in the extremities and by flaccid paralysis.

p., progressive hypertrophic. A rare familial disease beginning in childhood and characterized by increased size of peripheral nerves due to multiplication and hypertrophy of cells of the sheath of Schwann.

polyneuroradiculitis (pŏl″ē-nū″rō-ră-dĭk″ū-lī′tĭs) [″ + ″ + *radix,* root, + *itis,* inflammation]. Inflammation of the nerve roots, the peripheral nerves, and spinal ganglia.

polynuclear (pŏl″ē-nū′klē-ăr) [″ + L. *nucleus,* a kernel]. Possessing more than one nucleus. SYN: *multinuclear.*

polynucleate (pŏl″ē-nū′klē-āt). Having many nuclei.

polynucleotidase (pŏl″ē-nū″klē-ō′tĭ-dās). An enzyme present in intestinal mucosa and intestinal juice that catalyzes the breakdown of nucleic acid to nucleotides.

polynucleotide (pŏl″ē-nū′klē-ō-tīd). Nucleic acid composed of two or more nucleotides.

polyodontia (pŏl″ē-ō-dŏn′shē-ă) [″ + *odous,* tooth]. State of having supernumerary teeth.

polyomavirus (pŏl″ē-ō-mă-vī′rŭs). A virus of the papovavirus family that produces malignancies in lower animals

polyonychia (pŏl″ē-ō-nĭk′ē-ă) [″ + *onyx,* nail]. Having supernumerary nails.

polyopia, polyopsia (pŏl″ē-ō′pē-ă, -ŏp′sē-ă) [″ + *opsis,* vision]. Multiple vision; perception of more than one image of the same object.

polyorchidism (pŏl″ē-or′kĭ-dĭzm) [″ + *orchis,* testicle, + *-ismos,* condition]. Condition of having more than two testicles.

polyorchis (pŏl″ē-or′kĭs). An individual with more than two testicles.

polyorchism (pŏl″ē-or′kĭzm) [″ + *orchis,* testicle, + *-ismos,* condition]. Having more than two testicles.

polyostotic (pŏl″ē-ŏs-tŏt′ĭk) [″ + *osteon,* bone]. Concerning many bones.

polyotia (pŏl″ē-ō′shē-ă) [″ + *ous,* ear]. State of having more than two ears.

polyovulatory (pŏl″ē-ŏv′ū-lă-tō″rē) [″ + L. *ovulum,* little egg]. Releasing several ova in a single ovulatory cycle.

polyoxyl stearate (pŏl″ē-ŏks′ĭl). Any of several polyoxyethylene stearates. They have varying lengths of the polymer chain, e.g., polyoxyl 8 stearate (trade name Myrj 45) and polyoxyl 40 stearate (trade name Myrj 52) have polymer lengths of 8 and 40 respectively. They are nonionic surface-active agents that are useful emulsifiers. SYN: *polyoxy-*

ethylene stearate.

polyp (pŏl′ĭp) [″ + *pous,* foot]. A tumor with a pedicle. Commonly found in vascular organs such as the nose, uterus, and rectum. Polyps bleed easily; if there is a possibility that they will become malignant, they should be removed surgically. SYN: *polypus.*

p., adenomatous. Benign neoplastic tissue originating in glandular epithelium.

p., bleeding. Angioma of the nasal mucous membrane.

p., cardiac. A pedunculated tumor attached to the inside of the heart. If situated close to a valve, it may cause blockage of the valve intermittently.

p., cervical. A fibrous or mucous polyp of the cervical mucosa.

p., choanal. Nasal polyp that extends into the pharynx.

p., fibrinous. Polyp containing fibrin and blood, and located in the uterine cavity.

p., fleshy. A submucous myoma in the uterus.

p., gelatinous. 1. A polyp made up of loose swollen edematous tissue. 2. Myxoma.

p., Hopmann's. A papillary growth of the nasal mucosa.

p., hydatid. A cystic polyp.

p., juvenile. A benign rounded mucosal hamartoma of the large bowel. They may be present in an infant in large numbers and are commonly associated with rectal bleeding.

p., laryngeal. Polyp attached to the vocal cords and extending to the air passageway.

p., lymphoid. Benign lymphoma of the rectum.

p., mucous. A polyp of soft or jellylike consistency and exhibiting mucoid degeneration.

p., nasal. A pedunculated polyp of the nasal mucosa.

p., placental. A polyp composed of retained placental tissue.

p., retention. P., juvenile, q.v.

p., vascular. A pedunculated angioma.

polypapilloma (pŏl″ē-păp″ĭ-lō′mă) [Gr. *polys,* many + L. *papilla,* nipple, + Gr. *oma,* tumor]. Yaws, q.v.

polyparesis (pŏl″ē-pă-rē′sĭs) [″ + *paresis,* relaxation]. General progressive paralysis of paralytic dementia.

polypathia (pŏl″ē-păth′ē-ă) [″ + *pathos,* disease]. In the same person, the presence of several diseases at one time.

polypectomy (pŏl″ĭ-pĕk′tō-mē) [″ + *pous,* foot, + *ektome,* excision]. Surgical removal of a polyp.

polypeptidase (pŏl″ē-pĕp′tĭ-dās). An enzyme that catalyzes the hydrolysis of peptides.

polypeptide (pŏl″ē-pĕp′tīd) [″ + *peptein,* to digest]. A union of two or more amino acids. SEE: *peptide.*

polypeptidemia (pŏl″ē-pĕp″tĭ-dē′mē-ă) [″ + ″ + *haima,* blood]. Presence of polypeptides in the blood.

polypeptidorrhachia (pŏl″ē-pĕp″tĭ-dō-rā′kē-ă) [″ + ″ + *rhachis,* spine]. Presence of polypeptides in the cerebrospinal fluid.

polyphagia (pŏl″ē-fā′jē-ă) [Gr. *polys,* many, + *phagein,* to eat]. Eating abnormally large amounts of food at a meal.

RS: acoria; anorexia; bulimia; parorexia; taste.

polyphalangism (pŏl″ē-fă-lăn′jĭzm) [″ + *phalanx,* phalanx, + *-ismos,* condition]. An extra number of phalanges on a hand or foot.

polypharmacy (pŏl″ē-făr′mă-sē) [″ + *pharmakon,* drug]. 1. Excessive use of drugs or overdose of a drug. 2. Prescription of many dugs given at one time.

polyphenoloxidase (pŏl″ē-fē″nŏl-ŏk′sĭ-dās). An enzyme present in bacteria, fungi, and some plants that catalyzes the oxidation of polyphenols, but not monophenols such as tyrosine, to quinones.

polyphobia (pŏl″ē-fō′bē-ă) [Gr. *polys,* many, + *phobos,* fear]. Excessive or abnormal fear of a number of things.

polyphrasia (pŏl″ē-frā′zē-ă) [″ + *phrasis,* speech]. Excessive talkativeness, a manifestation of insanity.

polyphyletic (pŏl″ē-fī-lĕt′ĭk) [″ + *phyle,* tribe]. Having more than one origin. Opposed to monophyletic.

polyphyodont (pŏl″ē-fī′ō-dŏnt) [″ + *phyein,* to produce, + *odous,* tooth]. Developing more than two sets of teeth at intervals during a lifetime.

polypiform (pō-lĭp′ĭ-form) [″ + *pous,* foot, + L. *forma,* form]. Resembling a polyp.

polyplastic (pŏl″ē-plăs′tĭk) [″ + *plastos,* formed]. 1. Having had many evolutionary modifications. 2. Having many substances in cellular composition.

polyplastocytosis (pŏl″ē-plăs″tō-sī-tō′sĭs) [″ + ″ + *kytos,* cell, + *osis,* condition]. Increase in formation of blood platelets.

polyplegia (pŏl″ē-plē′jē-ă) [″ + *plege,* stroke]. Paralysis affecting several muscles.

polyploid (pŏl′ē-ployd). 1. Characterized by polyploidy. 2. An individual in which the chromosome number is two or more times the normal haploid number.

polyploidy (pŏl′ē-ploy″dē). Condition in which the chromosome number is two or more times the normal haploid number found in gametes.

polypnea (pŏl″ĭp-nē′ă) [″ + *pnoia,* breath]. Very rapid breathing. SYN: *panting.*

polypodia (pŏl″ē-pō′dē-ă) [″ + *pous,* foot]. Possession of more than the normal number of feet.

polypoid (pŏl′ē-poyd) [″ + ″ + *eidos,* like]. Like a polyp.

polyporous (pŏl-ĭp'ō-rŭs) [" + *poros,* pore]. Possessing many small openings or pores.

polyposia (pŏl"ē-pō'zē-ă) [Gr. *polys,* many, " + *posis,* drinking]. Sustained ingestion of large amounts of fluid.

polyposis (pŏl"ē-pō'sĭs) [" + *pous,* foot, + *osis,* condition]. The presence of numerous polyps.

p. coli. Polyposis of the large intestine.

p., familial. A rare familial condition in which the mucosa of the colon is covered with polyps. This causes rectal bleeding, and the passage of polyps that come loose. These may become infected, and cause chronic intussusception of the colon. The polyps may become malignant.

p. ventriculi. Presence of numerous polyps in the stomach, sometimes involving entire mucosa, accompanied by chronic atrophic gastritis.

polypotome (pŏl-ĭp'ō-tōm) [" + " + *tome,* incision]. Instrument for excision of polyps.

polypotrite (pō-lĭp'ō-trīt) [" + " + L. *terere,* to crush]. A device for crushing polyps.

polypsychotropia (pŏl"ē-sī-kō-trō'pē-ă). The simultaneous use of two or more psychotropic drugs. SEE: *psychotropic drugs.*

polyptychial (pŏl"ē-tī'kē-ăl) [" + *ptyche,* fold]. Arranged in several layers as is the case in some glands.

polypus (pŏl'ĭ-pŭs) [L.]. (pl. *polypi*) A polyp.

polyradiculitis (pŏl"ē-ră-dĭk"ū-lī'tĭs) [" + L. *radix,* root, + Gr. *itis,* inflammation]. Inflammation of nerve roots, esp. those of spinal nerves.

polyradiculoneuritis (pŏl"ē-ră-dĭk"ū-lō-nū-rī'tĭs) [" + " + Gr. *neuron,* nerve, + *itis,* inflammation]. Inflammation of the peripheral nerves and spinal ganglia.

polyradiculoneuropathy (pŏl"ē-ră-dĭk"ū-lō-nū-rŏp'ă-thē) [" + " + " + *pathos,* disease]. Guillain-Barré syndrome, q.v.

polyribosome (pŏl"ē-rī'bō-sōm). A cluster or group of ribosomes, q.v. They are important in transmitting genetic information and in protein synthesis. SYN: *polysome.*

polyrrhea, polyrrhoea (pŏl"ē-rē'ă) [" + *rhoia,* flow]. Excessive secretion of fluid.

polysaccharide (pŏl"ē-săk'ă-rīd) [" + Sanskrit *sarkara,* sugar]. One of a group of carbohydrates that upon hydrolysis yield more than two molecules of simple sugars. They are complex carbohydrates of high molecular weight, usually insoluble in water, but, when soluble, they form colloidal solutions. Their basic formula is $(C_6H_{12}O_6)_x$. They include two groups: starch (Ex.: starch, inulin, glycogen, dextrin) and cellulose (Ex.: cellulose and hemicelluloses). The hemicelluloses include the pentosans (Ex.: gum arabic), hexosans (Ex.: agar-agar), and hexopentosans (Ex.: pectin). SEE: *carbohydrates; disaccharide; monosaccharide.*

p.'s, immune. Polysaccharides in bacteria, esp. in the cell wall, that are antigenic.

polysaccharose (pŏl"ē-săk'ă-rōs). A polysaccharide.

polyscelia (pŏl"ē-sē'lē-ă) [" + *skelos,* leg]. Condition of having more than the normal number of legs.

polyscelus (pŏ-lĭs'ĕ-lŭs). One having polyscelia, q.v.

polyserositis (pŏl"ē-sē-rō-sī'tĭs) [" + L. *serum,* whey, + *itis,* inflammation]. Familial Mediterranean fever.

p., familial paroxysmal. SEE: *familial Mediterranean fever.*

polysialia (pŏl"ē-sī-ā'lē-ă) [" + *sialon,* saliva]. Ptyalism, q.v.

polysinusitis, polysinuitis (pŏl"ē-sī"nŭs-ī'tĭs, -nū-ī'tĭs) [" + L. *sinus,* a hollow, + Gr. *itis,* inflammation]. Inflammation of several sinuses simultaneously.

polysomaty (pŏl"ē-sō'mă-tē) [" + *soma,* body]. Having reduplicated chromatin in the nucleus.

polysome. Polyribosome.

polysomia (pŏl"ē-sō'mē-ă) [" + *soma,* body]. Having more than one body, as in the doubling of the body of a fetus.

polysorbates (pŏl"ē-sor'bāts). Nonionic surface-active agents composed of polyoxyethylene esters of sorbitol. They usually contain associated fatty acids. The series include polysorbates 20, 40, 60, and 80, which are used in preparing pharmaceuticals. These polysorbates have the trade names of Tween 20, Tween 40, etc.

polyspermia (pŏl"ē-spĕr'mē-ă) [Gr. *polys,* many, + *sperma,* seed]. 1. Excessive secretion of seminal fluid. 2. Entrance of several spermatozoa into one ovum. SYN: *polyspermism.*

polyspermism (pŏl"ē-spĕrm'ĭzm). Polyspermia.

polyspermy (pŏl"ē-spĕr'mē). Fertilization of an ovum by multiple spermatozoa.

polystichia (pŏl"ē-stĭk'ē-ă) [" + *stichos,* a row]. Condition in which there are two or more rows of eyelashes.

polystomatous (pŏl"ē-stō'mă-tŭs) [" + *stoma,* mouth]. Possessing many mouths or openings.

polystyrene (pŏl"ē-stī'rēn). A synthetic resin produced by the polymerization of styrene from ethylene and benzene. The formula is $(CH_2CHC_6H_5)_n$. It is used in the plastics industry.

polysynaptic (pŏl"ē-sĭ-năp'tĭk) [" + *synapsis,* point of contact]. Pert. to nerve pathways involving multiple synapses.

polysyndactyly (pŏl"ē-sĭn-dăk'tĭl-ē) [" + *syn,* together, + *daktylos,* digit]. Multiple syndactyly.

polytendinitis (pŏl″ē-tĕn″dī-nī′tĭs) [″ + L. *tendo*, tendon, + Gr. *itis*, inflammation]. Inflammation of several tendons.

polytene (pŏl′ĕ-tēn) [″ + *tainia*, band]. Composed of many filaments of chromatin.

polyteny (pŏl″ĕ-tē′nē) [″ + *tainia*, band]. Multiple lateral duplication of the chromosome. This produces a giant chromosome.

polythelia (pŏl″ē-thē′lē-ă) [″ + *thele*, nipple, + *-ismos*, condition]. Presence of more than one nipple on a mamma. SYN: *polythelism*.

polythelism (pŏl″ē-thē′lĭzm). Polythelia.

polythiazide (pŏl″ē-thī′ă-zīd). USP. A diuretic drug. Trade name is Renese.

polytocous (pō-lĭt′ō-kŭs) [″ + *tokos*, birth]. Producing several offspring at one time.

polytrichia (pŏl″ē-trĭk′ē-ă) [Gr. *polys*, many, + *thrix*, hair]. Hypertrichosis.

polytrichosis (pŏl″ē-trĭ-kō′sĭs) [″ + ″ + *osis*, condition]. Excessive growth of hair. SYN: *hypertrichosis*.

polytrophia (pŏl″ē-trō′fē-ă) [″ + *trophe*, nourishment]. Excessive or abundant nutrition. SYN: *polytrophy*.

polytrophy (pō-lĭt′rō-fē). Polytrophia.

polytropic (pŏl″ē-trŏp′ĭk) [″ + *trope*, a turning]. Affecting more than one type of cell, said of viruses, or affecting more than one type of tissue, said of certain poisons.

polyunguia (pŏl″ē-ŭng′gwē-ă) [″ + L. *unguis*, nail]. Polyonychia, q.v.

polyunsaturated. In chemistry, rel. to long-chain carbon compounds, esp. fats that have many carbon atoms joined by double or triple bonds.

polyuria (pŏl″ē-ū′rē-ă) [″ + *ouron*, urine]. Excessive secretion and discharge of urine. The urine does not, as a rule, contain abnormal constituents. Several liters in excess of normal may be voided each day. The urine is virtually colorless. Sp. gr. 1.000 to 1.002 and higher in diabetes.

ETIOL: Occurs in diabetes insipidus; diabetes mellitus; chronic nephritis; nephrosclerosis; following edematous states, esp. those induced by heart failure treated with diuretics; in hyperthyroidism; and following excessive intake of liquids.

polyvalent (pŏl″ē-vā′lĕnt, pō-lĭv′ă-lĕnt) [″ + L. *valere*, to be strong]. Multivalent; having a combining power of more than two atoms of hydrogen.

polyvalent serum. Serum with antibodies produced by injecting several strains of microorganisms of the same species, or by injecting different species.

polyvalent vaccine. Vaccine produced from cultures of a number of strains of the same species.

polyvinyl alcohol (pŏl″ē-vī′nĭl). USP. A water-soluble synthetic resin used in preparing medicines, esp. ophthalmic solutions.

polyvinyl chloride. ABBR: PVC. A thermoplastic polymer formed from vinyl chloride. It is used in the manufacture of many products such as rainwear, garden hoses, phonograph records, and floor tiles.

NOTE: Exposure to toxic fumes of PVC can cause respiratory arrest due to oxygen deprivation. The reaction to PVC is delayed from 6 to 24 hrs. after exposure. Patients with suspected exposure should be closely monitored.

polyvinylpyrrolidone (pŏl″ē-vī″nĭl-pĕr-rŏl′ĭ-dōn). ABBR: PVP. Previously used name for povidone, q.v.

pomade (pō-mād′) [Fr. *pommade*]. A perfumed ointment, esp. one for the hair. SYN: *pomatum*.

pomatum (pō-mā′tŭm). A medicinal ointment, esp. one used on the hair. SYN: *pomade*.

Pompe's disease. Glycogen storage disease, type II, q.v.

pompholyx. Dyshidrosis, q.v.

pomphus (pŏm′fŭs) [L.]. (pl. *pomphi*) A blister or a circumscribed elevation on the skin; a wheal.

POMR. *problem-oriented medical record.*

pomum (pō′mŭm) [L.]. An apple.

p. adami. Prominence in the middle line of the throat, caused by junction of two lateral wings of the thyroid cartilage. SYN: *Adam's apple*.

ponderal (pŏn′dĕr-ăl) [L. *pondus*, weight]. Rel. to weight.

ponderal index. The ratio of an individual's height to the cube root of his weight; used to determine body mass. Expressed as:

$$\frac{\text{height (in inches)}}{\sqrt[3]{\text{weight (in pounds)}}}$$

SEE: *Quatelet index*.

Pondimin. Trade name for fenfluramine hydrochloride.

ponograph (pō′nō-grăf) [Gr. *ponos*, pain, fatigue, + *graphein*, to write]. Device for measuring and registering sensitiveness to pain or fatigue.

ponopalmosis (pŏn″ō-păl-mō′sĭs) [″ + *palmos*, palpitation, + *osis*, condition]. Palpitation of the heart produced by slight exertion SYN: *neurocirculatory asthenia*.

ponophobia (pŏ″nō-fō′bē-ă) [″ + *phobos*, fear] 1. Abnormal distaste for exerting oneself. 2 Dread of pain.

pons (pŏnz) [L., bridge]. (pl. *pontes*) 1. A process of tissue connecting two or more parts. 2. [NA] Pons varolii.

p. cerebelli. Pons varolii.

p. hepatis. Part of liver sometimes present that extends from the quadrate lobe to the left lobe across the umbilical fissure.

p. varolii. [Costanzo Varolio, It. anatomist, 1544–1575] A rounded eminence on the ventral surface of the brain stem. It lies between the medulla and cerebral peduncles, and appears externally as a broad band of transverse fibers. It is connected to the cerebellum by the midcerebellar peduncle or brachium pontis. It contains fiber tracts connecting the medulla oblongata and cerebellum with upper portions of the brain. The origins of the abducens, facial, trigeminal, and cochlear divisions of the 8th (vestibulocochlear) nerves are at the borders of the pons. SYN: *pons* (def. 2) [NA]; *p. cerebelli.*

Ponstel. Trade name for mefenamic acid.

pontic (pŏn'tĭk) [L. *pons, pontis,* bridge]. An artifical tooth set in a bridge.

ponticulus (pŏn-tĭk'ū-lŭs) [L., little bridge]. An obsolete term for a little ridge.

pontile (pŏn'tēl). Pert. to the pons varolii.

pontile hemiplegia. Hemiplegia due to lesion of the pons. The arm and leg on one side and the opposite side of the face are affected.

pontile nuclei. The gray matter in the pons.

pontine (pŏn'tēn). Pert. to the pons varolii.

pontobulbar (pŏn"tō-bŭl'bar). Pert. to the pons and the medulla oblongata.

Pontocaine. Trade name for tetracaine.

Pontocaine Hydrochloride (pŏn'tō-kān). A trade name for tetracaine hydrochloride. Is available in several forms for use as a topical or spinal anesthetic.

pool. 1. To mix blood from several donors. 2. Accumulation of blood in a body site.

p., abdominal. The accumulation of blood in the visceral organs of the abdominal cavity. This may occur during shock.

p., gene. The sum of the genetic material in the members of a specified population.

p., metabolic. All of the chemical compounds included in metabolic processes in the body.

p., vaginal. The mucus and cells that are present in the posterior fornix of the vagina when the patient is in a supine position. Material obtained from this site is used in cancer detection and in evaluating the character of the vaginal fluid in investigating infertility problems.

poples (pŏp'lēz) [L., ham]. The popliteal or posterior region of the knee.

popliteal (pŏp"lĭt-ē'ăl, pŏp-lĭt'ē-ăl) [L. *poples,* ham]. Concerning the posterior surface of the knee.

popliteus (pŏp-lĭt'ē-ŭs, -lĭt-ē'ŭs). Muscle located in hind part of the knee joint that flexes the leg and aids it in rotating. SEE: *Muscles* in *Appendix.*

poppy. Any of the several plants of the genus Papaver. Opium is obtained from the juice of the unripe pods of Papaver somniferum.

population of world. A variable depending upon the rate at which the number of people on earth increases. The number of people on earth has never been known with any degree of accuracy due to the difficulty of obtaining accurate census data. It is estimated that there were 250,000,000 people on earth in the year A.D. 1; 500,000,000 by the early 17th century; 3,200,000,000 by 1964; and 5,800,000,000 in 1975. It is estimated there will be 6,182,000,000 people on earth by the year 2000. It is also estimated that the world population increases by 120,000,000 each year, and the U.S. population will be 262,500,000 by the year 2000.

POR. *problem-oriented record.*

poradenitis (por"ăd-ĕ-nī'tĭs [Gr. *poros,* pore, + *aden,* gland, + *itis,* inflammation]. Formation of small abscesses in the iliac glands.

porcelain (por'sĕ-lĭn). A hard, translucent ceramic made by fusing clay. It is colored by glazing with fusible pigments. It is used in dentistry.

porcelaneous, porcelanous (por"sĕ-lā'nē-ŭs, -sĕl'ăn-ŭs) [Fr. *porcelaine*]. Translucent or white like porcelain, as the skin.

porcine (por'sīn) [L. *porcus,* pig]. Pig-like.

pore (por) [L. *porus,* a pore]. 1. A minute opening, esp. one on an epithelial surface. SYN: *porus* [NA]. 2. Opening of the excretory duct of a sweat gland. SEE: *skin; stoma; sweat glands.*

p., alveolar. A minute opening that is thought to exist between adjacent alveoli of the lung.

p., gustatory. P., taste.

p., taste. The external opening of a taste bud. SYN: *p., gustatory.* SEE: *taste.*

porencephalia, porencephaly (por"ĕn-sĕf-ā'lē-ă, por"ĕn-sĕf'ă-lē) [L. *porus,* pore, + *enkephalos,* brain]. An anomalous condition in which the ventricles of the brain are connected with the subarachnoid space.

porencephalitis (por"ĕn-sĕf"ă-lī'tĭs) [" + " + *itis,* inflammation]. Inflammation of the brain with development of cavities communicating with the subarachnoid space.

porencephalous. Pert. to porencephalia.

pori. Pl. of porus.

poriomania [Gr. *poreia,* walking, + *mania,* madness]. Morbid desire to wander from home.

porion (pō'rē-ŏn) [Gr. *poros,* pore]. The midpoint of the upper margin of the auditory meatus.

pornography (por-nŏg'ră-fē) [Gr. *porne,* prostitute, + *graphein,* to write]. Written or graphic forms of communication that either are intended to, or may, incite sexual interest.

porocele (pō'rō-sēl) [Gr. *poros,* callus, + *kele,* hernia]. A herniation into the scrotal sac. This causes hardening and thickening of the scrotum.

porocephaliasis, porocephalosis (pō″rō-sĕf″ă-lī′ă-sĭs, -lō′sĭs) [Gr. *poros,* pore, + *kephale,* head]. Infection with a species of Porocephalus.

Porocephalus (pō″rō-sĕf′ă-lŭs). A genus of wormlike arthropods found commonly in snakes. The young sometimes infest mammals, including man.

porokeratosis (pō″rō-kĕr″ă-tō′sĭs) [″ + *keras,* a horn, + *osis,* condition]. A rare skin disease marked by thickening of the stratum corneum in linear arrangement, followed by its atrophy. Porokeratosis appears on smooth areas. It is irregular in form and size with a circumscribed outline and affects hands and feet, forearms and legs, the face, neck, and scalp.

poroma (pō-rō′mă) [Gr.]. 1. A collosity. 2. A tumor of cells lining the opening of the sweat glands.

p., eccrine. A tumor arising from the duct of an eccrine gland. It usually occurs on the palm or sole.

p., cerebral. At postmortem examination, the presence of cavities in the brain substance due to gas-forming bacteria.

porosis (pō-rō′sĭs) [Gr. *poros,* pore, + *osis,* condition]. Formation of callus in repair of fractured bone. SEE: *callus.*

porosity (pō-rŏs′ĭ-tē) [Gr. *poros,* pore]. The state of being porous.

porotomy (pō-rŏt′ō-mē) [″ + *tome,* incision]. Incision of the urethral meatus.

porous (pō′rŭs). Full of pores; able to admit passage of a liquid.

porphin (por′fĭn). The basic ring structure forming the framework of all porphyrins. Consisting of four pyrrole rings united by methene, $-CH_2-$, couplings.

porphobilinogen (por″fō-bī-lĭn′ō-jĕn). An intermediate product in heme synthesis sometimes found in the urine of patients with acute porphyria. The urine may appear to be normal when fresh, but will change to a Burgundy wine color or even to black when heated with dilute hydrochloric acid to 100° C.

porphyria (por-fī′rē-ă, por-fĭr′ē-ă) [Gr. *porphyra,* purple]. A group of disorders that result from a disturbance in porphyrin metabolism, causing increased formation and excretion of porphyrin or its precursors.

p., acute intermittent. A rare metabolic disorder characterized by excessive excretion of porphyrins, acute abdominal pain, and neurological disturbances, inherited as an autosomal dominant trait. Sometimes precipitated by excessive use of sulfonamides, barbiturates, or other drugs. Sensitivity to light is characteristic.

p., congenital erythropoietic. A rare condition characterized by severe skin lesions, hemolytic anemia, and splenomegaly. Inherited as an autosomal recessive trait.

p. cutanea tarda hereditaria. Porphyria inherited as an autosomal dominant characteristic. Onset of symptoms usually occurs between the ages of 10 and 30.

p. erythropoietica. Mild form of porphyria characterized by cutaneous lesions and excess protoporphyrin in erythrocytes and feces.

p. hepatica. Porphyria due to disturbance in liver metabolism such as occurs following hepatitis, poisoning by heavy metals, certain anemias, and other conditions.

p., South African genetic. P., variegate, q.v.

p., variegate. A form of hepatic porphyria in which there are recurrent episodes of abdominal pain and neuropathy. The skin is especially fragile.

porphyrin (por′fĭ-rĭn) [Gr. *porphyra,* purple]. Any of a group of nitrogen-containing organic compounds that occur in protoplasm and form the basis of animal and plant respiratory pigments, obtained from hemoglobin and chlorophyll.

porphyrinuria (por″fĭ-rĭ-nū′rē-ă) [″ + *ouron,* urine]. The excretion of an increased amount of porphyrin in the urine. SYN: *porphyruria.*

porphyrization (por″fĭr-ĭ-zā′shŭn). Process of pulverizing.

porphyruria (por″fĭr-ū′rē-ă) [″ + *ouron,* urine]. Excretion of an increased amount of porphyrin in urine. SYN: *porphyrinuria.*

Porro's operation (por′ōz). [Eduardo Porro, It. obstetrician, 1842–1902] Cesarean section followed by removal of the uterus, the ovaries, and tubes. SYN: *cesarean hysterectomy.*

porta [L., gate]. (pl. *portae*) The point of entry of nerves and vessels into an organ or part.

p. hepatis. [NA] The fissure of the liver where the portal vein and hepatic artery enter and the hepatic duct leaves.

p. lienis. Hilus of the spleen where vessels enter.

p. pulmonis. Pulmonary hilus for entry and exit of the bronchi, nerves, and vessels.

p. renis. Hilus of the kidney for entry of the vessels.

portacaval (por″tă-kā′văl). Concerning the portal vein and the vena cava.

portacaval shunt. Surgical joining of the portal vein and the inferior vena cava.

portal [L. *porta,* gate]. 1. An entryway. 2. Concerning a porta or entrance to an organ, esp. that through which the blood is carried to the liver.

p., intestinal. The opening of the midgut or yolk sac into the foregut or hindgut of an embryo.

p. of entry. The avenue by which infectious organisms gain access to the body.

portal circulation. The circulation of blood into the liver by the portal vein and out by the hepatic vein.

portal hypertension. Increased pressure in the portal vein as a result of obstruction of the flow of blood through the liver.

portal system. The portal vein and its branches by which blood is collected from abdominal viscera and conveyed to the sinusoids of the liver, from which it passes through the hepatic veins to the inferior vena cava.

portal vein. Vein formed by the veins of the splanchnic area that conveys its blood into the liver. It is made of the combined superior and inferior mesenteric, splenic, gastric, and cystic veins.

portio (por'shē-ō) [L.]. (pl. *portiones*) [NA] A part. In anatomy, it designates a certain portion of a structure or organ.

p. dura. The seventh cranial nerve; the facial nerve.

p. intermedia. Nerve, intermedius, q.v.

p. vaginalis. The part of the cervix within the vagina.

portogram (por'tō-grăm) [L. *porta,* gate, + Gr. *gramma,* mark]. Roentgenogram of the portal vein.

portography (por-tŏg'ră-fē) [" + Gr. *graphein,* to write]. Roentgenography of the portal vein while an opaque medium is in it.

p., portal. Portography after injection of opaque material into the superior mesenteric vein. This is usually done during laparotomy.

p., splenic. Roentgenography of the splenic and portal veins after injection of opaque material into the spleen.

portosystemic (por"tō-sĭs-tĕm'ĭk). Joining the portal and systemic venous circulation.

port-wine mark, stain. A superficial purplish-red birthmark. SYN: *nevus flammeus.*

porus (pō'rŭs) [L.]. (pl. *pori*) A meatus or foramen; a tiny aperture in a structure; a pore.

p. acusticus externus. [NA] The outer opening of the external acoustic meatus.

p. acusticus internus. [NA] The opening of the internal acoustic meatus into the cranial cavity.

p. gustatorius. The small taste pore openings in the taste buds of the tongue.

p. lactiferous. Opening of a lactiferous duct on the tip of the nipple of the mammary gland.

p. opticus. Opening in center of the optic disk through which retinal vessels (central artery and vein) reach retina through the lamina cribrosa of the sclera.

p. sudoriferus. [NA] Opening of a sweat gland.

posiomania (pō"sē-ō-mā'nē-ă) [Gr. *posis,* drinking, + *mania,* madness]. Addiction to alcoholic drinks. SYN: *dipsomania.*

position (pō-zĭsh'ŭn) [L. *positio*]. 1. Place in which a thing is put. 2. Manner in which a body is arranged, as by the nurse or physician for examination. 3. In obstetrics, the relation of some arbitrarily chosen portion of the child in the pelvis to the right or left side of the mother, the occiput, chin, sacrum, and scapula being the points of reference that are most commonly used. SEE: table; *presentations of fetus* for illus.

p., anatomic. Position assumed when a person is standing erect with arms at the sides, palms forward. SYN: *p., orthograde.*

p., Bonner's. In inflammation of the hip joint, flexion, abduction, and outward rotation of the thigh, which produces relief.

Positions of Fetus in Utero

VERTEX PRESENTATION (point of designation—occiput):	
Left occiput anterior	LOA
Right occiput posterior	ROP
Right occiput anterior	ROA
Left occiput posterior	LOP
Right occiput transverse	ROT
Occiput anterior	OA
Occiput posterior	OP
BREECH PRESENTATION (point of designation—sacrum):	
Left sacroanterior	LSA
Right sacroposterior	RSP
Right sacroanterior	RSA
Left sacroposterior	LSP
Sacroanterior	SA
Sacroposterior	SP
Left sacrotransverse	LST
Right sacrotransverse	RST
FACE PRESENTATION (point of designation—chin [mentum]):	
Left mentoanterior	LMA
Right mentoposterior	RMP
Right mentoanterior	RMA
Left mentoposterior	LMP
Mentoposterior	MP
Mentoanterior	MA
Left mentotransverse	LMT
Right mentotransverse	RMT
TRANSVERSE PRESENTATION (point of designation—scapula of presenting shoulder):	
Left scapuloanterior	LScA
Right scapuloposterior	RScP
Right scapuloanterior	LScA
Left scapuloposterior	LScP

p., Bozeman's. The knee-elbow position wherein the patient is strapped to supports.

p., Brickner. A method of obtaining traction, abduction, and external rotation of the shoulder by tying the patient's wrists to the head of the bed.

p., centric. The most posterior position of the mandible in relation to the maxilla; the constant position into which the patient will close the jaws, which may be true centric or his or her convenience relationship.

p., decubitus. Position of the patient on a flat surface. The exact position is indicated by which surface of the body is closest to the flat surface, i.e., in left or right lateral decubitus, the patient is flat on the left or right side, respectively; and in dorsal or ventral decubitus, the patient is on the back or abdomen, respectively.

p., dorsal. Position in which the patient is on back. SYN: *supine*.

p., dorsal elevated. Position with patient lying on back with head and shoulders elevated at an angle of 30° or more. Employed in digital examination of genitalia and in bimanual examination.

p., dorsal recumbent. Position of patient on back with lower extremities moderately flexed and rotated outward. Employed in application of obstetrical forceps, repair of lesions following parturition, vaginal examination, and bimanual palpation. SEE: illus.

p., dorsosacral. P., lithotomy. SEE: illus.

p., Edebohl's. P., Simon's.

p., Elliott's. Position in which supports are placed under the small of the patient's back so that patient resembles a double inclined plane.

p., English. P., left lateral recumbent.

p., Fowler's. Position where the head of the patient's bed is raised about 1½ ft. (46 cm.), and knees are elevated. SEE: illus.

p., genucubital. Position with patient on knees, thighs upright, body resting on elbows, head down on hands. Employed when it is not possible to use the classic knee-chest position. SYN: *p., knee-elbow.*

p., genupectoral. Position with patient on knees, thighs upright, head and upper part of chest resting on table, arms crossed above head. Employed in displacement of prolapsed fundus, dislodgment of impacted head of fetus, management of transverse presentation, replacement of retroverted uterus or displaced ovary, or flushing of intestinal canal. SYN: *p., knee-chest.* SEE: illus.

p., horizontal. Position with patient lying supine with feet extended. Employed in palpation, in auscultation of fetal heart, and in operative procedures.

p., horizontal abdominal. Position with patient flat on abdomen, feet extended. Employed in examination of back and spinal column.

p., jackknife. Position with patient on back, shoulders elevated, legs flexed on thighs, thighs at right angles to abdomen. Employed when passing urethral sound. SYN: *p., reclining.*

p., knee-chest. P., genupectoral. SEE: illus.

p., knee-elbow. P., genucubital.

p., laterosemiprone. P., Sims'.

p., left lateral recumbent. Position with patient on left side, right knee and thigh drawn up. Employed in vaginal examination.

p., lithotomy. Position with patient on back, thighs flexed on abdomen, legs on thighs, thighs abducted. Employed in operation on genital tract, in vaginal hysterectomy, and diagnosis and treatment of diseases of urethra and bladder. SYN: *p., dorsosacral.* SEE: illus.

p., Noble's. Position in which the patient is standing, leaning forward, and supporting the upper body by bracing the arms against the wall or a chair. This position is useful in examining the kidney.

p., obstetrical. P., left lateral recumbent.

p., orthograde. P., anatomic.

p., orthopneic. Sitting erect or propped up in bed by use of pillows or bed angulation. Position is for those who have difficulty breathing.

p., physiologic rest. In dentistry, position of the mandible at rest when the patient is sitting upright and the condyles are in an unstrained position. The jaw muscles are relaxed.

p., prone. Position in which patient is lying face downward. SEE: illus.

p., reclining. P., jackknife.

p., rest. In dentistry, the position of the mandible when the jaws are at rest. The masticatory musculature is relaxed, and the teeth are slightly separated.

p., Rose's. In repairing a laceration of the upper lip or mouth; the patient's head is extended and hangs over the end of the table. This permits blood to flow down and not into the patient's mouth.

p., side, semiprone. P., Sims'.

p., Simon's. Exaggerated lithotomy position. Patient flat on back, legs flexed on thighs, thighs on abdomen, hips somewhat elevated, thighs strongly abducted. Employed in vaginal operations.

p., Sims'. Position with patient on left side, right knee and thigh drawn well up above left, left arm back of patient and hanging over edge of table, chest inclined forward so that patient rests upon it. Employed in curettement of uterus, intrauterine irrigation after labor, tamponade of vagina, rectal exploration, and operations on cervix. SYN: *p., laterosemiprone; p., side, semiprone*. SEE: illus.

p., Trendelenburg. Dorsal position in which patient's body is supine on a bed tilted at about 45° angle with the head low. Employed in abdominal surgery to favor gravitation upward of abdominal viscera and in treating cardiovascular shock. SEE: illus.

p., unilateral recumbent. Position in which patient is on right side, used in acute pleurisy, lobar pneumonia of the right side, and in a greatly enlarged liver; position in which patient is on left side, used in lobar pneumonia, pleurisy on that side, and in large pericardial effusions. SEE: illus.

p., Walcher. Position in which patient's hips are on edge of table and lower extremities hanging down.

positioner (pō-zĭsh'ŭn-ĕr). Apparatus for holding or placing the body or part, esp. the head, in a certain position.

positive (pŏz'ĭ-tĭv) [L. *positivus,* ruling]. 1. Definite; affirmative; opposed to negative. 2. Indicating an abnormal condition in examination and diagnosis. 3. Having a value greater than zero.

Often in laboratory findings and mathematical expressions, positive is indicated by a plus (+) sign.

positive end-expiratory pressure. ABBR: PEEP. In respiratory medicine, a method of holding alveoli open during expiration. This is done by gradually increasing the expiratory pressure. When PEEP is used, it is important that pulmonary capillary wedge pressure be monitored by use of a Swan-Ganz catheter in the pulmonary artery. The goal is to achieve adequate arterial oxygenation without using toxic levels of inspired oxygen, and without compromising cardiac output.

CAUTION: The patient must be carefully monitored during the therapy to ensure compliance and to observe for undesired side effects such as pneumomediastinum, subcutaneous emphysema, and pneumothorax.

positron (pŏz'ĭ-trŏn). A particle having the same mass as a negative electron, but possessing a positive charge.

posological (pŏ"sō-lŏj'ĭ-kăl) [Gr. *posos,* how much, + *logos,* a study]. Concerning dosage of medicines.

posology (pō-sŏl'ō-jē). Branch of scientific study dealing with dosage of medicines.

possessed. Obsessed, or as if controlled by an outside spirit or force.

possession (pō-zĕsh'ŭn) [ME. *possessen*]. Psychological state of being dominated by an idea, a passion, or a mental obsession.

possession, demoniacal. Belief of being controlled by an evil spirit or demon.

Possum (pŏs'ŭm). [*p*atient *o*perated *s*elector *m*echanism]. A device that permits a disabled individual to control and operate various machines such as switches, telephones, and typewriters by breathing into the master control of the apparatus.

post. In dentistry, a dowel.

post- [L.]. A prefix meaning behind, after, or posterior.

postabortal (pōst"ă-bor'tăl) [L. *post,* after, + *abortus,* abortion]. Happening subsequent to abortion.

postacetabular (pōst"ăs-ĕ-tăb'ū-lăr) [" + *acetabulum,* a little saucer for vinegar]. Behind the acetabulum.

postadolescent (pōst"ăd-ō-lĕs'ĕnt) [" + *adolescens,* adolescence]. An individual who has passed adolescence.

postanal (pōst-ā'năl) [" + *anus,* anus]. Located behind the anus.

postanesthetic (pōst"ăn-ĕs-thĕt'ĭk) [" + *an-,* not, + *aisthesis,* sensation]. Pert. to the period following anesthesia.

postapoplectic (pōst"ăp-ō-plĕk'tĭk) [" + Gr. *apoplessein,* to cripple by a stroke]. Pert. to the period immediately following a stroke or apoplexy.

postaxial (pōst-ăk'sē-ăl) [" + Gr. *axon,* axis]. Situated or happening behind an axis.

postbrachial (pōst-brā'kē-ăl) [" + *brachiolis,* arm]. Pert. to the posterior portion of the upper arm.

postcapillary (pōst-kăp'ĭl-lā-rē). A terminal vessel of a capillary network that leads to a venule. SYN: *capillary, venous.*

postcardial (pōst-kăr'dē-ăl) [" + Gr. *kardia,* heart]. Behind the heart.

postcardiotomy (pōst-kăr"dē-ŏt'ō-mē) [" + " + *tome,* incision]. The period after open-heart surgery.

postcava (pōst-kā'vă) [L. *post,* after, + *cavus,* a hollow]. The ascending or inferior vena cava.

postcaval. Concerning the postcava.

postcentral (pōst-sĕn'trăl) [" + Gr. *kentron,* center]. 1. Situated or happening behind a center. 2. Located behind the fissure of Rolando.

postcibal (pōst-sī'băl) [" + *cibum,* food]. Occurring after meals.

postclavicular (pōst"klă-vĭk'ū-lăr) [" + *clavicula,* a little key]. Located or occurring behind the clavicle.

postclimacteric (pōst"klī-măk-tĕr'ĭk, -măk'tĕr-ĭk) [L. *post,* after, + Gr *klimakter,* rung of a ladder]. Occurring after the menopause.

postcoital (pōst-kō'ĭt-ăl) [" + *coitio,* a coming together]. Subsequent to sexual intercourse.

postconnubial (pōst"kŏn-ū'bē-ăl) [" + *con-*

POSITIONS

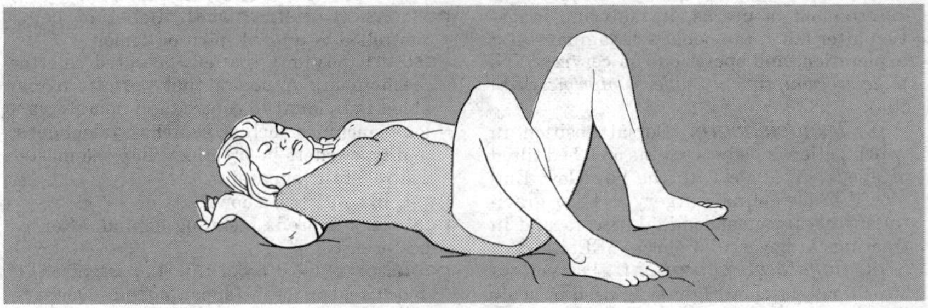

DORSAL RECUMBENT POSITION

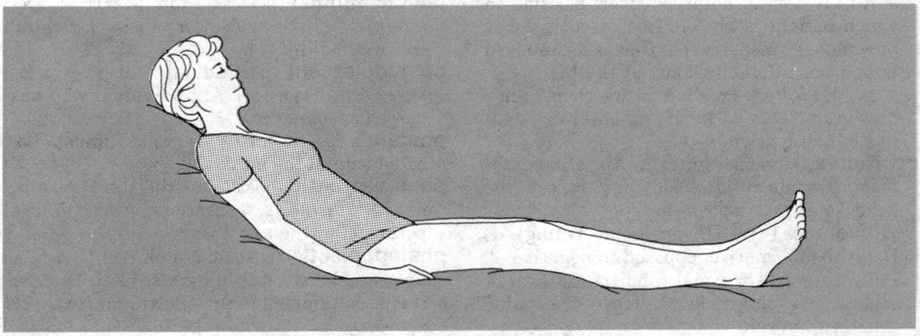

FOWLER'S POSITION

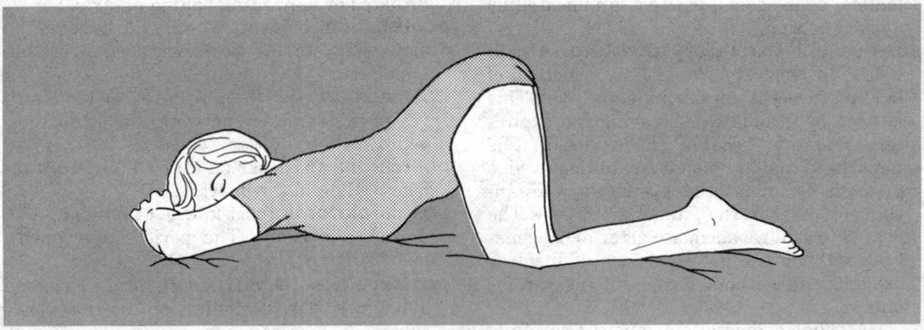

KNEE-CHEST OR GENUPECTORAL POSITION

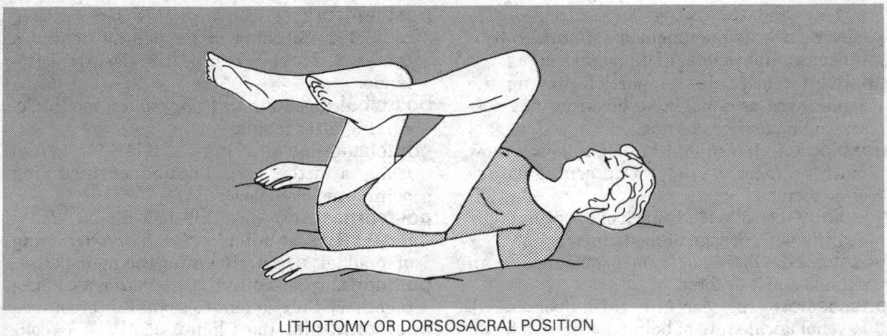

LITHOTOMY OR DORSOSACRAL POSITION

POSITIONS

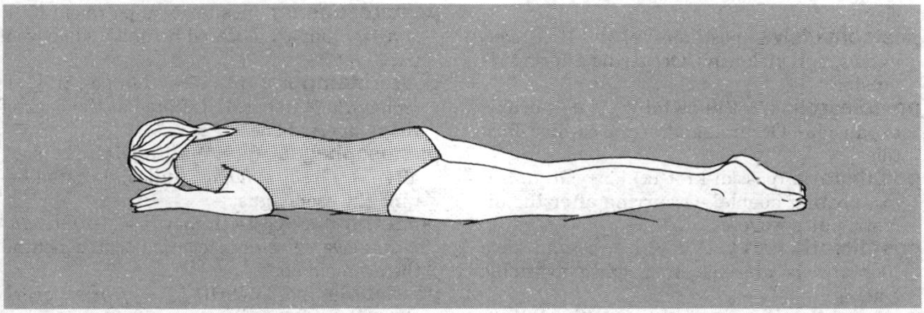

PRONE POSITION

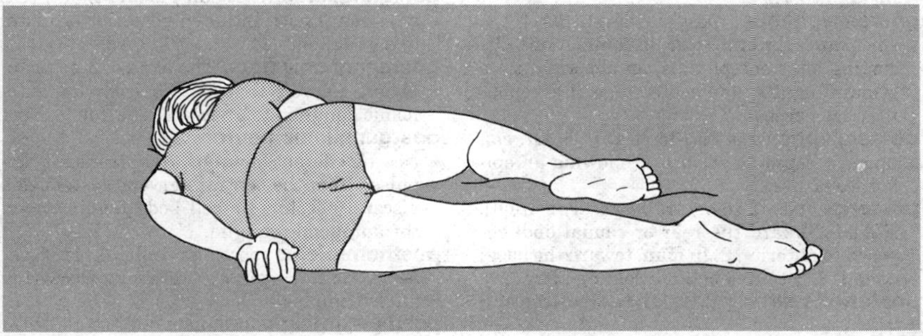

SIMS' POSITION

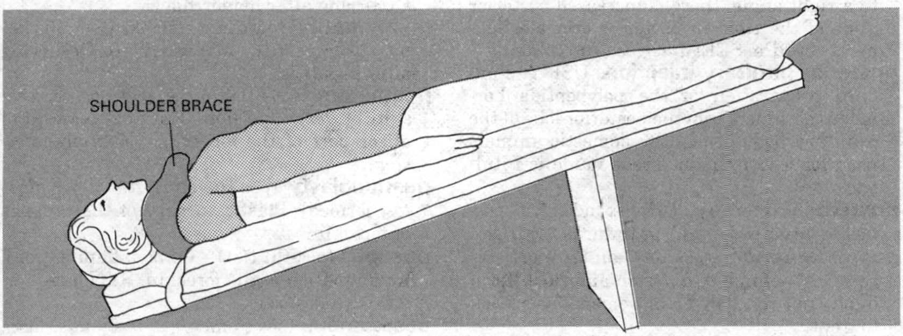

TRENDELENBURG POSITION

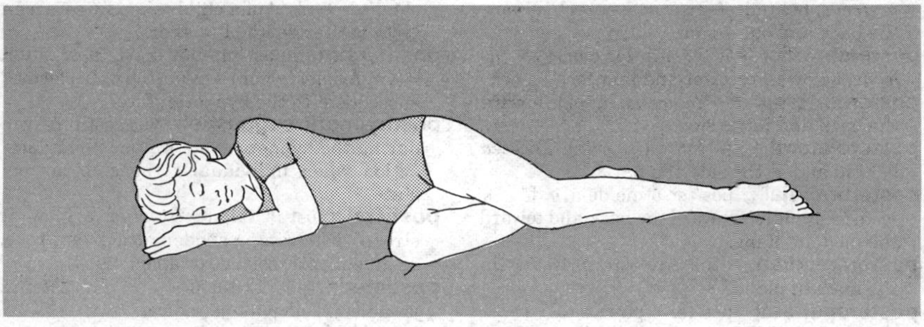

RIGHT LATERAL RECUMBENT POSITION

nubium, marriage]. Occurring after marriage.

postconvulsive (pōst″kŏn-vŭl′sĭv) [″ + *convulsus,* pull violently]. Occurring after a convulsion.

postdiastolic (pōst″dī-ăs-tŏl′ĭk) [″ + *diastole,* expansion]. Occurring after the cardiac diastole.

postdicrotic (pōst″dī-krŏt′ĭk) [″ + Gr. *dikrotos,* beating double]. Occurring after the dicrotic pulse wave.

postdicrotic wave. A recoil or second wave (not always present) in a sphygmographic tracing.

postdiphtheritic (pōst″dĭf-thĕr-ĭt′ĭk). Following diphtheria.

postencephalitis (pōst″ĕn-sĕf-ă-lī′tĭs) [″ + *enkephalos,* brain, + *itis,* inflammation]. Occurring after encephalitis; an abnormal state remaining after the acute stage of encephalitis has passed.

postepileptic (pōst″ĕp-ĭ-lĕp′tĭk) [″ + Gr. *epi,* upon, + *lepsis,* a seizure]. Following an epileptic seizure.

posterior (pŏs-tē′rē-or) [L. *posterus,* behind]. [NA] 1. Toward the rear or caudal end; opposed to anterior. 2. In man, toward the back; dorsal. 3. Situated behind; coming after.

posterior central gyrus. Gyrus, postcentral, q.v.

posterior drawer sign. With the knee flexed to a right angle, there is increased posterior glide of the tibia in posterior cruciate ligament rupture. SEE: *anterior drawer sign.*

posterior pituitary injection. USP. A standard preparation of the polypeptide hormones obtained from the posterior lobe of the pituitary body of healthy domestic animals used for food by man. Trade name is Pituitrin.

postero- (pŏs′tĕr-ō) [L.]. Prefix indicating posterior, situated behind, or towards the back.

posteroanterior (pŏs″tĕr-ō-ăn-tēr′ē-or) [L. *posterus,* behind, + *anterior,* anterior]. Term indicating the flow or movement from back to front.

posteroexternal (pŏs″tĕr-ō-ĕks-tĕr′năl) [L. *posterus,* behind, + *externus,* outer]. Toward the back and outer side.

posteroinferior (pŏs″tĕr-ō-ĭn-fēr′ē-or) [″ + *inferus,* below]. Posterior and inferior.

posterointernal [″ + *internus,* inner]. Toward the back and inner side.

posterolateral [″ + *lateralis,* side]. Located behind and at the side of a part.

posteromedial (pŏs″tĕr-ō-mē′dē-ăl) [″ + *medius,* middle]. Toward the back and toward the median plane.

posteromedian. Situated posteriorly and in the median plane.

posteroparietal (pŏs″tĕr-ō-pă-rī′ĕ-tăl) [″ + *paries,* a wall]. Located at the back of the parietal bone.

posterosuperior (pŏs″tĕr-ō-sū-pē′rē-or) [″ + *superior,* upper]. Located behind and above a part.

posterotemporal (pŏs″tĕr-ō-tĕm′pō-răl) [″ + *temporalis,* temporal]. Located at the back of the temporal bone.

postesophageal (pōst″ē-sŏf″ă-jē′ăl) [L. *post,* after, + Gr. *oisophagos,* gullet]. Located behind the esophagus.

postethmoid (pōst-ĕth′moyd) [″ + Gr. *ethmos,* sieve, + *eidos,* form]. Located behind the ethmoid bone.

postfebrile (pōst-fē′brĭl) [″ + *febris,* fever]. Occurring after a fever.

postganglionic (pōst″găn-glē-ŏn′ĭk) [″ + Gr. *ganglion,* knot]. Situated posterior or distal to a ganglion.

postganglionic fiber. The axon of a postganglionic neuron that passes from an autonomic ganglion to a visceral effector.

postganglionic neuron. The second of a series of efferent neurons that transmit impulses from the central nervous system to a visceral effector. Its cell body lies in one of the autonomic ganglia.

posthemiplegic (pōst″hĕm-ĭ-plē′jĭk) [″ + Gr. *hemi,* half, + *plege,* a stroke]. Occurring after hemiplegia.

posthemorrhagic (pōst-hĕm″ō-răj′ĭk) [″ + Gr. *haima,* blood, + *rhegnynai,* to burst forth]. Occurring after hemorrhage.

posthepatitic (pōst″hĕp-ă-tĭt′ĭk) [″ + Gr. *hepar,* liver, + *itis,* inflammation]. Occurring after hepatitis.

posthetomy (pŏs-thĕt′ō-mē) [Gr. *posthe,* foreskin, + *tome,* incision]. Surgical removal of all or part of the foreskin. SYN: *circumcision.*

posthioplasty (pŏs′thē-ō-plăs″tē) [″ + *plastos,* formed]. Plastic surgery of the prepuce or foreskin.

posthitis (pŏs-thī′tĭs) [″ + *itis,* inflammation]. Inflammation of the foreskin. SYN: *acrobystitis; acroposthitis.*

posthumous (pŏs′tū-mŭs) [L. *postumus,* last]. 1. Occurring after death. 2. Born after death of father. 3. Said of a child taken by cesarean section after death of mother.

posthypnotic (pōst″hĭp-nŏt′ĭk) [L. *post,* after, + Gr. *hypnos,* sleep]. Occurring or performed subsequent to the hypnotic state.

posthypnotic suggestion. Suggestion given during the hypnotic state influencing a later action when individual returns to normal state.

postictal (pōst-ĭk′tăl) [″ + *ictus,* a blow or stroke]. Following a sudden attack or stroke, as an epileptic seizure or apoplexy.

posticteric (pōst″ĭk-tĕr′ĭk) [″ + Gr. *ikteros,* jaundice]. Following jaundice.

postmalarial (pōst″mă-lā′rē-ăl) [″ + It. *ma-*

laria, bad air]. Occurring after malaria.

postmature (pōst″mă-tūr′) [″ + *maturus,* ripe]. 1. Pert. to an infant born after the calculated due date. 2. Pert. to an infant born after 42 weeks of gestation.

postmaturity (pōst″mă-tū′rĭ-tē) [″ + *maturus,* ripe]. Overdevelopment, as in a postmature infant.

postmediastinal (pōst″mē-dē-ăs′tĭ-năl) [″ + *mediastinum,* in the middle]. Behind the mediastinum.

postmenopausal (pōst″mĕn-ō-paw′zăl) [″ + Gr. *men,* month, + *pausis,* cessation]. Occurring after the menopause.

post mortem [L.]. After death.

postmortem [L.]. Occurring or performed after death.

postmortem examination. Examination of the organs and tissue of a body to determine the cause of death or pathological conditions. SYN: *autopsy.*

postnasal (pōst-nā′zăl) [L. *post,* after, + *nasus,* nose]. Located behind the nose.

postnatal [″ + *natus,* birth]. Happening after birth.

postnecrotic (pōst″nē-krŏt′ĭk) [″ + Gr. *nekros,* dead]. After death of a tissue or a part.

postneuritic (pōst″nū-rĭt′ĭk) [″ + *neuron,* nerve, + *itis,* inflammation]. Occurring after neuritis.

postocular (pōst-ŏk′ū-lar) [″ + *oculus,* eye]. Behind the eye.

postocular neuritis. Inflammation of the optic nerve behind the eyeball.

postolivary (pōst-ŏl′ĭ-vā-rē) [″ + *oliva,* olive]. Behind the olivary body; back of the anterior pyramid of the medulla.

postoperative care [L. *post,* after, + *operatus,* work]. Care after or following a surgical operation.

NURSING IMPLICATIONS: Prior to discharge from the recovery room, the following criteria should be met: recovery from the effects of anesthesia; stable vital signs; no excessive drainage from any site or body cavity; satisfactory level of consciousness; essential orders must be completed; adequate urine output (30 ml. per hour); and notification of the nursing unit receiving the patient of his or her status and essential equipment needed to care for the patient.

Throughout the postoperative period, the nurse must monitor vital signs at indicated intervals, obtain necessary equipment and supplies, observe patient for adequate circulatory function, provide for adequate nutrition and elimination, maintain fluid and electrolyte balance, check wounds and tubes for drainage, administer analgesics as prescribed, provide comfort by properly positioning the patient. If guard rails are indicated, be certain they are in place; also, all electrical devices used must be properly grounded. Provide sufficient rest periods, provide wound care, establish range of motion exercises progressing to ambulation as indicated, prevent and recognize postoperative complications and prepare patient and family for discharge with pertinent discharge instruction.

postoperculum (pōst-ō-pŭr′kū-lŭm) [″ + *operculum,* a cover]. The fold covering the insula that is formed of part of the superior temporal gyrus of the brain.

postoral (pōst-or′ăl) [″ + *os,* mouth]. Behind, or in the posterior part of, the mouth.

postorbital (pōst-or′bĭ-tăl) [″ + *orbita,* track]. Behind the orbit of the eye.

postpalatine (pōst-păl′ă-tīn) [″ + *palatum,* palate]. Behind the palate.

postpallium (pōst-păl′ē-ŭm) [″ + *pallium,* cloak]. That part of the cerebral cortex behind the fissure of Rolando.

postpaludal (pōst-păl′ū-dăl) [″ + *palus,* swamp]. After a malarial attack.

postparalytic (pōst″păr-ă-lĭt′ĭk) [″ + *para,* beside, + *lyein,* to loosen]. Subsequent to an attack of paralysis.

post partum (pōst-păr′tŭm) [L. *post,* after, + *partus,* birth]. After childbirth.

postpartum. Occurring after childbirth.

postpartum blues. The "let-down" feeling experienced during the postpartum period for no apparent reason. The mother becomes tearful and irritable, loses her appetite, and finds sleeping difficult. This temporary state may occur during the hospital stay or after. It is thought to be due to hormonal changes as well as emotional needs during this period. This occurs in 70 to 80% of mothers.

postpartum depression. The most common neurotic reaction during the puerperal period is depression. The symptoms are tearfulness, despondency, a feeling of hopelessness, inadequacy, inability to cope with infant care, mood swings, extreme anxiety over the baby, guilt of not loving the baby enough, irritability, fatigue, loss of normal interests, and insomnia. This depression occurs in about 3% of women.

postpartum hemorrhage. Hemorrhage that occurs after childbirth.

NURSING IMPLICATIONS: During the first postpartum hour, the chance of hemorrhage is the greatest, and to prevent hemorrhage, check the mother's fundus every 5 minutes or less and massage it. Check the mother's vital signs and vaginal discharge at least every 15 minutes.

If hemorrhage begins, the first measure is to massage the uterus through the abdominal wall until it becomes hard. If softness begins to occur, massage is immediately reinstituted. A hand is kept on the uterus during the treatment of hemorrhage in order to assess its condition and to massage it as indicated. Overmassage is contraindicated. The mother's bladder should be kept empty. I.V. oxytocic drugs, plasma, or blood may be prescribed by the physician.

It is important to provide support and comfort for these patients, who are understandably quite apprehensive. Assure her that during this period the newborn is well taken care of.

postpartum pituitary necrosis. Sheehan's syndrome, q.v.

postpartum psychosis. A psychosis that develops during the six months following childbirth, the highest incidence being in the third to sixth day after delivery through the first month postpartum. The symptoms and signs include: hallucinations, delusions, preoccupation with death, self-mutilation, infanticide, distorted reality, extreme dependency, and a demanding attitude. This psychosis may become a chronic condition but for most women it becomes an isolated event in their lives.

postpharyngeal (pōst-fă-rĭn′jē-ăl) [L. *post,* after, + Gr. *pharynx,* pharynx]. Behind the pharynx.

postpneumonic (pōst″nū-mŏn′ĭk) [″ + *pneumon,* lung]. Occurring after pneumonia.

postpontile (pōst-pŏn′tĭl) [″ + *pons,* bridge]. Situated behind the pons varolii.

postprandial (pōst-prăn′dē-ăl). Following a meal.

postpubertal (pōst-pū′bĕr-tăl) [″ + *pubertas,* puberty]. Concerning the period following puberty.

postpuberty (pōst-pū′bĕr-tē). The period after puberty.

postpubescent (pōst″pū-bĕs′ĕnt) [″ + *pubescens,* becoming hairy]. Following puberty.

postpyramidal (pōst-pĭ-răm′ĭd-ăl). Behind a pyramidal tract.

postpyramidal nucleus. Mass of gray matter in posterior column of the medulla. SYN: *nucleus funiculi gracilis.*

postradiation (pōst″rā-dē-ā′shŭn). Occurring after exposure to ionizing radiation.

postsacral (pōst-sā′krăl) [″ + *sacrum,* sacred]. Below the sacrum.

postscapular (pōst-skăp′ū-lăr) [″ + *scapula,* shoulder blade]. Below or behind the scapula.

postscarlatinal (pōst″skăr-lă-tī′năl) [″ + *scarlatina,* scarlet fever]. Following scarlet fever.

postsphygmic (pōst-sfĭg′mĭk) [″ + Gr. *sphygmos,* pulse]. Following the pulse wave.

postsplenic (pōst-splĕn′ĭk) [″ + Gr. *splen,* spleen]. Behind the spleen.

poststenotic (pōst″stĕ-nŏt′ĭk) [″ + Gr. *stenosis,* narrowing]. Distal to a stenosed or constricted area, esp. of an artery.

postsynaptic (pōst″sĭ-năp′tĭk) [″ + Gr. *synapsis,* point of contact]. Located distal to a synapse.

post-tarsal (pōst-tăr′săl) [″ + Gr. *tarsos,* a broad, flat surface]. Behind the tarsus.

post-term infant. An infant born after the beginning of the 42nd week of gestation as counted from the first day of the last normal menstrual period.

post-tibial (pōst-tĭb′ē-ăl) [″ + *tibia,* shin bone]. Behind the tibia.

post-transfusion syndrome. Condition of fever, splenomegaly, atypical lymphocytes, abnormal liver function tests, and occasionally a skin rash that develops following blood transfusion or perfusion of an organ during surgery. The syndrome appears three to five weeks after transfusion or perfusion with fresh (less than 24-hour old) blood, usually in large quantities. The causative agent is thought to be cytomegalovirus.

post-traumatic (pōst″traw-măt′ĭk) [″ + *traumatikos,* traumatic]. Following an injury.

postulate (pŏs′tū-lāt) [L. *postulare,* to request]. A supposition or view, usually self-evident, that is assumed without proof. SEE: *Koch's law.*

postural (pŏs′tū-răl) [L. *postura,* position]. Pert. to or affected by posture.

postural drainage. Drainage of secretions from the bronchi or a cavity in the lung by having the patient positioned so that gravity will allow drainage of the particular lobe or lobes of the lung involved. Used in bronchiectasis and before operation for lobectomy. The position aggravates coughing, resulting in expectoration of much sputum, 5 to 10 oz. (148 to 296 ml.) in severe cases. Five to 10 minutes morning and evening is recommended. High-protein diet to replace protein lost. SEE: illus.

NURSING IMPLICATIONS: Assess necessity for procedure, and if it is to be used, evaluate patient's physical tolerance, teach and assist the patient in the procedure by positioning for effective drainage, encouraging the patient to mechanically remove secretions with forceful cough, and caution the patient not to perform procedure after meals, in order to prevent aspiration.

postural hypotension. Decrease in blood pressure upon assuming erect posture. This is normal, but may be of such degree as to cause fainting, esp. in persons who first stand up after having been flat in bed for several days. SEE: *blackout.* SYN: *orthostatic hypotension.*

posture (pŏs′tŭr) [L. *postura*]. Attitude or position of the body.

p., coiled. Body on one side with legs drawn up to meet the trunk. Noted in cerebral diseases and in hepatic, intestinal, and renal colic.

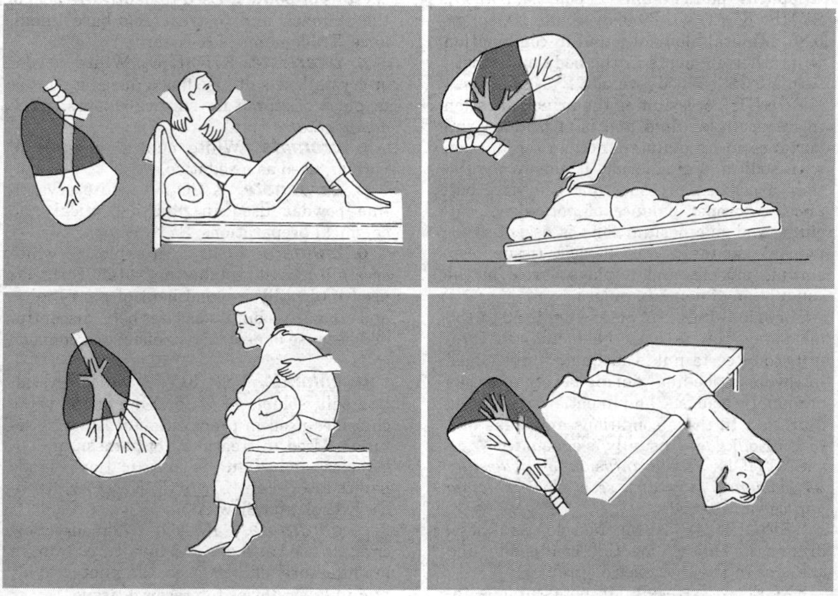

DRAINAGE OF APICAL SEGMENTS OF RIGHT UPPER LOBE
DRAINAGE OF LATERAL SEGMENTS OF RIGHT MIDDLE LOBE
DRAINAGE OF APICAL SEGMENTS OF LEFT LOWER LOBE
DRAINAGE OF TRACHEA

POSTURAL DRAINAGE OF LUNGS

p., dorsal rigid. Patient on back with both legs drawn up. Seen in peritonitis, meningitis, ascites, tympanites. In appendicitis the right leg is drawn up. Also occurs in pelvic inflammation or peritonitis of right side, renal calculus in right ureter, and in psoas abscess.

p., orthopnea. Patient sitting upright, hands or elbows resting upon some support. Seen in spasmodic asthma, emphysema, dyspnea, ascites, effusions into the pleural and pericardial cavities, and in late stages of diseases of the heart.

p., orthotonos. Neck and trunk extended rigidly in straight line; seen in tetanus, strychnine poisoning, rabies, or meningitis.

p., prone. Posture assumed after abdominal colic or because of tuberculosis of the spine, eroded vertebrae, abdominal pain, or gastric ulcer.

p., semireclining. Posture used for patients with diseases of heart and interference with respiration in asthma and pleural effusions.

postuterine (pōst-ū'tĕr-ĭn) [L. *post,* after, + *uterus,* womb]. Situated behind the uterus.

postvaccinal (pōst-văk'sĭ-năl) [" + *vaccinus,* pert. to cows]. Following vaccination for smallpox.

potable (pō'tă-bl) [L. *potabilis*]. Suitable for drinking.

Potain's apparatus (pō-tănz'). [Pierre C. E. Potain, Fr. physician, 1825–1901] A form of aspirator.

Potain's sign. In dilatation of the aorta, there will be dullness on percussion over the area extending from the manubrium sterni toward the third costal cartilage on the right, and to the base of the sternum.

potamophobia (pŏt"ă-mō-fō'bē-ă) [Gr. *potamos,* river, + *phobos,* fear]. A morbid fear of large bodies of water.

potash (pŏt'ăsh). Potassium carbonate.

p., caustic. Potassium hydroxide.

p., sulfurated. Liver-colored or greenish-yellow substance made up of potassium thiosulfate and potassium polysulfides and containing 12.8% sulfur as a sulfide. A principal ingredient of white lotion.

potassemia (pŏt-ă-sē'mē-ă) [L. *potassa,* potash, + Gr. *haima,* blood]. Presence of excessive quantity of potassium in the blood.

potassic (pō-tăs'ĭk). Composed of or containing potash.

potassium (pō-tăs'ē-ŭm) [L. *potassa,* potash]. SYMB: K. At. wt. 39.098; at. no. 19; sp. gr. 0.86. Mineral element found in combination with other elements in the body and constituting 0.35% of body weight. SYN: *kalium.*

FUNCT: Potassium is the principal cation in intracellular fluid and is of primary importance in its maintenance. In conjunction with sodium and chloride, it aids in regulation of osmotic pressure and acid-base balance. A proper balance of potassium, calcium, and magnesium ions is essential for normal excitability of muscle tissue, esp. cardiac muscle, and it plays a role in the conduction of nerve impulses.

The usual intake of potassium is 50 to 150 mEq./day. Intake must be monitored carefully to be certain it is adequate in prolonged intravenous feeding, during severe diarrhea or diabetic acidosis, and in patients receiving diuretics. In these conditions an intake of 1 to 3 mEq./kg./day usually is adequate.

CAUTION: *Rapid infusion of potassium intravenously may cause severe hyperkalemia and cardiac arrest.*

DEFICIENCY SYM: Muscle weakness, dizziness, thirst, mental confusion, and changes in the electrocardiogram.

EXCESS: Extracellular potassium is increased in renal failure; in destruction of cells with release of intracellular potassium in burns, crushing injuries, or severe infection; in adrenal insufficiency; in overtreatment with potassium salts; and in metabolic acidosis. This causes weakness and paralysis, impaired electrical conduction in the heart and eventually ventricular fibrillation and death. Hyperkalemia can be treated by withholding potassium and by using drugs such as sodium polystyrene sulfonate, a cation exchange resin, to lower the potassium concentration in cells; and calcium gluconate to counteract the effects on the heart.

SOURCES: Found in most foods. Excellent sources are cereals, dried peas and beans, fresh vegetables, fresh or dried fruits, fruit juices such as orange or prune, sunflower seeds, watermelon, nuts, molasses, cocoa, fresh fish, beef, ham, and poultry.

p. acetate. USP. CH_3COOK. A white powder or crystalline flakes. Used to replenish potassium.

p. alum. Aluminum potassium sulfate; strongly astringent, used topically as a styptic. SEE: *alum.*

p. aminosalicylate. Para-aminosalicylic acid, q.v.

p. arsenite solution. An arsenical solution containing 0.95 to 1.4 gm. of arsenic trioxide in each 100 ml. of solution. SYN: *Fowler's solution.*

p. bicarbonate. USP. $KHCO_3$. White crystals or powder. Used to neutralize acid of the stomach and to treat acid-base imbalance. Trade name is K-Lyte.

p. bitartrate. $KHC_4H_4O_6$. White powder or crystalline salt, used as a dusting powder in place of starch for surgical gloves. SYN: *cream of tartar.*

p. bromide. White cubical crystals of powder, used as a sedative.

p. carbonate. K_2CO_3. A white crystalline powder used in pharmaceutical and chemical preparations. SYN: *potash.*

p. chlorate. $KClO_3$. An explosive white crystalline salt, soluble in water. Formerly used internally in treatment of pharyngitis and stomatitis but its use has been discontinued because of destructive effect on red blood cells.

p. chloride. USP. KCl. A white crystalline salt, soluble in water. One of the three chlorides used in preparation of Ringer's solution. Used in treatment of potassium deficiencies and digitalis intoxication. Trade names are K-Lor, K-Lyte/Cl, Kaochlor, Kaon-Cl, K Ciel, and Slow-K.

p. chromate. K_2CrO_4. Lemon-yellow crystals used as a dye and furniture stain, in manufacture of batteries, in photography, and in laboratories to preserve tissue.

p. citrate. USP. Transparent prismatic crystals. Used as an alkalizer.

INCOMPAT: Caffeine sodium benzoate.

p. cyanide. KCN. A highly poisonous compound used as a fumigant.

p. gluconate. USP. A drug used orally to replenish loss of potassium ion. Trade name is Kaon.

p. guaicosulfonate. USP. Medicine used in some expectorants.

p. hydroxide. KOH. Grayish-white compound used in preparation of soap and as a chemical reagent. SYN: *potash, caustic.*

p. iodide. Colorless or white crystals having a faint odor of iodine. Used as an expectorant.

p. nitrite. Medicine formerly used as a diuretic.

p. permanganate. USP. $KMnO_4$. Crystals of dark purple prisms, odorless, with sweet taste. Used as a topical astringent and antiseptic, as an oxidizing agent, and as an antidote in phosphorus poisoning. Concentrated solutions irritate and even corrode the skin and, when swallowed, induce gastroenteritis. The solutions have considerable power as disinfectants, because their oxidizing ability destroys bacteria. They fail to penetrate deeply in an active form and this renders them of less value than many other disinfectants, except for use in very superficial infections.

p. phosphate, dibasic. USP. A drug used to treat calcium imbalance.

p. sodium tartrate. USP. A saline cathartic.

p. sulfate. K_2SO_4. Has been used as a laxative, but because of its irritant qualities it is not recommended.

p. tartrate. A medicine used as a cathartic.

potassium chlorate poisoning. Large doses cause abdominal discomfort, vomiting, diarrhea, hematuria with nephritis, and disturbances of the blood. Stomach should be washed out, other treatment symptomatic.

CAUTION: Do not induce vomiting.

potassium chromate poisoning. May be contracted by inhalation or from touching the nose with contaminated fingers, causing deep indolent ulcers.

SYM: When taken by mouth has a disagreeable taste, causes cramping, pain, vomiting, diarrhea, slow respiration; may affect liver and kidneys.

NURSING IMPLICATIONS: For ingestion, treat as if poisoned with a strong acid. Dilute with water and milk. BAL or penicillamine may be used.

CAUTION: Do not induce vomiting.

potassium hydroxide poisoning. Characterized by nausea, soapy taste and burning pain in mouth; bloody, slimy vomitus; abdominal cramping; bloody purging and prostration.

NURSING IMPLICATIONS: The patient will require hospitalization, morphine for pain, and most probably treatment for shock. If airway has been burned, then tracheostomy may be required. Corticosteroids and antibiotics will also be given.

CAUTION: Do not induce vomiting.

potbelly. Slang term for the selective deposition of adipose tissue in the abdominal subcutaneous tissue. This usually occurs in middle-aged persons who have sedentary occupations. The condition is accentuated by weakening of the anterior abdominal musculature and lumbar lordosis.

TREATMENT: Weight reduction; exercises to strengthen abdominal muscles; and therapy for lordosis.

potency (pō′tĕn-sē) [L. *potentia,* power]. 1. Strength; force; power. 2. Strength of a medicine. 3. Ability of male to perform coitus.

potent (pō′tĕnt) [L. *potens,* powerful]. 1. Powerful. 2. Highly effective medicinally. 3. Having power of procreation.

potentia coeundi (pō-tĕn′shē-ă kō-ē-ŭn′dī) [L.]. Ability to perform sexual intercourse in a normal manner.

potential. 1. Latent; existing in possibility. 2. In electricity, voltage or electrical pressure; a condition in which a state of tension or pressure exists capable of doing work. When two electrically charged bodies of different potentials are brought together, an electric current passes from the body of high potential to that of low.

p., action. ABBR: A.P. The change in electrical potential of nerve or muscle fiber when stimulated.

p., after. The period occurring subsequent to the spike potential, q.v.

p., demarcation. The difference in potential between an intact longitudinal surface and the injured end of a muscle or nerve. SYN: *p., injury.*

p., injury. P., demarcation.

p., membrane. The electrical charge or potential difference between the inside and the outside of a cell membrane.

p., resting. The potential difference in electrical charge between the inside and outside of a cell at rest.

p., spike. A change in potential that occurs when a cell membrane is stimulated.

potentiate (pō-tĕn′shē-āt). To augment or increase the potency or action.

potentiation (pō-tĕn″shē-ā′shŭn). The synergistic action of two substances, such as hormones or drugs, in which the total effects are greater than the sum of the independent effects of the two substances.

potentiometer (pō-tĕn″shē-ŏm′ĕ-tĕr). A voltmeter.

potion (pō′shŭn) [L. *potio,* draft]. A drink or draught; a dose of poison or liquid medicine.

Pott's disease. [Percivall Pott, Brit. surgeon, 1713–1788] Caries or osteitis of the vertebrae, usually of tuberculous origin; tubercular inflammation of bodies of the vertebrae. The disease is primarily a disease of children and of adults up to age 40. Destruction and compression of affected vertebrae often results in kyphosis with resulting compression of spinal cord and nerves. Often infection spreads to paravertebral tissues giving rise to paravertebral abscesses. SYN: *spondylitis, tuberculous.* SEE: *kyphosis.*

SYM: Child will complain of pain in region supplied by the nerves arising from affected segment of the cord—if disease is lumbar, pains are abdominal and apt to be associated with vesical irritability; if dorsal, pains are epigastric or intercostal and respiration sometimes irregular and hurried from failure of respiratory muscles to take the full share in the work; if cervical, neuralgic pain or numbness in hands, a tickling cough, and difficult swallowing. Pains apt to be symmetrical.

Increase of pain on jumping, flexing, or rotating spine is extremely significant. If child can jump painlessly from chair to floor it is almost certain that inflammation of the body of a vertebra is not present. If vertebrae are compressed by pressure on head or shoulders while the patient sits or stands or while he lies face downward across the knees of the surgeon, pain is much increased. If patient is placed in traction, so spine is elongated, relief is obtained.

Involuntary immobilization of spine, as a result of pain on movement, gives a very characteristic military attitude. If child is asked to look at something behind him, he turns his whole trunk. If requested to pick up something from the floor, he stoops by bending the thighs upon the trunk and knees upon the thighs, never by flexing the spinal column in the usual way.

In walking, the patient moves as if on ice, sliding or shuffling along so as to avoid the jar of successive steps. In standing, he fixes the upper portion of the column by aid of the trapezii and other scapular muscles, action of which at the same time raises shoulders and throws arms out from sides. In standing or sitting, there is an involuntary transfer of the weight of head and shoulders and parts above diseased area to the pelvis, by means of the upper extremities. Hands placed upon the hips and arm muscles are tense. In walking about the room, he holds on to furniture for aid. Spinal abscess occurs later, location varying with seat of caries. Paralysis may occur, always motor at first, not affecting sensation at all.

TREATMENT: Endeavor to secure resolution of the tuberculous osteitis. Limit destruction of tissue and resulting deformity. Promote ankylosis if indicated. Evacuate abscess. Remove a sequestrum or the focus of carious bone. Rest in bed in recumbent position. Adequate diet and exercise care to prevent development of decubitus ulcers. Chemotherapy as for pulmonary tuberculosis.

Pott's fracture. Fracture of the lower end of the fibula and medial malleolus of the tibia with dislocation of foot outward and backward. After reduction, foot and leg are put in plaster in which a walking iron is incorporated. The patient is able to walk, and plaster is removed in about 6 weeks.

pouch (powch) [ME. *pouche*]. Any pocket or sac.

p., abdominovesical. The pouch formed by the extension of the peritoneum from the abdominal wall to the distended bladder.

p., branchial. P., pharyngeal.

p., Broca's. A sac in tissues of the labia majora.

p., Heidenhain. A small, surgically constructed pouch of the stomach that is denervated and separated from the stomach and drained to the outside of the body. Used to study the physiology of the stomach.

p., laryngeal. Blind pouch of mucosa entering the ventral portion of the ventricle of the larynx.

p. of Douglas. P., rectouterine.

p., Pavlov. A stomach pouch formed surgically for the experimental study of gastric secretion. A section of the stomach is separated from the main stomach except for the vagal nerves. Named after I. P. Pavlov, who devised the pouch in order to investigate gastric function and conditioned reflexes.

p., pharyngeal. One of a series of five pairs of entodermal outpocketings that develop in lateral walls of the pharynx of the embryo. SYN: *p., branchial.*

p., Prussak's. The anterior recess of the tympanic membrane.

p., Rathke's. An outpocketing of the roof of embryonic stomodeum. Gives rise to the anterior lobe of the hypophysis cerebri.

p., rectouterine. Pouch between anterior rectal wall and posterior uterine wall. SYN: *cul-de-sac; p. of Douglas.*

p., rectovesical. A fold of peritoneum that in the male extends downward between bladder and rectum.

poudrage (pū-drăzh′) [Fr.]. Application of an irritating, but otherwise nontoxic, powder to the pleural space of the lung in order to produce pleural adhesions.

poultice (pōl′tĭs) [L. *pultes,* thick paste]. A hot, moist mass of linseed, mustard, or soap and oil between two pieces of muslin applied to the skin to relieve congestion or pain, to stimulate absorption of inflammatory products, and to act as a counterirritant. SEE: *plaster.*

pound (pownd) [L. *pondus,* weight]. SYMB: lb. A measure of weight of the avoirdupois and the apothecaries systems that is equal to 16 ounces. SEE: *Weights and Measures* in *Appendix.*

p., avoirdupois. Sixteen ounces, equal to 453.59 gm.

p., foot-. Work expended when one pound is moved a distance of one foot in the direction of the force.

p., troy. Twelve ounces, 5760 grains, and equal to 373.242 gm.

Poupart's ligament (pū-părz′). [François Poupart, Fr. anatomist, 1616–1708] The ligament forming the lower border of aponeurosis of external oblique muscle between anterosuperior spine of the ilium and spine of the pubis. SYN: *inguinal ligament.*

Povan. Trade name for pyrvinium pamoate, USP.

poverty. The condition of having an inadequate supply of money, resources, or means of subsistence. Poverty is sometimes defined on the basis of income and sometimes on

budget for an urban family's modest but adequate standard of living. Poverty levels are used to establish eligibility for federal and state aid, such as aid to dependent children, supplemental security income, or food stamps.

povidone (pō'vĭ-dōn). USP. A synthetic polymer used as a dispersing and suspending agent in manufacturing drugs. The name previously used was polyvinylpyrrolidone. Trade name is Pladone.

povidone-iodine. USP. A complex of iodine with povidone. It contains not less than 9% and not more than 12% available iodine. This iodophor is used in dilute concentration as a surgical scrub, aerosol spray, in vaginal douche solutions, and in ointments and gels. Trade names are Betadine and PVP-Iodine.

powder [ME. *poudre*]. 1. Aggregation of fine particles of one or more substances that may be passed through fine meshes. 2. A dose of such a powder, contained in a paper.

power [ME. *power*]. 1. Rate at which work is done. 2. Capacity for action. 3. In optics, the degree to which a lens or optical instrument magnifies. 4. In microscopy, the number of times the diameter of an object is magnified, indicated by placing an × after the number. Ex.: 10× indicates magnification of ten times. 5. In mathematics and in scientific nomenclature, the number of times a value is to be multiplied times itself, i.e., $10^2 = 10 \times 10 = 100$; $10^3 = 10 \times 10 \times 10 = 1000$. A negative power, e.g., 10^{-2}, indicates the reciprocal of that value. For example, $10^{-2} = 1/10^2 = 1/100$.

pox (pŏks) [ME. *pokkes*, pits]. 1. An eruptive, contagious disease. 2. A papular eruption that becomes pustular. SEE: *chickenpox; smallpox.*

poxvirus (pŏks'vī-rŭs). One of a group of DNA viruses that produce characteristic spreading vesicular lesions, often called pocks. It is the largest of the true viruses and includes viruses responsible for smallpox, vaccinia, molluscum contagiosum, and orf. Lower animals are also susceptible to the poxvirus.

P.P. *punctum proximum,* near point of accommodation (in vision).

ppb. *parts per billion.*

P.P.D. *purified protein derivative,* substance used in intradermal test for tuberculosis.

P.P.F. *pellagra preventive factor* in vitamin B.

PPLO. *pleuropneumonia-like organisms,* now called Mycoplasma. SEE: *mycoplasmas.*

ppm. *parts per million.*

Ppt. *precipitate; prepared.*

ppt. *parts per trillion.*

Pr. 1. *presbyopia.* 2. Chem. symb. for praseodymium.

P.R. *punctum remotum,* far point of visual accommodation.

practical nurse. Nurse, licensed practical.

practice (prăk'tĭs) [Gr. *praktike,* business]. The use, by a health care professional, of knowledge and skill to provide a service in the prevention of illness, diagnosis and treatment of illness, and the maintenance of health.

practitioner (prăk-tĭsh'ŭn-ĕr). One who has met the professional and legal requirements necessary to provide a health care service, such as a physician, nurse, dentist, or physical therapist.

prae-. SEE: words beginning with *pre-*.

praecox (prē'kŏks) [L.]. Early.

praevia, praevius (prē'vē-ă, prē'vē-ŭs) [L.]. Going before in time or place

pragmatagnosia (prăg"măt-ăg-nō'zē-ă) [Gr. *pragma,* object, + *agnosia,* lack of recognition]. Inability to recognize objects once familiar.

pragmatamnesia (prăg"măt-ăm-nē'zē-ă) [" + *amnesia,* forgetfulness]. Inability to recall the appearance of an object.

p., visual. Name for the mental condition making possible pragmatamnesia.

pragmatic (prăg-măt'ĭk) [Gr. *pragma,* a thing done]. Pert. to, or concerned with, the practical side of anything.

pragmatism (prăg'mă-tĭzm) [" + *-ismos,* condition]. A belief that the practical application of a principle should be the determining factor.

pragmatist (prăg'mă-tĭst). One who believes that practical application should be the determining factor of a principle.

pralidoxime chloride (prăl"ĭ-dŏks'ēm). USP. A cholinesterase reactivator used in treating poisoning due to certain pesticides or drugs with anticholinesterase activity. Trade name is Protopam Chloride.

pramoxine hydrochloride (prăm-ŏk'sēn). USP. A topical anesthetic. It is too irritating to be used on the eye or in the nose. Trade names are Tronolane and Tronothane Hydrochloride.

prandial (prăn'dē-ăl) [L. *prandium,* breakfast]. Rel. to a meal.

Prantal. Trade name for diphemanil methylsulfate.

praseodymium (prā"sē-ō-dĭm'ē-ŭm) [Gr. *prasios,* leek-green, + *didymium*]. SYMB: Pr. At. wt. 140.907; at. no. 59. A metallic element obtained from rare earth.

Prausnitz-Küstner reaction (prows'nĭts-kĭst'nĕr). [Carl W. Prausnitz, Ger. hygienist, b. 1876; Heinz Küstner, Ger. gynecologist, b. 1897] Intracutaneous injection of the hypersensitive patient's serum into a nonallergic person; then 24–48 hours later, the suspected antigen is applied to the injected site. If a wheal and flare occur, then this is evidence that the suspected antigen is causing the hypersensitivity. Because of the danger of transmitting viral hepatitis, this test is no longer used.

praxinoscope (prăk-sĭn′ō-skōp) [Gr. *praxis,* action, + *skopein,* to examine]. Contrivance for studying the larynx.

praxiology (prăk″sē-ŏl′ō-jē) [″ + *logos,* study]. Study of behavior.

praxis (prăk′sĭs) [Gr., action]. The ability to plan and execute coordinated movement.

-praxis [Gr., action]. Combining form indicating: 1. Act or activity. 2. Practice, use.

Prayer of Maimonides. [Rabbi Moses ben Maimon, Jewish philosopher and physician in Egypt, 1135–1204] A prayer used at graduation ceremonies by some medical schools.

"Thy eternal providence has appointed me to watch over the life and health of Thy creatures. May the love for my art actuate me at all times; may neither avarice nor miserliness, nor thirst for glory, or for a great reputation engage my mind; for the enemies of truth and philanthropy could easily deceive me and make me forgetful of my lofty aim of doing good to Thy children.

"May I never see in the patient anything but a fellow creature in pain.

"Grant me strength, time, opportunity always to correct what I have acquired, always to extend its domain; for knowledge is immense and the spirit of man can extend indefinitely to enrich itself daily with new requirements.

"Today he can discover his errors of yesterday and tomorrow he can obtain a new light on what he thinks himself sure of today. Oh, God, Thou has appointed me to watch over the life and death of Thy creatures; here am I ready for my vocation and now I turn unto my calling." SEE: *Declaration of Geneva; Declaration of Hawaii; Hippocratic oath; Nightingale Pledge.*

prazepam (pră′zē-păm). An anti-anxiety medicine. Trade names are Centrax and Verstran.

praziquantel. A broad-spectrum antischistosomal drug that is very useful in treating infections with helminths such as Hymenolepis nana, and Taenia saginata. It is also quite effective in treating infections with Diphyllobothrium latum. Trade names are Biltricide and Droncit.

prazosin hydrochloride. Drug used in treating hypertension. It acts as an alpha-adrenergic receptor blocker.

pre- [L. *prae,* before]. Prefix indicating before or in front of.

preadmission certification. Review of the need for proposed inpatient services prior to the time of admission to an institution.

preagonal (prē-ăg′ō-năl) [L. *prae,* before, + Gr. *agonia,* agony]. Pert. to condition immediately before death agony.

prealbuminuric (prē″ăl-bū″mĭn-ū′rĭk) [″ + *albumen,* white of egg]. Before the appearance of albuminuria.

preanal (prē-ā′năl) [″ + *anus,* anus]. In front of the anus.

preanesthesia (prē″ăn-ĕs-thē′zē-ă). A light anesthesia produced by medication given prior to the anesthesia.

preanesthetic (prē″ăn-ĕs-thĕt′ĭk) [L. *prae,* before, + Gr. *anaisthesia,* lack of sensation]. Preliminary drug given to facilitate induction of general anesthesia.

preantiseptic (prē″ăn-tĭ-sĕp′tĭk) [″ + Gr. *anti,* against, + *sepsis,* decay]. Before the adoption of antisepsis in surgery.

preaortic (prē″ā-or′tĭk) [″ + Gr. *aorte,* aorta]. Located in front of the aorta.

preataxic (prē-ă-tăk′sĭk) [″ + Gr. *ataxia,* disorder]. Before the onset of ataxia.

preauricular (prē″aw-rĭk′ū-lăr) [″ + *auricula,* little ear]. Located in front of the ear.

preaxial (prē-ăk′sē-ăl) [L. *prae,* before, + Gr. *axon,* axis]. In front of the axis of a limb or of the body.

precancer (prē′kăn-sĕr) [″ + L. *cancer,* crab]. A condition that tends to become malignant.

precancerous (prē-kăn′sĕr-ŭs) [″ + *cancer,* crab]. Said of a growth that is not yet, but probably will become, cancerous.

precapillary [″ + *capillaris,* hairlike]. An arterial capillary; one that branches from an arteriole or venule. SYN: *metarteriole.*

precava (prē-kā′vă) [″ + *cavus,* hollow]. The descending or superior vena cava. SEE: *vena cava superior* [NA].

precentral (prē-sĕn′trăl) [″ + Gr. *kentron,* center]. In front of a center, as the central fissure of the brain.

precentral convolution. The ascending frontal convolution of the brain.

prechordal (prē-kor′dăl) [″ + Gr. *chorde,* cord]. In front of the notochord.

precipitable (prē-sĭp′ĭ-tă-b'l). Capable of being precipitated.

precipitant (prē-sĭp′ĭ-tănt) [L. *praecipitare,* to cast down]. A substance bringing about precipitation.

precipitate (prē-sĭp′ĭ-tāt). 1. A deposit separated from a suspension or solution by precipitation, the reaction of a reagent that causes the deposit to fall to the bottom or float near the top. 2. To separate as a precipitate. 3. Occurring suddenly or unexpectedly.

precipitation (prē-sĭp″ĭ-tā′shŭn) [L. *praecipitatio*]. 1. Process of a substance being separated from a solution by action of a reagent so that a precipitate forms. 2. The sudden and unprepared-for delivery of an infant. SEE: *delivery, precipitate.*

precipitation test. Test in which positive reaction is indicated by formation of a precipitate in the solution being tested.

precipitin (prē-sĭp'ĭ-tĭn). An antibody formed in the blood serum of an animal due to presence of a soluble antigen, usually a protein. When added to a solution of the antigen, it brings about precipitation. The injected protein is called the antigen and the antibody produced is the precipitin. It was originally thought that these antibodies were members of a unique class, but most antibodies are capable of precipitating when combined with their antigens. SEE: *autoprecipitin; precipitinogen.*

precipitinogen (prē-sĭp"ĭ-tĭn'ō-jĕn). Any protein that, acting as an antigen, stimulates the production of a specific precipitin.

precipitinoid (prĕ-sĭp'ĭt-ĭn-oyd). Precipitin that can no longer cause precipitation when mixed with its antigen, but that retains its affinity to the antigen.

precipitin reaction, test. The formation of a precipitate in a solution containing a soluble antigen upon addition of serum containing the specific precipitin. The reaction is specific. The test is used for identification of unknown proteins; determination of types of pneumococci and meningococci; and determination of types of blood stains, whether human or animal.

precipitophore (prē-sĭp'ĭt-ō-for"). The part of a precipitin that produces the actual precipitation. SEE: *haptophore.*

precipitum (prē-sĭp'ĭ-tŭm). The precipitate produced by action of a precipitin.

preclinical (prē-klĭn'ĭ-kăl) [L. *prae,* before, + Gr. *klinike,* medical treatment in bed]. Occurring before diagnosis of a definite disease is possible.

preclinical (dental) training. Study and mastery of the theory and techniques related to the various dental procedures required prior to treating human patients.

preclinical technique. In dentistry, the use of manikins, mechanical articulator, artificial or extracted teeth, and the variety of dental instruments and materials to study and master the techniques necessary to do clinical dentistry.

preclival (prē-klī'văl) [" + *clivus,* slope]. In front of the cerebellar clivus.

precocious (prē-kō'shŭs) [L. *praecox,* ripening]. Either mental or physical development earlier than would be expected.

precocity (prē-kŏs'ĭ-tē) [L. *praecox,* ripening early]. Premature development of physical or mental traits.

p., sexual. Premature genital maturation; precocious sexual maturity.

precognition (prē"kŏg-nĭsh'ŭn) [L. *prae,* before, + *cognoscere,* to know]. Prior knowledge that an event will occur even though there is no rational explanation of why one would have that knowledge.

precoital (prē-kō'ĭ-tăl) [" + *coitio,* a going together]. Prior to sexual intercourse.

precoma (prē-kō'mă) [" + Gr. *koma,* a deep sleep]. The mental state immediately prior to a coma.

preconscious (prē-kŏn'shŭs) [" + *conscius,* aware]. Not present in consciousness but able to be recalled as desired.

preconvulsive (prē"kŏn-vŭl'sĭv) [" + *convulsio,* pulling together]. Before a convulsion.

precordia (prē-kor'dē-ă) [L. *praecordia*]. The precordium.

precordial (prē-kor'dē-ăl). Pert. to the precordium or epigastrium.

precordialgia (prē"kor-dē-ăl'jē-ă) [L. *praecordia,* precordia, + Gr. *algos,* pain]. Pain in the chest or precordial area.

precordium (prē-kor'dē-ŭm). The area on the anterior surface of the body overlying the heart and the lower part of the thorax. SYN: *antecardium; precordia.*

precornu (prē-kor'nū) [L. *prae,* before, + *cornu,* horn]. Anterior horn of lateral ventricle of the brain.

precostal (prē-kŏs'tăl) [" + *costa,* rib]. In front of the ribs.

precritical (prē-krĭt'ĭ-kăl) [" + Gr. *kritikos,* critical]. Prior to the occurrence of a crisis.

precuneus (prē-kū'nē-ŭs) [" + *cuneus,* wedge]. [NA] The division of the mesial surface of a cerebral hemisphere between the cuneus and the paracentral lobule.

precursor. A substance that precedes another substance.

predentin. Uncalcified dentinal matrix.

prediabetes (prē-dī"ă-bē'tēz) [" + Gr. *diabetes,* passing through]. The condition prior to the development of clinical diabetes.

prediastole (prē"dī-ăs'tō-lē) [" + Gr. *diastellein,* to expand]. The period in the cardiac cycle immediately prior to diastole.

prediastolic (prē"dī-ă-stŏl'ĭk) [" + Gr. *diastole,* expansion]. Before the diastole, or interval in the cardiac cycle that precedes it.

predicrotic (prē"dī-krŏt'ĭk) [" + Gr. *dikrotos,* beating double]. Preceding the dicrotic wave of the sphygmographic tracing.

predigestion (prē"dĭ-jĕs'chŭn) [" + *digestio,* carrying apart]. Artificial proteolysis or digestion of proteins and amylolysis of starches before ingestion.

predisposing (prē"dĭs-pōz'ĭng) [" + *disponere,* to dispose]. Indicating a tendency to, or susceptibility to, disease.

predisposition (prē"dĭs-pō-zĭsh'ŭn). The potential to develop a certain disease or condition in the presence of specific environmental stimuli.

prednisolone (prĕd-nĭs'ō-lōn). USP. A glucocorticosteroid drug. It is available in a variety of dosage forms. Trade names are Delta-Cortef, Hydeltra, Metiderm, and Sterane.

prednisone (prĕd'nĭ-sōn). USP. A steroid hormone with the same effects as cortisone. Trade names are Deltasone, Meticorten, Orasone, and SK-Prednisone.

predormition (prē-dor-mĭ'shŭn) [" + *dormire,* to sleep]. State of unconsciousness immediately preceding actual sleep.

pre-eclampsia (prē"ē-klămp'sē-ă) [" + Gr. *ek,* out, + *lampein,* to flash]. A toxemia of pregnancy characterized by increasing hypertension, headaches, albuminuria, and edema of the lower extremities. If this condition is neglected or not treated properly, the patient may develop true eclampsia. SEE: *eclampsia.*

pre-eruptive (prē"ē-rŭp'tĭv) [" + *eruptio,* a breaking out]. Before an eruption.

pre-excitation (prē-ĕk"sī-tā'shŭn) [" + *excitare,* to arouse]. Premature excitation of the ventricle by an impulse that traveled a path other than through the atrioventricular node. This produces a short P-R interval.

pre-existing condition. Any injury, disease, or physical condition occurring prior to an arbitrary date; usually used in reference to the issuance of a health insurance policy. This often results in an exclusion from coverage for costs resulting from the injury, disease, or condition.

Prefrin Liquifilm. Trade name for phenylephrine hydrochloride, USP.

prefrontal (prē-frŏn'tăl) [" + *frons,* front]. 1. The middle portion of the ethmoid bone. 2. In anterior part of the frontal lobe of the brain.

preganglionic (prē"găng-lē-ŏn'ĭk) [" + Gr. *ganglion,* knot]. Situated in front of or anterior to a ganglion.

preganglionic fiber. The axon of a preganglionic neuron.

preganglionic neuron. The first of a series of two efferent neurons that transmit impulses to visceral effectors. Its cell body lies in the central nervous system. Its axon terminates in an autonomic ganglion.

pregenital (prē-jĕn'ĭ-tăl) [" + *genitalia,* genitals]. In psychology, rel. to that period when erotic interest in the reproductive organs and functions is not yet organized.

pregnancy (prĕg'năn-sē) [L. *praegnans*]. The condition of carrying a developing embryo in the uterus. SEE: Pregnancy Table for Expected Date of Delivery.

SYM AND SIGNS: Presumptive signs are amenorrhea, nausea and vomiting, inordinate appetite, pigmentation of the areola of the breasts, the development of Montgomery's tubercles around the nipple, changes in the cervix and uterus (softening and progressive enlargement), vaginal and cervical discoloration, and frequent urination.

Positive signs are hearing and counting the fetal heartbeat, detection of movements of the fetus, and use of ultrasound to detect the fetal outline. There are various immunodiagnostic tests for pregnancy and these are 90 to 95% accurate. These tests are based on various methods of detecting human chorionic gonadotropin (HCG) in the urine or serum.

The duration of pregnancy is approximately 280 days. To estimate the day of delivery, count back 3 months from the day of onset of the last menstrual period and then add 7 days. For example, if the last menstrual period began the 10th of June, subtracting 3 months leaves March 10th and adding 7 days indicates the expected day of delivery would be March 17 of the next year. This method assumes all months have the same number of days; thus the date determined will not agree exactly with that found by using the Pregnancy Table.

PHYSICAL CHANGES: *Uterus:* Changes shape, size, and consistency; lining undergoes changes; peritoneal covering enlarges; muscle mass increases enormously.

Vaginal Canal: Elongation caused by rising of uterus in pelvis; mucosa thickens; secretion increased; increased vascularity and elasticity; cervix, vagina, and vulva become softer.

Abdominal: Growing distention and flattened navel; striae gravidarum.

Breasts: Enlarged and tender; skin thin and sensitive; nipple erectile and areola enlarged and darker; escape of colostrum; tingling sensation.

Endocrine Glands: Thyroid increases in size and activity; parathyroids enlarge and secretion increases; pituitary increases its activity; placenta produces hormones, affecting ovaries and corpus luteum.

Circulatory System: Increased activity; increased blood volume; blood pressure should be normal; varicose veins may be present.

Skeletal: Pelvic joints soften; pelvic joints more movable; bones and teeth affected.

Respiratory: Lungs impeded in late pregnancy; breathing is deeper and more frequent.

Digestive Tract: Nausea and vomiting in early pregnancy; appetite affected; loss of weight in early pregnancy with slight anemia; basal metabolism raised in later pregnancy; constipation frequent.

Liver: Displaced in late pregnancy.

Skin: Sudoriparous and sebaceous glands very active; deposit of brown pigment on face (mask of pregnancy); linea nigra.

Weight: In normal-size individuals, the weight gain is 2 to 3 pounds (907 to 1361 grams) per month of pregnancy. Weight gain above 30 pounds (13.6 kg.) is not desired.

Pregnancy Table for Expected Date of Delivery

Find the date of the last menstrual period in the top line (light-face type) of the pair of lines.
The dark number (bold-face type) in the line below will be the expected day of delivery.

Jan.	1	2	3	4	5	6	7	8	9	10	11	12	13	14	15	16	17	18	19	20	21	22	23	24	25	26	27	28	29	30	31	
Oct.	8	9	10	11	12	13	14	15	16	17	18	19	20	21	22	23	24	25	26	27	28	29	30	31	(1	2	3	4	5	6	7	Nov.
Feb.	1	2	3	4	5	6	7	8	9	10	11	12	13	14	15	16	17	18	19	20	21	22	23	24	25	26	27	28				
Nov.	8	9	10	11	12	13	14	15	16	17	18	19	20	21	22	23	24	25	26	27	28	29	30	(1	2	3	4	5				Dec.
Mar.	1	2	3	4	5	6	7	8	9	10	11	12	13	14	15	16	17	18	19	20	21	22	23	24	25	26	27	28	29	30	31	
Dec.	6	7	8	9	10	11	12	13	14	15	16	17	18	19	20	21	22	23	24	25	26	27	28	29	30	31	(1	2	3	4	5	Jan.
April	1	2	3	4	5	6	7	8	9	10	11	12	13	14	15	16	17	18	19	20	21	22	23	24	25	26	27	28	29	30		
Jan.	6	7	8	9	10	11	12	13	14	15	16	17	18	19	20	21	22	23	24	25	26	27	28	29	30	31	(1	2	3	4		Feb.
May	1	2	3	4	5	6	7	8	9	10	11	12	13	14	15	16	17	18	19	20	21	22	23	24	25	26	27	28	29	30	31	
Feb.	5	6	7	8	9	10	11	12	13	14	15	16	17	18	19	20	21	22	23	24	25	26	27	28	(1	2	3	4	5	6	7	Mar.
June	1	2	3	4	5	6	7	8	9	10	11	12	13	14	15	16	17	18	19	20	21	22	23	24	25	26	27	28	29	30		
Mar.	8	9	10	11	12	13	14	15	16	17	18	19	20	21	22	23	24	25	26	27	28	29	30	31	(1	2	3	4	5	6		April
July	1	2	3	4	5	6	7	8	9	10	11	12	13	14	15	16	17	18	19	20	21	22	23	24	25	26	27	28	29	30	31	
April	7	8	9	10	11	12	13	14	15	16	17	18	19	20	21	22	23	24	25	26	27	28	29	30	(1	2	3	4	5	6	7	May
Aug.	1	2	3	4	5	6	7	8	9	10	11	12	13	14	15	16	17	18	19	20	21	22	23	24	25	26	27	28	29	30	31	
May	8	9	10	11	12	13	14	15	16	17	18	19	20	21	22	23	24	25	26	27	28	29	30	31	(1	2	3	4	5	6	7	June
Sept.	1	2	3	4	5	6	7	8	9	10	11	12	13	14	15	16	17	18	19	20	21	22	23	24	25	26	27	28	29	30		
June	8	9	10	11	12	13	14	15	16	17	18	19	20	21	22	23	24	25	26	27	28	29	30	(1	2	3	4	5	6	7		July
Oct.	1	2	3	4	5	6	7	8	9	10	11	12	13	14	15	16	17	18	19	20	21	22	23	24	25	26	27	28	29	30	31	
July	8	9	10	11	12	13	14	15	16	17	18	19	20	21	22	23	24	25	26	27	28	29	30	31	(1	2	3	4	5	6	7	Aug.
Nov.	1	2	3	4	5	6	7	8	9	10	11	12	13	14	15	16	17	18	19	20	21	22	23	24	25	26	27	28	29	30		
Aug.	8	9	10	11	12	13	14	15	16	17	18	19	20	21	22	23	24	25	26	27	28	29	30	31	(1	2	3	4	5	6		Sept.
Dec.	1	2	3	4	5	6	7	8	9	10	11	12	13	14	15	16	17	18	19	20	21	22	23	24	25	26	27	28	29	30	31	
Sept.	7	8	9	10	11	12	13	14	15	16	17	18	19	20	21	22	23	24	25	26	27	28	29	30	(1	2	3	4	5	6	7	Oct.

Posture: Changes as enlargement of abdomen advances; sacroiliac joints and symphysis pubis more movable; painful locomotion and backache; gait may be altered.

Urinary Tract: Increased kidney activity; failure of kidneys produces nephritic toxemia; ureters, esp. right one, dilated; pressure on bladder; frequent urination in late pregnancy; bladder lifted into abdomen and pressure diminished. Bladder later pressed upon by presenting part; urinary output varies; presence of albumin abnormal.

DISORDERS OF: *Nausea and vomiting:* May be noted when stomach is empty, but may occur at any time. Four or five small meals per day may control this.

Constipation and flatulence: Pressure of uterus on intestines may be a cause; stool softeners and an increase in fiber content of diet may help; intestinal stasis may cause flatulence; gas-forming foods should be avoided.

Muscular cramps: Rest between periods of standing. Tetany may ensue because of deficient calcium supply; calcium and vitamin D supplement indicated.

Pressure edema: May occur at end of pregnancy with condition better in morning and worse at night. Frequent rest and elevation of limbs indicated. May be due to calcium deficiency. Toxemia must be considered. The blood pressure and weight should be recorded, and a urinalysis done at each prenatal visit. All of these will help to alert the physician to the possible development of toxemia of pregnancy.

Headache: Cause may be sinusitis or toxemia.

Toothache: May be due to caries induced by deficient calcium. Frequent dental examinations desirable.

Backache: Abnormal balance caused by protruding abdomen; proper shoes indicated. Intra-abdominal pressure may be a cause; flatulence aggravates; enemas may help.

Dyspnea: Pressure of uterus upward on transverse colon and stomach; aggravated by flatulence, esp. when lying down. Alkalies may help; pillows under head and shoulder indicated; reexamination of heart indicated.

Vaginal discharge: Routine perineal hygiene but douches are not indicated. Foul, blood-tinged, or profuse discharge should be reported.

Pruritus: Breasts, abdomen, and vulva may be affected; stretching of skin of abdomen a cause in that area. If general, a toxic or nervous origin may be cause. Sugar in urine may cause pruritus of vulva.

Heartburn: Hyperacidity or nervous tension may be responsible. Sedation, frequent small meals, no highly seasoned foods.

Varicose veins: Aggravated by pregnancy. May occur in pelvis, vulva, and legs. Avoid round garters, tight clothing, and standing. Rest and support stockings indicated; elevation of lower limbs while sleeping; Sims' position, pillow under hips to shift uterus.

Hemorrhoids: Avoid constipation. Ointments, wet compresses, suppositories on doctor's orders; surgical therapy may be required.

p., abdominal. Pregnancy with implantation of the ovum in the abdominal cavity. SYN: *p., extrauterine; p., ectopic.*

p., ampullar. Pregnancy in the ampulla of the uterine tube.

p., bigeminal. Pregnancy with twins in utero.

p., cervical. Pregnancy with implantation of the ovum in the cervical canal.

p., cornual. Pregnancy in one of the horns of the bicornuate uterus.

p., ectopic. Pregnancy where ovum develops outside the uterus. SEE: illus.

p., extrauterine. Pregnancy where ovum develops outside the uterine cavity. SYN: *p., ectopic.*

p., false. P., phantom.

p., heterotopic. Combined intrauterine and extrauterine pregnancies.

p., hydatid. Pregnancy giving rise to a hydatidiform mole. SEE: *hydatid mole.*

p., interstitial. Pregnancy that occurs in the uterine wall where the oviduct is formed. SYN: *p., intramural.*

p., intraligamentary. Pregnancy that occurs within the broad ligament.

p., intramural. P., interstitial.

p., mask of. Area of brown pigmentation sometimes appearing on the face during pregnancy. SYN: *chloasma gravidarum.*

p., membranous. Pregnancy in which the amniotic sac ruptures and fetus comes to lie in direct contact with the uterine wall.

p., mesenteric. P., tuboligamentary.

p., molar. Pregnancy in which instead of the ovum developing into an embryo, it develops into a mole.

p., multiple. State of having more than one fetus in the uterus during the same pregnancy.

p., mural. P., interstitial, q.v.

p., ovarian. Implantation of the fertilized ovum in the substance of the ovary.

p., phantom. Enlargement of the abdomen simulating pregnancy. SYN: *p., false; pseudopregnancy.* SEE: *pseudocyesis.*

p., tubal. A form of ectopic pregnancy in which the embryo develops in the fallopian tube.

p., tuboabdominal. Pregnancy in which part of the fetus is in the uterine tube and part in the abdominal cavity.

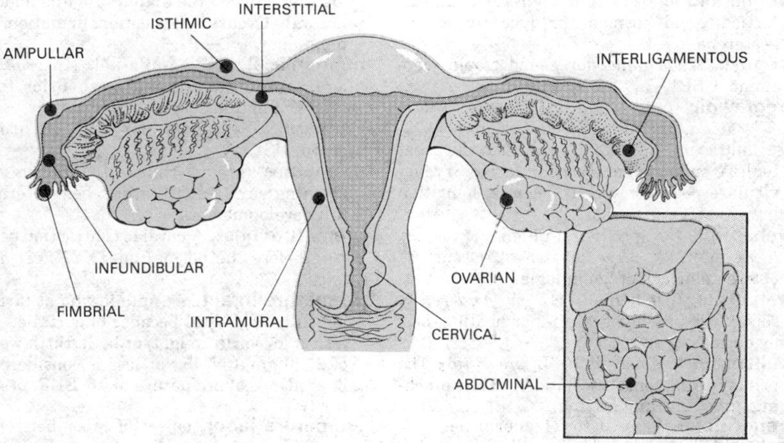

VARIOUS SITES OF ECTOPIC PREGNANCY

p., tuboligamentary. Pregnancy occurring in the uterine tube and extending into the broad ligament. SYN: *p., mesenteric.*

p., tubo-ovarian. Pregnancy in which development of the fetus occurs in both the uterine tube and the ovary.

p., uteroabdominal. Twin pregnancy with one embryo in the uterus and the other in the abdominal cavity.

pregnancy-specific β_1 glycoprotein. A protein that is found in 97% of women who have been pregnant for 6 to 8 weeks and in 100% at later stages of pregnancy. The function of this protein is not known, but it may be useful in estimating the quality of placental function.

pregnancy test. In addition to the clinical signs and symptoms of pregnancy, almost none of which are reliable within the first several weeks of pregnancy, there are chemical tests for pregnancy that are quite accurate by as early as the time the first menstrual period is missed. There are also test kits that are available for purchase without a prescription. If that type of test is used, it is very important to follow the directions carefully.

A major class of pregnancy tests is those using immunodiagnostic procedures. They are: hemagglutination inhibition test, which requires a sample of urine (trade name is Pregnosticon); agglutination inhibition test, which requires a sample of urine (trade name is Gravindex); radioreceptor assay, which requires blood from the patient; radioimmunoassay, which requires a blood sample; and monoclonal antibody determination, which requires a sample of urine. In general, these tests are accurate beginning the 40th day following the first day of the last menstrual period; the monoclonal antibody test is somewhat more sensitive. Reliability of the test methods increases as pregnancy continues.

pregnane (prĕg′nān). The organic compound that is a precursor of two series of steroid hormones: the progesterones and several adrenal cortical hormones.

pregnanediol (prĕg″nān-dī′ŏl). $C_{21}H_{36}O_2$. The inactive end product of metabolism of progesterone present in the urine. Amount in urine increases during premenstrual or luteal phase of menstrual cycle and during pregnancy.

pregnanetriol (prĕg″nān-trī′ŏl). A metabolite of progesterone. Its presence in the urine is increased in those who have congenital adrenal hyperplasia.

pregnant (prĕg′nănt) [L. *praegnans*]. Having conceived; with child. SYN: *gravid.*

pregnene (prĕg'nēn). A steroid that forms the nucleus of progesterone.

pregneninolone (prĕg"nēn-ĭn'ō-lōn). A progestin, ethisterone.

pregnenolone (prĕg-nĕn'ō-lōn). A synthetic corticosteroid hormone produced from progesterone.

Pregnyl. Trade name for gonadotropin, chorionic, USP.

pregravidic (prē-gră-vĭd'ĭk) [L. *prae,* before, + *gravida,* pregnant]. Before pregnancy.

prehallux (prē-hăl'ŭks) [" + *hallux,* the great toe]. A supernumerary bone, accessory naviculare pedis, or sometimes a prolongation inward of it on the foot.

prehemiplegic (prē"hĕm-ĭ-plē'jĭk) [" + Gr. *hemi,* half, + *plege,* a stroke]. Occurring before an attack of hemiplegia.

prehensile (prē-hĕn'sĭl) [L. *prehendere,* to seize]. Adapted for grasping or holding, esp. by encircling an object.

prehension (prē-hĕn'shŭn) [L. *prehensio*]. The primary function of the hand; includes pinching, grasping, and seizing.

prehormone. A precursor of a hormone.

prehyoid (prē-hī'oyd) [L. *prae,* before, + Gr. *hyoeides,* U-shaped]. In front of the hyoid bone.

prehypophysis (prē"hī-pŏf'ĭ-sĭs) [" + Gr. *hypophysis,* an undergrowth]. Anterior lobe of the pituitary gland.

preictal (prē-ĭk'tăl) [" + *ictus,* stroke]. The period just prior to a stroke or convulsion.

preicteric (prē-ĭk-tĕr'ĭk) [" + *ikteros,* jaundice]. In liver disease, the period prior to the appearance of jaundice.

preimmunization (prē-ĭm"ū-nĭ-zā'shŭn) [L. *prae,* before, + *immunis,* safe]. Immunization produced artificially in very young infants.

preinvasive (prē"ĭn-vā'sĭv) [" + *in,* into, + *vadere,* to go]. A stage of development of a malignancy in which the neoplastic cells have not invaded adjacent tissues.

Preiser's disease (prī'zĕrz). [Georg K.F. Preiser, Ger. orthopedic surgeon, 1879–1913] Osteoporosis caused by trauma and affecting the scaphoid bone of the wrist.

preleukemia. A group of nondiagnostic physical and blood abnormalities that may indicate leukemia will develop later. These include unexplained anemia, purpura, susceptibility to infections, or slow healing of skin and mucous membrane lesions. Possible laboratory findings are anemia, neutropenia, sometimes a relative lymphopenia, and marked monocytosis. In general, the diagnosis of preleukemia is made in retrospect because all of the findings and signs may be reversible abnormalities that occur in patients with various other illnesses.

Preludin. Trade name for phenmetrazine hydrochloride.

prelum (prē'lŭm) [L.]. Pressure or compression.

p. abdominale. Squeezing of abdominal viscera between the diaphragm and abdominal wall. Occurs in defecation, urination, and pregnancy.

premaniacal (prē"mā-nī'ă-kăl) [L. *prae,* before, + Gr. *mania,* madness]. Prior to an attack of mania.

Premarin. Trade name for estrogens, conjugated, USP.

premature (prē-mă-chūr') [L. *praematurus,* ripening early]. Not mature; before term or full development.

premature beat. A cardiac contraction occurring before the normal one. SYN: *extrasystole.*

premature infant. An infant who at birth is not fully developed because of curtailed gestation, low birth weight, or both. Birth weight of 2500 gm. (5.5 lb.) or less is considered to be evidence of premature birth. SEE: *prematurity.*

premature labor. Onset of labor before full term.

prematurity. The state of an infant born any time prior to completion of the 37th week of gestation. The normal gestation period for the human being is 40 weeks. Because of the difficulty of obtaining accurate and objective data concerning the exact length of gestation, a birth weight of 2500 gm. (5.5 lb.) or less has been accepted internationally as the clinical criterion of prematurity regardless of the period of gestation. Other measures suggestive of prematurity are crown-heel length (47 cm. or less), crown-rump length (32 cm. or less), occipitofrontal circumference (33 cm. or less), occipitofrontal diameter (11.5 cm. or less), and ratio of the thorax circumference to the head circumference (less than 93%).

The use of a single-criterion measure (birth weight) imposes limitations in accurately identifying those infants born before adequate development of body organs and systems has been achieved; it can easily include mature infants who are of low birth weight for reasons other than a shortened gestation period. The Expert Committee on Prematurity of the World Health Organization (1961) has recommended that the concept of prematurity in the international definition be replaced by that of low birth weight. This term, low birth weight, more accurately describes infants weighing less than 2500 gm. at birth than does the term prematurity; the latter should be reserved for those neonates within the low birth weight group with evidence of incomplete development.

In the United States approx. 7.1% white

Percentage Distribution and Survival of Low–Birth Weight Infants

Birth Weight Group	Total Live Births* (percent)	Low–Birth Weight Infants Only* (percent)	Approximate Survival of Low–Birth Weight Infants** (percent)
Under 1000 grams	0.5	6.25	10
1001–1500 grams	0.7	8.75	50
1501–2000 grams	1.5	18.75	85
2001–2500 grams	5.3	66.25	95
Total 2500 grams or less:	8.0	100.00	85***
Total 2500 grams or over:	92.0		
Total Live Births:	100.0		

*U.S. National Vital Statistics 1962.
**New York City Infant Mortality Rates 1962.
***Weighted average.

liveborn and 13.4% nonwhite infants weighed 2500 gm. or less. Chances of survival depend upon degree of maturity achieved, general condition, and quality of care received. SEE: Percentage Distribution and Survival of Low–Birth Weight Infants table.

Prematurity is the leading cause of death in the neonatal period; mortality among infants weighing less than 2500 gm. at birth is seventeen times greater than among infants with birth weight above 2500 gm. Chief causes of mortality are abnormal pulmonary ventilation, infection, intracranial hemorrhage, abnormal blood conditions, and congenital anomalies.

ETIOL: The incidence of neonates of low birth weight is more frequent among the female sex, nonwhite races, plural births, and the first- and fifth- (and over) born infants. Delivery of infants of low birth weight is reported to be more frequent among women with one or more of the following characteristics: who have their children at either a very young age or between age 45 and 49; being unmarried; having children closely spaced, i.e., less than 2 to 4 years between births; living in a large urban area.

Another factor associated with low birth weight is the socioeconomic status of the family as measured by the mother's educational attainment. The proportion of infants of low birth weight born to mothers with 16 years or more of education was half of that of infants born to mothers with less than 9 years of education. Low birth weight is also associated with generally elevated risk of infant mortality, congenital malformations, mental retardation, and various other physical and neurological impairments.

COMPLICATIONS: Frequently, premature infants are handicapped by a number of anatomical and physiological limitations. These limitations vary in direct proportion to the degree of immaturity present. Limitations include weakness of the sucking and swallowing reflexes, small capacity of stomach, impairment of renal function, incomplete development of capillaries of medulla and lungs, immature alveoli of the lungs, weakness of the cough and gag reflexes, weakness of the thoracic cage muscles and muscles used in respiration, inadequate regulation of body temperature, incomplete or poorly developed enzyme systems, hepatic immaturity, and deficient placental transfer and antenatal storage of minerals, vitamins, and immune substances.

NURSING IMPLICATIONS: Perform a physical assessment that is correlated with expected maturation at the fetal age; this will include neurological evaluation; perform Apgar rating; provide: a proper environmental temperature, proper fluid and caloric intake, appropriate parental bonding and support; assess laboratory reports; monitor intake and output; notify the nursery of the birth of the possible premature infant; weigh infant daily without clothing and on the same scale and at the same time; monitor oxygen concentration at frequent intervals; hold and cuddle infant during feedings; cover sufficiently when removing infant from isolette; and provide adequate time for feeding.

Care of low–birth weight infants: Care of low–birth weight infants should be individualized and reflect the needs of the developing organism in relation to the presence of anatomical and physiological handicaps. Evaluation for degree of immaturity present and the identification of special problems appearing after birth will dictate care required by these infants. In general, care revolves around the prevention of infection, stabilization of body temperature, maintenance of respiration, provision for adequate nutrition and hydration, and conservation of energy.

Aseptic technique is practiced to prevent infection. An incubator or heated bed provides a suitable environment for maintenance of body temperature. A high-humidity environment may be of value in respiratory difficulties. Gentle nasal and pharyngeal suctioning will aid to keep airways clear. Use of oxygen should be restricted to those minimal amounts required for survival of infant. Because of the danger of retrolental fibroplasia, the oxygen concentration should not exceed 30%.

Depending upon the ability of the infant to suck and swallow, gavage feedings may be necessary. Some of these infants may not be given anything by mouth for as long as 72 hours following birth. Caloric and fluid intakes are gradually increased until 100–120 Cal./kg. and 140–150 ml./kg., respectively, in 24 hr. are reached. The time required to achieve these intakes depends upon the size and condition of the newborn baby. Small, frequent feedings may be needed to cope with the small capacity of the stomach, to prevent vomiting and distention, and to meet caloric and fluid requirements of the body. Overfeeding should be avoided. During early days of life, clyses sometimes are administered to maintain adequate hydration.

The infant should not be allowed to become fatigued either from excessive handling, prolonged feeding procedures, or too much crying. Body position should be changed every 2 to 4 hours. Minimal handling regimen should not be used indiscriminately; gentle handling, rather than minimal handling, should be practiced. It is essential that the newborn and infant be cuddled at least several times a day.

premaxilla (prē″măk-sĭl′ă) [L. *prae,* before, + *maxilla,* upper jaw]. A separate element, derived from the median nasal process embryologically, that fuses with the maxilla in man; formerly called the incisive bone.

premaxillary (prē-măk′sĭ-lĕr″ē). Located before the maxilla.

premedication (prē″mĕd-ĭ-kā′shŭn) [″ + *medicari,* to heal]. Induction of unconsciousness by internal drugs prior to administration of inhalation anesthesia. SYN: *prenarcosis.*

premenarchal (prē″mĕ-năr′kăl) [″ + Gr. *men,* month, + *arche,* beginning]. The time prior to the first menstrual period, i.e., prior to menarche.

premenstrual (prē-mĕn′stroo-ăl) [″ + *menstruare,* to menstruate]. Before menstruation.

premenstrual (tension) syndrome. A syndrome that occurs several days prior to the onset of menstruation. Characterized by one or more of the following: irritability, emotional tension, anxiety, mood changes, esp. depression, headache, breast tenderness with or without swelling, water retention, which may be sufficient enough to cause edema. The symptoms subside close to the onset of menstruation.

ETIOL: Not completely understood, but related to the alterations in estrogen and progesterone during the menstrual cycle.

TREATMENT: Depends on the severity of symptoms. Mild analgesics may be helpful, but in severe cases restriction of salt intake and use of a diuretic to control fluid retention are indicated.

premenstruum (prē-mĕn′stroo-ŭm) [″ + *menstruum,* monthly fluid]. The period of time prior to menstruation.

premolar (prē-mō′lĕr) [″ + *moles,* a mass]. 1. One of the permanent teeth occurring between the canine and the molar on each side of the jaw. SEE: *dentition.* 2. Before a molar tooth.

premonition (prĕm″ĕ-, prē-mĕ-nĭsh′ŭn) [L. *praemonere,* to warn beforehand]. A feeling of an impending event.

premonitory (prē-mŏn′ĭ-tō-rē) [LL. *praemonitorius*]. Giving a warning, as an early symptom.

premonocyte (prē-mŏn′ō-sīt) [L. *prae,* before, + Gr. *monos,* alone, + *kytos,* cell]. An embryonic cell transitional in development prior to a monocyte.

premorbid (prē-mor′bĭd) [″ + *morbidus,* sick]. Prior to the development of disease.

premunition (prē″mū-nĭsh′ŭn) [″ + *munitio,* a fortification]. Immunity depending upon existence of a long-continued latent infection.

premyeloblast (prē-mī′ĕ-lō-blăst) [″ + Gr. *myelos,* marrow, + *blastos,* germ]. A precursor of the mature myeloblast.

premyelocyte (prē-mī′ĕl-ō-sīt) [″ + ″ + *kytos,* cell]. The cell that is the immediate precursor of a myelocyte.

prenarcosis (prē-năr-kō′sĭs) [″ + Gr. *narkosis,* stuporous condition]. Induction of unconsciousness by drugs before administration of a general inhalation anesthetic. SYN: *premedication.*

prenares (prē-nā′rēz) [″ + *naris,* nostril]. The nostrils.

prenatal (prē-nā′tl) [″ + *natalis,* birth]. Before birth.

prenatal care. Care of the woman during the period of gestation. This consists of periodic examinations for determination of blood pressure, weight, changes in the size of the uterus, condition of the fetus; urinalysis; instruction in nutritional requirements, preparation for labor and delivery, care of the newborn; and provision of suggestions and support to deal with the discomforts of pregnancy.

Scheduled visits at regular intervals offer the opportunity to detect any untoward changes in the condition of the mother so that necessary treatment can be instituted.

prenatal diagnosis. A great number of pathological conditions can be diagnosed prenatally by use of tests such as ultrasound, amniocentesis, q.v., and fetoscopy. Thus the sex of the child and information provided by study of the physical and chemical characteristics of the placenta, fetus, and inherited characteristics can be determined in the early months of pregnancy. If the results of these tests indicate a treatable disease is present, then the indicated therapy can sometimes be instituted prenatally and, if needed, on the first day of life. If the tests indicate an incurable condition, genetic counseling is advisable.

preneoplastic (prē″nē-ō-plăs′tĭk) [″ + *neos,* new, + *plassein,* to form]. Prior to the development of a tumor.

preoperative care (prē-ŏp′er-ă-tĭv) [″ + *operatus,* work]. Care preceding an operation.

NURSING IMPLICATIONS: Instruct the patient to cough, breathe deeply (splinting incision as necessary), turn, and exercise extremities at frequent intervals. Prepare the operative site as prescribed; prepare the gastrointestinal tract as indicated (restrict food and fluids as ordered); promote rest and sleep; review laboratory results; administer preoperative medications as prescribed after the patient has voided. Have patient perform oral hygiene; and remove dentures. Remove jewelry and make-up, apply a patient gown, and verify proper identification is present on the patient identification bracelet. If patient is menstruating, be certain appropriate chart notation is made concerning type of menstrual protection used and be certain that tampons or pads are changed, at least every 4 to 6 hours in the case of tampons.

preoptic area. The anterior portion of the hypothalamus. It is above the optic chiasma and on the sides of the third ventricle.

preoral (prē-ō′răl) [L. *prae,* before, + *os,* mouth]. In front of the mouth.

prep (prĕp) [*prepare; preparation*]. Used esp. when referring to preparation for surgery. SEE: *preoperative care.*

prepalatal (prē-păl′ă-tăl) [L. *prae,* before, + *palatum,* plate]. Located in front of the teeth.

preparalytic (prē″păr-ă-lĭt′ĭk) [″ + Gr. *para,* at the side, + *lyein,* to loosen]. Before the appearance of paralysis.

preparation (prĕp-ă-rā′shŭn) [L. *praeparatio*]. 1. The making ready, esp. of a medicine for use. 2. A specimen set up for demonstration in anatomy, pathology, or histology. 3. A medicine made ready for use.

p., corrosion. In anatomical and pathology investigations, hollow organs and structures such as vessels are filled with a liquid substance that hardens. Then the surrounding tissues are dissolved by use of suitable chemicals. This leaves a cast of the structures.

p., heart-lung. In animal studies and in open-heart surgery, the use of devices that take over the function of the heart and lungs while those organs are being treated or possibly replaced.

p.'s, rectal. *Chloral hydrate:* 0.5 to 1.0 gm. dissolved in 90 ml. of warmed olive oil, or 90 ml. of very warm milk, or 90 ml. of thin, boiled cornstarch water. This makes a good preparation or a base in which to hold the medicine in suspension. The patient's pulse should be taken 5 minutes before and 5 minutes after the administration. If adverse effects are noticed, action may be taken to prevent further absorption.

Paraldehyde: 1 to 4 ml. may be mixed with water in the proportion of 1:8 and in this ratio it may be mixed with thin starch water for rectal medication. There should be about 90 ml. of starch water.

prepatellar (prē″pă-tĕl′ăr) [L. *prae,* before, + *patella,* pan]. In front of the patella.

prepatellar bursitis. Inflammation of the bursa in front of the patella. SYN: *housemaid's knee.* SEE: *bursitis.*

prepatent. Before becoming evident or manifest.

prepatent period. Period between the time of introduction of parasitic organisms into the body and their appearance in the blood or tissues.

preperception (prē″pĕr-sĕp′shŭn) [″ + L. *percepitio,* to perceive]. The anticipation of a perception. This intensifies the response to the perception.

preperitoneal (prē″pĕr-ĭ-tō-nē′ăl) [″ + Gr. *peritonaion,* peritoneum]. Located in front of the peritoneum.

preplacental (prē″plă-sĕn′tăl) [″ + *placenta,* flat cake]. Occurring prior to formation of the placenta.

prepotent (prē-pō′tĕnt) [″ + *potentia,* power]. Pert. to the greater power of one parent to transmit inherited characteristics to the offspring.

preprandial (prē-prăn′dē-ăl) [″ + *prandium,*

breakfast]. Prior to a meal.

prepuberal, prepubertal (prē-pū'bĕr-ăl, -tăl) [" + *pubertas,* puberty]. Prior to puberty.

prepubescent (prē"pū-bĕs'ĕnt) [" + *pubescens,* becoming hairy]. Pert. to the period just prior to puberty.

prepuce (prē'pūs) [L. *praeputium,* prepuce]. The foreskin or fold of skin over the glans penis in the male. Excision constitutes circumcision, a common religious practice, but also performed in cases of phimosis and for hygienic purposes. A sebaceous secretion under the prepuce is called smegma.

RS: acroposthitis; aposthia; circumcision; frenulum; penis; phimosis; smegma; urethra.

p. of clitoris. Fold of the labia minora that covers the clitoris. SEE: *clitoris.*

preputial (prē-pū'shăl). Concerning the prepuce.

preputial glands. Small sebaceous glands of the corona of the penis that secrete an odoriferous discharge. SYN: *Tyson's glands.*

preputiotomy (prē-pū"shē-ŏt'ō-mē) [" + Gr. *tome,* incision]. Incision of the prepuce of the penis to relieve phimosis.

preputium (prē-pū'shē-ŭm) (pl. *preputia*) [NA] The fold of skin that covers the glans penis. SYN: *prepuce.*

p. clitoridis. [NA] Prepuce of the clitoris, a fold overhanging the glans clitoridis formed by the union of the two labia minora.

p. penis. [NA] Fold of skin covering the glans penis. SYN: *foreskin.*

prepyloric (prē"pī-lor'ĭk). Anterior to, or preceding, the pylorus of the stomach.

prerectal (prē-rĕk'tăl) [L. *prae,* before, + *rectus,* straight]. Located in front of the rectum.

prerenal (prē-rē'năl) [" + *ren,* kidney]. 1. Located in front of the kidney. 2. Occurring prior to reaching the kidney, such as changes in consistency of the blood prior to its flow to the kidney.

preretinal (prē-rĕt'ĭ-năl) [" + *retina,* retina]. In front of the retina of the eye.

presacral (prē-sā'krăl) [" + *sacrum,* sacred]. In front of the sacrum.

Presamine. Trade name for imipramine hydrochloride, USP.

Pre-Sate. Trade name for chlorphentermine hydrochloride.

presbyacusia, presbyacousia (prĕz"bē-ă-kū'sē-ă) [Gr. *presbys,* old, + *akousis,* hearing]. Progressive loss of hearing ability due to the normal aging process. SYN: *presbycusis.*

presbyatrics, presbyatry (prĕz-bē-ăt'rĭks, prĕz'bē-ăt-rē) [" + *iatrikos,* healing]. That branch of medicine dealing with the diseases of old age. SYN: *geriatrics; presbytiatrics.*

presbycardia (prĕz-bĭ-kăr'dē-ă) [" + *kardia,* heart]. Disease or decreased functional capacity of the heart associated with aging.

presbycusis, presbykousis (prĕz-bĭ-kū'sĭs) [" + *akousis,* hearing]. Impairment of hearing in old age. SYN: *presbyacusia.*

presbyope (prĕs'bē-ōp) [" + *ops,* eye]. A person who is presbyopic.

presbyopia (prĕz-bē-ō'pē-ă) [" + *ops,* eye]. Defect of vision in advancing age involving loss of accommodation or recession of near point. Due to loss of elasticity of crystalline lens. The onset usually occurs between 40 and 45 years of age. SEE: *farsightedness.*

presbyopic (prĕs"bē-ŏp'ĭk). Concerning presbyopia.

presbytiatrics (prĕz"bĭ-tē-ăt'rĭks) [" + *iatrikos,* healing]. Science of old age and its treatment. SYN: *geriatrics; presbyatrics; presbyatry.*

prescribe (prē-skrīb') [L. *praescriptio,* prescription]. To indicate the medicine to be administered. This can be done orally but is usually done by writing a prescription or an order in the patient's hospital chart.

prescription (prē-skrĭp'shŭn) [L. *praescriptio*]. A written direction or order for dispensing and administering drugs. It is signed by a physician, dentist, or other practitioner licensed by law to prescribe such a drug. A prescription consists of four main parts.

Superscription: Represented by the symbol Rx, which signifies Recipe, from the Latin *recipere,* meaning to take.

Inscription: Containing the ingredients. This is generally constructed of four parts: the basis or principal drug; the adjuvant, which assists the action of the basis; the corrective, which diminishes unpleasant taste or pain or griping, etc.; the vehicle to hold the drugs either in solution or suspension.

Subscription: Directions to the dispenser as to the manner of preparation of the drugs.

Signature: Directions to the patient with regard to the manner of taking, dosage; finally the physician's signature, address, telephone number, date, and whether or not the prescription may be refilled. When applicable, the physician's narcotics registry number must be included. Also, some states require that the prescriber indicate on the prescription whether or not a generic drug may be substituted for the trade name equivalent.

p., shotgun. Indiscriminate prescription for a large number of drugs in the hope that at least one of them will accomplish the desired effect.

prescription drug. A drug available to the public only upon prescription written by a physician, dentist, or other practitioner licensed to do so.

prescription writing. Modern practice is to write prescriptions entirely in the language of the country in which written (as English in the United States) and to use few, if any, abbreviations. All drug quantities should be shown by using the metric system of weights and measures (grams, milligrams, liters, milliliters, etc.). SEE: *prescription writing, abbreviations,* in *Appendix.*

The following classical presentation of the art of prescription writing is included primarily for its historical interest: An official Latin name is in the nominative case. Drugs are written in the genitive case because the prescription is an order, meaning "take thou." The word "of" is not written in Latin but is indicated by the ending of a word: *quinina* means *quinine,* but changing the termination to "ae" we have *quininae,* meaning *of quinine.*

ALKALOIDS: Written the same as in English, except that the final "e" is changed to "a" to form the nominative case, as *quinina,* for the English quinine. To form the genitive case, the final "e" is changed to "ae," as *quininae.*

ACTIVE PRINCIPLES: These, such as glucosides, resinoids, and others, add "um" to the nominative and "i" to the genitive, so that Strophanthin becomes *strophanthinum* to form the Latin nominative, and *strophanthini,* to form the Latin genitive.

ACIDS: The names of these are formed in the same way as those of alkaloids, except that the adjective is formed in the same way and follows the nominative, as *acidum hydrochloricum,* or the genitive, *acidi hydrochlorici.*

METALS: Latin names of metals, except those of a few known to the ancients, are the same as English forms ending in "um," as in *sodium,* forming the Latin nominative, but ending in "i" to form the genitive, *sodii.*

SALTS: Written first with the name of the base in its genitive form, next the acid radical in the nominative, followed by the qualitative adjective in the nominative, as *ferri sulfas exsiccatus,* exsiccated sulfate of iron.

NAMES OF PREPARATIONS: Show the class to which it belongs first, the name of the ingredient next, and the qualifying adjective last, as *syrupus scillae compositus* (compound syrup of squills). First and last words are in nominative case and middle one in genitive.

DRUGS WITH TWO NAMES: Both should be in the genitive, as *liquor potassi arsenitis.* (-ate endings): The Latin nominative ends in "as," as *sulfas,* for sulfate; and the genitive in "atis," as *sulfatis.* (-ite endings): If the English word ends in "ite," as *sulfite,* the Latin nominative ends in "is," as *sulfis,* and the genitive in "itis," as *sulfitis.* (-ide endings): If an English word has this ending, as "bromide," the Latin nominative ends in "um," dropping the final "e" in the English form, as *bromidum;* the genitive dropping the "um" to add "i," as *bromidi.* (-a, -us -um endings): English words with these endings are the same in the Latin nominative, but the genitive is formed by changing "a" to "ae," or the "us" or "um" to "i." (-in endings): An English word having this ending adds "um" (usually) to form the Latin nominative as benzoin and *benzoinum,* the genitive being formed by merely adding "i," as *benzoini.* (-ol endings): The Latin nominative is the same as the English, as in phenol, but "is" is added to form the genitive, as *phenolis.* (-al endings): To form the Latin nominative, "um" is added, as chloral and *chloralum.* To form the genitive, "i" is added to the English form, as *chlorali.*

There are, of course, exceptions to the foregoing. Many Latin words have the same form as in English.

RS: active principle; antidotes; dosage; drug action; drugs and their administration; names of individual drugs in alphabetical order; names of poisons; poison; poisoning; preparations often given rectally.

presenile (prē-sē′nīl) [L. *prae,* before, + *senilis,* old]. Premature old age as judged by mental or physical condition but usually the former.

presenium (prē-sē′nē-ŭm) [″ + *senium,* old age]. Just prior to the onset of senility.

presentation (prē″zĕn-tā′shŭn) [L. *praesentatio*]. 1. In obstetrics, term applied to the manner of the fetus presenting itself to the examining finger in the vagina or rectum. Thus longitudinal (normal) and transverse (pathological) presentation. 2. Relationship of the long axis of fetus to that of mother; also called *lie.* SEE: illus.; Positions of Fetus in Utero (table).

p., breech. When buttocks of fetus present. Breech presentation is of three types: complete breech, when the thighs of the fetus are flexed on the abdomen and the legs flexed upon the thighs; frank breech, when the legs of the fetus are extended over the anterior surface of the body; and footling, when a foot or feet present. Footling can be single, double, or if the leg remains flexed, knee presentation. SEE: illus.

p., brow. When the brow of the fetus presents. SEE: illus.

p., cephalic. Presentation of the head of the fetus in any position.

p., compound. A prolapsed limb that is alongside the main presenting part.

p., face. When the head of the fetus is sharply extended so that the face presents. SEE: illus.

p., footling. A fetus presenting feet first. SEE: *p., breech.*

p., funic; p., funis. Appearance of the

PRESENTATIONS OF FETUS

ATTITUDES OF THE FETUS

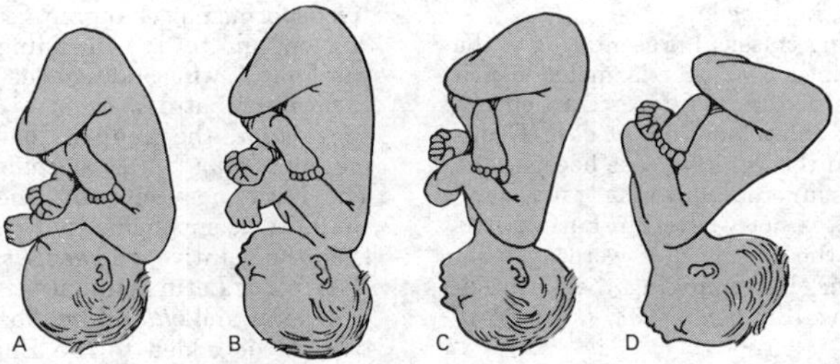

A—VERTEX PRESENTATION; B—SINCIPUT PRESENTATION;
C—BROW PRESENTATION; D—FACE PRESENTATION*

BROW PRESENTATION

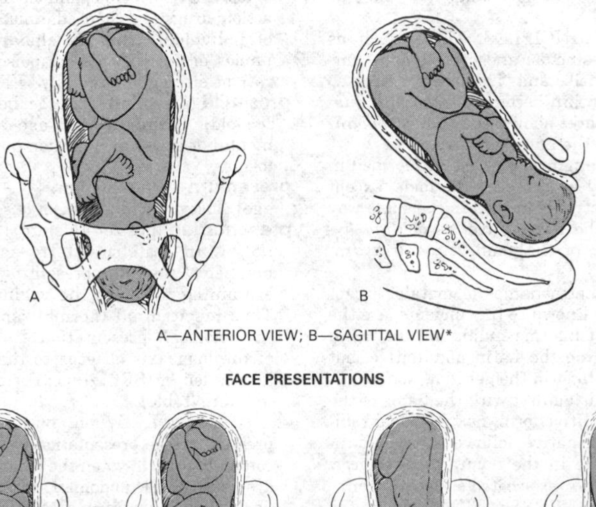

A—ANTERIOR VIEW; B—SAGITTAL VIEW*

FACE PRESENTATIONS

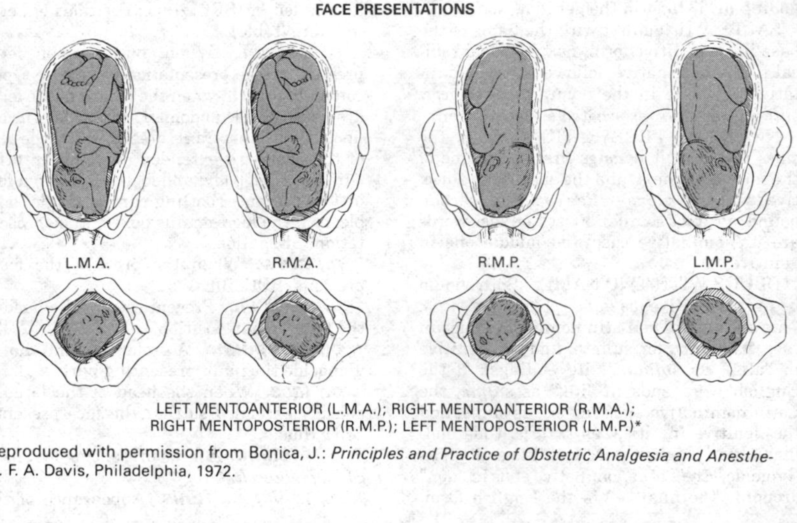

LEFT MENTOANTERIOR (L.M.A.); RIGHT MENTOANTERIOR (R.M.A.);
RIGHT MENTOPOSTERIOR (R.M.P.); LEFT MENTOPOSTERIOR (L.M.P.)*

*Reproduced with permission from Bonica, J.: *Principles and Practice of Obstetric Analgesia and Anesthesia.* F. A. Davis, Philadelphia, 1972.

PRESENTATIONS OF FETUS

TYPES OF BREECH PRESENTATIONS

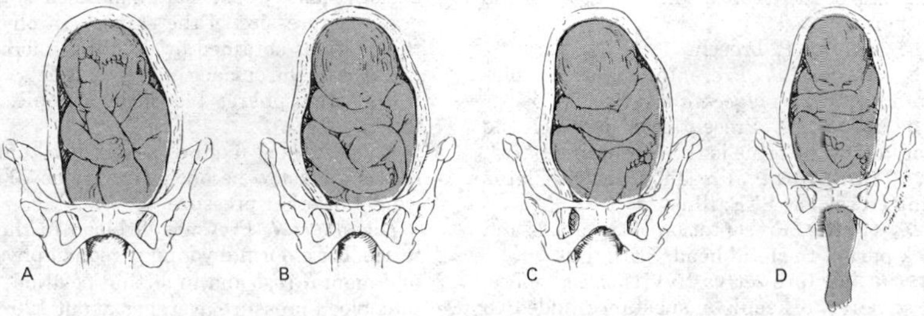

A—FRANK; B—COMPLETE; C—INCOMPLETE; D—FOOTLING*

TRANSVERSE PRESENTATION

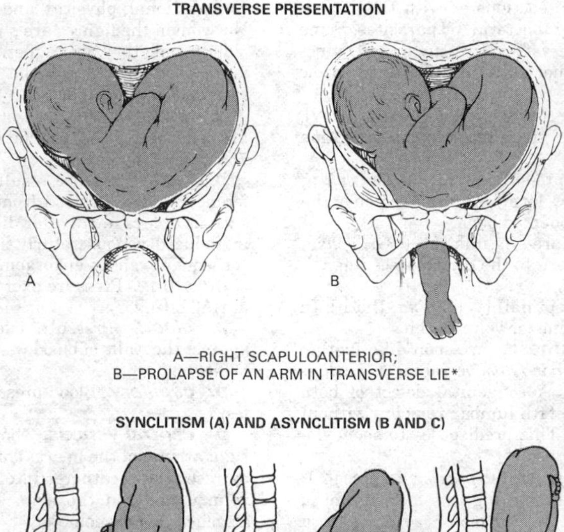

A—RIGHT SCAPULOANTERIOR;
B—PROLAPSE OF AN ARM IN TRANSVERSE LIE*

SYNCLITISM (A) AND ASYNCLITISM (B AND C)

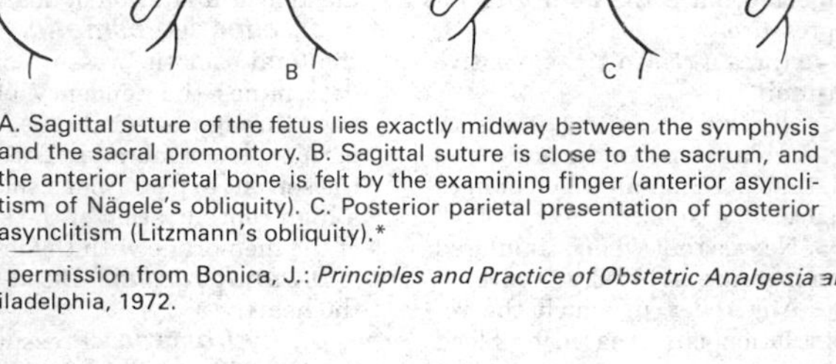

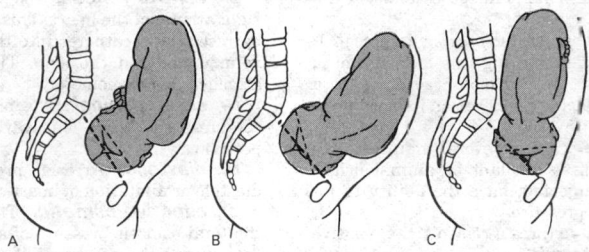

A. Sagittal suture of the fetus lies exactly midway between the symphysis and the sacral promontory. B. Sagittal suture is close to the sacrum, and the anterior parietal bone is felt by the examining finger (anterior asynclitism of Nägele's obliquity). C. Posterior parietal presentation of posterior asynclitism (Litzmann's obliquity).*

*Reproduced with permission from Bonica, J.: *Principles and Practice of Obstetric Analgesia and Anesthesia.* F. A. Davis, Philadelphia, 1972.

umbilical cord during labor.

p., longitudinal. Presentation in which the long axis of the fetus is parallel to the long axis of the mother.

p., oblique. Presentation in which the long axis of the fetus is oblique to that of the mother.

p., pelvic. P., breech.

p., placental. Presentation of the placenta first. SYN: *placenta previa.*

p., shoulder. Presentation in which the shoulder of the fetus is the presenting part.

p., transverse. Presentation with fetus lying crosswise. SEE: illus.

p., vertex. Presentation of the upper and back part of the fetal head. SEE: illus.

preservative (prē-zĕr'vă-tĭv) [L. *prae,* before, + *servare,* to keep]. A substance added to medicines or foods to prevent them from spoiling. It may act by interfering with certain chemical reactions or with the growth of molds, fungi, bacteria, or parasites. Some common preservatives are sugar, salt, vinegar, ethyl alcohol, sulfur dioxide, and benzoic acid.

presomite (prē-sō'mīt) [" + Gr. *soma,* body]. The embryonic stage prior to the formation of somites.

presphenoid (prē-sfē'noyd) [" + Gr. *sphen,* wedge, + *eidos,* form]. Anterior region of the body on the sphenoid bone.

presphygmic (prē-sfĭg'mĭk) [" + Gr. *sphygmos,* pulse]. Pert. to the period preceding the pulse wave.

prespinal (prē-spī'năl) [" + *spina,* thorn]. In front of the spine, or ventral to it.

prespondylolisthesis (prē-spŏn"dĭl-ō-lĭs-thē'sĭs) [" + Gr. *spondylos,* vertebra, + *olisthanein,* to slip]. A congenital defect of both pedicles of the fifth lumbar vertebra without displacement. This predisposes to spondylolisthesis.

pressor (prĕs'or) [O. Fr. *presser,* to press]. 1. Stimulating, increasing the activity of a function, esp. of vasomotor activity, as a nerve. 2. Inducing an elevation in blood pressure.

pressor base. One of several amines or nitrogenous bases of plant or animal origin that, when injected, have the ability to increase blood pressure.

pressoreceptive (prĕs"ō-rē-sĕp'tĭv). Sensitive to pressure stimuli.

pressoreceptor (prĕs"ō-rē-sĕp'tōr). Sensory nerve ending, such as those in the aorta and carotid sinus, that is stimulated by changes in blood pressure.

pressor nerves. Nerves that when stimulated bring about an increase in blood pressure.

pressor reflex. Any reflex in which the response to stimulation is increased by blood pressure.

pressosensitive (prĕs"ō-sĕn'sĭ-tĭv). Pressoreceptive, q.v.

pressure (prĕsh'ŭr) [L. *pressura*]. 1. A compression. 2. Stress or force exerted on a body, as by tension, weight, or pulling. 3. In psychology, quality of sensation aroused by moderate compression of the skin. 4. In physics, the quotient obtained by dividing a force by the area of the surface on which it acts.

RS: atmosphere; blood; hypertonic; isotonic.

p., after-. A feeling of pressure that remains for a few seconds after removal of a weight or other pressure.

p., arterial. Pressure of blood in the arteries. For a normal young person at physical and mental rest and in sitting position, systolic blood pressure averages about 120 mm. Hg; diastolic pressure about 80 mm. Hg. There is a wide range of normal variation due to constitutional, physical, and psychic factors. For women the figures are slightly lower. For older people they are higher. Normally there is little difference in the blood pressure recorded in the two arms.

p., atmospheric. Pressure of weight of atmosphere; at sea level it averages about 760 mm. of mercury.

p., back. Pressure resulting from interference in flow of blood from the ventricles, such as occurs in valvular disorders. Results in reduced venous return to the heart and consequent venous engorgement.

p., biting. Pressure exerted on the teeth during biting.

p., blood. Pressure exerted by blood against the walls of blood vessels. SEE: *blood pressure.*

p., capillary. Blood pressure in capillaries.

p., central venous. The pressure in the right atrium of the heart. This is determined by inserting a catheter into the heart via a vein, usually in the arm. The catheter is attached to a manometer.

p., cerebrospinal. The pressure of the cerebrospinal fluid. This varies with body position.

p., diastolic. Arterial pressure during diastole or dilatation of heart chambers.

p., effective osmotic. That portion of the total osmotic pressure of a solution that determines the tendency of the solvent to pass through a membrane, usually a semipermeable membrane. The tendency is for the solvent to pass from a solution containing a high concentration of the solute to the side of the membrane with the low concentration.

p., endocardiac. Blood pressure within the heart.

p., hydrostatic. Pressure exerted by a fluid within a closed system.

p., intra-abdominal. Pressure within the abdominal cavity, such as that caused by descent of the diaphragm.

p., intracranial. Pressure of the cerebrospinal fluid in the subarachnoid space between the skull and the brain. The pressure is normally the same as that found during lumbar puncture.

p., intraocular. Normal tension within the eyeball, equal to approximately 12 to 20 mm. of mercury.

p., intrathoracic. Pressure within the thorax.

p., intraventricular. Pressure within the ventricles of the heart during different phases of diastole and systole.

p., negative. Any pressure less than that of the atmosphere, or less than that pressure to which the initial pressure is being compared.

p., occlusal. P., biting, q.v.

p., oncotic. The osmotic pressure exerted by colloids in a solution.

p., osmotic. The force with which a solvent, usually water, passes through a semipermeable membrane separating solutions of different concentrations. It is measured by determining the hydrostatic (mechanical) pressure that must be opposed to the osmotic force to bring the passage to a standstill.

p., partial. In a gas containing several different components, the pressure exerted by each component.

p., positive. Pressure greater than atmospheric or greater than the pressure to which the initial pressure is being compared.

p., positive end-expiratory. ABBR: PEEP. The application of slight positive pressure at the end of expiration while intermittent positive pressure is being used. This increases the amount of air remaining in the lungs at the end of expiration.

p., pulse. The difference between systolic and diastolic pressures.

p., solution. The pressure that tends to dissolve a solid present in a solution.

p., systolic. Arterial pressure at time of the contraction of the ventricles, or the ventricular systole.

p., venous. Pressure of the blood within the veins. It is highest near the periphery, diminishing progressively from capillaries to the heart. Near the heart the pressure may be below zero (negative pressure) due to negative intrathoracic pressure.

p., wedge. The pressure determined by use of a fluid-filled catheter wedged in the distal end of a branch of the pulmonary artery. This provides an indirect measurement of the pressure in the left atrium of the heart.

pressure of speech. Loud and emphatic speech that is increased in amount, accelerated, and usually difficult or impossible to interrupt. The speech is not in response to a stimulus and may continue even though no one is listening. May be present in manic episodes, organic brain disease, depression with agitation, psychotic disorders, and sometimes as an acute reaction to stress.

pressure palsy. Temporary paralysis due to pressure on a nerve trunk.

pressure paralysis. Paralysis due to pressure on the spinal cord.

ETIOL: Injury, tumor, gummata.

pressure points. Areas for exerting pressure to control bleeding. For control of hemorrhage, pressure above bleeding point when an artery passes over a bone may be sufficient. Principal pressure points follow.

Common carotid artery, 2 in. (5 cm.) above clavicle, press backwards against spine. *Temporal artery,* at side of face in front of ear. *Occipital artery,* behind mastoid process. *Subclavian artery,* behind clavicle, pressing down onto first rib. *Axillary artery,* by compression in axilla. *Brachial artery,* compressed by pressure at inner edge of biceps muscle halfway down arm and also above bend of elbow before artery divides into radial and ulnar arteries. *Radial artery,* press on thumb side of wrist against radius. *Ulnar artery,* press on little finger side of wrist against ulna. *Deep palmar arch,* in thumb opposite root of abducted thumb. *Abdominal artery,* may be compressed against lumbar vertebrae to left of middle line when patient lies on back. *Femoral artery,* by abduction and external rotation of thigh, bringing head of femur forward into groin and compressing artery against it. *Popliteal artery,* in popliteal space over artery. *Anterior tibial artery,* at front of bend of ankle. *Posterior tibial artery,* behind internal malleolus as it passes into foot. SEE: *bleeding* for table (Arrest of Arterial Bleeding).

pressure sore. A sore caused by pressure from a splint or other appliance, or from the body itself when it has remained immobile in bed for extended periods of time. SYN: *bedsore; decubitus ulcer.*

presternum (prē-stĕr'nŭm) [L. *prae,* before, + Gr. *sternon,* chest]. The upper part of the sternum. SYN: *manubrium sterni* [NA].

presuppurative (prē-sŭp'ū-rā"tĭv) [" + *sub,* under, + *puris,* pus]. Rel. to period of inflammation before suppuration.

presylvian fissure (prē-sĭl'vē-ăn). The anterior division of the sylvian fissure.

presymptomatic (prē"sĭmp-tō-măt'ĭk). The state of health prior to the clinical appearance of the signs and symptoms of a disease.

presynaptic (prē"sĭ-năp'tĭk) [" + Gr. *synapsis,* point of contact]. Located before the nerve synapse.

presystole (prē-sĭs'tō-lē) [L. *prae,* before, + Gr. *systole,* contraction]. The period in the heart's cycle just before the systole. SYN: *perisystole.*

presystolic (prē-sĭs-tŏl'ĭk). Before the systole of the heart.

pretarsal (prē-tăr'săl) [" + Gr. *tarsos,* tarsus]. In front of the tarsus.

preterm. In obstetrics, events occurring prior to the 37th week of gestation.

pretibial (prē-tĭb'ē-ăl) [" + *tibia,* shin]. In front of the tibia.

pretibial fever. A form of leptospirosis caused by one of the several serotypes of the autumnalis serogroup. It is characterized by fever, rash on legs, prostration, splenomegaly, and respiratory disturbances. SYN: *Fort Bragg fever.*

pretympanic (prē"tĭm-păn'ĭk) [" + *tympanon,* a drum]. Located in front of the tympanic membrane.

preurethritis (prē"ū-rē-thrī'tĭs) [" + Gr. *ourethra,* urethra, + *itis,* inflammation]. Inflammation around the urethral orifice of the vaginal vestibule.

prevalence (prĕv'ă-lĕns) [L. *praevalens,* prevail]. The number of cases of a disease present in a specified population at a given time. SEE: *incidence.*

preventive (prē-vĕn'tĭv) [ME. *preventen,* to anticipate]. Hindering the occurrence of something, esp. disease. SYN: *prophylactic.*

preventive dentistry. That phase of dentistry concerned with the maintenance of the normal masticatory apparatus by teaching good oral hygiene and dietary practice, and preserving dental health by early restorative procedures.

preventive medicine. The branch of medicine concerned with preventing the occurrence of both mental and physical illness and disease.

There are three levels of preventive effort. Primary preventive medicine is concerned with preventing the development of disease in a susceptible or potentially susceptible population. These efforts include general promotion of health and specific protection such as immunization. Secondary preventive medicine involves early diagnosis and prompt therapy to shorten duration of illness, reduce the severity of disease, reduce possibility of contagion, and limit sequelae. Tertiary preventive medicine is important in limiting the degree of disability and promoting rehabilitation in chronic and irreversible diseases.

preventive nursing. The nurse is an essential part of the health care team and has the opportunity and status to emphasize and indeed implement health care services, the purpose of which are to promote health and prevent disease. Nursing expertise and general professional competence can also be utilized in supporting community action at all levels for promoting public health measures. There are three levels of preventive nursing:

A. Primary. The goals of primary prevention are general health promotion. This incudes whatever intervention is required to provide a health-promoting environment at home, in the schools, and in the workplace by ensuring good nutrition, adequate clothing and shelter, rest and recreation, and health education, including sex education and for the aging realistic plans for retirement. Areas of emphasis are specific protective measures such as immunizations, environmental sanitation, accident prevention, and protection from occupational hazards. Behavior modification, though difficult, must be attempted with respect to those areas known to represent major health risk factors, i.e., smoking, obesity, improper diet, alcohol and drug abuse, and major efforts to prevent automobile accidents.

B. Secondary. Nursing care aimed at early recognition and treatment of disease and includes general nursing interventions and teaching of early signs of disease conditions. Disease such as infectious diseases, glaucoma, and cancer *in situ* fall in this category.

C. Tertiary. Nursing care for incurable diseases, and patient instruction concerning how to manage those conditions and diseases. Parkinson's disease, multiple sclerosis, and diabetes are conditions that lend themselves to tertiary prevention. The goal is to prevent further deterioration of physical and mental function, and to have each such patient utilize whatever residual function is available for maximum enjoyment of and participation in life's activities. Rehabilitation is of course an essential part of tertiary prevention.

prevertebral (prē-vĕr'tē-brăl) [L. *prae,* before, + *vertebra,* vertebra]. In front of a vertebra.

prevertebral ganglia. Ganglia of the sympathetic division of the autonomic nervous system, located near origins of the celiac and mesenteric arteries. These include the celiac and mesenteric ganglia. SYN: *collateral ganglia.*

prevertiginous (prē-vĕr-tĭj'ĭ-nŭs) [" + *vertigo,* dizziness]. Having a tendency to fall forward.

prevesical (prē-vĕs'ĭ-kl) [" + *vesica,* bladder]. Located in front of the bladder.

previa, praevia (prē'vē-ă) [L.]. Appearing before or in front of.

previable. Pert. to a fetus not sufficiently mature to survive outside the uterus.

prevocational evaluation. In rehabilitation,

the assessment of a patient's ability to perform those component tasks necessary for engagement in a selected vocation.

prezonular. Pert. to the posterior chamber of the eye, the space between the iris and ciliary zonule (suspensory ligament).

prezygotic (prē-zī-gŏt'ĭk) [" + *zygotos,* yoked]. Happening prior to fertilization of the ovum.

priapism (prī'ă-pĭzm) [L. *priapismus*]. Abnormal, painful, and continued erection of the penis due to disease, and usually without sexual desire. SEE: *erection; gonorrhea.*

ETIOL: May be due to lesions of the cord above the lumbar region, or turgescence of the corpora cavernosa without erection may exist. It may be reflex from peripheral sensory irritants, from organic irritation of nerve tracts or nerve centers when libido may be lacking. Sometimes seen in patients with acute leukemia.

priapitis (prī-ă-pī'tĭs) [Gr. *priapos,* phallus, + *itis,* inflammation]. Inflammation of the penis.

priapus (prī'ă-pŭs) [Gr. *priapos*]. The penis.

prickle cell (prĭk'l). A cell with rod-shaped processes, intercellular bridges connecting with similar adjoining cells.

prickly heat. Noncontagious cutaneous eruption of red pimples with itching and tingling of the affected parts, seen usually in hot weather. SYN: *lichen tropicus; miliaria.*

ETIOL: Inflammation of skin around sweat glands.

Priessnitz compress (prēs'nĭtz). [Vincent Priessnitz, Silesian farmer, 1799–1851] A cold wet compress.

prilocaine hydrochloride (prĭl'ō-kān). USP. A local anesthetic. It may cause methemoglobinemia. Trade name is Citanest.

primal scene. In psychiatry, the term for a child's first observation of sexual intercourse.

primaquine phosphate (prĭm'ă-kwĭn). USP. An antimalarial drug.

primary (prī'mă-rē) [L. *primarius,* principal]. First in time or order. SYN: *principal.*

primary amputation. Amputation performed before inflammation has set in.

primary bubo. Inflamed lymph node that represents the initial lesion following exposure to a veneral disease, esp. to syphilis. ALSO: *bubon d'emblée.*

primary care. Basic or general health care provided at the person's first contact with the health care system. Usually this contact is for common illnesses. The primary health care provider assumes ongoing responsibility for health maintenance and therapy for illness, including consultation with specialists.

primary cell. In physical therapy, a device consisting of a container, two solid conducting elements, and an electrolyte for the production of electric current by chemical energy.

primary hemorrhage. Bleeding at time of an injury.

primary lesion. 1. An original lesion from which a second one originates. 2. Lesion of syphilis, a chancre, q.v.

primary nursing. The nursing practice system in which the entire nursing care of a patient is managed and coordinated by one nurse for a 24-hour period. The nurse is involved in, manages, and coordinates all aspects of the patient's case in that period. This includes scheduling of activities, tests, and procedures.

primary physician. The physician to whom a family or individual goes initially for medical care and the management of their care even if eventually referred to other physicians.

primary radiation. That radiation being emitted directly to the patient from the x-ray source.

primary sore. The initial sore or hard chancre of syphilis.

primate (prī'māt) [L. *primus,* first]. A member of the order Primates.

Primatene Mist. Trade name for epinephrine, USP.

Primates (prī-mā'tēz). An order of vertebrates belonging to the class Mammalia, subclass Theria. Includes the lemurs, tarsiers, monkeys, apes, and man. This order is most highly developed with respect to the brain and nervous system.

prime (prīm) [L. *primus,* first]. 1. Period of greatest health and strength. 2. To give an initial treatment in preparation for either a larger dose of the same medicine, or a different medicine.

primidone (prĭm'ĭ-dōn). USP. An anticonvulsive drug used in treating epilepsy. Trade name is Mysoline.

primigravida (prī-mĭ-grăv'ĭ-dă) [" + *gravida,* pregnant]. A woman during her first pregnancy.

primipara (prī-mĭp'ă-ră) [" + *parere,* to bear offspring]. A woman who has produced one infant of 500 grams (or of 20 weeks gestation) regardless of whether it is alive or dead.

primiparity (prī"mĭ-păr'ĭ-tē). Condition of having given birth to only one infant of 500 grams (or 20 weeks gestation) regardless of its viability.

primiparous (prī-mĭp'ă-rŭs). Pert. to a primipara.

primitiae (prī-mĭsh'ē-ē) [L. *primus,* first]. Liquor amnii appearing just before birth of the fetus. SEE: *amnion; bag of waters; labor; liquor amnii.*

primitive (prĭm'ĭ-tĭv) [L. *primitivus*]. Original; early in point of time; embryonic.

primitive groove. The longitudinal depression in the dorsum of the embryonic area.

primitive streak. A dark, thickened longitudinal band that forms at caudal end of the embryonic disk, consisting of a surface layer of ectoderm overlying a thickened mass of mesoderm cells. It marks the future longitudinal axis of the embryo.

primordial (prī-mor′dē-ăl) [L. *primordialis*]. 1. Existing first. 2. Existing in an undeveloped, primitive, or early form.

primordium (prī-mor′dē-ŭm) [L., origin]. (pl. *primordia*) The first accumulation of cells in an embryo that constitutes the beginning of a future tissue, organ, or part. SYN: *anlage.*

primum non nocere (prī″mŭm nōn nō′sĕ-rā) [L.]. "First do no harm." No one's condition should be made worse because of having visited a physician.

princeps (prĭn′sĕps) [L., chief]. 1. Original; first. 2. The name of certain arteries. Ex.: princeps cervicis. 3. Chief, principal.

principal (prĭn′sĭ-păl). 1. Chief. 2. Outstanding.

principal fibers of the periodontal ligament. ABBR: PDL. The oriented bundles of collagen fibers that by their attachments and position within the periodontal ligament space are recognized as specific parts of the alveolodental ligament; bundles of PDL fibers named according to orientation and attachment.

Principen/N. Trade name for ampicillin sodium, USP.

principle (prĭn′sĭ-pl) [L. *principium*, foundation]. 1. A constituent of a compound representing its essential properties. 2. A fundamental truth. 3. An established rule of action.

p., active. The portion of a pharmaceutical preparation that produces the therapeutic action.

p., antianemic. A substance stored in the liver that is essential for the normal development of red blood cells in the bone marrow. It is formed in the stomach and intestine by the interaction of an extrinsic factor, vitamin B_{12}, and an intrinsic factor present in gastric juice. It is used in the treatment of pernicious anemia. SYN: *factor, antianemic.*

p., antidiuretic. The antidiuretic hormone (ADH) present in extracts of the posterior lobe of the pituitary gland.

p.′s, gastrointestinal. Substances, secreted by mucosa of stomach and intestine, that are absorbed by the blood and act as hormones. SEE: *cholecystokinin; gastrin; secretin.*

p., oxytocic. A hormone in extracts of the posterior lobe of the hypophysis that stimulates contraction of uterine muscle.

p., pleasure. In psychoanalysis, the idea that unconsciously the individual is striving to attain pleasure and avoid painful situations.

p., proximate. A substance that may be extracted from its complex form without destroying or altering its chemical properties.

p., purpura-producing. A toxic substance produced when pneumococci are autolyzed. This causes dermal and internal hemorrhages when injected into rabbits.

p., reality. In psychoanalysis, the idea that the striving for pleasure is balanced by the situations produced by the real world.

Prinzmetal's angina. [Myron Prinzmetal, U.S. cardiologist, b. 1908] An unusual and uncommon form of angina where pain is experienced at rest and sometimes while in bed rather than during activity. The electrocardiogram taken during an attack will indicate S-T segment elevation rather than depression. Nitroglycerin and drugs that influence calcium metabolism by the myocardium are of benefit. SYN: *angina, variant.*

Priscoline Hydrochloride. Trade name for tolazoline hydrochloride.

prism (prĭzm) [Gr. *prisma*]. A transparent solid three sides of which are parallelograms. The bases, perpendicular to the three sides, are triangles. A transverse section of the solid is a triangle. Light rays going through a prism are deflected toward the base of the triangle and at the same time are split into the primary colors.

p., enamel. A minute rod of calcareous material deposited at the end of an ameloblast in the formation of the enamel of a tooth.

p., Maddox. Two base-together prisms used in testing for cyclophoria or torsion of the eyeball.

p., Nicol. A prism made by splitting a prism of Icelandic spar and rejoining the cut surfaces. This causes the light passing through to be split. Ordinary light rays are reflected by the joined surfaces and polarized light is transmitted.

p., Risley's rotary. Prism mounted in a device that allows it to be rotated. This is used in testing eye muscle imbalance.

prismatic (prĭz-măt′ĭk). 1. Shaped like a prism. 2. Produced by a prism.

prismoid (prĭz′moyd) [″ + *eidos*, form]. Resembling a prism.

prismoptometer (prĭz-mŏp-tŏm′ĕ-tĕr) [″ + *opsis*, vision, + *metron*, measure]. Device for estimating abnormal refraction of the eye by using prisms.

private patient. A patient whose care is the responsibility of one identifiable health care professional, usually a physician. The health care professional is either paid directly by the patient or by the patient's insurer.

private practice. Practice by a health care professional, usually a physician or dentist, in a setting in which the practice and the practitioner are independent of external policy control other than ethics of the professional and state licensing laws.

privileged communication. Confidential information furnished (in order to facilitate diagnosis and treatment) by the patient to a professional authorized by law to care for him. In some states the person who has received this communication may not be made to divulge it. When this is the case, communication between the patient and the recipient is classed as privileged.

Privine Hydrochloride. Trade name for naphazoline hydrochloride, USP.

p.r.n. L. *pro re nata,* as circumstance may require; as necessary. Frequently used in prescription and order writing.

pro- [L., Gr. *pro,* before]. Prefix indicating for, in front of, before, from, in behalf of, on account of.

proaccelerin. The fifth factor (Factor V) in blood coagulation. Present in normal plasma but deteriorates rapidly at room temperature. Its function in blood coagulation is unclear. SEE: *coagulation factors.*

proactinomycin (prō-ăk″tĭ-nō-mī′sĭn). An antibiotic obtained from Nocardia gardneri. Effective against gram-positive bacteria.

proactivator (prō-ăk′tĭ-vā″tor). A substance that contains a portion that can be split off; and when it is, the fragment activates another chemical substance.

proagglutinoid (prō″ă-gloo′tĭ-noyd). An agglutinoid having a greater affinity for the agglutinogen than that possessed by the agglutinin.

proal (prō′ăl) [Gr. *pro,* before]. Concerning forward movement.

proamnion (prō-ăm′nē-ŏn) [Gr. *pro,* before, + *amnion,* amnion]. A region anterior to the head in a vertebrate embryo in which mesoderm is lacking.

proantithrombin (prō″ăn-tĭ-thrŏm′bĭn). A substance present in blood plasma or serum which, through the action of heparin, is converted into antithrombin.

proatlas (prō-ăt′lăs) [″ + *atlas,* a support]. A rudimentary vertebra in front of the atlas of small animals. It may be present as an anomaly in the understructure of the occipital bone in man.

probability. The ratio that expresses the likelihood of the occurrence of a specific event. The probability of a tossed coin landing head side up is one half or 50%, as is the probability of the tail side landing up. This 50% probability remains the same each time a coin is tossed. Probability ratios based on sophisticated techniques are used for estimating the chance of occurrence of diseases in a population and are used in projecting vital statistics such as birth and death rates.

proband [L. *probare,* to test]. The initial subject presenting a mental or physical disorder, who causes a study of his or her heredity in order to determine if other members of the family have had the same disease or carry it. SYN: *propositus.*

probang (prō′băng). A slim, flexible rod with a sponge or similar material attached to the end. Used for determining the location of strictures in the larynx or esophagus; and for removing objects from the trachea. Medicines may also be applied to these areas by use of this device.

Pro-Banthine. Trade name for propantheline bromide, USP.

probationary (prō-bā′shŭn-ăr-ē) [L. *probatio,* probation]. One who is in a trial period waiting, as for admission or for a test.

probationer (prō-bā′shŭn-ĕr). A person working during a trial period, as a student nurse just after entering training.

probe (prōb) [L. *probare,* to test]. An instrument, usually flexible, for exploring the depth and direction of a wound or sinus.

p., dental. A sharp, pointed hand instrument used to examine the surface features of teeth and dental restorations for irregularities, cracks, and soft or carious enamel. SYN: *dental explorer.*

p., periodontal. A fine-caliber probe calibrated in millimeters designed and used to measure the depth and extent of the gingival sulcus and periodontal pockets present.

probenecid. USP. A benzoic acid derivative useful in treating gout. In large doses it prevents reabsorption of uric acid by the kidney and retards the excretion of penicillin in the urine. Trade name is Probenecid.

problem-oriented medical record. ABBR: POMR. Method of establishing and maintaining the patient's medical record so that the problems are clearly stated, usually in order of importance, and a rational plan for dealing with these problems is stated. These data are kept at the front of the chart and are evaluated as frequently as indicated with respect to recording changes in the patient's problems as well as progress made in solving these problems. The use of this system has the potential of bringing a degree of comprehensiveness to total patient care that might not be possible with conventional medical records.

problem-oriented record. ABBR: POR. SEE: *problem-oriented medical record.*

probucol (prō′bū-kōl). An antihypercholesteremic drug. Trade name is Lorelco.

procainamide hydrochloride. USP. A drug used in treating cardiac arrhythmias, particularly those that originate in the ventricle.

procaine hydrochloride (prō′kān). USP. White, colorless, crystalline compound. Trade names are Neocaine and Novocain.

ACTION AND USES: A safe, local anesthetic, less toxic than cocaine. Used in infiltration anesthesia, nerve block, and spinal anesthesia. Its effect is prolonged by simultaneous injection of epinephrine.

Procan. Trade name for procainamide hydrochloride, USP.

procarbazine hydrochloride (prō-kăr′bă-zēn). USP. A cytotoxic drug used in treating Hodgkin's disease and certain other neoplastic diseases. Trade name is Matulane.

procarboxypeptidase (prō″kăr-bŏk″sē-pĕp′tĭ-dās). Inactive precursor of carboxypeptidase. Trypsin activates it.

procaryote (prō-kăr′ē-ōt) [Gr. *pro,* before, + *karyon,* nucleus]. Prokaryote, q.v.

procatarctic (prō″kă-tărk′tĭk) [″ + *katarchein,* to begin]. Predisposing or inciting, as the cause of a disease.

procatarxis (prō″kă-tărk′sĭs). Inception of a disease through a predisposing cause.

procedure (prō-sē′dūr) [L. *procedere,* to proceed]. A particular way of accomplishing a desired result.

procelous (prō-sē′lŭs) [Gr. *pro,* before, + *koilos,* hollow]. Concave anteriorly.

procentriole (prō-sĕn′trē-ōl). The early form of the centrioles and ciliary basal bodies in the cell. SEE: *centriole.*

procephalic (prō″sē-făl′ĭk) [″ + *kephale,* a head]. Of, or relating to, the anterior part of the head.

procercoid (prō-sĕr′koyd). The first larval stage in the development of certain cestodes belonging to the order Pseudophillidea. It is an elongated structure that develops in crustaceans.

procerus muscle. [NA] A muscle that arises in the skin over the nose and is connected to the forehead. It acts to draw the eyebrows down.

process (prŏs′ĕs) [L. *processus,* going before]. 1. A method of action. 2. State of progress of a disease. 3. A projection or outgrowth of bone or tissue. SYN: *processus* [NA]. 4. Series of steps or events that lead to achievement of specific results.

p., acromion. The acromion.

p., alar. A process of cribriform plate of the ethmoid bone that articulates with the frontal bone.

p., alveolar. 1. The inferior border of the maxilla containing sockets for upper teeth. 2. The superior border of body of mandible containing sockets for lower teeth.

p., articular, of vertebra. One of four processes (two superior and two inferior) by which vertebrae articulate with each other.

p., basilar. Narrow part of the base of the occipital bone, in front of the foramen magnum, articulating with the sphenoid bone. SYN: *pars basilaris ossis occipitalis.*

p., caudate. Process of the caudate lobe of the liver extending under the right lobe.

p., ciliary. One of about 70 prominent meridional ridges projecting from the corona ciliaris of the choroid coat of the eye to which the suspensory ligament of the lens is attached.

p., clinoid. The three processes of the sphenoid bone: anterior, middle, and posterior clinoid.

p., condyloid. Posterior process on the superior border of the ramus of the mandible that articulates with the temporal bone.

p., coracoid. A beak-shaped process extending upward and laterally from the neck of the scapula.

p., coronoid. 1. Process extending upward from the anterior portion of the ramus of the mandible. 2. Sharp projection forming the anterior and lower border of the semilunar notch of the ulna.

p., ensiform. The xiphoid process of the sternum.

p., ethmoidal. Small process on superior border of the inferior concha that articulates with the uncinate process of the ethmoid.

p., falciform. An extension of the posterior edge of the sacrotuberous ligament to the ramus of the ischium.

p., frontal. Upward projection of maxilla that articulates with the frontal bone. Forms part of the orbit and nasal fossa.

p., frontonasal. In the area of the primitive mouth of the embryo, a median swelling that is the anlage of the nose, upper lip, and front part of the palate.

p., frontosphenoidal. Upward projecting process of the zygomatic bone.

p., head. An axial strand of cells in vertebrate embryos extending forward from the primitive knot. Forms primitive axis about which the embryo differentiates. SYN: *notochordal plate.*

p., infraorbital. Medially projecting process of the zygomatic bone that articulates with the maxilla. Forms inferior lateral margin of orbit.

p., jugular. Process of occipital bone lying lateral to the occipital condyle.

p., lacrimal. A short process of inferior concha that articulates with the lacrimal bone.

p., lenticular. A knob on the malleus in the ear that articulates with the stapes.

p., malar. The projection from the maxilla that articulates with the zygomatic bone.

p., mandibular. Posterior portion of the first branchial arch from which the lower jaw develops.

p., mastoid. Projection of the mastoid portion of the temporal bone.

p., maxillary. 1. Anterior portion of the first branchial arch, which, with medial nasal processes, forms the upper jaw. 2. Process of inferior nasal concha extending laterally and covering the orifice of the antrum. 3. Process on the anterior border of the perpendicular portion of the palatine bone.

p., nursing. The entire process for the practice of nursing, including the step-by-step approach to the nurse's delivering patient care. In doing this, the nurse and the nursing staff utilize all of their skills for organization, administration, and actually carrying out the details of providing nursing care for patients. The systematic approach to the nursing process involves assessment of the patient's situation and conditions in the context of the nursing diagnosis. Correlating the patient's needs with those special family conditions created by the patient's illness will need to be done in analyzing and formulating a plán for caring for the patient. Implementation of the medical care plan will, of course, determine how successful the nursing care process has been; and this can only be determined by a continuing evaluation of the process as judged by the results. The nursing process will in individual situations need to be modified, altered, perhaps changed in emphasis as the patient's condition begins to be resolved or to worsen.

p., odontoid. Toothlike process extending upward from the axis and about which the axis rotates. SYN: *dens.*

p., olecranon. The olecranon, q.v., an extension at the proximal end of the ulna.

p., orbital. 1. Process at tip of the perpendicular portion of the palatine bone directed upward and backward. 2. Process of the zygomatic bone that forms the anterior boundary of the temporal fossa.

p., palatine. Process extending transversely from the medial surface of the maxilla. With the corresponding process from the other side, it forms the major portion of the hard palate.

p., postglenoid. Process of the temporal bone separating the mandibular fossa from the external acoustic meatus.

p., pterygoid. Process of sphenoid bone extending downward from junction of the body and great wing. Consists of the lateral and medial pterygoid plates.

p., spinous, of vertebrae. The posterior-most part of a vertebra. This spine projects back and serves as a point of attachment for muscles of the back.

p., styloid. Styloid process.

p., transverse. Process extending laterally and dorsally from the arch of a vertebra.

p., uncinate, of ethmoid bone. A sickle-shaped bony process on the medial wall of the ethmoidal labyrinth below the concha.

p., vermiform. Vermiform appendix.

p., vocal. Process of arytenoid cartilage that serves for attachment of the vocal ligament.

p., xiphoid. Thin, elongated process extending caudally from the body of the sternum. SYN: *p., ensiform.*

p., zygomatic. SEE: *zygomatic process.*

processus (prō-sĕs′ŭs) [L.]. (pl. *processus*) [NA] Process, q.v., or processes.

p. cochleariformis. [NA] Curved portion of a thin plate of bone separating the eustachian tube from the canal for the tensor tympani muscle over which the tendon of the muscle passes before insertion into the manubrium of the malleus.

p. retromandibularis. Wedge-shaped portion of the parotid gland that projects medially toward the pharynx.

p. uncinatus. [NA] 1. Curved process of ethmoid labyrinth projecting from the lateral wall of the middle meatus that forms the inferior border of hiatus semilunaris. 2. A hooklike portion of the head of the pancreas that curves around the superior mesenteric vessels.

procheilon (prō-kī′lŏn) [Gr. *pro,* before, + *cheilon,* lip]. Prominence in central portion of the upper lip.

prochlorperazine (prō″klor-pĕr′ă-zēn). USP. A phenothiazine-type drug used in treating nausea and vomiting. Trade name is Compazine.

prochondral (prō-kŏn′drăl) [″ + *chondral,* cartilage]. Preceding the formation of cartilage.

prochordal (prō-kor′dăl) [″ + *chorde,* cord]. In front of the notochord.

procidentia (prō″sĭ-dĕn′shē-ă) [L.]. A complete prolapse, esp. of the uterus to such an extent that the uterus lies outside of the vulva with everted vaginal walls.

ETIOL: Generally due to relaxation of the tissues that provide support for the pelvic organs.

procollagen (prō-kŏl′ă-jĕn) [″ + *kolla,* glue, + *gennan,* to produce]. Precursor of collagen.

proconvertin (prō″kŏn-vĕr′tĭn). Coagulation factor VII, q.v.

procreate [L. *procreare*]. To beget; to bring forth young.

procreation (prō″krē-ā′shŭn). The act or state of bringing forth young. SYN: *reproduction.*

procreative (prō′krē-ā′tĭv). Concerning procreation.

proctagra (prŏk-tăg′ră) [Gr. *proktos,* anus, + *agra,* seizure]. Sudden rectal pain.

proctalgia (prŏk-tăl′jē-ă) [″ + *algos,* pain]. Pain in or about the anus and rectum.

p. fugax. Rectal pain that occurs usually

nocturnally. The pain is usually of short duration and even though its cause is unknown, it is not considered to be due to organic disease. In some individuals, having orgasm or a bowel movement will alleviate the pain.

proctatresia (prŏk″tă-trē′zē-ă) [″ + *atresis,* imperforation]. Imperforation of the anus.

proctectasia (prŏk″tĕk-tā′sē-ă) [″ + *ektasis,* dilatation]. Dilatation of the anus or rectum.

proctectomy (prŏk-tĕk′tō-mē) [″ + *ektome,* excision]. Excision of the rectum or anus. SYN: *rectectomy.*

proctenclisis (prŏk″tĕn-klī′sĭs) [″ + *enkleiein,* to shut in]. Stricture of the anus or rectum.

procteurynter (prŏk′tū-rĭn″tĕr) [″ + *eurynein,* to widen]. Instrument for dilation of the anus or rectum.

proctitis [″ + *itis,* inflammation]. Inflammation of rectum and anus. It may be acute or chronic with rectal discomfort and repeated urge to evacuate the rectum accompanied by inability to pass feces. Mucus, blood, or pus may be present in the stools and there may be tenesmus. SYN: *rectitis.*

ETIOL: Infectious organisms; trauma; radiation injury; drugs, esp. broad-spectrum antibiotics; allergy.

p., diphtheritic. Proctitis in which a diphtheritic and albuminous membrane forms over the surface of mucous membrane. There is headache with roaring in ears; constipation, gas, and bloating; neurasthenia.

p., dysenteric. Proctitis resulting from ordinary diarrhea, affects upper part the most. May produce ulcers and scarring of the rectum and anus.

p., gonorrheal. Gonorrheal infection around the rectum and anus.

p., traumatic. Proctitis with pain, pressure as if bowels were going to move; irritable; mucous membrane red, eroded. Surface tissues sensitive to touch. Chronic constipation.

procto-, proct- [Gr. *proktos,* anus]. Combining forms indicating relationship to the anus and rectum.

proctocele (prŏk′tō-sēl) [″ + *kele,* hernia]. A protrusion of the rectal mucosa into the vagina. SYN: *rectocele.*

proctoclysis (prŏk-tŏk′lĭ-sĭs) [″ + *klysis,* a washing out]. A continuous infusion into the rectum and colon in which the solution is introduced drop by drop. SEE: *enteroclysis.*

THERAP. EFFECT: To supply fluid in postoperative cases when fluids cannot be taken otherwise; to supply the body with fluid as in hemorrhage, vomiting, or diarrhea; to relieve thirst as in persistent vomiting; to lower body temperature by giving ice water enemas.

SOLUTIONS: The fluid usually consists of a normal saline solution, a sodium bicarbonate solution, or plain tap water at body temperature. Normal salt solution half strength frequently is used. This need not be a sterile solution unless so ordered. Sodium bicarbonate of 2%–5% strength or a glucose solution of 2%–5%, but no stronger, may be used. A combination of these may also be ordered as a normal saline with glucose and sodium bicarbonate, 5% and 2%, respectively, or other combinations may be used.

NURSING IMPLICATIONS: A cleansing enema is given prior to beginning proctoclysis; when the bowel is completely evacuated, fluid at body temperature is introduced through a lubricated rectal catheter inserted to approx. 4 in. (10 cm.). The liquid is given at a rate of 40–60 drops/min. If given faster, the bowel will be stimulated. Do not give more than 6 oz. (180 ml.) in a single continuous proctoclysis. Turn the patient frequently during the treatment. If rectal gas needs to be passed, clamp the tube temporarily. Discontinue if pain or distention develops.

proctococcypexia, proctococcypexy (prŏk″tō-kŏk-sĭ-pĕk′sē-ă, -kŏk′sĭ-pĕk″sē) [″ + *kokkyx,* coccyx, + *pexis,* fixation]. Suture of rectum to the coccyx.

proctocolitis (prŏk″tō-kō-lī′tĭs) [″ + *kolon,* colon, + *itis,* inflammation]. Inflamed condition of colon and rectum.

proctocolonoscopy (prŏk″tō-kō″lŏn-ŏs′kō-pē) [″ + ″ + *skopein,* to examine]. Examination of interior of rectum and lower colon.

Proctocort. Trade name for hydrocortisone, USP.

proctocystoplasty (prŏk″tō-sĭs′tō-plăs″tē) [″ + *kystis,* bladder, + *plastos,* formed]. Plastic surgery involving the rectum and bladder.

proctocystotomy (prŏk″tō-sĭs-tŏt′ō-mē) [Gr. *proktos,* anus, + *kystis,* bladder, + *tome,* incision]. Incision into the bladder through the rectum.

proctodeum (prŏk-tō-dē′ŭm) [″ + *hodaios,* a way]. An ectodermal depression located caudally that, upon rupture of the cloacal membrane, forms the anal canal.

Proctodon. Trade name for diperodone monohydrate.

proctodynia (prŏk″tō-dĭn′ē-ă) [″ + *odyne,* pain]. Pain in the rectum or about the anus.

proctologic (prŏk″tō-lŏj′ĭk) [″ + *logos,* study]. Concerning proctology.

proctologist (prŏk-tŏl′ō-jĭst) [″ + *logos,* study]. One who specializes in diseases of the colon, rectum, and anus.

proctology (prŏk-tŏl′ō-jē). Phase of medicine dealing with treatment of diseases of the colon, rectum, and anus.

proctoparalysis (prŏk″tō-păr-ăl′ĭ-sĭs) [″ +

para, at the side, + *lyein,* to loosen]. Paralysis of the anal sphincter muscle. SYN: *proctoplegia.*

proctoperineoplasty (prŏk″tō-pĕr″ĭ-nē′ō-plăs″tē) [″ + *perinaion,* perineum, + *plassein,* to form]. Plastic surgery of the anus and rectum.

proctoperineorrhaphy (prŏk″tō-pĕr″ĭ-nē-or′ă-fē) [″ + ″ + *rhaphe,* a sewing]. Proctoperineoplasty, q.v.

proctopexia, proctopexy (prŏk-tō-pĕk′sē-ă, prŏk′tō-pĕk″sē) [″ + *pexis,* fixation]. Suture of the rectum to some other part.

proctophobia (prŏk″tō-fō′bē-ă) [″ + *phobos,* fear]. Abnormal apprehension in those suffering from rectal disease.

proctoplasty (prŏk′tō-plăs″tē) [″ + *plastos,* formed]. Plastic surgery of the anus or rectum.

proctoplegia (prŏk″tō-plē′jē-ă) [″ + *plege,* a stroke]. Paralysis of the anal sphincter. SYN: *proctoparalysis.*

proctopolypus (prŏk″tō-pŏl′ĭ-pŭs) [″ + *polys,* many, + *pous,* foot]. Polyp of the rectum.

proctoptosis (prŏk″tŏp-tō′sĭs) [″ + *ptosis,* a dropping]. Prolapse of the anus and rectum. SEE: *procidentia.*

proctorrhagia (prŏk″tō-rā′jē-ă) [Gr. *proktos,* anus, + *rhegnynai,* to burst forth]. Bleeding from the rectum.

proctorrhaphy (prŏk-tor′ă-fē) [″ + *rhaphe,* a sewing]. Suturing of rectum or anus.

proctorrhea (prŏk-tō-rē′ă) [″ + *rhoia,* flow]. Mucous discharge from the anus.

proctoscope [″ + *skopein,* to examine]. Instrument for inspection of the rectum.

proctoscopy (prŏk-tŏs′kō-pē). Instrumental inspection of the rectum.

proctosigmoidectomy (prŏk″tō-sĭg″moy-dĕk′tō-mē) [″ + *sigma,* Gr. letter S, + *eidos,* form, + *ektome,* excision]. Surgical removal of the anus, rectum, and sigmoid flexure of the colon.

proctosigmoiditis (prŏk″tō-sĭg″moyd-ī′tĭs) [″ + ″ + *eidos,* form, + *itis,* inflammation]. Inflamed condition of the rectum and sigmoid.

proctosigmoidoscopy (prŏk″tō-sĭg-moyd-ŏs′kō-pē). Visual examination of the rectum and sigmoid colon by use of a sigmoidoscope.

proctospasm [″ + *spasmos,* a contracting]. Rectal spasm.

proctostasis (prŏk″tō-stā′sĭs) [″ + *stasis,* stoppage]. Constipation resulting from failure of rectum to respond to defecation stimulus.

proctostenosis (prŏk″tō-stĕn-ō′sĭs) [″ + *stenosis,* narrowing]. Stricture of the anus or rectum.

proctostomy (prŏk-tŏs′tō-mē) [″ + *stoma,* mouth]. Surgical creation of a permanent opening into the rectum.

proctotome (prŏk′tō-tōm) [″ + *tome,* incision]. Knife for incision into rectum.

proctotomy (prŏk-tŏt′ō-mē). Incision of the rectum or anus.

NURSING IMPLICATIONS: Assess the dressing at frequent intervals for the presence and amount of bleeding and drainage, and record. Dressings should be changed or reinforced as prescribed by the physician. Application of a T bandage is advantageous to ensure proper dressing placement.

proctotoreusis (prŏk″tō-tō-roo′sĭs) [″ + *toreusis,* boring]. Surgical procedure for correcting an imperforate anus.

proctotresia (prŏk-tō-trē′sē-ă) [″ + *tresis,* a perforation]. Surgical correction of an imperforate anus.

proctovalvotomy (prŏk″tō-văl-vŏt′ō-mē) [″ + L. *valva,* valve, + Gr. *tome,* incision]. Incision of the rectal valves.

procumbent [L. *procumbens,* lying down]. Lying face down. SYN: *prone.*

procursive (prō-kŭr′sĭv) [L. *procursivus*]. Having an involuntary tendency to run forward.

procurvation (prō″kŭr-vā′shŭn) [L. *procurvare,* to bend forward]. A bending forward.

procyclidine hydrochloride (prō-sī′klĭ-dēn). USP. An antiparkinsonism drug. Trade name is Kemadrin.

prodromal (prō-drō′măl) [Gr. *prodromos,* running before]. Pert. to the initial stage of a disease; the interval between the earliest symptoms and the appearance of the rash or fever.

prodromal rash. A rash that precedes the true rash of an infectious disease.

prodrome. (pl. *prodromes, prodromata*) A symptom indicative of an approaching disease.

prodromic (prō-drō′mĭk). Prodromal, q.v.

prodrug. A newly developed group of chemicals that exhibit their pharmacologic activity after biotransformation.

product (prŏd′ŭkt) [L. *productum*]. Anything that is made naturally or artificially.

production (prō-dŭk′shŭn). Development or formation of a substance.

productive (prō-dŭk′tĭv). Forming, esp. new tissue.

productive inflammation. Inflammation producing new tissue with or without an exudate.

proencephalus (prō″ĕn-sĕf′ă-lŭs) [Gr. *pro,* before, + *enkephalos,* brain]. A deformed fetus in which the brain protrudes through a fissure in the frontal area of the skull.

proenzyme (prō-ĕn′zīm) [Gr. *pro,* before, + *en,* in, + *zyme,* a leaven]. The inactive form of an enzyme found within a cell, which, upon leaving the cell, is converted into the active form such as pepsinogen.

proerythroblast (prō″ĕ-rĭth′rō-blăst) [″ + *erythros,* red, + *blastos,* germ]. The earliest cells that show differentiation in the direction of erythrocyte formation.

proestrus (prō-ĕs′trŭs). The period preceding estrus in females, characterized by development of ovarian follicles and uterine endometrium.

proferment [Gr. *pro,* before, + L. *fermentum,* leaven]. An inactive precursor of a ferment. SYN: *proenzyme.*

professional (prō-fĕsh′ŭn-ăl) [ME. *profession,* sacred vow]. Pert. to a profession.

professional liability. The obligation of health care providers or their insurers to pay for damages resulting from the providers' acts of omission or commission in treating patients.

Professional Standards Review Organization. ABBR: PSRO. Peer review at the local level required by Public Law 92-603 of the U.S. for the services provided under the Medicare, Medicaid, and maternal and child health programs funded by the federal government.

profibrinolysin (prō″fī-brĭ-nō-lī′sĭn) [Gr. *pro,* before, + L. *fibra,* fiber, + Gr. *lysis,* dissolution]. The inactive precursor of the proteolytic enzyme fibrinolysin.

Profilate. Trade name for antihemophilic factor, USP.

profile (prō′fīl) [L. *pro,* forward, + *filare,* to draw a line]. 1. An outline of the side view of an object, esp. the human head. 2. A summary, graph, or table presenting a subject's or thing's most notable characteristics and achievements.

profluvium (prō-floo′vē-ŭm) [L.]. An excessive flow or discharge; a flux.

p. lactis. Excessive flow of milk.

p. seminis. Flow of semen from the vagina deposited during coition.

profondometer (prō″fŏn-dŏm′ĕ-tĕr) [L. *profundus,* deep, + Gr. *metron,* a measure]. Device for locating a foreign body with the fluoroscope.

profunda [L.]. Deep seated; term applied to certain deeply located blood vessels.

profundus (prō-fŭn′dŭs) [L.]. Located deeper than the indicated reference point.

progastrin (prō-găs′trĭn). The inactive precursor of gastrin.

progenitor (prō-jĕn′ĭ-tor) [L.]. An ancestor.

progeny (prŏj′ĕ-nē) [ME. *progenie*]. Offspring.

progeria (prō-jē′rē-ă) [Gr. *pro,* before, + *geras,* old age]. Premature senility occurring in childhood.

ETIOL: Unknown.

SYM AND SIGNS: Small stature, face looks old and wizened, skin is dry and thin, hair is scanty, and sex organs are infantile.

progestational (prō″jĕs-tā′shŭn-ăl). Concerned with the luteal phase of the menstrual cycle at which time, by the action of the hormone progesterone, q.v., the endometrium is further prepared for implantation of the fertilized ovum.

progestational agent. Any one of several chemical substances that have the effect of progesterone. They are usually synthetic, and are used in birth control pills. SYN: *progestin.*

progesterone (prō-jĕs′tĕr-ōn). USP. $C_{21}H_{30}O_2$, a steroid hormone obtained from the corpus luteum and placenta. It is responsible for changes in uterine endometrium in the second half of the menstrual cycle preparatory for implantation of the blastocyst, development of maternal placenta after implantation, and development of mammary glands.

USES: In treatment of menstrual disorders (amenorrhea, dysmenorrhea) and threatened abortion.

progestin (prō-jĕs′tĭn). 1. A corpus luteum hormone that prepares the endometrium for implantation of the fertilized ovum. SYN: *progesterone.* 2. This word is now used to cover a large group of synthetic drugs that have a progesteronelike effect on the uterus.

progestogen (prō-jĕs′tō-jĕn). Any natural or synthetic hormonal substance that produces effects similar to those due to progesterone, q.v.

proglossis (prō-glŏs′ĭs) [Gr.]. Tip of the tongue.

proglottid. Proglottis.

proglottis (prō-glŏt′tĭs) [Gr. *pro,* before, + *glossa,* tongue]. (pl. *proglottides*) A segment of a tapeworm, containing both male and female reproductive organs. SEE: *Cestoda; tapeworm.*

Proglycem. Trade name for diazoxide.

prognathic (prŏg-nā′thĭk) [″ + *gnathos,* jaw]. Prognathous, q.v.

prognathism (prŏg′nă-thĭzm) [″ + *gnathos,* jaw + *-ismos,* condition]. Projection of jaws beyond projection of forehead.

prognathous (prŏg′nă-thŭs). Having jaws projecting forward beyond rest of the face.

prognose (prŏg-nōs′). To predict the course of disease.

prognosis (prŏg-nō′sĭs) [Gr., foreknowledge]. Prediction of course and end of disease, and the estimate of chance for recovery.

p. anceps. Doubtful prognosis.

p. fausta. Favorable prognosis.

p. infausta. Unfavorable prognosis.

prognostic. Rel. to prediction of outcome of a disease.

prognosticate (prŏg-nŏs′tĭ-kāt) [Gr. *prognostikon,* knowing before]. To make a statement on the probable outcome of an illness.

prognostician (prŏg″nŏs-tĭsh′ăn). One skilled in making prognoses.

progonoma (prō″gō-nō′mă) [Gr. *pro,* before,

+ *gonos,* sperm, + *oma,* tumor]. A tumor that develops from displacement of embryonic cells that resemble ancestral forms of the species. An example is a hairy mole.

progranulocyte (prō-grăn'ū-lō-sīt) [" + L. *granula,* granule, + Gr. *kytos,* cell]. A promyelocyte.

progravid (prō-grăv'ĭd) [" + L. *gravidus,* pregnant]. Before or preceding pregnancy.

progression (prō-grĕsh'ŭn) [L. *progressus*]. Advancing or moving forward.

progressive (prō-grĕs'ĭv). Advancing, as a disease from bad to worse.

progressive muscular atrophy. Gradual advancing atrophy of groups of muscles due to spinal cord degeneration. SYN: *paralysis, wasting.* SEE: *atrophy, muscular.*

progressive ossifying myositis. Tendency to bony deposits in the muscles with chronic inflammation.

progressive resistive exercise. ABBR: PRE. A form of active resistive exercise based on a principle of gradual increases in the amount of resistance in order to achieve maximum strength.

progress notes. Notes made on the chart by those involved in caring for the patient. Thus physicians, nurses, consultants, and therapists may record their notes concerning the progress or lack of progress made by the patient in the interim between the previous note and the time of the most recent note. In patients who are not critically ill, a note concerning progress might be made daily or less frequently; in critical care situations, notes could be made hourly.

prohormone (prō-hor'mōn). Precursor of a hormone.

proinsulin. A precursor of insulin produced in the beta cells of the pancreas.

projectile vomiting. Vomiting in which the stomach contents are ejected with great force.

projection (prō-jĕk'shŭn) [Gr. *pro,* before, + *jacere,* to throw]. 1. The act of throwing forward. 2. A part extending beyond the level of its surroundings. 3. The mental process by which sensations are referred to the sense organs or receptors stimulated, or outside the body to the object that is the stimulus. 4. Distortion of a perception as a result of its repression, resulting in such a phenomenon as hating without cause one who has been dearly loved, or attributing to others one's own undesirable traits. Characteristic of the paranoid reaction.

prokaryon (prō-kăr'ē-ŏn) [" + *karyon,* nucleus]. 1. Nuclear material that is spread throughout the cell cytoplasm and is not bounded by a membrane. 2. Prokaryote, q.v.

prokaryote (prō-kăr'ē-ōt) [" + *karyon,* nucleus]. Organism with a single, circular chromosome, without a nuclear membrane, or membrane-bound organelles, i.e., mitochondria and lysosomes. Included in this classification are bacteria and blue-green algae. SEE: *eukaryote.*

Proketazine. Trade name for carphenazine maleate.

Proklar. Trade name for sulfamethizole.

prolabium (prō-lā'bē-ŭm) [" + *labium,* lip]. The entire central portion of the upper lip.

prolactin (prō-lăk'tĭn) [" + *lac,* milk]. A hormone produced by the pituitary gland. In humans, prolactin in association with estrogen and progesterone stimulates breast development and the formation of milk during pregnancy. The act of sucking is an important stimulus for the production of prolactin in the postpartum period. Some of the metabolic effects of prolactin resemble those of growth hormone. Hyperprolactinemia may be associated with amenorrhea in women and reduced sexual potency in men. Stress of all kinds can stimulate prolactin release.

prolamin(e) (prō-lăm'ĭn, prō'lă-mĭn). Any one of a class of proteins found in seeds.

prolapse (prō-lăps') [L. *prolapsus*]. A falling or dropping down of an organ or internal part, such as the uterus or rectum. SYN: *procidentia; ptosis.*

p. of anus. Protrusion of lower portion of the digestive tract through external sphincter of anus.

p. of cord. Expulsion of umbilical cord prematurely. SEE: *labor.*

p. of iris. Protrusion of iris through an injury in the cornea.

p. of rectum. Protrusion of rectal mucosa through the anus.

p. of uterus. Downward displacement of uterus, the cervix sometimes protruding from the vaginal orifice.

prolapsus [L.]. A falling or downward displacement of some part of the body, as the uterus. SYN: *prolapse.*

prolepsis [Gr. *pro,* before, + *lepsis,* a seizure]. Return of paroxysmal attacks at successively shorter intervals.

proleptic. Recurring before the time expected, said of paroxysms.

proleukocyte (prō-lū'kō-sīt) [" + *leukos,* white, + *kytos,* cell]. An undeveloped leukocyte.

proliferate (prō-lĭf'ĕr-āt) [L. *proles,* offspring, + *ferre,* to bear]. To increase by reproduction of similar forms.

proliferation (prō-lĭf"ĕr-ā'shŭn). 1. Reproduction rapidly and repeatedly of new parts, as by cell division. 2. Process or result of rapid reproduction.

proliferous. 1. Multiplying, as by formation of new tissue cells. 2. Bearing offspring.

proliferous cyst. Cyst with epithelial lining, proliferating and projecting from its inner surface.

prolific [L. *prolificus*]. Fruitful; reproductive. SYN: *fertile*.

prolinase. An enzyme found in animal tissues and yeast that hydrolyzes proline peptides to simpler peptids and proline.

proline (prō'lēn). An important amino acid, C_4H_8NCOOH, formed by decomposition of protein.

Prolixin Enanthate. Trade name for fluphenazine enanthate, USP.

Proloid. Trade name for thyroglobulin.

Proloprim. Trade name for trimethoprim.

prolymphocyte (prō"lĭmf'ō-sīt) [" + L. *lympha*, water, + Gr. *kytos*, cell]. A cell intermediate between a lymphoblast and lymphocyte.

Promapar. Trade name for chlorpromazine hydrochloride, USP.

promazine hydrochloride (prō'mă-zēn). USP. An antipsychotic drug. Trade name is Sparine.

promegakaryocyte (prō-mĕg"ă-kăr'ē-ō-sīt) [" + *megas*, big, + *karyon*, nucleus, + *kytos*, cell]. Cell from which a megakaryocyte develops.

promegaloblast (prō-mĕg'ă-lō-blast") [" + " + *blastos*, germ]. A cell of the erythrocyte series preceding the megaloblast.

prometaphase (prō-mĕt'ă-fāz) [" + *meta*, change, + *phasis*, to appear]. Stage of mitosis in which the nuclear membrane disintegrates, and the chromosomes move toward the equatorial plate.

promethazine hydrochloride (prō-mĕth'ă-zēn). USP. An antihistamine drug. Trade names are Anergan 25, Ganphen, and Remsed.

promethium (prō-mē'thē-ŭm). SYMB: Pm. At. wt. 144.9128; at. no. 61. A radioactive element of the rare earth series.

promine. A tissue extract that promotes growth of certain tumors in mice.

prominence (prŏm'ĭ-nĕns) [L. *prominens*, project]. A projection or protrusion. SEE: *prominentia* [NA].

prominentia (prŏm"ĭ-nĕn'shē-ă) [L.]. (pl. *prominentiae*) [NA] A projection.

p. laryngea. [NA] The laryngeal prominence; Adam's apple. SYN: *pomum adami*.

p. spiralis. [NA] A small ridge extending entire length of the cochlea located on inner surface of spiral ligament. It projects slightly into cochlear canal and contains blood vessels including the vas prominens.

promonocyte (prō-mŏn'ō-sīt) [Gr. *pro*, before, + *monos*, single, + *kytos*, cell]. In the development of white blood cells, the precursor of the monocyte. It is between the monoblast and monocyte.

promontory (prŏm'ŏn-tor"ē) [L. *promontorium*]. A projecting process or part.

p. of sacrum. The anterior projecting portion of the pelvic surface of the base of the sacrum. With the 5th lumbar vertebra, it forms the sacrovertebral angle.

p. of tympanic cavity. Projection on medial wall of the tympanic cavity produced by first turn of the cochlea.

promoter (prō-mō'tĕr). A substance that assists a catalyst to act.

promyelocyte (prō-mī'ĕl-ō-sīt) [Gr. *pro*, before, + *myelos*, marrow, + *kytos*, cell]. 1. A large mononuclear myeloid cell seen in the blood in leukemia. 2. Cell development between myeloblast and a myelocyte, resembling a myeloblast.

pronate (prō'nāt). To place in a prone position.

pronation (prō-nā'shŭn) [L. *pronus*, prone]. 1. The act of lying prone or face downward. 2. The act of turning the hand so the palm faces downward or backward. SEE: *supination*.

pronator. A muscle that pronates. SEE: *Muscles* in *Appendix*.

pronator syndrome. A neurological disorder caused by entrapment of the median nerve at the elbow. Symptoms and signs include aching pain in the wrist with a subjective feeling of poor coordination; paresthesias extending into the hand; paresis of the thumb muscles; pain on pronation of the forearm and flexion of the wrist against resistance; and tenderness in the proximal thenar muscles. A positive Tinel's sign over the pronator teres muscles may be present. The disease usually affects the dominant arm of males. Corticosteroid injection into the site is usually effective.

pronaus, pronaeus (prō-nā'ŭs) [Gr. *pro*, before, + *naos*, temple]. The vagina or vestibule of the vagina.

prone (prōn) [ME.]. 1. Lying horizontal with face downward. 2. Denoting the hand with the palm turned downward. Opposite of supine.

pronephric (prō-nĕf'rĭk) [Gr. *pro*, before, + *nephros*, kidney]. Pert. to the pronephros.

pronephric duct. Duct that connects posteriorly to the cloaca and to which pronephric tubules are connected.

pronephric tubules. Several pairs of segmentally arranged tubules that open into the cranial portion of the pronephric duct. They communicate with coelom through a ciliated funnel-shaped nephrostome. They are vestigial in higher vertebrates.

pronephros, pronephron (prō-nĕf'rŏs, -rŏn). The earliest and simplest type of excretory organ of vertebrates, functional in simpler forms (cyclostomes), and serving as a provisional kidney in some fishes and amphibians. In reptiles, birds, and mammals, it appears in the embryo as a temporary, functionless structure.

Pronestyl. Trade name for procainamide hydrochloride, USP.

prong (prŏng). A conically shaped body such as the root of a tooth.

pronograde (prō′nō-grād) [L. *pronus,* prone, + *gradus,* a step]. Walking on hands and feet or resting with the body in a horizontal position. Opposite of orthograde.

pronometer (prō-nŏm′ĕ-tĕr) [″ + Gr. *metron,* a measure]. Device for showing amount of pronation or supination of forearm.

pronormoblast (prō-nor′mō-blăst) [Gr. *pro,* before, + L. *norma,* rule, + Gr. *blastos,* germ]. An early precursor of the red blood cell.

pronucleus (prō-nū′klē-ŭs) [Gr. *pro,* before, + *nucleus,* little kernel]. Nucleus of the ovum (the female pronucleus) or of the spermatozoon (the male pronucleus) after fertilization of the ovum.

prootic (prō-ŏt′ĭk, -ō′tĭk) [″ + *ous,* ear]. In front of the ear.

propagation (prŏp-ă-gā′shŭn) [L.]. Act of reproducing or giving birth. SYN: *generation; reproduction.*

propagative (prŏp′ă-gā″tĭv). Pert. to or taking part in reproduction.

propalinal (prō-păl′ĭ-năl) [Gr. *pro,* before, + *palin,* back]. Applied to a backward and forward movement, as of the jaws.

propane (prō′pān). A hydrocarbon, C_3H_8, that is present in natural gas. It is odorless and colorless. When it is to be used in dwellings, as a fuel, to produce heat, or in hot air balloon, an odoriferous substance is added so that a leak that could go undetected would be obvious because of the odor.

propantheline bromide (prō-păn′thĕ-lēn). USP. An anticholinergic drug that acts like belladonna. Trade name is Pro-Banthine.

proparacaine hydrochloride (prō-păr′ă-kān). USP. A topical anesthetic drug used in ophthalmology. Trade names are Alcaine, Ophthaine, and Ophthetic.

propepsin (prō-pĕp′sĭn). Pepsinogen.

propeptone (prō-pĕp′tōn) [″ + *peptein,* to digest]. An intermediate product in the digestive conversion of protein into peptone. SYN: *hemialbumose.*

propeptonuria (prō″pĕp-tō-nū′rē-ă) [″ + ″ + *ouron,* urine]. Excretion of propeptone in the urine. SYN: *hemialbumosuria.*

properdin (prō-pĕrd′ĭn). A serum protein that, in the presence of magnesium ions and complement, has the ability to help destroy various bacteria and viruses. SEE: *complement.*

prophase (prō′fāz) [″ + *phasis,* phase of the moon]. First stage of indirect cell division. SEE: *centriole; metaphase; mitosis.*

prophylactic (prō-fĭ-lăk′tĭk) [Gr. *prophylaktikos,* guarding]. 1. Any agent or regimen that contributes to the prevention of infection and disease. 2. Popular term for a condom.

prophylaxis (prō-fĭ-lăk′sĭs, prō-fĭl-ăks′ĭs) [Gr. *prophylassein,* to guard against]. Observance of rules necessary to prevent disease.

p., oral. The removal of calculus and stains from the exposed and unexposed surfaces of the teeth by scaling and polishing as a preventive measure for the control of local irritational factors.

propiolactone (prō″pē-ō-lăk′tōn). A disinfectant used in preparing certain viral and bacterial vaccines. Trade name is Betaprone. SYN: β-*propiolactone,* or *beta-propiolactone.*

propiomazine hydrochloride (prō″pē-ō-mā′zēn). USP. A sedative drug. Trade name is Largon.

propionic acid. Methylacetic acid, C_2H_5COOH, which is present in sweat.

Propitocaine Hydrochloride. Previously used trade name for prilocaine hydrochloride.

proplasmacyte (prō-plăz′mă-sīt) [Gr. *pro,* before, + *plasma,* a thing formed, + *kytos,* cell]. The precursor of the plasma cell.

proplastid (prō-plăs′tĭd). The cytoplasmic body from which a plastid is formed.

Proplex. Trade name for Factor IX complex.

propositus (prō-pŏz′ĭ-tŭs) [L. *proponere,* to put on view]. The initial individual whose condition led to investigation of an hereditary disorder. SYN: *index case; proband.*

propoxycaine hydrochloride (prō-pŏk′sē-kān). USP. A local anesthetic drug. Trade names are Blockaine Hydrochloride and Ravocaine Hydrochloride.

propoxyphene hydrochloride (prō-pŏk′sē-fēn). USP. An analgesic drug available in a variety of dosage forms and combinations. Trade names are Darvon, Dolene, Proxagesic, and SK 65.

propranolol hydrochloride. USP. A β-adrenergic blocking agent used in treating hypertension; for prevention of angina pectoris; and for treating certain cardiac arrhythmias, esp. those caused by overdose of digitalis. Trade name is Inderal. CAUTION: Persons with asthma should not be treated with this drug.

proprietary medicine (prō-prī′ĕ-tar″ē) [L. *proprietarius,* pert. to property]. Any chemical, drug, or similar preparation used in the treatment of diseases, if such article is protected against free competition as to name, product, composition, or process of manufacture by secrecy, patent or copyright, or by another means. SEE: *nonproprietary name; patent medicine.*

proprioception (prō″prē-ō-sĕp′shŭn) [L. *proprius,* one's own, + *capio,* to take]. The awareness of posture, movement, and changes in equilibrium and the knowledge of position, weight, and resistance of objects in relation to the body.

proprioceptive (prō″prē-ō-sĕp′tĭv). Pert. to proprioception.

proprioceptive impulses. Afferent impulses arising in a proprioceptor, q.v.

proprioceptive sense. The correlation of unconscious sensations from the skin and joints that allows conscious appreciation of the position of the body.

proprioceptor (prō″prē-ō-sĕp′tor) [″ + *ceptor,* a receiver]. A receptor that responds to stimuli originating within the body itself, esp. those responding to pressure, position, or stretch.

Ex.: muscle spindles, pacinian corpuscles, and labyrinthine receptors.

propriospinal (prō″prē-ō-spī′năl) [″ + *spina,* thorn]. Concerned exclusively with the spinal cord.

proptometer (prŏp-tŏm′ĕ-tĕr) [Gr. *proptosis,* protrusion, + *metron,* a measure]. An instrument for measuring extent of exophthalmos.

proptosis (prŏp-tō′sĭs). A downward displacement such as the uterus or the eyeball in exophthalmic goiter or in inflammatory conditions of the orbit.

propulsion (prō-pŭl′shŭn) [L. *propulsus,* driven forward]. 1. A tendency to push or fall forward in walking. 2. A condition seen in paralysis agitans. SEE: *festination.*

propyl (prō′pĭl). The radical of propyl alcohol or propane, $CH_3-CH_2-CH_2-$.

propylene glycol (prŏp′ĭ-lēn). USP. A demulcent agent used as a solvent for medicines, and in cosmetics.

propylhexedrine (prō″pĭl-hĕk′sĕ-drēn). USP. A sympathomimetic drug usually dispensed in an inhaler to produce nasal decongestion. Trade name is Benzedrex.

propyliodone (prō″pĭl-ī′ō-dōn). USP. A radiopaque dye used in x-ray studies of the bronchi.

propylparaben (prō″pĭl-păr′ă-bĕn). Propyl *p*-hydroxybenzoate, $C_{10}H_{12}O_3$, a chemical used as an antifungal agent and as a preservative in pharmaceuticals.

propylthiouracil (prō″pĭl-thī″ō-ū′ră-sĭl). USP. Antithyroid drug used in treatment of hyperthyroidism, thyroiditis, and thyrotoxicosis. Also employed for preoperative therapy and in cases where surgery is contraindicated.

pro re nata (prō rē nā′tă) [L.]. ABBR: p.r.n. According to the circumstances; as necessary.

prorrhaphy (prō′ră-fē) [Gr. *pro,* before, + *rhaphe,* suture]. Surgical movement of a muscle or tendon insertion to a point farther away. Done to change the action of a muscle. SYN: *advancement.*

prorsad (pror′săd). In a forward direction.

prorubricyte (prō-roo′brĭ-sīt). A basophilic normoblast.

prosecretin (prō″sē-krē′tĭn) [″ + *secretio,* a secretion]. Substance present in the duodenal mucosa that, when acted on by hydrochloric acid in chyme, is converted into secretin. SEE: *secretin.*

prosection (prō-sĕk′shŭn) [″ + L. *sectio,* cutting]. Dissection for the purpose of demonstrating anatomic structure.

prosector (prō-sĕk′tor) [L.]. One who prepares cadavers for dissection or dissects for demonstration.

prosencephalon (prŏs″ĕn-sĕf′ă-lŏn) [Gr. *proso,* before, + *enkephalos,* brain]. The embryonic forebrain, which gives rise to the telencephalon and diencephalon, q.v.

proso- [Gr. *proso,* forward]. Combining form indicating forward or anterior.

prosodemic (prŏs″ō-dĕm′ĭk) [″ + *demos,* people]. Spread by individual contact; said of a disease. SEE: *epidemic.*

prosopagnosia (prŏs″ō-păg-nō′sē-ă) [Gr. *prosopon,* face, + *a-,* not, + *gnosis,* recognition]. Inability to recognize faces, even one's own face.

prosopalgia (prŏs″ō-păl′jē-ă) [″ + *algos,* pain]. Neuralgic pain in the trigeminal nerve and its branches. SYN: *prosopodynia; prosoponeuralgia; tic douloureux.*

prosopectasia (prŏs″ō-pĕk-tā′zē-ă) [″ + *ektasis,* dilatation]. Enlarged size of the face.

prosopic (prō″sŏp′ĭk). Pert. to face or facial skeleton that is convex anteriorly.

prosoplasia (prŏs″ō-plā′sē-ă) [Gr. *proso,* forward, + *plassein,* to form]. Progressive transformation of cells until they develop into cells with a higher degree of function.

prosopoanoschisis (prŏs″ō-pō″ă-nŏs′kĭ-sĭs) [Gr. *prosopon,* face, + *ana,* up, + *schisis,* cleft]. Oblique facial cleft, a slanting furrow extending from mouth to eye.

prosopodiplegia (prŏs″ō-pō-dī-plē′jē-ă) [″ + *dis,* double, + *plege,* a stroke]. Paralysis on both sides of the face.

prosopodynia (prŏs″ō-pō-dĭn′ē-ă) [″ + *odyne,* pain]. Pain in the face. SYN: *prosoponeuralgia; tic douloureux.*

prosoponeuralgia (prŏs″ō-pō-nū-răl′jē-ă) [″ + *neuron,* sinew, + *algos,* pain]. Facial neuralgia. SYN: *prosopalgia; tic douloureux.*

prosopopagus (prŏs″ō-pŏp′ă-gŭs) [″ + *pagos,* a thing fixed]. Unequal conjoined twins in which the parasite is attached to some part of the face other than the jaw.

prosopoplegia (prŏs″ō-pō-plē′jē-ă) [″ + *plege,* stroke]. Facial paralysis. SYN: *facioplegia.*

prosoposchisis (prŏs-ō-pŏs′kĭ-sĭs) [Gr. *prosopon,* face, + *schisis,* a cleft]. Congenital cleft of the face.

prosopospasm (prŏs′ō-pō-spăzm) [″ + *spasmos,* a spasm]. Facial spasm.

prosopothoracopagus (prŏs″ō-pō-thō″ră-kŏp′ă-gŭs) [″+ *thorax,* chest, + *pagos,* a thing fixed]. Conjoined twins joined in the frontal area between the face and the chest.

prosopotocia (prŏs″ō-pō-tō′shē-ă) [″ + *tokos,* birth]. Presentation of the face in parturition.

prosopus varus (prŏs′ō-pŭs vă′rŭs) [Gr. *prosopon,* face, + L. *varus,* crooked]. Congenital obliquity of the face due to atrophy of one side of the head.

prospective study. A clinical or epidemiological investigation of patients or health subjects with respect to the medical, social, and environmental factors encountered from the time of the beginning of the study until the investigation is terminated. SEE: *retrospective study.*

prostaglandins (prŏs′tă-glănd-ĭns). A group of fatty acid derivatives present in many tissues including prostate gland, menstrual fluid, brain, lung, kidney, thymus, seminal fluid, and pancreas. They are synthesized in the body from unsaturated fatty acids. There are a great number of prostaglandins. They are extremely active biological substances that affect many tissues and organs. Certain prostaglandins have a marked effect on the uterus and have been used as abortifacients due to their oxytocic effects. Their general use for these purposes is limited by a great number of undesired side effects. Prostaglandins are being studied intensively for their effects on the cardiovascular, gastrointestinal, and respiratory systems.

Prostaphlin. Trade name for oxacillin sodium, USP.

prostatalgia (prŏs-tă-tăl′jē-ă) [Gr. *prostates,* prostate, + *algos,* pain]. Pain of the prostate gland.

prostate (prŏs′tāt) [Gr. *prostates*]. A gland that surrounds the neck of the bladder and the urethra in the male. It is partly muscular and partly glandular, with ducts opening into the prostatic portion of the urethra. Consists of a median lobe and two lateral lobes. About 2 × 4 × 3 cm., and weighing about 20 gm., it is enclosed in a fibrous capsule containing smooth muscle fibers in its inner layer. Muscle fibers also separate the glandular tissue and encircle the urethra. The gland secretes a thin, opalescent, slightly alkaline fluid that forms part of the seminal fluid.

PATH: Inflammation of the prostate may occur, often the result of gonorrheal urethritis. Enlargement of the prostate is common, esp. after middle age. This results in urethral obstruction, impeding urination and sometimes leading to retention. Benign and malignant tumors, calculi, and nodular hyperplasia are common, particularly in men past 60.

prostatectomy (prŏs″tă-tĕk′tō-mē) [Gr. *prostates,* prostate, + *ektome,* excision]. Excision of part or all of the prostate gland. The operation may be performed through an incision in the perineum (perineal prostatectomy), into the bladder (suprapubic prostatectomy), or through the urethra (transurethral prostatectomy). After prostatectomy, the libido is unaffected but during ejaculation sperm enters the bladder rather than the urethra. This prevents fertilization.

COMPLICATIONS: Retention of urine, hematuria, cystitis, infection of kidney, pyelitis, infective nephritis, renal failure.

prostathelcosis (prŏs″tă-thĕl-kō′sĭs) [″ + *helkosis,* ulceration]. Ulceration of the prostate gland.

prostatic (prŏs-tăt′ĭk) [Gr. *prostates,* prostate]. Concerning the prostate gland.

prostatic calculus. A stone in the prostate.

prostatic hypertrophy. Enlargement of the prostate gland due to the aging process rather than inflammation or neoplasm. The condition is benign, but if enlargement progresses to cause obstruction of the urethra, surgical intervention is required.

prostatic plexus. 1. Veins around the base and neck of the bladder and prostate gland. 2. Nerves from the pelvic plexus to the prostate gland, erectile tissue of the penis, and the seminal vesicles.

prostatic syncope. Fainting during examination of the prostate. This is a rare occurrence that usually can be avoided by examining the patient in the lateral recumbent position.

prostatic urethra. That part of the urethra surrounded by the prostate gland.

prostatism (prŏs′tă-tĭzm) [″ + *-ismos,* condition]. Any condition of the prostate gland that interferes with the flow of urine from the bladder.

ETIOL: Benign hypertrophy, carcinoma, prostatitis, nodular hyperplasia.

SYM: Frequent uncomfortable urination, nocturia. Retention of urine may occur with development of uremia.

prostatitis (prŏs″tă-tī′tĭs) [″ + *itis,* inflammation]. Inflamed condition of the prostate gland. May be a complication of gonorrheal infection.

p., acute. Discomfort and pain in the perineal area. Frequent urination; later, retention of urine. If severe, marked malaise, rise of temperature, constipation, chills, and vomiting.

p., chronic. Dull, aching pain in perineal region. Discharge from the penis.

p., chronic bacterial. ABBR: CBP. Inflammation of the prostate due to long-standing bacterial infection. Clinical symptoms of fever, pain, and dysuria may be relatively mild as compared with the acute infection.

Therapy depends upon the causative organism and in addition to antibiotics may involve treatment of prostatic hypertrophy.

prostatocystitis (prŏs″tă-tō-sĭs-tī′tĭs) [Gr. *prostates,* prostate, + *kystis,* bladder, + *itis,* inflammation]. Inflammation of the prostatic urethra involving the bladder.

prostatocystotomy (prŏs″tă-tō-sĭs-tŏt′ō-mē) [″ + ″ + *tome,* incision]. Surgical incision of the prostate and bladder.

prostatodynia (prŏs″tă-tō-dĭn′ē-ă) [″ + *odyne,* pain]. Pain in the prostate gland. SYN: *prostatalgia.*

prostatography (prŏs″tă-tŏg′ră-fē) [″ + *graphein,* to write]. Radiographic examination of the prostate gland after introduction of a contrast medium.

prostatolith (prŏs-tăt′ō-lĭth) [″ + *lithos,* stone]. A calculus of the prostate gland.

prostatolithotomy (prŏs-tăt″ō-lĭ-thŏt′ō-mē) [″ + ″ + *tome,* incision]. Incision of the prostate in order to remove a calculus.

prostatomegaly (prŏs″tă-tō-mĕg′ă-lē) [″ + *megas,* large]. Enlargement of the prostate gland.

prostatomy (prŏs-tăt′ō-mē) [″ + *tome,* incision]. Incision into the prostate. SYN: *prostatotomy.*

prostatomyomectomy (prŏs″tă-tō-mī″ō-mĕk′tō-mē) [″ + *mys,* muscle, + *ektome,* excision]. Surgical excision of a prostatic myoma.

prostatorrhea (prŏs″tă-tō-rē′ă) [″ + *rhoia,* flow]. Abnormal discharge from the prostate gland.

prostatosis (prŏs″tă-tō′sĭs) [″ + *osis,* condition]. General term indicating nonmalignant and noninflammatory disorders of the prostate gland.

prostatotomy (prŏs″tă-tŏt′ō-mē) [″ + *tome,* incision]. Incision into the prostate gland.

prostatovesiculectomy (prŏs″tă-tō-vē-sĭk″ū-lĕk′tō-mē) [Gr. *prostates,* prostate, + L. *vesiculus,* a little sac, + Gr. *ektome,* excision]. Removal of the prostate gland and seminal vesicles.

prostatovesiculitis (prŏs″tă-tō-vē-sĭk″ū-lī′tĭs) [″ + ″ + Gr. *itis,* inflammation]. Inflammation of the seminal vesicles and prostate gland.

prosternation (prō″stĕr-nā′shŭn) [Gr. *pro,* before, + *sternon,* chest]. Deformity characterized by habitual flexion of the trunk forward when the individual is erect. SYN: *camptocormia.*

prostheon (prŏs′thē-ŏn) [Gr. *prosthios,* foremost]. The alveolar point; midpoint of lower border of upper alveolar arch of the jaw.

prosthesis (prŏs′thē-sĭs) [Gr. *prosthesis,* an addition]. (pl. *prostheses*) 1. Replacement of a missing part by an artificial substitute, such as an artificial extremity. SEE: *Boston arm.* 2. An artificial organ or part. 3. Device to augment performance of a natural function such as a hearing aid.

Advances in bioengineering have enabled scientists to develop artificial extremities including arms, hands, and portions of legs. SEE: *Boston arm.*

p., dental. Replacement of a tooth or of a section of teeth by partial or full dentures.

p., maxillofacial. Repair and artificial replacement of face and jaw missing because of disease or injury.

prosthetic group (prŏs-thĕt′ĭk). The nonamino acid component of a conjugated protein. Usually that portion of an enzyme which is not an amino acid. SEE: *apoenzyme; holoenzyme.*

prosthetics (prŏs-thĕt′ĭks). The branch of surgery dealing with replacement of missing parts.

prosthetist (prŏs′thĕ-tĭst). 1. Specialist in artificial dentures. 2. Maker of artificial limbs.

prosthetosclerokeratoplasty (prŏs″thĕ-tō-sklē″rō-kĕr′ă-tō-plăs″tē). Surgical procedure for replacement of diseased scleral and corneal tissue with a transparent prosthesis.

prosthion (prŏs′thē-ŏn) [Gr. *prosthios,* foremost]. The lowest joint on the alveolar process of the maxilla.

prosthodontics (prŏs″thō-dŏn′tĭks) [″ + *odous,* tooth]. Branch of dentistry dealing with construction of artificial appliances for the mouth. To replace one or more missing teeth and related tissues; usually considered in three main areas of specialization, removable prosthodontics, fixed prosthodontics, and maxillofacial prosthodontics.

prosthodontist (prŏs″thō-dŏn′tĭst). A dentist who specializes in the mechanics of making and fitting artificial teeth.

prosthokeratoplasty (prŏs″thō-kĕr′ă-tō-plăs″tē) [″ + *keras,* horn, + *plassein,* to form]. Surgical replacement of diseased or scarred corneal tissue with a transparent prosthesis.

Prostigmin. Trade name for neostigmine bromide, USP.

Prostin E_2. Trade name for dinoprostone.

Prostin F_2 Alpha. Trade name for dinoprost.

Prostin/15M. Trade name for carboprost; and carboprost tromethamine.

prostitute (prŏs′tĭ-tūt) [L. *prostituere,* to prostitute]. 1. A person who solicits or accepts payment for sexual relations. 2. To sell oneself basely, such as to prostitute one's talents.

prostitution (prŏs″tĭ-tū′shŭn). Act or practice of prostituting. Prostitution is a major cause of the spread of venereal disease.

prostrate (prŏs′trāt) [Gr. *pro,* before, + L. *sternere,* stretch out]. 1. Lying with body extended. 2. To deprive of strength or to exhaust.

prostrated. Depleted of strength; exhausted.

prostration (prŏs-trā′shŭn). Absolute exhaustion.

p., heat. Exhaustion resulting from exposure to excessive heat.

p., nervous. General physical and nervous exhaustion. SYN: *neurasthenia.*

protactinium (prō″tăk-tĭn′ē-ŭm). SYMB: Pa. At. wt. 231; at. no. 91. A radioactive element.

protal (prō′tăl) [Gr. *protos,* first]. Existing from time of birth or before. SYN: *congenital.*

protamine (prō′tă-mĭn). 1. One of a class of simple proteins that are strongly basic, noncoagulable in heat, and yield diamino acids when hydrolyzed. 2. An amine, $C_{16}H_{32}O_2N_9$, isolated from spermatozoa and spawn of fish. Found in fish sperm and named from the fish from which it is derived. SEE: *salmine; sturine.*

p. insulin. Preparations of insulin that are more slowly dissolved and absorbed by body tissues than ordinary insulin. Acts longer than ordinary insulin and lowers the blood sugar for 20 to 24 hours.

p. sulfate. USP. A purified form of protamine used to neutralize the anticogulant action of heparin.

protanope (prō′tă-nōp) [Gr. *protos,* first, + *an-,* not, + *opsis,* vision]. A person with protanopia, q.v.

protanopia (prō-tăn-ō′pē-ă) [″ + ″ + *opsis,* vision]. Red blindness; color blindness in which there is a defect in the perception of red. SEE: *color blindness.*

protean (prō′tē-ăn). [Gr. *Proteus,* a god who changed shapes at will] Having ability to change form, as the ameba. Variable.

protease (prō′tē-ās) [Gr. *protos,* first, + *-ase,* enzyme]. A protein-splitting enzyme.

protective (prō-tĕk′tĭv) [L. *protectus,* shielding]. 1. Covering, preventing infection, providing immunity. 2. An agent that will mechanically protect the part to which applied such as collodion or plaster. SYN: *dressing.*

protective isolation. Isolation in which the patient is being protected from potentially harmful bacteria in the environment. This is particularly important in caring for immunodeficient patients such as those undergoing transplantation surgery.

proteidogenous (prō″tē-ĭd-ŏj′ĕn-ŭs). Producing proteins.

protein (prō′tē-ĭn, prō′tēn) [Gr. *protos,* first]. One of a class of complex nitrogenous compounds that occur naturally in plants and animals and yield amino acids when hydrolyzed. Proteins provide the amino acids essential for the growth and repair of animal tissue.

COMP: Proteins, composed of carbon, hydrogen, oxygen, nitrogen, phosphorus, sulfur, and iron, make up the greater part of plant and animal tissue. Amino acids represent the basic structure of proteins. Foods containing protein consist of different numbers and kinds of amino acids. A complete protein is one that contains all the essential amino acids (tryptophan, lysine, methionine, valine, leucine, isoleucine, phenylalanine, threonine, arginine, and histidine). These are necessary for growth and maintenance of body weight.

FUNCT: Proteins are a source of heat and energy to the body. They are essential for growth, the building of new tissue, and the repair of injured or broken-down tissue. They form an integral part of the protoplasm of every cell. When they are oxidized in the body, heat is liberated. One gm. supplies 4 Cal.

Infants and children require from 2 to 2.2 gm. of protein per kilogram of body weight per day. This should be calculated on the basis of ideal, rather than actual, weight of the child. Age also is a factor in determining protein requirements, the amount decreasing with age. Physical work, menstruation, pregnancy, lactation, and convalescence require increased protein intake. Excess protein in the diet results in increased nitrogen excretion in the urine.

SOURCES: Milk, eggs, cheese, meat, fish, and some vegetables such as soybeans are the best sources. Proteins are found in both vegetable and animal sources of food. Many "incomplete" proteins are found in vegetables; they contain some but not all the essential amino acids. A vegetarian diet can make up for this by combining vegetable groups that complement each other in their basic amino acid groups. This provides the body with complete protein.

Principal animal proteins are ovalbumin in eggs; lactalbumin in milk; serumalbumin in serum; myogen or myosinogen in striated muscle tissue; fibrinogen in blood; ovoglobulin in eggs; lactoglobulin in milk; serum globulin in serum; myosin in striated muscle tissue; thyroglobulin in thyroid; globin in blood; thymus histones in thymus; collagen and gelatin in connective tissue; elastin; and keratin. Nucleoprotein is found in the thymus, pancreas, liver, animal cells, and glands; chondroprotein is found in tendons and cartilage; mucin and mucoids are found in various secreting glands and animal mucilaginous substances; caseinogen in milk; vitellin in egg yolk; hemoglobin in blood; and lecithoprotein in blood, brain, and bile.

p., Bence Jones. An abnormal protein that occurs in urine. Its presence is symptomatic of certain pathologic conditions: multiple myeloma, lymphosarcoma, leukemia, or Hodgkin's disease.

p.'s, blood. Proteins present in blood

include hemoglobin in red blood cells and serum proteins. Normal values are: hemoglobin, 13–18 gm./dl. in men and 12–16 gm./dl. in women; albumin, 3.5-5.0 gm./dl. of serum; globulin, 2.3-3.5 gm./dl. of serum. The amount of albumin in relation to the amount of globulin is referred to as the albumin-globulin (A/G) ratio, which is normally 1.5 to 2.5:1.

p., carrier. A protein that has the ability to elicit an immune response when coupled with a hapten.

p., complete. Protein containing all the essential amino acids.

p., conjugated. Proteins containing the protein molecule with some other molecule or molecules. *Chromoproteins:* Ex.: hemoglobin. *Glycoproteins:* Ex.: mucin. *Lecithoproteins:* Compounds of lecithins or similar substances with the protein molecule. *Nucleoproteins. Phosphoproteins:* Ex.: casein.

p., C-reactive. SEE: *C-reactive protein.*

p., denatured. Protein whose amino acid composition and stereochemical structure have been altered by physical or chemical means.

p., derived. Derivatives of protein molecules obtained by the action of chemical alteration or a physical agent such as heat.

p.'s, immune. Proteins that serve to protect the body against antigens. Immunoglobulins are immune proteins.

p., incomplete. Protein lacking one or more of the essential amino acids.

p., native. A protein in its natural state; one that has not been denatured.

p.'s, plasma. Proteins present in blood plasma, such as albumin or globulin.

p., serum. Proteins present in the serum part of the blood.

p., simple. Those proteins that produce alpha amino acids on hydrolysis. *Albumins:* Soluble in water and coagulated by heat. Ex.: egg albumin. *Globulins:* Insoluble in water, soluble in salt solutions, coagulated by heat. Ex.: edestin from hemp seed. *Glutelins, Prolamines:* alcohol-soluble proteins. Ex.: gliadin from wheat. *Albuminoids:* Ex.: keratin from corn. *Histones, Protamines:* Ex.: salmine from the ripe sperm of salmon.

proteinaceous (prō″tē-ĭn-ā′shŭs). Concerning or resembling proteins.

proteinase (prō′tē-ĭn-ās) [Gr. *protos,* first, + *ase,* enzyme]. A proteolytic enzyme; an enzyme that catalyzes the breakdown of native proteins.

protein balance. Equilibrium between protein intake and anabolism, and protein catabolism and elimination of nitrogenous products. SEE: *nitrogen equilibrium.*

protein-calorie malnutrition. Malnutrition usually seen in infants and young children whose diets are deficient in both proteins and calories. Clinically the condition may be precipitated by other factors such as infection or intestinal parasites. SEE: *kwashiorkor.*

proteinemia (prō″tē-ĭn-ē′mē-ă) [″ + *haima,* blood]. An excess of protein in the blood.

protein hydrolysate injection. USP. A sterile solution of amino acids and short-chain peptides. They represent the approximate nutritive equivalent of casein, lactalbumin, plasma, fibrin, or other suitable proteins from which the hydrolysate is derived by acid, enzymatic, or other method of hydrolysis. It may contain alcohol, dextrose, or other carbohydrate suitable for intravenous infusion. It is used intravenously in the treatment of hypoproteinemia in patients who are unable to eat or absorb food. Trade names are Aminosol and Travamin.

proteinic (prō″tē-ĭn′ĭk). Rel. to protein.

protein-losing enteropathy. Abnormal loss of protein into the gastrointestinal tract. May be due to any disease that causes extensive ulceration of the intestinal mucosa.

proteinogenous (prō″tē-ĭn-ŏj′ĕn-ŭs) [″ + *gennan,* to produce]. Developing from a protein.

proteinophobia (prō″tē-ĭn-ō-fō′bē-ă) [″ + *phobos,* fear]. Aversion to foods containing protein.

proteinosis (prō″tē-ĭn-ō′sĭs) [″ + *osis,* condition]. Accumulation of excess proteins in the tissues.

p., lipoid; p., lipid. A rare hereditary condition resulting from an undefined metabolic defect. Yellow deposits of a mixture of protein and lipoid occur, esp. on the mucous surface of the mouth and tongue. Nodules may appear on the face, extremities, and on the epiglottis and vocal cords. This latter abnormality produces hoarseness.

p., pulmonary alveolar. SEE: *pulmonary alveolar proteinosis.*

protein sensitization. Condition in which a patient is hypersensitive to foreign proteins, so that a severe reaction occurs when they are administered.

protein sparer. A substance in the diet such as carbohydrate or fat that prevents the utilization of protein for energy needs.

proteinuria (prō″tē-ĭn-ū′rē-ă) [″ + *ouron,* urine]. Protein, usually albumin, in the urine. SYN: *albuminuria.*

p., orthostatic. Appearance of protein in the urine when the patient has been standing but not while reclining.

p., postural. Protein in the urine in relation to bodily position.

Protenate. Trade name for plasma protein fraction.

proteoclastic (prō″tē-ō-klăs′tĭk) [Gr. *protos,* first, + *klasis,* a breaking]. Splitting up proteins.
proteolipid (prō″tē-ō-lĭp′ĭd). A lipid-protein complex that is insoluble in water. It is found principally in the brain.
proteolysin (prō″tē-ŏl′ĭ-sĭn) [″ + *lysis,* dissolution]. A specific substance causing decomposition of proteins.
proteolysis (prō″tē-ŏl′ĭ-sĭs). The hydrolysis of proteins, usually by enzyme action, into simpler substances.
proteolytic (prō″tē-ō-lĭt′ĭk). Hastening the hydrolysis of proteins.
proteometabolism (prō″tē-ō-mĕ-tăb′ō-lizm) [″ + *metabole,* change, + *-ismos,* condition]. Digestion, absorption, and assimilation of proteins.
proteopepsis (prō″tē-ō-pĕp′sĭs). The digestion of proteins.
proteopeptic (prō″tē-ō-pĕp′tĭk) [″ + *peptein,* to digest]. Pert. to the digestion of protein.
proteopexic (prō-tē-ō-pĕks′ĭk) [″ + *pexis,* fixation]. Pert. to fixation of proteins within the organism.
proteopexy (prō″tē-ō-pĕks′ē). The fixation of proteins within the body.
proteose (prō′tē-ōs) [Gr. *protos,* first]. One of the class of intermediate products of proteolysis between protein and peptone.

p., primary. First products formed during proteolysis of proteins.

p., secondary. Protein resulting from further hydrolysis of primary proteoses.

proteosuria (prō″tē-ōs-ū′rē-ă) [″ + *ouron,* urine]. Proteose in urine. SYN: *albumosuria.*
proteuria (prō″tē-ū′rē-ă). Proteins in the urine. SYN: *proteinuria.*
Proteus (prō′tē-ŭs) [Gr. Proteus, a god who could change his form]. A genus of enteric bacilli, found in intestines and decaying material, causing protein decomposition.

P. morganii. Species that may cause urinary tract infections and acute enteritis.

P. vulgaris. An essentially saprophytic species that may produce urinary tract infections.

prothrombin. A chemical substance existing in circulating blood that, through the medium of thrombokinase, interacts with calcium salts to produce thrombin. SEE: *coagulation factors.*
prothrombinase. An enzyme important in blood coagulation. In a reaction with factors X_a (activated factor X) and factor V in the presence of calcium, prothrombinase catalyzes the conversion of prothrombin to thrombin.
prothrombinemia (prō-thrŏm″bĭn-ē′mē-ă) [Gr. *pro,* before, + *thrombos,* a clot, + *haima,* blood]. Presence of prothrombin in the blood.
prothrombinogenic (prō-thrŏm″bĭ-nō-jĕn′ĭk) [″ + ″ + *gennan,* to produce] Promoting the formation of prothrombin.
prothrombinopenia (prō-thrŏm″bĭ-nō-pē′nē-ă) [″ + ″ + *penia,* poverty]. Deficiency of prothrombin in the blood. SYN: *hypoprothrombinemia.*
prothrombin time. A test of clotting time made by determining the time for clotting to occur after thromboplastin and calcium are added to decalcified plasma. Test is used to evaluate the effect of administration of anticoagulant drugs.
protide (prō′tīd). Protein.
protist (prō′tĭst). Any member of the Protista kingdom.
Protista (prō-tĭs′tă) [LL., simplest organisms]. Term applied to kingdom of organisms including the simpler unicellular animals and plants. Includes bacteria, some algae, spirochetes, protozoa, and other forms not easily classified as being either plants or animals. SEE: *eukaryote, prokaryote*
protistologist (prō-tĭs-tŏl′ō-jĭst) [″ + *logos,* study]. One who studies the Protista, the unicellular organisms.
protistology (prō-tĭs-tŏl′ō-jē). The science of Protista or unicellular plants and microorganisms. SYN: *microbiology.*
protium (prō′tē-ŭm). Hydrogen with atomic weight of one.
proto- [Gr. *protos,* first]. 1. Prefix signifying first. 2. The lowest of a series of compounds having the same elements
protobiology (prō″tō-bī-ŏl′ō-jē) [″ + *bios,* life, + *logos,* study]. The phase of science dealing with life forms more minute than bacteria, i.e., the ultraviruses and bacteriophages.
protoblast (prō′tō-blăst) [″ + *blastos,* a germ]. 1. A naked cell with no cell wall yet formed. 2. Blastomere of segmenting ovum that is parent cell of a part or organ.
protoblastic (prō″tō-blăs′tĭk). Pert. to a protoblast.
protocol (prō′tō-kŏl) [Gr. *protokollon,* first notes glued to manuscript]. 1. A clinical report from first notes taken. 2. Minutes of a meeting. 3. Description of steps to be taken in an experiment.
protodiastole (prō″tō-dī-ăs′tō-lē) [Gr. *protos,* first, + *diastole,* expansion]. The first of four phases of ventricular diastole characterized by drop in intraventricular pressure and closure of semilunar valves. Occurs immediately after second heart sound.
protoduodenum (prō″tō-dū-ō-dē′nŭm) [″ + L. *duodeni,* twelve]. The upper half of the duodenum. It is derived from the embryonic foregut.
protogaster (prō″tō-găs′tĕr) [″ + *gaster,* belly]. The archenteron or gastrocele; the cavity in a gastrula or developing embryo from which the digestive tract develops.

protokylol hydrochloride (prō″tō-kī′lŏl). A sympathomimetic drug used for its bronchodilator activity. Trade name is Ventaire.

protoleukocyte (prō″tō-lū′kō-sīt) [″ + *leukos,* white, + *kytos,* cell]. A minute lymphoid cell in red bone marrow and in the spleen.

Protomastigida (prō″tō-măst-ĭj′ĭ-dă) [″ + *mastix,* whip, + *eidos,* form]. An order of flagellate protozoa. It contains several pathogenic forms including Leishmania and Trypanosoma.

proton (prō′tŏn) [Gr. *protos,* first]. A positively charged particle forming the nucleus of hydrogen and present in the nuclei of all elements, the atomic number of the element indicating the number of protons present. Its mass is 1836 times that of an electron. SEE: *atom; atomic theory; electron; element.*

protoneuron (prō″tō-nū′rŏn) [″ + *neuron,* nerve]. The initial neuron in a reflex arc.

Protopam Chloride. Trade name for pralidoxime chloride, USP.

protopathic [″ + *pathos,* suffering]. Primitive, undiscriminating, esp. with respect to sensing and localizing pain stimuli. SEE: *sensibility.*

protoplasia (prō-tō-plā′zē-ă) [″ + *plassein,* to form]. The primary formation of tissue.

protoplasm (prō′tō-plăzm) [″ + *plasma,* a thing formed]. A thick, viscous colloidal substance that consitutes the physical basis of all living activities, exhibiting the properties of assimilation, growth, motility, secretion, irritability, and reproduction. It is a complex mixture of heterogeneous substances surrounded by a chemically active membrane that regulates the interchange of substances with the surrounding medium. It possesses the physical properties of a colloidal mass, the medium of dispersion being water. SEE: *cell; cytoplasm; nucleus.*

Protoplasm consists of inorganic substances (water, mineral compounds) and organic substances (proteins, carbohydrates, and lipids). The principal elements present are oxygen, carbon, hydrogen, nitrogen, calcium, and phosphorus, which comprise about 99% of protoplasm. Others present in small amounts are potassium, sulfur, chlorine, sodium, magnesium, and iron, together with trace elements (copper, cobalt, manganese, zinc, and others).

protoplasmic (prō-tō-plăz′mĭk). Pert. to protoplasm, or composed of it.

protoplast (prō′tō-plăst) [″ + *plassein,* to form]. In bacteriology, the sphere remaining after gram-positive bacteria have had their cell contents lysed. The bacterial cell wall constituents are absent. In gram-negative organisms these spheres retain an outer wall layer and are called spheroplasts.

protoporphyria (prō″tō-por-fĭr′ē-ă). Porphyria, erythropoietic, q.v.

protoporphyrin (prō″tō-por′fĭ-rĭn). A derivative of hemoglobin containing four pyrrole nuclei; $C_{34}H_{34}N_4O_4$. Formed from heme (ferriprotoporphyrin) by deletion of an atom of iron. Occurs naturally.

protoporphyrinuria (prō″tō-por″fĭ-rĭn-ū′rē-ă). Protoporphyrin in the urine.

protoproteose (prō″tō-prō′tē-ōz). A primary proteose that, upon further digestion, is converted to deuteroproteose.

protospasm (prō′tō-spăzm) [Gr. *protos,* first, + *spasmos,* a spasm]. A spasm beginning in one area and extending to other parts.

prototroph (prō′tō-trōf). An organism with the same nutritional requirements as its ancestors.

prototrophic (prō″tō-trō′fĭk) [″ + *trophe,* nourishment]. Requiring simple inorganic elements as food.

prototype (prō′tō-tīp). An original or initial model or type from which subsequent types arise.

protovertebra (prō″tō-vĕr′tĕ-bră) [″ + L. *vertebra,* vertebra]. Primitive vertebra in the notochord.

protoxide (prō-tŏk′sīd). Of the series of oxides of a metal, the one with the least amount of oxygen.

Protozoa [″ + *zoon,* animal]. The phylum of the animal kingdom that includes the simplest animals. Most are unicellular, although some are colonial. Reproduction usually asexual by fission, although conjugation and sexual reproduction occur.

protozoa. Pl. of protozoon.

protozoacide (prō-tō-zō′ă-sīd) [″ + *zoon,* animal, + L. *cidus,* kill]. Destructive to, or that which kills, protozoa.

protozoal (prō″tō-zō′ăl). Pert. to protozoa, unicellular organisms.

protozoal diseases. Diseases produced by single-celled organisms, such as amebic dysentery, sleeping sickness, and malaria. SEE: Table of Pathogenic Protozoa.

protozoan (prō″tō-zō′ăn) [″ + *zoon,* animal]. Concerning protozoa.

protozoiasis (prō″tō-zō-ī′ă-sĭs) [″ + ″ + *-iasis,* condition]. A disease caused by protozoa.

protozoology (prō″tō-zō-ŏl′ō-jē) [Gr. *protos,* first, + *zoon,* animal, + *logos,* study]. Phase of science dealing with study of protozoa.

protozoon. (pl. *protozoa*) Unicellular organism. SEE: *Protozoa.*

protozoophage (prō″tō-zō′ō-fāj) [″ + *zoon,* animal, + *phagein,* to eat]. A phagocyte that ingests protozoa.

protraction (prō-trăk′shŭn) [″ + L. *protractus,* dragged out]. The extension forward or drawing forward of a part of the body such as the mandible.

protractor (prō-trăk′tor) [L. *protractus,* dragged

Table of Pathogenic Protozoa

Subphylum	Genus and Species	Disease Caused
Mastigophora	Borrelia recurrentis	Relapsing fever
Locomotion by flagella	Borrelia duttonii	Relapsing fever
	Borrelia bronchialis	Bronchial infection
	Borrelia vincentii	Vincent's disease
	Leptospira icterohaemorrhagiae	Weil's disease
	Leishmania donovani	Kala-azar
	Leishmania braziliensis	American leishmaniasis
	Leishmania tropica	Oriental sore
	Giardia lamblia	Gastroenteritis
	Trypanosoma gambiense	Sleeping sickness
	Trypanosoma rhodesiense	Sleeping sickness
	Trypanosoma cruzi	Chagas' disease
Sarcodina	Entamoeba histolytica	Amebic dysentery
Locomotion by pseudopodia	Dientamoeba fragilis	Diarrhea, fever
Sporozoa	Plasmodium malariae	Quartan malaria
No locomotion in adult stage	Plasmodium falciparum	Malignant tertian malaria
	Plasmodium vivax	Benign tertian malaria
	Plasmodium ovale	Ovale malaria
Ciliophora	Balantidium coli	Balantidiasis
Possess cilia in some stage of life cycle		

out]. 1. Instrument for removing foreign bodies from wounds. 2. A muscle that draws a part forward. Opposed to retractor.

protriptyline hydrochloride (prō-trĭp′tĭ-lēn). USP. An antidepressant drug. Trade names are Triptil and Vivactil.

protrude [L. *protrudere*]. To project; to extend beyond a border or limit.

protrusion (prō-troo′zhŭn). State or condition of being thrust forward or projecting. In dentistry, particularly related to the position of the mandible, as opposed to retrusion.

protuberance (prō-tū′bĕr-ăns) [Gr. *pro,* before, + L. *tuber,* bulge]. A part that is prominent beyond a surface, like a knob.

protuberantia (prō-tū″bĕr-ăn′shē-ă). A protuberance, eminence, or projection.

proud flesh. A mass of excessive granulation formed when a wound shows no other sign of healing or tendency to cicatrization.

Provera. Trade name for medroxyprogesterone acetate, USP.

provertebra (prō-vĕr′tĕ-bră). Protovertebra, q.v.

provirus (prō-vī′rŭs). The precursor of a virus.

provisional (prō-vĭzh′ŭn-ăl) [L. *provisio,* provision]. Serving a temporary use pending permanent arrangements.

provitamin (prō-vī′tă-mĭn) [L. *pro,* before, + *vita,* life, + *amine*]. An inactive substance that can be transformed in the body to a corresponding active vitamin and thus function as a vitamin.

p. A. Carotene, the precursor of vitamin A.

Proxagesic. Trade name for propoxyphene hydrochloride, USP.

proximad (prŏk′sĭm-ăd) [L. *proximus,* next, + *ad,* toward]. Toward the proximal or central point.

proximal (prŏk′sĭm-ăl). Nearest the point of attachment, center of the body, or point of reference. Opposite of distal.

proximalis (prŏk″sĭ-mā′lĭs). Proximal.

proximate (prŏk′sĭm-āt). Closely related with respect to space, time, or sequence. Next to, or nearest.

proximoataxia (prŏk″sĭ-mō-ă-tăk′sē-ă) [″ + Gr. *ataxia,* lack of order]. Lack of coordination in muscles of the proximal area of an extremity, as the arm, forearm, thigh, or leg.

proximobuccal (prŏk″sĭ-mō-bŭk′ăl) [″ + *bucca,* cheek]. Concerning the proximal and buccal surfaces of a tooth.

proximolabial (prŏk″sĭ-mō-lā′bē-ăl) [″ + *labialis,* pert. to the lips]. Concerning the proximal and labial surfaces of a tooth.

proximolingual (prŏk″sĭ-mō-lĭng′gwăl) [″ + *lingua,* tongue]. Concerning the proximal and lingual surfaces of a tooth.

prozone. That portion of the low dilution range of a homologous serum that fails to agglutinate bacteria that are agglutinated by the same serum in a higher dilution.

prozymogen (prō-zī′mō-jĕn) [Gr. *pro,* before, + *zyme,* leaven, + *gennan,* to produce]. An intranuclear substance that is a precursor of zymogen.

prune (proon) [L. *pruna*]. A dried plum, rich in carbohydrate. Contains a substance that is useful in stimulating the bowel, esp. for those who suffer from chronic constipation. The ability of prunes and prune juice to exert a laxative effect is due to the presence of dihydroxyphenyl isatin.

prune-belly defect. A nonstandard, but descriptive, term for children with congenital absence of abdominal muscles.

pruriginous (proo-rĭj′ĭ-nŭs) [L. *prurigo,* itch]. Pert. to, or of the nature of, prurigo.

prurigo (proo-rī′gō) [L., the itch]. This term is used by dermatologists throughout the world, but it has not received a universally acceptable definition. Prurigo is a chronic skin disease marked by constantly recurring, discrete, pale, deep-seated, intensely itchy papules on extensor surfaces of limbs. Superimposed exanthematous manifestations may mask the true nature.

ETIOL: Exciting cause unknown.

PROG: Guarded. Prurigo begins in childhood and may last a lifetime.

TREATMENT: Constitutional and local. Hygienic regimen. Antipruritics locally.

p. agria. A severe type of prurigo that starts in childhood and persists. The skin becomes thickened and pigmented. Because of the severe itching and scratching, secondary pustules, boils, and abscesses may develop.

p. estivalis. A form of polymorphic light eruption characterized by prurigo and photodermatitis. Recurring every summer and continuing during hot weather.

p., Hebra's. P. mitis, q.v.

p. mitis. Mild prurigo.

p. nodularis. Eruption in skin of hard nodules with great itching. Occurs most commonly in middle-aged women. Etiology is unknown.

p., pregnancy. A form that usually has its onset in the middle trimester of pregnancy or later. The lesions occur on the proximal portion of the limbs and upper part of the trunk. The skin lesions usually improve spontaneously before term or rapidly after delivery.

p., simple acute. Simple form of prurigo with recurring tendency. Thought to be caused by reaction to bites in sensitive subjects.

p. simplex. Urticaria papulosa, q.v.

pruritogenic (proo″rĭ-tō-jĕn′ĭk) [L. *pruritus,* itching, + *gennan,* to produce]. Causing pruritus.

pruritus (proo-rī′tŭs) [L., itching]. Severe itching. May be a symptom of a disease process such as allergic response, or be due to emotional factors.

ETIOL: Predisposing factor is cutaneous hyperesthesia. Localized causes are present in pruritus ani, pruritus vulvae, intestinal parasites (pinworms), and mycotic infection.

TREATMENT: Exciting or contributory cause located and removed. Hygienic regimen. In anal and vulvar pruritus, examination by competent gynecologist or proctologist before cutaneous therapy is instituted. In bath avoid too sudden changes of temperature. For dry skins, avoid frequent soap and water bathing. Soft, nonirritating underclothing and soothing lotions are of benefit.

p. ani. Itching about the anus. May be due to pinworms; fistula in anus, hemorrhoids; contact with soap or detergents that remain in underclothing following improper washing; or irritation.

p., essential. Pruritus without apparent skin lesion.

p. estivalis. Pruritus with prickly heat occurring in hot weather.

p. hiemalis. Pruritus that occurs in cold weather and is provoked by cooling of the skin.

p. senilis. Pruritus in aged with degenerative skin changes.

p., symptomatic. Pruritus as a symptom of some other disorder.

p. vulvae. Disorder marked by severe itching of external female genitalia. Often an early sign of diabetes mellitus. May be sign of vaginitis.

Prussak's space (proo′săks). [Alexander Prussak, Russ. otologist, 1839–1897] Tiny space in middle ear between Shrapnell's membrane laterally and neck of malleus medially.

prussic acid (prŭs′ĭk). A rapidly acting poison. SYN: *acid, hydrocyanic.*

psalterium (săl-tē′rē-ŭm) [Gr. *psalterion,* harp].

1. Omasum, or third division of the stomach of a ruminant. 2. Commissure of the fornix of the brain.

psammoma (săm-ō'mă) [Gr. *psammos*, sand, + *oma*, tumor]. A small tumor of the brain, the choroid plexus, and other areas, containing calcareous particles.

psammoma bodies. Laminated concretions often found in the pineal body. SYN: *brain sand; corpora arenacea.*

psammosarcoma (săm"ō-săr-kō'mă) [" + *sarx*, flesh, + *oma*, tumor]. A sarcoma in which psammoma bodies are present.

psammotherapy (săm"ō-thĕr'ă-pē) [" + *therapeia*, treatment]. The application of sand baths in treatment.

psammous (săm'ŭs). Sandy, gritty.

pselaphesia, pselaphesis (sĕl-ă-fē'zē-ă, -sĭs) [Gr. *pselaphesis*, touch]. 1. Sense of touch. 2. Plucking at bedclothes with the fingers, a sign observed in delirium. SYN: *carphology.*

psellism, psellismus (sĕl'ĭzm, sĕl-ĭz'mŭs) [Gr. *psellisma*, stammer]. Defective pronunciation, stuttering, or stammering.

p. mercurialis. Jerking, hurried, unintelligible speech present as part of the tremor that accompanies mercury poisoning.

pseudacousma (sū"dă-kooz'mă) [Gr. *pseudes*, false, + *akousma*, a thing heard]. Condition in which all sounds are heard falsely, seeming to be altered in quality of pitch, or imaginary sounds are heard. SYN: *pseudacusis.*

pseudacusis (sū"dă-kū'sĭs). State in which sounds are heard falsely or imagined. SYN: *pseudacousma.*

pseudagraphia (sū"dă-grăf'ē-ă) [" + *a-*, not, + *graphein*, to write]. A form of agraphia in which a person is unable to write independently, but is able to copy words or letters. SYN: *pseudoagraphia.*

pseudarthritis (soo"dăr-thrī'tĭs) [" + *arthron*, joint, + *itis*, inflammation]. A condition that imitates arthritis.

pseudarthrosis (sū"dăr-thrō'sĭs) [" + *arthron*, joint, + *osis*, condition]. A false joint developing after a fracture that has not united.

pseudencephalus (soo"dĕn-sĕf'ă-lŭs) [" + *enkephalos*, brain]. A congenital deformity in which the cranium is open and contains poorly organized vascular tissue.

pseudesthesia (sū"dĕs-thē'zē-ă) [" + *aisthesis*, sensation]. 1. An imaginary or false sensation, as that felt in the lost part after amputation. 2. Sense of feeling not caused by external stimulation. SEE: *paraphia.*

pseudo- (sū'dō) [Gr. *pseudes*, false]. A prefix meaning false.

pseudoacanthosis nigricans (soo"dō-ăk"ăn-thō'sĭs) [" + *akantha*, thorn, + *osis*, condition]. Velvety, pigmented thickening of the flexural surfaces. This occurs in dark-skinned obese persons.

pseudoacephalus (soo"dō-ā-sĕf'ă-lŭs) [" + *a-*, not, + *kephale*, head]. A parasitic twin that has a rudimentary cranium.

pseudoagglutination (sū"dō-ă-glū"tĭ-nā'shŭn). The clumping together of red blood cells as in the formation of rouleaux, but differing from true agglutination in that they can be dispersed by shaking

pseudoagraphia. Pseudagraphia.

pseudoalbinism (sū"dō-ăl'bĭ-nĭzm) [" + L. *albus*, white, + Gr. *-ismos*, condition]. Loss of pigment of the skin, as occurs in leukopathia or vitiligo.

pseudoalleles (soo"dō-ă-lēlz") [" + *allelon*, of one another]. A set of genes that seem to be present in the same locus in certain conditions and in closely situated loci in other conditions.

pseudoanemia (sū"dō-ă-nē mē-ă) [" + *an-*, not, + *haima*, blood]. Pallor of mucous membranes and skin without other signs of true anemia.

pseudoangina (sū"dō-ăn'jĭ-nă, -ăn-jī'nă) [" + L. *angina*, a choking]. False symptoms of nervous origin, resembling angina pectoris.

SYM: Functional attacks in cardiac region but not associated with any disease of the heart or its vessels.

pseudoaneurysm (soo"dō-ăn'ū-rĭzm) [" + *aneurysma*, a widening]. A dilation or tortuosity in a vessel that gives the impression of an aneurysm.

pseudoankylosis (soo"dō-ăng"kĭ-lō'sĭs) [" + *ankyle*, stiff joint, + *osis*, condition]. A false joint.

pseudoapoplexy (sū"dō-ăp'ō-plĕk"sē). A mild condition simulating apoplexy, but not accompanied by cerebral hemorrhage. SYN: *parapoplexy.* SEE: *transient ischemic attack.*

pseudoataxia (sū"dō-ă-tăk'sē-ă) [" + *ataxia*, lack of order]. Condition resembling ataxia, but not due to tabes dorsalis.

pseudoblepsia, pseudoblepsis (sū"dō-blĕp'sē-ă, -sĭs) [" + *blepsis*, sight]. False or imaginary vision. SYN: *parablepsia; pseudopsia.*

pseudobulbar paralysis (sū"dō-bŭl'bĕr) [" + *bolbos*, a swollen end]. Paralysis resembling bulbar paralysis, but due to lesion of cortical centers.

pseudocartilaginous (sū"dō-kăr"tĭ-lăj'ĭ-nŭs) [" + L. *cartilago*, gristle]. Pert. to, or formed of, a substance resembling cartilage.

pseudocast (sū'dō-kăst) [" + ME. *casten*, a throwing off]. A sediment in urine resembling a true cast; a false cast.

pseudocele (sū'dō-sēl) [" + *koilos*, hollow]. The cavity of the septum pellucidum, the so-called 5th ventricle. SYN: *pseudocoele.*

pseudochancre (soo"dō-shăng'kĕr) [Gr. *pseudes*, false, + Fr. *chancre*, ulcer]. A lesion resembling the chancre produced by syphilis.

pseudocholesteatoma (soo″dō-kō″lĕs-tē-ă-tō′mă) [″ + *chole,* bile, + *steatos,* fat, + *oma,* tumor]. Hard epithelium present as a mass in the tympanic cavity in association with chronic inflammation of the middle ear.

pseudocholinesterase (sū″dō-kō″lĭn-ĕs′tĕr-ās). A nonspecific cholinesterase that hydrolyzes noncholine esters as well as acetylcholine. Found in blood serum and pancreatic tissue.

pseudochorea (sū″dō-kō-rē′ă) [″ + *choreia,* a dance]. Hysterical state resembling chorea.

pseudochromesthesia (sū″dō-krō″mĕs-thē′zē-ă) [″ + *chroma,* color, + *aisthesis,* sensation]. A condition in which sounds, esp. of the vowels, seem to induce a sensation of a distinct visual color. SEE: *phonism; photism; synesthesia.*

pseudochromidrosis (sū″dō-krō″mĭd-rō′sĭs) [″ + ″ + *hidros,* perspiration, + *osis,* condition]. Appearance of colored sweat, in which the sweat acquires its color after it is excreted.

pseudocirrhosis (sū″dō-sĭr-ō′sĭs) [″ + *kirros,* orange yellow, + *osis,* disease]. A condition with symptoms of cirrhosis of liver, due to any process that causes obstruction of venous flow from the liver. Constrictive pericarditis can cause this condition.

SYM: Cyanosis, ascites, dyspnea.

pseudocoele (sū′dō-sēl) [″ + *koilos,* hollow]. The 5th ventricle of the brain. SYN: *pseudocele.*

pseudocolloid (soo″dō-kŏl′oyd) [″ + *kollodes,* glutinous]. A mucoid substance present in various locations and in ovarian cysts.

p. of lips. Fordyce's spots, q.v.

pseudocoloboma (sū″dō-kŏl-ō-bō′mă) [″ + *koloboma,* imperfection]. A scarcely noticeable scar on the iris from an embryonic fissure.

pseudocoxalgia (soo″dō-kŏk-săl′jē-ă) [″ + L. *coxa,* hip, + Gr. *algos,* pain]. Osteochondrosis of the head of the femur, in children. SYN: *Legg-Calve-Perthes' disease.*

pseudocrisis (sū-dō-krī′sĭs) [″ + *krisis,* crisis]. A false crisis; a temporary fall of body temperature, which may be followed by a rise.

pseudocroup (sū-dō-kroop′). False croup. SYN: *laryngismus stridulus.*

pseudocyesis (sū″dō-sī-ē′sĭs) [″ + *kyesis,* pregnancy]. A condition in which a patient has nearly all of the usual signs and symptoms of pregnancy such as enlargement of abdomen, weight gain, cessation of menses, and morning sickness, but is not pregnant. Usually seen in women who either are very desirous of having children or wish to avoid pregnancy.

Treatment usually is done by psychiatric means. Pseudocyesis also occurs in men. SYN: *phantom pregnancy; pseudopregnancy.*

pseudocylindroid (soo″dō-sĭ-lĭn′droyd) [″ + *kylindros,* cylinder, + *eidos,* form]. A shred of mucus in the urine that resembles a cast.

pseudocyst (sū′dō-sĭst) [″ + *kystis,* bladder]. A dilatation resembling a cyst.

pseudodementia (sū″dō-dē-mĕn′shē-ă) [″ + L. *de-,* negative, + *mens,* mind]. Exaggerated indifference to environment without impairment of mental capacity.

pseudodiphtheria (sū″dō-dĭf-thē′rē-ă) [″ + *diphthera,* membrane]. A condition resembling diphtheria, but not due to Corynebacterium diphtheriae.

pseudoedema (sū″dō-ē-dē′mă) [Gr. *pseudes,* false, + *oidema,* a swelling]. A puffy condition of the skin simulating edema.

pseudoemphysema (sū″dō-ĕm-fĭ-zē′mă) [″ + *emphysema,* an inflation]. A bronchial condition simulating emphysema, due to temporary blockage of the bronchi.

pseudoencephalitis (sū″dō-ĕn-sĕf″ă-lī′tĭs) [″ + *enkephalos,* brain, + *itis,* inflammation]. A false encephalitis due to profuse diarrhea.

pseudoephedrine hydrochloride (soo″dō-ĕ-fĕd′rĭn). USP. A sympathomimetic drug, an isomer of ephedrine, that has actions similar to ephedrine. Trade names are Sudafed, Novafed, and Besan.

pseudoerysipelas (sū″dō-ĕr-ĭ-sĭp′ĕ-lăs) [″ + *erythros,* red, + *pella,* skin]. An inflammation of subcutaneous cellular tissue simulating erysipelas.

pseudoesthesia (sū″dō-ĕs-thē′zē-ă) [″ + *aisthesis,* sensation]. An imaginary sensation or a false one. SYN: *pseudesthesia.*

pseudofracture (sū″dō-frăk′chūr). A ribbon-like zone of decalcification seen in certain types of osteomalacia.

pseudoganglion (sū″dō-găn′glē-ŏn) [″ + *ganglion,* knot]. A slight thickening of a nerve, resembling a ganglion.

pseudogeusesthesia (sū″dō-gūs″ĕs-thē′zē-ă) [″ + *geusis,* taste, + *aisthesis,* sensation]. A sense of taste stimulated by one of the other senses.

pseudogeusia (sū″dō-gū′sē-ă). A subjective sensation of taste not produced by external stimulus.

pseudoglanders (soo″dō-glăn′dĕrz). Melioidosis, q.v.

pseudoglioma (sū″dō-glī-ō′mă) [″ + *glia,* glue, + *oma,* tumor]. Inflammatory changes curring in the vitreous body that simulate glioma of retina, but due to iridochoroiditis.

pseudoglobulin (sū″dō-glŏb′ū-lĭn) [″ + L. *globulus,* little globe]. One of a class of globulins characterized by being soluble in salt-free water. SEE: *euglobulin.*

pseudoglottis (sū″dō-glŏt′ĭs) [″ + *glottis,* glottis]. Area between false vocal cords.

pseudogout (sū′dō-gowt″). Chronic recurrent

arthritis clinically similar to gout. The crystals found in synovial fluid are calcium pyrophosphate dihydrate and not urate crystals. Also, the most commonly involved joint is the knee and not small joints as in gout. SYN: *chondrocalcinosis.*

TREATMENT: Joint aspiration, phenylbutazone or salicylates.

pseudogynecomastia (soo"dō-jĭn"ĕ-kō-măs'tē-ă) [Gr. *pseudes,* false, + *gyne,* woman, + *mastos,* breast]. Excess adipose tissue in the male breast, but with no increase in glandular tissue.

pseudohematuria (soo"dō-hē"mă-tū'rē-ă) [" + *haima,* blood, + *ouron,* urine]. A red pigment in the urine that makes the urine appear to have blood in it.

pseudohemophilia (soo"dō-hē"mō-fĭl'ē-ă) [" + " + *philos,* to love]. Von Willebrand's disease, q.v.

pseudohemoptysis (sū"dō-hē-mŏp'tĭ-sĭs) [" + *haima,* blood, + *ptyein,* to spit]. Spitting of blood that does not arise from the bronchi or the lungs.

pseudohermaphrodite (soo"dō-hĕr-măf'rō-dīt). An individual having the sex glands of only one sex but having some of the physical appearances of an individual of the opposite sex.

pseudohermaphroditism (sū"dō-hĕr-măf'rō-dīt"ĭzm) [" + *Hermaphroditos,* mythical two-sexed god, + Gr. *-ismos,* condition]. A congenital abnormality of the external genitalia and of the body in which one possesses sex glands of one sex but the genitalia of the opposite sex. SYN: *hermaphroditism, false.* SEE: *intersex.*

p., female. Condition in a female marked by a large clitoris, resembling the penis, and hypertrophied labia majora, resembling the scrotum, thus resembling a male. Can be caused by disease of the adrenal gland.

p., male. Condition in a male marked by a small penis, perineal hypospadias, and scrotum without testes, thereby resembling the vulva. Can be due to disease of the adrenal or condition of feminizing tumor of the undescended testis.

pseudohernia (soo"dō-hĕr'nē-ă) [" + L. *hernia,* hernia]. Inflammation in the scrotal area resembling a hernia.

pseudohypertrophic (sū"dō-hī-pĕr-trō'fĭk) [" + *hyper,* above, + *trophe,* nourishment]. Pert. to a false hypertrophy.

pseudohypertrophy (sū"dō-hī-pĕr'trō-fē). Increase in size of an organ or structure due to hypertrophy or hyperplasia of tissue other than parenchyma. Often accompanied by diminution of function.

pseudohypoparathyroidism (sū"dō-hī"pō-păr"ă-thī'royd-ĭzm). Hereditary disease resembling hypoparathyroidism but caused by an inadequate response to parathyroid hormone rather than a deficiency of the hormone. Some, but not all, of the patients will be obese with short, stocky build and moon-faced. Mental deficiency may be present along with cataracts, strabismus, tetany, stridor, convulsions, and muscular cramps.

pseudoicterus (soo"dō-ĭk'tĕr-ŭs) [" + *ikteros,* jaundice]. Pseudojaundice.

pseudoisochromatic (sū"dō-ī"sō-krō-măt'ĭk) [" + *isos,* equal, + *chroma,* color]. Seemingly of the same color; colors used in charts testing for color blindness.

pseudojaundice (soo"dō-jawn'dĭs) [" + Fr. *jaune,* yellow]. Pigment in the skin, such as in carotenemia, that resembles jaundice, but is not due to jaundice. SEE: *carotenemia.*

pseudologia (sū-dō-lō'jē-ă) [Gr. *pseudes,* false, + *logos,* a study]. Falsification in writing or in speech, a form of pathological lying.

p. fantastica. Pathological lying; one of the forms of the psychopathic state.

pseudomania (sū-dō-mā'nē-ă) [" + *mania,* madness]. 1. A psychosis in which patients falsely accuse themselves of crimes that they think they have commited. 2. Pathological lying.

pseudomasturbation (sū"dō-măs-tŭr-bā'shŭn) [" + L. *manus,* hand, + *stuprare,* to rape]. A nervous habit of pulling at the penis. SYN: *peotillomania.*

pseudomelanosis (sū"dō-mĕl-ă-nō'sĭs) [" + *melas,* black, + *osis,* condition]. Discoloration of tissues after death.

pseudomembrane (sū"dō-mĕm'brān) [" + L. *membrana,* membrane]. A false membrane, as in diphtheria.

pseudomembranous (sū"dō-mĕm'bră-nŭs). Pert. to, or marked by, false membranes.

pseudomeningitis (sū"dō-mĕn-ĭn-jī'tĭs) [" + *meninx,* membrane, + *itis,* inflammation]. A condition resembling symptoms of meningitis without lesions of meningeal inflammation.

pseudomenstruation (sū"dō-mĕn"strū-ā'shŭn) [" + L. *menstruare,* menstruate]. Bleeding from the uterus not accompanied by the usual changes in the endometrium.

pseudomnesia (sū"dŏm-nē'zē-ă) [" + *mnesis,* memory]. A memory perversion in which patient remembers that which never occurred.

Pseudomonas (sū-dō-mō'năs) [" + *monas,* single]. A genus of small, motile, gram-negative bacilli with polar flagella. Most are saprophytic, living in soil and decomposing organic matter. Some produce blue and yellow pigments.

P. aeruginosa. A species that is sometimes pathogenic for man. May cause urinary tract infections or otitis externa.

P. mallei. Species that causes glanders in

horses.

P. pseudomallei. Species that causes melioidosis, q.v., in man and animals.

pseudomucin (sū-dō-mū'sĭn) [" + L. *mucus,* mucus]. A variety of mucin found in ovarian cysts.

pseudomyopia (soo"dō-mī-ō'pē-ă) [" + *myein,* to shut, + *ops,* eye]. Persons whose defective vision causes them to hold objects close in order to see them but who do not have myopia.

pseudomyxoma (sū"dō-mĭk-sō'mă) [" + *myxa,* mucus, + *oma,* tumor]. A peritoneal tumor resembling a myxoma and containing a thick viscid fluid.

p. peritonei. A type of tumor that develops in the peritoneum from implantation metastases resulting from rupture of ovarian cystadenoma or cells escaping during surgical removal. Numerous papillomas develop attached to the abdominal wall and intestine, and the peritoneal cavity becomes filled with mucuslike fluid.

pseudoneoplasm (sū-dō-nē'ō-plăsm) [" + *neos,* new, + *plasma,* something formed]. A false or phantom tumor. A temporary swelling that simulates a tumor, usually of an inflammatory nature.

pseudoneuritis (soo"dō-nū-rī'tĭs) [Gr. *pseudes,* false, + *neuron,* nerve, + *itis,* inflammation]. Reddening and blurring of the optic disk that resembles optic neuritis.

pseudoneuroma (sū"dō-nū-rō'mă) [" + " + *oma,* tumor]. A mass of interlacing, coiled fibers, cells of Schwann, and fibrous tissue forming a mass at end of amputation stump. Also called amputation or traumatic neuroma. It is not a true neuroma. SYN: *neurofibroma.*

pseudonucleolus (sū"dō-nū"klē-ōl'ŭs) [" + L. *nucleus,* a nut]. The false nucleolus or karyosome.

pseudopapilledema (soo"dō-păp"ĭ-lĕ-dē'mă) [" + *papilla,* nipple, + *oidema,* swelling]. Swelling of the optic nerve head that is not caused by optic neuritis.

pseudoparalysis (sū"dō-pă-răl'ĭ-sĭs) [" + *para,* at the side, + *lyein,* to loosen]. A loss of muscular power not due to lesion of the nervous system. SYN: *pseudoplegia.*

pseudoparaplegia (sū"dō-păr-ă-plē'jē-ă) [" + " + *plege,* a stroke]. Seeming paralysis of the lower extremities without impairment of the reflexes.

pseudoparasite (sū"dō-păr'ă-sīt) [" + " + *sitos,* food]. 1. Anything resembling a parasite. 2. Organism that can live as a parasite, although it is normally not one. SEE: *parasite, facultative.*

pseudoparesis (sū"dō-păr-ē'sĭs, -păr'ĕ-sĭs) [" + *paresis,* relaxation]. A condition simulating paresis but unlike the ordinary forms and due to hysteria.

pseudopelade (soo"dō-pē'lād) [" + Fr. *pelade,* to remove hair]. A type of alopecia, of unknown etiology, associated with scarring.

Pseudophyllidea (sū"dō-fĭ-lĭd'ē-ă). An order belonging to the class Cestoidea, subclass Cestoda. Includes tapeworms with scolex bearing two lateral (or one terminal) sucking grooves (bothria). Includes Diphyllobothrium latum, the fish tapeworm of man.

pseudoplegia (sū"dō-plē'jē-ă) [" + *plege,* a stroke]. Paralysis of hysterical origin. SYN: *pseudoparalysis.*

pseudopod (sū'dō-pŏd) [" + *pous,* foot]. Temporary protruding protoplasmic process in protozoa for the purpose of taking up food and aiding in locomotion. SYN: *pseudopodium.*

pseudopodia. Pl. of pseudopodium.

pseudopodium (sū"dō-pō'dē-ŭm). (pl. *pseudopodia*) 1. A temporary protruding process of a protozoan or ameboid cell, such as a leukocyte, that aids in locomotion and the engulfing of food particles or foreign substances, as in phagocytosis. SYN: *pseudopod.* 2. An irregular projection at the edge of a wheal.

pseudopolyp (soo"dō-pŏl'ĭp) [" + *polys,* many, + *pous,* foot]. A hypertrophied area of mucous membrane resembling a polyp.

pseudopolyposis (soo"dō-pŏl"ĭ-pō'sĭs) [" + " + " + *osis,* condition]. A large number of pseudopolyps in the colon due to chronic inflammation.

pseudopregnancy (sū"dō-prĕg'năn-sē) [Gr. *pseudes,* false, + L. *praegnans,* with child]. 1. Condition occurring in lower animals following sterile matings in which anatomical and physiological changes occur simlar to those of pregnancy. 2. Pseudocyesis.

pseudo-pseudohypoparathyroidism (soo"dō-soo"dō-hī"pō-păr"ă-thī'royd-ĭzm) [" + *pseudes,* false, + *hypo,* under, + *para,* beside, + *thyreos,* shield, + *eidos,* form, + *-ismos,* condition]. Pseudohypoparathyroidism in which most of the clinical but none of the biochemical changes are present.

pseudopsia (sū-dŏp'sē-ă) [" + *opsis,* vision]. Visual hallucinations or false perceptions. SYN: *pseudoblepsis.*

pseudopterygium (soo"dō-tĕr-ĭj'ē-ŭm) [" + *pterygion,* wing]. A scar on the conjunctiva of the eye that is firmly attached to the underlying tissue.

pseudoptosis (sū-dō-tō'sĭs) [" + *ptosis,* fall]. Apparent ptosis of the eyelid, resulting from a fold of skin or fat projecting below the edge of the eyelid.

pseudorabies (soo"dō-rā'bē-ēz) [" + L. *rabere,* to rage]. A rabies-like disease in animals that is due to a type of herpesvirus. It causes death within several days.

pseudoreaction (sū″dō-rē-ăk′shŭn). A false reaction. A response to injection of a test substance into the tissues due to presence of an allergen other than one for which test is made.

pseudorickets (soo″dō-rĭk′ĕts). Rickets, renal, q.v.

pseudoscarlatina (sū″dō-skăr-lă-tē′nă). A septic febrile condition with rash resembling scarlatina.

pseudosclerosis (sū″dō-sklē-rō′sĭs) [″ + *sklerosis,* a hardening]. A condition with the symptoms, but without the lesions, of multiple sclerosis of the nervous system.

p., Westphal-Strümpell. Hepatolenticular degeneration, q.v.

pseudosmia (sū-dŏz′mē-ă) [″ + *osme,* smell]. An olfactory hallucination or perversion of the sense of smell.

pseudostoma (sū-dŏs′tō-mă) [″ + *stoma,* a mouth]. An apparent aperture between endothelial cells that have been stained.

pseudostratified (sū-dō-străt′ĭ-fīd) [″ + L. *strata,* sheets]. Apparently composed of layers.

pseudostratified epithelium. Epithelium in which basal ends of all cells rest on basement membrane but distal ends may or may not reach the surface. Their nuclei lie at different levels, giving the appearance of being stratified.

pseudosyphilis (sū″dō-sĭf′ĭ-lĭs). A nonspecific condition resembling syphilis.

pseudotabes (sū″dō-tā′bēz) [Gr. *pseudes,* false, + L. *tabes,* a wasting]. A neural disease simulating tabes dorsalis.

pseudotetanus (sū″dō-tĕt′ă-nŭs) [″ + *tetanos,* tension]. Persistent muscular contractions resembling tetanus.

pseudotruncus arteriosus (soo″dō-trŭnk′ŭs ăr-tē″rē-ō′sŭs). The severest form of tetralogy of Fallot.

pseudotuberculosis (sū″dō-tū-ber″kū-lō′sĭs) [″ + L. *tuberculus,* tubercle, + Gr. *osis,* condition]. A group of diseases that resemble tuberculosis but are due to an organism other than the tubercle bacillus. In man the most common cause is Yersinia pseudotuberculosis, a gram-negative organism.

pseudotumor cerebri (sū″dō-tū′mor sĕr′ĕ-brī). Benign intracranial hypertension. This diagnosis is made after exclusion of tumors, obstruction of the ventricles, intracranial infection, and vascular hypertensive encephalopathy. The cause may be due to a variety of disorders, but in most cases the etiology is unknown. The prognosis is for spontaneous recovery.

pseudotympany (sū″dō-tĭm′pă-nē) [″ + *tympanon,* drum]. Flattening of arch of diaphragm and swelling of abdomen with increased respiration. It disappears under anesthesia and is of purely nervous origin.

pseudoxanthoma (sū″dō-zăn-thō′mă) [″ + *xanthos,* yellow, + *oma,* tumor]. Condition resembling xanthoma.

p. elasticum. Chronic degenerative cutaneous disease marked by yellow patches and stretching of skin. Associated with hypertension and degeneration of elastic coat of arteries. Angioid streaks in retina are common.

p.s.i. *pounds per square inch.*

psilocin (sī′lō-sĭn). A hallucinogen similar to psilocybin.

psilocybin (sī″lō-sī′bĭn). A hallucinogen obtained from a particular mushroom.

psi phenomena. Occurrences, events, or actions that have no logical explanation.

Ex.: extrasensory perception, clairvoyance, precognition, psychokinesis, and telepathy.

psittacosis (sĭt-ă-kō′sĭs) [Gr. *psittakos,* parrot, + *osis,* condition]. An infectious disease, caused by Chlamydia psittaci, of parrots and other birds that may be transmitted to man. Tetracyclines, erythromycin, and penicillin are effective in treatment. SYN: *ornithosis; parrot fever.* SEE: *Chlamydia.*

SYM AND SIGNS (in man): Headache, epistaxis, nausea, chill followed by fever, constipation, sometimes pulmonary disorders.

psoas (sō′ăs) [Gr. *psoa*]. One of two muscles of the loins. SEE: *Muscles* in *Appendix.*

psoas abscess. A cold abscess in sheath of the psoas major muscle. It follows the sheath of this muscle until it reaches the surface and points. Generally it occurs above Poupart's ligament in the iliac fossa or near the attachment of the psoas muscle to the femur.

ETIOL: Usually tuberculous disease of vertebrae accompanied by pus.

psoitis (sō-ī′tĭs) [Gr. *psoa,* muscle of the loin, + *itis,* inflammation]. Inflammation of the psoas muscles or of the area of the loins.

psomophagia (sō″mō-fā′jē-ă) [Gr. *psomos,* morsel, + *phagein,* to eat]. The habit of swallowing food without thoroughly chewing it.

psora (sō′ră) [Gr., itch]. 1. An itching disease of the skin. SYN: *scabies.* 2. An erythematous, scaling, cutaneous eruption. SYN: *psoriasis.*

psoralen. A group of substances derived from plants, some of which are capable of causing a phototoxic dermatitis when applied to the skin and exposed to sunlight or artificial ultraviolet wavelengths. Methoxsalen, USP, is a psoralen, and trioxsalen, USP, is a synthetic psoralen. SEE: *psoriasis; PUVA therapy; vitiligo.*

psorelcosis (sō″rĕl-kō′sĭs) [″ + *helkosis,* ulceration]. Ulceration occurring as a result of scabies.

psorenteritis (sō″rĕn-tĕr-ī′tĭs) [″ + *enteron,* intestine, + *itis,* inflammation]. Inflammation of the intestines seen in Asiatic cholera.

psoriasis (sō-rī′ă-sĭs) [Gr., an itching]. A common, genetically determined dermatitis consisting of discrete pink or dull-red lesions surmounted by characteristic silvery scaling. Lesions may become confluent. Although they come and go, they usually are chronic. A specific type of arthritis frequently is associated with psoriasis.

ETIOL: Unknown.

SYM: May begin at any age as flat-topped papule covered with thin, grayish-white scale spreading peripherally; lesions coalescing; centers regressing, forming circinate lesions. Under the dry scales are red bleeding points (papillae).

TREATMENT: General and nonspecific measures are utilized to give comfort to the patient as well as to help control the disease.

Methotrexate is the drug of choice in severe psoriasis not controlled by the usual nonspecific topical agents.

CAUTION: It is essential to monitor renal, hepatic, and hematologic function when this drug is used.

The use of an oral psoralen with long-wave ultraviolet light in severe and extensive psoriasis has been used experimentally. Psoralen methoxsalen has been used in this manner.

p. annularis. Circular or ring-like lesions of psoriasis.

p. arthropica. Psoriasis associated with arthritis. SYN: *psoriatic arthropathy.*

p. buccalis. Leukoplakia of the oral mucosa.

p., elephantine. A rare, but persistent, psoriasis that occurs on the back, thighs, and hips in thick scaling plaques.

p., guttate. Psoriasis characterized by small distinct lesions that generally occur over the body. Appear particularly in the young after acute streptococcal infections.

p., nummular. The most common form of psoriasis with discs and plaques of varying sizes on the extremities and trunk. There may be a great number of lesions or a solitary lesion.

p., pustular. Psoriasis in which small sterile pustules form, dry up, and then form a scab.

p., rupioid. Psoriasis with hyperkeratotic lesions on the feet.

p. universalis. Severe generalized psoriasis.

psorophthalmia (sō″rŏf-thăl′mē-ă) [Gr.]. Marginal inflammation of the eyelids with ulceration.

psorous (sō′rŭs) [Gr. *psoros*]. Rel. to, or affected with, itch.

P.S.P. *phenolsulfonphthalein;* a substance used to test kidney function.

PSRO. *Professional Standards Review Organization.*

psychagogy (sī″kă-gō′jē) [Gr. *psyche,* soul, mind, + *agein,* to lead]. A psychotherapeutic re-educational procedure that stresses proper social adjustment of the individual.

psychalgia (sī-kăl′jē-ă) [″ + *algos,* pain]. 1. Pain of hysterical origin. 2. Mental distress characterized by auditory and visual hallucinations, often associated with melancholia. SYN: *phrenalgia.*

psychanalysis (sī-kăn-ăl′ĭ-sĭs) [″ + *analysis,* breaking apart]. Discovery of the pathogenic links between the objective and subjective consciousness by a system of recall. SYN: *psychoanalysis.*

psychanopsia (sī-kăn-ŏp′sē-ă) [″ + *an-,* not, + *opsis,* vision]. Condition in which the patient sees objects but perceives an erroneous concept of their size and three-dimensional relationships. SYN: *psychic blindness.*

psychataxia (sī″kă-tăk′sē-ă) [″ + *ataxia,* lack of order]. Disordered power of concentration.

psychauditory (sĭk-aw′dĭ-tor-ē) [″ + L. *auditorius,* hearing]. Pert. to the perception and interpretation of sounds.

psyche (sī′kē) [Gr. *psyche,* soul, mind]. All that constitutes the mind and its processes.

psychedelic (sī″kē-dĕl′ĭk) [″ + *delos,* manifest]. Originally used in 1963 to mean mind-manifesting. Now used by lay persons to describe some of the subjective aspects of intoxication, particularly with a drug such as lysergic acid diethylamide (LSD), or other drugs that produce visual hallucinations.

psychiatric (sī-kē-ă′trĭk) [″ + *iatrikos,* healing]. Pert. to psychiatry, the science concerned with the study, diagnosis, and prevention of mental illness.

psychiatrist (sī-kī′ă-trĭst). A physician who specializes in study, treatment, and prevention of mental disorders.

psychiatry (sī-kī′ă-trē). The branch of medicine that deals with diagnosis, treatment, and prevention of mental illness.

p., descriptive. A system of psychiatry concerned with the readily observable external factors that influence the mental state of an individual. SEE: *p., dynamic.*

p., dynamic. The study of the origin, influence, and control of emotions. This involves investigating the factors both from within and without that alter emotions and motivation. Such analysis provides a basis for judging regression or progression.

p., forensic. Use of psychiatry in legal matters, esp. in determining social adaptability of an individual suspected of insanity; or the presence or absence of insanity, esp. at the time the individual committed a crime.

p., orthomolecular. The concept that mental illness may be treated by determining and treating abnormalities of body chemistry.

psychiatry and neurology, words pert. to: aberration; abreaction; abulia; acathisia; affect; agnosia; agraphia; agoraphobia; akinesia; alcoholism; alexia, alienation; alliteration; allotropic; Alzheimer's disease; ambivalence; amentia; amnesia; amok; amusia; anal erotism; anhedonia; anomia; anorexia; apathy; aphasia; aphonia; aphrasia; aphrenia; apraxia; apsychosis; association; astereognosis; asyllabia; asymbolia; asynesia; atactilia; atavism; ataxaphasia; ataxia; ateliosis; athymia; attitude; autism; autistic child; automatism; autoecholalia; autophagia; autophobia; autopsychosis; autosuggestion; blocking; bradylalia; bradylexia; catatonia; catharsis; cenesthesia; chorea; claustrophilia; claustrophobia; complex; compulsion; conation; condensation; confabulation; conflict; coprolagnia; coprolalia; coprophilia; cretinism; deafness; delire de toucher; delirium; delusion; dementia; depersonalization; depression; dereistic; determinism; disorientation; displacement; dissociation; distractibility; dysbulia; dyscinesia; dyslexia; dysmnesia; echolalia; echomimia; ego; egocentric; electroconvulsive therapy; electroencephalogram; emotion; emotivity; empathy; erethism; ergasiomania; ergasiophobia; eroticism; erotomania; erythrophobia; exhibitionism; extrovert; fabrication; fastidium; fear; fixation; folie; free association; fugue; furor; Ganser's syndrome; geophagia; hallucination; hallucinosis; hebephrenia; heterolalia; holergasia; hyperhedonia; hyperprosexia; hypersthenia; hyperthymia; hypnagogic; hypnogenic zones; hypnosis; hypnotic; hypnotism; hypochondria; hypochondriac; hypochondriasis; hysteria; idea; illusion; image; imago; incoherence; incompetent; infantilism; inhibition; insanity; instinct; integration; intelligence; intrapsychic; introjection; introversion; introvert; kinesthesia; Korsakoff's syndrome; latent content; lethargy; malingerer; masochism; melancholia; mental deficiency; mesmerism; mind; narcissism; negativism; neologism; neurology; neurosis; noctambulism; non compos mentis; nymphomania; object choice; obsession; oligopnea; organic psychoses; orthopsychiatry; overtone; paragraphia; paralexia; paralogia; paramimia; paramnesia; paranoia; paranomia; parapathia; paraphasia; paraphonia; parent fixation; paresis; pathergasia; pedophilia; periphrastic; perseveration; personality; phantasia; phantasm; phantasy; phantom; phoneme; pica; pleasure principle; pragmatism; preconscious; rationalization; reaction; reactive depression; reading disorders; reality principle; recapitulation theory; repression; resistance; restraint; retardation; Rorschach; sadism; satyriasis; schizoid; schizophrenia; stereotypy; stupor; subconscious; subjective; sublimation; subliminal; suggestion; surrogate; sycophancy; symbiosis; symbol; symbolism; syntonic; transfer; transvestism; trend; twilight state; tyrannism; unconscious; verbigeration; vigil; vision; voice; word blindness; words beginning with "psyche-" or "neuro-".

psychic (sī'kĭk) [Gr. *psychikos*]. 1. Concerning the mind or psyche. 2. One said to be endowed with semisupernatural powers, such as the ability to read the minds of others, or to foresee coming events; one apparently sensitive to nonphysical forces.

psychic blindness. Sight without recognition of that which is seen. SYN: *psychanopsia.*

psychic contagion. Communication of another's nervous disorder by imitation, as a tic.

psychic deafness. Inability to recognize sounds heard.

psychic determinism. The theory that mental processes are determined by conscious or unconscious motives, and are never irrelevant.

psychic force. Force generated apart from physical energy.

psycho-, psych- [Gr. *psyche*, mind]. Combining form indicating relationship to the mind or mental processes.

psychoactive (sī"kō-ăk'tĭv) [" + L. *actio*, action]. Affecting the mental state, such as a drug that has that action.

psychoanaleptic (sī"kō-ăn'ă-lĕp'tĭk) [" + *analepsis*, a taking up]. Having a stimulating effect upon the mind.

psychoanalysis (sī"kō-ă-năl'ĭ-sĭs) [" + *analysis*, a loosening apart]. Method of obtaining a detailed account of past and present mental and emotional experiences and repressions in order to determine the source and to eliminate or diminish the undesirable effects of unconscious conflicts by making the patient aware of their existence, origin, and inappropriate expression in emotions and behavior. It is largely a system that was the creation of Sigmund Freud, q.v., and was originally the outgrowth of his observations of neurotics. Frequently the term is used synonymously with freudianism, but more commonly it is used for a more extensive system of psychological fact and theory applying both to normal and abnormal groups.

Psychoanalysis is based upon the theory that abnormal phenomena are caused by repression of painful or undesirable past experiences that, although totally forgotten, later manifest themselves in various abnormal ways. Psychoanalysis includes a study of the ego in relationship to reality, and more particularly the herd and the conflicting goals so created. This conflict is solved by repressing one component. This repressed or censored emotion-laden complex of ideas exists in the subconscious, manifesting itself in the hidden content of dreams, in neuroses, and tension states. Anger outbursts, rationalization of unfair attitudes, or slips of the tongue occur because the patient is unaware of the influence of the subconscious.

Repressed material is largely sexual and the peculiar conditioning of the patient is chiefly determined by emotional experiences of earlier years. Reactions of inferiority may result in a compensatory reaction of goodness or ambition. Sublimation is the escape of creative interest on levels not socially taboo. Therefore psychoanalysis makes an effort to bring forgotten memories into the conscious mind. The patient thus is enabled to view the occurrence in its true perspective, and to minimize its harm.

In addition to the freudian method, other schools of thought or disciplines utilized in analysis of the psyche include analytical psychology (Jung), psychobiology (Meyer), and individual psychology (Adler).

psychoanalyst (sī″kō-ăn′ă-līst) [Gr. *psyche,* mind, + *analysis,* breaking apart]. One who practices psychoanalysis.

psychobiology (sī″kō-bī-ŏl′ō-jē) [″ + *bios,* life, + *logos,* a study]. 1. The study of the biology of the psyche, including the anatomy, physiology, and pathology of the mind. SYN: *biopsychology.* 2. A method of psychoanalysis employing distributive analysis, which includes a study of all mental and physical factors involved in the growth and development of an individual.

p., objective. Psychobiology in which special emphasis is placed on the relationship of the individual to his environment.

psychocatharsis (sī″kō-kă-thăr′sĭs) [″ + *katharsis,* purging]. The bringing of so-called traumatic experiences and their affective associations into consciousness by interview, hypnosis, or by use of drugs such as sodium amytal. SEE: *catharsis.*

psychochrome (sī′kō-krōm) [″ + *chroma,* color]. Color impression resulting from sensory stimulation of a part other than the visual organ.

psychochromesthesia (sī″kō-krōm″ĕs-thē′zē-ă) [″ + ″ + *aisthesis,* sensation]. Color sensation produced by the stimulus of a sense organ other than that of vision. SEE: *pseudochromesthesia.*

psychocoma (sī″kō-kō′mă) [Gr. *psyche,* mind, + *koma,* stupor]. Condition of mental stupor.

psychocortical (sī″kō-kor′tĭ-kăl) [″ + L. *cortex,* rind]. Pert. to the cerebral cortex as the seat of sensory, motor, and psychic functions.

psychodiagnosis (sī″kō-dī″ăg-nō′sĭs) [″ + *diagignoskein,* to discern]. Use of psychological tests to assist in diagnosing diseases, esp. mental illness.

psychodiagnostics (sī″kō-dī″ăg-nŏs′tĭks). The use of psychological testing as an aid in diagnosing mental disorders.

Psychodidae (sī″kŏd′ĭ-dē). A family of the order Diptera, characterized by minute size, long legs, and hairy bodies and wings. Includes moth flies, owl midges, and sandflies. SEE: *Phlebotomus.*

psychodometry (sī″kō-dŏm′ĕ-trē) [″ + *hodos,* way, + *metron,* measure]. Measurement of rate of mental activity.

psychodrama (sī′kō-drăm′ă) [″ + L. *drama,* drama]. A form of group psychotherapy. Patients act out assigned roles and, in so doing, are able to gain insight into their own mental disturbances.

psychodynamics (sī″kō-dī-năm′ĭks) [″ + *dynamis,* power]. The scientific study of mental action or force.

psychoepilepsy (sī″kō-ĕp″ĭ-lĕp′sē) [″ + *epilepsia,* seizure]. A form of hysterical neurosis accompanied by movements resembling those of epilepsy.

psychogalvanic reflex. Variation in the electrical resistance of the skin in response to emotional stimuli.

psychogalvanometer (sī″kō-găl″vă-nŏm′ĕ-tĕr) [″ + *galvanism* + Gr. *metron,* measure]. Device for determining the changes in the electrical resistance of the skin in response to emotional stimuli.

psychogenesis (sī″kō-jĕn′ĕ-sĭs) [″ + *genesis,* formation]. 1. The origin and development of mind; the formation of mental traits. 2. Origination within the mind or psyche.

psychogenetic (sī″kō-jĕn-ĕt′ĭk). 1. Originating in the mind, as a disease. 2. Concerning formation of mental traits.

psychogenic (sī-kō-jĕn′ĭk) [″ + *gennan,* to produce]. 1. Of mental origin. 2. Concerning the development of the mind. SYN: *psychogenetic.*

psychogeusic (sī″kō-gū′sĭk) [″ + *geusis,* taste]. Pert. to perception of taste.

psychogram (sī′kō-grăm) [Gr. *psyche,* mind, + *gramma,* a mark]. A subjective visualization of a mental concept.

psychograph (sī′kō-grăf) [″ + *graphein,* to write]. 1. A chart that lists personality traits. 2. A history of the personality of an individual.

psychokinesis (sī″kō-kĭ-nē′sĭs) [″ + *kinesis,* motion]. 1. Explosive or impulsive maniacal action caused by defective inhibition. 2. In parapsychology, influence exerted on a physical object by a subject without any intermediate physical energy or instrumentation. SEE: *psi phenomena.*

psycholagny (sī″kō-lăg′nē) [″ + *lagneia,* lust]. Sexual excitation brought about by mental imagery; psychic or mental masturbation.

psycholepsy (sī″kō-lĕp′sē) [″ + *lepsis,* a seizure]. Sudden alteration of moods in which mental inertia and hopelessness are manifested. SYN: *paralepsy.*

psycholeptic (sī″kō-lĕp′tĭk). Concerning sudden shifting of moods, particularly to one marked by hopelessness and mental inertia.

psycholinguistics (sī″kō-lĭng-gwĭs′tĭks). The study of linguistics as it relates to human behavior.

psychological (sī″kō-lŏj′ĭ-kăl) [″ + *logos,* a study]. Pert. to study of the mind in all of its relationships, normal and abnormal.

psychologist (sī-kŏl′ō-jĭst). One who is trained in methods of psychological analysis, therapy, and research.

psychology (sī-kŏl′ō-jē) [″ + *logos,* a study]. The science dealing with mental processes, both normal and abnormal, and their effects upon behavior. There are two main approaches to the study: introspective, looking inward or self-examination of one's own mental processes, and objective, i.e., studying the minds of others. SEE: words beginning with *psych-.*

p., abnormal. The study of deviational behavior and the mental phenomena associated with such.

p., analytic. Psychoanalysis based on the concepts of Carl Jung, de-emphasizing sexual factors in motivation and emphasizing the "collective unconscious" and "psychological types" (introvert and extrovert).

p., animal. The study of animal behavior.

p., applied. The application of the principles of psychology to special fields, such as clinical, industrial, educational, nursing, or pastoral applications.

p., clinical. That branch of psychology concerned with diagnosing and treating mental disorders.

p., criminal. The branch of psychology concerned with the behavior and therapy of criminals.

p., dynamic. The psychology of motivation; that which seeks the causes of mental phenomena.

p., experimental. Study of mental acts by tests and experiments.

p., genetic. The branch of psychology concerned with the evolution of and inheritance of psychological characteristics.

p., gestalt. Psychology that emphasizes the wholeness of psychological processes and behavior, maintaining that such cannot be adequately explained by breaking down into constituent parts.

p., individual. A system of psychological thinking developed by Alfred Adler in which an individual is regarded as having three life goals: physical security, sexual satisfaction, and social integration. Self-evaluations lead to feelings of inferiority and inadequacy, which often lead to over-compensation or a striving for superiority.

p., physiologic. Psychology that deals with the structure and function of the nervous system and other bodily organs and their relationship to behavior.

p., social. The branch of psychology concerned with study of groups and their influence on the individual's actions and mental processes.

psychometrician (sī″kō-mĕ-trĭsh′ăn) [Gr. *psyche,* mind, + *metron,* measure]. 1. A person skilled in psychometry, q.v. 2. A person skilled in the application of statistical analysis to psychological data.

psychometry (sī-kŏm′ĕ-trē) [″ + *metron,* a measure]. The measurement of psychological variables, such as intelligence, aptitude, behavior, and emotional reactions.

psychomotor (sī″kō-mō′tor) [″ + L. *motor,* a mover]. Concerning or causing physical activity associated with mental processes.

psychomotor and physical development of infant. It is important that all concerned with the care of the newborn through infancy have guidelines for comparing the growth and development of an individual with normal standards. The charts provided will be of assistance in this.

Certain activities of infants serve as general indicators of normal psychomotor development. The average ages for certain of these activities are shown in the accompanying table.

Appearance and loss of certain reflexes and reactions: The Moro reflex is present at birth and disappears by 3 months; the stepping, and placing reflexes are present at birth and are no longer obtainable by 6 weeks; the tonic neck reflex is usually present at 2 months and is gone by 6 months; neck righting appears at 4–6 months and is gone by 24 months; the parachute reaction is present at 9 months and persists; sucking and rooting are present at birth and are usually gone by 4 months if tested while awake and by 7 months if tested while the infant is asleep; palmar grasp is present from birth to 6 months; plantar grasp is present from birth to 10 months.

psychomotor epilepsy. Epilepsy, temporal lobe, q.v.

psychoneurosis (sī″kō-nū-rō′sĭs) [″ + *neuron,* sinew, + *osis,* condition]. Emotional maladaptation due to unresolved unconscious conflicts. This leads to disturbances in thought, feelings, attitudes, and behavior. There is little, if any, loss of contact with

Psychomotor and Physical Development
Birth to One Year

Physical Development

Birth		Length Range		Weight Range	
boys	in.	18¼–21½	lbs.	5½–9¼	
	cm.	46.4–54.4	kg.	2.54–4.15	
girls	in.	17¾–20¾	lbs.	5¼–8½	
	cm.	45.4–52.9	kg.	2.36–3.81	
One Month					
boys	in.	19¾–23	lbs.	7–11¾	
	cm.	50.4–58.6	kg.	3.16–5.38	
girls	in.	19¼–22½	lbs.	6½–10¾	
	cm.	49.2–56.9	kg.	2.97–4.92	
Three Months					
boys	in.	22¼–25¾	lbs.	9¾–16¼	
	cm.	56.7–65.4	kg.	4.43–7.37	
girls	in.	21¾–25	lbs.	9¼–14¾	
	cm.	55.4–63.4	kg.	4.18–6.74	
Six Months					
boys	in.	25–28½	lbs.	13¾–20¾	
	cm.	63.4–72.3	kg.	6.20–9.46	
girls	in.	24¼–27¾	lbs.	12¾–19¼	
	cm.	61.8–70.2	kg.	5.79–8.73	
Nine Months					
boys	in.	26¾–30¼	lbs.	16½–24	
	cm.	68.0–77.1	kg.	7.52–10.93	
girls	in.	26–29½	lbs.	15½–22½	
	cm.	66.1–75.0	kg.	7.0–10.17	
Twelve Months					
boys	in.	28¼–32	lbs.	18½–26½	
	cm.	71.7–81.2	kg.	8.43–11.99	
girls	in.	27½–31¼	lbs.	17¼–24¾	
	cm.	69.8–79.1	kg.	7.84–11.24	

reality, but the patient's effectiveness in performing his or her usual responsibilities is handicapped. Psychoneurosis is a major category in classifying mental illness and is classified according to the symptoms that predominate. The patient usually recognizes that the altered thoughts and feelings are abnormal; and indeed unwelcome. This is in contrast to the patient with a psychosis or character disorder. SYN: *neurosis*.

p., anxiety reaction. Anxiety with apprehension out of proportion to any obvious external cause. SEE: *anxiety neurosis*.

p., conversion reaction. Psychoneurosis wherein unacceptable unconscious impulses are converted into hysterical somatic symptoms. Although the symptoms have a specific symbolic meaning to the patient, their interpretation is different in each individual.

p., depressive reaction. Psychoneurosis marked by depression out of proportion to any obvious cause.

p., dissociated reaction. Psychoneurosis characterized by dissociated behavior such as amnesia, fugue, sleepwalking, and dream states. Important to differentiate from schizophrenia, q.v.

p., obsessive-compulsive reaction.

Psychomotor and Physical Development Birth to One Year *(Continued)*

Psychomotor Development

Birth Through First Month	Ability to suck, and swallow, gag, cry, and maintain eye contact with a person. The head needs to be supported. Loud noises may cause a startle reflex.
Second Month	May turn to either side when they are on their back; will follow moving objects; able to lift head but not for a sustained period; begin to smile, frown, and turn away.
Third Month	Greater movement and vocal response to stimuli; notices own hands and sucks on them; head will be steady while in a supported position.
Fourth and Fifth Months	Able to lift head higher when lying on stomach; will reach for objects and may be able to encircle a bottle with both hands; may drool a lot; attempts to put all kinds of objects in mouth.
Sixth to Ninth Month	Develop ability to grasp and pick up food; are able to pull themselves up to a sitting position and eventually will crawl; they begin to make noises that sound like words and to recognize certain words; will play peek-a-boo.
Ninth to Eleventh Month	Develop ability to handle food, and to drink from a cup; may imitate sounds and say certain words; crawl by pulling body along with arms and pull themselves to a standing position; they will point at objects and throw things; they want to feed themselves and to help with dressing and undressing; they will walk while holding a person's hand.
Twelve Months	Can eat food alone and drink from a cup with assistance; able to move around easily, and crawl up stairs, and out of crib.

Persistent, repetitive impulses to perform certain acts or rituals, such as handwashing, touching something, or counting.

p., phobic reaction. Irrational fear of any of a variety of situations, persons, or objects.

psychoneurotic (sī″kō-nū-rŏt′ĭk) [Gr. *psyche,* mind, + *neuron,* sinew]. 1. Pert. to a functional disorder of mental origin. 2. A person suffering from a psychoneurosis.

psychoparesis (sī″kō-pă-rē′sĭs, -păr′ĕ-sĭs) [″ + *paresis,* relaxation]. Weakness or enfeeblement of the mind.

psychopath (sī′kō-păth) [″ + *pathos,* disease]. Individual with a psychopathic personality. SEE: *personality, psychopathic.*

psychopathia. Psychopathy.

psychopathic (sī″kō-păth′ĭk). 1. Concerning or characterized by a mental disorder. 2. Concerning treatment of mental disorders. 3. Abnormal.

psychopathology (sī″kō-păth-ŏl′ō-jē) [″ + *pathos,* disease, + *logos,* a study]. The study of the causes and nature of mental disease or abnormal behavior.

psychopathy (sī-kŏp′ă-thē). Any mental disease, esp. one characterized by defective character or personality. SEE: *personality, psychopathic.*

psychopharmacology (sī″kō-făr″mă-kŏl′ō-jē). The science of drugs having an effect on psychomotor behavior and emotional states.

psychophysical (sī″kō-fĭz′ĭ-kăl) [″ + *physikos,* natural]. Concerning the relationship of the physical and the mental. SEE: *childbirth natural; psychoprophylactic childbirth.*

psychophysics (sī″kō-fĭz′ĭks). 1. The study of mental processes in relationship to physical processes. 2. The study of stimuli in relationship to the effects they produce.

psychophysiologic (sī″kō-fĭz-ē-ō-lŏ′jĭk). Pert. to psychophysiology, q.v.

psychophysiologic disorders. Term applied to a large number of disorders of organs and viscera innervated by the autonomic nervous system in which emotional factors are a primary contributing factor. Formerly called psychosomatic disease or disorder.

psychophysiology (sī″kō-fĭz″ē-ŏl′ō-jē). Physiology of the mind; science of the correlation of body and mind.

psychoplegic (sī″kō-plē′jĭk) [″ + *plege,* a stroke]. An agent reducing excitability of the mental processes.

psychoprophylactic childbirth. Mental and

physical training of the mother in preparation for delivery. The goals of the preparation are the dispelling of the fear of pain and the delivery of a healthy child. SEE: *Lamaze; childbirth, natural.*

psychoprophylaxis (sī″kō-prō″fĭ-lăk′sĭs). In obstetrics, a method of mental and physical preparation for natural childbirth. SEE: *childbirth, natural; Lamaze.*

psychorhythmia (sī″kō-rĭth′mē-ă) [″ + *rhythmos,* rhythm]. Mental condition in which involuntary repetition of previous voluntary actions occurs.

psychorrhea (sī″kō-rē′ă) [″ + *rhoia,* flow]. A mental condition characterized by an incoherent stream of thought resulting in vague and often bizarre theories and ideas.

psychosensory (sī″kō-sĕn′sō-rē) [″ + L. *sensorius,* sensation]. 1. Understanding and interpreting sensory stimuli. 2. Concerning perceptions not arising in sensory organs, as hallucinations.

psychosexual (sī″kō-sĕks′ū-ăl) [Gr. *psyche,* soul, mind, + L. *sexus,* sex]. Concerning the emotional components of sexual instinct.

psychosexual development. Evolution of personality through infantile and pregenital periods to sexual maturity.

psychosexual disorders. Disorders of sexual function not due to organic causes. Included are gender identity disorders, transsexualism, paraphilias, transvestism, zoophilia, pedophilia, exhibitionism, voyeurism, and sexual sadism.

psychosine (sī′kō-sēn). A cerebroside present in brain tissue.

psychosis (sī-kō′sĭs) [″ + *osis,* condition]. (pl. *psychoses*) A term formerly applied to any mental disorder, but now generally restricted to those disturbances of such magnitude that there is personality disintegration and loss of contact with reality. The disturbances are of psychogenic origin, or without clearly defined physical cause or structural change in the brain. They usually are characterized by delusions and hallucination, and hospitalization generally is required.

This condition is manifest in the behavior, emotional reaction, and ideation of the patient, who fails to mirror reality as it is, reacts erroneously to it, and builds up false concepts regarding it. Behavior responses are peculiar, abnormal, inefficient, or definitely antisocial.

All this does not include amentia because defective intelligence merely lessens comprehension of reality but does not distort it. The psychopathic personality reacts badly because of intrinsic emotional differences playing upon an undistorted world of reality.

p., alcoholic. Psychosis resulting from chronic alcoholism. SEE: *delirium tremens; Korsakoff's syndrome.*

p., depressive. Psychosis characterized by extreme depression, melancholia, and feelings of unworthiness.

p., drug. A psychosis caused by ingestion of a drug.

p., exhaustion. Acute state of confusion and delirium that occurs in relation to extreme fatigue, chronic illness, prolonged sleeplessness, or tension.

p., functional. Psychosis that is not due to an organic disease.

p., gestational. Psychosis that occurs during pregnancy.

p., involutional. Psychosis occurring during involutional period of bodily and intellectual decline. In women from ages 40 to 55 and in men from 50 to 65.

p., Korsakoff's. Korsakoff's syndrome, q.v.

p., manic-depressive. Ordinarily a series of periods of psychotic depression or excessive well-being, appearing in any sequence and alternating with longer periods of relative normalcy. Though intensity may vary greatly, the manic shows an elated though unstable mood, a flight of ideas, and great physical activity. In primary depression, the victim finds all exertion exhausting; there is difficulty in thinking or acting, and the victim is very unhappy.

p., organic. Psychosis resulting from a pathological condition of the central nervous system, such as paresis.

p., polyneuritic. Korsakoff's syndrome, q.v.

p., postinfectious. Psychosis following an infectious disease such as meningitis, pneumonia, typhoid fever.

p., postpartum. Psychosis occurring in the period following childbirth. SEE: *postpartum psychosis.*

p., puerperal. Postpartum psychosis, q.v.

p., senile. Psychosis due to old age.

p., situational. Psychosis due to excessive stress in an unbearable environmental situation.

p., toxic. Psychosis resulting from toxic agents.

p., traumatic. Psychosis resulting from head injuries and belonging to the organic group.

psychosocial (sī″kō-sō′shăl). Related to both psychological and social factors.

psychosomatic (sī″kō-sō-măt′ĭk) [Gr. *psyche,* mind, + *soma,* body]. Pert. to the relationship of the mind and body.

Disorders that have a physiological component but are thought to originate in the emotional state of the patient are termed psychosomatic. When so used the impression is created that the mind and body are separate entities and that a disease may be purely somatic in its effect or entirely emotional.

This partitioning of the human being is not possible; thus no disease is limited to only the mind or the body. A complex interaction is always present even though in specific instances a disease might on superficial examination appear to involve only the body or the mind. SEE: *psychophysiologic disorders.*

psychosomatic medicine. Branch of medicine that recognizes the importance of mind-body interrelationships in all illnesses and in which therapy and management are based on this fact.

psychosurgery (sī″kō-sur′jĕr-ē) [″ + L. *chirurgia,* surgery]. Surgical intervention for mental disorders, esp. for certain types of violent or antisocial behavior.

psychotechnics (sī″kō-tĕk′nĭks) [″ + *techne,* art]. Use of psychological methods in the study of economic and social problems.

psychotherapeutic drugs. Drugs that are used because of the effects they have in ameliorating the principal symptoms that occur in mentally disturbed persons, such as anxiety, depression, and psychosis. SEE: table.

psychotherapy (sī-kō-thĕr′ă-pē) [Gr. *psyche,* mind, + *therapeia,* treatment]. A method of treating disease, esp. nervous disorders, by mental means rather than physical.

Ex.: suggestion, re-education, hypnotism, psychoanalytic therapy.

psychotic (sī-kŏt′ĭk). Pert. to or affected by psychosis.

psychotogenic (sī-kŏt″ō-jĕn′ĭk) [″ + *gennan,* to produce]. Producing a psychosis, usually temporary and due to certain powerful drugs.

psychotomimetic (sī-kŏt″ō-mĭ-mĕ′tĭk) [″ + *mimetikos,* imitative]. A hallucinogen producing weird illusions and phantasms.

psychotropic drugs [″ + *trope,* a turning]. Drugs that affect psychic function, behavior, or experience. Many drugs can be classed as being intentionally psychotropic, but many other drugs also occasionally may produce undesired psychotropic side effects.

psychroalgia (sī″krō-ăl′jē-ă) [Gr. *psychros,* cold, + *algos,* pain]. Painful sensation of cold.

psychroesthesia (sī″krō-ĕs-thē′zē-ă) [″ + *aisthesis,* sensation]. A sensation of cold in a part of the body, although it is warm.

psychrometer (sī-krŏm′ĕ-tĕr) [″ + *metron,* measure]. Device for measuring relative humidity of the atmosphere. Calculations are made utilizing the readings of two thermometers, one with a dry bulb and one with a wet bulb.

psychrophilic (sī-krō-fĭl′ĭk) [″ + *philein,* to love]. Preferring cold, as bacteria that thrive at low temperatures, between 0° and 30° C. (32° and 86° F.).

Psychotherapeutic Drugs and Agents

Indication	Drugs	Clinical Use	Note
Antianxiety	Benzodiazepines Monoamine oxidase inhibitors Tricyclic antidepressants Sedatives	Anxiety Nervousness Psychoneuroses Insomnia	Patients may become tolerant to the drug, or abuse the drug and become addicted. Use may delay definitive therapy.
Antidepressants	Tricyclic compounds Lithium carbonate (for manic phase of manic-depressive disorders; not to be used in patients on a salt-free diet) Electroconvulsive therapy	Depression	Patient must be closely monitored with respect to the possibility of self-destruction (suicide) while waiting for medicines to have their effect.
Antipsychotics	Phenothiazines (chlorpromazine, thioridazine, trifluoperazine) Thioxanthenes Butyrophenones Dihydroindolone Dibenzoxazepine	Schizophrenic reactions Excitement Chronic brain syndromes Mental retardation	May have long-term undesired side effects on the autonomic nervous system and extrapyramidal tract.

psychrophobia (sī-krō-fō'bē-ă) [" + *phobos,* fear]. Abnormal aversion or sensitiveness to cold.

psychrophore (sī'krō-for) [" + *phorein,* to carry]. A double-lumen catheter for applying cold to the urethra, or any canal.

psychrotherapy (sī"krō-thĕr'ă-pē) [" + *therapeia,* treatment]. Treatment of disease by use of cold.

psyllium seed (sĭl'ē-ŭm). The dried ripe seed of the psyllium plant, grown in France, Spain, and India. Used as a mild laxative.

PT. *prothrombin time.*

Pt. Chem. symb. for platinum.

pt. *pint.*

PTA. *plasma thromboplastin antecedent.*

ptarmic (tăr'mĭk) [Gr. *ptarmikos,* causing to sneeze]. 1. Causing sneezing. 2. Agent that causes sneezing. SYN: *sternutatory.*

ptarmus (tar'mŭs). Spasmodic sneezing.

PTC. 1. *plasma thromboplastin component.* 2. *phenylthiocarbamide.*

pterion (tē'rē-ŏn) [Gr. *pteron,* wing]. Point of suture of frontal, parietal, temporal, and sphenoid bones.

pternalgia (tĕr-năl'jē-ă) [Gr. *pterna,* heel, + *algos,* pain]. Pain in the heel.

pteroylglutamic acid. Folic acid.

pterygium (tĕr-ĭj'ē-ŭm) [Gr. *pterygion,* wing]. Triangular thickening of bulbar conjunctiva extending from inner canthus to border of the cornea with apex toward pupil.

p. colli. A congenital band of fascia extending from the mastoid process of the temporal bone to the clavicle.

p., progressive. Stage in which the growth extends toward center of cornea.

p., stationary. Stage in which the head of the pterygium remains permanently attached to the same point on the cornea.

TREATMENT: Surgical.

pterygoid (tĕr'ĭ-goyd) [Gr. *pterygodes*]. Wing shaped. SYN: *alate.*

pterygoid process. One of two large processes of the sphenoid bone extending downward from the junction of the body and great wings, each consisting of lateral and medial pterygoid plates.

pterygomandibular (tĕr"ĭ-gō-măn-dĭb'ū-lăr) [" + L. *mandibula,* lower jawbone]. Concerning the pterygoid process of the sphenoid bone and the mandible.

pterygomaxillary (tĕr"ĭ-gō-măk'sĭ-lĕr"ē) [" + L. *maxillaris,* upper jaw]. Concerning the pterygoid process and the upper jaw.

pterygopalatine (tĕr"ĭ-gō-păl'ă-tĭn) [" + L. *palatinus,* palate]. Rel. to the pterygoid process and the palate bone.

PTH. *parathyroid hormone.*

ptilosis (tī-lō'sĭs) [Gr.]. Loss of eyelashes.

ptomaine (tō'mān, tō-mān') [Gr. *ptoma,* dead body]. One of a class of nitrogenous organic bases formed in the action of putrefactive bacteria on proteins and amino acids.

Ex.: cadaverine, $NH_2(CH_2)_5NH_2$.

ptosed (tōst). Having ptosis.

ptosis (tō'sĭs) [Gr. *ptosis,* a dropping]. Dropping or drooping of an organ or part, as the upper eyelid from paralysis, or the visceral organs from weakness of the abdominal muscles.

p., abdominal. Sagging of the transverse colon, sometimes almost to the pelvic floor.

ETIOL: Obesity or lack of abdominal muscle tone.

TREATMENT: A properly adjusted abdominal belt may help. This is contraindicated if the patient shows dependence upon belt instead of exercising and developing abdominal muscles.

p., morning. Difficulty in raising the eyelids upon awakening.

p., waking. P., morning, q.v.

ptotic (tŏt'ĭk). Concerning ptosis.

ptyalagogue (tī-ăl'ă-gŏg) [Gr. *ptyalon,* saliva, + *agogos,* leading]. Causing, or that which causes, a flow of saliva. SYN: *sialogogue.*

ptyalectasis (tī"ă-lĕk'tă-sĭs) [" + *ektasis,* dilation]. Surgical dilation of a salivary duct.

ptyalin (tī'ă-lĭn). A salivary enzyme that hydrolyzes starch and glycogen to maltose and a small amount of glucose. The optimum pH for ptyalin activity is 6.9. SYN: *amylase, salivary.* SEE: *enzyme; ptyalism; saliva.*

ptyalism (tī'ă-lĭzm) [" + *-ismos,* condition]. Excessive secretion of saliva. SYN: *salivation.* SEE: *xerostomia.*

ETIOL: May be due to pregnancy, stomatitis, rabies, exophthalmic goiter, menstruation, epilepsy, hysteria, nervous conditions, and gastrointestinal disorders. May be induced by mercury, iodides, pilocarpine, and other drugs.

ptyalith (tī'ă-lĭth) [" + *lithos,* stone]. A calculus in a salivary gland.

ptyalocele (tī-ăl'ō-sēl) [" + *kele,* hernia]. A salivary cystic tumor or cystic dilatation of a salivary duct.

ptyalogenic (tī"ăl-ō-jĕn'ĭk) [Gr. *ptyalon,* saliva, + *gennan,* to produce]. Of salivary origin.

ptyalogogue (tī"ăl'ō-gŏg) [" + *agogos,* leading]. An agent that causes the flow of saliva. SYN: *sialogogue.*

ptyalography (tī-ăl-ŏg'ră-fē) [" + *graphein,* to write]. Roentgenography of the salivary glands and ducts. SYN: *sialography.*

ptyalolith (tī'ă-lō-lĭth) [" + *lithos,* stone]. A salivary concretion.

ptyalolithiasis (tī"ă-lō-lĭ-thī'ă-sĭs). Presence of a concretion in a salivary gland or duct.

ptyalolithotomy (tī"ăl-ō-lĭ-thŏt'ō-mē) [Gr. *ptyalon,* saliva, + *lithos,* stone, + *tome,* incision]. Surgical removal of a concretion from a salivary duct or gland.

ptyaloreaction (tī″ă-lō-rē-ăk′shŭn). A reaction occurring in saliva.

ptyalorrhea (tī″ă-lō-rē′ă) [″ + *rhoia,* flow]. An excessive flow of saliva.

ptyocrinous (tī-ŏk′rĭ-nŭs). A type of glandular secretion in which the contents of the cell are discharged.

ptysis (tī′sĭs) [Gr.]. Spitting; the ejection of saliva from the mouth.

ptysmagogue (tīz′mă-gŏg) [″ + *agogos,* leading]. An agent that induces the flow of saliva.

Pu. Chem. symb. for plutonium.

pubarche (pū-băr′kē) [L. *puber,* grown up, + Gr. *arkhe,* beginning]. 1. The beginning of puberty. 2. Beginning development of pubic hair.

puber (pū′bĕr) [L., grown up]. One at onset of puberty.

puberal (pū′bĕr-ăl) [L. *pubertas,* puberty]. Concerning puberty.

pubertal. Pert. to puberty.

pubertas (pū′bĕr-tăs) [L.]. Puberty.

p. praecox. Precocious puberty or puberty at an early age.

puberty (pū′bĕr-tē). Period in life at which one of either sex becomes functionally capable of reproduction. A period of rapid change in boys and girls. It occurs between the ages of 13 and 15 in boys and from 9 to 16 in girls, and ends in the attainment of sexual maturity.

p., onset of. *Boys:* Between the ages of 13 and 15 there is a relatively rapid increase in height and weight with broadening of the shoulders and increase in size of the penis and testicles. Pubic hair and the beard begin to grow. Endocrine and sebaceous gland activity is increased. Nocturnal emissions usually occur. Young boys should be assured that the size of the penis is not related to the degree of masculinity and is not an important factor in experiencing or providing sexual gratification.

Girls: Between the ages of 9 and 16, a marked increase in growth rate is accompanied by breast enlargement and appearance of pubic hair. Within one to two years after these changes, underarm hair grows and the normal whitish vaginal secretion (physiological leukorrhea) characteristic of the adult female is noticed. Several months later the first menstrual period (menarche) occurs. Each individual will vary somewhat from this schedule. The young girl should be told prior to puberty about menstruation and the technique of menstrual protection through use of perineal pads or tampons. In addition, she should be told that a certain amount of intermenstrual vaginal discharge (leukorrhea) is normal but if the secretion is malodorous or causes irritation of the vulva, a physician should be consulted. SEE: *menstruation.*

p., precocious. Onset of puberty at an age much earlier than normal.

pubes (pū′bēz) [L., grown up] (sing. *pubis*) 1. Anterior part of innominate bone. SYN: *os pubis* [NA]. 2. The pubic region. 3. [NA] Hair of the pubic region.

pubescence (pū-bĕs′ĕns) [L. *pubescens,* becoming hairy]. 1. Puberty or its approach. 2. Covering of fine, soft hairs on the body. SYN: *lanugo.*

pubescent (pū-bĕs′ĕnt). 1. Reaching puberty. 2. Covered with downy hair.

pubetrotomy (pū″bĕ-trŏt′ō-mē) [L. *pubes,* grown up, + Gr. *etron,* belly, + *tome,* incision]. Section through the os pubis and lower abdominal wall.

pubic (pū′bĭk) [L. *pubes,* grown up]. Concerning the pubes.

pubic bone. The lower anterior part of the innominate bone. SYN: *os pubis* [NA].

pubic hair. Hair over the pubes, which appears at onset of sexual maturity. The distribution is somewhat different in men as compared with women.

pubio-, pubo- [L. *pubes,* grown up]. Combining form meaning the pubic hair or the pubic bone or region.

pubiotomy (pū-bē-ŏt′ō-mē) [″ + *tome,* a cutting]. Incision across the pubis in order to enlarge the pelvic passage, facilitating the delivery of the fetus when pelvis is malformed. SYN: *hebosteotomy; hebotomy.*

pubis (pū′bĭs) [L., grown up] (pl. *pubes*) Pubic bone; os pubis.

public health. The science of providing protection and promotion of community health through organized community effort.

Public Health Service Act. One of the principal laws of Congress giving the authority for federal health activities. First enacted July 1, 1944, it provided a complete codification of all the federal public health laws. Many of the health laws since 1944 have actually been amendments to the PHS act that have revised, extended, or given new authority to the act.

pubococcygeal (pū″bō-kŏk-sĭj′ē-ăl) [L. *pubis,* grown up, + Gr. *kokkyx,* coccyx]. Concerning the pubis and coccyx.

pubofemoral (pū″bō-fĕm′or-ăl) [″ + *femur,* thigh bone]. Pert. to the os pubis and the femur.

puboprostatic (pū″bō-prŏs-tăt′ĭk) [″ + Gr. *prostates,* prostate]. Rel. to the os pubis and prostate gland.

puborectal (pū″bō-rĕk′tăl) [″ + *rectus,* straight]. Concerning the pubis and rectum.

pubovaginal device. Apparatus that is fitted for use in the vagina to help prevent urinary incontinence.

pubovesical (pū″bō-vĕs′ĭ-kl) [L. *pubis,* grown up, + *vesiculus,* a little sac]. Pert. to the os pubis and bladder.

pudenda (pū-dĕn′dă) [L.]. (sing. *pudendum*) The external genitalia, esp. of the female. SYN: *vulva.*

pudendagra (pū″dĕn-dăg′ră) [″ + Gr. *agra,* seizure]. Pain in the external genitals.

pudendal (pū-dĕn′dăl) [L. *pudenda,* external genitals]. Rel. to the external genitals of the female. SYN: *pudic.*

pudendum (pū-dĕn′dŭm) [L.]. (pl. *pudenda*) The external genitals, esp. those of the female. SYN: *vulva.*

p. feminium. Vulva, q.v.

p. muliebre. External genitals of the female.

pudic (pū′dĭk) [L. *pudicus,* modest]. Concerning external female genitalia. SYN: *pudendal.*

puerile (pū′ĕ-rĭl) [L. *puerilis*]. Concerning a child; childlike.

puerilism (pū′ĕr-ĭl-ĭzm) [″ + Gr. *-ismos,* condition]. Childlishness; second childhood.

puerpera (pū-ĕr′pĕr-ă) [L. *puer,* child, + *parere,* to bear]. A woman during puerperium.

puerperal (pū-ĕr′pĕr-ăl) [L. *puerperalis*]. Concerning puerperium.

puerperal eclampsia. Convulsions and eclampsia during puerperium.

puerperal fever. Septicemia following childbirth. SYN: *childbed fever; puerperal sepsis.*

puerperalism (pū-ĕr′pĕr-ăl-ĭzm) [L. *puer,* child, + *parere,* to bear, + Gr. *-ismos,* condition]. Pathological condition accompanying childbirth.

puerperal period. Period immediately following childbirth.

puerperal sepsis. Any infection of the genital tract occurring during the puerperium or as a complication of abortion. This disease is presumed to be present when the temperature is 38° C. (100.4° F.) on any two consecutive days, exclusive of the first 24 hours postpartum, if no other causes of fever are apparent. The causative organisms, which are usually Streptococci or Clostridia, are introduced from the outside in the majority of cases. The establishment of careful techniques of asepsis and hygiene in maternity wards has effectively reduced the importance of this disease as a cause of death in the puerperium.

DIAG: Made on the basis of clinical findings consistent with infection of the genital tract, including fever and pain and tenderness of the lower abdominal area and genital tract.

TREATMENT: Appropriate antibiotic, incision and drainage if abscess forms, and supportive therapy.

puerperant (pū-ĕr′pĕr-ănt). A woman in labor, or one who recently has been delivered.

puerperium (pū″ĕr-pē′rē-ŭm) [L.]. The period of 42 days following childbirth and expulsion of the placenta and membranes. The generative organs usually return to normal during this time.

puerperous (pū-ĕr′pĕr-ŭs) [″ + *parere,* to bear]. In the period following childbirth. SYN: *puerperal.*

PUFA. *polyunsaturated fatty acids.* SEE: *acid, fatty.*

puff. A soft, short, blowing sound heard on auscultation.

Pulex (pū′lĕks) [L., flea]. A genus of fleas belonging to the order Siphonaptera.

P. irritans. The human flea, which also infests dogs, hogs, and other mammals. May serve as intermediate host of the tapeworms Dipylidium caninum and Hymenolepis diminuta. SEE: *flea.*

pulicatio (pū″lĭ-kā′tē-ō). Infested with fleas.

Pulicidae (pū-lĭs′ĭ-dē). A family of fleas belonging to the order Siphonaptera. Pulicidae includes the genera Pulex, Echidnophaga, Ctenocephalides, and Xenopsylla. SEE: *flea.*

pulicide (pū′lĭ-sīd) [L. *pulex,* flea, + *caedere,* to kill]. An agent that kills fleas.

pullulate (pŭl′ū-lāt) [L. *pullulare,* to sprout]. To bud or germinate.

pullulation (pŭl″ū-lā′shŭn). The act of budding or germinating, as seen in yeast plant.

pulmo- (pŭl′mō-, pool′mō-) [L. *pulmo,* lung]. Combining form meaning lung.

pulmoaortic (pŭl″mō-ā-or′tĭk) [″ + Gr. *aorte,* aorta]. 1. Concerning the lungs and the aorta. 2. Rel. to the pulmonary artery and aorta.

pulmometer (pŭl-mŏm′ĕ-tĕr) [″ + Gr. *metron,* measure]. Device for measuring lung capacity. SYN: *spirometer.*

pulmometry (pŭl-mŏm′ĕ-trē). Determination of capacity of the lungs.

pulmonary (pŭl′mō-nĕ-rē) [L. *pulmonarius*]. Concerning or involving the lungs.

pulmonary alveolar proteinosis. Disease of unknown cause in which eosinophilic material is deposited in the alveoli. Principal symptom is dyspnea. Death from pulmonary insufficiency may occur but complete recovery has been observed. There is no specific treatment but general supportive measures and bronchopulmonary lavage have helped.

pulmonary arterial webs. Weblike deformities seen in pulmonary angiograms at the site of previous pulmonary thromboembolism.

pulmonary artery. The artery leading from the right ventricle of the heart to the lungs.

pulmonary artery wedge pressure. Pressure measured in the pulmonary artery at its capillary end. The pressure is determined during cardiac catheterization by pushing the catheter from the right atrium into the pulmonary artery. This provides an indication of left ventricular pressure at the end of diastole and the average pressure in the left atrium. SEE: *Swan-Ganz catheter.* SYN: *wedge pressure.*

pulmonary circulation. Passage of blood from the heart to the lungs for purification and the return to the heart. The blood flows from the right cardiac ventricle through to the lungs; there to be oxygenated; then back to the left cardiac atrium. SEE: *circulation, pulmonary; circulation* for illus.

pulmonary edema. Lung, edema of, q.v.

pulmonary embolism. Embolism, pulmonary, q.v.

pulmonary emphysema. SEE: *emphysema* (def. 2).

pulmonary function tests. A number of different tests used to determine the ability of the lungs to exchange oxygen and carbon dioxide. These are done by measuring the amount of air that can be maximally exhaled after a maximum inspiration and the time required for that expiration; and by determining the ability of the alveolar capillary membrane to transport oxygen into the blood and carbon dioxide from the blood into the expired air. SEE: FEV_1.

pulmonary insufficiency. Failure of the pulmonary valve to close properly.

pulmonary mucociliary clearance. The removal of inhaled particles, endogenous cellular debris, and excessive secretions from the tracheobronchial tree by the action of the ciliated cells that live in the respiratory tract. The cilia of these cells beat and are therefore able to propel mucus and debris upward and out of the tracheobronchial tree. This action is one of the most important defenses of the respiratory tract.

pulmonary stenosis. Narrowing of the opening into the pulmonary artery from the right cardiac ventricle.

pulmonary surfactant. A phospholipid substance important in controlling the surface tension of the air-liquid emulsion that is present in the lungs. Abnormalities in this surfactant have been noted in prematurity, respiratory distress syndrome, and pulmonary edema.

pulmonary valve. The valve between the right ventricle and the opening into the pulmonary artery.

pulmonary vein. The vein draining the lungs and returning the blood to the left atrium of the heart.

pulmonectomy (pŭl″mō-nĕk′tō-mē) [L. *pulmonis,* lung, + Gr. *ektome,* excision]. Removal of part or all of a lung's tissue. SYN: *pneumonectomy.*

pulmonic (pŭl-mŏn′ĭk). 1. Concerning the lungs. 2. Concerning the pulmonary artery.

pulmonitis (pŭl-mō-nī′tĭs) [″ + Gr. *itis,* inflammation]. Inflamed condition of the lung. SYN: *pneumonia.*

pulmotor (pŭl′mō-tor) [″ + *motor,* mover]. Apparatus for inducing artificial respiration by forcing oxygen into the lungs and allowing the removal of carbon dioxide.

pulp [L. *pulpa,* flesh]. 1. The soft part of fruit. 2. The soft part of an organ. 3. Mass of partly digested food passed from stomach to duodenum. SYN: *chyme.* 4. In dentistry, the soft vascular portion of the center of a tooth.

p., coronal. That portion of the dental pulp in the crown of the pulp cavity.

p., dead. Devitalized or necrotic dental pulp.

p., dental. The connective tissues that fill the pulp cavity enclosed by dentin of the tooth; it includes a vascular and nerve network, a peripheral layer of odontoblasts involved with dentin formation, and other cellular and fibrous components.

p., digital. Elastic, soft prominence on the palmar or plantar surface of the last phalanx of a finger or toe.

p., enamel. Cells forming a stellate reticulum lying between outer and inner layers of the enamel organ of a tooth.

p., exposed. Pulp that due to disease is exposed to the air and saliva in the mouth.

p., nonvital. P., dead.

p., putrescent. Dead pulp that has a foul odor due to the action of putrefactive bacteria.

p., radicular. Pulp that is in the root canal of a tooth.

p., red. The portion of splenic pulp consisting of venous sinuses plus pulp cords.

p., splenic. Soft spongelike tissue-forming substance of the spleen.

p., vertebral. Nucleus pulposus, q.v., of the intervertebral disk.

p., vital. Dental pulp that is alive and thus normal.

p., white. Portion of splenic pulp consisting of a compact type of lymphatic tissue that forms a sheath about certain arteries.

pulpa (pŭl′pă) [L., flesh]. Pulp.

pulpal (pŭl′păl). Rel. to pulp.

pulpalgia (pŭl-păl′jē-ă) [″ + Gr. *algos,* pain]. Pain in the pulp of a tooth.

pulp amputation. The technique of removing the coronal portion of an exposed or involved vital pulp in an effort to retain the radicular pulp in a healthy, vital condition.

pulp capping. The technique and material for covering and protecting from external conditions a vital, exposed pulp while the pulp heals and secondary or tertiary dentin forms to cover it.

pulpectomy (pŭl-pĕk′tō-mē) [″ + Gr. *ektome,* excision]. Pulp extirpation q.v.

pulpefaction (pŭl-pĭ-făk′shŭn) [L. *pulpa,* pulp, + *facere,* to make]. Conversion into pulpy substance.

pulp extirpation. The complete removal of the pulp tissue from the pulp chamber and root canal, irrespective of the state of health of the pulp.

pulpitis (pŭl-pī′tĭs) [″ + *itis,* inflammation]. (pl. *pulpitides*) Inflammation of the pulp of a tooth.

pulpotomy (pŭl-pŏt′ō-mē) [″ + Gr. *tome,* incision]. Pulp amputation, q.v.

pulpy (pŭl′pē). Resembling pulp; flabby. SYN: *pultaceous.*

pulsate (pŭl′sāt) [L. *pulsare*]. To throb or beat in rhythm.

pulsatile (pŭl′să-tĭl). Pulsating; characterized by a rhythmic beat. SYN: *throbbing.*

pulsation (pŭl-sā′shŭn) [L. *pulsatio,* a beating]. The rhythmic beat, as of the heart and blood vessels; a throbbing. SEE: *pulse.*

ABNORMAL CENTERS OF PULSATION: *Epigastric:* May result from forceful action of heart from any cause; enlargement of right ventricle; pulsating aorta noted in certain anxious persons and in anemic patients; aortic aneurysm; tumors of left lobe of liver resting on the aorta. *Left axillary region:* May result from enlargement of heart; a tense purulent effusion in left pleural sac (pulsating empyema); aneurysm; chronic disease of left lung and pleura associated with retraction of the lung. *Carotids:* May result from strong heart beat from any cause; exophthalmic goiter; anemia; valvular disease, esp. aortic regurgitation; aneurysm or dilatation of the vessels; unnatural elasticity of the vessels noted in certain nervous and anemic patients. *Jugular:* Often becomes distended in forced expiration and coughing; sometimes noted in adherent pericardium. A true rhythmical venous pulsation usually results from tricuspid regurgitation. A pulsation may be transmitted to the jugular vein from the underlying carotid, but this false pulsation will continue when light pressure is made on the vein of the neck, while the true venous pulse will cease.

pulse (pŭls) [L. *pulsus,* beating]. 1. Rate, rhythm, condition of arterial walls, compressibility and tension, and size and shape of the wave. 2. Rhythmical throbbing. 3. Throbbing caused by the regular contraction and alternate expansion of an artery as the wave of blood passes through the vessel; the periodic thrust felt over arteries in time with the heartbeat.

A tracing of this is called a sphygmogram and consists of a series of waves in which the upstroke is called the anacrotic limb and the downstroke (on which is normally seen the dicrotic notch) the catacrotic limb.

Normal pulse rate of the adult is 70 to 72 in men and 78 to 82 in women. It is usually felt in the radial artery of the wrist.

POINTS TO BE OBSERVED: Hour, frequency, pressure, regularity, force. Temperature and respiration are of clinical importance to the physician. Right and left radial arteries are usually tested and differences, if any, or absence of either should be noted. If pressure of finger on artery is too great the vessel will be collapsed and the pulse will not be discernible. The thumb should not be used because the examiner may be counting the pulse in his or her own thumb rather than patient's. Count for at least half a minute.

The rate of the pulse depends upon sex, age, exertion, position of body, and state of general health. It is higher in children and increases with very old age. It is slower in tall persons than it is in short persons. It is 10 to 12 beats more frequent during standing than sitting. Physical exertion will increase it normally to as much as 200 beats per minute in young healthy persons. Eating and drinking likewise increase heart action. Pulse rate decreases during sleep, relaxation, and rest.

p., abdominal. A palpable pulse in the abdominal area. This is produced by the pulse of the abdominal aorta.

p., accelerated. A common symptom in most fevers. The pulse of the adult rarely exceeds 150 beats per minute even in acute inflammatory infections; when it exceeds 170, it may portend a fatal outcome. If such an acceleration does not diminish within a short time, it is esp. unfavorable. When quick and bounding, it indicates acute fever or inflammation, or it may result from a toxic goiter; organic heart disease; pressure at the base of the brain sufficient to paralyze the phrenic nerve as in clot, tumor, and advanced meningitis; shock; rheumatoid arthritis; or the use of certain drugs such as belladonna, nitrites, or alcohol. SYN: *p., rapid; tachycardia.*

p., alternating. Pulse with alternating weak and strong pulsations.

p., anacrotic. Pulse showing a secondary wave on ascending limb of the main wave.

p., anadicrotic. A pulse wave with two small notches on the ascending portion.

p., asymmetrical radial. Pulse in which beats vary in force. SYN: *p., unequal.*

p., bigeminal. Pulse in which two regular beats are followed by a longer pause. It has the same significance as an irregular pulse.

p., bounding. Pulse that reaches a higher intensity than normal, then disappears quickly. Best detected when arm is held aloft. Due to shortened ventricular systole and reduced peripheral pressure. SYN: *p., collapsing*.

p., brachial. Pulse felt in the brachial artery.

p., capillary. Alternating redness and pallor of capillary region, as in the matrices beneath the nails, occurring chiefly where an excessive cardiac impulse coincides with general arterial narrowing. SYN: *p., Quincke's*.

p., carotid. Pulse felt in the carotid artery.

p., catacrotic. Pulse showing one or more secondary waves on descending limb of the main wave.

p., catadicrotic. A pulse wave with two small notches on the descending portion.

p., central. Pulse recorded near the origin of the carotid or subclavian arteries.

p., collapsing. Pulse feebly striking the finger, then subsiding abruptly and completely. SYN: *p., bounding*.

p., Corrigan's. Short, forceful, bounding pulse characteristic of aortic insufficiency. SEE: *p., waterhammer*.

p., coupled. P., bigeminal, q.v.

p., deficit. Condition in which the number of pulse beats counted at the wrist is less than those counted in the same period of time at the heart. Seen in atrial fibrillation.

p., dicrotic. A pulse with a double beat, one heartbeat for two arterial pulsations, or a seemingly weak wave between the usual heartbeats. This weak wave should not be counted as a regular beat. It is indicative of low arterial tension and is noted in fevers.

p., dorsalis pedis. Pulse felt over the dorsalis pedis artery of the foot.

p., entoptic. Intermittent subjective sensations of light that accompany the heartbeat.

p., febrile. A full, bounding pulse at onset of fever, becoming feeble and weak when fever subsides.

p., femoral. Pulse felt over the femoral artery.

p., filiform. P., thready.

p., formicant. A small, feeble pulse.

p., full. A distended pulse in an artery, giving a tense feeling. Observed in inflammation.

p., hard. Pulse with sensation of hardness due to changes in the arterial wall or to vascular distention.

p., hepatic. Pulse due to expansion of veins of the liver at each ventricular contraction.

p., high-tension. Pulse in which force of beat is relatively increased. The force may be roughly estimated by noting the amount of pressure of the fingers that is required to arrest the beat. It is observed in many conditions: cardiac diseases, such as hypertrophy; chronic nephritis; cerebral affections; high fever; irritation of the vasomotor center as in apoplexy, tumors, and beginning meningitis; after the use of certain drugs such as digitalis, ergot, and alcoholic stimulants; chills; angina pectoris; epileptic and hysterical seizures; gout; and uremia.

p., incident. Pulse with second beat weaker than first, the third weaker than the fourth, followed by a stroke as strong as the first.

p., intermediate. Pulse recorded in proximal portions of carotid, femoral, and brachial arteries.

p., intermittent. Pulse in which occasional beats are skipped. Caused by an apparent drop of a heartbeat. It is not inconsistent with health, yet it is commonly an indication of disease, frequently from gastric, hepatic, uterine, and renal causes. It is common in fatty degeneration of the heart and is habitual in certain people after exercise, eating, or excitement.

p., irregular. Pulse with a variation in force and frequency. Has same significance as intermittent pulse. Common in myocarditis and valvular diseases, esp. in mitral regurgitation. Heart trouble may be noted by long-continued irregular pulse.

p., jerky. Pulse characteristic of aortic regurgitation, because from a state of emptiness, the artery is suddenly filled with blood.

p., jugular. Venous pulse felt in the jugular vein.

p., Kussmaul's. P., paradoxical, q.v.

p., long. Pulse in which duration of the systolic wave is comparatively long.

p., low-tension. Pulse with sudden onset, short duration, and rapid decline, esp. noted in heart failure, collapse, debility, and fevers.

p., monocrotic. Pulse in which the sphygmogram shows a simple ascending and descending uninterrupted line and no dicrotism.

p., nail. Visible pulsation in the capillaries under the nails.

p., paradoxical. Pulse that is more or less suppressed at close of each full inspiration. Thought to be due to compression of the great vessels by inflammatory adhesions, the latter being stretched during act of inspiration. Frequently noted in adherent pericarditis.

p., peripheral. Pulse recorded in arteries (radial or pedal) in distal portion of limbs.

p., pistol-shot. Pulse resulting from rapid distention and collapse of an artery as occurs in aortic regurgitation.

p., plateau. Pulse associated with an increase in pressure that slowly rises but is maintained.

p., popliteal. Pulse felt over the popliteal artery.

p., Quincke's. P., capillary.

p., radial. Pulse felt over the radial artery.

p., rapid. P., accelerated.

p., regular. Pulse felt when the force and frequency are the same, i.e., when the length of beat and number of beats per minute and the strength are the same.

p., respiratory. Alternate dilatation and contraction of the large veins of the neck occurring simultaneously with inspiration and expiration.

p., Riegel's. Diminution of the pulse during expiration.

p., running. A weak, rapid pulse with one wave continuing into the next.

p., senile. Pulse characteristic of the aged. The sphygmogram shows a high position of the secondary waves in descent with increased amplitude of the first secondary wave as compared with the second.

p., short. Pulse with a short, quick systolic wave.

p., slow. A very slow pulse, fully accentuated, often found among the aged. It is a habitual rate among those inclined to be slow and easy in their actions and is found in the highly conditioned athlete. Such a pulse rate ranges between 40 and 60 beats per minute.

p., soft. Pulse that may be stopped by moderate digital compression.

p., tense. A full but not bounding pulse.

p., thready. A fine, scarcely perceptible pulse. SYN: *p., filiform.*

p., tremulous. Pulse in which a series of oscillations is felt with each beat.

p., tricrotic. Pulse with three separate expansions during each heartbeat.

p., trigeminal. Pulse in which a pause follows three regular beats.

p., triphammer. P., Corrigan's, q.v.

p., undulating. Pulse that seems to have several successive waves.

p., unequal. Pulse in which beats vary in force. SYN: *p., asymmetrical radial.*

p., vagus. A slow pulse resulting from vagus inhibition of the heart.

p., venous. Pulse in a vein, esp. one of the large veins near the heart, such as the internal and external jugular. Normally is undulating and scarcely palpable. In conditions such as tricuspid regurgitation, it is pronounced.

p., vermicular. A small, frequent pulse with a wormlike feeling.

p., waterhammer. Pulse characterized by a short, powerful, jerky beat that suddenly collapses. The peculiar pulsation may be distinctly visible, not only in the carotids but throughout the brachial artery. It is diagnostic of aortic regurgitation during the period of compensation, and its force is due to excessive ventricular hypertrophy and to the large amount of blood expelled with each systole; its sudden recession is due to the incompetent valves failing to support the column of blood. SYN: *p., Corrigan's.*

p., wiry. A tense pulse that feels like a wire or firm cord.

pulse, words pert. to: acrotic; acrotism; Adams-Stokes syndrome; anacrotic; arrhythmia; artery; asphyctic; bisferious; bradycrotic; diastole; diastolic pressure; dicrotic; heart; hemisystole; murmur; phlebogram; pulsate; pulsation; pulsus; respiration; sphygmomanometer; systole; systolic pressure; thermometry; vein.

pulse generator. Device for producing an intermittent electrical discharge in order to serve as a cardiac pacemaker.

pulseless disease. Progressive arterial disease that obliterates the arteries leading to the brain and the arms. This causes absent pulses in the carotid and brachial arteries and ischemia of the areas supplied. SYN: *Takayasu's arteritis.*

pulse pressure. The difference between the systolic and the diastolic pressure. This is really expressive of the tone of the arterial walls. Ex.:

systolic pressure is	120
diastolic pressure is	100
pulse pressure is	20

systolic pressure is	130
diastolic pressure is	90
pulse pressure is	40

Normal pulse pressure: The systolic pressure is normally about 40 points greater than the diastolic. *Abnormal pulse pressure:* A pulse pressure over 50 points or under 30 points is considered abnormal.

pulse wave. A wave in the blood column and the arterial walls that is initiated by the ejection of blood from the left ventricle into the aorta. The velocity in the aorta may be as high as 500 cm./sec.; and as low as 0.07 cm./sec. in capillaries.

pulsimeter (pŭl-sĭm′ĕt-ĕr) [L. *pulsus,* a beat, + Gr. *metron,* measure]. Device for measuring frequency and force of the pulse. SYN: *sphygmometer.*

pulsing electromagnetic field. ABBR: PEMF. The production of a pulsing electromagnetic field applied to a fractured bone in order to induce healing. The electric field is applied externally to the affected leg and does not involve invasion of the tissue. This treatment is esp. useful in treating fractures that have previously failed to heal. Direct-current stimulation has also been used in treating these conditions.

pulsion (pŭl′shŭn). Driving or propelling in any direction.

p., lateral. Movement, particularly walking as if pulled to one side.

pulsus (pŭl′sŭs) [L.]. Pulse.

p. alternans. A weak pulse alternating with a strong one.

p., bigeminus. Pulse, bigeminal, q.v.

p. celer. Quick pulse that rises and falls suddenly.

p. differens. Condition in which the pulses on either side of the body are of unequal intensity.

p. paradoxus. Pulse, paradoxical, q.v.

p. parvus et tardus. Pulse that is small and rises and falls slowly.

p. tardus. An abnormally slow pulse.

pultaceous (pŭl-tā′shŭs) [L. *pultaceus*]. Resembling a poultice. SYN: *pulpy.*

pulv. [L.]. *pulvis,* powder.

pulverization (pŭl″vĕr-ī-zā′shŭn) [L. *pulvis,* powder]. The crushing of any substance to powder or tiny particles.

pulverulent (pŭl-vĕr′ū-lĕnt). Of the nature of, or resembling, powder.

pulvinar (pŭl-vī′năr) [L., cushioned seat]. [NA] Part of the thalamus comprising a portion of the posterior nuclei. Projects posteriorly and medially partially overlying midbrain.

pulvinate (pŭl′vĭ-nāt) [L. *pulvinus,* cushion]. Convex; shaped like a cushion.

pulvis [L.]. Powder.

pumice (pŭm′ĭs). USP. A substance derived from volcanic material. It contains chiefly complex silicates of aluminum, potassium, and sodium. Used as an abrasive, esp. in dental prophylaxis.

pump [ME. *pumpe*]. 1. Apparatus that transfers fluids or gases by pressure or suction. 2. To force air or fluid along a certain pathway, as the heart pumps blood.

p., air. Device for forcing air in or out of a chamber.

p., blood. Device for pumping blood. It is attached to an extracorporeal circulation system.

p., breast. Apparatus for removing milk from the breasts.

p., dental. Apparatus for removing saliva from the mouth during operation on teeth or jaws.

p., sodium. The biological system that permits the flow or transport of sodium across a membrane even though the sodium concentration is higher on the side of the membrane to which the sodium is flowing.

p., stomach. Apparatus for removing contents from the stomach.

pump-oxygenator. A device that pumps blood and oxygenates it.

puna (poo′nă). Mountain sickness.

punch. An instrument for making a small circular hole in material or tissue, esp. the skin.

punchdrunk. 1. A concussion syndrome present in persons who have boxed and experienced multiple episodes of trauma to the head. If severe, both the cognitive and memory functions of the brain are affected. At autopsy, there is evidence of multiple scars of the cerebral tissue. 2. One who is punchdrunk.

punched out. Appears as if holes have been made; used to describe appearance of bones (as seen on x-ray film) in certain pathological states.

puncta (pŭnk′tă) [L.]. (sing. *punctum*) Points.

punctate (pŭnk′tāt) [L. *punctum,* point]. Having pinpoint punctures or depressions on the surface; marked with dots.

punctate keratoses. Discrete yellow-to-brown firm keratotic papules of the palms and soles. Most probably due to the performing of manual labor.

punctate pits. Depressed areas of the skin, esp. of the palmar creases of the hands and soles.

punctate rash. Rash with minute red points.

punctiform (pŭnk′tĭ-form) [″ + *forma,* shape]. 1. Formed like a point. 2. In bacteriology, referring to pinpoint colonies of less than 1 mm. in diameter.

punctio (pŭnk′shē-ō) [L. *punctura,* a point]. The act of puncturing or pricking.

punctograph (pŭnk′tō-grăf) [″ + Gr. *graphein,* to write]. Device employing radiography for localization of foreign bodies in the tissues.

punctum (pŭnk′tŭm) [L.]. (pl. *puncta*) Point.

p. caecum. Spot in fundus of the eyeball where the optic nerve enters. SYN: *blind spot.*

puncta dolorosa. Painful points in the course of, or at the exit of, nerves affected by neuralgia.

p. lacrimale. [NA] Outlet of lacrimal canaliculus.

p. nasale inferius. Lower portion of suture joining the nasal bones. SYN: *rhinion.*

p. proximum. ABBR: P.P. Visual accommodation near-point.

p. remotum. ABBR: P.R. Visual accommodation far-point.

p. saliens. First trace of the embryonic heart.

p. vasculosa. Minute red areas that mark the cut surface of white central substance of the brain, caused by blood escaping from divided blood vessels.

puncture (pŭnk′chūr) [L. *punctura,* a point]. 1. A hole or wound made by a sharp pointed instrument. 2. To make a hole with such an instrument.

p., cisternal. Puncture of the cerebromedullary cisterna by introducing a needle through the suboccipital tissue. This is done in order to obtain a sample of cerebrospinal fluid.

p., diabetic. Puncture in floor of the 4th ventricle, which results in glycosuria.

p., exploratory. Piercing of a cavity or cyst for purpose of examining fluid or pus removed.

p., lumbar. Puncture of the lumbar spinal membranes to relieve dropsy or for examination of spinal fluid. SEE: *cerebrospinal fluid; cisternal puncture; lumbar puncture.*

p., Quincke's. P., lumbar, q.v.

p., spinal. P., lumbar, q.v.

p., sternal. Puncture of the manubrium sternum by use of a needle, the purpose of which is to obtain a bone marrow specimen.

p., ventricular. Puncture of a ventricle of the brain for purpose of withdrawing fluid or introducing air for ventriculography.

puncture wound. A wound made by piercing with a sharp instrument. SEE: *wound, puncture; Wounds* in *Appendix.*

pungency (pŭn′jĕn-sē) [L. *pungens,* prick]. Quality of being sharp, strong, or bitter, as an odor or taste.

pungent (pŭn′jĕnt). Acrid or sharp, as applied to an odor or taste.

P.U.O. *pyrexia of unknown origin.*

pupa (pū′pă) [L., girl]. Stage in complete metamorphosis of an insect that follows the larva and precedes the adult or imago. The insect does not feed in this stage and usually is inactive.

pupil (pū′pĭl) [L. *pupilla*]. The contractile opening at the center of the iris of the eye. It contracts when exposed to strong light and when the focus is on a near object. It dilates in the dark and when the focus is on a distant object. Average diameter is 4 to 5 mm. The pupils should be equal.

DIFF. DIAG: Constriction of the pupil occurs in old age and in photophobia. It is induced by morphine, pilocarpine, physostigmine, eserine, and other miotic drugs.

Dilation of the pupil may occur in blindness or deficient sight from any cause; from distress or strong emotion; in fevers, comatose states, oculomotor nerve paralysis, and glaucoma. May be induced by belladonna (atropine), cocaine, homatropine, hyoscine (scopolamine), and other mydriatic drugs.

RS: accommodation; adaptation; anisocoria; ciliospinal center; corectasia; eye; hippus; iris; iridoplegia; isocoria; miosis; miotic; mydriasis; mydriatic; myosis; reflex; seclusio pupillae.

p., Adie's. SEE: *Adie's syndrome.*

p., Argyll Robertson. Pupil that reacts to accommodation but not to light. Seen occasionally in diseases affecting the midbrain.

p., artificial. Pupil made by iridectomy when normal pupil is occluded.

p., bounding. Rapid dilatation of pupil alternating with contraction.

p., Bumke's. Dilation of the pupil due to psychic stimulus.

p., cat's-eye. Pupil that is narrow and slitlike.

p., cornpicker's. Dilated pupils found in agricultural workers who are exposed to dust from Jimson weed. The dust contains stramonium, a mydriatic.

p., fixed. A pupil that does not react to stimuli.

p., Hutchinson's. Condition in which one pupil is dilated and the other is not. The pupil on the side of the lesion is dilated and the other is contracted. This is usually due to compression of the third cranial nerve in meningitis.

p., keyhole. A pupil with an artificial coloboma at the pupillary margin.

p., occlusion of. Pupil with opaque membrane shutting off the pupillary area.

p., pinhole. Pupil of minute size; one excessively constricted. Seen after use of miotics, in opium poisoning, and in certain brain disorders.

p., stiff. P., Argyll Robertson, q.v.

p., tonic. Pupil that reacts slowly in accommodation-convergence reflexes.

pupilla (pū-pĭl′ă) [L., pupil]. Pupil of the eye.

pupillary (pū′pĭ-lĕr-ē) [L. *pupilla,* pupil]. Concerning the pupil.

pupillary reflex. 1. Constriction of pupil upon stimulation of retina by light. 2. Constriction of pupil upon accommodation for near vision, and dilatation upon accommodation for far vision. SYN: *accommodation reflex.* 3. Constriction of pupil of one eye in response to stimulation of the other by light. SYN: *consensual light reflex.* 4. Constriction of pupil upon attempted closure of eyelids that are held apart. SEE: *ciliospinal reflex; hippus.*

pupillometer (pū-pĭl-ŏm′ĕ-tĕr) [″ + Gr. *metron,* measure]. Device for measurement of diameter of a pupil.

pupillometry (pū″pĭl-lŏm′ĕ-trē) [″ + *metron,* measure]. Measurement of the diameter of the pupil.

pupillomotor reflex. Purkinje phenomenon, q.v.

pupilloplegia (pū″pĭ-lō-plē′jē-ă) [″ + *plege,* stroke]. Slow reaction of the pupil of the eye.

pupilloscopy (pū-pĭl-ŏs′kō-pē) [″ + Gr. *sko-*

pein, to examine]. 1. Measurement of eye refraction by effect of light and shadow on the retina. SYN: *retinoscopy; skiascopy.* 2. Examination of the pupil.

pupillostatometer (pū″pĭl-ō-stă-tŏm′ĕ-tĕr) [″ + Gr. *statos,* placed, + *metron,* measure]. Device for measuring distance between centers of the pupils.

pure (pūr) [ME.]. Free from pollution; uncontaminated.

pure line. 1. The progeny of a single homozygous individual obtained by self-fertilization. 2. The progeny of an individual reproducing asexually by simple fission, or by buds, runners, stolons, etc. 3. The progeny of two homozygous individuals reproducing sexually.

purgation (pŭr-gā′shŭn) [L. *purgatio*]. 1. Cleansing. 2. Evacuation of bowels by action of a purgative medicine. SYN: *catharsis.*

purgative (pŭr′gă-tĭv) [L. *purgativus*]. 1. Cleansing. 2. An agent that will cause watery evacuation of the intestinal contents such as castor oil or magnesium sulfate. SEE: *cathartic; cathartic.*

p., cholagogue. Purgative that stimulates flow of bile, producing green stools.

p., drastic. Purgative that produces violent action of bowels with cramps and griping.

p., saline. Purgative that produces copious watery discharges.

p., simple. Purgative that produces free discharge from bowels with some griping.

purgative enema. A strong, high colonic purgative that is used when other enemas fail. SEE: *enema.*

purge (pŭrj) [L. *purgare,* to cleanse]. 1. To evacuate the bowels by means of a cathartic. 2. A drug that causes evacuation of the bowels.

puriform (pū′rĭ-form) [L. *pus,* pus, + *forma,* shape]. Resembling pus. SYN: *puruloid.*

purinase (pū′rĭ-nās). An enzyme that catalyzes purine metabolism.

purine (pū′rēn″) [L. *purum,* pure, + *uricus,* uric acid]. Parent compound of purine bases, as adenine, guanine, xanthine, caffeine, and uric acid. Purines are the end products of nucleoprotein digestion. They may be synthesized in the body. They break down to form uric acid. SEE: *aminopurine; oxypurine; methylpurine.*

p., endogenous. Purine originating from nucleoproteins within the tissues.

p., exogenous. Purine present in, or derived from, foods. SEE: table.

purine base. Xanthine base, q.v.

purine-free diet. Diet that excludes the following: meat, esp. sweetbreads, liver, kidney; poultry; fish; condiments; alcohol; concentrated sweets, rich pastries, and fried foods.

Purines in Food

Group A: High concentration (150 to 1000 mg. per 100 gm.)	
Liver	Sardines (in oil)
Kidney	Meat extracts
Sweetbreads	Consomme
Brains	Gravies
Heart	Fish roes
Anchovies	Herring
Group B: Moderate amounts (50 to 150 mg. per 100 gm.)	
Meat, game, and fish other than those mentioned in Group A	
Fowl	Asparagus
Lentils	Cauliflower
Whole grain cereals	Mushrooms
Beans	Spinach
Peas	
Group C: Very small amounts. Need not be restricted in diet of persons with gout.	
Vegetables other than those mentioned above	
Fruits of all kinds	Coffee
Milk	Tea
Cheese	Chocolate
Eggs	Carbonated beverages
Refined cereals, spaghetti, macaroni	Tapioca
Butter, fats, nuts, peanut butter*	Yeast
Sugars and sweets	
Vegetable soups	

*Fats interfere with the urinary excretion of urates and thus should be limited when attempting to promote excretion of uric acid.

purine-low diet. Diet that excludes foods such as meat, fish, fowl, spinach, lentils, mushrooms, peas, asparagus.

purinemia (pū″rĭ-nē′mē-ă) [*purine* + Gr. *haima,* blood]. Purine in the blood.

Purinethol. Trade name for mercaptopurine, USP.

Purkinje, Johannes E. von (pŭr-kĭn′jē). Bohemian anatomist and physiologist, 1787–1869.

P. cells. Large neurons that have dendrites extending to the molecular layer of the cerebellar cortex and into the white matter of the cerebellum.

P. fibers. Atypical muscle fibers lying beneath the endocardium. They form the electrical impulse–conducting system of the heart.

P. figures. Shadows of blood vessels perceived when light is projected out of focus or obliquely onto the retina.

P. network. Fibrous network of large muscle cells found in cardiac muscle beneath the endocardium.

P. phenomenon. A phenomenon of adjustment of the pupil of the eye to light intensity. When the eye adapts from light to dark conditions, the maximum pupillary movement is caused by green instead of yellow light. SYN: *pupillomotor reflex.*

P.-Sanson images. [Louis J. Sanson, Fr. physician, 1790–1841] Three images of the same object. They are produced by reflections from the surface of the cornea and the anterior and posterior surfaces of the lens. For the most part, the viewer adapts to this phenomenon and ignores these normal images.

P. vesicle. The nuclear portion of an ovum. SYN: *germinal vesicle.*

Purodigin. Trade name for digitoxin, USP.

purohepatitis (pū″rō-hĕp″ă-tī′tĭs) [L. *pus,* pus, + Gr. *hepar,* liver, + *itis,* inflammation]. Purulent inflammation of the liver.

puromucous (pū″rō-mū′kŭs) [″ + *mucus,* phlegm]. Mucopurulent, containing both mucus and pus.

purple. Color formed by mixing red with blue.

p., visual. Rhodopsin.

purposeful movement. Motor activity requiring the planned and consciously directed involvement of the patient. It is hypothesized that evoking cortical involvement in movement patterns during sensorimotor rehabilitation will enhance the development of coordination and voluntary control.

purpura (pŭr′pū-ră) [L., purple]. A condition with various manifestations and diverse causes, characterized by hemorrhages into the skin, mucous membranes, internal organs, and other tissues. Hemorrhage into the skin shows red, darkening into purple, then brownish-yellow and finally disappearing in 2 to 3 weeks. Areas of discoloration do not disappear under pressure. SYN: *peliosis.*

p., allergic. A group of purpuras due to a variety of agents including bacteria, drugs, and food.

p., anaphylactoid. P., Schönlein-Henoch, q.v.

p. annularis telangiectodes. Eruption of ring-shaped spots on lower limbs with pronounced telangiectasia. SYN: *Majocchi's disease.*

p., fibrinolytic. Purpura resulting from excess fibrinolytic activity of blood.

p. fulminans. A rapidly progressing form of purpura occurring principally in children; of short duration and frequently fatal.

p., hemorrhagic. P., idiopathic thrombocytopenic, q.v.

p., Henoch. P., Schönlein-Henoch, q.v., with acute vomiting, diarrhea, and renal colic, but without joint involvement.

p., idiopathic thrombocytopenic. ABBR: ITP. A hemorrhagic disorder in which there is a pronounced reduction in circulating blood platelets, due to presence in blood plasma of a substance that agglutinates platelets. Primary cause unknown.

SYM: Bleeding from mouth and skin upon slight injury. Bleeding may also occur from mucous membranes, in serous membranes, and sometimes into brain. Increased bleeding time and reduced platelet count. Clot is nonretractile, but the coagulation time is normal.

p. nervosa. P., Henoch, q.v.

p., nonthrombocytopenic. P., allergic.

p. rheumatica. Purpura with joint pain, colic, bloody stools and vomiting of blood.

p., Schönlein-Henoch. Purpura due to vasculitis. It was first described by William Heberden prior to 1800, by Schönlein in 1830, and by Henoch in the 1870s. The skin lesions are obvious but the visceral lesions are difficult to diagnose, but are very serious. The cause is unknown, but allergy or drug sensitivity is important in some cases. There is no specific treatment unless a specific allergen can be proven and then removed.

p., senile. Purpura occurring in debilitated and aged persons with ecchymoses and petechiae on legs.

p. simplex. Purpura that is not associated with systemic illness.

p., thrombocytopenic. P., idiopathic thrombocytopenic.

p., thrombopenic. P., idiopathic thrombocytopenic, q.v.

p., thrombotic thrombocytopenic. A rare disease characterized by embolism and thrombosis of the small blood vessels of the brain. Shifting neurological signs such as aphasia, blindness, and convulsions are present. Therapy has been of little value, but adrenal corticosteroids in large doses have been tried. Exchange transfusions have been of some help in treating this disease.

purpureaglycosides A and B (pŭr-pū″rē-ă-glī′kō-sīds). True cardiac glycosides present in the leaves of Digitalis purpurea, foxglove.

purpuric (pŭr-pū′rĭk) [L. *purpura,* purple]. Pert. to, resembling, or suffering from purpura.

purpurin (pŭr′pū-rĭn). 1. An acid dye used to stain nuclei. 2. A red pigment sometimes present in urine. SYN: *uroerythrin.*

purpurinuria (pŭr″pū-rĭn-ū′rē-ă) [″ + Gr. *ouron,* urine]. Purpurin in urine.

purring thrill. Thrill or vibration, like a cat's purring, due to mitral stenosis, aneurysm, or valvular disease of the heart; felt by palpation over the precordium.

purulence (pūr'ū-lĕns) [L. *purulentia*]. The state of containing pus. SYN: *suppuration.*

purulency (pūr'ū-lĕn"sē). Purulence.

purulent (pūr'ū-lĕnt) [L. *purulentus*]. Suppurative; forming or containing pus. SEE: *sputum.*

puruloid (pūr'ū-loyd) [L. *pus*, pus, + Gr. *eidos*, form]. Like pus. SYN: *puriform.*

pus (pŭs) [L.]. Liquid product of inflammation composed of albuminous substances, a thin fluid, and leukocytes; generally yellowish in color. If red, it suggests rupture of small vessels. If blue or green, it indicates presence of Pseudomonas aeruginosa.

ETIOL: Streptococci, staphylococci, gonococci, pneumococci, and other species of bacteria.

p., blue. Purulence with a blue tint; usually associated with infection due to Pseudomonas aeruginosa.

p., cheesy. Very thick pus.

p., concrete. Fibropurulent coagula seen in infective endocarditis.

p., ichorous. Pus that is thin with shreds of sloughing tissue. It may have a fetid odor.

p., sanious. Ichorous pus colored by blood.

pus, words pert. to: cell; empyema; pyemia; resorption; suppurate; suppuration; "pyo-" words.

pus cells. Leukocytes that are dead or show degenerative changes. Found in suppurative inflammation.

pus in urine. Condition in which there are more than the normal number of white blood cells in the urine. It may be due to cystitis, pyelitis, urethritis, tuberculosis of the kidney, infection of the genitourinary tract, or trauma. Freshly passed urine may be cloudy due to presence of phosphates or pus. If the former, the addition of acid will cause it to clear; if pus is present, it will not clear but may become gelatinous. SYN: *pyuria.*

pustula (pŭs'tū-lă) [L., blister]. Pustule.

pustulant (pŭs'tū-lănt) [L. *pustula*, blister]. 1. Causing pustules. 2. Agent that produces the formation of pustules.

pustular (pŭs'tū-lĕr). Pert. to, or characterized by, pustules.

pustulation (pŭs"tū-lā'shŭn). The development of pustules.

pustule (pŭs'tūl) [L. *pustula*, blister]. Small elevation of skin filled with lymph or pus. Pustules may be circumscribed, flat, rounded, or umbilicated. They occur in eczema pustulosum, acne vulgaris, dermatitis herpetiformis, impetigo simplex, ecthyma, varicella, syphilis, and smallpox. SEE: *pus; pustulant.*

pustulocrustaceous (pŭs"tū-lō-krŭs-tā'shŭs) [" + *crusta*, shell]. Characterized by formation of pustules and crusts.

pustulosis (pŭs"tū-lō'sĭs) [" + Gr. *osis*, condition]. A generalized eruption of pustules.

putamen (pū-tā'mĕn) [L., shell]. [NA] The darker outer layer of the lenticular nucleus.

Putnam-Dana syndrome (pŭt'năm-dā'nă). [James J. Putnam, U.S. neurologist, 1846–1918; Charles L. Dana, U.S. neurologist, 1852–1935] Subacute combined degeneration of the spinal cord that may be present in patients with untreated pernicious anemia.

putrefaction (pū"trĕ-făk'shŭn) [L. *putrefactio*]. Decomposition of animal matter, esp. protein associated with malodorous and poisonous products such as the ptomaines, mercaptans, and hydrogen sulfide, caused by certain kinds of bacteria and fungi. Decomposition occurring spontaneously in sterile tissue after death is called autolysis. SEE: *sepsis.*

putrefactive (pū"trĕ-făk'tĭv) [L. *putrefacere*, to putrefy]. 1. Causing, or pert. to, putrefaction. 2. Agent promoting putrefaction.

putrefy (pū'trĕ-fī) [L. *putrefacere*, to putrefy]. To undergo putrefaction.

putrescence (pū-trĕs'ĕns) [L. *putrescens*, grow rotten]. Decay; rottenness.

putrescine (pū-trĕs'ĭn). A poisonous polyamine formed by bacterial action on the amino acid arginine.

putrid (pū'trĭd) [L. *putridus*]. Decayed; rotten; foul.

PUVA therapy [*p*soralen + *u*ltraviolet *A*]. Therapy of psoriasis by use of a psoralen and high-intensity long-wave ultraviolet light. SEE: *psoralen; psoriasis.*

PVC. *polyvinyl chloride.*

PVP. *polyvinylpyrrolidone.*

PVP-iodine. *povidone-iodine*

pyarthrosis (pī"ăr-thrō'sĭs) [Gr. *pyon*, pus, + *arthron*, joint, + *osis*, condition]. Pus in the cavity of a joint.

pycnemia (pĭk-nē'mē-ă) [Gr *pyknos*, thick, + *haima*, blood]. Thickening of the blood. SYN: *pyknemia.*

pycno- (pĭk'nō) [Gr. *pyknos*, thick]. Combining form meaning dense or thick. SEE: words beginning with *pykno-*.

pyecchysis (pī-ĕk'ĭ-sĭs) [Gr *pyon*, pus, + *ek*, out, + *chein*, to pour]. An effusion of pus.

pyelectasia, pyelectasis (pī"ĕ-lĕk-tā'zē-ă, -lĕk'tă-sĭs) [Gr. *pyelos*, pelvis, + *ektasis*, dilatation]. Dilatation of the renal pelvis.

pyelitic (pī"ĕ-lĭt'ĭk). Rel. to or affected with, pyelitis.

pyelitis (pī"ĕ-lī'tĭs) [Gr. *pyelos*, pelvis, + *itis*, inflammation]. Inflammation of the pelvis of the kidney and its calices.

p., calculous. Pyelitis resulting from a calculus.

p. cystica. Pyelitis associated with multiple small cysts in the mucosa of the renal pelvis.

pyelo- [Gr. *pyelos*, pelvis]. Combining form

meaning the pelvis.

pyelocaliectasis (pī″ĕ-lō-kăl″ē-ĕk′tă-sĭs) [″ + *kalyx,* cup, + *ektasis,* dilation]. Dilation of the pelvis and calyces of the kidney.

pyelocystitis (pī″ĕ-lō-sĭs-tī′tĭs) [″ + *kystis,* bladder, + *itis,* inflammation]. Inflamed condition of the renal pelvis and bladder.

pyelocystostomosis (pī″ĕ-lō-sĭs″tō-stō-mō′sĭs) [″ + ″ + *stoma,* mouth, + *osis,* condition]. Establishment of surgical communication between the kidney and the bladder.

pyelogram (pī′ĕ-lō-grăm) [Gr. *pyelos,* pelvis, + *gramma,* a mark]. A roentgenogram of the ureter and renal pelvis.

p., intravenous. Pyelogram in which a radiopaque material is given intravenously. A roentgenogram of the urinary tract taken while the material is excreted provides important information about the structure and function of the kidney, ureter, and bladder. Any blockage along this tract will be readily detected by this examination.

pyelography (pī″ĕ-lŏg′ră-fē) [″ + *graphein,* to write]. Roentgenography of the renal pelvis and ureter.

pyelolithotomy (pī″ĕ-lō-lĭth-ŏt′ō-mē) [″ + *lithos,* stone, + *tome,* incision]. Removal of calculus from the pelvis of a kidney through an incision.

pyelometer (pī″ĕ-lŏm′ĕ-ter) [″ + *metron,* measure]. Device to measure the pelvic diameters. SYN: *pelvimeter.*

pyelometry (pī″ĕ-lŏm′ĕ-trē). 1. Measurement of the kidney's pelvis. 2. Measurement of the diameters of the pelvis. SYN: *pelvimetry.*

pyelonephritis (pī″ĕ-lō-nĕ-frī′tĭs) [″ + *nephros,* kidney, + *itis,* inflammation]. Inflammation of kidney substance and pelvis.

ETIOL: Usually due to bacteria that have ascended from the bladder after entering through the urethra.

SYM: Sudden onset of chilliness and fever with dull pain in the flank over either or both kidneys. There is tenderness when the kidney is palpated. Usually there are signs of cystitis, i.e., urgency with burning and frequency of urination. White blood cells will be present in the urinary sediment.

PROG: Depends upon character and virulence of infection, accessory etiological factors, drainage of kidney, presence or absence of complications, and general physical condition.

TREATMENT: Recognition and removal of cause; measures to increase resistance of patient; bedrest. Avoidance of drugs irritating to kidney, and alcohol. Apply heat to flanks; administer antipyretic drugs and an appropriate antibiotic. Surgery if necessary (nephrotomy, nephrectomy, pyelotomy).

pyelonephrosis (pī″ĕ-lō-nĕ-frō′sĭs) [Gr. *pyelos,* pelvis, + *nephros,* kidney, + *osis,* condition]. Disease of the pelvis of the kidney.

pyelopathy (pī″ĕ-lŏp′ăth-ē) [″ + *pathos,* disease]. Any disease of the pelvis of the kidney. SYN: *pyelonephrosis.*

pyeloplasty (pī′ĕ-lō-plăs″tē) [″ + *plastos,* formed]. Reparative surgery on the pelvis of the kidney.

pyeloplication (pī″ĕ-lō-plĭ-kā′shŭn) [″ + L. *plicare,* to fold]. Shortening of the wall of a dilated renal pelvis by taking tucks in it.

pyeloscopy (pī″ĕl-ŏs′kō-pē) [″ + *skopein,* to examine]. Examination of the pelvis of the kidney using fluoroscopy.

pyelostomy (pī″ĕ-lŏs′tō-mē) [″ + *stoma,* mouth]. Creation of an opening into the renal pelvis.

pyelotomy (pī″ĕ-lŏt′ō-mē) [″ + *tome,* incision]. Incision of renal pelvis.

NURSING IMPLICATIONS: Secure all catheters to the patient to prevent dislodgement. Assess and record the appearance of the urine, including color, consistency, and amount. Catheter drainage tubing must be kept free of kinks. Catheters should never be clamped. Monitor and record intake and output.

pyemesis (pī-ĕm′ĭ-sĭs) [Gr. *pyon,* pus, + *emesis,* vomiting]. Vomiting of pus.

pyemia (pī-ē′mē-ă) [″ + *haima,* blood]. A form of septicemia due to presence of pus-forming organisms in the blood, manifested by formation of multiple abscesses of a metastatic nature.

SYM: High intermittent temperature with recurrent chills; metastatic processes in various parts of the body, esp. in lungs; septic pneumonia, empyema. May be fatal.

TREATMENT: Antibiotics. Prophylactic treatment consists in prevention of suppuration.

p., arterial. Pyemia resulting from dissemination of emboli from a thrombus in cardiac vessels.

p., cryptogenic. Pyemia the origin of which is hidden in the deeper tissues.

p., metastatic. Multiple abscesses resulting from infected pyemic thrombi.

p., portal. Suppurative inflammation of the portal vein.

pyemic (pī-ē′mĭk) [Gr. *pyon,* pus, + *haima,* blood]. Rel. to, or affected with, blood poisoning.

Pyemotes (pī-ĕ-mō′tĕz). A genus of mites parasitic on the larvae of insects.

P. ventricosus. A mite present in the straw of some cereals. Contact with it causes a vesiculopapular dermatitis in man. This is called grain itch.

pyencephalus (pī″ĕn-sĕf′ă-lŭs) [″ + *enkephalos,* brain]. A brain abscess with suppuration within the cranium. SYN: *pyocephalus.*

pyesis (pī-ē′sĭs). Formation of pus. SYN: *sup-*

puration.

pygal (pī′găl) [Gr. *pyge,* rump]. Concerning the buttocks. SEE: *steatopygia.*

pygalgia (pī-găl′jē-ă) [″ + *algos,* pain]. Pain in the rump or buttocks.

pygmalionism (pĭg-mā′lē-ŏn-ĭzm). [named for Pygmalion, a sculptor and king in Gr. mythology, who fell in love with a figure he carved] Psychopathic condition in which a person is in love with a creation of his own.

pygmy (pĭg′mē). A very small person, a dwarf.

pygo- [Gr. *pyge,* rump]. Combining form meaning the rump.

pygoamorphus (pī″gō-ă-mor′fŭs) [″ + *a-,* not, + *morphe,* form]. Conjoined twins in which the parasite, jointed to the buttocks, is an amorphous mass of tissue, or a teratoma.

pygodidymus (pī″gō-dĭd′ĭ-mŭs) [″ + *didymos,* twin]. Conjoined twins with fusion of the cephalothoracic area, but with doubling of the pelvis and extremities.

pygomelus (pī-gŏm′ĕ-lŭs) [″ + *melos,* limb]. Unequal conjoined twins with the parasite represented by an accessory limb attached to the pelvic area.

pyin (pī′ĭn) [Gr. *pyon,* pus]. A substance of albuminous nature sometimes present in pus.

pyknemia. Pycnemia, q.v.

pyknic (pĭk′nĭk) [Gr. *pyknos,* thick]. Pert. to a body type characterized by roundness of the extremities, stockiness, large chest and abdomen, and tendency to obesity.

pykno- [Gr. *pyknos,* thick]. Combining form meaning thick, compact, dense, frequent. SEE: words beginning with *pycn-.*

pyknocardia (pĭk-nō-kăr′dē-ă) [″ + *kardia,* heart]. Rapid pulse. SYN: *tachycardia.*

pyknocyte (pĭk′nō-sīt) [″ + *kytos,* cell]. A form of spiculed red cell. SEE: *spiculed red cell.*

pyknodysostosis (pĭk″nō-dĭs″ŏs-tō′sĭs) [″ + *dys,* bad, + *osteon,* bone, + *osis,* condition]. An autosomal recessive disease that affects bones and resembles osteopetrosis, but the disease is mild and not associated with hematologic or neurologic abnormalities. The children have short stature, open fontanels, frontal bossing, hypoplastic facial bones, and dental abnormalities. There may be double rows of malformed teeth. The only treatment is surgical correction of deformities and fractures.

pyknometer (pĭk-nŏm′ĕ-tĕr) [″ + *metron,* measure]. Device for determining specific gravity of liquids.

pyknomorphous (pĭk″nō-morf′ŭs) [″ + *morphe,* form]. Characterized by compact arrangement of the stainable portions, said esp. of certain nerve cells.

pyknophrasia (pĭk″nō-frā′zē-ă) [″ + *phrasis,* speech]. Thickness of words uttered in speech.

pyknosis (pĭk-nō′sĭs) [″ + *osis,* condition]. Thickness, esp. shrinking of cells through degeneration. SYN: *inspissation.*

pyle- [Gr. *pyle,* gate]. Combining form meaning orifice, esp. that of the portal vein.

pylemphraxis (pī″lĕm-frăk′sĭs) [″ + *emphraxis,* stoppage]. Occlusion of the portal vein.

pylephlebectasia, pylephlebectasis (pī″lē-flē-bĕk-tā′zē-ă, -bĕk′tă-sĭs) [″ + *phleps,* vein, + *ektasis,* dilatation]. Distention of the portal vein.

pylephlebitis (pī″lē-flē-bī′tĭs) [″ + ″ + *itis,* inflammation]. Inflamed condition of the portal vein, generally suppurative.

p., adhesive. Thrombosis of the portal vein.

p. obturans. Pylephlebitis with obstructed flow in the portal vein.

pylethrombophlebitis (pī″lē-thrŏm″bō-flē-bī′tĭs) [″ + *thrombos,* clot, + *phleps,* vein, + *itis,* inflammation]. Thrombosis and inflammation of the portal vein.

pylethrombosis (pī″lē-thrŏm-bō′sĭs) [Gr. *pyle,* gate, + *thrombos,* a clot, + *osis,* condition]. Occlusion of portal vein by a thrombus.

pylon (pī′lŏn). A temporary artificial leg.

pyloralgia (pī″lō-răl′jē-ă) [Gr. *pyloros,* gatekeeper, + *algos,* pain]. Pain around the pylorus, distal aperture of the stomach.

pylorectomy (pī″lō-rĕk′tō-mē) [″ + *ektome,* excision]. Surgical removal of the pylorus.

pyloric (pī-lor′ĭk) [Gr. *pyloros,* gatekeeper]. Pert. to the opening between the stomach and duodenum.

pyloric antrum. The first part of the pyloric portion of the stomach; portion leading to pyloric canal.

pyloric canal. The narrow constricted region of the pyloric portion of the stomach that opens through the pylorus into the duodenum.

pyloric cap. First part of the duodenum.

pyloric gland. A gland of the stomach near the pylorus.

pyloric obstruction and dilatation. Pyloric obstruction increases the resistance offered to the expulsion of food from the stomach. In its efforts to overcome this, the stomach first becomes hypertrophied, then dilated. Causes of dilatation are pyloric obstruction, laxness of walls from simple atony, or excessive ingestion of food or drink.

SYM: The general symptoms of dyspepsia and the following symptoms relating to vomiting. Vomiting occurs long after eating, sometimes several hours or days. Amount is often excessive, sometimes several quarts; it is sour and fermented, and on standing it separates into a sediment of undigested food and a turbid, frothy liquid. Ejected fluid is rich in torulae and sarcinae, forms of bacteria. Obstinate constipation.

SIGNS: Bulging over epigastrium; in thin subjects, the outline of stomach may be visible. Palpation gives a splashing fremitus. In percussion there is an increased area of gastric tympany. In auscultation, splashing sounds often are audible at some distance. Ordinarily an esophageal sound may be inserted a distance of 60 cm. from the teeth. After dilatation may be inserted 65 to 70 cm.

PROG: Guarded but depends upon the cause. More favorable in dilatation without obstruction.

TREATMENT: Diet light, nutritious, not bulky, and should be given in small amounts at frequent intervals.

pyloric orifice. Opening or passage between the stomach and duodenum.

pyloric stenosis. Narrowing of the pyloric orifice. May be due to excessive thickening of the circular muscle of the pylorus (hypertrophic pyloric stenosis) or hypertrophy and hyperplasia of mucosa and submucosa.

TREATMENT: Surgical section of the thickened muscle around the pylorus.

NURSING IMPLICATIONS: *Pre-op:* Position the infant to prevent aspiration; feed and observe; obtain accurate daily weights; observe and record vomitus; provide pacifier as needed; monitor and record administration of parenteral fluids; chart intake and output and instruct parents concerning surgery.

Post-op: Administer parenteral fluids as prescribed; continue nothing by mouth for 12 to 24 hours; instruct parents concerning deep-breathing exercises; turn and position at scheduled intervals. Increase oral feedings gradually; position infant in upright position for one hour after feeding to prevent aspiration; include instruction for the parents in the care of the infant; provide visual stimulation for infant; and promote comfort. Implement discharge teaching to prepare parents adequately to meet infant's needs at home, and establish home referral for follow-up.

pyloristenosis (pī-lor″ĭ-stĕn-ō′sĭs) [Gr. *pyloros,* gatekeeper, + *stenosis,* a narrowing]. Constriction of the pylorus.

pyloritis (pī″lō-rī′tĭs) [″ + *itis,* inflammation]. Inflamed condition of the pylorus.

pyloro- [Gr. *pyloros,* gatekeeper]. Combining form meaning gatekeeper; applied to the pylorus.

pylorodiosis (pī-lō″rō-dī-ō′sĭs) [″ + *diosis,* pushing under]. Dilation of the pylorus of the stomach.

pyloroduodenitis (pī-lor″ō-dū″ō-dē-nī′tĭs) [″ + L. *duodeni,* twelve, + Gr. *itis,* inflammation]. Inflammation of the mucosa of the pyloric outlet of the stomach and duodenum.

pylorogastrectomy (pī-lor″ō-găs-trĕk′tō-mē) [″ + *gaster,* belly, + *ektome,* excision]. Excision of pyloric portion of the stomach.

pyloromyotomy (pī-lor″ō-mī-ŏt′ō-mē) [Gr. *pyloros,* gatekeeper, + *mys,* muscle, + *tome,* incision]. Incision and suture of the pyloric sphincter.

pyloroplasty (pī-lor′ō-plăs″tē) [″ + *plassein,* to form]. Operation to repair the pylorus, esp. one to increase the caliber of the pyloric opening by stretching.

p., Finney. Surgical procedure for enlarging the opening from the stomach to the duodenum.

p., Heineke-Mikulicz. Surgical procedure for correcting a pyloric stricture. The stricture is incised longitudinally and closed transversely.

pyloroptosia (pī-lō″rŏp-tō′sē-ă) [″ + *ptosis,* a dropping]. Displacement downward of the pyloric end of the stomach.

pyloroschesis (pī″lor-ō-shē′sĭs). Obstruction of the pyloric orifice.

pyloroscopy (pī-lō-rŏs′kō-pē) [Gr. *pyloros,* gatekeeper, + *skopein,* to examine]. Fluoroscopic examination of the pylorus.

pylorospasm (pī-lor′ō-spăzm) [″ + *spasmos,* a spasm]. Spasmodic contraction of the pyloric orifice. Usually due to a disturbance in the motor mechanism of the pylorus. May occur secondary to lesions of the stomach and duodenum near the pylorus.

pylorostenosis (pī-lor″ō-stĕn-ō′sĭs) [″ + *stenosis,* narrowing]. Abnormal narrowing or stricture of the pyloric orifice. SEE: *pyloric stenosis.*

pylorostomy (pī-lor-ŏs′tō-mē) [″ + *stoma,* opening]. Formation of an opening through the abdominal wall into the pylorus.

pylorotomy (pī-lor-ŏt′ō-mē) [″ + *tome,* incision]. Incision of the pyloric submucosa to relieve hypertrophic stenosis.

pylorus (pī-lor′ŭs) [Gr. *pyloros,* gatekeeper]. The lower orifice of the stomach opening into the duodenum. The pylorus is closed most of the time but opens at intervals permitting acid chyme to enter the duodenum. The primary factor in the opening of the pylorus is elevation of gastric pressure over duodenal pressure.

pyo-, py- [Gr. *pyon,* pus]. Combining forms meaning pus.

pyocele (pī′ō-sēl) [Gr. *pyon,* pus, + *kele,* hernia]. A hernia or distended cavity containing pus.

pyocelia (pī″ō-sē′lē-ă) [″ + *koilia,* cavity]. Pus formation in the abdominal cavity.

pyocephalus (pī″ō-sĕf′ă-lŭs) [″ + *kephale,* head]. Effusion of purulent nature within the cranium.

p., circumscribed. Brain abscess.

p., external. Suppuration of the meninges.

p., internal. Pus in the cerebrospinal fluid.

pyochezia (pī″ō-kē′zē-ă) [Gr. *pyon,* pus, +

chezein, to defecate]. Pus in the feces.

pyococcus (pī″ō-kŏk′ŭs) [″ + *kokkos*, berry]. A micrococcus that causes pus formation, such as Streptococcus pyogenes.

pyocolpocele (pī″ō-kŏl′pō-sēl) [″ + *kolpos*, vagina, + *kele*, mass]. A vaginal tumor containing pus. SEE: *pyocolpos*.

pyocolpos (pī″ō-kŏl′pōs). Accumulation of pus in the vagina.

pyoculture (pī′ō-kŭl″chūr) [″ + L. *cultura*, growth]. Comparative tests for cultivation of pus from a wound, a portion being left in the collecting tube and a portion being cultivated on artificial media.

pyocyanase (pī″ō-sī′ă-nāz). An antibiotic obtained from Pseudomonas aeruginosa. Active principally against gram-positive organisms, on which it has a lytic action.

pyocyanic (pī″ō-sī-ăn′ĭk) [″ + *kyanos*, dark blue]. Pert. to pyocyanin or blue pus.

pyocyanin (pī″ō-sī′ă-nĭn). An antibiotic obtained from Pseudomonas aeruginosa. Active principally against gram-positive organisms, on which it has a lytic action.

pyocyst (pī′ō-sĭst) [″ + *kystis*, sac]. A cyst containing pus.

pyoderma (pī-ō-dĕr′mă) [″ + *derma*, skin]. Any acute, inflammatory, purulent bacterial dermatitis.

p. gangrenosum. Pyoderma usually associated with ulcerative colitis or any severe chronic disease that leads to wasting. Occurs principally on the trunk.

pyodermatitis (pī″ō-dĕr″mă-tī′tĭs) [″ + ″ + *itis*, inflammation]. Pyogenic infection of the skin causing a dermatitis.

pyodermatosis (pī″ō-dĕr″mă-tō′sĭs) [″ + ″ + *osis*, condition]. Any skin condition of pyogenic origin. SYN: *pyodermia*.

pyodermia (pī″ō-dĕr′mē-ă). Any suppurative skin disease.

pyofecia (pī″ō-fē′sē-ă) [Gr. *pyon*, pus, + L. *faeces*, feces]. Pus in the stools.

pyogenesis (pī″ō-jĕn′ĕ-sĭs) [″ + *genesis*, formation]. The formation of pus. SYN: *pyopoiesis; suppuration*.

pyogenic (pī-ō-jĕn′ĭk) [″ + *gennan*, to produce]. Producing pus.

pyogenic microorganisms. Microorganisms that form pus. The principal ones are Staphylococcus aureus, Staphylococcus epidermidis, Streptococcus hemolyticus, Bacillus anthracis, B. subtilis, Clostridium perfringens, Pseudomonas aeruginosa, and Neisseria gonorrhoeae.

pyohemia (pī″ō-hē′mē-ă) [″ + *haima*, blood]. Pyemia.

pyohemothorax (pī″ō-hē″mō-thō′răks) [″ + *haima*, blood, + *thorax*, chest]. Pus and blood in the pleural cavity.

pyoid (pī′oyd) [″ + *eidos*, like]. Resembling pus.

pyolabyrinthitis (pī″ō-lăb″ĭ-rĭn-thī′tĭs) [″ + *labyrinthos*, a maze, + *itis*, inflammation]. Inflammation with suppuration of the labyrinth of the ear.

pyometra (pī″ō-mē′tră) [″ + *metra*, uterus]. Retained pus accumulation in the uterine cavity.

pyometritis (pī″ō-mē-trī′tĭs) [″ + ″ + *itis*, inflammation]. Purulent inflammation of the uterus.

pyonephritis (pī″ō-nĕf-rī′tĭs) [″ + *nephros*, kidney, + *itis*, inflammation]. Inflammation of the kidney, suppurative in character.

pyonephrolithiasis (pī″ō-nĕf″rō-lĭth-ī′ă-sĭs) [″ + ″ + *lithos*, stone, + -iasis, condition]. Pus and calculi in the kidney.

pyonephrosis (pī″ō-nĕf-rō′sĭs) [″ + ″ + *osis*, condition]. Pus accumulation in the pelvis of the kidney.

pyoovarium (pī″ō-ō-vā′rē-ŭm) [″ + L. *ovarium*, ovary]. Abscess formation in an ovary.

Pyopen. Trade name for carbenicillin disodium, USP.

pyopericarditis (pī″ō-pĕr″ĭ-kăr-dī′tĭs) [″ + *peri*, around, + *kardia*, heart, + *itis*, inflammation]. Pericarditis with suppuration.

pyopericardium (pī″ō-pĕr″ĭ-kăr′dē-ŭm). Pus formation in the pericardium.

pyoperitoneum (pī″ō-pĕr″ĭ-tō-nē′ŭm) [Gr. *pyon*, pus, + *peritonaion*, peritoneum]. Pus formation in the peritoneal cavity.

pyoperitonitis (pī″ō-pĕr″ĭ-tō-nī′tĭs) [″ + ″ + *itis*, inflammation]. Purulent inflammation of the lining of peritoneum.

pyophagia (pī″ō-fā′jē-ă) [″ + *phagein*, to eat]. Swallowing of purulent substance.

pyophthalmia (pī″ŏf-thăl′mē-ă) [″ + *ophthalmos*, eye]. Suppurative inflamed condition of the eye. SYN: *pyophthalmitis*.

pyophthalmitis (pī″ŏf-thăl-mī′tĭs) [″ + ″ + *itis*, inflammation]. Suppurative inflamed condition of the eye. SYN: *pyophthalmia*.

pyophylactic (pī″ō-fĭ-lăk′tĭk) [″ + *phylaxis*, protection]. Protective against formation of pus.

pyophylactic membrane. Lining membrane of an abscess cavity separating it from healthy tissue.

pyophysometra (pī″ō-fī″sō-mē′tră) [″ + *physa*, air, + *metra*, uterus]. Pus and gas accumulation in the uterus.

pyoplania (pī″ō-plā′nē-ă) [″ + *planos*, wandering]. Spreading of pus by infiltration into other tissue.

pyopneumocholecystitis (pī″ō-nū″mō-kō-lē-sĭs-tī′tĭs) [″ + *pneuma*, air, + *chole*, bile, + *kystis*, sac, + *itis*, inflammation]. Distention of the gallbladder with air and pus.

pyopneumocyst (pī″ō-nū′mō-sĭst) [″ + ″ + *kystis*, bladder]. A cyst enclosing pus and gas.

pyopneumohepatitis (pī″ō-nū″mō-hĕp″ă-tī′tĭs)

[" + *pneuma*, air, + *hepar*, liver, + *itis*, inflammation]. Liver abscess with gas in the abscess cavity.

pyopneumopericardium (pī"ō-nū"mō-pĕr"ĭ-kăr'dē-ŭm) [" + " + *peri*, around, + *kardia*, heart]. Pus and air or gas in the pericardium.

pyopneumoperitoneum (pī"ō-nū"mō-pĕr"ĭ-tō-nē'ŭm) [" + " + *peritonaion*, peritoneum]. Peritonitis with gas and pus in the peritoneal cavity.

pyopneumoperitonitis (pī"ō-nū"mō-pĕr"ĭ-tō-nī'tĭs) [" + " + " + *itis*, inflammation]. Pus and air in the peritoneal cavity complicating peritonitis.

pyopneumothorax (pī"ō-nū"mō-thō'răks) [" + " + *thorax*, chest]. Presence of pus and gas in the pleural cavity.

pyopoiesis (pī"ō-poy-ē'sĭs) [" + *poiein*, to make]. Formation of pus. SYN: *pyogenesis; suppuration*.

pyopoietic (pī"ō-poy-ĕt'ĭk). Pert. to formation of pus. SYN: *suppurative*.

pyoptysis (pī-ŏp'tĭ-sĭs) [" + *ptysis*, spitting]. Spitting of pus.

pyopyelectasis (pī"ō-pī"ĕ-lĕk'tă-sĭs) [" + *pyelos*, pelvis, + *ektasis*, dilation]. Purulent fluid in the dilated renal pelvis.

pyorrhagia (pī-or-ă'jē-ă) [" + *rhegnynai*, to burst forth]. Profuse flow of pus, as when an abscess ruptures.

pyorrhea (pī"ō-rē'ă) [" + *rhoia*, flow]. A discharge of purulent matter.

p. alveolaris. A periodontal disease characterized by inflammatory or degenerative changes of the periosteum, alveolar bone, and tooth cementum. Resorption of alveolar bone occurs, resulting in loosening of teeth and recession of gums. SYN: *periodontitis; periodontoclasia*.

pyosalpingitis (pī"ō-săl"pĭn-jī'tĭs) [Gr. *pyon*, pus, + *salpinx*, tube, + *itis*, inflammation]. Retained pus in the oviduct with inflammation.

pyosalpingo-oophoritis (pī"ō-săl-pĭn"gō-ō"ŏf-ō-rī'tĭs) [" + " + *oon*, ovum, + *phoros*, a bearer, + *itis*, inflammation]. Inflammation of ovary and oviduct with suppuration.

pyosalpinx (pī"ō-săl'pĭnks). Pus in the fallopian tube.

pyospermia (pī"ō-spĕr'mē-ă) [Gr. *pyon*, pus, + *sperma*, seed]. Pus in the semen.

pyostatic (pī"ō-stăt'ĭk) [" + *statikos*, halting]. 1. Preventing pus formation. 2. Agent preventing the development of pus.

pyotherapy (pī"ō-thĕr'ă-pē) [" + *therapeia*, treatment]. Treatment of disease with pus.

pyothorax (pī"ō-thō'răks) [" + *thorax*, chest]. Pus in the pleural cavity. SYN: *empyema*.

pyotorrhea (pī"ō-tō-rē'ă) [" + *ous*, ear, + *rhoia*, flow]. Purulent discharge from the ear.

pyotoxinemia (pī"ō-tŏk"sĭ-nē'mē-ă) [" + *toxikon*, poison, + *haima*, blood]. Infection from toxic products of bacterial organisms in the blood.

pyoturia (pī"ō-tū'rē-ă) [" + *ouron*, urine]. Pus cells in the urine. SYN: *pyuria*.

pyourachus (pī"ō-ū'ră-kŭs) [" + *ourachos*, fetal urinary canal]. Accumulation of pus in the urachus, q.v.

pyoureter (pī"ō-ū-rē'tĕr) [" + *oureter*, ureter]. Pus collection in the ureter.

pyovesiculosis (pī"ō-vĕ-sĭk"ū-lō'sĭs) [" + L. *vesiculus*, a small vessel, + Gr. *osis*, condition]. Pus collection in the seminal vesicles.

pyoxanthin(e) (pī"ō-zăn'thĭn) [" + *xanthos*, yellow]. A yellow pigment resulting from oxidation of pyocyanin. Sometimes present in pus.

pyramid (pĭr'ă-mĭd) [Gr. *pyramis*, a pyramid]. 1. A solid on the base with three or more triangular sides that meet at an apex. 2. Any part of the body resembling a pyramid. 3. A compact bundle of nerve fibers in the medulla oblongata. 4. Petrous portion of temporal bone. SYN: *pyramis*.

p., malpighian. P., renal.

p. of cerebellum. A median ventral projection of vermis of cerebellum lying between tuber and uvula.

p. of light. The triangular-shaped light reflex from the typanic membrane of the ear.

p. of medulla. A pair of elongated tapering prominences on the anterior surface of the medulla oblongata, composed of descending corticospinal fibers.

p. of temporal bone. The pyramis or petrous portion of the temporal bone.

p. of thyroid. A conical process sometimes present, extending cephalad from the isthmus of the thyroid gland.

p. of tympanum. A hollow projection on the inner wall of the tympanum through which passes the stapedius muscle.

p., renal. One of a number of cone-shaped structures comprising the medulla of the kidney along with renal columns. Each pyramid has an external base in the kidney's boundary with an apex that projects as a renal papilla into the renal sinus. The pyramids converge. SYN: *pyramid, malpighian*.

pyramidal (pĭ-răm'ĭ-dăl) [L. *pyramidalis*]. In the shape of a pyramid.

pyramidal cell. Pyramid-shaped cell of cerebral cortex.

pyramidalis (pĭ-răm"ĭ-dăl'ĭs) [L.]. The muscle that arises from the crest of the pubis and is inserted into the linea alba upward about halfway to the navel.

p. auriculae. Small muscle inserted into the auricle of the ear. It is often absent.

pyramidal tract. One of three descending tracts (lateral, ventral, ventrolateral) of the spinal cord. Consists of fibers arising from giant pyramidal cells of Betz present in the motor area of the cerebral cortex. SYN: *corticospinal tract.*

pyramidotomy (pĕr″ăm-ĭ-dŏt′ō-mē) [Gr. *pyramis,* a pyramid, + *tome,* incision]. Excision of the pyramidal tracts of the spinal cord in order to alleviate involuntary muscular movements.

pyramis (pĭr′ă-mĭs) [Gr., a pyramid]. (pl. *pyramides*) A general term for a structure resembling a pyramid.

pyran (pī′răn). A chemical, C_5H_6O, the ring structure of which consists of five carbon atoms and one oxygen atom.

pyranose (pī′ră-nōs). A cyclic sugar or glycoside with a structure similar to a pyran, q.v.

pyrantel pamoate (pĭ-răn′tĕl). USP. A drug used in treating the parasitic diseases ascariasis and enterobiasis, as well as those caused by Ancylostoma, Necator americanus, and Trichostrongylus. Trade names are Antiminth, and Combantrin.

pyrazinamide (pī″ră-zĭn′ă-mĭd). USP. A drug used in treating tuberculosis. It is used in treating persons who are resistant to usually effective agents.

pyrectic (pī-rĕk′tĭk). Concerning fever.

pyrenemia (pī″rĕ-nē′mē-ă) [Gr. *pyren,* fruit stone, + *haima,* blood]. Condition in which there are nucleated red cells in the blood.

pyretherapy (pī″rĕ-thĕr′ă-pē) [Gr. *pyr,* fever, + *therapeia,* treatment]. Artificial fever treatment. SEE: *pyretotherapy.*

pyrethrins (pī-rē′thrĭnz). General name of substances derived from pyrethrum flowers (chrysanthemums). Used as insecticides.

pyretic (pī-rĕt′ĭk) [Gr. *pyretos,* fever]. Concerning fever.

pyretic therapy. Treatment of disease by artificial induction of fever, either by heat or by the inoculation of malarial organisms.

pyreticosis (pī-rĕt″ĭ-kō′sĭs) [″ + *osis,* condition]. Any condition characterized by fever.

pyreto- (pī-rĕt′ō) [Gr. *pyretos,* fever]. Prefix indicating relationship to fever.

pyretogen (pī-rĕt′ō-jĕn) [″ + *gennan,* to produce]. A substance producing fever.

pyretogenesia, pyretogenesis (pī″rĕ-tō-jĕn-ē′zē-ă, -jĕn′ĕ-sĭs) [″ + *genesis,* production]. Origin and production of fever.

pyretogenic (pī″rĕt-ō-jĕn′ĭk). Producing or causing fever.

pyretogenic bacteria. Pathogenic bacteria causing fever.

pyretogenic stage. Period in a fever when it is rising slowly.

pyretogenous (pī″rĕ-tŏj′ĕn-ŭs). 1. Producing or causing fever. 2. Caused by fever.

pyretolysis (pī″rĕ-tŏl′ĭ-sĭs) [″ + *lysis,* dissolution]. 1. Reduction of fever. 2. Lysis of symptoms of disease process that is accelerated by fever.

pyretotherapy (pī″rĕ-tō-thĕr′ă-pē) [″ + *therapeia,* treatment]. 1. Treatment by artificially raising the patient's temperature. 2. Treatment of fever.

pyretotyphosis (pī″rĕ-tō-tī-fō′sĭs) [″ + *typhosis,* delirium]. The delirious or stuporous condition characteristic of high fever.

pyrexia (pī-rĕk′sē-ă) [Gr. *pyressein,* to be feverish]. Condition in which the temperature is above normal. SYN: *fever*

Some classify it as:

Low	99°–101° F.	(37.2°–38.3° C.)
Moderate	101°–103° F.	(38.3°–39.4° C.)
High	103°–105° F.	(39.4°–40.6° C.)

pyrexial (pī-rĕk′sē-ăl). Concerning fever.

pyrexin (pī′rĕks′ĭn). A substance extracted from inflammatory exudates that induces fever.

Pyribenzamine Hydrochloride. Trade name for tripelennamine hydrochloride, USP.

pyridine (pĕr′ĭ-dēn). A colorless, volatile liquid with a charred odor. It is obtained by dry distillation of nitrogen-containing organic matter. It is used as an industrial solvent.

Pyridium. Trade name for phenazopyridine hydrochloride.

pyridostigmine bromide (pĕr″ĭ-dō-stĭg′mēn). USP. An anticholinesterase drug used in treating myasthenia gravis. Trade names are Mestinon and Regonol.

pyridoxal 5-phosphate. A derivative of pyridoxine. It serves as a coenzyme of certain amino-acid decarboxylases in bacteria, and in animal tissues of 3,4-dihydroxyphenyalanine (dopa) decarboxylase.

pyridoxamine (pĭr″ĭ-dŏks′ă-mĭn). One of the vitamin B_6 group; a 4-aminoethyl analog of pyridoxine.

4-pyridoxic acid (pĭr″ĭ-dŏks′ĭk). The principal end product of pyridoxine metabolism excreted in human urine.

pyridoxine hydrochloride (pī-rĭ-dŏks′ēn). USP. One of a group of substances, including pyridoxal and pyridoxamine, that make up vitamin B_6. Trade names are Hexa-Betalin and Beesix. SEE: *vitamin B_6* in *Vitamins* in *Appendix.*

pyriform (pĭr′ĭ-form) [L. *pirum,* pear, + *forma,* shape]. Shaped like a pear. Also spelled piriform.

pyrilamine maleate (pĕr-ĭl′ă-mēn). USP. A histamine antagonist drug used in treating certain allergic diseases. Trade names are Dorantamin, Enrumay, Histan, Paraminyl Maleate, and Stamine.

pyrimethamine (pĕr″ĭ-mĕth′ă-mēn). USP. An antimalarial drug used in prophylaxis against malaria rather than in treatment of an acute attack. Trade name is Daraprim.

pyrimidine (pī-rĭm′ĭd-ĭn). The parent of a group of heterocyclic nitrogen compounds,

$C_4H_4N_2$, including uracil, cytosine, and thymine, some of which are components of nucleic acid.

pyrithiamine (pĭr″ĭ-thī′ă-mĭn). A synthetic analog of thiamine that acts as an antithiamine substance. When administered, it produces many of the symptoms of thiamine deficiency.

pyro- (pī′rō) [Gr. *pyr,* fire]. Prefix meaning heat or fire.

pyrogallol (pī″rō-găl′ōl). A toxic chemical, $C_6H_6O_3$, derived from gallic acid.

pyrogen (pī′rō-jĕn) [Gr. *pyr,* fire, + *gennan,* to produce]. Any substance that produces fever.

CAUTION: Do not give fluids intravenously that have been opened previously and allowed to stand, even though the top may have been closed tightly, because pyrogens will have formed.

p., leukocytic. A substance found in blood during fever that acts upon the thermoregulatory centers of the hypothalamus.

pyrogenic (pī″rō-jĕn′ĭk) [Gr. *pyr,* fire, + *gennan,* to produce]. Producing fever.

pyroglobulinemia (pī″rō-glŏb″ū-lĭ-nē′mē-ă) [″ + *globulus,* globule, + *haima,* blood]. Presence of an abnormal globulin in the blood of patients with multiple myeloma and certain other diseases. The globulin is irreversibly precipitated when heated to 56° C.

pyrolagnia (pī″rō-lăg′nē-ă) [″ + *lagneia,* lust]. Insane desire to see or produce fires; accompanied by sexual gratification. SEE: *pyromania.*

pyrolysis (pī-rŏl′ĭ-sĭs) [″ + *lysis,* dissolution]. Decomposition of organic matter when there is a rise in temperature.

pyromania (pī″rō-mā′nē-ă) [″ + *mania,* madness]. Fire madness; mania for setting fires or seeing them.

pyrometer (pī-rŏm′ĕ-tĕr) [Gr. *pyr,* fire, + *metron,* measure]. Device for measuring temperature.

pyronine (pī′rō-nĭn). A histologic stain used to demonstrate the presence of RNA and DNA.

pyronyxis (pī″rō-nĭk′sĭs) [″ + *nyxis,* a piercing]. Treatment or cauterization by puncturing a part with hot needles. SYN: *ignipuncture.*

pyrophobia (pī″rō-fō′bē-ă) [″ + *phobos,* fear]. Abnormal fear of fire.

pyrophosphatase (pī″rō-fŏs′fă-tās). An enzyme that catalyzes splitting of phosphoric groups.

pyrophosphate (pī″rō-fŏs′fāt). Any salt of phosphoric acid.

pyroptothymia (pī″rŏp-tō-thī′mē-ă) [″ + *ptoein,* to scare, + *thymos,* mind]. A psychosis in which one imagines himself surrounded by flames.

pyropuncture (pī″rō-pŭnk′chūr) [″ + L. *punctura,* piercing]. Treatment by puncture of a part with hot needles. SEE: *counterirritation.*

pyrosis (pī-rō′sĭs) [Gr. *pyrosis,* burning]. A burning sensation in the epigastric and sternal region with raising of acid liquid from stomach. SYN: *heartburn.*

NURSING IMPLICATIONS: Assess what the term means to the patient, exact location, time of occurrence in relation to food intake, duration, if position changes exaggerate discomfort, precipitating factors (such as type and amount of food), modality of relief, and factors that aggravate the discomfort.

pyrotic (pī-rŏt′ĭk) [Gr. *pyrotikos*]. 1. Caustic; burning. 2. Pert. to pyrosis.

pyrotoxin (pī″rō-tŏk′sĭn) [Gr. *pyr,* fire, + *toxikon,* poison]. A toxin produced during a febrile disease.

pyroxylin (pī-rŏk′sĭ-lĭn). USP. A substance obtained by the action of a mixture of nitric and sulfuric acids on cotton. It consists chiefly of cellulose tetranitrate. It is combined with ether and alcohol to form collodion, q.v. SYN: *gun cotton.*

CAUTION: Dry pyroxylin and collodion are exceedingly flammable.

pyrrobutamine phosphate (pĕr″rō-bū′tă-mēn). USP. An antihistamine drug. Trade name is Pyronil.

pyrrol cells. Cells of the reticuloendothelial system so called because of their ability to ingest colloidal dyes (pyrrol blue). SYN: *histiocytes.*

pyrrole (pĕr′ōl). A heterocyclic substance that provides the building blocks for a large number of vital compounds such as hemoglobin, chlorophyll, and bile acids. It is a colorless liquid with the odor of chloroform.

pyrrolidine (pĭ-rŏl′ĭ-dĭn). Tetramethylamine, $(CH_2)_4NH$. It may be obtained from pyrrole or tobacco, which contains pyrrole.

pyruvate (pī′roo-vāt). A salt or ester of pyruvic acid.

pyruvic acid (pī-roo′vĭk). $CH_3CO{\bullet}COOH$, an organic acid that plays an important role in Krebs cycle, q.v. It is an intermediate product in the metabolism of carbohydrates, fats, and amino acids. It increases in quantity in the blood and tissues in thiamine deficiency because thiamine is essential for its oxidation.

pyrvinium pamoate (pĭr-vĭn′ē-ŭm). USP. A cyanine dye drug used in treating pinworms. Trade name is Povan.

pythogenesis (pī″thō-jĕn′ĕ-sĭs) [Gr. *pythein,* to rot, + *genesis,* production]. Originating in decaying matter.

pyuria (pī-ū′rē-ă) [Gr. *pyon,* pus, + *ouron,* urine]. Pus in the urine; evidence of renal disease. Condition in which there are more than the normal number of pus or white blood cells in the urine. Freshy passed urine may be cloudy due to presence of phosphates or pus. If the former, the addition of acid will cause it to clear; it pus is present, it will not clear but may become gelatinous.

ETIOL: Lesion of urethra, ureters, bladder, kidneys, infection.

RS: cystitis; kidney; pye itis, ureteritis; urethritis.

PZI. *protamine zinc insulin*. SEE: *insulin*.

Q

Q. 1. quantity. 2. Symb. for coulomb.
Q angle. Obtuse angle formed by patellar tendon and patellar ligament.
Qco_2. Number of microliters of CO_2 given off per milligram of dry weight of tissue per hour.
q.d. L. *quaque die,* every day.
Q disk. A dark, doubly refractile, anisotropic band of a striated muscle myofibril. SYN: *disk, anisotropic.*
Q fever [Q is for *query* because its etiology was unknown]. An acute infectious disease characterized by headache, fever, malaise, myalgia, and anorexia. Caused by the rickettsial organism, Coxiella burnetii. Contracted by inhaling infected dusts, drinking unpasteurized milk from infected animals, or by handling infected animals such as goats, cows, or sheep. Transmission by human contact is rare but has occurred. An effective vaccine is available for prevention of infection in persons who have a good chance of being exposed to the disease. Tetracyclines are effective in treating Q fever.
q.h. L. *quaque hora,* every hour.
q.i.d. L. *quater in die,* four times a day.
q.l. L. *quantum libet,* as much as one pleases.
Q law. As temperature decreases, chemical activity decreases.
q.m. L. *quaque matin,* every morning.
q.n. L. *quaque nox,* every night.
Qo_2. Number of microliters of O_2 taken up per milligram of dry weight of tissue per hour.
q.q.h. *quaque quarta hora,* every four hours.
QRS complex. The Q, R, and S waves or deflections of an electrocardiogram produced during the transmission of the excitation wave through the conductile tissue of the heart. Consists of an initial downward deflection (Q wave), a large upward deflection (R wave), and a second downward deflection (S wave) that represents the spread of the electrical impulse from the Purkinje fibers to the ventricular muscle. This initiates ventricular depolarization. Normal duration is 0.06 to 0.08 seconds.
QRST complex. The Q, R, S, and T waves of an electrocardiogram. Duration is approx. same as that of mechanical systole. The T wave, which follows the QRS complex, reflects ventricular depolarization. During the T wave, the ventricles are in their recovery period. Between the QRS complex and the T wave is the ST segment, which represents the completion of depolarization and the beginning of repolarization of the ventricles; this being the time of ventricular contraction. SEE: *electrocardiogram* for illus.
q.s. L. *quantum sufficit,* as much as necessary.
qt. *quart.*
Quaalude. Trade name for methaqualone hydrochloride. Because of the illegal and abused use of this drug, it is no longer distributed in the United States.
quack (kwăk) [D. *kwaksalven,* to peddle salve]. One who pretends to have knowledge or skill in medicine. SYN: *charlatan.*
quad. Medical "shorthand" for quadriceps, quadrilateral, quadrant, quadriplegia.
quadrangular (kwŏd-răng′ū-lĕr) [L. *quadri,* four, + *angulus,* angle]. Having four angles.
quadrangular lobe. A region forming the superior portion of each cerebellar hemisphere.
quadrangular membrane. The upper portion of the elastic membrane of the larynx. Extends from the aryepiglottic folds above to the level of the ventricular folds below.
quadrant (kwŏd′rănt) [L. *quadrans,* a fourth]. 1. The quarter or fourth of a circle. 2. One of four corresponding regions, as of the abdomen, divided for descriptive and diagnostic purposes.
quadrantanopia (kwŏd″rănt-ă-nō′pē-ă) [″ + Gr. *an-,* not, + *opsis,* vision]. Blindness or diminished visual acuity in one quarter of the visual field.
quadrantanopsia (kwŏd″rănt-ăn-ŏp′sē-ă) [″ + ″ + *opsis,* vision]. Loss of sight in approximately one fourth of the visual field.
quadrate (kwŏd′rāt) [L. *quadratus,* squared]. Square, or having four equal sides.
quadrate lobe. A small lobe of liver located on the visceral surface and lying in contact with the pylorus and duodenum.
quadrate lobule. The square lobule of the upper surface of the cerebellum.
quadri-, quadr- [L. *quattuor,* four]. Combining forms meaning having four or consisting of four.
quadribasic (kwŏd″rĭ-bā′sĭk). Having four replaceable atoms of hydrogen.
quadriceps (kwŏd′rĭ-sĕps) [″ + *caput,* head]. Four-headed, as a quadriceps muscle.
quadriceps femoris. A large muscle on the anterior surface of the thigh composed of four muscles: rectus femoris, vastus lateralis, vastus medialis, and vastus intermedius. These muscles are inserted by a common tendon on the tuberosity of the tibia. Quadriceps femoris is an extensor of the leg. SEE: *Muscles* in *Appendix.*
quadricepsplasty (kwŏd″rĭ-sĕps′plăs-tē) [″ + ″ + Gr. *plassein,* to form]. Plastic surgery for adhesions and scars around the quadriceps femoris muscle in order to restore function.
quadriceps reflex. Extension of the leg following contraction of the quadriceps muscle

resulting from a quick tap of the patellar tendon. SYN: *knee-jerk reflex; patellar reflex.* SEE: *Jendrassik's maneuver.*

quadricuspid (kwŏd″rĭ-kŭs′pĭd) [″ + *cuspis,* point]. Having four cusps, as a heart valve or a tooth.

quadridigitate (kwŏd″rĭ-dĭj′ĭ-tāt). Having only four fingers on a hand or four toes on a foot.

quadrigemina (kwŏd″rĭ-jĕm′ĭn-ă) [″ + *geminus,* twin]. The corpora quadrigemina. SEE: *colliculus inferior; colliculus superior.*

quadrigeminal (kwŏd″rĭ-jĕm′ĭn-ăl). Fourfold; having four symmetrical parts. Pert. to the corpora quadrigemina, q.v.

quadrigeminum (kwŏd″rĭ-jĕm′ĭ-nŭm). One of the four quadrigeminal bodies of the brain.

quadrigeminus (kwŏd″rĭ-jĕm′ĭ-nŭs). Composed of four parts.

quadrilateral (kwŏd″rĭ-lăt′ĕr-ăl) [″ + *latus,* side]. Having four sides.

quadrilocular (kwŏd″rĭ-lŏk′ū-lăr) [″ + *loculus,* a small space]. Having four chambers, cavities, or spaces.

quadripara (kwŏd-rĭp′ă-ră) [″ + *parere,* to bear]. A woman who has had four pregnancies that have continued beyond the 20th week of gestation. SYN: *quartipara.* SEE: *para.*

quadripartite (kwŏd″rĭ-păr′tīt) [″ + *partire,* to divide]. Divided into four parts.

quadriplegia (kwŏd″rĭ-plē′jē-ă) [″ + Gr. *plege,* stroke]. Paralysis of all four extremities and usually the trunk.

ETIOL: Injury to the spinal cord, usually at the level of the 5th or 6th cervical vertebra. The injury may be higher, but death occurs when damage is above the level of the 3rd cervical vertebra.

EMERGENCY CARE: When a fracture of a cervical vertebra is suspected, the injured patient's head and neck should be held steady with applied traction during transportation.

TREATMENT: Initial treatment includes immobilization with the use of Crutchfield tongs and antibiotic therapy. When the fracture has healed, physical and occupational therapy are instituted.

NURSING IMPLICATIONS: Initially establish and maintain a patent airway and immobilize the patient's head and neck. Observe patient closely for signs of spinal shock. The nursing concern includes adequate nutrition, skin care, elimination (regulation of both urinary bladder and bowel), positioning and exercise schedule, emotional and psychological support to patient, and respiratory toiletry regimen. Long-term nursing implications must be directed toward prevention of complications. Prompt institution of rehabilitation measures is of utmost importance. Assist in making long-term plans for the rehabilitation program.

quadripolar (kwŏd″rĭ-pō′lăr). Pert. to a cell having four poles.

quadrisect (kwŏd′rĭ-sĕkt) [″ + *sectio,* a cutting]. To divide into four parts.

quadrisection (kwŏd″rĭ-sĕk′shŭn). Dividing into four sections or parts.

quadritubercular (kwŏd″rĭ-tū-bĕr′kū-lĕr) [″ + *tuberculum,* a tubercle]. Having four tubercles or cusps.

quadrivalent (kwŏd″rĭ-vā′lĕnt) [″ + *valens,* powerful]. Having ability to replace four atoms of hydrogen in a compound, i.e., a chemical valence of four.

quadruped (kwŏd′roo-pĕd″) [″ + *pes,* foot]. 1. Four-footed animal. 2. Assuming a position with hands and feet on floor.

quadrupedal reflex (kwŏd-roop′ĕd-ăl). Extension of flexed arm on assuming quadrupedal posture.

quadruplet (kwŏd′roo-plĕt, kwŏ-droo′plĕt) [L. *quadruplus,* fourfold]. One of four children born of the same mother in the same confinement. SEE: *Hellin's law.*

quale (kwā′lē) [L. *qualis,* of what kind]. The quality of anything, esp. of a sensation.

qualimeter (kwŏl-ĭm′ĕt-ĕr) [″ + Gr. *metron,* measure]. Device for measuring the quality of roentgen rays. SEE: *penetrometer.*

qualitative (kwŏl′ĭ-tā″tĭv) [L. *qualitativus*]. Referring to the quality of anything.

qualitative analysis. In chemistry, an analysis that determines the nature of the elements of a compound, or the identity of the components of a mixture. SEE: *quantitative.*

quality (kwŏl′ĭ-tē) [L. *qualitas,* quality]. That which constitutes or characterizes a thing; the natural character.

quality assurance. Activities and programs designed to achieve a desired degree or grade of care in a defined medical, nursing, or health care setting or program. The quality assurance program must include evaluation and educational components to identify and correct problems. Such programs are required for funding by the Public Health Act.

The Quality Assurance Program for Medical Care in the Hospital (QAP) is a guide developed by the American Hospital Association for development of such programs by hospital administrators and medical staffs.

quanta (kwŏn′tă) [L.]. Pl. of quantum.

quantimeter (kwŏn-tĭm′ĕt-ĕr) [L. *quantus,* how great, + Gr. *metron,* measure]. Device for measuring quantity of roentgen rays to which a subject is exposed.

quanti-Pirquet (kwŏn″tĭ-pēr-kā′). [Clemens Pirquet, Austrian physician, 1874–1929] Quantitative cutaneous test of amount of sensitiveness to tuberculin by use of graduated dilutions.

quantitative (kwŏn″tĭ-tā′tĭv) [LL. *quantitativus*]. Concerning quantity.

quantitative analysis. Analysis that determines the proportionate parts of elements in a compound, or the percentage of components of a mixture. SEE: *qualitative.*

quantity (kwŏn′tĭ-tē) [L. *quantitas,* quantity]. Amount; portion.

quantivalence. The number of hydrogen atoms with which an element or radical will combine.

quantum (kwŏn′tŭm) [L., how much]. (pl. *quanta*) 1. A definite amount. 2. A unit of radiant energy.

quantum theory. Theory stating that radiation is an intermittent, not continuous, emission of energy in varying multiples of quanta action.

quantum libet (kwŏn′tŭm lī′bĕt) [L.]. ABBR: q.l. As much as desired.

quantum sufficit (kwŏn′tŭm sŭf′fĭ-sĭt) [L.]. ABBR: q.s. As much as needed.

quarantine (kwor′ăn-tēn″) [It. *quarantina,* 40 days]. 1. The period of debarring from entrance to a country, or the isolation of persons exposed to infectious diseases—formerly 40 days. 2. Period of isolation from public communication following onset of a contagious disease.

Complete quarantine is limitation of freedom of movement of healthy persons or domestic animals that have been exposed to a communicable disease for a period of time equal to the longest incubation period of the disease, in such a manner as to prevent effective contact with those not so exposed. SEE: *contagious; isolation.*

quart (kwort) [L. *quartus,* a fourth]. ABBR: qt. A unit of fluid or dry measure; one-fourth part of a gallon or two pints; one-eighth part of a peck; 946 ml.

quartan (kwor′tăn) [L. *quartana,* of the fourth]. 1. Occurring every fourth day. 2. Malarial fever with a paroxysm every fourth day, figuring from and including the first day of paroxysm. SEE: *fever; malaria.*

q., double. Malaria in which there are two concurrent cycles resulting in fever occurring on two successive days.

q., triple. Malaria in which there are three concurrent cycles resulting in fever occurring every day.

quartile (kwor′tīl) [L. *quartus,* a fourth]. One of the two middle values of each half of a series of variables.

quartipara (kwor-tĭp′ă-ră) [″ + *parere,* to bear]. A woman who has had four pregnancies that have continued beyond the 20th week of gestation. SYN: *quadripara.* SEE: *para.*

quartisect (kwor′tĭ-sĕkt) [″ + *sectio,* a cutting]. To cut into four parts.

quartz (kwărts) [Ger. *quarz*]. Silicon dioxide, the principal ingredient of sandstone (crystallized silica; rock crystal). When crystal is clear and colorless, it permits the passage of large amounts of ultraviolet radiations.

quartz applicator. Quartz rod of various shapes and angles to conduct, by total internal reflection, ultraviolet radiation from a water-cooled mercury arc quartz lamp.

quartz glass. Crystalline quartz is used for prisms and lenses; fused quartz for windows, through which ultraviolet radiations are freely transmitted.

Quarzan. Trade name for clidinium bromide.

quassation (kwă-sā′shŭn) [L. *quassatio*]. A beating, a shaking; breaking up of crude materials into small pieces.

quassia (kwŏsh′ă, kwŏsh′ē-ă) [*Quassi,* Surinam inhabitant who discovered its medicinal value]. The wood of a tree, Quassia amara, grown in tropical America. Once considered valuable as a bitter tonic, and in an enema for certain intestinal parasites.

quassin (kwŏs′ĭn). $C_{22}H_{30}O_6$, a bitter principle extracted from the wood of quassia.

Quatelet index. An index for estimating obesity. The weight in kilograms is divided by the height in meters squared, i.e., $\frac{W}{H^2}$. SYN: *body mass index.* SEE: *ponderal index.*

quater in die (kwŏ′tĕr ĭn dē′ā) [L.]. ABBR: q.i.d. Four times a day.

quaternary (kwŏ-tĕr′nă-rē) [L. *quaternarius,* of four]. 1. The fourth in order. 2. Composed of four elements.

Queckenstedt's sign (kwĕk′ĕn-stĕts). [Hans Queckenstedt, Ger. physician, 1887–1918] Upon compression of the veins of the neck, unilaterally or bilaterally, cerebrospinal fluid pressure rises rapidly in healthy persons; this disappears when pressure is released. In vertebral canal block, the pressure is scarcely affected by this procedure.

quenching (kwĕnch′ĭng). 1. Cooling something that is hot; or decreasing the radioactive energy released. 2. In toxicology, the effect of a material to decrease the toxicity of some of the chemical or chemicals in the compound.

q., fluorescence. A technique for investigating antigen-antibody reactions by measuring the light absorbed by antigen mixed with fluorescent-labeled antibody.

querulent (kwĕr′ū-lĕnt) [L. *querulus,* complaining]. 1. Complaining; fretful. 2. One who is dissatisfied, complaining, and suspicious.

Quervain's disease (kār′vănz). [Fritz de Quervain, Swiss surgeon, 1868–1940] Chronic tenosynovitis of the abductor pollicis longus and extensor pollicis brevis muscles.

Questran. Trade name for cholestyramine resin, USP.

quick (kwĭk) [ME. *quicke,* alive]. 1. A part

susceptible to keen feeling, esp. part of a finger or toe to which nail is attached. 2. Pregnant and experiencing fetal movements.

quickening (kwĭk′ĕn-ĭng). First movements of the fetus felt in utero. Occurs from 18th to 20th week of pregnancy. Movements have been felt as early as the tenth week and in rare cases are not felt during the entire pregnancy.

quicklime. CaO. Calcium oxide, unslaked lime. Forms calcium hydroxide when water is added to it.

quicksilver [ME. *quicke,* alive, + *silver,* silver]. The metal mercury.

Quick's test (kwĭks). [Armand J. Quick, U.S. physician, b. 1894] 1. A liver function test that measures the amount of hippuric acid excreted after a dose of sodium benzoate is given. 2. A test for the amount of prothrombin present in blood plasma.

Quide. Trade name for piperacetazine.

Quiess. Trade name for hydroxyzine hydrochloride.

quinacrine hydrochloride. USP. An agent used in the treatment of malaria. Also used in infestations of Giardia lamblia, a parasite. Trade name is Atabrine.

Quinaglute. Trade name for quinidine gluconate, USP.

Quincke's disease (kwĭnk′ēz). [Heinrich I. Quincke, Ger. physician, 1842–1922]. Angioneurotic edema of skin; urticaria; giant hives.

Quincke's pulse. A sign of aortic insufficiency, seen under fingernails and indicated by alternate reddening and blanching. SYN: *pulse, capillary.*

Quincke's puncture. Lumbar puncture to determine tension of spinal fluid, or to remove some of the spinal fluid.

Quine. Trade name for quinine sulfate, USP.

quinestrol (kwĭn-ĕs′trōl). USP. An estrogen. Trade name is Estrovis.

quinethazone (kwĭn-ĕth′ă-zōn). USP. A diuretic. Trade name is Hydromox.

quingestanol acetate (kwĭn-jĕs′tă-nōl). A progestational drug. SEE: *progestational agents.*

quinic acid. A substance present in some plants, including cinchona bark, and berries.

Quinidex. Trade name for quinidine sulfate, USP.

quinidine sulfate (kwĭn′ĭ-dēn). USP. The sulfate of an alkaloid obtained from cinchona bark; a white, crystalline substance with a bitter taste. Trade names are Quindex, Quincardine, Cin-Quin, and SK-Quinidine Sulfate.

ACTION AND USES: To regulate heart rhythm, esp. to prevent fibrillation.

quinine (kwī′nīn″, kwĭ-nēn′) [Sp. *quina*]. Bitter white crystalline alkaloid derived from cinchona bark.

USES: Analgesic, antipyretic, antimalarial. Usually administered in the form of its salts.

q. bisulfate. The acid sulfate of quinine. Used the same as quinine sulfate, but has greater solubility. Trade names are Coco-Quinine, Quinamine, and Quine.

q. dihydrochloride. The dihydrochloride of quinine, freely soluble in water, 1 gm. dissolving in 0.6 ml. of water. Suitable for intravenous injection.

q. hydrochloride. The hydrochloride of quinine. Used in treatment of malaria.

q. sulfate. USP. The sulfate of an alkaloid obtained from cinchona. Antipyretic and specific in malaria.

q. tannate. A nearly tasteless and odorless compound of quinine and tannic acid. A means of administering quinine to young children.

quinine and urea hydrochloride. Combination used, in dilute solutions, as a sclerosing agent for injection treatment of hemorrhoids and varicose veins.

quininism (kwī′nĭn-ĭzm, kwĭ-nēn′ĭzm) [Sp. *quina,* quinine, + Gr. *-ismos,* condition]. Poisoning by cinchona or its alkaloids. SYN: *cinchonism.*

quinoline (kwĭn′ō-lēn″). C_9H_7N, a tertiary amine derived from coal tar. It is a solvent and antiseptic and many of its salts are used medicinally as antipyretics, analgesics, and in the treatment of amebic dysentery and other infections.

quinone (kwĭn′ōn). 1. Yellow crystalline oxidation product of quinic acid. 2. Class of organic compounds in which two atoms of hydrogen are replaced by two oxygen atoms.

quinqu- [L. *quinque*]. Combining form meaning five.

Quinquaud's disease (kăn-kōz′). [Charles E. Quinquaud, Fr. physician, 1841–1894] Purulent inflammation of the hair follicles of the scalp, resulting in bald patches.

quinquetubercular (kwĭn″kwē-tū-bĕr′kū-lăr). Having five cusps or tubercles.

quinquevalent (kwĭng″kwĕ-vā′lĕnt). Pert. to a radical or element with a valence of five.

quinquina (kwĭn-kwī′nă, kĭn-kē′nă). Cinchona.

quinsy (kwĭn′zē) [ME. *quinesye,* sore throat]. Abscess of tonsil capsule due to bacterial inflammation. Abscess may rupture spontaneously; if not, surgical incision may be required. SYN: *abscess, peritonsillar.*

quintan (kwĭn′tăn) [L. *quintanus,* of a fifth]. 1. Occurring every fifth day. 2. Intermittent fever, the paroxysms occurring every fifth day with intermission of three days.

quinti- [L. *quintus,* fifth]. Combining form meaning fifth.

quintipara (kwĭn-tĭp'ă-ră) [" + *parere,* to bear]. A woman who has had five pregnancies that have continued beyond the 20th week of gestation. SEE: *para.*

quintuplet (kwĭn'tū-plĕt, kwĭn-tŭp'lĕt) [LL. *quintuplex,* fivefold]. One of five children born of one mother during the same confinement. SEE: *Hellin's law.*

Quotane. Trade name for dimethisoquin hydrochloride.

quotidian (kwō-tĭd'ē-ăn) [L. *quotidianus,* daily]. Occurring daily.

quotidian fever. A malarial fever characterized by daily paroxysms.

quotient (kwō'shĕnt) [L. *quotiens,* how many times]. Number of times one number is contained in another.

q., achievement. A percentile rating of a child's score on a test with respect to age, level of education, and peer performance.

q., intelligence. Division of the patient's mental age by the actual age.

q., respiratory. The result of dividing amount of carbon dioxide in expired air by the oxygen inhaled, normally 0.9.

q.v. *quantum vis,* as much as you like; *quod vide,* which see.

Q wave. A downward or negative wave of an electrocardiogram following the P wave. It is usually not prominent and may be absent without significance.

R

R. 1. *respiration; right; roentgen.* 2. In chem., a radical.

R–. Abbr. used in organic chemistry to indicate part of a molecule.

–R. Rinne negative. SEE: *Rinne's test.*

+R. Rinne positive. SEE: *Rinne's test.*

℞. Symb. for L. *recipe,* to take prescription, treatment.

RA. *rheumatoid arthritis.*

Ra. Chem. symb. for radium.

rabbetting (răb′ĕt-ĭng) [Fr. *raboter,* to plane]. Interlocking of the jagged edges of a fractured bone.

rabbit fever. Tularemia.

rabbit pox. An acute viral disease of laboratory rabbits.

rabiate (rā′bē-āt) [L. *rabies,* rage]. Suffering from rabies. SYN: *rabid.*

rabic (răb′ĭk). Concerning rabies.

rabicidal (răb-ĭ-sī′dăl) [L. *rabies,* rage, + *cidus,* kill]. Destructive to causative virus of rabies.

rabid (răb′ĭd). Pert. to, or affected with, rabies. SYN: *rabiate.*

rabies (rā′bēz) [L. *rabere,* to rage]. An acute infectious disease of warm-blooded mammals, esp. carnivores. Wildlife, esp. bats, skunks, foxes, and raccoons, have been found to have rabies; dogs, cats, and cattle are the domestic animals particularly susceptible. Characterized by involvement of central nervous system, resulting in paralysis and finally death. May be communicated to man through the bite of a rabid animal. The virus can also be transmitted to man or other animals from bats without a direct bite. It is assumed this transmission is by inhalation of infectious aerosols. SYN: *hydrophobia; lyssa.*

INCUBATION: Usually 4 to 6 weeks but may be as short as 6 days or as long as a year, depending on depth of laceration and site of wound. The virus moves along nerve axons passively at about 3 millimeters per hour. It is not known how or where the virus remains during prolonged incubation periods.

ETIOL: A neurotropic filtrable virus present in saliva of rabid animals.

SYM: The site of the bite is painful, tingles, and is sensitive to changes in temperature. Attempts to drink water produce laryngeal spasm. Behavior is restless and abnormal, and convulsions may be produced by sensory stimuli. Excess thick saliva is produced.

DIAG: Specific fluorescent-antibody staining of brain tissue or by virus isolation in mouse or tissue culture systems. Presumptive diagnosis may be made by specific fluorescent-antibody staining of frozen skin sections, corneal impressions, or mucosal scrapings.

PREVENTION: Thoroughly clean all bites or scratches made by any animal with strong (20%) medicinal soap solution. Deep puncture wounds should be opened to permit access of solution.

NURSING IMPLICATIONS: Administer the immunizations, antibiotics, and other drug therapy as prescribed. Cleanse and dress the wound, changing bandages as needed. Observe the cardiac and pulmonary function closely. Keep the room quiet and dark. Maintain strict isolation techniques throughout the duration of the illness.

TREATMENT: If the attack by the animal was unprovoked, the animal not caught, and rabies is present in that species in the geographic area, then give rabies immune globulin and vaccine immediately. If the animal is available and the owner and the health authorities agree, the animal may be killed and the brain examined by fluorescent-antibody technique to determine the need for antirabies treatment. Valuable or loved animals may be confined and observed for 10 days. If this is done, the decision to treat the patient is based on the behavior of the animal while observed, the presence of rabies in the area, and the circumstances of the bite.

The wound should be treated as soon as possible with virus-destroying solutions such as soap and water, alcohol, iodine, and quaternary-ammonium disinfectants. The wound should be sutured only if absolutely required. Tetanus prophylaxis is included in the treatment as is the use of antibiotics when indicated.

Human diploid cell rabies (HDVC) vaccine and rabies immune globulin (RIG) are available. These should be given as soon as possible after exposure to the bite of an animal known to be rabid. Some of the RIG is infiltrated around the bite and the rest is given intramuscularly. If the animal is not caught and rabies is known to be present in the area, start HDVC and RIG immediately, following the schedule enclosed in the vaccine package.

rabies immune globulin. USP. ABBR: RIG. A standardized preparation of globulins derived from the blood plasma or serum from selected human donors who have been immunized with rabies vaccine and have developed high titers of rabies antibody. It is used to produce passive immunity in persons bitten by animals. Trade name is Hyperab. SEE: *rabies.*

rabies virus group. A genus of virus the official designation of which is Lyssa virus. The virus that causes human rabies is included in this group.

rabiform (rā'bĭ-form) [" + *forma,* shape]. Resembling rabies.

race (rās) [Fr.]. 1. A distinct ethnic group characterized by traits that are transmitted through the offspring. 2. A group of individuals with the same characteristics who originated from a common ancestor. 3. A taxonomic classification of individuals within the same species who show distinct genetic characteristics.

racemase (rā'sē-mās). An enzyme that catalyzes racemization, i.e., the production of an optically active compound.

racemate (rā'sē-māt). A racemic compound.

racemic (rā-sē'mĭk). A mixture that is optically inactive.

racemization (rā"sē-mī-zā'shŭn). The production of a racemic form of an optically active compound.

racemose (răs'ĕ-mōs) [L. *racemosus,* full of clusters]. Resembling a clustered bunch of grapes, as a gland, divided and subdivided, ending in a bunch of follicles.

rachi-, rachio- [Gr. *rhachis,* spine]. Combining forms indicating spine.

rachial (rā'kē-ăl) [Gr. *rhachis,* spine]. Concerning the spine. SYN: *rachidial.*

rachialbuminimeter (rā"kē-ăl-bū"mĭn-ĭm'ĕt-ĕr) [" + L. *albumen,* white protein, + Gr. *metron,* measure]. Device for determining the amount of albumin in the cerebrospinal fluid.

rachialbuminimetry (rā"kē-ăl-bū"mĭn-ĭm'ĕt-rē). Determination of the amount of albumin in the cerebrospinal fluid.

rachialgia (rā-kē-ăl'jē-ă) [" + *algos,* pain]. Pain in the spine. SYN: *rachiodynia.*

rachianalgesia (rā"kē-ăn-ăl-jē'zē-ă) [" + *analgesia,* lack of pain]. Spinal anesthesia. SYN: *rachianesthesia.*

rachianesthesia (rā"kē-ăn-ĕs-thē'zē-ă) [" + *an-,* negative, + *aisthesis,* sensation]. Spinal anesthesia.

rachicele (rā'kĭ-sēl) [" + *kele,* hernia]. Protrusion of contents of spinal canal in spina bifida.

rachicentesis (rā"kĭ-sĕn-tē'sĭs) [" + *kentesis,* puncture]. Puncture into the spinal canal.

rachidial (rā-kĭd'ē-ăl). Concerning the spine.

rachidian (rā-kĭd'ē-ăn). Rel. to the spinal column.

rachigraph (rā'kĭ-grăf) [" + *graphein,* to write]. Device for outlining the curves of the spine.

rachilysis (rā-kĭl'ĭ-sĭs) [" + *lysis,* dissolution]. Mechanical treatment of lateral curvature of the spine through traction and pressure.

rachiocampsis (rā-kē-ō-kămp'sĭs) [" + *kampsis,* a bending]. Curvature of spine.

rachiocentesis (rā"kē-ō-sĕn-tē'sĭs) [" + *kentesis,* puncture]. Lumbar puncture.

rachiochysis (rā-kē-ŏk'ĭ-sĭs) [" + *chysis,* a pouring]. Accumulation of fluid within the spinal canal.

rachiodynia (rā-kē-ō-dĭn'ē-ă) [" + *odyne,* pain]. Painful condition of the spinal column. SYN: *rachialgia.*

rachiometer (rā-kē-ŏm'ĕ-tĕr) [" + *metron,* measure]. Instrument for measuring a curvature of the spine.

rachiomyelitis (rā"kē-ō-mī"ĕ-lī'tĭs) [" + *myelos,* marrow, + *itis,* inflammation.] Inflammation of the spinal cord.

rachiopagus (rā"kē-ŏp'ă-gŭs) [" + *pagos,* thing fixed]. A conjoined twin deformity in which the two are joined at the vertebral column.

rachiopathy (rā"kē-ŏp'ă-thē) [" + *pathos,* disease]. Disease of the spine.

rachioplegia (rā-kē-ō-plē'jē-ă) [" + *plege,* a stroke]. Paralysis due to a lesion in the spinal cord.

rachioscoliosis (rā"kē-ō-skō"lē-ō'sĭs) [" + *skoliosis,* bending]. Lateral curvature of the spine.

rachiotome (rā'kē-ō-tōm") [" + *tome,* incision]. Instrument for dividing the vertebrae.

rachiotomy (rā"kē-ŏt'ō-mē). Surgical cutting of the vertebral column.

rachis (rā'kĭs) [Gr. *rhachis*]. (pl. *rachises*) The spinal column.

rachischisis (rā-kĭs'kĭ-sĭs) [" + *schisis,* cleft]. Congenital spinal column fissure. SYN: *spina bifida.*

r., posterior. Spina bifida.

rachitic (ră-kĭt'ĭk). Pert. to, or affected with, rickets.

rachitis (ră-kī'tĭs) [" + *itis,* inflammatory]. 1. Inflammation of the spine. 2. Rickets.

r. fetalis annularis. Congenital enlargement of epiphyses of long bones.

r. fetalis micromelica. Congenital shortness of the bones.

rachitism (răk'ĭ-tĭsm). Tendency to rickets.

rachitogenic (ră-kĭt"ō-jĕn'ĭk) [" + *genesis,* production]. Causing or inducing development of rickets.

rachitome (răk'ĭ-tōm") [" + *tome,* incision]. Instrument employed for opening spinal canal.

rachitomy (ră-kĭt'ō-mē) [" + *tome,* incision]. Rachiotomy, q.v.

raclage (ră-klŏzh') [Fr.]. Destruction and removal of a soft growth by scraping or rubbing. SEE: *curettage.*

rad. *radiation absorbed dose.*

radectomy (rā-dĕk'tō-mē) [L. *radix,* root, + Gr. *ektome,* excision]. Surgical removal of all or a portion of the root of a tooth.

radiability (rā"dē-ă-bĭl'ĭ-tē) [L. *radius,* ray, + *habilitas,* able]. Capability of being penetrated readily by roentgen ray.

radiad (rā′dē-ăd) [L. *radialis,* radial, + *ad,* toward]. In direction of the radial side.

radial (rā′dē-ăl). 1. Radiating out from a given center. 2. Pert. to the radius.

radialis (rā″dē-ā′lĭs) [L.]. Concerning the radius bone.

radial reflex. Flexion of forearm resulting when lower end of radius is percussed.

radian (rā′dē-ăn). 1. A unit of angular measurement equivalent to 57.295 degrees. It is subtended at the center of a circle by an arc the length of the radius of a circle. 2. In ophthalmometry, a lens of one radian would have one plane surface equal in length to the radius of curvature of the curved surface.

radiant (rā′dē-ănt) [L. *radians*]. 1. Emitting beams of light. 2. Transmitted by radiation. 3. Emanating from a common center. SEE: *energy; heat; radiation.*

radiate (rā′dē-āt) [L. *radiatus*]. To spread from a common center.

radiatio (rā-dē-ā′shē-ō) [L.]. An anatomical structure, esp. a neurological one, that by means of radiating fibers forms interconnections between parts.

radiation (rā-dē-ā′shŭn) [L. *radiatio*]. 1. Process by which energy is propagated through space or matter. 2. Emission of rays in all directions from a common center. 3. Ionizing radiation used for diagnostic or therapeutic purposes. 4. A general term for any form of radiant energy emission or divergence, as of energy in all directions from luminous bodies, roentgen ray tubes, radioactive elements, and fluorescent substances. 5. In neurology, a group of fibers that diverge from a common origin.

r., acoustic. R., auditory.

r., auditory. A band of fibers that connect auditory areas of cerebral cortex with the medial geniculate body of the thalamus. SYN: *r., acoustic.*

r., corpuscular. Radiation composed of discrete elements or particles such as elements of atomic nuclei, i.e., alpha, beta, neutron, positron, or proton particles.

r., electromagnetic. Rays that travel at the speed of light. They exhibit both magnetic and electrical properties. SEE: *electromagnetic spectrum* for table.

r., heterogeneous. Radiation containing waves of various wavelengths.

r., homogeneous. Radiation containing waves of only one wavelength.

r., infrared. Invisible heat rays beyond the red end of the spectrum. Near or short infrared extends from 7200 to 14,000 Angstrom units (A.U.); far or long infrared extends from 15,000 to 120,000 A.U. SEE: *infrared rays.*

r., interstitial. Radiation accomplished by insertion of radium or radon directly into tissues.

r., ionizing. Radiation that either directly or indirectly induces ionization of radiation-absorbing material. SEE: *radiation injury, ionizing.*

r., irritative. Overdose of ultraviolet irradiation resulting in erythema and, in exceptional cases, blister formation.

r., occipitothalamic. R., optic.

r. of corpus callosum. Total of fibers radiating from corpus callosum into each cerebral hemisphere.

r., optic. A system of fibers extending from the lateral geniculate body of the thalamus through the sublenticular portion of the internal capsule to the calcarine occipital cortex (striate area). SYN: *geniculocalcarine tract; r., occipitothalamic.*

r., photochemical. From a therapeutic standpoint, the electromagnetic spectrum is divided into photothermal and photochemical radiations. Photochemical radiations penetrate tissues only fractions of a mm., are absorbed by protoplasm, and cause physical and biological changes. Photothermal radiation does not penetrate the skin but causes surface heating. A heating pad provides photothermal, i.e., infrared, heat

r., pyramidal. Radiation of fibers from the cerebral cortex to the pyramidal tract.

r., solar. Radiations of the sun, 60% in infrared region and 40% visible and ultraviolet.

r., striomesencephalic. Fibers originating in corpus striatum and terminating principally in substantia nigra of midbrain.

r., striosubthalamic. A system of fibers consisting of three groups emerging from medial aspect of lentiform nucleus and entering subthalamic region, most terminating there but some continuing into the midbrain. SYN: *ansa lenticularis.*

r., striothalamic. Groups of fibers connecting the corpus striatum with the thalamus and subthalamus.

r., thalamic. Groups of fibers that connect thalamus with cerebral hemispheres. Include frontal, centroparietal, occipital, and optic radiations.

r., ultraviolet. Radiant energy extending from 3900 to 200 Angstrom units (A.U.) Divided into near ultraviolet, which extends from 3900 to 2900 A.U., and far ultraviolet, which extends from 2900 to 200 A.U.

r., visible. Visible spectrum may be broken up into different wavelengths representing different colors:

Violet, 3900–4550 Angstrom units (A.U.)
Blue, 4550–4920 A.U.
Green, 4920–5770 A.U.
Yellow, 5770–5970 A.U.
Orange, 5970–6220 A.U.
Red, 6220–7700 A.U.

SEE: *heliotherapy; helium; spectrum*.

radiation absorbed dose. The quantity of ionizing radiation that is absorbed by any material per unit mass of matter.

radiation accidents, emergency handling of. As the field of nuclear energy expands into industry, medicine, and university studies, it is to be expected that there will be a rise in contamination accidents. The U.S. Atomic Energy Commission in cooperation with the American Medical Association in 1969 printed an order of procedures to be followed in case of radiation accidents. These rules are adapted from *Industrial Medicine and Surgery,* 39:(No. 1) 87, 1970.

The U.S. Energy Research and Development Administration has regional offices for information and assistance on radiological emergencies. Contacts may be made in person or by phone. SEE: *Radiologic Assistance* in *Appendix*.

Emergency handling of radiation exposure or radioactive contamination cases should not be feared. The handling of these cases is a matter involving common sense, cleanliness, and good housekeeping. Radiation accident problems have parallels in other conditions handled frequently by emergency rooms and rescue squads.

Radiation can be detected and measured by a simple instrument, a survey meter. Your hospital or your medical team can be involved by following these simple rules.

There are four types of radiation accident patients. The first type is the individual who has received whole or partial external body radiation and may have received a lethal dose of radiation, but is no hazard to attendants, other patients, or the environment. This patient is no different from the radiation therapy or diagnostic x-ray patient.

The second type is the individual who has received internal contamination by inhalation or ingestion. This patient also is no hazard to attendants, other patients, or the environment. Following cleansing of minor amounts of contaminated material deposited on the body surface during airborne exposure, this individual is similar to the patient with chemical poisoning, such as lead. Body wastes should be collected and saved for measurements of the amount of nuclides to assist in determination of appropriate therapy.

External contamination of body surface and clothing by liquids or by dirt particles presents a third type, with problems similar to vermin infestation. Surgical isolation technique to protect attendants and cleansing to protect other patients and the hospital environment must take place to confine and remove a potential hazard.

In the fourth type, when external contamination is complicated by a wound, care must be taken not to cross-contaminate surrounding surfaces from the wound and vice versa. The wound and surrounding surfaces are cleansed separately and sealed off when clean. When crushed dirty tissue is involved, early preliminary wet debridement following wound irrigation may be indicated. Further debridement and more definitive therapy can await sophisticated measurement and consultant guidance.

STANDING ORDERS FOR EMERGENCY HANDLING: If the ambulance or rescue squad that picks up the radiation accident case has a radio or telephone, the crew should alert the Emergency Room to expect a patient who may have had radiation exposure or radioactive contamination.

It is the responsibility of the senior person on duty in the hospital Emergency Room (nurse or physician) on receipt of notification of the momentary arrival of a case involving radiation exposure or contamination, to take the following steps:

1. Notify responsible staff physician or nurse and aides (trained health physicists or technicians from the nuclear medicine or x-ray department).

2. Get appropriate survey meter, if one is on hand in the hospital. If the hospital has no meter, notify the hospital administrator or responsible hospital official so that a survey meter and other pertinent equipment may be obtained by calling the police department.

3. Notify the hospital administrator so he or she may seek *expert professional consultation* for technical management of the case.

4. Prepare separate space if contamination is suspected, using either isolation room or cubicle if available. Some hospitals use the morgue, since the autopsy table lends itself to washing. The morgue entrance would then be used rather than the Emergency Room. When the morgue is used, the patient and family must be reassured of why that space is used. If no separate space is available, cover a floor area immediately adjacent to the entrance way to the Emergency Room with absorbent paper—the area to be adequate for stretcher-cart, disposal hampers, and working space for professional attendants. Mark and close off this area. If dust is involved, be prepared to shut off the air-circulation system to prevent spread of contamination.

Upon arrival of the ambulance, the responsible physician or nurse in the Emergency Room should:

1. Check patient on stretcher for contamination (preferably as stretcher is removed from the ambulance) by use of a survey meter.

2. If patient is seriously injured, give emergency lifesaving assistance immediately.

3. Handle contaminated patient and wound as one would a surgical procedure, with gown, gloves, cap, and mask.

4. If possible external contamination is involved, save all clothing and bedding from ambulance, blood, urine, stool, vomitus, and all metal objects (such as jewelry, belt buckles, dental plates). Label with name, body location, time, and date. Save each in appropriate containers; mark containers clearly, "Radioactive—Do Not Discard."

5. Start decontamination, if physical status permits, with cleansing and scrubbing the area of highest contamination first. If an extremity alone is involved, clothing may serve as an effective barrier and the affected limb alone may be scrubbed and cleansed. Initial cleansing should be done with soap and warm water. If the body as a whole is involved or clothing generally permeated by contaminated material, showering and scrubbing will be necessary. Pay special attention to hair-covered areas, body orifices, and body folds. Remeasure radiation contamination and record measurement after each washing or showering.

If a wound is involved, prepare and cover the wound with self-adhering disposable surgical drape. Cleanse neighboring surfaces of skin. Seal off cleansed areas with self-adhering disposable surgical drapes. Remove wound covering and irrigate wound with sterile water, catching the irrigating fluid in a basin or can to be marked and handled as described in rule 4 above. Each step in the decontamination should be preceded and followed by monitoring and recording of the location and extent of contamination.

6. Save physicians', nurses', and attendants' scrub or protective clothing, as described in rule 4 for patients' clothing. Doctors, nurses, and attendants must follow the same monitoring and decontamination routine as the patients.

7. If the Emergency Room staff is confronted with a grossly contaminated wound with dirt particles and crushed tissue, they should be prepared to do a preliminary simple wet debridement. Further measurements may necessitate sophisticated wound counting detection instruments supplied by the consultant who will advise if further definitive debridement is necessary.

When the accident has occurred at a plant, university, or medical group regularly working with nuclear material, the health physicist, supervisor, coworker, and the patient should be able to inform the rescue squad of the nature of the accident, type of radiation exposure or radioactive contamination involved, and possible body areas that may be affected.

radiation exposure limit. Recommended limit of accumulated exposure of an individual to ionizing radiation to prevent excess exposure. The National Council of Radiation and Protection and Measurements recommends that radiation exposure to the whole body, active blood-forming organs, gonads, or ocular lens accumulated at any age shall not exceed 5 rems multiplied by the number of years beyond age 18 and that exposure in any 13 consecutive weeks shall not exceed 3 rems. This can be expressed by the formula MPL = 5 (N − 18) rems. MPL is the maximum permissible accumulated exposure in dose equivalents (rems) and N is the individual's age in years. These limits apply to persons who are designated radiation workers. Members of the general population should be allowed only 10% of these limits.

Both patients and those who work where they may be exposed to ionizing radiation should be prevented from excess exposure. Nurses caring for patients treated with radioisotopes are exposed to the radiation given off by the isotope present in the patient's body and in the patient's excreta and bandages. Hospital personnel working with radioisotopes should wear a device for monitoring their exposure to radiation. These devices should be calibrated as often as necessary to ensure their accuracy. SEE: *radiation accidents, emergency handling of; radiation protection.*

radiation injury, ionizing. Injury to cell life because of therapeutic radiation. Ionizing radiation has the ability to penetrate cells and deposit energy within them in a random fashion, unaffected by the usual cellular barriers. This form of energy, when sufficiently intense, kills cells by inhibiting their division. The sensitivity of cells to ionizing radiation varies considerably in different stages of cell life. Because of this effect of ionizing radiation, the amount of exposure to all forms of it, including x-rays, radioisotopes, and other radioactive sources, is limited to a certain amount each year and to a specific total lifetime dose. SEE: *radiation accidents, emergency handling of; radiation exposure limit.*

radiation protection. There is no substitute for prevention. The only effective preventive measures are shielding the source and the operator or handlers, maintaining appropriate distance from the source, and limiting the time and amount of exposure. In general the use of drugs to protect against radiation is not practical because of their toxicity. An exception is the use of orally administered potassium iodide to protect the thyroid from radioactive iodine. SEE: *radiation exposure limit.*

radiation sickness. Radiation syndrome.

radiation symbol. A universal symbol used

to indicate radioactive sources, containers for radioactive materials, and areas where radioactive materials are stored and used. Presence of the symbol notes the need for caution in order to prevent contamination with or undue exposure to atomic radiation. The symbol consists of a purple propeller on a yellow field. SEE: illus.

radiation syndrome. 1. Illness resulting from exposure of body tissue to ionizing radiations from radioactive substances (radium, radon) or roentgen rays. Mild acute illness is manifested by anorexia, headache, nausea, vomiting, and diarrhea. Delayed effects resulting from repeated or prolonged exposure may result in amenorrhea, sterility, disturbances in blood cell formation, cataract formation, carcinogenesis, and leukemia. 2. Illness resulting from effects of explosion of an atomic bomb. Effects include destruction of lymphatic tissue, extensive hemorrhages, aplastic bone marrow, prolonged clotting and bleeding times, loss of hair and teeth, and possible genetic changes. In massive exposure to radiation such as would occur in persons close to the center of an atomic bomb explosion, death may occur within several weeks if the individual is not fortunate enough to die immediately from the physical effects of the explosion. SYN: *radiation sickness.*

radiation therapy. SEE: *Radiation Therapy* in *Appendix.*

radiator (rā′dē-ā″tor) [L. *radiatus,* radiate]. Device for radiating heat or light.

r., infrared. Device for transmitting infrared rays.

radical (răd′ĭ-kăl) [L. *radicalis*]. 1. In chemistry, a group of atoms acting as a single unit, passing without change from one compound to another, but not able to exist in a free state. 2. Oriented toward the origin or root. 3. A foundation or principle.

UNIVERSAL RADIATION SYMBOL

(PURPLE PROPELLER ON A YELLOW BACKGROUND)

r., acid. The electronegative portion of a molecule when the acid hydrogen is removed.

r., alcohol. The portion of an alcohol molecule left when the hydrogen of the OH group is removed.

r., color. Any group that when introduced into an organic compound causes it to become colored.

r., free. In chemistry, an atom or group of atoms that has an unpaired electron and thus is not, while in that state, bound to another chemical compound. They are highly reactive and participate in very brief reactions in living systems.

radical treatment. A treatment that seeks an absolute cure, as radical surgery; not palliative. Opposite of conservative treatment.

radices (răd′ĭ-sēz) [L.]. Pl. of radix.

radiciform. Resembling a root.

radicle (răd′ĭ-kl) [L. *radicula,* little root]. A structure resembling a rootlet, as a radical of a nerve or vein.

radicotomy (răd″ĭ-kŏt′ō-mē) [L. *radix,* root, + Gr. *tome,* incision]. Section of spinal nerve roots. SYN: *rhizotomy.* SEE: *radiculectomy.*

radicula (ră-dĭk′ū-lă) [L.]. Radicle, q.v.

radiculalgia (ră-dĭk″ū-lăl′jē-ă) [L. *radix,* root, + Gr. *algos,* pain]. Neuralgia of roots of nerves.

radicular (rā-dĭk′ū-lăr) [L. *radix,* root]. Concerning a root or radicle.

radiculectomy (ră-dĭk″ū-lĕk′tō-mē) [″ + Gr. *ektome,* excision]. 1. Excision of a spinal nerve root. 2. Resection of posterior spinal nerve root. SEE *radicotomy.*

radiculitis (ră-dĭk″ū-lī′tĭs) [L. *radicula,* radicle, + Gr. *itis,* inflammation]. Inflammation of spinal nerve roots, accompanied by pain and hyperesthesia.

radiculoganglionitis (ră-dĭk″ū-lō-găng″glē-ō-nī′tĭs) [″ + Gr. *ganglion,* knot, + *itis,* inflammation]. Inflammation of posterior spinal roots and their ganglia.

radiculomedullary (ră-dĭk″ū-lō-mĕd′ū-lĕr″ē) [″ + *medullaris,* marrow]. Concerning the nerve roots and the spinal cord.

radiculomeningomyelitis (ră-dĭk″ū-lō-mĕ-nĭn″gō-mī-ĕl-ī′tĭs) [″ + Gr. *meninx,* membrane, + *myelos,* marrow, + *itis,* inflammation]. Inflamed condition of nerve roots, meninges, and spinal cord.

radiculomyelopathy (rā-dĭk″ū-lō-mī″ĕ-lŏp′ă-thē) [″ + Gr. *myelos,* marrow, + *pathos,* disease]. Any diseased condition involving the spinal cord and roots of spinal nerves.

radiculoneuritis (ră-dĭk″ū-lō″nū-rī′tĭs) [L. *radicula,* radicle, + Gr. *neuron,* sinew, + *itis,* inflammation]. Inflammation of roots of spinal nerves.

radiculoneuropathy (ră-dĭk″ū-lō-nū-rŏp′ă-thē) [″ + ″ + *pathos,* disease]. Pathological condition of the nerve roots and nerve.

radiculopathy (rā-dĭk″ū-lŏp′ă-thē) [″ + Gr. *pathos,* disease]. Any diseased condition of roots of spinal nerves.

radiectomy (rā″dē-ĕk′tō-mē) [L. *radix,* root, + Gr. *ektome,* excision]. Surgical removal of the root of a tooth.

radiferous (rā-dĭf′ĕr-ŭs). Containing radium.

radii (rā′dē-ī) [L.]. Plural of radius.

radio- [L. *radius,* ray]. 1. Combining form indicating relationship to radiant energy or radioactive substances. 2. As a prefix to a chemical element indicating a radioactive isotope.

radioactinium (rā″dē-ō-ăk-tĭn′ē-ŭm). A radioactive product formed from disintegration of the element actinium.

radioactive (rā″dē-ō-ăk′tĭv) [L. *radius,* ray, + *activus,* acting]. Capable of emitting radiant energy.

radioactive decay. The decrease with passage of time in the number of radioactive atoms in a radioactive substance. This occurs when the nuclei disintegrate spontaneously by emitting radiant energy.

radioactive patient. An individual who originally was treated or accidentally contaminated with radioactive materials and who continues to be radioactive. If still emitting radiation when discharged from the hospital, the patient should be told how long to avoid close contact with children and pregnant women. SEE: *radiation accidents, emergency handling of.*

radioactive tracer. An atom that has been made radioactive so that its course may be followed in the body. SEE: *tagging.*

radioactivity (rā″dē-ō-ăk″tĭv′ĭ-tē). The ability of a substance to emit rays or particles (alpha, beta, gamma) from its nucleus.

r., artificial. Radioactivity resulting from bombardment of a substance with high-energy particles in a cyclotron, betatron, or other apparatus.

r., induced. Temporary radioactivity of a substance that has been within the sphere of influence of a radioactive element.

r., natural. Radioactivity possessed by a number of elements that are continuously disintegrating and emitting alpha particles (helium nuclei) or beta particles (electrons) atom by atom. Radium is an example.

radioallergosorbent test (rā″dē-ō-ăl″ĕr-gō-sor′bĕnt). ABBR: RAST. Blood test for allergy. It is capable of measuring minute quantities of immunoglobulin E (IgE) in blood. Persons who are allergic to foreign substances will develop antibodies that can be detected by use of this test.

radioanaphylaxis (rā″dē-ō-ăn″ă-fĭ-lăk′sĭs) [″ + Gr. *ana,* away from, + *phylaxis,* protection]. Abnormal sensitivity to radiation.

radioautogram (rā″dē-ō-aw′tō-grăm) [″ + Gr. *autos,* self, + *gramma,* mark]. Autoradiogram, q.v.

radioautograph (rā″dē-ō-aw′tō-grăf) [L. *radius,* ray, + Gr. *autos,* self, + *graphein,* to write]. A photograph of a histologic section of a tissue showing the distribution of radioactive substances in the tissue.

radioautography (rā″dē-ō-aw-tŏg′ră-fē). Autoradiography, q.v.

radiobicipital (rā″dē-ō-bī-sĭp′ĭ-tăl). Concerning the radius and biceps muscle of the arm.

radiobiology (rā″dē-ō-bī-ŏl′ō-jē). Branch of biology that deals with the effects of ionizing radiations on living organisms.

radiocalcium (rā″dē-ō-kăl′sē-ŭm). A radioisotope of calcium; ^{45}Ca and ^{47}Ca are used in medical studies.

radiocarbon (rā″dē-ō-kăr′bŏn). Radioactive isotope of carbon; ^{11}C and ^{14}C are used in medical studies.

radiocardiogram (rā″dē-ō-kăr′dē-ō-grăm) [″ + Gr. *kardia,* heart, + *gramma,* mark]. The record or film obtained during radiocardiography.

radiocardiography (rā″dē-ō-kăr″dē-ŏg′ră-fē) [″ + ″ + *graphein,* to write]. The investigation of the anatomy and function of the heart by obtaining a record or film of a radioactive substance as it travels through the heart.

radiocarpal (rā″dē-ō-kăr′păl) [″ + Gr. *karpos,* wrist]. Concerning the radius and carpus.

radiochemistry [″ + Gr. *chemeia,* chemistry]. The phase of chemistry dealing with radioactive phenomena.

radiochroism (rā″dē-ō-krō′ĭzm) [″ + Gr. *chroa,* color]. The ability of a substance to absorb radioactive rays.

radiochrometer (rā″dē-ō-krŏm′ĕ-tĕr) [″ + Gr. *chroma,* color, + *metron,* measure]. Device for measuring penetrating powers of x-rays and the character of roentgen tubes. SEE: *penetrometer.*

radiocinematograph (rā″dē-ō-sĭn″ĕ-măt′ō-grăf) [″ + Gr. *kinema,* motion, + *graphein,* to write]. Simultaneous recording of the picture provided during fluoroscopy of organs of the body.

radiocurable (rā″dē-ō-kūr′ă-bl) Curable by use of radiation therapy.

radiocystitis (rā″dē-ō-sĭs-tī′tĭs) [″ + Gr. *kystis,* bladder, + *itis,* inflammation]. Inflammation of the bladder following treatment by radium or roentgen rays.

radiode (rā′dē-ōd) [″ + Gr. *hodos,* way]. Metal container for radium used in therapeutic application.

radiodermatitis (rā″dē-ō-dĕr″mă-tī′tĭs) [″ + Gr. *derma,* skin, + *osis,* condition]. Inflammation of the skin caused by exposure to roentgen rays or radioactive elements.

radiodiagnosis (rā″dē-ō-dī″ăg-nō′sĭs) [″ + Gr. *dia,* through, + *gnosis,* knowledge]. Diagnosis by means of roentgen rays.

radiodigital (rā″dē-ō-dĭg′ĭ-tăl). Concerning the

radius of the arm and the fingers.

radiodontia (rā″dē-ō-dŏn′shē-ă) [″ + Gr. *odous,* tooth]. Roentgenography of the teeth.

radioecology (rā″dē-ō-ē-kŏl′ō-jē) [″ + Gr. *oikos,* house, + *logos,* study]. Investigation of the effect of radiation on the living organisms in the environment.

radioelectrocardiogram (rā″dē-ō-ē-lĕk″trō-kăr′dē-ō-grăm). The record obtained by radioelectrocardiography.

radioelectrocardiography (rā″dē-ō-ē-lĕk″trō-kăr″dē-ŏg′ră-fē) [L. *radius,* ray, + Gr. *elektron,* amber, + *kardia,* heart, + *graphein,* to write]. Recording of changes in heartbeats by radio wave from subject to receiver without direct attachment of apparatus, thus allowing recordings to be made during normal life activities of the patient. SEE: *telemetry.*

radioelement (rā″dē-ō-ĕl′ĕ-mĕnt) [″ + *elementum,* element]. Any of the elements possessing power of radioactivity.

radioencephalogram (rā″dē-ō-ĕn-sĕf′ă-lō-grăm″) [″ + Gr. *enkephalos,* brain, + *gramma,* mark]. The record obtained when a radioactive tracer passes through the cerebral blood vessels.

radioencephalography (rā″dē-ō-ĕn-sĕf″ă-lŏg′ră-fē) [″ +″ + *graphein,* to write]. The recording of radio waves transmitted from the brain to a receiver but without use of electrodes placed on the scalp.

radioepidermitis (rā″dē-ō-ĕp″ĭ-dĕr-mī′tĭs) [″ + Gr. *epi,* upon, + *derma,* skin, + *itis,* inflammation]. Destructive changes in the skin caused by radioactive rays.

radioepithelitis (rā″dē-ō-ĕp″ĭ-thē-lī′tĭs) [″ + ″ + *thele,* nipple, + *itis,* inflammation]. Disintegration of epithelium due to exposure to irradiation.

radiofrequency electrophrenic respiration. Method of stimulating respiration in cases of respiratory paralysis from injury of the spinal cord at the cervical level. Electrical stimuli to the phrenic nerves are supplied by a radiofrequency transmitter implanted subcutaneously. The diaphragmatic muscles contract in response to intermittent electrical stimuli.

radiogenesis (rā″dē-ō-jĕn′ĕ-sĭs) [″ + Gr. *genesis,* production]. Production of radiant energy.

radiogenic (rā″dē-ō-jĕn′ĭk) [″ + *gennan,* to produce]. 1. Producing radiation. 2. Caused by radiation. SYN: *actinogenic.*

radiogold (rā′dē-ō-gōld). A radioisotope of gold.

radiogram (rā′dē-ō-grăm) [″ + Gr. *gramma,* a writing]. X-ray picture, esp. of internal organs. SYN: *roentgenogram.*

radiograph (rā′dē-ō-grăf) [″ + Gr. *graphein,* to write]. 1. A record produced on a photographic plate, film, or paper by the action of roentgen rays or radium; specifically an x-ray photograph. 2. To make a radiograph.

r., dental. R., periapical, q.v.

r., lateral cephalometric. A film of the entire head, taken from the side with the head in a known, fixed position for the purpose of making definitive observations or measurements.

r., panoramic. A type of extra-oral body-section radiograph that shows the entire upper and lower jaws in a continuous single film.

r., periapical. An intra-oral film that depicts the tooth and surrounding tissues extending to the apical region. SYN: *r., dental.*

radiographer (rā″dē-ŏg′ră-fĕr). A person skilled in making roentgenograms or radiographs.

radiography (rā-dē-ŏg′ră-fē). The making of x-ray pictures. SYN: *roentgenography.*

radiohumeral (rā″dē-ō-hū′mĕr-ăl) [″ + *humerus,* humerus]. Concerning the radius and humerus.

radioimmunity (rā″dē-ō-ĭ-mū′nĭ-tē) [″ + *immunitas,* immunity]. Apparent decreased sensitivity to radiation that may follow repeated radiation therapy.

radioimmunoassay (rā″dē-ō-ĭm″ū-nō-ăs′ā). ABBR: RIA. A very sensitive method of determining the concentration of substances, particularly the protein-bound hormones, in blood plasma. The procedure is based on the competitive inhibition of binding of radioactively-labeled hormones to a specific antibody. Concentrations of protein in the picogram (10^{-12} gm.) range can be measured by using this technique.

radioimmunodiffusion (rā″dē-ō-ĭm″ū-nō-dĭf-fū′zhŭn) [″ + ″ + *dis,* apart, + *fundere,* to pour]. Study of antigen-antibody interaction by use of radioisotope-labeled antigens or antibodies diffused through a gel.

radioimmunoelectrophoresis (rā″dē-ō-ĭm″ū-nō-ē-lĕk″trō-fō-rē′sĭs) [″ + ″ + Gr. *elektron,* amber, + *phoresis,* bearing]. Electrophoresis involving the use of radioisotope-labeled antigen or antibody. An autoradiograph is taken of the electrophoretic pattern produced.

radioiodine (rā″dē-ō-ī′ō-dīn). A radioactive isotope of iodine. Used in the diagnosis and treatment of thyroid disorders. The most commonly used isotope is ^{131}I.

radioiron (rā″dē-ō-ī′ĕrn). A radioactive isotope of iron; ^{55}Fe and ^{59}Fe are used in medical studies.

radioisotopes (rā″dē-ō-ī′sō-tōps). Radioactive forms of elements.

radiolead (rā″dē-ō-lĕd′). A radioactive isotope of lead.

radiolesion (rā″dē-ō-lē′zhŭn). A lesion or injury caused by radiation.

radioligand (rā″dē-ō-lī′gănd, răd″dē-ō-lĭg′ănd). A molecule, esp. an antigen or antibody, with a radioactive tracer attached to it.

radiological emergency assistance. For list of addresses and phone numbers of U.S. Energy Research and Development Administration's Regional Coordinating Offices for Radiological Emergency Assistance, SEE: *Radiologic Assistance Directory* in *Appendix.*

radiologic technologist, technician. An individual who maintains and safely uses equipment and supplies necessary to produce images of the human body on x-ray film or fluoroscopic screen for diagnostic purposes. This individual may also supervise or teach others. Radiologic technology programs approved by the American Medical Association Council on Medical Education are conducted in hospitals, medical schools, and colleges with hospital affiliations.

radiologist (rā-dē-ŏl′ō-jĭst) [L. *radius,* ray, + Gr. *logos,* study]. A physician who practices diagnosis and treatment by use of radiant energy.

radiology (rā-dē-ŏl′ō-jē). The branch of medicine concerned with radioactive substances, including x-rays, radioactive isotopes, and ionizing radiations, and the application of this information to prevention, diagnosis, and treatment of disease.

radiolucency (rā″dē-ō-lū′sĕn-sē) [″ + *lucere,* to shine]. Property of being partly or wholly permeable to radiant energy.

radiolucent (rā″dē-ō-lū′sĕnt) [″ + *lucere,* to shine]. Allowing x-rays to pass through.

radiolus (rā-dē′ō-lŭs) [L., a little ray]. A sound or probe.

radiometer (rā-dē-ŏm′ĕ-tĕr) [″ + Gr. *metron,* measure]. Instrument for measuring intensity of radiation.

radiomicrometer (rā″dē-ō-mī-krŏm′ĕ-tĕr) [″ + Gr. *mikros,* small, + *metron,* measure]. An instrument for measuring small changes in radiation.

radiomimetic (rā″dē-ō-mĭm-ĕt′ĭk) [″ + Gr. *mimetikos,* imitation]. Imitating the biological effects of radiation. Alkylating agents are examples of substances with this property. SEE: *alkylating agent.*

radiomuscular (rā″dē-ō-mŭs′kū-lăr). Concerning the radius or radial artery and muscles of the arm.

radion (rā′dē-ŏn) [″ + Gr. *on,* being]. One of the radioactive particles given off by radioactive matter.

radionecrosis (rā″dē-ō-nĕ-krō′sĭs) [″ + Gr. *nekrosis,* death]. Disintegration of tissue due to exposure to radiant energy.

radioneuritis (rā″dē-ō-nū-rī′tĭs) [″ + Gr. *neuron,* sinew, + *itis,* inflammation]. Neuritis caused by exposure to radioactive substance.

radionitrogen (rā″dē-ō-nī′trō-jĕn). A radioisotope of nitrogen.

radionuclides (rā″dē-ō-nū′klīds). Atoms that disintegrate by emission of electromagnetic radiation.

radiopacity (rā″dē-ō-păs′ĭ-tē). The condition of being radiopaque.

radiopaque (rā-dē-ō-pāk′) [″ + *opacus,* dark]. Impenetrable to the x-ray or other forms of radiation.

radioparency (rā″dē-ō-păr′ĕn-sē). The condition of being radiolucent or radioparent.

radioparent (rā′dē-ō-păr′ĕnt) [″ + *parere,* to appear]. Penetrable by radioactive rays.

radiopathology (rā″dē-ō-pă-thŏl′ō-jē) [″ + Gr. *pathos,* disease, + *logos,* study]. Study of pathological changes induced by radiation.

radiopelvimetry (rā″dē-ō-pĕl-vĭm′ĕt-rē) [″ + *pelvis,* basin, + Gr. *metron,* measure]. Measurement of the pelvis by roentgen ray.

radiopharmaceuticals (rā″dē-ō-fărm″ă-sū′tĭ-kăls). Radioactive chemicals either in the form of individual elements or elements attached to other substances called carriers. They are used in testing the location, size, outline, or function of tissues, organs, vessels, or body fluids. The presence and location of radiopharmaceutical substances in the body are detected by special methods or apparatus that record or take an x-ray picture of the radioactivity produced. These compounds may also be used to treat certain diseases.

CAUTION: Radiopharmaceuticals must be handled in accordance with prescribed methods in order to prevent the patient or those treating the patient from being exposed to unnecessary ionizing radiation. SEE: table.

radiophobia (rā″dē-ō-fō′bē-ă) [″ + Gr. *phobos,* fear]. Abnormal fear of x-rays and radiation.

radiophosphorus (rā″dē-ō-fŏs′fō-rŭs). A radioactive isotope of phosphorus; ^{32}P is used in medical studies.

radiopotassium (rā″dē-ō-pō-tăs′ē-ŭm). A radioactive isotope of potassium; ^{42}K is used in medical studies.

radiopotentiation (rā″dē-ō-pō-tĕn″shē-ā′shŭn) [″ + *potentia,* power]. The action of potentiating the effect of radiation. This may be produced by certain drugs, and by oxygen.

radiopraxis (rā″dē-ō-prăk′sĭs) [L. *radius,* ray, + Gr. *praxis,* practice]. Diagnosis or treatment by use of some radioactive substance.

radioprotective drugs. Drugs that protect man against the damaging or lethal effects of ionizing radiation. Example: Lugol's solution or a saturated solution of potassium iodide will block the uptake of inhaled or ingested radioactive iodine by the thyroid.

radiopulmonography (rā″dē-ō-pŭl″mō-nŏg′ră-fē) [″ + *pulmo,* lung, + Gr. *graphein,* to write]. Use of radioactive materials to measure the flow of (or lack of) gases through the lung during respiration.

radioreaction (rā″dē-ō-rē-ăk′shŭn). The reac-

Clinical Uses of Radiopharmaceuticals*

Use	Isotope	Half-Life		Carrier
Thyroid Studies	^{131}I	8.08	days	sodium iodide, thyroxine, liothyronine
Kidney Studies	^{131}I	8.08	days	iodohippurate sodium
	^{197}Hg	65	hours	chlormerodrin
	^{203}Hg	46	days	chlormerodrin
Liver Studies	^{131}I	8.08	days	rose bengal sodium
	^{198}Au	64.8	hours	gold colloid
Gastrointestinal Tract Studies	^{131}I	8.08	days	triolein, oleic acid, tolpovidone
	^{57}Co	270	days	vitamin B_{12}
	^{53}Cr	27.8	days	sodium chromate
Blood Studies	^{131}I	8.08	days	serum albumin
	^{51}Cr	27.8	days	sodium chromate
	^{59}Fe	44.5	days	ferric chloride, ferrous citrate, ferrous sulfate
Brain Studies	^{131}I	8.08	days	serum albumin
	^{74}As	17.9	days	sodium arsenate
	^{197}Hg	65	hours	chlormerodrin
	^{99m}Tc	6	hours	albumin
Eye Studies	^{32}P	14.3	days	sodium phosphate
Electrolyte Studies	^{22}Na	2.58	years	sodium chloride
	^{42}K	12.5	hours	potassium chloride
	^{45}Ca	165	days	calcium chloride
	^{47}Ca	4.56	days	calcium chloride
Cancer Therapy	^{131}I	8.08	days	sodium iodide
	^{131}I	8.08	days	ethiodized oil
	^{198}Au	64.8	hours	gold colloid
	^{32}P	14.3	days	chromic phosphate
Thyroid Therapy	^{131}I	8.08	days	sodium iodide
Blood Disease Therapy	^{32}P	14.3	days	sodium phosphate

*Adapted from *Radioisotopes in Medicine*, 1970. Abbott Laboratories/Radiopharmaceutical Products Division, P.O. Box 68, Abbott Park, Chicago, Ill. 60064.

tion of the body to radiation.

radioreceptor (rā″dē-ō-rē-sĕp′tor). Something that receives radiant energy such as light, heat, or x-ray.

radioresistant. Resistant to the action of radiation, esp. said of a tumor that cannot be destroyed by treatment with radiation.

radioresponsive (rā″dē-ō-rē-spŏn′sĭv). Radiosensitive, q.v.

radioscopy (rā-dē-ŏs′kō-pē) [L. *radius*, ray, + Gr. *skopein*, to examine]. Inspection and examination of the inner structures of the body by means of roentgen rays. SYN: *fluoroscopy.*

radiosensibility. Radiosensitivity, q.v.

radiosensitivity (rā″dē-ō-sĕn″sĭ-tĭv′ĭ-tē). Reactiveness or responsiveness of a cell to radiation.

radiosodium (rā″dē-ō-sō′dē-ŭm). A radioisotope of sodium; ^{24}Na and ^{22}Na are used in medical studies.

radiostrontium (rā″dē-ō-strŏn′shē-ŭm). A radioisotope of strontium.

radiosulfur (rā″dē-ō-sŭl′fŭr). A radioisotope of sulfur.

radiosurgery (rā″dē-ō-sŭr′jĕr-ē) [″ + Gr. *cheirurgia,* handwork]. The use of high-energy protons and alpha particles in the form of beams as an atomic knife in treating diseases such as cancer or in selectively destroying an overactive endocrine gland.

radiotelemetry (rā″dē-ō-tĕl-ĕm′ĕ-trē) [″ + Gr. *tele,* at a distance, + *metron,* measure]. Transmission of data, including biological data, via radio from a patient to a remote monitor or recording device for storage, analysis, and interpretation.

radiotherapeutics (rā″dē-ō-thĕr″ă-pū′tĭks). 1. Radiotherapy. 2. Study of radiotherapeutic agents.

radiotherapist (rā″dē-ō-thĕr′ă-pĭst) [″ + Gr. *therapeia,* treatment]. One trained in use of radiant energy for therapeutic purposes.

radiotherapy (rā″dē-ō-thĕr′ă-pē). The treatment of disease by application of roentgen rays, radium, ultraviolet, and other radiations.

radiothermy (rā″dē-ō-thĕr′mē) [″ + Gr. *therme,* heat]. 1. Use of radiant heat or heat from radioactive substances for therapeutic purposes. 2. Short-wave diathermy.

radiothorium (rā″dē-ō-thō′rē-ŭm). A radioisotope of thorium.

radiotoxemia (rā″dē-ō-tŏk-sē′mē-ă) [″ + Gr. *toxikon,* poison, + *haima,* blood]. Toxemia produced by exposure to radioactive substance.

radiotransparent (rā″dē-ō-trăns-păr′ĕnt) [″ + *trans,* across, + *parere,* to appear]. Penetrable by radiation.

radiotropic (rā″dē-ō-trŏp′ĭk) [″ + Gr. *tropos,* turning]. Affected by radiation.

radioulnar (rā″dē-ō-ŭl′năr) [″ + *ulna,* arm]. Concerning the radius and ulna.

radium (rā′dē-ŭm) [L. *radius,* ray]. SYMB: Ra. There are more than a dozen isotopes, but radium with a half-life of 1622 years and an atomic weight of 226 is the most common. At. no. 88. A metallic element found in very small quantities in pitchblende. It is radioactive and fluorescent.

Radiation is of three kinds: alpha (α-rays); beta (β-rays); and gamma (γ-rays), which are analogous to x-rays. SEE: words beginning with *actin-*.

radium needles. Slender containers for radium. These are inserted into tissue in order to kill malignant cells.

radium therapy [″ + Gr. *therapeia,* treatment]. The treatment of disease by means of radium or radon, its emanation, or its active deposit. SYN: *radiotherapy.*

radius [L., ray]. (pl. *radii*) 1. A line extending from a circle's center point to its circumference. 2. [NA] The outer and shorter bone of the arm, which revolves partially about the ulna. Its head articulates with the capitulum of the humerus. Its lower portion articulates by the ulnar notch with the ulna, and by another articulation with the navicular and lunate bones of the wrist.

r., fracture of. A fracture and dislocation of the lower end of the radius, generally caused by falling on the outstretched hand. SEE: *Colles' fracture.*

radix (rā′dĭks) [L., root]. (pl. *radices*) [NA] 1. The root portion of a cranial or spinal nerve. 2. The root of a plant.

radon (rā′dŏn) [L. *radius,* ray]. SYMB: Rn. At. wt. 222; at. no. 86. A radioactive gaseous element resulting from disintegration of radium.

raffinose (răf′ĭ-nōs). A trisaccharide, melitose, present in certain plants, cereals, and fungi. Hydrolysis yields fructose and melibiose.

rage (rāj′) [ME.]. Violent anger.

r., sham. A rage reaction produced by stimuli to decorticated animals.

ragsorters' disease. A febrile pulmonary disease that may occur in persons who sort paper and rags. It is caused by the anthrax bacillus.

ragweed. One of several species of the genus Ambrosia whose pollen is an important allergen. Pollen-producing period of grasses is, in temperate zones, from middle of August to the first hard frost, usually the middle of October. SEE: *allergy.*

Raillietina (rī″lē-ĕ-tī′nă). A genus of tapeworms belonging to family Davaineidae.

R. demerariensis. A species that infests humans, reported from several S. American countries, esp. Ecuador.

railway sickness. Motion sickness resulting from riding on a train.

Raimeste's phenomenon. An associated reaction in hemiplegia whereby resistance to hip abduction or adduction in the non-involved extremity evokes the same motion in the involved extremity.

raised (rāzd) [ME. *reisen,* to rise]. In bacteriology, having a thick elevated growth with terraced edges.

rale (răl) [Fr., rattle]. An abnormal sound heard on auscultation of the chest, produced by passage of air through bronchi that contain secretion or exudate or that are constricted by spasm or a thickening of their walls. May be heard on inspiration or expiration.

CLASSIFICATION: There is no general agreement as to classification of the sounds. They are designated moist and dry. Moist rales are also called crackling and these in turn, coarse, medium, or dry. If loud and sharp, they are consonating. Dry rales are sometimes designated musical and may be tinkling, sonorous, snoring, or low pitched, or they may be whistling, piping, and high pitched.

r., amphoric. The musical sound heard by auscultation of the chest when a fluid-containing cavity communicates with a bronchus.

r., atelectatic. Transitory rale that disappears upon deep breathing or coughing.

r., bronchiectatic. Rale heard over bronchiectatic cavities filled with accumulated secretion. Disappears with expectoration.

r., bubbling. Rale heard in inspiration and expiration, produced by passage of air through mucus in the larger tubes. May be classified as small or medium.

r., cavernous. Rale heard in inspiration and expiration, produced by passage of air through a small cavity with flaccid walls that collapse with expiration. Hollow and metallic.

r., clicking. Rale heard in inspiration only, produced by passage of air through softening material in smaller bronchi. Small, sticky. Heard in pulmonary tuberculosis, early stage.

r., coarse. Rale that originates in the larger bronchi.

r., consonating. A loud, sharp rale sounding close to the ear. Usually associated with consolidation of tissues about bronchial tubes.

r., crackling. Rale heard chiefly in inspiration, produced by fluid in the finer bronchi. May be classified as small or medium. Heard in softening of the tubercular deposit or pneumonic exudation.

r., crepitant. Rale heard at end of inspiration, produced by passage of air into collapsed vesicles containing fibrinous exudation, usually at base of lungs. Heard in early-stage edema of lungs, and in hypostatic pneumonia. It is localized in pulmonary tuberculosis. SYN: *r., vesicular.*

r., dry. Rale heard in inspiration and expiration, produced by narrowing of the bronchial tubes from thickening of their mucous lining, from spasmodic contraction of the muscular coat, viscid mucus within, or pressure from without. Large and sonorous, small, hissing or whistling. Heard in bronchitis, asthma, and localized in beginning pulmonary tuberculosis.

r., gurgling. Heard in inspiration and expiration, produced by passage of air through fluid in cavities of large bubbles. Heard in pulmonary tuberculosis after formation of cavities.

r., moist. Rale produced by passage of air through bronchi containing fluid.

r. redux. Rale heard in inspiration and expiration, produced by passage of air through fluid in bronchial tubes. Crackling, unequal. Heard in pneumonia in the stage of resolution.

r., sibilant. High-pitched, whistling, and frequent rale heard at the end of inspiration.

r., sonorous. Low snoring rale that continues during inspiration.

r., subcrepitant. Rale heard in inspiration and expiration, produced by passage of air through mucus in the capillary bronchial tubes. Small, moist. Heard in capillary bronchitis.

r., vesicular. R., crepitant.

ramal (rā′măl) [L. *ramus,* branch]. Concerning a ramus.

rami (rā′mī) [L.]. Pl. of ramus.

ramicotomy (răm″ĭ-kŏt′ō-mē) [L. *ramus,* branch, + Gr. *tome,* incision]. Ramisection, q.v.

ramification (răm″ĭ-fĭ-kā′shŭn) [L. *ramificare,* to make branches]. 1. Process of branching. 2. A branch. 3. Arrangement in branches.

ramify (răm′ĭ-fī). To branch; to spread out in different directions.

ramisection (răm′ĭ-sĕk″shŭn) [L. *ramus,* branch, + *sectio,* a cutting]. Surgical division of a ramus communicans between a spinal nerve and a ganglion of the sympathetic trunk.

ramisectomy (răm-ĭs-ĕk′tō-mē) [″ + Gr. *ektome,* excision]. Excision of a ramus, specifically ramus communicans. SEE: *ramisection.*

ramitis (răm-ī′tĭs) [″ + Gr. *itis,* inflammation]. Inflammation of a ramus.

ramollissement (ră″mŏl-ēs-mŏn′) [Fr.]. Pathological softening of some organ or tissue, esp. of brain.

ramose (rā′mōs) [L. *ramus,* branch]. Branching; having many branches.

ramulus [L.]. (pl. *ramuli*) A small branch or ramus.

ramus (rā′mŭs) [L., branch]. (pl. *rami*) [NA] A branch; one of the divisions of a forked structure.

r., anterior. A primary division of a spinal nerve that supplies the lateral and ventral portions of body wall, the limbs, and perineum.

r., bronchial. Collateral branches of each primary bronchus.

r. communicans. [NA] One of the primary branches of a spinal nerve that connects with a sympathetic ganglion. Each consists of a white portion (white ramus communicans) of myelinated preganglionic sympathetic fibers and a gray portion (gray ramus communicans) composed of unmyelinated postganglionic fibers.

r., meningeal. One of the primary branches of a spinal nerve that re-enters the vertebral foramen and supplies meninges and vertebral column.

r., posterior. One of the primary branches of a spinal nerve that supplies muscles and skin of the back.

rancid (răn′sĭd) [L. *rancidus*]. Offensive; having a disagreeable smell or taste from partial decomposition, esp. of a fatty substance.

rancidify (răn-sĭd′ĭ-fī). To make rancid.

rancidity (răn-sĭd′ĭ-tē). Condition of being rancid.

random controlled trial. An experimental study for assessing the effects of a particular variable (such as a drug or treatment) in which subjects are assigned on a random basis to either of two groups, experimental or control. The experimental group receives the drug or procedure while the control group does not. Laboratory tests or clinical evaluations are performed on both groups (usually using the double-blind technique) to determine the effects of the drug or procedure.

randomization. In research, a method used to assign subjects to experimental groups. Prior to this step every attempt is made to ensure that the subjects are as equivalent as possible. Then by some random method such as tossing a coin or using a list of numbers each individual in the study is assigned to either a treatment or nontreatment group. Use of this technique helps to prevent inadvertent selection bias in the study. SEE: *clinical trial; technique, double-blind.*

range [ME., series]. The difference between the highest and lowest in a set of variables or in a series of values or observations.

range of accommodation. Difference between least and greatest distance of distinct vision. SEE: *accommodation.*

range of motion. ABBR: ROM. The range of movement of a joint. SEE: *goniometer.*

range of motion exercise. SEE: *exercise, range of motion.*

ranine (rā'nīn) [L. *rana,* a frog]. 1. Pert. to a ranula, or to the region beneath the tip of the tongue. 2. Branch of the lingual artery supplying that area. 3. Pert. to frogs.

ranula (răn'ū-lă) [L., little frog]. A large cystic tumor seen on underside of tongue on either side of the frenum; a retention cyst of the submandibular or sublingual ducts. The swelling may be small or large.

SYM: Semitranslucent; soft, large, dilated veins coursing over it. Fullness and discomfort. Usually no pain. Contains clear glairy fluid, due to dilatation of ducts of salivary glands and to obstruction of those of sublingual mucous glands.

TREATMENT: Periodic emptying of sac by careful needle aspiration will provide temporary relief. Surgical intervention is required for complete removal.

r., pancreatic. Cystic disease of pancreas due to obstruction of its ducts.

Ranvier's nodes (rŏn-vē-āz'). [Louis A. Ranvier, Fr. pathologist, 1835–1922] Constrictions in the medullary substance of a nerve fiber at more or less regular intervals. SEE: *nerve fiber.*

rape (rāp) [L. *rapere,* to snatch]. Heterosexual or homosexual intercourse against the will of the victim. Complete penetration of the vagina (or other body orifice) by the penis or emission of seminal fluid is not necessary to constitute rape. Most rapes include force or violence but acquiescence due to verbal threats indicates lack of consent.

NURSING IMPLICATIONS: Provide sensitive care, esp. psychological support. Remain with the patient and encourage verbalization. Assist with the physical examination, pelvic and rectal examinations, and diagnostic tests. Obtain a history of the assault and sexual history; discover whether or not the female rape victim was menstruating, and if so, the type of menstrual protection used.

Perform prescribed treatments on associated injuries. Administer prescribed prophylactic medications for venereal disease. Offer services of crisis intervention for emotional expression by the victim. Provide antipregnancy measures if indicated. Provide cleansing measures if patient desires. Assist patient in explaining situation to his or her family. Provide follow-up services and written and verbal instructions for prescribed medications, including actions and possible side effects. Arrange for escort home.

r., statutory. Sexual intercourse with an individual younger than the legal age of consent.

rape and sexual assault prevention. The situation of rape usually means the victim is confronted with a mentally ill person who may also be a criminal, thus rational behavior in attempting to prevent rape may be of no avail, which is not to say that such behavior should not even be considered. In the suggestions provided, it is assumed that the potential victim is a female who is being forced to have sexual intercourse or participate in other sexual acts. Preventive measures should be directed to as much as possible being, night or day, in a well-secured area close to persons who can be called for assistance. If the latter isn't possible, have emergency police number available and call for help without delay if you become suspicious that your apartment or home is being illegally entered. When preparing to enter your car or home, be constantly alert for the presence of a stranger hidden in the dark. Once you have decided that entering the car or apartment is safe, enter quickly—do not place yourself in the situation of having to fumble for a key. Immediately after entering, bolt the door, or lock the car doors. If you are entering a house or apartment that has been left unattended, be certain no one is hiding in it. This same precaution applies to entering a car, but look in car prior to opening the door. On the streets, avoid unlighted or dimly lit streets and walk in the street if traffic permits. Insist that strangers provide appropriate identification prior to allowing them to enter your home. If in doubt, refuse admission and phone for help.

If assaulted or confronted, immediately attempt to evaluate the person. It may be possible to distract him by a stream of talk, bizarre acts, or feigning illness or menstruation. If it is at all possible, flee to the nearest possible source of assistance. If you feel your life is in danger, do anything possible to offer resistance; if he is wearing glasses, try to remove or break them, spit, bite, scream, gouge eyes, claw his face, and attempt to kick him in the groin as hard as possible. If you are able to break free, run, and scream fire! (It is most probably true that persons who could aid you will respond more quickly to a scream of fire than to a call for help.)

If forced to participate in oral sex, i.e., fellatio, and you feel your life is in danger, then a vigorous, quick, and forceful attempt to amputate the penis by biting could completely demotivate the rapist because of extreme pain. You should immediately flee at that time. It would, of course, be inadvisable to do this if the rapist is threatening to shoot you or hit you in the head with a weapon during fellatio.

If raped, attempt to remember all details of the attacker: his clothes; size; race; accent; color of hair; identifying marks, scars, mustache; vehicle used; evidence of drug use.

rapeseed [L. *rapa,* turnip]. Seed of Brassica campestris and other species. Rape oil, which is used in foods and industry, is obtained from this seed.

raphania (ră-fā'nē-ă) [Gr. *rhaphanos,* radish]. A spasmodic disease caused by eating seeds of the wild radish; allied to ergotism, q.v. SYN: *rhaphania.*

raphe (rā'fē) [Gr. *rhaphe*]. [NA] A crease, ridge, or seam noting union of the halves of a part.

r., abdominal. Linea alba.

r., buccal. Raphe on cheek indicating line of fusion of maxillary and mandibular processes.

r. of penis. [NA] A median ridge on the posterior surface of the penis, a continuation of the raphe of the scrotum.

r. of scrotum. A ridge in the midline of the scrotum.

r. of tongue. A median groove on the dorsum of the tongue.

r., palatine. A line or ridge in the median line of the palate.

r., perineal. A line or ridge in the midline of the perineum.

r., pterygomandibular. A tendinous line of fusion between the buccinator and superior pharyngeal constrictor muscles that passes between the pterygoid process and the mandible, serving as an important landmark in dental anesthesia.

rapport (ră-por') [Fr. *rapporter,* to bring back]. A relationship of mutual trust and understanding, esp. between the patient and physician, nurse, or other health care provider.

raptus (răp'tŭs) [L.]. A sudden seizure or attack.

r. hemorrhagicus. A sudden massive hemorrhage.

r. maniacus. A sudden maniacal attack.

r. melancholicus. A sudden attack of agitation occurring during melancholia.

rarefaction (răr"ĕ-făk'shŭn) [L. *rarefacere,* to make thin]. Process of decreasing density and weight, as of air. The farther from the surface of the earth, the less dense the atmosphere becomes.

r. of bone. The process of making bone more porous because of absorption of mineral substances.

ETIOL: Disturbed calcium-phosphorus metabolism possibly resulting from excess parathyroid hormone. SEE: *osteoporosis; parathyroid.*

rarefy (rār'ĕ-fī). To make less dense, or to increase porosity of.

rarefying osteitis. Chronic bone inflammation marked by development of granulation tissue in marrow spaces with absorption of surrounding hard bone.

RAS. *reticular activating system.*

rash (răsh) [O. Fr. *rasche*]. General term applied to any eruption of the skin, esp. those associated with communicable diseases. Usually temporary. The rash usually is a shade of red, which varies with disease. SYN: *exanthema.* SEE: *eruption; lesion; roseola.*

NURSING IMPLICATIONS: Assess the location, size, and characteristics such as color, height and diameter of lesion. Obtain history of pruritus and allergies. Apply ointments and dressings as prescribed by the physician.

r., butterfly. Skin rash of both cheeks joined by an extension across the bridge of the nose. Seen in systemic lupus erythematosus, esp. after the patient's face has been exposed to sunlight. Also seen in seborrheic dermatitis, tuberous sclerosis, q.v., and dermatomyositis, q.v. SEE: *lupus erythematosus; butterfly* for illus.

r., cable. An acneiform eruption caused by contact with chlorinated waxes, which are used to lubricate cables.

r., diaper. Inflammation of skin of infants in the diaper area due to one or more diverse primary irritants. Improperly processed diapers and metabolic by-products of wastes are probable irritant sources.

r., drug. Rash caused by use of certain drugs, such as bromide or iodine. SYN: *dermatitis medicamentosa.* SEE: *drug rashes; idiosyncrasy.*

r., ecchymotic. R., hemorrhagic.

r., gum. A red, papular eruption of the

chin and anterior chest area of children seen during teething. A form of miliaria due to excess saliva coming in contact with the skin. SYN: *r., red; strophulus.*

r., heat. Miliaria rubra.

r., hemorrhagic. A rash consisting chiefly of hemorrhages or ecchymoses.

r., mulberry. Rash seen in typhus fever; dusky in color.

r., nettle. Smooth, elevated, itchy, white patches. SYN: *hives; urticaria.*

r., red. R., gum.

r., rose. Any rose-colored rash. SYN: *roseola.*

r., serum. Rash accompanying serum sickness resulting from injection of a foreign serum. SEE: *serum sickness.*

r., tooth. R., gum.

r., wandering. Condition of tongue marked by numerous denuded patches on the dorsal surface coalescing into freeform shapes similar to geographic presentations on maps. SYN: *geographic tongue.*

rasion (rā′zhŭn) [L. *rasio*]. Grating of drugs by use of a file.

raspatory (răs′pă-tō″rē) [L. *raspatorium*]. File used in surgery, esp. for trimming surfaces of bone. SYN: *xyster.*

RAST. *radioallergosorbent test.*

rasura (ră-sū′ră) [L. *rasura,* a scraping]. 1. Process of scraping or shaving. 2. Scrapings or filings. SYN: *rasure.*

rat [ME]. A rodent of the genus Rattus, found in and around human habitations. In addition to causing economic loss due to crop destruction, rats are of primary importance in the spread of human and animal diseases. They serve as hosts of various protozoans, flukes, tapeworms, and threadworms; reservoirs of amebiasis, murine and scrub typhus, and plague (bubonic, septicemic, pneumonic). The plagues are transmitted to man principally through arthropods (rat flea). Rats also transmit rat-bite fever, q.v. SEE: *flea; vector.*

rat-bite fever. Either of two infectious diseases transmitted by the bite of a rat. One is caused by Streptobacillus moniliformis, characterized by skin inflammation, headache, vomiting, and back and joint pain; the other is caused by Spirillum minus. Associated with it are ulceration, rash, and recurrent fever. The latter disease is rare in the U.S.A.

rate (rāt) [L. *rata,* calculated]. The speed or frequency of occurrence of an event. Usually expressed with respect to time or some other known standard.

r., attack. The rate of occurrence of new cases of a disease.

r., basal metabolic. SEE: *basal metabolic rate.*

r., birth. The number of live births in a given year.

r., case. R., morbidity, q.v.

r., case fatality. The ratio of the number of deaths caused by a disease to the total number of people who contract the disease.

r., death. The number of deaths in a specified population. Usually expressed as number of deaths per 100,000 population.

r., dose. The quantity of medicine administered per unit of time

r., erythrocyte sedimentation. ABBR: ESR. SEE: *sedimentation rate.*

r., glomerular filtration. The rate of filtrate formation as the blood passes through the glomeruli of the kidneys.

r., growth. The rate of growth of an individual, tissue, or organ. This may be expressed as rate per arbitrary unit of time such as hours, days, months, or years.

r., heart. The number of heart contractions per unit of time.

r., morbidity. The number of cases per year of certain diseases in relation to the population in which they occur.

r., mortality. The frequency of all deaths over a period of time, usually a year, in relation to the population (sick and well) in which the deaths occur. SYN: *r., death.*

r., pulse. The number of contractions of the heart per unit of time that can be detected by palpating a peripheral artery.

r., respiration. The number of breaths per unit of time.

r., sedimentation. Sedimentation rate, q.v.

Rathke's pouch (răth′kĕz). [Martin H. Rathke, Ger. anatomist, 1793–1860.] A depression in the mouth of the embryo. It is just anterior to the buccopharyngeal membrane. The anterior lobe of the pituitary arises from this structure.

ratio (rā′shē-ō) [L., computation]. Relationship in degree or number between two things.

r., A-G. R., albumin-globulin.

r., albumin-globulin. Ratio of albumin to globulin in blood plasma or serum. Normally 1.3:1 to 3.0:1.

r., arm. In chromosomes, the relation of the length of the long arm of the mitotic chromosome to the short arm.

r., body-weight. Body weight in grams divided by body height in centimeters.

r., cardiothoracic. The relation of the overall diameter of the heart to the widest part of the inside of the thoracic cavity. Usually the heart diameter is one half or less than that of the thoracic cavity.

r., curative. R., therapeutic.

r., dextrose-nitrogen. Ratio of dextrose to nitrogen in urine.

r., lecithin-sphingomyelin. ABBR: L/S

ratio. The ratio of lecithin in the amniotic fluid to sphingomyelin. This is used to determine fetal maturity. The ratio increases as the pregnancy approaches term, so that by the time of delivery, it is two or more to one.

r., sex. Ratio of males to females in a given population. Usually expressed as number of males per 100 females.

r., therapeutic. Ratio obtained by dividing effective therapeutic dose by minimum lethal dose. SYN: *r., curative.*

ration (rā'shŭn). Fixed allowance of food and drink for a certain period.

rational (răsh'ŭn-ăl) [L. *rationalis,* reasoning]. 1. Of sound mind. SYN: *sane.* 2. Reasonable or logical; employing treatments based on reasoning or general principles, opposed to empiric.

rationale (răsh"ŭn-ăl') [L.]. The logical or fundamental reason for a course of action or procedure.

rationalization (răsh"ŭn-ăl-ĭ-zā'shŭn). In psychology, a justification for an unreasonable or illogical act or idea to make it appear reasonable.

rattle (răt'l) [ME. *ratelen*]. A sound or rale heard on auscultation.

r., death. A gurgling sound or subcrepitant rale heard in the trachea of the dying.

rattlesnake. A poisonous snake of the genus Crotalid. It has articulated cuticular extensions at the tip of the tail. These produce a characteristic rattle. SEE: *snake.*

raucous (raw'kŭs) [L. *raucus*]. Hoarse, harsh, as the sound of a voice.

Raudixin. Trade name for rauwolfia serpentina, USP.

Rauscher leukemia virus. Virus known to cause leukemia in mice.

Rau-Sed. Trade name for reserpine, USP.

Rauserpa. Trade name for rauwolfia serpentina, USP.

Rauwiloid. Trade name for alseroxylon.

rauwolfia serpentina (raw-wŏlf'ē-ă). [Leonhard Rauwolf, Ger. botanist, died 1596] USP. The dried roots of Rauwolfia serpentina. Extracts are potent hypotensive agents and sedatives with low toxicity. Derivatives are serpentine, serpentinine, and reserpine, q.v. Trade names are Raudixin and Rauserpa.

rave (rāv) [ME. *raven,* to be delirious]. To talk irrationally, as in delirium.

raving. 1. Irrational utterance. 2. Talking irrationally.

ray (rā) [L. *radius,* ray]. 1. One of a number of lines diverging from a common center. 2. Line of propagation of any form of radiant energy, esp. light or heat; loosely, any narrow beam of light.

RS: energy; energy, radiant; fluorescence; heat; radiation; "roentgen-" words; spectrum; x-ray.

r., actinic. A solar ray of the spectrum, capable of producing chemical changes. SYN: *r., chemical.*

r., alpha. Ray composed of positively charged particles of helium derived from atomic disintegration of radioactive elements. Velocity is one tenth the speed of light. Alpha rays are completely absorbed by a thin sheet of paper and possess powerful fluorescent, photographic, and ionizing properties. They are less penetrative than beta rays.

r., antirachitic. Ultraviolet ray from 2700 to 3020 A.U.

r., bactericidal. Ray between 1850 and 2600 A.U., which is strongly destructive to bacteria.

r.'s, Becquerel's. Rays emitted from radium, uranium, and other radioactive substances.

r.'s, beta. Negatively charged electrons expelled from atoms of disintegrating radioactive elements.

r.'s, border. R., grenz.

r.'s, cathode. Negatively charged electrons discharged by the cathode through a vacuum, moving in a straight line and, upon hitting solid matter, producing roentgen rays.

r.'s, characteristic. Secondary roentgen rays, the wavelengths of which are determined by the chemical constitution of the object that emits, transmits, or scatters them.

r., chemical. R., actinic.

r.'s, cosmic. Electromagnetic waves (radiation) coming from sources in outer space. Cosmic rays have a short wavelength and exceptionally high velocity and penetrative power. SYN: *r.'s, Millikan.*

r.'s, delta. Highly penetrative waves given off by radioactive substances.

r., erythema-producing. Ray between 1800 and 4000 A.U., which produces erythema, with those around 2540 and between 2050 and 3100 A.U. being most effective.

r.'s, fluorescent roentgen. Secondary rays whose wavelengths are characteristic of the substance that emits them.

r., gamma. Heterogeneous vibrations caused by electronic disturbance in atoms of radioactive elements during their disintegration. They appear identical with roentgen rays except that the wavelengths range from about 1.4 to 0.01 A.U. and they derive from the nucleus rather than from the orbit of the element. They have high velocity and penetrative power.

r.'s, grenz. Soft roentgen ray with an average wavelength of 2 A.U. (range from 1 to 3 A.U.); obtained with peak voltage of less than 10 kilovolts. They lie between ultraviolet and roentgen rays.

r.'s, hard. X-rays of short wavelength and

great penetration.

r.'s, heat. Visible rays from 3900 to 7700 A.U. and infrared rays from 7700 to 14,000 A.U. The heating effect of visible rays on deeper tissue is proportionately stronger than that of infrared rays, because the visible rays have greater penetrating power. SEE: *heat.*

r.'s, Hertzian. Electromagnetic waves used in radio communication.

r.'s, infrared. Radiations just beyond the red end of the spectrum. Their wavelengths range between 7700 and 500,000 A.U. The therapeutic range extends from about 7700 to about 14,000 A.U.

r., luminous. Visible rays of the spectrum.

r., medullary. One of many slender processes composed of straight tubules that project into the cortex from the bases of renal pyramids. SYN: *pars radiata.*

r.'s, Millikan. R.'s, cosmic.

r.'s, monochromatic. Rays characterized by a definite wavelength, as secondary rays.

r.'s, pigment-producing. Rays at 2500 and 3000 A.U. are most effective in stimulating the production of pigment in the skin. This is due to a local response to irritation of cutaneous prickle cells.

r.'s, positive. Rays of positively charged ions that, in a discharge tube, move from the anode toward the cathode.

r., primary. Ray discharged directly from a radioactive substance, as the alpha, beta, and gamma rays.

r.'s, roentgen. X-rays discovered by Wilhelm Konrad Roentgen. They have a penetrative power through opaque substances; used for photographing internal organs and parts, and for diagnostic and therapeutic purposes.

r.'s, scattered. Roentgen rays or gamma rays that, in their passage through a substance, have been deflected and changed by an increase in wavelength.

r.'s, Schumann. Rays in the region bounded between 1220 and 1850 A.U.

r.'s, secondary. Roentgen rays emitted in all directions by any matter irradiated with roentgen rays.

r.'s, ultraviolet. Invisible rays of the spectrum that are beyond the violet rays, and of varying wavelengths. They may be refracted, reflected, and polarized, but will not traverse many substances impervious to the rays of the visible spectrum. They rapidly destroy the vitality of bacteria. They produce photochemical and photographic effects.

r.'s, x-. R.'s, roentgen.

Raynaud's disease (rā-nōz'). [Maurice Raynaud, Fr. physician, 1834–1881] A peripheral vascular disorder found most frequently in females between the ages of 18 and 30. It is characterized by abnormal vasoconstriction of the extremities upon exposure to cold or emotional stress. A history of symptoms for at least 2 years is necessary for diagnosis.

SYM: Intermittent attacks of pallor or cyanosis of the digits (usually fingers) associated with cold or emotional disturbance, pallor or cyanosis that is bilateral or symmetrical, normal radial and ulnar pulse. No evidence of occlusive disease is present; gangrene may occur but is limited to the skin of the tips of the digits.

PROG: Attacks persist but can be controlled. No serious disability develops, but this condition is sometimes associated with the development of rheumatoid arthritis or scleroderma.

TREATMENT: Maintenance of warmth of extremities by wearing wool gloves, socks, avoidance of contact with cold materials, avoidance of use of tobacco. Vasodilators and tranquilizers may be helpful.

Raynaud's phenomenon. Intermittent attacks of pallor followed by cyanosis, then redness of digits, before return to normal. Initiated by exposure to cold or emotional disturbance. Numbness, tingling, and burning may occur during the attacks. Secondary to such conditions as occlusive arterial disease, systemic scleroderma, thoracic outlet syndrome, pulmonary hypertension, myxedema, or trauma.

TREATMENT: Based on recognition and treatment of the underlying condition.

rayon, purified. USP. A fibrous form of regenerated cellulose manufactured by the viscose process, desulfured, washed, and bleached. It is used in surgical dressings and bandages.

Rb. Chem. symb. for rubidium.

RBC, rbc. *red blood cell; red blood count.*

R.B.E. *relative biological effectiveness.*

R.C.D. *relative cardiac dullness.*

R.C.P. *Royal College of Physicians.*

R.C.S. *Royal College of Surgeons.*

R.D.A. *right dorsoanterior,* presentation position of the fetus.

R.D.P. *right dorsoposterior,* presentation position of the fetus.

RDS. *respiratory distress syndrome.*

R.E. *radium emanation; right eye; reticuloendothelium.*

Re. Chem. symb. for rhenium.

re- [L.]. Prefix meaning back or again.

reabsorb (rē"ăb-sorb'). To absorb again.

reabsorption (rē"ăb-sorp'shŭn). The process of absorbing again. This occurs in the kidney when some of the materials filtered out of the blood by the glomerulus are reabsorbed as the filtrate passes through the nephron.

reacher. Adapted device permitting extended reach for persons with limited upper extremity range of motion. SYN: *reaching tongs.*

react (rē-ăkt′) [L. *re,* again, + *agere,* to act]. 1. To respond to a stimulus. 2. To participate in a chemical reaction.

reactant (rē-ăk′tănt). A chemical or substance taking part in a chemical reaction.

reaction (rē-ăk′shŭn) [LL. *reactus,* reacted]. 1. Response of an organism, or part of it, to a stimulus. 2. In chemistry, a chemical process or change; transformation of one substance into another in response to a stimulus. 3. An opposing action or counteraction. 4. Emotional and mental state created by a situation.

r., alarm. The first stage in the general adaptation syndrome, q.v., which includes changes occurring in the body when subjected to stressful stimuli. Physiological changes that occur are direct results of damage and/or shock, or reactions of the body to defend itself against shock.

r., allergic. A reaction resulting from hypersensitivity to an antigen.

r., anamnestic. The reappearance of antibodies that may occur when an antigen is injected a considerable time after the first injection.

r., anaphylactic. Reaction that follows injection or administration of a foreign substance to an animal that has been sensitized to it. SYN: *anaphylaxis.*

r., antigen-antibody. The combination of molecules of an antigen with one or more molecules of its specific antibody.

r., anxiety. In current psychiatric terminology, this condition is classed as an anxiety disorder, q.v.

r., Arias-Stella. Decidual changes in the endometrial epithelium. These changes consist of hyperchromatic cells with large nuclei; they may be associated with ectopic pregnancy.

r., biuret. 1. A test for measuring proteins in serum. 2. A chemical test for urea.

r., chain. A self-renewing reaction in which the initial stage causes the next reaction, which in turn causes the next reaction, etc.

r., complement-fixation. The reaction seen when the complement enters into combinations formed between soluble or particulate antigens and antibody. Used for diagnosis of certain diseases, esp. syphilis. SEE: *complement; fixation, complement.*

r., consensual. 1. An involuntary action. 2. A crossed reflex.

r., conversion. A conversion type of hysterical neurosis in which there is loss of or alteration in physical functioning suggesting a physical disorder but instead representing the expression of a psychological conflict or need. The disturbance is not under voluntary control and cannot be explained by a disease process; it is not limited to pain or sexual dysfunction.

r., cross. A reaction between an antibody and an antigen that is not specific for the antibody but is closely allied to the one that is.

r., defense. A mental response the purpose of which is to protect the ego.

r., delayed. Reaction occurring a considerable time after a stimulus, esp. a reaction such as inflammation of the skin occurring hours or days after exposure to the allergen.

r., dissociative. A sudden, temporary alteration in the normal functions of consciousness, identity, or motor behavior. Thus the individuals may temporarily forget their identity; or important personal events cannot be recalled; or the persons may wander as if in a dream-state.

r., false-negative. A test result that is inaccurate in that it was negative when in reality it should have been positive.

r., false-positive. A positive reaction in a test, esp. test for syphilis, that is due to faulty technique or to presence of another disease.

r., hemianopic. In some forms of homonymous hemianopia, the pupils of both eyes fail to react to a thin pencil of light from the blind side, but react normally to light from the normal side.

r., hemiopic pupillary. A reaction in certain cases of hemianopia in which light from one side will cause the iris to contract but light from the other side will not cause the contraction.

r., immune. A reaction that demonstrates the presence of antibodies in the blood. Indicative of a high degree of immunity.

r., leukemic or leukemoid. Changes in the blood smear of peripheral blood that are consistent with those present in leukemia. This may occur in patients with an infection or tumor but who do not have leukemia.

r., local. Reaction occurring at point of stimulation or injection of exciting substances.

r., myasthenic. Gradual decrease and eventual cessation of muscle contractions when a muscle is stimulated repeatedly by direct current.

r., neutral. In chemistry, a reaction indicating absence of acid or alkaline properties. Expressed as pH 7.0.

r. of degeneration. The change in muscle reactivity to electricity, seen in lower motor neuron paralysis.

r., ophthalmic. Local reaction of conjunctiva to introduction of toxins of tuberculosis and typhoid fever; more severe in those having the diseases.

r., Prausnitz-Kustner. SEE: *Prausnitz-Kustner reaction.*

r., quellung. The swelling of capsules of bacteria when mixed with their specific immune serum.

r., transfusion. Reaction following transfusion of incompatible blood, which causes agglutination and hemolysis of the recipient's or donor's red blood cells or both.

r., wheal and flare. The response within 10–15 minutes to an antigen injected into the skin. The area demonstrates an elevated blanched irregular wheal surrounded by erythema.

reaction time. The time required to respond to a stimulus.

reactivate. To make active again, esp. the process of returning activity to immune serum that has lost its potency by the addition of fresh normal serum, thus restoring the complement, which had become inactive through age, heat, or other factors.

reactive depression. In psychology, a psychosis resulting from bereavement, sadness, or a situation causing such emotions, lasting longer and more marked than the normal reaction.

reactivation (rē-ăk″tĭ-vā′shŭn). To make something or some process active again.

reactivity (rē″ăk-tĭv′ĭ-tē). The action of reacting to a stimulus.

reading. Interpreting or perusing written or printed characters or material. Reading may or may not include comprehension of the material.

r., lip. Interpretation of what is being spoken by watching movements of the speaker's lips.

reading disorders. Conditions that interfere with or prevent comprehension of written or printed material. A term used esp. in reference to children. The condition seen in some adults may have developed due to injury to the brain or may have persisted from infancy. SEE: *dyslexia.*

reagent (rē-ā′jĕnt) [L. *reagere,* to react]. 1. A substance involved in a chemical reaction. 2. A substance used to detect the presence of another substance. 3. Subject of a psychological experiment, esp. one reacting to a stimulus.

reagin (rē′ă-jĭn). A type of immunoglobulin gamma E (IgGE) present in the serum of atopic individuals. Reagin does not cross the placental barrier.

reaginic (rē′ă-jĭn-ĭk). Concerning reagin.

reality principle (rē-ăl′ĭ-tē). Awareness of external demands and adjustment in a manner that meets these demands, yet assures continued self-gratification.

reality testing. The attempt by the individual to evaluate and understand the real world and his or her relation to it.

reality therapy. A psychiatric treatment based on the concept that some patients deny the reality of the world around them. Therapy is directed to assist patient to recognize and accept the present situation. The main technique is confrontation; the therapist consistently confronts the client with the reality of the situation. Illness or pathology is viewed as a defense against the real world. The purpose of the confrontation is to minimize distortion.

reamer (rē′mĕr). A small instrument used in dentistry for enlarging the root canal of a tooth.

reanimate (rē-ăn′ĭ-māt) [L. *re,* again, + *animare,* fill with life]. To reactivate, restore to life, revive, resuscitate.

reapers' keratitis (rēp′ĕrs kĕr-ă-tī′tĭs). Inflammation of the cornea caused by dust from grain. SEE: *keratitis.*

reasonable care. Those acts performed or omitted that an ordinary prudent medical practitioner or health care professional would have or have not done. A measure against which a defendant's malpractice conduct is compared.

reasonable charge. The reimbursement for any service provided for health care. Under Medicare this is the lowest customary charge by a particular physician for a service or the prevailing charge of other physicians in that area for the same service.

reasonable cost. The amount a third party (usually the medical insurer) will actually reimburse for health care based on the cost to the provider for delivering that service.

reattachment (rē″ă-tăch′mĕnt). 1. Recementing a dental crown. 2. Re-embedding periodontal ligament fibers into the cementum of a tooth that has become dislodged. 3. Rejoining parts that have been separated, as a finger that has been traumatically detached.

rebase (rē-bās′). To refit a denture by replacing the base material without altering the occlusal characteristics.

rebound [ME. *rebounden,* to leap back]. Response even in reflexes in which sudden withdrawal of stimulus is followed by fresh activity, such as a strong contraction following a moderate one, marked relaxation following moderate relaxation, or contraction replacing inhibition.

rebound phenomenon. When a limb or a part is acting against a resistance and the resistance is suddenly removed, the limb will move forcibly in the direction toward which effort was being directed. This is indicative of a cerebellar lesion.

recalcification (rē″kăl-sĭ-fĭ-kā′shŭn) [L. *re,* again, + *calx,* lime, + *facere,* to make]. The restoration of calcium salts to tissues from which they have been withdrawn.

recall [" + AS. *ceallian,* to call]. Act of bringing back to mind that which has been previously learned or experienced.

recapitulation theory (rē″kă-pĭt-ū-lā′shŭn) [" + *capitulum,* a section]. The theory that an individual in its development from the ovum to maturity passes through successive stages that approximate the series of adult ancestors from which that organism has descended. Summarized in the statement, "ontogeny recapitulates phylogeny."

receiver (rē-sēv′ĕr) [" + *capere,* to take]. 1. Container for holding a gas or a distillate. 2. Apparatus for receiving electrical waves or current, such as a radio receiver.

receptaculum (rē″sĕp-tăk′ū-lŭm) [L.]. (pl. *receptacula*) A vessel or cavity in which a fluid is contained.

r. chyli. Inferior, pear-shaped, expanded portion of the lower end of the thoracic duct, near 1st and 2nd lumbar vertebrae, into which the right and left lumbar trunks, an intestinal trunk, and some thoracic vessels empty. SYN: *cisterna chyli.*

receptor (rē-sĕp′tor) [L., a receiver]. 1. In pharmacology, a cell component that combines with a drug or hormone to alter the function of the cell. SEE: *Ehrlich's side-chain theory.* 2. Various sensory nerve endings.

r., adrenergic. The area in certain cells that is thought to be the site of action of adrenergic stimulation whether produced by the body or drugs. There are two types of receptors. Some act in response to sympathomimetic or adrenergic stimuli or drugs. These are called alpha-adrenergic receptors. Some react to inhibit the action of sympathomimetic or adrenergic stimuli, and these are called beta-adrenergic receptors. Epinephrine is a powerful activator of alpha-adrenergic receptors; and isoproterenol is a powerful activator of beta-adrenergic receptors.

r., auditory. The hair cells in the organ of Corti in cochlea of the ear.

r., cell. SEE: *r., drug.*

r., cholinergic. Sites in nerve synapses or effector cells that respond to the effect of acetylcholine.

r., contact. A receptor that gives rise to a sensation such as touch, temperature, or pain that can be localized in or on the surface of the body.

r., cutaneous. Receptor that is located in the skin.

r., distance. A receptor that responds to stimuli originating at a distance from the body. Includes visual, auditory, and olfactory sense organs. SYN: *teleceptor.*

r., drug. Constituents of cells, including chemicals, protein, and portions of a membrane, that serve to sense extracellular signals and to translate them into intracellular physiological or metabolic events. In the case of drugs, the receptors sense the presence of the pharmacologically active agent and produce the effects of the drug on the cell. There may be thousands of such receptors in *each* cell.

r.'s, gravity. Macula hair cells of utricle and saccule, which respond to changes in position of the head and linear acceleration.

r.'s, olfactory. The olfactory cells, bipolar nerve cells, found in olfactory epithelium, whose axons form fibers of olfactory nerve.

r.'s, optic. The rods and cones of the retina.

r.'s, proprioceptive. Muscle and tendon spindles, the receptors of the muscle or kinesthetic, or position, sense.

r.'s, rotary. The hair cells in the cristae of the ampulla of semicircular ducts of the ear, which are stimulated by angular acceleration or rotation.

r., sensory. A sensory nerve-ending, a cell or group of cells, or a sense organ that, when stimulated, gives rise to an afferent or sensory impulse.

CLASSIFICATION: *Exteroreceptors:* those located on or near the surface that respond to stimuli of the outside world. Include eye and ear (receptors for remote stimuli) and touch, temperature, and pain receptors (contact receptors). *Interoceptors:* those in mucous linings of alimentary and digestive tracts that respond to internal stimuli; also called visceroceptors. *Proprioceptors:* those responding to stimuli arising within body tissues.

Receptors also are classified on the basis of nature of stimuli to which they respond: *chemoreceptors,* those that respond to chemical substances (taste buds, olfactory cells, receptors in aortic and carotid bodies); *pressoreceptors,* those that respond to pressure (receptors in aortic arch and carotid sinus); *photoreceptors,* those that respond to light (rods and cones); *tangoreceptors,* those that respond to touch (Meissner's corpuscle).

r.'s, stretch. Neuromuscular and neurotendinar spindles and organs of Golgi, which are stimulated by stretch. SEE: *proprioceptor.*

r.'s, taste. The gustatory cells of the taste buds.

r.'s, temperature. Krause's end-bulbs (receptors of cold) and Ruffini's corpuscles (receptors for warmth).

r.'s, touch. Merkel's disks, Meissner's corpuscles, and nerve plexus about the roots of hairs.

r., universal. SEE: *universal recipient.*

recess (rē′sĕs) [L. *recessus,* receded]. A small indentation, depression, or cavity. SYN: *recessus.*

r., cochlear. A small concavity lying between the two limbs of the vestibular crest in vestibule of ear that lodges the beginning of the cochlear duct.

r., elliptical. A small concavity lying superiorly and posteriorly on medial wall of vestibule that lodges the utricle of the ear.

r., epitympanic. That portion of the tympanic cavity that lies above the level of tympanic membrane. It contains the head of the malleus and short limb of the incus. SYN: *attic.*

r., infundibular. A small projection of the third ventricle that extends into the infundibular stalk of hypophysis.

r., lateral, of fourth ventricle. One of two lateral extensions of the 4th ventricle, forming narrow pockets on each side and around upper portions of the restiform bodies.

r., nasopalatine. A small depression on the floor of the nasal cavity near the nasal septum. Lies immediately over the incisive foramen.

r., omental. One of three pocket-like extensions of the omental bursa. The superior recess extends upward behind the caudate lobe of the liver; the inferior recess extends downward into the great omentum; and the lineal recess extends laterally to the hilus of the spleen.

r., optic. A pocket of the 3rd ventricle lying anterior to the infundibular recess. It is bound inferiorly by the optic chiasma.

r., pharyngeal. Recess in the lateral wall of the nasal pharynx lying above and behind the opening to the auditory tube. SYN: *fossa, Rosenmüller's.*

r., pineal. A recess of the roof of the 3rd ventricle extending into the stalk of the pineal body.

r., piriform. A deep depression in the wall of the laryngeal pharynx lying lateral to the orifice of the larynx. It is bounded laterally by thyroid cartilage and medially by cricoid and arytenoid cartilages. It is a common site for lodgement of foreign objects.

r., sphenoethmoidal. Small space in the nasal fossa lying above the superior concha. Lies between the ethmoid bone and the anterior surface of the body of the sphenoid bone and posteriorly receives the opening of the sphenoidal sinus.

r., spherical. Recess on medial wall of the vestibule of the inner ear that accommodates the saccule.

r., suprapineal. A posterior extension of roof of the 3rd ventricle forming a small cavity above the pineal body.

r., tympanic membrane. One of two pouches of tympanic mucous membrane (anterior and posterior) lying between the tympanic membrane and anterior and posterior malleolar folds.

r., umbilical. A dilatation on the left main branch of the portal vein that marks the position where the umbilical vein was originally attached.

recession (rē-sĕsh′ŭn) [L. *recessus,* recess]. The withdrawal of a part from its normal position. In dentistry, the shrinkage of gingival tissue in a direction toward the root of the tooth. This allows exposure of more of the tooth structure. SEE: *periodontitis.* SYN: *ulatrophia.*

recessive. Tending to recede or go back; lacking control; not dominant.

recessive gene. A gene that, in the presence of its dominant allele, does not express itself.

recessus (rē-sēs′ŭs) [L.]. A small hollow or recess.

recidivation (rē-sĭd″ĭ-vā′shŭn) [L. *recidivus,* falling back]. 1. The relapse of a disease or recurrence of a symptom. 2. The return to criminal activity.

recidivism. Habitual criminality; repetition of antisocial acts.

recidivist. 1. A confirmed criminal. 2. A patient, esp. one with mental illness who has repeated relapses, esp. a mentally ill patient who relapses into behavior marked by antisocial acts.

recidivity. Tendency to relapse, or to return to a former condition.

recipe (rĕs′ĭ-pē) [L., take]. 1. Take, indicated by the sign ℞. 2. A prescription or formula for a medicine. SEE: *prescription.*

recipient (rē-sĭp′ē-ĕnt) [L. *recipiens,* receiving]. One who receives anything, esp. those who receive blood, tissues, or organs provided by a donor, as in a blood transfusion or kidney transplant. SEE: *donor.*

recipiomotor (rē-sĭp″ē-ō-mō′tor) [″ + *motor,* mover]. Concerning the reception of motor stimuli.

reciprocal (rē-sĭp′rō-kăl) [L. *reciprocus,* alternate]. Interchangeable in character.

reciprocal inhibition. Inhibition of muscles antagonistic to those being facilitated; this is essential for coordinated movement.

reciprocation (rē-sĭp″rō-kā′shŭn) [L. *reciprocare,* to move backward and forward]. The condition of one action countering another reaction. In dentistry, the action of one part of a dental device to counter the effect of another part.

reciprocity. The recognition by one state of the license to practice granted to a health care professional by another state.

Recklinghausen, Friedrich D. von (rĕk′lĭng-how″zĕn). German pathologist, 1833–1910.

R.'s canals. Rootlets of the lymphatics, minute spaces in connective tissue. SYN: *von Recklinghausen's canals.*

R.'s disease. Multiple neurofibromata of nerve sheaths. They occur along peripheral nerves, where they are quite obvious, and on spinal and cranial nerve roots. Extremely variable in size, number, and shape. Area over tumor may be hyperpigmented. Symptoms may be completely absent or may be those of pain due to pressure on spinal cord or on the brain. SYN: *neurofibromatosis; von Recklinghausen's disease.*

TREATMENT: Surgical as required to relieve symptoms.

R.'s tumor. An adenoleiomyofibroma on wall of the fallopian tube or posterior uterine wall. SYN: *von Recklinghausen's tumor.*

reclination (rĕk″lĭ-nā′shŭn) [L. *reclinatio,* lean back]. The turning of the eye lens covered with a cataract over into the vitreous to remove it from line of vision. SYN: *couching.*

recline (rē-klīn′) [L. *reclinare*]. To be in recumbent position; to lie down.

Reclus' disease (rā-klooz′). [Paul Reclus, Fr. surgeon, 1847–1914] Multiple, benign, cystic growths in the breast.

recombinant DNA. Artificial manipulation of segments of DNA from one organism into the DNA of another organism. Using a technique known as gene splicing, it is possible to join genetic material of unrelated species. When the host's genetic material is reproduced, the transplanted genetic material is also copied. This technique permits isolating and examining the properties and action of specific genes. SEE: *plasmid; gene splicing.*

Studies in this area must be done in a carefully controlled environment. Levels of containment have been defined and are designated as P-1 for the lowest level and P-4 for the highest. The P-4 level is for experiments involving animal virus DNA that contains potentially lethal genes. Experiments using DNA from pathogenic organisms, cancer-causing viruses, and viruses associated with certain toxins are prohibited in the U.S.A.

recombination (rē″kŏm-bĭ-nā′shŭn). 1. Joining together again. 2. In genetics, the joining together of gene combinations in the offspring that were not present in the parents.

recomposition [L. *re,* again, + *composer,* to place together]. The recombining of constituents or parts.

recompression [″ + LL. *compressare,* press together]. Resubjecting a person to increased atmospheric pressure, a procedure used in the treatment of caisson disease (bends).

recon (rē′kŏn). In genetics, the smallest unit that can enter into recombination.

reconstitution (rē″kŏn-stĭ-tū′shŭn). Returning a substance, previously altered for preservation and storage, to its approximate original state, as is done with dried blood plasma.

record (rĕk′ord). 1. A written account of something. SEE: *problem-oriented medical record.* 2. In dentistry, a registration of jaw relations in a malleable material or on a device.

r., functional chewing. A record of the natural chewing action of the mandible made on an occlusion rim by the teeth or scribing studs.

r., interocclusal. A record of the positional relationship of teeth or jaws to each other. This is made by placing a plastic material that hardens between the teeth prior to biting down on the material.

recover (rē-kŭv′ĕr) [O. Fr. *recoverer*]. To regain health after illness; to regain a former state of health. To regain a normal state as to recover from fright.

recovery (rē-kŭv′ĕr-ē). The process or act of becoming well or returning to a state of health.

recovery room. Area provided with equipment and nurses needed to care for patients who have just come from surgery. Patients remain there until they regain consciousness and are no longer drowsy and stuporous from the effects of anesthesia. SEE: *postoperative care.*

recrement (rĕk′rē-mĕnt) [L. *recrementum,* sifted again]. Secretion, such as the saliva or part of the bile, that, after having performed its function, is reabsorbed by the body.

recrementitious (rĕk″rē-mĕn-tĭsh′ŭs). Of the nature of a secretion that, having performed its function, is reabsorbed by the body.

recrudescence (rē″kroo-dĕs′ĕns) [L. *recrudescere,* to get worse]. Return of symptoms after a remission. SYN: *relapse.*

recrudescent (rē″kroo-dĕs′ĕnt). Assuming renewed activity after dormant or inactive period.

recruitment (rē-kroot′mĕnt) [O. Fr. *recrute,* new growth]. 1. Condition in which response in a reflex action increases to a maximum when a stimulus is prolonged, even though strength of stimulus is unchanged; due to activation of increasingly greater numbers of motor neurons. Ex.: If, while testing the patellar reflex, the normal patient clasps his hands together and attempts to pull them apart, the intensity of the reflex response will be increased. SEE: *Jendrassik's maneuver.* 2. In audiology, an increase in the perceived intensity of a sound out of proportion to the actual increase in the sound level.

recruitment of end-organs. Increase in discharge from sensory end-organs, resulting from increase in number of end-organs discharging and increase in frequency in discharge from each.

rectal (rĕk'tăl) [L. *rectus,* straight]. Pert. to the rectum.
rectal alimentation. Rectal feeding.
rectal anesthesia. Introduction of anesthetic into rectum for local desensitization, used esp. in labor.
rectal crisis. Tenesmus and rectal pain in locomotor ataxia.
rectal feeding. The introduction of nutrients in fluid form into the colon through the rectum. SYN: *enema, nutrient; nutritive enema.*
rectalgia (rĕk-tăl'jē-ă) [L. *rectus,* straight, + Gr. *algos,* pain]. Pain in rectum.
rectal reflex. The normal desire to evacuate feces present in rectum.
rectectomy (rĕk-tĕk'tō-mē) [" + Gr. *ektome,* excision]. Excision of the rectum or anus. SYN: *proctectomy.*
rectification (rĕk"tĭ-fĭ-kā'shŭn) [" + *facere,* to make]. 1. The process of refining or purifying a substance. 2. Act of straightening or correcting. 3. Process of changing an alternating current into a direct current.
rectified (rĕk'tĭ-fīd). Made pure or straight. Set right.
rectifier (rĕk'tĭ-fī"ĕr) [L. *rectum,* straight, + *-ficare,* to make]. In electricity, a device for transforming an alternating current into a direct one.
rectitis (rĕk-tī'tĭs) [" + Gr. *itis,* inflammation]. Inflamed condition of the rectum. SYN: *proctitis.*
recto- [L. *rectum,* straight]. Combining form meaning straight or the rectum.
rectoabdominal (rĕk"tō-ăb-dŏm'ĭ-năl) [" + *abdomen,* belly]. Concerning the rectum and abdomen.
rectocele (rĕk'tō-sēl) [" + Gr. *kele,* hernia]. Protrusion or herniation of posterior vaginal wall with anterior wall of rectum through the vagina. SEE: *cystocele.*
rectoclysis (rĕk-tŏk'lĭ-sĭs) [" + Gr. *klysis,* a washing out]. Slow introduction of fluid into rectum.
rectococcygeal (rĕk-tō-kŏk-sĭj'ē-ăl) [" + Gr. *kokkyx,* coccyx]. Concerning the rectum and the coccyx.
rectococcypexia (rĕk"tō-kŏk-sĭ-pĕks'sē-ă) [" + " + *pexis,* fixation]. Fixation of rectum by suturing it to coccyx.
rectocolitis (rĕk"tō-kō-lī'tĭs) [" + Gr. *kolon,* colon, + *itis,* inflammation]. Inflamed condition of rectum and colon. SYN: *proctocolitis.*
rectocystotomy (rĕk"tō-sĭs-tŏt'ō-mē) [" + Gr. *kystis,* bladder, + *tome,* incision]. Incision of the bladder through rectum, usually to remove a calculus.
rectolabial (rĕk"tō-lā'bē-ăl) [" + *labium,* lip]. Concerning the rectum and a labium of the vaginal introitus.
rectoperineorrhaphy (rĕk"tō-pĕr"ĭ-nē-or'ă-fē). Surgical repair of the anus and perineum. SYN: *proctoperineoplasty.*
rectopexy (rĕk'tō-pĕk-sē) [" + Gr. *pexis,* fixation]. Fixation of rectum by suturing to another part. SYN: *proctopexy.*
rectophobia (rĕk"tō-fō'bē-ă) [" + Gr. *phobos,* fear]. Acute anxiety concerning the possibility of having cancer in those patients with rectal disease.
rectoplasty (rĕk'tō-plăs"tē) [" + Gr. *plassein,* to form]. Plastic surgery on the anus and rectum. SYN: *proctoplasty.*
rectorrhaphy (rĕk-tor'ă-fē) [L. *rectum,* straight, + Gr. *rhaphe,* a sewing]. Suture of rectum and anus. SYN: *proctorrhaphy.*
rectoscope (rĕk'tō-skōp) [" + Gr. *skopein,* to examine]. A speculum to examine the rectum.
rectoscopy (rĕk-tŏs'kō-pē). Proctoscopy.
rectosigmoid (rĕk"tō-sĭg'moyd) [" + Gr. *sigma,* letter S, + *eidos,* form]. Upper part of rectum and adjoining portion of the sigmoid colon.
rectosigmoidectomy (rĕk"tō-sĭg"moy-dĕk'tō-mē) [" + " + *ektome,* excision]. Surgical removal of the rectum and sigmoid colon.
rectostenosis (rĕk"tō-stĕn-ō'sĭs) [" + Gr. *stenosis,* a narrowing]. Stricture of the rectum.
rectostomy (rĕk-tŏs'tō-mē) [" + Gr. *stoma,* a mouth]. Creation of an artificial opening into the rectum to relieve stricture. SYN: *proctostomy.*
rectotomy (rĕk-tŏt'ō-mē) [" + Gr. *tome,* an incision]. Incision for stricture of the rectum or other purposes. SYN: *proctotomy.*
rectourethral (rĕk"tō-ū-rē'thrăl) [" + Gr. *ourethra,* urethra]. Concerning the rectum and urethra.
rectouterine (rĕk"tō-ū'tĕr-ĭn) [" + *uterus,* womb]. Concerning the rectum and uterus.
rectovaginal (rĕk"tō-văj'ĭ-năl) [" + *vagina,* sheath]. Concerning the rectum and vagina.
rectovesical (rĕk"tō-vĕs'ĭ-kăl) [" + *vesica,* a small vessel]. Concerning the rectum and bladder.
rectovestibular (rĕk"tō-vĕs-tĭb'ū-lăr) [" + *vestibulum,* vestibule]. Concerning the rectum and the vestibule of the vagina.
rectovulvar (rĕk"tō-vŭl'văr) [" + *vulva,* covering]. Concerning the rectum and the vulva.
rectum (rĕk'tŭm) [L., straight]. Lower part of large intestine, about 5 in. (12.7 cm.) long, between sigmoid flexure and the anal canal. The centers for the defecation reflex are located in the medulla and 2nd, 3rd, and 4th sacral segments. SEE: *color* for illus.

PREPARATIONS SOMETIMES GIVEN BY RECTUM: *Chloral Hydrate:* Prescribed dose dissolved in 3 oz. (90 ml.) of warm olive oil; 3 oz. (90 ml.) of very warm milk; or 3 oz. (90 ml.) of thin boiled cornstarch water. This makes a good preparation or base to hold the medicine in suspension. If adverse effects are noticed, as indicated by a sudden change in vital signs, action should be taken to prevent further absorption. A cleansing enema will accomplish this. SEE: *enema.*

Paraldehyde: Prescribed dose may be mixed with water in the proportion of 1:8, and in this ratio it may be mixed with thin starch water for rectal medication. There should be about 3 oz. (90 ml.) of starch water.

Sodium Bicarbonate: Four grams to 500 ml., or 1 pt. of water aids in the expulsion of the bowel content. The neutralizing action on the acidity of the bowel content brought about by the sodium bicarbonate solution leaves the bowel soothed and with a bland reaction.

RS: anorectal; anus; archocele; archoptosis; archorrhagia; archostenosis; cloaca; colon; enema; feeding, rectal; hemorrhoid; sigmoid; "proct-" or "rect-" words.

rectus (rĕk'tŭs) [L.]. Straight; not crooked.

rectus muscles. 1. Two external abdominal muscles, one on each side, from pubic bone to the ensiform cartilage and 5th, 6th, and 7th ribs. 2. Four short muscles of the eye: exterior, interior, superior, and inferior.

recumbency (rē-kŭm'bĕn-sē) [L. *recumbens,* lying down]. State of leaning or reclining.

recumbent. 1. Lying down. SEE: *left lateral recumbent position; position, unilateral recumbent; prone.* 2. Inactive, idle.

recuperation (rē-kū"pĕr-ā'shŭn) [L. *recuperare,* to recover]. Restoration to normal health.

recurrence (rē-kŭr'ĕns) [L. *re,* again, + *currere,* to run]. Return of symptoms after a period of quiescence, as in recurrent fever and in yellow fever. SYN: *relapse.*

recurrent (rē-kŭr'ĕnt) [L. *recurrens,* returning]. Returning at intervals, as a fever.

recurvation (rē"kŭr-vā'shŭn) [L. *recurvus,* bent back]. The act of bending backward.

recurve (rē-kŭrv'). Bend backward.

red (rĕd) [AS. *read*]. A primary color of the spectrum.

r., Congo. An odorless reddish-brown powder used as an indicator in testing for free hydrochloric acid in gastric fluids. Also used in testing for amyloid. In polarized light, amyloid treated with Congo red produces a green fluorescence.

r., cresol. An indicator of pH. It is yellow below pH of 7.4 and red above 9.0.

r., methyl. An indicator of pH. It is red at pH 4.4 and yellow at 6.2.

r., neutral. An indicator of pH. It is red at pH 6.8 and yellow at 8.0.

r., phenol. Phenolsulfonphthalein, a chemical used in testing renal function. It is also an indicator of pH. It is yellow at pH 6.8 and red at 8.4.

r., scarlet. An azo dye used in staining tissues for microscopic examination.

r., vital. A stain used in preparing tissues for microscopic examination.

red blindness. Inability to see red hues. The most frequent type of color blindness.

red blood cell. Blood corpuscle containing hemoglobin. SYN: *erythrocyte.*

r.b.c., spiculed. Spiculed red cell, q.v.

red cross. A red cross on a white background is an internationally recognized sign of a medical installation or of medical personnel. It is also the emblem of the American Red Cross.

redia (rē'dē-ă). [Francesco Redi, It. naturalist, 1626–1698] (pl. *rediae*) Stage in life cycle of a trematode following the sporocyst. The organisms are sac-like structures, possessing an oral sucker and a blind gut. They arise parthenogenetically from germ masses within the sporocyst and in turn give rise to second- or third-generation rediae or to cercaria.

redifferentiation (rē"dĭf-ĕr-ĕn"shē-ā'shŭn). The resuming of the characteristics of mature cells by malignant cells.

red. in pulv. L. *reductus in pulverum,* reduced to powder.

redintegration (rĕd-ĭn"tē-grā'shŭn) [L. *redintegratio*]. 1. Restitution of a part. 2. Restoration to health. 3. Recall by mental association.

Redisol. Trade name for cyanocobalamin, USP.

red lead. Lead tetroxide, Pb_3O_4. Also called minium.

red nucleus. Gray matter in the tegmentum of the midbrain. SYN: *nucleus ruber,* q.v.

red-out (rĕd'owt). A term used in aerospace medicine to describe what happens to the vision and central nervous system, i.e., seeing red and perhaps experiencing unconsciousness, when the aircraft is doing part or all of an outside loop at high speed, or any other maneuver that causes the pilot to experience a negative force of gravity. The condition is due to engorgement of the vessels of the head including those of the retina.

redox. Combined form indicating oxidation-reduction system or reaction.

red precipitate. Red mercuric oxide. Poisoning symptoms are similar to those of mercuric chloride, q.v.

redressement (rĕ-drĕs-mŏn') [Fr.]. 1. Correction of a deformity. 2. Dressing of a wound more than once.

reduce (rē-dūs') [L. *re,* again, + *ducere,* to lead]. 1. To restore to usual relationship, as the ends of a fractured bone. 2. To weaken, as a solution. 3. To diminish, as in bulk or weight.

reducible (rē-dūs'ĭ-bl). Capable of being replaced in a normal position, as a dislocated bone or a hernia.

reducing agent. A substance that loses electrons easily, hence causes other substances to be reduced.

Ex.: hydrogen sulfide; sulfur dioxide.

reductant (rē-dŭk'tănt). The atom that is oxidized in an oxidation-reduction reaction.

reductase (rē-dŭk'tās) [" + *ducere,* to lead, + *ase,* enzyme]. An enzyme accelerating process of reduction of chemical compounds.

reduction (rē-dŭk'shŭn) [L. *reductio,* leading back]. 1. Restoration to normal position, as a fractured bone or a hernia. 2. In chemistry, a type of reaction in which a substance gains electrons and positive valence is decreased. SEE: *oxidation.*

r. of fractures, closed. Treatment of fractures of bones by placing the bones in proper position, i.e., reducing the fragments without the use of surgery.

r. of fractures, open. Treatment of fractures of bones by the use of surgery to place the bones in proper position, i.e., reducing the fragments.

reduction division. Cell division occurring in gametogenesis following synapsis in which diploid number of chromosomes is reduced to the haploid number (one half the diploid number). SYN: *meiosis.*

redundant (rē-dŭn'dĕnt) [L. *redundare,* to overflow]. More than necessary.

reduplicated (rē-dū'plĭ-kā"tĕd) [L. *re,* again, + *duplicare,* to double]. 1. Doubled. 2. Bent backward upon itself, as a fold.

reduplication (rē-dū"plĭ-kā'shŭn). 1. A doubling, as of the heart sounds in some morbid conditions. 2. A fold.

Reduviidae (rē"dū-vī'ĭ-dē). A family of the order Hemiptera, including the assassin bugs.

Reduvius (rē-dū'vē-ŭs). A genus of true bugs belonging to the family Reduviidae.

R. personatus. A species that normally feeds on other insects, but sometimes attacks man, inflicting painful bites about the face. In some individuals, these bugs may cause severe allergic symptoms. SYN: *kissing bug.*

Reed-Sternberg cell. [Dorothy Reed, U.S. pathologist, b. 1874; Karl Sternberg, Viennese pathologist, b. 1872] A giant connective tissue cell with one or two large nuclei that is characteristic of Hodgkin's disease.

re-education (rē"ĕd-ū-kā'shŭn) [L. *re,* again, + *educare,* to educate]. 1. Training to partially restore lost competence to a disabled or mentally ill person. 2. Physical means for restoring muscular tone and activity.

reef (rēf). A fold or a tuck, usually taken in redundant tissue.

re-entry (rē-ĕn'trē). In cardiology, the diversion of a repolarization wave going in one direction where it is blocked to another where it is not blocked. The wave then goes back up the pathway that was blocked but is no longer blocked to produce a contraction. This leads to a continuing series of premature beats.

refection (rē-fĕk'shŭn) [L. *reficere*]. 1. Act of restoring. 2. In the laboratory rat, recovery from symptoms of vitamin B-complex deficiency on a diet deficient in vitamin B. Thought to be due to bacterial synthesis of vitamins by intestinal bacteria.

reference man. Concept used in nutritional investigation and surveys. A man 22 years of age, weight 70 kg., living in an environment with a mean temperature of 20°C., wearing clothing compatible with thermal comfort, engaged in light physical activity, and with an estimated caloric intake of 2800 kcal./day.

reference woman. A hypothetical model used in nutritional references, described the same as reference man, q.v., except in weight (58 kg.) and caloric intake (2000 kcal./day).

referred pain. Pain felt in a part removed from its point of origin. Referred pain is usually the result of visceral pain and it is usually referred to areas distant from the viscus. Pain from the heart, angina pectoris, may be referred to either arm, but most commonly the left, or to the ear, jaw, back, or teeth.

refine (rē-fīn') [L. *re,* again, + ME. *fin,* finished]. To purify or render free from foreign material.

reflection (rē-flĕk'shŭn) [L. *reflexio,* a bending back]. 1. Condition of being turned back upon itself, as when the peritoneum passes from wall of a body cavity to and around an organ and back to the body wall. 2. The throwing back of a ray of radiant energy from a surface not penetrated. 3. Mental consideration of some previous subject matter.

reflector (rē-flĕk'tor) [L. *re,* again, + *flectere,* to bend]. Device or surface that reflects waves of radiant energy or sound.

reflex (rē'flĕks) [L. *reflexus,* bent back]. An involuntary response to a stimulus; a reflex action. Reflexes are specific and predictable and are usually purposeful and adaptive. Reflexes depend upon an intact neural pathway between point of stimulation and responding organ (muscle or gland). This pathway is called reflex arc. In a simple reflex this includes a sensory receptor, afferent or sensory neuron, reflex center in brain or spinal cord, one or more efferent neurons, and an effector organ (muscle or gland). Most reflexes, however, are more complicated and include internuncial or associative neurons intercalated between afferent and efferent neurons. SEE: *arc, reflex,* for illus.

RS: Achilles jerk; areflexia; chemoreflex; chin jerk; conditioned reflex; consensual; intestinal reflex; jaw jerk reflex; jerk; reaction; reinforcement reflex; Setchenov's inhibitory centers; and reflexes under individual names.

r., abdominal. SEE: *abdominal reflexes.*

r., abdominocardiac. A change in heart

rate, usually a slowing, resulting from mechanical stimulation of abdominal viscera.

r., accommodation. The changes that take place when the eye adjusts to bring light rays from an object to focus on the retina. This involves change in the size of the pupil, convergence or divergence of the eyes, and either a decrease or increase in the convexity of the lens depending upon the previous condition of the lens.

r., Achilles. SEE: *Achilles tendon reflex.*

r., acquired. R., conditioned.

r., after-discharge of. Reflex activity that persists for a time after cessation of the stimulus.

r.'s, allied. Reflexes initiated by several stimuli originating in widely separated receptors whose impulses follow the final common path to effector organ and reinforce one another.

r., anal. SEE: *anal reflex.*

r., ankle. SEE: *ankle jerk.*

r.'s, antagonistic. Two or more reflexes initiated simultaneously in different receptors that involve the same motor center but produce opposite effects. The most important or adaptive response takes place.

r., auditory. SEE: *auditory reflex.*

r., autonomic. Any reflex involving the response of a visceral effector (cardiac muscle, smooth muscle, glands). Such reflexes always involve two efferent neurons (a preganglionic and postganglionic).

r., autonomic, true. A visceral response in which afferent impulses do not pass through central nervous system, but instead enter prevertebral ganglia where connections are made with efferent neurons.

r., axon. A reflex that does not involve a complete reflex arc, hence is not a true reflex. The afferent and efferent limbs of the reflex are branches of a single nerve fiber, the axon (axonlike dendrite) of a sensory neuron. An example is vasodilation resulting from stimulation of skin.

r., Babinski's. SEE: *Babinski's reflex.*

r., biceps. Flexion of forearm upon percussion of tendon of biceps brachii.

r., Brain's. SEE: *Brain's reflex.*

r., carotid sinus. Pressure in the area of the neck over the carotid sinus causes reflex slowing of the heart.

r., cat's eye. A pupillary flash or reflection from the eye that may be momentary, may be white, yellow, or pinkish, and is best seen under diminished natural illumination. This reflex, which may be noticed first by a child's parent, may be caused by a variety of conditions, the most important of which is retinoblastoma. Also observed in tuberous sclerosis, inflammatory diseases of the eye, and certain congenital malformations of the eye. SEE: *retinoblastoma.*

r., Chaddock's. SEE: *Chaddock's reflexes.*

r., chain. A reflex initiated by several separate serial reflexes each of which was activated by the preceding one.

r., chin. SEE: *chin reflex.*

r., ciliary. SEE: *ciliary reflex.*

r., ciliospinal. SEE: *ciliospinal reflex.*

r., clasp-knife. Quick inhibition of the stretch reflex when extensor muscles are forcibly stretched by flexing the limb. SYN: *reaction, lengthening.*

r., conditioned. A reflex acquired as a result of training in which the cerebral cortex is an essential part of the neural mechanism. Any reflex not inborn or inherited.

r., conjunctival. SEE: *conjunctival reflex.*

r., consensual. R., crossed.

r., convulsive. Condition in which a weak stimulus will induce a convulsion resulting in widespread uncoordinated and purposeless actions. Seen in strychnine poisoning.

r., corneal. SEE: *corneal reflex.*

r., cough. SEE: *cough reflex.*

r., cranial. Any reflex whose center lies in the brain.

r., cremasteric. SEE: *cremasteric reflex.*

r., crossed. Reflex in which stimulation of one side of the body results in response on the opposite side. SYN: *r., consensual; r., indirect.*

r., crossed extension. Extension of the opposite side lower extremity when a painful stimulus is applied to the skin.

r., deep. Reflex caused by stimulation of parts beneath skin, like tendons or bones, as the jaw, elbow, wrist, triceps, knee, and ankle jerk reflexes.

r., delayed. Reflex not taking place until some seconds after application of stimulus.

r., digital. SEE: *digital reflex.*

r., elbow. R., triceps.

r., elementary. A typical reflex common to all vertebrates. Includes postural, flexion, stretch, and extensor thrust reflexes.

r., embrace. SEE: *embrace reflex.*

r., extensor thrust. A quick and brief extension of a limb upon application of pressure to plantar surface.

r., flexor withdrawal. Flexion of the lower extremity when the foot receives a painful stimulus.

r., gag. SEE: *gag reflex.*

r., gastrocolic. SEE: *gastrocolic reflex.*

r., gastroileal. SEE: *gastroileal reflex.*

r., grasp. Grasping reaction of the fingers and toes when stimulated.

r., Hering-Breuer. SEE: *Hering-Breuer reflex.*

r., Hoffman's. Flicking of the tip of the

nail of either the ring, middle, or index finger produces flexion of the terminal phalanx of the thumb and the second and third phalanges of another finger.

r., inborn. An unconditioned reflex; an innate or inherited reflex.

r., indirect. R., crossed.

r.'s, inhibition of. Prevention of a reflex action, as inhibiting a sneeze by pressure on facial nerve as it passes just under the upper lip

r., intersegmental. Reflex in which several segments of spinal cord are involved.

r., intestinal. R., myenteric.

r., intrasegmental. Reflex that involves only a single segment of the spinal cord.

r.'s, irradiation of. The spreading of reflexes through the central nervous system whereby impulses entering the cord in one segment activate motor neurons located in many segments.

r., jaw. Chin reflex, q.v.

r., kinetic. R., labyrinthine.

r., knee-jerk. Extension of the leg resulting from percussion of patellar tendon. This is an example of a myotatic or stretch reflex of importance in the maintenance of posture. The reflex is diminished or abolished in lesions of the nerve supplying the muscle and tendon, lesions of posterior roots involving a sensory pathway as in tabes dorsalis, lesions of anterior root involving motor pathways, or lesions of lower motor neurons in anterior horns of gray matter of spinal cord, as in poliomyelitis. If, however, the upper motor neuron is destroyed, muscle tone and the motor response are greatly increased. So-called pathologic reflexes under these conditions may appear. Reflexes are also modified by higher centers, e.g., emotional tension increases the knee jerk (and muscle tension generally). SEE: *Babinski's reflex; Jendrassik's maneuver.*

r., labyrinthine. A reflex, esp. a postural reflex, resulting from stimulation of receptors in semicircular ducts, utricle, and saccule of inner ear. SYN: *r., kinetic.*

r., light. SEE: *light reflex.*

r., local. Reflex that does not involve the central nervous system.

Ex.: the myenteric reflex, which occurs even though extrinsic nerves to intestine have been cut.

r., long. Reflex involving many segments of the spinal cord.

r., lung. Dilatation of the lung tissue under the area of the skin that is irritated by percussion or cold.

r., Magnus-de Kleijn. In decerebrate rigidity, extension of the limbs on the side to which the chin is turned by rotating the head. There is flexion of the limbs of the opposite side.

r., mass. Condition following a section of spinal cord in which a weak stimulus through radiation brings about widespread responses due to release from inhibition of higher cortical centers.

r., Mayer's. Downward pressure on the index finger is followed by opposition and adduction of the thumb, flexion at the metacarpophalangeal joint, and extension at the interphalangeal joint.

r., Mendel-Bechtereu. Plantar flexion of the toes in response to percussion of the dorsum of the foot.

r., monosynaptic. Reflex involving only two neurons, an afferent and efferent.

r., Moro. SEE: *Moro reflex.*

r., myenteric. Reflex caused by distention of the intestine, resulting in contraction above the point of stimulation, and relaxation below it. SYN: *r., intestinal.*

r., myotatic. R., stretch

r., near. R., accommodation.

r., neck-righting. In the infant, rotation of the trunk in the same direction in response to the direction the head of the supine infant is turned. This reflex appears at age 4 to 6 months and is no longer obtainable by age 2 years.

r., nociceptive. A reflex initiated by a painful stimulus.

r., optical righting. Use of visual stimuli to maintain the normal position of the body and head.

r., palatal. SEE: *palatal reflex.*

r., palmar grasp. The lightly stimulated palm grasps the stimulating object. This reflex is present at birth and is gone by the age of 6 months.

r., palm-chin. Vigorous stroking or scratching of the thenar eminence, producing contraction of the skin and lower lip muscles on the same side.

r. (reaction), parachute. Extension of the arms, hands, and fingers when the infant is suspended in the prone position and dropped a short distance onto a soft surface. This reaction appears at 9 months of age and persists.

r., patellar. R., knee-jerk.

r., pathologic. Abnormal reflex due to disease; the reflex is seen as one of the symptoms of the disease.

r., pharyngeal. SEE: *pharyngeal reflex.*

r., pilomotor. SEE: *pilomotor reflex.*

r., placing. The infant is held erect and the dorsum of one foot is dragged along the under-edge of a table top. The response is flexion of that leg and then extension. This reflex is present at birth and is no longer present by age 6 weeks.

r., plantar. SEE: *plantar reflex; Babin-*

ski's reflex.

r., plantar grasp. Light stimulation of the sole of the foot produces a grasp reflex of the foot. This reflex is present at birth and is gone by the age of 10 months.

r., postural. Any reflex that is concerned with maintenance of posture.

r., pressor. A reflex that results in elevation of blood pressure brought about by constriction of arterioles.

r., proprioceptive. Reflexes initiated by movement of the body to maintain the position of the moved part. Any reflex initiated by stimulation of a proprioceptor.

r., psychogalvanic. Decreased electric resistance of the skin in response to emotional stress or stimuli.

r., pupillary. Reflex that occurs when a beam of light strikes the retina, causing the pupil to contract (protective against excessive stimulation). The same effect results with accommodation to near objects.

r., quadriceps. R., knee-jerk, q.v.

r., quadrupedal extensor. Brain's reflex, q.v.

r., red. The red light reflection seen when examining the eye by use of the ophthalmoscope.

r., righting. Any of the reflexes that enable an animal to maintain the body in a definite relationship to the head and thus maintain its body right side up.

r., rooting. Stroking the cheek of the infant causes turning of the mouth toward the stimulus. This reflex is present at birth; by 7 months of age it is gone if done while the infant is asleep; and is gone by 4 months if done while the infant is awake.

r., Rossolimo's. SEE: *R.'s reflex.*

r.'s, sexual. Reflexes concerned with sexual activities, esp. erection and ejaculation.

r., short. Reflex involving one or a few segments of spinal cord.

r., somatic. Reflex induced by stimulation of somatic sensory nerve endings.

r., spinal. A reflex whose center is in the spinal cord.

r., startle. R., Moro's, q.v.

r., static. Reflex concerned with establishment and maintenance of posture when body is at rest.

r.'s, statokinetic. Reflexes occurring when body is moving, e.g., walking or running.

r., stepping. Movements of progression elicited when the infant is held upright, inclined forward, as the soles of the feet are touching a flat surface. This reflex is present at birth and is gone by 6 weeks of age.

r., stretch. Contraction of a muscle as a result of stretching the same muscle. SYN: *r., myotatic.*

r., sucking. Sucking movements of the infant produced by stroking the lips.

r., superficial. Cutaneous reflex caused by irritation of the skin or areas depending upon the spinal cord as a motor center, such as the scapular, epigastric, abdominal, cremasteric, gluteal, and plantar reflexes, or upon centers in the medulla, such as conjunctival, pupillary, and palatal reflexes.

r., swallowing. Production of the succession of reflexes and muscular activity concerned with swallowing when the palate is stimulated by food.

r., tendon. Deep reflex obtained by sharply tapping skin over tendon of a muscle. It is exaggerated in disease of an upper neuron and diminished or lost in disease of lower neuron.

r., tonic neck. In the infant, forcibly turning the head causes extension of one or both extremities on the side to which the head is turned. There is flexion of the extremities on the other side.

r., tonic neck, asymmetrical. Presence of the tonic neck reflex in which the reflex is abnormal on one side. SEE: *r., tonic neck.*

r., triceps. Sharp extension of forearm resulting from tapping of triceps tendon while arm is held loosely in bent position. SYN: *r., elbow.*

r., triceps surae. Achilles tendon reflex, q.v.

r., unconditioned. A natural or inherited reflex action; one not acquired.

r., vascular. R., vasomotor, q.v.

r., vasomotor. Constriction or dilatation of a blood vessel in response to a stimulus, as in becoming pale from fright. SYN: *r., vascular.*

r., visceral. Any reflex induced by stimulation of visceral nerves.

r., visceromotor. Contraction or tenseness of skeletal muscles resulting from painful stimuli originating in visceral organs.

reflex action. An involuntary response to a stimulus; a reflex.

reflex arc. The neural pathway or circuit between the point of stimulation and the responding organ in a reflex action. SEE: *arc, reflex,* for illus.

reflex center. A region, usually in the brain or spinal cord, where impulses from an afferent limb of a reflex arc initiate impulses in the efferent limb.

reflexogenic (rē-flĕks″ō-jĕn′ĭk) [L. *reflexus,* bent back, + Gr. *gennan,* to produce]. Causing a reflex action.

reflexogenous (rē″flĕks-ŏj′ĕ-nŭs). Reflexogenic, q.v.

reflexograph (rē-flĕks′ō-grăf) [″ + Gr. *graphein,* to write]. Device for recording and graphing a reflex, esp. one produced by muscular activity.

reflexology (rē"flĕk-sŏl'ō-jē) [" + Gr. *logos,* study]. Study of reflexes.

reflexometer (rē"flĕks-ŏm'ĕ-tĕr) [" + Gr. *metron,* measure]. Instrument for measuring force of the tap required to produce a reflex.

reflexophil (rē-flĕks'ō-fĭl) [L. *reflexus,* reflex, + Gr. *philein,* to love]. Characterized by activity of reflexes or by exaggerated reflexes.

reflexotherapy (rē-flĕks"ō-thĕr'ă-pē) [" + Gr. *therapeia,* treatment]. Treatment by manipulation, anesthetizing, or cauterizing an area distant from seat of the disorder. SEE: *spondylotherapy.*

reflux (rē'flŭks) [L. *re,* back, + *fluxus,* flow]. A return or backward flow. SEE: *regurgitation.*

r., hepatojugular. Pressure on the liver in patients with congestive heart failure causes increased pressure in the cervical venous pressure.

r., vesicoureteral. Reflux of urine up the ureter during micturition.

refract (rē-frăkt') [L. *refractus,* broken away]. 1. To turn back; to deflect. 2. To detect errors of refraction in the eyes and to correct them.

refracta dosi (rē-frăk'tă dō'sē) [L.]. In divided doses, denoting a definite amount of a drug taken within a given time in a number of fractional equal parts.

refraction (rē-frăk'shŭn) [L. *refractio,* break back]. 1. Deflection from a straight path, as of light rays as they pass through media of different densities; the change of direction of a ray when it passes from one medium to another of a different density. 2. Determination of amount of ocular refractive errors and their correction.

RS: ametropia; anisometropia; astigmatism; emmetropia; hypermetropia; myopia; presbyopia.

r., angle of. The angle formed by a refracted ray of light with a line perpendicular to surface at point of refraction.

r., coefficient of. The quotient or sine of angle of incidence divided by sine of angle of refraction.

r., double. Possessing more than one refractive index, resulting in a double image. SEE: *birefringent.*

r., dynamic. Static refraction of the eye plus that accomplished by accommodation; the reciprocal of the near-point distance.

r., errors of. Condition in which parallel rays of light are not brought to a focus upon the retina because of a defect in shape of the eyeball or in refracting media of the eye. SYN: *ametropia.*

r., index of. 1. Ratio of angle made by incident ray with the perpendicular (angle of incidence) to that made by emergent ray (angle of refraction). 2. The ratio of speed of light in air to its speed in another medium. The refractive index of water is 1.33; of crystalline lens of the eye it is 1.413.

r., ocular. R. of eye.

r. of eye. Ocular refraction brought about by refractive media of the eye (cornea, aqueous humor, crystalline lens, vitreous body).

r., static. Refraction of the eye when accommodation is at rest or paralyzed.

refractionist (rē-frăk'shŭn-ĭst) [L. *refractio,* break back]. One skilled in determining and correcting ocular refractive errors by use of appropriate glass lenses.

refractive (rē-frăk'tĭv) [L. *refractus*]. Concerning refraction.

refractive power. The degree to which a transparent body deflects a ray of light from a straight path. SEE: *diopter.*

refractivity (rē"frăk-tĭv'ĭ-tē). The quality of being refractive; the ability to refract.

refractometer (rē-frăk-tŏm'ĕt-ĕr) [" + Gr. *metron,* measure]. Device for measuring refractive power, as of the eye.

refractometry (rē"frăk-tŏm'ĕ-trē). Measurement of refractive power of lenses.

refractory (rē-frăk'tō-rē) [L. *refractarius*]. 1. Obstinate, stubborn. 2. Resistant to ordinary treatment. 3. Resistant to stimulation, said of muscle or nerve.

refractory period, relative. Brief period of relaxation of a muscle during which excitability is depressed. If stimulated, it will respond, but a stronger stimulus is required and response is less.

refracture (rē-frăk'chūr) [L. *refractus,* broken away]. 1. To break again, as a bone set wrongly. 2. Rebreaking of a fracture united in a malaligned or incorrect position.

refrangible (rē-frăn'jĭ-bl) [L. *re,* again, + ME. *frangible,* breakable]. Capable of being refracted.

refresh (rē-frĕsh') [O. Fr. *refreschir,* to renew]. 1. To restore strength; to relieve from fatigue; to renew; to revive. 2. To scrape epithelial covering from two opposing surfaces of a wound to facilitate the healing and joining together.

refrigerant (rē-frĭj'ĕr-ănt) [L. *refrigerans,* to make cold]. 1. Cooling. 2. Agent that produces coolness or reduces fever. SYN: *algefacient.*

refrigerant gases. A number of these gases are used in ordinary household refrigerators; poisoning due to leaks, faulty connections or breakage, and gas dissipated into atmosphere may occur.

refrigeration (rē-frĭj"ĕr-ā'shŭn) [L. *refrigeratio*]. Cooling; reduction of heat.

refrigeration anesthesia. Anesthesia resulting from cold, such as that produced in a limb by immersion in cold water.

refringent. Refractive.

Refsum's disease (rĕf'soomz). [S. Refsum, contemporary Norwegian physician] An inherited metabolic disease due to inability to metabolize phytanic acid. Clinically there are visual disturbances, ataxia, and heart disease. Diets low in animal fat and milk products may relieve some of the symptoms.

refusion (rē-fū'zhŭn) [L. *refusus,* poured back]. The return of blood into the same circulatory system from which it was removed.

regainer (rē-gān'ĕr). 1. A device that ameliorates or restores that which was lost. 2. A device that applies pressure between teeth on either side of the space left by a missing tooth. This is done to push the teeth away from the edentulous space.

regel [Ger.]. Menstruation.

r. Kleine. Slight bloody discharge from the uterus at time of ovulation.

regeneration (rē-jĕn"ĕr-ā'shŭn) [L. *re,* again, + *generare,* to produce]. Repair, regrowth, or restoration of a part, as tissues. Opposite of degeneration.

regimen (rĕj'ĭ-mĕn) [L., rule]. A systematic plan of activities and regulation of diet, sleep, and exercise designed to improve or maintain health or to keep a certain condition under control.

regio (rē'jē-ō) [L.]. Region.

region (rē'jŭn) [L. *regio,* boundary line]. A portion of the body with natural or arbitrary boundaries.

RS: abdomen; epigastrium; inguinal region; Kiesselbach's area; temple.

regional (rē'jŭn-ăl). Concerning a region.

register [LL. *registra,* list]. 1. An official recording of names or facts. 2. The compass or range of a voice. 3. A series of tones of like quality or character, as low or high register, chest or head register.

registered nurse. A nurse who has graduated from a school of nursing, passed the State Board Examination administered by a State Board of Nursing Examiners, and is granted the right to practice for hire. The nurse is registered and licensed to practice.

registrant (rĕj'ĭs-trănt) [L. *registrans,* registering]. A nurse who is named on the books of a registry as being "on call" or available to be called for duty.

registrar (rĕj'ĭs-trăr) [O. Fr. *registreur*]. The official manager of a registry.

registration [L. *registratio*]. The act of recording information such as births or deaths; or the recording of those who are registered or licensed to practice within a state.

registry (rĕj'ĭs-trē) [LL. *registra,* list]. An office or book where a list of nurses ready for duty is kept; a placement bureau for nurses.

Regitine Hydrochloride. Trade name for phentolamine hydrochloride.

Reglan. Trade name for metoclopramide hydrochloride.

Regonol. Trade name for pyridostigmine bromide, USP.

regression (rē-grĕsh'ŭn) [L. *regressio,* a going back]. 1. A turning back or return to a former state. 2. A return of symptoms. 3. Retrogression. 4. In psychology, an abnormal return to earlier reaction, characterized by mental state and behavior inappropriate to the situation. Regression may occur as a result of frustration or in states of fatigue, dreams, hypnosis, intoxication, illness, and in certain psychoses (schizophrenia). 5. In statistics, a procedure used to predict one variable on the basis of data about one or more other variables.

r., filial. In biology, tendency of offspring to deviate less from the average of a population than their parents.

regressive (rē-grĕs'ĭv). Concerning or marked by regression.

regressive resistive exercise. ABBR: RRE. A form of active resistive exercise that advocates gradual reduction in the amount of resistance as muscles fatigue.

regular (rĕg'ū-lăr) [L. *regula,* rule]. 1. Conforming to rule or custom. 2. Methodical, steady in course, as pulse. SYN: *normal; typical.*

regulation. 1. State of being controlled or directed. 2. The ability of an individual, such as a developing embryo, to develop normally in spite of experimental modifications.

regulation development. In embryology, condition in which a single blastomere, or a portion of an embryo, can give rise to a whole embryo. Opposite of mosaic development.

regulative. Pert. to regulation.

regulator. A device for adjusting or controlling the rate of flow or administration of fluids, oxygen, or blood.

regurgitant (rē-gŭr'jĭ-tănt) [L. *re,* again, + *gurgitare,* to flood]. Throwing back or flowing in a direction opposite to the normal.

regurgitation (rē-gŭr"jĭ-tā'shŭn). A backward flowing, as in the return of solids or fluids to the mouth from the stomach or the backward flow of blood through a defective heart valve.

r., aortic. Backflow of blood into the left ventricle as a result of incompetent aortic valves.

r., cardiac. Backward flow of blood through the aortic, mitral, or tricuspid valves due to incomplete closure.

r., duodenal. Return flow of chyme from the duodenum to stomach.

r., functional. Regurgitation not due to valvular disorder but to dilatation of ventricles, the great vessels, or valve rings.

r., mitral. Backflow of blood from the left ventricle into the left atrium, resulting from imperfect closure of the mitral or bicuspid valve.

r., pulmonic. Backflow of blood from the pulmonary artery into the right ventricle.

r., tricuspid. Backflow of blood from the right ventricle into the right atrium.

r., valvular. Flow of blood back through a valve, esp. a heart valve, that is not, as it would normally be, completely closed.

Regutol. Trade name for docusate sodium.

rehabilitation (rē″hă-bĭl″ĭ-tā′shŭn) [L. *rehabilitare*]. The processes of treatment and education that lead the disabled individual to attainment of maximum function, a sense of well-being, and a personally satisfying level of independence. The need for rehabilitation may be due to any disease that causes the person to be impaired either mentally or physically. The post-coronary patient, the post-trauma patient, and the post-surgical patient all need and can benefit from rehabilitation efforts. The individual who is recovering from a mental disorder is also in need of rehabilitative support. The combined efforts of the individual, family, friends, medical, nursing, allied health personnel, and community resources are essential in order to make rehabilitation possible.

rehabilitee (rē″hă-bĭl′ĭ-tē). A person rehabilitated.

rehalation (rē″hă-lā′shŭn) [L. *re*, again, + *halare*, to breathe]. Rebreathing process occasionally employed in anesthesia.

rehydration (rē″hī-drā′shŭn) [″ + Gr. *hydor*, water]. Restoration of fluid volume in a person who has been dehydrated. This may be done by use of fluids orally or parenterally.

Reichert's cartilage (rī′kĕrts). [Karl B. Reichert, Ger. anatomist, 1811–1884] The second branchial arch of the embryo, which gives rise to stapes, styloid process, stylohyoid ligament, and lesser cornua of hyoid bone.

Reid's base line (rēdz). [Robert W. Reid, Scottish anatomist, 1851–1938] Line extending from lower edge of the orbit to center of aperture of external auditory canal backward to center of occipital bone.

Reil's island (rīlz). [Johann C. Reil, Ger. anatomist, 1759–1813] Three or more small convolutions at bottom of fissure of Sylvius in the brain. SYN: *insula* [NA]; *island of Reil.*

reimplantation (rē″ĭm-plăn-tā′shŭn) [L. *re*, again, + *in*, into, + *plantare*, to set]. Replacement of a part from where it has been taken out, as a tooth, finger, hand, or arm.

reinfection (rē″ĭn-fĕk′shŭn) [″ + *infectus*, infect]. A second infection by the same organism. SEE: *superinfection*.

reinforcement (rē″ĭn-fors′mĕnt) [″ + *inforce*, enforce]. Strengthening; augmentation of force. Part of the fundamental process of learning, along with motivation, stimulation and action. The reward for the appropriate response in a learning situation.

reinforcement of reflex. Strengthening of the response to one stimulus by concurrent action of another; the exaggeration of a reflex by nervous activity elsewhere. Thus, during the raising of a heavy weight the knee jerk is stronger. SEE: *Jendrassik's maneuver.*

reinforcer (rē″ĭn-fors′ĕr). That which produces reinforcement.

reinfusion (rē″ĭn-fū′zhŭn) [″ + *infusio*, to pour in]. The reinjection of blood serum or cerebrospinal fluid.

reinnervation (rē″ĭn-ĕr-vā′shŭn) [″ + *in*, into, + *nervus*, nerve]. 1. Anastomosis of a paralyzed part with a living nerve. 2. Grafting of a fresh nerve for restoration of function in a paralyzed muscle.

reinoculation (rē″ĭn-ŏk″ū-lā′shŭn) [″ + *in*, into, + *oculus*, bud]. A second inoculation with the same virus or organism. SEE: *reinfection*.

reintegration. In psychology, the resumption of normal behavior and mental functioning following disintegration of personality in mental illness.

reinversion (rē″ĭn-vĕr′shŭn) [″ + *in*, into, + *versio*, turning]. Correction of an inverted organ, as of an inverted uterus by pressure on the fundus.

Reissner's membrane (rīs′nĕrz). [Ernest Reissner, Ger. anatomist, 1824–1878] Delicate membrane separating the cochlear canal from the scala vestibuli.

Reiter's syndrome (rī′tĕrz). [Hans Reiter, Ger. bacteriologist, 1881–1969] Syndrome consisting of urethritis, arthritis, and conjunctivitis. Urethritis usually appears first. Occurs mainly in young men.

ETIOL: Unknown.

PROG: Generally good; however recurrences are common.

TREATMENT: There is no specific therapy. Broad-spectrum antibiotics are used for urethritis. Arthritis is treated symptomatically. No treatment is necessary for the conjunctivitis.

rejection [L. *rejicere*, to throw back]. 1. Refusal to accept or to show affection for. In lower animals the young may be ignored or driven away by their mother. 2. In transplantation of tissues and organs, destruction of transplanted material at the cellular level by the host's immune mechanism.

r., acute. Early destruction of grafted or transplanted material; usually begins a week after implantation. May be reversed by increased use of immunosuppressive agents.

r., chronic. Slow destruction of grafted or transplanted material. This may occur over a period of months or years.

r., hyperacute. Immediate, intense, and

irreversible destruction of grafted material due to preformed antibodies.

rejuvenation (rē-jū″vĕ-nā′shŭn) [L. *re,* again, + *juvenis,* young]. A return to youthful conditions or to the normal.

rejuvenescence (rē-jū″vĕ-nĕs′ĕns) [″ + *juvenescere,* to become young]. The renewal of youth or return to earlier stage of existence.

Rela. Trade name for carisoprodol.

relapse (rē-lăps′) [L. *relapsus*]. Recurrence of a disease or symptoms after apparent recovery.

relapsing. Recurring after apparent recovery.

relapsing fever. An infectious disease marked by intermittent attacks of high fever.

ETIOL: Several species of spirochetes belonging to genus Borrelia and transmitted by head lice, body lice, and ticks of the genus Ornithodorus.

TREATMENT: A single dose of either tetracycline, erythromycin, or procaine penicillin G and symptomatic treatment.

relation (rē-lā′shŭn) [L. *relatio,* a carrying back]. The condition, connection, or state of one thing compared to another.

r., jaw. Any relation of the position of the maxilla to the mandible.

r., occlusal jaw. Relation of the mandibular teeth to the maxillary teeth when the teeth are in contact.

r., unstrained jaw. Position of the jaw when normal tonus of all of the jaw muscles is present.

relative biological effect. Comparison of the effectiveness of types of radiation compared with that of x-rays or gamma rays.

relax [L. *relaxare,* to loosen]. To decrease tension or intensity, or to be rid of strain, anxiety, and nervousness.

relaxant (rē-lăk′sănt). 1. Rel. to or producing relaxation. 2. A drug that reduces tension. 3. A laxative.

r., muscle. A drug or therapeutic treatment that specifically relieves muscular tension.

relaxation (rē-lăk-sā′shŭn). 1. A lessening of tension or activity in a part. 2. Phase or period in a single muscle-twitch following contraction in which tension decreases, fibers lengthen, and muscle returns to resting position.

r., general. Relaxation of the entire body.

r., local. Relaxation limited to a particular muscle group, or to a certain part.

relaxation response. The physiological reaction that is sought and produced by sitting quietly and alone in a quiet place with eyes closed and arms and hands relaxed; paying careful attention to respiration; and repeating a brief word or phrase at each respiratory cycle. This is done for 15 to 30 minutes at a time, twice daily.

This approach to quiet meditation is found in the practices of many religions, and in Transcendental Meditation.

The relaxation response has been used by some physicians to produce therapeutic alteration in control of stress, as indicated by a reduction in blood pressure in hypertensive patients.

relaxed movement. Form of bodily movement that the operator carries through without the assistance or resistance of the patient. SYN: *passive exercise.*

relaxin (rē-lăk′sĭn). A polypeptide hormone secreted in the corpus luteum during pregnancy. Obtained commercially from ovaries of pregnant sows. In certain rodents, relaxin produces relaxation of the symphysis, inhibition of uterine contractions, and softening of the cervix.

releasing hormone. Hormone, releasing, q.v.

relief (rē-lēf′) [ME.]. Alleviation or removal of a distressing or painful symptom.

relieve [L. *relever*]. To provide relief.

reline (rē-līn′). Replacing or resurfacing the lining of a denture.

REM. *rapid eye movement.* Cyclic movement of the closed eyes observed or recorded during sleep. SEE: *sleep, stages and states of.*

rem. *roentgen equivalent* (in) *man.*

Remak's axis cylinder (rā′măks). [Robert Remak, Ger. neurologist, 1815–1865] The conducting part of a nerve.

Remak's band. The axis cylinder of a neuron.

Remak's fibers. The nonmedullated nerve fibers.

Remak's ganglion. A group of nerve cells in coronary sinus near its entry into the right atrium.

Remak's sign. [Ernest Julius Remak, Ger. neurologist, 1849–1911] A sign or symptom pertaining to perception of stimuli. It can be one of two types: one in which a single stimulus is perceived as if it were several stimuli applied in separate locations (polyesthesia) or one in which there is a delay in perception of stimuli. Both are seen in tabes dorsalis.

remedial (rē-mē′dē-ăl) [L. *remedialis*]. Curative; intended for a remedy.

remedy (rĕm′ĕd-ē) [L. *remedium,* medicine]. 1. To cure or relieve a disease. 2. Anything that relieves or cures a disease.

r., local. Agent to relieve a local condition, as a sore.

r., systemic. Agent to relieve or cure a disease affecting the entire organism.

remineralization (rē-mĭn″ĕr-ăl-ĭ-zā′shŭn). Therapeutic replacement of the mineral content of the body after it has been disrupted by disease or improper diet.

remission (rē-mĭsh′ŭn) [L. *remissio,* remit]. 1. Lessening of severity or abatement of symptoms. 2. The period during which symptoms abate.

remittance (rē-mĭt'ĕns). Temporary but not permanent abatement of symptoms.

remittent (rē-mĭt'ĕnt) [L. *remittere,* to send back]. Alternately abating and returning at certain intervals. SEE: *fever.*

remittent fever. A fever alternately abating and returning, without intervals of afebrility. SEE: *malaria.*

remnant radiation. Ionizing radiation that passes through the part being examined to make the radiographic image.

Remsed. Trade name for promethazine hydrochloride, USP.

ren (rĕn) [L.]. (pl. *renes*) [NA] The kidney.

r. amyloidens. Amyloid degeneration of the kidneys.

r. mobilis. Movable kidney.

r. unguliformis. Horseshoe kidney.

renal (rē'năl) [LL. *renalis*]. 1. Pert. to the kidney. SYN: *nephric.* SEE: *kidney* and *urinary tract* for illus. 2. Shaped like a kidney.

renal clearance test. One of several kidney function tests based on the ability of the kidney to eliminate a given substance in a standard time. Urea, phenolsulfonphthalein (PSP), iodopyracet, and other substances are employed.

renal failure, acute. Acute failure of the kidney to perform its essential functions. May be due to trauma; any condition that impairs the flow of blood to the kidneys; certain toxic substances such as compounds of mercury, carbon tetrachloride, or ethylene glycol; bacterial toxins; glomerulonephritis; acute obstruction of the urinary tract.

NURSING IMPLICATIONS: Assist in identifying the cause and in its removal. Instruct patient regarding dietary restrictions including fluid limitations; implement dietary restrictions. Promote prevention of infection. Instruct patient concerning activity restrictions due to metabolic alterations; implement restrictions.

Monitor fluid and electrolyte balance. Promote skin care and oral hygiene. Assess the patient for bleeding tendencies and anemia.

Provide psychological support to the patient and the family. Explain the dialysis procedure if utilized. Promote independence. Initiate seizure precautions. Observe patient closely for drug toxicity. Assess blood values.

Refer patient for sexual and vocational counseling. Establish learning plan for the patient and the family. Provide follow-up care and evaluation.

TREATMENT: Specific therapy for primary disease; either peritoneal dialysis or hemodialysis.

renal insufficiency. The reduced capacity of the kidney to perform its functions.

renal papillary necrosis. Destruction of the papillae of the kidney. May be caused by a variety of conditions including diabetes mellitus, acute pyelonephritis, urinary obstruction, sickle cell trait, and repeated use of phenacetin. Management consists of ureteral catheter irrigation of renal pelvis to remove obstruction; appropriate antibiotics; and adequate hydration.

renal pelvis. SEE: *pelvis, renal.*

renal scanning. Method of determining renal function and shape of the kidney. A radioactive substance that concentrates in the kidney is given intravenously. The irradiation emitted from the substance as it accumulates in the kidneys is recorded on a suitable photographic film.

renal transplantation. Surgical implantation of a donor kidney to replace one removed from a patient.

renal tubule. A nephron.

Rendu-Osler-Weber disease (rŏn-dū'ōs'lĕr-wĕb'ĕr). [Henri L. M. Rendu, Fr. physician, 1844–1902; Sir William Osler, Canadian-born physician, 1849–1919; Frederick P. Weber, Brit. physician, 1863–1962] Polycythemia vera, q.v.

Renese. Trade name for polythiazide.

reniculus (rĕ-nĭk'ū-lŭs) [L.]. A lobule of the kidney.

renifleur (rā-nĭ-flūr') [Fr.]. One stimulated sexually by certain odors esp. by the urine of others.

reniform (rĕn'ĭ-form) [L. *ren,* kidney, + *forma,* shape]. Shaped like a kidney. SYN: *nephroid.*

renin (rĕn'ĭn). An enzyme, produced by the kidney, that acts on angiotensin to form a pressor substance, angiotensin I. Renin is elevated in some forms of hypertension.

renin substrate. Alpha-2-globulin of the plasma. SYN: *hypertensinogen.*

renipelvic (rĕn″ĭ-pĕl'vĭk) [″ + *pelvis,* basin]. Concerning the pelvis of the kidney.

reniportal (rĕn″ĭ-por'tăl) [″ + *porta,* gate]. 1. Concerning the "hilum" of the kidney. 2. Concerning the renal and portal circulations.

renipuncture (rĕn″ĭ-pŭnk'chūr) [L. *ren,* kidney, + *punctura,* a piercing]. Surgical puncture of the capsule of the kidney.

rennet (rĕn'ĕt) [ME.]. 1. An infusion of inner coat of calf's stomach. 2. A fluid containing rennin, a coagulating enzyme, used for making junket or cheese.

rennin (rĕn'ĭn). An enzyme that coagulates milk. Present in the gastric juice of ruminants. It is not present in the human stomach.

renninogen (rĕn-ĭn'ō-jĕn) [ME. *rennet,* rennet, + Gr. *gennan,* to produce]. Antecedent or zymogen from which rennin is formed. The inactive form of rennin.

renocutaneous (rē″nō-kū-tā'nē-ŭs) [″ + *cu-*

tis, skin]. Concerning the kidneys and the skin.

renogastric (rē″nō-găs′trĭk) [L. *ren,* kidney, + Gr. *gaster,* belly]. Concerning the kidney and stomach.

renogram (rē′nō-grăm) [″ + Gr. *gramma,* a mark]. Record of rate of removal from the blood by the kidneys of an intravenously injected dose of radioactive iodine (^{131}I).

renography (rē-nŏg′ră-fē) [″ + Gr. *graphein,* to write]. Radiography of the kidney.

renointestinal (rē″nō-ĭn-tĕs′tĭn-ăl) [″ + *intestinum,* intestine]. Concerning the kidney and the intestine.

renopathy (rē-nŏp′ă-thē) [″ + Gr. *pathos,* disease]. Any pathological condition of the kidneys.

renoprival (rē″nō-prī′văl). The condition of loss of kidney function.

Renoquid. Trade name for sulfacytine.

renotrophic (rē″nō-trŏf′ĭk) [″ + Gr. *trophe,* nourishment]. Having the ability to induce hypertrophy of the kidney.

renotropic (rē″nō-trŏp′ĭk) [″ + *trope,* a turn]. Having a special affinity for kidney tissue.

Renshaw cells (rĕn′shaw). Small cells with short axons that serve to connect motor nerve axons with each other. The process functions to inhibit motor neurons.

reovirus (rē″ō-vī′rŭs) [*r*espiratory *e*nteric *o*rphan *virus*]. Viruses found in the respiratory and digestive tracts of apparently healthy persons. Their exact importance in producing disease is not known. The group of viruses was formerly classed as ECHO virus, type 10.

rep. L. *repetator,* let it be repeated.

repair (rē-păr′) [L. *reparare,* to prepare again]. To remedy, replace, or heal, as a wound or a lost part.

r., plastic. Utilization of plastic surgery to repair tissue.

repellance [L. *repellere,* drive back]. Condition in which certain individuals are relatively immune to bites of arthropods.

repellent. An agent that repels noxious organisms such as insects, ticks, and mites. Repellents may be applied to surface of body as a liquid, spray, or dust, or they may be used to impregnate clothing.

repercolation (rē″pĕr-kō-lā′shŭn) [L. *re,* again, + *percolare,* to filter]. Repeated percolation using same materials.

repercussion (rē-pĕr-kŭsh′ŭn) [L. *repercussio,* rebound]. 1. Reciprocal action. 2. Action involved in causing subsidence of a swelling, tumor, or eruption. 3. In obstetrics, diagnosis of pregnancy by insertion of a finger into the vagina to push the uterus, causing embryo to rise and fall. SYN: *ballottement.*

repercussive (rē″pĕr-kŭs′ĭv). 1. Causing repercussion. 2. An agent that repels; a repellent.

replacement. The act of replacing.

replantation [L. *re,* again, + *planto,* to plant]. Surgical reimplantation of that which has been removed from the body, esp. the surgical procedure of rejoining a hand, arm, or leg to the body after its having been removed as a result of an accident. In dentistry, replacement of a tooth that has been removed from its socket.

repletion (rē-plē′shŭn) [L. *repletio,* a filling up]. Condition of being full or satisfied.

replication (rĕp″lĭ-kā′shŭn). 1. A doubling back of tissue. 2. In medical investigations, the repetition of an experiment. 3. In genetics, the process of duplication of genetic material.

replicon (rĕp′lĭ-kŏn). Any genetic element that behaves as an autonomous unit of DNA replication. The element is able to replicate under its own control.

Repoise. Trade name for butaperazine.

repolarization. Re-establishment of the electrical polarized state in a muscle or nerve fiber following contraction or conduction of a nerve impulse.

report. The account of the nursing staff going off duty to the oncoming staff. The purpose is to provide continuity of care despite the change in staff. The report is usually verbal. Obviously the information provided is of the utmost importance in caring for the critically ill.

reportable diseases. Diseases that must be reported by the physician to the health authorities. The communicable diseases required by International Health Regulations to be reported universally are the internationally quarantinable diseases: plague, cholera, yellow fever, and smallpox. Other diseases that require such a report are the diseases under surveillance by the World Health Organization. They are louse-borne typhus fever, relapsing fever, paralytic poliomyelitis, malaria, and influenza.

Special notification is required of all outbreaks or epidemics of diseases not listed above. Even a single case of a communicable disease long absent from a population or not previously recognized in that area is sufficient reason to require immediate reporting and institution of a full field investigation.

reposition (rē″pō-zĭsh′ŭn) [L. *repositio,* a replacing]. Restoration of an organ or tissue to its correct or original position.

repositioning (rē″pō-zĭsh′ŭn-ĭng). The placement of a part in its original place.

r., jaw. The changing of the position of the mandible in relation to the maxilla by altering occlusion of the teeth.

r., muscle. Surgical placement of a muscle to another attachment point in order to enhance function.

repositor. Instrument for restoring a tissue or an organ to its normal position.

r., inversion. Instrument for replacement of an inverted uterus.

r., uterine. A lever for replacement of the uterus when out of normal position.

repression (rē-prĕsh'ŭn) [L. *repressus,* press back]. In psychology, refusal to entertain distressing or painful ideas, thus submerging them in the unconscious, where they continue to exert their influence upon the individual. Psychoanalysis seeks to discover and to release these repressions.

r., coordinate. Simultaneous reduction of the levels of enzymes of a metabolic pathway.

r., enzyme. An enzyme that interferes with a metabolic pathway, usually the same pathway that produced the enzyme.

repressor (rē-prĕs'or) [L. *repressus,* press back]. Something, esp. an enzyme, that inhibits or interferes with the initiation of protein synthesis by genetic material.

reproduction (rē-prō-dŭk'shŭn) [L. *re,* again, + *productio,* production]. 1. Process by which plants and animals give rise to offspring. SEE: *ovary* for illus. 2. The creation of a similar structure or situation; the act of duplicating.

r., asexual. Reproduction in which sex cells are not involved, as by fission or budding.

r., cytogenic. Reproduction by means of asexual single germ cells.

r., sexual. Reproduction by means of sexual or germ cells. Usually a male cell (spermatozoon) fuses with a female cell (egg or ovum). SYN: *syngamy.* SEE: *parthenogenesis.*

r., somatic. Asexual reproduction by budding of somatic cells.

reproductive (rē"prō-dŭk'tĭv). Concerning, or employed in, reproduction.

repullulation (rē-pŭl"ū-lā'shŭn) [" + *pullulare,* to sprout]. Renewed growth by budding or sprouting.

repulsion (rē-pŭl'shŭn) [L. *repulsio,* a thrusting back]. 1. Act of driving back. 2. The force exerted by one body on another to cause separation. Opposite of attraction.

required services. Those services that must be included in a health program for it to qualify for federal funds.

RES. *reticuloendothelial system.*

rescinnamine (rē-sĭn'ă-mĭn). An antihypertensive drug derived from species of Rauwolfia. Trade name is Moderil.

research (rĭ-sĕrch', rē'sĕrch) [O. Fr. *recerche,* research]. Scientific and diligent study, investigation, or experimentation in order to establish facts and analyze their significance. Inherent in such study is an orderly approach with accurate record-keeping. A hallmark of acceptable research is that it is conducted and described so that other scientists may read the report and have sufficient information concerning the design and methods to repeat it.

r., clinical. Research based mainly on bedside observation of the patient, rather than through laboratory work.

r., laboratory. Research done principally in the laboratory.

r., medical. Research concerned with any phase of medical science.

resect (rē-sĕkt') [L. *resectus,* cut off]. To cut off, or to cut out, a portion of a structure or organ, as to cut off the end of a bone or to remove a segment of the intestine.

resectable (rē-sĕk'tă-bl). Able to be removed, esp. by surgical means. Usually used in reference to malignant growths that can be removed completely by use of surgery.

resection (rē-sĕk'shŭn) [L. *resectio,* a cutting off]. Partial excision of a bone or other structure.

r., gastric. Surgical resection of a part of the stomach.

r., transurethral. Surgical removal of the prostate by use of an instrument introduced through the urethra.

r., wedge. Surgical removal of a wedge-shaped piece of tissue, esp. from the ovary as a means of treating polycystic ovaries. SEE: *ovaries, polycystic.*

r., window. Resection of a portion of the nasal septum after reflection of a flap of mucous membrane.

resectoscope (rē-sĕk'tō-skōp) [L. *resectus,* cut off, + Gr. *skopein,* to examine]. An instrument for resection of the prostate gland through the urethra.

resectoscopy (rē"sĕk-tŏs'kō-pē). Resection of the prostate through the urethra.

reserpine (rē-sĕr'pĭn). USP. A chemically pure derivative of the plant Rauwolfia serpentina. A folk medicine used in India for centuries for snake bite, mental illness, and anxiety states. It lowers blood pressure and acts as a tranquilizer. Trade names are Rau-Sed, Reserpoid, Sandril, and Serpasil.

Reserpoid. Trade name for reserpine, USP.

reserve (rē-zĕrv') [L. *reservare,* to keep back]. 1. That which is held back for future use. 2. Self-control of one's feelings and thoughts.

r., alkali. Alkali content of body available for neutralization of acid.

r., cardiac. The ability of the heart to increase cardiac output to meet the needs of the body as energy output increases.

reserve air. Additional amount of air that can be expelled from the lungs over the normal quantity, which is 1200 to 1600 cc.

reservoir (rĕz'ĕr-vwor) [Fr.]. A place or cavity

for storage of fluids.

reservoir of infection. A source of supply of an infectious agent or disease. These may be man, animals, plants, or organic matter that will allow an infectious agent to live. For example, the reservoir for tuberculosis usually is man, but may also occur in the milk from tubercular cows.

residency. A period of at least one year and often 3 to 4 years of on-the-job training, usually postgraduate, that is part of the formal educational program for health care professionals.

resident. A physician who is obtaining further clinical training after internship. Usually this is done as a member of the house staff of a hospital.

residual (rē-zĭd′ū-ăl) [L. *residuum,* remaining]. 1. Rel. to that which is left as a residue. 2. In psychology, any aftereffect of experience influencing later behavior.

residual function. The functional capacity remaining after an illness or injury.

residual urine. Urine left in bladder after urination. This occurs in cases of enlarged prostate.

residue (rĕz′ĭ-dū). The remainder of something after a part is removed.

residue diet, high-. A diet with increased amounts of cellulose (fiber) and water.

residue diet, low-. A diet that includes solid food, but in which residue is reduced to a minimum. SEE: *nonlaxative diet.*

residue-free diet. Diet without cellulose or roughage. Semisolid and bland foods are included.

residuum (rē-zĭd′ū-ŭm) [L.]. (pl. *residua*) Residue; the remainder.

resilience (rē-zĭl′ē-ĕns) [L. *resiliens,* leaping back]. The quality of coming back to normal shape after straining, as a stretched rubberband when released. SYN: *elasticity.*

resilient (rē-zĭl′ē-ĕnt). Elastic; coming back to normal shape after straining.

resin (rĕz′ĭn) [L. *resina*]. 1. An amorphous, nonvolatile solid or soft-solid substance, a natural exudation from plants. It is practically insoluble in water, but soluble in alcohol. SEE: *rosin.* 2. Any of a class of solid or soft organic compounds of natural or synthetic origin. They have no definite melting point, they are usually of high molecular weight, and most are polymers. Included are polyvinyl, polyethylene, and polystyrene. These are combined with chemicals such as epoxides, plasticizers, pigments, fillers, and stabilizers to form plastics.

r., ion-exchange. Ionizable synthetic substances, which may be acid or basic, used accordingly to remove either acid or basic ions from solutions. Thus anionic-exchange resins may be used to absorb acid in the stomach. Cationic-exchange resins have the ability to remove basic (alkaline) ions from solutions.

resina (rē-zī′nă) [L.]. Resin.

resinoid (rĕz′ĭ-noyd) [″ + Gr. *eidos,* form]. Resembling a resin.

resinous (rĕz′ĭ-nŭs). Of the nature of, or pert. to, resin.

res ipsa loquitur [L.]. The thing that speaks for itself. In malpractice this concept is used for cases where an injury occurs to the plaintiff in a situation solely under the control of the defendant. If the injury would not have occurred if the defendant exercised due care the defendant is judged negligent. In medicine the classic example of this situation is when an object such as a sponge or clamp has been left in a patient's body after a surgical procedure.

resistance (rē-zĭs′tăns) [L. *resistens,* standing back]. 1. Opposition to, or the ability to oppose, anything, such as the power of a fluid to retard that which is passing through it; of the air; or opposition of the body to passage of an electric current. 2. The sum total of body mechanisms that interpose barriers to the progress of invasion, multiplication of infectious agents, or damage by their toxic products. Immunity is resistance associated with the presence of antibodies having a specific action on infectious microorganisms. Inherent resistance is the ability to resist disease independently of antibodies. 3. The force exerted to penetrate the unconcious or to submerge memories in the unconscious. 4. In psychoanalysis, condition in which the ego avoids bringing into consciousness conflicts and unpleasant events responsible for neurosis; reluctance of subject to give up old patterns of thought and behavior. It may take a variety of forms such as silence, failure to remember dreams, forgetfulness, and undue annoyance with trivial aspects of the treatment situation.

r., peripheral. The resistance of the arterial vascular system, esp. the arterioles and capillaries, to the flow of blood.

resistance transfer factor. A genetic factor in bacteria that controls resistance to certain antibiotic drugs. The factor is spread by bacteria to bacteria. This makes it possible for nonpathogenic bacteria to become resistant to antibiotics and to transfer that resistance to pathogens, thereby establishing a potential source for an epidemic.

resolution (rĕz-ō-lū′shŭn) [L. *resolutio,* a relaxing]. 1. Decomposition; absorption or breaking down of the products of inflammation. 2. Cessation of inflammation without suppuration. The return to normal. 3. The ability of the eye or series of lenses to distinguish fine detail.

resolve (rē-zŏlv') [L. *resolvere,* to release]. 1. To return to normal as after a pathological process. 2. To separate into component parts.

resolvent (rē-zŏl'vĕnt) [ME. *resolven,* releasing]. 1. Promoting disappearance of inflammation. 2. That which reduces inflammation or swelling.

resonance (rĕz'ō-năns) [L. *resonantia,* resound]. 1. Quality or act of resounding. 2. Quality of the sound heard on percussion of a hollow structure such as the chest or abdomen. Absence of resonance is termed *flatness* and diminished resonance *dullness.* 3. In physics, modification of sound due to vibrations of a body that are set up by waves of another vibrating body. 4. In electricity, state in which two electrical circuits are in tune with each other.

r., amphoric. Sound similar to that produced when blowing across mouth of an empty bottle.

r., bandbox. Pulmonary resonance heard in percussion of chests of patients with emphysema.

r., bell-metal. Sound heard in pneumothorax in auscultation when coin is held against the chest wall and it is struck by another coin.

r., cracked-pot. A sound having a peculiar clinking quality sometimes heard on percussion of chest in cases of advanced tuberculosis when cavities are present.

r., normal. Normal pulmonary resonance.

r., skodaic. Increased percussion sound over upper lung when there is pleural effusion in lower part.

r., tympanic. The sound, low-pitched and drum-like, heard upon percussing over a large air-containing space.

r., tympanitic. Resonance obtained by percussion of a hollow structure, such as the stomach or colon, when moderately distended with air.

r., vesicular. Normal pulmonary resonance.

r., vocal. In auscultation the vibrations of the voice transmitted to the ear, normally more marked over the right apex of the lung. Abnormally increased in pneumonic consolidation, in lungs infiltrated with tuberculosis, or in cavities that freely communicate with a bronchus.

Vocal resonance is diminished or absent in pleural effusion (air, pus, serum, lymph, or blood); emphysema; pulmonary collapse; pulmonary edema; egophony, a modified bronchophony characterized by a trembling, bleating sound usually heard above the upper border of dullness of pleural effusions and occasionally heard in beginning pneumonia.

r., whispering. Auscultation sound heard when patient whispers.

resonant (rĕz'ō-nănt). Producing a vibrating sound on percussion.

resonating [L. *resonantia,* resound]. Vibrating sympathetically with a source of sound or electrical oscillations.

resonating cavities. The resonator of the human voice. Includes upper portion of the larynx, pharynx, nasal cavity, paranasal sinuses, and mouth cavity.

resonator (rĕz'ō-nā"tĕr). 1. A structure that is capable of being set into sympathetic vibration when sound waves of the same frequency from another vibrating body strike it. 2. In electricity, an apparatus consisting of an electrical circuit in which oscillations of a certain frequency are set up by oscillations of the same frequency in another circuit.

resorb (rē-sorb', rē-zorb') [L. *resorbere,* to suck in]. 1. To undergo resorption. 2. To absorb again.

resorbent (rē-sor'bĕnt) [L. *resorbens,* sucking in]. An agent that promotes the absorption of abnormal matter, as exudates or blood clots.

Ex.: potassium iodide, ammonium chloride.

resorcin (rĕ-zor'sĭn). Resorcinol.

resorcinol (rĕ-zor'sĭ-nŏl). USP. An agent with keratolytic, fungicidal, and bactericidal actions. It is used in treating certain skin diseases.

resorcinolphthalein (rē-zor"sĭ-nŏl-thăl'ē-ĭn). Fluorescein.

resorption (rē-sorp'shŭn) [L. *resorbere,* to suck in]. 1. Act of removal by absorption, as resorption of an exudate or pus. 2. Removal of enamel and other calcific portions of a tooth as a result of lysis and other pathological processes.

respirable (rē-spīr'ă-bl, rĕs'pĕr-ă-bl) [L. *respirare,* breathe again]. Fit or adapted for respiration.

respiration (rĕs"pĭr-ā'shŭn) [L. *respiratio,* breathing]. 1. The interchange of gases between an organism and the medium in which it lives. More specifically the taking in of oxygen, its utilization in the tissues, and the giving off of carbon dioxide. 2. The act of breathing, i.e., inhaling and exhaling during which the lungs are provided with air, and the carbon dioxide is removed by exhaling. It is, of course, not possible to have normal respiratory exchange of oxygen and carbon dioxide in the lungs unless the pulmonary tissue is adequately perfused with blood. There are various abnormal forms of respiration: jerking, spasmodic, stertorous, stridulous, whistling, wavy, lack of evenness, abdominal, and thoracic. SEE: *ventilation; diaphragm* for illus.

SOUNDS: *Friction:* These are produced by the rubbing together of roughened pleural surfaces; may be heard both in inspiration and expiration. Often resemble subcrepitant rales, but are more superficial and localized than the latter, and are not modified by cough or deep inspiration.

Metallic tinkling: Silvery bell-like sounds heard at intervals over a pneumohydrothorax or large cavity. Speaking, coughing, and deep breathing usually induce them. Must not be confounded with similar sound produced by liquids in the stomach.

Rales: Abnormal bubbling sounds heard in air cells or bronchial tubes.

Succussion-splash or hippocratic succussion: A splashing sound produced by the presence of air and liquid in the chest, may be elicited by gently shaking the patient while auscultating. Nearly always indicates either a hydro- or a pyopneumothorax, although it has been detected over very large cavities. Air and liquid in stomach produce similar sounds.

AUSCULTATION: *Normal breath sounds:* In the normal person, breath sounds are low-pitched and have a frequency of 200–400 cycles per second (cps) and rarely greater than 500 cps. These are produced by the air passing in and out of the alveoli, and are called vesicular breath sounds.

Bronchial and tracheal breath sounds: These are produced by the air passing over the walls of the bronchi and trachea. These sounds are normally heard only over the bronchi and trachea. The vesicular sounds are heard over most of the lungs. These sounds are high-pitched and loud compared to vesicular sounds. Normally the inspiratory phrase of respiration lasts longer than the expiratory.

Amphoric and cavernous breathing: These two are almost identical. Sounds are loud and the expiration is prolonged and hollow. Pitch of amphoric breathing is a little higher than cavernous type. May be imitated by blowing over the mouth of an empty jar. Heard in bronchiectatic cavities or pneumothorax when the opening to the lung is patulous; in the area of consolidation near a large bronchus; sometimes over a lung compressed by a moderate effusion.

METHOD OF COUNTING: With the hand in the same position as when taking the pulse, watch the patient's chest, without his or her knowledge if possible because breathing is controlled by both the voluntary and involuntary muscles. Count each inspiration and expiration as one breath. Observe for one full minute by watching rise and fall of chest or upper abdomen. When the movements are scarcely perceptible, place the hand gently but firmly on the chest or back and count in this manner. Note hour, frequency, and any abnormal condition, such as pain associated with breathing. SEE: Rate of Respiration table.

Total lung capacity (T.L.C.): In normal adult males, depending upon their size, T.L.C. range is 3.6 to 9.4 liters. In females, 2.5 to 6.9 liters.

r., abdominal. Respiration where chiefly the diaphragm exerts itself, while walls of chest are nearly at rest. Utilized in normal, quiet breathing, esp. by males, and in pathological conditions as in pleurisy, pericarditis, and fracture of ribs. SYN: *r., diaphragmatic.*

r., absent. Respiration in which respiratory sounds are suppressed.

r., accelerated. Respiration occurring at a rate that is faster than normal. Considered accelerated when it exceeds 25 per minute in the adult. Increased frequency may result from exercise, physical exertion, or mental disturbances, and frequently occurs in disease. It is present in many disorders of the lungs, such as pneumonia, bronchiectasis, advanced pulmonary tuberculosis, consolidation or compression of a lobe or of the entire lung, congestion, asthma, emphysema, abscess, tumors, aneurysms, diseases of the chest wall, hernia of the diaphragm, and partial obstruction to the entrance of air into the lungs. It may be seen in diseases of the blood, such as the anemias; in kidney troubles; febrile disease; diseases of the heart; and as a result of drugs or nervous conditions such as anxiety, panic, and hysteria.

r., aerobic. Respiration in which air or free oxygen is utilized.

r., amphoric. Respiration having amphoric resonance. SEE: *resonance, amphoric.*

r., anaerobic. Respiration in which oxygen is obtained from chemical reactions not involving the liberation of free oxygen.

r., apneustic. Breathing characterized by prolonged inspiration unrelieved by attempts to expire. Seen in patients who have had the upper part of the pons of the brain removed or damaged.

r., artificial. Artificial methods to restore

Rate of Respiration

Premature infant	40–90/min.
Newborn	30–80/min.
1st year	20–40/min.
2nd year	20–30/min.
5th year	20–25/min.
15th year	15–20/min.
Adult	15–20/min.

respiration in cases of suspended breathing. For specific methods, SEE: *artificial respiration; cardiopulmonary resuscitation.*

r., Biot's. Breathing with irregularly alternating periods of apnea and hyperpnea. Occurs in meningitis and disorders of the brain that cause increased intracranial pressure.

r., cell. The combination of oxygen with various substances within cells resulting in formation of CO_2 and H_2O and release of energy. There are many intermediary reactions in which substances other than oxygen act as oxidizing agents, i.e., hydrogen or electron acceptors. Reactions are catalyzed by respiratory enzymes, which include the flavoproteins, cytochromes, and other enzymes. Certain vitamins (nicotinamide, riboflavin, thiamine, pyridoxine, and pantothenic acid) are essential in the formation of components of various enzyme systems.

r., Cheyne-Stokes. A common and bizarre breathing pattern characterized by a period of apnea lasting 10 to 60 seconds followed by gradually increasing and then decreasing respirations. It accompanies depression of frontal lobe and diencephalic dysfunction. Postulated to be due to an abnormality in the neurological respiration center. SEE: illus.

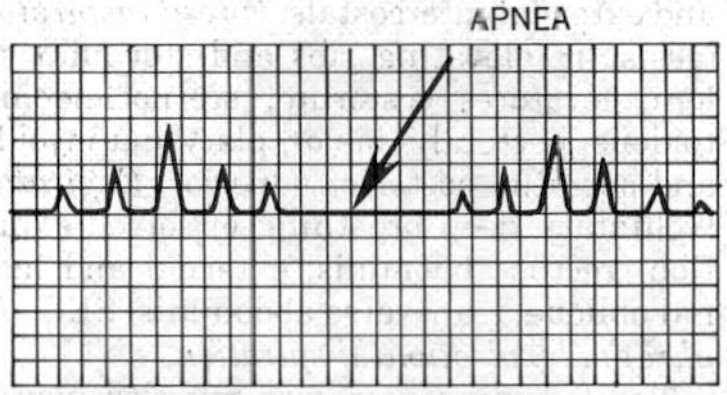

GRAPH OF RESPIRATORY MOVEMENTS IN CHEYNE-STOKES BREATHING

r., cogwheel. R., interrupted.

r., costal. Respiration in which the chest cavity is enlarged by raising the ribs.

r., decreased. Occurs in uremia, diabetic coma, most conditions that cause increased intracranial pressure, shock, hysteria, stenosis of the larynx, poisoning with opium or its derivatives, and approaching death.

r., diaphragmatic. R., abdominal.

r., direct. Respiration in which an organism, such as a one-celled ameba, secures its oxygen and gives up carbon dioxide directly to the surrounding medium.

r., electrophrenic. Application of intermittent electrical stimuli to cutaneous electrodes over the phrenic nerves in the neck to stimulate respiration rhythmically. Used in patients whose respiratory center has been damaged. SEE: *radiofrequency electrophrenic respiration.*

r., external. The processes involved in ventilating the lungs (breathing) and the exchange of gases (O_2 and CO_2) between the air in lungs and the blood within capillaries in the walls of alveoli.

Inspiration or drawing in of air is accomplished by expansion of the thoracic cavity. This is brought about by contraction of the diaphragm and raising the ribs and sternum. Expiration or the expulsion of air may be active or passive. In ordinary breathing it is passive, no muscular effort being needed to bring the chest wall back to normal position. In forced or labored respiration, muscular effort is involved.

If the aspiration of air is accomplished chiefly by contraction of the diaphragm, the abdomen will bulge with each inspiration because the diaphragm, forming at once the floor of the thorax and the roof of the abdominal cavity, is dome-shaped with its concavity downward. In contracting, it pushes the abdominal viscera down. This type of respiration is called diaphragmatic or abdominal. Its opposite is the thoracic type, in which the ribs and sternum must be raised, and which is seen when the abdomen is confined by tight clothing.

r., fetal. Exchange of gases in the placenta between blood of fetus and maternal blood. SYN: *r., placental.*

r., forced. Voluntary hyperpnea (increase in rate and depth of breathing).

r., internal. The passage of oxygen from the blood into the cells, its utilization by the cells, and the passage of carbon dioxide from cells into the blood. Oxygen is carried in combination with hemoglobin. Oxyhemoglobin gives arterial blood its red color; reduced hemoglobin gives venous blood its blue color. Carbon dioxide is carried in combination with metallic elements in the blood as bicarbonates and also as carbonic acid. Normally the partial pressure of oxygen in the blood is 75 to 100 mm. of mercury, depending upon age; and for CO_2 it is 35 to 45 mm. SEE: *r., cell.*

r., interrupted. Respiration in which inspiration or expiration sounds are not continuous. SYN: *r., cogwheel.*

r., intrauterine. Respiration by fetus before birth. SEE: *r., fetal.*

r., Kussmaul's. Deep, gasping respiration characteristic of air hunger or diabetic coma.

r., labored. Dyspnea or difficult breathing; respiration that involves active participation of accessory inspiratory and expiratory muscles.

r., muscles of. *Inspiration:* diaphragm and external intercostals. *Forced inspiration:* (assist in elevating ribs and sternum) scaleni, levatores costorum, sternocleidomastoideus, pectoralis major, platysma myoides, and serratus posterior superior. *Expiration:* (voluntary deep breathing or forced expiration) rectus abdominis, external and internal oblique, transverse abdominis. SEE: *diaphragm; expiration; inspiration.*

The following accessory muscles may assist in depressing the ribs: internal intercostals, serratus posterior inferior, quadratus lumborum.

r., paradoxical. 1. A type of respiratory activity seen in pneumothorax. The affected side bulges out on expiration and caves in on inspiration. 2. Condition seen in paralysis of diaphragm in which diaphragm ascends during inspiration.

r., periodic. Breathing of uneven rhythm as in Cheyne-Stokes respiration, q.v.

r., placental. R., fetal.

r., slow. Breathing in which there are fewer than 12 respirations each minute. Generally result of some structural or functional derangement of the nervous system. Observed in apoplexy, increased intracranial pressure and hemorrhage, uremia, and in most of the circumstances that occasion coma. It may be induced by carbon monoxide, and opium or its derivatives.

r., stertorous. Respiration characterized by rattling or bubbling sounds.

r., stridulous. A high-pitched crowing or barking sound heard during inspiration caused by an obstruction in vicinity of glottis or in respiratory passageway.

r., thoracic. Respiration performed entirely by expansion of the chest when abdomen does not move. Observed when peritoneum or diaphragm is inflamed, when abdominal cavity is physically restricted by tight bandages or clothes, or during abdominal surgery.

r., tissue. R., internal, q.v.

respiration, words pert. to: air; anapnea; apnea; asphyxia; Biot's breathing; Bouchut's respiration; chest; Cheyne-Stokes respiration; diaphragm; dyspnea; eupnea; hyperpnea; hypopnea; infant; inspiration; oligopnea; orthopnea; polypnea; respirator; respiratory; stridor; stridulous; tachypnea; thermometry.

respirator (rĕs′pĭ-rā″tor) [L. *respirare,* to breathe]. A machine for prolonged artificial respiration. Mechanical methods of assisting respiration usually include the capability of producing either intermittent or continuous positive pressure in the lungs. SEE: *Drinker respirator; ventilation, continuous positive-pressure; ventilation, intermittent positive-pressure.*

respiratory (rē-spīr′ă-tō-rē, rĕs′pĭ-ră-tō″rē) [L. *respiratio,* breathing]. Pert. to respiration.

respiratory anemometer. A form of respirometer used in investigating pulmonary function. The passage of air through the mask or mouthpiece drives a vane so that it rotates. This motion is recorded by use of a clockwise mechanism that permits measurement of the amount of air passed through the system.

respiratory center. A region in the medulla oblongata of the brain stem that regulates movements of respiration. Consists of an inspiratory center, located in the rostral half of the reticular formation overlying the olivary nuclei, and an expiratory center, located dorsal to the inspiratory center. A pneumotaxic center, located in the pons, also is concerned with respiratory movements.

respiratory distress syndrome. ABBR: RDS. A condition formerly known as hyaline membrane disease. It accounts for more than 25,000 infant deaths per year in the U.S.A. Clinical signs, including delayed onset of respiration and low Apgar score, are usually present at birth.

ETIOL: Delivery of an infant who has not matured to the point where the lungs can manufacture the lecithin-rich pulmonary surfactant. This results in collapse of the alveoli with consequent cyanosis and hypoxia.

SYM: Dyspnea, rapid breathing, expiratory grunt, cyanosis, limpness, cardiac failure, respiratory disease, and cardiac arrest.

TREATMENT: No specific therapy. Supportive measures include administering oxygen while maintaining positive airway pressure continuously during expiration, correction of dehydration and acid-base imbalance, control of humidity and temperature of environment.

PROG: Good if the arterial blood oxygen content increases when the patient breathes 100% oxygen. If death occurs, it is almost always within the first three days.

r.d.s., adult. SEE: *adult respiratory distress syndrome.*

respiratory failure, acute. Inability of the lungs to perform their ventilatory function. This may be due to impairment of gas exchange in the lung or obstruction of the free flow of air to the lung.

TREATMENT: If due to obstruction, remove the cause. If due to impaired gas exchange, positive-pressure ventilation is indicated. If the combination of ventilation and perfusion of the lung does not maintain the arterial oxygen concentration (Pao_2) of 50–55 mm. Hg or greater, then supplemental oxygen will be required.

respiratory failure, chronic. Any disease process that interferes with ventilation and perfusion of the lungs will cause pulmonary insufficiency. The degree will depend on the severity and duration of the disease process. A great number of diseases can cause chronic pulmonary insufficiency. Examples are: airway obstruction due to asthma, emphysema, chronic bronchitis, or cystic fibrosis; chronic diseases of the pulmonary interstitial tissue such as sarcoidosis, pneumoconiosis, disseminated carcinoma, radiation sickness, and leukemia.

respiratory insufficiency. Inability of the respiratory system to function adequately.

respiratory myoclonus. Leeuwenhoek's disease.

respiratory quotient. The relation of CO_2 produced and O_2 consumed. SEE: *quotient, respiratory.*

respiratory syncytial virus. A virus that induces formation of syncytial masses in infected cell cultures. It is a major cause of acute respiratory disease in children.

respiratory system. The organs involved in the interchange of gases between an organism and the atmosphere. In the human, consists of the nose, pharynx, larynx, trachea, bronchi, and lungs. SEE: *lung* for illus.

respiratory therapist. Person who by training and background is qualified to provide respiratory therapy.

respiratory therapy. Treatment to preserve or improve pulmonary function.

respirometer (rĕs″pĭr-ŏm′ĕt-ĕr) [L. *respirare,* to breathe, + Gr. *metron,* a measure]. Instrument to ascertain character of respirations. Several devices are available for measuring specific respiratory qualities such as minute and tidal volume. SEE: *respiratory anemometer.*

response [L. *respondere,* reply]. 1. A reaction, such as contraction of a muscle or secretion of a gland, resulting from a stimulus. SEE: *reaction.* 2. The sum total of reactions of an individual to specific conditions, e.g., the response (favorable or unfavorable) of a patient to a certain treatment.

r., anamnestic. The rapid production of an antibody response after the injection of an antigen that had previously produced an immune response in the individual.

r., conditioned. SEE: *reflex, conditioned.*

r., galvanic skin. The measurement of the change in the electrical resistance of the skin in response to emotional stimuli.

r., immune. SEE: *immune response.*

r., reticulocyte. The increase in reticulocyte production in response to administration of a hematinic agent.

r., triple. Three phases of vasomotor reactions occurring when a pointed instrument is drawn across the skin. Includes, in order of appearance, red reaction, flare or spreading flush, and wheal.

r., unconditioned. An inherent response rather than one that is learned. SEE: *conditioned response.*

rest (rĕst) [AS. *raest*]. 1. Repose of body due to sleep. 2. Freedom from activity, as of mind or body. 3. To lie down; to cease from motion. 4. A remnant of embryonic tissue that persists in the adult.

restenosis (rē″stĕ-nō′sĭs) [L. *re,* again, + Gr. *stenosis,* a narrowing]. The reoccurrence of a stenosis condition as in a heart valve or vessel.

restiform (rĕs′tĭ-form) [L. *restis,* rope, + *forma,* shape]. Ropelike; rope-shaped.

restiform body. One of the inferior cerebellar peduncles of the brain. They are along the lateral border of the 4th ventricle. The nerve fibers contained in these bodies connect the medulla oblongata and spinal cord with the cerebellum.

resting. Inactive, motionless, at rest.

resting cell. 1. A cell not in the process of dividing. SEE: *interphase.* 2. A cell that is not performing its normal function, i.e., a nerve cell that is not conducting an impulse or a muscle cell that is not contracting.

resting pan splint. Splint designed to position fingers and stabilize hand in a functional position with the fingers held in opposition. Also: *resting hand splint.*

resting potential. The potential difference that exists across a cell membrane between the outside and the inside of a resting cell.

restitutio integrum (rĕs″tĭ-tū′shē-ō ĭn-tĕ′grŭm) [L.]. Complete restoration to health.

restitution (rĕs″tĭ-tū′shŭn) [L. *restitutio*]. 1. A return to a former status. 2. The act of making amends. 3. The turning of a fetal head to the right or left after it has completely emerged through the vagina.

restless legs. A condition of unknown etiology characterized by an intolerable creeping and internal itching sensation occurring in the lower extremities. Symptoms are worse at the end of the day when patient is either seated or in bed. Patient is compelled to move legs and this brings relief. This symptom is sometimes associated with the onset of renal colic due to the attempt to pass or actual passage of a renal stone.

restoration (rĕs″tō-rā′shŭn) [L. *restaurare,* to fix]. 1. To return anything to its previous state. 2. In dentistry, any treatment, material, or device that restores a tooth surface, or replaces a tooth or all of the teeth and adjacent tissues.

r., temporary. The use of zinc oxide and eugenol or some plastic material to provide a temporary filling of a tooth cavity.

restorative (rē-stor′ă-tĭv) [L. *restaurare*, to fix]. 1. Pert. to restoration. 2. An agent that is effective in the regaining of health and strength.

restraint (rē-strānt′) [O. Fr. *restrainte*]. 1. The process of confining from any action, mental or physical. 2. State of being hindered. 3. That which hinders or restricts; device or method used to keep a patient from injuring himself. Various states have laws concerning methods to be used in restraining patients.

r. in bed. If a proper bed is not available, the following may be used as a makeshift alternative. Move bed against wall, place straight-backed chairs along open side of bed. Tie them into place by interlacing with rope and then tying to foot and head of bed, or place a wide board the length of bed on either side and fasten through three or four holes bored near ends of the boards. Fold sheet lengthwise to width of one foot. Place under patient's back and cross in front below armpits. At sides secure hem ends to side bar or springs of bed. This allows some freedom for turning from side to side. The hands and feet may be restrained by a clove hitch of wide bandage around wrists and ankles and tied to side or foot of bed.

r., mechanical. Restraint by physical devices, esp. restraint of insane.

r., medicinal. Restraint of violent mentally ill patients through use of narcotics or sedatives.

r. of lower extremities. Tie a sheet across knees and tie feet together with a figure-of-eight bandage. Start loop under ankles, cross between feet, bring ends around feet, and tie on top. CAUTION: Restraint should not interfere with the circulation of blood to the legs.

resuscitation (rē-sŭs″ĭ-tā′shŭn) [L. *resuscitatio*]. Revival after apparent death. SYN: *anabiosis*. SEE: *artificial respiration*.

r., cardiopulmonary. SEE: *cardiopulmonary resuscitation*.

r., heart-lung. SEE: *cardiopulmonary resuscitation*.

r., oral. SEE: *artificial respiration*.

resuscitator (rē-sŭs′ĭ-tā″tor) [L. *resuscitare*, to revive]. An automatic breathing-assist machine that forces oxygen into the lungs under pressure of 4 oz. per sq. in. (1.4 mm. Hg) when back pressure of 3 oz. (about 1 mm. Hg) trips the machine for exhalation.

ret. *roentgen equivalent therapy*. It is analogous to rem, q.v., used in describing radiation protection or exposure.

retainer (rē-tān′ĕr). 1. Any device or attachment for retaining or keeping something in place. 2. In dentistry, a device used in orthodontia for maintaining the teeth and jaws in position.

retardate (rē-tăr′dāt) [L. *retardare*, to delay]. One who is mentally retarded.

retardation (rē″tăr-dā′shŭn) [L. *retardare*, to delay]. 1. A holding back or slowing down; delay. 2. Delayed mental or physical response due to pathological conditions. SEE: *mental retardation*.

r., mental. SEE: *mental retardation*.

retch (rĕch) [AS. *hraecan*, to cough up phlegm]. Involuntary attempt to vomit, q.v.

retching (rĕch′ĭng). Involuntary attempting to vomit.

rete (rē′tē) [L.]. (pl. *retia*) [NA] A network. A plexus of nerves or blood vessels.

r., arterial; r. arteriosum. A vascular, arterial network just prior to the point where arteries become capillaries.

r., articular. Rete about a joint, esp. a deep anastomosis at knee joint.

r., cutaneum. A network of blood vessels at junction of the corium and superficial fascia.

r., malpighian. Stratum germinativum, q.v.

r. mirabile. [NA] A plexus formed by sudden division of a vessel into small twigs that unite again to form one vessel, as in the glomeruli of the kidneys.

r. olecrani. A network of vessels at back of elbow formed by divisions of the recurrent ulnar arteries.

r. ovarii. A layer of cells lying in the broad ligament and mesovarium of the ovary. They are homologous to rete testes in male.

r. patellae. [NA] A superficial network of vessels lying about the patella. Formed by branches of genicular arteries.

r. subpapillare. A network of vessels between papillary and reticular layers of the dermis.

r. testis. [NA] A network of tubules in mediastinum testis that receives sperm through the tubuli recti from the seminiferous tubules. From the rete testis, efferent ducts convey sperm to the epididymis.

r., venosum. Venous network.

r., vertebral. Two plexuses within the vertebral canal that extend from the foramen magnum to the coccyx. They lie posteriorly and laterally to the dura and between the dura and arches of the vertebrae.

retention (rē-tĕn′shŭn) [L. *retentio*, a holding back]. Retaining in the body that which does not belong there, or which should be excreted, as urine, feces, or perspiration.

retention cyst. Cyst caused by retention of a secretion in a gland, due to closure of the gland's duct.

retention defect. Inability to recall a name, number, or fact shortly after the subject was requested to remember it.

retention enema. Enema to be retained to provide nourishment, medicate the mucosa, or act as anesthetic. SEE: *enema*.

retention of urine. Inability to empty bladder. This may be due to a number of causes, such as loss of muscle tone of the bladder from anemia, old age, exposure to cold, or prolonged operation; lesions involving nervous pathways to and from the bladder; lesions involving reflex centers in brain and spinal cord; obstruction of the urethra, which may result from inflammation, stricture, stones, diverticula, cysts, tumors, or pressure from the outside as in cases of hypertrophy of the prostate; psychogenic factors; and medication such as morphine or certain antihistamines.

retention with overflow. Spasm of sphincter, causing failure to empty the bladder at one voiding, with only overflow dribbling away; due to same causes as urine retention.

retia (rē'tē-ă) [L.]. Pl. of rete.

retial (rē'tē-ăl). Concerning a rete.

reticula (rē-tĭk'ū-lă) [L.]. Pl. of reticulum.

reticular (rē-tĭk'ū-lăr) [L. *reticula,* net]. Meshed, or in the form of a network.

reticular activating system. ABBR: RAS. The alerting system of the brain consisting of the reticular formation, subthalamus, hypothalamus, and medial thalamus. It extends from central core of the brain stem to all parts of the cerebral cortex. This system is essential in initiating and maintaining wakefulness and introspection, and in directing attention. Some of the tranquilizing drugs act on this system to depress it.

reticular cells. 1. Phagocytic cells present in lymphatic and myeloid tissues. 2. The cells of reticular connective tissue. SEE: *reticular tissue.*

reticular fibers. Extremely fine argyrophilic (i.e., silver-staining) fibers found in reticular tissue, q.v.

reticular formation. Groups of cells and fibers arranged in a diffuse network throughout the brain stem. These both fill the spaces and connect the tracts that ascend and descend through the area. They are important in controlling or influencing alertness, waking, sleeping, and various reflexes.

reticular layer. Layer of connective tissue forming deeper portion of dermis. Lies beneath papillary layer.

reticular membrane. Membrane formed by cuticular plates of distal ends of supporting cells in the organ of Corti of the ear.

reticular tissue. A form of connective tissue consisting of a network of reticular fibers and cells. Cells are stellate with protoplasmic processes anastomosing with adjacent cells. Protoplasm also encloses and extends along the fibers. Found principally in bone marrow and lymphatic organs (lymph nodes). Also found in various organs (liver, kidney), in tissue underlying mucous membranes, and in walls of blood vessels.

reticulate (rē-tĭk'ū-lāt). Of the nature of a network.

reticulate substance. Reticular formation.

reticulated (rē-tĭk'ū-lā"tĕd) [L. *reticula,* net]. Netlike; pert. to a reticulum.

reticulation (rē-tĭk"ū-lā'shŭn). The formation of a network mass.

reticulin (rē-tĭk'ū-lĭn) [L. *reticula,* net]. An albuminoid or scleroprotein substance in the connective tissue framework of reticular tissue.

reticulocyte (rĕ-tĭk'ū-lō-sīt) [" + Gr. *kytos,* cell]. A red blood cell containing a network of granules or filaments representing an immature stage in development. Normally comprise about 1% of circulating red blood cells.

reticulocytopenia (rē-tĭk"ū-lō-sī"tō-pē'nē-ă) [" + " + *penia,* poverty]. Lowering of the number of the reticulocytes of the blood.

reticulocytosis (rē-tĭk"ū-lō-sī-tō'sĭs) [" + " + *osis,* condition]. Increase in number of reticulocytes in circulating blood. Indicative of active erythropoiesis in red bone marrow. Occurs after hemorrhage; during acclimatization to high altitude; and following treatment for pernicious anemia.

reticuloendothelial (rē-tĭk"ū-lō-ĕn"dō-thē'lē-ăl) [L. *reticula,* net, + Gr. *endon,* within, + *thele,* nipple]. Pert. to the reticuloendothelial system.

reticuloendothelial cell. A phagocytic cell of the reticuloendothelial system. SYN: *histiocyte; macrophage.*

reticuloendothelial system ABBR: RES. Term applied to those cells scattered throughout the body that have the power to ingest (phagocytose) particulate matter (bacteria, colloidal particles). Includes macrophages (histiocytes, clasmatocytes, or resting wandering cells) of loose connective tissue; reticular cells of lymphatic organs and myeloid tissues; Kupffer cells of the liver; cells lining blood sinuses of spleen, bone marrow, adrenal cortex, and hypophysis; microglia of central nervous system; adventitial cells about blood vessels; and dust cells of the lungs. The above types of cells are called fixed reticuloendothelial cells. Under certain conditions, esp. inflammatory stimuli, fixed cells may become wandering reticuloendothelial cells, i.e., they become actively motile. Monocytes of the blood also are included in this group. Reticuloendothelial cells function in elimination of worn out cells, esp. red blood cells; in repair of injured tissue; and in defense mechanisms, both local and general, of the body.

Diseases of the reticuloendothelial system

include lymphosarcoma, reticulum cell sarcoma, Hodgkin's disease, follicular lymphoma, mycosis fungoides, Gaucher's disease, and Niemann-Pick's disease.

reticuloendothelioma (rĕ-tĭk″ū-lō-ĕn″dō-thē-lē-ō′mă) [″ + ″ + ″ + *oma,* tumor]. A neoplasm composed of reticuloendothelial tissue.

reticuloendotheliosis (rē-tĭk″ū-lō-ĕn″dō-thē-lē-ō′sĭs) [″ + ″ + *thele,* nipple, + *osis,* condition]. Hyperplasia of reticuloendothelium.

reticuloendothelium (rē-tĭk″ū-lō-ĕn″dō-thē′lē-ŭm). Tissue of the reticuloendothelial system, q.v. SEE: *reticuloendothelial system.*

reticulohistiocytoma (rē-tĭk″ū-lō-hĭs″tē-ō-sī-tō′mă) [L. *reticula,* net, + Gr. *histion,* little web, + *kytos,* cell, + *oma,* tumor]. A giant cell granulomacytosis involving the skin, mucous membranes, and synovial membranes of the long bones.

reticulohistiocytosis (rē-tĭk″ū-lō-hĭs″tē-ō-sī-tō′sĭs) [″ + ″ + ″ + *osis,* condition]. Reticuloendotheliosis, q.v.

reticuloid (rĕ-tĭk′ū-loyd) [″ + Gr. *eidos,* form]. Resembling reticulosis.

reticuloma (rĕ-tĭk″ū-lō′mă) [″ + Gr. *oma,* tumor]. Neoplasm composed of reticuloendothelial cells.

reticulopenia (rĕ-tĭk″ū-lō-pē′nē-ă) [″ + Gr. *penia,* lack]. Decreased number of reticulocytes in the blood.

reticulopodium (rĕ-tĭk″ū-lō-pō′dē-ŭm). Rhizopodium, q.v.

reticulosarcoma (rĕ-tĭk″ū-lō-săr-kō′mă) [″ + Gr. *sarx,* flesh, + *oma,* tumor]. A neoplasm composed of large monocytic cells that originated in the reticuloendothelium of the lymph and other glands.

reticulosis (rē-tĭk-ū-lō′sĭs) [″ + Gr. *osis,* condition]. Reticulocytosis.

r., familial histiocytic. A severe and fatal type of lymphoma characterized by anemia; granulocytopenia; enlargement of the spleen, liver, and the lymph nodes; and phagocytosis of red blood cells.

reticulum (rē-tĭk′ū-lŭm) [L., a little net]. (pl. *reticula*) A network.

r., endoplasmic. SEE: *endoplasmic reticulum.*

r. of nucleus. A fine network of linin threads on which are arranged masses of chromatin.

r., sarcoplasmic. The network of fine tubules, similar to endoplasmic reticulum, present in muscle tissues.

r., stellate. The enamel pulp of a developing tooth, consisting of stellate cells lying between inner and outer epithelial layers.

retiform (rĕt′ĭ-form) [L. *rete,* net, + *forma,* shape]. Resembling a network. SYN: *reticular.*

Retin-A. Trade name for tretinoin, USP.

retina (rĕt′ĭ-nă) [L.]. (pl. *retinae*) [NA] Innermost or third tunic of the eye, which receives image formed by the lens and is the immediate instrument of vision. SEE: illus.

The retina is a light-sensitive structure upon which light rays come to a focus. It extends from the point of entrance of the optic nerve anteriorly to the margin of the pupil, completely lining the interior of the eye. It consists of three parts: pars optica, the nervous or sensory portion extending from the optic disk forward to the ora serrata, a wavy line immediately behind the ciliary process; pars ciliaris, the part lining the inner surface of the ciliary process; and pars iridica, the part forming the posterior surface of the iris. Slightly lateral to the posterior pole of the eye is a small, oval, yellowish spot, the macula lutea, in the center of which is a depression, the fovea centralis. This region contains only cones and is the region of most acute vision. About 3.5 mm. nasally from the fovea is the optic papilla (optic disk), the point at which nerve fibers from the retina make their exit and form the optic nerve. This region is devoid of rods and cones and is insensitive to light, hence named the blind spot.

The layers of the retina from without inward are layer of pigment epithelium, layer of rods and cones, external limiting membrane, external nuclear layer, external plexiform layer, internal nuclear layer, internal plexiform layer, layer of ganglion cells, layer of nerve fibers, and internal limiting membrane.

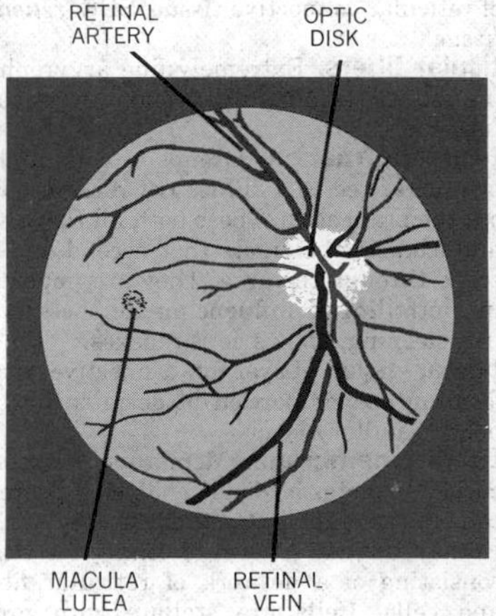

RETINA OF RIGHT EYE

COLOR: Normally a purplish-red tint, varying with complexion. It is colorless in severe anemia or in ischemia, and is reddened in hyperemia.

VESSELS: The arteries shown in the illustration are branches of a single central artery, a branch of the ophthalmic artery. The central artery enters at the center of the optic papilla, and it supplies the inner layers of retina. The outer layers, including rods and cones, are nourished by capillaries of the choroid layer. The veins lack muscular coats. They parallel the arteries, blood leaving by a central vein that leads to the superior ophthalmic vein.

r., coarctate. Condition in which there is an effusion of fluid between the retina and choroid, giving the retina a funnel shape.

r., detachment of. Complete or partial separation of the retina from the choroid. May follow trauma, choroidal hemorrhages, or tumors. May also be associated with diabetes mellitus. SEE: illus.

r., shot-silk. Retina having an opalescent appearance, sometimes seen in young persons.

r., tigroid. Retina having a spotted or striped appearance seen in retinitis pigmentosa.

retinaculum (rĕt″ĭ-năk′ū-lŭm) [L., halter]. (pl. *retinacula*) [NA] A band or membrane holding any organ or part in its place. Thickenings of the deep fascia in distal portions of limbs that hold tendons in position when muscles contract, called retinaculum tendinum.

r. cutis. [NA] A fibrous band connecting the corium with underlying fascia.

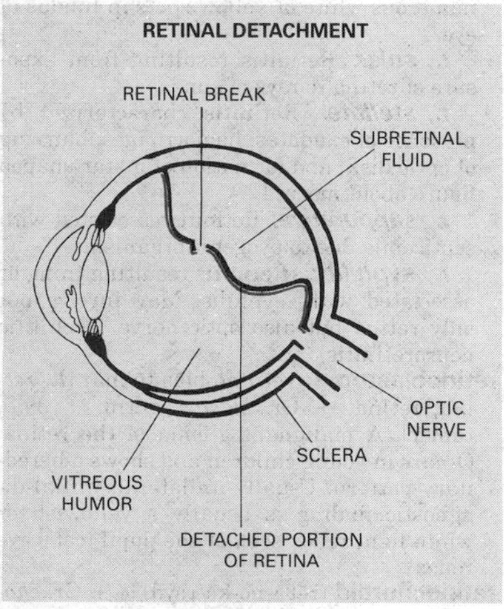

r., extensor, of ankle. 1. The superior extensor retinaculum, a band that crosses the extensor tendons of the foot and is attached to the lower portion of the tibia and fibula. 2. The inferior extensor retinaculum, a band located on dorsum of foot. Consists of two limbs having common origin on the lateral surface of the calcaneum. The upper limb is attached to the medial malleolus; the lower limb curves around the instep and is attached to the fascia of the abductor hallucis on the medial side of the foot.

r., extensor, of wrist. An oblique band attached medially to the styloid process of the ulna, hammate bone, and medial ligament of the wrist joint. Laterally it is attached to the anterior border of the radius. Contains six separate compartments for passage of extensor tendons to hand.

r., flexor, of ankle. Retinaculum extending from the medial malleolus to the medial tubercle of the calcaneum.

r., flexor, of hand. The fascial band that holds down the flexor tendons of the digits.

r., flexor, of wrist. Retinaculum extending from the trapezium and scaphoid bones laterally to the hammate and pisiform bones medially.

r. mammae. Strands of connective tissue in the mammary gland extending from glandular tissue through fat toward the skin, where they are attached to deep fascia. Over the cephalic portion of mammae, they are well developed and called suspensory ligaments of Cooper.

r. of hip joint. Any one of three flat bands lying along the neck of the femur and continuous with the capsule of the hip joint.

r., patellar. Two fibrous bands (medial and lateral) lying on either side of the knee joint and forming part of the joint capsule. They are extensions of the insertions of the medial and lateral vastus muscles.

r., peroneal. Two fibrous bands on lateral side of the foot that contain tendons of peroneus longus and brevis muscles. The superior peroneal retinaculum extends from the lateral malleolus to the lateral surface of the calcaneum; the inferior peroneal retinaculum is attached below to the calcaneum and above to the lower border of the inferior extensor retinaculum.

r. tendinum. The annular band of the wrist or ankle.

retinal (rĕt′ĭ-năl) [L. *retina*, retina]. Concerning the retina.

retinal breaks. A break in the continuity of the retina. Usually caused by trauma to the eye. Detachment of the retina may follow appearance of the break.

retinal correspondence. Condition in which

simultaneous stimulation of points in the retinas of both eyes results in formation of a single visual sensation. Such points are called corresponding points. These lie in the foveas of the two retinas, or in the nasal half of one retina and the temporal half of the other. Abnormal correspondence results in double vision (diplopia) and usually is the result of imbalance of ocular muscles. SEE: *strabismus*.

retinal detachment. Separation of the inner sensory layer of the retina from the outer pigment epithelium, leading to loss of retinal function. Usually caused by a hole or break in the inner sensory layer that permits fluid to accumulate between the two layers. SEE: *retina, detachment of,* for illus.

retine (rĕt′ēn). A tissue extract that inhibits growth of certain tumors in mice.

retinene (rĕt′ĭ-nēn). An orange-yellow carotenoid pigment formed in the retina as a result of the action of light on rhodopsin; an aldehyde of vitamin A. In dark adaptation, rhodopsin is regenerated from retinene. SYN: *xanthopsin*.

retinitis (rĕt-ĭ-nī′tĭs) [L. *retina,* retina, + Gr. *itis,* inflammation]. Inflamed condition of the retina.

SYM: Diminished vision, contractions of fields or scotomata, alteration in size of objects, photophobia.

TREATMENT: Absolute rest of eyes, protection from light, treatment of underlying cause.

r., actinic. Retinitis due to exposure to intense light or other forms of radiant energy.

r., albuminuric. Retinitis associated with chronic kidney disease and malignant hypertension. General signs of retinitis are present; it is distinguished by white patches in the fundus, esp. surrounding the papilla and in the macular region.

r., apoplectic. Retinitis associated with hemorrhaging of retinal vessels.

r., circinate. Retinitis in which there is a circle of white spots about the macula.

r., circumpapillar. Retinitis in which there is a proliferation of outer layers of retina about the optic disk.

r., diabetic. Retinitis occurring in diabetes, esp. that of long duration. Characterized by aneurysmal dilatation of blood vessels, hemorrhages, and waxy and cottonwool exudates.

r., disciform. Retinitis accompanied by degeneration of retina in region of macula.

r., exogenous purulent. Retinitis following introduction of infectious organisms into eye as a result of perforating wound or ulcer.

r., external exudative. Condition in which large masses of white and yellow crystals occur beneath retina as a result of organization of hemorrhages.

r., exudative. Chronic inflammation of the retina with elevated areas around the optic disk.

r., hemorrhagic. Retinitis with pronounced hemorrhage into the retina.

r., metastatic. Acute purulent retinitis resulting from lodgement of infective emboli in retinal vessels.

r. of prematurity. SEE: *retrolental fibroplasia.*

r. pigmentosa. A chronic progressive disease, which has its onset in early childhood, characterized by degeneration of retinal epithelium, esp. rods; atrophy of the optic nerve; and widespread pigmentary changes in the retina. A degenerative condition without inflammation. An early event is defective night vision followed by constricted field of vision.

ETIOL: Unknown but a hereditary tendency is suspected.

TREATMENT: No specific therapy, but professional and vocational guidance and genetic counseling can be provided.

r. proliferans. Vascularized masses of connective tissue that project from the retina into the vitreous. End result of recurrent hemorrhage from retina into the vitreous.

r. punctata albescens. A nonprogressive, degenerative, familial disease, characterized by presence of innumerable minute white spots scattered over entire retina, and without pigmentary changes. Usually starts early in life.

r., punctate. Retinitis characterized by numerous white or yellow spots in fundus of eye.

r., solar. Retinitis resulting from exposure of retina to rays of sun.

r., stellate. Retinitis characterized by presence of exudates, hemorrhages, blurring of optic disk, and formation of a star-shaped figure about macula.

r., suppurative. Retinitis associated with septicemia due to pyogenic organisms.

r., syphilitic. Retinitis resulting from, or associated with, syphilis. May involve not only retina but also optic nerve (syphilitic neuroretinitis).

retinoblastoma (rĕt″ĭ-nō-blăs-tō′mă) [L. *retina,* retina, + Gr. *blastos,* germ, + *oma,* tumor]. A malignant glioma of the retina. Occurs in young children and shows a hereditary pattern. Usually unilateral. Initial diagnostic finding is usually a yellowish or white light reflex seen at the pupil (cat's eye reflex).

retinochoroid (rĕt″ĭ-nō-kō′royd) [″ + Gr. *chorioeides,* skinlike]. Concerning the retina and the choroid of the eye.

retinochoroiditis (rĕt″ĭ-nō-kō-royd-ī′tĭs) [″ + ″ + *itis,* inflammation]. Inflamed condition of retina and choroid.

r. juxtapapillaris. Retinochoroiditis close to the optic nerve.

retinocystoma (rĕt″ĭ-nō-sĭs-tō′mă) [″ + Gr. *kystis,* sac, + *oma,* tumor]. Glioma of the retina.

retinodialysis (rĕt″ĭ-nō-dī-ăl′ĭ-sĭs) [″ + Gr. *dialysis,* separation]. Detachment of the retina at its periphery. SYN: *disinsertion.*

retinoid (rĕt′ĭ-noyd). 1. [L. *retina,* retina, + Gr. *eidos,* resemblance] Like the retina. 2. [Gr. *rhetine,* resin, + *eidos,* resemblance] Resembling a resin; resinous.

retinol (rĕt′ĭ-nŏl). Vitamin A_1, the mammalian form of vitamin A.

retinopapillitis (rĕt″ĭ-nō-pă″pĭl-ī′tĭs) [L. *retina,* retina, + *papilla,* nipple, + Gr. *itis,* inflammation]. Inflamed condition of retina and optic papilla. SYN: *papilloretinitis.*

retinopathy (rĕt″ĭn-ŏp′ă-thē) [″ + Gr. *pathos,* disease]. Any disorder of the retina.

r., arteriosclerotic. Retinopathy accompanying generalized arteriosclerosis and moderate hypertension.

r., circinate. A ring of degenerated white exudative area of the retina around the macula of the eye.

r., diabetic. Retinopathy occurring in diabetics.

r., hypertensive. Retinopathy associated with hypertension, toxemia of pregnancy, or glomerulonephritis.

r., solar. Pathological changes in the retina after looking directly at the sun. Seen frequently following an eclipse of the sun during which time the individual looks directly at the sun.

r., syphilitic. Retinopathy occurring in later stages of syphilis.

retinoschisis (rĕt″ĭ-nŏs′kĭ-sĭs) [″ + Gr. *schisis,* division]. Splitting of the retina into two layers with cyst formation between the layers.

retinoscope (rĕt′ĭ-nō-skōp) [″ + Gr. *skopein,* to examine]. An instrument used in performing retinoscopy.

retinoscopy (rĕt″ĭn-ŏs′kō-pē). Objective method of determining refractive errors of the eye. The examiner projects light into eyes and judges error of refraction by movement of reflected light rays. SYN: *skiascopy.*

retinosis (rĕt″ĭ-nō′sĭs) [″ + Gr. *osis,* condition]. Any degenerative process of the retina not associated with inflammation.

retisolution (rĕt″ĭ-sō-lū′shŭn) [L. *rete,* net, + *solutio,* dissolution]. Dissolution of the Golgi structures.

retispersion (rĕt″ĭ-spĕr′zhŭn) [″ + *spersio,* a scattering]. Transference of Golgi structures to periphery of the cell.

retoperithelium (rē″tō-pĕr″ĭ-thē′lē-ŭm) [L. *rete,* net, + Gr. *peri,* around, + *thele,* nipple]. Epithelium covering a reticulum.

retort (rē-tort′) [L. *retortus,* bent back]. A flasklike, long-necked vessel used in distillation.

retothelium (rē″tō-thē′lē-ŭm) [L. *rete,* net, + Gr. *thele,* nipple]. Cellular layers covering reticular tissue. SYN: *reticuloendothelium.*

retract (rē-trăkt′) [L. *retractus*]. To draw back.

retractile (rē-trăkt′ĭl) [L. *retractilis*]. Capable of being drawn back or in.

retraction (rē-trăk′shŭn). A shortening; the act of drawing backward or state of being drawn back.

r., clot. The shrinking of the clot that forms when blood is allowed to stand. The contraction is due to the fibrin network formed in the clot.

r., uterine. The process by which muscular fibers of the uterus remain permanently shortened to a small degree following each contraction or labor pain.

retraction ring. A ridge sometimes felt on uterus above the pubes, marking line of separation between upper contractile and lower dilatable segments of the uterus. SEE: *Bandl's ring.*

retractor 1. Instrument for holding back the margins of a wound. 2. Muscle that draws in any organ or part.

retrad (rē′trăd) [L. *retro,* backward]. Toward the posterior part of the body.

retreat (rē-trēt′) [ME. *retret,* draw back]. Act of retiring or withdrawing from difficult life situations. May be direct, as in physical flight, or indirect, as in malingering, illness, abnormal preoccupation, and self-deception.

retrenchment [Fr. *retrencher,* to cut back]. Procedure used in plastic surgery to remove excess tissue.

retrieval (rē-trē′văl). In psychology, the process of bringing remembered information back to the conscious level.

retro- [L.]. Prefix meaning backward.

retroaction (rĕt″rō-ăk′shŭn). Action in a reverse direction.

retroauricular (rĕt″rō-aw-rĭk′ū-lăr) [L. *retro,* backward, + *auricula,* ear] Behind the auricle or ear.

retrobuccal (rĕt″rō-bŭk′ăl) [″ + *bucca,* cheek]. Concerning the back part of the mouth or area behind the mouth.

retrobulbar (rĕt″rō-bŭl′băr) [″ + Gr. *bulbus,* bulb]. 1 Behind the eyeball. 2. Posterior to the medulla oblongata.

retrocecal (rĕt″rō-sē′kăl) [″ + *caecum,* cecum]. Back of or pert. to the area posterior to the cecum.

retrocedent (rĕt″rō-sē′dĕnt) [L. *retrocedere*]. 1. Going backward; returning. 2. A condition affecting some interior organ and disappearing from the surface.

retrocervical (rĕt″rō-sĕr′vĭ-kăl) [L. *retro,* backward, + *cervix,* neck]. Back of the cervix uteri.

retrocession (rĕt″rō-sĕsh′ŭn) [L. *retrocessio,* going back]. 1. A going back; a relapse. 2. Metastasis of a condition from the surface to an internal organ. 3. An abnormal position of the uterus; backward displacement.

retroclusion (rĕt″rō-kloo′zhŭn) [″ + *claudere,* to close]. A method of stopping arterial bleeding. A needle is placed through the tissues over a severed artery and then turned around and down so that it is passed back through the tissues under the artery. This causes compression of the vessel.

retrocolic (rĕt″rō-kŏl′ĭk) [L. *retro,* backward, + Gr. *kolon,* colon]. Back of the colon.

retrocollic (rĕt″rō-kŏl′ĭk) [″ + *collum,* neck]. Concerning the back of the neck.

retrocollic spasm. Wryneck with spasms affecting posterior muscles of neck.

retrocollis (rĕt″rō-kŏl′ĭs). Spasm of posterior muscles of the neck with drawing of the head backward. SEE: *torticollis.*

retrocursive (rĕt″rō-kŭr′sĭv) [L. *retro,* backward, + *curro,* to run]. Stepping or turning backward.

retrodeviation (rē″trō-dē″vē-ā′shŭn) [″ + *deviare,* to turn aside]. Backward displacement, as of an organ.

retrodisplacement (rē″trō-dĭs-plās′mĕnt) [″ + Fr. *desplacer,* displace]. Displacement backward of a part.

retroesophageal (rĕt″rō-ē-sŏf″ă-jē′ăl) [L. *retro,* backward, + Gr. *oisophagos,* gullet]. Located behind the esophagus.

retrofilling (rĕt″rō-fĭl′ĭng). Placement of filling material in a root canal by using an opening made in the apex of the tooth.

retroflexed (rĕt′rō-flĕkst″) [″ + *flexus,* bent]. Bent backward.

retroflexion (rĕt″rō-flĕk′shŭn). A bending or flexing backward.

retroflexion of uterus. A condition of the womb in which its body is bent backward at an angle with the cervix, whose position usually remains unchanged.

retrogasserian (rĕt″rō-găs-sē′rē-ăn). Referring to the posterior root of the gasserian ganglion.

retrognathia (rĕt″rō-năth′ē-ă) [″ + Gr. *gnathos,* jaw]. Location of the mandible back of the frontal plane of the maxilla.

retrognathism (rĕt″rō-năth′ĭzm) [″ + Gr. *gnathos,* jaw]. Having retrognathia.

retrograde (rĕt′rō-grād, rē′trō-grād) [L. *retro,* backward, + *gradi,* to step]. Moving backward; degenerating from better to worse state.

retrograde amnesia. Loss of memory for events and situations just preceding the time of patient's illness.

retrograde aortography. Roentgenography of the aorta by injecting a contrast medium into one of its branches, against the direction of blood flow.

retrograde flow. The flow of fluid in a direction opposite to that which is considered normal.

retrograde pyelography. Pyelography wherein the radiopaque dye is injected into the kidneys from below, via the ureters.

retrography (rē-trŏg′ră-fē) [″ + Gr. *graphein,* to write]. Mirror writing, a symptom of certain brain diseases.

retrogression (rĕt″rō-grĕsh′ŭn) [L. *retrogressus,* go backward]. A going backward as in the involution, degeneration, or atrophy of a tissue or structure.

retroiridian (rē″trō-ī-rĭd′ē-ăn) [″ + Gr. *iridos,* colored circle]. Posterior to the iris.

retroinfection (rē″trō-ĭn-fĕk′shŭn) [L. *retro,* backward, + *infectio,* infection]. Infection communicated by the fetus in utero to the mother.

retroinsular (rĕt″rō-ĭn′sū-lăr) [″ + *insula,* island]. Situated behind the island of Reil in the brain.

retrojection (rĕt″rō-jĕk′shŭn) [″ + *jacio,* to throw]. Washing out a cavity from within by injection of a fluid.

retrolabyrinthine (rē″trō-lăb″ĭ-rĭn′thĭn) [″ + Gr. *labyrinthos,* a maze]. Situated behind the labyrinth of the ear.

retrolental. Behind the crystalline lens.

retrolental fibroplasia. ABBR: RLF. A bilateral disease of the retinal vessels present in premature infants some of whom were exposed to high postnatal oxygen concentrations. High oxygen concentration used in treating premature infants, esp. those weighing less than 1500 grams, causes vasoconstriction of the immature retinal vessels and eventually occlusion of the vessels. This may be followed by fibrous proliferation and invasion of the vitreous. Retinal detachment may occur at that time or many years later. Blindness develops within several weeks. Other factors can have an important role in the pathogenesis of RLF. Apnea, asphyxia, sepsis, nutritional deficiencies, and a large number of blood transfusions given over a short period of time have all been related to RLF.

Prevention is possible by using only the lowest possible effective oxygen concentration in treating premature infants. Thus the lowest level possible without endangering the life of the infant is used. Too severe restriction of oxygen will increase the likelihood of hyaline membrane disease, and neurologic disorders. All premature infants treated with supplemental oxygen should have careful examination by an ophthalmologist prior to discharge from the hospital. Once blindness develops there is no effective treatment. SYN: *retinopathy of prematurity.*

retrolenticular (rē″trō-lĕn-tĭk′ū-lăr) [″ + *lenticularis,* pert. to a lens]. Retrolental, q.v.

retrolingual (rĕt″rō-lĭng′gwăl) [L. *retro,* backward, + *lingua,* tongue]. Behind the tongue.

retromammary (rĕt″rō-măm′mă-rē) [″ + *mamma,* breast]. Located behind the mammary gland.

retromandibular (rē″trō-măn-dĭb′ū-lăr) [″ + *mandibulum,* jaw]. Located behind the lower jaw.

retromastoid (rē″trō-măs′toyd) [L. *retro,* backward, + Gr. *mastos,* breast, + *eidos,* like]. Situated behind the mastoid process.

retromorphosis (rē″trō-mor′fō-sĭs) [″ + Gr. *morphe,* form, + *osis,* condition]. 1. Change in shape accompanying a transition from a higher to a lower type of structure. 2. Retrogressive changes within cells or tissues. SYN: *catabolism.*

retronasal (rĕt″rō-nā′zăl) [″ + *nasus,* nose]. Rel. to, or situated at, the back part of the nose.

retroocular (rĕt″rō-ŏk′ū-lar) [″ + *oculus,* eye]. Located behind the eye.

retroparotid (rē″trō-pă-rŏt′ĭd) [″ + Gr. *para,* beside, + *ous,* ear]. Behind the parotid gland.

retroperitoneal (rē″trō-pĕr″ĭ-tō-nē′ăl) [″ + Gr. *peritonaion,* peritoneum]. Located behind the peritoneum and outside the peritoneal cavity, such as the kidneys.

retroperitoneal fibrosis. Development of a mass of fibrotic tissue in the retroperitoneal space. This may lead to physical compression of the ureters, and even the vena cava and aorta. This disease may be associated with taking methysergide for migraine and other drugs. SYN: *Ormond's syndrome.*

retroperitoneum (rē″trō-pĕr-ĭ-tō-nē′ŭm). The space behind the peritoneum.

retroperitonitis (rē″trō-pĕr″ĭ-tō-nī′tĭs). Inflammation behind the peritoneum.

retropharyngeal (rē″trō-făr-ĭn′jē-ăl) [″ + Gr. *pharynx,* pharynx]. Behind the pharynx.

retropharyngitis (rē″trō-făr″ĭn-jī′tĭs) [″ + ″ + *itis,* inflammation]. Inflammation of the retropharyngeal tissue.

retropharynx (rē″trō-făr′ĭnks) [″ + Gr. *pharynx,* pharynx]. Posterior portion of the pharynx.

retroplacental (rē″trō-plă-sĕn′tăl) [″ + *placenta,* a flat cake]. Behind the placenta, or behind both the placenta and the uterine wall.

retroplasia (rē″trō-plā′zē-ă) [″ + Gr. *plassein,* to form]. Degenerative change of a cell or tissue into a more primitive form.

retroposed (rē-trō-pōsd′) [″ + *positus,* placed]. Displaced backward.

retroposition (rē″trō-pō-zĭsh′ŭn). Backward displacement of a tissue or organ.

retropulsion (rē″trō-pŭl′shŭn) [″ + *pulsio,* a thrusting]. 1. Pushing back of any part, as of the fetal head in labor. 2. A walking or running backward involuntarily, seen in some nervous disorders.

retrospective study. A clinical study in which the patients or their records are investigated after they have experienced the disease or condition. SEE: *prospective study.*

retrospondylolisthesis (rĕt′rō-spŏn″dĭ-lō-lĭs-thē′sĭs) [″ + Gr. *spondylos,* vertebra, + *olisthesis,* a slipping]. Posterior displacement of a vertebra.

retrosternal (rē″trō-stĕr′năl) [″ + Gr. *sternon,* chest]. Behind the sternum.

retrosternal pulse. Venous pulse felt over the suprasternal notch.

retrotarsal (rē″trō-tăr′săl) [″ + Gr. *tarsos,* edge of eyelid]. Located behind the tarsus of the eye.

retrouterine (rē″trō-ū′tĕr-ĭn) [L. *retro,* backward, + *uterus,* womb]. Located behind the uterus.

retrovaccination (rē″trō-văk″sĭ-nā′shŭn). Vaccination with virus obtained from a calf inoculated with smallpox virus obtained from a human.

retroversioflexion (rē″trō-vĕr″sē-ō-flĕk′shŭn) [″ + *versio,* a turning, + *flexio,* flexion]. Retroversion and retroflexion of the uterus.

retroversion (rĕt″rō-vĕr′shŭn, rē″trō-vĕr′shŭn) [″ + *versio,* turning]. A turning, or state of being turned back, esp. an entire organ being tipped.

retroversion of uterus. Displacement of the uterus backward with the cervix pointing forward toward the symphysis pubis. Normally, the cervix points toward the lower end of the sacrum with the fundus toward the suprapubic region.

retroviruses (rē″trō-, rĕt″rō-vī′rŭs-ĕs). The common name for the family of Retroviridae; RNA-containing tumor viruses some of which are oncogenic and induce sarcomas, leukemias, lymphomas, and mammary carcinomas in lower animals. These viruses contain reverse transcriptase.

retrude (rē-trood′) [L. *re,* back, + *trudere,* to shove]. To force inward or backward.

retrusion (rē-troo′shŭn). 1. Process of forcing backward, esp. with reference to teeth. 2. Condition in which teeth are retroposed.

Retzius, lines of (rĕt′zē-ŭs). [Magnus Gustav Retzius, Swedish anatomist, 1842–1919] Brownish, concentric lines in the enamel of a tooth.

Retzius, space of (rĕt′zē-ŭs). [Anders Adolf Retzius, Swedish anatomist, 1796–1860] Space in lower portion of abdomen between bladder and pubic bones and bounded superiorly by peritoneum. Contains areolar tissue, fat, and a plexus of veins.

Retzius, veins of. [A. A. Retzius] Veins forming communications between the mesenteric veins and inferior vena cava.

reunient (rē-ūn′yĕnt) [L. *re,* again, + *unire,* to unite]. 1. To connect tissues. 2. The ductus reuniens, q.v.

Reuss, August R. von (roys). Austrian ophthalmologist, 1841–1924.

R.'s color charts. Colored letters printed on a colored background for use in testing color vision. To a color-blind person, the letters will appear to be the same color as the background.

R.'s test. Test for atropine, employing sulfuric acid and an oxidizing agent.

revaccination (rē″văk-sĭ-nā′shŭn). Vaccination for a second time.

revascularization (rē-văs″kū-lăr-ī-zā′shŭn). Restoration of blood flow to a part. This may be done by using surgical means or by removing the obstruction from the original vessels.

revellent (rē-vĕl′ĕnt) [L. *re,* back, + *vellere,* to draw]. 1. Producing revulsion, the diversion of disease or blood from one part of the body to another. 2. Agent producing revulsion.

reverberation (rē″vĕr-bĕr-ā′shŭn) [L. *reverberare,* to cause to rebound]. 1. Process by which closed chains of neurons, when excited by a single impulse, will continue to discharge impulses from collaterals of their cells. 2. The repeated echoing of a sound.

Reverdin's needle (rā-vĕr-dănz′). [Jacques L. Reverdin, surgeon in Geneva, 1842–1929] A special needle with an eye at the tip that can be opened and closed by use of a lever.

reversal (rē-vĕr′săl) [L. *reversus,* revert]. 1. A change, or turning in the opposite direction. 2. In psychology, a change in an instinct to its opposite, as from love to hate.

r., sex. The process of changing an individual's sexual identity to that of the opposite sex. SEE: *sex reassignment.*

reversible (rē-vĕr′sĭ-bl). Able to change back and forth.

reversion (rē-vĕr′zhŭn). 1. Return to a previously existing condition. 2. In genetics, the appearance of traits possessed by a remote ancestor. SEE: *atavism.*

revertant. An organism that has reverted to a less advanced type by mutation.

review of systems. ABBR: ROS. In the process of examining and questioning a patient, esp. a patient not previously seen or examined, it is important to ask questions concerning each organ and region of the body. To fail to do this is to invite overlooking something in the history that is essential to the diagnosis of the disease process. This review is done in an orderly and systematic manner and is recorded. In general, it is true that if the examining person's findings are not recorded in the chart, then they might as well have not been done—at least with respect to being available for others involved in the patient's care.

In asking questions, keep in mind the possible differences between the examiner and the patient with respect to economic values, social and cultural mores, and life experiences. Thus questions concerning those areas generally considered to be personal, private, and confidential such as neuropsychiatric, sexual, and marital history must be tactful and done in a nonjudgmental manner. Also important is for the examiner to be aware constantly that the patient's vocabulary most probably does not include complex or abstruse medical, anatomical, and chemical terms. Most individuals who know slang terms for urine, feces, and sexual intercourse are unaware of the usual medical terms. It is sometimes useful to do the ROS during the physical examination. The ROS outline that follows should not be used slavishly for each patient. Obviously the questions asked of an adolescent will reasonably be less detailed than those asked of an elderly patient.

The systems and regions and questions include but are not restricted to the following:

General. History of fatigue, weight loss, travel to other climates or countries, recent weight change, chills, fever, and lifestyle change. Has individual ever been refused for life insurance or military service? How many persons occupy the patient's dwelling? Hobbies, outside interests. Religious activities, if any. History of exposure to animal pets and the health of those pets. Obtain history of military service and in what locations.

Skin. Rash, itching, sunburn, change in size of moles, vesicles, hair loss.

Head, face, and neck. Headache, migraine, vertigo, trauma, stiffness, pain, swelling.

Eyes. Are glasses worn and when were eyes last examined concerning visual acuity and glaucoma? Pain, diplopia, scotomata, itch, discharge, redness, infection.

Ears. Acute or chronic loss of hearing, pain, discharge, tinnitus, vertigo, does ear wax collect and periodically need to be removed, history of failure to adjust to descending from altitude.

Nose. Dryness, crust formation, bleeding, pain, discharge, obstruction, acuity of smell, malodor, sneezing, do nose hairs have to be trimmed to prevent irritation?

Mouth and teeth. Soreness, ulcers, pain, dryness, infection, hoarseness, bleeding gums, swallowing difficulty, condition of teeth either real or false, bruxism, temporomandibular syndrome.

Breasts. Pain, swelling, tenderness, lumps, bleeding from nipple, infection, change in ability of nipples to become erect.

Respiratory. Cough, pain, sputum production, character of sputum, hemoptysis, exposure to persons with contagious diseases such as tuberculosis. History of occupational or other exposure to asbestos, silica, chickens, parrots, or dusty environment. Dyspnea, cyanosis, tuberculosis, pneumonia, pleurisy. If pulmonary function tests were done, the date(s). Extent and duration of use of tobacco.

Cardiac. Angina, dyspnea, orthopnea, palpitations, heart murmur, heart failure, cardiac infarction, surgical procedures on coronary arteries or heart valves, history of stress test results and how recently done, hypertension, rheumatic fever, cardiac arrhythmias, exercise tolerance, history of athletic participation including jogging and running and are these current activities, the date(s) of EKG if ever taken.

Vascular. Claudication, history of cold intolerance esp. of extremities, history of frostbite, phlebitis, ulcers esp. of lower extremities.

Gastrointestinal. Appetite, history of recent gain or loss of weight, and has patient been on a particular diet for gaining or losing weight? Is patient a vegetarian? Difficulty in swallowing. Anorexia, nausea, vomiting and character of vomitus, diarrhea and possible explanation such as foreign travel or food "poisoning," belching, constipation, change in bowel habits, melena, hemorrhoids and history of surgery for this condition, use of laxatives or antacids, jaundice, hepatitis, other liver disease, use of injected "street" drugs.

Renal and urinary and genital tract. History and if positive time of last kidney or bladder stone, dysuria, hematuria, pyuria, nocturia, frequency, incontinence, urgency, history of antibiotics used for urinary tract infections, history of bedwetting, history of sexually transmitted diseases, sexual preference, penile or urethral discharge, marital history, frequency of sexual activity.

In females, vulval pruritus, vaginal discharge, vaginal malodor, history of menarche, frequency and duration of menstrual periods, amount of flow, type of menstrual protection devices used, type(s) of contraception used, total number of pregnancies, abortions, miscarriages, normal deliveries; number, sex, and ages of living children. Vaginal, cervical, uterine infections, pelvic inflammatory disease, tubal ligation, D & C, hysterectomy, dyspareunia.

In males, vasectomy, wet dreams, scrotal pain or swelling, prostate trouble.

Musculoskeletal. Muscle twitches, pain, heat, tenderness, swelling, loss of range of motion or strength, cramps, sprains, strains, trauma, fractures, stiffness, backache, osteoporosis, and character with respect to time of day of onset and duration esp. with respect to effect of exercise, backache, osteoporosis.

Hematological. Anemia, bleeding, bruising, hemarthrosis, history of hemophilia, sickle cell disease or trait, recent loss of blood, history of transfusions received and blood donation. Was patient ever turned down as a blood donor?

Endocrine. History of sexual maturation and development or lack of weight change, tolerance to heat or cold esp. with respect to other persons in the same environment, dryness of hair and skin, hair loss, voice change. In men, change in rate of beard growth, development of facial hair in the female, increase in or loss of libido, polyuria, polydipsia, polyphagia, pruritus, diabetes, exophthalmos, goiter, unexplained flushing, and sweating.

Nervous system. Recent change in ability to control muscular activity syncope, stroke ("shock"), seizures, tremor, coordination, sensory disturbance, pain, change in memory, dizziness, tremor.

Emotional and psychological status. History of psychiatric illness, anxiety, depression, overactivity, mania, lassitude, change in sleep pattern, insomnia, hypersomnia, nightmares, sleepwalking, hallucinations, feeling of unreality, paranoia, phobias, obsessions, compulsions, criminal behavior, increase in or loss of libido, satyriasis, nymphomania, suicidal thoughts, satisfaction with occupation and life in general, marital and divorce record, family discord, employment history and recent job changes, educational history and achievement, self-image.

revivescence (rē″vī-vĕs′ĕns) Revivification, q.v.

revivification (rē-vĭv″ĭ-fĭ-kā′shŭn) [L. *re,* again, + *vivere,* to live, + *facere,* to make]. 1. Attempt to restore life to those apparently dead; restoration to life or consciousness. Also restoring life in local parts, as a limb after freezing. 2. Paring of surfaces to facilitate healing, as in a wound.

revulsant (rē-vŭl′sănt) [L. *revulsio,* pulling back]. 1. Causing transfer of disease or blood from one part of the body to another. 2. Counterirritant that draws blood to an inflamed part.

revulsion (rē-vŭl′shŭn). 1. Act of driving backward, as diverting disease from one part to another by a quick withdrawal of the blood from that part. 2. In physical therapy, circulatory changes obtained by sudden and intense reactions to heat and cold. SEE: *counterirritation.*

revulsive (rē-vŭl′sĭv). 1. Causing revulsion. 2. A counterirritant.

Reye's syndrome (rīz). [R. D. K. Reye, 20th-cent. Australian pathologist] A syndrome first recognized in 1963, characterized by acute encephalopathy and fatty infiltration of the liver and possibly of the pancreas, heart, kidney, spleen and lymph nodes. Seen in children under 18 years of age after an acute viral infection.

ETIOL: Unknown, but usually occurs after acute infection with influenza B.

SYM: Upper respiratory infection (viral) followed in about 6 days by pernicious nausea and vomiting and a change in mental status (disorientation, agitation, coma, seizures), hepatomegaly without jaundice in 40% of cases.

PROG: Outcome is related to severity of the central nervous system involvement.

NURSING IMPLICATIONS: Perform a neurological assessment at frequent intervals. Monitor temperature and perform prescribed measures to alleviate hyperthermia. Implement seizure precautions. Monitor intake and output carefully. Observe for impaired hepatic function such as signs of bleeding. Instruct the parent or guardian not to administer aspirin to a child experiencing chicken pox or influenza, because use of aspirin in those conditions may induce Reye's syndrome.

TREATMENT: Supportive care including I.V. administration of fluids and electrolytes.

RF, Rf. *rheumatoid factor.*

Rf. Chem. symb. for rutherfordium.

R.F.A. *right fronto-anterior* fetal position.

R. factor. Resistance transfer factor.

R.F.P. *right fronto-posterior* fetal position.

R.F.T. *right fronto-transverse* fetal position.

RH. *releasing hormone.*

Rh. 1. Chem. symb. for rhodium. 2. *rhesus,* a monkey (Macaca rhesus) in which the Rh factor was first identified.

Rhabditis (răb-dī′tĭs) [Gr. *rhabdos,* rod]. A genus of small nematode worms, some of which are parasitic.

rhabdo- [Gr. *rhabdos,* rod]. Combining form meaning rod.

rhabdoid (răb′doyd) [″ + *eidos,* form]. Resembling a rod.

rhabdomyoblastoma (răb″dō-mī″ō-blăs-tō′mă) [″ + ″ + *blastos,* germ, + *oma,* tumor]. Rhabdomyosarcoma.

rhabdomyolysis (răb″dō-mī-ŏl′ĭ-sĭs) [″ + ″ + *lysis,* dissolution]. An acute, sometimes fatal disease characterized by destruction of skeletal muscle.

rhabdomyoma (răb″dō-mī-ō′mă) [″ + *mys,* muscle, + *oma,* tumor]. A striated muscular tissue tumor. SYN: *myoma striocellulare.*

rhabdomyosarcoma (răb″dō-mī″ō-săr-kō′mă) [″ + ″ + *sarx,* flesh, + *oma,* tumor]. An extremely malignant neoplasm originating in skeletal muscle.

rhabdophobia (răb-dō-fō′bē-ă) [″ + *phobos,* fear]. Abnormal fear of being hit or beaten with a stick or rod.

rhabdosarcoma (răb″dō-săr-kō′mă) [″ + *sarx,* flesh, + *oma,* tumor]. Rhabdomyosarcoma.

rhabdovirus (răb″dō-vī′rŭs) [″ + L. *virus,* poison]. Any of a group of rod-shaped RNA viruses with one important member, the rabies virus, pathogenic to man. The virus has a predilection for tissue of mucus-secreting glands and the central nervous system. All warm-blooded animals are susceptible to infection with these viruses.

rhachialgia (rā″kē-ăl′jē-ă) [Gr. *rhachis,* spine, + *algos,* pain]. Pain in the spine.

rhachiocampsis (rā″kē-ō-kămp′sĭs) [″ + *kampsis,* a bending]. Curvature of spine.

rhachioplegia (rā″kē-ō-plē′jē-ă) [″ + *plege,* a stroke]. Spinal paralysis.

rhachioscoliosis (rā″kē-ō-skō″lē-ō′sĭs) [″ + *skoliosis,* bending]. Curvature of the spine laterally.

rhachis (rā′kĭs) [Gr.]. Spinal column.

rhachischisis (rā-kĭs′kĭ-sĭs) [″ + *schisis,* fissure]. A congenital cleft in the spinal column.

rhachitis (rā-kī′tĭs) [″ + *itis,* inflammation]. Constitutional disease of infancy marked by faulty nutrition and bone deformity. SYN: *rachitis; rickets.*

rhacoma (rā-kō′mă) [Gr. *rhakoma,* rags]. 1. Ragged, irregular abrasion, usually of the skin. 2. Relaxation of integument of scrotum.

rhagades (răg′ă-dēz) [Gr., tears]. Linear fissures appearing in skin, esp. at the corner of the mouth or anus, causing pain. If due to syphilis, they form a radiating scar on healing.

rhagadiform (rā-găd′ĭ-form) [Gr. *rhagas,* tear, + L. *forma,* shape]. Fissured; having cracks.

-rhage, -rhagia [Gr. *rhegnynai,* to burst forth]. Suffix meaning bleeding, profuse discharge.

Rh antiserum. Human serum that contains Rh antibodies.

rhaphania (ră-fā′nē-ă) [Gr. *raphanos,* radish]. Spasmodic disease caused by eating the seeds of wild radish; allied to ergotism. SYN: *raphania.*

rhaphe (rā′fē) [Gr.]. A seam or ridge. SYN: *raphe.*

-rhaphy [Gr. *rhaphe*]. Suffix meaning joining in a seam, or suturation.

Rh blood group. A blood group discovered on the surface of erythrocytes of the rhesus monkey. It is present to a variable degree in human populations. When present, an individual is designated Rh^+ (Rh positive). In those without the factor (Rh^- or Rh negative) it causes, when injected, the formation of anti-Rh agglutinin. Subsequent transfusions of Rh^+ blood may result in serious transfusion reactions (agglutination and hemolysis of red blood cells). A pregnant woman who is Rh negative may become sensitized by blood of an Rh^+ fetus. In subsequent pregnancies, if the fetus is Rh^+, Rh antibodies produced in maternal blood may cross the placenta and destroy fetal cells, giving rise to erythroblastosis fetalis, q.v.

-rhea [Gr. *rhoia,* flow]. Suffix meaning to flow.

rhegma (rĕg′mă) [Gr. *rhegma,* a tear]. Rupture, fracture, or rent.

rhegmatogenous (rĕg″mă-tŏj′ĕ-nŭs) [″ + *gennan,* to produce]. Originating or due to a rhegma.

rhembasmus (rĕm-băs′mŭs) [Gr. *rhembasmos*]. Wandering of mind; indecision.

rhenium (rē′nē-ŭm). SYMB: Re. At. wt. 186.2; at. no. 75. A metallic element similar to manganese.

rheo- [Gr. *rheos,* current]. Combining form indicating current, stream, or to flow.

rheobase (rē′ō-bās) [″ + *basis,* step]. In unipolar testing with the galvanic current using negative as active pole, the minimal voltage required to produce a stimulated response. This is the rheobase or threshold of excitation. SEE: *chronaxie.*

rheobasic (rē″ō-bā′sĭk). Concerning rheobase.

rheology (rē-ŏl′ō-jē) [″ + *logos,* study]. Study of the deformation and flow of materials.

Rheomacrodex. Trade name for dextran 40.

rheometer (rē-ŏm′ĕt-ĕr) [″ + *metron,* measure]. 1. Instrument for qualitative determination of presence of an electric current. SYN: *galvanometer.* 2. Device for measuring rapidity of the blood current.

rheostat (rē′ō-stăt) [″ + *statos,* standing]. A device maintaining fixed or variable resistance for controlling the amount of electrical current entering a circuit.

rheostosis (rē-ŏs-tō′sĭs) [″ + *osteon,* bone]. A hypertrophying and condensing osteitis occurring in streaks, involving long bones.

rheotachygraphy (rē″ō-tă-kĭg′ră-fē) [″ + *tachys,* swift, + *graphein,* to write]. Graphic recording of variation of electromotive force in a muscle.

rheotaxis (rē″ō-tăk′sĭs) [″ + *taxis,* arrangement]. Reaction to a current of fluid, causing the part acted upon to move against the current.

rheotropism (rē-ŏt′rō-pĭzm) [″ + *trope,* a turn, + *-ismos,* condition]. Rheotaxis, q.v.

rheum, rheuma (room, room′ă) [Gr. *rheuma,* discharge]. Any catarrhal or watery discharge.

rheumatic (roo-măt′ĭk) [Gr. *rheumatikos*]. Pert. to rheumatism.

rheumatic fever. A systemic, febrile disease that is inflammatory and nonsuppurative in nature and variable in severity, duration, and sequelae. It is frequently followed by serious heart or kidney disease.

ETIOL: Unknown, but its onset follows a preceding infection with a strain of group A streptococci. Attacks usually occur in childhood; an individual is esp susceptible to subsequent attacks.

SYM: Sometime following a streptococcal infection the patient will experience the sudden occurrence of fever and joint pain; this is the most common type of onset. Other symptoms include fever, migratory polyarthritis, pain upon motion, abdominal pain, chorea, cardiac involvement (pericarditis, myocarditis, and endocarditis). Later gives rise to precordial discomfort and development of heart murmurs. Skin manifestations include erythema marginatum or circinatum, and development of subcutaneous nodules. Epistaxis is common.

Rheumatic fever may occur without any sign or symptom of joint involvement.

NURSING IMPLICATIONS: Ensure maintenance of bedrest by informing the patient of the significance of compliance. Monitor temperature frequently for elevation; institute appropriate nursing measures for fever reduction. Monitor pulse and notify the physician if an arrhythmia occurs. Instruct the patient concerning altered lifestyle and permitted activities. Instruct the patient concerning the prescribed bland, high-protein and high-carbohydrate diet. Force fluids unless the cardiac status contraindicates this, in which case the diet should also include salt restriction. Administer prescribed medications and provide drug information to the patient and family. The drug information should include action, frequency of use, and possible side effects.

TREATMENT: Enforced bedrest until signs of active rheumatic fever have disappeared. Salicylates for symptomatic relief. Penicillin administered to eradicate streptococci. Complications, esp. those involving heart, require special treatment.

PROPHYLAXIS: Prompt and adequate treatment of streptococcal infections with penicillin preferably, or erythromycin in appropriate dose, for a minimum of 10 days. Following an attack of rheumatic fever, individuals should receive continuous prophylaxis with penicillin or sulfonamide for an indefinite period.

Patients known to have carditis who must undergo major dental procedures should receive additional antibiotic coverage on the day of the treatment and for several days thereafter.

rheumatid (roo′mă-tĭd). Skin lesion associated with rheumatic disease

rheumatism (roo′mă-tĭzm) [Gr. *rheumatismos*]. A general term for acute and chronic conditions characterized by inflammation, soreness and stiffness of muscles, and pain in joints and associated structures. It includes arthritis (infectious, rheumatoid, gouty); arthritis due to rheumatic fever or trauma; degenerative joint disease; neurogenic arthropathy; hydroarthrosis; myositis; bursitis; fibromyositis; and many other conditions. SEE: *arthritis; rheumatic fever.*

r., acute articular. Rheumatic fever.

r., chronic. Rheumatism associated with a joint disorder, such as rheumatoid arthritis, gout, or degenerative joint disease, usually resulting in deformity of the joint.

r., gonorrheal. Arthritis resulting from gonorrheal infection. SEE: *gonorrhea.*

r., muscular. Term applied to a number of muscular conditions characterized by tenderness, soreness, pain, and local spasm. Includes such conditions as fibromyositis, myositis, myalgia, and torticollis, q.v.

r., palindromic. Intermittent joint pain with tenderness, heat, and swelling that lasts from a few hours to as long as a week. The knee is most often involved but the disease does not necessarily return to the same joint(s). Between attacks there is no evidence of the disease. The cause is unknown, and there is no specific treatment.

r., psychogenic. Rheumatism of psychic origin, esp. that occurring under emotional stress.

r., soft tissue. General term for a variety of localized and generalized conditions that cause pain around joints but that are not related to or caused by joint disease. Included in this general classification are bursitis, tennis elbow, tendinitis, perichondritis, stiff man syndrome, and Tietze's disease.

rheumatismal (roo″mă-tĭz′măl). Concerning or related to rheumatism.

rheumatoid (roo′mă-toyd) [Gr. *rheuma,* discharge, + *eidos,* like]. Of the nature of rheumatism; resembling rheumatism.

rheumatoid arthritis. Form of arthritis with inflammation of the joints, stiffness, swelling, cartilaginous hypertrophy, and pain. SEE: *arthritis, rheumatoid.*

rheumatoid factor. An immunoglobulin present in serum of 50 to 95% of adults with rheumatoid arthritis. This factor, though not specific for rheumatoid arthritis, is quite helpful in diagnosing and investigating the disease.

rheumatologist (roo″mă-tŏl′ō-jĭst). A physician who specializes in rheumatic diseases.

rheumatology (roo″mă-tŏl′ō-jē). The division of medicine concerned with rheumatic diseases.

rhexis (rĕk′sĭs) [Gr., rupture]. Rupture of any organ, blood vessel, or tissue.

Rh factor. SEE: *Rh blood group.*

Rh genes. A series of eight allelic genes that are responsible for the various Rh blood types and designated by Wiener as R^1, R^2, R^0, R^z, r, r′, r″, and r_y. Genes represented by small r's are responsible for Rh-negative (Rh^-) persons; those by large R's for Rh-positive (Rh^+) persons.

rhicnosis (rĭk-nō′sĭs) [Gr. *rhytis,* wrinkle, + *osis,* condition]. Wrinkling of the skin due principally to atrophy of subcutaneous tissue, esp. elastic fibers.

rhigosis (rī-gō′sĭs) [Gr. *rhigosis,* shivering]. Perception of cold.

Rh immune globulin. A solution of gamma globulin containing anti-Rh. Given to the mother within 72 hours after delivery of an Rh-positive infant to an Rh-negative mother, it acts to prevent and suppress the Rh immune response. Also indicated in abortion done on an Rh-negative mother.

rhinal (rī′năl) [Gr. *rhis,* nose]. Concerning the nose. SYN: *nasal.*

rhinalgia (rī-năl′jē-ă) [″ + *algos,* pain]. Pain in the nose; nasal neuralgia.

rhinedema (rī″nĕ-dē′mă) [″ + *oidema,* swelling]. Edema of the nose.

rhinencephalon (rī-nĕn-sĕf′ă-lŏn) [″ + *enkephalos,* brain]. Portion of brain concerned with reception and integration of olfactory impulses. Includes olfactory bulb, olfactory tract and striae, intermediate olfactory area, pyriform area, paraterminal area, hippocampal formation, and fornix. It constitutes the paleopallium and archipallium.

rhinencephalus (rī″nĕn-sĕf′ă-lŭs) [″ + *enkephalos,* brain]. Rhinocephalus.

rhinesthesia (rī-nĕs-thē′zē-ă) [″ + *aisthesis,* sensation]. The sense of smell.

rhineurynter (rĭn″ū-rĭn′tĕr) [″ + *eurynein,* to dilate]. Elastic bag used for dilating the nostrils.

rhinion (rĭn′ē-ŏn) [Gr.]. Lower end of the suture between nasal bones; a craniometric point. SYN: *punctum nasale inferius.*

rhinism (rī′nĭzm) [Gr. *rhis,* nose, + *-ismos,* condition]. Nasal quality of the voice.

rhinitis (rī-nī′tĭs) [″ + *itis,* inflammation]. Inflammation of the nasal mucosa. SEE: *endorhinitis; ozena.*

r., acute. Acute congested condition of the nose with increased secretion of mucus. SYN: *coryza.*

TREATMENT: No specific treatment is known. General measures include rest, adequate fluids, well-balanced diet. Analgesics and antipyretics may be used to make patient comfortable. Sulfonamides and antibiotics are of no value and should not be administered. Antihistamines may relieve early symptoms but do not abort or alter course. Vasoconstrictors in form of inhalants, nasal sprays, or drops may give temporary relief. Their use helps prevent the development of middle ear infections by helping to maintain the patency of the eustachian tubes.

r., allergic. Rhinitis due to sensitivity of nasal mucosa to an allergen. SYN: *hay fever; r., vasomotor.*

r., atrophic. Chronic inflammation with marked atrophy of mucous membrane and with considerable dry crusting and disturbance in the sense of smell. Usually accompanied by ozena. The throat is dry and, as a rule, contains crusts. A husky voice or hoarseness often is common.

SYM: Fetid odor from nose and throat with considerable crusting.

TREATMENT: Irrigation of nose with warm alkalinized saline solution twice daily. General hygienic measures. Correction of any associated disorders. Surgical treatment seldom helpful.

r. caseosa. Rhinitis characterized by accumulation of offensive cheeselike masses in nose and sinuses and accompanied by a seropurulent discharge.

r., chronic hyperplastic. Chronic inflammation of mucous membrane accompanied by polypoid formation and underlying sinus pathology. SEE: *sinus.*

r., chronic hypertrophic. Inflammation of the mucous membrane of the nose characterized by hypertrophy of the mucous membrane of the turbinates and the septum.

SYM: Those of nasal obstruction, postnasal discharge, and recurrent head colds.

TREATMENT: Consists in surgical removal of hypertrophic or mulberry ends of inferior turbinates and cauterization of mucosa of inferior turbinates and septum.

r., fibrinous. Rhinitis characterized by formation of a false membrane in nasal cavities.

r., hypertrophic. Rhinitis characterized by thickening and swelling of the nasal mucosa.

r., membranous. Chronic rhinitis accompanied by a fibrinous exudate.

r., perennial. Rhinitis that is nonseasonal, but continues indefinitely with variations in severity.

r., periodic. R., allergic.

r., pseudomembranous. R., fibrinous.

r., purulent. Chronic rhinitis accompanied by pus formation.

r., vasomotor. Rhinitis with rhinorrhea due to increased secretion of mucus from the nasal mucosa. May be caused by allergy or neurovascular imbalance.

rhino- [Gr. *rhis*]. Combining form indicating the nose.

rhinoanemometer (rī″nō-ăn″ĕ-mŏm′ĕ-tĕr). Device that determines the presence of nasal obstruction by measuring the rate of flow of air through the nasal passages.

rhinoantritis (rī″nō-ăn-trī′tĭs) [″ + *antron,* cavity, + *itis,* inflammation]. Inflamed condition of the nasal cavities and one or both maxillary antra.

rhinobyon (rī-nō′bē-ŏn) [″ + *byein,* to plug]. A tampon or plug for the nose.

rhinocanthectomy (rī″nō-kăn-thĕk′tō-mē) [Gr. *rhis,* nose, + *kanthos,* canthus, + *ektome,* excision]. Excision of inner corner of the eye. SYN: *rhinommectomy.*

rhinocele (rī′nō-sēl) [″ + *koilia,* hollow]. The ventricle or hollow of the olfactory lobe or rhinoencephalon.

rhinocephalus (rī″nō-sĕf′ă-lŭs) [″ + *kephale,* head]. An individual with rhinocephaly.

rhinocephaly (rī″nō-sĕf′ă-lē) [″ + *kephale,* head]. A congenital deformity in which the eyes are fused and the nose present as a fleshy protuberance above the eyes.

rhinocheiloplasty (rī″nō-kī′lō-plăs″tē) [″ + *cheilos,* lip, + *plastos,* formed]. Plastic surgery of the nose and upper lip.

rhinocleisis (rī-nō-klī′sĭs) [Gr. *rhis,* nose, + *kleisis,* closure]. Nasal obstruction. SYN: *rhinostenosis.*

rhinodacryolith (rī″nō-dăk′rē-ō-lĭth) [″ + *dakryon,* tear, + *lithos,* stone]. A nasal calculus.

rhinodynia (rī″nō-dĭn′ē-ă) [″ + *odyne,* pain]. Nasal pain. SYN: *rhinalgia.*

Rhinoestrus (rī-nĕs′trŭs). A genus of flies belonging to the family Oestridae. Larvae may be deposited in eye, nasal, or buccal cavities of mammals.

R. purpureus. Russian gadfly, whose larvae sometimes cause nasomyiasis and ophthalmomyiasis in man.

rhinogenous (rī-nŏj′ĕn-ŭs) [″ + *gennan,* to produce]. Originating in the nose.

rhinokyphosis (rī″nō-kī-fō′sĭs) [″ + *kyphos,* hump, + *osis,* condition]. A deformity of the bridge of the nose.

rhinolalia (rī″nō-lā′lē-ă) [″ + *lalia,* speech]. Nasal quality of the voice. SEE: *rhinolalia.*

r. aperta. Rhinolalia caused by undue patency of posterior nares.

r. clausa. Rhinolalia caused by closure of nasal passages.

rhinolaryngitis (rī″nō-lăr″ĭn-jī′tĭs) [″ + *larynx,* larynx, + *itis,* inflammation]. Simultaneous inflammation of mucosa of nose and larynx.

rhinolith (rī′nō-lĭth) [″ + *lithos,* stone]. Nasal concretion.

rhinolithiasis (rī″nō-lĭth-ī′ă-sĭs). The formation of nasal calculi.

rhinologist (rī-nŏl′ō-jĭst) [″ + *logos,* study]. A specialist in diseases of the nose.

rhinology (rī-nŏl′ō-jē). Science of the nose and

its diseases.

rhinomanometer (rī″nō-măn-ŏm′ĕt-ĕr) [Gr. *rhis,* nose, + *manos,* thin, + *metron,* a measure]. A device for measuring the amount of nasal obstruction.

rhinomanometry (rī″nō-mă-nŏm′ĕ-trē). Measurement of the air flow through and air pressure in the nose.

rhinometer (rī-nŏm′ĕt-ĕr). Device for measurement of the nose or its cavities.

rhinomiosis (rī″nō-mī-ō′sĭs) [″ + *meiosis,* a lessening]. Surgical reduction in size of the nose.

rhinommectomy (rī″nŏm-mĕk′tō-mē) [″ + *omma,* eye, + *ektome,* excision]. Surgical excision of the inner canthus of the eye. SYN: *rhinocanthectomy.*

rhinomycosis (rī″nō-mī-kō′sĭs) [″ + *mykes,* fungus, + *osis,* condition]. Fungi in mucous membranes and secretions of the nose.

rhinonecrosis (rī″nō-nē-krō′sĭs) [″ + *nekrosis,* death]. Necrosis of the nasal bones.

rhinopathy (rī-nŏp′ă-thē) [″ + *pathos,* disease]. Any nasal disease.

rhinopharyngeal (rī″nō-fă-rĭn′jē-ăl). Concerning the nasopharynx.

rhinopharyngitis (rī″nō-făr-ĭn-jī′tĭs) [″ + *pharynx,* pharynx, + *itis,* inflammation]. Inflamed condition of the nasopharynx.

rhinopharyngocele (rī″nō-făr-ĭn′gō-sēl) [″ + ″ + *kele,* mass]. A nasopharyngeal tumor.

rhinopharyngolith (rī″nō-făr-ĭn′gō-lĭth) [″ + ″ + *lithos,* stone]. Concretion in the nasal pharynx.

rhinopharynx (rī″nō-făr′ĭnks). Upper portion of pharynx continuous with the nasal passages. SYN: *nasopharynx.*

rhinophonia (rī″nō-fō′nē-ă) [″ + *phone,* voice]. A nasal tone in speaking.

rhinophycomycosis (rī″nō-fī″kō-mī-kō′sĭs) [″ + *phykos,* seaweed, + *mykes,* fungus, + *osis,* condition]. A fungus infection that may occur in man or animals. It affects the nasal and paranasal sinuses and may spread to the brain. It is caused by the phycomycete Entomophthora coronata.

rhinophyma (rī-nō-fī′mă) [″ + *phyma,* growth]. Lobular hypertrophy of nose, with red coloration, congestion, and retention of sebum. SYN: *acne rosacea.*

rhinoplasty (rī′nō-plăs″tē) [″ + *plastos,* formed]. Plastic surgery of the nose.

rhinopneumonitis (rī″nō-nū″mō-nī′tĭs) [Gr. *rhis,* nose, + *pneumon,* lung, + *itis,* inflammation]. Inflammation of the nasal and pulmonary mucous membranes.

rhinopolypus (rī″nō-pŏl′ĭ-pŭs) [″ + *polys,* many, + *pous,* foot]. Polypus of the nose.

rhinorrhagia (rī″nō-rā′jē-ă) [″ + *rhegnynai,* to burst forth]. Profuse hemorrhage from the nose. SYN: *epistaxis; nosebleed.*

rhinorrhea (rī″nō-rē′ă) [″ + *rhoia,* a flow]. Thin watery discharge from the nose.

r., cerebrospinal. Discharge of spinal fluid from the nose due to a defect in or trauma to the cribriform plate.

r., gustatory. Flow of a thin watery material from the nose while eating.

rhinosalpingitis (rī″nō-săl″pĭn-jī′tĭs) [″ + *salpinx,* tube, + *itis,* inflammation.]. Inflammation of the mucosa of the nose and eustachian tube.

rhinoscleroma (rī″nō-sklē-rō′mă) [″ + *skleros,* hard, + *oma,* tumor]. A chronic, infectious disease involving nose and upper portions of respiratory tract in which growths of almost stony hardness develop, sometimes leading to marked deformity.

ETIOL: Klebsiella rhinoscleromatis, a gram-negative encapsulated bacillus.

SYM: The disease presents a hard, nodular growth, which usually begins at anterior end of nose and spreads to the lower respiratory tract. There usually is no pain and no tendency to ulceration.

TREATMENT: Surgical, in combination with streptomycin.

rhinoscope (rī′nō-skōp) [″ + *skopein,* to examine]. Instrument for examination of the nose.

rhinoscopic (rī″nō-skŏp′ĭk). Concerning rhinoscopy.

rhinoscopy (rī-nŏs′kō-pē). Examination of nasal passages.

r., anterior. Examination through anterior nares.

r., posterior. Examination through posterior nares, usually with a small mirror in the nasopharynx.

rhinosporidiosis (rī″nō-spō-rĭd″ē-ō′sĭs) [″ + *sporidion,* little seed, + *osis,* condition]. Condition caused by a fungus, Rhinosporidium seeberi, characterized by development of pedunculated polyps on mucous membranes of nose, larynx, eyes, penis, vagina, and sometimes skin of various parts of body. Disease is contracted from cattle. Found in India, Ceylon, and other parts of the world.

Rhinosporidium (rī″nō-spō-rĭd′ē-ŭm). A genus of fungi that is pathogenic to man.

R. seeberi. Causative agent of rhinosporidiosis.

rhinostenosis (rī″nō-stĕn-ō′sĭs) [″ + *stenosis,* a narrowing]. Obstruction of the nasal passages. SYN: *rhinocleisis.*

rhinotomy (rī-nŏt′ō-mē) [″ + *tome,* incision]. Incision of the nose for drainage purposes.

rhinotracheitis (rī″nō-trā″kē-ī′tĭs) [″ + *tracheia,* trachea, + *itis,* inflammation]. Inflammation of the nasal mucous membranes and the trachea.

rhinovaccination (rī″nō-văk-sĭn-ā′shŭn) [″ + L. *vaccinus,* pert. to a cow]. Vaccine applied to the mucosa of the nose.

rhinovirus (rī″nō-vī′rŭs). One of a subgroup of picornaviruses, q.v., that causes the common cold in man. There are probably more than 100 rhinoviruses and they occur worldwide. There is no specific therapy. Viruses other than rhinoviruses also cause the syndrome diagnosed as a cold. These include the A21 coxsackievirus and coronaviruses.

Rhipicephalus (rī″pĭ-sĕf′ă-lŭs) [Gr. *rhipis,* fan, + *kephale,* head]. A genus of ticks belonging to the family Ixodidae. Several species, esp. R. sanguineus, serve as vectors for the organisms of spotted fever, boutonneuse fever, and other rickettsial diseases.

rhitidectomy (rĭt″ĭ-dĕk′tō-mē) [Gr. *rhytis,* wrinkle, + *ektome,* excision]. Removal of wrinkles by plastic surgery. SYN: *rhytidectomy.*

rhitidosis (rĭt-ĭ-dō′sĭs) [Gr. *rhytidosis*]. Wrinkling of the cornea, indicating its disintegration. One of the signs of approaching death. SYN: *rhytidosis.*

rhizo- [Gr. *rhiza*]. Combining form meaning root.

rhizodontropy (rī″zō-dŏn′trō-pē) [Gr. *rhiza,* root, + *odous,* tooth, + *trope,* a turning]. Process of attaching an artificial crown upon the root of a tooth.

rhizodontrypy (rī″zō-dŏn′trĭ-pē) [″ + ″ + *trype,* a hole]. Puncture of root of a tooth.

rhizoid (rī′zoyd) [″ + *eidos,* form]. 1. Rootlike. 2. A rootlike structure, usually one-celled, occurring in lower forms of plant life. 3. In bacteriology, term applied to a colony showing an irregular rootlike system of branching.

rhizome (rī′zōm) [Gr. *rhizoma,* mass of roots]. A rootlike stem growing horizontal along or below the ground and sending out roots and shoots.

rhizomelic (rī″zō-mĕl′ĭk) [Gr. *rhiza,* root, + *melos,* limb]. Concerning the hip joint and shoulder joint.

rhizomeningomyelitis (rī″zō-mē-nĭn″gō-mī″ĕ-lī′tĭs) [″ + *meninx,* membrane, + *myelos,* marrow, + *itis,* inflammation]. Radiculomeningomyelitis, q.v.

Rhizopoda (rī-zŏp′ō-dă) [″ + *pous,* foot]. A subclass of the class Sarcodina, phylum Protozoa, characterized by possession of lobose pseudopodia and lacking a central filament. Includes the amebae and foraminifera.

rhizotomy (rī-zŏt′ō-mē) [″ + *tome,* incision]. Section of a root, as of a nerve or tooth.

r., anterior. Section of the ventral root of the spinal nerve.

r., posterior. Section of the dorsal root of the spinal nerve for the relief of pain.

Rh_o (D) immune globulin (human). USP. Immune globulin prepared from the plasma of persons with a high concentration of Rh antibodies. Administration of the gamma globulin to an Rh-negative mother within 72 hours after delivery of an Rh-positive infant usually prevents isoimmunization and thus prevents hemolytic disease of the newborn in subsequent pregnancies. The dose must be repeated after each delivery. It is also given on the same schedule after an Rh-negative mother has an abortion and the fetus is Rh positive. Trade name is RhoGAM. SEE: *erythroblastosis fetalis.*

rhodium (rō′dē-ŭm). SYMB: Rh. At. wt. 102.905; at. no. 45. A rare metallic element.

rhodo- (rō′dō) [Gr. *rhodon,* rose]. Combining form meaning red.

rhodogenesis (rō″dō-jĕn′ĕ-sĭs) [″ + *genesis,* formation]. Regeneration of visual purple that has been bleached by light.

rhodophane (rō′dō-fān) [″ + *phainein,* to show]. A red pigment found in retinal cones of birds and fishes.

rhodophylaxis (rō″dō-fĭ-lăk′sĭs) [″ + *phylaxis,* protection]. Ability of the retinal epithelium to regenerate visual purple that has been bleached by light.

rhodopsin (rō-dŏp′sĭn) [″ + *opsis,* vision]. Visual purple, a pigment in outer segment of retinal rods.

RhoGAM. Trade name for Rh_o(D) immune globulin, USP.

rhombencephalon (rŏm″bĕn-sĕf′ă-lŏn) [Gr. *rhombos,* rhomb, + *enkephalos,* brain]. [NA] A primary division of the embryonic brain that gives rise to metencephalon and myelencephalon. Includes the pons, cerebellum, and medulla oblongata. SYN: *hindbrain.*

rhombocele (rŏm′bō-sēl) [″ + *koilos,* a hollow]. The cavity of the rhombencephalon.

rhomboid (rŏm′boyd) [″ + *eidos,* shape]. An oblique parallelogram.

rhomboideus (rŏm-bō-ĭd′ē-ŭs) [L.]. One of two muscles beneath the trapezius muscle. SEE: *Muscles* in *Appendix; muscles* for illus.

rhomboid fossa. The 4th ventricle of the brain.

rhombomere (rŏm′bō-mēr) [Gr. *rhombos,* rhomb, + *meros,* part]. Neuromere, q.v.

rhoncal, rhonchial (rŏng′kăl, rŏng′kē-ăl) [Gr. *rhonchos,* a snore]. Pert. to, or produced by, a rattle in the throat.

rhonchi. Plural of rhonchus.

rhonchus (rŏng′kŭs). (pl. *rhonchi*) A rale or rattling in the throat, esp. when it resembles snoring.

rhopheocytosis (rō″fē-ō-sī-tō′sĭs) [Gr. *rhophein,* gulp down, + *kytos,* cell, + *osis,* condition]. Mechanism of transfer of ferritin from one cell in the bone marrow to another. SEE: *pinocytosis.*

rhotacism (rō′tă-sĭzm) [Gr. *rhotakizein,* to overuse letter "r"]. Overuse or improper utterance of "r" sounds, with too much emphasis upon this letter.

rhubarb (roo'bărb) [ME. *rubarbe*]. Extract made from roots and rhizome of Rheum officinale, R. palmatum, and other species. Used as a cathartic and astringent. High in oxalic acid. Of little food value, but desirable for its mineral content.

Rhus (rŭs) [L.]. A genus of trees and shrubs, some of which are poisonous, i.e., poison ivy (R. toxicodendron) and poison sumac (R. venenata), and which produce a severe dermatitis.

rhyostomaturia (rī"ō-stō"mă-tū'rē-ă) [Gr. *rhyas*, fluid, + *stoma*, mouth, + *ouron*, urine]. The elimination of urinary elements by the salivary glands.

rhyparia (rī-pā'rē-ă) [Gr., filth]. Foul substance that collects in the mouth during some fevers. SYN: *sordes*.

rhypophagy (rī-pŏf'ă-jē) [Gr. *rhypos*, filth, + *phagein*, to eat]. The eating of filth. SYN: *scatophagy*.

rhypophobia (rī"pō-fō'bē-ă) [" + *phobos*, fear]. Abnormal disgust at the act of defecation, feces, or filth.

rhythm (rĭth'ŭm) [Gr. *rhythmos*, measured motion]. 1. A measured time or movement; regularity of occurrence of action or function. 2. In electroencephalography, the regular occurrence of an impulse.

r., alpha. In electroencephalography, oscillations in electric potential occurring at a rate of 8½ to 12 per second.

r., atrioventricular. Rhythmic discharges of impulses from atrioventricular (A-V) node that occur when activity of sinoatrial (S-A) node is depressed or abolished. SYN: *r., nodal*.

r., beta. In electroencephalography, waves ranging in frequency from 15 to 30 per second and of lower voltage than alpha waves. More pronounced in frontomotor leads.

r., bigeminal. The coupling of extrasystoles with previously normal beats of the heart. SEE: *bigeminal pulse*.

r., biological. Regular occurrence of certain phenomena in living organisms. SEE: *circadian; clock, biological*.

r., cantering. R., gallop.

r., circadian. The recurrence of certain biological activities approximately every 24 hours regardless of environmental influences.

r., coupled. Rhythm in which every other heartbeat produces no pulse at the wrist.

r., delta. In electroencephalography, slow waves with a frequency of 4 or fewer per second and of relatively high voltage (20 to 200 microvolts). May be found over the area of a gross lesion such as a tumor or hemorrhage.

r., ectopic. A cardiac rhythm originating outside the sinoatrial node.

r., escape. The heart rhythm when the supraventricular rate set by the sinoatrial node rhythm is completely blocked.

r., gallop. Abnormal heart rhythm with three sounds in each cycle, resembling the gallop of a horse. SYN: *r., cantering*.

r., gamma. The 50/second rhythm seen in the electroencephalogram.

r., idioventricular. Rhythm of ventricles occurring in heart block resulting from establishment of a new center of rhythmicity in ventricular myocardium, usually in bundle of His.

r., nodal. R., atrioventricular.

r., nyctohemeral. Day and night rhythm.

r., pendulum. Rhythm with the two heart sounds alike, similar to the sound of a ticking clock.

r., sinus. Normal cardiac rhythm proceeding from the sinoatrial node.

r., theta. The 4 to 7/second rhythm seen in the electroencephalogram.

r., tic-tac. A state of cardiac distress in which the first and second heart sounds are the same quality. SYN: *embryocardia*.

r., ventricular. Very slow ventricular contractions in heart block.

rhythmic [Gr. *rhythmos*]. Rhythmical; pert. to, or marked by, rhythm.

rhythmicity (rĭth-mĭs'ĭ-tē). Characterized by rhythmic activity.

rhytidectomy (rĭt"ĭ-dĕk'tō-mē) [Gr. *rhytis*, wrinkle, + *ektome*, excision]. Excision of wrinkles by plastic surgery.

rhytidoplasty (rĭt'ĭ-dō-plăs"tē) [" + *plassein*, to form]. Elimination of facial wrinkles by use of plastic surgery.

rhytidosis (rĭt"ĭ-dō'sĭs) [" + *osis*, condition]. Wrinkling of cornea. Occurs in cases of great diminution in tension of eyeball, particularly after the escape of aqueous or vitreous humor, usually near death. SYN: *rhitidosis*.

RIA. *radioimmunoassay*.

rib (rĭb) [AS. *ribb*]. One of a series of 12 pairs of narrow, curved bones extending laterally and anteriorly from sides of thoracic vertebrae and forming a part of the skeletal thorax. With the exception of the floating ribs, they are connected to the sternum by means of costal cartilages.

r., abdominal. False rib.

r.'s, asternal. R.'s, false.

r., bicipital. Irregular condition resulting from fusion of two ribs, usually involving the first rib.

r., cervical. A supernumerary rib sometimes developing in connection with a cervical vertebra, usually the lowest.

r.'s, false. Five ribs on each side that are not directly attached to the sternum. SYN: *r.'s, asternal*.

r.'s, floating. Lower two ribs that are not

attached to the sternum.

r., lumbar. A rudimentary rib that develops in relation to a lumbar vertebra.

r., slipping. A rib in which the costal cartilage is repeatedly dislocating.

r., sternal. R., true.

r.'s, true. The upper seven ribs on each side, which join the sternum by separate cartilages.

r., vertebral. R., floating, q.v.

r., vertebrocostal. The upper three false ribs on each side.

r., vertebrosternal. True rib.

ribbon (rĭb'ŭn). A ribbon or band-shaped structure.

riboflavin (rī"bō-flā'vĭn). USP. $C_{17}H_{20}N_4O_6$. A water-soluble vitamin of the B complex group. It is an orange-yellow crystalline powder comparatively stable to heat and air but unstable to light. SYN: *vitamin* B_2.

SOURCES: Milk and milk products, leafy green vegetables, liver, beef, fish, dry yeast. Also synthesized by bacteria in body.

DAILY REQUIREMENT: Adults: 0.55 mg./1000 Cal. of food intake. Infants, children, and pregnant and lactating women require increased amounts.

DEFICIENCY SYM: Eye disorders, cheilosis, glossitis, seborrheic dermatitis, esp. of face and scalp.

FUNCT: It is a constituent of certain flavoproteins that function as coenzymes in cellular oxidations. Essential for tissue repair.

ribonuclease (rī"bō-nū'klē-ās). ABBR: RNase. An enzyme that catalyzes the depolymerization of ribonucleic acid (RNA) with formation of mononucleotides.

ribonucleic acid (rī"bō-nū"klē'ĭk). A nucleic acid that controls protein synthesis in all living cells, and takes the place of DNA in certain viruses. It differs from DNA in that its sugar is ribose and the pyrimidine uracil rather than thymine is present. RNA occurs in several forms that are determined by the number of nucleotides. SEE: *deoxyribonucleic acid.*

Messenger RNA (mRNA) carries the code for specific amino acid sequences from the DNA to the cytoplasm for protein synthesis.

Transfer RNA (tRNA) carries the amino acid groups to the ribosome for protein synthesis.

Ribosomal RNA exists within the ribosomes and is thought to assist in protein synthesis.

ribonucleoprotein (rī"bō-nū"klē-ō-prō'tē-ĭn). A compound containing both protein and ribonucleic acid.

ribonucleotide (rī"bō-nū'klē-ō-tīd). A nucleotide in which the sugar ribose is combined with the purine or pyrimidine base.

ribose (rī'bōs). $C_5H_{10}O_5$, a pentose sugar present in ribonucleic acids, riboflavin, and some nucleotides.

ribosome (rī'bō-sōm). An extremely small portion of the submicroscopic structure of a cell. It contains ribonucleoprotein and functions to synthesize protein. Ribosomes may be single units or in clusters called polyribosomes or polysomes.

ribosyl (rī'bō-sĭl). The compound glycosyl, $C_5H_9O_4$, formed from ribose.

rice, polished. Rice that has been milled to produce the white product commercially available in Western countries. This treatment removes the hull, which contains the majority of the vitamin B_1.

ricin (rī'sĭn). A white, amorphous, highly toxic protein (albumin) present in the seed of the castor bean, Ricinus communis.

ricinine (rĭs'ĭn-ĕn, -īn). A poisonous alkaloid present in the leaves and seeds of castor bean plant, Ricinus communis.

ricinoleic acid. 12-hydroxy-9-octadecenoic acid. An unsaturated hydroxy acid comprising about 80% of fatty acids in the glycerides of castor oil. Has a strong laxative action.

rickets (rĭk'ĕts). A deficiency condition in children that results in inadequate deposition of lime salts in developing cartilage and newly formed bone, causing abnormalities in shape and structure of bones. SYN: *osteomalacia; rachitis.*

ETIOL: Due primarily to vitamin D deficiency, which affects the absorption of calcium and phosphorus from the intestine and the reabsorption of phosphorus by the renal tubules. May also result from inadequate intake or excessive loss of calcium.

SYM: Restlessness and slight fever at night (101 to 102° F. or 38.3 to 38.9° C.); free perspiration about head; diffuse soreness and tenderness of body; pallor; slight diarrhea; enlargement of liver and spleen; delayed dentition and eruption of badly formed teeth; head large and more or less square in outline; craniotabes or skull bones often so thin they crackle like parchment.

Sides of thorax flattened; sternum prominent; nodules can be felt at sternal end of ribs, forming rachitic rosary. Deformity may be kyphosis, lordosis, or scoliosis. Liver and spleen may be considerably enlarged; long bones are curved and prominent at their extremities.

PROG: Serum phosphatase studies are helpful in making diagnosis and prognosis. Usually favorable. Deformity disappears in 90% of cases.

PROPHYLAXIS AND TREATMENT: *Prevention:* Exposure to ultraviolet light (sunlight or artificial light) and administration of vitamin D in quantities to provide 400

I.U. of vitamin D activity per day.

Active rickets: Careful regulation of diet to meet nutritive requirements of the child, plus administration of 2200 I.U. of vitamin D per day usually is effective. Some bone deformities may require surgery.

CAUTION: Excessive use of vitamin D (in infants, over 20,000 I.U. daily; in adults over 100,000 I.U. daily) is to be avoided because of danger of hypervitaminosis D.

r., adult. Softening of bones, osteomalacia, occurring in adult life. It resembles rickets.

r., late. Rickets that has its onset in older children.

r., renal. A disturbance in epiphyseal growth during childhood due to severe chronic renal insufficiency resulting in persistent acidosis. Dwarfism and failure of gonadal development result. Prognosis is poor.

TREATMENT: Diet low in meat, milk, cheese, and egg yolk. Administration of calcium lactate or calcium gluconate in large doses.

r., vitamin D–resistant. Defect of renal tubular function that causes excessive loss of phosphorus and calcium and results in rickets poorly responsive to vitamin D therapy.

Rickettsia (rĭ-kĕt′sē-ă). [Howard T. Ricketts, U.S. pathologist, 1871–1910] Name of a genus applied to a group of microorganisms, family Rickettsiaceae, order Rickettsiales, that occupy a position intermediate between viruses and bacteria. They differ from bacteria in that they are obligate parasites requiring living cells for growth, and differ from viruses in that they are retained by the Berkefeld filter. They are the causative agents of many diseases, and are usually transmitted by arthropods (lice, fleas, ticks, mites), which serve as vectors. SEE: *rickettsial disease; rickettsialpox; rickettsiosis.*

R. typhi. The agent that causes flea-borne murine (endemic) typhus.

rickettsia (rĭ-kĕt′sē-ă). (pl. *rickettsiae*) Term applied to any of the microorganisms belonging to the genus Rickettsia.

rickettsial disease. A disease caused by an organism of the genus Rickettsia. The most common types are the spotted-fever group (Rocky Mountain spotted fever or rickettsialpox), epidemic typhus, endemic typhus, Brill's disease, Q fever, scrub typhus, and trench fever.

rickettsialpox (rĭ-kĕt′sē-ăl-pŏks″). An acute, febrile, self-limited disease caused by Rickettsia akari. It is transmitted from the house mouse to man by a small colorless mite, Allodermanyssus sanguineus.

rickettsicidal (rĭ-kĕt″sĭ-sī′dăl). Lethal to rickettsiae.

rickettsiosis (rĭ-kĕt″sē-ō′sĭs). Infection with rickettsiae.

rickettsiostatic (rĭ-kĕt″sē-ō-stăt′ĭk). Preventing or slowing the growth of rickettsiae.

riders' bone. Bony formation in the adductor muscle of the leg. Seen in those who ride horses extensively. SYN: *cavalry bone.*

riders' sprain. Sprain of adductor muscles of the thigh.

ridge (rĭj) [ME. *rigge*]. An elongated projecting structure or crest.

r., alveolar. The bony process of the maxillae or mandible that contains the alveoli or tooth sockets; the alveolar process without teeth present.

r., carotid. A sharp ridge between the carotid canal and the jugular fossa.

r., dental. Any elevation on the crown of a tooth.

r., dermal. The ridges on the surface of the fingers. These make up the fingerprints. SYN: *cristae cutis.*

r., epicondylic. One of two ridges for muscular attachments on the humerus.

r., gastrocnemial. A ridge on the posterior femoral surface for attachment of gastrocnemius muscles.

r., genital. Ridge that develops on the ventromedian surface of the urogenital ridge and gives rise to gonads.

r., gluteal. A ridge extending obliquely downward from the great trochanter of the femur for the attachment of the gluteus maximus muscle.

r., interosseous. A ridge on the fibula for attachment of the interosseous membrane.

r., interureteric. A ridge between the openings of the ureters in the bladder.

r., mammary. In the embryo of mammals, a ridge extending from the axilla to the groin. The breasts arise from this ridge. In the human, only one breast normally remains on each side. SYN: *milk line.*

r., mesonephric. Ridge that develops on the lateral surface of the urogenital ridge and gives rise to mesonephros. SYN: *r., wolffian.*

r., pronator. Oblique ridge on the anterior surface of the ulna, providing attachment to the pronator quadratus.

r., pterygoid. Ridge at angle of junction of temporal and infratemporal surface of great wing of the sphenoid bone.

r., superciliary. Curved ridge of the frontal bone over supraorbital arch.

r., supracondylar. One of two ridges (lateral and medial) on the distal end of the humerus extending upward from the lateral to medial epicondyles.

r., tentorial. Ridge on upper inner surface of the cranium to which is attached the tentorium.

r., trapezoid. An oblique ridge on the upper surface of the clavicle giving attachment to the trapezoid ligament.

r., urogenital. Ridge on dorsal wall of coelom that gives rise to genital and mesonephric ridges. SYN: *urogenital fold.* SEE: *r., genital; r., mesonephric.*

r., wolffian. R., mesonephric.

ridgel (rĭj'ĕl). A male animal, esp. a horse, with only one testicle, or only one descended testicle.

Riedel's lobe (rē'dĕlz). [Bernhard M. C. L. Riedel, Ger. surgeon, 1846–1916] A tongue-shaped process of liver, frequently found protruding over the gallbladder in cases of chronic cholecystitis.

Rifadin. Trade name for rifamycin.

rifampin (rĭf'ăm-pĭn). USP. An antibiotic synthesized from rifamycin B, which in turn is produced by fermentation of Streptomyces mediterranei. It is used in treating Mycobacterium tuberculosis and carriers of Neisseria meningitidis. Trade names are Rimactane and Rifadin.

rifamycin (rĭf"ă-mī'sĭn). An antibiotic produced by certain strains of Streptomyces mediterranei.

Riga-Fede's disease (rē'gă fā'dāz). [Antonio Riga, It. physician, 1832–1919; Francesco Fede, It. physician, 1832–1913] Ulceration of frenum of the tongue with membrane formation. Occurs after abrasion by the lower central incisors.

Riggs' disease. Periodontitis, q.v.

right (rīt) [AS. *riht*]. ABBR: R; rt. Pert. to the right side of the body; the side that on most persons is the stronger or preferred. SYN: *dexter.*

right-handed. Voluntary preference for use of the right hand. SYN: *dextrality.* SEE: *sinistrality.*

rigid (rĭ'jĭd) [L. *rigidus*]. Stiff, hard, unyielding.

rigidity (rĭ-jĭd'ĭ-tē). 1. Tenseness; immovability; stiffness; inability to bend or be bent. 2. In psychiatry, refers to one who is excessively resistant to change.

r., cadaveric. Rigor mortis.

r., cerebellar. Stiffness of body and extremities resulting from lesion of middle lobe of cerebellum.

r., clasp-knife. Passive flexion of the joint causes increased resistance of the extensors. This gives way abruptly if the pressure to produce flexion is continued.

r., cogwheel. Condition noted upon passively stretching a hypertonic muscle in which resistance is jerky.

r., decerebrate. Sustained contraction of extensor muscles of limbs resulting from a lesion in the brain stem between superior colliculi and vestibular nuclei.

rigor (rĭg'or) [L. *rigor,* stiffness]. 1. A sudden, paroxysmal chill with high temperature, called the cold stage, followed by a sense of heat and profuse perspiration, called the hot stage. 2. A state of hardness and stiffness, as in a muscle.

r. mortis. The stiffness that occurs in dead bodies. SEE: *Nysten's law.*

rim. An edge or border.

r., bite. R., occlusion, q.v.

r., occlusion. Occluding surfaces built on denture bases in order to make maxillomandibular relation records and for arranging teeth.

rima (rī'mă) [L., a slit]. (pl. *rimae*) [NA] A slit, fissure, or crack.

r. cornealis. Groove in the sclera holding edge of the cornea.

r. glottidis. [NA] An elongated slit between the vocal folds. SYN: *r. vocalis.*

r. oris. [NA] Aperture of the mouth.

r. palpebrarum. [NA] Slit between the eyelids.

r. pudendi. [NA] Space between the labia majora, through which urethra and vagina open.

r. respiratoria. Space behind the arytenoid cartilages.

r. vestibuli. [NA] Space between the false vocal cords.

r. vocalis. R. glottidis.

Rimactane. Trade name for rifampin.

rimose (rī'mōs, rī-mōs') [L. *rimosus*]. Fissured or marked by cracks.

rimula (rĭm'ū-lă) [L.]. (pl. *rimulae*) A minute fissure or slit, esp. of the spinal cord or brain.

rind (rīnd) [AS.]. A thick or firm outer coating of an organ, plant, or animal.

ring (rĭng) [AS. *hring*]. 1. Any round area, organ, or band around a circular opening. SEE: *annulus.* 2. In chemistry, a collection of atoms chemically bound in a circular form.

r., abdominal. Apertures in the abdominal wall. SEE: *abdominal rings.*

r., Albl's. A curved thin shadow seen on roentgenogram of an intracranial aneurysm.

r., Bandl's. R., pathologic retraction, q.v.

r., benzene. The closed ring of six carbon atoms.

r., Cannon's. A contracted band of muscles in the transverse colon near the hepatic flexure.

r., ciliary. Portion of the ciliary body consisting of a bandlike zone lying directly anterior to the ora serrata. SYN: *orbiculus ciliaris.*

r., conjunctival. A narrow ring at the junction of the edge of the cornea with the conjunctiva. SYN: *anulus conjunctiva.*

r., constriction. A stricture of the body of the uterus. A circular area of the uterus contracts around a part of the fetus.

r., femoral. The superior aperture of the femoral canal.

r., inguinal, abdominal. The abdominal opening of the inguinal canal. SEE: *abdominal rings.*

r., inguinal, deep. The inguinal canal's opening deep inside the abdominal wall.

r., inguinal, subcutaneous. The external opening of the inguinal canal. SEE: *abdominal rings.*

r., inguinal, superficial. The opening of the superficial end of the inguinal canal.

r., Kayser-Fleischer. SEE: *Kayser-Fleischer ring; Wilson's disease.*

r., pathologic retraction. During delivery, a prolonged contraction of the ring formed by the junction of the body and isthmus of the uterus.

r., physiologic retraction. A normal contraction of the ring formed by the junction of the body and isthmus of the uterus.

r., Schwalbe's. The thickened peripheral margin of the Descemet's membrane of the cornea of the eye. It is formed by a circular bundle of connective tissue.

r., tympanic. A band of bone formed by three elements (squamous, petromastoid, and tympanic) that develop into the tympanic plate.

r., umbilical. The opening in the linea alba of the embryo. The umbilical vessels pass through this ring.

r., vascular. An anomalous ring of vascular structures around the trachea and esophagus.

ring, removal from swollen finger. Technique for removal of ring from an injured or swollen finger. Pass one end of a length of string under the ring. Push the ring as far away from the swollen area toward the hand as is possible; wrap the string on the side of the swollen area around the finger for a dozen turns or so. Grasp the end of the string that extends under the ring and while holding it firmly unwind the string from the hand side of the ring. This will move the ring toward the free end of the finger. Continue this until the ring is free.

Ringer, Sydney (rĭng'ĕr). British physiologist, 1835–1910.

R.'s injection, lactated. USP. A sterile solution of specified amounts of calcium chloride, potassium chloride, sodium chloride, and sodium lactate in water for injection. It is used intravenously to replace electrolytes.

R.'s irrigation. USP. A solution of recently boiled distilled water containing 8.6 gm. sodium chloride, 0.3 gm. potassium chloride, and 0.33 gm. calcium chloride per liter. For topical use only. Previously used name was *Ringer's solution.*

ringworm (rĭng'wŭrm). Popular term for a dermatomycosis due to various species of fungi belonging to the genera Microsporum and Trichophyton. Ringworm of the scalp is called tinea capitis; of the body, tinea corporis; of the beard, tinea barbae; of the nails, tinea unguium; of the feet, athlete's foot. SEE: *tinea.*

SYM: Red-ringed patch of vesicles, itching, pain, scaling.

TREATMENT: Griseofulvin may be helpful in certain types. At the same time, treatment with topical fungistatic preparations is important.

Rinne's test (rĭn'nēz). [Heinrich A. Rinne, Ger. otologist, 1819–1868] Use of tuning fork to compare bone conduction hearing with air conduction. The vibrating fork is held by its stem on the mastoid process of the ear until it is no longer heard by the patient. Then it is held close to the external auditory meatus. If the subject still hears the vibrations this is called a positive Rinne test. If the fork is not heard by air conduction the test is repeated; but first air conduction is tested until the sound is no longer heard, then the stem of the fork is placed on the mastoid process of the ear. If the sound is still heard, this is called a negative Rinne test. SEE: *Weber's test.*

Riolan's arch (rē"ō-lănz'). [Jean Riolan, Fr. anatomist, 1580–1657] Arch formed by the mesentery of the transverse colon.

Riolan's bouquet. Two ligaments and three muscles attached to styloid process of temporal bone.

Riolan's muscle. Ciliary portion of orbicularis oculi.

Riopan. Trade name for magaldrate, USP.

ripa (rī'pă) [L., bank]. Any line of reflection of the ependyma of the brain from the ventricular wall to the choroid plexus.

Ripault's sign (rē-pōz'). [Louis H. A. Ripault, Fr. physician, 1807–1856] Change in shape of pupil produced by unilateral (external) pressure upon eyeball.

ripening. 1. Softening and dilatation of the uterine cervix during labor. 2. Maturation of a cataract.

risk factors. Factors in the environment, or chemical, psychological, physiological, or genetic elements that are thought to predispose an individual to the development of a disease.

Ex.: Known risk factors for coronary artery disease include: hypertension, high circulating blood lipids and cholesterol, obesity, cigarette smoking, diabetes mellitus, inability to cope with stress, physical inactivity, and a family history of atherosclerosis.

risorius (rī-sŏ'rē-ŭs) [L., laughing]. Muscular fibrous band arising over masseter muscle and inserted into tissues at the corner of the mouth. SEE: *Muscles* in *Appendix*.

ristocetin (rĭs″tō-sē′tĭn). An antibiotic obtained from cultures of Nocardia lurida.

risus (rī′sŭs) [L.]. Laughter; a laugh.

r. sardonicus. A peculiar grin, as seen in tetanus, caused by acute spasm of facial muscles.

Ritalin Hydrochloride. Trade name for methylphenidate hydrochloride, USP.

Ritter's disease (rĭt′ĕrz). [Gottfried Ritter von Rittershain, Ger. physician, 1820–1883] A generalized form of impetigo of the newborn.

Ritter-Valli law (rĭt″ĕr-văl′ē). [Johann Wilhelm Ritter, Ger. physicist, 1776–1810; Eusebio Valli, It. physiologist, 1726–1810] Increased irritability from center outward, if a nerve is cut off from its center or if the center is destroyed. Irritability is lost.

ritual (rĭch′ū-ăl). 1. A routine the individual feels is essential and should not fail to be carried out. 2. In psychiatry, any activity that is performed compulsively in an attempt to relieve anxiety.

ritualistic surgery. Surgical procedures without scientific justification. Performed in primitive societies without direction toward treatment or prevention of disease. Included in this are alterations of the skin, ears, lips, teeth, genitalia, and head. In some cases, even in nonprimitive societies, surgical procedures without rational justification are considered to be ritualistic.

rivalry (rī′văl-rē). Competition between two individuals, groups, or systems seeking to attain the same goal.

r., binocular. The continuous alternation in the conscious perception of visual stimuli to the two eyes.

r., retinal. R., binocular, q.v.

r., sibling. The competition between children for attention and affection of others, but esp. their parents.

rivalry strife. Alternate sensations of color and shape when the fields of vision of the two eyes cannot combine in one visual image.

Rivinus' canals (rē-vē′nŭs). [August Quirinus Rivinus, Ger. anatomist, 1652–1723] Ducts of the sublingual glands.

Rivinus' glands. Sublingual glands.

Rivinus' incisore. The tympanic notch in the upper part of the tympanic portion of the temporal bone. It extends from the lesser to the greater tympanic spines and is occupied by the pars flaccida of the tympanic membrane.

Rivinus' ligament. Small portion of the tympanic membrane in the notch of Rivinus. SYN: *Shrapnell's membrane.*

rivus lacrimalis (rī′vŭs) [L. *rivus,* little stream, + *lacrima,* tear]. The pathway under the eyelids for the tears to travel from their source in the lacrimal glands to the punctum lacrimale.

riziform (rĭz′ĭ-form) [Fr. *riz,* rice, + L. *forma,* form]. Resembling rice grains.

R.L.E. *right lower extremity.*

RLF. *retrolental fibroplasia.*

R.L.L. *right lower lobe* of the lung.

RLQ. *right lower quadrant* (of abdomen).

R.M.A. *right mentoanterior presentation* (of the fetal face).

R.M.P. *right mentoposterior presentation* (of the fetal face).

R.M.T. *right mentotransverse* fetal position.

R.N. *registered nurse.*

Rn. Chem. symb. for radon.

RNA. *ribonucleic acid.*

RNase. *ribonuclease.*

R.O.A. *right occipitoanterior* fetal position.

Robalate. Trade name for dihydroxyaluminum aminoacetate.

Robamox. Trade name for amoxicillin.

Robaxin. Trade name for methocarbamol.

Robert's pelvis (rō′bārts). [Heinrich L. F. Robert, Ger. gynecologist, 1814–1874] Transverse contraction of the pelvis due to osteoarthritis of the sacroiliac joints.

Robertson's pupil. Argyll Robertson pupil.

Robicillin-VK. Trade name for penicillin V potassium, USP.

Robimycin. Trade name for erythromycin, USP.

Robinul. Trade name for glycopyrrolate.

Robitet. Trade name for tetracycline hydrochloride.

Robitussin. Trade name for guaifenesin.

Rocaltrol. Trade name for calcitriol.

Rochelle salt (rō-shĕl′). Potassium sodium tartrate; a colorless, transparent powder having a cooling and saline taste and used as a saline cathartic.

rocker knife. Adapted device for persons with limited upper extremity function. Allows one-handed stabilization and cutting of food.

Rocky Mountain spotted fever. An infectious disease caused by the parasite Rickettsia ricketsii transmitted by the wood tick Dermacentor andersoni or Dermacentor variabiles. Originally thought to exist only in the western U.S., it can occur anywhere that the tick vector is present.

The organism causes vasculitis, giving rise to fever, headache, myalgia, and a characteristic rash. The rash appears several days after other symptoms, first erupting on the wrists and ankles, then on the palms and soles. It is nonpruritic and macular, and spreads to legs, arms, trunk, and face. Tetracycline is the drug of choice. SEE: *tick fever.*

Rocky Mountain spotted fever vaccine. USP. A standardized preparation of inactivated Rickettsia rickettsii.

rod (rŏd) [AS. *rodd,* club]. 1. A slender, straight bar. 2. One of the slender, long, sensory bodies in the retina, which respond to faint light. 3. Bacterium shaped like a rod.

r., Corti's. Pillar cells, q.v.

r.'s, enamel. Minute calcareous rods or prisms laid down by ameloblasts and forming enamel of a tooth.

r., retinal. Visual cells in the eye that are the light-sensing elements of the retina, along with the cones.

rodenticide (rō-dĕn′tĭ-sīd) [L. *rodens,* gnawing, + *caedere,* to kill]. An agent that kills rodents.

rodent ulcer (rō′dĕnt) [″ + *ulcus,* ulcer]. A slowly growing, gnawing cancer that slowly destroys soft tissues and bones, causing great destruction. Usual sites are on outer angle of the eye, near side and on tip of nose, and on edges of the scalp. SYN: *Jacob's ulcer.*

rodonalgia (rō-dō-năl′jē-ă) [Gr. *rhodon,* rose, + *algos,* pain]. Vasomotor condition marked by redness and neuralgic pain of the extremities, swelling, and fever. SYN: *erythromelalgia.*

rods and cones. The light-sensitive portions of rod and cone visual cells of the retina. They form the second layer lying between the external limiting membrane and the pigment epithelium. The rods contain visual purple (rhodopsin), which is essential for vision in dim light.

Roentgen, Wilhelm Konrad (rĕnt′gĕn). German physicist, 1845–1923, who discovered roentgen rays in 1895 and won the Nobel prize in physics in 1901.

roentgen (rĕnt′gĕn). ABBR: R. Unit for describing exposure dose of x- or γ-radiation. One unit is sufficient to liberate enough electrons and positrons to produce, in air, ions carrying positive and negative charges of 2.58×10^{-4} coulomb per kilogram of air.

roentgenkymogram (rĕnt″gĕn-kī′mō-grăm) [*roentgen* + Gr. *kyme,* wave, + *gramma,* mark]. A record in the form of a tracing of the heart's action as determined by use of x-ray.

roentgenkymograph (rĕnt″gĕn-kī′mō-grăf) [″ + ″ + *graphein,* to write]. The device for recording the movements of the heart and attached large vessels on a single x-ray film.

roentgenkymography (rĕnt″gĕn-kī-mŏg′ră-fē). Recording of heart movements by use of a roentgenkymograph.

roentgenocinematography (rĕnt″gĕn-ō-sĭn″ĕ-mă-tŏg′ră-fē) [″ + Gr. *kinema,* motion, + *graphein,* to write]. Moving picture photography of x-ray studies.

roentgenogram (rĕnt-gĕn′ō-grăm, rĕnt′gĕn-ō-grăm″). Film produced by roentgenography. SYN: *radiogram.* Preferred term is *radiograph.*

roentgenography (rĕnt″gĕn-ŏg′ră-fē) [*roentgen* + Gr. *graphein,* to write]. The process of obtaining pictures by use of roentgen rays. Preferred term is *radiography.*

r., body section. Tomography, q.v.

r., mucosal relief. X-ray of the intestinal mucosa after ingested barium has been removed, and air under slight pressure has been injected. This leaves a light coat of barium on the mucosa and permits x-ray pictures of the fine detail of the mucosa.

r., serial. Taking repeated x-rays of an area at defined but arbitrary intervals.

r., spot-film. X-ray picture taken of a small area during the course of fluoroscopy.

roentgenologist (rĕnt″gĕn-ŏl′ō-jĭst) [″ + Gr. *logos,* study]. A physician skilled in roentgen diagnosis, roentgentherapy, or both. Preferred term is *radiologist.*

roentgenology (rĕnt″gĕn-ŏl′ō-jē). The science of applying roentgen rays for diagnostic and therapeutic purposes. Preferred term is *radiology.*

roentgenometer (rĕnt″gĕ-nŏm′ĕ-tĕr) [″ + Gr. *metron,* measure]. Radiometer, q.v.

roentgenoscope (rĕnt-gĕn′ō-skōp) [″ + Gr. *skopein,* to examine]. A fluoroscope, q.v.

roentgenoscopy (rĕnt″gĕ-nŏs′kō-pē). Fluoroscopy.

roentgenotherapy, roentgentherapy (rĕnt″gĕn-ō-thĕr′ăp-ē) [*roentgen* + Gr. *therapeia,* treatment]. The treatment of disease by exposure of the patient to roentgen rays. Preferred term is *radiotherapy.*

roentgen ray. X-ray, q.v.

roeteln, roetheln (rĕt′ĕln) [Ger.]. German measles, rubella.

Roger's disease (rō-zhāz′). [Henri L. Roger, Fr. physician, 1809–1891] Ventricular septal defect.

Rokitansky's disease (rō″kĭ-tăn′skēz). [Karl Freiherr von Rokitansky, Austrian pathologist, 1804–1878] Acute yellow atrophy of the liver.

Rolaids. Trade name for dihydroxyaluminum sodium carbonate.

Rolando's area (rō-lăn′dōz). [Luigi Rolando, It. anatomist, 1773–1831] Motor area in the cerebral cortex.

Rolando's fissure. Fissure between the parietal and frontal lobes. SYN: *sulcus centralis.*

role (rōl) [O. Fr. *rolle,* roll of paper on which a part is written]. The characteristic social behavior of an individual in relationship to the group.

role model. The demonstration of the behavior associated with a particular position or profession that serves as an example for others.

role playing. The assignment and acting out of a role in a treatment setting to provide individuals the opportunity to see themselves as others do. Also used as a method of teaching such skills as interviewing, taking history, and doing a physical examination.

rolfing. [Ida Rolf, U.S. physiotherapist, 1897–1979] Deep massage of the tissues around muscles. The purpose is to increase the range of motion of the joints and to enhance suppleness.

rolitetracycline (rō″lē-tĕt″ră-sī′klēn). USP. An antibiotic drug. Trade name is Syntetrin.

roll. A usually solid, cylindrical structure.

r., ileal. A sausage-shaped mass in the left ileac fossa. It is due to a collection of feces in or induration of the walls of the sigmoid colon.

r., scleral. Spur, scleral, q.v.

roller (rōl′ĕr) [O. Fr., roll]. 1. Strip of muslin or other cloth rolled up in cylinder form for surgeon's use. 2. A roller bandage. SEE: *bandage.*

R.O.M. *range of motion.* SEE: *exercise, range of motion.*

Roman numerals. Letters used by the ancient Romans for numeration in contradistinction to the Arabic numerals that we now use. In Roman notations, values are increased either by adding one or more symbols to the initial symbol or by subtracting a symbol from one or more to the right of it. Ex.: V is 5, IV is 4, and VI is 6. Thus, since X is 10, IX is 9 and XI is 11. SEE: *Roman numerals* in *Appendix.*

romanopexy (rō-măn′ō-pĕk″sē) [L. *romanum,* the sigmoid, + Gr. *pexis,* fixation]. Fixation of the sigmoid flexure for prolapse of the rectum. SYN: *sigmoidopexy.*

romanoscope (rō-măn′ō-skōp) [″ + Gr. *skopein,* to examine]. Instrument for examining the sigmoid flexure.

rombergism (rŏm′bĕrg-ĭzm). While standing, tendency to fall when the eyes are closed. SEE: *Romberg's sign.*

Romberg's sign (rŏm′bĕrgs). [Maritz Heinrich Romberg, Ger. physician, 1795–1873] Inability to maintain the body balance when the eyes are shut and the feet close together. The sign is positive if the patient sways and falls when the eyes are closed. Seen in sensory ataxia.

Rondomycin. Trade name for methacycline hydrochloride.

rongeur (rŏn-zhŭr′) [Fr., to gnaw]. A gouge forceps, an instrument for removing tiny fragments of bone.

Roniacol. Trade name for nicotinyl alcohol.

roof nucleus. Small mass of gray matter in white substance of vermis of the cerebellum.

room [AS. *rum*]. An area or space in a building, partitioned off for occupancy or available for specific procedures.

r., clean. A room, particularly one housing delicate electronic medical instruments, that is constructed so as to be isolated from the free entry of air. Air that enters is filtered, and personnel wear special clothing to prevent particles from their bodies from becoming freely dispersed in the room.

r., delivery. A room to which an obstetric patient is taken for childbirth.

r., dustfree. A type of room designed to eliminate or reduce particulate matter, including airborne microorganisms, from circulating. This kind of room is useful in housing burn patients, in removing allergens from the air, in transplantation surgery, and in preparing drugs and solutions for intravenous use.

r., intensive therapy. Intensive care room wherein patients who need close medical attention and use of various medical devices such as resuscitation equipment are treated.

r., labor. Room in which an obstetric patient is placed during the first stage of labor, prior to being taken to the delivery room.

r., operating. A room in a hospital used for surgical procedures.

r., postdelivery. The room where patients are kept following childbirth.

r., recovery. Recovery room, q.v.

rooming-in. The placing of infants in the same hospital room as their mothers, beginning immediately following birth.

root (rūt) [AS. *rot*]. 1. The part of a plant that is underground. 2. Proximal end of a nerve. 3. Portion of an organ implanted in tissues. SYN: *radix* [NA]. 4. The part of the human tooth covered by cementum, and designated by location, i.e., mesial, distal, buccal, lingual.

r., anterior. One of two roots by which a spinal nerve is attached to the spinal cord. Contains efferent nerve fibers.

r., dorsal. Radix dorsalis or sensory root of each spinal nerve.

r., motor. The anterior and motor division of a spinal nerve.

r., posterior. One of two roots by which a spinal nerve is attached to the spinal cord. Contains afferent nerve fibers.

r., sensory. R., dorsal, q.v.

r., ventral. R., motor, q.v.

root arteries. Arteries accompanying nerve roots into the spinal cord.

root canal. Pulp cavity of root of a tooth.

rooting reflex. SEE: *reflex, rooting.*

root resorption of teeth. Condition of the roots of teeth caused by endocrine imbalance or excessive pressure of orthodontic appliances. X-ray photographs demonstrate roots that appear to be sawed off or shortened.

root sheath. 1. Epithelium covering the hair follicle. 2. The epithelial covering that induces root formation in teeth. Also: *Hertwig's root sheath.*

root zone. Burdach's column of the spinal cord. Outer tract of posterior funiculus or white column of the cord. SYN: *fasciculus cuneatus*.

R.O.P. *right occipitoposterior* fetal presentation, in which the occiput of the fetus is in relationship to the right sacroiliac joint of the mother.

Rorschach test (ror′shăk). [Hermann Rorschach, Swiss psychiatrist, 1884–1922] A psychological test consisting of 10 different inkblot designs. The subject is asked to interpret each design individually. This may reveal disturbances in personality.

rosa (rō′ză) [L.]. Rose.

rosacea (rō-zā′sē-ă) [L. *rosaceus,* rosy]. A syndrome of unknown cause associated with varying degrees of papules, pustules, and hyperplasia of the sebaceous glands. Predominantly on the face. The onset is usually between 30 and 50 years of age but may be as early as 10 or occur first in old age. In adults, it occurs three times as often in females as in males.

TREATMENT: Symptomatic. Tetracyclines in small doses may help. If sunlight makes the disease worse, chloroquine for six weeks should be tried. Firm massage, using a bland oil as a lubricant, repeatedly moving the fingers from the nose to the edge of the face for five to ten minutes each evening, is the single most effective measure.

rosaniline (rō-zăn′ĭ-lĭn). A basic dye used in preparing other dyes.

rosary (rō′ză-rē). Something that resembles a string of beads.

r., rachitic. Palpable areas at the site of joining of the ribs to their cartilages. This is seen in conjunction with rickets.

Rose, Frank A. (rōz). British surgeon.

R.'s position. The patient's head in a fully extended position is allowed to hang over the end of the operating room table. This prevents aspiration of blood during surgery on the mouth and lips.

rose bengal sodium I 131 (injection). USP. A standardized preparation of radioactive iodine and rose bengal used in photoscanning the liver and to test liver function. Trade name is Robengatope I-131.

rose fever. Summer or June cold; hay fever of early summer attributed to inhaling rose pollen. SEE: *hay fever.*

Rosenbach, Ottomar (rō′zĕn-bŏk). German physician, 1851–1907.

R.'s sign. 1. Fine rapid tremor of closed eyelids. Seen in hyperthyroidism. 2. In hysteria, inability to obey command to close eyes. 3. Absence of abdominal skin reflex in intestinal inflammation or hemiplegia.

R.'s test. A test for bile in the urine. Urine is passed several times through the same filter paper. After the paper has dried, a drop of nitric acid is added to it. If bile is present, a play of colors is produced.

Rosenmüller, Johann Christian (rō′zĕn-mĭl″ ĕr). German anatomist, 1771–1820.

R.'s body. A rudimentary structure located in the mesosalpinx. Consisting of a longitudinal duct (duct of Gartner) and 10 to 15 transverse ducts, it is the remains of the upper portion of the mesonephros and is the homologue of the head of the epididymis in the male. SYN: *epoophoron; parovarium.*

R.'s cavity. Slitlike depression in the pharyngeal wall behind the opening of the eustachian tube.

roseo- [L. *roseus,* rosy]. 1. Combining form meaning rose-colored. 2. A prefix in chemical terms.

roseola (rō-zē′ō-lă, rō″zē-ō′lă) [L. *roseus,* rosy]. Skin condition marked by maculae or red spots of varying sizes on the skin; any rose-colored rash.

r. idiopathica. Macular eruptions not associated with any well-defined symptoms.

r. infantum. A noninfectious roseola occurring in infants. Characterized by high fever, splenomegaly, and a rash that appears just as the fever subsides. SYN: *exanthem subitum.*

r. symptomatica. Macular eruption occurring in well-defined disease.

roseolous (rō-zē′ō-lŭs) [L. *roseus,* rosy]. Resembling or pert. to roseola.

rosette [Fr., small rose]. 1. Something that resembles a rose. 2. A spherical group of fine red vacuoles surrounding cytocentrum of a monocyte.

rose water. Saturated aqueous solution of the oil of rose. Used to impart agreeable odor to lotions.

rose water ointment. USP. An emollient used to soften the skin. It contains waxes, almond oil, sodium borate, rose water, rose oil, and purified water.

rosin (rŏz′ĭn) [L. *resina*]. USP. Substance distilled from species of pine and used as a stiffening agent in preparing plasters.

Ross' bodies. [Edward Halford Ross, Brit. pathologist, 1875–1928] Copper-colored, round bodies showing dark granules. Found in blood and tissue fluids in syphilis. Sometimes they exhibit ameboid movements.

Rossolimo's reflex (rŏs″ō-lē′mōz). [Gregorij I. Rossolimo, Russian neurologist, 1860–1928] Plantar flexion of second to fifth toes in response to percussion of plantar surface of the toes.

rostellum (rŏs-tĕl′lŭm) [L., little beak]. (pl. *rostella*) A fleshy protrusion on anterior end of scolex of tapeworms bearing one or more rows of spines or hooks.

rostral (rŏs′trăl) [L. *rostralis*]. 1. Resembling a beak. 2. Toward the front or cephalic end of the body.

rostrate (rŏs′trāt) [L. *rostratus,* beaked]. Having a beak or hook formation.

rostriform (rŏs′trĭ-form) [″ + *forma,* shape]. Shaped like a beak.

rostrum (rŏs′trŭm) [L., beak]. (pl. *rostrums, rostra*) Any hooked or beaked structure.

rosulate (rŏs′ū-lāt) [L. *rosulatus,* like a rose]. Shaped like a rosette.

R.O.T. *right occipitotransverse* fetal position.

rot (rŏt) [ME. *roten*]. To decay or decompose.

r., jungle. Common term for certain fungus diseases of the skin that occur in the tropics.

rotameter (rō-tăm′ĕ-tĕr). Device for measuring the flow of gas or a liquid.

rotate (rō′tāt) [L. *rotare,* to turn]. To twist or revolve.

rotating tourniquet. SEE: *tourniquet, rotating.*

rotation (rō-tā′shŭn) [L. *rotatio,* a turning]. Process of turning on an axis.

r., fetal. Twisting of the fetal head as it follows the curves of the birth canal downward.

rotator (rō-tā′tor). (pl. *rotatores*) A muscle revolving a part on its axis.

rotaviruses (rō′tă-vī″rŭs-ĕs) [L. *rota,* wheel, + *virus,* poison]. A group of viruses that are a major cause of sporadic acute enteritis in infants and small children, and epidemic acute gastroenteritis.

röteln, rötheln (rĕt′ĕln) [Ger. *rot,* red]. German measles. SYN: *roeteln; rubella.*

rotenone (rō′tĕ-nōn). A poisonous chemical, $C_{23}H_{22}O_6$, used as an insecticide.

Roth's spots. [Moritz Roth, Swiss physician and pathologist, 1849–1914] Small white spots in the retina close to the optic disk. They are often surrounded by areas of hemorrhage.

ETIOL: Systemic infection, particularly cases of acute infective endocarditis.

rotoxamine tartrate (rō-tŏks′ă-mēn). An antihistamine drug.

Rouget's cells (roo-zhāz′). [Charles M. B. Rouget, Fr. physiologist, 1824–1904] Contractile cells that surround the capillaries, observed in frogs and salamanders.

rough (rŭf). Not smooth.

roughage (rŭf′ĭj) [AS. *ruh,* rough]. Indigestible fiber of fruits, vegetables, and cereals, that acts as a stimulant to aid intestinal peristalsis. Plenty of water should be added to consumption of roughage. Should not be used in colitis or in intestinal irritation. SYN: *fiber, dietary.* SEE: *cellulose.*

rouleau (roo-lō′) [Fr., roll]. (pl. *rouleaux*) A group of red blood corpuscles arranged like a roll of coins.

round (rownd) [O. Fr. *ronde*]. 1. Circular in shape. 2. Spherical, globular.

round ligament. 1. Curved fibrous cord attached to the center of articular surface of the head of the femur. 2. Two round cordlike structures passing from front of the body of the uterus in anterior wall of broad ligament, below the fallopian tubes, outward through the inguinal canals to soft tissues of the labia majora. 3. Fibrous cord that is the remnant of the umbilical vein.

roundworm. Any member of the phylum Nemathelminthes (Aschelminthes), esp. one belonging to the class Nematoda, q.v. SYN: *threadworm.*

Roux-en-Y. Anastomosis of the distal divided end of the small bowel to another organ such as the stomach or esophagus. The proximal end is anastomosed to the small bowel below the anastomosis.

Roven's IMDC. [Milton D. Roven, contemporary U.S. podiatrist] A new procedure for intramedullary metatarsal decompression performed through a small dorsal incision. It is less traumatic than previous procedures, allowing immediate ambulation and minimal postoperative pain and edema.

RPF. *renal plasma flow.*

rpm. *revolutions per minute.*

RPS. *renal pressor substance.* SEE: *renin.*

R.Q. *respiratory quotient.*

-rrhagia (rā′jē-ă) [Gr. *rhegnynai,* to burst forth]. Combining form indicating abnormal discharge, hemorrhage.

rRNA. *ribosomal RNA.*

R.S.A. *right sacroanterior* fetal position.

R.Sc.A. *right scapuloanterior* fetal position.

R.Sc.P. *right scapuloposterior* fetal position.

R.S.P. *right sacroposterior* fetal position.

R.S.T. *right sacrotransverse* fetal position.

R.S.V. *Rous sarcoma virus.*

R.T. *reading test; registered technician; registered technologist.*

R.T.N. *registered technologist—nuclear medicine.*

R.T.R. *registered technologist radiographer.*

R.U. *rat unit.*

Ru. Chem. symbol for ruthenium.

rub. Friction of one surface moving over another. In auscultation, a roughened surface moving over another causes a characteristic sound.

r., pericardial. The sound heard by use of auscultation with each heart beat when the inflamed pericardial surface moves over the heart.

rubber-dam. Thin rubber tissue used by dentists to seal off the tooth from saliva in the mouth during dental treatment.

rubefacient (roo″bĕ-fā′shĕnt) [L. *rubefaciens,* making red]. 1. Causing redness, as of the skin. 2. Agent that reddens the skin, producing a local congestion, the vessels becoming dilated and the supply of blood increased. Rubefacients include mustard, turpentine, capsicum, flaxseed, arnica, and liniments.

rubella (roo-bĕl′lă) [L. *rubellus,* reddish]. Acute infectious disease resembling both scarlet fever and measles, but differing from these in its short course, slight fever, and freedom from sequelae. SYN: *German measles; roeteln; röteln.*

INCUBATION: 14 to 21 days. Rubella produces a maculopapular rash that desquamates and vanishes in from 2 to 3 days.

SYM: Prodromes, slight or altogether absent. Drowsiness, slight fever, sore throat. Eruption first or second day. In some cases rash composed of pale red, scarcely elevated papules, more or less discrete rubella morbilliforme; in others rash is bright red and diffuse like that of scarlet fever, rubella scarlatiniforme. Rash begins on face, spreads rapidly over whole body, but fades so rapidly that face may be clear before extremities are affected. Slight desquamation frequently present, though not always. Superficial cervical and posterior auricular glands more swollen than in measles. Duration is 3 to 5 days.

COMPLICATIONS: Rubella in pregnant women, esp. in first two or three months of gestation, is serious in that it may give rise to fetal anomalies, esp. congenital cataract.

TREATMENT: Nonspecific. Local antipruritics for itching; rest; liquid diet; sponging with tepid water.

PROG: Good.

rubella titer. Serology test to determine immune status to rubella.

rubella virus vaccine, live. USP. A standardized preparation of live rubella virus. Used to immunize against rubella. Trade name is Meruvax.

rubeola (roo-bē′ō-lă, roo″bē-ō′lă) [L., reddish]. 1. Acute contagious disease marked by fever, catarrhal symptoms, and a typical cutaneous eruption. SYN: *measles.* 2. Term occasionally applied to acute infectious disease with mild symptoms and rose-colored macular eruption. SYN: *rubella.*

rubeosis iridis. A condition in which new blood vessels form on the anterior surface of the iris, associated with vascular disease that affects the retinal vein of the eye. Seen most frequently in diabetics although it is not limited to these patients. Leads to painful, hemorrhagic glaucoma.

ruber (roo′bĕr) [L.]. Red.

rubescent (roo-bĕs′ĕnt) [L. *rubescere,* to grow red]. Growing red; flushing.

rubidium (roo-bĭd′ē-ŭm) [L. *rubidus,* red]. SYMB: Rb. At. wt. 85.47; at. no. 37. A soft, silvery metal that decomposes water with violence and bursts into flame spontaneously in air. Its salts are used medicinally.

rubiginous (roo-bĭj′ĭ-nŭs) [L. *rubiginosus*]. Rusty or rust-colored.

rubigo (roo-bī′gō) [L., rust]. Rust; mildew.

Rubin's test (roo′bĭns). [Isidor Clinton Rubin, U.S. physician, 1883–1958] Transuterine insufflation with carbon dioxide of the fallopian tubes to test their patency. SEE: *sterility.*

Rubner's test (roob′nĕrz). [Max Rubner, Ger. physiologist, 1854–1932] 1. A test for lactose or glucose in the urine. 2. A test for carbon monoxide in blood.

rubor (roo′bor) [L.]. Discoloration or redness caused by inflammation. It is one of the four classical symptoms of inflammation. The others are calor (heat), dolor (pain), and tumor (swelling).

Rubramin PC. Trade name for cyanocobalamin, USP.

rubriblast (roo′brĭ-blăst) [L. *ruber,* red, + Gr. *blastos,* germ]. Pronormoblast.

rubric (roo′brĭk) [L. *ruber,* red]. Concerning or being red.

rubricyte (roo′brĭ-sīt) [″ + Gr. *kytos,* cell]. Polychromatic normoblast.

rubrospinal (roo″brō-spī′năl) [L. *ruber,* red, + *spina,* thorn]. A descending tract consisting of a small bundle of nerve fibers in lateral funiculus of spinal cord. Fibers arise in cells of the red nucleus of midbrain and terminate in ventral horn of gray matter.

rubrothalamic (roo″brō-thăl-ăm′ĭk) [″ + Gr. *thalamos,* chamber]. Concerning the red nucleus of the brain and thalamus.

rubrum (roo′brŭm) [L., red]. Reddish nucleus of gray matter in crus cerebri near optic thalamus.

r. scarlatinum. Scarlet red, a substance used as a healing agent and stain.

ructus (rŭk′tŭs) [L.]. Belching of air from stomach. SYN: *eructation.*

rudiment (roo′dĭ-mĕnt) [L. *rudimentum,* beginning]. 1. That which is undeveloped. 2. In biology, a part just beginning to develop. 3. Remains of a part functional at an earlier stage of an individual or in his ancestors.

rudimentary (roo″dĭ-mĕn′tă-rē). 1. Elementary. 2. Undeveloped; not fully formed; remaining from an earlier stage. SYN: *vestigial.*

rudimentum (roo″dĭ-mĕn′tŭm) [L.]. Rudiment.

Ruffini's corpuscles (roo-fē′nēz). [Angelo Ruffini, It. anatomist, 1864–1929] Encapsulated sensory nerve endings found in subcutaneous tissue, thought to mediate sense of warmth. SYN: *organ of Ruffini.*

rufous (roo′fŭs) [L. *rufus,* red]. Ruddy; having a ruddy complexion and reddish hair.

ruga (roo′gă) [L.]. (pl. *rugae*) A fold or crease, esp. one of the folds of mucous membrane seen on internal surface of the stomach.

rugae of vagina. Small ridges on inner surface of the vagina extending laterally and upward from the columna rugarum (long ridges on anterior and posterior walls).

Ruggeri's reflex. Increase in pulse rate when eyes are strongly converged on a near object.

rugine (roo-zhēn'). 1. Periosteal elevator. 2. A raspatory.

rugose, rugous (roo'gōs, -gŭs) [L. *rugosus,* wrinkled]. Having many wrinkles or creases.

rugosity (rū-gŏs'ĭ-tē) [L. *rugositas*]. 1. Condition of being folded or wrinkled. 2. A ridge or wrinkle.

R.U.L. *right upper lobe* of lung.

rule (rool) [ME. *riule*]. A guide or principle based on experience or observation.

r. of nines. Formula for estimating percentage of body surface areas. It is particularly helpful in judging the portion of skin that has been burned. The head represents 9%; each upper extremity 9%; the back of the trunk is 18%, and the front is 18%; each lower extremity represents 18%; and the perineum makes up the remaining 1%. SEE: *burns* for illus.

ruminant (roo'mĭ-nănt). An animal that regurgitates food in order to chew it again. This is called chewing the cud.

rumination (roo"mĭ-nā'shŭn) [L. *ruminatio*]. 1. Regurgitation, esp. with rechewing, of previously swallowed food. 2. In psychiatry, obsessional preoccupation of the mind by a single idea or a set of thoughts, and inability to dismiss or dislodge them.

rump (rŭmp) [ME. *rumpe*]. Posterior end of the back, the gluteal region, or buttocks.

Rumpf's symptom (roompfs). [Heinrich Theodor Rumpf, Ger. physician, b. 1851] 1. In neurasthenia, quickening of the pulse when pressure is exerted over a painful spot. 2. Twitching after strong faradization, in traumatic neuroses.

run [AS. *rinnan,* run]. To exude pus or mucus.

runaround, runround. Superficial infection encircling the fingernail. SYN: *whitlow.*

rupia (roo'pē-ă) [Gr. *rhypos,* filth]. A cutaneous eruption, usually of tertiary syphilis, that manifests itself at first by large elevations of the epidermis filled with a clear or blood-stained serum, soon becoming turbid and purulent. The bulla bursts and allows some fluid to escape. As it desiccates, it is covered with a crust that dries, accumulates new layers, and becomes covered with greenish-brown scales, sometimes to depth of ½ in. (13 mm.). Thickest of all syphilides and presents most extensive ulcerations.

TREATMENT: Antisyphilitic antibiotics.

rupioid (roo'pē-oyd) [" + *eidos,* form]. Resembling rupia.

rupophobia (roo"pō-fō'bē-ă) [" + *phobos,* fear]. Abnormal dislike for dirt or filth. SYN: *rhypophobia.*

rupture (rŭp'chūr) [L. *ruptura,* breaking]. 1. A breaking apart of an organ or tissue. 2. Hernia.

r. of membranes. Rupture of amniotic sac as normal result of dilation of the cervix uteri in labor.

r. of perineum. Rupture of perineum in labor, a condition that can be prevented by episiotomy, q.v. More frequent in primiparae.

r. of tubes. Rupture of a fallopian tube, a serious event in extrauterine pregnancy. May occur without the woman's knowledge of her pregnancy.

r. of uterus. Rare rupture due to unrelieved obstructed labor.

RUQ. *right upper quadrant* of abdomen.

rush. 1. A strong contraction wave that moves down the small intestine. 2. The first surge of pleasure produced by a drug, esp. a narcotic drug.

Russell bodies (rŭs'ĕl). [William Russell, Brit. physician, 1852–1940] Small spherical hyaline bodies in cancerous and simple inflammatory growths.

Russell's viper venom (rŭs'ĕlz). [Patrick Russell, Irish physician who worked in India, 1727–1805] The venom from Russell's viper. It is used in investigating defective blood coagulation due to a deficiency of Factor X.

Russian bath. Hot vapor bath followed by friction and a plunge in cold water.

Rust's disease (rŭsts). [Johann N. Rust, Ger. surgeon, 1775–1840] Tuberculosis of cervical vertebrae and their articulations.

rusts. Members of an order of parasitic fungi (Uredinales), all of which are parasitic on plants. Many are allergens.

rusty (rŭst'ē) [AS. *rustig*]. Reddish in color. Resembling, or containing, rust. SYN: *rubiginous.*

rut (rŭt) [O. Fr. *ruit,* roaring of deer]. In lower male animals, seasonal period of sexual excitement during which mating usually takes place. SEE: *estrus; heat.*

rut-formation. In psychology, loss of interest in environment, fixation upon a single object, and concentration of emotional or other interests in a groove or rut.

ruthenium (roo-thē'nē-ŭm). SYMB: Ru. At. wt. 101.07; at. no. 44. A hard, brittle, metallic element of platinum group.

rutherford. [Ernest Rutherford, Brit. physicist, 1871–1937] ABBR: rd. A unit of radioactivity representing 10^6 disintegrations per second.

rutherfordium (rŭth"ĕr-ford'ē-ŭm). SYMB: Rf. A radioactive element with atomic weight of 261 and atomic number of 104.

rutidosis (roo"tĭ-dō'sĭs) [Gr. *rhytis,* wrinkle]. Contraction or puckering of cornea just before death. SYN: *rhytidosis; rytidosis.*

rutilizm (roo'tĭl-ĭzm) [L. *rutilis,* red, + Gr. *-ismos,* condition]. Having red or auburn-colored hair.

rutin (roo'tĭn). A crystalline glucoside of quercetin, closely related to hesperidin. Derived from buckwheat but present in many plants.

R.V. *residual volume.*

℞. Symb. for *recipe; take.* SEE: *prescription.*

rye (rī) [AS. *ryge*]. A cereal grass that produces a grain used in food and beverage production. When rye grain is infected with a certain fungus, ergot is produced.

rytidosis (rĭt″ĭ-dō'sĭs) [Gr. *rhytis,* a wrinkle, + *osis,* condition]. Wrinkling or contraction of cornea preceding death. SYN: *rhytidosis; rutidosis.*

S

σ. Sigma, the eighteenth letter of the Greek alphabet. In statistics, the symbol for standard deviation.

Σ. Capital of the Greek sigma. In statistics, the symbol for summation.

S. *signa,* mark, or let it be written, term used in prescription writing to indicate the instructions to the patient that the pharmacist will place on the dispensed medicine; *smooth,* description of bacterial colonies; *spherical* or *spherical lens; subject* (pl. *Ss*), participant in an experiment; chem. symb. for sulfur.

s. *semis,* half; *sinister,* left.

s̄, s. Symb. for (L.) *sine,* without; used as a form of shorthand in hospital charts and clinical records.

S1, S2, etc. *first sacral nerve, second sacral nerve.*

S-A, SA, S.A. *sinoatrial.*

S.A.B. *Society of American Bacteriologists.*

saber shin. Anterior border of the tibia marked with sharp convexity, found in hereditary syphilis.

Sabin vaccine. [Albert B. Sabin, contemporary American virologist] An oral vaccine for poliomyelitis. SYN: *live oral poliovirus vaccine.* SEE: *poliomyelitis.*

sabulous (săb'ū-lŭs) [L. *sabulosus,* sand]. Gritty; sandy.

saburra (să-bŭr'ră) [L., sand]. Foulness of stomach or mouth due to decayed food. SYN: *sordes.*

saburral (să-bŭr'ăl). 1. Pert. to foulness of mouth or stomach due to accumulation of decayed food. 2. Pert. to sand, as in application of a hot sand bath for relief from pain, as in muscular rheumatism.

sac (săk) [L. *saccus,* pouch]. A baglike part of an organ, a cavity or pouch, sometimes containing fluid. SYN: *saccus.* SEE: *cyst.*

s., air. An alveolar cell in the lung. SEE: *s., alveolar.*

s., allantoic. The expanded end of the allantois, well developed in birds and reptiles.

s., alveolar. The terminal portion of an air passageway within the lung. Its wall contains pocketlike structures (alveoli) and each alveolar sac is connected to a respiratory bronchiole by an alveolar duct.

s., amniotic. A thin membrane, containing a serous fluid, enclosing the embryo. SYN: *amnion.*

s., chorionic. Saclike structure, consisting of chorion, that encloses the developing embryo.

s., conjunctival. The cavity, lined with conjunctiva, that lies between the eyelids and anterior surface of the eye.

s., dental. The mesenchymal tissue surrounding a developing tooth.

s., endolymphatic. The expanded distal end of the endolymphatic duct.

s., heart. Pericardium.

s., hernial. A saclike protrusion of the peritoneum containing a herniated organ. SEE: *hernia; hernial sac.*

s., lacrimal. Upper dilated portion of the nasolacrimal duct.

s., lesser peritoneal. A cavity within the layers of the peritoneum forming the great omentum. Its opening into the main peritoneal cavity is via the epiploic foramen. SYN: *omental bursa.*

s., vitelline. S., yolk.

s., yolk. An extra-embryonic membrane that encloses the yolk in reptiles, birds, and monotremes. It is formed of an inner layer of entoderm invested by splanchnic mesoderm. In marsupials and placental mammals that lack a yolk mass, the yolk sac is a rudimentary vesicle lying within the chorionic sac.

saccades (să-kāds') [Fr. *saccade,* jerk]. Fast, involuntary movements of the eyes as they change from one point of gaze to another.

saccadic (să-kăd'ĭk) [Fr. *saccade,* jerk]. Pert. to rapid intermittent movements, esp. of the eye. This type of eye movement is important when the fovea follows a moving target. SEE: *nystagmus; vergence.*

saccate (săk'āt) [L. *saccatus,* baglike]. 1. Pert. to, like, or enclosed in a sac. SYN: *encysted.* 2. In bacteriology, marking a sac-shaped form, as in a type of liquefaction.

saccharase (săk'ă-rās) [Sanskrit *sarkara,* sugar]. An enzyme that catalyzes the breakdown of disaccharides to monosaccharides, esp. the hydrolysis of sucrose to dextrose. Ex.: sucrase; invertase.

saccharated (săk'ă-rāt"ĕd). Containing sugar.

saccharephidrosis (săk"ăr-ĕ-"ĭ-drō'sĭs) [" + Gr. *ephidrosis,* a sweating]. Presence of sugar in sweat.

saccharic acid. A dibasic acid, COOH-$(CHOH)_4$CO·OH, formed by the action of nitric acid on dextrose.

saccharide (săk'ă-rīd). A group of carbohydrates including sugars. The group is divided into the following classifications: monosaccharides, disaccharides, trisaccharides, and polysaccharides.

sacchariferous (săk"ă-rĭf'ĕr-ŭs) [Sanskrit *sarkara,* sugar, + L. *ferre,* to carry]. Producing or containing sugar.

saccharification (săk"ăr-ĭ-fĭ-kā'shŭn) [" + L. *facere,* to make]. Conversion into sugar.

saccharin (săk'ă-rĭn). $C_7H_5NO_3S$. A sweet, white, powdered, synthetic product derived from coal tar, 300 to 500 times as sweet as sugar. Used as artificial sweetener. Its use is now restricted because of its ability to cause cancer in experimental animals.

saccharine (săk′ă-rĭn, -rīn) [L. *saccharinus*]. Of the nature of, or having the quality of, sugar. SYN: *sweet.*

saccharo- [Sanskrit *sarkara,* sugar]. Combining form meaning sugar.

saccharogalactorrhea (săk″ă-rō-gă-lăk″tō-rē′ă) [″ + Gr. *gala,* milk, + *rhoia,* flow]. Excessive lactose secreted in milk.

saccharolytic (săk″ă-rō-lĭt′ĭk) [″ + Gr. *lysis,* dissolution]. Able to split up sugar.

Saccharomyces (săk″ă-rō-mī′sēz) [Sanskrit *sarkara,* sugar, + Gr. *mykes,* fungus]. (pl. *saccharomycetes*) A genus of fungi, reproducing by budding. SYN: *yeasts.*

saccharomycosis (săk″ă-rō-mī-kō′sĭs) [″ + ″ + *osis,* condition]. Any disease or pathological condition due to yeasts or saccharomycetes.

saccharorrhea (săk″ă-rō-rē′ă) [Sanskrit *sarkara,* sugar, + Gr. *rhoia,* flow]. Presence of sugar in the body fluids, as in urine or perspiration. SEE: *diabetes mellitus; glycosuria.*

saccharose (săk′ă-rōs). 1. Sucrose; cane, beet, or maple sugar. 2. One of the group of carbohydrates having the same chemical formula, $C_{12}H_{22}O_{11}$.

saccharosuria (săk″ă-rō-sū′rē-ă) [Sanskrit *sarkara,* sugar, + Gr. *ouron,* urine]. Saccharose in the urine.

saccharum (săk′ă-rŭm) [L., sugar]. Sugar.

s. album. White crystallized sugar.

s. canadense. Maple sugar.

s. candidum. Rock candy.

s. lactis. Sugar of milk. SYN: *lactose.*

s. ustum. Burnt sugar; caramel.

saccharuria (săk″ă-roo′rē-ă) [Sanskrit *sarkara,* sugar, + Gr. *ouron,* urine]. Sugar in the urine.

sacciform (săk′sĭ-form) [L. *saccus,* pouch, + *forma,* shape]. Bag-shaped or like a sac. SYN: *saccate.*

saccular (săk′ū-lăr) [L. *sacculus,* a little bag]. Having the shape of or resembling a sac.

sacculated (săk′ū-lāt″ĕd) [L. *sacculatus,* baglike]. Consisting of small sacs or saccules.

sacculation (săk″ū-lā′shŭn). 1. Formation into a sac or sacs. 2. Group of sacs, collectively.

saccule (săk′ūl) [L. *sacculus,* a little bag]. 1. A small sac. 2. The smaller of two sacs comprising the portion of the membranous labyrinth occupying the vestibule of the inner ear. It communicates with the utricle, cochlear duct, and endolymphatic duct, all of which are filled with endolymph. In its wall is the macula sacculi, a sensory area.

s., laryngeal. A small diverticulum extending ventrally from the laryngeal ventricle lying between the ventricular fold and the thyroarytenoid muscle. SYN: *ventricular appendix.*

sacculocochlear (săk″ū-lō-kŏk′lē-ăr) [″ + Gr. *kokhlos,* land snail]. Concerning the saccule and cochlea of the ear.

sacculus (săk′ū-lŭs) [L., a small bag]. (pl. *sacculi*) A saccule or little sac.

s. laryngis. A blind sac extending up from the laryngeal ventricle to between the vestibular fold and the inner surface of the thyroid cartilage.

saccus (săk′ŭs) [L., a bag]. (pl. *sacci*) [NA] A sac or pouch.

s. endolymphaticus. [NA] Dilated, blind end of the ductus endolymphaticus.

s. lacrimalis. [NA] The lacrimal sac, into which empty the two lacrimal ducts.

sacrad (sā′krăd) [L. *sacrum,* sacred, + *ad,* toward]. In the direction of the sacrum.

sacral (sā′krăl) [L. *sacralis*]. Rel. to the sacrum.

sacral bone. A triangular bone made up of five fused vertebrae just above the coccyx. SYN: *sacrum.*

sacral canal. Continuation of the vertebral canal in the sacrum.

sacral flexure. Rectal curve in front of the sacrum.

sacralgia (sā-krăl′jē-ă) [L. *sacrum,* sacred, + Gr. *algos,* pain]. Pain in the sacrum. SYN: *hieralgia.*

sacral index. Sacral breadth multiplied by 100 and divided by sacral length.

sacralization (sā″krăl-ī-zā′shŭn). Fusion of the sacrum and the 5th lumbar vertebra.

sacral nerves. Five pairs of spinal nerves, the upper four of which emerge through the posterior sacral foramina, the fifth pair through the sacral hiatus (termination of sacral canal). All are mixed nerves (motor and sensory).

sacral plexus. Plexus of sacral nerves from which sciatic nerve originates. It is a part of the lumbosacral plexus.

sacral vertebra. Fused vertebrae forming the sacrum.

sacra media (sā′kră mē′dē-ă) [L.]. Middle sacral artery.

sacrectomy (sā-krĕk′tō-mē) [L. *sacrum,* sacred, + Gr. *ektome,* excision]. Excision of part of the sacrum.

sacro- (sā′krō) [L. *sacrum,* sacred]. Prefix indicating relationship to the sacrum.

sacroanterior (sā″krō-ăn-tē′rē-or) [″ + *anterior,* before]. Denoting intrauterine fetal position in which the fetal sacrum is directed anteriorly.

sacrococainization (sā″krō-kō-kăn″ī-zā′shŭn). Injection of cocaine through the sacrolumbar space into the spinal cord.

sacrococcygeal (sā″krō-kŏk-sĭj′ē-ăl) [″ + Gr.

kokkyx, coccyx]. Concerning the sacrum and coccyx.

sacrococcygeus (săk″rō-kŏk-sĭj′ē-ŭs). One of two small muscles (anterior and posterior) extending from the sacrum to coccyx.

sacrocoxalgia (sā″krō-kŏks-ăl′jē-ă) [″ + *coxa,* hip, + Gr. *algos,* pain]. Pain in the sacroiliac joint, usually due to inflammation. SEE: *sacrocoxitis.*

sacrocoxitis (sā″krō-kŏks-ī′tĭs) [″ + ″ + Gr. *itis,* inflammation]. Inflammation of the sacroiliac joint.

sacrodynia (sā″krō-dĭn′ē-ă) [″ + *odyne,* pain]. Pain in the region of the sacrum.

sacroiliac (sā″krō-ĭl′ē-ăk) [″ + *iliacus,* hipbone]. Of, or pert. to, the sacrum and ilium.

sacroiliac joint. The articulation between the hipbone and sacrum. It is a diarthrodial joint with a narrow cavity. Joint movement is limited because of interlocking of articular surfaces.

sacroiliitis (sā″krō-ĭl″ē-ī′tĭs) [″ + ″ + Gr. *itis,* inflammation]. Inflammation of the sacroiliac joint.

sacrolisthesis (sā″krō-lĭs-thē′sĭs) [″ + Gr. *olisthesis,* slipping]. A deformity wherein the sacrum is in front of the last lumbar vertebra.

sacrolumbar (sā″krō-lŭm′băr) [″ + *lumbus,* loin]. Of, or concerning, the sacrum and lumbar area.

sacrolumbar angle. Angle formed by articulation of the last lumbar vertebra and the sacrum.

sacroposterior (sā″krō-pŏs-tē′rē-or) [″ + *posterior,* coming after]. Denoting intrauterine fetal position in which the fetal sacrum is directed posteriorly.

sacrosciatic (sā″krō-sī-ăt′ĭk) [″ + *sciaticus,* hipjoint]. Concerning the sacrum and ischium.

sacrospinal (sā″krō-spī′năl) [″ + *spina,* thorn]. Concerning the sacrum and the spine.

sacrospinalis [″ + *spina,* thorn]. A large muscle lying on either side of the vertebral column extending from the sacrum to the head. Its two chief components are the iliocostalis and longissimus muscles. SEE: *Muscles* in *Appendix.*

sacrotomy (sā-krŏt′ō-mē) [L. *sacrum,* sacred, + Gr. *tome,* incision]. Surgical excision of the lower part of the sacrum.

sacrouterine (sā″krō-ū′tĕr-ĭn) [″ + *uterus,* womb]. Concerning the sacrum and uterus.

sacrovertebral (sā″krō-vĕr′tĕ-brăl) [″ + *vertebra,* vertebra]. Concerning the sacrum and the spinal column.

sacrovertebral angle. Angle formed by the base of the sacrum and 5th lumbar vertebra.

sacrum (sā′krŭm) [L., sacred]. The triangular bone situated dorsal and caudal from the two ilia between the 5th lumbar vertebra and the coccyx. It is formed of five united vertebrae and is wedged between the two innominate bones, its articulations forming the sacroiliac joints. It forms the base of the vertebral column and, with the coccyx, forms the posterior boundary of the true pelvis. The sacrum in a male is narrower and more curved than in a female. SYN: *vertebra magnum.* SEE: illus.

sactosalpinx (săk″tō-săl′pĭnks) [Gr. *saktos,* stuffed, + *salpinx,* tube]. Dilated fallopian tube due to retention of secretions, as in pyosalpinx or hydrosalpinx.

saddle. A surface or structure that resembles a seat used to ride a horse. The base of artificial dentures is often referred to as a saddle.

saddle area. The portion of the buttocks, perineum, and thighs that would come in contact with the seat of the saddle when riding a horse.

saddle back. Term applied to an exaggerated curve of the lower back, lordosis, q.v.

saddle block anesthesia. Type of anesthesia produced by introducing the anesthetic agent

SACRUM AND COCCYX
(ANTERIOR VIEW)

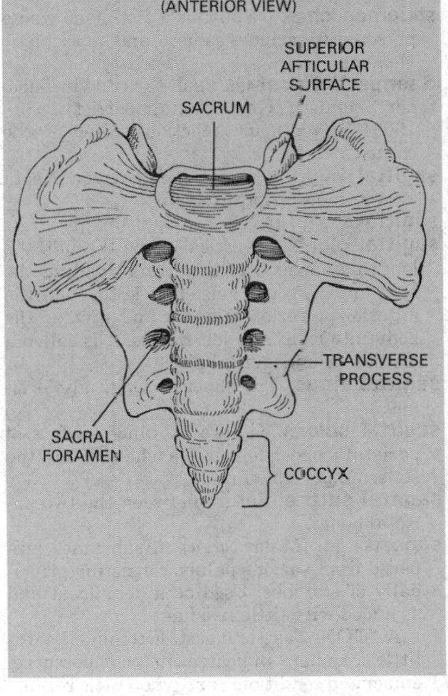

into the 4th lumbar interspace. This anesthetizes the perineum and buttocks area.

saddle joint. Joint with articulating surfaces convex in one direction and concave in the other.

Ex.: carpometacarpal joint of the thumb.

saddle nose. A nose with a depressed bridge due to congenital absence of bony or cartilaginous support or due to a disease such as leprosy or congenital syphilis.

sadism (sā'dĭzm, săd'ĭzm). [Comte Donatien Alphonse François de Sade, Marquis de Sade, 1740–1814] Conscious or unconscious sexual pleasure derived from inflicting mental or physical pain on others. SEE: *algolagnia; masochism.*

sadist (sā'dĭst, săd'ĭst). One who practices sadism.

sadness. A normal emotional feeling of dejection or melancholy. A result of an unhappy event or situation that warrants a change in the emotional state. Not to be confused with depression, in which the person is melancholy for no apparent reason or in which the degree of depression is out of proportion to the cause for sadness.

sadomasochism (sā″dō-măs'ĕ-kĭzm, săd″ō-măs'ĕ-kĭzm). Sexual pleasure related to both sadism and masochism.

sadomasochist (sā″dō-măs'ĕ-kĭst). One whose personality includes sadistic and masochistic elements.

Saemisch's ulcer (sā'mĭsh-ĕs). [Edwin Theodor Saemisch, Ger. ophthalmologist, 1833–1909] Serpiginous infectious ulcer of the cornea.

sagittal (săj'ĭ-tăl) [L. *sagittalis*]. Arrowlike; in an anteroposterior direction.

sagittalis (săj″ĭ-tā'lĭs) [L.]. Sagittal, q.v.

sagittal plane. A vertical plane through the longitudinal axis of the trunk dividing the body into two portions. If it is through the anterior-posterior midaxis and divides the body into right and left halves, it is called a median or midsagittal plane.

sagittal sinus. The superior longitudinal sinus.

sagittal sulcus. Groove on inner surface of parietal bones, forming a channel for the superior sagittal sinus.

sagittal suture. Suture between the two parietal bones.

sago (sā'gō) [Malay *sagu*]. A substance prepared from various palms, consisting principally of starches. Used as a demulcent and as a food with little residue.

ACTION: Easy to digest. Fattening. Leaves little residue. Indicated in convalescence, emaciated conditions, and when little residue is desired. SEE: *carbohydrates; starch.*

Saint Anthony's fire. Any of certain inflammations or gangrenous skin conditions, esp. erysipelas, hospital gangrene, and ergotism, q.v.

St. Joseph's Cough Syrup for Children. Trade name for dextromethorphan hydrobromide.

Saint's triad. Hiatus hernia, diverticula of the colon, and cholelithiasis.

Saint Vitus' dance. Nervous disease with involuntary jerking motions. SYN: *chorea, Sydenham's.*

sal (săl) [L.]. Salt; or a substance resembling salt.

s. ammoniac. Chloride of ammonia.

s. soda. Sodium carbonate.

s. volatile. Ammonium carbonate.

salaam convulsion (sŭ-lŏm') [Arabic *salam,* peace]. Clonic spasm of the sternomastoid muscles resulting in a bowing movement. SYN: *nodding spasm.*

salacious (sĕ-lā'shŭs) [L. *salax,* lustful]. Lustful or inciting to lust.

Sal-Hepatica. Trade name for sodium phosphate, USP.

salicylamide (săl″ĭ-sĭl-ăm'ĭd). The amide of salicylic acid, $C_7H_7NO_2$. An analgesic drug.

salicylanilide (săl″ĭ-sĭl-ăn'ĭ-lĭd). An antifungal drug.

salicylate (săl″ĭ-sĭl'āt, săl-ĭs'ĭl-āt). Any salt of salicylic acid.

s., methyl. The principal constituent of oil of wintergreen. It is applied externally as a counterirritant.

s., sodium. White crystalline substance with disagreeable taste, in some cases even nauseating. Used to reduce pain and temperature. SEE: *acetylsalicylic acid.*

salicylated (săl-ĭs'ĭl-āt-ĕd). Impregnated with salicylic acid.

salicylate poisoning. SEE: *aspirin poisoning.*

salicylazosulfapyridine (săl″ĭ-sĭl″ă-zō-sŭl″fă-pĭr'ĭ-dēn). Previously used name for sulfasalazine, q.v.

salicylic acid (săl″ĭ-sĭl'ĭk). USP. $C_7H_6O_3$. A white crystalline acid derived from phenol.

USES: In making aspirin, as a preservative and flavoring agent, and in external treatment of certain skin conditions.

salicylism (săl'ĭ-sĭl″ĭzm). Toxic condition caused by an overdose of salicylic acid or its derivatives.

salicylsulfonic acid test. Test for albumin in urine. SEE: *albumin.*

salicyluric acid (săl″ĭ-sĭ-lū'rĭk). Acid found in urine after an individual takes salicylic acid or its derivatives.

salifiable (săl″ĭ-fī'ă-bl) [L. *sal,* salt, + *fieri,* to be made]. Capable of forming a salt by combining with an acid.

salify (săl'ĭ-fī) [″ + *fieri,* to be made]. To convert to salt.

salimeter (săl-ĭm'ĕ-ter) [″ + Gr. *metron,* a

measure]. Device for testing strength of saline solutions.

saline (sā'līn, sā'lēn) [L. *salinus,* of salt]. Containing or pert. to salt; salty.

saline cathartic. A salt, such as Epsom salts, used to produce evacuation of the bowel.

saline enema. An enema consisting of a salt solution, used to induce peristalsis and evacuation. The salt solutions most frequently used are physiological saline; 1 teaspoonful (4 gm.) table salt (sodium chloride) dissolved in 1 pint (500 ml.) of warm water (115° F or 46.1° C); and Epsom salts (magnesium sulfate) 15 to 113 grams in a sufficient quantity of warm water to dissolve the salt.

saline solution. A solution of sodium chloride and distilled water. A 0.9% solution of sodium chloride is considered isotonic to the body. A normal saline solution (one having an osmolality similar to blood serum) consists of 0.85% salt solution, which is necessary to maintain osmotic pressure and the stimulation and regulation of muscular activity. SEE: *physiological salt solution.*

salinometer (săl″ĭ-nŏm'ĕ-tĕr) [L. *salinus,* of salt, + *metron,* measure]. An instrument for determining the salt content of a solution.

saliva (să-lī'vă) [L.]. Salivary gland and oral mucous gland fluid, the secretion that begins the process of digesting food.

CHARACTER: It is normally tasteless, clear, odorless, viscid, and weakly alkaline, being neutralized after being acted upon by gastric acid in the stomach. Sp. gr. 1.002–1.006. The amount secreted in 24 hours is estimated to be 1500 ml. The flow varies from 0.2 ml. per minute from resting glands to 4.0 ml. per minute with maximum secretion.

COMP: Inorganic substances: 99.5% water; salts (chlorides, carbonates, phosphates, sulfates); gases in solution; and sometimes abnormal substances being excreted from the body, i.e., acetone. Organic substances include enzymes (ptyalin, maltase, lysozyme); proteins (serum albumin and globulin, mucin); and small amounts of urea, uric acid, creatine, and amino acids. Cellular elements include epithelial cells and leukocytes.

FUNCT: To moisten food, facilitating mastication and deglutition; to moisten and lubricate mouth parts; to act as a solvent for excretion of waste products; to initiate digestion of starches; to assist in regulation of water balance.

RS: aptyalism; parotid; ptyalin; ptyalism; salivary digestion; salivary glands; sialagogue.

s., artificial. A solution that is useful in treating excessive dryness of the mouth (xerostomia). One such formula is 20 ml. of a 4% solution of methylcellulose, 10 ml. of glycerin, sufficient normal saline to make 90 ml., and one drop of lemon oil.

salivant (săl'ĭ-vănt) [L. *saliva,* saliva]. Something that stimulates the flow of saliva.

salivary (săl'ĭ-vĕr-ē) [L. *salivarius*]. Pert. to, producing, or formed from saliva.

salivary corpuscles. Nucleated spherical bodies in saliva thought to be modified leukocytes from lymphatic tissue.

salivary digestion. Digestion occurring in the mouth resulting from action of salivary enzymes. Ptyalin, a salivary enzyme, is an amylase that initiates the breakdown of starch and glycogen to maltose and a small amount of glucose. Oral digestion is limited because of the short time food remains in the mouth, but digestion continues in the stomach until food becomes acidified by gastric juice. The optimum pH for ptyalin activity is 6.9. SEE: *digestion.*

salivary glands. The glands of the oral cavity whose secretions form saliva. These glands are the parotid, one on each side of the face below the ear; submaxillary, principally in the floor of the mouth; sublingual, principally in the floor of the mouth; and buccal, scattered beneath the mucous membrane of the lips and cheeks.

Salivary secretion is under nervous control, being reflexly initiated by mechanical, chemical, or radiant stimuli acting on taste buds (gustatory receptors) in the mouth, olfactory receptors, visual receptors (eyes), or other sense organs. Secretion may also occur as a result of conditioned reflexes, as when one thinks about food or hears a dinner bell.

NERVE SUPPLY: Facial and glossopharyngeal nerves and from the autonomic nervous system.

BLOOD SUPPLY: Branches from the external carotid artery.

salivation (săl″ĭ-vā'shŭn) [L. *salivatio*]. 1. The act of secreting saliva. 2. Excessive secretion of saliva. SYN: *ptyalism.*

salivatory (săl'ĭ-vă-tor″ē). Producing secretion of saliva.

salivolithiasis (să-lī″vō-lĭ-thī'ă-sĭs) [L. *saliva,* saliva, + Gr. *lithos,* stone, + *-iasis,* condition]. Sialolithiasis, q.v.

Salk vaccine (sŏlk). [Jonas E. Salk, U.S. microbiologist, b. 1914] First successful poliomyelitis vaccine; a vaccine that contains three types of formalin-inactivated poliomyelitis viruses and induces immunity against the disease. SEE: *poliomyelitis.*

sallow (săl'ō) [AS. *salo*]. Of a sickly, yellowish color, usually said of complexion or skin.

salmin(e) (săl'mēn, -mĭn) [L. *salmo,* salmon]. $C_{30}H_{57}N_{14}O_6$. A toxic protamine obtained from spermatozoa of salmon. SEE: *protamine; protein.*

Salmonella (săl″mō-nĕl'ă) [L.]. [Daniel E.

Salmon, U.S. pathologist, 1850–1914] A genus of bacteria belonging to the family Enterobacteriaceae. Salmonella are gram-negative, usually motile, rods. Several species are pathogenic, some producing mild gastroenteritis, others producing a severe and often fatal food poisoning. SEE: *salmonellosis.*

S. choleraesuis. A species often found to be the cause of septicemia.

S. enteritidis. Species causing gastroenteritis and food poisoning in man.

S. paratyphi. A group of Salmonella, types A, B, and C, that causes paratyphoid fever.

S. schottmülleri. Species causing paratyphoid fever, type B.

S. typhimurium. A species frequently isolated from persons having acute gastroenteritis.

S. typhosa. Species causing typhoid fever in man only.

salmonellosis (săl-mō-nĕ-lō'sĭs). Infestation with bacteria of genus Salmonella. There are three forms of salmonella infection that occur in man: enteric fever (typhoid fever); septicemia, which usually is caused by Salmonella choleraesuis; and acute gastroenteritis, which can be caused by a variety of species of salmonella. More than 1400 species of Salmonella have been classified.

salmon patch. Salmon-colored areas of the cornea in syphilitic keratitis. SYN: *Hutchinson's patch.*

salpingectomy (săl″pĭn-jĕk'tō-mē) [Gr. *salpinx,* tube, + *ektome,* excision]. Surgical removal of the fallopian tube.

salpingemphraxis (săl″pĭn-jĕm-frăk'sĭs) [″ + *emphraxis,* a stoppage]. Obstruction of the eustachian tube.

salpingian (săl-pĭn'jē-ăn). Concerning the eustachian tube or fallopian tube.

salpingion (săl-pĭn'jē-ŏn). A point at the inferior surface of the apex of the petrous portion of the temporal bone.

salpingitis (săl″pĭn-jī'tĭs) [Gr. *salpinx,* tube, + *itis,* inflammation]. Inflammation of the fallopian tube.

ETIOL: The condition may be acute, subacute, or chronic. The organisms most often associated with salpingitis are the gonococcus, staphylococcus, streptococcus, colon bacillus, and tubercle bacillus.

s., eustachian. Inflammation of the eustachian tube. SYN: *eustachitis.*

salpingo- [Gr. *salpinx,* tube]. Combining form indicating eustachian or fallopian tube.

salpingocatheterism (săl-pĭng″gō-kăth'ĕt-ĕr-ĭzm) [″ + *katheter,* catheter, + *-ismos,* process]. Catheterization of the eustachian tube.

salpingocele (săl-pĭng'gō-sēl) [″ + *kele,* hernia]. Hernial protrusion of a fallopian tube.

salpingocyesis (săl-pĭng″ō-sī-ē'sĭs) [Gr. *salpinx,* tube, + *kyesis,* pregnancy]. Pregnancy in which fetus begins to develop in a fallopian tube; tubal pregnancy.

salpingography (săl″pĭng-gŏg'ră-fē) [″ + *graphein,* to write]. X-ray study of the fallopian tubes into which a radiopaque dye has been introduced. Used in testing for patency of the tubes in investigating infertility.

salpingolithiasis (săl-pĭng″gō-lĭ-thī'ă-sĭs) [″ + *lithos,* stone, + *-iasis,* condition]. Presence of calculi in the fallopian tube.

salpingolysis (săl″pĭng-gŏl'ĭ-sĭs) [″ + *lysis,* dissolution]. Surgical disruption of adhesions in the fallopian tube.

salpingo-oophorectomy (săl-pĭng″gō-ō″ŏf-ō-rĕk'tō-mē) [″ + *oon,* egg, + *phoros,* a bearer, + *ektome,* excision]. Excision of an ovary and fallopian tube. SYN: *salpingo-ovariectomy.*

salpingo-oophoritis (săl-pĭng″ō-ō″ŏf-ō-rī'tĭs) [″ + ″ + ″ + *itis,* inflammation]. Inflammation of a fallopian tube and ovary. SYN: *salpingo-oothecitis.*

salpingo-oophorocele (săl-pĭng″gō-ō-ŏf'or-ō-sēl) [Gr. *salpinx,* tube, + *oon,* egg, + *phoros,* a bearer, + *kele,* hernia]. Hernia enclosing the ovary and fallopian tube.

salpingo-oothecitis (săl-pĭng″gō-ō″ō-thē-sī'tĭs) [″ + ″ + *theke,* box, + *itis,* inflammation]. Inflammation of a fallopian tube and ovary. SYN: *salpingo-oophoritis.*

salpingo-oothecocele (săl-pĭng″gō-ō″ō-thē'kō-sēl) [″ + ″ + ″ + *kele,* hernia]. Hernia of ovary and fallopian tube.

salpingo-ovariectomy (săl-pĭng″gō-ō″văr-ē-ĕk'tō-mē) [″ + L. *ovarium,* ovary, + Gr. *ektome,* excision]. Surgical removal of an ovary and fallopian tube. SYN: *salpingo-oophorectomy.*

salpingoperitonitis (săl-pĭng″gō-pĕr″ĭ-tō-nī'tĭs) [″ + *peritonaion,* peritoneum, + *itis,* inflammation]. Inflammation of the serosal covering of the fallopian tubes.

salpingopexy (săl-pĭng'ō-pĕk″sē) [″ + *pexis,* fixation]. Fixation of a fallopian tube.

salpingopharyngeal (săl-pĭng″gō-fă-rĭn'jē-ăl) [″ + *pharynx,* pharynx]. Concerning the eustachian tube of the ear and the pharynx.

salpingopharyngeus (săl-pĭng″gō-făr-ĭn'jē-ŭs) [″ + *pharynx,* pharynx]. The muscle arising near the opening of the eustachian tube. Raises the nasopharynx.

salpingoplasty (săl-pĭng'gō-plăs″tē) [″ + *plassein,* to form]. Plastic surgery of the fallopian tube. Used in treating female infertility. SYN: *tuboplasty.*

salpingorrhaphy (săl″pĭng-gor'ă-fē) [″ + *rhaphe,* a seam]. Suture of a fallopian tube.

salpingosalpingostomy (săl-pĭng″gō-săl″pĭng-gŏs'tō-mē) [″ + *salpinx,* tube, + *stoma,* a mouth]. The operation of attaching one fallopian tube to the other.

salpingoscope (săl-pĭng'gō-skōp") [" + *skopein,* to see]. Device for examining the nasopharynx and eustachian tube.

salpingostenochoria (săl-pĭng"gō-stĕn"ō-kor'ē-ă) [" + *stenosis,* stenosis, + *choreia,* dance]. Stenosis or stricture of the eustachian tube.

salpingostomatomy (săl-pĭng"gō-stō-măt'ō-mē) [" + *stoma,* a mouth, + *tome,* incision]. Creation of an artificial opening in a fallopian tube after it has been occluded as a result of inflammation and scarring.

salpingostomy (săl-pĭng-ŏs'tō-mē). Surgical opening of a fallopian tube that has been occluded, or for drainage purposes.

salpingotomy (săl-pĭng-ŏt'ō-mē) [" + *tome,* incision]. Incision of a fallopian tube.

salpingo-ureterostomy (săl-pĭng"gō-ūr-ēt"ĕr-ŏs'tō-mē) [" + *oureter,* ureter, + *stoma,* opening]. Surgical connection of the ureter and the fallopian tube.

salpingysterocyesis (săl"pĭng-jĭs"tĕr-ō-sī-ē'sĭs) [" + *hystera,* uterus, + *kyesis,* pregnancy]. Pregnancy in which the embryo is located at the entrance of the fallopian tube into the uterus; ectopic pregnancy.

salpinx (săl'pĭnks) [Gr., tube]. (pl. *salpinges*) The fallopian or eustachian tube.

salt [AS. *sealt*]. 1. White crystalline compound occurring in nature, known chemically as sodium chloride, NaCl. 2. Containing, or treated with salt. 3. To treat with salt. 4. In the plural, any mineral salt or saline mixture used as an aperient or cathartic, esp. Epsom salts or Glauber's salt. 5. In chemistry, a compound consisting of a positive ion other than hydrogen, and a negative ion other than hydroxyl. 6. A chemical compound resulting from the interaction of an acid and a base.

Salts and water are the inorganic or mineral constituents of the body. They play specific roles in the functions of cells and are indispensable for life. The principal salts are chlorides, carbonates, bicarbonates, sulfates, and phosphates, combined with sodium, potassium, calcium, or magnesium.

In general, salts serve the following roles in the body: maintenance of proper osmotic conditions; maintenance of water balance and regulation of blood volume; maintenance of proper acid-base balance; provision for essential constituents of tissue, esp. bones and teeth; maintenance of normal irritability of muscle and nerve cells; maintenance of condition for coagulation of the blood; provision for essential components of certain enzyme systems, respiratory pigments, and hormones; regulation of cell membrane and capillary permeability.

RS: chloride; low-salt diet; normal; sal; saline; salt-free diet; salt glow; secretion.

s., acid. A salt in which one or more hydrogen atoms remain unreplaced by the hydroxyl (OH) radical.

s., basic. A salt in which the ability to react with an acid radical still remains.

s., bile. The salt of glycocholic and taurocholic acid present in bile.

s., buffer. A salt that fixes excess amounts of acid or alkali without a change in hydrogen-ion concentration.

s., double. Any salt formed from two other salts.

s., Epsom. Magnesium sulfate.

s., Glauber's. Sodium sulfate.

s., haloid. Any salt of a halogen, i.e., chloride, iodide, bromide, or fluoride.

s., iodized. Salt containing 1 part sodium or potassium iodide to 10,000 parts of sodium chloride. An important source of iodine in the diet. The use of this form of salt will prevent goiter.

s., neutral. Any salt that contains no replaceable hydrogen or hydroxyl groups. SYN: *s., normal.*

s., Rochelle. Potassium sodium tartrate, used as a saline cathartic.

s., rock. Native sodium chloride.

s., smelling. Aromatized ammonium carbonate.

saltation (săl-tā'shŭn) [L. *saltatio,* leaping]. 1. Act of leaping or dancing, as in chorea. 2. Abrupt variation in character of a species. SYN: *mutation.*

saltatory (săl'tă-tō"rē). Marked by dancing or leaping.

saltatory conduction. Skipping from node to node, said of movement of the potential along myelinated neurons.

saltatory spasm. Tic of muscles of lower extremity, causing convulsive leaping upon attempt to stand. SEE: *Jumping Frenchmen of Maine; miryachit; palmus.*

salt-free diet. It is impractical to attempt to maintain a diet absolutely free of sodium chloride. Thus salt-free means a low-sodium diet that allows 500 mg. (0.5 gm.) or less of salt per day. On this diet, table salt should not be added to the food. Also, it is important to know the amount of salt in the drinking water and in commonly used beverages such as beer, because some areas have water containing a large amount of sodium. Some medicines (for example, sodium salicylate) are quite high in sodium content. Exclusion of sodium-containing medicines is important in attempting to regulate the amount of sodium consumed. SEE: *salt.*

salt glow. Name given to a rub of the entire body with moist salt for stimulation.

salting out. A method of separating a specific

protein from a mixture of proteins by the addition of a salt, e.g., ammonium sulfate.

salt-losing syndrome. The condition of greatly increased loss of sodium from the body due to renal disease, adrenal cortical insufficiency, or gastrointestinal disease.

saltpeter, saltpetre (sawlt-pē'tĕr) [L. *sal,* salt, + *petra,* rock]. A common name for potassium nitrate.

s., Chile. A common name for sodium nitrate, $NaNO_3$. Crystalline powder, saline in taste and soluble in water.

salt-poor diet. Diet where all food is prepared and served without the addition of salt, including salt-free bread and butter. Milk intake is limited.

salts. Pl. of salt.

salt solution, normal. Salt solution, physiological.

salt solution, physiological. A sterile solution containing 0.9% of sodium chloride in chemically pure distilled water (9 gm. sodium chloride in 1000 ml. or 1 liter of distilled water).

salubrious (să-lū'brē-ŭs) [L. *salubris*]. Promoting or favorable to health; wholesome.

saluresis (săl"ū-rē'sĭs) [L. *sal,* salt, + Gr. *ouresis,* urination]. The excretion of sodium chloride in the urine.

saluretic (săl"ū-rĕt'ĭk). Something that promotes excretion of sodium chloride in the urine.

Saluron. Trade name for hydroflumethiazide.

salutary (săl'ū-tā"rē) [L. *salutaris*]. Healthful; promoting health; curative.

salvarsan (săl'văr-săn) [L. *salvus,* safe, + Gr. *arsen,* arsenic]. An arsenical, yellowish powder preparation developed by Ehrlich for treatment of syphilis. Since the development of penicillin, there has been little need for salvarsan. SYN: *arsphenamine.*

salve (săv) [AS. *sealf*]. 1. An ointment applied to wounds. 2. In pharmacology, any ointment or cerate made with a base of a fat, oil, petrolatum, or resin.

samarium (să-mā'rē-ŭm). SYMB: Sm. or Sa. At. wt. 150.35; at. no. 62; sp. gr. approx. 7.50. A very rare metallic element.

sample. 1. A piece or portion of a whole that will demonstrate the characteristics or quality of the whole, such as a specimen of blood. 2. In research, a portion of a population selected to represent the entire population.

sampling. The process of selecting a portion or part to represent the whole.

s., random. One of several ways of selecting a sample of a population. This method involves using a listing of the entire population and a table of random numbers to select the sample.

sanative (săn'ă-tĭv) [L. *sanare,* to heal]. Of a healing nature. SYN: *curative.*

sanatorium (săn"ă-tō'rē-ŭm) [L. *sanatorius,* healing]. An establishment for preservation of health, or for the treatment of the chronically sick. SYN: *sanitarium.*

sanatory (săn'ă-tō"rē). Curative; conducive to health.

sand (sănd) [AS.]. Fine grains of disintegrated rock.

s., auditory. Calcareous concretion in labyrinth of the ear. SYN: *ear dust; otoconium; otolith.*

s., brain. Concretion of matter near base of the pineal gland. SYN: *acervulus cerebri.*

sandflies. Flies of the order Diptera belonging to the genus Phlebotomus. They transmit sandfly fever, Oroya fever, and various types of leishmaniasis.

sandfly fever. A mild virus disease that clinically resembles influenza, except for absence of respiratory symptoms. The causative organism, any one of three species of arboviruses, is transmitted by the common sandfly Phlebotomus papatasii, a small hairy bloodsucking midge that bites at night and has a limited flight range. The disease occurs in tropical and subtropical areas that experience long periods of hot, dry weather. There is no specific therapy. SYN: *pappataci fever; phlebotomus fever.*

Sandhoff's disease. A rare form of Tay-Sachs disease, q.v., in which two essential enzymes (hexosaminidase A and B) for metabolizing ganglioside are absent. In Tay-Sachs disease only one enzyme, hexosaminidase A, is absent.

Sandril. Trade name for reserpine, USP.

Sandwith's bald tongue (sănd'wĭths). [Fleming M. Sandwith, Br. physician, 1777–1843] Abnormally clean tongue seen in late stages of pellagra.

sane (sān) [L. *sanus*]. Sound of mind; mentally normal.

Sanfilippo's disease. [S. J. Sanfilippo, contemporary U.S. pediatrician] A hereditary disease transmitted as an autosomal recessive. Characterized by severe progressive mental retardation and mild dwarfism, skeletal defects, and hepatosplenomegaly. SYN: *mucopolysaccharidosis III.*

sanguicolous (săng-gwĭk'ō-lŭs) [L. *sanguis,* blood, + *colere,* to dwell]. Inhabiting the blood, as a parasite.

sanguifacient (săng-gwĭ-fā'shĕnt) [" + *facere,* to make]. Making blood.

sanguiferous (săng-gwĭf'ĕr-ŭs) [" + *ferre,* to carry]. Conducting or containing blood, as the circulatory organs.

sanguification (săng"gwĭ-fĭ-kā'shŭn) [" + *facere,* to make]. Conversion into, or production of, blood. SYN: *hematopoiesis.*

sanguimotor, sanguimotory (săng"gwĭ-mō'tor, -tō-rē) [" + *motor,* a mover]. Pert. to blood circulation.

sanguine (săng′gwĭn) [L. *sanguineus,* bloody]. 1. Optimistic; cheerful. 2. Plethoric, bloody; marked by abundant and active blood circulation, particularly a ruddy complexion. 3. Pert. to, or consisting of, blood.

sanguineous (săng-gwĭn′ē-ŭs) [L. *sanguineus,* bloody]. 1. Bloody; rel. to blood. 2. Having an abundance of blood. SYN: *plethoric.*

sanguinolent (săng-gwĭn′ō-lĕnt) [L. *sanguinolentus*]. Containing, or tinged with, blood.

sanguinopoietic (săng″gwĭn-ō-poy-ĕt′ĭk) [L. *sanguis,* blood, + *poiein,* to form]. Forming or making blood. SYN: *hematopoietic; sanguifacient.*

sanguinopurulent (săng″gwĭ-nō-pū′rū-lĕnt) [″ + *purulentus,* purlulent]. Concerning or containing blood and pus.

sanguinous (săng′gwĭ-nŭs) [L. *sanguineus,* bloody]. Sanguineous, q.v.

sanguirenal (săng″gwĭ-rē′năl) [L. *sanguis,* blood, + *ren,* kidney]. Pert. to the blood supply of the kidneys.

sanguis (săng′gwĭs) [L.]. [NA] Blood.

sanguisuga (săng-gwĭ-sū′gă) [″ + *sugere,* to suck]. A leech or bloodsucker. SEE: *Hirudo.*

sanguivorous (săng-gwĭv′ō-rŭs) [″ + *vorare,* to eat]. Blood eating.

sanies (sā′nē-ēz) [L.]. A thin, fetid, greenish discharge from a wound or ulcer, presenting appearance of pus tinged with blood.

saniopurulent (sā″nē-ō-pū′roo-lĕnt) [L. *sanies,* diseased blood, + *purulentus,* full of pus]. Having characteristics of sanies and pus; pert. to a fetid, serous, blood-tinged discharge containing pus.

sanioserous (sā″nē-ō-sē′rŭs) [″ + *serum,* whey]. Composed of sanies and serum.

sanitarian (săn″ĭ-tā′rē-ăn) [L. *sanitarius,* sanitary]. A person who by training and experience is skilled in sanitation and public health.

sanitarium (săn-ĭ-tā′rē-ŭm) [L. *sanatorius,* healing]. Institution for treatment and recuperation of persons having physical or mental disorders; occasionally limited to place where conditions are prophylactic rather than therapeutic. SYN: *sanatorium.*

sanitary (săn′ĭ-tā″rē) [L. *sanitarius*]. 1. Promoting or pertaining to conditions that are conducive to good health. 2. Clean, free of dirt.

sanitary napkin. Perineal pad, esp. one used for absorbing menstrual fluid.

sanitation (săn″ĭ-tā′shŭn) [L. *sanitas,* health]. The formulation and application of measures to promote and establish conditions favorable to health, esp. public health. SEE: *hygiene.*

sanitization (săn″ĭ-tĭ-zā′shŭn) [L. *sanitas,* health]. The act of making sanitary.

sanitize (săn′ĭ-tīz). To make sanitary.

sanitizer. An agent that reduces the number of bacterial contaminants to safe levels as judged by public health requirements. Usually used to describe agents applied to eating and drinking utensils and dairy equipment.

sanity (săn′ĭ-tē). Soundness of health or mind; normal mentality.

San Joachim valley fever. Coccidioidomycosis, q.v.

Sanorex. Trade name for mazindol.

Sansert. Trade name for methysergide maleate, USP.

santonin (săn′tō-nĭn). A colorless, crystalline substance obtained from the unexpanded flower heads of species of the plant Artemisia cina.

ACTION AND USES: A vermifuge against the roundworm. Because of its toxicity, it is not used.

sap (săp) [AS. *saep*]. 1. Any fluid essential to life and vitality of a living structure. 2. To cause gradual exhaustion or weakness, as to sap one's strength.

s., cell. The fluid portion of protoplasm. SYN: *hyaloplasm.*

s., nuclear. Liquid portion of a cell nucleus. SYN: *karyolymph.*

saphena (să-fē′nă) [Gr. *saphenes,* manifest]. (pl. *saphenae*) Either of two large superficial veins of the leg. The great saphenous vein is the longest vein in the body and the small saphenous vein is the large superficial vein of the back of the leg. SEE: *saphenous.*

saphenectomy (săf″ĕ-nĕk′tō-mē) [″ + *ektome,* excision]. Surgical removal of the saphenous vein.

saphenous (să-fē′nŭs). Pert. to, or associated with, a saphenous vein or nerve in the leg.

saphenous nerve. A deep branch of the femoral nerve. In the lower leg, it follows the long saphenous vein that supplies the medial side of the leg, ankle, and foot.

saphenous opening. An aperture in the fascia, oval in shape, in inner and upper part of the thigh, transmitting the saphenous vein below Poupart's ligament. SYN: *fossa ovalis.*

saphenous veins. Two superficial veins, the great and small, passing up the leg. The great saphenous vein extends from the foot to the saphenous opening; the small vein runs behind the outer malleolus up the back of the leg, joining the popliteal vein. SYN: *saphenae.* SEE: *vein.*

sapid (săp′ĭd) [L. *sapidus,* tasty]. Savory; tasty; opposed to insipid.

sapo (sā′pō) [L.]. Soap prepared from pure olive oil and sodium hydroxide.

saponaceous (sā″pō-nā′shŭs) [L. *saponaceus,* soapy]. Soapy; resembling soap in feel or quality.

saponatus (să″pō-nā′tŭs) [L.]. Mixed with soap.

saponification (să-pŏn″ĭ-fĭ-kā′shŭn) [L. *sapo,* soap, + *facere,* to make]. 1. Conversion into soap; chemically, the hydrolysis or the splitting of fat by an alkali yielding glycerol and three molecules of alkali salt of the fatty acid, the soap. 2. In chemistry, hydrolysis of an ester into corresponding alcohol and acid (free or in form of a salt).

saponification number. In analysis of fats, the number of milligrams of potassium hydroxide needed to saponify 1 gm. of oil or fat.

saponify (să-pŏn′ĭ-fī). To convert into a soap, as when fats are treated with an alkali to produce a free alcohol plus the salt of the fatty acid. Thus, stearin, saponified with sodium hydroxide, yields the alcohol glycerol plus the soap sodium stearate.

saponin (săp′ō-nĭn) [Fr. *saponine,* soap]. Unabsorbable glucoside contained in the roots of some plants forming a lather in an aqueous solution. Saponins cause hemolysis of red blood cells even in high dilutions. When taken orally, they can produce diarrhea and vomiting.

sapophore (săp′ō-for) [L. *sapor,* taste, + Gr. *phoros,* bearing]. The component of a molecule that imparts taste to it.

saporific (săp″ō-rĭf′ĭk) [L. *saporificus,* producing taste]. Imparting a taste or flavor.

sapphism (săf′ĭzm) [Sappho, Gr. poetess, 7th-century B.C.]. Female homosexuality. SYN: *lesbianism.*

sapremia (să-prē′mē-ă) [Gr. *sapros,* rotten, + *haima,* blood]. A toxic condition caused by the absorption into the blood of toxins or poisons produced by saprophytes or putrefactive bacteria. SYN: *septicemia.*

sapro- [Gr. *sapros,* rotten]. Combining form meaning putrid or rotten.

saprobes (să′prōbs) [Gr. *sapros,* rotten, + *bios,* life]. Organisms that live as parasites because, in the case of fungi, they do not possess photosynthetic pigments.

saprodontia (săp″rō-dŏn′shē-ă) [″ + *odous,* tooth]. Caries of the teeth; tooth decay.

saprogen (săp′rō-jĕn) [″ + *gennan,* to produce]. Any microorganism causing or produced by putrefaction.

saprogenic (săp″rō-jĕn′ĭk). Causing putrefaction, or resulting from it.

saprophilous (săp-rŏf′ĭl-ŭs) [Gr. *sapros,* rotten, + *philein,* to love]. Living on decaying or dead substances, as a microorganism. SYN: *saprophytic.*

saprophyte (săp′rō-fīt) [″ + *phyton,* plant]. Any organism living on decaying or dead organic matter. Most of the higher fungi are saprophytes. SEE: *parasite.*

saprophytic (săp″rō-fĭt′ĭk). Living or growing in decaying or dead matter; characteristic of a saprophyte. SYN: *metatrophic; saprophilous.*

saprozoic (săp″rō-zō′ĭk) [″ + *zoon,* animal]. Living on decaying or dead organic matter.

sarapus (săr′ă-pŭs) [Gr. *sarapous*]. A person having flat feet.

Sarcina (săr′sĭ-nă) [L., bundle]. A genus of spherical saprophytic bacteria of the family Micrococcaceae. The individual organisms remain adherent to each other after splitting in two or three perpendicular directions. This process yields square tetrads or cubical packets.

sarcina (săr′sĭ-nă). (pl. *sarcinas* or *sarcinae*) Any organism of the genus Sarcina. SEE: *bacteria* for illus.

sarcitis (săr-sī′tĭs) [Gr. *sarx,* flesh, + *itis,* inflammation]. Inflammation of muscle tissue. SYN: *myositis.*

sarco- [Gr. *sarx,* flesh]. Combining form indicating flesh.

sarcoadenoma (săr″kō-ăd″ĕn-ō′mă) [″ + *aden,* gland, + *oma,* tumor]. A fleshy tumor of a gland. SYN: *adenosarcoma.*

sarcobiont (săr″kō-bī′ŏnt) [″ + *bioun,* to live]. A microorganism that lives on flesh.

sarcoblast (săr′kō-blăst) [″ + *blastos,* a germ]. Embryonic cell that develops into a muscle cell. SYN: *myoblast.*

sarcocarcinoma (săr″kō-kăr″sĭn-ō′mă) [″ + *karkinos,* crab, + *oma,* tumor]. A malignant tumor of sarcomatous and carcinomatous types.

sarcocele (săr′kō-sēl) [″ + *kele,* a mass]. A fleshy tumor of the testicle.

sarcocyst (săr′kō-sĭst) [″ + *kystis,* bladder]. An elongated tubular body produced by Sarcocystis.

Sarcocystis (săr″kō-sĭs′tĭs) [″ + *kystis,* bladder]. A genus of sporozoons found in the muscles of higher vertebrates (reptiles, birds, and mammals).

S. lindemanni. A species infesting the muscles of man.

Sarcodina (săr-kō-dī′nă) [″ + *eidos,* form]. A class of Protozoa characterized by absence of a thick pellicle and movement by pseudopodia. Sarcodina are typically holozoic and reproduce principally by asexual methods. Includes the families Amoebidae and Endamoebidae, the latter including many forms parasitic and pathogenic in man.

sarcogenic (săr″kō-jĕn′ĭk) [″ + *gennan,* to produce]. Producing flesh or muscle.

sarcoid (săr′koyd) [″ + *eidos,* form]. 1. Resembling flesh. 2. A small epithelioid tubercle-like lesion characteristic of sarcoidosis.

s., Boeck's. SEE: *Boeck's sarcoid.*

sarcoidosis (săr″koyd-ō′sĭs) [″ + ″ + *osis,* condition]. A disease of unknown etiology characterized by widespread granulomatous lesions that may affect any organ or tissue of the body. The liver is frequently affected, as are the skin, lungs, lymph nodes, spleen, eyes, and small bones of the hands and feet. Formerly called Boeck's sarcoid.

sarcolemma (săr"kō-lĕm'ă) [" + *lemma,* a rind]. A delicate membrane surrounding each striated muscle fiber.

sarcology (săr-kŏl'ō-jē) [" + *logos,* a study]. Branch of medicine dealing with study of the soft tissues of the body.

sarcolysis (săr-kŏl'ĭ-sĭs) [" + *lysis,* a dissolution]. Decomposition of the soft tissues or flesh.

sarcolytic (săr"kō-lĭt'ĭk). Decomposing flesh.

sarcoma (săr-kō'mă) [" + *oma,* tumor]. (pl. *sarcomas, -mata*) Cancer arising from connective tissue such as muscle or bone. May affect the bones, bladder, kidneys, liver, lungs, parotids, and spleen.

s., alveolar soft part. Malignant neoplasm composed of a reticular stroma of connective tissue surrounding clumps of large round cells.

s., botryoid. Sarcoma of the uterus composed of a polypoid mass of soft edematous tissues. Most often seen in infants or children.

s., chondro-. Sarcoma composed of masses of cartilage.

s., endometrial. Malignant neoplasm of the endometrial stroma.

s., Ewing's. A diffuse endothelioma or endothelial myeloma forming a fusiform swelling on a long bone.

s., fibro-. A malignant tumor with fibrous tissue, many spindle cells, and dilated vessels.

s., giant cell. Sarcoma from cancellous bone tissue with large cells with many nuclei. A special type called an epulis is seen in the jaw. SYN: *s., myeloid.*

s., Kaposi's. Kaposi's sarcoma, q.v.

s., lipo-. A rare tumor of bone containing cells of various types with small vacuoles of fat.

s., lymphangio-. Sarcoma arising from endothelium of lymph vessels in a lymph gland.

s., myeloid. S., giant cell.

s., myxo-. A benign tumor of mucoid tissue, such as that of the umbilical cord. SYN: *myxoma.*

s., osteogenic. Sarcoma composed of osseous tissue containing variously shaped cells.

s., reticulum cell. A variety of malignant lymphoma involving the lymph nodes and other lymphatic tissue.

s., rhabdomyo-. An embryonal tumor of striated muscle containing multinucleated cells with a striated cytoplasm.

s., spindle cell. Sarcoma consisting of small and large spindle-shaped cells.

sarcomatoid (sar-kō'mă-toyd) [Gr. *sarx,* flesh, + *oma,* tumor, + *eidos,* form]. Resembling a sarcoma.

sarcomatosis (săr"kō-mă-tō'sĭs) [" + " + *osis,* condition]. Condition marked by presence and spread of a sarcoma; sarcomatous degeneration.

sarcomatous (săr-kō'mă-tŭs). Of the nature of, or like, a sarcoma.

sarcomere (săr'kō-mēr) [" + *meros,* a part]. The portion of a striated muscle fibril lying between two adjacent dark lines called Krause's membranes.

sarcomphalocele (săr"kŏm-făl'ō-sēl) [" + *omphalos,* umbilicus, + *kele,* mass]. Fleshy tumor of the umbilicus.

sarcomyces (săr"kō-mī'sēz) [" + *mykes,* fungus]. A fleshy growth having the appearance of a fungus.

Sarcophagidae (săr"kō-făj'ĭ-dē) [Gr. *sarx,* flesh, + *phagein,* to eat]. The family of the order Diptera that includes the flesh flies. Females deposit their eggs or larvae on decaying flesh of dead animals. Larvae of two genera, Sarcophaga and Wohlfahrtia, frequently infest open sores and wounds of man giving rise to cutaneous myiasis.

sarcophagy (săr-kŏf'ă-jē). Practice of eating flesh.

sarcoplasm (săr'kō-plăzm) [" + *plasma,* a thing formed]. Semifluid interfibrillary substance of striated muscle cells. The cytoplasm of muscle cells.

sarcoplasmic (săr"kō-plăz'mĭk). Concerning or containing sarcoplasm.

sarcopoietic (săr"kō-poy-ĕt'ĭk) [" + *poiein,* to form]. Forming muscle or flesh.

Sarcoptes (săr-kŏp'tēz). A genus of Acarina that includes the mites that infest man and animals. Sarcoptes scabiei causes scabies in man.

Sarcoptidae (săr-kŏp'tĭ-dē). A family of mites of the order Acarina, class Arachnida, which includes Sarcoptes scabiei, the causative agent of scabies or itch in man and mange and scab in other animals.

sarcosis (săr-kō'sĭs) [" + *osis,* condition]. 1. The development of multiple fleshy tumors. 2. Abnormal formation of flesh.

sarcosome (săr'kō-sōm) [" + *soma,* body]. Term previously used for mitochondria, particularly of muscle cells.

Sarcosporidia (săr"kō-spō-rĭd'ē-ă) [" + *sporos,* a seed]. An order of protozoa belonging to the class Sporozoa that are parasitic in the muscles of higher vertebrates. Includes the genus Sarcocystis.

sarcosporidiosis (săr"kō-spō-rĭd"ē-ō'sĭs) [" + " + *osis,* condition]. Infestation with Sarcosporidia or condition produced by them.

sarcostosis (săr"kŏs-tō'sĭs) [" + *osteon,* bone, + *osis,* condition]. Ossification of fleshy or muscular tissue.

sarcostyle (săr′kō-stīl) [″ + *stylos,* a column]. Any one of the fine longitudinal fibrillae of a striated muscle fiber.

sarcotic (săr-kŏt′ĭk) [Gr. *sarx,* flesh]. 1. Producing or pert. to flesh formation. 2. Agent producing growth of flesh.

sarcotubules (săr″kō-tū′būlz). A continuous membranous tubule system present in striated muscle.

sarcous (săr′kŭs) [Gr. *sarkos,* flesh]. Concerning flesh or muscle.

sardonic laugh. Old term for a spasmodic affection of facial muscles that gives the appearance of laughter. SYN: *risus sardonicus.*

sartorius (săr-tō′rē-ŭs) [L. *sartor,* tailor]. A long, ribbon-shaped muscle of the thigh. The longest muscle in the body, it aids in flexing the knee. So called from its use in crossing the legs, as tailors do. SEE: *Muscles* in *Appendix.*

SAS-500. Trade name for sulfasalazine.

sat. *saturated.*

satellite (săt′l-īt) [L. *satelles,* attendant]. A small structure attached to a larger one, esp. a minute body attached to a chromosome by a slender chromatin filament.

s., bacterial. A bacterial colony that grows best when close to a colony of another microorganism.

satellite cells. 1. Flat epithelium-like cells forming the inner portion of a double-layered capsule which covers a neuron. 2. Neuroglial cells enclosing the cell bodies of neurons in spinal ganglia.

satellitosis (săt″l-ī-tō′sĭs) [″ + Gr. *osis,* condition]. The accumulation of satellite cells about neurons of the central nervous system, seen in certain degenerative and inflammatory conditions.

satiety (sā-tī′ĕt-ē) [L. *satietas,* sufficiency]. Being full to satisfaction, esp. with food.

saturated (săt′ū-rā″tĕd) [L. *saturatio*]. Holding all that can be absorbed, received, or combined, as a solution in which no more of a substance can be dissolved. Term is applied to hydrocarbons in which the maximum number of hydrogen atoms is present and there are no double or triple bonds between the carbon atoms.

saturated compound. An organic compound with all carbon bonds filled. It does not contain double or triple bonds. SEE: *unsaturated compound.*

saturated hydrocarbon. A carbon-hydrogen compound with all carbon bonds filled so there are no double or triple bonds. SEE: *polyunsaturated.*

saturated solution. Solution containing as much of the solid drug material as can be dissolved.

saturation (săt″ū-rā′shŭn). 1. State where all of a substance that can be is dissolved in a solution. Adding more of the substance will not increase the concentration. 2. In organic chemistry, to have all available carbon atom valences satisfied so that there are no double or triple bonds between the carbon atoms.

s., oxygen. The ratio of amount of oxygen present in a known volume of blood to amount of oxygen that could be carried by that volume of blood.

saturation index. In hematology, the amount of hemoglobin present in a known volume of blood compared to the normal.

saturation time. Time required for arterial blood of a person inhaling pure oxygen to become saturated.

Saturday night paralysis. Paralysis, occurring often in alcoholics, from lying immobile with arm pressed against a projecting surface so that the musculospiral nerve is compressed. SYN: *paralysis, musculospiral.*

saturnine (săt′ŭr-nīn) [L. *saturnus,* lead]. Concerning or produced by lead.

saturnine breath. Sweet breath produced by lead poisoning.

saturnine gout. Goutlike symptoms produced by lead poisoning.

saturnism (săt′ŭr-nĭzm) [″ + Gr. *-ismos,* condition]. Lead poisoning. SYN: *plumbism.*

satyriasis (săt-ī-rī′ă-sĭs) [LL.]. Excessive, and often uncontrollable, sexual drive in men. SEE: *nymphomania.*

satyromania (săt″ī-rō-mā′nē-ă). Satyriasis, q.v.

saucerization (saw″sĕr-ī-zā′shŭn). Surgical creation of a shallow area in tissue; or the production of such a depression due to trauma.

savory (sā′vō-rē) [O. Fr. *savoure,* tasty]. Having a pleasant or appetizing taste or odor.

saw [AS. *sagu*]. A cutting instrument with an edge of sharp toothlike projections; used esp. for cutting bone in surgery.

saxifragant (săks-ĭf′ră-gănt) [L. *saxum,* rock, + *frangere,* to break]. Dissolving or breaking calculi, esp. in the bladder.

saxitoxin (săk″sĭ-tŏk′sĭn). A toxin obtained from some forms of marine life, including mussels, clams, and plankton.

Sayre's jacket (sārz). [Lewis Albert Sayre, U.S. surgeon, 1820–1900] A jacket of plaster of Paris worn to support the spine in vertebral diseases.

Sb. Chem. symb. for antimony.

$SbCl_3$. Antimony trichloride.

Sb_2O_5. Antimonic oxide; antimony pentoxide.

Sb_4O_6. Antimonious oxide.

Sc. Chem. symb. for scandium.

s.c. *subcutaneously.*

scab (skăb) [ME. *scabbe*]. 1. Crust of a cutaneous sore, wound, ulcer, or pustule formed by drying up of the discharge. 2. To become covered with a crust.

scabicide (skā′bĭ-sīd). An agent that kills mites, esp. the causative agent of scabies.

scabies (skā′bē-ēz, -bēz) [L. *scabies,* itch]. A highly communicable skin disease caused by an arachnid, Sarcoptes scabiei, the itch mite. SEE: illus. SYN: *itch* (def. 2).

SYM: Papules, vesicles, pustules, burrows, and intense itching resulting in eczema. The impregnated females live in burrows that appear as slightly discolored lines several millimeters to several centimeters in length. Eggs deposited within the tunnel hatch within 4 to 8 days. Parts most commonly affected are hands, between fingers, wrists, axillae, genitalia, beneath the mammae, and inner aspect of the thighs.

PROG: Favorable.

TREATMENT: 1% gamma benzene hexachloride, 25% benzyl benzoate cream or lotion, or 10% crotamiton applied to the entire body, except the eyes, nose, and mouth, after the patient has taken a prolonged hot bath or shower. The affected areas are scrubbed thoroughly and then the medicine is applied. A second application is made the following morning.

s., Norwegian. A rare form of scabies in which the mites are present in great number.

scabietic (skā″bē-ĕt′ĭk) [L. *scabies,* itch]. Concerning scabies.

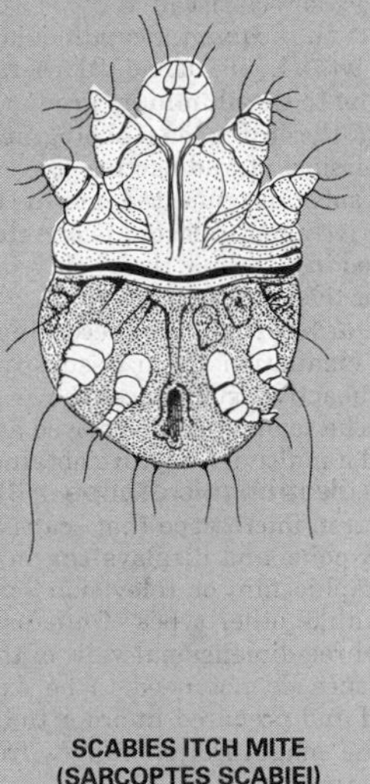

SCABIES ITCH MITE (SARCOPTES SCABIEI)

scabieticide (skā″bē-ĕt′ĭ-sīd) [″ + *cidus,* killing]. Scabicide.

scabiphobia (skă″bĭ-fō′bē-ă) [L. *scabies,* itch, + Gr. *phobos,* fear]. Abnormal fear of acquiring scabies.

scabrities (skā-brĭsh′ē-ēz) [L. *scaber,* rough]. 1. Scaly, roughened condition of the skin. 2. A morbid roughness of inner surface of eyelids causing sensation as if sand were in eyes.

s. unguium. Morbid degeneration of the nails making them rough, thick, distorted, and separated from the flesh at the root. Symptomatic of syphilis and leprosy.

scala (skā′lă) [L. *scalae,* stairs]. Any one of the three spiral passages of the cochlea.

s. media. The cochlear duct that lies between the scala tympani and scala vestibuli. Its floor contains the spiral organ of Corti. It extends from the saccule to the tip of the cochlea and is filled with endolymph.

s. tympani. The cochlear duct filled with perilymph lying below the spiral lamina. Extends from tip of the cochlea to the round cochlear window.

s. vestibuli. The cochlear duct forming the upper portion of the osseous canal. It lies above the spiral lamina and extends from the floor of the vestibule to the tip of the cochlea, where it communicates with the scala tympani through an aperture, the helicotrema.

scald (skōld) [LL. *excaldare,* wash in hot water]. 1. Burn to skin or flesh caused by moist heat and hot vapors, as steam. 2. To cause a burn with hot liquid or steam.

When the heat applied is approximately equivalent, a scald is deeper than a burn from dry heat and should be treated as a burn, q.v. Healing is slower and scar formation greater. Emergency treatment of a scalded area should be the immediate application of cold in the most readily available form, i.e., ice packs or immersion of the part in very cold water. This should be continued for at least an hour.

scalded skin syndrome. Necrosis of the epidermal layer of the skin with very little damage to underlying dermis. As much as 80% of the skin may be affected.

ETIOL: Staphylococcal infection.

TREATMENT: Appropriate antibiotic.

scale (skāl). 1. [O. Fr. *escale,* husk] A small, thin, dry exfoliation shed from upper layers of skin. Shedding of scales from skin in small amounts is normal. More shedding is seen in cutaneous disorders such as squamous eczema, seborrhea sicca, psoriasis, ichthyosis, syphilis, lupus erythematosus, pityriasis rosea, and tinea tonsurans. SEE: *macule; rash.* 2. Film of tartar encrusting the teeth. 3. To remove a film of tartar from the teeth. 4. To form a scale on. 5. To shed scales. 6. [ME. *scole,* balance] An instrument for weighing. 7. [L. *scala,* ladder] A graduated or proportioned measure, a series of tests, or an instrument for measuring quantities or for rating, e.g., individual intelligence.

s., absolute. A scale used for indicating low temperatures based on absolute zero. SEE: *absolute temperature; absolute zero.*

s., Baumé. Scale for indicating the specific gravity of liquids.

s., Celsius. SEE: *Celsius scale.*

s., centigrade. Celsius scale.

s., Fahrenheit. Scale in which the freezing point of water is 32° and the boiling point is 212°. SEE: *Fahrenheit scale; thermometer* for table.

s., French. SEE: *French scale.*

s., Kelvin. SEE: *Kelvin scale.*

s. of contrast. The range of densities on a radiograph, the number of tonal grays that are visible.

scalene (skā-lēn') [Gr. *skalenos,* uneven]. 1. Having unequal sides and angles, said of a triangle. 2. Designating a scalenus muscle.

s. tubercle. Tubercle on upper surface of the first rib, the insertion of the scalenus anticus muscle. SYN: *tubercle, Lisfranc's.*

scalenectomy (skā″lĕ-nĕk'tō-mē) [″ + *ektome,* excision]. Resection of any of the scalenus muscles.

scaleniotomy (skā-lēn″ē-ŏt'ō-mē) [″ + *tome,* incision]. Incision of scalenus muscles near their insertion to check expansive movements in tuberculosis of the apex of the lung.

scalenotomy (skā″lĕ-nŏt'ō-mē) [″ + *tome,* incision]. Surgical division of one or more of the scalenus muscles.

scalenus (skā-lē'nŭs) [L., uneven]. One of three deeply situated muscles on each side of the neck, extending from the tubercles of the transverse processes of the 3rd through 6th cervical vertebrae to the 1st or 2nd rib. Known as scalenus anterior (anticus), medius, and posterior. SEE: *Muscles* in *Appendix.*

scalenus syndrome. A symptom complex characterized by brachial neuritis with or without vascular or vasomotor disturbance in the upper extremities. Also called *scalenus anticus syndrome.*

SYM: Not clearly defined but pain, tingling, and numbness may occur anywhere from shoulder to fingers. Atrophy of small muscles of the hand or even the deltoid or other muscles of arm.

TREATMENT: Correction of posture, and sometimes immobilization of arm and shoulder. When relief is not obtained, surgical correction may be required.

scaler (skā'lĕr) [O. Fr. *escale,* husk]. 1. A dental instrument used in the procedure of removing calculus from the teeth. 2. A device for counting pulses detected by a radiation detector.

scaling (skāl'ĭng) [O. Fr. *escale,* husk]. Removal of calculus from teeth.

scall (skawl) [Norse *skalli,* baldhead]. Dermatitis of the scalp producing a crusted scabby eruption.

scalp (skălp) [ME.]. The hairy integument of the head. In anatomy, includes skin, dense subcutaneous tissue, occipitofrontalis muscle with the galea aponeurotica, loose subaponeurotic tissue, and the cranial periosteum.

scalpel (skăl'pĕl) [L. *scalpellum,* little knife]. A small, straight surgical knife with a convex edge and thin keen blade. SEE: illus.

scalpriform (skăl'prĭ-form) [L. *scalper,* knife, + *forma,* shape]. Shaped like a chisel.

scalprum (skăl'prŭm) [L.]. (pl. *scalpra*) 1. A toothed instrument for removal of carious bone or for trephining. 2. A large scalpel. 3. Cutting edge of an incisor tooth.

scalp tourniquet. Tourniquet applied to the scalp during I.V. administration of antineoplastic drugs to restrict blood flow to the hair-bearing portion of the scalp. This procedure is helpful in preventing the cranial alopecia that may accompany chemotherapy used in treating certain types of cancer.

scaly (skā'lē) [O. Fr. *escale,* husk]. Resembling or characterized by scales.

scan. Short for scintiscan, q.v.

scandium [L. *Scandia,* Scandinavia]. SYMB: Sc. At. wt. 44.956; at. no. 21. A rare metal belonging to the aluminum group.

scanning. Recording, on a photographic plate, the emission of radioactive waves from a specific substance injected into the body. The radioactive agent selected is one that is concentrated in a specific tissue such as thyroid, brain, or liver.

s., radioisotope. The recording of radioisotope emanations from tissues into which the radioactive substances have been injected. The scanner can be moved around the site and a multiview picture obtained.

scanning electron microscope. ABBR: SEM. An electron microscope that scans an image point-by-point and displays the image on a photographic film or television screen. The SEM, unlike other types of microscopes, allows a three-dimensional view of the tissues and tissues do not need to be extensively handled and prepared in order to be visualized. The magnification ranges from 20 to 100,000 times.

scanning speech. Pronunciation of words in syllables, or slowly and hesitatingly; a symptom of disseminated sclerosis, q.v. SEE:

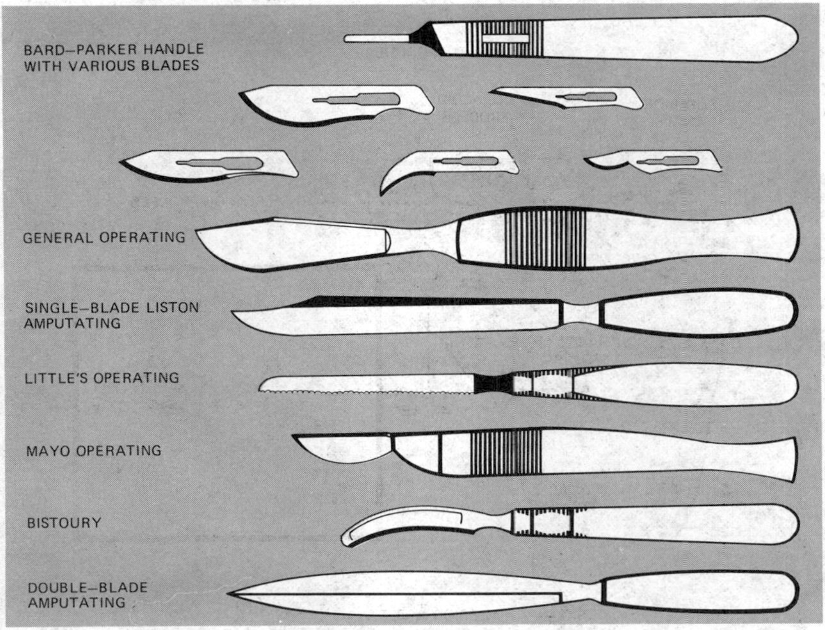

SCALPELS

speech.

scanty (skăn′tē) [ME. *skant,* short]. Not abundant; insufficient, as a secretion.

scapha (skā′fă) [L., skiff]. [NA] Elongated depression of the ear between the helix and anthelix. SYN: *scaphoid fossa.*

scapho- [Gr. *skaphe,* skiff]. Combining form meaning boat.

scaphocephalic (skăf″ō-sĕf-ăl′ĭk) [″ + *kephale,* head]. Having a deformed head, projecting like a boat's keel.

scaphocephalism (skăf″ō-sĕf′ăl-ĭzm) [″ + ″ + *-ismos,* condition]. Condition of having a deformed head, projecting like the keel of a boat.

scaphocephalous (skăf″ō-sĕf′ă-lŭs) [″ + *kephale,* head]. Scaphocephalic.

scaphocephaly (skăf″ō-sĕf′ă-lē) [″ + *kephale,* head]. Scaphocephalism.

scaphohydrocephaly (skăf″ō-hī″drō-sĕf′ă-lē) [″ + *hydor,* water, + *kephale,* head]. Hydrocephalus combined with scaphocephalism.

scaphoid (skăf′oyd) [Gr. *skaphe,* skiff, + *eidos,* resemblance]. 1. Boat-shaped, navicular, hollowed. 2. A proximal boat-shaped bone of the carpus or the tarsus. SYN: *os scaphoideum.*

scaphoid fossa. Scapha, q.v.

scaphoiditis (skăf″oyd-ī′tĭs) [″ + ″ + *itis,* inflammation]. Inflamed condition of the scaphoid bone.

scapula [L.]. (pl. *scapulae*) [NA] The large, flat, triangular bone that forms the posterior part of the shoulder. It articulates with the clavicle and the humerus. SYN: *shoulder blade.* SEE: illus.; *triceps.*

s., winged. Condition in which the medial border of the scapula is prominent, usually the result of paralysis of serratus anterior or trapezius muscles. SYN: *angel's wing.*

RS: acromial; acromial angle; acromioclavicular joint; acromiocoracoid; acromion; glenoid cavity.

scapulalgia (skăp-ū-lăl′jē-ă) [L. *scapula,* shoulder blade, + Gr. *algos,* pain]. Pain in the region of the shoulder blade.

scapular (skăp′ū-lăr). Of, or pert. to, the shoulder blade.

scapular reflex. Muscular contraction following percussion or stimulus between the scapulae.

scapulary (skăp′ū-lā-rē). A shoulder bandage for keeping a body bandage in place. A broad roller bandage is split in half. The undivided section of the roller bandage is fastened in front with the two ends passing over the shoulders and attached to the back of the body bandage.

SCAPULA

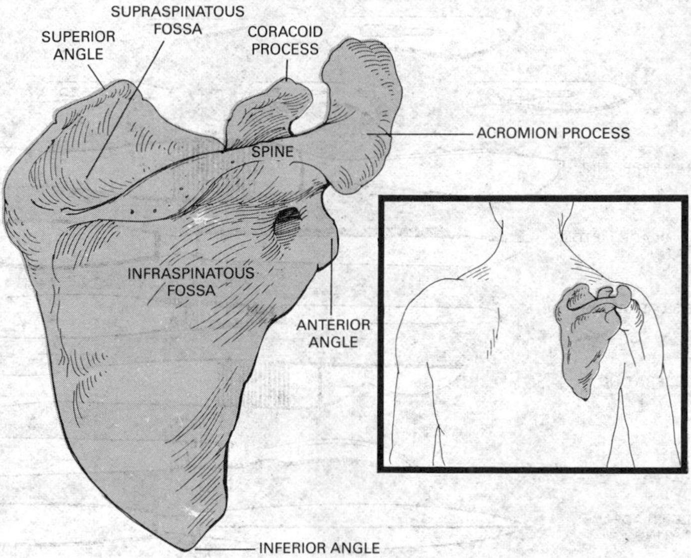

scapulectomy (skăp″ū-lĕk′tō-mē) [L. *scapula,* shoulder blade, + Gr. *ektome,* excision]. Surgical excision of the scapula.

scapulo- [L. *scapula,* shoulder blade]. Combining form meaning shoulder.

scapuloclavicular (skăp″ū-lō-klă-vĭk′ū-lar) [″ + *clavicula,* a little key]. Concerning the scapula and the clavicle.

scapulodynia (skăp″ū-lō-dĭn′ē-ă) [″ + *odyne,* pain]. Inflammation and pain in the shoulder muscles.

scapulohumeral (skăp″ū-lō-hū′mĕr-ăl) [″ + *humerus,* shoulder]. Concerning the scapula and the humerus.

scapulohumeral reflex. Reflex where the upper arm is adducted and rotated outward when vertebral border of scapula is percussed.

scapulopexy (skăp″ū-lō-pĕk′sē) [″ + Gr. *pexis,* fixation]. Fixation of the scapula to the ribs.

scapulothoracic (skăp″ū-lō-thō-răs′ĭk) [″ + Gr. *thorax,* chest]. Concerning the scapula and the thorax.

scapus (skā′pŭs) [L. *scapus,* stalk]. (pl. *scapi*) A shaft or stem.

s. penis. Shaft of penis.

s. pili. [NA] Major portion of a hair, esp. that section that extends beyond the outer scalp. SYN: *shaft, hair.* SEE: *hair.*

scar (skăr) [Gr. *eskhara,* scab caused by a burn]. Mark left in skin or internal organ by healing of a wound, sore, or injury because of replacement by connective tissue of the injured tissue. Scars may result from wounds that have healed, lesions of diseases, or surgical operations. When first developed a scar is red or purple, later whitish and glistening. SYN: *cicatrix.* SEE: *keloid.*

s., cicatricial. A scar or cicatrix with considerable contraction. It may be necessary to divide the scar and graft on new skin, as in burns.

s., keloid. A red, raised, smooth scar containing blood vessels, often irritable.

s., painful. Scar that is painful because of involvement of a nerve during healing. The end of the nerve may become bulbous.

TREATMENT: Dissection of scar or excision of nerve.

scarabiasis (skăr″ă-bī′ă-sĭs) [L. *scarabaeus,* scarab, + Gr. *-iasis,* condition]. Condition in which the intestine is invaded by the dung beetle. Occurs principally in children.

scarification (skăr″ĭ-fĭ-kā′shŭn) [Gr. *skariphismos,* scratching up]. Making of numerous superficial incisions in the skin.

scarificator (skăr′ĭf-ĭ-kā″tor) Instrument for making small incisions in the skin. SYN:

scarifier.

scarifier. Scarificator, q.v.

scarlatina (skăr″lă-tē′nă) [L.]. Scarlet fever.

s. anginosa. A severe form of scarlatina with extensive necrosis and ulceration of the pharynx, and in some cases peritonsillar abscess.

s. hemorrhagica Scarlatina with hemorrhage into the skin and mucous membranes.

s. maligna. A fulminant and usually lethal form of scarlatina.

scarlatinal (skăr″lă-tē′năl). Concerning or due to scarlatina.

scarlatinella (skăr-lăt″ĭ-nĕl′ă) [L.]. A mild disease resembling measles and scarlet fever.

scarlatiniform (skăr-lă-tĭn′ĭ-form) [L. *scarlatina,* scarlatina, + *forma,* shape, + Gr. *eidos,* form]. Resembling scarlatina or its rash.

scarlatinoid (skăr-lăt′ĭ-noyd) [″ + Gr. *eidos,* form]. Resembling scarlet fever.

scarlet fever [L. *scarlatum,* red]. An acute contagious disease characterized by sore throat, strawberry tongue, fever, punctiform scarlet rash, and rapid pulse. SYN: *scarlatina.*

ETIOL: Many strains (over 40) of Type A hemolytic, toxin-producing streptococci have been recovered from scarlet fever patients. The erythema-producing toxin was discovered by Dick and Dick (1924–1925). SEE: *Dick method.*

INCUBATION: Probably never less than 24 hr. May be 1 to 3 days, rarely longer.

SYM: Onset is sudden, rarely with a chill, but sometimes with a convulsion in very young children. As a rule, begins with sore throat, temperature from 101° to 105° F. (38.3° to 40.6° C.), frequent vomiting; followed within 12 to 36 hours by a rash, first on the neck and chest, rapidly extending over body, finally involving the extremities. Face is flushed and circumoral pallor may be present. The punctiform rash on the remainder of the body is seldom seen on face.

With first eruption, the throat is markedly injected, tonsils are swollen, tongue is heavily coated, and the papillae are enlarged, projecting through it; the tongue is described as a strawberry tongue. In the mild or average case, duration of rash is 2 to 3 days. By the end of the third day, the coating has disappeared from tongue though the papillae are still enlarged, the remainder of tongue presenting a deep red appearance. In this stage, the tongue may be referred to as the raspberry tongue.

With disappearance of the rash in an uncomplicated case, the temperature closely approaches normal and recovery is uneventful. Extremely mild cases occur in which the rash is very faint and of very short duration, possibly not exceeding 24 hours. Scarlet fever may actually occur without any rash whatsoever. In any form, a leukocytosis is to be expected in the average case. Number of leukocytes may range from 10,000 to 20,000 with 75 to 90% neutrophils.

SPECIFIC TREATMENT: Penicillin is the agent of choice. Penicillin should be given for a minimum of 10 days no matter how mild the infection in order to prevent the subsequent development of complications such as rheumatic fever and acute glomerulonephritis.

GENERAL TREATMENT: Isolation from time of diagnosis until one day after beginning antibiotic therapy. Patients with uncomplicated scarlet fever should be kept in bed during the acute phase of the illness.

scarlet rash. A rose-colored rash, specifically that of German measles, q.v.

scarlet red. An azo dye, of the color its name suggests. Used to stimulate healing of indolent ulcers, burns, wounds, etc., or in histology, as a stain. SYN: *rubrum scarlatinum.*

Scarpa's fascia (skăr′păs). [Antonio Scarpa, It. anatomist, 1747–1832]. Deep layer of superficial abdominal fascia around edge of the subcutaneous inguinal ring.

Scarpa's fluid. Fluid in membranous labyrinth of the ear. SYN: *endolymph.*

Scarpa's foramina. Bony passages opening into the incisor canal for passage of the nasopalatine nerves.

Scarpa's ganglion. The vestibular ganglion. SEE: *ganglion, vestibular.*

Scarpa's membrane. Membrane that closes the fenestra rotunda of the tympanic cavity.

Scarpa's triangle. Triangular space bounded laterally by the inner edge of the sartorius, above by Poupart's ligament, and medially by the adductor longus.

SCAT. *sheep cell agglutination test.*

scatacratia (skăt″ă-krā′shē-ă) [Gr. *skatos,* dung, + *akratia,* lack of control]. Fecal incontinence.

scatemia (skă-tē′mē-ă) [″ + *haima,* blood]. Toxemia from absorption of material present in the intestines.

scato- [Gr. *skatos,* dung]. Combining form denoting relationship to dung or fecal matter.

scatologic (skăt″ō-lŏj′ĭk). Concerning fecal matter.

scatology (skă-tŏl′ō-jē) [″ + *logos,* study]. 1. Scientific study and analysis of the feces. SYN: *coprology.* 2. Interest in obscene things, esp. literature.

scatoma (skă-tō′mă) [″ + *oma,* tumor]. Mass of inspissated feces in colon or rectum resembling an abdominal tumor. SYN: *fecaloma; stercoroma.*

scatophagy (skă-tŏf′ă-jē) [″ + *phagein,* to

eat]. The eating of excrement. SYN: *coprophagy; rhypophagy.*

scatoscopy (skă-tŏs′kō-pē) [″ + *skopein,* to examine]. Examination of excreta for diagnostic purposes.

scatter (skăt′ĕr). The diffusion of x-rays when they strike an object.

s., back-. The scattering of x-rays back to the source after they have been reflected by striking an object.

scattered radiation. X-rays that have changed direction because of a collision with matter.

scattergram (skăt′ĕr-grăm). Display of data on a chart so that each value is indicated by a symbol. The symbols are not connected by a line.

scavenger cell (skăv′ĕn-jer) [ME. *skawager,* toll collector]. A phagocytic cell, such as a macrophage or a neutrophil leukocyte, that functions in the removal of disintegrating tissues.

Sc.D. *Doctor of Science* (degree).

scent (sĕnt). An emanation from living or dead tissues, or materials that stimulate the olfactory sense.

Schafer's method of artificial respiration. [Sir Edward A. Sharpey-Schafer, Brit. physiologist, 1850–1935] A method of artificial respiration in which the subject lies prone with both arms extended forward, with one flexed so that hand rests under cheek and mouth. Operator kneels astride one or both thighs and places palms of hands on back over lower ribs. Operator rhythmically applies pressure with hands on the patient's back at a rate of 12 times per minute. This method, which is of little if any benefit, has been replaced by mouth-to-mouth breathing technique. SEE: *artificial respiration; cardiopulmonary resuscitation.*

Schäffer's reflex (shā′fĕrs). [Max Schäffer, Ger. neurologist, 1852–1923] Dorsiflexion of toes and flexion of foot resulting when middle portion of Achilles tendon is pinched.

Scheie's syndrome. [H. G. Scheie, U.S. physician, b. 1909] An inherited metabolic disease that becomes clinically apparent at about ten years of age. Stiff joints of the hands and feet, corneal clouding, generalized hypertrichosis, and valvular heart disease develop. The mouth is abnormally broad. Intelligence is slightly impaired or not affected. Patients may survive until the fifth decade of life. SYN: *mucopolysaccharidosis V.*

schema (skē′mă) [Gr., form, shape]. Shape, plan, or outline.

schematic (skē-măt′ĭk) [L. *schematicus,* planned]. Pert. to a diagram or model; showing part for part in a diagram.

scheroma (shē-rō′mă). A condition caused by lack of lacrimal fluid. SYN: *xerophthalmia.*

Schick test (shĭk). [Béla Schick, U.S. pediatrician, 1877–1967] Test to determine degree of immunity to diphtheria. Injection intradermally of 0.1 ml. of dilute diphtheria toxin, 1/50 MLD. (MLD: minimum lethal dose, the amount of diphtheria toxin that would kill a small guinea pig in four days.)

Results are obtained 3 to 4 days later. Susceptibility (positive test) is indicated by the development of a red inflamed area at point of injection, which slowly disappears after a few days. A negative test (little or no reaction) indicates the presence of antibodies sufficient to neutralize the toxin; hence the person is immune. SEE: *diphtheria.*

Schick test control. USP. Inactivated diphtheria toxin for Schick test. It is used in the Schick test as a control.

Schilder's disease (shĭl′dĕrs). [Paul Ferdinand Schilder, Austrian-U.S. neurologist, 1886–1940] A rare but invariably fatal disease of the central nervous system characterized by adrenal atrophy and diffuse cerebral demyelination. This leads to mental deterioration and blindness. SYN: *adrenoleukodystrophy.*

Schiller's test (shĭl′ĕrs). [Walter Schiller, Austrian-U.S. pathologist, b. 1887] Test for superficial cancer, esp. of the cervix uteri. The tissue is painted with solution of iodine. Cancer cells not containing glycogen fail to stain, thus revealing their presence.

Schilling's classification. [Victor Schilling, Ger. hematologist, 1883–1960] Method of classifying polymorphonuclear neutrophils into four categories according to number and arrangement of the nuclei in the cells.

Schilling test. [Robert F. Schilling, U.S. hematologist, b. 1919] A test, utilizing radioactive vitamin B_{12}, for gastrointestinal absorption of vitamin B_{12}. For diagnosis of primary pernicious anemia.

schindylesis (skĭn″dĭ-lē′sĭs) [Gr. *schindylesis,* a splintering]. A form of wedge and groove suture in which a crest of one bone fits into a groove of another.

Schirmer's test. Use of a piece of absorbent paper placed so that it hangs out of the conjunctival sac. The rate and amount of wetting of the paper provide an estimate of tear production.

schisto- (skĭs′tō) [Gr. *schistos,* split]. Combining form meaning split or cleft.

schistocelia (skĭs″tō-sē′lē-ă) [″ + *koilia,* belly]. Congenital abdominal fissure.

schistocephalus (skĭs″tō-sĕf′ă-lŭs) [″ + *kephale,* head]. Fetus with a cleft head.

schistocormia (skĭs″tō-kor′mē-ă) [″ + *kormos,* trunk]. Fetus with a cleft trunk.

schistocystis (skĭs″tō-sĭs′tĭs) [″ + *kystis,* bladder]. Fissure of the bladder.

schistocyte (skĭs′tō-sīt) [″ + *kytos,* a cell]. A fragmented segment of a red blood cell. Seen in patients with hemolytic anemia.

schistocytosis (skĭs″tō-sī-tō′sĭs) [″ + ″ + *osis,* condition]. Schistocytes in the blood.

schistoglossia (skĭs″tō-glŏs′ē-ă) [Gr. *schistos,* split, + *glossa,* tongue]. A cleft tongue.

schistomelus (skĭs-tŏm′ĕ-lŭs) [″ + *melos,* limb]. Fetus with a cleft in a limb.

schistoprosopia (skĭs″tō-prō-sō′pē-ă) [″ + *prosopon,* face]. Congenital fissure of the face.

schistorrhachis (skĭs-tor′ă-kĭs) [″ + *rhachis,* spine]. Protrusion of membranes through a congenital cleft in the lower vertebral column. SYN: *spina bifida.*

Schistosoma (skĭs″tō-sō′mă) [″ + *soma,* body]. A genus of blood flukes belonging to the family Schistosomatidae, class Trematoda. Adults live in blood vessels of visceral organs. Eggs make their way into the bladder or intestine and are discharged in urine or feces. Eggs hatch into miracidia, which enter snails and transform into sporocysts. These develop daughter sporocysts, which give rise to fork-tailed cercaria. These leave the snail and enter the final host directly through the skin or through mucous membrane.

S. haematobium. A species common in Africa and southwestern Asia. Adults infest pelvic veins of vesicle plexus. Eggs work their way through the bladder wall and are discharged through urine. Cause of urinary schistosomiasis.

S. japonicum. A species common in many parts of the Orient. Adults live principally in branches of the superior mesenteric vein. Eggs work their way through the intestinal wall into the lumen and are discharged with feces. Cause of Oriental schistosomiasis.

S. mansoni. A species occurring in many parts of Africa and tropical America, including the West Indies. Adults live in branches of the inferior mesenteric veins. Eggs discharged through either the intestine or bladder. Cause of bilharzial dysentery or Manson's intestinal schistosomiasis.

schistosome dermatitis (skĭs′tō-sōm). Dermatitis resulting from penetration of skin of humans by cercariae of non–human blood flukes. Common in lake region of northern U.S. It is not associated with visceral schistosomiasis. SYN: *seabather's eruption; swimmer's itch.*

schistosomia (skĭs″tō-sō′mē-ă) [″ + *soma,* body]. Deformed fetus with a fissure in the abdomen; the limbs are rudimentary if present.

schistosomiasis (skĭs″tō-sō-mī′ăs-ĭs) [Gr. *schistos,* split, + *soma,* body, + *-iasis,* infection]. A parasitic disease due to infestation with blood flukes belonging to the genus Schistosoma, q.v. The disease is endemic throughout Asia, Africa, and tropical America. Infestation occurs by wading or bathing in water containing cercariae that have issued from snails. SYN: *bilharziasis.*

schistosomicide (skĭs″tō-sō′mĭ-sīd) [″ + ″ + L. *cidus,* killing]. Something that destroys schistosomes.

schistosternia (skĭs″tō-stĕr′nē-ă) [″ + *sternon,* sternum]. Schistothorax.

schistothorax (skĭs″tō-thō′răks) [″ + *thorax,* chest]. Fissure of the thorax.

schistotrachelus (skĭs″tō-tra-kē′lŭs). Fetus with a cleft in the neck.

schizamnion (skĭz-ăm′nē-ŏn) [Gr. *schizein,* to divide + *amnion,* lamb]. An amnion formed by development of a cavity in the inner cell mass.

schizaxon (skĭz-ăk′sŏn) [″ + *axon,* axle]. An axon that divides in two equal, or nearly equal, branches.

schizencephaly (skĭz″ĕn-sĕf′ă-lē) [″ + *enkephalos,* brain]. Deformed fetus with a longitudinal cleft in the skull.

schizo- (skĭz′ō) [Gr. *schizein,* to divide]. Combining form indicating division.

schizoblepharia (skĭz″ō-blĕf′ă-rē″ă) [″ + *blepharon,* eyelid]. Fissure of an eyelid.

schizocyte (skĭz′ō-sīt) [″ + *kytos,* cell]. Schistocyte.

schizocytosis (skĭz″ō-sī-tō′sĭs) [″ + ″ + *osis,* condition]. Schistocytosis.

schizogenesis (skĭz″ō-jĕn′ĕs-ĭs) [Gr. *schizein,* to divide, + *genesis,* production]. Reproduction by fission.

schizogony (skĭz-ŏg′ō-nē) [″ + *gone,* seed]. Reproduction by multiple asexual fission characteristic of sporozoans, esp. the lifecycle of the malarial parasite.

schizogyria (skĭz″ō-jī′rē-ă) [″ + *gyros,* a circle]. A cleft in the cerebral convolutions.

schizoid (skĭz′oyd) [Gr. *schizein,* to split, + *eidos,* resemblance]. Resembling schizophrenia.

schizoid personality. The type of person characterized by seclusiveness, inability to develop close emotional attachments to others, reduced initiative, morbid introspection, and oftentimes queer behavior. The so-called shut-in type.

schizomycete (skĭz″ō-mī-sēt) [″ + *mykes,* fungus]. Any organism belonging to the class Schizomycetes.

Schizomycetes (skĭz″ō-mī-sē′tēz) [″ + *mykes,* fungus]. Class of plant microorganisms or fungi that multiplies by fission. Includes the bacteria.

schizont (skĭz′ŏnt) [″ + *ontos,* being]. 1. A stage appearing in the life cycle of a sporozoan protozoon resulting from multiple division or schizogony. 2. Stage in asexual phase of life cycle of Plasmodium found in red blood cells. By schizogony, each gives rise to from 12 to 24 or more merozoites. An early schizont is called a presegmenter; a mature schizont is called a rosette or segmenter.

schizonticide (skĭ-zŏn'tĭ-sīd) [" + " + L. *cidus,* killing]. Something that destroys schizonts.

schizonychia (skĭz"ō-nĭk'ē-ă) [Gr. *schizein,* to split, + *onyx,* nail]. Split condition of the nails.

schizophasia (skĭz"ō-fā'zē-ă) [" + *phasis,* speech]. Muttered and incomprehensible speech of the schizophrenic.

schizophrenia (schizophrenic disorders). A less than well understood group of mental disorders that include psychotic features. The disorders usually represent a deterioration from a previous level of function and the onset is prior to age 45. The disorders are not due to affective disorders or organic mental disorder. At some time during the course of the disorders, a patient will have delusions, hallucinations, or thought disturbances. These individuals are usually impaired in daily functions such as work, social relations, and personal care. Treatment includes pharmacologic and psychiatric.

s., catatonic. A schizophrenic disorder dominated by any of the following: catatonic stupor or mutism; catatonic negativism; catatonic rigidity; catatonic excitement; catatonic posturing. The patients need careful attention to prevent hurting themselves or others, and to treat malnutrition, exhaustion, hyperpyrexia, or injury.

s., paranoid. A type of schizophrenic disorder wherein there are delusions of persecution, grandiosity, jealousy, or hallucinations with persecutory or grandiose content.

s., undifferentiated. A type of schizophrenic disorder characterized by delusions, incoherence, or grossly disorganized behavior; and that does not meet the criteria for some other type of schizophrenic disorder.

schizophrenic (skĭz"ō-frĕn'ĭk) [Gr. *schizein,* to split, + *phren,* mind]. Afflicted with, or person afflicted with, schizophrenia.

schizoprosopia (skĭz"ō-prō-sō'pē-ă) [" + *prosopon,* face]. Fissure of the face, such as harelip or cleft palate.

schizotonia (skĭz"ō-tō'nē-ă) [" + *tonos,* tension]. Uneven tone of muscle groups.

schizotrichia (skĭz"ō-trĭk'ē-ă) [" + *thrix,* hair]. Splitting of the tips of the hair.

schizozoite (skĭz"ō-zō'īt) [" + *zoon,* animal]. Merozoite.

Schlatter-Osgood disease (shlăt'ĕr-ŏz'good). Osgood-Schlatter disease, q.v.

Schlemm, canal of (shlĕm). [Friedrich S. Schlemm, Ger. anatomist, 1795–1858] Irregular space or spaces in the sclerocorneal region of the eye. It receives the aqueous humor from the anterior chamber of the eye.

Schmorl's disease. [Christian G. Schmorl, Ger. pathologist, 1861–1932] Herniation of the nucleus pulposus.

Schmorl's nodules. Schmorl's disease, q.v.

schneiderian membrane (shnī-dē'rē-ăn). [Conrad Victor Schneider, Ger. physician, 1610–1680] The nasal mucosa.

Schönlein's disease (shān'līnz). [Johann Lukas Schönlein, Ger. physician, 1793–1864] An allergic or anaphylactic purpura occurring in individuals, esp. children, with drug sensitivities, serum sickness, and other allergic disorders. It is usually accompanied by pains in joints and abdomen. SYN: *purpura, idiopathic thrombocytopenic.*

Schönlein-Henoch purpura. SEE: *Henoch-Schönlein purpura.*

Schüffner's dots (shĭf'nĕrz). [Wilhelm P. A. Schüffner, Ger. pathologist, 1867–1949] Minute granules present in red blood cells infected by Plasmodium vivax.

Schüller's disease. SEE: *Hand-Schüller-Christian disease.*

Schultz reaction. [Werner Schultz, Ger. physician, 1878–1947] A test that demonstrates the ability of muscle tissues from an animal that has been made anaphylactic to contract when re-exposed to the antigen. Either guinea pig uterine muscles or intestines are used. The test is very specific, as unrelated antigens will not cause the sensitized muscle to contract. Sir Henry Dale demonstrated the same phenomenon independent of Schultz's work. SYN: *Dale reaction.*

Schultze's bundle (shooltz'ĕs). [Max Johann Schultze, Ger. biologist, 1825–1874] Longitudinal mass of descending fibers, shaped like a comma, in the fasciculus cuneatus of spinal cord.

Schultze's cells. Olfactory cells.

Schultze's granule masses. Fine, granular masses formed by breaking up of plaques in the blood.

Schwabach test (shvă'băk). [Dagobert Schwabach, Ger. otologist, 1846–1920] A test for hearing using five tuning forks, each of a different tone.

Schwalbe's ring (shvăl'bĕz). [Gustav A. Schwalbe, Ger. anatomist, 1844–1917] The peripheral edge of Descemet's membrane of the eye. Also: *Schwalbe's line.*

Schwann's cells (shvŏnz). [Theodor Schwann, Ger. anatomist, 1810–1882] Cells of ectodermal origin that comprise the neurilemma.

schwannoma (shwŏn-nō'mă). A benign tumor of the neurilemma or sheath of Schwann of a nerve.

schwannosis (shwŏn-nō'sĭs). Hypertrophy of the sheath of Schwann of a nerve.

Schwann's sheath. The neurilemma of a nerve fiber. SYN: *neurilemma.*

Schwann's white substance. Myelin of a medullated nerve fiber.

sciage (sē-ăzh′) [Fr., a sawing]. A movement of the hand in massage resembling that in sawing.

sciatic (sī-ăt′ĭk) [L. *sciaticus*]. 1. Pert. to the hip or ischium. 2. Pert. to, due to, or afflicted with sciatica, q.v. SYN: *ischiac; ischiatic.*

sciatica (sī-ăt′ĭ-kă) [L.]. Severe pain in the leg along the course of the sciatic nerve felt at back of thigh running down the inside of the leg. SEE: *meralgia; sciatic nerve.*

ETIOL: 1. Compression or trauma of the sciatic nerve or its roots, esp. that resulting from ruptured intervertebral disk or osteoarthrosis of lumbosacral vertebrae. 2. Inflammation of sciatic nerve resulting from metabolic, toxic, or infectious disorders. 3. Pain referred to sciatic nerve from other parts of body.

SYM: May begin abruptly or gradually and is characterized by a sharp shooting pain running down back of thigh. Movement of limb generally intensifies the suffering. Pain may be uniformly distributed along the limb, but frequently there are certain spots where it is more intense; numbness, tingling; nerve may be extremely sensitive to touch. Symptoms grow worse at night and on approach of stormy weather. Duration of attack varies from few days to several months. In long-standing cases, muscles grow atrophied and rigid.

PROG: Recovery follows in majority of cases when treatment is instituted early and is carried out persistently.

TREATMENT: Surgical intervention if due to ruptured intervertebral disk. In acute stage, rest is essential. Hot dressings may alleviate pain to some extent. Morphine or meperidine may be required to control pain, but the danger of habituation must be kept in mind. In arthritic patients, full doses of salicylates are useful. In chronically ill patients, prolonged rest. Improve general health; good, nourishing diet; hot applications often help to provide relief. Some patients are relieved by spraying ethyl chloride over course of the nerve, nerve stretching by pulling the affected leg, or a lift in the shoe of the affected limb.

sciatic nerve. Largest nerve in the body, arising from the sacral plexus on either side, passing from the pelvis through the greater sciatic foramen, down the back of the thigh, where it divides into tibial and peroneal nerves. Lesions cause paralysis of flexion and extension of toes; abduction and adduction of toes; rotation inward and adduction of foot; plantar flexion and lowering of ball of foot; anesthesia in cutaneous distribution (external popliteal nerve); paralysis of dorsiflexion and adduction of foot; rotation of ball of foot outward and of raising external border of foot and of extension of toes; also anesthesia in cutaneous distribution. SEE: *Nerves* in *Appendix.*

sciatic nerve, small. The posterior femoral cutaneous nerve, a cutaneous nerve supplying skin of buttocks, perineum, popliteal region, and back of thigh and leg.

scieropia (sī-ĕr-ō′pē-ă) [Gr. *skieros,* shadow, + *opsis,* vision]. Abnormal vision in which things appear to be in a shadow.

scintigram (sĭn′tĭ-grăm). The record produced by a scintiscan, q.v.

scintillascope (sĭn-tĭl′ă-skōp) [L. *scintilla,* spark, + Gr. *skopein,* to examine]. Device for viewing the effect of ionizing radiation, alpha particles, on a fluorescent screen.

scintillation (sĭn″tĭ-lā′shŭn) [L. *scintillatio*]. 1. Sparkling; a subjective sensation, as of seeing sparks. 2. The emissions that come from radioactive substances

scintiphotography (sĭn″tĭ-fō-tŏg′ră-fē). Photographing the scintillations emitted by radioactive substances injected into the body. Used to determine the outline and function of organs and tissues in which the radioactive substance collects or is secreted.

scintiscan (sĭn′tĭ-skăn). Use of scintiphotography to produce a map of scintillations produced when a radioactive substance is introduced into the body. The intensity of the record indicates the differential accumulation of a substance in the various parts of the body.

scintiscanner (sĭn″tĭ-skăn′ĕr). The device used in doing a scintiscan.

scirrho- [Gr. *skirrhos,* hard]. Combining form meaning hard, or indicating relationship to a hard tumor or scirrhus.

scirrhoid (skĭr′oyd) [″ + *edios,* form]. Pert. to, or like, a hard carcinoma or scirrhus.

scirrhoma (skĭr-ō′mă) [″ + *oma,* tumor]. A hard carcinoma or scirrhus.

scirrhosarca (skĭr″ō-săr′kă) [″ + *sarx,* flesh]. Hardening of the flesh, esp. of the newly born. SYN: *sclerema neonatorum.*

scirrhous (skĭr′rŭs) [L. *skirrhosus*]. Hard, like a scirrhus.

scirrhus (skĭr′ŭs) [Gr. *skirrhos*]. A hard, cancerous tumor due to overgrowth of fibrous tissue.

scission (sĭzh′ŭn) [L. *scindere,* to split]. Dividing, cutting, or splitting.

scissor gait. Crossing the legs in walking. SEE: *gait.*

scissor leg. Abnormal tendency of the legs to cross due to contraction of thigh adductor muscles.

scissors (sĭz′ors) [LL. *cisorium*]. A cutting instrument composed of two opposed cutting blades with handles, held together by a central pin. This allows the cutting edge to be opened and closed.

scissura (sĭ-sū′ră) [L.]. (pl. *scissurae*) A fissure or cleft; a splitting.

sclera (sklē′ră) [Gr. *skleros*, hard]. (pl. *sclerae*) [NA] A tough white fibrous tissue that covers the so-called white of the eye. It extends from the optic nerve to the cornea. SYN: *sclerotica*.

s., blue. Abnormal degree of blueness of the sclera. This may be a sign of osteogenesis imperfecta.

scleradenitis (sklē″răd-ĕn-ī′tĭs) [″ + *aden*, gland, + *itis*, inflammation]. Inflammation and induration of a gland.

scleral (sklē′răl) [Gr. *skleros*, hard]. Concerning the sclera.

scleratogenous (sklē″ră-tŏj′ĕ-nŭs). Sclerogenous, q.v.

sclerectasia (sklē″rĕk-tā′zē-ă) [″ + *ektasis*, dilatation]. Protrusion of the sclera.

sclerectoiridectomy (sklĕ-rĕk″tō-ĭr″ĭ-dĕk′tō-mē) [″ + *iris*, iris, + *ektome*, excision]. Formation of a filtering cicatrix in glaucoma by combined sclerectomy and iridectomy.

sclerectoiridodialysis (sklĕ-rĕk″tō-ĭr″ĭd-ō-dī-ăl′ĭ-sĭs) [″ + ″ + *dialysis*, a loosening]. Sclerectomy and iridodialysis for relief of glaucoma.

sclerectomy (sklĕ-rĕk′tō-mē) [″ + *ektome*, excision]. 1. Excision of a portion of the sclera. 2. Removal of adhesions in chronic otitis media.

scleredema (sklē″rĕ-dē′mă) [″ + *oidema*, a swelling]. A condition usually following an acute infection characterized by edema and induration of the skin. It is a benign self-limited disease occurring more frequently in females than males. It is often confused with scleroderma, q.v.

s. adultorum. S., Buschke's, q.v.

s., Buschke's. Generalized non-pitting edema that begins on the head or neck and spreads to the body. This lasts a year or less and leaves no sequelae. The cause is unknown.

s. neonatorum. Sclerema, q.v.

sclerema (sklē-rē′mă) [Gr. *skleros*, hard]. Hardening of the skin. SYN: *scleroderma*.

s. adiposum. S. neonatorum.

s. adultorum. Scleroderma.

s. neonatorum. Progressive hardening of the skin in the newborn; usually fatal.

sclerencephalia (sklē″rĕn-sĕ-fā′lē-ă) [″ + *enkephalos*, brain]. Sclerosis of the brain.

scleriasis (sklē-rī′ă-sĭs) [Gr. *skleriasis*]. 1. Progressive hardening of the skin. 2. Hardening of the eyelid.

scleriritomy (sklē″rĭ-rĭt′ō-mē) [″ + *iris*, iris, + *tome*, incision]. Incision of the iris and sclera.

scleritis (sklē-rī′tĭs) [″ + *itis*, inflammation]. Superficial and deep inflammation of the sclera. SYN: *sclerotitis*. SEE: *episcleritis*.

s., annular. Inflammation limited to the area surrounding the limbus of the cornea. A complete ring is formed.

s., anterior. Scleritis of the area adjacent to the limbus of the cornea.

s., posterior. Scleritis limited to the posterior half of the globe of the eye.

scleroblastema (sklē″rō-blăs-tē′mă) [Gr. *skleros*, hard, + *blastema*, a sprout]. The embryonic tissue from which formation of bone takes place.

scleroblastemic (sklē″rō-blăs-tĕm′ĭk). Rel. to or derived from scleroblastema.

sclerocataracta (sklē″rō-kăt-ă-răk′tă) [″ + *katarraktes*, a pouring down]. A hard cataract.

sclerochoroiditis (sklē″rō-kō″royd-ī′tĭs) [″ + *chorioeides*, skinlike, + *itis*, inflammation]. Inflammation of the sclera and choroid coat of the eye.

s., posterior. Myopic choroiditis, posterior staphyloma.

scleroconjunctival (sklē″rō-kŏn″jŭnk-tī′văl) [″ + L. *conjunctivus*, to bind together]. Pertaining to the sclera and conjunctiva.

sclerocornea (sklē′rō-kor′nē-ă) [″ + L. *cornu*, a horn]. The sclera and cornea together considered as one coat.

sclerodactylia (sklē″rō-dăk-tĭl′ē-ă) [″ + *daktylos*, a finger]. Induration of the skin of the fingers and toes. SYN: *acroscleroderma*.

scleroderma (sklē″rō-dĕr′mă) [Gr. *skleros*, hard, + *derma*, skin]. A chronic disease of unknown etiology that occurs four times as frequently in women as in men. It causes sclerosis of the skin and certain organs including the gastrointestinal tract, lungs, heart, and kidneys. The skin is taut, firm, and edematous and is firmly bound to subcutaneous tissue; it feels tough and leathery, may itch, and later becomes hyperpigmented. The skin changes usually, but not always, precede the development of signs of visceral involvement. For a limited period the only findings may be the CREST syndrome: calcinosis, Raynaud's phenomenon, esophageal dysfunction, sclerodactyly, and telangiectasia. SYN: *progressive systemic sclerosis*. SEE: *collagen diseases*.

PROG: Variable and unpredictable with respect to rate of pathological changes. Progress is worse in white males than in white females and is worse in black females than in black males. When the onset of the disease is later in life the prognosis is poor.

TREATMENT: There is no specific therapy. General supportive therapy is indicated. A great number of drugs including corticosteroids, vasodilators, D-penicillamine, and immunosuppressive agents have been tried. Physical therapy will help in maintaining muscular strength but will not influence the course of joint disease.

s., circumscribed. Localized patches of linear sclerosis of the skin. There is no systemic involvement and the course of the disease is usually benign.

s. neonatorum. Hardness and tightness of the skin in early infancy. SYN: *sclerema neonatorum.*

sclerodermatitis (sklē"rō-dĕr-mă-tī'tĭs) [Gr. *skleros,* hard, + *derma,* skin, + *itis,* inflammation]. Inflammation of the skin accompanied by thickening and hardening.

sclerodermatous (sklē"rō-dĕr'mă-tŭs) [" + *derma,* skin]. Concerning scleroderma.

sclerogenic (sklē"rō-jĕn'ĭk) [" + *gennan,* to produce]. Sclerogenous, q.v.

sclerogenous (sklē-rŏj'ĕ-nŭs) [" + *gennan,* to produce]. Causing sclerosis or hardening of tissue.

scleroid (sklē'rŏyd) [" + *eidos,* form]. Having a hard or firm texture.

scleroiritis (sklē"rō-ī-rī'tĭs) [" + *iris,* iris, + *itis,* inflammation]. Inflammation of both the sclera and iris.

sclerokeratitis (sklē"rō-kĕr-ă-tī'tĭs) [" + *keras,* horn, + *itis,* inflammation]. Cellular infiltration with inflammation of the sclera and cornea.

sclerokeratoiritis (sklē"rō-kĕr"ă-tō-ī-rī'tĭs) [" + " + *iris,* iris, + *itis,* inflammation]. Inflamed condition of the sclera, cornea, and iris.

sclerokeratosis (sklē"rō-kĕr"ă-tō'sĭs) [" + " + *osis,* condition]. Sclerokeratitis.

scleroma (sklē-rō'mă) [Gr. *skleroma,* induration]. Indurated, circumscribed area of granulation tissue in mucous membrane or skin. SEE: *sclerosis.*

scleromalacia (sklē"rō-mă-lā'sē-ă) [Gr. *skleros,* hard, + *malakia,* a softening]. Softening of the sclera.

s. perforans. Scleromalacia accompanied by perforation.

scleromere (sklē'rō-mēr) [" + *meros,* a part]. 1. Any segment or metamere of the skeleton. 2. The caudal half of a sclerotome, q.v.

scleromyxedema (sklē"rō-mĭk"sē-dē'mă) [" + *myxa,* mucus, + *oidema,* swelling]. A type of lichen myxedematosis wherein the skin under the papules is greatly thickened.

scleronychia (sklē"rō-nĭk'ē-ă) [" + *onyx,* nail]. Thickening and hardening of the nails.

scleronyxis (sklē-rō-nĭk'sĭs) [Gr. *skleros,* hard, + *nyxis,* a piercing]. Surgical puncture of the sclera.

sclero-oophoritis (sklē"rō-ō-ŏf"ō-rī'tĭs) [" + *oon,* egg, + *phoros,* a bearer, + *itis,* inflammation]. Induration and inflammation of the ovary.

sclerophthalmia (sklē"rŏf-thăl'mē-ă) [" + *ophthalmos,* eye]. Congenital condition in which opacity of the sclera advances over the cornea.

scleroplasty (sklē'rō-plăs"tē) [" + *plassein,* to form]. Plastic surgery of the sclera.

scleroprotein (sklē"rō-prō'tē-ĭn) [" + *protos,* first]. A group of proteins noted for their insolubility in most chemicals. Found in skeletal tissue, cartilage, hair, nails, and in animal claws and horns.

sclerosal (sklē-rō'săl). Sclerous.

sclerosant (sklē-rō'sănt) [Gr. *skleros,* hard]. Something that produces sclerosis.

sclerose (sklē-rōs') [Gr. *skleros,* hard]. To become hardened.

sclerosed (sklē-rōsd', sklē'rōsd) [Gr. *skleros,* hard]. Having sclerosis; hardened. SYN: *indurated.*

sclerosing (sklē-rōs'ĭng). Causing or developing sclerosis.

sclerosis (sklē-rō'sĭs) [Gr. *sklerosis,* a hardening]. 1. A hardening or induration of an organ or tissue, esp. that due to excessive growth of fibrous tissue. 2. Hardening within the nervous system, esp. of the brain and spinal cord, resulting from degeneration of nervous elements, as the myelin sheath. SYN: *cerebrosclerosis.* 3. Thickening and hardening of the layers in the wall of an artery. SEE: *arteriosclerosis; atherosclerosis.*

RS: cerebrosclerosis; Charcot-Marie-Tooth disease; scleritis.

s., Alzheimer's. Hyaline degeneration affecting small blood vessels of the brain.

s., amyotrophic lateral. Progressive muscular atrophy resulting from disease conditions, degenerative in nature, involving anterior horn cells and the pyramidal tracts. It is rapidly progressive, usually ending in bulbar paralysis.

s., annular. Sclerosis in which hardened substance forms a band about the spinal cord.

s., arterial. Hardening of the coats of the arteries. SYN: *arteriosclerosis.*

s., arteriolar. Sclerosis of arterioles.

s., diffuse. Sclerosis affecting large areas of the brain and spinal cord.

s., disseminated. S., multiple.

s., hyperplastic. S., medial.

s., insular. S., multiple.

s., intimal. Atherosclerosis.

s., lateral. Sclerosis of the lateral column of the spinal cord. SEE: *s., amyotrophic lateral.*

s., lobar. Sclerosis of the cerebrum resulting in mental disturbances.

s., medial. Sclerosis involving the tunica media of arteries, usually the result of involutional changes accompanying aging. SYN: *s., hyperplastic.*

s., multiple. A chronic, slowly progressive disease of the central nervous system characterized by development of disseminated demyelinated glial patches called plaques. Symptoms and signs are numerous, but common early symptoms include paresthesias and visual disturbances and, in later stages, those of Charcot's triad (nystagmus, scanning speech, and intention tremor) are common. Occurs in the form of many clinical syndromes, the most common being the cerebral, brain stem-cerebellar, and spinal. A history of remissions and exacerbations is diagnostic. Etiological factors are unknown and there is no specific therapy. SYN: *s., disseminated.*

s., neural. Sclerosis with chronic inflammation of a nerve trunk with branches.

s., renal. Nephrosclerosis.

s., tuberous. SEE: *tuberous sclerosis.*

s., vascular. Sclerosis of the walls of blood vessels; arterial and venous sclerosis.

s., venous. Phlebosclerosis.

scleroskeleton (sklē″rō-skĕl′ĕ-tŏn) [Gr. *skleros,* hard, + *skeleton,* skeleton]. Skeletal changes resulting from ossification of fibrous structures, such as ligaments, fasciae, and tendons.

sclerostenosis (sklē″rō-stĕ-nō′sĭs) [″ + *stenosis,* a narrowing]. Contraction and induration of tissues, esp. those about an orifice.

s. cutanea. Induration of the skin. SYN: *scleroderma.*

sclerostomy (sklē-rŏs′tō-mē) [″ + *stoma,* an opening]. Surgical formation of an opening in the sclera.

sclerotherapy (sklē″rō-thĕr′ă-pē) [″ + *therapeia,* treatment]. Use of sclerosing agents in treating diseases, esp. hemorrhoids.

sclerothrix (sklē′rō-thrĭks) [″ + *thrix,* hair]. Brittleness of the hair.

sclerotic (sklē-rŏt′ĭk) [L. *scleroticus,* hard]. Pert. to or affected with sclerosis.

sclerotica (sklē-rŏt′ĭ-kă) [L. *scleroticus,* hard]. The exterior white coat of the eye. SYN: *sclera.*

sclerotic acid. An amorphous, brown powder from ergot. A hemostatic and oxytocic.

sclerotic dentin. Areas of dentin where the tubules have been filled by mineralization producing a more dense, radiopaque dentin; it is often produced in response to caries, attrition, and abrasion.

scleroticectomy (sklē-rŏt″ĭ-sĕk′tō-mē) [″ + Gr. *ektome,* excision]. Excision of a part of the sclera. SYN: *sclerectomy.*

scleroticochoroiditis (sklē-rŏt″ĭ-kō-kō″roy-dī′tĭs) [″ + Gr. *chorioeides,* skinlike, + *itis,* inflammation]. Inflammation of sclerotic and choroid coats of the eye. SYN: *sclerochoroiditis.*

scleroticonyxis (sklē-rŏt″ĭ-kō-nĭk′sĭs) [″ + Gr. *nyxis,* a piercing]. Surgical puncture of the sclera. SYN: *scleronyxis.*

scleroticopuncture (sklē-rŏt″ĭ-kō-pŭnk′tūr) [″ + *punctura,* a piercing]. Surgical puncture of the sclera. SYN: *scleronyxis; scleroticonyxis.*

scleroticotomy (sklē-rŏt″ĭ-kŏt′ō-mē) [″ + Gr. *tome,* incision]. Incision of the sclerotic coat of the eye. SYN: *sclerotomy.*

sclerotic teeth. Teeth that are hard and highly resistant to caries.

sclerotitis (sklē-rō-tī′tĭs) [Gr. *skleros,* hard, + *itis,* inflammation]. Inflammation of the sclera. SYN: *scleritis.*

sclerotium (sklē-rō′shē-ŭm). Hardened mass formed by growth of certain fungi. That formed by ergot on rye is of medical importance.

sclerotome (sklē′rō-tōm) [″ + *tome,* incision]. 1. Knife used in incision of the sclera. 2. One of a series of segmentally arranged masses of mesenchymal tissue lying on either side of the notochord. They give rise to the vertebrae and ribs.

sclerotomy (sklē-rŏt′ō-mē). Surgical incision of sclera. SYN: *scleroticotomy.*

s., anterior. Incision made at angle of the anterior chamber of the eye in glaucoma.

s., posterior. Incision through the sclera into the vitreous for detached retina, or removal of a foreign body.

sclerotrichia (sklē-rō-trĭk′ē-ă) [Gr. *sclerosis,* hard, + *thrix,* hair]. Hardness and brittleness of the hair.

sclerous (sklē′rŭs). Hard; indurated.

scobinate (skō′bĭn-āt) [L. *skobina,* rasp]. Having a rough, uneven, nodular surface.

scoleciasis (skō-lĕ-sī′ă-sĭs) [Gr. *skolex,* worm, + *-iasis,* condition]. Presence of larval forms of butterflies or moths in the body.

scoleciform (skō-lĕs′ĭ-form) [″ + L. *forma,* form]. Resembling a scolex.

scolecoid (skō′lĕ-koyd) [″ + *eidos,* form] Resembling a worm.

scolecology (skō″lĕ-kŏl′ō-jē) [″ + *logos,* study]. Helminthology.

scolex (skō′lĕks) [Gr. *skolex,* worm]. (pl. *scolices*) The portion of a tapeworm, the so-called head, by which it attaches itself to the wall of the intestine. Scolices usually possess organs such as hooks, suckers, or grooves (bothria) for attachment.

scoliokyphosis (skō″lē-ō-kī-fō′sĭs) [Gr. *skolios,* twisted, + *kyphosis,* humpback]. Combined scoliosis and kyphosis.

scoliometer (skō″lē-ŏm′ĕt-ĕr) [″ + *metron,* measure]. Device for measuring curves, esp. lateral ones of the spine.

scoliorachitic (skō″lē-ō-ră-kĭt′ĭk) [″ + *rhachis,* spine]. Pert. to, or afflicted with, spinal curvature from rickets.

scoliosiometry (skō″lē-ō-sē-ŏm′ĕ-trē) [″ + *metron,* a measure]. Measurement of degree of spinal curvature. SYN: *scoliosometry.*

scoliosis (skō″lē-ō′sĭs) [Gr. *skoliosis,* curvature]. Lateral curvature of the spine. Usually consists of two curves, the original abnormal curve and a compensatory curve in the opposite direction.

NURSING IMPLICATIONS: Make provisions to assist the adolescent and family to meet the psychosocial needs associated with the illness. Teach the patient and family concerning treatment modality (cast, brace, or traction), exercises, activity level, skin care, prevention of complications, and breathing exercises. Provide preoperative teaching when necessary, including anesthetic, breathing exercises, apparatus that will be used postoperatively (such as a Stryker frame or Circ-O-Lectric bed), exercises, diet, and analgesics.

s., cicatricial. Scoliosis due to cicatricial contraction resulting from necrosis.

s., congenital. Scoliosis present at birth, usually the result of defective embryonic development of the spine.

s., coxitic. Scoliosis in the lumbar spine due to tilting of the pelvis in hip disease.

s., empyematic. Scoliosis following empyema and retraction of one side of the chest.

s., habit. Scoliosis due to habitually assumed improper position.

s., inflammatory. Scoliosis due to disease of the vertebrae.

s., ischiatic. Scoliosis due to hip disease.

s., myopathic. Scoliosis due to weakening of spinal muscles. SYN: *s., osteopathic.*

s., ocular. Scoliosis from tilting of the head because of visual defects of extraocular muscle imbalance.

s., osteopathic. S., myopathic.

s., paralytic. Scoliosis due to paralysis of muscles.

s., rachitic. Scoliosis due to rickets.

s., rheumatic. Scoliosis due to rheumatism of dorsal muscles.

s., sciatic. Scoliosis due to sciatica.

s., static. Scoliosis due to difference in length of legs.

scoliosometry (skō″lē-ō-sŏm′ĕt-rē) [″ + *metron,* measure]. Determination of degree of spinal curvature. SYN: *scoliosiometry.*

scoliotic (skō-lē-ŏt′ĭk). Suffering from, or related to, scoliosis.

scoliotone (skō′lē-ō-tōn) [Gr. *skolios,* twisted, + *tonos,* tension]. An apparatus for correcting the curve in scoliosis by stretching the spine.

scombrine (skŏm′brĭn). A protamine present in mackerel sperm.

scombroid. Fish of the suborder Scombroidea. Included in this group are mackerels, tuna, bonitos, albacores, and skipjacks.

scombroid poisoning. Intoxication due to eating raw or inadequately cooked fish of the suborder Scombroidea. Certain bacteria act on the fish to produce a histamine-like toxin.

SYM: Nausea, vomiting, abdominal cramps, diarrhea, flushing, headache, urticaria, and a burning sensation in the mouth. The incubation period varies from 15 minutes to 3 hours and averages 45 minutes. Symptoms last approximately 8 hours.

TREATMENT: There is no specific therapy.

scoop (skoop) [ME., a ladle]. Spoon-shaped surgical instrument.

s., bone. Instrument for scraping or removing necrosed bone or contents of suppurative tracts.

s., bullet. Instrument for dislodging bullets.

s., cataract. Instrument for removing fluids or foreign growths.

s., ear. Instrument for removing middle ear granulations.

s., lithotomy. Instrument for dislodging encysted calculi or removing stones, debris, etc.

s., mastoid. Instrument used in mastoid operations.

s., renal. Instrument to dislodge or remove small stones from pelvis of kidney.

scoparius (skō-pā′rē-ŭs). The fresh or dried tops of broom, Cysticus scoparius. It acts as a diuretic and emetic.

-scope [Gr. *skopein,* to examine]. Combining form meaning an instrument or device for viewing or examining.

scopolamine hydrobromide (skō-pŏl′ă-mēn hī″drō-brō′mīd). USP. The hydrobromide of alkaloids obtained from plants of the nightshade family.

ACTION AND USES: As a sedative; locally as a mydriatic; and with morphine and pentobarbital in labor to produce "twilight" sleep. SYN: *hyoscine hydrobromide.*

scopometer (skō-pŏm′ĕ-tĕr) [Gr. *skopein,* to examine, + *metron,* measure]. Instrument for measuring the density of a suspension.

scopophilia (skō″pō-fĭl′ē-ă) [Gr. *skopos,* a watcher, + *philein,* to love]. Sexual pleasure derived from visual sources such as nudity and obscene pictures. SEE: *voyeur.*

scopophobia (skō″pō-fō′bē-ă) [″ + *phobos,* fear]. Abnormal fear of being seen.

scopophobiac (skō″pō-fō′bē-ăk). One who is afraid of being seen.

-scopy [Gr. *skopein,* to examine]. Combining form meaning examination.

scoracratia (skor″ă-krā′shē-ă) [Gr. *skor,* dung, + *akratia,* lack of control]. Inability to retain the feces. SYN: *scatacratia.*

scorbutic (skor-bū′tĭk) [L. *scorbuticus*]. Concerning or affected with scurvy.

scorbutigenic (skor-bū″tĭ-jĕn′ĭk) [L. *scorbutus,* scurvy, + Gr. *gennan,* to produce]. Something that causes scurvy.

scorbutus (skor-bū'tŭs) [L., scurvy]. A deficiency disease due to lack of vitamin C in the diet. SYN: *scurvy*. SEE: *vitamin C*.

scordinema (skor-dĭ-nē'mă) [Gr. *skordinema*, yawning]. Yawning and stretching with fatigue and heaviness of the head, a prodromal symptom of an infectious disease.

score (skor). 1. A rating or grade as compared to a standard of other individuals esp. in a competitive event. 2. To mark the skin with lines in order to have landmarks available, as in plastic surgery.

s., Apgar. SEE: *Apgar score*.

scoretemia (skor-ĕ-tē'mē-ă) [Gr. *skor*, dung, + *haima*, blood]. Scatemia.

scorpion (skor'pē-ŏn) [Gr. *skorpios*]. An arachnid belonging to the order Scorpionida confined principally to warm countries. Scorpions are capable of inflicting a dangerous and sometimes fatal sting by means of an erectile tail equipped with a stinger. The venom contains neurotoxins, hemolysins, cardiac toxins, and agglutinins. SEE: *spider, black widow*.

scorpion sting. Symptoms resemble those of a black widow spider bite or of strychnine poisoning. Severity of symptoms depends on age of victim. Stings often are fatal to children under 3 years of age; adults usually recover.

TREATMENT: Same as a black widow spider bite. Apply tourniquet with caution. Apply ice or freeze with ethyl chloride to slow dissemination of venom. Specific antivenin should be administered if available. In Southwest U.S.A., it can be secured from Poisonous Animals Research Laboratory, Arizona State College, Tempe, Arizona; or contact the local Poison Control Center to obtain the nearest source of the antivenin. SEE: *Poison Control Centers* in *Appendix*.

scoto- (skō'tō) [Gr. *skotos*, darkness]. Combining form indicating a relation to darkness.

scotochromogen (skō"tō-krō'mō-jĕn) [" + *chroma*, color, + *gennan*, to produce]. Any microorganism that produces a chromogen when grown in light or darkness.

scotodinia (skō"tō-dĭn'ē-ă) [" + *dinos*, whirl]. Vertigo with black spots before the eyes and faintness of vision.

scotogram, scotograph (skō'tō-grăm, -grăf) [" + *gramma*, mark; " + *graphein*, to write]. Any radiation effect recorded in the dark on a photographic plate.

scotoma (skō-tō'mă) [Gr. *skotoma*, darkness]. (pl. *scotomata*) Islandlike blind gap in the visual field.

s., absolute. An area in the visual field in which there is absolute blindness.

s., annular. A scotomatous zone that encircles the point of fixation like a ring, not always completely closed, but leaving the fixation point intact.

s., arcuate. Scotoma that is arc-shaped and near the blind spot of the eye. It is caused by a nerve bundle defect on the temporal side of the optic disk.

s., central. An area of depressed vision involving the point of fixation, seen in lesions of the macula.

s., centrocecal. Defect in vision that is oval-shaped and includes the fixation point and the blind spot of the eye.

s., color. Colorblindness in a limited portion of the visual field.

s., eclipse. An area of blindness in the visual field due to having looked directly at the sun during an eclipse.

s., flittering. S., scintillating.

s., negative. Scotoma not perceptible by the patient, being a blind spot in the visual field.

s., peripheral. A defect in vision removed from the point of fixation of the vision.

s., physiological. Blind spot due to absence of rods and cones where the optic nerve enters the retina.

s., positive. Area that patient perceives in the visual field as a dark spot.

s., relative. Scotoma in which perception of the object is impaired but not completely lost.

s., ring. SEE: *s., annular*.

s., scintillating. An irregular outline around a luminous patch in the visual field following mental or physical labor, eyestrain, or in migraine. SYN: *s., flittering*.

scotomagraph (skō-tō'mă-grăf) [Gr. *skotoma*, darkness, + *graphein*, to write]. Device for recording scotomata.

scotomata (skō-tō'mă-tă) [Gr.]. Pl. of scotoma.

scotomatous (skō-tŏm'ă-tŭs) [Gr. *skotoma*, darkness]. Rel. to, of the nature of, or afflicted with scotoma.

scotometer (skō-tŏm'ĕt-ĕr) [" + *metron*, a measure]. Device for detecting and measuring scotomata in the visual field.

scotometry (skō-tŏm'ĕ-trē). The locating and measurement of scotomata.

scotomization (skō"tō-mī-zā'shŭn) [Gr. *skotoma*, darkness]. Development of blind spots, particularly mental ones, wherein the patient denies, or fails to be aware of, that which his or her ego finds unpleasant.

scotophilia (skō"tō-fĭl'ē-ă) [" + *philein*, to love]. Preference for darkness or for the night. SYN: *nyctophilia*.

scotophobia (skō"tō-fō'bē-ă) [" + *phobos*, fear]. Abnormal dread of darkness. SYN: *noctiphobia; nyctophobia*.

scotopia (skō-tō'pē-ă) [" + *ops*, eye]. Adjustment of the eye for vision in dim light. Opposite of photopia.

scotopic (skō-tŏp′ĭk). Pert. to scotopia.

scotopic vision. Dark adaptation; the adjustment of the eyes for vision in dark or dim light. SYN: *night vision.*

scotopsin (skō-tŏp′sĭn). The protein portion of the rods of the retina of the eye. It combines with retinal to form rhodopsin.

scotoscopy (skō-tŏs′kō-pē) [Gr. *skotos,* darkness, + *skopein,* to examine]. Examination of internal organs by use of the fluoroscope. SYN: *skiascopy.*

scout film. In radiology, an x-ray, esp. of the abdomen, for detecting abnormalities. These films are of assistance in excluding or including certain diseases being considered as diagnostic possibilities.

scr. *scruple.*

scratch (skrăch) [ME. *cracchen*]. 1. A mark or superficial injury produced by scraping with the nails on a rough surface. 2. To make a thin, shallow cut with a sharp instrument. 3. To rub the skin, esp. with fingernails, to relieve itching.

scratch test. Placement of an appropriate dilution of a test material, suspected of being an allergen, in a lightly scratched area of the skin. If the material is an allergen, a wheal will develop within 15 minutes.

screatus (skrē-ā′tŭs) [L. *screatus,* a hawking]. A neurosis characterized by paroxysmal fits of hawking or snorting.

screen [O. Fr. *escren*]. 1. A flat area upon which movies or slides are viewed, or suitable for visualizing x-ray pictures. 2. To make a fluoroscopic examination. 3. To examine systemically to determine the presence of a certain disease or characteristics. 4. A structure or substance used to protect, guard, or shield from a damaging influence such as x-rays or sun rays. 5. A system used to select or reject personnel. 6. In psychiatry, the blocking of one memory with another.

s., Bjerrum. [P. J. Bjerrum, Danish ophthalmologist, 1827–1872] A one-meter square planar surface viewed from a distance of one meter. It is used to plot the physiological blind spot, scotomata, and other visual field defects. SYN: *s., tangent.*

s., fluorescent. A flat screen covered with a material that in a darkened room will light up when x-rays pass through it. Used in studying the image produced on the screen during fluoroscopy.

s., intensifying. An apparatus for intensifying the image produced by x-ray pictures.

s., tangent. SEE: *s., Bjerrum.*

screening. 1. The testing, usually using one diagnostic tool, of large groups of people to determine the presence of a particular disease or of certain risk factors known to be associated with that disease.

Ex.: chest x-ray or tuberculin test for tuberculosis, urinalysis for diabetes, serum cholesterol for potential arteriosclerosis, intraocular pressure for glaucoma. 2. In psychiatry, the initial examination to determine the mental status of an individual and the appropriate initial therapy.

s., multiphasic. The use of many diagnostic tests to determine the presence of one or more diseases.

scrobiculate (skrō-bĭk′ū-āt) [L. *scrobiculatus*]. Having shallow depressions; pitted.

scrobiculus (skrō-bĭk′ū-lŭs) [L., a little pit]. A small groove or pit.

s. cordis. Pit of the stomach; precordial or epigastric depression.

scrofula (skrŏf′ū-lă) [L. *scrofula,* a breeding sow]. A variety of tuberculous adenitis that is most frequently encountered. It is thought to be a secondary involvement of cervical lymph nodes as a result of a localized hematogenous spread from a pulmonary lesion. Most common in childhood.

TREATMENT: Responds to specific antituberculosis chemotherapy.

scrofulid(e) (skrŏf′ū-lĭd, -līd). Scrofuloderma.

scrofuloderma (skrŏf″ū-lō-dĕr′mă) [L. *scrofula,* a breeding sow, + Gr. *derma,* skin]. A skin manifestation of tuberculous origin, usually secondary to scrofula. Marked by ulcers usually resulting from a tuberculous sinus. Occurs most commonly on chest, neck, and in the axillae and groins, esp. in children and adolescents. Now very rare.

TREATMENT: Responds to ultraviolet light treatments and specific chemotherapy for tuberculosis.

scrofulosis (skrŏf″ū-lō′sĭs [″ + Gr. *osis,* condition]. Scrofula.

scrofulous (skrŏf′ū-lŭs) [L. *scrofula,* a breeding sow]. Of the nature of, or afflicted with, scrofula.

scrotal (skrō′tăl) [L. *scrotum,* a bag]. Concerning the scrotum.

scrotal reflex. Slow vermicular contraction of scrotal muscle when perineum is stroked or cold applied.

scrotectomy (skrō-tĕk′tō-mē) [″ + Gr. *ektome,* excision]. Excision of part of the scrotum.

scrotitis [″ + Gr. *itis,* inflammation]. Inflamed condition of the scrotum.

scrotocele (skrō′tō-sēl) [″ + Gr. *kele,* hernia]. Hernia in the scrotum.

scrotoplasty (skrō′tō-plăs″tē) [″ + Gr. *plassein,* to form]. Plastic surgery on the scrotum.

scrotum (skrō′tŭm) [L., a bag]. (pl. *scrota, -ums*) [NA] The double pouch of the male, which contains the testicles and part of the spermatic cord, found in most mammals. Constituent parts of the scrotum are skin; a network of nonstriated muscular fibers called dartos; cremasteric, spermatic, and infundibuliform fasciae; cremasteric muscle; and tunica vaginalis.

RS: chimney-sweeps' cancer; chyloderma; dartos; oscheal; oscheitis; oscheoncus; rhacoma; urocele; varicocoele.

scrubbing [MD. *schrubben*]. Term applied to washing the hands, fingernails, and lower arms in preparation for performing surgery. The precise procedure to follow usually is posted in a special area where the washing is done.

METHOD: Scrubbing with soap and water and a nail brush, immersion in a mild germicidal solution, and the wearing of sterilized rubber gloves, cap, gown, and mask.

scrub nurse. Term applied to operating room nurse who hands instruments to the surgeon; and who has previously scrubbed his or her hands and wears a mask, sterile rubber gloves, and gown.

scrub typhus. An acute febrile illness caused by Rickettsia tsutsugamushi transmitted by several species of mites, including Trombicula akamushi and T. deliensis. Common in the Asiatic-Pacific area. If untreated, fever lasts for about 14 days. Fatality rate varies in untreated cases from 1 to 4%. SYN: *tsutsugamushi disease*.

TREATMENT: Tetracycline or chloramphenicol.

scruple (skrū'pl) [L. *scrupulus*, a small stone]. ABBR: scr. SYMB: ℈. Twenty grains in apothecaries' weight; 1.296 gm.

scultetus bandage (skŭl-tē'tŭs). [Johann Schultes (Scultetus), Ger. surgeon, 1595–1645] A many-tailed bandage or binder, applied around the abdomen so the ends overlap each other as if they were roof shingles. The binder is used to hold dressings in place and to support abdominal muscles postoperatively. SEE: *binder, scultetus*, for illus.

scultetus position. Position in which head is low and the body on an inclined plane.

scum (skŭm) [ME. *scume*]. Slimy floating islands of bacteria or impurities on the surface of a culture; an interrupted pellicle of bacterial growth.

scurf [AS. *scurf*]. A branny desquamation of the epidermis, esp. on the scalp. SEE: *dandruff*.

scurvy (skŭr'vē) [L. *scorbutus*]. A deficiency disease characterized by hemorrhagic manifestations and abnormal formation of bones and teeth.

ETIOL: Deficiency of vitamin C usually resulting from lack of fresh fruits and vegetables in diet.

SYM: Preceded by period of ill health characterized by sallow complexion; loss of energy; pains in legs, limbs, and joints. Anemia; great weakness; spongy, bleeding gums; fetor of breath; loosening of teeth; subcutaneous hemorrhages and hemorrhages from mucous membranes; painful, brawny indurations of muscles characterize overt symptoms.

PROG: Favorable in early stages.

TREATMENT: For infants, 300 mg. of vitamin C (ascorbic acid) daily for 1 week, then 150 mg. daily for 1 month, or 4 to 8 oz. (52 to 104 ml.) of orange juice or 12 to 24 oz. (155 to 311 ml.) of tomato juice daily. For adults, 300 to 500 mg. of ascorbic acid daily until symptoms have disappeared.

s., infantile. A form of scurvy that sometimes follows the prolonged use of condensed milk, sterilized milk, or proprietary foods that do not contain supplementary vitamin C. SYN: *Barlow's disease*.

SYM: Anemia, immobility of legs, pseudoparalysis, extreme tenderness, swelling without pitting, thickening of bones from subperiosteal hemorrhage, ecchymoses, and tendency toward fractures of epiphyses of bones.

scute (skūt) [L. *scutum*, shield]. 1. A thin plate or scale, esp. the horny plates found on the carapace of turtles. 2. Term formerly applied to the tegmen tympani.

scutiform (skū'tĭ-form) [" + *forma*, a shield]. Shield-shaped.

scutular (skū'tū-lăr) [L. *scutulum*, a little shield]. Having small indented crusts of the skin.

scutulum (skū'tū-lŭm) [L., a little shield]. (pl. *scutula*) Lesion of the scalp caused by the fungus Trichophyton schoenleini. A yellow cup-shaped crust consisting of a dense mass of mycelia and epithelial debris. The cup faces up and its center is pierced by the hair around which it has developed. SEE: *favus*.

scutum (skū'tŭm) [L., shield]. Plate of bone resembling a shield.

scybalous (sĭb'ă-lŭs) [Gr. *skybalon*, dung]. Of the nature of hard fecal matter.

scybalum (sĭb'ă-lŭm). (pl. *scybala*) A hard rounded mass of fecal matter.

scypho- [Gr. *skyphos*, cup]. Combining form meaning cup.

scyphoid (sī'foyd) [" + *eidos*, like]. Cup-shaped.

S.D. *skin dose; standard deviation*.

SDA. 1. *specific dynamic action*. 2. Abbreviation for Latin *sacrodextra anterior*. The right sacroanterior fetal position.

S.E. *standard error*.

Se. Chem. symb. for selenium.

seabather's eruption. Itching red papules that may appear on the skin within a few hours of swimming in the sea. The lesions progress to form crusted papules and disappear spontaneously in 7 to 10 days. Treatment is symptomatic. Caused by a form of schistosome found in coastal and inland waters of North America. SYN: *schistosome dermatitis; swimmer's itch.*

seal. 1. To firmly close. 2. A material such as an adhesive or wax used to make an airtight closure.

s., border. The edge of a denture that contacts the tissues in order to close the area under the denture to entrance by food, air, or liquids.

s., posterior palatal. The seal at the posterior border of a denture.

s., velopharyngeal. The seal between the oral and nasopharyngeal cavities.

searcher (sĕrch'ĕr) [ME. *serchen*]. Instrument for locating opening of ureter previous to inserting catheter or exploring sinuses, and esp. for detecting stones in the bladder. SYN: *sound.*

seasickness [AS. *sae,* sea, + *seocness,* illness]. Disorder due to motion of a boat, or riding in cars, trains, and elevators. A similar condition affects some air travelers. SYN: *motion sickness.*

ETIOL: Motion affects the middle ear, and the vomiting center in the brain stem is stimulated. There is wide individual variation in susceptibility.

SYM: Giddiness, vomiting, headache, nausea, and often extreme drowsiness, retching, prostration.

PREVENTION: Select position in craft where up-and-down motion is least; avoid dietary and alcoholic excesses; avoid reading or unusual visual stimuli; assume a supine or recumbent position.

TREATMENT: 50 mg. of Dramamine (dimenhydrinate) every four hours as necessary. This medicine causes some people to experience drowsiness; those individuals should not operate a motor vehicle or dangerous machinery. Sedatives and supportive therapy, such as intravenous fluids, may be required in severe and prolonged cases. Generally, antinausea pills should not be given to pregnant women during early pregnancy.

seat. The structure upon which another structure rests or is supported.

s., basal. Tissues in the mouth that support a denture.

s., rest. An area upon which a denture or restoration rests.

Seattle foot [after the city Seattle, Washington, U.S.A., where it was developed]. An artificial foot that has a spring-back quality that makes it feel like a real foot. Use of this device allows single- or double-foot amputees to run and engage in other sports.

seatworm. A species of nematode worms, Enterobius vermicularis, that commonly infest man. Adult worms inhabit large intestine in region of cecum and appendix. Gravid females migrate nightly to anus where they deposit eggs in the perianal region. Movement of the worms about anus causes intense itching. SYN: *pinworm.*

sebaceous (sē-bā'shŭs) [L., fatty]. Containing, or pert. to, sebum, an oily, fatty matter secreted by the sebaceous glands.

sebaceous cyst. A cyst filled with sebum from a distended sebaceous gland. These cysts are sometimes known as wens. They frequently form on the scalp and consist of a small sac, containing sebaceous matter, that may grow to a large size. They may result from impairment of localized circulation and closure of sebaceous glands or ducts. Drainage does not remove them permanently because they will recur unless entirely extirpated. Extirpation, q.v., should be done with an electric current or cutting knife. One should never attempt to drain such a cyst without taking every precaution against infection.

sebaceous gland. Oil-secreting gland of the skin. The glands are simple or branched alveolar glands, most of which open into hair follicles. They are holocrine glands, their secretion, sebum, arising from disintegration of cells filling the alveoli. Most but not all sebaceous glands have a hair follicle associated with them.

sebastomania (sē-băs"tō-mā'nē-ă) [Gr. *sebastos,* reverend, + *mania,* madness]. Religious insanity. SYN: *theomania.*

sebiferous (sē-bĭf'ĕr-ŭs) [L. *sebum,* tallow, + *ferre,* to carry]. Producing fatty or sebaceous matter. SYN: *sebiparous.*

sebiparous (sē-bĭp'ă-rŭs) [" + *parere,* to produce]. Producing sebum or sebaceous matter. SYN: *sebiferous.*

sebolite, sebolith (sĕb'ō-īt, -lĭth) [" + Gr. *lithos,* a stone]. Concretion in a sebaceous gland. SYN: *sebolith.*

seborrhagia (sĕb"ō-rā'jē-ă [" + Gr. *rhegnynai,* to burst forth]. Excessive secretion of sebaceous glands. SYN: *seborrhea.*

seborrhea (sĕb-or-ē'ă) [" + Gr. *rhoia,* flow]. Functional disease of the sebaceous glands marked by increase in the amount, and often alteration of the quality, of the sebaceous secretion.

TREATMENT: Mild dandruff may be treated with a shampoo containing selenium sulfide or sulfur. If severe, a lotion or cream containing corticosteroids, preferably in the form of hydrocortisone, is rubbed into the affected areas two or three times a day.

s. capiti. Seborrhea of the scalp.

s. congestiva. Facial form of seborrhea with elevated patches with red borders and covered with crusts and scars. SYN: *lupus erythematosus.*

s. corporis. Seborrhea of the trunk.

s. faciei. Seborrhea of the face.

s. furfuracea. Dermatitis seborrheica.

s. nigricans. Dark-colored crusts occurring in seborrhea.

s. oleosa. Seborrhea in which fat elements predominate. Shows shiny skin with widely dilated follicular orifices, many of which contain comedones.

s. sicca. Seborrhea with grayish-brown or yellow scale and crust formation in addition to abnormal oiliness. Differentiation from seborrheic dermatitis is difficult. This form most frequently observed on scalp and constitutes what is popularly called dandruff. Examination reveals an encrustation composed of thin yellowish-gray scales. In uncomplicated cases the skin is pale but often becomes hyperemic or inflamed from irritation. When allowed to continue, nutrition of hair is interfered with, and baldness results.

On the body, seborrhea sicca appears as yellowish-gray, slightly elevated patches covered with greasy scales. Outlets of follicles are often dilated. There is generally more or less redness of the skin from hyperemia (seborrheal eczema).

seborrheic (sĕb″ō-rē′ĭk) [L. *sebum,* tallow, + Gr. *rhoia,* flow]. Afflicted with or like seborrhea.

seborrheid (sĕb″ō-rē′ĭd) [″ + Gr. *rhoia,* flow]. Seborrheic dermatitis.

seborrhoic (sĕb″ō-rō′ĭk). Suffering from or like seborrhea. SYN: *seborrheic.*

sebum (sē′bŭm) [L., tallow]. A fatty secretion of the sebaceous glands of the skin. It varies in different parts of the body. Sebum from the ears is called cerumen, q.v.; that from the foreskin is called smegma, q.v.

s. palpebrale. Lema, q.v.

secernent (sē-sĕr′nĕnt) [L. *secernens,* secreting]. 1. Secreting. 2. A secreting organ.

seclusion of pupil. Shutting off of the pupil due to adherence of iris to the lenticular capsule. SYN: *synechia, annular.*

seclusio pupillae siderosis bulbi. Deposit of iron pigment within the eyeball. Seen in cases of iron foreign bodies retained in the eye.

secobarbital. USP. A barbiturate used for its sedative and hypnotic effects. Trade name is Seconal.

s. sodium. USP. A hypnotic and sedative drug. Trade name is Seconal Sodium.

secodont (sē′kō-dŏnt) [L. *secare,* to cut, + Gr. *odous,* tooth]. Having molar teeth with cutting edges on the cusps.

Seconal. Trade name for secobarbital, USP.

Seconal Sodium. Trade name for secobarbital sodium, USP.

secondary. 1. Next to or following; second in order. 2. Produced by a primary cause.

secondary areola. Pigmentation around the nipples during pregnancy. SEE: *areola.*

secondary care. Health care beyond the primary. Included are more sophisticated diagnostic methods and techniques, and laboratory facilities. This level of care is more nearly available in medical care institutions serving a large population. SEE: *primary care; tertiary care.*

secondary hemorrhage. 1. Hemorrhage appearing more than 24 hours after an injury or operation that is due to sepsis and septic ulceration into a blood vessel. 2. Uterine bleeding due to septic infection or from infant's umbilicus due to same cause.

secondary nursing care. Nursing care aimed at early recognition and treatment of disease. It includes general nursing intervention and teaching of early signs of disease conditions so that prompt medical care can be obtained.

secondary radiation. X-rays that are produced by the interaction between primary radiation and the substance being examined.

second cranial nerve. A sensory nerve that conveys visual impulses from eye to thalamus. The two optic nerves undergo partial decussation at the optic chiasma. SEE: *cranial nerves; Cranial Nerves* in *Appendix.*

second intention. Healing by granulation or indirect union. Granulation tissue is formed to fill the gap between the edges of the wound with a thin layer of fibrinous exudate. It bars bacteria and aids in checking bleeding by the coagulation of the blood. Connective tissue cells support the new capillaries. This form of healing is slower than that by first intention and its grayish-red surface may become pale and flabby if the healing is too long delayed. If the granulations show above the surface they may have to be removed with caustics. If the granulations first form at the top instead of the bottom of the wound, it may have to be kept open with drainage. SEE: *intention; resolution.*

second sight. Alteration in refractive powers of the lens so that reading is possible again without glasses in incipient cataract.

second stage of labor. Period in labor between complete dilation of the cervix and delivery of the child. During this stage involuntary contractions of the uterus become quite strong. This stage normally lasts 2 to 4 hours in primiparae and about 1 hour in multiparae. SEE: *labor.*

second wind. Condition occurring following strenuous exercise in which the feeling of subjective breathlessness subsides.

secreta (sē-krē′tă) [L.]. The products of secretion.

secretagogue (sē-krē′tă-gŏg) [L. *secretum,* secretion, + Gr. *agogos,* leading]. 1. That which stimulates secreting organs. 2. An agent that causes secretion. SYN: *secretogogue.*

secrete (sē-krēt′) [L. *secretio,* separation]. To separate from the blood, living organism, or gland; more specifically, to form a secretion.

secretin (sē-krē′tĭn). A hormone that stimulates pepsinogen secretion by the stomach and inhibits the secretion of acid by the stomach. It is also important in stimulating the secretion of bicarbonate (HCO_3) from both the pancreas and the liver. SEE: *cholecystokinin.*

secretinase (sē-krē′tĭ-nās). An enzyme in blood that inactivates secretin.

secretion [L. *secretio,* separation]. 1. The process whereby cells of glandular organs produce certain materials from the blood. 2. The substance produced by glandular organs.

If the material flows out through a duct (e.g., saliva) it is called an external secretion; if it is returned to the blood or lymph (e.g., insulin) it is called an internal secretion.

FLUIDS OF BODY: *Blood:* Composed of 79% water, 21% solids, including the cellular elements of blood. *Bile:* Emulsifies fats and precipitates soluble peptones, 20–24 oz. (259–311 ml.) are produced daily. Sp. gr. 1.026–1.032. Reaction alkaline. *Chyle:* Absorbed by lacteals, the lymphatics of the small intestines. Contains fat absorbed from food. *Chyme:* Food that has undergone gastric digestion only. *Gastric juice:* Clear, acid, watery secretion of the glands of the stomach. Principal ingredients are hydrochloric acid, mucus, and pepsin. *Intestinal juice:* Has combined action of saliva and gastric and pancreatic juices. Starch and complex sugars are converted into monosaccharides. Reaction alkaline. *Lymph:* Characteristics vary with site of origin. If derived from a limb, it may be clear and have less than 1 gm. of protein/100 ml. If derived from gut, protein is increased and fluid may have milky appearance. *Menstrual:* Menstrual flow. Average 60 ml. during each period. Consists of blood, cellular tissue, and mucus. Blood clots are not usually abnormal. *Pancreatic juice:* Contains enzymes that act on fats, proteins or products of protein digestion, and carbohydrates. Approx. 2000 ml. of a fluid of pH 7.5–8.0 secreted daily. *Perspiration:* The secretion of sweat glands. From 100–1000 ml./day under normal conditions. May be many times that amount in extremely hot and dry conditions. *Saliva:* Composition varies with particular glands, being watery if from parotid and viscous from submandibular glands. Approx. 1500 ml. secreted/day. Serves to lubricate food and break down starch and glycogen. *Urine:* 1000–2500 ml./24 hours, but highly variable. Sp. gr. 1.003–1.025. Reaction acid. Contains 50–70 gm. of solids, 12–20 gm./day of urea nitrogen, and chlorides 110–250 nmol./liter depending upon chloride intake. SEE: *urine.*

s., apocrine. Secretion in which the apical end of a secreting cell is broken off and its contents extruded, as in the mammary gland.

s., external. A secretion that passes through a duct and is discharged upon an epithelial surface, either internal or external.

s., holocrine. Secretion in which the entire cell and its contents are extruded as a part of the secretory product, as in sebaceous glands.

s., internal. Secretion imparted to the blood instead of being eliminated by a duct.

s., merocrine. Secretion in which the product is elaborated within cells and discharged through the cell membrane, the cell itself remaining intact.

s., paralytic. Continuous abundant watery secretion from a gland after section of its secretory nerves.

secretion, words pert. to: acrinia; amyxia; apolepsis; asteatosis; athyreosis; athyroidism; cerumen; ceruminal; ceruminosis; ceruminous; choleresis; chromocrinia; crinogenic; diacrisis, errhine; exsiccant; hormone; interstitial; saliva; sebum; secretagogue; secrete; secretin; semen; smegma; succorrhea.

secretogogue (sē-krē′tō-gŏg) [L. *secretio,* separation, + Gr. *agogos,* leading]. 1. Causing secretion. 2. That which stimulates secretion. SYN: *secretagogue.*

secretoinhibitory (sē-krē″tō-ĭn-hĭb′ĭ-tō″rē). Inhibiting secretion.

secretomotor (sē-krē″tō-mō′tor). Something, esp. a nerve, that stimulates secretion.

secretor (sē-krē′tor) [L. *secretio,* separation]. A person who secretes ABO blood group substances into mucous secretions such as saliva or gastric juice.

secretory (sē-krē′tō-rē, sē′krē-tō″rē). Pert. to or promoting secretion; secreting.

secretory capillaries. Very small canaliculi receiving secretion discharged from gland cells.

secretory fibers. Centrifugal nerve fibers that excite secretion.

sectarian (sĕk-tā′rē-ăn) [L. *sectus,* having cut]. A medical practitioner who follows a dogma, tenet, or principle based on some unscientific belief to the exclusion of scientific demonstration.

sectile (sĕk′tĭl) [L. *sectilis*]. Capable of being cut.

sectio (sĕk′shē-ō) [L., a cutting]. Section or cut.

section [L. *sectio,* a cutting]. 1. Process of cutting. 2. A division or segment of a part. 3. A surface made by cutting.

s., abdominal. Any incision through the abdomen. SYN: *laparotomy.*

s., cesarean. Incision of the uterus for delivery of a fetus through the abdominal wall.

s., coronal. S., frontal.

s., frontal. Section dividing the body into two parts, dorsal and ventral. SYN: *s., coronal.*

s., frozen. A thin section of the body, an organ, or a piece of tissue that has been frozen before being sectioned and then studied microscopically.

s., midsagittal. Section that divides the body into right and left halves.

s., paraffin. A section of a tissue that has been infiltrated with paraffin.

s., perineal. External incision into the urethra to relieve stricture.

s., Pitres'. One of the series of sections made through the brain for postmortem examination.

s., sagittal. A section cut parallel to the median plane of the body.

s., serial. Microscopic sections made and arranged in consecutive order.

s., vaginal. Incision into the abdominal cavity through the vagina.

sectioning [L. *sectio,* a cutting]. The slicing of thin sections of tissue for examination under the microscope. SEE: *microtome.*

s., ultrathin. The cutting of sections extraordinarily thin (less than 1 micron in thickness), esp. for use in electron microscopy.

sector (sĕk'tor) [L., cutter]. The area of a circle included between two radii and an arc.

sectorial (sĕk-tō'rē-ăl). Having cutting edges, as teeth.

secundigravida (sē-kŭn"dĭ-grăv'ĭd-ă) [L. *secundus,* second, + *gravida,* pregnant]. A woman in her second pregnancy.

secundina (sē"kŭn-dī'nă) [L., from *secundinus,* following]. That which follows.

secundines (sĕk'ŭn-dīnz, sĭ-kŭn'dīnz) [LL. *secundinae*]. The placenta, umbilical cord, and fetal membranes expelled during the third stage of labor. SYN: *afterbirth.*

secundipara (sē"kŭn-dĭp'ă-ră) [L. *secundus,* second, + *parere,* to give birth]. A woman who has produced two infants at separate times that have weighed 500 grams or more, regardless of their viability. SEE: *gravida; para.*

secundiparity (sē-kŭn"dĭ-păr'ĭ-tē). The condition of being a secundipara.

secundum artem (sē-kŭn'dŭm ăr'tĕm) [L.]. In an approved manner; according to rule or science.

S.E.D. *skin erythema dose.*

sedation (sē-dā'shŭn) [L. *sedatio,* from *sedare,* to calm]. 1. Process of allaying nervous excitement. 2. State of being calmed.

sedative (sĕd'ă-tĭv) [L. *sedativus,* calming]. 1. Quieting. 2. An agent that exerts a soothing or tranquilizing effect. Sedatives may be general, local, nervous, or vascular.

s., cardiac. Sedative that decreases the heart's force.

s., nervous. Sedative affecting nervous system.

sedentary (sĕd'ĕn-tā"rē) [L. *sedentarius*]. 1. Sitting. 2. Pert. to an occupation or mode of living requiring minimal physical exercise.

sediment (sĕd'ĭ-mĕnt) [L. *sedimentum,* a settling]. The substance settling at bottom of a liquid. SYN: *hypostasis.* SEE: *precipitate.*

sedimentation (sĕd"ĭ-mĕn-tā'shŭn). Formation or depositing of sediment.

sedimentation rate. ABBR: ESR (erythrocyte sedimentation rate). Laboratory test of speed at which erythrocytes settle. In this test, blood to which an anticoagulant has been added is placed in a long, narrow tube, and the distance the red cells fall in one hour is the rate, ESR. Normally, in males, it is less than 10 mm./hr.; and is slightly higher in females.

The speed at which the cells settle depends upon the size of the clumps into which the red cells aggregate, and the size of the clumps appears to depend upon the amount of fibrinogen in the blood. The sedimentation rate is a nonspecific indicator of disease, esp. inflammatory conditions, and a great number of other abnormal conditions in which it is usually elevated. Some conditions retard sedimentation. These include polycythemia, congenital heart disease, and hypochromic microcytic anemia.

sedimentator (sĕd"ĭ-mĕn-tā'tor). A centrifuge.

seed (sēd) [AS. *saed*]. 1. The ripened ovule of a spermatophyte plant usually consisting of the embryo (germ), and a supply of nutrient material enclosed within the seed coats. It is a resting sporophyte. 2. Sperm; semen. 3. Capsule containing radon or radium for use in treatment of cancer. 4. Offspring. 5. To introduce microorganisms into a culture medium.

Seessel's pouch (zā'sĕlz). [Albert Seessel, U.S. embryologist and neurologist, 1850–1910] In the embryo, a small ectodermal diverticulum of the foregut close to the buccopharyngeal membrane. It disappears in man.

segment (sĕg'mĕnt) [L. *segmentum,* a portion]. 1. A part or section, esp. a natural one, of an organ or body. 2. One of the serial divisions of an animal.

s., bronchopulmonary. A small subdivision of the lobes of the lung.

s.'s, hepatic. Subdivision of the lobes of the liver.

s., interannular. Portion of a neuron between two nodes of Ranvier.

s., mesodermal. A somite.

s.'s, uterine. The segments of the uterus during labor. The upper portion becomes thicker and the lower segment is thinned-out.

segmental (sĕg-mĕn'tăl). Pert. to, resembling, or composed of segments.

segmental reflex. A reflex action in which afferent impulses enter the cord in the same segment or segments from which the efferent impulses emerge.

segmental static reactions. Postural reflexes in which movements of one extremity result in a movement in an opposite extremity.

segmentation (sĕg"mĕn-tā'shŭn) [L. *segmentum,* a portion]. 1. Division into similar parts. 2. The division of a fertilized egg into many smaller cells or blastomeres. SYN: *cleavage.* SEE: *blastomere; cleavage; embryo.*

s., rhythmic. Division of the intestine and the chyme within it into segments by contraction of circular muscle fibers.

segmenter. Stage in development of the malarial organism (Plasmodium) in which the organism is undergoing schizogony. SYN: *rosette.* SEE: *schizont.*

segmentum (sĕg-mĕn'tŭm) [L.]. A portion or part of a structure.

segregation [L. *segregare,* to separate]. 1. Setting apart, separating. 2. In genetics, the process that takes place in the formation of germ cells (gametogenesis) in which each gamete (egg or sperm) receives only one of each pair of genes.

segregator. Instrument composed of two ureteral catheters for securing urine from each kidney separately.

Séguin's signal symptom (sā-gănz'). [Edouard Séguin, 1812–1880] Involuntary contractions of muscles just before an epileptic attack.

Seidlitz powder (sĕd'lĭts, sĭd'lĭtz). [Seidlitz, village in Bohemia] Effervescent cathartic composed of tartaric acid, sodium bicarbonate, and sodium and potassium tartrate.

seisesthesia (sīz"ĕs-thē'zē-ă) [Gr. *seisis,* concussion, + *aisthesis,* sensation]. Perception of a concussion.

seismesthesia (sīz"mĕs-thē'zē-ă) [Gr. *seismos,* earthquake, + *aisthesis,* sensation]. Perception of vibrations.

seismotherapy (sīz"mō-thĕr'ă-pē) [" + *therapeia,* treatment]. Treatment of disease by vibratory massage. SYN: *sismotherapy.*

seizure (sē'zhŭr) [O. Fr. *seisir,* to take possession of]. A sudden attack of pain, of a disease, or of certain symptoms.

s., absence. Petit mal epilepsy attack in which there is a brief, less than 30-second, loss of consciousness but there is no fall. The eyes flutter and the patient stops all other activity. Normalcy returns and the patient makes no notice of this absence. SEE: *epilepsy.*

s., convulsive. 1. A convulsion. 2. An attack of epilepsy. SEE: *epilepsy.*

s., grand mal. SEE: *epilepsy.*

s., jacksonian. SEE: *jacksonian epilepsy.*

s., larval. A seizure indicated by abnormal brain waves in an electroencephalogram but not evidenced by clinical symptoms.

s., petit mal. SEE: *epilepsy.*

Seldinger technique. Method for introducing a catheter into a vein or artery. The vessel is located with a special needle that contains a wire; the needle is removed. The catheter is threaded into the vein while being guided by the wire over which it is moving. The wire is then removed from the catheter.

selection [L. *selectus,* having chosen]. 1. Choice; the process of choosing or selecting. 2. In biology, the factors that determine the reproductive ability of a certain genotype.

s., artificial. Process by which man selects desirable characteristics in animals and breeds for these phenotypes.

s., natural. Mechanism of evolution proposed by Darwin stating that the genotypes best adapted to their environment have a tendency to survive and reproduce.

s., sexual. A theory originated to account for differences in secondary sex characteristics between males and females. It assumes that individuals preferentially mate with individuals of the opposite sex who possess these characteristics.

selenium (sē-lē'nē-ŭm) [Gr. *selene,* moon]. SYMB: Se. At. wt. 78.96; at. no. 34. A chemical element resembling sulfur. It is poisonous to certain animals that feed on plants grown on soil that contains an excess of selenium.

s. sulfide. USP. A drug used in treating dandruff and tinea versicolor. Trade names for preparations including selenium sulfide are Exsel, Selsun, and Selsun Blue.

selenoid cells. SEE: *achromocytes.*

selenomethionine Se 75 injection (sĕl"ĕn-ō-mĕ-thī'ō-nēn). USP. Radioactive L-selenomethionine wherein the sulfur atom in the methionine has been replaced by selenium. The compound is used intravenously to investigate methionine metabolism.

self. In immunology, an individual's own antigenic make-up.

self-differentiation. The differentiation of tissues even though they are isolated.

self-digestion. Destruction or disintegration of a cell or tissue by its own juice, as that of the walls of the stomach by the gastric juice occurring in certain diseases of that organ. SYN: *autodigestion.*

self-hypnosis. Hypnotizing oneself.
self-infection. Autoinfection.
self-limited disease. Disease that, without treatment, runs a definite course within a limited time.
self-tolerance. In immunology, tolerance to self-antigens.
sellar (sĕl'ăr). Concerning the sella turcica.
sella turcica (sĕl'ă tŭr'sĭ-kă) [L., Turkish saddle]. [NA] A concavity on superior surface of body of sphenoid bone that houses the hypophysis cerebri (pituitary gland). SEE: *empty-sella*.
Selsun. Trade name for selenium sulfide, USP.
Selsun Blue. Trade name for selenium sulfide, USP.
semantics (sē-măn'tĭks) [Gr. *semantikos*, significant]. The area of linguistics concerned with meaning.
semeiography (sē"mē-ŏg'ră-fē) [Gr. *semeion*, sign, + *graphein*, to write]. Description of the signs and symptoms of a disease.
semeiology (sē"mī-ŏl'ō-jē) [" + *logos*, study]. The branch of medicine dealing with the study of symptoms. SYN: *symptomatology*.
semeiosis (sē"mī-ō'sĭs) [" + *osis*, condition]. Study of disease by symptoms.
semeiotic (sē"mī-ŏt'ĭk) [Gr. *semeiotikos*]. Of or pert. to symptoms. SYN: *symptomatic*.
semeiotics (sē"mī-ŏt'ĭks). 1. Branch of medical science concerning symptoms. SYN: *semiotics; symptomatology*. 2. Symptoms of a disease in a particular case considered as a whole.
semelincident (sĕm"ĕl-ĭn'sĭ-dĕnt) [L. *semel*, once, + *incidens*, falling upon]. Occurring only once in a person.
semen (sē'mĕn) [L., seed]. (pl. *semina*) A thick, opalescent, viscid secretion discharged from the urethra of the male at the climax of sexual excitement (orgasm). Contains the spermatozoa. Semen is the mixed product of various glands (prostate and bulbourethral) plus the spermatozoa, which, having been produced in the testicles, are stored in the seminal vesicles.

Normal values for the seminal fluid ejaculate: volume, 2–5 ml.; pH, 7.8–8.0; leukocytes, absent or only an occasional one seen per high-power field; sperm count, 60–150 million/ml.; motility, 80% or more should be motile; morphology, 80–90% should be normal.

RS: aspermatism; azoospermia; bradyspermatism; coitus; copulation; ejaculation; emission; erection; fertilization; insemination; libido; orgasm; penis; prostate; sexual intercourse; sperm; vesicle, seminal.

s., frozen. Semen stored in a bank for future use in insemination. It offers a supply of donors in small communities where it would be impossible to maintain anonymity of local donors. However, in artificial insemination the number of successful pregnancies is lower with frozen semen than with fresh.
semenuria (sē"mĕn-ū'rē-ă) [L. *semen*, seed, + Gr. *ouron*, urine]. Excretion of semen in the urine. SYN: *seminuria; spermaturia*.
semi- [L. *semis*, half]. Prefix meaning half.
semicanal (sĕm"ē-kăn-ăl') [" + *canalis*, passage]. A duct open on one side.
semicanalis (sĕm"ē-kă-nā'lĭs) [L., semicanal]. A channel that is open on one side.

s. musculi tensoris tympani. Semicanal of tensor tympani muscle in the temporal bone.

s. tubae auditivae. Semicanal of the auditory tube.
semicartilaginous (sĕm"ē-kăr"tĭ-lăj'ĭ-nŭs) [" + *cartilago*, gristle]. Partially cartilaginous.
semicircular (sĕm"ē-sŭr'kū-lăr) [" + *circulus*, a ring]. In the form of a half circle.
semicircular canals. Superior, posterior, and inferior passages forming part of inner ear.
semicoma (sĕm"ē-kō'mă) [" + Gr. *koma*, lethargy]. Mild degree of impaired consciousness from which it is possible to arouse the patient.
semicomatose (sĕm"ē-kō'măt-ōs). In a condition of impaired consciousness from which patient may be aroused. SEE: *consciousness*.
semicrista (sĕm"ē-krĭs'tă) [L.]. A small or rudimentary crest.

s. incisiva. The nasal crest of the maxilla.
semidecussation (sĕm"ē-dē"kŭs-sā'shŭn) [" + *decussare*, to make an X]. Incomplete crossing of nerve fibers.
semierection (sĕm"ē-ē-rĕk'shŭn) [" + *erigere*, to erect]. An incomplete erection.
semiflexion (sĕm"ē-flĕk'shŭn) [" + *flexio*, bending]. Halfway between flexion and extension of a limb.
semi-Fowler's position. Semisitting position with knees flexed and supported by pillows on the bed.
semilunar (sĕm"ē-lū'năr) [L. *semis*, half, + *luna*, moon]. Shaped like a crescent.
semilunar bone. Half-moon-shaped bone of carpus.
semilunar cartilages. Two crescentic cartilages (medial and lateral) in the knee joint between the femur and tibia.
semilunar cusps. The three segments of the aortic valve between the left ventricle and the ascending aorta.
semilunare (sĕm"ē-lū-nā'rē) [L.]. The lunate bone of the wrist.
semilunar ganglion. The ganglion associated with the sensory root of the 5th cranial nerve. SYN: *Gasserian ganglion; trigeminal ganglion*.
semilunar line. SEE: *line, semilunar*.
semilunar lobe. Lobe on upper surface of the

cerebellum.

semilunar notch. A notch at the proximal end of the ulna for articulation with trochlea of the humerus.

semilunar valves. The heart valves between the ventricles and the vessels leaving the ventricles, i.e., the pulmonary artery and the aorta.

semiluxation (sĕm″ē-lŭk-sā′shŭn) [″ + *luxatio,* dislocation]. Subluxation.

semimembraneous (sĕm″ē-mĕm′bră-nŭs) [″ + L. *membrana,* membrane]. Composed partly of a membrane.

semimembranosus (sĕm″ē-mĕm″brăn-ō′sŭs) [L.]. Large muscle of inner and back part of thigh. SEE: *Muscles* in *Appendix.*

seminal (sĕm′ĭ-năl) [L. *seminalis*]. Concerning the semen or seed.

seminal duct. Any duct that conveys sperm, esp. the ductus deferens and the ejaculatory duct. SYN: *spermatic duct.*

seminal emission. Discharge of semen.

seminal filament. Male seed. SYN: *spermatozoon.*

seminal fluid. Semen.

seminal vesicle. One of two saclike structures in the male, lying behind the bladder close to the prostate and connected to the ductus deferens on each side. They secrete a thick viscous fluid that forms a part of the semen.

semination (sĕm-ĭ-nā′shŭn) [L. *seminatio,* a begetting]. Introduction of semen into the female genital tract. Occurs during sexual intercourse or may be introduced artificially. SYN: *insemination.*

s., artificial. Introduction of semen into the vagina or uterus by artificial means. SYN: *artificial insemination.*

seminiferous (sĕm-ĭn-ĭf′ĕr-ŭs) [L. *semen,* seed, + *ferre,* to produce]. Producing or conducting semen, as the tubules of the testes.

seminoma (sĕm″ĭ-nō′mă) [″ + Gr. *oma,* tumor]. A tumor of the testis.

seminormal (sĕm″ē-nor′măl) [L. *semis,* half, + *norma,* rule]. One half the normal standard.

seminormal solution. Solution having half the quantity of the substance in the normal solution. Indicated thus: 0.5 N or N/2.

seminose (sĕm′ĭ-nōs). Mannose.

seminuria (sē″mĭn-ū′rē-ă) [L. *semen,* seed, + Gr. *ouron,* urine]. Semen in the urine. SYN: *semenuria; spermaturia.*

semiology (sē″mē-ŏl′ō-jē) [Gr. *semeion,* sign, + *logos,* a study]. Phase of medicine dealing with study of symptoms. SYN: *semeiology; symptomatology.*

semiorbicular (sĕm″ē-or-bĭk′ū-lăr) [L. *semis,* half, + *orbiculus,* a small circle]. Semicircular.

semiotic (sē″mē-ŏt′ĭk) [Gr. *semeiotikos*]. Like or pert. to symptoms of disease. SYN: *semeiotic; symptomatic.*

semiotics (sē″mē-ŏt′ĭks). Scientific study of symptoms as a whole, or in one particular case. SYN: *semeiotics; symptomatology.*

semipenniform (sĕm″ē-pĕn′ĭ-form) [L. *semis,* half, + *penna,* feather, + *forma,* shape]. Penniform on one side.

semipermeable (sĕm″ē-per′mē-ă-bl) [″ + *per,* through, + *meare,* to pass]. Half permeable; said of a membrane that will allow fluids but not the dissolved substance to pass through it. SEE: *membrane; osmosis.*

semipronation (sĕm″ē-prō-nā′shŭn) [″ + *pronus,* prone]. A semiprone position.

semiprone (sĕm-ē-prōn′) [″ + *pronus,* prone]. In a position on left side and chest, with both thighs flexed on abdomen, the right higher than the left, and left arm back. SYN: *Sims′ position.*

semirecumbent (sĕm″ē-rē-kŭm′bĕnt) [″ + *recumbere,* to lie down]. Reclining, but not fully recumbent.

semis (sē′mĭs) [L.]. ABBR: ss. Half.

semisideratio, semisideration (sĕm″ē-sĭd-ĕr-ā′shē-ō, -ā′shŭn) [″ + *sideratio,* a blight]. Paralysis on one side of the body. SYN: *hemiplegia.*

semisopor (sĕm″ē-sō′por) [″ + *sopor,* deep sleep]. Light coma from which patient can be roused. SYN: *semicoma.*

semispinalis (sĕm″ē-spī-năl′ĭs) [L.]. Deep layer of muscle of back on either side of spinal column, divided into three parts. SEE: *Muscles* in *Appendix.*

semisulcus (sĕm″ē-sŭl′kŭs) [L *semis,* half, + *sulcus,* furrow]. A small sulcus or channel in a structure. It usually joins with another small channel to form a complete sulcus.

semisupination (sĕm″ē-sū-pĭn-ā′shŭn) [″ + *supinus,* bent back]. A position halfway between supination and pronation.

semisupine (sĕm″ē-sū′pīn) [″ + *supinus,* lying on the back]. Not completely supine.

semisynthetic (sĕm″ē-sĭn-thĕt′ĭk) [″ + Gr. *synthetikos,* synthetic]. Chemical alteration of a portion of a natural substance.

semitendinosus (sĕm″ē-tĕn″dĭn-ō′sŭs) [L.]. Fusiform muscle of posterior and inner part of thigh. SEE: *Muscles* in *Appendix.*

semitendinous (sĕm″ē-tĕn′dĭ-nŭs) [L. *semis,* half, + *tendinosus,* tendinous]. Being partially tendon.

senescence (sē-nĕs′ĕns) [L. *senescens,* growing old]. 1. The process of growing old. 2. The period of old age.

Sengstaken-Blakemore tube (sĕngz′tā-kĕn-blāk′mor). [Robert W. Sengstaken, U.S. neurosurgeon, b. 1923; Arthur H. Blakemore, U.S. surgeon, b. 1897] A three-lumen tube used to treat bleeding esophageal varices. One tube leads to the stomach; another to a balloon at the gastric end—it is used to inflate the balloon after the tube is in place; the third lumen leads to an inflatable cuff around a portion of the entire tube. This latter lumen allows the cuff to be inflated and provide pressure against the varices. The gastric balloon permits the balloon to resist being inadvertently removed and to keep the entire tube in place.

senile (sē′nīl, sĕn′īl) [L. *senilis,* old]. Pert. to growing old and the mental or physical weakness with which it is sometimes associated.

senilism (sē′nĭl-ĭzm, -nĭl-ĭzm) [″ + Gr. *ismos,* condition]. Old age, particularly when premature. SEE: *progeria.*

senility (sē-nĭl′ĭ-tē) [L. *senilis,* old]. Mental or physical weakness that may be associated with old age.

s., premature. Onset of senile characteristics before old age, as early as 40 years.

s., psychosis of. Mental disorder in old age.

senium (sē′nē-ŭm) [L.]. Old age, esp. its debility.

senna (sĕn′ă) [Arabic *sana*]. USP. The dried leaves of the plant Cassia acutifolia and C. angustifolia. Used as a cathartic.

sennosides A and B (sĕn′ō-sīdz). USP. Anthraquinone glucosides present in senna that are used as cathartics. Trade name is Glysennid.

senopia (sĕn-ō′pē-ă, sē-nō′-) [L. *senilis,* old, + Gr. *ops,* eye]. Improvement in near vision of old people. Usually precedes the development of nuclear cataract. SYN: *gerontopia.*

sensation (sĕn-sā′shŭn) [L. *sensatio*]. A feeling or awareness of conditions within or without the body resulting from the stimulation of sensory receptors.

s., cincture. S., girdle.

s., cutaneous. Sensation arising from receptors of the skin.

s., delayed. Sensation not experienced immediately following a stimulus.

s., epigastric. A sinking feeling in the stomach.

s., external. Effect upon the mind of stimuli produced from a source outside the body.

s., girdle. A painful sensation, as a bandage tightened about a limb or the trunk as in spinal disease. SYN: *zonesthesia.*

s., gnostic. One of the more finely developed senses such as touch, tactile discrimination, position sense, and vibration.

s., internal. S., subjective.

s., palmesthetic. Sensation felt in the skin from vibration.

s., primary. The sensation that results from a direct stimulus.

s., proprioceptive. Proprioceptive sensation. This use is inappropriate because this sense rarely is at the conscious level.

s., referred. Sensation that seems to arise from a source other than the actual one. SYN: *s., reflex.*

s., reflex. S., referred.

s., somesthetic. Sense, proprioception.

s., subjective. Sensation that does not result from any external stimulus and is perceptible only by the subject. SYN: *s., internal.*

s., tactile. Sensation produced through the sense of touch.

sense (sĕns) [L. *sensus,* a feeling]. 1. To perceive through a sense organ. 2. The general faculty by which conditions outside or inside the body are perceived. 3. Any special faculty of sensation connected with a particular organ. 4. Normal power of understanding.

The most important of the senses are sight, hearing, smell, taste, touch and pressure, temperature, weight, resistance and tension (muscle sense), pain, position, proprioception, visceral and sexual sensations, equilibrium, and hunger and thirst.

s., color. The perception of various colors.

s., kinesthetic. S., muscular.

s., light. Perception of degree of light.

s., muscular. Consciousness of muscular movement required in a given act. SYN: *s., kinesthetic.*

s., posture. Ability through muscle sense to differentiate positions of the body or its structures.

s., pressure. Faculty of feeling various degrees of pressure on the body surface. SYN: *baresthesia.*

s., proprioception. The correlation of unconscious sensations from the skin and joints that allows conscious appreciation of the position of the body.

s., sixth. General feeling of normal functioning of the body in general. SYN: *cenesthesia.*

s., space. That sense by which we recognize objects in space, their relationship, and dimensions.

s.'s, special. The five senses of sight, hearing, smell, touch, and taste.

s., static. The sense that makes it possible to maintain equilibrium.

s., stereognostic. Ability to judge consistency and shape of objects held in the fingers.

s., temperature. Ability to detect differences of temperature.

s., time. Ability to detect differences in time intervals.

s., tone. Ability to distinguish between different tones.

s., visceral. Subjective perception of the

sensations of the internal organs.

sensibility (sĕn″sĭ-bĭl′ĭ-tē) [L. *sensibilitas*]. Capacity to receive and respond to stimuli.

s., deep. 1. The sensibility existing after an area of the skin is made anesthetic. 2. Sensation by which the position of a limb and estimation of difference in weight and tension are apparent.

s., mesoblastic. S., deep.

s., palmesthetic. The sensibility existing in the skin to vibration.

sensibilization (sĕn″sĭ-bĭl-ĭz-ā′shŭn). 1. The process of making sensitive; sensitization. 2. Production of hypersusceptibility to a foreign substance by injecting it into the body. SYN: *sensitization.*

sensible (sĕn′sĭ-bl) [L. *sensibilis,* feeling]. 1. Capable of being perceived by the senses; perceptible. 2. Capable of receiving sensations. SYN: *sensitive.* 3. Having reason.

sensiferous (sĕn-sĭf′ĕr-ŭs) [L. *sensus,* a feeling, + *ferre,* to bear]. Causing, conducting, or transmitting sensations.

sensigenous (sĕn-sĭj′ĕn-ŭs) [″ + Gr. *gennan,* to produce]. Causing or starting a sensory impulse.

sensimeter (sĕn-sĭm′ĕ-tĕr) [″ + Gr. *metron,* measure]. Machine for recording the degree of sensitiveness of various areas of the body.

sensitinogen (sĕn″sĭ-tĭn′ō-jĕn) [″ + Gr. *gennan,* to produce]. The collective of antigens which sensitize the body.

sensitive (sĕn′sĭ-tĭv) [L. *sensitivus*]. 1. Capable of transmitting a sensation. 2. Able to feel a sensation. 3. Subject to destructive action of a complement. 4. Susceptible to suggestions, as a hypnotic. 5. Abnormally susceptible to a substance, as a drug or foreign protein. SEE: *allergy.*

sensitivity tests, antimicrobial. Laboratory method of determining the susceptibility of the patient's bacterial infection to antibiotics or antibacterials. The specimen obtained from the patient is cultured in various liquid dilutions of the drugs or on solid media containing various concentrations of the drugs in disks placed on the surface of the media. The disk-type test is not completely reliable.

sensitivity training. A form of group therapy wherein individuals are given the opportunity to relate verbally and physically with complete candor and honesty with other members of the group. The goals of therapy are to increase self-awareness, learn constructive ways of dealing with conflicts, establish a better sense of inner direction, and to relate to persons with warmth and affection.

sensitization (sĕn″sĭ-tĭ-zā′shŭn). 1. A condition of being made sensitive to a specific substance (i.e., antigen) such as a protein or pollen. 2. Process of making a person susceptible to a substance by repeated injections of it.

s., active. Sensitization produced by injecting an antigen into a susceptible person.

s., autoerythrocyte. A syndrome characterized by spontaneous appearance of painful ecchymoses, usually at a site of a bruise. The areas itch and burn. The lesions may come and go, and in general, they are benign. The cause is assumed to be due to autosensitivity to a component of the red blood cell membrane. There is no specific therapy.

s., passive. The production of sensitization in a normal person by injecting the person with the serum from a sensitized animal or man.

s., protein. Sensitization as a result of previous injection of a foreign protein into the body.

sensitized (sĕn′sĭ-tīzd). Made susceptible to a specific substance.

sensitized vaccine. A live culture that has been mixed with its antiserum before introduction.

sensitizer (sĕn′sĭ-tī″zĕr) [L. *sensitivus,* feeling]. In allergy and dermatology, a substance that makes the susceptible individual react to the same or other irritants.

sensitometer (sĕn″sĭ-tŏm′ĕt-ĕr) [″ + Gr. *metron,* a measure]. Device for determining the penetrating power of light.

sensomobile (sĕn″sō-mō′bĭl) [L. *sensus,* sense, + *mobilis,* mobile]. Movement in response to a stimulus.

sensomobility (sĕn″sō-mō-bĭl′ĭ-tē) [″ + *mobilitas,* mobility]. The capacity for movement in response to a stimulus.

sensomotor. Sensorimotor, q.v.

sensorial (sĕn-sō′rē-ăl) [L. *sensorialis*]. Pert. to the sensorium, the seat of sensation.

sensoriglandular (sĕn″sō-rē-glănd′dū-lăr) [L. *sensus,* sense, + *glandula,* little acorn]. Concerning glandular excretion in response to stimulation of a nerve.

sensorimetabolism (sĕn″sō-rē-mĕ-tăb′ō-lĭzm) [″ + Gr. *metaballein,* to alter, + *-ismos,* condition]. Metabolic activity in response to sensory nerve stimulation.

sensorimotor (sĕn″sō-rē-mō′tor) [L. *sensus,* sense, + *motor,* motion]. Both sensory and motor. SYN: *sensomotor.*

sensorimuscular (sĕn″sō-rē-mŭs′kū-lăr) [″ + *muscularis,* muscular]. Muscular activity in response to a sensory stimulus.

sensorineural (sĕn″sō-rē-nū′răl) [″ + *neuralis,* neural]. Concerning a sensory nerve.

sensorium (sĕn-sor′ē-ŭm) [L., organ of sensation]. (pl. *sensoriums, sensoria*) 1. That portion of the brain that functions as a center of sensations. 2. The sensory apparatus of the body taken as a whole.

sensorivasomotor (sĕn″sō-rē-văs″ō-mō′tor) [L. *sensus,* sense, + *vas,* vessel, + *motor,* a mover]. Vascular changes induced by sensory nerve stimulation.

sensory (sĕn′sō-rē) [L. *sensorius*]. 1. Conveying impulses from sense organs to the reflex or higher centers. SYN: *afferent.* 2. Pert. to sensation.

sensory amusia. Musical deafness; inability to comprehend music or musical sounds.

sensory aphasia. Inability to understand written or spoken words.

sensory area. Any area of the cerebral cortex in which sensations are perceived.

s.a., somesthetic. Area occupying the postcentral gyrus of the cerebral cortex and extending into adjacent areas in which sensations of general somatic sensibility are perceived.

sensory deprivation. Enforced absence of usual and accustomed sensory stimuli. Ex.: patients whose eyes are bandaged for extended periods following eye surgery, patients in respirators, astronauts, those who are isolated as would be the case of a sailor adrift alone following an accident, or those imprisoned in completely dark and soundproof cells. The absence of normal stimuli will, if continued, lead to severe mental changes including auditory and visual hallucinations, anxiety, depression, and insanity.

In psychological experimentation, sensory deprivation is achieved by confining a volunteer in a small soundproof room while wearing gloves, an eye mask, and ear muffs. Deprivation may also be produced by immersing an individual equipped for underwater breathing in a tank of water that is devoid of stimuli except for the sound of breathing.

sensory ending. A termination of an afferent nerve fiber that upon stimulation gives rise to a sensation. SEE: *receptor, sensory.*

sensory epilepsy. Disturbances of sensation that replace epileptic convulsions.

sensory integration. Skill and performance required in the development and coordination of sensory input, motor output, and sensory feedback. Includes sensory awareness, visual spatial awareness, body integration, balance, bilateral motor coordination, visual-motor integration, praxis, and other components.

sensory nerve. An afferent nerve conveying sensory impulses to the sensorium, or one composed of sensory fibers.

sensory unit. A single sensory nerve fiber with all its branches and their terminal nerve endings.

sensual (sĕn′shū-ăl) [L. *sensus,* sense]. Concerning or consisting in the gratification of the senses; indulgence of the appetites; not spiritual or intellectual; carnal, worldly.

sensualism (sĕn′shū-ăl-ĭzm). State or condition of being sensual; condition in which one's actions are dominated by emotions.

sensuous (sĕn′shū-ŭs) [L. *sensus,* sense]. 1. Pert. to or affecting the senses. 2. Susceptible to influence through the senses.

sentient (sĕn′shē-ĕnt) [L. *sentiens,* perceive]. Capable of perceiving sensation. SYN: *sensitive.*

sentiment (sĕn′tĭ-mĕnt) [L. *sentio,* to feel]. Feeling, sensibility, esp. susceptibility to tender feelings; an emotional attitude toward an object or a group of objects.

sentinel node. An enlarged supraclavicular lymph node. This may be the initial sign of cancer of the upper gastrointestinal tract, esp. of the stomach.

separation. The process of disconnecting, disuniting, or severing.

separator [L. *separator*]. 1. Anything that prevents two substances from mingling. 2. Any device or instrument used for bringing about a separation of two substances such as cream from milk.

separatorium (sĕp″ă-ră-tō′rē-ŭm) [L.]. Instrument for separating the pericranium from the skull.

sepsis (sĕp′sĭs) [Gr. *sepsis,* putrefaction]. Pathologic state, usually febrile, resulting from the presence of microorganisms or their poisonous products in the bloodstream. May be manifested as cellulitis (local dissemination of infection), lymphangitis or lymphadenitis (dispersion along lymphatic channels), or bacteremia (widespread dissemination by way of the bloodstream). The latter is commonly called blood poisoning. SYN: *bacteremia; septicemia.*

s., puerperal. Infection of the genital tract following childbirth. The infection may occur through exogenous or endogenous means. The organisms most commonly associated with this type of infection are streptococci, staphylococci, and Escherichia coli. SYN: *childbed fever.*

PATH: In minor cases of ulceration, the vaginal tract is covered by a dirty membrane. In streptococcal and staphylococcal infections, the endometrium is smooth and the lymphatics are congested with the invading organisms. As a rule, the uterine cavity is filled with very little lochia. The uterus shows poor involution. In the event that the infection extends further than the uterus, the parametrium or cellular tissues show edema, inflammation, and in some cases purulent infiltration. Extension of the process to the veins produces infectious thrombi, which in turn produce localized abscesses in other parts of the body.

SYM: Onset may be gradual or sudden. Patient begins to have general malaise, headache, chilly sensations or shaking chills, and rise in temperature. The uterus is tender and there is some abdominal distention.

COURSE: Early diagnosis and appropriate therapy will effectively control the course of the infection in most cases.

TREATMENT: Appropriate antibiotic and general measures include absolute bedrest, light or liquid diet, maintenance of fluid balance by parenteral injections if necessary, and analgesics for pain.

septa (sĕp'tă) [L. *saeptum,* a partition]. Pl. of septum.

septal (sĕp'tăl) [L. *saeptum,* a partition]. Concerning a septum.

septan (sĕp'tăn) [L. *septem,* seven]. Recurring every seventh day, as the paroxysms of malarial fever.

septate (sĕp'tāt) [L. *saeptum,* a partition]. Having a dividing wall.

septectomy (sĕp-tĕk'tō-mē) [" + Gr. *ektome,* excision]. Excision of a septum, esp. the nasal septum or a part of it.

septemia (sĕp-tē'mē-ă). Septicemia.

septic (sĕp'tĭk) [Gr. *septikos,* putrefying]. 1. Pert. to sepsis. 2. Pert. to pathogenic organisms or their toxins.

septicemia (sĕp-tĭ-sē'mē-ă) [" + *haima,* blood]. Presence of pathogenic bacteria in the blood. If allowed to progress, the organisms may multiply and cause an overwhelming infection and death. Symptoms and signs usually include chills and fever, petechiae, purpuric pustules, and abscesses. SYN: *blood poisoning.*

s., bronchopulmonary. Septicemia following entry, usually by aspiration, of infected material into the bronchi.

s., cryptogenic. Septicemia in which no primary focus of infection can be found.

s., fungal. Presence of pathogenic fungi in the blood. May be seen as a complication of parenteral hyperalimentation. SYN: *fungemia.*

s., puerperal. Septicemia occuring following prolonged and difficult labor or incomplete abortion. SYN: *puerperal sepsis.*

septicemic (sĕp-tĭ-sē'mĭk). Relating to, resulting from, or of the nature of septicemia.

septic fever. Fever or infection due to presence of pathogenic organisms or their products in the blood. SYN: *septicemia.*

septicophlebitis (sĕp"tĭ-kō-flē-bī'tĭs) [Gr. *septikos,* putrefying, + *phleps,* vein, + *itis,* inflammation]. Septic inflammation of a vein.

septicopyemia (sĕp"tĭ-kō-pī-ē'mē-ă) [" + *pyon,* pus, + *haima,* blood]. Septicemia and pyemia together.

septic shock. SEE: *shock, septic.*

septic sore throat. Streptococcal inflammation of the throat with fever and marked prostration.

septigravida (sĕp"tĭ-grăv'ĭ-dă) [L. *septem,* seven, + *gravida,* pregnant]. A woman pregnant for the seventh time.

septimetritis (sĕp"tĭ-mē-trī'tĭs) [Gr. *septos,* putrid, + *metra,* uterus, + *itis,* inflammation]. Inflammation of uterus due to sepsis.

septipara (sĕp-tĭp'ă-ră) [L. *septem,* seven, + *parere,* to bring forth]. A woman who has given birth seven times to an infant, alive or dead, weighing 500 gm. or more.

septivalent (sĕp-tĭ-vā'lĕnt, -tĭv'ă-lĕnt) [" + *valere,* to be strong]. Having a valence of seven or combining with or replacing seven hydrogen atoms.

septomarginal (sĕp"tō-măr'jĭ-năl) [L. *saeptum,* a partition, + *marginalis,* border]. Pert. to the margin or the border of a septum.

septometer (sĕp-tŏm'ĕ-ter). 1. [L. *saeptum,* a partition, + Gr. *metron,* measure] Calipers for measuring the width of the nasal septum. 2. [Gr. *sepsis,* putrefaction, + *metron,* a measure] Device for determining bacterial contamination of air.

septonasal (sĕp-tō-nā'zăl) [L. *saeptum,* a partition, + *nasus,* nose]. Concerning the nasal septum.

septoplasty (sĕp"tō-plăs'tē) [" + Gr. *plassein,* to form]. Plastic surgery of the nasal septum.

septostomy (sĕp-tŏs'tō-mē) [" + Gr. *stoma,* mouth]. Surgical formation of an opening in a septum.

septotome (sĕp'tō-tōm) [L. *saeptum,* a partition, + Gr. *tome,* incision]. An instrument for cutting or removing a section of the nasal septum.

septotomy (sĕp-tŏt'ō-mē) [" + Gr. *tome,* incision]. Incision of a septum, esp. the nasal septum.

septula (sĕp-tū'lă) [L.]. Pl. of septulum.

s. testis. [NA] Thin partition extending inward from mediastinum testis and separating testis into the lobuli testis.

septulum (sĕp'tū-lŭm) [L.]. (pl. *septula*) A small partition or septum.

septum (sĕp'tŭm) [L. *saeptum,* a partition]. (pl. *septa*) A wall dividing two cavities.

s., atrial. A wall between the atria of the heart.

s. atriorum cordis. A wall between the atria of the heart. SYN: *s., interatrial.*

s., atrioventricular. The septum that separates the right and left atria of the heart from the respective ventricles.

s., crural. S., femoral.

s., femoral. Connective tissue that closes the femoral ring.

s., interatrial. S. atriorum cordis.

s., intermuscular. 1. A connective tissue septum that separates two muscles, esp. one from which muscles may take their origin. 2. One of two connective tissue septa that separate the muscles of the leg into anterior, posterior, and lateral groups.

s., interventricular. S., ventricular.

s., lingual. A sheet of connective tissue separating the halves of the tongue.

s. lucidum. 1. A translucent septum, the interior boundary of lateral ventricles of the brain. SYN: *s. pellucidum* [NA]. 2. The stratum corneum layer of the epidermis.

s., mediastinal. Mediastinum.

s., nasal. The partition that divides the nasal cavity into two nasal fossae. Bony portion formed by the perpendicular plate of ethmoid and the vomer bone; cartilaginous portion formed by septal and vomeronasal cartilages and medial crura of greater alar cartilages.

s., orbital. A fibrous sheet extending partially across the anterior opening of the orbit and partially closing it.

s. pectiniforme. Comblike partition that separates the corpora cavernosa.

s. pellucidum. [NA] A thin triangular sheet of nervous tissue consisting of two laminae attached to the corpus callosum above and the fornix below. It forms the medial wall of the lateral ventricles. SYN: *s. lucidum.*

s. primum. In the primitive, embryonic heart, a septum between the right and left chambers.

s., rectovaginal. Partition between the rectum and the vagina.

s., rectovesical. The membraneous septum between the rectum and vagina.

s. scroti. [NA] Partition dividing the chambers of the scrotum.

s., ventricular. Partition between the ventricles of the heart. SYN: *s., interventricular.*

septuplet (sĕp'tŭ-plĕt) [L. *septuplum,* a group of seven]. One of seven children born from the same gestation.

sequel (sē'kwĕl) [L. *sequela,* sequela]. Sequela.

sequela (sē-kwē'lă) [L. *sequela,* sequel]. (pl. *sequelae*) A condition following and resulting from a disease.

sequence (sē'kwĕns) [L.]. The order or occurrence of a series of related events.

sequester (sē-kwĕs'tĕr) [L. *sequestrare,* to separate]. 1. To isolate. 2. A piece of necrosed bone separated from surrounding tissue. SYN: *sequestrum.*

sequestra (sē-kwĕs'tră) [L.]. Pl. of sequestrum.

sequestral (sē-kwĕs'trăl). Concerning a sequestrum.

sequestration (sē"kwĕs-trā'shŭn) [L. *sequestratio,* a separation]. 1. The formation of sequestrum. 2. Isolation of a patient for treatment or quarantine. 3. Reduction of hemorrhage of head or trunk by temporarily stopping the return of blood from the extremities by applying tourniquets to the thighs and arms.

s., pulmonary. A nonfunctioning area of the lung that receives its blood supply from the systemic circulation.

sequestrectomy (sē"kwĕs-trĕk'tō-mē) [" + Gr. *ektome,* excision]. Excision of a necrosed piece of bone.

sequestrotomy (sē"kwĕs-trŏt'ō-mē) [" + Gr. *tome,* incision]. Operation for removal of a sequestrum, a fragment of necrosed bone. SYN: *sequestrectomy.*

sequestrum (sē-kwĕs'trŭm) [L., something set aside]. (pl. *sequestra*) Fragment of a necrosed bone that has become separated from surrounding tissue. Designated primary if piece is entirely detached, secondary if still loosely attached, and tertiary if it is partially detached but still remaining in place.

sera (sē'ră) [L.]. Pl. of serum.

seralbumin (sēr-ăl-bū'mĭn) [L. *serum,* whey, + *albumen,* white of egg]. Albumin of the blood.

Serax. Trade name for oxazepam.

serendipity (sĕr"ĕn-dĭp'ĭ-tē). The gift of finding, by chance and wisdom, valuable or agreeable things not sought for. In medical research an unexpected reaction or result may produce new insights into some area totally unrelated to that which prompted the investigation.

Serenium. Trade name for ethoxazene hydrochloride.

Serentil. Trade name for mesoridazine besylate.

serial (sē'rē-ăl) [L. *series,* a succession]. In numerical order, in continuity or sequence, as in a series.

sericeps (sĕr'ĭ-sĕps) [L. *sericus,* silken, + *caput,* head]. Silk sac used in making traction on fetal head.

series (sēr'ēz) [L. *series,* a succession]. 1. Arrangement of objects in succession or in order. 2. In electricity, batteries or mode of arranging the parts of a circuit by connecting them successively end to end to form a single path for the current. The parts so arranged are said to be "in series."

s., aliphatic. Chemical compounds with a structure of an open chain of carbon atoms.

s., aromatic. Any series of organic compounds containing the benzene ring.

s., erythrocytic. The group of immature cells that develop into mature erythrocytes.

s., fatty. Aliphatic series, esp. those similar to methane.

s., granulocytic. The immature cells in

the bone marrow that develop into mature granular leukocytes.

s., homologous. In chemistry, compounds that proceed from one to the next by some constant such as a CH_2 group.

s., leukocytic. S., granulocytic, q.v.

s., monocytic. The immature cells that proceed to develop into the mature monocyte.

s., thrombocytic. The immature cells that proceed to develop into platelets.

serine. Two-amino-3-hydroxypropionic acid; an amino acid present in many proteins including casein, vitellin, and others. Found in the urine of normal human beings.

seriscission (sĕr-ĭ-sĭsh'ŭn) [L. *sericum,* silk, + *scindere,* to cut]. Division of soft tissues, as a pedicle, by tying a silk ligature around it.

sero- [L.]. Combining form pert. to serum.

seroalbuminuria (sē"rō-ăl-bū"mĭn-ū'rē-ă) [L. *serum,* whey, + *albumen,* white of egg, + Gr. *ouron,* urine]. Serum albumin in the urine.

serocolitis (sē"rō-kō-lī'tĭs) [" + Gr. *kolon,* colon, + *itis,* inflammation]. Inflammation of serous coat of the colon. SYN: *pericolitis.*

seroconversion. Development of evidence of antibody response to a disease or vaccine.

seroculture (sē'rō-kŭl-chūr) [L. *serum,* whey, + *cultura,* cultivation]. A bacterial culture on blood serum.

serocystic (sē"rō-sĭs'tĭk) [" + Gr. *kystis,* a cyst]. Composed of cysts containing serous fluid.

serodermatosis (sē"rō-der-mă-tō'sĭs) [" + Gr. *derma,* skin, + *osis,* condition]. Skin disease with serous effusion into tissues of the epidermis.

serodiagnosis (sē"rō-dī-ăg-nō'sĭs) [" + Gr. *dia,* through, + *gnosis,* knowledge]. Diagnosis by observing the reactions of blood serum.

seroenteritis (sē"rō-ĕn-tĕr-ī'tĭs) [" + Gr. *enteron,* intestine, + *itis,* inflammation]. Inflammation of serous covering of the intestine.

serofast (sē'rō-făst"). Serum-fast, q.v.

serofibrinous (sē"rō-fī'brĭn-ŭs) [" + *fibra,* fiber]. 1. Composed of both serum and fibrin. 2. Denoting a serofibrinous exudate.

serofibrous (sē"rō-fī'brŭs) [" + *fibra,* fiber]. Concerning serous and fibrous surfaces.

seroflocculation (sē"rō-flŏk"ū-lā'shŭn) [" + *flocculus,* little tuft]. Flocculation produced in serum by an antigen.

serohepatitis (sē"rō-hĕp-ă-tī'tĭs) [" + Gr. *hepar,* liver, + *itis,* inflammation]. Inflammation of the peritoneal covering of the liver.

seroimmunity (sē"rō-ĭ-mū'nĭ-tē) [" + *immunitas,* immunity]. Immunity produced by the administration of an antiserum.

serolipase (sē"rō-lĭp'ās) [" + Gr. *lipos,* fat, + *ase,* enzyme]. Lipase found in blood serum.

serologic, serological (sē-rō-lŏj'ĭk, -ăl) [" + Gr. *logos,* a study]. Pert. to or the study of sera.

serologist (sē-rŏl'ō-jĭst) [" + Gr. *logos,* a study]. One who has special knowledge and ability in serology.

serology (sē-rŏl'ō-jē) [L. *serum,* whey, + Gr. *logos,* a study]. The scientific study of serum.

serolysin (sē-rŏl'ĭs-ĭn) [" + Gr. *lysis,* dissolution]. A bactericidal substance or lysin found in the blood serum.

seroma (sēr-ō'mă) [" + Gr. *oma,* tumor]. A localized collection of serum that resembles a tumor.

seromembranous (sē"rō-mĕm'brăn-ŭs) [" + *membrana,* membrane]. Both serous and membranous; rel. to a serous membrane.

seromucous (sē"rō-mū'kŭs) [" + *mucus,* mucus]. Pert. to or composed of both serum and mucus.

seromuscular (sē"rō-mŭs'kū-lăr) [" + *muscularis,* muscular]. Concerning the serous and muscular coats of the intestines.

seronegative (sē"rō-nĕg'ă-tĭv). Producing a negative reaction to serological tests.

seroperitoneum (sē"rō-pĕr"ĭ-tō-nē'ŭm) [" + Gr. *peritonaion,* peritoneum]. Fluid in the peritoneum. SYN: *ascites; hydroperitoneum.*

seropositive (sē"rō-pŏz'ĭ-tĭv). Producing a positive reaction to serological tests.

seroprevention. Seroprophylaxis.

seroprognosis (sē"rō-prŏg-nō'sĭs) [" + Gr. *pro,* before, + *gnosis,* knowledge]. Prognosis of disease determined by seroreactions.

seroprophylaxis (sē"rō-prō-fĭ-lăks'ĭs) [" + Gr. *pro,* before, + *phylaxis,* protection]. Prevention of a disease by injection of serum. SYN: *seroprevention.*

seropurulent (sē"rō-pū'roo-lĕnt) [" + *purulentus,* full of pus]. Composed of serum and pus, as an exudate.

seropus (sē"rō-pŭs') [" + *pus,* pus]. A collection of serum and pus.

seroreaction (sē"rō-rē-ăk'shŭn) [" + *re,* back, + *actio,* action]. 1. Any reaction taking place in or involving serum. 2. Reaction to an injection of serum marked by rash, fever, pain, etc.

seroresistance (sē"rō-rē-zĭs tăns). Failure of a serum reaction to become negative or be reduced in titer following treatment.

seroresistant (sē"rō-rē-zĭs'tănt). The serum becoming positive after exposure to a pathogen and after being treated

serosa (sē-rō'să) [L. *serum,* whey]. A serous membrane. Examples are the peritoneum, pleura, and pericardium.

serosamucin (sē-rō"să-mū'sĭn) [L. *serosus,* serous, + *mucus,* mucus]. A mucinlike substance in ascitic fluid from inflamed sites.

serosanguineous (sē"rō-săn-gwĭn'ē-ŭs) [L. *serum,* whey, + *sanguineus,* bloody]. Containing or of the nature of serum and blood.

seroserous (sē″rō-sē′rŭs) [L. *serosus,* serous, + *serum,* whey]. Pert. to two serous surfaces.

serositis (sē″rō-sī′tĭs) [″ + Gr. *itis,* inflammation]. (pl. *serositides*) Inflamed condition of a serous membrane.

serosity (sē-rŏs′ĭ-tē) [Fr. *serosite*]. The quality of being serous.

serosynovial (sē″rō-sĭ-nō′vē-ăl) [L. *serum,* whey, + Gr. *syn,* with, + *oon,* egg]. Concerning serous and synovial material.

serosynovitis (sē″rō-sĭn″ō-vī′tĭs) [″ + Gr. *syn,* with, + *oon,* egg, + *itis,* inflammation]. Synovitis with increase of synovial fluid.

serotherapy (sē″rō-thĕr′ă-pē) [″ + Gr. *therapeia,* treatment]. The treatment of disease by the injection of blood serum, either human or animal, containing antibodies. This type of therapy is concerned with producing temporary artificial immunity in a person by injecting the blood serum of an animal that has acquired active immunity to the disease in question. SYN: *orotherapy.*

serotonin (sĕr″ō-tōn′ĭn). A chemical, 5-hydroxytryptamine (5-HT), present in platelets, gastrointestinal mucosa, mast cells, and in carcinoid tumors. Serotonin is a potent vasoconstrictor. It is thought to be involved in neural mechanisms important in sleep and sensory perception. SEE: *carcinoid syndrome.*

serotype (sē′rō-tīp). A microorganism determined by the kinds and combinations of constituent antigens present in the cells.

serous (sĕr′ŭs) [L. *serosus*]. 1. Having the nature of serum. 2. Producing a serous secretion, or containing serum or a serumlike substance.

serous cavity. A cavity lined by a serous membrane, specifically the pleural, peritoneal, and pericardial cavities.

serous cell. A cell that secretes a thin, watery, albuminous secretion.

serous effusion. Escape of serum into tissues or a body cavity.

serous exudate. Exudate consisting mostly of serum.

serous fluids. Liquids of the body, similar to blood serum, that are in part secreted by serous membranes.

serous glands. A gland secreting a watery, albuminous fluid, as the parotid gland.

serous inflammation. Inflammation of a part with serous exudate, or inflammation of a serous membrane.

serous membrane. A membrane lining a serous cavity.

serovaccination. A process with combined injection of serum, to secure immediate passive immunity, and bacterial vaccine, to acquire subsequent active immunity.

serovar. Subdivision of a species on the basis of its antigenic character. Previously called serotype.

serozymogenic (sē″rō-zī″mō-jĕn′ĭk) [L. *serum,* whey, + Gr. *zyme,* ferment, + *gennan,* to produce]. Pert. to a serous fluid and enzymes.

serpiginous (sĕr-pĭj′ĭ-nŭs) [L. *serpere,* to creep]. Creeping from one part to another.

serpigo (sĕr-pī′gō) [ME.]. Any creeping eruption, esp. ringworm, herpes, or tinea.

serrate (sĕr′āt) [L. *serratus,* toothed]. Notched; toothed. SYN: *dentate.*

Serratia (sĕr-ā′shē-ă). [Serafino Serrati, 18th-century It. physicist] A genus of bacteria of the family Enterobacteriaceae.

S. marcescens. Formerly called Chromobacterium prodigiosum, and erroneously believed to be nonpathogenic to man. Causes septicemia and pulmonary disease, esp. in immunocompromised patients. Found in water, soil, milk, and stools.

serration (sĕr-ā′shŭn) [L. *serratio,* a notching]. 1. Formation with sharp projections like the teeth of a saw. 2. A single tooth or notch in a serrated edge.

serratus muscle. Any of several muscles arising from the ribs or vertebrae by separate slips. SEE: *Muscles* in *Appendix.*

serrefine (sār-fēn′) [Fr.]. A small wire spring forceps for compressing bleeding vessels.

serrenoeud (sār-nŭd′) [Fr. *serrer,* to squeeze, + *noeud,* knot]. Device for tightening ligatures, esp. those placed on vessels in a deep cavity out of reach of fingers.

serrulate (sĕr′ū-lāt) [L. *serrulatus*]. Finely notched or serrated.

Sertoli's cells (sĕr-tō′lēz). [Enrico Sertoli, It. histologist, 1842–1910] Supporting elongated cells of seminiferous tubules that nourish spermatids.

serum (sē′rŭm) [L., whey]. (pl. *serums, sera*) 1. Any serous fluid, esp. the fluid that moistens the surfaces of serous membranes. 2. The watery portion of the blood after coagulation; a fluid found when clotted blood is left standing long enough for the clot to shrink. 3. Serum from an animal rendered immune against a pathogenic organism, to be injected into a patient with the disease resulting from the same organism. It consists of plasma minus fibrinogen.

s. albumin. A protein found in blood serum. SEE: *blood; protein, simple.*

s., anticrotalus. Serum used in treating rattlesnake poison.

s., antidiphtheritic. Serum used to counteract the effects of diphtheria.

s., antilymphocytic. ABBR: ALS. Serum used to reduce host rejection response to transplanted tissues. Produced by inoculating animals with certain tissues from other species.

s., antimeningococcus. Serum antagonistic to meningococcal infection.

s., antipneumococcus. Serum used in treating pneumococcal infection.

s., antitetanic. Serum given to counteract tetanus toxin.

s., antitoxic. Serum containing antitoxin.

s., antityphoid. Serum containing antibodies of the typhoid bacillus.

s., bactericidal. Serum having no effect on toxins but destructive to bacteria.

s., bacteriolytic. A serum containing a lysin that destroys certain bacteria.

s., blood. The clear liquid portion of blood without its fibrin and corpuscles. SEE: *plasma.*

s., convalescent. Blood serum from a person convalescing from an infection, the serum to be used in treating others having the same disease.

s., foreign. Serum from one animal injected into another animal of another species, or into man.

s., immune. A serum containing antibodies for specific antigens.

s., polyvalent. Serum containing antibodies to several types of the same bacterial species.

s., pooled. Mixed blood serum from several persons.

s., pregnancy. Blood serum from pregnant women.

s., pregnant mare's. Serum derived from the blood of pregnant mares; source of hormones, esp. chorionic gonadotrophin.

serum, words pert. to: agglutinin; agglutinogen; antigen; antitropin; antivenin; autoserodiagnosis; autoserotherapy; autoserous; autoserum; complement; icteric index; isohemagglutinin; opsonic index; opsonin; serology; serous.

serumal (sĕ-roo′măl) [L. *serum,* whey]. Rel. to serum.

serum-fast. Capable of resisting the destructive forces present in serum.

serum glutamic oxaloacetic transaminase. ABBR: SGOT. An intracellular enzyme involved in amino acid and carbohydrate metabolism. It is present in high concentrations in muscle, liver, and brain. An increased level of this enzyme in the blood indicates necrosis or disease in these tissues. SYN: *aspartate aminotransferase.*

serum glutamic pyruvic transaminase. ABBR: SGPT. An intracellular enzyme involved in amino acid and carbohydrate metabolism. It is present in high concentrations in muscle, liver, and brain. An increased level of this enzyme in the blood indicates necrosis or disease in these tissues. SYN: *alanine aminotransferase.*

serum protein. Any protein in blood serum. Serum protein forms weak acids mixed with alkali salts; this increases the buffer effects of the blood but to a lesser extent than cell protein.

serum rash. Rash first seen at site of an injection of serum. It remains thickest there, but it may invade other parts of the body. It resembles a combination of urticarial, morbilliform, and scarlatiniform rashes.

SYM: Severe irritation; marked swelling of skin, esp. of the face; malaise; and constitutional symptoms.

serum sickness. A hypersensitivity reaction that may occur from several days to 2 to 3 weeks after administration of antisera or following certain drug therapy.

SYM: Fever, enlarged lymph nodes and spleen, skin rash, and painful joints.

TREATMENT: Symptomatic and adrenal cortical hormones if needed.

servomechanism (sŭr″vō-mĕk′ă-nĭzm). In biology and physiology, a control mechanism that operates by negative or positive feedback. For example, when in the normal person the blood glucose level rises, the pancreas responds by releasing insulin, which enables the glucose to be metabolized. The level of hormones is also regulated by this mechanism when the anterior pituitary responds to the levels of hormones circulating in the blood.

SES. *socioeconomic status.*

sesame oil. Oil obtained from the seeds of Sesamum indicum. It is used as a pharmaceutical aid and as a cooking oil.

sesamoid (sĕs′ă-moyd) [L. *sesamoides*]. Resembling a grain of sesame in size or shape.

sesamoid bone. An oval nodule of bone or fibrocartilage in a tendon playing over a bony surface. The patella is the largest one.

sesamoid cartilage. One or more small cartilage plates present in fibrous tissue between the lateral nasal and greater alar cartilages of the nose.

sesamoiditis (sĕs″ă-moy-dī′tĭs) [″ + Gr. *itis,* inflammation]. Inflammation of a sesamoid bone.

sesqui- [L.]. Prefix meaning one and a half.

sesquihora (sĕs″kwĭ-hō′ră) [L.]. Every hour and a half.

sesquioxide (sĕs″kwē-ŏk′sīd). Any oxide in which three parts of oxygen combine with two atoms of another element.

sessile (sĕs′l) [L. *sessilis,* low]. Having no peduncle but attached directly by a broad base.

set. 1. To fix firmly in place, as to set a bone in reduction of a fracture. 2. To allow an amalgam or plaster to harden. 3. In psychology, a group of conditions or attitudes that favor the occurrence of a certain response.

seta (sē′tă) [L.]. (pl. *setae*) A stiff bristlelike

structure. SEE: *vibrissae.*

setaceous (sē-tā′shŭs) [L. *setaceus*]. Bristly, hairy; resembling a bristle.

Setchenov's inhibitory centers (sĕtch′en-ŏfs). [Ivan M. Setchenov, Russian neurologist, 1829–1905] Centers in the spinal cord and medulla oblongata involved in reflex inhibition of muscular and visceral activity.

setiferous (sē-tĭf′ĕr-ŭs) [L. *seta,* bristle, + *ferre,* to bear]. Having bristles.

setigerous (sē-tĭj′ĕr-ŭs) [″ + *gerere,* to carry]. Setiferous.

seton (sē′tŏn) [L. *seta,* a thread]. A thread or threads drawn through a fold of skin to act as a counterirritant or as a guide for instruments.

setose (sē′tōs). Having bristlelike appendages.

setup. The arrangement of teeth on a trial denture base.

seven-year itch. Scabies.

seventh cranial nerve. Facial nerve; nervus facialis. SEE: *cranial nerves.*

sevum (sē′vŭm) [L.]. Tallow or suet.

sewer gas. Gas produced by biodegradation of sewage. Contains methane and hydrogen sulfide. May be used for fuel. SEE: *carbon monoxide.*

sex [L. *sexus*]. 1. The characteristics that differentiate males and females in most plants and animals. 2. Motivation, both psychological and physiological, for behavior associated with procreation and erotic pleasure.

s., chromosomal. The sex as determined by the presence of the female XX or male XY genotype in somatic cells.

s., morphological. The sex of an individual as determined by the form of the external genitalia.

s., nuclear. The genetic sex of an individual determined by the absence or presence of sex chromatin in the body cells, particularly blood cells.

s., psychological. The individual's self-image of his or her gender. This may be at variance with the anatomical or morphological sex.

sex chromatin. Mass seen within the nuclei of normal female somatic cells. According to the Lyon hypothesis, one of the two X chromosomes in each somatic cell of the female is genetically inactivated. The sex chromatin represents the inactivated X chromosome. SYN: *Barr body.*

sex chromosomes. Chromosomes associated with determination of sex. In humans, these are the X (female) and Y (male) chromosomes. The normal female has two X chromosomes and the normal male has one X and one Y chromosome. SEE: *Barr body.*

sex clinic. Clinic for diagnosis and treatment of an individual or couple with sexual problems.

sexdigital (sĕks-dĭj′ĭ-tăl) [L. *sex,* six, + *digitus,* digit]. Having six fingers and toes.

sexduction (sĕks-dŭk′shŭn). Process of transfer of bacterial genes from one cell to another by means of the sex factors within which they are incorporated.

sexism. All of the actions and attitudes that relegate individuals of either sex to a secondary and inferior status in society.

sexivalent (sĕks″ĭ-vā′lĕnt, -ĭv′ăl-ĕnt) [″ + *valere,* to be strong]. Capable of combining with six atoms of hydrogen.

sex-limited. Expression of a genetic character or trait in one sex only.

sex-linked. A character that is controlled by genes on the sex chromosomes.

sexology [L. *sexus,* sex, + Gr. *logos,* study]. Scientific study of sexuality.

sex ratio. Ratio of females to males. Used in defining proportion of births of the two sexes or in the representation by sexual distribution in certain diseases.

sex surrogate. In sex therapy, the use of a surrogate sexual partner to assist in the therapeutic process.

sextan (sĕks′tăn) [L. *sextanus,* of the sixth]. Occurring every sixth day.

sextigravida (sĕks″tĭ-grăv′ĭd-ă) [L. *sextus,* six, + *gravida,* a pregnant woman]. A woman pregnant for the sixth time.

sextipara (sĕks-tĭp′ă-ră) [″ + *parere,* to bear a child]. A woman who has had six pregnancies that produced infants of 500 g. (or 20 weeks' gestation) regardless of their viability.

sextuplet (sĕks′tū-plĕt) [L. *sextus,* six]. One of six children born of a single gestation.

sexual (sĕks′ū-ăl) [L. *sexualis*]. 1. Pert. to sex. 2. Having sex.

sexual intercourse. Sexual union between a male and a female. SYN: *coition; coitus; copulation.*

RS: clitoris; coitus interruptus; dyspareunia; ejaculation; emission; excitation; orgasm; penis; semen; vagina.

s.i., homosexual. Sexual union between persons of the same sex.

sexuality (sĕks-ū-ăl′ĭ-tē) [L. *sexus,* sex]. 1. State of having sex; the collective characteristics that mark the differences between the male and the female. 2. Constitution and life of individual as related to sex; all the dispositions related to the love life whether associated with the sex organs or not.

sexually transmitted disease. Disease acquired as a result of sexual intercourse with an infected individual. A more inclusive term than venereal disease, including conditions such as syphilis, gonorrhea, lymphogranuloma venereum, chancroid, granuloma inguinale, and other conditions such as trichomoniasis, genital candidiasis, genital herpes, genital warts, and nonspecific urethritis, due to chlamydiae. SEE: *acquired immune deficiency syndrome; Reiter's syndrome; venereal disease.*

sexual reassignment. Legal, surgical, or social action or decision to assign the appropriate sexuality to an individual who has been considered previously to be of the opposite sex.

sexual reflex. Erection and ejaculation resulting from direct genital stimulation or indirectly from emotion, whether asleep or awake.

Sézary cell. [A. Sézary, Fr. dermatologist, 1880–1956] A cell, probably a lymphocyte, that contains an abundance of vacuoles filled with a mucopolysaccharide. Present in the blood of patients with Sézary syndrome.

Sézary syndrome. Skin disease characterized by infiltration with atypical Sézary cells. The exfoliative dermatitis is considered a variant form of mycosis fungoides.

SGA. *small for gestational age.*

S.G.O. *Surgeon-General's Office.*

SGOT. *serum glutamic-oxalacetic transaminase.* SEE: *transaminase, aspartate.*

SGPT. *serum glutamic pyruvic transaminase.* SEE: *transaminase, alanine.*

SH. *serum hepatitis.*

shadow [AS. *sceaduwe*]. A hemolyzed erythrocyte. SYN: *ghost corpuscle; phantom corpuscle.*

shadow-casting. A technique to increase the definition of the material being examined by use of electron microscopy. The object is sprayed from an oblique angle with a heavy metal.

shadowgram, shadowgraph [" + Gr. *graphein,* to write]. A print on a photographic plate exposed to x-rays.

shaft [AS. *sceaft*]. 1. The principal portion of any cylindrical body. 2. The diaphysis of a long bone.

s., hair. The keratinized portion of a hair that extends from a hair follicle beyond the surface of the epidermis. SEE: *hair.*

shakes (shāks) [AS. *sceacen*]. 1. Shivering caused by a chill, esp. in intermittent fever. 2. Colloquial term for state of tremulousness and extreme irritability often seen in chronic alcoholics. SYN: *jitters.*

shaking. A passive movement in Swedish massage.

shaking palsy. A basal ganglion disease with progressive rigid tremulousness, peculiar gait, muscular contraction, and weakness. SYN: *paralysis agitans; Parkinson's disease.*

shaman (shă′mŭn, shŏ′-) [Russ., ascetic]. One who heals or attempts to heal by the use of magic; one acting as both priest and doctor. SYN: *medicine man.* SEE: *shamanism.*

shamanism (shă′mŭn-ĭsm, shŏ′-). 1. Primitive religion of certain peoples of northern Asia who believe good and evil spirits pervade the world and can be influenced only by shamans acting as mediums. 2. Any similar form of primitive spiritualism, such as practiced among American Indian tribes.

shank (shăngk) [AS. *sceanca*]. The tibia or portion of leg from knee to ankle. SYN: *shin.*

shape (shāp) [AS. *sceapan*]. 1. To mold to a particular form. 2. Outward form; contour.

RS: aliform; arcate; arc form; arcuation; asteroid; bilateralism; bosselated; bosselation; bulbiform; calculus; caudate; circle; circumvallate.

sharkskin. Condition seen in pellagra (nicotinic acid deficiency) in which openings of sebaceous glands become plugged with a dry yellowish material.

Sharpey's intercrossing fibers (shăr′pēz). [William Sharpey, Scot. physiologist, 1802–1880] Fibers forming the lamellae constituting the walls of the haversian canals in bone.

Sharpey's perforating fibers. 1. Fibers extending from the periosteum into the lamellae of bone. 2. Fibers extending from the periodontal membrane into the cementum of a tooth.

shear (shēr). A force applied parallel to the planes of an object but opposite in direction to whatever force was present.

sheath (shēth) [AS. *sceath*]. A covering structure of connective tissue, usually of an elongated part, such as the membrane covering a muscle.

s., arachnoid. Delicate partition between pial sheath and dural sheath of the optic nerve.

s., axon. The myelin sheath or neurilemma. SEE: *s., myelin.*

s., carotid. Portion of cervical or pretracheal fascia enclosing the carotid artery, interior jugular vein, and vagus nerve.

s., crural. Fascial covering of femoral vessels.

s., dentinal. An obsolete term that was used when less complete microscopic information was available; no such sheath exists in dentin. It is an interface between peritubular and intertubular dentin that is apparent because of differing degrees of mineralization of the two areas, but it is of no significance and is not named. SYN: *s. of Neumann.*

s., dural. A fibrous membrane or external investment of the optic nerve.

s., femoral. The fascial covering of femoral vessels.

s., lamellar. Connective tissue sheath covering a bundle of nerve fibers. SYN: *s., nerve; perineurium.*

s., medullary. SEE: *s., myelin.*

s., myelin. Layers of lipid and protein substances that form a semifluid covering of nerves. The layers are an extension of the plasma membrane of the Schwann cell. The sheath is relatively insensitive to the action of temperature and electrolytes. SEE: *nerve fiber; neuron.*

s., nerve. S., lamellar.

s. of Henle. Sheath of Key and Retzius.

s. of Key and Retzius, connective tissue. Delicate reticular fibrils around individual nerve fibers.

s. of Neumann. An obsolete term. SEE: *s., dentinal.*

s. of Schwann. Membranous covering of myelin sheath of a nerve fiber.

s. of Schweigger-Seidel. The thickened wall of a sheathed artery of the spleen.

s., pial. Extension of the pia, closely investing surface of the optic nerve.

s., root. The layers of a hair follicle derived from the epidermis. Includes the outer root sheath, which is a continuation of the stratum germinativum, and the inner root sheath, which consists of three layers of cells closely investing the root of the hair. SEE: *hair.*

s., synovial. A double-walled tubelike bursa that encloses a tendon. Consists of an inner visceral layer lying upon and adhering to a tendon and an outer parietal layer, the two being separated by a space filled with synovial fluid. Found esp. in the hands and feet where tendons are confined to osteofibrous canals or pass over bony surfaces.

s., tendon. A dense fibrous sheath that confines a tendon to an osseous groove converting it into an osteofibrous canal. Found principally in the wrist and ankle. SEE: *s., synovial.*

shedding [ME. *sheden,* shed]. 1. The loss of deciduous teeth. 2. Casting off of surface layer of the epidermis. 3. Loss of bacteria from the skin.

Sheehan's syndrome. Hypopituitarism resulting from an infarct of the pituitary following postpartum shock or hemorrhage. Damage to the anterior pituitary gland causes partial to complete loss of thyroid, adrenocortical, and gonadal function.

sheep cell agglutination test. ABBR: SCAT. A test for rheumatoid factor in serum. Sheep erythrocytes sensitized with rabbit antisheep erythrocyte immune globulin will be agglutinated if serum containing the rheumatoid factor is added.

sheet (shēt) [AS. *sciete,* cloth]. Linen or cotton bedcovering next to the sleeper.

s., draw. A sheet folded under a patient so it may be withdrawn without lifting the patient. This is accomplished by turning the patient to the side of the bed to allow one side of the sheet to be removed and replaced with a clean one. The patient is then turned to the other side of the bed. The soiled sheet is removed and placement of the clean one is completed. SEE: *draw sheet.*

s., lift. A sheet folded under a patient over the bottom sheet to assist with moving the patient up in bed.

shelf. Any shelf-like structure.

s., dental. The epithelial invagination formed by the dental ridge. The dental papillae are formed beneath this shelf.

shelf-life. The time a food may be kept on a store shelf and still be considered safe to eat.

shell. A hard covering, as that for an egg or turtle.

shellac (shĕ-lăk'). A refined resinous substance obtained from plants that contain the secretions of certain insects. It is used in paints, varnishes, and as a coating for pills.

shell shock. An obsolete term used during World War I to designate a wide variety of psychotic and neurotic disorders associated with the stress of combat. SEE: *hysteria.*

Shenton's line (shĕn'tŏnz). [Thomas Shenton, Brit. radiologist] A radiographic line used to determine the relationship of the head of the femur to the acetabulum. The line follows the inferior border of the ramus of the pubic bone and continued outward follows the curve down the medial border of the neck of the femur.

shield (shēld) [AS. *scild,* shield]. 1. Any protecting device. 2. In biology, a protective plate or hard outer covering.

s., embryonic. The two-layered blastoderm or blastodisk from which a mammalian embryo develops. SYN: *disk, embryonic.*

s., nipple. A cover to protect sore nipples of a nursing woman.

s., phallic. An antiseptic covering for the male genitals during operations.

shift [AS. *sciftan,* to arrange]. A change in position or direction.

s., chloride. The shift of chloride ions from the plasma into red blood cells upon the addition of carbon dioxide from the tissues and the reverse movement when carbon dioxide is released in the lungs. It is a mechanism for maintaining constant pH of the blood.

s. to the left. Arneth's term for an increase in the number of young polymorphonuclear leukocytes in the blood. SEE: *Arneth's classification of neutrophils.*

s. to the right. Arneth's term for an increase in the number of older polymorphonuclear leukocytes in the blood. SEE: *Arneth's classification of neutrophils.*

Shiga's bacillus (shē'găs). [Kiyoshi Shiga, Japanese physician, 1870–1957] The bacillus causing a form of dysentery. SYN: *Shigella dysenteriae.*

Shigella (shĭ-gĕl'lă). [Kiyoshi Shiga] A genus of non-lactose-fermenting, nonmotile, gram-negative rods belonging to the family Enterobacteriaceae. It contains a number of species that cause digestive disturbance ranging from mild diarrhea to a severe and often fatal dysentery. SEE: *dysentery, bacillary.*

S. boydii. The name of a species that causes acute diarrhea in man. SYN: *Group C dysentery bacilli.*

S. dysenteriae. Shiga's bacillus, a virulent form isolated during a severe epidemic of dysentery in Japan in 1896.

S. flexneri. The name of a species that is a frequent cause of acute diarrhea in man. SYN: *Group B dysentery bacilli.*

S. sonnei. The name of a species that is a frequent cause of bacillary dysentery. SYN: *Group D dysentery bacilli.*

shigellosis (shĭ″gĕl-lō′sĭs) [*Shigella* + *osis,* condition]. The disease produced by infection with Shigella.

shin (shĭn) [AS. *scinu,* shin]. Anterior edge of tibia, portion of leg between the ankle and knee. SYN: *shank.*

s., saber. Condition seen in congenital syphilis in which anterior edge of tibia is extremely sharp.

shin-splints. Pain in the anterior compartment of the tibia. It usually follows strenuous exercise. The cause is ischemia of the muscles in the compartment and minute tears in the tissues.

shin spots. Hyperpigmented and retracted scars of the skin on the anterior lower legs. Condition is usually, but not always, associated with diabetes.

shingles (shĭng′lz) [L. *cingulus,* a girdle]. Eruption of acute, inflammatory, herpetic vesicles on the trunk of the body along a peripheral nerve; occasionally elsewhere. SYN: *herpes zoster,* q.v.

ship fever. A general term indicating a fever due to unhygienic conditions aboard ship, usually typhus fever and occasionally yellow fever.

Shirodkar operation. [Shirodkar, contemporary Indian physician] Surgical placement of a purse-string suture around an incompetent cervical os to attempt to prevent premature onset of labor. The suture material used for this cerclage procedure is nonabsorbable and must be removed prior to delivery.

shiver (shĭv′ĕr) [ME. *chiveren*]. 1. A slight tremor of the skin, as from cold or fear. 2. To tremble or shake.

shock (shŏk) [ME. *schokke*]. A clinical syndrome in which the peripheral blood flow is inadequate to return sufficient blood to the heart for normal function, particularly transport of oxygen to all organs and tissues. Shock may be caused by a variety of conditions including hemorrhage infection, drug reaction, trauma, poisoning myocardial infarction, and dehydration. Every injury is accompanied by some degree of shock and should be treated promptly. Syncope is caused by insufficient blood supply to the brain in certain persons and the clinical picture resembles shock. SEE: *catalepsy; insulin shock; septic shock; toxic shock syndrome.*

SYM: The most outstanding symptoms are marked paleness of the skin; evidence of decreased oxygenation of the skin as shown by cyanosis as the process continues; the face is pinched and without expression; there may be a staring of the eyes, which often lose their characteristic luster, and the pupils may be dilated; the pulse is weak and rapid; the breathing rate is increased and is shallow; the blood pressure is decreased and may be unobtainable; there may be urinary retention and incontinence of feces; occasionally there is an unusual restlessness or excitement; and very often the patient expresses an extreme thirst. If conscious, the patient seems quite disinterested in the surroundings and complains little of pain even though he or she may be groaning.

F.A.: Depends on diagnosis. In general, treat specific etiological factor and maintain body heat by warm but not hot blankets or water bottles. Keep body either flat or with head lower than feet. Do not move patient except to transport to a medical care facility. Give fluids sparingly but, in case of head injuries or suspected internal bleeding, do not give stimulants. Call a physician immediately.

TREATMENT: Maintain circulation by keeping patient lying down with head lower than body. The lower extremities can be slightly elevated by placing the lower half of the body on pillows, or by elevating the foot of the bed.

Patient should be kept comfortably warm, but application of external heat is not advisable. Avoid unnecessary questions and noises. Do not move patient unnecessarily.

Even though thirst is present, give fluids by mouth sparingly in order to reduce the possibility of vomiting and aspirating vomitus. If bleeding is present, it should be controlled. If internal hemorrhage is suspected or head injuries are present, no stimulants are permissible.

The use of hypodermics and intramuscular and intravenous injections such as epinephrine or ephedrine may be recommended by the doctor. Oxygen may be necessary. Blood transfusion or even artificial respiration may be required, depending on the seriousness of the condition.

Relieve pain by splints, posture, supporting bandages, and drugs. Morphine is valuable. Blood transfusions may be lifesaving. If blood is not available, artificial substances for increasing plasma volume may be used.

Respiration may be aided by administration of oxygen preferably mixed with 4 to 10% carbon dioxide as a respiratory stimulant. Constant, kindly, tactful encouragement and extreme gentleness in all procedures are of importance.

CAUTION: The shock syndrome is a serious life-endangering medical emergency and requires very careful therapy and monitoring. If the shock does not respond at once it is essential that the patient be treated and monitored in the best facility available, such as an intensive care unit. It is important that the ECG, arterial and central venous blood pressures, blood gases, core and skin temperatures, pulse rate, blood volume, blood glucose, hematocrit, cardiac output, urine flow rate, changes in size, shape, and reaction of pupils, and mental state be monitored as frequently as needed. An electroencephalogram may be required.

Artificial blood has been used experimentally in treating shock due to blood loss.

s., anaphylactic. Shock resulting from injection of protein substance to which patient is sensitized. SEE: *anaphylaxis.*

s., anesthesia. Shock due to an overdose of anesthesia. This calls for the immediate cessation of anesthesia. Artificial respiration, oxygen, and appropriate stimulants should be given at once. The condition is manifested by a weak rapid pulse, a fall or drop in blood pressure, cold clammy skin, and shallow respirations.

s., cardiogenic. Shock resulting from failure to maintain blood supply to the circulatory system and tissues because of inadequate cardiac output.

s., deferred. Late manifestation of shock following injury or burns. May appear in 3 to 30 hours and may be due to transportation, emotional stress, hemorrhage, dehydration, acidosis, or toxemia. SYN: *s., secondary.*

s., electric. Shock resulting from the passage of electric current through any part of the body.

s., endotoxin. Septic shock due to toxins from gram-negative bacteria. SEE: *s., septic.*

s., epigastric. Shock resulting from a blow or other trauma (surgery) in upper abdomen.

s., insulin. Shock resulting from an overdosage of insulin with subsequent hypoglycemia.

F.A.: Give orange juice, glucose, candy, lump of sugar. If unconscious, inject glucose intravenously. SEE: *insulin shock therapy.*

s., mental. Shock due to emotional stress or to seeing an injury or accident. SEE: *s., psychic.*

s., peptone. Shock reaction resulting from parenteral administration of a protein.

s., psychic. Shock due to excessive fear, joy, anger, grief. SEE: *s., mental.*

s., secondary. S., deferred.

s., septic. Shock caused by bacteria, esp. gram-negative bacteria, within the body. Generally seen in pelvic procedures that are not performed in a sterile manner, and in severe systemic infections. The client may appear cold and clammy as in "typical shock" or "hot and flushed." Hyperthermia generally develops.

s., serum. Shock occurring as part of a reaction to injection of serum.

s., spinal. Immediate flaccid paralysis and loss of all sensation and voluntary and involuntary reflex activity below the level of injury in acute transverse spinal cord injury.

s., surgical. Shock following operations and including traumatic shock. SEE: *shock, traumatic.*

s. syndrome, toxic. SEE: *toxic shock syndrome.*

s., traumatic. Shock due to injury or surgery. May occur as the result of abdominal injury from any cause. Shock is proportional to the extent of injury. Esp. severe in upper abdomen and more marked when viscera are damaged. If prolonged, indicates hemorrhage or peritonitis or both.

Cerebral injury: Concussion of brain or skull fracture. May come on immediately or later from edema or intracranial hemorrhage.

Chemical injury: Shock due to pain from the effect of chemicals, esp. corrosives.

Crushing injury: The greater the extent of injury the more severe the degree of shock.

Fracture: Esp. in compound fracture. Often extensive blood loss into tissues and hence circulation is impaired.

Heart damage: As in angina pectoris, myocardial infarctions, pericarditis, or myocarditis.

Inflammation: As acute general peritonitis or fulminating sepsis anywhere in the body.

Intestinal obstruction: Shock is present when obstruction is acute.

Nerve injury: Contusion of highly sensitive parts, as testicle, solar plexus, eye, urethra.

Operations: May occur even after minor operations, as paracentesis and catheterization.

Perforation or rupture of viscera: As in acute pneumothorax, ruptured aneurysm, perforated peptic ulcer, perforation in appendicitis, ectopic pregnancy.

Strangulation: As in hernia, intussusception, volvulus.

Thermal injury: As burns, frostbite, heat exhaustion.

Torsion of viscera: As of an ovary, testicle.

shock therapy. Form of treatment in mental illness. In electric shock therapy, convulsions are induced by passage of electric current through the brain, used chiefly in depression.

shoemakers' cramp. Spasm of muscles of hand and arm occurring in shoemakers.

Shohl's solution. A sterile solution of 140 gm. of citric acid and 90 gm. of sodium citrate dihydrate in one liter of water. Used in treating electrolyte disturbances, esp. in renal tubular acidosis.

shortsightedness (short-sīt'ĕd-nĕs). A condition of not being able to see very far, due to light rays coming to a focus in front of the retina. SYN: *myopia; nearsightedness.*

shotgun prescription. Prescription containing many drugs given with hope that one of them may prove effective. Not a recommended approach to the treatment of disease.

shoulder (shōl'dĕr) [AS. *sculdor*]. The junction of the clavicle and scapula where the arm meets the trunk. SEE: *scapula.*

s., dislocation of. Displacement of shoulder joint. Because dislocation of the shoulder is frequently accompanied by a fracture, surgeons advise making an x-ray examination of affected bones. Attempts to reduce dislocations without knowledge of fractures is very dangerous, sometimes resulting in serious paralysis of the entire upper extremity or grave damage to the large blood vessels in the armpit.

CAUSES: Usually the result of a fall on an outstretched arm or a blow to the arm in some unusual position. It is very common among athletes, esp. football and basketball players. A patient with a dislocated shoulder usually has a hollow in place of the normal bulge of the shoulder. There seems to be a slight depression at the outer end of the clavicle, and such patients cannot place their hand at their opposite shoulder while their elbow is on their chest. Always compare both sides.

F.A.: Send for a physician as soon as possible. Lay the patient on the back, with a pillow (or folded pad) between the shoulders. Place a large, soft pad under the elbow on the affected side, then bind the forearm horizontally across the chest using an open sling that is reinforced by a broad cravat bandage, and apply cold applications to the affected shoulder. Treat for shock if present.

shoulder blade. The scapula.

shoulder girdle. The two scapulae and two clavicles attaching the bones of the upper extremities to the axial skeleton i.e., the vertebrae of the backbone.

shoulder joint. Joint formed by humerus and glenoid cavity of the scapula

show (shō) [AS. *sceawian,* to look at]. The sanguinoserous discharge from the vagina during the first stage of labor or just preceding menstruation.

Shrapnell's membrane (shrăp'nĕls). [Henry J. Shrapnell, Brit. anatomist, 1761–1841] A small triangular portion of the tympanic membrane lying above the malleolar folds. It is thin and lax and attached directly to the petrous bone at the tympanic notch (notch of Rivinus) SYN: *pars flaccida*

shreds (shrĕds) [AS. *screade*]. Slender strands of mucus seen in freshly voided urine, indicative of inflammation of the urinary tract or associated organs.

shrink [from *headshrinker*]. Slang term for psychiatrist.

shudder [ME. *shuddren*]. A temporary convulsive tremor resulting from fright, horror, or aversion.

shunt (shŭnt) [ME. *shunten,* to avoid]. 1. To turn away from; to divert. 2. Anomalous passage or one artificially constructed to divert flow from one main route to another. 3. Electric conductor connecting two points in a circuit to form a parallel circuit through which a portion of the current may pass.

s., arteriovenous. An abnormal connection between an artery and the venous system.

s., cardiovascular. An abnormal connection between the cavities of the heart or between the systemic and pulmonary vessels.

s., left-to-right. Passage of blood from the left side of the heart to the right side through an abnormal opening, as in patent ductus arteriosus.

s., portacaval. Surgical creation of a connection between the portal vein and the vena cava.

s., postcaval. S., portacaval.

s., reversed. SEE: *s., right-to-left.*

s., right-to-left. Passage of blood from the right side of the heart to the left side through some abnormal opening such as a septal defect. The shunted blood has no opportunity to become oxygenated because of having failed to pass through the lungs.

Shy-Drager syndrome. [G. M. Shy, U.S. neurologist, 1919–1967; G. A. Drager, U.S. physician, 1917–1967]. Chronic orthostatic hypotension due to primary autonomic nervous system insufficiency.

SI. *Système International;* International System of Measurement. SEE: *SI Units* in *Appendix.*

Si. Chem. symb. for silicon.

siagonantritis (sī"ăg-ŏn-ăn-trī'tĭs) [Gr. *siagon,* jawbone, + *antron,* cavity, + *itis,* inflammation]. Inflammation of the maxillary sinus.

sial(o)- (sī'ă-lō) [Gr. *sialon,* saliva]. Combining form meaning saliva.

sialaden (sī-ăl'ă-dĕn) [" + *aden,* gland]. A salivary gland.

sialadenitis (sī"ăl-ăd"ĕ-nī'tĭs) [" + " + *itis,* inflammation]. Inflamed condition of a salivary gland.

sialadenoncus (sī"ăl-ăd"ĕ-nŏng'kŭs) [" + " + *onkos,* tumor]. Tumor of salivary gland.

sialagogue (sī-ăl'ă-gŏg) [Gr. *sialon,* saliva, + *agogos,* leading]. Agent increasing flow of saliva. Also spelled sialogogue.

sialaporia (sī"ăl-ă-pō'rē-ă) [" + *aporia,* lack]. Deficiency in secretion of saliva.

sialectasia, sialectasis (sī"ăl-ĕk-tā'sē-ă, sī"ă-lĕk'tă-sĭs) [" + *ektasis,* dilation]. Hypertrophy or swelling of the salivary glands.

sialemesis (sī"ăl-ĕm'ĕs-ĭs) [" + *emesis,* vomiting]. Vomiting of saliva or vomiting caused by an excessive secretion of saliva.

sialic (sī-ăl'ĭk). Concerning or resembling saliva.

sialine (sī'ă-līn) [Gr. *sialon,* saliva]. Concerning the saliva.

sialism, sialismus (sī'ăl-ĭzm, sī-ăl-ĭz'mŭs) [" + *-ismos,* condition]. An excessive secretion of saliva. SYN: *ptyalism; salivation.*

sialitis (sī"ă-līt'tĭs) [" + *itis,* inflammation]. Inflammation of a salivary gland.

sialoadenitis (sī"ă-lō-ăd"ĕ-nī'tĭs) [" + *aden,* gland, + *itis,* inflammation]. Inflammation of a salivary gland. SYN: *sialadenitis.*

sialoadenotomy (sī"ă-lō-ăd"ĕ-nŏt'ō-mē) [" + " + *tome,* incision]. Incision of a salivary gland.

sialoaerophagy (sī"ă-lō-ā"ĕr-ŏf'ă-jē) [" + *aer,* air, + *phagein,* to eat]. Constant swallowing, thus taking saliva and air into the stomach.

sialoangiectasis (sī"ă-lō-ăn"jē-ĕk'tă-sĭs) [Gr. *sialon,* saliva, + *angeion,* vessel, + *ektasis,* dilation]. Dilation of a salivary gland duct.

sialoangiography (sī"ă-lō-ăn"jē-ŏg'ră-fē) [" + " + *graphein,* to write]. Sialography.

sialoangitis, sialoangiitis (sī"ă-lō-ăn-jī'tĭs, -ăn"jē-ī'tĭs) [" + " + *itis,* inflammation]. Inflamed condition of the salivary ducts.

sialocele (sī'ă-lō-sēl) [" + *kele,* tumor]. Cyst or tumor of a salivary gland.

sialodochitis (sī"ă-lō-dō-kī'tĭs) [" + *doche,* receptacle, + *itis,* inflammation]. Inflamed condition of salivary ducts.

s. fibrinosa. Sialodochitis with duct obstructed by a fibrinous exudate.

sialodochoplasty (sī"ă-lō-dō'kō-plăs"tē) [" + " + *plassein,* to form]. Plastic surgery of a salivary gland.

sialoductitis (sī"ă-lō-dŭk-tī'tĭs) [" + L. *ductus,* duct, + Gr. *itis,* inflammation]. Inflamed condition of Stensen's duct.

sialogenous (sī"ă-lŏj'ĕ-nŭs) [" + *gennan,* to produce]. Forming saliva.

sialogogic (sī"ă-lō-gŏj'ĭk). Producing or promoting a secretion of saliva.

sialogogue (sī-ăl'ō-gŏg) [" + *agogos,* leading]. 1. An agent that stimulates the secretion of saliva. 2. Producing or promoting the secretion of saliva. Also spelled sialagogue. SYN: *ptyalagogue.*

sialogram (sī-ăl'ō-grăm) [" + *gramma,* mark]. A radiographic record of sialography, q.v.

sialography (sī"ă-lŏg'ră-fē) [" + *graphein,* to write]. Examination of salivary ducts and glands with x-rays. SYN: *ptyalography.*

sialolith (sī-ăl'ō-lĭth) [" + *lithos,* a stone]. A salivary concretion or calculus.

sialolithiasis (sī"ă-lō-lĭ-thī'ă-sĭs). Presence of salivary calculi.

sialolithotomy (sī"ă-lō-lĭ-thŏt'ō-mē) [Gr. *sialon,* saliva, + *lithos,* a stone, + *tome,* incision]. Removal of a calculus from a salivary gland or duct.

sialoncus (sī"ă-lŏng'kŭs) [" + *onkos,* mass]. A tumor under the tongue caused by obstruction of a salivary gland or duct.

sialoporia (sī"ă-lō-pō'rē-ă) [" + *aporia,* lack]. Deficient secretion of saliva.

sialorrhea (sī"ă-lō-rē'ă) [" + *rhoia,* a flow]. Excessive flow of saliva. SYN: *sialism.* SEE: *transtympanic neurectomy.*

sialoschesis (sī"ă-lŏs'kĕ-sĭs) [" + *schesis,* suppression]. Suppression or retention of saliva.

sialosemeiology (sī"ă-lō-sē"mī-ŏl'ŏ-jē) [" + *semeion,* sign, + *logos,* a study]. Diagnosis based upon examination of the saliva.

sialosis (sī-ă-lō'sĭs) [" + *osis,* condition]. The flow of saliva.

sialostenosis (sī"ă-lō-stĕ-nō'sĭs) [" + *stenosis,* a narrowing]. Closure of a salivary duct.

sialosyrinx (sī"ă-lō-sī'rĭnks) [" + *syrinx,* a pipe]. 1. Fistula into the salivary gland. 2. A syringe for washing out salivary ducts. 3. Drainage tube for a salivary duct.

sialotic (sī"ă-lŏt'ĭk) [Gr. *sialon,* saliva]. Concerning the flow of saliva.

Siamese twins (sī-ă-mēz'). [After Chang and Eng (1811–1874), joined Chinese twins born in Siam] Congenitally united twins. In some cases the individuals are joined in a small area and are capable of activity, but the extent of union may be so great that survival is impossible. Nevertheless, modern surgical techniques have made it possible to separate infants who would not in the past have been expected to survive and have a good prognosis. SEE: *twin.*

sib [AS. *sibb,* kin]. 1. A brother or sister. SYN: *sibling.* 2. A blood relative.

sibilant (sĭb'ĭ-lănt) [L. *sibilans,* hissing]. Hissing or whistling, as a sound heard in a certain rale, q.v.

sibilation. Pronunciation in which the hissing

sound is predominant.

sibilismus. A hissing sound.

s. aurium. Tinnitus.

sibilus (sĭb'ĭ-lŭs) [L. *sibilans*, hissing]. A hissing rale.

sibling (sĭb'lĭng) [AS. *sibb*, kin, + *-ling*, having the quality of]. One of two or more children of same parents; a brother or sister.

s., half. A half brother or sister.

sibship. Brothers and sisters of a single family.

siccant (sĭk'ănt) [L. *siccus*, dry]. Drying.

siccative (sĭk'ă-tĭv) [L. *siccativus*, drying]. Drying or that which dries. SYN: *siccant*.

sicchasia (sī-kā'shē-ă) [Gr. *sikchasia*, loathing]. Nausea.

siccolabile (sĭk"ō-lā'bĭl) [L. *siccus*, dry, + *labilis*, unstable]. Altered or destroyed by drying.

siccostabile (sĭk"ō-stā'bĭl) [" + *stabilis*, stable]. Resistant to drying.

siccus (sĭk'ŭs) [L.]. Dry.

sick (sĭk) [AS *seoc*, ill]. 1. Not well. SYN: *ill*. 2. Mentally ill or disturbed. 3. Nauseated.

sickle cell. Abnormal red blood corpuscle that has a crescent shape. SYN: *meniscocyte*.

sickle cell anemia. A hereditary chronic form of anemia in which abnormal sickle or crescent-shaped erythrocytes are present. Due to the presence of abnormal type of hemoglobin, hemoglobin S, in the red blood cells. The frequency of the gene that causes this disease is high in Mediterranean and African populations. SEE: *anemia; hemoglobin*.

sickle cell crisis. The sickled cells interfere with oxygen transport, obstruct capillary blood flow, and cause fever and severe pain in joints and the abdomen. The abdominal pain may simulate that caused by appendicitis or other indications for surgical intervention. The crisis is precipitated by decreased ambient oxygen as can occur during flying at high altitude without use of supplemental oxygen.

sicklemia (sĭk-lē'mē-ă) [AS. *sicol*, sickle, + Gr. *haima*, blood]. Sickle cells in the blood.

sickling. Tendency of red blood cells to be sickle shaped. SEE: *sickle cell anemia*.

sickness [AS. *seoc*, ill]. State of being unwell. SYN: *illness*.

s., bleeding. Abnormal tendency to bleed. SYN: *hemophilia*.

s., car. Nausea and malaise from riding in vehicles such as trains or automobiles. SYN: *motion sickness*.

s., falling. Epilepsy.

s., green. Form of anemia with greenish pallor. SYN: *chlorosis*.

s., morning. Nausea of early pregnancy.

s., motion. Nausea and vomiting caused by a variety of motions, such as those experienced on boats, airplanes, trains, automobiles, or rides in amusement parks.

s., mountain. Nausea and dyspnea caused by insufficient oxygen at high altitudes.

s., sea. Sickness caused by motion of a vessel while at sea.

s., serum. Sickness following injection of serum.

s., sleeping. 1. Infection with genus of Trypanosomes with involvement of central nervous system and ultimately continuous sleeping. The disease is transmitted by the bite of an infected Glossina, the tsetse fly. The disease can be transmitted congenitally. SYN: *trypanosomiasis*. 2. Acute infectious disease with increasing lethargy. SYN: *encephalitis lethargica*.

sick sinus syndrome. ABBR: SSS. Several electrocardiographic abnormalities due to malfunction of the sinoatrial node of the heart. These may include persistent sinus bradycardia that may alternate with tachyarrhythmias; sinoatrial block; and sinus arrest for brief or prolonged periods.

SYM: Lightheadedness, dizziness, fainting, dyspnea, fatigue, and angina pectoris.

TREATMENT: Insertion of a pacemaker; and anticoagulant therapy may be required to prevent thromboembolism.

S.I.D. *Society for Investigative Dermatology*.

side (sīd) [AS. *side*]. 1. Left or right part of trunk of the body. 2. An outer portion considered as facing in a particular direction.

side effect. The action or effect of a drug other than that desired. Commonly this is an undesirable effect such as nausea, headache, insomnia, acute toxic reaction, or drug interaction. SEE: *Drug Interactions* in *Appendix*.

side position. Position where patient is lying on one side, thighs flexed, with underarm behind back. SYN: *Sims' position*. SEE: *position* for illus.

sideration (sĭd-ĕr-ā'shŭn) [L. *siderari*, to be struck by a star]. 1. Therapeutic application of electric sparks. 2. A sudden stroke of disease, as in apoplexy. 3. Lightning stroke.

siderism, siderismus (sĭd'ĕr-ĭzm, sĭd-ĕr-ĭz'mŭs) [Gr. *sideros*, iron, + *-ismos*, condition]. Therapeutic application of metals to the skin. SYN: *metallotherapy*.

sidero- (sĭd'ĕr-ō) [Gr. *sideros*, iron]. Combining form meaning iron or steel.

sideroblast (sĭd'ĕr-ō-blăst") [" + *blastos*, germ]. A ferritin-containing normoblast in the bone marrow. They comprise from 20 to 90% of normoblasts in the marrow. The ferritin gives a positive Prussian-blue reaction, indicating the iron is ionized and not bound to the heme protein.

siderocyte (sĭd'ĕr-ō-sīt) [" + *kytos*, cell]. A red blood cell containing iron in a form other than hematin.

sideroderma (sĭd"ĕr-ō-dĕr'mă) [" + *derma*, skin]. Bronzed coloration of the skin from disordered hemoglobin disintegration.

siderodromophobia (sĭd″ĕr-ō-drō″mō-fō′bē-ă) [″ + *dromos,* a way, + *phobos,* fear]. Morbid fear of railway travel.

siderofibrosis (sĭd″ĕr-ō-fī-brō′sĭs) [″ + L. *fibra,* fiber, + Gr. *osis,* condition]. Fibrosis associated with deposits of iron.

siderogenous (sĭd″ĕr-ŏj′ĕ-nŭs) [″ + *gennan,* to produce]. Producing or forming iron.

sideropenia (sĭd″ĕr-ō-pē′nē-ă) [″ + *penia,* poverty]. Iron deficiency; deficiency of iron in the blood.

sideropenic (sĭd″ĕr-ō-pē′nĭk). Characterized by deficiency of iron in the blood.

siderophil (sĭd′ĕr-ō-fĭl). A cell that has affinity for iron.

siderophilin (sī′dĕr-ŏf″ĭ-lĭn). Transferrin, q.v.

siderophilous (sĭd″ĕr-ŏf′ĭ-lŭs) [″ + *philein,* to love]. Having a tendency to absorb iron, as the red blood corpuscles.

siderophone (sĭd′ĕr-ō-fōn). A telephone-like device used to detect intraocular, iron-containing foreign bodies.

siderophore (sĭd′ĕr-ō-for) [″ + *phoros,* bearing]. A macrophage that contains hemosiderin.

sideroscope (sĭd′ĕr-ō-skōp) [″ + *skopein,* to examine]. Instrument for finding particles of iron in the eye.

siderosis (sĭd″ĕr-ō′sĭs) [″ + *osis,* condition]. A form of pneumoconiosis resulting from inhalation of dust or fumes containing iron particles. SYN: *arc-welder's disease.* SEE: *hemosiderosis.*

s., hepatic. Accumulation of an abnormal amount of iron in the liver.

s., urinary. Hemosiderin granules in the urine.

siderosome (sĭd″ĕr-ō-sōm′) [″ + *soma,* body]. A reticulocyte in which iron-containing granules are present.

siderotic (sĭd″ĕr-ŏt′ĭk). Concerning siderosis.

SIDS. *sudden infant death syndrome.*

siemens (sē′mĕnz). The SI unit of electrical conductivity, the symbol for which is *mho,* i.e., ohm spelled backward.

Siemens' syndrome. [H.W. Siemens, Ger. physician, b. 1891] Ichthyosis congenita.

sieve (sĭv). A device consisting of a mesh with holes of uniform size. Used to separate particles above a certain size from solutions or powders.

s., molecular. A type of sieve in which the molecular material present in the gel or crystal will adsorb certain sized molecules and let others pass.

sig. An abbreviation for the Latin *signa,* meaning in prescription writing to label it.

Sigault's operation (sē-gōz′). [Jean René Sigault, Fr. obstetrician, b. 1740] Division of the symphysis pubis to facilitate childbirth by enlarging the pelvic outlet. SYN: *symphysiotomy.*

sigh [AS. *sican*]. A deep inspiration followed by a slow audible expiration.

sight (sīt) [AS. *sihth*]. 1. Power or faculty of seeing. 2. Range of sight. 3. A thing or view seen. SYN: *vision.*

s., day. Night blindness. SYN: *nyctalopia.*

s., far. Rays of light focusing behind the retina. SYN: *hypermetropia; hyperopia.*

s., near. Rays of light focusing before the retina. SYN: *myopia.*

s., night. Day blindness. SYN: *hemeralopia.*

s., old. Loss of accommodation of near point. SYN: *presbyopia.*

s., second. Alteration in refractive powers of the lens of the eye so that reading is again possible without glasses. May be caused by incipient cataract. SYN: *senopia.*

sight, words pert. to: achromatopsia; afterimage; alexia; amaurosis; amblyopia; ametropia; aniseikonia; anisocoria; anisoiconia; anisometropia; anorthopia; aprosexia; asthenopia; astigmatism; blindness; brachymetropia; cataract; gerontopia; hemeralopia; hypermetropia; hyperopia; myopia; night blindness; nyctalopia; -phoria words; photophobia; presbyopia; squint.

sigma (sĭg′mă). The eighteenth letter, Σ or σ, in the Greek alphabet.

sigmatism (sĭg′mă-tĭzm) [Gr. *sigma,* letter S, + *-ismos,* condition]. Excessive or defective use of "s" sounds in speech.

sigmoid (sĭg′moyd) [Gr. *sigmoeides*]. 1. Shaped like the capital Greek letter sigma, Σ. 2. Pert. to the sigmoid flexure of the colon.

sigmoidectomy (sĭg″moyd-ĕk′tō-mē) [″ + *ektome,* excision]. Removal of all or part of the sigmoid flexure.

sigmoid flexure. The lower part of the descending colon, between the iliac crest and the rectum, shaped like the letter S. SEE: *cecosigmoidostomy; colon.*

sigmoiditis (sĭg″moyd-ī′tĭs) [″ + *itis,* inflammation]. Inflammation of the sigmoid flexure of the colon.

sigmoidopexy (sig-moy′dō-pĕk″sē) [″ + *pexis,* fixation]. Fixation of the sigmoid to an abdominal incision for prolapse of the rectum.

sigmoidoproctostomy (sĭg-moy″dō-prŏk-tŏs′tō-mē) [Gr. *sigmoeides,* shaped like Gr. letter S, + *proktos,* rectum, + *stoma,* passage]. Establishment of artificial passage by anastomosis of the sigmoid flexure with the rectum.

sigmoidorectostomy (sĭg-moy″dō-rĕk-tŏs′tō-mē) [″ + L. *rectus,* straight, + Gr. *stoma,* passage]. Anastomosis of sigmoid flexure with the rectum to establish an artificial passage. SYN: *sigmoidoproctostomy.*

sigmoidoscope (sĭg-moy′dō-skōp) [″ + *sko-*

pein, to examine]. Tubular speculum for examination of sigmoid flexure.

sigmoidoscopy (sĭg″moy-dŏs′kō-pē) [″ + *skopein,* to examine]. Use of a sigmoidoscope to inspect the sigmoid colon.

sigmoidosigmoidostomy (sĭg-moy″dō-sĭg-moy-dŏs′tō-mē) [″ + *sigmoeides,* sigmoid, + *stoma,* mouth]. Surgical creation of a connection between two segments of the sigmoid colon.

sigmoidostomy (sĭg-moyd-ŏs′tō-mē) [″ + *stoma,* passage]. Creation of an artificial anus in the sigmoid flexure.

sigmoidotomy (sĭg-moyd-ŏt′ō-mē) [″ + *tome,* incision]. Incision of the sigmoid.

sigmoidovesical (sĭg-moy″dō-vĕs′ĭ-kăl) [″ + L. *vesica,* bladder]. Concerning a connection between the sigmoid colon and the urinary bladder.

sign (sīn) [L. *signum*]. 1. Symbol or abbreviation, esp. one used in pharmacy. 2. Any objective evidence or manifestation of an illness or disordered function of the body. Signs are more or less definitive and obvious, and apart from the patient's impressions, in contrast to symptoms, which are subjective. SEE: *symptom.*

s., objective. In physical diagnosis, a sign that can be seen, heard, measured, or felt by the diagnostician. Finding of such a sign(s) can be used to confirm or deny the diagnostician's impressions of the disease suspected of being present. SYN: *s., physical.*

s., physical. S., objective.

s.'s, vital. Those physical signs concerning functions essential to life, i.e., pulse, rate of respiration, blood pressure, and temperature.

signa (sĭg′nă) [L. *signa*]. ABBR: S or sig. A term used in writing prescriptions, q.v., meaning to label the subscription according to the dose and frequency of medication.

signature (sĭg′nă-tūr) [L. *signatura*]. The part of a prescription, q.v., giving instructions to the patient.

significant (sĭg-nĭf′ĭ-kănt). Important. In statistics, a difference is said to be statistically significant if the analysis indicates the results have little probability of having occurred due to chance.

significant others. Persons with whom a patient or client has a close relationship.

sign language. Representing words by signs made with the position and movement of the fingers and hand. SEE: *Sign Alphabet* in *Appendix.*

Silain. Trade name for simethicone, USP.

Silastic. Trade name for a silicone material that because of its inertness and compatibility with biological tissues is used in plastic surgery to help form body structures.

silent. Free from noise; mute; still.

silent disease. A disease that produces no clinically obvious symptoms or signs.

silent period. Period in a tendon reflex that immediately follows the contraction of the responding muscles during which the motor neurons do not respond to afferent impulses entering the reflex center.

silica (sĭl′ĭ-kă) [L. *silex,* flint]. SiO_2. Silicon dioxide.

silicate (sĭl′ĭ-kāt) [L. *silicus,* flintlike]. A salt of silicic acid.

siliceous, silicious (sĭ-lĭsh′ŭs). Containing silica.

silicic (sĭl-ĭs′ĭk). Pert. to silica or silicon.

silicoanthracosis (sĭl″ĭ-kō-ăn″thră-kō′sĭs) [L. *silex,* flint, + Gr. *anthrax* coal, + *osis,* condition]. Silicosis combined with anthracosis, in coal miners.

silicofluoride (sĭl″ĭ-kō-floo′ō-rīd). A compound of silicon, fluorine, and the fluoride of a metal.

silicon (sĭl′ĭ-kŏn) [L. *silex,* flint]. SYMB: Si. At. wt. 28.086; at. no. 14; sp. gr. 2.33. A nonmetallic element found in the soil. Silicon comprises approximately 25% of the earth's crust, being exceeded only by oxygen. It occurs in traces in skeletal structures (bones and teeth). Silicon is commonly combined with oxygen to form silicon dioxide, SiO_2, which occurs in many forms, both crystalline and amorphous. In a pure state it forms quartz or rock crystal. It is present in many abrasive materials and is the principal constituent of glass.

silicone (sĭl′ĭ-kōn″). 1. An organic compound in which carbon has been replaced by silicon. 2. Any of a group of polymeric organic silicon compounds. Used in adhesives, lubricants, synthetic rubber, and prostheses.

s., injectable. Medical-grade silicone compounds suitable for implantation in the body. Used in plastic surgery. Use of nonmedical-grade silicone for cosmetic breast augmentation has produced unfortunate results.

silicosiderosis (sĭl″ĭ-kō-sĭd″ĕr-ō′sĭs) [″ + Gr. *sideros,* iron, + *osis,* condition]. A type of pneumonoconiosis in which the inhaled particles contain silicates and iron.

silicosis (sĭl-ĭ-kō′sĭs) [″ + Gr. *osis,* condition]. A form of pneumoconiosis resulting from inhalation of silica (quartz) dust, characterized by formation of small discrete nodules. In advanced cases, a dense fibrosis and emphysema with impairment of respiratory function may develop.

silicotic (sĭl-ĭ-kŏt′ĭk). 1. Relating to silicosis. 2. One affected with silicosis.

silicotuberculosis (sĭl″ĭ-kō-tū-bĕr-kū-lō′sĭs) [″ + *tuberculus,* a tubercle, + Gr. *osis,* condition]. Silicosis associated with pulmonary tuberculosis.

siliquae olivae (sĭl′ĭ-kwē ŏl′ĭ-vē) [L.]. Fibers

that appear to encircle the olive of the brain.

siliquose (sĭl'ĭ-kwōs) [L. *siliqua*, pod]. Resembling a two-valve capsule or a pod.

siliquose cataract. Cataract with a dry, wrinkled capsule.

siliquose desquamation. Shedding of dried vesicles from the skin.

silo-filler's disease. Damage to the lungs produced in silo workers wherein they are exposed to nitrogen dioxide and nitric acid. These gases are produced by the fermenting organic matter in the silo.

Silvadene. Trade name for silver sulfadiazine.

silver (sĭl'vĕr) [AS. *siolfor*]. SYMB: Ag. At. wt. 107.870; at. no. 47; sp. gr. 10.5. A white, soft, ductile malleable metal, its salts being widely used in medicine for their caustic, astringent, and antiseptic effects. SEE: *argyria.*

s. chloride. SYMB: AgCl. An insoluble salt of silver.

s., colloidal. Silver preparations in which the particles of silver or silver proteinate are suspended in the solution rather than being dissolved in it.

s. nitrate. USP. $AgNO_3$. A toxic preparation made from silver. Most of its former uses have passed out of vogue, but it remains important as a germicide and local astringent.

INCOMPAT: Aspirin, sodium chloride. SEE: *silver nitrate poisoning.*

s. nitrate, toughened. USP. A mixture of silver nitrate and silver chloride used as a caustic on wounds and granulation tissue, and in treating warts.

s. picrate. A compound of silver and picric acid, containing 30% silver. Useful as an antiseptic, similar to other preparations of silver.

s. protein. A combination of silver and protein, containing from 7.5 to 8.5% (strong) silver.

s. sulfadiazine. A medicine used topically in treating burns of the skin. It is composed of silver and sulfadiazine. Trade name is Silvadene.

silver fork deformity. Deformity in Colles' fracture of wrist and hand resembling curve on back of a fork.

silver nitrate poisoning. When taken by mouth, silver nitrate causes a grayish discoloration of mucous membranes.

SYM: Burning in throat and stomach; rather prompt vomiting. When small amounts of silver are taken over a long period, as in nose or eye drops, patient develops argyria, a peculiar bluish discoloration of all the exposed tissues of body including the gingiva.

F.A.: Large volumes of ordinary table salt in water precipitate the silver as a slightly soluble chloride; follow with egg whites, oils, and other demulcents.

Silvester's method. [Henry Robert Silvester, Brit. physician, 1829–1908] A method of artificial respiration in which the patient lies on his or her back, with arms raised to the sides of the head, held there temporarily, then brought down and pressed against the chest. Movement repeated 16 times per minute. This method is no longer the preferred or effective method of producing artificial respiration. SEE: *artificial respiration; cardiopulmonary resuscitation.*

simesthesia (sĭm-ĕs-thē'zē-ă) [Gr. *aisthesis*, sensation]. Sensibility felt in a bone.

simethicone (sī-mĕth'ĭ-kōn). USP. A mixture of liquid dimethylpolysiloxanes that because of its antifoaming properties is used in treating intestinal gas. Trade names are Mylicon and Silain.

simian crease. A crease on the palm of the hand, so termed because of its similarity to the transverse flexion crease found in some monkeys. Normally the palm of the hand at birth contains several flexion creases, two of which are separate and approx. transverse. When these two appear to fuse and thus form a single transverse crease, it is termed simian crease. The crease may be present in a variety of developmental abnormalities including Down's syndrome, rubella syndrome, Turner's syndrome, Klinefelter's syndrome, q.v., pseudohypoparathyroidism, q.v., and gonadal dysgenesis, q.v. SEE: illus.

similia similibus curantur (sĭ-mĭl'ē-ă sĭ-mĭl'ĭ-bŭs kū-răn'tūr) [L., likes are cured by likes]. The homeopathic doctrine that a drug producing pathological symptoms in those who are well will cure such symptoms in disease states.

similimum (sĭ-mĭl'ĭ-mŭm) [L., most like]. A medicine that causes a symptom quite similar to that produced by the disease. This therapeutic concept and practice is used in homeopathic medicine.

Simmonds' disease (sĭm'mŏnds). [Morris Simmonds, Hamburg physician, 1855–1925] Condition in which complete atrophy of the pituitary body causes loss of function of the thyroid, adrenals, and gonads, premature se-

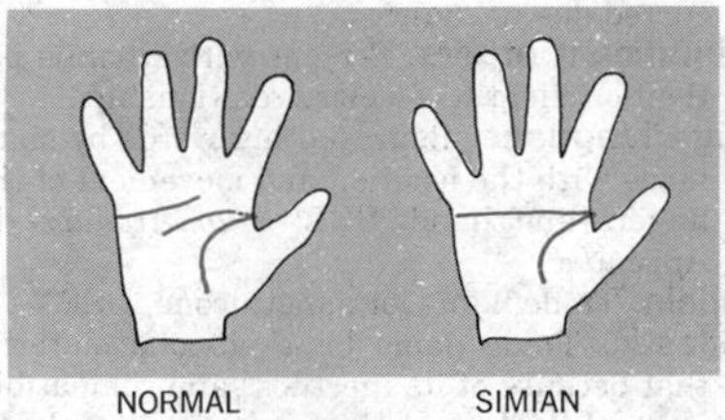

SIMIAN AND NORMAL PALMAR CREASES

nility, psychic symptoms, and cachexia. SYN: *cachexia, pituitary.*

Simon's position (zē'mōns). [Gustav Simon, Ger. surgeon, 1824–1876] An exaggerated lithotomy position in which the hips are somewhat elevated with thighs strongly abducted. Employed in operations on the vagina.

simple (sĭm'pl) [L. *simplex*]. 1. Not complex; not compound. 2. A medicinal plant.

simple fracture. Fracture without rupture of ligaments and skin.

simple inflammation. Inflammation without pus or other inflammatory exudates.

simple reflex. A reflex in which only two or possibly three neurons are interposed between receptor and effector organs.

Sims' position (sĭmz) [J. Marion Sims, U.S. gynecologist, 1813–1883] A semiprone position with patient on left side, right knee and thigh drawn well up, left arm along patient's back, and chest inclined forward so patient rests upon it. It is the position of choice for administering enemas, because the sigmoid and descending colon are located on the left side of the body. Fluid is readily accepted in this position. Also employed in curettement of uterus, intrauterine irrigation after labor, and rectal examination.

simul (sī'mŭl, sĭm'ŭl) [L.]. At once or at the same time; term used in signature of prescription.

simulation (sĭm-ū-lā'shŭn) [L. *simulatio*, imitation]. 1. Pretense of having a disease; feigning of illness. SEE: *malingerer.* 2. Imitation of symptoms of one disease by another.

simulator (sĭm"ū-lā'tor). Any situation or device that creates a condition or situation similar to one that might be encountered. This technique is useful in teaching.

Simulium (sī-mū'lē-ŭm). A genus of insects of the order Diptera that includes the black flies (buffalo gnats), which are important annoyers of domestic animals and man. The females are vicious blood suckers.

S. damnosum. Species that serves as intermediate host of a filarial worm Onchocerca volvulus.

S. venustum. A very annoying species common in North America.

Sinapis (sĭn-ā'pĭs) [Gr. *sinapi*, mustard]. A genus of plants, the mustard plant.

sinapiscopy (sĭn-ă-pĭs'kō-pē) [" + *skopein*, to examine]. Use of mustard in testing for sensory disturbance.

sinapism (sĭn'ă-pĭzm) [Gr. *sinapismos*]. A mustard plaster used to produce counterirritation by applying it to the skin. Enough water is added to flour to make a paste in these proportions: Adult: 3 to 4 parts wheat flour to 1 of mustard flour; child: 8 to 10 parts wheat flour to 1 of mustard flour; and infant: 10 to 12 parts wheat flour to 1 of mustard flour.

sinapized (sĭn'ă-pīzd) [Gr. *sinapi*, mustard]. Containing mustard.

sincipital (sĭn-sĭp'ĭ-tăl) [L. *sinciput*, half a head]. Concerning the sinciput.

sinciput (sĭn'sĭp-ŭt) [L. *sinciput*, half a head]. [NA] 1. Fore and upper part of the cranium. 2. Upper half of the skull. SYN: *calvaria.*

Sinemet. Trade name for a combination of levodopa and carbidopa.

Sinequan. Trade name for doxepin hydrochloride.

sinew (sĭn'ū) [AS. *sinu*]. A tendon.

s., weeping. A ganglion cyst that contains synovial fluid.

sing. L. *singulorum*, of each.

singer's node. A swelling between the arytenoid cartilages of singers. SYN: *chorditis nodosa.*

singleton. One of something described, esp. a single infant rather than a twin.

singultation (sĭng"gŭl-tā'shŭn) [L. *singultus*, a hiccup]. A hiccup.

singultus (sĭng-gŭl'tŭs) [L.]. Hiccup.

sinister (sĭn-ĭs'tĕr) [L.]. In anatomy, left; or present on the left-hand side of the body.

sinistrad (sĭn'ĭs-trăd) [L. *sinister*, left, + *ad*, toward]. Toward the left.

sinistral (sĭn'ĭs-trăl) [L.]. 1. Pert. to or showing preference for the left hand, eye, or foot in certain actions. 2. On the left side.

sinistrality (sĭn"ĭs-trăl'ĭ-tē). Left-handedness.

sinistraural (sĭn-ĭs-traw'răl) [" + *auris*, ear]. Having better hearing with the left ear.

sinistro- (sĭn'ĭs-trō) [L. *sinister*, left]. Combining form meaning left.

sinistrocardia (sĭn"ĭs-trō-kăr'dē-ă) [" + Gr. *kardia*, heart]. Displacement of the heart to left of the medial line; opposed to dextrocardia.

sinistrocerebral (sĭn"ĭs-trō-sĕr'ĕ-brăl) [" + *cerebrum*, brain]. Located in the left cerebral hemisphere.

sinistrocular (sĭn-ĭs-trŏk'ū-lar) [" + *oculus*, eye]. Having stronger vision in the left eye.

sinistrocularity (sĭn"ĭs-trŏk"ū-lăr'ĭ-tē). Condition of having better vision in the left eye.

sinistrogyration (sĭn"ĭs-trō-jī-rā'shŭn) [" + Gr. *gyros*, a circle]. Inclination to the left.

sinistromanual (sĭn"ĭs-trō-măn'ū-ăl) [" + *manus*, hand]. Left-handed.

sinistropedal (sĭn-ĭs-trŏp'ĕd-ăl) [" + *pes*, foot]. Left-footed.

sinistrotorsion (sĭn"ĭs-trō-tor'shŭn) [" + *torsio*, a turning]. A twisting or turning toward the left.

sinistrous (sĭn'ĭs-trŭs). Awkward, clumsy, unskilled, the opposite of dextrous.

sinoatrial (sĭn"ō-ā'trē-ăl). Pertaining to the sinus venosus and the atrium. SYN: *sinoauricular.*

sinoatrial node. Node at junction of superior vena cava with right cardiac atrium, regarded as starting point of the heartbeat.

sinoauricular (sī″nō-aw-rĭk′ū-lar). Sinoatrial. The preferred term is sinoatrial.

sinobronchitis (sī″nō-brŏng-kī′tĭs) [L. *sinus,* a curve, + *bronchus,* bronchus, + Gr. *itis,* inflammation]. Paranasal sinusitis with bronchitis.

sinogram (sī′nō-grăm″) [L. *sinus,* a curve, + Gr. *gramma,* a mark]. Roentgenogram of a sinus injected with a radiopaque dye to determine the range and course of the sinus.

sinter (sĭn′tĕr). 1. The calcium or silica deposits formed from water obtained from mineral springs. 2. To reduce material to a solid form by heating without melting.

sinuitis (sī-nū-ī′tĭs) [″ + Gr. *itis,* inflammation]. Inflammation of a sinus. SYN: *sinusitis.*

sinuotomy (sĭn-ū-ŏt′ō-mē) [″ + Gr. *tome,* incision]. Surgical incision into a sinus. SYN: *sinusotomy.*

sinuous (sĭn′ū-ŭs) [L. *sinuosus,* winding]. Winding; wavy; tortuous.

sinus (sī′nŭs) [L. *sinus,* a curve, hollow]. (pl. *sinuses, sinus*) 1. A canal or passage leading to an abscess. 2. A cavity within a bone. 3. Dilated channel for venous blood. 4. Any cavity having a relatively narrow opening.

RS: antritis; antronasal; antrotympanic; antrum; cephalhematocele; lateral sinus; sinusitis; transillumination.

s.'s, accessory nasal. The paranasal sinuses: frontal, maxillary, ethmoidal, and sphenoidal. Anterior group: frontal, maxillary, and anterior ethmoids. Posterior group: posterior ethmoids and sphenoid.

Sinuses develop embryologically from nasal cavities, are lined with the same type of epithelium, are filled with air, and communicate with nasal cavities through their various ostia. Function of sinuses not definitely known. Various theories give them the same function as nasal cavities, namely, warming, moistening, and filtering the air.

s., anal. The sac-like recesses behind the anal columns.

s., aortic. A dilatation of the aorta or pulmonary artery opposite the segment of the semilunar valve. SYN: *sinus of Valsalva.*

s., basilar. S., transverse.

s., carotid. SEE: *carotid sinus.*

s., cavernous. A large sinus from the sphenoidal fissure to the apex of the petrous portion of the temporal bone.

s., cerebral. Any ventricle of the brain.

s., circular. A venous sinus around the pituitary body, communicating on each side with the cavernous sinus.

s., coccygeal. A sinus in the midline of the natal cleft just over the coccyx. SEE: *cleft, pilonidal.*

s., coronary, of heart. A vein in the transverse groove between the left cardiac atrium and ventricle.

s.'s, cranial. Venous canals between folds of the dura.

s., dermal. A congenital sinus tract connecting the surface of the body with the spinal canal.

s.'s, ethmoidal. Air cavities in the ethmoid bone.

s., frontal. An irregular cavity in the frontal bone on each side of the midline above the nasal bridge. One may be larger than the other. A duct carries secretions to the upper part of the nostrils.

s., genitourinary. S., urogenital.

s., hair. The sinus formed when hair is embedded in the skin and acts as a foreign body.

s., inferior longitudinal. A venous sinus along the posterior half of the lower border of the falx cerebri.

s., inferior petrosal. A large venous sinus from the cavernous sinus, running along the lower margin of the petrous portion of the temporal bone.

s., inferior sagittal. A venous sinus in the inferior margin of the falx cerebri.

s.'s, intercavernous. The anterior and posterior halves of the circular sinus.

s., lateral. One of two large venous sinuses in inner side of skull passing near the mastoid antrum and emptying into the jugular vein.

s.'s, lymph. Small spaces throughout the parenchyma of a lymphatic gland.

s., marginal. 1. A large venous sinus around part of the margin of the placenta. 2. Small bilateral venous sinuses of the dura mater at the edge of the foramen magnum. 3. A venous sinus around a portion of the white pulp of the spleen.

s., maxillary. A cavity in the maxillary bone communicating with the middle meatus of the nasal cavity. SYN: *antrum of Highmore.*

s., occipital. A small venous sinus in the attached margin of the falx cerebelli extending to the margin of the foramen magnum.

s. of the pulmonary trunk. One of the dilatations in the pulmonary trunk, across from a cusp of the pulmonary valve of the heart.

s. of spleen. A venous sinusoid in the reticulum of the spleen.

s. of Valsalva. A dilatation of the aorta or pulmonary artery opposite the segment of the semilunar valve. SYN: *s., aortic.*

s. of venal canal; s. venarum cavarum. The portion of the right atrium of the heart posterior and to the left of the crista terminalis. The inferior and superior vena caval veins empty into it.

s.'s, paranasal. Accessory nasal sinuses.

s., pilonidal. SEE: *pilonidal fistula.*

s.'s, pleural. Spaces in the pleural sac along the lower and inferior portions of the lung that the lung does not occupy.

s. pocularis. Lacuna in prostatic part of the urethra. SYN: *s. prostaticus.*

s. prostaticus. S. pocularis.

s. rectus. Venous sinus at the junction of the falx cerebri and the cerebellar tentorium. SYN: *s. of the dura mater, straight; straight sinus.*

s., renal. The area in the kidney composed of the renal pelvis, renal calices, vessels, nerves, and fatty tissue.

s., rhomboid. The fourth cranial ventricle.

s., sigmoid. Continuation, on both sides, of the transverse sinuses down along the posterior border of the petrous part of the temporal bone to the jugular foramen to the jugular veins.

s.'s, sphenoidal. Air sinuses that occupy the body of the sphenoid bone and connect with the nasal cavity.

s., sphenoparietal. 1. A venous sinus uniting the cavernous sinus and a meningeal vein. 2. The portion of the cavernous sinus below the ensiform process.

s., straight. SEE: *s. rectus.*

s., superior longitudinal. A triangular sinus along the upper edge of the falx cerebri.

s., superior petrosal. A venous canal running in a groove in the petrous portion of the temporal bone.

s., superior sagittal. Large venous sinus along the attached border of the falx cerebri from the crista galli to the internal occipital protuberance where it joins either the right or left transverse sinuses or both. SYN: *s. of the dura mater, superior sagittal.*

s., tarsal. A tunnel between the calcaneus and talus of the ankle.

s., tentorial. SEE: *s. rectus.*

s., terminal. A vein encircling the vascular area of the blastoderm.

s., transverse. 1. Sinus that unites the two inferior petrosal sinuses. 2. Venous network in the dura over the basilar process of the occipital bone. SYN: *s., basilar.*

s., transverse, of the dura mater. Large, bilateral venous sinuses along the attached margin of the cerebellar tentorium. They receive the superior sagittal and straight sinuses and drain into the sigmoid sinuses and then to the jugular veins.

s., transverse, of the pericardium. A channel posterior to the aorta and the pulmonary trunk but in front of the atria.

s., tympanic. A deep recess in the labyrinthine wall of the tympanic cavity. It opens into the fenestra of the cochlea.

s., urogenital. 1. Duct into which, in the embryo, the wolffian ducts and bladder empty; it opens into the cloaca. 2. The common receptacle of the genital and urinary ducts. SYN: *s., genitourinary.*

s., uterine. Venous channels in the walls of the uterus during pregnancy.

s.'s, uteroplacental. Slanting venous channels from the placenta serving to convey the maternal blood from the intervillous lacunae back into the uterine veins.

s., venous. A sinus conveying venous blood.

s., venous, of the dura mater. Venous channels between the two layers of the dura mater. They drain the venous blood from the brain.

s., venous, of sclera. A circular channel at the sclero-corneal junction in the sclera. It drains into the anterior ciliary vein. Aqueous humor leaves the eye via this sinus. SYN: *Schlemm's canal.*

sinus arrhythmia. Cardiac irregularity characterized by an increased heart rate during inspiration and decrease in heart rate on expiration. This arrythmia has no clinical significance except in older patients, in which case it may occur in coronary artery disease.

sinusitis (sī-nŭs-ī'tĭs) [L. *sinus,* a curve, a hollow, + Gr. *itis,* inflammation]. Inflammation of a sinus, esp. a paranasal sinus. SYN: *sinuitis.*

ETIOL: A number of causative agents including viruses, bacteria, or allergy.

PREDISPOSING FACTORS: Inadequate drainage, which may result from presence of polyps, enlarged turbinates, or deviated septum; chronic rhinitis; general debility; or dental abscess in maxillary bone.

s., acute catarrhal. Inflammation accompanying a similar process in the nose.

s., acute suppurative. Purulent inflammation with symptoms of pain over the sinus, fever, chills, and headache.

TREATMENT: Conservative. Shrinkage in the nasal mucosa to facilitate ventilation and drainage of the sinus. Rest in bed, force fluids, decongestants, hot packs. If inflammation is due to bacterial infection, antibiotic therapy is indicated.

s., chronic hyperplastic. Polyps present in sinuses and nose and underlying osteitis of sinus walls.

TREATMENT: Surgical. Conservative, removal of polyps and intranasal opening into sinuses for adequate ventilation and drainage, and radical, complete removal of sinus mucosa either through external or intranasal route.

s., chronic hypertrophic. Inflammation found in conjunction with chronic hypertrophic rhinitis. Living in a climate where the temperature fluctuations are not extreme may be beneficial.

sinusoid (sī'nŭs-oyd) [" + Gr. *eidos,* like]. 1. Resembling a sinus. 2. A minute blood vessel found in such organs as the liver, spleen, adrenal glands, and bone marrow. It is slightly larger than a capillary and has a lining of reticuloendothelium.

sinusoidal (sī-nŭs-oyd'ăl). Pert. to a sinusoid.

sinusoidal current. Alternating induced electric current, the two strokes of which are equal.

sinusoidalization (sī"nŭ-soy"dăl-ī-zā'shŭn) [L. *sinus,* a hollow, a curve, + Gr. *eidos,* like]. Use of a sinusoidal current.

sinusotomy (sī-nŭs-ŏt'ō-mē) [" + Gr. *tome,* incision]. The operation of incising a sinus.

sinus rhythm. The normal cardiac rhythm commencing at the sinoatrial node.

SiO_2. Silicon dioxide.

Sioux alarm. Native American Indians of the Sioux tribe learned, after carefully controlled experiments, that they could use a full urinary bladder as a kind of alarm clock. By drinking a certain amount of fluids at bedtime, they found they would awaken in a specific number of hours. Were they to increase the amount of fluid taken, they would awaken earlier; and if they took less, they would awaken later.

siphon (sī'fŏn) [Gr. *siphon,* tube]. A tube bent at an angle to form two unequal lengths for transferring liquids from one container to another by atmospheric pressure. One container must be higher than the other for this to work.

siphonage (sī'fŭn-ĭj). Use of a siphon to drain a body cavity such as the stomach or bladder.

Siphonaptera (sī"fō-năp'tĕr-ă) [" + *apteros,* wingless]. An order of insects commonly called fleas. They are wingless, undergo complete metamorphosis, and have piercing and sucking mouth parts, their food being the blood of birds and mammals. The body is compressed laterally and their legs are adapted for leaping. In addition to being annoying pests, they transmit the causative organisms of several diseases (bubonic plague, endemic or murine typhus, and among rodents, tularemia). They also serve as intermediate hosts of certain tapeworms. SEE: *flea.*

siphonoma (sī-fŏn-ō'mă) [" + *oma,* tumor]. A tumor made up of fine tubes.

Sippy diet (sĭp'ē). [Bertram W. Sippy, U.S. physician, 1866–1924] Treatment of gastric ulcer by diet, neutralizing acidity of gastric juice. Small amounts of milk and cream every hour and alkaline powders every half hour. This diet is no longer in general use.

Average mixture: 1½ oz. (44.4 ml.) each of cream and milk given once each hour for a total of 13 feedings during the day. For the next 3 to 4 days continue these feedings but substitute an egg and fine cereal for one feeding in the morning and one at night. The next day, 3 oz. (85 gm.) soft cereal added to afternoon feeding; another egg the next day; and finally 3 servings of cereal and 3 eggs per day added to the milk and cream. Purée, custards, and toast added the next week. Decreased feedings as amount of each feeding is increased until six feedings are given per day. Each feeding replaces the scheduled milk and cream.

This schedule is monotonous, deficient in vitamins, and provides no feeding at night. It is usually modified to compensate for these deficiencies.

sirenomelia (sī"rĕn-ŏm-ē'lē-ă) [Gr. *seiren,* mermaid, + *melos,* limb]. Congenital anomaly in which the lower extremities are fused.

siriasis (sĭ-rī'ă-sĭs) [Gr. *seirian,* to be hot]. Sunstroke, q.v.

-sis. Gr. suffix indicating condition or state. Depending upon the preceding vowel, it may appear in the form of -asis, -esis, -iasis, or -osis.

sismotherapy (sĭs"mō-thĕr'ă-pē) [Gr. *seismos,* a shake, + *therapeia,* treatment]. Therapeutic employment of vibration. SYN: *seismotherapy.*

sister. A term used by the British for nurse, esp. a senior or head nurse.

site [L. *situs,* place]. Position or location.

sitieirgia (sĭt-ē-īr'jē-ă) [Gr. *sition,* food, + *eirgein,* to bar out]. Hysterical refusal to take food.

sitio-, sito- [Gr. *sition, sitos,* food]. Combining forms meaning bread or made from grain; food.

sitiology (sĭt-ē-ŏl'ō-jē) [" + *logos,* a study]. Science of nutrition. SYN: *sitology.*

sitiomania (sĭt"ē-ō-mā'nē-ă) [" + *mania,* madness]. Periodic abnormal appetite or craving for food. SYN: *sitomania.*

sitology (sī-tŏl'ō-jē) [" + *logos,* a study]. Science of nutrition and food. SYN: *sitiology.*

sitomania (sī"tō-mā'nē-ă) [" + *mania,* madness]. 1. Periodic abnormal craving for food. 2. Periodic abnormality of appetite. SYN: *sitiomania.*

sitophobia (sī"tō-fō'bē-ă) [" + *phobos,* fear]. Psychoneurotic abhorrence of food, or morbid dread of or repugnance to food, whether generally or only to specific dishes.

sitosterols (sī-tŏs'tĕr-ōls). 1. A group of similar organic compounds that occur in plants. They contain the steroid nucleus, perhydrocyclopentanophenanthrene, q.v. 2. A pharmaceutical compound that contains several sitosterols. Used in treating hypercholesterolemia.

sitotaxis (sī"tō-tăk'sĭs) [" + *taxis,* arrangement]. Sitotropism, q.v.

sitotherapy (sī"tō-thĕr'ă-pē) [" + *therapeia,* treatment]. The therapeutic use of food.

sitotoxin (sī"tō-tŏk'sĭn) [" + *toxikon,* poison].

Units of the International System of Units

Basic Quantity	Basic Unit	Symbol
Length	meter	m
Mass	kilogram	kg
Time	second	s
Electric current	ampere	A
Thermodynamic temperature	kelvin	K
Luminous intensity	candela	cd
Amount of substance	mole	mol

Prefixes and Their Symbols Used to Designate Decimal Multiples and Submultiples in SI Units

Prefix	Symbol	Factor
tera	T	10^{12} = 1 000 000 000 000
giga	G	10^{9} = 1 000 000 000
mega	M	10^{6} = 1 000 000
kilo	k	10^{3} = 1 000
hecto	h	10^{2} = 100
deka	da	10^{1} = 10
deci	d	10^{-1} = 0.1
centi	c	10^{-2} = 0.01
milli	m	10^{-3} = 0.001
micro	μ	10^{-6} = 0.000 001
nano	n	10^{-9} = 0.000 000 001
pico	p	10^{-12} = 0.000 000 000 001
femto	f	10^{-15} = 0.000 000 000 000 001
atto	a	10^{-18} = 0.000 000 000 000 000 001

Any poison developed in food, esp. one produced by bacteria growing in a cereal or grain product.

sitotoxism (sī″tō-tŏks′ĭzm) [″ + ″ + *-ismos,* condition]. Poisoning by vegetable foods infested with molds or bacteria.

sitotropism (sī-tŏt′rō-pĭzm) [″ + *tropos,* a turning, + *-ismos,* condition]. Response of cells to the attraction or repulsion of food elements.

situation. 1. A set of circumstances. 2. The location of an entity in relation to other objects, e.g., between a rock and a hard object.

situs (sī′tŭs) [L.]. A position.

s. inversus viscerum. Abnormal displacement of viscera to opposite side of the body.

s. perversus. Malposition of any visceral structure.

sitz bath (sĭtz). Bath to sit in with water above and covering the hips. The tub or fixture is usually shaped to allow the legs to be out of the water.

SI units. *International System of Units,* from Fr. *Systeme Internationale d'Unites.* ABBR: SI. SEE: tables; *SI Units* in *Appendix.*

sixth cranial nerve. Abducens nerve that supplies the external rectus of the eye. SEE: *cranial nerves.*

Sjögren's syndrome. Syndrome occurring in postmenopausal women including rheumatoid arthritis, xerostomia, and keratoconjunctivitis sicca. It is thought to be a form of collagen disease.

SK-65. Trade name for propoxyphene hydrochloride, USP.

SK-Apap. Trade name for acetaminophen, USP.

skateboard. A therapeutic device used for upper extremity rehabilitation. It consists of a forearm platform mounted on ball-bearing rollers. It assists the patient in making coordinated movements.

skatol(e) (skăt′ōl) [Gr. *skatos,* dung]. Betamethyl indole, C_9H_9N, a malodorous, solid, heterocyclic nitrogen compound found in feces, formed by protein decomposition in the intestines and giving them their odor.

skatoxyl (skă-tŏk′sĭl). A derivative of skatole.

SK-Bamate. Trade name for meprobamate, USP.

SK-Chloral Hydrate. Trade name for chloral hydrate, USP.

SK-Chlorothiazide. Trade name for chlorothiazide, USP.

SK-Dexamethasone. Trade name for dexamethasone, USP.

SK-Digoxin. Trade name for digoxin, USP.

SK-Diphenhydramine. Trade name for diphenhydramine.

skein (skān). A continuous tangled thread. SYN: *spireme.*

skelalgia (skē-lăl′jē-ă) [Gr. *skelis,* leg, + *algos,* pain]. Pain in the leg.

Skelaxin. Trade name for metaxalone.

skeletal (skĕl′ĕ-tăl) [Gr. *skeleton,* a dried-up body]. Pert. to the skeleton.

skeletal muscle. Muscle fibers that with few exceptions are attached to parts of the skeleton and involved primarily in movements of the parts of the body. SYN: *striated muscle; voluntary muscle.*

skeletal survey. Procedure in which entire skeleton is radiographed to determine the presence of pathology.

skeletal traction. Pulling force applied directly to the bone through surgically applied pins and tongs.

NURSING IMPLICATIONS: Place the patient on a firm mattress and in supine position while in traction. Care must be taken to keep the insertion points of pins and tongs on the skin clean and free of infection. Infection at the insertion sites can lead to osteomyelitis of the bone. Prevent such infection by assessing the area for odor and other signs of infection and cleansing the area utilizing aseptic technique, applying prescribed medication and a sterile dressing. Perform daily skin inspection for signs of pressure or friction, and institute appropriate nursing measures to alleviate any pressure or friction. Maintain proper traction alignment at all times; adjust as necessary. Establish exercise regimen for unaffected extremities. Assess any patient complaint without delay. Implement respiratory toiletry regimen to prevent pulmonary complications. Administer analgesics as prescribed. Promote adequate nutrition and fluid intake for tissue healing and repair. Prevent constipation and fecal impaction by dietary and medical management. Assess affected extremity daily or more frequently if necessary for complications such as phlebitis, nerve or circulatory impairment, and foot drop. Promote social and diversional activities. Teach the patient the use of a trapeze, exercises, and activity limitations. Establish discharge plan and follow-up.

skeletization (skĕl″ĕt-ī-zā′shŭn). 1. Excessive emaciation. 2. Removal of soft parts of the body leaving only the skeleton.

skeleto- [Gr. *skeleton*]. Combining form meaning skeleton.

skeletogenous (skĕl-ĕ-tŏj′ĕ-nŭs) [″ + *gennan,* to produce]. Forming skeletal structures or tissues.

skeletology (skĕl″ĕ-tŏl′ŏ-jē) [″ + *logos,* study]. The special division of anatomy and biomechanics concerned with the skeleton.

skeleton (skĕl′ĕt-ŏn) [Gr., a dried-up body]. The bony framework of the body consisting of 206 bones: 80 axial or trunk and 126 of the limbs. This number does not include teeth or sesamoid bones other than the patella. The various bones follow. SEE: illus.

AXIAL (80 Bones)
- Head (29 Bones)
  - Cranial (8)
    - frontal—1
    - parietal—2
    - occipital—1
    - temporal—2
    - sphenoid—1
    - ethmoid—1
  - Facial (14)
    - maxilla—2
    - mandible—1
    - zygoma—2
    - lacrimal—2
      - nasal—2
      - turbinate—2
      - vomer—1
      - palate—2
    - Hyoid (1)
    - Auditory ossicles (6)
      - malleus—2
      - incus—2
      - stapes—2
- Trunk (51 Bones)
  - Vertebrae (26)
    - cervical—7
    - dorsal—12
    - lumbar—5
    - sacrum—1
    - coccyx—1
  - Ribs (24)
    - true rib—14
    - false rib—6
    - floating rib—4
  - Sternum (1)

LIMBS (126 Bones)
- Upper Extremities (64 Bones)
  - Arms and Shoulders (10)
    - clavicle—2
    - scapula—2
    - humerus—2
    - radius—2
    - ulna—2
  - Wrists (16)
    - navicular or scaphoid—2
    - lunate—2
    - triquetrum—2
    - pisiform—2
    - trapezium—2
    - trapezoid—2
    - capitate—2
    - hamate—2

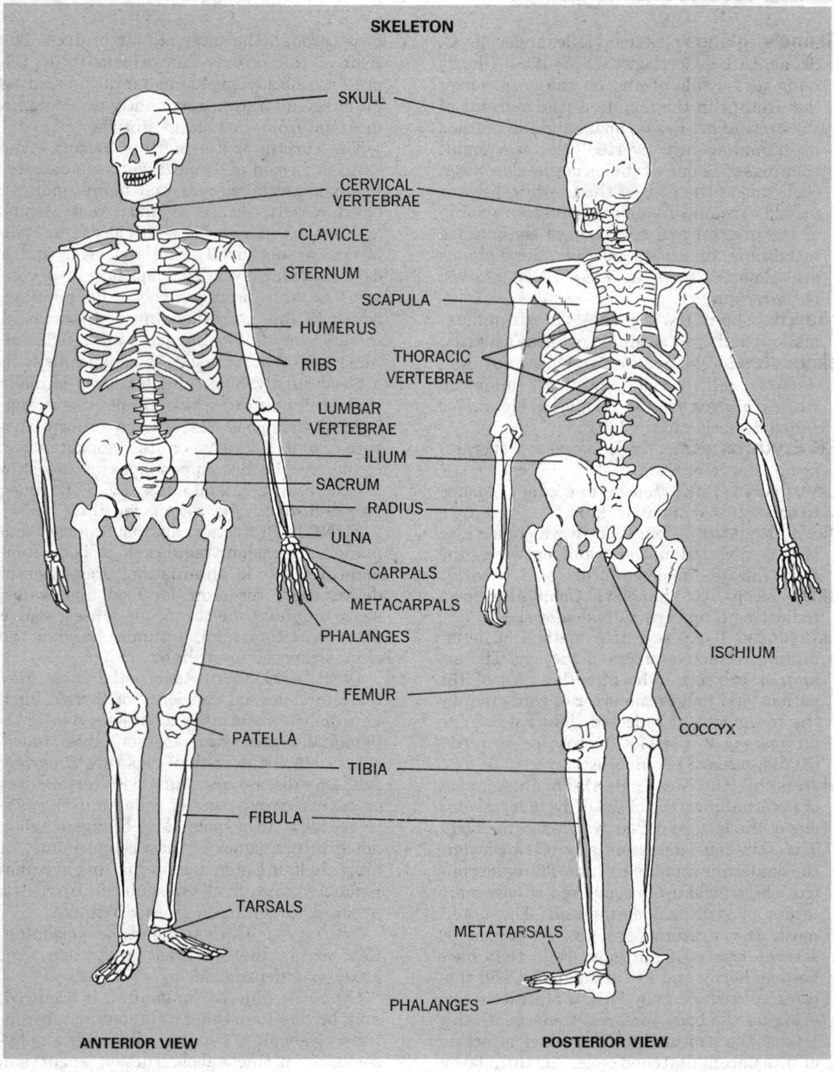

Hands (38)
metacarpal—10
phalanx (finger bones)—28
Lower Extremities (62 Bones)
Legs and Hips (10)
hip bone—2
femur—2
tibia—2
fibula—2
patella (knee cap)—2
Ankles (14)
astragaloid—2
heel bone—2
scaphoid—2
cuboid—2
cuneiform, internal—2
cuneiform, middle—2
cuneiform, external—2
Feet (38)
metatarsal—10
phalanx (toe bones)—28

s., axial. Bones of the head and trunk.

s., cartilaginous. Structure from which the bones have been formed through ossification.

Skene's glands (skēns). [Alexander J. C. Skene, U.S. gynecologist, 1838–1900] Glands lying just inside of and on the posterior of the urethra in the female. If the margins of the urethra are drawn apart and the mucous membrane gently everted, the two small openings of Skene's tubules or glands, one on each side of the floor of the urethra, become visible. Trauma frequently causes a gaping of the urethra and ectropion of the mucous membrane. In acute gonorrhea, these glands are almost always infected. SYN: *glands, paraurethral.*

skenitis (skē-nī′tĭs) [*Skene* + Gr. *itis,* inflammation]. Inflamed condition of Skene's glands.

skeocytosis (skē″ō-sī-tō′sĭs) [Gr. *skaios,* left, + *kytos,* cell, + *osis,* condition]. Immature white corpuscles in the peripheral blood; also called deviation to the left.

SK-Erythromycin. Trade name for erythromycin stearate, USP.

skew (skyū) [ME. *skewen,* to escape]. Turned to one side; asymmetrical.

skew deviation. Condition in which one eyeball is directed upward and outward, the other inward and downward.

skia- (skī′ă) [Gr., shadow]. Combining form indicating a concern with shadows.

skiascopy. 1. An objective method of determining refractive errors of the eye. The examiner projects light into the eyes of the patient and judges the error of refraction by the movement of reflected light rays. SYN: *retinoscopy.* 2. Use of a fluoroscope for medical diagnosis. SYN: *fluoroscopy.*

skin (skĭn) [Old Norse *skinn*]. The integument or external covering of the body. It represents one of the largest organ systems in the body. The skin consists essentially of two layers, the epidermis and the corium. The epidermis (cuticle, scarfskin) is composed of four main layers of stratified epithelium. The outermost, the stratum corneum, is formed by several layers of flattened cells that have become horny and lost their nuclei and that contain keratin. They form a protective covering for the body surfaces. Underneath this layer is the stratum lucidum, which is formed of translucent flattened cells. The third layer, the stratum granulosum, consists of two or three layers of flattened cells containing granules of eleidin, the precursor of keratin. The fourth and last layer is the stratum germinativum (stratum mucosum, stratum Malpighi). The cells in the upper portion of this layer are cuboidal; those nearest the corium are columnar. Cells of this layer possess well-defined intercellular bridges that appear as spines projecting from the surface; hence these cells are often called prickle cells and the entire layer, stratum spinosum. These cells contain peculiar fibrils, tonofibrils, which pass through the intercellular bridges. The color of the skin is due principally to the presence of a pigment, melanin, present as granules in stratum germinativum. Melanin is absent from the skin in albinism.

The corium (cutis, dermis, derma, true skin) is formed of connective tissue containing lymphatics, nerves and nerve endings, blood vessels, sebaceous and sweat glands, and elastic fibers. It is divided into two layers, a superficial papillary layer and a deep reticular layer. The papillary layer contains conical protuberances, the papillae, which fit into corresponding depressions in the epidermis. Within each papilla is a capillary loop that furnishes the epidermis with a blood supply. The reticular layer is made up in the main of white fibrous tissue supporting the blood vessels and other structures in it. It rests on the subcutaneous connective tissue. Appendages of the skin are the hair, q.v., and nails, q.v. SEE: illus.; *hair* and *strata of epidermis* for illus.

FUNCT: Protection against injuries and parasitic invasion; regulation of body temperature; aids in elimination; prevention of dehydration; reservoir for food and water; sense organ for the cutaneous senses; source of antirachitic vitamin (vitamin D) when the skin is exposed to sunlight.

DIFF. DIAGNOSIS: *Abnormal dryness:* May indicate abnormal deficiency of thyroid function, diabetes, and other conditions. *Ashy:* Malignant diseases, severe anemia, cancer, tuberculosis, chronic interstitial nephritis. *Bronzing:* Addison's disease, poisoning with certain dyes or metals, early stages of pellagra. *Brownish-yellow spots* (liver spots): May be due to aging; noted in pregnancy (chloasma uterinum), in exophthalmic goiter, and uterine and liver malignancies; also freckles, sunburn, cosmetics, mustard, turpentine, and other irritants.

Cherry red: Carbon monoxide poisoning. *Cold sweats:* Indicate great prostration, fear, anxiety, or depression.

Cyanosis: May be congenital; if acquired, may be due to asthma, pulmonary tuberculosis, whooping cough, advanced emphysema, croup, tracheal obstruction, aneurysm, goiter, flushing (hyperemia), emotion, febrile disorders, pulmonary tuberculosis, convulsions, large ovarian tumor, plethora, polycythemia. *Cyanosis alternating with pallor:* Cerebrospinal diseases, typhoid, vasomotor disturbances, menopause, argyria associated with ingestion of silver salts. May be noted in lips, mucous membranes, fingertips, and external ear. If extreme, entire body shows dusky, leaden tint. Indicates lack of oxygen and excess of carbon dioxide in blood. May be due to inflammation or abscess of pharynx and larynx, Ludwig's angina, croup, and dis-

VIEW OF SKIN AND UNDERLYING TISSUES

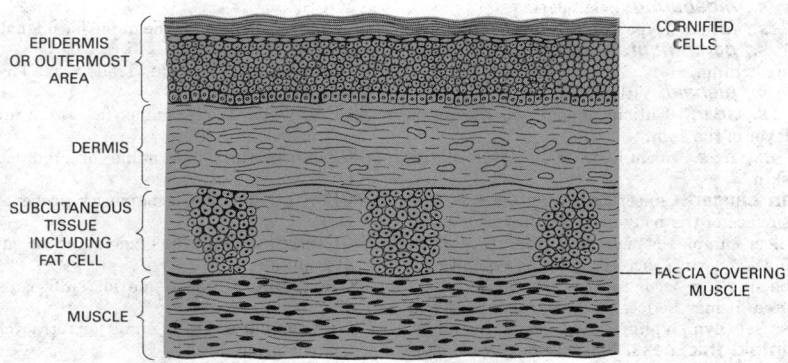

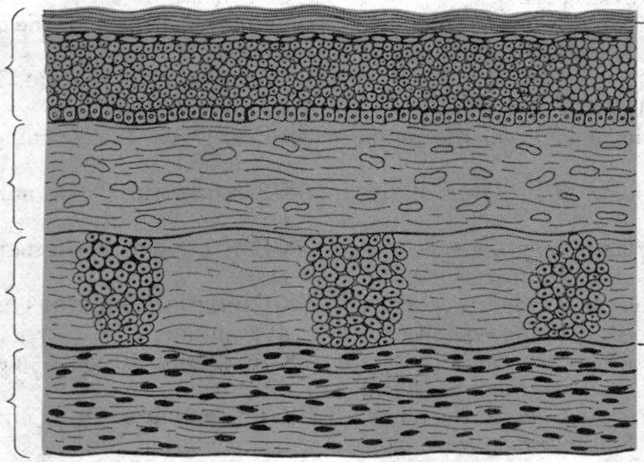

orders affecting respiration. Also to overdose of drugs or asphyxiation by gas.

Discolorations: Seen in icterus, chlorosis, leprosy, administration of silver nitrate, jaundice, carotenemia, vitiligo, albinism, malignant diseases, and asphyxia from gas. *Edema:* Seen in anemia, hydremia, obstruction, inflammation, and cardiac, circulatory and renal decompensation. If local, may be due to obstruction of return circulation or heart failure, in which case it will be evident in ankles and often legs, esp. at night. May also be due to renal diseases. *Emphysema:* Due to free air or gas in subcutaneous tissue. *Hot and dry:* Indicates fever, mental excitement, or excessive salt intake. *Moist:* Increased perspiration (hyperhidrosis) may be due to fevers, such as malarial, rheumatic, relapsing, or septic fever; pneumonic crisis; pulmonary tuberculosis; Graves' disease; neuralgia; migraine; drugs; hot drinks; exercise. Lack of moistness noted in dehydration and in ichthyosis.

Paleness: Nervous prostration, dropsy, paralysis, malnutrition. *Pallor:* Occurs in those living an indoor life, esp. in prisoners and night workers. May be due to anemia. Temporary pallor occurs in syncope, chills, shock, rigors, and some vasomotor instability. If sudden and persistent, may be sign of internal hemorrhage. Also seen in lead poisoning. If it gradually becomes permanent, may indicate chronic febrile disease, chronic gastrointestinal disease, cancer, arsenical poisoning, chronic suppuration, chronic mercurial poisoning, hemorrhages, leukemia, cachexia, nephrosis, nephritis, syphilis, parasitic diseases, tuberculosis, or malaria. *Purplish:* Interference of circulation common in asthma and typhus.

Rashes: SEE: *rash. Redness:* Local redness seen in inflammation, skin diseases, chronic alcoholism, vasomotor disturbances, and pyrexia. Local redness with pain indicates inflammation. Sunburn (actinic dermatitis). *Sallowness:* Cachexia, syphilis, chronic gallbladder disease, arthritis deformans, constipation, some anemias, gastric, pancreatic, enteric, or hepatic disorders.

Temperature: Usually correlates with internal temperature, unless raised by local applications of heat or exposure to cold. If generally cold, may be due to poor circulation or obstruction of same, vasomotor spasms, venous or arterial thrombosis, exposure to cold. General abnormal heat seen in febrile disorders, although in some of them a cold and clammy skin is present. *Wrinkling:* If permanent, may be due to aging; temporary due to prolonged immersion in water or dehydration. *Yellow:* May be due to increased carotene intake; jaundice, liver disease. If jaundiced, plethoric, hyperemic, or pigmented, it should be noted.

Miscellaneous: Rashes, scars, and their cause are also diagnostic. Texture and temperature of skin are important signs. Undue moisture, cold or hot spots on body, dryness of skin are other points to look for in diagnosis. SEE: *anemia, pernicious; biliousness; endocarditis; face; liver.*

s., alligator. Severe scaling of the skin with formation of thick plates resembling hide of an alligator. SEE: *ichthyosis.*

s., deciduous. Shedding of the epidermis. SYN: *keratolysis.*

s., elastic. Skin that has property of great elasticity.

s., glossy. Shining atrophy of the skin.

s., hidebound. Scleroderma.

s., loose. Hypertrophy of the skin.

s., parchment. Atrophy of the skin with stretching.

s., piebald. Vitiligo.

s., scarf. Cuticle, epidermis, the outer layer of the skin.

s., true. Corium or inner layer of the skin.

skin cancer. Cancer that may arise on the surface of the body and manifest as a small ulcer, pimple, or mole. It may be red, brown, black, or white, according to the type. It may be single or occur in a group, open or ulcerated. It may be localized or invade the blood vessels, lymph glands, and connecting ducts.

skinfold thickness. Measurement with calibrated calipers of thickness of a fold of skin at a selected body site. The sites usually are upper arm or triceps, subscapular region, and upper abdomen. The measurements are used in evaluating nutritional status by estimating the amount of subcutaneous fat.

skin graft. Using the skin from another part of the body, or from a donor, to repair a defect or trauma of the skin. SEE: *graft; Thiersch's graft.*

skin-marking. Application of nontoxic paints or dyes to the skin to provide landmarks during plastic surgery or to permit accurate alignment of the wound edges at the time the skin is closed.

Skinner box (skĭn'ĕr). [Burrhus F. Skinner, U.S. psychologist, b. 1904] A device used in experimental psychology. It is designed so that an animal presses a lever or button and thus is rewarded by receiving food.

skin rash. A usually temporary eruption of the skin covering a small area, a portion of the body, or the entire body. The rash may consist of macules, papules, vesicles, or pustules and is usually red or reddish-blue. It may be itchy. A rash is often indicative of a systemic disease such as measles or lupus or it may indicate a local irritation such as contact dermatitis or diaper rash.

skin test. Any test in which a suspected allergen or sensitizer is applied to the skin.

sklero- [Gr.]. SEE: words beginning with *sclero-.*

SK-Lygen. Trade name for chlordiazepoxide hydrochloride, USP.

skodaic (skō-dā'ĭk). Concerning Josef Skoda. SEE: *Skoda's resonance.*

Skoda's rales (skō'dăs). [Josef Skoda, Austrian physician, 1805–1881] Bronchial rales heard through consolidated tissue of the lungs in pneumonia.

Skoda's resonance. Tympanic resonance above the line of fluid in pleuritic effusion, or above consolidation in pneumonia.

SK-Penicillin VK. Trade name for penicillin V, USP.

SK-Phenobarbital. Trade name for phenobarbital, USP.

SK-Potassium Chloride. Trade name for potassium chloride, USP.

SK-Pramine. Trade name for imipramine hydrochloride, USP.

SK-Prednisone. Trade name for prednisone, USP.

SK-Probenecid. Trade name for probenecid, USP.

SK-Quinidine Sulfate. Trade name for quinidine sulfate, USP.

SK-Soxazole. Trade name for sulfisoxazole, USP.

SK-Tetracycline. Trade name for tetracycline hydrochloride, USP.

SK-Tolbutamide. Trade name for tolbutamide, USP.

skull (skŭl) [ME. *skulle,* bowl]. The bony framework of the head, composed of eight cranial bones, the 14 bones of the face, and the teeth. SYN: *calvaria; cranium.* SEE: illus.; *skeleton.*

s., fracture of. Classified according to whether the fracture is in the vault or the base, but from the point of view of treatment, a more useful classification is as follows:

Simple uncomplicated fractures: Not common.

Compound fractures: If in vault of skull, the bone is depressed and driven inward with possible damage to brain. Treatment is operative.

skull cap. Upper round portion of skull covering the brain.

slant. Tube of solid culture medium that is slanted to increase the surface area of the medium. Used in culturing bacteria.

slave. A device that allows the body movements to be transferred to a machine either directly or by remote control.

Ex.: apparatus for lifting, squeezing, and turning laboratory equipment containing radioactive materials. The remote "hands" are controlled by the operator from sufficient distance and proper shielding to prevent exposure to radiation or other highly toxic materials. Artificial arms and legs equipped to respond to physical or electrical stimulation have been developed.

SLE. *systemic lupus erythematosus.*

sleep (slēp) [AS. *slaep*]. Period of rest where physiological activities and consciousness are diminished and voluntary physical activity is absent. It is easily differentiated from the lessened consciousness of stupor in that nor-

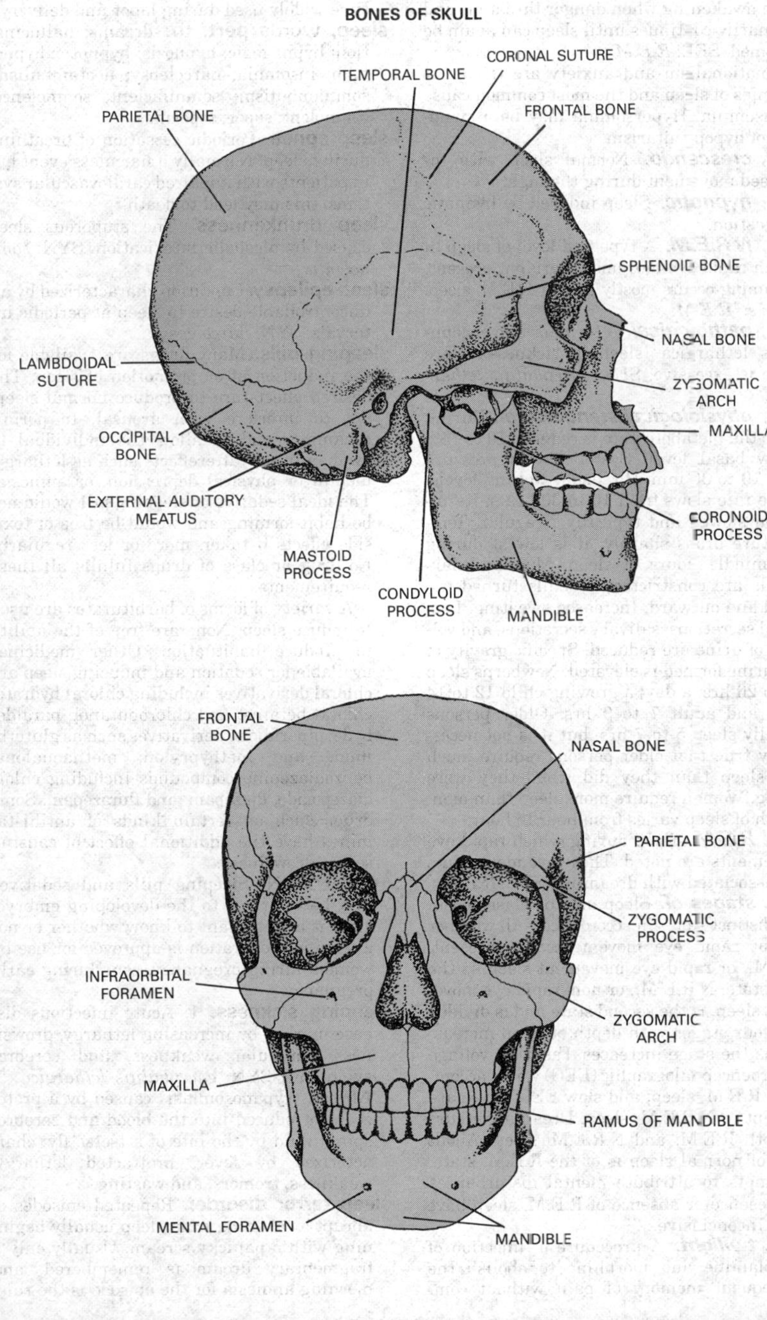
BONES OF SKULL
CORONAL SUTURE
TEMPORAL BONE
PARIETAL BONE
FRONTAL BONE
SPHENOID BONE
NASAL BONE
LAMBDOIDAL SUTURE
ZYGOMATIC ARCH
OCCIPITAL BONE
MAXILLA
EXTERNAL AUDITORY MEATUS
CORONOID PROCESS
MASTOID PROCESS
CONDYLOID PROCESS
MANDIBLE
FRONTAL BONE
NASAL BONE
PARIETAL BONE
ZYGOMATIC PROCESS
INFRAORBITAL FORAMEN
ZYGOMATIC ARCH
MAXILLA
RAMUS OF MANDIBLE
MENTAL FORAMEN
MANDIBLE

mal awareness can completely reassert itself upon awakening when danger threatens and ordinarily continues until sleep can again be resumed. SEE: *R.E.M.*

Emotionalism and anxiety are the great enemies of sleep and the most common cause of insomnia. Hypersomnia may be a symptom of hypopituitarism.

s., crescendo. Normal sleep with increased movement during the night.

s., hypnotic. Sleep induced by hypnotic suggestion.

s., N.R.E.M. A type and level of sleep in which rapid eye movements are not present. Dreaming occurs mostly during R.E.M. sleep. SEE: *s., R.E.M.*

s., pathological. A term used in encephalitis lethargica (sleeping sickness). Here sleep is excessive. SEE: *encephalitis lethargica.*

s., physiological standards of. During sleep the metabolic rate is reduced 10 to 15% below basal level. Systolic blood pressure falls 10 to 30 mm. Hg. below waking levels. Pulse rate slows from 10 to 30 beats. Respiration slowed and typically irregular. Temperature drops sharply; it is lowest during the middle hours of sleep. Muscles relax. Pupils are constricted, eyeballs turned upward and outward. Increased sweating. Lacrimal secretions, salivary secretions, and volume of urine are reduced. Specific gravity of the urine formed is elevated. Newborns sleep 18 to 20 hrs. a day; a growing child 12 to 14 hrs., and adult 7 to 9 hrs. Older persons usually sleep 5 to 7 hrs. but it is not necessarily true that older persons require much less sleep than they did when they were young. Women require more sleep than men. Depth of sleep varies from hour to hour.

s., R.E.M. Sleep during which rapid eye movements are noted. These eye movements are associated with dreaming. SEE: *R.E.M.*

s., stages of. Sleep may be classified in two distinct states in accordance with whether or not rapid eye movements are present. R.E.M., or rapid eye movement sleep, is the first state. N.R.E.M., or non–rapid eye movement sleep, is the second state and is divided into four stages with depth of sleep increasing as the stage increases. Fast, low-voltage electroencephalographic (EEG) waves accompany R.E.M. sleep; and slow EEG waves are present in N.R.E.M. sleep. Dreaming occurs in both R.E.M. and N.R.E.M. sleep. About 25% of normal sleep is of the R.E.M. state. Attempts to attribute mental disturbances to presence or absence of R.E.M. sleep have been inconclusive.

s., twilight. A procedure of injection of scopolamine and morphine to abolish the subsequent memory of pain without completely abolishing pain at the time. At one time widely used during labor and delivery.

sleep, words pert. to: dreams; hallucination; hypnagogic; hypnosis; hypnotic; hypnotism; insomnia; narcolepsy; noctambulism; somnambulism; somnifacient; somnolence; somnolent; sopor; soporific.

sleep apnea. Periodic cessation of breathing during sleep. Normally a harmless event but in patients with impaired cardiovascular systems, this may lead to death.

sleep drunkenness. The stuporous sleep caused by alcoholic intoxication. SYN: *somnolentia.*

sleep epilepsy. Condition characterized by an uncontrollable desire to sleep at periodic intervals. SYN: *narcolepsy.*

sleeping pills. Many drugs are available for the induction of or promotion of sleep. The desired effects are to produce normal sleep, not to interfere with arousal, to permit dreaming, and to allow the individual to awaken free of aftereffects such as lethargy, mental or physical depression, or amnesia. The ideal sedative or sleeping pill would not be habit-forming and would be free of toxic side effects if taken more or less regularly. No drug or class of drugs fulfills all these requirements.

A variety of forms of barbiturates are used to induce sleep. None are free of the ability to produce habituation. Other medicines available for sedation and inducing sleep are chloral derivatives including chloral hydrate, chloral betaine, and chlorobutanol; paraldehyde; piperidione derivatives such as glutethimide and methyprylon; methaqualone; benzodiazepine compounds including chlordiazepoxide, diazepam, and flurazepam. Some drugs such as certain kinds of antihistamines have the additional effect of causing severe drowsiness.

CAUTION: Sleeping pills and sedatives may be injurious to the developing embryo. Thus it is important to know whether or not a specific preparation is approved for use by women during pregnancy, esp. during early pregnancy.

sleeping sickness. 1. Acute infectious disease marked by increasing lethargy, drowsiness, muscular weakness, and cerebral symptoms. SYN: *encephalitis lethargica.* 2. African trypanosomiasis caused by a protozoon introduced into the blood and cerebrospinal fluid by the bite of a tsetse fly; characterized by fever, protracted lethargy, weakness, tremors, and wasting.

sleep terror disorder. Repeated episodes of abrupt awakening from sleep usually beginning with a panicky scream. Usually only a fragmentary dream is remembered, and morning amnesia for the episode is the rule.

This condition is seen mostly in children and young adults. SYN: *pavor nocturnus*.

sleep-wake disorders. A general classification of conditions that are concerned with hypersomnia, i.e., excessive sleepiness; insomnia; parasomnias; and disorders of the sleep-wake schedule.

Hypersomnia includes obstructed sleep apnea syndrome associated with micrognathia, tonsillar hypertrophy, and obesity hypoventilation syndrome; narcolepsy; and hypersomnia associated with menstruation.

Insomnia includes disorders of initiating and maintaining sleep. It is caused by psychiatric disorders; a syndrome in which environmental and cognitive stimuli lead to a conditioned arousal response at sleep onset; drug and alcohol dependency; sleep-related myoclonus and restless legs syndrome; and sleep apnea syndromes.

Sleep-wake schedule disorders include delayed sleep-phase syndrome wherein the 24-hour temperature rhythm is usually phase-delayed three or more hours relative to conventional bedtimes and wake times.

Parasomnias consist of disturbing phenomena that either occur only in sleep or are exacerbated by sleep. Included are snoring; difficulty breathing; swallowing; choking and seizures associated with sleep. In some cases parasomnia causes the individual no difficuty but a bedmate or family member brings the condition to a physician's attention.

sleep walking. Walking in one's sleep. SYN: *somnambulism*.

slide. 1. A thin glass plate on which an object is placed for microscopic examination. 2. A photograph prepared so that it may be used in a film slide projector.

slime mold. A primitive mold that is not easily classified. It has been claimed by both the zoologists and the botanists.

slimy (slī'mē) [AS. *slim*, smooth]. Resembling slime or a viscid substance; of a growth, adhering to needle so it can be drawn out as a long thread.

sling (slĭng) [AS. *slingan*, to wind]. A support for an injured upper extremity: SEE: *bandage; triangular bandage* for illus.

s., clove-hitch. Make clove hitch in center of roller bandage. Fit to hand and carry ends over shoulder. Tie beside neck with square knot, making longer ends. They may be carried over and behind the shoulders, brought under each axilla, and tied over chest.

s., counterbalanced. A rehabilitation device to assist upper extremity motion; it suspends the arm by way of an overhead frame and pulley and weight system. Also called *deltoid aid*.

s., cravat. The center of cravat is placed under wrist or forearm and ends tied around neck.

s., folded cravat. In this lesser arm sling, place broad fold in position on chest with one end over affected shoulder and other hanging down in front of chest. Flex arm as desired across sling. Bring lower end up over sound shoulder and secure with a knot located where it will not press on the affected shoulder.

s., open. The point of the triangle is placed at tip of elbow. The ends are brought around at back of neck and tied. The point should be brought forward and pinned or tied in a single knot, forming a cup to prevent elbow from slipping out.

s., simple figure-of-eight roller arm. Flex arm on chest in desired position, then fix bandage with single turn toward uninjured side around arm and chest, crossing elbow just above external epicondyle of humerus. Make second turn overlapping two thirds of first and bring bandage forward under tip of elbow, then upward along flexed forearm to root of neck of sound side. Then bring downward over scapula and cross chest and arm horizontally, overlapping, turn above, and continue as in progressive figure-of-eight.

s., St. John's. Apply triangle with point downward under elbow, upper end over sound shoulder. Flex arm acutely on chest. Bring lower end under affected arm and around back to knot with upper end on sound shoulder. Bring point up over elbow and fasten to base. Support is wholly for injured shoulder.

s., swathe arm or cravat. Use wide cravat or folded muslin band. Place center under acutely flexed elbow, carry front and upward across the forearm and over affected shoulder. Proceed obliquely across back to sound axilla. Bring other end around front of arm and across body to sound axilla, where it is pinned to other end, continuing around back to part of sling surrounding affected elbow and pinned again.

s., triangular. With suspension from uninjured side (brachioscapular sling). Place triangle on chest with one end over sound shoulder, the point under affected extremity, and fold the base. Flex injured arm outside of triangle. Carry lower end upward under axilla of injured side, back of shoulder, and tie with upper end behind back. Bring point of triangle anteriorly and medially around back of elbow and fasten to body of bandage. This bandage changes point of carrying and also relieves the clavicle on injured side of the load. SEE: *triangular bandage* for illus.

s., triangular, reversed. Apply with one end over injured shoulder, point toward the sound side, base vertical under injured elbow. Flex arm acutely over triangle. Lower end is brought upward over front of arm and over sound shoulder. Pull ends taut and tie over sound shoulder. The point is pulled taut over forearm and fixed to anterior and posterior layers between forearm and arm. Holds elbow more acutely flexed—the weight is supported by the elbow.

slit [ME. *slitte*]. A narrow opening.

s., vestibular. The opening between left and right ventricular folds of the larynx.

slit-lamp. SEE: *lamp, slit.*

slope. 1. An inclined plane or surface. 2. Tube of solid culture medium that is slanted to increase the surface area of the medium. Used in culturing bacteria. SYN: *slant.*

s., lower ridge. The slope of the crest of the mandibular residual ridge from the third molar forward as viewed in profile.

Slo-Phyllin. Trade name for theophylline, USP.

slough (slŭf) [ME. *slughe,* a skin]. 1. Dead matter or necrosed tissue separated from living tissue or an ulceration. 2. To separate in the form of dead or necrosed parts from living tissue. 3. To cast off, as dead tissue. SEE: *escharotic.*

sloughing (slŭf′ĭng). The formation of a slough; separation of dead from living tissue.

slow (slō) [AS. *slaw,* dull]. 1. Mentally dull. 2. Exhibiting retarded speed, as the pulse. 3. Said of a morbid condition or of a fever when it is not acute. SEE: words beginning with *brady-*.

Slow K. Trade name for potassium chloride, USP.

slow-reacting substance of anaphylaxis. ABBR: SRS-A. A substance released by certain tissues including the lungs during anaphylaxis. It causes slow contraction of smooth muscle tissue and may be of major importance in allergic bronchospasm.

slows (slōz). A condition resulting from ingestion of plants such as snakeroot (Eupatorium urticaefolium) or jimmey weed (Aploppus heterophyllus). Common in domestic animals and may occur in humans as a result of ingesting the plants or, more commonly, from drinking milk or eating the meat of poisoned animals. Symptoms are weakness; anorexia; nausea and vomiting; prostration; and possibly death. SYN: *trembles.*

slow virus infection. An infection caused by a virus that remains dormant in the body for a prolonged period prior to causing signs and symptoms of illness. Such viruses may require years to incubate prior to causing such diseases as scrapie in sheep or kuru in man. Diseases of a chronic degenerative nature that are now suspected to be due to slow viruses include subacute sclerosing panencephalitis and progressive multifocal leukoencephalopathy.

sludge (slŭjh). Under the Resource Conservation and Recovery Act of 1976, sludge is defined as any solid, semisolid, or liquid waste generated from a municipal, commercial, or industrial wastewater treatment plant, or air pollution control facility, or any such waste having similar characteristics or effects.

sludged blood. Condition of the blood in certain abnormal states such as tissue injury or shock in which volume of plasma is reduced and the cells show a pronounced tendency to agglutinate and form large clumps or masses that move slowly through the vessels and sometimes clog the smaller vessels.

slurry (slŭr′ē) [ME. *slory*]. A thin, watery mixture.

Sm. Chem. symb. for samarium.

SMA-12. Trade name of device that does 12 blood chemistry tests on a single blood sample.

small-for-gestational age. Term describing an infant whose stage of maturity at birth is less than would be considered normal for the length of the calculated gestation period.

smallpox (smawl′pŏks) [AS. *smael,* tiny, + *poc,* pustule]. An acute, contagious, febrile disease, the constitutional symptoms of which are followed by the appearance of an eruption. SEE: table. For complete description SEE: *variola.* SYN: *variola.*

NOTE: Smallpox is considered to have been eradicated.

smallpox vaccine. USP. A standardized preparation of the living virus of vaccinia. It was used in immunizing against smallpox, but its use is no longer thought to be necessary since smallpox is considered to have been eradicated worldwide. Trade name is Dryvax.

smear (smēr) [AS. *smerian,* to anoint]. 1. In bacteriology, material spread on a surface, as a microscopic slide or a culture medium. 2. Material obtained from infected matter spread over solid culture media.

s., blood. A thin film of blood on a glass slide. Blood is prepared in this manner for staining and microscopic examination.

s., Pap; s., Papanicolaou. SEE: *Papanicolaou test.*

smegma (smĕg′mă) [Gr. *smegma,* soap]. Secretion of sebaceous glands, specifically, the thick, cheesy, odoriferous secretion found under the labia minora about the glans clitoridis and under the male prepuce from Tyson's glands.

s. clitoridis. Odoriferous secretion of the glands of the clitoris.

s. embryonum. Vernix caseosa.

s. praeputii. Cheesy odoriferous substance collecting under prepuce in the male.

smegmatic (smĕg-măt′ĭk). Pert. to or made up of smegma.

smegmolith (smĕg′mō-lĭth) [Gr. *smegma,* soap,

Differential Diagnosis of Smallpox and Chickenpox

	Smallpox	Chickenpox
General symptoms	May be severe, with pyrexia, backache, prostration for 3 to 4 days before appearance of eruption	Mild Appear at same time as rash
Eruption	About 4th day of illness	First day
Type	Papules before vesicles; deep, often "shotty"	Maculopapular for few hours, then vesicular
Appearance	All spots at same stage of development	Successive crops; therefore, all stages present at the same time
	Pustules appear on the 8th day	Pustules on 3rd or 4th day
Distribution	Maximum on distal parts, not in axillae or groins	Maximum on trunk, present in axillae

+ *lithos,* a stone]. Calcareous mass in the smegma.

smell (smĕl) [ME. *smellen,* to reek]. 1. To perceive by stimulation of the olfactory nerves. 2. To emit an odor, pleasant or offensive. 3. A chemical sense dependent upon end-organs on the surface of the upper part of the nasal septum and the superior nasal concha. 4. Property of a thing affecting the olfactory organs, pleasant or unpleasant. SYN: *odor.*

The sense of smell may be affected by many conditions, some of which are the following:

Anosmia: A loss of the sense of smell. It may be a local and a temporary condition resulting from acute and chronic rhinitis, mouth breathing, nasal polyps, dryness of the nasal mucous membrane, pollens, or very offensive odors. It may also result from disease or injury of the olfactory tract, bone disease near the olfactory nerve, disease of the nasal accessory sinuses, basal meningitis, or tumors or gumma affecting the olfactory nerve. It is sometimes found in locomotor ataxia, and frequently in hysteria and neurasthenia. Disease of one cranial hemisphere or of one nasal chamber may account for anosmia. SYN: *anodmia; anosphrasia.*

Hyperosmia: An increased sensitivity to odors.

Kakosmia: The perception of bad odors where none exist; it may be due to head injuries or occur in hallucinations in certain psychoses. SYN: *cacosmia.*

Parosmia: A perverted sense of smell. Odors that are considered agreeable are assumed to be offensive and disagreeable odors may be found pleasant to those suffering from certain functional derangements and in some catarrhs. SYN: *parosphresia.* SEE: *cacosmia.*

smell, words pert. to: anodmia; anosmia; anosphrasia; aroma; aromatic; cacosmia; dysosmia; hyperosmia; jumentous; kakosmia; odor; odoriferous; olfaction; olfactory; organoleptic tests; osmesthesia; osphresis; oxyosphresia.

Smith's fracture. [Robert W. Smith, Irish physician, 1807–1873] Fracture of the lower end of the radius, with forward displacement of the lower fragment.

Smith-Peterson nail. [Marius N. Smith-Peterson, U.S. orthopedic surgeon, 1886–1953] A special nail that on cross-section has three flanges, used for stabilizing fractures of the neck of the femur.

Smith-Strang disease. An inherited disease due to malabsorption of methionine and in which the urine has a characteristic oasthouse odor. The patients have white hair, mental retardation, convulsions, diarrhea, and increased respiratory rate. SYN: *oasthouse disease.*

smog [blend of *smoke* and *fog*]. Dense fog combined with smoke and other forms of air pollution.

smoker's cancer. Cancer of the lip, throat, or lung caused by irritation from excessive smoking.

SMON. *subacute myelo-optic neuropathy.*

smooth muscle. SEE: *muscle, smooth.*

smudging (smŭj'ĭng). A speech defect in which difficult consonants are omitted.

Sn [L. *stannum*]. Chem. symb. for tin.

snail [ME.]. A small mollusk having a spiral shell and belonging to the class Gastropoda. They are important as intermediate hosts of many species of parasitic flukes.

snake [ME.]. A creeping reptile possessing scales and lacking limbs, external ears, and functional eyelids.

s., poisonous. A venom-producing snake. Venom is produced in a poison gland, which is connected by a tube or groove to a poison fang, one of two sharp elongated teeth present in upper jaw. The following are poisonous snakes of the U.S.: coral snake, copperhead, water moccasin (cottonmouth), and rattlesnake, of which there are 15 species. All except the coral snake belong to a group known as pit vipers because of presence of a

SNAKES

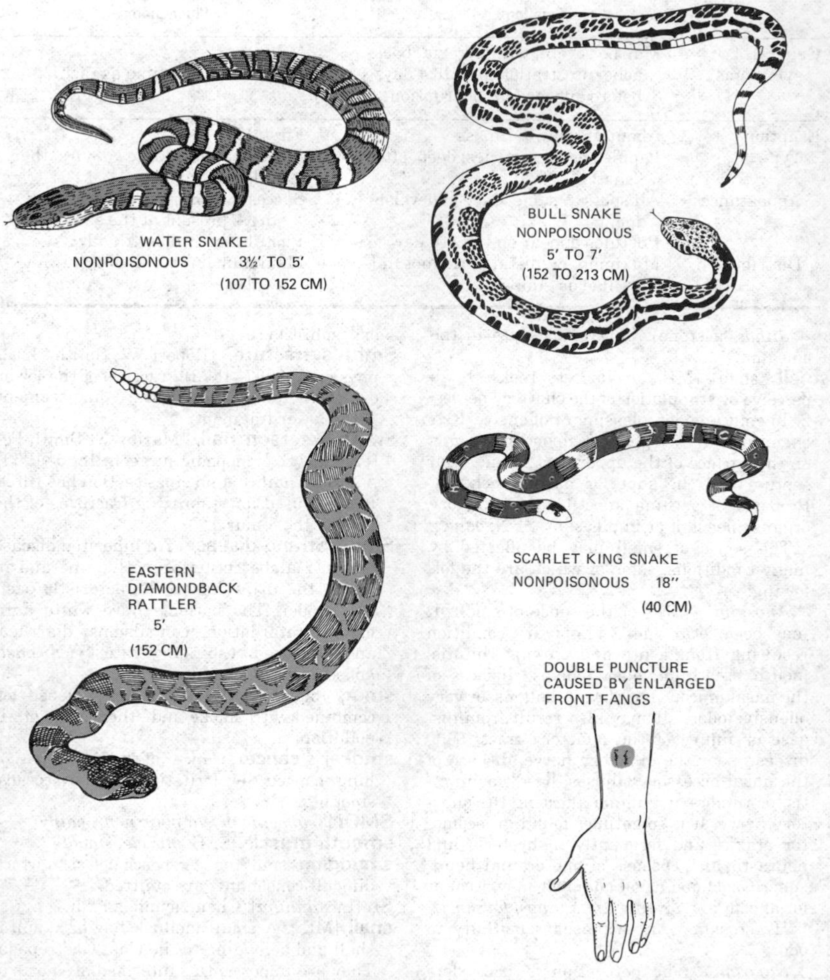

distinct pit between eye and nostril. SEE: illus.; *venom, snake.*

A polyvalent antivenin serum for bites by pit vipers is prepared by Wyeth Lab. Inc., Philadelphia, Pa. Antivenin for coral snake bite is available from the Florida State Dept. of Health, Jacksonville, Fla.

Information concerning the nearest source of antivenin may be obtained from the National Institutes of Health, Bethesda, Md.; the Reptile Institute, Silver Springs, Fla.; or from large zoos.

RS: antivenin; ophidism; ophiotoxemia; venenation; venene; veneniferous; venom.

snake bite. All snakes should be considered poisonous, although there are only a few that secrete an amount of venom sufficient to inoculate poison deeply into the tissues.

F.A.: Apply tourniquet just tight enough to stop venous return of blood, but it should not be tight enough to prevent arterial circulation. Application of cold to the area will impede spread of the venom. Then incise and induce bleeding. Immobilize patient immediately in order to delay spread of venom. If swelling persists, incise again. This may need to be done frequently. Inject antivenin. If the type of snake cannot be determined, use mixed antivenin. Release tourniquet cautiously for 90 seconds every 10 minutes and observe effect. At the same time, cooling of the entire limb or area is effective in preventing transfer of the venom from the area to the general circulation.

CAUTION: A tourniquet should not be applied too tight or remain on too long. Alcoholic stimulants must not be taken and nothing should be done to increase circulation. Do not cauterize with strong acids or depend upon home remedies. Antibiotics and tetanus prophylaxis are essential.

snap. A sharp cracking sound.

s., closing. The intense first heart sound heard in mitral stenosis.

s., opening. A sharp sound of increased pitch heard in early systole. It is associated with opening of the abnormal valve in mitral stenosis.

snapping finger. A snapping sound or feeling produced by bending the finger. In adults it is usually caused by tenosynovitis; in children by the sliding of tendons out of a cramped space when the finger is extended.

snapping hip. Slipping of the hip joint with a snap due to displacement over the great trochanter of a tendinous band.

snare (snār) [AS. *sneare,* noose]. Device for excision of polyps or tumors by tightening wire loops around them.

sneeze (snēz) [AS. *fneosan,* to pant]. 1. To expel air forcibly through the nose and mouth by spasmodic contraction of muscles of expiration due to irritation of nasal mucosa. The sneeze reflex may be produced by a great number of stimuli. Placing a foot on a cold surface will provoke a sneeze in some people, while looking at a bright light or sunlight will cause it in others. Firm pressure applied to the middle of the upper lip and just under the nose will sometimes prevent a sneeze that is about to occur. SEE: *photic sneezing; ptarmus.* 2. The act of sneezing. SEE: *sternutation; sternutatory.*

Snellen's chart (snĕl'ĕns). [Herman Snellen, Dutch ophthalmologist, 1834–1908] Chart imprinted with lines of black letters graduating in size from smallest on the bottom to largest on top used for testing visual acuity.

Snellen's reflex. Congestion of ear on same side upon stimulation of the distal end of the divided auriculotemporal nerve. SYN: *auriculocervical nerve reflex.*

Snellen's test. Test for visual acuity where the patient reads Snellen's chart at a certain distance with one eye, then with the other eye, and then with both eyes.

snore (snor) [AS. *snora*]. 1. To breathe noisily during sleep, due to vibration of the uvula and soft palate. 2. Noisy breathing in sleep or coma. SYN: *stertor.*

snoring rale (snor'ĭng răl). A sonorous rale, low in pitch, resembling a snore.

snow, carbon dioxide. SEE: *carbon dioxide solid therapy.*

snow blindness. Irritation of the conjunctiva caused by reflection of the sun on the snow.

SYM: Photophobia, blepharospasm, burning pain in the eyes, hyperemia, or temporary blindness.

SNS. *Society of Neurological Surgeons.*

snuff. 1. A medicinal powder inhaled through the nose. 2. A powdered form of tobacco inhaled through the nose, or placed in the posterior part of the buccal cavity on one side.

snuffbox, anatomical. Triangular area of the dorsum of the hand at the base of the thumb. When the thumb is extended, the tendons of the long and short extensor muscles of the thumb bound this area, which appears as a depression. When snuff was used, a small pinch could be placed in this "box" and snuffed up into the nose from that site. Tenderness in this area may be present when the navicular bone is fractured.

snuffles (snŭf'ls) [D. *snuffelen,* to snuff]. Obstructed nasal breathing with discharge from the nasal mucosa, esp. in infants, chiefly in congenital syphilis.

SOAP. Acronym for an organized structure for keeping progress notes in the chart. Each entry contains date, number and title of the patient's particular problem, followed by the SOAP headings: Subjective findings; Objective findings; Assessment, the documented resolution of the findings; and Plan for further diagnostic or therapeutic action. If the patient has multiple problems, a SOAP entry on the chart is made for each problem.

soap (sōp) [AS. *sape*]. A cleansing chemical compound formed by an alkali acting on a fatty acid, such as sodium stearate, $NaC_{18}H_{35}O_2$. Castile soap is made by saponifying olive oil with sodium hydroxide, and contains mainly sodium oleate, $NaC_{18}H_{33}O_2$. SEE: *detergent; saponification.*

s., green. S., soft medicinal.

s., soft medicinal. A liquid soap made by saponification of vegetable oils excluding coconut oil and palm kernel oil and without removal of glycerin. Used in the treatment of skin diseases. SYN: *s., green.*

soap liniment. A solution of soap and camphor in alcohol and water. Used as a stimulant and rubefacient.

soap-suds enema. Enema given so that the irritating action of the soap will stimulate the bowel. Less harsh forms of enema are preferred. SEE: *enema.*

S.O.B. *short of breath.*

sob [ME. *sobben,* to catch breath]. 1. To weep with convulsive movements of the chest. 2. A cry or wail resulting from a sudden convulsive inspiration accompanied by spasmodic closure of the glottis. SEE: *sigh*.

socialization (sō″shă-lĭ-zā′shŭn). The process of adapting an individual to the social customs of society; in the process he or she becomes a useful member of the society.

socioacusis (sō″sē-ō-ă-kū′sĭs) [L. *socius*, companion, + Gr. *akoustikos*, hearing]. The long-range ill effects of environmental noise on auditory acuity.

sociobiology (sō″sē-ō-bī-ŏl′ō-jē) [″ + Gr. *bios*, life, + *logos*, study]. The branch of biology concerned with the biological and genetic determinants of social behavior.

socioeconomic status. The combined social and economic level of individuals or groups. Such classification is useful in studying the relationship of income and living conditions on the prevalence and incidence of various diseases.

sociology (sō-sē-ŏl′ō-jē) [″ + Gr. *logos*, a study]. Study of human social behavior and the origins, institutions, and functions of human groups and societies.

sociomedical. Pert. to sociology and medicine, esp. the interrelationships between the two.

sociometry (sō″sē-ŏm′ĕ-trē) [″ + Gr. *metron*, measure]. The science concerned with measuring social behavior.

sociopath (sō′sē-ō-păth) [″ + Gr. *pathos*, disease]. An individual with antisocial personality disorder, q.v.

sociopathic personality. SEE: *personality, antisocial*.

sociopathy (sō″sē-ŏp′ă-thē) [″ + Gr. *pathos*, disease]. The condition of being antisocial.

socket (sŏk′ĕt) [ME. *soket*, a spearhead]. 1. A hollow in a joint or part for another corresponding organ, as a bone socket or an eye socket. SEE: *acetabulum*. 2. The proximal portion of a prosthesis, into which the stump of an amputated extremity is fitted.

s., dry. Alveolitis following tooth extraction characterized by extreme pain but without suppuration.

s., tooth. A dental alveolus of the maxilla or mandible; a cavity that contains the root of a tooth.

soda (sō′dă) [Medieval L., headache]. 1. Term loosely applied to various salts of sodium, esp. to caustic soda (sodium hydroxide) and baking soda (sodium bicarbonate). SEE: *sodium*. 2. Short for soda water, which is water charged with carbon dioxide.

s. ash. Commercial sodium carbonate.

s., baking. Sodium bicarbonate.

s., caustic. Sodium hydroxide.

s. lime. A white granular substance consisting of a mixture of calcium hydroxide and sodium hydroxide or potassium hydroxide or both. Used to absorb carbon dioxide.

s., lye. Sodium hydroxide.

s., niter. Nitrate of soda.

Soda Mint. Trade name for sodium bicarbonate, USP.

soda water. A solution of carbon dioxide under pressure; carbonic acid.

Sodestrin. Trade name for estrogens, conjugated.

sodic (sō′dĭk). Relating to or containing soda or sodium.

sodio-. Combining form denoting a compound containing sodium.

sodium (sō′dē-ŭm) [LL.]. SYMB: Na. At. wt. 22.9898; at. no. 11; sp. gr. 0.971. Sodium constitutes approximately 0.15% of elements of the body. Sodium (Na^+), K^+, Ca^{++}, and Mg^{++} constitute the principal cations of the body, their relative concentration determining the integrity of cell membranes and the bioelectric potentials of tissues. Na^+ is the principal cation found in extracellular fluids.

FUNCT: Sodium salts are found in the fluids of the body, serum, blood, and lymph, and in the tissues, the concentration being lower in the tissues. They are necessary to preserve a balance between calcium and potassium to maintain normal heart action and the equilibrium of the body. They regulate osmotic pressure in the cells and fluids, act as an ion balance in tissues, produce a buffer action in the blood, and guard against an excessive loss of water from the tissues.

DEFICIENCY SYM: Weakness, nerve disorders, loss of weight, "salt hunger," miner's cramps, disturbed digestion.

s. acetate. USP. A chemical compound that is used to alkalize the urine, and is used in kidney dialysis solutions.

s. alginate. A purified carbohydrate product extracted from certain species of seaweed. It is used as a food additive and as a pharmaceutic aid.

s. amytal. The monosodium salt of isoamylethylbarbituric acid.

ACTION AND USES: Sedative and hypnotic in control of insomnia; preliminary to surgical anesthesia and in labor.

s. ascorbate. USP. The sodium salt of ascorbic acid, vitamin C. It may be used in solution when parenteral administration of vitamin C is required.

s. benzoate. A white, odorless powder with sweet taste. Used as a food preservative.

s. bicarbonate. USP. White odorless powder with saline taste. $NaHCO_3$.

ACTION AND USES: Orally as an antacid. Effectiveness for this purpose is questionable. Externally, mild alkaline wash.

INCOMPAT: Acids, acid salts, ammonium chloride, lime water, ephedrine hydrochloride, iron chloride.

s. biphosphate, monobasic. USP. Chemical substance that is used as a cathartic.

s. bisulfite. Granular or crystalline powder, sulfurous taste and odor, soluble in water. Used as an antioxidant in industry.

s. borate. Borax. Used as a detergent and water softener and as an ingredient of certain pharmaceutical preparations for external use.

s. caprylate. An antifungal drug.

s. carbonate. Na_2CO_3. White crystalline powder (washing soda). Used as an alkali employed chiefly in alkaline baths.

s. carboxymethyl cellulose. USP. The sodium salt of carboxymethyl cellulose, q.v.

s. chloride. USP. NaCl. Common table salt.

ACTION AND USES: In preparation of normal saline solution, emetic, and to add flavor to foods.

INCOMPAT: Silver nitrate.

In aqueous solution sodium chloride, a neutral salt, is a strong electrolyte, being almost completely ionized. The sodium and chlorine ions are important in maintaining the proper electrolyte balance in body fluids. The kidneys control excretion of sodium chloride in the urine. This control mechanism is complex but the hormones vasopressin and aldosterone are essential to the process. Sodium chloride is also present in sweat, milk, and intestinal juices.

s. citrate. USP. White granular powder, saline in taste and soluble in water. Used as an anticoagulant for blood in transfusion.

s. cyclamate. A nonnutritive sweetener.

s. fluoride. USP. NaF. White crystalline powder, saline in taste, soluble in 25 parts of water.

ACTION AND USES: In drinking water and in solution for local application to teeth for prevention of dental caries. Commercially, in etching glassware, for eradication of rats, insects, ants, and other pests. SEE: *fluoridation; sodium fluoride poisoning.*

s. fluoride and phosphoric acid topical solution. USP. A preparation used for direct application to teeth when incorporated into toothpaste.

s. glucosulfone. A drug used in treating leprosy.

s. glutamate. The monosodium salt of L-glutamate. It is used in treating hepatic coma.

s. hydroxide. NaOH. A whitish solid; soluble in water, making a clear solution. SYN: *soda, caustic; soda, lye.*

USES: Antacid and caustic. In the laundry and in commercial compounds, in cleaning sink traps, toilets, etc., and in the preparation of soap.

CAUTION: Use great care in handling it as it rapidly destroys organic tissues. Protective glasses should be worn while working with this chemical. If splashed in eye, may cause blindness.

s. hypochlorite solution. USP. An antiseptic used in root canal therapy. CAUTION: This solution is not suitable for application to wounds.

s. hyposulfite. S. thiosulfate.

s. iodide. USP. NaI. A salt resembling in appearance and action potassium iodide.

s. lactate injection. USP. Sodium salt of inactive lactic acid. In one sixth or one fourth molar solution it is used I.V. to control electrolyte disturbances, esp. acidosis.

s. lauryl sulfate. An anionic surface-active agent that is used as a pharmaceutic acid.

s. monofluorophosphate. USP. An agent suitable for topical application to teeth to prevent dental caries.

s. morrhuate injection. USP. The sodium salt of the fatty acids, found in cod liver oil. Used as a sclerosing agent for the obliteration of varicose veins.

s. nitrate. The chemical $NaNO_3$, used in industrial chemical processes.

s. nitrite. USP. $NaNO_2$. White crystalline powder. Antidote for cyanide poisoning.

s. nitroprusside. USP. A powerful vasodilator used when rapid reduction in blood pressure is required.

s. perborate. USP. An antiseptic agent used in certain topical drugs and solutions.

s. peroxide. Sodium oxide, Na_2O_2, used as a bleaching agent.

s. phosphate, dibasic. USP. Chemical that is used as a cathartic.

s. phosphate P32 solution. USP. A standardized preparation of radioactive phosphorus (^{32}P).

s. polystyrene sulfonate. USP. A cation-exchange resin used to lower the potassium in the body.

s. propionate. A pharmaceutic aid that also has antifungal action.

s. psylliate. A sclerosing agent.

s. salicylate. USP. $C_7H_5NaO_3$. White powder or scales with sweet saline taste. Used as an analgesic and antipyretic.

INCOMPAT: Caffeine citrate, caffeine sodium benzoate.

s. sulfate. USP. A salt used as a saline cathartic and diuretic. Also has some uses in veterinary medicine. SYN: *Glauber's salt.*

s. tetradecyl sulfate. An anionic surfactant that is used for its sclerosing action.

s. thiosulfate. USP. White crystalline substance, having a cooling taste. Used externally to remove stains of iodine and intravenously as an antidote for cyanide poisoning.

sodium fluoride poisoning. Symptoms include conjunctivitis, retching, vomiting, nausea, eventual cardiac weakness, kidney disturbances, and interference with coagulation of blood.

F.A.: In addition to washing affected areas, precipitate by addition of soluble calcium salts such as lime water, calcium gluconate, or calcium lactate. Give emetics and soothing drinks such as milk, cream, or egg whites.

Sodium Versenate. Trade name for edetate disodium, USP.

sodokosis (sŏd-ō-kō′sĭs) [Jap. *sodoku,* rat poison + Gr. *osis,* condition]. Sodoku, q.v. SEE: *rat-bite fever.*

sodoku (sō-dō′koo). Infectious febrile disease due to Spirillum minus transmitted by rat bite. SEE: *rat-bite fever.* SYN: *rat-bite fever; sodokosis.*

sodomist, sodomite (sŏd′ō-mĭst, -mīt) [LL. *Sodoma,* Sodom]. A person who practices sodomy.

sodomy (sŏd′ō-mē) [LL. *Sodoma,* Sodom]. Anal intercourse, usually between males.

Soemmering's bone (sĕm′ĕr-ĭngz). [Samuel T. von Soemmering, German anatomist, 1755–1830] Marginal process of malar (zygomatic) bone.

Soemmering's foramen. The fovea centralis retinal.

Soemmering's ring. Annular swelling of the periphery of the lens capsule.

Soemmering's spot. The macula lutea of the retina.

soft (sŏft) [AS. *softe*]. Not hard, firm, or solid.

soft diet. A diet consisting of nothing but soft or semi-solid foods or liquids. Includes fish, egg, and cheese dishes, chicken, cereals, bread, toast, and butter. No red meats or vegetables or fruits having seeds or thick skins. No cellulose, raw fruits, or salads. SYN: *convalescent diet.*

soft palate. The posterior portion of the roof of the mouth, partly separating the mouth and the pharynx. SYN: *velum palatinum.*

soft sore. A highly infectious nonsyphlitic venereal ulcer caused by Ducrey's bacillus. SYN: *chancroid,* q.v.

softening (sŏf′ĕn-ĭng) [AS.]. Process of becoming soft. SYN: *malacia; mollities.*

s., anemic. White softening of the brain from lack of blood.

s., colliquative. The liquefying of tissues.

s., gray. Softening of the brain with absorption of fat following yellow softening.

s., hemorrhagic. S., red.

s., mucoid. Myxomatous degeneration.

s. of bones. Osteomalacia.

s. of brain. Paresis with progressive dementia. SYN: *encephalomalacia.*

s. of heart. Myomalacia cordis.

s. of stomach. Gastromalacia.

s., red. Softening of the brain with bleeding into necrosed portions. SYN: *s., hemorrhagic.*

s., white. S., anemic.

sol (sŏl, sōl) [Gr. *sole,* salt water]. State of a colloid system in which the dispersion medium or solvent forms a continuous phase in which the particles of the solute are dispersed, forming a fluid mass. It is called a hydrosol if dispersion medium is a liquid and aerosol if a gas. SEE: *gel.*

sol. Solution.

solace. An object or resource that does or seems to soothe pain or mental stress. In children a teddy bear or a "security" blanket may provide solace. In later life, one's spouse, a friend, or a hobby may be a source of solace.

Solanaceae (sōl″ă-nā′sē-ē). A family of herbs, shrubs, and trees from which several important drugs such as scopolamine and belladonna are derived. The potato is one of the species.

solanaceous (sōl″ă-nā′shŭs): Concerning the family Solanaceae.

solanine (sō′lă-nēn). A poisonous narcotic alkaloid obtained from potato sprouts and tomatoes. SEE: *poisoning, potato.*

solar (sō′lăr) [L. *solaris*]. 1. Pert. to the sun or its rays. 2. The solar plexus.

solarium (sō-lā′rē-ŭm) [L. *solarium,* terrace]. 1. A room or porch exposed to the sun. 2. A room designed for heliotherapy or for the application of artificial light. 3. Day or recreational room for patients; often used as a waiting area for family or visitors.

solar plexus. The celiac plexus, behind the stomach and between the suprarenal glands and consisting of two large ganglia, the celiac and superior mesenteric ganglia, from which sympathetic fibers pass to visceral organs.

solar therapy. Treatment with the sun's rays. SYN: *heliotherapy.*

solation (sō-lā′shŭn). In colloidal chemistry, the transformation of a gel into a sol.

solder (sŏd′ĕr). Any fusible alloy usually made of tin and lead used to join metal parts. The alloy is applied in a melted state.

sole (sōl) [AS. *sole*]. 1. Underpart of the foot. SYN: *planta.* 2. The portion of a motor endplate at termination of a motor nerve fiber that is directly adjacent to the contractile substance of a muscle fiber. A large number of muscle nuclei are usually aggregated here. SEE: *antithenar; thenar.*

solenoid (sōl′lĕ-noyd). A coil of insulated wire in which a magnetic force is created in the long axis of the coil when an electric current flows through the wire. This may be used to activate switches.

sole reflex. Plantar flexion of the foot muscles when tickling the sole. SYN: *plantar reflex.*

soleus (sō'lē-ŭs) [L. *solea,* sole of foot]. A flat, broad muscle of the calf of the leg. SEE: *Muscles* in *Appendix.*

Solfoton. Trade name for phenobarbital, USP.

Solganal. Trade name for aurothioglucose, USP.

solid (sŏl'ĭd) [L. *solidus*]. 1. Not gaseous, hollow, or liquid. 2. A substance not gaseous, liquid, or hollow.

solipsism (sŏl'ĭp-sĭzm) [L. *solus,* alone, + *ipse,* self]. The theory that the self may know only its own feelings and changes and there is then only subjective reality.

solitary (sŏl'ĭ-tăr-ē) [L. *solitarius*]. Alone; single or existing separately.

solitary lymph nodules. Small spherical lymphatic nodules found in the lamina propria of the small and large intestine.

solo practitioner. A physician, dentist, or other practitioner who practices alone rather than with a group or partner.

solubility (sŏl"ū-bĭl'ĭ-tē) [L. *solubilis,* soluble]. Capability of being dissolved.

soluble (sŏl'ū-bl). Able to be dissolved.

Solu-Cortef. Trade name for hydrocortisone sodium succinate, USP.

Solu-Medrol. Trade name for methylprednisolone sodium succinate, USP.

solum tympani (sō'lŭm tĭm'pă-nē) [L.]. The floor of the tympanic cavity.

solute (sŏl'ūt) [L. *solutus,* solution]. The substance that is dissolved in a solution.

solutio (sō-lū'shē-ō) [L. *solutus,* solution]. Solution.

solution (sō-lū'shŭn) [L. *solutus*]. 1. Liquid containing dissolved substance. 2. Process by which a solid is homogeneously mixed with a fluid or a solid or gas so that the dissolved substances cannot be distinguished from the resultant fluid. 3. Mixture formed by dissolution of substances.

The liquid in which the substances are dissolved is called the solvent, q.v., and the substance dissolved, the solute, q.v.

s., aqueous. A solution that contains water as the solvent.

s., buffer. A solution of a weak acid and its salt (e.g., carbonic acid, sodium bicarbonate) of importance in maintaining a constant pH, esp. of the blood.

s., colloidal. A solution in which the solute is suspended and not dissolved, such as gelatin or albumin.

s., contrast. A solution that contains a radiopaque substance. These solutions are used to facilitate x-ray examination of body cavities.

s., hyperbaric. A solution with a specific gravity greater than one, or greater than the solution to which it is being compared. This is important in injecting medicines or anesthetic agents into the spinal canal.

s., hypertonic. A solution having a greater osmotic pressure than that of cells or body fluids; a solution that draws water out of cells, thus inducing plasmolysis.

Ex.: A concentrated solution of sodium chloride.

s., hypotonic. A solution having an osmotic pressure less than that of cells or body fluids; a solution that will cause water to enter cells, thus inducing turgor and possibly hemolysis.

Ex.: A sodium chloride solution containing less than 0.9 gm. of NaCl in each 100 ml. of water.

s., iodine. A solution of iodine and potassium iodine used as a source of iodine.

s., isobaric. A solution with a specific gravity equal to one or equal to the solution with which it is being compared. SEE: *s., hyperbaric.*

s., isohydric. A solution having the same hydrogen ion concentration or pH as another.

s., isosmotic. S., isotonic.

s., isotonic. A solution that has the same osmotic pressure as that of body cells or fluids.

Ex.: A sodium chloride solution containing 0.9 gm. of NaCl in each 100 ml. of water. SYN: *s., isosmotic.*

s., Locke-Ringer's. A buffered isotonic solution containing 9.0 gm. sodium chloride, 0.42 gm. potassium chloride, 0.24 gm. calcium chloride, 0.5 gm. sodium bicarbonate, 0.2 gm. magnesium chloride, 0.5 gm. dextrose, and distilled water to make 1000 ml.

s., molar. Solution containing a gram molecular weight or mole of the reagent dissolved in one liter (1000 ml.) of solution. Designated 1M.

s., normal. Solution containing one gram equivalent weight of reagent in one liter (1000 ml.) of solution. Designated 1N.

s., normal saline. An isotonic saline solution. SEE: *s., isotonic.*

s., ophthalmic. A sterile preparation suitable for instillation in the eye.

s., physiological saline. An isotonic solution of sodium chloride. SEE: *s., isotonic.*

s., repair. Any solution given intravenously to treat an electrolyte or metabolic disturbance.

s., Ringer's. A solution containing chlorides of sodium, calcium, and potassium in most favorable concentration It contains 8.6 gm. sodium chloride, 0.3 gm. calcium chloride, 0.3 gm. potassium chloride, and distilled water to make one liter (1000 ml.).

s., saline. A solution of a salt, usually sodium chloride.

s., saturated. A solution that contains

all the solute it can dissolve. This limit is called the saturation point.

s., sclerosing. An irritating substance that produces sclerosis when applied to tissues or injected into a vein.

s., seminormal. ABBR: 0.5N or N/2. A solution containing one half of a gram equivalent weight of reagent in one liter (1000 ml.) of solution.

s., standard. A solution containing a definite amount of a substance as a normal solution. Used for comparison or analysis.

s., supersaturation. Solution in which the saturation point is reached, but when heated, it is possible to dissolve more of the solute.

s., test. A reagent solution, one used in performing a particular test.

s., Tyrode's. A modified Ringer's solution containing, in addition, a small amount of magnesium chloride and acid and sodium phosphates.

s., volumetric. A standard solution containing a definite amount (1/2, 1/10, etc.) gram equivalent of a substance in one liter (1000 ml.) of solution. Used in volumetric analysis.

solv. L. *solve,* dissolve.

solvate (sŏl'vāt). A compound formed by reaction between solvent and solute.

solvation (sŏl-vā'shŭn). The formation of a solvate.

solvent (sŏl'vĕnt) [L. *solvens*]. 1. Producing a solution, dissolving. 2. A liquid holding another substance in solution. 3. A liquid that reacts with a solvent bringing it into solution.

solvolysis (sŏl-vŏl'ĭ-sĭs). General term for reactions involving decomposition by hydrolysis, ammonolysis, and sulfolysis.

Soma. Trade name for carisoprodol.

soma (sō'mă) [Gr. *soma,* body]. 1. The body as distinct from the mind. 2. All of the body cells except the germ cells. 3. The body exclusive of the extremities.

somasthenia (sōm"ăs-thē'nē-ă) [" + *astheneia,* weakness]. A condition of chronic bodily weakness. SYN: *somatasthenia.*

somat(o)- (sō'mă-tō) [Gr. *soma,* body]. Combining form indicating a relationship to the body.

somatasthenia (sō"măt-ăs-thē'nē-ă). Chronic bodily weakness usually with low blood pressure, but not neurasthenia. SYN: *somasthenia.*

somatalgia (sō"mă-tăl'jē-ă) [" + *algos,* pain]. Pain in the body due to organic causes.

somatesthesia (sō"măt-ĕs-thē'zē-ă) [" + *aisthesis,* sensation]. The consciousness of the body; bodily sensation.

somatic (sō-măt'ĭk) [Gr. *soma,* body]. 1. Pert. to nonreproductive cells or tissues. 2. Pert. to the body. 3. Pert. to structures of the body wall, e.g., skeletal muscles (somatic musculature) in contrast to structures associated with the viscera, e.g., visceral muscles (splanchnic musculature).

somaticosplanchnic (sō-măt"ĭ-kō-splănk'nĭk) [" + *splanchna,* viscera]. Somaticovisceral, q.v.

somaticovisceral (sō-măt"ĭ-kō-vĭs'ĕr-ăl) [" + L. *viscera,* body organs]. Concerning the body and the viscera.

somatist (sō'mă-tĭst) [Gr. *soma,* body]. One who believes mental disorders have an organic basis.

somatization (sō"mă-tī-zā'shŭn). The process of expressing a mental condition as a disturbed bodily function.

somatization disorder. Condition of recurrent and multiple somatic complaints of several years' duration for which medical attention has been sought but no physical basis for the disorder has been found. The age of onset is usually prior to 30. The somatic complaints may be related to virtually any organ system.

somatoceptors (sō-măt"ō-sĕp'tors). Term applied to proprioceptors and exteroceptors collectively.

somatochrome (sō-măt'ō-krōm) [" + *chroma,* color]. A nerve cell in which the nucleus is completely surrounded by cytoplasm.

somatogenic (sō"mă-tō-jĕn'ĭk) [" + *gennan,* to produce]. Originating in the body. SEE: *psychogenic.*

somatology (sō"mă-tŏl'ō-jē) [" + *logos,* a study]. Comparative study of structure, functions, and development of the human body.

somatome (sō'mă-tōm) [" + *tome,* incision]. 1. A device for cutting the body of the fetus. 2. A somite.

somatomedin. Substance important in regulating growth by its action on the effect of growth hormone on cartilage and bone. Its synthesis in the liver is influenced by the growth hormone.

somatomegaly (sō"mă-tō-mĕg'ă-lē) [" + *megas,* large]. Abnormally large size of the body.

somatometry (sō"mă-tŏm'ĕ-trē) [" + *metron,* measure]. Measurement of the body.

somatopagus (sō"mă-tŏp'ă-gŭs) [" + *pagos,* thing fixed]. A deformed twin fetus with the trunks merged.

somatopathic (sō"mă-tō-păth'ĭk) [" + *pathos,* disease]. Organically ill, as distinguished from neuropathic or psychopathic diseases.

somatoplasm (sō-măt'ō-plăzm) [Gr. *soma,* body, + *plasma,* a thing formed]. The protoplasm of all the body cells as distinguished from that of the germ plasm.

somatopleural (sō"mă-tō-ploor'ăl). Concerning somatopleure.

somatopleure (sō-măt′ō-ploor) [″ + *pleura,* a side]. The lateral and ventral body wall of an embryo consisting of the outer ectoderm and a layer of somatic mesoderm underlying it. It continues beyond the embryo as the amnion and chorion.
somatopsychic (sō″măt-ō-sī′kĭk) [″ + *psyche,* mind]. Pert. to both body and mind.
somatopsychosis (sō″mă-tō-sī-kō′sĭs) [″ + ″ + *osis,* condition]. Any mental disorder that is a symptom of a bodily disease.
somatoschisis (sō″mă-tŏs′kĭ-sĭs) [″ + *schistos,* split]. A deformed fetus with a cleft in the trunk.
somatoscopy (sō-mă-tŏs′kō-pē) [″ + *skopein,* to examine]. Physical examination of the body.
somatosexual (sō″mă-tō-sĕks′ū-ăl) [″ + L. *sexus,* sex]. Concerning the body and sexual characteristics.
somatostatin (sō-măt′ō-stăt″ĭn). A hormone that inhibits the release of somatotropin. It is a hypothalamic peptide that also inhibits the secretion of insulin and gastrin.
somatotonia (sō″mă-tō-tō′nē-ă) [″ + L. *tonus,* tone]. A personality type, described by the anthropologist Sheldon, in which there is a predominance of physical assertiveness and activity.
somatotopic (sō″mă-tō-tŏp′ĭk) [″ + *topos,* place]. Concerning the correspondence between a particular part of the body and a particular area of the brain.
somatotrophic (sō″mă-tō-trŏf′ĭk) [″ + *tropos,* a turning]. 1. Having selective attraction for or influence on body cells. 2. Stimulating growth.
somatotrophin (sō″mă-tō-trō′fĭn) [″ + *trophe,* nourishment]. Growth hormone, somatotropin.
somatotropic (sō″mă-tō-trŏp′ĭk) [″ + *trope,* a turn]. Influencing the body or body cells.
somatotropin (sō″măt-ō-trō′pĭn) [″ + *tropos,* a turning]. The anterior pituitary lobe's growth-stimulating principle. In the human, this is called human growth hormone (HGH).
somatotype (sō-măt′ō-tīp). A particular build or type of body, based on physical characteristics. SEE: *ectomorph; endomorph; mesomorph.*
Sombulex. Trade name for hexobarbital.
somesthesia (sŏm-ĕs-thē′sē-ă) [″ + *aisthesis,* sensation]. Awareness of bodily sensations. SYN: *somatesthesia.*
somesthetic (sō-mĕs-thĕt′ĭk). Pert. to sensations and sensory structures of the body.
somesthetic area. The region in the cortex in which lie the terminations of the axons of general sensory conduction paths.
somesthetic path. General sensory conduction path leading to the cortex.
somite (sō′mīt) [Gr. *soma,* body]. Embryonic blocklike segment formed on either side of the neural tube and its underlying notochord. Each somite gives rise to a muscle mass supplied by a spinal nerve and each pair gives rise to a vertebra.
somnambulance (sŏm-năm′bū-lăns) [L. *somnus,* sleep, + *ambulare,* to walk]. Somnambulism.
somnambule. A person who walks while asleep.
somnambulism (sŏm-năm′bū-lĭzm) [L. *somnus,* sleep, + *ambulare,* to walk]. Sleepwalking, an affection that prompts the sleeping person to perform, unconsciously, acts that naturally belong to the waking state.
somnambulist (sŏm-năm′bū-lĭst). One who is subject to sleepwalking.
somnifacient (sŏm-nĭ-fā′shĕnt) [″ + *facere,* to make]. 1. Producing sleep. SYN: *hypnotic.* 2. A medicine producing sleep. SYN: *soporific.*
somniferous (sŏm-nĭf′ĕr-ŭs) [″ + *ferre,* to bear]. Sleep-producing; pert. to that which promotes sleep.
somnific (sŏm-nĭf′ĭk). Producing sleep.
somniloquence (sŏm-nĭl′ō-kwĕns) [″ + *loqui,* to speak]. Somniloquism, q.v.
somniloquism (sŏm-nĭl′ō-kwĭzm) [″ + ″ + *-ismos,* condition]. Talking in one's sleep.
somniloquist (sŏm-nĭl′ō-kwĭst) [″ + *loqui,* to speak]. One who talks in his sleep.
somniloquy (sŏm-nĭl′ō-kwē) [″ + *loqui,* to speak]. Act of talking during sleep or in a hypnotic condition.
somnipathist (sŏm-nĭp′ă-thĭst) [″ + Gr. *pathos,* disease]. 1. One who is susceptible to hypnosis, or who is under the influence of hypnosis. 2. A person who experiences somnipathy.
somnipathy (sŏm-nĭp′ă-thē) [″ + Gr. *pathos,* disease]. 1. Any disorder of sleep. 2. Hypnotism.
somnocinematograph (sŏm″nō-sĭn-ĕ-măt′ō-grăf) [″ + Gr. *kinema,* motion, + *graphein,* to write]. Device for recording motions of those who are asleep.
somnolence (sŏm′nō-lĕns) [L. *somnolentia,* sleepiness]. Prolonged drowsiness or a condition resembling trance that may continue for a number of days; sleepiness.
somnolent (sŏm′nō-lĕnt) [L. *somnolentus*]. Sleepy; drowsy.
somnolentia (sŏm″nō-lĕn′shē-ă) [L.] 1. Drowsiness. 2. The sleep of drunkenness in which the faculties are only partially depressed.
somnolism (sŏm′nō-lĭzm) [″ + *-ismos,* condition]. Condition of being in a hypnotic trance.
Somophyllin. Trade name for theophylline, USP.
Sonazine. Trade name for chlorpromazine hydrochloride, USP.

sone (sōn) [L. *sonus,* sound]. A unit of loudness; the loudness of a pure tone of 1000 cycles per second, 40 decibels above the listener's threshold of audibility.

sonicate (sŏn'ĭ-kāt) [L. *sonus,* sound]. To expose to sound waves.

sonication (sŏn"ĭ-kā'shŭn). Exposure to sound waves.

sonic boom (sŏn'ĭk) [L. *sonus,* sound]. Noise caused by shock waves from an airborne object traveling at a speed in excess of the speed of sound. When the waves hit the ground they may break windows and also affect the hearing.

Sonilyn. Trade name for sulfachlorpyridazine.

sonitus (sŏn'ĭ-tŭs) [L.]. Subjective noises in the ear. SYN: *tinnitus aurium.*

sonogram (sō'nō-grăm) [L. *sonus,* sound, + Gr. *gramma,* mark]. The record obtained by use of ultrasonography.

sonography (sō-nŏg'ră-fē) [" + Gr. *graphein,* to write]. Ultrasonography.

sonolucent (sō"nō-loo'sĕnt). In ultrasonography, the condition of not reflecting the ultrasound waves back to their source.

sonometer (sō-nŏm'ĕ-tĕr) [" + Gr. *metron,* a measure]. Device to cause sound for production of anesthesia; used by dentists.

sonorous (sō-nō'rŭs) [L.]. Giving forth a loud and rounded sound.

sonorous rale. A dry or low-pitched rale often caused by vibration of mucous secretion in a bronchus.

sophistication (sō-fĭs"tĭ-kā'shŭn) [Gr. *sophistikos,* deceitful]. In medicine, the adulteration of any substance.

sophomania (sŏf"ō-mā'nē-ă) [Gr. *sophos,* wise, + *mania,* madness]. Unrealistic belief in one's own wisdom.

sopor (sō'por) [L.]. Deep, lethargic sleep. SYN: *stupor.*

soporiferous (sō"pō-rĭf'ĕr-ŭs) [" + *ferre,* to bring]. Promoting sleep.

soporific (sō-pō-rĭf'ĭk) [" + *facere,* to make]. 1. Inducing sleep. 2. Narcotic; a drug producing sleep.

soporose, soporous (sō'por-ōs, -ŭs) [L.]. Marked by or resembling sound sleep or coma.

sorbefacient (sor"bē-fā'shĕnt) [L. *sorbere,* to suck, + *facere,* to make]. Causing or that which causes or promotes absorption.

sorbitan (sor'bĭ-tăn). The anhydride of sorbitol, $C_6H_8O(OH)_4$.

sorbitol. A crystalline alcohol, $CH_2OH(CHOH)_4CH_2OH$, present in some berries and fruits.

sordes (sor'dēz) [L. *sordere,* to be dirty]. Foul brown crusts or accumulations on the teeth and about the lips from foul stomach or secretions of the mouth in low forms of fever.

NURSING IMPLICATIONS: The nurse's main goal is prevention. Good oral hygiene must be provided for the debilitated person at regular intervals. The nurse may prescribe and administer hydrogen peroxide mouthwash (one part hydrogen peroxide to three parts water) to remove crust formations.

sore (sor) [AS. *sar,* sore]. 1. Tender; painful. 2. Any type of tender or painful ulcer or lesion of the skin or mucous membrane.

s., bed. Gangrene of skin due to pressure. For detailed description, SEE: *bedsore.* SYN: *decubitus; pressure sore.*

s., canker. A small lesion of the mucous membrane of the mouth. They often accompany a number of systemic conditions. Cause is unknown. SEE: *stomatitis, aphthous.*

s., cold. Blister on the lips. SEE: *herpes simplex.*

s., Delhi. Cutaneous leishmaniasis.

s., desert. An ulcer of the skin associated with being in the desert.

s., hard. Syphilitic chancre, q.v., primary lesion of syphilis.

s., Oriental. Cutaneous leishmaniasis.

s., pressure. A bedsore.

s., soft venereal. Soft nonsyphilitic venereal sore occurring on the genitalia. SYN: *chancroid; s., venereal.*

s., tropical. S., oriental.

s., venereal. S., soft venereal.

sore throat. Any inflammation of the tonsils, pharynx, or larynx.

s.t., diphtheritic. Croupous tonsillitis.

s.t., quinsy. Peritonsillar abscess. SEE: *quinsy.*

s.t., septic. Severe, epidemic, pseudomembranous inflammation of fauces and tonsils caused by the hemolytic streptococcus.

soroche (sō-rō'chā) [Sp.]. Mountain sickness, esp. that occurring in the Andes.

sororiation (sō-ror-ē-ā'shŭn) [L. *sororiare,* to increase together]. Growth of the breasts at puberty.

sorption (sorp'shŭn) [L. *sorbere,* to suck in]. The condition of being absorbed.

s.o.s. L. *si opus sit,* if necessary or required.

sotalol hydrochloride (sō'tă-lōl). An antiadrenergic medicine.

soterenol hydrochloride (sō-tĕr'ĕ-nōl). An adrenergic medicine used as a bronchodilator.

souffle (soof'fl) [Fr. *souffler,* to puff]. A soft blowing sound heard in auscultation; a bruit; an auscultatory murmur.

s., cardiac. Heart murmur.

s., fetal. The soft blowing sound heard over the location of the umbilical cord of the fetus in utero and synchronous with the fetal heartbeat during late pregnancy. SYN: *s., funic.*

s., funic. S., fetal.

s., placental. SEE: *placental souffle.*

s., splenic. Sound heard over spleen in malaria.

s., uterine. Sound caused by blood entering dilated arteries of the uterus in last months of pregnancy; synchronous with maternal pulse. It is more frequent than the fetal souffle and is heard as a loud blowing murmur along left side of uterus, and frequently all over it. An enlarged uterus may cause it. That of pregnancy is variable, whereas other forms are constant.

sound (sownd) [L. *sonus,* sound]. 1. Auditory sensations produced by vibrations; noise. It is measured in decibels, which is the logarithm of the intensity of sound; thus 20 d. represents not twice 10 d., but ten times as much. Exposure to excessively loud noises, esp. in certain frequencies, if repeated will cause permanent injury to the hearing. SEE: *decibel; noise; sonic boom.* 2. A form of vibrational energy that gives rise to auditory sensations. SEE: *cochlea; ear; organ of Corti; sonic boom.* 3. Healthy, not diseased. 4. Heart sounds. SEE: *diastole; systole.* 5. [Fr. *sonder,* to probe] Instrument for introduction into a cavity or canal for exploration. SYN: *searcher.*

s., anasarcous. Moist sound heard on auscultation when skin is edematous.

s., blowing. Organic murmur as of air from an aperture expelled with moderate force.

s., bottle. Noise as of fluid in a bottle. SEE: *amphoric.*

s.'s, breath. Respiratory sounds heard on auscultation of the chest. In a normal chest, they are classified as vesicular, tracheal, and bronchovesicular.

s., bronchial. Sound not heard in normal lung but occurring in pulmonary disease, indicating infiltration and solidification of lung.

s.'s, bronchovesicular. A mixture of bronchial and vesicular sounds.

s., cracked-pot. A tympanic resonance heard over pulmonary cavities.

s., ejection. High-pitched clicking sound heard just after the first heart sound.

s., fetal heart. Sound made by the fetal heart.

s., friction. Sound produced by rubbing together two inflamed mucous surfaces.

s.'s, heart. The two sounds "lubb" and "dupp" resulting from closure of atrial, pulmonic, mitral, and tricuspid valves. Third and fourth heart sounds may be present in some conditions. SEE: *heart.*

s., Korotkoff. SEE: *Korotkoff sounds.*

s., percussion. SEE: *percussion.*

s.'s, physiological. The sound perceived when the auditory canals are closed. The sound is produced by the blood flowing through adjacent vessels.

s., respiratory. Any sound heard over the lungs, bronchi, or trachea.

s., succussion. Splashing sound heard over a cavity with fluid in it.

s., to-and-fro. Rasping friction sounds of pericarditis.

s., tracheal. Sound normally heard over the trachea or larynx.

s., tubular. Sound heard over the trachea or large bronchi.

s., urethral. A device suitable for use in exploring the urethra.

s., vesicular. Sound heard over the entire lung during inspiration resulting from distention of alveoli with air.

s., white. Sound made up of all audible frequencies.

sound, words pert. to: amphoric; aspirate; auscultation; capotement; clang; clapotage; heart; hyperacusis; murmur; rale; resonance; souffle; stridulous; succussion.

Souque's phenomenon. Finger extension on the involved side of a hemiplegic patient when the extremity is raised to a position above 90° of shoulder flexion or abduction.

source-skin distance. In radiation therapy, the distance from the radiographic source to the skin of the patient.

soybean oil. USP. The refined oil obtained from seeds of the soya plant.

sp. L. *spiritus,* spirit; *species.*

spa (spă) [Spa, a Belgium resort town]. A mineral spring, esp. one having healing properties.

space (spās) [L. *spatium,* space]. 1. An area, region, or segment. 2. A cavity of the body. SYN: *spatium* [NA]. 3. The expanse in which the solar system, stars, and galaxies exist; outside the Earth's atmosphere.

s., axillary. The axilla or space beneath the arm.

s., circumlental. Space between the equator of the lens and the ciliary body.

s., dead. 1. In respiratory physiology, the space between the nose and bronchioles that does not exchange oxygen and carbon dioxide. 2. Unobliterated space remaining after closure of a surgical wound. This space favors the accumulation of blood, and eventually infection.

s., epidural. Space between the dura mater and vertebral periosteum, or between the bones of the cranium and the dura mater, assumed to be lymph spaces.

s., intercostal. The interval between ribs.

s., interfascial. S., Tenon's.

s., interpleural. The mediastinum.

s., interproximal. The space between the surfaces of adjacent teeth in the dental arch; it is divided into the septal space, gingival to the contact point of the teeth and occupied normally by the interdental papilla of the gingiva, and the embrasure, the space occlusal to the contact point of the teeth.

s., interradicular. The area between the roots of a multirooted tooth, which contains an alveolar bony septum and the periodontal ligament.

s., intervillous. Space in the placenta that develops from early chorionic trophoblast. It forms a blood sinus in which chorionic villi of fetus are bathed in maternal blood received from uterine vessels.

s., lymph. Any space occupied by lymph tissue.

s., Meckel's. Cavum trigeminale, q.v.

s., mediastinal. The mediastinum.

s., medullary. The marrow-containing area of cancellous bone.

s., Nuel's. Space between outer hair cells and rods in the organ of Corti.

s.'s of Fontana. Spaces in scleral meshwork in angle of the iris through which aqueous humor passes from the anterior chamber to the canal of Schlemm.

s., palmar. The mid-palmar and thenar spaces of the hand.

s., parasinoidal. Lateral spaces in the dura mater adjacent to the superior sagittal sinus that receive meningeal and diploic veins.

s., perforated. Space pierced by blood vessels at base of brain. SYN: *substantia perforata.*

s.'s, perivascular. Space within adventitia of larger blood vessels of the brain. They communicate with subarachnoid space.

s., personal. In psychiatry, an individual's personal area and the surrounding space. This space is important in interpersonal relations. SEE: *proxemics.*

s., plantar. One of four spaces between the fascial layers of the foot. When the foot is infected, pus may be found there.

s., pneumatic. Air-containing spaces in bone, esp. those in the paranasal sinuses.

s., popliteal. Space back of the knee joint, containing the popliteal artery and vein and small sciatic and popliteal nerves.

s., prezonular. The anterior portion of the posterior chamber of the eye.

s., Prussak's. Space in tympanum behind Shrapnell's membrane.

s., retroperitoneal. The potential space outside the parietal peritoneum of the abdominal cavity.

s., retropharyngeal. Space behind pharynx separating prevertebral from visceral fascia. SYN: *retropharyngeal fascial cleft.*

s.'s, subarachnoid. Spaces between the pia mater and arachnoid containing the cerebrospinal fluid. The spaces, esp. in the cranium, are traversed by numerous trabeculae.

s., subdural. Narrow space between the dura and the arachnoid.

s., subphrenic. Space between the diaphragm and the abdominal organs.

s., suprasternal. Triangular space immediately above the sternum between layers of deep cervical fascia.

s., Tenon's. Lymph space between the sclera and Tenon's capsule. SYN: *s., interfascial.*

s., thenar. A deep fascial space in the hand lying anterior to the adductor pollicis muscle.

s., tissue. Any space within tissues not lined with epithelium and containing tissue fluid.

s.'s, zonular. Spaces within the zonule (suspensory ligament of lens).

space maintainer. An appliance placed within the dental arch to prevent adjacent teeth from moving into the space left by a missing tooth; it is a temporary placement until the permanent tooth erupts into the space, or until a bridge is placed to replace the missing permanent tooth.

space medicine. Branch of medical science concerned with the physiological and pathological problems encountered by humans who are projected into the area beyond the Earth's atmosphere. Included in space medicine are investigation of effects of weightlessness (zero gravity), sensory deprivation, motion sickness, enforced inactivity during lengthy travels in space, and the heat and decelerative forces encountered at the time of reentry into the Earth's atmosphere. SEE: *aerospace medicine.*

spagyrism (spăj'ĭ-rĭzm). The obsolete paracelsian theory of medicine.

spallation (spawl-lā'shŭn). 1. The process of breaking into very small parts. The term may be applied to gross structures or to atomic particles. 2. The release of inert particles into the bloodstream. An example would be splintering of bits of plastic from the pump used in hemodialysis.

span. The distance from one fixed point to another, as the distance, when the hand is fully expanded, from the tip of the thumb to the tip of the little finger. Each individual should know that measurement of his or her own hand so that it may be used in estimating the size of objects.

Spanish fly. A strong rubefacient and blistering agent produced from these beetles. Believed by laymen to be an aphrodisiac, which it is not. SYN: *cantharides.*

spanogyny (spăn'ō-jĭn"ē) [Gr. *spanos,* scarce, + *gyne,* a woman]. More males than females; decrease in female births.

sparer (spār'ĕr) [AS. *sparian,* to refrain]. A substance destroyed by catabolism but that, nevertheless, lessens catabolic action upon other substances.

s., protein. Carbohydrates and fats, so designated because their presence in diet prevents tissue proteins from being utilized as a source of energy.

sparganosis (spăr″gă-nō′sĭs). Infestation with a variety of Sparganum.

Sparganum (spăr′gă-nŭm) [Gr. *sparganon,* swathing band]. (pl. *spargana*) The plerocercoid larva of tapeworms, esp. those of the genus Dibothriocephalus.

S. mansoni. An elongated plerocercoid species, 3 to 14 in. (7.6 to 35 cm.) in length, found in muscles and connective tissue, esp. that around the eye. Common in the Far East.

S. mansonoides. Species occasionally occurring in U.S. The adult form is unknown.

S. proliferum. Minute species infesting man and producing acne-like nodules. It is thought to proliferate by means of budlike outgrowths.

sparge (spărj) [L. *spargere,* to scatter]. To introduce air or gas into a liquid.

spargosis (spăr-gō′sĭs) [Gr. *spargosis,* swelling]. 1. Distention of the female breasts with milk. 2. Swelling or thickening of the skin. SYN: *elephantiasis.*

Sparine. Trade name for promazine hydrochloride.

spark coil. Coil consisting of primary and secondary coils with an interrupted current passing through them.

spark gap. 1. Arrangement of opposed points or surfaces between which an electric spark may jump. 2. An adjustable gap between needle points or between spheres used to measure high potentials.

s.g., quenched. A multiple spark gap with numerous electrodes about 0.3 mm. apart and equipped with a copper air-cooling device.

spasm (spăzm) [Gr. *spasmos,* a convulsion]. An involuntary sudden movement or convulsive muscular contraction. Spasms may be clonic (characterized by alternate contraction and relaxation) or tonic (sustained). They may involve either visceral (smooth) muscle or skeletal (striated) muscle. When contractions are strong and painful, they are called cramps. The effect depends upon the part affected. Asthma is assumed to be due to spasm of muscular coats of smaller bronchi, renal colic to spasm of muscular coat of the ureter.

TREATMENT: General measures to reduce tension, induce muscle relaxation, and improve circulation. Specific measures include analgesics for relief of pain and physiotherapy (heat, diathermy, electrical therapy). Special orthopedic supports or braces are sometimes effective. For vascular spasm, chemical sympathectomy may give relief.

s., Bell's. Convulsive tic of the face.

s., bronchial. Contraction of the muscle fibers around bronchial tubes. This occurs in asthma.

s., choreiform. Spasmodic movements resembling chorea.

s., clonic. Intermittent contractions and relaxation of muscles.

s., habit. Spasm due to habit.

s., nodding. A psychogenic condition in adults, causing nodding of the head from clonic spasms of the sternomastoid muscles. A similar nodding in babies with head turning from side to side.

s. of esophagus. Paroxysmal dysphagia (inability to swallow), often associated with a sense of constriction in the chest. Characterized by intense dyspnea and occurs in spasmodic croup, true croup, ulceration of larynx, laryngismus stridulus, whooping cough, tetany, hysteria, hydrophobia, laryngeal crises of locomotor ataxia, when foreign bodies have lodged in larynx, and when aneurysms or mediastinal tumors press on the recurrent laryngeal nerve and irritate it.

PROG: Indefinite regarding duration, not threatening to life.

TREATMENT: Search for exciting cause and remove. Treatment largely dietetic, hygienic, and psychologic. Dilation by passage of a bougie may be of great value.

s., saltatory. Term employed to designate a condition allied to hysteria in which a violent spasm seizes the muscles of the leg as soon as the feet touch the ground and, as a result, patient is thrown violently in the air.

s., tetanic. Spasm in which contractions continue for a time without interruption.

s., tonic. Continued involuntary contractions.

s., torsion. Spasm characterized by a turning of a part, esp. the turning of the body at the pelvis.

s., toxic. Spasm due to poison.

s., winking. Spasmus nictitans.

spasm, words pert. to: campospasm; cardiospasm; carpopedal; child crowing; chirospasm; Chvostek's sign; clonic; clonospasm; clonus; face; habit; hypertonus; mobile; Raynaud's disease; spasticity; tetanus; tetany; tic douloureux; tonic spasm; torticollis; trismus; vaginismus.

spasmatic (spăz-măt′ĭk) [Gr. *spasmos,* a convulsion]. Pert. to, like, or marked by spasm. SYN: *spasmodic.*

spasmatic asthma. Asthma caused by spasm of the bronchioles.

spasmatic croup. Laryngismus stridulus.

spasmatic stricture. Temporary narrowing

of any canal, as the urethra, due to localized spasmodic muscular contraction of its coat.

spasmodic (spăz-mŏd′ĭk) [Gr. *spasmos,* a convulsion]. Concerning spasms.

spasmogen (spăz′mō-jĕn) [″ + *gennan,* to produce]. Something that causes spasms.

spasmology (spăz-mŏl′ō-jē) [″ + *logos,* a study]. The study of spasms, their nature and cause.

spasmolygmus (spăz-mō-lĭg′mŭs) [″ + *lygmos,* a sob]. 1. Spasmodic hiccup. 2. Spasmodic sobbing.

spasmolysin (spăz-mŏl′ĭ-sĭn). Something that abolishes spasms.

spasmolytic (spăz-mō-lĭt′ĭk) [″ + *lysis,* dissolution]. Arresting spasms or that which acts as an antispasmodic.

spasmophemia (spăz-mō-fē′mē-ă) [″ + *pheme,* speech]. A spasmodic disorder of speech. SYN: *stuttering.*

spasmophilia (spăz-mō-fĭl′ē-ă) [″ + *philein,* to love]. A tendency to tetany and convulsions; almost always associated with rickets.

spasmous (spăz′mŭs) [Gr. *spasmos,* convulsion]. Of the nature of a spasm.

spasmus (spăz′mŭs) [Gr. *spasmos,* convulsion]. A spasm.

s. agitans. Paralysis agitans.

s. bronchialis. Bronchial asthma.

s. caninus. Spasm of face causing a constant grin. SYN: *risus sardonicus.*

s. coordinatus. Imitative or compulsive movements, as mimic tics or festination.

s. cynicus. Spasmodic contraction of muscles on both sides of the mouth.

s. Dubini. Rhythmic contractions, in rapid succession, of a group or groups of muscles, starting at an extremity or half of the face, and covering a large part or all of the body. Usually fatal.

s. glottidis. Spasm of larynx. SYN: *laryngismus stridulus.*

s. nictitans. A winking movement of the eyelid.

s. nutans. Nodding spasm.

spastic (spăs′tĭk) [Gr. *spastikos,* convulsive]. 1. Resembling or of the nature of spasms or convulsions. 2. Produced by spasms. 3. One afflicted with spasms.

spastic colon. A syndrome of disordered motility of the small and large intestines accompanied by pain, usually in the lower abdominal area, and constipation alternating with diarrhea. For complete description and treatment, SEE: *colon, irritable.*

spastic gait. A stiff movement with toes seeming to catch together and to drag.

spastic hemiplegia. Partial hemiplegia with spasmodic muscular contractions.

spasticity (spăs-tĭs′ĭ-tē). Increased tone or contractions of muscles causing stiff and awkward movements: the result of upper motor neuron lesion.

spastic paralysis. Muscular rigidity accompanying partial paralysis. Usually due to a lesion involving upper motor neurons.

spastic paraplegia. Paraplegia due to transverse lesions of the cord or sclerosis.

spatial (spā′shăl). Pertaining to space.

spatial discrimination. Ability to perceive as separate points of contact the two blunt points of a compass when applied to the skin.

spatium (spā′shē-ŭm) [L.]. (pl. *spatia*) [NA] A space.

spatula (spăt′ū-lă) [L. *spatula,* blade]. Instrument for spreading or mixing semisolids. It is usually flat, thin, somewhat flexible, and shaped like a knife.

s., eye. Blades for separating lips of corneal wounds, arresting hemorrhage, or for making pressure; made of sheet metal or rubber.

s., nasal. Device for holding mucous flaps in place or to guard against burning from cautery.

spatulate (spăch′ŭ-lāt). To mix something by use of a spatula. In dentistry, to mix or manipulate certain dental materials with a spatula to achieve a uniform, homogenous mass.

spay, spaying (spā, spā′ĭng) [Gael. *spoth,* castrate]. Surgical removal of ovaries, usually said of animals. SEE: *castration.*

SPCA. 1. *serum prothrombin conversion accelerator.* 2. *Society for the Prevention of Cruelty to Animals.*

specialist (spĕsh′ăl-ĭst) [L. *specialis*]. A dentist, nurse, physician, or other health professional who has advanced education and training in one clinical area of practice such as internal medicine, pediatrics, maternal and child health, or cardiology. When a certifying board exists this individual has met the criteria for such certification.

specialization (spĕsh″ăl-ī-zā′shŭn). The limitation of one's practice to a particular branch of medicine, surgery, dentistry, or nursing. This is customarily done after having received postgraduate training in the area of specialization.

specialty (spĕsh′ăl-tē). The branch of medicine, surgery, dentistry, or nursing in which a specialist practices.

speciation (spē″sē-ā′shŭn) [L. *species,* a kind]. The evolutionary process by which new species of living organisms are formed.

species (spē′shēz) [L. *species,* a kind]. In biology, a category of classification for living organisms. This group is just below genus and is usually capable of interbreeding.

species-specific. The characteristics of a species, esp. the immunological nature that differentiates that species from another.

species type. The original species that served

as the basis for identifying a new genus or subgenus.

specific (spĕ-sĭf'ĭk) [L. *specificus,* pert. to a kind]. 1. A remedy having a curative effect on a particular disease or symptom. 2. Pert. to a species. 3. A disease always caused by the same organism. 4. Restricted, explicit; not generalized.

specific dynamic action. ABBR: SDA. The increase in metabolic rate resulting from absorption of food. For protein it amounts to about 30%, for carbohydrates, 7%, and for fats, 4%. After a general meal the increase would be 10 to 15%. This effect lasts for 4 to 6 hours.

specific gravity. Weight of a substance compared with an equal volume of water. Water is used as a standard and considered to have a specific gravity of one (1.000).

specificity (spĕ-sĭ-fĭs'ĭ-tē). State of being specific; having a relation to a definite result or to a particular cause.

specillum (spē-sĭl'lŭm) [L. *specere,* to look]. (pl. *specilla*) 1. Lens. 2. Button-shaped silver probe.

specimen (spĕs'ĭ-mĕn) [L. *specere,* to look]. A part of a thing intended to show kind and quality of the whole, as a specimen of urine.

spectacles (spĕk'tăk-lz) [L. *spectare,* to see]. Two lenses supported by a nose bridge and side pieces passing over the ears. Used to aid vision or protect the eyes. SYN: *glasses.*

spectinomycin hydrochloride, sterile. USP. A sterile preparation of the antibiotic spectinomycin hydrochloride. When diluted with the appropriate amount of sterile water for injection, the medicine may be used intramuscularly.

spectral (spĕk'trăl) [L. *spectrum,* image]. Concerning a spectrum.

spectro- [L. *spectrum,* image]. Combining form meaning appearance, image, form, spectrum.

spectrocolorimeter (spĕk-trō-kŭl-or-ĭm'ĕ-tĕr) [" + *color,* color, + Gr. *metron,* measure]. Device for detecting colorblindness by isolating a single spectral color.

spectrofluorometer (spĕk"trō-floo"or-ŏm'ĕ-tĕr). An instrument for measuring degree of fluorescence.

spectrograph (spĕk'trō-grăf) [" + Gr. *graphein,* to write]. An instrument designed to photograph spectra on a sensitive photographic plate.

spectrometer (spĕk-trŏm'ĕt-ĕr) [" + Gr. *metron,* a measure]. A spectroscope so constructed that angular deviation of a ray of light produced by a prism or by a diffraction grating thus indicates the wavelength.

spectrometry (spĕk-trŏm'ĕ-trē) [" + Gr. *metron,* measure]. The process of determining the wavelength of light rays by use of a spectrometer.

spectrophotometer (spĕk"trō-fō-tŏm'ĕt-ĕr) [" + Gr. *photos,* light, + *metron,* a measure]. Device for measuring amount of color in a solution by comparison with the spectrum.

spectrophotometry (spĕk"trō-fō-tŏm'ĕt-rē) Estimation of coloring matter in a solution by use of the spectroscope or spectrophotometer.

spectropolarimeter (spĕk"trō-pō'lăr-ĭm'ĕ-tĕr) [" + *polaris,* pole, + *metron,* measure]. Device for measuring the rotation of light rays of a specific wavelength by passage through a translucent solid.

spectropyrheliometer (spĕk"trō-pīr-hē-lē-ŏm'ĕ-tĕr) [" + Gr. *pyr,* fire, + *helios,* sun, + *metron,* measure]. Instrument to measure solar radiation.

spectroscope (spĕk'trō-skōp) [" + Gr. *skopein,* to examine]. An instrument for separating radiant energy into its component frequencies or wavelengths by means of a prism or grating to form a spectrum for inspection.

spectroscopic (spĕk"trō-skŏp'ĭk). Concerning a spectroscope.

spectroscopy (spĕk-trŏs'kō-pē). The branch of physical science that treats the phenomena observed with the spectroscope, or those principles on which its action is based; also, the art of using the spectroscope.

spectrum (spĕk'trŭm) [L., image]. (pl. *spectra*) Charted band of wavelengths of electromagnetic vibrations obtained by refraction and diffraction of ray of white light.

s., absorption. The spectrum recorded after light rays have passed through a substance that is capable of absorbing some of the wavelengths passing through. This spectrum is specific for various chemicals.

s., broad. A term that refers to antibiotics effective against a variety of microorganisms.

s., chromatic. That portion of the spectrum that produces visible light. Wavelengths of about 7700 to 3900 Ångström units are visible.

s., invisible. Spectral portion either below the red (infrared) or above the violet (ultraviolet), which is invisible to the eye, the waves being too long or too short to affect the retina. The invisible spectrum includes rays less than 3900 Ångström units (A.U.) in length (ultraviolet, roentgen or X, gamma, and cosmic rays) and those exceeding 7700 A.U. in length (infrared, high-frequency oscillations used in short- and long-wave diathermy, radio, hertzian, and very long waves). These range in length from 7700 A.U. to 5,000,000 meters.

s., visible. Portion of spectrum that is visible The visible spectrum consists of the colors from red to violet with wavelengths of 3900 A.U. to 7700 A.U. When white light is passed through a prism, the various colors, because of different wavelengths, are refracted to various degrees giving rise to the diverse colors of the rainbow. These are in order from the shortest wavelength to the longest violet, indigo, blue, green, yellow, orange, and red.

s., visible electromagnetic. The complete range of wavelengths of electromagnetic radiation.

speculum (spĕk'ū-lŭm) [L., a mirror]. (pl. *specula*) 1. Instrument for examination of canals. 2. Membrane separating anterior cornua of lateral ventricles of brain. SYN: *septum pellucidum*.

s., ear. Short, funnel-shaped tubes, tubular or bivalve; former preferable.

s., eye. Device for separating eyelids. Plated steel wire, plain, Von Graefe's, Steven's, and Luer's are most common.

s., vaginal. A speculum, usually with two opposing portions that, after being inserted, can be pushed apart, for examining the vagina and cervix.

NOTE: A vaginal speculum should be warmed prior to use.

speech [AS. *spaec*]. 1. Verbal expression of one's thought. 2. The act of uttering articulate words or sounds. 3. Words that are spoken.

It is thought that certain crude sounds served as warnings or threats in much the same way as did facial and bodily expressions. As sounds became highly differentiated, each became associated and gradually identified with a certain idea. These word-symbols are a most valuable tool in ideation, and thinking is very largely dependent on this internal speech. Further identifications have made possible visual symbols (written language), though primitive written language was entirely unrelated—a series of pictures and crude representations.

External speech requires the coordination of larynx, mouth, lips, chest, and abdominal muscles. These have no special innervation for speech but the upper neurons respond to complex motor pattern fields that convert the idea into suitable motor stimuli.

s., aphonic. Whispering.

s., ataxic. Defective speech resulting from muscular incoordination usually the result of cerebellar disorder.

s., clipped. S., scamping.

s., echo. Parrotlike repetition of words spoken by others. SYN: *echolalia*.

s., esophageal. In persons who have had laryngectomies, the modulation of air expelled from the esophagus to produce sound that can be used in speech. The mouth, tongue, and pharynx all participate in this.

s., explosive. Sudden loud sounds produced by persons with organic brain disease or mental disorders.

s., interjectional. Speech characterized by inarticulate sounds.

s., mirror. Speech characterized by reversing the order of syllables of a word.

s., scamping. Speech characterized by omission of consonants or syllables when unable to pronounce them. SYN: *s., clipped*.

s., scanning. A staccato-like speech with pauses between syllables.

s., slurring. Slovenly articulation of letters difficult to pronounce.

s., staccato. Slow and laborious speech with each syllable pronounced separately, as in multiple sclerosis.

speech abnormalities. Speech failure results in motor aphasia, in which the patient is speechless but there is no paralysis of muscles of articulation. Although unable to express thoughts in words, the patient can still understand what he or she hears and reads.

Labialism is the excessive use of labial sounds.

Absence of speech or hoarseness may be part of a hysteria.

Word-deafness is the condition when a word is heard but the patient has no idea of its meaning. Similarly, word-blindness means that the written symbol might as well be a foreign word. This is sometimes called alexia, q.v. Aphasia, q.v., in right-handed patients is classically referable to left-sided brain lesions, but the concept of centers for internal speech esp. is rather misleading. It is probably a diffuse cortical activity and countless minor distortions occur in addition to those mentioned. Chief of those not enumerated is the slurring speech of paresis, q.v., where letters and syllables are omitted without recognition of defect, and this further identifies the abnormality. Dysarthria, q.v., describes any defect of articulation; muscular tone disturbances as seen in cerebellar disease, chorea, paralysis agitans, lenticular degeneration, or multiple sclerosis, producing jerky, monotonous, or scanning speech.

Paralysis due to bilateral medullary pathology results in indistinct enunciation (mouthful speech) often entirely unintelligible. Pseudobulbar palsy (as in cases of double hemiplegia) adds a slow spastic characteristic. Peripheral nerve lesions, cleft palate, adenoids, and myasthenia gravis merely suggest the many possible modifications.

Stammering and stuttering are usually psychogenic.

Emotional values may be added to speech qualities; tremulousness and tension may render the voice high-pitched, irritating, or unsustained and broken. Emotional flattening may occur in the neuroses and psychoses. In the latter, diagnostic changes may occur in the stream of talk.

Slowing is common in all depressed states. When complete (mutism), it suggests the negativism esp. likely to occur in schizophrenia. Aphonic-like aphasia patients will find some means of communication.

Excessive talk flow is generally seen in mania and excited states. When merely voluble but relevant, it constitutes circumstantiality. If the goal ideal is lost, irrelevancy is associated with a "flight of ideas"—in extreme form a "word salad." The manner of speech often mirrors the mood.

Neologisms are words created by the patient, often of no apparent significance.

Stereotyped speech is constant repetition of a word or phrase. It should be distinguished from perseveration in which the repetition is against the intention or wishes of the patient.

Amentia, q.v., invariably delays speech appearance and its faulty development is of diagnostic value. Its delayed or non-appearance may be referable to deafness (deaf-mutism). Childish indistinctness (e.g., "r's" replaced by "w's") may persist in feebleminded adults.

speech pathologist. An individual who is prepared by education and training to plan, direct, and conduct programs to improve communicative skills of children and adults with language and speech impairments arising from physiologic disturbances, defective articulation, or dialect. This individual can evaluate programs and perform research related to speech and language problems.

speech therapy. The study, diagnosis, and treatment of defects and disorders of the voice and of spoken and written communication.

speech, words pert. to: alliteration; alogia; aphasia; aphonia; aphrasia; area, Broca's; articulation; bradyarthria; bradylalia; deaf-mute; dyslalia; dyslexia; dysphasia; dysphonia; egophony; monophasia; mute; mutism; onomatomania; onomatopoiesis; perseveration; scanning speech; stammering; stutter; tachyphasia; Wernicke's syndrome.

sperm (spĕrm) [Gr. *sperma,* seed]. 1. The ejaculate from the male; contains spermatozoa. SYN: *semen.* 2. Spermatozoa. SEE: illus.

sperma (spĕr′mă) [Gr.]. 1. Testicular secretion containing the male reproductive cells, spermatozoa. SYN: *semen.* 2. Individual male germ cell. 3. Also used as a combining form.

spermacrasia (spĕr″măk-rā′zē-ă) [Gr. *sperma,* seed, + *akrasia,* bad mixture]. Lack of spermatozoa in the semen. SYN: *aspermia.*

sperm agglutination. Agglutination of spermatozoa.

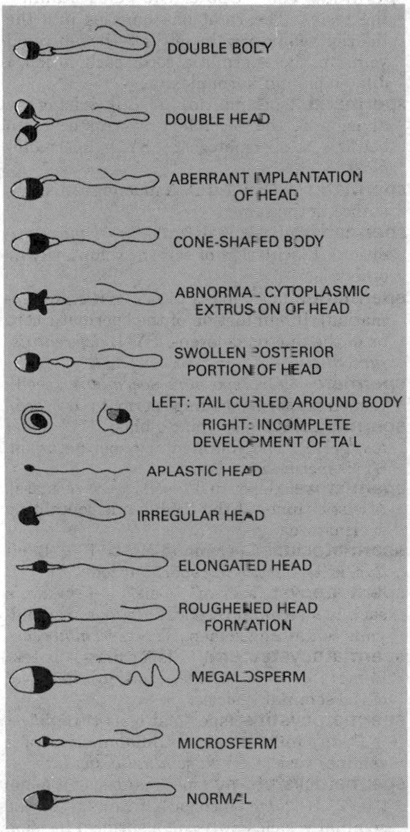

NORMAL AND ABNORMAL SPERM

spermatemphraxis (spĕr″măt-ĕm-frăk′sĭs) [″ + *emphraxis,* stoppage]. An obstruction to emission of semen.

spermatic (spĕr-măt′ĭk) [Gr. *sperma,* seed]. Pert. to semen or sperm.

spermatic arteries. Two long slender vessels, branches of the abdominal aorta, following each spermatic cord to the testes.

spermatic cord. The cord suspending the testis composed of veins, arteries, lymphatics, nerves, and the ductus deferens. SEE: *cord, spermatic; infundibulum; varicocele.*

spermatic duct. Canal for passage of semen, esp. the ductus deferens and the ejaculatory duct. SYN: *seminal duct.*

spermaticidal (spĕrm″ăt-ĭ-sīd′ăl) [Gr. *sperma,* seed, + L. *cidus,* kill]. Destructive to or causing the death of spermatozoa.

spermatic vein. One of two veins draining the testes. The right one empties into the inferior vena cava, the left into the left renal vein. In the spermatic cord, each forms a dilated pampiniform plexus.

spermatid (spĕr′mă-tĭd). A cell arising by division of the secondary spermatocyte to become a spermatozoon. SYN: *spermatoblast.*

spermatin (spĕrm′ă-tĭn). A mucilaginous substance in the semen.

spermatism (spĕr′mă-tĭzm) [″ + *-ismos,* condition]. Ejaculation of semen, voluntarily or otherwise.

spermatitis (spĕr″mă-tī′tĭs) [″ + *itis,* inflammation]. Inflammation of the spermatic cord or of the ductus deferens. SYN: *deferentitis; funiculitis.*

spermato- [Gr. *sperma, spermatos,* seed]. Combining form meaning sperm, to sow seed.

spermatoblast (spĕr-măt′ō-blăst) [″ + *blastos,* germ]. The rudimentary spermatozoon. SYN: *spermatid.*

spermatocele (spĕr-măt′ō-sēl) [″ + *kele,* mass]. A cystic tumor of the epididymis containing spermatozoa.

spermatocidal (spĕr″mă-tō-sī′dăl) [″ + L. *cidus,* kill]. Destroying spermatozoa.

spermatocyst (spĕr-măt′ō-sĭst) [″+ *kystis,* a sac]. 1. A seminal vesicle. 2. Tumor of epididymis containing semen. SYN: *spermatocele.*

spermatocystectomy (spĕr″măt-ō-sĭs-tĕk′tō-mē) [″ + ″ + *ektome,* excision]. Removal of the seminal vesicles.

spermatocystitis (spĕr″măt-ō-sĭs-tī′tĭs) [″ + ″ + *itis,* inflammation]. Inflammation of a seminal vesicle. SYN: *seminal vesiculitis.*

spermatocystotomy (spĕr″mă-tō-sĭs-tŏt′ō-mē) [″ + ″ + *tome,* incision]. Drainage of the seminal vesicles by use of a surgical incision into the vesicle.

spermatocytal (spĕr″mă-tō-sī′tăl) [″ + *kytos,* cell]. Concerning spermocytes.

spermatocyte (spĕr-măt′ō-sīt) [″ + *kytos,* cell]. A cell originating from a spermatogonium that forms by division the spermatids, which give rise to spermatozoa.

s., primary. Cell arising by growth and development from a spermatogonium.

s., secondary. Cell arising from primary spermatocyte by a meiotic division. It undergoes a second meiotic division, giving rise to two spermatids with haploid, q.v., number of chromosomes.

spermatocytogenesis (spĕr″mă-tō-sī″tō-jĕn′ĕ-sĭs) [″ + ″ + *genesis,* production]. The initial stage of sperm formation.

spermatogenesis (spĕr″măt-ō-jĕn′ĕ-sĭs) [″ + *genesis,* production]. The formation of mature functional spermatozoa. In the process, undifferentiated spermatogonia become primary spermatocytes, each of which divides to form two secondary spermatocytes. Each of these divide to form two spermatids, which transform into functional motile spermatozoa. In the process the chromosome number is reduced from the diploid to the haploid number. SEE: *gametogenesis; maturation; meiosis.*

spermatogenic (spĕr″mă-tō-jĕn′ĭk). Producing sperm.

spermatogenous (spĕr″mă-tŏj′ĕ-nŭs). Spermatogenic.

spermatogeny (spĕr″mă-tŏj′ĕ-nē). Spermatogenesis.

spermatogonium (sper″măt-ō-gō′nē-ŭm) [″ + *gone,* generation]. (pl. *spermatogonia*) A large unspecialized germ cell that in spermatogenesis gives rise to a primary spermatocyte. SYN: *spermatospore.* SEE: *spermatogenesis.*

spermatoid (spĕr′mă-toyd) [″ + *eidos,* form]. Resembling a spermatozoon.

spermatology (spĕr″mă-tŏl′ō-jē) [″ + *logos,* a study]. The study of the seminal fluid.

spermatolysin (spĕr″măt-ŏl′ĭ-sĭn) [″ + *lysis,* dissolution]. A lysin destroying spermatozoa.

spermatolysis (spĕr″măt-ŏl′ĭ-sĭs) [″ + *lysis,* dissolution]. Dissolution or destruction of spermatozoa.

spermatolytic (spĕr″măt-ō-lĭt′ĭk). Destroying spermatozoa.

spermatopathia (spĕr″mă-tō-păth′ē-ă) [Gr. *spermatos,* seed, + *pathos,* disease]. Disease of sperm cells or their secreting glands or ducts.

spermatopathy (spĕr-mă-tŏp′ă-thē). Spermatopathia.

spermatophobia (spĕr″mă-tō-fō′bē-ă) [″ + *phobos,* fear]. Abnormal fear of being afflicted with spermatorrhea, involuntary loss of semen.

spermatopoietic (spĕr″măt-ō-poy-ĕt′ĭk) [″ + *poiein,* to make]. Promoting the formation and secretion of semen.

spermatorrhea (spĕr″mă-tō-rē′ă) [″ + *rhoia,* flow]. Abnormally frequent involuntary loss of semen without orgasm.

spermatoschesis (spĕr″măt-ŏs′kĕ-sĭs) [″ + *schesis,* checking]. Suppression of the semen.

spermatospore (spĕr-măt′ō-spor) [″ + *sporos,* a seed]. A primitive cell from which spermatozoa arise. SYN: *spermatogonium.*

spermatotoxin (spĕr″mă-tō-tŏk′sĭn) [″ + *toxikon,* poison]. A toxin that destroys spermatozoa. SYN: *spermatoxin.*

spermatovum (spĕr″măt-ō′vŭm) [″ + L. *ovum,* egg]. A fecundated or impregnated ovum.

spermatoxin (spĕr″mă-tŏks′ĭn) [″ + *toxikon,* poison]. A toxin that causes destruction of spermatozoa. It is formed by injecting spermatozoa from an animal of another species.

spermatozoa (spĕr″măt-ō-zō′ă). Pl. of spermatozoon.

spermatozoal (spĕr″mă-tō-zō′ăl) [″ + *zoon,* life]. Concerning spermatozoa.

spermatozoicide (spĕr″mă-tō-zō′ĭ-sīd) [″ + ″ + L. *cidus,* kill]. Spermicide.

spermatozoon (spĕr″măt-ō-zō′ŏn) [″ + *zoon,* life]. (pl. *spermatozoa*) The mature male sex or germ cell formed within the seminiferous tubules of the testes. The spermatozoon has a broad oval flattened head with a nucleus and a protoplasmic neck or middle piece and tail. It is about 51 microns in length and resembles a tadpole. It has the power of self-propulsion by means of a flagellum. Develops after puberty from the spermatids in the testes in enormous quantities. The head pierces the envelope of the ovum and loses its tail when fusion of the two cells takes place. This process is called fertilization. SEE: *fertilization; sperm* for illus.

RS: acrosome; contraception; fertilization; gamete; ovum; semen; sperm; zygote.

spermaturia (spĕr″mă-tū′rē-ă) [″ + *ouron,* urine]. Semen discharged with the urine.

spermectomy (spĕr-mĕk′tō-mē) [″ + *ektome,* excision]. Resection of a portion of the spermatic cord and duct.

spermic (spĕr′mĭk). Concerning sperm, male reproductive cells.

spermicidal (spĕr″mĭ-sī′dăl) [″ + L. *cidus,* kill]. Killing spermatozoa.

spermicide (spĕr′mĭ-sīd). An agent that kills spermatozoa.

spermidine (spĕr′mĭ-dĭn). An amine present in semen.

spermiduct (spĕr′mĭ-dŭkt) [″ + L. *ductus,* a duct]. The ejaculatory duct and ductus deferens considered as one.

spermine (spĕr′mĭn). An amine present in semen and other animal tissues.

spermiogenesis (spĕr″mē-ō-jĕn′ĕ-sĭs). The processes involved in the transformation of a spermatid to a functional spermatozoon.

spermiogram (spĕr′mē-ō-grăm) [″ + *gramma,* mark]. Record of examining and classifying sperm in a semen sample.

spermoblast (spĕr′mō-blăst) [″ + *blastos,* a germ]. A cell developing into a spermatozoon. SYN: *spermatid; spermatoblast.*

spermolith (spĕr′mō-lĭth) [″ + *lithos,* stone]. A calculus in the seminal vesicle or spermatic duct.

spermolysin (spĕr-mŏl′ĭ-sĭn). A cytolysin formed following the inoculation of spermatozoa.

spermolytic (spĕr-mō-lĭt′ĭk) [″ + *lysis,* dissolution]. Causing the destruction of spermatozoa.

spermoneuralgia (spĕr″mō-nū-răl′jē-ă) [″ + *neuron,* nerve, + *algos,* pain]. Neuralgic pain in the testicles and spermatic cord.

spermophlebectasia (spĕr″mō-flē″bĕk-tā′zē-ă) [″ + *phleps,* vein, + *ektasis,* dilatation]. Varicosity of the spermatic veins.

spermoplasm (spĕr′mō-plăzm) [″ + *plasma,* a thing formed]. The protoplasm of a male germ cell.

spermosphere (spĕr′mō-sfēr) [″ + *sphaira,* a circle]. Mass of spermatoblasts derived from spermatogonia.

spermospore (spĕr′mō-spor) [″ + *sporos,* seed]. A primitive cell from which spermatozoa originate. SYN: *spermatogonium.*

spermotoxin (spĕr″mō-tŏk′sĭn) [″ + *toxikon,* poison]. Something that destroys sperm.

sp. gr. *specific gravity.*

sph. *spherical.*

sphacelate (sfăs′ĕl-āt) [Gr. *sphakelos,* gangrene]. 1. To affect with gangrene. 2. Gangrenous. SYN: *mortified; necrosed.*

sphacelation (sfăs″ĕl-ā′shŭn). Mortification; formation of a mass of gangrenous tissue. SYN: *gangrene; necrosis.*

sphacelism (sfăs′ĕl-ĭzm) [″ + *-ismos,* condition]. Condition of being affected with sphacelus or gangrene. SYN: *necrosis.*

sphaceloderma (sfăs″ĕl-ō-dĕr′mă) [″ + *derma,* skin]. Gangrene of the skin, esp. when symmetrical. SEE: *Raynaud's disease.*

sphacelotoxin (sfăs″ĕl-ō-tŏk′sĭn) [″ + *toxikon,* poison]. Poisonous principle obtained from ergot used to produce abortion.

sphacelous (sfăs′ĕl-ŭs) [Gr. *sphakelos,* gangrene]. Pert. to a slough or patch of gangrene. SYN: *gangrenous; necrosed; necrotic.*

sphacelus (sfăs′ĕl-ŭs). 1. A necrosed mass of tissue. SYN: *slough.* 2. Process of becoming gangrenous. SYN: *gangrene; mortification; necrosis.*

sphagiasmus (sfă″jē-ăz′mŭs) [Gr. *sphagiasmos,* a slaying]. Spasm of neck muscles occurring in an epileptic seizure.

sphagitis (sfă-jī′tĭs) [Gr. *sphage,* throat, + *itis,* inflammation]. Inflammation of the throat.

sphenethmoid (sfĕn-ĕth′moyd) [Gr. *sphen,* wedge, + *ethmoid,* sieve]. Sphenoethmoid, q.v.

sphenion (sfē′nē-ŏn) [Gr. *sphen,* wedge]. (pl. *sphenia*) Point at apex of the sphenoidal angle of the parietal bone.

spheno- [Gr. *sphen,* wedge]. Combining form meaning a wedge, the sphenoid bone.

sphenobasilar (sfē″nō-băs′ĭ-lăr) [″ + L. *basilaris,* basal]. Concerning the sphenoid bone and the basilar portion of the occipital bone.

sphenoccipital (sfē″nŏk-sĭp′ĭ-tăl) [″ + L. *occipitalis,* occipital]. Concerning the sphenoid and occipital bones.

sphenocephalus (sfē″nō-sĕf′ă-lŭs) [″ + *kephale,* head]. A deformed fetus in which the head is wedge-shaped.

sphenoethmoid (sfē″nō-ĕth′moyd) [″ + *ethmos,* sieve, + *eidos,* form]. Pert. to the sphenoid and the ethmoid bones.

sphenoethmoid recess. Groove back and above the superior concha, or turbinate bone.
sphenofrontal (sfē″nō-frŭn′tăl) [″ + L. *frontalis,* frontal]. Concerning the sphenoid and frontal bones.
sphenoid (sfē′noyd) [″ + *eidos,* form]. Cuneiform or wedge-shaped.
sphenoidal (sfē-noy′dăl). Concerning the sphenoid bone.
sphenoid bone. Large bone at base of skull between occipital and ethmoid in front, and the parietal and temporal bones at the side.
sphenoid fissure. Fissure in sphenoid and frontal bones for nerves and blood vessels.
sphenoiditis (sfē″noy-dī′tĭs) [″ + ″ + *itis,* inflammation]. 1. Inflammation of the sphenoidal sinus. 2. Necrosis of the sphenoid bone.
sphenoidostomy (sfē″noy-dŏs′tō-mē) [″ + ″ + *stoma,* mouth]. Surgically producing an opening into the sphenoid sinus.
sphenoidotomy (sfē″noyd-ŏt′ō-mē) [″ + ″ + *tome,* incision]. Incision into the sphenoid bone.
sphenomalar (sfē″nō-mā′lăr) [″ + L. *mala,* cheek]. Concerning the sphenoid and malar bones.
sphenomaxillary (sfē″nō-măk′sĭ-lā-rē) [″ + L. *maxilla,* jaw]. Concerning the sphenoid and the maxilla.
spheno-occipital (sfē″nō-ŏk-sĭp′ĭ-tăl) [″ + L. *occipitalis,* occipital]. Concerning the sphenoid and occipital bones.
sphenopalatine (sfē″nō-păl′ă-tēn) [″ + L. *palatum,* palate]. Concerning the sphenoid and palatine bones.
sphenoparietal (sfē″nō-pă-rī′ĕ-tăl) [″ + L. *paries,* a wall]. Concerning the sphenoid and parietal bones.
sphenorbital (sfē″nor′bĭ-tăl) [″ + L. *orbita,* track]. Concerning the sphenoid bone and the orbits.
sphenosis [Gr., wedging]. Condition in which fetus becomes wedged in the pelvis.
sphenosquamosal (sfē″nō-skwā-mō′săl) [Gr. *sphen,* wedge, + L. *squamosa,* scaly]. Concerning the sphenoid bone and the squamous portion of the temporal bone.
sphenotemporal (sfē″nō-tĕm′pō-răl) [″ + L. *temporalis,* temporal]. Concerning the sphenoid and temporal bones.
sphenotic (sfē-nŏt′ĭk) [Gr. *sphen,* wedge, + *eidos,* form]. A fetal bone that becomes part of the sphenoid bone.
sphenotresia (sfē″nō-trē′zē-ă) [Gr. *sphen,* wedge, + *tresis,* boring]. Perforating of the basal part of the fetal skull in craniotomy.
sphenotribe (sfē′nō-trīb) [″ + *tribein,* to crush]. Instrument for breaking up basal part of the fetal cranium.
sphenoturbinal (sfē″nō-tŭr′bĭ-năl) [″ + *turbo,* whirl]. A thin curved bone anterior to each of the lesser wings of the sphenoid.
sphenovomerine (sfē″nō-vō′mĕr-ĭn) [″ + L. *vomer,* plowshare]. Concerning the sphenoid and vomer bones.
sphenozygomatic (sfē″nō-zī″gō-măt′ĭk) [″ + *zygoma,* cheekbone]. Concerning the sphenoid and zygomatic bones.
sphere (sfēr) [Gr. *sphaira,* a globe]. 1. A ball or globelike structure. 2. The environment one controls or in which one lives and works.
s., attraction. A clear region in cytoplasm close to nucleus and usually containing a centriole or diplosome (a divided centriole).
s., segmentation. The segmented ovum or morula.
spheresthesia (sfēr″ĕs-thē′zē-ă) [″ + *aisthesis,* sensation]. A morbid sensation, as of a ball or lump ascending from stomach to throat. Seen in hysteria and other neuroses. SYN: *globus hystericus.*
spherical (sfĕr′ĭ-kăl) [Gr. *sphairikos*]. Having the form of, or pert. to, a sphere. SYN: *globular.*
spherocylinder (sfē″rō-sĭl′ĭn-dĕr) [Gr. *sphaira,* globe, + *kylindros,* cylinder]. A lens with a spherical surface and a cylindrical surface.
spherocyte (sfē′rō-sīt) [″ + *kytos,* cell]. An erythrocyte that assumes a spheroid shape.
spherocytosis (sfē″rō-sī-tō′sĭs) [″ + ″ + *osis,* condition]. Condition in which erythrocytes assume a spheroid shape. Occurs in certain hemolytic anemias.
s., hereditary. An inherited chronic disease characterized by hemolysis, anemia, spherocytosis, jaundice, and splenomegaly. The only effective treatment is splenectomy.
spheroid (sfē′royd) [″ + *eidos,* form]. 1. A body shaped like a sphere. 2. Sphere-shaped.
spheroidal (sfē-roy′dăl). Shaped like a sphere.
spherolith (sfē′rō-lĭth) [″ + *lithos,* stone]. A minute concretion in the kidney of the newborn.
spheroma (sfē-rō′mă) [″ + *oma,* tumor]. A tumor of spherical form.
spherometer (sfē-rŏm′ĕt-ĕr) [″ + *metron,* measure]. Device to ascertain curvature of a surface.
spheroplast (sfĕr′ō-plăst). In bacteriology, the cell wall remaining after gram-negative organisms have been lysed. Spheroplasts may be formed when synthesis of the cell wall is prevented by the action of certain chemicals while cells are growing. SEE: *protoplast.*
spherospermia (sfē″rō-spĕr′mē-ă) [″ + *sperma,* seed]. Round spermatozoa without tails.
spherule (sfĕr′ūl) [LL. *sphaerula,* little globe]. 1. A very small sphere. 2. A minute granule found in the center of a centromere of a chromosome. 3. The structures present in tissues infected with Coccidioides immitis. These spherules contain up to hundreds of

endospores.

sphincter (sfĭnk′tĕr) [Gr. *sphinkter,* a binder]. Circular muscle constricting an orifice. In normal contraction, it closes the orifice.

s. ampullae. Delicate network of fibers about papilla of Vater, occasionally present in adults, a part of sphincter of Oddi.

s. ani. Sphincter that closes the anus, the external one being of striated muscle, the internal one, of plain muscle.

s., bladder. Plain muscle about opening of bladder into the urethra.

s., cardiac. Plain muscle about the esophagus at cardiac opening into the stomach.

s. choledochus. Smooth muscle investing common bile duct just before its junction with pancreatic duct; a part of sphincter of Oddi.

s., ileocecal. Plain muscle about the ileum at its opening into the cecum.

s. of Oddi. Contracted region in common bile duct at papilla of Vater.

s. pancreaticus. Smooth muscle encircling pancreatic duct just before it joins the ampulla.

s., pyloric. A thickening of the muscular wall around the pyloric orifice.

sphincteral (sfĭngk′tĕr-ăl). Concerning a sphincter.

sphincteralgia (sfĭnk″tĕr-ăl′jē-ă) [Gr. *sphinkter,* a binder, + *algos,* pain]. Pain in the sphincter ani muscles.

sphincterectomy (sfĭnk″tĕr-ĕk′tō-mē) [″ + *ektome,* excision]. 1. Excision of any sphincter muscle. 2. Excision of part of the iris′ pupillary border.

sphincteric (sfĭngk-tĕr′ĭk). Concerning a sphincter.

sphincterismus (sfĭnk″tĕr-ĭz′mŭs) [″ + *-ismos,* condition]. Spasm of sphincter ani muscles.

sphincteritis (sfĭnk″tĕr-ī′tĭs) [″ + *itis,* inflammation]. Inflammation of any sphincter muscle.

sphincterolysis (sfĭnk″tĕr-ŏl′ĭ-sĭs) [″ + *lysis,* dissolution]. Freeing of the iris from the cornea in anterior synechia affecting only the pupillary border.

sphincteroplasty (sfĭnk′tĕr-ō-plăs″tē) [″ + *plassein,* to form]. Plastic operation upon any sphincter muscle.

sphincteroscope (sfĭnk′tĕr-ō-skōp″) [″ + *skopein,* to examine]. Instrument for inspection of the anal sphincter.

sphincteroscopy (sfĭnk″tĕr-ŏs′kō-pē). Inspection of the internal anal sphincter.

sphincterotome (sfĭngk′tĕr-ō-tōm″) [″ + *tome,* incision]. Surgical instrument for cutting a sphincter.

sphincterotomy (sfĭnk″tĕr-ŏt′ō-mē) [″ + *tome,* incision]. Cutting of a sphincter muscle.

sphingolipid (sfĭng″gō-lĭp′ĭd) [Gr. *sphingein,* to bind, + *lipos,* fat]. Lipid containing one of several long-chain bases such as sphingosine, q.v., or dihydrosphingosine, q.v., or bases of similar chemical structure but containing longer chains.

sphingolipidosis [″ + ″ + *osis,* condition]. Any disease characterized by defective metabolism of sphingolipids. These genetically determined errors of metabolism include Sandhoff′s disease, Fabry′s disease, Tay-Sachs disease, Kufs′ disease, Gaucher′s disease, Krabbe′s leukodystrophy, and Niemann-Pick disease. They are characterized by neurological deterioration, usually beginning a few months after birth, eventually leading to death except in the adult form of Gaucher′s disease. These diseases can be detected by examining fluid obtained by amniocentesis.

sphingolipodystrophy (sfĭng″gō-lĭp″ō-dĭs′trō-fē) [″ + *dys,* bad, + *trophe,* nutrition]. A group of diseases caused by defective sphingolipid metabolism.

sphingomyelins (sfĭng″gō-mī′ĕl-ĭns). A major group of phosphorus-containing sphingolipids, q.v. They are found primarily in nervous tissue and in lipids in the blood. They are derived from choline phosphate and a ceramide.

sphingosine (sfĭng′gō-sĭn). A long-chain base, $C_{18}H_{37}O_2N$, present in sphingolipids. SEE: *dihydrosphingosine; sphingolipid.*

sphygmic (sfĭg′mĭk) [Gr. *sphygmikos*]. Rel. to the pulse.

sphygmo- [Gr. *sphygmos,* pulse]. Combining form indicating pulse.

sphygmobolometer (sfĭg″mō-bō-lŏm′ĕ-tĕr) [″ + *bolos,* mass, + *metron,* a measure]. Device to measure force of the pulse rather than the blood pressure.

sphygmocardiogram (sfĭg″mō-kăr′dē-ō-grăm) [″ + *kardia,* heart, + *gramma,* mark]. A tracing made by a sphygmocardiograph of the heartbeat and radial pulse.

sphygmocardiograph (sfĭg″mō-kăr′dē-ō-grăf) [″ + ″ + *graphein,* to write]. Device for simultaneous recording of the radial pulse and the heartbeat.

sphygmocardioscope (sfĭg″mō-kăr′dē-ō-skōp) [″ + ″ + *skopein,* to examine]. Device for recording the action of the pulse and heart. SYN: *sphygmocardiograph.*

sphygmochronograph (sfĭg″mō-krō′nō-grăf) [″ + *chronos,* time, + *graphein,* to write]. A sphygmograph graphically recording time between the heartbeat and the pulse.

sphygmogram (sfĭg′mō-grăm) [″ + *gramma,* mark]. A tracing of the pulse made by using the sphygmograph.

sphygmograph (sfĭg′mō-grăf) [″ + *graphein,* to write]. Instrument for recording the shape and force of the pulse wave. SYN:

polygraph.

sphygmography (sfĭg-mŏg′ră-fē). Recording the arterial pulse by use of a sphygmograph.

sphygmoid (sfĭg′moyd) [Gr. *sphygmos,* pulse, + *eidos,* form]. Resembling the pulse.

sphygmology (sfĭg-mŏl′ō-jē) [″ + *logos,* a study]. Scientific study of the pulse.

sphygmomanometer (sfĭg″mō-măn-ŏm′ĕt-ĕr) [″ + *manos,* thin, + *metron,* measure]. Instrument for determining arterial blood pressure indirectly. The two types are aneroid and mercury. SEE: *blood pressure.*

s., random-zero. A special type of sphygmomanometer that allows the blood pressure to be taken without the observer knowing where zero pressure is on the device. After the pressure is obtained, the mercury comes to rest at a point. The observed pressure is then corrected by subtracting the at-rest value on the device from the pressure obtained. Used to prevent subjective bias in determining blood pressure.

sphygmometer (sfĭg-mŏm′ĕt-ĕr) [″ + *metron,* measure]. Instrument for measuring the pulse. SYN: *sphygmograph.*

sphygmopalpation (sfĭg″mō-păl-pā′shŭn) [″ + L. *palpatio,* palpation]. Palpating the pulse.

sphygmophone (sfĭg′mō-fōn) [Gr. *sphigmos,* pulse, + *phone,* voice]. Instrument for hearing the pulse beat.

sphygmoplethysmograph (sfĭg″mō-plĕth-ĭz′mō-grăf) [″ + *plethysmos,* increase, + *graphein,* to write]. Device that traces the pulse with its curve of fluctuation in volume.

sphygmoscope (sfĭg′mō-skōp) [″ + *skopein,* to examine]. Instrument for showing the heart's movements or pulsations of arteries and veins.

sphygmosystole (sfĭg″mō-sĭs′tō-lē) [Gr. *sphigmos,* pulse, + *systole,* contraction]. The segment of the sphygmogram that corresponds to the heart's systole.

sphygmotonograph (sfĭg″mō-tō′nō-grăf) [″ + *tonos,* tension, + *graphein,* to write]. An instrument for simultaneous recording and timing of arterial blood pressure, jugular or carotid pulse, and the brachial pulse.

sphygmotonometer (sfĭg″mō-tō-nŏm′ĕt-ĕr) [″ + ″ + *metron,* measure]. Instrument for ascertaining elasticity of walls of an artery.

sphygmus (sfĭg′mŭs) [Gr. *sphygmos*]. A pulse or pulsation.

sphyrectomy (sfī-rĕk′tō-mē) [Gr. *sphyra,* malleus, + *ektome,* excision]. Surgical excision of the malleus of the foot.

sphyrotomy (sfī-rŏt′ō-mē) [″ + *tome,* incision]. Surgical excision of a portion of the malleus of the foot.

spica (spī′kă) [L., ear of grain]. A reverse spiral bandage, the turn of which crosses like the letter V. SEE: *bandage, spica.*

spica hip cast. A cast containing the lower torso and extending to one or both lower extremities. If only one lower extremity is included, it is called a single hip spica; if two are included, it is called a double hip spica. These are used for treating pelvic and femoral fractures.

spicular (spĭk′ū-lar) [L. *spiculum,* a dart]. Pert. to or resembling a spicule; dartlike.

spicule (spĭk′ūl). A small, needle-shaped body.

s., bony. A needle-shaped fragment of bone.

spiculed red cell. Crenated red blood cells with surface projections. In most instances, this is a normal variation in red cell equilibrium, and is reversible.

spiculum (spĭk′ū-lŭm) [L., a dart]. (pl. *spicula*) A sharp, small spike. SYN: *spicule.*

spider (spī′dĕr). 1. An arachnid, belonging to the order Araneae, subclass Arachnida, class Arachnoidea, phylum Arthropoda. The body is divided into cephalothorax and abdomen joined by a narrow waist. A spider usually possesses four pairs of legs as well as poison fangs. It often possesses spinnerets. 2. Anything resembling a spider in appearance.

s., black widow. The female of Latrodectus mactans. It is glossy black in color with a brilliant red or yellow spot, usually shaped like an hourglass or two triangles, on undersurface of the abdomen. Its bite causes excruciating pain and may prove fatal.

SYM: Initially the sensation resembles the prick of a pin. This pain usually lasts for a short period of time, subsides, and later the abdominal muscles become rigid. Within a half hour severe abdominal cramps begin. The venom, which is neurotoxic, causes an ascending motor paralysis. Because of the extreme abdominal pain, the patient may be suspected of having an acute condition requiring abdominal surgery.

TREATMENT: Avoid all stimulants. Suction is of little value as the toxin is rapidly absorbed. Calcium gluconate intravenously often gives relief from pain. Large doses of morphine, repeated when necessary, given slowly by vein, also control pain. Apply heat either locally or by using a hot tub bath, and forcing fluids also recommended. A specific antivenin Latrodectus mactans is available. This horse serum–containing preparation should be given intramuscularly as soon as the diagnosis is made provided the patient is not sensitive to horse serum. SEE: *bites or stings.*

s., brown recluse. Loxosceles reclusa, a small, three-eighth in. (10 mm.) long spider native to North America. Its venom is quite toxic and is capable of causing death. The venom produces a large area of necrosis at the site of the bite. Treatment is symptomatic.

spider bites or poisoning. Not all spider bites are dangerous.

SYM: Local symptoms include slight burning followed in about half an hour by severe radiating pains, often extending long distances from puncture. Sloughing at site and along lymphatics may occur. Collapse, unconsciousness, convulsions, and death sometimes follow.

spider-burst. An area on the leg in which capillaries radiate from a central point. The veins though dilated are not varicosities.

spider cells. Branching cells in neuroglia. SYN: *Deiters' cells; cells, neuroglia,* q.v.

spider fingers. Abnormally long phalanges of the hands. SYN: *arachnodactyly.* SEE: *Marfan's syndrome.*

spider nevus. A branched growth of dilated capillaries on the skin resembling a spider. SYN: *nevus araneus.*

Spielmeyer-Vogt disease. Late juvenile cerebral sphingolipidosis.

spigelian line (spī-jē'lē-ăn). [Adrian van der Spieghel, Flemish anatomist, 1578–1625] Line on abdomen lying parallel to median line and marking edge of rectus abdominis muscle. SYN: *linea semilunaris; semilunar line.*

spigelian lobe. A small lobe behind right lobe of liver.

spike. The main peak in an oscillographic record of the action potential.

spikeboard. Adapted device for persons with limited upper extremity or one-handed function that allows for stabilization of food while it is being prepared.

spill (spĭl) [AS. *spillan,* to squander]. An overflow.

s., cellular. Dissemination of cells through lymph or the blood resulting in metastasis.

s., radioactive. Massive leak of radioactive materials from any source of radioactive materials. SEE: *radiation accidents, emergency handling of.*

spillway (spĭl'way). The contour of the teeth that allows food to escape from the cusps during mastication.

spiloma, spilus (spī-lō'mă, spī'lŭs) [Gr. *spiloma, spilos,* spot]. A mole or discoloration of skin. SYN: *nevus.*

spiloplania (spī"lō-plā'nē-ă) [" + *plane,* a wandering about]. Transient and wandering erythema of the skin.

spiloplaxia (spī"lō-plăk'sē-ă) [" + *plax,* plate]. A red spot appearing in leprosy.

spina (spī'nă) [L., thorn]. (pl. *spinae*) [NA] 1. Any spinelike protuberance. 2. The spine.

s. bifida. Congenital defect in walls of the spinal canal caused by lack of union between the laminae of the vertebrae. Lumbar portion is section chiefly affected. SYN: *rachischisis.*

SYM: As result of this deficiency, the membranes of the cord are pushed through the opening, forming a tumor known as *spina bifida,* due to condition of spine that gives rise to the deformity, and *hydrorrhachis* caused by the fluid contained in the tumor.

s. bifida occulta. Failure of vertebrae to close without hernial protrusion.

s. ventosa. Tuberculosis of the bone. The bone is expanded and the cortex thins.

spinal (spī'năl) [L. *spinalis*]. Pert. to the spine or spinal cord.

spinal accessory nerve. Accessory nerve, q.v.

spinal anesthesia. Anesthesia produced by an anesthetic injected into the spinal canal. SYN: *narcosis, medullary.*

spinal canal. Canal of the vertebral column that contains the spinal cord.

spinal column. The vertebral column enclosing the spinal cord and consisting of 33 vertebrae: 7 cervical, 12 dorsal or thoracic, 5 lumbar, 5 sacral fused to form 1 bone, and 4 in the coccyx fused to form 1 bone. The number is sometimes increased by an additional vertebra in one region, and sometimes one may be absent in another. SEE: illus.

spinal cord. An ovoid column of nervous tissue about 44 cm. long, flattened anteroposteriorly, extending from the medulla to the 2nd lumbar vertebra in the spinal canal. All nerves to the trunk and limbs are issued from the spinal cord, and it is the center of reflex action containing the conducting paths to and from the brain. In cross section, it does not fill the vertebral space, being surrounded by the pia mater, the cerebrospinal fluid, the arachnoid, and the dura mater, which fuses with the periosteum of the inner surfaces of the vertebrae.

The gray substance approximates the shape of an "H," there being a posterior and anterior horn in either half. The anterior horn is composed of motor cells from which the fibers making up the motor portions of the peripheral nerves arise. Sensory neurons enter posteriorly. The "H" also divides the surrounding white matter into posterior, lateral, and anterior bundles. These serve to connect brain and cord in both directions (i.e., with efferent and afferent nerves) as well as various portions of the cord itself.

spinal curvature. Abnormal curvature of the spine, frequently constitutional in children. It may be angular, lateral (scoliosis), or anteroposterior (kyphosis, q.v., lordosis, q.v.).

spinal curvature, angular. Caries of the spine. SYN: *Pott's disease.*

spinal curvature, lateral. Deviation of spine to one side or the other causing a twist of the spine.

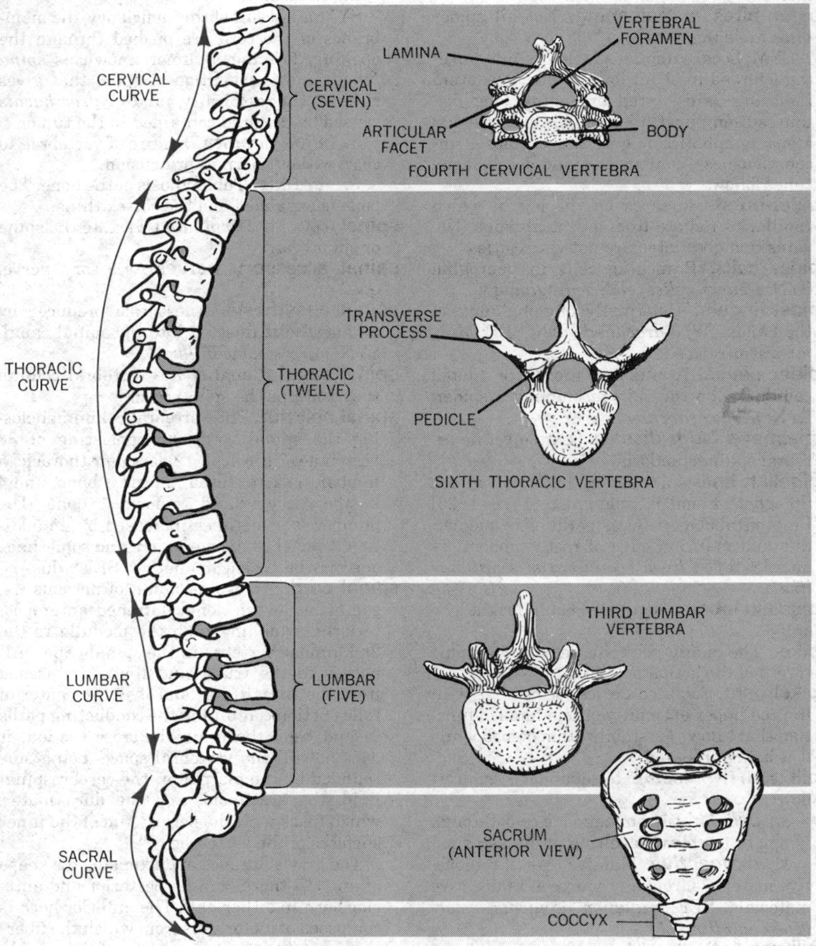

SPINAL COLUMN

INDICATING INDIVIDUAL VERTEBRAE AT VARIOUS LEVELS

spinal fluid. Cerebrospinal fluid. When normal, it contains 50 to 75 mg. of sugar per 100 ml. The sugar content is lower than that in the blood.

DIAG: *Cell count:* If normal, 0 to 5 mononuclear cells per ml. Increased in all diseased states, several hundred or thousands in meningitis, when fluid becomes opaque. *Lymphocytes:* Found in encephalitis and tuberculous meningitis; polymorphonuclears predominate in septic meningitis and epidemic meningitis. *Bloody fluid:* Brain hemorrhages due to arteriosclerosis, high blood pressure, tumors, and other causes. Spinal fluid may contain blood due to needle having punctured a small blood vessel. *Encephalitis:* Sugar content is increased, fluid clear, cell count 100 plus. *Globulin:* Its presence is abnormal.

Microorganisms: Meningococci, streptococci, pneumococci, tubercle bacilli, and influenza bacilli may be present, any of which may be indicative of meningitis. Epidemic meningitis indicated by gram-negative, intracellular diplococcus, biscuit-shaped microorganisms. Typhoid bacilli may produce meningeal symptoms in typhoid fever. Streptococci enter the meninges through the ear; the invading point of pneumococci, influenza bacilli, and pneumobacilli is the lungs. All these may be found in smears though sometimes missed and found in cultures. *Meningitis:* Lower spinal fluid sugar than sugar content of blood; 25 to 15 mg. If suppurative meningitis, spinal fluid is puslike and turbid, but it is clear in tuberculous meningitis, encephalitis, and poliomyelitis. *Poliomyelitis:* Same as encephalitis.

RS: anhydromyelia; calcinorrhachia; cerebrospinal fluid; meningitis; poliomyelitis.

spinal fusion. After removal of herniated disks, the adjacent vertebrae are immobilized by surgical procedure. SEE: *spondylosyndesis.*

spinal ganglion. Enlargement on dorsal or posterior root of a spinal nerve composed principally of cell bodies of somatic and visceral afferent neurons.

spinal nerves. Nerves arising from the spinal cord: 31 pairs, consisting 8 cervical, 12 thoracic, 5 lumbar, 5 sacral, and 1 coccygeal, corresponding with the spinal vertebrae. Each spinal nerve is attached to the spinal cord by two roots: a dorsal or posterior sensory root and a ventral or anterior root. The former consists of afferent fibers conveying impulses to the cord; the latter of efferent fibers conveying impulses from the cord. A typical spinal nerve, on passing through the intervertebral foramen, divides into four branches, a recurrent branch, a dorsal ramus or posterior primary division, a ventral ramus or anterior primary division, and two rami communicantes (white and gray), which pass to ganglia of the sympathetic trunk.

spinal puncture. Puncture of the spinal cavity with a needle to extract the spinal fluid for diagnostic purposes, to introduce anesthetic agents into the spinal canal, or to remove fluid so other fluids such as radiopaque substances may be injected. SEE: *Queckenstedt's test.*

SITE OF PUNCTURE: To prevent injury of the nerve fibers, the puncture is usually made at the juncture between the 3rd and 4th lumbar vertebrae. A line drawn posteriorly from the crest of one ilium over the crest of the other will usually pass over the tip of the spinous process of the 4th lumbar vertebra. The point for the needle injection is directly above this line (i.e., toward the head).

NURSING IMPLICATIONS: Assess the patient's understanding of the procedure and correct any misinterpretations. Obtain permission or consent if necessary. Procure the equipment needed to perform the procedure. Have the patient void and defecate if possible. Provide privacy and position the patient properly. Assist as necessary during the procedure, and provide verbal and nonverbal reassurance to the patient. Send specimens to the laboratory as requested. Instruct patient concerning the need to remain flat, preferably in a prone position for the first several hours immediately following the procedure. This will help to prevent post–spinal puncture headache. Document the specimens that were sent as well as the patient's response to the procedure.

CAUTION: If the cerebrospinal fluid pressure is elevated, it may be dangerous to perform spinal puncture.

spinal reflex. Any reflex centering in the spinal cord.

spinal shock. Effects resulting from transverse section of the spinal cord and that occur in segments below level of section. Principal effects are anesthesia, paralysis, loss of muscle tone, and suppression of reflexes, both visceral and somatic.

spinalgia (spī-năl′jē-ă) [L. *spina,* thorn, + Gr. *algos,* pain]. Pain in a vertebra under pressure.

spinalis (spī-nā′lĭs) [L.]. A muscle attached to the spinal process of a vertebra. SEE: *Muscles* in *Appendix.*

spinate (spī′nāt). Having spines or shaped like a thorn.

spindle (spĭn′dl) [AS. *spinel*]. 1. A fusiform-shaped body. 2. The portion of the achromatic apparatus seen in mitosis consisting of a bundle of delicate fibrils that connect the two centrosomes or asters. The chromosomes arrange themselves on the spindle in an equatorial plate.

s., aortic. A dilatation of the aorta following the aortic isthmus.

s., enamel. A tubular hypomineralized structure extending a short distance from the dentinoenamel junction into enamel, seen in ground sections of teeth.

s., muscle. A nerve receptor present in voluntary muscle tissues. This specialized tissue is involved in the stretch and myotatic reflexes.

s., neuromuscular. A complex sensory nerve ending consisting of muscle fibers enclosed within a capsule and supplied by an afferent nerve fiber. It mediates proprioceptive sensations and reflexes.

s., neurotendinous A proprioceptive nerve ending found in a tendon, in muscle septa or sheaths, in a muscle tissue, or at junction of a muscle or tendon. SYN: *organ of Golgi.*

s., sleep. Specific waves that appear in

the electroencephalogram during sleep.

spine (spīn). 1. A sharp process of bone. 2. The spinal column, consisting of 33 vertebrae: 7 cervical, 12 thoracic, 5 lumbar, 5 sacral, 4 coccygeal. The bones of the sacrum and coccyx are ankylosed in adult life and counted as one each. SYN: *backbone.*

RS: cephalorhachidian; cord, spinal; cramp; curvature; rachialgia; rachilysis, "rach-" words; scoliosis.

s., alar. Spinous process of the sphenoid bone.

s., anterior nasal. Projection formed by anterior prolongation of the inferior border of the nasal notch of the maxilla.

s., bifid. Spina bifida.

s., fracture of. A fractured spine often is treated in a plaster jacket with the spine hyperextended to reduce the fracture after essential treatment with skeletal traction. A window is cut over the abdomen. If the fracture is high the neck is included in the jacket, which must be short enough to allow flexion of the thighs. The patient is allowed to walk in the jacket, which is left on for 3 or 4 months. A vest is put on under this plaster, and the prominences are padded with felt. The muscles of the back are exercised by carrying weight on the head.

Traction, Balkan, and Stryker frames are used if the fracture involves the cord with paralysis below the injury. Bedsores and cystitis must be prevented. An enema is given when needed.

s., frontal. Sharp-pointed medial process extending downward from nasal process of frontal bone. SYN: *s., nasal.*

s., hemal. That part of the hemal arch of a typical vertebra that closes it in.

s., Henle's. S., suprameatal.

s., iliac. One of four spines of the ilium, namely the anterior and posterior inferior spines and the anterior and posterior superior spines.

s., ischial. Spine of the ischium, a pointed eminence on its posterior border. SYN: *s., sciatic.*

s., mental. Small process on the inner surface of mandible at back of the symphysis formed of one or more small projections (genial tubercles).

s., nasal. A sharp process descending in the middle line from the inferior surface of the frontal bone between the superior maxillae.

s., neural. Spinous process of a vertebra. The posterior projection of the neural arch.

s. of pubes. A prominent tubercle on upper border of the pubis.

s. of scapula. An osseous plate projecting from the posterior surface of the scapula.

s. of sphenoid. Spinous process of the greater sphenoid wing.

s., pharyngeal. Ridge under the basilar process of the occipital bone.

s., posterior nasal. Spine formed by medial ends of the horizontal processes of the palatine bones.

s., sciatic. S., ischial.

s., suprameatal. A small spine at junction of superior and posterior walls of the external auditory meatus. SYN: *s., Henle's.*

s., typhoid. Acute arthritis due to infection causing spinal ankylosis during or following typhoid fever.

spinifugal (spī-nĭf'ū-găl) [L. *spina,* thorn, + *fugare,* to flee]. Moving away from the spinal cord.

spinipetal (spī-nĭp'ĕ-tăl) [" + *petere,* to seek]. Conducting nerve impulse toward the spinal cord.

spinnbarkheit (spĭn'băr-kīt) [Ger.]. The elasticity of cervical mucus. Useful in choosing a day for artificial insemination. The cervical secretion is aspirated and placed on a slide. Spinnbarkheit (SBK) is measured by pulling upward on the secretion with a forceps. Before ovulation there is no elasticity. On the day of ovulation there is good elasticity, measuring 12 to 24 cm. or more. The day after ovulation, elasticity diminishes.

Not all women have SBK changes that are clear-cut. Therefore this test is used in conjunction with other signs of ovulation. SEE: *basal temperature chart; fern pattern; mittelschmerz; mucorrhea.*

spinobulbar (spī"nō-bŭl'băr) [" + Gr. *bulbos,* a bulb]. Concerning the spinal cord and medulla oblongata.

spinocostalis (spī"nō-kŏs-tā'lĭs) [" + *costa,* rib]. The combination of the superior and inferior serratus muscles.

spinocellular (spī"nō-sĕl'ū-lăr) [" + *cellula,* a little chamber]. Pert. to or like prickle cells.

spinocerebellar (spī"nō-sĕr-ĕ-bĕl'ăr) [" + *cerebellum,* little brain]. Concerning spinal cord and cerebellum.

spinocortical (spī"nō-kor'tĭ-kăl) [" + *cortex,* rind]. Pert. to the spinal cord and cerebral cortex. SYN: *corticospinal.*

spinoglenoid (spī"nō-glĕn'oyd) [" + Gr. *glene,* cavity, + *eidos,* form]. Rel. to the spine of the scapula and the glenoid cavity.

spinoglenoid ligament. Ligament joining the spine of the scapula to the border of the glenoid cavity.

spinose (spī'nōs) [L. *spina,* thorn]. Spinous.

spinotectal (spī"nō-tĕk'tăl) [" + *tectum,* roof]. Pert. to the spinal cord and the tectum, the dorsal portion (corpora quadrigemina) of the midbrain.

spinous (spī'nŭs) [L. *spina,* thorn]. Pert. to or resembling a spine.

spinous point. Spot over a spinous process

very sensitive to pressure.

spinous process. Prominence at posterior part of each vertebra.

spintherism (spĭn'thĕr-ĭzm) [Gr. *spintherizein,* to emit sparks]. Sensation of sparks before the eyes.

spintheropia (spĭn"thĕr-ō'pē-ă) [Gr. *spinther,* spark, + *ops,* eye]. Subjective sensation of sparks before the eyes.

spiradenitis (spī"răd-ĕn-ī'tĭs) [Gr. *speira,* coil, + *aden,* gland, + *itis,* inflammation]. A funiculus beginning in coil of a sweat gland. SEE: *hidrosadenitis.*

spiradenoma (spī"răd-ĕn-ō'mă) [" + " + *oma,* tumor]. Benign tumor of the sweat glands.

spiral (spī'răl) [L. *spiralis*]. Coiling around a center like the thread of a screw.

s., Curschmann's. SEE: *Curschmann's spirals.*

spiral bandage. Roller bandage to be applied spirally.

spiral canal of cochlea. The bony cochlea enclosing the scala tympani, scala vestibuli, and cochlear duct.

spiral canal of modiolus. Canal that runs spirally around the modiolus and contains the spiral ganglion.

spiral lamina. A thin, bony plate projecting from the modiolus into the cochlear canal, dividing it into two portions, the upper scala vestibuli and lower scala tympani. SYN: *lamina spiralis.*

spiral organ of Corti. Structure in floor of cochlear duct resting on basilar membrane. It contains hair cells, the receptors of stimuli produced by sound. SEE: *Corti, organ of.*

spirilla (spī-rĭl'ă) [L.]. Pl. of spirillum.

spirillicidal (spī-rĭl"ĭ-sīd'ăl) [L. *spirillum,* coil, + *cidus,* kill]. Destroying spirochetes or spirilla.

spirillicide (spī-rĭl'ĭ-sīd). Destructive to spirilla.

spirillolysis (spī"rĭ-lŏl'ĭ-sĭs) [" + Gr. *lysis,* dissolution]. The destruction of spirilla.

spirillosis (spī-rĭl-ō'sĭs) [" + Gr. *osis,* condition]. A disease caused by presence of spirilla in the blood.

spirillotropic (spī"rĭ-lō-trŏp'ĭk) [" + Gr. *trope,* a turning]. Having an attraction to spirilla.

spirillotropism (spī"rĭ-lŏt'rō-pĭzm) [" + " + *-ismos,* condition]. The ability to attract spirilla.

Spirillum (spī-rĭl'ŭm) [L., coil]. (pl. *Spirilla*) A genus of spiral-shaped motile microorganisms belonging to the family Pseudomonadaceae, tribe Spirilleae. Found in freshwater and saltwater.

S. minus. Species found in the blood of rats and mice. The causative agent of one form of ratbite fever.

spirillum. (pl. *spirilla*) A flagellated aerobic bacterium with an elongated spiral shape, of the genus Spirillum. SEE: *bacteria* for illus.

spirit (spĭr'ĭt) [L. *spiritus,* breath]. 1. A solution of essential or volatile liquid. 2. Any distilled or volatile liquid. 3. Alcoholic beverage.

s. of ammonia. A pungent solution of approximately 4% ammonium carbonate in 70% alcohol flavored with lemon, lavender, and myristica oil. It is used to elicit reflex stimulation of respiration and as smelling salts to stimulate patients who have fainted.

s. of bitter almond. A mixture of oil of bitter almond, almond, and distilled water, employed as a flavoring agent.

s. of camphor. A mixture of camphor and alcohol, employed locally as a counterirritant.

s. of juniper. A mixture of oil of juniper and alcohol.

s. of lavender. A mixture of oil of lavender flowers and alcohol, employed as a flavoring agent.

s. of mustard. A solution of volatile oil of mustard in alcohol, employed as a counterirritant.

s. of peppermint. A mixture of oil of peppermint, peppermint, and alcohol, employed as a carminative.

spiritual therapy [L. *spiritus,* breath, + Gr. *therapeia,* treatment]. The application of spiritual knowledge in the treatment of mental and physical disorders. Based upon the assumption that man is a spiritual being living in a spiritual universe, that in proportion to his acceptance of this idea and in proportion to his success in demonstrating it, he may control the body and the material elements in harmony with a divine plan.

spirituous (spĭr'ĭt-ū-ŭs") [L. *spiritus,* breath]. 1. Pert. to alcohol. 2. An alcoholic.

spiritus (spĭr'ĭ-tŭs) [L., breath]. Alcoholic solution of a volatile substance. Usually, 5 to 10% strength. SYN: *spirit*

s. frumenti. Whiskey.

s. juniperi. Gin.

s. myrciae. Bay rum.

s. vini gallici. Brandy.

Spirochaeta (spī"rō-kē'tă) [Gr. *speira,* coil, + *chaite,* hair]. A genus of slender, spiral, motile microorganisms belonging to the family Spirochaetaceae, order Spirochaetales.

S. icterohaemorrhagiae. Species found in Weil's disease or acute febrile jaundice. SYN: *Leptospira icterohaemorrhagiae.*

S. pallida. The microorganism that causes syphilis. SYN: *Treponema pallidum.*

Spirochaetales (spī"rō-kē-tā'lēs). An order of slender spiral organisms belonging to the class Schizomycetes. It includes the families Spirochaetaceae and Treponemataceae.

spirochetal (spī"rō-kē'tăl) [" + *chaite,* hair]. Pert. to spirochetes, esp. infections caused by them.

spirochetalytic (spī″rō-kē″tă-lĭt′ĭk) [″ + ″ + *lysis,* dissolution]. Destructive of spirochetes.

spirochete (spī′rō-kēt). Any member of the order Spirochaetales.

spirochetemia (spī″rō-kē-tē′mē-ă) [″ + *chaite,* hair, + *haima,* blood]. Spirochetes in the blood.

spirocheticidal (spī″rō-kē″tĭ-sī′dăl) [″ + ″ + L. *cidus,* kill]. Destructive to spirochetes.

spirocheticide (spī″rō-kē′tĭ-sīd). Anything that destroys spirochetes.

spirochetolysis (spī″rō-kē-tŏl′ĭ-sĭs) [″ + *chaite,* hair, + *lysis,* dissolution]. The destruction of spirochetes by specific antibodies, chemotherapy, or lysins.

spirochetosis (spī″rō-kē-tō′sĭs) [″ + ″ + *osis,* condition]. Any infection caused by spirochetes.

spirochetotic (spī″rō-kē-tŏt′ĭk). Pert. to or marked by spirochetosis.

spirocheturia (spī″rō-kē-tū′rē-ă) [Gr. *speira,* coil, + *chaite,* hair, + *ouron,* urine]. Spirochetes in the urine.

spirogram (spī′rō-grăm″) [L. *spirare,* to breathe, + Gr. *gramma,* a mark]. A record made by a spirograph indicating respiratory movements.

spirograph (spī′rō-grăf) [″ + Gr. *graphein,* to write]. Graphic record of respiratory movements.

spiroid (spī′royd) [Gr. *speira,* coil, + *eidos,* form]. Resembling a spiral.

spirokinesis (spī″rō-kĭn-ē′sĭs) [″ + *kinesis,* motion]. The tendency of motile organisms, including man, to veer or move in a spiral direction when deprived of external reference points.

spiroma (spī-rō′mă) [″ + *oma,* tumor]. Multiple, benign, cystic epithelioma of the sweat glands. SYN: *spiradenoma.*

spirometer (spī-rŏm′ĕt-ĕr) [L. *spirare,* to breathe, + Gr. *metron,* measure]. An apparatus consisting of a cylindrical bell immersed in water and so equipped with outlets that gases can be exhaled into it or inhaled out of it while measurements of volume are made. The following are typical measurements made on normal men by using the spirometer:

Complemental air (inspiratory reserve volume): 1600 cc., the amount that a subject can still inhale by special effort after a normal inspiration.

Dead space air: 150 cc., the air inhaled through the nose that gets only as far as nasopharynx, bronchi, bronchioles, and trachea and does not reach the lungs.

Functional residual air (functional residual capacity): About 2600 cc., the sum of the supplemental and residual air.

Minimal air: Less than 1000 cc., that which remains in the lungs after complete collapse as in pneumothorax.

Reserve air: Supplemental air.

Residual air (residual volume): 1000 cc. that are left in the lungs after a complete expiration.

Supplemental air (expiratory reserve volume): 1600 cc. that can still be exhaled after a normal exhalation.

Tidal volume: 500 cc., the amount exhaled or inhaled during normal respiration.

spirometry (spī-rŏm′ĕ-trē) [L. *spirare,* to breathe, + Gr. *metron,* measure]. Measurement of air capacity of the lungs.

spironolactone (spī-rō″nō-lăk′tōn). USP. A diuretic drug that blocks the action of aldosterone on the renal tubules. It acts to decrease potassium loss in the urine. Trade name is Aldactone.

spissated (spĭs′āt-ĕd) [L. *spissatus*]. Thickened. SYN: *inspissated.*

spissitude (spĭs′ĭ-tūd) [L. *spissitudo*]. Condition of being inspissated, as a fluid thickened by evaporation almost to a solid; thickness.

spit (spĭt) [AS. *spittan*]. 1. Saliva. SYN: *expectoration; spittle; sputum.* 2. To expectorate spittle.

spittle [AS. *spatl*]. The digestive fluid of the mouth. SYN: *saliva.*

splanchna (splăngk′nă) [Gr.]. The intestines or the viscera.

splanchnapophysis (splăngk″nă-pŏf′ĭ-sĭs) [Gr. *splanchnos,* viscus, + *apophysis,* offshoot]. 1. Any skeletal element connected with the alimentary canal, as the lower jaw. 2. Outgrowth of a vertebra on opposite side of a vertebral axis, enclosing some viscus.

splanchnectopia (splăngk″nĕk-tō′pē-ă) [″ + *ektopos,* out of place]. Dislocation of a viscus or of the viscera.

splanchnemphraxis (splăngk″nĕm-frăk′sĭs) [″ + *emphraxis,* stoppage]. Obstruction of any internal organ, particularly of the intestine.

splanchnesthesia (splăngk″nĕs-thē′zē-ă) [″ + *aisthesis,* sensation]. Visceral sensation.

splanchnesthetic (splăngk″nĕs-thĕt′ĭk). Rel. to visceral consciousness or sensation.

splanchnic (splăngk′nĭk) [Gr. *splanchnikos*]. Pert. to the viscera.

splanchnicectomy (splănk″nē-sĕk′tō-mē) [Gr. *splanchnos,* viscus, + *ektome,* excision]. Resection of the splanchnic nerves.

splanchnic nerves. Three nerves from the thoracic sympathetic ganglia distributed to the viscera.

splanchnicotomy (splăngk″nĭ-kŏt′ō-mē) [″ + *tome,* incision]. Section of a splanchnic nerve.

splanchnoblast (splăngk′nō-blăst) [″ + *blastos,* germ]. Incipient rudiment of a viscus. SEE: *anlage; proton.*

splanchnocele (splăngk′nō-sēl). 1. [″ + *koilos,* a hollow]. That part of the coelom persisting in the adult, giving rise to the visceral cavities. SYN: *splanchnocoele.* 2. [″ + *kele,* hernia]. Protrusion of any abdominal viscus.

splanchnocoele (splăngk′nō-sēl) [″ + *koilos,* a hollow]. Rudimentary embryonic cavity from which the visceral cavities arise.

splanchnocranium (splănk″nō-krā′nē-ŭm) [″ + *kranion,* upper part of head]. The portion of the skull derived from the visceral or branchial skeleton.

splanchnodiastasis (splăngk″nō-dī-ăs′tă-sĭs) [″ + *diastasis,* separation]. Displacement or separation of any viscus.

splanchnodynia (splăngk-nō-dĭn′ē-ă) [Gr. *splanchnos,* viscus, + *odyne,* pain]. Pain in the abdominal region.

splanchnography (splăngk-nŏg′ră-fē) [″ + *graphein,* to write]. Descriptive treatise on anatomy of the viscera.

splanchnolith (splăngk′nō-lĭth) [″ + *lithos,* stone]. An intestinal calculus.

splanchnology (splăngk-nŏl′ō-jē) [″ + *logos,* a study]. The study of the viscera.

splanchnomegaly (splănk″nō-mĕg′ă-lē) [″ + *megas,* large]. Visceromegaly, q.v.

splanchnomicria (splănk″nō-mĭk′rē-ă) [″ + *mikros,* small]. The condition of having small splanchnic organs.

splanchnopathia (splăngk″nō-păth′ē-ă) [″ + *pathos,* disease]. Pathological conditions of the viscera.

splanchnopleural (splănk″nō-ploor′ăl) [″ + *pleura,* side]. Concerning the splanchnopleure.

splanchnopleure (splăngk′nō-plūr) [″ + *pleura,* side]. The embryonic layer formed by the union of the visceral layer of the mesoderm with the entoderm. SEE: *somatopleure.*

splanchnoptosia, splanchnoptosis (splăngk″nō-tō′sē-ă, -sĭs) [″ + *ptosis,* a dropping]. Prolapse of the viscera. SYN: *ptosis, abdominal; enteroptosis; visceroptosis.*

splanchnosomatic (splănk″nō-sō-măt′ĭk) [″ + *soma,* body]. Viscerosomatic, q.v.

splanchnosclerosis (splăngk″nō-sklĕr-ō′sĭs) [″ + *sklerosis,* a hardening]. Hardening of any of the viscera through overgrowth or infiltration of connective tissue.

splanchnoscopy (splăngk-nŏs′kō-pē) [″ + *skopein,* to examine]. Examination of the viscera with aid of roentgen rays or transillumination.

splanchnoskeleton (splăngk″nō-skĕl′ĕ-tŏn) [″ + *skeleton,* skeleton]. 1. In primitive vertebrates such as fishes, the cartilaginous or bony arches (branchial) that encircle pharyngeal portion of digestive tract. 2. In higher vertebrates, the bones derived from the branchial arches, which include the maxilla, mandible, malleus, incus, stapes, hyoid bone, and cartilages of the larynx.

splanchnotomy (splăngk-nŏt′ō-mē) [″ + *tome,* incision]. Dissection of the viscera.

splanchnotribe (splăngk′nō-trīb) [″ + *tribein,* to crush]. A crushing instrument for temporarily closing the lumen of the intestine prior to resection.

splayfoot [ME. *splayen,* to spread out, + AS. *fot,* foot]. A flatfoot or the deformity flatfoot. SYN: *pes planus; talipes valgus.*

spleen (splēn) [Gr. *splen*]. The largest collection of reticuloendothelial cells in the body; an elongated, dark red, ovoid body lying in upper left quadrant of abdomen posterior and inferior to the stomach. It is composed of spongelike tissue (splenic pulp) consisting of lymphatic tissue differentiated into white pulp and pulp infiltrated with red blood cells (red pulp). It is enclosed by a dense capsule from which trabeculae extend into substance of the spleen. On one side is the hilus through which the splenic vessels and nerves enter and exit. SYN: *lien* [NA]. SEE: *abdominal quadrants* for illus.

FUNCT: *Blood formation:* In the embryo, all types of blood cells are formed by the spleen but in the adult, only lymphocytes and monocytes. In the adult, if bone marrow is damaged, the spleen can function to produce various blood cells. *Blood storage:* Smooth muscle and elastic tissue fibers in the capsule and trabeculae enable the spleen to contract and discharge blood cells into circulation. *Blood filtration:* By which bacteria and particulate matter, esp. aged, non-functioning red blood cells, are removed from circulation. The spleen also removes inclusion bodies such as Heinz bodies and the nuclei of immature red blood cells from circulating red blood cells.

DISORDERS OF: Acute and chronic infections and certain infectionlike states, hypersplenism, primary splenic thrombocytopenia, primary splenic neutropenia, Felty's syndrome, Banti's disease, congestive splenomegaly, tumors. SEE: *thrombosis.*

s., accessory. Splenic tissue nodules near the spleen.

s., floating. An enlarged movable spleen that is not protected by the ribs.

s., lardaceous. Enlargement of spleen due to fatty tissue. SEE: *degeneration, amyloid.*

s., sago. Spleen having appearance of grains of sago, q.v.

splenadenoma (splēn″ăd-ē-nō′mă) [Gr. *splen,* spleen, + *aden,* gland, + *oma,* tumor]. Enlargement of the spleen caused by hyperplasia of its pulp.

splenalgia (splē-năl'jē-ă) [" + *algos,* pain]. Neuralgic pain in the spleen. SYN: *splenodynia.*

splenceratosis (splēn"sĕr-ă-tō'sĭs) [" + *keras,* horn, + *osis,* condition]. Induration of the spleen.

splenectasia, splenectasis (splē"nĕk-tā'zē-ă, splē-nĕk'tă-sĭs) [" + *ektasis,* dilatation]. Enlargement of the spleen.

splenectomy (splē-nĕk'tō-mē) [" + *ektome,* excision]. Surgical excision of the spleen.

splenectopia, splenectopy (splē"nĕk-tō'pē-ă, -nĕk'tō-pē) [" + *ektopos,* out of place]. Displacement or mobility of the spleen. SYN: *spleen, floating.*

splenelcosis (splē"nĕl-kō'sĭs) [" + *helkosis,* ulceration]. Ulceration or abscess of the spleen.

splenemia (splē-nē'mē-ă) [Gr. *splen,* spleen, + *haima,* blood]. 1. Splenic congestion with blood. 2. Leukemia with splenic hypertrophy.

splenemphraxis (splē"nĕm-frăk'sĭs) [" + *emphraxis,* stoppage]. Congested condition of the spleen.

spleneolus (splē-nē'ō-lŭs). Accessory spleen.

splenepatitis (splē"nĕp-ă-tī'tĭs) [" + *hepar,* liver, + *itis,* inflammation]. Inflammation of both spleen and liver.

splenetic (splē-nĕt'ĭk). 1. Pert. to the spleen. 2. Suffering with chronic disease of the spleen. 3. Surly, fretful, impatient.

splenetic cords. Poorly defined cords of red pulp of the spleen.

splenetic flexure. Junction of transverse and descending colon, making a bend on the left side near the spleen.

splenetic nodule. A concentrated mass of white pulp in the spleen. SYN: *malpighian body* (def. 2).

splenetic sinus. One of a series of wide channels with thin walls forming an anastomosing plexus throughout red pulp of spleen. SYN: *terminal veins.*

splenetic vein. Vein carrying blood from spleen to the portal vein.

splenial (splē'nē-ăl) [Gr. *splen,* spleen]. Concerning the spleen.

splenic (splĕn'ĭk) [Gr. *splenikos*]. Splenetic.

splenicterus (splē-nĭk'tĕr-ŭs) [Gr. *splen,* spleen, + *ikteros,* jaundice]. Inflammation of the spleen associated with jaundice.

splenification (splē"nĭ-fĭ-kā'shŭn) [" + L. *facere,* to make]. Change in a structure whereby it resembles splenic tissue. SYN: *splenization.*

spleniform (splĕn'ĭ-form) [" + L. *forma,* form]. Resembling the spleen.

splenitis (splē-nī'tĭs) [" + *itis,* inflammation]. Inflamed condition of the spleen. Comprises acute and chronic hypertrophy, proliferative splenitis, and suppurative inflammation, the result of acute infectious disease.

SYM: Indefinite or absent. Usually little pain or tenderness unless perisplenitis exists. Considerable enlargement may be attended by sense of weight, tension, or distress in left hypochondrium, accompanied perhaps by slight dyspnea, sudden pain appearing in gastric region followed by vomiting of pus and blood in course of infectious disease, which may be due to abscess of spleen.

PROG: Depends upon systemic condition.

splenium (splē'nē-ŭm) [Gr. *splenion,* bandage]. 1. A compress or bandage. 2. A structure resembling a bandaged part.

s. corporis callosi. [NA] The thickened posterior end of the corpus callosum.

splenius (splē'nē-ŭs). A flat muscle on either side of back of neck and upper thoracic area. SEE: *muscles* for illus.; *Muscles* in *Appendix.*

splenization (splē"nĭ-zā'shŭn). The change in a tissue, as of the lung, when it resembles splenic tissue.

splenocele (splē'nō-sēl) [Gr. *splen,* spleen, + *kele,* hernia]. 1. A hernia of the spleen. 2. A splenic tumor.

splenoceratosis (splē"nō-sĕr"ă-tō'sĭs) [" + *keras,* horn, + *osis,* condition]. Induration of the spleen.

splenocleisis (splē"nō-klī'sĭs) [" + *kleisis,* closure]. Friction on the surface of the spleen or wrapping with gauze in order to induce the formation of fibrous tissue.

splenocolic (splē"nō-kŏl'ĭk) [" + *kolon,* colon]. Pert. to the spleen and colon or reference to a fold of peritoneum between the two viscera.

splenocyte (splē'nō-sīt) [" + *kytos,* cell]. A unicellular leukocyte or lymphocyte of the spleen. It probably originates elsewhere in the body.

splenodynia (splē"nō-dĭn'ē-ă) [" + *odyne,* pain]. Pain in the spleen. SYN: *splenalgia.*

splenogenic, splenogenous (splē"nō-jĕn'ĭk, splē-nŏj'ĕn-ŭs) [" + *gennan,* to produce]. Originating in the spleen.

splenography (splē-nŏg'ră-fē) [" + *graphein,* to write]. A treatise on, or a description of, the spleen.

splenohemia (splē"nō-hē'mē-ă) [Gr. *splen,* spleen, + *haima,* blood]. Congestion of the spleen with blood. SYN: *splenemia.*

splenohepatomegaly (splē"nō-hĕp"ă-tō-mĕg'ă-lē) [" + *hepar,* liver, + *megas,* large]. Enlargement of spleen and liver.

splenoid (splē'noyd) [" + *eidos,* resemblance]. Resembling the spleen.

splenokeratosis (splē"nō-kĕr"ă-tō'sĭs) [" + *keras,* horn, + *osis,* condition]. Induration of the spleen.

splenolaparotomy (splē"nō-lăp"ă-rŏt'ō-mē) [" + *lapara,* flank, + *tome,* incision]. Incision through the abdominal wall into the spleen.

splenology (splē-nŏl'ō-jē) [" + *logos*, study]. The study of functions and diseases of the spleen.

splenolymphatic (splē"nō-lĭm-făt'ĭk) [" + L. *lympha*, lymph]. Concerning the spleen and lymph nodes.

splenolysin (splē-nŏl'ĭ-sĭn) [" + *lysis*, dissolution]. An antibody that destroys splenic tissue.

splenolysis (splē-nŏl'ĭ-sĭs). Destruction of splenic tissue.

splenoma (splē-nō'mă) [" + *oma*, tumor]. (pl. *splenomas, -mata*) A tumor of the spleen. SYN: *splenocele.*

splenomalacia (splē"nō-mă-lā'shē-ă) [" + *malakia*, softening]. Softening of the spleen.

splenomedullary (splē"nō-mĕd'ū-lĕr"ē) [" + L. *medulla*, marrow]. Concerning the spleen and bone marrow, or originating in the spleen and bone marrow.

splenomegalia, splenomegaly (splē"nō-mē-gā'lē-ă, -mĕg'ă-lē) [" + *megas*, large]. Enlargement of the spleen.

s., congestive. A syndrome consisting of anemia, splenic enlargement, hemorrhages, and ultimately cirrhosis of the liver. SYN: *Banti's syndrome.*

s., hemolytic. Enlargement of the spleen in association with hemolytic disease of the blood.

splenometry (splē-nŏm'ĕ-trē) [" + *metron*, measure]. Determining the size of the spleen.

splenomyelogenous (splē"nō-mī"ĕ-lŏj'ĕ-nŭs) [" + *myelos*, marrow, + *gennan*, to produce]. Splenomedullary, q.v.

splenomyelomalacia (splē"nō-mī"ĕl-ō-mă-lā'shē-ă) [" + " + *malakia*, softening]. Abnormal softening of the spleen and bone marrow.

splenoncus (splē-nŏng'kŭs) [Gr. *splen*, spleen, + *onkos*, tumor]. Tumor of the spleen.

splenonephric (splē"nō-nĕf'rĭk) [" + *nephros*, kidney]. Rel. to the spleen and the kidney. SYN: *lienorenal.*

splenonephroptosis (splē"nō-nĕf"rŏp-tō'sĭs) [" + " + *ptosis*, a dropping]. Downward displacement of the spleen and kidney.

splenopancreatic (splē"nō-păn"krē-ăt'ĭk) [" + *pankreas*, pancreas]. Rel. to the spleen and pancreas.

splenopathy (splē-nŏp'ă-thē) [" + *pathos*, disease]. Any disorder of the spleen.

splenopexy (splē'nō-pĕk"sē) [" + *pexis*, fixation]. Artificial fixation of a movable spleen.

splenophrenic (splĕn-ō-frĕn'ĭk) [" + *phren*, diaphragm]. Concerning the spleen and diaphragm.

splenopneumonia (splē"nō-nū-mō'nē-ă) [" + *pneumonia*, inflammation of lung]. Pneumonia with splenization, q.v., of the lung.

splenoportography (splē"nō-por-tŏg'ră-fē) [" + L. *porta*, gate, + Gr. *graphein*, to write]. X-ray study of the spleen and portal vein after injection of a radiopaque dye into the spleen.

splenoptosis (splē"nŏp-tō'sĭs) [" + *ptosis*, a dropping]. Downward displacement of the spleen.

splenorenal (splē"nō-rē'năl). Pert. to the spleen and kidney.

splenorenal shunt. Anastomosis of splenic vein to renal vein to enable blood from portal system to enter general venous circulation. Performed in cases of portal hypertension.

splenorrhagia (splē"nō-rā'jē-ă) [" + *rhegnynai*, to burst forth]. Hemorrhage from a ruptured spleen.

splenorrhaphy (splē-nor'ă-fē) [" + *rhaphe*, suture]. Suture of wound of the spleen.

splenotomy (splē-nŏt'ō-mē) [" + *tome*, incision]. Incision of the spleen.

splenotoxin (splē"nō-tŏks'ĭn) [" + *toxikon*, poison]. Cytotoxin having specific action on splenic cells. SYN: *lienotoxin.*

splenulus (splĕn'ū-lŭs) [L., a little spleen]. A rudimentary or accessory spleen.

splenunculus (splē-nŭng'kū-lŭs). Accessory spleen.

splint (splĭnt) [MD. *splinte*, a wedge]. An appliance made of bone, wood metal, or plaster of Paris, used for the fixation, union, or protection of an injured part of the body. It may be movable or immovable.

s., Agnew's. A splint used in fractures of the patella and metacarpus.

s., airplane. An appliance usually used on ambulatory patients in the treatment of fractures of the humerus. It takes its name from the elevated (abducted) position in which it holds the arm suspended in air.

s., anchor. A splint for fracture of the jaw, with metal loops fitting over the teeth and held together by a rod.

s., Ashhurst's. A bracketed splint of wire with a footpiece to cover the thigh and leg after excision of the knee joint.

s., Balkan. Splint used for continuous extension in fracture of the femur.

s., banjo traction. Splint made out of a steel rod bent to resemble the shape of a banjo. Used for the treatment of contractures and fractures of the fingers.

s., Bavarian. An immovable dressing in which the plaster is applied between two layers of flannel.

s., blow-up. Tubular material that fits around the injured extremity. It contains compartments that can be inflated. These immobilize the injured part when filled with air.

s., Bond's. A splint used for fracture of the lower end of the radius.

s., Bowlby's. A splint used for fracture of the shaft of the humerus.

s., bracketed. A splint composed of two pieces of metal or wood united by brackets.

s., Cabot's. A splint composed of a metal structure placed posterior to the thigh and leg.

s., Carter's intranasal. A steel bridge with wings connected by a hinge. Used for operation of depressed nasal bridge.

s., coaptation. Small splint adjusted about a fractured part to prevent overriding of the fragments of bones. Usually covered by a longer splint for fixation of entire section.

s., dental. A rigid or flexible device or compound used to support, protect, or immobilize teeth that have been loosened, replanted, fractured, or subjected to surgical procedures.

s., Dupuytren's. A splint used to prevent eversion in Pott's fracture, q.v.

s., dynamic. A splint that assists in movements initiated by the patient.

s., Fox's. A splint used for fractured clavicle.

s., functional. S., dynamic, q.v.

s., Gibson walking. A splint that is a modification of Thomas splint.

s., Gordon's. A side splint used for the arm and hand in Colles' fracture, q.v.

s., inflatable. Inflatable device for immobilizing part or all of an extremity. The hollow tubular device is placed around the part and then inflated. SEE: *s., blow-up.*

CAUTION: Do not inflate tightly enough to prevent flow of blood to and from the extremity. If the patient is to be transported by air, an inflatable splint should not be used without carefully monitoring the pressure.

s., Jones' nasal. A splint used for fracture of nasal bones.

s., Kanavel. Splint used for stiffened hands.

s., Levis'. A splint of perforated metal extending from below the elbow to the end of the palm; shaped to fit the arm and hand.

s., McIntire's. A splint shaped like a double inclined plane, used as a posterior splint for leg and thigh.

s., Sayre's. One of three varieties of splint: ankle, knee, and hip joint disease.

s., Stromeyer's. A splint with two hinged sections that can be set at any angle, used esp. for the knee.

s., Thomas. A long wire splint with a proximal ring. The ring fits over the lower extremity and is placed as far as it will go toward the hip. Used in emergency treatment of femoral fracture.

s., Thomas' knee. A rigid metal used to remove pressure of body weight from a weak knee joint by transferring weight to the ischium and perineum.

s., Thomas' posterior. SEE: *Thomas splint.*

s., Volkmann's. Splint used for fracture of lower extremity, consisting of a footpiece and two lateral supports.

splinter (splĭn'tĕr) [MD. *splinte,* a wedge]. 1. A fragment from a fractured bone. 2. A slender, sharp piece of material piercing or imbedded in the skin.

splinter hemorrhage. Small linear hemorrhage under the finger- or toenails. May be due to subacute bacterial endocarditis.

splinter skill. Any trained, developed, or learned skill that is acquired in an intermittent or inconsistent pattern and is unrelated to any variety or integration of skills a person possesses.

splinting. Fixation of a dislocation or fracture with a splint.

split (splĭt) [D. *splitten,* to divide]. 1. A longitudinal fissure. 2. Characterized by a deep fissure.

split foot. Congenital deformity, the division of the toes extending into the metatarsal region.

split hand. Congenital deformity, the division between the fingers extending into the metacarpal region. SYN: *cleft hand.*

split pelvis. Congenital failure of pubic bones to form a union at the symphysis.

splitting (splĭt'ĭng) [D. *splitten,* to divide]. In chemistry, the breaking up of complex molecules into two or more simpler compounds.

split tongue. A cleft or bifid tongue resulting from developmental arrest.

spodogenous (spō-dŏj'ĕn-ŭs) [Gr. *spodos,* ashes, + *gennan,* to produce]. Caused by waste material.

spodophagous (spō-dŏf'ă-gŭs) [" + *phagein,* to eat]. Destroying the waste matters in the body; said of scavenger cells.

spondee (spŏn-dē). Two-syllable words that receive equal stress on each syllable.

spondyl- (spŏn'dĭl) [Gr. *spondylos,* vertebra]. Combining form for vertebra.

spondylalgia (spŏn"dĭl-ăl'jē-ā) [" + *algos,* pain]. Painful condition of a vertebra.

spondylarthritis (spŏn"dĭl-ăr-thrī'tĭs) [" + *arthron,* joint, + *itis,* inflammation]. Inflammation of a vertebra; arthritis of the spine.

spondylarthrocace (spŏn"dĭl-ăr-thrŏk'ă-sē) [" + " + *kake,* badness]. Tuberculous condition of the vertebrae.

spondylexarthrosis (spŏn"dĭl-ĕks"ăr-thrō'sĭs) [" + *exarthrosis,* dislocation]. Dislocation of a vertebra.

splondylitic (spŏn"dĭ-lĭt'ĭk) [" + *itis,* inflammation]. 1. A person with spondylitis. 2. Concerning spondylitis.

spondylitis (spŏn-dĭl-ī'tĭs) [" + *itis,* inflammation]. Inflammation of one or more vertebrae; esp. tuberculous disease of the vertebrae, Pott's disease, q.v.

s., ankylosing. S., rheumatoid.

s. deformans. Inflammation of the vertebral joints resulting in the outgrowth of bonylike deposits on the vertebrae, which may fuse and cause rigid and distorted spine.

s., hypertrophic. Condition occurring in most people over 50 in which bodies of vertebrae hypertrophy. Bony changes such as slipping at bases, and the development of bony outgrowths on articular processes occur.

s., Kummell's. Traumatic spondylitis in which symptoms do not appear until some time after the injury.

s., Marie-Strumpell. S., rheumatoid.

s., rheumatoid. A chronic progressive disease involving the joints between articular processes, costovertebral joints, and sacroiliac joints. Bilateral sclerosis of sacroiliac joints is a diagnostic sign. Changes occurring in joints are similar to those seen in rheumatoid arthritis. Ankylosis may occur, giving rise to stiff back (poker spine). SYN: *s., ankylosing.*

s. tuberculosis. SEE: *Pott's disease.*

spondylizema (spŏn″dĭl-ĭ-zē′mă) [Gr. *spondylos,* vertebra, + *izema,* depression]. Downward displacement of a vertebra caused by the disintegration of the one below it.

spondylo- [Gr. *spondylos,* vertebra]. Combining form meaning a vertebra.

spondylocace (spŏn″dĭ-lŏk′ă-sē) [″ + *kake,* badness]. Tuberculosis of the vertebrae. SYN: *spondylarthrocace.*

spondylodiagnosis (spŏn″dĭ-lō-dī″ăg-nō′sĭs) [″ + *dia,* through, + *gnosis,* knowledge]. Diagnosis by means of visceral reflexes obtained by percussion of the vertebrae.

spondylodymus (spŏn″dĭ-lŏd′ĭ-mŭs) [″ + *didymos,* twin]. Twin fetuses joined at the vertebrae.

spondylodynia (spŏn″dĭ-lō-dĭn′ē-ă) [″ + *odyne,* pain]. Pain in a vertebra.

spondylolisthesis (spŏn″dĭ-lō-lĭs″thē′sĭs) [″ + *olisthesis,* a slipping]. Forward subluxation of the lower lumbar vertebrae on the sacrum.

spondylolisthetic (spŏn″dĭ-lō-lĭs-thĕt′ĭk). Concerning spondylolisthesis.

spondylolysis (spŏn″dĭ-lŏl′ĭ-sĭs) [″ + *lysis,* a dissolution]. The breaking down of a vertebral structure.

spondylomalacia (spŏn″dĭ-lō-mă-lā′shē-ă) [″ + *malakia,* softness]. Softening of the vertebrae.

spondylopathy (spŏn″dĭl-ŏp′ă-thē) [″ + *pathos,* disease]. Any disorder of the vertebrae.

spondyloptosis (spŏn″dĭ-lō-tō′sĭs) [″ + *ptosis,* a dropping]. Spondylolisthesis, q.v.

spondylopyosis (spŏn″dĭ-lō″pī-ō′sĭs) [″ + *pyosis,* suppuration]. Suppuration with inflammation of a vertebra.

spondyloschisis (spŏn″dĭ-lŏs′kĭ-sĭs) [″ + *schisis,* cleft]. Congenital fissure of one or more of the vertebral arches SYN: *rhachioschisis.*

spondylosis (spŏn″dĭ-lō′sĭs) [Gr. *spondylos,* vertebra, + *osis,* condition]. Vertebral ankylosis.

s., cervical. Degenerative arthritis, osteoarthritis, of the cervical vertebrae and related tissues. If severe, it may cause pressure on nerve roots with subsequent pain or paresthesia in the arms.

s., rhizomelic. Ankylosis interfering with movements of hips and shoulders.

spondylosyndesis (spŏn″dĭ-lō-sĭn′dĕ-sĭs) [″ + *syndesis,* a binding together]. Surgical formation of an ankylosis between vertebrae.

spondylotherapy (spŏn″dĭl-ō-thĕr′ă-pē) [″ + *therapeia,* treatment]. Spinal therapeutics; spinal manipulation in the treatment of disease.

spondylotomy (spŏn″dĭl-ŏt′ō-mē) [″ + *tome,* incision]. Removal of part of the vertebral column to correct a deformity or facilitate delivery of a fetus. SYN: *rachitomy.*

spondylous (spŏn′dĭ-lŭs) [Gr. *spondylos,* vertebra]. Concerning a vertebra.

sponge (spŭnj) [Gr. *sphongos,* sponge]. 1. Elastic, porous mass forming internal skeleton of certain marine animals; or rubber or synthetic substance that resembles sponge in properties and appearance. Used to hold liquids for washing or mopping up spillage. 2. An absorbent pad made of gauze and cotton used to absorb fluids and blood in surgery or to dress wounds. 3. Short term for sponge bath. 4. To moisten, clean, or wipe with a sponge.

s., abdominal. Flat sponges from ½ to 1 in. (1.27–2.54 cm.) thick, 3 to 6 in. (7.62–15.24 cm.) in diameter, used as packing, to prevent closing or obstruction by intrusion of viscera, as covering to prevent tissue injury, and as absorbents.

s., gelatin. Spongy substance prepared from gelatin. It is a nonantigenic, readily absorbable material used esp. to stop internal bleeding. Sold under trade name of Gelfoam.

sponge graft. Sponge placed in an ulcer to cause granulation.

spongia (spŏn′jē-ă) [Gr. *sphongos,* sponge]. Sponge.

spongiform (spŭn′jĭ-form) [Gr. *sphongos,* sponge, + L. *forma,* shape]. Having the appearance or quality of a sponge.

spongioblast (spŭn′jē-ō-blăst) [″ + *blastos,* germ]. Cell that develops from embryonic neural tube and serves as forerunner of ependymal cells and astrocytes.

spongioblastoma (spŭn″jē-ō-blăs-tō′mă) [″ + ″ + *oma,* tumor]. A glioma of the brain derived from spongioblasts.

spongiocyte (spŭn′jē-ō-sīt″) [″ + *kytos,* cell]. A neuroglial cell.

spongioid (spŭn′jē-oyd) [″ + *eidos,* resemblance]. Resembling a sponge. SYN: *spongiform.*

spongioplasm (spŭn′jē-ō-plăzm) [Gr. *sphongos,* sponge, + *plasma,* a thing formed]. Fibrillar network supporting protoplasm. SYN: *cytoreticulum.*

spongiosis (spŭn″jē-ō′sĭs) [″ + *osis,* condition]. Intercellular edema of the spongy layer of the skin.

spongiositis (spŭn″jē-ō-sī′tĭs) [″ + *itis,* inflammation]. Inflammation of the corpus spongiosum of the urethra.

spongy (spŭn′jē). Resembling a sponge in texture.

spontaneous (spŏn-tā′nē-ŭs) [L.]. Occurring unaided or without apparent cause; voluntary.

spontaneous fracture. Fracture of a demineralized bone as in osteoporosis. This type of fracture may be painless.

ETIOL: Fragilitas ossium; nerve conditions such as tabes; secondary malignant growths; osteoporosis of bones of the aged.

spontaneous version. The unaided conversion of a transverse presentation of a fetus into a vertex or breech presentation.

spoon [AS. *spon,* a chip]. Instrument consisting of a small bowl on a handle, used in scooping out tissues, tumors, or in measuring quantities.

spoon nail. A toenail or fingernail having a concave outer surface.

sporadic (spō-răd′ĭk) [Gr. *sporadikos*]. Occurring occasionally or in scattered instances, as a disease. SEE: *endemic; epidemic; pandemic.*

sporangiophore (spō-răn′jē-ō-for) [Gr. *sporos,* seed, + *angeion,* vessel, + *phoros,* a bearer]. In bacteriology, the supporting stalk for a spore sac of certain fungi.

sporangium (spō-răn′jē-ŭm). A sac enclosing spores, seen in certain fungi.

spore (spor) [Gr. *sporos,* seed]. 1. A reproductive cell, usually unicellular, produced by plants and some protozoons. Usually spores are asexual, but certain fungi form sexual spores (oospores, zygospores, or ascospores). Spores usually possess a thick wall enabling the cell to withstand unfavorable environmental conditions.

Sporing is an asexual method of reproduction in many unicellular animals and plants. Certain bacteria also form spores, but more in the nature of a defensive mechanism than for reproduction. The spores of bacteria are difficult to destroy because they are very resistant to heat and require prolonged exposure to high temperatures to destroy them.

sporicidal (spor-ĭ-sī′dăl) [″ + L. *cidus,* kill]. Destructive to spores.

sporicide (spor′ĭ-sīd). An agent that destroys bacterial and mold spores. Because spores are more difficult to kill than vegetative cells, a sporicide also acts as a sterilizing agent.

sporiferous (spor-ĭf′ĕr-ŭs) [″ + L. *ferre,* to bear]. Producing spores.

spork. Adapted utensil for persons with limited upper extremity function. Distal end may swivel to allow food to remain level due to gravitational force.

sporoblast (spor′ō-blăst) [″ + *blastos,* germ]. Structure within the oocyst of certain parasitic protozoons (Eimeria and Isospora) that gives rise to a sporocyst and eventually a spore.

sporocyst (spor′ō-sĭst) [″ + *kystis,* sac]. 1. Any sac containing spores or reproductive cells. 2. Sac secreted around a sporoblast by certain protozoons prior to spore production. 3. Stage in life cycle of a trematode worm usually found in tissues of first intermediate host, a mollusk. It develops from a miracidium and is essentially a germinal sac containing germ cells. It gives rise to daughter sporocysts or redia.

sporogenesis (spor″ō-jĕn′ĕ-sĭs) [Gr. *sporos,* seed, + *genesis,* production]. The production or formation of spores.

sporogenic (spor″ō-jĕn′ĭk) [″ + *gennan,* to produce]. Having the ability of developing into spores.

sporogenous (spor-ŏj′ĕ-nŭs) [″ + *gennan,* to produce]. Concerning sporogenesis.

sporgeny (spor-ŏj′ĕ-nē). Sporogenesis.

sporogony (spor-ŏg′ō-nē) [″ + *goneia,* generation]. Reproducing by development of spores. SYN: *sporogenesis.*

sporophore (spor′ō-for) [″ + *phoros,* bearing]. The spore-bearing portion of an organism.

sporophyte (spor′ō-fīt) [″ + *phyton,* plant]. The spore-bearing stage of a plant exhibiting alternation of generation.

sporoplasm (spor′ō-plăzm) [″ + *plasmos,* a thing formed]. The cell protoplasm of spores.

Sporothrix (spor′ō-thrĭks). A genus of fungi of the family Moniliaceae.

S. schenckii. Causative agent of sporotrichosis.

sporotrichin (spor-ŏ′trĭ-kĭn). Antigenic substance derived from Sporothrix and used for diagnostic purposes.

sporotrichosis (spor″ō-trī-kō′sĭs) [″ + *thrix,* hair, + *osis,* condition]. A chronic granulomatous infection usually involving the skin and superficial lymph nodes characterized by formation of abscesses, nodules, and ulcers. It is caused by the fungus Sporotrichum schenckii, q.v

Sporotrichum (spō-rŏt′rĭ-kŭm). (pl. *Sporotri-*

cha) A yeastlike genus of microorganisms, one of which is the causative agent of sporotrichosis.

S. schenckii. Former name for the species that is the causative agent of sporotrichosis.

Sporozoa (spor″ō-zō′ă) [″ + *zoon,* animal]. A subphylum of the phylum Protozoa that includes a miscellaneous assortment of organisms that are parasitic, usually with complicated life cycles including sexual and asexual forms and lacking locomotor organs in the adult forms. The medically important genera are Isospora, Plasmodium, and Toxoplasma.

sporozoan. 1. Pert. to the sporozoa. 2. Sporozoon.

sporozoite (spor″ō-zō′īt) [″ + *zoon,* animal]. 1. An animal spore. 2. An elongated sickle-shaped cell that develops from a sporoblast within the oocyst in the life cycle of the malaria organism. Upon bursting of oocyst, sporozoites are released into body cavity and make their way to salivary gland. They are introduced into human blood by a mosquito and almost immediately enter tissue cells. Here they go through two schizogonic divisions and then reenter bloodstream and infect erythrocytes.

sporozoon. (pl. *sporozoa)* A protozoon belonging to the subphylum Sporozoa.

sport [ME. *sporten,* to divert]. A sudden permanent variation in a gene that is not characteristic of previous generations. SYN: *mutation.*

sports medicine. The application of medical knowledge and science to the physiological and pathological aspects of all persons who indulge in sports and athletics. This includes not only prevention and treatment of injuries but also scientific investigation of training methods and practices.

sporular (spor′ū-lăr) [L. *sporula,* little spore]. Concerning a spore.

sporulation (spor-ū-lā′shŭn) [L. *sporula,* little spore]. Production of spores, a method of reproduction of unicellular organisms.

spot (spŏt) [MD. *spotte*]. A small area of surface differing from surrounding parts in appearance. SYN: *loculus; macula; papule; pustule.*

s., blind. The optic disk where the optic nerve enters the retina. SEE: *scotoma.*

s., blue. S., mongolian.

s., cherry-red. Red spot occurring on retina in cases of Tay-Sachs disease.

s., cold. An area on surface of skin that, when stimulated, gives rise to sensation of coldness.

s., corneal. An opaque area on the cornea. SYN: *leukoma.*

s., genital. Area on nasal mucosa that tends to bleed during menstruation. SEE: *menstruation, vicarious.*

s., hot. S., warm.

s., hypnogenic. A point that, when pressed, will throw a susceptible person into hypnosis or sleep.

s.'s, Koplik's. Minute white or bluish-white spots on mucous membrane of mouth before appearance of the rash of measles.

s., liver. Popular term for pigmentary skin discolorations, usually in yellowish brown patches. SEE: *chloasma; lentigo.*

s., milk. 1. A thickened and opaque area seen on epicardium at autopsy. 2. A dense area of macrophages in the omentum.

s., mongolian. Bluish or mulberry-colored spots usually located in the sacral region. May be present at birth in Oriental, American Indian, Black, and Southern European infants. It usually disappears during childhood. SYN: *s., blue.*

s.'s, rose. Rose-colored maculae occurring on abdomen or loins in eruption of typhoid fever.

s., ruby. A tumor consisting of a compressible mass of blood vessels. SYN: *angioma, senile.*

s., temperature. A cutaneous spot that responds to temperature changes. SEE: *s., cold; s., warm.*

s., warm. Areas on surface of skin that, when stimulated, give rise to sensation of warmth. SYN: *s., hot.*

s., white. Light-colored, elevated areas of various sizes occurring on ventricular surface of anterior leaflet of mitral valve.

s., yellow. Area surrounding and including the fovea centralis in the retina. SYN: *macula lutea retinae.*

spotted fever. General and imprecise name for various eruptive fevers: typhus, tick fever, and rickettsial fevers. SEE: *Rocky Mountain spotted fever.*

spotting. Appearance of blood-tinged discharge from the vagina, usually between menstrual periods or at onset of labor.

spp. *Species.*

sprain (sprān) [O. Fr. *espraindre,* to wring]. Trauma to a joint that causes pain and disability depending upon degree of injury to ligaments. In severe sprain, ligaments may be completely torn. The ankle joint is the most often sprained. SEE: *fracture; strain.*

SYM: The signs of a sprain are rapid swelling, heat, and disability; often discoloration and limitation of function.

TREATMENT: During the first 24 to 48 hours, use cold compresses, bandage, and elevate the joint. After initial treatment with cold, apply heat. If recovery proves slow, immobilization of the joint is indicated followed by careful massage.

s. of back. Overstretching of muscles, ligaments, or other spinal structures, often associated with small fractures.

SYM: Pain, esp. on extreme movements; tenderness; muscle spasm.

F.A.: Have patient lie down on rigid support; do not allow to sit up or walk until fracture is ruled out. Intermittent heat, rest, with adhesive strapping, brace, etc.

s. of foot. Tearing of the ligaments of the foot or ankle.

SYM: Pain, tenderness, swelling, discoloration.

TREATMENT: Sprain is best treated as a fracture by complete immobilization until proven otherwise by x-ray examination.

s., riders'. Sprain of the adductor longus muscles of the thigh, resulting from strain in riding horseback.

sprain fracture. The separation of a tendon or ligament from its insertion, taking with it a piece of the bone.

spray (sprā) [MD. *spraeyen,* to sprinkle]. 1. A jet of fine medicated vapor applied to a diseased part or discharged into the air. 2. A pressurized container. SYN: *atomizer.* 3. To discharge fluid in a fine stream.

spray tube. Device for converting liquid into a spray.

spreader (sprĕd'ĕr). 1. An instrument for distributing something evenly over a tissue or culture plate. 2. A bacterial culture that as it grows spreads over the surface of the culture medium.

s., bladder-neck. An instrument used to expose the bladder neck and prostatic cavity while doing a retropubic prostatectomy.

s., root-canal. In dentistry, an instrument that is pointed and of variable diameter and taper. It is used to apply force to the material used in filling a root canal.

spreading (sprĕd'ĭng) [AS. *spraedan,* to strew]. Term indicating a growth on a bacterial culture, extending much (several millimeters or more) beyond the site of inoculation.

spreading factor. A substance produced by staphylococci that increases the permeability of connective tissue. SYN: *hyaluronidase.*

spring [AS. *springan,* a rising]. 1. The season of the year that comes after winter and before summer. SYN: *vernal season.* 2. A flying back of a body to its original position through its elasticity.

spring conjunctivitis. A form of conjunctivitis recurring each year in the spring but disappearing with the first frost. SYN: *vernal conjunctivitis.*

spring fever. A feeling of lassitude, rejuvenation, or increased sex drive that affects some people in the spring.

spring finger. Arrested movement of a finger in flexion or extension followed by a jerk. SYN: *trigger finger.*

spring ligament. Interior calcaneoscaphoid ligament of the sole of the foot. It joins the os calcis to the scaphoid bone.

sprue (sproo) [D. *sprouwe*]. 1. A disease endemic in many tropical regions and occurring sporadically in temperate countries, characterized by weakness, loss of weight, steatorrhea, and various digestive disorders, esp. impaired absorption of glucose, fats, and vitamins. It occurs in two forms, tropical and idiopathic or nontropical sprue. Its cause is unknown. 2. In dentistry, the wax, metal, or plastic used to form the aperture(s) through which molten gold or resin will pass to make a casting; also the part of the casting that later fills the sprue hole.

spud (spŭd) [ME. *spudde,* short knife]. Short, flattened, spadelike blade to dislodge a foreign substance.

spur [AS. *spura,* a pointed instrument]. 1. A sharp or pointed projection. 2. A sharp horny outgrowth of the skin.

s., calcaneal. An exostosis of the heel, often painful and resulting in disability.

s., femoral. Spur sometimes present on medial and underside of neck of femur.

s., scleral. A pointed portion of sclera that projects into the deeper part of cornea immediately behind canal of Schlemm at angle of iris.

spurious (spū'rē-ŭs) [L. *spurius*]. Not true or genuine; adulterated; false.

sputum (spū'tŭm) [L.]. (pl. *sputa*) Substance expelled by coughing or clearing the throat. It may contain a variety of material from the respiratory tract including one or more of the following: cellular debris, mucus, blood, pus, caseous material, and microorganisms. SEE: *Charcot-Leyden crystals.*

DIFF. DIAG: *Amount:* Copious; seen in chronic inflammations of lower respiratory tract. Scanty; in all pulmonary bronchial acute inflammations and the early stages of lobar pneumonia and beginning bronchopneumonia.

Color: This varies with the origin, cause, and amount of decomposition.

Conditions: Anthracosis (coal dust): sputum is black. *Bronchiectasis:* sputum is mucopurulent and foul if expectoration is infrequent. *Bronchial asthma:* scanty sputum and frothy, later becoming purulent and grayish, containing eosinophils. *Bronchitis:* sputum is mucous, later purulent, and in chronic cases, greenish-yellow and thick. *Bronchopneumonia:* frothy, mucoid, thin, mucopurulent, copious often with blood, or prune juice in color. *Calcinosis:* shows a sputum containing particles of lime or chalky deposits such as plaster of Paris. *Empyema:* if accompanied by perforations the sputum resembles that of pulmonary abscess. *Gangrene of lung and putrid bronchitis:* sputum has an obnoxious odor and is purulent, separates on standing into three layers containing pus cells, hematoidin crystals, and leukocytes. *Lobar pneumonia:* scanty and viscid, yellowish, and somewhat mucopurulent during early stages; in later stages, rusty, bloody, tenacious and viscid, esp. near or soon after crisis. *Pulmonary abscess:* usually purulent and fetid with many pus cells and pieces of lung tissue. *Pulmonary tuberculosis:* in early stages, scanty, whitish, or grayish-yellow, frothy, and expectorated in small quantities during coughing; later when consolidation takes place, it becomes more copious, tenacious, and yellowish-gray; and in the late stages, it becomes mucopurulent, musty and fetid, containing fibers and tubercle bacilli, sometimes blood-tinged or mixed with blood. *Pneumonoconiosis:* depends upon character of inhaled dust that produced the disease. *Siderosis:* contains particles of iron or other metals and resembles sputum of chronic bronchitis. It also contains alveolar cells. *Silicosis:* contains particles of silica or other stone dusts.

NURSING IMPLICATIONS: Provide appropriate disposal equipment. Instruct the patient on the proper use of the disposal equipment to prevent contamination and to wash hands after disposing of sputum. Instruct the patient how to expectorate to prevent air contamination. The nurse should turn his or her own head away when the patient is coughing. Wash hands after handling items containing sputum. Wear a face mask if the patient is suspected of having a contagious disease that can be spread through the air.

Keep the patient clean and comfortable. Promote frequent mouth and nose care to minimize mouth and breath odors and eliminate unpleasant taste. Hard candy may be sucked on to freshen mouth between meals. Administer prescribed medications to loosen secretions and alleviate irritation. Encourage cessation of smoking to increase ciliary action and decrease inflammation. Auscultate the lungs for signs of consolidation of secretions. Observe respirations at regular intervals and document abnormalities. Promote adequate hydration of the patient to liquefy the secretions. Use disposable equipment whenever possible.

s., bloody. This occurs most often in hemorrhages, although sputum can be blood-tinged from vigorous coughing. If the blood is mixed with the sputum, the hemorrhage is in the finer bronchioles. Large quantities of blood indicate rupture of a larger vessel. SYN: *hemoptysis.*

s., nummular. Round, coin-shaped, flat forms that sink in water; seen in bronchiectasis and advanced pulmonary tuberculosis.

s., prune juice. Thin, reddish, bloody sputum seen in gangrene, cancer of the lung, and certain pneumonias.

s., rusty. Sputum seen in lobar pneumonia.

s., septicemia. Sputum acquired from inoculation with organisms in saliva or sputum.

sputum specimen. A specimen of material expectorated from the mouth. If produced after a cough, it may contain, in addition to saliva, material from the throat and bronchi. The physical and bacterial character of the sputum will depend upon the disease process involved and the ability of the patient to cough up material. Some bronchial secretions are quite tenacious and difficult to cough up.

NURSING IMPLICATIONS: Explain the procedure to the patient. Have the patient rinse the mouth to remove food particles. Provide the appropriate collection container. Encourage deep coughing. Have the patient collect the specimen in the early morning prior to ingesting food or drink if possible. Examine the specimen to differentiate between sputum and saliva. Document characteristics (color, viscosity, odor) and volume. If the patient is unable to produce a specimen, heated aerosol may be prescribed to induce expectoration. If the specimen is to be sterile, give the patient explicit instructions on the usage of the container. Send the specimen to the laboratory immediately or refrigerate. Treat all sputum specimens as infective until proven otherwise. Thus specimens are handled by using appropriate isolation procedures.

sq. *subcutaneous.*

squalene (skwăl′ēn). An unsaturated carbohydrate present in shark-liver oil and some vegetable oils. It is an intermediate in the biosynthesis of cholesterol.

squama (skwā′mă) [L.]. (pl. *squamae*) 1. [NA] A thin plate of bone. 2. A scale from the epidermis.

squamate (skwā′māt) [L. *squama,* scale]. Scaly; squamous.

squamatization (skwā″mă-tī-zā′shŭn) [L. *squama,* scale]. The changing of cells into squamous cells.

squame (skwām) [L. *squama,* scale]. Squama.

squamocellular (skwā″mō-sĕl′ū-lar) [L. *squama,* scale, + *cellula,* cell]. Rel. to or having squamous cells.

squamofrontal (skwā″mō-frŏn′tăl) [″ + *frontalis,* frontal]. Concerning or belonging to the orbital palate.

squamomastoid (skwā″mō-măs′toyd) [″ + Gr. *mastos,* breast, + *eidos,* form]. Concerning the squamous and mastoid portions of the temporal bone.

squamo-occipital (skwā″mō-ŏk-sĭp′ĭ-tăl) [″ + *occipitalis,* occipital]. Concerning the squamous portion of the occipital bone.

squamoparietal (skwā″mō-pă-rī′ĕ-tăl) [″ + *paries,* wall]. Rel. to the squamous and parietal bones.

squamopetrosal (skwā″mō-pē-trō′săl) [″ + *petrosus,* stony]. Concerning the squamous and petrosal portions of the temporal bone.

squamosa (skwā-mō′să) [L., scaly]. The squamous part of temporal bone.

squamosal (skwā-mō′săl) [L. *squama,* scale]. Squamous.

squamosphenoid (skwā″mō-sfē′noyd) [″ + Gr. *sphen,* wedge, + *eidos,* form]. Concerning the squamous portion of the temporal bone and the sphenoid bone.

squamous (skwā′mŭs) [L. *squamosus*]. Scalelike.

squamous bone. Upper anterior portion of temporal bone.

squamous cell. Flat, scaly, epithelial cell.

squamous epithelium. Flat form of epithelial cells.

squamous suture. Line uniting squamosa and parietal bone.

squamozygomatic (sqwā″mō-zī″gō-măt′ĭk) [″ + *zygoma,* cheekbone]. Concerning the squamous part and the zygomatic part of the temporal bone.

square knot. Double knot in which ends and standing parts are together and parallel to each other. This knot is used universally because it holds well. It is quite easy to tie but may be very difficult to untie. SEE: *knot* for illus.

Hold one end in each hand, carry right end over left end and make a simple knot. Now reverse by carrying left end over right end and again tying, thus forming a simple symmetrical knot. If this is not done correctly a false or granny knot results, a type of knot that usually slips. To untie, steady the knot, take one end and draw it over knot, and then continue pulling in this direction until knot slips or jumps and forms two half hitches that may be slipped off.

square lobe. 1. The quadrate lobe of the liver. 2. A lobe on upper surface of the cerebellum.

squarrose, squarrous (skwăr′ōs, -ŭs) [L. *squarrosus*]. Scurfy or scaly; full of scabs or scales.

squatting position. Position in which person crouches with legs drawn up closely in front of, or beneath, body; sitting on one's haunches and heels.

squeeze-bottle. Bottle made of a flexible, semirigid material that can be deformed by applying hand pressure to it. Used to contain irrigating solutions, esp. those required in ophthalmology.

squill (skwĭl) [Gr. *skilla*]. A drug derived from a liliaceous plant that was once popular as an expectorant and diuretic.

squint (skwĭnt) [ME. *asquint,* sidelong glance]. 1. Abnormality in which the right and left visual axes do not bear toward an objective point simultaneously. SYN: *strabismus.* 2. To close the eyes partly as in excess light. 3. To be unable to direct both eyes simultaneously toward a point.

s., convergent. Condition existing when eyes are turned toward the medial line. SYN: *esotropia.*

s., divergent. Condition existing when eyes are turned outward. SYN: *exotropia.*

s., external. S., divergent.

s., internal. S., convergent.

SR. *sedimentation rate.*

Sr. Chem. symb. for strontium.

SRF. *somatotropin releasing factor.*

sRNA. *soluble ribonucleic acid.*

SRS, SRS-A. *slow-reacting substance.*

SS. *saliva sample; soap suds; sterile solution.*

Ss. *subjects,* as in Ss of an experiment or clinical study.

ss. *semis,* half.

SSD. *source-skin distance.*

sse. *soapsuds enema.*

SSS. *sterile saline soak.*

ST. *sedimentation time.*

ST-37. Proprietary germicide and disinfectant. SYN: *hexylresorcinol.*

stab (stăb) [ME. *stob,* stick]. 1. To pierce with a knife. 2. Wound produced by piercing with a knife or pointed instrument. 3. A stab culture.

stab culture. Bacterial culture in which organism is introduced into a solid gelatin medium with a wire or needle.

stabile (stā′bĭl) [L. *stabilis,* stable]. Not moving; fixed.

stabilization (stā″bĭl-ī-zā′shŭn) [L. *stabilis,* stable]. To make something such as a structure or chemical reaction stable.

stable (stā′bl). Firm; steady.

staccato speech (stă-kă′tō) [It. *staccare,* to detach]. Jerky pronunciation with words and syllables separated by pauses. SYN: *scanning speech.* SEE: *speech.*

stactometer (stăk-tŏm′ĕt-ĕr) [Gr. *staktos,* dropping, + *metron,* measure]. Instrument for measuring fluid in drops.

stadium (stā′dē-ŭm) [Gr. *stadion,* alteration]. A stage or period in the progress of a disease. SEE: *fastigium.*

s. acmes. The height of a disease.

s. augmenti. Period of rising temperature or other symptoms.

s. caloris. The hot stage in a fever or disease.

s. decrementi. Period of defervescence or decrease of symptoms.

s. florescentiae. Stage of eruption in an exanthematous disease.

s. frigoris. Cold shivering stage in intermittent fevers, as malaria.

s. incrementi. Period of increase of fever or symptoms.

s. invasionis. Incubation period of an infectious disease.

s. sudoris. Sweating stage of a paroxysm of malaria.

s. vitimum. Last stage of a febrile disease.

Stadol. Trade name for butorphanol tartrate.

staff (stăf) [AS. *staef,* a stick]. 1. An instrument to be introduced into the urethra and bladder as a guide to a surgical knife. 2. The medical, nursing, and other personnel attached to a hospital.

s., attending. The group of physicians and surgeons who are in regular attendance at a hospital.

s., consulting. Physicians and surgeons attached to a hospital who may be consulted by members of the attending staff.

s., house. SEE: *house staff.*

s. of Wrisberg. Prominence of the cuneiform cartilage seen in the normal larynx during examination.

stage (stāj) [O. Fr. *estage*]. 1. A period in the course of a disease or in the life history of an organism. SYN: *stadium.* 2. The platform of a microscope on which the slide is placed.

s., algid. Period of chilliness at the beginning of a fever.

s., amphibolic. Stage that intervenes between acme of a disease and its outcome, at a time when the outcome is unknown.

s., asphyxial. Preliminary stage of Asiatic cholera.

s., cold. Chill or rigor of a malarial paroxysm.

s., defervescent. Period in which temperature is declining.

s., eruptive. Period in which an exanthem appears.

s., expulsive, of labor. Stage of dilatation of the cervix uteri during which the child is expelled from uterus; second stage of labor, q.v.

s., first, of labor. Period when the fetal head is molded and the cervix dilated.

s., hot. Febrile stage in a malarial paroxysm.

s. of invasion. Period in which the causative agent is present in the body prior to the onset of a disease.

s. of latency. The incubation period of an infectious disorder.

s., placental, of labor. Period of labor during which placenta and fetal membranes are discharged; third stage of labor, q.v.

s., preeruptive. Stage following infection and before appearance of eruption.

s., pyrogenetic. Stage of onset in a febrile disease.

s., resting. A stage of relative inactivity between periods of activity as in a cell between mitotic divisions; a dormant stage.

s., second, of labor. Expulsive stage of labor.

s., sweating. The third or terminal stage of malaria during which sweating occurs.

s., third, of labor. S., placental.

staggers (stăg'ĕrz). Vertigo and confusion that occur in decompression illness.

staging. Process of classifying tumors, esp. malignant tumors, with respect to their degree of differentiation, to their potential for responding to therapy, and to the patient's prognosis.

stagnation (stăg-nā'shŭn) [L *stagnans,* stagnant]. 1. Cessation of motion. 2. In pathology, a stoppage of motion of any fluid in the body, as blood. SYN: *stasis.*

stain (stān) [O. Fr. *desteindre,* deprive of color]. 1. Any discoloration. SEE: *anti-stain formulary.* 2. A pigment or dye used in coloring microscopic objects and tissues. 3. To apply pigment to a tissue or microscopic object.

s., acid. Stain in which the color-bearing ion (chromatophore) is the anion.

Ex.: eosin, commonly used for staining the cytoplasmic or basic elements of cells.

s., acid-fast. A stain used in bacteriology, esp. for staining Mycobacterium tuberculosis. A special solution of carbolfuchsin is used, which the organism retains in spite of washing with the decolorizing agent acid alcohol. SEE: *Ziehl-Neelsen method.*

s., basic. Stain in which the color-bearing ion is the cation.

Ex.: methylene blue, commonly used to stain the nucleic or acidic elements of cells.

s., Commission Certified. A stain that has been certified by the Biological Stain Commission.

s., contrast. Stain used to color one part of a tissue or cell unaffected when another part is stained by another color.

s., counter. A stain, usually a contrast stain, that is used following the staining of specific elements of a tissue.

s., dental. A discoloration accumulating on the surface of teeth, denture, or denture base material, most often attributed to use of tea, coffee, or tobacco.

s., differential. In bacteriology, a stain such as Gram's stain that enables one to differentiate between different types of bacteria.

s., double. A mixture of two contrasting dyes, usually an acid and a basic stain.

s., Giemsa. A stain that contains Azur II-eosin and Azur II. It is used in staining tissues including blood cells, Negri bodies, and chromosomes.

s., Gram's. SEE: *Gram's stain.*

s., hematoxylin-eosin. A widely used method of staining tissues for microscopic examination. It stains nuclei deep blue-black, and cytoplasm pink.

s., intravital. A nontoxic dye that, when introduced into an organism, selectively stains certain cells or tissues. SYN: *s., vital.*

s., inversion. A basic stain that when under the influence of a mordant, acts as an acid stain.

s., metachromatic. A stain with which the constituents of cells or tissues develop a color different from the stain itself.

s., neutral. A combination of an acid and a basic stain.

s., nuclear. A basic stain affecting nuclei.

s., port-wine. Nevus flammeus, q.v.

s., substantive. A stain that is directly absorbed by the tissues when they are immersed in the staining solution.

s., supravital. A stain that will color living cells or tissues that have been removed from the body.

s., tumor. In arteriography, an abnormally dense area in an x-ray caused by the collection of contrast medium in the vessels. This may be a sign of neoplastic growth.

s., vital. S., intravital.

s., Wright's. A polychrome stain used for staining blood smears. SEE: *Wright's technique.*

staining (stān′ĭng) [O. Fr. *desteindre*]. Process of impregnating a substance, esp. a tissue, with pigments so that its component parts may be visible under a microscope. SEE: *Wright's technique.*

staircase phenomenon. The effect exhibited by skeletal and heart muscle when subjected to rapidly repeated maximal stimuli following a period of rest. In the resulting series of contractions each is greater than the preceding one until a state of maximum contraction is reached. SYN: *treppe.* SEE: *stress test.*

stalagmometer (stăl-ăg-mŏm′ĕ-tĕr) [Gr. *stalagmos,* dropping, + *metron,* a measure]. Instrument for measuring number of drops in a given amount of fluid.

stalk (stawk) [ME.]. An elongated structure usually serving to attach or support an organ or structure.

s., belly. Structure in embryo that develops into umbilical cord.

s., body. A bridge of mesoderm that connects the caudal end of embryo with chorion. Into it grow the allantois and embryonic blood vessels, the latter forming the umbilical arteries and vein, which connect the embryo with the placenta.

s., cerebellar. One of the cerebellar peduncles that connect the cerebellum with brain stem.

s., infundibular. Stalk that connects the diencephalon with the neural lobe of the hypophysis. SYN: *infundibulum.*

s., optic. Structure that connects the optic vesicle or cup to the forebrain.

s., yolk. The narrow constricted portion by which the yolk sac is connected to the midgut of the embryo. SYN: *vitelline duct.*

stamina (stăm′ĭ-nă) [L., thread of the warp, thread of human life]. Inherent force; constitutional energy; strength; endurance.

stammering (stăm′ĕr-ĭng) [AS. *stamerian*]. Hesitant or faltering speech disorder. May be due to hesitation, mispronunciation, transposing the letters l, r, or s, or repetition. SYN: *anarthria literalis; spasmophemia; stuttering.*

s. of bladder. Interrupted and irregular flow of urine, the muscles which control micturition acting spasmodically.

standard [O. Fr. *estandard,* marking rallying place]. That which is established by custom or authority as a model, criterion, or rule for comparison of measurement.

s., biological. The standardization of drugs or biological products (vitamins, hormones, antibiotics) by testing their effects upon animals. Utilized when chemical analysis is impossible or impracticable.

standard deviation. SYMB: σ. ABBR: S.D. In statistics, commonly used measure of dispersion or variability in a distribution. The square root of the variance, q.v.

standard error. ABBR: S.E. A measure of variability that could be expected of a statistical constant following the taking of random samples of a given size in a particular set of observations. An important standard error is that of the difference between the means of two samples.

standardization. The process of standardizing, esp. that of determining the strength or scale value of a substance or device by comparing with some standard, as standardization of solutions or thermometers.

standards of practice. The criteria against which one measures one's practice, for example, the American Nurses' Association Standards of Practice.

standing orders. Orders, rules, regulations, or procedures prepared by the professional staff of a hospital or clinic. Used as guidelines in preparation for and carrying out medical and surgical procedures. Standing orders serve to assure that such procedures are carried out correctly without being dependent upon an individual's fallible memory.

standstill. A cessation of activity.

s., atrial. Cessation of atrial contractions.

s., cardiac. Cessation of contractions of the heart.

s., inspiratory. Temporary cessation of inspiration normally following each inspiration resulting from stimulation of proprioceptors in alveoli of lungs. SEE: *Hering-Breuer reflex.*

s., respiratory. Cessation of respiratory movements.

s., ventricular. Cessation of ventricular contractions.

stannic (stăn'ĭk) [L. *stannum,* tin]. 1. Resembling or containing tin. 2. In chemistry, containing tetravalent tin.

stannous (stăn'ŭs) [L. *stannum,* tin]. 1. Resembling or containing tin. 2. In chemistry, containing divalent tin.

stannous fluoride. USP. A fluoride compound used in toothpaste to prevent dental caries.

stannum (stăn'ŭm) [L.]. Tin.

stanolone (stăn'ō-lōn). An anabolic steroid drug.

stanozolol (stăn'ō-zō-lŏl"). USP. An anabolic steroid. Trade name is Winstrol.

Stanton's disease. Melioidosis, q.v.

stapedectomy (stā"pē-dĕk'tō-mē) [L. *stapes,* stirrup, + Gr. *ektome,* excision]. Excision of the stapes in the ear in order to improve hearing, esp. in cases of otosclerosis. The stapes is replaced by a prosthesis.

During the first 24 hours following surgery the patient remains flat in bed, head movements are kept to a minimum, and the patient is instructed to refrain from blowing his or her nose or sneezing (if possible). In the second 24 hours the patient moves or arises only if assisted. The patient should not allow the ear to get wet for at least ten days postoperatively. For 30 days following surgery, the patient should not fly, climb to high altitudes, or be exposed to loud sounds such as those produced by jet aircraft. Sudden movements, even in elevators, should be avoided.

stapedial (stā-pē'dē-ăl). Rel. to the stapes.

stapediotenotomy (stā-pē"dē-ō-tĕn-ŏt'ō-mē) [" + Gr. *tenon,* tendon, + *tome,* incision]. Division of the tendon of the stapedius muscle.

stapediovestibular (stā-pē"dē-ō-vĕs-tĭb'ū-lar) [" + *vestibulum,* an antechamber]. Rel. to the stapes and vestibule of the ear.

stapedius (stā-pē'dē-ŭs) [L. *stapes,* stirrup]. A small muscle of the middle ear inserted in the stapes. SEE: *Muscles* in *Appendix.*

stapes (stā'pēz) [L., stirrup]. [NA] Ossicle in the middle ear that articulates with the incus. Commonly called stirrup. The footplate of the stapes fits into the oval window. SEE: *ear.*

Staphcillin. Trade name for methicillin sodium, USP.

staphylagra (stăf"ĭ-lā'gră) [Gr. *staphyle,* a bunch of grapes, + *agra,* a way of catching]. An instrument for holding the uvula.

staphyle (stăf'ĭ-lē) [Gr. *staphyle,* a bunch of grapes]. Pendulous, fleshy mass hanging from the soft palate. SYN: *cion; uvula.*

staphylectomy (stăf"ĭ-lĕk'tō-mē) [" + *ektome,* excision]. Amputation of the uvula. SYN: *staphylotomy* (def. 1); *uvulotomy.*

staphyledema (stăf"ĭl-ē-dē'mă) [" + *oidema,* swelling]. Swelling of the uvula.

staphyline (stăf'ĭ-līn) [Gr. *staphyle,* a bunch of grapes]. 1. Resembling a bunch of grapes. SYN: *botryoid.* 2. Rel. to the uvula. SYN: *uvular.*

staphylion (stăf-ĭl'ē-ŏn) [Gr., little grape]. 1. Craniometric point at median line of posterior border of hard palate. 2. Uvula. 3. A nipple or teat.

staphylitis (stăf"ĭl-ī'tĭs) [Gr. *staphyle,* a bunch of grapes, + *itis,* inflammation]. Inflammation of the uvula.

staphylo- [Gr. *staphyle,* a bunch of grapes]. Combining form indicating the uvula, pert. to or resembling a bunch of grapes, or pert. to Staphylococcus.

staphyloangina (stăf"ĭl-ō-ăn'jĭ-nă) [" + L. *angina,* sore throat]. Sore throat due to staphylococcus.

staphylococcal (stăf"ĭl-ō-kŏk'ăl) [" + *kokkos,* berry]. Pert. to or caused by staphylococci.

staphylococcal actinophytosis. Botryomycosis, a condition characterized by granulomatous lesions resembling those of actinomycoses; however, when organisms recovered from the lesions are cultured, they grow as staphylococci.

staphylococcal food poisoning. Poisoning by food containing a heat-stable enterotoxin produced by certain strains of staphylococci. When ingested, the toxin causes nausea, vomiting, diarrhea, intestinal cramps, and in severe cases prostration and shock. Attack usually lasts three to six hours. Fatalities are rare.

staphylococcemia (stăf"ĭl-ō-kŏk-sē'mē-ă) [" + " + *haima,* blood]. The presence of staphylococcus in the blood.

staphylococci (stăf"ĭl-ō-kŏk'sē). Pl. of staphylococcus.

Staphylococcus (stăf"ĭl-ō-kŏk'ŭs) [Gr. *staphyle,* bunch of grapes, + *kokkos,* berry]. A genus of micrococci belonging to the family Micrococcaceae, order Eubacteriales. They are gram-positive and on agar produce white, yellow, or orange-colored colonies. Some species are pathogenic, causing suppurative conditions and elaborating endotoxins destructive to tissue cells. Some produce enterotoxins and are the cause of a common type of food poisoning.

S. aureus. A species commonly present

on skin and mucous membranes, esp. those of nose and mouth, characterized by production of a golden-yellow pigment. They are gram-positive, coagulase-positive anaerobes. A cause of suppurative conditions such as boils, carbuncles, and internal abscesses in man. Various strains of this species produce toxins including those that cause food poisoning, staphylococcal scalded skin syndrome, and toxic shock syndrome. Some strains also produce hemolysins and staphylokinase.

S. epidermidis. A species of low pathogenicity characterized by formation of white colonies. Previously termed *S. albus*.

S. saphrophyticus. A newly recognized species. It can cause urinary tract infections.

staphylococcus (stăf″ĭl-ō-kŏk′ŭs). (pl. *staphylococci*) Term applied loosely to any pathogenic micrococci. SEE: *bacteria* for illus.; *Staphylococcus*.

staphyloderma (stăf″ĭ-lō-dĕr′mă) [″ + *derma*, skin]. Cutaneous infection with staphylococci.

staphylodermatitis (stăf″ĭl-ō-derm″ă-tī′tĭs) [″ + ″ + *itis*, inflammation]. A dermatitis caused by staphylococci.

staphylodialysis (stăf″ĭ-lō-dī-ăl′ĭ-sĭs) [″ + *dialysis*, a loosening]. Relaxed and elongated condition of the uvula.

staphylohemia (stăf″ĭ-lō-hē′mē-ă) [″ + *haima*, blood]. Staphylococci in the blood. SYN: *staphylococcemia*.

staphylokinase (stăf″ĭ-lō-kī′nās). Material produced by some strains of Staphylococcus aureus that can convert plasminogen to plasmin.

staphylolysin (stăf″ĭ-lŏl′ĭ-sĭn) [″ + *lysis*, dissolution]. A hemolysin produced by staphylococci.

staphyloma (stăf″ĭl-ō′mă) [Gr.]. A protrusion of the cornea or sclera of the eye.

s., anterior. Globular enlargement of anterior part of the eye. SYN: *keratoglobus*.

s., ciliary. Staphyloma in region of the ciliary body.

s. corneae. Thinning and bulging of the cornea.

s., equatorial. Staphyloma in equatorial region of the eye.

s., intercalary. Staphyloma in the region of union of the sclera with periphery of the iris.

s., partial. Staphyloma that extends in one direction displacing the pupil; the remainder of the cornea is clear.

s., posterior. Bulging of sclera backward.

s., total. Opaque, protuberant cicatrix found in place of the cornea.

ETIOL: Perforation of cornea resulting in poor vision, increased tension, rupture of thin scar.

TREATMENT: Prophylaxis, incision, excision, ablation.

s. uveale. Protrusion of any portion of the uvea through the sclera.

staphylomatous (stăf″ĭ-lŏm′ă-tŭs). Concerning or similar to a staphyloma.

staphyloncus (stăf″ĭ-lŏng′kŭs) [Gr. *staphyle*, a bunch of grapes, + *onkos*, tumor]. A tumor or enlargement of the uvula.

staphylopharyngeus (stăf″ĭ-lō-făr-ĭn′jē-ŭs) [″ + *pharynx*, pharynx]. Muscle of soft palate narrowing fauces and occluding nasopharynx. SYN: *palatopharyngeus*.

staphylopharyngorrhaphy (stăf″ĭ-lō-făr″ĭn-gor′ă-fē) [″ + ″ + *rhaphe*, suture]. Term used to describe several different operations on the soft palate and uvula.

staphyloplasty (stăf′ĭ-lō-plăs″tē) [″ + *plassein*, to form]. Plastic surgery of the uvula or soft palate.

staphyloptosia, staphyloptosis (stăf″ĭ-lŏp-tō′sē-ă, -sĭs) [″ + *ptosis*, a dropping]. Relaxation or elongation of the uvula. SYN: *staphylodialysis*.

staphylorrhaphy (stăf″ĭl-or′ă-fē) [″ + *rhaphe*, suture]. Suture of a cleft palate.

staphyloschisis (stăf″ĭ-lŏs′kĭ-sĭs) [″ + *schisis*, a fissure]. Fissure of the uvula. SYN: *cleft palate*.

staphylotome (stăf′ĭ-lō-tōm) [″ + *tome*, incision]. Instrument for cutting the uvula.

staphylotomy (stăf″ĭ-lŏt′ō-mē). 1. [″ + *tome*, incision] Amputation or any incision of the uvula. 2. [Gr. *staphyloma*, corneal protrusion, + *tome*, incision] Excision of a staphyloma.

staphylotoxin (stăf″ĭ-lō-tŏk′sĭn) [Gr. *staphyle*, a bunch of grapes, + *toxikon*, poison]. A toxin elaborated by one of the staphylococci, esp. S. aureus. Among some of the toxins produced are an enterotoxin, a cause of food poisoning, and exotoxins, including a hematoxin that lyses red blood cells, a dermonecrotic toxin, and leukocidins.

staple food. Any food that supplies a substantial part, at least 25 to 35%, of the caloric requirement and is regularly consumed by a certain population.

stapling. In surgery, a means of fastening tissues together by using special staples compatible with tissues. The staples are U-shaped lengths of wire that are pushed through the tissues. The ends are then bent over on an anvil.

star [AS. *steorra*]. Any structure resembling a star. SYN: *aster*.

s., lens. A starlike structure developing in the lens of the eye as a result of unequal growth of lens fibers.

s.'s of Verheyen. Star-shaped masses of veins on the surface of the kidney. SYN: *venulae stellatae; stellate veins*.

Classification of Starches

Groups	Examples
I. Potato Group	Canna, potato, arrowroot
II. Leguminous Group	Beans, peas, lentils
III. Wheat Group	Wheat, barley, rye
IV. Sago Group	Sago, cassava, arum
V. Rice Group	Rice, maize, oats

Starches

Name	From
1. Cornflour	Maize or corn
2. Arrowroot	Maranta
3. Cassava	Brazilian arrowroot
4. Curcuma	East Indian arrowroot
5. Arum	Portland arrowroot
6. Tous-les-mois	Canna (West India)
7. Sago	Palm (East India)
8. Inulin	Dahlia tubers
9. Lichen	Iceland moss
10. Glycogen	Animal livers

NOTE: Starch is soluble at 150° F. (65.6° C.). Only slightly so in cold water.
IODINE acting on starch paste gives a deep blue.
BROMINE acting on starch paste gives an orange-yellow.

The Percentage of Starch in Various Foods

Article	Percent	Article	Percent
Arrowroot	23	Oatmeal (uncooked), dry	68
Bananas	22	Peanuts, roasted and salted	19
Barley	79	Peas, dried	60
Beans, common	61	Peas, green, canned, drained solids	17
Beans, green	26	Potatoes (uncooked)	17
Bread fruit, raw	26	Potatoes, sweet (uncooked)	26
Buckwheat flour	72	Rice, white, uncooked	80
Chestnuts, dried	79	Rye flour, light	78
Corn grits (degermed, dry)	78	Soybeans (dry, uncooked)	34
Corn meal (degermed, dry)	78	Wheat flour, all purpose	76
Lentils, raw	60		

starch [AS. *stercan*]. Noncrystalline carbohydrate of the polysaccharide group found in plants. Included are vegetable starches, pectins, dextrins, and gums. All are rather easily decomposed, have high molecular weights, and yield monosaccharides on complete hydrolysis. Those that the body is able to hydrolyze into hexoses are useful as concentrated energy-giving foods. All are reduced to simple sugars before they are absorbed. In some fruits the starch is changed to sugar when they ripen, while some vegetables (peas and corn) change sugar into starch as their seeds develop. SEE: table.

The amylases of saliva and pancreatic juice hydrolyze starches to dextrins and maltose. These in turn are hydrolyzed to glucose, which is absorbed into the bloodstream. Glucose not immediately needed for energy is converted into glycogen, a form of starch that is stored in the liver or in muscle tissue.

Pure starches, having the formula $(C_6H_{10}O_5)_n$, if normally metabolized, leave no residue and give rise only to carbon dioxide and water.

s., animal. Glycogen.

s., corn. Starch obtained from ordinary corn or maize (Zea mays). It is used as a dusting powder and an absorbent and is a constituent in many pastes and ointments. It is widely used in industry and as a food.

starch glycerite. A combination of starch, benzoic acid, purified water, and glycerin. Used as an emollient in formulations for external use.

stare (stār) [AS. *starian*]. To gaze fixedly at anyone or anything.

Starling's law of heart. [Ernest Henry Starling, Brit. physiologist, 1866–1927] The force of the heartbeat is determined primarily by the length of the fibers comprising its muscular wall, i.e., an increase in diastolic filling increases force of heartbeat.

Starling's law of intestine. A stimulus within the intestine, i.e., the presence of food, initiating a band of constriction on proximal side and relaxation on distal side. This results in a peristaltic wave.

starter. A pure culture of bacteria or other microorganism used to initiate a particular fermentation as in the making of cheese.

starvation [AS. *steorfan,* to die]. 1. The condition of being without food for a long period of time. When everything but air and water is withheld, the sequence of events is as follows: (1) Hunger, beginning about four hours after the last meal, accompanied by special activity of the stomach and general restlessness, becoming more acute periodically, esp. at times when meals were customarily taken; (2) loss of weight; (3) utilization of glycogen stored in liver and muscles; (4) utilization of stored fat; (5) spells of nausea and diminishing acuteness of the sensation of hunger; (6) destruction of body protein. The greatest loss of weight is in the fatty tissues, spleen, and liver. 2. Condition in which the supply of a specific food is below minimum bodily requirements, such as protein starvation. SEE: *kwashiorkor.* 3. Condition resulting from failure of the body to digest and absorb essential foodstuffs. SEE: *deficiency disease; diet; dietetics.*

stasibasiphobia (stā″sĭ-bā″sĭ-fō′bē-ă) [Gr. *stasis,* a standing, + *basis,* step, + *phobos,* fear]. Delusion of one's inability to stand or walk, or fear to make the attempt.

stasimorphia, stasimorphy (stā″sĭ-mor′fē-ă, -fē) [″ + *morphe,* form]. Deformity due to failure to develop and grow.

stasiphobia (stā″sĭ-fō′bē-ă) [″ + *phobos,* fear]. Delusion of one's inability to stand erect or hesitation to make the attempt.

stasis (stā′sĭs) [Gr. *stasis,* standing still]. Stagnation of normal flow of fluids, as of the blood, urine, or of the intestinal mechanism.

s., diffusion. Stasis with diffusion of lymph or serum.

s., intestinal. Condition in which peristaltic movements fail to move food along the intestine.

s., venous. Stasis of blood caused by venous congestion.

stat [L.]. *statim,* immediately.

state [L. *status,* condition]. 1. A condition. 2. A mode or condition of being.

s., anxiety. A condition characterized by more or less continuous anxiety and apprehension. SEE: *neurosis, anxiety.*

s., central excitatory. ABBR: C.E.S. A condition of increased excitability in the central nervous system, esp. in the spinal cord, following an excitatory stimulus.

s., central inhibitory. ABBR: C.I.S. A condition of decreased excitability in the central nervous system, esp. in the spinal cord, resulting from an inhibitory stimulus.

s., dream. A state of diminished consciousness in which the surroundings are perceived as if in a dream.

s., excited. The new state produced when energy is added to a nucleus, atom, or molecule. The energy is added by the absorption of photons or by collisions with other particles.

s., fatigue. Nervous exhaustion, commonly following depressed states. SYN: *neurasthenia.*

s., ground. The state of the lowest energy of a system such as an atom or molecule.

s., refractory. The condition of reduced ability to be excited just after a muscle and nerve have been stimulated.

s., steady. In physiology, the condition of the metabolic needs of a system such as the muscles being supplied with nutrients at the same rate the energy is expended. Dynamic equilibrium.

static (stăt′ĭk) [Gr. *statikos,* standing]. At rest; in equilibrium; not in motion.

static electricity. Electricity produced by friction.

static equilibrium. Equilibrium concerned with recognition of position of head in relation to gravity. Opposite of dynamic equilibrium.

static reflex. A reflex action having to do with maintenance of posture or maintenance of muscle tone.

statics (stăt′ĭks). Study of matter at rest and forces bringing about equilibrium. SEE: *dynamics.*

static splint. Any orthosis without movable parts used for positioning, stability, protection, or support.

statim (stăt′ĭm) [L.]. ABBR: stat. Immediately; at once.

station (stā′shŭn) [L. *statio,* standing]. 1. The manner of standing. 2. A stopping place.

s., aid. Site in the army for collecting the wounded in battle.

s., dressing. A temporary station for wounded soldiers in the field.

s., rest. A temporary relief station for the sick on a military road or railway.

stationary (stā′shŭn-ĕr-ē) [L. *stationarius,* belonging to a station]. Remaining in a fixed condition.

statistical (stă-tĭs′tĭ-kăl). Pert. to statistics.

statistics (stă-tĭs′tĭks) [LL. *statisticus*]. The systematic collection, organization, analysis, and interpretation of numerical data pert. to any subject.

s., medical. Statistics pert. to medical

sciences, esp. data pert. to human disease.

s., morbidity. Statistics pert. to sickness.

s., vital. Statistics dealing with births, deaths and marriages.

statoacoustic (stăt″ō-ă-koo′stĭk) [Gr. *statos,* placed, + *akoustikos,* acoustic]. Concerning balance and hearing.

statoconia (stăt″ō-kō′nē-ă) [″ + *konos,* dust]. Minute bits of calcium adhering to the hair cells of the maculae of the utricle and saccule of the middle ear. These are important in sensing the orientation to gravity.

statokinetic (stăt″ō-kĭn-ĕt′ĭk) [″ + *kinetikos,* moving]. Pert. to reactions of the body produced by movement.

statokinetic reflexes. Reactions that are the result of movement of the body (positive or negative acceleration) or movements of the head. SYN: *accelerator reflexes; reflexes, kinetic.*

statolith (stăt′ō-lĭth) [″ + *lithos,* stone]. Statoconia, q.v.

statometer (stă-tŏm′ĕt-ĕr) [″ + *metron,* a measure]. Instrument for measuring amount of abnormal protrusion of eyeball.

statosphere (stăt′ō-sfēr) [″ + *sphaira,* a globe]. Centrosome.

stature (stăt′ūr) [L. *statura*]. Height of the body in a standing position.

status (stā′tŭs) [L.]. (pl. *statuses*) A state or condition.

s. anginosus. A sustained attack of angina pectoris.

s. arthriticus. Predisposition to having attacks of gout.

s. asthmaticus. Persistent and intractable asthma.

s. dysgraphicus. Condition resulting from imperfect closure of neural tube of embryo.

s. dysmyelinisatus of Vogt. Condition marked by demyelination of the globus pallidus and various nuclei of the brain, esp. the hypothalamic nuclei and dentate nucleus of the cerebellum.

s. epilepticus. Rapid succession of epileptic attacks without regaining consciousness during the intervals.

s. parathyreoprivus. Condition resulting from loss of parathyroid tissue.

s. praesens. The state of a patient at time observed.

s. raptus. A state of ecstasy.

s. verrucosus. Defective development of the cerebral gyri with many small gyri. This gives a warty appearance to the surface of the brain.

s. vertiginosus. Persistent condition of vertigo.

statuvolence (stăt-ū′vō-lĕns) [″ + *volens,* willing]. Self-induced hypnotism.

staunch (stŏnch) [O. Fr. *estanche,* firm]. To stop the flow of blood from a wound.

staurion (staw′rē-ŏn) [Gr. *stauros,* little cross]. Craniometric point where transverse palatine suture crosses the median one.

stauroplegia (staw″rō-plē′jē-ă) [″ + *plege,* stroke]. Alternate hemiplegia.

S.T.D. 1. *skin test dose.* SEE: *Dick test.* 2. *sexually transmitted disease.*

steal (stēl). The deviation of blood flow from its normal course or rate of flow.

s., subclavian. SEE: *subclavian steal syndrome.*

steam (stēm) [AS. *steam,* vapor]. 1. Invisible vapor into which water is converted at boiling point by heat. 2. Mist formed by condensation of water vapor. 3. Any vaporous exhalation.

steam tent. A device that permits inhalation of vapors. If no tent is available, a makeshift tent may be improvised. It is important that the method used does not burn the patient.

SOLUTIONS: Approx. a quart (a liter) of boiling water to which is added a teaspoonful (5 ml.) of compound tincture of benzoin or a teaspoonful (5 ml.) of tincture of benzoin (this does not contain aloe), a few crystals of menthol or camphor, or a few drops of methyl salicylate. These ingredients are pleasant to smell but have relatively little therapeutic effect. Most of the value is in the water vapor.

steapsin (stē-ăp′sĭn) [Gr. *stear,* fat, + *pepsis,* digestion]. A lipolytic enzyme present in pancreatic juice that hydrolyzes fats to fatty acid and glycerine. The bile salts prepare the fats for the action of steapsin by emulsifying them. SYN: *lipase, pancreatic.* SEE: *enzyme; pancreas.*

stearate (stē′ă-rāt). An ester or salt of stearic acid.

stearic acid (stē-ăr′ĭk) [Gr. *stear,* fat]. A white, fatty acid found in solid animal fats and a few vegetable fats.

steariform (stē-ăr′ĭ-form) [″ + L. *forma,* shape]. Resembling fat.

stearin (stē′ă-rĭn) [Gr. *stear,* fat]. A white, crystalline solid in animal and vegetable fats; $C_3H_5(C_{18}H_{35}O_2)_3$; any of the esters of glycerol and stearic acid, specifically glyceryl tristearate. One of the commonest fats in the body, esp. the solid ones. It breaks down into stearic acid and glycerol.

stearodermia (stē″ă-rō-dĕr′mē-ă) [″ + *derma,* skin]. Disease of the sebaceous glands of the skin.

stearopten(e) (stē″ă-rŏp′tēn) [″ + *ptenos,* volatile]. The more solid portion of a volatile oil as distinguished from the more fluid portion or eleoptene. Ex.: menthol, thymol.

stearrhea (stē″ă-rē′ă) [Gr. *stear,* fat, + *rhoia,* flow]. Excessive secretion of sebum or fat. SYN: *seborrhea oleosa.*

s. flavescens. Stearrhea with yellow sebaceous matter deposited on the skin.

s. nigricans. Stearrhea with black sweat due to presence of indican. SEE: *chromidrosis; chromodermatosis.*

s. simplex. Excessive discharge of sebum.

steatadenoma (stē-ăt"ăd-ĕ-nō'mă) [Gr. *steatos,* fat, + *aden,* gland, + *oma,* tumor]. Tumor of the sebaceous glands.

steatite (stē'ă-tīt). Talc.

steatitis (stē"ă-tī'tĭs) [" + *itis,* inflammation]. Inflammation of adipose tissue.

steato- [Gr. *steatos,* fat]. Prefix meaning fatty.

steatocele (stē-ăt'ō-sēl, stē'ăt-ō-sēl) [" + *kele,* tumor]. Fatty tumor within the scrotum.

steatocryptosis (stē"ă-tō-krĭp-tō'sĭs) [" + *krypte,* a sac, + *osis,* condition]. Any disease of sebaceous glands. SEE: *stearodermia.*

steatocystoma multiplex. A skin disorder characterized by development of many sebaceous cysts.

steatogenous (stē"ă-tŏj'ĕn-ŭs) [Gr. *steatos,* fat, + *gennan,* to produce]. 1. Causing fatty degeneration. 2. Producing any sebaceous gland disease.

steatolysis (stē"ă-tŏl'ĭ-sĭs) [" + *lysis,* dissolution]. 1. The process by which fats are first emulsified and then hydrolyzed to fatty acids and glycerine preparatory to absorption. 2. The decomposition of fat. SYN: *lipolysis.*

steatolytic (stē"ă-tō-lĭt'ĭk). Concerning steatolysis.

steatoma (stē"ă-tō'mă) [" + *oma,* tumor]. 1. Sebaceous cyst. SYN: *wen.* 2. Benign tumor composed of fat cells. SYN: *lipoma.*

Smooth, shiny, globular, cutaneous or subcutaneous tumor from pea to orange size arising from sebaceous glands, single or multiple, usually on neck, scalp, back, or scrotum.

ETIOL: Duct occlusion is causative in some.

PROG: Prolonged irritation may cause suppuration.

TREATMENT: Surgical excision by dissection without perforating sac. Packing in suppurative cases.

steatomatous (stē"ă-tō'mă-tŭs). Presence of multiple sebaceous cysts.

steatonecrosis (stē"ă-tō-nē-krō'sĭs) [" + *nekros,* dead, + *osis,* condition]. Necrosis of fatty tissue in small patches.

steatopathy (stē-ă-tŏp'ă-thē) [" + *pathos,* disease]. Disease of the sebaceous glands of the skin.

steatopygia (stē"ă-tō-pĭj'ē-ă) [" + *pyge,* buttock]. Abnormal fatness of the buttocks seen more frequently in women. Seen in some tropical areas of Africa. Location of this excess fat accumulation in the buttocks may represent an adaptation to a very hot climate. If the fat present in the buttocks were evenly spread throughout the subcutaneous tissue it is thought that normal cooling of the skin would be severely limited.

steatopygous (stē"ă-tŏp'ĭ-gŭs) [" + *pyge,* buttock]. Concerning or having steatopygia.

steatorrhea (stē"ă-tō-rē'ă) [Gr. *steatos,* fat, + *rhoia,* flow]. 1. Increased secretion of sebaceous glands. SYN: *seborrhea.* 2. Fatty stools, as seen in pancreatic diseases.

s., idiopathic. Term applied to gastrointestinal disorders characterized by impaired absorption. SYN: *sprue.*

s. simplex. Excessive secretion of sebaceous glands of the face.

steatosis (stē"ă-tō'sĭs) [" + *osis,* condition]. 1. Fatty degeneration. 2. Disease of the sebaceous glands.

stege (stē'jē) [Gr. *stegos,* roof]. The internal pillar of the organ of Corti of the ear.

stegnosis (stĕg-nō'sĭs) [Gr. *stegnosis,* obstruction]. 1. Checking of a secretion or discharge. 2. Closing of a passage. SYN: *stenosis.* 3. Constipation. SYN: *costiveness.*

stegnotic (stĕg-nŏt'ĭk). Bringing about stegnosis. SYN: *astringent; constipating.*

Stegomyia (stĕg"ō-mī'ē-ă). A subgenus of mosquito of the genus Aedes, family Culicidae, suspected of transmitting the causative organism of yellow fever.

Steinert's disease (stīn'ĕrts). [Hans Steinert, 19th-century Ger. physician] A hereditary disease characterized by muscular wasting, myotonia, and cataract. SYN: *myotonia atrophica.*

Stein-Leventhal syndrome (stīn-lĕv'ĕn-thăl). [Irving F. Stein, Sr., U.S. gynecologist, b. 1887; Michael L. Leventhal, U.S. obstetrician and gynecologist, b. 1901] The polycystic ovary syndrome characterized by normal growth and development with or without hirsutism. Menses may or may not be regular, but later oligomenorrhea develops and then amenorrhea, but infrequently ovulation will occur. Infertility is usually persistent but may be treated with clomiphene, gonadotropins, or wedge resection of the ovary. SYN: *polycystic ovary syndrome.*

Steinmann's extension (stīn'mănz). [Fritz Steinmann, Bern surgeon, 1872–1932] Traction applied to a limb by applying weight to a pin placed through the bone at right angles to the direction of pull of the traction force.

Steinmann's pin. A sturdy pin placed in the distal end of a long bone so that a weight may be attached in order to apply traction.

Stelazine. Trade name for trifluoperazine hydrochloride.

stella [L.]. (pl. *stellae*) Star.

s. lentis hyaloidea. Posterior pole of the crystalline lens of the eye.

s. lentis iridica. Anterior pole of the crystalline lens of the eye.

stellate [L. *stellatus*]. Star-shaped; arranged with parts radiating from a center.

stellate bandage. Bandage that is wrapped on the back, crossways.

stellate cell. Any cell that appears star-shaped.

Ex.: neurons of molecular layer of cerebellum; Kupffer's cells of the liver sinusoids; astrocytes.

stellate fracture. Fracture with numerous fissures radiating from central point of injury.

stellate ganglion. A sympathetic ganglion formed by the fusion of inferior cervical and first thoracic ganglions.

stellate ligament. One of the anterior costovertebral ligaments.

stellate veins. Venous plexuses beneath the kidney's capsule. SYN: *stars of Verheyen.*

stellectomy (stĕl-lĕk'tō-mē) [" + *ektome,* excision]. Surgical removal of the stellate ganglion.

Stellwag's sign (stĕl'văgs). [Carl Stellwag von Carion, Austrian oculist, 1823–1904] Widening of palpebral aperture with absence or lessened frequency of winking, seen in Graves' disease.

stem. 1. [AS. *stemn,* tree trunk] Any stalklike structure. 2. Offspring. 3. To derive from or originate in. 4. [ME. *stemmen*] To check, stop, or hold back.

s., brain. The lower portion of the brain excluding the cerebrum and cerebellum. Includes the medulla oblongata, pons, midbrain, and diencephalon.

stem cell. A cell that gives rise to a specific type of cell as in hematopoiesis.

stenion (stĕn'ē-ŏn) [Gr. *stenos,* narrow]. Craniometric point at extremities of the smallest transverse diameter in the temporal region.

steno- [Gr. *stenos,* narrow]. Combining form meaning narrow or short.

stenobregmatic (stĕn"ō-brĕg-măt'ĭk) [" + *bregma,* front of head]. Term applied to a skull with narrowing of the upper and frontal portion of the skull.

stenocardia (stĕn"ō-kăr'dē-ă) [" + *kardia,* heart]. Angina pectoris.

stenocephaly (stĕn"ō-sĕf'ă-lē) [" + *kephale,* head]. Narrowness of the cranium in one or more diameters.

stenochoria (stĕn"ō-kō'rē-ă) [" + *choros,* space]. Partial constriction, esp. of the lacrimal duct. SYN: *stenosis.*

stenocompressor (stĕn"ō-kŏm-prĕs'or) [" + L. *compressor,* that which presses together]. An instrument for compressing Stensen's ducts to stop the flow of saliva.

stenocoriasis (stĕn"ō-kō-rī'ă-sĭs) [" + *kore,* pupil, + *-iasis,* state]. Narrowing of pupil of the eye.

stenocrotaphia (stĕn"ō-krō-tā'fē-ă) [" + *krotaphos,* the temple]. Abnormal narrowness of the temporal area of the head.

stenopaic, stenopeic (stĕn-ō-pā'ĭk, -pē'ĭk) [Gr. *stenos,* narrow, + *ope,* opening]. Provided with a narrow opening or slit, esp. denoting optical devices to protect against snow blindness.

stenosal (stē-nō'săl) [Gr. *stenos,* narrow]. Stenotic.

stenosed (stē-nōst', stĕn'ōzd). Characterized by stenosis; constricted.

stenosis (stē-nō'sĭs) [Gr.]. Constriction or narrowing of a passage or orifice. SYN: *stricture.*

ETIOL: May result from embryonic maldevelopment, hypertrophy and thickening of a sphincter muscle, inflammatory disorders, or excessive development of fibrous tissue. It may involve almost any tube or duct.

s., aortic. Constriction of the aortic orifice at cardiac base, or narrowing of the aorta.

s., cardiac. A narrowing or constriction of any of the orifices leading into or from the heart or between chambers of the heart.

s., cicatricial. Stenosis resulting from any contracted cicatrix.

s., mitral. Stenosis of mitral valve or orifice of heart, or of both. Usually the result of rheumatic heart disease.

s., pulmonary. SEE: *pulmonary stenosis.*

s., pyloric. Obstruction caused by hypertrophy of walls of the pyloric orifice.

s., subaortic. Congenital constriction of aortic tract below aortic valves.

s., tricuspid. Narrowing of the opening to the tricuspid valve.

stenostomia (stĕn"ō-stō'mē-ă) [Gr. *stenos,* narrow, + *stoma,* mouth]. Narrowing of the mouth.

stenothermal (stĕn"ō-thĕr'măl) [" + *therme,* heat]. Resisting only a small change of temperature.

stenothorax (stĕn"ō-thō'răks) [" + *thorax,* chest]. An unusually narrow thorax.

stenotic [Gr. *stenosis,* a narrowing]. Produced by or characterized by stenosis.

Stensen's duct (stĕn'sĕns) [Niels Stensen, Danish anatomist, 1638–1686] The excretory duct of the parotid gland.

Stensen's foramina. Incisive foramina of the hard palate, transmitting anterior branches of the descending palatine vessels.

stent. [Charles R. Stent, 19th-century Brit. dentist] 1. Originally a compound used in making dental molds. 2. Any material used to hold tissue in place or to provide a support for a graft or anastomosis while healing is taking place.

stentorophonic (stĕn"tō-rō-fŏn'ĭk). [Stentor, loud-voiced herald in the *Iliad*] Speaking or sounding very loud.

step. A series of rests for the foot in ascending or descending.

s., Rönne's. A step-like defect in the visual field.

stephanion (stĕ-fā'nē-ŏn) [Gr. *stephanos,* crown]. Point at intersection of the superior temporal ridge and coronal suture.

steppage gait. The high-stepping gait seen in diabetic neuritis of the peroneal nerve. Patient lifts the foot very high in walking to raise the drooping toes from the ground or floor.

stepping reflex. SEE: *reflex, stepping.*

steradian (stē-rā'dē-ăn). The unit of measurement of solid angles. It encloses an area on the surface of a sphere equal to the square of the radius of the sphere.

Sterane. Trade name for prednisolone, USP.

sterco- [L. *stercus,* dung]. Combining form indicating a relationship to feces.

stercobilin (stĕr"kō-bī'lĭn) [" + *bilis,* bile]. A brown pigment derived from the bile giving the characteristic color to feces. SEE: *urobilin.*

stercobilinogen (stĕr"kō-bī-lĭn'ō-jĕn). A colorless substance derived from urobilinogen. It is present in the feces and turns brown on oxidation.

stercolith (stĕr'kō-lĭth) [" + Gr. *lithos,* stone]. A fecal calculus.

stercoraceous (stĕr"kō-rā'shŭs) [L. *stercoraceus*]. Having the nature of, pert. to, or containing feces.

stercoral (stĕr'kō-răl) [L. *stercus,* dung]. Pert. to feces. SYN: *stercoraceous.*

stercorin (stĕr'kō-rĭn). A sterol, $C_{27}H_{47}OH$, in feces.

stercorolith (stĕr'kō-rō-lĭth) [" + Gr. *lithos,* stone]. A fecal concretion. SYN: *coprolith; fecalith.*

stercoroma (stĕr"kō-rō'mă) [" + Gr. *oma,* tumor]. A fecal tumorlike mass in the rectum. SYN: *coproma; fecaloma; scatoma.*

stercorous (stĕr'kō-rŭs) [L. *stercorosus*]. Resembling excrement. SYN: *stercoral; stercoraceous.*

stercus (stĕr'kŭs) [L.]. (pl. *stercora*) Feces. SYN: *excreta; excrement.*

stere (stēr, stār) [Gr. *stereos,* solid]. A measure of volume equal to one cubic meter.

stereo- [Gr. *stereos,* solid]. Combining form meaning solid or indicating three-dimensional.

stereoagnosis (stĕr"ē-ō-ăg-nō'sĭs) [" + *a-,* not, + *gnosis,* knowledge]. Astereognosis, q.v.

stereoanesthesia (stĕr"ē-ō-ăn"ĕs-thē'zē-ă) [" + *an-,* not, + *aisthesis,* sensation]. Inability to recognize objects by feeling their form.

stereoarthrolysis (stĕr"ē-ō-ăr-thrŏl'ĭ-sĭs) [" + *arthron,* joint, + *lysis,* dissolution]. Surgical formation of a movable new joint in bony ankylosis.

stereoauscultation (stĕr"ē-ō-aws"kŭl-tā'shŭn) [" + L. *auscultare,* listen to]. Auscultation by use of a stethoscope with two ends on it so each may be placed on different parts of the chest. One tube of each instrument is inserted into an ear while the other is squeezed shut by the fingers.

stereocampimeter (stĕr"ē-ō-kăm-pĭm'ĕ-tĕr) [" + L. *campus,* field, + Gr. *metron,* measure]. A device for measuring the visual field of both eyes simultaneously.

stereochemical (stĕr"ē-ō-kĕm'ĭ-kăl) [" + *chemeia,* chemistry]. Concerning stereochemistry.

stereochemistry (stĕr"ē-ō-kĕm'ĭs-trē). That branch of chemistry dealing with atoms in their space relationship; and the effect of such relationship on the action and effects of the molecule.

stereocilia (stĕr"ē-ō-sĭl'ē-ă). (sing. *stereocilium*) Nonmotile protoplasmic projections from free surfaces of cells of ductus epididymis and ductus deferens.

stereocinefluorography (stĕr"ē-ō-sĭn"ē-flū"or-ŏg'ră-fē). Motion picture photography of the images produced by stereofluorography. This provides a three-dimensional visualization.

stereoencephalotomy (stĕr"ē-ō-ĕn-sĕf"ă-lŏt'ō-mē) [" + *enkephalos,* brain, + *tome,* incision]. Surgical incision by use of stereotaxis.

stereognosis (stĕr"ē-ŏg-nō'sĭs) [" + *gnosis,* knowledge]. Ability to recognize form of solid objects by touch.

stereogram (stĕr'ē-ō-grăm) [" + *gramma,* mark]. Stereoscopic roentgenogram.

stereoisomer (stĕr"ē-ō-ī'sō-mĕr). A substance exhibiting stereoisomerism.

stereoisomerism (stĕr"ē-ō-ī-sō'mĕr-ĭzm). Condition in which two or more substances may have the same empirical formula, but a different structural formula, structural formulas being mirror images of each other.

Ex.: dextrose and levulose differ in optical activity with regard to their effect on a plane of polarized light.

stereology (stĕr"ē-ŏl'ō-jē) [Gr. *stereos,* solid, + *logos,* study]. Study of three-dimensional aspects of objects.

stereometer (stĕr"ē-ŏm'ĕ-tĕr) [" + *metron,* measure]. An instrument used in stereometry.

stereometry (stĕr"ē-ŏm'ĕ-trē) [" + *metron,* a measure]. The measurement of a solid body or the cubic contents of a hollow body.

stereo-ophthalmoscope (stĕr"ē-ō-ŏf-thăl'mō-skōp) [" + *ophthalmos,* eye, + *skopein,* to examine]. An ophthalmoscope that is designed to permit the fundus to be seen simultaneously by both eyes of the examiner.

stereo-orthopter (stĕr"ē-ō-or-thŏp'tĕr) [" + *orthos,* straight, + *opsis,* vision]. A mirror-reflecting device for treatment of strabismus.

stereophantoscope (stĕr″ē-ō-făn′tō-skōp) [″ + *phantos,* visible, + *skopein,* to examine]. A stereoscopic device with rotating disks for testing vision.

stereophorometer (stĕr″ē-ō-for-ŏm′ĕ-tĕr) [″ + *phoros,* a bearer, + *metron,* a measure]. A prism-refracting device for use in correcting defective vision.

stereophotography (stĕr″ē-ō-fō-tŏg′ră-fē) [″ + *phos,* light, + *graphein,* to write]. Photography that produces effect of solidity or depth in the pictures.

stereophotomicrograph (stĕr″ē-ō-fō″tō-mī′krō-grăf) [″ + ″ + *mikros,* tiny, + *graphein,* to write]. A photograph showing solidity or depth of a microscopic subject.

stereopsis (stĕr″ē-ŏp′sĭs) [″ + *opsis,* vision]. Stereoscopic vision.

stereoradiography (stĕr″ē-ō-rā″dē-ŏg′ră-fē) [″ + L. *radius,* ray, + Gr. *graphein,* to write]. Taking roentgenograms from two slightly different angles so that when they are viewed through a stereoscope, there will be a stereoscopic effect.

stereoroentgenography (stĕr″ē-ō-rĕnt″gĕn-ŏg′ră-fē) [″ + *roentgen* + Gr. *graphein,* to write]. Stereoradiography.

stereoscope (stĕr′ē-ō-skōp) [″ + *skopein,* to see]. Instrument that creates an impression of solidity or depth of objects seen by combining images of two pictures.

stereoscopic, stereoscopical. Pert. to the stereoscope or its use.

stereoscopic vision. Vision in which things have the appearance of solidity and relief as though seen in three dimensions. Binocular vision produces this effect.

stereospecific (stĕr″ē-ō-spĕ-sĭf′ĭk). Specific for only one of the possible receptors on a cell.

stereotactic (stĕr″ē-ō-tăk′tĭk). Stereotaxic, q.v.

stereotaxic (stĕr″ē-ō-tăk′sĭk) [″ + *taxis,* arrangement]. Concerning stereotaxis.

stereotaxis (stĕr″ē-ō-tăk′sĭs) [Gr. *stereos,* solid, + *taxis,* arrangement]. A method of precisely locating areas in the brain; use of this technique is essential in certain neurosurgical procedures.

stereotropic (stĕr″ē-ō-trŏp′ĭk) [″ + *trope,* a turn]. Concerning stereotropism.

stereotropism (stĕr″ē-ŏt′rō-pĭzm) [″ + *tropos,* a turning, + *-ismos,* condition]. A response toward (positive stereotropism) or away from (negative stereotropism) a solid object. SYN: *thigmotropism.*

stereotypy (stĕr-ē-ō-tī′pē) [″ + *typos,* type]. Persistent repetition of words, posture, or movement without meaning; seen in catatonic partial stupors.

steric (stē′rĭk). Concerning the spatial arrangement of atoms in a chemical compound.

sterid (stĕr′ĭd). Steroid.

sterile (stĕr′ĭl) [L. *sterilis,* barren]. 1. Free from living microorganisms. Solutions that have passed through certain filters are called sterile solutions because bacteria, fungi, and their spores have been removed. However, viruses can pass through some filters, and the term sterile is incorrectly used in this context. 2. Not fertile; unable to reproduce young. SYN: *barren.* SEE: *sterility.*

sterility (stĕr-ĭl′ĭ-tē) [L. *sterilitas,* barrenness]. 1. Condition of being free from living microorganisms. 2. Inability of the female to become pregnant or for the male to impregnate a female.

Investigation into the cause of sterility includes investigation of both partners. A routine examination for sterility in the female includes a study of the vaginal secretions, a bimanual pelvic examination, visualization of the cervix, in some cases a test for patency of the fallopian tubes, and a record of basal body temperature. A history of pelvic disorder in the female is of great importance. The male should have the seminal fluid examined for the number, motility, viability, and normality of the spermatozoa.

TREATMENT: Treatment of sterility depends upon the finding and correction of any or all causes of the condition. A high percentage of couples who have an infertility problem in the first year of marriage will, without treatment, produce offspring within two to three years.

s., absolute. Complete and incurable inability to produce offspring as a result of anatomical or physiological factors that prevent production of functional germ cells, conception, or normal development of a zygote.

s., acquired. The failure of further conception after once having given birth to a child.

s., female. The inability of the woman to conceive.

ETIOL: *Congenital abnormalities:* Absence or maldevelopment of the uterus, tubes, or ovaries; infantile uterus. *Acquired local conditions: Vagina:* Inflammation. *Cervix:* Narrowing of the internal os; acute and chronic endocervicitis; polyps occluding the cervical canal; cervical mucus that, due to either its chemical or physical qualities, is hostile to sperm. *Body of the uterus:* Fibroids of the uterus that block the canal; diseased endometrium, particularly endometritis. *Fallopian tube:* Chronic salpingo-oophoritis with closure of the tubal ostium and where the ovary is embedded in adhesions. *Ovarian dysfunction:* Congenital conditions, or secondary to endocrine disorders, infections, trauma, neoplasms, x-ray or surgical castration, or effects of toxic agents. Psychological and emotional disturbances, coital difficulties, and dietary deficiencies may also result in sterility.

s., male. Inability of a male either to produce sperm or to produce viable sperm. This results in inability to fertilize the ovum.

ETIOL: May result from congenital factors such as cryptorchidism or maldevelopment of testicular ducts or testis; acquired factors; lack of libido or impotence.

s., primary. Sterility resulting from failure of the testis or ovary to produce functional germ cells.

s., relative. Sterility due to causes other than defect of sex organs.

sterilization (stĕr″ĭl-ī-zā′shŭn) [L. *sterilis,* barren]. 1. Process of completely removing or destroying all microorganisms on a substance by exposure to chemical or physical agents, exposure to ionizing radiation, or by filtering gas or liquids through porous materials that remove microorganisms. A substance cannot be properly described as being partially sterile. SEE: *sterile.* 2. Process of rendering barren. Can be accomplished by surgical removal of testes or ovaries (castration) or inactivation by irradiation, or by tying off or removal of a portion of reproductive ducts (ductus deferens or uterine tubes). SEE: *vasectomy; salpingectomy; tubal ligation.*

s., dry heat. Sterilization of microorganisms accomplished by subjection to high heat (165° to 170° C.) for 2 to 3 hours in ovens.

s., fractional. Sterilization of microorganisms in which heating is done at separated intervals, so that spores can develop into bacteria and be destroyed. Usually accomplished by subjecting organisms to free-flowing steam for 15 min. for three or four successive days. SYN: *s., intermittent.*

s., gas. Exposure to gases such as formaldehyde or ethylene oxide that destroy microorganisms.

s., intermittent. S., fractional.

s., laparoscopic. Sterilization by use of a laparoscope.

s., steam. Sterilization by exposure of microorganisms at 212° F. (100° C.) to flowing steam in an unsealed receptacle or by exposure of microorganisms to steam under pressure in an autoclave.

sterilize (stĕr′ĭ-līz) [L. *sterilis,* barren]. 1. To free from microorganisms. 2. To make incapable of reproduction.

sterilizer (stĕr′ĭ-lī″zĕr). Oven or appliance for sterilizing.

s., steam. An autoclave that sterilizes by steam under pressure at temperatures above 100° C.

sternad (stĕr′năd) [Gr. *sternon,* sternum]. Toward the sternum.

sternal (stĕr′năl) [Gr. *sternalis*]. Rel. to the sternum or breastbone.

sternalgia (stĕr-năl′jē-ă) [Gr. *sternon,* sternum, + *algos,* pain]. Pain in the sternum. SYN: *sternodynia.*

sternal puncture. Use of a large-bore needle to obtain a specimen of marrow from the sternum.

Sternberg-Reed cells. SEE: *Reed-Sternberg cells.*

sternebra (stĕr′nē-bră) [″ + L. *vertebra,* vertebra]. Parts of the sternum prior to fusion.

sternen (stĕr′nĕn) [Gr. *sternon,* sternum]. Concerning the sternum and no other structures.

sterno- [Gr. *sternon*]. Combining form meaning sternum.

sternoclavicular (stĕr″nō-klă-vĭk′ū-lăr) [″ + L. *clavicula,* a little key]. Concerning the sternum and clavicle.

sternocleidal (stĕr″nō-klī′dăl) [″ + *kleis,* key]. Sternoclavicular.

sternocleidomastoid (stĕr″nō-klī″dō-măs′toyd) [″ + *kleis,* clavicle, + *mastos,* breast, + *eidos,* like]. One of two muscles arising from the sternum and inner part of the clavicle. SEE: *Muscles* in *Appendix.*

sternocostal (stĕr″nō-kŏs′tăl) [″ + L. *costa,* rib]. Rel. to sternum and ribs.

sternodymia (stĕr″nō-dĭm′ē-ă) [″ + *didymos,* twin]. Condition in which deformed twin fetuses are joined at the sternum.

sternodynia (stĕr″nō-dĭn′ē-ă) [″ + *odyne,* pain]. Pain in the sternum. SYN: *sternalgia.*

sternohyoid (stĕr″nō-hī′oyd) [″ + *hyoeides,* U-shaped]. Muscle from the medial end of the clavicle and sternum to the hyoid bone. SEE: *Muscles* in *Appendix.*

sternoid (stĕr′noyd) [″ + *eidos,* resemblance]. Resembling the breastbone.

sternomastoid (stĕr″nō-măs′toyd) [″ + *mastos,* breast, + *eidos,* form]. Pert. to the sternum and mastoid process of the temporal bone.

sternomastoid region. Wide area on lateral region of the neck covered by sternocleidomastoid muscle.

sternopagia (stĕr″nō-pā′jē-ă) [″ + *pagos,* a thing fixed]. Sternodymia, q.v.

sternopericardial (stĕr″nō-pĕr″ĭ-kăr′dē-ăl) [″ + *peri,* around, + *kardia,* heart]. Concerning the sternum and pericardium.

sternoschisis (stĕr-nŏs′kĭ-sĭs) [″ + *schisis,* cleft]. A cleft or fissured sternum.

sternothyroid (stĕr″nō-thī′royd) [″ + *thyreos,* shield, + *eidos,* like]. Muscle extending beneath the sternohyoid that depresses thyroid cartilage. SEE: *Muscles* in *Appendix.*

sternotomy (stĕr-nŏt′ō-mē) [″ + *tome,* incision]. The operation of cutting through the

STERNUM

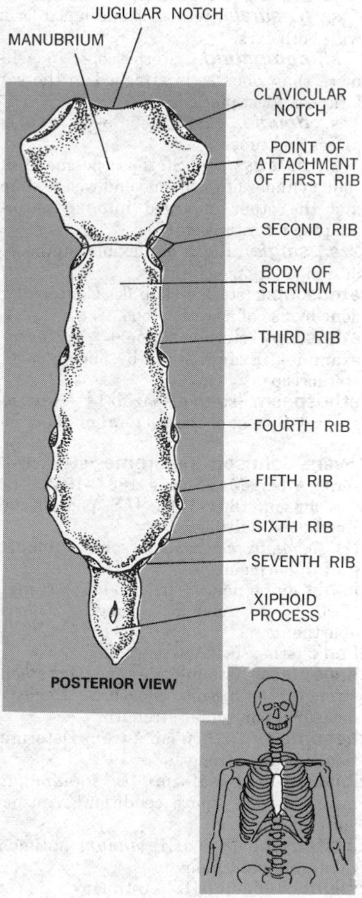

sternum.

sternotracheal (stĕr″nō-trā′kē-ăl) [″ + *tracheia,* trachea]. Concerning the sternum and trachea.

sternotrypesis (stĕr″nō-trī-pē′sĭs) [″ + *trypesis,* a boring]. Surgical perforation of the sternum.

sternovertebral (stĕr″nō-vĕr′tē-brăl) [″ + L. *vertebra,* vertebra]. Concerning the sternum and vertebrae.

sternum (stĕr′nŭm) [L.]. [NA] The narrow, flat bone in the median line of the thorax in front. It consists of three portions distinguished as the manubrium, the gladiolus, and the ensiform or xiphoid process. SEE: illus.

RS: breast, chicken; chondrosternal; cleft; ensiform; gladiolus; manubrium; xiphoid process.

s., cleft. Congenital fissure of the sternum.

sternutament (stĕr-nū′tăm-ĕnt) [L. *sternutare,* to sneeze]. A substance causing sneezing.

sternutatio (stĕr-nū-tā′shē-ō) [L.]. Sneezing.

s. convulsiva. Paroxysmal sneezing as in hay fever.

sternutation (stĕr-nū-tā′shŭn). Act of sneezing.

s., convulsive. Spasmodic or paroxysmal sneezing with profusion of watery secretion from the nose.

sternutator (stĕr′nū-tā″tor) [L. *sternutatorius,* causing sneezing]. An agent, such as a war gas, that induces sneezing.

sternutatory (stĕr-nū′tă-tō″rē). Causing sneezing.

steroid (stĕr′oyd). 1. An organic compound containing in its chemical nucleus the perhydrocyclopentanophenanthrene ring. SEE: *perhydrocyclopentanophenanthrene; steroid hormones* for illus. 2. Term applied to any one of a large group of substances chemically related to sterols. Includes sterols, D vitamins, bile acids, certain hormones, saponins, glucosides of digitalis, and certain carcinogenic substances.

steroid hormones. The sex hormones and hormones of the adrenal cortex. SEE: illus.

STEROID HORMONE NUCLEUS

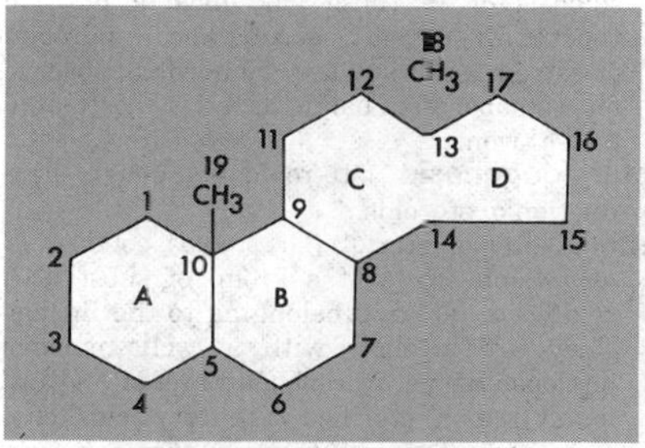

PERHYDROCYCLOPENTANOPHENANTHRENE, THE BASIC STRUCTURE OR "BUILDING BLOCK" OF STEROID HORMONES.
CARBON ATOMS ARE NUMBERED.

steroid hormone therapy. Treatment with various steroid hormones, esp. those from the adrenal cortex. If therapy is continued for longer than a few days, the following general precautions should be observed: low-salt diet; high-protein diet; control gastric acidity; adequate potassium intake; determine need for covering antibiotic such as isoniazid in sarcoidosis or in those who have a positive tuberculin test; nitrogen balance (androgen or estrogen therapy may be needed); observe for osteoporosis, particularly in postmenopausal women.

steroidogenesis (stē-roy″dō-jĕn′ĕ-sĭs). Production of steroids.

sterol (stĕr′ŏl, stēr′ŏl) [Gr. *stereos,* solid, + L. *oleum,* oil]. One of a group of substances related to fats and belonging to the lipoids. They are alcohols with a cyclic nucleus (cyclopentanoperhydrophenanthrene) and are found free or esterified with fatty acids (cholesterides). They are found in animals (zoosterols) or in plants (phytosterols). Generally colorless, crystalline compounds, nonsaponifiable and soluble in certain organic solvents.

Ex.: cholesterol.

stertor (stĕr′tor) [L. *stertor*]. Snoring or laborious breathing due to obstruction of air passages in the head, seen in certain diseases such as apoplexy.

stertorous (stĕr′tō-rŭs). Pert. to laborious breathing provoking a snoring sound.

stethalgia (stĕth-ăl′jē-ă). Pain in the chest.

stetho- [Gr. *stethos,* chest]. Combining form indicating the chest.

stethocyrtograph (stĕth″ō-sĕr′tō-grăf) [″ + *kyrtos,* bent, + *graphein,* to write]. Stethokyrtograph.

stethogoniometer (stĕth″ō-gō″nē-ŏm′ĕt-ĕr) [″ + *gonia,* angle, + *metron,* measure]. Device for measuring the curvature of the chest.

stethogram (stĕth′ō-grăm) [″ + *gramma,* a mark]. A record of heart sounds. The record may be stored for later comparison with subsequent heart sounds. SYN: *phonocardiogram.*

stethograph (stĕth′ō-grăf) [″ + *graphein,* to write]. Device to record chest movements in respiration.

stethokyrtograph (stĕth″ō-kĭr′tō-grăf) [″ + *kyrtos,* bent, + *graphein,* to write]. Device for measuring and recording the dimensions and amount of curves of the chest.

stethometer (stĕth-ŏm′ĕt-ĕr) [″ + *metron,* measure]. Device for measuring the chest's expansion during respiration.

stethomyitis, stethomyositis (stĕth″ō-mī-ī′tĭs, -mī″ō-sī′tĭs) [″ + *mys,* muscle, + *itis,* inflammation]. Inflammation of the muscles of the chest.

stethoparalysis (stĕth″ō-pă-răl′ĭ-sĭs) [″ + *paralyein,* to paralyze]. Paralysis of the muscles of the chest.

stethophonometer (stĕth″ō-fō-nŏm′ĕt-ĕr) [″ + *phone,* voice, + *metron,* measure]. Instrument for determining intensity of sound emitted in auscultation.

stethoscope (stĕth′ō-skōp) [″ + *skopein,* to examine]. Instrument used to mediate sounds produced in the body. Ordinarily consists of rubber tubing in a Y shape.

s., binaural. Stethoscope designed for use with both ears.

s., compound. Stethoscope in which more than one set is attached to the same fork and chest piece.

s., double. Stethoscope with two earpieces and tubes.

s., percussion. Stethoscope made of a solid cylinder of wood, one end wedge shaped and the other enlarged into an earpiece adapted for intercostal use.

s., single. Rigid or flexible stethoscope designed for one ear only.

stethoscopic (stĕth″ō-skŏp′ĭk). Concerning or done by use of a stethoscope.

stethoscopy (stĕth-ŏs′kō-pē) [″ + *skopein,* to examine]. Examination by means of the stethoscope.

stethospasm (stĕth′ō-spăzm) [″ + *spasmos,* spasm]. Spasm of the pectoral or chest muscles.

Stevens-Johnson syndrome (stē′vĕnz-jŏn′sŏn). [Albert M. Stevens, 1884–1945, Frank C. Johnson, 1894–1934, U.S. pediatricians] Erythema multiforme, q.v.

STH. *somatotropic hormone;* somatotropin, the growth hormone.

sthenia (sthē′nē-ă) [Gr. *sthenos,* strength]. Normal or unusual strength. Opposite of asthenia.

sthenic (sthĕn′ĭk). Active; strong.

sthenometer (sthĕn-ŏm′ĕ-tĕr) [Gr. *sthenos,* strength, + *metron,* measure]. Device for measuring muscular strength.

sthenometry (sthĕn-ŏm′ĕ-trē). Determination of bodily strength.

stibialism (stĭb′ē-ăl-ĭzm) [L. *stibium,* antimony, + Gr. *-ismos,* condition]. Antimony poisoning.

stibiated (stĭb′ē-āt″ĕd) [L. *stibium,* antimony]. Containing antimony.

stibium (stĭb′ē-ŭm) [L.]. Antimony.

stibophen (stĭb′ō-fĕn). A trivalent antimony compound, used in treating schistosomiasis, and granuloma inguinale.

stichochrome (stĭk′ō-krōm) [Gr. *stichos,* row, + *chroma,* color]. A nerve cell in which the stainable bodies (Nissl bodies) are arranged in parallel rows.

stiff [AS. *stif*]. Rigid, firm, inflexible.

stiff joint. Joint with reduced mobility.

stiff man syndrome. Intermittent aching, tightness, and stiffness of the muscles, which progresses to permanent stiffness to the extent of limiting voluntary movement. Etiology is unknown. Improvement with diazepam has been reported.

stiff neck. Rigidity of neck resulting from spasm of neck muscles. It is a symptom of many disorders. SYN: *torticollis; wryneck.*

stiff-neck fever. 1. Dengue. 2. Cerebrospinal meningitis.

stigma (stĭg′mă) [Gr., mark]. (pl. *stigmata, -mas*) 1. A mark or spot on the skin; lesions or sores of hands and feet that resemble crucifixion wounds. 2. Spot on ovarian surface where rupture of a graafian follicle will occur. 3. Mental or physical mark characterizing a specific disease. There is often shame and embarrassment because of a stigmatizing condition; there is often some mental anguish since one has a condition that marks one as being different.

s., hysterical. Any of the peculiar marks or symptoms of hysteria such as spots on the skin or impairment of sensory functions.

s. of degeneration. Any of the developmental variations from the normal. Formerly thought to be associated with mental degeneracy.

DEGENERATIVE CHANGES: *Face:* May be unusually hairy in the female and abnormally smooth in the male. *Fingers and toes:* May be an extra one, or adherent or webbed. *Forehead:* May be sloping and very low. *Eyes:* May be different in color or set at different levels. *Ears:* Unusual in many ways. *Jaws:* Either one may project unusually. *Head:* May be unusually large or small. *Teeth:* May be irregular or project. *Roof of mouth:* May be high and pointed or unusually narrow. Only several of these irregularities may be considered as indicative of defective mentality.

s., psychic. Mental state characterized by susceptibility to suggestion.

stigmatic (stĭg-măt′ĭk) [Gr. *stigma,* mark]. Pert. to or marked with a stigma.

stigmatism. 1. Condition characterized by possession of stigmata. 2. Condition in which the rays of light are accurately focused on the retina. SEE: *astigmatism.*

stigmatization (stĭg″mă-tĭ-zā′shŭn). The formation of stigmata, esp. hysterical stigmata on the skin.

stigmatometer (stĭg″mă-tŏm′ĕ-tĕr) [″ + *metron,* measure]. Device for testing eye refraction. SYN: *astigmatometer.*

stilbestrol (stĭl-bĕs′trŏl). Diethylstilbestrol, q.v.

stilet, stilette (stĭ-lĕt′) [Fr. *stilette*]. 1. Small, sharp-pointed instrument for probing. 2. Wire used to pass through or stiffen a flexible catheter.

stillbirth [AS. *stille,* quiet, + ME. *burth,* birth]. Birth of a dead fetus.

stillborn [″ + *boren,* to bring forth]. Dead at birth.

Still's disease. Arthritis, juvenile rheumatoid, q.v.

stillicidium (stĭl″ĭ-sĭd′ē-ŭm) [L. *stilla,* drop, + *cadere,* to fall]. A dribbling or flowing, drop by drop.

s. lacrimarum. Watering of the eye. SYN: *epiphora.*

s. narium. Watery mucus discharged at onset of coryza.

s. urinae. Urinary incontinence from a distended bladder. SYN: *strangury.*

Stilphostrol. Trade name for diethylstilbestrol diphosphate.

stimulant (stĭm′ū-lănt) [L. *stimulans,* goading]. Any agent temporarily increasing functional activity. Stimulants may be classified according to the organ upon which they act as follows: cardiac, bronchial, gastric, cerebral, intestinal, nervous, motor, vasomotor, respiratory, and secretory.

stimulate (stĭm′ū-lāt) [L. *stimulare,* to goad on]. To increase functional activity of an organ or structure.

stimulation (stĭm″ū-lā′shŭn). 1. Process of being stimulated. 2. Irritating action of agents on muscles, nerves, or sensory end-organs by which activity in a part is evoked.

stimulator (stĭm″ū-lā′tor). Something that stimulates.

s., long-acting thyroid. A substance present in the blood of persons with hyperthyroidism that stimulates the thyroid. It is an immune gamma globulin.

stimulus (stĭm′ū-lŭs) [L., a goad]. (pl. *stimuli*) 1. Any agent or factor able to influence living protoplasm directly, as one capable of causing muscular contraction or secretion in a gland, or of initiating an impulse in a nerve. 2. A change of environment of sufficient intensity to evoke a response in an organism. 3. An excitant or irritant.

s., adequate. 1. Any stimulus capable of evoking a response, i.e., an environmental change possessing a certain intensity, acting for a certain length of time, and occurring at a certain rate. 2. A stimulus capable of initiating a nerve impulse in a specific type of receptor.

s., chemical. A chemical substance (liquid, gaseous, or solid) that is capable of evoking a response.

s., conditioned. A stimulus that gives rise to a conditioned response. SEE: *reflex, conditioned.*

s., electric. Stimulus resulting from initiation of or cessation of a flow of electrons as from a battery, induction coil, or generator.

s., homologous. A stimulus that acts only on specific sensory end-organs.

s., iatrotropic. The stimulus or event that makes a person seek or receive medical attention; also called the sick person's chief complaint. However there are many reasons why medical care is voluntarily sought by apparently healthy people, e.g., an Armed Forces draft examination, pre-employment or premarital examination, or in a health screening survey. Thus it is possible for disease to be discovered prior to the time when the disease would ordinarily make itself known to the individual.

s., liminal. S., threshold.

s., mechanical. A stimulus produced by a physical change such as contact with objects or changes in pressure.

s., minimal. S., threshold.

s., nociceptive. A painful and usually injurious stimulus.

s., subliminal. A stimulus that is weaker than a threshold stimulus.

s., thermal. Stimulus produced by a change in temperature of the skin, a rise giving sensations of warmth, a fall giving sensations of coldness.

s., threshold. The least or weakest stimulus that is capable of initiating a response or giving rise to a sensation. SYN: *s., liminal.*

s., unconditioned. Any stimulus that elicits an unconditioned response, i.e., a response that was inherently present rather than one that was learned.

sting [AS. *stingan*]. 1. Sharp, smarting sensation, as of a wound or astringent. 2. A puncture wound made by an insect. SEE: *bites and stings.*

stingray. A group of rays of the family Dasyatidae. A number of species are found in the coastal waters of the United States. It is flat with wide pectoral fins that resemble wings. A venomous spine runs along the top of its whip-like tail, with which it can inflict severe injuries.

TREATMENT: Pain relievers, debridement of wound, irrigation with removal of foreign material and stinger if it is present, and injection of site with local anesthetic. Soak area in hot water (45 to 60° C.) 30 to 60 min. to inactivate venom.

S-T interval. The interval in an electrocardiogram that represents the initial and final ventricular complexes. SEE: *QRST complex; electrocardiogram* for illus.

stippling (stĭp′lĭng) [Dutch *stippelen,* to spot]. A spotted condition, as in the retina in certain ocular diseases or in basophilic red corpuscles.

s., gingival. An orange-peel appearance of the attached gingiva in health, believed to be due to the enlargement of the underlying connective tissue papillae in response to massage and tooth brushing; the indent lies between the bulging pupillae where the epithelia grow downward as rete ridges.

stirrup, stirrup bone (stĭr′ŭp) [AS. *stigrap,* a stirrup]. Stapes of the ear. SEE: *ear.*

stitch (stĭch) [AS. *stice,* a pricking]. 1. A local sharp, lancinating, or spasmodic pain. 2. A single loop of suture material passed through skin or flesh by a needle, to facilitate healing of a wound. 3. To unite skin or flesh with a needle and suture material. Stitches made of nonabsorbable materials are removed after a few days and other types are absorbed by the body. SYN: *suture.*

stitch abscess. Abscess developing in a suture; due to infection.

stochastic model (stō-kăs′tĭk) [Gr. *stokastikos,* skillful in guessing]. A statistical model that attempts to reproduce that sequence of events which would be expected to occur in a real-life situation. This technique has some usefulness in predicting the importance and extent of disease in a specified population.

stock (stŏk) [AS. *stocc,* tree trunk]. The original individual, race, or tribe from which others have descended.

stock culture. Permanent culture of a microorganism reinforced from time to time by fresh media.

stockinet. Tubular woven material of uniform size that is open at both ends. Used to hold bandages in place or to place uniform pressure on a leg, finger, arm, or other part of an extremity.

stocking. Snug covering for the foot and leg. A stocking made of elastic material will place firm, even pressure on the extremity, which is useful in preventing thrombophlebitis of the leg in bedfast patients and in treating varicose veins.

stoichiology (stoy″kē-ŏl′ō-jē) [Gr. *stoicheion,* element, + *logos,* study]. The study of cell physiology.

stoichiometry (stoy″kē-ŏm′ĕ-trē) [″ + *metron,* measure]. Study of the mathematics of chemistry and chemical reactions; chemical calculations.

stoke (stōk). [Sir George Stokes, Brit. physicist, 1819–1903] A unit of viscosity equal to 10^{-4} square meters per second (10^{-4}m. s^{-1}).

Stokes-Adams syndrome (stōks-ăd′ăms). [William Stokes, Ir. physician, 1804–1878; Robert Adams, Ir. physician, 1791–1875] Altered state of consciousness caused by decreased flow of blood to brain. Caused by any transient interference with cardiac output such as incomplete or complete heart block. The patient may be lightheaded or become completely unconscious and have convulsions.

TREATMENT: Intracardiac epinephrine, a sharp blow to the precordium, or use of an external electric pacemaker.

Stokes' disease (stōks). [William Stokes] Exophthalmic goiter. SEE: *hyperthyroidism.*

Stokes' law (stōks). [William Stokes] A muscle lying above an inflamed serous or mucous membrane may be paralyzed.

Stokes' lens. [George Stokes] Device used to diagnose astigmatism.

stoma (stō'mă) [Gr., mouth]. (pl. *stomata, -mas*) 1. A mouth, small opening, or a pore. 2. Artificially created opening between two passages or body cavities or between a cavity or passage and the body's surface. 3. A minute opening between cells of certain epithelial membranes, esp. peritoneum and pleura.

stomach (stŭm'ăk) [Gr. *stomachos*]. A dilated, saclike, distensible portion of the alimentary canal below the esophagus and below the diaphragm to right of spleen, partly under the liver. It is composed of a fundus or round part, a body or middle portion, and pyloric portion, which is the small, distal end.

It has two openings: the upper cardiac orifice opens into the esophagus and the lower pyloric orifice opens into the duodenum. The stomach is composed of four layers; the outer serous coat covers almost all of the organ. The muscular layer just beneath is formed of three layers of smooth muscle fibers: an outer longitudinal layer, a medial circular layer, and an inner oblique layer. Submucous layer is a connecting medium between the muscular and mucous layer, the inner lining of the stomach.

The cardiac, fundic (parietal or oxyntic), and pyloric glands of the stomach are composed of columnar and tubular cells that secrete gastric juice containing hydrochloric acid and pepsin. SEE: illus.

FUNCT: The stomach secretes gastric juice and converts proteins into peptones. In addition to its basic function of serving as an organ of digestion, the stomach also serves in the following ways: it regulates the passage of food to the remainder of the gut, acting as a reservoir; its acid kills a large proportion of the microbes present in most food; it has limited ability to absorb; it is important in the acid-base equilibrium of the body, particularly when electrolytes are removed from the body during vomiting; it can excrete some drugs, administered parenterally, into the gastric juice; it acts as a kind of receptor for chemical and nervous mechanisms by which secretion and movement are stimulated in lower parts of the gastrointestinal tract; it forms a hematinic principle (antianemic factor), effective in prevention of pernicious anemia, by the action of an intrinsic factor (present in gastric juice) on an extrinsic factor (vitamin B_{12}) present in foods.

DIET IN SOME DISORDERS: *Atony and hypomotility:* Food is retained longer than normal and decomposition may occur if hydrochloric acid is deficient. Liquids are retained longer than solids. Therefore diet should consist of quickly and easily digested foods—soft-cooked vegetables, chicken, fish, strained beef, and moderate amount of skim milk. Avoid liquids, pastries, and rich gravies. *Hypermotility:* The stomach empties too rapidly; therefore, diet should be liquid, soft, in small amounts, and in frequent feedings. Fats delay the emptying of the stomach. *Hyperacidity:* Give protein to combine with acid. Frequent small feedings are advisable.

s., bilocular. S., hourglass.

s., cardiac. Fundus of the stomach.

s., cascade. A form of hourglass stomach in which there is a constriction between cardiac and pyloric portions. Cardiac portion fills first and then contents cascade into pyloric portion.

s., cow horn. A high, transversely placed stomach.

s., foreign bodies in. In the average case foreign bodies pass through the alimentary tract without disturbance. However, these patients should be under a doctor's care. Usually symptoms are absent, but the patient may be alarmed. Give nothing by mouth. Under no circumstances should salts, cathartics, and enemas be used as they can make the condition worse.

s., hourglass. Stomach resembling an hourglass, caused by constriction from a band of fibrous tissue. SYN: *s., bilocular.*

s., leather-bottle. A condition of the stomach caused by hypertrophy of the stomach walls or their infiltration with malignant tissue.

s., thoracic. Condition in which stomach lies above the diaphragm. May result from an embryonic anomaly in which the stomach fails to descend, or from hernia of diaphragm. The latter results in so-called upside-down stomach.

s., water-trap. Stomach with the pylorus situated unusually high, causing slow emptying.

stomach, words pert. to: abdominal cavity; absorption; achylia gastrica; acidity; anachlorhydria; atony; cardialgia; cardiopyloric; cardiospasm; chlorhydria; cholangiogastrostomy; clapotage; digestion; ectasia; feeding, artificial; gastric digestion; gastric juice; gastric lavage; "gastr-" words; gavage; hourglass stomach; hunger; lavage; linitis; pylorus; secretagogue; ulcer; ventriculus.

stomach ache. Pain in the stomach. SYN: *gastralgia; gastrodynia.*

stomachal (stŭm'ă-kăl) [Gr. *stomachos*, stomach]. 1. Rel. to the stomach. 2. A gastric tonic.

stomachalgia [" + *algos*, pain]. Pain in the stomach.

stomach cancer. May be carcinoma, lymphoma, or sarcoma.

SYM: General symptoms of dyspepsia with following characteristic symptoms: continued pain, often tenderness vomiting of par-

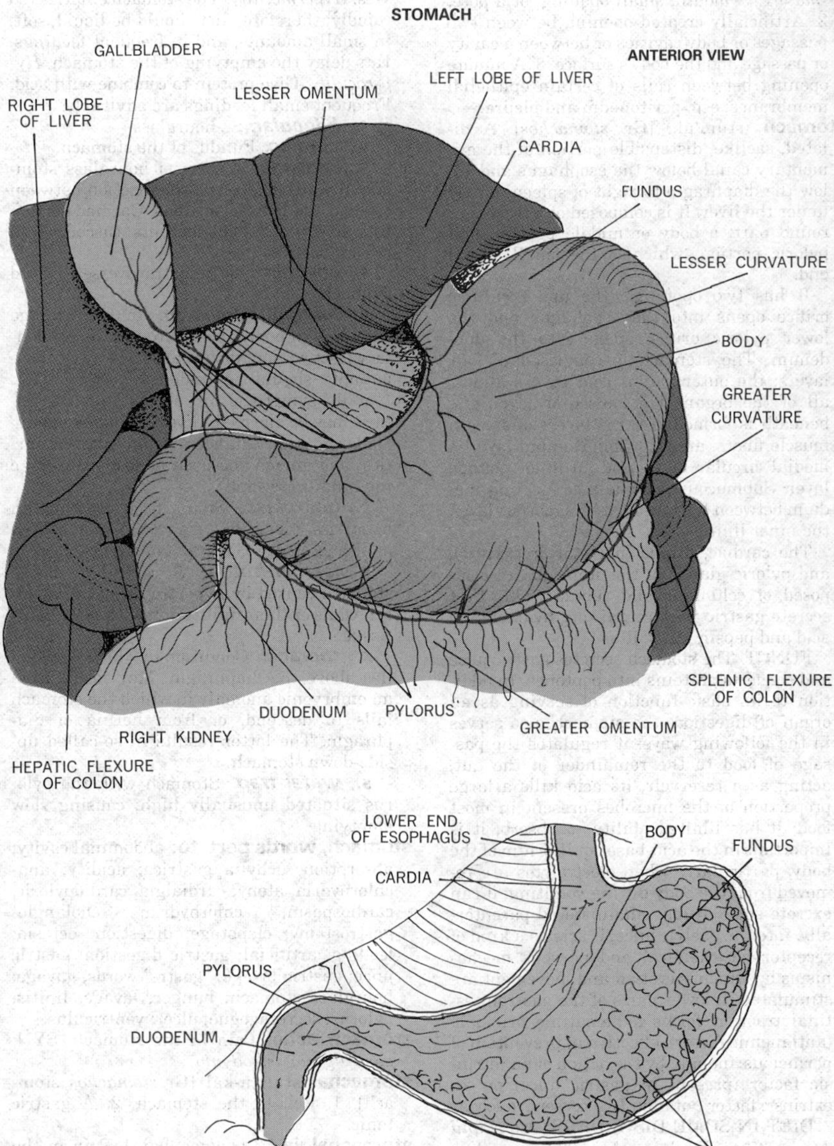
STOMACH
ANTERIOR VIEW
GALLBLADDER
RIGHT LOBE OF LIVER
LESSER OMENTUM
LEFT LOBE OF LIVER
CARDIA
FUNDUS
LESSER CURVATURE
BODY
GREATER CURVATURE
SPLENIC FLEXURE OF COLON
DUODENUM
PYLORUS
GREATER OMENTUM
RIGHT KIDNEY
HEPATIC FLEXURE OF COLON
LOWER END OF ESOPHAGUS
BODY
FUNDUS
CARDIA
PYLORUS
DUODENUM
RUGAE
INSIDE VIEW

tially digested food; absence of free hydrochloric acid in gastric juice; hematemesis or blood in stools, slight in amount and blood-altered so it has a coffee-grounds appearance; presence of tumor; loss of weight and strength; extreme anemia; involvement of superficial lymph glands. When the pylorus is involved, symptoms of gastric dilatation will be added.

PROG: Very poor.

TREATMENT: Early treatment. Surgery; liquid or semiliquid diet; rest.

stomachic (stō-măk'ĭk). 1. Concerning the stomach. 2. Medicine that stimulates the action of the stomach.

stomach intubation. Passage of a tube into the stomach to obtain gastric contents for examination, for prophylaxis and treatment of ileus, or to remove ingested poisons.

stomachoscopy [" + *skopein,* to inspect]. Examination of the stomach. SYN: *gastroscopy.*

stomach pump. Device for removing contents of the stomach through a tube inserted through the mouth.

stomach tooth. A lower canine tooth during first dentition.

stomach tube. Tube used to wash out or to introduce food or liquids into the stomach.

stomal (stō'măl) [Gr. *stoma,* mouth]. Concerning a stoma.

stomata. Pl. of stoma.

stomatal (stō'mă-tăl) [Gr. *stoma,* mouth]. Concerning stomata.

stomatalgia (stō"mă-tăl'jē-ă) [Gr. *stoma,* mouth, + *algos,* pain]. Pain in the mouth. SYN: *stomatodynia.*

stomatic. Pert. to or rel. to the mouth.

stomatitis (stō"mă-tī'tĭs) [" + *itis,* inflammation]. Inflammation of the mouth. SEE: *gangrene; noma; thrush.*

SYM: Heat, pain, increased flow of saliva, fetor of breath, restlessness, languor, disinclination to nurse in infants, sometimes fever.

ETIOL: Stomatitis may be caused by many factors or conditions. Among them are pathogenic organisms, including bacteria and viruses; mechanical trauma; irritants such as alcohol, tobacco, hot foods, spices; sensitization to chemical substances in toothpastes or mouthwashes; nutritional deficiencies, esp. avitaminoses; blood disorders; poisoning by drugs, esp. heavy metals; certain skin disorders; systemic infections such as measles, scarlet fever, syphilis. There are also several forms with unknown etiology.

s., aphthous. Formation of tiny ulcers (canker sores) on mucosa of the mouth. SYN: *s., follicular; s., vesicular.*

SYM: General symptoms of stomatitis and on inspection numerous small, round vesicles on cheeks, lips, and tongue, which soon break and leave little shallow ulcers with red areola.

ETIOL: Mechanical injury to the oral mucosa by hard-bristled toothbrushes, sharp food, or objects that can scrape or cut the mucosa; iron or vitamin deficiencies, esp. folic acid and vitamin B_{12}; and nutritional deficiencies. In addition, there seems to be a familial component.

PROG: Good.

TREATMENT: For infants, sterilize milk. Nurse at regular intervals. Wash mouth with clean linen cloth. In adults, correct gastric disturbance or other cause.

s., catarrhal. Simple stomatitis.

SYM: General symptoms of stomatitis with diffuse red swelling of mucous membrane.

TREATMENT: Good hygienic conditions; cleanse mouth with weak solution of boric acid as a wash.

s., corrosive. Stomatitis resulting from intentional or accidental exposure to corrosive substances.

s., diphtheritic. Diphtheria of mucous membranes of the gums or cheeks.

s., follicular. S., aphthous.

s., herpetic. Stomatitis characterized by cold sores (fever blisters).

s., membranous. Stomatitis accompanied by the formation of a false or adventitious membrane.

s., mercurial. A form of stomatitis seen in those who work with mercury; after the administration of very large doses of mercurials; and after small doses in individuals who have a high susceptibility to mercury.

SYM: Early symptoms are tenderness of gums, redness near insertion of teeth, metallic taste, and increase of saliva. Later symptoms include profuse salivation and fetor of breath; redness, swelling, and tenderness of gums. Tongue may be similarly affected and protrude from mouth. In severe cases ulceration of mucous membrane, loss of teeth, and necrosis of jaw result.

TREATMENT: If due to acute poisoning, early administration of dimercaprol (British antilewisite) will be helpful. If chronic, remove patient from source of poison and treat symptomatically.

s., mycotic. Fungus infection of the mouth or throat, esp. in infants and young children. Characterized by formation of white patches and ulcers, frequently with fever and gastrointestinal inflammation. SYN: *thrush.*

s. parasitica. Stomatitis caused by a yeastlike fungus, Candida albicans. SEE: *thrush.*

SYM: Those of general stomatitis with milk-white elevations on tongue and mouth, which on removal leave a raw surface. Disease may extend to pharynx, esophagus, and larynx. Microscopic examination reveals fungus.

PROG: Good.

TREATMENT: Correct hygiene. Treat any gastric disturbance; locally, milk alkaline mouthwash. Diluted gentian violet mouthwash is effective also. Topical application of diluted nystatin solution may be necessary.

s., simple. Erythematous inflammation of the mouth occurring in patches on the mucous membranes.

s., traumatic. Stomatitis resulting from mechanical injury as from ill-fitting dentures, sharp jagged teeth, or biting cheek.

s., ulcerative. Thought by some to be an infectious disease, as it often occurs in epidemics and attacks both children and adults when congregated and unable to practice good oral hygiene. SYN: *trench mouth; Vincent's angina.*

SYM: Gums of lower jaw chiefly affected, are swollen, red, and spongy. Linear ulcers soon form and may extend to cheek; gland under jaw swollen. In severe cases, loosening of teeth and necrosis of jaw may follow.

PROG: Guardedly favorable.

TREATMENT: Correct hygiene; antiseptic mouthwashes such as hydrogen peroxide; no smoking.

s., vesicular. S., aphthous.

s., Vincent's. S., ulcerative.

stomato- [Gr. *stoma,* mouth]. Combining form indicating mouth.

stomatodynia (stō″mă-tō-dĭn′ē-ă) [Gr. *stoma,* mouth, + *odyne,* pain] Pain in the mouth. SYN: *stomatalgia.*

stomatogastric (stō″mă-tō-găs′trĭk) [″ + *gaster,* belly]. Concerning the stomach and mouth.

stomatognathic (stō″mă-tŏg-năth′ĭk) [″ + *gnathos,* jaw]. Indicating the mouth and jaws together.

stomatologist (stō″mă-tŏl′ō-jĭst) [″ + *logos,* a study]. Specialist in treatment of diseases of the mouth.

stomatology (stō″mă-tŏl′ō-jē). Science of the mouth and teeth and their diseases.

stomatomalacia (stō″mă-tō-mă-lā′shē-ă) [″ + *malakia,* softening]. Pathological softening of any structures of the mouth.

stomatomenia (stō″mă-tō-mē′nē-ă) [″ + *meniaia,* menses]. Bleeding from the mouth at the time of menstruation.

stomatomy (stō-măt′ō-mē) [″ + *tome,* incision]. Surgical nicking of the edges of the os uteri to facilitate delivery.

stomatomycosis (stō″mă-tō-mī-kō′sĭs) [″ + *mykes,* fungus, + *osis,* condition]. Any disease of the mouth caused by fungi.

stomatonecrosis (stō″mă-tō-nē-krō′sĭs) [″ + *nekrosis,* death]. Gangrenous ulcerative inflammation of the mouth. SYN: *cancrum oris; noma; stomatitis, gangrenous; stomatonoma.*

stomatonoma (stō″mă-tō-nō′mă) [″ + *nome,* a spreading]. Gangrenous inflammation of the mouth. SYN: *cancrum oris; noma; stomatitis, gangrenous; stomatonecrosis.*

stomatopathy (stō″mă-tŏp′ă-thē) [″ + *pathos,* disease]. Any mouth disease.

stomatoplasty (stō′mă-tō-plăs″tē) [″ + *plassein,* to form]. Plastic surgery or repair of the mouth.

stomatorrhagia (stō″mă-tō-rā′jē-ă) [″ + *rhegnynai,* to burst forth]. Hemorrhage from the mouth or gums.

stomatoscope (stō-măt′ō-skōp) [″ + *skopein,* to examine]. Instrument for examining the mouth.

stomatosis (stō″mă-tō′sĭs) [″ + *osis,* condition]. Any disease of the mouth.

stomatotomy (stō″mă-tŏt′ō-mē) [″ + *tome,* incision]. Stomatomy, q.v.

stomion (stō′mē-ŏn) [Gr., dim. of *stoma,* mouth]. A landmark used in physical anthropology. It is the central point in the oral fissure when the lips are together.

stomocephalus (stō″mō-sĕf′ă-lŭs) [Gr. *stoma,* mouth, + *kephale,* head]. Deformed fetus with very small head and neck.

stomodeal (stō″mō-dē′ăl). Concerning the stomodeum.

stomodeum (stō″mō-dē′ŭm) [″ + *hodaios,* a way]. An external depression lined with ectoderm and bounded by frontonasal, mandibular, and maxillary processes of the embryo. It forms the anterior portion of the oral cavity. Its floor, the pharyngeal membrane, separates the stomodeum from the foregut.

stone [AS. *stan*]. 1. Hardened mineral matter, as a gallstone or a kidney stone. SYN: *calculus.* 2. In Britain, a unit of weight, 14 pounds avoirdupois.

stool (stool) [AS. *stol,* a seat]. 1. Evacuation of the bowels. 2. Waste matter discharged from the bowels. SYN: *feces.*

COLOR: Iron and bismuth turn the stool black, and certain vegetables and berries darken it or produce a distinct color. Pathological stools are usually grayish or a whitish glistening color, and tarry in hemorrhage or show fresh blood.

CHARACTER: *Fatty stools:* These are observed in obstructive jaundice, cancer of the pancreas, pancreatic calculi, and in indigestion or overfeeding in infants.

Frothy poorly-formed stools: They may indicate a spastic colon, the presence of gas, or intestinal inflammation.

Lienteric stools: These contain much undigested food and are noted in inflammatory conditions of the stomach and upper bowel.

Tarry stools: They may indicate gastric hemorrhage, swallowed blood from the nose or lungs, bleeding ulcers of the gastrointes-

tinal tract, hepatic cirrhosis, or cancer.

Membranous shreds: They may exist in cancer of the colon, dysentery, relapsing fever, acute proctitis, and in sloughing of intestinal mucosa.

Mucous stools: Exist in catarrhal or inflamed conditions of the intestines or rectum, in dysentery, enterocolitis, proctitis, impaction, and ulcerative colitis.

SHAPE: *Cylindrical:* If of small caliber, they may be indicative of prolapsus ani, annular rectal stricture, or intestinal spasms.

Ribbon-shaped: Indicative of stricture or cancer of the rectum; possibly enlargement of the prostate in males, hemorrhoids, spasm of the lower bowel and anus, prostatic abscess, and prolapse of the uterus.

Scybala: Rounded masses or balls of fecal matter or hardened feces, the result of habitual constipation, atony or sacculation (diverticulum) of the colon, gastric ulcer, dilation, rectal cancer, or dysentery.

s., bilious. Yellowish or yellowish-brown discharges in diarrhea becoming darker on exposure.

s., fatty. Fat in the feces, as in pancreatic disease.

s., lienteric. Stool containing undigested food.

s., pea soup. Liquid stools characteristic of typhoid.

s., rice water. Watery serum stools with detached epithelium, as in cholera.

stool softeners. Substances that act as wetting agents and thus promote soft malleable bowel movements. They are not laxatives and therefore are not indicated for constipation caused by decreased or absent peristaltic activity. Docusate sodium or docusate calcium may be used to soften stools.

stopcock (stŏp'kŏk). A valve, usually made of glass if used in chemistry, that regulates the flow of fluid from a container.

stop needle. A needle with an eye at the tip and a disk on the shaft to prevent penetration deeper than desired.

stoppage (stŏp'ăj) [AS. *stoppian*]. Obstruction of an organ. SEE: *cholestasia.*

storax (stō'răks). USP. A balsam obtained from the scarred trunk of Liquidamber orientalis. It has been used as an expectorant. It is a component of tincture of benzoin.

storm [AS.]. A sudden outburst or exacerbation of symptoms of a disease.

s., renal. A sudden attack of renal symptoms accompanying a neurosis sometimes occurring in patients suffering from aortic regurgitation.

s., thyroid. A complication of thyrotoxicosis that, if untreated, is almost always fatal. Consists of abrupt onset of fever, sweating, tachycardia, pulmonary edema or congestive heart failure, tremulousness, and restlessness. Occurs in patients with untreated or poorly treated thyrotoxicosis. Usually precipitated by infection, trauma, or a surgical emergency.

stout (stowt) [O. Fr. *estout*, bold]. 1. Having a bulky body. SYN: *corpulent.* 2. Strong, dark beer.

Stoxil. Trade name for idoxuridine, USP.

STP. *standard temperature and pressure.*

STPD. *standard temperature, and pressure, dry.* Gas volume at 0° C. 760 mm. of mercury total pressure and partial pressure of water of zero, i.e., dry.

Str. *Streptococcus.*

strabismal (stră-bĭz'măl) [Gr. *strabismos*, a squint]. Strabismic, q.v.

strabismic (stră-bĭz'mĭk) [Gr. *strabismos*, a squint]. Pert. to or afflicted with strabismus.

strabismometer (stră-bĭz-mŏm'ĕt-ĕr) [" + *metron*, a measure]. Instrument for determining amount of strabismus.

strabismus (stră-bĭz'mŭs) [Gr. *strabismos*, a squinting]. Disorder of eye in which optic axes cannot be directed to same object. The squinting eye always deviates to the same extent when the eyes are carried in different directions: *unilateral* when same eye always deviates; *alternating* when either deviates, the other being fixed; *constant* when the squint remains permanent; *periodic* when eyes are occasionally free from it. Strabismus can result from reduced visual acuity, unequal ocular muscle tone, or an oculomotor nerve lesion. SYN: *heterotropia; squint.* SEE: *microstrabismus.*

s., accommodative. Strabismus due to disorder of ocular accommodation. SYN: *s., bilateral.*

s., alternating. Strabismus affecting either eye alternately.

s., bilateral. S., accommodative.

s., concomitant. Strabismus in which both eyes move freely but retain false relationship to each other.

s., convergent. Strabismus where the deviating eye turns inward.

s. deorsum vergens. Vertical strabismus, the deviating eye turning downward. SYN: *hypotropia.*

s., divergent. Strabismus in which the deviating eye turns outward.

s., horizontal. Strabismus in which the deviation of the visual axis is in the horizontal plane.

s., intermittent. Strabismus recurring at intervals.

s., monocular. Strabismus in which the same eye habitually deviates.

s., monolateral. Strabismus with the squinting eye always the same.

s., nonconcomitant. Strabismus of an

eye that varies in degree with the change in direction the eye moves.

s., paralytic. Strabismus that is due to paralysis of a muscle. The deviation is present only in the sphere of action of the paralyzed muscle. In paralytic squint, the secondary deviation is greater than the primary. This condition is due to paralysis of one or more ocular muscles and may point to grave cerebral disease or to the presence of some constitutional disease. This form of strabismus is recognized by the fact that if a light or the finger of the examiner is carried from right to left before the face of the patient, the deviating eye fails to follow to its proper limit. This response leads the physician to look for lesions of the 6th nerve in failure of external rectus, of the 3rd nerve in failure of internal rectus of either side, and of the 4th nerve in impairment of superior oblique muscles. In adults this usually is caused by syphilis involving the nerve centers or trunks.

PROG: In general, guarded.

TREATMENT: Directed to the cause. Eyeglasses or contact lenses; miotics; corrective surgery.

s., spastic. Strabismus due to contraction of an ocular muscle.

s. sursum vergens. Vertical upward squint. SYN: *hypertropia*.

ETIOL: Defects of fusion faculty, errors of refraction, poor vision in one eye, anisometropia.

TREATMENT: Refraction with prescribing of correcting lenses, orthoptic training (training of fusion), operative.

s., vertical. Strabismus in which the eye turns upward. The vision is double (diplopia) unless there is unconscious suppression of the image in the squinting eye. Expression of face is bizarre. Vertical strabismus usually is the result of ametropia in childhood, or of central nervous system disease in adult life.

strabometer (stră-bŏm′ĕt-ĕr) [Gr. *strabos,* squinting, + *metron,* a measure]. Instrument to ascertain the degree of strabismus.

strabotome (stră′bō-tōm) [″ + *tome,* incision]. A knife for performing strabotomy.

strabotomy (stră-bŏt′ō-mē) [″ + *tome,* incision]. Operation for strabismus.

strain (strān). 1. [AS. *streon,* offspring]. A stock, said of bacteria or protozoa from a specific source and maintained in successive cultures or animal inoculation. 2. Hereditary streak or tendency. 3. [O. Fr. *estreindere,* to draw tight]. To pass through, as a filter. 4. To injure by making too strong an effort or by excessive use. 5. Excessive use of a part of the body so that it is injured. 6. Trauma to the muscle or the musculotendinous unit from violent contraction or excessive forcible stretch. May be associated with failure of synergistic action of muscles. SEE: *sprain.* 7. To make a great effort as in straining to have a bowel movement. This is done by means of the Valsalva maneuver, which increases intra-abdominal pressure and helps to expel feces.

strainer (strān′ĕr). Device used for retaining solid pieces while liquid passes through. SYN: *filter.*

strain x-ray. X-ray picture taken with the part, usually a bone or joint, under static force or tension. Used to better demonstrate the pathological change, which might be inapparent if this technique were not employed.

strait (strāt) [O. Fr. *estreit,* narrow]. A constricted or narrow passage.

s., inferior. The lower outlet of the pelvic canal.

s.'s of pelvis. The inferior and superior openings of the true pelvis.

s., superior. The upper opening or inlet of the pelvic canal.

straitjacket. Shirt with long sleeves laced on patient and fastened to restrain the arms. SYN: *camisole.*

stramonium (stră-mō′nē-ŭm) [L.]. Jamestown weed, jimsonweed. The dried leaves of Datura stramonium.

USES: An ingredient in asthma powder used for its antispasmodic effect.

stramonium poisoning. Caused in children by accidental ingestion of medicine or by self-administered overdose. Related to atropine. SEE: *atropine sulfate poisoning.*

strand. A single thread or fiber.

strangalesthesia (străng″găl-ĕs-thē′zē-ă) [Gr. *strangalizein,* to choke, + *aisthesis,* sensation]. A girdlelike sensation of constriction. SYN: *zonesthesia.*

strangle (străng′gl) [L. *strangulare*]. To choke or suffocate or be choked from compression of the trachea.

strangulated (străng′ū-lā″tĕd). Constricted so that air or blood supply is cut off, as a strangulated hernia.

strangulation (străng″ū-lā′shŭn) [L. *strangulare*]. Compression or constriction of a part, as the bowel or throat, causing suspension of breathing or of passage of contents; congestion accompanies condition.

s., internal. Slipping of a coil of the intestine through the diaphragm or an abnormal opening.

strangury (străng′gū-rē) [Gr. *stranx,* a drop, + *ouron,* urine]. Painful and interrupted urination in drops produced by spasmodic muscular contraction of urethra and bladder.

strap (străp) [Gr. *strophos,* a cord]. 1. A band, as one of adhesive plaster, used to hold dressings in place or to approximate surfaces of a

wound. 2. To bind with strips of adhesive plaster.

s., Montgomery's. SEE: *Montgomery straps.*

strapping (străp′ĭng). 1. Adhesive plaster or other substance used to bind surfaces together or hold dressings in place. 2. Application of adhesive plaster strips on a part so as to give it support or compress it.

stratification (străt″ĭ-fĭ-kā′shŭn) [L. *stratificare,* to arrange in layers]. Arranged in layers.

stratified (străt′ĭ-fīd) [L. *stratificare,* to arrange in layers]. Arranged in the form of layers.

stratified epithelium. Epithelium in superimposed layers with differently shaped cells in the various layers.

stratiform (străt′ĭ-form) [L. *stratum,* layer, + *forma,* shape]. Arranged in layers, as manner of liquefaction of gelatin stab culture, in which there is liquefaction to the walls of the tube at the top and then downward horizontally.

stratum (strā′tŭm, străt′ŭm) [L.]. (pl. *strata*) A layer.

s. basale. The innermost or deepest layer of the endometrium of the uterus.

s. compactum. The superficial or outermost layer of the endometrium.

s. corneum. The outermost horny layer of the epidermis. SEE: illus.

s. disjunction. The outermost layer of the stratum corneum, which is being shed constantly.

s. germinativum. Innermost layer of epidermis. A row of columnar cells that divide to replace the rest of the epidermis as it wears away. SYN: *s. malpighii.* SEE: illus.; *prickle cell layer.*

s. granulosum. A layer of cells containing deeply staining granules of keratohyalin found in the epidermis of skin lying between stratum germinativum and stratum lucidum. SEE: illus.

s. lucidum. A translucent layer of the epidermis lying between stratum corneum and stratum granulosum. It is frequently absent. SEE: illus.

s. malpighii. Inner layer of the epidermis. SYN: *s. germinativum.*

s. mucosum. S. malpighii.

s. papillare. The papillary layer of the corium lying adjacent to the epidermis.

s. reticulare. The recticular layer of the corium lying just beneath the papillary layer.

s. spinosum. S. malpighii.

s. spongiosum. Middle layer of decidua.

s. submucosum. Layer of smooth muscle fibers of the myometrium lying contiguous with the endometrium.

STRATA OF EPIDERMIS

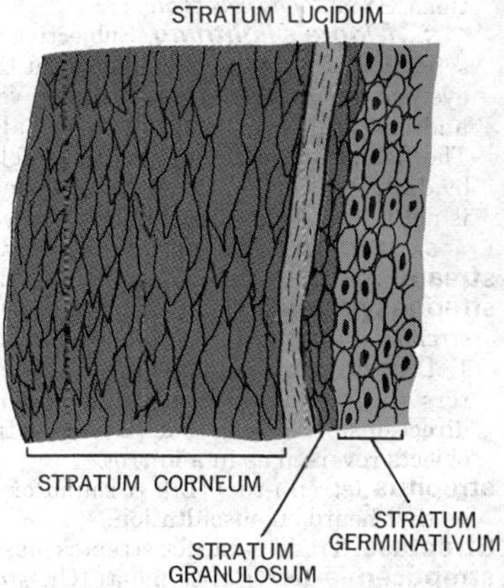

STRATUM CORNEUM OF SKIN

GREATLY THICKENED IN AREA OF CALLUS FORMATION

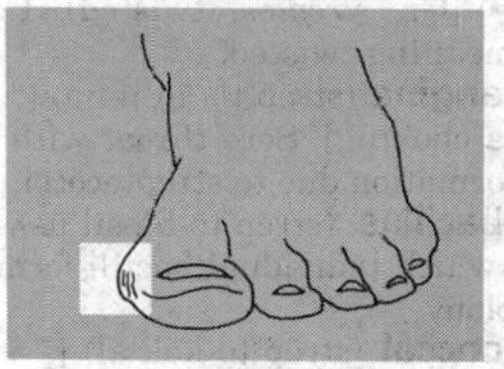

s. subserosum. Layer of smooth muscle fibers of myometrium that lies immediately under the serous coat.

s. supravasculare. A layer of circular and longitudinal muscle fibers lying between stratum subserosum and stratum vasculare.

s. vasculare. A layer of smooth muscles in myometrium lying between stratum submucosum and stratum supravasculare.

strawberry mark. A soft, nodular, vascular nevus usually present on face or neck, occurring at birth or shortly afterward. SEE: *nevus flammeus.*

strawberry tongue. The peculiar red, papillated tongue characteristic of scarlatina, q.v. SEE: *tongue.*

straw itch. A skin condition accompanied by itching due to working in straw or sleeping on a straw mattress.

streak (strēk) [AS. *strica*]. A line or stripe. SYN: *stric.*

s., angioid. A dark streak seen in the retina in individuals with pseudoxanthoma elasticum and sickle cell anemia.

s., medullary. Deep longitudinal groove on dorsal surface of the embryo that becomes the medullary tube.

s., meningitic. A red line across the skin formed by drawing a pointed article across it; seen in meningitis and nerve center affections. SYN: *tache cérébrale.*

s., Moore's lightning. Subjective visual sensation of lightning-like flashes at time of eye movements. They are usually vertical and on the lateral part of the visual field. The flashes are accompanied by or followed by dark spots before the eyes. This condition is not related to significant eye disease.

s., primitive. SEE: *primitive streak.*

stream (strēm). A steady flow of a liquid.

strephosymbolia (strĕf″ō-sĭm-bō′lē-ă) [Gr. *strephein,* to twist, + *symbolon,* symbol]. 1. Difficulty in distinguishing between letters that are similar but face in opposite directions. Ex.: p-q, b-d. 2. Perception of objects reversed as in a mirror.

strepitus (strĕp′ĭ-tŭs) [L.]. A sound or noise, as that heard on auscultation.

Streptase. Trade name for streptokinase.

strepticemia (strĕp″tĭ-sē′mē-ă) [Gr. *streptos,* twisted, + *haima,* blood]. Streptococci present in the blood causing infection. SYN: *streptococcemia.*

strepto- [Gr. *streptos,* twisted]. Combining form meaning twisted.

streptoangina (strĕp″tō-ăn′jĭ-nă) [″ + L. *angina,* a choking]. Sore throat with membranous formation due to streptococci.

streptobacillus (strĕp″tō-bă-sĭl′ŭs). A bacillus in which individual bacilli form a chain-like colony.

streptococcal (strĕp″tō-kŏk′ăl) [″ + *kokkos,* berry]. Caused by or pert. to streptococci.

streptococcemia (strĕp″tō-kŏk-sē′mē-ă) [″ + ″ + *haima,* blood]. Presence of streptococci in the blood causing infection. SYN: *strepticemia.*

streptococci (strĕp″tō-kŏk′sī). Pl. of streptococcus. SEE: *Streptococcus.*

streptococcic (strĕp″tō-kŏk′sĭk) [″ + *kokkos,* berry]. Resembling, produced by, or pert. to streptococci.

streptococcicosis (strĕp″tō-kŏk″sĭ-kō′sĭs) [″ + ″ + *osis,* condition]. Any streptococcal infection.

streptococcolysin (strĕp″tō-kŏk-kŏl′ĭ-sĭn) [″ + ″ + *lysis,* dissolution]. A lysin produced by streptococci.

Streptococcus (strĕp″tō-kŏk′ŭs) [″ + *kokkos,* berry]. (pl. *streptococci*) ABBR: Str. A genus of bacteria belonging to the family Lactobacillaceae, tribe Streptococceae. They are gram-positive cocci occurring in chains. Most species are harmless saprophytes, but some are among the most common and dangerous pathogens of man. They are differentiated on the basis of their reactions on blood-agar plates into three types: alpha (α), beta (β), and gamma (γ). Those of the alpha type (viridans group) form a greenish coloration about colonies and partially hemolyze blood; those of the beta or hemolytic type form clear zones about colonies and completely hemolyze blood (Str. pyogenes); those of the gamma type are nonhemolytic and produce a grayish coloration about colonies (Str. faecalis). SEE: *scarlet fever; rheumatic fever.*

Str. pneumoniae. Former name of Diplococcus pneumoniae.

Str. pyogenes. Any of the hemolytic streptococci causing suppurative processes. The causative agent of scarlet fever, erysipelas, septic sore throat, puerperal sepsis, and various pyogenic infections.

Str. thermophilus. Streptococcus found in dairy products.

Str. viridans. A group of α-hemolytic streptococci that are normally present in the upper respiratory tract. Minor trauma such as vigorous chewing may result in their being admitted to the bloodstream. Thus when heart valves are damaged, these organisms are the ones that most frequently colonize on them. When this occurs, subacute bacterial endocarditis has an excellent chance of developing.

streptococcus (strĕp″tō-kŏk′ŭs). (pl. *streptococci*) An organism of the genus Streptococcus. SEE: *bacteria* for illus.

s., β-hemolytic. Streptococci that, when grown on blood-agar, produce hemolysis around each colony. The hemolysis is complete and a clear zone is present at the site. Group A β-hemolytic streptococci are the type pathogenic for man.

streptocolysin (strĕp″tō-kŏl′ĭ-sĭn) [″ + *lysis,* dissolution]. A hemolysin produced by streptococci. SYN: *streptococcolysin; streptolysin.*

streptodermatitis (strĕp″tō-dĕr″mă-tī′tĭs) [″ + *derma,* skin, + *itis,* inflammation]. Inflammation of the skin caused by streptococci.

streptodornase (strĕp″tō-dor′nās). One of the enzymes (streptokinase is another) produced by certain strains of hemolytic streptococci that is capable of liquefying fibrinous and purulent exudates. SEE: *streptokinase.*

streptokinase (strĕp″tō-kī′nās). Enzyme produced by certain strains of streptococci that is capable of converting plasminogen to plasmin. SEE: *streptodornase.*

streptokinase-streptodornase. A mixture of these two enzymes. They are produced by hemolytic streptococci, and are used topically and in body cavities to remove clotted blood and purulent material.

streptoleukocidin (strĕp″tō-lū″kō-sī′dĭn) [″ + *leukos,* white, + L. *cidus,* to kill]. A toxin produced by streptococci, destructive to leukocytes.

streptolysin (strĕp-tŏl′ĭ-sĭn). A hemolysin produced by streptococci. SYN: *streptococcolysin; streptocolysin.*

s. O. A streptolysin that is inactivated by oxygen.

s. S. A streptolysin that is inactivated by heat or acid, but not by oxygen.

streptomycin sulfate (sterile) (strĕp″tō-mī′sĭn). USP. An antibiotic derived from a soil microbe, Streptomyces griseus. Trade name is Isoject-Streptomycin.

streptomycosis (strĕp″tō-mī-kō′sĭs) [″ + *mykes,* fungus, + *osis,* condition]. Infection caused by microorganisms of the genus Streptomyces.

streptosepticemia (strĕp″tō-sĕp″tĭ-sē′mē-ă) [″ + *septikos,* putrid, + *haima,* blood]. Septicemia resulting from streptococcus infection. SYN: *streptococcemia; streptomycosis.*

streptothricin (strĕp-tō-thrī′sĭn). An antibiotic biosynthesized by Streptomyces lavendulae. It is effective against both gram-negative and gram-positive bacteria and some fungi. Because of its toxicity, it is of limited usefulness.

streptothricosis (strĕp″tō-thrĭ-kō′sĭs) [Gr. *streptos,* twisted, + *thrix,* hair, + *osis,* condition]. Infection caused by a species of Streptothrix. Produces a chronic suppurative inflammation. SEE: *actinomycosis.*

stress (strĕs) [O. Fr. *estresse,* narrowness]. In medicine, the result produced when a structure, system, or organism is acted upon by forces that disrupt equilibrium or produce strain. In health care, the term denotes the physical (gravity, mechanical force, pathogen, injury) and psychological (fear, anxiety, crisis, joy) forces that are experienced by individuals. It is generally believed that biological organisms require a certain amount of stress in order to maintain their well-being. However when stress occurs in quantities that the system cannot handle, it produces pathological changes. This biological concept of stress was developed by the late Hans Selye, who intended originally for stress to indicate cause rather than effect. But through a linguistic error, he gave the term stress to effect and then later had to use the word *stressor* for the cause. SEE: *general adaptation syndrome.*

stress-breaker. A device incorporated into a removable denture. It is designed to relieve abutting teeth from excessive stress during chewing.

stress fracture. A fracture, usually of a hairline type, that develops gradually in response to repeated and prolonged stress.

stressor. An agent or condition capable of producing stress.

s., systemic. Stress that produces generalized systemic responses.

s., topical. Stress that causes mild inflammation or local damage.

stress radiography. Strain x-ray, q.v.

stress test. Method of evaluating cardiovascular fitness. While exercising, usually on a treadmill or a bicycle ergometer, the individual is subjected to steadily increasing levels of work. At the same time the amount of oxygen consumed is being determined and an electrocardiogram is being monitored. If abnormalities are noted in the ECG, the test is terminated.

stress ulcer. Peptic ulcer caused by acute or chronic stress such as cerebral trauma, burns, surgery, or acute infection.

stretch (strĕch) [AS. *streccan,* extend]. To draw out or extend to full length.

stretcher (strĕch′er). A litter for carrying the sick, injured, or dead.

stretching of contractures. Process performed to loosen contracted ligaments, muscles, and adhesions in stiff joints. There should be a slow, steady, and gradually increasing pull by the operator or with gradually increasing weights.

stretch marks. Stria, q.v.

stretch receptor. A proprioceptor located in a muscle or tendon that is stimulated by a stretch or pull.

stretch reflex. The contraction of a muscle as a result of a pull exerted upon the tendon of the responding muscle. Stretch reflexes are of primary importance in maintenance of posture. SYN: *myotactic reflex.*

stria (strī′ă) [L., a channel]. (pl. *striae*) [NA] A line or band elevated above or depressed below surrounding tissue, or differing in color and texture. SYN: *streak.*

s. acusticae. Horizontal white stripes on floor of the 4th ventricle of the brain. SYN: *stria medullares.*

s. atrophica. A fine pinkish-white or gray line, usually 14 cm. in length, seen in parts of body where skin has been stretched. Commonly seen on thighs, abdomen, and breasts of women who are or have been pregnant; in persons whose skin has been stretched by obesity, tumor, or dropsy; or in persons who have taken adrenocortical hormones for a prolonged period. SYN: *stria distensae; stria gravidarum.*

s. cerebellares. S. acusticae.

s. distensae. S. atrophica.

s. gravidarum. S. atrophica.

s. longitudinalis lateralis. One of the longitudinal bands of gray matter, slightly elevated on upper part of the corpus callosum.

s. medullares. S. acusticae.

s. terminalis. A band of fibers in roof of inferior horn running to floor of body of the lateral ventricle.

striatal (strī-ā′tăl) [L. *striatus,* striped]. Concerning the corpus striatum.

striate, striated (strī′āt, strī′ā-tĕd) [L. *stria-*

tus]. Striped; marked by streaks or striae.

striated arteries. Branches of the middle cerebral artery that supply basal nuclei of brain.

striated body. Mass of gray and white bands in each cerebral hemisphere. SYN: *corpus striatum.*

striated muscle. Skeletal muscle, consisting of fibers marked by cross striations. SEE: *muscle.*

striated veins, inferior. Branches of basal vein that drain corpus striatum.

striation (strī-ā'shŭn) [L. *striatus,* striped]. 1. State of being striped or streaked. 2. One of a series of streaks. SYN: *stria.*

striatum (strī-ā'tŭm) [L., grooved]. The caudate and lentiform nuclei of the brain considered as one. SYN: *corpus striatum.*

stricture (strĭk'chŭr) [L. *strictura,* contraction]. A narrowing or constricture of the lumen of a tube, duct, or hollow organ such as the esophagus, ureter, or urethra. Strictures may be congenital or acquired. Acquired strictures may result from infection, trauma, fibrosis resulting from mechanical or chemical irritation, muscular spasm, or pressure from adjacent structures or tumors. They may be temporary or permanent, depending on cause.

s., annular. Ringlike obstruction of an organ involving entire circumference of structure.

s., anorectal. Fibrotic narrowing of the anorectal canal.

s., bridle. Stricture caused by a band of membrane stretched across a tube, partially occluding it.

s., cicatricial. Stricture resulting from a scar or wound.

s., functional. Stricture due to muscular spasm. SYN: *s., spasmodic.*

s., impermeable. Stricture closing the lumen of a tube or canal so that an instrument cannot pass through it.

s., irritable. Stricture causing pain when an instrument is passed.

s. of urethra. Partial or complete narrowing of the urethra. Occurs most commonly in men.

SYM: Straining to pass urine, esp. at commencement of urination.

ETIOL: Spasm of urethral muscle, congestion of urethra, and fibrous formation.

s., spasmodic. S., functional.

stricturotome (strĭk'chūr-ō-tōm) [L. *strictura,* contraction, + Gr. *tome,* incision]. Instrument for cutting strictures.

stricturotomy (strĭk"chūr-ŏt'ō-mē). Operation of cutting strictures of the urethra.

stride length. The length of the stride. It is useful to measure the right and left leg stride lengths in attempting to determine a neuromuscular disease that affects only one leg.

strident (strī'dĕnt). Stridulous, q.v.

stridor (strī'dor) [L., a harsh sound]. Harsh sound during respiration; high pitched and resembling the blowing of wind, due to obstruction of air passages.

s., congenital laryngeal. Stridor present at birth or during first three weeks.

s. dentium. Noise from grinding of the teeth.

s. serraticus. Sound of respiration like that of sawing, produced by patient's tracheostomy tube.

stridulous (strĭd'ū-lŭs) [L. *stridulus*]. Making a shrill, grating sound.

string-of-pearls deformity. Fusiform enlargement of proximal and middle phalanges seen in rickets.

string sign. A greatly narrowed terminal ileum seen in roentgenological examination of abdomen in regional enteritis.

striocerebellar (strī"ō-sĕr"ĕ-bĕl'ăr) [L. *striatus,* striped, + *cerebellum,* little brain]. Concerning or affecting the corpus striatum and the cerebellum.

strip (strĭp) [AS. *striepan,* to plunder]. To remove all contents from, esp. by gentle pressure, as to strip the seminal vesicles.

strobila (strō-bī'lă) [Gr. *strobilos,* anything twisted up]. The adult form of a tapeworm.

strobiloid (strō'bĭ-loyd) [" + *eidos,* form]. Resembling a twisted chain. Tapeworm segments have this appearance.

stroboscope (strō'bō-skōp) [Gr. *strobos,* whirl, + *skopein,* to examine]. A device that produces an interrupted light. The light is shown on moving or vibrating objects. This makes it appear to be stationary. This provides the opportunity for taking a film of the various stages of the moving event.

stroke (strōk) [ME.]. 1. A sharp blow. 2. To rub gently in one direction, as in massage. 3. Gentle movement of the hand across a surface. 4. Sudden loss of consciousness followed by paralysis caused by hemorrhage into brain, formation of an embolus or thrombus that occludes an artery, or rupture of an extracerebral artery causing subarachnoid hemorrhage. SYN: *apoplexy; cerebrovascular accident.*

SYM: Onset acute. Unconsciousness. Stertorous breathing due to paralysis of portion of the soft palate; expiration puffs out the cheeks and mouth. Pupils sometimes unequal, the larger one being on the side of the hemorrhage. Paralysis usually involves one side of the face, arm and leg of one side, with eyeballs turned away from the side of the body paralysis, skin covered with clammy sweat, the surface temperature of which is often subnormal; speech disturbances. Onset more gradual if caused by a thrombosis, q.v.

F.A.: Keep patient quiet and sitting up or lying down with head and shoulders elevated. Do not give stimulants. Apply cooling applications to head and neck. Do not transport unless absolutely imperative, and then very carefully.

PROG: Depends upon symptoms. Often grave.

NURSING IMPLICATIONS: The nurse's chief concern is to maintain a patent airway. Position the patient in lateral or semiprone position with the head elevated slightly to decrease cerebral venous pressure. Use pharyngeal and tracheal suction as necessary to remove secretions and maintain a patent airway.

Initiate a neurological flow sheet to monitor signs at frequent intervals. Orient the patient at frequent intervals. Provide support to the aphasic patient. Maintain body temperature by providing appropriate nursing measures as necessary. Prescribe elimination regimen for both bowel and bladder. Maintain fluid and electrolyte balance. Initiate appropriate nursing measures to prevent the occurrence of complications of bedrest. Monitor blood pressure and administer antihypertensives as prescribed. Observe for seizure activity and initiate precautions.

Begin rehabilitation after the acute phase has subsided. Prevent deformities through exercises, proper positioning, and supportive devices such as a foot board, and splints. Provide quiet and adequate rest periods. Encourage the patients to participate in and perform their own personal hygiene and to establish independence in activities of daily living. Establish an educational program for the patient and family members that includes activity, diet, and drugs. Support the family members in their acceptance of the patient's disabilities and help them to develop realistic expectations. Provide counseling resources for the patient and family. Establish communication process for the aphasic patient. Provide positive reinforcement.

s., heat. An acute and dangerous reaction to heat exposure. The basic defect is failure of the heat-regulating mechanisms of the body. SEE: *heat hyperpyrexia.*

s., paralytic. Sudden onset of paralysis resulting from injury to brain or spinal cord. SEE: *stroke* (def. 4).

stroke volume. The amount of blood ejected by the left ventricle at each beat. Amount varies with age, sex, and exercise. SYN: *systolic discharge.*

stroking. Technique of tactile stimulation used to facilitate muscular responses in neurophysiological rehabilitation.

stroma (strō'mă) [Gr., mattress]. (pl. *stromata*) [NA] 1. Foundation-supporting tissues of an organ. Opposite of parenchyma. 2. Spongy, colorless framework of an erythrocyte.

stromal, stromatic (strō'măl, strō-măt'ĭk). Concerning or resembling the stroma of an organ.

stromatolysis (strō"mă-tŏl'ĭ-sĭs) [" + *lysis,* dissolution]. Destruction of the stroma of a cell.

stromatosis (strō"mă-tō'sĭs) [" + *osis,* condition]. Presence of mesenchymal-like tissue throughout the endometrium of the uterus.

Stromeyer's splint (strō'mī-ĕrz). [Georg F. L. Stromeyer, Ger. surgeon, 1804–1876] A hinged splint for a joint, which can be fixed at an angle.

stromuhr (strō'moor) [Ger. *strom,* stream, + *uhr,* clock]. Device for measuring velocity of blood flow. SYN: *rheometer.*

Strongyloides (strŏn"jĭ-loy'dēz). A genus of roundworms that infect man.

S. stercoralis. A roundworm that infrequently causes infection in man. It may be fatal. In the U.S.A., S. stercoralis is found mainly in the rural South. The ova hatch in the intestines of the host and rod-shaped larvae are passed in the stool. In the soil these may develop into adults and continue their life cycle or may metamorphose into filiform larvae that can infect man. The filiform larvae enter the skin, pass through the venous system to the lungs, where they migrate upward and are swallowed. A rash or pneumonia may accompany their migration. The rod-shaped larvae have the ability to metamorphose into the filiform larvae in the human intestine. This form then enters the circulation, migrates to the lungs, and begins the cycle again.

This life cycle allows for a massive infection sufficient to cause overwhelming systemic infection with fever, severe abdominal pain, shock, and possibly death. Severe reactions are more likely to occur in immunosuppressed patients or patients with diseases that alter their immune status.

TREATMENT: Thiabendazole or mebendazole are the drugs of choice. Repeated courses of treatment may be required.

strongyloidosis (strŏn"jĭ-loy-dō'sĭs) [Gr. *strongylos,* compactly formed, + *osis,* condition]. Infestation with Strongyloides.

strongylosis (strŏn"jĭ-lō'sĭs). Infestation with Strongylus.

Strongylus (strŏn'jĭ-lŭs). A genus of parasitic nematodes.

strontium (strŏn'shē-ŭm). [Strontian, mining village in Scotland] SYMB: Sr. At. wt. 87.62; at. no. 38; sp. gr. 2.6. A dark yellowish metal. Medically it is of interest because its radioactive isotope ^{90}Sr constitutes a radioactive hazard in fallout from atom bombs. The isotope has a half-life of 28 years and is stored in bone when ingested.

Strophanthus (strō-făn'thŭs) [Gr. *strophos,* twisted cord, + *anthos,* flower]. Plant yielding a poisonous, white, crystalline glucoside; used chiefly in the form of alkaloid; strophanthin. Used as a heart stimulant.

strophocephaly (strŏf"ō-sĕf'ă-lē) [" + *kephale,* head]. Distortion of the head and face due to a developmental anomaly.

strophulus (strŏf'ū-lŭs) [L.]. Papular urticaria; but the term has been used to indicate other skin conditions such as prickly heat. Because of its lack of precise meaning, this term is rarely used.

structural (strŭk'tū-răl) [L. *structura,* structure]. Pert. to organic structure.

structure (strŭk'chŭr). The arrangement of the component parts of an organism.

s., denture-supporting. The tissues that support a partial or complete denture.

struma (stroo'mă) [L. *struma,* a mass]. Enlargement of the thyroid gland. SYN: *goiter.*

s. aberranta. Struma of the accessory thyroid glands.

s., cast iron. Chronic thyroiditis accompanied by extreme development of fibrous tissue.

s. congenita. Goiter present at birth.

s. lingualis. Presence of thyroid tissue in tongue in region of foramen cecum.

s. lymphomatosa. Rare form involving a diffuse and extensive infiltration of the entire thyroid gland. SYN: *Hashimoto's struma.*

s. maligna. Carcinoma of the thyroid gland.

s. ovarii. A form of ovarian teratoma in which mass is composed of typical thyroid follicles filled with colloid.

s., Riedel's. A form of chronic thyroiditis in which the gland becomes enlarged, hard, and adherent to adjacent tissues. Follicles become atrophic and fibrosis occurs.

strumectomy (stroo-mĕk'tō-mē) [" + *ektome,* excision]. Removal of a goiter.

strumiprivous (stroo"mĭ-prī'vŭs) [" + *privus,* deprived]. Rel. to or caused by removal of the thyroid gland.

strumitis (stroo-mī'tĭs) [" + Gr. *itis,* inflammation]. Inflammation of a thyroid gland with goiter. SYN: *thyroiditis.*

strumous (stroo'mŭs) [L. *strumosus*]. 1. Affected with scrofula. SYN: *scrofulous.* 2. Affected with goiter.

Strümpell's disease (strĭm'pĕlz). Strümpell-Marie disease, q.v.

Strümpell-Marie disease. [Adolf von Strümpell, Ger. physician, 1853–1925; Pierre Marie, Fr. neurologist, 1853–1940] Ankylosing or rheumatoid spondylitis. SEE: *spondylitis, rheumatoid.*

Strümpell's sign (strĭm'pĕls). Dorsiflexion of foot when thigh is flexed on abdomen.

struvite. Crystals of magnesium ammonium phosphate. Sometimes found as a harmless ingredient of canned food, where the crystals may be mistaken for glass. Struvite crystals will dissolve in vinegar. This simple test will distinguish struvite from glass.

strychnine (strĭk'nĭn, -nēn, -nĭn) [Gr. *strychnos,* nightshade]. A poisonous alkaloid obtained from plants, as nux vomica. It has no therapeutic usefulness but has been used as an experimental tool in neuropharmacology.

strychnine poisoning. SEE: *Poisons and Poisoning* in *Appendix.*

strychninism (strĭk'nĭn-ĭzm) [" + *-ismos,* condition]. Chronic strychnine poisoning.

strychnism (strĭk'nĭzm). Poisoning from use of strychnine.

Stryker frame. A frame on which canvas is stretched, and one frame is on each side of the body. These may be secured together and thus the patient can be turned around the long axis. SEE: illus.

STS. *serological test for syphilis.*

STU. *skin test unit.*

Stuart factor. The 10th factor (Factor X) in blood coagulation. It is present in plasma and serum and is essential for blood coagulation. SYN: *thrombokinase.*

stump. The distal portion of an amputated extremity.

stump hallucination. Sensation of still possessing a limb after its amputation. SYN: *phantom limb.*

stun (stŭn) [O. Fr. *estoner,* a blow]. To render unconscious or stupefied by a blow.

stupe (stūp) [L. *stupa,* tow]. A counterirritant for topical use. It is prepared by adding a small amount of an irritant such as turpentine to a hot liquid.

stupefacient (stū"pĕ-fā'shĕnt) [L. *stupefaciens,* stupefying]. Causing or that which causes stupor. SYN: *narcotic; soporific.*

stupefactive (stū"pĕ-făk'tĭv) [L. *stupefaciens,* stupefying]. Producing narcosis or stupor.

stupemania (stū"pĕ-mā'nē-ă) [L. *stupor,* numbness, + Gr. *mania,* madness]. Insanity with symptoms of numbness.

stupor (stū'por) [L.]. 1. Condition of unconsciousness, torpor, or lethargy with suppression of sense or feeling. 2. In psychiatry, a state of lessened responsiveness. Stupor occurs in visceral and infectious diseases, melancholia, catatonia, epilepsy, paresis, poisonings, and hysteria. A benign form is seen in manic-depressive psychosis.

RS: carotic; catatonia; collapse; coma; lethargy; syncope; unconsciousness.

s., anergic. Stupor accompanied with immobility seen in certain psychoses.

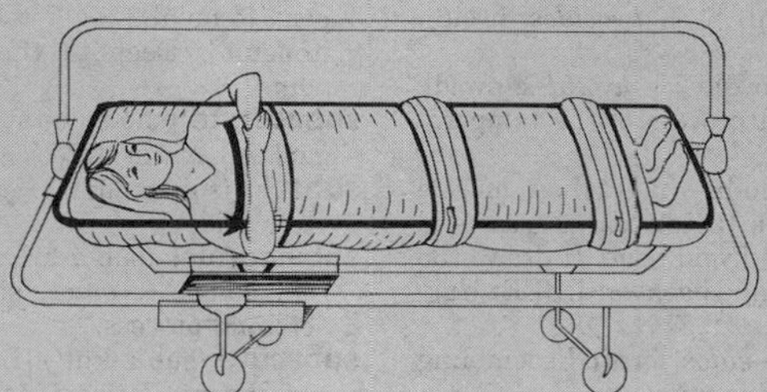

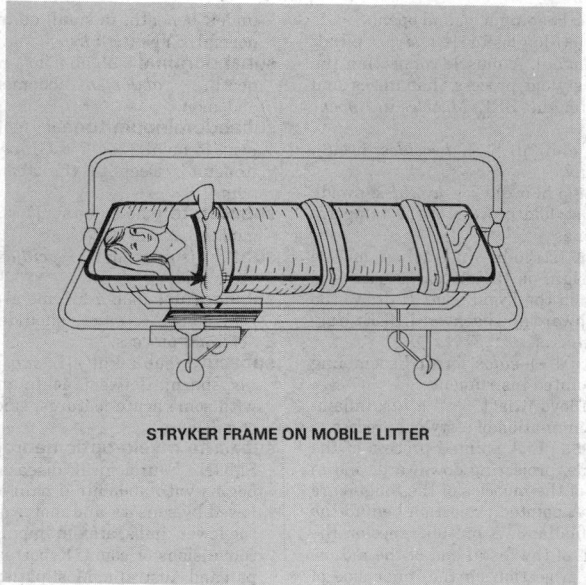

STRYKER FRAME ON MOBILE LITTER

s., delusional. Stupor accompanied by delusions.

s., epileptic. Stupor sometimes following an attack of epilepsy.

s., lethargic. Stupor accompanied by lethargy. SEE: *trance.*

s. melancholicus. Stupor associated with mental depression.

stuporous. Affected with stupor.

stuporous depression. An extremely depressed phase of manic-depressive psychosis typified by extreme psychomotor retardation and unresponsiveness to surrounding conditions.

Sturge-Weber syndrome. Congenital syndrome characterized by port-wine nevi along the distribution of the trigeminal nerve, angiomas of leptomeninges and choroid, intracranial calcifications, mental retardation, epileptic seizures, and glaucoma. SYN: *amentia, nevoid.*

sturine (stū′rĭn) [L. *sturio,* sturgeon]. Protamine obtained from sperm of sturgeon. SEE: *protamine, salmine.*

stutter (stŭt′ĕr) [ME. *stutten,* to stutter]. To hesitate and repeat or stumble spasmodically in speaking. Due to a variety of causes, among them difficulty in pronouncing initial consonants caused by spasm of lingual and palatal muscles.

stuttering (stŭt′ĕr-ĭng). Defect in speech in which there is stumbling and spasmodic repetition of the same syllable. SYN: *anarthria literalis; spasmophemia; stammering.* SEE: *lallation; mogilalia; speech.*

s., urinary. Irregular, spasmodic urination. SYN: *stammering of bladder.*

sty(e) (stī) [AS. *stigan,* to rise]. (pl. *styes; sties*) A localized circumscribed inflammatory swelling of one of several sebaceous glands of the eyelid. Caused by a bacterial infection. External styes are superficial and affect Zeis' glands or glands of Moll at the edge of the lid. Internal styes concern the meibomian or tarsal glands under the eyelid and are more severe. SYN: *hordeolum.* SEE: *chalazion.*

SYM: General edema of lid, pain, localized conjunctivitis. As the internal sty progresses, an abscess that can be seen through the conjunctiva will form.

TREATMENT: Frequent application of hot packs usually brings about drainage and resolution. Incision and drainage if not resolved. Topical antibiotics will prevent spread of infection.

s., meibomian. Inflammation of a meibomian gland.

s., zeisian. Inflammation of one of Zeis' glands.

style, stylet (stīl, stī′lĕt) [Gr. *stylos,* pillar]. 1. A slender, solid or hollow, plug of metal for making a canal permanent after operation or for stiffening or clearing a cannula or catheter. 2. A thin probe.

styliform (stī′lĭ-form) [″ + L. *forma,* form]. Long and pointed.

styliscus (stī-lĭs′kŭs) [Gr. *styliskos,* a pillar]. A slender, cylindrical plug for dilating a channel or for keeping a wound open.

styloglossus (stī-lō-glŏs′ŭs) [Gr. *stylos,* pillar, + *glossa,* tongue]. A muscle connecting the tongue and styloid process that raises and retracts the tongue. SEE: *Muscles* in *Appendix.*

stylohyal (stī″lō-hī′ăl) [″ + *hyoeides,* hyoid]. Stylohyoid, q.v.

stylohyoid (stī-lō-hī′oyd) [″ + *hyoeides,* hyoid]. Pert. to the styloid process of the temporal and hyoid bones.

stylohyoideus (stī″lō-hī-oyd′ē-ŭs). A muscle having its origin on the styloid process and its insertion on the hyoid bone. It draws the hyoid bone upward and backward. SEE: *Muscles* in *Appendix.*

styloid (stī′loyd) [″ + *eidos,* form]. Resembling a stylus or pointed instrument.

styloiditis (stī″loyd-ī′tĭs) [″ + ″ + *itis,* inflammation]. Inflammation of a styloid process.

styloid process. 1. A pointed process of the temporal bone, projecting downward, and to which some of the muscles of the tongue are attached. 2. A pointed projection behind the head of the fibula. 3. A protuberance on the outer portion of the distal end of the radius. 4. An ulnar projection on the inner side of the distal end.

stylomandibular (stī″lō-măn-dĭb′ū-lar) [″ + L. *mandibula,* lower jaw]. Concerning the styloid process of the temporal bone and the mandible.

stylomastoid (stī″lō-măs′toyd) [″ + *mastos,* breast, + *eidos,* form]. Concerning the styloid and mastoid processes of the temporal bone.

stylopharyngeus (stī″lō-făr-ĭn′jē-ŭs) [″ + *pharynx,* pharynx]. Muscle connecting the styloid process and pharynx that elevates and dilates the pharynx. SEE: *Muscles* in *Appendix.*

stylostaphyline (stī″lō-stăf′ĭ-līn) [″ + *staphyle,* bunch of grapes]. Concerning the styloid process of the temporal bone and the uvula.

stylosteophyte (stī-lŏs′tē-ō-fīt). A peg-shaped outgrowth from bone.

stylus (stī′lŭs) [Gr. *stylos,* a pillar]. 1. A probe or slender wire for stiffening or clearing a canal or catheter. 2. Pointed medicinal preparation in stick form for external application.

stype (stīp) [Gr. *stype,* tow]. A pledget or tampon of cotton or other material.

stypsis (stĭp′sĭs) [Gr., contraction]. Astringency or the use of an astringent.

styptic (stĭp′tĭk) [Gr. *styptikos,* contracting]. 1. Contracting a blood vessel; stopping a hemorrhage by astringent action. 2. Anything that stops a hemorrhage such as alum, ferrous sulfate, or tannic acid. SYN: *astringent; hemostat.*

sub- [L. *sub,* under]. Combining form meaning under, beneath, in small quantity, less than normal. SYN: [Gr.] *hypo-.*

subabdominal (sŭb″ăb-dŏm′ĭ-năl) [L. *sub,* beneath, + *abdomen,* abdomen]. Below the abdomen.

subabdominoperitoneal (sŭb″ăb-dŏm″ĭ-nō-pĕr″ĭ-tō-nē′ăl) [″ + ″ + Gr. *peritonaion,* peritoneum]. Deep to the abdominal peritoneum.

subacetate (sŭb-ăs′ĕ-tāt) [″ + *acetum,* vinegar]. A basic acetate.

subacid (sŭb-ăs′ĭd) [″ + *acidus,* sour]. Moderately acid.

subacromial (sŭb-ă-krō′mē-ăl) [″ + Gr. *akron,* point, + *omos,* shoulder]. Under the acromial process.

subacute (sŭb″ă-kūt′) [L. *sub,* under, + *acutus,* sharp]. Between acute and chronic, but with some acute features, said of the course of a disease.

subacute myelo-optic neuropathy. ABBR: SMON. Neurological disease that usually begins with abdominal pain or diarrhea followed by sensory and motor disturbances in the lower limbs, ataxia, impaired vision, and convulsions or coma. Reported mostly in Japan and Australia. Most patients survive but neurological disability remains. Many of those who have the disease have a history of taking drugs of the halogenated oxyquinoline group, but a cause-and-effect relationship has not been established.

subacute sclerosing panencephalitis. ABBR: SSPE. A cerebral degenerative disease thought to be secondary to entrance of the measles virus into the brain. The first signs are due to a progressive decrease in higher cerebral functions, usually manifested as failure to progress in school. There are personality changes, emotional instability, and generalized myoclonic jerks. In late stages dementia and generalized rigidity occur. There is no treatment and most patients die of the disease. SYN: *panencephalitis.*

subalimentation (sŭb″ăl-ĭ-mĕn-tā′shŭn) [″ + *alimentum,* food]. A state of insufficient nourishment.

subanal (sŭb-ā′năl) [″ + *analis,* anal]. Below the anus.

subanconeus (sŭb″ăn-kō′nē-ŭs) [″ + Gr. *ankon,* elbow]. 1. Below the elbow. 2. Muscle beneath the elbow that contracts its posterior ligament. SEE: *Muscles* in *Appendix.*

subapical (sŭb-ăp′ĭ-kăl) [″ + *apex,* tip]. Below the apex.

subaponeurotic (sŭb″ăp-ō-nū-rŏt′ĭk) [″ + Gr. *apo,* from, + *neuron,* tendon]. Below an aponeurosis.

subarachnoid (sŭb″ă-răk′noyd) [″ + Gr. *arachne,* spider, + *eidos,* form]. Between the arachnoid membrane and the pia mater.

subarachnoid cisternae. Spaces at the base

of the brain where the arachnoid becomes widely separated from the pia, giving rise to large cavities.

subarachnoid space. Space between the pia proper and arachnoid containing the cerebrospinal fluid.

subarcuate (sŭb-ăr'kū-āt) [L. *sub,* beneath, + *arcuatus,* arched]. Slightly arched.

subarcuate fossa. Depression that extends backward as a blind tunnel under the superior semicircular canal of the temporal bone.

subareolar (sŭb"ă-rē'ō-lăr) [" + *areola,* a small space]. Below the areola.

subastragalar (sŭb-ăs-trăg'ă-lăr) [" + Gr. *astragalos,* ball of the ankle joint]. Beneath the astragalus.

subastringent (sŭb"ăs-trĭn'jĕnt) [" + *astringere,* to contract]. Mildly astringent.

subatomic (sŭb"ă-tŏm'ĭk) [" + Gr. *atomos,* indivisible]. Less than the size of an atom.

subaural (sŭb-aw'răl) [" + *auris,* ear]. Below the ear.

subauricular (sŭb"aw-rĭk'ū-lăr) [" + *auricula,* little ear]. Below an auricle, esp. of the ear.

subaxial (sŭb-ăk'sē-ăl) [" + *axis,* axis]. Below an axis.

subaxillary (sŭb-ăk'sĭ-lĕr"ē) [" + *axilla,* armpit]. Below the axilla, or armpit.

subbrachycephalic (sŭb"bră-kē-sĕ-făl'ĭk) [" + Gr. *brachys,* short, + *kephale,* head]. Having a cephalic index of 78 to 79.

subcalcarine (sŭb-kăl'kăr-īn) [" + *calca,* spur]. Below the calcarine sulcus.

subcapsular (sŭb-kăp'sū-lăr) [" + *capsula,* a little box]. Below any capsule, esp. the capsule of the brain, or a capsular ligament.

subcarbonate (sŭb-kăr'bō-nāt) [" + *carbo,* coal]. A basic carbonate; one having proportion of carbonic acid radical less than the normal carbonate.

subcartilaginous (sŭb"kăr-tĭ-lăj'ĭn-ŭs) [" + *cartilago,* cartilage]. 1. Located beneath a cartilage. 2. Cartilaginous in part.

subception (sŭb-sĕp'shŭn). Subliminal perception.

subchondral (sŭb-kŏn'drăl) [" + *chondrus,* cartilage]. Below or under a cartilage.

subchoroidal (sŭb"kō-roy'dăl) [" + Gr. *chorioeides,* skinlike]. Below the choroid.

subchronic (sŭb-krŏn'ĭk) [" + Gr. *chronos,* time]. Noting a condition between subacute and chronic; almost chronic.

subclass (sŭb'klăs). In taxonomy, between a class and an order.

subclavian (sŭb-klā'vē-ăn) [" + *clavis,* a key]. Under the clavicle or collarbone. SYN: *subclavicular.*

subclavian artery. Large artery at base of neck that supplies blood to arm. The right subclavian artery branches from the innominate artery; the left subclavian artery branches from the aortic arch.

subclavian steal syndrome. Shunting of blood, which was destined for the brain, away from the cerebral circulation. This occurs when the subclavian artery is occluded. Blood then flows from the opposite vertebral artery across to and down the vertebral artery on the side of the occlusion.

SYM: Signs of insufficient blood flow to the brain. Symptoms are transient and are aggravated by exercise. Usually the blood pressure in the arm on the affected side will be significantly lower than in the other arm.

subclavian triangle. Triangle-shaped part of the neck formed by the clavicle and the omohyoid and sternomastoid muscles.

subclavian vein. Large vein draining arm. It unites with the interior jugular to form the innominate vein.

subclavicular (sŭb"klă-vĭk'ū-lăr) [L. *sub,* beneath, + *clavicula,* a little key]. Beneath the clavicle. SYN: *subclavian.*

subclavius (sŭb-klā'vē-ŭs) [" + *clavis,* a key]. A tiny muscle from the first rib to the undersurface of the clavicle. SEE: *Muscles* in *Appendix.*

subclinical (sŭb-klĭn'ĭ-kăl) [" + Gr. *klinikos,* pert. to a bed]. Pert. to a period before appearance of typical symptoms of a disease or to a disease or condition that does not present clinical symptoms. Some infections may not produce characteristic symptoms, but can be demonstrated by antigenic reactions.

subcollateral (sŭb-kō-lăt'ĕr-ăl) [" + *con,* with, + *latus,* side]. Below the collateral fissure, indicating a cerebral convolution.

subconjunctival (sŭb"kŏn-jŭnk-tī'văl) [" + *conjunctiva,* a joining]. Beneath the conjunctiva.

subconsciousness (sŭb-kŏn'shŭs-nĕs) [" + *conscius,* aware]. 1. The state of being partially unconscious. 2. The condition in which mental processes take place without the individual's being aware of their occurrence. SEE: *subliminal.*

subcontinuous (sŭb"kŏn-tĭn'ū-ŭs) [" + *continuus,* holding together]. Almost continuous; with periods of abatement.

subcontinuous fever. Fever with periods of remission and exacerbation. SYN: *remittent fever.*

subcoracoid (sŭb-kor'ă-koyd) [" + Gr. *korakoeides,* crowlike]. Beneath the coracoid process.

subcortex (sŭb-kor'tĕks) [" + *cortex,* rind]. White substance of the brain underlying the cortex.

subcortical (sŭb-kor'tĭ-kăl). Pert. to the region beneath the cerebral cortex.

subcostal (sŭb-kŏs'tăl) [" + *costa,* rib]. Beneath the ribs.

subcostalgia (sŭb"kŏs-tăl'jē-ă) [" + " + Gr.

algos, pain]. Pain in region over the subcostal nerve.

subcranial (sŭb-krā′nē-ăl) [″ + Gr. *kranion,* skull]. Beneath or below the cranium.

subcrepitant (sŭb-krĕp′ĭ-tănt) [″ + *crepitare,* to rattle]. Partially crepitant or crackling in character; noting a rale.

subcrureus (sŭb-kroo-rē′ŭs) [″ + *crus,* leg]. Small muscle between anterior surface of femoral shaft and synovial membrane of knee joint. SEE: *Muscles* in *Appendix.*

subculture (sŭb-kŭl′chūr) [″ + *cultura,* cultivation]. To make a culture of bacteria with material derived from another culture.

subcutaneous (sŭb″kū-tā′nē-ŭs) [″ + *cutis,* skin]. Beneath or to be introduced beneath the skin. SYN: *hypodermic.*

subcutaneous surgery. Operation performed through a small opening in the skin.

subcutaneous wound. A wound with only a small opening through the skin.

subcuticular (sŭb″kū-tĭk′ū-lăr) [L. *sub,* beneath, + *cuticula,* little skin]. Beneath the cuticle or epidermis. SYN: *subepidermal.*

subcutis (sŭb-kū′tĭs). The layer of connective tissue beneath the skin.

subdelirium (sŭb″dē-lĭr′ē-ŭm) [″ + *de,* away from, + *lira,* track]. A mild or partial state of delirium.

subdeltoid (sŭb-dĕl′toyd) [″ + Gr. *delta,* letter d, + *eidos,* form]. Beneath the deltoid muscle.

subdental (sŭb-dĕn′tăl) [″ + *dens,* tooth]. Beneath the teeth, or a tooth.

subdermal [″ + Gr. *derma,* skin]. Below the skin.

subdiaphragmatic (sŭb″dī-ă-frăg-măt′ĭk) [″ + Gr. *dia,* across, + *phragma,* wall]. Beneath the diaphragm. SYN: *subphrenic.*

subdorsal (sŭb-dor′săl) [″ + *dorsum,* back]. Below the dorsal area.

subduct (sŭb-dŭkt′) [″ + *ducere,* to lead]. To draw down.

subdural (sŭb-dū′răl) [″ + *durus,* hard]. Beneath the dura mater.

subdural space. Space between the arachnoid and dura mater.

subendocardial (sŭb″ĕn-dō-kăr′dē-ăl) [″ + Gr. *endon,* within, + *kardia,* heart]. Below the endocardium.

subendothelial (sŭb″ĕn-dō-thē′lē-ăl) [″ + Gr. *endon,* within, + *thele,* nipple]. Beneath the endothelium.

subendothelium (sŭb″ĕn-dō-thē′lē-ŭm) [″ + Gr. *endon,* within, + *thele,* nipple]. Beneath the endothelium.

subependymal (sŭb″ĕp-ĕn′dĭ-măl) [″ + Gr. *ependyma,* ependyma]. Beneath the ependyma.

subepidermal (sŭb″ĕp-ĭ-dĕr′măl) [″ + Gr. *epi,* upon, + *derma,* skin]. Beneath the epidermis. SYN: *subcuticular.*

subepithelial (sŭb″ĕp-ĭ-thē′lē-ăl) [″ + ″ + *thele,* nipple]. Beneath the epithelium.

suberosis (sū″bĕr-ō′sĭs) [L. *suber,* cork, + Gr. *osis,* condition]. Pulmonary hypersensitivity reaction in workers exposed to cork. The antigen is present in a mold in the cork.

subfamily (sŭb-făm′ĭ-lē). In taxonomy, between a family and a tribe.

subfascial (sŭb-făsh′ē-ăl) [L. *sub,* beneath, + *fascia,* band]. Beneath a fascia.

subfebrile (sŭb-fē′brĭl) [″ + *febris,* fever]. Mild fever, usually considered to be less than 101° F. (38.3° C.).

subfertility (sŭb″fĕr-tĭl′ĭ-tē) [″ + *fertilis,* fertile]. Not as fertile as would be considered normal.

subflavous (sŭb-flā′vŭs) [″ + *flavus,* yellow]. Yellowish.

subflavous ligament. Yellowish ligament connecting the laminae of the vertebrae.

subfolium (sŭb-fō′lē-ŭm) [″ + *folium,* leaf]. A leaf-like division of the cerebellar folia.

subfrontal (sŭb-frŏn′tăl) [″ + *frons,* forehead]. Below a frontal convolution or lobe of the brain.

subgenus (sŭb-jē′nŭs). In taxonomy, between a genus and species.

subgingival (sŭb-jĭn′jĭ-văl) [″ + *gingiva,* gum]. Beneath the gingiva. Related to a point or area apical to the margin of the free gingiva, usually within the confines of the gingival sulcus, e.g., subgingival calculus, or subgingival margin of a restoration.

subglenoid (sŭb-glē′noyd) [″ + Gr. *glene,* cavity, + *eidos,* form]. Below the glenoid fossa or glenoid cavity.

subglossal (sŭb-glŏs′ăl) [″ + Gr. *glossa,* tongue]. Under the tongue. SYN: *hypoglossal; sublingual.*

subglossitis (sŭb-glŏs-sī′tĭs) [″ + ″ + *itis,* inflammation]. Inflammation of the undersurface or tissues of the tongue.

subglottic (sŭb-glŏt′ĭk) [″ + Gr. *glottis,* back of tongue]. Beneath the glottis.

subgranular (sŭb-grăn′ū-lăr) [″ + *granulum,* little grain]. Not completely granular.

subgrondation, subgrundation (sŭb-grŏn-dā′shŭn, -grŭn-dă′shŭn) [Fr.]. Depression of one fragment of a broken bone beneath the other, as of the cranium.

subhepatic (sŭb″hĕ-păt′ĭk) [L. *sub,* beneath, + Gr. *hepar,* liver]. Beneath the liver.

subhyaloid (sŭb-hī′ă-loyd) [″ + Gr. *hyalos,* glass, + *eidos,* form]. Located beneath the hyaloid membrane.

subhyoid (sŭb-hī′oyd) [″ + Gr. *hyoeides,* U-shaped]. Beneath the hyoid bone.

subicteric (sŭb″ĭk-tĕr′ĭk) [″ + Gr. *ikteros,* jaundice]. Mildly jaundiced.

subicular (sŭ-bĭk′ū-lăr). Concerning the uncinate gyrus.

subiliac (sŭb-ĭl′ē-ăk) [″ + *iliacus,* pert. to the

hip]. 1. Below the ilium. 2. Pert. to the subilium.

subilium (sŭb-ĭl'ē-ŭm). The lowest part of the ilium.

subincision. Production of a fistula of the penile urethra. May interfere with conception. Used by some primitive groups, esp. Australian aborigines.

subinfection (sŭb"ĭn-fĕk'shŭn) [" + *infectio,* a putting into]. Mild infection with minimal clinical signs or symptoms.

subinflammation [" + *inflammatio,* a setting on fire]. Very mild inflammation. SYN: *irritation.*

subinflammatory (sŭb"ĭn-flăm'ă-tō-rē). Very mildly inflammatory.

subintimal (sŭb-ĭn'tĭ-măl) [" + *intima,* innermost]. Beneath the intima.

subintrant (sŭb-ĭn'trănt) [L. *subintrans,* stealing into]. Having cycles or paroxysms in such rapid succesion that they intermingle and thus overlap. SYN: *proleptic.*

subintrant fever. Intermittent fever in which the paroxysms occur so rapidly that one comes on before the previous one has disappeared.

subinvolution (sŭb"ĭn-vō-lū'shŭn) [L. *sub,* beneath, + *involutio,* a turning into]. Imperfect involution; incomplete return of a part to normal dimensions after physiological hypertrophy, as when the uterus fails to reduce to normal size following childbirth. SEE: *uterus.*

subjacent (sŭb-jā'sĕnt) [" + *jacere,* to lie]. Lying underneath.

subject (sŭb'jĕkt) [L. *subjectus,* brought under]. 1. A patient undergoing treatment, observation, or investigation; a well person participating in a medical or scientific investigation. 2. A body used for dissection. 3. To have a liability to develop attacks of a particular disease. 4. To submit to a procedure or to the action of another.

subjective [L. *subjectivus*]. Arising from or concerned with the individual; not perceptible to an observer. Opposite of objective.

subjective sensation. A sensation occurring when stimuli due to internal causes excite the nervous system; one not of objective origin.

subjective symptoms. Those symptoms that are of internal origin and evident only to the patient.

subjugal (sŭb-jū'găl) [L. *sub,* beneath, + *jugum,* yoke]. Below the malar bone or os zygomaticum.

sublatio (sŭb-lā'shē-ō) [L.]. Removal, elevation, or detachment of a part.

s. retinae. Detachment of the retina.

sublation (sŭb-lā'shŭn) [L. *sublatio,* elevation]. The displacement, elevation, or removal of a part.

sublesional (sŭb-lē'shŭn-ăl) [L. *sub,* beneath, + *laesio,* wound]. Beneath a lesion.

sublethal (sŭb-lē'thăl) [" + Gr. *lethe,* oblivion]. Less than lethal; almost fatal.

sublethal dose. Dose containing not quite enough of a toxin or noxious substance to cause death.

sublimate (sŭb'lĭ-māt) [L. *sublimare,* to elevate]. 1. A substance obtained or prepared by sublimation. 2. To cause a solid or gas to change state without becoming a liquid during transition. Ex.: Ice may evaporate without first becoming a liquid. 3. An ego defense mechanism by which one diverts unwanted aggressive or sexual drives into socially acceptable activities.

sublimation (sŭb"lĭ-mā'shŭn) [L. *sublimatio*]. 1. Altering the state of a gas or solid without first changing it into a liquid. 2. Conversion of unwanted aggressive or sexual drives into socially acceptable channels. A freudian term pert. to unconscious mental processes of ego defense whereby unwanted sexual or aggressive drives find an outlet through creative mental work.

Sublimaze. Trade name for fentanyl citrate, USP.

sublime (sŭb-līm') [L. *sublimis,* to the limit]. To evaporate a substance directly from the solid into the vapor state and condense it again. Thus metallic iodine on heating does not liquefy, but forms directly a violet gas.

subliminal (sŭb-lĭm'ĭn-ăl). 1. Below the threshold of sensation; too weak to arouse sensation or muscular contraction. 2. Below the normal consciousness.

subliminal self. In psychiatry, part of the normal individual's personality in which mental processes function without consciousness under normal waking conditions.

sublimis (sŭb-lī'mĭs) [L.]. Near the surface.

sublingual (sŭb-lĭng'gwăl) [L. *sub,* under, + *lingua,* tongue]. Beneath or concerning the area beneath the tongue.

sublingual gland. The smallest of the salivary glands, located between side of tongue and the mandible, one on each side. It has about 20 ducts, most of which open directly above the gland.

sublinguitis (sŭb"lĭng-gwī'tĭs) [" + " + Gr. *itis,* inflammation]. Inflammation of the sublingual gland.

sublobular (sŭb-lŏb'ū-lăr) [" + *lobulus,* a lobule]. Beneath a lobule.

sublumbar (sŭb-lŭm'băr) [" + *lumbus,* loin]. Below the lumbar region.

subluxation (sŭb"lŭks-ā'shŭn) [" + *luxatio,* dislocation]. 1. A partial or incomplete dislocation. 2. In dentistry, it also means injury to supporting tissues that results in abnormal loosening of teeth without displacement, or when loosely applied to the temporomandibular joint, refers to the relaxation or stretching of the capsule and ligaments that results in popping noises during movement or partial dislocation of the mandible forward.

submammary (sŭb-măm′ă-rē) [″ + *mamma,* breast]. Below the mammary gland.

submandibular [″ + *mandibula,* lower jaw bone]. Beneath the mandible or lower jaw.

submandibular gland. One of the salivary glands, a mixed tubuloalveolar gland about the size of a walnut that lies in digastric triangle beneath the mandible. Its main duct (Wharton's duct) opens at the side of the frenulum linguae.

submandibularitis. Inflammation of or mumps affecting the submandibular gland.

submarginal (sŭb-măr′jĭn-ăl) [″ + *marginalis,* margin]. Close to or next to a margin or border of a part. In dentistry, pert. to a deficiency in material or contour at the margin of a restoration in a tooth.

submedial, submedian (sŭb-mē′dē-ăl, -ăn) [″ + *medium,* middle]. Below or close to the middle.

submembranous (sŭb-mĕm′bră-nŭs) [″ + *membrana,* membrane]. Containing partly membranous material.

submental [″ + *mentum,* chin]. Under the chin.

submerge (sŭb-mĕrj′) [″ + *mergere,* to immerse]. To place under water.

submetacentric (sŭb″mĕt-ă-sĕn′trĭk) [″ + Gr. *meta,* beyond, + *kentron,* center]. Concerning a chromosome in which the centromere is within the two central quarters but away from the middle.

submicron [″ + Gr. *mikros,* tiny]. A particle smaller than 10^{-5} cm. in diameter. Visible only with an ultramicroscope. SEE: *micron.*

submicroscopic [″ + ″ + *skopein,* to examine]. Too minute to be seen through a microscope. SYN: *amicroscopic.*

submorphous (sŭb-mor′fŭs) [″ + Gr. *morphe,* form]. Neither completely amorphous nor crystalline, as some calculi.

submucosa (sŭb″mū-kō′să) [L. *sub,* beneath, + *mucosus,* mucous]. The layer of areolar connective tissue under a mucous membrane.

submucous (sŭb-mū′kŭs) [″ + *mucus,* mucus]. Beneath a mucous membrane.

submucous resection. Removal of tissue below the mucosa, esp. excision of cartilaginous tissue beneath the mucosal tissue of the nose.

subnarcotic (sŭb-năr-kŏt′ĭk) [″ + Gr. *narkotikos,* numb]. Mildly narcotic.

subnasal [″ + *nasus,* nose]. Under the nose.

subnasale (sŭb″nā-sā′lē) [″ + *nasus,* nose]. The base of the anterior nasal spine.

subnasal point. Craniometric point at base of the nasal spine.

subnasion (sŭb-nā′zē-ŏn) [″ + *nasus,* nose]. Subnasal.

subneural (sŭb-nū′răl) [″ + Gr. *neuron,* nerve]. Beneath the neural axis or the central nervous system.

subnormal (sŭb-nor′măl) [″ + *norma,* rule]. Less than normal or average.

subnormality (sŭb″nor-măl′ĭ-tē) [″ + *normalis,* normal]. Being subnormal.

subnucleus (sŭb-nū′klē-ŭs) [″ + *nucleus,* a nut]. One of the secondary nuclei into which a nucleus of the central nervous system may be divided.

suboccipital (sŭb″ŏk-sĭp′ĭ-tăl) [″ + *occiput,* back of head]. Situated below the occiput or occipital bone.

suboperculum (sŭb″ō-pĕr′kū-lŭm) [″ + *operculum,* covering]. Portion of occipital convolution overlapping the insula. SEE: *operculum.*

suboptimal (sŭb-ŏp′tĭ-măl) [″ + *optimum,* best]. Less than optimum.

suborbital (sŭb-or′bĭ-tăl) [″ + *orbita,* track]. Beneath the orbit.

suborder (sŭb-or′dĕr). In taxonomy, between an order and a family.

suboxides (sŭb-ŏk′sīdz). In a series of oxides, ones that contain the smallest amount of oxygen.

subpapular (sŭb-păp′ū-lăr) [″ + *papula,* pimple]. Very slightly papular, as papules elevated being scarcely more than macules.

subparietal (sŭb″pă-rī′ĕ-tăl) [″ + *paries,* wall]. Below the parietal bone, or lobe.

subpatellar (sŭb″pă-tĕl′ăr) [″ + *patella,* a pan]. Beneath the patella.

subpectoral (sŭb-pĕk′tor-ăl) [″ + *pectus,* chest]. Below the pectoral area; beneath the pectoral muscles.

subpeduncular (sŭb″pē-dŭn′kū-lăr) [″ + *pedunculus,* a stem]. Below a peduncle.

subpeduncular lobe. Tiny lobe on undersurface of either cerebellar hemisphere. SYN: *flocculus.*

subpelviperitoneal (sŭb-pĕl″vē-pĕr″ĭ-tō-nē′ăl) [L. *sub,* beneath, + *pelvis,* basin, + Gr. *peritonaion,* peritoneum]. Beneath the pelvic peritoneum.

subpericardial (sŭb″pĕr-ĭ-kăr′dē-ăl) [″ + Gr. *peri,* around, + *kardia,* heart]. Beneath the pericardium.

subperiosteal (sŭb″pĕr-ē-ŏs′tē-ăl) [″ + ″ + *osteon,* bone]. Beneath the periosteum.

subperitoneal (sŭb″pĕr-ĭ-tō-nē′ăl) [″ + Gr. *peritonaion,* peritoneum]. Beneath the peritoneum.

subperitoneoabdominal (sŭb″pĕr-ĭ-tō-nē″ō-ăb-dŏm′ĭ-năl) [″ + ″ + L. *abdomen,* abdomen]. Subperitoneal.

subpharyngeal (sŭb″făr-ĭn′jē-ăl) [″ + Gr. *pharynx,* pharynx]. Beneath the pharynx.

subphrenic (sŭb-frĕn′ĭk) [″ + Gr. *phren,* diaphragm]. Beneath the diaphragm. SYN: *subdiaphragmatic.*

subphrenic abscess. Collection of pus beneath the diaphragm.

subphylum (sŭb-fī′lŭm). In taxonomy, between a phylum and a class.

subpial (sŭb-pī′ăl) [″ + *pia*, soft]. Beneath the pia.

subplacenta (sŭb″plă-sĕn′tă) [″ + *placenta*, a flat cake]. During pregnancy the endometrium that lines the entire uterine cavity except at the site of the implanted blastocyst. SYN: *decidua parietalis* [NA].

subpleural (sŭb-plū′răl) [″ + Gr. *pleura*, a side]. Beneath the pleura.

subpontine (sŭb-pŏn′tĭn, -tīn) [″ + *pons*, bridge]. Below the pons.

subpreputial (sŭb″prē-pū′shăl) [″ + *praeputium*, prepuce]. Under the prepuce.

subpubic (sŭb-pū′bĭk) [″ + *pubes*, pubis]. Beneath the pubic arch, as a ligament, or performed beneath the pubic arch.

subpulmonary (sŭb-pŭl′mō-nă-rē) [″ + *pulmon*, lung]. Below the lung.

subpyramidal (sŭb″pī-răm′ĭ-dăl) [″ + Gr. *pyramis*, a pyramid]. Beneath a pyramid of the kidney.

subretinal (sŭb-rĕt′ĭ-năl) [″ + *rete*, a net]. Beneath the retina.

subscapular (sŭb-skăp′ū-lăr) [″ + *scapula*, shoulder]. Below the scapula.

subscleral (sŭb-sklē′răl) [″ + Gr. *skleros*, hard]. Beneath the sclera of the eye.

subsclerotic (sŭb-sklē-rŏt′ĭk) [″ + Gr. *skleros*, hard]. 1. Subscleral. 2. Not completely sclerosed.

subscription (sŭb-skrĭp′shŭn) [L. *subscriptas*, written under]. That part of a prescription that contains directions for compounding ingredients.

subserous (sŭb-sē′rŭs) [L. *sub*, beneath, + *serum*, whey]. Beneath a serous membrane.

subsibilant (sŭb-sĭb′ĭ-lănt) [″ + *sibilans*, hissing]. Having the sound of a muffled whistle.

subsidence (sŭb-sīd′ĕns) [L. *subsidere*, to sink down]. The gradual disappearance of symptoms or manifestations of a disease.

subspecies (sŭb′spē-sēz). In taxonomy, subordinate to a species.

subspinale (sŭb″spī-nā′lē) [″ + *spina*, thorn]. The deepest point between the nasal spine and the crest of the maxilla.

subspinous (sŭb-spī′nŭs) [″ + *spina*, thorn]. 1. Beneath any spinous process. 2. Anterior to or beneath the spinal column.

subspinous dislocation. Dislocation with head of the humerus resting below spine of the scapula.

substage (sŭb′stāj) [″ + O. Fr. *estage*, position]. That part of the microscope below the stage by which attachments are held in place.

substance (sŭb′stăns) [L. *substantia*]. Material of which any organ or tissue is composed; matter.

s., anterior perforated. Portion of rhinencephalon lying immediately anterior to optic chiasma. It is perforated by numerous small arteries.

s., anterior pituitary–like. Chorionic gonadotrophin. SEE: *gonadotrophin*.

s., black. Substantia nigra.

s., chromophilic. Substance found in the cytoplasm of certain cells that stains similar to chromatin with basic dyes. Includes Nissl bodies of neurons and granules in serozymogenic cells.

s., colloid. Jellylike substance in colloid degeneration.

s., gray. Gray matter of the brain and spinal cord.

s., ground. The matrix or intercellular substance in which the cells of an organ or tissue are embedded.

s., ketogenic. A substance that, in its metabolism, gives rise to ketone bodies.

s., medullary. The soft inner material of any part such as a bone or organ.

s., Nissl. Chromatophilic substance of nerve cells. SEE: *Nissl bodies*.

s., posterior perforated. A triangular area forming floor of the interpeduncular fossa. It lies immediately behind the corpora mammillaria and contains numerous openings for blood vessels.

s., pressor. A substance that elevates arterial blood pressure.

s., reticular. The skein of threads present in some red blood cells. These are visible only when the cells are appropriately stained.

s., slow-reacting. SEE: *slow-reacting substance*.

s., specific soluble. ABBR: SSS. A polysaccharide hapten obtained from the capsules of pneumococci.

s., threshold, high. A substance such as glucose or sodium chloride present in the blood and excreted by the kidney only when its concentration exceeds a certain level.

s., threshold, low. A substance such as urea or uric acid that is excreted by the kidney from the blood almost in its entirety. It occurs in the urine in high concentrations.

s., transmitter. Neurotransmitter.

s., white. White matter of brain and spinal cord.

s., white, of Schwann. A nerve fiber's medullary sheath.

substandard. Failing to meet the usual or accepted standard.

substantia (sŭb-stăn′shē-ă) [L.]. Material of which any organ or tissue is composed; matter. SYN: *substance*.

s. alba. [NA] White substance of the brain. SEE: *matter, white*.

s. cinerea. Gray substance of brain and

spinal cord.

s. ferruginea. [NA] Elongated mass of pigmented cells in the locus ceruleus.

s. gelatinosa. [NA] Gray matter of the cord surrounding central canal and capping head of posterior horns of spinal cord.

s. grisea. [NA] Gray matter of the spinal cord. SEE: *matter, gray.*

s. nigra. [NA] Black substance in a section of the crus cerebri. SYN: *locus niger.*

s. propria membranae tympani. Fibrous middle layer of drum membrane.

substernal (sŭb-stĕr′năl) [L. *sub,* beneath, + Gr. *sternon,* chest]. Situated beneath the sternum.

substernomastoid (sŭb″stĕr-nō-măs′toyd) [″ + ″ + Gr. *mastos,* breast, + *eidos,* form]. Beneath the sternomastoid muscle.

substitute (sŭb′stĭ-tūt). Something that may be used in place of another.

s., blood. A fluid used to expand the plasma volume, but not a true substitute for the blood. Artificial substances capable of functioning as blood are being investigated.

s., plasma. SEE: *s., blood.*

substitution (sŭb-stĭ-tū′shŭn) [L. *substitutio,* replacing]. 1. Displacing an atom (or more than one) of an element in a compound by atoms of another element of equal valence. 2. In psychiatry, the ego defense mechanism of turning from an obstructed desire to one whose gratification is socially acceptable. 3. The turning from an obstructed form of behavior to a more primitive one, as a substitution neurosis. 4. The replacement of a substance by another. 5. In pharmacy, the replacement of one drug by another drug in dispensing. Usually a generic drug is substituted for a proprietary one.

substitution products. Compounds formed by an element or a radical replacing another element or radical in a compound.

substitution therapy. The use in treatment of a substance such as a product of glandular secretion (hormone or enzyme) to replace natural substance in body. This method is employed when glands fail to secrete properly or substance secreted is unavailable to tissues.

substitutive (sŭb′stĭ-tū″tĭv) [L. *substitutivus*]. Causing a change or substitution of characteristics.

substitutive therapy. Treatment to overcome an inflammation of a specific character by exciting an acute nonspecific inflammation.

substrate, substratum (sŭb′strāt, sŭb-strā′tŭm) [L. *substratum,* to lie under]. 1. An underlying layer or foundation. 2. A base, as of a pigment. 3. The substance acted upon, as by an enzyme. SYN: *zymolyte.* SEE: *enzyme.*

substructure (sŭb′strŭk-chŭr). The underlying structure of supporting material.

subsultus (sŭb-sŭl′tŭs) [L., springing up]. Any tremor or twitching.

s. tendinum. Involuntary twitchings of muscles, esp. of arms and feet, causing movement of tendons. Observed in certain febrile conditions.

subsylvian (sŭb-sĭl′vē-ăn). Below the fissure of Sylvius.

subtarsal (sŭb-tăr′săl) [L. *sub,* beneath, + Gr. *tarsos,* tarsus]. Below the tarsus.

subtentorial. Located beneath the tentorium.

subterminal (sŭb-tĕr′mĭ-năl) [″ + *terminus,* boundary]. Close to the end of an extremity.

subtetanic (sŭb″tē-tăn′ĭk) [″ + Gr. *tetanikos,* tetanic]. Moderately tetanic.

subthalamic (sŭb″thă-lăm′ĭk) [″ + Gr. *thalamos,* chamber]. Located below the thalamus.

subthalamic nucleus. An elliptical mass of gray matter lying in the ventral thalamus above the cerebral peduncle and rostral to substantia nigra. It receives fibers from the globus pallidus.

subthalamus. Portion of the diencephalon lying below the thalamus and above the hypothalamus. SEE: *thalamus.*

subtile, subtle (sŭb′tĭl, sŭt′l) [L. *subtilis,* fine]. 1. Very fine or delicate. 2. Very acute. 3. Mentally acute or crafty or piercing, as sharp. 4. Causing injury without attracting attention, as subtle poisons or early symptoms of a disease.

subtilin (sŭb′tĭl-ĭn). An antibiotic biosynthesized by Bacillus subtilis. It is of low toxicity and effective against gram-positive organisms.

subtotal (sŭb-tō′tăl) [L. *sub,* beneath, + *totus,* whole]. Less than total, as partial removal of a gland.

subtraction. Process by which undesired, overlying structures can be removed from a radiographic image.

subtrapezial (sŭb″tră-pē′zē-ăl) [″ + Gr. *trapezion,* a little table]. Beneath the trapezius muscle.

subtribe (sŭb′trīb). In taxonomy, between a genus and a tribe.

subtrochanteric (sŭb″trō-kăn-tĕr′ĭk) [″ + Gr. *trochanter,* a runner]. Below a trochanter.

subtrochlear (sŭb-trŏk′lē-ăr) [″ + Gr. *trokhileia,* trochlea]. Beneath the trochlea.

subtuberal (sŭb-tū′bĕr-ăl) [″ + *tuber,* a knot]. Located under a tuber.

subtympanic (sŭb-tĭm-păn′ĭk) [″ + Gr. *tympanon,* drum]. Below the tympanum.

subumbilical (sŭb″ŭm-bĭl′ĭ-kăl) [″ + *umbilicus,* navel]. Below the umbilicus.

subumbilical space. Space within the body cavity below the navel resembling a triangle in shape.

subungual, subunguial (sŭb-ŭng′gwăl, -gwē-ăl) [″ + *unguis,* nail]. Situated beneath the nail of a finger or toe.

subungual hematoma. Collection of blood under the nail as a result of trauma. Condition may be treated by heating the end of a paper clip and then placing its point against the nail. This permits a small hole to be melted painlessly in the nail. The blood is then permitted to escape from under the nail.

suburethral (sŭb"ū-rē'thrăl) [" + Gr. *ourethra,* urethra]. Below the urethra.

subvaginal (sŭb-văj'ĭn-ăl) [" + *vagina,* sheath]. 1. Below the vagina. 2. On inner side of any tubular sheathing membrane.

subvertebral (sŭb-vĕr'tĕ-brăl) [" + *vertebra,* vertebra]. Beneath or on ventral side of the vertebral column or of a vertebra.

subvirile (sŭb-vĭr'ĭl, -vī'rĭl) [" + *virilis,* male]. Deficient in, or lacking, virility.

subvitrinal (sŭb-vĭt'rĭn-ăl) [" + *vitrina,* vitreous body]. Located beneath the vitreous body.

subvolution (sŭb"vō-lū'shŭn) [" + *volutus,* turning]. Method of turning over a flap surgically to prevent adhesions.

subwaking (sŭb-wāk'ĭng). Between waking and sleeping.

subzonal (sŭb-zō'năl). Beneath a zone.

subzygomatic (sŭb"zī-gō-măt'ĭk) [" + Gr. *zygoma,* cheekbone]. Beneath the zygomatic bone.

succagogue (sŭk'ă-gŏg) [L. *succus,* juice, + Gr. *agogos,* leading]. 1. To stimulate glandular secretion. 2. A substance that stimulates glandular secretion.

succedaneous (sŭk"sē-dā'nē-ŭs) [L. *succedaneus,* substituting]. Acting as a substitute or relating to one. In dentistry, it refers to the secondary or permanent set of teeth, which follow an earlier deciduous set.

succedaneum (sŭk"sē-dā'nē-ŭm) [L. *succedaneus,* substituting]. Something that may be used as a substitute.

succenturiate (sŭk"sĕn-tū'rē-āt) [L. *succenturiare,* to substitute]. Acting as a substitute.

succi. Pl. of succus.

succinate (sŭk'sĭ-nāt). Any salt of succinic acid.

succinic acid. SEE: *acid, succinic.*

succinylcholine chloride (sŭk"sĭ-nĭl-kō'lēn). USP. A drug used for its neuromuscular blocking effect. It is used as an adjuvant in surgical anesthesia, and to prevent trauma in electroconvulsive shock therapy. Trade names are Anectine, Sucostrin Chloride, and Sux-Cert.

CAUTION: This drug should be used only by physicians who have had extensive training in its use and in a setting where facilities for respiratory and cardiovascular resuscitation are immediately at hand.

succinylsulfathiazole (sŭk"sĭ-nĭl-sŭl"fă-thī'ă-zōl). 2-(N_4-succinylsulfanilamido) thiazole. Because of lack of evidence of its clinical efficacy, the drug is no longer used.

succorrhea (sŭk-kō-rē'ă) [L. *succus,* juice, + Gr. *rhoia,* flow]. Unnatural increase in secretion of any juice, esp. of a digestive fluid.

succubus (sŭk'ū-bŭs) [L.]. 1. A nightmare. 2. An evil demon thought to have sexual intercourse with men during sleep.

succus (sŭk'kŭs) [L. *succus,* juice]. (pl. *succi*) A juice or fluid secretion.

s. entericus. The intestinal juice. It is alkaline. The secretion of the minute glands lining the small intestine.

s. gastricus. The gastric juice.

s. pyloricus. An alkaline secretion by the pyloric end of the stomach.

succussion (sŭ-kŭsh'ŭn) [L. *succussio,* a shaking]. Shaking of a person to detect the presence of fluid in the body cavity by listening for a splashing sound, esp. in the thorax.

suck [AS. *sucan,* to suck]. 1. To draw fluid into the mouth, as from the breast. 2. To exhaust air from a tube and thus siphon fluid from a container. 3. That which is drawn into the mouth by sucking.

sucking pad. Mass of fat in cheeks, esp. well developed in an infant, aiding it to suck.

suckle. To nurse at the breast.

Sucostrin Chloride. Trade name for succinylcholine chloride, USP.

sucrase (sū'krās) [Fr. *sucre,* sugar]. An enzyme in the intestinal juice that splits cane sugar into glucose and fructose, the two being absorbed into the portal circulation. SYN: *invertase.*

sucrose (sū'krōs) [Fr. *sucre,* sugar]. NF. A saccharose, $C_{12}H_{22}O_{11}$, obtained from sugar cane, sugar beet, and other sources. It is hydrolyzed in the intestine to glucose and fructose by sucrase present in intestinal juice.

ACTION: Only a little is retained by the stomach, and it is all absorbed in the intestines. The lack of residue tends to cause constipation. Sucrose is stored by the hepatic cells of the liver after it is made into glycogen, for future use.

RS: carbohydrates; disaccharose; fructose; galactose; glucose; lactose; levulose; maltose.

sucrosemia (sū"krō-sē'mē-ă) [" + Gr. *haima,* blood]. Sucrose in the blood.

sucrosuria (sū"krō-sū'rē-ă) [" + Gr. *ouron,* urine]. Sucrose in the urine.

suction [LL. *suctio,* sucking]. The act of, or capacity for, sucking up by reduction of air pressure over part of the surface of a substance. SEE: *aspiration.*

s., post-tussive. Suction sound over a lung cavity heard on auscultation after a cough.

suction abortion. Removing the products of conception from the uterus by using a device that sucks the tissues away from the lining of the uterus.

suction biopsy. Obtaining tissue by use of a device that applies suction to the area from which tissue is desired. This technique is used in obtaining tissue from the mucosa of the stomach and intestines.

suctorial (sŭk-tō′rē-ăl) [LL. *suctio,* sucking]. 1. Concerning sucking. 2. Equipped for sucking.

Sudafed. Trade name for pseudoephedrine hydrochloride.

sudamen (sū-dā′mĕn) [L., sweat]. (pl. *sudamina*) Noninflammatory eruption from sweat glands characterized by whitish vesicles caused by the retention of sweat in corneous layer of the skin, appearing after profuse sweating or in certain febrile diseases, disappearing by absorption.

sudamina (sū-dăm′ĭn-ă). Pl. of sudamen.

sudaminal (sū-dăm′ĭ-năl) [L. *sudamen,* sweat]. Concerning sudamina, q.v.

Sudan (sū-dăn′). One of a number of related biological stains for which fats have a special affinity. Includes Sudan II, Sudan III (G), Sudan IV, and Sudan R.

sudanophil (sū-dăn′ō-fĭl) [*sudan* + Gr. *philein,* to love]. A leukocyte that stains readily with Sudan III, indicative of fatty degeneration.

sudanophilia (sū-dăn″ō-fĭl′ē-ă). Affinity for Sudan stains.

sudanophilic (sū-dăn″ō-fĭl′ĭk). Staining easily with Sudan stain.

sudation (sū-dā′shŭn) [L. *sudatio*]. 1. The act of sweating. 2. Excessive perspiration.

sudatoria (sū″dă-tō′rē-ă) [L.]. (sing. *sudatorium*) Excessive sweating. SYN: *ephidrosis; hyperhidrosis.*

sudatorium (sū″dă-tō′rē-ŭm) [L. *sudatorium,* a sweating room]. (pl. *sudatoria*) 1. A hot air bath or any bath to induce perspiration. 2. A room used to induce sweat baths.

sudden infant death syndrome. ABBR: SIDS. The completely unexpected and unexplained death of an apparently well, or virtually well, infant. The most common cause of death between the second week and first year of life. This worldwide syndrome has been of a constant rate over the years. Occurs more frequently in the third and fourth months of life, in premature infants, in males, and in infants living in poverty. The deaths usually occur during sleep and are more likely to happen in winter than in summer. SYN: *crib death.* SEE: *apnea; apnea alarm mattress.*

ETIOL: The cause is uncertain. In 10 to 15% of cases, autopsies show an unsuspected abnormality of the heart or brain, or evidence of overwhelming infection. Other findings are minimal but suggest that an agonal episode of motor activity had occurred and was accompanied by increased negative intrathoracic pressure.

Further information can be obtained from the National SIDS Foundation, Suite 1910, 310 South Michigan, Chicago, Ill. 60604.

Sudeck's disease or atrophy (soo′dĕks). [Paul H. M. Sudeck, Hamburg surgeon, 1866–1938] Acute atrophy of the bone at the site of an injury. SYN: *traumatic osteoporosis.*

sudokeratosis (sū″dō-kĕr″ă-tō′sĭs) [L. *sudor,* sweat, + Gr. *keras,* horn, + *osis,* condition]. Circumscribed horny overgrowths that obstruct the sweat ducts.

sudomotor (sū″dō-mō′tor) [″ + *motor,* a mover]. Pert. to stimulating the secretion of sweat; noting certain nerves.

sudor (sū′dor) [L.]. Secretion from the sweat glands. SYN: *perspiration; sweat.*

RS: anhidrosis; bromidrosis; chromidrosis; hematidrosis; hydrosis; perspiration; pore; skin; sudorific; sweat; uridrosis.

s. cruentus. Blood-tinged sweat. SYN: *hematidrosis.*

sudoral (sū′dor-ăl). Pert. to, caused by, or marked by perspiration.

sudoresis (sū″dō-rē′sĭs) [L.]. Profuse sweating. SYN: *diaphoresis.*

sudoriferous (sū-dor-ĭf′ĕr-ŭs) [″ + *ferre,* to bear]. Conveying or producing sweat.

sudoriferous glands. Sweat-secreting glands of the skin.

sudorific (sū″dor-ĭf′ĭk) [L. *sudorificus*]. 1. Secreting or promoting the secretion of sweat. 2. Agent that produces sweating. SYN: *diaphoretic.*

sudoriparous (sū″dor-ĭp′ă-rŭs) [L. *sudor,* sweat, + *parere,* to produce]. Secreting sweat. SYN: *sudoriferous.*

suet (sū′ĕt) [Fr. *sewet,* suet]. Hard fat from cattle's or sheep's kidneys and loins. Used as the base of certain ointments and as an emollient.

suffocate (sŭf′ō-kāt) [L. *suffocare*]. To impair respiration; to smother, asphyxiate.

suffocation (sŭf″ō-kā′shŭn). 1. State of being choked by obstruction of air passages by drowning, smothering, throttling, or inhalation of noxious gases. SYN: *asphyxiation.* SEE: *asphyxia; resuscitation; unconsciousness.* 2. Act of obstructing the air passages.

SYM: Insensibility, breathing slight, face purple and swollen, livid lips. Symptoms not always present.

TREATMENT: Dash cold water in face. Slap chest. Apply ammonia to nostrils. Artificial respiration. Tracheotomy may be required.

suffusion (sŭ-fū′zhŭn) [L. *suffusio,* a pouring over]. 1. Spreading of a bodily fluid into surrounding tissues. SYN: *extravasation*. 2. Pouring of a fluid over the body as treatment.

sugar [O. Fr. *zuchre*]. A sweet-tasting carbohydrate belonging to the monosaccharose and disaccharose groups. Crystalline carbohydrates of comparatively low molecular weight and generally having a sweet taste. SEE: *carbohydrates*.

CLASSIFICATION: They are classified in two ways: the number of atoms of simple sugars yielded on hydrolysis by a molecule of the given sugar and the number of carbon atoms in the molecules of the simple sugars so obtained. Thus, dextrose, q.v., is a monosaccharide because it cannot be hydrolyzed to a simpler sugar; it is a hexose because it contains six carbon atoms per molecule. Sucrose is a disaccharide because on hydrolysis it yields two molecules, one of dextrose and one of levulose.

s., beet. Sucrose obtained from sugar beets.

s., blood. The carbohydrate present in the blood; principally glucose.

s., brain. Galactose.

s., cane. Sucrose obtained from sugar cane.

s., diabetic. Glucose in the urine of diabetics.

s., fruit. Levulose or fructose.

s., grape. Glucose.

s., invert. Mixture consisting of one molecule of glucose and one of fructose resulting from the hydrolysis of sucrose.

s., liver. Glycogen.

s., malt. Maltose.

s., milk. Lactose.

s., muscle. Inositol; it is not a true sugar.

s., starch. Dextrin, a carbohydrate but not a true sugar.

s., wood. Xylose.

sugar, words pert. to: aglycosuric; blood; carbohydrates; dextrose; disaccharide; fructose; galactose; glucide; hypoglycemia; invert; invertase; lactose; levulose; mannitol; melitemia; monosaccharide; pentose; pentosuria; polysaccharide; sucrose; xylose; words beginning with "gluco-," "glyco-," and "sacchar-."

suggestibility (sŭg-jĕs″tĭ-bĭl′ĭ-tē) [L. *suggestus*, suggested]. A condition in which a person responds readily to suggestions or opinions of another. SYN: *sympathism*.

suggestible (sŭg-jĕs′tĭ-bl). Very susceptible to the opinions or suggestions of others.

suggestion (sŭg-jĕs′chŭn) [L. *suggestio*]. 1. Imparting an idea indirectly; to imply. 2. The idea so conveyed. 3. The psychological process of having an individual adopt or accept an idea without argument or persuasion.

s., auto-. Self-suggestion as distinguished from that coming from another person, esp. in hypnotic state.

s., hypnotic. Suggestion placed in the mind of a person while under the influence of hypnosis.

s., posthypnotic. Suggestion made to a subject while under hypnosis. After emerging from the hypnotic state, the person usually performs the suggested act.

suggestive (sŭg-jĕs′tĭv). Stimulating or pert. to suggestion.

suggestive medicine. Therapy by suggestion either during consciousness or hypnosis.

suggestive therapeutics. The practice of treating disease by hypnotic suggestion.

suggillation (sŭg-jĭl-ā′shŭn) [L. *suggillatio*]. A bruise or black and blue mark. SYN: *ecchymosis*.

suicide (sū′ĭ-sīd) [L. *sui*, of oneself, + *caedere*, to kill]. Act or instance of taking one's own life voluntarily.

MENTAL STATES CONDUCIVE TO: Depression; delusions of persecution, being ruined, or voices. In melancholia, schizophrenia, epilepsy, confusional states, and alcoholism. In those who act on sudden impulse or those suffering from an incurable disease. Through accidents causing acute delirium, mania, or general paralysis.

METHODS: Hanging; drowning; poisoning; cutting an artery; burning; jumping from heights; overdose of various medications; inhalation of toxic gases such as carbon monoxide; bombs; deliberately crashing vehicles or airplanes. Instruments used may be harmless articles such as sheets, suspenders, belts, nail files, spoons or potentially dangerous items as knives, razor blades, or glass. All must be removed from the room if patient is inclined to harm self or others.

suicidology (soo″ĭ-sīd-ŏl′ō-jē) [″ + ″ + Gr. *logos*, study]. The science of suicide including its cause prediction of those susceptible, and prevention.

suint (swĭnt). The crude potash soap obtained from lamb's wool. Lanolin is obtained from this substance.

suit. An outer garment.

s., anti-G. SEE: *anti-G suit*.

sulcal (sŭl′kăl) [L.]. Pert. to a sulcus.

sulcal artery. A tiny branch of the anterior spinal artery.

sulcate, sulcated (sŭl′kāt, -ĕd) [L. *sulcatus*]. Furrowed or grooved.

sulciform (sŭl′sĭ-form) [L. *sulcus*, groove, + *forma*, form]. Resembling a sulcus.

sulculus (sŭl′kū-lŭs) [L.]. A small sulcus.

sulcus (sŭl′kŭs) [L., groove]. (pl. *sulci*) A furrow, groove, slight depression, or fissure, esp. of the brain.

s., alveololingual. The space in the floor

of the mouth between the base of the tongue and the alveolar ridge, on each side extending from the frenum of the tongue back to the retromolar wall.

s., calcarine. A deep horizontal fissure on the medial surface of the occipital lobe of the brain.

s. centralis. Fissure dividing the frontal and parietal lobes of each cerebral hemisphere. SYN: *fissure, Rolando's.*

s., collateral. A sulcus on the tentorial surface of the brain. It bounds the inferior lingual gyrus and is parallel to the calcarine and postcalcarine sulci.

sulci cutis. The ridges on the skin of the palmar surface of the fingers and toes. These comprise the fingerprints.

s., gingival. The space or crevice between the free gingiva and the tooth surface; the depth of the sulcus varies according to the state of oral hygiene, deepening to become a periodontal pocket.

s., hippocampal. A sulcus on the medial side of the hippocampal gyrus.

s., intraparietal. Groove that separates the inferior from the superior parietal bones and lobes.

s. precentralis. [NA] An interrupted sulcus generally parallel with the fissure of Rolando and anterior to it.

s. pulmonalis. [NA] Depression on either side of the vertebral column.

s. spiralis cochleae. Groove between the labium tympanicum and labium vestibulare.

Sulf-10 Ophthalmic. Trade name for sulfacetamide sodium, USP, 10%.

sulfacetamide (sŭl″fă-sĕt′ă-mīd). An antibacterial sulfonamide that is highly soluble. It is particularly useful for topical application to the eye.

s., sodium. USP. A very soluble sulfonamide used in solution to treat infections of the cornea and conjunctiva. Trade names are Bleph-20 Liquifilm, Sulamyd Sodium, and Isopto Cetamide.

sulfadiazine (sŭl″fă-dī′ă-zēn). USP. One of a group of diazine derivatives of sulfanilamide. Because it readily penetrates the blood-brain barrier, it has been used extensively in treating meningococcal meningitis. Some strains of meningococci have become resistant to sulfadiazine.

s., silver. USP. SEE: *silver sulfadiazine.*

sulfadimethoxine (sŭl″fă-dī″mĕ-thŏks′ēn). A sulfonamide drug.

sulfa drugs. Drugs of the sulfonamide group possessing bacteriostatic properties. SEE: *sulfonamides.*

sulfaethidole (sŭl″fă-ĕth′ĭ-dōl). A sulfonamide drug.

sulfaguanidine (sŭl″fă-gwăn′ĭ-dēn). A sulfonamide drug that is poorly absorbed from the gastrointestinal tract. Because of its lack of demonstrated effectiveness, it is no longer used.

sulfamerazine (sŭl″fă-mĕr′ă-zēn). USP. An antibacterial sulfonamide that is more readily absorbed than sulfadiazine, from which it is derived. SEE: *sulfadiazine.*

sulfameter (sŭl′fă-mē″tĕr). A sulfonamide drug.

sulfamethazine (sŭl″fă-mĕth′ă-zēn). USP. An antibacterial sulfonamide similar to sulfadiazine.

sulfamethizole (sŭl″fă-mĕth′ĭ-zōl). USP. A sulfonamide used in treating urinary tract infections. Trade names are Bursul, Microsul, Proklar, and Thiosulfil.

sulfamethoxazole (sŭl″fă-mĕth-ŏks′ă-zōl). USP. A sulfonamide used in treating urinary tract infections. Usually used in combination with trimethoprim. Trade name is Gantanol. SEE: *trimethoprim.*

sulfamethoxypyridazine (sŭl″fă-mĕth-ŏk′sē-pī-rĭd′ă-zēn). A sulfonamide drug.

Sulfamylon. Trade name for mafenide.

sulfanilamide (sŭl″făn-ĭl′ă-mīd). Para-aminobenzenesulfonamide. White, slightly bitter, crystalline substance from coal tar, the parent of the azo dyes. Formerly it was widely used in the treatment of a number of infections, but because of its toxic reactions it has been superseded by more effective and less toxic sulfonamides.

sulfapyridine (sŭl″fă-pĭr′ĭ-dēn). USP. A sulfonamide that is used only in treating dermatitis herpetiformis.

s. sodium monohydrate. A soluble salt of sulfapyridine for intravenous use only.

sulfarsphenamine (sŭlf″ăr-sfĕn′ă-mēn). A sulfur compound, containing 19% arsenic; effective in treating syphilis.

sulfasalazine (sŭl″fă-săl′ă-zēn). USP. A sulfonamide that is poorly absorbed from the gastrointestinal tract. It is used in treating ulcerative colitis. Trade names are Azulfidine and SAS-500.

sulfatase (sŭl′fă-tās). An enzyme that hydrolyzes sulfuric acid esters.

sulfate (sŭl′fāt) [L. *sulphas*]. A salt or ester of sulfuric acid.

s., cupric. USP. The penta hydrate salt of copper, $CuSO_4 \cdot 5H_2O$, used as an antidote in treating phosphorus poisoning.

s., ferrous. USP. An iron compound used in treating iron-deficiency anemia.

s., iron. Green vitriol; copperas. Fatal in large dosage. SEE: *ferrous sulfate; copper salts* in *Poisons and Poisoning* in *Appendix.*

s., magnesium. Magnesium sulfate.

sulfathiazole (sŭl″fă-thī′ă-zōl). A rapidly absorbed and excreted sulfanilamide compound. Largely replaced by less toxic sulfonamides.

sulfatide (sŭl′fă-tīd). Any cerebroside with a sulfate radical esterified to the galactose.

sulfhemoglobin (sŭlf″hēm-ō-glō′bĭn). Substance formed by action of hydrogen sulfide on blood. SYN: *sulfmethemoglobin*.

sulfhemoglobinemia (sŭlf″hēm-ō-glō″bĭn-ē′mē-ă). Persistent cyanotic condition due to sulfhemoglobin in blood.

sulfhydryl (sŭlf-hī′drĭl). The univalent radical, SH, of sulfur and hydrogen.

sulfide (sŭl′fīd). Any compound of sulfur with an element or base.

sulfinpyrazone (sŭl″fĭn-pī′ră-zōn). USP. A drug used to promote excretion of uric acid in the urine. Trade name is Anturane.

sulfisoxazole (sŭl″fĭ-sŏk′să-zōl). USP. A sulfonamide used for treating certain bacterial infections, esp. certain urinary tract infections. Trade names are SK-Soxazole, Gantrisin, and Sulfizin.

Sulfizin. Trade name for sulfisoxazole, USP.

sulfmethemoglobin (sŭlf″mĕt-hē″mō-glō′bĭn). The greenish hemoglobin compound formed when hemoglobin and hydrogen sulfide are combined. SYN: *sulfhemoglobin*.

sulfo-. A combining form usually indicating the presence of divalent sulfur or of the sulfo-group, $-SO_3OH$.

sulfobromophthalein (sŭl″fō-brō″mō-thăl′ē-ĭn). USP. A drug administered intravenously in testing liver function.

sulfonamides. A group of compounds consisting of amides of sulfanilic acid derived from their parent compound sulfanilamide. They are bacteriostatic, their action on bacteria resulting from interference with functioning of enzyme systems necessary for normal metabolism, growth, and multiplication.

sulfone (sŭl′fōn). An oxidation product of sulfur compound in which the $=SO_2$ is united to two hydrocarbon radicals.

sulfourea (sŭl″fō-ū-rē′ă). Urea with oxygen replaced by sulfur. SYN: *thiourea*.

sulfoxide (sŭl-fŏk′sīd). The divalent radical $=SO$.

sulfoxone sodium (sŭl-fŏks′ŏn). USP. A drug used in treating leprosy and dermatitis herpetiformis. The leprosy bacillus has, in some areas, become resistant to this drug. Trade name is Diasone Sodium.

sulfur (sŭl′fŭr) [L.]. SYMB: S. At. wt. 32.06, at. no. 16; sp. gr. 2.07. A pale yellow, crystalline element that burns with a blue flame, producing sulfur dioxide.

The amount of sulfur excreted in urine varies with amount of protein in diet but more or less parallels the amount of nitrogen excreted, as both are derived from protein catabolism. The S:N ratio is approx. 1:14, i.e., for each gm. of sulfur excreted, 14 gm. of nitrogen are excreted. The amount of sulfur excreted daily is about 1 gm. It is oxidized to sulfate and required for the synthesis of body proteins as cystine, cysteine, or their combination.

DEFICIENCY SYM: Dermatitis, imperfect development of hair and nails. Deficiency of cystine or cysteine proteins in diet restricts growth and may be fatal. Tissue oxidation of cystine forms inorganic sulfate if the protein intake is sufficient.

s. dioxide. An irritating gas used in industry to manufacture acids. Also used in mechanical refrigerators. A bactericide and important disinfectant.

s., precipitated. USP. A form of sulfur used in various skin diseases including scabies. Its keratolytic effect helps to make it effective in those disorders.

s., sublimed. USP. A form of sulfur used in various skin diseases. Its keratolytic effect helps to make it effective in those disorders.

sulfurated potash. USP. A mixture composed chiefly of potassium polysulfides and potassium thiosulfate. It is used as a parasiticide.

sulfurated, sulfureted (sŭl′fū-rā″tĕd, -rĕt″ĕd). Combined or impregnated with sulfur.

sulfurated hydrogen. H_2S, a colorless, inflammable gas of disagreeable odor resulting from decomposition of organic matter containing sulfur; used as a chemical reagent. SYN: *hydrogen sulfide*.

sulfuric acid (sŭl-fū′rĭk). A colorless odorless liquid of heavy, oily consistency. It is extremely caustic and corrosive. It is widely used in manufacturing. SYN: *vitriol, oil of*.

s.a., dilute. An aqueous 10% solution of H_2SO_4. Used as an astringent and for gastric hypoacidity.

sulfuric acid poisoning. Sulfuric acid is sometimes accidentally taken by mouth, as it resembles syrup or glycerin. SEE: *nitrous fumes* in *Poisons and Poisoning* in *Appendix*.

SYM: Local effects. Burning, with destruction of skin. If it strikes eye it may result in blindness. If taken by mouth, intense pain extending from mouth to esophagus and down to stomach, causing marked, excruciating pain; swelling of affected tissues; salivation; painful swallowing; often gasping for breath, and hoarse voice. Mucous membrane has a grayish-white coating. There is persistent, painful vomiting. Patient quickly goes into shock.

TREATMENT: Dilute acid with large volumes of water. Neutralize acid with milk of magnesia, baking soda, or other well-diluted alkalies. Follow by soothing substances, as raw eggs.

CAUTION: Do not attempt gastric lavage by using a stomach tube if poisoning has occurred more than an hour previously.

sumac (soo'măk). General term applied to several species of Rhus.

s., poison. A type of sumac that causes a contact dermatitis. SEE: *poison sumac.*

summation (sŭm-ā'shŭn) [L. *summatio,* adding]. Cumulative action or effect, as of stimuli. Thus an organ reacts to two or more weak stimuli as if they were a single strong one.

summer (sŭm'ĕr) [AS. *sumer*]. The warmest season of the year, occurring between spring and autumn.

Sumycin. Trade name for tetracycline hydrochloride, USP.

sunburn [AS. *sunne,* sun, + *bernan,* to burn]. Dermatitis due to excessive exposure to the actinic rays of the sun. SEE: *burn.*

Sunday morning paralysis. Radial nerve palsy, sometimes the indirect result of acute alcoholism resulting from stuporous patient lying immobile with arm pressed over a projecting surface. SYN: *Saturday night paralysis.*

sunflower eyes. Slang term for the appearance of the eyes of patients with Wilson's disease. Deposits of copper around the edge of the cornea (Kayser-Fleischer rings) cause this condition.

sunscreen. Substance used to protect the skin from ultraviolet rays of the sun. Usually applied as an ointment or cream.

sunstroke (sŭn'strōk) [AS. *sunne,* sun, + *strake,* a blow]. An acute and dangerous reaction to heat exposure. Characterized by high body temperature, usually above 105°F. (40.6°C.); cessation of sweating; headache; numbness; tingling and confusion prior to sudden delirium or coma; fast pulse; rapid respiratory rate; usually elevated blood pressure. The basic defect is failure of the heat-regulating mechanisms of the body. SYN: *heatstroke.*

TREATMENT: Effective therapy may save the patient's life. Without delay, the nude patient should be placed in a bathtub filled with ice water. This will not cause pain, shock, or cutaneous vasoconstriction. The patient's temperature will need to be monitored carefully. Remove from bath when temperature falls to 103°F. (39.4°C.). If ice water and a bathtub are not available, place wet sheets on nude body, fan vigorously, and massage the skin. The use of sedatives may be required to control convulsions. Careful observation of patient for signs of fluid imbalance and renal failure will be required for several days.

super- [L.]. Combining form meaning above, beyond, superior.

superabduction (soo"pĕr-ăb-dŭk'shŭn) [L. *super,* above, + *abducens,* drawing away from]. Pronounced or extreme abduction.

superacidity (soo"pĕr-ă-sĭd'ĭ-tē). Excess acidity.

superacromial (soo"pĕr-ă-krō'mē-ăl). Supra-acromial.

superactivity (soo"pĕr-ăk-tĭv'ĭ-tē). Hyperactivity.

superacute (soo"pĕr-ă-kūt') [" + *acutus,* sharp]. Markedly acute.

superalimentation (soo"pĕr-ăl"ĭ-mĕn-tā'shŭn) [" + *alimentum,* food]. Therapeutic administration of food in excess of body needs or appetite. SYN: *hyperalimentation.*

superalkalinity (soo"pĕr-ăl"kă-lĭn'ĭ-tē) [" + *alkalinus,* alkaline]. Excessive alkalinity.

superciliary (soo"pĕr-sĭl'ē-ă-rē) [L. *supercilium,* eyebrow]. Pert. to or in the region of an eyebrow.

supercilium (soo"pĕr-sĭl'ē-ŭm) [L.]. (pl. *supercilia*) 1. [NA] Eyebrow. 2. A hair of the eyebrow.

superclass (soo'pĕr-klăs). In taxonomy, between a phylum and a class.

superduct (soo"pĕr-dŭkt') [" + *ducere,* to lead]. To elevate.

superego (soo"pĕr-ē'gō) [L. *super,* above, + *ego,* I; later translators of Freud's writings feel the word *uber-ich* should have been translated to over-I or upper-I and not to superego]. In freudian psychoanalytical theory, the portion of the personality associated with ethics, self-criticism, and the moral standard of the community. It is formed in infancy by the individual's adopting as his or her personal standards the values of the significant persons with whom he or she identifies. This serves to help form the conscience. The superego functions to protect and to reward when the ego-ideal of behavior or thought is satisified; and to criticize, punish, and evoke a sense of guilt when the reverse is true. In neuroses, symptoms develop when instinctual drives conflict with those dictated by the superego. SEE: *ego.*

superexcitation (soo"pĕr-ĕk"sī-tā'shŭn) [" + *excitatio,* excitation]. Excess excitement.

superextension (soo"pĕr-ĕks-tĕn'shŭn) [" + *extensio,* extension]. Excess extension.

superfamily (soo"pĕr-făm'ĭ-lē). In taxonomy, between an order and a family.

superfecundation (soo"pĕr-fē"kŭn-dā'shŭn) [" + *fecundare,* to fertilize]. Successive fertilization by two or more separate instances of sexual intercourse of two or more ova formed during the same menstrual cycle. Fertilization may be by the same or two different males.

superfemale. A female having three X chromosomes.

superfetation (soo"pĕr-fē-tā'shŭn) [" + *fetus,* fetus]. Fertilization of two ova in the same uterus at different menstrual periods within a short interval. SYN: *hypercyesis.*

superficial (soo″pĕr-fĭsh′ăl) [L. *superficialis*]. 1. Confined to the surface. 2. Not thorough; cursory.

superficialis (soo″pĕr-fĭsh-ē-ā′lĭs) [L.]. Superficial; noting a structure such as an artery, vein, or nerve, that is near the surface.

superficial reflex. Reflex induced by very light stimulus, such as stroking skin lightly with soft cotton wad.

superficies (soo″pĕr-fĭsh′ē-ēz) [L.]. An outer surface.

superflexion (soo″pĕr-flĕk′shŭn) [L. *super,* above, + *flexio,* flexion]. Excess flexion.

supergenual (soo″pĕr-jĕn′ū-ăl) [″ + *genu,* knee]. Above the knee.

superimpregnation (soo″pĕr-ĭm″prĕg-nā′shŭn) [″ + *impregnatio,* impregnation]. Conception during pregnancy; fertilization from two different ovulations. SEE: *superfecundation; superfetation.*

superinduce (soo″pĕr-ĭn-dūs′) [″ + *in,* into, + *ducere,* to lead]. To bring on, over, or above an already existing condition or situation.

superinfection (soo″pĕr-ĭn-fĕk′shŭn) [″ + *infectio,* a putting into]. A new infection caused by an organism different from that which caused the initial infection. The microbe responsible is usually resistant to the treatment given for the initial infection.

superinvolution (soo″pĕr-ĭn-vō-lū′shŭn) [″ + *involutus,* a turning]. Excessive reduction of the uterus to less than its normal size following childbirth. SYN: *hyperinvolution.*

superior (soo-pē′rē-or) [L. *superus,* upper]. 1. [NA] Higher than; situated above something else. 2. Better than. 3. One in charge of others.

superiority complex. An exaggerated conviction of one's own superiority; a pretense of superiority in order to compensate for one's feeling of inferiority.

superjacent (soo″pĕr-jā′sĕnt). Immediately above.

superlactation (soo″pĕr-lăk-tā′shŭn) [L. *super,* above, + *lactare,* to suckle]. Oversecretion of milk, or continuance of lactation beyond normal time.

superlethal (soo″pĕr-lē′thăl) [″ + *lethum,* death]. A dose of a drug, or exposure to trauma, greater than that required to produce death.

supermedial (soo″pĕr-mē′dē-ăl) [″ + *medium,* middle]. Above the middle.

supermoron (soo″pĕr-mō′rŏn) [″ + Gr. *moros,* stupid]. One only slightly mentally deficient.

supermotility (soo″pĕr-mō-tĭl′ĭ-tē) [″ + *motilis,* able to move]. Excessive motility in any part. SYN: *hyperkinesia.*

supernatant (soo″pĕr-nā′tănt) [″ + *natare,* to float]. 1. Floating on surface, as oil on water. 2. The clear liquid remaining at the top after a precipitate settles.

supernate (soo′pĕr-nāt). A supernatant fluid.

supernumerary (soo″pĕr-nū′mĕr-ăr″ē) [L. *supernumerarius*]. Exceeding the regular number.

supernumerary teeth. More than the usual number of teeth. Extra teeth develop in approx. 2% of the population, with almost all of them involving maxillary incisors or mesiodens, q.v Cleft palate or other developmental disturbances disrupt the dental lamina and often result in palatal supernumerary teeth.

supernutrition (soo″pĕr-nū-trĭ′shŭn) [L. *super,* above, + *nutritio,* nourishment]. More than normal nutrition.

superolateral (soo″pĕr-ō-lăt′ĕr-ăl) [″ + *latus,* side]. Above and to the side.

superovulation (soo″pĕr-ŏv″ū-lā′shŭn) [″ + *ovulum,* little egg]. Increased frequency of ovulation or production of a greater number of ova at one time. This is usually caused by the administration of gonadotropins.

superoxide. A highly reactive form of oxygen ($\bar{O}_2^{\cdot}$), the superoxide anion, produced when oxygen is reduced by a single electron. Superoxide is produced during the normal catalytic function of certain enzymes, by the oxidation of hemoglobin to methemoglobin, and when ionizing radiation passes through water. Superoxide is produced when granulocytes phagocytose bacteria. Superoxide is destroyed by the enzyme superoxide dismutase, which catalyzes the conversion of two molecules of superoxide anion to one molecule of oxygen and one of hydrogen peroxide: $\bar{O}_2^{\cdot} + \bar{O}_2^{\cdot} + 2H^+ \leftrightarrow H_2O_2 + O_2$.

superoxide dismutase. Enzyme that destroys superoxide. One form of the enzyme contains manganese and another contains copper and zinc.

superparasite (soo″pĕr-păr′ă-sīt) [″ + Gr. *parasitos,* fellow guest]. 1. A parasite that is parasitic on another parasite. 2. A parasite involved in superparasitism.

superparasitism (soo″pĕr-păr′ă-sī″tĭzm) [″ + ″ + *-ismos,* condition]. Condition in which the host is infested or infected with a greater number of parasites than can be supported.

superphosphate (soo″pĕr-fŏs′fāt). Acid phosphate.

supersaturate. To add more of a substance to a solution than can be dissolved permanently.

superscription (soo″pĕr-skrĭp′shŭn) [L. *super,* above, + *scriptio,* a writing]. The beginning of a prescription noted by the sign ℞, signifying (L.) *recipe,* take.

supersecretion (soo″pĕr-sē-krē′shŭn) [″ + *secretio,* a separating]. An excess of any secretion.

supersensitiveness (soo″pĕr-sĕn′sĭ-tĭv″nĕs) [″ + *sensitivus,* sensitive]. Excessive susceptibility to a foreign protein or other antigenic substance. SYN: *hypersensitiveness.*

supersoft (soo″pĕr-sŏft′) [″ + AS. *softe,* soft]. Exceptionally soft; noting roentgen rays of extremely long wavelength and low penetrating power.

supersonic (soo″pĕr-sŏn′ĭk) [″ + *sonus,* sound]. 1. Pert. to vibrations of sound space waves of frequencies above 20,000 cycles per second, which are inaudible to the human ear. SYN: *ultrasonic.* 2. Used to describe speeds greater than that of sound. At sea level, in air at 0° C., the speed of sound is about 331 meters, or 1087 feet per second (741 miles per hour).

superstructure (soo″pĕr-strŭk′chŭr). The visible portion of a structure, esp. those parts external to the main structure.

supertension (soo″pĕr-tĕn′shŭn) [″ + *tensio,* a stretching]. Extremely high tension.

supervenosity (soo″pĕr-vē-nŏs′ĭ-tē). Abnormally decreased oxygen in the venous blood.

supervention (soo″pĕr-vĕn′shŭn) [L. *superventio,* a coming over]. The development of an additional condition as a complication to an existing disease.

supervirulent (soo″pĕr-vĭr′ū-lĕnt) [″ + *virulentus,* poisonous]. More virulent than usual.

supervisor (soo′pĕr-vīz″ĕr) [L. *supervisus,* having looked over]. One who directs and evaluates the performance of others. In a health care setting, the supervisor has the knowledge and skills to provide the same service as those being directed, such as supervisor of the pharmacy, physical therapy, or maternity nursing.

supervitaminosis. Excess accumulation of vitamins in the body due to administration of an excess dose. SYN: *hypervitaminosis.*

supervoltage (soo′pĕr-vŏl″tĭj). A term applied to x-rays produced by very high voltage.

supinate (sū′pĭ-nāt) [L. *supinatus,* bent backward]. 1. To turn the forearm or hand so that the palm faces upward. 2. To rotate the foot and leg outward. 3. To cause to assume, or to assume, a position of supination.

supination (sū″pĭn-ā′shŭn) [L. *supinatio*]. 1. Turning of the palm or foot upward. 2. Act of lying flat upon the back. 3. Condition of being on the back or having the foot or palm facing upward.

supinator (sū″pĭn-ā′tor) [L.]. A muscle producing the motion of supination of the forearm. SEE: *Muscles* in *Appendix.*

supinator longus reflex. Flexion of the forearm caused by tapping of the tendon of the supinator longus.

supine (sū-pīn′) [L. *supinus,* lying on the back]. 1. Lying on the back or with the face upward. 2. Noting position of the hand or foot with the palm or foot facing upward. Opposite of prone.

suppedania (sŭp″ĕ-dā′nē-ă) [L. *sub,* under, + *pes,* foot]. Applications to the soles of the feet.

supplemental (sŭp″lĕ-mĕn′tăl) [L. *supplementum,* an addition]. Referring to something added to supply a need or to reinforce.

supplemental air. The air that by the most forcible effort can be expelled after an ordinary expiration that has followed a normal inspiration. In adult males, it averages about 1500 cc. SYN: *reserve air.*

support (sŭp-port′). That which assists in maintaining something in place.

suppository (sŭ-pŏz′ĭ-tō-rē) [L. *suppositorium,* something placed underneath]. (pl. *suppositories*) A semisolid substance for introduction into the rectum, vagina, or urethra, where it dissolves. It often serves as a vehicle for medicines to be absorbed. Commonly shaped like cylinder or cone and made of soap, glycerinated gelatin, or cocoa butter (oil of theobroma).

NURSING IMPLICATIONS: Provide privacy. Instruct the patient to retain suppository for approximately 20 minutes for effectiveness. Position the patient appropriately. Lubricate prior to insertion, and be certain the appropriate orifice is used. For neurological rehabilitation, a rectal suppository may be utilized by the patient after the patient has been taught bowel management. Check with the patient for effectiveness and document.

suppression (sŭ-prĕsh′ŭn) [L. *suppressio,* a pressing under]. 1. Repression of the external manifestation of a morbid condition. 2. Complete failure of natural production of a secretion or excretion, as distinguished from retention, in which normal secretion occurs but the discharge is retained within the organ or body. 3. In psychoanalysis, the freudian ego defense mechanism of conscious inhibition of an idea or desire, as distinguished from repression, which is considered an unconscious process.

suppression of menses. 1. Amenorrhea in which menstruation ceases after once being established and from some cause other than pregnancy or menopause. 2. Any suppression of the menses.

suppurant (sŭp′ū-rănt) [L. *suppurans*]. 1. Producing, tending to produce, or characterized by pus formation. 2. Agent causing pus formation. SYN: *suppurative.*

suppurate (sŭp′ū-rāt) [L. *suppurare*]. To form or generate pus.

suppuration (sŭp-ū-rā′shŭn) [L. *suppuratio*]. 1. The process of pus formation. SYN: *pyogenesis; pyopoiesis.* 2. The discharge produced by suppuration. SYN: *purulence; pus.*

Inflammation is caused by the presence of certain microorganisms called pyogenic (pus-forming) bacteria. Suppuration does not always develop even though microorganisms are present in the affected part, as may be the case in erysipelas and acute joint affections where exudate is serous. Liquefaction of tissues and formation of pus will continue so long as the microorganisms are alive. They cause the death of the leukocytes (white cells) and the cells of the part, liquefying the tissue so that the area becomes filled with a liquid containing the dead and dying cells. This fluid is called pus. An abscess may form because of the accumulation of this liquid. The abscess is indicated by redness, swelling, heat, and pain. It will show fluctuation, which may be felt by palpating it with two fingers. When the abscess reaches the surface, it will burst and discharge its contents. In most cases it is advisable to surgically incise the abscess rather than to wait for it to burst spontaneously.

RS: abscess; gangrene; infection; inflammation; purulent; pus; pustulant; pustule; pyogenic.

suppurative (sŭp'ū-rā"tĭv, -ră-tĭv) [L. *suppuratus*]. 1. Producing or associated with generation of pus. 2. Agent producing pus formation.

suppurative fever. Pus in the blood resulting in fever; a form of septicemia. SYN: *pyemia.*

supra- [L.]. Combining form meaning above.

supra-acromial (soo"pră-ă-krō'mē-ăl) [L. *supra,* above, + Gr. *akron,* point, + *omos,* shoulder]. Located above the acromion.

supra-anal (soo-pră-ā'năl) [" + *analis,* anal]. Located above the anus.

supra-auricular (soo"pră-ŏ-rĭk'ū-lăr) [" + *auricula,* ear]. Located above the auricle.

supra-axillary (soo"pră-ăk'sĭ-lĕr"ē) [" + *axilla,* underarm]. Located above the axilla.

suprabuccal (soo"pră-bŭk'ăl) [" + *bucca,* cheek]. Located above the buccal area.

suprabulge (soo'pră-bŭlj). The part of the crown of a tooth that curves toward the occlusal surface.

supracerebellar (soo"pră-sĕr"ĕ-bĕl'ăr) [" + *cerebellum,* little brain]. On or above the upper surface of the cerebellum.

suprachoroid (soo"pră-kō'royd) [" + Gr. *chorioeides,* skinlike]. Situated upon or above the choroid layer of the eyeball.

suprachoroidea (soo"pră-kō-roy'dē-ă). Outermost layer of the choroid. SYN: *suprachoroid lamina.*

suprachoroid lamina. The superficial layer of the choroid consisting of thin transparent layers, the outermost adhering to the sclera. SYN: *lamina suprachoroidea.*

supraciliary (soo"pră-sĭl'ē-ĕr"ē) [L. *supra,* above, + *cilia,* hairs]. Superciliary, q.v.

supraclavicular (soo"pră-klă-vĭk'ū-lar) [" + *clavicula,* a little key]. Located above the clavicle.

supraclavicular fossa. Depression on either side of the neck reaching down behind the clavicle.

supraclavicular point. A stimulation point over the clavicle at which contraction of arm muscles may be produced.

supracondylar (soo"pră-kŏn'dĭ-lăr) [" + Gr. *kondylos,* knuckle]. Above a condyle.

supracostal (soo"pră-kŏs'tăl) [" + *costa,* rib]. Above the ribs.

supracotyloid (soo"pră-kŏt'ĭ-loyd) [" + Gr. *kotyloeides,* cup-shaped]. Above the acetabulum.

supradiaphragmatic (soo"pră-dī"ă-frăg-măt'ĭk) [" + Gr. *dia,* across, + *phragma,* wall]. Above the diaphragm.

supraduction (soo"pră-dŭk'shŭn) [" + *ducere,* to lead]. Turning upwards of the eye.

supraepicondylar (soo"pră-ĕp"ĭ-kŏn'dĭ-lăr) [" + Gr. *epi,* upon, + *kondylos,* condyle]. Located above an epicondyle.

supraglenoid (soo"pră-glē'noyd) [" + Gr. *glene,* cavity, + *eidos,* form]. Above the glenoid cavity or fossa.

supraglenoid tuberosity. A rough surface of the scapula above the glenoid cavity to which is attached the long head of the biceps muscle.

supraglottic (soo"pră-glŏt'ĭk). Located above the glottis.

suprahepatic (soo"pră-hē-păt'ĭk) [" + Gr. *hepar,* liver]. Located above the liver.

suprahyoid (soo"pră-hī'oyd) [" + *hyoeides,* U-shaped]. Located above the hyoid bone; denoting accessory thyroid glands within the geniohyoid muscle.

suprahyoid muscles. The digastric, geniohyoid, mylohyoid, and stylohyoid muscles.

suprainguinal (soo"pră-ĭn'gwĭn-ăl) [" + *inguinalis,* pert. to the groin]. Above the groin.

supraintestinal (soo"pră-ĭn-tĕs'tĭ-năl) [" + *intestinum,* intestine]. Overlying the intestine.

supraliminal (soo"pră-lĭm'ĭ-năl) [L. *supra,* above, + *limen,* threshold]. 1. Above the threshold of consciousness; conscious. 2. Exceeding the stimulus threshold. SEE: *subliminal.*

supralumbar (soo"pră-lŭm'băr) [" + *lumbus,* loin]. Above the lumbar region.

supramalleolar (soo"pră-mă-lē'ō-lăr) [" + *malleolus,* little hammer]. Located above either malleolus.

supramammary (soo"pră-măm'ă-rē) [" + *mamma,* breast]. Located above the breast.

supramandibular (soo"pră-măn-dĭb'ū-lăr) [" + *mandibula,* mandible]. Located above the mandible.

supramarginal (soo"pră-măr'jĭn-ăl) [" + *margo,* margin]. Above any border.

supramarginal convolution. A cerebral convolution on lateral surface of the parietal lobe above the posterior part of the sylvian fissure.

supramastoid (soo″pră-măs′toyd) [″ + *mastos,* breast, + *eidos,* like]. Above the mastoid process of the temporal bone.

supramastoid crest. A ridge on the temporal bone. SYN: *temporal line.*

supramaxilla (soo″pră-măk-sĭl′ă) [″ + *maxilla,* jaw]. The upper jawbone. SYN: *maxilla.*

supramaxillary (soo″pră-măk′sĭ-lĕr-ē). 1. Rel. to the upper jaw. 2. Located above the upper jaw.

suprameatal (soo″pră-mē-ā′tăl) [″ + *meatus,* passage]. Above a meatus, esp. the exterior auditory meatus, noting the spine of Henle, a small bony projection at the posterosuperior margin of the external auditory meatus.

suprameatal spine. Small bony projection at the posterosuperior margin of the external auditory meatus marking the anterosuperior apex of the suprameatal triangle, q.v. SYN: *spine, Henle's.*

suprameatal triangle. Triangular space bordered by the posterior wall of the external auditory meatus and the posterior root of the zygomatic process of the temporal bone.

supramental (soo″pră-mĕn′tăl) [L. *supra,* above, + *mentum,* chin]. Located above the chin.

supranasal (soo″pră-nā′zăl) [″ + *nasus,* nose]. Located above the nose.

supranuclear (soo″pră-nū′klē-lăr) [″ + *nucleus,* little kernel]. Concerning nerve fibers located above a nucleus in the brain.

supraoccipital (soo″pră-ŏk-sĭp′ĭ-tăl) [″ + *occiput,* back of head]. Lying above or in upper portion of the occiput.

supraocclusion (soo″pră-ō-kloo′zhŭn) [″ + *occlusio,* occlusion]. The condition of teeth that are beyond the occlusal plane.

supraorbital (soo″pră-or′bĭ-tăl) [″ + *orbita,* circuit]. Located above the orbit.

supraorbital neuralgia. Neuralgia of the supraorbital nerve. SYN: *hemicrania* (def. 1).

supraorbital notch. A notch in the superior margin arch of the orbit for transmitting supraorbital vessels and nerve.

supraorbital reflex. Contraction of orbicularis oculi muscle with closure of lids resulting from percussion above the supraorbital nerve.

suprapatellar (soo″pră-pă-tĕl′ăr) [″ + *patella,* kneecap]. Above the patella.

suprapelvic (soo″pră-pĕl′vĭk) [″ + *pelvis,* basis]. Located above the pelvis.

suprapontine (soo″pră-pŏn′tĭn) [″ + *pons,* bridge]. Located above the pons varolii.

suprapubic (soo″pră-pū′bĭk) [″ + *pubis,* pubis]. Above the pubic arch.

suprapubic aspiration of urine. Use of a sterile needle and syringe to obtain urine from the bladder. There is less chance of introducing bacteria into the bladder with this method than during routine catherization.

TECHNIQUE: Patient is instructed to drink fluids and not to urinate. When the bladder is palpable, the suprapubic area is cleaned with alcohol and a 21-gauge sterile needle is inserted through the skin into the bladder. Urine is then aspirated. Local anesthetic may not be required.

CAUTION: The needle may pierce a loop of bowel that is lying over the anterior surface of the bladder.

suprapubic catheter. Catheter inserted through a suprapubic incision into the bladder to drain urine. Generally used when unable to insert through the urethra due to obstruction or there is a need to allow the urethra and bladder sphincter to heal.

NURSING IMPLICATIONS: Observe for hemorrhage or prolonged hematuria. Maintain catheter patency and a closed drainage system. Utilize aseptic technique during dressing changes and equipment change. Perform bladder irrigation as prescribed. Observe patient for signs of local or systemic infection. Administer prescribed medications such as analgesics, antispasmodics, and bowel stimulants. Evaluate the patient's ability to micturate. Monitor and record intake and output. Force fluids in order to ensure passage of dilute urine.

suprapubic cystotomy. Surgical opening of the bladder from just above the symphysis pubis.

suprapubic reflex. Deflection of linea alba toward stroked side when abdomen is stroked above Poupart's ligament.

suprarenal (soo″pră-rē năl) [L. *supra,* above, + *ren,* kidney]. 1. Above the kidney. 2. Pert. to the tiny gland above each kidney. SYN: *adrenal.*

suprarenalectomy (soo″pră-rē″năl-ĕk′tō-mē) [″ + ″ + Gr. *ektome,* excision]. Adrenalectomy.

suprarenal gland. An endocrine gland lying adjacent to and in a superior and medial position to the kidney. SYN: *adrenal gland.* SEE: *ACTH; adrenalin; corticosterone; cortisone; endocrine gland; epinephrine; norepinephrine.*

suprarenalopathy (soo″pră-rē-năl-ŏp′ă-thē) [″ + ″ + Gr. *pathos,* disease]. A disorder due to abnormal functioning of the adrenal glands.

suprascapular (soo″pră-skăp′ū-lăr) [″ + *scapula,* shoulder]. Located above the scapula.

suprascleral (soo″pră-sklē′răl) [″ + Gr. *skleros,* hard]. On the surface of the sclera.

suprasegmental [″ + *segmentum,* segment]. Above the segmented portion.

suprasegmental brain. The cerebrum, midbrain, and cerebellum as distinguished from the segmental portion (pons and medulla oblongata).

suprasellar (soo″pră-sĕl′ăr) [″ + *sella,* saddle]. Above or over the sella turcica.

suprasonic, supersonic (soo″pră-sŏn′ĭk) [″ + *sonus,* sound]. Noting sound with frequencies of vibration above 20,000 cycles per second. SEE: *supersonic.*

supraspinal (soo″pră-spī′năl) [″ + *spina,* a thorn]. Above a spine.

supraspinous. Above any spinous process.

supraspinous fossa. A groove above the spine of the scapula.

suprastapedial (soo″pră-stă-pē′dē-ăl) [″ + *stapes,* stirrup]. Above the stapes of the inner ear.

suprasternal (soo″pră-stĕr′năl) [L. *supra,* above, + Gr. *sternon,* chest]. Above the sternum. SYN: *episternal.*

suprasterol (soo″pră-stĕr′ŏl). Substance related to ergosterol produced by excessive irradiation of vitamin D.

suprasylvian (soo″pră-sĭl′vē-ăn). Above the sylvian fissure of the brain.

supratemporal (soo″pră-tĕm′pō-răl) [″ + *temporalis,* temporal]. Above the temporal bone or fossa.

supratentorial (soo″pră-tĕn-tō′rē-ăl). Located above the tentorium.

suprathoracic (soo″pră-thō-răs′ĭk) [″ + Gr. *thorax,* chest]. Above the thorax.

supratonsillar (soo″pră-tŏn′sĭ-lăr) [″ + *tonsilla,* almond]. Above the tonsil.

supratrochlear (soo″pră-trŏk′lē-ăr) [″ + *trochlea,* pulley]. Above a trochlea, esp. that of the humerus.

supratympanic (soo″pră-tĭm-păn′ĭk) [″ + *tympanon,* drum]. Above the tympanic membrane of the ear.

supravaginal (soo″pră-văj′ĭ-năl) [″ + *vagina,* sheath]. Above the vagina or any sheathing membrane.

supraventricular (soo″pră-vĕn-trĭk′ū-lăr) [″ + *ventriculus,* a little belly]. Above the ventricle, esp. the heart ventricles.

supravergence (soo″pră-vĕr′jĕns) [″ + *vergere,* to be inclined]. Condition in which one eye moves upward in the vertical plane while the other does not.

supraversion (soo″pră-vĕr′zhŭn) [″ + *versio,* a turning]. 1. A turning upward. 2. In dentistry, a tooth out of occlusal line.

sura (sū′ră) [L.]. [NA] Calf of the leg; muscular posterior portion of lower leg.

sural (sū′răl). Rel. to the calf of the leg.

suralimentation (sŭr″ăl-ĭ-mĕn-tā′shŭn) [Fr. *sur,* above, + L. *alimentum,* nourishment]. Treatment by overfeeding. SYN: *hyperalimentation; superalimentation.*

suramin sodium (soo′ră-mĭn). A urea derivative used in treating trypanosomiasis. It is available only from the Parasitic Disease Division of the Centers for Disease Control (CDC), Atlanta, Georgia 30333, U.S.A.

surditas (sŭr′dĭ-tăs) [L.]. Deafness.

surdity (sŭr′dĭ-tē) [L. *surditas,* deafness]. Inability to hear. SYN: *deafness.*

surdomute (sŭr′dō-mūt″) [L. *surdus,* deaf, + *mutus,* dumb]. 1. A deaf-mute. 2. Deaf and dumb.

surface (sŭr′fĕs) [Fr. *sur,* above, over, + L. *facies,* face]. 1 The exterior boundary of an object 2. The external or internal exposed portions of a hollow structure, as the outer or inner surfaces of the cranium or stomach. 3. The face or faces of a body such as a bone.

s., body. SEE: *body surface area.*

surface tension. Condition at the surface of a liquid in contact with a gas or another liquid that causes its surface to act as a stretched rubber membrane. It is the result of mutual attraction of the molecules to each other, thus producing a cohesive state that causes liquids to assume a shape presenting the smallest surface area to the surrounding medium. This accounts for the spherical shape assumed by fluids, such as drops of oil or water.

surfactant (sŭr-făk′tănt). An agent that lowers surface tension.

Ex.: oils and various forms of detergents.

s., pulmonary. A phospholipid substance important in controlling the surface tension of air-liquid emulsion that is present in the lungs. Abnormalities in this surfactant have been noted in prematurity, hyaline membrane disease, and pulmonary edema.

Surfak. Trade name for docusate calcium.

surfer's knots. Nodular swelling and possibly bone changes of area of lower leg and foot exposed to pressure and trauma while on a surfboard. Nodules may be painful.

surgeon (sŭr′jŭn) [L. *chirurgia*]. A medical practitioner who specializes in surgery.

s., dental. A dentist whose training and skills are in the area of surgery of the mouth and teeth. SYN: *stomatologist.*

Surgeon-General. The chief medical officer in one of the armed forces of the U.S.A. or the U.S. Public Health Service.

surgery (sŭr′jĕr-ē) [L. *chirurgia*]. 1. Branch of medicine dealing with manual and operative procedures for correction of deformities and defects, repair of injuries, and diagnosis and cure of certain diseases. SYN: *chirurgery, chirurgia.* 2. Surgeon's operating room. 3. Treatment or work performed by a surgeon. SYN: *operation.*

s., aseptic. Operative procedures carried on under aseptic conditions or in the absence of pathogenic organisms.

s., aural. Surgery of the ear.

s., conservative. Surgery in which as much as possible of a part or structure is retained. Opposite of radical surgery.

s., cosmetic. Surgery done to revise or change the texture, configuration, or relationship of contiguous structures of any feature of the human body that would be considered by the average observer to be within the broad range of normal and acceptable variation for age and ethnic origin and, in addition, is performed for a condition that is judged by competent medical opinion to be without potential for jeopardy to physical or mental health. (Adapted from official A.M.A. definition, 1974.) SEE: *s., plastic.*

s., major. Important and serious operations involving a risk to life.

s., minor. Simple operations not considered to involve a risk to life.

s., oral. Operative procedures pert. to the mouth and associated structures, esp. the teeth and jaws.

s., orthopedic. Surgery for correction of deformities and treatment of chronic joint diseases.

s., plastic. Surgery concerned with the repair or restoration of defective or missing structures, frequently involving the transference of tissue from a part or person to another part or person. SEE: *s., cosmetic.*

s., radical. Surgery involving extensive extirpation to remove diseased tissues or adjoining areas of lymphatic drainage in an attempt to obtain complete cure. Opposite of conservative surgery.

surgical (sŭr'jĭ-kăl). Of the nature of or pert. to surgery.

surgical diathermy. The use of high-frequency electrical oscillations in such a way that animal tissues are destroyed.

surgical dressing. Sterile protective covering of gauze or other substance applied to an operative wound.

surgical fever. Fever following an operation or injury.

surgical neck. Constricted part of shaft of humerus below the tuberosities; commonly the seat of fracture.

surgical resident. A physician who has graduated from medical school and is in a hospital-based training program in order to complete the requirements for certification as a board-qualified surgeon.

surgical suture, absorbable. Suture, absorbable surgical, q.v.

surgical suture, nonabsorbable. Suture, nonabsorbable surgical, q.v.

Surgicel. Trade name for oxidized cellulose.

Surital. Trade name for thiamylal sodium.

Surmontil. Trade name for trimipramine.

surrogate (sŭr'ō-gāt) [L. *surrogatus,* substituted]. 1. Something or someone replacing another; a substitute, esp. an emotional substitute for another. 2. In psychoanalysis, the representation of one whose identity is concealed from conscious recognition as in a dream; a figure of importance may represent one's loved one.

s., sex. SEE: *sex surrogate.*

sursumduction (sŭr"sŭm-dŭk'shŭn) [L. *sursum,* upward, + *ducere,* to lead]. Elevation, as the power or act of turning an eye upward independently of the other one.

sursumvergence (sŭr"sŭm-vĕr'jĕns) [" + *vergere,* to turn]. An upward turning, as of the eyeballs.

sursumversion (sŭr"sŭm-vĕr'zhŭn) [" + *versio,* turning]. Process of turning upward; simultaneous movement of both eyes upward.

surveillance (sŭr-vāl'ăns). The monitoring or controlling of something.

s., immunological. The idea that the body defenses recognize alien materials or malignant cells and destroy them when they appear.

survivor guilt. The feeling of guilt present in some persons who have survived an experience in which others have lost their lives, e.g., a war, ship sinking, holocaust, or prison camp.

susceptibility (sŭs-sĕp"tĭ-bĭl'ĭ-tē). Being susceptible.

susceptible (sŭ-sĕp'tĭ-bl) [L. *susceptibilis,* capable of receiving]. 1. Having little resistance to a disease or foreign protein. 2. An individual with little resistance to an infectious disease or who is not known to have become immune to one. 3. Easily impressed or influenced.

suscitate (sŭs'ĭ-tāt) [L. *suscitare,* to rouse]. To arouse to increased activity; to stimulate.

suscitation (sŭs"ĭ-tā'shŭn) [L. *suscitatio,* arousal]. Act of stimulating to greater activity. SYN: *excitation.*

suspended (sŭs-pĕnd'ĕd) [L. *suspendere,* to hang up]. 1. Hanging. 2. Temporarily inactive.

suspension (sŭs-pĕn'shŭn) [L. *suspensio,* a hanging]. 1. A condition of temporary cessation, as of any vital process. 2. Treatment by immobilization of a part or whole by hanging from a suspension in desired position. 3. State of a solid when its particles are mixed with, but not dissolved in, a fluid or another solid; also a substance in this state.

s., cephalic. Supported suspension of a patient by the head to extend the vertebral column.

s., colloid. A colloidal solution in which particles of the dispersed phase are relatively large.

s., tendon. Fixation of a tendon. SYN: *tenodesis.*

suspensoid (sŭs-pĕn'soyd) [" + Gr. *eidos,* form]. A colloid solution in which the dispersed particles are solid, as distinguished from emulsoid. SYN: *colloid suspension.*

suspensory (sŭs-pĕn'sō-rē) [L. *suspensorius,* hanging]. 1. Supporting a part, as a muscle, ligament, or bone. 2. A structure of the body that supports a part. 3. Bandage or sac for supporting or compressing a part, esp. the scrotum.

suspensory bandage. A sling for support of the testicles.

suspensory ligament. Any one of a number of ligaments that support a specific organ or structure. SEE: *ligament.*

Sus-Phrine. Trade name for epinephrine hydrochloride.

suspiration (sŭs″pĭr-ā′shŭn) [L. *suspiratio*]. A sigh or the act of sighing.

suspirious (sŭs-pī′rē-ŭs) [L. *suspirare,* to sigh]. Breathing with apparent effort; sighing.

sustentacular (sŭs″tĕn-tăk′ū-lăr) [L. *sustentaculum,* support]. Supporting; upholding.

sustentacular cell. A supporting cell such as those found in the acoustic macula, organ of Corti, olfactory epithelium, taste buds, or testes. SEE: *Sertoli's cells.*

sustentacular fibers of Müller. Fibers forming the supporting framework of the retina.

sustentaculum (sŭs″tĕn-tăk′ū-lŭm) [L.]. (pl. *sustentacula*) A supporting structure.

s. hepatis. A fold of peritoneum upon which rests the right margin of the liver.

s. lienis. Phrenocolic ligament that apparently supports the spleen.

s. tali. [NA] A process of the calcaneum that supports part of the astragalus.

susurrus (sū-sŭr′ŭs) [L., a whisper]. A murmur.

sutilains (soo′tĭ-lāns). USP. Proteolytic enzymes derived from the bacterium Bacillus subtilis. Calculated on the dry basis, it contains not less than 2,500,000 USP casein units. It is used in ointment form to debride necrotic lesions. Trade name is Travase.

CAUTION: Keep away from the eyes.

Sutton's disease (sŭt′ŏnz). 1. [Richard L. Sutton, Sr., U.S. dermatologist, 1878–1952] A halo nevus. 2. [Richard L. Sutton, Jr., U.S. dermatologist, b. 1908] Granuloma fissuratum.

Sutton's law. [Willie Sutton, contemporary bank robber] Originally the concept that a bank robber robs banks because "that is where the money is." Applied to medicine, the law indicates one should look for diseases where they are most likely to be. Ex.: malaria in tropical areas that harbor Anopheles mosquitoes; atherosclerosis in patients who are middle-aged or older.

sutura (sū-tū′ră) [L., a seam]. (pl. *suturae*) 1. [NA] A kind of fibrous union found only in the skull; one in which bony surfaces are closely united by a thin fibrous membrane that does not permit movement. SYN: *synarthrosis.* 2. Suture of any kind.

s. dentata. Sutura with interlocking of bony processes resembling the teeth of a saw.

s. harmonia. Simple apposition of two contiguous bones.

s. limbosa. Beveled suture in which opposing margins fit in parallel ridges as between parietal and frontal bones.

s. notha. A false suture with ill-defined projections.

s. serrata. [NA] Suture with deeper and more irregular indentations than a dental suture.

s. squamosa. [NA] Suture formed by overlapping of contiguous bones by broad beveled edges as in suture between squamous portion of temporal and parietal bones.

s. vera. A true suture in which no movement of united bones can occur.

sutural (sū′tū-răl) [L. *sutura,* a seam]. Rel. to a suture.

sutural joint. Articulation between two bones.

sutural ligament. Fibers uniting opposed bones forming a cranial suture.

suturation (sū″tū-rā′shŭn). Application of sutures; stitching.

suture (sū′chūr) [L. *sutura,* a seam]. 1. Line of union in an immovable articulation, as those between the skull bones; also such an articulation itself. SYN: *sutura; synarthrosis.* SEE: *raphe.* 2. Operation of uniting parts by stitching them together. 3. The thread or wire or other material used in the operation of stitching parts of the body together. 4. The seam or line of union formed by surgical stitches. 5. To unite by stitching.

s., absorbable surgical. USP. A sterile strand prepared from collagen derived from healthy mammals or from synthetic polymer. This type of suture is absorbed and thus does not need to be removed.

s., apposition. Suture in the superficial layers of the skin in order to produce precise apposition of the edges.

s., aproximation. A deep suture for joining the deep tissues of a wound.

s., basilar. Suture between the occipital bone and sphenoid bone.

s., bifrontal. Suture between the frontal and parietal bones.

s., biparietal. Suture between the two parietal bones.

s.'s, buried. Sutures placed so they are completely covered by skin.

s., button. Suture in which the threads are passed through buttons on the surface and tied to prevent the suture material from cutting into the skin.

s., catgut. Material used in suturing, made from a portion of the small intestine of sheep. It can be sterilized. Eventually it is absorbed by body fluids.

s., coaptation. Superficial suture for cutaneous wounds.

s., cobbler's. A suture in which the

thread has a needle at each end.

s., continuous. The closure of a wound by means of one continuous thread, usually by transfixing first one lip and then the other alternately from within outward. SYN: *s., uninterrupted.*

s., coronal. Suture between the frontal and parietal bones. SYN: *s., frontoparietal.*

s.'s, cranial. Sutures between the bones of the skull.

s., dentate. A suture consisting of long and toothlike processes.

s., ethmoidofrontal. Suture between the ethmoid and frontal bones.

s., ethmoidolacrimal. Suture between the ethmoid and lacrimal bones.

s., ethmosphenoid. Suture between the ethmoid and sphenoid bones.

s., false. Any form of suture in which one surface is smooth.

s., figure-of-eight. Suture that has shape of the figure eight.

s., frontal. An occasional suture in the frontal bone from the sagittal suture to root of the nose. SYN: *s., mediofronta; s., metopic.*

s., frontolacrimal. Suture between the frontal and lacrimal bones.

s., frontomalar. Suture between the frontal and malar bones.

s., frontomaxillary. Suture between the frontal bone and superior maxilla.

s., frontonasal. The suture between the frontal bone and the alae of the sphenoid bone.

s., frontoparietal. S., coronal.

s., frontotemporal. Suture between the frontal and temporal bones.

s., glover's. A continuous suture in which the needle is passed through the loop of the preceding stitch.

s., harmonic. Suture in which there is simple apposition of bone.

s., implanted. A suture formed by placing pins opposite each other on the two sides of a wound, and approximating the lips by winding thread or other similar material about the pins.

s., intermaxillary. Suture between the superior maxillae.

s., internasal. Suture between the nasal bones.

s., interparietal. S., sagittal.

s., interrupted. A suture formed by single stitches inserted separately, the needle usually being passed through one lip from without inward, and through the other from within outward.

s., lambdoid. Suture between the parietal bones and the two superior borders of the occipital bone. SYN: *s., occipital; s., occipitoparietal.*

s., longitudinal. S., sagittal.

s., maxillolacrimal. Suture between the maxilla and lacrimal bone.

s., mediofrontal. S., frontal.

s., metopic. S., frontal.

s., nasomaxillary. Suture between the nasal bone and superior maxilla.

s., nonabsorbable. Suture made from a material that is not absorbed by the body such as silk, silkworm gut, horsehair, certain synthetic materials, and wire.

s., nonabsorbable surgical. USP. A sterile or nonsterile strand of material that is suitably resistant to the action of living mammalian fluids and tissue. This suture should be used only in those applications where it may eventually be removed or where its staying in the tissues will cause no harm.

s., occipital. S., lambdoid.

s., occipitomastoid. Suture between the occipital bone and mastoid portion of temporal bone. SYN: *s., temporo-occipital.*

s., occipitoparietal. S., lambdoid.

s., palatine. Suture between the palatine bones.

s., palatine transverse. Suture between the palatine processes and superior maxilla.

s., parietal. S., sagittal.

s., parietomastoid. Suture between the parietal bone and mastoid portion of the temporal bone.

s., petro-occipital. Suture between the petrus portion of the temporal bone and occipital bone.

s., petrosphenoidal. Suture between the petrous portion of the temporal bone and ala magna of the sphenoid bone.

s., purse-string. Suture entering and exiting around the periphery of a circular opening, closing when drawn taut.

s., quilled. An interrupted suture in which a double thread is passed deep into the tissues below the bottom of the wound, needle being so withdrawn as to leave a loop hanging from one lip and the two free ends of the thread from the other. A quill, or more commonly a piece of bougie, is passed through the loops, which are tightened upon it, and the free ends of each separate thread are tied together over a second quill. Purpose of quilled suture is prevention of tearing when tension becomes greater.

s., relaxation. A suture that may be loosened to relieve excessive tension.

s., relief. A row of supplementary sutures including the tissues to the extent of 1 to 1½ in. (2.5 to 3.8 cm.) on each side of a fistula or a deep wound, for the purpose of lessening the strain on the coaptation sutures.

s., right-angled. A suture used in sewing intestine. The needle is passed in the same direction as the long axis of the incision and the process repeated on the opposite side of the incision, the suture being continuous.

s., sagittal. Suture between the two parietal bones. SYN: *s., interparietal; s., longitudinal; s., parietal.*

s., serrated. An articulation by suture in which there is an interlocking of bones by small, fine, and delicate projections and indentations.

s., shotted. A suture in which both ends of a wire or silkworm gut are passed through a perforated shot that is then compressed tightly over them.

s., silk. Type of suture made of silk. May be twisted, braided, or floss.

s., silkworm gut. Type of suture that causes little friction, is pliable, does not curl or twist, and is less liable to produce irritation.

s., sphenoparietal. Suture between the pariteal bone and ala magna of the sphenoid bone.

s., sphenosquamous. Articulation of the great wing of the sphenoid with squamous portion of the temporal bone.

s., sphenotemporal. Suture between the sphenoid and temporal bones.

s., squamoparietal. Suture between the parietal and squamous portion of the temporal bone.

s., squamosphenoidal. Suture between the squamous portion of the temporal bone and great wing of the sphenoid.

s., squamous. A suture between flat overlapping bones.

s., subcuticular. A buried continuous suture in which the needle is passed horizontally under the epidermis into the cutis vera, emerging at the edge of the wound but beneath the skin, then in a similar manner passed through the cutis vera of the opposite side of the wound, and so on until the other angle of the wound is reached.

s., temporo-occipital. S., occipitomastoid.

s., temporoparietal. Suture between the temporal and parietal bones.

s., twisted. A suture in which pins are passed through the opposite lips of a wound. and material is wound about the pins, crossing them first at one end and then at the other in a figure-of-eight fashion, thus holding the lips of the wound firmly together.

s., uninterrupted. S., continuous.

s., vertical mattress. An interrupted suture in which a deep stitch is taken and the needle inserted upon the same side as that from which it emerged, and passed back through both lips of the wound. The suture is then tied to the free end on the side the needle originally entered. This suture is particularly useful in holding together thick fragile tissues.

s., wire. Type of suture adapted for cases where there is tension or resection, or for uniting ends of bones. Usually stainless steel or silver wire is used.

suxamethonium chloride (sŭk″să-mē-thō′nē-ŭm). Succinylcholine chloride, USP.

Sux-Cert. Trade name for succinylcholine chloride, USP.

SV 40 virus. Simian virus 40, which is a member of the papovavirus family. The virus will produce sarcomas after subcutaneous inoculation into newborn hamsters.

swab (swăb) [Dutch *swabbe,* mop]. 1. Cotton or gauze on end of slender stick used for cleansing cavities, applying remedies, or for obtaining a piece of tissue or secretion for bacteriological examination. 2. To wipe with a swab.

s., test tube. Swab for cleansing tubes.

s., urethral. A slender rod for holding cotton used in examinations with the speculum, in treating ulcers or removing secretions. The male urethral swab is a rod about 7 in. (17.8 cm.) long.

s., uterine. A slender flattened wire, plain rod, or one with coarse thread on the distal end for absorbing or wiping away discharges.

swaddling. Restraining an infant by wrapping with strips of cloth. A historic practice that has been used experimentally in modern times.

swage (swāj). 1. To shape metal, esp. around something in order to make a close fit. 2. Fusing a suture to a needle.

swallow (swăl′ō) [AS. *swelgan*]. To cause or enable the passage of something from the mouth through the throat and esophagus into the stomach by muscular action. SYN: *deglutition.*

swallowing (swăl′ō-ĭng). A complicated act, usually initiated voluntarily but always completed reflexively, whereby food is moved from the mouth through the pharynx and esophagus to the stomach. It occurs in the following three stages.

In the *first stage,* food is placed on the surface of the tongue. The tip of the tongue is placed against the hard palate; then elevation of the larynx and backward movement of the tongue forces food through the isthmus of the fauces in the pharynx.

In the *second stage,* the food passes through the pharynx. This involves constriction of the walls of the pharynx, backward bending of the epiglottis, and an upward and forward movement of the larynx and trachea. This may be observed externally with the bobbing of the Adam's apple. Food is kept from entering the nasal cavity by elevation of the soft palate and from entering the larynx by closure of the glottis and backward inclination of the epiglottis. During this stage, respiratory movements are inhibited by reflex.

In the *third stage,* food moves down the esophagus and into the stomach. This movement is accomplished by momentum from the second stage, peristaltic contractions, and gravity. With the body in upright position, liquids pass rapidly and do not require assistance from the esophagus. However, second stage momentum and peristaltic contractions are sufficient to allow liquids to be drunk even when the head is lower than the stomach.

Difficulty in swallowing is called dysphagia, q.v. It may be caused by congenital defects such as cleft palate or esophageal obstruction; neural and psychogenic disturbances; muscular dysfunction; or local conditions such as presence of tumors, abscesses, and inflammation. SYN: *deglutition.*

RS: aglutition; aphagia; choking; Heimlich maneuver.

s., air. Introduction of air into the stomach or intestines while eating, drinking, chewing gum, or smoking. May be habitual on part of the patient or brought on by hysteria. SYN: *aerophagia.*

s., tongue. Condition in which the tongue has a tendency to fall backward and obstruct the openings to the larynx and esophagus. The tongue is not swallowed and the term is inaccurate; nevertheless, it is commonly used. The condition is due to excessive flaccidity of tongue during unconsciousness. Control of this requires forceful elevation of the chin and extension of the head during artificial respiration in order to help provide an airway. The tongue may also be pulled forward in order to clear the airway.

swallow's nest. Cerebral depression between the uvula and the posterior velum. SYN: *nidus hirundinis.*

Swan-Ganz catheter. [Harold James Swan, contemporary U.S. physician, b. 1922; William Ganz, contemporary U.S. physician, b. 1919] A soft, flexible catheter that contains a balloon near its tip. The sterile catheter is passed through the vein to the right heart, being carried along by the blood returning to the heart. The balloon then helps, without the use of fluoroscopy, to guide the catheter to the pulmonary artery. Once in the pulmonary artery, the balloon is inflated sufficiently to block the flow of blood from the right heart to the lung. This allows the back pressure in the pulmonary artery distal to the balloon to be recorded. This pressure reflects the pressure transmitted back from the left atrial chamber of the heart.

A catheter similar to the Swan-Ganz was originally developed in 1953 and used in dogs by the contemporary U.S. physiologists Michael Lategola and Hermann Rahn.

Swan neck deformity. Hand deformity frequently seen in rheumatoid arthritis characterized by hyperextension of the proximal interphalangeal joints and flexion of the distal interphalangeal joints due to tight interossei.

swarming (sworm'ĭng). The spread of bacteria over a culture medium.

sway-back (swā'băk). Lordosis.

sweat (swĕt) [AS. *sweatan*]. 1. The secretion of the sudoriparous glands of the skin. SYN: *perspiration; sudor.* SEE: *glands, Moll's.* 2. Condition of perspiring or of being made to perspire freely, as to order a sweat for a patient. 3. To emit moisture through the skin's pores. SYN: *perspire.* 4. To cause to emit moisture through the pores.

Perspiration is a colorless, slightly turbid, salty, aqueous fluid, although that from the sweat glands in the axillae, around the anus, and of the ceruminous glands has an oil consistency. It contains urea, fatty substances, and sodium chloride. This salty, watery fluid is difficult to collect without contamination with sebum, q.v. SEE: *perspiration, insensible; perspiration, sensible.*

FUNCT: To cool the body by evaporation and to rid it of what waste may be expressed through the pores of the skin. The amount per day is about a liter; this figure is subject to extreme variation according to muscular activity and atmospheric conditions, and in extreme conditions may be as much as 10 to 15 liters in 24 hours.

PHYS: Perspiration is controlled by the sympathetic nervous system through true secretory fibers supplying sweat glands.

s., bloody. Sweat tinged with blood. SYN: *hematidrosis.*

s., colliquative. Profuse, clammy sweat.

s., colored. Sweat tinged with a pigment. SYN: *chromidrosis.*

s., fetid. Sweat with a foul odor. SYN: *bromidrosis.*

s., night. Sweating during the night; may be a symptom of pulmonary tuberculosis.

s., profuse. Excessive perspiration. SYN: *hyperhidrosis.*

s., scanty Abnormally small amount or lack of sweat. SYN: *anhidrosis.*

sweat centers. Principal centers controlling perspiration located in the hypothalamus; secondary centers are present in the spinal cord.

sweat glands. Simple, coiled, tubular glands found on all body surfaces except margin of lips, glans penis, and inner surface of prepuce. The coiled secreting portion lies in the corium or subcutaneous portion of skin; the

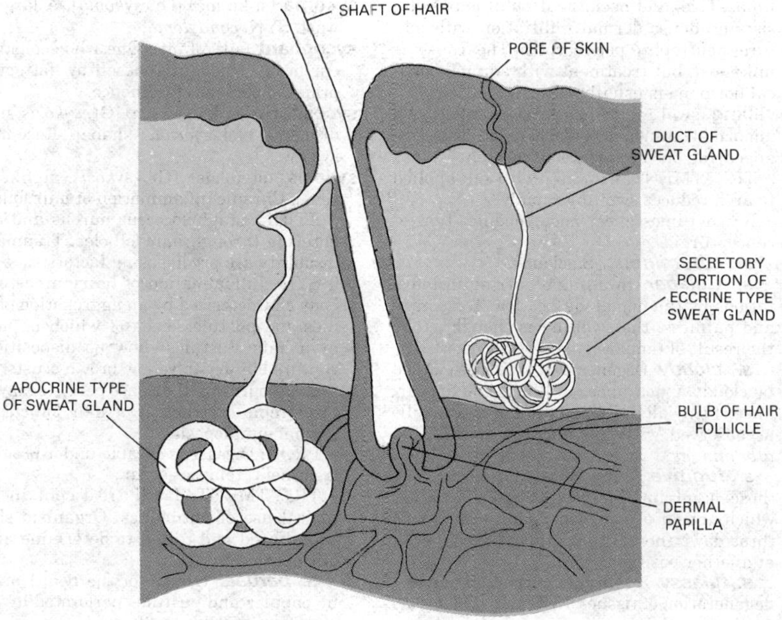

ECCRINE AND APOCRINE SWEAT GLANDS

excretory duct follows a straight or oblique course through the dermis, but becomes spiral in passing through the epidermis to its opening, a sweat pore.

Most sweat glands are merocrine; those of the axilla, areola, mammary gland, labia majora, and circumanal region are apocrine. Sweat glands are most numerous on the palms of the hands and soles of the feet. SEE: illus.; *glands, eccrine; glands, apocrine.*

sweat, words pert. to: bromidrosis; chromidrosis; diaphoresis; diaphoretic; dyshidria; dysidrosis; hidradenitis; hidrorrhea; hidrosis; hydradenitis; hydradenoma; hyperhidrosis, hyphidrosis; melanidrosis; perspiration; sudor; sudorific; sudoriparous; uridrosis.

sweating (swĕt'ĭng) [AS. *swat,* sweat]. 1. Act of exuding sweat. 2. Emitting sweat. 3. Causing profuse sweat.

To induce sweat in a localized area, paint 2 in. (5.1 cm) square of skin under each axilla with mixture of equal parts of olive oil and guaiacol solution. Cover with several layers of gauze, then flannel, and hold with adhesive tape. Wrap patient in warm blankets.

s., deficiency of. Diminished or complete absence of secretion of sweat. Seen in profuse diarrhea, polyuria, vomiting, hemorrhage, diabetes insipidus, myxedema, general anasarca, ichthyosis, and in high temperature. SYN: *anhidrosis.*

s., excessive Overabundance of secretion of sweat. Seen in rheumatic, malarial, and relapsing fever, septic fevers, pneumonia at crisis, pulmonary tuberculosis, hyperthyroidism, migraine, neuralgia. Locally of hands and feet in hysteria, neurasthenia, vagotonia, nervous irritability, exophthalmic goiter, fright, and other emotions. SYN: *hyperhidrosis.*

s., urinous. Presence of urea in the sweat. Often found in uremia. SYN: *uridrosis.*

RS: anhidrosis; bromidrosis; chromidrosis; hidrosis; perspiration; pores; skin; sudor; sudorific; sweat; uridrosis.

Swedish gymnastics. System of active and passive exercise of the various muscles and joints of the body without using apparatus.

Swedish massage. Massage combined with Swedish gymnastics.

sweet [AS. *swete,* sweet]. 1. Pleasing to the taste or smell. SEE: *taste.* 2. Containing or derived from sugar. 3. Free from excess of acid, sulfur, or corrosive salts.

Sweet's syndrome. [R. D. Sweet, contemporary Brit. physician] A condition characterized by fever; raised painful plaques on the limbs, face, and neck; neutrophil leukocytosis; and dense dermal infiltration with mature neutrophil polymorphs. The cause is unknown, but treatment with adrenal cortical hormone is usually effective.

swelling (swĕl'ĭng) [AS. *swellan*, swollen]. An abnormal transient enlargement, esp. one appearing on the surface of the body.

TREATMENT: Ice water with salt applied to area reduces swelling rapidly.

RS: detumescence; node; nodule; turgescence; turgid.

s., albuminous. S., cloudy.

s., Calabar. Swelling occurring in infestations by the nematode Loa loa. Temporary and painless, the swelling is thought to be the result of temporary sensitization.

s., cloudy. Degeneration of tissues marked by cloudy appearance, swelling, and appearance of tiny albuminoid granules in the cells as observed with the microscope. SYN: *s., albuminous.*

s., fugitive. Temporary swellings such as those occurring in infestations of Loa loa which appear at one place, persist for two or three days, then disappear, possibly to recur at another position.

s., glassy. Swelling occurring in amyloid degeneration of tissues. SEE: *amyloid degeneration; erythredema.*

s., white. Swelling seen in tuberculous arthritis, esp. of the knee.

Swift's disease. Acrodynia.

swimmer's ear. A type of external otitis seen in persons who swim for a considerable period of time or fail to completely dry their ear canals after swimming. If excess cerumen is not present, the condition can be prevented by placing a few drops of 70% alcohol in the ear canals at the end of each swimming session.

swimmer's itch. Appearance of papules resembling insect bites on the skin of persons who swim in water containing the cercariae of certain schistosomes. Usually present only on exposed surfaces of the skin. The papules appear from 4 to 13 days after exposure. Disease is self-limited; thus treatment is symptomatic. SYN: *dermatitis, cercarial.* SEE: *dermatitis, schistosome; seabather's eruption.*

switch (swĭch) [MD. *swijch*, bough]. In physical therapy, device used to break or open an electrical circuit or to divert current from one conductor to another.

s., foot. A switch whereby the operator, using both hands in application of surgical high-frequency currents, may use a foot to start or break the current.

s., pole-changing. A switch by which the polarity of a circuit may be reversed.

swoon [AS. *swogan*, to suffocate]. 1. A fainting spell. SYN: *syncope.* 2. To faint.

sycoma (sī-kō'mă) [Gr. *sykoma*]. A large soft wart. SYN: *condyloma.*

sycophant (sĭk'ō-fănt). One who seeks to incur favor or advance oneself by flattery and praise of persons of influence.

sycosiform (sī-kō'sĭ-form) [Gr. *sykosis*, figlike disease, + L. *forma*, shape]. Resembling sycosis.

sycosis (sī-kō'sĭs) [Gr. *sykosis*, figlike disease]. Chronic inflammation of hair follicles.

ETIOL: Staphylococcus aureus and albus entering through hair follicles. Trauma and disability are predisposing factors.

SYM: Inflammation of hairy areas of the body characterized by an aggregation of papules and pustules, each of which is pierced by a hair. Pustules show no disposition to rupture but dry to yellow-brown crusts. Itching and burning. If disease persists may lead to extreme destruction of hair follicles and permanent alopecia.

PROG: Disease is curable under prolonged treatment; relapses occur.

TREATMENT: Local treatment includes topical use of antibiotics. Organism should be cultured and tested to determine antibiotic of choice.

s. barbae. Sycosis of the beard marked by papules and pustules perforated by hairs and surrounded by infiltrated skin.

s., lupoid. Pustular lesions of the hair follicles of the beard.

s. vulgaris. S. barbae, q.v.

Sydenham's chorea (sĭd'ĕn-hămz). [Thomas Sydenham, Brit. physician, 1624–1689] A disease of childhood commonly occurring between 5 and 15 years of age; more females than males are affected. Usually associated with rheumatic fever. Characterized by involuntary purposeless contractions of the muscles of the trunk and extremities; anxiety; impairment of memory and sometimes of speech.

PROG: Recovery usually in course of 6 to 10 weeks. Relapses not infrequent, esp. in pregnancy. A possible sequel is chronic chorea. Rare complication is death from heart disease.

TREATMENT: Rest of body and mind. Remove child from school; place under favorable hygienic conditions. Protection against injury if chorea severe. Sedation is indicated in some cases.

syllabic utterance (sĭ-lăb'ĭk) [Gr. *syllabikos*]. A staccato accentuation of syllables, slowly but separately, observed in multiple sclerosis. SYN: *scanning speech.*

syllable stumbling (sĭl'ă-bl) [Gr. *syllabe*, syllable]. Hesitating utterance (dysphasia) with difficulty in pronouncing certain syllables.

syllabus (sĭl'ă-bŭs) [Gr. *syllabos*, table of contents]. Abstract of a lecture or outline of a course of study or of a book.

syllepsis (sĭl-ĕp'sĭs) [Gr. *syllepsis,* conception]. Conception, impregnation, or pregnancy.

sylvatic plague. Bubonic plague that is endemic among wild rodents. The causative organism is transmitted by fleas. SEE: *plague.*

sylvian aqueduct (sĭl'vē-ăn). [Jacobus Sylvius, Fr. anatomist, 1478–1555] A narrow canal from 3rd to 4th ventricle.

sylvian artery. [François Sylvius, Fr. anatomist, 1614–1672] Middle cerebral artery in the fissure of Sylvius.

sylvian fissure. [François Sylvius] The fissure separating the temporal lobe from the frontal and parietal lobes.

sylvian line. [François Sylvius] Line on exterior of the cranium, marking direction of the sylvian fissure.

sym- [Gr. *syn,* together]. Combining form meaning with, along, together with, beside.

symballophone (sĭm-băl'ō-fōn) [" + *ballein,* to throw, + *phone,* sound]. A special stethoscope with two chest pieces. Use of this device assists in locating a lesion in the chest by comparing the different sounds detected by the two chest pieces.

symbion, symbiont (sĭm'bē-ŏn, -bē-ŏnt) [Gr. *syn,* together, + *bios,* life]. An organism that lives with another in a state of symbiosis, q.v. SYN: *commensal.*

symbiosis (sĭm"bē-ō'sĭs) [Gr.]. The living together in close association of two organisms of different species. If neither organism is harmed, such is referred to as commensalism; if the association is beneficial to both, it is mutualism; if one is harmed and the other benefited, it constitutes parasitism.

symbiote (sĭm'bī-ōt) [Gr. *syn,* together, + *bios,* life]. An organism symbiotic with another.

symbiotic (sĭm"bī-ŏt'ĭk). Concerning symbiosis.

symblepharon (sĭm-blĕf'ă-rŏn) [" + *blepharon,* eyelid]. Adhesion between conjunctivae of lid and eyeball due to injuries, esp. burns from lime or acids. Also seen in trachoma, pemphigus, and following operations.

SYM: Interference with movement of eyeball, conjunctival irritation.

TREATMENT: Division of cicatricial bands and keeping raw surfaces separated. Mucous membrane grafts.

symblepharopterygium (sĭm-blĕf"ă-rō-tĕr-ĭj'ē-ŭm) [" + " + *pterygion,* wing]. Abnormal joining of the eyelid to the eyeball.

symbol (sĭm'bŏl) [Gr. *symbolon,* a sign]. 1. An object or sign that represents an idea or quality by association, resemblance, or convention. SEE: *Prescription Writing* and *Symbols* in *Appendix.* 2. In psychology, an object used as an unconscious substitute that is not connected consciously with the libido, but into which the libido is concentrated. 3. A mark or letter representing an atom or an element in chemistry. SEE: *Physical Constants of Elements* in *Appendix.*

s., phallic. An object that bears some resemblance to the penis.

symbolia (sĭm-bō'lē-ă). Ability to identify or recognize an object by the sense of touch.

symbolism (sĭm'bŏl-ĭzm) [" + *-ismos,* condition]. 1. Unconscious substitutive expression of subconscious thoughts of sexual significance in terms recognized by the objective consciousness. 2. An abnormal condition in which everything that occurs is interpreted as a symbol of the patient's own thoughts.

symbolization. An unconscious process by which an object or idea comes to represent another object or idea on the basis of similarity or association.

symbolophobia (sĭm"bŏl-ō-fō'bē-ă) [" + *phobos,* fear]. Hesitancy in expressing one's self in words or action for fear that it may be interpreted as possessing a symbolic meaning.

symbrachydactyly (sĭm-brăk"ē-dăk'tĭ-lē) [" + *brachys,* short, + *daktylos,* finger]. Webbing of fingers that are abnormally short.

Syme's operation (sīmz). [James Syme, Scottish surgeon, 1799–1870] 1. Amputation of the foot at the ankle joint with removal of the malleoli. 2. Excision of the tongue. 3. External urethrotomy.

symmelia (sĭm-mē'lē-ă) [Gr. *syn,* together, + *melos,* limb]. Fusion of limbs.

symmelus, symelus (sĭm'ĕ-lŭs, -ē-lŭs) [" + *melos,* limb]. Sirenomelia, q.v.

Symmetrel. Trade name for amantadine hydrochloride.

symmetromania (sĭm"ĕ-trō-mā'nē-ă) [Gr. *symmetria,* symmetry, + *mania,* madness]. An abnormal impulse to make symmetrical motions such as moving both arms instead of one.

symmetry (sĭm'ĕt-rē). Correspondence in shape, size, and relative position of parts on opposite sides of a body.

s., bilateral. Symmetry of an organism or body whose right and left halves are mirror images of each other or in which a median longitudinal section divides the organism or body into equivalent right and left halves.

s., radial. Symmetry of an organism whose parts radiate from a central axis.

sympathectomize (sĭm"pă-thĕk'tō-mīz). To perform a sympathectomy.

sympathectomy (sĭm"pă-thĕk'tō-mē) [Gr. *sympathetikos,* sympathy, + *ektome,* excision]. Excision of a portion of the sympathetic division of the autonomic nervous system. It may include a nerve, plexus, ganglion, or a series of ganglia of the sympathetic trunk.

s., chemical. The use of chemicals to destroy or temporarily inactivate part of the sympathetic nerve.

s., periarterial. Removal of sheath of an artery in which sympathetic nerve fibers are located; used in trophic disturbances.

sympatheoneuritis (sĭm-păth″ē-ō-nū-rī′tĭs) [″ + *neuron,* nerve, + *itis,* inflammation]. Inflammation of the sympathetic nerve.

sympathetic (sĭm″pă-thĕt′ĭk). 1. Pert. to sympathetic nervous system. 2. Caused by or pert. to sympathy.

sympatheticalgia (sĭm″pă-thĕt″ĭ-kăl′jē-ă) [″ + *algos,* pain]. Pain in the cervical sympathetic ganglion.

sympathetic irritation. Irritation of one structure caused by irritation of another related structure.

sympathetic nervous system. A large part of the autonomic nervous system. It consists of ganglia, nerves, and plexuses that supply the involuntary muscles. Most of the nerves of the system are motor, but some are sensory. SEE: *nervous system; parasympathetic nervous system; autonomic nervous system* for illus.

sympatheticoparalytic (sĭm″pă-thĕt″ĭ-kō-păr″ă-lĭt′ĭk) [″ + *paralysis,* a loosening at the sides]. Resulting from paralysis of the sympathetic nervous system.

sympatheticopathy (sĭm″pă-thĕt″ĭ-kŏp′ă-thē) [″ + *pathos,* disease]. Any condition resulting from disorder of the sympathetic nervous system.

sympathetic ophthalmia. Inflammation of the uveal tract in one eye due to similar inflammation in the other eye.

sympatheticotonia (sĭm″pă-thĕt″ĭ-kō-tō′nē-ă) [″ + *tonos,* tension]. Condition characterized by excessive tone of the sympathetic nervous system with unusually high blood pressure and tendency to vascular spasm. SYN: *sympathicotonia.*

sympatheticotonic (sĭm″pă-thĕt″ĭ-kō-tŏn′ĭk). Marked by increased arterial tone or vasoconstriction due to overaction of the sympathetic nervous system.

sympatheticotripsy. Sympathicotripsy, q.v.

sympathetic plexuses. Plexuses formed at intervals by the sympathetic nerves and ganglia.

sympathetoblast (sĭm″pă-thĕt′ō-blăst) [Gr. *sympathetikos,* sympathy, + *blastos,* germ]. Sympathoblast, q.v.

sympathic (sĭm-păth′ĭk) [Gr. *sympathetikos,* sympathy]. Sympathetic.

sympathicectomy (sĭm-păth″ĭ-sĕk′tō-mē) [″ + *ektome,* excision]. Excision of part of the sympathetic nervous pathways. SYN: *sympathectomy.*

sympathicoblast (sĭm-păth′ĭ-kō-blăst) [″ + *blastos,* a germ]. A primitive sympathetic nerve cell. SEE: *sympathoblast.*

sympathicoblastoma (sĭm-păth″ĭ-kō-blăs-tō′mă) [″ + ″ + *oma,* tumor]. A tumor made up of sympathicoblasts.

sympathicolytic (sĭm-păth″ĭ-kō-lĭt′ĭk) [″ + *lytikos,* dissolving]. Interfering with, opposing, inhibiting, or destroying impulses from the sympathetic nervous system. SYN: *sympatholytic.*

sympathicomimetic (sĭm-păth″ĭ-kō-mĭm-ĕt′ĭk) [″ + *mimetikos,* imitating]. Producing effects resembling those resulting from stimulation of the sympathetic nervous system, such as effects following the injection of epinephrine. SYN: *sympathomimetic.*

sympathiconeuritis (sĭm-păth″ĭ-kō-nū-rī′tĭs) [″ + *neuron,* nerve, + *itis,* inflammation]. Inflammation of the sympathetic nerves.

sympathicopathy (sĭm-păth″ĭ-kŏp′ă-thē) [″ + *pathos,* disease]. Disease or disordered function due to malfunction of the autonomic nervous system.

sympathicotonia (sĭm-păth″ĭ-kō-tō′nē-ă) [″ + *tonos,* tension]. Increased tonus of the sympathetic system with marked tendency to vascular spasm and heightened blood pressure. Opposite of vagotonia. SYN: *sympatheticotonia.*

sympathicotripsy (sĭm-păth″ĭ-kō-trĭp′sē) [″ + *tripsis,* a crushing]. Crushing of the superior cervical ganglion. SYN: *sympatheticotripsy.*

sympathicotropic (sĭm-păth″ĭ-kō-trŏp′ĭk) [″ + *tropos,* a turning]. Having a special affinity for the sympathetic nerve.

sympathicus (sĭm-păth′ĭ-kŭs). The sympathetic nervous system.

sympathism (sĭm′pă-thĭzm) [″ + *-ismos,* condition]. Condition of susceptibility to the suggestions and opinions of others. SYN: *suggestibility.*

sympathist (sĭm′pă-thĭst) [″ + *-ismos,* condition]. One susceptible to sympathism.

sympathoadrenal (sĭm″păth-ō-ă-drē′năl) [″ + L. *ad,* to, + *ren,* kidney]. Concerning the sympathetic part of the autonomic nervous system and the adrenal medulla.

sympathoblast (sĭm-păth′ō-blăst) [″ + *blastos,* germ]. A primitive cell from which arises a sympathetic ganglion cell. SYN: *sympathicoblast.*

sympathoblastoma (sĭm″păth-ō-blăs-tō′mă) [″ + ″ + *oma,* tumor]. A malignant tumor made up of sympathetic nerve cells.

sympathoglioblastoma (sĭm″păth-ō-glī″ō-blăs-tō′mă) [Gr. *sympathetikos,* sympathy, + *glia,* glue, + *blastos,* germ, + *oma,* tumor]. A tumor made up primarily of sympathoblasts with scattered neuroblasts and spongioblasts.

sympathogonia (sĭm″pă-thō-gō′nē-ă) [″ +

gone, seed]. Primitive cells from which sympathetic cells are derived.

sympathogonioma (sĭm″pă-thō-gō″nē-ō′mă) [″ + ″ + *oma,* tumor]. A tumor containing sympathogonia.

sympatholytic. Opposing or inhibiting adrenergic nerve function.

sympathoma [″ + *oma,* tumor]. A tumor composed of tissue similar to that of the sympathetic nervous system.

sympathomimetic (sĭm″pă-thō-mĭm-ĕt′ĭk) [″ + *mimetikos,* imitating]. Sympathicomimetic.

sympathy (sĭm′pă-thē) [Gr. *sympatheia*]. 1. Relationship between two organs or parts through which one unaffected part is affected or becomes disordered from disease in the other part without actual transmission of the causative agent. 2. An affective reaction to, and like that of, another person. It may be imitative sympathy in which the reaction is like that of another person as perceived or thought (weeping because another person is weeping); or reflective sympathy in which the reaction is like that of another person as his or her situation is understood. 3. Feeling as another feels. SEE: *empathy.*

sympexion (sĭm-pĕks′ē-ŏn) [Gr. *sympexis,* concretion]. A concretion in certain sites such as the prostate or seminal vesicles.

sympexis (sĭm-pĕks′ĭs). Arrangement of red blood cells due to the effect of surface tension.

symphalangism (sĭm-făl′ăn-jĭzm) [Gr. *syn,* together, + *phalanx,* phalanx]. 1. Ankylosis of joints of the fingers or toes. 2. Web-fingered or web-toed condition.

symphyogenetic (sĭm″fē-ō-jĕ-nĕt′ĭk) [Gr. *syn,* together, + *phyein,* to grow, + *gennan,* to produce]. Concerning the combined effect of heredity and environment upon the development and function of an organism.

symphyseal (sĭm-fĭz′ē-ăl) [Gr. *symphysis,* growing together]. Pert. to symphysis.

symphyseotomy (sĭm-fĭz″ē-ŏt′ō-mē) [″ + *tome,* incision]. Section of symphysis pubis to enlarge the pelvic diameters during delivery. SYN: *hebosteotomy; hebotomy; pelvioplasty; pubiotomy; symphysiectomy; symphysiotomy.*

symphysiectomy (sĭm-fĭz″ē-ĕk′tō-mē) [″ + *ektome,* excision]. Resection of the symphysis pubis to facilitate delivery.

symphysion (sĭm-fĭz′ē-ŏn) [Gr. *symphysis,* growing together]. Most anterior point of the alveolar process of the lower jaw.

symphysiorrhaphy (sĭm-fĭz″ē-or′ă-fē) [″ + *rhaphe,* suture]. Surgical repair of a divided symphysis.

symphysiotome (sĭm-fĭz′ē-ō-tōm) [″ + *tome,* incision]. An instrument for dividing a symphysis.

symphysiotomy (sĭm-fĭz″ē-ŏt′ō-mē) [″ + *tome,* incision]. Section of the symphysis pubis to facilitate childbirth by enlarging the pelvic outlet.

symphysis (sĭm′fĭ-sĭs) [Gr., growing together]. (pl. *symphyses*) 1. A line of fusion between two bones that are separate in early development, as symphysis of mandible. 2. [NA] A form of synchondrosis in which the bones are separated by a disk of fibrocartilage, as in joints between bodies of vertebrae or between pubic bones. SEE: *intervertebral disk.*

s. cartilaginosum. A synchondrosis.

s. ligamentosa. Syndesmosis.

s. mandibulae. S. menti.

s. menti. The symphysis of the chin or the ridge marking the line of union of the two halves of the mandible. SYN: *symphysis mandibulae.*

s. of jaw. An anterior, median, vertical ridge upon outer surface of lower jaw representing line of union of its halves.

s. pubis. The junction of the pubic bones on midline in front; the bony eminence under the pubic hair. SEE: *disk, interpubic.*

symphysodactyly (sĭm″fĭ-sō-dăk′tĭ-lē) [″ + *daktylos,* finger]. Fusion of the fingers or toes. SYN: *syndactylism.*

symplasm (sĭm′plăzm) [Gr. *syn,* together, + *plasmos,* a thing formed]. Living nucleated material lacking in cellular structure.

sympodia (sĭm-pō′dē-ă) [″ + *pous,* foot]. Condition in which lower extremities are united.

symporter (sĭm-por′tĕr). Mechanism for carrying two different molecules or ions in the same direction through a membrane.

symptom (sĭm′tŭm, sĭmp-) [Gr. *symptoma,* occurrence]. Any perceptible change in the body or its functions that indicates disease or the kind or phases of disease. Symptoms may be classified as objective, subjective, cardinal, and sometimes as constitutional. However, another classification considers all symptoms as being subjective, with objective indications being called signs, q.v. Some of the symptoms affecting different parts follow.

Aspects of general symptom analysis include the following. *Onset:* date, manner (gradual or sudden), precipitating factors. *Characteristics:* character, location, radiation, severity, timing, aggravating or relieving factors, associated symptoms. *Course since onset:* incidence, progress, effects of therapy.

ABDOMEN: May be distended, rigid, flat, flabby, adipose, tympanitic, shiny, enlarged, or bulging in certain areas, certain discolorations, stripings, or markings. Muscles may be tensed and little affected by pressure. May be cold areas. Various sounds may be heard such as splashings, roarings, and rumblings (borborygmus, also known as intestinal flatus).

Pain is closely associated with abdominal symptoms. Locate exact area affected and note nature, time of duration, time when it arises, and any causes that might be responsible. Also the effect of movement or pressure on the pain; and the alteration in the pain if the pressure is suddenly released. SEE: *tenderness, rebound.*

Emesis is another condition associated with symptoms pert. to the abdominal region. Emesis may be watery, clear, or contain mucus or undigested food; may be stertorous, bilious, frothy, profuse, purulent, colored from food or medication, and contain blood (hematemesis). If blood is present in large quantity and has been acted on by gastric juices it may resemble coffee grounds. Emesis may be sour, have odor of feces or garlic, may be ammoniacal, or have odor characteristic of some food or drug.

The patient may complain of abdominal distention, gas, and pain caused by gas, crowding in the region of the heart, and interference with respiration. Heartburn may be present, or gastritis and regurgitation. Pain may be felt when food enters the stomach, or relieved by eating or shortly after eating, or by changing body position. Distention after eating as well as desire to eructate or to expel flatus from the stomach should be noted. Colicky pains in the abdomen may be accompanied by pain in the shoulder. Pain at pit of stomach and in lower right quadrant may be indicative of appendicitis. When pains are over the lower right ribs or a little below, disease of the gallbladder may be suspected. SEE: *abdomen; emesis.*

BACK: The dorsal side of the body may reveal edema, deformities, irregularities of the spine, discolorations, eruptions, impaired motion, decubitus, or any condition affecting the skin. SEE: *backache.*

BREATH: May have a fecal odor, a sweet (acetone) odor, one of wet hay, an odor of fish, ammonia, urine, blood, or pus. Respiration may be abdominal or thoracic and show dyspnea, orthopnea, apnea, or it may be normal (eupnea). SEE: *apnea; breath; dyspnea; orthopnea.*

CHEST: The chest may show abnormalities and deformities. Coughing may be whooping, hacking, crowing, hoarse, dry, rasping, or hysterical. There may or may not be expectoration. A cough may be spasmodic or occur on awakening; during deep sleep it may awaken patient; it may or may not produce sputum; it may occur when swallowing food, when in a horizontal position, or when subjected to change of temperatures. If hiccupping is present, note when it occurs. Sputum may be mucoid, yellowish, thick, tenacious, ropy, gelatinous, dark green, offensive in odor, copious, streaked with bright (brick red) or dark blood (hemoptysis), or it may resemble cheesy lumps. It may be clear and watery, scanty, or profuse.

Frequency of coughing and clearing throat should be noted. Patient's respirations may be shallow; dyspnea may be present, or inability to expand the lungs, complaints of irritation, sticking pains, or catchy pains on inspiration. There may be an accumulation of phlegm in the air passages or a tickling in the throat. Patient may not be able to take deep inspirations or may be constantly yawning. There may be migrating, knifelike pains in region of heart or throughout chest. Heart-consciousness may be present, or a fluttering feeling about the heart, or cardiac pain. Queer sensations, the loud beating of the heart, and heaviness in cardiac region are other symptoms. SEE: *apnea; chest; cough; dyspnea; hiccough; sputum.*

DEFECATION: Symptoms to observe are the frequency of defecation; the presence of constipation; hemorrhoids; the nature of the feces such as formation (ribbon-shaped, soft, semiformed, hard or scybala, cylindrical) and whether watery, liquid, or semiliquid; the color, whether dark brown, light brown, clay-colored, green, yellowish, black, bloody; and whether lienteric, serous, mucous, purulent, tarry, or containing membranous shreds, calculi, or foreign substances. The amount should be noted, as small, medium, large, or copious. The odor may be characteristic of various conditions: sour, putrid, offensive, or fetid. The nature of the evacuation should be noted, as natural, difficult, involuntary, or painful. SEE: *feces; stool.*

DENTITION: Teeth may be irregular, missing, misshapen, or affected by caries. There may be a partial or complete denture. Dental hygiene may be good or poor. There may be a loosening of teeth, a film over them, or they may show the presence of sordes.

EARS: Tinnitus aurium, q.v., (ringing in the ears) occurs in certain diseases. Pain in or about ears, or swelling under either or both should be noted. Impacted cerumen, foreign bodies, or insects may be present in auditory canals. SEE: *ear.*

EYES: May be staring, have an excited look, or expressionless. Nystagmus, strabismus, and coma vigil, q.v., may be present. Pupils may be contracted or dilated, or one pupil affected. Patient may keep eyes closed constantly, or keep one open and the other closed. Eyes may be sunken or protruding. Lacrimation may be present. Eyelids may be edematous, and eyeball soft to the touch. Accommodation may be faulty. Nictitating, squinting, or tremor of the eyelids should always be recorded. Blurring of vision usually is associated with other symptoms. Patient may complain of specks dancing before the eyes (muscae volitantes). These may be colorless or colored. SEE: *eye*.

GAIT: May be faltering, scissors, festinating, unsteady, staggering, weakened, swaying, or movements may be stiff, awkward, or unusual. May be total disability or immobility. SEE: *gait*.

GENERAL APPEARANCE: The face may show an expression of anxiety, have a pinched look or a drawn expression. Patient may have air of apathy, a distorted or a blank look, an emotional expression, a risus sardonicus, or sudden lack of all expression (masklike).

GENERAL SYM: Burning sensations may be complained of in various parts of the body, as in the head, throat, arms, chest, or abdomen. They may or may not be accompanied by tenderness. The complaint may be of feeling too hot or too cold without apparent cause, or of having a general feeling of distress.

Anorexia and nausea upon taking food, at the thought of food, or with no reference to food are significant and should be noted; also when nausea occurs: on awakening, when taking fluids, after eating, when changing a position, when taking medication, or in the presence of odors. There always should be an explanation for nausea, either somatic or psychiatric.

Fear of death (angor animi), anxiety, agitation, or panic may be present.

LIMBS: The symptoms pert. to the skin, of course, apply to skin of the limbs. Note if there are deformities, abnormalities, impaired motion, discolorations, sensitivity, varicosities.

LIPS: May be pale, dry, cyanotic, edematous, drawn, deformed, out of proportion, motionless and expressionless, flushed, fissured, or show other lesions or growths. SEE: *lip*.

MOUTH AND GUMS: May be pale or ulcerated, highly inflamed and red, infected, discolored, edematous, or abnormally shaped. Pyorrhea or edema may be present. Patient may complain of certain tastes such as bitter, sweet, salty, sour, fishy, or flat tastes, or an absence of taste. Medication may have much to do with temporary disorders of taste. SEE: *gum; mouth*.

NOSE: May appear deformed, discolored, edematous, or enlarged. Nostrils may discharge or show obstruction. May be inability to breathe through one or both nostrils. Patient may complain of odors not usually manifested as objective symptoms, or for which there is no known cause. SEE: *nose*.

PAIN: The exact area affected must be ascertained, and the wording of the patient's complaint of pain must be charted or reported. Note if pain is in nature of a cramp or spasm, if it is dull, superficial, deep, remittent, shifting, shooting, lancinating, gnawing, fixed, sharp, inflammatory; or if there is an absence of pain, esp. in conditions in which pain usually occurs. Note whether pain is relieved or increased by pressure, heat, cold, change of body position or environment, or other causes. When is pain experienced, how often does the same type of pain recur, and does it awaken the patient from sleep, esp. at night? Observe the facial expression during an attack of pain and listen carefully to the patient's description.

The patient may locate a *headache* around the eyes and nose, in the center of the forehead, above the nose, in one or both temples accompanied by throbbing, at the top of the head, or at the base of the brain. It may be felt as a tight, bandlike sensation around the head above the eyes. It may be in the center of the forehead above the eyebrow line, in the upper region of the center forehead, all over the top of the head, over one or both ears, or back of both ears. Pain may be sharp, dull, or shifting. It may accompany head noises, or a roaring in the head may be experienced without pain. Vertigo or a sensation of fainting may be present. Pulsations may be felt in the occiput or in the temporal region. A patient may be very sensitive to light and sound, and headaches may be accompanied by nausea, vomiting, the sensation of flashing lights, and chills. Tenderness or soreness may be associated with rigidity. SEE: *headache; pain*.

POSITIONS AND POSTURES: An inability to lie down; to arise; or to lie on one side, on the back, or in any special position reveals much to the doctor. Whether lying on the affected or unaffected side is also important to observe. The left leg may be flexed or the right one, or both, or there may be an inclination to lie with the arms above the head. SEE: *posture*.

SKIN: May appear pale, flushed all over or in spots; may be cyanotic, jaundiced, shiny, erupted, burned, blistered, sunburned, wrinkled, lacerated, nodular, bruised; or exhibit dermographia, lesions, growth, or deformities; or be puffy and edematous, ashy, gray, wet with perspiration, or discolored. SEE: *skin*.

THROAT: May show abnormalities, discoloration, inflammation, diseased tonsils and presence of adenoids. Dysphagia and hoarseness or aphonia and other conditions affecting the voice may be present. A lump in the throat (globus hystericus), or a dry, scratchy irritation or fullness or pulsations may be present.

TONGUE: May be coated, clean, smooth, atrophic, shiny, dry on top and moist on the sides or dry all over; may look like raw beef or appear furry, glossy, tremulous, or sharp pointed. It may be edematous or abnormal in size; there may be fissures; the papillae may have disappeared; there may be a strawberry tongue, or it may have various colors. SEE: *tongue*.

URINE: It may be blue, milky, pale, lemon, smoky, brick-colored, clear, amber, straw-colored, orange, or almost any other color. Hematuria may be present. Polyuria or oliguria may be indicated, or there may be frequent urination of small amounts. The odors may be ammoniacal, aromatic, stercorous, or like that of new-mown hay, ripe apples, or violets. There may be retention, suppression, or dribbling, and urination may be painful. SEE: *urine*.

s., accessory. A minor symptom, or one that is not pathognomonic.

s., accidental. Symptom occurring incidentally during course of a disease, but having no relationship to the disease.

s., assident. S., accessory.

s., cardinal. A principal symptom in the diagnosis of a disease.

s., concomitant. Symptom occurring along with the essential symptoms of a disease.

s., constitutional. Symptom caused by or indicating disease of the whole body. SYN: *s., general*.

s., delayed. Symptom appearing sometime after the precipitating cause.

s., direct. Symptom resulting from direct effects of the disease.

s., dissociation. Anesthesia to heat, cold, and pain without loss of tactile sensibility. Seen in syringomyelia.

s., equivocal. Symptom that may occur in several diseases.

s., focal. Symptom at a specific location.

s., general. S., constitutional.

s., indirect. Symptom occurring secondarily as a result of a disease.

s., labyrinthine. A group of symptoms, such as tinnitus, vertigo, or nausea, indicating a disease or lesion of the inner ear.

s., local. Symptom indicating the specific location of the pathological process.

s., negative pathognomonic. Symptom that never occurs in a certain disease or condition; hence its occurrence rules out the existence of that disease.

s., objective. Symptom apparent to the observer. SEE: *sign*.

s., passive. S., static.

s., pathognomonic. Symptom that unmistakably points out presence of a particular disease.

s., presenting. The symptom that led the patient to seek medical care.

s.'s, prodromal. Symptoms that indicate an approaching disease. SYN: *prodrome*.

s., rational. Symptom apparent only to the patient. SYN: *s., subjective*.

s., signal. A symptom that is premonitory of an impending condition such as the aura that precedes an attack of epilepsy or migraine.

s., static. Symptom pert. to the condition of a single organ or structure without reference to remainder of body. SYN: *s., passive*.

s., subjective. Symptom apparent only to the patient. SYN: *s., rational*.

s., sympathetic. A symptom for which there is no specific inciting cause and usually occurring at a point more or less remote from the point of disturbance. SEE: *sympathy* (def. 1).

s.'s, withdrawal. Those symptoms following sudden withdrawal of a substance to which a person has become addicted.

symptomatic (sĭmp″tō-măt′ĭk) [Gr. *symptomatikos*]. Of the nature of or concerning a symptom.

symptomatology (sĭmp″tō-mă-tŏl′ō-jē) [Gr. *symptoma,* symptom, + *logos,* a study]. 1. Science of symptoms and indications. SYN: *semeiology*. 2. All of the symptoms of a given disease as a whole.

symptomatolytic (sĭmp″tō-măt″ō-lĭt′ĭk) [″ + *lysis,* destruction]. Causing the removal of symptoms.

symptom complex. A group of symptoms that occur together and thus characterize a specific disease. SYN: *syndrome*.

symptomolytic (sĭmp″tō-mō-lĭt′ĭk) [″ + *lysis,* destruction]. Pert. to the removal of symptoms. SYN: *symptomatolytic*.

symptosis (sĭmp-tō′sĭs) [Gr. *syn,* together, + *ptosis,* fall]. Emaciation; wasting away of the body or an organ.

sympus (sĭm′pŭs) [″ + *pous,* foot]. A deformed fetus fused at the lower limbs.

syn- [Gr., together]. Prefix meaning joined, together. SEE: words beginning with *con-*.

synache. Inflammation of the throat that obstructs the airway.

synactosis (sĭn″ăk-tō′sĭs) [Gr. *syn,* together, + L. *actio,* function, + Gr. *osis,* condition]. Malformation resulting from the abnormal fusion of parts.

synadelphus (sĭn″ă-dĕl′fŭs) [″ + *adelphos,* brother]. A deformed fetus with eight limbs.

Synalar. Trade name for fluocinolone acetonide, USP.

synalgia (sĭn-ăl′jē-ă) [″ + *algos,* pain]. Referred or reflex pain felt in a part distant from the site of its origin.

synalgic (sĭn-ăl′jĭk). Pert. to or characterized by referred pain.

Synamol. Trade name for fluocinolone acetonide, USP.

synapse (sĭn′ăps) [Gr. *synapsis,* point of contact]. The point of junction between two neurons in a neural pathway, where the termination of the axon of one neuron comes into close proximity with the cell body or dendrites of another. At this point, where the relationship of the two neurons is one of contact only, the impulse traveling in the first neuron initiates an impulse in the second neuron. Synapses are polarized, i.e., the impulses pass in one direction only. They are susceptible to fatigue, offer a resistance to the passage of impulses, and are markedly susceptible to the effects of oxygen deficiency, anesthetics, and other agents, including therapeutic drugs and toxic chemicals.

s., axodendritic. Connection between an axon of one neuron and the dendrites of another.

s., axodendrosomatic. Connection between the axon of one neuron and the dendrites and body of another.

s., axosomatic. Connection between the axon of one neuron and the body of another.

synapsis (sĭn-ăp′sĭs) [Gr., point of contact]. 1. Synapse. 2. The process of first maturation division in gametogenesis in which there is conjugation of pairs of homologous chromosomes forming double or bivalent chromosomes. In the resulting meiotic division, the chromosome number is reduced from the diploid to the haploid number. It is at this stage that crossing over occurs.

RS: crossing over; meiosis; oogenesis; spermatogenesis.

synaptic. Pert. to a synapse or synapsis.

synaptic field. A field in the cerebral cortex, cerebellar cortex, and retina where large numbers of contacts between neurons can take place.

synaptolemma (sĭn-ăp″tō-lĕm′ă). The membrane at a synapse separating two neurons.

synaptology (sĭn″ăp-tŏl′ō-jē) [″ + *logos,* study]. Study of the synapse.

synarthrodia (sĭn″ăr-thrō′dē-ă) [Gr. *syn,* together, + *arthron,* joint, + *eidos,* form]. Type of immovable cartilaginous joint without a joint cavity in which bones are separated by only a connective tissue membrane; a fixed articulation. SYN: *synarthrosis*. SEE: *joint*.

synarthrodial. Pert. to an immovable articulation between bones.

synarthrophysis (sĭn″ăr-thrō-fī′sĭs) [″ + *arthron,* joint, + *physis,* growth]. Progressive ankylosis of joints.

synarthrosis [″ + *arthrosis,* joint]. (pl. *synarthroses*) A type of joint in which the skeletal elements are united by a continuous intervening substance (cartilage, fibrous tissue, or bone). Movement is absent or limited and a joint cavity is lacking. It includes the synchondrosis, suture, and syndesmosis types of joints. SYN: *synarthrodia*.

Synasal. Trade name for phenylephrine hydrochloride, USP.

syncanthus (sĭn-kăn′thŭs) [″ + *kanthos,* angle]. Adhesion of the eyeball to the structures of the orbit.

syncaryon (sĭn-kăr′ē-ŏn). Synkaryon, q.v.

syncephalus (sĭn-sĕf′ă-lŭs) [″ + *kephale,* head]. A deformed fetus with one head, one face, and four ears.

synchilia (sĭn-kī′lē-ă) [″ + *cheilos,* lip]. Congenital adhesions of the lips or atresia of the mouth.

synchiria (sĭn-kī′rē-ă) [″ + *cheir,* hand]. Disorder of sensibility in which stimulus applied to one side of the body is felt on both sides. SEE: *achiria; allochiria; dyschiria*.

synchondroseotomy (sĭn″kŏn-drō″sē-ŏt′ō-mē) [″ + *chondros,* cartilage, + *tome,* incision]. An operation of cutting through the sacroiliac ligaments and closing the arch of the pubes in congenital absence of the anterior wall of the bladder (exstrophy).

synchondrosis (sĭn″kŏn-drō′sĭs) [″ + ″ + *osis,* condition]. An immovable joint having surfaces between the bones connected by cartilages. This may be temporary, in which case the cartilage eventually becomes ossified, or permanent.

synchondrotomy (sĭn-kŏn-drŏt′ō-mē) [″ + ″ + *tome,* incision]. 1. Division of articulating cartilage of a synchondrosis. 2. Section of the symphysis pubis to facilitate childbirth. SEE: *symphyseotomy*.

synchorial (sĭn-kō′rē-ăl) [″ + *chorion,* chorion]. Pert. to multiple fetuses that share a single placenta.

synchronism (sĭn′krō-nĭzm) [″ + *chronos,* time, + *-ismos,* condition]. Simultaneous occurrence of acts or events.

synchronous (sĭn′krō-nŭs). Occurring simultaneously.

synchrotron (sĭn′krō-trŏn). An apparatus that accelerates atomic particles around a circular path by use of electrostatic forces.

synchysis (sĭn′kĭs-ĭs) [Gr., confound]. Fluid state of vitreous of the eye.

s. scintillans. Bright flashes of light resulting from presence of crystals of cholesterol or fat substances in vitreous body.

syncinesis (sĭn″sĭn-ē′sĭs) [″ + *kinesis,* motion]. An involuntary movement produced in association with a voluntary one. SYN: *synkinesis*.

s., imitative. Involuntary movement occurring on sound side when movement is attempted on paralyzed side.

s., spasmodic. Syncinesis occurring on paralyzed side when muscles of opposite side are voluntarily moved.

synciput (sĭn′sĭ-pŭt). Anterior upper half of the cranium. SYN: *sinciput*.

synclinal (sĭn-klī′năl) [Gr. *synklinein,* to lean

together]. Inclined in the same direction toward a point.

synclitism (sĭn'klĭt-ĭzm) [Gr. *synklinein,* to lean together, + *-ismos,* condition]. Parallelism between the planes of the fetal head and those of the maternal pelvis.

synclonus (sĭn'klō-nŭs) [" + *klonos,* turmoil]. 1. Clonic contraction of several muscles together. 2. A disease marked by muscular spasms.

s. ballismus. Paralysis agitans.

s. tremens. Generalized tremor.

syncopal (sĭn'kō-păl) [Gr. *synkope,* fainting]. Rel. to or marked by syncope.

syncope (sĭn'kŭ-pē) [Gr. *synkope,* fainting]. A transient loss of consciousness due to inadequate blood flow to the brain. SYN: *fainting; swoon.* SEE: illus.; *unconsciousness.*

ETIOL: Syncope or fainting may be due to deficient blood flow resulting from peripheral circulatory failure, cerebral vascular accident (stroke), cardiac arrhythmia or transient cardiac standstill in Stokes-Adams syndrome, q.v., or altered blood chemistry as in hyperventilation or hypoglycemia. Predisposing factors include fatigue, prolonged standing, nausea, pain, emotional disturbances, anemia, dehydration, poor ventilation, and many others.

F.A.: It is important to have the person in a horizontal position, preferably with the head low in order to facilitate blood flow to the brain. At the same time, be certain there is a clear airway. The clothing must be loose, esp. if a tight collar was being worn. Fainting usually is of short duration and is counteracted by the individual's being in a supine position. Nevertheless it is important to attempt to establish the cause of the faint prior to dismissing the episode as being of no consequence. If recovery from fainting is not prompt, then it is important to move the patient to a hospital.

s. anginosa. Syncope occurring with anginal pain.

s., cardiac. Syncope of cardiac origin as in Stokes-Adams syndrome, aortic stenosis, tachycardia, bradycardia, or myocardial infarction.

s., carotid sinus. Syncope resulting from pressure on, or hypersensitivity of, carotid sinus. May result from turning head to one side or from too tight a collar.

s., cough. Syncope that occurs during a coughing spell.

s., hysterical. Syncope resulting from anxiety.

s., laryngeal. Brief unconsciousness following coughing and tickling in the throat. SYN: *vertigo, laryngeal.*

s., local. Numbness of a part with sudden blanching, as of the fingers; a symptom of Raynaud's disease or of local asphyxia.

s., vasovagal. Syncope resulting from fall in blood pressure due to failure of peripheral resistance with concomitant reduced venous return, or due to slowing of the heart. May be caused by emotional stress, pain, acute loss of blood, fear, or by assuming an upright position after having been in bed for a prolonged period.

syncopic (sĭn-kŏp'ĭk) [Gr. *synkope,* fainting]. Syncopal.

syncretio (sĭn-krē'shē-ō) [L.]. Development of adhesions between opposing inflamed surfaces.

Syncurine. Trade name for decamethonium bromide.

syncytial (sĭn-sĭ'shăl). Of the nature of a syncytium.

syncytiolysin (sĭn"sĭt-ē-ŏl'ĭ-sĭn) [Gr. *syn,* together, + *kytos,* cell, + *lysis,* destruction]. A cytolysin that is formed from injections of emulsions of placental tissue.

syncytioma (sĭn"sĭt-ē-ō'mă) [" + " + *oma,* tumor]. A tumor of the chorion. SYN: *chorioma; deciduoma.*

s. benignum. A mole.

s. malignum. A tumor formed of cells from the syncytium and chorion, occurring frequently after abortion or during puerperium at site of placenta.

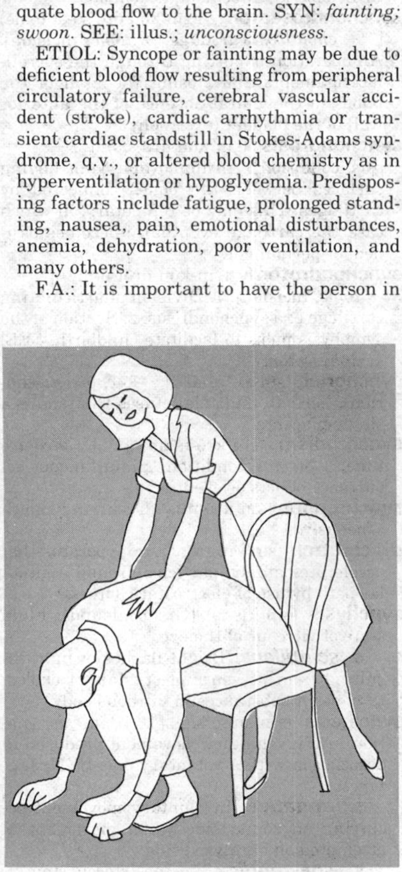

SYNCOPE

POSITION TO ASSIST PATIENT TO REGAIN CONSCIOUSNESS

syncytiotrophoblast (sĭn-sĭt″ē-ō-trō′fō-blăst) [″ + ″ + *trophe,* nourishment, + *blastos,* germ]. The outer layer of cells covering the chorionic villi of the placenta. These cells are in contact with the maternal blood or decidua. SYN: *syntrophoblast.*

syncytium (sĭn-sĭt′ē-ŭm) [″ + *kytos,* cell]. 1. A multinucleated mass of protoplasm such as a striated muscle fiber. 2. A group of cells in which the protoplasm of one cell is continuous with that of adjoining cells such as the mesenchyme cells of the embryo. SYN: *coenocyte.*

syndactylism (sĭn-dăk′tĭl-ĭzm) [″ + *daktylos,* digit, + *-ismos,* condition]. A fusion of two or more toes or fingers.

syndactylous (sĭn-dăk′tĭ-lŭs) [″ + *daktylos,* digit]. Concerning syndactyly.

syndectomy (sĭn-dĕk′tō-mē) [″ + *dein,* to bind, + *ektome,* excision]. Excision of a circular strip of the conjunctiva around the cornea to relieve pannus. SYN: *peritomy* (def. 1).

syndesis (sĭn-dē′sĭs) [″ + *desis,* binding]. 1. Condition of being bound together. 2. Surgical fixation or ankylosis of a joint.

syndesmectomy (sĭn″dĕs-mĕk′tō-mē) [Gr. *syndesmos,* ligament, + *ektome,* excision]. Excision of a section of a ligament.

syndesmectopia (sĭn″dĕs-mĕk-tō′pē-ă) [″ + *ektopos,* out of place]. Abnormal position of a ligament.

syndesmitis (sĭn″dĕs-mī′tĭs) [″ + *itis,* inflammation]. 1. Inflammation of a ligament or ligaments. 2. Inflammation of the conjunctiva.

syndesmochorial (sĭn″dĕs″mō-kor′ē-ăl). Pert. to a type of placenta found in ungulates (Ex.: sheep and goats) in which there is destruction of surface layer of uterine mucosa, thus allowing chorionic villi to come into direct contact with maternal blood vessels.

syndesmography (sĭn-dĕs-mŏg′ră-fē) [Gr. *syndesmos,* ligament, + *graphein,* to write]. Treatise on the ligaments.

syndesmologia (sĭn″dĕs-mō-lō′jē-ă) [″ + *logos,* study]. A term concerned with the articulations of joints and their related ligaments.

syndesmology (sĭn″dĕs-mŏl′ō-jē) [″ + *logos,* a study]. Study of the ligaments, joints, their movements, and their disorders.

syndesmoma (sĭn″dĕs-mō′mă) [″ + *oma,* tumor]. A connective tissue tumor.

syndesmopexy (sĭn-dĕs′mō-pĕk″sē) [″ + *pexis,* fixation]. Joining of two ligaments or fixation of a ligament in a new place, used in correction of a dislocation.

syndesmophyte (sĭn-dĕs′mō-fīt) [″ + *phyton,* plant]. 1. A bony bridge formed between adjacent vertebrae. 2. A bony outgrowth from a ligament.

syndesmoplasty (sĭn-dĕs′mō-plăs″tē) [″ + *plassein,* to form]. Plastic surgery on a ligament.

syndesmorrhaphy (sĭn″dĕs-mor′ă-fē) [″ + *rhaphe,* suture]. Repair or suture of a ligament.

syndesmosis (sĭn″dĕs-mō′sĭs) [Gr. *syndesmos,* ligament, + *osis,* condition]. (pl. *syndesmoses*) [NA] Articulation in which the bones are united by ligaments. Ex.: the distal tibiofibular articulation.

syndesmotomy (sĭn″dĕs-mŏt′ō-mē) [″ + *tome,* incision]. Surgical section of ligaments.

syndrome (sĭn′drōm) [Gr., a running together]. A group of signs and symptoms that collectively characterize or indicate a particular disease or abnormal condition; the sum of signs associated with any pathological process. For syndromes not listed here, see the adjectives. SYN: *symptom complex.*

s., Adair-Dighton. A familial condition characterized by fragility of bones, deafness, and blue sclerae. SEE: *osteogenesis imperfecta.*

s., adiposogenital. S., Fröhlich's.

s., adrenogenital. Syndrome characterized by pubertas praecox in children, overmasculinization in adults, virilism, and hirsutism, due to excess production of adrenocortical hormones. SEE: *Cushing's syndrome.*

s., Angelucci's. Palpitation, excitable temperament, and vasomotor disturbance in some of those who experience spring conjunctivitis.

s., dumping. Symptom complex that may follow partial or complete gastrectomy. Appears to be related to rapid emptying of the gastric pouch. Occurs immediately after eating. Consists of weakness, varying degrees of syncope, nausea, sweating, and palpitation, and sometimes diarrhea and sensation of warmth. Usually lying down affords some relief.

s., Fröhlich's. Syndrome characterized by increase in fat, atrophy of the genitals, transition to feminine type due to lesions of the pituitary and hypothalamus. SYN: *dystrophy, adiposogenital.*

s., Gilles de la Tourette's. SEE: *Gilles de la Tourette's syndrome.*

s., Gradenigo's. Paralysis of the external rectus muscle with severe temporoparietal pain and suppurative otitis media on affected side. Caused by infection in petrous portion of the temporal bone involving the 6th nerve.

s., Horner's. Contracted pupil, ptosis, enophthalmos, and dry, cool face on affected side produced by paralysis of sympathetic nerves. Caused by tumors in neck, trauma, apical tuberculosis, tabes, syringomyelia, and neuritis of cervical plexus.

s., Korsakoff's. A psychosis, ordinarily due to chronic alcoholism, with polyneuritis, disorientation, insomnia, muttering delirium, hallucinations, and a bilateral wrist or foot drop.

s., Marfan's. A hereditary syndrome characterized by disorders of connective tissue, bones, eyes, muscles, ligaments, and skeletal structures.

s., skin-eye. Syndrome consisting of deposits on the anterior surface of the lens and posterior cornea, and skin pigmentation. Due to extensive medication with some of the phenothiazine-type tranquilizers. SEE: *iatrogenic disorder.*

s., sick sinus. SEE: *sick sinus syndrome.*

s., Stokes-Adams. Syndrome of bradycardia and intermittent convulsive seizures with loss of consciousness due to decreased flow of blood to the brain. Caused by partial or complete heart block.

s., toxic shock. SEE: *toxic shock syndrome.*

s., Weber's. Paralysis of hypoglossal nerve on one side and of oculomotor nerve on other with paralysis of limbs due to lesion of a cerebral peduncle.

syndromic (sĭn-drŏm'ĭk) [Gr. *syndrome,* a running together]. Pert. to or occurring as a syndrome.

synechia (sĭn-ĕk'ē-ă) [Gr. *synecheia,* continuity]. (pl. *synechiae*) Adhesion of parts, esp. adhesion of iris to lens and cornea.

s., annular. Adhesion of the iris to the lens throughout its entire pupillary margin.

s., anterior. Adhesion of iris to cornea.

s., posterior. Adhesion of iris to capsule of lens.

s., total. Adhesion of entire surface of iris to lens.

s. vulvae. Fusion of the vulvae, usually congenital.

synechotome (sĭn-ĕk'ō-tōm) [" + *tome,* incision]. An instrument for cutting synechia.

synechotomy (sĭn"ĕk-ŏt'ō-mē) [" + *tome,* incision]. Division of a synechia or adhesion.

synechtenterotomy (sĭn"ĕk-tĕn"tĕr-ŏt'ō-mē) [" + *enteron,* intestine, + *tome,* incision]. Division of an intestinal adhesion.

synecology (sĭn"ē-kŏl'ō-jē) [Gr. *syn,* together, + *oikos,* house, + *logos,* a study]. The study of organisms in relationship to their environment in group form.

Synemol. Trade name for fluocinolone acetonide, USP.

synencephalocele (sĭn"ĕn-sĕf'ă-lō-sēl") [" + *enkephalos,* brain, + *kele,* hernia]. Encephalocele with adhesions to adjacent structures.

syneresis (sĭn-ĕr'ĕ-sĭs) [Gr. *synairesis,* drawing together]. Contraction of a gel resulting in its separation from the liquid, as a shrinkage of fibrin when blood clots.

synergetic (sĭn"ĕr-jĕt'ĭk) [Gr. *syn,* together, + *ergon,* work]. Exhibiting cooperative action, said of certain muscles; working together. SYN: *synergic.*

synergia (sĭn-ĕr'jē-ă). The association and correlation of the activity of synergetic muscle groups.

synergic (sĭn-ĕr'jĭk) [" + *ergon,* work]. Rel. to or exhibiting cooperation, as certain muscles. SYN: *synergetic.*

synergism (sĭn'ĕr-jĭzm) [" + " + *-ismos,* condition]. The harmonious action of two agents, such as drugs or organs, producing an effect that neither could produce alone or an effect that is greater than the total effects of each agent operating by itself.

synergist (sĭn'ĕr-jĭst). 1. A remedy that acts to enhance the action of another. SYN: *adjuvant.* 2. A muscle or organ functioning in cooperation with another, as the flexor muscles. Opposite of antagonist.

synergistic (sĭn"ĕr-jĭs'tĭk). 1. Concerning synergy. 2. Acting together.

synergy (sĭn'ĕr-jē) [Gr. *synergia*]. Action of two or more agents or organs working with each other; cooperation. Combined action; coordinated action. SEE: *synergism.*

synesthesia (sĭn"ĕs-thē'zē-ă) [Gr. *syn,* together, + *aisthesis,* sensation]. 1. A sensation in one area from a stimulus applied to another part. 2. A subjective sensation of another sense than the one being stimulated. Hearing a sound may also produce the sensation of smell. SEE: *phonism.*

s. algica. Painful synesthesia.

synesthesialgia (sĭn"ĕs-thē-zē-ăl'jē-ă) [" + " + *algos,* pain]. A painful sensation giving rise to a subjective one of different character. SEE: *synesthesia.*

synezesis (sĭn"ĕ-zē'sĭs) [Gr. *synizesis,* a sitting together]. Closure of the pupil.

Syngamus (sĭn'gă-mŭs). A genus of nematode worms parasitic in the respiratory tract of birds and mammals.

S. laryngeus. Species normally parasitic in ruminants, but sometimes accidentally infesting man.

syngamy (sĭn'gă-mē) [Gr. *syn,* together, + *gamos,* marriage]. 1. Sexual reproduction. 2. Cell union as of gametes in fertilization.

syngeneic. Term used to describe individuals or cells without detectable tissue incompatibility. Strains of mice that are inbred for a great number of generations become syngeneic. Identical twins are also syngeneic.

syngenesioplasty (sĭn"jĕ-nē"zē-ō-plăs'tē) [" + *genesis,* origin, + *plassein,* to form]. Indicating transplantation of tissue from one individual to one related and of the same species.

syngenesious (sĭn"jĕ-nē'shŭs) [" + *genesis,* origin]. Derived from an individual of the same species, said of tissue transplants.

syngenesis (sĭn-jĕn′ĕ-sĭs) [″ + *genesis*, origin]. Arising from the germ cells derived from both parents, rather than from a single cell from one parent.

syngnathia (sĭn-nā′thē-ă) [″ + *gnathos*, jaw]. Congenital adhesions between the jaws.

synhidrosis (sĭn″hī-drō′sĭs) [″ + *hidrosis*, a sweating]. Sweating, esp. excessive sweating associated with another condition.

synizesis (sĭn″ĭ-zē′sĭs) [Gr. *synizesis*]. 1. An occlusion, or shutting. 2. Clumping of nuclear chromatin during prophase of mitosis.

s. pupillae. Closure of the pupil of the eye with loss of vision.

synkaryon (sĭn-kăr′ē-ŏn) [Gr. *syn*, together, + *karyon*, kernel]. A nucleus resulting from fusion of two pronuclei.

synkinesis (sĭn″kĭ-nē′sĭs) [″ + *kinesis*, motion]. An involuntary movement of one part occurring simultaneously with reflex or voluntary movement of another part.

s., imitative. An involuntary movement in a healthy or normal muscle accompanying an attempted movement of a paralyzed muscle on the opposite side.

synnecrosis (sĭn″nĕ-krō′sĭs) [″ + *nekrosis*, deadness]. The condition of association between groups or individuals that causes mutual inhibition or death.

synonym (sĭn′ō-nĭm) [Gr. *synonymon*]. ABBR: syn. A word that has the same or very similar meaning; an additional or substitute name for the same disease, sign, symptom, or anatomical structure.

synophrys (sĭn-ŏf′rĭs) [Gr. *syn*, together, + *ophrys*, eyebrow]. Condition in which the two eyebrows grow together.

synophthalmus (sĭn″ŏf-thăl′mŭs) [″ + *ophthalmos*, eye]. Cyclops.

synopsia (sĭn′ŏp-sē-ă) [″ + *opsis*, vision]. Condition in which there is congenital fusion of the eyes.

synopsis (sĭn-ŏp′sĭs) [Gr.]. A summary; a general review of the whole.

synoptophore (sĭn-ŏp′tō-for) [″ + *ops*, sight, + *phoros*, bearing]. Apparatus for diagnosing and treating strabismus.

synoptoscope (sĭn-ŏp′tō-skōp) [″ + ″ + *skopein*, to examine]. An instrument for diagnosis and treatment of strabismus. SYN: *synoptophore*.

synorchidism, synorchism (sĭn-or′kĭd-ĭzm, -kĭzm) [″ + *orchis*, testicle, + *-ismos*, condition]. Union or partial fusion of the testicles.

synoscheos (sĭn-ŏs′kē-ŏs) [″ + *oscheon*, scrotum]. Adhesions between the penis and scrotum.

synosteology (sĭn″ŏs-tē-ŏl′ō-jē) [″ + ″ + *logos*, study]. The branch of medical science concerned with joints and articulations.

synosteosis (sĭn″ŏs-tē-ō′sĭs). Synostosis.

synosteotomy (sĭn″ŏs-tē-ŏt′ō-mē) [″ + *osteon*, bone, + *tome*, incision]. Dissection of joints.

synostosis (sĭn″ŏs-tō′sĭs) [″ + ″ + *osis*, condition]. (pl. *synostoses*) 1. [NA] Articulation by osseous tissue of adjacent bones. 2. Union of separate bones by osseous tissue.

synostotic (sĭn″ŏs-tŏt′ĭk) [″ + ″ + *osis*, condition]. Concerning synostosis.

synotia (sĭn-ō′shē-ă) [″ + *ous*, ear]. The union of, or approximation of, the ears occurring in embryonic development, usually associated with absence of, or incomplete development of, the lower jaw.

synotus (sī-nō′tŭs) [″ + *ous*, ear]. A fetus with synotia.

synovectomy (sĭn″ō-vĕk′tō-mē) [L. *synovia*, joint fluid, + Gr. *ektome*, excision]. Excision of synovial membrane.

synovia (sĭn-ō′vē-ă) [L.]. [NA] A colorless, viscid, lubricating fluid of joints, bursae, and tendon sheaths secreted within synovial membranes. It contains mucin, albumin, fat, and mineral salts. SYN: *synovial fluid*. SEE: *asynovia; joint* for illus.

synovial (sĭn-ō′vē-ăl). Pert. to synovia, the lubricating fluid of the joints.

synovial bursa. A cavity in connective tissue between muscles, tendons, ligaments, and bones lined by a synovial membrane and containing synovia. SYN: *bursa*.

synovial crypt. Diverticulum of a synovial membrane of a joint.

synovial cyst. Accumulation of synovia in a bursa, synovial crypt, or sac of a synovial hernia, causing a tumor.

synovial fluid. Clear lubricating fluid secreted by the synovial membrane of a joint. SYN: *synovia*. SEE: *joint* for illus.

synovial folds. Smooth folds of synovial membrane on inner surface of the joint capsule. SYN: *plica synoviales* [NA].

synovial hernia. Protrusion of a portion of synovial membrane through a tear in the stratum fibrosum of a joint capsule.

synovialis (sĭ-nō″vē-ā′lĭs) [L.]. Synovial.

synovial membrane. Membrane lining the capsule of a joint. SYN: *synovium*.

synovialoma (sĭ-nō″vē-ă-lō′mă) [L. *synovia*, joint fluid, + Gr. *oma*, tumor]. Synovioma.

synovial tendon sheaths. Sheaths that develop in osteofibrous canals through which tendons pass. Each is a double-layered tube, the space between the two layers being occupied by synovial fluid. SYN: *vagina mucosa tendinis*.

synovial villi. Slender avascular processes on the free surface of a synovial membrane projecting into the joint cavity.

synovioma (sĭn″ō-vē-ō′mă) [L. *synovia*, joint fluid, + Gr. *oma*, tumor]. A tumor arising from a synovial membrane.

synoviparous (sĭn″ō-vĭp′ă-rŭs) [″ + *parere,* to produce]. Forming synovia.

synovitis (sĭn″ō-vī′tĭs) [″ + Gr. *itis,* inflammation]. Inflammation of a synovial membrane.

ETIOL: Simple inflammation may be the result of an aseptic wound, a subcutaneous injury (contusion or sprain), irritation produced by damaged cartilage, or exposure to cold and dampness.

SYM: The joint is painful, much more so on motion, esp. at night. Swollen, tense; may be fluctuating. In synovitis of the knee, patella is floated up from condyles, and it can be readily depressed, to rise again when pressure is taken off. The part is never in full extension, as this increases the pain. Skin, which is very sensitive to pressure only at certain points, is neither thickened nor reddened. After a few days, when pain lessens and swelling diminishes as the effusion and extravasated blood are absorbed, the limb takes its natural position and recovery follows.

s., chronic. Synovitis in which active congestion appears, but an undue amount of fluid remains in the cavity and the membrane itself is edematous. Later if disease does not subside, membrane and articular structures become irregularly thickened by plastic exudation and formation of fibrous tissue. Joint is weak but not esp. painful, except on pressure and sometimes not even then. Movements, esp. in extension, are restricted, and generally attended by some grating or creaking. Symptoms are well marked when there is great accumulation of liquid. Fluid, which is straw-colored, somewhat viscid, sometimes flocculent, and may or may not be blood stained, can be drawn off with the hypodermic needle.

s., dendritic. Synovitis with villous growths developing in the sac.

s., dry. Synovitis with little or no effusion. SYN: *s. sicca.*

s., purulent. Synovitis with purulent effusion within the sac. SYN: *arthritis, suppurative.*

s., serous. Synovitis with nonpurulent, copious effusion.

s. sicca. S., dry.

s., simple. Synovitis with effusion only slightly turbid, if not clear.

s., tendinous. Inflammation of a tendon sheath.

s., vaginal. S., tendinous.

s., vibration. Synovitis resulting from a wound near a joint.

synovium (sĭn-ō′vē-ŭm) [L. *synovia,* joint fluid]. A synovial membrane.

syntactic (sĭn-tăk′tĭk). Concerning or affecting syntax.

syntasis (sĭn-tā′sĭs) [Gr. *syn,* together, + *teinein,* to stretch]. Stretching.

syntaxis (sĭn-tăk′sĭs) [″ + *taxis,* arrangement]. A junction between two bones. SYN: *articulation.*

syntectic (sĭn-tĕk′tĭk). Concerning syntexis.

syntexis (sĭn-tĕk′sĭs) [Gr.]. Wasting or cachexia.

synthermal (sĭn-thĕr′măl) [″ + *therme,* heat]. Having the same temperature.

synthesis (sĭn′thĕs-ĭs) [Gr.]. In chemistry, the union of elements to produce compounds; the process of building up. In general, the process or processes involved in the formation of a complex substance from simpler elements or compounds, as the synthesis of proteins from amino acids. Opposite of decomposition.

synthesize (sĭn″thĕ-sīz′). To produce by synthesis.

synthetase (sĭn′thĕ-tās). Ligase, q.v.

synthetic (sĭn-thĕt′ĭk) [Gr. *synthetikos*]. Rel. to or made by synthesis; artificially prepared.

synthorax (sĭn-thō′răks) [Gr. *syn,* together, + *thorax,* chest]. Thoracopagus, q.v.

Synthroid. Trade name for levothyroxine sodium, USP.

Syntocinon. Trade name for oxytocin injection.

syntone (sĭn′tōn) [″ + *tonos,* tension]. An individual whose personality indicates a stable responsiveness to the environment and its social demands. SEE: *syntonic.*

syntonic (sĭn-tŏn′ĭk). Pert. to a personality characterized by an even temperament, a normal emotional responsiveness to life situations. Opposite of schizoid. Syntonic type is exaggerated in manic states or in depression. SEE: *syntone.*

syntonin (sĭn′tō-nĭn). An acid albumin formed by the action of dilute hydrochloric acid on muscle during gastric digestion.

syntoxoid (sĭn-tŏk′soyd) [Gr. *syn,* together, + *toxikon,* poison, + *eidos,* form]. A toxoid having the same degree of affinity for an antitoxin as that possessed by the toxin.

syntripsis (sĭn-trĭp′sĭs) [Gr., destruction]. A comminuted fracture or act causing it.

syntrophism (sĭn′trōf-ĭzm) [″ + *trophe,* nourishment, + *-ismos,* condition]. Stimulation of an organism to grow by mixing with or closeness of another strain.

syntrophoblast (sĭn-trŏf′ō-blăst) [″ + ″ + *blastos,* germ]. The outer syncytial layer of the trophoblast. SEE: *trophoblast.*

syntropic (sĭn-trŏp′ĭk) [″ + *trope,* a turn]. Concerning syntropy.

syntropy (sĭn′trō-pē) [″ + *trope,* a turn]. Turning or pointing in the same direction.

synulosis (sĭn″ū-lō′sĭs) [Gr. *synoulosis*]. Formulation of scar tissue

synulotic (sĭn″ū-lŏt′ĭk). 1. Promoting cicatrization. 2. An agent stimulating cicatrization.

syphilelcosis (sĭf-ĭl-ĕl-kō′sĭs) [*syphilis* + Gr. *helkosis,* ulceration]. Syphilitic ulceration.

syphilelcus (sĭf″ĭl-ĕl′kŭs) [″ + Gr. *helkos,* ulcer]. A syphilitic ulcer or chancre.

syphilid(e) (sĭf″ĭl-ĭd) [Fr.]. (pl. *syphilides*) Skin eruption caused by secondary syphilis.

syphilionthus (sĭf″ĭl-ē-ŏn′thŭs) [″ + Gr. *ionthos,* eruption]. A copper-colored, branny-scaled syphilide.

syphiliphobia (sĭf″ĭl-ĭ-fō′bē-ă) [″ + Gr. *phobos,* fear]. Morbid fear of syphilis. SYN: *syphilophobia.*

syphilis (sĭf′ĭ-lĭs). [*Syphilis,* shepherd having the disease in a Latin poem] An infectious, chronic, venereal disease characterized by lesions that may involve any organ or tissue. It usually exhibits cutaneous manifestations, relapses are frequent, and it may exist without symptoms for years. SYN: *lues.*

ETIOL: Treponema pallidum, a spirochete that is transmitted by direct contact between humans, contact with freshly contaminated material, transfusion of infected blood or plasma, or in utero by passage of the organism from mother to fetus. The organism may enter through any broken place in skin or mucous membrane.

SYM: *Primary stage:* Initial lesion appears 2 to 4 weeks after inoculation, changing from a small red papule to a small ulcer to a hard chancre. Usually upon prepuce or vulva but may be on any skin or mucous membrane site. Lymph nodes enlarge about two weeks after appearance of lesion.

Secondary stage: Symptoms appear about 6 weeks after appearance of primary lesion, principally in the form of lesions of the skin and mucous membranes. The character of the skin lesions is protean, syphilis often being called the "great imitator." Systemic symptoms such as headache, fever, and malaise are common but may be absent. Enlargement and induration of regional lymph nodes occur. Eruptions of skin, maculae (roseola), syphilide, reddish-brown coppery spots continuing for a week or two and possibly recurring later.

Tertiary stage: The heart and blood vessels (cardiovascular syphilis) and the central nervous system (neurosyphilis) are frequently involved. Tabes dorsalis, paresis (general paralysis of the insane), and various types of psychoses may result.

DIAG: Laboratory tests for syphilis are based on three procedures: *microscopic,* darkfield demonstration of spirochetes in material taken from a chancre or other early lesion; *biopsy,* examination of cerebrospinal fluid; *serologic tests for syphilis* (S.T.S.) done on blood and spinal fluid. These include complement-fixation techniques (Wassermann test and its modifications). The VDRL (Venereal Disease Research Laboratory), Treponema pallidum immobilization (TPI), and fluorescent treponemal antibody (FTA) tests also are useful in diagnosing syphilis and distinguishing it from biological false-positive serologic reactions.

CAUTION: A person who contracts gonorrhea also may have been exposed to syphilis at the same time. Because the clinical signs and symptoms of gonorrhea develop several weeks prior to those of syphilis, the patient may be treated for that disease. The treatment for gonorrhea may be sufficient to mask or delay the signs of syphilis, but insufficient to rid the patient of the spirochetes. When this occurs, syphilis will develop and may be unnoticed by the patient. It is therefore of vital importance either to treat each case of gonorrhea as if syphilis had also been contracted, or to test the patient for serologic evidence of syphilis each month for at least four months following the treatment for gonorrhea.

NURSING IMPLICATIONS: Teach the patient about the illness and the importance of locating all contacts, treatment, and the significance of follow-up care. Administer penicillin as prescribed or alternative antibiotic if patient is allergic to penicillin. Encourage follow-up care. Refer to public health agency to assist in identification of contacts. Teach methods of prevention. Provide supportive counseling. Report disease to infection control authorities as prescribed by local health agency. Utilize caution when handling laboratory specimens. Instruct patient to avoid sexual contact with anyone until he or she has completed therapy; and to avoid sexual contact with previous partners who have not received adequate investigation for the possible presence of syphilis, and treatment if indicated. Employ secretory precautions if the patient has skin or mucous membrane lesions for 24 hours after the initiation of proper antibiotic therapy.

TREATMENT: Penicillin is the treatment of choice for all types and stages. Should allergic reactions occur, other antibiotics (oxytetracycline, chlortetracycline, or erythromycin) may be substituted. The use of arsenicals, bismuth, and mercurials has been almost completely supplanted by antibiotics.

s., cardiovascular. Syphilis involving the heart and great blood vessels, esp. the aorta. Saccular aneurysms of the aorta and aortic insufficiency frequently result.

s., congenital. Syphilis transmitted from the mother to the fetus in utero. SYN: *s., prenatal.*

s., extragenital. Syphilis in which the primary chancre is located elsewhere than on genital organs.

s. innocentium. Syphilis not contracted through coition.

s., latent. Phase of syphilis in which symptoms are absent, and the disease can be diagnosed only by serological tests.

s., meningovascular. A form of neurosyphilis in which the meninges and vascular structures of the brain and spinal cord are involved. May be localized or general.

s., neuro-. Involvement of the nervous system by syphilis.

s., nonvenereal. An acute disease confined to certain geographical areas. It begins with an eruption of the skin and mucous membrane, usually without being preceded by a primary lesion. The disease is caused by Treponema pallidum and resembles syphilis, but it is transmitted by nonsexual body contact; and the central nervous system and cardiovascular system are rarely involved. Penicillin is effective therapy.

s., prenatal. *S.*, congenital.

s., visceral. Syphilis in which visceral organs are involved.

syphilitic (sĭf″ĭ-lĭt′ĭk) [L. *syphiliticus*]. Rel. to, caused by, or affected with syphilis.

syphilitic fever. Rise in temperature in early stage of secondary syphilis.

syphilitic macules. Small red eruptions manifested in secondary syphilis, often covering the entire body.

SYM: Associated with chancre or scar, alopecia, pain in bones, swollen glands, and sore throat.

syphiloderm, syphiloderma (sĭf′ĭl-ō-dĕrm″, sĭf″ĭl-ō-dĕr′mă) [″ + Gr. *derma*, skin]. A syphilitic cutaneous disorder.

syphilogenesis, syphilogeny (sĭf″ĭl-ō-jĕn′ĕ-sĭs, sĭf″ĭl-ŏj′ĕn-ē) [″ + Gr. *genesis*, production]. The development or origin of syphilis.

syphilographer (sĭf″ĭl-ŏg′ră-fĕr) [″ + Gr. *graphein*, to write]. One who writes about syphilis.

syphilography (sĭf″ĭl-ŏg′ră-fē). A treatise on syphilis.

syphiloid (sĭf′ĭ-loyd) [″ + Gr. *eidos*, form]. Resembling syphilis.

syphilology (sĭf″ĭl-ŏl′ō-jē). The study of syphilis and its treatment.

syphiloma (sĭf″ĭl-ō′mă) [″ + Gr. *oma*, tumor]. A syphilitic tumor; a gumma, q.v.

syphilomania (sĭf″ĭl-ō-mā′nē-ă) [″ + Gr. *mania*, madness]. Morbid fear of syphilis or inference that one is suffering with it. SYN: *syphilophobia*.

syphilopathy (sĭf″ĭ-lŏp′ă-thē) [″ + Gr. *pathos*, disease]. Any syphilitic disorder.

syphilophobia (sĭf″ĭl-ō-fō′bē-ă) [″ + Gr. *phobos*, fear]. 1. Morbid fear of syphilis. 2. Delusion of having syphilis.

syphilophobic (sĭf″ĭl-ō-fō′bĭk). Pert. to or affected with syphilophobia.

syphilophyma (sĭf″ĭl-ō-fī′mă) [″ + Gr. *phyma*, a growth]. 1. Any growth or excrescence due to syphilis. 2. Syphiloma of the epidermis.

syphilosis (sĭf″ĭ-lō′sĭs) [″ + Gr. *osis*, disease]. Generalized syphilitic disease.

syphilotherapy (sĭf″ĭl-ō-thĕr′ă-pē) [″ + Gr. *therapeia*, treatment]. Treatment of syphilis.

syphilotropic (sĭf″ĭl-ō-trŏp′ĭk) [″ + Gr. *tropos*, a turning]. Esp. susceptible to syphilis.

syphilous (sĭf′ĭl-ŭs). Of the nature of or pert. to syphilis. SYN: *syphilitic*.

syphionthus (sĭf″ē-ŏn′thŭs) [″ + Gr. *ionthos*, eruption]. Copper-colored patches of the skin seen in syphilis.

syr. *syrupus*, syrup.

syrigmophonia (sĭr″ĭg-mō-fō′nē-ă) [Gr. *syrigmos*, a whistle, + *phone*, voice]. 1. A sibilant rale. 2. A whistling sound in pronunciation of "s" due to a denture peculiarity.

syrigmus (sĭr-ĭg′mŭs) [Gr. *syrigmos*, a whistle]. A subjective sound such as a hissing or ringing heard in the ears.

syringadenoma (sĭr-ĭng″ă-dē-nō′mă) [Gr. *syrinx*, pipe, + *aden*, gland, + *oma*, tumor]. Tumor of a sweat gland.

syringe (sĭr-ĭnj′, sĭr′ĭng) [Gr. *syrinx*, pipe]. 1. Instrument for injecting fluids into cavities or vessels. SEE: *needle* for illus. 2. To wash out or introduce fluid with a syringe.

s., hypodermic. Syringe, fitted with a needle, used to administer drugs by injecting them into the subcutaneous tissue.

s., oral. A syringe made of plastic or glass. It is not fitted with a needle. It is graduated and is used to dispense liquid medication to children. The tip is constructed to prevent its breaking in the child's mouth.

syringectomy (sĭr″ĭn-jĕk′tō-mē) [″ + *ektome*, excision]. Removal of the walls of a fistula.

syringitis (sĭr″ĭn-jī′tĭs) [″ + *itis*, inflammation]. Inflammation of eustachian tube.

syringoadenoma (sĭ-rĭng″gō-ăd″ĕ-nō′mă) [″ + *aden*, gland, + *oma*, tumor]. Syringocystadenoma, q.v.

syringobulbia (sĭr-ĭn″gō-bŭl′bē-ă) [″ + *bulbos*, a bulb]. A chronic progressive disease characterized by development of cavities in the medulla oblongata. SEE: *syringomyelia*.

syringocarcinoma (sĭ-rĭng″gō-kăr″sĭ-nō′mă) [″ + *karkinos*, cancer, + *oma*, tumor]. Carcinoma of the sweat gland.

syringocele (sĭr-ĭn′gō-sēl) [″ + *koilia*, a hollow]. 1. The central canal of the myelon or spinal cord. 2. A form of meningomyelocele that contains a cavity in the ectopic spinal cord.

syringocystadenoma (sĭr-ĭn″gō-sĭs″tă-dĕ-nō′mă) [″ + *kystis*, a bladder, + *aden*, gland, + *oma*, tumor]. Adenoma of sweat glands characterized by tiny, hard, papular formations.

syringocystoma (sĭr-ĭn″gō-sĭs-tō′mă) [″ + ″ + *oma,* tumor]. Cystic tumor having its origin in ducts of the sweat gland.

syringoencephalomyelia (sĭ-rĭng″gō-ĕn-sĕf″ ă-lō-mī-ē′lē-ă) [″ + *enkephalos,* brain, + *myelos,* marrow]. Condition of cavities in the brain and spinal cord.

syringoid (sĭr-ĭn′goyd) [Gr. *syrinx,* pipe, + *eidos,* form]. Resembling a tube; fistulous.

syringoma (sĭr″ĭn-gō′mă) [″ + *oma,* tumor]. Tumor of the sweat glands.

syringomeningocele (sĭr-ĭn″gō-mĕn-ĭn′gō-sēl) [″ + *meninx,* membrane, + *kele,* hernia]. Meningocele that is similar to a syringomyelocele.

syringomyelia (sĭr-ĭn″gō-mī-ē′lē-ă) [″ + *myelos,* marrow]. A chronic progressive disease of the spinal cord characterized by the development of cavities and gliosis of surrounding tissue. Usually begins before age of 30 and is more common among males. Its cause is unknown.

SYM: Cavitation occurs in cervical and lumbar regions and soon involves pathways of the cord that carry impulses of pain and temperature sensations, resulting in dissociated sensory loss. Destruction of lateral and anterior gray matter causes muscular atrophy and weakness.

TREATMENT: There is no satisfactory treatment. Sudden enlargement of cavity may warrant surgical intervention with decompression of cavity. Persistent pain may necessitate chordotomy or medullary tractotomy for relief.

syringomyelitis (sĭr-ĭn″gō-mī″ĕ-lī′tĭs) [″ + *myelos,* marrow, + *itis,* inflammation]. Inflammation coincident with abnormal dilation of the central canal of the spinal cord.

syringomyelocele (sĭr-ĭn″gō-mī′ĕl-ō-sēl) [″ + ″ + *kele,* tumor]. A form of spina bifida in which the cavity of the projecting portion communicates with the central canal of the spinal cord.

syringomyelus (sĭr-ĭn″gō-mī′ĕl-ŭs). Abnormal dilatation of the central canal of the spinal cord.

syringopontia (sĭr-ĭn″gō-pŏn′shē-ă) [″ + L. *pons,* bridge]. Cavities in the pons varolii similar to syringomyelia.

syringosystrophy (sĭr-ĭn″gō-sĭs′trō-fē) [″ + *systrophe,* a twist]. Twisting of the oviduct.

syringotome (sĭr-ĭn′gō-tōm) [″ + *tome,* incision]. Instrument for incision of a fistula.

syringotomy (sĭr″ĭn-gŏt′ō-mē). Operation for incision of a fistula.

syrinx (sĭr′ĭnks) [Gr., pipe]. 1. The eustachian tube. 2. Pathological cavity in the spinal cord or brain. 3. A fistula.

syrup (sĭr′ŭp) [L. *syrupus*]. ABBR: syr. Concentrated solution of sugar in water. Usually specific medicinal substances are added. Syrup usually does not represent a very high percentage of the active drug. Some syrups are used principally to give a pleasant odor and taste to solutions.

s., simple. A combination of purified water and sucrose.

syssarcosis (sĭs″ăr-kō′sĭs) [Gr. *syn,* together, + *sarkosis,* fleshy growth]. The union of bones by muscles; a muscular articulation such as the hyoid and patella.

systaltic (sĭs-tăl′tĭk) [Gr. *systaltikos,* contracting]. Contracting and dilating alternately; having a systole. SYN: *pulsating.*

system (sĭs′tĕm) [Gr. *systema,* a composite whole]. 1. An organized grouping of related structures or parts. 2. A group of structures or organs related to each other and functioning together in the performance of certain functions such as the digestive system. 3. A group of cells or aggregations of cells that perform a particular function such as the reticuloendothelial, cardiovascular, respiratory, and central nervous systems.

s., alimentary. S., digestive, q.v.

s., autonomic nervous. That portion of the peripheral nervous system that innervates all smooth muscle, cardiac muscle, and glands, the activities of which are involuntary. It includes the craniosacral (parasympathetic) and thoracolumbar (sympathetic) divisions, each of which provides fibers for most of the visceral structures or organs. SYN: *system, vegetative nervous.*

s., cardiovascular. The heart and blood vessels (aorta, arteries, arterioles, capillaries, venules, veins, venae cavae).

s., centimeter-gram-second. ABBR: CGS. A system of measurement in units of length, mass, and time. SYN: *metric system.*

s., central nervous. That portion of the nervous system consisting of the brain and spinal cord.

s., chromaffin. The mass of tissue forming paraganglia and medulla of suprarenal glands, which secretes epinephrine and stains readily with chromium salts. Similar tissue is found in the organs of Zuckerkandl, and in the liver, testes, ovary, and heart.

s., circulatory. System concerned with circulation of body fluids. It includes the cardiovascular and lymphatic systems. SYN: *s., vascular.*

s., conduction, of the heart. The pathway of excitation of the cardiac muscle beginning with the sinoatrial node, atrioventricular node and bundle, and the Purkinje fibers.

s., cytochrome. Cytochrome oxidase and three hemochromogen-like pigments (cytochromes a, b, and c) that make molecular oxygen available for the oxidation of hydrogen liberated from cellular metabolites.

s., digestive. The alimentary canal

(mouth, teeth, tongue, pharynx, esophagus, stomach, small and large intestines) and accessory glands (salivary glands, liver, pancreas). SEE: *digestion; digestive system* for illus.

s., endocrine. The ductless glands or the glands of internal secretion, which include the pituitary, pineal body, pancreas, paraganglia, thyroid, parathyroid, and the adrenal glands. SEE: *endocrine gland.*

s., extrapyramidal motor. Functional system including all descending fibers arising in cortical and subcortical motor centers that reach the medulla and spinal cord by pathways other than recognized pyramidal tracts. The system is important in maintenance of equilibrium and muscle tone.

s., genital. S., reproductive.

s., genitourinary. The organs of reproduction combined with the urinary organs. SEE: *genitalia* for illus.

s., haversian. Architectural unit of bone consisting of a central tube (haversian canal) with alternate layers of intercellular material (matrix) surrounding it in concentric cylinders. Alternating layers of matrix and cells are called haversian lamellae.

s., hematopoietic. The blood-forming tissues and organs of the body. Includes the bone marrow, spleen, and lymphatic tissue.

s., heterogeneous. Any system the components of which may be separated by mechanical means.

s., homogeneous. Any system the components of which cannot be separated by mechanical means.

s., hypophyseoportal. The series of vessels that lead from the hypothalamus to the anterior lobe of the pituitary. The releasing factors are carried to the pituitary through this system.

s., impulse-conducting. A system of atypical muscle fibers (Purkinje fibers) within the heart that conducts impulses regulating contractions of the atria and ventricles. Includes S-A and A-V nodes and bundle of His.

s., integumentary. The skin and its derivatives (hair, nails).

s., lymphatic. System concerned with the circulation of lymph. Includes lymph vessels and ducts and lymphatic organs (lymph nodes, tonsils, thymus, spleen). SEE: *lymph; lymphatic.*

s., metric. A system of weights and measures based on the meter (39.37 in.) as the unit of linear measure; the gram (15.432 gr.) as the unit of weight; the liter (1.057 qt.) as the unit of volume. SEE: *Metric System* in *Appendix.*

s., muscular. System that includes all the muscles (smooth, cardiac, striated, or skeletal) of the body. SEE: *muscle.*

s., nervous. System that includes the brain, spinal cord, ganglia, and nerves.

S. of Units, International. ABBR: SI. The modern version of the metric system. SEE: *SI units* in *Appendix.*

s., osseous. The bony structures of the body; the skeleton. SEE: *skeleton.*

s., parasympathetic nervous. SEE: *parasympathetic nervous system.*

s., peripheral nervous. That part of the nervous system outside the central nervous system.

s., portal. A system of vessels where blood passes through a capillary network, a large vessel, and then another capillary network before returning to the systemic circulation, as the circulation of blood through the liver.

s., reproductive. The gonads and their associated structures and ducts. In the female this includes the ovaries, uterine tubes (oviducts), uterus, vagina, and vulva. In the male this includes the testes, efferent ducts, epididymis, ductus deferens, ejaculatory duct, urethra and accessory glands (bulbourethral, prostate, seminal vesicles), and penis. SYN: *s., genital.* SEE: *genitalia* for illus.

s., respiratory. The air passageways and organs (nasal cavities, oral cavity, pharynx, larynx, trachea, and lungs, including bronchi, bronchioles, alveolar ducts, and alveoli). SEE: *lung* for illus.

s., reticuloendothelial. ABBR: RES. Collectively, all the phagocytic cells of the body excepting the leukocytes. Includes macrophages, histiocytes, Kupffer's cells of the liver, reticular cells of lymphatic organs, microglia of the brain, and many others.

s., skeletal. The bony framework of the body. SEE: *skeleton.*

s., sympathetic nervous. The thoracolumbar or sympathetic division of the autonomic nervous system.

s., urinary. The kidneys, ureters, bladder, and urethra.

s., urogenital. The urinary and reproductive systems combined. SEE: *genitalia* for illus.

s., vascular. System of all vessels of the body (heart, blood vessels, and lymphatics). SYN: *s., circulatory.*

s., vasomotor. The part of the nervous system that controls the size of the vascular system vessels.

s., vegetative nervous. S., autonomic nervous.

s., visceral efferent. System that includes all efferent nerve fibers conveying impulses to the visceral organs; the autonomic nervous system, q.v.

systema (sĭs-tē′mă) [Gr., a composite whole]. System.

systematic (sĭs″tē-măt′ĭk). Concerning a system or organized according to a system.

systematization (sĭs-tĕm″ă-tī-zā′shŭn). The process of organizing something according to a plan.

systemic (sĭs-tĕm′ĭk). Pert. to a whole body rather than to one of its parts; somatic.

systemic circulation. The blood flow from the left ventricle through the aorta and all its branches (arteries) to the capillaries of the tissues and its return to the heart through veins and the venae cavae, which empty into the right atrium.

systemic remedies. Remedies that will act on the body as a whole.

systemoid (sĭs′tĕ-moyd) [″ + *eidos,* form]. 1. Resembling a system. 2. Pert. to tumors made up of several types of tissues.

systems theory. As used in clinical medicine, an approach that considers the human being as a whole as opposed to his or her parts. Human beings are considered open systems constantly exchanging information, matter, and energy with the environment. There are three levels of reference for systems: the system-level on which one is focusing, such as man; the suprasystems-level above the focal system, such as man's family, the community, and the culture; and subsystem, the level below the focal system, such as the bodily systems and the cell. Nursing must view persons as being affected constantly by supra- and subsystems. Nursing care, in the systems approach, transcends the idea of treating illness and addresses the larger issue of attaining and maintaining health through assessment and intervention of the total person.

systole (sĭs′tō-lē) [Gr., contraction]. That part of the heart cycle in which the heart is in contraction, i.e., the myocardial fibers are tightening and shortening. Occurs in the interval between first and second heart sound during which blood is surged through the aorta and pulmonary artery. SEE: *diastole; murmur; presystole.*

s., aborted. A premature cardiac systole in which arterial pressure is increased little if at all because of inadequate filling of ventricles due to shortening of preceding diastole.

s., anticipated. Systole that is aborted because it occurs before the ventricle is filled.

s., arterial. The rebound or recoil of the stretched elastic walls of the arteries following ventricular systole.

s., atrial. The contraction of the atria. Precedes the ventricular systole.

s., electrical. The total duration of the QRST complex in an electrocardiogram. Approximately the same as that of the mechanical systole.

s., extra. A premature systole occurring in addition to the fundamental rhythm.

s., premature. Systole slightly preceding a normal systole. SYN: *extrasystole.*

s., ventricular. Ventricular contraction.

systolic (sĭs-tŏl′ĭk) [Gr. *systole,* contraction]. Pert. to the systole.

systolic discharge. The amount of blood ejected by the heart at each systole.

systolic murmur. A cardiac murmur during systole.

systolic pressure. Maximum blood pressure. This occurs during contraction of the ventricle. SEE: *blood pressure; diastolic pressure; pulse; pulse pressure.*

systremma (sĭs-trĕm′ă) [Gr. *systremma,* anything twisted together]. Cramp in calf of the leg, the muscles assuming form of a hard knot.

Sytobex. Trade name for cyanocobalamin, USP.

Sytobex-H. Trade name for hydroxocobalamin.

syzygial (sĭ-zĭj′ē-ăl) [Gr. *syzygia,* conjunction]. Pert. to a syzygium.

syzygiology (sĭ-zĭj″ē-ŏl′ō-jē) [″ + *logos,* a study]. Study of interdependence or interrelationship of the whole as opposed to that of isolated functions or separate parts.

syzygium (sĭ-zĭj′ē-ŭm) [Gr. *syzygia,* conjunction]. Fusion of two parts or structures without loss of identity of the parts.

syzygy (sĭz′ĭ-jē). Fusion of organs, each remaining distinct.

T

T. *temperature; time; intraocular tension.*

t. *temporal;* L. *ter,* three times.

$t_{1/2}$, $T_{1/2}$. In nuclear medicine, the symbol of half-life of a radioactive substance.

T_3. Triiodothyronine. SEE: *thyroid function tests.*

T_4. Tetraiodothyronine. SEE: *thyroid function tests.*

T-1824. Evans blue dye.

T-250. Trade name for tetracycline hydrochloride, USP.

T.A. *toxin-antitoxin.*

Ta. Chem. symb. for tantalum.

tabacism (tăb′ă-sĭzm) [L. *tabacum,* tobacco, + Gr. *-ismos,* condition]. Chronic tobacco poisoning. SYN: *tabacosis.*

tabacosis (tăb″ă-kō′sĭs) [″ + Gr. *osis,* condition]. Chronic tobacco poisoning or pneumoconiosis from inhaling tobacco dust.

tabacum (tă-bā′kum, tăb′ă-kum) [L.]. Tobacco.

tabagism (tăb′ă-jĭzm) [″ + Gr. *-ismos,* condition]. Poisoning from excessive use of tobacco or nicotine. SYN: *nicotinism.*

tabanid (tăb′ă-nĭd) [L. *tabanus,* horsefly]. A member of the dipterous family Tabanidae, q.v.

Tabanidae (tă-băn′ĭ-dē) [L. *tabanus,* horsefly]. A family of insects belonging to the order Diptera. It includes horseflies, gadflies, deer flies, and mango flies, all bloodsucking insects that attack man and other warm-blooded animals. Tabanidae is of medical importance in that flies serve in the transmission of the filaria worm, Loa loa, tularemia, anthrax, and other diseases. Their bites are extremely painful and heal with difficulty.

Tabanus (tă-bā′nŭs) [L., horsefly]. A genus of flies of the family Tabanidae, q.v.

tabardillo (tăb″ăr-dē′lyō) [Sp.]. Spanish term for epidemic louse-borne typhus fever that occurs in parts of Mexico. SEE: *typhus.*

tabatiere anatomique (tă-bă″tē-ār′ ă-nă″tō-mēk′) [Fr., anatomical snuffbox]. Depression at base of thumb in back when thumb is extended. Triangular area of the dorsum of the hand at the base of the thumb. When the thumb is extended the tendons of the long and short extensor muscles of the thumb bound this area, which appears as a depression. When snuff was used, a small pinch could be placed in this box and snuffed up into the nose from that site. SYN: *snuffbox, anatomical.*

tabella (tă-bĕl′ă) [L., tablet]. (pl. *tabellae*) A medicated mass of material formed into a small disk. SEE: *lozenge; tablet; troche.*

tabes (tā′bēz) [L., wasting away]. A gradual, progressive wasting in any chronic disease.

t., diabetic. Peripheral neuritis affecting diabetics. May affect spinal cord and simulate tabes caused by syphilis.

t. dorsalis. Sclerosis of the posterior columns of the spinal cord. SYN: *ataxia, locomotor.* SEE: *syphilis.*

ETIOL: Infection of central nervous system with Treponema pallidum, the causative agent of syphilis.

SYM: Postural instability, esp. when eyes are closed, and a staggering wide-base gait are characteristic; hence the name locomotor ataxia. Pains and paresthesias are common, esp. lightning pains, described as sharp, stabbing, and paroxysmal. Ankle and knee reflexes are diminished or lost. Many symptoms characteristic of syphilis such as pupillary changes, optic atrophy, bladder disturbances, and development of trophic ulcers, esp. on feet, make diagnosis certain.

TREATMENT: Antiluetic treatment. Special measures should be taken to relieve severe pains. Rehabilitation measures are often essential for those with disturbed gait. SEE: *syphilis.*

t. ergotica. Tabes resulting from the use of ergot.

t. mesenterica. Emaciation and general disorder of the functions of nutrition due to engorgement and tubercular degeneration of the mesenteric glands.

tabescent (tă-bĕs′ĕnt) [L. *tabes,* wasting away]. Progressive withering or wasting away.

tabetic (tă-bĕt′ĭk) [L. *tabes,* wasting away]. Pert. to or afflicted with tabes.

tabetic crises. Paroxysms of pain or other acute manifestations of episodic character in tabes due to syphilis.

tabetic foot. Twisted foot in locomotor ataxia.

tabetiform (tă-bĕt′ĭ-form) [″ + *forma,* shape]. Resembling or characteristic of tabes.

tabic (tăb′ĭk). Tabetic.

tabid (tăb′ĭd). Tabetic.

tablature (tăb′lă-chūr). The formation of the cranial bones into two outer hard layers and a spongy center, the diploë.

table (tā′bl) [L. *tabula,* a board]. 1. A flat-topped structure, as an operating table. 2. A thin flat plate, as of bone.

t.'s of skull. Inner and outer condensed layers of the cranial bone separated by diploë (cancellous bony tissue).

t., periodic. SEE: *periodic table.*

t., tilt. A table that may be tilted. A person is secured to it and the circulatory response to various angles of tilt from flat to perpendicular is observed and recorded. It is useful in studying postural hypotension.

t., vitreous. The inner cranial table.

t., water. The level at which rock or any underground stratum is saturated with water. This overlies an impervious stratum. SYN: *groundwater level.*

tablespoon (tā'bl-spoon). ABBR: tbsp. A rough measure utilizing a household spoon. When instructed to administer a tablespoon of medicine, give 15 ml. of the substance.

tablet (tăb'lĕt) [O. Fr. *tablete,* a small table]. A small, disklike mass of medicinal powder.

t., buccal. Tablet designed to be placed in the mouth and held between the cheek and gum until dissolved and absorbed through the buccal mucosa.

t., coated. Type of tablet usually made by coating compressed tablets with sugar or chocolate.

t., compressed. Tablet made by forcibly compressing the powdered substances into the desired shape; usually made to contain from 65 to 650 mg. of the active drug. Frequently they are very hard and not readily soluble.

t., dispensing. A tablet that contains a comparatively large amount of the active drug. Used by pharmacists and dispensing physicians to avoid the necessity of weighing small amounts of a potent drug in filling prescriptions.

t., enteric-coated. Tablet with an outer layer that is resistant to dissolution by gastric juices.

t., hypodermic. A tablet that frequently contains, in addition to the active drug, some agents that produce chemical action when water is added, thus causing a rapid disintegration of the mass. Used to form injectable solutions.

t., sublingual. A small, flat, oval tablet placed beneath the tongue to permit direct absorption of the active substance.

t., triturate. A tablet made by moistening the powder with a volatile liquid, such as alcohol, and then molding into shape and allowing the liquid to evaporate. Such tablets seldom contain more than 65 mg. of the active agent. They usually disintegrate readily and are a very desirable form for administering certain drugs.

tablier (tă-blyā') [Fr., apron]. Pudendal apron; enlarged vulvae.

taboo [Polynesian *tabu, tapu,* inviolable]. An act, object, or social custom separated or set aside as being sacred or profane, thus forbidden for general use.

taboparalysis (tā"bō-păr-ăl'ĭ-sĭs) [L. *tabes,* a wasting, + Gr. *paralyein,* to disable]. Tabes associated concurrently with general paralysis. SYN: *taboparesis.*

taboparesis (tā"bō-păr-ē'sĭs, -păr'ĕ-sĭs) [" + Gr. *paresis,* relaxation]. General paralysis in combination with tabes. SYN: *taboparalysis.*

tabophobia (tā"bō-fō'bē-ă) [" + Gr. *phobos,* fear]. A morbid fear of being afflicted with tabes, a common symptom of neurasthenia.

tabular (tăb'ū-lăr) [L. *tabula,* a table]. 1. Resembling a table. 2. Set up in columns, as a tabulation.

tabular bone. A flat bone, or one with two compact bonelike parts with cancellous tissue between them.

Tacaryl Hydrochloride. Trade name for methdilazine hydrochloride.

Tace. Trade name for chlorotrianisene.

tache (tŏsh) [Fr., spot]. A colored spot or macule on the skin, as a freckle.

t. blanche. A white spot on the liver in some infectious diseases.

t. bleuatre. A blue spot on the skin, usually due to bite of cutaneous parasites. SYN: *macula caerulea.*

t. cérébrale. The red line that occurs in meningitis and other nervous disorders when the fingernail is drawn across the skin.

t. motrice. The motor endplate of a striated muscle fiber.

t. noire. A small round or oval ulcer covered by a black scab; the primary lesion of boutonneuse fever and rickettsialpox.

tachetic (tăk-ĕt'ĭk) [Fr. *tache,* spot]. Marked by purple or reddish blue patches (taches).

tachistoscope (tă-kĭs'tō-skōp) [Gr. *tachistos,* swiftest, + *skopein,* to view]. A device used to determine the speed of visual perception. The time of exposure can be adjusted so that the length of time needed for detection of the viewed object can be measured.

tachogram (tăk'ō-grăm) [Gr. *tachos,* speed, + *gramma,* mark]. A graphic tracing of rate of flow of blood.

tachography (tăk-ŏg'ră-fē) [" + *graphein,* to write]. The recording of the speed of the blood circulation.

tachy- [Gr. *tachys,* swift]. Combining form meaning swift.

tachyarrhythmia (tăk"ē-ă-rĭth'mē-ă) [" + *a,* not, + *rhythmos,* rhythm]. Irregularity of heartbeat combined with rapid rate.

tachyauxesis (tăk"ē-awk-sē'sĭs) [" + *auxesis,* increase]. Condition in which a part of an organism grows more rapidly than the whole.

tachycardia (tăk"ē-kăr'dē-ă) [" + *kardia,* heart]. Abnormal rapidity of heart action, usually defined as a heart rate over 100 beats per minute.

t., atrial. Rapid heart rate usually less than 200 beats per minute. The beats arise from an atrial focus.

t., ectopic. Rapid heart beat due to stimuli arising from outside the sino-atrial node.

t., essential. Rapid persistent heart action due to functional disturbance.

t., nodal. Tachycardia resulting from an increase in rhythmicity of A-V node over the

S-A node. May be the result of digitalis therapy.

t., paroxysmal atrial. Atrial tachycardia beginning and ending suddenly. Rate is usually from 150 to 240 beats per minute.

t., paroxysmal nodal. Tachycardia due to increased activity of the A-V junctional focus. Rate is usually 120 to 180 beats per minute.

t., paroxysmal ventricular. Ventricular tachycardia beginning and ending suddenly.

t., polymorphic ventricular. Very rapid ventricular tachycardia characterized by a gradually changing QRS complex in the ECG. It is usually self-limiting but may change into ventricular fibrillation. SYN: *Torsade des pointes.*

t., reflex. Tachycardia resulting from stimuli outside the heart, reflexly accelerating heart rate or depressing vagal tone.

t., sinus. Uncomplicated tachycardia when sinus rhythm is faster than 100 beats per minute, as that due to exercise. Causes other than exercise include hyperthermia, thyrotoxicosis, hemorrhage, anoxia, infections, cardiac failure, and certain drugs such as atropine, epinephrine, and nicotine.

TREATMENT: Tachycardia sometimes ceases following procedures that cause vagal stimulation. Among these are pressure on one or both carotid sinuses, pressure on eyeballs, induction of gagging or vomiting, attempted expiration with glottis closed, lying down with feet in air, and bending over. If above procedures when employed singly are unsuccessful, two or more combined may produce desirable results. If these general measures are ineffective, specific therapy based on etiological factors will be required.

t. strumosa exophthalmica. Tachycardia occurring as a symptom of exophthalmic goiter.

t., ventricular. A series of at least three beats arising from a ventricular focus at a rate greater than 100 beats per minute. The beats usually arise from a single focus and are at a rate of 150 to 200 beats per minute.

tachycardiac (tăk"ē-kăr'dē-ăk) [Gr. *tachys,* swift, + *kardia,* heart]. Pert. to or afflicted with tachycardia.

tachylalia (tăk"ē-lā'lē-ă) [" + *lalein,* to speak]. Rapid speech.

tachymeter (tăk-ĭm'ĕ-tĕr) [" + *metron,* measure]. Instrument for estimating the speed of any body in motion.

tachyphagia (tăk"ē-fā'jē-ă) [" + *phagein,* to eat]. Rapid eating.

tachyphasia (tăk"ē-fā'zē-ă) [" + *phasis,* speech]. Very rapid or voluble speech. SYN: *tachyphrasia.*

tachyphemia (tăk"ē-fē'mē-ă) [" + *pheme,* speech]. Tachyphrasia, q.v.

tachyphrasia (tăk"ē-frā'zē-ă) [" + *phrasis,* speech]. Excessive volubility or rapidity of speech, as seen in mental disorders. SYN: *tachyphasia.*

tachyphrenia (tăk"ē-frē'nē-ă) [" + *phren,* mind]. Abnormally rapid mental activity.

tachyphylaxis (tăk"ē-fĭ-lăk'sĭs) [" + *phylaxis,* protection]. Rapid immunization to a toxic dose of a substance by previously injecting tiny doses of the same substance.

tachypnea (tăk"ĭp-nē'ă) [" + *pnoia,* breath]. Abnormal rapidity of respiration.

t., nervous. Respiratory rate of 40 or more per minute. It occurs in hysteria, neurasthenia, etc. If prolonged, this will cause excess loss of CO_2 and the hyperventilation syndrome will develop. SEE: *alkalosis, respiratory; hyperventilation.*

tachyrhythmia (tăk"ē-rĭth'mē-ă) [" + *rhythmos,* rhythm]. 1. Rapid heart action. SYN: *tachycardia.* 2. Increase in frequency of brain waves in electroencephalography up to 12 to 50/sec.

tachysterol (tă-kĭs'tĕ-rōl). One of the isomers of ergosterol, q.v., obtained by irradiation.

tachysystole (tăk"ē-sĭs'tō-lē) [" + *systole,* contraction]. Abnormally rapid systole. SEE: *extrasystole.*

tachytrophism (tăk"ē-trō'fĭzm) [" + *trophe,* nourishment, + *-ismos,* condition]. Accelerated metabolism.

tactile (tăk'tĭl) [L. *tactilis*]. Perceptible to the touch.

tactile corpuscles. Minute elongated bodies enclosing the endings of several afferent nerve fibers and serving as the receptor for slight pressure or touch. They are located in dermal papillae just beneath the epidermis and are most numerous on fingertips, toes, soles, palms, lips, nipples, and tip of tongue. SYN: *Meissner's corpuscles.*

tactile defensiveness. A defense reaction due to sensitivity to being touched.

tactile discrimination. The ability to localize two points of pressure on the surface of the skin and to identify them as discrete sensations.

tactile disk. Tiny expanded end of a sensory nerve fiber found in epidermis and in epithelial root sheath of a hair.

tactile system. That portion of the nervous system concerned with the sensation of touch. Includes sensory nerve endings (Meissner's corpuscles, Merkel's tactile disks, hair-root endings), afferent nerve fibers, conducting pathways in the cord and brain, and sensory (somesthetic) area of cerebral cortex.

taction (tăk'shŭn) [L. *tactio*]. 1. Sense of touch. 2. Touching.

tactometer (tăk-tŏm'ĕt-ĕr) [L. *tactus,* touch, + Gr. *metron,* measure]. Instrument for determining acuity of tactile sensitiveness.

tactor (tăk'tor). Any tactile organ.

tactual (tăk'tū-ăl) [L. *tactus,* touch]. Rel. to the sense of touch. SYN: *tactile.*

tactus (tăk'tŭs) [L.]. Touch.

t. eruditus. Sensitiveness of touch acquired by long practice.

taedium vitae (tē'dē-ŭm wē"tī) [L.]. Weariness of life with suicidal inclination.

Taenia (tē'nē-ă) [L., tape]. A genus of parasitic flatworms belonging to the class Cestoda, phylum Platyhelminthes. They are elongated ribbonlike worms consisting of a scolex, usually armed, and a chain of segments (proglottids). Adults live as intestinal parasites of vertebrates; larvae parasitize both vertebrates and invertebrates, which serve as intermediate hosts. SEE: *taeniasis; tapeworm.*

T. echinococcus. Echinococcus granulosus, q.v.

T. lata. The broad or fish tapeworm. The adult lives in the intestine of fish-eating mammals including man. It is the largest human tapeworm and may reach a length of 50 to 60 feet (15.2 to 18.3 meters). The eggs develop into ciliated larvae called coracidia, which are eaten by certain species of copecids in which each becomes an onchosphere, which develops into a procercoid. Further development occurs in a fish, where the procercoid develops into a wormlike plerocercoid or sparganum larva. Infection of the final host occurs following ingestion of improperly cooked fish. Pathological effects are abdominal pain, loss of weight, digestive disorders, progressive weakness, and a severe type of anemia that is clinically identical to pernicious anemia. SYN: *Diphyllobothrium latum; tapeworm, fish.*

T. saginata. Tapeworm whose larval stages live in cattle, the adult living in the intestine of man. Humans acquire it by eating insufficiently cooked beef infested with the encysted larval form (cysticercus or bladderworm). Adult worms may reach a length of 15 to 20 ft. (4.6 to 6.1 meters) or longer. SYN: *tapeworm, beef.*

T. solium. Tapeworm whose larval stages live in hogs, the adult living in the intestine of man. Humans acquire it by eating insufficiently cooked pork infested with larval form. Infected pork containing the bladderworm (Cysticercus cellulosae) is called measly pork. The cysticerci may also develop in humans, infection occurring from self-infection with eggs from contaminated hands or by hatching of eggs liberated in the intestine. SYN: *tapeworm, pork.*

taenia (tē'nē-ă) [L., tape]. 1. Any bandlike structure. SYN: *tenia* [NA]. 2. A tapeworm.

t. coli. One of three bands of the large intestines into which muscular fibers are collected. They are taenia mesocolica (mesenteric insertion), taenia libera (opposite mesocolic band), and taenia omentalis (at place of adhesion of omentum to transverse colon).

t. fimbriae. The folded or recurved lateral edge of the fimbria to which the epithelium covering the choroid plexus of the inferior horn of the lateral ventricle is attached.

t. pontis. One or two small transverse bands of fiber at rostral border of the pons.

t. semicircularis. Stria terminalis.

t. thalami. Structure separating the superior surface from the lateral surface of the thalamus, its lateral portion containing the stria medullaris.

t. ventriculi tertii. The taenia of the third ventricle.

taeniacide (tē'nē-ă-sīd) [L. *taenia,* tapeworm, + *cidus,* kill]. An agent that kills tapeworms.

taeniafuge (tē'nē-ă-fūj") [" + *fugere,* to put to flight]. Anything that expels tapeworms.

taeniasis (tē-nī'ă-sĭs) [" + Gr. *-iasis,* condition]. Condition of being infested with tapeworms of the genus Taenia. SEE: *tapeworm.*

taeniform (tē'nĭ-form) [" + *forma,* shape]. Having the structure of, or resembling, a tapeworm.

taenifuge (tē'nĭ-fūj) [" + *fuga,* flight]. An agent that expels tapeworms.

taeniophobia (tē"nē-ō-fō'bē-ă) [" + Gr. *phobos,* fear]. Morbid fear of becoming infested with tapeworms.

tag. 1. A small polyp or growth. 2. A label or tracer; or application of a label or tracer.

t., radioactive. A radioactive isotope that is incorporated into a chemical or organic material to allow its detection in metabolic or chemical processes.

t., skin. A small outgrowth of skin, usually occurring on the neck, axilla, and groin. SEE: *acrochordon.*

Tagamet. Trade name for cimetidine.

tagliacotian operation (tă-lē-ă-kō'shē-ăn). [Gasparo Tagliacozzi, It. surgeon, 1546–1599] Plastic operation on the nose in which skin is used from another part of the body.

tail (tāl) [AS. *taegel*]. Posterior, long, flexible terminus, as the extremity of the spinal column. SEE: *cauda* [NA].

tailgut (tāl'gŭt). A transient diverticulum of the entodermal cloaca of the embryo. It extends into the tail.

tailor's cramp. An occupational syndrome characterized by spasm of the muscles of the arms and hands.

taint (tānt) [O. Fr. *teint,* color, tint]. To spoil or cause putrefaction, as in tainted meat.

Takayasu's arteritis (pulseless disease). [Michishige Takayasu, Japanese physician, b. 1872] An inflammatory disease of the aorta that occludes one or more of the large branches of the aortic arch. This decreases the flow of blood to the areas supplied by these branches, which in turn leads to a lack of pulse in those areas. Dr. Takayasu noted the lack of pulse in the arteries of the eye, thus the name pulseless disease. The etiology is unknown and the only effective treatment is to implant vascular grafts to bypass the occluded vessels.

talalgia (tăl-ăl'jē-ă) [L. *talus,* heel, + Gr. *algos,* pain]. Pain in the heel or ankle.

talar (tā'lăr) [L. *talaris,* of the ankle]. Pert. to the talus, the ankle.

talbutal (tăl'bū-tăl). USP. A barbiturate that acts as a hypnotic and sedative. Trade name is Lotusate.

talc (tălk) [Persian *talk*]. Powdered soapstone; a soft, soapy powder; native hydrous magnesium silicate used as a dusting powder.

CAUTION: Talc should not contain asbestos fibers.

talcosis (tăl-kō'sĭs) [Persian *talk,* talc, + Gr. *osis,* condition]. Disease due to inhalation or implantation of talc in the body.

talcum (tălk'ŭm) [L.]. Talc.

tali (tā'lī). Pl. of talus.

talipedic (tăl″ĭ-pē'dĭk) [L. *talus,* ankle, + *pes,* foot]. Clubfooted. SEE: *talipes.*

talipes (tăl'ĭ-pēz) [L. *talus,* ankle, + *pes,* foot]. Any of a number of deformities of the foot, esp. those occurring congenitally; a nontraumatic deviation of the foot in the direction of one or the other of the four lines of movement, or of two of these combined. SYN: *clubfoot.*

t. arcuatus. Talipes in which there is an exaggerated normal arch of the foot. SYN: *talipes cavus.*

t. calcaneus. Talipes in which the foot is flexed and the heel alone touches the ground, causing the patient to walk on the inner side of the heel. Often follows infantile paralysis of the muscle of Achilles tendon.

t. cavus. T. arcuatus.

t. equinus. Talipes in which the foot is extended and the person walks on the toes.

t. percavus. Talipes in which there is excessive plantar curvature.

t. valgus. Talipes in which the heel and foot are turned outward.

t. varus. Talipes in which the heel is turned inward, away from the midline.

talipomanus (tăl″ĭp-ŏm'ăn-ŭs) [L. *talus,* ankle, + *pes,* foot, + *manus,* hand]. Deformity of the hand in which it is twisted out of position. SYN: *clubhand.*

tallow (tăl'ō). Fat obtained from suet, the solid fat of certain ruminants.

talocalcaneal (tā″lō-kăl-kā'nē-ăl) [″ + *calcaneum,* heel bone]. Pert. to the talus and calcaneus, bones of the tarsus.

talocrural (tā″lō-kroo'răl) [″ + *crus,* leg]. Pert. to the talus and leg bones.

talocrural articulation. The ankle joint, a ginglymus or hinge joint.

talofibular (tā″lō-fĭb'ū-lăr) [″ + *fibula,* pin]. Concerning the talus and fibula.

talon (tăl'ŏn) [L.]. The portion of the claw of a bird, esp. a bird of prey, that projects posteriorly.

t. noir. Minute intracutaneous black areas of the heels, toes, or hands. They are thought to be areas of hemorrhage caused by trauma.

talonavicular (tā″lō-nă-vĭk'ū-lăr) [L. *talus,* ankle, + *navicula,* boat]. Concerning the talus and the navicular bones.

talonid (tăl'ō-nĭd) [ME. *talon,* heel]. The crushing region, the posterior or heel part, of a lower molar tooth.

taloscaphoid (tā″lō-skăf'oyd) [L. *talus,* ankle, + Gr. *skaphe,* skiff, + *eidos,* form]. Talonavicular.

talotibial (tā″lō-tĭb'ē-ăl) [″ + *tibia,* shinbone]. Concerning the talus and tibial bones.

talus (tā'lŭs) [L., ankle]. (pl. *tali*) [NA] The ankle bone articulating with the tibia, fibula, calcaneus, and navicular bone. Formerly called astragalus.

Talwin (tăl'wĭn). Trade name for pentazocine, USP.

tambour (tăm-boor') [Fr., drum]. A shallow, drum-shaped appliance used in transmitting and registering arterial pulsations, blood pressure, respiratory movements, peristaltic contractions, and other slight movements.

tamoxifen citrate (tă-mŏks'ĭ-fĕn). An antiestrogen drug used in treating carcinoma of the breast. Trade name is Nolvadex.

tampon (tăm'pŏn) [Fr., plug]. A roll or pack made of various absorbent substances, such as cotton, rayon, wool, and gauze, used to arrest hemorrhage or absorb secretions from a wound or body cavity.

t., menstrual. An absorbent material suitably shaped and prepared to provide a hygienic means of absorbing menstrual fluid in the vagina. A cord is attached and this remains outside the vagina to facilitate removal. These tampons are made for self-insertion.

t., Mikulicz's. A large-scale capillary drain. It consists of a square piece of iodoform gauze of requisite size, placed in a cavity and filled with narrow strips of plain gauze until the necessary degree of compression is secured. Used where there is parenchymatous oozing. Serves as a tampon to arrest bleeding and also acts as a capillary drain. SYN: *Mikulicz's drain.*

t., nasal. Soft rubber bulb dilated with compressed air, used in plugging nostrils to stop hemorrhage from the nose.

tamponade (tăm'pŏn-ăd') [Fr., plug]. 1. To use or make use of a tampon. SYN: *tamponage.* 2. Pathologic compression of a part.

t., balloon. Producing pressure against some object by use of a catheter surrounded by an elongated balloon. Often used in the esophagus to arrest bleeding from varices. The Sengstaken-Blakemore tube is most frequently used. This is a three-lumen tube: one lumen is used to administer fluids to the patient or to provide gastric suction, another goes to a balloon inserted in the stomach to hold the tube in place and the third is attached to the balloon for application of pressure to the esophageal walls. SEE: *varicose veins.*

NURSING IMPLICATIONS: After balloon insertion, monitor vital signs, electrolyte status, and changes in the blood and differential counts. Because balloon prevents swallowing, administer fluids and tube feedings as prescribed. Instruct the patient to expectorate saliva, and provide emesis basin for oral secretions. Aspirate secretions as necessary. If patient is comatose, continuous drainage of the esophagus above the balloon will be required.

t., cardiac. Pathological condition resulting from accumulation of excess fluid in the pericardium. May result from pericarditis or injuries to the heart or great blood vessels, with accumulation of blood.

NURSING IMPLICATIONS: Question patient for history of trauma. Perform physical assessment, including measurement of arterial pressure, if possible. Administer oxygen as prescribed. Explain cardiac pericardiocentesis to the patient. Obtain the necessary supplies and equipment and place them at bedside. Assist the physician with the procedure. The patient will be in the intensive care unit. Administer blood and intravenous fluids as prescribed. Maintain and care for thoracotomy tubes if they are inserted.

tamponage (tăm′pŏn-ŏj) [Fr., plug]. Tamponade.

tamponing, tamponment (tăm′pŏn-ĭng, tăm-pŏn′mĕnt). Tamponade, q.v.

Tandearil. Trade name for oxyphenbutazone.

Tangier disease (tăn-jēr′). [Tangier Island, in Chesapeake Bay, where the disease was first discovered] A rare disease caused by familial high-density lipoprotein deficiency. Symptoms and signs include polyneuropathy, lymphadenopathy, orange-yellow discoloration of enlarged tonsillar tissue, hepatosplenomegaly, and a marked decrease in high-density lipoproteins. There is no specific therapy.

tank, Hubbard. SEE: *Hubbard tank.*

tannase (tăn′ās). An enzyme that is capable of hydrolysing tannins. It is present in certain plants and is produced by cultures of various microorganisms, esp. molds.

tannate (tăn′āt). Any salt or ester of tannic acid.

tannic acid. SEE: *acid, tannic.*

tannin (tăn′ĭn) [Fr. *tanin*]. 1. Acid substance found in bark of certain plants and trees or their products, usually from nutgall. Found in coffee and to a greater extent in tea. 2. Any of several substances containing tannin.

ACTION AND USES: Astringent, antidote for various poisons, for burns, and as a hemostatic. It is constipating. It is partly eliminated in the urine as gallic acid.

tantalum (tăn′tă-lŭm). SYMB: Ta. At. wt. 180.947; at. no. 73. A rare metallic element derived from tantalite. Because it is noncorrosive and malleable, it has been used to repair cranial defects, as a wire suture, and in prostheses.

tantrum (tăn′trŭm). Display of great anger, which may or may not include violent action. SEE: *temper tantrums.*

Tao. Trade name for troleandomycin.

tap (tăp). 1. [AS. *taeppa*]. To puncture or to empty a cavity of fluid. SEE: *lumbar puncture; paracentesis; thoracentesis.* 2. [O. Fr. *taper*]. A light blow.

Tapar. Trade name for acetaminophen, USP.

Tapazole (tăp′ă-zŏl). Trade name for methimazole, USP.

tape (tāp) [AS. *taeppe*]. 1. A long, flexible, narrow strip of linen, cotton, paper, or plastic such as adhesive tape. 2. To wrap a part with a long bandage made of adhesive or other type of material.

t., adhesive. USP. A fabric, film, or paper, one side of which is coated with an adhesive substance, that remains in place after application to the skin. SYN: *plaster, adhesive.*

tapeinocephaly (tăp″ĭ-nō-sĕf′ă-lē) [Gr. *tapeinos*, low-lying, + *kephale*, head]. A flattened head in which the vertical index of the skull is less than 72.

tapeinocephalic (tăp″ĭ-nō-sĕ-făl′ĭk). Pert. to tapeinocephaly.

tapetum (tă-pē′tŭm) [LL., a carpet]. A layer of fibers from the corpus callosum forming roof and lateral walls of inferior and posterior horns of lateral ventricles of the brain. Fibers pass to temporal and occipital lobes.

t. choroideae. T. lucidum, q.v.

t. lucidum. A layer of tissue in the choroid of the eye between the vascular and capillary layers in some animals, but not in man. This membrane reflects light shown into the animal's eyes. This produces a green reflex and is readily seen in cats. SYN: *t. choroideae.*

tapeworm [AS. *taeppe*, a narrow band, + *wyrm*, worm]. Any of the species of parasitic worms belonging to the class Cestoda, phylum Platyhelminthes. A typical tapeworm consists of a scolex with hooks and suckers for attachment, and a series of segments or proglottids that vary in number from a few to several thousand. New proglottids are budded off of the scolex, so that a worm is actually a linear colony consisting of immature, mature, and ripe or gravid proglottids. Adults live as endoparasites in the intestine. The terminal ripe proglottids containing the ova break off and pass out with the feces. The eggs develop into minute six-hooked oncospheres, which when ingested by the proper intermediate host (usually another vertebrate) develop in muscle tissues into an encysted larva known as a cysticercus. Infestation occurs when uncooked meat containing encysted larvae is eaten. These larvae develop into the mature adult in the primary host.

Species of medical importance are: Diphyllobothrium latum, Echinococcus granulosus, Hymenolepis nana, H. diminuta, Taenia saginata, and T. solium, q.v. SEE: *cysticercosis; cysticercus; hydatid; taeniasis.*

SYM: Often absent. If numerous, may cause intestinal obstruction. Occasionally mild systemic symptoms may occur from absorption of metabolic wastes. Sometimes there are dyspeptic symptoms.

t., armed. Taenia solium, the pork tapeworm, whose scolex possesses a row of hooks about the rostellum.

t., beef. Taenia saginata.

t., broad. Diphyllobothrium latum, q.v.

t., dog. Dipylidium caninum.

t., dwarf. Hymenolepis nana.

t., fish. Diphyllobothrium latum.

t., hydatid. Echinococcus granulosus, q.v.

t., mouse. Hymenolepis nana.

t., pork. Taenia solium.

t., rat. Hymenolepis nana.

t., unarmed. Taenia saginata.

taphephobia (tăf″ĕ-fō′bē-ă) [Gr. *taphos,* grave, + *phobos,* fear]. Abnormal fear of being buried alive.

taphophilia (tăf″ō-fĭl′ē-ă) [″ + *philos,* love]. Abnormal attraction for graves.

Tapia syndrome (tā′pē-ă). [A. G. Tapia, Sp. physician, 1875–1950] Paralysis of the pharynx and larynx on one side and atrophy of the tongue on the opposite side. Caused by a lesion affecting the accessory (tenth) and hypoglossal (twelfth) cranial nerves on the side in which the pharynx is affected.

tapinocephalic (tăp″ĭn-ō-sĕf-ăl′ĭk) [Gr. *tapeinos,* lying low, + *kephale,* head]. Pert. to flatness of top of cranium.

tapinocephaly (tăp″ĭn-ō-sĕf′ă-lē). Flatness of top of the skull.

tapiroid (tā′pĭr-oyd) [AmerInd. *tapira,* tapir, + Gr. *eidos,* form]. Resembling a tapir's snout; said of an elongated cervix uteri.

tapotement (tă-pōt-mŏn′) [Fr.]. Percussion in massage. It is divided into *beating* with the clenched hand, used for sciatica and muscular atrophy; *clapping* performed with the palm of the hand, used to reach superficial nerves; *hacking* with the ulnar border of the hand, used principally around a nerve center and upon the muscles; *punctuation* with the tips of the fingers, used principally around the heart and upon the head.

The strength of the manipulations is an essential factor in the massage treatment, and care must be taken not to bruise the patient. As a rule, begin with moderate pressure, ascertaining from the patient his sensation. White petrolatum or some other oleaginous substance should be used to avoid abrading the skin. SEE: *massage.*

tapping (tăp′ĭng). 1. [O. Fr. *taper,* of imitative origin]. Percussion in massage. SYN: *tapotement.* 2. [AS. *taeppa,* tap]. Removal of fluid from a cavity. SYN: *paracentesis.*

tar. A term applied to a dark, viscid mass of complex chemicals obtained by destructive distillation of coal, shale, and organic matter, esp. wood from pine and juniper trees.

t., coal. Coal tar, USP, q.v.

t., juniper. USP. Material obtained from destructive distillation of oil obtained from the wood of the juniper tree, Juniperus oxycedrus. It is used in certain medicines applied topically in treating certain skin diseases.

t., pine. Pine tar, USP, q.v.

Taractan. Trade name for chlorprothixene.

tarantism (tăr′ăn-tĭzm) [It. *taranto,* tarantula, + Gr. *-ismos,* condition]. A nervous affection marked by stupor, melancholy, and uncontrollable dancing mania. Popularly attributed to bite of the tarantula.

tarantula (tă-răn′tū-lă). A large venomous spider feared by many people; however, its bite is comparable in severity to a bee sting. SEE: *spider bites or poisoning.*

Tardieu's spots (tăr-dyūz′). [Auguste A. Tardieu, Fr. physician, 1818–1879] Subpleural spots of ecchymosis following death by strangulation.

tardive (tăr′dĭv) [Fr.]. Characterized by lateness, esp. pert. to a disease wherein the characteristic sign or symptom appears late in the course of the disease.

tare (tăr). The weight of an empty container. That weight is subtracted from the total weight of the vessel and substance added to it in order to determine the precise amount of the material that is weighed out.

tared. A container of known and predetermined tare, q.v.

tarentism (tăr′ĕn-tĭzm). Tarantism.

target (tăr′gĕt) [O. Fr. *targette,* light shield]. 1. A structure or organ that something is directed to. SEE: *target organ.* 2. The electrode on which cathode rays within an x-ray tube are focused and from which roentgen rays are emitted; usually of a heavy metal such as tungsten.

target cell. An abnormal erythrocyte with a rounded central area, which stains deeply, surrounded by a lightly staining area, which in turn is surrounded by denser cytoplasm at the periphery of the cell, the whole somewhat resembling a target with a bull's eye. Found in certain types of anemia and after splenectomy.

target organ. The organ or structure toward which the effects of a drug, hormone, or therapeutic agent are primarily directed.

tarichatoxin (tăr″ĭk-ă-tŏk′sĭn). A neurotoxin from the Taricha newt.

Tarnier's sign (tăr-nē-āz′). [Etienne Stéphene Tarnier, Fr. obstetrician, 1828–1897] A sign of impending abortion; the disappearance of the angle between upper and lower uterine segments in pregnancy.

tarsadenitis (tăr″săd-ĕn-ī′tĭs) [Gr. *tarsos,* a broad flat surface, + *aden,* gland, + *itis,* inflammation]. Inflammation of the tarsal or meibomian glands of the eyelid.

tarsal (tăr′săl) [Gr. *tarsalis*]. 1. Pert. to the tarsus or supporting plate of the eyelid. 2. Pert. to the ankle or tarsus.

tarsal arches. Two branches, superior and inferior, of the median palpebral artery supplying the eyelid.

tarsal bones. The seven bones of the ankle.

tarsal cartilages. The dense connective tissue of the tarsus of the eyelid. It is not true cartilage.

tarsalgia (tăr-săl′jē-ă) [Gr. *tarsos,* a broad flat surface, + *algos,* pain]. Pain in tarsus or ankle. May be due to flatfoot, shortening of Achilles tendon, or other causes.

tarsal glands. Branched sebaceous alveolar glands embedded in the tarsus and opening on the margin of the eyelid. SYN: *meibomian glands.*

tarsalia (tăr-sā′lē-ă) [L.]. (sing. *tarsale*) The tarsal bones.

tarsalis (tăr-sā′lĭs) [L.]. One of the tarsal muscles. SEE: *Muscles* in *Appendix.*

tarsal lacrimal glands. Accessory lacrimal glands located on the inner surface of the eyelids, esp. the upper lid.

tarsal tunnel. In the ankle, the bony-fibrous passage for the posterior tibial vessels, tibial nerve, and flexor tendons.

tarsal tunnel syndrome. Neuropathy of the distal portion of the tibial nerve at the ankle due to chronic pressure on the nerve at the point it passes through the tarsal tunnel. This causes pain in and numbness of the sole of the foot and weakness of plantar flexion of the toes.

tarsectomy (tar-sĕk′tō-mē) [″ + *ektome,* excision]. 1. Excision of tarsus or a tarsal bone. 2. Removal of tarsal plate of an eyelid.

tarsectopia (tăr″sĕk-tō′pē-ă). Dislocation of the tarsus.

tarsi. Pl. of tarsus.

tarsitis (tăr-sī′tĭs) [″ + *itis,* inflammation]. 1. Inflammation of tarsus of the foot. 2. Inflammation of the margin of an eyelid. SYN: *blepharitis.*

tarso- [Gr. *tarsos,* a broad flat surface]. Combining form meaning the flat of the foot, or the edge of the eyelid.

tarsocheiloplasty (tăr″sō-kī′lō-plăs″tē) [″ + *cheilos,* lip, + *plassein,* to form]. Plastic surgery of borders of the eyelid.

tarsoclasia, tarsoclasis (tăr″sō-klā′sē-ă, tăr-sŏk′lăs-ĭs) [″ + *klasis,* a breaking]. Surgical fracture of the tarsus for correction of clubfoot.

tarsomalacia (tăr″sō-mă-lā′sē-ă) [″ + *malakia,* a softening]. Softening of the tarsal cartilages of the eyes.

tarsomegaly (tăr″sō-mĕg′ă-lē) [″ + *megas,* large]. Enlargement of the heel bone, calcaneus.

tarsometatarsal (tăr″sō-mĕt″ă-tăr′săl) [″ + *meta,* between, + *tarsos,* flat of the foot]. Pert. to the tarsus and the metatarsus.

tarso-orbital (tăr″sō-or′bĭ-tăl) [″ + L. *orbita,* track]. Concerning the tarsus of the eyelid and the orbit.

tarsophalangeal (tăr″sō-fă-lăn′jē-ăl) [″ + *phalanx,* closely knit row]. Concerning the tarsus of the foot and the phalanges of the toes.

tarsophyma (tăr″sō-fī′mă) [″ + *phyma,* a growth]. Any tarsal tumor of the eyelid. SYN: *hordeolum; sty*

tarsoplasia, tarsoplasty (tăr″sō-plā′zē-ă, tăr′sō-plăs″tē) [″ + *plassein,* to form]. Plastic surgery of margin of the eyelid. SYN: *blepharoplasty.*

tarsoptosis (tăr″sŏp-tō′sĭs) [″ + *ptosis,* falling]. Flat foot; fallen arch of the foot.

tarsorrhaphy (tăr-sor′ă-fē) [″ + *rhaphe,* a seam]. The operation of uniting the edges of the lids at the outer commissure for the purpose of reducing the width of the palpebral fissure.

tarsotarsal (tăr″sō-tăr′săl) [″ + *tarsos,* a broad, flat surface]. Concerning the articulation between two rows of tarsal bones.

tarsotibial (tăr″sō-tĭb′ē-ăl) [″ + L. *tibia,* shinbone]. Concerning the tarsus and the tibia of the foot.

tarsotomy (tăr-sŏt′ō-mē) [″ + *tome,* incision]. 1. Incision of tarsal cartilage of an eyelid. 2. Any surgical incision of the tarsus of the foot.

tarsus (tăr′sŭs) [Gr. *tarsos,* a broad flat surface]. (pl. *tarsi*) 1. The ankle with its seven bones located between bones of the lower leg and metatarsus. It forms the proximal portion of the foot. It consists of the following bones: calcaneus (os calcis), talus (astragalus), cuboid (os cuboideum), navicular (scaphoid), and first, second, and third cuneiform bones. The talus articulates with the tibia and fibula, the cuboid and cuneiform bones with the metatarsals. SEE: *foot; skeleton;* names of individual bones. 2. A curved plate of dense white fibrous tissue forming the supporting structure of the eyelid. Also: *tarsal plates.*

t. inferior palpebrae. The firm layer of connective tissue that provides internal support for the lower eyelid.

t. superior palpebrae. The firm layer of connective tissue that provides internal support for the upper eyelid.

tartar [Gr. *tartaron,* dregs]. 1. An acid compound found in the juice of grapes and deposited on the sides of casks during winemaking. 2. Calcareous matter deposited upon the teeth. SYN: *calculus; plaque, dental.*

t., cream of. Potassium bitartrate.

t. emetic. Antimony potassium tartrate. Used as an emetic.

tartaric acid (tăr-tăr'ĭk). Any one of four isomers of an organic compound, $C_4H_6O_6$. Used in making potassium bitartrate, which is cream of tartar.

tart cells. Certain cells containing altered nuclear material appearing along with L.E. cells in suspensions of leukocytes or bone marrow cells.

tartrate. A salt of tartaric acid.

taste (tāst) [O. Fr. *taster,* to feel, to taste]. 1. To attempt to determine the flavor of a substance by touching it with the mouth. 2. A chemical sense dependent upon sense organs on the surface of the tongue. These organs, called taste buds, when appropriately stimulated, produce one or a combination of the four fundamental taste sensations: sweet, bitter, sour, and salty. The nervous impulses are carried to the brain by the lingual (from the anterior two thirds of the surface) and the glossopharyngeal (from the posterior third) nerves. Loss of taste may be due to bilateral disease of chorda tympani nerve and of gustatory fibers of the glossopharyngeal nerve.

RS: ageusia; agnosia; appetite; degustation; dysgeusia; gustation; gustatory; hypogeusia.

t., after. The persistence of a taste sensation after removal of original stimulus.

taste area. Area in cerebral cortex at lower end of somesthetic area.

taste blindness. Inability to taste certain substances such as phenylthiocarbamide (PTC). This inability is due to a hereditary factor that is transmitted as an autosomal recessive trait.

taste buds. Sensory end-organs that mediate the sensation of taste. They are oval structures located on the surface of the tongue, esp. the sides of the circumvallate papillae, on soft palate, epiglottis, and portions of the pharynx. Each contains sensory and gustatory (taste) cells and supporting (sustentacular) cells. When stimulated by chemical stimuli, they give rise to sense of taste. SEE: *chemoreceptor, taste cells.*

taste cells. Neuroepithelial cells within a taste bud that serve as receptors for the sense of taste. Each possesses on the free surface a short taste hair that projects through the inner taste pore. SYN: *cell, gustatory.*

taster (tās'tĕr). 1. A person capable of detecting a particular substance by using the taste sense. SEE: *phenylthiocarbamide.* 2. An individual who tastes food prior to its being approved for ingestion by a person whom others might wish to poison.

TAT. *thematic apperception test.*

T.A.T. *tetanus antitoxin; toxin-antitoxin.*

tattooing (tă-too'ĭng) [Tahitian *tatau*]. Indelible marking of the skin produced by introducing minute amounts of pigments into the skin. Tattooing is usually done to produce a certain design, picture, or name. When done commercially, sterile procedures are rarely used and infectious hepatitis virus may be transmitted to the customer. The technique may also be used to conceal a corneal leukoma, to mask pigmented areas of skin, or to color skin to look like the areola in mammoplasty.

taurine (taw'rĭn). A derivative of cysteine. it is present in bile, as taurocholic acid, in combination with bile acid.

taurocholate (taw"rō-kō'lāt). A salt of taurocholic acid.

taurocholemia (taw"rō-kō-lē'mē-ă) [Gr. *tauros,* a bull, + *chole,* bile, + *haima,* blood]. Taurocholic acid in the blood.

taurocholic acid. A substance occurring in bile and yielding cholic acid and taurine on hydrolysis.

taurodontism (taw"rō-dŏn'tĭzm) [" + *odous,* tooth, + *-ismos,* condition]. Condition in which teeth have greatly enlarged pulp chambers that are deepened. In that shape, the pulp chamber encroaches on the roots of the teeth.

Taussig-Bing syndrome (taw'sĭg-bĭng). [Helen B. Taussig, U.S. pediatrician, b. 1898; Richard J. Bing, U.S. surgeon, b. 1909] Congenital deformity of the heart in which the aorta arises from the right ventricle and the pulmonary artery arises from both ventricles. An intraventricular septal defect is present.

tauto- [Gr. *tautos,* identical]. Prefix meaning

the same.

tautomenial (taw″tō-mē′nē-ăl) [″ + *meniaia,* menses]. Concerning the same menstrual period.

tautomer (taw′tō-mĕr) [″ + *meros,* a part]. A chemical that is capable of tautomerism.

tautomeral, tautomeric (taw-tŏm′ĕr-ăl, -tō-mĕr′ĭk) [″ + *meros,* a part]. Noting certain neurons that send processes to the white matter on the same side of the spinal cord.

tautomerase (taw-tŏm′ĕr-ās) [″ + ″ + *-ase,* enzyme]. An enzyme that catalyzes tautomeric reactions.

tautomerism (taw-tŏm′ĕr-ĭzm) [″ + ″ + *-ismos,* condition]. Phenomenon in which two formulae are possible and exist in dynamic equilibrium so that as the amount of one substance is altered, the second is changed into the other form in order to maintain the equilibrium. SEE: *isomerism.*

tautorotation (taw″tō-rō-tā′shŭn) [″ + L. *rotare,* to turn round]. A change in specific rotation that occurs when a solution of certain sugars stands a while.

Tavist. Trade name for clemastine fumarate.

taxis (tăk′sĭs) [Gr., arrangement]. 1. Manual replacement or reduction of a hernia or dislocation. 2. The response of an organism to its environment; a turning toward (positive taxis) or away from (negative taxis) a particular stimulus. SEE: *chemotaxis.*

t., bipolar. Replacing of a retroverted uterus by applying traction on the cervix while the uterus is pushed upward by manipulating it through the rectum.

taxon (tăk′sŏn) [Gr. *taxis,* arrangement]. A taxonomic group.

taxonomic (tăk″sō-nŏm′ĭk). Concerning taxonomy.

taxonomy (tăks-ŏn′ō-mē) [″ + *nomos,* law]. Laws and principles of classification of animals and plants. Also used for classification of learning objectives.

Taylor brace (tā′lĕr). [C. F. Taylor, U.S. surgeon, 1827–1899] Brace with two rigid posterior oblique portions and soft straps crossed anteriorly over the chest.

Tay-Sachs disease. [Warren Tay, Brit. physician, 1843–1927; Bernard Sachs, U.S. neurologist, 1858–1944] An inherited disease transmitted as an autosomal recessive. The rate of occurrence in Ashkenazi Jews in the U.S.A. is estimated to be 400 per million births. SYN: *G_{M2} gangliosidosis.*

ETIOL: Because of the lack of a specific enzyme, hexosaminidase A, important in metabolizing sphingolipids, they accumulate in the cells, esp. those of nerves and the brain.

SYM: Neurological deterioration characterized by mental and physical retardation, blindness, cherry-red spots on the macula, an exaggerated startle response, spasticity, convulsions, and enlargement of the head may be present.

PROG: Death usually occurs prior to the age of 4.

TREATMENT: There is no specific therapy.

PREVENTION: Carriers of the trait can be accurately detected by assay of hexosaminidase A. It is possible to detect affected embryos by measurement of hexosaminidase A in amniotic fluid.

Tay's spot. Spot, cherry-red, q.v.

TB. Colloquialism for *tuberculosis.*

Tb. Chem. symb. for terbium.

T.b. *tubercle bacillus; tuberculosis.*

T bandage. Bandage resembling the letter T, used for the head and the perineum.

TBP. *thyroxine-binding protein.*

tbsp. *tablespoon.*

Tc. Chem. symb. for technetium.

T cells. Lymphocytes migrate to the thymus, where they develop into T cells and begin to mature. From the thymus they go to a particular area of the peripheral lymphoid tissues and from there they circulate between blood and lymph. Three subpopulations of T cells are known: helper or cooperator cells, which enhance the production of antibody-forming cells from B lymphocytes; cytotoxic or killer T cells, which are formed after mature T cells interact with some antigens present on foreign cells—these cells cause graft rejection and kill foreign cells in vitro; suppressor T cells, which suppress production of antibody-forming cells from B lymphocytes.

$TCID_{50}$. *Tissue culture infective dose* that will produce a cytopathic effect in *50%* of the cultures inoculated.

t.d.s. L. *ter die sumendum,* to be taken three times a day.

Te. Chem. symb. for tellurium.

tea (tē). 1. An infusion of a medicinal plant. 2. Leaves of plant Thea chinensis, from which a beverage is made by steeping the leaves in boiling hot water.

COMP: The principal ingredients are caffeine, tannin, and a volatile oil that gives the beverage prepared from tea leaves the characteristic taste and aroma. Caffeine, which comprises 1 to 4% of tea leaves, is the only medically important ingredient in the beverage. The caloric content is negligible until sugar and milk are added to the beverage.

t., black. Tea made from leaves that have been fermented before they are dried.

t., green. Tea prepared by heating leaves in open trays.

t., Paraguay copper. A tea made from the leaves and stems of the Ilex paraguayensis. It is a stimulating drink and contains volatile oil, tannin, and caffeine.

TEAB. *tetraethylammonium bromide.*

TEAC. *tetraethylammonium chloride.*

tear (tăr) [AS. *taer*]. 1. To separate or pull apart by force. 2. The liquid excreted into the eyes by the lacrimal glands.

tear duct, test of patency of. This can be easily done by placing several drops of a weak solution of sugar in the eye. If the person detects a sweet taste in the mouth, then the duct is patent.

Tear-Efrin. Trade name for phenylephrine hydrochloride, USP.

tears (tērs) [AS. *tear*]. 1. The watery saline solution secreted by the lacrimal glands, q.v. They lubricate the surfaces between the eyeball and eyelids, i.e., the conjunctiva. 2. Hardened lumps or tearlike drops of any gummy or resinous material.

t., crocodile. Crocodile tears, q.v.

tease (tēz) [AS. *taesan,* to pluck]. To separate a tissue into minute parts with a needle to prepare it for the microscope.

teaspoon (tē′spoon). ABBR: tsp. A household measure equal to approximately 5 ml. Teaspoons used in the home vary from 3 to 6 ml. Since household measures are not accurate, when a teaspoon dose is prescribed or ordered, give 5 ml. of the substance.

teat (tēt) [ME. *tete,* from AS. *tit,* teat]. 1. The nipple of the mammary gland. SYN: *papilla mammae.* SEE: *nipple; breast.* 2. Any protuberance resembling a nipple.

teatulation (tēt″ū-lā′shŭn) [AS. *tit,* teat]. The development of a nipplelike elevation.

technetium (tĕk-nē′shē-ŭm). SYMB: Tc. At. wt. of the isotope with the longest life 98; at. no. 43. A synthetic metallic chemical element.

technetium^{99m}. SYMB: ^{99m}Tc. A radioisotope of technetium that emits gamma rays. Used in determining blood flow to certain organs by use of scanning technique. It has a half-life of six hours.

technetium Tc 99m albumin aggregated injection. USP. A radioactive isotope with a half-life of 2×10^5 years. It is used intravenously for scanning the lung.

technic (tĕk′nĭk) [Gr. *techne,* art]. SEE: *technique.*

technical (tĕk′nĭ-kăl) [Gr. *tekhnikos,* skilled]. Requiring technique or special skill.

technician (tĕk-nĭsh′ăn) An individual who has the knowledge and skill required to carry out specific technical procedures. This individual usually has a diploma from a specialized school or an associate degree from a community college.

t., biomedical engineering. A technician who assembles, repairs, and adapts medical equipment used for the delivery of health care and assists in the development and maintenance of these systems.

t., cardiopulmonary. A technician who performs a wide range of tests related to the functions and therapeutic care of the heart and lung system. This includes operating and maintaining a heart-lung machine, assisting in cardiac catheterization, cardiac resuscitation, postoperative monitoring, and in care and treatment of patients who have undergone heart or lung surgery.

t., dental. A technician who constructs complete and partial dentures, makes orthodontic appliances, and fixes bridgework, crowns, and other dental restorations as authorized by dentists.

t., dialysis. A technician who operates and maintains an artificial kidney machine following approved methods to provide dialysis treatment for patients with kidney disorders.

t., dietetic. A technician who works with the food service manager and dietitian in a health care facility assisting with planning, implementing, and evaluating food programs, and may train and supervise dietary aides.

t., electrocardiographic. A technician who operates and maintains electrocardiographic machines, records the heart's electrical activity, and provides data for diagnosis and treatment of heart ailments by physicians.

t., electroencephalographic. A technician who operates and maintains electroencephalographic machines.

t., electromyographic. A technician who assists the physician in recording and analyzing bioelectric potentials that originate in muscle tissue. This includes the operation of various electronic devices, maintenance of electronic equipment, assisting with patient care during testing, and record keeping.

t., emergency medical. A technician who responds to medical emergency calls, evaluates the nature of the emergency, and carries out specific diagnostic measures and emergency treatment procedures under the standing orders or specific directions of a physician.

t., environmental health. A technician who assists in the survey of environmental hazards and performs technical duties under professional supervision in areas such as pollution control, radiation protection, and sanitation.

t., health physics. A technician who monitors radiation levels, gives instructions in radiation safety, labels radioactive materials, and assists the health physicist in conducting experimental studies in radiation.

t., histologic. A technician who works under the supervision of a pathologist in sectioning, staining, and mounting human and animal tissue and fluid for microscopic study.

t., medical laboratory. A technician who performs biological and chemical tests requiring limited independent judgment or correlation competency under the supervision of a medical technologist, pathologist, or physician.

t., medical record. A technician who assists the medical record administrator by coding, analyzing, and preserving patients' medical records and compiling reports, disease indices, and statistics in health care institutions.

t., operating room. A technician who works as a general assistant on the surgical team by arranging supplies and instruments in the operating room, maintaining antiseptic conditions, and assisting the surgeon during the operation.

t., orthopedic. A technician who sets up traction rooms, applies all types of traction, makes casts, and applies splints.

t., pharmacy. A technician who assists the pharmacist in certain activities such as medication profile reviews for drug incompatibilities, typing prescription labels, prescription packaging, handling purchase records, inventory control, and may, where state law and hospital policy permit, dispense drugs to patients under the supervision of a registered pharmacist.

t., psychiatric. A technician who works under the supervision of a professional in the care of mentally ill patients in a psychiatric care facility; assists in carrying out the prescribed treatment plan and assigned individual and group activities with patients.

t., radiologic. A technician who maintains and safely uses equipment and supplies necessary to demonstrate portions of the human body on x-ray film or fluoroscopic screens for diagnostic purposes.

t., respiratory therapy. A technician who routinely treats patients requiring noncritical respiratory care and who recognizes and responds to a limited number of specified respiratory emergencies.

technique (tĕk-nēk') [Fr., Gr. *technikos*]. 1. Systematic procedure or methods by which an involved or scientific task is completed. 2. The skill in performing details of a procedure or operation.

techno- [Gr. *techne,* art]. Combining form meaning art or skill.

technologist (tĕk"nŏl'ō-jĭst). An individual who has studied a specific aspect of a profession or science. A technologist usually has a baccalaureate degree.

t., circulation. A technologist who designs and operates circulation devices and monitoring instruments that provide circulatory support to the patient. These include heart-lung machines, dialysis machines, and artificial organs.

t., medical. A technologist who works in conjunction with pathologists, physicians, and scientists in all general areas of the clinical laboratory. Independent and correlational judgements are made in a wide range of complex procedures. A medical technologist may teach and supervise laboratory personnel.

t., radiation therapy. A technologist who administers x-rays and electron beam therapy to treat disease and assists in preparing and handling radioactive materials for therapeutic purposes.

technology (tĕk-nŏl'ō-jē) [" + *logos,* study]. 1. The application of scientific knowledge. 2. The entire scientific knowledge used in solving or approaching problems and situations. 3. The entire body of knowledge available to a civilization.

tectocephalic (tĕk"tō-sĕ-făl'ĭk). Concerning tectocephaly.

tectocephaly (tĕk-tō-sĕf'ăl-ē) [L. *tectum,* roof, + Gr. *kephale,* head]. Possession of a boat-shaped cranium. SYN: *scaphocephalism.*

tectorial (tĕk-tō'rē-ăl) [L. *tectum,* roof]. Pert. to a roof or covering. SYN: *tegmental.*

tectorium (tĕk-tō'rē-ŭm) [L. *tectorium,* a covering]. (pl. *tectoria*) 1. Any rooflike structure. SYN: *tectum; tegmentum; tegument.* 2. Corti's membrane.

tectospinal (tĕk"tō-spī'năl) [L. *tectum,* roof, + *spina,* thorn]. From the tectum mesencephali to the spinal cord.

tectospinal tract. A tract of white fibers of the spinal cord passing from the tectum of the midbrain and going down through the medulla to the spinal cord. It begins on one side and crosses to the other.

tectum (tĕk'tŭm) [L., roof]. 1. Any structure serving as, or resembling, a roof. 2. The dorsal portion of the midbrain consisting of the superior and inferior colliculi (corpora quadrigemina). SYN: *tegmentum.*

t. mesencephali. Roof of the midbrain including the corpora quadrigemina.

T.E.D. *threshold erythrema dose.*

teenage. Pert. to those who are thirteen through nineteen years of age. SYN: *adolescent.*

teeth (tēth) [AS. *toth,* tooth]. (sing. *tooth*) Hard bony projections in jaws serving as organs of mastication, there being 32 permanent teeth, 16 in each jaw. They include the following types: incisors, canines (cuspids), premolars (bicuspids), and molars. An average child should have 6 teeth at 1 year, 12 at 18 months, 16 at 2 years, and 20 at 2½ years. A child may be born with teeth, and in other cases the teeth may not appear until 16 months. SEE: *dentition* for illus.

t., anterior. Teeth located close to the midline of the dental arch on either side of the jaw, including the incisors and canine.

t., auditory. Minute toothlike projections along the free margin of the labium vestibulare of the cochlea. SYN: *Huschke's auditory teeth.*

t., charting and numbering. The various systems developed for designating teeth in a chart system include numbers, letters, or symbols and are not uniformly accepted; widely used is a two-digit system of Federation Dentaire Internationale (FDI system) and the American system, which numbers the permanent teeth consecutively from upper right third molar as #1 through the maxillary teeth to #16, and then to left mandibular third molar as #17 and through the mandibular teeth to the right third molar as #32.

t., deciduous. Teeth comprising the first dentition, which are shed and replaced by the permanent teeth. SYN: *teeth, milk; teeth, temporary.* SEE: illus.

t., Hutchinson's. Condition where lateral incisors of the upper jaw are pegged and central incisors of same jaw have convex sides and crescentic notches on their cutting edges; noted only on permanent teeth, sometimes indicating hereditary syphilis.

t., malacotic. Teeth that are esp. prone to decay, soft in structure and white in color.

t., milk. T., deciduous.

t., permanent. Teeth of the second dentition, replacing the deciduous teeth. SEE: illus.

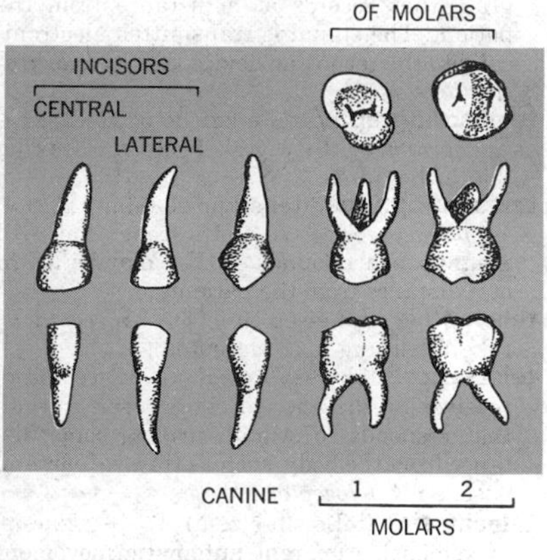

DECIDUOUS TEETH
LEFT SIDE

t., sclerotic. Yellowish teeth that are naturally hard and not subject to ready decay.

t., secondary. T., permanent.

t., temporary. T., deciduous.

t., wisdom. The third molar teeth of the permanent dentition, which are the last to erupt.

teething (tēth'ĭng) [AS. *toth,* tooth]. Eruption of the teeth. SEE *dentition.*

tegmen (tĕg'mĕn) [L. *tegmen,* covering]. (pl. *tegmina*) A structure that covers a part.

t. mastoidem. Bony roof of mastoid cells.

t. tympani. [NA] Roof of tympanum separating middle ear from cranial cavity.

t. ventriculi quarti. [NA] The roof of the 4th ventricle.

tegmental (tĕg-mĕn'tăl) [L. *tegmentum,* covering]. Relating to a tegument or tegmentum; a covering. SYN: *tentorial.*

tegmental nuclei. Several masses of gray matter lying in the tegmentum of the midbrain and upper portion of the pons. Include the dorsal, pedunculopontile, reticular, and ventral nuclei.

tegmentum (tĕg-mĕn'tŭm) [L. *tegmentum,* covering]. 1. A roof or covering. SYN: *tectorium; tegument.* 2. The dorsal portion of the cruri cerebri of the midbrain. It contains the red nucleus and nuclei and roots of the oculomotor nerve. SYN: *tectum.*

Tegopen (tĕg'ō-pĕn). Trade name for cloxacillin sodium, USP.

tegument (tĕg'ū-mĕnt). 1. The skin; the covering of the body. SYN: *integument.* 2. A covering structure.

tegumental, tegumentary (tĕg″ū-mĕn'tăl, -tă-rē). Concerning the skin or tegument; covering.

teichopsia (tī-kŏp'sē-ă) [Gr. *teichos,* wall, + *opsis,* vision]. Zigzag lines bounding a luminous area appearing in the visual field. This causes temporary blindness in that portion of the field of vision. This condition is sometimes associated with migraine headaches, or mental or physical strain. SYN: *scotoma, scintillating.*

teinodynia (tī″nō-dĭn'ē-ă) [Gr. *tenon,* tendon, + *odyne,* pain]. Pain in the tendons. SYN: *tenalgia; tenodynia.*

tela (tē'lă) [L. *tela,* web]. (pl. *telae*) Any weblike structure.

t. choroidea. Part of the pia mater covering roof of the 3rd and 4th cerebral ventricles.

t. conjunctiva. Connective tissue.

t. elastica. Elastic tissue.

t. subcutanea. Subcutaneous connective tissue; superficial fascia.

t. submucosa. The submucosa of the intestine.

telalgia (tĕl-ăl'jē-ă) [Gr. *tele,* far away, +

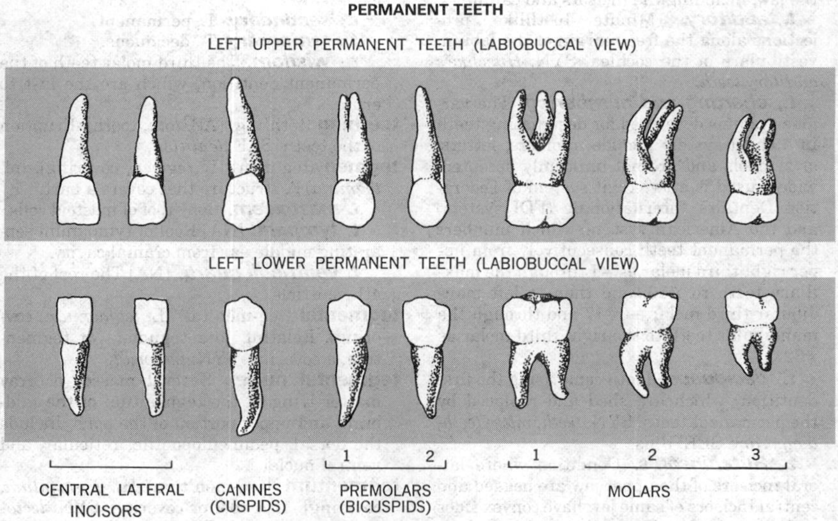

algos, pain]. Pain felt at a distance from its stimulus. SYN: *referred pain.*

telangiectasia, telangiectasis (tĕl-ăn″jē-ĕk-tā′zē-ă, -ĕk′tă-sĭs) [Gr. *telos,* end, + *angeion,* vessel, + *ektasis,* dilatation]. A vascular lesion formed by dilatation of a group of small blood vessels. It may appear as a birthmark or become apparent in young children. May occur anywhere on the skin but is seen most frequently on the face and the thighs.

t., hereditary hemorrhagic. A hereditary disease characterized by thinness of walls of blood vessels of nose, skin, and digestive tract and tendency to hemorrhage. SYN: *Osler-Weber-Rendu disease.*

t. lymphatica. Tumor composed of dilated lymph vessels.

t., spider. A stellate angioma (nevus araneus).

telangiectatic (tĕl-ăn″jē-ĕk-tăt′ĭk). Concerning telangiectasia.

telangiectodes (tĕl-ăn″jē-ĕk-tō′dēz). Tumors that have telangiectasia.

telangiitis (tĕl-ăn″jē-ī′tĭs) [″ + ″ + *itis,* inflammation]. Inflammation of the capillaries.

telangioma (tĕl-ăn″jē-ō′mă) [Gr. *telos,* end, + *angeion,* vessel, + *oma,* tumor]. A tumor made up of dilated capillaries or arterioles.

telangion (tĕl-ăn′jē-ŏn) [″ + *angeion,* vessel]. A capillary or terminal arteriole.

telangiosis (tĕl″ăn-jē-ō′sĭs) [″ + ″ + *osis,* condition]. Disease of capillary vessels.

Teldrin. Trade name for chlorpheniramine maleate, USP.

tele-, tel-. 1. [Gr. *telos,* end] Combining form meaning the end. 2. [Gr. *tele,* distant] Combining form meaning at a distance or far off.

telecanthus (tĕl″ĕ-kăn′thŭs) [Gr. *tele,* distant, + *kanthos,* canthus]. Increased distance between the inner canthi of the eyelids.

telecardiogram (tĕl″ĕ-kăr′dē-ō-grăm) [″ + *kardia,* heart, + *gramma,* mark]. A cardiogram that records at a distance from the patient. The signal is transmitted electronically to the recording device. SYN: *telelectrocardiogram.*

telecardiography (tĕl″ĕ-kăr″dē-ŏg′ră-fē) [″ + ″ + *graphein,* to write]. Process of taking telecardiograms.

telecardiophone (tĕl″ĕ-kăr′dē-ō-fōn) [″ + ″ + *phone,* voice]. A stethoscope that will magnify heart sounds so they may be heard at a distance from the patient.

teleceptive (tĕl-ĕ-sĕp′tĭv) [″ + L. *ceptivus,* take]. Relating to a teleceptor.

teleceptor (tĕl′ĕ-sĕp″tor) [″ + L. *ceptor,* a receiver]. A distance receptor; a sense organ that responds to stimuli arising some distance from the body, such as the eye, ear, and nose. SYN: *teloceptor.*

telecinesia (tĕl″ĕ-sĭn-ē′zē-ă) [″ + *kinesis,* movement]. Apparent automatic movement of an object produced without contact with any stimulus or power.

telecurietherapy (tĕl-ĕ-kū″rē-thĕr′ă-pē) [″ +

curie + Gr. *therapeia,* treatment]. Application of radiation therapy from a source distant from the lesion or patient.

teledendrite, teledendron (tĕl-ĕ-dĕn′drīt, -dĕn′drŏn) [Gr. *telos,* end, + *dendron,* a tree]. The terminal processes of an axon. SYN: *telodendron.*

telediagnosis (tĕl″ĕ-dī″ăg-nō′sĭs) [Gr. *tele,* distant, + *diagignoskein,* to discern]. Diagnosis made on the basis of data transmitted electronically to the physician's location.

telediastolic (tĕl″ē-dī-ă-stŏl′ĭk) [Gr. *telos,* end, + *diastole,* a dilatation]. Concerning the last phase of the diastole.

telelectrocardiogram (tĕl″ē-lĕk″trō-kăr′dē-ō-grăm) [Gr. *tele,* distant, + *elektron,* amber, + *kardia,* heart, + *gramma,* mark]. An electrocardiogram taken with a galvanometer attached to the patient by a wire some distance from the instrument. SYN: *telecardiogram.*

telefluoroscopy (tĕl″ĕ-floo″or-ŏs′kō-pē). Transmission of fluoroscopic images by electronic means.

telekinesis (tĕl″ĕ-kī-nē′sĭs) [″ + *kinesis,* movement]. Willful movement of articles without touching them. Some practitioners of the occult claim to have this ability. Be skeptical.

telemeter (tĕl-ĕ-mē′tĕr) [″ + *metron,* measure]. To transmit information to a distant point by using electronic devices.

telemetry (tĕ-lĕm′ĕ-trē). The transmission of data electronically to a distant location.

telemnemonic (tĕl″ĕ-nĕ-mŏn′ĭk) [″ + *mnemonikos,* pert. to memory]. Becoming aware of the content of the memory of another person.

telencephalic (tĕl″ĕn-sĕf-ăl′ĭk) [Gr. *telos,* end, + *enkephalos,* brain]. Pert. to the endbrain (telencephalon).

telencephalization (tĕl″ĕn-sĕf″ăl-ī-zā′shŭn). The evolutionary degree of control over functions previously mediated by lower nerve centers.

telencephalon (tĕl-ĕn-sĕf′ă-lŏn) [″ + *enkephalos,* brain]. The embryonic endbrain or posterior division of the prosencephalon from which the cerebral hemispheres, corpora striata, and rhinencephalon develop.

teleneurite (tĕl″ĕ-nū′rīt) [″ + *neuron,* nerve]. The branching end of an axon.

teleneuron (tĕl″ĕ-nū′rŏn) [″ + *neuron,* nerve]. A nerve ending.

teleo- [Gr. *teleos,* complete]. Combining form meaning perfect or complete.

teleological (tē″lē-ō-lŏj′ĭ-kăl). Concerning teleology.

teleology (tĕl-ē-ŏl′ō-jē) [″ + *logos,* a study]. The belief that everything is directed toward some final purpose. The doctrine of final causes.

teleomitosis (tĕl″ē-ō-mī-tō′sĭs) [″ + *mitos,* thread, + *osis,* condition]. Mitosis that is complete.

teleonomic (tĕl″ē-ō-nŏm′ĭk). Concerning teleonomy.

teleonomy (tĕl″ē-ŏn′ō-mē) [″ + *nomos,* law]. The concept that, in an organism or animal, the existence of a structure, capability, or function indicates it had a survival function.

teleopsia (tĕl-ē-ŏp′sē-ă) [Gr. *tele,* distant, + *ops,* eye]. A visual disorder in which objects perceived in space have excessive depth or close objects appear far away.

teleorganic (tĕl″ē-or-găn′ĭk) [Gr. *teleos,* complete, + *organon,* organ]. Necessary to organic life. SYN: *vital.*

teleotherapeutics (tĕl″ē-ō-thĕr-ă-pū′tĭks) [Gr. *tele,* distant, + *therapeutike,* treatment]. The use of hypnotic suggestion in the treatment of disease. SYN: *suggestive therapeutics.*

Telepaque (tĕl′ĕ-pāk). Trade name for iopanoic acid, USP.

telepathist (tĕ-lĕp′ă-thĭst) [″ + *pathos,* feeling]. One who claims the ability to read the mind of others.

telepathy (tĕ-lĕp′ă-thē). Supposed communication of one mind with another at a distance without any physical or psychological explanation. SYN: *telesthesia.*

teleradiography (tĕl″ĕ-rā-dē-ŏg′ră-fē) [Gr. *tele,* distant, + L. *radius,* ray, + Gr. *graphein,* to write]. Radiography with the radiation source about 2 meters (6½ ft.) from the body. Done to minimize distortion by having rays virtually parallel at that distance. SYN: *teleroentgenography.*

teleradium (tĕl″ĕ-rā′dē-ŭm). A radium source distant from the area being treated.

telergy (tĕl′ĕr-jē) [″ + *ergon,* work]. 1. Action without conscious exercise of the will. SYN: *automatism.* 2. Hypothetical action of one individual's thoughts upon brain of another by transmission of some unknown form of energy.

teleroentgenogram (tĕl″ĕ-rĕnt-gĕn′ō-grăm) [″ + *roentgen* + Gr. *gramma,* mark]. An x-ray picture obtained by teleroentgenography.

teleroentgenography (tĕl″ĕ-rĕnt″gĕn-ŏg′ră-fē) [″ + ″ + Gr. *graphein,* to write]. Radiography in which the radiation source is about 2 meters (6½ ft.) from the body. SYN: *teleradiography.*

telesthesia (tĕl-ĕs-thē′zē-ă) [″ + *aisthesis,* sensation]. 1. An impression received at a distance without normal operation of organs of sense. 2. Distance perception. SYN: *telepathy.*

telesystolic (tĕl″ĕ-sĭs-tŏl′ĭk) [Gr. *telos,* end, + *systole,* contraction]. Pert. to the termination of the cardiac systole.

teletactor (tĕl″ĕ-tăk′tor) [″ + L. *tactus,* touch]. A device used by the deaf to receive vibrations through the skin.

teletherapy (tĕl-ĕ-thĕr′ă-pē) [Gr. *tele,* distant, + *therapeia,* treatment]. Treatment of disease by telepathy.

teletypewriter. ABBR: TTY. A typewriter that may be connected to a telephone. Use of this device permits deaf persons to communicate by sending and receiving typewritten messages.

telluric (tĕ-lūr′ĭk) [L. *tellus,* earth]. Of or rel. to the earth.

tellurism (tĕl′ū-rĭzm) [″ + Gr. *-ismos,* condition]. The concept that emanations from the earth cause disease.

tellurium (tĕl-ū′rē-ŭm) [L. *tellus,* earth]. SYMB: Te. At. wt. 127.60; at. no. 52; sp. gr. 6.24. A nonmetallic element used as an electric rectifier and in coloring glass.

tellurium poisoning. Characterized by a garlic odor of all secretions and excretions. A disagreeable odor to the breath with suppression of perspiration and saliva, resulting in dry skin and mouth. Anorexia, nausea, drowsiness, and weakness.

TREATMENT: Give saline cathartics; increase fluid intake; induce perspiration; otherwise treatment is symptomatic.

telocentric (tĕl″ō-sĕn′trĭk) [Gr. *telos,* end, + *kentron,* center]. Location of the centromere in the extreme end of the replicating chromosome so that there is only one arm on the chromosome.

teloceptor. Teleceptor.

telodendron (tĕl-ō-dĕn′drŏn) [Gr. *telos,* end, + *dendron,* a tree]. The more or less diffuse arborizations at the end of an axon or its collaterals. SYN: *teledendrite.*

telogen (tĕl′ō-jĕn) [″ + *genesis,* production]. Resting stage of hair growth cycle. SEE: *anagen; catagen.*

teloglia (tĕl-ŏg′lē-ă). Cells that cover the outer surface of the motor endplate.

telolecithal. Concerning an egg in which the large yolk mass is concentrated at one pole.

telolemma (tĕl″ō-lĕm′mă) [″ + *lemma,* rind]. The membrane covering the motor endplate in a striated muscle fiber.

telomere (tĕl′ō-mēr) [″ + *meros,* part]. The end of an arm of a chromosome.

telophase (tĕl′ō-fāz) [″ + *phasis,* a phase]. The final phase or stage of mitosis (karyokinesis) during which reconstruction of the daughter nuclei takes place and the cytoplasm of the cell divides, giving rise to two daughter cells.

telophragma (tĕl″ō-frăg′mă) [″ + *phragmos,* a fencing in]. The Z line or disk in striated muscle. SEE: *Z disk.*

telosynapsis (tĕl″ō-sĭ-năp′sĭs) [″ + *synapsis,* conjunction]. End-to-end union of pairs of homologous chromosomes during gametogenesis.

telotism (tĕl′ō-tĭzm) [″ + *-ismos,* process]. The entire performance of a function, as that of one of the senses.

TEM. *triethylene melamine.* SEE: *nitrogen mustards.*

Temaril (tĕm′ă-rĭl). Trade name for trimeprazine tartrate, USP.

tempeh. A wheat-soy bean food developed as an excellent inexpensive source of protein for children. It is used in economically depressed countries. Quality of protein in tempeh is almost equal to casein.

temper [AS. *temprian,* to mingle]. State of the individual's mood, disposition, or mind. For example, even-tempered, or foul-tempered.

temperament (tĕm′pĕr-ă-mĕnt) [L. *temperamentum,* mixture]. The combination of intellectual, emotional, ethical, and physical characteristics of a specific individual.

temperate (tĕm′pĕr-ĭt). Moderate; not excessive.

temperature (tĕm′pĕr-ă-tūr) [L. *temperatura,* proportion]. 1. Degree of heat of a living body. 2. Degree of hotness or coldness of a substance.

Body temperature varies with the body area in which it is measured and with the time of day. The temperature in the liver may be 105° F. (40.6° C.), while that under the tongue is 98.6° F. (37° C.); the rectal temperature is likely to be 0.5 to 1.0° F. (0.28° to 0.56° C.) above the oral.

One of the mechanisms for raising temperature is muscular work (as in shivering); one for lowering it is sweating.

Body temperature may be measured by a clinical thermometer placed in the mouth, rectum, or under the arm. Rectal temperature usually is from 0.5 to 1.0° F. (0.28° to 0.56° C.) higher than by mouth; axillary temperature about 0.5° F. (0.28° C.) lower than by mouth. Oral temperature may be inaccurate if taken just after the patient has ingested cold substances or has been breathing with the mouth open.

Body temperature is the result of the balance between heat production and heat loss. Eighty-five percent of body heat is lost through the skin, the remainder via lungs and through fecal and urinary excretions. Regulation of body temperature is accomplished principally through thermoregulatory centers located in the hypothalamus. Elevation of temperature above normal is designated fever (pyrexia), and subnormal temperature is hypothermia.

t., absolute. Temperature measured from absolute zero, which is −273.15° C.

t., ambient. The surrounding temperature or that present in the place, site, or location indicated.

t., axillary. Temperature obtained by

placing thermometer in apex of the axilla with arm pressed closely to side of body. Temperature obtained by this method is usually 0.5 to 1.0° F. (0.28° to 0.56° C.) lower than oral.

t., body. Temperature of the body.

t. chart, basal. SEE: *basal temperature chart.*

t., core. Core temperature, q.v.

t., critical. The temperature below which a gas may be converted to liquid form by pressure.

t., inverse. Condition in which body temperature is higher in the morning than in the evening.

t., maximum. Temperature above which bacterial growth will not take place.

t., mean. The average temperature for a stated period in a given locality.

t., minimum. In bacteriology, temperature below which bacterial growth will not take place.

t., normal. Temperature of the body, taken orally, in a healthy individual; 98.6° F. (37° C.) in man.

t., optimum. Temperature at which a procedure is best carried out, as the culture of a given organism or the action of an enzyme.

t., oral. Temperature obtained by placing a thermometer under the patient's tongue with lips closed for three minutes. It should not be taken for at least 10 minutes after ingestion of hot or cold liquids. It is not advisable for infants, mouth-breathers, comatose patients, or those extremely ill.

t., rectal. Temperature obtained by inserting the thermometer into the anal canal a depth of at least 1½ in. (3.8 cm.) and allowed to remain 3 to 5 minutes. Do not take following a rectal operation or if rectum is diseased. Rectal temperature is more accurate than either oral or axillary temperature. It averages about 1° F. (0.56° C.) higher than the oral temperature.

t., room. Temperature between 65 and 80° F. (18.3° and 26.7° C.).

t., subnormal. Temperature below the normal of 98.6° F. (37° C.).

temperature, words pert. to: algid; algid stage; algogenic; chauffage; cold; frigid; frigidity; frigorific; hardening; heat; infant; myothermic; pseudocrisis; respiration; temperature scale; "therm-" words.

temperature senses. The sensations of warmth resulting from raising the temperature of the skin and that of cold aroused by lowering it. The sensation of warmth is mediated by Ruffini's corpuscles, that of cold by end-bulbs of Krause. These receptors are distributed so as to form cold and warm sensing spots on the skin. Afferent impulses from receptors, on reaching the thalamus, may give rise to crude uncritical temperature sensations; on being relayed to the somesthetic area of the cortex, they result in discrete and fairly well localized sensations of heat and cold. Adaptation is rapid.

temper tantrums. A stage of anger and reaction in which the individuals, esp. children, are no longer in control of themselves and they are unaware of how their condition appears to others. The parents or associates need to realize that it is not possible to talk the child out of this behavior or reaction. The child needs to be separated, at that time, from the person who the child thinks caused the incident. The parents or those involved should not demean the child or make fun of him or her during the episode. The child will eventually learn that control of anger is important and that at times, controlled anger is an appropriate response to certain situations.

template (těm′plāt). A pattern, mold, or form used as a guide in duplicating a shape, structure, or device.

temple (těm′pl) [O. Fr. from L. *tempora,* pl. of *tempus,* temple]. The region of the head in front of the ear and over the zygomatic arch.

tempolabile (těm″pō-lā′bl) [L. *tempus,* time, + *labilis,* unstable]. Becoming altered spontaneously within a definite time.

tempora (těm′pō-ră) [L. pl. of *tempus,* time]. The temples.

temporal (těm′por-ăl) [L. *temporalis*]. 1. Pert. to or limited in time. 2. Rel. to the temples.

temporal bone. A bone on both sides of the skull at its base. Composed of squamous, mastoid, and petrous portions, the latter enclosing the organ of hearing. SYN: *os temporale.* SEE: *Arnold's canal; mastoid; petrosa; styloid process.*

temporalis (těm″pō-rā′lĭs) [L.]. Muscle in temporal fossa that elevates the mandible. SEE: *Muscles* in *Appendix.*

temporal line. One of two lines on lateral surface of the frontal and parietal bones that mark upper limit of temporal fossa.

temporal lobe. Lobe of the cerebrum located laterally and below the frontal and occipital lobes. Contains auditory receptive areas.

temporo- [L *tempora*]. Combining form meaning temples of the head.

temporoauricular (těm″pō-rō-aw-rĭk′ū-lăr) [″ + *auricula,* little ear]. Concerning the temples and auricular areas.

temporohyoid (těm″pō-rō-hī′oyd) [″ + Gr. *hyoeides,* U-shaped]. Concerning the temporal and hyoid bones.

temporomalar (těm″pō-rō-mā′lăr) [″ + *mala,* cheek]. Temporozygomatic, q.v.

temporomandibular (těm″pō-rō-măn-dĭb′ū-lăr) [″ + *mandibula,* lower jaw]. Pert. to the temporal and mandible bones; esp. important in dentistry because of the articulation of the bones, of the temporomandibular joint.

temporomandibular joint(s). The encapsulated, double, synovial joints between the condyles of the mandible and the temporal bones of the skull. SYN: *craniomandibular joints.*

temporomaxillary (tĕm″pō-rō-măk′sĭ-lĕr-ē) [″ + *maxilla,* jawbone]. Pert. to the temporal and maxillary bones.

temporo-occipital (tĕm″pō-rō-ŏk-sĭp′ĭ-tăl) [″ + *occipitalis,* pert. to the occiput]. Pert. to the temporal and occipital bones or their regions.

temporoparietal (tĕm″pō-rō-pă-rī′ĕ-tăl) [″ + *paries,* wall]. Concerning the temporal bone and the parietal bones.

temporopontine [″ + *pons,* a bridge]. Concerning or situated between the temporal lobe of the brain and the pons.

temporosphenoid (tĕm″pō-rō-sfē′noyd) [″ + Gr. *sphen,* wedge, + *eidos,* form]. Pert. to the temporal and sphenoid bones.

temporozygomatic (tĕm″pō-rō-zī″gō-măt′ĭk) [″ + Gr. *zygoma,* cheekbone]. Concerning the temporal and zygomatic bones.

tempostabile (tĕm″pō-stā′bĭl) [L. *tempus,* time, + *stabilis,* stable]. Descriptive of something, esp. a chemical compound, that remains stable with the passage of time.

Tempra. Trade name for acetaminophen, USP.

tenacious (tĕ-nā′shŭs) [L. *tenax*]. Adhering to; adhesive; retentive.

tenacity (tĕ-năs′ĭ-tē). The condition of being tough, stubborn, or obstinate.

tenaculum (tĕn-ăk′ū-lŭm) [L., a holder]. Sharp, hooklike, pointed instrument with slender shank for grasping and holding a part, as an artery.

tenalgia (tĕn-ăl′jē-ă) [Gr. *tenon,* tendon, + *algos,* pain]. Pain in a tendon. SYN: *tenodynia.*

t. crepitans. Inflammation of a tendon sheath that on movement results in a crackling sound. SYN: *tendosynovitis crepitans; tenosynovitis crepitans.*

tenderizers. Preparations, containing proteolytic enzymes such as papain or bromelin, used to make meat more tender.

tenderness (tĕn′dĕr-nĕs). Sensitiveness to pain upon pressure.

t., rebound. Production of or intensification of pain when pressure is released.

tendinitis (tĕn″dĭn-ī′tĭs) [L. *tendo,* tendon, + Gr. *itis,* inflammation]. Inflammation of a tendon. SYN: *tenonitis; tenontitis.*

tendinoplasty (tĕn′dĭ-nō-plăs″tē) [″ + Gr. *plassein,* to form]. Plastic surgery of tendons. SYN: *tendoplasty; tenontoplasty; tenoplasty.*

tendinosuture (tĕn″dĭn-ō-sū′tŭr) [″ + *sutura,* sewing]. The suturing of a divided tendon. SYN: *tenorrhaphy.*

tendinous (tĕn′dĭ-nŭs) [L. *tendinosus*]. Pert. to, composed of, or resembling tendons.

tendinous synovitis. Inflammation of a tendon's synovial sheath.

tendo [L.]. (pl. *tendines*) [NA] A tendon.

tendolysis (tĕn-dŏl′ĭ-sĭs) [″ + Gr. *lysis,* a loosening]. The process of freeing a tendon from adhesions.

tendon (tĕn′dŭn) [L. *tendo,* tendon]. Fibrous connective tissue serving for the attachment of muscles to bones and other parts. SYN: *sinew.*

t., Achilles. The large tendon at lower end of the gastrocnemius muscle, inserted into the os calcis. It is the strongest and thickest tendon in the body.

t., calcaneous. T., Achilles.

t., central. The central portion of the diaphragm consisting of a flat aponeurosis in which fibers of the diaphragm are inserted.

t. of Zinn. Portion of the fibrous ring (annulus tendineus communis) from which inferior rectus muscle of eye originates.

t., superior, of Lockwood. Portion of fibrous ring from which the superior oblique muscle of the eye originates.

tendon cells. Fibroblasts of white fibrous connective tissue of tendons arranged in parallel rows.

tendonitis [″ + Gr. *itis,* inflammation]. Inflammation of a tendon.

tendon reflex. Reflex act in which a muscle contracts when its tendon is percussed.

t.r., patellar. Slight extension of the leg when tendon of quadriceps muscle is tapped immediately below the patella. Tested with leg slightly bent at the knee if patient is in bed. May be tested while leg hangs free when patient is sitting on edge of bed. SYN: *knee jerk; patellar reflex.* SEE: *Jendrassik maneuver.*

tendon spindle. Fusiform nerve ending in a tendon.

tendoplasty (tĕn′dō-plăs″tē) [″ + Gr. *plassein,* to mold]. Reparative surgery of an injured tendon. SYN: *tendinoplasty; tenontoplasty; tenoplasty.*

tendosynovitis (tĕn″dō-sĭn″ō-vī′tĭs) [″ + *syn,* with, + *ovum,* egg, + Gr. *itis,* inflammation]. Inflammation of a sheath of a tendon or the tendon. SYN: *tendovaginitis; tenosynovitis.*

t. crepitans. Tendosynovitis accompanied by a crackling sound on movement. SYN: *tenalgia crepitans; tenosynovitis crepitans.*

tendotome (tĕn′dō-tōm) [″ + Gr. *tome,* incision]. Instrument for severing a tendon. SYN: *tenotome.*

tendotomy (tĕn-dŏt′ō-mē). Division of a tendon. SYN: *tenotomy.*

tendovaginal (tĕn″dō-văj′ĭ-năl) [L. *tendo,* tendon, + *vagina,* sheath]. Rel. to a tendon and its sheath.

tendovaginitis (tĕn″dō-văj″ĭn-ī′tĭs) [″ + ″ + Gr. *itis,* inflammation]. Inflamed condition of a tendon and its sheath. SYN: *tenosynovitis.*

Tenebrio (tĕ-nĕb′rē-ō). A genus of beetles including the species of T. molitor, which serves as intermediate host of helminth parasites of vertebrates.

tenectomy [″ + *ektome,* excision]. Excision of a lesion of a tendon or tendon sheath; removal of a ganglion or xanthoma.

t., graduated. Partial division of a tendon.

tenesmic (tĕn-ĕz′mĭk). Pert. to or like tenesmus.

tenesmus (tĕ-nĕz′mŭs) [Gr. *teinesmos,* a stretching]. Spasmodic contraction of anal or vesical sphincter with pain and persistent desire to empty the bowel or bladder, with involuntary ineffectual straining efforts.

teni-. SEE: words beginning with *taeni-.*

tenia (tē′nē-ă) [L. *taenia,* tape]. A flat band or strip of soft tissue.

teniasis (tē-nī′ă-sĭs) [L. *taenia,* tapeworm, + Gr. *-iasis,* a condition]. Presence of tapeworms in the body.

tenicide (tĕn′ĭ-sīd) [″ + *cidus,* killing]. Taeniacide, q.v.

tenifuge (tĕn′ĭ-fūj) [″ + *fuga,* flight]. Causing or that which causes expulsion of tapeworms.

tennis elbow. Condition characterized by pain over lateral epicondyle of humerus radiating to outer side of arm and forearm and aggravated by dorsiflexion and supination of wrist. Weakness of wrist and difficulty in grasping objects. Usually caused by strain, as in playing tennis.

TREATMENT: In mild cases, immobilization by a splint or adhesive strapping, supplemented by heat or diathermy. In long continued cases, surgical intervention may be indicated.

teno- [Gr. *tenon*]. Combining form indicating tendon.

tenodesis (tĕn-ŏd′ĕ-sĭs) [″ + *desis,* a binding]. Surgical fixation of a tendon. Usually a tendon is transferred from its initial point of origin to a new origin in order to restore muscle balance to a joint, to restore lost function, or to increase active power of joint motion.

tenodesis splint. Orthosis fabricated to allow pinch and grasp movements through use of wrist extensors. Also called *wrist-driven flexor hinge hand splint.*

tenodynia (tĕn″ō-dĭn′ē-ă) [″ + *odyne,* pain]. Pain in a tendon. SYN: *tenalgia.*

tenofibril (tĕn′ō-fī″brĭl) [″ + *fibrilla,* little fiber]. A fine thread present in the cytoplasm of epithelial cells.

tenolysis (tĕn-ŏl′ĭ-sĭs) [″ + *lysis,* dissolution]. Tendolysis, q.v.

tenomyoplasty (tĕn″ō-mī′ō-plăs″tē) [″ + *mys,* muscle, + *plassein,* to form]. Reparative operation upon a tendon and muscle. SYN: *tenontomyoplasty.*

tenomyotomy (tĕn″ō-mī-ŏt′ō-mē) [″ + ″ + *tome,* incision]. Excision of lateral portion of a tendon or muscle.

tenonectomy (tĕn″ō-nĕk′tō-mē) [″ + *ektome,* excision]. Excision of a portion of a tendon.

tenonitis (tĕn″ō-nī′tĭs) [″ + *itis,* inflammation]. 1. Inflammation of a tendon. SYN: *tenontitis.* 2. Inflammation of Tenon's capsule.

tenonometer (tĕn″ō-nŏm′ĕ-tĕr) [Gr. *teinein,* to stretch, + *metron,* measure]. Device for measuring degree of intraocular tension.

Tenon's capsule (tē′nōns). [Jacques R. Tenon, Fr. surgeon, 1724–1816] A thin connective tissue envelope of the eyeball behind the conjunctiva.

Tenon's space. Space between the posterior surface of the eyeball and Tenon's capsule.

tenontitis (tĕn′ŏn-tī′tĭs) [Gr. *tenontos,* tendon, + *itis,* inflammation]. Inflammation of a tendon SYN: *tendinitis; tenositis.*

tenontodynia (tĕn″ŏn-tō-dĭn′ē-ă) [″ + *odyne,* pain]. Pain in a tendon. SYN: *tenalgia; tenodynia*

tenontography (tĕn″ŏn-tŏg′ră-fē) [″ + *graphein,* to write]. A treatise on the tendons.

tenontolemmitis (tĕn-ŏn″tō-lĕm-mī′tĭs) [″ + *lemma,* rind, + *itis,* inflammation]. Tenosynovitis, q.v.

tenontology (tĕn″ŏn-tŏl′ō-jē) [″ + *logos,* a study]. Study of tendons.

tenontomyoplasty (tĕn-ŏn″tō-mī′ō-plăs″tē) [″ + *mys,* muscle, + *plassein,* to form]. Plastic surgery, including muscle and tendon repair, in treatment of hernia. SYN: *myotenontoplasty; tenomyoplasty.*

tenontomyotomy (tĕn-ŏn″tō-mī-ŏt′ō-mē) [″ + ″ + *tome,* incision]. Cutting of the principal tendon of a muscle with excision of the muscle in part or in whole. SYN: *myotenotomy.*

tenontoplasty (tĕn-ŏn′tō-plăs″tē) [″ + *plassein,* to form]. Plastic surgery of defective or injured tendons. SYN: *tenoplasty.*

tenontothecitis (tĕn-ŏn″tō-thē-sī′tĭs) [″ + *theke,* sheath, + *itis,* inflammation]. Inflammation of a tendon and its sheath. SYN: *tendosynovitis; tendovaginitis; tenosynovitis.*

t. stenosans. A chronic form of tenontothecitis with narrowing of the sheath.

tenophyte (tĕn′ō-fīt) [″ + *phyton,* a growth]. A cartilaginous or osseous growth on a tendon.

tenoplastic (tĕn″ō-plăs′tĭk). Concerning tenoplasty.

tenoplasty (tĕn′ō-plăs″tē) [″ + *plassein,* to

form]. Reparative surgery of tendons. SYN: *tendinoplasty; tenontoplasty.*

tenoreceptor (tĕn″ō-rē-sĕp′tor) [″ + L. *receptor,* receiver]. Proprioceptive nerve ending in a tendon.

tenorrhaphy (tĕn-or′ă-fē) [″ + *rhaphe,* suture]. Suturing of a tendon.

tenositis (tĕn″ō-sī′tĭs) [″ + *itis,* inflammation]. Inflammation of a tendon. SYN: *tenontitis.*

tenostosis (tĕn″ŏs-tō′sĭs) [Gr. *tenon,* tendon, + *osteon,* bone, + *osis,* condition]. Conversion of a tendon into bony tissue.

tenosuspension (tĕn″ō-sŭs-pĕn′shŭn) [″ + L. *suspensio,* a hanging under]. In surgery, use of a tendon to support a structure.

tenosuture (tĕn″ō-sū′chūr) [″ + L. *sutura,* sewing]. Reunion of a divided tendon. SYN: *tenorrhaphy.*

tenosynovectomy (tĕn″ō-sĭn″ō-vĕk′tō-mē) [″ + *syn,* with, + L. *ovum,* egg, + Gr. *ektome,* excision]. Excision of a tendon sheath.

tenosynovitis (tĕn″ō-sĭn″ō-vī′tĭs) [″ + ″ + ″ + Gr. *itis,* inflammation]. Inflammation of a tendon sheath.

t. crepitans. Inflammation of a tendon sheath in which a crackling sound is heard on motion. Most commonly affects flexor tendons.

ETIOL: May follow puncture wounds, contusions, and lacerations, or be caused by lymphatic extension from an abrasion.

SYM: Pain, excessive tenderness.

TREATMENT: Early drainage, rest.

t. hyperplastica. Painless swelling of extensor tendons over the wrist joint.

tenotome (tĕn′ō-tōm) [″ + *tome,* incision]. Instrument for section of a tendon.

tenotomist (tĕn-ŏt′ō-mĭst). Specialist in tenotomy.

tenotomy (tĕn-ŏt′ō-mē). Surgical section of a tendon.

tenovaginitis (tĕn″ō-văj″ĭn-ī′tĭs) [″ + L. *vagina,* sheath, + Gr. *itis,* inflammation]. Inflammation of a tendon sheath. SYN: *tendosynovitis; tenontothecitis; tenosynovitis.*

tense (tĕns). Tight, rigid, anxious, under mental stress.

Tensilon. Trade name for edrophonium chloride, USP.

tensiometer (tĕn″sē-ŏm′ĕ-tĕr) [L. *tensio,* a stretching, + Gr. *metron,* measure]. A device for determining the surface tension of liquids.

tension (tĕn′shŭn) [L. *tensio,* a stretching]. 1. Process or act of stretching; state of being strained or stretched. 2. Pressure, as arterial tension. 3. Expansive force of a gas or vapor. 4. Mental, emotional, or nervous strain.

t., arterial. Tension resulting from the force exerted by the blood pressure on the walls of arteries.

t., intraocular. The pressure of the fluid within the eyeball. SEE: *tonometry.*

t., intravenous. Force exerted by the blood pressure on the walls of a vein.

t., muscular. Condition of a muscle in which fibers tend to shorten and thus perform work or liberate heat.

t., premenstrual. Condition occurring periodically in some individuals a few days before menstruation; characterized by varying degrees of nervousness and irritability, emotional instability, headaches, and sometimes depression. Usually disappears a short time after onset of menstrual flow. SEE: *premenstrual syndrome.*

t., surface. Molecular property of film on surface of a liquid to resist rupture, the particles tending to pull inward.

t., tissue. The theoretical state of equilibrium between the cells of a tissue.

tension headache. Headache caused by sustained tension of muscles of the face, neck, and scalp.

tension of gases. Gas pressure usually measured in millimeters of mercury (mm. Hg).

tension pneumothorax. Pneumothorax, valvular, q.v.

tension suture. Suture used to reduce pull of the edges of a wound.

tensometer (tĕn-sŏm′ĕ-tĕr) [L. *tensio,* a stretching, + Gr. *metron,* measure]. A device for testing the tensile strength of materials.

tensor (tĕn′sor) [L., a stretcher]. Any muscle that makes a part tense. SEE: *Muscles* in *Appendix.*

tent (tĕnt) [O. Fr. *tente,* from L. *tenta,* stretched out]. 1. A plug of soft material used to maintain or dilate the opening to a sinus, canal, or body cavity. A variety of cylindrically shaped materials may be used. 2. A portable covering or shelter composed of fabric.

t., oxygen. A tent that can be placed over a bed for the continuous administration of oxygen.

t., sponge. A plug made of compressed sponge.

tentacle (tĕn′tă-k′l). A slender projection of invertebrates. It is used for prehension, tactile purposes, or feeding.

tentative (tĕn′tă-tĭv) [L. *tentativus*]. Noting a diagnosis subject to change because of insufficient data.

tenth cranial nerve. Nerve supplying most of the abdominal viscera, the heart, lungs, and esophagus. SYN: *vagus nerve.* SEE: *cranial nerves.*

tentorial (tĕn-tō′rē-ăl). Pertaining to a tentorium.

tentorial notch. An arched cavity formed by

the anterior and inner border of the tentorium cerebelli.

tentorial pressure cone. Projection of a portion of the temporal lobe of the cerebrum through the incisure of the tentorium due to increased intracranial pressure.

tentorium (těn-tō'rē-ŭm) [L., tent]. (pl. *tentoria*) A tentlike structure or part.

t. cerebelli. [NA] The process of the dura mater between the cerebrum and cerebellum supporting the occipital lobes.

Tenuate. Trade name for diethylpropion hydrochloride.

Tepanil. Trade name for ethylpropion hydrochloride.

tephromalacia (tĕf"rō-măl-ā'shē-ă) [Gr. *tephros,* gray, + *malakia,* softening]. Softening of the gray substance of brain or spinal cord.

tephromyelitis (tĕf"rō-mī"ĕl-ī'tĭs) [" + *myelos,* marrow, + *itis,* inflammation]. Inflammation of the gray matter of the spinal cord.

tephrosis (tĕf-rō'sĭs) [" + *osis,* condition]. Incineration; cremation.

tephrylometer (tĕf"rĭ-lŏm'ĕ-tĕr) [" + *hyle,* matter, + *metron,* measure]. Device for measuring the thickness of the cerebral cortex, the gray matter of brain.

tepid (tĕp'ĭd) [L. *tepidus,* lukewarm]. Slightly warm; lukewarm.

tepidarium (tĕp"ĭd-ā'rē-ŭm) [L.]. A place for a warm bath.

tepor (tē'por) [L., lukewarmness]. Moderate heat.

TEPP. *tetraethylpyrophosphate.*

ter- [L., thrice]. Combining form meaning three times.

teracurie (tĕr"ă-kū'rē). A unit of radioactivity, 10^{12} curies.

teramorphous (tĕr-ă-mor'fŭs) [Gr. *teras,* monster, + *morphe,* form]. Similar to, or of the nature of, a congenitally deformed fetus, infant, or child.

teras (tĕr'ăs) [L., Gr.]. (pl. *terata*) A severely deformed fetus.

teratic (tĕr-ăt'ĭk) [Gr. *teratikos,* monstrous]. Pert. to a severely malformed fetus.

teratism (tĕr'ă-tĭzm) [Gr. *teratisma*]. An anomaly or structural abnormality either inherited or acquired.

t., acquired. Abnormality resulting from a prenatal environmental influence.

t., atresic. Teratism in which natural openings such as the mouth or anus fail to form.

t., casemic. Teratism in which a normal union of parts fails to occur.

t., ectogenic. Condition in which parts are absent or defective.

t., ectopic. Abnormality in which a part becomes displaced.

t., hypergenetic. Teratism in which a part is exceptionally large.

t., symphysic. Teratism in which parts that are normally separate are fused.

terato- [Gr. *teratos,* monster]. Combining form indicating a severely malformed fetus.

teratoblastoma (tĕr"ă-tō-blăs-tō'mă) [" + *blastos,* germ, + *oma,* tumor]. A tumor containing embryonic material but that is not representative of all three germinal layers. SEE: *teratoma.*

teratocarcinoma (tĕr"ă-tō-kăr"sĭ-nō'mă) [" + *karkinos,* cancer, + *oma,* tumor]. A carcinoma that has developed from the epithelial cells of a teratoma.

teratogen (tĕr-ăt'ō-jĕn) [" + *gennan,* to produce]. Anything that causes teratogenesis. SEE: table.

teratogenesis (tĕr"ă-tō-gĕn'ĕ-sĭs) [" + *genesis,* production]. The development of abnormal structures in an embryo resulting in a severely deformed fetus.

teratogenetic (tĕr"ă-tō-jĕ-nĕt'ĭk) [" + *genesis,* production]. Concerning teratogenesis.

teratogenous (tĕr"ă-tŏj'ĕ-nŭs) [" + *gennan,* to produce]. Developed from severely deformed fetal parts.

teratogeny (tĕr"ă-tŏj'ĕ-nē). Teratogenesis.

teratoid (tĕr'ă-toyd) [Gr. *teratos,* monster, + *eidos,* form]. Resembling a severely malformed fetus.

teratoid tumor. Tumor of embryonic remains from all germinal layers. SYN: *teratoma.*

teratologic (tĕr"ă-tō-lŏj'ĭk). Concerning teratology.

teratology (tĕr-ă-tŏl'ō-jē) [" + *logos,* a study]. Branch of science dealing with the study of congenitally deformed fetuses.

teratoma (tĕr-ă-tō'mă) [" + *oma,* tumor]. Congenital tumor containing embryonic elements of all three primary germ layers such as hair and teeth. SYN: *dermoid cyst.* SEE: *fetus in fetu.*

teratomatous (tĕr"ă-tō'mă-tŭs). Pert. to or resembling a teratoma.

teratophobia (tĕr"ă-tō-fō'bē-ă) [" + *phobos,* fear]. Abnormal fear of giving birth to a malformed fetus or of being in contact with one.

teratosis (tĕr"ă-tō'sĭs) [" + *osis,* condition]. A deformed fetus.

teratospermia (tĕr"ă-tō-spĕr'mē-ă) [" + *sperma,* seed]. Malformed sperm in semen.

terbium (tĕr'bē-ŭm). SYMB: Tb. At. wt. 158.9254; at. no. 65; sp. gr. 8.272. A metal of the rare earths.

terchloride (tĕr-klō'rīd). Trichloride.

terebrant (tĕr'ĕ-brănt). Piercing pain.

terebration (tĕr"ĕ-brā'shŭn) [L. *terebratio*]. 1. Boring, trephination. 2. A boring pain.

terbutaline sulfate. USP. A synthetic sympathomimetic amine used in treating asthma.

Teratogenic and Fetotoxic Drugs

Maternal Medication	Fetal or Neonatal Effect
Established Teratogenic Agents	
Antineoplastic agents Antimetabolites (amethopterin, fluorouracil, DON, 6-azauridine, etc.) Alkylating agents (cyclophosphamide, etc.) Antibiotics (amphotericin B, mitomycin, etc.)	Multiple anomalies, abortion
Estrogens	Vaginal adenocarcinoma in daughter in later years*
Other sex hormones (androgens, progestogens)	Masculinization, advanced bone age
Thalidomide	Fetal death or phocomelia; deafness; cardiovascular, gastrointestinal, or genitourinary abnormalities
Organic mercury	Cerebral palsy
Polychlorinated biphenyls (PCBs) (contaminants in manufacture of rice, cooking oil)	"Cola"-colored neonates with other developmental defects
Possible Teratogens	
Insulin (shock or hypoglycemia)	Anomalies
LSD	"Fractured chromosomes," anomalies
Sulfonylurea derivatives	Anomalies

*FDA Drug Bulletin (Nov) 1971: Diethylstilbestrol contraindicated in pregnancy.

It is an effective bronchodilator. Trade names are Brethine and Bricanyl.

teres (tē′rēz) [L., round]. Round and smooth; cylindrical. Used to describe certain muscles and ligaments.

tergal (tĕr′găl) [L. *tergum*, back]. Concerning the back or dorsal surface.

tergum (tĕr′gŭm) [L.]. The back.

ter in die (tĕr ĭn dē′ă) [L.]. Three times a day. ABBR: t.i.d.

term [L. *terminus*, a boundary]. 1. A limit or boundary. 2. A definite period of duration such as the normal period of pregnancy, approx. nine calendar months.

terminal (tĕr′mĭ-năl) [L. *terminalis*]. Pert. to or placed at the end.

terminal arteriole. Arteriole with no branches; but it splits into capillaries.

terminal bars. Minute bars of dense intercellular cement that occupy and close spaces between epithelial cells and bind them together.

terminal ganglia. Ganglia of the parasympathetic division of the autonomic nervous system that are located in or close to walls or visceral structures such as heart or intestines.

terminal illness. An illness that because of its nature can be expected to cause the patient to die. Usually a chronic disease for which there is no known cure.

terminal infection. Infection appearing in the late stage of another disease; often fatal.

terminal veins. One of two veins (anterior and posterior) draining portions of the brain and emptying into interior cerebral veins.

terminatio (tĕr″mĭ-nā′shē-ō) [L.]. The termination or ending.

termination [L. *terminatio*, limiting]. 1. The distal end of a part. 2. The cessation of anything.

terminology (tĕr-mĭ-nŏl′ō-jē) [L. *terminus*, term, + Gr. *logos*, word]. The vocabulary of scientific and technical terms used in specific arts, trades, or professions. SYN: *nomenclature*.

terminus (tĕr′mĭ-nŭs) [L.]. An ending.

ternary (tĕr′nă-rē) [L. *ternarius*, triple]. 1. Threefold; triple; third. 2. Chemical substance containing three different elements or radicals.

teroxide (tĕr-ŏk′sīd). Trioxide.

Teratogenic and Fetotoxic Drugs (Continued)

Maternal Medication	Fetal or Neonatal Effect
Vitamin D	Cardiopathies
Fetotoxic Drugs	
Analgesics, narcotics	
Heroin, morphine	Neonatal death or convulsions, tremors
Salicylates (excessive)	Neonatal bleeding
Cardiovascular drugs	
Ammonium chloride	Acidosis
Hexamethonium	Neonatal ileus
Reserpine	Nasal congestion, drowsiness
Coumarin anticoagulants	Fetal death or hemorrhage
Poliomyelitis immunization (Sabin)	Death or neurologic damage
Sedatives, hypnotics, tranquilizers	
Meprobamate	Retarded development
Phenobarbital (excessive)	Neonatal bleeding
Phenothiazines	Hyperbilirubinemia
Smallpox vaccination	Death or fetal vaccinia
Tetracyclines	Dental discoloration and abnormalities
Thiazides	Thrombocytopenia
Tobacco smoking	Undersized babies
Vitamin K (excessive)	Hyperbilirubinemia

From Krupp, M.A. and Chatton, M.J. (eds.): Current Medical Diagnosis & Treatment. Lange Medical Publications, Los Altos, CA, 1982.

terpene (tĕr′pēn). Any member of the family of hydrocarbons of the formula $C_{10}H_{16}$.

terpin hydrate (tĕr′pĭn hī′drāt). NF. White crystalline substance with a turpentine taste; made by the interaction of rectified spirits of turpentine, alcohol, and nitric acid.

ACTION AND USES: In the form of an elixir; used as an expectorant.

terra (tĕr′ă) [L.]. Earth; soil.

t. alba. White clay.

t. fullonica. Fuller's earth.

terracing (tĕr′ăs-ĭng) [O. Fr. *terrasse*]. Suturing in several rows through thick tissues in closing a wound.

Terramycin (tĕr″ă-mī′sĭn). A trade name for the oxy derivative of tetracycline. An antibiotic biosynthesized by Streptomyces rimosus. It is a broad-spectrum antibiotic effective against both gram-negative and gram-positive bacteria, rickettsias, and some viruses. SEE: *oxytetracycline; tetracycline.*

territoriality (tĕr″ĭ-tor″ē-ăl′ĭ-tē). The tendency of animals and human groups to defend a particular area or region.

terror [L.]. Very great fear.

t., night. Nightmare, esp. of children.

tertian (tĕr′shŭn) [L. *tertianus,* the third]. Occurring every third day. Usually pertaining to malarial fever.

tertiary (tĕr′shē-ār-ē) [L. *tertiarius*]. Third in order or stage.

tertiary alcohol. Alcohol containing the trivalent group ≡COH.

tertiary care. A level of medical care that would be available only in large medical care institutions. Included would be techniques and methods of therapy and diagnosis involving equipment and personnel that would not be economically feasible to have in a smaller institution because of the lack of utilization. SEE: *primary care; secondary care.*

tertiary syphilis. Third and most advanced stage of syphilis.

tertigravida (tĕr″shē-grăv′ĭ-dă) [″ + *gravida,* pregnant]. A woman pregnant for the third time.

tertipara (tĕr-shĭp′ă-ră) [L. *tertius,* third, + *parere,* to bring forth]. A woman who has had three pregnancies terminating after the twentieth week of gestation or has produced three infants of at least 500 grams of weight, regardless of their viability.

Teslac. Trade name for testolactone, USP.

Tessalon. Trade name for benzonatate.

tessellated (tĕs′ĕ-lā″tĕd) [L. *tessella,* a square]. Composed of little squares.

test [L. *testum,* earthen vessel]. 1. An examination. 2. Method to determine the presence or nature of a substance or the presence of a disease. 3. A chemical reaction. 4. A reagent or substance used in making a test.

t., acetic acid. A test for albumin in urine. Adding a few drops of acetic acid to urine that has been boiled causes a white precipitate if albumin is present.

t., acetone. Test for presence of acetone in the urine; made by adding a few drops of sodium nitroprusside to the urine along with strong ammonia water. Presence of acetone causes formation of a magenta ring at outline of contacts.

t., agglutination. A widely used test in which adding an antiserum containing antibodies to cells or bacteria causes them to agglutinate.

t., alkali denaturation. A test for hemoglobin F (fetal hemoglobin) in the blood. Spectrophotometry is used in this test.

t., Allen-Doisy. Test to determine amount of estrogen content in female blood serum by its reaction on secretions of mice.

t., aptitude. Test used to determine an individual's capability in various areas, esp. specific occupations.

t., Aschheim-Zondek. Test for pregnancy by injecting the patient's urine subcutaneously into immature female mice. If the patient is pregnant, the ovaries of the mouse begin to mature prematurely.

t., association. Test used to determine an individual's response to word stimuli. The nature of the response and time required may provide insight into the subject's personality and previous experiences.

t., autohemolysis. A test of the rate of hemolysis of sterile defibrinated whole blood incubated at 37° C. Normal cells hemolyze at a certain rate and blood cells from persons with certain types of disease hemolyze at a faster rate.

t., biuret. Test to determine the presence of proteins or urea.

t., challenge. Administering a substance in order to determine its ability to cause a response, esp. the giving of an antigen and observing or testing for the antibody response.

t., chromatin. A test for genetic sex wherein blood or tissue cells are examined for presence or absence of Barr bodies, q.v.

t., coin. A test for pneumothorax. A metal coin is placed flat on the chest and struck with another coin. The chest is auscultated at the same time. If a pneumothorax is present, a sharp, metallic ringing sound is heard.

t., complement-fixation. SEE: *complement fixation.*

t., concentration. A kidney function test based on the ability of the person to produce concentrated urine under conditions that would normally cause such production, as in intentional dehydration.

t., conjunctival. An allergy test in which the suspected antigen is placed in the conjunctival sac; if it is allergenic for that patient, the conjunctiva becomes red, itches, and lacrimates.

t., creatinine clearance. A test of glomerular function of the kidney. The amount of creatinine present in a timed volume of urine is compared with the plasma creatinine value.

t., double-blind. SEE: *double-blind technique.*

t., finger-nose. A test of cerebellar function wherein the patient is asked to, while keeping the eyes open, touch the nose with the finger and remove the finger, and repeat this rapidly. The test is done by using a finger of each hand successively or in concert. How fast and well this is done is recorded.

t., Friedman. Test for pregnancy by injecting urine of the patient into unmated mature female rabbits, a positive reaction being indicated by formation of corpora lutea and corpora haemorrhagica.

t., galactose tolerance. A test of the ability of the liver to metabolize galactose. A standard dose of galactose is administered to the fasting patient and the amount of galactose excreted in the urine in the next five hours is determined. If the liver is damaged, the galactose is not metabolized to glycogen, but is instead excreted in the urine.

t., Gellé's. Test for ear lesions by employing rubber tubing and a tuning fork.

t., glucose tolerance. SEE: *glucose tolerance test.*

t., guaiac. A test for occult blood in the feces. An alcoholic solution of guaiac resin and hydrogen peroxide is mixed with the specimen. The appearance of a blue color indicates a positive test.

t., histamine. 1. Injection of histamine subcutaneously in order to stimulate gastric secretion of hydrochloric acid. 2. A test for vasomotor headache; a histamine injection precipitates the onset of a headache in persons with this disease.

t., Huhner. Aspiration of vagina within an hour after coitus, to investigate sperm activity.

t., human repeated patch insult. The test material is applied fresh to the same skin site every other day for 10 applications. Each application remains on for 48 hours.

Then after a rest period of about two weeks, the test material is applied again for 48 hours to a different skin site than that originally used. This area is examined daily for the next four days for evidence of irritation. The test measures the ability of the test substance to cause sensitization or irritation reactions or both.

t., intracutaneous. Injection of an antigen intracutaneously and observing the response.

t., Kahn. Precipitation test for syphilis.

t., McMurray. A test for torn muscles of the knee. The supine patient flexes the knees completely. One foot is slowly rotated outward by the examiner as the knee is slowly extended. If a painful click occurs, the medial meniscus of that knee is torn; if as the foot is rotated inward a click is felt, then the lateral meniscus is torn.

t., multiple-puncture. Any skin test, but esp. a tuberculin test, in which the material is placed on the skin and multiple superficial punctures are produced under the material, thus allowing the material to enter the skin.

t., neutralization. A test of the ability of an antibody to neutralize the toxic effects of an antigen.

t., patch. A skin test wherein a test substance, usually a suspected skin sensitizer, is held in contact with the skin for up to two days. If the material being tested is a sensitizer, the skin under it wil be reddened. It is important to use nonallergenic adhesive tape in holding the test material on the skin.

t., precipitin. An antigen-antibody test wherein a specific antigen is added to a solution. If the solution contains the antibody to that antigen, a precipitate is formed.

t., pregnancy. SEE: *pregnancy test.*

t., prothrombin consumption. A test for amount of thromboplastin present in the plasma that reacts with prothrombin. This is determined by quantitating the prothrombin that remains in the serum after coagulation is complete.

t., Rubin. Test for patency of the fallopian tubes by insufflation with carbon dioxide; used in investigating the cause of sterility.

t., Schiller's. Test for detection of cancer of the cervix by painting the tissue with iodine solution; areas that contain glycogen are stained by the iodine. Those sites that do not stain, but become white or yellow, are assumed to be abnormal. Tissue is taken from those areas for microscopic examination.

t., Schwabach. Test for hearing using tuning forks.

t., scratch. An allergy test wherein the antigen is applied to skin that has been lightly scratched.

t., serologic. Any test done on serum.

t., sickling. A test for the ability of red cells to sickle. This is done by placing the red cells in an atmosphere of reduced oxygen tension. If the red cells contain hemoglobin S, they will sickle.

t., thematic apperception. A projective test in which the subject is shown life situations in pictures that could be interpreted in several ways. The subject is asked to provide a story of what the picture represents. The results may provide insights into the subject's personality.

t., three-glass. Upon awakening, the patient urinates sequentially into three glasses. The amount of cellular debris visible to the naked eye in the glasses helps to locate the site of urinary infection, i.e., whether it is in the anterior urethra, posterior urethra, or prostate. If the first glass is turbid and the other two are clear, the anterior urethra is inflamed but the rest of the urinary tract is clear. If the initial specimen is clear and the second and third ones are turbid, the posterior urethra or prostate is inflamed. If only the third specimen is turbid, then only the prostate is inflamed.

t., tine. SEE: *tine test.*

t., tolerance. A test of the ability of the patient or subject to endure the medicine given or exercise taken.

t., tourniquet. A test for capillary fragility. A blood pressure cuff is inflated sufficiently to occlude venous return from the arm. This is kept in place for a set time. After the cuff is removed, the skin distal to the cuff is examined for petechiae.

t., tuberculin. SEE: *tuberculin test.*

t., urea balance. Test of kidney function by measuring intake and output of urea.

t., Wassermann. Diagnostic test for syphilis based on principle of fixation of complement.

testa (tĕs'tă) [L.]. A shell.

testalgia (tĕs-tăl'jē-ă) [L. *testis,* testicle, + Gr. *algos,* pain]. Pain in the testicle.

Testate. Trade name for testosterone enanthate, USP.

testectomy (tĕs-tĕk'tō-mē) [" + Gr. *ektome,* excision]. 1. Removal of a testicle. SYN: *castration.* 2. Removal of a corpus quadrigeminum.

testes (tĕs'tēs) [L.]. Pl. of testis.

testicle (tĕs'tĭ-kl) [L. *testiculus,* a little testis]. A testis.

testicond (tĕs'tĭ-kŏnd) [L. *testis,* testicle, + *condere,* to hide]. The condition of having the testicles remain undescended. This is abnormal in man and in many but not all animals.

testicular (tĕs-tĭk'ū-lăr). Rel. to a testicle.

testis (tĕs′tĭs) [L.]. (pl. *testes*) [NA] The male gonad. One of two reproductive glands located in the scrotum that produce the male reproductive cells or spermatozoa and the male hormone, testosterone. Each is an ovoid body about 4.0 cm. long and 2 to 2.5 cm. in width and thickness enclosed within a dense inelastic fibrous tunica albuginea. The testis is divided into numerous lobules separated by septa, each lobule containing one to three seminiferous tubules within which the spermatozoa arise. The lobules lead to straight ducts that join a plexus, the rete testis, from which 15 to 20 efferent ducts lead to the epididymis. The epididymis leads to the ductus deferens, through which sperm are conveyed to the urethra. Between the seminiferous tubules are located the interstitial cells (cells of Leydig), which are considered to be the source of the male hormone.

The testes are suspended from the body by the spermatic cord, a structure extending from the inguinal ring to the testis. It contains the ductus deferens, testicular vessels (spermatic artery, vein, lymph vessels), and nerves. SYN: *testicle.*

Hyperfunction (hypergonadism) may cause early maturity such as dentition, large sexual organs with early functional activity, and growth of hair.

Hypofunction (hypogonadism) is indicated by undeveloped testes, absence of body hair, high-pitched voice, sterility, smooth skin, loss of sexual desire, low metabolism, and eunuchoid or eunuch type.

t., descent of. Change in position of the testis from abdominal cavity to scrotum during fetal life.

t., displaced. A testis located abnormally within the inguinal canal or pelvis.

t., femoral. An inguinal testis that is near or over the femoral ring.

t., inverted. A testis reversed in the scrotum so that the epididymis attaches to the anterior instead of the posterior part of the gland.

t., perineal. Testis that is located in the perineal region outside the scrotum.

t., undescended. Testis remaining in the inguinal canal or abdominal cavity at birth.

testis compression reflex. Contraction of abdominal muscles following moderate compression of testis.

testitis (tĕs-tī′tĭs) [L. *testis,* testicle, + Gr. *itis,* inflammation]. Inflammation of a testis. SYN: *orchitis.*

testitoxicosis (tĕs″tĭ-tŏk-sĭ-kō′sĭs) [″ + Gr. *toxikon,* poison, + *osis,* condition]. A toxic state sometimes following ligation of the ductus deferens.

test meal. A meal usually small and of definite quality and composition, given to aid in chemical analysis of the stomach contents or x-ray diagnosis of the stomach.

testoid (tĕs′toyd). Resembling a testis.

testolactone (tĕs-tō-lăk′tōn). USP. An anabolic steroid used in treating carcinoma of the breast. Trade name is Teslac.

testopathy (tĕs-tŏp′ă-thē) [″ + Gr. *pathos,* disease]. Any disease of the testes.

testosterone (tĕs-tŏs′tĕr-ōn) [L. *testis,* testicle]. USP. An androgen isolated from the testes of a number of animals including man and considered to be the principal testicular hormone produced in man. It is a steroid produced by the interstitial cells of Leydig of the testicles. This hormone is also normally produced by the adrenal cortex of both human males and females. It has been prepared synthetically by conversion of other sterols, esp. cholesterol.

ACTION: It accelerates growth in tissues upon which it acts and stimulates blood flow. It stimulates and promotes the growth of secondary sexual characteristics and is essential for normal sexual behavior and the occurrence of erections. It is essential for normal growth and development of the male accessory sexual organs. It is responsible for deepening of the male voice at puberty, greater muscular development in men, development of beard and pubic hair, and distribution of fat in adult men. It also affects many metabolic activities.

Testostroval. Trade name for testosterone enanthate, USP.

Testred. Trade name for methyltestosterone, USP.

test tube baby. A baby born to a mother whose ovum was removed, fertilized outside her body, and then implanted in her uterus.

test type. Letters or figures of various size printed on paper. These are used in testing visual acuity.

tetanic (tĕ-tăn′ĭk) [Gr. *tetanikos*]. 1. Pert. to or producing tetanus. 2. Any agent producing tetanic spasms.

tetanic convulsion. A tonic convulsion with constant muscular contraction.

tetaniform (tĕ-tăn′ĭ-form) [Gr. *tetanos,* tetanus, + L. *forma,* shape]. Resembling tetanus.

tetanigenous (tĕt″ă-nĭj′ĕ-nŭs) [″ + *gennan,* to produce]. Causing tetanus or tetanic spasms.

tetanilla (tĕt″ă-nĭl′ă) [L.]. 1. Mild form of tetany, q.v., without rigidity. 2. Twitchings of a limited group of muscular fibers with clonic paroxysmal contractions.

tetanism (tĕt′ă-nĭzm) [″ + *-ismos,* condition]. Persistent muscular hypertonicity resembling tetanus, esp. in infants.

tetanization (tĕt″ă-nī-zā′shŭn) [Gr. *tetanos,*

tetanus]. 1. Production of tetanus or tetanic spasms by induction of the disease. 2. Induction of tetanic contractions in a muscle by electrical stimuli.

tetanize (tĕt'ă-nīz). To induce tonic muscular spasms.

tetanode (tĕt'ă-nōd) [" + *eidos,* form]. In tetany the quiet period between spasms.

tetanoid (tĕt'ă-noyd) [" + *eidos,* form]. Resembling tetanus. SYN: *tetaniform.*

tetanoid paraplegia. Paralysis of lower extremities due to lateral sclerosis of the spinal cord. SYN: *paraplegia, spastic.*

tetanolysin (tĕt"ă-nŏl'ĭ-sĭn). A hemolytic component of the toxin produced by Clostridium tetani, causative organism of tetanus.

tetanomotor (tĕt"ăn-ō-mō'tor) [" + L. *motor,* a mover]. Appliance for the production of tetanic motor spasms mechanically by electrical stimulation of a nerve.

tetanophil, tetanophilic (tĕt'ăn-ō-fĭl, tĕt"ăn-ō-fĭl'ĭk) [" + *philein,* to love]. Possessing an affinity for tetanus toxin.

tetanospasmin (tĕt"ă-nō-spăs'mĭn) [" + L. *spasmus,* spasm]. A component of the toxin produced by tetanus bacillus that is responsible for tetanic convulsions.

tetanus (tĕt'ă-nŭs) [Gr. *tetanos,* tetanus]. 1. An acute infectious disease due to the toxin of tetanus bacillus, Clostridium tetani, growing anaerobically at the site of injury. There is a state of more or less persistent painful tonic spasm of some of the voluntary muscles. 2. A state of sustained contraction of a muscle, esp. that induced experimentally.

Tetanus usually begins gradually but may begin suddenly, may be of brief duration or last some weeks. The first sign is stiffness of the jaw, and esophageal muscles, and some of the muscles of the neck. Soon the jaws become rigidly fixed (trismus or lockjaw), the voice is altered, and muscles of the face contract producing a wild excited expression, a compound of bitter laughter and crying (risus sardonicus). The muscles of back and extremities become tetanic.

If the patient is bent back in a bow, the condition is termed opisthotonos; if bent to the side, pleurothotonos; if bent forward, emprosthotonos.

The paroxysms are reflex and are excited by noises, currents of air, and irritation of bedclothes. The temperature usually rises and may become extremely high. The pain is great; the patient also suffers from hunger, thirst, and want of sleep. The mind is clear. This disease is usually, but not always, fatal, the patient expiring from asphyxia or exhaustion.

TREATMENT: The patient is treated in an intensive care unit. Debride the wound and give penicillin if wound is infected. Give tetanus immune globulin intramuscularly. If this is unavailable, give 10,000 units of tetanus antitoxin intravenously after testing for horse serum sensitivity. Antiserum does not neutralize toxin fixed to central nervous system cells and is of little use in patients with symptoms present at time of hospitalization. It is esp. beneficial if administered early in mild to moderately severe cases. The muscle spasms are treated with sedatives, muscle relaxants, or neuromuscular blocking agents. Tracheostomy is an important treatment and reduces the risk of aspiration when laryngospasm prevents respiration. The use of hyperbaric oxygen in treating tetanus is experimental.

RS: emprosthotonos; lockjaw; opisthotonos; pleurothotonos; posture; risus sardonicus.

t. anticus. Form of tetanus in which the body is bowed forward.

t., artificial. Tetanus produced by a drug such as strychnine.

t., ascending. Tetanus in which muscle spasms occur first in lower part of body and then spread upward, finally involving muscles of head and neck.

t., cephalic. Form of tetanus due to a wound of the head, esp. one near the eyebrow. It is marked by trismus, facial paralysis on one side, and pronounced dysphagia; resembles rabies; often fatal. SYN: *t., hydrophobic.*

t., cerebral. A form of tetanus produced by inoculating the brain of animals with tetanus antitoxin, marked by epileptiform convulsions and excitement.

t., chronic. 1. A latent infection in a healed wound, reactivated upon opening the wound. 2. A form of tetanus in which onset and progress of the disease are slower and more prolonged and symptoms less severe.

t., descending. Tetanus in which muscle spasms occur first in head and neck and later are manifested in other muscles of the body.

t. dorsalis. Tetanus in which the body is bent backward.

t., extensor. Tetanus that affects the extensor muscles especially.

t., hydrophobic. T., cephalic.

t., idiopathic. Tetanus that occurs without any visible lesion.

t., imitative. Hysteria that simulates tetanus.

t. infantum. T. neonatorum.

t., intermittent. Tetany.

t. lateralis. Form of tetanus in which the body is bent sideways.

t., local. Tetanus characterized by spasticity of a group of muscles near the wound. Trismus, tonic contraction of jaw muscles, usually is absent.

t. neonatorum. Tetanus of very young infants, usually due to infection of the navel caused by using nonsterile technique in ligating the umbilical cord.

t. paradoxus. Cephalic tetanus in which condition is combined with paralysis of the facial or other cranial nerve.

t., postoperative. Tetanus that follows an operation.

t., puerperal. Tetanus that occurs following childbirth.

t., rheumatic. Form of tetanus due to exposure to cold and wet.

t., Ritter's. Tetanic contractions at opening of a constant current that has been passing along a nerve for some time; seen in tetany.

t., toxic. Tetanus produced by overdose of nux vomica or strychnine.

t., traumatic. Tetanus following a wound.

tetanus antitoxin. 1. An antibody that develops in the blood of man or other animals (horse) as a result of infection by the tetanus organism (Clostridium tetani) or inoculation with tetanus toxin or toxoid. 2. An antitoxin derived from the blood of horses or cattle immunized against tetanus toxin. It is used to produce passive immunity to prevent the development of tetanus and in the treatment of active tetanus. Prophylactic dose is 1500 units injected subcutaneously; for active tetanus, 5000 to 20,000 units injected intravenously or subcutaneously.

tetanus immune globulin. USP. Immune globulin from human blood for use in persons not previously immunized against tetanus whose wound would indicate the need for tetanus prophylaxis. Tetanus immune globulin (human) will produce fewer side effects than will tetanus antitoxin produced from horse serum.

tetanus toxoid. Tetanus toxin modified so that its toxicity is greatly reduced but its capacity to promote active immunity has been retained.

tetany (tĕt'ă-nē) [Gr. *tetanos,* tetanus]. A nervous affection characterized by intermittent tonic spasms that are usually paroxysmal and involve the extremities; most frequent in the young; frequently associated with pregnancy or lactation.

ETIOL: Tetany is induced by changes in pH and extracellular calcium that increase nervous and muscular excitability. Causative factors are parathyroid deficiency or inadvertent operative removal of parathyroids during thyroidectomy, alkalosis, vitamin D deficiency, or hyperventilation.

SYM: Characterized by nervousness, irritability and apprehension, numbness and tingling of the extremities, cramps of the various muscles, particularly those of the hands producing a typical accoucheur type of hand such as carpopedal spasm, and extreme extension of the feet. Bilateral tonic spasms in arms and legs with jaws rarely involved. Contractions usually paroxysmal and are attended with pain. Electrocontractility of muscles greatly exaggerated. May be slight edema. Sensation not disturbed; mind clear; fever slight or absent.

SIGNS: Characteristic diagnostic signs are Trousseau's sign, Chvostek's sign, and the peroneal sign. Prolongation of the isoelectric phase of the ST segment of the ECG usually is indicative of low calcium. SEE: *Chvostek's sign; hyperventilation; Trousseau's sign.*

PROG: Usually favorable. Attacks following thyroidectomy sometimes fatal.

t., alkalotic. Tetany resulting from respiratory alkalosis, as in hyperventilation, or from metabolic alkalosis induced by excessive intake of sodium bicarbonate or excessive loss of chlorides by vomiting, gastric lavage, or suction.

t., duration. Continuous contraction, esp. in degenerated muscles, in response to a continuous electric current.

t., epidemic. A form of tetany occurring in Europe, esp. in the winter season. It is of short duration and seldom fatal. SEE: *tetanus, rheumatic.*

t., gastric. Severe tetany from stomach disorders accompanied by tonic, painful spasms of the extremities.

t., hyperventilation. Tetany caused by continued hyperventilation.

t., hypocalcemic. Tetany due to low serum calcium and high serum phosphate levels. May be due to lack of vitamin D, factors that interfere with calcium absorption such as steatorrhea or infantile diarrhea, or defective renal excretion of phosphorus.

t., latent. Tetany that requires mechanical or electrical stimulation of nerves to show characteristic signs of excitability.

t., manifest. Tetany in which the characteristic symptoms such as carpopedal spasm, laryngospasm, and convulsions are present. Opposite of latent tetany.

t., parathyroid. Tetany resulting from excision of the parathyroid gland or from hyposecretion of the parathyroid gland as a result of disease or disorders of the gland. SEE: *hypoparathyroidism.*

t., rachitic. Tetany due to hypocalcemia accompanying vitamin D deficiency.

t., thyreoprival. Tetany resulting from removal of the thyroid gland accompanied by removal of parathyroid glands.

tetarcone (tĕt'ăr-kōn) [Gr. *tetartos,* fourth, + *konos,* cone]. Fourth or distolingual cusp of an upper premolar tooth. SYN: *tetartocone.*

tetartanopia, tetartanopsia (tĕt"ăr-tăn-ō'pē-ă, -ŏp'sē-ă) [" + *opsis,* vision]. Symmetrical blindness in the same quadrant of each visual field. SYN: *quadrantanopsia.*

tetartocone (tĕt-ăr'tō-kōn) [" + *konos,* cone]. The distolingual cusp of an upper premolar tooth. SYN: *tetarcone.*

tetra-, tetr- [Gr. *tetras,* four]. Combining forms meaning four.

tetrabasic (tĕt"ră-bā'sĭk) [" + *basis,* base]. Having four replaceable hydrogen atoms, said of an acid or acid salt.

tetrablastic (tĕt"ră-blăs'tĭk) [" + *blastos,* germ]. Having four germinal layers: the ectoderm, endoderm, and two mesodermic layers.

tetrabrachius (tĕt"ră-brā'kē-ŭs) [" + *brachion,* arm]. A deformed fetus with four arms.

tetrabromofluorescein (tĕt"ră-brōm"ō-flū-or-ĕs'ĭn, -ē-ĭn). A dye, $C_{20}H_8Br_4O_5$, obtained from action of bromine on fluorescein, used as a stain in microscopy. SYN: *eosin.*

tetracaine hydrochloride. USP. A local anesthetic agent used topically, and by infiltration. Trade name is Pontocaine hydrochloride.

tetrachirus (tĕt"ră-kī'rŭs) [" + *cheir,* hand]. A deformed fetus with four hands.

tetrachlorethylene (tĕt"ră-klor-ĕth'ĭ-lēn). USP. A clear, colorless liquid with a characteristic odor, used as an anthelmintic.

tetrachloride (tĕt"ră-klō'rīd). A radical with four atoms of chlorine.

tetracid (tĕ-trăs'ĭd) [" + L. *acidus,* sour]. 1. Able to react with four molecules of a monoacid or two of a diacid to form a salt or ester, said of a base or alcohol; term disapproved by some authorities. 2. Having four hydrogen atoms replaceable by basic atoms or radicals, said of acids.

Tetracoccus (tĕt"ră-kŏk'ŭs) [" + *kokkos,* berry]. Genus of micrococcus arranged in groups of four by division into two planes.

tetracrotic (tĕt"ră-krŏt'ĭk) [" + *krotos,* beat]. Noting a pulse or pulse tracing with four upward strokes in the descending limb of the wave.

tetracycline (tĕt"ră-sī'klēn). USP. A member of the tetracycline group of broad-spectrum antibiotics having similar pharmacological activity (i.e., tetracycline, chlortetracycline, oxytetracycline). Esp. effective in treatment of Q fever, typhus fever, psittacosis, acute brucellosis, and granuloma inguinale. Trade names are Tedracyn, Robitet, and SK-Tetracycline.

tetrad (tĕt'răd) [Gr. *tetras,* four]. 1. A group of four things with something in common. 2. An element having a valence or combining power of four. 3. A group of four similar bodies. 4. A group of four parts, said of cells produced by division in two planes, or of a chromosome in four parts in preparation for two mitotic divisions in maturation.

tetradactyly (tĕt"ră-dăk'tĭ-lē) [" + *daktylos,* finger] Having four digits on a hand or foot.

tetraethylammonium chloride (tĕt-ră-ĕth-ĭl-ăm-ō'nē-ŭm klō'rīd). A quaternary ammonium compound used as a ganglionic blocking agent in diagnosis and treatment of circulatory diseases. ABBR: TEAC.

tetraethylpyrophosphate (tĕt-ră-ĕth"ĭl-pī-rō-fŏs'fāt). A powerful cholinesterase inhibitor used as an insecticide; poisonous to man. Has had some use in treatment of myasthenia gravis The antidote is atropine. ABBR: TEPP.

tetragenous (tĕt-răj'ĕn-ŭs) [Gr. *tetras,* four, + *gennan,* to produce]. Pert. to organisms, esp. bacteria, that divide into groups of four.

tetrahydrocannabinol (tĕt"ră-hī"drō-kă-năb'ĭ-nŏl). A chemical, $C_{21}H_{30}O_2$, that is the principal active component in cannabis, or marijuana.

tetrahydrozoline hydrochloride (tĕt"ră-hī-drō'zō-lēn). USP. A vasoconstrictor agent used as a nasal decongestant and ophthalmic vasoconstrictor. Trade name is Iyzine.

tetraiodothyronine (tĕt"ră-ī"ō-dō-thī'rō-nēn). One of the principal hormones secreted by the thyroid gland. Chemically it is 3,5,3',5'-tetraiodothyronine. ABBR: T_4. SEE: *thyroid; thyroid function tests; triiodthyronine.* SYN: *thyroxine.*

tetralogy. The combination of four symptoms or elements.

t. of Fallot. An anomaly of the heart consisting of pulmonary stenosis, interventricular septal defect, dextroposed aorta that receives blood from both ventricles, and hypertrophy of the right ventricle.

tetramastia, tetramazia (tĕt"ră-măs'tē-ă, tĕt"ră-mā'zē-ă) [" + *mastos, mazos,* breast]. Condition characterized by presence of four breasts.

tetramastigote (tĕt"ră-măs'tĭ-gōt) [" + *mastix,* lash]. Having four flagella.

tetrameric, tetramerous (tĕt"ră-mĕr'ĭk, tĕt-răm'ĕr-ŭs) [" + *meros,* a part]. Having four parts.

tetranopsia (tĕt"ră-nŏp'sē-ă) [" + *an-,* not, + *opsis,* vision]. Obliteration of one quarter of the visual field.

tetraotus (tĕt"ră-ō'tŭs) [Gr. *tetras,* four, + *otos,* ear]. Tetrotus, q.v.

tetraparesis (tĕt"ră-păr'ĕ-sĭs) [" + *paresis,* relaxation]. Muscular weakness of all four extremities.

tetrapeptide (tĕt"ră-pĕp'tīd). A peptide that yields four amino acids when it is hydrolyzed.

tetraplegia (tĕt"ră-plē'jē-ă) [" + *plege,* a stroke]. Paralysis of both arms and legs. SYN: *quadriplegia.*

tetraploid (tĕt'ră-ployd) [" + *ploos,* a fold, + *eidos,* form]. 1. Concerning tetraploidy. 2. Having four sets of chromosomes.

tetrapus (tĕt'ră-pŭs) [″ + *pous,* foot]. A deformed fetus having four feet.
tetrasaccharide (tĕt″ră-săk'ă-rīd). A carbohydrate composed of four monosaccharides.
tetrascelus (tĕt-răs'ē-lŭs) [″ + *skelos,* leg]. A deformed fetus having four legs.
tetrasomic (tĕt-ră-sō'mĭk) [″ + *soma,* body]. Possessing four instead of the usual two of a pair of chromosomes in an otherwise diploid cell, that is, having a chromosome number of 2n + 2.
tetraster (tĕt-răs'tĕr) [″ + *aster,* star]. A mitotic figure in which there are four asters instead of the usual two; occurring abnormally in mitosis.
tetrastichiasis (tĕt″ră-stĭ-kī'ă-sĭs) [″ + *stichos,* row, + *-iasis,* conditon]. A deformed fetus having four rows of eyelashes.
tetratomic (tĕt″ră-tŏm'ĭk) [″ + *atomos,* indivisible]. Having four atoms.
tetravalent (tĕt″ră-vā'lĕnt). Having a valence or combining power of four. SYN: *quadrivalent.*
Tetrex. Trade name for tetracycline phosphate complex.
tetrodotoxin (tĕt″rō-dō-tŏks'ĭn). A powerful nerve poison found in the eggs of the California newt and in certain puffer fish in Japan. In concentrated form it is more toxic than cyanide.
tetrotus (tĕt-rō'tŭs) [″ + *otos,* ear]. A deformed fetus with two faces, four eyes, and four ears.
tetroxide (tĕ-trŏk'sīd). A chemical compound containing four oxygen atoms.
tetter (tĕt'ĕr) [AS. *teter*]. Obsolete term for various vesicular cutaneous diseases such as herpes, ringworm, or eczema.
texis (tĕk'sĭs) [Gr. *tiktein,* to give birth]. Childbearing.
textiform (tĕks'tĭ-form) [L. *textum,* something woven, + *forma,* shape]. Resembling a network, web, or mesh.
textoblastic (tĕks″tō-blăs'tĭk) [L. *textus,* tissue, + Gr. *blastos,* germ]. Forming adult tissue; regenerative.
textural (tĕks'tū-răl) [L. *textura,* weaving]. Concerning the texture or constitution of a tissue.
texture (tĕks'tūr) [L. *textura*]. The organization of a tissue or structure.
textus (tĕks'tŭs) [L.]. Tissue.
T fracture. Fracture in which bone splits both longitudinally and transversely.
T-group. Group of individuals who meet in sensitivity training sessions in order to become more sensitive to themselves and others.
Th. Chem. symbol for thorium.
thalamencephalon (thăl″ă-mĕn-sĕf'ă-lŏn) [Gr. *thalamos,* chamber, + *enkephalos,* brain]. [NA] The part of the diencephalon that includes the thalamus, pineal body, and geniculate bodies. SYN: *diencephalon.*
thalamic (thăl-ăm'ĭk) [Gr. *thalamos,* inner chamber]. Pert. to the thalamus.
thalamic syndrome. Vascular lesions of the thalamus causing disturbances of sensation and partial or complete paralysis of one side of the body. An extremely severe, sharp, boring-type pain may occur spontaneously. There also is a tendency to over-respond to a sensory stimulus and to be aware of the stimulus long after it has ceased.

ETIOL: Optic thalamus lesion.

thalamo- [Gr. *thalamos,* chamber]. 1. Combining form meaning chamber, part of brain at which a nerve originates. 2. Pert. to the thalamus.
thalamocele, thalamocoele (thăl'ăm-ō-sēl) [″ + *koilia,* a hollow]. The 3rd ventricle of the brain.
thalamocortical (thăl'ăm-ō-kor'tĭ-kăl) [″ + L. *cortex,* rind]. Pert. to the optic thalamus and the cerebral cortex.
thalamolenticular (thăl″ăm-ō-lĕn-tĭk'ū-lăr) [″ + L. *lenticula,* a small lentil]. Concerning the optic thalamus and the lenticular nucleus.
thalamotomy (thăl-ă-mŏt'ō-mē) [″ + *tome,* incision]. Destruction by one of several methods of a portion of the thalamus in order to treat psychosis or intractable pain.
thalamus (thăl'ă-mŭs) [L.]. (pl. *thalami*) [NA] The largest subdivision of the diencephalon on either side, consisting chiefly of an ovoid gray nuclear mass in the lateral wall of the 3rd ventricle. Each consists of a number of nuclei (anterior, medial, lateral, and ventral), the medial and lateral geniculate bodies, and the pulvinar.

FUNCT: All sensory stimuli, with the exception of olfactory, are received by the thalamus. These are associated, synthesized, and then relayed through thalamocortical radiations to specific cortical areas. Impulses are also received from the cortex, hypothalamus, and corpus striatum and relayed to visceral and somatic effectors. The thalamus is also the center for appreciation of primitive uncritical sensations of pain, crude touch, and temperature.

thalassemia (thăl-ă-sē'mē-ă) [Gr. *thalassa,* sea, + *haima,* blood]. A group of hereditary anemias occurring in populations bordering the Mediterranean and in Southeast Asia. Anemia is produced by either a defective production rate of the alpha or beta hemoglobin polypeptide chain or a decreased synthesis of the beta chain. Heterozygotes are usually asymptomatic. The severity in homozygotes varies according to the complexity of the inheritance pattern, but may be fatal. SEE: *anemia, sickle cell.*

t. major. The homozygous form of deficient beta chain synthesis, which is very severe and presents during childhood. Characterized by fatigue, splenomegaly, severe anemia, enlargement of the heart, slight jaundice, leg ulcers, and cholelithiasis. Increased bone marrow activity causes thickening of the cranial bones and increased malar eminences. Prognosis varies; however, the younger the child when the disease appears, the more unfavorable the outcome. SYN: *Cooley's anemia.*

t. minor. Heterozygosity for either β or α chain produces a mild disease that may be completely asymptomatic. Usually revealed by chance or as a result of study of the family of an individual having thalassemia major. Prognosis is excellent.

thalassophobia (thăl-ăs″ō-fō′bē-ă) [Gr. *thalassa,* sea, + *phobos,* fear]. Abnormal fear of the sea.

thalassoposia (thăl-lăs″sō-pō′zē-ă) [″ + *posis,* drinking]. Ingestion of sea water.

thalassotherapy (thăl-ăs″sō-thĕr′ă-pē) [″ + *therapeia,* treatment]. Treatment of disease by living at the seaside, by sea bathing, sea voyages, or sea air.

thalidomide (thă-lĭd′ŏ-mīd). A chemical substance, α (N-phthalimido) glutarimide, used extensively as a sedative and sleeping pill in Europe in the early 1960s. Its use was discontinued when it was discovered to cause severe malformation in limbs of developing fetuses exposed to the drug in their very early intrauterine life.

thallinization (thăl″ĭn-ĭ-zā′shŭn). Treatment with doses of thalline or its salts.

thallitoxicosis (thăl″ĭ-tŏk″sĭ-kō′sĭs). Poisoning by accidental ingestion of thallium sulfate–containing pesticides. SEE: *thallium* in *Poisons and Poisoning* in *Appendix.*

thallium (thăl′ē-ŭm) [Gr. *thallos,* a young shoot]. SYMB: Tl. At. wt. 204.383; at. no. 81; sp. gr. 11.85. A metallic element. Its salts are poisonous.

t. sulfate. A chemical used as a rodenticide. It is also quite toxic to humans.

thallium poisoning. Characterized by severe abdominal pain, vomiting, diarrhea, tremors, delirium, convulsions, paralysis, coma, and death. SEE: *Poisons and Poisoning* in *Appendix.*

thallotoxicosis (thăl″ō-tŏk″sĭ-kō′sĭs). Thallitoxicosis, q.v.

THAM. Trade name for tromethamine.

thamuria (thă-mū′rē-ă) [Gr. *thamys,* often, + *ouron,* urine]. Abnormally frequent urination.

thanato- [Gr. *thanatos,* death]. Combining form meaning death.

thanatobiological (thăn″ă-tō-bī-ō-lŏj′ĭ-kăl) [Gr. *thanatos,* death, + *bios,* life, + *logos,* study]. Rel. to the processes of life and death

thanatognomonic (thăn″ăt-ŏg-nō-mŏn′ĭk) [″ + *gnomonikos,* knowing]. Indicative of the approach of death.

thanatoid (thăn′ă-toyd) [″ + *eidos,* form]. Resembling death.

thanatology (thăn″ă-tŏl′ō-jē) [Gr. *thanatos,* death, + *logos,* science]. The science of death.

thanatomania (thăn″ă-tō-mā′nē-ă) [″ + *mania,* madness]. Condition of homicidal or suicidal mania.

thanatometer (thăn″ă-tŏm′ĕt-er) [″ + *metron,* measure]. Instrument for determining occurrence of death by internal temperature.

thanatophidia (thăn″ă-tō-fĭd′ē-ă) [″ + *ophis,* snake]. Venomous snakes.

thanatophobia (thăn″ă-tō-fō′bē-ă) [″ + *phobos,* fear]. Morbid fear of death. SYN: *necrophobia.*

thanatophoric (thăn″ă-tō-for′ĭk) [″ + *pherein,* to bear]. Lethal.

thanatophoric dwarfism. Dwarfism caused by generalized failure of endochondral bone formation. Characterized by large head, prominent forehead, hypertelorism, saddle nose, and short limbs extending straight out from the trunk. Most of these infants die soon after birth. SEE: *dwarf, micromelic.*

thaumato- [Gr. *thauma,* wonder]. Combining form meaning wonder, marvel.

thaumaturgic [″ + *ergon,* work]. To work miracles or magic.

Thayer-Martin medium. A special medium used for growing the causative organism of gonorrhea, Neisseria gonorrhoeae.

theaism (thē′ă-ĭzm) [L. *thea,* tea, + Gr. *-ismos,* condition]. Chronic poisoning from excessive tea drinking.

thebaic (thē-bā′ĭk) [L. *Thebaicus,* Theban, from Thebes, where opium was once prepared]. Concerning opium.

thebaine (thē-bā′ĭn). An alkaloid present in opium.

thebesian foramina (thē-bē′zē-ăn). [Adam Christian Thebesius, Ger. physician, 1686–1732] Orifices of the thebesian veins, opening into the right auricle of the heart.

thebesian valve. An endocardial fold at entrance of the coronary sinus into right auricle.

thebesian veins. Venules conveying blood from the myocardium to the atria or ventricles.

theca (thē′kă) [Gr. *theke,* sheath]. (pl. *thecae*) A sheath of investing membrane.

t. cordis. Pericardium that sheaths the heart.

t. folliculi. [NA] Outer wall of a graafian follicle, consisting of an inner vascular layer (theca interna) and outer fibrous layer (theca externa).

thecal (thē′kăl) [Gr. *theke,* sheath]. Pert. to a sheath.

thecitis (thē-sī′tĭs) [″ + *itis,* inflammation]. Inflammation of the sheath of a tendon.
theco- [Gr. *theke,* sheath]. Combining form meaning sheath, case, or receptacle.
thecodont (thē′kō-dŏnt) [″ + *odous,* tooth]. Having teeth that are inserted in sockets.
thecoma (thē-kō′mă) [″ + *oma,* tumor]. A tumor of the ovary usually occurring during or following the menopause. Only rarely is it malignant.
thecomatosis (thē″kō-mă-tō′sĭs) [″ + ″ + *osis,* condition]. Increased connective tissue in the ovary.
thecostegnosia, thecostegnosis (thē″kō-stĕg-nō′sē-ă, -nō′sĭs) [″ + *stegnosis,* a narrowing]. Constriction of a tendon sheath.
Theelin. Trade name for estrone.
theine (thē′ĭn). Caffeine.
theinism (thē′ĭn-ĭzm). Theaism, q.v.
thelalgia (thē-lăl′jē-ă) [Gr. *thele,* nipple, + *algos,* pain]. Pain in the nipples.
thelarche (thē-lăr′kē) [″ + *arche,* beginning]. The beginning of breast development at puberty.
thelasis (thē-lăs′ĭs) [″ + *-asis,* condition]. The act of sucking.
Thelazia (thē-lā′zē-ă) [Gr. *thelazo,* to suck]. A genus of nematodes that inhabits the conjunctival sac and lacrimal ducts of various species of vertebrates. Occasionally Thelazia are found in man.
thelaziasis (thē″lā-zī′ă-sĭs) [″ + *-iasis,* condition]. Condition of being infested by worms of the genus Thelazia.
theleplasty (thē′lĕ-plăs″tē) [Gr. *thele,* nipple, + *plassein,* to form]. Plastic surgery of the nipple. SYN: *mammilliplasty.*
thelerethism (thēl-ĕr′ĕ-thĭzm) [″ + *erethisma,* stimulation]. Erection of the nipple.
thelitis (thē-lī′tĭs) [″ + *itis,* inflammation]. Inflammation of the nipples. SYN: *acromastitis.*
thelium (thē′lē-ŭm) [L.]. (pl. *thelia*) 1. A papilla. 2. A nipple. 3. A cellular layer.
theloncus (thē-lŏn′kŭs) [″ + *onkos,* mass]. A tumor of a nipple.
thelophlebostemma (thē″lō-flĕb″ō-stĕm′mă) [″ + *phleps,* vein, + *stemma,* wreath]. A dark or venous circle of veins about the nipple.
thelorrhagia (thē″lō-rā′jē-ă) [″ + *rhegnynai,* to burst forth]. Hemorrhage from a nipple.
thelothism (thē′lō-thĭzm) [″ + *erethisma,* stimulation]. Erection of a nipple brought about by contraction of smooth muscle fibers. SEE: *thelerethism.*
thelygenic (thē″lē-jĕn′ĭk) [Gr. *thelys,* female, + *gennan,* to produce]. Producing only female children.
thenad (thē′năd) [Gr. *thenar,* palm, + L. *ad,* toward]. Toward the palm or thenar eminence.
thenal (thē′năl) [Gr. *thenar,* palm]. Pert. to the palm or thenar eminence.
thenal aspect. Outer side of the palm.
thenal eminence. Ball of the thumb.
thenar (thē′năr) [Gr. *thenar,* palm]. 1. Palm of hand or sole of foot. 2. Fleshy eminence at base of thumb. 3. Concerning the palm.
thenar cleft. A fascial cleft of the palm overlying volar surface of adductor pollicis muscle.
thenar eminence. A prominence at the base of the thumb.
thenar fascia. A thin membrane covering the short muscles of the thumb.
thenar muscles. Abductor and flexor muscles of the thumb.
theobromine (thē-ō-brō′mēn) [Gr. *theos,* god, + *broma,* food]. A white powder obtained from Theobroma cacao.

ACTION AND USES: Dilates blood vessels in the heart and peripherally. Used as a mild stimulant and as a diuretic.

theomania (thē-ō-mā′nē-ă) [Gr. *theos,* god, + *mania,* madness]. Religious insanity; esp. that in which the patient thinks he is a deity or has divine inspiration.
theophobia (thē″ō-fō′bē-ă) [″ + *phobos,* fear]. Abnormal fear of the wrath of God.
theophylline (thē″ō-fĭl′ēn, -ĭn) [L. *thea,* tea, + Gr. *phyllon,* plant]. USP. A white crystalline powder with action resembling caffeine and theobromine. Trade names include Elixophyllin, Elixophyllin Sr, and Slo-Phyllin.

t. olamine. USP. A smooth muscle relaxant. A theophylline preparation available only as a solution for rectal administration.

t. sodium glycinate. USP. A smooth muscle relaxant.

t. ethylenediamine. Previously used name for aminophylline, USP.

theorem (thē′ō-rĕm) [Gr. *theorema,* principle arrived at by speculation]. A proposition that can be proved by use of logic, or by argument, from information previously accepted as being valid.

t., Bayes. SEE: *Bayes theorem.*

theory (thē′ō-rē) [Gr. *theoria,* speculation as opposed to practice]. A supposition or an assumption based on certain evidence or observations but lacking scientific proof. When a theory becomes generally accepted and firmly established, it is a doctrine or principle.

t., cell. The proposition that living things are composed of cells capable of life.

t., clonal selection, of immunity. A theory formulated by the Australian Nobel prize winner F. M. Burnett, in 1959, that mesenchymal cells, precursors of the cells that form antibodies, are made up of innumerable clones. The clones capable of reacting with "self" components, i.e., the individual's own cells, are eliminated or suppressed in the prenatal period. Those clones not eliminated or suppressed that are specific for foreign substances react with the antigen fitting to the receptor, and this leads to the proliferation of that clone.

t., germ. The proposition that infectious diseases are due to microorganisms.

t., quantum. The proposition that energy can be emitted in discrete quantities (quanta); and that atomic particles can exist only in certain energy states. Quanta are measured by multiplying the frequency of the radiation, *v*, times *h*, Planck's constant. SYN: *Planck's theory.*

t., recapitulation. The theory that during development an individual organism goes through the same progressive stages as did the species in developing from lower to higher forms of life. Referred to as ontogeny recapitulates phylogeny.

theotherapy (thē″ō-thĕr′ă-pē) [Gr. *theos,* god, + *therapeia,* treatment]. Treatment of disease by spiritual and religious methods.

theque (tĕk) [Fr., a box]. A nest of nevus cells or other cells in the epidermis.

Theralax. Trade name for bisacodyl, USP.

therapeusis (thĕr″ă-pū′sĭs). Therapeutics.

therapeutic (thĕr-ă-pū′tĭk) [Gr. *therapeutikos,* treating]. 1. Pert. to results obtained from treatment. 2. Having medicinal or healing properties. 3. A healing agent.

therapeutic exercise. Scientific supervision of exercise for the purpose of preventing muscular atrophy, restoring joint and muscle function, increasing muscular strength, and improving efficiency of cardiovascular and pulmonary function.

therapeutics (thĕr″ă-pū′tĭks) [Gr. *therapeutike,* treatment]. That branch of medicine concerned with the application of remedies and the treatment of disease. SYN: *therapy.*

therapia sterilisans magna (thĕr″ă-pē′ă stē-rĭl′ĭ-săns măg′nă) [L.]. Ehrlich's method of administering a chemical agent that would destroy in one large dose all the parasites in a patient without causing serious injury to the patient.

therapist (thĕr′ă-pĭst) [Gr. *therapeia,* treatment]. A person skilled in giving therapy. Usually in a specific field of health care.

t., physical. A person trained in physical medicine and is capable of administering physical therapy. SYN: *physiotherapist.*

t., respiratory. A person skilled in managing the techniques and equipment used in treating those with acute and chronic respiratory diseases.

t., speech. A person skilled in assisting patients who have speech and language difficulties.

therapy (thĕr′ă-pē) [Gr. *therapeia,* treatment]. Treatment of a disease or pathological condition. SEE: *treatment.*

t., anticoagulant. The use of anticoagulants to decrease the tendency of the blood to coagulate and cause thrombosis.

t., aversion. Aversion therapy, q.v.

t., collapse. Production of a pneumothorax on one side in order to treat pulmonary tuberculosis. This allows the lung on that side to be at rest.

t., electroconvulsive. SEE: *electroconvulsive therapy.*

t., fever. Therapy involving artificially produced fever. This is accomplished by exposure to high environmental temperature or by the injection of foreign proteins.

t., group. SEE: *group therapy.*

t., immunosuppressive. SEE: *immunosuppressive agent.*

t., inhalation. Administration of medicines, water vapor, gases (such as oxygen, carbon dioxide, or helium), or anesthetics by inhalation. The medicines usually are nebulized by using an aerosol or spray apparatus, SEE: *intermittent positive-pressure breathing.*

t., insulin shock. SEE: *insulin shock therapy.*

t., light. Treatment with radiation from the visible spectrum.

t., milieu. Treatment of mental illness by altering the patient's immediate social and environmental circumstances in order to facilitate whatever other therapy is being used.

t., nonspecific. Use of injections of foreign proteins or bacterial vaccines in treatment of infection to stimulate general cellular activity. SEE: *t., specific.*

t., occupational. SEE: *occupational therapy.*

t., opsonic. Use of bacterial vaccines to elevate the opsonic index of the blood. SYN: *t., vaccine.*

t., physical. Use of physical agents in the treatment of disease, as massage, heat, hydrotherapy, radiation, electricity, and exercise.

t., radiation. The treatment of diseases by the use of ionizing radiation.

t., replacement. The therapeutic use of a medicine to substitute for the natural substance that is either absent or diminished, e.g., insulin and thyroid hormone.

t., serum. Use of injections of blood serum from immunized animals or persons in the treatment of disease. SYN: *serotherapy.*

t., shock. SEE: *shock therapy.*

t., specific. Administration of a remedy acting directly against the cause of a disease, as arsphenamine or mercury for syphilis, or quinine for malaria.

t., speech. SEE: *speech therapy.*

t., spiritual. SEE: *spiritual therapy.*

t., substitution. Administration of a substance that the body normally produces such as a hormone.

t., vaccine. Injection of bacteria or their products to produce active immunization against a disease. SYN: *t., opsonic.*

therapy putty. Generic name for malleable plastic material used as a therapeutic modality to provide resistance in various hand exercises. Trade name is Theraplast.

therm [Gr. *therme,* heat]. Term used to indicate a variety of quantities of heat. SEE: MET.

thermacogenesis (thĕr″mă-kō-jĕn′ĕs-ĭs) [Gr. *therme,* heat, + *genesis,* production]. Production of an increase of body temperature by drug therapy.

thermaerotherapy (thĕr-mā″ĕr-ō-thĕr′ă-pē) [″ + *aer,* air, + *therapeia,* treatment]. Therapeutic application of hot air.

thermal (thĕr′măl) [Gr. *therme,* heat]. Pert. to heat.

thermal death point. In bacteriology, the degree of heat that will kill organisms in a fluid culture in 10 minutes.

thermalgesia (thĕr″măl-jē′zē-ă) [″ + *algesis,* sense of pain]. Pain caused by heat.

thermalgia (thĕr-măl′jē-ă) [″ + *algos,* pain]. Neuralgia accompanied by intense burning sensation, pain, redness, and sweating of the area involved. SYN: *causalgia.*

thermal luminescence dosimeter. A personal monitoring device consisting of a small crystal in a plastic container taped to the patient. It stores energy caused by X radiation. When heated, it gives off light proportional to the radiation exposure received by the patient.

thermal radiation. Heat radiation.

thermal sense. Capacity for recognition of heat. SYN: *thermesthesia.*

thermanalgesia (thĕrm″ăn-ăl-jē′zē-ă) [″ + *an-,* not, + *algesis,* pain]. Inability to experience reaction to heat because of a cerebral lesion.

thermanesthesia (thĕrm″ăn-ĕs-thē′zē-ă) [″ + ″ + *aisthesis,* sensation]. Inability to recognize sensations of heat and cold; insensibility to heat changes. It sometimes occurs in syringomyelia. SYN: *thermoanesthesia.*

thermatology (thĕr-mă-tŏl′ō-jē) [Gr. *therme,* heat, + *logos,* science]. The study of heat in treatment of disease.

thermelometer (thĕr″mĕl-ŏm′ĕ-tĕr) [″ + *elektron,* amber, + Gr. *metron,* a measure]. An electric thermometer used to indicate temperature changes too slight to be measured on an ordinary thermometer.

thermesthesia (thĕr″mĕs-thē′zē-ă) [″ + *aisthesis,* sensation]. Capability of perceiving heat and cold; temperature sense. SYN: *thermoesthesia.*

thermesthesiometer (thĕrm″ĕs-thē-zē-ŏm′ĕt-ĕr) [″ + *aisthesis,* sensation, + *metron,* a measure]. Device for determining sensibility to heat.

thermhyperesthesia (thĕrm″hī-pĕr-ĕs-thē′zē-ă) [″ + Gr. *hyper,* above, + *aisthesis,* sensation]. Excessive sensitivity to heat.

thermhypesthesia (thĕrm″hī-pĕs-thē′zē-ă) [″ + *hypo,* under, + *aisthesis,* sensation]. Lessened sensibility of the temperature sense. SYN: *thermohypesthesia.*

thermic (thĕr′mĭk) [Gr. *therme,* heat]. Pert. to heat.

thermic sense. The temperature sense; ability to react to heat stimuli.

thermistor (thĕr-mĭs′tor). An apparatus for quickly determining very small changes in temperature. Materials that alter their resistance to the flow of electricity as the temperature changes are used in these devices.

thermo- [Gr. *therme,* heat]. Combining form indicating hot or heat.

thermoalgesia (thĕr″mō-ăl-jē′zē-ă) [Gr. *therme,* heat, + *algesis,* pain]. Condition in which pain is caused by application of moderate heat. SYN: *thermalgesia.*

thermoanalgesia (thĕr″mō-ăn″ăl-jē′zē-ă) [″ + *an,* not, + *algesis,* pain]. Loss of heat sensation. SYN: *thermanalgesia.*

thermoanesthesia (thĕr″mō-ăn″ĕs-thē′zē-ă) [″ + ″ + *aisthesis,* sensation]. 1. Inability to distinguish between heat and cold. 2. Insensibility to heat or temperature changes.

thermobiosis (thĕr″mō-bī-ō′sĭs) [″ + *biosis,* way of life]. Ability to withstand high temperature.

thermobiotic (thĕr″mō-bī-ŏt′ĭk) [″ + *bios,* life]. Able to exist at high temperature.

thermocauterectomy (thĕr″mō-kaw-tĕr-ĕk′tō-mē) [″ + *kauterion,* branding iron, + *ektome,* excision]. Excision by thermocautery.

thermocautery (thĕr″mō-kaw′tĕr-ē). 1. Cautery by application of heat. 2. Cauterizing iron.

thermochemistry (thĕr″mō-kĕm′ĭs-trē). The branch of science concerned with the interrelationship of heat and chemical reactions.

thermochroism (thĕr-mŏk′rō-ĭzm) [″ + *chroa,* color]. Property of a substance reflecting or transmitting portions of thermal radiation and absorbing or altering others.

thermochroic (thĕr″mō-krō′ĭk) [″ + *chroa,* color]. Concerning thermochroism.

thermocoagulation (thĕr″mō-kō-ăg-ū-lā′shŭn) [″ + L. *coagulare,* to clot]. The use of high-frequency currents to produce coagulation to destroy tissue.

thermocouple (thĕr′mō-kŭ″pl) [″ + L. *copula,* a bond]. Device for measuring slight temperature changes. SYN: *thermopile.*

thermocurrent (thĕr″mō-kŭr′ĕnt). An electric current produced by thermoelectric means.

thermode. A device for heating or cooling a part of the body. Thermodes have been used in studying the effect on body function when temperature of some organ or tissue is changed.

thermodiffusion (thĕr″mō-dĭ-fū′zhŭn). Increased diffusion of a substance as a result of increased heat.

thermodilution (thĕr″mō-dī-lū′shŭn). Use of an injected cold liquid such as sterile saline into the bloodstream and measuring the temperature change downstream. This has been used in determining cardiac output.

thermoduric (thĕr″mō-dū′rĭk) [″ + L. *durus,* resistant]. Able to live in high temperatures. SEE: *thermophylic.*

thermodynamics (thĕr″mō-dī-năm′ĭks) [″ + *dynamis,* power]. The branch of physics concerned with the laws that govern heat production, changes, and conversion into other forms of energy.

thermoelectric (thĕr″mō-ē-lĕk′trĭk). Concerning thermoelectricity.

thermoelectricity (thĕr″mō-ē-lĕk-trĭs′ĭ-tē). Electricity generated by heat.

thermoesthesia (thĕr″mō-ĕs-thē′zē-ă) [Gr. *therme,* heat, + *aisthesis,* sensation]. Ability to recognize temperature differences. SYN: *thermesthesia.*

thermoexcitory (thĕr″mō-ĕk-sī′tor-ē) [″ + L. *excitare,* to irritate]. Stimulating the production of heat in the body.

thermogenesis (thĕr″mō-jĕn′ĕ-sĭs) [″ + *genesis,* production]. The production of heat, esp. in the body.

thermogenics (thĕr″mō-jĕn′ĭks). The study of and science of heat production.

thermogram (thĕr′mō-grăm). A graphic record of variation in heat.

thermograph (thĕr′mō-grăf) [″ + *graphein,* to write]. Device for registering variations of heat.

thermography. In medicine, the use of a device that detects and records the heat present in very small areas of the part being studied. When these multiple readings are accumulated, the relatively hot and cold spots on the body surface are revealed. The technique has been used to study blood flow to limbs, and to detect cancer of the breast.

thermohyperalgesia (thĕr″mō-hī″pĕr-ăl-jē′zē-ă) [″ + *hyper,* above, + *algesis,* pain]. Unbearable pain upon the application of heat.

thermohyperesthesia (thĕr″mō-hī″pĕr-ĕs-thē′zē-ă) [″ + *hyper,* above, + *aisthesis,* sensation]. Exceptional sensitiveness to heat.

thermohypesthesia (thĕr″mō-hī″pĕs-thē′zē-ă) [″ + *hypo,* under, + *aisthesis,* sensation]. Diminished perception of heat.

thermohypoesthesia (thĕr″mō-hī″pō-ĕs-thē′zē-ă) [″ + ″ + *aisthesis,* sensation]. Thermohypesthesia, q.v.

thermoinhibitory (thĕr″mō-ĭn-hĭb′ĭ-tor″ē) [″ + L. *inhibere,* to restrain]. Arresting or impeding the generation of body heat.

thermolabile (thĕr″mō-lā′bĭl) [″ + *labilis,* unstable]. Destroyed or changed easily by heat; unstable. SEE: *heat; heat, latent.*

thermolamp (thĕr′mō-lămp) [″ + *lampe,* torch]. Lamp used for providing heat.

thermology (thĕr-mŏl′ō-jē) [″ + *logos,* study]. The science of heat.

thermolysis (thĕr-mŏl′ĭ-sĭs) [″ + *lysis,* dissolution]. 1. Loss of heat from the body, as by evaporation. 2. Chemical decomposition by heat.

thermolytic (thĕr″mō-lĭt′ĭk) [″ + *lytikos,* dissolving]. Promoting thermolysis.

thermomassage (thĕr″mō-mă-săzh′). Massage by use of heat.

thermometer (thĕr-mŏm′ĕ-tĕr) [″ + *metron,* measure]. An instrument for indicating the degree of heat or cold. First mention of a thermometer in diagnosis of disease was given by It. physician, Sanctorius, in 1626. The instrument used today is little different from the one he used.

t., alcohol. Thermometer containing alcohol.

t., Celsius. Thermometric scale generally used in scientific notation. Temperature of boiling water at sea level 100° C. and freezing point 0° C., with 100° between. SEE: tables

t., centigrade. T., Celsius.

Comparative Thermometric Scale

	Celsius*	Fahrenheit
Boiling point of water	100°	212°
	90	194
	80	176
	70	158
	60	140
	50	122
	40	104
Body temperature	37°	98.6°
	30	86
	20	68
	10	50
Freezing point of water	0°	32°
	−10	14
	−20	−4

CONVERSION: *Fahrenheit to Celsius:* Subtract 32 and multiply by 5/9. *Celsius to Fahrenheit:* Multiply by 9/5 and add 32.

*Also called Centigrade.

Thermometric Equivalents (Celsius and Fahrenheit)

C°	F°	C°	F°	C°	F°	C°	F°
0	32	27	80.6	54	129.2	81	177.8
1	33.8	28	82.4	55	131	82	179.6
2	35.6	29	84.2	56	132.8	83	181.4
3	37.4	30	86.0	57	134.6	84	183.2
4	39.2	31	87.8	58	136.4	85	185
5	41	32	89.6	59	138.2	86	186.8
6	42.8	33	91.4	60	140	87	188.6
7	44.6	34	93.2	61	141.8	88	190.4
8	46.4	35	95	62	143.6	89	192.2
9	48.2	36	96.8	63	145.4	90	194
10	50	37	98.6	64	147.2	91	195.8
11	51.8	38	100.4	65	149	92	197.6
12	53.6	39	102.2	66	150.8	93	199.4
13	55.4	40	104	67	152.6	94	201.2
14	57.2	41	105.8	68	154.4	95	203
15	59	42	107.6	69	156.2	96	204.8
16	60.8	43	109.4	70	158	97	206.6
17	62.6	44	111.2	71	159.8	98	208.4
18	64.4	45	113	72	161.6	99	210.2
19	66.2	46	114.8	73	163.4	100	212
20	68	47	116.6	74	165.2		
21	69.8	48	118.4	75	167		
22	71.6	49	120.2	76	168.8		
23	73.4	50	122	77	170.6		
24	75.2	51	123.8	78	172.4		
25	77	52	125.6	79	174.2		
26	78.8	53	127.4	80	176		

t., clinical. Thermometer for measuring temperature of the body; one in which the mercury remains stationary at the registration point until shaken down. SEE: *clinical thermometer.*

t., differential. Thermometer recording slight variations of temperature.

t., Fahrenheit. Thermometric scale used in English-speaking countries. Boiling point 212° F., freezing point 32° F. SEE: tables.

t., gas. Thermometer filled with gas, such as air, helium, or oxygen. SEE: *t., air.*

t., Kelvin. Thermometric scale in which absolute zero is zero degrees Kelvin; the freezing point of water is 273.15°; the boiling point of water is 373.15°. Thus one degree on the Kelvin scale is exactly equivalent to one degree on the Celsius scale.

t., mercury. Thermometer containing mercury for measurement of temperature.

t., recording. A device with a suitable sensor that continuously monitors and records temperature.

t., rectal. Thermometer that is inserted into the rectum for determining body temperature.

t., self-registering. Thermometer recording variations of temperature.

t., spirit. Thermometer filled with alcohol instead of mercury for registering low temperatures.

t., surface. Thermometer for indicating temperature of the body's surface.

t., wet-and-dry-bulb. A device for determining relative humidity consisting of two thermometers, the bulb of one being kept saturated with water vapor. The difference in temperatures between the two is dependent upon relative humidity.

thermometer, disinfection of. Disinfection of a thermometer with a substance that is able to kill ordinary bacteria and Mycobacterium tuberculosis as well as viruses. A variety of chemical solutions are used but the effectiveness of these agents can be greatly diminished if the thermometer is not washed thoroughly prior to being disinfected.

thermometric (thĕr″mō-mĕt′rĭk) [Gr. *therme,* heat, + *metron,* measure]. Pert. to heat measurement or a thermometer.

thermometry (thĕr-mŏm′ĕ-trē). Measurement of temperature.

t., clinical. Oral temperature of the healthy body ranges between 96.6° and 100° F. (35.9° and 37.8° C.). During a 24-hour period, a person's body temperature may vary from 0.5° to 2.0° F. (0.28° to 1.1° C.). It is highest in late afternoon and lowest during sleep in early hours of the morning. Slightly increased by eating, exercising, and external heat; reduced about 1.5° F. (0.8° C.) during sleep. In disease the temperature of the body deviates several degrees above and below the average of health.

In facial erysipelas, acute meningitis, pneumonia, scarlatina, typhus, smallpox, and intermittent fever, body temperature sometimes rises as high as 106° to 107° F. (41.1° to 41.7° C.). In other febrile diseases, it rarely reaches 104° F. (40° C.). However, temperature may reach as high as 110° F. (43.3° C.) in sunstroke, with patient recovering. The lowest extreme of temperature is found sometimes in the cold stage of cholera when temperature may be very low (90° to 85° F. or 32.2° to 29.4° C.) for several days.

Subnormal temperatures, below 98° F. (36.7° C.) are observed in the following conditions: during convalescence from certain febrile conditions, after pneumonia and typhoid fever; in collapse resulting from shock, hemorrhage, or rupture of a viscus, as the bowel in typhoid or the stomach in perforating ulcer.

In general, for every degree of fever the pulse rises 10 beats per minute, but elevation of temperature to 99.5° F. (37.5° C.) provides greater evidence of disease than a pulse rate increase from 70 to 90 beats per minute. If temperature remains above normal after general symptoms denote convalescence, the patient is in danger of a relapse or the supervention of some other disease. The range of the increase of heat in different febrile diseases extends to 110° F. (43.3° C.) or more and as a rule the amount of increase is a criterion of the intensity of the disease.

Artificial fever induced through diathermy, continuous hot bath, or malarial injections was formerly utilized in treating some diseases but is seldom used in modern medicine.

thermoneurosis (thĕr″mō-nū-rō′sĭs) [Gr. *therme,* heat, + *neuron,* nerve, + *osis,* condition]. Elevation of body temperature in hysteria and other nervous conditions.

thermonuclear (thĕr″mō-nū′klē-ăr). Concerning thermonuclear reactions.

thermopenetration (thĕr″mō-pĕn-ĕ-trā′shŭn) [″ + L. *penetrare,* to penetrate]. Application of heat to the deeper tissues of the body by diathermy. SYN: *thermoradiotherapy.*

thermoperiodicity (thĕr″mō-pĕr-ē-ō-dĭs′ĭ-tē). Condition in which an organism grows better when exposed to alternating high and low temperatures.

thermophagy (thĕr-mŏf′ă-jē) [″ + *phagein,* to eat]. Eating of extremely hot food.

thermophilic (thĕr″mō-fĭl′ĭk) [″ + *philein,* to love]. Preferring or thriving best at high temperatures, said of bacteria that thrive best at temperatures between 40° and 70° C. (104° and 158° F.).

thermophils (thĕr′mō-fĭlz). Organisms that grow best at elevated temperatures, i.e., 40° to 70° C.

thermophobia (thĕr″mō-fō′bē-ă) [″ + *phobos,* fear]. Abnormal dread of heat.

thermophore (thĕr′mō-for) [″ + *phoros,* a bearer]. Apparatus for applying heat to a part, consisting of water heater and tubes conveying water to a coil and returning to heater, or salts that produce heat when moistened.

thermophylic (thĕr″mō-fĭ′lĭk) [″ + *phylake,* guard]. Resistant to destruction by heat, characteristic of certain bacteria.

thermopile (thĕr′mō-pīl) [″ + L. *pila,* pile]. In physical therapy, a thermoelectric battery used in measuring small variations in the degree of heat. It consists of a number of connected dissimilar metallic plates. Under the influence of heat, these produce an electric current.

thermoplacentography (thĕr″mō-plăs″ĕn-tŏg′ră-fē) [″ + L. *placenta,* placenta, + Gr. *graphein,* to write]. Use of thermography for determining the location of placental attachment.

thermoplastic (thĕr″mō-plăs′tĭk). Concerning or being softened or made malleable by heat.

thermoplegia (thĕr″mō-plē′jē-ă) [″ + *plege,* a stroke]. Heatstroke.

thermopolypnea (thĕr″mō-pŏl-ĭp-nē′ă) [″ + *polys,* many, + *pnoia,* breath]. Quickened breathing caused by high fever or great heat.

thermoradiotherapy (thĕr″mō-rā″dē-ō-thĕr′ă-pē) [″ + L. *radius,* ray, + Gr. *therapeia,* treatment]. Application of heat to deep tissues by diathermy. SYN: *thermopenetration.*

thermoreceptor (thĕr″mō-rē-sĕp′tor) [″ + L. *receptor,* receiver]. A sensory receptor that is stimulated by a rise of body temperature.

thermoregulation (thĕr″mō-rĕg″ū-lā′shŭn). Heat regulation.

thermoregulatory (thĕr″mō-rĕg′ū-lă-tor″ē). Pert. to the regulation of temperature, esp. body temperature.

thermoregulatory centers. Centers in the hypothalamus that regulate heat production and heat loss, esp. the latter, so that a normal body temperature is maintained. They are influenced by nervous impulses from cutaneous receptors and by the temperature of the blood flowing through them.

thermoresistant (thĕr″mō-rē-zĭs′tănt) [″ + L. *resistentia,* resistance]. Ability to survive in relatively high temperature. Characteristic of some types of bacteria.

thermostabile (thĕr″mō-stā′bl) [″ + L. *stabilis,* stationary]. Not changed or destroyed by heat.

thermostasis (thĕr″mō-stā′sĭs) [″ + *stasis,*

standing]. The maintenance of body temperature.

thermostat (thĕr′mō-stăt) [″ + *statos,* standing]. An automatic device for regulating the temperature.

thermosteresis (thĕr″mō-stĕ-rē′sĭs) [″ + *steresis,* deprivation]. The deprivation or loss of heat.

thermosterilization. Bacterial sterilization by use of heat.

thermosystaltic (thĕr″mō-sĭs-tăl′tĭk) [Gr. *therme,* heat, + *systellein,* to contract]. Pert. to contraction of the muscles under stimulus of heat.

thermotactic, thermotaxic (thĕr″mō-tăk′tĭk, -tăks′ĭk) [″ + *taktikos,* regulating]. Rel. to regulation of the body temperature.

thermotaxis (thĕr″mō-tăks′ĭs) [″ + *taxis,* arrangement]. 1. Regulation of bodily temperature. 2. Reaction of organisms or of protoplasm in the living body to heat. 3. The movement of certain organisms or cells toward (positive thermotaxis) or away from (negative thermotaxis) heat. SYN: *thermotropism.*

thermotherapeutics (thĕr″mō-thĕr-ă-pū′tĭks) [″ + *therapeutike,* treatment]. Use of heat in treatment of disease. SYN: *thermotherapy.*

thermotherapy (thĕr″mō-thĕr′ă-pē) [″ + *therapeia,* treatment]. The therapeutic application of heat. Heat may be applied locally by radiant heating devices that give off infrared rays and by conductive heating that utilizes hot water bottles, paraffin baths, and hot packs. The temperature of the body may be increased by artificial fever, by raising environmental temperature, or by preventing heat loss from the body. SEE: *heat; hyperthermia.*

thermotics (thĕr-mŏt′ĭks). The science of heat.

thermotolerant (thĕr″mō-tŏl′ĕr-ănt) [″ + L. *tolerare,* to tolerate]. Able to live normally in high temperature.

thermotonometer (thĕr″mō-tō-nŏm′ĕ-tĕr) [″ + *tonos,* tension, + *metron,* measure]. Device for measuring muscle contraction caused by heat stimuli.

thermotoxin (thĕr″mō-tŏks′ĭn) [″ + *toxikon,* poison]. A poison formed in the tissues as a result of excessive heat.

thermotropism (thĕr-mŏt′rō-pĭzm) [″ + *trope,* turning, + *-ismos,* condition]. Thermotaxis.

theroid (thē′royd) [Gr. *theriodes,* beast-like]. Having animal instincts and characteristics.

thesaurismosis (thē-să″rĭs-mō′sĭs) [Gr. *thesauros,* treasure, + *-osis,* condition]. Abnormal or excessive storage of substances in certain cells. Usually due to a metabolic disease such as lipoidosis.

thesaurosis (thē″saw-rō′sĭs) [Gr. *thesauros,* treasure, + *osis,* condition]. Accumulation of foreign or normal substances in the body.

thiabendazole (thī″ă-bĕn′dă-zŏl). USP. An antihelmintic drug used in treating cutaneous larva migrans and strongyloidiasis. Trade name is Mintezol.

thiaminase (thī-ăm′ĭ-nās). An enzyme that hydrolyses thiamine.

thiamine hydrochloride. $C_{12}H_{17}ClN_4OSHCl$. A white crystalline compound occurring naturally and produced synthetically. It is widely distributed in various animal and plant foods, dry yeast and wheat germ being the richest natural resources. It is present in the outer layers of seeds and in nuts, legumes, most vegetables, and in some meats (pork, muscle, liver, heart, and kidneys). SYN: *vitamin* B_1.

FUNCT: It is essential for the normal metabolism of carbohydrates and fats. It acts as a coenzyme of carboxylases in the carboxylation of pyruvic acid, hence is essential for the liberation of energy and disposal of pyruvic acid.

DEFICIENCY SYM: Moderate deficiency results in impaired functioning of nervous, circulatory, digestive, and endocrine systems. Neurasthenia, neurological disorders, and cardiac and gastrointestinal symptoms may result. Loss of appetite, fatigue, muscle tenderness, and increased irritability are symptoms. Severe and prolonged deficiency results in beriberi, q.v.

DAILY REQUIREMENTS: For children and adults 0.5 mg. per 1000 Cal. of food intake.

thiamine mononitrate. USP. Thiamine in which the chloride has been replaced by nitrate.

thiamine pyrophosphate. An enzyme important in carbohydrate metabolism. It is the active form of thiamine. SYN: *cocarboxylase.*

thiamylal sodium for injection (thī-ăm′ĭ-lăl). USP. An ultra-short-acting barbiturate. Trade name is Surital.

thiemia (thī-ē′mē-ă) [Gr. *theion,* sulfur, + *haima,* blood]. An excess of sulfur in the blood.

Thiersch's graft (tērsh′ĕz). [Karl Thiersch, Ger. surgeon, 1822–1895] A method of skin grafting using epidermis and a portion of the dermis.

thiethylperazine malate (thī-ĕth″ĭl-pĕr′ă-zēn). USP. An antiemetic drug. Trade name is Torecan.

thigh (thī) [AS. *theoh*]. The proximal portion of the lower extremity; the portion lying between the hip joint and the knee. SEE: *femur; hip; pectineus; sartorius.*

thigmesthesia (thĭg″mĕs-thē′zē-ă) [Gr. *thigma,* touch, + *aisthesis,* sensation]. Sensitivity to touch.

thigmotaxis (thĭg″mō-tăks′ĭs) [″ + *taxis,* arrangement]. The negative or positive response of certain motile cells to touch.

thigmotropism (thĭg-mŏt′rō-pĭzm) [″ + *tropos,* a turning, + *-ismos,* condition]. The response of certain motile cells to move toward something that touches them.

thimerosal (thī-mĕr′ō-săl). USP. An organic mercurial antiseptic used topically and as a preservative in pharmaceutical preparations. Trade name is Merthiolate.

thinking. The process of mentation and reasoning that occurs in the human mind.

thin-layer chromatography. ABBR: TLC. Chromatography involving the adsorption and partitioning of compounds on a thin porous solid applied as a thin layer on a glass plate.

thio- [Gr. *theion,* sulfur]. Prefix denoting the presence of sulfur replacing oxygen.

thiocyanate (thī″ō-sī′ă-nāt). Any compound containing the radical —SCN.

thiogenic (thī″ō-jĕn′ĭk) [Gr. *theion,* sulfur, + *gennan,* to produce]. Able to convert hydrogen sulfide into higher sulfur compounds, said of bacteria in the water of some mineral springs.

thioglucosidase (thī″ō-glū-kō′sĭ-dās). An enzyme that catalyzes the hydrolysis of thioglycoside to a thiol and a sugar.

thioguanine (thī″ō-gwă′nēn). USP. An antimetabolite used in treating certain types of leukemia. It also acts as an immunosuppressant.

Thiomerin. Trade name for mercaptomerin sodium, USP.

thioneine (thī′ō-nēn) [″ + *neos,* new]. Thiolhistidine-betaine, compound containing crystalline sulfur, found in ergot and red blood cells. Also: *ergthioneine.*

thionic (thī′ō-nĭk). Concerning sulfur.

thiopectic, thiopexic (thī-ō-pĕk′tĭk, -pĕks′ĭk) [″ + *pexis,* fixation]. Pert. to the fixation of sulfur.

thiopental sodium (thī″ō-pĕn′tăl). USP. An ultra-short-acting barbiturate used as an adjuvant in surgical anesthesia. Trade name is Pentothal Sodium.

thiopexy (thī″ō-pĕks′ē). The fixation of sulfur.

thiophil, thiophilic (thī′ō-fĭl, thī″ō-fĭl′ĭk) [Gr. *theion,* sulfur, + *philein,* to love]. Thriving in the presence of sulfur or its compounds, as some bacteria.

thioridazine hydrochloride (thī″ō-rĭd′ă-zēn). USP. An antipsychotic drug. Trade name is Mellaril Hydrochloride.

thiosulfate (thī″ō-sŭl′fāt). Any salt of thiosulfuric acid.

Thiosulfil. Trade name for sulfamethizole.

Thiotepa. Trade name for thiotepa, USP.

thiotepa (thī″ō-tē′pă). USP. An alkylating agent that is cytotoxic. It is used in treating certain types of neoplasms. Trade name is Thiotepa. CAUTION: Great care should be taken to prevent inhaling particles of thiotepa or exposing the skin to it.

thiothixene (thī″ō-thĭks′ēn). USP. An antipsychotic drug. Trade name is Navane Hydrochloride.

thiouracil (thī″ō-ū′ră-sĭl). An antithyroid drug that is little used now. SEE: *propylthiouracil.*

thiourea (thī″ō-ūr-ē′ă) [Gr. *theion,* sulfur, + *ouron,* urine]. Colorless crystalline compound of urea in which sulfur replaces the oxygen. SYN: *sulfourea.*

thiram (thī′răm). An antifungal agent.

thiram poisoning. Toxic exposure may occur in those engaged either in manufacturing or applying this compound in agricultural work. SEE: *Poisons and Poisoning* in *Appendix.*

third cranial nerve. Oculomotor nerve. SEE: *cranial nerves.*

third intention. Healing of a wound by filling with granulations. SEE: *healing.*

third ventricle. Third ventricle of the brain, a narrow cavity between the two optic thalami. It communicates anteriorly with the lateral ventricles and posteriorly, via the cerebral aqueduct of Sylvius, with the 4th ventricle. SYN: *ventriculus tertius.*

thirst [AS. *thurst*]. 1. Desire for fluid, esp. for water. This may occur in fevers and certain other maladies, or it may be entirely lacking in some conditions. The nurse should note whether the intake of fluids allays the patient's thirst. 2. The sensation resulting from the lack of or the need of water. Thirst may result from drying of mucous membranes, esp. those of the pharynx, or from reduced salivary secretion. It also results from general dehydration as may occur following hemorrhage, profuse sweating, vomiting, or excessive loss of urine as in diabetes mellitus or insipidus. SEE: *adipsia; anadipsia; aposia.*

Thiry's fistula (tē′rēz). [Ludwig Thiry, Austrian physiologist, 1817–1897] An artificial fistula placed in a dog's intestines for obtaining intestinal juices for experimental purposes.

Thiuretic. Trade name for hydrochlorothiazide, USP.

thixolabile (thĭk″sō-lā′bĭl). Especially susceptible to being changed by shaking.

thixotropy (thĭks-ŏt′rō-pē) [Gr. *thixis,* a touching, + *trope,* turning]. The property of certain gels in which they liquefy when agitated and revert to a gel upon standing.

thlipsencephalus (thlĭp″sĕn-sĕf′ă-lŭs) [Gr. *thlipsis,* pressure, + *enkephalos,* brain]. A deformed fetus with a malformed or absent skull.

Thomas splint. [Hugh O. Thomas, Brit. orthopedic surgeon, 1834–1891] A splint originally developed to treat hip-joint disease. It is now used mainly to place traction on the leg in its long axis. It is used in treating fractures of the upper leg. It consists of a proximal ring that fits around the upper leg and to which two long rigid slender steel rods are attached. These extend down to another smaller ring distal to the foot.

Thomsen's disease (tŏm'sĕnz). [Asmus Julius Thomsen, Danish physician, 1815–1896] Myotonia congenita, q.v.

thoracalgia (thō"răk-ăl'jē-ă) [Gr. *thorakos,* chest, + *algos,* pain]. Pain in the chest wall. SYN: *pleurodynia.*

thoracectomy (thō"ră-sĕk'tō-mē) [" + *ektome,* excision]. Incision of the chest wall with resection of a portion of rib.

thoracentesis (thō"ră-sĕn-tē'sĭs) [" + *kentesis,* a puncture]. Surgical puncture of the chest wall for removal of fluids. Usually done by using a large-bore needle. SYN: *pleurocentesis; thoracocentesis.*

NURSING IMPLICATIONS: Before thoracentesis, determine whether a chest x-ray was done, and make sure a consent form was signed. Explain the procedure to the patient. Identify allergies to topical anesthetics, and administer prescribed sedatives. Position the patient appropriately and comfortably. Assist the physician and reassure the patient during the procedure. Check the patient every 10 to 15 minutes for dizziness, faintness, rapid pulse rate, shortness of breath, chest pain, cough, shock, chills, nausea, pallor, cyanosis, weakness, diaphoresis, and blood-tinged sputum. Ensure that a chest x-ray is performed after the procedure to rule out pneumothorax. Document the procedure and the patient's response.

thoracic (thō-răs'ĭk) [Gr. *thorax,* chest]. Pert. to the chest or thorax.

thoracic cage. The bony structure surrounding the thorax.

thoracic cavity. The space lying above the diaphragm and enclosed within the walls of the thorax; the space occupied by the thoracic viscera. It includes the pleural cavities occupied by the lungs and the mediastinum, the space between the lungs occupied by the heart lying within the pericardium, the thoracic aorta, pulmonary artery and veins, vena cava, thymus gland, lymph nodes, trachea, bronchi, esophagus, and thoracic duct. It is separated from the abdominal cavity by the diaphragm. SEE: *lymphatic drainage* for illus.

RS: chyle; cisterna chyli; lacteal; lymphatic; lymphatic system.

thoracic duct. The main lymph duct of the body having its origin at the cisterna chyli on the abdomen. It passes upward through the diaphragm into the thorax, continuing upward alongside the aorta and esophagus to the neck where it turns to the left and enters the left subclavian vein near its junction with the left internal jugular vein. It receives lymph from all parts of the body except the right side of the head, neck, and thorax and right upper extremity.

thoracic limbs. Upper extremities.

thoracicoabdominal (thō-răs"ĭ-kō-ăb-dŏm'ĭ-năl). Concerning the thorax and abdomen.

thoracicohumeral (thō-răs"ĭ-kō-hū'mĕr-ăl). Concerning the thorax and humerus bone.

thoracic outlet compression syndrome. A symptom complex characterized by brachial neuritis with or without vascular or vasomotor disturbance in the upper extremities. SYN: *scalenus syndrome.*

thoracic squeeze. A rare occurrence in divers who are skilled enough to go approx. 80 to 100 ft. (24.4 to 30.5 meters) deep while holding their breath. The lungs become compressed sufficiently to cause rupture of alveolar capillaries.

TREATMENT: Immediate removal from the water; artificial respiration preferably with an apparatus that will deliver increased oxygen concentration rather than just air.

thoracic surgery. Surgery involving the rib cage and structures contained within the thoracic cage.

thoraco- [Gr. *thorakos,* chest]. Combining form meaning chest or chest wall.

thoracoacromial (thō"ră-kō-ă-krō'mē-ăl). Concerning the thorax and the acromion.

thoracobronchotomy (thō"răk-ō-brŏn-kŏt'ō-mē) [" + *bronchos,* windpipe, + *tome,* incision]. Incision through the thoracic wall into the bronchus.

thoracocautery (thō"răk-ō-kaw'tĕr-ē) [" + *kauterion,* branding iron]. The use of cautery in breaking up pulmonary adhesions to collapse the lung.

thoracoceloschisis (thō"răk-ō-sē-lŏs'kĭ-sĭs) [Gr. *thorakos,* chest, + *koilia,* belly, + *schisis,* a fissure]. Congenital fissure of the thoracic and abdominal cavities.

thoracocentesis (thō"răk-ō-sĕn-tē'sĭs) [" + *kentesis,* a puncture]. Surgical entry into the thoracic cavity in order to remove fluid. Usually done by using a needle. SYN: *thoracentesis.*

thoracocyllosis (thō"răk-ō-sĭl-ō'sĭs) [" + *kyllosis,* crippling]. Deformity of the chest.

thoracocyrtosis (thō"răk-ō-sĭr-tō'sĭs) [" + *kyrtosis,* curvature]. Excessive curvature of the chest.

thoracodelphus (thō"ră-kō-dĕl'fŭs) [" + *adelphos,* brother]. A deformed fetus with a single head and thorax, but four legs.

thoracodidymus (thō"ră-kō-dĭd'ĭ-mŭs) [" + *didymos,* twin]. Conjoined twins united at the thorax.

thoracodynia (thō"răk-ō-dĭn'ē-ă) [" + *odyne,* pain]. Pain in the thorax.

thoracogastroschisis (thō"răk-ō-găs-trŏs'kĭ-sĭs) [" + *gaster,* belly, + *schisis,* a fissure].

Congenital fissure of abdomen and thorax.

thoracograph (thō-răk'ō-grăf) [" + *graphein,* to write]. A device for plotting and recording the contour of the thorax and its change during inspiration and expiration.

thoracolaparotomy (thō"ră-kō-lăp"ă-rŏt'ō-mē) [" + *lapara,* loin, + *tome,* incision]. Surgical incision of the thoracic wall and the diaphragm in order to gain access to adjacent areas.

thoracolumbar (thō"răk-ō-lŭm'bar) [" + L. *lumbus,* loin]. Pert. to the thoracic and lumbar parts of the spine; noting their ganglia and the fibers of the sympathetic nervous system.

thoracolysis (thō"răk-ŏl'ĭ-sĭs) [" + *lysis,* dissolution]. The freeing of a lung that is attached to the chest wall. SYN: *pneumonolysis.*

thoracomelus (thō"ră-kŏm'ē-lŭs) [" + *melos,* limb]. A deformed fetus with an extra leg attached to the thorax.

thoracometer (thō"ră-kŏm'ĕ-tĕr) [Gr. *thorakos,* chest, + *metron,* measure]. A device for measuring the expansion of the chest.

thoracometry (thō"ră-kŏm'ĕt-rē) [" + *metron,* measure]. The measurement of the thorax.

thoracomyodynia (thō"ră-kō-mī"ō-dĭn'ē-ă) [" + *mys,* muscle, + *odyne,* pain]. Pain in chest muscles.

thoracopagus (thō"ră-kŏp'ă-gŭs) [" + *pagos,* fixed]. Two malformed fetuses joined at the thorax.

thoracoparacephalus (thō"ră-kō-păr"ă-sĕf'ă-lŭs) [" + *para,* beside, + *kephale,* head]. Thoracopagus twins in which a rudimentary head is attached to the smaller twin.

thoracopathy (thō"răk-ŏp'ă-thē) [" + *pathos,* disease]. Any disease of the thorax, thoracic organs, or tissues.

thoracoplasty (thō'ră-kō-plăs"tē, thō-ră'kō-plăs"tē) [" + *plassein,* to form]. A plastic operation upon the thorax; removal of portions of the ribs in stages to collapse diseased areas of the lung. SEE: *empyema.*

thoracopneumoplasty (thō"ră-kō-nū'mō-plăs-tē) [" + *pneumon,* lung, + *plassein,* to form]. Plastic surgery involving the chest and lung.

thoracoschisis (thō"ră-kŏs'kĭ-sĭs) [" + *schisis,* fissure]. Congenital fissure of the chest wall.

thoracoscope (thō-ră'kō-skōp, -răk'ō-skōp) [" + *skopein,* to examine]. 1. Instrument for inspection of the thoracic cavity. It has an electric light and is inserted through an intercostal space. 2. An instrument used in auscultation to convey the sounds of the chest to the ear. SYN: *stethoscope.*

thoracoscopy (thō"ră-kŏs'kō-pē). Diagnostic examination of the pleural cavity with an endoscope.

thoracostenosis (thō"ră-kō-stĕn-ō'sĭs) [" + *stenosis,* a contraction]. Narrowness of the thorax due to atrophy of trunk muscles. SYN: *wasp waist.*

thoracostomy (thō"răk-ŏs'tō-mē) [" + *stoma,* mouth]. Resection of chest wall to allow room for enlarged heart or for drainage.

thoracotomy (thō"răk-ŏt'ō-mē) [" + *tome,* incision]. Surgical incision of the chest wall.

thorax (thō'răks) [Gr.]. (pl. *thoraces, thoraxes*) [NA] That part of the body between the base of the neck superiorly and the diaphragm inferiorly.

The surface of the thorax is divided into regions as follows: *Anterior surface:* supraclavicular, above the clavicles; suprasternal, above the sternum; clavicular, over the clavicles; sternal, over the sternum; mammary, the space between the 3rd and 6th ribs on either side; inframammary, below the mamma and above the lower border of the 12th rib on either side. *Posterior surface:* scapular, over the scapulae; interscapular, between the scapulae; infrascapular, below the scapulae. *On sides:* axillary, above the 6th rib. SYN: *chest.* SEE: illus.

RS: acromiothoracic; cholohemothorax; "thorac-" words.

t., barrel-shaped. A malformed chest rounded like a barrel seen in advanced pulmonary emphysema.

t. paralyticus. The long, flat chest of patients with constitutional visceroptosis.

t., Peyrot's. A chest that has an obliquely oval deformed shape, seen with large pleural effusions.

Thorazine. Trade name for chlorpromazine hydrochloride. It is a central nervous system depressant, and it is employed as a sedative and antiemetic. It potentiates the effects of sedatives and general anesthetics and is of value in quieting severely excited psychiatric patients.

Thorel's bundle (tō'rĕlz). [Christen Thorel, Ger. physician, 1880–1935] A muscle bundle in the heart that connects the sinoatrial and atrioventricular nodes, and passes medial to the orifice of the inferior vena cava.

thorium (thō'rē-ŭm). SYMB: Th. At. wt. 232.038; at. no. 90. A metallic element that is radioactive. At one time it was used to outline blood vessels in roentgenography.

Thorn test. [George W. Thorn, U.S. physician, b. 1906] Administration of corticotrophin, which causes a decrease in circulating eosinophils of a normal person, but does not cause a decrease if given to patients with adrenal insufficiency.

thoron (thō'rŏn). SYMB: Tn. At. wt. 220; at. no. 86. A radioactive isotope of radon. It has a half-life of 51.5 seconds.

thread (thrĕd). 1. Any thin filamentous structure, e.g., a stringy substance present in the

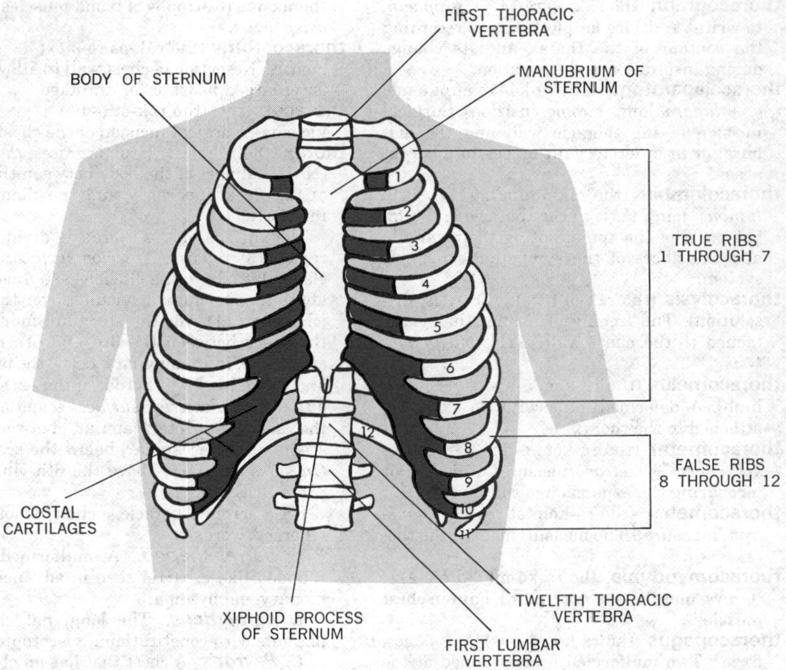

THORAX

urine in some infectious diseases of the urinary tract. 2. Suture material.

threadworm. Common name applied to the pinworm, Enterobius vermicularis.

three-day fever. A viral disease transmitted by the sandfly, Phlebotomus papatasii. The disease resembles dengue but is less severe. SYN: *sandfly fever.*

thremmatology (thrĕm″ă-tŏl′ō-jē) [Gr. *thremma,* nursling, + *logos,* science]. Scientific breeding of plants and animals.

threonine (thrē′ō-nĭn). Alpha-amino-beta-hydroxy butyric acid. One of the essential amino acids.

threshold (thrĕsh′ōld) [AS. *therscold*]. 1. Point at which a psychological or physiological effect begins to be produced. 2. A measure of the sensitivity of an organ or function that is obtained by finding the lowest value of the appropriate stimulus that will give the response.

t., absolute. The lowest amount or intensity of a stimulus that will give rise to a sensation or a response.

t., auditory. Minimum audible sound perceived.

t., differential. The lowest limit at which two stimuli can be differentiated from each other.

t., erythema. Stage in which erythema of the skin due to radiation just begins.

t., ketosis. The lower limit at which ketone bodies (acetoacetic acid, hydroxybutyric acid, and acetone), upon their accumulation in the blood, are excreted by the kidney. At that point ketone bodies are being produced faster by the liver than the body can oxidize them.

t. of consciousness. In psychoanalysis, point at which a stimulus is just barely perceived.

t., renal. The concentration at which a substance in the blood normally not excreted by the kidney begins to appear in the urine. The renal threshold for glucose is 160–180 mg./dl.

t., sensory. The minimal stimulus for any sensory receptor that will give rise to a sensation.

t. stimulus. The least or minimal stimulus that will give rise to a sensation or bring about a response such as a muscle contraction. SYN: *liminal stimulus*. SEE: *rheobase*.

threshold dose. Minimum dose that will produce an effect on the patient.

threshold substance. A substance present in the blood that, on being filtered through glomeruli of the kidney, is reabsorbed by the tubules up to a certain limit, that being the upper limit of the concentration of the substance in normal plasma. High-threshold substances are those that are entirely or almost entirely reabsorbed. Ex.: chlorides; glucose. Low-threshold substances are those that are reabsorbed in limited quantities. Ex.: phosphates; urea. No-threshold substances are those excreted in their entirety. Ex.: creatinine sulfate.

thrill (thrĭl) [ME. *thrillen,* to pierce]. 1. Abnormal tremor accompanying a vascular or cardiac murmur felt on palpation. SYN: *fremitus*. 2. A tingling or shivering sensation of tremulous excitement as from pain, pleasure, or horror.

t., aneurysmal. Thrill felt on palpation of an aneurysm.

t., aortic. Thrill heard over aortic aperture on lesions of valves.

t., arterial. Thrill heard over an artery.

t., diastolic. Thrill felt over the heart during diastole of the ventricle.

t., hydatid. Peculiar tremor felt on palpation of a hydatid cyst.

t., presystolic. Thrill sometimes felt over apex of the heart preceding ventricular contraction.

t., systolic. A thrill felt during systole over the precordium. It may be associated with aortic or pulmonary stenosis, or interventricular septal defect.

thrix. Hair.

t. annulata. A hair with light and dark segments alternating along the shaft.

-thrix [Gr. *thrix,* hair]. A word ending indicating hair.

throat (thrōt) [AS. *throte*]. 1. The pharynx and the fauces. 2. Cavity from the arch of the palate to the glottis and superior opening of the esophagus. 3. The anterior portion of the neck. 4. Any narrow orifice.

throat, foreign bodies in. Symptoms depend somewhat on the location and size of the foreign body, and vary from simple discomfort to distressing coughing, difficulty in breathing, retching, and cyanosis. If not relieved, suffocation results in unconsciousness.

If the symptoms are relieved but it is not known that the foreign body has been removed, then it is important to seek medical attention in case the object has moved farther down the respiratory tract.

F.A.: The Heimlich maneuver should be performed. This consists of (1) wrapping your arms around victim's waist from behind; (2) making a fist with one hand and placing it against the victim's abdomen between the navel and rib cage; (3) clasping your fist with your free hand pressing in with a quick forceful upward thrust. Repeat several times if necessary. SEE: *Heimlich maneuver* for illus.

throb (thrŏb) [ME. *throbben,* of imitative origin]. 1. A beat or pulsation, as of the heart. 2. To pulsate.

throbbing (thrŏb'ĭng). Pulsation; a beating rhythmic movement.

Throckmorton's reflex (thrŏk'mor"tŭnz). [Thomas Bentley Throckmorton, U.S. neurologist, b. 1885] Extension of great toe and flexion of others when dorsum of foot is percussed in metatarsophalangeal region.

throe (thrō) [AS. *thruwe,* paroxysm]. A severe spasm of pain.

thrombase (thrŏm'bās). Thrombin.

thrombasthenia (thrŏm"băs-thē'nē-ă) [Gr. *thrombos,* clot, + *astheneia,* weakness]. A hemorrhagic disorder due to abnormal platelet function characterized by abnormal clot retraction, prolonged bleeding time, and lack of aggregation of the platelets on a blood smear.

thrombectomy (thrŏm-bĕk'tō-mē) [" + *ektome,* excision]. Excision of a thrombus.

thrombi (thrŏm'bī). Pl. of thrombus.

thrombin (thrŏm'bĭn) [Gr. *thrombos,* clot]. 1. An enzyme formed in shed blood from prothrombin, which reacts with soluble fibrinogen converting it to fibrin, which forms the basis of a blood clot. SEE: *coagulation*. 2. USP. A sterile plasma protein substance prepared from prothrombin of bovine origin. Used topically to control capillary oozing during surgical procedures. Used alone it is not capable of controlling arterial bleeding.

thrombinogen (thrŏm-bĭn'ō-jĕn). An obsolete term for prothrombin.

thrombo- [Gr.]. Combining form meaning clot of blood; a thrombus.

thromboangiitis (thrŏm"bō-ăn"jē-ī'tĭs) [Gr. *thrombos,* clot, + *angeion,* vessel, + *itis,* inflammation]. Inflammation of inner coat of a blood vessel with clot formation. SEE: *thrombosis*.

t. obliterans. Chronic recurring inflammatory occlusive disease, chiefly of the peripheral arteries and veins. It has a high incidence in young Jewish males. SYN: *Buerger's disease*.

SYM: Occlusion; thrombosis; excruciating pain in leg or foot that is worse at night; cyanotic, clammy, cold extremity; diminished sense of heat and cold; gangrene of toes or foot may develop.

thromboarteritis (thrŏm″bō-ăr-tĕ-rī′tĭs) [″ + *arteria,* artery, + *itis,* inflammation]. Inflammation of an artery in connection with thrombosis.

thromboclasis (thrŏm-bŏk′lă-sĭs) [″ + *klasis,* a breaking]. The breaking up or lysis of a thrombus. SYN: *thrombolysis.*

thromboclastic (thrŏm″bō-klăs′tĭk). Pert. to or producing the dissolution of a thrombus. SYN: *thrombolytic.*

thrombocyst (thrŏm′bō-sĭst) [Gr. *thrombos,* clot, + *kystis,* a sac]. A membranous sac enveloping a thrombus. Also: *thrombocystis.*

thrombocyte (thrŏm′bō-sīt) [″ + *kytos,* cell]. An old term for a blood platelet.

thrombocythemia (thrŏm″bō-sī-thē′mē-ă) [″ + ″ + *haima,* blood]. An absolute increase in the number of platelets in the blood.

thrombocytocrit (thrŏm″bō-sī′tō-krĭt) [″ + ″ + *krinein,* to separate]. Device for estimating the platelet content of the blood.

thrombocytolysis (thrŏm″bō-sī-tŏl′ĭ-sĭs) [″ + ″ + *lysis,* dissolution]. Dissolution of thrombocytes.

thrombocytopathy (thrŏm″bō-sī-tŏp′ă-thē) [″ + ″ + *pathos,* suffering]. Deficient function of platelets.

thrombocytopenia (thrŏm″bō-sī″tō-pē′nē-ă) [″ + ″ + *penia,* lack]. Abnormal decrease in number of the blood platelets. SYN: *thrombopenia.*

NURSING IMPLICATIONS: Watch for signs of internal hemorrhage, esp. cerebral, and handle the patient gently to prevent hemorrhage. Observe carefully for signs of hemorrhage such as hematuria, bleeding gums, abdominal distention, melena, prolonged menstruation, epistaxis, and ecchymosis. Control bleeding by applying pressure to bleeding sites. Promote bedrest to prevent excessive activity and exhaustion. Advise the patient to avoid constipation and straining and to avoid exposure to upper respiratory infections, which may cause sneezing and coughing. Instruct the patient to prevent injury by using a soft toothbrush. If the patient shaves, an electric razor should be used. Monitor platelet count, and administer platelet transfusions and steroids as prescribed, and observe for side effects. If a splenectomy is performed, provide preoperative and postoperative nursing care.

thrombocytopoiesis (thrŏm″bō-sī″tō-poy-ē′sĭs) [″ + ″ + *poiesis,* production]. The formation of blood platelets.

thrombocytosis (thrŏm″bō-sī-tō′sĭs) [″ + *kytos,* cell]. Increase in number of blood platelets.

thromboembolism (thrŏm″bō-ĕm′bō-lĭzm) [″ + L. *embolismus,* obstruction]. An embolism; the blocking of a blood vessel by a thrombus that has become detached from its site of formation.

thromboendarterectomy (thrŏm″bō-ĕnd″ăr-tĕr-ĕk′tō-mē) [″ + *endon,* within, + *arteria,* artery, + *ektome,* excision]. Surgical removal of a thrombus from an artery; and removal of the diseased intima of the artery.

thromboendarteritis (thrŏm″bō-ĕnd-ăr″tĕr-ī′tĭs) [″ + ″ + ″ + *itis,* inflammation]. Thromboarteritis.

thromboendocarditis (thrŏm″bō-ĕn″dō-kăr-dī′tĭs) [″ + *endon,* within, + *kardia,* heart, + *itis,* inflammation]. Formation of a clot on inflamed surface of a heart valve.

thrombogenesis (thrŏm″bō-jĕn′ĕ-sĭs) [″ + *genesis,* production]. The formation of a blood clot.

thrombogenic (thrŏm″bō-jĕn′ĭk) [″ + *gennan,* to produce]. Producing or tending to produce a clot.

thromboid (thrŏm′boyd) [″ + *eidos,* form]. Resembling a thrombus or clot.

thrombokinase (thrŏm″bō-kĭn′ās) [″ + *kinesis,* motion]. Obsolete term for the tenth blood coagulation factor (Factor X) or Stuart factor, q.v.

thrombokinesis (thrŏm″bō-kĭ-nē′sĭs) [″ + *kinesis,* motion]. The coagulation of the blood.

thrombolymphangitis (thrŏm″bō-lĭm″făn-jī′tĭs) [″ + L. *lympha,* lymph, + Gr. *angeion,* vessel, + *itis,* inflammation]. Inflammation of a lymphatic vessel due to obstruction by thrombus formation.

thrombolysis (thrŏm-bŏl′ĭ-sĭs) [″ + *lysis,* destruction]. The breaking up of a thrombus. SYN: *thromboclasis.*

thrombolytic (thrŏm″bō-lĭt′ĭk). Pert. to or causing the breaking up of a thrombus.

thrombon (thrŏm′bŏn) [Gr. *thrombos,* a clot]. The portion of the hematopoietic system concerned with platelet formation.

thrombopathy (thrŏm-bŏp′ă-thē) [″ + *pathos,* disease]. A defect in the coagulation apparatus of the blood.

thrombopenia (thrŏm-bō-pē′nē-ă) [″ + *penia,* lack]. Lessening of the number of blood platelets.

thrombophilia (thrŏm-bō-fĭl′ē-ă) [″ + *philein,* to love]. A tendency to the occurrence of clot formation.

thrombophlebitis (thrŏm″bō-flē-bī′tĭs) [″ + *phleps,* vein, + *itis,* inflammation]. Inflammation of a vein in conjunction with the formation of a thrombus. Usually occurs in an extremity, most frequently a leg. SYN: *phlebitis; phlegmasia alba dolens.*

NURSING IMPLICATIONS: Promote bedrest. Apply warm, moist compresses at regular intervals. Elevate the foot of the bed approx. 6 inches (15 cm.). Administer heparin as prescribed, and observe for side effects.

Apply elastic stockings and administer analgesics as ordered. Instruct the patient not to rub or massage extremities. Assess the neurovascular status of the extremity frequently.

TREATMENT: The therapeutic goal is to prevent a thrombus from becoming an embolus that may reach the lung. The anticoagulant heparin is used but requires careful monitoring of the patient's response. Therapy may also include ligation of the vein proximal to the thrombus to prevent pulmonary embolism.

t. migrans. Recurring attacks of thrombophlebitis in various sites.

t., postpartum, iliofemoral. Thrombophlebitis of the iliofemoral artery that occurs during the postpartum period.

thromboplastic (thrŏm″bō-plăs′tĭk) [″ + *plassein,* to form]. Pert. to or causing acceleration of clot formation in the blood.

thromboplastid (thrŏm″bō-plăs′tĭd). A blood platelet.

thromboplastin (thrŏm″bō-plăs′tĭn) [″ + *plassein,* to form]. The third blood coagulation factor (Factor III). A substance found in both blood and tissues. Tissue thromboplastin is found in most parts of the body as an intracellular substance. A substance with thromboplastic activity is also present in red blood cells. Even though these two substances are separate and act in different manners, both are able to accelerate the clotting of blood.

thromboplastinogen (thrŏm″bō-plăs-tĭn′ō-jĕn). Blood clotting factor VIII. SEE: *coagulation factors.*

thrombopoiesis (thrŏm″bō-poy-ē′sĭs) [″ + *poiesis,* production]. The formation of blood platelets.

thrombosed (thrŏm′bōzd) [Gr. *thrombos,* a clot]. 1. Coagulated; clotted. 2. Denoting a vessel containing a thrombus.

thrombosinusitis (thrŏm″bō-sī-nŭs-ī′tĭs) [″ + L. *sinus,* cavity, + Gr. *itis,* inflammation]. Thrombus formation of a dural sinus.

thrombosis (thrŏm-bō′sĭs) [″ + *osis,* condition]. The formation, development, or existence of a blood clot or thrombus within the vascular system. This is a life-saving process when it occurs during hemorrhage. It is a life-threatening event when it occurs at any other time because the clot can occlude a vessel and stop the blood supply to an organ or a part. The thrombus, if detached, becomes an embolus and occludes a vessel at a distance from the original site; for example, a clot in the leg may break off and cause a pulmonary embolus.

ETIOL: Trauma, esp. following an operation and parturition; cardiac and vascular disorders, obesity, heredity, increasing age, an excess of erythrocytes and of platelets, an overproduction of fibrinogen, and sepsis are predisposing causes.

SYM: *Lungs:* Obstruction of smaller vessels in the lungs causes an infarct manifested by sudden pain in the side of the chest, similar to pleurisy; also the spitting of blood, a pleural friction rub, and signs of consolidation. *Kidneys:* Blood appears in the urine, and small hemorrhagic spots in the skin. *Spleen:* Pain is felt in the left upper abdomen. *Extremities:* If a large artery in one of the extremities, such as the brachial, is suddenly obstructed, the part becomes cold, pale, bluish, and the pulse disappears below the obstructed site. Gangrene of the digits or of the whole limb may ensue. Same symptoms may be present with an embolism, q.v.

If the limb is swollen, watch for pressure sores. Guard against burning with hot water bottle or electric pad. Prolonged bedrest may be necessary depending on the condition of the patient.

TREATMENT: Anticoagulant therapy is necessary. When a thrombus or embolus is large, surgical removal may be necessary.

RS: angina pectoris; embolus; "thromb-" words.

t., cardiac. Thrombosis of an artery supplying the heart muscle (myocardium).

t., coagulation. Thrombosis due to coagulation of fibrin in a blood vessel.

t., compression. Thrombosis due to compression between a thrombus and the heart.

t., coronary. Thrombosis of a coronary artery. A common cause of myocardial infarction.

SYM: Sudden onset of severe and prolonged substernal oppression and pain, the pain arising over the precordium and being referred to the upper and middle sternum and often radiating to the left and sometimes right arm and into the neck or back. Blood pressure usually falls, pulse becomes rapid, fever and leukocytosis are usually observed within 24 hours. Erythrocyte sedimentation rate becomes elevated and electrocardiographic changes occur.

Certain enzyme tests are very helpful in diagnosing myocardial infarction. The serum level of creatine phosphokinase (CPK) is elevated in the first 24 hours following the infarction; the degree of elevation is proportional to the amount of cardiac muscle damaged. The CPK level may also be elevated if skeletal muscle damage is present. In that case other enzyme tests such as aspartate aminotransferase or lactic dehydrogenase (LDH) will be helpful in diagnosis.

TREATMENT: Complete physical and

mental rest for a variable length of time depending upon severity. This is sometimes best accomplished by allowing the patient to rest in a reclining chair rather than a bed; and to use a bedside toilet instead of having to strain to use a bedpan. Special nursing care is desirable. Prompt and complete relief from pain by use of intravenous morphine sulfate; oxygen administration sometimes necessary. Vasopressor drugs to elevate blood pressure; digitalis when there is evidence of congestive heart failure; treatment of cardiac arrhythmias, esp. tachycardia; anticoagulants. Treatment in coronary care unit is usually mandatory.

DIET: As regulated by patient but restrict caloric intake to 1000 to 1500 Cal. Restrict salt intake and maintain record of fluid intake and output.

COMPLICATIONS: Shock; acute pulmonary edema; pulmonary embolism; paroxysmal ventricular tachycardia; congestive heart failure; aneurysm of the ventricle.

Most patients will develop some form of cardiac arrhythmia. This can be simple sinus tachycardia; bradycardia; atrial fibrillation; ventricular tachycardia; ventricular fibrillation; or cardiac arrest. The latter two are life-threatening and require prompt and diligent therapeutic intervention. Depending on the cause, the arrhythmia will be treated with one or more of the following: atropine, lidocaine, digitalis, defibrillation, or a pacemaker.

t., embolic. Thrombosis caused by an embolus obstructing a vessel.

t., infective. Thrombosis in which there is bacterial infection.

t., marasmic. Thrombosis due to wasting diseases of infancy and old age.

t., placental. Thrombi in the placenta and veins of the uterus.

t., plate. Thrombus formed from an accumulation of blood platelets.

t., puerperal. Coagulation in veins following labor.

t., sinus. Formation of a blood clot in a venous sinus.

t., traumatic. Thrombosis due to a wound or injury of a part.

t., venous. Thrombosis of a vein.

thrombostasis (thrŏm-bŏs′tă-sĭs) [″ + *stasis,* a standing still]. Stasis of blood in a part causing or due to formation of thrombus.

thrombosthenin (thrŏm″bō-sthē′nĭn) [″ + *sthenos,* strength]. A contractile protein present in the platelets. Because of this protein that is active in clot retraction, the platelets have been characterized as being muscle cell.

thrombotic (thrŏm-bŏt′ĭk) [Gr. *thrombos,* clot]. Related to, caused by, or of the nature of, a thrombus.

thrombus (thrŏm′bŭs) [Gr. *thrombos*]. A blood clot that obstructs a blood vessel or a cavity of the heart. Anticoagulants are being used in prevention and treatment of this condition.

t., annular. Thrombus whose circumference is attached to the walls of a vessel, an opening still remaining in the center.

t., antemortem. A clot formed in the heart or large vessels before death.

t., ball. A round clot in the heart, esp. in the atria.

t., hyaline. Thrombus having a glassy appearance usually occurring in smaller blood vessels.

t., Laennec's. A globular thrombus that forms in the heart, usually in cases of fatty degeneration.

t., lateral. T., mural.

t., milk. A curdled milk tumor in the female breast due to obstruction in a lactiferous duct.

t., mural. Thrombus attached to the wall of a vessel or the heart. SYN: *t., parietal.*

t., obstructing. Thrombus completely occluding the lumen of a vessel.

t., occluding. A thrombus that completely closes the vessel.

t., parietal. A thrombus attached to the wall of a vessel.

t., progressive. Thrombus that increases in size.

t., stratified. Thrombus composed of layers.

t., white. A pale thrombus in any site. Made up principally of platelets.

through and through drainage. Irrigation and drainage of a cavity or an organ such as the bladder by having two perforated tubes, drains, or catheters into the area. A solution is instilled through one tube, usually by continuous drip, and the other tube is attached to either straight or gravity drainage or a suction machine.

through illumination. Passage of light through the walls of an organ or cavity for medical examination. SYN: *transillumination.*

thrush (thrŭsh) [D. *troske,* rotten wood]. Infection, caused by Candida albicans of mouth, or throat, esp. in infants and young children, characterized by formation of white patches and ulcers, frequently fever and gastrointestinal inflammation. SEE: *aphtha; sprue; stomatitis.*

thrypsis (thrĭp′sĭs) [Gr., breaking in pieces]. A fracture in which the bone is splintered or crushed.

thulium (thū′lē-ŭm). SYMB: Tm. At. wt. 168.934; at. no. 69. A rare metallic element found in combination with minerals.

thumb (thŭm) [AS. *thuma,* thumb]. The short thick first finger on the radial side of the hand, having two phalanges and being opposable to the other four digits. SYN: *pollex* [NA]. SEE: *hand* for illus.

t., tennis. Calcification and inflammation of the tendon of the flexor pollicis longus muscle due to repeated irritation and stress while playing tennis.

thumb sign. Protrusion of the thumb across the palm and beyond the clenched fist. Seen in children with Marfan's syndrome.

thumb sucking. The habit of sucking one's own thumb. Intermittent thumb sucking is not abnormal, but prolonged and intensive thumb sucking past the time the first permanent teeth erupt at five or six years of age can lead to a misshapen mouth and displaced teeth. If the habit persists, combined dental and psychological therapy should be instituted.

thus (thŭs) [L.]. Frankincense, the oleoresin obtained as an exudate from trees of the Pinus species. Genuine frankincense is obtained from the bark of trees of the genus Boswellia.

thylacitis (thī″lă-sī′tĭs) [Gr. *thylax,* pouch, + *itis,* inflammation]. Inflammation of the sebaceous glands of the skin.

thylakoid (thī′lă-koyd) [Gr. *thylakon,* a small sac, + *eidos,* form]. Part of the lamellae of chloroplasts. They contain photosynthetic pigments and catalytic enzymes for light-dependent reactions.

thymectomize (thī-mĕk′tō-mīz). Surgical removal of the thymus gland.

thymectomy (thī-mĕk′tō-mē) [Gr. *thymos,* thymus, + *ektome,* excision]. Surgical removal of the thymus gland.

thymelcosis (thī″mĕl-kō′sĭs) [″ + *helkosis,* ulceration]. Ulceration of the thymus gland.

-thymia [Gr. *thymos,* mind]. A word ending indicating a state of the mind.

thymic (thī′mĭk) [L. *thymicus*]. Rel. to the thymus gland.

thymicolymphatic (thī″mĭ-kō-lĭm-făt′ĭk). Rel. to the thymus and lymph glands.

thymidine (thī′mĭ-dēn). A nucleoside present in deoxyribonucleotide. It is formed from the condensation product of thymine and deoxyribase.

thymine (thī′mĭn). A base 5-methyl uracil present in deoxyribonucleic acid.

thymion (thĭm′ē-ŏn) [Gr.]. A wart.

thymitis (thī-mī′tĭs) [Gr. *thymos,* thymus, + *itis,* inflammation]. Inflammation of the thymus gland.

thymo-. 1. [Gr. *thymos,* thymus] Combining form indicating relationship to the thymus. 2. [Gr. *thymos,* mind, spirit] Combining form indicating relationship with the soul or emotions.

thymocyte (thī′mō-sīt) [Gr. *thymos,* thymus, + *kytos,* cell]. A thymus gland–derived cell.

thymokesis (thī″mō-kē′sĭs). Abnormal enlargement of the thymus in the adult.

thymokinetic (thī″mō-kĭ-nĕt′ĭk) [″ + *kinesis,* movement]. Stimulating the thymus gland.

thymol (thī′mōl) [Gr. *thumon,* thyme, + L. *oleum,* oil]. White crystals obtained from oil of thyme. Formerly used in treatment of hookworm.

t. iodide. An antifungal and antibacterial agent.

thymolysis (thī-mŏl′ĭ-sĭs) [Gr. *thymos,* thymus, + *lysis,* dissolution]. Dissolution of thymus tissue.

thymolytic (thī-mō-lĭt′ĭk). Destructive to thymus tissue.

thymoma (thī-mō′mă) [″ + *oma,* tumor]. A tumor originating in epithelial tissues of the thymus gland.

thymopathy (thī-mŏp′ă-thē). Disease of the thymus.

thymopexy (thī″mō-pĕks′ē) [″ + *pexis,* fixation]. Fixation of an enlarged thymus in a new position.

thymopoietin (thī″mō-poy′ĕ-tĭn). A substance produced by the thymus that stimulates differentiation of thymocytes.

thymoprivic (thī″mō-prĭv′ĭk) [″ + L. *privus,* deprived of]. Concerning or caused by removal of the thymus.

thymotoxic (thī″mō-tŏks′ĭk) [″ + *toxikon,* poison]. Poisonous to thymus tissue.

thymus (thī′mŭs) [Gr. *thymos*]. An unpaired organ located in the mediastinal cavity anterior to and above the heart. It consists of two flattened symmetrical lobes each enclosed in a capsule, from which trabeculae extend into the gland dividing each lobe into many lobules, each consisting of a cortex and medulla. The cortex is composed of dense lymphoid tissue containing many cells (thymocytes) closely packed together. The medulla also contains thymocytes but they are less numerous. It also contains characteristic thymic (Hassall's) corpuscles.

At birth the average weight of the thymus is 13 gm. Growth is rapid during the first two years, then slow, attaining a weight of about 30 gm. at puberty, after which it begins to undergo involution and the thymic tissue is replaced with adipose and connective tissue.

FUNCT: Important in development of immune response in newborn. Its removal during early childhood has been associated with an increased susceptibility to acute infectious diseases at a later time.

The thymus is essential to the maturation of the thymic lymphoid cells, called T cells. When the T cells enter the circulation they are the small and medium-sized lymphocytes; they may survive for up to 5 years. These cells are important in the body's cellular immune response.

PATH: Sometimes it is much larger than it should be and is then known as an enlarged thymus. Children having these enlarged structures were routinely irradiated in the past. This practice has been discontinued because of the high incidence of cancer of the thyroid in these individuals when they reached adulthood. It is recommended that anyone who has undergone thymus irradiation be examined for possible thyroid cancer. SEE: *asthma, thymic; status thymicolymphaticus.*

t., accessory. A lobule isolated from the mass of the thymus gland.

t. persistens hyperplastica. A thymus persisting into adulthood, sometimes hypertrophying.

thymusectomy (thī″mŭs-ĕk′tō-mē) [Gr. *thymos,* thymus, + *ektome,* excision]. Surgical excision of the thymus.

thyreo-, thyro- [Gr. *thyreos,* shield]. Combining forms meaning oblong, shield, or thyroid.

thyreoplasia. Defective functioning of the thyroid gland due to abnormal development.

thyroadenitis (thī″rō-ăd-ĕ-nī′tĭs) [″ + *aden,* gland, + *itis,* inflammation]. Inflammation of the thyroid gland.

thyroaplasia (thī″rō-ă-plā′zē-ă) [″ + *a-,* not, + *plasis,* a molding]. Imperfect development of the thyroid gland.

thyroarytenoid (thī″rō-ă-rĭt′ĕn-oyd) [″ + *arytaina,* ladle + *eidos,* form]. Rel. to the thyroid and arytenoid cartilages.

thyrocalcitonin (thī″rō-kăl″sĭ-tō′nĭn). Calcitonin, q.v.

thyrocardiac (thī″rō-kăr′dē-ăk) [″ + *kardia,* heart]. 1. Pert. to the heart and thyroid gland. 2. A person suffering from thyroid disease complicated by heart disorder.

thyrocele (thī′rō-sēl) [″ + *kele,* mass]. Enlarged condition of the thyroid gland. SYN: *goiter.*

thyrochondrotomy (thī″rō-kŏn-drŏt′ō-mē) [″ + *chondros,* cartilage, + *tome,* incision]. Surgical incision of thyroid cartilage.

thyrocolloid (thī″rō-kŏl′oyd). Colloid contained in the thyroid gland.

thyrocricotomy (thī″rō-krī-kŏt′ō-mē) [″ + *krikos,* ring, + *tome,* incision]. Division of the cricothyroid membrane.

thyroepiglottic (thī″rō-ĕp″ĭ-glŏt′ĭk) [″ + *epi,* upon, + *glottis,* glottis]. Rel. to the thyroid and epiglottis.

thyroepiglottic muscle. Muscle arising on inner surface of thyroid cartilage. It extends upward and backward and is inserted on the epiglottis. It depresses the epiglottis.

thyroepiglottideus (thī″rō-ĕp″ĭ-glŏt-ĭd′ē-ŭs) Muscle in the thyroid cartilage that depresses the epiglottis.

thyrofissure (thī″rō-fĭsh′ŭr). Surgical creation of an opening through the thyroid cartilage in order to expose the inside of the larynx.

thyrogenic, thyrogenous (thī-rō-jĕn′ĭk, thī-rŏj′ĕ-nŭs) [″ + *gennan,* to produce]. Having its origin in the thyroid.

thyroglobulin (thī″rō-glŏb′ū-lĭn) [″ + L. *globulus,* a tiny sphere]. 1. An iodine-containing protein secreted by the thyroid gland and stored within its colloid substance. 2. USP. A substance obtained by the fractionation of thyroid glands from the hog, Sus scrofa. Trade name is Proloid.

thyroglossal (thī″rō-glŏs′săl) [″ + *glossa,* tongue]. Pert. to the thyroid gland and the tongue.

thyroglossal duct. A duct that in the embryo connects the thyroid diverticulum with the tongue. It eventually disappears, its point of origin being indicated as a pit, the foramen cecum. It sometimes persists as an anomaly.

thyrohyal (thī″rō-hī′ăl). Concerning the thyroid cartilage and the hyoid bone.

thyrohyoid (thī″rō-hī′oyd) [″ + *hyoeides,* U-shaped]. Rel. to thyroid cartilage and hyoid bone.

thyroid (thī′royd) [″ + *eidos,* form]. 1. A gland of internal secretion in the neck, anterior to and partially surrounding the thyroid cartilage and upper rings of the trachea. SEE: *thyroid gland.* 2. USP. The cleaned, dried, and powdered thyroid gland of animals slaughtered for food, usually pigs. The preparation is free of fat and connective tissue.

ACTION AND USES: Used in cases of deficient action of the gland (hypothyroidism) or following thyroidectomy.

ADM: Tablet form by mouth. The maximum effect will not be obtained for at least 7 to 10 days. It is advisable to start with a small dose and increase it gradually until the proper dose is determined.

thyroid cachexia. Exophthalmic goiter. SEE: *hyperthyroidism.*

thyroid cartilage. The principal cartilage of the larynx consisting of two broad laminae united anteriorly to form a V-shaped structure. It forms a subcutaneous projection called the laryngeal prominence or Adam's apple. SEE: *thyroid gland* for illus.

thyroid crisis. Thyroid storm.

thyroidea accessoria; thyroidea ima (thī-roy′dē-ă). Accessory thyroid.

thyroidectomized (thī″roy-dĕk′tō-mīzd) [″ + *eidos,* form, + *ektome,* excision]. With the thyroid gland removed.

thyroidectomy (thī″royd-ĕk′tō-mē). Excision of the thyroid gland.

NURSING IMPLICATIONS: Postoperatively, assess the patient frequently for signs of respiratory distress. Keep an emergency tracheotomy tray at the bedside. Elevate the head of the bed, support the patient's head with pillows, and observe the posterior dressing for signs of bleeding. Administer oral fluids initially as tolerated, then progress to soft diet as tolerated. Observe the patient for laryngeal nerve damage by noting any voice changes. Encourage voice rest immediately after surgery. Assess for signs of tetany. Watch for signs of thyroid storm, such as altered consciousness, tachycardia, and elevated temperature. Administer analgesics as prescribed. Teach the patient how to support the weight of the head and neck. After the sutures have been removed, begin an active exercise regimen for head and neck. Inform the patient to apply a lubricant to the incision site daily to minimize scarring. Instruct the patient concerning medications, and make follow-up appointments. Counsel the patient concerning rest, relaxation, and nutrition. Provide emotional support, and assist in emotional readjustment in the home environment to reduce emotional tension.

thyroid function tests. Tests for evidence of increased or decreased thyroid function including clinical physical examination, which is usually reliable, and a variety of reliable laboratory tests. Some of the more common tests are based on direct or indirect determination of the two thyroid hormones, and triiodothyronine (T_3) and tetraiodothyronine (T_4). Also frequently used are tests on radioactive iodine uptake by the thyroid.

Most thyroid function tests are unreliable in certain circumstances. They may be influenced by the patient's having been exposed to organic or inorganic iodides or to drugs that interfere with the binding capacity of serum proteins.

thyroid gland. A gland of internal secretion located in the base of the neck on both sides of the lower part of the larynx and upper part of trachea. It consists of two lateral lobes connected by an isthmus. Sometimes a third medial or pyramidal lobe extends upward from the isthmus. Histologically it consists of a large number of closed vesicles called follicles that contain a homogeneous substance called colloid, which contains the thyroglobulin, which in turn contains various active substances such as thyroxine. The thyroid gland is enlarged in goiter and it may pulsate. SEE: illus.

RS: endocrine gland; hormone; hyperthyroidism; hypothyroidism; iodine; struma; thyrotropic hormone; thyroxine.

thyroidism (thī′royd-ĭzm). Disease caused by hyperactivity of the thyroid gland.

thyroiditis (thī″royd-ī′tĭs) [″ + *eidos*, form, +

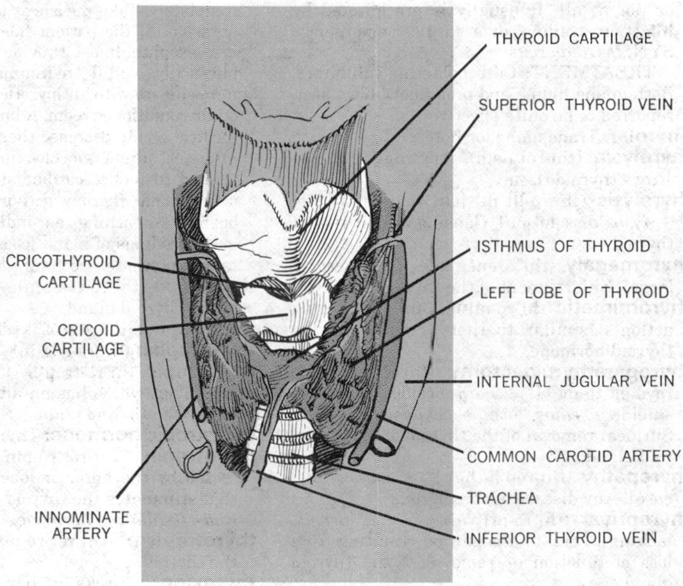

THYROID GLAND AND RELATED STRUCTURES

itis, inflammation]. Inflammation of the thyroid gland. SEE: *struma, Riedel's.*

t., giant cell. Thyroiditis characterized by presence of giant cells, round-cell infiltration, fibrosis, and destruction of follicles.

t., Hashimoto's. A form of autoimmune thyroiditis that affects women eight times more often than men. Clinically there is an enlarged thyroid and hypothyroidism. The treatment is life-long replacement therapy with thyroid hormone.

thyroidomania (thī″royd-ō-mā′nē-ă) [″ + ″ + *mania,* frenzy]. Mental disorder associated with hyperthyroidism.

thyroidotomy (thī″royd-ŏt′ō-mē) [″ + ″ + *tome,* incision]. Incision of the thyroid gland.

thyroidotoxin (thī″royd-ō-tŏk′sĭn). A substance that is specifically toxic for cells of the thyroid gland.

thyroid-stimulating hormone. ABBR: TSH. Hormone secreted by the anterior lobe of the pituitary that stimulates the thyroid gland. SYN: *thyrotropin.*

thyroid storm. A complication of thyrotoxicosis that if untreated is almost uniformly fatal. Consists of abrupt onset of fever, sweating, tachycardia, pulmonary edema or congestive heart failure, tremulousness, and restlessness. Occurs in a patient in whom existing thyrotoxicosis has been treated poorly or not at all. It usually is precipitated by infection, trauma, or a surgical emergency. SYN: *thyroid crisis.*

TREATMENT: Catecholamine inhibitors. Both guanethidine and propranolol have been reported to be quite effective.

Thyrolar. Trade name for liotrix.

thyrolysin (thī-rŏl′ĭ-sĭn). Anything that destroys thyroid tissue.

thyrolytic (thī″rō-lĭt′ĭk) [Gr. *thyreos,* shield, + *lysis,* dissolution]. Causing destruction of thyroid tissue.

thyromegaly (thī″rō-mĕg′ă-lē) [″ + *megas,* large]. Enlargement of the thyroid gland.

thyromimetic (thī″rō-mĭ-mĕt′ĭk). Concerning action(s) similar to that produced by the thyroid hormone.

thyroparathyroidectomy (thī″rō-păr″ă-thī″royd-ĕk′tō-mē) [″ + *para,* beside, + *thyreos,* shield, + *eidos,* form, + *ektome,* excision]. Surgical removal of the thyroid and parathyroid glands.

thyropathy (thī-rŏp′ă-thē) [″ + *pathos,* disease]. Any disease of the thyroid.

thyroprival (thī″rō-prī′văl) [″ + L. *privus,* lacking]. Pert. to a condition resulting from loss of function or removal of the thyroid gland.

thyroprivia (thī″rō-prĭv′ē-ă) [″ + L. *privus,* without]. Hypothyroidism due to deficient action of or removal of the thyroid.

thyroptosis (thī″rŏp-tō′sĭs) [″ + *ptosis,* a dropping]. Downward displacement of the thyroid into the thorax.

thyrosis (thī-rō′sĭs) [″ + *osis,* condition]. Any condition due to abnormal function of the thyroid.

thyrotherapy (thī″rō-thĕr′ă-pē) [″ + *therapeia,* treatment]. Treatment with thyroid gland extracts.

thyrotome (thī′rō-tōm) [″ + *tome,* incision]. Knife for cutting the thyroid cartilage.

thyrotomy (thī-rŏt′ō-mē). 1. The splitting of the thyroid cartilage anteriorly in midline in order to expose laryngeal structures. 2. Surgery on the thyroid gland.

thyrotoxic (thī″rō-tŏks′ĭk) [″ + *toxikon,* poison]. Pert. to, affected by, or marked by toxic activity of the thyroid gland.

thyrotoxicosis (thī″rō-tŏks″ĭ-kō′sĭs) [″ + ″ + *osis,* condition]. Toxic condition due to hyperactivity of the thyroid gland. SYN: *goiter, exophthalmic.*

SYM: Rapid heart action; tremors; elevated basal metabolism; enlarged gland; exophthalmos; nervous symptoms; and loss of weight.

NURSING IMPLICATIONS: Place the patient in semi-Fowler's position to enhance venous return and decrease orbital swelling. Synthetic tear preparations may be used to lubricate the eyes if the patient is unable to close them completely. Take measures to prevent corneal abrasions if the patient has protruding eyes, i.e., exophthalmos. Provide a mentally and physically restful environment. Reduce body temperature with antipyretic agents, ice packs, or air-conditioned room. Administer prescribed medications to decrease thyroxine output. Administer adrenergic blocking agents as prescribed to reduce cardiac symptoms. Provide occupational therapy activities. Perform preoperative teaching as indicated. Offer frequent feedings of bland foods. Reduce salt intake to prevent periorbital edema.

thyrotoxin (thī″rō-tŏk′sĭn). A toxin produced in the thyroid gland.

thyrotrophic (thī″rō-trōf′ĭk). Thyrotropic, q.v.

thyrotrophin (thī″rō-trōf′ĭn). Thyrotropin, q.v.

thyrotropic (thī″rō-trŏp′ĭk) [″ + *trope,* a turning]. That which has an affinity for or stimulates the thyroid gland.

thyrotropic hormone. Thyrotropin.

thyrotropin (thī-rŏt′rō-pĭn). Hormone secreted by the anterior lobe of the pituitary that stimulates the thyroid gland. SYN: *thyroid-stimulating hormone.*

thyrotropism (thī-rŏt′rō-pĭzm). Affinity for the thyroid.

thyroxine (thī-rŏks′ĭn) [Gr. *thyreos,* shield]. 3,5,3′,5′-Tetraiodothyronine, a hormone produced by the thyroid gland. Used in the treatment of hypothyroidism. SYN: T_4.

Ti. Chem. symb. for titanium.

TIA. *transient ischemic attack.*

tibia (tĭb'ē-ă) [L., *tibia,* shinbone]. The inner and larger bone of the leg between the knee and ankle articulating with the femur above and with the talus below.

t., saber-shaped. A deformity of the tibia due to gummatous periostitis (syphilitic) in which it curves outward.

t. valga. A bulging of the lower legs in which the convexity is inward. SYN: *genu valgum.*

t. vara. A bowing of the lower legs in which the convexity is outward. SYN: *genu varum.*

tibiad (tĭb'ē-ăd) [" + *ad,* to]. Toward the tibia.

tibial (tĭb'ē-ăl) [L. *tibialis*]. Concerning the tibia.

tibialgia (tĭb"ē-ăl'jē-ă) [" + Gr. *algos,* pain]. Pain in the tibia.

tibialis (tĭb"ē-ā'lĭs) [L.]. [NA] Pert. to the tibia.

tibioadductor reflex (tĭb"ē-ō-ăd-dŭk'tor) [L. *tibia,* shinbone, + *adducere,* to lead to]. Adduction of either the stimulated leg or the opposite one when the tibia is percussed on the inner side.

tibiocalcanean (tĭb"ē-ō-kăl-kā'nē-ăn). Concerning the tibia and calcaneus bones.

tibiofemoral (tĭb"ē-ō-fĕm'or-ăl) [" + L. *femur,* thigh]. Rel. to the tibia and femur.

tibiofibular (tĭb"ē-ō-fĭb'ū-lăr) [" + L. *fibula,* buckle]. Rel. to the tibia and fibula.

tibionavicular (tĭb"ē-ō-nă-vĭk'ū-lăr). Concerning the tibia and navicular bones.

tibioperoneal (tĭb"ē-ō-pĕr"ō-nē'ăl). Tibiofibular.

tibioscaphoid (tĭb"ē-ō-skăf'oyd). Tibionavicular.

tibiotarsal (tĭb"ē-ō-tăr'săl) [" + Gr. *tarsos,* broad flat surface]. Rel. to the tibia and tarsus.

tic (tĭk) [Fr.]. A spasmodic muscular contraction, most commonly involving the face, head, neck, or shoulder muscles. The spasms may be tonic, q.v., or clonic, q.v. The movement appears purposeful, is often repeated, is involuntary, and can be inhibited for a short time only to burst forth with increased severity. SYN: *habit spasm.* SEE: *neuralgia.*

ETIOL: Certain of these cases are due to structure changes, many psychogenic, or the expression of frustration and its correlated muscular tension. The former group is most commonly encountered in patients who have suffered from lethargic encephalitis.

t., convulsive. Spasm of muscles of face supplied by the seventh cranial nerve.

t. douloureux. Degeneration of or pressure on the trigeminal nerve, resulting in neuralgia of that nerve. The pain comes on in severe lightning-like stabs and radiates from the angle of the jaw along one of the involved branches. If it is the first branch, a shocklike pain is felt along the eye and back over the forehead. If it is the middle fiber, the upper lip, nose, and cheek under the eye are affected. If it is the third branch, pain is in the lower lip and outer border of the tongue on the affected side. Pain is momentary but may occur repetitively for as long as 20 seconds. Paroxysms may last for hours and then subside for weeks or months. SYN: *prosopalgia; neuralgia, trigeminal.*

TREATMENT: Injection of the nerve with alcohol. Anticonvulsants may be helpful to shorten attacks or cause remission. Surgical therapy may be required.

t., facial. Tic of the facial muscles.

t., habit. Habitual repetition of a grimace or muscular action.

t. rotatoire. Spasmodic torticollis in which head and neck are forcibly rotated or turned from one side to the other.

t., spasmodic. Tonic contractions and paralysis of muscles of one or both sides of the face.

Ticar. Trade name for ticarcillin disodium, USP.

ticarcillin disodium, sterile (tī"kăr-sĭl'ĭn). USP. A semisynthetic penicillin esp. effective against Pseudomonas aeruginosa. Trade name is Ticar.

tick (tĭk) [ME. *tyke*]. Any of the numerous bloodsucking acarids of the order Acarida. Ixodidae is the hard tick family and Argasidae the soft. They transmit specific diseases to man and lower animals. SEE: illus.

tick bite. Ticks can be vectors for several diseases including Rocky Mountain spotted fever, Q fever, tularemia, borreliosis, human babesiosis, and Lyme disease, but the bite itself usually produces a mildly itching papule. If the tick is incompletely removed, the retained mouth parts may cause a pruritic nodule. The nodule should be surgically excised. Removal of a tick should not be done by crushing but by either gentle traction or application of Vaseline, oil, or nail polish to the tick, which will facilitate removal.

tick-borne rickettsiosis. A variety of tick-borne rickettsial diseases similar to Rocky Mountain spotted fever. They are caused by a rickettsial organism (Rickettsia rickettsii) transmitted by Ixodid ticks.

tickle (tĭk'l) [ME. *tikelen*]. 1. Peculiar sensation caused by titillation or touching, esp. in certain regions, resulting in reflex muscular movements, laughter, or hysteria. 2. To arouse such a sensation by touching a surface lightly.

tickling (tĭk'lĭng). Gentle stimulation of a sensitive surface and its reflex effect, such as involuntary laughter. SYN: *titillation.*

t.i.d. L. *ter in die,* three times a day.

tidal (tī'dăl). Periodically rising and falling, increasing and decreasing.

DORSAL VIEW FEMALE

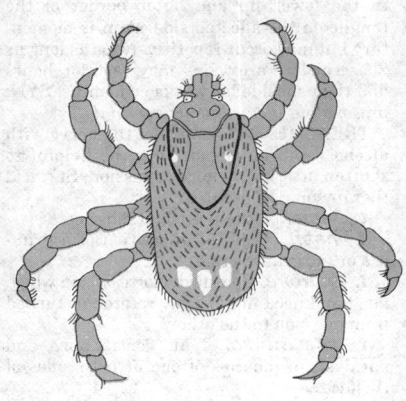

TICK
(MARGAROPUS REIDI)

tidal air. Air that is inhaled and exhaled during normal quiet breathing. SEE: *air; respiration.*

tidal drainage. The drainage of a paralyzed bladder by use of an automatic irrigation apparatus.

tide [AS. *tid,* time]. Alternate rise and fall; a space of time.

t., acid. A temporary increase in acidity of urine due to increased secretion of alkaline substances into the duodenum or after fasting.

t., alkaline. Temporary decrease in acidity of urine following awakening and after meals. The former results from hyperpnea, in which excess CO_2 is eliminated; the latter results from increase of base in the blood following the secretion of HCl into gastric juice.

t., fat. Increased fat in the lymph and blood after a fatty meal.

Tietze's syndrome (tēt'sĕz). [Alexander Tietze, Ger. surgeon, 1864–1927] Inflammation of the costochondral cartilages. A self-limiting disease of unknown etiology. Pain may be confused with that of myocardial infarction. There is no specific therapy, but some relief will be provided by injecting the area with procaine and corticosteroids.

T-I-Gammagee. Trade name for tetanus immune globulin, USP.

Tigan. Trade name for trimethobenzamide hydrochloride.

tigering [Gr. *tigris,* tiger]. Tiger-like striped appearance of heart muscle due to irregular areas of fatty degeneration. Seen in conditions that cause severe anoxemia such as anemia.

tigretier (tē-grĕt″ē-ā′) [Fr.]. A dancing mania or form of tarantism due to bite of a poisonous spider, occurring in Tigré, Abyssinia.

tigroid (tī′groyd) [Gr. *tigroeides,* tiger-spotted]. Striped, spotted, or marked like a tiger.

tigroid bodies. Masses of chromophil substance present in the cell bodies of neurons. SYN: *Nissl bodies.*

tigrolysis (tĭg″rŏl′ĭ-sĭs). Dissolution and disappearance of chromophil substance of a nerve cell. May occur following injury to an axon (retrograde degeneration) or subsequent to direct injury to a nerve cell. SYN: *chromatolysis.*

tilmus (tĭl′mŭs) [Gr. *tilmos,* a plucking]. Delirious picking at the bedclothes by the patient. SYN: *carphology.*

tiltometer (tĭl-tŏm′ĕ-tĕr). A device for measuring the degree of tilt of a bed or operating table. Used when spinal anesthesia has been given in order to know which end of the spinal canal is lower.

timbre (tĭm′bĕr, tăm′br) [Fr., a bell to be struck with a hammer]. Resonance quality of a sound by which it is distinguished, other than pitch or intensity, depending upon the number and character of vibrating body's overtones.

time (tīm) [AS. *tima,* time]. Interval between beginning and ending; measured duration.

t., bleeding. Time required for bleeding from a small wound to cease. Usually tested by puncturing the lobe of the ear. Normal time is 1 to 3 minutes. SEE: *bleeding time.*

t., clot retraction. Time required following withdrawal of blood for a clot to completely contract and express the serum entrapped within the fibrin net. Normal time is about 1 hour. Clot retraction is dependent upon the number of platelets in the specimen.

t., coagulation. Time required for clotting to occur in whole blood that has been placed in tubes coated with silicone. Time required is somewhat different for each laboratory but will usually vary from 20 to 60 minutes.

t., prothrombin. Time needed for oxalated plasma to clot, measured in seconds, after adding thromboplastin and recalcifying.

t., reaction. Period between application of a stimulus and the response.

t., thermal death. Time required to kill a bacterium at a certain temperature.

time frame. The limits of time for any event or occurrence.

timer (tĭm'ĕr). A device for measuring, signaling, recording, or regulating time. Various forms of timers are used in x-ray, surgical, and laboratory work.

Timoptic Solution. Trade name for timolol maleate.

tin (tĭn) [AS.]. SYMB: Sn. At. wt. 118.69; at. no. 50. A metallic element used in various industries, and in making certain tissue stains. SEE: *tin poisoning*.

Tinactin. Trade name for tolnaftate, USP.

tinct. *tincture*.

tinctable (tĭnk'tă-bl). Stainable.

tinction (tĭnk'shŭn) [L. *tingere*, to dye]. 1. The process of staining. 2. A stain.

tinctorial (tĭnk-tō'rē-ăl) [L. *tinctorius*, dyeing]. Rel. to staining or color.

tinctura (tĭnk-tū'ră) [L., a dyeing]. (pl. *tincturae*) Tincture.

tincturation (tĭnk"tū-rā'shŭn). Making a tincture from an appropriate drug.

tincture (tĭnk'chūr). An alcoholic extract of vegetable or animal substances. Simple alcoholic solutions of pure substances such as iodine and quinine are no longer called tinctures. The name of material contained in the tincture other than alcohol is added to the name of the tincture.

This class of preparations usually contains tannic acid, so, in most instances, cannot be employed with agents that are incompatible with that drug. Those tinctures that contain much resinous matter or oils will precipitate with water. Some examples are tinctures of belladonna, ginger, benzoin, and guaiac. Tinctures of the most potent drugs usually represent 10% of the crude drug, as tinctures of opium and digitalis. Where more than a teaspoon of a 10% tincture would have to be taken to get a dose of the drug, the tincture is usually made to represent 20%, or more, of the agent.

tincture of iodine. Obsolete term for simple alcoholic solution of iodine.

tincture of iodine poisoning. This commonly used antiseptic is sometimes taken by mouth either accidentally or for the purpose of suicide.

SYM: Very strong irritation of mouth, esophagus, and stomach. Stains membranes dark brown or black. Pain is intense and leads to early vomiting and purging; extreme thirst, often collapse.

TREATMENT: Give large amounts of water, milk and starchy paste; gruels, as boiled rice or cream of wheat. Gastric lavage with either one to 10% starch solution, or sodium thiosulfite or protein solution such as egg white or milk. Control pain, circulatory collapse, and fluid and electrolyte balance with appropriate therapy. Tracheotomy may be required.

Tindal. Trade name for acetophenazine maleate.

tinea (tĭn'ē-ă) [L., worm]. Any fungus skin disease occurring on various parts of the body, the name indicating the part affected. Ex.: tinea barbae (beard), tinea corporis (body). Commonly called ringworm. SEE: *dermatomycosis*.

SYM: Of two types. Superficial symptoms are marking by scaling; slight itching; reddish or grayish patches; dry, brittle hair that is easily extracted with hair shaft. The deep type is characterized by flat, reddish, kerion-like tumors, the surface studded with dead or broken hairs or by gaping follicular orifices. Nodules may be broken down in center, discharging pus through dilated follicular openings.

TREATMENT: Griseofulvin, given orally for all types of true trichophyton infections. Local treatment alone is of little benefit in ringworm of the scalp, nails, and in most cases the feet. Topical preparations containing fungicidal agents are useful in treatment of tinea cruris and tinea pedis.

Personal hygiene is important in controlling these two common diseases. The use of antiseptic foot baths to control tinea pedis does not prevent spread of the infection from person to person. Persons affected should not allow their personal items, such as clothes, towels and sports equipment, to be used by others.

Tinea of the scalp, tinea capitis, is particularly resistant if due to Microsporum audouini. Do not treat topically. Griseofulvin is quite effective.

t. amiantacea. Pityriasis amiantacea, q.v.

t. barbae. A fungus skin disease of the bearded portions of neck and face. SYN: *barber's itch*.

t. capitis. A fungal infection of the scalp. May be due to one of several types of Microsporum or Trichophyton tonsurans.

t. corporis. Tinea of the body. Begins with red, slightly elevated scaly patches that on examination reveal minute vesicles or papules. New patches spring from the periphery while central portion clears up. Often considerable itching.

t. cruris. A fungus skin disease of surfaces of contact in the scrotal, crural, anal, and genital areas. SYN: *dhobie itch*.

t. imbricata. Chronic tinea caused by Trichophyton concentricum. It is present in tropical regions. The annular lesions have scales at their periphery.

t. kerion. Kerion, q.v.

t. nigra. An asymptomatic superficial fungal infection that affects the skin of the palms. Characterized by deeply pigmented, macular, non-scaly patches. SYN: *pityriasis* *nigra.*

ETIOL: Cladosporium werneckii or C. mansonii.

t. nodosa. Sheathlike nodular masses in hair of beard and mustache from growth of either Piedraia hortai, which causes black piedra, or Trichosporon beigelii, which causes white piedra. The masses surround the hairs, which become brittle; hairs may be penetrated by fungus and thus split. SYN: *piedra.*

t. pedis. A fungus skin infection of the foot. SYN: *athlete's foot; dermatophytosis.*

t. profunda. A rare type of tinea characterized by indolent nodules and plaques. These skin lesions may ulcerate.

t. sycosis. T. barbae, q.v.

t. unguium. Onychomycosis.

t. versicolor. Fungus infection of skin producing branny patches that are yellow or fawn-colored. Topically applied acrisorcin cream is effective in treating the causative agent, the fungus Malassezia furfur. SYN: *pityriasis versicolor.*

Tinel's sign (tĭn-ĕlz'). [Jules Tinel, Fr. neurologist, 1879–1952] Cutaneous tingling sensation produced by pressing on or tapping the nerve trunk that has been damaged or is regenerating following trauma.

tine test. A skin test for tuberculosis. The tuberculin is on metal tines that are barely pressed into the skin. The test is read in 48 and 72 hours. The unit is sterile and disposable and therefore is very useful in mass surveys. SEE: *tuberculin test.*

tingibility (tĭn"jĭ-bĭl'ĭ-tē). The property of being stainable.

tingible (tĭn'jĭ-bl) [L. *tingere,* to stain]. Capable of being stained by a dye.

tingle (tĭng'gl). A prickling or stinging sensation. May be caused by cold or nerve injury.

tinnitus (tĭn-ī'tŭs) [L., a jingling]. A subjective ringing or tinkling sound in the ear.

t. aurium. Ringing, tinkling, buzzing, or other sounds in the ear. Found in certain diseases of the exterior, middle, or inner ear. SYN: *sonitus.*

ETIOL: Impacted cerumen; myringitis; otitis media; labyrinthitis; Ménière's symptom complex; otosclerosis; hysteria. Also follows overdosage of drugs such as quinine and salicylates including aspirin.

tin poisoning. Tin in soldered containers has occasionally been responsible for poisoning. This is exceedingly rare.

SYM: Metallic taste in mouth, gastrointestinal irritation, nausea, vomiting, cramping, and diarrhea.

TREATMENT: Wash out stomach and administer bland or soothing drinks.

tintometer (tĭn-tŏm'ĕ-ter) [L. *tinctus,* a dyeing, + Gr. *metron,* a measure]. A scale of different shades of color to determine by comparison the intensity of color of the blood or other fluid.

tintometric (tĭn"tō-mĕt'rĭk). Rel. to tintometry.

tintometry (tĭn-tŏm'ĕ-trē). Estimation of color by comparison with a scale of colors.

tip (tĭp) [ME]. A point or apex of a part.

"tipped uterus." In the past, malposition of the uterus has been invoked as the cause of a great number of conditions including pelvic pain, backache, abnormal uterine bleeding, infertility, and emotional difficulties. Simple malposition of the uterus without evidence of a specific disease condition that accounts for the malposition is felt to be harmless and virtually symptomless. It is essential therefore that individuals who have been told that a "tipped uterus" is the cause of their symptoms be carefully examined in order to attempt to find a specific organic cause for the symptoms. If in the absence of other findings a vaginal pessary relieves symptoms associated with a retrodisplaced uterus and these symptoms return when the pessary is removed, then surgical suspension of the uterus is indicated. If surgery is not acceptable to the patient, then the pessary may be worn intermittently.

tipping (tĭp'ĭng). Angulation of a tooth about its long axis.

tiqueur (tĭ-kĕr') [Fr.]. One afflicted with a tic.

tire (tīr) [AS. *teorian,* to tire]. 1. Exhaustion; fatigue. 2. To exhaust or fatigue. 3. To become fatigued.

tirefond (tēr-fŏn') [Fr.]. Appliance like a corkscrew for raising depressed portions of bone or for removing foreign bodies.

tires (tīrz). Condition marked by constipation, vomiting, muscular tremors, and pain. SYN: *trembles.*

tiring (tīr'ĭng). Fastening wire around the fragments of a bone.

tissue (tĭsh'ū) [O. Fr. *tissu,* from L. *texere,* to weave]. A group or collection of similar cells and their intercellular substance that act together in the performance of a particular function. The primary tissues are epithelial, connective, skeletal, muscular, glandular, and nervous.

t., adenoid. Lymphoid tissue.

t., adipose. Areolar tissue containing aggregations of densely packed fat cells. SYN: *fat.*

t., areolar. A form of loose connective tissue consisting of interlacing collagenous and elastic fibers embedded in a semifluid matrix together with fibroblasts, histiocytes, mast cells, plasma cells, and other cellular elements. It is widely distributed forming the interstitial tissue of most organs, the membranes surrounding blood vessels and nerves, and constituting the principal portion of fascia.

t., bony, bone. Bone in its usual or abnormal site, i.e., in calcified tissue.

t., brown adipose, brown fat. A special type of fat in which brown pigment and small fat droplets are present. This occurs in some mammals, esp. between the scapulae of hibernating animals.

t., cancellous. Spongy bone with many marrow cavities. It is present at the ends of long articular bones and in the interior of most flat bones.

t., cartilage. The dense connective tissue of cartilage consisting of cells embedded in a matrix.

t., chondroid. Embryonic cartilage.

t., chordal. Tissue of the notochord or derived therefrom. The nucleus pulposus is derived from the notochord.

t., chromaffin. Tissues containing cells that give the chromaffin reaction. Found in the adrenal medulla and ganglia of the parasympathetic nervous system. SEE: *chromaffin system.*

t., chromophil. Those tissues that give a chromophil reaction; found in the medulla and sympathetic ganglia.

t., cicatricial. The thick fibrous tissue formed as part of the healing process in soft tissue wounds.

t., connective. Tissue that supports and connects other tissues and parts of the body. The cells of connective tissue are comparatively few in number, the bulk of the tissue consisting of intercellular substance or matrix, the nature of which gives each type of connective tissue its particular properties. Connective tissues are highly vascular with the exception of cartilage. Connective tissue proper includes the following types: mucous, fibrous (areolar, white fibrous, yellow fibrous, or elastic), reticular, and adipose. Dense connective tissue includes cartilage and bone (osseous tissue).

t., elastic. A form of connective tissue in which yellow elastic fibers predominate. Found in certain ligaments and the walls of blood vessels, esp. the larger arteries.

t., embryonic. T., mucous.

t., endothelial. Endothelium, q.v.

t., epithelial. A form of tissue composed of cells arranged in a continuous sheet consisting of one or several layers. It forms the epidermis of skin, covers surfaces of organs, lines cavities and canals, and forms tubes and ducts and secreting portions of glands. SYN: *epithelium.*

t., erectile. Spongy tissue, the spaces of which fill with blood, causing it to harden and expand. Found in the penis, clitoris, and nipples.

t., extracellular. All of the tissue and fluids outside of the cells of the body. Included are plasma, serum, lymph, aqueous and vitreous humors, and connective tissue such as collagen, cartilage, and some bone.

t., fatty. T., adipose.

t., fibrous. Connective tissue consisting principally of fibers. Includes three types: areolar or loose connective, white fibrous, and yellow fibrous or elastic.

t., gelatinous. Tissue from which gelatin may be obtained by treating it with hot water.

t., glandular. A group of epithelial cells capable of producing secretions.

t., granulation. The newly formed vascular and cellular tissue produced in the early stages of wound healing.

t., indifferent. Tissue composed of undifferentiated cells as in embryonic tissue.

t., interstitial. Connective tissue that forms a network with the cellular elements of an organ.

t., lymphadenoid. Lymphoid tissue present in various sites including the liver, spleen, and bone marrow.

t., lymphoid. A collection of developing and mature lymphocytes mingled with a supporting lattice of connective tissue. Such collections are present in the adenoids, tonsils, and in Peyer's patches in the intestines.

t., mesenchymal. The embryonic mesenchyme.

t., myeloid. The red bone marrow in which most blood cells are formed.

t., mucous. Jelly-like tissue from which connective tissue is derived. SYN: *t., embryonic.*

t., muscular. The material composing the muscles. *Voluntary:* Striped or striated tissue principally connected with the bony framework. In animals it is known as lean meat or flesh. It is a cross-striped muscular tissue, the fibers like a long cylinder with flattened sides and conical ends, enveloped in a delicate sheath, the sarcolemma. *Involuntary:* Smooth or unstriped, or nonstriated, not under control of the will. Principally found in walls of hollow organs, tubes, arteries, and veins. SEE: *muscle.*

t., nerve, nervous. All of the tissue of the central and peripheral nervous systems.

t., osseous. Connective tissue with intercellular substance impregnated with phosphate and carbonate of calcium, the mineral substances being two thirds of the bone's dry weight. SYN: *bony tissue.*

t., reticular. A type of connective tissue consisting of delicate fibers forming interlacing networks. Fibers stain selectively with silver stains and are called argyrophil fibers. It supports lymph nodes and is found in muscular tissue and bone marrow, the spleen, liver, lungs, kidneys, and mucous membranes of the gastrointestinal tract.

t., scar. T., cicatricial, q.v.

t., sclerous. Firm connective tissues such as bone and cartilage.

t., skeletal. The bones, cartilages, and connective tissues that comprise the skeleton.

t., splenic. The highly vascular splenic pulp.

t., subcutaneous. Areolar tissue under and becoming part of the corium.

t., subcutaneous adipose. Adipose tissue within subcutaneous tissue.

t., white fibrous. Connective tissue with white inelastic fibers, forming tendons, ligaments, and resistant membranes.

t., white nervous. Nervous tissue of medullated nerve fibers.

tissue culture. Growth of tissue in vitro on artificial media for experimental research.

tissue macrophage. A large, wandering, uninucleated cell with many branches. A fixed macrophage of loose connective tissue. It is capable of ingesting particulate material and has the property of selectively storing certain dyes in colloidal solution. In inflammatory conditions, it becomes actively ameboid and is important in providing protection against local invasion by bacteria, which it ingests. SYN: *clasmatocyte.*

tissue typing. Techniques utilized in determining the histocompatibility of tissues to be used in grafts and transplants with the recipient's tissues and cells. SEE: *transplantation.*

tissular (tĭsh'ū-lăr). Concerning living tissues.

titanium (tī-tā'nē-ŭm) [L. *titan,* the sun]. SYMB: Ti. At. wt. 47.88; at. no. 22; sp. gr. 4.54. A metallic element found in combination with minerals.

t. dioxide. USP. A chemical used to protect the skin from the sun. It is also used in industrial applications to produce a white color in paints and plastics.

titer (tī'tĕr) [F. *titre,* standard]. Standard of strength per volume of a volumetric test solution.

t., agglutination. The highest dilution of a serum that will cause clumping or agglutination of the bacteria being tested.

titillation (tĭt"ĭl-ā'shŭn) [L. *titillatio,* a tickling]. 1. Act of tickling, as in the throat. 2. State of being tickled. 3. Sensation produced by tickling.

titrate (tī'trāt). To determine or estimate by titration.

titration (tī-trā'shŭn) [Fr. *titre,* a standard]. 1. Estimation of the concentration of a chemical solution by adding known amounts of standard reagents until alteration in color or electrical state occurs. 2. Determination of quantity of antibody in an antiserum.

titre. Titer.

titrimetric (tī"trĭ-mĕt'rĭk) [" + Gr. *metron,* a measure]. Employing the process of titration.

titrimetry (tī-trĭm'ĕ-trē) [*titration* + Gr. *metron,* measure]. To analyze something by using titration.

titubation (tĭt"ū-bā'shŭn) [L. *titubatio,* a staggering]. A staggering gait, seen in diseases of the cerebellum.

t., lingual. Stuttering, stammering.

Tl. Chem. symb. for thallium.

TLC. 1. *thin-layer chromatography.* SEE: *chromatography, thin-layer.* 2. *tender loving care.* The concept of administering medical and nursing care and attention to a patient in a kindly, compassionate, and humane manner as distinguished from a cold technical approach. This is particularly important in intensive care units where patients are dependent on electronic monitors and devices for their care. 3. *total lung capacity.*

T.L.R. *tonic labyrinthine reflex.*

Tm. 1. Chem. symb. for thulium. 2. Symb. for maximal tubular excretory capacity of the kidneys.

Tn. Symb. for normal intraocular tension.

TNM classification. Method of classifying malignant tumors with respect to primary *t*umor, involvement of regional lymph *n*odes, and presence or absence of *m*etastases. SEE: *cancer.*

TNT. *trinitrotoluene.*

TO. *old tuberculin* (also abbr. OT).

toadskin (tōd'skĭn). Condition characterized by excessive dryness, wrinkling, and scaling of skin sometimes seen in vitamin deficiencies. SEE: *phrynoderma.*

toadstool (tōd'stool). Any of various fungi with an umbrella-shaped cap; popularly a poisonous mushroom.

toadstool poisoning. Symptoms appear from a few minutes to 15 hours after ingestion, characterized by marked abdominal pain, vomiting, and intense diarrhea associated with blood and mucus. Profound weakness comes early and remains. Sometimes perspiration and lacrimation present and occasionally convulsions or coma.

F.A.: Absolute bedrest. Empty stomach and bowels promptly and completely with gastric lavage and quick-acting cathartic and enemas. Atropine is especially helpful and may be given by any route. Fluid, and sodium chloride and high carbohydrate intake should be maintained intravenously if required. Excitement, hypotension, convulsions, pain, and fever are treated symptomatically. Dialysis has been used in treating poisoning due to Amanita phalloides.

tobacco (tō-băk'ō) [Sp. *tabaco*]. Dried leaves

of Nicotiana tabacum and other species. It contains nicotine, pyridine, picoline, and collidin. Widely used in forms of cigars, cigarettes, pipe tobacco, snuff, and chewing. During its combustion, various products are given off, the most important being nicotine, q.v., and certain compounds that have an adverse effect on the lungs. For this reason, the use of tobacco products may be injurious to health.

tobramycin (tō″bră-mī′sĭn). USP. An antibiotic drug.

toco- [Gr. *tokos,* birth]. Prefix indicating a relationship to childbirth.

tocodynagraph (tō″kō-dī′nă-grăf) [″ + *dunamis,* power, + *graphein,* to write]. A device for measuring the intensity of uterine contractions.

tocodynamometer (tō″kō-dī″năm-ŏm′ĕ-tĕr) [″ + *dunamis,* power, + *metron,* a measure]. Device for estimating force of uterine contractions in childbirth. SYN: *tocometer.*

tocograph (tŏk′ō-grăf) [″ + *graphein,* to write]. A device for estimating and recording the force of uterine contractions.

tocography (tō″kŏg′ră-fē). Recording the intensity of uterine contractions.

tocology (tō-kŏl′ō-jē) [″ + *logos,* science]. Science of parturition and obstetrics.

tocometer (tō-kŏm′ĕt-ĕr) [″ + *metron,* a measure]. Device for estimating force of contractions of the uterus during labor. SYN: *tocodynamometer.*

tocopherol (tō-kŏf′ĕr-ŏl) [″ + *pherein,* to carry, + L. *oleum,* oil]. Generic term for vitamin E (alpha tocopherol) and a number of chemically related compounds, most of which have the biological activity of vitamin E.

tocophobia (tō″kō-fō′bē-ă) [″ + *phobos,* fear]. Abnormal fear of childbirth.

tocus (tō′kŭs) [L.]. Parturition; childbirth.

toe (tō) [AS. *ta*]. A digit of the foot. SYN: *digit.* SEE: *foot* for illus.

RS: acroataxia; acrodynia; bunion; camptodactylia; clavus; corn; dactylus; gout; hallux; metatarsus.

t., claw. Hammertoe.

t., dislocations of. Treated essentially same as dislocations of the fingers. SEE: *finger, dislocation of.*

t.'s., fanning of. Spreading of toes, esp. when sole is stroked.

t., hammer. Condition of dorsal flexion of the first phalanx and plantar flexion of the second and third phalanges.

t., Morton's. Metatarsalgia.

t., pigeon. Walking with the toes turned inward.

t.'s, webbed. Toes joined by webs of skin.

toe clonus. Contraction of the big toe due to sudden extension of the first phalanx.

toe drop. Inability to lift the toes.

toenail (tō′nāl). Unguis.

toe reflex. Reflex where strong flexion of the great toe flexes all muscles below the knee.

Tofranil. Trade name for imipramine hydrochloride, USP.

Togaviridae [L. *toga,* coat, + *virus,* poison]. A family of arthropod-borne viruses comprising the genera Alphavirus (arbovirus group A) and Flavivirus (arbovirus group B) of importance in humans. These viruses cause a great number of diseases characterized by symptoms such as encephalitis, headache, hepatitis, and myalgia. These diseases are controlled by eradicating the arthropod vectors.

toilet (toy′lĕt) [Fr. *toilette,* a little cloth]. 1. Cleansing of a wound after operation, or cleansing of an obstetrical patient. 2. An apparatus for use during defecation and urination to collect and dispose of these waste products. The disposal may be immediate by flushing with water, by chemical digestion, or by incineration.

toilet training. Teaching the child to control urination and defecation until placed on a toilet. The bowel movements of an infant may establish the habit of occurring at the same time each day very early in life but it is not advisable to begin to train the child until the end of the second year. Close to that time, placing the child on a small potty chair for a short period of time at regular intervals may allow the child to stay dry. First the diapers are removed while the child is awake. Later they are removed during naps and the child is told he or she should be able to stay dry. This schedule may need to be interrupted for a period if the child does not remain dry. Later on there will be no need for diapers during the day or night. To protect the bed a rubber sheet should be used during the training period. Children who are unsuccessful in remaining dry or training their bowel habits should not be punished. To do this promotes the later development of enuresis or constipation.

toko-. Toco-, q.v.

tokodynagraph (tō″kō-dī′nă-grăf) [Gr. *tokos,* birth, + *dunamis,* power, + *graphein,* to write]. Tocodynagraph, q.v.

tolazamide (tŏl-ăz′ă-mīd). USP. An oral hypoglycemia agent of the sulfonylurea class. Trade name is Tolinase.

CAUTION: This drug should be used only in patients with diabetes of the insulin-independent type who cannot be treated with diet alone and who are unwilling or unable to take insulin if weight reduction and dietary control fail.

tolazoline hydrochloride (tŏl-ăz′ō-lēn). USP. An α-adrenergic blocking agent used to produce peripheral vasodilation. Trade name is Priscoline Hydrochloride.

tolbutamide (tŏl-bū′tă-mīd). USP. An oral

hypoglycemic agent of the sulfonylurea class. Trade name is Orinase.

CAUTION: This drug should be used only in patients with diabetes of the insulin-independent type who cannot be treated with diet alone and who are unwilling or unable to take insulin if weight reduction and dietary control fail.

Tolectin. Trade name for tolmetin sodium.

tolerance (tŏl′ĕr-ăns) [L. *tolerantia,* tolerance]. Capacity for enduring a large amount of a substance (food, drug, or poison) without an adverse effect and to show a decreased sensitivity to subsequent doses of the same substance.

t., drug. Progressive decrease in effectiveness of a drug.

t., exercise. The amount of physical activity that can be done before exhaustion under supervision.

t., glucose. The ability of the body to absorb and utilize glucose. SEE: *glucose tolerance test.*

t., immunologic. A state of immunologic inactivity or diminution so that an antigen that would ordinarily induce an immune response does not.

tolerant. Capable of enduring or withstanding drugs without experiencing ill-effects.

tolerogen (tŏl′ĕr-ō-jĕn). That which causes immunological tolerance or failure of the body to react to an antigen by forming an antibody. The mechanism of formation of this specific unresponsive state is poorly understood.

tolerogenic (tŏl″ĕr-ō-jĕn′ĭk). Producing immunological tolerance.

Toleron. Trade name for ferrous fumarate, USP.

Tolinase. Trade name for tolazamide, USP.

tollwut (tŏl-voot′) [Ger.]. Rabies.

tolnaftate (tŏl-năf′tāt). USP. A synthetic antifungal agent used topically in treating various forms of tinea. Trade name is Tinactin.

tolu balsam. USP. A balsam obtained from Myroxylon balsamum. It is used as an expectorant.

toluene. A hydrocarbon derived from coal tar.

toluene poisoning. SEE: *benzene* in *Poisons and Poisoning* in *Appendix.*

toluidine (tŏl-ū′ĭ-dĭn). Aminotoluene, $CH_3{\cdot}C_6H_4{\cdot}NH_2$, a derivative of toluene.

tomatine (tō′mă-tēn). A substance derived from tomato plants affected by wilt. It has antifungal action.

-tome [Gr. *tome,* incision]. Combining form meaning cutting, or cutting instrument.

tomo- [Gr. *tome,* incision]. A combining form indicating a section or layer.

tomogram (tō′mō-grăm) [″ + *gramma,* mark]. The x-ray picture obtained by use of tomography.

tomograph (tō′mō-grăf) [″ + *graphein,* to write]. A special type of x-ray apparatus that demonstrates the organ or tissue at a particular depth.

tomography (tō-mŏg′ră-fē). Any of several noninvasive special techniques of roentgenography designed to show detailed images of structures in a selected plane of tissue by blurring images of structures in all other planes.

t., computerized axial. ABBR: CAT. Tomography where transverse planes of tissue are swept by a pinpoint radiographic beam and a computerized analysis of the variance in absorption produces a precise reconstructed image of that area. This technique has a greater sensitivity in showing the relationship of structures than conventional radiography and has been used most successfully in diagnostic studies of the brain.

tomomania (tō″mō-mā′nē-ă) [Gr. *tome,* incision, + *mania,* madness]. 1. Tendency of a surgeon to resort to unnecessary surgical operations. 2. Abnormal desire to be operated upon.

-tomy. A word ending indicating a cutting or an incision.

tonaphasia (tō″nă-fā′sē-ă) [L. *tonus,* a stretching, + *a-,* not, + *phasis,* speech]. Inability to remember a tune due to cerebral lesion.

tone (tōn) [L. *tonus,* a stretching]. 1. That state of a body or any of its organs or parts in which the functions are healthy and normal. In a more restricted sense, the resistance of muscles to passive elongation or stretch. 2. Normal tension or responsiveness to stimuli, as of arteries or muscles, seen particularly in involuntary muscle (such as the sphincter of the urinary bladder). SYN: *tonicity.* 3. A musical or vocal sound.

t., muscular. Condition in which a muscle is in a steady state of contraction; the ability of a muscle to resist a force for a considerable period of time without change in length.

tone deafness. Inability to detect differences in musical sounds. SYN: *amusia.*

tongue (tŭng) [AS. *tunge*]. A freely movable muscular organ lying partly in the floor of the mouth and partly in the pharynx. Its function is manipulation of food in mastication and deglutition, speech production, and taste. Its surface is covered with mucous membrane. SYN: *lingua.* SEE: illus.

ANAT: The tongue consists of a body and root and is attached by muscles to the hyoid bone below, the mandible in front, the styloid process behind, and the palate above, and by mucous membrane to the floor of the mouth, the lateral walls of the pharynx, and the epiglottis. A median fold, the frenulum lin-

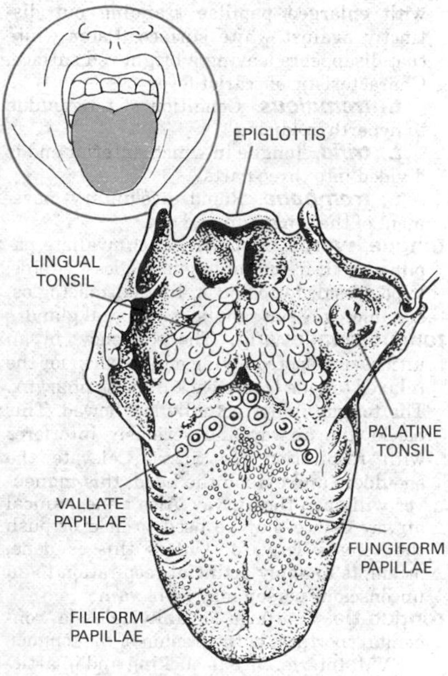

SURFACE OF TONGUE

guae, connects the tongue to the floor of the mouth. The surface of the tongue bears numerous papillae of three types: filiform, fungiform, and vallate. Taste buds are present on the surfaces of many of the papillae, esp. the vallate papillae. Mucous and serous glands (lingual glands) are present, their ducts opening on the surface. Lymphoid tissue comprising the lingual tonsils is present in the posterior third of the tongue. A median fibrous septum extends the entire length of the tongue.

Arteries: Lingual, exterior maxillary, and ascending pharyngeal. *Muscles:* Extrinsic muscles include genioglossus, hypoglossus, and styloglossus. Intrinsic muscles consist of four groups: superior, inferior, transverse, and vertical lingualis muscles. *Nerves:* Lingual nerve (containing fibers from trigeminal and facial nerves), glossopharyngeal, vagus, and hypoglossal.

DIFF. DIAG: *Pain:* Occurs in local lesions; fissures; glossitis; malignancies; and pernicious anemia. *Protrusion and movement:* This occurs with very sick patients, as in advanced typhoid fever and toxemia. The tongue is tremulous in early typhoid and in meningitis. In chorea it is thrust out suddenly and at once withdrawn. If it is protruded very slowly or if left exposed after being shown, it is a sign of great exhaustion, vascular congestion, or disorder of the nerve supply. If the tongue when protruded points to the right or left involuntarily then a central or peripheral lesion of the nerve supply is present. Some persons have the ability to curl the tongue along its long axis. This ability is genetically determined. *Thrust to one side:* Indicates hemiplegia if continually held in this position. *Scars:* These may be the result of injury or bulbar palsy causing ulceration and resulting in scars. *Sharp-pointed:* Observed in irritation and inflammation of the brain, smoker's tongue, leukoplakia. *Spasm:* Occurs in multiple sclerosis, general paresis, melancholia, and in stuttering. *Tremors:* Noted in asthenia, alcoholism, bulbar palsy, and Graves' disorder. In hemiplegia it is turned toward the paralyzed side if the face is affected. If turned toward the unaffected side, it denotes a lesion of the medulla. *Tremulous:* In all acute diseases but no particular significance in chronic nervous disorders.

Colored: The tongue may be temporarily discolored by a variety of colored medicines, foods, and liquids. *Black coating:* Glossophytia; may be due to stain or presence of microphytes. In dysentery, indicates exhaustion, mortification, death. In jaundice, denotes organic disease of liver. Onset of jaundice is usually first detectable in the yellowish discoloration of the area seen under the tongue when its tip is placed against the roof of the mouth. *Bluish:* Denotes impaired circulation, interference with respiration, heart disease, asthma, cyanosis. *Dark brown:* Addison's disease. *Black hairy:* SEE: *t., black hairy. Pale:* Indicates severe anemia; the tongue appears smaller than normal. *Red:* An early sign in typhoid fever. *Bright red:* Indicates glossitis or stomatitis. *Clean red:* With papillae prominent, or a white-coated tongue with papillae projecting through the fur, indicates scarlatina. *Red tip and edges,* or having red dry streak in center typical of typhoid. *Strawberry:* White fur through which project bright red and prominent papillae. Seen in early stage of scarlet fever. *Yellow:* With thick fur covering the tongue, indicates jaundice.

Macroglossia: large tongue, generally congenital, or may result from inflammation, Ludwig's angina, glossitis, actinomycosis, acromegaly, myxedema. If localized, may be due to gumma, carcinoma, or local trauma. *Microglossia:* small tongue, observed in anemia, emaciation, convalescence from typhoid. These conditions are temporary.

t., bifid. Tongue with a cleft at its anterior end. SYN: *t., forked.*

t., black hairy. Condition in which tongue possesses a brown furlike area on its dorsum.

The area is composed of hypertrophied filiform papillae pigment and possibly microorganisms. Sometimes results from excessive use of oxygen-liberating mouthwashes or antibiotic therapy. SYN: *lingua nigra*.

t., burning. Burning sensation of the tongue. SYN: *glossopyrosis*.

t., cleft. T., bifid.

t., coated. Tongue covered with layer of whitish or yellowish material consisting of desquamated epithelium, bacteria, or food debris. Significance is difficult to interpret. May mean only that patient slept with mouth open or has not eaten because of loss of appetite. If darkly coated, it may indicate a fungus infection.

t., deviation of. Marked turning of tongue from the midline when protruded. Indicative of lesions of the hypoglossal nerve.

t., dry. Tongue that is dry and shriveled, usually indicative of dehydration. May also be the result of mouth breathing.

t., fern-leaf. Tongue possessing a prominent central furrow and lateral branches.

t., filmy. Tongue possessing symmetrical whitish patches.

t., fissured. Tongue bearing deep furrows in its epithelium. May be normal. Causes are obscure. If deep and inflamed, may be due to syphilitic infection, dissecting glossitis, a broken tooth, chronic dysentery, hepatic disease, or diabetes mellitus.

t., forked. T., bifid.

t., furred. Coated tongue on which surface epithelium appears as a coat of white fur. Seen in nearly all fevers. Unilateral furring may result from disturbed innervation, as in condition affecting the 2nd and 3rd branches of the 5th nerve. Has been noted in neuralgia of those branches and in fractures of the skull involving the foramen rotundum. Yellow fur indicates jaundice.

t., geographic. Tongue possessing white raised areas resembling mountain ranges on a relief map. Areas consist of heaped-up epithelium surrounding areas of atrophy.

t., magenta. Magenta-colored tongue seen in cases of riboflavin deficiency.

t., parrot. A dry shriveled tongue, seen in typhus.

t., raspberry. T., strawberry, q.v.

t., scrotal. Furrowed and fissured tongue, resembling skin of scrotum. SEE: *t., fissured*.

t., smoker's. Condition of tongue characterized by white opaque patches of thickened epithelium later thickening and becoming fissured. SYN: *leukoplakia*.

t., smooth. Condition of tongue resulting from atrophy of papillae. Characteristic of many conditions such as anemia and malnutrition.

t., strawberry. Tongue that first has a white coat except at tip and along edges, with enlarged papillae standing out distinctly against white surface. Later white coat disappears leaving a bright red surface. Characteristic of scarlet fever.

t., tremulous. Condition of tongue due to hyperthyroidism.

t., trifid. Tongue in which anterior end is divided into three parts.

t., trombone. Rapid involuntary movement of the tongue in and out.

tongue, words pert. to:. circumvallate papillae; cleft; frenulum linguae; "gloss-" words; hypoglossal; hypoglottis; lingua; macroglossia; microglossia; ranula; sublingual gland.

tongue-swallowing. The tendency, in an unconscious person lying on the back, for the relaxed tongue to slip back into the pharynx. The tongue is not actually swallowed. This blocks the airway and seriously interferes with respiration. To correct, elevate the shoulders and extend the head; this maneuver will open the airway. Also a mechanical airway device may be used to hold or push the tongue forward. Unless this is done, attempts to apply artificial respiration to an unconscious person may be in vain.

tongue-tie. Lay term for ankyloglossia, congenital shortness of the frenum of the tongue.

SYM: Interference in sucking and in articulation.

TREATMENT: Minor surgery.

tonic (tŏn′ĭk) [Gr. *tonikos*, pert. to tone]. 1. Pert. to or characterized by tension or contraction, esp. muscular tension. 2. Restoring tone. 3. A medicine that increases strength and tone. They are subdivided according to action such as cardiac or general. Ex.: iron; digitalis.

tonicity (tō-nĭs′ĭ-tē) [Gr. *tonos*, tone]. 1. Property of possessing tone, esp. muscular tone. 2. State of normal tension or partial contraction of muscle fibers while at rest. SYN: *tone*.

tonic labyrinthine reflex. In animals, the postural reflex. In decerebrate humans, this reflex manifests as extension of the four extremities when the head is placed in the normal erect position.

tonic neck reflex. Reflex, tonic neck, q.v.

tonicoclonic (tŏn″ĭ-kō-klŏn′ĭk). Tonoclonic.

tonic spasm. A persistent, involuntary, firm or violent muscular contraction. SEE: *clonic spasm*.

tonoclonic (tŏn″ō-klŏn′ĭk) [″ + *klonos*, tumult]. Both tonic and clonic, said of muscular spasms.

tonofibril (tŏn′ō-fī″brĭl). Tenofibril, q.v.

tonofilament (tŏn″ō-fĭl′ă-mĕnt). A filament of a tonofibril.

tonogram (tō′nō-grăm) [″ + *gramma*, mark]. The record produced by a tonograph.

tonograph (tō'nō-grăf) [" + *graphein*, to write]. A recording tonometer.

tonography (tō-nŏg'ră-fē). The recording of changes in intraocular pressure.

tonometer (tōn-ŏm'ĕ-tĕr) [" + *metron*, a measure]. Instrument for measuring tension or pressure, esp. intraocular pressure.

tonometry (tōn-ŏm'ĕ-trē). The measurement of tension of a part, as intraocular tension. This test is extremely useful in detecting glaucoma.

t., digital. Determining intraocular pressure by use of the fingers.

t., non-contact. The intraocular pressure is determined by measuring the alteration in the cornea produced by a puff of air.

tonoplast (tŏn'ō-plăst) [" + *plassein*, to form]. The membrane surrounding an intracellular vacuole.

tonsil (tŏn'sĭl) [L. *tonsilla*, almond]. 1. A mass of lymphatic tissue located in depressions of the mucous membrane of fauces and pharynx. 2. A rounded mass on the inferior surface of the cerebellum lying lateral to the uvula.

FUNCT: Acts as a filter to protect body from invasion of bacteria, and aids in the formation of white cells.

t., cerebellar. One of a pair of cerebellar lobules on either side of the uvula, q.v., projecting from the inferior surface of the cerebellum.

t., faucial. T., palatine.

t., lingual. A mass of lymphoid tissue located in the root of the tongue.

t., Luschka's. T., pharyngeal.

t., nasal. Lymphoid tissue on the nasal septum.

t., palatine. A mass of lymphoid tissue that lies in tonsillar fossa on each side of oral pharynx between glossopalatine and pharyngopalatine arches. The free surface of each tonsil is covered with stratified squamous epithelium that forms deep indentations or crypts extending into the substance of the tonsil. The lateral surface of each tonsil is covered with a firm fibrous capsule. Efferent lymph vessels convey lymph from the tonsil. No afferent vessels are present.

t., pharyngeal. Lymphoid tissue on the roof of the posterior wall of the pharynx. SYN: *t., Luschka's*. SEE: *adenoid*.

t., tubal. Lymphatic tissue present in mucous membrane of the auditory tube near its opening into the pharynx.

tonsilla (tŏn-sĭl'ă) [L.]. General anatomic term for a small, discrete, rounded mass of tissue.

tonsillar (tŏn'sĭ-lăr). Pert. to a tonsil, esp. the faucial or palatine tonsil.

tonsillar area. Area composed of the palatine arch, tonsillar fossa, glossopalatine sulcus, and posterior faucial pillar.

tonsillar crypt. A deep indentation into the pharyngeal surface of a tonsil. It is lined with stratified epithelium.

tonsillar fossa. A depression between the glossopalatine and pharyngopalatine arches in which the palatine tonsil is situated.

tonsillar ring. The almost complete ring of tonsillar tissue encircling the pharynx. Includes the palatine, lingual, and pharyngeal tonsils.

tonsillar sinus. Space lying between the plica triangularis and the anterior surface of the palatine tonsil.

tonsillectomy (tŏn-sĭl-ĕk'tō-mē) [L. *tonsilla*, almond, + Gr. *ektome*, excision]. Surgical removal of the tonsils.

NURSING IMPLICATIONS: Until the patient is reactive after anesthesia, place patient in semiprone position to promote drainage; observe for bleeding. When patient is reactive, place in semi-Fowler's position. Monitor and record vital signs and assess for signs of shock, such as restlessness, extensive bleeding, tachycardia, and pallor. Give fluids and soft foods as tolerated. Instruct the patient to rest the throat by not speaking, coughing, or clearing the throat, as these may precipitate bleeding. Provide alkaline mouthwash to remove thick sputum. Apply ice pack to throat area, and administer analgesics as prescribed. Discharge instructions should include soft diet, avoidance of overactivity, and assessment for bleeding for one week.

tonsillith (tŏn'sĭ-lĭth) [" + Gr. *lithos*, stone]. Tonsillolith.

tonsillitis (tŏn-sĭl-ī'tĭs) [" + Gr. *itis*, inflammation]. Inflammation of a tonsil, esp. the faucial tonsil.

t., acute. Inflammation of the lymphatic tissue of the pharynx, esp. the palatine or faucial tonsils. May occur sporadically or in epidemic form. SEE: *rheumatic fever*.

ETIOL: May be caused by a variety of organisms. If due to group A beta-hemolytic streptococci, sequelae such as rheumatic fever, carditis, and nephritis must be considered.

SYM: Onset is sudden, usually accompanied by chills. Temperature may reach 105° F. (40.6° C.). Malaise; headache; pains and aches in back and extremities; pain in tonsils, esp. when swallowing, may be present. Tonsils appear enlarged and red with yellowish exudate projecting from crypts.

PROG: Usually self-limited but serious complications may occur such as sinusitis, otitis media, mastoiditis, or peritonsillar abscess

TREATMENT: *General:* Bedrest; liquid diet; antipyretics; hot saline or 30% glucose gargles or throat irrigations. *Specific:* Procaine penicillin or tetracycline drugs.

If the disease is thought to be due to group A beta-hemolytic streptococci, the throat should be cultured and then penicillin therapy instituted for a full ten-day course. If therapy was instituted prior to the report of the culture and the report is negative for these organisms, the penicillin therapy may be discontinued when clinical signs of infection have subsided.

If throat culture technique is not available and infection with group A beta-hemolytic streptococci is suspected, then a full ten-day course of penicillin should be given. This regimen will prevent the streptococci from elaborating the toxic substances that cause rheumatic fever, rheumatic heart disease, and certain kidney diseases. Administration of penicillin for less than ten days when tonsillitis is due to group A beta-hemolytic streptococci is not advisable, even though clinical signs of infection may disappear within the first several days of treatment.

t., follicular. Tonsillitis in which the crypts are affected.

t., parenchymatous, acute. Tonsillitis in which the entire tonsil is affected.

tonsilloadenoidectomy (tŏn″sĭl-ō-ăd″ĕ-noy-dĕk′tō-mē). Excision of the tonsils and adenoids of the pharynx.

tonsillolith (tŏn′sĭl-ō-lĭth) [″ + Gr. *lithos,* stone]. A concretion within a tonsil. SYN: *amygdalolith.*

tonsillopathy (tŏn″sĭ-lŏp′ă-thē). Any disease of the tonsil.

tonsilloscopy (tŏn″sĭl-lŏs′kō-pē) [″ + Gr. *skopein,* to examine]. Inspection of the tonsils.

tonsillotome (tŏn-sĭl′ō-tōm). Surgical instrument used in tonsillectomy.

tonsillotomy (tŏn″sĭl-ŏt′ō-mē) [″ + Gr. *tome,* incision]. Incision of the tonsils.

tonus (tō′nŭs) [L., tone]. That partial steady contraction of muscle which determines tonicity or firmness. Opposite of clonus. SYN: *tone; tonicity.*

tooth [AS. *toth*]. (pl. *teeth*) One of the conical hard structures used for mastication in the upper and lower jaws. A tooth consists of a crown or portion above the gum, a root, portion embedded in socket (alveolus) of jaw bones, and neck or cervix, constricted region between crown and root which is covered by the gum or gingiva. The major portion of a tooth consists of dentin, an ivorylike substance harder than bone, which surrounds the pulp cavity. A layer of enamel covers the crown and cementum covers the dentin of the root. A periodontal membrane surrounds the root and holds the tooth firmly in its socket. The pulp cavity contains dental pulp consisting of connective tissue, capillaries, lymph vessels, and nerve endings. SEE: illus.; *dentition; teeth;* words beginning with *odonto-.*

t., accessional. The third molar.

t., impacted. A tooth that fails to or is unable to erupt.

toothache. Pain in a tooth or the region about a tooth. SYN: *odontalgia; odontodynia.*

top-, topo-. Combining form meaning place or locale.

topagnosis (tŏp″ăg-nō′sĭs) [Gr. *topos,* place, + *a,* not, + *gnosis,* recognition]. Loss of ability to localize site of tactile sensations.

topalgia (tō-păl′jē-ă) [″ + *algos,* pain]. Pain in a localized site.

topectomy (tō-pĕk′tō-mē) [″ + *ektome,* excision]. A modified form of frontal lobotomy in which small incisions are made through the thalamofrontal tracts. A psychosurgical procedure used in the treatment of certain mental diseases.

topesthesia (tŏp″ĕs-thē′zē-ă) [″ + *aisthesis,* sensation]. Ability through tactile sense to determine any part that is touched. SYN: *topognosia.*

tophaceous (tō-fā′shŭs) [L. *tophaceus,* sandy]. 1. Relating to a tophus. 2. Sandy or gritty.

tophus (tō′fŭs) [L., porous stone]. (pl. *tophi*) 1. Deposit of sodium biurate in tissues near a joint, in the ear, or in bone in gout. 2. A salivary calculus. 3. Tartar on the teeth.

tophyperidrosis (tŏf″ĭ-pĕr″ĭ-drō′sĭs) [Gr. *topos,* place, + *hyper,* above, + *hidros,* perspiration]. Excessive sweating in local areas.

topical [Gr. *topos,* place]. Pert. to a definite area; local.

Topicort. Trade name for desoximetasone.

Topicycline. Trade name for tetracycline hydrochloride, USP.

topoalgia (tō″pō-ăl′jē-ă) [″ + *algos,* pain]. Localized pain; common in neurasthenia following emotional upsets.

topoanesthesia (tō″pō-ăn″ĕs-thē′zē-ă) [″ + *an-,* not, + *aisthesis,* sensation]. Loss of ability to recognize the location of a tactile sensation.

topognosia, topognosis (tō″pŏg-nō′sē-ă, -sĭs) [″ + *gnosis,* knowledge]. Recognition of the location of a tactile sensation. SYN: *topesthesia.*

topographic (tŏp″ō-grăf′ĭk) [″ + *graphein,* to write]. Pert. to description of special regions.

topographic anatomy. A study of all the structures and their relationships in a given region, for example, the axilla.

topography (tō-pŏg′ră-fē). Description of a part of the body.

topology (tō-pŏl′ō-jē). 1. Topographic anatomy, q.v. 2. In obstetrics, the relationship of the presenting fetal part to the pelvic outlet. 3. In mathematics, the study of the properties of geographic configurations, both solid and plane.

toponarcosis (tō″pō-năr-kō′sĭs) [″ + *narko-*

STRUCTURE OF TOOTH

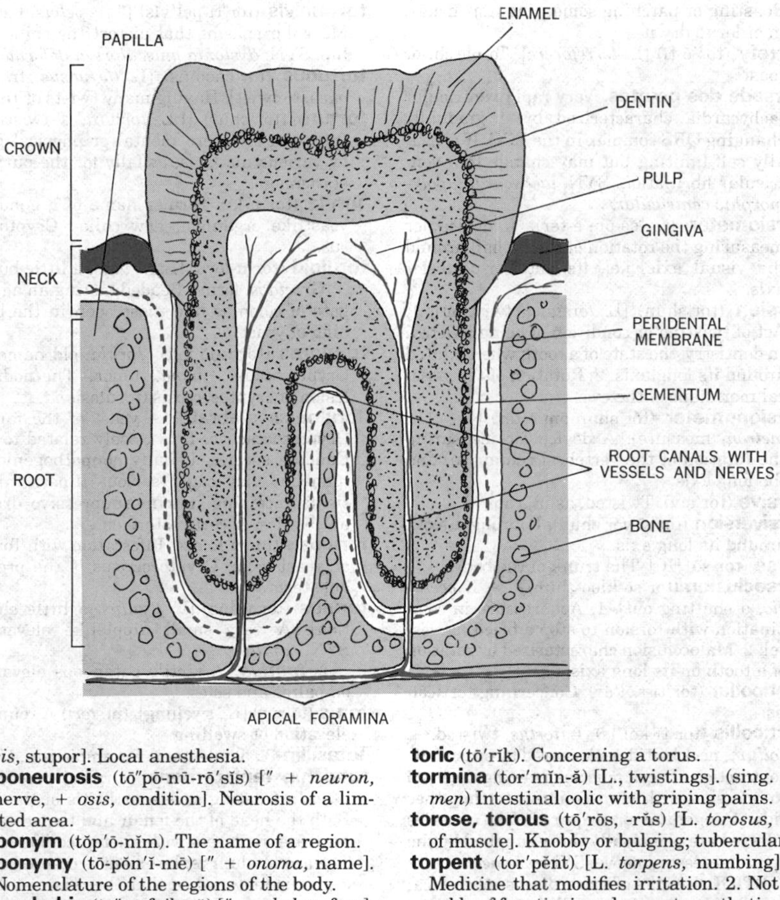

sis, stupor]. Local anesthesia.

toponeurosis (tō″pō-nū-rō′sĭs) [″ + *neuron,* nerve, + *osis,* condition]. Neurosis of a limited area.

toponym (tŏp′ō-nĭm). The name of a region.

toponymy (tō-pŏn′ĭ-mē) [″ + *onoma,* name]. Nomenclature of the regions of the body.

topophobia (tō″pō-fō′bē-ă) [″ + *phobos,* fear]. A fear of psychoneurotic origin in relation to a particular locality.

topothermesthesiometer (tŏp″ō-thĕr″ mĕs-thē-zē-ŏm′ĕ-ter) [″ + *therme,* heat, + *aisthesis,* sensation, + *metron,* measure]. Device for measuring local temperature sense.

TOPS. Acronym for an organization that assists obese persons to *T*ake *O*ff *P*ounds *S*ensibly.

Topsyn. Trade name for fluocinonide.

TOPV. *trivalent oral polio vaccine.* SEE: *poliovirus vaccine, trivalent oral.*

torcular Herophili (tor′kū-lăr). The confluence of sinuses at the internal occipital protuberance of the skull.

Torecan. Trade name for thiethylperazine.

toric (tō′rĭk). Concerning a torus.

tormina (tor′mĭn-ă) [L., twistings]. (sing. *tormen*) Intestinal colic with griping pains.

torose, torous (tō′rōs, -rŭs) [L. *torosus,* full of muscle]. Knobby or bulging; tubercular.

torpent (tor′pĕnt) [L. *torpens,* numbing]. 1. Medicine that modifies irritation. 2. Not capable of functioning; dormant, apathetic, torpid.

torpid (tor′pĭd) [L. *torpidus,* numb]. Not acting vigorously; sluggish.

torpidity (tor-pĭd′ĭ-tē). Sluggishness; inactivity.

torpor [L. *torpor,* numbness]. Abnormal inactivity; dormancy; numbness; apathy.

t. intestinorum. Constipation.

t. peristalticus. Atonic constipation.

t. retinae. Reduced sensitivity of retina to light stimuli.

torque (tork) [L. *torquere,* to twist]. A force producing rotary motion. In dentistry, applying force to rotate a tooth around its long axis.

torr (tor). The pressure of 1 mm. of mercury

under standard conditions of temperature and atmospheric pressure.

torrefaction (tor″ĕ-făk′shŭn) [L. *torrefactio*]. Roasting or parching something, esp. drugs, in order to dry it.

torrefy (tor′ĕ-fī) [L. *torrefacere*]. To parch, or roast.

Torsade des pointes. Very rapid ventricular tachycardia characterized by a gradually changing QRS complex in the ECG. It is usually self-limiting but may change into ventricular fibrillation. SYN: *tachycardia, polymorphic ventricular.*

torsiometer (tor″sē-ŏm′ĕ-tĕr). A device for measuring the rotation of the eyeball around the visual axis, i.e., its anterior-posterior axis.

torsion (tor′shŭn) [L. *torsio,* a twisting]. 1. Act of twisting or condition of being twisted. In dentistry, the state of a tooth when rotated around its long axis. 2. Rotation of the vertical meridians of the eye.

torsionometer (tor″shŭn-ŏm′ĕ-tĕr) [″ + Gr. *metron,* measure]. A device for measuring the rotation of the vertebral column around the long axis.

torsive (tor′sĭv). Twisted, as in a spiral.

torsiversion (tor″sĭ-vĕr′zhŭn). Rotating a tooth around its long axis.

torso (tor′sō) [It.]. The trunk of the body.

torsoclusion (tor″sō-kloo′zhŭn) [″ + L. *occlusio,* a shutting out]. 1. Acupressure in combination with torsion to stop a bleeding vessel. 2. Malocclusion characterized by rotation of a tooth on its long axis.

torticollar (tor″tĭ-kŏl′ăr). Concerning torticollis.

torticollis (tor″tĭ-kŏl′ĭs) [L. *tortus,* twisted, + *collum,* neck]. Stiff neck caused by spasmodic contraction of neck muscles drawing the head to one side with chin pointing to the other side. Congenital or acquired. The muscles affected are principally those supplied by the spinal accessory nerve. SYN: *wryneck.*

ETIOL: Results of scars; disease of cervical vertebrae; adenitis; tonsillitis; rheumatism; enlarged cervical glands; retropharyngeal abscess; cerebellar tumors. It may be spasmodic (clonic) or permanent (tonic). The latter type may be due to Pott's disease (tuberculosis of the spine).

t., fixed. Abnormal position of head due to organic shortening of the muscles.

t., intermittent. T., spasmodic.

t., ocular. Torticollis from inequality in sight of the two eyes.

t., rheumatic. T., symptomatic.

t., spasmodic. Torticollis with recurrent but transient contractions of muscles of the neck and esp. of the sternocleidomastoid. SYN: *t., intermittent.*

t., spurious. Torticollis from caries of the cervical vertebrae.

t., symptomatic. Rheumatic stiff neck. SYN: *t., rheumatic.*

tortipelvis (tor″tĭ-pĕl′vĭs) [″ + *pelvis,* basin]. Muscular spasms that distort the spine and hip. SYN: *dystonia musculorum deformans.*

tortuous (tor′choo-ŭs) [L. *tortuosus,* fr. *torqueo,* to twist]. Having many twists or turns.

torture (tor′chūr) [LL. *tortura,* a twisting]. Infliction of severe mental or physical pain by various methods, usually for the purpose of coercion.

Torula (tor′ū-lă). Former name of a genus of yeastlike organism, now called Cryptococcus.

toruloid (tor′ū-loyd) [L. *torulus,* a little bulge, + Gr. *eidos,* form]. Beaded; noting an aggregate of colonies like those seen in the budding of yeast.

toruloma (tor-ū-lō′mă) [*Torula,* old name for Cryptococcus, + *oma,* tumor]. The nodular lesion of cryptococcosis (torulosis).

Torulopsis glabrata. A yeast of the family Cryptococcaceae. It is closely related to the Candida species. Usually nonpathogenic for man but may cause serious illness in patients receiving immunosuppressive drugs, antibiotics, or corticosteroids.

torulosis (tor-ū-lō′sĭs). Infestation with Torula or yeast cells. Cryptococcosis is the preferable term.

torulus (tor′ū-lŭs) [L. *torulus,* a little elevation]. A very small nipplelike elevation. SYN: *papilla.*

t. tactilis. A tactile cutaneous elevation on palms and soles.

torus (tō′rŭs) [L., swelling]. (pl. *tori*) A rounded elevation or swelling.

Totacillin-N. Trade name for ampicillin, USP.

total hip replacement. Surgical procedure used in treating severe arthritis of the hip. Both the head of the femur and the acetabulum are replaced with metal components. The acetabulum replacement is covered with a plastic material so that there is metal-to-plastic contact rather than metal-to-metal. SEE: *arthroplasty.*

NURSING IMPLICATIONS: Preoperatively, establish a plan of instruction that includes mobility regimen, respiratory toiletry, exercises, hip abduction methods, and use of a bedpan or urinal in the recumbent position. Explain balanced suspension traction and use of the trapeze. Administer anticoagulants and prophylactic antibiotics as prescribed. Perform preoperative procedures and explain their significance, e.g., antiseptic skin scrub. Encourge the patient to express and discuss anxiety and apprehension.

Postoperatively, check dressings frequently for hemorrhage. Examine under the patient's buttocks for bleeding. Sterile technique during dressing changes is necessary to prevent postoperative infections. Monitor traction alignment daily at regular intervals. Turn patient frequently and position with pillows to maintain hip abduction. Assess nerve function and circulation frequently for the first 24 to 48 hours and then as patient status warrants. Start a quadriceps-setting exercise program in conjunction with the physical therapist. Observe the incision site for drainage and signs of infection. Prevent skin breakdown over bony prominences. Assess for complications such as thrombophlebitis, embolus, and dislocation. Apply elastic stockings as ordered. Avoid prolonged hip flexion by placing the patient in a recumbent position several times a day. Consult with the physician regarding the type and amount of exercise that can be done on the affected leg. Before ambulation, the extent of weight-bearing on the affected extremity must be determined. Leg crossing and internal rotation tend to enhance dislocation of the prosthesis; therefore, they should be avoided both in the hospital and after discharge. Discharge planning should include a progressive exercise regimen and discussion of activity limitations.

totipotency (tō″tē-pō′tĕn-sē) [L. *totus,* all, + *potentia,* power]. The ability of a cell to develop into a great number of different tissues.

totipotent (tō-tĭp′ō-tĕnt) [L. *totus,* all, + *potentia,* power]. A cell capable of differentiating into a large variety of cells. The fertilized ovum has this ability.

touch (tŭch) [O. Fr. *tochier*]. 1. To perceive by the tactile sense; to feel with the hands, to palpate. 2. The sense by which pressure on the skin or mucosa is perceived; the tactile sense. 3. Examination with the hand. SYN: *palpation.*

Various disorders may disturb or impair the tactile sense or the ability to feel normally. There are a number of words and suffixes pert. to sensation and its modifications, a few of the more important ones being listed as follows: algesia; -algia; anesthesia; dysesthesia; -dynia; esthesia; esthesioneurosis; hyperesthesia; paresthesia; synesthesia.

t., abdominal. Palpation of the abdomen. SEE: *abdominal examination.*

t., after. Persistence of the sensation of touch after contact with stimulus has ceased.

t., double. Vaginal and rectal examination made at the same time.

t., rectal. Digital examination of the rectum.

t., vaginal. Digital examination of the vagina.

t., vesical. Digital examination of the bladder.

touch, words pert. to: astereognosis; atopognosis; delire de toucher; hallucination; haptic; polyesthesia; stereognosis; tactile.

tour de maitre (toor″ dĕ mā-tr′) [Fr., the master's turn]. A method of introducing a catheter or sound into the male bladder or into the uterus. This involves very carefully turning and angulating the device so as to follow the curvature of the canal.

Tourette's syndrome, disorder. SEE: *Gilles de la Tourette's syndrome.*

Tournay's sign (tūr-nāz′). [Auguste Tournay, Fr. ophthalmologist] Dilatation of the pupil of the eye on unusually strong lateral fixation.

tourniquet (toor′nĭ-kĕt) [Fr., a turning instrument]. Any constrictor used on an extremity to apply pressure over an artery and thereby control bleeding; also used to distend veins to facilitate venipuncture or intravenous injections. Tourniquets are made more effective by placing a firm object such as a padded stone or a padded piece of wood over an artery to concentrate pressure at that point.

Arterial hemorrhage: Apply tourniquet between the wound and the heart, close to the wound, placing a hard pad over point of pressure. Should be discontinued as soon as possible and a tight bandage substituted under the loosened tourniquet.

Venous hemorrhage: Place tourniquet below bleeding point, but close to the wound. The tourniquet should remain in place with periodic momentary loosening until released by a physician.

CAUTION: Tourniquet should never be left in place too long. Ordinarily, it should be released from 12 to 18 minutes after application to determine whether bleeding has ceased. If it has, leave tourniquet loosely in place so that it may be retightened if necessary. If bleeding has not ceased, retighten at once. In general, a tourniquet should not be used if steady firm pressure over the bleeding site will stop the flow. SEE: *bleeding, arterial,* for Arrest of Arterial Bleeding table.

t., rotating. In certain types of medical emergencies such as acute pulmonary edema, it is essential to reduce the return of blood to the heart. This is accomplished by applying blood pressure cuffs to three extremities; the patient is placed in a head-high position (Fowler's). The pressure is kept midway between systolic and diastolic. Every 10 minutes the cuffs are deflated and when inflated, the previously free extremity is now used. This allows each extremity to be free of a tourniquet for 10 minutes out of each 40-minute cycle. Obviously, a cuff would not be applied to an extremity into which an intravenous infusion is running.

tourniquet paralysis. Injury to a nerve due

to a tourniquet's having been applied for too long a period or too tightly.

tourniquet test. Test for determining the ability of capillaries to withstand increased pressure.

Touton cells (toot'ŏn). [Karl Touton, Ger. dermatologist, b. 1858] Giant multinucleated cells found in lesions of xanthomatosis.

towelette (tow"ĕl-ĕt') [ME. *towelle,* towel]. A small towel for surgical or obstetrical use.

tox-, toxi-, toxo-. Combining forms indicating toxic, poison.

toxanemia (tŏks"ă-nē'mē-ă) [L. *toxicum,* poison, + Gr. *an-,* not, + *haima,* blood]. Anemia due to a hemolytic toxin.

toxemia (tŏks-ē'mē-ă) [" + Gr. *haima,* blood]. Distribution throughout the body of poisonous products of bacteria growing in a focal or local site, thus producing generalized symptoms.

SYM: Fever; diarrhea; vomiting; pulse and respiration quickened or depressed; shock. In tetanus, the nervous system is esp. affected; in diphtheria, nerves and muscles.

t., alimentary. Illness due to absorption of bacterial or other toxins from the gastrointestinal tract.

t., eclamptogenic. Toxemia of pregnancy. SEE: *eclampsia.*

t. of pregnancy. SEE: *eclampsia.*

toxenzyme (tŏks-ĕn'zīm) [" + Gr. *en,* in, + *zyme,* leaven]. A poisonous enzyme.

toxic (tŏks'ĭk) [L. *toxicum,* poison]. Pert. to, resembling or caused by poison. SYN: *poisonous.*

toxic-allergic syndrome. A disease characterized by toxic-allergic pneumonopathy, with respiratory distress, fever, headache, nausea, myalgia, abdominal pains, rash, hepatosplenomegaly, and eosinophilia.

ETIOL: Ingestion of rapeseed oil adulterated with aniline and containing acetanilide.

TREATMENT: There is no specific therapy, but mechanically assisted respiratory therapy and corticosteroids are helpful.

toxicant (tŏks'ĭ-kănt) [L. *toxicans,* poisoning]. 1. Poisonous; toxic. 2. Any poison.

toxicemic. Toxemic.

toxic erythema. Redness of skin or a rash resulting from toxic agents such as drugs.

toxicide (tŏks'ĭ-sīd) [L. *toxicum,* poison, + *cidus,* kill]. 1. Destructive to toxins. 2. A chemical antidote for poisons.

toxicity (tŏks-ĭs'ĭ-tē). The extent, quality, or degree of being poisonous.

toxico- [Gr. *toxikon,* poison]. Combining form meaning poisonous.

Toxicodendron (tŏk"sĭ-kō-dĕn'drŏn). A genus of plants that includes poison ivy and poison oak. Previously called Rhus.

toxicoderma (tŏks"ĭ-kō-dĕr'mă) [" + *derma,* skin]. Any skin disease resulting from a poison.

toxicodermatitis (tŏks"ĭ-kō-dĕrm-ă-tī'tĭs) [" + " + *itis,* inflammation]. Inflammation of the skin due to a poison.

toxicodermatosis (tŏks"ĭ-kō-dĕrm-ă-tō'sĭs) [" + " + *osis,* condition]. Toxicoderma.

toxicogenic (tŏks"ĭ-kō-jĕn'ĭk) [" + *gennan,* to produce]. Caused by, or producing, a poison.

toxicoid (tŏks'ĭ-koyd) [" + *eidos,* resemblance]. Of the nature of a poison.

toxicologist (tŏks"ĭ-kŏl'ō-jĭst) [" + *logos,* study]. A specialist in the field of poisons or toxins.

toxicology (tŏks"ĭ-kŏl'ō-jē). Division of medical and biological science concerned with toxic substances, detecting them, studying their chemistry and pharmacological actions, and establishing antidotes and treatment of toxic manifestations, prevention of poisoning, and methods for controlling exposure to harmful substances.

toxicomania (tŏks"ĭ-kō-mā'nē-ă) [" + *mania,* madness]. Abnormal craving for narcotics, intoxicants, or poisons.

toxicopathic (tŏks"ĭ-kō-păth'ĭk) [" + *pathos,* disease]. Pert. to any condition caused by a poison.

toxicopathy (tŏks"ĭ-kŏp'ă-thē) [" + *pathos,* disease]. Any disease caused by a poison.

toxicopexy (tŏk'sĭ-kō-pĕk"sē) [" + Gr. *pexis,* fixation]. Neutralization of a toxin or poison in the body.

toxicophidia (tŏk"sĭ-kō-fĭd'ē-ă) [" + Gr. *ophis,* snake]. Poisonous snakes. SYN: *thanatophidia.*

toxicophobia (tŏks"ĭ-kō-fō'bē-ă) [" + *phobos,* fear]. Abnormal fear of being poisoned by any medium: food, gas, water or drugs.

toxicosis (tŏks"ĭ-kō'sĭs) [" + *osis,* condition]. A diseased condition resulting from poisoning.

t., endogenic. Disease due to poisons generated within the body. SYN: *autointoxication.*

t., exogenic. Any toxic condition resulting from a poison not generated in the body.

t., retention. Toxicosis from retained products that normally are excreted as formed.

toxic shock syndrome. ABBR: TSS. A rare and sometimes fatal disease apparently caused by a toxin or toxins produced by certain strains of the bacterium Staphylococcus aureus. The diagnosis is made when the following criteria are met: Fever of 102° F. (38.9° C.) or greater; diffuse macular erythematous rash followed in one or two weeks by desquamation, particularly of the palms and soles; hypotension or orthostatic syncope; and involvement of three or more of the following organ systems: gastrointestinal (vomiting or diarrhea at onset of illness); muscular (severe myalgia); mucous membrane (vaginal, oropharyngeal, or conjunctival hyperemia);

renal; hepatic; hematologic (platelets less than 100,000/cubic millimeter); central nervous system (disorientation or alteration in consciousness without focal neurologic signs when fever and hypotension are absent). In addition, negative results on the following tests if obtained: blood, throat, or cerebrospinal fluid culture, but blood culture may be positive for Staphylococcus aureus; and no rise in titer to tests for Rocky Mountain spotted fever, leptospirosis, or rubeola.

The disease has occurred principally in young menstruating women, most of whom were using vaginal tampons for menstrual protection. The disease has been reported in increasing numbers in young boys, men, and non-menstruating women. The recurrence rate has been reported to be up to 30% but recurrences are usually milder than the original.

CAUTION: Anyone who develops these symptoms and signs should seek medical attention immediately and if a tampon is being used, it should be removed at once.

TREATMENT: Beta-lactamase-resistant antimicrobials and immediate therapy to combat shock and renal failure if present.

toxidermitis (tŏks″ĭ-dĕr-mī′tĭs) [″ + *derma,* skin, + *itis,* inflammation]. Any inflammatory skin disease due to poisoning. SYN: *toxicodermatitis.*

toxiferous (tŏks-ĭf′ĕr-ŭs) [″ + L. *ferre,* to carry]. Containing a poison. SYN: *poisonous.*

toxigenic (tŏks″ĭ-jĕn′ĭk) [″ + *gennan,* to produce]. Producing toxins or poisons.

toxigenicity (tŏks″ĭ-jĕn-ĭs′ĭ-tē). The virulence of a toxin-producing pathogenic organism.

toxignomic (tŏks″ĭg-nŏm′ĭk) [″ + *gnomikos,* knowing]. Having the toxic action peculiar to a poison.

toxin (tŏks′ĭn) [L. *toxicum,* poison]. A poisonous substance of animal or plant origin. SEE: *antitoxin; phytotoxin; toxoid.*

t., bacterial. Toxin produced by bacteria. Includes exotoxins, which diffuse from bacterial cells into surrounding medium, and endotoxins, which are liberated only when the bacterial cell is destroyed. SEE: *bacteria.*

t., botulinus. Toxin produced by Clostridium botulinum, the causative organism for botulism. Seven types of the toxin have been identified.

t., dermonecrotic. Any one of a group of different toxins that can cause necrosis of the skin. Coagulase-positive staphylococci aureus produce several such toxins. SEE: *Kawasaki disease; scalded skin syndrome; toxic shock syndrome.*

t., Dick. An erythrogenic toxin produced by some streptococci.

t., diphtheria. The specific toxin produced by Corynebacterium diphtheriae.

t., dysentery. The exotoxin of various species of Shigella.

t., erythrogenic. T., Dick, q.v.

t., extracellular. A toxin produced and excreted by microorganisms; an exotoxin, q.v.

t., fatigue. An alleged toxin present in the body due to muscular fatigue.

t., intracellular. A toxin produced in the bacterial cell, but retained therein; an endotoxin, q.v.

t., plant. Any toxin produced by a plant; a phytotoxin.

toxin-antitoxin (tŏks′ĭn-ăn″tĭ-tŏks′ĭn) [L. *toxicum,* poison, + Gr. *anti,* against, + L. *toxicum,* poison]. ABBR: T.A.T. Diphtheria toxin with its antitoxin in a nearly neutral mixture, the diphtheria toxin being about 85% neutralized. Used for immunization against diphtheria.

toxinicide (tŏks-ĭn′ĭs-ĭd) [″ + *cidus,* kill]. That which is destructive to toxins.

toxinology (tŏk″sĭn-ŏl′ō-jē) [″ + Gr. *logos,* study]. The branch of science concerned with toxins.

toxinosis (tŏk″sĭ-nō′sĭs) [″ + Gr. *osis,* condition]. Any disease or condition caused by a toxin.

toxipathic. Concerning toxipathy.

toxipathy (tŏks-ĭp′ă-thē) [″ + Gr. *pathos,* disease]. Any disease due to poison.

toxiphobia (tŏks″ĭ-fō′bē-ă) [″ + Gr. *phobos,* fear]. Abnormal fear of being poisoned.

toxisterol (tŏk-sĭs′tĕr-ŏl). Toxic derivative obtained by radiating ergosterol.

toxitabellae (tŏks″ĭ-tăb-ĕl′ē) [″ + *tabella,* tablet]. Poisonous tablets. Usually designated by having an angular shape or by having the word "poison" or the skull and crossbones symbol stamped upon them.

toxitherapy (tŏks″ĭ-thĕr′ă-pē) [″ + Gr. *therapeia,* treatment]. Use of toxins in treatment of disease.

toxituberculid (tŏks″ĭ-tū-bĕr′kū-lĭd). A skin lesion resulting from action of toxin of tuberculosis organism.

toxoalexin (tŏks″ō-ăl-ĕks′ĭn) [″ + *alexein,* to ward off]. An alexin that counteracts bacterial toxins.

toxocariasis (tŏks″ō-kăr-ī′ă-sĭs) [″ + *kara,* head, + *-iasis,* condition]. A self-limiting disease due to infection with nematode worms Toxocara canis or T. cati. In man, the eggs penetrate the bowel wall and enter the circulation. Larvae may be carried to any part of the body where the blood vessel is large enough to accommodate them. They may end up in the brain, retinal vessels, liver, lung, or heart. The larvae cause hemorrhage, inflammation, and necrosis in these tissues. Thus the patient may have myocarditis, endophthalmitis, epilepsy, or encephalitis. Diagnosis is made by immunological tests and by presence of larvae in tissue obtained by liver biopsy. It is important that toxocariasis be considered in cases diagnosed as retinoblastoma. SYN: *larva migrans, visceral.*

toxogenin (tŏks-ŏj'ĕn-ĭn) [Gr. *toxikon,* poison, + *gennan,* to produce]. Hypothetical substance in the blood caused by injection of antigens, innocuous in itself, but causing anaphylaxis upon addition of fresh antigen.

toxoid (tŏks'oyd) [" + *eidos,* form]. A toxin that has been treated to destroy its toxicity, but is still capable of inducing formation of antibodies on injection. SYN: *anatoxin.*

t., alum-precipitated. Toxoid of diphtheria or tetanus precipitated with potash alum.

t., diphtheria. Diphtheria toxin detoxified by formaldehyde treatment.

t., tetanus. Tetanus toxoid, q.v.

toxolecithin (tŏks"ō-lĕs'ĭ-thĭn) [" + *lekithos,* yolk of egg]. A compound of lecithin with a toxin such as certain snake venoms.

toxolysin (tŏks-ŏl'ĭ-sĭn) [" + *lysis,* dissolution]. Substance destroying toxins. SYN: *antitoxin; toxicide.*

toxomucin (tŏks"ō-mū'sĭn) [" + L. *mucus,* mucus]. Specific toxic albuminoid from cultures of tubercle bacilli.

toxonosis (tŏks"ō-nō'sĭs) [" + *osis,* condition]. A disease caused by poisoning. SYN: *toxicosis.*

toxopeptone (tŏks"ō-pĕp'tōn) [" + *pepton,* digesting]. A protein derivative produced by action of a toxin on peptones.

toxophil(e) (tŏks'ō-fĭl, -fīl) [" + *philein,* to love]. Having a special affinity for toxins.

toxophilic (tŏk"sō-fĭl'ĭk) [" + Gr. *philein,* to love]. Concerning a toxophile.

toxophore (tŏks'ō-for) [" + *phoros,* a bearer]. That portion of a toxin which gives to a toxin its poisonous qualities.

toxophore group. Poison-bearing group of a toxin.

toxophorous (tŏk-sŏf'ō-rŭs). Concerning a toxophore.

toxophylaxin (tŏks"ō-fī-lăks'ĭn) [" + *phylax,* guard]. A substance that neutralizes bacterial toxins.

Toxoplasma (tŏks"ō-plăs'mă). A genus of protozoa.

T. gondii. The causative agent of toxoplasmosis.

toxoplasmin (tŏk"sō-plăs'mĭn). An antigen obtained from mouse peritoneal fluid infected with Toxoplasma gondii.

toxoplasmosis (tŏks-ō-plăs-mō'sĭs). A disease due to infection with the protozoa Toxoplasma gondii. The organism is found in many mammals and birds. Symptoms may be so mild as to be barely noticeable or may be more severe with lymphadenopathy, malaise, muscle pain, and little if any fever. In the severe disseminated form, there are pneumonitis, hepatitis, and encephalitis. In the congenital form, destructive lesions of the central nervous system, jaundice, anemia, and generalized lymphadenopathy usually are present.

DIAG: By identification of culture of the organism and by serologic test.

TREATMENT: Even though treatment is not entirely satisfactory, pyrimethamine with triple sulfonamides and folinic acid is indicated.

T.P.I. test. *Treponema pallidum immobilizing test* (for syphilis).

TPN. 1. *triphosphopyridine nucleotide.* 2. *total parenteral nutrition.*

t.p.r. *temperature, pulse, respiration.*

tr. L. *tinctura,* tincture.

trabecula (tră-bĕk'ū-lă) [L., a little beam]. (pl. *trabeculae*) [NA] Fibrous cord of connective tissue that serves as supporting fiber by forming a septum that extends into an organ from its wall or capsule.

trabeculae carneae cordis. [NA] Thick muscular tissue bands attached to inner walls of the ventricles of the heart.

trabecular (tră-bĕk'ū-lăr). Concerning a trabecula.

trabecularism (tră-bĕk'ū-lăr-ĭzm). Condition of having a trabecular structure.

trabeculate (tră-bĕk'ū-lāt). Having trabeculae.

trabs (trăbz) [L., a beam]. (pl. *trabes*) A supporting band.

t. cerebri. Arched band of white fibers connecting the cerebral hemispheres. SYN: *corpus callosum* [NA].

trace (trās) [O. Fr. *tracier*]. 1. A very small quantity. 2. A visible mark or sign.

t., primitive. Pale white streak in germinal area indicating beginning of development of the blastoderm. SYN: *primitive streak.*

trace elements. Organic elements normally found in minute quantities in foods and tissues.

Ex.: aluminum, bromine, cobalt, copper, fluorine, manganese, nickel, silicon, zinc, and other physiologically rare minerals.

tracer. A radioactive isotope, capable of being incorporated into compounds, that when introduced into the body "tags" a specific portion of the molecule so that its course may be traced. Used in absorption and excretion studies, for identifying intermediary products of metabolism, and determination of distribution of various substances in the body. Radioactive carbon (^{14}C), calcium (^{42}Ca), and iodine (^{131}I) are examples of tracers commonly used.

trachea (trā'kē-ă) [Gr. *tracheia,* rough]. (pl. *tracheae*) [NA] A cylindrical cartilaginous tube, 4½ inches (11.3 cm.) long, from the larynx to the bronchial tubes. It extends from the 6th cervical to the 5th dorsal vertebra. Here it divides at a point called the carina into two bronchi, one leading to each lung. It is lined with mucous membrane and its inner surface is lined with ciliated epithelium. SYN: *windpipe*. SEE: *bronchi*.

tracheaectasy (trā″kē-ă-ĕk′tă-sē) [Gr. *tracheia*, trachea, + *ektasis*, dilatation]. Dilatation of the trachea.

tracheal (trā′kē-ăl). Pert. to the trachea.

tracheal tugging. Pulsation of the larynx or downward pull of the trachea, symptomatic of thoracic aneurysm.

trachealgia (trā″kē-ăl′jē-ă) [″ + *algos*, pain]. Pain in the trachea.

trachealis (trā″kē-ā′lĭs) [L.]. A muscle composed of smooth muscle fibers that extends between the ends of the tracheal rings. Its contraction reduces the size of the lumen.

tracheitis (trā″kē-ī′tĭs) [Gr. *tracheia*, trachea, + *itis*, inflammation]. An inflammation of the trachea. It may be acute or chronic and may be associated with bronchitis and laryngitis.

NURSING IMPLICATIONS: Promote bedrest to prevent pulmonary complications. Monitor and record pulse and temperature frequently. Place a cool vaporizer at the patient's bedside. Make sure an emergency tracheotomy tray is available in case of airway obstruction.

trachelagra (trā″kĕl-ăg′ră) [Gr. *trachelos*, neck, + *agra*, seizure]. Rheumatism or gout of neck muscles resulting in torticollis.

trachelectomopexy (trā″kē-lĕk′tŏm-ō-pĕk″sē) [″ + *ektome*, excision, + *pexis*, fixation]. Fixation of uterine neck with partial excision.

trachelectomy (trā″kĕl-ĕk′tō-mē) [″ + *ektome*, excision]. Amputation of the cervix uteri.

trachelematoma (trā″kĕl-ĕm″ă-tō′mă) [″ + *haima*, blood, + *oma*, tumor]. A hematoma situated on the neck.

trachelism, trachelismus (trā′kē-lĭzm, trā-kē-lĭz′mŭs) [″ + *-ismos*, condition]. Backward spasm of the neck, sometimes preceding an epileptic attack.

trachelitis (trā-kē-lī′tĭs) [″ + *itis*, inflammation]. Inflammation of mucous membrane of the cervix uteri. SYN: *cervicitis*.

trachelo- [Gr. *trachelos*]. Combining form, meaning neck.

trachelobregmatic (trā″kē-lō-brĕg-măt′ĭk) [″ + *bregma*, front of the head]. Pert. to the neck and the bregma.

trachelocele (trăk′ē-lō-sēl) [″ + *kele*, hernia]. Tracheocele.

trachelocyrtosis (trā″kē-lō-sĭr-tō′sĭs) [″ + *kyrtos*, curved, + *osis*, condition]. Trachelokyphosis.

trachelocystitis (trā″kĕl-ō-sĭs-tī′tĭs) [″ + *kystis*, bladder, + *itis*, inflammation]. Inflammation of the neck of the bladder.

trachelodynia (trā″kē-lō-dĭn′ē-ă) [″ + *odyne*, pain]. Pain in the neck.

trachelokyphosis (trā″kĕl-ō-kī-fō′sĭs) [″ + *kyphosis*, humpback]. Excessive anterior curvature of cervical portion of spine.

trachelology (trā″kē-lŏl′ō-jē) [″ + *logos*, study]. Scientific study of the neck, its diseases and injuries.

trachelomastoid (trā″kē-lō-măs′toyd) [″ + *mastos*, breast, + *eidos*, form]. A muscle of the neck. SEE: *Muscles* in *Appendix*.

trachelomyitis (trā″kē-lō-mī-ī′tĭs) [″ + *mys*, muscle, + *itis*, inflammation]. Inflammation of muscles of the neck.

trachelopexy (trā′kĕl-ō-pĕks″ē) [″ + *pexis*, fixation]. Surgical fixation of the cervix uteri to an adjacent part.

tracheloplasty (trā′kĕl-ō-plăs″tē) [″ + *plassein*, to form]. Surgical repair or plastic surgery of the neck of the uterus.

trachelorrhaphy (trā″kĕl-or′ă-fē) [″ + *rhaphe*, seam]. Suturing of a torn cervix uteri.

tracheloschisis (trā″kē-lŏs′kĭ-sĭs) [″ + *schisis*, fissure]. Congenital opening or fissure in the neck.

trachelotomy (trā″kĕl-ŏt′ō-mē) [″ + *tome*, incision]. Incision of the cervix of the uterus.

tracheo- [Gr. *tracheia*, rough]. Combining form meaning trachea or windpipe.

tracheoaerocele (trā″kē-ō-ā′ĕr-ō-sēl) [Gr. *tracheia*, trachea, + *aer*, air, + *kele*, hernia]. Hernia or cyst of trachea containing air.

tracheobronchial (trā″kē-ō-brŏng′kē-ăl). Concerning the trachea and bronchus.

tracheobronchomegaly (trā″kē-ō-brŏng″kō-mĕg′ă-lē). Congenitally enlarged size of the trachea and bronchi.

tracheobronchoscopy (trā″kē-ō-brŏng-kŏs′kō-pē) [″ + *bronkhos*, windpipe, + *skopein*, to examine]. Inspection of the trachea and bronchi through a bronchoscope.

tracheocele (trā′kē-ō-sēl) [″ + *kele*, hernia]. Protrusion of mucous membrane through the wall of the trachea.

tracheoesophageal (trā″kē-ō-ē-sŏf″ă-jē′ăl) [″ + *oisophagos*, esophagus]. Pert. to the trachea and esophagus.

tracheolaryngeal (trā″kē-ō-lăr-rĭn′jē-ăl). Concerning the trachea and larynx.

tracheolaryngotomy (trā″kē-ō-lăr″ĭn-gŏt′ō-mē) [″ + *larynx*, larynx, + *tome*, incision]. Incision into larynx and trachea.

tracheomalacia. Softening of the cartilage of the trachea.

tracheopathia, tracheopathy (trā″kē-ō-păth′ē-ă, -ŏp′ă-thē) [″ + *pathos*, disease]. Diseased condition of the trachea.

tracheopharyngeal (trā″kē-ō-făr-ĭn′jē-ăl) [″

+ *pharynx,* pharynx]. Pert. to both the trachea and pharynx.

tracheophonesia (trā″kē-ō-fōn-ē′zē-ă) [″ + *phonesis,* a sounding]. Cardiac auscultation at the sternal notch.

tracheophony (trā″kē-ŏf′ō-nē) [″ + *phone,* a sound]. Sound heard over the trachea in auscultation.

tracheoplasty (trā′kē-ō-plăs″tē) [″ + *plassein,* to form]. Plastic operation on the trachea.

tracheopyosis (trā″kē-ō-pī-ō′sĭs) [″ + *pyon,* pus, + *osis,* condition]. Tracheitis with suppuration.

tracheorrhagia (trā″kē-ō-rā′jē-ă) [Gr. *tracheia,* trachea, + *rhegnynai,* to burst forth]. Tracheal hemorrhage.

tracheoschisis (trā″kē-ŏs′kĭs-ĭs) [″ + *schisis,* a cleft]. Fissure of the trachea.

tracheoscopy (trā″kē-ŏs′kō-pē) [″ + *skopein,* to examine]. Inspection of interior of trachea, by means of reflected light.

tracheostenosis (trā″kē-ō-stĕn-ō′sĭs) [″ + *stenosis,* a narrowing]. Contraction or narrowing of lumen of the trachea.

tracheostoma (trā″kē-ŏs′tō-mă). Opening into the trachea, via the neck.

tracheostomize (trā″kē-ŏs′tō-mīz). To perform a tracheostomy.

tracheostomy (trā″kē-ŏs′tō-mē) [″ + *stoma,* opening]. Operation of incising the skin over the trachea and making a surgical wound in the trachea in order to permit an airway during tracheal obstruction.

NURSING IMPLICATIONS: Monitor vital signs frequently after surgery. Administer warmed, humidified oxygen. Place patient in semi-Fowler's position to enhance drainage and promote ease of breathing. Provide a restful environment. Establish range-of-motion exercises and physical therapy of the chest to promote aeration of the lung. Administer analgesics, antibiotics, and other prescribed medications. Monitor and record intake and output; provide adequate fluids and nutrition. Perform suctioning of secretions and tracheostomy care, q.v., as necessary. Change the dressing frequently during the first 24 hours postoperative, and observe for excessive bleeding. Encourage coughing and deep breathing at regular intervals. Establish a learning plan for the patient; this should include stoma care, consisting of cleansing, removing crusts, and filtering air with a suitable filter. Be alert for signs of infection. Instruct the patient to avoid crowds, to continue coughing and deep-breathing regimen, to take adequate fluids and nutrition, and to avoid smoking. Activities may gradually be increased to include non-contact sports, but should not include swimming. Showering may be permitted if the patient wears a protective plastic bib or uses the hand to cover the stoma. Reassure the patient that secretions will decrease and that taste and smell will gradually return. Stress the importance of follow-up care.

tracheostomy care. Suction as often as necessary to remove secretions. Before suctioning, aerate the patient well; this can be accomplished by using an Ambu bag attached to a source of oxygen. Maintain sterile technique throughout the procedure. Before suctioning, test the patency of the suction catheter by aspirating sterile normal saline through it. Insert the catheter without applying suction until the patient coughs. Apply suction intermittently and withdraw the catheter in a rotating motion. Assess the airway by auscultating the lungs; repeat suctioning procedure until the airway is clear. Each suctioning episode should take no longer than 15 seconds, and the patient should be allowed to rest and breathe between suctioning episodes. Cleanse the suction catheter with sterile normal saline solution and cleanse the oral cavity if necessary. The inner cannula should be cleansed or replaced after each aspiration. Metal cannulas should be cleansed with sterile water.

Keep an emergency tracheotomy set at the bedside at all times. Also keep a Kelly clamp at the bedside to hold open the tracheostomy site in an emergency. Cuffed tracheostomy tubes must be inflated if the patient is on positive-pressure ventilation unless ordered otherwise. In other cases, keep the cuff deflated if the patient has problems with aspiration. Using aseptic technique, change dressing and tape every 8 hours. Tracheostomies should always be covered with a dressing to prevent skin breakdown. To apply neck tapes, obtain two lengths of twill tape approx. 10 inches (25 cm.) long; fold the end of each and make a slit ½ inch (1.3 cm) long about 1 inch (2.5 cm.) from the fold; slip the slit end under the neck plate, and pull the other end of the tape through the slit; repeat for the other side; wrap the tape around the neck and secure it with a square knot on the side. Neck tapes should be left in place until new tapes are attached. Culture tracheal secretions every three days; observe and record their color, viscosity, amount, and abnormal odor, if any. Inspect site daily for bleeding, hematoma formation, subcutaneous emphysema, and signs of infection. Provide appropriate skin care. Help to alleviate the patient's anxiety and apprehension, and provide a communication process. Document patient response.

tracheotome (trā′kē-ō-tōm) [″ + *tome,* incision]. Instrument used in opening of the trachea.

tracheotomy (trā″kē-ŏt′ō-mē). Incision of the trachea through the skin and muscles of the neck overlying the trachea. SEE: *tracheostomy.*

trachitis (trā-kī′tĭs) [″ + *itis,* inflammation]. Inflammation of the trachea. SYN: *tracheitis.*

trachoma (trā-kō′mă) [Gr., roughness]. A chronic contagious form of conjunctivitis, noted by hypertrophy of conjunctiva and formation of follicles with subsequent cicatricial changes. The disease affects 400,000,000 people, mostly in Asia and Africa; but is also seen in the southwestern part of the United States. Approximately 20,000,000 persons have been blinded by this disease. SYN: *ophthalmia, Egyptian; conjunctivitis, granular.*

ETIOL: The causative agent was previously considered a virus but is now classified as a strain of Chlamydia trachomatis, an organism closely related to bacteria and rickettsia. Chlamydial organisms are responsible for psittacosis, inclusion conjunctivitis, lymphogranuloma venereum, and possibly catscratch fever. The disease is readily transmitted, esp. in early stages. Transmission occurs by direct contact with trachomatous material or indirectly through contaminated articles such as towels or handkerchiefs.

COMPLICATIONS: Pannus, ptosis, corneal ulcers.

SEQUELAE: Blindness; corneal opacities; ectropion; entropion; staphyloma; symblepharon; trichiasis.

TREATMENT: Tetracycline or erythromycin used topically or systemically is effective. Surgery may be necessary when lid deformities occur.

t., brawny. Trachoma with general lymphoid infiltration without granulation of the conjunctiva.

t. deformans. Vulvitis with cicatricial contractions.

t., diffuse. Trachoma with large granulations.

trachomatous (tră-kō′mă-tŭs). Concerning trachoma.

trachychromatic (trā″kĭ-krō-măt′ĭk) [Gr. *trachys,* rough, + *chroma,* color]. Pert. to a nucleus with very deeply staining chromatin.

trachyphonia (trā″kĭ-fō′nē-ă) [″ + *phone,* voice]. Roughness of the voice.

tracing (trā′sĭng). 1. A graphic record of some event that changes with time such as respiratory movements, electrical activity of the heart or brain. 2. In dentistry, a graphic display of movements of the mandible.

tract (trăkt) [L. *tractus,* extent]. 1. A course or pathway. 2. A group or bundle of nerve fibers within the spinal cord or brain that constitutes an anatomical and functional unit. SEE: *fasciculus.* 3. A group of organs or parts forming a continuous pathway.

t., afferent. T., ascending.

t., alimentary. The canal or passage from the mouth to the anus. SYN: *t., digestive.*

t., ascending. White fibers in the spinal cord that carry nerve impulses toward the brain. SYN: *t., afferent.*

t., biliary. SEE: *biliary tract.*

t., descending. Fibers in the spinal cord that carry nerve impulses from the brain.

t., digestive. T., alimentary.

t., dorsolateral. A spinal cord tract superficial to the tip of the dorsal horn. It is made up of short pain and temperature fibers that are processes of neurons having their cell bodies in the dorsal root ganglion. SYN: *Lissauer's tract.*

t., extrapyramidal. SEE: *system, extrapyramidal.*

t., gastrointestinal. The stomach and intestines.

t., genitourinary. The genital and urinary pathways.

t., iliotibial. A thickened area of fascia lata extending from the lateral condyle of the tibia to the iliac crest.

t., intestinal. The small and large intestines.

t., motor. Descending pathway that conveys motor impulses from the brain to lower portions of the spinal cord.

t., olfactory. A narrow white band that extends from the olfactory bulb to the anterior perforated substance of the brain.

t., optic. A band of fibers that extends from the optic chiasma to the lateral geniculate body of the thalamus. Some fibers of the tract continue on to the midbrain and hypothalamus.

t., pyramidal. Any of the columns of "motor" fibers in the spinal cord that are continuations of pyramids in the medulla.

t., respiratory. The respiratory organs in continuity.

t., rubrospinal. A descending tract of fibers arising from cell bodies located in red nucleus of the midbrain. Fibers terminate in gray matter of the spinal cord.

t., supraopticohypophyseal. A tract consisting of fibers arising from cell bodies located in supraoptic and paraventricular nuclei of the hypothalamus and terminating in the posterior lobe of the hypophysis.

t., urinary. The urinary passageway from kidney to the outside of the body. Includes the pelvis of the kidney, ureter, bladder, and urethra.

t., uveal. The vascular and pigmented tissues that comprise the middle coat of the eye. Included are the iris, ciliary body, and choroid.

tractellum (trăk-tĕl'ŭm) [L.]. An anterior flagellum of a protozoan. It propels the body by traction.

traction (trăk'shŭn) [L. *tractio*]. Process of drawing or pulling.

t., axis. Traction in line with the long axis of a course through which a body (fetus) is to be drawn.

t., elastic. Traction exerted by elastic devices such as rubber bands.

t., head. Traction applied to the head as in the treatment of injuries to cervical vertebrae.

t., weight. Traction exerted by means of weights.

tractor (trăk'tor) [L., drawer]. Any device or instrument for applying traction.

tractotomy (trăk-tŏt'ō-mē). Surgical section of a fiber tract of the central nervous system. Sometimes resorted to for relief of intractable pain.

tractus (trăk'tŭs) [L.]. (pl. *tractus*) A tract, q.v., or path.

tragacanth (trăg'ă-kănth) [Gr. *tragakantha,* a goat thorn]. The dried gummy exudation from the plant Astragalus gummifer and related species, grown in Asia. Used in the form of mucilage as a greaseless lubricant, and as an application for chapped skin.

tragal (trā'găl) [Gr. *tragos,* goat]. Relating to the tragus.

tragi (trā'jī). Pl. of tragus.

tragicus (trăj'ĭk-ŭs) [L.]. Muscle on the outer surface of the tragus. SEE: *Muscles* in *Appendix.*

tragion (trăj'ē-ŏn). An anthropometric point at the upper margin of the tragus of the ear.

tragomaschalia (trăg"ō-măs-kāl'ē-ă) [Gr. *tragos,* goat, + *maschale,* the armpit]. Odorous perspiration (bromidrosis) of the axilla.

tragophonia, tragophony (trăg"ō-fō'nē-ă, -ŏf'ŏ-nē) [" + *phone,* voice]. A bleating sound heard in auscultation at level of fluid in hydrothorax. SYN: *egophony.*

tragopodia (trăg"ō-pō'dē-ă) [" + *pous,* foot]. Knock-knee.

tragus (trā'gŭs) [Gr. *tragos,* goat]. (pl. *tragi*) [NA] Cartilaginous projection in front of the exterior meatus of the ear. SYN: *antilobium.*

train (trān). To participate in a special program of instruction in order to attain competence in a certain occupation or profession.

trainable (trān'ă-bl). 1. A mentally retarded individual who is capable of being trained. 2. To have the ability to be instructed and to learn from being taught. In classifying severity of mental retardation or brain damage it is important to know to what extent individuals may be trainable in various areas such as safety, personal care, or self-feeding.

training. An organized system of instruction.

t., assertive. A type of behavior modification therapy wherein the patient is taught to respond in a more positive and assertive manner to the normal stimuli encountered in daily activities. The goal is to have the patient become capable of expressing his or her true feelings, be they positive or negative. The use of role playing in group therapy may be used to teach this to patients.

trait (trāt). A distinguishing feature; a characteristic or property of an individual.

t., acquired. Trait that is not inherited; one resulting from effects of environment.

t., inherited. Trait due to genes transmitted through germ cells.

trajector (tră-jĕk'tor) [L. *trajectus,* thrown across]. Device for determining approximate location of a bullet in a wound.

Tral. Trade name for hexocyclium methylsulfate.

tramazoline hydrochloride (tră-măz'ō-lēn). An adrenergic drug.

trance (trăns) [L. *transitus,* a passing over]. A sleeplike state, as in deep hypnosis, appearing also in hysteria and in some spiritualistic mediums, with limited sensory and motor contact with the ordinary surroundings, and with subsequent amnesia of what has occurred during the state.

t., death. Trance simulating death.

t., induced. Trance caused by some external event such as hypnosis.

Trancopal. Trade name for chlormezanone.

tranquilizer (trăn"kwĭ-līz'ĕr) [L. *tranquillus,* calm]. A drug that acts to reduce mental tension and anxiety without interfering with normal mental activity. This ideal state of tranquilization is difficult to attain. Thus patients taking these medicines may find that their reactions are slowed. The use of tranquilizers has facilitated the treatment of severely disturbed psychiatric patients. Among the drugs in use are chlordiazepoxide (Librium), chlorpromazine (Thorazine), diazepam (Valium), meprobamate (Miltown, Equanil), promazine (Sparine), and reserpine (Serpasil).

Side effects, particularly from chlorpromazine and reserpine, have included jaundice, nausea, rashes, and in some surprising instances severe mental depression. The U.S. Public Health Service has warned of "a significant incidence of severe depression, with suicidal tendencies in some instances," in persons under heavy reserpine dosage.

CAUTION: Some tranquilizers may be injurious to the developing embryo. Therefore, prior to prescribing one, it is important to know whether it is approved for use during pregnancy, esp. during early pregnancy.

trans- [L.]. Prefix meaning across, over, beyond, through.

transabdominal (trăns″ăb-dŏm′ĭ-năl). Through or across the abdomen or abdominal wall.

transacetylation (trăns-ăs″ĕ-tĭl-ā′shŭn). Transfer of an acetyl group,

$$CH_3-\underset{\underset{O}{\|}}{C}-$$

in a chemical reaction.

transamidination (trăns-ăm″ĭ-dĭn-ā′shŭn). The transfer of an amidine group from one amino acid to another.

transaminase (trăns-ăm′ĭn-ās). An enzyme that catalyzes transamination.

t., glutamic-oxalacetic. ABBR: GOT, or SGOT for serum GOT. Enzyme present in the serum and body tissue; the highest concentration being in the heart and the liver. Tissue injury stimulates its release in the bloodstream and measurement of serum levels can indicate myocardial infarction or hepatic cell damage. Previously used name for aspartate aminotransferase, q.v.

t., glutamic-pyruvic. ABBR: GPT, or SGPT for serum GPT. Enzyme present in the serum and many tissues; the highest concentration is found in the liver. Injury of hepatic cells liberates the enzyme into the bloodstream. Thus measurement of the level in the serum (SGPT) provides a valuable test for hepatic cell injury. Previously used name for alanine aminotransferase, q.v.

transamination (trăns″ăm-ĭ-nā′shŭn). The transfer of an amino group from one compound to another or the transposition of an amino group within a single compound.

transanimation (trăns″ăn-ĭ-mā′shŭn) [L. *trans,* across, + *anima,* breath]. Resuscitation by mouth-to-mouth breathing. SEE: *artificial respiration.*

transaortic (trăns″ā-or′tĭk). Done through the aorta, e.g., a surgical procedure.

transatrial (trăns-ā′trē-ăl). Done through the atrium, e.g., a surgical procedure.

transaudient (trăns-aw′dē-ĕnt) [″ + *audire,* to hear]. Permeable to sound waves.

transaxial (trăns-ăk′sē-ăl). Across the long axis of a structure or part.

transcalent (trăns-kā′lĕnt) [″ + *calere,* to be hot]. Permeable by heat rays. SYN: *diathermal.*

transcapillary (trăns″kăp′ĭl-lă-rē) [″ + *capillaris,* relating to hair]. Across the endothelial wall of a capillary.

transcapillary exchange. The passage of substances between blood and tissue (interstitial) fluid.

transcervical (trăns-sĕr′vĭ-kăl). Done through the cervical os of the uterus.

transcortical (trăns-kor′tĭ-kăl). Joining two parts of the cerebral cortex.

transcortin (trăns-kor′tĭn). A corticosteroid-binding globulin.

transcriptase (trăns-krĭp′tās). A polymerase that performs transcription by converting a DNA base sequence into its complementary RNA base sequence.

transcription (trăn-skrĭp′shŭn). In synthesizing genes and proteins, the necessary process of duplication or copying of information from certain aspects of the chemical compound deoxyribonucleic acid (DNA). Messenger ribonucleic acid (mRNA) is synthesized by copying information from DNA and bringing that information to ribosomes, which are particles containing RNA.

transcutaneous electrical nerve stimulation (TENS). Application of mild electrical stimulation to skin electrodes placed over a painful area. This causes interference with transmission of painful stimuli.

transdermal infusion system. A method of delivering medicine by placing it in a special gel-like matrix that is applied to the skin. The medicine is absorbed through the skin at a fixed rate. Each application will provide medicine for from one to several days. Nitroglycerin and scopolamine are examples of medicines that have been prepared for use in this type of system.

transducer (trăns-dū′sĕr) [L. *trans,* across, + *ducere,* to lead]. A device that converts one form of energy to another. Used in medical electronics to receive the energy produced by sound or pressure and relay it as an electrical impulse to another transducer, which can either convert the energy back into its original form or make a record of it on a recording device. The telephone is an example of this.

transduction (trăns-dŭk′shŭn). A phenomenon causing genetic recombination in bacteria in which DNA is carried from one bacterium to another by bacteriophage. SEE: *transformation.*

transection (trăn-sĕk′shŭn) [″ + *sectio,* cutting]. A cutting made across a long axis; a cross section.

transfection (trans-fĕk′shŭn). The infection of bacteria by purified phage DNA after pretreatment with calcium ions or conversion to spheroplasts.

transfer, transference (trăns′fer, trăns-fĕr′ĕns) [″ + *ferre,* to bear]. 1. The mental process whereby a person transfers patterns of feelings and behavior that had previously been experienced with important figures such as parents or siblings to another person. Quite often these feelings are shifted to the psychiatrist. 2. State in which the symptoms of one area are transmitted to a similar area.

transferase (trăns′fĕr-ās). An enzyme that catalyzes the transfer of atoms or groups of atoms from one chemical compound to another.

transfer board. Device used to bridge the space between a wheelchair and a bed, toilet, or carseat. Used to facilitate independent or assisted transferring. Also: *sliding board.*

transfer factor. In immunology, a factor present in lymphocytes that have been sensitized to antigens, which can, in man, be transferred to a nonsensitized recipient. Thus the recipient will react to the same antigen that was originally used to sensitize the lymphocytes of the donor. In man the factor can be transferred by injecting the recipient with either intact lymphocytes or extracts of disrupted cells.

transferrin (trăns-fĕr′rĭn). A globulin in the blood that binds and transports iron.

transferring. The act of moving a person with limited function from one location to another. May be accomplished by the patient or with assistance.

transfix (trăns-fĭks′) [″ + *figere,* to fix]. To pierce through or impale with a sharp instrument.

transfixion (trăns-fĭk′shŭn). Maneuver in performing an amputation in which a knife is passed into the soft parts and cutting is from within outward.

transforation (trăns″for-ā′shŭn) [″ + *forare,* to pierce]. The perforation of the fetal skull at the base in craniotomy.

transforator (trăns′for-ā″tor). Instrument for perforating fetal skull.

transformation (trăns″for-mā′shŭn) [″ + *formatio,* a forming]. 1. Change of shape or form. SYN: *metamorphosis.* 2. In oncology, the change of one tissue into another. SEE: *metastasis.* 3. A type of mutation occurring in bacteria. It results from DNA of a bacterial cell penetrating the host cell and becoming incorporated into the genotype of the host.

transformer (trăns-form′er) [″ + *formare,* to form]. A stationary induction apparatus to change electrical energy at one voltage and current to electrical energy at another voltage and current through the medium of magnetic energy, without mechanical motion.

t., step-down. A transformer that changes electricity to a lower voltage.

t., step-up. A transformer that changes electricity to a higher voltage.

transfusion (trăns-fū′zhŭn) [″ + *fusio,* a pouring]. 1. The injection of blood or a blood component into the bloodstream. SEE: *blood transfusion.* 2. Injection of saline or other solutions into a vein for a therapeutic purpose.

t., cadaver blood. Transfusion using blood obtained from a cadaver within a short time after death.

t., direct. Transfer of blood directly from one person to another.

t., exchange. Transfusion and withdrawal of small amounts of blood repeated until blood volume is almost entirely exchanged. Used in infants born with hemolytic disease and in patients with uremia.

t., indirect. Transfusion of blood from a donor to a suitable storage container and then to the patient.

t., replacement. T., exchange.

t., single unit. Administration of a single unit of blood. In general it is believed that this is not indicated. However, attempts to regulate transfusion resulted in administration of two units, an amount not always necessary. Therefore the Committee on Blood of the A.M.A. proposed that the appropriate amount of blood always be administered.

transfusion reactions. A variety of reactions can occur as a result of blood transfusions. The most serious is the response of the recipient when incompatible blood is administered. In that case, massive intravascular clumping and lysis of red cells occur. Other causes of hemolytic reactions are: administering hemolyzed or fragile red blood cells due to the age of the blood or to its having been stored at an inappropriate temperature or having come in contact with incompatible I.V. solutions. If the reaction is severe, the patient will experience a bursting feeling in the head, face flushing, pain in the neck and lumbar area, vomiting, and shock. If the blood contains something to which the patient is allergic, then the symptoms of urticaria, edema, wheezing, and headache will be present. Infrequently, anaphylactic shock will occur. Some patients with compromised cardiovascular systems will experience heart failure, shock, pulmonary edema, and cyanosis if too much blood is administered. The transfusion should be stopped when these symptoms and signs appear. Such patients should not receive whole blood.

Prevention of these types of reactions is dependent upon meticulous attention to detail and accuracy in labeling the patient's blood sample for typing and cross-matching; doubly checking this at the time of transfusion; and starting the blood flow very slowly during the first 15 minutes and observing carefully for reactions. To prevent allergic reactions in persons with a history of allergies, an antihistamine may be administered orally or intramuscularly just before the transfusion is started.

transfusion syndrome, multiple. Development of hemorrhagic tendency caused by multiple transfusions with blood low in platelets and by increased fibrinolytic activity in the blood. SEE: *post-transfusion syndrome.*

TREATMENT: Transfuse with blood that is only a few hours old and give fibrinogen.

Transgrow. Proprietary name of a special medium for culturing Neisseria gonorrhoeae. The specimen may be placed in the medium and then shipped to the laboratory. The bacteria will remain viable even though they were not incubated while being transported.

transient ischemic attack. ABBR: TIA. Temporary interference with blood supply to the brain. The symptoms of neurological deficit may last for only a few moments or several hours. After the attack no evidence of residual brain damage or neurological damage remains. It is not necessarily true that individuals who have experienced transient ischemic attacks will within the predictable future develop a full vascular occlusion and have a stroke. SEE: *stroke.*

ETIOL: Insufficient blood flow to the brain due to decreased cardiac output, hypotension, overmedication with antihypertensive agents, or cerebrovascular spasm. Intravascular microembolization is suspected of causing some cases.

SYM: Usually abrupt onset of giddiness or light-headed sensation. The specific signs and symptoms will depend upon the portion of the brain affected. Thus, any one or a combination of several of the following may be present: fleeting monocular blindness, hemiparesis, hemiplegia, aphasia, astereognosis, dizziness, staggering, numbness, difficulty in swallowing, or paresthesias.

transiliac (trăns-ĭl′ē-ăk) [L. *trans,* across, + *iliacus,* pert. to a haunch bone]. Extending between the two ilia.

transilient (trăns-sĭl′ē-ĕnt). Jumping across or passing over as occurs when nerve fibers in the brain link nonadjacent convolutions.

transillumination (trăns″ĭl-lū″mĭ-nā′shŭn) [″ + *illuminare,* to enlighten]. Inspection of a cavity or organ by passing a light through its walls. When pus or lesion is present, the transmission of light is diminished or absent.

transinsular (trăns-ĭn′sū-lăr). Across the insula of the brain.

transischiac (trăns-ĭs′kē-ăk). Across or between the ischia of the pelvis.

transisthmian (trăns-ĭs′mē-ăn). Across an isthmus.

transition (trăn-zĭ′shŭn) [L. *transitio,* a going across]. Passage from one state or position to another, or from one part to another part.

transitional (trăn-zĭsh′ŭn-ăl). Marked by or relating to change.

translation (trăns-lā′shŭn) [L. *trans,* across, + *latus,* borne]. 1. The synthesis of proteins under the direction of ribonucleic acid. 2. To change to another place or to convert into another form.

translocation (trăns″lō-kā′shŭn) [″ + *locus,* place]. The alteration of a chromosome either by transfer of a portion of it to another chromosome or to another portion of the same chromosome. The latter is called shift or intrachange. When two chromosomes interchange material, it is called reciprocal translocation.

translucent (trăns-lū′sĕnt) [″ + *lucens,* shining]. Not transparent but permitting passage of light.

transmethylase (trăns-mĕth′ĭ-lās). Methyltransferase.

transmethylation (trăns″mĕth-ĭ-lā′shŭn). Process in the metabolism of amino acids in which a methyl group is transferred from one compound to another; for example, the conversion in the body of homocysteine to methionine. In this case the methyl group is furnished by choline or betaine.

transmigration (trănz″mī-grā′shŭn) [″ + *migratio,* migration]. Wandering across or through, especially the passage of white blood cells through capillary membranes into the tissues.

t., external. Transfer of an ovum from an ovary to an opposite tube through the pelvic cavity.

t., internal. Transfer of an ovum through the uterus to the opposite oviduct.

transmissible (trăns-mĭs′ă-bl) [L. *transmissio,* a sending across]. Capable of being carried from one person to another, as an infectious disease.

transmission (trăns-mĭsh′ŭn). Transfer of anything, as a disease or hereditary characteristics.

t., biological. Condition in which the organism that transmits the causative agent of a disease plays an essential role in the life history of a parasite or germ.

t., duplex. Passage of impulses through a nerve trunk in both directions.

t., mechanical. The passive transfer of causative agents of disease, esp. by arthropods. May be indirect, as when flies pick up organisms from excreta of a man or animals and deposit them on food, or direct, as when they pick up organisms from body of a diseased individual and directly inoculate them into body of another individual by bites or through open sores. SEE: *vector.*

t., neuromyal. The transmission of excitation from a motor neuron to a muscle fiber at a neuromyal (myoneural) junction.

t., placental. The transmission of substances in the mother's blood to the blood of the fetus by way of the placenta.

t., synaptic. The mechanism by which an impulse in one neuron gives rise to an impulse in another neuron.

t., transovarial. The transmission of causative agents of disease to offspring following invasion of ovary and infection of eggs. Occurs in ticks and mites.

transmural (trăns-mū'răl) [L. *trans,* across, + *murus,* wall]. Across the wall of an organ or structure, as in transmural myocardial thrombosis, in which the tissue in the entire thickness of a portion of the cardiac wall is affected.

transmutation (trăns"mū-tā'shŭn) [L. *transmutatio,* a changing across]. A transformation or change, as the evolutionary change of one species into another.

transocular (trăns-ŏk'ū-lăr) [" + *oculus,* eye]. Across the eye.

transonance (trăns'ō-năns) [L. *trans,* across + *sonans,* sounding]. Transmission of sounds through an organ, as heart sounds through the lungs and chest wall.

transorbital (trăns-or'bĭ-tăl) [" + *orbita,* track]. Passing through the orbit of the eye.

transovarial passage (trăns-ō-vā'rē-ăl). The passage of infectious or toxic agents into the ovary. A process that might invade and infect the oocytes.

transparent (trăns-păr'ĕnt) [" + *parere,* to appear]. 1. Transmitting light rays so that objects are visible through the substance. 2. Pervious to radiant energy. SEE: *clearing agent.*

transparietal (trăns"pă-rī'ĕ-tăl) [" + *paries,* wall]. Through a parietal region or wall.

transpeptidase (trăns-pĕp'tĭ-dās). An enzyme that catalyzes the transfer of a peptide from one compound to another.

transperitoneal (trăns"pĕr-ĭ-tō-nē'ăl). Across or through the peritoneum.

transphosphorylase (trăns-fŏs-for'ĭ-las). An enzyme that catalyzes the transfer of a phosphate group from one compound to another.

transphosphorylation (trăns-fŏs"for-ĭ-lā'shŭn). The exchange of phosphate groups from one compound to another.

transpirable (trăns-pī'ră-bl) [" + *spirare,* to exhale]. Permitting excretion through the skin or membranes, as perspiration.

transpiration (trăns"pī-rā'shŭn) [" + *spiratio,* exhalation]. 1. Act of exhaling water, gas, or vapor through the skin or a membrane. SEE: *perspiration.* 2. Substance exhaled.

t., cutaneous. Giving off sweat from pores of the skin. SYN: *perspiration.*

t., pulmonary. Escape of watery vapor from the blood to the air in the lungs.

transplacental (trăns"plă-sĕn'tăl). Through the placenta, esp. penetration of the placenta by a toxin, chemical, or organism that would affect the fetus.

transplant [" + *plantare,* to plant]. 1. (trăns-plănt') To transfer tissue or an organ from one part to another as in grafting or plastic surgery. 2. (trăns'plănt) A piece of tissue or organ used in transplantation, q.v.

transplantar (trăns-plăn'tăr) [" + *planta,* sole]. Across the sole of the foot.

transplantation (trăns"plăn-tā'shŭn). 1. The grafting of living tissue from its normal position or from another person to a similar tissue at another site. SEE: *autotransplantation; graft; replantation.* 2. In dentistry, the transfer of a tooth from one alveolus to another.

t., autoplastic. Transplantation of tissue from one part to another part of the same body. SYN: *t., homoplastic.*

t., heteroplastic. The transplantation of a part from one individual to another individual of the same or a closely related species.

t., heterotopic. Transplantation in which transplant is placed in a different location in host than it had in donor.

t., homoplastic. T., autoplastic.

t., homotopic. Transplantation in which transplant occupies the same location in the host as it had in the donor.

t., tenoplastic. Transplantation of tissue between individuals belonging to different genera.

transpleural (trăns-ploor'răl). Through the pleura.

transport. Movement or transfer of substances in a biological system, esp. movement of electrolytes, nutrients, and liquids across cell membranes. Transport may occur actively, passively, or with the assistance of a carrier.

t., active. Transfer of a substance across a membrane even though its concentration may be higher on the side toward which the movement is taking place.

transportation of the injured. *Carrying in arms:* Patient is picked up in both arms, as a child.

One-arm assist: Patient's arm is placed about neck of bearer and bearer's arm is placed about waist, thus assisting patient to walk.

Chair carry, chair stretcher: Any ordinary firm chair may be used. Patient is seated upon the tilted-back chair. One bearer grasps back of the chair and the other the legs of the chair (either the front or rear, depending on the construction of the chair). Both bearers face in the same direction. Patient's head rests either on chest or back of the head bearer.

Fireman's drag: Patient's wrists are crossed and tied with a belt or rope. Bearer kneels astride patient, with head under patient's wrists, and walks on all fours dragging patient beneath him.

Fireman's lift: Bearer grasps patient's left wrist with right hand; bearer's head is placed under patient's left armpit drawing patient's body over his left shoulder. Bearer's left arm should encircle both thighs, then lift patient. Patient's wrist is transferred to bearer's left hand, thus leaving one hand free to remove obstacles or to open doors.

Four-handed basket seat: Each of two bearers grasps own wrist and then grasps partner's free wrist. Patient sits upon this support.

Pack-strap carry: Patient is supported along bearer's back. Patient's right arm is brought over bearer's right shoulder and held by bearer's left hand. Left arm is brought over left shoulder and held by bearer's right hand. Patient is thus carried on the back with arms resembling pack straps.

Piggyback carry: Patient is supported along bearer's back with knees raised to sides of bearer's torso. This leaves patient practically in a sitting position astride bearer's back with arms around the bearer's neck or trunk.

Six- or eight-person carry: This is done as the three-person carry, q.v., except three or four bearers are on each side of patient, thus dividing weight more uniformly.

Three-handed basket seat: Bearer grasps own wrist, partner grasps the free wrist and leaves one arm free for supporting patient.

Three- or four-person carry: The litter-type carry used by emergency squads. Three persons kneel on one side of patient, place their hands under patient and lift up. The head bearer supports the patient's head and shoulders, center bearer lifts waist and hips, and third bearer lifts both lower extremities. A fourth person, if available, should help steady patient while patient is being lifted.

Two-handed seat: Bearers kneel on either side of patient. Each passes one arm around back (under armpits) and other arm under knees and lifts patient carefully in a sitting position.

Wheel chair, improvised: Fasten the legs of a chair, preferably with arms, to parallel boards and attach skates or casters to the bottom of the boards. A footrest can be made by attaching a broom handle or stick across the parallel boards in front of the chair.

Vehicles: If an ambulance is not available stretchers can be improvised with ropes and chairs, ladders or poles. The patient should always be tied to the stretcher during transportation. Several bearers will be necessary to assist entering and leaving the vehicle.

transposition (trănz″pō-zĭ′shŭn) [L. *trans,* across, + *positio,* a placing]. 1. A transfer of position from one spot to another. SYN: *metathesis.* 2. Displacement of an organ, esp. a viscus, to the opposite side. 3. Transplantation of a flap of tissue without severing it entirely from its original position until it has united in the new position.

transposition of great vessels. A fetal deformity of the heart in which the aorta arises from the right ventricle and the pulmonary artery arises from the left ventricle.

transposon (trănz-pō′zŏn). A genetic unit such as a DNA sequence that is transferred from one cell's genetic material to another.

transsection (trăns-sĕk′shŭn). Transection.

transsegmental (trăns″sĕg-mĕn′tăl) [″ + *segmentum,* a cutting]. Extending across or beyond a segment, as of a limb.

transseptal (trăns-sĕp′tăl) [″ + *saeptum,* partition]. Across a septum.

transsexual (trăns-sĕks′ū-ăl) [″ + *sexus,* sex]. 1. An individual who has an overwhelming desire to be the opposite sex. 2. An individual who has had his or her external sex changed by surgery.

transsexualism (trăns-sĕks′ū-ă-lĭzm). The condition of being of a certain definite sex, i.e., male or female, but feeling and acting as if a member of the opposite sex. In some instances the desire to alter this situation leads individuals to seek medical and surgical assistance in order to alter anatomical characteristics so that their anatomy would more nearly match their feelings about their true sexuality. The success of this therapy is controversial.

transsexual surgery. Surgical therapy for alteration of the anatomical sex of an individual whose psychological gender is not consistent with the anatomical sexual characteristics.

transsphenoidal (trăns″sfē-noy′dăl). Done through the sphenoid bone.

transtemporal (trăns-tĕm′pō-răl) [″ + *temporalis,* pert. to a temple]. Crossing the temporal lobe or the cerebrum.

transthalamic (trăns″thăl-ăm′ĭk) [″ + Gr. *thalamos,* chamber]. Passing across the optic thalamus.

transthermia (trăns-thĕr′mē-ă) [″ + Gr. *therme,* heat]. Production of heat in the deep tissues by electric currents. SYN: *diathermy; thermopenetration.*

transthoracic (trăns″thō-răs′ĭk) [″ + Gr. *thorax,* chest]. Across the thorax.

transthoracotomy (trăns″thō-ră-kŏt′ō-mē) [″ + Gr. *thorax,* chest, + *tome,* incision]. The operation of incising across the thorax.

transtympanic neurectomy. Surgical interruption of the parasympathetic nerve supply to the parotid and submandibular glands by bilateral sectioning of the tympanic and chorda tympani nerves. The technique is used in treating sialorrhea in mentally retarded children.

transubstantiation (trăn″sŭb-stăn″shē-a′shŭn) [″ + *substantia,* substance]. The process of replacing one tissue by another.

transudate (trăns′ū-dāt) [″ + *sudare,* to sweat]. The fluid that passes through a membrane, esp. that which passes through capillary walls. Compared to an exudate, q.v., a transudate has fewer cellular elements and is of a lower specific gravity.

transudation (trăns-ū-dā'shŭn). Oozing of a fluid through pores or interstices, as of a membrane.

transureteroureterostomy (trăns"ū-rē"tĕr-ō-ū-rē"tĕr-ŏs'tō-mē). Section of one ureter and joining both ends to the opposite ureter.

transurethral (trăns"ū-rē'thrăl) [" + Gr. *ourethra,* urethra]. Pert. to an operation performed through the urethra.

transvaginal (trăns-văj'ĭn-ăl) [" + *vagina,* sheath]. Through the vagina or across its wall as in a surgical procedure.

transvector (trăns-vĕk'tor). An animal that transmits a toxin that it does not produce and by which it is itself unaffected, i.e., as is the case when a bivalve mollusc, such as the oyster, filters viruses out of the water and transmits them to those who ingest the mollusc.

transversalis (trăns"vĕr-să'lĭs) [" + *vertere,* to turn]. A structure occurring at right angles to the long axis of the body.

transversalis fascia. A thin membrane forming the peritoneal surface of the transversus muscle and its aponeurosis.

transverse (trăns-vĕrs') [L. *transversus*]. Lying at right angles to the long axis of the body; crosswise.

transversectomy (trăns"vĕr-sĕk'tō-mē) [" + Gr. *ektome,* excision]. Excision of a transverse vertebral process.

transverse foramen. Canal in each transverse process of a cervical vertebra for the arteries and veins.

transverse plane. Plane that divides the body into a top and bottom portion.

transversion (trăns-vĕr'zhŭn). The eruption of a tooth at the site of another tooth. The end result is that the two teeth are transposed.

transversocostal (trăns-vĕr"sō-kŏs'tăl). Costotransverse, q.v.

transversospinalis (trăns-vĕr"sō-spī-nā'lĭs) [L. *transversus,* turned across, + *spina,* thorn]. Semispinalis capitis, semispinalis cervicis. SEE: *Muscles* in *Appendix*.

transversourethralis (trăns-vĕr"sō-ū"rē-thrā'lĭs). The transverse fibers of the sphincter urethrae muscle.

transversus (trăns-vĕr'sŭs) [L.]. 1. Any of several small muscles. SEE: *Muscles* in *Appendix*. 2. Lying across the long axis of a part or organ.

transvesical (trăns-vĕs'ĭ-kăl). Across or through the bladder.

transvestism, transvestitism (trăns-vĕst'ĭzm, -ĭ-tĭzm) [L. *trans,* across, + *vestitus,* clothed, + Gr. *-ismos,* condition]. The desire to dress in the clothes of and be accepted as a member of the opposite sex. SEE: *eonism*.

transvestite (trăns-vĕs'tīt). An individual who practices transvestism.

Trantas' dots (trăn'tăs). [Alexios Trantas, Gr. ophthalmologist, b. 1867] Chalky concretions of the conjunctiva around the limbus. These are associated with vernal conjunctivitis.

Tranxene. Trade name for chlorazepate dipotassium.

tranylcypromine (trăn"ĭl-sī'prō-mēn). USP. An antidepressant drug. Trade name is Parnate.

trapeze bar. Triangular device suspended above a bed to facilitate transferring and positioning the patient. Also called *swivel trapeze bar*.

trapezial (tră-pē'zē-ăl). Concerning the trapezium.

trapeziform (tră-pĕz'ĭ-form). Shaped like a trapezoid.

trapeziometacarpal (tră-pē"zē-ō-mĕt"ă-kăr'păl). Concerning or connecting the trapezium and the metacarpus of the thumb.

trapezium (tră-pē'zē-ŭm) [Gr. *trapezion,* a little table]. 1. A four-sided, single-plane geometric figure in which none of the sides are parallel. 2. The os trapezium, the first bone on the radial side of the distal row of the bones of the wrist. It articulates with the base of the metacarpal bone of the thumb. SYN: *multangular bone, greater*.

trapezius (tră-pē'zē-ŭs). A flat, triangular muscle covering posterior surface of neck and shoulder. SEE: *Muscles* in *Appendix*.

trapezoid (trăp'ĕ-zoyd) [Gr. *trapezoeides,* table-shaped]. A four-sided figure having two parallel sides and two divergent sides.

trapezoid body. A bundle of transverse fibers in the ventral portion of tegmentum of pons. SYN: *corpus trapezoideum* [NA].

trapezoid bone. The second bone in the distal row of carpal bones. It lies between the greater multangular and capitate bones. SYN: *multangular bone, lesser*.

trapezoid ligament. The lateral portion of the coracoclavicular ligament.

trauma (traw'mă) [Gr. *trauma,* wound]. (pl. *traumata* or *traumas*) 1. A physical injury or wound caused by external force or violence. 2. An emotional or psychological shock that may produce disordered feelings or behavior.

t., birth. Injury to the fetus during the birthing process.

t., psychic. A painful emotional experience that may cause anxiety.

traumatic (traw-măt'ĭk) [Gr. *traumatikos*]. Caused by or relating to an injury.

traumatic fever. Fever following an injury.

traumatic psychosis. Psychosis resulting from physical injuries or emotional shock.

traumatism (traw'mă-tĭzm) [Gr. *traumatismos*]. Morbid condition of system due to an injury or wound.

traumato-. A combining form indicating a relationship to trauma.

traumatology (traw-mă-tŏl'ō-jē) [Gr. *trauma,* wound, + *logos,* study]. The branch of surgery dealing with wounds and their care.

traumatonesis (traw"mă-tō-nē'sĭs). Repair of a wound by use of sutures.

traumatopathy (traw"mă-tŏp'ă-thē) [" + *pathos,* disease]. Pathological state caused by trauma.

traumatophilia (traw"mă-tō-fĭl'ē-ă) [" + *philein,* to love]. The enjoyment of or unconscious desire to be traumatized, either mentally or physically. SEE: *masochism.*

traumatopnea (traw"mă-tŏp-nē'ă) [" + *pnoia,* breath]. Passage of air in and out of a wound in the chest wall.

traumatopyra (traw"mă-tō-pī'ră) [" + *pyr,* fever]. Fever caused by trauma.

traumatotherapy (traw"mă-tō-thĕr'ă-pē). Treatment of injury.

Travad. Trade name for barium sulfate, USP.

travail (tră-vāl'). The labor during childbirth.

Travase. Trade name for sutilains.

tray (trā). A flat surface with raised edges.

Treacher Collins syndrome. [Edward Treacher Collins, Brit. ophthalmologist, 1862–1919] Mandibulofacial dysostosis.

treacle (trē'kl) [Gr. *theriaka*]. A thick molasses-like residue that remains when sugar is refined.

treatment (trēt'mĕnt) [ME. *treten,* to handle]. 1. Medical, surgical, or psychiatric management of a patient. 2. Any specific procedure used for the cure or the amelioration of a disease or pathological condition. SEE: *therapy.*

t., active. Treatment directed specifically toward cure of a disease.

t., causal. Treatment directed toward removal of the cause of the disease.

t., conservative. 1. The withholding of administration of medicine or utilization of operative procedures until such procedures are clearly indicated. 2. In surgical cases, the preservation of the organ or part if at all possible with the least possible mutilation.

t., dietetic. Treatment of disease based on regulation of diet.

t., electric shock. Electroshock therapy, shock therapy, q.v.

t., empiric. Treatment based on observation and experience rather than having a scientific basis.

t., expectant. Relief of symptoms as they arise, i.e., not directed at the specific cause.

t., Kenny. Treatment of acute poliomyelitis by use of wet hot pack applications to the affected muscles. SEE: *Kenny treatment.*

t., palliative. Treatment designed for the relief of symptoms of the disease rather than curing the disease.

t., preventive. Treatment directed to prevention of disease.

t., rational. Treatment based on scientific principles.

t., shock. Shock therapy.

t., specific. Treatment directed to the cause of a disease.

t., starvation. 1. Treatment employed in which food is withheld as in cases of bacillary dysentery following hemorrhage. 2. The treatment of diabetes in which there are days of fasting followed by a restricted and carefully controlled diet.

t., supportive. Special measures employed to supplement specific therapy.

t., surgical. Treatment by means of operation.

t., symptomatic. Treatment directed toward constitutional symptoms such as pyrexia, shock, and pain.

treatment plan. In dentistry, the projected series and sequence of restorative procedures necessary to restore the oral health of the patient, based on oral diagnosis and a complete evaluation of the patient.

Trecator SC. Trade name for ethionamide, USP.

tree. A structure that resembles a tree.

t., bronchial. The right or left bronchus with its branches and their terminal arborizations.

t., tracheobronchial. The trachea, bronchi, and their branches.

trehala (trē-hă'lă). A sweet substance secreted by the insect Larinus maculatus.

trehalase (trē-hă'lās). An enzyme that hydrolyzes trehalose to form two molecules; D-glucose.

trehalose (trē-hă'lōs). A disaccharide of trehala, q.v. It is also present in certain fungi.

Trematoda (trĕm"ă-tō'dă) [Gr. *trematodes,* pierced]. A class of flatworms commonly called flukes belonging to the phylum Platyhelminthes. It includes two orders: Monogenea, which are external or semi-external parasites having direct development with no asexual multiplication, and Digenea, internal parasites with asexual generation in their life cycle. The Digenea usually require two or more hosts, the hosts alternating. SEE: *fluke.*

trematode (trĕm'ă-tōd). A fluke, a parasitic flatworm belonging to the class Trematoda. SEE: *cercaria; fluke.*

trematodiasis (trĕm"ă-tō-dī'ă-sĭs). Infestation with a trematode.

tremble (trĕm'bl) [O. Fr. *trembler*]. 1. An involuntary quivering or shaking. 2. To shiver, quiver, or shake.

trembles (trĕm'blz). A condition resulting from ingestion of plants such as snakeroot (Eupatorium urticaefolium) or jimmey weed (Aploppus heterophyllus). Common in domestic animals and may occur in humans as a result of ingesting the plants or more commonly from drinking milk or eating the meat of poisoned animals. Symptoms are weakness; anorexia; nausea and vomiting; prostration; and possibly death. In humans, the illness is called milk sickness.

tremelloid, tremellose (trĕm′ĕ-loyd, -lōs). Jelly-like.

tremetol (trĕm′ĕ-tŏl). A poisonous substance occurring in snakeroot, rayless goldenrod, and other plants that may cause trembles in animal or man. SEE: *trembles*.

Tremin. Trade name for trihexyphenidyl hydrochloride, USP.

tremogram (trĕm′ō-grăm) [L. *tremere,* to shake, + Gr. *gramma,* a mark]. Graphic representation made by a tremograph.

tremograph (trĕm′ō-grăf) [″ + Gr. *graphein,* to write]. Device for recording tremors.

tremolabile (trē″mō-lā′bl) [″ + *labilis,* unsteady]. Easily destroyed or inactivated by shaking; said of a ferment.

tremophobia (trē″mō-fō′bē-ă) [″ + Gr. *phobos,* fear]. Abnormal fear of trembling.

tremor (trĕm′or, trē′mor) [L. *tremor,* a shaking]. 1. A quivering, esp. continuous quivering of a convulsive nature. 2. An involuntary movement of a part or parts of the body resulting from alternate contractions of opposing muscles.

Tremors may be classified as involuntary, static, dynamic, kinetic, hereditary, and hysteric. Pathologic tremors are independent of the will. The trembling may be fine or coarse, rapid or slow, may appear on movement (intention tremor) or improve when the part is employed. Often due to organic disease; trembling may express an emotion (e.g., fear). SEE: *subsultus.*

t., alcoholic. The visible tremor exhibited by alcoholics.

t., coarse. Tremor in which oscillations are relatively slow.

t., continuous. Tremor that resembles tremors of paralysis agitans.

t., essential. A benign tremor, usually of the head, chin, outstretched hands, and occasionally in the voice, that needs to be differentiated from the tremor of parkinsonism. Essential tremor, which is made worse by anxiety or action, is usually eight to ten cycles per second and that of parkinsonism four to five. There is usually a family history of essential tremor but not in parkinsonism. The medicines that are effective in treating parkinsonism have no effect on essential tremor.

t., fibrillary. Tremor caused by consecutive contractions of separate muscular fibrillae rather than of a muscle or muscles.

t., fine. A rapid tremor.

t., flapping. Coarse tremor of a muscle group. The supported part momentarily loses its support and there is an attempt to regain the support. When seen in the outstretched arm and hand, the part flaps like a wing. Seen in hepatic coma and other diseases that cause encephalopathy. SYN: *asterixis.*

t., forced. Tremor continuing after voluntary motion has ceased.

t., Hunt's. A tremor associated with all voluntary movements. It is present in certain cerebellar lesions.

t., hysterical. A fine tremor occurring in hysteria. May be limited to one extremity or generalized.

t., intention. Tremor when voluntary motion is attempted.

t., intermittent. Tremor common to paralyzed muscles in hemiplegia when attempting voluntary movement.

t., muscular. Slight oscillating muscular contractions in rhythmical order.

t., physiologic. A transient tremor occurring in normal individuals, resulting from excessive physical exertion, excitement, hunger, fatigue, or other causes.

t., rest. Tremor present when the involved part is at rest but absent or diminished when active movements are attempted. SYN: *t., static.*

t., senile. A tremor occurring in old age.

t., static. T., rest.

t., volitional. Trembling of limbs or of body when making a voluntary effort. Seen in multiple sclerosis and other nervous diseases.

tremorgram (trĕm′or-grăm). Tremogram.

tremulor (trĕm′ū-lor). A device for administering vibratory massage.

tremulous (trĕm′ū-lŭs) [L. *tremulus*]. Trembling or shaking.

trench fever. A nonfatal, febrile disease of diverse signs, symptoms, and severity. Usually present are headache, malaise, pain, tenderness esp. in the shins, splenomegaly, and sometimes a transient macular rash. The causative organism Rickettsia quintana may be cultured from the blood. Even though man is the host for the organism, the disease is not directly transmitted from person to person. The body louse, Pediculus humanus humanus, is the intermediate host. It begins to excrete infectious feces five to twelve days after ingesting blood from an infected human.

TREATMENT: The causative organism is sensitive *in vitro* to antibiotics such as tetracyclines and chloramphenicol, but there is no evidence that they are clinically effective.

trench foot. A condition resembling frostbite

affecting feet of soldiers who are obliged to stand in cold water for long periods of time.

trench mouth. Painful pseudomembranous ulceration of the mucous membranes of the mouth and pharynx. SYN: *gingivitis, necrotizing ulcerative.*

trend [ME. *trenden,* to revolve]. The inclination to proceed in a certain direction or at a certain rate. Used to describe the prognosis or course of a symptom or disease.

Trendelenburg position (trĕn-dĕl'ĕn-bŭrg). [Friedrich Trendelenburg, Ger. surgeon, 1844–1925] Position where the patient's head is low and the body and legs are on an elevated and inclined plane. This may be accomplished by having the patient flat on a bed and elevating the foot of the bed. In this position, the abdominal organs are pushed up toward the chest by gravity. The foot of the bed may be elevated by resting upon blocks. This position is used in abdominal surgery. In treating shock, this position is usually used, but if there is an associated head injury, the head should not be kept lower than the trunk.

trepan (trē-păn') [Gr. *trypanon,* a borer]. 1. To perforate the skull with a trepan to relieve the brain from pressure. 2. An instrument resembling a carpenter's bit for incision of the skull. SYN: *trephine.*

trepanation (trĕp"ă-nā'shŭn) [L. *trepanatio*]. Surgery utilizing a trepan.

t., corneal. Keratoplasty.

trephination (trĕf"ĭn-ā'shŭn) [Fr. *trephine,* a bore]. Process of cutting out a piece of bone with the trephine.

trephine (trē-fīn'). 1. To perforate with a trephine. 2. A cylindrical saw for cutting circular piece of bone out of skull. SYN: *trepan.*

trephining. 1. The process of cutting bone with a trephine. 2. The removal of a piece of cornea for the relief of glaucoma.

trephocyte (trĕf'ō-sīt) [Gr. *trephein,* to feed, + *kytos,* cell]. Trophocyte, q.v.

trepidant (trĕp'ĭ-dănt) [L. *trepidans,* trembling]. Marked by tremor.

trepidatio (trĕp"ĭ-dā'shē-ō) [L.]. Trepidation.

t. cordis. Palpitation of the heart.

trepidation (trĕp"ĭ-dā'shŭn) [L. *trepidatio,* a trembling]. 1. Fear, anxiety. 2. Trembling movement, esp. when involuntary.

Treponema (trĕp"ō-nē'mă) [Gr. *trepein,* to turn, + *nema,* thread]. A genus of spirochetes, parasitic in man, with undulating or rigid bodies. They belong to the family Treponemataceae. SEE: *bacteria* for illus.

T. carateum. The causative agent of pinta, an infectious disease of the skin.

T. pallidum. Causative organism of syphilis. SYN: *Spirochaeta pallida.*

T. pertenue. Causative organisms of yaws (frambesia).

Treponemataceae (trĕp"ō-nē"mă-tā'sē-ē). A family of spiral organisms belonging to the order Spirochaetales. Includes the genera Borrelia, Leptospira, and Treponema.

treponematosis (trĕp"ō-nē-mă-tō'sĭs). Infection with Treponema.

treponeme (trĕp'ō-nēm). Any organism of the genus Treponema.

treponemiasis (trĕp"ō-nē-mī'ă-sĭs) [" + *nema,* thread, + *-iasis,* condition]. Infestation with Treponema.

treponemicidal (trĕp"ō-nē"mĭ-sī'dăl) [" + " + L. *cidus,* to kill]. Destructive to Treponema.

trepopnea (trĕp-ŏp'nē-ă) [" + *pnoia,* breath]. Condition of being able to breathe with less difficulty when in a certain position.

treppe (trĕp'ĕ) [Ger., staircase]. Increase in height of contractions when the heart or a muscle is stimulated rapidly at regular intervals. SYN: *staircase phenomenon.* SEE: *stress test.*

tresis (trē'sĭs) [Gr. *tresis,* perforation]. Perforation.

tretinoin (trĕt'ĭ-noyn). USP. All-transretinoic acid. It is a keratolytic agent used topically in treating acne. Trade name is Retin-A.

TRF. *thyrotropin releasing factor.*

TRH. *thyrotropin releasing hormone.*

tri- [Gr. *treis,* three]. Combining form meaning three.

triacetate (trī-ăs'ĕ-tāt). Any acetate that contains three acetic acid groups.

triacetin (trī-ăs'ĕ-tĭn). USP. An antifungal agent used topically. Trade name is Enzactin. Previously used name was glyceryl triacetate.

triacetyloleandomycin (trī-ăs"ĕ-tĭl-ō"lē-ăn"dō-mī'sĭn). Previously used name for troleandomycin.

triad (trī'ăd) [Gr. *trias,* group of three]. 1. Any three things having something in common. 2. A trivalent element. 3. Trivalent.

t., Hutchinson's. Syndrome characteristic of prenatal syphilis consisting of notched teeth, interstitial keratitis, and eighth-nerve deafness due to meningeal involvement.

triage (trē-ăzh') [Fr., sorting]. The screening and classification of sick, wounded, or injured persons during war or other disasters to determine priority needs for efficient use of medical and nursing manpower, equipment, and facilities. It is also done in emergency rooms and in acute care clinics to determine priority of treatment. Use of triage is essential if the maximum number of lives is to be saved during an emergency situation that produces many more sick and wounded than the available medical care facilities and personnel can possibly handle.

NURSING IMPLICATIONS: For each patient, the emergency room staff must obtain a brief history, perform a rapid physical assessment including vital signs, perform first aid if necessary, assist in determining the severity of illness, and transfer the patient to the appropriate place of care. The triage nurse must know the ABCs of triage and treat patients promptly and appropriately. The ABCs of triage are airway, bleeding, consciousness, digestive organs, excretory organs, and fractures. Reassess patients frequently, and alter prescribed care as necessary.

triakaidekaphobia (trī″ă-kī″dĕk-ă-fō′bē-ă) [Gr. *treis,* three, + *kai,* and, + *deka,* ten, + *phobos,* fear]. Superstition regarding the number 13. SYN: *triskaidekaphobia.*

triamcinolone (trī″ăm-sĭn′ō-lōn). USP. A synthetic glucosteroid drug. Trade names are Aristocort, Kenacort, and SK-Triamcinolone.

triamterene (trī-ăm′tĕr-ēn). USP. A diuretic drug of the potassium-sparing type. Trade name is Dyrenium.

triangle (trī′ăng-gl) [L. *triangulum*]. A figure or area formed by three angles and three sides.

t., anal. Triangle with its base between the two ischial tuberosities and its apex at the coccyx.

t., anterior, of neck. The space bounded by the middle line of the neck, the anterior border of the sternocleidomastoid muscle, and a line running along the lower border of the mandible and continued to the mastoid process of the occipital bone.

t., carotid, inferior. The space bounded by the middle line of the neck, the sternomastoid muscle, and the anterior belly of the omohyoid muscle. SYN: *t., muscular.*

t., carotid, superior. The space bounded by the anterior belly of the omohyoid muscle, the posterior belly of the digastricus muscle, and the sternomastoid muscle. SYN: *t., omohyoid.*

t., cephalic. A triangle on the anteroposterior plane of the skull formed by lines joining the occiput and forehead and chin, and a line uniting the occiput and the chin.

t., digastric. Triangular region of the neck. Its borders are the mandible, stylohyoid muscle, and the anterior belly of the digastric muscle. SYN: *trigonum submandibulare.*

t., facial. A triangle bounded by lines uniting the basion and the alveolar and nasal points, and one uniting the nasal and basion.

t., femoral. Triangle on the inner part of the thigh, bounded by sartorius and adductor longus muscles and above by the inguinal ligament. SYN: *t., inguinal; t., Scarpa's.*

t., frontal. A triangle bounded by the maximum frontal diameter and lines joining its extremities and the glabella.

t., Hesselbach's. The interval in the groin bounded by Poupart's ligament, the edge of the rectus muscle, and the deep epigastric artery.

t., inferior occipital. Area having the bimastoid diameter for its base and the inion for its apex.

t., inguinal. T., femoral.

t., Lesser's. Triangle bounded below by anterior and posterior bellies of the digastric muscle and above by the hypogastric nerve.

t., lumbocostoabdominal. The triangle bounded in front by the obliquus abdominis externus, above by the lower border of the serratus posticus inferior and the point of the 12th rib, behind by the outer edge of the erector spinae, and below by the obliquus abdominis internus.

t., muscular. T., carotid, inferior.

t., mylohyoid. The triangular space formed by the mylohyoid muscle and the two bellies of the digastric muscle.

t., occipital, of the neck. The triangle bounded by the sternocleidomastoid, the trapezius, and the omohyoid muscles.

t. of elbow. The area in front of the elbow bounded by the brachioradialis and the pronator teres muscles on the sides and the base is toward the humerus.

t. of necessity. T., carotid, inferior, q.v.

t. of Petit. The space above the hip bone between the exterior oblique muscle, the latissimus dorsi, and the interior oblique muscle.

t., omoclavicular. T., subclavian.

t., omohyoid. T., carotid, superior.

t., posterior cervical. The triangle bounded by the upper border of the clavicle, the posterior border of the sternocleidomastoid muscle, and the anterior border of the trapezius muscle.

t., pubourethral. A triangular space in the perineum bounded externally by the ischiocavernous muscle, internally by the bulbocavernous muscle, and posteriorly by the transversus perinei muscle.

t., Scarpa's. T., femoral.

t., subclavian. A triangular space bounded by the posterior belly of the omohyoid, the upper border of the clavicle, and the posterior margin of the sternocleidomastoid. SYN: *t., omoclavicular; t., supraclavicular.*

t., submandibular. The triangular region of the neck, bounded by the inferior border of the mandible, the stylohyoid muscle and the posterior belly of the digastric muscle, and the anterior belly of the digastric muscle; it is one of three triangles included in the anterior triangle of the neck. Formerly called submaxillary triangle.

t., suboccipital. Triangle bounded by the

obliquus inferior and superior muscles on two sides and the rectus capitis posterior major muscle on the third side. The floor contains the posterior arch of the atlas bone and the vertebral artery. It is covered by the semispinalis capitis muscle.

t., supraclavicular. T., subclavian.

t., suprameatal. Triangle slightly above and behind the exterior auditory meatus. It is bounded above by the root of the zygoma and anteriorly by the posterior wall of the exterior auditory meatus.

t., urogenital. Triangle with its base formed by a line between the two ischial tuberosities and its apex just below the symphysis pubis.

t., vesical. The triangular space at the base of the bladder. SYN: *trigone.*

triangular. Having three sides; shaped like a triangle.

triangular bandage. A bandage folded diagonally. When folded, the several thicknesses afford support. SEE: illus.

triangularis (trī-ăng″gū-lā′rĭs) [L.]. A muscle of the chin. SEE: *Muscles* in *Appendix.*

triangular ligament. One of two ligaments, right and left, connecting posterior portions of the right and left lobes of the liver with corresponding portions of the diaphragm.

triangular nucleus of Schwalbe. The chief or dorsal nucleus of the vestibular division of the 8th cranial nerve. Located in the pons and occupying most of the area acoustica of the rhomboid fossa.

Triatoma (trī-ăt′ō-mă). A genus of bloodsucking bugs belonging to the order Hemiptera, family Reduviidae. Commonly called cone-nosed bugs or assassin bugs. It includes the species T. braziliensis, T. dimidiata, T. infestans, T. protracta, T. recurva, T. rubida, and others. They are house-infesting pests and some species, especially T. infestans, serve to transmit Trypanosoma cruzi, causative agent of Chagas' disease.

triatomic (trī″ă-tŏm′ĭk). Composed of three atoms.

tribadism (trĭb′ăd-ĭzm) [Gr. *tribein,* to rub, + *-ismos,* condition]. A relationship in which women attempt to imitate heterosexual intercourse with each other.

tribasic (trī-bā′sĭk) [Gr. *treis,* three, + L. *basis,* base]. Composed of three replaceable hydrogen atoms.

tribasilar (trī-băs′ĭl-ăr) [″ + L. *basilaris,* base]. Having three bases.

tribasilar synostosis. Condition resulting from premature fusion of three skull bones—the occipital, sphenoid, and temporal. Results in arrested cerebral development and mental deficiency.

tribe (trīb) [L. *tribus,* division of the Roman people]. In taxonomy, an occasional subdivision of a family; often equal to or below subfamily and superior to genus.

tribology (trī-bŏl′ō-jē). Study of the effect of friction on the body, esp. the articulating joints.

triboluminescence (trī″bō-lū″mĭ-nĕs′ĕns) [Gr. *tribein,* to rub, + L. *lumen,* light, + O. Fr. *escence,* continuing]. Luminescence or sparks

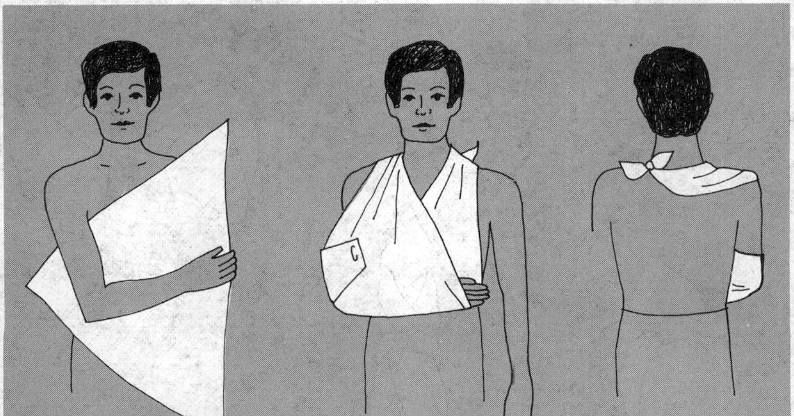

TRIANGULAR BANDAGE

STEPS IN MAKING SLING FOR ARM

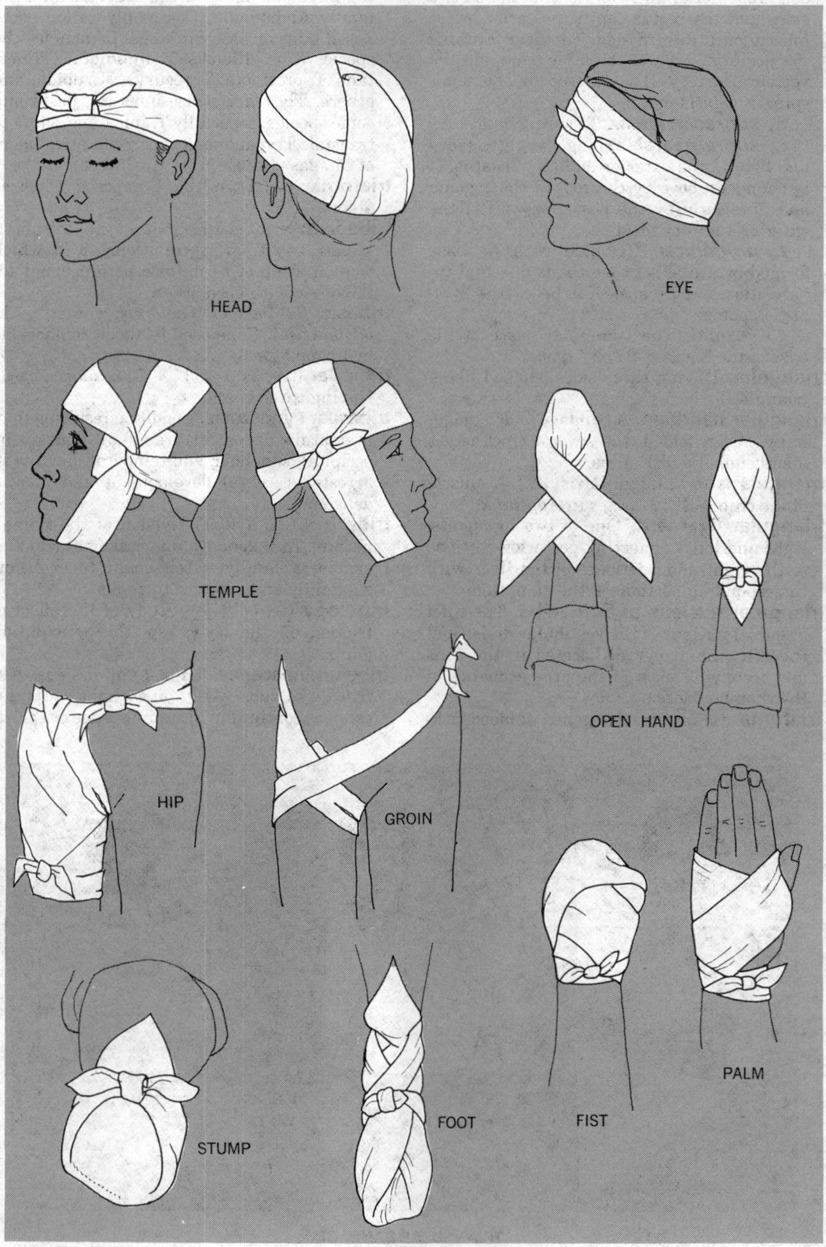

TRIANGULAR BANDAGES

produced by friction or mechanical force applied to certain chemicals. Has been observed when wintergreen mints are broken by the teeth in the dark.

tribrachia (trī-brā'kē-ă). Condition of having three arms.

tribrachius (trī-brā'kē-ŭs). Deformed fetus, usually conjoined twins, exhibiting three arms.

tribromide (trī-brō'mīd) [Gr. *treis,* three, + *bromos,* stench]. A compound having three atoms of bromine in the molecule.

tribromoethanol (trī-brō"mō-ĕth'ă-nŏl). A white crystalline substance that is used in anesthesia.

TRIC agents. Acronym for *tr*achoma and *in*clusion *c*onjunctivitis. SEE: *Chlamydia.*

tricarboxylic acid cycle. A complicated series of reactions in the body involving the oxidative metabolism of pyruvic acid and liberation of energy. It is the main pathway of terminal oxidation in the utilization of carbohydrates, fats, and proteins. SYN: *citric acid cycle; Krebs cycle.* SEE: *Krebs cycle* for illus.

tricellular (trī-sĕl'ū-lăr). Three-celled.

tricephalus (trī-sĕf'ă-lŭs) [Gr. *treis,* three, + *kephale,* head]. A deformed fetus having three heads.

triceps (trī'sĕps) [" + L. *caput,* head]. A muscle arising by three heads with a single insertion. SEE: *Muscles* in *Appendix.*

triceps reflex. Sharp extension of forearm resulting from tapping of triceps tendon while arm is held loosely in bent position.

Tricercomonas (trī"sĕr-cŏm-ō'năs). Genus of very small protozoa considered identical to Enteromonas. SEE: *Enteromonas hominis.*

trichangiectasia, trichangiectasis (trĭk"ăn-jē-ĕk-tā'zē-ă, -ĕk'tă-sĭs) [Gr. *thrix,* hair, + *angeion,* vessel, + *ektasis,* dilatation]. Dilatation of capillaries. SYN: *telangiectasia.*

trichatrophia (trĭk"ă-trō'fē-ă) [" + *atrophia,* atrophy]. Brittleness of hair resulting from atrophy of the root.

trichauxe, trichauxis (trĭk-awk'sē, -sĭs) [" + *auxe,* increase]. Excessive growth of hair. SYN: *hypertrichosis.*

trichi-, tricho- [Gr. *thrix*]. Combining forms meaning hair.

trichiasis (trĭk-ī'ă-sĭs) [Gr. *trichiasis,* hair condition]. Inversion of eyelashes so that they rub against the cornea, causing a continual irritation of the eyeball.

SYM: Photophobia, lacrimation, and feeling of foreign body in the eye.

TREATMENT: Epilation, electrolysis, and operation, such as correcting the underlying entropion with which this condition is usually associated.

trichilemmoma (trĭk"ĭ-lĕm-ō'mă). A benign tumor of the outer root sheath epithelium of a hair follicle.

Trichina (trĭk-ī'nă) [Gr. *trichinos,* of hair]. Trichinella, q.v.

trichina (trĭ-kī'nă). (pl. *trichinae*) A larval worm of the genus Trichinella.

Trichinella (trĭk"ĭ-nĕl'lă). A genus of nematode worms belonging to the suborder Trichurata. They are parasitic in humans, hogs, rats, and many other mammals.

T. spiralis. The species of Trichinella that commonly infests man, causing trichinosis. Infection occurs when raw or improperly cooked meat, particularly pork, containing cysts is eaten. Larvae encyst in the duodenum and invade mucosa of small intestine, becoming adults in five to seven days. After fertilization, each female deposits 1000 to 2000 living larvae, which enter blood or lymph vessels and are circulated to various parts of the body where they encyst in striated muscle. SEE: *trichinosis.*

trichinelliasis (trĭk"ĭ-nĕl-lī'ă-sĭs). Trichinosis.

trichinellosis (trĭk"ĭ-nĕl-lō'sĭs) [Gr. *trichinos,* of hair, + *osis,* condition]. Disease caused by Trichinella spiralis. SYN: *trichinosis.*

trichiniasis (trĭk"ĭ-nī'ă-sĭs). Trichinosis.

trichiniferous (trĭk"ĭ-nĭf'ĕr-ŭs) [" + L. *ferre,* to bear]. Containing trichinae.

trichinization (trĭk"ĭn-ĭ-zā'shŭn). Infestation with trichinae.

trichinophobia (trĭk"ĭn-ō-fō'bē-ă) [Gr. *trichinos,* of hair, + *phobos,* fear]. Abnormal fear of developing trichinosis.

trichinosis (trĭk"ĭn-ō'sĭs) [" + *osis,* condition]. Disease caused by the ingestion of Trichinella spiralis into the system through eating raw or insufficiently cooked pork.

SYM: Sometimes lacking. When large numbers have been ingested, gastrointestinal symptoms develop in a few days. These are pain, nausea, vomiting, and serous diarrhea. In one to two weeks muscular symptoms develop. Muscles become swollen, firm, and extremely painful. Movement is inhibited and dyspnea results from involvement of respiratory muscles. Edema, esp. of the face, is a prominent symptom. Profuse sweating is observed sometimes and high fever is usually present. Blood shows an eosinophilia.

In the third to sixth week of the disease, signs and symptoms of encephalitis and meningitis with visual and auditory symptoms may develop.

PROG: Depends on number of worms ingested. Majority of patients recover.

TREATMENT: For acute stage, thiabendazole may be helpful. In later stages after worms have involved muscles, muscle pains should be relieved by analgesics. Treatment is in general symptomatic and supportive to enable patient to survive the acute toxemia following invasion of muscles. After encystment, the only symptom is vague muscular pains, which may persist for weeks.

trichinous (trĭk'ĭn-ŭs) [Gr. *trichinos*, of hair]. Infested with trichinae.

trichinous myositis. Myositis trichinosa, q.v.

trichion (trĭk'ē-ŏn) [Gr.]. The anthropometric point at which the midsagittal plane of the head intersects the hairline.

trichitis (trĭk-ī'tĭs) [Gr. *thrix*, hair, + *itis*, inflammation]. Inflammation of hair bulbs.

trichloride (trī-klō'rīd). A compound containing three atoms of chlorine.

trichlormethiazide (trī-klor"mĕ-thī'ă-zīd). USP. A diuretic drug of the thiazide type. Trade names are Metahydrin and Naqua.

trichloroacetic acid. USP. A drug used as a caustic to destroy certain types of warts, condylomata, keratoses, and hyperplastic tissue.

trichloroethylene (trī"klor-ō-ĕth'ĭl-ēn). A colorless clear volatile liquid with a specific gravity of 1.47 at 59° F. (15° C.). It is inhaled and used as an analgesic and anesthetic agent to supplement the action of nitrous oxide. It is a halogenated hydrocarbon having the chemical formula CCl_2:CHCl. Marketed under the trade names Trilene and Trimar. It should not be used with epinephrine.

CAUTION: Should never be used in a system that requires soda lime. The heat generated in this type of system by the action of CO_2 and the lime will break trichloroethylene down to form the toxic gas phosgene and hydrochloric acid. Also in the presence of alkali the toxic and flammable substance dichloroacetylene is formed.

tricho- [Gr. *thrix, trichos*, hair]. A prefix denoting a relationship to hair.

trichoanesthesia (trĭk"ō-ăn"ĕs-thē'zē-ă). Loss of ability to sense stimulation of the hair.

trichobacteria (trĭk"ō-băk-tē'rē-ă) [" + *bakterion*, rod]. 1. Filamentous bacteria. 2. Bacteria possessing flagella.

trichobezoar (trĭk"ō-bē'zor) [" + Arabic *bazahr*, protecting against poison]. A hair ball or concretion in the intestine or stomach.

trichocardia (trĭk-ō-kăr'dē-ă) [" + *kardia*, heart]. Pericardial inflammation with elevations resembling hair. SYN: *heart, hairy; pericardium, shaggy.*

trichoclasia, trichoclasis (trĭk"ō-klā'zē-ă, -ŏk'lăs-ĭs) [" + *klasis*, a breaking]. Brittleness of the hair. SYN: *trichorrhexis.*

trichocryptosis (trĭk"ō-krĭp-tō'sĭs) [" + *kryptos*, concealed]. Any disease of the hair follicles.

trichocyst (trĭk'ō-sĭst) [" + *kystis*, bladder]. 1. A cell structure derived from cytoplasm. 2. In some single-celled organisms, a vesicle equipped with a thread that can be thrust out for the purposes of defense or attack.

Trichodectes (trĭk"ō-dĕk'tēz) [" + *dektes*, biter]. A genus of lice of the suborder Mallophaga. It does not bite man.

trichoepithelioma (trĭk"ō-ĕp"ĭ-thē-lē-ō'mă) [" + *epi*, upon, + *thele*, nipple, + *oma*, tumor]. A benign skin tumor originating in the hair follicles.

trichoesthesia (trĭk"ō-ĕs-thē'zē-ă) [" + *aisthesis*, sensation]. 1. Sensation felt when a hair is touched. 2. A paresthesia causing a sensation of the presence of a hair on a mucous membrane or on the skin.

trichoesthesiometer (trĭk"ō-ĕs-thē"zē-ŏm'ĕ-ter) [" + " + *metron*, a measure]. Device for testing sensibility of the scalp by means of the hair.

trichogen (trĭk'ō-jĕn) [" + *gennan*, to produce]. An agent stimulating growth of hair.

trichogenous (trĭk-ŏj'ĕn-ŭs). Promoting hair growth.

trichoglossia (trĭk"ō-glŏ'sē-ă) [" + *glossa*, tongue]. Hairy condition of the tongue.

trichohyalin (trĭk"ō-hī'ă-lĭn) [" + *hyalin*]. The hyaline of the hair.

trichoid (trĭk'oyd) [" + *eidos*, resemblance]. Hairlike.

trichokryptomania (trĭk"ō-krĭp"tō-mā'nē-ă) [" + *kryptos*, hidden, + *mania*, madness]. Abnormal desire to break off the hair or beard with the fingernail. SYN: *trichorrhexomania.*

tricholith (trĭk'ō-lĭth) [" + *lithos*, stone]. 1. A hairy nodule on the hair. Seen in piedra. 2. A calcified intestinal bezoar that contains hair.

trichologia (trĭk"ō-lō'jē-ă) [" + *legein*, to pick out]. Trichotillomania, q.v.

trichology (trĭk-ŏl'ō-jē) [" + *logos*, a study]. Study of the hair and its care and treatment.

trichoma (trĭk-ō'mă) [Gr., hairiness]. 1. Inversion of one or more eyelashes. SYN: *entropion.* 2. Matted, verminous, encrusted state of the hair. SYN: *plica polonica.*

trichomadesis (trĭk"ō-mă-dē'sĭs). The falling out of hair.

trichomatosis (trĭk"ō-mă-tō'sĭs) [" + *osis*, condition]. Entangled matted hair due to fungus disease of the scalp and lack of cleanliness. SYN: *plica polonica.*

trichomatous (trĭ-kŏm'ă-tŭs). Of the nature of, or affected with trichoma.

trichome (trī'kōm) [Gr. *trichoma*, a growth of hair]. 1. A hair or other appendage of the skin. 2. A colony of blue-green algae that grows end-to-end in chain-like fashion.

trichomegaly (trĭk"ō-mĕg'ă-lē) [Gr. *trichos*, hair, + *megas*, large]. Long, coarse eyebrows.

trichomonacide (trĭk"ō-mō'nă-sīd). Anything that is lethal to trichomonads.

trichomonad (trĭ-kŏm'ō-năd). Related to or resembling the genus of flagellate Trichomonas.

Trichomonas (trĭk-ŏm′ō-năs) [″ + *monas,* unit]. Genus of flagellate parasitic protozoa.

T. hominis. Species in human intestines sometimes causing diarrhea and bacillary dysentery.

T. tenax. A benign trichomonas that may be present in the mouth. SYN: *T. buccalis.*

T. vaginalis. Species found in the vagina that produces discharge. A fairly common condition in women, esp. during pregnancy or following vaginal surgery. It is sometimes found in the male urethra and is communicated through intercourse.

SYM: Persistent burning and itching of the vulvar tissue associated with a profuse white frothy discharge. Occasionally T. vaginalis is present but asymptomatic.

TREATMENT: Metronidazole (Flagyl) taken orally by the female and her partner. Alcohol should not be consumed during metronidazole therapy.

trichomoniasis (trĭk″ō-mō-nī′ă-sĭs) [″ + ″ + *-iasis,* infection]. Infestation with a parasite of genus Trichomonas.

trichomycosis (trĭk″ō-mī-kō′sĭs) [″ + *mykes,* fungus, + *osis,* condition]. Any disease of the hair due to a fungus.

t. axillaris. An affection of the axillary region and sometimes pubic hairs caused by Nocardia tenuis.

t. nodosa. Disease marked by nodule formations on the hair shafts. SYN: *piedra.*

trichonodosis (trĭk″ō-nō-dō′sĭs). Trichorrhexis nodosa, q.v.

trichonosis, trichonosus (trĭk-ō-nō′sĭs, -ŏn′ō-sŭs) [Gr. *trichos,* hair, + *nosos,* disease]. Any diseased condition of the hair.

trichopathic (trĭk″ō-păth′ĭk). Concerning disease of the hair.

trichopathophobia (trĭk″ō-păth″ō-fō′bē-ă) [″ + *pathos,* disease, + *phobos,* fear]. Morbid fear of hair on the face experienced by women, or any abnormal anxiety regarding hair.

trichopathy (trĭk-ŏp′ă-thē) [″ + *pathos,* disease]. Any disease of the hair.

trichophagia, trichophagy (trĭk-ō-fā′jē-ă, -ŏf′ă-jē) [″ + *phagein,* to eat]. The habit of eating hair.

trichophobia (trĭk″ō-fō′bē-ă) [″ + *phobos,* fear]. Abnormal dread of hair or of touching it.

trichophytic (trĭk″ō-fĭt′ĭk) [″ + *phyton,* plant]. 1. Relating to Trichophyton. 2. Promoting hair growth.

trichophytic granulosa (trĭk″ō-fĭt′ĭk). Tinea profunda, q.v.

trichophytid (trī-kŏf′ĭ-tĭd). A skin disorder considered to be an allergic reaction to fungi of the genus Trichophyton.

trichophytin (trī-kŏf′ĭ-tĭn). An extract prepared from cultures of the fungi of the genus Trichophyton. Used as an antigen for skin tests and for the treatment of certain trichophytid infections.

trichophytobezoar (trĭk-ō-fī″tō-bē′zor) [″ + *phyton,* plant, + Arabic *bazahr,* protecting against poison]. A hair ball found in the stomach or intestine composed of hair, vegetable fibers, and miscellaneous debris.

Trichophyton (trĭk-ŏf′ĭt-ŏn). A genus of parasitic fungi that lives in or on the skin or its appendages (hair and nails) and is the cause of various dermatomycoses and ringworm infections. Species that produce spores arranged in rows on the outside of the hair are designated ectothrix; if spores are within the hair, endothrix.

T. mentagrophytes. Species, one form of which, called granulare, is parasitic on several mammals including horses, dogs, and rodents can also affect man; another variety, called interdigitale, is associated with tinea pedis.

T. schoenleinii. Causative agent of favus of the scalp. SEE: *favus.*

T. tonsurans. The most frequent cause of ringworm of the scalp. SEE: *tinea capitis.*

T. violaceum. Causative agent of some forms of ringworm of the scalp, beard, or nails.

trichophytosis (trĭk″ō-fī-tō′sĭs) [″ + *phyton,* plant, + *osis,* condition]. Infestation with Trichophyton fungi.

trichoptilosis (trĭk″ŏp-tĭl-ō′sĭs) [″ + *ptilon,* feather, + *osis,* condition]. 1. The splitting of hairs at their ends, giving them a featherlike appearance. 2. Disease of hair marked by development of nodules along the hair shaft at which point it splits off. SYN: *trichorrhexis nodosa.*

trichorrhea (trĭk-or-ē′ă) [″ + *rhoia,* a flow]. Rapid loss of hair.

trichorrhexis (trĭk″ō-rĕks′ĭs) [″ + *rhexis,* a breaking]. Condition in which the hair splits. SYN: *trichoschisis.*

t. nodosa. Sparse, brittle hairs with bamboo-like nodes. These apparent nodes are actually partial fractures of the hair shaft. This is caused by an atrophic condition of the hair. SYN: *hair, bamboo.*

trichorrhexomania (trĭk″ō-rĕks″ō-mā′nē-ă) [″ + ″ + *mania,* madness]. The abnormal habit of breaking off the hair with the fingernails.

trichoschisis (trĭ-kŏs′kĭs-ĭs) [″ + *schisis,* a fissure]. Splitting of the hairs.

trichoscopy (trĭk-ŏs′kō-pē) [″ + *skopein,* to examine]. Inspection of the hair.

trichosiderin (trĭk″ō-sĭd′ĕr-ĭn) [″ + *sideros,* iron]. An iron-containing pigment normally present in red hair.

trichosis (trī-kō′sĭs) [″ + *osis,* condition]. Any disease of the hair or its abnormal growth or development in an abnormal place.

t. decolor. Any abnormal coloring or lack

of coloring of the hair. SYN: *canities.*

t. setosa. Coarse hair.

Trichosporon (trĭ-kŏs'pō-rŏn) [" + *sporos,* a seed]. A genus of fungi that grows on hair and causes piedra.

T. beigelii. The causative agent of white piedra. SEE: *piedra.*

trichosporosis (trĭk"ō-spō-rō'sĭs) [" + " + *osis,* condition]. Infestation of the hair with Trichosporon.

trichostasis spinulosa (trĭ-kŏs'tă-sĭs spĭn"ū-lō'să) [" + *stasis,* a standing]. A congenital condition in which the hair follicle is plugged with keratin and fine, lanugo hairs.

trichostrongyliasis (trĭk"ō-strŏn-jĭ-lī'ă-sĭs). Infestation with the intestinal parasite Trichostrongylus. A rare disease in the U.S.A.

trichostrongylosis (trĭk"ō-strŏn"jĭ-lō'sĭs). Infestation with Trichostrongylus.

Trichostrongylus (trĭk"ō-strŏn'jĭ-lŭs). A genus of nematode worms of the family Trichostrongylidae. These worms are of economic importance because of the damage they cause to domestic animals and birds.

Trichothecium (trĭk"ō-thē'sē-ŭm) [" + *theke,* a box]. A genus of mold fungi causing disease of the hair.

T. roseum. A species of mold fungus found in certain cases of inflammation of the eardrum (mycomyringitis).

trichotillomania (trĭk"ō-tĭl"ō-mā'nē-ă) [" + *tillein,* to pull, + *mania,* madness]. The unnatural impulse to pull out one's own hair.

trichotomous (trī-kŏt'ō-mŭs) [Gr. *tricha,* threefold, + *tome,* incision]. Divided into three.

trichotomy (trī-kŏt'ō-mē) [Gr. *tricha,* threefold, + *tome,* incision]. Divided into three parts.

trichotoxin (trĭk"ō-tŏks'ĭn) [Gr. *trichos,* hair, + *toxikon,* poison]. An antibody or cytotoxin that destroys ciliated epithelial cells.

trichotrophy (trĭ-kŏt'rō-fē) [" + *trophe,* nourishment]. Nutrition of the hair.

trichroic (trī-krō'ĭk) [Gr. *treis,* three, + *chroa,* color]. Presenting three different colors when viewed along each of three different axes.

trichroism (trī'krō-ĭzm) [" + " + *-ismos,* condition]. Quality of showing a different color when viewed along each of three axes.

trichromatic (trī"krō-măt'ĭk) [" + *chroma,* color]. Rel. to or able to see the three primary colors; denoting normal color vision. SYN: *trichromic.*

trichromatism (trī-krō'mă-tĭzm). Trichoism.

trichromatopsia (trī"krō-mă-tŏp'sē-ă). Normal color vision.

trichromic (trī-krō'mĭk). Pert. to normal color vision or ability to see the three primary colors. SYN: *trichromatic.*

trichterbrust (trĭch'tĕr-broost) [Ger.]. Funnel chest.

trichuriasis (trĭk"ū-rī'ă-sĭs) [Gr. *trichos,* hair, + *oura,* tail, + *-iasis,* condition]. Presence of worms of genus Trichuris in the colon or in the ileum.

Trichuris (trĭ-kū'rĭs). Parasitic nematode worms that belong to the class Nematoda.

T. trichiura. Species of Trichuris that infects man when the ova that have undergone incubation in the soil are ingested. The larvae develop into adults, which inhabit the large intestine. If the infection is heavy, the patient will develop diarrhea and abdominal pain. Rectal prolapse may occur if a great number of worms are present. It is not definitely known that infection with Trichuris causes intestinal blood loss. SYN: *whipworm.*

TREATMENT: Mebendazole is the drug of choice.

tricipital (trī-sĭp'ĭ-tăl) [Gr. *treis,* three, + L. *caput,* head]. Three-headed, as the triceps muscle.

tricitrates oral solution. A solution of sodium citrate, potassium citrate, and citric acid in a suitable aqueous medium. The sodium and potassium ion contents of the solution are approximately one mEq. per ml.

triclofos sodium (trī'klō-fōs). A sedative-hypnotic drug. Trade name is Triclos.

Triclos. Trade name for triclofos sodium.

tricornic (trī-kor'nĭk) [" + L. *cornu,* horn]. Having three horns or cornua. SYN: *tricornute.*

tricornute (trī-kor'nūt) [" + L. *cornutus,* horned]. Having three horns.

tricrotic (trī-krŏt'ĭk) [Gr. *trikrotos,* rowed with a triple stroke]. Condition in which three accentuated waves or notches occur on a sphygmograph tracing from one beat of the pulse.

tricrotism (trī'krŏt-ĭzm) [" + *-ismos,* condition]. Condition of being tricrotic.

tricuspid (trī-kŭs'pĭd) [Gr. *treis,* three, + L. *cuspis,* a point]. 1. Pert. to the tricuspid valve. 2. Having three points or cusps.

tricuspid area. Lower portion of the body of the sternum where sounds of the right atrioventricular orifice are best heard.

tricuspid atresia. Stenosis of the tricuspid valve. A fairly uncommon congenital malformation that causes cyanosis and clubbing.

SYM: Paroxysmal dyspnea; difficulty in feeding.

tricuspid murmur. Murmur caused by stenosis of the tricuspid valve or by its incompetency.

tricuspid orifice. Right atrioventricular cardiac aperture.

tricuspid tooth. Tooth with a crown that has three cusps.

tricuspid valve. Right atrioventricular valve. SYN: *valvula tricuspidalis.*

trident, tridentate (trī'dĕnt, trī-dĕn'tāt) [L. *tres, tria,* three, + *dens,* tooth]. Having three prongs.

tridermic (trī-dĕr'mĭk) [Gr. *treis,* three, + *derma,* skin]. Developed from the ectoderm, endoderm, and mesoderm.

tridermoma (trī"dĕr-mō'mă) [" + " + *oma,* tumor]. A teratoid growth containing all three germ layers.

Tridesilon. Trade name for desonide.

tridihexethyl chloride (trī"dī-hĕks-ĕth'ĭl). USP. An anticholinergic drug that acts similarly to belladonna. Trade name is Pathilon.

Tridione. Trade name for trimethadione, USP.

tridymite (trĭd'ĭ-mīt). A crystalline form of silica, SiO_2, that may be obtained by heating quartz.

trielcon (trī-ĕl'kŏn) [" + *helkein,* to draw]. Instrument with three branches for removing bullets or other foreign substances from wounds.

triencephalus (trī"ĕn-sĕf'ă-lŭs) [" + *enkephalos,* brain]. A deformed fetus lacking organs of sight, hearing, and smell.

triethanolamine (trī"ĕth-ă-nōl'ā-mēn). Previously used name for trolamine, q.v.

triethylenemelamine (trī-ĕth"ĭ-lēn-mĕl'ă-mēn). ABBR: TEM. One of the nitrogen mustard compounds. SEE: *nitrogen mustards.*

triethylenethiophosphoramide (trī-ĕth"ĭ-lēn-thī"ō-fŏs-for'ă-mīd). An alkylating agent used in treating certain types of malignancies. SYN: *thiotepa.*

trifacial (trī-fā'shăl) [L. *trifacialis*]. Pert. to the fifth cranial nerve. SYN: *trigeminal.*

trifacial neuralgia. Neuralgia of one of the branches of the fifth cranial nerve; often severe. SYN: *tic douloureux.*

trifid (trī'fĭd) [L. *trifidus,* split thrice]. Split into three; having three clefts.

trifluoperazine hydrochloride (trī"floo-ō-păr'ă-zēn). USP. An antipsychotic drug. Trade name is Stelazine.

triflupromazine (trī"floo-prō'mă-zēn). USP. An antipsychotic drug that is also used in treating nausea and vomiting.

trifurcation (trī"fŭr-kā'shŭn) [Gr. *treis,* three, + L. *furca,* fork]. Division into three branches.

trigastric (trī-găs'trĭk) [Gr. *treis,* three, + *gaster,* belly]. Having three bellies, as certain muscles.

trigeminal (trī-jĕm'ĭn-ăl) [L. *tres, tria,* three, + *geminus,* twin]. Pert. to the trigeminus or fifth cranial nerve.

trigeminal cough. A reflex cough from irritation of the trigeminal terminations in respiratory upper passages.

trigeminal nerve. A large mixed nerve arising superficially from the side of the pons near its superior border. It is attached to the brain stem by two roots: a large sensory root and a small motor root. The sensory root bears an enlargement, the semilunar gasserian ganglion, from which three large branches arise. These are *ophthalmic,* purely sensory, from skin of upper part of head, mucous membranes of nasal cavity and sinuses, cornea and conjunctiva; *maxillary,* purely sensory, from dura mater, gums and teeth of upper jaw, upper lip, and orbit; *mandibular,* the largest division, containing sensory fibers from tongue, gums and teeth of lower jaw, skin of cheek, lower jaw and lip, and motor fibers supplying principally muscles of mastication. SYN: *fifth cranial nerve; nervus trigeminus.*

trigeminal neuralgia. Facial neuralgia. SYN: *tic douloureux.* SEE: *neuralgia, trigeminal.*

NURSING IMPLICATIONS: Observe and record characteristics of attack. Encourage the patient to maintain independence and social activities. Administer analeptic drugs as prescribed and observe for side effects. Inform the patient receiving alcohol injections that pain will return with nerve regeneration and to notify physician of pain recurrence. Before surgery, eliminate causative factors such as extreme temperatures of foods and jarring of the bed. Instruct the patient to use a cotton pad to cleanse the face and a blunt-toothed comb to comb the hair.

After surgery, assess sensory deficits to prevent trauma to the face and affected areas. Instruct the patient who has had an ophthalmic branch resection to examine the eye with a hand mirror every hour for foreign substances, as they cannot be felt, and to wear protective glasses to minimize entry of foreign substances in the eye. Instruct the patient who has had a mandibular or maxillary branch resection to be careful when eating. Teach the patient to chew food on the unaffected side so as to be aware of inner cheek injury. Tell the patient to have frequent dental examinations to detect any abnormalities that the patient cannot feel. Care for the patient who undergoes an intracranial surgical approach is similar to that for any patient undergoing intracranial surgery. Provide emotional support.

trigeminal pulse. Pulse with longer or shorter interval after each three beats because the third beat is an extrasystole.

trigeminus (trī-jĕm'ĭ-nŭs). The fifth cranial nerve. SYN: *trigeminal nerve.* SEE: *Cranial Nerves* in *Appendix.*

trigeminy (trī-jĕm'ĭ-nē). Occurring in threes, esp. three pulse beats in rapid succession.

trigenic (trī-jĕn'ĭk) [Gr. *treis,* three, + *gennan,* to produce]. In genetics, condition in which three alleles are present at any particular locus on the chromosome.

trigger (trĭg'ĕr) [D. *trekker,* something pulled]. 1. An event or impulse that initiates other actions or events. SYN: *stimulus.* 2. To initiate or start with suddenness.

trigger action. A physiological process or a pathological change initiated by a sudden stimulus.

trigger finger. State in which flexion or extension of a digit is arrested temporarily but finally completed with a jerk.

trigger point or zone. Any place on the body that when stimulated causes in a specific area a sudden pain, esp. a type of pain previously felt spontaneously at the same location.

trigger substance. A chemical substance that initiates a function or action.

trigger zone. 1. An area that when stimulated will initiate an attack of neuralgia. 2. An area of cerebral cortex that when stimulated produces abnormal reactions similar to those in acquired epilepsy. SEE: *epileptogenic zone.*

triglycerides (trī-glĭs′ĕr-īds). Combinations of glycerol with three of five different fatty acids. A large portion of the fatty substances, i.e., lipids, in the blood is triglycerides. Because these lipids are insoluble in water, they are transported in combination with proteins (lipoproteins). About one or two grams of triglycerides per kilogram of body weight are ingested daily in the usual diet in the U.S.A. In addition, triglycerides are produced in the liver from carbohydrates. SEE: *hyperlipoproteinemia.*

trigonal (trĭg′ō-năl) [Gr. *trigonon,* a three-cornered figure]. Triangular; pert. to a trigone.

trigone (trī′gōn). A triangular space, esp. one at the base of the bladder. SYN: *trigonum; triangle, vesical.*

t., carotid. The triangular area in the neck bounded by the posterior belly of the digastric muscle, the sternocleidomastoid muscle, and the midline of the neck.

t. of bladder. A triangular area at the base of the bladder. It is between the two openings of the ureters and the urethra.

t., olfactory. A small triangular eminence at the root of the olfactory peduncle and anterior to the anterior perforated space of the base of the brain.

t., vesical. T. of bladder.

trigonectomy (trī″gōn-ĕk′tō-mē) [″ + *ektome,* excision]. Excision of the base of the bladder.

trigonid (trī-gō′nĭd). The first three cusps of a lower molar tooth.

trigonitis (trĭg″ō-nī′tĭs) [″ + *itis,* inflammation]. Inflammation confined to mucous membrane of the trigone of the bladder.

trigonocephalic (trī″gō-nō-sĕ-făl′ĭk) [″ + *kephale,* head]. Having a head shaped like a triangle.

trigonocephalus (trĭg″ō-nō-sĕf′ă-lŭs). A fetus exhibiting trigonocephaly.

trigonocephaly (trī-gō″nō-sĕf′ă-lē). The condition of the head of the fetus being shaped like a triangle.

trigonum (trī-gō′nŭm) [L.]. (pl. *trigona*) Any triangular area. SYN: *trigone.*

t. lumbale. Petit's triangle, q.v.

trihexyphenidyl hydrochloride (trī-hĕk″sē-fĕn′ĭ-dĭl). USP. An anticholinergic drug, used in treating parkinsonism. Trade names are Antitrem, Artane, Pipanol, and Tremin.

trihybrid (trī-hī′brĭd) [Gr. *treis,* three, + L. *hybrida,* mongrel]. In genetics, the offspring of a cross between two individuals differing in three unit characters.

tri-iniodymus (trī″ĭn-ē-ŏd′ĭ-mŭs) [″ + *inion,* nape of the neck, + *didymos,* twin]. A deformed fetus with a single body and three heads joined at the occiput.

triiodothyronine (trī″ī-ō″dō-thī′rō-nēn). One of two forms of the principal hormone secreted by the thyroid gland. Chemically it is 3,5,3′-triiodothyronine (liothyronine). ABBR: T_3. SEE: *tetraiodothyronine; thyroid-function tests.*

trikates. USP. A solution of potassium acetate, potassium bicarbonate, and potassium citrate. Used in treating electrolyte deficiencies.

trilabe (trī′lāb) [Gr. *treis,* three, + *labe,* a handle]. Three-pronged forceps for removing foreign substances from the bladder. SEE: *lithotrite.*

Trilafon. Trade name for perphenazine.

trilaminar (trī-lăm′ĭ-năr). Composed of three layers.

trilateral (trī-lăt′ĕr-ăl) [″ + L. *latus,* side]. Concerning three sides.

trill (trĭl) [It. *trillare,* probably imitative]. A tremulous sound, esp. in vocal music.

trilobate (trī-lō′bāt) [″ + L. *lobus,* lobe]. Having three lobes.

trilocular (trī-lŏk′ū-lăr) [″ + L. *loculus,* cell]. Having three compartments.

trilogy (trĭl′ō-jē). A series of three events.

trimanual (trī-măn′ū-ăl) [″ + *manualis,* by hand]. Performed with three hands, as an obstetrical maneuver.

trimensual (trī-mĕn′shū-ăl) [″ + *mensualis,* monthly]. Occurring quarterly or every three months.

trimeprazine tartrate hydrochloride (trī-mĕp′ră-zēn). USP. A drug used for its antipruritic action. Trade name is Temaril.

trimester (trī-mĕs′tĕr). A three-month period.

t., first. The first three months of pregnancy.

t., second. The second and middle three months of pregnancy.

t., third. The third and final three months of pregnancy.

trimethadione (trī″mĕth-ă-dī′ōn). USP. An anticonvulsive agent used in treating certain forms of epilepsy. Trade name is Tridione.

trimethaphan camsylate (trī-mĕth′ă-făn). USP. A ganglionic blocking agent used to diminish blood pressure in acute hypertensive crisis. Trade name is Arfonad.

trimethidinium methosulfate (trī-mĕth″ĭ-dĭn′ē-ŭm). An antihypertensive drug.

trimethobenzamide hydrochloride (trī-mĕth″ō-bĕn′ză-mīd). USP. An antiemetic drug. Trade name is Tigan.

trimethoprim (trī-mĕth′ō-prĭm). USP. An antibacterial drug usually used in combination with sulfamethoxazole because they act to interfere with two sequential steps in the metabolism of certain bacteria. The combination is useful in treating various bacterial infections. Trade names are Proloprim and Trimpex. SEE: *sulfamethoxazole.*

trimethylene (trī-mĕth′ĭ-lēn). Cyclopropane, q.v.

trimorphous (trī-mor′fŭs) [″ + *morphe,* form]. 1. Having three different forms as the larva, pupa, and adult of certain insects. 2. Having three different forms of crystals.

Trimox. Trade name for amoxicillin trihydrate.

Trimpex. Trade name for trimethoprim, USP.

trinitroglycerol (trī-nī″trō-glĭs′ĕr-ŏl). Nitroglycerin.

trinitrophenol (trī″nī-trō-fē′nōl). A yellow crystalline powder that precipitates proteins. Used as a dye and as a reagent. SYN: *acid, picric.*

trinitrotoluene (trī″nī-trō-tŏl′ū-ēn). An explosive compound. SYN: *TNT.*

triocephalus (trī″ō-sĕf′ă-lŭs) [″ + *kephale,* head]. A deformed fetus with a rudimentary head without eyes, nose, or mouth.

triolein. Olein, q.v.

triolism (trī′ō-lĭzm). A sexual activity involving two persons of one sex and the other of the opposite sex.

triophthalmos (trī″ŏf-thăl′mŏs) [″ + *ophthalmos,* eye]. A deformed fetus with three eyes.

triopodymus (trī″ō-pŏd′ĭ-mŭs) [″ + *ops,* face, + *didymos,* twin]. A deformed fetus with three fused heads and three faces.

triorchid, triorchis (trī-or′kĭd, -kĭs) [″ + *orchis,* testicle]. Person who has three testicles.

triorchidism (trī-or′kĭd-ĭzm) [″ + ″ + *-ismos,* condition]. The condition of having three testicles.

triose (trī′ōs). A monosaccharide having three carbon atoms in its molecule.

triotus (trī-ō′tŭs) [″ + *ous,* ear]. A person with a third ear.

trioxsalen (trī-ŏk′să-lĕn). USP. An agent used to promote repigmentation in vitiligo. Trade name is Trisoralen. SEE: *psoralen; vitiligo.*

trip (trĭp). A slang term used to refer to hallucinations produced by various drugs including LSD, mescaline, and some narcotics.

tripara (trĭp′ă-ră) [L. *tres, tria,* three, + *parere,* to bear]. A woman who has had three pregnancies that have lasted beyond 20 weeks or have produced an infant of 500 grams. Designated Para III. SYN: *tertipara.*

tripelennamine citrate (trī″pĕ-lĕn′ă-mĭn). USP. An antihistamine drug. Trade name is Pyribenzamine Citrate.

tripeptide (trī-pĕp′tīd) [Gr. *treis,* three, + *pepton,* digested]. Product of combination of three amino acids formed during proteolytic digestion.

triphalangia (trī″fă-lăn′jē-ă) [″ + *phalanx,* phalanx]. Deformity marked by presence of three phalanges in a thumb or great toe.

triphasic (trī-fā′sĭk) [″ + *phasis,* phase]. Consisting of three phases or stages, said of electric currents.

triphenylmethane (trī-fĕn″ĭl-mĕth′ān). A coal tar–derived chemical that serves as the basis of some dyes and stains.

Tripier's amputation (trĭp-ē-āz′). [Léon Tripier, Fr. surgeon, 1842–1891] Amputation of a foot with part of the calcaneus removed.

triple (trĭp′l) [L. *triplus,* threefold]. Consisting of three; threefold; treble.

triple response. The three reactions of the skin to injury: a red reaction along line of injury; a red area (flare or erythema) about injury; and an elevated area (welt or wheal) resulting from localized edema.

triplegia (trī-plē′jē-ă) [″ + *plege,* stroke]. Hemiplegia with paralysis of one limb on the other side of the body.

triplet (trĭp′lĕt) [L. *triplus,* threefold]. 1. One of three children produced in one gestation and one birth. SEE: *Hellin's law.* 2. A combination of three of a kind.

triplex (trī′plĕks, trĭp′lĕks) [Gr. *triploos,* triple]. Triple; threefold.

triploblastic (trĭp″lō-blăst′ĭk) [″ + *blastos,* germ]. Consisting of three germ layers: ectoderm, entoderm, and mesoderm.

triploid (trĭp′loyd). Concerning triploidy.

triploidy (trĭp′loy-dē). In the human, having three sets of chromosomes.

triplokoria (trĭp″lō-kor′ē-ă) [″ + *kore,* pupil]. Possessing three pupillary openings in one eye.

triplopia (trĭp-lō′pē-ă) [″ + *ope,* vision]. Condition in which three images of the same object are seen.

tripod (trī′pŏd) [Gr. *treis,* three, + *pous,* foot]. A stand having three supports, usually legs.

t., Haller's. Truncus celiacus, q.v.

t., vital. The three essentials for life-support: brain, lungs, and heart.

tripodia (trī-pō′dē-ă). Having three feet.

tripoding (trī′pŏd-ĭng). Use of three bases for support, e.g., two legs and a cane, or one leg and two crutches.

triprolidine hydrochloride (trī-prō′lĭ-dēn). USP. An antihistamine drug. Trade name is Actidil.

triprosopus (trī″prō-sō′pŭs) [″ + *prosopon,* face]. A deformed fetus with three faces.

tripsis (trĭp′sĭs) [Gr. *tripsis,* rubbing]. 1. The

process of trituration. 2. Massage.

-tripsy (trĭp′sē) [Gr. *tripsis,* rubbing]. A word ending indicating intentional crushing of something.

triquetral (trī-kwĕt′răl) [L. *triquetrous*]. Triangular.

triquetral bone. 1. The third carpal bone in the proximal row, enumerated from radial side. 2. Any wormian bone. SYN: *cuneiform bone.*

triquetrous (trī-kwē′trŭs) [L. *triquetrus,* triangular]. Triangular.

triquetrum (trī-kwē′trŭm) [L.]. Three-cornered.

triradial, triradiate (trī-rā′dē-ăl, -āt) [Gr. *treis,* three, + L. *radiatus,* rayed]. Having three rays; radiating in three directions.

triradius (trī-rā′dē-ŭs). In classifying fingerprints, the point of convergence of dermal ridges coming from three directions.

trisaccharide (trī-săk′ă-rīd). A carbohydrate that upon hydrolysis yields three molecules of simple sugars (monosaccharides).

triskaidekaphobia (trĭ-skī-dĕk-ă-fō′bē-ă) [Gr. *triskaideka,* thirteen, + *phobos,* fear]. Superstition concerning the number 13. SYN: *triakaidekaphobia.*

trismic (trĭz′mĭk). Concerning trismus.

trismoid (trĭz′moyd) [Gr. *trismos,* trismus, + *eidos,* form]. 1. Of the nature of trismus. 2. A form of trismus nascentium; once thought to be due to pressure on occiput during delivery.

trismus (trĭz′mŭs) [Gr. *trismos,* grating]. Tonic contraction of the muscles of mastication. May occur in mouth infections, encephalitis, inflammation of salivary glands, and tetanus. SYN: *ankylostoma; lockjaw.*

t. nascentium. In the newborn, inability to open the mouth.

trisomic (trī-sōm′ĭk). In genetics, an individual possessing 2n + 1 chromosomes, that is, one set of chromosomes contains an extra (third) chromosome. SEE: *chromosome; karyotype.*

trisomy (trī′sō-mē). In genetics, having three homologous chromosomes per cell instead of two.

t. 13. Trisomy of chromosome 13, which causes severe congenital deformation and mental retardation. These children usually do not survive past the first year of life. They have a large broad nose, widely spaced small eyes (hypertelorism), low-set ears, and poorly formed lower jaw.

t. 18. Trisomy of chromosome 18, which causes severe deformity and mental retardation. These children usually do not survive beyond the first year of life. Characterized by prominent occiput, overlapping of index finger over third finger, frequent facial abnormalities, straight nose coming off sharply from the forehead, low-set ears, and cleft palate and lip.

t. 21. A variety of congenital moderate-to-severe mental retardation. Marked by sloping forehead, presence of epicanthal folds causing an Oriental appearance of eyes, gray or very light yellow spots at periphery of iris (Brushfield's spots), short broad hand with a single palmar crease (simian crease), a flat nose or absent bridge, low-set ears, and generally dwarfed physique. SYN: *Down's syndrome; trisomy G.*

t. G. Down's syndrome, q.v.

trisplanchnic (trī-splănk′nĭk) [Gr. *treis,* three, + *splanchna,* viscera]. Pert. to the three large body cavities: the skull, thorax, and abdomen.

tristichia (trī-stĭk′ē-ă) [″ + *stichos,* row]. The presence of three rows of eyelashes.

tristimania (trĭs″tĭ-mā′nē-ă) [L. *tristis,* sad, + Gr. *mania,* madness]. Melancholia.

trisulcate (trī-sŭl′kāt) [L. *tres, tria,* three, + *sulcus,* groove]. Having three grooves or furrows.

trisulfapyrimidines oral solution (trī-sŭl″fă-pī-rĭm′ĭ-dēnz). USP A combination of sulfadiazene, sulfamerazine, and sulfamethazine. This antimicrobial combination was developed in order to reduce the precipitation of crystals of the sulfonamides in the urinary tract. Trade names are Neotrizine, Terfonyl, Triple-Sulfas, Sulfose, and Sulfonsol.

trisulfate (trī-sŭl′fāt). A chemical compound containing three sulfate, SO_4, groups.

trisulfide (trī-sŭl′fīd). A chemical compound containing three sulfur atoms.

tritanomalopia (trī″tă-nŏm′ă-lō-pē-ă) [Gr. *tritos,* third, + *anomalos,* irregular, + *ope,* sight]. Color vision defect similar to tritanopia, q.v., but the defect is less pronounced.

tritanomaly (trī″tă-nŏm′ă-lē). Tritanomalopia.

tritanopia (trī″tă-nō′pē-ă) [Gr. *tritos,* third, + *an-,* not, + *ope,* vision]. Blue blindness; color blindness in which there is a defect in the perception of blue. SEE: *color blindness.*

Triten. Trade name for dimethindene maleate.

tritiate (trĭt′ē-āt). To treat with tritium.

triticeous (trĭt-ĭsh′ŭs) [L. *triticeus,* of wheat]. Shaped like a grain of wheat.

t. cartilage. A cartilaginous nodule in the thyrohyoid ligament.

tritium (trĭt′ē-ŭm, trĭsh′ē-ŭm) [Gr. *tritos,* third]. The mass three isotope of hydrogen; triple-weight hydrogen.

triturable (trĭt′ū-ră-bl) [L. *triturare,* to pulverize]. Capable of being powdered.

triturate (trĭt′ū-rāt). 1. To reduce to a fine powder by rubbing. 2. A finely divided substance made by rubbing.

trituration (trĭt-ū-rā′shŭn) [LL. *triturare,* to pulverize]. 1. The act of reducing to a powder. 2. A finely ground and easily mixed powder. 3. The creation of a homogenous mixture of metal alloy particles and mercury to form dental amalgam. SYN: *amalgamation.*

trivalence (trĭv'ă-lĕns). Condition of being trivalent.

trivalent (trī-vā'lĕnt, trĭv'ăl-ĕnt) [Gr. *treis,* three, + L. *valens,* powerful]. Combining with or replacing three hydrogen atoms.

trivalve (trī'vălv). Having three valves.

trivial name. A nonsystematic or semisystematic name and qualifying term used to name drugs. These names do not provide assistance in determining the chemical structure or biological function of the drug. Examples are aspirin, caffeine, and belladonna.

trizonal (trī-zō'năl). Having three zones or layers.

tRNA. *transfer RNA.*

Trobicin. Trade name for spectinomycin dihydrochloride.

trocar (trō'kăr) [Fr. *trois quarts,* three quarters]. A sharply pointed surgical instrument contained in a metal cannula. Used for aspiration or removal of fluids from cavities.

troch. Troche.

trochanter (trō-kăn'tĕr) [Gr. *trokhanter,* a runner]. Either of the two bony processes below the neck of the femur.

t., greater. T. major.

t., lesser. T. minor.

t. major. [NA] A thick process at upper end of the femur projecting upward externally to union of neck and shaft. SYN: *t., greater.*

t. minor. [NA] A conical tuberosity upon inner and posterior surface of upper end of femur, at junction of shaft and neck. SYN: *t., lesser.*

t. tertius. [NA] The gluteal ridge of the femur when it is unusually prominent.

t., third. T. tertius.

trochanterian, trochanteric (trō"kăn-tē'rē-ăn, trō-kăn-tĕr'ĭk). Rel. to a trochanter.

trochanterplasty (trō-kăn'tĕr-plăs"tē). Plastic surgery of the neck of the femur.

trochantin (trō-kăn'tĭn). Trochanter minor.

trochantinian (trō"kăn-tĭn'ē-ăn). Concerning the lesser trochanter of the femur.

troche (trō'kē, trōk') [Gr. *trokhiskos,* a small wheel]. Solid, discoid, or cylindrical mass consisting chiefly of medicinal powder, sugar, and mucilage. Troches are intended to be used by placing them in the mouth and allowing them to remain until, through slow solution or disintegration, their purpose of mild medication is effected. SYN: *lozenge.*

trochiscus (trō-kĭs'kŭs) [L., Gr. *trochiskos,* a small disk]. A medicated tablet or troche.

trochlea (trŏk'lē-ă) [Gr. *trokhileia,* system of pulleys]. (pl. *trochleae*) 1. A structure having the function of a pulley; a ring or hook through which a tendon or muscle projects. 2. The articular smooth surface of a bone upon which glides another bone.

trochlear (trŏk'lē-ăr). 1. Of the nature of a pulley. 2. Pert. to a trochlea.

trochlear fovea. A depression on the orbital plate of the frontal bone for attachment of the cartilaginous pulley of the superior oblique muscle.

trochleariform (trŏk"lē-ăr'ĭ-form). Pulley-shaped.

trochlearis (trŏk"lē-ā'rĭs) [L.]. Superior oblique muscle of the eye. SEE: *Muscles* in *Appendix.*

trochlear nerve. A small mixed nerve making its exit from the dorsal surface of the midbrain. It contains efferent motor fibers to the superior oblique muscle of the eye and afferent sensory fibers conveying proprioceptive impulses from the same muscle. SYN: *nerve trochlearis; fourth cranial nerve.* SEE: *Cranial Nerves* in *Appendix.*

trochocardia (trō"kō-kăr'dē-ă) [Gr. *trokhos,* a wheel, + *kardia,* heart]. Rotary displacement of the heart on its axis.

trochocephalia, trochocephaly (trō"kō-sē-fā'lē-ă, -sĕf'ă-lē) [" + *kephale,* head]. Roundheadedness, a deformity due to premature union of the frontal and parietal bones.

trochoid (trō'koyd) [Gr. *trokhos,* a wheel, + *eidos,* form]. Rotating or revolving, noting an articulation resembling a pivot or pulley. SEE: *joint, pivot.*

trochoides (trō-koy'dēz). A pivot or rotary joint.

Trocinate. Trade name for thiphenamil hydrochloride.

Troglotrematidae (trŏg"lō-trē-măt'ĭ-dē). A family of flukes that includes Paragonimus (human lung fluke) and Troglotrema nanophyetus, the fluke associated with salmon poisoning in dogs.

Troisier's node (trwă-zē-āz'). [Charles E. Troisier, Fr. physician, 1844–1919] Sentinel node, q.v.

trolamine (trō'lă-mēn). An alkalizing agent. Previously used name is triethanolamine.

troland (trō'lănd). A unit of visual stimulation to the retina of the eye. It is one equal to the illumination received per square millimeter of pupil from a source of one lux brightness.

troleandomycin (trō"lē-ăn-dō-mī'sĭn). An antibacterial drug. Previously used name is triacetyloleandomycin.

trolnitrate phosphate (trŏl-nī'trāt). A vasodilator drug. Trade name is Metamine.

Trombicula (trŏm-bĭk'ū-lă). A genus of mites belonging to the Trombiculidae. The larvae called redbugs or chiggers are annoying pests causing an irritating dermatitis and rash. They may serve as vectors of various diseases.

T. akamushi. Species of mites that transmits the causative agent of scrub typhus.

trombiculiasis (trŏm-bĭk"ū-lī'ă-sĭs). Infestation with Trombiculidae.

Trombiculidae (trŏm-bĭk′ū-lī″dē). A family of mites; only the genus Trombicula is of medical significance.

tromethamine (trō-mĕth′ă-mēn). USP. A drug used intravenously to correct acidosis. It should not be used longer than one day. Trade names are THAM and Tris Amino.

tromomania (trŏm″ō-mā′nē-ă) [Gr. *tromos,* a trembling, + *mania,* madness]. Delirium tremens.

Tronothane Hydrochloride. Trade name for pramoxine hydrochloride.

troph-, tropho- [Gr. *trophe*]. Combining forms meaning nourishment.

trophectoderm (trŏf-ĕk′tō-dĕrm) [Gr. *trophe,* nourishment, + *ectoderm*]. Trophoblast.

trophedema (trŏf″ē-dē′mă) [Gr. *trophe,* nourishment, + *oidema,* a swelling]. Localized edema due to congenital hypoplasia of lymphatic vessels or resulting secondarily from obstruction to lymph flow by external pressure. Repeated low-grade infection may also obstruct the flow of lymph.

trophic (trŏf′ĭk) [Gr. *trophikos*]. Concerned with nourishment. Applied particularly to a type of efferent nerves believed to control the growth and nourishment of the parts they innervate. SEE: *autotrophic; center, trophic.*

trophism (trŏf′ĭzm). Nutrition.

trophoblast (trŏf′ō-blăst) [Gr. *trophe,* nourishment, + *blastos,* germ]. The outermost layer of the developing blastocyst (blastodermic vesicle) of a mammal. It differentiates into two layers, the cytotrophoblast and syntrophoblast, the latter coming into intimate relationship with the uterine endometrium, with which it establishes nutrient relationships. SEE: *fertilization* for illus.

trophoblastic (trŏf″ō-blăs′tĭk). Concerning trophoblasts.

trophoblastoma (trŏf″ō-blăs-tō′mă) [″ + ″ + *oma,* tumor]. A neoplasm due to excessive proliferation of chorionic epithelium. SYN: *chorioepithelioma.*

trophocyte (trŏf′ō-sīt). A cell, Sertoli cell, of the testicle, that supports and nourishes the developing spermatozoa.

trophoderm (trŏf′ō-dĕrm) [Gr. *trophe,* nourishment, + *derma,* skin]. Term applied to the trophoblast and its underlying layer of mesoderm. It is homologous to the serosa of birds, reptiles, and lower mammals.

trophodynamics (trŏf″ō-dī-năm′ĭks). Study of the forces and factors concerned with nutrition.

trophology (trō-fŏl′ō-jē) [″ + *logos,* a science]. The science of nutrition.

trophoneurosis (trŏf″ō-nū-rō′sĭs) [″ + *neuron,* nerve, + *osis,* condition]. Any trophic disorder due to defective function of the nerves concerned with nutrition of the part.

t., disseminated. Thickening and hardening of the skin. SYN: *sclerema; scleroderma.*

t., facial. Progressive facial atrophy.

t., muscular. Muscular changes in connection with nervous disorders.

trophoneurotic (trŏf″ō-nū-rŏt′ĭk). Rel. to a trophoneurosis.

trophonosis (trŏf″ō-nō′sĭs) [″+ *nosos,* disease]. Trophopathia.

trophonucleus (trŏf′ō-nū′klē-ŭs) [″ + L. *nucleus,* kernel]. Protozoan nucleus concerned with vegetative functions in metabolism and not reproduction.

trophopathia (trŏf″ō-păth′ē-ă) [″ + *pathos,* disease]. 1. Any disorder of the nutrition. 2. A trophic disease.

trophopathy (trŏf-ŏp′ă-thē). Trophopathia.

trophotaxis (trŏf″ō-tăks′ĭs) [″ + *taxis,* arrangement]. The movement of cells away from or toward nutrients. SYN: *trophotropism.*

trophotherapy (trŏf″ō-thĕr′ă-pē). Nutritional therapy of disease.

trophotonos (trŏf-ŏt′ŏn-ŏs) [″ + *tonos,* tension]. A rigid state of contractile tissue resulting from trophic disorder.

trophotropism (trŏf-ŏt′rō-pĭzm) [″ + *tropos,* a turning, + *-ismos,* condition]. Attraction and repulsion of cells to nutritive substances; positive and negative trophotropism respectively. SYN: *trophotaxis.*

trophozoite (trŏf″ō-zō′īt) [″ + *zoon,* animal]. A sporozoan nourished by its hosts during its growth stage.

tropia (trō′pē-ă) [Gr. *trope,* turn]. Deviation of the eye or eyes away from the visual axis. Observed with the eyes open and uncovered. Esotropia indicates inward or nasal deviation; exotropia, outward; hypertropia, upward; hypotropia, downward. SYN: *manifest squint; strabismus.* SEE: *phoria.*

tropical (trŏp′ĭ-kăl) [Gr. *tropikos,* turning]. Pert. to the tropics.

tropical immersion foot. Syndrome with severe wrinkling and maceration of the soles of the feet and marked lowering of the threshold of pain. Due to prolonged exposure of the feet to warm water as would occur in the tropics. May be prevented by allowing feet to dry thoroughly each night and by protecting the feet with silicone grease.

tropical lichen. Acute inflammation of the sweat glands. SYN: *prickly heat.*

tropicamide (trō-pĭk′ă-mīd). USP. An anticholinergic drug used to produce mydriasis and cycloplegia in treating eye conditions. Trade name is Mydriacyl.

-tropin [Gr. *tropos,* a turn]. Suffix indicating the stimulating effect of a substance, esp. a hormone, on its target organ.

tropine (trō′pĭn). An alkaloid, $C_8H_{15}NO$, that smells like tobacco. It is present in certain plants.

tropism (trō′pĭzm) [Gr. *trope,* a turn, + *-ismos,* condition]. 1. Reaction of living organisms involuntarily toward or away from light, darkness, heat, cold, or other stimuli. 2. The involuntary response of an organism as a bending, turning, or movement toward (positive tropism) or away from (negative tropism) an external stimulus. SYN: *taxis.* SEE: *chemotropism; galvanotropism; phototropism.*

-tropism. Combining form meaning a response to or a turning toward or away from an external stimulus.

tropocollagen (trō″pō-kŏl′ă-jĕn) [″ + *collagen*]. The basic molecular unit of collagen fibrils, composed of three polypeptide chains.

tropometer (trŏp-ŏm′ĕ-ter) [″ + *metron,* a measure]. 1. Device for measuring the rotation of the eyeballs. 2. Instrument for measuring torsion in long bones.

tropomyosin (trō″pō-mī′ō-sĭn). A muscle protein that is involved in the formation of cross-bridges during muscle contraction.

troponin (trō′pō-nĭn). A muscle protein that attaches to both actin and tropomyosin. It is concerned with calcium binding and inhibiting cross-bridge formation.

trough (trŏf). A groove or channel.

t., gingival. Gingival sulcus, q.v.

t., synaptic. The depression in a muscle fiber that is occupied by the axon termination in a motor endplate.

Trousseau's sign (troo-sōz′). [Armand Trousseau, Fr. physician, 1801–1867] Muscular spasm resulting from pressure applied to nerves and vessels of the upper arm. It is indicative of latent tetany. Also occurs in osteomalacia. SEE: *tetany.*

Trousseau's spots. Streaking of the skin with the fingernail, seen in meningitis and other cerebral diseases.

Trousseau's symptom. Spasmodic muscular contractions produced by pressing the principal vessel and nerve of the limb. Presence of this symptom is a sign of tetany.

troxidone (trŏk′sĭ-dōn). Trimethadione, USP.

Troy weight. A system of weighing gold, silver, precious metals, and jewels in which 5760 grains equal 1 pound; one grain equals 0.0648 grams. SEE: *Weights and Measures* in *Appendix.*

true (troo) [AS. *treowe,* faithful]. Not false; real; genuine.

true conjugate diameter of pelvic inlet. The distance from the posterior surface of the symphysis pubis to the promontory of the sacrum (about 11 cm. in female).

true pelvis. Portion of the pelvis that falls below the iliopectineal line.

true ribs. The seven upper ribs on each side with cartilages articulating directly with the sternum. SYN: *costa vera.* SEE: *rib.*

truncal (trŭng′kăl) [L. *truncus,* trunk]. Rel. to the trunk.

truncate (trŭng′kāt) [L. *truncare,* to cut off]. 1. Having a square end as if it were cut off; lacking an apex. 2. To shorten by amputation of a part of the entity.

truncus (trŭng′kŭs). Trunk.

t. arteriosus. The arterial trunk from the embryonic heart.

t. brachiocephalicus. The initial branch of the arch of the aorta.

t. celiacus. The trunk arising from the abdominal artery. Most of the blood supply for the liver, stomach, spleen, gallbladder, pancreas, and duodenum comes from this trunik.

t. pulmonalis. The vessel arising from the right ventricle. It transports venous blood to the lungs.

trunk (trŭnk) [L. *truncus,* trunk]. 1. The body exclusive of the head and limbs. SYN: *torso.* 2. Main stem of a lymphatic vessel, nerve, or blood vessel.

t., celiac. Truncus celiacus, q.v.

t., lumbosacral. Truncus pulmonalis, q.v.

t., sympathetic. The two long chains of ganglia, connected by sympathetic nerve fibers, that extend along the vertebral column from the skull to the coccyx.

trusion (troo′zhŭn) [L. *trudere,* to show]. Malposition of a tooth or teeth.

truss (trŭs) [ME. *trusse,* a bundle]. 1. Device for holding a hernia in its place. 2. To tie or bind as with a cord or string.

truth serum. One of several hypnotic drugs supposedly having the effect of causing a person upon questioning to talk freely and without inhibition.

try-in The temporary placement of a dental restoration or device to determine its fit and comfortableness.

trypanocide, trypanocidal (trĭp-ăn′ō-sīd, trĭp″ ăn-ō-sī′dăl) [Gr. *trypanon,* a borer, + L. *cide,* kill]. 1. Destructive to trypanosomes. 2. An agent that kills trypanosomes. SYN: *trypanosomicide.*

trypanolysis (trĭp-ăn-ŏl′ĭ-sĭs) [″ + *lysis,* dissolution]. The dissolution of trypanosomes.

Trypanoplasma (trī″păn-ō-plăz′mă) [″ + *plasma,* a thing formed]. A genus of protozoan parasites resembling trypanosomes.

Trypanosoma (trī″păn-ō-sō′mă) [″ + *soma,* a body]. A genus of parasitic, flagellate protozoa found in the blood of many vertebrates including man. They are transmitted by insect vectors.

T. brucei. The causative agent of trypanosomiasis in horses and other domestic animals. Nonpathogenic in man.

T. cruzi. The causative agent of American trypanosomiasis in many animals and specifically Chagas' disease in humans. It is transmitted by blood-sucking insects (triatomids) belonging to the family Reduviidae.

T. gambiense. The causative agent of African sleeping sickness. It is transmitted by the tsetse fly.

T. rhodesiense. An organism parasitic in wild game and domestic animals of portions of Africa. May cause East African sleeping sickness in humans.

trypanosomal (trī-păn-ō-sō'măl). Pert. to trypanosomata.

trypanosome (trī'păn-ō-sōm). Any protozoan belonging to the genus Trypanosoma.

trypanosomiasis (trī-păn"ō-sō-mī'ă-sĭs) [" + *soma,* body, + *-iasis,* infection]. Any of the several diseases occurring in man and domestic animals caused by a species of Trypanosoma. SEE: *sleeping sickness.*

t., African. African sleeping sickness, caused by Trypanosoma gambiense.

t., American. Trypanosomiasis in the western hemisphere. In man it is caused by Trypanosoma cruzi transmitted by blood-sucking triatomids. SYN: *Chagas' disease.*

trypanosomic (trī-păn"ō-sō'mĭk). Concerning trypanosomes.

trypanosomicide. Trypanocide, q.v.

trypanosomid (trī-păn'ō-sō-mĭd). A skin eruption in any disease caused by a trypanosome.

tryparsamide (trĭp-ărs'ă-mĭd, -mīd). An arsenic compound containing about 25% arsenic. Used chiefly in sleeping sickness.

trypsin (trĭp'sĭn) [Gr. *tripsis,* a rubbing]. 1. A proteolytic enzyme formed in the intestine from the action of enterokinase of the intestinal juice (succus entericus) on trypsinogen secreted by the pancreas and present in pancreatic juice. It catalyzes the hydrolysis of peptide bonds in partly digested proteins and some native proteins, the final products being amino acids and various polypeptides. 2. USP. Proteolytic enzyme crystallized from an extract of the pancreas gland of an ox. SEE: *chymotrypsin; digestion; enzyme; pancreas.*

t., crystallized. USP. A standardized preparation of the proteolytic enzyme trypsin. It is extracted from the pancreas of the ox, Bos taurus.

trypsinized (trĭp'sĭ-nīzd). Subjected to action of trypsin, thus having antitryptic power abolished.

trypsinogen (trĭp-sĭn'ō-jĕn) [" + *gennan,* to produce]. The proenzyme, or inactive form of trypsin found in pancreatic juice. Activated when mixed in the intestine with the enterokinase of the succus entericus.

Tryptar. Trade name for trypsin, crystallized.

tryptic (trĭp'tĭk). Rel. to trypsin.

tryptolysis (trĭp-tŏl'ĭ-sĭs) [" + *lysis,* dissolution]. The hydrolysis of proteins or their derivatives by trypsin.

tryptone (trĭp'tōn). A peptide produced by the action of trypsin on a protein.

tryptophan (trĭp'tō-făn). USP. An essential amino acid present in high concentrations in animal and fish protein. It is necessary for normal growth and development. Tryptophan is a precursor of serotonin, a chemical important in the transmission of nerve impulses across nerve cell connections. Tryptophan has been used experimentally in the treatment of insomnia. In high doses it may cause nausea and vomiting.

tryptophanase (trĭp'tō-făn-ās). An enzyme that catalyzes the splitting of tryptophan into indole, pyruvic acid, and ammonia.

tryptophanuria (trĭp"tō-fă-nū'rē-ă) [*tryptophan* + Gr. *ouron,* urine]. Tryptophan in the urine.

T/S. *thyroid:serum* (thyroid to serum iodine ratio).

T.S. *test solution; triple strength.*

TSD. *target skin distance.*

tsetse fly (tsĕt'sē) [S. African]. One of several species of blood-sucking flies belonging to the genus Glossina, order Diptera, confined to Africa south of the Sahara Desert. It is an important transmitter of trypanosomes, the causative agents of African sleeping sicknesses in man, and nagana and other diseases of cattle and game animals. SEE: *Trypanosoma; trypanosomiasis.*

TSH. *thyroid-stimulating hormone.*

TSH-RF. *thyroid-stimulating hormone releasing factor.*

tsp. *teaspoon.*

TSTA. *tumor-specific transplantation antigens.*

tsutsugamushi disease (soot"soo-gă-moosh'ĭ) [Japanese, dangerous bug]. Scrub typhus.

TT. *transit time* of blood through heart and lungs.

T-tube. A device inserted into the biliary duct after removal of the gallbladder. It allows for drainage of the gallbladder and also introduction of contrast medium for postoperative cholangiography.

T.U. *toxid unit; toxin unit.*

tuaminoheptane sulfate (too-ăm"ĭ-nō-hĕp'tān). USP. A sympathomimetic drug used to produce vasoconstriction of the nasal mucosa or the conjunctiva. It is prepared in an appropriate solution and applied topically. Trade name is Tuamine Sulfate.

tub (tŭb) [ME. *tubbe*]. 1. A receptacle for bathing. 2. The use of the cold bath. 3. To treat by using a cold bath.

tuba (too'bă) [L., trumpet]. Tube.

tubal (tū'băl) [L. *tuba,* tube]. Pert. to a tube, esp. the fallopian tube.

tubal nephritis. Inflammation of kidney tubules.

tubal pregnancy. Pregnancy in one of the oviducts.

tubatorsion (tū″bă-tor′shŭn) [″ + *torsio,* a twisting]. The twisting of an oviduct.

tubba, tubboe (tŭb′ă, -ō). Yaws that attacks the palms and soles.

tube (tūb) [L. *tubus,* a tube]. A long, hollow, cylindrical structure.

t., auditory. Eustachian tube, q.v.

t., Cantor. T., intestinal decompression.

t., cathode-ray. A vacuum tube with a thin window at the end opposite the cathode to allow the cathode rays to pass outside. More generally, any discharge tube in which the vacuum is fairly high.

t., Coolidge. A kind of hot cathode tube that is so highly exhausted that the residual gas plays no part in the production of the cathode stream, and that is regulated by variable heating of the cathode filament.

t., Crookes'. Vacuum tube used in producing roentgen rays.

t., drainage. A glass or rubber tube that, when inserted into a cavity, drains away its fluid contents.

t., endobronchial. A double-lumen tube used in anesthesia. One tube may be used to aerate a portion of the lung while the other is occluded in order to deflate the other lung or a portion of it. SYN: *Carlen's catheter.*

t., endotracheal. A catheter inserted into the trachea for the purpose of providing an airway.

t., esophageal. T., stomach.

t., eustachian. The tube passing from the throat to the middle ear.

t., fallopian. One of two oviducts leading from the peritoneal cavity into the uterine cavity.

t., fermentation. A U-shaped tube open only at one end. Bacteria cultured in media in the upright tubes will if they produce gas cause the level of fluid to decrease in the tube with the closed end.

t., hot-cathode. A vacuum tube in which the cathode is electrically heated to incandescence and in which the supply of electrons depends on the temperature of the cathode.

t., hot cathode roentgen-ray. A vacuum roentgen-ray tube in which the electron stream is supplied by a heated cathode. The cathode stream may be regulated by varying the current through the cathode filament.

t., intestinal decompression. A tube placed in the intestinal tract, usually via the nose and esophagus, in order to relieve gas pressure produced when paralytic ileus or intestinal obstruction is present. Tubes may be plain, made of rubber, plastic, or silicone; or they may be equipped with a mercury-filled tip to facilitate passage into the intestinal tract. The latter is called a Cantor tube. The tubes are impregnated with a radiopaque substance in order to allow x-ray visualization of their location.

t., intubation. A tube for passing into the larynx to facilitate breathing. SEE: *intubation.*

t., Levin A tube passed via the nose into the gastrointestinal tract.

t., Miller-Abbott. A double-channel intestinal tube used to relieve intestinal distention. Inserted through a nostril, the tube is passed through the stomach into the small intestine.

t., nasogastric. A tube passed via the nose into the gastrointestinal tract for the purpose of instilling liquid foods into the stomach.

t., neural. SEE: *neural tube.*

t., otopharyngeal. Eustachian tube, q.v.

t., Sengstaken-Blakemore. A three-element nasogastric tube used in treating esophageal bleeding. One tube is for aspiration, another for feeding, and the third is attached to an elongated balloon that surrounds the tubes. The balloon is inflated after the tube is inserted. This causes the bleeding areas to be compressed.

t., Southey's. Very small tube pushed into tissue to help drain edema fluid. Used in severe congestive heart failure to relieve edema of the legs.

t., stomach. A rubber tube for introducing food into the stomach or for washing out the stomach. SYN: *t., esophageal.*

t., test. A glass tube closed at one end. It is used in chemistry to hold chemicals and materials being tested.

t., thoracostomy. Tube inserted into the pleural space via the chest wall in order to remove air or fluid present in the space.

t., tracheotomy. A tube for inserting into the trachea.

t., uterine. Fallopian tube, q.v.

t., Wangensteen. Tube used in Wangensteen method, q.v.

tubectomy (too-bĕk′tō-mē). Surgical removal of all or part of a tube, esp. the fallopian tube.

tube feeding. Providing the patient's fluids and nutritional requirements by instilling foods into the stomach via a nasogastric tube.

tuber (tū′bĕr) [L., a swelling]. (pl. *tubers, tubera*) A swelling or enlargement.

t. cinereum. A part of the base of the hypothalamus bordered by mammillary bodies, the optic chiasma, and on either side by the optic tract. It is connected by the infundibulum with the posterior lobe of the pituitary.

tubercle (tū′bĕr-kl) [L. *tuberculum,* a little swelling]. 1. A small rounded elevation or eminence on a bone. 2. A small nodule, esp. a circumscribed solid elevation of the skin or mucous membrane. 3. The characteristic lesion resulting from infection by tubercle bacilli. It consists typically of three parts: a central giant cell, a midzone of epithelioid cells, and a peripheral zone of nonspecific structure. SYN: *tuberculum.* SEE: *tuberculosis.*

t., adductor. Tubercle of the femur to which is attached the tendon of the adductor magnus.

t., articular. Tubercle at the base of the zygomatic arch to which is attached the temporomandibular ligament; lateral to the articular eminence of the glenoid fossa, with which it is often confused. SYN: *t., zygomatic.*

t., deltoid. Tubercle on the clavicle for attachment of the deltoid muscle.

t., fibrous. Fibrous tissue that has replaced a previously inflamed area.

t., genial. Tubercle on either side of the lower jawbone.

t., genital. The embryonic structure that becomes the clitoris or the penis.

t., lacrimal. Tubercle on the upper jawbone.

t., laminated. The cerebellar nodule.

t., Lisfranc's. Tubercle for attachment of the scalenus anticus muscle on the first rib.

t., mental. A small tubercle on either side of the midline of the chin.

t., miliary. A small tubercle resembling a millet seed; the lesion of tuberculosis.

t., pubic. A small projection at the crest at the lateral end of the crest of the pubic bone. The inguinal ligament attaches to it.

t., supraglenoid. A rough, elevated area just above the glenoid cavity of the clavicle. The long head of the biceps muscle of the arm attaches to this tubercle.

t., zygomatic. Tubercle on the zygoma at the junction of the anterior root.

tubercula (tū-bĕr′kū-lă). Pl. of tuberculum.

tubercular (tū-bĕr′kū-lăr) [L. *tuberculum,* a little swelling]. Relating to or marked by nodules. SYN: *torose.*

tuberculate, tuberculated (tū-bĕr′kū-lāt, -lāt″ĕd) [L. *tuberculum,* a small swelling]. Covered with nodules. SYN: *tubercular.*

tuberculation (tū-bĕr″kū-lā′shŭn). The formation of tubercles.

tuberculid(e) (tū-bĕr′kū-lĭd, -līd) [L. *tuberculum,* a little swelling]. A tuberculous cutaneous eruption due to toxins of tuberculosis. SYN: *tuberculoderma.*

t., follicular. A cutaneous eruption characterized by presence of groups of follicular lesions, esp. on the trunk.

t., papulonecrotic. Form of tuberculid characterized by symmetrically distributed bluish papules, esp. on extremities. These undergo central necrosis and, on healing, leave deep scars.

tuberculigenous (tū-bĕr-kū-lĭj′ĕn-ŭs) [″ + Gr. *gennan,* to produce]. Causing or predisposing to tuberculosis.

tuberculin (tū-bĕr′kū-lĭn) [L. *tuberculum,* a little swelling]. 1. A soluble cell substance prepared from the tubercle bacillus, usually the human type, which is used to determine the presence of a tuberculosis infection. Among the types of tuberculin used are Koch's original or old tuberculin (ABBR: OT or TO) and tuberculin purified protein derivative (ABBR: PPD). 2. USP. The tuberculin used for diagnostic tests of the ability of the skin to react to the intradermal injection of tuberculin. Trade names are Aplisol and Aplitest.

t., new. A suspension of tubercle bacilli fragments from which the soluble materials have been removed and to which glycerine has been added. Tuberculin, USP, is now used in place of this prepration.

t., old. The tuberculin originally prepared by Koch from cultures of Mycobacterium tuberculosis.

t., purified protein derivative. A purified tuberculin obtained by the same technique as that used for Old Tuberculin except a synthetic broth is used to culture the Mycobacterium tuberculosis.

tuberculin test. A test to determine the presence of a tuberculosis infection based on positive reaction of subject to tuberculin. Tests commonly used are: Mantoux test, intradermal injection of tuberculin; von Pirquet test, rubbing tuberculin on scarified skin; and Vollmer patch test, the application to skin of a piece of gauze impregnated with dried tuberculin. In all three tests a local inflammatory reaction is observed in infected persons after 48 to 96 hours. Tests do not reveal whether infection is active or inactive.

tuberculin tine test. Tuberculin test performed by using a special disposable instrument that contains multiple sharp points or prongs for piercing the skin. These tines penetrate the skin and introduce the tuberculin that has been applied to them. The test is read in 48 to 72 hours.

tuberculitis (tū″bĕr-kū-lī′tĭs). Inflammation of a tubercle.

tuberculocele (tū-bĕr′kū-lō-sēl″) [″ + *kele,* tumor]. Tuberculosis of the testis.

tuberculocidal (tū-bĕr″kū-lō-sī′dăl). Anything that destroys Mycobacterium tuberculosis.

tuberculoderma (tū-bĕr″kū-lō-dĕr′mă) [″ + Gr. *derma,* skin]. A tuberculous lesion of the skin. SYN: *tuberculide.*

tuberculofibroid (tū-bĕr″kū-lō-fī'broyd) [″ + *fibra,* fiber, + Gr. *eidos,* form]. Denoting fibroid degeneration of tubercles.

tuberculofibrosis (tū-bĕr″kū-lō-fī-brō'sĭs) [″ + ″ + Gr. *osis,* condition]. 1. Chronic pulmonary inflammation with formation of fibrous tissue. 2. Interstitial pneumonia.

tuberculoid (tū-bĕr'kū-loyd) [L. *tuberculum,* a little swelling, + Gr. *eidos,* resemblance]. Resembling tuberculosis or a tubercle.

tuberculoma (tū-bĕr-kū-lō'mă) [″ + Gr. *oma,* tumor]. 1. A tuberculous abscess. 2. Any tuberculous neoplasm.

tuberculophobia (tū-bĕr″kū-lō-fō'bē-ă) [″ + Gr. *phobos,* fear]. An abnormal fear of being infected with tuberculosis.

tuberculoprotein (tū-bĕr″kū-lō-prō'tē-ĭn). A protein derived from tubercle bacilli.

tuberculosilicosis (tū-bĕr″kū-lō-sĭl″ĭ-kō'sĭs). Silicosis and pulmonary tuberculosis at the same time.

tuberculosis (tū-bĕr″kū-lō'sĭs) [″ + Gr. *osis,* disease]. An infectious disease caused by the tubercle bacillus, Mycobacterium tuberculosis, and characterized pathologically by inflammatory infiltrations, formation of tubercles, caseation, necrosis, abscesses, fibrosis, and calcification. It most commonly affects the respiratory system but other parts of the body such as gastrointestinal and genitourinary tracts, bones, joints, nervous system, lymph nodes, and skin may become infected. Fish, amphibians, birds, and mammals (esp. cattle) are subject to the disease. Three types of the tubercle bacillus exist, namely human, bovine, and avian. Man may become infected by any of the three types but in the U.S.A., the human type predominates. Infection usually is acquired from contact with an infected person or an infected cow or through drinking contaminated milk.

Tuberculosis may occur in an acute generalized form (miliary tuberculosis) or in a chronic localized form. In man, the primary infection usually consists of a localized lesion and regional adenitis, these constituting the primary complex. From this state, lesions may heal by fibrosis and calcification and the disease exist in an arrested or inactive stage. Reactivation or exacerbation of the disease or reinfection gives rise to the chronic progressive form.

NOTE: Many varieties of Mycobacteria that previously were thought to be nonpathogenic for man have been found to cause chronic progressive pulmonary disease closely resembling pulmonary tuberculosis. These organisms have been termed anonymous or atypical Mycobacteria. They have been classified into four groups: photochromogens, scotochromogens, nonphotochromogens, and rapid growers.

TREATMENT: Hospital care is recommended for active cases; however, recent developments in chemotherapy have greatly altered time-honored views concerning the need for strict isolation and prolonged bedrest. In advanced cases, bedrest, adequate well-balanced diet, relief from emotional tension, collapse therapy (pneumoperitoneum, pneumothorax, phrenemphraxis), and, in some cases, surgery (thoracoplasty) may be required. Among chemotherapeutic drugs, several are widely used: streptomycin, para-amino-salicylic acid (PAS), rifampin, and isoniazid. Kanamycin and ethambutol are useful in cases where the tubercle bacillus has become resistant to the usual drugs. Symptomatic treatment is necessary for cough, hemoptysis, chest pain, and other symptoms. SEE: *tuberculosis chemotherapy, short course.*

CAUTION: When isoniazid is used, it is important to determine the plasma level of the drug. The rate of inactivation of isoniazid is genetically determined and individuals may be slow or fast inactivators of the drug. A larger dose than normal will be required in order to achieve the desired plasma concentration in patients who are fast inactivators of isoniazid.

RS: mycobacterium; tubercle; tubercle bacillus; tuberculin; tuberculin test; tuberculin tine test.

t., avian. Tuberculosis of birds due to Mycobacterium avium.

t., bovine. Tuberculosis of cattle due to Mycobacterium tuberculosis.

t., endogenous. Tuberculosis originating in a tubercle in another body site.

t., exogenous. Tuberculosis originating from a source outside the body.

t., hematogenous. Spread of tuberculosis from a primary site to another site via the bloodstream.

t., open. Tuberculosis in which the tubercle bacilli are present in bodily secretions that leave the body.

t. verrucosa. Tuberculosis of the skin or mucous membranes characterized by formation of warty lesions.

tuberculosis chemotherapy, short course. The U.S. Public Health Service has conducted trials that indicate that isoniazid (INH) and rifampin (RIF) given for 20 weeks followed by daily INH and ethambutol (EMB) until sputum cultures have remained negative for one year is an extremely effective and well-tolerated treatment schedule. Patients who have difficulty in adhering to self-administered treatment schedules must be carefully supervised.

tuberculostatic (tū-bĕr″kū-lō-stăt'ĭk). Arresting the growth of the tubercle bacillus.

tuberculotic (tū-bĕr″kū-lŏt'ĭk). Concerning

tuberculosis.

tuberculous (tū-bĕr'kū-lŭs) [L. *tuberculum,* a little swelling]. Relating to or affected with tuberculosis, or conditions marked by infiltration of a specific tubercle, as opposed to the term tubercular, referring to nonspecific tubercle.

tuberculum (tū-bĕr'kū-lŭm) [L. *tuberculum,* a little swelling]. (pl. *tubercula*) A small knot or nodule; a tubercle.

t. acusticum. Dorsal nucleus of the cochlear nerve.

t. majus humeri. [NA] Larger tuberosity of the humerus at upper end of its lateral surface giving attachment to infraspinatus, supraspinatus, and teres minor muscles.

t. minus humeri. [NA] The projection at the proximal end of the anterior humerus providing attachment to the subscapularis muscle.

tuberin (tū'bĕr-ĭn) [L. *tuber,* a swelling]. A simple protein; a globulin in potatoes.

tuberosis (tū"bĕr-ō'sĭs). A condition in which nodules develop; a nonspecific term that indicates no specific disease process.

tuberositas (tū-bĕr-ŏs'ĭt-ăs) [L.]. (pl. *tuberositates*) A projection, nodule, or prominence.

tuberosity (tū-bĕr-ŏs'ĭ-tē) [L. *tuberositas,* tuberosity]. 1. An elevated round process of a bone. 2. A tubercle or nodule.

tuberous (tū'bĕr-ŭs). Pert. to tubers.

tuberous sclerosis. A syndrome manifested by convulsive seizures, progressive mental disorder, adenoma sebaceum, and tumors of the kidneys and brain with projections into the cerebral ventricles.

tubo- [L. *tubus*]. Combining form meaning tube.

tuboabdominal (tū"bō-ăb-dŏm'ĭn-ăl) [L. *tubus,* tube, + *abdominalis,* pert. to the abdomen]. Pert. to the fallopian tubes and the abdomen.

tuboabdominal pregnancy. Ectopic gestation with embryo partly in tube and partly in the abdominal cavity.

tubocurarine chloride (tū"bō-kū-ră'rĭn klō'rīd). USP. Drug used to produce skeletal muscle relaxation during anesthesia and convulsive states, and in treating poisoning due to black widow spider bites. Tubocurarine was originally obtained from the Indian arrow poison, curare, q.v.

CAUTION: Tubocurarine should be administered only by those who have the proper equipment and are fully capable of providing artificial ventilation, tracheal intubation, appropriate antidotes, and additional therapy in case of overdose.

tuboligamentous (tū"bō-lĭg-ă-mĕn'tŭs) [" + *ligamentum,* a band]. Pert. to the fallopian tube and broad ligament of the uterus.

tubo-ovarian (tū"bō-ō-vā'rē-ăn) [" + *ovarium,* egg holder]. Pert. to the fallopian tube and the ovary.

tubo-ovariotomy (tū'bō-ō-vā-rē-ŏt'ō-mē) [" + *ovarium,* egg holder, + Gr. *tome,* incision]. Excision of ovaries and oviducts. SYN: *salpingo-oothecotomy.*

tubo-ovaritis (tū"bō-ō"vă-rī'tĭs) [" + " + Gr. *itis,* inflammation]. Inflammation of the ovary and fallopian tube.

tuboperitoneal (tū"bō-pĕr-ĭ-tō-nē'ăl) [" + Gr. *peritonaion,* peritoneum]. Rel. to the oviduct and peritoneum.

tuboplasty (tū'bō-plăs"tē). 1. Plastic repair of any tube. 2. Plastic repair of fallopian tube or tubes in an attempt to restore patency so that fertilization of the ovum may occur.

tuborrhea (tū-bor-rē'ă) [" + Gr. *rhoia,* a flow]. Discharge from the eustachian tube.

tubotorsion (tū"bō-tor'shŭn). The act of twisting a tube.

tubotympanal (tū"bō-tĭm'pă-năl) [" + Gr. *tympanon,* a drum]. Rel. to the tympanum of the ear and the eustachian tube.

tubouterine (tū"bō-ū'tĕr-ĭn) [" + *uterinus,* pert. to the uterus]. Rel. to the oviduct and the uterus.

tubovaginal (tū"bō-văj'ĭ-năl). Concerning the fallopian tube and the vagina.

tubular (tū'bū-lăr) [L. *tubularis,* like a tube]. Rel. to or having the form of a tube or tubule.

tubule (tū'būl) [L. *tubulus,* a tubule]. A small tube or canal.

t., collecting. Tubule in the renal medulla that is part of the discharging tubule.

t., convoluted, of kidney. The convoluted tubules of the nephron unit of the kidney that, along with the loop of Henle, the distal convoluted tubule, and the collecting tubule, provide a passageway for the glomerular filtrate to reach the renal pelvis. SEE: *kidney; nephron.*

t., convoluted seminiferous. The tubules present in each lobe of the testes.

t., dentinal. Very small canals in the dentin. They extend from the pulp cavity of the tooth to the enamel.

t., excretory. The uriniferous tubules in medullary portion of the kidneys.

t., galactophorous. The lactiferous ducts of the breast. They provide a channel for the milk formed in the lobes of the breast to pass to the nipple.

t., Henle's. Henle's loop, q.v.

t., junctional. Short part of a uriniferous tubule connecting with a collecting tubule.

t., lactiferous. T., galactophorous, q.v.

t., mesonephric. The tubes that make up the temporary kidney of amniotes (animals that form amnions).

t., metanephritic. The tubes that make up the permanent kidneys of amniotes.

t., renal. The tubules that connect the glomeruli to the renal pelvis. Included, in order, are the proximal convoluted tubules, loop of Henle, distal convoluted tubules, and the collecting tubules. SEE: *kidney; nephron.*

t.'s, seminiferous. Very small channels of the testes in which spermatozoa develop and through which they leave the testes.

t., uriniferous. Minute canals forming the glandular substance of the kidney, originating in Bowman's capsules and emptying into the pelvis of the kidney.

tubulin (tū'bū-lĭn). A protein present in the microtubules of cells.

tubulization (too"bū-lī-zā'shŭn). A method of repairing severed nerves in which the nerve ends are placed in a tube of absorbable material.

tubuloalveolar. Consisting of tubes and alveoli, as in a tubuloalveolar salivary gland.

tubulocyst (too'bū-lō-sĭst). The cystic dilatation of a functionless duct or canal.

tubulodermoid (tū"bū-lō-dĕr'moyd) [" + Gr. *derma,* skin, + *eidos,* form]. A dermoid tumor due to the persistent embryonic tubular structure.

tubuloracemose (too"bū-lō-răs'ĕ-mōs). Pert. to a gland that has tubular and racemose characteristics.

tubulorrhexis (too"bū-lō-rĕk'sĭs) [" + *rhexis,* a breaking]. Focal ruptures of renal tubules.

tubulous (too'bū-lŭs). Containing tubules.

tubulus (tū'bū-lŭs) [L.]. (pl. *tubuli*) [NA] A tubule; a small tube.

tubus (too'bŭs) [L.]. Tube.

t. digestorius. The alimentary canal.

tuft. A small clump, cluster, or coiled mass.

t., enamel. Abnormal structure formed in development of enamel consisting of poorly calcified twisted rods.

t., malpighian. The renal glomerulus.

tugging. A dragging or pulling.

t., tracheal. An indication of thoracic aneurysm.

SYM: A sense of downward pulling of larynx with cardiac systole when thyroid cartilage is gently raised between the finger and thumb.

tularemia (tū-lăr-ē'mē-ă) [*Tulare,* part of California where disease was first discovered]. An acute plague-like infectious disease caused by Francisella tularensis (formerly classed as Pasteurella tularensis). Transmitted to man by the bite of an infected tick or other bloodsucking insect; by direct contact with infected animals; by eating inadequately cooked meat or by drinking water that contains the organism. SYN: *deer fly fever; rabbit fever.*

SYM: May appear from 1 to 10 days but averaging 3 days after infection, headache, chilliness, vomiting, aching pains, and fever develop. Site of infection develops into an ulcer. Glands at elbow or in armpit become enlarged, tender, and painful; later [illegible] velop into an abscess. Sweating, loss of w[illegible] and debility.

TREATMENT: Streptomycin and tetracyclines are effective.

tumbu fly. Species of fly belonging to the genus Cordylobia in Africa and the genus Dermatobia in tropical America. Their larvae develop in the skin of wild and domesticated animals, and man is frequently attacked.

tumefacient (tū-mĕ-fā'shĕnt) [L. *tumefaciens,* producing swelling]. Producing or tending to produce swelling; swollen.

tumefaction (tū"mĕ-făk'shŭn) [L. *tumefactio,* a swelling]. 1. A swelling. 2. Act of swelling or the state of being swollen. SYN: *intumescence.*

tumentia (tū-mĕn'shē-ă) [L.]. Swelling.

t., vasomotor. Irregular swellings in lower extremities associated with vasomotor disturbances.

tumescence (tū-mĕs'ĕns). 1. Condition of being swollen or tumid. 2. A swelling.

tumid (tū'mĭd) [L. *tumidus*]. Swollen.

tumor (tū'mor) [L. *tumor,* a swelling]. 1. A swelling or enlargement. 2. Swelling, one of the four classical signs of inflammation. The others are calor (heat), dolor (pain), and rubor (redness). 3. A spontaneous new growth of tissue forming an abnormal mass. It is with few exceptions of unknown cause, noninflammatory, and develops independent of, and unrestrained by normal laws of growth and morphogenesis. SYN: *neoplasm.* SEE: *cancer.*

TYPES: *Myeloid sarcomata* or *giant-celled sarcomata:* Consist of elements formed chiefly of protoplasm containing two or more nuclei, up to 20 or even 50; with a varying number of round, spindle, or mixed cells. Vary in consistency from that of jelly to that of muscle. More frequently occurs on lower jaw, femur, and tibia. *Round-celled sarcomata:* Usually soft, vascular, rapidly growing, become large, and give rise to metastatic deposits in distant parts and in viscera. Occur in periosteum, bone, lymphatic glands, subcutaneous tissue, testicle, eye, ovary, uterus, lung, and kidneys although they may occur wherever fibrous tissue exists. *Glioma:* Grows from the connective tissue of nerve centers and its basic substance resembles that structure. Occurs in retina and brain. *Melanotic sarcoma:* In cells may be of either round or spindle variety. This type of tumor is extremely malignant. *Spindle-cell sarcoma:* Cells vary much in size, from small oat-shaped cells to greatly elongated bodies with long, fine, tapering extremities. Chiefly in bones. *Endotheliomata:* Occur, in different forms, in the testicle, pia mater, pleura, and peritoneum.

Acinous or spheroidal-celled carcinoma: Occurs in two forms: (1) hard, spheroidal-celled (scirrhus or chronic carcinoma) and (2) soft, spheroidal-celled (encephaloid or acute carcinoma). It resembles brain tissue in appearance and consistency. Occurs in testicle, liver, bladder, kidney, ovary, fundus oculi, and more rarely in the breast. SEE: *scirrhus*. *Colloid carcinoma:* One of preceding varieties that has undergone mucoid degeneration and so distended the alveoli that they may be seen by the naked eye. Occurs in stomach, intestine, omentum, and ovary. *Epithelial carcinoma:* (1) The squamous-celled epitheliomata that always spring from skin or mucous membranes or their glands, esp. at junctions of mucous and cutaneous surfaces. Are not encapsulated. Commence as wart-like growth, flattened tubercle, or fissure, ulceration in all these forms setting in early. (2) Cylindrical or columnar-celled. Less common form of carcinoma. Originates from either the cylindrical surface epithelium of a mucous membrane or its glands, closely imitating these structures in microscopic appearance. These growths form indurated infiltrating masses in the walls of organs attacked, producing considerable stenosis of lumen of hollow viscera; as rectum and small intestinal obstruction. Occur in uterus and intestinal tract.

Warty or villous growth (papillomata): Resemble in their structure hypertrophied papillae of skin or mucous membrane. These include condylomata and mucous tubercles. Occur about the anus and genitals or in the mouth and throat. Warts and warty growths on skin of hands and genitalia and mucous surface of larynx. Villous growths, bladder, rectum, and larynx. *Teratoma:* Tumors containing bone, hair, or teeth, usually situated in ovaries or testicles but may also be present in other tissues.

t., carotid body. A benign tumor of the carotid body, q.v.

t., connective tissue. Any tumor of connective tissue such as fibroma, lipoma, chondroma, or sarcoma.

t., desmoid. A tumor of the fibrous connective tissue.

t., erectile. A tumor composed of erectile tissue.

t., Ewing's. Malignant tumor of bone.

t., false. An enlargement due to hemorrhage into tissue or extravasation of fluid into a space but not due to a neoplastic growth.

t., fibroid. Benign fibrous tissue tumor of the myometrium.

t., giant cell, of bone. Tumor of bone that may be benign or malignant in which the cells are multinucleated and surrounded by cellular spindle cell stroma.

t., giant cell, of tendon sheath. Localized nodular tenosynovitis.

t., granulosa, granulosa cell. An estrin-secreting tumor of the granulosa cells of the ovary.

t., granulosa-theca cell. An estrogen-secreting tumor of the ovary made up of either granulosa or theca cells.

t., heterologous. A tumor the tissue of which is different from the tissue in which it is growing.

t., homoeiotypic, homologous. A tumor the tissue of which resembles the tissue in which it is growing.

t., Hürthle cell. A benign or malignant tumor of the thyroid gland. The cells are large and acidophilic.

t., islet cell. Tumor of the islets of Langerhans of the pancreas.

t., Krukenberg's. A tumor of the ovary due to metastases from a tumor in the gastrointestinal tract.

t., lipid cell, of the ovary. A masculinizing tumor of the ovary. It may be malignant.

t., mast cell. A benign nodular accumulation of mast cells.

t., melanotic neuroectodermal. A benign tumor of the jaw. It occurs mostly during the first year of life.

t., mesenchymal mixed. A tumor comprised of tissue that resembles mesenchymal cells.

t. of pregnancy. The abdominal swelling produced by the growing conceptus of pregnancy.

t., phantom. Gaseous distention of the intestinal tract.

t., sand. Psammoma, q.v.

t., turban. Multiple cutaneous cylindromata that cover the scalp like a turban.

t., Wilms. SEE: *Wilms tumor*.

tumoraffin (tū′mor-ăf-ĭn) [L. *tumor*, a swelling, + *affinis*, related]. Having an affinity for tumor cells. SYN: *oncotropic*.

tumor angiogenesis factor. ABBR: T.A.F. A protein present in animal and human cancer tissue that in experimental studies appears to be essential to growth of the cancer. The substance is thought to act by stimulating the growth of new blood capillaries for supplying the tumor with nutrients and removing waste products.

tumoricidal (too″mor-ĭ-sī′dăl). Lethal to neoplastic cells.

tumorigenesis (too″mor-ĭ-jĕn′ĕ-sĭs). Producing tumors.

tumorigenic (tū″mor-ĭ-jĕn′ĭk) [″ + Gr. *genesis*, origin]. To produce tumors, esp. malignancies. SYN: *oncogenic*. SEE: *carcinogenic*.

tumor markers, serum. Certain substances in blood serum that indicate the possible presence of a malignancy. None of these is perfectly reliable, but they do serve the purpose of monitoring response to therapy and estimating prognosis. Examples of the markers and the malignancies concerned are: carcinoembryonic antigen (ABBR: CEA) for tumors of the colon, lung, breast, and ovary; beta-chorionic gonadotropin for trophoblastic and testicular tumors; alpha-fetoprotein for testicular teratocarcinoma and primary hepatocellular carcinoma; and prostatic acid phosphatase for prostatic malignancy.

tumorous (too'mor-ŭs). Tumor-like.

tumor viruses. Viruses that cause malignant neoplasms. This is known to occur in a variety of species including some primates, but conclusive proof that any human tumor is virus-induced is lacking. Viruses that are suspected of being oncogenic, i.e., tumor-inducing, in man are Epstein-Barr virus linked to African Burkitt's lymphoma; hepatitis B virus with primary hepatocellular carcinoma; herpes simplex type 2 with carcinoma of the cervix; and cytomegalovirus with Kaposi's sarcoma.

tumultus (tū-mŭl'tŭs) [L.]. Excessive or agitated activity.

t. cordis. Irregular heart action with palpitation.

t. sermonis. Extreme stuttering due to pathologic cause.

Tunga (tŭng'ă). A genus of fleas of the family Hectopsyllidae.

T. penetrans. A small flea common in tropical regions. It infests man, cats, dogs, rats, pigs, and other animals. They produce a severe local inflammation frequently liable to secondary infection.

tungiasis (tŭng-gī'ă-sĭs). Infestation of the skin with Tunga penetrans.

tungsten (tŭng'stĕn). SYMB: W (for wolfram). At. wt. 183.85; at. no. 74. A metallic element.

tunic (tū'nĭk) [L. *tunica,* a sheath]. An investing membrane.

t., Bichat's. Tunica intima, q.v.

tunica (tū'nĭ-kă) [L. *tunica,* a sheath]. (pl. *tunicae*) An enveloping or covering membrane.

t. adventitia. [NA] Outer coat of an artery or any tubular structure.

t. albuginea. The white fibrous coat of the eye, testicle, ovary, or spleen. SEE: *testis* for illus.

t. conjunctiva. Conjunctiva, q.v.

t. dartos. [NA] The muscular, contractile tissue beneath the skin of the scrotum.

t. externa. Outer coat of an artery.

t. interna. T. intima.

t. intima. Lining coat of an artery. SYN: *t. interna.*

t. media. Middle muscular coat of an artery.

t. mucosa. Mucous membrane lining of various structures.

t. muscularis. The muscular tissue around structures such as the bronchi, intestines, and blood vessels.

t. propria. Most superficial portion of the corium containing loose connective tissue and small blood vessels, nerves, glands, and hair follicles. SYN: *lamina propria.*

t. serosa. The mesothelial lining of the external walls of the body cavities such as the pleural, peritoneal, and pericardial.

t. vaginalis. Serous membrane surrounding the front and sides of the testicle. SEE: *testis* for illus.

t. vasculosa. Any vascular layer.

tunicin (too'nĭ-sĭn). A cellulose-like substance found in the covering of some lower vertebrates.

tuning fork. Device that when struck at the forked end vibrates and thus can be heard and felt. It is used in testing the sensations of hearing, including bone conduction and vibration. A fork that vibrates at 256 cycles per second is suitable for use in these tests.

tunnel (tŭn'ĕl). A narrow channel or passageway.

t., carpal. The canal in the wrist bounded by osteofibrous material through which the flexor tendons and the median nerve pass.

t., flexor. T., carpal, q.v.

t., inner. Triangular canal lying between the inner and outer pillars of Corti in the organ of Corti of inner ear.

t., tarsal. The osteofibrous canal in the tarsal area bounded by the flexor retinaculum and tarsal bones. The posterior tibial vessels, tibial nerve, and flexor tendons pass through this tunnel.

tunnel vision. 1. A condition seen in hysteria wherein the field of vision is the same regardless of distance from the visual screen. 2. Severe constriction of the visual field due to advanced chronic glaucoma. 3. A figure of speech indicating an individual has a very narrow view or perspective of a situation or condition.

turbid (tŭr'bĭd) [L. *turba,* a tumult]. Cloudy; not clear. SEE: *turbidity.*

turbidimeter (tŭr-bĭ-dĭm'ĕ-ter) [L. *turbidus,* disturbed, + Gr. *metron,* a measure]. Device for estimating degree of turbidity of a fluid.

turbidimetry (tŭr-bĭ-dĭm'ĕ-trē) [" + Gr. *metron,* a measure]. Estimation of the turbidity of a liquid.

turbidity (tŭr-bĭd'ĭ-tē) [L. *turbiditas,* turbidity]. 1. Quality of not having translucent appearance of liquid due to growth of microorganisms. 2. Having flaky or granular particles suspended in a clear liquid giving it a cloudy appearance. SEE: *clarificant.*

turbinal, tubinate (tŭr'bĭ-năl, -nāt) [L. *turbinalis,* fr. *turbo,* a child's top]. Shaped like an inverted cone.

turbinated (tŭr'bĭ-nā"tĕd) [L. *turbo,* whirl]. Top- or cone-shaped. SEE: *concha.*

turbinectomy (tŭr-bĭn-ĕk'tō-mē) [" + Gr. *ektome,* excision]. Excision of a turbinated bone.

turbinotome (tŭr-bĭn'ō-tōm) [" + Gr. *tome,* incision]. Instrument for excision of a turbinated bone.

turbinotomy (tŭr-bĭn-ŏt'ō-mē) [" + Gr. *tome,* incision]. Surgical incision of a turbinated bone.

turgescence (tŭr-jĕs'ĕns) [L. *turgescens,* swelling]. Swelling or enlargement of a part.

turgescent (tŭr-jĕs'ĕnt) [L. *turgescens,* swelling]. Swollen; inflated.

turgid (tŭr'jĭd) [L. *turgidus,* swollen]. Swollen; bloated.

turgometer (tŭr-gŏm'ĕ-tĕr) [L. *turgor,* swelling, + Gr. *metron,* measure]. Device for measuring turgescence.

turgor [L., a swelling]. 1. Normal tension in a cell. 2. Distention, swelling.

t., skin. The resistance of the skin to deformation, esp. to being grasped between the fingers. The skin of the healthy person may, on the back of the hand, be grasped between the fingers and upon release either re-form immediately to its normal appearance or it may gently and relatively slowly settle back into its normal appearance. Which of these reactions occurs depends on several factors, including state of hydration of the skin but most importantly age. In the skin of the older person, the skin returns much more slowly to its normal position after having been pinched between the fingers of the examiner.

t. vitalis. Normal fullness of the capillaries and blood vessels.

turista (tū-rēs'tă) [Sp.]. One of the many names applied to travelers' diarrhea, q.v., esp. that which occurs in tourists in Mexico.

Turner's syndrome. [H. H. Turner, U.S. physician, b. 1892] Congenital endocrine disorder caused by failure of the ovaries to respond to pituitary hormone stimulation. Clinically there is amenorrhea, failure of sexual maturation, and usually short stature. About a third of these patients have webbing of the neck and may have marked cubitus valgus. Intelligence may be impaired. These patients usually have only 45 chromosomes, the second X chromosome being absent. SYN: *gonadal dysgenesis.* SEE: *karyotype.*

turning [AS. *turnian,* to turn]. Process of manually changing position of fetus in utero to permit normal delivery. SYN: *version.*

turpentine (tŭr'pĕn-tīn) [Gr. *terebinthos,* turpentine tree]. Oleoresin obtained from various species of pine trees. A mixture of terpenes and other hydrocarbons obtained from pine trees used externally in liniments and counterirritants. It is the source of oil of turpentine or spirits of turpentine.

turpentine poisoning. Usually contracted by inhalation. SEE: *Poisons and Poisoning* in *Appendix.*

SYM: Warm or burning sensation in the gullet and stomach, followed by cramping, vomiting, and diarrhea. Pulse and respiration become weak, slow, and irregular; irritation of urinary tract and central nervous system resembling alcoholic intoxication.

F.A.: Gastric lavage, soothing drinks, and stimulants. Increase fluid intake.

turricephaly (tŭr"ĭ-sĕf'ă-lē). Oxycephaly.

turunda (tū-rŭn'dă) [L.]. 1. A surgical tent, drain, or tampon. 2. A suppository.

tussal (tŭs'ăl) [L. *tussis,* cough]. Rel. to a cough. SYN: *tussive.*

Tusscapine. Trade name for noscapine.

tussicular (tŭ-sĭk'ū-lăr) [L. *tussis,* cough]. Pertaining to a cough.

tussiculation (tŭ-sĭk"ū-lā'shŭn). A short, dry cough.

tussis (tŭs'ĭs) [L.]. A cough.

t. convulsiva. Pertussis or whooping cough.

t. stomachalis. Reflex cough from irritation of the mucosa forming the lining of the stomach.

tussive (tŭs'ĭv) [L. *tussis,* cough]. Relating to a cough. SYN: *tussal.*

tutamen (tū-tā'mĕn) [L.]. Any tissue that has a protective action.

t. oculi. The structures around the eye that protect it: the eyebrows, eyelids, and eyelashes.

tutin (too'tĭn). A highly poisonous glycoside present in the New Zealand toot plant.

T.V.R. *tonic vibration reflex.* A polysynaptic reflex believed to depend on spinal and supraspinal pathways.

T wave. Portion of the electrocardiogram that is due to repolarization of the ventricles. The wave may be positive or negative depending upon the lead involved in recording the ECG and whether or not the electrical activity of the heart is within normal limits. SEE: *electrocardiogram; QRST complex.*

twelfth cranial nerve. One of a pair of cranial nerves distributing to the base of the tongue. SEE: *cranial nerves; hypoglossal nerve; Nerves* in *Appendix.*

twig. The final branch of a structure such as a nerve or vessel.

twilight sleep. A state of partial anesthesia and hypoconsciousness in which pain sense has been greatly reduced by the injection of morphine and scopolamine. Patient responds to pain, but afterward memory of pain is dulled or effaced. SEE: *labor.*

twilight state. One in which consciousness is disordered, making possible actions subsequently forgotten. Evidenced in hysteria and epilepsy.

twin (twĭn) [AS. *twinn*]. One of two children developed within the uterus at the same time from the same impregnation. SEE: illus.; *fetus papyraceus; Hellin's law.*

t.'s, biovular. Dizygotic twins.

t.'s, conjoined. Twins that are united. SEE: *Siamese twins.*

t.'s, dizygotic. Twins from two separate ova fertilized at the same time. SYN: *t.'s, biovular; t.'s, fraternal.* SEE: *t.'s, monozygotic.*

t.'s, enzygotic. T.'s, monozygotic.

t.'s, fraternal. T.'s, dizygotic.

t.'s, identical. T.'s, monozygotic.

t.'s, impacted. Twins so entwined in utero as to prevent normal delivery.

t.'s, interlocked. Twins in which the neck of one becomes interlocked with the head of the other, making vaginal delivery impossible.

t.'s, monozygotic. Twins that develop from a single fertilized ovum. Twins of this type have the same genetic makeup and, consequently, are of the same sex and resemble each other strikingly in physical, physiological, and mental traits. They develop within a common chorionic sac and have a common placenta. Each usually develops its own amnion and umbilical cord. Such twins may result from development of two inner cell masses within a blastocyst, development of two embryonic axes on a single blastoderm, or the division of a single embryonic axis into two centers. SYN: *t.'s, enzygotic; t.'s, identical; t.'s, true; t.'s, uniovular.*

t., parasitic. The smaller of a pair of conjoined twins, when there is a marked disparity in size.

t.'s, Siamese. Symmetrically conjoined twins. SEE: *Siamese twins.*

t.'s, true. T.'s, monozygotic.

t.'s, unequal. Twins, one of which is underdeveloped.

t.'s, uniovular. T.'s, monozygotic.

twinge (twĭnj) [AS. *twengan,* to pinch]. A sudden keen pain.

twinning (twĭn′ĭng). Delivery of or producing twins.

twitch (twĭch) [ME. *twicchen*]. 1. A simple, quick, spasmodic contraction of a muscle. SEE: *myokymia; myopalmus.* 2. To jerk convulsively.

twitching (twĭtch′ĭng). Repeated contractions of portions of muscles.

two-point discrimination test. Test of cu-

TWIN PREGNANCIES

SEPARATE PLACENTAS

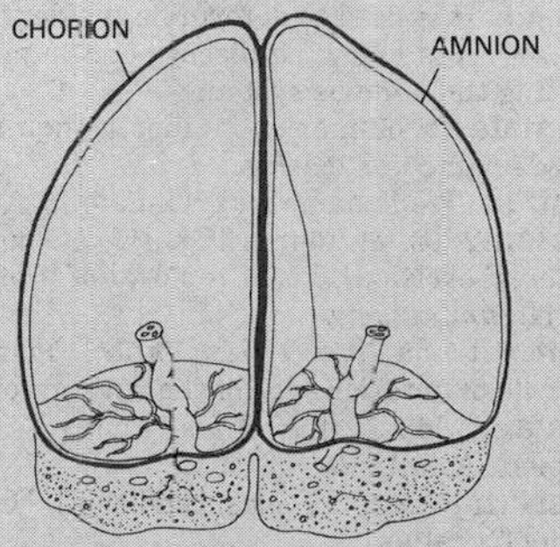

TWO PLACENTAS, TWO AMNIONS, TWO CHORIONS (DIZYGOTIC TWINS, OR MONOZYGOTIC TWINS WITH CLEAVAGE OF ZYGOTE DURING FIRST 3 DAYS AFTER FERTILIZATION)

SINGLE PLACENTA

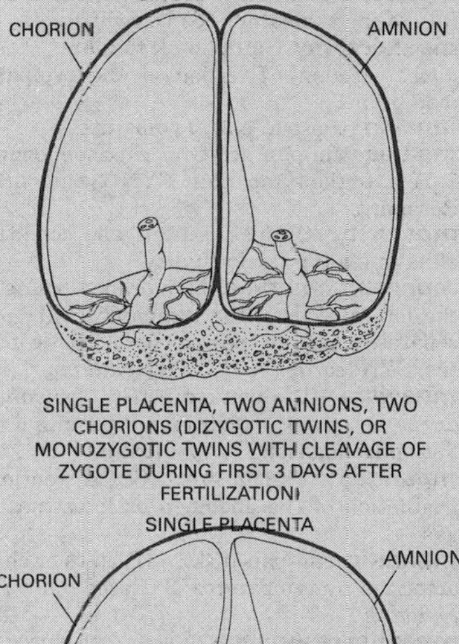

SINGLE PLACENTA, TWO AMNIONS, TWO CHORIONS (DIZYGOTIC TWINS, OR MONOZYGOTIC TWINS WITH CLEAVAGE OF ZYGOTE DURING FIRST 3 DAYS AFTER FERTILIZATION)

SINGLE PLACENTA

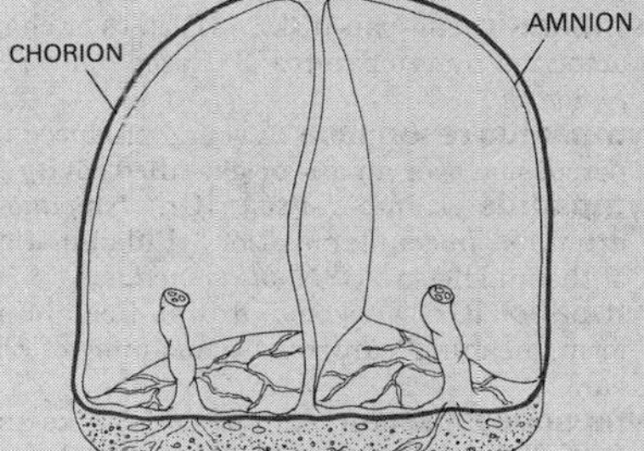

SINGLE PLACENTA, SINGLE CHORION, TWO AMNIONS (MONOZYGOTIC TWINS WITH CLEAVAGE OF ZYGOTE FROM 4TH TO 8TH DAY AFTER FERTILIZATION)

taneous sensation involving determination of the ability of the patient to detect that the skin is being touched by two pointed objects at once. It is used to determine the degree of sensory loss following disease or trauma affecting the nervous system.

tybamate (tī'bă-māt). A minor tranquilizer. Trade name is Tybatran.

Tybatran. Trade name for tybamate.

tylectomy (tī-lĕk'tō-mē) [Gr. *tylos,* knot, + *ektome,* excision]. Local removal of a lesion. SYN: *lumpectomy.*

tylion (tĭl'ē-ŏn) [Gr. *tyleion,* knot]. Point at middle of anterior edge of the optic groove.

tyloma (tī-lō'mă) [Gr. *tylos,* knot, + *oma,* tumor]. A callosity.

tylosis (tī-lō'sĭs) [" + *osis,* condition]. Formation of a callus.

tyloxapol (tī-lŏks'ă-pōl). USP. A nonionic liquid polymer of the alkyl aryl polyether alcohol type. It is a detergent used to reduce the viscosity of bronchopulmonary secretions. Trade name is Superinone.

tympanal (tĭm'păn-ăl) [Gr. *tympanon,* drum]. Rel. to the tympanum. SYN: *tympanic.*

tympanectomy (tĭm"păn-ĕk'tō-mē) [" + *ektome,* excision]. Excision of the tympanic membrane.

tympania (tĭm-păn'ē-ă). Tympanites.

tympanic (tĭm-păn'ĭk) [Gr. *tympanon,* drum]. 1. Pert. to the tympanum. SYN: *tympanal.* 2. Resonant.

tympanicity (tĭm"pă-nĭs'ĭ-tē). The condition of having a tympanic quality.

tympanic membrane. Membrane serving as the lateral wall of the tympanic cavity and separating it from the external acoustic meatus. SYN: *eardrum.* SEE: *tympanum.*

tympanism (tĭm'păn-ĭzm) [Gr. *tympanon,* drum, + *-ismos,* condition]. Abdominal inflation from gas. SYN: *tympanites.*

tympanites (tĭm-păn-ī'tēz) [Gr., distention]. Distention of the abdomen or intestines by gas.

tympanitic (tĭm-păn-ĭt'ĭk). 1. Pert. to or characterized by tympanites. 2. Resonant. SYN: *tympanic.*

tympanitic resonance. A sound produced by percussion over an air- or gas-filled cavity.

tympanitis (tĭm-păn-ī'tĭs) [Gr. *tympanon,* drum, + *itis,* inflammation]. Inflammation of the middle ear. SYN: *otitis media.*

tympano- [Gr. *tympanon,* drum]. Combining form meaning eardrum, tympanum of the ear.

tympanoeustachian (tĭm"pă-nō-ū-stā'kē-ăn). Concerning the tympanic cavity and the eustachian tube.

tympanography. Radiographic examination of the eustachian tubes and middle ear after introduction of a contrast medium.

tympanohyal (tĭm"pă-nō-hī'ăl). Concerning the tympanic cavity and the hyoid arch.

tympanomalleal (tĭm"pă-nō-măl'ē-ăl). Concerning the tympanic membrane and the malleus.

tympanomandibular (tĭm"pă-nō-măn-dĭb'ū-lăr). Concerning the middle ear and the mandible.

tympanomastoiditis (tĭm"păn-ō-măs"toy-dī'tĭs) [" + *mastos,* breast, + *eidos,* form, + *itis,* inflammation]. Inflammation of the tympanum and mastoid cells.

tympanometry (tĭm"pă-nŏm'ĕ-trē). Procedure for objective evaluation of the mobility and patency of the eardrum.

tympanoplasty (tĭm"păn-ō-plăs'tē) [" + *plassein,* to form]. Any one of several surgical procedures designed either to cure a chronic inflammatory process in the middle ear or to restore function to the sound-transmitting mechanism of the middle ear.

tympanosclerosis (tĭm"pă-nō-sklĕ-rō'sĭs). Infiltration by hard fibrous tissue around the ossicles of the middle ear.

tympanosis (tĭm-pă-nō'sĭs) [" + *osis,* condition]. Tympanites.

tympanosquamosal (tĭm"pă-nō-skwă-mō'săl). Concerning the pars tympanica and pars squamosa of the temporal bone.

tympanostapedial (tĭm"pă-nō-stă-pē'dē-ăl). Concerning the tympanic cavity and the stapes.

tympanotemporal (tĭm"pă-nō-tĕm'pō-răl). Concerning the tympanic cavity and the area of the temporal bone.

tympanotomy (tĭm"păn-ŏt'ō-mē) [" + *tome,* incision]. Incision of the membrana tympani. SYN: *myringotomy.*

tympanous (tĭm'păn-ŭs) [Gr. *tympanon,* a drum]. Marked by abdominal distention with gas.

tympanum (tĭm'păn-ŭm) [L.; Gr. *tympanon*]. The middle ear or tympanic cavity. SYN: *cavum tympani; eardrum.* SEE: *ear, middle.*

tympany (tĭm'pă-nē). 1. Abdominal distention with gas. 2. Tympanic resonance on percussion. It is a clear hollow note like that of a drum having no vesicular quality. It indicates a pathological condition of the lung or of a cavity.

type (tīp) [Gr. *typos,* mark]. The general character of a person, a disease, or substance.

t., asthenic. Having a thin, flat, long-chested body build with poor muscular development.

t., athletic. Having broad shoulders, deep chest, flat abdomen, thick neck, and excellent muscular development.

t., blood. SEE: *blood groups.*

t., phage. Distinguishing subgroups of bacteria by the type of bacteriophage associated with that specific bacterium.

t., pyknic. Having a rounded body, large

chest, thick shoulders, broad head, thick neck, and usually short stature.

typhlectasis (tĭf-lĕk'tă-sĭs) [Gr. *typhlon,* cecum, + *ektasis,* dilatation]. Cecal distention.

typhlectomy (tĭf-lĕk'tō-mē) [" + *ektome,* excision]. Excision of the cecum. SYN: *cecectomy.*

typhlenteritis (tĭf"lĕn-tĕr-ī'tĭs) [" + *enteron,* intestine, + *itis,* inflammation]. Inflammation of the cecum. SYN: *typhlitis.*

typhlitis (tĭf-lī'tĭs) [" + *itis,* inflammation]. Inflammation of the cecum.

typhlo-. 1. Combining form indicating a relationship to the cecum. 2. Combining form indicating a relationship to blindness.

typhlodicliditis (tĭf"lō-dĭk-lĭ-dī'tĭs) [" + *diklis,* door, + *itis,* inflammation]. Inflammation of the ileocecal valve.

typhloempyema (tĭf"lō-ĕm-pī-ē'mă) [" + *en,* in, + *pyon,* pus, + *haima,* blood]. An abdominal abscess following appendicitis.

typhloenteritis (tĭf"lō-ĕn-tĕr-ī'tĭs) [" + *enteron,* intestine, + *itis,* inflammation]. Inflammation of the cecum. SYN: *typhlenteritis; typhlitis.*

typhlolexia (tĭf"lō-lĕk'sē-ă) [Gr. *typhlos,* blind, + *lexis,* speech]. Alexia.

typhlolithiasis (tĭf"lō-lĭ-thī'ă-sĭs) [Gr. *typhlon,* cecum, + *lithos,* stone, + *-iasis,* condition]. Formation of a concretion in the cecum.

typhlology (tĭf-lŏl'ō-jē) [Gr. *typhlos,* blind, + *logos,* study]. Study of blindness, its causes and effects.

typhlomegaly (tĭf"lō-mĕg'ă-lē) [Gr. *typhlon,* cecum, + *megas,* large]. Abnormally large cecum.

typhlon (tĭf'lŏn) [Gr.]. The cecum.

typhlopexy (tĭf'lō-pĕks"ē) [Gr. *typhlon,* cecum, + *pexis,* fixation]. Suturing of a movable cecum to the abdominal wall.

typhlorrhaphy (tĭf-lor'ă-fē). Surgical repair of the cecum.

typhlosis (tĭf-lō'sĭs) [Gr. *typhlos,* blind, + *osis,* condition]. Blindness.

typhlospasm (tĭf'lō-spăsm). Spasm of the cecum.

typhlostenosis (tĭf"lō-stĕn-ō'sĭs) [Gr. *typhlon,* cecum, + *stenosis,* a narrowing]. Stenosis or stricture of the cecum.

typhlostomy (tĭf-lŏs'tō-mē) [" + *stoma,* opening]. Establishment of a permanent cecal fistula.

typhlotomy (tĭf-lŏt'ō-mē) [Gr. *typhlon,* cecum, + *tome,* incision]. Incision of the cecum.

typhloureterostomy (tĭf"lō-ū-rē"tĕr-ŏs'tō-mē) [" + *oureter,* ureter, + *stoma,* opening]. Implantation of a ureter in the cecum.

typho- [Gr. *typhos,* stupor arising from fever]. Combining form pert. to fever or to typhoid.

typhobacillosis (tī"fō-băs-ĭl-ō'sĭs) [" + L. *bacillus,* little stick, + Gr *osis,* condition]. Poisoning due to toxins produced by the typhoid bacillus.

typhohemia (tī"fō-hē'mē-ă) [" + *haima,* blood]. Degeneration of the blood due to presence of bacilli.

typhoid (tī'foyd) [Gr. *typhos,* stupor, + *eidos,* form]. Resembling typhus.

typhoidal (tī-foy'dăl). Resembling typhoid.

typhoid carrier. An individual who has recovered from typhoid fever but who harbors the bacteria, usually in the gallbladder, and who excretes the organism in urine and feces.

typhoid fever. An acute infectious disease characterized by definite lesions in Peyer's patches, mesenteric glands, and spleen accompanied by fever, headache, and abdominal pain.

ETIOL: Causative organism Salmonella typhi (S. typhi), a gram-negative, motile bacillus. It may be transmitted by infected water or milk supplies. Human carriers, particularly when food handlers, may be responsible for spread of infection. Body discharges from active or convalescent cases may be the means of infecting others.

INCUBATION: Average two weeks; varies from one to three weeks.

SYM: Early symptoms are headache, general weakness, indefinite pains, and nosebleed. Constipation may occur. Within a few days to a week the temperature may reach a maximum of 104° to 105° F. (40° to 40.6° C.) and during this time, or up to the 10th day, rose spots can usually be seen, particularly on the abdomen, though they may be observed on the chest and back. They usually come out in crops during a period of several days. They will blanch upon pressure. Abdominal tenderness develops and with it, generally, distention. Splenomegaly will be found in more than half of the cases by the end of the first week.

During following weeks fever is characterized by marked daily remissions, evening temperature being from 1° to 3° F. (0.56° to 1.7° C.) higher than the morning. In the young the temperature often rises very abruptly. When the diurnal remissions are slight, a protracted case is forecast. As defervescence advances, the temperature becomes more irregular. Remissions are more decided and not infrequently a higher temperature is recorded in the morning. Rapid respiratory rate, slight cough, and bronchial rales are common. Pulse is usually slow in comparison with the temperature rise and is dicrotic. Heart sounds are often feeble, expression dull and heavy, cheeks somewhat flushed, conjunctivae clear, pupils dilated.

Tongue tremulous; at first red at tip and

edges, and covered posteriorly with a whitish fur. In severe cases, tongue becomes dry, brown and fissured, and sordes collect on teeth. Gastric symptoms not common but when present they are obstinate. Vomiting sometimes develops and becomes a serious complication. Abdomen is tympanitic and there is tenderness on palpation, esp. in the iliac fossa. Diarrhea generally present though not a constant symptom. Bowel movements vary from three to six or more a day; thin, offensive, yellowish. Stupor, muttering, delirium, twitching of the muscles, carphologia, and coma vigil may be present. Proteinuria and retention of urine is common. White blood count demonstrates a leukopenia. Convalescence marked by anemia, loss of hair, often desquamation. The patient gives evidence of having suffered from a protracted illness that has produced general mental and physical debilitation.

COMPLICATIONS: These occur in approximately 25% of untreated cases and account for the majority of deaths. The most frequent and dangerous complications are intestinal hemorrhage and intestinal perforation. An abrupt fall of several degrees in temperature is suggestive of intestinal hemorrhage or perforation. Usually occurs during 3rd or 4th week.

DIFF. DIAG: Paratyphoid, pneumonia, dysentery, meningitis, smallpox, appendicitis. Diagnostic points of value will be the presence of rose spots, splenomegaly, leukopenia, the Widal serological test, blood culture, and examination of feces for presence of causative organism.

PROG: Should always be guarded, no matter how mild the case appears to be. Fatality rate varies in different epidemics. Hemorrhages in any form, together with excessive diarrhea, are unfavorable signs.

PROPHYLAXIS: Immunity can ordinarily be established by administering two injections of vaccine several weeks apart. SEE: *typhoid vaccine*.

TREATMENT: General care, isolation of patient, and disinfection of all discharges are of primary importance. Those caring for the typhoid patient should be immunized against the disease. All precautions applicable to such infections must be adopted. Articles in contact with the patient must be sterilized or disinfected before being handled by persons other than the immediate attendant. It is necessary to guard against development of bedsores. Since delirium is not infrequent, patient may require constant watching to prevent his or her leaving the bed. The mouth should be kept as clean as possible to prevent development of sordes. Ampicillin is the drug of choice, but chloramphenicol may be required in severe cases.

Ice bags and cold sponging are little used at the present time. On the other hand, sponging with tepid water, or with alcohol, is sometimes used when the temperature has reached unusual heights. Surgical intervention will be necessary if antibiotics and bowel decompression fail to control severe hemorrhage or if intestinal perforation occurs.

NURSING IMPLICATIONS: Offer emotional support. Administer drugs as prescribed, and observe for complications such as bacteremia and intestinal bleeding. During the acute phase, monitor temperature and initiate appropriate antipyretic measures, cleanse the incontinent patient, and encourage high fluid intake. Watch for bladder distention, and monitor intake and output. Watch for constipation and institute appropriate measures to relieve it. Observe enteric precautions until three consecutive stool cultures are negative for S. typhi. Maintain adequate nutrition. Inform the patient of the importance of follow-up care and examination to be certain of being or not being a carrier.

Charting: A four-hour chart should be kept of temperature, pulse, and respiration, although the pulse should be taken much more frequently than this. In the 3rd week, the temperature should be taken every two hours. A sudden drop in temperature indicates hemorrhage.

Disinfection: The usual methods of disinfection should be observed in handling all excreta and secretions, linens, and utensils. Disinfection for the nurse is also very important.

typhoid vaccine. A vaccine containing killed Salmonella typhi. Even though its effectiveness in preventing typhoid fever is limited to protecting only those who have experienced a small infecting dose of Salmonella typhi, its use is advisable in persons who will be exposed to typhoid bacilli.

typholysin (tī-fŏl′ĭ-sĭn) [″ + *lysis,* dissolution]. A lysin destructive to typhoid bacilli.

typhomalarial (tī″fō-mă-lā′rē-ăl) [″ + It. *malaria,* bad air]. Having symptoms of both typhoid and malarial fever.

typhomania (tī-fō-mā′nē-ă) [″ + *mania,* madness]. Muttering delirium characteristic of typhoid fever and typhus.

typhopneumonia (tī″fō-nū-mō′nē-ă) [″ + *pneumonia,* inflammation of lungs]. 1. Pneumonia occurring in typhoid fever. 2. Pneumonia with typhoid symptoms.

typhous (tī′fŭs) [Gr. *typhos,* stupor]. Pert. to typhus fever.

typhus (tī′fŭs) [Gr. *typhos,* stupor arising from fever]. Any of a group of acute infectious diseases characterized by great prostration, severe headache, generalized maculopapular rash, sustained high fever, and usually progressive neurologic involvement, ending in a crisis in 10 to 14 days.

Three diseases are included in the group: epidemic (louse-borne) typhus, caused by Rickettsia prowazekii; Brill-Zinsser disease (recrudescent typhus), caused by Rickettsia prowazekii; and murine (flea-borne) typhus, caused by Rickettsia typhi. Although clinically and pathologically similar, they differ in intensity of symptoms, severity, and mortality rate.

Epidemic typhus is particularly prevalent amid unsanitary conditions. It often develops on shipboard, in army camps, and where living conditions are unfavorable and congestion is marked. The disease is rare in the U.S.A.

INCUBATION: One to two weeks except for Brill-Zinsser disease, which may recur years after the initial attack.

SYM: Onset sudden. Severe headache, pain in back and limbs, extreme prostration. Fever rises rapidly, often reaching 104° to 105° F. (40° to 40.6° C.) in two to three days. Remains high for about 10 days, when it falls by crisis. Pulse rapid, weak, often dicrotic. Tongue tremulous, may be covered with whitish fur; in severe cases becomes black and rolled up like a ball in back of mouth. Face dusky, conjunctivae injected, pupil contracted, headache, stupor, delirium, muscle twitching, picking at the bedclothes (carphologia).

From 4th to 5th day, bluish spots appear over body, esp. on abdomen. These are petechial in character and do not disappear on pressure. The extent of eruption is indicative of severity of attack. Sometimes there is a diffuse, dark red, subcuticular mottling. Bowels are constipated, urine is scanty, high-colored, and often albuminous.

COMPLICATIONS: Bronchopneumonia occurs more frequently than lobar. Hypostatic congestion of lungs, nephritis, and parotid abscess.

DIFF. DIAG.: Typhoid fever, hemorrhagic smallpox, Henoch's purpura, epidemic meningitis of fulminating type, and ulcerative endocarditis may have to be considered.

PROG: Variable. Mortality may be quite high in epidemic typhus and almost nonexistent in murine typhus. Broad-spectrum antibiotics will be life-saving if given early enough.

TREATMENT: *Preventive:* Absolute cleanliness, sterilization of clothing, and the use of apparel to prevent infestation by the body louse. Patient must be isolated. Absolute rest necessary, and liquid diet. *Specific:* Broad-spectrum antibiotics, such as the tetracyclines and chloramphenicol, give excellent results.

t., classic. T., epidemic.

t., endemic. T., murine.

t., epidemic. An infectious disease caused by Rickettsia prowazekii and transmitted by human body louse (Pediculus humanus humanus). SYN: *t., classic.*

t., flea-borne. T., murine.

t., Mexican. A louse-borne epidemic typhus present in certain portions of Mexico. SYN: *tabardillo.*

t., mite-borne. Tsutsugamushi disease or scrub typhus.

t., murine. A disease caused by Rickettsia mooseri and occurring in nature as a mild infection of rats and transmitted from rat to rat by the rat-louse or flea. Humans may acquire it by being bitten by infected rat fleas or ingesting food contaminated by rat urine or flea feces. SYN: *t., endemic; t., flea-borne; t., shop.*

t., recrudescent. A recurrence or recrudescence of a preceding attack of epidemic typhus after initial attack.

t., rural. T., scrub.

t., scrub. A self-limited febrile disease of two weeks' duration caused by Rickettsia tsutsugamushi and transmitted by two species of mites (chiggers) of the genus Trombicula. Occurs principally in Pacific-Asiatic area. SYN: *t., mite-borne; t., rural; tsutsugamushi disease.*

t., shop. T., murine.

t., urban. T., epidemic.

typhus vaccine. USP. A sterile suspension of the killed rickettsial organism of a strain or strains of epidemic typhus rickettsiae.

typical (tĭp'ĭ-kăl) [Gr. *typikos,* pert. to type]. Having the characteristics of, pert. to, or conforming to, a type or condition or group.

typing (tīp'ĭng). Identification of type.

t., bacteriophage. Determination of the subdivision of a bacterial species using a type-specific bacteriophage.

t., blood. Determination of the specific blood group of an individual. SEE: *blood transfusion.*

t., tissue. Determination of the histocompatibility of tissues to be used in grafts and transplants. SEE: *transplantation.*

typo- [Gr. *typos*]. Combining form meaning a type.

typoscope (tī'pō-skōp) [" + *skopein,* to examine]. A reading aid device for patients with amblyopia or cataract.

typus (tī'pŭs) [L.]. Type.

tyramine (tī'ră-mēn). Intermediate product in the conversion of tyrosine to epinephrine. Tyramine is found in most cheeses and in beer, broad bean pods, yeast, wine, and chicken liver. When persons taking certain types of antidepressant monoamine oxidase inhibitors also eat these foods, they may experience severe hypertension, headache, palpitation, neck pain, and perhaps intracranial hemorrhage. This is due to the tyramine's not being inactivated by monoamine oxidation. This has been called the "cheese reaction."

tyrannism (tĭr'ăn-ĭzm) [Gr. *tyrannos,* tyrant, + *-ismos,* condition]. Abnormal tendency to exercise cruelty. SYN: *sadism.*

tyrogenous (tī-rŏj'ĕn-ŭs) [Gr. *tyros,* cheese, + *gennan,* produce]. Having origin in or produced by cheese.

Tyroglyphus (tī-rŏg'lĭ-fŭs) [Gr. *tyros,* cheese, + *glyphein,* to carve]. A genus of sarcoptoid mites commonly known as cheese mites. They infest cheese and dried vegetable food products and occasionally infest man causing a pruritus. Contains species causing grocer's itch, vanillism, and copra itch.

tyroid (tī'royd) [" + *eidos,* form]. Caseous; cheesy.

tyroma (tī-rō'mă). A tumor containing cheese-like material.

tyromatosis (tī"rō-mă-tō'sĭs) [" + *oma,* tumor, + *osis,* condition]. Conversion of necrotic tissue into a granular amorphous mass resembling cheese. SYN: *caseation.*

tyrosinase (tī-rō'sĭn-ās) [Gr. *tyros,* cheese]. An enzyme that acts on tyrosine to produce melanin.

tyrosinemia (tī"rō-sĭ-nē'mē-ă). A disease of tyrosine metabolism due to a deficiency of the enzyme tyrosine aminotransferase. In addition to an accumulation of tyrosine in the blood, mental retardation, keratitis, and dermatitis are present. Treatment consists of controlling the phenylalanine and tyrosine intake.

tyrosine (tī'rō-sĭn). USP. An amino acid present in many proteins, esp. casein. It serves as a precursor of epinephrine, thyroxine, and melanin. Two vitamins, ascorbic acid and folic acid, are essential for its metabolism.

tyrosinosis (tī"rō-sĭn-ō'sĭs) [" + *osis,* condition]. Condition resulting from faulty metabolism of tyrosine, whereby its oxidation products appear in the urine.

tyrosinuria (tī"rō-sĭn-ū'rē-ă) [" + *ouron,* urine]. Tyrosine in the urine.

tyrosis (tī-rō'sĭs) [" + *osis,* condition]. 1. Curdling of milk. 2. Vomiting of cheesy substance by infants. 3. Cheesy degeneration. SYN: *tyromatosis.*

tyrosyluria (tī"rō-sĭl-ū'rē-ă). Increased tyrosine-derived products in the urine.

tyrothricin (tī"rō-thrī'sĭn). An antibacterial drug.

tyrotoxism (tī"rō-tŏks'ĭzm) [" + *toxikon,* a poison, + *-ismos,* condition]. Poisoning produced by a milk product or by cheese.

Tyrrell's fascia (tĭr'rĕlz). [Frederick Tyrrell, Brit. anatomist, 1797–1843] An ill-defined fibromuscular layer from the middle aponeurosis of the perineum, behind the prostate gland.

Tyson's glands (tī'sŭnz). [Edward Tyson, Brit. physician and anatomist, 1649–1708] Modified sebaceous glands located on neck of penis and inner surface of prepuce. Their secretion is one of the components of smegma. SYN: *preputial glands.*

tysonitis (tī"sŏn-ī'tĭs). Inflammation of Tyson's glands.

tyvelose (tī'vĕl-ōs). A carbohydrate, 3-6-dideoxy-D-mannose, derived from certain strains of Salmonella. It is a somatic antigen.

Tyzine. Trade name for tetrahydrozoline hydrochloride, USP.

Tzank test (tsănk). [Arnault Tzank, Russ. dermatologist in Paris, 1886–1954] Examination of tissue from the lower surface of a lesion in vesicular disease to determine the cell type.

tzetze (sĕt'sē). Tsetse.

U

U. 1. *unit.* 2. Chem. symb. for uranium.

[235]U. Isotope of uranium with mass number 235.

UAO. *upper airway obstruction.*

uberous (ū'bĕr-ŭs) [L. *uber,* udder]. Prolific; fruitful; fertile.

uberty (ū'bĕr-tē) [L. *uber,* udder]. Fruitfulness; fertility.

ubiquinol (ū-bĭk'wĭ-nŏl). Coenzyme QH_2, the reduced form of ubiquinone, q.v.

ubiquinone (ū-bĭk'wĭ-nōn) [*ubi*quitous + coenzyme *quinone*]. Coenzyme Q, a lipid-soluble quinone present in virtually all cells. It is a collector of reducing equivalents during intracellular respiration. It is converted to its reduced form, ubiquinol, while involved in this process.

udder (ŭd'ĕr). The mammary gland of animals such as cows and goats.

UDP. *uridine diphosphate.*

Uffelmann's test (oof'ĕl-mănz). [Jules Uffelmann, Ger. physician, 1837–1894] Test for determination of lactic acid in gastric juice.

U-Gencin. Trade name for gentamicin sulfate, USP.

Uhthoff's sign (oot'hŏfs). [Wilhelm Uhthoff, Ger. ophthalmologist, 1853–1927] The nystagmus that occurs in multiple disseminated sclerosis.

ulaganactesis (ū-lăg"ă-năk'tē-sĭs) [Gr. *oulon,* gum, + *aganektesis,* irritation]. Disagreeable sensations or irritation in or about the gums.

ulalgia (ū-lăl'jē-ă) [" + *algos,* pain]. Pain in the gums.

ulatrophia (ū-lă-trō'fē-ă) [" + *atrophos,* ill-nourished]. Shrinking of gums; recession of the gums.

ulcer (ŭl'sĕr) [L. *ulcus,* ulcer]. An open sore or lesion of the skin or mucous membrane accompanied by sloughing of inflamed necrotic tissue. If the sore becomes infected, pus is discharged. Simple ulcers may result from trauma, caustics, intense heat or cold, or arterial or venous stasis. They may occur as a complication of varicose veins due to stasis of blood leading to inflammation, necrosis, and sloughing of tissue. Ulcers of the mucous membrane of the stomach or duodenum are caused by the effect of gastric acid and pepsin. The sores of acquired syphilis are caused by blockage of small vessels. The secretion from these sores contains the causative agent Treponema pallidum.

RS: abscission; anabrosis; anthracosis; aphtha; argema; carcinelcosis; carcinomelcosis; dieresis; phagedena; slough; stomach.

u., amputating. Ulcer that destroys tissue to the bone by encircling the part.

u., atonic. A chronic ulcer.

u., callous. A chronic ulcer with indurated, elevated edges and no granulations, which does not heal.

u., chronic leg. Any long-standing slow-to-heal ulcer of the lower extremity, esp. one due to occlusive disease of the arteries or veins, or varicose veins.

u., Curling's. Peptic ulcer that sometimes occurs following severe burns to the body. A form of stress ulcer.

u., decubitus. Ischemic necrosis and ulceration of tissue, esp. over a bony prominence. Due to pressure from prolonged confinement in bed or from a cast or splint. SYN: *bedsore.* SEE: *decubitus ulcer.*

u., duodenal. An ulcer on the mucosa of the duodenum, due to the action of the gastric juice.

u., follicular. A tiny ulcer having its origin in a lymph follicle and affecting a mucous membrane.

u., fungus. Ulcer in which the granulations protrude above edges of the wound and bleed easily.

u., gastric. An ulcer of the gastric mucosa. SEE: *peptic ulcer.*

u., Hunner's. A painful, slow-to-heal ulcer of the urinary bladder.

u., indolent. Nearly painless ulcer usually found on the leg, characterized by an indurated and elevated edge and a nongranulating base.

u., peptic. An ulcer of the mucosa of the duodenum or stomach. SEE: *peptic ulcer.*

u., perforating. An ulcer that permeates the entire thickness of the part, as the foot or intestine.

u., phagedenic. An ulcer that spreads rapidly and disintegrates the tissues, producing a slough and discharge.

u., rodent. A deeply infiltrating ulcer that slowly destroys bones and soft tissues; commonly affects the upper part of the face. SYN: *Jacob's ulcer.*

u., serpiginous. A creeping ulcer that heals in one part and extends to another.

u., simple. A local ulcer with no severe inflammation or pain.

u., specific. An ulcer caused by a specific disease, as syphilis or lupus.

u., stercoral. 1. Ulcer caused by pressure from impacted feces. 2. Ulcer through which feces escape.

u., stress. Peptic ulcer due to acute or chronic stress such as may be present with cerebral trauma, burns, surgery, acute infection, prolonged adrenal corticosteroid therapy, or central nervous system disease.

u., trophic. An ulcer due to failure of supply of nutrients to a part.

u., tropical. 1. An indolent ulcer, usually of the lower extremity, that occurs in persons living in hot, humid areas. The etiology may or may not be known, and it may be due to a combination of bacterial, environmental, and nutritional factors. 2. The tropical sore caused by leishmaniasis.

u., varicose. An ulcer, esp. of the lower extremity, associated with varicose veins.

u., venereal. An ulcer caused by a venereal disease, i.e., chancre, or chancroid.

ulcera. Pl. of ulcus.

ulcerate (ŭl'sĕr-āt) [L. *ulcerare*]. To produce or become affected with an ulcer.

ulcerated (ŭl'sĕr-ā"tĕd). Of the nature of an ulcer or affected with one.

ulcerated tooth. Suppuration of the alveolar periosteum with ulceration of gum surrounding the decaying root of a tooth.

ulceration (ŭl"sĕr-ā'shŭn). Suppuration taking place on a free surface, as on the skin or on a mucous membrane, to form an ulcer.

ulcerative (ŭl'sĕr-ā-tĭv) [L. *ulcerare,* to form ulcers]. Pert. to or causing ulceration.

ulcerogangrenous (ŭl"sĕr-ō-găng'grĕ-nŭs). An ulcer that contains gangrenous tissue.

ulcerogenic drugs. Medicines that, because of their systemic rather than local effects, may cause peptic ulcers.

ulceromembranous (ŭl"sĕr-ō-mĕm'brăn-ŭs) [" + *membrana,* membrane]. Pert. to ulceration and formation of a fibrous pseudomembrane.

ulceromembranous tonsillitis. Tonsillitis that ulcerates and develops a membranous film.

ulcerous (ŭl'sĕr-ŭs). Pert. to or affected with an ulcer.

ulcus (ŭl'kŭs) [L.]. (pl. *ulcera*) Ulcer.

u. cancrosum. Cancerous ulcer that eats away the tissues. SYN: *rodent ulcer.*

u. induratum. A chancre, q.v.

u. vulvae acutum. Acute erosive ulcers on the female external genitalia. The cause is unknown but the ulcers may appear in association with acute infectious diseases such as typhoid fever, viral pneumonia, or brucellosis, or may appear as a variant of Behçet's syndrome, q.v. The disease may be confused with herpes simplex and ulcers caused by trauma.

ulectomy (ū-lĕk'tō-mē). 1. [Gr. *oule,* scar, + *ektome,* excision]. Excision of scar tissue, esp. in secondary iridectomy. 2. [Gr. *oulon,* gum, + *ektome,* excision]. Removal of gum tissue, as in pyorrhea alveolaris. SYN: *gingivectomy.*

ulegyria (ū"lē-jī'rē-ă) [Gr. *oule,* scar, + *gyros,* ring]. Condition in which gyri of the cerebral cortex are abnormal due to scar tissue from injuries usually occurring in early development.

ulemorrhagia (ū"lĕm-ō-rā'jē-ă) [Gr. *oulon,* gum, + *rhegnynai,* to burst forth]. Bleeding from the gums.

ulerythema (ū-lĕr-ĭ-thē'mă) [Gr. *oule,* scar, + *erythema,* redness]. An erythematous disorder with atrophic scar formation.

u. ophryogenes. Folliculitis of eyebrows characterized by falling out of hair and scarring.

u. sycosiforme. Inflammation of the hair follicles of the beard with alopecia in the affected area.

uletic (ū-lĕt'ĭk) [Gr. *oulon,* gum]. Pert. to the gums.

uletomy (ū-lĕt'ō-mē) [Gr. *oule,* scar, + *tome,* incision]. Incision of a scar to relieve tension. SYN: *cicatricotomy.*

uliginous (ū-lĭj'ĭ-nŭs) [L. *uliginosus,* wet]. Muddy; slimy.

ulitis (ū-lī'tĭs) [Gr. *oulon,* gum, + *itis,* inflammation]. Inflammation of the gums. SYN: *oulitis.*

u., interstitial. Inflammation of connective tissue of gums about the necks of the teeth.

ulna (ŭl'nă) [L., elbow]. The inner and larger bone of the forearm, between the wrist and the elbow, on the side opposite that of the thumb. It articulates with the head of the radius and humerus above and with the radius below.

RS: coronoid process; cubital; cubitus; elbow; olecranon; skeleton.

ulnad (ŭl'năd) [" + *ad,* toward]. In the direction of the ulna.

ulnar (ŭl'năr) [L. *ulna,* elbow]. 1. Rel. to the ulna, or to nerve or artery named from it. 2. Cuneiform carpal bone.

ulnaris (ŭl-nā'rĭs). 1. Ulnar. 2. Concerning the ulna.

ulnocarpal (ŭl"nō-kăr'păl) [" + Gr. *karpos,* wrist]. Relating to the carpus and ulna, or to the ulnar side of the wrist.

ulnoradial (ŭl"nō-rā'dē-ăl) [" + *radius,* spoke of a wheel]. Rel. to the ulna and radius, as their ligaments and articulations.

Ulo. Trade name for chlophedianol hydrochloride.

ulocace (ū-lŏk'ă-sē) [Gr. *oulon,* gum, + *kake,* badness]. Ulcerative inflammation of the gums.

ulocarcinoma (ū"lō-kăr-sĭn-ō'mă) [" + *karkinos,* cancer, + *oma,* tumor]. Carcinoma of the gums.

ulodermatitis (ū"lō-dĕrm-ă-tī'tĭs) [Gr. *oule,* scar, + *derma,* skin, + *itis,* inflammation]. Dermatitis with scar tissue formation.

uloglossitis (ū"lō-glŏs-ī'tĭs) [Gr. *oulon,* gum, + *glossa,* tongue, + *itis,* inflammation]. Inflammation of the gums and tongue.

uloid (ū'loyd) [Gr. *oule,* scar, + *eidos,* resemblance]. 1. Scarlike. 2. A scarlike lesion caused by subcutaneous degeneration.

uloncus (ū-lŏn′kŭs) [Gr. *oulon,* gum, + *onkos,* mass]. Swelling or tumor of the gums. SEE: *epulis.*

ulorrhagia (ū-lor-ā′jē-ă) [″ + *rhegnynai,* to burst forth]. Bleeding from the gums. SYN: *oulorrhagia.*

ulorrhea (ū″lor-rē′ă) [″ + *rhoia,* a flow]. Slow bleeding from the gums.

ulosis (ū-lō′sĭs) [Gr. *oule,* scar, + *osis,* condition]. Formation of scar tissue. SYN: *cicatrization.*

ulotic (ū-lŏt′ĭk) [Gr. *oule,* scar]. Causing cicatrization. SYN: *cicatricial.*

ulotomy (ū-lŏt′ō-mē). 1. [″ + *tome,* incision]. The cutting of scar tissue to relieve deformity or tension. 2. [Gr. *oulon,* gum, + *tome,* incision]. Incision of the gums.

ulotrichous (ū-lŏt′rĭk-ŭs) [Gr. *oulos,* woolly, + *thrix,* hair]. Having short woolly hair, characteristic of some races.

ulotripsis (ū″lō-trĭp′sĭs) [Gr. *oulon,* gum, + *tripsis,* massage]. Stimulation of the gums by massage.

ultimate (ŭl′tĭm-āt) [L. *ultimus,* last]. Final or last.

ultimobranchial bodies (ŭl″tĭ-mō-brăng′kē-ăl). Two embryonic pharyngeal pouches usually considered as rudimentary fifth pouches. They become separated from the pharynx and incorporated into substance of the thyroid gland, where they give rise to parafollicular cells that secrete calcitonin, a hormone used to regulate blood calcium level.

ultra- [L.]. Prefix meaning beyond, excess.

ultrabrachycephalic (ŭl″tră-brăk″ĭ-sē-făl′ĭk) [L. *ultra,* beyond, + Gr. *brachys,* short, + *kephale,* head]. Having a cephalic index of 90 or over.

ultracentrifugation (ŭl″tră-sĕn-trĭf″ū-gā′shŭn). To treat or prepare substances by use of the ultracentrifuge.

ultracentrifuge (ŭl-tră-sĕn′trĭ-fūj) [″ + *centrum,* center, + *fugere,* to flee]. A high-speed centrifuge capable of producing centrifugal forces more than 100,000 times gravity. Used in the study of proteins, viruses, etc.

ultradian (ŭl-trā′dē-ăn) [″ + *dies,* day]. Concerning biologic rhythms that occur less frequently than every 24 hours.

ultrafilter (ŭl-tră-fĭl′tĕr). A filter by which colloidal particles may be separated from their dispersion medium or from crystalloids.

ultrafiltration (ŭl″tră-fĭl-trā′shŭn) [″ + *filtrum,* a filter]. Filtration of a colloidal substance in which the dispersed particles, but not the liquid, are held back.

ultraligation (ŭl″tră-lī-gā′shŭn) [″ + *ligare,* to bind]. Ligation of a blood vessel beyond the origin of a branch.

ultramicrobe (ŭl″tră-mī′krōb) [″ + Gr. *mikros,* tiny, + *bios,* life]. A microorganism too small to be visible by the ordinary microscope.

ultramicroscope (ŭl″tră-mī′krō-skōp) [″ + ″ + *skopein,* to examine]. Microscope by which objects invisible through an ordinary microscope may be seen by means of powerful side illumination. SYN: *microscope, darkfield.*

ultramicroscopy (ŭl″tră-mī-krŏs′kō-pē). The use of the ultramicroscope.

ultramicrotome (ŭl″tră-mī′krō-tōm). A microtome that makes extremely thin slices of tissue.

ultrasonic (ŭl-tră-sŏn′ĭk) [″ + *sonus,* sound]. Pertaining to sounds of frequencies above approx. 20,000 cycles per second. They are inaudible to the human ear. SEE: *supersonic; ultrasound; ultrasonography.*

ultrasonic cleaning. Use of ultrasonic energy to clean objects, including medical and surgical instruments.

ultrasonics (ŭl-tră-sŏn′ĭks). The division of acoustics that studies inaudible sounds with frequencies greater than 20,000 cycles per second. Biological effects may result depending on intensity of beams. Heating effects are produced by beams of low intensity, paralytic effects by those of moderate intensity, and lethal effects by those of high intensity. The lethal action of ultrasonics is primarily the result, either directly or indirectly, of cavitation of tissues. Ultrasonics are utilized clinically for therapeutic and diagnostic purposes. SEE: *ultrasound.*

ultrasonogram (ŭl″tră-sŏn′ō-grăm). The image produced by use of ultrasonography.

ultrasonography (ŭl-tră-sŏn-ŏg′ră-fē). Use of ultrasound to produce an image or photograph of an organ or tissue. Ultrasonic echoes are recorded as they strike tissues of different densities.

ultrasound. Inaudible sound in the frequency range of approx. 20,000 to 10,000,000,000 cycles per second. Ultrasound has different velocities in tissues that differ in density and elasticity from others. This property permits the use of ultrasound in outlining the shape of various tissues and organs in the body. Use of ultrasound for diagnostic and therapeutic purposes requires special equipment. SEE: *ultrasonography.*

ultrastructure (ŭl′tră-strŭk″chŭr). The fine structure of tissues. It is visible only by use of electron microscopy.

ultraviolet (ŭl″tră-vī′ō-lĕt) [″ + *viola,* violet]. Beyond the visible spectrum at its violet end, said of rays between the violet rays and roentgen rays. SEE: *infrared rays.*

ultraviolet rays. Invisible rays emitted by very hot bodies and ionized gases with wavelengths between 3900 and 1800 angstroms. From a therapeutic standpoint, physiological effects include erythema production, pigmentation of skin, antirachitic effect through production of vitamin D, bactericidal effects, and various effects on metabolism. In clinical practice, dosage is measured in terms of minimum erythema dose (M.E.D.).

ultraviolet therapy. Treatment with ultraviolet radiation. SEE: *heliotherapy; light therapy.*

ululation (ŭl″ū-lā′shŭn) [L. *ululare,* to howl]. The crying and screaming of mentally ill persons.

umbilical (ŭm-bĭl′ĭ-kăl) [L. *umbilicus,* navel]. Pert. to the umbilicus.

umbilical artery catheter. Catheter placed in the umbilical artery of the infant in order to facilitate administration of medicines parenterally or to do an exchange transfusion.

umbilical cord. The attachment connecting the fetus with the placenta. It contains two arteries and one vein surrounded by a gelatinous substance, Wharton's jelly, q.v. The embryo receives nourishment from the blood supplied by the arteries of the umbilical cord, which go from the placenta to the fetus. SEE: illus.

The umbilical cord is surgically severed after the birth of the child. In order to give the infant a better blood supply, the cord should not be cut or tied until umbilical vessels have ceased pulsating. The stump of severed cord atrophies and leaves a depression on the abdomen of the child, called a navel or umbilicus.

umbilical fissure. Portion of hepatic longitudinal fissure in which the umbilical vein is lodged.

umbilical hernia. A hernia in the region of the umbilicus.

umbilical souffle. A hissing sound said to arise from the umbilical cord.

umbilical vesicle. That part of the embryonic yolk sac leading from the umbilicus.

umbilicate (ŭm-bĭl′ĭ-kāt) [L. *umbilicatus,* dimpled]. Pert. to or shaped like the navel, noting a bacterial colony with a central depression resembling an umbilicus.

umbilication (ŭm-bĭl-ĭ-kā′shŭn) [L. *umbilicatus,* dimpled]. 1. A depression resembling a navel. 2. Formation at apex of a pustule or vesicle of a pit or depression.

umbilicus (ŭm-bĭ-lī′kŭs, -bĭl′ĭ-kŭs) [L., a pit]. (pl. *umbilici*) [NA] A depressed point in the middle of the abdomen; the scar that marks the former attachment of the umbilical cord to the fetus.

RS: funic souffle; funiculus; funis; hydromphalus; mesogastrium; navel; "omphal-" words; umbilical cord; varicomphalus.

umbo (ŭm′bō) [L., boss]. Projecting center of

UMBILICAL CORD

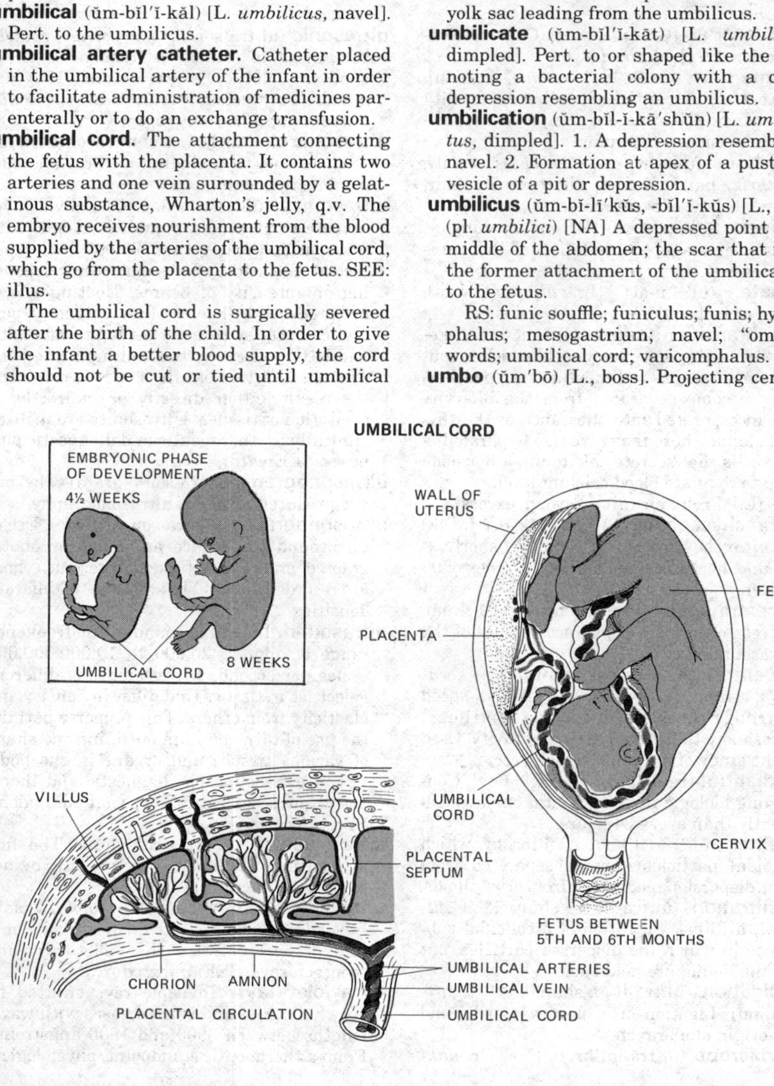

a round surface.

u. of tympanic membrane. The central depressed portion of the concavity on the lateral surface of the tympanic membrane. It marks the point where the handle (manubrium of malleus) is attached to the inner surface.

umbrella filter. Filter placed in a blood vessel in order to prevent emboli from passing that point. Has been used in the vena cava to prevent emboli in the veins from reaching the lungs.

UMP. *uridine monophosphate.*

un- [AS. *un-*, against]. Prefix meaning back, reversal, annulment of, and not.

uncal (ŭng'kăl). Concerning the uncus of the brain.

uncal herniation. Herniation, transtentorial, q.v.

unciform (ŭn'sĭ-form) [L. *uncus,* hook, + *forma,* shape]. Hook-shaped.

unciform bone. Hook-shaped bone on ulnar side of distal row of the carpus. SYN: *os hamatum* [NA].

unciforme (ŭn"sĭ-for'mē) [L.]. Uncinate, q.v.

unciform fasciculus. Bundle of fibers connecting frontal cerebral lobes with the temporosphenoid lobes.

unciform process. 1. Long thin lamina of bone from orbital plate of the ethmoid articulating with the inferior turbinate. 2. Hook at anterior end of the hippocampal gyrus. 3. Hooked end of unciform bone.

uncinariasis (ŭn"sĭn-ă-rī'ă-sĭs). Condition of being infested with hookworms, i.e., worms of the genus Uncinaria.

uncinate (ŭn'sĭn-āt) [L. *uncinatus,* hooked]. Hook-shaped; hooked.

uncinate bundle of Russell. Fibers that arise in the fastigial superior cerebellar peduncle and pass inferiorly to the vestibular nuclei and reticular formation by which impulses are carried to muscles, esp. those of the neck and body.

uncinate convolution. Uncinate gyrus.

uncinate epilepsy. Form of epilepsy occurring in disease of uncinate area of the temporal lobe.

uncinate fasciculus. Bundle of fibers connecting orbital gyri of frontal lobe with rostral portion of temporal lobe. They curve sharply as they pass over lateral fissure of cerebrum.

uncinate fits. Episodic attacks characterized by olfactory and gustatory hallucinations, usually disagreeable, a sense of unreality, and sometimes convulsions and temporary loss of senses of taste and smell. Associated with lesions of uncinate gyrus.

uncinate gyrus. A gyrus of the temporal lobe of the brain consisting of recurved rostral portion of hippocampal gyrus. SYN: *uncinate convolution; uncus.*

uncinatum (ŭn"sĭ-nā'tŭm) [L.]. Hooked.

uncipressure (ŭn'sĭ-prĕsh"ŭr) [L. *uncus,* hook, + *pressura,* pressure]. Pressure applied with the use of a blunt hook to arrest bleeding.

uncomplemented (ŭn-kŏm'plē-mĕnt"ĕd). Not joined or associated with complement and thus inactive.

unconditioned reflex. An inborn or natural reflex; one not dependent upon previous experience or training.

unconscious (ŭn-kŏn'shŭs) [AS. *un,* not, + L. *conscius,* aware]. 1. Insensible; lacking in awareness of the environment. State in which a person experiences no sensory impressions and has no subjective experiences. SEE: *unconsciousness.* 2. In freudian psychiatry, that part of our personality consisting of a complex of feelings and drives of which we are unaware and that are not available to our consciousness.

unconsciousness (ŭn-kŏn'shŭs-nĕs) [AS. *un,* not, + L. *conscius,* aware]. State of being insensible or without conscious experiences. Unconsciousness physiologically occurs in sleep; pathologically it may occur temporarily as in syncope (fainting) or be prolonged and vary in depth from stupor (semiconsciousness) to coma (profound unconsciousness). SEE: *Glasgow coma scale.*

CAUSES: Anoxia; alcohol, barbiturate and bromide intoxication; brain tumor; carbon monoxide poisoning; cardiac decompensation; cerebral accident (hemorrhage, thrombosis, embolism), concussion; diabetes; eclampsia; epilepsy; fear; fracture of skull; fright; heat stroke; hemorrhage (especially subarachnoid); hypertensive encephalopathy; meningitis; neurosyphilis, opium poisoning; overdose of insulin; pneumonia; severe infections; subdural hematoma; uremia.

SYM: Patient is unable to swallow; eyes do not react and patient is insensible to surroundings.

TREATMENT: If the face is flushed or if hemorrhage is present or suspected, do not lower head and do not give stimulants. In other instances, it is desirable to lower head and shoulders, loosen clothing, and keep patient comfortably warm but not hot. Turn head to one side to prevent vomitus, if any, from being inhaled. Provide artificial respiration, if necessary. Look for evidence of blows to the head, and for fractures and paralysis. Test pulse, respiration, odor of breath, condition of skin, and pupils of eyes. It is important to diagnose the cause of unconsciousness prior to instituting specific therapy.

CAUTION: The patient should be examined for a Medic Alert bracelet or pendant or a medical record card indicating chronic illness, critical medications, or allergy to drugs.

NURSING IMPLICATIONS: In the initial approach, follow the ABCs of emergency care, i.e., airway, bleeding, consciousness, digestive organs, excretory organs, and fractures. Establish adequate circulation and ventilation. Assess the patient for other health problems and treat them if they are of immediate concern. Implement safety measures to prevent further trauma. Re-examine the patient, and if the patient is conscious, obtain a history. Maintain fluid and electrolyte balance, assess level of consciousness frequently, and initiate a neurological flowsheet. Have blood drawn for determination of levels of glucose and drugs of abuse. Turn and position the patient often to allow drainage of secretions. Aspirate when necessary. Administer oxygen as prescribed. Perform eye care. Insert Foley catheter if patient is incontinent. Monitor intake and output. Perform mouth care frequently. Monitor temperature and implement appropriate antipyretic measures.

MOVING UNCONSCIOUS PATIENT, STRETCHER TO BED: *Method I:* Fold draw sheet in half lengthwise and place it across center of stretcher, pleating the excess and tucking the ends under for about 6 in. before patient is put on stretcher. (This sheet should be under the buttocks when patient is on stretcher.) Place stretcher parallel with bed and as close as possible to it. Get three other people to help you. Have one person at patient's head, one at feet, one at side, and one at far side of bed. The people at the sides take firm hold of the ends of the draw sheet and all four lift together, the person at the far side pulling the draw sheet toward the bed.

Method II: This movement requires three people. Place stretcher at right angles to the foot of the bed with patient's head at end of bed nearest stretcher. Standing side by side the three people put their arms under the patient, lift and swing the patient around onto the bed.

unconsciousness, words pert. to: apoplexy; asphyctic; asphyxial; asphyxia; catalepsy; collapse; coma; fainting; shock; sleep; stupor; syncope; trance; twilight sleep.

unco-ossified (ŭn″kō-ŏs′ĭ-fīd). Not ossified into one bone.

uncovertebral (ŭn″kō-vĕr′tĕ-brăl). Concerning the uncinate process of a vertebra.

unction (ŭnk′shŭn) [L. *unctio,* ointment]. 1. The application of an ointment. 2. Substance used for anointing. SYN: *unguent.*

unctuous (ŭnk′chū-ŭs) [L. *unctus,* an ointment]. Oily; greasy.

uncus (ŭn′kŭs) [L. *uncus,* hook]. 1. Any structure that is hook-shaped. 2. Hooked anterior end of hippocampal gyrus.

undecylenic acid. USP. An antifungal drug used topically to treat tinea pedis.

undercut (ŭn′dĕr-kŭt). A condition of having overhanging tissue as could be the case in preparing a dental cavity for restoration. Undercutting helps to keep the filling material in place.

undernutrition (ŭn″dĕr-nū-trĭsh′ŭn) [AS. *under,* beneath, + LL. *nutritio,* nourish]. Inadequate nutrition from any cause.

SYM: Loss of body weight representing at first mostly loss of body fat; then loss of protein manifested by atrophy of muscles, weakness, and edema.

undertoe (ŭn′dĕr-tō) [″ + *ta,* toe]. Condition of displacement of the great toe underneath the others.

underweight (ŭn′dĕr-wāt″). Condition in which body weight is at least 10% less than what would be considered within normal limits for a particular individual. It is an imprecise term.

undifferentiation (ŭn-dĭf″ĕr-ĕn-shē-ā′shŭn) [AS. *un,* not, + L. *differens,* bearing apart]. Alteration in cell character to a more embryonic type or toward a malignant state. SYN: *anaplasia.*

undine (ŭn′dīn) [L. *unda,* wave]. A small glass flask used for irrigating the eye.

undinism (ŭn′dĭn-ĭzm). Awakening of the libido by running water, as by urination or at sight of urine.

undulant (ŭn′dū-lănt) [L. *undulatio,* wavy]. Rising and falling like waves, or moving like them.

undulant fever (ŭn′dū-lănt). Brucellosis, q.v.

undulate (ŭn′dū-lāt) [L. *undulatio,* wavy]. Wavy; having a wavy border with shallow sinuses, said of bacterial colonies.

undulation (ŭn-dū-lā′shŭn). A continuous wavelike motion or pulsation.

u., jugular. A venous pulse.

u., respiratory. Fluctuation in blood pressure due to respiratory movements.

ung. [L.]. *unguentum,* ointment.

ungual (ŭng′gwăl) [L. *unguis,* nail]. Pert. to or resembling the nails. SYN: *unguinal.*

ungual phalanx. Terminal phalanx of each finger and toe.

ungual tuberosity. Spatula-shaped extremity of the terminal phalanx that supports the nails of fingers and toes.

unguent (ŭng′gwĕnt) [L. *unguentum,* ointment]. A lubricant or salve for sores or burns. SYN: *ointment.*

unguentum (ŭn-gwĕn′tŭm). 1. Fatty, soft, solid preparation intended to be applied to the skin by inunction. 2. Simple ointment. SYN: *ointment.*

unguiculate (ŭng-gwĭk′ū-lāt). Having nails or claws rather than hooves.

unguinal. Ungual, q.v.

unguis (ŭng'gwĭs) [L., nail]. (pl. *ungues*) 1. [NA] A fingernail or toenail. SYN: *onyx.* 2. The lacrimal bone. 3. A white prominence on floor of the posterior horn of the lateral ventricle. SYN: *hippocampus minor.*

u. incarnatus. An ingrowing nail, esp. a toenail.

ungula (ŭn'gū-lă) [L., claw]. Instrument for removal of dead fetus from the uterus.

uni- [L. *unus*]. Combining form meaning one.

uniarticular (ū"nē-ăr-tĭk'ū-lăr) [L. *unus,* one, + *articulus,* joint]. Pertaining to a single joint.

uniaxial (ū"nē-ăk'sē-ăl) [" + *axis,* axis]. Having a single axis.

unibasal (ū"nē-bā'săl) [" + *basis,* base]. Having a single base.

unicameral (ū"nĭ-kăm'ĕr-ăl) [" + *camera,* chamber]. Having a single cavity.

unicentral (ū"nĭ-sĕn'trăl) [" + *centrum,* center]. Having a single center.

unicellular (ū"nĭ-sĕl'ū-lăr) [" + *cellula,* a little box]. Having only one cell.

uniceps (ū'nĭ-sĕps) [" + *caput,* head]. Having a single head or origin, as in muscles.

unicorn (ū'nĭ-korn) [" + *cornu,* horn]. Having a single cornu or horn.

unicornous (ū-nĭ-kor'nŭs). Having but one horn or cornu.

unicuspid (ū"nĭ-kŭs'pĭd). Having a single cusp.

uniflagellate (ū"nĭ-flăj'ĕ-lāt). Having a single flagellum.

uniforate (ū"nĭ-fō'rāt) [" + *foratus,* pierced]. Having a single opening.

unigerminal (ū"nĭ-jĕr'mĭ-năl). Concerning a single ovum or germ.

uniglandular (ū"nĭ-glăn'dū-lăr). Concerning one gland.

unigravida (ū"nĭ-grăv'ĭ-dă) [" + *gravida,* pregnant]. Woman who is pregnant for the first time.

unilaminar (ū"nĭ-lăm'ĭ-năr). Having a single layer.

unilateral (ū"nĭ-lăt'ĕr-ăl) [" + *latus,* side]. Affecting or occurring on only one side. SEE: *contralateral; homolateral; ipsilateral.*

unilobar (ū"nĭ-lō'băr). Having a single lobe.

unilocular (ū"nĭ-lŏk'ū-lăr) [" + *loculus,* a little place]. Having but one cavity.

uninuclear (ū"nĭ-nū'klē-ăr) [" + *nucleus,* a kernel]. Having only one nucleus.

uninucleated (ū"nĭ-nū'klē-āt"ĕd). Having a single nucleus.

uniocular (ū"nē-ŏk'ū-lăr) [" + *oculus,* eye]. Pert. to or having only one eye.

uniovular (ū"nē-ŏv'ū-lăr) [" + *ovum,* egg]. Monozygotic, as in the case of twins that develop from a single ovum.

union (ūn'yŭn) [L. *unio*]. 1. Act of joining two or more things into one part, or the state of being so united. 2. Growing together of severed or broken parts, as of bones or lips of a wound. SEE: *healing.*

u., non-. Failure to unite, as a fractured bone that fails to heal completely.

u., secondary. A healing by second intention with adhesion of granulating surfaces. SEE: *healing.*

u., vicious. Union of ends of a broken bone in such a way as to cause deformity.

unioval (ū"nē-ō'văl) [L. *unus,* one, + *ovum,* egg]. Developed from one ovum, as identical twins.

unipara (ū-nĭp'ă-ră) [" + *parere,* to bring forth]. A woman who has had one pregnancy over 20 weeks or has produced a fetus of 500 grams, regardless of the viability of the fetus. SYN: *primipara.*

uniparous (ū-nĭp'ă-rŭs) [" + *parere,* to bring forth]. 1. Giving birth to one offspring at a time. 2. Having produced one child of 500 grams or having a pregnancy lasting 20 weeks, regardless of the viability of the fetus.

Unipen. Trade name for nafcillin sodium, USP.

unipolar (ū"nĭ-pō'lăr) [" + *polus,* pole]. 1. Having or pert. to one pole. 2. Having a single process, as a unipolar neuron.

unipotent, unipotential (ū-nĭp'ō-tĕnt, ū"nĭ-pō-tĕn'shăl). Concerning a cell that can only develop in a specific way to produce a certain end-result.

uniseptate (ū"nē-sĕp'tāt). Having only one septum.

Unisom. Trade name for doxylamine succinate.

unit (ū'nĭt) [L. *unus,* one]. 1. One of anything. 2. ABBR: u. A determined amount adopted as a standard of measurement.

u., amboceptor. The smallest amount of amboceptor required in the presence of which a given quantity of red blood corpuscles will be hemolyzed by an excess of complement.

u., Angström. ABBR: Å or A.U. An internationally adopted unit of measurement of wavelength, 1/10,000,000 of a millimeter, or 1/254,000,000 of an inch.

u., antigen. Smallest quantity of antigen required to fix one unit of complement.

u., antitoxic. A unit for expressing the strength of an antitoxin. Originally the various units were defined biologically but now are compared to a weighed standard specified by the U.S. Public Health Service and the World Health Organization. SYN: *immunizing unit.*

u., atomic mass. ABBR: AMU. One-twelfth of the mass of a neutral carbon atom. This is equal to 1.657×10^{-24} gram.

u., Bodansky. In clinical chemistry, a unit of alkaline phosphatase equal to that which will liberate 1 mg. of phosphorus as inorganic phosphate after one hour of incubation with a buffered substrate containing sodium β-glycerophosphate. SEE: *phosphatase, alkaline.*

u., British thermal. ABBR: BTU. The amount of heat necessary to raise the temperature of one pound of water from 39° F. to 40° F.

u., cat. The amount of drug per kg. of body weight just sufficient to kill a cat when injected intravenously slowly and continuously.

u., complement. Smallest quantity of complement required for hemolysis of a given amount of red blood corpuscles with one amboceptor unit present.

u., electrostatic. ABBR: ESU or ESE (from the German *elektrostatische einheit*). Any static electricity unit based on the unit electrostatic charge expressed in the centimeter-gram-second system of measurement.

u., hemolytic. The amount of inactivated immune serum that causes complete hemolysis of 1 ml. of a 5% emulsion of washed red blood corpuscles in the presence of complement.

u., International. Unit defined and adopted by the International Conference for Unification of Formulae. Used for measurement of hormones, enzymes, and some vitamins.

u., light. A foot-candle, or the amount of light one ft. from a standard candle. SEE: *candela; lumen.*

u., Mache. ABBR: M.U. Unit of measurement of radium emanation.

u., motor. The unit that provides motor activity. It consists of a somatic neuron cell and the muscles innervated by it.

u., mouse. Least amount of estrogen that induces, in a spayed mouse, a characteristic desquamation of the vaginal epithelium.

u. of capacity. Capacity of a condenser that gives a difference of potential of one volt when charged with one coulomb. SYN: *curie; farad.*

u., rat. Greatest dilution of estrogen that will cause desquamation and cornification of vaginal epithelium during first day, if given to a mature spayed rat in three injections, every four hours.

u., SI. Any of the units specified by the International System of Units adopted by an International Conference of Weights and Measures in 1960. SEE: *SI units* for tables; *SI units* in *Appendix.*

u., Todd. In a test of inhibition hemolysis by enzymes such as antistreptolysin O, the reciprocal of the highest dilution that inhibits hemolysis.

u., USP. Any unit specified by the U.S. Pharmacopeia.

unitarian (ū-nĭ-tā′rē-ăn) [L. *unitarius*]. Composed of a single unit.

unitary (ū′nĭ-tā-rē). Rel. to a single unit.

unit dose. A dose form in which individual doses of medicine are prepared in each packet. This saves time in dispensing medicines esp. to hospitalized patients.

United States Adopted Names. ABBR: USAN. Names of nonproprietary drugs approved by the USAN Council, an organization sponsored by the American Medical Association, the U.S. Pharmacopeial Convention, and the American Pharmaceutical Association. The purpose is to have nonproprietary names assigned to new drugs in accordance with established principles. SEE: *USAN and the USP Dictionary of Drug Names.*

United States Pharmacopeia. ABBR: USP followed by the edition number expressed in Roman numerals. USP XX was published in 1980. The official pharmacopeia of the United States. SEE: *pharmacopeia, United States.*

Unitensen. Trade name for cryptenamine acetates.

uniterminal (ū″nĭ-tĕr′mĭn-ăl) [L. *unus,* one, + *terminus,* end]. Having only one terminal. SEE: *monoterminal.*

univalence (ū″nĭ-vā′lĕns). The condition of having but one valence.

univalent (ū″nĭ-vā′lĕnt, ū-nĭv′ă-lĕnt) [″ + *valens,* to be powerful]. 1. Possessing the power of combining or replacing one atom of hydrogen. SYN: *monovalent.* 2. Single, noting a chromosome that lacks or fails to unite with a synaptic mate.

universal (ū″nĭ-vĕr′săl) [L. *universalis,* combined into one whole]. General or applicable or common to all situations or conditions.

universal antidote. Antidote used in poisoning where specific antidote is unknown or not available. Two parts activated charcoal; one part tannic acid; one part magnesium oxide. Give orally a paste of 5 heaping tsp. of the mixture dissolved in a glass of water. After the patient has swallowed the antidote, the stomach contents should then be removed by gastric lavage.

universal cuff. An adapted device fitted around the palm of the hand to permit attachment of self-care tools when normal grasp is absent.

universal donor. A person belonging to blood group O whose blood as a rule may be transfused without danger of untoward reactions into persons belonging to any of the other ABO blood groups.

NOTE: Because there are multiple blood type factors in addition to those of ABO, it would be dangerous to assume that group O blood could, without further tests of compatibility, be given to persons of different blood type.

universal dressing. A large flat bandage that

may be folded several times to make a relatively large dressing or folded several more times to make a smaller and thicker bandage. This process can be continued until the unit is suitable for use as a cervical collar. SEE: *dressing, universal,* for illus.

universal recipient. A person belonging to blood group AB, whose serum will not agglutinate the cells of the other ABO blood groups.

unmedullated (ŭn-mĕd′ū-lāt″ĕd). A nerve that does not contain a myelin sheath.

unmyelinated (ŭn-mī′ĕ-lĭ-nāt″ĕd). A nerve that does not contain a myelin sheath.

Unna's paste (oo′năz). [Paul G. Unna, Ger. dermatologist, 1850–1929] A combination of 15% zinc oxide in a glycogelatin base.

Unna's (paste) boot. A boot-like dressing of the lower extremity made of layers of gauze and Unna's paste. It is used in treating chronic ulcers, usually due to varicosities, of the leg.

unofficial (ŭn-ō-fĭsh′ăl) [AS. *un,* not, + L. *officialis,* doing work]. Indicates a drug not listed by the U.S. Pharmacopeia or National Formulary.

unorganized (ŭn-or′găn-īzd) [″ + L. *organizare,* to form a structure]. 1. Not organized into an organic structure. 2. Without characteristics of a living organism; inorganic.

unphysiological (ŭn-fĭz-ē-ō-lŏj′ĭk-ăl). Contrary to physiological principles.

unrest. Turbulence, instability, or irregularity.

unsaturated (ŭn-săt′ū-rāt″ĕd) [″ + L. *saturare,* to sate]. 1. Capable of dissolving or absorbing to a greater degree. 2. Not combined to the greatest possible extent.

unsaturated compound. An organic compound having double or triple bonds between the carbon atoms.

unsex (ŭn-sĕks′) [″ + L. *sexus,* sex]. 1. To castrate; to spay or excise the ovaries. 2. To deprive of sexual character.

unstriated (ŭn-strī′āt-ĕd) [″ + *striatus,* striped]. Unstriped, as smooth muscle fiber.

Unverricht's disease, syndrome (oon′fĕr-ĭkts). [Heinrich Unverricht, Ger. physician, 1853–1912] A rare, fatal disease inherited as an autosomal recessive. It is characterized by the onset in later childhood of myoclonic epilepsy, tetraplegia, and dementia. Also: *Unverricht-Lafora disease.*

unwell [″ + *wel,* well]. Sick; ill; indisposed.

upper airway obstruction. ABBR: UAO. Condition of the respiratory system in which it has the capability of functioning but is prevented from doing so by an obstruction in the upper portion of the airway, such as the main bronchus, larynx, mouth, or nose. SEE: *cardiopulmonary resuscitation; tracheostomy.*

upper G.I. *upper gastrointestinal.* Radiographic and fluoroscopic examinations of the stomach and duodenum after the ingestion of a contrast medium.

upper motor neuron lesion. Neurological condition resulting from damage to corticospinal or pyramidal tract in the brain or spinal cord. Results in hemiplegia, paraplegia, or quadriplegia, depending upon the location and extent of the lesion. Clinical signs include loss of voluntary movement, spasticity, sensory loss, and pathological reflexes.

upper respiratory infection. ABBR: URI. An imprecise term for almost any kind of infectious disease process involving the nasal passages, pharynx, and bronchi. The etiological agent may be bacterial or viral and is rarely accurately known.

upsiloid (ŭp′sĭ-loyd) [Gr. *upsilon,* letter U, + *eidos,* form]. Shaped like the letter U or V.

uptake (ŭp′tāk). The absorption of a nutrient, chemicals including radioactive materials, and medicines by tissues or an entire organism.

urachal (ū′ră-kăl) [Gr. *ourachos,* fetal urinary canal]. Rel. to the urachus.

urachus (ū′ră-kŭs) [Gr. *ourachos,* fetal urinary canal]. An epithelioid cord surrounded by fibrous tissue extending from the apex of the bladder to the umbilicus. In the embryo it is continuous with the allantoic stalk; postnatally it forms the middle umbilical ligament of the bladder.

u., patent. Condition in which the urachus remains as a hollow tube that connects the vertex of the bladder with the umbilicus, resulting in an umbilical urinary fistula.

uracil (ū′ră-sĭl). $C_4H_4N_2O_2$. A pyrimidine base found in ribonucleic acids.

uracil mustard. USP. An alkylating type of cytotoxic drug used in treating certain types of malignant tumors. CAUTION: Handle this drug with exceptional care. It must be handled in a well-ventilated hood, using a protective mask, protective glasses, and gloves. Thoroughly clean the work area afterward and then rinse hands in water for several minutes followed by washing with soap and water.

uracrasia (ū-ră-krā′sē-ă) [Gr. *ouron,* urine, + *akrasia,* bad mixture]. 1. A disordered condition of urine. 2. Inability to retain the urine. SEE: *enuresis; incontinence, urinary stress.*

uracratia (ū-ră-krā′shē-ă) [″ + *akratia,* incontinence]. Incontinence of the urine.

uragogue (ū′ră-gŏg) [″ + *agogos,* leading]. Increasing the secretion of urine. SYN: *diuretic.*

uraniscotitis (ū-răn-ĭs″kŏn-ī′tĭs) [Gr. *ouraniskos,* palate, + *itis,* inflammation]. Inflammation of the palate.

uraniscoplasty (ū-răn-ĭs′kō-plăs″tē) [″ + *plassein,* to form]. Operation for repair of *cleft palate. SYN: uranoplasty; uranorrhaphy.*

uraniscorrhaphy (ū″răn-ĭs-kor′ră-fē) [″ + *rhaphe,* a seam]. Operation for suturing of a cleft palate. SYN: *uraniscoplasty.*

uraniscus (ū-răn-ĭs′kŭs) [Gr. *ouraniskos,* palate]. Palate, or roof of mouth.

uranium (ū-rā′nē-ŭm) [LL., planet Uranus]. SYMB: U. At. wt. 238.029; at. no. 92. A radioactive element, the parent of radium and other radioelements. Uranium ore contains the isotopes ^{238}U, ^{235}U, and ^{234}U.

uranoplasty (ū′răn-ō-plăs″tē) [Gr. *ouranos,* palate, + *plassein,* to form]. Operation for cleft palate. SYN: *uraniscoplasty.*

uranoplegia (ū″ră-nō-plē′jē-ă) [″ + *plege,* stroke]. Paralysis of muscles of the soft palate.

uranorrhaphy (ū-răn-or′ră-fē) [″ + *rhaphe,* a seam]. Operation for suture of a cleft palate. SYN: *uraniscorrhaphy.*

uranoschisis (ū-răn-ŏs′kĭs-ĭs) [″ + *schisis,* a fissure]. Cleft palate.

uranostaphyloplasty (ū″răn-ō-stăf′ĭl-ō-plăs″tē) [″ + *staphyle,* uvula, + *plassein,* to form]. Operation for correction of a defect of the soft and hard palates.

uranostaphylorrhaphy (ū″răn-ō-stăf-ĭl-or′ă-fē) [″ + ″ + *rhaphe,* a seam]. Operation for repair of cleft of hard and soft palates.

uranostaphyloschisis (ū″ră-nō-stăf″ĭ-lŏs′kĭ-sĭs). Cleft of the hard and soft palate.

uranyl (ū′ră-nĭl). The bivalent uranium radical UO^{++}. It forms salts with many acids. An example is uranyl nitrate, $UO_2 (NO_3)_2 \cdot 6H_2O$.

urapostema (ū″ră-pŏs-tē′mă) [Gr. *ouron,* urine, + *apostema,* abscess]. An abscess containing urine.

uraroma (ū-ră-rō′mă) [″ + *aroma,* spice]. Aromatic spicy odor of the urine.

urarthritis (ū″răr-thrī′tĭs). Arthritis due to gout.

urase (ū′rās). Urease.

urate (ū′rāt) [Gr. *ouron,* urine]. Combination of uric acid with a base; a salt of uric acid. Urates are normally present in urine.

uratemia (ū″ră-tē′mē-ă) [″ + *haima,* blood]. Urates, esp. sodium urate, in the blood.

uratic (ū-răt′ĭk). Concerning urates or gout.

uratoma (ū″ră-tō′mă). Concretions of urates around joints caused by gout; a tophus.

uratosis (ū″ră-tō′sĭs). Any condition leading to deposition of urates in tissues.

uraturia (ū″ră-tū′rē-ă) [Gr. *ouron,* urine]. Excess of urates in the urine. SYN: *lithuria.*

urceiform (ŭr-sē′ĭ-form) [L. *urceus,* pitcher, + *forma,* shape]. Pitcher shaped.

urceolate (ŭr-sē′ō-lāt). Urceiform, q.v.

ur-defense(s) (ŭr″dē-fĕns′) [Gr. *Ur,* ultimate, + *defense*]. Basic beliefs such as religious or scientific that are essential to man's emotional well-being.

urea (ū-rē′ă) [Gr. *ouron,* urine]. The diamide of carbonic acid, a crystalline solid having the formula $CO(NH_2)_2$; found in blood, lymph, and urine. It is formed in the liver from ammonia derived from amino acids by deamination. It may also be formed directly from arginine.

Urea is the chief nitrogenous constituent of urine and along with CO_2 the final product of protein metabolism in the body. In normal conditions, urea represents 80 to 90% of the total urinary nitrogen. It is without odor and colorless, appearing as white prismatic crystals, and forming salts with acids. Its excess is one of the signs of uremia, q.v. The amount of urea excreted varies directly with the amount of protein in the diet. Excretion is increased in fever, diabetes, or increased activity of the adrenal gland.

USES: As a diuretic.

u., sterile. USP. A standardized preparation of urea that when appropriately diluted may be used intravenously as a diuretic. Trade name is Ureaphil.

urea cycle. The complex cyclic chemical reactions in some (ureotelic) animals, including man, that produces urea from the metabolism of nitrogen-containing foods. This cycle provides a method of excreting the nitrogen produced by the metabolism of amino acids as urea. The cycle was first described by Sir Hans Krebs [1900–1981].

urea frost. White flaky deposits of urea seen on skin in patients with advanced uremia.

ureagenetic (ū-rē″ă-jĕn-ĕt′ĭk) [″ + *genesis,* production]. Pert. to or producing urea.

ureal (ū-rē′ăl). Rel. to or containing urea.

ureameter (ū-rē-ăm′ĕt-er) [″ + *metron,* a measure]. Device for determining amount of urea in urine. SYN: *ureometer.*

ureametry (ū-rē-ăm′ĕt-rē). Determination of amount of urea in urine.

urea nitrogen. ABBR: BUN. The nitrogen of urea as distinguished from nitrogen in blood proteins.

Ureaphil. Trade name for urea, USP.

ureapoiesis (ū-rē″ă-poy-ē′sĭs) [*urea* + Gr. *poiesis,* forming]. Production of urea.

urease (ū′rē-ās) [Gr. *ouron,* urine]. An enzyme that accelerates hydrolysis of urea into ammonium carbonate and hippuric acid into glycocoll and benzoic acid. It is found in alkaline fermentation of urine, is produced by many microorganisms, and is also found in jack beans and soybeans. It is used in determining the amount of urea in blood or in urine.

urecchysis (ū-rĕk′ĭs-ĭs) [″ + *ekchysis,* a pouring out]. Effusion of urine into tissues.

Urecholine. Trade name for bethanechol chloride.

uredema (ū-rē-dē′mă) [″ + *oidema,* a swelling]. Urine in the subcutaneous tissues, thus distending them.

ureide (ū'rē-īd) [Gr. *ouron,* urine]. Any compound of urea in which acid radicals have taken the place of one or more of its hydrogen atoms.

urelcosis (ū-rěl-kō'sĭs) [" + *helkosis,* ulceration]. Ulceration of the urinary tract.

uremia (ū-rē'mē-ă) [" + *haima,* blood]. Toxic condition associated with renal insufficiency produced by the retention in the blood of nitrogenous substances normally excreted by the kidney. SEE: *azotemia; coma, uremic.*

ETIOL: Result of disturbed kidney function seen in nephritis and due to suppression or deficient secretion of urine from any cause.

SYM: Nausea, vomiting, headache, dizziness, dimness of vision, coma or convulsions, urinous odor of breath and perspiration. Stupor, stertorous respiration. No change in pupillary reaction; dry skin; hard rapid pulse; elevated blood pressure; scanty urine containing casts and albumin. There is a reduction of urea in the urine. Tube casts are present in uremic coma. Urea retention is 150 to 500 mg. or more per decaliter of blood.

TREATMENT: Dialysis.

u., extrarenal. U., prerenal.

u., prerenal. Uremia occurring not as a result of primary renal disease but due to other conditions such as disturbances in circulation, fluid balance, or metabolism arising in other parts of the body.

uremic (ū-rē'mĭk). Pert. to or caused by uremia.

uremigenic (ū-rē"mĭ-jěn'ĭk) [Gr. *ouron,* urine, + *haima,* blood, + *gennan,* to produce]. Caused by or producing uremia.

ureogenesis (ūr"ē-ō-jěn'ĕ-sĭs) [" + *genesis,* production]. Formation of urea.

ureometer (ū"rē-ŏm'ĕt-ĕr) [" + *metron,* a measure]. Appliance used to determine the amount of urea in urine. SYN: *ureameter.*

ureometry (ū-rē-ŏm'ĕt-rē). Estimation of amt. of urea in urine.

ureotelic (ū"rē-ō-těl'ĭk) [*urea* + Gr. *telikos,* belonging to the completion]. Concerning animals that excrete amino nitrogen in the form of urea. Included in this group are most terrestrial vertebrates and sharks. SEE: *ammonotelic; urea cycle; uricotelic.*

uresiesthesia, uresiesthesis (ū-rē"sē-ĕs-thē'zē-ă, -sĭs) [Gr. *ouresis,* urination, + *aisthesis,* sensation]. The normal inclination to void urine.

uresis (ū-rē'sĭs) [Gr. *ouresis*]. The passage of urine. SYN: *urination.*

ureter (ū'rĕ-ter, ū-rē'tĕr) [Gr. *oureter*]. The tube that carries urine from the kidney to the bladder. The ureter originates in the pelvis of the kidney and terminates in the base of the bladder. Each kidney has one ureter measuring from 28 to 34 cm. long, the right being slightly shorter than the left. The diameter varies from 1 mm. to 1 cm. The wall consists of three layers: the mucosal, muscular, and fibrous coats. SEE: *kidney; urethra.*

ureteral (ū-rē'tĕr-ăl). Concerning the ureter.

ureteralgia (ū"rē-tĕr-ăl'jē-ă) [" + *algos,* pain]. Pain in the ureter.

uretercystoscope (ū-rē"tĕr-sĭs'tō-skōp) [" + *kystis,* bladder, + *skopein,* to examine]. A cystoscope combined with a ureteral catheter.

ureterectasis (ū-rē"tĕr-ĕk'tă'sĭs) [" + *ektasis,* dilatation]. Dilatation of the ureter.

ureterectomy (ū-rē"tĕr-ĕk'tō-mē) [" + *ektome,* excision]. Excision of a ureter.

ureteric (ū"rĕ-tĕr'ĭk). Ureteral, q.v.

ureteritis (ū-rē"tĕr-ī'tĭs) [" + *itis,* inflammation]. Inflammation of the ureters.

ureterocele (ū-rē'tĕr-ō-sēl) [" + *kele,* hernia]. Cystlike dilatation of the ureter near its opening into the bladder. Usually a result of congenital stenosis of ureteral orifice.

ureterocelectomy (ū-rē"tĕr-ō-sē-lĕk'tō-mē) [" + " + *ektome,* excision]. Surgical removal of a ureterocele.

ureterocervical (ū-rē"tĕr-ō-sĕr'vĭ-kăl) [" + L. *cervicalis,* pert. to cervix]. Concerning the ureter and the cervix uteri.

ureterocolostomy (ū-rē"tĕr-ō-kō-lŏs'tō-mē) [" + *kolon,* colon, + *stoma,* passage]. The implantation of the ureter into the colon.

ureterocystanastomosis (ū-rē"tĕr-ō-sĭs"tă-năs"tō-mō'sĭs) [Gr. *oureter,* ureter, + *kystis,* bladder, + *anastomosis,* opening]. Ureteroneocystostomy, q.v.

ureterocystoneostomy (ū-rē"tĕr-ō-sĭst"ō-nē-ŏs'tō-mē) [" + *kystis,* bladder, + *neos,* new, + *stoma,* passage]. Ureteroneocystostomy.

ureterocystoscope (ū-rē"tĕr-ō-sĭs'tō-skōp) [" + " + *skopein,* to view]. Uretercystoscope, q.v.

ureterocystostomy (ū-rē"tĕr-ō-sĭs-tŏs'tō-mē) [" + " + *stoma,* passage]. Ureteroneocystostomy.

ureterodialysis (ū-rē"tĕr-ō-dī-ăl'ĭ-sĭs) [" + *dialysis,* a separation]. Rupture of a ureter. SYN: *ureterolysis.*

ureteroenterostomy (ū-rē"tĕr-ō-ĕn-tĕr-ŏs'tō-mē) [" + *enteron,* intestine, + *stoma,* passage]. Formation of a passage between a ureter and the intestine.

ureterography (ū-rē"tĕr-ŏg'ră-fē) [" + *graphein,* to write]. Radiography of the ureter after injection of a radiopaque substance into it.

ureteroheminephrectomy (ū-rē"tĕr-ō-hĕm"ĭ-nĕ-frĕk'tō-mē) [" + *hemi-,* half, + *nephros,* kidney, + *ektome,* excision]. In cases of reduplication of the upper urinary tract on one side, surgical removal of the reduplicated portion.

ureterohydronephrosis (ū-rē″tĕr-ō-hī″drō-nĕ-frō′sĭs) [″ + *hydor,* water, + *nephros,* kidney, + *osis,* condition]. Dilatation of ureter and pelvis of the kidney resulting from a mechanical or inflammatory obstruction in the urinary tract.

ureteroileostomy (ū-rē″tĕr-ō-ĭl″ē-ŏs′tō-mē) [″ + *ileum,* ileum, + *stoma,* passage]. Surgical anastomosis of a ureter to an isolated segment of the ileum. The ileum is connected to an abdominal stoma so that urine leaves the body via that opening.

ureterolith (ū-rē′tĕr-ō-lĭth) [″ + *lithos,* stone]. A stone or calculus in the ureter.

ureterolithiasis (ū-rē″tĕr-ō-lĭth-ī′ăs-ĭs) [″ + ″ + *iasis,* condition]. Development of a calculus in the ureter.

ureterolithotomy (ū-rē″tĕr-ō-lĭth-ŏt′ō-mē) [″ + ″ + *tome,* incision]. Surgical incision for removal of a calculus from the ureter.

ureterolysis (ū-rē″tĕr-ŏl′ĭ-sĭs) [″ + *lysis,* loosening]. 1. Rupture of the ureter. 2. Paralysis of the ureter. 3. The process of loosening adhesions around the ureter.

ureteroneocystostomy (ū-rē″tĕr-ō-nē″ō-sĭs-tŏs′tō-mē) [″ + *neos,* new, + *kystis,* bladder, + *stoma,* passage]. Surgical formation of a new passage between a ureter and the bladder. SYN: *ureterocystoneostomy; ureterocystostomy.*

ureteroneopyelostomy (ū-rē″tĕr-ō-nē″ō-pī-ĕ-lŏs′tō-mē) [″ + ″ + *pyelos,* pelvis, + *stoma,* passage]. Excision of a portion of the ureter with attachment of the severed end of the lower portion to a new aperture in the renal pelvis. SYN: *ureteropyeloneostomy.*

ureteronephrectomy (ū-rē″tĕr-ō-nĕf-rĕk′tō-mē) [″ + *nephros,* kidney, + *ektome,* excision]. Removal of a kidney and its ureter.

ureteropathy (ū-rē″tĕr-ŏp′ă-thē) [″ + *pathos,* disease]. Any diseased condition of the ureter.

ureteropelvioplasty (ū-rē″tĕr-ō-pĕl′vē-ō-plăs″tē) [Gr. *oureter,* ureter, + L. *pelvis,* basin, + Gr. *plassein,* to mold]. Plastic surgery of the junction of the ureter and the pelvis of the kidney.

ureterophlegma (ū-rē″tĕr-ō-flĕg′mă) [″ + *phlegma,* phlegm]. Accumulation of mucus in the ureter.

ureteroplasty (ū-rē′tĕr-ō-plăs″tē) [″ + *plassein,* to form]. Plastic surgery of the ureter.

ureteroproctostomy (ū-rē″tĕr-ō-prŏk-tŏs′tō-mē) [″ + *proktos,* anus, + *stoma,* passage]. Formation of a passage from the ureter to the lower rectum.

ureteropyelitis (ū-rē″tĕr-ō-pī-ĕl-ī′tĭs) [″ + *pyelos,* pelvis, + *itis,* inflammation]. Inflammation of the pelvis of the kidney and a ureter.

ureteropyeloneostomy (ū-rē″tĕr-ō-pī″ĕl-ō-nē-ŏs′tō-mē) [″ + ″ + *neos,* new, + *stoma,* passage]. Ureteroneopyelostomy.

ureteropyelonephritis (ū-rē″tĕr-ō-pī″ĕl-ō-nĕf-rī′tĭs) [″ + ″ + *nephros,* kidney, + *itis,* inflammation]. Inflammation of the renal pelvis and the ureter.

ureteropyeloplasty (ū-rē″tĕr-ō-pī′ĕl-ō-plăs″tē) [″ + ″ + *plassein,* to mold]. Plastic surgery of the ureter and renal pelvis.

ureteropyelostomy (ū-rē″tĕr-ō-pī″ĕ-lŏs′tō-mē) [″ + ″ + *stoma,* passage]. Ureteropyeloneostomy.

ureteropyosis (ū-rē″tĕr-ō-pī-ō′sĭs) [″ + *pyon,* pus, + *osis,* condition]. Suppurative inflammation within a ureter.

ureterorectostomy (ū-rē″tĕr-ō-rĕk-tŏs′tō-mē) [″ + L. *rectum,* straight, + Gr. *stoma,* passage]. Ureteroproctostomy.

ureterorrhagia (ū-rē″tĕr-or-rā′jē-ă) [″ + *rhegnynai,* to burst forth]. Hemorrhage from the ureter.

ureterorrhaphy (ū-rē″tĕr-or′ră-fē) [″ + *rhaphe,* a seam]. Suture of the ureter, as for fistula.

ureterosigmoidostomy (ū-rē″tĕr-ō-sĭg-moyd-ŏs′tō-mē) [″ + *sigma,* letter S, + *eidos,* shape, + *stoma,* passage]. Surgical implantation of the ureter into the sigmoid flexure.

ureterostegnosis (ū-rē″tĕr-ō-stĕg-nō′sĭs). Ureterostenosis.

ureterostenosis (ū-rē″tĕr-ō-stĕn-ō′sĭs) [″ + *stenosis,* a narrowing]. Stricture of a ureter.

ureterostoma (ū″rē-tĕr-ŏs′tō-mă) [Gr. *oureter,* ureter, + *stoma,* passage]. The orifice through which the ureter enters the urinary bladder.

ureterostomy (ū-rē″tĕr-ŏs′tō-mē) [″ + *stoma,* passage]. Formation of a permanent fistula for drainage of a ureter.

u., cutaneous. Surgical implantation of the ureter into the skin. This allows urine to drain via the ureter to the outside of the body by going through the stoma.

ureterotomy (ū-rē″tĕr-ŏt′ō-mē) [″ + *tome,* incision]. Incision or surgery of the ureter.

ureterotrigonoenterostomy (ū-rē″tĕr-ō-trī-gō″nō-ĕn″tĕr-ŏs′tō-mē) [″ + *trigonon,* three-sided figure, + *enteron,* intestine, + *stoma,* passage]. Surgical removal of the trigone of the bladder with one or both of the ureteral openings and implanting it into the intestine.

ureteroureteral (ū-rē″tĕr-ō-ū-rē′tĕr-ăl) [″ + *oureter,* ureter]. Concerning two parts of the same ureter or the union of one ureter with the other.

ureteroureterostomy (ū-rē″tĕr-ō-ū-rē″tĕr-ŏs′tō-mē) [″ + ″ + *stoma,* passage]. 1. Formation of a connection from one ureter to the other. 2. Reestablishment of a passage between the ends of a divided ureter.

ureterouterine (ū-rē″tĕr-ō-ū′tĕr-ĭn) [″ + L. *uterus,* womb]. Concerning the ureter and the uterus or a fistula between them.

ureterovaginal (ū-rē″tĕr-ō-văj′ĭ-năl) [″ + L. *vagina,* sheath]. Relating to a ureter and the vagina, noting a fistula connecting them.

ureterovesical (ū-rē″tĕr-ō-vĕs′ĭ-kăl) [″ + L. *vesica,* bladder]. Pert. to a connection between the ureter and the bladder.

ureterovesicostomy (ū-rē″tĕr-ō-vĕs″ĭ-kŏs′tō-mē) [″ + ″ + Gr. *stoma,* passage]. Reimplantation of a ureter into the bladder.

urethan(e) (ū′rĕ-thăn, -thān). An antineoplastic and hypnotic drug previously called ethyl carbamate.

urethra (ū-rē′thră) [Gr. *ourethra*]. A canal for the discharge of urine extending from the bladder to the outside. In the female its orifice lies in the vestibule between the vagina and clitoris; in the male the urethra traverses the penis, opening at the tip of the glans penis. In the male it serves as the passage for semen as well as urine. Its inner lining, the mucosa, is thrown into folds and contains openings of lacunae into which the glands of Littre open. Surrounding the mucosa is a lamina propria containing many elastic fibers and blood vessels, outside of which is an indefinite muscular layer. SEE: *penis.*

u. muliebris. The female urethra.

u. virilis. The male urethra.

urethra, words pert. to: aerourethroscopy; anaspadias; ankylurethria; atreturethria; bulb; bulbourethral glands; corpus spongiosum; gleet; habenula urethralis; hypospadias; meatus urinarius; Skene's glands; urelcosis; "urethr-" words.

urethral (ū-rē′thrăl) [Gr. *ourethra,* urethra]. Relating to the urethra.

urethralgia (ū-rē-thrăl′jē-ă) [″ + *algos,* pain]. Urethral pain; pain in the urethra.

urethral syndrome. SEE: *acute urethral syndrome.*

urethrascope (ū-rē′thră-skōp). Urethroscope.

urethratresia (ū-rē″thră-trē′zē-ă) [″ + *atresis,* imperforation]. Occlusion, or imperforation of the urethra.

urethrectomy (ū-rē-thrĕk′tō-mē) [″ + *ektome,* excision]. Surgical excision of the urethra or part of it.

urethremphraxis (ū″rē-thrĕm-frăk′sĭs) [″ + *emphraxis,* obstruction]. Urethral obstruction. SYN: *urethrophraxis.*

urethreurynter (ū-rēth″rūr-ĭn′tĕr) [″ + *eurynein,* to dilate]. Appliance for dilating the urethra.

urethrism, urethrismus (ū′rē-thrĭzm, ū″rē-thrĭz′mŭs) [″ + *-ismos,* condition]. Irritability or spasm of the urethra.

urethritis (ū″rē-thrī′tĭs) [″ + *itis,* inflammation]. Inflammation of the urethra.

u., anterior. Inflammation of that portion of the urethra anterior to the anterior layer of the triangular ligament.

u., gonococcal. Urethritis caused by gonococcus.

u., nongonococcal. ABBR: NGU. U., nonspecific, q.v.

u., nonspecific. ABBR: NSU. Inflammation and irritation of the urethra that in the past was not directly attributable to a specific organism. It is now known that about half of the cases are due to Chlamydia trachomatis.

TREATMENT: Both tetracyclines and erythromycin are of benefit. The latter drug should be used if the patient is pregnant. Test for syphilis before and after initiating therapy. Abstain from sexual intercourse until cured.

u., posterior. Inflammation of membranous and prostatic portions of the urethra.

u., specific. Urethritis due to a specific organism, usually gonococcus.

urethro- [Gr. *ourethra*]. Combining form meaning urethra.

urethrobulbar (ū-rē″thrō-bŭl′băr). Concerning the urethra and the bulbar penis.

urethrocele (ū-rē′thrō-sēl) [″ + *kele,* hernia]. 1. Pouchlike protrusion of the urethral wall in the female. 2. Thickening of connective tissue around the urethra in the female.

urethrocystitis (ū-rē″thrō-sĭs-tī′tĭs) [″ + *kystis,* bladder, + *itis,* inflammation]. Inflammation of the urethra and bladder.

urethrocystopexy (ū-rē″thrō-sĭs′tō-pĕk″sē) [″ + *kystis,* bladder, + *pexis,* fixation]. Plastic surgery of the urethral-bladder junction in order to relieve urinary stress incontinence.

urethrodynia (ū-rē″thrō-dĭn′ē-ă) [″ + *odyne,* pain]. Urethralgia.

urethrograph (ū-rē′thrō-grăf). Device for recording the caliber of the urethra.

urethrography (ū-rē-thrŏg′ră-fē) [″ + *graphein,* to write]. Roentgenography of the urethra after the injection of a radiopaque substance into it.

u., voiding. Radiographic examination of the urethra during micturition after the introduction of a contrast medium.

urethrometer (ū-rē-thrŏm′ĕt-ĕr) [Gr. *ourethra,* urethra, + *metron,* a measure]. Instrument for measuring diameter of the urethra or lumen of a stricture.

urethropenile (ū-rē″thrō-pē′nīl) [″ + L. *penis,* penis]. Relating to the urethra and penis.

urethroperineal (ū-rē″thrō-pĕr-ĭ-nē′ăl) [″ + *perinaion,* perineum]. Rel. to the urethra and perineum.

urethroperineoscrotal (ū-rē″thrō-pĕr-ĭ-nē″ō-skrō′tăl) [″ + ″ + L. *scrotum,* pouch]. Relating to the urethra, perineum, and scrotum.

urethropexy (ū-rē′thrō-pĕks-ē) [″ + Gr. *pexis,* fixation]. Surgical fixation of the urethra.

urethrophraxis (ū-rē-thrō-frăks′ĭs) [″ + *phrassein,* to obstruct]. Urethral obstruction.

SYN: *urethremphraxis.*

urethrophyma (ū-rē-thrō-fī'mă) [" + *phyma,* growth]. A neoplasm in the urethra.

urethroplasty (ū-rē'thrō-plăs"tē) [" + *plassein,* to mold]. Reparative surgery of the urethra.

urethroprostatic (ū-rē"thrō-prŏs-tăt'ĭk). Concerning the urethra and the prostate.

urethrorectal (ū-rē"thrō-rĕk'tăl) [Gr. *ourethra,* urethra, + L. *rectus,* straight]. Rel. to the urethra and the rectum.

urethrorrhagia (ū-rē"thror-ā'jē-ă) [" + *rhegnynai,* to burst forth]. Hemorrhage from the urethra.

urethrorrhaphy (ū-rē-thror'ăf-ē) [" + *rhaphe,* a seam]. Suture of the urethra, as a urethral fistula.

urethrorrhea (ū-rē"thror-ē'ă) [" + *rhoia,* a flow]. Abnormal discharge from the urethra.

u. ex libidine. The discharge of normal glandular secretions resulting from sexual stimulation, esp. that preceding sexual intercourse. SEE: *Cowper's glands.*

urethroscope (ū-rē'thrō-skōp) [" + *skopein,* to examine]. Device for examining the interior of the urethra.

urethroscopic (ū-rē"thrō-skŏp'ĭk) [" + *skopein,* to examine]. Relating to the urethroscope or urethroscopy.

urethroscopy (ū-rē-thrŏs'kō-pē). An examination of the mucous membrane of the urethra with a urethroscope.

urethrospasm (ū-rē'thrō-spăzm) [" + *spasmos,* a spasm]. Spasmodic stricture of the urethra.

urethrostaxis (ū-rē"thrō-stăks'ĭs) [" + *staxis,* a dropping]. Oozing of blood from the urethral mucous membrane.

urethrostenosis (ū-rē"thrō-stĕn-ō'sĭs) [" + *stenosis,* a narrowing] Stricture of the urethra.

urethrostomy (ū-rē-thrŏs'tō-mē) [" + *stoma,* opening]. Formation of a permanent fistula opening into the urethra by perineal section and fixation of membranous urethra in the perineum.

urethrotome (ū-rē'thrō-tōm) [" + *tome,* incision]. An instrument for incision of urethral stricture.

urethrotomy (ū-rē-thrŏt'ō-mē). Incision of a urethral stricture.

urethrotrigonitis (ū-rē"thrō-trī"gō-nī'tĭs) [" + *trigonon,* three-sided figure, + *itis,* inflammation]. Inflammation of the urethra and the trigone of the bladder.

urethrovaginal (ū-rē"thrō-văj'ĭ-năl) [" + L. *vagina,* sheath]. Pert. to the urethra and vagina.

urethrovesical (ū-rē"thrō-vĕs'ĭ-kăl) [" + L. *vesicula,* little bladder]. Concerning the urethra and the bladder.

urhydrosis (ūr"hī-drō'sĭs) [Gr. *ouron,* urine, + *hidros,* sweat]. Excretion of urea in sweat.

URI. *upper respiratory infection.*

uric (ū'rĭk) [Gr. *ourikos,* urine]. Of or pert. to urine.

uric acid. $C_5H_4N_4O_2$. A crystalline acid occurring as an end product of purine metabolism. It is formed from purine bases derived from nucleoproteins. It is a common constituent of urinary and renal calculi and of gouty concretions.

OUTPUT: Between 0.5 and 1 gm. per day if patient is on ordinary mixed diet. Uric acid must be excreted because it cannot be destroyed within the body.

Increased elimination is observed in ingestion of proteins and nitrogenous foods, after exercise, and in gout, leukemia, and acute articular rheumatism. *Decreased elimination* is observed in nephritis, chlorosis, lead poisoning, and protein-free diet.

u.a., endogenous. Uric acid derived from purines undergoing metabolism from the nucleoprotein of body tissues.

u.a., exogenous. Uric acid derived from those purines from food made up of free purines and nucleoproteins. SEE: *urate; uraturia.*

uricacidemia (ū"rĭk-ăs-ĭd-ē'mē-ă) [Gr. *ourikos,* urine, + L. *acidus,* sour, + Gr. *haima,* blood]. Excess uric acid in the blood.

uricaciduria (ū"rĭk-ăs-ĭd-ū'rē-ă) [" + " + Gr. *ouron,* urine]. Excessive amount of uric acid in the urine.

uricase (ū'rĭ-kāz) [" + *-ase,* enzyme]. An enzyme present in the liver and kidneys of most mammals, but not man. This enzyme is capable of oxidizing uric acid into allantoin and carbon dioxide.

uricemia (ū-rĭ-sē'mē-ă) [" + *haima,* blood]. Excess uric acid in the blood. SYN: *uricacidemia.*

uricocholia (ū"rĭ-kō-kō'lē-ă) [" + *chole,* bile]. Uric acid in the bile.

uricolysis (ū-rĭ-kŏl'ĭ-sĭs) [" + *lysis,* dissolution]. The decomposition of uric acid.

uricolytic (ū"rĭ-kō-lĭt'ĭk). Decomposing uric acid.

uricometer (ū"rĭk-ŏm'ĕ-ter) [" + *metron,* a measure]. Apparatus for quantitative estimation of uric acid in the urine.

uricopoiesis (ū"rĭ-kō-poy-ē'sĭs) [" + *poiesis,* formation]. Producing uric acid.

uricosuria (ū"rĭ-kō-sū'rē-ă) [" + *ouron,* urine]. The excessive excretion of uric acid in the urine.

uricosuric (ū"rĭ-kō-sū'rĭk). Potentiating the excretion of uric acid in the urine.

uricosuric agent. A drug (such as probenecid) that increases the urinary excretion of uric acid, thereby reducing the concentration of uric acid in the blood. Used in treatment of gout.

NURSING IMPLICATIONS: Instruct the patient to consume at least 8 glasses (240 ml. each) of fluid a day to facilitate renal elimination of excess uric acid. Encourage activity to prevent urinary stasis. To prevent stagnation of urine, encourage the patient to void when the urge is experienced. Instruct the patient to consume an alkaline-ash diet. Request a visit from the dietitian to promote patient understanding of the dietary requirements.

uricotelic (ū″rĭ-kō-tĕl′ĭk) [″ + *telikos,* belonging to the completion]. Concerning animals that excrete amino nitrogen in the form of uric acid. Included in this group are birds, snakes, and lizards. SEE: *ammonotelic; urea cycle; ureotelic.*

uricoxidase (ū″rĭk-ŏks′ĭ-dās) [″ + *oxys,* sharp, + *-ase,* enzyme]. An enzyme capable of oxidizing uric acid.

uridine (ūr′ĭ-dĭn). A nucleoside that is one of the four main riboside components of ribonucleic acid. It consists of uracil and D-ribose.

u. diphosphate. A uridine-containing nucleotide important in certain metabolic reactions, in which it transports sugars such as glucose and galactose.

uridrosis (ū-rĭ-drō′sĭs) [″ + *hidrosis,* a sweating]. The presence of urea in the sweat. Evaporation may show white scales, the crystals of urea.

u. crystallina. White powder of uric acid deposited on the skin. SYN: *urea frost.*

uriesthesis (ū-rē-ĕs-thē′sĭs) [″ + *aisthesis,* sensation]. Normal desire to void urine.

urina (ū-rī′nă) [L.]. Urine.

u. cibi. Urine voided after a full meal.

u. galactodes. Urine of a milky color.

u. hysterica. Pale, watery urine following hysteria.

u. jumentosa. Cloudy urine.

urinaccelerator (ū″rĭn-ăk-sĕl′ĕr-ā″tor). Musculus bulbospongiosus.

urinal (ū′rĭn-ăl) [L. *urina,* urine]. A container into which one urinates. Also a toilet or bathroom fixture for receiving urine and flushing it away.

urinalysis (ū″rĭ-năl′ĭ-sĭs) [″ + Gr. *ana,* apart, + *lysis,* a loosening]. Analysis of the urine.

urinary (ū′rĭ-năr″ē) [L. *urina,* urine]. Pert. to, secreting, or containing urine.

urinary bladder. Receptacle for urine excreted by the kidneys. SEE: *bladder.*

urinary calculi. Concretions formed in the urinary passages. They vary in composition but may contain urates, calcium, oxalate, calcium carbonate, phosphates, and cystine.

NURSING IMPLICATIONS: Allow the patient to verbalize anxieties and concern related to severe pain. Administer pain relief measures such as analgesics, antispasmodics, and warm, moist heat. Strain all urine, watch for stone passage, and send calculus for analysis. Observe for hematuria. Test for specific gravity on voided specimens. Monitor vital signs; if temperature is elevated, institute appropriate antipyretic measures. Force fluids to enhance dilution of urine, and monitor intake and output. Promote activity to prevent urinary stasis. Be alert for complications such as infection, stasis, and retention. Catheterize as ordered. Monitor renal function studies. Dietary management is based on the composition of the stone. If calcium stones are present, dietary calcium generally should be reduced and foods that acidify the urine, such as cereals and cranberry and grape juices, should be encouraged. If phosphate stones are present, acid-ash foods such as cereals, eggs, meat, and cranberry and grape juices should be given. Persons prone to uric acid stones are advised to consume an alkaline-ash diet of green vegetables and fruits. To minimize urinary infection, esp. for female patient, teach the patient adequate perineal hygiene, and emphasize that increased fluid intake is essential.

urinary casts. Casts of kidney tubules passed in the urine.

urinary incontinence. SEE: *incontinence.*

urinary infection. Infection of the urinary tract with microorganisms.

NURSING IMPLICATIONS: Administer the prescribed antimicrobial that is specific for the causative organism. Obtain urine culture to validate the effectiveness of drug therapy. Administer antispasmodics as prescribed to relieve bladder irritation. Force fluids to 3 liters a day to dilute the bacterial concentration. Monitor and record intake and output. Encourage the patient to void every 2 hours to empty the bladder and excrete the bacteria. Measure specific gravity of voided specimens. Provide relief from urgency by administering analgesics, sitz baths, and warm tub baths. Monitor vital signs every 4 hours; if temperature is elevated, administer appropriate antipyretic medications. Since urinary infections recur frequently in females, teach the patient the following: wear cotton pants; drink large amounts of fluids; avoid bubble baths; cleanse the perineum from front to back after elimination; take a shower rather than a bath; void immediately after sexual intercourse and take prescribed single dose of antimicrobial after intercourse. If symptoms persist after taking prescribed course of antibiotics, notify the physician.

urinary organs. The structures concerned with the secretion and excretion of urinary products, consisting of the two kidneys, two ureters, the bladder, and the urethra.

urinary pigments. Urochrome, urobilin, uroerythrin, and hematoporphyrin.

urinary reflex. Desire to void resulting from accumulation of urine in the bladder.

urinary sediments. Substances found in standing urine, i.e., bacteria, mucus, phosphates, uric acid, calcium oxalate, calcium carbonate, calcium phosphate, magnesium and ammonium phosphate; more rarely, cystine, tyrosine, xanthine, hippuric acid, hematoidin.

urinary stammering. Temporary interruptions in voiding urine.

urinary system. Kidneys, ureters, bladder, and urethra.

urinary tract. Organs and ducts participating in secretion and elimination of urine. SEE: illus.

urinate (ū'rĭ-nāt) [L. *urinare,* to discharge urine]. To pass the urine from the bladder. SYN: *micturate.*

urination (ū″rĭ-nā'shŭn) [L. *urinatio,* a discharging of urine]. The act of voiding urine. Although this act is somewhat under voluntary control, it is accomplished chiefly by the action of involuntary muscles. The musculus sphincter vesicae relaxes, while the general musculature of the wall of the urinary bladder contracts to force out its contents. SYN: *micturition; uresis.*

DIFF. DIAG: *Increased frequency* is seen in polyuria; nervous excitement; irritation of bladder, urethra, or urinary meatus; disease of spinal cord; enlarged prostate in male; pregnancy in female; beer drinking; interstitial nephritis; diabetes; phimosis. *Decreased frequency* occurs after sweating, diarrhea, or bleeding; in anuria, oliguria, uremia, brain disease, drug poisoning, coma, and parenchymatous nephritis. SEE: *urine.*

urination, words pert. to: anisuria; bacilluria; bladder; bradyuria; catheterization; diuresis; diuretic; dysuria; enuresis; kidney; melanuria; micturate; micturition; nocturia; nycturia; oliguria; polyuria; strangury; uracratia; urea; "uret-" words; uric acid; "urin-" words; void.

urine (ū'rĭn) [L. *urina;* Gr. *ouron,* urine]. The fluid secreted from the blood by the kidneys, stored in the bladder, and discharged, usually voluntarily, through the urethra. It is conveyed to the bladder by two ureters, one from each of the kidneys. SEE: Significance of Changes in Urine table.

In healthy persons, urine is of amber color with a slightly acid reaction, has a peculiar odor with a bitter saline taste, frequently deposits a precipitate of phosphates when fresh, but esp. on standing. It has a specific gravity that varies from 1.005 to 1.030.

The greater the amount of urine excreted, the lower the specific gravity. The normal amount of nonprotein nitrogen is from 25 to 35 mg. per 100 ml. of blood. The amount of this substance present in the blood is related to how well the kidneys are functioning. The daily output is equally variable, being adapted to the amount of water taken in and to the amount lost by evaporation from the skin in expired air.

COMP: Urine consists of approx. 95% water and 5% solids. Solids amount to 30 to 70 gm. per liter and include the following (values are in grams per 24 hours unless otherwise noted): *Organic substances:* urea, uric acid (20 to 40), creatine (0 to 40 mg./d. in men and 0 to 80 in women), creatinine (15 to 25 mg./kg. of body weight/day), ammonia (0.5 to 1.3). *Inorganic substances:* chlorides (110 to 250 nmol./liter depending upon chloride intake), calcium (0.1 to 0.2), magnesium (3 to 5 nmol./d.), phosphorus (0.4 to 1.3).

In addition to the above, many other substances may be present depending on the diet and state of health of the individual. Among component substances indicating pathological states are albumin, glucose, ketone bodies, blood, pus, casts, and bacteria.

Collection of urine: For a routine urinalysis, a voided specimen of urine in a clean container is usually sufficient. For culture, either a clean-catch or a catheterized specimen is required. For a clean-catch specimen the individual cleanses the perineum or glans penis with soap and water or an antiseptic solution such as benzalkonium chloride prior to voiding. A midstream specimen of urine is then collected in a sterilized container. A catheterized specimen is obtained by passing a catheter into the bladder using sterile technique.

DIAG: *Color:* Normal urine is amber in color, resulting from the presence of urobilin, q.v., a pigment mainly derived from bilirubin, q.v., in the bile. This pigment is found in excessive quantities in fever and it may be indicative of excess destruction of red blood cells. The effect of food and medication must be considered before concluding that the color of the urine is abnormal. *Black:* Melanuria, malignant pigmented tumor, melanotic cancer, or carbolic acid poisoning. *Bile-colored:* Seen in jaundice. *Blue:* May result from methylene blue or the presence of indigo. *Colorless:* This is known as achromaturia and is usually due to the urine's being extremely dilute. *Milky:* May be due to chyluria, lipuria, or pus. *Orange-red:* May indicate the presence of pyridine dyes. *Pale:* Indicates an excess of water; it is found in conditions causing polyuria. *Red or reddish color:* May be due to the presence of blood in the urine, hematuria, or to senna or rhubarb, which may color the urine either brown or orange.

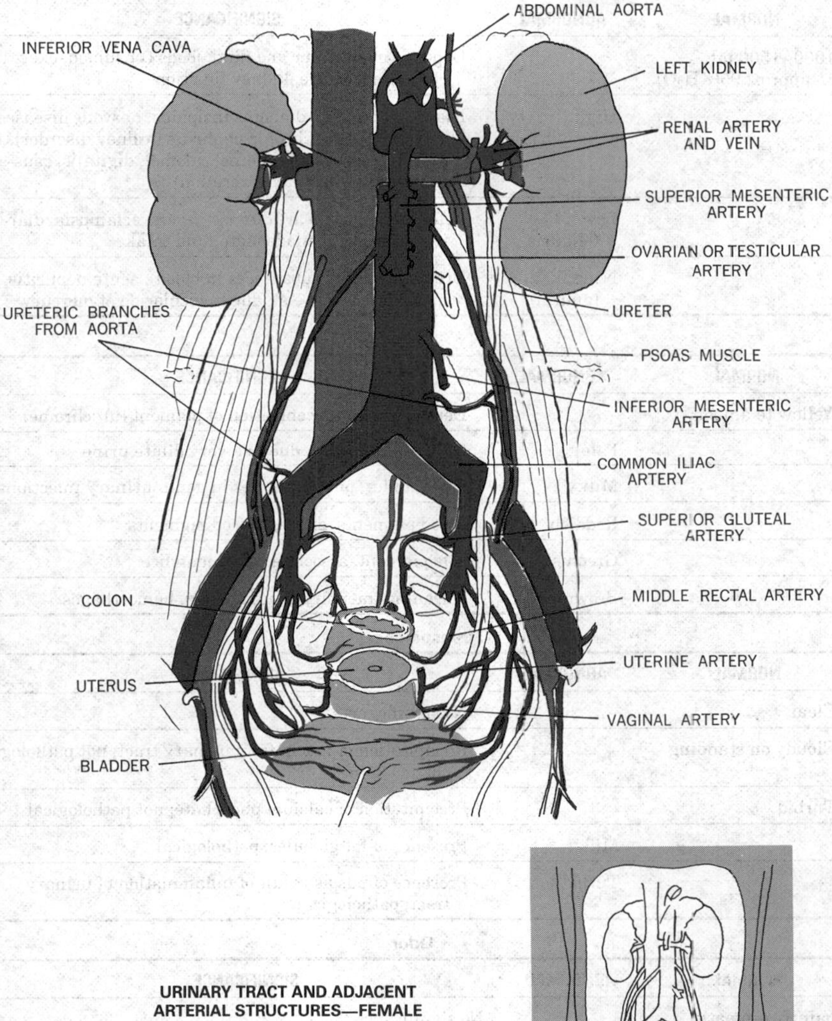

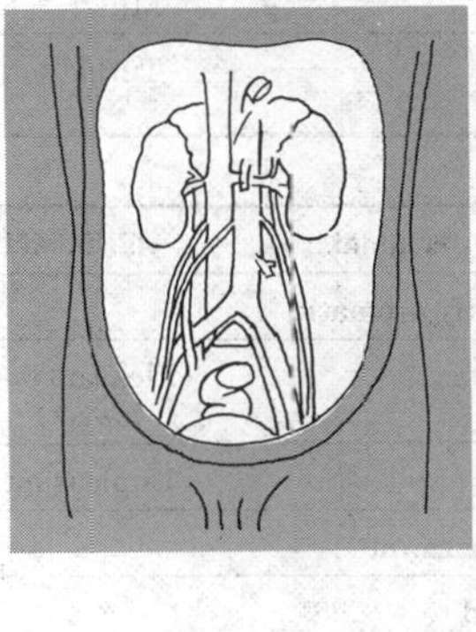

URINARY TRACT AND ADJACENT ARTERIAL STRUCTURES—FEMALE

Significance of Changes in Urine

Quantity

NORMAL	ABNORMAL	SIGNIFICANCE
1000–1500 ml. (approx. 95% H_2O)		Depends upon water and fluid, foods consumed, exercise, temperature, kidney function
	High (polyuria)	Diabetes mellitus, diabetes insipidus, nervous diseases, certain types of chronic nephritis (kidney disorder), diuretics (drugs as caffeine, calomel, digitalis, causing increased urinary excretion)
	Low (oliguria)	Acute nephritis, heart disease, fevers, eclampsia, diarrhea, vomiting, inadequate fluid intake
	None (anuria)	Uremia (urinary substances in blood), acute nephritis, metal poisoning, e.g., due to bichloride of mercury

Color

NORMAL	ABNORMAL	SIGNIFICANCE
Yellow to amber		Depends upon concentration of pigment (urochrome)
	Pale	Diabetes insipidus, due to a very dilute urine
	Milky	Fat globules, pus corpuscles in genitourinary infections
	Reddish	Blood pigments, drugs, or food pigments
	Greenish	Bile pigment, associated with jaundice
	Brown-black	Poisoning (mercury, lead, phenol), hemorrhages

Transparency

NORMAL	ABNORMAL	SIGNIFICANCE
Clear		No significance
Cloudy on standing		Precipitation of mucin from urinary tract; not pathological
Turbid		Precipitation of calcium phosphate; not pathological
	Milky	Presence of fat globules; pathological
	Turbid	Presence of pus as result of inflammation of urinary tract; pathological

Odor

NORMAL	ABNORMAL	SIGNIFICANCE
Faintly aromatic		No significance
	Pleasant (sweet)	Acetone, associated with diabetes mellitus
	Unpleasant	Decomposition or ingestion of certain drugs or foods
Peppermint		Menthol ingestion
Acrid		Asparagus in diet
Spicy		Ingestion of sandalwood oil or saffron

Significance of Changes in Urine (*Continued*)

Proteinuria

NORMAL	ABNORMAL	SIGNIFICANCE
Albumin and globulin		Excretion of 10–100 mg. each 24 hr. is normal but this amount is not detected by usual tests
	Albumin	Evidence of altered renal function, which may be due to renal pathology or a systemic disease such as diabetes
	Globulin	Bence Jones proteins are associated with multiple myeloma and diseases of globulin metabclism. Other types of globulins may be present in acute and chronic pyelonephritis

Specific Gravity

NORMAL	ABNORMAL	SIGNIFICANCE
1.010 to 1.025 sp. gr.		Ordinarily, sp. gr. inversely proportional to volume
	Low	Dilution if volume is large; otherwise nephritis
	High	Acute nephritis; concentrated if volume is small; otherwise if volume is large and light colored, diabetes mellitus

Acidity

NORMAL	ABNORMAL	SIGNIFICANCE
Acid (slight)		Diet of acid-forming foods (meats, eggs, prunes, wheat) overbalancing the base-forming foods (vegetables and fruits)
	High acidity	Acidosis, diabetes mellitus, many pathological disorders (fevers, starvation)
	Alkaline	Putrefying bacteria change urea into ammonium carbonate; infection or ingestion of alkaline compounds

Odor: Ammoniacal: May result from decomposition products. *Aromatic:* This is the odor of a normal urine. *Fecal:* Due to fistulous communications between the intestinal and urinary tracts. *Fishy:* Cystitis. *New-mown hay:* Indicative of diabetes. *Overripe apple:* Indicative of acetonuria or the presence of acetone bodies in the urine. *Violet:* May be caused by turpentine.

NOTE: Some foods but esp. asparagus cause the urine to have a characteristic odor. This is a transient phenomenon.

Products in Disease: Acidic: May be found in acidosis and pyelonephritis. *Alkaline:* May show a white sediment. *Albumin:* Due to nephritis and inflammation of mucous membrane of any portion of the urinary apparatus. *Acetone:* Represents the by-products of excessive fat metabolism excreted by the kidneys and known as ketonuria. *Animal parasites:* Rare, found as result of contamination. *Bacteria:* Usually regarded as being of little importance if fewer than 100,000 can be cultured from each ml. of urine. Appears cloudy. *Bile:* Bile in the urine indicates abnormal retention of bile. *Blood:* Shows a smoky sediment and is reddish-brown. Indicates hemorrhagic nephritis, calculi, congestion of a kidney, renal carcinoma, tuberculosis of kidney, chronic infections, or trauma. *Casts:* These indicate renal disease. A few hyaline casts in the aged denote slight damage to the kidneys. Casts are found in large numbers in nephritis. The less acute the disease, the finer are the granular casts. *Crystals:* Calcium oxalate and uric acid crystals will be present in acid urine; crystals of ammonium biurate and phosphates will be present in alkaline urine. Crystals have little significance except leucine and tyrosine crystals, which may indicate liver disease. *Cylindroids:* No special significance. *Acetoacetic acid:* Deficient carbohydrate metabolism of an advanced stage; it is preceded by the presence of acetone. *Epithelial cells* (squamous): If in large numbers from urinary bladder and ureters, they indicate inflammation of these parts; renal epithelial cells of kidney indicate serious damage to the same. *Fat droplets:* Fatty degeneration of kidneys and lipemia. *Froth:* Indicates presence of bile. *Indican:* Small significance but is seen in intestinal putrefaction. *Mucus:* If visible and in quantity, urethritis is indicated. No special significance in women if the quantity is small. *Mucous threads:* Mucoid ribbonlike structures of no great significance. *Pus:* This is mucoid and shows a white sediment. It is found in bacterial infections of the urinary tract. The presence of the occasional pus cell may be normal per high-power field; if accompanied by red cells, pus cells indicate inflammation. *Red blood cells:* Stones or inflammation of kidney or urinary tract. No significance if due to contamination by menstrual fluid. *Sediment:* Pinkish due to excess of urates; white, caused by phosphates. In order to obtain sediment, the examination should be made quickly after urine is voided by centrifuging for 3 min. *Sugar* (glucose): Denotes faulty carbohydrate metabolism as seen in diabetes mellitus. *Urea:* Principal end product of protein metabolism. *Yeasts and molds:* Result of contamination.

Conditions: Difficult urination (dysuria): Found in urethral stricture, enlarged prostate, atony and impairment of the bladder's muscular power, and in gonorrhea and other inflammatory conditions involving the urethra, bladder or lower ureter. *Diminished* (oliguria): Diminished in disease of the liver and in low protein intake. Scanty in all fevers unless fluid intake is increased. Accompanies cardiac failure; acute, chronic, and parenchymatous nephritis; obstruction of return venous circulation of kidney; thrombosis of renal vein or inferior vena cava; loss of fluids through hemorrhages, vomiting, or diarrhea; inadequate fluid intake; obstruction or pressure upon ureter; lead poisoning.

Incontinence (enuresis, q.v.): Inability to retain urine because of paralysis or relaxation of sphincters or contraction of longitudinal muscular layer of bladder; incontinence and dribbling are results. This can occur in all forms of coma, during an epileptic seizure, shock, typhoid, and typhus. It may also occur in conjunction with injuries to or tumors of the spinal cord; transverse myelitis, spinal meningitis, locomotor ataxia, paralysis, and reflex excitability of nervous system. Other causes include local irritation of the bladder, cystitis, phimosis, vesical calculus, contracted meatus, ascarides, and very concentrated urine.

Increased (polyuria): In fevers, esp. if weight is lost; after pregnancy; during parturition; after the intake of large quantities of liquid. May be indicative of chronic interstitial nephritis; diabetes mellitus or insipidus; amyloid disease of kidney; reabsorption of effusions; functional disease of nervous system as hysteria, neurasthenia, migraine. Persistent in bulbar, cerebellar, and spinal tumors, locomotor ataxia, and meningitis. *Obstructive:* Result of occlusion of one or both ureters. *Painful:* Dysuria, q.v., vesical tenesmus. There is a persistent desire to urinate. *Residual:* That remaining in bladder after urination; usually indicative of a pathological condition such as prostatic disease or cystocele. *Retention* (ischuria): Inability to urinate; almost same diseases and injuries of cord that produce incontinence. All forms of coma; typhoid; peritonitis; hysteria; atony; prostatic enlargement; urethral stricture; urethritis, cystitis; tumors of bladder; calculus in urethra. *Strangury:* Painful and spasmodic. May be indicative of cystitis; neuralgia; acute nephritis; tuberculosis; cancer or ulceration of bladder; urethritis; urethral stricture; hypertrophied, cancerous, or inflamed prostate; prolapsus uteri; pelvic peritonitis and abscess; vesical tenesmus. Pain and burning often caused by concentrated or acid urine. *Suppression:* Failure of kidneys to secrete urine. May be complete (anuria) or partial (oliguria). Failure of kidneys to secrete the urine or failure of urine to reach the bladder if secreted may be found in acute nephritis or congestion, renal abscess, last stages of chronic nephritis. Renal damage caused by patient's having received a blood transfusion with incompatible blood.

u., residual. Residual urine, q.v.

urine, words pert. to: acetoaectic acid; acetone; acetone bodies; acetone in urine, tests for; acetonuria; achromaturia; acidaminuria; albuminuria; alkalinuria; alkaptone; alkaptonuria; allantoinuria; alloxuria; aminuria; ammoniuria; amylosuria; amyluria; anisuria; antidiuretic; anuria; arabinosuria; azoturia; Bence Jones albumose; Benedict's test for sugar; bilirubinuria; bladder, stammering of; bladder, urinary; calcariuria; cast; ceramuria; cerebrosuria; chloride, test for, in urine; chloriduria; chondroituria; chromaturia; chyluria; enuresis; epithelium; galactosuria; galacturia; glucose; glycosuria; Heller's test; hemoglobinuria; hippuria; hyaline casts; hydruria; incontinence; ischuria; ketonuria; ketosis; kidney; lactosuria; lipuria; lithuria; litmus paper; melanuria; mucus; myosinuria; nocturia; oliguresis; oxaluria; pentosuria; pus; pyuria; residual urine; retention of urine; secretion; tyrosinuria; uraturia; urea; uredema; uremia; ureter; uric acid; urinalysis; urolagnia; "uro-" words.

urinemia (ū″rĭ-nē′mē-ă) [L. *urina*, urine, + Gr. *haima*, blood]. Accumulation in the blood of substances such as urea, which are normally excreted in the urine. SYN: *uremia*.

uriniferous (ū-rĭ-nĭf′ĕr-ŭs) [″ + *ferre*, to bear]. Carrying urine.

urinific (ū″rĭ-nĭf′ĭk). Uriniparous.

uriniparous (ū-rĭ-nĭp′ă-rŭs) [″ + *parere*, to bear]. Producing or secreting urine.

urinogenital (ū″rĭ-nō-jĕn′ĭ-tăl) [″ + *genitalia*, genitals]. Pert. to the genital and urinary organs. SYN: *urogenital*.

urinogenous (ū″rĭ-nŏj′ĭ-nŭs) [″ + Gr. *gennan*, to produce]. 1. Producing urine. 2. Originating in urine. SYN: *urogenous*.

urinology (ū″rĭ-nŏl′ō-jē). Urology.

urinoma (ū″rĭ-nō′mă) [″ + Gr. *oma*, mass]. A cyst containing urine.

urinometer (ū″rĭ-nŏm′ĕ-tĕr) [″ + Gr. *metron*, a measure]. Device for determining specific gravity of urine.

urinometry (ū″rĭ-nŏm′ĕt-rē). Determination of specific gravity of the urine.

urinophil (ū′rĭ-nō-fĭl) [″ + Gr. *philein*, to love]. Capable of existing in the urine, as bacteria that grow best in urine.

urinoscopy (ū″rĭ-nŏs′kō-pē). Uroscopy.

urinose, urinous (ū′rĭ-nōs, ū′rĭ-nŭs) [L. *urina*, urine]. Having the characteristics of or containing urine.

urinosexual (ū″rĭ-nō-sĕks′ū-ăl). Urogenital.

uriposia (ū″rĭ-pō′zē-ă) [″ + *posis*, drinking]. Drinking of urine.

urisolvent (ū″rĭ-sŏl′vĕnt) [″ + *solvens*, dissolving]. Dissolving uric acid or causing it to be dissolved.

Urispas. Trade name for flavoxate hydrochloride.

uro- [Gr. *ouron*]. Combining form meaning pert. to urine.

uroammoniac (ū″rō-ă-mō′nē-ăk). Containing urine and ammonia.

uroanthelone (ū″rō-ăn′thĕ-lōn). Urogastrone.

urobilin (ū″rō-bī′lĭn) [″ + L. *bilis*, bile]. A brown pigment formed by the oxidation of urobilinogen, a decomposition product of bilirubin. Urobilin may be formed from the urobilinogen in stools or in urine after exposure to air.

urobilinemia (ū″rō-bī″lĭn-ē′mē-ă) [″ + ″ + Gr. *haima*, blood]. Urobilin in blood.

urobilinicterus (ū″rō-bī-lĭn-ĭk′tĕr-ŭs) [″ + L. *bilis*, bile, + Gr. *ikteros*, jaundice]. Jaundice resulting from urobilinemia.

urobilinogen (ū″rō-bī-lĭn′ō-jĕn) [″ + ″ + Gr. *gennan*, to produce]. A colorless derivative of bilirubin, from which it is formed by the action of intestinal bacteria.

urobilinogenemia (ū″rō-bī″lĭn-ō-jĕn-ē′mē-ă) [″ + ″ + ″ + *haima*, blood]. Urobilinogen in the blood.

urobilinuria (ū″rō-bī″lĭn-ū′rē-ă) [″ + ″ + Gr. *ouron*, urine]. Excess of urobilin in the urine.

urocele (ū′rō-sēl) [″ + *kele*, hernia]. Escape of urine into the scrotum.

urocheras (ū-rŏk′ĕr-ăs) [″ + *cheras*, gravel]. Gravel or calcareous sediment in the urine.

urochesia (ū-rō-kē′zē-ă) [″ + *chezein*, to defecate]. A discharge of urine in the feces.

urochrome (ū′rō-krōm) [″ + *chroma*, color]. The pigment that gives urine its characteristic color. It is derived from urobilin.

uroclepsia (ū-rō-klĕp′sē-ă) [″ + *kleptein*, judge]. Involuntary urination without being aware of it.

urocrisia (ū″rō-krĭz′ē-ă) [″ + *krinein*, to judge]. Diagnosis by examining the urine.

urocyanin (ū-rō-sī′ă-nĭn) [″ + *kyanos*, blue]. A blue pigment present in the urine in certain diseases, esp. scarlet fever.

urocyanogen (ū″rō-sī-ăn′ō-jĕn) [″ + *kyanos*, blue, + *gennan*, to produce]. A blue pigment in urine, esp. in cholera patients.

urocyanosis (ū″rō-sī-ăn-ō′sĭs) [″ + ″ + *osis*, condition]. Blue discoloration of the urine. May be due to presence of indigo blue from oxidation of indican, or from ingestion of drugs such as methylene blue. SYN: *indicanuria*.

urocyst (ū′rō-sĭst) [Gr. *ouron*, urine, + *kystis*, bladder]. The urinary bladder.

urocystic (ū″rō-sĭs′tĭk). Concerning the urinary bladder.

urocystis (ū″rō-sĭs′tĭs). The urinary bladder.

urocystitis (ū″rō-sĭs-tī′tĭs). Inflammation of the urinary bladder.

urodynamics (ū″rō-dī-năm′ĭks). Study of the holding or storage of urine in the bladder; the facility with which it empties; and the rate of movement of urine out of the bladder during micturition.

urodynia (ū″rō-dĭn′ē-ă) [″ + *odyne*, pain]. Pain associated with urination.

uroedema (ū″rō-ē-dē′mă) [′ + *oidema*, a swelling]. Extravasation of urine distending the tissues. SYN: *uredema*.

uroenterone (ū″rō-ĕn′tĕr-ōn). Urogastrone.

uroerythrin (ū″rō-ĕr′ĭth-rĭn) [″ + *erythros*, red]. A reddish pigment sometimes present in urine. SYN: *purpurin*.

uroflavin (ū″rō-flā′vĭn). A fluorescent compound present in the urine of persons taking riboflavin.

urofuscin (ū″rō-fŭs′ĭn) [″ + L. *fuscus*, tawny]. A reddish-brown pigment sometimes found in samples of urine, esp. in cases of porphyrinuria.

urofuscohematin (ū″rō-fŭs″kō-hĕm′ăt-ĭn) [″ + ″ + Gr. *haima,* blood]. A reddish-brown pigment in urine in some diseases.

urogastrone (ū″rō-găs′trōn) [″ + *gaster,* belly]. A polypeptide present in urine that has an inhibitory effect on gastric secretion.

urogenital (ū″rō-jĕn′ĭ-tăl) [″ + L. *genitalia,* genitals]. Pert. to the urinary and reproductive organs. SYN: *urinogenital.*

urogenital fold. Ridge, urogenital, q.v.

urogenous (ū-rŏj′ĕn-ŭs) [″ + *gennan,* to produce]. 1. Producing urine. 2. Originating in urine. SYN: *urinogenous.*

uroglaucin (ū″rō-glaw′sĭn) [″ + *glaukos,* green]. Urocyanin.

urogram (ū′rō-grăm) [″ + *gramma,* a mark]. A roentgenogram of any part of the urinary tract.

urography (ū-rŏg′ră-fē) [Gr. *ouron,* urine, + *graphein,* to write]. Roentgenography of any part of the urinary tract after introduction of a radiopaque substance.

u., ascending; u., cystoscopic. Urography in which the radiopaque dye is injected into the bladder during cystoscopy.

u., descending; u., excretion; u., excretory; u., intravenous. Urography in which an injected dye is excreted by the kidney and studied by x-ray during excretion.

u., retrograde. U., ascending, q.v.

urohematin (ū″rō-hĕm′ăt-ĭn) [″ + *haima,* blood]. Pigment in urine, considered as identical with hematin, q.v., that alters color of urine in proportion to degree of oxidation.

urohematonephrosis (ū″rō-hĕm″ă-tō-nē-frō′sĭs) [″ + ″ + *nephros,* kidney]. Pathological condition of the kidney in which the pelvis is distended with blood and urine.

urohematoporphyrin (ū″rō-hĕm″ă-tō-por′fĭr-ĭn) [″ + ″ + *porphyra,* purple]. Iron-free hematin in urine when hemolysis occurs.

urokinase (ū-rō-kī′nās). An enzyme obtained from human urine. Used experimentally for dissolving venous thrombi and pulmonary emboli. It is administered intravenously.

urokinetic (ū″rō-kĭ-nĕt′ĭk) [″ + *kinesis,* movement]. Resulting reflexly from stimulation of the urinary organs.

urolagnia (ū-rō-lăg′nē-ă) [″ + *lagneia,* lust]. Sexual excitation associated with urine or urination.

urolith (ū′rō-lĭth) [″ + *lithos,* stone]. A concretion in the urine.

urolithiasis (ū″rō-lĭ-thī′ă-sĭs) [″ + ″ + *-iasis,* condition]. Formation of urinary calculi and the illness associated with the presence of calculi in the urinary tract. SEE: *calculus, renal.*

urolithic (ū″rō-lĭth′ĭk). Concerning urinary calculi.

urolithology (ū″rō-lĭ-thŏl′ō-jē) [″ + ″ + *logos,* study]. Science dealing with urinary calculi.

urologic (ū-rō-lŏj′ĭk) [″ + *logos,* study]. Pert. to urology.

urologist (ū-rŏl′ō-jĭst). A physician who specializes in the practice of urology.

urology (ū-rŏl′ō-jē) [″ + *logos,* a study]. The branch of medicine concerned with the urinary tract in both sexes and the genital tract in the male. SYN: *uronology.*

urolutein (ū-rō-lū′tē-ĭn) [″ + L. *luteus,* yellow]. A yellow pigment seen in the urine.

uromancy (ūr′ō-măn″sē) [″ + *manteia,* a divination]. Use of urinalysis for diagnosis of disease.

uromelanin (ū-rō-mĕl′ăn-ĭn) [″ + *melas,* black]. A black pigment occurring in urine resulting from the decomposition of urochrome.

uromelus (ū-rŏm′ē-lŭs) [Gr. *oura,* tail, + *melos,* limb]. Congenitally deformed fetus in which the lower extremities are fused. SYN: *sirenomelus.*

urometer (ū-rŏm′ĕt-ĕr) [Gr. *ouron,* urine, + *metron,* a measure]. Instrument for determining specific gravity of urine. SYN: *urinometer.*

uroncus (ū-rŏn′kŭs) [″ + *onkos,* a mass]. A swelling or cyst containing urine.

uronephrosis (ū″rō-nĕf-rō′sĭs) [″ + *nephros,* kidney, + *osis,* condition]. Dilatation of renal structures from obstruction of urinary flow. Distention of renal pelvis and tubules with urine. SYN: *hydronephrosis.*

uronology (ū-rō-nŏl′ō-jē) [″ + *logos,* a study]. The science of urine and genitourinary diseases. SYN: *urology.*

uronophile (ū-rŏn′ō-fīl) [″ + *philein,* to love]. Developing best in a culture containing urine, noting a microorganism.

uropathogen (ū″rō-păth′ō-jĕn) [″ + *pathos,* disease, + *gennan,* to produce]. A microorganism capable of causing disease of the urinary tract.

uropathy (ū-rŏp′ă-thē) Any disease affecting the urinary tract.

u., obstructive. Any disease resulting from obstruction of the urinary tract.

uropenia (ū-rō-pē′nē-ă) [″ + *penia,* a lack]. Lack of urinary secretion.

uropepsin (ū″rō-pĕp′sĭn). The end product of pepsin metabolism. It is excreted in the urine.

urophanic (ū-rō-făn′ĭk) [″ + *phainein,* to appear]. Appearing in the urine.

urophein (ū″rō-fē′ĭn) [″ + *phaios,* gray]. Gray pigment in urine said to cause its characteristic odor. Also spelled urophaein.

urophosphometer (ū″rō-fŏs-fŏm′ĕ-tĕr) [″ + L. *phosphas,* phosphorus]. Device for estimating amount of phosphorus in the urine.

uroplania (ū″rō-plā′nē-ă) [″ + *plane,* a wandering]. Condition in which urine is present or discharged from parts other than the urinary organs.

uropoiesis (ū″rō-poy-ē′sĭs) [Gr. *ouron,* urine, + *poiesis,* production]. Formation of urine by the kidneys.

uropoietic (ū″rō-poy-ĕt′ĭk) [″ + *poiein,* to form]. Concerned in the formation of urine or in uropoiesis.

uroporphyria (ū″rō-por-fĭr′ē-ă). Porphyria in which an excess amount of uroporphyrin is excreted in the urine.

uroporphyrin (ū″rō-por′fĭ-rĭn). A reddish pigment present in the urine and feces in cases of porphyria. May also be present in the urine of persons taking certain drugs.

uroporphyrinogen (ū″rō-por″fĭ-rĭn′ō-jĕn). Any one of several porphyrins that are the precursors of uroporphyrins.

u. I. An abnormal isomer of a precursor of protoporphyrin, which accumulates in one form of porphyria. It causes the urine to be red; the teeth to fluoresce brightly in ultraviolet light; and the skin to be abnormally sensitive to sunlight. This is congenital erythropoietic porphyria.

uropsammus (ū″rō-săm′ŭs) [″ + *psammos,* sand]. Gravel or calcareous sediment in the urine.

uropyonephrosis (ū″rō-pī-ō-nĕf-rō′sĭs) [″ + *pyon,* pus, + *nephros,* kidney, + *osis,* condition]. Urine and pus in the renal pelvis.

uropyoureter (ū″rō-pī″ō-ū-rē′tĕr) [″ + ″ + *oureter,* ureter]. Accumulation of urine and pus in the ureter.

urorosein (ū″rō-rō′zē-ĭn) [″ + L. *roseus,* rosy]. A rose-colored pigment in urine, which is increased in certain diseases. SYN: *urorrhodin.*

urorrhagia (ū-rō-ră′jē-ă) [″ + *rhegnynai,* to burst forth]. Excessive secretion of urine. SYN: *polyuria.*

urorrhea (ū-rō-rē′ă) [″ + *rhoia,* a flow]. Involuntary flow of urine. SYN: *enuresis.*

urorrhodin (ū-rō-rō′dĭn) [″ + *rhodon,* rose]. A rose-colored pigment in the urine in certain infectious diseases such as typhoid fever and tuberculosis.

urorrhodinogen (ū″rō-rō-dĭn′ō-jĕn) [Gr. *ouron,* urine, + *rhodon,* rose, + *gennan,* to produce]. A chromogen of the urine that, when decomposed, forms urorrhodin.

urorubin (ū-rō-roo′bĭn) [″ + L. *ruber,* red]. A red pigment obtained from urine by treatment with hydrochloric acid.

urorubrohematin (ū″rō-rū″brō-hĕm′ă-tĭn) [″ + ″ + Gr. *haima,* blood]. A reddish pigment occasionally found in the urine in some chronic diseases.

urosacin (ū-rō′sā-sĭn). A red pigment in the urine. SYN: *urorrhodin.*

uroscheocele (ū-rŏs′kē-ō-sēl) [″ + *oscheon,* scrotum, + *kele,* mass]. Swelling of the scrotum from extravasation of urine into the scrotal sac. SYN: *urocele.*

uroschesis (ū-rŏs′kĕs-ĭs) [″ + *schesis,* a holding]. 1. Suppression of urine. 2. Retention of the urine.

uroscopy (ū-rŏs′kō-pē) [″ + *skopein,* to examine]. 1. Examination of the urine. 2. Diagnosis by examination of the urine.

urosepsis (ū-rō-sĕp′sĭs). Septic poisoning due to retention and absorption of urinary products in the tissues.

urospectrin (ū-rō-spĕk′trĭn) [″ + L. *spectrum,* image]. A pigment derived from normal urine; seen when urine is shaken with acetic ether.

urostealith (ū″rō-stē′ă-lĭth) [″ + *stear,* fat, + *lithos,* stone]. A fatty substance in some urinary calculi.

urotoxia (ū″rō-tŏk′sē-ă) [″ + *toxikon,* poison]. The toxicity of the urine.

urotoxicity (ū″rō-tŏks-ĭs′ĭ-tē) [″ + *toxikon,* poison]. The toxic character of the urine.

urotoxin (ū″rō-tŏk′sĭn). Toxic substances in the urine.

uroureter (ū″rō-ū′rĕ-tĕr, ū″rō-ū-rē′tĕr) [″ + *oureter,* ureter]. Distention of the ureter with urine due to stricture or obstruction.

urous (ū′rŭs) [Gr. *ouron,* urine]. Having the nature of urine.

uroxanthin (ū″rō-zăn′thĭn) [″ + *xanthos,* yellow]. Yellow pigment of the urine; an indigo-forming substance.

uroxin (ū-rŏk′sĭn) [″ + *oxys,* sharp]. Alloxantin, a derivative of alloxan.

urtica (ŭr-tī′kă) [L., a stinging nettle]. (pl. *urticae*) A wheal.

urticant (ŭr′tĭ-kănt). That which causes an urticarial reaction in the skin.

urticaria (ŭr-tĭ-kā′rē-ă) [L. *urtica,* nettle]. A vascular reaction of the skin characterized by the eruption of pale evanescent wheals, which are associated with severe itching. SYN: *hives; nettle rash.* SEE: *allergy; angioneurotic edema.*

ETIOL: Contact with an external irritant such as the nettle, physical agents, foods, insect bites, serum sickness, pollens, drugs, or neurogenic factors.

SYM: Sudden general eruption of papules or wheals associated with intense itching.

TREATMENT: *General measures.* Because the skin manifestation is an allergic reaction, identify and remove the antigenic offender if possible. Check diet for common offenders such as wheat, milk, eggs, chocolate, and other food allergens. Avoid unnecessary medications, as drugs are often causative factors. *Specific measures.* Antihistaminic drugs often give quick relief. Injection of epinephrine (subcutaneous). Ephedrine may be used. In severe cases ACTH or cortisone used with caution has proved effective. Locally, antipruritic lotions and baths are frequently beneficial.

u., aquagenic. Urticaria caused by exposure of the skin to ordinary water.

u. bullosa. Eruption of temporary vesicles with infusion of fluid under the epidermis.

u., cold. Cold-induced urticarial eruption that may progress to angioedema.

u. factitia. Urticaria following slight irritation of the skin. SYN: *dermatographia.*

u. gigantea. Angioneurotic edema.

u. haemorrhagica. Urticaria with lesions infiltrated with blood.

u. maculosa. A chronic form of urticaria with red-colored lesions.

u. maritima. Urticaria due to salt water bathing.

u. medicamentosa. Urticaria due to certain drugs.

u. papulosa. In this form of urticaria, the wheal is followed by a lingering papule that is attended by considerable itching. Most commonly observed in debilitated children. SYN: *lichen urticatus; prurigo simplex.*

u. pigmentosa. Mastocytosis in which clumps of mast cells are present in the corium of the skin. These appear as brown areas that itch.

u. pigmentosa juvenilis. A form of urticaria pigmentosa that begins in infancy.

u. solaris. Urticaria occurring in certain individuals following exposure to sunlight.

urticarial (ŭr″tĭ-kā′rē-ăl) [L. *urtica,* a nettle]. Pert. to urticaria. SYN: *urticarious.*

urticate (ŭr′tĭ-kāt). 1. To produce urticaria. 2. Marked by the appearance of wheals.

urtication (ŭr-tĭ-kā′shŭn). 1. Flogging of a part with nettles to induce counterirritation. 2. Burning or itching sensation. 3. Eruption of itching wheals. SYN: *urticaria.*

urushiol (ū-roo′shē-ŏl″) [Jap. *urushi,* lac, + L. *oleum,* oil]. The principal toxic irritant substance of plants (Toxicodendron) such as poison ivy that produce the characteristic severe dermatitis upon contact.

U.S. AEC. *U.S. Atomic Energy Commission.*

USAN. *United States Adopted Names* (for drugs).

USAN and the USP Dictionary of Drug Names. A dictionary of nonproprietary names, brand names, code designations, and Chemical Abstracts Service registry numbers for drugs. The 1983 edition was cumulative for U.S. adopted names (USAN) from June 15, 1961, through June 15, 1982.

USP, U.S. Phar. *United States Pharmacopeia.*

U.S.P.H.S. *United States Public Health Service.*

ustilaginism (ŭs-tĭl-ăj′ĭn-ĭzm) [L. *ustulatus,* scorched, + Gr. *-ismos,* condition]. Poisoning resulting from eating corn infected with smut fungus, Ustilago maydis.

Ustilago (ŭs-tĭl-ā′gō). A moldlike fungus, Ustilago maydis, commonly called smut.

ustion (ŭs′chŭn) [L. *ustio,* a burning]. Cauterization with actual cautery.

ustulation (ŭs-tū-lā′shŭn) [L. *ustulare,* to scorch]. Roasting, parching, or drying of a moist drug.

ustus (ŭs′tŭs) [L.]. Burned. SEE: *calcination.*

uta (ū′tă). Infection with Leishmania braziliensis involving the nasopharyngeal and mucocutaneous membranes. Common in Central and South America. SYN: *leishmaniasis, American.*

ut dict. L. *ut dictum,* as directed.

utend. L. *utendus,* to be used.

uter-, utero- [L. *uterus,* womb]. Combining forms denoting relationship to the uterus.

uteralgia (ū″tĕr-ăl′jē-ă) [L. *uterus,* womb, + Gr. *algos,* pain]. Uterine pain.

uterectomy (ū″tĕr-ĕk′tō-mē) [″ + Gr. *ektome,* excision]. Removal of uterus through the abdomen or vagina. SYN: *hysterectomy.*

uterine (ū′tĕr-ĭn, -īn) [L. *uterinus*]. Pert. to the uterus.

uterine bleeding. Bleeding from the uterus. Physiologic bleeding via the vagina occurs in normal menstruation. Abnormal forms include excessive menstrual flow (hypermenorrhea, menorrhagia) or too frequent menstruation (polymenorrhea). Nonmenstrual bleeding is called metrorrhagia. Pseudomenstrual or withdrawal bleeding may occur following estrogenic therapy. Breakthrough bleeding is the term used for intermenstrual bleeding that sometimes occurs in women who take progestational agents such as birth control pills. SEE: *menstruation; tampon, menstrual.*

uterine glands. The tubular glands in the endometrium.

uterine milk. A milky white substance between the gravid uterus and the placental villi.

uterine souffle. A vascular sound that may be heard in the pregnant uterus by using a stethoscope.

uterine subinvolution. Failure of the uterus to return to normal size after childbirth. A uterus that weighs more than 100 gm. is considered to be enlarged.

uterine tube. One of two small tubes attached to either side of the uterus and leading from the region of the ovary. SYN: *fallopian tube.*

uteroabdominal (ū″tĕr-ō-ăb-dŏm′ĭ-năl) [L. *uterus,* womb, + *abdominalis,* pert. to abdomen]. Pert. to both the uterus and abdomen.

uterocele (ū-tĕr′ō-sēl) [″ + Gr. *kele,* hernia]. Hernia containing the uterus.

uterocervical (ū″tĕr-ō-sĕr′vĭ-kăl) [″ + *cervix,* neck]. Rel. to the uterus and the cervix.

uterocystostomy (ū″tĕr-ō-sĭs-tŏs′tō-mē) [″ + Gr. *kystis,* bladder, + *stoma,* mouth]. Formation of a passage between the uterine cervix and the bladder.

uterofixation (ū″tĕr-ō-fĭks-ā′shŭn) [″ + *fixatio,* a fixing]. Fixation of a displaced uterus. SYN: *hysteropexy.*

uterogenic (ū″tĕr-ō-jĕn′ĭk). Formed in the uterus.

uterogestation (ū″tĕr-ō-jĕs-tā′shŭn) [″ + *gestatio,* a carrying]. Pregnancy in the uterus; normal pregnancy.

uterography (ū″tĕr-ŏg′ră-fē) [″ + Gr. *graphein,* to write]. Roentgenography of the uterus.

uterolith (ū′tĕr-ō-lĭth) [″ + Gr. *lithos,* stone]. A uterine concretion.

uterometer (ū″tĕr-ŏm′ĕt-er) [″ + Gr. *metron,* measure]. Device for measuring the uterus and for determining its position.

uteroovarian (ū″tĕr-ō-ō-vā′rē-ăn) [″ + *ovarium,* ovary]. Rel. to the uterus and ovary.

uteropexia, uteropexy (ū″tĕr-ō-pĕks′ē-ă, ū′tĕr-ō-pĕks″ē) [″ + Gr. *pexis,* fixation]. Fixation of the uterus to the abdominal wall. SYN: *hysteropexy.*

uteroplacental (ū″tĕr-ō-plă-sĕn′tăl) [″ + *placenta,* a flat cake]. Rel. to the placenta and uterus.

uteroplasty (ū″tĕr-ō-plăs′tē) [″ + Gr. *plassein,* to form]. Plastic surgery of the uterus.

uterorectal (ū″tĕr-ō-rĕk′tăl). Concerning the uterus and rectum.

uterosacral (ū″tĕr-ō-sā′krăl) [″ + *sacralis,* pert. to the sacrum]. Rel. to the uterus and sacrum.

uterosalpingography (ū″tĕr-ō-săl-pĭng-ŏg′ră-fē) [″ + Gr. *salpinx,* tube, + *graphein,* to write]. Visualization of the interior of the uterus and fallopian tubes by roentgenography.

uteroscope (ū′tĕr-ō-skōp) [″ + Gr. *skopein,* to examine]. Device for viewing the uterine cavity.

uterotome (ū′tĕr-ō-tōm) [″ + Gr. *tome,* incision]. An instrument used for uterotomy.

uterotomy (ū-tĕr-ŏt′ō-mē). Incision of the uterus.

uterotonic (ū″tĕr-ō-tŏn′ĭk) [L. *uterus,* womb, + Gr. *tonos,* tone]. Giving muscular tone to the uterus.

uterotractor (ū″tĕr-ō-trăk′tor) [″ + *tractor,* a drawer]. An instrument for applying traction to the cervix uteri.

uterotubal (ū″tĕr-ō-tū′băl) [″ + *tuba,* tube]. Relating to the uterus and the oviducts.

uterotubography (ū″tĕr-ō-tū-bŏg′ră-fē) [″ + ″ + Gr. *graphein,* to write]. Hysterosalpingography.

uterovaginal (ū″tĕr-ō-văj′ĭ-năl) [″ + *vagina,* sheath]. Rel. to the uterus and vagina.

uteroventral (ū″tĕr-ō-vĕn′trăl). Uteroabdominal, q.v.

uterovesical (ū″tĕr-ō-vĕs′ĭ-kăl) [″ + *vesica,* bladder]. Rel. to the uterus and bladder.

uterus (ū′tĕr-ŭs) [L.]. [NA] An organ of the female reproductive system for containing and nourishing the embryo and fetus from the time the fertilized egg is implanted to the time of birth of the fetus. SYN: *womb.* SEE: *genitalia, female,* for illus.; *pregnancy test.*

ANAT: A muscular, hollow, pear-shaped structure. It is partly covered by peritoneum and the cavity is lined by a mucous membrane, the endometrium.

The uterus consists of three areas: the body or expanded upper portion, the isthmus or constricted central area, and the cervix, the lowermost cylindrical portion that joins the uterus to the upper end of the vagina. The rounded portion of the body lying above the openings of the two uterine tubes is the fundus. The uterus is situated in the midpelvis approximately halfway between the sacrum and the symphysis pubis. It is supported in this position by the pelvic diaphragm, supplemented by two broad ligaments, two round ligaments, and two uterosacral ligaments, as well as other lesser ligaments. The upper part of the body is called the fundus and the lateral borders of the fundus to which the tubes are attached are called the cornual ends. The cavity of the uterus, a potential space, is triangular in shape with the base of the triangle in the fundal portion. The canal of the cervix is long and narrow and is constricted at the upper end by the internal os and at the lower end by the external os.

The largest portion of the uterus is made up of musculature that is longitudinal and circular. The outer covering of the uterus is peritoneum, with the exception of that part upon which the bladder rests and the vaginal portion of the cervix. The inner lining of the body of the uterus varies in form and histological structure with the period of life in which it is studied, the prepuberty stage, the actively menstruating stage, and the menopausal stage, each having its own characteristics. The uterus is normally anteflexed. The blood supply of the uterus is derived from the uterine and ovarian arteries.

POSITIONS: Anteflexion: bending forward. Anteversion: forward displacement of fundus toward pubis, while cervix is tilted up toward sacrum. Retroflexion: bending backward at junction of body and cervix. Retroversion: inclination backward with retention of normal curve; opposite of anteversion.

AUSCULTATION: After the fourth month of gestation, if the uterus contains a living fetus, three distinct sounds may be heard. *Fetal heart sounds:* Consist of a succession of short, rapid, double pulsations varying in frequency from 120 to 140 per minute. First sound is short, feeble, and obscure, while the second, the one usually heard, is loud and distinct; sounds like ticking of a watch wrapped in a napkin. Sound is usually transmitted over a space of 3 or 4 in. (7.6 to 10.2 cm.) square. Location is determined by the position of the fetus. Generally, when maximum intensity is on the level of or above the umbilicus, it is a breech presentation. During labor, examinations, if made, should be between uterine contractions. In protracted labors the fetal heart sound is of value in indicating the time for manual or instrumental interference to save life of child. Irregularity and feebleness of sound are indicative of a life-threatening situation for the fetus.

Funic souffle: The soft blowing sound heard over the location of the umbilical cord of the fetus in utero and synchronous with the fetal heartbeat during late pregnancy.

Uterine bruit: This sound is single, intermittent in character, and a combination of blowing and hissing sounds. Increases in intensity up to the period of labor. Believed to depend upon rapid passage of blood from the arteries into the distended venous sinuses of the uterus. Synchronous with maternal pulse, subject to same variations, and is always heard before the pulsations of the fetal heart. The area over which it is audible varies, with the greatest point of intensity in a median line a little above the pubes.

PALPATION: During pregnancy in third month, if walls of abdomen are not too thick, palpate by placing patient upon her back with head raised and thighs flexed, and pressing points of fingers gently downward and backward above the pubes. A hard round mass will be found beneath the median line, rising out of the pelvis. Two or four weeks later the increase is marked. As pregnancy advances the mass loses its hardness and becomes more elastic, like a cyst filled with water. In doubtful cases where decided enlargement of abdomen is present, a standard hormonal test for pregnancy should be done.

By vaginal examination one may be able to diagnose the stage of gestation, stage of parturition, or if the woman is near term, the progress of labor, the presentation and position of the child, and the position of the uterus. The sensation of the tip of the cervix of an unimpregnated uterus to the touch is like that imparted to the finger by touching the tip of the nose, i.e., firm and cartilaginous; of the impregnated, like that of touching the lips and is soft like velvet, but deeper, beyond the softness, is a hardness, as of board.

PERCUSSION: The nonpregnant uterus is inaccessible to touch externally or to percussion. In pregnancy at end of second month a dull sound on percussion just above the pubes indicates the enlarging uterus; later, as uterus increases in volume and rises into abdomen, one is able, by oval tumor felt in hypogastrium and by circumscribed area of dullness corresponding to situation of the tumor, to establish strong presumptive evidence of pregnancy. This presumption becomes strengthened if the area of dullness increases with the regularity proper to gestation. Palpation and percussion, however, are not sufficient to determine whether the enlargement is due to pregnancy or to some other form of new growth. After the fifth month, both these methods are inferior to auscultation.

u. acollis. Uterus without a cervix.

u. arcuatus. Uterus with a depressed arched fundus.

u. bicornis. Uterus in which the fundus is divided into two parts.

u. biforis. Uterus in which the external os is divided into two parts by a septum.

u. bilocularis. Uterus in which the cavity is divided into two parts by a partition. SYN: *uterus septus.*

u., bipartite. Uterus in which body is partially divided by a median septum.

u., cancer of. Malignant neoplasm of the uterus. Detected by size, intermittent bleeding, purulent discharge, vaginal or Papanicolau smear, or cervical or endometrial biopsy. May produce sterility, abortion, hemorrhage, sepsis. Extremely rare in pregnancy; however, growth of a tumor usually will increase during pregnancy.

u. cordiformis. A heart-shaped uterus.

u. didelphys. Double uterus.

u. duplex. A double uterus resulting from failure of union of mullerian ducts.

u., fetal. Uterus that is retarded in development and possesses an extremely long cervical canal.

u., gravid. Pregnant uterus.

u. masculinus. The prostatic utricle. *SEE: utricle, prostatic.*

u. parvicollis. Normal uterus with disproportionately small vaginal portion.

u., prolapse of. Downward displacement of uterus, the cervix sometimes protruding from the vaginal orifice. SEE: *descensus uteri.*

u., pubescent. An adult uterus that resembles a uterus of a prepubertal female.

u., rupture of, in pregnancy. Rare but serious. May be spontaneous or traumatic. Child and amniotic sac may be expelled into peritoneal cavity.

ETIOL: Obstruction, weakness of uterine wall. Scars may cause weakness.

SYM. AND SIGNS: Obstruction usually precedes symptoms. Abdominal pains, shock, hemorrhage. Child easily palpated. However, spontaneous rupture may occur without warning.

TREATMENT: Combat shock and hemorrhage and surgically remove fetus from peritoneal cavity.

u. septus. U. bilocularis.

u., subinvolution of. The lack of involution of the uterus following childbirth. It is manifested by a large uterus and a continuation of lochia rubra beyond the usual time. The factors in its causation are usually puerperal infection, multiparity, overdistention of the uterus by multiple pregnancy or polyhydramnios, lack of lactation, malposition of the uterus, and retained secundines. Involution is aided by being certain that the placenta is intact at the time of delivery, and the use of ecbolics, q.v., to cause contraction of the uterus.

u., tipped. SEE: *tipped uterus.*

u., tumors of. May cause sterility, abortion, or obstruct labor; may become infected or twisted on their attachments. Myomata (fibroids) are possible but not common in young women; fibroids are more common beyond age 30 and in black women. Subserous tumors do not affect pregnancy, may impede labor or may disappear following labor. Interstitial and submucous type may interfere with pregnancy and produce abortion.

EFFECTS UPON LABOR: Tumors usually have no effect. If low, may cause malpresentation or impossible labor; labor pains may be weak and inefficient. Often severe pains and rupture of uterus. Submucous tumors may protrude before or after birth. Placenta may be retained. Tumor may be infected postpartum. Knee-chest position helps patient if tumor is in pelvis. If in fundus, delivery is through vagina; if not, cesarean section may be needed. Control hemorrhage by packing.

u. unicornis. Uterus that possesses only one lateral half and usually having only one uterine tube.

Utibid. Trade name for oxolinic acid.

Uticillin VK. Trade name for penicillin V potassium, USP.

Uticort. Trade name for betamethasone benzoate.

utilization review. Evaluation of the necessity, quality, effectiveness or efficiency of medical services, procedures, and facilities. In regard to a hospital, the review includes appropriateness of admission, services ordered and provided, length of stay, and discharge practices.

Utimox. Trade name for amoxicillin.

utricle (ū'trĭk'l) [L. *utriculus,* a little bag]. 1. One of two sacs of the membranous labyrinth in the bony vestibule of the inner ear. The utricle communicates with the semicircular ducts by five openings on posterior wall and with the sacculus and endolymphatic duct by an opening on anterior wall. On its inner surface is an area of sensory epithelium, the macula utriculi, containing cells that respond to movement of otoliths due to changes in position. 2. Any small sac.

u. of urethra. The prostatic vesicle of the male.

u. of vestibule. Vestibular cavity connecting with the semicircular canals.

u., prostatic. A small blind pouch of the urethra extending into substance of prostate gland. It is a remnant of the embryonic mullerian duct. SYN: *uterus masculinus.*

utricular (ū-trĭk'ū-lăr) [L. *utriculus,* a little bag]. 1. Pert. to the utricle. 2. Like a bladder.

utriculitis (ū-trĭk-ū-lī'tĭs) [" + Gr. *itis,* inflammation]. Inflammation of the utricle, either that of the vestibule or the prostatic utricle.

utriculoplasty (ū-trĭk'ū-lō-plăs"tē) [" + Gr. *plassein,* to form]. Surgical reduction of the size of the uterus by excision of a longitudinal wedge-shaped section.

utriculosaccular (ū-trĭk"ū-lō-săk'ū-lăr) [" + *sacculus,* a small cavity]. Pert. to the utricle and saccule of the labyrinth.

utriculosaccular duct. A duct uniting the utricle and saccule.

utriculus (ū-trĭk'ū-lŭs) [L., a little bag]. A utricle.

u. masculinus. Utricle, prostatic.

u. prostaticus. Utricle, prostatic.

utriform (ū'trĭ-form) [L. *uter,* a skin bag, + *forma,* shape]. Having a shape like a bottle.

uva (ū'vă) [L., grape]. The dried fruit of the grapevine; the raisin.

uvea (ū'vē-ă) [L. *uva,* grape]. The second or vascular coat of the eye lying immediately beneath the sclera. It consists of the iris, ciliary body, and choroid, and forms the pigmented layer.

uveal (ū'vē-ăl). Pert. to the middle coat of the eye, or uvea.

uveitic (ū-vē-ĭt'ĭk) [" + Gr. *itis,* inflammation]. Marked by or pert. to uveitis.

uveitis (ū-vē-ī'tĭs). Inflammation of the iris, ciliary body, and choroid, or the entire uvea.

u., heterochromic. Chronic uniocular iridocyclitis with abnormal pigmentation of the iris, inflammation of the uvea, and opacities in the vitreous.

u., sympathetic. Severe, bilateral uveitis that started as inflammation of the uveal tract of one eye resulting from a puncture wound. The injured eye is termed the "exciting eye." If the affected eye is not removed within 10 days of the accident that caused the wound, then blindness will be the outcome.

uveoparotitis (ū"vē-ō-păr-ō-tī'tĭs) [" + Gr. *para,* near, + *ous,* ear, + *itis,* inflammation]. Inflammation of the parotid gland and uveitis.

uveoplasty (ū′vē-ō-plăs″tē) [″ + Gr. *plassein,* to form]. Reparative operation of the uvea.

uveoscleritis (ū″vē-ō-sklē-rī′tĭs). Inflammation of the sclera in which the infection has spread from the uvea.

uviform (ū′vĭ-form) [″ + *forma,* form]. Shaped like a grape.

uviofast (ū′vē-ō-făst). Unaffected by ultraviolet radiation.

uviol (ū′vē-ŏl). Glass that is unusually transparent to ultraviolet rays.

uviolize (ū′vē-ō-līz). To use ultraviolet rays therapeutically.

uviometer (ū″vē-ŏm′ĕ-tĕr). An instrument for measuring the intensity of ultraviolet light.

uvioresistant (ū″vē-ō-rē-zĭs′tănt). Resistant to effects of ultraviolet rays. SYN: *uviofast.*

uviosensitive (ū″vē-ō-sĕn′sĭ-tĭv). Sensitive to effects of ultraviolet rays.

uvula (ū′vū-lă) [L. *uvula,* a little grape]. Small, soft structure hanging from free edge of soft palate in midline above the root of the tongue. It is composed of muscle, connective tissue, and mucous membrane. SYN: *cion; staphyle.*

u. fissa. A cleft uvula.

u. of cerebellum. A small lobule of the cerebellum lying on inferior surface of inferior vermis, anterior to the pyramis.

u. patula. Uvula.

u. vermis. A small, triangular elevation on the vermis of the cerebellum of the brain.

u. vesicae. A median projection of mucous membrane of the urinary bladder located immediately anterior to the orifice of the urethra.

uvulaptosis (ū″vū-lăp-tō′sĭs) [″ + Gr. *ptosis,* a dropping]. A relaxed condition of the uvula. SYN: *uvuloptosis.*

uvular (ū′vū-lăr) [L. *uvula,* little grape]. Pert. to the uvula.

uvularis (ū-vū-lā′rĭs) [L.]. The azygos uvulae muscle. SEE: *Muscles* in *Appendix.*

uvulatome (ū′vū-lă-tōm) [″ + Gr. *tome,* incision]. Instrument for removal of the uvula.

uvulatomy (ū-vū-lăt′ō-mē). Excision of the uvula.

uvulectomy (ū″vū-lĕk′tō-mē) [″ + Gr. *ektome,* excision]. Surgical removal of the uvula.

uvulitis (ū″vū-lī′tĭs) [″ + Gr. *itis,* inflammation]. Inflammation of the uvula.

uvuloptosis (ū″vū-lŏp-tō′sĭs) [″ + Gr. *ptosis,* a dropping]. Relaxed and pendulous condition of the palate.

uvulotome (ū′vū-lō-tōm) [L. *uvula,* little grape, + Gr. *tome,* incision]. Instrument for performing uvulotomy. SYN: *uvulatome.*

uvulotomy (ū-vū-lŏt′ō-mē). Amputation of the uvula.

U wave. In the electrocardiogram, a low-amplitude deflection that follows the T wave. Its significance is unknown and its absence does not indicate abnormality. SEE: *QRST complex; electrocardiogram.*

V

V. 1. *Vibrio; vision; visual acuity.* 2. Chem. symb. for vanadium.

v. L. *vena, vein; volt.*

vaccigenous (văk-sĭj′ĕn-ŭs) [L. *vaccinus,* pert. to cows, + Gr. *gennan,* to produce]. Producing vaccine. SYN: *vaccinogenous.*

vaccina (văk-sī′nă). Vaccinia, q.v.

vaccinable (văk-sĭn′ă-b′l). Capable of being successfully vaccinated.

vaccinal (văk′sĭn-ăl). Rel. to vaccine or to vaccination.

vaccinate (văk′sĭn-āt) [L. *vaccinus,* pert. to cows]. To inoculate with vaccine to produce immunity against disease.

vaccination (văk″sĭ-nā′shŭn) [L. *vaccinus,* pert. to cows]. 1. Inoculation with any vaccine to establish resistance to a specific infectious disease. 2. A scar left on the skin by inoculation of a vaccine.

vaccinator (văk′sĭ-nā″tor). One who vaccinates.

vaccine (văk′sēn, văk-sēn′) [L. *vaccinus,* pert. to cows]. A suspension of infectious agents or some part of them, given for the purpose of establishing resistance to an infectious disease. SEE: table.

Vaccines are of four general classes:

(1) Those containing living attenuated infectious organisms. Ex.: BCG vaccine for tuberculosis and vaccines for smallpox and yellow fever.

(2) Those containing infectious agents killed by physical or chemical means. Ex.: vaccines used to protect human beings against typhoid fever, rabies, and whooping cough. Vaccines for use in preventing cholera, dysentery, undulant fever, and plague are available but they are less reliable than the former vaccines.

(3) Those containing soluble toxins of microorganisms, sometimes used as such, but generally forming toxoids. Ex.: toxoid used in the prevention of diphtheria and tetanus.

(4) Those containing substances extracted from infectious agents. Ex.: capsular polysaccharides extracted from pneumococci.

FUNCT: To stimulate the development of specific defensive mechanisms in the body that result in more or less permanent protection against a disease. An attack of smallpox or diphtheria, for example, usually leaves the recovered patient permanently immune to those diseases. As a result of infection, the body succeeds in building up its own defenses, so that a new infection causes no illness. A successful vaccine does the same thing without risk of illness.

v., aqueous. Vaccine employing physiological salt solution as the vehicle.

v., autogenous. Bacterial vaccine prepared from lesions of the individual to be inoculated. SYN: *v., homologous.*

v., bacterial. A suspension of bacteria, killed or attenuated, in saline solution. Used for injection into body to induce development of active immunity to the same organism.

v., BCG. Bacille Calmette-Guérin, a preparation of a dried, living culture of Mycobacterium tuberculosis. It is used in prophylactic vaccination of infants against tuberculosis. Virulence of the bacillus has been reduced by repeated cultures on glycerinated ox bile.

v., cholera. Vaccine prepared from killed Vibrio cholerae. It is effective for only a few months.

v., DTP. A preparation of diphtheria and tetanus toxoids and killed pertussis vaccine that is used in active immunization. It is administered intramuscularly.

v., epidemic typhus fever. Vaccine made of killed Rickettsia prowazekii for treating epidemic typhus fever.

v., heterologous. Vaccine prepared from organisms obtained from a source other than the person to be inoculated.

v., homologous. V., autogenous.

v., human diploid cell rabies (HDCV). An inactivated virus vaccine prepared from fixed rabies virus grown in human diploid cell tissue culture.

v., humanized. Vaccine obtained from vaccinia vesicles in human beings.

v., influenza. A polyvalent vaccine containing inactivated antigenic variants of the influenza virus for use in areas expected to have epidemics. Its use is particularly helpful to the aged and chronically ill.

v., killed. Vaccine prepared from dead microorganisms. This type of vaccine is used for strains that have a high virulence.

v., measles virus, inactivated. Vaccine prepared from inactivated measles virus. Protection provided is short-lived. This preparation should be used only when there are contraindications to the use of live attenuated measles vaccine, q.v.

v., measles virus, live attenuated. Vaccine prepared from live strains of measles virus. This type of measles vaccine is the preferred form except in patients who have one of the following: lymphoma, leukemia, or other generalized malignancy; radiation therapy; pregnancy; active tuberculosis; egg sensitivity; prolonged treatment with drugs that suppress the immune response; administration of gamma globulin, blood, or plasma. SEE: *vaccine, measles virus, inactivated.*

Vaccines

Name	Age Administered	Booster Schedule	Comments
Cholera	see Comments	Every 6 mos. for those who remain in endemic areas	Only those traveling to countries where cholera is present need to be vaccinated
DTP (diphtheria, tetanus, pertussis)	Given routinely beginning as early as 3 mos., a total of 3 inoculations at 4–6 wk. intervals. A 4th dose is given a yr. later. Administered I.M.	Repeat inoculation at time of entering school. After that children need *only* tetanus and diphtheria immunization every 10 yrs.	Tetanus booster may be required following a wound even though all routine and booster immunizations have been received. Booster of diphtheria toxoid should be given if child under six is exposed to diphtheria
Hepatitis B	All ages of persons at risk of contracting the virus, e.g., dialysis patients	Every 6 to 12 months	The vaccine is expensive and should be given only to those at high risk of developing the disease who do not show evidence of immunity to the virus
Influenza (flu)	All ages	Variable depending upon strain of virus predicted to cause the next influenza epidemic	Recommended for those who may become seriously ill if they develop flu, i.e., the elderly and those of any age who have chronic diseases of the heart or lungs or metabolic diseases such as diabetes
Measles (live attenuated rubeola)	15 mos. but may be given as early as 6 mos. during an epidemic	If vaccinated before 10 mos. of age, should be revaccinated within a yr.	Vaccine will usually prevent measles if given within 2 days after a child has been exposed to the disease. Not given to adults. Contraindicated in those known to be hypersensitive to eggs, chicken, chicken feathers, or neomycin
Mumps	Any age after 15 mos.	Not indicated	Particularly valuable for children approaching puberty, adolescents, and adults who have never had mumps. Contraindicated in those known to be hypersensitive to eggs, chicken, chicken feathers, or neomycin
Plague	see Comments	see Comments	Recommended for those traveling to SE Asia; persons who work closely with wild rodents in plague areas; and laboratory personnel working with Yersinia pestis organisms

Vaccines (*Continued*)

Name	Age Administered	Booster Schedule	Comments
Pneumococcal vaccine, polyvalent	Do not give to children under age two; or pregnant women	None	Vaccine is effective against the 23 most prevalent types of pneumococci. Administered to those who have an increased risk of developing pneumococcal pneumonia. Included are those who have chronic diseases; are recovering from an acute illness; are in chronic care facilities; or are over 50 years of age
Polio (live oral trivalent vaccine)	6–8 wks. for 1st dose; 2nd given 6 wks. later; 3rd, 2 mos. later; 4th at 15–18 mos. of age	At time of entering school	Administration is postponed in those with persistent vomiting, diarrhea, or acute illness
Rabies	see Comments	see Comments	Each exposure to rabies needs to be evaluated on an individual basis by the physician. The use of human diploid cell rabies vaccine is the treatment of choice for those never previously immunized against rabies. SEE: *rabies*
Rh immune globulin	1 dose 72 hrs. after delivery, abortion, or accidental transfusion of Rh-positive blood to Rh-negative patient	None	Should be given to Rh-negative women who give birth to Rh-positive infants and to Rh-negative women who have abortions
Rocky Mountain spotted fever	see Comments	see Comments	Vaccine is recommended only for laboratory personnel working with the causative organism, Rickettsia rickettsii; or for those who come in contact with ticks in their work or recreation
Rubella (German measles)	No earlier than 1 yr. of age	Not indicated	Object is to prevent infection of the fetus. Because the major source of virus dissemination is from children in elementary school, all children regardless of their previous experience with rubella should be vaccinated. CAUTION: Pregnant women should not be given rubella vaccine

Vaccines (*Continued*)

Name	Age Administered	Booster Schedule	Comments
Smallpox	see Comments	see Comments	Because smallpox is considered to have been completely eradicated world-wide, the vaccine is no longer administered.
Typhoid	see Comments	see Comments	Immunization is indicated when a person has come into contact with a known typhoid carrier; if there is an outbreak of typhoid fever; or prior to traveling to an area where typhoid is endemic
Typhus	see Comments	see Comments	Needed only for special high-risk groups such as those working in laboratories involved with Rickettsia prowazekii investigations; missionaries and others living in areas where typhus is endemic; and medical personnel caring for patients with typhus
Viral hepatitis	see Comments	see Comments	Immune serum globulin is recommended for those living in the same house or otherwise in close contact with someone who has viral hepatitis due to hepatitis A. Hepatitis B immune globulin is available for persons exposed to blood positive for B virus antigen, and to infants born of B virus antigen–positive mothers. SEE: *Hepatitis B* in this table.
Yellow fever	see Comments	Every 10 years	Vaccine should be given to persons 6 mos. or older traveling in or living in areas where yellow fever is present

v., mixed. Vaccine prepared from more than one infectious agent or from more than one strain of an infectious agent.

v., multivalent. V., polyvalent.

v., mumps. A live attenuated vaccine used to prevent mumps. Its use should be governed by the same restrictions listed for live attenuated measles virus vaccine.

v., plague. Vaccine made from a crude fraction of killed plague bacilli for immunizing against plague.

v., pneumococcal, polyvalent. A vaccine effective against the 23 most prevalent types of pneumococci. Do not give to children under two years of age or to pregnant women.

v., poliovirus, live oral trivalent. Oral vaccine prepared from three types of attenuated poliovirus. SEE: *v., Sabin.*

v., polyvalent. Vaccine made from several strains of the same species of bacterium or virus. SYN: *v., multivalent.*

v., rabies. Vaccine prepared from killed, fixed virus of rabies, used prophylactically following bite by a rabid animal. SEE: *v., human diploid cell rabies (HDCV); rabies.*

v., Sabin. Oral vaccine prepared from live attenuated poliovirus. SEE: *poliomyelitis.*

v., sensitized. Vaccine prepared from bacteria treated with their specific immune serum.

v., smallpox. Vaccine made from lymph of cowpox vesicles obtained from healthy vaccinated bovine animals. NOTE: This vaccine is no longer used because smallpox has been eradicated world-wide.

v., TAB. A mixture of typhoid, paratyphoid A, and paratyphoid B vaccines.

v., triple. Vaccine prepared from cultures of three different microorganisms.

v., typhoid. Vaccine made of killed Salmonella typhosa organisms for immunizing against typhoid. May not be effective if person receives unusually large doses of the live organism at time of exposure.

v., yellow fever. Vaccine made from a live attenuated strain of yellow fever virus.

vaccinia (văk-sĭn'ē-ă) [L. *vaccinus,* pert. to cows]. A contagious disease of cattle, produced in humans by inoculation with cowpox virus to confer immunity against smallpox. Papules form about third day after vaccination, changing to umbilicated vesicles about the fifth day, and at end of first week becoming umbilicated pustules surrounded by a red areola. They dry and form scabs which fall off about the second week, leaving a white pitted depression. SYN: *cowpox.* SEE: *vaccination; varicella; variola.*

v. necrosum. Spreading necrosis at the site of smallpox vaccination. May be accompanied by similar necrotic areas elsewhere on the body.

vaccinia immune globulin. USP. Hyperimmune gamma globulin. The therapeutic agent of choice for dermal complications of vaccination for smallpox, i.e., eczema vaccinatum and progressive vaccinia. May be obtained commercially or by contacting one of the designated consultants listed by the Regional Blood Centers of the American Red Cross. NOTE: There is no longer a need for this material because smallpox has been eradicated world-wide.

vaccinial (văk-sĭn'ē-ăl). Resembling vaccinia.

vacciniform (văk-sĭn'ĭ-form) [L. *vaccinus,* pert. to cows, + *forma,* shape]. Of the nature of vaccinia or cowpox.

vacciniola (văk"sĭn-ē-ō'lă) [L., little cows]. Secondary general eruption after local eruption from vaccine.

vaccinogen (văk-sĭn'ō-jĕn). A source of vaccine.

vaccinogenous (văk"sĭn-ŏj'ĕn-ŭs) [L. *vaccinus,* pert. to cows, + Gr. *gennan,* to produce]. Producing vaccine or pert. to its production.

vaccinoid (văk'sĭn-oyd) [" + Gr. *eidos,* form]. 1. Resembling vaccinia. 2. Modified or spurious vaccinia.

vaccinostyle (văk-sĭn'ō-stīl). A pointed stylus used in vaccination.

vaccinotherapeutics (văk"sĭn-ō-thĕr"ă-pū'tĭks). Treatment by injection of bacterial vaccines.

vaccinum (văk-sī'nŭm) [L.]. Vaccine.

vacuolar (văk'ū-ō-lăr) [L. *vacuum,* vacuum]. Pert. to or possessing vacuoles.

vacuolar degeneration. Swelling of cells with increase in number and size of vacuoles. SYN: *cloudy swelling.*

vacuolated (văk'ū-ō-lāt"ĕd). Possessing or containing vacuoles.

vacuolation (văk"ū-ō-lā'shŭn). Formation of vacuoles. SYN: *vacuolization.*

vacuole (văk'ū-ōl) [L. *vacuum,* vacuum]. A clear space in cell protoplasm filled with fluid or air.

v., autophagic. A vacuole that contains recognizable fragments of the ribosomes or mitochondria.

v., contractile. A cavity filled with fluid in the cytoplasm of a protozoan. The cavity is emptied by sudden contraction of its walls.

v., heterophagous. A vacuole that contains substances that come from outside the cell.

v., plasmocrin. A vacuole present in cytoplasm of secretory cell that is filled with crystalloid material.

v., rhagiocrin. A vacuole present in cytoplasm of secretory cell that is filled with colloid material.

vacuolization (văk"ū-ō-lĭ-zā'shŭn) [L. *vacuum,* vacuum]. Vacuolation.

vacuome (văk'ū-ōm). A system of vacuoles in cells that stain in the living cell with neutral red.

vacuum (văk'ū-ŭm) [L., empty]. A space exhausted of its air content.

vacuum aspiration. Removal of uterine contents by using a hollow curet or catheter to which a suction apparatus is attached. Used prior to 12th week of pregnancy.

vacuum extractor. Device, using a suction cup attached to the fetal head, for applying traction to the fetus during delivery. Its use may be hazardous except in the hands of experts.

vacuum tube. A vessel of insulating material (usually glass) that is sealed and has a vacuum sufficiently high to permit the free flow of electrons between the electrodes that extend into the tube from the outside. In England, it is called a vacuum valve.

vade mecum (wā"dē mē'kŭm) [L., go with me]. A useful object that a person has available with him at all times. A dictionary or handbook.

vagabond's disease. Discoloration of skin caused by exposure and scratching due to presence of lice. SEE: *pediculosis corporis.*

vagal (vā'găl) [L. *vagus,* wandering]. Pert. to the vagus nerve.

vagal attack. A condition of dyspnea with cardiac distress and a fear of impending death. A sinking sensation assumed to be the result of vasomotor spasm.

vagal escape. Condition in which one or more beats of the heart occurs even though the vagus nerve is being continuously stimulated. Stimulation of the vagus normally inhibits heartbeat.

vagal substance. Substance liberated at termination of vagus nerve fibers in the heart. SEE: *acetylcholine.*

vagal tone. Condition in which impulses over the vagus nerve exert a continuous inhibitory effect upon the heart.

vagi (vā'gī). Pl. of vagus.

vagina (vă-jī'nă) [L., sheath]. (pl. *vaginae, vaginas*) 1. A sheathlike part. 2. [NA] A musculomembranous tube that forms the passageway between the cervix uteri and the vulvae.

ANAT: In the uppermost part, the cervix divides the vagina into four fornices: the two lateral, the anterior, and the posterior. The bladder is situated adjacent to the anterior wall of the vagina and the rectum is behind the posterior wall. The vagina represents a potential space, the walls of which are in contact with each other. Close to the cervix uteri the walls form a horizontal crescent shape, at the midpoint an H shape, and close to the vulva the shape of a vertical slit. The vagina is lined by mucous membrane made up of squamous epithelium. It is surrounded by fascias that allow for easy distensibility. The blood supply of the vagina is furnished from the inferior vesical, inferior hemorrhoidal, and uterine arteries.

FUNCT: A passage for the intromission of the penis, for the reception of semen, and for the discharge of the menstrual flow; and the passageway through which the fetus is delivered.

v., bulb of. Small erectile body on each side of the vaginal vestibule. SYN: *Bartholin's glands; bulbi vestibuli.*

v. fibrosa tendinis. A fibrous sheath surrounding a tendon that usually confines it to an osseous groove.

v. masculinus. The prostatic utricle. SEE: *utricle, prostatic.*

v. mucosa tendinis. A synovial sheath that develops about a tendon.

v., septate. Congenital condition in which the vagina is divided longitudinally into two parts. Division may be partial or complete.

vagina, words pert. to: bulbus vestibuli; coitus; "colp-" words; cystocele; "elytr-" words; endocolpitis; enterocele; fistula; fornix; fourchette; gynatresia; hematocolpometra; hydrocolpos; hymen; leukorrhea; paravaginal; pronaus; rectocele; supravaginal; transvaginal; "vagin-" words.

vaginal (văj'ĭn-ăl) [L. *vagina,* sheath]. Pert. to the vagina or to any enveloping sheath.

vaginalectomy (văj"ĭn-ăl-ĕk'tō-mē) [" + Gr. *ektome,* excision]. Excision of the tunica vaginalis. SYN: *vaginectomy* (def. 1).

vaginal hysterectomy. Surgical removal of uterus through the vagina.

vaginalitis (văj-ĭn-ăl-ī'tĭs) [" + Gr. *itis,* inflammation]. Inflammation of tunica vaginalis testis.

vaginapexy (văj"ĭn-ă-pĕk'sē) [" + Gr. *pexis,* fixation]. Repair of a relaxed and prolapsed vagina. SYN: *colpopexy; vaginofixation.*

vaginate (văj'ĭn-āt) [L. *vaginatus*]. Forming or enclosed in a sheath.

vaginectomy (văj-ĭn-ĕk'tō-mē) [L. *vagina,* sheath, + Gr. *ektome,* excision]. 1. Resection of tunica vaginalis. 2. Excision of the vagina or a part of it.

vaginismus (văj"ĭn-ĭz'mŭs) [L.]. Painful spasm of vagina from contraction of the muscles surrounding the vagina. May interfere with coitus. May be due to extraordinary hyperesthesia of nerve supply to mucous membrane of vagina at or near site of the hymen, resulting in spasmodic constriction of sphincter vaginae muscle, preventing coitus. May also be due to local trauma, ulceration, lack of physiological lubrication, vaginitis, menopausal involution, congenital malformation, or neurotic aversion to coitus.

SYM: Extreme sensitiveness. Spasmodic tension of tissues surrounding the vagina on slightest touch.

TREATMENT: Correction of primary causative factors; education correcting misinformation and fear; psychotherapy.

v., deep. Vaginismus caused by spasm of the levator ani muscle.

v., mental. Vaginismus resulting from aversion to sexual intercourse.

v., posterior. Vaginismus due to contraction of the levator ani muscle.

vaginitis (văj-ĭn-ī'tĭs) [L. *vagina,* sheath, + Gr. *itis,* inflammation]. 1. Inflammation of a sheath. 2. Inflammation of the vagina. SYN: *colpitis; kysthitis.*

ETIOL: May be caused by microorganisms such as gonococci, chlamydia, staphylococci, streptococci, spirochetes; chemical irritation from use of strong chemicals in douching; fungus infection (candidiasis) caused by Candida albicans; protozoan infection (Trichomonas vaginalis); irritation from foreign bodies (pessaries); vitamin deficiency as in pellagra; conditions involving vulva and surrounding area, as uncleanliness or intestinal parasites.

SYM: Free purulent vaginal discharge, sometimes malodorous and occasionally stained with blood. There is irritation and itching of the vulvae and perineum, increased frequency of micturition, and smarting pain on the passage of urine. The vaginal mucous membrane is reddened and there may be superficial ulceration.

TREATMENT: Specific therapy as indicated. Improve perineal hygiene by instructing in proper method of cleaning anus after a bowel movement, proper use of menstrual protection materials, and necessity of drying vulvae following urination. Douching is not essential to the maintenance of vaginal health or cleanliness.

v. adhaesiva. Inflammation of the vagina causing adhesions between its walls.

v., atrophic. Natural or artificial vaginitis following the menopause. SYN: *v., postmenopausal; v., senile.*

v., diphtheritic. Vaginitis with membranous exudate caused by infection with Corynebacterium diphtheriae.

v., emphysematous. Vaginitis with gas-bubble formation in connective tissues.

v., Gardnerella vaginalis. SEE: *Gardnerella vaginalis vaginitis.*

v., granular. Vaginitis with cellular infiltration and enlargement of papillae.

v., nonspecific. In the past, a term used to describe virtually all cases of vaginitis in which no specific etiological agent could be identified. It is now known that the majority of cases are caused by either Gardnerella vaginalis or Trichomonas vaginalis organisms.

DIAG: A fresh specimen diluted with normal saline will upon microscopic examination reveal Trichomonas organisms; if short motile rods are seen to cover vaginal epithelial cells (so-called "clue" cells), then Gardnerella organisms are the cause. The vaginal aspirate is usually acid and will when mixed with a 10% potassium hydroxide solution emit a characteristic offensive (fishy) odor.

TREATMENT: For Trichomonas use metronidazole; for Gardnerella tetracycline is used. If both are present, use both drugs simultaneously.

v., postmenopausal. V., atrophic.

v., senile. V., atrophic.

v. testis. Inflammation of the tunica vaginalis of the testis.

v., Trichomonas vaginalis. Vaginitis associated with, or caused by, infection by Trichomonas vaginalis, a flagellate protozoon. T. vaginalis may be present in the vagina without causing disease in the host. Because the causative organism may be spread by direct contact during sexual intercourse, T. vaginalis vaginitis is classified as a sexually transmitted disease.

vaginoabdominal (văj″ĭn-ō-ăb-dŏm′ĭn-ăl) [L. *vagina,* sheath, + *abdominalis,* abdominal]. Rel. to the vagina and abdomen.

vaginocele (văj′ĭn-ō-sēl) [″ + Gr. *kele,* hernia]. Vaginal hernia. SYN: *colpocele.*

vaginodynia (văj″ĭn-ō-dĭn′ē-ă) [″ + Gr. *odyne,* pain]. Pain in the vagina.

vaginofixation (văj″ĭn-ō-fĭks-ā′shŭn) [″ + *fixatio,* a fixing]. 1. Process of rendering the vagina immovable. 2. Attachment of uterus to vaginal peritoneum.

vaginogenic (văj″ĭn-ō-jĕn′ĭk) [″ + Gr. *gennan,* to produce]. Developed from or originating in the vagina.

vaginography (văj-ĭn-ŏg′ră-fē) [″ + Gr. *graphein,* to write]. Roentgenography of the vagina.

vaginolabial (văj′ĭn-ō-lā′bē-ăl) [″ + *labium,* lip]. Rel. to the vagina and the labia. SYN: *vaginovulvar; vulvovaginal.*

vaginometer (văj-ĭn-ŏm′ĕ-tĕr) [″ + Gr. *metron,* measure]. Device for measuring the length and expansion of the vagina.

vaginomycosis (văj″ĭn-ō-mī-kō′sĭs) [″ + Gr. *mykes,* fungus, + *osis,* condition]. A fungus infection (mycosis) of the vagina.

vaginopathy (văj″ĭ-nŏp′ă-thē) [″ + Gr. *pathos,* disease]. Any disease of the vagina.

vaginoperineal (văj″ĭn-ō-pĕr-ĭ-nē′ăl) [″ + Gr. *perinaion,* perineum]. Rel. to the vagina and perineum.

vaginoperineorrhaphy (văj″ĭn-ō-pĕr″ĭ-nē-or′ăf-ē) [″ + ″ + *rhaphe,* a sewing]. Repair of a laceration involving both the perineum and vagina. SYN: *colpoperineorrhaphy.*

vaginoperineotomy (văj″ĭn-ō-pĕr″ĭn-ē-ŏt′ō-mē) [″ + ″ + *tome,* incision]. Surgical incision of the vagina and perineum. Usually done in order to facilitate childbirth.

vaginoperitoneal (văj″ĭn-ō-pĕr″ĭ-tō-nē′ăl). Rel. to the vagina and peritoneum.

vaginopexy (vă-jī′nō-pĕk″sē) [″ + Gr. *pexis,* fixation]. Fixation of the vagina. SYN: *colpopexy.*

vaginoplasty (vă-jī′nō-plăs″tē) [″ + Gr. *plassein,* to form]. Plastic surgery on the vagina.

vaginoscope (văj′ĭn-ō-skōp) [″ + Gr. *skopein,* to examine]. Instrument for inspection of the vagina. May be a speculum or an optical instrument.

vaginoscopy (vă″jĭn-ŏs′kō-pē). Visual examination of the vagina.

vaginotome (văj-ĭ′nō-tōm) [″ + Gr. *tome,* incision]. An instrument for making an incision in the vaginal walls.

vaginotomy (văj″ĭ-nŏt′ō-mē) [″ + Gr. *tome,* incision]. Incision of the vagina.

vaginovesical (văj″ĭ-nō-vĕs′ĭ-kăl) [″ + *vesica,* bladder]. Rel. to the vagina and bladder. SYN: *vesicovaginal.*

vaginovulvar (văj″ĭn-ō-vŭl′văr) [″ + *vulva,* a covering]. Pert. to the vulva and vagina. SYN: *vaginolabial; vulvovaginal.*

vagitis (vă-jī′tĭs) [L. *vagus,* wandering, + Gr. *itis,* inflammation]. Inflammation of the vagal nerve.

vagitus (vă-jī′tŭs) [L. *vagire,* to squall]. First cry of newly born infant.

v. uterinus. Crying of the fetus before birth while still in the uterus.

v. vaginalis. Cry of an infant with head still in the vagina.

vagolysis (vā-gŏl′ĭ-sĭs) [L. *vagus,* wandering,

+ Gr. *lysis,* dissolution]. Surgical destruction of the vagus nerve.

vagolytic (vā″gō-lĭt′ĭk). 1. Concerning vagolysis. 2. An agent, surgical or chemical, that prevents function of the vagus nerve.

vagomimetic (vā″gō-mĭ-mĕt′ĭk) [″ + Gr. *mimetikos,* imitating]. Resembling action caused by stimulation of the vagus nerve.

vagosympathetic (vā″gō-sĭm-pă-thĕt′ĭk) [″ + Gr. *sympathetikos,* suffering with]. The cervical sympathetic and the vagus nerves considered together.

vagotomy (vā-gŏt′ō-mē) [″ + Gr. *tome,* incision]. Section of the vagus nerve.

v., medical. Administration of drugs to prevent function of the vagus nerve.

vagotonia (vā″gō-tō′nē-ă) [″ + Gr. *tonos,* tension]. Hyperirritability of the parasympathetic nervous system. SEE: *sympatheticotonia.*

vagotonic (vā″gō-tŏn′ĭk). Pert. to vagotonia.

vagotropic (vā″gō-trŏp′ĭk) [″ + Gr. *tropos,* a turning]. Acting upon the vagus nerve.

vagotropism (vā-gŏt′rō-pĭzm) [″ + ″ + *-ismos,* condition]. Affinity for the vagus nerve, as a drug.

vagovagal (vā″gō-vā′găl). Reflex activity mediated entirely through the vagus nerve, i.e., via efferent and afferent impulses transmitted through the vagus nerve.

vagrant (vā′grănt) [L. *vagrans*]. Wandering from place to place without a fixed home.

vagus (vā′gŭs) [L., wandering]. (pl. *vagi*) The pneumogastric or 10th cranial nerve. It is a mixed nerve, having motor and sensory functions and a wider distribution than any of the other cranial nerves. SEE: illus.; *cranial nerves.*

vagus pulse. Decreased heart rate due to the slowing action of stimuli from the vagus

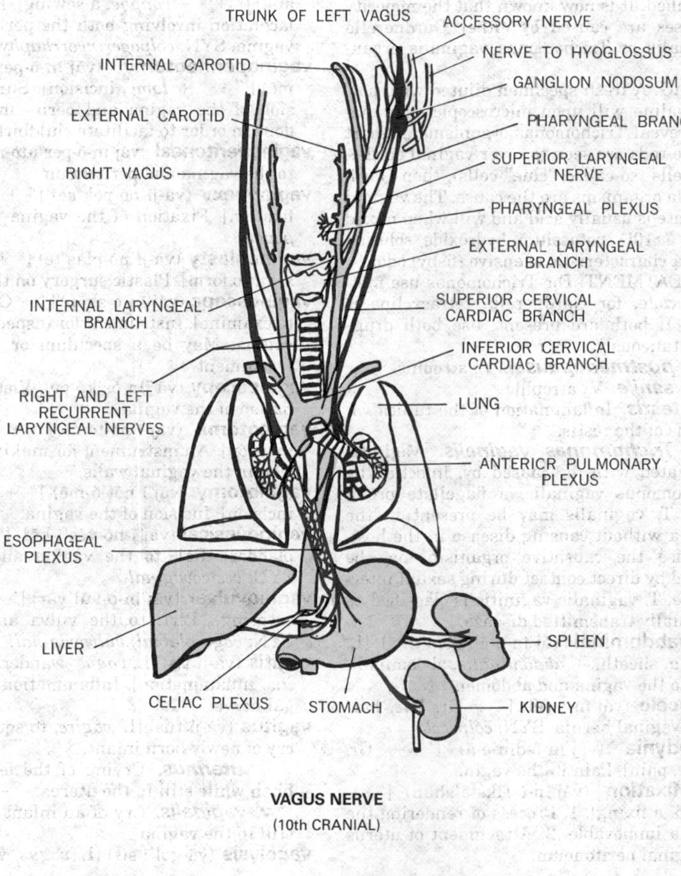

VAGUS NERVE
(10th CRANIAL)

nerve. SEE: *vagotomy; vagotonia.*

vagusstoff (vā′gŭs-stŏf) [″ + Ger. *Stoff,* substance]. Acetylcholine.

Valadol. Trade name for acetaminophen, USP.

valence, valency (vā′lĕns, -lĕn-sē) [L. *valens,* powerful]. 1. Property of an atom or group of atoms causing them to combine in definite proportion with other atoms or groups of atoms. Valency may be as high as 8 and is determined by the number of electrons in the outer orbit of the atom. 2. Degree of the combining power or replacing power of an atom or group of atoms, the hydrogen atom being the unit of comparison. The number indicates how many atoms of hydrogen can unite with one atom of another element.

Valentin's ganglion (văl′ĕn-tēnz). [Gabriel Gustav Valentin, Ger. physician, 1810–1883] A small ganglion at junction of the middle and posterior branches of the superior dental plexus.

valethamate bromide (văl-ĕth′ă-māt). An anticonvulsant drug.

valetudinarian (văl″ē-tū″dĭn-ā′rē-ăn) [L., *valetudinarius*]. Chronically ill; an invalid.

valgus (văl′gŭs) [L., bowlegged]. A term denoting position, meaning bent outward or twisted, applied esp. to deformities in which a part is bent outward and away from the midline of the body, as talipes valgus, q.v., or hallux valgus, q.v.

validity (vă-lĭd′ĭ-tē). 1. The degree to which data or results of a study are correct or true. 2. The extent to which a situation as observed reflects the true situation.

valine (văl′ēn, vā′lēn). $C_5H_{11}NO_2$, an amino acid derived from digestion of proteins. It is essential for normal growth in infants and for nitrogen balance in adults.

valinemia (văl″ĭ-nē′mē-ă). Increased valine in the blood.

Valisone. Trade name for betamethasone valerate.

Valium. Trade name for diazepam, USP.

vallate (văl′āt) [L. *vallatus,* walled]. Having a rim around a depression.

vallate papilla. A circumvallate papilla; one of a group of papillae forming a V-shaped row on posterior dorsal surface of tongue.

vallecula (văl-lĕk′ū-lă) [L., a depression]. [NA] A depression or crevice.

v. cerebelli. [NA] A deep fissure on inferior surface of the cerebellum. SYN: *valley of cerebellum.*

v. epiglottica. [NA] Depression lying lateral to the median epiglottic fold and separating it from the pharyngoepiglottic fold.

v. ovata. A depression in the liver in which rests the gallbladder.

v. sylvii. A depression marking beginning of the fissure of Sylvius.

v. unguis. Fold of skin in which the proximal and lateral edges of the nails are embedded.

Valleix's points (văl-lāz′). [François L. I. Valleix, Fr. physician, 1807–1855] In neuralgia, distinct painful points along the course of the affected nerve.

valley fever. Coccidioidomycosis, q.v.

valley of cerebellum. Hollow on inferior surface of cerebellum. SYN: *vallecula cerebelli* [NA].

vallis (văl′ĭs) [L., valley]. Vallecula cerebelli.

vallum unguis (văl′ŭm ŭng′gwĭs). [NA] Fold of skin overlapping the nail.

Valmid. Trade name for ethinamate.

Valpin. Trade name for anisotropine methylbromide.

Valsalva's maneuver (văl-săl′văz). [Antonio Maria Valsalva, It. anatomist, 1666–1723] Attempt to forcibly exhale with the glottis, nose, and mouth closed. If the eustachian tubes are not obstructed, the pressure on the tympanic membranes will be increased. Maneuver can also be done with just the glottis closed, but only intrathoracic pressure will be increased. This causes increased intrathoracic pressure, slowing of the pulse, decreased return of blood to the heart, and increased venous pressure.

Valsalva's sinuses. Three dilatations in wall of the aorta behind the flaps of the three aortic semilunar valves.

value (văl′ū) [ME. from L. *valere,* to be of value]. 1. The amount of a specific substance or the magnitude of an entity. 2. Something that is cherished or held dear.

valva (văl′vă) [sing. of L. *valvae,* folding door]. Valve.

valvate (văl′vāt) [L. *valva,* valve]. Pert. to or provided with valves. SYN: *valvular.*

valve (vălv) [L. *valva,* a fold]. Any one of various membranous structures in a hollow organ or passage that temporarily closes in order to permit flow of fluid in one direction only.

v., aortic. Valve between the left ventricle and the ascending aorta. Composed of 3 segments (semilunar cusps). The aortic valve prevents regurgitation at the entrance of the aorta to the heart.

v., atrioventricular, left. The biscuspid or mitral valve of the heart.

v., atrioventricular, right. The tricuspid valve of the heart.

v., bicuspid. Valve that closes the orifice between the left cardiac atrium and the left ventricle. SYN: *v., mitral.*

v., cardiac. The four valves that control the flow of blood into, through, and out of the heart. In order of the entry of the venous blood into the right atrium, they are: right atrioventricular, pulmonary, left atrioventricular, and aortic.

v., coronary. The coronary sinus valve at the entrance of the coronary sinus into the right atrium.

v., Houston's. Mucosal folds of the rectum. SYN: *plicae transversales recti.*

v., ileocecal. Valve between the ileum and large intestine that prevents regurgitation of intestinal contents. It is composed of two membranous folds. SYN: *v. of Varolius; valvula coli.*

v., mitral. V., bicuspid.

v. of Varolius. V., ileocecal.

v., pulmonary. Valve composed of three cusps, separating the pulmonary artery and right ventricle.

v., pyloric. Prominent circular membranous fold at pyloric orifice of the stomach.

v., semilunar. Valve between heart and the aorta and valve between the heart and the pulmonary artery.

v., thebesian. V., coronary, q.v.

v., tricuspid. Valve between the right cardiac atrium and right ventricle.

valvotomy (văl-vŏt'ō-mē) [" + Gr. *tome,* incision]. Incision into a valve.

valvula (văl'vū-lă) [L., a tiny fold]. (pl. *valvulae*) [NA] A valve, specifically a small valve.

v. bicuspidalis. Valve between the left cardiac atrium and left ventricle. SYN: *valve, bicuspid.*

v. coli. Valve between ileum and large intestine. SYN: *valve, ileocecal.*

v. pylori. Prominent mucosal fold at pyloric entrance of the stomach. SYN: *valve, pyloric.*

v. semilunaris. [NA] Valve separating heart and aorta and heart and pulmonary artery. SYN: *valve, semilunar.*

v. tricuspidalis. Valve between the right atrium and right ventricle of the heart. SYN: *valve, tricuspid.*

valvulae (văl'vū-lē). Pl. of valvula.

v. conniventes. Circular membranous folds that project into the lumen of the small intestine; they do not disappear on distention of the bowel. They act by retarding passage of food along the bowel and provide a greater absorbing area. SYN: *plica circularis.*

valvular (văl'vū-lăr) [L. *valvula,* a small fold]. Rel. to or having a valve. SYN: *valvate.*

valvulitis (văl"vū-lī'tĭs) [" + Gr. *itis,* inflammation]. Inflammation of a valve, esp. a cardiac valve.

valvuloplasty (văl'vū-lō-plăs"tē). Plastic or restorative surgery on a valve, esp. a cardiac valve.

valvulotome (văl'vū-lō-tōm) [" + Gr. *tome,* incision]. An instrument for incising a valve.

valvulotomy (văl"vū-lŏt'ō-mē). Process of cutting through a valve, as a rectal fold that is too rigid. SYN: *valvotomy.*

vanadium (vă-nā'dē-ŭm) [*Vanadis,* a Scandinavian goddess]. SYMB: V. At. wt. 50.941; at. no. 23. A light gray metallic element.

vanadiumism (vă-nā'dē-ŭm-ĭzm). Toxicity due to chronic exposure to vanadium. The symptoms include bronchitis, pneumonitis, conjunctivitis, and anemia.

van Buren's disease (văn bū'rĕnz). [William Holme van Buren, U.S. surgeon, 1819–1883] Induration of the corpora cavernosa. SYN: *Peyronie's disease.*

Vanceril. Trade name for beclomethasone dipropionate.

Vancocin Hydrochloride. Trade name for vancomycin hydrochloride, USP.

vancomycin hydrochloride (văn'kō-mī"sĭn). USP. An antibacterial drug. Trade name is Vancocin Hydrochloride.

van den Bergh's test (văn"dĕn bŭrgz'). [A. A. Hymans van den Bergh, Dutch physician, 1869–1943] A test to detect the presence of bilirubin in blood serum or plasma.

van der Hoeve's syndrome. [J. van der Hoeve, Dutch ophthalmologist, 1878–1952] Conductive deafness due to otosclerosis-like changes in the temporal bone. Blue sclerae and osteogenesis imperfecta are also present.

van der Waals forces. [Johannes D. van der Waals, Dutch physicist, 1837–1923] The definite but weak forces of attraction between the nuclei of atoms of compounds. These forces do not exist on the basis of ionic attraction, hydrogen bonding, or sharing of electrons.

vanilla (vă-nĭl'ă) [Sp. *vainilla,* little sheath]. Any one of a group of tropical orchids. The cured seed pods of Vanilla planifolia contain an aromatic substance, also called vanilla, that is used as a flavoring substance.

vanillin. A crystalline compound found in vanilla pods or produced synthetically used for flavoring foods and in pharmaceuticals.

vanillism (vă-nĭl'ĭzm). Irritation of the skin, mucous membranes, and conjunctiva sometimes experienced by workers handling raw vanilla. It is caused by a mite.

vanillylmandelic acid. ABBR: VMA. 3-methoxy-4-hydroxymandelic acid. Approx. 90% of the catecholamines epinephrine and norepinephrine are metabolized to VMA and are secreted in the urine. Persons with pheochromocytoma produce excess amounts of catecholamines; thus VMA is present in their urine in increased amount.

van't Hoff's rule. [Jacobus Henricus van't Hoff, Dutch chemist, 1852–1911] The speed of chemical reactions is doubled, at least, for each 10° C. rise in temperature.

Vapo-Iso. Trade name for isoproterenol hydrochloride, USP.

vapor (vā'por) [L., steam]. 1. Gaseous state of any substance. 2. Medicinal substance for administration by inhalation.

vaporium (vā-pō′rē-ŭm) [L.]. Apparatus for applying hot, cold, or medicated vapors.

vaporization (vā″por-ī-zā′shŭn) [L. *vapor,* steam]. 1. The conversion of a liquid or solid into vapor. 2. Therapeutic use of a vapor.

vaporize (vā′por-īz). To change a material to a vapor form.

vaporizer (vā′por-ī″zer). Device for converting liquids into a vapor spray.

vaporous (vā′por-ŭs) [L. *vapor,* steam]. Consisting of, pert. to, or producing vapors.

vapotherapy (vā″pō-thĕr′ă-pē). Therapeutic use of vapors.

Vaquez's disease (vă-kāz′). [Louis Henri Vaquez, Fr. physician, 1860–1936] Polycythemia vera.

variability (văr″ē-ă-bĭl′ĭ-tē). Condition of being variable.

variable (vā′rē-ă-b'l) [L. *variare,* to change]. 1. Anything that is not constant but can and does change in different circumstances. In statistics, it is often possible to graph the relationship of one variable to another, e.g., the increase in height and weight in the growing child. 2. Changing form, or structure, behavior, or physiology.

variance (văr′ē-ăns) [L. *variare,* vary]. In statistics, the square of the standard deviation.

variant (văr′ē-ănt). That which is different from the characteristics of the other organisms or entities in a particular classification, esp. a disease, species, or physical appearance.

variate (vā′rē-āt). Variable.

variation (vā″rē-ā′shŭn). Differences between individuals of a certain species or class.

v., continuous. Variation in which the difference between successive groups or individuals is quite small.

v., meristic. Variation in number as opposed to kind.

varication (văr″ĭ-kā′shŭn). 1. Formation of a varix. 2. The condition of a varicosity.

variced. Concerning a varix.

varicella (văr″ĭ-sĕl′ă) [L., a tiny spot]. An acute, highly contagious viral disease characterized by an eruption that makes its appearance in successive crops, and passes through stages of macules, papules, vesicles, and crusts. SYN: *chickenpox.*

ETIOL: Varicella-zoster virus, which also is the causative agent of herpes zoster. May occur at any age, though far less common in adults than in children. Epidemics most frequent in winter and spring and in temperate zones. Approx. 75% of all children will contract varicella by age 15.

INCUBATION: From 2 to 3 weeks; usually 13 to 17 days.

SYM: There may be a slight elevation of temperature at onset, followed within 24 hr. by appearance of the eruption, after which time temperature usually rises still further. Eruption first appears on back and chest, crops continuing to make their appearance for a period of from 2 to 3 days on an average. Each crop requires about 36 hr. to pass through the several stages. Because of this, macules, papules, vesicles, and crusts may be found side by side in the same general locality. Lesions are superficial and rupture very easily. They have a tendency to be ovoid. On the chest their distribution is often particularly marked along the course of the intercostal nerves. Some, though possibly few, scars nearly always remain as evidence of a varicella attack. The extremities are relatively free as compared with the trunk.

COMPLICATIONS: Secondary infections due to scratching, which may result in abscess formation; at times development of erysipelas or even septicemia. Occasionally lesions in the vicinity of the larynx may cause edema of the glottis and threaten the life of the patient. Encephalitis is a rare complication. Varicella may be fatal in children taking adrenocortical steroids.

PREVENTION: Administration of varicella-zoster immune globulin (VZIG) within 72 hours of exposure will prevent clinical varicella in susceptible, normal children. The following conditions should alert one to the possible need for use of VZIG: immunocompromised children; newborns of mothers who develop varicella in the period 5 days before to 48 hours after delivery; postnatal exposure of newborn infants (esp. those who are premature) to varicella; normal adults who are susceptible to varicella and who have been exposed; pregnant women who have no history of having had varicella and who have had significant exposure. Use of VZIG in pregnant women will not prevent fetal infection or congenital varicella syndrome.

DIFF. DIAG: Confusion between this disease and smallpox is responsible for the chief importance given varicella. Impetigo, dermatitis herpetiformis, herpes zoster, and furunculosis may require consideration.

PROG: Always favorable except in a very severe type, which is described as varicella gangrenosa. In this variety, gangrene may develop about the site of the lesions.

TREATMENT: Isolation. Restrain the hands in the case of infants or young children in order that the lesions may not be scratched. Use of calamine lotion locally may alleviate irritation. Keep the skin, bedclothes, and sheets clean to help prevent skin infections. Also keep patient's fingernails well trimmed. The usual duration of the disease is from 2 to 3 weeks. Cases usually classed as contagious from 5 days prior to the skin eruption until not more than 6 days after the first crop of vesicles.

v. gangrenosa. Varicella in which necrosis occurs around the vesicles, resulting in gangrenous ulceration.

varicella-zoster immune globulin. ABBR: VZIG. An immune globulin obtained from the blood of normal persons found to have high antibody titers to varicella-zoster. For indications for its use, SEE: PREVENTION under *varicella*.

varicelliform (văr″ĭ-sĕl′ĭ-form). Resembling varicella.

varicelloid (văr″ĭ-sĕl′oyd) [″ + Gr. *eidos*, form]. Resembling varicella.

varices (văr′ĭ-sēz) [L.]. Pl. of varix.

variciform (văr-ĭs′ĭ-form) [L. *varix*, a twisted vein, + *forma*, shape]. Resembling a varix. SYN: *varicose*.

varicoblepharon (văr″ĭ-kō-blĕf′ă-rŏn) [″ + Gr. *blepharon*, eyelid]. Varicose tumor of the eyelid.

varicocele (văr′ĭ-kō-sēl) [″ + Gr. *kele*, hernia]. Enlargement of the veins of the spermatic cord (pampiniform plexus), commonly occurring on the left side in adolescent males; these seldom require treatment.

SYM: Vessels on affected side of scrotum are full, feeling like a bundle of worms, sometimes purplish in color. Dull ache along the cord. Slight dragging sensation in groin.

TREATMENT: Dragging sensation from exceptionally large varicocele may be relieved by a suspensory. Surgery is required for persistent symptomatic varicocele.

v., ovarian. Varicosity of veins of the ovarian or pampiniform plexus of the broad ligament.

v., utero-ovarian. Varicosity of the veins of the ovarian (pampiniform) plexus and uterine plexus of the broad ligament.

varicocelectomy (văr″ĭ-kō-sē-lĕk′tō-mē) [L. *varix*, twisted vein, + Gr. *kele*, hernia, + *ektome*, excision]. Excision of portion of scrotal sac with ligation of the dilated veins to relieve varicocele.

varicography (văr″ĭ-kŏg′ră-fē) [″ + Gr. *graphein*, to write]. Roentgenography of varicose veins.

varicoid (văr′ĭ-koyd) [″ + Gr. *eidos*, form]. Resembling a varix.

varicole (văr′ĭ-kōl). Varicocele.

varicomphalus (văr″ĭ-kŏm′fă-lŭs) [″ + Gr. *omphalos*, navel]. Varicose tumor of the navel.

varicophlebitis (văr″ĭ-kō-flē-bī′tĭs) [″ + Gr. *phleps*, vein, + *itis*, inflammation]. Phlebitis combined with varicose veins.

varicose (văr′ĭ-kōs) [L. *varicosus*]. Pert. to varices; distended, swollen, knotted veins.

varicose veins. Enlarged, twisted superficial veins. May occur in almost any part of the body but are most commonly observed in the lower extremity and in the esophagus.

ETIOL: Incompetent venous valves that may be acquired or congenital. The development of varicose veins is promoted and aggravated by pregnancy, obesity, and occupations that require prolonged standing. Esophageal varices are caused by portal hypertension that accompanies cirrhosis of the liver.

SYM: Pain in feet and ankles, swelling, ulcers on skin. Severe bleeding if a vein is injured.

F.A.: In hemorrhage, elevation of extremity and gentle but firm pressure over wound will stop bleeding. The use of a tourniquet is undesirable. Sterile dressing should be held in place with a firm bandage. Patient should not be permitted to walk for some time. The Sengstaken-Blakemore tube is used to control bleeding due to hemorrhage from esophageal varices. SEE: *tamponade, balloon*.

NURSING IMPLICATIONS: Teach the patient to avoid anything that impedes venous return, such as wearing garters and tight girdles, crossing the legs at the knees, and prolonged sitting. Apply support hose after the legs have been elevated for 10 to 15 minutes. Instruct the patient not to sit in a chair for longer than 1 hour at a time. Encourage ambulation for at least 5 minutes every hour. Elevate legs whenever possible, but no less than twice a day for 30 minutes each time. Instruct the patient to avoid prolonged standing. Teach the patient the signs of thrombophlebitis, a common complication of varicose veins; these are heat, local pain, and a positive Homan's sign, q.v. If surgery is performed, postoperatively apply elastic stockings and elevate the foot of the bed above the level of the heart. Encourage the overweight patient to lose weight.

TREATMENT: In general, consists of rest, elevation of extremity, and use of an external support. The use of elastic stockings is much preferred to elastic bandages. Unna's paste boots recommended for elderly or debilitated persons. Injection of sclerosing solutions may be utilized for small varicosities. High ligation and removal of vein by stripping may be necessary for major varicosities.

varicose ulcers. Ulcers that form as a result of varicose veins. When thrombophlebitis develops in varicose veins, this leads to venous stasis and eventually edema and ulcer formation.

NURSING IMPLICATIONS: Maintain patient on bedrest. Continuously apply warm, moist compresses to relieve discomfort and infection. Use aseptic technique when applying dressings.

varicosis (văr″ĭ-kō′sĭs) [L.]. Varicose condition

of veins.

varicosity (văr″ĭ-kŏs′ĭ-tē) [L. *varix,* twisted vein]. 1. Condition of being varicose. 2. A swollen, twisted vein. SYN: *varix.*

varicotomy (văr″ĭ-kŏt′ō-mē) [″ + Gr. *tome,* incision]. Excision of a varicose vein.

varicula (văr-ĭk′ū-lă) [L., a tiny dilated vein]. A small varix, esp. of the conjunctiva.

variety (vă-rī′ĕ-tē) [L. *varietas,* variety]. A term used in classifying individuals in a subpopulation of a species.

variola (vă-rī′ō-lă) [L., pustule]. An acute, contagious, systemic, viral disease characterized by a prodromal stage during which the constitutional symptoms usually are severe, followed by an eruption that passes through the successive stages of macules, papules, vesicles, pustules, and crusts. SYN: *smallpox.*

NOTE: This disease is considered to have been completely eradicated world-wide. Cultures of the virus are kept in only one or two research laboratories.

v. minor. Mild form of smallpox with sparse rash and low-grade fever.

variolar (văr-ī′ō-lăr) [L. *variola,* pustule]. Pert. to smallpox.

variolate (văr′ē-ō-lāt). 1. To vaccinate with smallpox virus. 2. Having lesions like those of smallpox.

variolation, variolization (văr″ē-ō-lā′shŭn, văr″ē-ō-lĭ-zā′shŭn) [L. *variola,* pustule]. Inoculation with smallpox.

variolic (văr″ē-ŏl′ĭk). Variolar.

varioliform (vă″rē-ŏl′ĭ-form). Resembling smallpox.

varioloid (văr′ē-ō-loyd) [″ + Gr. *eidos,* form]. 1. Resembling smallpox. 2. Pert. to varioloid. 3. A mild but contagious type of smallpox in those who have had smallpox or have been vaccinated.

variolous (vă-rī′ō-lŭs). Rel. to smallpox.

varix (vā′rĭks) [L., a twisted vein]. (pl. *varices*) 1. A tortuous dilatation of a vein. SEE: *varicose veins.* 2. Less commonly, dilatation of an artery or lymph vessel.

v., aneurysmal. A direct communication between an artery and a varicose vein without an intervening sac.

v., arterial. 1. A varicosity or dilation of an artery. 2. A connection between an artery and a vein as in an arteriovenous fistula.

v., chyle. A varix of a lymphatic vessel that conveys chyle.

v., esophageal. Varicosities of the veins of the esophagus. These are associated with increased portal vein pressure, usually secondary to cirrhosis of the liver.

v., lymphaticus. Dilatation of a lymphatic vessel.

v., turbinal. Permanent dilatation of veins of turbinate bodies.

varnish (văr′nĭsh). A solution of gums and resins in a solvent. When these are applied to a surface, the solvent evaporates and leaves a hard more-or-less flexible film. In dentistry, varnishes are used to protect sensitive tooth areas such as the pulp.

varolian (vă-rō′lē-ăn). [Costanzo Varolio, It. surgeon, 1543–1575] Rel. to the pons varolii.

varolian bend. Anterior extension of hindgut on its ventral surface in the fetus.

varus (vā′rŭs) [L.]. 1. Turned inward. 2. A condition in which a clubfooted person walks on outer border of the foot. SYN: *talipes varus.* SEE: *valgus.*

vas (văs) [L., vessel]. (pl. *vasa*) [NA] A vessel or duct.

v. aberrans. 1. A narrow tube varying in length from 1½ to 14 in. (3.8 to 35.6 cm.), occasionally found connected with the lower part of the canal of the epididymis or with the commencement of the vas deferens. 2. Vestige of the biliary ducts sometimes found in the liver.

v. afferens. [NA] An afferent vessel of a lymph node.

v. afferens glomeruli. [NA] The afferent arteriole that conveys blood to the glomerulus of a renal corpuscle.

v. capillare. [NA] A capillary blood vessel.

v. deferens. The excretory duct of the testis, the continuation of the canal of the epididymis. This slim, muscular tube approximately 18 in. (45.7 cm.) in length transports the sperm from each testis to the prostatic urethra. SYN: *ductus deferens* [NA]. SEE: *testis* for illus.

RS: ampullitis; cord; deferentitis; spermatic.

v. lymphaticum. [NA] One of the vessels carrying the lymph.

v. prominens. [NA] Blood vessel on the cochlea's accessory spiral ligament.

v. spirale. A large blood vessel beneath the tunnel of Corti in the basilar membrane.

vasa (vā′sā) [L. *vas,* vessel]. Pl. of vas.

v. afferentia. [NA] The lymphatic vessels entering a lymph node.

v. brevia. Branches of the splenic artery going to greater curvature of the stomach.

v. efferentia. 1. Lymphatics that leave a lymph node. 2. Excretory ducts of the testis to the head of the epididymis.

v. praevia. The blood vessels of the umbilical cord presenting before the fetus.

v. recta. 1. Tubules that become straight prior to entering the mediastinum testis. 2. Straight collecting tubules of the kidney.

v. vasorum. [NA] Tiny blood vessels which are distributed to the walls of the larger veins and arteries.

v. vorticosa. Stellate veins of the choroid, carrying blood to the superior ophthalmic vein.

Vasal. Trade name for papaverine hydrochloride.

vasal (vā'săl) [L. *vas,* vessel]. Rel. to a vas or vessel.

vasalgia (vă-săl'jē-ă). Pain in a vessel of any kind.

vascular (văs'kū-lăr) [L. *vasculum,* a small vessel]. Pert. to or composed of blood vessels.

vascularity (văs"kū-lăr'ĭ-tē). State of being vascular.

vascularization (văs"kū-lăr-ī-zā'shŭn) [L. *vasculum,* a small vessel]. Development of new blood vessels in a structure.

vascularize (văs'kū-lăr"īz) [L. *vasculum,* a small vessel]. To become vascular by development of new blood vessels.

vascular reflex. Constriction or dilation of vascular trunk or area resulting from mental or physical irritation.

vascular system. The heart, blood vessels, lymphatics, and their parts considered collectively. It includes the pulmonary and portal systems.

vascular tuft. One of the vascular processes on the chorion in the fetus at an early stage of development. SYN: *chorionic villi.*

vascular tumor. Tumor containing dilated blood vessels. SYN: *angioma; telangioma.*

vasculature (văs'kū-lă-tūr"). The arrangement of blood vessels in the body or any part of it, including their relationship and functions.

vasculitis (văs"kū-lī'tĭs) [" + *itis,* inflammation]. Inflammation of a blood or lymph vessel. SYN: *angiitis.*

vasculogenesis (văs"kū-lō-jĕn'ĕ-sĭs) [" + Gr. *genesis,* production]. Development of the vascular system.

vasculomotor (văs"kū-lō-mō'tor). Vasomotor.

vasculopathy (văs"kū-lŏp'ă-thē). Any disease of blood vessels.

vasculum (văs'kū-lŭm) [L.]. A tiny vessel.

vasectomy (văs-ĕk'tō-mē) [L. *vas,* vessel, + Gr. *ektome,* excision]. Removal of all or a segment of the vas deferens. Usually done bilaterally to produce sterility in the male.

NOTE: Persons who have had this surgical procedure ejaculate in a normal manner but the ejaculate does not contain sperm. There are no anatomical or physiological reasons for sterilization by this method to alter the sex drive or libido.

Vaseline. Trade name for petrolatum.

vasifactive (văs"ĭ-făk'tĭv) [" + *facere,* to make]. Forming new vessels. SYN: *vasofactive; vasoformative.*

vasiform (văs'ĭ-form) [" + *forma,* shape]. Resembling a tubular structure or vas.

vasitis (vă-sī'tĭs). Inflammation of the ductus deferens of the testicle.

vaso- [L. *vas*]. Combining form meaning a vessel, as a blood vessel.

vasoactive (văs"ō-ăk'tĭv). Affecting blood vessels.

vasoconstrictive (văs"ō-kŏn-strĭk'tĭv) [" + *constrictus,* bound]. Causing constriction of the blood vessels.

vasoconstriction (văs"ō-kŏn-strĭk'shŭn). Decrease in the caliber of blood vessels.

vasoconstrictor (văs"ō-kŏn-strĭk'tor) [" + *constrictor,* a binder]. 1. Causing constriction of blood vessels. 2. That which constricts or narrows the caliber of blood vessels, as a drug or a nerve.

vasodentin (văs"ō-dĕn'tĭn) [" + *dentinus,* pert. to a tooth]. Modified dentin provided with blood capillaries. Present in fishes but seldom seen in other animals.

vasodepression (văs"ō-dē-prĕsh'ŭn) [" + *depressio,* a pushing down]. Vasomotor depression or collapse.

vasodepressor (văs"ō-dē-prĕs'or) [" + *depressor,* that which pushes down]. 1. Having a depressing influence on the circulation, lowering blood pressure by dilatation of blood vessels. 2. An agent that decreases circulation.

Vasodilan. Trade name for isoxsuprine hydrochloride.

vasodilatation (văs"ō-dīl-ă-tā'shŭn) [" + *dilatare,* to widen]. Dilatation of blood vessels, esp. small arteries and arterioles.

v., antidromic. Vasodilatation resulting from stimulation of dorsal root of a spinal nerve.

v., reflex. Blood vessel dilation due to stimulation of its dilator nerves or inhibition of its constrictor substance or nerves. This can be done by stimulating the sensory reflex arc.

vasodilation (văs"ō-dī-lā'shŭn). Increase in the caliber of blood vessels.

vasodilative (văs"ō-dī'lā-tĭv). Causing dilation of the blood vessels.

vasodilator (văs"ō-dī-lā'tor) [" + *dilatare,* to widen]. 1. Causing relaxation of the blood vessels. 2. A nerve or drug that dilates the blood vessels.

vasoepididymostomy (văs"ō-ĕp"ĭ-dĭd-ĭ-mŏs'tō-mē) [" + Gr. *epi,* upon, + *didymos,* testicle, + *stoma,* passage]. Formation of a passage between the vas deferens and the epididymis.

vasofactive (văs"ō-făk'tĭv) [" + *facere,* to make]. Forming new blood vessels. SYN: *vasifactive; vasoformative.*

vasoformative (văs"ō-for'mă-tĭv) [" + *formare,* to form]. Forming new blood vessels. SYN: *vasifactive; vasofactive.*

vasoganglion (văs"ō-găng'glē-ŏn). Any mass of blood vessels.

vasography (văs-ŏg'ră-fē) [" + Gr. *graphein,*

to write]. Roentgenography of the blood vessels.

vasohypertonic (văs″ō-hī″pĕr-tŏn′ĭk) [″ + Gr. *hyper,* over, + *tonikos,* pert. to tension]. Causing or that which causes constriction of blood vessels. SYN: *vasoconstrictor.*

vasohypotonic (văs″ō-hī″pō-tŏn′ĭk) [″ + Gr. *hypo,* under, + *tonikos,* pert. to tension]. Relaxing or that which relaxes blood vessels. SYN: *vasodilator.*

vasoinhibitor (văs″ō-ĭn-hĭb′ĭ-tor) [″ + *inhibere,* to restrain]. An agent that decreases the action of vasomotor nerves.

vasoinhibitory (văs″ō-ĭn-hĭb′ĭ-tor-ē). Restricting vasomotor activity.

vasoligation (văs″ō-lī-gā′shŭn) [″ + *ligare,* to bind]. Ligation of a vessel, specifically the vas deferens.

vasomotion (văs″ō-mō′shŭn) [″ + *motio,* movement]. Change in caliber of a blood vessel.

vasomotor (văs″ō-mō′tor) [″ + *motor,* a mover]. Pert. to the nerves having muscular control of the blood vessel walls. The circularly arranged fibers of the muscles of arteries and veins can contract or relax; the affected region is accordingly either blanched or flushed. The former effect can commonly be produced by stimulating sympathetic fibers, and is consequently called vasoconstrictor; certain other nerves on stimulation cause vasodilation, examples being the nervus chorda tympani and the nervi erigentes. A vasomotor reflex is one in which the stimulus, such as a horrifying sight, results in a change in vasomotor tone, e.g., pallor. SYN: *angiokinetic.* SEE: *vasoconstrictor; vasodilator.*

vasomotor epilepsy. Epilepsy with vasomotor changes in the skin.

vasomotor spasm. Spasm of smaller arteries.

vasomotory (văs″ō-mō′tor-ē). Controlling changes in the size of the blood vessels. SYN: *vasomotor.*

vasoneuropathy (văs″ō-nū-rŏp′ă-thē). Disease due to the combined effect of vascular and neurologic effects.

vasoneurosis (văs″ō-nū-rō′sĭs) [L. *vas,* vessel, + Gr. *neuron,* nerve, + *osis,* condition]. A neurosis affecting blood vessels; a disorder of the vasomotor system. SEE: *angioneurosis.*

vaso-orchidostomy (văs″ō-or″kĭd-ŏs′tō-mē) [″ + Gr. *orchis,* testicle, + *stoma,* mouth]. Surgical connection of the epididymis to the severed end of the vas deferens.

vasoparesis (văs″ō-păr-ē′sĭs) [″ + Gr. *paresis,* relaxation]. Partial paralysis or weakness of the vasomotor nerves.

vasopressin (văs″ō-prĕs′ĭn). A hormone formed in supraoptic and paraventricular nuclei of hypothalamus and transported to posterior lobe of hypophysis through the hypothalamo-hypophyseal tract. It has an antidiuretic, and a pressor effect that elevates blood pressure. This drug should not be used as an agent to increase blood pressure because of its effect of reducing coronary artery blood flow. Trade name is Pitressin. SYN: *antidiuretic hormone* (ABBR: ADH). SEE: *oxytocin.*

vasopressin injection. USP. A sterile solution, in a suitable diluent, of material containing the polypeptide hormone having the properties of causing the contraction of vascular and other smooth muscle, and of diuresis. Trade name is Pitressin.

vasopressor (văs″ō-prĕs′or). 1. Causing contraction of the muscles of capillaries and arteries. This increases resistance to the flow of blood and thus elevates blood pressure. 2. Agents that stimulate contraction of muscles of capillaries and arteries.

vasopuncture (văs′ō-pŭnk″chūr) [″ + *punctura,* a piercing]. Puncture of the vas deferens.

vasoreflex (văs″ō-rē′flĕx). A reflex that alters the caliber of blood vessels.

vasorelaxation (văs″ō-rē-lăks-ā′shŭn) [″ + *relaxare,* to loosen]. Lessening of vascular pressure.

vasorrhaphy (văs-or′ă-fē) [″ + Gr. *rhaphe,* a seam]. Surgical suture of the vas deferens.

vasosection (văs″ō-sĕk′shŭn) [″ + *sectio,* a cutting]. Surgical division of the vasa deferentia.

vasosensory (văs″ō-sĕn′sō-rē) [″ + *sensorius,* pert. to sensation]. Rel. to sensation in the blood vessels.

vasospasm (văs′ō-spăzm) [″ + Gr. *spasmos,* a spasm]. Spasm of a blood vessel. SYN: *angiohypotonia; angiospasm; vasoconstriction.*

vasospastic (văs″ō-spăs′tĭk). Concerning or characterized by vasospasm.

vasostimulant (văs″ō-stĭm′ū-lănt) [L. *vas,* vessel, + *stimulare,* to goad]. Exciting vasomotor action.

vasostomy (vă-sŏs′tō-mē) [″ + Gr. *stoma,* mouth]. Surgical procedure of making an opening into the vas deferens.

vasotomy (văs-ŏt′ō-mē) [″ + Gr. *tome,* incision]. Incision of the vas deferens.

vasotonia (văs″ō-tō′nē-ă) [″ + Gr. *tonos,* tone]. The tone of blood vessels.

vasotonic (văs″ō-tŏn′ĭk) [″ + Gr. *tonikos,* pert. to tone]. 1. Pert. to the tone of a vessel. 2. Causing vasotonia.

vasotribe (văs′ō-trīb) [″ + Gr. *tribein,* to crush]. Pressure forceps used for controlling hemorrhages. SYN: *angiotribe.*

vasotripsy (văs′ō-trĭp″sē) [″ + Gr. *tripsis,* a crushing]. Arrest of hemorrhages with a strong forceps by crushing an artery. SYN: *angiotripsy.*

vasotrophic (văs″ō-trŏf′ĭk) [″ + Gr. *trophe,*

nourishment]. Concerned with the nutrition of blood vessels.

vasotropic (văs″ō-trŏp′ĭk). Affecting blood vessels.

vasovagal (văs″ō-vā′găl). Concerning the action of stimuli from the vagus nerve on blood vessels.

vasovagal syncope. Sudden faint due to hypotension induced by the response of the nervous system to abrupt emotional stress, pain, or trauma. This is accompanied by pallor, sweating, hyperventilation, and bradycardia. Vagal stimulation causes this reaction. Treatment consists of having the patient lie flat and being certain there is a clear airway; treat the underlying condition if indicated. Vomiting does not usually occur, but if it does, position patient to prevent aspiration of vomitus.

vasovasostomy (văs″ō-vă-sŏs′tō-mē) [″ + *vas,* vessel, + *stoma,* passage]. Rejoining of the previously severed ductus deferens of the testicle.

vasovesiculectomy (văs″o-vē-sĭk″ū-lĕk′tō-mē) [″ + *vesicula,* tiny sac, + Gr. *ektome,* excision]. Excision of the vas deferens and seminal vesicles.

vasovesiculitis (văs″ō-vē-sĭk″ū-lī′tĭs) [″ + *vesicula,* tiny sac, + Gr. *itis,* inflammation]. Inflammation of the vas deferens and seminal vesicles.

Vasoxyl. Trade name for methoxamine hydrochloride, USP.

vastus (văs′tŭs) [L., vast]. 1. Great, large, extensive. 2. One of three muscles of the thigh. SEE: *Muscles* in *Appendix.*

Vater's ampulla (fă′tĕrz). [Abraham Vater, Ger. anatomist, 1684–1751] Former name for papilla of Vater.

Vater's corpuscles. Ovoid end-organs of nerves supplying the skin. SYN: *pacinian corpuscles.*

Vater's papilla. The duodenal end of the drainage systems of the pancreatic and common bile ducts. Formerly called ampulla of Vater.

vault (vawlt). A part or structure resembling a dome or arched roof.

VC. *vital capacity.*

V-Cillin. Trade name for penicillin V, USP.

V-Cillin K. Trade name for penicillin V potassium, USP.

V.D. *venereal disease.*

V.D.H. *valvular disease of the heart.*

VDRL. *Venereal Disease Research Laboratories.*

vectis (vĕk′tĭs) [L., pole]. A curved lever for making traction on presenting part of fetus.

vection (vĕk′shŭn) [L. *vectio,* a carrying]. Transfer of disease agents by a vector from the sick to the well.

vector (vĕk′tor) [L., a carrier]. 1. Any force or influence that is a quantity completely specified by magnitude, direction, and sense, which can be represented by a straight line of appropriate length and direction. 2. A carrier, usually an arthropod or insect that transmits the causative organisms of disease from infected to noninfected individuals, esp. one in which the organism goes through one or more stages in its life cycle.

v., biological. An animal vector wherein the disease-causing organism multiplies or develops prior to becoming infective for a susceptible individual.

v., mechanical. A vector in or upon which growth and development of the infective agent do not occur.

vectorcardiogram (vĕk″tor-kăr′dē-ō-grăm). [″ + Gr. *kardia,* heart, + *gramma,* a mark]. A graphic record of the direction and magnitude of the electrical forces of the heart's action by means of a continuous series of vector loops. Analysis of the configuration of these loops permits certain statements to be made about the state of health or diseased condition of the myocardium. At any moment the electrical activity of the heart can be represented as an electrical vector with a specific direction and magnitude. This is called the instantaneous cardiac vector. A series of these vectors may be established for the entire cardiac cycle. By joining the tips of these vectors with a continuous line, the vectorcardiogram loop is formed. The configuration so obtained may be projected on the frontal plane or viewed as a three-dimensional loop. Three vectorcardiogram loops are formed during each cardiac cycle—one for the electrical activity of the atrium; one for ventricular depolarization; one for ventricular repolarization.

vectorcardiography. Analysis of the direction and magnitude of the electrical forces of the heart's action by a continuous series of loops (vectors) that represent the cardiac cycle.

vectorial (vĕk-tō′rē-ăl) [L. *vector,* a carrier]. Rel. to a vector.

Vectrin. Trade name for minocycline hydrochloride, USP.

VEE. *Venezuelan equine encephalitis.*

vegan (vĕj′ăn). An extreme vegetarian who omits all animal protein from the diet.

veganism (vĕj′ă-nĭzm). Strict vegetarianism in which one eats no food, including milk or cheese products, from an animal source.

vegetable (vĕj′ĕ-tă-bl). 1. Pert. to, of the nature of, or derived from plants. 2. A herbaceous plant, esp. one cultivated for food. 3. The edible part or parts of plants that are used as food, including the leaves, stems, seeds and seed pods, flowers, roots, tubers, and fruits.

Vegetables are important sources of minerals and vitamins; provide bulk, which stimulates intestinal motility; and are sources of energy. Caloric value is indirectly proportional to water content. Vegetables in general are valuable for their mineral content and for their cellulose. Copper is estimated at 1.2 mg./kg. for leafy vegetables, and 0.7 mg./kg. for nonleafy ones. They are deficient in fat, which can be corrected by adding milk, cream, or butter in their preparation.

Plant and vegetable proteins are nutritionally inferior to those from animal sources but by combining certain plants in the diet, a completely adequate and balanced mixture of essential amino acids can be provided. Corn is low in lysine but has adequate amounts of tryptophan; beans are adequate in lysine but low in tryptophan. Thus neither of these two foods contains adequate amounts of essential amino acids, but eaten in combination, they are adequate. Rice and soybeans eaten together provide adequate essential amino acids even though each is lacking in essential amino acids. SEE: *incaparina*.

All starches in vegetables must be changed to sugars before they can be absorbed. Dry heat changes starch to dextrin; heat and acid or a ferment change dextrin to dextrose. In germinating grain, starch is changed to dextrin and dextrose. Dextrose in fermentation turns to alcohol and carbon dioxide.

vegetal (vĕj'ĕ-tăl). 1. Pertaining to plants. 2. Tropic or nutritional, esp. with reference to that part of an ovum which contains the yolk. SEE: *pole, vegetal*.

vegetarian (vĕj-ĕ-tā'rē-ăn) [from *vegetable*, coined 1847 by Vegetarian Society]. One whose diet consists mainly of vegetables, sometimes also excluding dairy products.

vegetarianism (vĕj-ĕ-tā'rē-ăn-ĭzm) [" + Gr. *-ismos*, condition]. The belief and practice of eating vegetables and fruits only; may or may not exclude dairy products.

vegetate (vĕj'ĕ-tāt) [LL. *vegetare*, to grow]. 1. To grow luxuriantly with the production of fleshy or warty outgrowths such as a polyp. 2. To lead a passive existence either mentally or physically; to do little more than eat and maintain autonomic body functions.

vegetation (vĕj-ĕ-tā'shŭn). A morbid luxurious outgrowth on any part, esp. wartlike projections made up of collections of fibrin in which are enmeshed white and red blood cells; sometimes seen on denuded areas of the endocardium covering the valves of the heart.

v., adenoid. Fungus-like masses of lymphoid tissue in nasopharynx.

vegetative (vĕj'ĕ-tā"tĭv). 1. Having the power to grow, as plants. 2. Functioning involuntarily. 3. Quiescent, passive, noting a stage of development.

vegetoanimal (vĕj"ĕ-tō-ăn'ĭ-măl). Concerning plants and animals.

vehicle (vē'ĭ-kl) [L. *vehiculum*, that which carries]. A substance, usually inactive therapeutically, used in a medicinal preparation as the agent for carrying the active ingredient.

Ex.: a syrup in liquid preparations.

veil (vāl) [L. *velum*, a covering]. 1. Any veil-like structure. 2. A piece of the amniotic sac occasionally covering the face of a newborn infant. SYN: *caul*. 3. Slight alteration in the voice in order to disguise it.

vein (vān) [L. *vena*, vein]. Vessel carrying dark red (unaerated) blood to the heart, except for the pulmonary vein, which carries oxygenated blood. Veins have three coats: inner, middle, and outer. They differ from arteries in their larger capacity and greater number; also in their thinner walls, larger and more frequent anastomoses, and presence of valves that prevent backward circulation. They consist of two sets, superficial or subcutaneous, and the deep veins, with frequent communications between the two. The former do not usually accompany an artery, as do the latter. The systemic veins consist of three groups—those entering the heart through the superior vena cava, those through the inferior vena cava, and those through the coronary sinus. Blood from the capillary plexuses enters the right atrium of the heart. SEE: *circulation; Veins* in *Appendix; vena*.

vein, words pert. to: basilic vein; cephalic vein; innominate veins; intravenous; jugular veins; phlebectomy; phlebitis; phlebogram; phlebotomy; phlegmasia alba dolens; portal vein; thrombophlebitis; thrombus; "varic-" words; varix; vascular; vasoconstrictor; vasodilator; vasomotor; vasoparesis; vena; vena cava; venesection; venosity; venotomy; venous; venule.

velamen (vē-lā'mĕn) [L., veil]. (pl. *velamina*) Any covering membrane.

v. nativum. The skin covering the body.

v. vulvae. Abnormal elongation of the nymphae.

velamentous (vĕl"ă-mĕn'tŭs). Expanding like a veil, or sheet.

velamentum (vĕl"ă-mĕn'tŭm) [L., a cover]. (pl. *velamenta*) A membranous covering.

velar (vē'lăr) [L. *velum*, a veil]. Pert. to a velum or veil-like structure.

Velban. Trade name for vinblastine sulfate, USP.

Velcro. Trade name for fabric tape closures frequently used in orthotic fabrication and in adapting garments and devices for use by disabled persons with limited upper extremity function.

veliform (vĕl'ĭ-form). Velamentous.

vellication (vĕl-ĭk-ā′shŭn) [L. *vellicare,* to twitch]. Spasmodic twitching of muscular fibers.

vellus (vĕl′ŭs) [L., fleece]. The fine hair present on the body after the lanugo hair of the newborn is gone.

velopharyngeal (vĕl″ō-fă-rĭn′jē-ăl) [L. *velum,* veil, + Gr. *pharynx,* pharynx]. Concerning the soft palate and the pharynx.

velosynthesis (vĕl″ō-sĭn′thĕs-ĭs) [″ + Gr. *synthesis,* a placing together]. Suture of a cleft palate, particularly the soft palate. SYN: *staphylorrhaphy.*

Velpeau's bandage (vĕl-pōz′). [Alfred Velpeau, Fr. surgeon, 1795–1867] A special immobilizing roller bandage that incorporates the shoulder, forearm and arm. SEE: *bandage* for illus.

Velpeau's deformity. Deformity seen in Colles' fracture, q.v., in which lower fragment is displaced backward.

velum (vē′lŭm) [L., veil]. [NA] Any veil-like structure.

v. palatinum. [NA] The soft palate.

vena (vē′nă) [L.]. (pl. *venae*) A vein. SEE: *Veins* in *Appendix.*

v. cava inferior. [NA] The principal vein draining lower portion of the body. It is formed by junction of the two common iliac veins and terminates in the right atrium of the heart. SEE: *heart.*

v. cava superior. [NA] The principal vein draining the upper portion of the body. It is formed by the junction of the right and left innominate veins and empties into the right atrium of the heart. SEE: *heart.*

venacavography (vē″nă-kā-vŏg′ră-fē). The taking of x-ray pictures of the vena cava.

venae comitantes [L.]. Two or more veins accompanying an artery. They are usually present with the deep arteries of the extremities.

venation. The distribution of veins to an organ or structure.

venectasia (vē″nĕk-tā′zē-ă) [L. *vena,* a vein, + Gr. *ektasis,* dilation]. Dilation of a vein. SYN: *phlebectasia.*

venectomy (vē-nĕk′tō-mē) [″ + Gr. *ektome,* excision]. Phlebectomy.

venenation (vĕn″ē-nā′shŭn) [L. *venenum,* poison]. 1. Condition of being poisoned. 2. Act of poisoning.

venene (vē-nēn′). A mixture of venoms from poisonous snakes.

veneniferous (vĕn″ĕ-nĭf′ĕr-ŭs) [″ + *ferre,* to carry]. Transmitting or carrying poison.

venenific (vĕn″ĕ-nĭf′ĭk) [″ + *facere,* to make]. Producing poison.

venenosalivary (vĕn″ĕ-nō-săl′ĭ-vĕr″ē). Venomosalivary, q.v.

venenosity (vĕn″ĕ-nŏs′ĭ-tē). State of being venomous.

venenous (vĕn′ĕn-ŭs) [L. *venenum,* poison]. Poisonous.

venepuncture (vĕn′ē-pŭnk″chūr) [L. *vena,* vein, + *punctura,* a piercing]. Venipuncture.

venereal (vē-nē′rē-ăl) [L. *venereus*]. Pert. to or resulting from sexual intercourse.

venereal bubo. Enlarged lymph node in the groin, the result of a venereal disease.

venereal collar. Mottled condition of the neck seen occasionally in syphilis.

venereal disease. Disease acquired ordinarily as a result of sexual intercourse with an individual who is afflicted. The diseases are gonorrhea, nonspecific urethritis, chlamydiosis, syphilis, and chancroid. Trichomonas vaginalis vaginitis can be, but is not always, contracted through sexual intercourse. Genital candidiasis, lymphogranuloma venereum, granuloma inguinale, genital herpes, genital warts, balanoposthitis, and proctitis are also included in this classification. SYN: *sexually transmitted disease.* SEE: *acquired immune deficiency syndrome.*

venereal sore. Chancroid.

venereal urethritis. Urethritis occurring in gonorrhea.

venereal wart. Moist reddish elevation on genitals and anus. SYN: *condyloma; verruca acuminata.*

venereologist (vē-nĕr″ē-ŏl′ō-jĭst) [″ + Gr. *logos,* a study]. A doctor who specializes in the treatment of venereal diseases.

venereology (vē-nĕr″ē-ŏl′ō-jē). The scientific study and treatment of venereal diseases.

venereophobia (vē-nĕr″ē-ō-fō′bē-ă) [L. *venereus,* pert. to sexual intercourse, + Gr. *phobos,* fear]. Abnormal fear of venereal disease. SYN: *cypridophobia.*

venery (vĕn′ĕr-ē) [L. *venerus,* pert. to Venus]. Archaic term for indulgence in sexual activity.

venesection (vĕn″ĕ-sĕk′shŭn) [L. *vena,* vein, + *sectio,* a cutting]. Surgical opening of a vein for withdrawal of blood. SYN: *phlebotomy; venisection.*

venin(e) (vĕn′ĭn) [L. *venenum,* poison]. Toxic substance in snake venom. SYN: *venene.*

venin-antivenin (vĕn″ĭn-ăn″tĭ-vĕn′ĭn). Vaccine to counteract snake poison.

veniplex (vĕn′ĭ-plĕks) [L. *vena,* vein, + *plexus,* a braid]. A plexus of veins.

venipuncture (vĕn′ĭ-pŭnk″chūr) [″ + *punctura,* a piercing]. Puncture of a vein for any purpose.

venisection (vĕn″ĭ-sĕk′shŭn). Venesection.

venisuture (vĕn′ĭ-sū″chūr) [″ + *sutura,* a stitch]. Suture of a vein. SYN: *phleborrhaphy.*

venoatrial (vē″nō-āt′rē-ăl) [″ + *atrium,* corridor]. Rel. to the vena cava and the atrium. SYN: *venoauricular.*

venoauricular (vē″nō-aw-rĭk′ū-lăr) [″ + *au-*

ricula, little ear]. Venoatrial.

venoclysis (vē-nŏk′lĭ-sĭs) [″ + Gr. *klysis,* injection]. The continuous injection of medicinal or nutrient fluid intravenously. SYN: *phleboclysis.*

venofibrosis (vē″nō-fī-brō′sĭs). Phlebosclerosis.

venogram (vē′nō-grăm) [″ + Gr. *gramma,* a writing]. 1. A roentgenogram of the veins. SYN: *phlebogram.* 2. A tracing of the venous pulse.

venography (vē-nŏg′ră-fē) [″ + Gr. *graphein,* to write]. 1. Roentgenography of veins. 2. The making of a tracing of the venous pulse.

venom (vĕn′ŏm) [L. *venenum,* poison]. A poison excreted by some animals, such as insects or snakes, and transmitted by bites or stings.

v., Russell's viper. SEE: *Russell's viper venom.*

v., snake. The poisonous secretion of the labial glands of certain snakes. Venoms contain proteins, chiefly toxins and enzymes, which are responsible for their toxicity. They are classified as neurocytolysins, hemolysins, hemocoagulins, proteolysins, and cytolysins on the basis of the effects produced. SEE: *snake, poisonous.*

venomization (vĕn″ŭm-ī-zā′shŭn). Treatment of a material with snake venom.

venomosalivary (vĕn″ō-mō-săl′ĭ-vĕr″ē). Secreting saliva with venom in it.

venomotor (vē″nō-mō′tor) [L. *vena,* vein, + *motus,* moving]. Pert. to constriction or dilatation of veins.

venomous (vĕn′ō-mŭs). 1. Poisonous. 2. Pert. to animals or insects that have venom-secreting glands.

venomous snake. In the U.S.A., the coral snakes and pit vipers (copperhead, cottonmouth moccasin, and rattlesnake). SEE: *snake, poisonous.*

veno-occlusive (vē″nō-ŏ-kloo′sĭv). Concerning obstruction of veins.

venoperitoneostomy (vē″nō-pĕr″ĭ-tō″nē-ŏs′tō-mē) [L. *vena,* vein, + Gr. *peritonaion,* peritoneum, + *stoma,* passage]. Surgically inserting the cut end of the saphenous vein into the cavity of the peritoneum. This is done to allow ascitic fluid from the peritoneal cavity to drain into the vein.

venopressor (vē′nō-prĕs″or) [″ + *pressor,* that which squeezes]. Pert. to venous blood pressure.

venosclerosis (vē″nō-sklĕ-rō′sĭs) [″ + Gr. *sklerosis,* a hardening]. Sclerosis of veins. SYN: *phlebosclerosis.*

venose (vē′nōs). Having veins.

venosinal (vē″nō-sī′năl). Concerning the vena cava and the right atrium of the heart.

venosity (vē-nŏs′ĭ-tē) [L. *vena,* vein]. 1. Condition in which there is an excess of venous blood in a part causing venous congestion. 2. Deficient aeration of venous blood.

venospasm (vē nō-spăzm) [″ + Gr. *spasmos,* a convulsion]. Contraction of a vein. May follow infusion of cold or irritating substance into the vein.

venostasis (vē″nō-stā′sĭs) [″ + Gr. *stasis,* a standing]. The trapping of blood in an extremity by compression of veins, a method sometimes employed for reducing the amount of blood in circulation.

venostat (vē′nō-stăt) [″ + Gr. *statikos,* standing]. Appliance for performing venous compression.

venothrombotic (vē″nō-thrŏm-bŏt′ĭk). Having the property of inducing the formation of thrombi in veins.

venotomy (vē-nŏt′ō-mē) [″ + Gr. *tome,* incision]. Incision of a vein.

venous (vē′nŭs) [L. *vena,* vein]. Pert. to the veins or blood passing through them.

venous blood. The dark blood in the veins.

venous hum. Murmur heard upon auscultation over larger veins of the neck.

venous hyperemia. Excess of venous blood in a part. SYN: *venosity.*

venous return. The amount of blood returning to the atria of the heart.

venous sinus. A channel that carries venous blood. Important venous sinuses are those of the dura mater draining the brain and those of the spleen.

venous sinus of sclera. The canal of Schlemm. SEE: *canal, Schlemm's.*

venous thrombosis. SEE: *thrombosis, venous.*

venovenostomy (vē″nō-vē-nŏs′tō-mē) [″ + ″ + Gr. *stoma,* mouth]. Formation of an anastomosis of a vein joined to a vein.

vent (vĕnt) [O. Fr. *fente,* slit]. An opening in any cavity, esp. one for excretion.

v., alveolar. An opening between adjacent alveoli of the lung.

venter (vĕn′tĕr) [L., belly]. 1. A belly-shaped part. 2. The cavity of the abdomen. 3. [NA] The wide swelling part or belly of a muscle.

ventilation (vĕn″tĭ-lā′shŭn) [L. *ventilare,* to air]. 1. Circulation of fresh air in a room and withdrawal of foul air. 2. Oxygenation of blood. 3. In physiology, the amount of air inhaled per day. This can be estimated by spirometry, multiplying the tidal air by the number of respirations per day. An average figure is 10,000 liters. This must not be confused with the total amount of oxygen consumed, which is on the average only 360 liters per day. These volumes are more than doubled during hard physical labor.

v., continuous positive-pressure. Method of mechanically assisted pulmonary ventilation. A device administers air or oxygen to the lungs under a continuous pressure that never returns to zero.

v., intermittent positive-pressure. Mechanical method for assisting pulmonary ventilation employing a device that administers air or oxygen for the inflation of the lungs under positive pressure. Exhalation is usually passive. SYN: *breathing, intermittent positive-pressure.*

v., pulmonary. The inspiration and expiration of air from the lungs.

ventilation coefficient. The amount of air that must be respired for each liter of oxygen to be absorbed.

ventilation rate. ABBR: VR. The amount of air breathed in one minute.

ventilator. A mechanical device for artificial ventilation of the lungs. The mechanism may be hand operated or machine driven, and in the latter case may be automatic.

ventouse (vĕn-toos′) [Fr.]. A glass or glass-shaped vessel used in cupping, q.v.

ventrad (vĕn′trăd) [L. *venter,* belly, + *ad,* toward]. Toward the ventral aspect. Opposite of dorsad.

ventral (vĕn′trăl) [L. *ventralis,* pert. to the belly]. Pert. to the belly. Hence, in quadrupeds, pertaining to the lower or underneath side of the body; in man, pertaining to the anterior portion or the front side of the body. Opposite of dorsal.

ventral hernia. Hernia through the abdominal wall, esp. at points other than the umbilicus and groin.

ventralis (vĕn-trā′lĭs) [L.]. Anterior, or closer to the front.

ventricle (vĕn′trĭk-l) [L. *ventriculus,* a little belly]. 1. A small cavity. 2. Either of two lower chambers of the heart that when filled with blood contract to propel it into the arteries. The right ventricle forces blood into the pulmonary artery and thence into the lungs; the left pumps blood through the aorta into the arteries. 3. One of the cavities of the brain. SEE: *Arantius' body.*

v., aortic. Left ventricle of the heart.

v., fifth. Cavity of the septum lucidum of the brain. It is between the two laminae of the septum lucidum.

v., fourth. The cavity above the pons and medulla of the brain. It extends from the central canal of the upper end of the spinal cord to the aqueduct of the midbrain. Its roof is the cerebellum and the superior and inferior medullary vela. Its floor is the rhomboid fossa.

v., lateral. The cavity in each cerebral hemisphere that communicates with the third ventricle through the interventricular foramen. It consists of a triangular central body; and four horns, two inferior and two posterior.

v., left. The cavity of the heart that receives blood from the left atrium and pumps it out into the general circulation through the aortic valve.

v., Morgagni's. The recess in the lateral wall on each side of the larynx between the vestibular and vocal folds.

v. of Arantius. The terminal depression of the median sulcus of the fourth ventricle of the brain.

v. of larynx. The space between the true and false vocal cords.

v., pineal. The pineal recess of the third ventricle of the brain.

v., right. The cavity of the heart that receives blood from the right atrium and pumps it into the lungs via the pulmonary veins.

v., third. The median cavity in the brain bounded by the thalamus and hypothalamus on either side; anteriorly by the optic chiasma; the floor is made up of the tuber cinereum, mammillary body, the posterior perforated substance and tegmentum of the cerebral peduncle; the roof is the ependyma. Anteriorly, it communicates with the lateral ventricles and posteriorly, with the aqueduct of the midbrain.

ventricornu (vĕn″trĭ-kor′nū) [L. *venter,* belly, + *cornu,* horn]. The anterior ventral horn of gray matter of the spinal cord.

ventricose (vĕn′trĭ-kōs) [L. *ventricosus,* big-bellied]. 1. Inflated or distended. 2. Corpulent.

ventricular (vĕn-trĭk′ū-lăr) [L. *ventriculus,* a little belly]. Pert. to a ventricle.

ventricular folds. The false vocal cords or folds of mucous membrane parallel or above the true vocal cords.

ventricular ligament. A narrow band of fibrous tissue lying within each ventricular fold.

ventricular septal defect. A defect in the septum between the left and right ventricles of the heart. This permits blood to be shunted between the ventricles.

ventriculitis (vĕn-trĭk″ū-lī′tĭs) [″ + Gr. *itis,* inflammation]. Inflammation of a ventricle.

ventriculoatriostomy (vĕn-trĭk″ū-lō-ā″trē-ŏs′tō-mē) [″ + *atrium,* corridor, + Gr. *stoma,* passage]. Plastic surgery for the relief of hydrocephalus. Subcutaneous catheters are placed to connect a cerebral ventricle to the right atrium via the jugular vein. The catheters contain one-way valves so that cerebral spinal fluid can flow into the catheters but blood may not be pumped into the cerebral ventricle.

ventriculocisternostomy (vĕn-trĭk″ū-lō-sĭs″tĕr-nŏs′tō-mē) [″ + *cisterna,* cavity, + Gr. *stoma,* passage]. Plastic surgery to create an opening between the ventricles of the brain and the cisterna magna.

ventriculocordectomy (vĕn-trĭk″ū-lō-kor-dĕk′tō-mē) [″ + Gr. *khorde,* cord, + *ektome,* excision]. Surgery for relief of laryngeal stenosis. The ventricular floor is removed but the buccal processes are left in place.

ventriculogram (vĕn-trĭk′ū-lō-grăm) [″ + Gr. *gramma,* mark]. Roentgenogram of the cerebral ventricles.

ventriculography (vĕn-trĭk″ū-lŏg′ră-fē) [″ + Gr. *graphein,* to write]. 1. An x-ray process used for visualizing the size and shape of the cerebral ventricles by injecting air to display the cerebrospinal fluid that normally fills these cavities. 2. Visualization of ventricles of the heart by x-ray after injection of a contrast material.

ventriculometry (vĕn-trĭk″ū-lŏm′ĕ-trē) [″ + Gr. *metron,* a measure]. The measurement of the intraventricular cerebral pressure.

ventriculonector (vĕn-trĭk″ū-lō-nĕk′tor) [L. *ventriculus,* a little belly, + *nector,* a joiner]. The atrioventricular bundle.

ventriculopuncture (vĕn-trĭk′ū-lō-pŭnk″tūr) [″ + *punctura,* point]. Use of a needle to puncture a lateral ventricle of the brain.

ventriculoscopy (vĕn-trĭk″ū-lŏs′kō-pē) [″ + Gr. *skopein,* to examine]. Examination of the ventricles of the brain with an endoscope.

ventriculostomy (vĕn-trĭk″ū-lŏs′tō-mē) [″ + Gr. *stoma,* passage]. Plastic surgery in order to establish communication between the floor of the third ventricle of the brain and the cisterna interpeduncularis. This is done to treat hydrocephalus.

ventriculosubarachnoid (vĕn-trĭk″ū-lō-sŭb″ă-răk′noyd). Concerning the cerebral ventricles and the subarachnoid spaces.

ventriculotomy (vĕn-trĭk″ū-lŏt′ō-mē) [″ + Gr. *tome,* incision]. Surgical incision of a ventricle.

ventriculus (vĕn-trĭk′ū-lŭs) [L., a little belly]. [NA] 1. Ventricle. 2. The stomach. 3. A ventricle of the brain or heart.

v. tertius. Third ventricle, q.v.

ventricumbent (vĕn″trĭ-kŭm′bĕnt) [L. *venter,* belly, + *cumbere,* to lie]. Lying on the belly. SYN: *prone.*

ventriduct (vĕn′trĭ-dŭkt) [″ + *ductus,* leading]. To draw toward the abdomen.

ventriduction (vĕn″trĭ-dŭk′shŭn). Pulling or placing a part ventrad.

ventrimeson (vĕn″trĭ-mēs′ŏn) [″ + Gr. *mesos,* middle]. The median line on the ventral surface of the body.

ventripyramid (vĕn″trĭ-pĭr′ă-mĭd) [″ + Gr. *pyramis,* pyramid]. An anterior pyramid of the medulla oblongata.

ventro- [L. *venter,* belly]. Combining form denoting the abdomen or ventral (anterior) surface of the body.

ventrocystorrhaphy (vĕn″trō-sĭs-tor′ă-fē) [″ + Gr. *kystis,* sac, + *rhaphe,* a seam]. Suture of a cyst or the bladder to the abdominal wall.

ventrodorsal (vĕn″trō-dor′săl) [″ + *dorsum,* back]. In a direction from the front to the back.

ventrofixation (vĕn″trō-fĭks-ā′shŭn) [″ + *fixare,* to fix]. The suture of a displaced viscus to the abdominal wall.

ventrohysteropexy (vĕn″trō-hĭs′tĕr-ō-pĕks″ē) [″ + Gr. *hystera,* uterus, + *pexis,* fixation]. Attachment of the uterus to the abdominal wall.

ventroinguinal (vĕn″trō-ĭng′gwĭ-năl) [″ + *inguen,* groin]. Concerning the ventral and inguinal regions.

ventrolateral (vĕn″trō-lăt′ĕr-ăl) [″ + *latus,* side]. Both ventral and lateral.

ventromedian (vĕn″trō-mē′dē-ăn) [″ + *medianus,* median]. Both ventral and medial.

ventroptosia, ventroptosis (vĕn″trŏp-tō′sē-ă, -sĭs) [″ + Gr. *ptosis,* falling]. Downward displacement of the stomach. SYN: *gastroptosis.*

ventroscopy (vĕn-trŏs′kō-pē) [L. *venter,* belly, + Gr. *skopein,* to examine]. Examination of the abdominal cavity by illumination. SYN: *celioscopy.*

ventrose (vĕn′trōs). Having a swelling like a belly.

ventrosity (vĕn-trŏs′ĭ-tē). Having an enlarged belly; corpulence.

ventrosuspension (vĕn″trō-sŭs-pĕn′shŭn) [″ + *suspensio,* a hanging]. Fixation of displaced uterus to abdominal wall.

ventrotomy (vĕn-trŏt′ō-mē) [″ + Gr. *tome,* incision]. Incision into abdominal cavity. SYN: *celiotomy; laparotomy.*

ventrovesicofixation (vĕn″trō-vĕs″ĭ-kō-fĭks-ā′shŭn) [″ + *vesica,* bladder, + *fixare,* to fix]. Suture of uterus to abdominal wall and bladder. SYN: *hysterocystopexy.*

Venturi mask. A special mask for administering a controlled concentration of oxygen to a patient.

venturimeter (vĕn″tūr-ĭm′ĕ-ter). [Giovanni Battista Venturi, It. physicist, 1746–1822] Device for measuring flow of fluids through vessels.

venula (vĕn′ū-lă) [L., little vein]. Venule.

venule (vĕn′ūl) [L. *venula,* little vein]. A tiny vein continuous with a capillary.

Venus's collar (vē′nŭs). [L., the Roman goddess of love] Pigmentation around the neck in eruption due to syphilis.

Venus, crown of. An eruption around the hairline caused by syphilis.

Venus, mount of. The mons pubis or mons veneris, q.v.

Veracillin. Trade name for dicloxacillin sodium, USP.

verbigeration (vĕr-bĭj″ĕr-ā′shŭn) [L. *verbigerare,* to chatter]. Repetition of words that are either meaningless or have no significance.

verbomania (vĕr″bō-mā′nē-ă) [L. *verba,* word, + Gr. *mania,* madness]. The flow of talk in some forms of psychosis.

Vercyte. Trade name for pipobroman.

verdigris (vĕr′dĭ-grĭs) [O. Fr. *vert de Grece,* green of Greece]. 1. Mixture of basic copper acetates. 2. Deposit of copper carbonate upon copper and bronze vessels. These are of a greenish-gray color.

verdigris poisoning. Same as for copper sulfate. SEE: *copper salts* in *Poisons and Poisoning* in *Appendix.*

verdohemoglobin (vĕr″dō-hēm′ō-glōb″ĭn). A greenish pigment occurring as an intermediate product in the formation of bilirubin from hemoglobin.

Verga's ventricle (vĕr′găz). [Andrea Verga, It. neurologist, 1811–1895] Cleftlike space between the corpus callosum and the body of the fornix of the brain.

verge (vĕrj). An edge or margin.

v., anal. The transitional area between the smooth perianal area and the hairy skin.

vergence (vĕr′jĕns) [L. *vergere,* to bend]. A turning of one eye with reference to the other. May be horizontal (convergence or divergence) or vertical (infravergence or supravergence). SEE: *phoria.*

Verheyen's stars (fĕr-hī′ĕns). [Philippe Verheyen, Flemish anatomist, 1648–1710] Starlike venous plexuses on surface of the kidney below its capsule.

Veriloid. Trade name for alkavervir.

vermicidal (vĕr″mĭ-sī′dăl) [L. *vermis,* worm, + *cidus,* kill]. Destroying worms parasitic in the intestines.

vermicide (vĕr′mĭ-sīd). 1. Destroying worms. 2. An agent that will kill intestinal worms.

vermicular (vĕr-mĭk′ū-lăr) [L. *vermicularis*]. Resembling a worm.

vermicular movements. The wormlike movements of peristalsis.

vermicular pulse. Small rapid pulse resulting in wormlike feeling in the fingers.

vermiculation (vĕr-mĭk″ū-lā′shŭn) [L. *vermiculare,* to wriggle]. A wormlike motion, as in the intestines. SEE: *peristalsis.*

vermicule (vĕr′mĭ-kūl) [L. *vermiculus,* a small worm]. A small worm, or having a wormlike shape.

vermiculose, vermiculous (vĕr-mĭk′ŭ-lōs, vĕr-mĭk′ū-lŭs) [L. *vermicularis,* wormlike]. 1. Infested with worms or larvae. 2. Wormlike.

vermiform (vĕr′mĭ-form) [L. *vermis,* worm, + *forma,* shape]. Contoured like a worm.

vermiform appendix. A long, narrow, worm-shaped tube connected to the cecum. It varies in length from less than 1 to more than 8 in. (2.5 to 20.3 cm.) with an average of about 3 in. (7.6 cm.). Its distal end is closed. It is

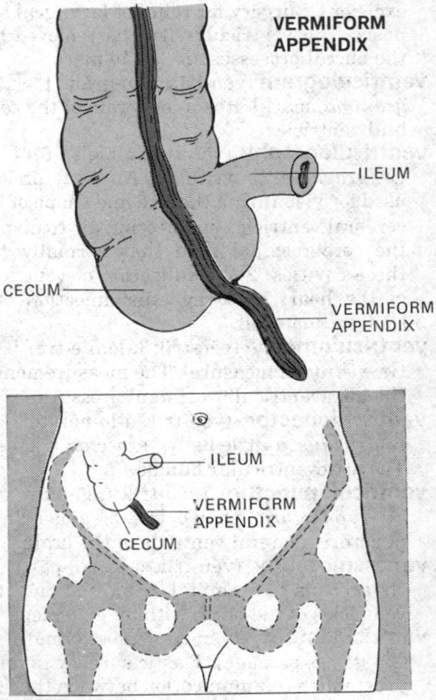

lined with mucosa similar to that of the large intestine. Inflammation of it is called appendicitis, q.v. SEE: illus.

vermifugal (vĕr-mĭf′ū-găl) [″ + *fugare,* to put to flight]. Expelling worms from the intestines.

vermifuge (vĕr′mĭ-fūj). Agent for expelling intestinal worms. SYN: *anthelmintic; vermicide.*

vermilion border. The junction of the pinkish red area of the lips with the surrounding skin.

vermilionectomy (vĕr-mĭl″yŏn-ĕk′tō-mē) [*vermilion border* + Gr. *ektome,* excision]. Surgical removal of the vermilion border of the lip.

vermin (vĕr′mĭn) [L. *vermis,* worm]. Small insects and animals such as mice, lice, or bedbugs that are annoying or cause destruction or disease.

verminal (vĕr′mĭ-năl). Concerning or caused by worms.

vermination (vĕr″mĭn-ā′shŭn). Vermin or worm infestation.

verminosis (vĕr″mĭn-ō′sĭs) [″ + Gr. *osis,* condition]. Infestation with vermin.

verminous (vĕr′mĭn-ŭs). Pert. to or infested with worms.

vermiphobia (vĕr″mĭ-fō′bē-ă) [″ + Gr. *pho-*

bos, fear]. An abnormal fear of being infested with worms.

vermis (vĕr'mĭs) [L. worm]. 1. A worm. 2. Vermis cerebelli.

v. cerebelli. [NA] Median connecting lobe of the cerebellum.

v., inferior. The anteroinferior portion of the vermis of the cerebellum. Includes the nodule, uvula, pyramis, and tuber.

v., superior. The posterior dorsal portion of the vermis. Includes the folium, declive, culmen, and central lobule.

Vermox. Trade name for mebendazole.

vernal (vĕr'năl) [L. *vernalis*, pert. to spring]. Occurring in or pert. to the spring.

Vernet's syndrome (vĕr-nāz'). [Maurice Vernet, Fr. physician, b. 1837] Paralysis of glossopharyngeal, vagus, and spinal accessory nerves on the opposite side of a lesion involving the jugular foramen.

vernix (vĕr'nĭks) [L.]. Varnish.

v. caseosa. A sebaceous deposit covering the fetus. It is protective during intrauterine life. Most abundant in creases and flexor surfaces. Consists of exfoliations of outer skin layer, lanugo, and secretions of sebaceous glands. It is not necessary to remove this after the fetus is delivered. SEE: *sebum*.

verruca (vĕr-roo'kă) [L., wart]. (pl. *verrucae*) Tumor of the epidermis of the skin. Produces a circumscribed elevated area of hypertrophy of the papillae. SYN: *wart*.

ETIOL: Caused by a papillomavirus.

PROG: Essentially benign and may disappear spontaneously, particularly in children and young adults. In elderly with longstanding dry seborrhea, lesions are potentially malignant.

TREATMENT: Removal with sharp spoon curet under local anesthesia. If elevated, clip off with sharp scissors and touch with iodine. Freezing with carbon dioxide snow or fulguration.

v. acuminata. A pointed, reddish, moist wart about the genitals and the anus. Develops near mucocutaneous junctures, forming pointed, tufted, or pedunculated pinkish or purplish projections of varying lengths and consistency. Venereal warts should be treated with applications of 25% podophyllum resin in compound tincture of benzoin followed by removal of the resin by washing with soap and water about six hours after application. SYN: *venereal wart*.

v. digitata. Form of verruca seen on face and scalp, possibly serving as starting point of cutaneous horns. Several filiform projections with horny caps are formed, closely grouped on a comparatively narrow base that in turn may be separated from skin surface by slightly contracted neck.

v. filiformis. Small threadlike growths on neck and eyelids covered with smooth and apparently normal epidermis.

v. gyri hippocampi. One of the small wartlike protuberances on the convex surface of the gyrus hippocampi.

v. plana. A flat or slightly raised wart.

v. plantaris. Warts on the soles of the feet. SYN: *plantar wart*.

v. vulgaris. Common warts, usually on backs of hands and fingers, but may occur anywhere on the skin.

verruciform (vĕ-roo'sĭ-form) [L. *verruca*, wart, + *forma*, shape]. Wartlike.

verrucose, verrucous (vĕr'roo-kōs, vĕr-roo'kŭs) [L. *verrucosus*, wartlike]. Wartlike, with raised portions.

verrucosis (vĕr'oo-kō'sĭs) [L. *verruca*, wart, + Gr. *osis*, condition]. The condition of having multiple warts.

verruga peruana (vĕ-roo'gă pĕr-wăn'ă) [Sp., Peruvian wart]. The eruptive second clinical stage of bartonellosis, q.v. Croya fever is the first or febrile stage.

Versapen. Trade name for hetacillin.

Versapen K. Trade name for hetacillin potassium.

versicolor (vĕr'sĭ-kŏl″or) [L., of changing colors]. 1. Having many shades or colors. 2. Changeable in color.

version (vĕr'zhŭn) [L. *versio*, a turning]. 1. Altering of position of the fetus in the uterus. May occur naturally or may be done mechanically by the physician in order to facilitate delivery. 2. Deflection of an organ such as the uterus from its normal position.

v., bipolar. Changing the position of the fetus by combined internal and external manipulation.

v., cephalic. Turning of fetus so that the head presents.

v., combined. Mechanical version by combined internal and external manipulation.

v., external. Version of the fetus through the abdominal wall.

v., internal. Version of the fetus with one hand inserted through the vagina.

v., pelvic. Version of a cross-presentation until it is changed to a pelvic presentation.

v., podalic. Version of fetus by the feet so that the breech presents.

v., spontaneous. Version of fetus by uterine muscular contraction without artificial assistance.

Verstran. Trade name for prazepam.

vertebra (vĕr'tĕ-bră) [L.]. (pl. *vertebrae*) [NA] Any one of the 33 bony segments of the spinal column. The spinal vertebrae are comprised of 7 cervical, 12 thoracic (dorsal), 5 lumbar, 5 sacral, and 4 coccygeal vertebrae. In adults, the five sacral vertebrae fuse to form a single bone, the sacrum, and the four rudimentary coccygeal vertebrae fuse to form the coccyx.

A typical vertebra consists of a ventral body and a dorsal or neural arch. In the thoracic region the body bears on each side two costal pits for reception of the head of the rib. The arch that encloses the vertebral foramen is formed of two roots or pedicles and two laminae. The arch bears seven processes: a dorsal spinous process, two lateral transverse processes, and four articular processes (two superior and two inferior). A deep concavity, inferior vertebral notch, on the inferior border of the arch provides a passageway for a spinal nerve. The successive vertebral foramina surround the spinal cord.

The bodies of successive vertebrae articulate with one another and are separated by intervertebral disks, disks of fibrous cartilage enclosing a central mass, the nucleus pulposus. The inferior articular processes articulate with the superior articular processes of the next succeeding vertebra in the caudal direction. Several ligaments (supraspinous, interspinous, anterior and posterior longitudinal, and the ligamenta flava) hold the vertebrae in position yet permit a limited degree of movement. SEE: *sacrum* for illus.

RS: acantha; anapophysis; anticlinal; atlas; axis; lamina; "spondyl-" words.

v., basilar. The lowest of the lumbar vertebrae.

v., cervical. The seven vertebrae of the neck.

v., coccygeal. The rudimentary vertebrae of the coccyx.

v. dentata. The second cervical vertebra. SYN: *axis* [NA]; *v., odontoid.*

v., false. The sacral and coccygeal vertebrae that fuse. SYN: *v., fixed.*

v., fixed. V., false.

v., flexion. All vertebrae except the atlas and axis.

v., lumbar. The five vertebrae between the thoracic vertebrae and the sacrum.

v. magnum. The sacrum.

v., odontoid. V. dentata.

v. prominens. [NA] The seventh cervical vertebra.

v., rotation. The first two cervical vertebrae, the atlas and axis.

v., sacral. The five fused vertebrae forming the sacrum. SEE: *sacrum* for illus.

v., sternal. The segments of the sternum.

v., thoracic. The 12 vertebrae that connect the ribs and form part of the posterior wall of the thorax. SEE: *spinal column* for illus.

v., true. The vertebrae that remain unfused through life: the cervical, thoracic, and lumbar.

vertebral (vĕr′tĕ-brăl) [L. *vertebra,* vertebra]. Pertaining to a vertebra or the vertebral column.

vertebral arch. The thoracic portion of a vertebra that encloses a vertebral foramen.

vertebral canal. Cavity of the spinal column that contains the spinal cord. SYN: *spinal canal.*

vertebral column. Spinal column.

vertebral foramen. The hollow space enclosed by a vertebral arch.

vertebral groove. Groove lying on either side of the spinous processes of the vertebrae.

vertebral notch. Notch on inferior surface of vertebral arch for transmission of a spinal nerve.

vertebral ribs. The lower two, or floating, ribs.

vertebrarium (vĕr″tĕ-brā′rē-ŭm) [L.]. The vertebral column.

Vertebrata (vĕr″tĕ-brā′tă). A subphylum of the phylum Chordata characterized by possession of segmented backbone or spinal column. They possess an axial notochord at some period of their existence. Includes the following classes: Agnatha (cyclostomes); Chondrichthyes (cartilaginous fishes); Osteichthyes (bony fishes); Amphibia; Reptilia; Aves; and Mammalia.

vertebrate (vĕr′tĕ-brāt) [L. *vertebra,* vertebra]. Having or resembling a vertebral column.

vertebrated (vĕr′tĕ-brāt″ĕd). Composed of jointed segments.

vertebrectomy (vĕr″tĕ-brĕk′tō-mē) [″ + Gr. *ektome,* excision]. Excision of a vertebra or part of one.

vertebroarterial (vĕr″tĕ-brō-ăr-tē′rē-ăl) [″ + Gr. *arteria,* artery]. Concerning the vertebral artery.

vertebrobasilar (vĕr″tĕ-brō-băs′ĭ-lăr) [″ + *basilaris,* basilar]. Concerning the vertebral and basilar arteries.

vertebrochondral (vĕr″tĕ-brō-kŏn′drăl) [″ + Gr. *chondros,* cartilage]. Denoting the vertebra and the costal cartilages.

vertebrocostal (vĕr″tĕ-brō-kŏs′tăl) [″ + *costa,* rib]. Pert. to a vertebra and a rib. SYN: *costovertebral.*

vertebrofemoral (vĕr″tĕ-brō-fĕm′or-ăl) [″ + *femur,* thigh]. Concerning the vertebrae and the femur.

vertebroiliac (vĕr″tĕ-brō-ĭl′ē-ăk) [″ + *iliacus,* pert. to ilium]. Concerning the vertebrae and the ilium.

vertebromammary (vĕr″tĕ-brō-măm′mă-rē) [″ + *mammarius,* pert. to a breast]. Pert. to the vertebral and mammary area.

vertebrosacral (vĕr″tĕ-brō-sā′krăl) [″ + *sacrum,* sacred]. Concerning the vertebrae and the sacrum.

vertebrosternal (vĕr″tĕ-brō-stĕr′năl) [″ + Gr. *sternon,* chest]. Pert. to a vertebra and the sternum.

vertex (vĕr′tĕks) [L., summit]. [NA] The top of the head. SYN: *corona capitis; crown.*

v. cordis. Apex of the heart.

vertical (vĕr′tĭ-kăl) [L. *verticalis,* summit]. 1. Pert. to or situated at the vertex. 2. Perpendicular to the plane of the horizon of the earth; upright.

verticalis (vĕr″tĭ-kā′lĭs) [L.]. Vertical. Indicating any plane that passes through the body parallel to the long axis of the body.

verticality. The ability to accurately perceive the vertical position in the absence of environmental cues.

verticillate (vĕr-tĭs′ĭl-āt, -tĭs-ĭl′āt) [L. *verticillus,* a little whirl]. Arranged like the spokes of a wheel or a whorl.

verticomental (vĕr″tĭ-kō-mĕn′tăl) [L. *vertex,* summit, + *mentum,* chin]. Concerning the crown of the head and the chin.

vertiginous (vĕr-tĭj′ĭ-nŭs) [L. *vertiginosus,* a turning around]. Pert. to or afflicted with vertigo.

vertigo (vĕr′tĭ-gō, vĕr-tī′gō) [L. *vertigo,* a turning round]. True vertigo is the sensation of moving around in space (subjective vertigo) or of having objects move about the person (objective vertigo) and is a result of a disturbance of equilibratory apparatus. Sometimes used as a synonym for dizziness, lightheadedness, and giddiness.

ETIOL: May be caused by a variety of entities including middle ear disease; toxic conditions such as those caused by salicylates, alcohol, or streptomycin; sunstroke; postural hypotension; or toxemia due to food poisoning or infectious diseases.

NURSING IMPLICATIONS: Assessment should include whether or not the patient experiences a turning or whirling sensation; direction of the sensation; whether it is intermittent or constant; time of day it occurs; whether or not it is related to position, drugs, occupation, or menses; is it associated with nausea and vomiting or with nystagmus and migraine. Implement safety measures such as use of siderails at all times. Ambulate gradually after a slow, assisted move from a sitting position. Have the call bell available at all times; make sure tissues, water, and other needed supplies are within easy reach and that furniture and other obstacles are removed from the path of ambulation. The patient who received a fenestration operation on the ear and is experiencing severe vertigo should be confined to bed for several days and then begin a gradual increase in activity.

v., auditory. Vertigo due to disease of the ear.

v., central. Vertigo caused by disease of the central nervous system.

v., cerebral. Vertigo due to brain disease.

v., epileptic. Vertigo attending an epileptic attack or following it.

v., essential. Vertigo from an unknown cause.

v., gastric. Vertigo associated with gastric disturbance.

v., hysterical. Vertigo accompanying hysteria.

v., labyrinthine. Vertigo due to disease of labyrinth of the ear. SYN: *Ménière's disease.*

v., laryngeal. Vertigo accompanying laryngeal spasm.

v., objective. Vertigo in which stationary objects appear to be moving.

v., ocular. Vertigo caused by disease of the eye.

v., organic. Vertigo due to a brain lesion.

v., peripheral. Vertigo due to disturbances in the peripheral areas of the central nervous system.

v., positional; v., postural. Vertigo that occurs when the head is in a specific position.

v., subjective. Vertigo in which the patient has the sensation of turning or rotating.

v., toxic. Vertigo from presence of a toxin in the body.

v., vestibular. Vertigo due to disease or malfunction of the vestibular apparatus.

verumontanitis (vĕr″ū-mŏn″tăn-ī′tĭs) [L. *verumontanum,* mountainous ridge, + Gr. *itis,* inflammation]. Inflammation of the verumontanum. SYN: *colliculitis.*

verumontanum (vĕr″ū-mŏn-tā′nŭm) [L. *verumontanum,* mountainous ridge]. An elevation on the floor of the prostatic portion of the urethra where the seminal ducts enter.

very low density lipoproteins. ABBR: VLDL. Plasma lipids bound to albumin consisting of chylomicrons and prelipoproteins. This class contains a greater ratio of lipid than low-density lipoproteins and are the least dense. SEE: *lipoproteins.*

vesalianum (vĕs-ā″lē-ā′nŭm). [Andreas Vesalius, Flemish anatomist and physician, 1514–1564] One of the sesamoid bones in the tendon of origin of the gastrocnemius muscle, and another on outer border of foot in the angle between the cuboid and fifth metatarsal.

Vesalius, foramen of (vĕs-ā′lē-ŭs). [Andreas Vesalius] Opening in base of the skull transmitting an emissary vein.

Vesalius, vein of. Small emissary vein from cavernous sinus passing through foramen of Vesalius and conveying blood to the pterygoid plexus.

vesica (vĕ-sī′kă) [L.]. [NA] A bladder.

v. fellea. [NA] The gallbladder.

v. prostatica. A minute pouch in the prostatic urethra, remnant of the müllerian duct. SYN: *utriculus prostaticus.*

v. urinaria. [NA] The urinary bladder.

vesical (vĕs′ĭ-kăl). Pert. to or shaped like a bladder.

vesical reflex. Inclination to urinate caused by moderate bladder distention.

vesicant (vĕs′ĭ-kănt) [L. *vesicare,* to blister]. 1. Blistering; causing or forming blisters. 2. Agent used to produce blisters. It is much less severe in its effects than escharotics. 3. A blistering gas used in chemical warfare. SEE: *gas, vesicant.*

vesication (vĕs″ĭ-kā′shŭn). 1. Process of blistering. 2. A blister.

vesicatory (vĕs′ĭ-kă-tor″ē). 1. Causing or pert. to blisters. 2. Agent causing blisters. SYN: *vesicant.*

vesicle (vĕs′ĭ-kl) [L. *vesicula,* a little bladder]. 1. A small sac or bladder containing fluid. 2. A blisterlike small elevation on the skin containing serous fluid.

Vesicles may vary in diameter from a few millimeters to a centimeter. They may be round, transparent, opaque, or dark elevations of the skin, sometimes containing seropurulent or bloody fluid. They are seen in sudamina as the result of sweat that cannot escape from the skin; in herpes, mounted on an inflammatory base, having no tendency to rupture but associated with burning pain. In herpes zoster they follow the line of the nerve trunks. They are seen in dermatitis venenata as the result of poison ivy or oak and accompanied by great itching; in dermatitis herpetiformis or multiformis. In impetigo contagiosa they occur especially in children in discrete form, flat and umbilicated, filled with straw-colored fluid with no tendency to break. They dry up, forming yellow crusts with little itching. They are also seen in vesicular eczema, molluscum contagiosa, miliaria (prickly heat or heat rash), chickenpox, smallpox, and scabies. SEE: *herpes; miliaria.*

v., allantoic. The hollow, enlarged part of the allantois, esp. in birds and reptiles.

v., auditory. That portion of the cerebral vesicle from which the exterior ear is formed.

v., blastodermic. Sac developed from the blastoderm.

v., brain. The five embryonic subdivisions of the brain.

v., brain, primary. The three earliest subdivisions of the embryonic neural tube.

v., cerebral. Expansion of neural embryonic canal from which the brain develops.

v., chorionic. The outer villus-covered layer of the early embryo. It encloses the embryo, amnion, umbilical cord, and yolk stalk.

v., compound. Multilocular vesicles.

v., encephalic. V., brain.

v., lens. The embryonic vesicle formed from the lens pit. It develops into the lens of the eye.

v., multilocular. Vesicles that contain multiple chambers.

v., optic. Hollow outgrowths from the lateral aspects of the embryonic brain. The retinae and optic nerves develop from these paired vesicles.

v., otic. V., auditory, q.v.

v., seminal. One of the two membranous sacculated tubes situated at the base of the bladder, between it and the rectum, serving as a reservoir for the semen and having a secretion of its own.

v., umbilical. Portion of embryonic yolk sac outside the body cavity.

vesico- (vĕs′ĭ-kō) [L. *vesica,* bladder]. Combining form meaning bladder.

vesicoabdominal (vĕs″ĭ-kō-ăb-dŏm′ĭ-năl) [″ + *abdomen,* abdomen]. Concerning the urinary bladder and the abdomen.

vesicocele (vĕs′ĭ-kō-sēl″) [L. *vesica,* bladder, + Gr. *kele,* hernia]. Hernia of the bladder into the vagina. SYN: *cystocele.*

vesicocervical (vĕs″ĭ-kō-sĕr′vĭ-kăl) [″ + *cervix,* neck]. Rel. to the urinary bladder and cervix uteri.

vesicoclysis (vĕs″ĭ-kŏk′lĭ-sĭs) [″ + Gr. *klysis,* a washing out]. Injection of fluid into the bladder.

vesicoenteric (vĕs″ĭ-kō-ĕn-tĕr′ĭk) [″ Gr. *enteron,* intestine]. Concerning the urinary bladder and the intestine.

vesicofixation (vĕs″ĭ-kō-fĭks-ā′shŭn) [L. *vesica,* bladder, + *fixatio,* a fixing]. Attachment of the uterus to the bladder or the bladder to the abdominal wall.

vesicointestinal (vĕs″ĭ-kō-ĭn-tĕs′tĭ-năl). Vesicoenteric.

vesicoprostatic (vĕs″ĭ-kō-prŏs-tăt′ĭk) [″ + Gr. *prostates,* prostate]. Relating to the bladder and prostate.

vesicopubic (vĕs″ĭ-kō-pū′bĭk) [″ + *pubis,* pubis]. Pert. to the bladder and the os pubis.

vesicopustule (vĕs″ĭ-kō-pŭs′tūl) [″ + *pustula,* blister]. A vesicle in which pus is developing.

vesicosigmoid (vĕs″ĭ-kō-sĭg′moyd) [″ + Gr. *sigmoid,* shaped like Gr. letter S]. Concerning the urinary bladder and the sigmoid colon.

vesicosigmoidostomy (vĕs″ĭ-kō-sĭg″moy-dŏs′tō-mē) [″ + ″ + *stoma,* passage]. Surgical creation of an anastomosis between the urinary bladder and the sigmoid colon.

vesicospinal (vĕs″ĭ-kō-spī′năl) [″ + *spina,* a thorn]. Relating to the urinary bladder and spinal cord.

vesicostomy (vĕs″ĭ-kŏs′tō-mē) [″ + Gr. *stoma,* passage]. Surgical production of an opening into the bladder.

vesicotomy (vĕs″ĭ-kŏt′ō-mē) [″ + Gr. *tome,* incision]. Incision of the bladder.

vesicoumbilical (vĕs″ĭ-kō-ŭm-bĭl′ĭ-kăl) [″ + *umbilicus,* a pit]. Concerning the urinary bladder and the umbilicus.

vesicoureteral (vĕs″ĭ-kō-ū-rē′tĕr-ăl) [″ + Gr. *oureter,* ureter]. Concerning the urinary bladder and a ureter.

vesicouterine (vĕs″ĭ-kō-ū′tĕr-ĭn) [″ + *uterinus,* pert. to the womb]. Pert. to the urinary bladder and the uterus.

vesicouterine pouch. Downward extension of the peritoneal cavity located between bladder and uterus.

vesicouterovaginal (vĕs″ĭ-kō-ū″tĕr-ō-văj′ĭ-năl) [″ + *uterus,* womb, + *vagina,* sheath]. Concerning the urinary bladder, the uterus, and the vagina.

vesicovaginal (vĕs″ĭ-kō-văj′ĭ-năl) [″ + *vagina,* a sheath]. Pert. to the urinary bladder and vagina.

vesicovaginorectal (vĕs″ĭ-kō-văj″ĭ-nō-rĕk′tăl) [″ + *vagina,* sheath, + *rectum,* straight]. Concerning the urinary bladder, the vagina, and the rectum.

vesicula (vĕ-sĭk′ū-lă) [L.]. (pl. *vesiculae*) [NA] A small bladder or vesicle.

v. seminalis. [NA] Tiny reservoir of semen at base of the bladder. SYN: *seminal vesicle.*

vesicular (vĕ-sĭk′ū-lăr). Pert. to vesicles or small blisters.

vesicular breathing. Murmur heard in normal breathing. SYN: *vesicular murmur.*

vesicular eczema. Eczema accompanied by formation of vesicles.

vesicular murmur. The normal sound of respiration heard on auscultation. SYN: *vesicular breathing.*

vesicular rale. The crepitant rale, a crackling sound heard at end of inspiration.

vesicular resonance. Percussion sound heard over the normal lung.

vesiculase (vĕ-sĭk′ū-lās). An enzyme in prostatic fluid said to coagulate semen.

vesiculated (vĕ-sĭk′ū-lāt″ĕd). Having vesicles present.

vesiculation (vĕ-sĭk″ū-lā′shŭn) [L. *vesicula,* a tiny bladder]. Formation of vesicles or state of having or forming them.

vesiculectomy (vĕ-sĭk″ū-lĕk′tō-mē) [″ + Gr. *ektome,* excision]. Partial or complete excision of a vesicle, particularly a seminal vesicle.

vesiculiform (vĕ-sĭk′ū-lĭ-form) [″ + *forma,* shape]. Having the shape of a vesicle.

vesiculitis (vĕ-sĭk″ū-lī′tĭs) [″ + Gr. *itis,* inflammation]. Inflammation of a vesicle, particularly the seminal vesicle.

vesiculobronchial (vĕ-sĭk″ū-lō-brŏng′kē-ăl) [″ + Gr. *bronchos,* windpipe]. Both vesicular and bronchial.

vesiculocavernous (vĕ-sĭk″ū-lō-kăv′ĕr-nŭs) [″ + *cavernosis,* hollow]. Vesicular and cavernous.

vesiculogram (vĕ-sĭk′ū-lō-grăm) [″ + Gr. *gramma,* a mark]. An x-ray picture of the seminal vesicles.

vesiculography (vĕ-sĭk″ū-lŏg′ră-fē) [″ + Gr. *graphein,* to write]. Roentgenography of the seminal vesicles.

vesiculopapular (vĕ-sĭk″ū-lō-păp′ū-lăr) [″ + *papula,* a pimple]. Composed of vesicles and papules.

vesiculopustular (vĕ-sĭk″ū-lō-pŭs′tū-lăr) [″ + *pustula,* pustule]. Having both vesicles and pustules.

vesiculotomy (vĕ-sĭk″ū-lŏt′ō-mē) [″ + Gr. *tome,* incision]. Surgical incision into a vesicle, as a seminal vesicle.

vesiculotubular (vĕ-sĭk″ū-lō-tū′bū-lăr) [″ + *tubulus,* a tube]. Sounds from auscultation of the chest that have both vesicular and tubular qualities.

vesiculotympanic (vĕ-sĭk′ū-lō-tĭm-păn′ĭk) [″ + Gr. *tympanon,* drum]. Having both vesicular and tympanic qualities.

Vesprin. Trade name for triflupromazine hydrochloride.

vessel (vĕs′ĕl) [O. Fr. from L. *vascellum,* a little vessel]. A tube, duct, or canal to convey the fluids of the body. SYN: *vas* [NA].

RS: anastomose; anastomosis; angiitis; angiodystrophia; arrosion; endothelial; intima; rhegma; vas; vascular.

v.'s, absorbent. The lacteals, lymphatics, and capillaries of the intestines.

v., blood. Any of the vessels carrying blood, i.e., arteries, veins, and capillaries.

v.'s, chyliferous. Vessels arising in the villi of the intestinal walls carrying chyle and terminating in the thoracic duct.

v., collateral. A vessel parallel to the vessel from which it arose.

v.'s, great. The large blood vessels entering and leaving the heart.

v., lacteal. A lymph vessel that collects chyle from the intestinal villi.

v.'s, lymphatic. Vessels conveying lymph.

v.'s, nutrient. Vessels supplying specific areas such as the interior of bones.

v., radicular. Branch of a vertebral artery supplying cerebral nerve root.

vestibular (vĕs-tĭb′ū-lăr) [L. *vestibulum,* vestibule]. Pert. to a vestibule.

vestibular bulbs. Two sacculated collections of veins, lying on either side of the vagina beneath the bulbocavernosus muscle, connected anteriorly by the pars intermedia, and through this strip of cavernous tissue communicating with the erectile tissue of the clitoris. The vestibular bulbs are the homologues of the male corpus spongiosum.

Injury during labor may give rise to troublesome bleeding. SEE: *Bartholin's glands; vagina; vestibule of vagina.*

vestibular nerve. A main division of the auditory nerve. Arises in the vestibular ganglion and is concerned with equilibrium.

vestibule (vĕs′tĭ-būl). A small space or cavity at the beginning of a canal, such as the aortic vestibule.

v., aortic; v. of aorta. The part of the left ventricle of the heart just below the aortic valve.

v. of ear. The middle part of the inner ear, behind the cochlea, and in front of the semicircular canals; it contains the utriculus and sacculus.

v. of larynx. The portion of the larynx above the vocal cords.

v. of mouth. The part of the oral cavity between the lips and the cheeks and between the teeth and the gums.

v. of nose. The anterior part of the nostrils, containing the vibrissae.

v. of pharynx. The space surrounded by the soft palate, base of the tongue, and the palatoglossal and palatopharyngeal arches.

v. of vagina. An almond-shaped space between the lines of attachment of the labia minora. At the anterior angle the clitoris is situated; the posterior boundary is the fourchette. The vestibule is approx. 4 to 5 cm. long and 2 cm. in greatest width when the labia minora are separated. Four major structures open into the vestibule: the urethra anteriorly, the vagina posteriorly, and the two excretory ducts of the glands of Bartholin laterally. The covering membranes are pink in color and constructed of delicate stratified squamous epithelium. Collections of cavernous tissue are disposed beneath the integument. SEE: *Bartholin's glands; vagina; vestibular bulbs.*

vestibulocochlear nerve (vĕs-tĭb″ū-lō-kŏk′lē-ăr) [L. *vestibulum,* vestibule, + *cochlea,* snail shell]. The 8th cranial nerve, which emerges from the brain behind the facial nerve between the pons and medulla oblongata. SYN: *acoustic nerve.* SEE: illus.

vestibuloplasty (vĕs-tĭb′ū-lō-plăs″tē) [″ + Gr. *plassein,* to mold]. Plastic surgery of the vestibule of the mouth.

vestibulotomy (vĕs-tĭb″ū-lŏt′ō-mē) [″ + Gr. *tome,* incision]. Surgical incision into the vestibule of the inner ear.

vestibulourethral (vĕs-tĭb″ū-lō-ū-rē′thrăl) [″ + Gr. *ourethra,* urethra]. Rel. to the vestibule of the vagina and urethra.

vestibulum (vĕs-tĭb′ū-lŭm) [L.]. (pl. *vestibula*) [NA] Vestibule.

vestige (vĕs′tĭj) [L. *vestigium,* footstep]. A small degenerate or incompletely developed structure that has been more fully developed in the embryo or in a previous stage of species.

vestigial (vĕs-tĭj′ē-ăl). Of the nature of a vestige. SYN: *rudimentary.*

vestigium (vĕs-tĭj′ē-ŭm) [L., a footstep]. (pl. *vestigia*) Vestige.

veta (vā′tă) [Sp.]. Mountain sickness, esp. that which occurs in the Andes.

veterinarian (vĕt″ĕr-ĭ-năr′ē-ăn). One who is trained and licensed to practice veterinary

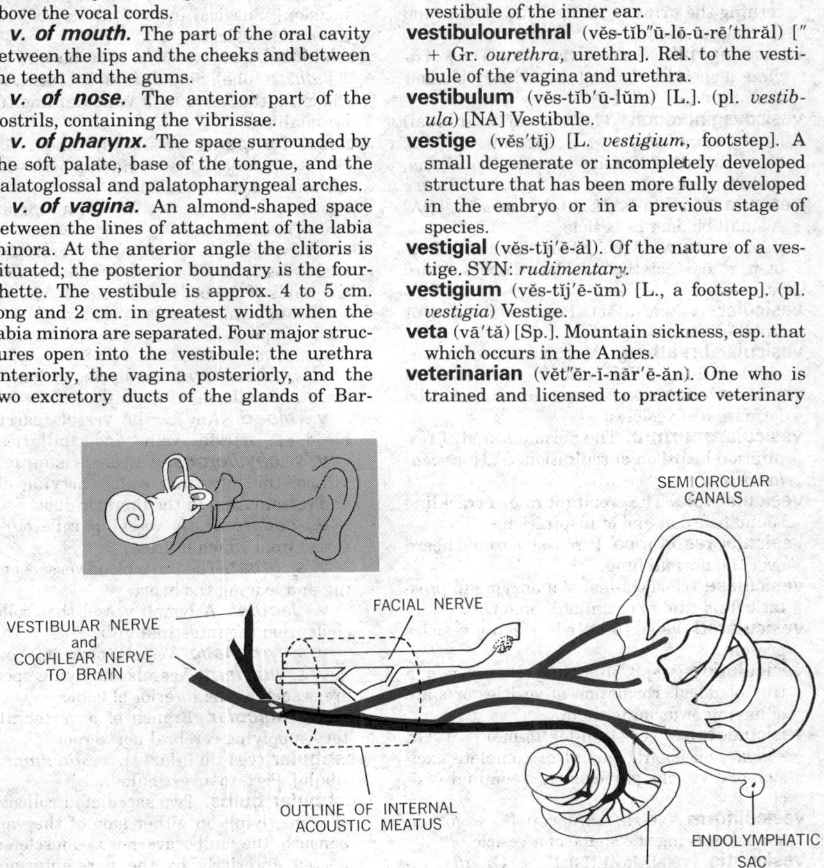

VESTIBULOCOCHLEAR NERVE
(8th CRANIAL)

medicine and surgery.

veterinary (vĕt′ĕr-ĭ-năr′ē). 1. Pert. to animals, their diseases and treatment. 2. A veterinarian.

veterinary medicine. That which deals with diseases of animals and their treatment.

V.F. *vocal fremitus.*

V.H. *viral hepatitis.*

via (vē′ă, vī′ă) [L.]. (pl. *viae*) Any passage in the body such as nasal, intestinal, or vaginal.

viability (vī″ă-bĭl′ĭ-tē) [L. *vita,* life, + *habilis,* fit]. Ability to live, grow, and develop.

viable (vī′ă-bl) [L. *vita,* life, + *habilis,* fit]. Capable of living, as a newborn or a fetus that has reached a stage, usually 28 weeks or older, that will permit it to live outside the uterus.

vial (vī′ăl) [Gr. *phiale,* a drinking cup]. A small glass bottle for medicines or chemicals.

vibex (vī′bĕks) [L. *vibix,* mark of a blow]. (pl. *vibices*) Narrow linear mark, as a line of blood in subcutaneous tissue.

Vibramycin. Trade name for doxycycline, USP.

vibrapuncture (vī″bră-pŭnk′tūr). Medical use of tattoo technique to introduce medicine into skin lesions. Multiple punctures are made into the skin by a needle that has passed through a small amount of the solution of medicine placed on the site.

Vibra Tabs. Trade name for doxycycline hyclate, USP.

vibratile (vī′bră-tĭl) [L. *vibrare,* to shake]. Adapted to or used in vibratory motion; moving to and fro. SEE: *vibratory.*

vibration (vī-brā′shŭn). 1. A to-and-fro movement. SYN: *oscillation.* 2. Therapeutic shaking of the body, a form of massage. Consists of a quick motion of the fingers or the hand vertical to the body or use of a mechanical vibrator.

vibrative (vĭb′ră-tĭv). 1. Vibratory. 2. Indicating sound produced by vibration of parts of the respiratory tract as air passes through.

vibrator (vī′brā-tor) [L. *vibrator,* a shaker]. Device for causing artificial vibration of body or its parts.

vibratory (vī′bră-tō″rē) [L. *vibrator,* a shaker]. Having a vibrating or oscillatory movement.

vibratory sense. The ability to perceive vibrations transmitted through the skin to deep tissues. Usually tested by placing a vibrating tuning fork over bony prominences.

Vibrio (vĭb′rē-ō). A genus of curved, motile, gram-negative bacilli. The only one pathogenic for man is V. cholerae. It is, in fresh culture, shaped like a comma.

V. cholerae. The etiological agent of cholera.

V. fetus. Old name for Campylobacter jejuni.

vibrio (vĭb′rē-ō). (pl. *vibrios*) An organism of the genus Vibrio. SEE: *bacteria* for illus.

vibriocidal (vĭb″rē-ō-sī′dăl). Destructive to vibrio organism.

vibrion (vē″brē-ŏn′) [Fr.]. A vibrio organism.

vibriosis (vĭb″rē-ō′sĭs). Condition of being infected with organisms of the genus Vibrio.

vibrissae (vī-brĭs′ē) [L. *vibrissa,* that which shakes]. (sing. *vibrissa*) Stiff hairs within the nostrils at the anterior nares.

vibromassage (vī″brō-mă-săj′). Massage given by a mechanical vibrator.

vibromasseur (vī″brō-mă-sūr′). Instrument used to produce vibratory massage of the ear.

vibrometer (vī-brŏm′ĕt-ĕr) [L. *vibrare,* to shake, + Gr. *metron,* a measure]. 1. Device that produces rapid vibrations of the membrana tympani. A form of massage treatment for deafness. 2. A device used to measure the vibratory sensation threshold. It is particularly useful in judging the progression or remission of peripheral neuropathy.

vibrotherapeutics (vī″brō-thĕr″ă-pū′tĭks) [″ + Gr. *therapeutike,* treatment]. The therapeutic application of vibration.

vicarious (vī-kā′rē-ŭs) [L. *vicarius,* substitute]. Acting as a substitute; pert. to assumption of the function of one organ by another.

vicarious menstruation. Blood loss during menstruation at some site other than the vagina, as hemorrhage from the nose, the breast, or eyes. SEE: *stigmata.*

vicarious respiration. Increased respiration in one lung when respiration in the other is lessened or abolished.

Vicq d'Azyr's tract (vĭk dă-zērz′). [Felix Vicq d'Azyr, Fr. anatomist, 1748–1794] A large myelinated bundle arising in mammillary nuclei and terminating in anterior thalamic nuclei of the brain.

vidarabine (vī-dăr′ă-bēn). USP. An antiviral agent effective against the herpes simplex and herpes zoster-varicella viruses. It has been successfully used in treating encephalitis due to herpes simplex. Trade name is Vira-A. SYN: *ara-A.*

videognosis (vĭd″ē-ŏg-nō′sĭs) [L. *videre,* to see, + Gr. *gnosis,* knowledge]. Diagnosis utilizing data and roentgenograms transmitted by use of television.

vidian artery (vĭd′ē-ăn). [Guido Guidi (L. *Vidius*), It. physician, 1500–1569] Artery passing through the pterygoid canal of the brain.

vidian canal. A canal in the medial pterygoid plate of the sphenoid bone for transmission of pterygoid (vidian) vessels and nerve. SYN: *pterygoid canal.*

vidian nerve. A branch from the sphenopalatine ganglion. SEE: *Nerves* in *Appendix.*

vigil (vĭj′ĭl) [L., awake]. Insomnia, wakefulness.

v., coma. Condition of muttering delirium in which patient is partially conscious and not completely comatose. SEE: *vigilambulism.*

vigilambulism (vĭj″ĭl-ăm′bū-lĭzm) [″ + *ambulare,* to walk, + Gr. *-ismos,* condition]. Automatism that occurs while the person is awake. Resembles somnambulism.

vigilance (vĭj′ĭ-lăns) [L. *vigilantia*]. Being attentive, alert, and watchful.

vigintinormal (vī-jĭn″tĭ-nor′măl) [L. *viginti,* twenty, + *norma,* rule]. Consisting of one-twentieth of what is normal, as a solution.

vigor (vĭg′or) [L.]. Active force or strength of body or mind.

Villaret's syndrome (vē-lăr-āz′). [Maurice Villaret, Fr. neurologist, 1877–1946] Ipsilateral paralysis of the ninth, tenth, eleventh, twelfth, and sometimes the seventh cranial nerves and the cervical sympathetic fibers. It is caused by a lesion in the posterior retroparotid space. The signs and symptoms include paralysis and anesthesia of the pharyngeal area with difficulty swallowing; loss of taste sensation in the posterior third of the tongue; paralysis of the vocal cords, sternocleidomastoid and trapezius muscles; and Horner's syndrome, q.v.

villi (vĭl′ī) [L.]. Pl. of villus.

v., chorionic. Tiny branching processes of the surface of chorion that become vascular and help to form the placenta.

villiferous (vĭl-ĭf′ĕr-ŭs) [″ + *ferre,* to bear]. Having villi or tufts of hair.

villoma (vĭ-lō′mă) [L. *villus,* tuft of hair + Gr. *oma,* tumor]. A villous tumor.

villose, villous (vĭl′ōs, vĭl′ŭs) [L. *villus,* tuft of hair]. Pert. to or furnished with villi or with fine hairlike extensions.

villositis (vĭl″ōs-ī′tĭs) [″ + Gr. *itis,* inflammation]. Inflammation of the placental villi.

villosity (vĭ-lŏs′ĭ-tē). Condition of being covered with villi.

villus (vĭl′ŭs) [L., tuft of hair]. (pl. *villi*) The short filamentous processes found on certain membranous surfaces.

v., arachnoid. A protrusion of the cerebral arachnoid into the dural wall of a venous sinus or its lacuna.

v., chorionic. Tiny vascular projections of the chorionic surface that help to form the placenta. SEE: *chorion.*

v., intestinal. Multiple, minute projections of the intestinal mucosa into the lumen of the small intestines. These serve to absorb fluids and nutrients. SEE: illus.

v., synovial. Thin projections of synovial membrane into the joint cavity.

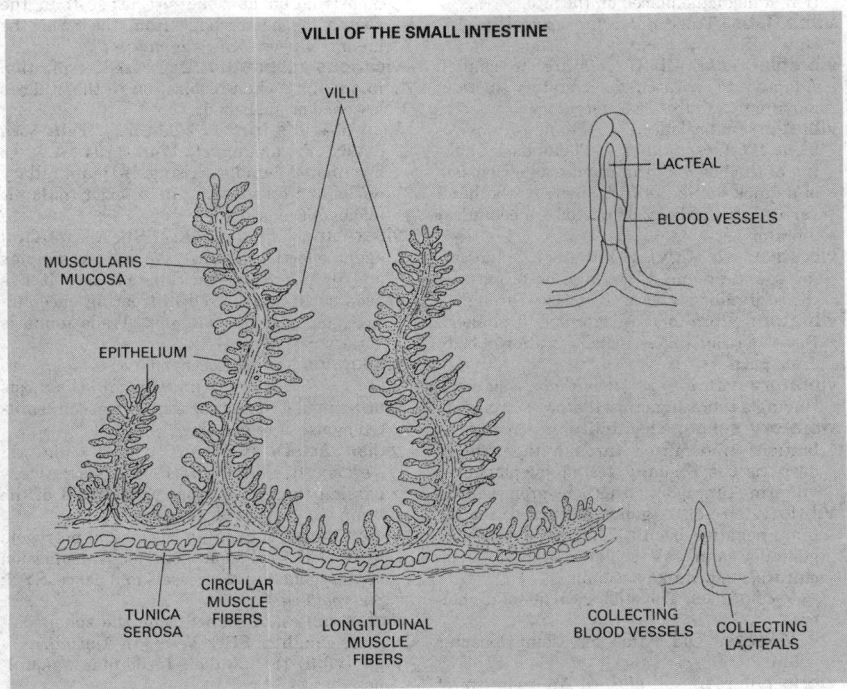

VILLI OF THE SMALL INTESTINE

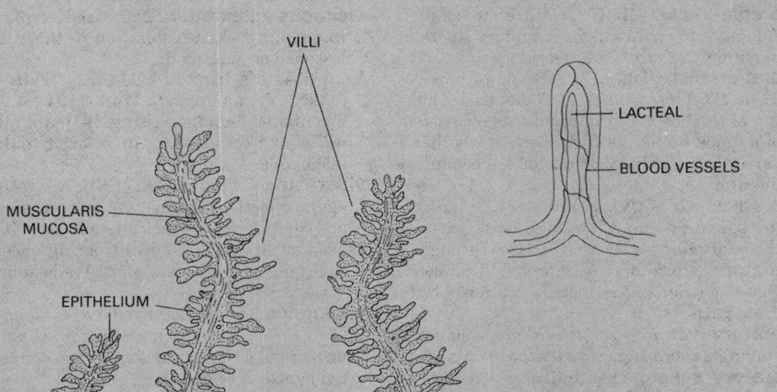

villusectomy (vĭl″ŭs-ĕk′tō-mē) [″ + Gr. *ektome,* excision]. Surgical removal of a synovial villus.

vinblastine sulfate (vĭn-blăs′tēn). USP. A fraction of an extract obtained from the periwinkle plant, Vinca rosea, a species of myrtle. It is a cytotoxic agent used in treating certain types of malignant tumors. CAUTION: Handle vinblastine sulfate with great care, since it is a potent cytotoxic agent. Trade name is Velban.

vinca (vĭn′kă). A genus of herbs including periwinkles, from which vincristine and vinblastine are obtained.

Vincent's angina (vĭn′sĕnts ăn-jī′nă). [Henri Vincent, Fr. physician, 1862–1950] Painful pseudomembranous ulceration of the gums, oral mucous membranes, pharynx, and tonsils. SYN: *gingivitis, Vincent's; trench mouth.* SEE: *Borrelia vincentii.*

ETIOL: Principally Bacteroides melaninogenicus but certain bacilli and spirilla may be involved. Poor oral hygiene, mental and physical stress, and nutritional deficiencies are important predisposing factors as are absorption of heavy metals, such as mercury and bismuth. Not considered to be a contagious disease.

SYM: Painful swelling of lymphatic nodes, inflammation of tonsils extending to floor of mouth. Pseudomembranous exudate, later ulceration; fever.

TREATMENT: In most cases institution of good dental hygiene, proper nutrition, debridement of sloughing gingival tissue by a dentist, discontinuing the use of tobacco, and relief of stress whether physical or emotional will effect a cure. Antibiotic therapy will facilitate recovery from the acute stage but proper nutrition and dental care are essential.

Vincent's disease, gingivitis. SEE: *Vincent's angina.*

vincristine sulfate (vĭn-krĭs′tēn). USP. A fraction of an extract obtained from the periwinkle plant, Vinca rosea, a species of myrtle. It is a cytotoxic agent used in treating certain types of malignant tumors. CAUTION: Handle vincristine sulfate with great care, since it is a potent cytotoxic agent. Trade name is Oncovin.

vinculum (vĭn′kū-lŭm) [L.]. (pl. *vincula*) A uniting band or bundle. SYN: *frenulum; frenum; ligament.*

v. tendinum. 1. Slender tendinous filaments connecting the phalanges with the flexor tendons. 2. The ringlike ligament of the ankle or wrist.

vinegar (vĭn′ĕ-găr) [ME. *vinegre,* from Fr. *vin,* wine, + *aigre,* sour]. The product of the oxidation of fermented alcoholic solutions such as beer or wine. A weak and impure solution of acetic acid. Usually contains 4 to 6% acetic acid. SEE: *condiment.*

vinic (vī′nĭk) [L. *vinum,* wine]. Concerning wine.

vinous (vī′nŭs) [L. *vinum,* wine]. Containing or of the nature of wine.

vinum (vī′nŭm) [L.]. Wine.

vinyl (vī′nĭl). The univalent ethenyl hydrocarbon molecule, $CH_2{=}CH{-}$.

v. chloride. Vinyl radical attached to a chlorine atom, $CH_2{=}CHCl$. Some individuals exposed to vinyl chloride have developed malignant tumors of the lung.

v. cyanide. A toxic liquid compound, $CH_2{=}CHCN$, used in making plastics. SYN: *acrylonitrile.*

v. ether. USP. An anesthetic agent that is virtually obsolete because it is explosive or flammable in the concentration required to produce anesthesia.

Vioform. Trade name for iodochlorhydroxyquin.

violaceous (vī″ĕ-lā′shŭs) [L. *violaceus*]. Having a purple discoloration, esp. of the skin.

violate (vī′ĕ-lāt″) [L. *violare,* to injure]. To harm or injure a person, especially to rape a female.

violence (vī′ō-lĕnts) [L. *violentia*]. 1. The use of force or physical compulsion to abuse or damage. 2. The act of violent behavior.

violet (vī′ō-lĕt) [ME. *violett,* from L. *viola,* violet]. One of the colors of the spectrum; similar to purple.

v., gentian. SEE: *gentian violet,* USP.

violet blindness. Inability to see violet tints.

viomycin (vī-ō-mī′sĭn). An antibiotic produced by strains of Streptomyces griseus.

viosterol (vī-ŏs′tĕr-ōl). A solution of irradiated ergosterol in vegetable oil. SYN: *calciferol.*

viper (vī′pĕr). Any venomous snake of the family Viperidae.

Vira-A. Trade name for vidarabine.

viraginity (vĭr″ă-jĭn′ĭ-tē) [L. *virago,* an amazon or manlike woman]. A condition in which a woman has the feeling she should be a male even though she is aware that her body is female. SEE: *transsexual.*

viral. Pert. to or caused by a virus.

viral interference. The inhibition of the multiplication of one type of virus by the presence of another virus in the same cell. SEE: *interferon.*

Virchow's node (vĕr′kōz). [Rudolf Virchow, Ger. pathologist, 1821–1902] Node, signal, q.v.

viremia (vī″rēm′ē-ă). Presence of viruses in the blood.

vires (vī′rēs). Pl. of vis.

virgin (vĕr′jĭn) [L. *virgo,* a maiden]. 1. A woman or man who has not had sexual intercourse. 2. Uncontaminated; fresh; new.

virginal (vĕr′jĭn-ăl) [L. *virgo,* a maiden]. Relating to a virgin or to virginity.

virginal membrane. The tissue surrounding the entrance to the vagina. Its absence cannot be regarded as proof that the individual has had sexual intercourse. SYN: *hymen.*

virginity (vĕr-jĭn′ĭt-ē) [L. *virginitas,* maidenhood]. The state of being a virgin; not having experienced sexual intercourse.

viricidal (vī-rĭ-sī′dăl) [L. *virus,* poison, + *cidus,* kill]. Destroying or neutralizing a virus. SYN: *virucidal.*

viricide (vĭr′ĭ-sīd). Destructive of viruses. SYN: *virucide.*

virile (vĭr′ĭl) [L. *virilis,* masculine]. Having characteristics of a mature male. SYN: *masculine.*

virile reflex. 1. Sudden downward movement of penis when the prepuce or gland of a completely relaxed penis is pulled upward. SYN: *bulbocavernous reflex.* 2. Contraction of bulbocavernous muscle on percussing dorsum of penis. 3. Contraction of bulbocavernous muscle resulting from compression of glans penis.

virilescence (vĭr-ĭl-ĕs′ĕns) [L. *virilis,* masculine]. The acquisition of secondary masculine characteristics in the female.

virilia (vĭr-ĭl′ē-ă) [L.]. The male sexual organs.

virilism (vĭr′ĭl-ĭzm) [″ + Gr. *-ismos,* condition]. Presence or development of male secondary characteristics in a woman.

virility (vĭr-ĭl′ĭ-tē) [L. *virilitas,* masculinity]. 1. The state of possessing masculine qualities. 2. Sexual potency in the male.

virilization (vĭr″ĭ-lī-zā′shŭn). Production of masculine secondary sex changes in the female. Included would be voice change, development of male-type baldness, clitoral enlargement, and increased growth of facial and body hair. This may be caused by one of several endocrine diseases that lead to excess production of testosterone, or by the female's taking anabolic steroids. In the latter case, this is often done in order to attempt to enhance muscular development.

virion (vī′rē-ŏn, vĭ′rē-ŏn). A complete virus particle; a unit of genetic material surrounded by a protective coat that serves as a vehicle for its transmission from one cell to another. SEE: *capsid.*

viripotent (vī-rĭp′ō-tĕnt) [L. *viripotens*]. 1. Sexually mature, as applied to a male. 2. Marriageable, as applied to a female.

viroids. Small, naked, infectious molecules of RNA. Viroids differ from viruses by the absence of a dormant phase and by genomes that are much smaller than those of known viruses.

virology (vī-rŏl′ō-jē) [L. *virus,* poison, + Gr. *logos,* study]. The study of viruses and viral diseases.

viropexis (vī″rō-pĕk′sĭs) [″ + Gr. *pexis,* fixation]. The fixation of a virus particle to a cell. This leads to the inclusion of the virus inside the cell.

Viroptic. Trade name for trifluridine.

virose, virous (vī′rōs, vī′rŭs) [L. *virus,* poison]. Having poisonous qualities or effects. SYN: *poisonous.*

virtual (vĕr′tū-ăl) [L. *virtus,* capacity]. Appearing to exist but not in actual fact or form.

virucidal (vĭr-ū-sī′dăl) [L. *virus,* poison, + *cidus,* to kill]. Destructive of a virus. SYN: *viricidal.*

virucide. An agent that destroys or inactivates a virus, esp. a chemical substance used on living tissue.

virulence (vĭr′ū-lĕns) [L. *virulentia,* a stench]. 1. Relative power and degree of pathogenicity possessed by organisms to produce disease. 2. Property of being virulent; venomousness, as of a disease. SEE: *attenuation.*

virulent (vĭr′ū-lĕnt) [L. *virulentus,* full of poison]. 1. Very poisonous. 2. Infectious; able to overcome the host's defensive mechanism.

viruliferous (vĭr-ū-lĭf′ĕr-ŭs) [L. *virus,* poison, + *ferre,* to bear]. Conveying or producing a virus.

viruria (vĭr-ūr′ē-ă) [″ + Gr. *ouron,* urine]. Presence of viruses in the urine.

virus (vī′rŭs) [L. *virus,* poison]. A minute organism not visible with ordinary light microscopy and a parasite dependent on nutrients inside cells for its metabolic and reproductive needs. Some bacteria share these properties but not the distinctive features of viruses such as their simple organization and composition and their mechanism of replication. Viruses can be seen by use of electron microscopy. They consist of a strand of either deoxyribonucleic acid (DNA) or ribonucleic acid (RNA) but not both, separated by a capsid, a covering of protein.

More than 300 viruses have been isolated from animals; some of these appear to be harmless to man. However, viruses cause a variety of important infectious diseases, among them the common cold, smallpox, yellow fever, most childhood diseases, and the majority of infections of the upper respiratory passages. Certain viruses cause cancer in laboratory animals, but evidence they cause cancer in man is inconclusive.

A virus was first synthesized in the laboratory in 1967. This was done by using natural virus DNA as a template for forming the synthetic virus DNA.

CLASSIFICATION: There are a variety of ways to classify viruses. Not all will be given here, but the more generally accepted types of classification follow. They may be broken down into two groups according to whether they contain DNA or RNA, with these groups further classified. They may be classed as to the host they dominate: bacteria (bacteriophages), animal, or plant.

They are also classified as to origin (reoviruses), mode of transportation (arboviruses), manifestation they produce in the host (polioviruses), and geographical site first located (coxsackievirus).

RS: adenovirus; arboviruses; capsid; coxsackievirus; deoxyribonucleic acid; ECHO virus; enterovirus; herpesvirus; microscope, electron; myxoviruses; papovaviruses; paramyxoviruses; picornaviruses; poliovirus; poxvirus; reovirus; rhabdovirus; rhinovirus; ribonucleic acid.

v., arbor. Former name for arboviruses, q.v.

v., attenuated. A virus with reduced pathogenicity due to treatment or repeated passage through hosts.

v., bacterial. A virus capable of inducing lysis or dissolution of certain bacterial cells. SYN: *bacteriophage.*

v., coxsackie. SEE: *coxsackievirus.*

v., cytomegalic. A member of herpesvirus family that is widely distributed and causes clinically detectable disease in infants up to 4 months of age. It is transmitted either transplacentally or at the time of birth to the fetus from a mother with a latent infection. The virus may also be transmitted by blood transfusion. SYN: *cytomegalovirus.*

v., defective. A virus particle that is because of lack of certain essential factors unable to replicate. Sometimes this can be overcome by the presence of a helper virus that provides the missing factor or factors.

v., EB. Epstein-Barr virus, q.v.

v., ECHO. [*E*nteric *C*ytopathogenic *H*uman *O*rphan] Virus that was accidentally discovered in human feces and not known to be associated with a disease, thus the name "orphan." Initially 33 ECHO virus serotypes were designated but numbers 10 and 28 have been reclassified. Various serotypes have been associated with aseptic meningitis, encephalitis, acute upper respiratory infection, enteritis, pleurodynia, and myocarditis.

v., enteric. Enterovirus, q.v.

v., enteric orphan. SEE: *v., ECHO.*

v., filtrable. A virus causing infectious disease, the essential elements of which are so tiny that they retain infectivity after passing through a filter of the Berkefeld type. SEE: *filter, Berkefeld.*

v. fixé, v., fixed. Rabies virus that was stabilized and modified but only partially attenuated by serial passage through rabbits.

v., helper. A virus that permits a defective virus present in the same cell to replicate. SEE: *v., defective.*

v., herpes. SEE: *herpesvirus.*

v., latent. Some viruses have the ability to infect the host initially but cause little or no signs of illness; but they persist for the lifetime of the infected individual. Later on, a specific triggering mechanism may cause the virus to produce a clinically apparent disease. This occurs with herpes simplex virus that remains latent in sensory ganglia and is reactivated by trauma to the skin supplied by the distal sensory nerves associated with these ganglia. After reactivation, the virus may cause localized or generalized lesions in the affected area and the central nervous system.

v., lytic. Any virus that after infecting a cell, lyses it.

v., masked. A virus that ordinarily occurs in the host in a noninfective state but is activated and demonstrated by indirect methods.

v., neurotropic. Viruses that reproduce in nervous tissue.

v.'s, orphan. Viruses that initially were thought not to be associated with pathogenicity. However, since then a number of them have been shown to be associated with disease. Includes enteroviruses and rhinoviruses.

v., parainfluenza. One of a group of viruses that affect infants and young children. Causes respiratory infections that may be mild or may progress to pneumonia. Most infections are so mild as to be clinically inapparent.

v., plant. Any virus that is pathogenic for plants.

v., pox. Poxvirus, q.v.

v., respiratory syncytial. A virus that is a major cause of lower respiratory tract disease during infancy and early childhood. It induces formation of large syncytial masses in cell cultures, and this led to its being so named. Attempts to develop an effective and safe vaccine have been in vain. Because it is difficult to recognize the disease early and inapparent cases are frequent, isolation and public health measures are not adequate to control the spread of the disease.

v., slow. SEE: *slow virus infection.*

v., street. Rabies virus obtained from an infected animal rather than from a laboratory strain.

v., tumor. Tumor viruses, q.v.

virusemia (vī″rŭs-ēm′ē-ă) [″ + Gr. *haima*, blood]. Virus in the blood. SYN: *viremia.*

virustatic (vīr″ŭ-stăt′ĭk) [″ + Gr. *statikos*, bringing to a standstill]. Stopping the growth of viruses.

vis (vĭs) [L.]. (pl. *vires*) Force, strength, energy, power.

v. afronte. Force that attracts.

v. formativa. Energy resulting in development of new tissue.

v. medicatrix naturae. The healing power of nature.

viscera (vĭs′ĕr-ă) [L.]. (sing. *viscus*) Internal organs enclosed within a cavity, esp. the abdominal organs. SEE: *celosomia; evisceration; splanchnic.*

viscerad (vĭs′ĕr-ăd) [″ + *ad,* toward]. Toward the viscera.

visceral (vĭs′ĕr-ăl) [L. *viscera,* body organs]. 1. Pert. to viscera. 2. Pert. to or derived from the gill arches of vertebrates.

visceral arches. Branchial arches.

visceral cavity. Body cavity containing the viscera.

visceral clefts. The fissures separating the visceral arches.

visceralgia (vĭs″ĕr-ăl′jē-ă) [″ + Gr. *algos,* pain]. Neuralgia of any of the viscera.

visceral skeleton. The pelvis, ribs, and sternum enclosing the viscera.

viscerimotor (vĭs″ĕr-ĭ-mō′tor) [″ + *motor,* mover]. A nerve supplying motor stimuli to a viscus. SYN: *visceromotor.*

viscero- (vĭs′ĕr-ō) [L. *viscera,* body organs]. Combining form meaning pertaining to the viscera.

viscerocranium (vĭs″ĕr-ō-krā′nē-ŭm). That portion of the skull derived from the pharyngeal arches.

viscerogenic (vĭs″ĕr-ō-jĕn′ĭk) [″ + Gr. *gennan,* to produce]. Originating in the viscera.

visceroinhibitory (vĭs″ĕr-ō-ĭn-hĭb′ĭ-tō-rē) [″ + *inhibere,* to restrain]. Checking the action of the viscera.

visceromegaly (vĭs″ĕr-ō-mĕg′ă-lē) [″ + Gr. *megalos,* great]. Generalized enlargement of the abdominal visceral organs.

visceromotor (vĭs″ĕr-ō-mō′tor) [L. *viscera,* body organs + *motor,* a mover]. Conveying motor impulses to the viscera.

visceromotor reflex. Increase in tonus of abdominal muscles resulting from painful stimuli originating in a viscus.

visceroparietal (vĭs″ĕr-ō-pă-rī′ĕ-tăl) [″ + *paries,* wall]. Rel. to the viscera and the abdominal wall.

visceroperitoneal (vĭs″ĕr-ō-pĕr″ĭ-tō-nē′ăl) [″ + Gr. *peritonaion,* peritoneum]. Rel. to the abdominal viscera and peritoneum.

visceropleural (vĭs″ĕr-ō-ploo′răl) [″ + Gr. *pleura,* a side]. Rel. to the thoracic viscera and the pleura. SYN: *pleurovisceral.*

visceroptosis (vĭs″ĕr-ŏp-tō′sĭs) [″ + Gr. *ptosis,* fall]. Downward displacement of a viscus.

visceroreceptors (vĭs″ĕr-ō-rē-sĕp′torz). A group of receptors that includes those located in visceral organs. Their stimulation gives rise to poorly localized and ill-defined sensations. In hollow visceral organs they are stimulated principally by excessive contraction or by distention.

viscerosensory (vĭs″ĕr-ō-sĕn′sō-rē) [″ + *sensorius,* sensory]. Pert. to sensations aroused by stimulation of visceroreceptors.

viscerosensory reflex. Pain or tenderness elicited in somatic structures (skin and muscle) due to visceral disorder. SEE: *referred pain.*

visceroskeletal (vĭs″ĕr-ō-skĕl′ĕt-ăl) [″ + Gr. *skeleton,* skeleton]. Rel. to the visceral skeleton.

viscerosomatic (vĭs″ĕr-ō-sō-măt′ĭk) [″ + Gr. *soma,* body]. Rel. to the viscera and the body.

viscerosomatic reaction. A reaction occurring in muscles of the body wall as a result of stimulation of visceroreceptors.

viscerotome (vĭs′ĕr-ō-tōm) [″ + Gr. *tome,* incision]. 1. An instrument used at autopsy for obtaining a specimen of the liver for microscopic examination. 2. That part of an abdominal organ that is supplied with afferent nerves from a single posterior root.

viscerotonia (vĭs″ĕr-ō-tōn′ē-ă) [″ + Gr. *tonos,* tension]. Personality traits characterized by predominance of social over intellectual and physical traits. Individual is sociable and convivial, exhibits gluttony for food, and loves company, affection, and social support.

viscerotrophic (vĭs″ĕr-ō-trŏf′ĭk) [″ + Gr. *trophe,* nourishment]. Pertaining to trophic conditions related to or associated with visceral conditions.

viscerotropic (vĭs″ĕr-ō-trŏp′ĭk) [″ + Gr. *tropos,* a turn]. Primarily affecting the viscera.

viscerovisceral reaction (vĭs″ĕr-ō-vĭs′ĕr-ăl). A reaction taking place in the viscera as a result of stimulation of visceral receptors. Such reactions are usually below the level of consciousness.

viscid (vĭs′ĭd) [L. *viscidus,* sticky]. Adhering, glutinous, sticky. In bacteriology, said of a colony that strings out by clinging to a needle when it is touched to the culture and withdrawn. The sediment rises in a coherent whirl when the liquid culture is shaken.

viscidity (vĭ-sĭd′ĭ-tē). The property of being viscid or sticky. SYN: *viscosity.*

viscometer (vĭs-kŏm′ĕ-tĕr). Viscosimeter.

viscosimeter (vĭs″kŏs-ĭm′ĕ-tĕr) [L. *viscosus,* sticky, + Gr. *metron,* a measure]. Device for estimating the viscosity of a fluid, esp. of blood.

viscosimetry (vĭs″kō-sĭm′ĕ-trē). Measurement of the viscosity of a substance.

viscosity (vĭs″kŏs′ĭ-tē) [L. *viscosus,* sticky]. 1. State of being sticky or gummy. 2. Resistance offered by a fluid to change of form or relative position of its particles due to attraction of molecules to each other.

v., specific. The internal friction of a fluid, measured by comparing the rate of flow of the liquid through a tube with that of some standard liquid, or by measuring the resistance to rotating paddles.

viscous (vĭs′kŭs). Sticky, gummy, gelatinous, with high viscosity.

viscus (vĭs′kŭs) [L., body organ]. (pl. *viscera*) Any internal organ enclosed within a cavity, such as the thorax or abdomen.

visibility (vĭz″ĭ-bĭl′ĭ-tē) [L. *visibilitas*]. Quality of being visible.

visible (vĭz′ĭ-bl) [L. *visibilis*]. Capable of being seen.

visile (vĭz′ĭl) [L. *visum,* seeing]. 1. Pert. to vision. 2. Readily recalling what is seen, more than that which is audible or motile.

vision (vĭzh′ŭn) [L. *visio,* a seeing]. 1. Act of viewing external objects. SYN: *sight.* 2. Sense by which light and color are apprehended. 3. An imaginary sight.

v., achromatic. Complete color blindness.

v., artificial. A technique, still in experimental stage, designed to make it possible for some blind persons to see. SEE: *Optacon.*

v., binocular. Visual sensation that is produced when the images perceived by each eye are fused to appear as one.

v., central. Vision resulting from rays falling on the fovea centralis.

v., day. Condition in which patient sees better during the day than at night, found in peripheral lesions of the retina such as retinitis pigmentosa.

v., dichromatic. A form of defective color vision in which only two of the primary colors are perceived.

v., double. Seeing of one object as two. SYN: *diplopia.*

v., field of. The space within which an object can be seen while the eye remains fixed on one point.

v., half. Blindness in one or both eyes for half of the visual field. SYN: *hemianopia.*

v., indirect. V., peripheral, q.v.

v., monocular. Vision utilizing only one eye.

v., multiple. Seeing of one object as two or more. SYN: *polyopia.*

v., night. Ability to see when illumination is reduced.

v., oscillating. Oscillopsia, q.v.

v., peripheral. Vision resulting from rays falling on the retina outside of the macular field.

v., phantom. An experience of visual sensations in an eye that has been surgically removed. Usually a transient condition.

v., tunnel. Tunnel vision, q.v.

vision, words pert. to: aberration; accommodation; aftercataract; afterimage; amblyopia; ametropia; anopsia; anotropia; asthenope; asthenopia; astigmatic; astigmatism; bifocal; blind; chloropsia; chromatic; chromatopsia; chromopsia; convergence; cyclophoria; diplopia; emmetropia; erythropsia; farpoint; farsightedness; glare; halation; hypermetropia; hypometropia; image; macropsia; metamorphosis; micropsia; muscae volitantes; myope; myopia; night blindness; night vision; nyctalopia; nyctamblyopia; nyctotyphlosis; ocular; oculist; scintillation; scotoma; second sight; strabismus; vergence; visile; visual; xanthopsia; words ending in "-phoria."

visit. An encounter between a patient or client and a health professional that requires either the client to travel from his home to the professional's usual place of practice (office visit) or vice versa (home visit).

visiting nurse association. A voluntary health agency that provides nursing services in the home, including health supervision, education and counseling, and maintenance of the medical regimen. Nurses and other personnel such as home health aides who are specifically trained for tasks of personal bedside care provide the services offered by the agency. These agencies had their origin in the visiting or district nurse service provided to the poor in their homes by voluntary agencies such as the New York City Mission, which existed in the 1870s. The first visiting nurse associations were established in Buffalo, Boston, and Philadelphia between 1886 and 1887.

Vistaril Pamoate. Trade name for hydroxyzine pamoate.

Vistaril Parenteral. Trade name for hydroxyzine hydrochloride.

visual (vĭzh′ū-ăl) [L. *visio,* a seeing]. 1. Pert. to vision. 2. One whose learning and memorizing processes are largely of a visual nature.

visual acuity. A measure of the resolving power of the eye. Usually determined by having the subject read letters of various sizes at a standard distance from the test chart. The result is expressed as a fraction. For example, 20/20 is normal vision. This means the subject's eyes have the ability to see from a distance of 20 feet (6.1 meters) what the normal eye would see at that distance. 20/40 means that a person sees at 20 feet (6.1 meters) what the normal eye could see at 40 feet (12.2 meters).

visual angle. Angle between line of sight and the extremities of object seen.

visual axis. The line of vision from object seen through the pupil's center to macula lutea.

visual cone. The cone whose vertex is at the eye and whose generating lines touch the boundary of a visible object.

visual field. The area within which objects may be seen when the eye is fixed. SEE: *perimetry.*

visualization (vĭzh″ū-ăl-ī-zā′shŭn). The act of viewing or sensing a picture of an object, esp. the picture of a body structure as obtained by x-ray study.
visualize (vĭzh′ū-ăl-īz). 1. To make visible. 2. To imagine or picture something in one's mind.
visual plane. The plane in which both optic axes lie.
visual point. Center of vision.
visual yellow. A pigment formed in the retina by the action of light on rhodopsin.
visuoauditory (vĭzh″ū-ō-aw′dĭ-tor″ē) [L. *visio,* a seeing, + *auditorius,* pert. to hearing]. Rel. to sight and hearing, as connecting nerve fibers between auditory and visual centers.
visuognosis (vĭzh″ū-ŏg-nō′sĭs) [″ + Gr. *gnosis,* knowledge]. The recognition and appreciation of what is seen.
visuopsychic (vĭzh″ū-ō-sī′kĭk) [″ + Gr. *psyche,* soul]. Both visual and psychic, applied to cerebral area involved in apprehension of visual sensations.
visuosensory (vĭzh″ū-ō-sĕn′sō-rē) [L. *visio,* a seeing, + *sensorius,* sensory]. Rel. to the recognition of visual impressions.
vitaglass (vī′tă-glăs) [L. *vita,* life + AS. *glaes,* glass]. Window glass containing quartz for transmitting the ultraviolet rays of sunlight.
vital (vī′tăl) [L. *vitalis,* pert. to life]. 1. Pert. to or characteristic of life. 2. Contributing to or essential for life.
vital capacity. Volume of air that can be expelled following full inspiration.
vital capacity, timed. Test of vital capacity of the lungs expressed with respect to the volume of air that can be quickly and forcibly breathed out in a certain amount of time. SEE: *FEV_1*.
vital center. Respiratory center in the medulla.
vitalism (vī′tăl-ĭzm) [″ + Gr. *-ismos,* condition]. The opinion that a force neither chemical nor mechanical is responsible for the phenomenon of life.
vitalist (vī′tăl-ĭst) [L. *vitalis,* pert. to life]. One who believes in vitalism.
vitalistic (vī-tăl-ĭs′tĭk). Relating to vitalism.
vitality (vī-tăl′ĭ-tē). 1. That which distinguishes living things from the nonliving. 2. Animation, action. 3. State of being alive.
vitalize (vī′tăl-īz). To instill life or force in anything.
vital signs. The traditional signs of life, i.e., heart beat, body temperature, respiration, and blood pressure.
vital statistics. Statistics relating to births (natality), deaths (mortality), marriages, health, and disease (morbidity). Vital statistics for the U.S.A. are published annually by the National Center for Health Statistics of the Department of Health and Human Services.
vitamer (vī′tă-mĕr). Any one of a number of compounds that have specific vitamin activity.
vitamin (vī′tă-mĭn) [L. *vita,* life, + *amine*]. Any of a group of organic substances other than proteins, carbohydrates, fats, minerals, and organic salts which are essential for normal metabolism, growth, and development of the body. Vitamins are not sources of energy nor do they contribute significantly to the substance of the body. They are indispensable for the maintenance of health. They are effective in minute quantities. They act principally as regulators of metabolic processes and play a role in energy transformations, usually acting as coenzymes in enzymatic systems.

Vitamins are extremely complex chemical substances, but the nature, chemical structure, and composition of most of them are known. Most have been isolated and some have been synthesized. In general, none of the vitamins can be formed in the body but must be obtained preformed from animal or plant sources. Exceptions to the above are the formation of vitamin A from its precursor, carotene, the formation of vitamin D by the action of ultraviolet light on the skin, and the formation of vitamin K by symbiotic bacteria of the intestines. Some vitamins are unstable, being readily destroyed by oxidation, heat, esp. in an alkaline medium, strong acids, light, and aging. SEE: *Vitamins* in *Appendix.*

There are several broad classifications of vitamins, for example, the fat-soluble vitamins (A, D, E, and K) and the water-soluble (B and C). This is of clinical importance in patients with diseases that interfere with digestion of fat, because they will eventually develop deficiencies of the fat-soluble vitamins, which are essential to body growth, development, and function. Certain vitamins cannot be manufactured by certain species. Man is one of the few species that cannot manufacture vitamin C.

A variety of conditions increase the need for vitamins above the usual recommended dose. These include lactation, pregnancy, use of certain drugs, excess use of alcohol or tobacco, and certain illnesses.

RS: avitaminosis; deficiency disease.

v., antiberiberi. Thiamine; vitamin B_1.
v., antidermatitis. Vitamin B_6.
v., antihemorrhagic. Vitamin K.
v., anti-infective. Vitamin A.
v., antineuritic. Thiamine (B_1).
v., antipellagra. Nicotinamide.
v., antirachitic. The vitamin D group.
v., antiscorbutic. Vitamin C.

v., antixerophthalmic. Vitamin A.
v., coagulation. Vitamin K.

vitamin A. USP. A fat-soluble vitamin formed in the body from precursors, yellow pigments of plants (alpha, beta, and gamma carotene). It is essential for normal growth and development, the integrity of epithelial tissues, and for normal tooth and bone development. It is stored in the liver. Trade names are Acon, Alphalin, and Aquasol. SYN: *retinol; vitamin, anti-infective*. SEE: *Vitamins* in *Appendix*.

ACTION: Essential to the normal function of epithelial cells and the formation of visual purple.

STABILITY: Resists boiling for some time if not exposed to oxidation. Quite stable to brief exposure to heat but not to continued high temperatures (above 100° C. or 212° F.). Vitamin A is present in fish liver oils, egg yolks, liver, butter, cream, green leafy vegetables, and yellow vegetables such as carrots.

DEFICIENCY DISORDERS: Interference with growth, reduced resistance to infections, interference with nutrition of cornea, conjunctiva, trachea, hair follicles, and renal pelvis. Thus these tissues have an increased susceptibility to infections. Interference with ability of eyes to adapt to darkness (night blindness). Visual acuity will also be impaired. Children will experience impaired growth and development. SEE: *Bitot's spots*.

SOURCES: Butter, butterfat in milk, egg yolks, and cod liver oil are rich sources. Liver; green leafy and yellow vegetables and some fruits: prunes, pineapples, oranges, limes, and cantaloupes.

vitamin A_1. Form of vitamin A found in fish liver oils.

vitamin A_2. A compound found in the livers of freshwater fish. Similar in properties to vitamin A but with different ultraviolet absorption spectra.

vitamin B complex. A group of water-soluble vitamins isolated from liver, yeast, and other sources. Only grain-made yeast that is dried at once preserves its potency. Among vitamins included are thiamine (B_1), riboflavin (B_2), niacin (nicotinic acid), pyridoxine (B_6), biotin, folic acid, and cyanocobalamin (B_{12}).

ACTION: Affects growth, appetite, lactation, and the gastrointestinal, nervous, and endocrine systems; aids in marasmus and lymphocytosis; stimulates appetite; reduces sugar content in diabetes; stimulates biliary action; aids in treating tuberculosis; and is necessary for carbohydrate metabolism.

B_1, thiamine, affects growth and nutrition and carbohydrate metabolism. B_2, riboflavin, affects growth and cellular metabolism. Nicotinic acid prevents pellagra.

Although not destroyed by ordinary cooking, B complex vitamins may be destroyed by excessive heating for 2 to 4 hours. Bicarbonate of soda used in cooking aids destruction. Riboflavin and nicotinic acid, more stable than thiamine, are not destroyed by heat or oxidation.

NOTE: Prolonged use of antibiotics may destroy the intestinal bacteria that normally produce some of the B vitamins. In those cases supplemental vitamins will be required.

DEFICIENCY DISORDERS: Beriberi, pellagra, digestive disturbances, enlargement of liver, disturbance of the thyroid, degeneration of sex glands, disturbance of the nervous system. Deficiency induces edema, affects the heart, liver, spleen, and kidneys, enlarges the adrenals, and causes dysfunction of the pituitary and salivary glands.

SOURCES: *Thiamine:* Whole grains, wheat embryo, brewer's yeast, legumes, nuts, egg yolk, fruits, and vegetables. *Riboflavin:* Brewer's yeast, liver, meat, esp. pork and fish, poultry, eggs, milk, and green vegetables. *Nicotinic acid:* Brewer's yeast, liver, meat, poultry, and green vegetables. *Pyridoxine:* Rice, bran, yeast. *Folic acid:* Leafy green vegetables, organ meats, lean beef and veal, wheat cereals.

STABILITY: Long-continued cooking or high-temperature cooking destroys vitamin B; bicarbonate of soda used in cooking aids its destruction. Ordinary cooking or heat does not destroy it.

vitamin B_1. Thiamine, or thiamine hydrochloride. Recommended daily allowance: 0.5 mg. per 1000 Cal. SEE: *Vitamins* in *Appendix*.

vitamin B_2. Riboflavin. SEE: *Vitamins* in *Appendix*.

vitamin B_6. Pyridoxine. Found in rice, bran, and yeast. SEE: *Vitamins* in *Appendix*.

vitamin B_{12}. A red crystalline substance extracted from liver that is essential for the formation of red blood cells. Its deficiency results in pernicious anemia. It is used for prophylaxis and treatment of these and other diseases in which there is defective red cell formation. Recommended daily requirement: 5 μg. per day for adults. SYN: *cyanocobalamin. SEE: Vitamins* in *Appendix*.

vitamin C. Ascorbic acid, a factor necessary for formation of intercellular substance of connective tissue and essential in maintenance of integrity of intercellular cement in many tissues, especially capillary walls. Deficiency leads to scurvy. SYN: *ascorbic acid*. SEE: *Vitamins* in *Appendix*.

NOTE: Large daily doses of vitamin C have been recommended for prevention and treatment of the common cold. Although the effectiveness of vitamin C for this purpose has not been established, it is felt that the vitamin may at least decrease the severity of symptoms of a cold.

STABILITY: Destroyed easily by heat in the presence of oxygen, as in open-kettle boiling. Less affected by heat in an acid medium; otherwise stable.

DEFICIENCY DISORDERS: Scurvy, imperfect prenatal skeletal formation, defective teeth, pyorrhea, anorexia, anemia, undernutrition injury to bone, cells, and blood vessels.

SOURCES: Raw cabbage, young carrots, orange juice, lettuce, celery, onions, tomatoes, radishes, and green peppers. Citrus fruits are especially rich in this vitamin. Strawberries are about as rich a source as tomatoes. Apples, pears, apricots, plums, peaches, and pineapples. Rutabagas are also rich in this vitamin.

vitamin D. One of several vitamins having antirachitic activity. The vitamin D group, which is fat-soluble, includes D_2 (calciferol), D_3 (irradiated 7-dehydrocholesterol), D_4 (irradiated 22-dihydroergosterol), and D_5 (irradiated dehydrositosterol). It is essential in calcium and phosphorus metabolism; consequently it is required for normal development of bones and teeth. SEE: *Vitamins* in *Appendix.*

ACTION: Related to utilization of calcium and phosphorus in blood and bone building. It is called the antirachitic vitamin because deficiency of it interferes with calcium and phophorus utilization, which in turn causes rickets, q.v. Exposure to the sun or ultraviolet radiation synthesizes this vitamin in the body. Necessary for most efficient absorption of calcium and phosphorus. A specific in treatment of infantile rickets, spasmophilia (infantile tetany), and softening of bone; valuable also in prevention of these conditions. Important in normal growth and mineralization of skeleton and teeth.

DEFICIENCY DISORDERS: Imperfect skeletal formation; bone diseases; rickets; caries.

SOURCES: Milk; cod liver oil; salmon and cod livers; egg yolk; butter fat. Ergosterol in the skin activated by sunlight or ultraviolet radiation possesses vitamin D potency.

STABILITY: Not affected by oxidation or by heat unless over 100° C. (212° F.) or long-continued cooking.

vitamin E. USP. An essential nutrient for man, although the exact biochemical mechanism whereby vitamin E functions in the body is unknown. Because of the amount of vitamin E present in foods, deficiency of this vitamin is absent in the general population. SYN: *alpha tocopherol.* SEE: *Vitamins* in *Appendix.*

vitamin K. An antihemorrhagic factor whose activity is associated with compounds derived from naphthoquinone. Vitamin K, which is fat-soluble, is present in alfalfa; vitamin K_2 in fishmeal; vitamin K_3 is synthesized as menadione sodium bisulfite. Vitamin K aids blood coagulation and is necessary for formation of prothrombin. Its deficiency prolongs blood-clotting time and causes hemorrhages. Vitamin K is not present in the digestive tract of newborn infants until food is ingested and bacteria produced in the intestines to synthesize vitamin K. Thus an intramuscular injection of 1 mg. of water-soluble vitamin K_1 (phytonadione) is recommended for all infants. SEE: *Vitamins* in *Appendix.*

ACTION: Helps to eliminate prolonged bleeding in operations and in biliary tract of jaundiced patients. Bile salts necessary for its absorption.

SOURCES: Found in fats, fishmeal, oats, wheat, rye, and alfalfa.

vitamin loss. Loss of vitamin content in food products because of vitamin instability, esp. in oxidation and during heating. Methods of preserving foods add to the loss of vitamins. Pickling, salting, curing, or fermenting processes usually cause complete loss of vitamin C. Commercial canning destroys from 50 to 85% of vitamin C contained in peas, lima beans, spinach and asparagus. Pasteurization, unless special precautions are observed, causes a loss of from 30 to 60% of vitamin C. Apple pie and freshly prepared applesauce retain only from 20 to 30% of the vitamin C value of the apple. Vitamin B_1 in wheat is lost though milling because the wheat embryo, rich in vitamin B_1, is removed in milling.

vitaminoid (vī′tă-mĭn-oyd) [*vitamin* + Gr. *eidos,* resemblance]. Of the nature of vitamin.

vitaminology (vī″tă-mĭn-ŏl′ō-jē). Study of vitamins.

vitellary (vĭt′ĕl-ā-rē) [L. *vitellus,* yolk of an egg]. Pert. to the vitellus. SYN: *vitelline.*

vitellin (vī-tĕl′ĭn). A protein that can be extracted from egg yolk and contains lecithin. SEE: *nucleoprotein; ovovitellin.*

vitelline (vī-tĕl′ēn). Pert. to the yolk of an egg or the ovum.

vitelline circulation. The embryonic circulation of blood to the yolk sac via vitelline arteries and its return to general circulation through the vitelline veins.

vitelline duct. The narrow duct connecting the yolk sac with the embryonic gut.

vitelline membrane. 1. The membrane forming the surface layer of an ovum. 2. In a chicken egg, the membrane forming the surface layer of the vitellus or yolk.

vitelline veins. Two veins conveying blood

from the yolk sac.

vitellogenesis (vī″tĕl-ō-jĕn′ĕ-sĭs). Production of yolk.

vitellointestinal (vī′tĕl-ō-ĭn-tĕs″tĭn-ăl). Concerning the embryonic yolk sac and the intestinal tract.

vitellolutein (vī″tĕl-ō-lū′tē-ĭn) [L. *vitellus,* yolk, + *luteus,* yellow]. Yellow pigment present in lutein.

vitellorubin (vī″tĕl-ō-rū′bĭn) [″ + *ruber,* red]. Red pigment present in lutein.

vitellose (vī-tĕl′ōs). A proteose present in vitellin.

vitellus (vī-tĕl′ŭs) [L.]. The yolk of an ovum, esp. the yolk of a hen's egg.

vitiation (vĭsh″ē-ā′shŭn) [L. *vitiare,* to corrupt]. Injury, contamination, impairment of use or efficiency.

vitiligines (vĭt″ĭ-lĭj′ĭ-nēz). Depigmented areas of skin. SEE: *vitiligo.*

vitiliginous (vĭt″ĭ-lĭj′ĭ-nŭs). Concerning vitiligo.

vitiligo (vĭt-ĭl-ī′gō) [L.]. An acquired cutaneous affection characterized by milk-white patches, surrounded by areas of normal pigmentation. More common in the tropics and in blacks. Cause unknown. SYN: *leukoderma; piebald skin.*

TREATMENT: Oral and topical synthetic trioxsalen, USP, and a natural psoralen, methoxsalen, USP, are used with exposure to long-wave ultraviolet light but the efficacy is doubtful. The lesions may be masked by use of cosmetic preparations. Vitiliginous areas should be protected from sunburn by applying a 5% aminobenzoic acid solution or gel to the affected areas.

v. capitis. Vitiligo of the scalp with depigmentation of the hairs of the affected area.

v. perinevoid. Vitiligo surrounding a nevus.

vitiligoidea (vĭt″ĭl-ĭg-oy′dē-ă) [″ + Gr. *eidos,* appearance]. Disease marked by formation of tiny yellow patches or nodules on the skin, as on the eyelids. SYN: *xanthoma.*

vitium (vĭsh′ē-ŭm) [L., fault]. (pl. *vitia*) A fault, defect, or vice.

v. cordis. An organic heart lesion.

vitrectomy (vĭ-trĕk′tō-mē) [L. *vitreus,* glassy, + Gr. *ektome,* excision]. Use of a special instrument in order to remove the contents of the vitreous chamber, and replacing them with a sterile physiological saline solution.

vitreocapsulitis (vĭt″rē-ō-kăp″sū-lī′tĭs) [L. *vitreus,* glassy, + *capsula,* capsule, + Gr. *itis,* inflammation]. Inflammation of the vitreous humor. SYN: *hyalitis.*

vitreodentin (vĭt″rē-ō-dĕn′tĭn). A particularly hard and brittle form of dentin.

vitreoretinal (vĭt″rē-ō-rĕt′ĭ-năl). Concerning the vitreous and the retina.

vitreous (vĭt′rē-ŭs) [L. *vitreus,* glassy]. 1. Glassy. 2. Pertaining to the vitreous body of the eye. 3. The vitreous body.

vitreous body. A transparent jellylike mass that fills the cavity of the eyeball, enclosed by the hyaloid membrane.

vitreous chamber. The portion of the cavity of the eyeball behind the lens.

vitreous degeneration. Retrogressive change of a part into a translucent shining substance, esp. of a blood vessel wall. SEE: *degeneration, hyaline.*

vitreous humor. The clear watery fluid filling the interstices of the stroma of the vitreous body.

vitreous membrane. 1. Inner membrane of the choroid. 2. The innermost layer of the connective tissue sheath surrounding a hair follicle.

vitreous table. The inner layer of compact tissue characteristic of most of the bones of the cranium.

vitrescence (vĭ-trĕs′ĕns). Becoming hard and transparent like glass.

vitreum (vĭt′rē-ŭm). The vitreous body of the eye.

vitriol (vĭt′rē-ōl) [L. *vitriolum*]. A sulfate of any of various metals.

v., blue. Copper sulfate.

v., green. Ferrous sulfate.

v., oil of. Sulfuric acid.

v., white. Zinc sulfate.

vitropression (vĭt″rō-prĕsh′ŭn) [L. *vitrum,* glass, + *pressio,* a squeezing]. Method of temporarily eliminating redness of the skin caused by hyperemia by pressure with a glass slide on the skin for purpose of studying any lesions or discolorations.

vitrum (vĭt′rŭm) [L.]. Glass.

Vi-Twel. Trade name for vitamin B_{12}.

Vivactil. Trade name for protriptyline hydrochloride.

vivi- (vĭv′ĭ) [L. *vivus*]. Combining form meaning alive.

vividialysis (vĭv″ĭ-dī-ăl′ĭ-sĭs). Dialysis through a living membrane.

vividiffusion (vĭv″ĭ-dĭf-ū′zhŭn) [L. *vivus,* alive, + *diffusio,* a pouring apart]. The process of removing diffusible substances from blood of a living animal by allowing it to flow through dialyzing membranes immersed in saline solution.

vivification (vĭv″ĭ-fĭ-kā′shŭn) [″ + *facere,* to make]. 1. Trimming of the surface layer of a wound to aid union of tissues. 2. Transformation of protein food through assimilation into the living matter of cellular organisms.

viviparity (vĭv″ĭ-păr′ĭ-tē). The ability to produce living young rather than by producing young by laying an egg and then having it hatch.

viviparous (vĭv-ĭp′ăr-ŭs) [″ + *parere,* to bear young]. Developing young within the body, the young being expelled and born alive, the opposite of oviparous.

vivisect (vĭv′ĭ-sĕkt) [L. *vivus,* alive, + *sectio,* a cutting]. To dissect a living animal for experimental purposes.

vivisection (vĭv″ĭ-sĕk′shŭn) [″ + *sectio,* a cutting]. Cutting of or operation upon a living animal for physiological investigation and the study of disease. The operations are usually performed upon an anesthetized animal under conditions similar to those encountered in an operating room of a hospital.

vivisectionist (vĭv″ĭ-sĕk′shŭn-ĭst). One who practices or believes in vivisection. SEE: *antivivisection.*

vivisector (vĭv-ĭs-ĕk′tor) [″ + *sector,* a cutting]. One who practices vivisection.

vivisepulture (vĭv″ĭ-sĕp′ŭl-tūr) [″ + *sepultura,* buried]. The practice or act of burying an individual alive.

VLDL. *very low density lipoprotein.*

Vlem-Dome. Trade name for sulfurated lime (topical solution).

Vleminckx's solution (flĕm′ĭnks). [Jean François Vleminckx, Belgian physician, 1800–1876] A solution of sulfurated lime used in various skin diseases.

VMA. *Vanillylmandelic acid.*

V.N.A. *Visiting Nurse Association.*

vocal (vō′kăl) [L. *vocalis,* talking]. Pert. to the voice.

vocal cords, false. The ventricular folds of the larynx.

vocal cords, true. Vocal folds.

vocal folds. The thin edges of the vocal lips of the larynx, each of which encloses the vocal ligament. They form the edges of the rima glottidis, and are involved in the production of sound. SYN: *vocal cords.*

vocal fremitus. Chest-wall vibration felt on palpation while patient is speaking.

vocal ligament. A strong band of elastic tissue lying within the vocal fold.

vocal lips. Two shelflike projections of the lateral walls of the larynx. Their edges bear the vocal folds, q.v.

vocal muscle. The inner portion of the thyroarytenoid muscle, which lies in the vocal lip lateral to and in contact with the vocal ligament.

vocal process. The area of the arytenoid cartilage to which are attached the vocal cords.

vocal resonance. Sound heard in auscultation of lung while patient is speaking.

vocal signs. Indication of disease by changes in the voice.

voces (vō-sēz) [L.]. Pl. of vox.

voice (voys) [L. *vox*]. Sound uttered by human beings produced by vibration of the vocal cords.

v., amphoric. V., cavernous, q.v.

v., cavernous. The quality of the voice as heard during auscultation of the chest over an area underneath that is a cavity. SEE: *amphoric.*

v., eunuchoid. The characteristic high-pitched voice of a male in whom the normal sexual development has not occurred or in a male who was castrated prior to puberty.

voice, words pert. to: amphoriloquy; arytenoid; heterophonia; hoarseness; paraphonia; phonation; resonance; rhinolalia; rhinophonia; trachyphonia.

voiceprint. Technique for depicting graphically the characteristics of an individual's speech pattern. Because voiceprints, like fingerprints, can be used to distinguish one person from another, the technique is useful in medicine and in identifying the voices of criminal suspects.

voices (voys′ĕz). In psychiatry, verbal-auditory hallucinations expressed as being heard by the patient.

void (voyd) [O. Fr. *voider,* to empty]. To evacuate the bowels or bladder.

vol. *volume.*

vol. %. *volume percent.*

vola, volar (vō′lă, vō′lăr) [L.]. Terms originally used to refer to the palm of the hand or sole of the foot. The preferred terms for reference to the palm of the hand are palmar or palmaris.

vola manus (vō′lă). Palm, q.v.

vola pedis. The sole of the foot.

volaris (vō-lā′rĭs). Volar.

volatile (vŏl′ă-tĭl) [L. *volatilis,* flying]. Easily vaporized or evaporated. Examples of volatile liquids are ether (boiling point, 34.5° C.) and ethyl chloride (b. p. 12.2° C.).

volatilization (vŏl″ă-tĭl-ĭ-zā′shŭn). Conversion of a solid or liquid into a vapor.

volatilize (vŏl′ă-tĭl-īz). To vaporize a liquid or solid.

vole (vōl). A mouse-like rodent of the genus Clethrionomys or Microtus.

volition (vō-lĭsh′ŭn) [L. *volitio,* will]. The act or power of willing or choosing.

volitional (vō-lĭsh′ŭn-ăl). Performed by volition.

Volkmann's canals (fōlk′mănz). [A. W. Volkmann, Ger. physiologist, 1800–1877] Vascular channels in compact bone. They are not surrounded by concentric lamellae as are the haversian canals.

Volkmann's contracture (fōlk′mănz). [Richard von Volkmann, Ger. surgeon, 1830–1899] Degeneration, contracture, fibrosis, and atrophy of a muscle resulting from injury to its blood supply. Usually seen in the hand. SYN: *paralysis, ischemic.*

volley (vŏl′ē) [L. *volare,* to fly]. The simultaneous or nearly simultaneous discharge of a number of nerve impulses from a center within the brain or spinal cord.

volsella (vŏl-sĕl'ă) [L., a tweezer]. Forceps with sharp, pointed hooks at end of each blade.

volt (vōlt). [Count Alessandro Volta, It. physicist, 1745–1827] An electrical unit of pressure, the electromotive force required to produce one ampere of current through a resistance of one ohm.

voltage (vōl'tĭj). Electromotive force or difference in potential expressed in volts.

voltaic (vŏl-tā'ĭk). Concerning electricity produced by a battery.

voltaism (vŏl'tă-ĭzm). Galvanism, q.v.

voltammeter (vōlt-ăm'mē-tĕr). A device for measuring both volts and amperes.

voltampere (vōlt-ăm'pēr). The value obtained by multiplying volts times amperes.

volubility (vŏl"ū-bĭl'ĭ-tē) [L. *volubilitas,* flow of discourse]. Excessive speech.

volume (vŏl'ūm). The space occupied by a substance. Usually expressed in cubic units.

v., expiratory reserve. The maximal amount of air that can be forced from the lungs after normal expiration.

v., inspiratory reserve. The maximal amount of air that can be inspired after the end of a normal inspiration.

v., mean corpuscular. ABBR: M.C.V. The mean volume of an average erythrocyte. Normal values range from 82 to 92 cubic microns.

v., minute. The amount of blood discharged from one ventricle in one minute.

v., packed cell. The volume of packed erythrocytes in a sample of centrifuged blood. Average volume equals 47% of blood volume in men, 42% in women. SYN: *hematocrit.*

v., residual. Volume of air remaining in the lungs after maximal expiration.

v., stroke. The amount of blood discharged by a ventricle in one contraction. Determined by dividing the minute volume by the number of heartbeats occurring in one minute.

v., tidal. The volume of air inspired and expired in one normal respiratory cycle.

volume index. A no longer used method of determining the size, i.e., volume, of red blood cells. SEE: *hematocrit; mean corpuscular volume.*

volumenometer (vŏl"ūm-nŏm'ĕ-tĕr). Volumometer.

volume percent. The number of cubic centimeters (milliliters) of a substance (usually O_2 or CO_2) contained in 100 cc. (or ml.) of another substance, e.g., blood. ABBR: vol.%.

volumetric (vŏl"ū-mĕt'rĭk) [L. *volumen,* a volume, + Gr. *metron,* a measure]. Pert. to measurement of volume.

volumometer (vŏl"ū-mŏm'ĕ-tĕr). A device for measuring volume.

voluntary (vŏl'ŭn-tĕr"ē) [L. *voluntas,* will]. Pert. to or under control of the will.

voluntary health agency. Any nonprofit, nongovernmental agency, governed by lay or professional individuals, organized on a national, state or local level, whose primary purpose is health related. This term applies to agencies supported mainly by voluntary public contributions. They are usually engaged in programs of service, education, and research related to a particular disability or group of diseases and disabilities; for example, the American Heart Association, American Cancer Society, National Foundation, National Lung Institute, and their state and local affiliates. The term can also be applied to such agencies as nonprofit hospitals, visiting nurse associations, and other local service organizations that have both lay and professional governing boards and are supported by both voluntary contributions and charges and fees for service provided.

voluntary muscle. Any muscle that is normally controlled by the will. They are generally attached to the skeleton and are innervated by myelinated nerves coming directly from the brain or spinal cord. Microscopically they consist of long cylindrical fibers bearing crosswise striations. The terms voluntary, striped, striated, cross-striated, and skeletal are practically synonymous when applied to muscle.

voluptuous (vō-lŭp'tū-ŭs) [L. *voluptas,* pleasure]. 1. Pert. to, arising from, or provoking consciously or otherwise, sensual desire, usually applied to the female sex. 2. Given to sensualism.

volupty (vŏl'ŭp-tē) [O. Fr. *volupte,* pleasure]. Sexual pleasure.

volute (vō-lūt') [L. *volutus,* rolled]. Spiral, rolled up. SYN: *convoluted.*

volvulosis (vŏl"vū-lō'sĭs). Onchocerciasis, q.v.

volvulus (vŏl'vū-lŭs) [L. *volvere,* to roll]. A twisting of the bowel upon itself causing obstruction. A prolapsed mesentery is the predisposing cause. Usually occurs at sigmoid and ileocecal areas of intestines.

vomer (vō'mĕr) [L., plowshare]. The plowshaped bone that forms the lower and posterior portion of the nasal septum, articulating with the ethmoid, sphenoid, the two palate bones, and two superior maxillary bones.

vomerine (vō'mĕr-ĭn). Pert. to the vomer.

vomerobasilar (vō"mĕr-ō-băs'ĭ-lăr). Concerning the vomer and the base of the skull.

vomeronasal (vō"mĕr-ō-nā'săl). Pert. to the vomer and nasal bones.

vomeronasal cartilages. Two narrow strips of cartilage lying along the anterior portion of the inferior border of the septal cartilage of the nose.

vomeronasal organ. A small tubular epithelial sac lying on the anteroinferior surface of the nasal septum. Rudimentary in man. SYN: *Jacobson's organ.*

vomica (vŏm'ĭ-kă) [L., ulcer]. (pl. *vomicae*) 1. A cavity in the lungs, as from suppuration. 2. Sudden and profuse expectoration of putrid purulent matter.

vomicose (vŏm'ĭ-kōs). Marked by many ulcers; ulcerous; purulent.

vomit (vŏm'ĭt) [L. *vomere,* to vomit]. 1. Material that is ejected from the stomach through the mouth. 2. To eject stomach contents through the mouth. SEE: *melena; nausea; vomitus.*

PHYS: The act is usually reflex involving coordinated activity of both voluntary and involuntary muscles. A certain position is assumed, the glottis is closed, the diaphragm and abdominal muscles contract, and the cardiac sphincter of the stomach relaxes while antiperistaltic waves course over the duodenum, stomach, and esophagus.

v., bilious. Bile forced back into the stomach and ejected with vomited matter.

v., black. Vomit containing blood acted on by the gastric juice. Seen in worst form of yellow fever.

v., coffee-ground. Vomit having the appearance and consistency of coffee grounds because of blood mixed with gastric contents. Occurs in any condition associated with hemorrhage into the stomach.

vomiting (vŏm'ĭt-ĭng) [L. *vomere,* to vomit]. Ejection through the mouth of the gastric contents, and, in cases of bowel obstruction, intestinal contents. It may result from toxins from ptomaines, drugs, uremia, and specific fevers; cerebral tumors and meningitis (often unaccompanied by nausea and does not relieve associated headache); diseases of the stomach such as ulcer, cancer, dilatation, dyspepsia; reflex from pregnancy, uterine or ovarian disease, irritation of the fauces, worms, biliary colic; intestinal obstruction; motion sickness; nervous affections such as hysteria and migraine. Vomiting may result from taking poisons such as arsenic, aconite, antimony, barium, colchicum, cantharides, copper, corrosive alkalis, acids, digitalis, iodine, mercury, phenol, phosphorus, veratrum, wood alcohol (methanol), food toxins or poisons, and zinc. Periodic vomiting may be in itself a neurosis or associated with the gastric crises of locomotor ataxia. Esophageal vomiting results from obstruction, and the vomitus, q.v., is alkaline in reaction. SYN: *emesis.* SEE: *anorexia nervosa.*

TREATMENT: Antinausea medicines by mouth if possible, otherwise intramuscularly or intravenously. Fluids may be given by mouth if patient will accept them. If vomiting continues, fluids and electrolytes intravenously will be required to replace those lost in the vomitus.

In pregnancy (hyperemesis gravidarum, q.v.): Fluid intake by mouth should be restricted but maintained by intravenous route. Frequent small feedings of more or less dry foods are advisable.

CAUTION: It is of utmost importance not to use medicines during pregnancy unless there is evidence that the drug being prescribed has been investigated and found to be harmless to the embryo and its development.

NURSING IMPLICATIONS: Assess causative factors such as drugs, food, disease entities, and psychological factors. Remove causative factor if possible. Assess frequency of vomiting, amount, time of occurrence, and characteristics of fluid. Provide an emesis basin and empty it as often as needed. Position patient to prevent aspiration, and have suction equipment available. Administer antiemetics as prescribed. Withhold food and fluids for several hours, and offer frequent mouth care. Prevent vomiting during or after surgery by restricting foods and fluids for approximately 8 hours before surgery. Use comfort measures such as a cool cloth to the face. Monitor serum electrolytes, and keep accurate intake and output records to ensure proper fluid replacement. Monitor vital signs and institute antipyretic measures if temperature is elevated. To prevent vomiting, encourage the patient to take deep breaths or to swallow. Promote a calm environment and provide distraction.

RS: anacatharsis; anorexia nervosa; antiemetic; emesis; emetic; hyperemesis; vomit; vomitus.

v., cyclic. Periodic and recurring attacks of vomiting occurring in patients with a nervous temperament. The condition is associated with acidosis.

v., dry. Nausea without vomitus.

v., epidemic. Sudden unexplained attacks of gastroenteritis characterized by nausea, vomiting, and sometimes diarrhea. Though not proven, the symptoms are believed to be due to a virus. Treatment is symptomatic.

v., incoercible. Uncontrollable vomiting.

v. of pregnancy. Vomiting of pregnancy, esp. morning sickness.

v., pernicious. Severe vomiting of pregnancy.

v., projectile. Ejection of vomitus with great force.

v., stercoraceous. Vomiting of fecal matter.

vomitive (vŏm'ĭ-tĭv). Emetic.

vomitory (vŏm'ĭ-tō-rē) [L. *vomitorius,* pert. to

vomit]. 1. Causing vomiting. 2. An agent inducing emesis. 3. A vessel to receive vomitus.

vomiturition (vŏm″ĭ-tū-rĭsh′ŭn) [L. *vomitus,* vomit]. Repeated involuntary and ineffective efforts to vomit. SYN: *retching.*

vomitus (vŏm′ĭ-tŭs). 1. Act of ejecting matter from the stomach through the mouth. 2. Material ejected from the stomach by vomiting.

CHARACTER: *Ammoniacal odor:* Indicates uremia. *Bilious:* Green or greenish-yellow, containing bile, appears after frequent and violent vomiting. *Fecal:* Indicative of intestinal obstruction, general peritonitis, and abnormal communication between the intestines and stomach. *Garlic odor:* Denotes phosphorus poisoning.

Hematemesis: The vomiting of blood. If bright and fluid, it has not been long in the stomach; otherwise, it has the appearance of coffee grounds, reddish-brown, or it forms in clots. Also, this may indicate rupture of an aneurysm into the stomach or esophagus or rupture of esophageal varicose veins; gastric ulcer; cirrhosis of liver; enlarged spleen; or carcinoma of the stomach. It is not necessarily fatal. Hematemesis may result from swallowed blood. It may occur in vicarious menstruation, gastritis, corrosive poisoning, in the presence of strong alkalies or acids, or it may result from anemia, leukemia, or Hodgkin's disease. Sometimes it is present in chronic nephritis, scurvy, purpura hemorrhagica, acute yellow atrophy of the liver, and in malaria.

Profuse: The ejection of large quantities of frothy fermented material is highly significant of gastric dilatation. *Purulent:* This may result from the rupture of an abscess into the esophagus or stomach. *Without nausea, distress, or other phenomena:* This may occur in certain neuroses of the stomach, in hysteria, uremia, brain disease as from a tumor, or as a precursor of apoplexy. The vomitus may be colored by certain fruits, by wine, coffee, cocoa, soups, and bile.

v., coffee-ground. Vomitus of dark red or black granular material (resembling coffee grounds), which is blood. The blood has been in the stomach or intestinal tract long enough to be changed from red to black by the action of gastric and intestinal juices. Occurs in conditions associated with hemorrhage into the stomach.

v. cruentus. Bloody vomit.

v. marinus. Seasickness.

v. matutinus. The vomiting of morning sickness.

von Gierke's disease (fŏn gēr′kĕz). [Edgar von Gierke, Ger. pathologist, b. 1877] Condition in which excessive amounts of glycogen are stored in tissues and the body is unable to use it. Results in excessive production of ketones. SYN: *glycogenosis; glycogen storage disease.*

von Graefe's sign (fŏn grā′fēz). [Albrecht von Graefe, Ger. ophthalmologist, 1828–1870] Failure of lid to move downward promptly with eyeball, the lid moving tardily and jerkily; seen in exophthalmic goiter.

von Hippel's disease. Hippel's disease, q.v.

von Jaksch's disease. A symptom complex consisting of anemia, hepatosplenomegaly, and infections that are associated with a number of chronic diseases such as tuberculosis and malnutrition.

von Pirquet's test (fŏn pēr′kāz). [Clemens Freiherr von Pirquet, Austrian pediatrician, 1874–1929] A diagnostic test for tuberculosis in which a small amount of tuberculin is applied to a scarified area of the skin of the arm. A positive reaction is seen if a red papillar eruption appears several days later at the site of inoculation.

von Recklinghausen's canals. Recklinghausen's canals, q.v.

von Recklinghausen's disease. Recklinghausen's disease, q.v.

von Recklinghausen's tumor. Recklinghausen's tumor, q.v.

Vontrol. Trade name for diphenidol.

von Willebrand's disease. [E. A. von Willebrand, Finnish physician, 1870–1949] A congenital bleeding disorder. The bleeding tendency manifests at an early age, usually as epistaxis and easy bruising but petechiae are rare. Bleeding in the intestinal tract during surgery and excess loss of blood during menstruation are common. The symptoms decrease in severity with age and during pregnancy.

ETIOL: Deficiency of factor VIII.

DIAG: Prolonged bleeding time and factor VIII deficiency.

TREATMENT: Administer factor VIII 24 to 48 hours prior to surgery or during attacks of bleeding.

Voorhees' bag (voor′ēz). [James Ditmors Voorhees, U.S. obstetrician, 1869–1929] An inflatable rubber bag for dilating the cervix uteri to induce labor.

voracious (vō-rā′shŭs) [L. *vorare,* to devour]. Having an insatiable or ravenous appetite.

Voranil. Trade name for clortermine hydrochloride.

vortex (vor′tĕks) [L., a whirlpool]. (pl. *vortices*) A structure having a spiral or whorled appearance.

v., coccygeal. The region over the coccyx where lanugo hairs of the embryo come to a point.

v. lentis. Spiral patterns on the surface of the lens due to concentric pattern of fiber growth.

v. of heart. Region at apex of heart where muscle fibers of the ventricles make a tight spiral and turn inward.

vortices (vor′tĭ-sēz) [L.]. Pl. of vortex.

v. pilorum. Hair whorls as in arrangement of hairs on the scalp.

vorticose (vor′tĭk-ōs) [L. *vortices,* whirlpools]. Whirling or having a whorled arrangement.

vorticose veins. Four veins (two superior and two inferior) that receive blood from all parts of the choroid of the eye. They empty into posterior ciliary and superior ophthalmic veins.

vox (vŏks) [L.]. (pl. *voces*) Voice.

v. abscissa. Loss of voice.

v. capitus. Falsetto voice or a voice in the upper register.

v. cholerica. The suppressed voice in last stages of cholera.

v. rauca. A hoarse voice.

voyeur (voy-yĕr′) [Fr., one who sees]. One who derives sexual pleasure from observing nude persons or the sexual activity of others.

voyeurism (voy′yĕr-ĭzm). The experiencing of sexual gratification by observing nude persons or the sexual activity of others.

V.R. *right vision; ventilation rate; vocal resonance.*

V.S. *vesicular sound; vital sign; volumetric solution.*

v.s. *vital signs.*

vuerometer (vū″ĕr-ŏm′ĕ-tĕr) [Fr. *vue,* sight, + Gr. *metron,* a measure]. Apparatus for measuring interpupillary distance of the eyes.

vulgaris (vŭl-gā′rĭs) [L.]. Ordinary, common.

vulnerable (vŭl′nĕr-ă-bl) [L. *vulnerare,* to wound]. Easily injured or wounded.

vulnerant (vŭl′nĕr-ănt). 1. Something that wounds or injures. 2. To inflict injury.

vulnerary (vŭl′nĕr-ār″ē). 1. Pert. to wounds. 2. An agent used to assist in wound healing.

vulnerate (vŭl′nĕr-āt). To wound.

vulnus (vŭl′nŭs) [L.]. (pl. *vulnera*) A wound or injury.

Vulpian-Heidenhain-Sherrington phenomenon. Contraction of denervated skeletal muscle by stimulating autonomic cholinergic fibers innervating its blood vessels.

vulsella, vulsellum (vŭl-sĕl′ă, vŭl-sĕl′ŭm) [L. *vulsella,* tweezers]. A forceps with a hook on each blade. SYN: *volsella.*

vulva (vŭl′vă) [L., a covering]. (pl. *vulvae*) That portion of the female external genitalia lying posterior to the mons veneris consisting of the labia majora, labia minora, clitoris, vestibule of the vagina, vaginal opening, and bulbs of the vestibule. SYN: *pudendum femininum* [NA].

v. connivens. Vulva in which the labia majora are in apposition.

v. hians. Vulva in which labia majora are gaping.

v., velamen. Abnormally elongated clitoris.

vulval, vulvar [L. *vulva,* covering]. Relating to the vulva.

vulvar leukoplakia. Condition characterized by diffuse or focal translucent thickening of the vulva. Often gives rise to carcinoma.

vulvectomy (vŭl-vĕk′tō-mē) [″ + Gr. *ektome,* excision]. Excision of the vulva.

vulvismus (vŭl-vĭz′mŭs) [″ + Gr. *-ismos,* condition]. Painful spasm of the vagina. SYN: *vaginismus.*

vulvitis (vŭl-vī′tĭs) [L. *vulva,* covering, + Gr. *itis,* inflammation]. Inflammation of the vulva.

v., acute nongonorrheal. Vulvitis resulting from chafing of opposed lips of vulva or from accumulated sebaceous material around the clitoris.

v., follicular. Inflammation of hair follicles of the vulva.

v., gangrenous. Necrosis and sloughing of areas of vulva, often a complication of infectious diseases such as diphtheria, scarlatina, herpes genitalis, or typhoid fever.

v., leukoplakic. A chronic atrophic vulvitis. SEE: *kraurosis vulvae.*

v., mycotic. Vulvitis caused by various fungi, most commonly by Candida albicans.

vulvo- [L. *vulva,* covering]. Combining form meaning a covering, or the vulva.

vulvocrural (vŭl″vō-kroo′răl) [″ + *cruralis,* pert. to the leg]. Rel. to the vulva and the thigh.

vulvopathy (vŭl-vŏp′ă-thē) [″ + Gr. *pathos,* disease]. Any disorder of the vulva.

vulvouterine (vŭl″vō-ū′tĕr-ĭn) [″ + *uterinus,* pert. to the uterus]. Rel. to the vulva and uterus.

vulvovaginal (vŭl″vō-văj′ĭ-năl) [″ + *vagina,* a sheath]. Pert. to the vulva and vagina. SYN: *vaginolabial; vaginovulvar.*

vulvovaginal glands. Small glands on either side of the vulvar orifice. SYN: *Bartholin's glands.*

vulvovaginitis (vŭl″vō-văj″ĭ-nī′tĭs) [″ + ″ + Gr. *itis,* inflammation]. Inflammation of both the vulva and vagina at the same time, or of the vulvovaginal glands.

v., diabetic. Mycotic vulvar infection commonly occurring with diabetes.

vv. *veins.*

v/v. Volume of dissolved substance per volume of solvent.

V.W. *vessel wall.*

v/w. Volume of a substance per unit of weight of another component.

W

W. Chem. symbol for tungsten.

w. *watt,* a unit of electric energy; *week; wife; with.*

Waardenberg syndrome. A congenital defect involving pigmentation. It consists of a white forelock, vitiligo, heterochromic irides, broad nasal root, dystopia canthorum (lateral displacement of the inner canthi), congenital deafness may or may not be present, deficient pigmentation of the fundus, synophrys (growing together of the two sets of eyebrows), and cutaneous hypopigmentation. The condition is inherited as an autosomal dominant.

Wachendorf's membrane (vŏk'ĕn-dorfs). [Eberhard J. Wachendorf, 18th-century Ger. anatomist] 1. A thin membrane occluding the pupil of the embryo. SYN: *membrana pupillaris.* 2. The outer membrane ensheathing a cell.

wafer (wā'fĕr) [Ger. *wafel*]. 1. A thin sheet of flour paste used to enclose a medicinal dose of powder. 2. A flat vaginal suppository.

Wagstaffe's fracture (wăg'stăfs). [William Warwick Wagstaffe, Brit. surgeon, 1843–1910] Fracture with separation of the internal malleolus of the ankle.

waist (wāst) [ME. *wast,* growth]. Small part of the human trunk between thorax and hips. SEE: *cincture sensation.*

wakeful (wāk'fŭl) [AS. *wacian,* to be awake, + *full,* complete]. Not able to sleep; sleepless.

Walcher's position (vŏl'kĕrz). [Gustav Adolf Walcher, Ger. gynecologist, 1856–1935] Position in which the patient assumes dorsal recumbent posture with hips at the edge of the bed and legs hanging down.

Wald, Lillian (wăld). U.S. nurse, 1867–1940, who founded the Henry Street Settlement in New York City, and one of the world's first visiting nurse associations.

Wald cycle. The transformations involved in the breakdown of resynthesis of rhodopsin.

Waldenström's disease (văl'dĕn-strĕmz). [Johann Henning Waldenström, Swedish surgeon, b. 1877] Osteochondritis deformans juvenilis, q.v.

Waldeyer's gland (vŏl'dī-ĕrz). [Wilhelm von Waldeyer, Ger. anatomist, 1836–1921] Sweat glands of the eyelids. Usually most prominent in the lower lid margin.

Waldeyer's neuron. The nerve cell and its processes.

Waldeyer's ring. The ring of tonsillar (lymphatic) tissue that encircles the nasopharynx and oropharynx. Consists of the two palatine tonsils, lingual and pharyngeal tonsils.

walk. 1. Method of locomotion of upright bipeds such as man. 2. The particular way an individual moves. SEE: *gait.*

walker. A mobile device used to assist a person in walking. It consists of a stable platform made of metal tubing that the patient grasps while taking a step. The walker is then moved forward and another step is taken. SEE: *crutch.*

walking [AS. *wealcan,* to roll]. Act of moving on foot; advancing by steps.

RS: abasia; acathisia; astasia; atremia; basophobia; claudication; dysbasia; gait.

w., sleep. Somnambulism.

walking cast. A cast that allows the patient to be ambulatory.

walking typhoid. Typhoid fever in which the symptoms are mild so that the patient is ambulatory.

walking well. Persons who are indeed ill, but still able to walk.

walking wounded. In military medicine, an ambulatory case.

wall [AS. *weall*]. The limiting or surrounding substance or material of a cell, vessel, or cavity such as an artery, vein, chest, or bladder.

Wallenberg's syndrome (vŏl'ĕn-bĕrgz). [Adolf Wallenberg, Ger. physician, 1862–1949] A complex of symptoms resulting from occlusion of the posteroinferior cerebellar artery or one of its branches supplying the lower portion of the brain stem. Dysphagia, muscular weakness or paralysis, impairment of pain and temperature senses, and cerebellar dysfunction are characteristic.

wallerian degeneration (wŏl-ē'rē-ăn). [Augustus Volney Waller, Brit. physician, 1816–1870] Degeneration of a nerve fiber (axon) that has been severed from its cell body. The myelin sheath also degenerates and is transformed into a chain of lipoid droplets that stains by the Marchi method, a method utilized in tracing the course of injured nerve fibers. The neurilemma does not degenerate but forms a tube that directs the growth of the regenerating axon.

walleye [ME. *wawil-eghed*]. 1. Eye in which iris is light-colored or white. 2. Leukoma or dense opacity of cornea. 3. Squint in which both visual axes diverge. SYN: *strabismus, divergent.*

Walthard's islets or inclusions. Nests or small cysts of embryological squamous epithelium-like cells in the superficial parts of the ovary, tubes, and uterine ligaments. They are thought to represent the beginning Brenner tumor.

wandering (wăn'dĕr-ĭng) [AS. *wandrian*]. Moving about; not fixed.

wandering abscess. Abscess that burrows and comes to the surface at a point distant from its origin.

wandering kidney. Dislocated floating kidney.

wandering mind. Daydream or reverie.

wandering spleen. Dislocated floating spleen.

Wangensteen's method (wăn′gĕn-stēnz). [Owen H. Wangensteen, U.S. surgeon, b. 1898] Technique for relieving postoperative abdominal distention, nausea, vomiting, and certain cases of mechanical bowel obstruction. It involves use of an intranasal catheter in combination with a suction siphonage apparatus. SEE: *decompression.*

Warburg apparatus. [Otto H. Warburg, Ger. biochemist, b. 1883] A capillary manometer used for determining oxygen consumption and CO_2 production of small bits of cellular tissue. Widely used in metabolism studies.

ward [AS. *weard,* watching over]. A large room in a hospital for the care of several patients, usually more than four.

w., accident. Ward reserved for accident cases.

w., psychiatric. Ward in a general hospital for mentally ill patients.

Wardrop's disease (wăr′drŏps). [James Wardrop, Brit. surgeon, 1782–1869] Acute inflammation of the nail bed with fetid ulceration and loss of the nail. SYN: *onychia maligna.*

Wardrop's operation. Ligation of an artery for aneurysm at a distance beyond the sac.

warehousemen's itch. Eczema of hands from touching irritating substances.

warfarin [name derived from initials of *W*isconsin *A*lumni *R*esearch *F*oundation]. An anticoagulant drug. Coumadin and Panwarfin are trade names.

NURSING IMPLICATIONS: Instruct the patient to observe for signs of bleeding such as epistaxis, bleeding gums, hematuria, melena, and skin trauma (ecchymosis, purpura, or petechia). Preventive measures should include gentle blowing of the nose, use of an electric razor and a soft-bristled toothbrush, gentle cleaning of the rectum, and avoidance of tight, constrictive clothing. Instruct the patient to avoid foods high in fat content, as they may precipitate formation of a thrombus. Stress the importance of having blood studies as prescribed by the physician and the significance of regular medical follow-up. Provide the patient with an identification card listing the prescribed drug, dosage, frequency of administration, and physician's name and phone number. Stress the importance of consulting with the physician before taking any over-the-counter medications. This is necessary because many drugs interact with anticoagulants.

w. potassium. USP. An anticoagulant drug. Trade name is Athrombin-K.

warfarin poisoning. Caused by accidental administration of an overdose of the drug, or by the cumulative effect of repeated administration of the drug. Warfarin is used as a rodenticide. Repeated ingestion of those materials by children may cause poisoning. SEE: *Poisons and Poisoning* in *Appendix.*

war gases. Any chemical substances, whether solid, liquid, or vapor, used to produce poisonous or irritant effects. SEE: *gas, war.*

wart (wort) [AS. *wearte*]. A circumscribed cutaneous elevation resulting from hypertrophy of the papillae and epidermis. It is caused by a papillomavirus. Also applied to benign conditions that resemble warts such as verruca.

RS: condyloma; keratosis, seborrheic; sycoma; venereal wart; verrucose.

w., fig. A growth of filiform projections usually occurring on genitalia. Frequently they are covered with a foul-smelling secretion. SYN: *venereal wart; verruca acuminata.*

w., plantar. Wart on pressure-bearing areas, esp. the sole of the foot. SYN: *verruca plantaris.*

w., seborrheic. Patch of corneous hypertrophy on face of the aged.

w., senile. W., seborrheic.

w., venereal. Vegetating growth upon skin, esp. on the mucocutaneous juncture of the genitals, having an offensive discharge. SYN: *verruca acuminata.*

wash (wăsh) [AS. *wacsan*]. 1. Act of cleaning, esp. a part or all of the body. 2. A medicinal preparation used in washing or coating.

w., eye. A lotion for the eyes. SYN: *collyrium.*

washerwoman's itch. Eczema of the hands of laundry workers.

wasp [AS. *waesp*]. Term sometimes applied to all insects belonging to the suborder Apocrita, order Hymenoptera (except the Formicidae or ants), but more generally restricted to the superfamilies Scolioidea, Vespoidea, and Specoidea. Members have the base of the abdomen constricted and females have a piercing ovipositor, which in many species is modified into a sting. Many are social, living in large colonies. Common representatives are yellow jackets and hornets.

wasp sting. The injection of wasp venom into the skin resulting in a painful wound and sometimes a mild systemic reaction. Multiple stings may be dangerous, esp. to sensitized individuals.

TREATMENT: Apply bicarbonate of soda paste, strong Epsom salt, or household ammonia solution locally. If pain is severe, infiltrate area with 2% procaine solution. Severe allergic reaction may require injection of epinephrine and cortisone. Application of cold to a large area around bite will slow absorption of the venom.

Wassermann-fast (wăs'ĕr-măn). [August Paul von Wassermann, Ger. bacteriologist, 1866–1925] Indicating a positive reaction shown by a Wassermann test that continues after adequate antisyphilitic medication.

Wassermann reaction. Serum complement-fixation test as a diagnosis of syphilis. A general term loosely applied to almost any serological test for syphilis. The results are designated as 1, 2, 3, and 4 plus, the intensity of the reaction usually corresponding to the severity of the infection. The disease may still exist with a negative reaction. Several negative Wasserman reactions a few years after treatment indicate the absence of syphilis.

waste (wāst) [L. *vastus,* empty]. 1. To shrink in physical bulk or strength, as from disease. SYN: *cachexia.* 2. Loss by breaking down of bodily tissue. 3. Refuse material no longer useful to an organism.

waste products. Carbon dioxide, organic and inorganic salts, urine, dead skin, hair, nails, undigested foods.

w.p., metabolic. Soluble salts in the form of nitrogenous salts (urea) and inorganic salts (sodium chloride), gas in form of carbon dioxide, and liquid in the form of water. They are excreta, removed by the process of elimination, q.v.

wasting (wāst'ĭng) [L. *vastare,* to devastate]. Enfeebling; causing loss of strength or size; emaciating. SEE: *marasmus.*

wasting palsy. Chronic disease marked by gradual atrophy of muscular tissue with paralysis. SYN: *progressive muscular atrophy.* SEE: *atrophy, muscular.*

water (wă'tĕr) [AS. *waeter*]. 1. H_2O, hydrogen combined with oxygen, forming a tasteless, clear, odorless fluid. 2. A solution of a volatile substance in water. 3. A lay term used to refer to urine or urinating.

Water freezes at 32° F. (0° C.) and boils at 212° F. (100° C.). It is the principal chemical constituent of the body, comprising approx. 65% of the body weight of an adult male and 55% of the adult female. It is distributed within the intracellular fluid and outside of the cells in the extracellular fluid. Water is indispensable for metabolic activities within cells as it is the medium in which chemical reactions can take place. Outside of cells, water is the principal transporting agent of the body. The following are properties of water that are of importance to living organisms: it is almost a universal solvent; it is a medium in which acids, bases, and salts ionize, and the concentrations of these substances (electrolytes) must be and are normally regulated quite precisely by the body; it possesses a high specific heat and has a high latent heat of vaporization, of importance in regulation and maintenance of a constant body temperature; it possesses a high surface tension; it is an important reacting agent and essential in all hydrolytic reactions.

Water is the principal constituent of all body fluids (blood, lymph, tissue fluid), of all secretions (salivary juice, gastric juice, bile, sweat), and all excretory fluids (urine). Intake of water is determined principally by the sense of thirst. Excessive intake may lead to water intoxication; excessive loss to dehydration. Humans can survive for only a short time without water intake. The exact length of survival time varies with ambient temperature, moisture in available food, and amount of physical activity.

w., bound. Water that in protoplasm is attached to organic substances. It is not available for metabolic processes.

w., deionized. Water that has been passed through a substance that removes cations and anions present as contaminants.

w., distilled. Water that has been purified by distillation, q.v. Used for pharmaceutical purposes.

w., emergency preparation of safe drinking. Water must be purified when only unclean water is available or if there is reason to believe that available drinking water has become contaminated. One of the following methods may be used: (1) Strain water through a clean cloth and boil water vigorously for 30 minutes. (2) Add three drops of alcoholic solution of iodine to each quart (approx. 1 liter) of water. Mix well and let it stand for 30 minutes prior to using. (3) Add either 10 drops of 1% chlorine bleach, or 2 drops of 4 to 6% chlorine bleach, or 1 drop of 7 to 10% chlorine bleach to each quart (liter) of water. Mix well and let stand for 30 minutes. If water is cloudy to begin with, use double the amount of chlorine.

w., hard. Water that contains dissolved salts of magnesium or calcium.

w., heavy. D_2O. An isotopic variety of water, esp. deuterium oxide, in which hydrogen has been displaced by its isotope, deuterium. Its properties differ from ordinary water in that heavy water has a higher freezing and boiling point and in the fact that it is incapable of supporting life.

w., lime. Calcium hydroxide solution.

w., purified. Water that is mineral free. Obtained by distillation, q.v., or deionization, q.v.

w., pyrogen-free. Water that has been rendered free of fever-producing proteins (bacteria and their metabolic products). SEE: *water for injection.*

w., soft. Water that contains very little, if any, dissolved salts of magnesium or calcium.

water bed. A rubber mattress partially filled with warm water (100° F. or 37.8° C.). If too full, the mattress will be hard. Used in preventing and treating bedsores.

water brash. Gastric burning pain with reflux of gastric acid into the esophagus. SYN: *heartburn; pyrosis.*

water cure. Use of water in treatment of a condition. SYN: *hydrotherapy.*

water for injection. Water for parenteral use that has been distilled and sterilized. Distilled, sterilized water that is stored in sealed containers will remain free of pyrogens and may be used after longer periods of storage.

water-hammer pulse. Pulse marked by a quick, powerful beat, collapsing suddenly. SYN: *pulse, Corrigan's.*

Waterhouse-Friderichsen syndrome. Acute adrenal insufficiency due to hemorrhage into the adrenal gland caused by meningococcal infection. SEE: *adrenal gland.*

water immersion. Immersion of the body in warm water in order to stimulate diuresis. This technique is used to induce or increase urine production in persons with nephrotic syndrome. The patient in a seated position is immersed in water up to the level of the neck. This is done daily for several hours at a time, at a temperature of 34° C. The loss of fluid due to sweating during this treatment is self-limiting because of hydromeiosis, a condition in which the epidermis swells and blocks the sweat ducts.

water intoxication. Excess water and sodium retention. Clinically, abdominal cramps, dizziness, lethargy, nausea, vomiting, convulsions, and coma may be present.

ETIOL: Excess ingestion of water, I.V. administration of hypotonic solutions, excess tap water enemas, hypothalamic tumors, cerebral concussion, or excess secretion of antidiuretic hormone. SEE: *brain edema.*

water on brain. Disease marked by abnormal increase in cerebrospinal fluid. SYN: *hydrocephalus.*

waters. Common term for the amniotic fluid surrounding the fetus.

Watson-Crick helix. [James Dewey Watson, U.S. biochemist, b. 1928; Francis Harry Comptom Crick, Brit. biochemist, b. 1916] A double helix named after the scientists who established its structure. Each half of the helix contains chemical compounds arranged in a specific sequence. Variation in the sequence of these compounds enables genetic information to be transmitted. The double helix is the structure of DNA (deoxyribonucleic acid).

Watson-Schwartz test (wŏt′sŏn-shwărts). [Cecil J. Watson, U.S. physician, b. 1901; Samuel Schwartz, U.S. physician, b. 1916] A test used in acute porphyria to differentiate porphobilinogen from urobilinogen.

watt. [James Watt, Scottish engineer, 1736–1819] Unit of electrical power. May be expressed as work at the rate of one joule per second. One watt is the power produced by one ampere of current flowing with a force or pressure, i.e., electromotive force, of one volt. SEE: *electromotive force.*

wattage (wŏt′ĭj). The electrical energy produced or consumed by an electrical device, expressed in watts.

wave (wāv) [ME. *wave*]. 1. A disturbance, usually orderly and predictable, observed as a moving ridge on the surface of a liquid. 2. An undulating or vibrating motion. 3. An oscillation seen in the recording of an electrocardiogram, electroencephalogram, or other graphic record of physiological activity. SEE: illus.

w., alpha. SEE: *rhythm, alpha.*

w., beta. SEE: *rhythm, beta.*

w., brain. The fluctuation, usually rhythmic, of electrical impulses produced by the brain. SEE: *electroencephalography.*

w., delta. SEE: *rhythm, delta.*

w., electromagnetic. A wave-form produced by simultaneous oscillation of electric and magnetic fields perpendicular to each other. The direction of propagation of the wave is perpendicular to the oscillations. The following waves are electromagnetic. They are listed in order of increasing frequency and decreasing wavelength: radio, television, microwave, infrared, visible light, ultraviolet, x-rays, and gamma rays. SEE: *electromagnetic spectrum* for table.

w., excitation. The excitatory impulse(s) that originate in the sinoatrial node of the heart and sweep through the musculature of the atria, stimulating the atrioventricular node and then continuing through the conductile tissue of the ventricles. They bring about the contraction of the chambers of the heart.

w., hertzian. Electromagnetic radiations used in radio and wireless transmission.

w., light. Electromagnetic waves that produce the sensation of visible light on the retina.

w., P. SEE: *electrocardiogram.*

w., pulse. The pressure wave originated

COMPONENTS OF WAVES

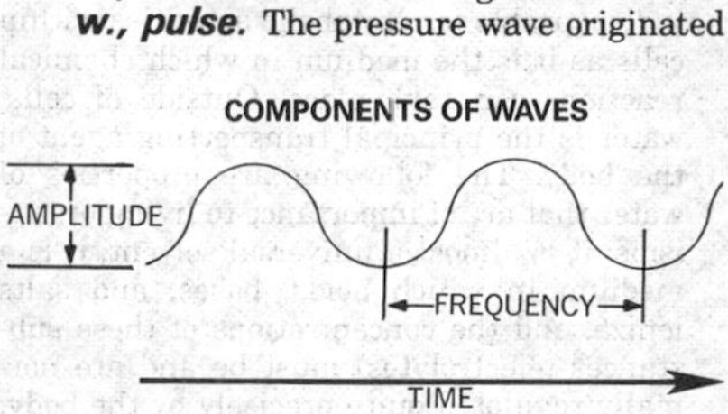

by the systolic discharge of blood into the aorta. It is not due to the passage of the ejected blood but is the result of the impact being transmitted through the arterial walls. Its speed of transmission varies with the nature of the arterial wall, increasing with age as the arteries become less resilient. Thus in arteriosclerosis, the velocity is increased over normal.

w., Q. SEE: *electrocardiogram.*

w., R. SEE: *electrocardiogram.*

w., radio. Electromagnetic waves between the frequencies of 10^{11} and 10^4 hertz.

w., S. SEE: *electrocardiogram.*

w.'s, sound. Vibrations of a vibrating medium that, upon stimulating sensory receptors of the cochlea, are capable of giving rise to sensations of sound. Velocity: in dry air 1087 ft. (331.6 meters) per sec. at 0° C.; in water, approx. 4 times faster than in air.

w., T. SEE: *electrocardiogram.*

w., theta. Brain waves present in the electroencephalogram. They have a frequency of about 4 to 7 hertz.

w., ultrashort. Arbitrary designation of radio waves of a wavelength of less than 1 meter.

w., ultrasonic. A sound wave of greater frequency than 20 kilohertz. These waves do not produce sound audible to the human ear.

wavelength (wāv'lĕngth). The distance between the beginning and end of a single wave cycle, usually measured from the top of one wave to the top of the next one.

wax [AS. *weax*]. 1. Beeswax, secreted by bees; a substance that is solid at room temperature. In medicine, a purified form, white wax, is used in making ointments and to stop bleeding from bones during surgery. 2. Any substance with the consistency of beeswax. 3. Earwax. SYN: *cerumen.*

w., dental. A variety of waxes compounded for their specific properties desired for dental procedures, e.g., baseplate wax, bone wax, boxing wax, burnout wax, casting wax, inlay wax, and pattern wax.

waxing-up. In dentistry, the shaping of wax around the contours of a trial denture.

waxy (wăks'ē) [AS. *weax,* wax]. Resembling or pert. to wax.

waxy cast. Dense, highly refractile urinary cast. Such casts have clean-cut contours, sometimes irregular curves and notches. Occurs in severe chronic renal disease.

waxy degeneration. Amyloid degeneration seen in wasting diseases.

W.B.C. *white blood cells; white blood count.*

weak (wēk) [Old Norse *veikr,* flexible]. 1. Lacking physical strength or vigor; infirm.

RS: asthenia; atony; cardiasthenia; enervation; ergasthenia; fatigue; lassitude.

2. Dilute, as in a weak solution; or weak tea.

wean (wēn) [AS. *wenian*]. To accustom an infant to discontinuation of breast milk by substitution of other nourishment.

weanling. A young child or infant recently changed from breast to formula feeding.

weanling diarrhea. Severe gastroenteritis that sometimes occurs in infants who recently have been weaned.

web. A tissue or membrane extending across a space.

w., esophageal. A tissue in the form of a web that extends across the esophageal lumen and thus interferes with the swallowing of food.

w., terminal. A web-like network, microscopic in size, that is beneath the microvilli of absorption cells of the intestines, and beneath the hair cells of the inner ear.

webbed (wĕbd) [AS. *webb,* a fabric]. Having a membrane or tissue connecting adjacent structures, as the toes of a duck's feet.

Weber-Christian disease (wĕb'ĕr-krĭs'chĕn). [Friedrich Weber, Brit. physician, 1863–1962; Henry A. Christian, U.S. physician, 1876–1951] Relapsing, febrile, nodular, nonsuppurative panniculitis, a generalized disorder of fat metabolism characterized by recurring episodes of fever and development of crops of subcutaneous fatty nodules.

Weber's glands (vā'bĕrz). [Moritz I. Weber, Ger. anatomist, 1795–1875] Mucous glands on the lateral borders of the lateral edges of the tongue.

Weber's paralysis (wĕb'ĕrz). [Sir Hermann David Weber, Brit. physician, 1824–1918] Paralysis of oculomotor nerve on one side with contralateral spastic hemiplegia.

ETIOL: Lesion of the crus cerebri.

Weber test. [Friedrich Eugen Weber, Ger. otologist, 1832–1891] A test for unilateral deafness. A vibrating tuning fork held against the midline of the top of the head is perceived as being so located by those with equal hearing ability in the ears; to persons with unilateral conductive-type deafness, the sound will be perceived as being more pronounced on the diseased side; in persons with unilateral nerve-type deafness, the sound will be perceived as being loudest in the good ear.

wedge pressure. Pulmonary artery wedge pressure, q.v.

WEE. *western equine encephalomyelitis.*

weeping [AS. *wepan,* to lament]. 1. Shedding tears. 2. Moist, dripping.

weeping eczema. Dermatitis with eruption of vesicles exuding serum.

weeping sinew. Circumscribed cystic swelling of a tendon sheath.

Wegener's granulomatosis or syndrome. A rare condition characterized by vasculitis, granulomatous lesions of the entire respiratory tract, and glomerulonephritis. The symptoms are fever, weakness, malaise, weight loss, purulent rhinitis, sinusitis, polyarthralgia, ulcerations of the nasal septum, and signs of severe progressive renal disease. If it is diagnosed early and treated with cyclophosphamide, the prognosis is very good; if it is not treated early, death is the outcome, usually within one year.

Weidel's reaction (vī'dĕlz). [Hugo Weidel, Austrian chemist, 1849–1899] Test for presence of xanthine bodies or uric acid.

Weigert's law (vī'gĕrts). [Karl Weigert, Ger. pathologist, 1843–1904] An observation that states that loss or destruction of tissue results in an excess of new tissue during repair.

weight (wāt) [AS. *gewiht*]. The measure of heaviness or the mass of something.

Weight of the body increases in pathological obesity and decreases in Addison's disease, cancer, chronic diarrhea, chronic suppurations, untreated Type I diabetes mellitus, hysteria, anorexia, fevers, lactation when prolonged, marasmus, obstruction of pylorus or thoracic duct, tuberculosis, and ulcer of the stomach.

Normal weight depends upon the frame of the individual. SEE: Height and Weight Tables for Men and Women According to Frame.

w., apothecaries'. SEE: *apothecaries' weights and measures*.

w., atomic. ABBR: at. wt. Weight of an atom of an element compared with that of oxygen which is taken as 16; the mean value of the isotopic weights of an element.

w., avoirdupois. SEE: *avoirdupois measure*.

w., equivalent. The weight of a chemical element that is equivalent to and will replace a hydrogen atom (1.008 grams) in a chemical reaction.

w., molecular. ABBR: mol. wt. The sum of all the atomic weights of all the elements in one molecule of a compound.

weightlessness. Condition of not being acted upon by the force of gravity. This is present when astronauts travel in areas so distant from the earth, moon, or planets that the force of gravity is virtually absent.

weights and measures. SEE: *Weights and Measures* in *Appendix*.

Weil-Felix reaction, test (vīl-fā'lĭks). [Edmund Weil, Ger. physician, 1880–1922; Arthur Felix, Ger. bacteriologist, 1887–1956] The agglutination of certain Proteus organisms due to the development of Proteus anti-

1983 Metropolitan Height and Weight Tables for Men and Women According to Frame, Ages 25–59

Men					Women				
Height (in Shoes)*		Weight in Pounds (In Indoor Clothing)†			Height (In Shoes)*		Weight in Pounds (In Indoor Clothing)†		
Ft.	In.	Small Frame	Medium Frame	Large Frame	Ft.	In.	Small Frame	Medium Frame	Large Frame
5	2	128–134	131–141	138–150	4	10	102–111	109–121	118–131
5	3	130–136	133–143	140–153	4	11	103–113	111–123	120–134
5	4	132–138	135–145	142–156	5	0	104–115	113–126	122–137
5	5	134–140	137–148	144–160	5	1	106–118	115–129	125–140
5	6	136–142	139–151	146–164	5	2	108–121	118–132	128–143
5	7	138–145	142–154	149–168	5	3	111–124	121–135	131–147
5	8	140–148	145–157	152–172	5	4	114–127	124–138	134–151
5	9	142–151	148–160	155–176	5	5	117–130	127–141	137–155
5	10	144–154	151–163	158–180	5	6	120–133	130–144	140–159
5	11	146–157	154–166	161–184	5	7	123–136	133–147	143–163
6	0	149–160	157–170	164–188	5	8	126–139	136–150	146–167
6	1	152–164	160–174	168–192	5	9	129–142	139–153	149–170
6	2	155–168	164–178	172–197	5	10	132–145	142–156	152–173
6	3	158–172	167–182	176–202	5	11	135–148	145–159	155–176
6	4	162–176	171–187	181–207	6	0	138–151	148–162	158–179

*Shoes with 1-inch heels.

†Indoor clothing weighing 5 pounds for men and 3 pounds for women.

Source of basic data: *Build Study, 1979,* Society of Actuaries and Association of Life Insurance Medical Directors of America, 1980.

bodies in certain rickettsial diseases.

Weil's disease (vīlz). [Adolf Weil, Ger. physician, 1848–1916] Severe leptospirosis caused by any one of several serotypes of Leptospira such as L. icterohemorrhagica, L. pomona, L. canicola, or L. autumnalis.

ETIOL: An organism found in rat urine and feces, and acquired by man through contaminated food or water or by contact of broken skin with an infected rat or its feces or urine. It is a specific infection accompanied by muscular pains, fever, jaundice, and enlargement of liver and spleen.

TREATMENT: Largely symptomatic because there is no specific therapeutic agent. Penicillin may shorten the course of the disease.

Weir Mitchell's treatment (wēr mĭt'chĕlz). [S. Weir Mitchell, U.S. neurologist, 1829–1914] Treatment for hysteria and neurasthenia that consists of rest in bed, massage, nourishing diet, and isolation.

weismannism (wīs'măn-ĭzm). [August F. L. Weismann, Ger. biologist, 1834–1914] The theory that acquired characteristics are not inherited.

Weitbrecht's foramen (vīt'brĕkts). [Josias Weitbrecht, Ger.-born Petrograd anatomist, 1702–1747] An opening in the articular cartilage of the shoulder joint.

Weitbrecht's ligament. The oblique cord connecting the ulna and radius.

Welch's bacillus (wĕlsh'ĕz). [William Henry Welch, U.S. pathologist, 1850–1934] Clostridium perfringens, the causative organism of gas gangrene. SEE: *gangrene, gas.*

welt [ME. *welte*]. An elevation on the skin produced by a lash, blow, or allergic stimulus. The skin is unbroken and the mark is reversible.

wen (wĕn) [AS.]. A cyst resulting from the retention of secretion in a sebaceous gland. SYN: *sebaceous cyst; steatoma.*

SYM: One or more rounded or oval elevations varying in size from a few millimeters to about 10 centimeters, slowly appear on scalp, face, or back; painless, rather soft, containing a yellowish-white caseous mass.

TREATMENT: Sac and contents should be carefully dissected in order to prevent its recurrence.

Wenckebach's period, pauses, or phenomenon (vĕn'kĕ-băks). [Karel F. Wenckebach, Dutch-born Vienna internist, 1864–1940] A form of incomplete heart block in which, as detected by electrocardiography, there is progressive lengthening of the P-R interval until there is not a ventricular response; and then the cycle of increasing P-R intervals begins again.

Werdnig-Hoffmann disease (vĕrd'nĭg-hŏf'măn). [Guido Werdnig, 19th-cent. Austrian neurologist; Johann Hoffmann, Ger. neurologist, 1857–1919] A hereditary, progressive, infantile form of muscular atrophy resulting from degeneration of anterior horn cells of the spinal cord. Characterized by early onset, hypotonia and wasting of muscles, complete flaccid paralysis, and death.

Werdnig-Hoffmann paralysis. Infantile muscular atrophy, considered by some to be identical with amyotonia congenita. SEE: *Hoffmann's syndrome.*

Werdnig-Hoffmann syndrome. SEE: *Hoffmann's syndrome.*

Werlhof's disease (vĕrl'hŏfs). [Paul G. Werlhof, Ger. physician, 1699–1767] Idiopathic thrombocytopenic purpura. SEE: *purpura, idiopathic thrombocytopenic.*

Wernicke's encephalopathy (vĕr'nĭ-kēz). [Karl Wernicke, Ger. neurologist, 1848–1905] Encephalopathy associated with thiamine deficiency. Usually associated with chronic alcoholism, gastric carcinoma, or hyperemesis gravidarum.

Wernicke's syndrome. Frequent condition of old age marked by loss of memory and disorientation with confabulation. SYN: *presbyophrenia.* SEE: *polioencephalitis, anterior superior.*

Westphal-Edinger nucleus. [Karl Westphal, Ger. neurologist, 1833–1890; Ludwig Edinger, Ger. neurologist, 1855–1918] Small group of nerve cells in rostral portion of nucleus of oculomotor nerve. Efferent fibers pass to ciliary ganglion conveying impulses destined for intrinsic muscles of the eye.

Westphal-Strümpell pseudosclerosis (vĕst'făl-strĭm'p'l). [K. Westphal; Ernst A. G. G. von Strümpell, Leipzig physician, 1853–1925] 1. Hepatolenticular degeneration. SEE: *Wilson's disease.* 2. Hysteria with symptoms of disseminated sclerosis but no pathological changes in the nervous system.

wet (wĕt) [AS. *waet*]. Soaked with moisture.

wet brain. Increased amount of cerebrospinal fluid with edema of the meninges, due to alcoholism.

wet cup. A cupping glass used after scarification.

wet dream. Nocturnal seminal emission.

wet-nurse. A woman who breastfeeds another's child.

wet pack. A form of bath given by wrapping patient in hot or cold wet sheets, covered with a blanket, used esp. to reduce fever.

Wetzel grid (wĕt'sĕl). [Norman C. Wetzel, U.S. pediatrician, b. 1897] A graph for use in evaluating growth and development in children aged 5 to 18 years.

Wharton's duct (hwăr'tŏnz). [Thomas Wharton, Brit. anatomist, 1614–1673] Duct of the submandibular salivary gland opening into the mouth at side of the frenum linguae.

Wharton's jelly. A gelatinous intercellular substance consisting of primitive connective tissue of the umbilical cord. It is rich in hyaluronic acid.

wheal (hwēl). 1. [AS. *hwele*]. More or less round and evanescent elevation of the skin, white in center with pale red periphery, accompanied by itching. Seen in urticaria, insect bites, anaphylaxis, angioneurotic edema. SYN: *pomphus*. 2. [ME. *wale,* a stripe]. An elongated mark or ridge. Such a ridge produced for intradermal injection or caused by injection or tests.

wheat (hwēt) [AS. *hwaete*]. Any of various cereal grasses, widely cultivated for its important edible grain used in making flour. Boiled whole wheat is an excellent food. SEE: *bread.*

STRUCTURE: Husk or outer coat, removed before grinding; bran coats, removed in making white flour and containing the mineral substances; gluten, contains the fat and protein; starch, center of the kernel.

Refined wheat products do not include the bran and germ, which contain B complex vitamins, phosphorus, and iron.

WHEAT PREPARATIONS AND PASTAS: Macaroni, vermicelli, and noodles are made from flour and water, molded, dried, and slightly baked. They are easy to digest and not over 10% of nitrogen content is lost.

wheatstone bridge. An electric circuit in which there are two branches each containing two resistors. These branches are joined to complete the circuit. If the resistance in three resistors is known, the resistance of the fourth and unknown one can be calculated.

wheelchair. A special chair equipped with large wheels for transporting patients. Especially useful in enabling partially paralyzed individuals to be mobile and have occupations that might otherwise be impossible.

Wheelchairs are made in a variety of sizes and weights to accommodate the patient and the type of injury. The universal wheelchair has larger wheels in the back and may be used indoors or outside. A wheelchair for amputees is available with rear wheels that are set farther back to compensate for the loss of weight of the amputated limbs. Power-driven wheelchairs should be used only for patients who cannot propel themselves.

wheeze (hwēz) [ME. *whesen*]. A whistling or sighing sound resulting from narrowing of the lumen of a respiratory passageway. Often only noted by use of stethoscope. Occurs in asthma, croup, hay fever, mitral stenosis, and pleural effusion. May result from presence of tumors, foreign obstructions, bronchial spasm, tuberculosis, obstructive emphysema, or edema.

wheezing. Production of whistling sounds during difficult breathing such as occurs in asthma, coryza, croup, and other respiratory disorders. SEE: *wheeze.*

whelk (hwĕlk) [AS. *hwylca*]. A wheal; a protuberance on the face as a nodule or tubercle.

whiff. 1. A slight gust or puff of air, esp. one conveying an odor. 2. A quick inhalation or exhalation, as of tobacco smoke.

whinolalia (wĭn″ō-lā′lē-ă) [AS. *whinan,* whine, + Gr. *lalein,* to talk]. Hypernasality and distortion of speech. Occurs in incompetent palate syndrome.

whiplash injury. Imprecise term for injury to the cervical vertebrae and adjacent soft tissues. Produced by a sudden jerking or relative backward or forward acceleration of the head with respect to the vertebral column. Injury may occur to those in a vehicle that is suddenly and forcibly struck from the rear.

Whipple's disease (hwĭp′ĕlz). [George Hoyt Whipple, U.S. pathologist, b. 1878] Intestinal lipodystrophy, characterized by fatty stools, loss of weight and strength, chronic arthritis, a distinctive lesion of the mucosa of the jejunum and ileum, and other signs of a malabsorption syndrome. This rare disease resembles idiopathic steatorrhea.

TREATMENT: Intensive antibiotic therapy with procaine penicillin followed by maintenance therapy with tetracycline provides good results.

whipworm. Common name for a roundworm often parasitic in the human intestines. SYN: *Trichuris trichiura.*

whirl (hwŭrl) [Old Norse *hvirfla*]. 1. To revolve rapidly. 2. To feel giddiness.

whirlbone. 1. The kneecap. SYN: *patella.* 2. The head of the femur.

whirlpool bath. SEE: *bath, whirlpool.*

whiskey, whisky (hwĭs′kē). A distilled alcoholic liquor made from grain. The alcohol present is ethyl alcohol.

CAUTION: Wood or methyl alcohol should never be used in alcoholic beverages intended for human consumption. It is extremely toxic and may cause death. In those who survive, blindness is a common occurrence.

whisper (hwĭs′pĕr) [AS. *hwisprian*]. 1. Speech with a low, soft voice, a low, sibilant sound. 2. To utter in a low sound.

w., cavernous. Direct transmission of a whisper through a cavity in auscultation.

whistle (hwĭs′ĕl). 1. A sound produced by pursing one's lips and blowing. 2. A tubular device driven by wind that produces a loud and usually shrill sound.

"whistling face syndrome." A congenital malformation with muscle dysfunction that produces a masklike "whistling face." Also present are hypoplastic nasal bones and clubfeet. The genetic transmission may be autosomal recessive.

white (hwīt) [AS. *hwit*]. 1. The achromatic color of maximum lightness that reflects all rays of the spectrum. 2. The color of milk or fresh snow; opposite of black.

white cell. The leukocyte.

white gangrene. Gangrene due to local anemia.

whitehead (hwīt′hĕd). Milium, q.v.

white leg. Phlebitis of femoral vein marked by white swelling of the leg. SYN: *phlegmasia alba dolens.*

white line. White tendinous attachment of abdominal oblique and transverse muscles. Visible in the midline of the skin covering the anterior wall of the abdomen. SYN: *linea alba.*

white lotion. USP. A combination of zinc sulfate, and sulfurated potash diluted in purified water, used in treating certain skin diseases.

white matter. Any nervous structure composed of white medullated nerve fibers.

white of egg. The albumin of an egg.

white of eye. Conjunctiva.

white ointment. USP. An ointment containing white wax and white petroleum.

whitepox (hwīt′pŏks). Variola minor.

white precipitate. A white amorphous powder used principally in ointments for external treatment of some skin diseases. SYN: *ammoniated mercury.*

white softening. Stage of softening of any substance in which the affected area has become white and anemic.

whitlow (hwĭt′lō) [ME. *whitflawe,* white flow]. Suppurative inflammation at the end of a finger or toe. It may be deep seated, involving the bone and its periosteum, or superficial, affecting parts of the nail. SYN: *felon; panaris; paronychia; runaround.*

Whitmore's disease. Melioidosis, q.v.

W.H.O. *World Health Organization.*

whole body counter. Instrument that detects the radiation present in the entire body.

wholism. Holism, q.v.

wholistic health. SEE: *holistic medicine.*

whoop (hoop) [AS. *hwopan,* to threaten]. The sonorous and convulsive inspiratory crow following a paroxysm of whooping cough.

whooping cough. An acute infectious disease caused by Bordetella pertussis with recurrent spasms of coughing ending in a whooping inspiration. SYN: *pertussis.*

whorl (hwŭrl) [ME. *whorle*]. 1. Spiral arrangement of cardiac muscular fibers. SYN: *vortex.* 2. A type of fingerprint in which the central papillary ridges turn through at least one complete circle. SEE: *fingerprint* for illus.

whortleberry (hwŭrt′tl-bĕr″ē). A sweet European blueberry. SEE: *blueberries.*

Widal's reaction or test (vē-dŏlz′). [Fernand Widal, Fr. physician, 1862–1929] An agglutination test for typhoid fever.

wild cherry. The dried bark of Prunus serotina, used principally in the form of syrup as a flavored vehicle for cough medicine.

will [AS.]. 1. The mental faculty used in choosing or deciding upon an act or thought. 2. Power of controlling one's actions or emotions.

Willis' circle (wĭl′ĭs). [Thomas Willis, Brit. anatomist, 1621–1675] An intercommunicating set of arteries that encircles the optic chiasma and hypophysis, from which the principal arteries supplying the brain are derived. It receives blood from the two internal carotid arteries and the basilar artery formed by union of the two vertebrals. SEE: illus.

Willis' cords. Cords crossing the superior longitudinal sinus transversely.

Wilms tumor (vĭlmz). [Marx Wilms, Ger. surgeon, 1867–1918] Rapidly developing tumor of the kidney that usually occurs in children. In the past, the mortality from this cancer was extremely high. Newer approaches to therapy have been very effective in controlling the tumor. SYN: *embryonal carcinosarcoma; nephroblastoma.*

Wilson's disease (wĭl′sŭnz). [Samuel A. K. Wilson, Brit. neurologist, 1765–1821] A hereditary syndrome transmitted as an autosomal recessive trait in which a decrease of ceruloplasmin, q.v., produces accumulation of copper in various organs (brain, liver, kidney, and cornea) associated with increased intestinal absorption of copper. A pigmented ring (Kayser-Fleischer ring) at the outer margin of the cornea is pathognomonic. Also characterized by degenerative changes in the brain, cirrhosis of the liver,

ARTERIES OF THE CIRCLE OF WILLIS

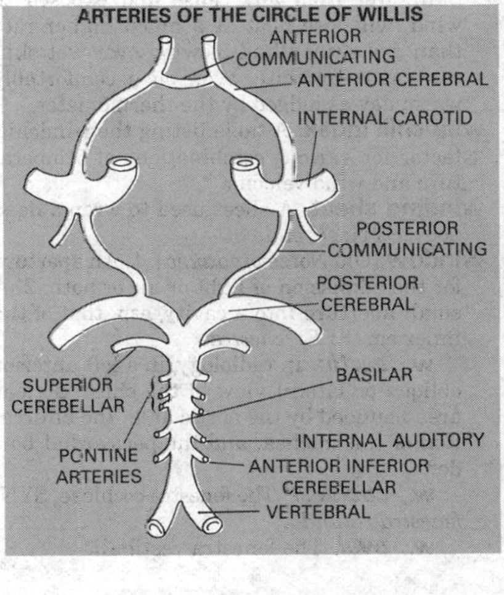

splenomegaly, tremor, muscular rigidity, involuntary movements, spastic contractures, psychic disturbances, dysphagia, and progressive weakness and emaciation. SYN: *hepatolenticular degeneration*.

Wilson-Mikity syndrome. A so-called pulmonary dysmaturity syndrome seen in premature infants. The symptoms are insidious onset of dyspnea, tachypnea, and cyanosis in the first month of life. Roentgenograms of the lungs reveal evidence of emphysema that develops into multicysts. Therapy is directed to the pulmonary insufficiency and cardiac failure. The death rate is about 25%.

Winckel's disease (vĭng'kĕlz). [Franz von Winckel, Ger. gynecologist, 1837–1911] A fatal disease of the newborn characterized by profuse hemorrhages, hematuria, jaundice, enlarged spleen, collapse, and convulsions.

windburn. Erythema, and irritation of the skin due to exposure to wind. Simultaneous exposure to the sun, moisture, wind, and cold may cause a severe dermatitis.

windchill. The cooling effect wind has on exposed human skin.

windchill factor. Loss of heat from exposure of skin to wind. Heat loss is proportional to the speed of the wind. Thus skin exposed to a wind velocity of 20 miles per hour (MPH) (32 kilometers per hour) when the temperature is 0° F. (−17.8° C.) will be cooled at the same rate it would be in still air at −46° F. (−43.3° C.). Similarly when the temperature is 20° F. (−6.7° C.) and the wind is 10, 20, or 35 MPH (16.1, 32.2, or 56.3 kilometers per hour), the equivalent skin temperature would be −4°, −18°, or −28° F. (−20°, −27.8°, or −33.3° C.), respectively.

Windchill factor is calculated for dry skin. Skin, wet from any cause and exposed to wind, will lose heat at a much higher rate than dry skin. Wind blowing over wet skin can cause frostbite, even on a comfortably warm day as judged by the thermometer.

windchill index. A table listing the windchill factor for various combinations of temperature and wind velocity.

winding sheet. A sheet used to wrap a dead body. SYN: *shroud*.

window [Old Norse *vindauga*]. 1. An aperture for the admission of light or air or both. 2. A small aperture into a cavity, esp. that of the inner ear. SEE: *fenestra*.

w., aortic. In radiology, in a left anterior oblique or lateral view of the chest, a clear area bounded by the aortic arch, the bifurcation of the trachea, and the pericardial border.

w., cochlear. The fenestra cochleae. SYN: *fenestra rotunda*.

w., oval. The fenestra vestibuli.

w., round. The fenestra cochleae. SYN: *fenestra rotunda*.

w., vestibular. The oval window. SYN: *fenestra vestibuli*.

windpipe. The tubular structure through which air passes from the larynx to the lungs. SYN: *trachea*.

wine (wīn) [L. *vinum*, wine]. 1. Fermented juice of any fruit, usually made from grapes and contains 10–15% alcohol. 2. Solution of a medicinal substance in wine. SYN: *vinum*.

wine glass. A fluid measure of approx. 2 fl. oz. (60 ml.).

wine sores. Slang term for superficial infected areas of the skin seen in alcoholics with poor personal hygiene. Erroneously thought to be due to specific action of the wine.

wing [Old Norse *vaengi*]. A structure resembling the wing of a bird, esp. the great and small wings of the sphenoid bone, q.v. SEE: *ala*.

wink [AS. *wincian*]. 1. To close and open the eyelids quickly. 2. Act of closing and opening the eyelids quickly.

Win-Kinase. Trade name for urokinase.

winking. Wink, def. 2, q.v.

w., jaw. Involuntary simultaneous closing of the eyelid as the jaw is moved.

w., jaw-, syndrome. Unilateral ptosis of the eye at rest; and rapid exaggerating elevation of the lid when the mandible is either depressed or moved to the opposite side of the ptosed lid. SYN: *Gunn's syndrome*.

Winslow, foramen of (wĭnz'lō). [Jacob B. Winslow, Fr. anatomist, 1669–1760] The epiploic foramen.

Winslow, ligament of. The oblique popliteal ligament located at back of knee.

Winslow, pancreas of. The processus uncinatus of the pancreas.

Winstrol. Trade name for stanozolol.

Wintergreen Oil. Trade name for methyl salicylate.

wintergreen oil. Methyl salicylate, a colorless, yellowish, or reddish liquid that has a characteristic taste and odor. It is used as a flavoring substance, and as a counterirritant applied topically in the form of salves, lotions, and ointments. SYN: *methyl salicylate; sweet birch oil*.

winter itch. Itching occurring only in cold weather. Probably due to drying of skin that is deficient in natural lubrication. SYN: *pruritus hiemalis*.

wire (wīr). 1. Metal drawn out into threads of varying thickness. 2. To join fracture fragments together by use of wire.

w., arch. In dentistry, application of wire around the dental arch in order to correct irregularities of position of the teeth.

w., Kirschner's. Steel wire placed through a long bone in order to apply traction to the bone.

w., ligature. Soft, thin wire used in orthodontics to anchor other dental devices to an arch wire.

w., separating. A soft wire used in dentistry to separate teeth prior to banding them.

wiring (wīr'ĭng). Fastening bone fragments together by use of wire.

w., circumferential. Method of treating a fractured mandible by passing wires around the bone and a splint in the oral cavity.

w., continuous loop. Forming wire loops on both mandibular and maxillary teeth in order to provide attachment sites for rubber bands. This is used in treating fractures of the mandible.

w., craniofacial suspension. Use of bones not contiguous with the oral cavity for attachment of wires that lead from those bones to the fractured jaw segments.

w., Gilmer. Wiring of single opposed teeth by use of wire passed circumferentially around the two teeth and the ends twisted together. Used to produce intermaxillary fixation.

w., Ivy loop. Placement of wire around adjacent teeth in order to provide an attachment of elastics.

w., perialveolar. Use of wires to fix a splint to the mandible. The wires are passed through the alveolar process from the buccal plate to the palate.

w., pyriform. Use of the nasal bones for stabilizing a fracture of the jaw. The wires are passed through the pyriform aperture of the nasal bone and then to the segment.

w., Stout's. W., continuous loop.

Wirsung, duct of (vēr'soong). [Johann Georg Wirsung, Ger. physician, 1600–1643] Excretory duct of the pancreas. SYN: *duct, pancreatic.*

wisdom tooth (wĭz'dŏm). The last molar tooth on each side of the jaw. These four molars may appear as late as the 25th year or may never erupt.

Wiskott-Aldrich syndrome. A sex-linked, recessive disorder with a defect in both T and B cell function. It is characterized by eczema, thrombocytopenia with bleeding tendency, and infections, esp. of the ears. Treatment consists of antibiotics, but the possibility of superinfection by viruses, fungi, and Pneumocystis carinii must be watched for. The use of transfer factor obtained from activated lymphocytes has been effective in about half of the cases. Because of the variable severity of the disease, some patients have lived into their teens, but death may occur at an earlier age.

witches' milk. Milk secreted by the newly born infant's breast, stimulated by the lactating hormone circulating in the mother.

withdrawal. Cessation of administration of a drug, esp. a narcotic, or alcohol to which the individual has become either physiologically or psychologically addicted. Withdrawal symptoms vary with the type of drug used. Neonates may exhibit withdrawal symptoms from drugs or alcohol ingested by the mother during pregnancy. SEE: *drug addiction.*

withdrawal syndrome. Partial collapse resulting from withdrawal of alcohol, stimulants, and some opiates. SYN: *abstinence syndrome.*

witkop (wĭt'kŏp) [Afrikaans, white scalp]. Matted crusts in the hair to produce a scalp-like structure. Seen in South African natives. SYN: *dikwakwadi; white head.*

witzelsucht (vĭt'sĕl-zookt). [M. Jastro Witz, Ger. physician, b. 1839] Condition produced by frontal lobe lesions characterized by self-amusement from poor jokes and puns. SEE: *moria.*

w., primary affective. A peculiar variety of witzelsucht characterized by teutonization of nomenclature.

Wohlfahrtia (vōl-făr'tē-ă). A genus of flies parasitic in animal tissue, belonging to the family Sarcophagidae, order Diptera.

W. magnifica. Species found in southeast Europe. The larvae may occur in human and animal wounds.

W. opaca. Species occurring in Canada, a common parasite of wild animals. Human infants may become infested.

W. vigil. Species found in Canada and northern United States.

wolffian body (wool'fē-ăn). [Kaspar Friedrich Wolff, Ger. anatomist, 1733–1794] An embryonic organ on each side of the vertebral column. SYN: *mesonephros.* SEE: *archinephron; embryo; paroophoron; parovarium.*

wolffian cyst. One of the broad ligaments of the uterus.

wolffian duct. Duct in the embryo leading from the mesonephros to cloaca. From it develop the ductus epididymis, ductus deferens, seminal vesicle, ejaculatory duct, ureter, and pelvis of kidney. SYN: *mesonephric duct.*

wolffian tubules. One of 30 to 34 tubules that develop within the mesonephros and empty into the mesonephric duct. Most are transitional, persisting for only a short time. Some persist in adult males as the efferent ductules of the testis; others persist only as vestigial structures. SYN: *mesonephric tubules.* SEE: *epoophoron; paradidymis; paroophoron.*

Wolff-Parkinson-White syndrome. [L. Wolff, U.S. physician, b. 1898; Sir John Parkinson, 19th-century Brit. physician; Paul Dudley White, U.S. cardiologist, 1886–1974] Abnormality of cardiac rhythm that manifests as supraventricular tachycardia. The diagnosis is made by use of electrocardiography. The PR interval is less than 0.12 seconds and the QRS complex contains an initial slur, called the delta wave, that broadens the complex.

Wolfina 50. Trade name for rauwolfia serpentina.

wolfram (wool'frăm). Tungsten.

wolfsbane (wŏlfs'bān). Old name for aconite root.

Wolhynian fever. Trench fever, q.v.

Wolman's disease. [M. Wolman, contemporary Israeli physician] An inherited metabolic disorder wherein infants develop hepatosplenomegaly, calcification of the adrenal glands, and foam cells in the bone marrow and other tissues.

womb (woom) [AS. *wamb*]. Female organ for protection and nourishment of the fetus. SYN: *uterus*.

wood alcohol. CH_3OH. Alcohol obtained by distillation from wood. It is a poisonous substance; its ingestion may cause death, and in those who survive, loss of eyesight. SEE: *methanol; methyl alcohol*.

Wood's rays. [Robert Williams Wood, U.S. physicist, 1868–1953] Ultraviolet rays. Used to detect fluorescent materials in the skin and hair in certain disease states such as tinea capitis. The terms Wood's light and Wood's lamp have become synonymous for Wood's rays, even though these are misnomers.

wood tick. Dermacentor andersoni, an important North American species of tick, which causes tick paralysis and transmits causative organisms of Rocky Mountain spotted fever and tularemia.

wool fat. Anhydrous lanolin, a fatty substance obtained from sheep's wool. Used as a base for ointments.

woolsorter's disease. A pulmonary form of anthrax that develops in those who handle wool contaminated with Bacillus anthracis.

word blindness. Inability to comprehend written words; a form of aphasia, q.v. SYN: *alexia*.

word salad. The use of words with no apparent meaning attached to them or to their relationship with one another. Usually found in schizophrenia.

work [Ger. *wirken*]. Mental or physical effort made in order to accomplish or produce something. SEE: *calorie; erg; unit*.

work-up. The process of obtaining all of the necessary data for diagnosing and treating a patient. This should be done in an orderly manner so that essential elements will not be overlooked. Included are retrieval of all previous medical records, the patient's family and personal medical history, social and occupational history, physical examination, laboratory studies, x-rays, and indicated diagnostic surgical procedures. The patient's work-up is an ongoing process wherein all hospital personnel cooperate in attempting to determine the correct diagnosis and effective therapy. SEE: *medical record, problem-oriented; nursing history form*.

World Health Organization. ABBR: W.H.O. The United Nations agency concerned with health. Its definition of health is as follows.

"Health is a state of complete physical and social well being, and not merely the absence of disease or infirmity. The enjoyment of the highest attainable standards of health is one of the fundamental rights of every human being without distinction of race, religion, political belief, economic or social condition. The health of all peoples is fundamental to the attainment of peace and security and is dependent upon the fullest cooperation of individuals and States. The achievement of any State in the promotion and protection of health is of value to all."

worm (wŭrm) [AS. *wyrm*]. 1. An elongated invertebrate belonging to one of the following phyla: Platyhelminthes (flatworms); Nemathelminthes or Aschelminthes (roundworms or threadworms); Acanthocephala (spinyheaded worms); and Annelida (Annulata) (segmented worms). SYN: *helminth*. SEE: individual worms by name. 2. Any small, limbless, creeping animal. 3. Median portion of the cerebellum. 4. Any wormlike structure.

wormian bones (wŭr'mē-ăn). [Olaus Worm, Dan. anatomist, 1588–1654] Small, irregular bones in the course of the cranial sutures.

wormseed (wĕrm'sēd). The dried, unexpanded capitula of several ragweeds, such as Artemisia santonica, A. maritima, or A. pauciflora, from which the vermifuge santonin is obtained.

w., American. Chenopodium.

wormwood (wĕrm'wood). A toxic substance, absinthium, obtained from Artemisia absinthium. It was used in certain alcoholic beverages (absinthe), but because of its toxicity, such use is prohibited in most countries.

worried well. Persons who are indeed well, but because of their anxiety or imagined illness, they frequent medical care facilities seeking reassurances concerning their health status.

wound (woond) [AS. *wund*]. Break in the continuity of soft parts of body structures caused by violence or trauma to tissues. In treating any wound, give the previously immunized patient a tetanus toxoid booster injection. If not previously immunized, the patient should be given tetanus immune globulin. If tetanus immune globulin is not available, the equine form may be used but the patient must be tested for hypersensitivity prior to administering the full dose.

w., abdominal. Frequently sustained and ordinarily involves structure of the abdominal wall. In such instances, the wound may be treated as an ordinary wound. Where a cavity has been opened, and esp. if viscera have been exposed, attempt to keep the area sterile and moist. This will help to prevent infection.

w., bullet. A puncture wound from a bullet. Usually there is a small point of entrance. If the bullet left the body, there is a larger point of exit; it is associated with injuries of bone, tendon, or blood vessels.

SYM: Depend on site, speed, and character of bullet.

TREATMENT: Tetanus booster injection or tetanus immune globulin. Antiseptic to wound and dressing. Treat complications, including hemorrhage, and shock.

w., cellulitis of. Local inflammation of a wound, occurring when wound has been closed without drainage, esp. in appendicitis.

SYM: Elevation of temperature from 4th to 7th day with an accompanying tenderness. Inspect dressing and chart findings.

TREATMENT: Evacuation of the abscess; hot, wet dressings; antibiotics.

w., contused. A bruise in which the skin is not broken. It may be caused by a blunt instrument. Injury of the tissues under the skin, leaving the skin unbroken, traumatizes the soft tissue. The blood vessels ruptured underneath the skin cause discoloration. If extravasated blood becomes encapsulated, it is termed hematoma; if it is diffused, an ecchymosis. SEE: *ecchymosis; hematoma.*

TREATMENT: Cold compresses, pressure, and rest. Elevation of injured area will help prevent or reduce swelling. When acute stage is over (24 to 48 hr.), continued rest, heat, and elevation are prescribed. Aseptic drainage may be indicated.

w., crushing. If wound is bleeding, apply cold cloths; if not, apply dressing and treat as an ordinary wound until patient can be given definitive surgical treatment. If bone is fractured, apply splint.

w., fishhook. Embedded fishhooks are difficult to remove. Push the hook through, then cut off barb with an instrument, and pull the remainder of the fishhook out by the route it entered. Antitetanus treatment as indicated. Frequently these injuries become infected, so carefully saturate with an antiseptic, cover with a dressing, and observe for several days.

w., incised. Any sharp cut in which the tissues are not severed; a clean cut caused by a keen cutting instrument. The wound may be either aseptic or infected, depending on circumstances that caused it.

An aseptic wound, one occurring under surgical conditions, should heal if conditions are favorable and no contaminations due to pathogenic organisms or foreign material enter into it. During the healing process, the area of the wound must be kept aseptic. The skin must be cleansed with plain soap and water, rinsed thoroughly, and covered securely with sterile dressings to keep the wound clean. A clean wound should be left alone. The dressings should be changed only often enough to keep the wound clean. There should be no squeezing or pulling of its edges.

w., lacerated. A torn wound with ragged edges; not a clean wound. It is a type of wound that provides many avenues for infection. May be caused by many kinds of implements, and the implement may be covered with any kind of pathogenic bacteria. Thus a variety of types of wound infections may be expected. Antitetanus and gas gangrene prophylaxis may be needed.

TREATMENT: The wound should be cleansed with mild soap and water and rinsed thoroughly. If wound edges are ragged, they will need to be trimmed and dead tissue removed. The patient should be given tetanus antitoxin or tetanus booster depending on previous history. The wound should never be sealed. It is best to hold the wound open with some form of drain.

w., nonpenetrating. Wound in which the surface of the skin remains intact.

w., open. Contusion where skin is also broken, such as a gunshot, incised, or lacerated wound.

w., ordinary. An uncomplicated wound of the skin that may or may not require repair by use of either suturing, debridement and suturing, or merely cleaning and application of a sterile "non-sticking" type of bandage.

w., penetrating. Wound in which the skin is broken and the agent causing the wound enters subcutaneous tissue or a deep-lying structure or cavity.

w., perforating. Wound in which the object that caused the wound entered the body and emerged, such as a bullet, projectile, or knife.

w., poisoned. This may be classed as a lacerated wound or a puncture wound, depending on tearing of tissue. The poisoned wound may be caused by a diseased animal such as a snake, dog, or a wild animal.

TREATMENT: A poisoned wound should be treated the same as a puncture wound. If possible, the animal should be put under observation for rabies, q.v.

w., puncture. Wound made by a sharp-pointed instrument such as a dagger, ice pick, or needle. The chief danger is from thrombosis and possible release of emboli. A puncture wound usually is collapsed. This provides ideal conditions for infection. Placement of a drain, antitetanus therapy or prophylaxis, and gas gangrene prophylaxis may be required. This will depend on the nature of the instrument that caused the injury.

w., subcutaneous. All wounds that are unaccompanied by a break in skin such as contusions.

w., tunnel. Wound having a small entrance and exit and of uniform diameter.

W-plasty. Technique used in plastic surgery to prevent contractures in straight-line scars. Each side of the edges of a wound is cut in the form of connected W's, and the edges are sutured together in a zig-zag fashion.

wreath (rēth). A structure that encircles something so that it resembles a circlet of leaves and branches (laurel) worn around the head.

Wright's stain. [James H. Wright, U.S. pathologist, 1871–1928] A combination of eosin and methylene blue used in studying blood cells and revealing malarial parasites. SEE: *Wright's technique.*

Wright's technique. Method of staining blood smears. Cover the dried blood smear with 5 to 10 drops of Wright's stain. Let stand 1 min. Add an equal amount of neutral distilled water to the stain. Let diluted stain stand for 3 to 10 min. A metallic sheen should appear. Remove stain by gently washing with distilled water. Stand slide on end and allow to dry. Mount in balsam or methacrylate. If staining results are good, red cells will have a pinkish or copper color, white cells will have densely stained blue nuclei, and the cytoplasmic granules will stain variously in the different types of leukocytes. SEE: *leukocyte.*

wrinkle (rĭng'kl) [AS. *gewrinclian,* to wind]. 1. A crevice, furrow, or ridge in the skin. 2. To make creases or furrows as in the skin by habitual frowning.

Wrisberg's cardiac ganglion (rĭs'bŭrgz). [Heinrich August Wrisberg, Ger. anatomist, 1739–1808] Wrisberg's ganglion, q.v.

Wrisberg's cartilages. The cuneiform cartilages of the larynx.

Wrisberg's ganglion. Ganglion of the superficial cardiac plexus. It is between the aortic arch and the pulmonary artery. SEE: *cardiac ganglia.* SYN: *Wrisberg's cardiac ganglion.*

Wrisberg's nerve. 1. The medial brachial cutaneous nerve, a branch of the medial cord of the brachial plexus. 2. The nervus intermedius (pars intermedia), a branch of the facial nerve lying between the motor root and the acoustic nerve.

wrist (rĭst) [AS]. The joint, or region, lying between the hand and the forearm.

wrist bones. The carpus consisting of eight bones. SEE: *skeleton; hand* for illus.

wrist drop. Condition in which hand is flexed at wrist and cannot be extended; due to injury of radial nerve or paralysis of extensor muscles of wrist and hand.

writer's cramp. A cramp affecting muscles of the thumb and two adjacent fingers after prolonged writing.

writing. The act of placing characters, letters, or words on a surface, usually paper, for the purpose of communicating ideas.

w., dextrad. Writing that progresses from left to right.

w., mirror. Writing so that letters and words are reversed and appear as in a mirror.

writing hand. Position of hand seen in paralysis agitans marked by contraction of muscle of the hand. The fingers assume the position similar to holding a pen.

wryneck (rī'nĕk). Contracted state of one or more muscles of the neck, producing an abnormal position of the head. Occasionally it is acute, due to cold or trauma; more commonly it is chronic, spastic in character, and dependent upon nerve irritation. Has been produced by habitual malposition of the head assumed because of existing ocular defect. May be congenital. When acute, it generally passes away under influence of rest, heat, and time. Chronic wryneck may require surgical therapy. SYN: *loxia; torticollis.*

w.s. *water soluble.*

wt. *weight.*

Wuchereria (voo″kĕr-ē'rē-ă). [Otto Wucherer, Ger. physician, 1820–1873] A genus of filarial worms belonging to the superfamily Filarioidea, class Nematoda. Common in warm regions of the world.

W. bancrofti. The causative agent of elephantiasis. Adults of the species live in lymph nodes and ducts of man. Females give birth to sheathed microfilariae, which remain in internal organs during the day but at night are in circulating blood, where they are sucked up by night-biting mosquitoes, in which they continue their development, becoming infective larvae in about two weeks. They are then passed on to the human when the mosquito bites. SYN: *Filaria bancrofti.*

W. malayi. Species occurring in Southeast Asia and largely responsible for lymphangitis and elephantiasis in that region. Closely resembles W. bancrofti.

wuchereriasis (voo″kĕr-ē-rī'ă-sĭs) Infestation with filaria worms of the genus Wuchereria. SYN: *elephantiasis; filariasis.*

w/v. *weight in volume.* It indicates the amount by weight of a solid substance dissolved in a measured quantity of liquid. Percent w/v expresses number of grams of an ingredient in 100 ml. of solution.

w/w. *weight in weight.* It indicates the amount by weight of a solid substance dissolved in a known amount (by weight) of liquid. Percent w/w expresses the number of grams of one ingredient in 100 grams of solution.

Wyamine Sulfate. Trade name for mephentermine sulfate.

Wyamycin S. Trade name for erythromycin stearate.

Wyamycin Liquid. Trade name for erythromycin ethylsuccinate, USP.

Wycillin. Trade name for penicillin G procaine, USP.

Wydase. Trade name for hyaluronidase (injection).

X

X. Symbol for Kienbock's unit of x-ray dose; symbol for xanthine.

xanchromatic (zăn″krō-măt′ĭk). Xanthochromic.

xanthelasma (zăn″thĕl-ăz′mă) [Gr. *xanthos,* yellow, + *elasma,* plate]. 1. Yellow. 2. Flat or slightly raised yellowish tumor occurring in elderly persons, found most frequently on the upper and lower lids, esp. near the inner canthus. SYN: *xanthoma.*

xanthelasmoidea (zăn″thĕl-ăz-moy′dē-ă) [″ + ″ + *eidos,* resemblance]. Chronic disease of childhood marked by wheals and followed by brownish-yellow patches. SYN: *urticaria pigmentosa.*

xanthematin (zăn-thĕm′ă-tĭn). A yellow-colored substance produced by the action of nitric acid on hematin.

xanthemia (zăn-thē′mē-ă) [″ + *haima,* blood]. Occurrence of yellow pigment in the blood. SYN: *carotenemia.*

xanthene (zăn′thēn). A crystalline compound, $O{=}(C_6H_4)_2{=}CH_2$, from which various dyes are formed, including rhodamine and fluorescein.

xanthic (zăn′thĭk) [Gr. *xanthos,* yellow]. 1. Yellow. 2. Pert. to xanthine.

xanthic calculus. A urinary concretion containing xanthine.

xanthine (zăn′thĭn, -thēn). A nitrogenous extractive contained in muscle tissue liver, spleen, pancreas, and other organs, and in the urine. It is formed during the metabolism of nucleoproteins. The three methylated xanthines are caffeine, theophylline, and theobromine.

x., dimethyl. Theobromine.

x., trimethyl. Caffeine.

xanthine base. A group of chemical compounds including xanthine, hypoxanthine, uric acid, and theobromine, which have a purine as their base. SYN: *purine base.*

xanthinuria (zăn″thĭn-ū′rē-ă) [″ + *ouron,* urine]. Excretion of large amounts of xanthine in the urine.

xanthiuria (zăn″thē-ū′rē-ă). Xanthinuria.

xanthochroia (zan″thō-krō′ē-ă) [″ + *chroia,* skin]. Yellowish discoloration of the skin.

xanthochromatic (zăn″thō-krō-măt′ĭk). Xanthochromic.

xanthochromia (zăn″thō-krō′mē-ă) [″ + *chroma,* color]. Yellow discoloration, as of the skin in patches or of the cerebrospinal fluid, resembling jaundice.

xanthochromic (zăn″thō-krō′mĭk). 1. Pert. to anything that is yellow. 2. Pert. to xanthochromia.

xanthochroous (zăn-thŏk′rō-ŭs) [Gr. *xanthochroos*]. Having a yellowish or light complexion.

xanthocyanopia, xanthocyanopsia (zăn″thō-sī-ăn-ŏ′pē-ă, -ŏp′sē-ă) [Gr. *xanthos,* yellow, + *kyanos,* blue, + *opsis,* sight]. A form of color blindness in which yellow and blue are distinguishable, but not red and green. SYN: *xanthokyanopy.*

xanthocyte (zăn′thō-sīt) [″ + *kytos,* cell]. A cell containing yellow pigment.

xanthoderma (zăn″thō-dĕr′mă) [″ + *derma,* skin]. Yellowness of the skin.

xanthodont, xanthodontous (zăn′thō-dŏnt, zăn″thō-dŏn′tŭs) [″ + *odous,* tooth]. Having yellow teeth.

xanthoerythrodermia perstans (zăn″thō-ē-rĭth″rō-dĕr′mē-ă). A rare symptomless disease requiring no treatment. It consists of persistent patches of erythema covered with fine scales, mostly on the trunk and limbs. SYN: *parapsoriasis.*

xanthogranuloma (zăn″thō-grăn″ū-lō′mă) [″ + L. *granulum,* grain, + *oma,* tumor]. A tumor having characteristics of both an infectious granuloma and a xanthoma.

x., juvenile. A skin disease that may be present at birth or develop in the first months of life. The firm dome-shaped yellow, pink, or orange papules from a few mm. to 4 cm. in size are usually present on the scalp, face, and upper trunk. Biopsy of these lesions reveals lipid-filled histiocytes, inflammatory cells, and Touton giant cells (multinucleated vacuolated cells with a wreath of nuclei and peripheral rim of foamy cytoplasm). Even though this illness is distressing, there is no need to attempt to treat the lesions because they regress spontaneously during the first years of life.

xanthokyanopy (zăn″thō-kī-ăn′ō-pē) [″ + *kyanos,* blue, + *opsis,* sight]. Partial blindness for color, only yellow and blue being discerned. SYN: *xanthocyanopia.*

xanthoma (zăn-thō′mă) [Gr. *xanthos,* yellow, + *oma,* tumor]. Flat, slightly elevated, soft rounded plaque or nodule, usually on the eyelids. May occur in patches of yellowish macule on orbital regions, confined to middle life or later, and to the female sex, consisting of a degenerative process involving fibers of the orbicularis muscle.

x., diabetic. Cutaneous disease associated with uncontrolled diabetes mellitus.

x. disseminatum. Condition characterized by presence of xanthoma throughout the body, esp. on the face, in tendon sheaths, and in mucous membranes. SYN: *Hand-Schüller-Christian disease.*

x. multiplex. Xanthomas all over the body.

x. palpebrarum. Xanthoma affecting the eyelids.

x. tuberosum. A form of xanthoma that may appear on the neck, shoulders, trunk, or extremities, consisting of small elastic and yellowish-colored nodules.

xanthomatosis (zăn″thō-mă-tō′sĭs) [″ + ″ + *osis,* condition]. Condition in which there is a deposition of lipid in tissues usually accompanied by hyperlipemia. Cholesterol may accumulate in tumor nodules (xanthoma) or in individual cells, esp. histiocytes and reticuloendothelial cells.

xanthomatous (zăn-thō′mă-tŭs). Concerning xanthoma.

xanthophose (zăn′thō-fōz) [″ + *phos,* light]. Any yellow phose. SEE: *phose.*

xanthophyll (zăn′thō-fĭl) [″ + *phyllon,* leaf]. A yellow pigment derived from carotene. It is present in some plants and egg yolk.

xanthoproteic (zăn″thō-prō-tē′ĭk) [″ + *protos,* first]. Derived from or pert. to xanthoprotein.

xanthoprotein (zăn″thō-prō′tē-ĭn). Yellowish substance produced by heating proteins with nitric acid.

xanthopsia (zăn-thŏp′sē-ă) [″ + *opsis,* sight]. Condition in which objects appear to be yellow.

xanthopsin (zăn-thŏp′sĭn). The visual purple produced by light acting on rhodopsin.

xanthopsis (zăn-thŏp′sĭs). Yellow pigmentation seen in certain cancers and degenerating tissue.

xanthorrhea (zăn″thō-rē′ă) [″ + *rhoia,* to flow]. Discharge of a yellow purulent substance from the vagina.

xanthosine (zăn′thō-sēn). 7-xanthine-D-ribose, a nucleoside formed by the deamination of guanosine.

xanthosis (zăn-thō′sĭs) [″ + *osis,* condition]. A yellowing of the skin seen in carotenemia resulting from ingestion of excessive quantities of carrots, squash, egg yolk, and other foods containing carotenoids. Condition usually harmless but it may indicate increase of lipochromes in blood due to other conditions such as hypothyroidism or diabetes.

xanthous (zăn′thŭs) [Gr. *xanthos,* yellow]. Yellow.

xanthurenic acid. 4,8-dihyroxyquinaldic acid, $C_{10}H_7NO_4$. It is excreted in the urine of pyridoxine-deficient animals after they are fed tryptophan.

xanthuria (zăn-thū′rē-ă) [″ + *ouron,* urine]. Excretion of an excess of xanthine in the urine. SYN: *xanthinuria.*

X chromosome. The chromosome that determines female sex characteristics. In the normal female there are two X chromosomes and in the male one X chromosome and one Y chromosome. SEE: *chromosome.*

x-disease. Poisoning caused by ingestion of peanuts or peanut products contaminated with Aspergillus flavus or other Aspergillus strains that produce aflatoxin, q.v. Farm animals and humans are susceptible to this toxicosis. SYN: *aflatoxicosis.*

Xe. Chem. symbol for xenon.

xeno- [Gr. *xenos,* stranger]. Combining form indicating strange or a foreign material.

xenobiotic (zĕn″ō-bī-ŏt′ĭk). An antibiotic chemical substance not produced by the body, and thus foreign to it.

xenogeneic (zĕn″ō-jĕn-ā′ĭk) [″ + *gennan,* to produce]. Tissues used for transplantation that are obtained from a species different from the recipient. SEE: *heterologous.*

xenogenesis (zĕn″ō-jĕn′ĕ-sĭs). Heterogenesis, q.v.

xenogenous (zĕn-ŏj′ĕn-ŭs) [Gr. *xenos,* stranger, + *gennan,* to produce]. 1. Caused by a foreign body. 2. Originating in the host, as a toxin resulting from stimuli applied to cells of the host.

xenograft (zĕn′ō-grăft) [″ + L. *graphium,* grafting knife]. Surgical graft of tissue from one species to an individual of a different species. SYN: *heterograft.*

xenology (zĕn-ŏl′ō-jē) [″ + *logos,* study]. The study of parasites and their relationships to one another, and their hosts.

xenomenia (zĕn-ō-mē′nē-ă) [″ + *meniaia,* menses]. Menstruation from a part of the body other than the normal one. SYN: *menstruation, vicarious.*

xenon (zē′nŏn) [Gr. *xenos,* stranger]. SYMB: Xe. At. wt. 131.29; at. no. 54. A gaseous element in the atmosphere.

xenon–133. USP. A radioactive isotope of xenon used in photoscanning studies of the lung. SYN: ^{133}*Xe.*

xenoparasite (zĕn″ō-păr′ă-sīt). An ectoparasite of a weakened animal, one that would not normally serve as a host.

xenophobia (zĕn″ō-fō′bē-ă) [″ + *phobos,* fear]. Abnormal dread of strangers.

xenophonia (zĕn″ō-fō′nē-ă) [″ + *phone,* voice]. Alteration in accent and intonation of a person's voice due to defect of speech.

xenophthalmia (zĕn″ŏf-thăl′mē-ă) [″ + *ophthalmia,* eye inflammation]. Inflammation of the eye caused by a foreign body.

Xenopsylla (zĕn″ŏp-sĭl′ă) [″ + *psylla,* flea]. A genus of fleas belonging to the family Pulicidae, order Siphonaptera.

X. cheopis. The rat flea, but other hosts include man and various animals. It is a vector for a number of pathogens including Hymenolepis nana, the dwarf tapeworm; Salmonella; and causative organisms of bubonic and sylvatic plague, and endemic typhus.

xenorexia (zĕn″ō-rĕk′sē-ă) [″ + *orexis,* appetite]. An abnormality of appetite marked by persistent swallowing of foreign objects.

xerantic (zē-răn′tĭk) [Gr. *xeros,* dry]. Causing dryness. SYN: *siccant; siccative.*

xerasia (zē-rā′sē-ă) [Gr. *xeros,* dry]. Disease of the hair in which there is abnormal dryness, brittleness, and eventual loss of hair.

xero- [Gr. *xeros*]. Prefix meaning dry.

xerocheilia (zē″rō-kī′lē-ă) [″ + *cheilos,* lip]. Dryness of the lips; a type of cheilitis.

xeroderma (zē″rō-dĕr′mă) [″ + *derma,* skin]. Roughness and dryness of the skin; mild ichthyosis.

x. pigmentosum. A rare disease of the skin starting in childhood marked by disseminated pigment discolorations, ulcers, cutaneous and muscular atrophy, and death. SYN: *Kaposi's disease; melanosis lenticularis.*

xerography (zē-rŏg′ră-fē). Xeroradiography, q.v.

xeroma (zē-rō′mă) [″ + *oma,* mass]. An abnormally dry state of the conjunctiva. SYN: *xerophthalmia.*

xeromammography (zē″rō-măm-mŏg′ră-fē). Xeroradiography of the breast.

xeromenia (zē″rō-mē′nē-ă) [″ + *meniaia,* menses]. The occurrence of the symptoms of menstruation without menstrual flow.

xeromycteria (zē″rō-mĭk-tē′rē-ă) [″ + *mykter,* nose]. Dryness of the nasal passages.

xeronosus (zē-rŏn′ō-sŭs) [″ + *nosos,* disease]. Dryness of the skin.

xerophagia (zē″rō-fā′jē-ă) [″ + *phagein,* to eat]. The eating of dry food only.

xerophagy (zē-rŏf′ă-jē). Eating of dry food exclusively.

xerophthalmia (zē-rŏf-thăl′mē-ă) [″ + *ophthalmos,* eye]. Conjunctival dryness with keratinization of epithelium following chronic conjunctivitis and in disease due to deficiency of vitamin A.

xerophthalmus (zē″rŏf-thăl′mŭs). Xerophthalmia.

xeroradiography (zē″rō-rā″dē-ŏg′ră-fē). Method of photoreproduction used in x-ray. It is a dry process involving the use of plates covered with a powdered substance, such as selenium, electrically and evenly charged. This is held between metal plates. The x-rays alter the charge or the substance to varying degrees dependent upon the tissues they have traversed. This produces the image.

xerosis (zē-rō′sĭs) [Gr.]. 1. Abnormal dryness of skin, mucous membranes, or of the conjunctiva. 2. Normal sclerosis of tissues in the aged.

xerostomia (zē″rō-stō′mē-ă) [″ + *stoma,* mouth]. Dryness of the mouth caused by the arresting of normal salivary secretion. It occurs in diabetes, hysteria, paralysis of facial nerve involving chorda tympani, acute infections, some types of neuroses, and is induced by certain drugs such as nicotine and atropine. SEE: *ptyalism.*

xerotes (zē′rō-tēz) [Gr.] Dryness.

xerotic (zē-rŏt′ĭk) [Gr. *xeros,* dry]. Dry; characterized by dryness.

xerotocia (zē″rō-tō′sē-ă) [″ + *tokos,* birth]. Dry labor due to diminished amount of amniotic fluid.

xerotripsis (zē″rō-trĭp′sĭs) [″ + *tripsis,* rubbing]. Dry friction.

xiphi-, xipho- [Gr. *xiphos,* sword]. Prefixes pert. to the xiphoid cartilage.

xiphisternum (zĭf″ĭ-stĕr′nŭm) [Gr. *xiphos,* sword, + *sternon,* chest]. The pointed process of the lower end of the sternum. SYN: *xiphoid process.*

xiphocostal (zĭf″ō-kŏs′tăl) [″ + L. *costa,* rib]. Rel. to the xiphoid cartilage and the ribs.

xiphocostal ligament. Ligament connecting the xiphoid cartilage to the cartilage of the 8th rib.

xiphodynia (zĭf″ō-dĭn′ē-ă) [″ + *odyne,* pain]. Pain in the ensiform cartilage.

xiphoid (zĭf′oyd) [Gr. *xiphos,* sword, + *eidos,* form]. Sword-shaped, ensiform.

xiphoid process. The lowest portion of the sternum; sword-shaped cartilaginous process supported by bone. It has no ribs attached to it, but some of the abdominal muscles are attached to it. It ossifies in the aged. SEE: *sternum* for illus.

xiphoiditis (zĭf″oyd-ī′tĭs) [″ + ″ + *itis,* inflammation]. Inflammation of the ensiform or xiphoid cartilage.

xiphopagotomy (zī-fŏp″ă-gŏt′ō-mē). Surgical separation of twins joined at the xiphoid process.

xiphopagus (zī-fŏp′ă-gŭs) [″ + *pagos,* thing fixed]. Symmetrical twins joined at the xiphoid process.

X-linked. Denoting characters that are transmitted by genes on the X chromosome. SEE: *choroideremic; hemophilia.*

X radiation. 1. Electromagnetic waves or energy composed of x-rays. 2. Treatment with or exposure to x-rays.

x-ray. A high-energy electromagnetic wave varying in length from 0.05 to 100 Angstrom units. X-rays are produced by bombarding a target in a vacuum tube with high-velocity electrons. Because of their ability to penetrate most solid matter to some extent and to act on photographic film they are used both in diagnosis and therapy. SYN: *roentgen ray.* SEE: *roentgenogram.*

x-r., bite-wing. Roentgenogram taken with the film holder held between the teeth and the film parallel to the teeth. This technique permits film to be taken of several upper and lower teeth at the same time.

x-r., strain. Roentgenogram taken with

the part, usually a bone or joint, under static force or tension. Used to better demonstrate the pathological change that might be inapparent if this technique were not employed.

x-ray dermatitis. Cutaneous inflammation due to exposure to x-rays.

xylene (zī'lēn, zī-lēn'). A mixture of isomeric hydrocarbons used in making lacquers and rubber cement.

xylene poisoning. SEE: *benzene* in *Poisons and Poisoning* in *Appendix*.

xylenin (zī'lē-nĭn) [Gr. *xylon,* wood]. A toxic substance extracted by xylene from tubercle bacilli.

xylenol (zī'lĕ-nŏl). General name for a series of dimethylphenols. They are in the pine-type coal tar disinfectants.

xylo- [Gr. *xylon,* wood]. Prefix pert. to wood.

Xylocaine. Trade name for lidocaine hydrochloride, USP.

xylol (zī'lŏl). Xylene.

xylometazoline hydrochloride (zī"lō-mĕt"ă-zō'lēn). USP. A vasoconstrictor drug used as a nasal decongestant. Trade names are Otrivin Hydrochloride and Dristan Long-Lasting Nasal Mist.

xylose (zī'lōs) [Gr. *xylon,* wood]. USP. Wood sugar, a crystalline, nonfermentable pentose.

xylulose (zī'lū-lōs). A pentose sugar present in nature as L-xylulose. It appears in the urine in essential pentosuria; and in the form of D-xylulose.

xylyl (zī'lĭl). A radical, $CH_3C_6H_4CH_2-$, derived by the removal of a hydrogen atom from xylene.

xyrospasm (zī'rō-spăzm) [Gr. *xyron,* razor, + *spasmos,* spasm]. Occupational neurosis of the fingers seen in barbers.

xysma (zĭz'mă) [Gr. *zysma,* filings]. Shreds of tissue sometimes seen in diarrhea stools.

xyster (zĭs'tĕr) [Gr., scraper]. File or rasp used in surgery. SYN: *raspatory.*

Y

Y. Chem. symb. for yttrium.
yard [AS. *gerd*, a rod]. A measure of 3 feet or 36 inches. Equal to 0.9144 meter. SEE: *Measures* in *Appendix*.
yaw (yaw). The primary lesion of yaws, q.v.
y., mother. The initial lesion of yaws, q.v., occurring at site of inoculation 3 to 4 weeks after infection. SYN: *frambesioma*.
yawn (yawn) [AS. *geonian*]. 1. To open the mouth involuntarily and usually take a deep breath as in drowsiness or fatigue. Yawning may stimulate observers to yawn. 2. Involuntary act of gaping, accompanied by attempts at inspiration, excited by drowsiness.
yawning (yawn'ĭng). Deep inspiration with mouth wide open; induced by drowsiness, boredom, or fatigue. SYN: *oscitation*. SEE: *pandiculation*.
yaws (yawz). An infectious nonvenereal disease caused by a spirochete, Treponema pertenue. Mainly found in humid, equatorial regions. SYN: *bouba; frambesia; tropica; parangi; pian*.
SYM: Febrile disturbances, rheumatism, eruption of tubercles with a caseous crust on hands, feet, face, and external genitals.
TREATMENT: Penicillin.
Yb. Chem. symb. for ytterbium.
Y cartilage. The cartilage that connects the pubis, ilium, and ischium and extends into the acetabulum.
Y chromosome. The chromosome that determines the male sex. Normal males possess one Y chromosome and one X chromosome; normal females possess two X chromosomes. SEE: *chromosome; Lyon hypothesis*.
yeast (yēst) [AS. *gist*]. 1. Any of several unicellular fungi of the genus Saccharomyces, which reproduce by budding. They are capable of fermenting carbohydrates. 2. A commercial product composed of meal impregnated with living yeast.
y., brewer's. Yeast obtained during the brewing of beer. May be used in the dried form as a good source of vitamin B.
y., dried. Dried yeast cells from strains of Saccharomyces cerevisiae. It is used as a source of proteins and vitamins, esp. B-complex.
yellow (yĕl'ō) [AS. *geolu*]. 1. One of the primary colors resembling that of a ripe lemon. 2. Colored yellow as the skin in disease.
y., visual. SEE: *visual yellow*.
yellow body. The corpus luteum.
yellow fever. An acute infectious disease characterized by jaundice, epigastric tenderness, vomiting, hemorrhages, and a febrile course consisting of two paroxysms.
Yellow fever is an endemic disease in certain tropical regions of South America and portions of tropical Africa adjacent to rain forests. Yellow fever has not been reported in Asia or the eastern coast of Africa.
ETIOL: The virus of yellow fever, a group B togavirus. It is transmitted by the bite of a female mosquito, Aedes aegypti. The incubation period is 3 to 6 days.
PROPHYLAXIS: Preventive measures include mosquito control by screening, spraying with nontoxic insecticides, and destruction of breeding areas. Preventive vaccines are available for those who plan to travel or live in areas where the disease is endemic.
SYM: *First Stage:* Disease begins with sudden onset of fever, sometimes accompanied by a chill, followed by pain in head, back, and limbs. Temperature rises rapidly till it reaches its maximum 103° to 105° F. (39.4° to 40.6° C.). Face flushed, conjunctivae injected, pupils small, gastroenteritis, urine scanty and albuminous. This stage lasts from a few hours to several days. It is followed by a marked fall in temperature and an improvement in general symptoms. At this time convalescence may begin or patient may pass into second febrile paroxysm. Jaundice rarely appears before the third day.
Second Stage, Period of Intoxication: Three to nine days. Fever rises to its original height, skin becomes yellow, vomiting persistent; vomitus may contain dark blood. Sometimes hemorrhages occur from other mucous membranes. Pulse rapid but not proportionate to the fever. Urine becomes very scanty and contains albumin and casts. Death frequently results from exhaustion or uremia, though recovery may follow the gravest symptoms.
PROG: Always grave. Mortality is 5% for natives of an area where the disease is endemic.
TREATMENT: There is no specific therapy. Absolute rest; cool, well-ventilated room; liquid diet; vitamin K and calcium gluconate for hemorrhagic tendency. Dehydration and electrolyte balance must be controlled by appropriate fluid replacement therapy. Parenteral fluids containing dextrose and saline should be given in cases of persistent vomiting. Transfusion may be required. Control fever by cool applications. Analgesics for pain.
yellow ointment. An ointment containing yellow wax and petrolatum.
yellow spot. 1. Yellowish nodule of anterior end of vocal cord. SYN: *macula flava laryngis*. 2. Center of the retina, the point of clearest vision. SYN: *macula lutea retinae*.
yellow vision. Condition in which objects seem yellow in color. SYN: *xanthopsia*.

yerba (yĕr′bă) [Sp.]. An herb.

y. maté. An herbal tea made from the dried leaves of maté, an evergreen tree. Popular in South America.

Yersin's serum (yĕr′sĭnz). [Alexandre Emil Jean Yersin, Swiss bacteriologist who worked in Paris, 1863–1943] An antitoxic serum for the plague.

Yersinia (yĕr-sĭn′ē-ă). [Yersin] A genus of gram-negative bacteria.

Y. enterocolitica. Species of large coccobacilli that are pathogenic for man. Clinical infections may be characterized by acute mesenteric lymphadenitis or enterocolitis. The disease may progress to a septicemic form in children and mortality may be as high as 50%. Therapy with ampicillin, kanamycin, or tetracycline is effective.

Y. pestis. Causative organism of plague, q.v. Formerly termed Pasteurella pestis.

Y. pseudotuberculosis. A gram-negative coccoid or ovoid organism that produces pseudotuberculosis in man.

yersiniosis (yĕr-sĭn″ē-ō′sĭs). Infection with yersinia.

yin-yang. The Chinese symbol of opposing but complementary entities or concepts such as light-dark; male-female; sun-moon. In Chinese philosophy and medicine, the goal is to have a proper balance of such biological forces. Applied to contemporary biology, this would embody a feedback type of control of physiological phenomena. SEE: illus.

-yl [Gr. *hyle,* matter, substance]. Suffix signifying a radical in chemistry.

-ylene. Suffix denoting a bivalent hydrocarbon radical in chemistry.

Y ligament. A y-shaped band covering the upper and anterior portions of the hip joint.

Yodoxin. Trade name for iodoquinol.

YIN-YANG

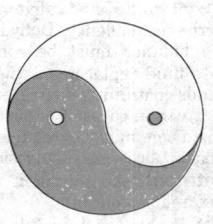

yoga [Sanskrit, union]. A system of beliefs and practices the goal of which is to attain a union of the individual self with Supreme Reality or the Universal Self. The term yoga as used in the Western world has been associated almost exclusively with physical postures and regulation of breathing. These are yoga exercises but not yoga in the spiritual sense.

yogurt, yoghurt (yōg′hŭrt) [Turkish]. A form of curdled milk, curdling caused by action of Lactobacillus bulgaricus. Extensive claims have been made concerning the therapeutic value of yogurt for various ailments. These have not been substantiated. SEE: *milk*.

yohimbine (yō-hĭm′bēn). A poisonous alkaloid derived from the bark of the tree Corynanthe yohimbi. It is an α-adrenergic blocking agent; and causes antidiuresis, increased blood pressure, tachycardia, irritability, tremor, sweating, nausea, and vomiting.

yoke (yōk). A tissue connecting two structures.

yolk (yōk) [AS. *geolca*]. The contents of the ovum; sometimes only the nutritive portion. SYN: *vitellus*. SEE: *zona pellucida*.

y. sac. Membranous sac surrounding food yolk in the embryo.

y. stalk. The umbilical duct connecting the yolk sac with the embryo.

Young-Helmholtz theory (yŭng-hĕlm′hōlts). [Thomas Young, Brit. physician, 1773–1829; H. L. F. Helmholtz, Ger. physician, 1821–1894] Theory that color vision depends on three different sets of retinal fibers responsible for perception of red, green, and violet. The loss of either red, green, or violet as color perceptive elements in the retina causes an inability to perceive a primary color or any color of which it forms a part.

Young's rule (yŭngz). [Thomas Young] A method for calculating the dose of medicine a child should receive. Divide the age by the age plus 12. The result represents the fraction of the adult dose suitable for the child.

Ex.: a child of 4 years of age requires the following fraction of the adult dose:

$$\frac{4}{4 + 12} = \frac{1}{4}$$

youth (yooth) [AS. *geoguth*]. Period between childhood and maturity.

ypsiliform (ĭp-sĭl′ĭ-form). Y-shaped.

y.s. *yellow spot* of the retina.

ytterbium (ĭ-tŭr′bē-ŭm). SYMB: Yb. At. wt. 173.04; at. no. 70. A rare metallic element.

yttrium (ĭt′rē-ŭm). SYMB: Y. At. wt. 88.905; at. no. 39. A metallic element.

yushi. Minamata disease, q.v.

Yutopar. Trade name for ritodrine hydrochloride.

Z

Z. 1. Ger. *Zuckung,* contraction. 2. Symb. for atomic number.

z. *zero; zone.*

Zaglas' ligament (ză'glŭs). The part of the posterior sacroiliac ligament from the posterosuperior spinous process of the ilium to the side of the sacrum.

Zahn's lines (zŏnz). [Frederick W. Zahn, Ger. pathologist, 1845–1904] Transverse whitish marks on the free surface of a thrombus made by the edges of the lamellae of blood platelets.

Zang's space (zăngz). [Christoph B. Zang, Ger. surgeon, 1772–1835] Space between the two lower tendons of the sternomastoid muscle in the supraclavicular fossa.

Zaroxolyn. Trade name for metolazone.

Z disk. A thin, dark disk that transversely crosses through and bisects the clear zone of a striated muscle and bisects the clear zone (isotropic disk) of a striated muscle fiber. The portion between two disks constitutes a sarcomere. SYN: *Krause's membrane.*

zeatin (zē'ă-tĭn). A cytotoxin that can be isolated from sweet corn.

zeaxanthin (zē"ă-zăn'thĭn). A carotenoid that is an isomer of xanthophyll. It is present in a great number of plants and animals.

zein (zē'ĭn) [Gr. *zeia,* a kind of grain]. A protein obtained from maize. It is deficient in tryptophan and lysine.

Zeis' glands. [Edourd Zeis, Ger. surgeon, 1807–1868] Sebaceous glands of the eyelid, close to the free edge of the lid. Each gland is associated with an eyelash. SEE: *Moll's glands.*

zeisian (zī'sē-ăn). Pert. to something originally described by Edourd Zeis.

zelotypia (zē"lō-tĭp'ē-ă) [Gr. *zelos,* zeal, + *typtein,* to strike]. 1. Morbid or monomaniacal zeal in the interest of any project or cause. 2. Insane jealousy.

zenkerism (zĕng'kĕr-ĭzm). Zenker's degeneration.

Zenker's degeneration (zĕng'kĕrz). [Friedrich A. Zenker, Ger. pathologist, 1825–1898] A glassy or waxy hyaline degeneration of skeletal muscles in acute infectious diseases, esp. in typhoid. SYN: *zenkerism.*

Zephiran. Trade name for benzalkonium chloride.

zero (zē'rō) [It.]. 1. Corresponding to nothing. SYMB: 0. 2. The point from which the graduation figures of a scale commence.

On the centigrade scale, zero (0°) is the temperature of melting ice, equivalent to 32° on the Fahrenheit scale. To obtain this fixed point, the thermometer is immersed in melting ice, and when the mercury column ceases to fall, the level at which it remains is fixed as 0° on the C. and as 32° on the F. scale. SEE: *thermometer.*

z., absolute. The temperature at which all atoms and molecules cease movement or at which all gases liquefy: −273.15° C. or −459.67° F.

z., limes. The greatest amount of toxin that, when mixed with one unit of antitoxin and injected into a guinea pig weighing 250 gm., will cause no local edema. SYMB: L0.

zero population growth. ABBR: ZPG. The demographic condition when in a given period of time the population neither increases nor decreases.

zestocausis (zĕs"tō-kŏw'sĭs) [Gr. *zestos,* boiling hot, + *kausis,* burning] Cauterization with a tube containing heated steam.

Zide. Trade name for hydrochlorothiazide, USP.

Ziehl-Neelsen method (zēl-nēl'sĕn). [Franz Ziehl, Ger. bacteriologist, 1857–1926; Friedrich K. A. Neelsen, 1854–1894] Method for staining Mycobacterium tuberculosis. A solution of carbolfuchsin is applied,which the organism retains after rinsing with acid alcohol.

Zieve's syndrome. [L. Zieve, U.S. physician, b. 1915] Hyperlipidemia, jaundice, hemolytic anemia, and abdominal pain following intake of a large amount of alcoholic beverages.

Zim jar opener. Adapted device allowing one-handed opening of bottles and jars.

zinc (zĭnk) [L. *zincum*]. SYMB: Zn. At. wt. 65.37; at. no. 30; sp. gr. 7.13. A bluish-white, crystalline metallic element that boils at 906° C. It is found as a carbonate and silicate, known as calamine, and as a sulfide (blende).

z. acetate. USP. White, pearly crystals.

ACTION AND USES: Astringent and antiseptic. Used chiefly in eye solutions, in a 0.1 to 0.5% solution.

z. bacitracin. SEE: *bacitracin zinc,* USP.

z. cadmium sulfide. Fluorescent material used in radiographic screens.

z. carbonate. A mild astringent used topically in dusting powders.

z. chloride. USP. White granular powder used as an antiseptic.

z. gelatin. USP. A combination of zinc oxide, glycerin, and purified water. This smooth jelly is placed between layers of gauze dressing to serve as a protective dressing and to support varicosities. It is removed by soaking in warm water. Trade names are Dome-Paste and Unna's Boot.

z. oxide. USP. Very fine white powder of zinc.

ACTION AND USES: Slightly antiseptic and astringent. Used chiefly in the form of ointment, 20%.

z. oxide and eugenol. Two substances that react together to produce a relatively hard mass, used in dentistry for impression material, cavity liners, temporary restorations, and cementing layers.

z. peroxide. A topical anti-infective agent, used in powder form.

z. salts. A bluish-white metal used to make various containers and also to galvanize iron to prevent rust. The most commonly used compounds are zinc oxide as a pigment for paints, in ointments, and in chloride and sulfate, which resemble Epsom salts and have been administered accidentally. The salts also are used as a wood preservative, in soldering, and in medicine to neutralize tissue, and in dilute solutions as an astringent and emetic. SEE: *zinc salts poisoning.*

z. stearate. USP. A very fine smooth powder used as a nonirritating antiseptic and astringent for burns, scalds, and abrasions.

z. sulfate. USP. Transparent white crystals used externally as an ophthalmic astringent. Trade names are Op-Thal-Zin and Verazine.

z. undecylenate. USP. An antifungal agent used in treating fungal infection of the skin. It is a component of Desenex ointment.

z. white. Z. oxide, USP.

zinc-eugenol cement. USP. A cement and protectant used in dentistry. SEE: *zinc oxide and eugenol.*

zinciferous (zĭng-kĭf'ĕr-ŭs). Containing zinc.

zincoid (zĭng'koyd) [L. *zincum,* zinc, + Gr. *eidos,* form]. Resembling or concerning zinc.

zinc ointment. An ointment consisting of 20% zinc oxide mixed with petrolatum and white ointment. Used topically in treating skin diseases.

zinc salts poisoning. Characterized by metallic taste with prompt burning of mouth, throat, esophagus, and stomach. Violent vomiting, often bloody; increased salivation; painful diarrhea; coma. If patient recovers, nervous complications are frequent. SEE: *Poisons and Poisoning* in *Appendix.*

F.A. Wash out stomach and treat as for sulfuric acid.

Zinn's ligament (zĭnz). [Johann G. Zinn, Ger. anatomist, 1727–1759] Connective tissue giving attachment to the rectus muscles of the eyeball. SEE: *zonule of Zinn.*

zirconium (zĭr-kō'nē-ŭm). SYMB: Zr. At. wt. 91.22; at. no. 40. A metallic element found only in combination.

Zn. Chem. symb. for zinc.

zoacanthosis (zō"ăk-ăn-thō'sĭs). Dermatitis due to foreign bodies such as bristles, hairs, or stingers from animals.

zoanthropy (zō-ăn'thrō-pē) [Gr. *zoon,* animal, + *anthropos,* man]. Delusion that one is an animal.

zoescope (zō'ĕ-skōp) [Gr. *zoe,* life, + *skopein,* to view]. Stroboscope.

zoetic (zō-ĕt'ĭk) [Gr. *zoe,* life]. Pert. to life. SYN: *vital.*

zoic (zō'ĭk). Concerning animal life.

Zollinger-Ellison syndrome. [Robert M. Zollinger, b. 1903, and Edwin H. Ellison, b. 1918, contemporary U.S. surgeons] Condition caused by non-insulin-secreting tumors of the pancreas, which secrete excess amounts of gastrin. This stimulates the stomach to secrete great amounts of hydrochloric acid and pepsin, which in turn leads to peptic ulceration of the stomach and small intestines. About 60% of the tumors are malignant.

TREATMENT: Total gastrectomy and local excision of pancreatic tumor if metastases have not appeared.

Zolyse. Trade name for chymotripsin, USP.

Zomax. Trade name for zomepirac sodium.

zona (zō'nă) [L., a girdle]. (pl. *zonae*) 1. A band or girdle. 2. An acute inflammatory disease, characterized by groups of small vesicles mounted on inflammatory bases, associated with neuralgic pain and following the distribution of certain nerve trunks. SYN: *herpes zoster.*

z. ciliaris. Ciliary processes combined.

z. facialis. Herpes zoster of the face.

z. fasciculata. The adrenal cortex.

z. glomerulosa. The outer layer of the adrenal cortex just inside the capsule.

z. ophthalmica. Old name for herpes zoster of the area supplied by the ophthalmic nerve.

z. pellucida. Inner, solid, thick, membranous envelope of the ovum. It is pierced by many radiating canals, giving it a striated appearance. SYN: *vitelline membrane; z. radiata.*

z. radiata. Z. pellucida.

z. reticularis. The inner layer of the cortex of the adrenal gland.

z. striata. Z. pellucida, q.v.

zonae. Pl. of zona.

zonal (zō'năl) [L. *zonalis*]. Pert. to a zone.

zonary (zō'năr-ē) [L. *zona,* a girdle]. Pert. to or shaped like a zone.

zonary placenta. Placenta arranged in the form of a broad ring around the chorion.

Zondek-Aschheim test (zŏn'dĕk-ăsh'hīm). [Berhardt Zondek, Ger. gynecologist, 1891–1966; Selmar Aschheim, Ger. gynecologist, 1878–1965] A test for pregnancy by injecting the patient's urine subcutaneously into immature female mice.

zone (zōn) [L. *zona,* a girdle]. An area or belt.

z., ciliary. The peripheral part of the anterior surface of the iris of the eye.

z., comfort. The range of temperature, humidity, and when applicable, the solar radiation and wind in which an individual doing work at a specified rate and in a certain specified garment is comfortable.

z., epileptogenic. Any area of the brain that after stimulation produces an epileptic seizure.

z., erogenous. An area of the body that may produce erotic desires when stimulated. These areas include the breasts, lips, genital and anal regions, buttocks, and sometimes the special senses that cause sexual excitation, such as certain odors.

z. hypnogenic, hypnogenous. Any area of the body that when pressed on induces a hypnotic state.

z. transitional. The area of the lens of the eye where the epithelial capsule cells change into lens fibers.

zonesthesia (zōn″ĕs-thē′zē-ă) [″ + *aisthesis,* sensation]. A sensation, as a cord constricting the body. SYN: *cincture sensation; girdle pain.*

zonifugal (zō-nĭf′ū-găl) [″ + *fugere,* to flee]. Passing outward from within any zone or area.

zoning. The occurrence of a stronger fixation of complement in a lesser amount of suspected serum; a phenomenon occasionally observed in diagnosing syphilis by complement-fixation method.

zonipetal (zō-nĭp′ĕt-ăl) [″ + *petere,* to seek]. Passing from without into a zone or area of the body.

zonoskeleton (zōn″ō-skĕl′ĕ-tŏn). Proximal bones to which limbs attach, such as the hip bone, scapula, and clavicle.

zonula (zōn′ū-lă) [L.]. A small zone. SYN: *zonule.*

z. ciliaris. [NA] Suspensory ligament of the crystalline lens. SYN: *zonule of Zinn.*

zonular (zōn′ū-lăr). Pert. to a zonula.

zonular cataract. Cataract with opacity limited to certain layers of the lens.

zonular fibers. Interlacing fibers of the zonula ciliaris.

zonular spaces. Spaces between fibers of ligaments of the lens.

zonule (zōn′ūl) [L. *zonula,* small zone]. A small band or area. SYN: *zonula.*

z. of Zinn. Suspensory ligament of the crystalline lens. SYN: *zonula ciliaris* [NA].

zonulitis (zōn-ū-lī′tĭs) [″ + Gr. *itis,* inflammation]. Inflammation of zonule of Zinn.

zonulolysis (zŏn″ū-lŏl′ĭ-sĭs) [″ + Gr. *lysis,* dissolution]. Use of enzymes to dissolve the zonula ciliaris of the eye.

zonulotomy (zŏn″ū-lŏt′ō-mē) [″ + Gr. *tome,* incision]. Surgical incision of the ciliary zonule.

zonulysis (zŏn″ū-lī′sĭs). Zonulolysis.

zoobiology (zō″ō-bī-ŏl′ō-jē) [Gr. *zoon,* animal, + *bios,* life, + *logos,* study]. The biology of animals.

zooblast (zō′ō-blăst) [″ + *blastos,* germ]. An animal cell, esp. an immature form.

zoochemistry (zō″ō-kĕm′ĭs-trē). Biochemistry of animals.

zoodermic (zō″ō-dĕr′mĭk) [″ − *derma,* skin]. Performed with the skin of an animal, said of a method of skin grafting.

zoodynamics (zō″ō-dī-năm′ĭks) [″ + *dynamis,* power]. Physiology of animals.

zooerasty (zō″ō-ē′răs-tē). Sexual intercourse with an animal. SYN: *bestiality.*

zoofulvin (zō″ō-fŭl′vĭn). A yellow pigment derived from certain animal feathers.

zoogenesis (zō″ō-jĕn′ĕ-sĭs). Zoogeny, q.v.

zoogenous (zō-ŏj′ĕn-ŭs) [″ + *gennan,* to produce]. Derived or acquired from animals.

zoogeny (zō″ŏj′ĕ-nē) [″ + *gennan,* to produce]. The development and evolution of animals.

zoogeography (zō″ō-jē-ŏg′ră-fē). Study of the distribution of animals on the earth.

zooglea (zō″ō-glē′ă) [″ + *gloios,* sticky]. A stage in development of certain organisms in which colonies of microbes are embedded in a gelatinous matrix.

zoogonous (zō-ŏg′ō-nŭs). Viviparous, q.v.

zoogony (zō-ŏg′ō-nē) [″ + *gone,* offspring]. 1. Production of living young from within the body. 2. Breeding of animals.

zoograft (zō′ō-grăft) [″ + L. *graphium,* a grafting knife]. A graft of tissue obtained from an animal.

zoografting (zō″ō-grăft′ĭng). Use of animal tissue in grafting on a human body.

zooid (zō′oyd) [″ + *eidos,* resemblance]. 1. Resembling an animal. 2. A form resembling an animal; an organism produced by fission. 3. An animal cell that can move or exist independently.

zoolagnia (zō″ō-lăg′nē-ă) [″ + *lagneia,* lust]. Sexual desire for animals.

zoologist (zō-ŏl′ō-jĭst) [″ + *logos,* a study]. A biologist who specializes in the study of animal life.

zoology (zō-ŏl′ō-jē). The science of animal life.

zoomania (zō″ō-mā′nē-ă) [Gr. *zoon,* animal, + *mania,* madness]. A morbid and excessive affection for animals.

zoonoses (zō-ō-nō′sēz) [″ + *nosos,* disease]. Diseases communicable from animals to man under natural conditions.

zoonotic (zō″ō-nŏt′ĭk). Concerning zoonoses.

zooparasite (zō″ō-păr′ă-sīt) [″ + *parasitos,* parasite]. An animal parasite.

zoopathology (zō″ō-păth-ŏl′ō-jē) [″ + *pathos,* disease, + *logos,* a study]. Science of the diseases of animals.

zoophagous (zō-ŏf′ă-gŭs) [″ + *phagein,* to eat]. Living upon animal food.

zoophile (zō′ō-fīl) [″ + *philein,* to love]. 1.

One who likes animals. 2. An antivivisectionist.

zoophilism (zō-ŏf'ĭl-ĭzm) [" + " + *-ismos,* condition]. Abnormal love of animals.

zoophobia (zō"ō-fō'bē-ă) [" + *phobos,* fear]. Abnormal fear of animals.

zoophyte (zō'ō-fīt) [" + *phyton,* plant]. A plantlike animal; any of numerous invertebrate animals resembling plants in appearance or mode of growth.

zooplankton (zō"ō-plănk'tŏn) [" + *planktos,* wandering]. Small animal organism present in natural waters. SEE: *phytoplankton.*

zooplasty (zō'ō-plăs"tē) [" + *plassein,* to form]. Transplantation of animal tissue to man.

zoopsia (zō-ŏp'sē-ă) [" + *opsis,* vision]. Hallucinations involving animals.

zoopsychology (zō"ō-sī-kŏl'ō-jē). Animal psychology.

zoosadism (zō"ō-sā'dĭzm). Being sadistic to animals.

zooscopy (zō-ŏs'kō-pē) [" + *skopein,* to view]. 1. Zoopsia. 2. Scientific observation of animals.

zoosmosis (zō"ŏs-mō'sĭs) [Gr. *zoe,* life, + *osmos,* impulsion]. Process of passage of living protoplasm into the tissues from blood vessels.

zoospore (zō'ō-spor) [" + *sporos,* seed]. A motile asexual spore that moves by means of one or more flagella.

zoosterol (zō"ō-stē'rŏl). Any sterol derived from animals.

zootechnics (zō"ō-tĕk'nĭks) [Gr. *zoon,* animal, + *techne,* art]. The complete care, management, and breeding of domestic animals.

zootic (zō-ŏt'ĭk). Concerning animals.

zootomy (zō-ŏt'ō-mē) [" + *tome,* incision]. Dissection of animals.

zootoxin (zō"ō-tŏks'ĭn) [" + *toxikon,* poison]. Any toxin or poison produced by an animal, as snake venom.

zootrophic (zō"ō-trŏf'ĭk) [" + *trophe,* nutrition]. Concerning animal nutrition.

zoster (zŏs'tĕr) [Gr. *zoster,* girdle]. Acute inflammatory disease with vesicles grouped in the course of cutaneous nerves. SYN: *herpes zoster; zona.*

z. auricularis. Herpes zoster of the ear.

z. ophthalmicus. Herpes zoster affecting the ophthalmic nerve.

zosteriform (zŏs-tĕr'ĭ-form) [" + L. *forma,* shape]. Resembling herpes zoster. SYN: *zosteroid.*

zosteroid (zŏs'tĕr-oyd) [" + *eidos,* form]. Resembling herpes zoster. SYN: *zosteriform.*

ZPG. *zero population growth.*

Z-plasty. A technique with a Z-shaped incision used in plastic surgery to relieve tension in scar tissue. The area under tension is lengthened at the expense of the surrounding elastic tissue. SEE: illus.

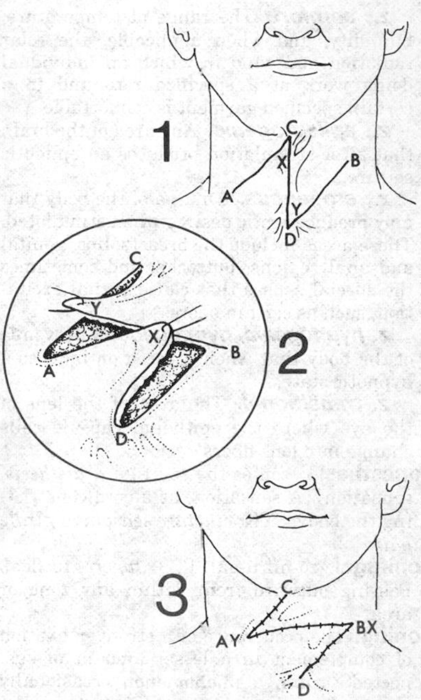

Z-PLASTY METHOD OF CORRECTING A DEFORMING SCAR

Zr. Chem. symb. for zirconium.

Z-track. Method of giving injections in order to prevent reflux of the injected material from seeping out by following the track of the needle after it is withdrawn. The needle is placed in the subcutaneous tissue a short distance and then the entire needle is moved laterally and then pulled further into the tissue. Next the needle is again moved laterally in a direction opposite of the first lateral movement. Then the needle is again pushed deeper into the tissue and the solution injected. This also helps to prevent tissue damage by injected medicine, which would, if allowed to reflux along the needle track, cause necrosis.

zwitterions (tsvĭt'ĕr-ī"ŏns). Dipolar ions that contain positive and negative charges of equal strength. They are therefore not attracted to either an anode or cathode. In a neutral solution amino acids function as zwitterions.

zygal (zī'găl) [Gr. *zygon,* yoke]. Concerning or shaped like a yoke.

zygapophyseal (zī"gă-pō-fĭz'ē-ăl). Concerning zygapophysis.

zygapophysis (zī"gă-pŏf'ĭ-sĭs) [" + *apo,* from, + *physis,* growth]. One of the articular processes of the neural arch of a vertebra.

zygion (zĭj'ē-ŏn) [Gr. *zygon,* yoke]. (pl. *zygia*) Craniometrical point on the zygoma at either end of the bizygomatic diameter.

zygocyte. Zygote, q.v.

zygodactyly (zī"gō-dăk'tĭl-ē) [" + *daktylos,* digit]. Fusion of two or more fingers or toes. SYN: *syndactylism.*

zygoma (zī-gō'mă) [Gr., cheekbone]. 1. The long arch that joins zygomatic processes of the temporal and malar bones on the sides of the skull. 2. The malar bone.

zygomatic (zī"gō-măt'ĭk). Pert. to the zygoma.

zygomatic arch. The formation on each side of the cheeks of the zygomatic process of each malar bone articulating with the zygomatic process of the temporal bone.

zygomatic bone. Bone on either side of the face below the eye. SYN: *malar bone.*

zygomaticoauricularis (zī"gō-măt"ĭ-kō-ăw-rĭk"ū-lā'rĭs) [L.]. Muscle that draws the pinna of the ear forward. SEE: *Muscles* in *Appendix.*

zygomaticofacial (zī"gō-măt"ĭ-kō-fā'shăl). Concerning the zygoma and the face.

zygomaticofrontal (zī"gō-măt"ĭ-kō-frŏn'tăl). Concerning the zygoma and the frontal bone of the face.

zygomaticomaxillary (zī"gō-măt"ĭ-kō-măk'sĭ-lĕr"ē). Concerning the zygoma and the maxilla.

zygomatico-orbital (zī"gō-măt"ĭ-kō-or'bĭ-tăl). Concerning the zygoma and the orbit of the eye.

zygomaticosphenoid (zī"gō-măt"ĭ-kō-sfē'noyd). Concerning the zygoma and the sphenoid bone.

zygomaticotemporal (zī"gō-măt"ĭ-kō-tĕm'por-ăl). Concerning the zygoma and the temporal bone.

zygomatic process. 1. A thin projection from the temporal bone bounding its squamous portion. 2. A part of the malar bone helping to form the zygoma.

zygomatic reflex. Movement of lower jaw toward percussed side when zygoma is percussed.

zygomaticum (zī"gō-măt'ĭ-kŭm) [L.]. The zygomatic bone.

zygomaticus (zī"gō-măt'ĭk-ŭs) [L.]. A muscle that draws the upper lip upward and outward. SEE: *Muscles* in *Appendix.*

zygomaxillary (zī"gō-măks'ĭl-ăr-ē) [Gr. *zygoma,* cheekbone, + L. *maxilla,* jaw]. Pert. to the cheekbone and upper jaw.

zygomaxillary point. A craniometrical point marked at the lower end of the zygomatic suture.

zygomycosis. A group of mycoses usually caused by fungi of the family Mucoraceae of the class Zygomycetes. These fungi have an affinity for blood vessels where they cause thrombosis and infarction. The disease in its form that affects the head and face usually causes paranasal sinus infections, esp. during periods of ketoacidosis in persons with diabetes mellitus. The pulmonary form of the disease causes infarcts of the lung; and in the gastrointestinal form, mucosal ulcers and gangrene of the stomach may occur. The disease is contracted by inhalation or ingestion of the fungus by susceptible individuals. Most persons have a natural resistance to the fungus and this accounts for the rarity of the disease. SYN: *mucormycosis.*

TREATMENT: Control of or prevention of diabetic acidosis, amphotericin B; and resection of necrotic tissue.

zygon (zī'gŏn) [Gr.]. The short cross-bar connecting the parallel limbs of a cerebral fissure.

zygopodium (zī"gō-pō'dē-ŭm). The intermediate-distal portion of a limb, i.e., the ulna and radius, and the tibia and fibula.

zygosis (zī-gō'sĭs) [Gr. *zygosis,* a balancing]. Sexual union of two unicellular animals.

zygosity (zī-gŏs'ĭ-tē) [Gr. *zygon,* yoke]. Concerning zygosis.

zygosperm (zī'gō-spĕrm). Zygospore.

zygospore (zī'gō-spor). A spore formed by fusion of morphologically identical structures.

zygote (zī'gōt) [Gr. *zygotos,* yoked]. Cell produced by union of two gametes. The fertilized ovum. SYN: *zygocyte.*

zygotene (zī'gō-tēn) [Gr. *zygotos,* yoked together]. The second stage of the prophase of the first meiotic division. During this stage, the homologous chromosomes pair side by side. SEE: *cell division.*

zygotic (zī-gŏt'ĭk). Concerning a zygote.

zygotoblast (zī-gō'tō-blăst) [" + *blastos,* germ]. Sporozoite, q.v.

zygotomere (zī-gō'tō-mēr) [" + *meros,* part]. Sporoblast, q.v.

Zyloprim. Trade name for allopurinol, USP.

zymase (zī'mās) [Gr. *zyme,* leaven, + *-ase,* enzyme]. Any of a group of enzymes that, in the presence of oxygen, convert certain carbohydrates into carbon dioxide and water or, in absence of oxygen, into alcohol and carbon dioxide or lactic acid. It is found in yeast, bacteria, and higher plants and animals. SEE: *enzyme, fermenting.*

zyme (zīm) [Gr. *zyme,* leaven]. 1. An enzyme or ferment. 2. An agent that produces an infectious disease.

zymic (zī'mĭk). Concerning enzymes.

zymogen (zī'mō-jĕn) [" + *gennan,* to produce]. A substance that develops into a chemical ferment or enzyme. It exists in an inactive form antecedent to the active enzyme. SYN: *proenzyme.* SEE: *pepsinogen; trypsinogen.*

zymogene (zī'mō-jēn). Microbe causing fermentation.

zymogen granules. Secretory granules of a

pre-enzyme substance seen in cells of synthetic organs such as salivary glands or pancreas.

zymogenic (zī″mō-jĕn′ĭk). 1. Causing a fermentation. 2. Pert. to or producing a zymogen.

zymogenous (zī-mŏj′ĕ-nŭs). Zymogenic.

zymogram (zī′mō-grăm). Electrophoretic graph of the separation of the enzymes in a solution.

zymohexase (zī″mō-hĕk′sās). The enzyme that is involved in splitting fructose 1,6-diphosphate into dihydroxy acetone phosphate and phosphoglyceric aldehyde.

zymohydrolysis (zī″mō-hī-drŏl′ĭ-sĭs) [″ + *hydor,* water, + *lysis,* dissolution]. Decomposition brought about by a ferment. SYN: *zymosis.*

zymoid (zī′moyd) [″ + *eidos,* form]. Resembling an enzyme.

zymologic (zī″mō-lŏ′jĭk) [″ + *logos,* a study]. Rel. to zymology.

zymologist (zī-mŏl′ō-jĭst). One who specializes in study of ferments.

zymology (zī-mŏl′ō-jē). The science of fermentation.

zymolysis (zī-mŏl′ĭ-sĭs) [Gr. *zyme,* leaven, + *lysis,* a dissolution]. Changes produced by an enzyme; action of enzymes. SYN: *fermentation; zymosis.*

zymolyte (zī′mō-līt″). Substance upon which a ferment acts. SYN: *substrate.*

zymolytic (zī″mō-lĭt′ĭk) [″ + *lytikos,* dissolved]. Causing fermentation; fermentative.

zymometer (zī-mŏm′ĕ-ter) [″ + *metron,* measure]. Device for measuring fermentation.

Zymonema (zī″mō-nē′mă) [″ + *nema,* thread]. A genus of fungi.

zymonematosis (zī″mō-nē″mă-tō′sĭs) [″ + ″ + *osis,* condition]. Infestation with Zymonema.

zymophore (zī′mō-for) [″ + *phoros,* a bearer]. Noting the atomic group bearing the ferment.

zymophoric, zymophorous (zī″mō-for′ĭk, zī-mŏf′or-ŭs). Having fermentative properties.

zymophyte (zī′mō-fīt) [″ + *phyton,* growth]. A microorganism causing fermentation.

zymoplastic (zī″mō-plăs′tĭk) [″ + *plassein,* to form]. Producing a ferment.

zymoprotein (zī″mō-prō′tē-ĭn). Any protein that also functions as an enzyme.

zymosan (zī′mō-săn). An anti-complement obtained from the walls of great cells.

zymoscope (zī′mō-skōp) [″ + *skopein,* to examine]. Device for determining zymotic power of yeast.

zymose (zī′mōs). An enzyme that changes a disaccharide into a monosaccharide, such as cane sugar into invert sugar. SYN: *invertin.*

zymosis (zī-mō′sĭs) [Gr. *zymosis,* fermentation]. 1. Fermentation. 2. Process by which an infectious disease is supposed to develop. 3. An infectious disease.

z. gastrica. Organic acid in the stomach due to action of yeasts.

zymosterol (zī-mŏs′tĕr-ŏl). A sterol obtained from yeast.

zymosthenic (zī-mŏs-thĕn′ĭk) [Gr. *zyme,* leaven, + *sthenos,* strength]. Increasing the power and activity of an enzyme.

zymotic (zī-mŏt′ĭk). Rel. to or produced by fermentation.

Z.Z.'Z.". Symb. for increasing strengths of contraction.

Appendices

Table of Contents for Appendices

Table of Contents for Appendices *(Continued)*

Index to Appendices

App. 1: Units of Measurement

Scientific Notation

Sometimes it is necessary to use very large and very small numbers. These can best be indicated and handled in calculations by use of scientific notation, which is to say by use of exponents. Use of scientific notation requires writing the number so that it is the result of multiplying some whole number power of 10 by a number between 1 and 10. Examples are:

$$1234 = 1.234 \times 10^3 \qquad 0.01234 = 1.234 \times \frac{1}{100} = 1.234 \times 10^{-2}$$

$$0.001234 = 1.234 \times \frac{1}{1000} = 1.234 \times 10^{-3}$$

To convert a number to its equivalent in scientific notation:

Place the decimal point to the right of the first non-zero digit. This will now be a number between 1 and 9.

Multiply this number by a power of 10, the exponent of which is equal to the number of places the decimal point was moved. The exponent is positive if the decimal point was moved to the left, and negative if it was moved to the right. For example:

$$\frac{1{,}234{,}000.0 \times 0.000072}{6000.0} = \frac{1.234 \times 10^6 \times 7.2 \times 10^{-5}}{6.0 \times 10^3}$$

Now, by simply adding or subtracting the exponents of ten, and remembering that moving an exponent from the denominator of the fraction to the numerator changes its sign,

$$= \frac{1.234 \times 10^6 \times 10^{-5} \times 10^{-3} \times 7.2}{6} = \frac{1.234 \times 10^{-2} \times 7.2}{6}$$

Now, dividing by 6,

$$= 1.234 \times 10^{-2} \times 1.2 = 1.4808 \times 10^{-2} = \frac{1.4808}{100} = 0.014808$$

The last operation changed 1.4808×10^{-2} into the final value, 0.014808, which is not expressed in scientific notation.

Metric System

Weights

Scale	Table		Grams		Grains
Kilo	1 Kilogram	=	1000.0	=	15,432.35
Hecto	1 Hectogram	=	100.0	=	1,543.23
Deca	1 Decagram	=	10.0	=	154.323
Unit	1 Gram	=	1.0	=	15.432
Deci	1 Decigram	=	0.1	=	1.5432
Centi	1 Centigram	=	0.01	=	0.15432
Milli	1 Milligram	=	0.001	=	0.01543
Micro	1 Microgram	=	10^{-6}	=	15.432×10^{-6}
Nano	1 Nanogram	=	10^{-9}	=	15.432×10^{-9}
Pico	1 Picogram	=	10^{-12}	=	15.432×10^{-12}
Femto	1 Femtogram	=	10^{-15}	=	15.432×10^{-15}
Atto	1 Attogram	=	10^{-18}	=	15.432×10^{-18}

Arabic numbers are used with weights and measures, as 10 gm., or 3 ml., etc. Portions of weights and measures are usually expressed decimally. 10^{-1} indicates 0.1; $10^{-6} = 0.000001$; etc. SEE: *Scientific Notation* in *Appendix*.

SI Units (Système international d'Units) or International System of Units

This system includes two types of units important in clinical medicine. The *base units* are shown in the first table, derived units in the second table, and derived units with special names in the third table.

SI Base Units

Quantity	Name	Symbol
Length	meter	m
Mass	kilogram	kg
Time	second	s
Electric current	ampere	A
Temperature	kelvin	K
Luminous intensity	candela	cd
Amount of a substance	mole	mol

Some SI Derived Units

Quantity	Name of Derived Unit	Symbol
Area	square meter	m^2
Volume	cubic meter	m^3
Speed, velocity	meter per second	m/s
Acceleration	meter per second squared	m/s^2
Density	kilogram per cubic meter	kg/m^3
Concentration of a substance	mole per cubic meter	mcl/m^3
Specific volume	cubic meter per kilogram	m^3/kg
Luminescence	candela per square meter	cd/m^2

SI Derived Names With Special Names

Quantity	Name	Symbol	Expressed in Terms of Other Units
Frequency	hertz	Hz	S^{-1}
Force	newton	N	$kg{\cdot}m{\cdot}s^{-2}$ or $kg{\cdot}m/s^2$
Pressure	pascal	Pa	$N{\cdot}m^{-2}$ or N/m^2
Energy, work, amount of heat	joule	j	N·m
Power	watt	W	j·s or j/s
Quantity of electricity	coulomb	C	A·s
Electromotive force	volt	V	W/A
Capacitance	farad	F	C/V
Electrical resistance	ohm	Ω	V/a
Conductance	siemens	S	A/V
Inductance	henry	H	Wϕ/A
Illuminance	lux	lx	ln/m^2
Absorbed (radiation) dose	gray	Gy	J/kg

Prefixes and Multiples Used in SI

Prefix	Symbol	Power	Multiple or Portion of a Multiple
tera	T	10^{12}	1,000,000,000,000
giga	G	10^{9}	1,000,000,000
mega	M	10^{6}	1,000,000
kilo	k	10^{3}	1,000
hecto	h	10^{2}	100
deca	da	10^{1}	10
unity			1
deci	d	10^{-1}	0.1
centi	c	10^{-2}	0.01
milli	m	10^{-3}	0.001
micro	μ	10^{-6}	0.000001
nano	n	10^{-9}	0.000000001
pico	p	10^{-12}	0.000000000001
femto	f	10^{-15}	0.000000000000001
atto	a	10^{-18}	0.000000000000000001

Tables of Data

Arabic numerals are used with weights and measures, as 10 gm., or 3 ml., etc. Portions of weights and measures are usually expressed decimally. For practical purposes, 1 cc. (cubic centimeter) is equivalent to 1 ml. (milliliter) and 1 drop (gtt) of water is equivalent to a minim (m).

Units of Length

Millimeters	Centimeters	Inches	Feet	Yards	Meters
1 mm. = 1.0	0.1	0.03937	0.00328	0.0011	0.001
1 cm. = 10.0	1.0	0.3937	0.03281	0.0109	0.01
1 in. = 25.4	2.54	1.0	0.0833	0.0278	0.0254
1 ft. = 304.8	30.48	12.0	1.0	0.333	0.3048
1 yd. = 914.40	91.44	36.0	3.0	1.0	0.9144
1 m. = 1000.0	100.0	39.37	3.2808	1.0936	1.0

1 μ = 1 mu = 1 **micrometer** = 0.001 millimeter. 1 mm. = 1000 μ.
1 km. = 1 kilometer = 1000 meters = 0.6215 mile.
1 mile = 5280 feet = 1.609 kilometers.

Units of Volume (fluid or liquid)

Milliliters	U.S. Fluid Drams	Cubic Inches	U.S. Fluid Ounces	U.S. Fluid Quarts	Liters
1 ml. = 1.0	0.2705	0.061	0.03381	0.00106	0.001
1 fl. ʒ = 3.697	1.0	0.226	0.125	0.00391	0.00369
1 cu. in. = 16.3866	4.4329	1.0	0.5541	0.0173	0.01639
1 fl. ℥ = 29.573	8.0	1.8047	1.0	0.03125	0.02957
1 qt. = 946.332	256.0	57.75	32.0	1.0	0.9463
1 L. = 1000.0	270.52	61.025	33.815	1.0567	1.0

1 gallon = 4 quarts = 8 pints = 3.785 liters.
1 pint = 473.16 ml.

Units of Weight

Grains	Grams	Apothecaries' Ounces	Avoirdupois Pounds	Kilograms
1 gr. = 1.0	0.0648	0.00208	0.0001429	0.000065
1 gm. = 15.432	1.0	0.03215	0.002205	0.001
1 ℥ = 480.0	31.1	1.0	0.06855	0.0311
1 lb. = 7000.0	453.5924	14.583	1.0	0.45354
1 kg. = 15432.358	1000.0	32.15	2.2046	1.0

1 γ = 1 gamma = 1 microgram = 0.001 milligram; 1000 γ = 1 mg.
1 mg. = 1 milligram = 0.001 gm.; 1000 mg. = 1 gm.
1 grain = 64.8 mg.; 1 mg. = 0.0154 grain.
NOTE: 1 microgram may also be expressed as 1 μg.

Weights* and Measures

Apothecaries' Weight

20 grains = 1 scruple
3 scruples = 1 dram
8 drams = 1 ounce
12 ounces = 1 pound

Avoirdupois Weight

27.343 grains = 1 dram
16 drams = 1 ounce
16 ounces = 1 pound
100 pounds = 1 hundredweight
2000 pounds = 1 short ton
2240 pounds = 1 long ton
1 oz. troy = 480 grains
1 oz. avoirdupois = 437.5 grains
1 lb. troy = 5760 grains
1 lb. avoirdupois = 7000 grains

Circular Measure

60 seconds = 1 minute
60 minutes = 1 degree
90 degrees = 1 quadrant
4 quadrants = 360 degrees = circle

Cubic Measure

1728 cubic inches = 1 cubic foot
27 cubic feet = 1 cubic yard
2150.42 cubic inches = 1 standard bushel
268.8 cubic inches = 1 dry (U.S.) gallon
1 cubic foot = about four-fifths of a bushel
128 cubic feet = 1 cord (wood)

Dry Measure

2 pints = 1 quart
8 quarts = 1 peck
4 pecks = 1 bushel

Liquid Measure

16 ounces = 1 pint
4 quarts = 1 gallon
2 barrels = 1 hogshead (U.S.)
1000 milliliters = 1 liter
31.5 gallons = 1 barrel (U.S.)
1 quart = 0.946 liters
4 gills = 1 pint
2 pints = 1 quart

Barrels and hogsheads vary in size. A U.S. gallon is equal to 0.8327 British gallon; therefore a British gallon is equal to 1.201 U.S. gallons.
1 liter is equal to 1.0567 quarts.

Linear Measure

1 inch = 2.54 centimeters
40 rods = 1 furlong
8 furlongs = 1 statute mile
12 inches = 1 foot
3 feet = 1 yard
5.5 yards = 1 rod
1 statute mile = 5280 feet
3 statute miles = 1 statute league

Troy Weight

24 grains = 1 pennyweight
20 pennyweights = 1 ounce
12 ounces = 1 pound

Used for weighing gold, silver, and jewels.

* For abbreviations and symbols of these weights, see *Symbols* in *Appendix*.

Household Measures* and Weights

Approximate Equivalents: 60 gtt. = 1 teaspoonful = 5 ml.
= 60 minims = 60 grains = 1 dram = $\frac{1}{8}$ ounce

1 teaspoon = $\frac{1}{8}$ fl. oz.; 1 dram
16 tablespoons (liquid) = 1 cup
3 teaspoons = 1 tablespoon
12 tablespoons (dry) = 1 cup
1 tablespoon = $\frac{1}{2}$ fl. oz.; 4 drams
1 cup = 8 fl. oz.
1 tumbler or glass = 8 fl. oz.; $\frac{1}{2}$ pint

* Household measures are not precise. For instance, household tsp. will hold from 3 to 5 ml. of liquid substances. Therefore, do not substitute household equivalents for medication prescribed by the physician.

Conversion Rules

To convert units of one system into the other, multiply the number of units in column I by the equivalent factor opposite that unit in column II.

Weight

I		II
1 milligram	=	0.015432 grain
1 gram	=	15.432 grains
1 gram	=	0.25720 apothecaries' dram
1 gram	=	0.03527 avoirdupois ounce
1 gram	=	0.03215 apothecaries' or troy ounce
1 kilogram	=	35.274 avoirdupois ounces
1 kilogram	=	32.151 apothecaries' or troy ounces
1 kilogram	=	2.2046 avoirdupois pounds
1 grain	=	64.7989 milligrams
1 grain	=	0.0648 gram
1 apothecaries' dram	=	3.8879 gram
1 avoirdupois ounce	=	28.3495 grams
1 apothecaries' or troy ounce	=	31.1035 grams
1 avoirdupois pound	=	453.5924 grams

Volume (air or gas)

I		II
1 cubic centimeter	=	0.06102 cubic inch
1 cubic meter	=	35.314 cubic feet
1 cubic meter	=	1.3079 cubic yard
1 cubic inch	=	16.3872 cubic centimeters
1 cubic foot	=	0.02832 cubic meter

Capacity (fluid or liquid)

I		II
1 milliliter	=	16.23 minims
1 milliliter	=	0.2705 fluid dram
1 milliliter	=	0.0338 fluid ounce
1 liter	=	33.8148 fluid ounces
1 liter	=	2.1134 pints
1 liter	=	1.0567 quart
1 liter	=	0.2642 gallon
1 fluid dram	=	3.697 milliliters
1 fluid ounce	=	29.573 milliliters
1 pint	=	473.166 milliliters
1 quart	=	946.332 milliliters
1 gallon	=	3.785 liters

To Convert Centigrade or Celsius Degrees to Fahrenheit Degrees*

Multiply the number of Centigrade degrees by $9/5$ and add 32 to the result.

Example: $55° C. \times 9/5 = 99 + 32 = 131° F.$

To convert Fahrenheit degrees to Centigrade degrees: Subtract 32 from the number of Fahrenheit degrees and multiply the difference by $5/9$.

Example: $243° F. - 32 = 211 \times 5/9 = 117.2° C.$

* SEE: *thermometry* for table.

Miscellaneous Conversion Factors

Pressure

to obtain	multiply	by
lb./sq. in.	atmospheres	14.696
lb./sq. in.	in. of water	0.03609
lb./sq. in.	ft. of water	0.4335
lb./sq. in.	in. of mercury	0.4912
lb./sq. in.	kg./sq. meter	0.00142
lb./sq. in.	kg./sq. cm.	14.22
lb./sq. in.	cm. of mercury	0.1934
lb./sq. ft.	atmospheres	2116.8
lb./sq. ft.	in. of water	5.204
lb./sq. ft.	ft. of water	62.48
lb./sq. ft.	in. of mercury	70.727
lb./sq. ft.	cm. of mercury	27.845
lb./sq. ft.	kg./sq. meter	0.20482
lb./cu. in.	gm./ml.	0.03613
lb./cu. ft.	lb./cu. in.	1728.0
lb./cu. ft.	gm./ml.	62.428
lb./U.S. gal.	gm./l.	8.345
in. of water	in. of mercury	13.60
in. of water	cm. of mercury	5.3543
ft. of water	atmospheres	33.95
ft. of water	lb./sq. in.	2.307
ft. of water	kg./sq. meter	0.00328
ft. of water	in. of mercury	1.133
ft. of water	cm. of mercury	0.4461
atmospheres	ft. of water	0.02947
atmospheres	in. of mercury	0.03342
atmospheres	kg./sq. cm.	0.9678
bars	atmospheres	1.0133
in. of mercury	atmospheres	29.921
in. of mercury	lb./sq. in.	2.036
mm. of mercury	atmospheres	760.0
gm./ml.	lb./cu. in.	27.68
gm./sq. cm.	kg./sq. meter	0.1
kg./sq. meter	lb./sq. in.	703.1
kg./sq. meter	in. of water	25.40
kg./sq. meter	in. of mercury	345.32
kg./sq. meter	cm. of mercury	135.95
kg./sq. meter	atmospheres	10332.0
kg./sq. cm.	atmospheres	1.0332

Flow Rate

To obtain	multiply	by
cu. ft./hr.	cc./min.	0.00212
cu. ft./hr.	L./min.	2.12
L./min.	cu. ft./hr.	0.472

Parts Per Million

Conversion of parts per million (ppm) to percent: 1 ppm = 0.0001%, 10 ppm = 0.001%, 100 ppm = 0.01%, 1000 ppm = 0.1%, 10,000 ppm = 1%, etc.

Miscellaneous Units of Measurement

Units of Time

1 millisecond = one thousandth (0.001) of a second
1 second = $\frac{1}{60}$ of a minute
1 minute = $\frac{1}{60}$ of an hour
1 hour = $\frac{1}{24}$ of a day

Units of Temperature

Given a temperature on the Fahrenheit scale; to convert it to Centigrade, subtract 32 and multiply by $\frac{5}{9}$. Given a temperature on the Centigrade scale; to convert it to Fahrenheit, multiply by $\frac{9}{5}$ and add 32. Celsius degrees are equivalent to Centigrade degrees.

Units of Energy

1 gram/centimeter = 980.665 dynes/centimeter
1 foot-pound = 13,558,200 ergs = 13,825.5 gram-centimeters
1 Joule = 0.2386 Calorie (kilocalorie)
1 Calorie = 4.26649×10^7 gram-centimeters = 3085.96 foot-pounds
1 Calorie (kilocalorie) = 1000 calories = 4184 Joules
A large Calorie, or kilocalorie, is always written with a capital C.

---

pH Table

The pH scale is simply a series of numbers stating where a given solution would stand in a series of solutions arranged according to acidity or alkalinity. At one extreme (i.e., high pH) lies an alkaline solution made by dissolving 4 gm. of sodium hydroxide in water to make a liter of solution; at the other is a solution containing 3.65 gm. of hydrogen chloride per liter. Halfway between lies purified water, which is neutral. All other solutions can be arranged on this scale, and their acidity or alkalinity can be stated by giving the numbers that indicate their relative positions.

Tenth-normal HCl	1.00	Litmus is red in this acid range.
Gastric juice	*1.4	
Urine	*6.0	
Water	7.00-Neutral	
Blood	7.35–7.45	Litmus is blue in this alkaline range.
Bile	*7.5	
Pancreatic juice	8.5	
Tenth-normal NaOH	13.00	

If one is told that the pH of a certain solution is 5.3, one knows at once that it falls between gastric juice and urine on the above scale, is moderately acid, and will turn litmus red.

* These body fluids vary rather widely in pH; typical figures have been used for simplicity. Urine samples obtained from healthy individuals may have pH's anywhere between 4.7 and 8.0.

Preparation of Percentage Solutions

When the metric system is used, the preparation of percentage solutions is simple: a 1% solution contains 1 gm. in 100 ml.; a 0.1% solution contains 0.1 gm. (or 100 milligrams) per 100 ml.

When the apothecaries' system is used the following are helpful: 4.55 grains to the ounce, or 2.5 drams to 32 ounces; or 3.25 drams to 40 ounces, all make a 1% solution.

To Prepare a Dilute Solution From One Which Is Stronger:

For example, to make 80% alcohol from 95%: Dilute 80 ml. of the 95% alcohol to 95 ml. with distilled water.

Rule: Dilute a volume equal to the percent desired to a volume equal to the percent used.

SEE: *dosage*.

Percentage Solution Tables

Weight-in-volume solutions are prescribed by the USP to be used in compounding prescriptions whenever gases or solids are dissolved in liquids, since most physicians have in mind a certain weight of substance in a definite volume of solution. Such solutions are defined by the USP as "the number of grams of an active constituent in 100 milliliters of solution" regardless of whether water or some other liquid is the vehicle.

For such weight-in-volume solutions, the following tables will afford a ready means of ascertaining the quantities (by weight) of substance required to prepare varying volumes of definite w/v percentage strength. The calculations are based on 1 fl. oz. (480 minims) of water = 455 grains (round number) in the Apothecaries table and 100 ml. of water = 100 gm. in the Metric table.

For example, if 8 fluid ounces of a 0.5% solution of salt in water (% weight in volume) is needed, add 18.2 grains of salt to 8 fluid ounces of water. In the metric system, if 500 ml. of a 0.5% solution of salt in water (% weight in volume) is required, add 2.5 grams of salt to 500 ml. of water.

APOTHECARIES

Strength of solution (% w/v)	*Grains* of substance required per given volume of solution										
	¼ fl oz	½ fl oz	1 fl oz	2 fl oz	3 fl oz	4 fl oz	6 fl oz	8 fl oz	10 fl oz	12 fl oz	16 fl oz
0.01	0.0114	0.023	0.046	0.091	0.137	0.182	0.273	0.364	0.455	0.546	0.728
0.02	0.023	0.046	0.091	0.182	0.273	0.364	0.546	0.728	0.910	1.092	1.456
0.04	0.046	0.091	0.182	0.364	0.546	0.728	1.092	1.456	1.820	2.184	2.912
0.05	0.057	0.114	0.2275	0.455	0.683	0.910	1.365	1.820	2.275	2.730	3.640
0.1	0.114	0.228	0.455	0.910	1.365	1.820	2.730	3.640	4.55	5.46	7.28
0.2	0.2275	0.455	0.910	1.820	2.730	3.640	5.460	7.28	9.10	10.92	14.56
0.25	0.284	0.569	1.138	2.275	3.413	4.55	6.83	9.10	11.38	13.65	18.20
0.5	0.569	1.138	2.275	4.55	6.83	9.10	13.65	18.20	22.75	27.3	36.4
1	1.138	2.275	4.55	9.10	13.65	18.2	27.3	36.4	45.5	54.6	72.8
2	2.275	4.55	9.10	18.20	27.30	36.4	54.6	72.8	91.0	109.2	145.6
3	3.413	6.83	13.65	27.30	40.95	54.6	81.9	109.2	136.5	163.8	218.4
4	4.55	9.10	18.20	36.40	54.60	72.8	109.2	145.6	182.0	218.4	291.2
5	5.69	11.37	22.75	45.50	68.25	91.0	136.5	182.0	227.5	273	364
10	11.38	22.75	45.50	91.0	136.50	182	273	364	455	546	728
15	17.06	34.13	68.25	136.5	204.75	273	409.5	546	682.5	819	1092
20	22.75	45.50	91.0	182	273	364	546	728	910	1092	1456
25	28.44	56.90	113.75	227.5	341.25	455	682.5	910	1137.5	1365	1820
30	34.13	68.25	136.5	273	409.5	546	819	1092	1365	1638	2184
40	45.5	91.0	182	364	546	728	1092	1456	1820	2184	2912

METRIC

Strength of solution (% w/v)	*Grams* of substance required per given volume of solution											
	10 ml	15 ml	25 ml	30 ml	60 ml	90 ml	100 ml	120 ml	150 ml	200 ml	500 ml	1000 ml
0.01	0.001	0.0015	0.0025	0.003	0.006	0.009	0.01	0.012	0.015	0.02	0.05	0.1
0.02	0.002	0.003	0.005	0.006	0.012	0.018	0.02	0.024	0.03	0.04	0.1	0.2
0.05	0.005	0.008	0.013	0.015	0.03	0.045	0.05	0.06	0.075	0.1	0.25	0.5
0.1	0.01	0.015	0.025	0.03	0.06	0.09	0.1	0.12	0.15	0.2	0.5	1.0
0.2	0.02	0.03	0.05	0.06	0.12	0.18	0.2	0.24	0.30	0.4	1.0	2.0
0.25	0.025	0.038	0.063	0.075	0.15	0.225	0.25	0.3	0.375	0.5	1.25	2.5
0.5	0.05	0.075	0.125	0.15	0.3	0.45	0.5	0.6	0.75	1.0	2.5	5.0
1	0.1	0.15	0.25	0.3	0.6	0.9	1.0	1.2	1.5	2.0	5.0	10.0
1.5	0.15	0.225	0.375	0.45	0.9	1.35	1.5	1.8	2.25	3.0	7.5	15.0
2	0.2	0.3	0.5	0.6	1.2	1.8	2.0	2.4	3.0	4.0	10.0	20.0
3	0.3	0.45	0.75	0.9	1.8	2.7	3.0	3.6	4.5	6.0	15.0	30.0
4	0.4	0.6	1.0	1.2	2.4	3.6	4.0	4.8	6.0	8.0	20.0	40.0
5	0.5	0.75	1.25	1.5	3.0	4.5	5.0	6.0	7.5	10.0	25.0	50.0
10	1.0	1.5	2.5	3.0	6.0	9.0	10.0	12.0	15.0	20.0	50.0	100.0
15	1.5	2.25	3.75	4.5	9.0	13.5	15.0	18.0	22.5	30.0	75.0	150.0
20	2.0	3.0	5.0	6.0	12.0	18.0	20.0	24.0	30.0	40.0	100.0	200.0
25	2.5	3.75	6.25	7.5	15.0	22.5	25.0	30.0	37.5	50.0	125.0	250.0
40	4.0	6.0	10.0	12.0	24.0	36.0	40.0	48.0	60.0	80.0	200.0	400.0

From *Merck Index*, ed. 10, Merck & Co., Rahway, NJ, with permission.

App. 2: Physical Constants of the Elements

Element	Symbol	Atomic number	Atomic weight
Actinium	Ac	89	227.0278*
Aluminum	Al	13	26.98154
Americium	Am	95	(243)
Antimony	Sb	51	121.75
Argon	Ar	18	39.948
Arsenic	As	33	74.9216
Astatine	At	85	(210)
Barium	Ba	56	137.33
Berkelium	Bk	97	(247)
Beryllium	Be	4	9.01218
Bismuth	Bi	83	208.9804
Boron	B	5	10.81
Bromine	Br	35	79.904
Cadmium	Cd	48	112.41
Calcium	Ca	20	40.08
Californium	Cf	98	(251)
Carbon	C	6	12.011
Cerium	Ce	58	140.12
Cesium	Cs	55	132.9054
Chlorine	Cl	17	35.453
Chromium	Cr	24	51.996
Cobalt	Co	27	58.9332
Copper	Cu	29	63.546
Curium	Cm	96	(247)
Dysprosium	Dy	66	162.50
Einsteinium	Es	99	(252)
Element 104		104	(261)
Element 105		105	(262)
Element 106		106	(263)
Erbium	Er	68	167.26
Europium	Eu	63	151.96
Fermium	Fm	100	(257)
Fluorine	F	9	18.998403
Francium	Fr	87	(223)
Gadolinium	Gd	64	157.25
Gallium	Ga	31	69.72
Germanium	Ge	32	72.59
Gold	Au	79	196.9665
Hafnium	Hf	72	178.49
Helium	He	2	4.00260
Holmium	Ho	67	164.9304
Hydrogen	H	1	1.0079
Indium	In	49	114.82
Iodine	I	53	126.9045
Iridium	Ir	77	192.22
Iron	Fe	26	55.847
Krypton	Kr	36	83.80
Lanthanum	La	57	138.9055
Lawrencium	Lr	103	(260)
Lead	Pb	82	207.2
Lithium	Li	3	6.941
Lutetium	Lu	71	174.967
Magnesium	Mg	12	24.305

Based on 1979 IUPAC Atomic Weights of the Elements.
A value given in parentheses denotes the mass number of the longest-lived isotope.
*Atomic weight of most commonly available long-lived isotope.

Physical Constants of the Elements *(Continued)*

Element	Symbol	Atomic number	Atomic weight
Manganese	Mn	25	54.9380
Mendelevium	Md	101	(258)
Mercury	Hg	80	200.59
Molybdenum	Mo	42	95.94
Neodymium	Nd	60	144.24
Neon	Ne	10	20.179
Neptunium	Np	93	237.0482*
Nickel	Ni	28	58.69
Niobium	Nb	41	92.9064
Nitrogen	N	7	14.0067
Nobelium	No	102	(259)
Osmium	Os	76	190.2
Oxygen	O	8	15.9994
Palladium	Pd	46	106.42
Phosphorus	P	15	30.97376
Platinum	Pt	78	195.08
Plutonium	Pu	94	(244)
Polonium	Po	84	(209)
Potassium	K	19	39.0983
Praseodymium	Pr	59	140.9077
Promethium	Pm	61	(145)
Protactinium	Pa	91	231.0359*
Radium	Ra	88	226.0254*
Radon	Rn	86	(222)
Rhenium	Re	75	186.207
Rhodium	Rh	45	102.9055
Rubidium	Rb	37	85.4678
Ruthenium	Ru	44	101.07
Samarium	Sm	62	150.36
Scandium	Sc	21	44.9559
Selenium	Se	34	78.96
Silicon	Si	14	28.0855
Silver	Ag	47	107.868
Sodium	Na	11	22.98977
Strontium	Sr	38	87.62
Sulfur	S	16	32.06
Tantalum	Ta	73	180.9479
Technetium	Tc	43	(98)
Tellurium	Te	52	127.60
Terbium	Tb	65	158.9254
Thallium	Tl	81	204.383
Thorium	Th	90	232.0381*
Thulium	Tm	69	168.9342
Tin	Sn	50	118.69
Titanium	Ti	22	47.88
Tungsten	W	74	183.85
Uranium	U	92	238.0289
Vanadium	V	23	50.9415
Xenon	Xe	54	131.29
Ytterbium	Yb	70	173.04
Yttrium	Y	39	88.9059
Zinc	Zn	30	65.38
Zirconium	Zr	40	91.22

Based on 1979 IUPAC Atomic Weights of the Elements.
A value given in parentheses denotes the mass number of the longest-lived isotope.
*Atomic weight of most commonly available long-lived isotope.

BLOOD, PLASMA OR SERUM VALUES

Determination	*Reference Range* Conventional	*Reference Range* SI	*Minimal ml. Required†*	*Note*
Acetoacetate plus acetone	0.3–2.0 mg/100 ml	3–20 mg/l	2-S	
Aldolase	1.3–8.2 mU/ml	12-75 nmol·s^{-1}l	2-S	Use fresh, unhemolyzed serum
Alpha amino nitrogen	3.0–5.5 mg/100 ml	2.1–3.9 mmol/l	5-P	Collect with heparin
Ammonia	80–110 μg/100 ml	47–65 μmol/l	2-B	Collect in heparinized tube, deliver *immediately* packed in ice.
Amylase	4–25 U/ml	4–25 arb. unit	3-S	
Ascorbic acid	0.4–1.5 mg/100 ml	23–85 μmol/l	7-B	Collect in heparin tube before any food is given.
Barbiturate	.0 Coma level: phenobarbital, approximately 10 mg/100 ml; most other drugs, 1–3 mg per 100 ml	0 μmol/l	5-S	
Bilirubin (van den Bergh test)	One minute: 0.4 mg/100 ml Direct: 0.4 mg/100 ml. Total: 1.0 mg/100 ml Indirect is total minus direct	up to 7 μmol/l up to 17 μmol/l	3-S	
Blood volume	8.5—9.0% of body weight in kg	80–85 ml/kg		
Bromide	0 Toxic level: 17 meq/l	0 mmol/l	3-S	
Bromsulphalein (BSP)	Less than 5% retention	<0.05 l	3-S	Inject intravenously 5 mg of dye/kg of body weight, draw blood 45 min. later
Calcium	8.5–10.5 mg/100 ml (slightly higher in children)	2.1–2.6 mmol/l	3-S	BSP dye interferes
Carbon dioxide content	24–30 meq/l 20–26 meq/l in infants (as HCO_3^-)	24–30 mmol/l	3-S	Draw without stasis under oil or fill tube to top
Carbon monoxide	Symptoms with over 20% saturation	0 (1)	5-B	Fill tube to top; tightly stopper; use anticoagulant

*From Scully, Robert E. (ed.): Case Records of the Massachusetts General Hospital, New England Journal of Medicine, vol. 302, pp. 37–48, Jan. 3, 1980.
†S = serum P = plasma B = blood

Carotenoids	0.8–4.0 μg/ml	1.5-7.4μmol/l	3-S	Vitamin A may be done on same specimen
Ceruloplasmin	27–37 mg/100 ml	1.8–2.5 μmol/l	2-S	
Chloride	100–106 meq/l	100–106 mmol/l	1-S	
Cholinesterase (pseudocholinesterase)	0.5 pH U or more/h	0.5 or more arb. unit	1-S	
	0.7 pH U or more/h for packed cells		1-S	
Copper	Total: 100–200 μg/100 ml	16–31 μmol/l	3-S	
Creatine phosphokinase (CPK)	Female 5–35 mU/ml Male 5–55 mU/ml	0.08–0.58 $\mu mol \cdot s^{-1}/l$	3-S	Immediately separate & freeze serum
Creatinine	0.6–1.5 mg/100 ml	60–130 μmol/l	1-S	
Doriden (Glutethimide)	0 mg/100 ml	0 μmol/l	5-S	
Ethanol	0.3–0.4%, marked intoxication; 0.4–0.5% alcoholic stupor; 0.5% or over, alcoholic coma	65–87 mmol/l 87–109 mmol/l >109 mmol/l	2-B	Collect in oxalate & refrigerate
Glucose	Fasting: 70–110 mg/100 ml	3.9–5.6 mmol/l	2-P	Collect with EDTA-fluoride mixture
Iron	50–150 μg/100 ml (higher in males)	9.0–26.9 μmol/l	5-S	Shows diurnal variation higher in a.m.
Iron-binding capacity	250–410 μg/100 ml	44.8–73.4 μmol/l	5-S	
Lactic acid	0.6–1.8 meq/l	0.6–1.8 mmol/l	2-B	Collect with oxalate fluoride mixture: deliver immediately packed in ice
Lactic dehydrogenase	60–120 U/ml	1.00–2.00 $\mu mol \cdot s^{-1}/l$	2-S	Unsuitable if hemolyzed
Lead	50 μg/100 ml or less	up to 2.4 μmol/l	2-B	Collect with oxalate fluoride mixture
Lipase	2 U/ml or less	up to 2 arb. unit	3-S	Fasting
Lipids				
Cholesterol	120–220 mg/100 ml	3.10–5.69 mmol/l	2-S	Fasting
Cholesterol esters	60–75% of cholesterol		2-S	Fasting
Phospholipids	9–16 mg/100 ml as lipid phosphorus	2.9–5.2 mmol/l	5-S	Fasting
Total fatty acids	190–420 mg/100 ml	1.9–4.2 g/l	10-S	Fasting
Total lipids	450–1000 mg/100 ml	4.5–10.0 g/l	5-S	Fasting
Triglycerides	40–150 mg/100 ml	0.4–1.5 g/l	2-S	
Lipoprotein electrophoresis (LEP)			2-S	Fasting; do not freeze serum
Lithium	Toxic level 2 meq/l	2 mmol/l	1-S	

BLOOD, PLASMA OR SERUM VALUES *(Continued)*

Determination	Reference range: Conventional	Reference range: SI	Minimal ml. Required	Note
Magnesium	1.5–2.0 meq/l	0.8–1.3 mmol/l	1-S	
Methanol	0		5-B	May be fatal as low as 115 mg per 100 ml; collect in oxalate
5′Nucleotidase	0.3–3.2 Bodansky U	30–290 nmol·s^{-1}/l	1-S	
Osmolality	285–295 mOsm/kg water	285–295 mmol/kg	5-S	
Oxygen saturation (arterial)	96–100%	0.96–1.00 l	3-B	Deliver in sealed heparinized syringe packed in ice
Pco_2	35–45 mm Hg	4.7–6.0 kPa	2-B	Collect and deliver in sealed heparinized syringe
pH	7.35–7.45	same	2-B	Collect without stasis in sealed heparinized syringe; deliver packed in ice
Po_2	75–100 mm Hg (dependent on age) while breathing room air	10.0–13.3 kPa	2-B	
	Above 500 mm Hg while on 100% O_2			
Phenylalanine	0–2 mg/100 ml	0–120 μmol/l	0.4-S	
Phenytoin (Dilantin)	Therapeutic level, 5–20 μg/ml	19.8–79.5 μmol/l	3-S	
Phosphatase (acid)	Male–Total: 0.13–0.63 Sigma U/ml	36–175 nmol·s^{-1}/l	1-S	Must always be drawn just before analysis or stored as frozen serum; avoid hemolysis
	Female—Total: 0.01–0.56 Sigma U/ml	2.8–156 nmol · s^{-1}/l		
	Prostatic: 0–0.7 Fishman-Lerner U/100 ml			
Phosphatase (alkaline)	13–39 IU/l; infants and adolescents up to 104 IU/l	0.22–0.65 μmol·s^{-1}/l up to 1.26 μmol·s^{-1}/l	1-S	BSP dye interferes For Bodansky U multiply IU/l by 0.15 up to 90 U; 0.13 to 256 U
Phosphorus (inorganic)	3.0–4.5 mg/100 ml (infants in 1st year up to 6.0 mg/100 ml)	1.0–1.5 mmol/l	2-S	Obtain blood in fasting state; serum must be separated promptly from cells.
Potassium	3.5–5.0 meq/l	3.5–5.0 mmol/l	2-S	Serum must be separated

				promptly from cells (within 1 hr)
Primidone (Mysoline)	Therapeutic level 4–12 μg/ml	18–55 μmol/l	3-S	
Protein: Total	6.0–8.4 g/100 ml	60–84 g/l	1-S	Patient should be fasting, avoid BSP dye
Albumin	3.5–5.0 g/100 ml	35–50 g/l	1-S	
Globulin	2.3–3.5 g/100 ml	23–35 g/l		Globulin equals total protein minus albumin
Electrophoresis	% of total protein		1-S	Quantitation by densitometry
Albumin	52–68	0.52–0.681		
Globulin:				
$Alpha_1$	4.2–7.2	0.042–0.072/l		
$Alpha_2$	6.8–12	0.068–0.12/l		
Beta	9.3–15	0.093–0.15/l		
Gamma	13–23	0.13–0.23/l		
Pyruvic acid	0–0.11 meq/l	0–0.11 mmol/l	2-B	Collect with oxalate fluoride, Deliver immediately packed in ice
Quinidine	Therapeutic: 1.5–3 μg/ml	4.6–9.2 μmol/l	1-S	
	Toxic: 5–6 μg/ml	15.4–18.5 μmol/l		
Salicylate:	0		5-P	Collect in heparin or EDTA
Therapeutic	20–25 mg/100 ml;	1.4–1.8 mmol/l		
	25–30 mg/100 ml to age 10 yrs. 3 h post dose	1.8–2.2 mmol/l		
Toxic	Over 30 mg/100 ml;	over 2.2 mmol/l		
	over 20 mg/100 ml after age 60	over 1.4 mmol/l		
Sodium	135–145 meq/l	135–145 mmol/l	2-S	
Sulfate	0.5–1.5 mg/100 ml	0.05–1.2 mmol/l	3-S	Avoid hemolysis
Sulfonamide	0 mg/100 ml	0 mmol/l	2-S,B	Value given as unconjugated unless total is requested
	Therapeutic: 5–15 mg 100/ml			
Thymol:				
Flocculation	Up to 1 + in 24 hr	up to 1 + arb. unit	1-S	Checked with phosphate buffer of higher molarity to rule out false-positive reaction
Turbidity	0–4 U	0–4 arb. unit	1-S	
Transaminase (SGOT)	10–40 U/ml	0.08–0.32 $\mu mol \cdot s^{-1}/l$	1-S	

BLOOD, PLASMA OR SERUM VALUES *(Continued)*

Determination	Reference range		Minimal ml. Required	Note
	Conventional	*SI*		
(aspartate aminotransferase)				
Urea nitrogen (BUN)	8–25 mg/100 ml	2.9–8.9 mmol/l	1-S,B	Urea = BUN×2.14. Use oxalate as anticoagulant
Uric acid	3.0–7.0 mg/100 ml	0.18–0.42 mmol/l	1-S	Serum must be separated from cells at once and refrigerated
Vitamin A	0.15–0.6 μg/ml	0.5–2.1 μmol/l	3-S	
Vitamin A tolerance test	Rise to twice fasting level in 3 to 5 h.		3-S	Samples taken fasting and at intervals up to 8 h after test dose

URINE VALUES

Determination	Reference Range		Minimal Quantity Required	Note
	Conventional	*SI*		
Acetone plus acetoacetate (quantitative)	0	0 mg/l	2 ml	Keep cold
Alpha amino nitrogen	64–199 mg/d; not over 1.5% of total nitrogen	4.6–14.2 mmol/d	24-h specimen	Preserve with thymol; refrigerate
Amylase	24–76 U/ml	24–76 arbitrary units		
Calcium	150 mg/d or less	3.8 or less mmol/d	24-h specimen	Collect in special bottle with 10 ml of concentrated HCl
Catecholamines	Epinephrine: under 20 μg/d Norepinephrine: under 100 μg/d	<55 nmol/d <590 nmol/d	24-h specimen	Should be collected with 12 ml of concentrated HCl (pH should be between 2.0 and 3.0)

Chorionic gonadotropin	0	0 arb. unit	1st morning voiding	Specific gravity should be at least 1.015
Copper	0–100 μg/d	0–1.6 μmol/d	24-h specimen	
Coproporphyrin	50–250 μg/d	80–380 nmol/d	24-h specimen	Collect with 5 g of sodium carbonate
	Children under 80 lb. 0–75 μg/d	0–115 nmol/d		
Creatine	Under 100 mg/d or less than 6% of creatinine. In pregnancy: up to 12%. In children under 1 yr.: may equal creatinine. In older children: up to 30% of creatinine	<0.75 nmol/d	24-h specimen	Also order creatinine
Creatinine	15–25 mg/kg of body weight/d	0.13–0.22 mmol · kg^{-1}/d	24-h specimen	
Creatinine clearance	150–180 l/d (104–125 ml/min) per 1.73 m^2 of body surface	1.7–2.1 ml/s	24-h specimen	Order serum creatinine also
Cystine or cysteine	0	0	10 ml.	Qualitative
Follicle-stimulating hormone:			24-h specimen	
Follicular phase	5–20 IU/d	same		
Mid-cycle	15–60 IU/d			
Luteal phase	5–15 IU/d			
Menopausal	50–100 IU/d			
Men	5–25 IU/d			
Hemoglobin and myoglobin	0		Freshly voided sample	Chemical examination with benzidine
Homogentisic acid	0		Freshly voided sample or 24-h sample kept cold	Must be refrigerated if not determined at once; test also measures gentisic acid and may be positive in patients on high doses of salicylates
5-Hydroxyindole acetic acid	2–9 mg/d (women lower than men)	10–45 μmol/d	24-h specimen	Collect in special bottle with 10 ml of concentrated HCl
Lead	0.08 μg/ml or 120 μg or less/d	0.39 μmol/l or less	24-h specimen	
Phenolsulfonphthalein (PSP)	At least 25% excreted by 15 min; 40% by 30 min; 60% by 120 min	0.25 l	Total output of urine collected 15, 30 and 120 min after injection	Inject 1 ml (6 mg) intravenously; BSP interferes
Phenylpyruvic acid	0	0	Freshly voided sample unless quantitation needed	

URINE VALUES *(Continued)*

Determination	Reference Range: Conventional			Reference Range: SI		Minimal ml. Required	Note
Phosphorus (inorganic)	Varies with intake; average 1 g/d			32 mmol/d		24-h specimen	Collect in special bottle with 10 ml of concentrated HCl
Porphobilinogen	0			0		10 ml	Use freshly voided urine
Protein:							
Quantitative	<150 mg/24 h			<0.15 g/d		24-h specimen	
Electrophoresis	(see blood protein)						
Steroids:							
17-Ketosteroids (per day)	*Age*	*Male*	*Female*	*μmol/d*	*μmol/d*	24-h specimen	Not valid if patient is receiving meprobamate
	10	1–4 mg	1–4 mg	3–14	3–14		
	20	6–21	4–16	21–73	14–56		
	30	8–26	4–14	28–90	14–49		
	50	5–18	3–9	17–62	10–31		
	70	2–10	1–7	7–35	3–24		
17-Hydroxysteroids	3–8 mg/d (women lower than men)			8–22 μmol/d as hydrocortisone		24-h specimen	Keep cold; chlorpromazine and related drugs interfere with assay
Sugar:							
Quantitative glucose	0			0 mmol/l		24-h or other timed specimen	Collect with toluene; refrigerate
Identification of reducing substances						50 ml	Use freshly voided urine; no preservatives
Fructose	0			0 mmol/l		50 ml	Use freshly voided urine; also quantitate total reducing substances
Pentose	0			0 mmol/l		50 ml	Use freshly voided urine
Titratable acidity	20–40 meq/d			20–40 mmol/d		24-h sample	Collect with toluene; refrigerate
Urobilinogen	Up to 1.0 Ehrlich U			to 1.0 arb. unit		2-h sample (1–3 p.m.)	
Uroporphyrin	0			0 nmol/d		See Coproporphyrin	
Vanillylmandelic acid (VMA)	Up to 9 mg/24 h			up to 45 μmol/d		24-h specimen	Collect as for catecholamines

SPECIAL ENDOCRINE TESTS
Steroid Hormones

Determination	Reference Range: Conventional	Reference Range: SI	Minimal ml. Required	Note
Aldosterone	Excretion: 5–19 μg/24 h	14–53 nmol/d	5/d	Keep specimen cold
	Supine: 48 ± 29 pg/ml	133 ± 80 pmol/l	3-S.P.	Fasting, at rest, 210 meq sodium diet
	Upright: (2 h) 65 ± 23 pg/ml	180 ± 64 pmol/l		Upright, 2 h, 210 meq sodium diet
	Supine: 107 ± 45 pg/ml	279 ± 125 pmol/l		Fasting, at rest, 110 meq sodium diet
	Upright: (2 h) 239 ± 123 pg/ml	663 ± 341 pmol/l		Upright, 2 h, 110 meq sodium diet
	Supine: 175 ± 75 pg/ml	485 ± 208 pmol/l		Fasting, at rest, 10 meq sodium diet
	Upright: (2 h) 531 ± 228 pg/ml	1476 ± 632 pmol/l		Upright, 2 h, 10 meq sodium diet
Cortisol	8 a.m.: 5–25 μg/100 ml	0.14—0.69 μmol/l	1-P	Fasting
	8 p.m.: Below 10 μg/100 ml	0–0.28 μmol/l	1-P	At rest
	4 h ACTH test: 30–45 μg/100 ml	0.83–1.24 μmol/l	1-P	20 U ACTH, IV per 4 h
	Overnight suppression test: Below 5 μg/100 ml	<0.14 nmol/l	1-P	8 a.m. sample after dexamethasone at midnight
	Excretion: 20–70 μg/24 h	55–193 nmol/d	2-d	Keep specimen cold
11-Deoxycortisol	Responsive: Over 7.5 μg/100 ml	>0.22 μmol/l	1-P	8 a.m. sample, preceded by 4.5 g of metyrapone PO per 24 h or by single dose of 2.5 g PO at midnight
Testosterone	Adult male: 300–1100 ng/100 ml	10.4–38.1 nmol/l	2-P	a.m. sample
	Adolescent male: Over 100 ng/100 ml	>3.5 nmol/l		
	Female: 25–90 ng/100 ml	0.87–3.12 nmol/l		

SPECIAL ENDOCRINE TESTS *(Continued)*

Steroid Hormones

Determination	Reference Range: Conventional	Reference Range: SI	Minimal ml. Required	Note
Unbound testosterone	Adult male:		2-P	a.m. sample
	3.06–24.0 ng/100 ml	106–832 pmol/l		
	Adult female:			
	0.09–1.28 ng/100 ml	3.1–44.4 pmol/l		

Polypeptide Hormones

Determination	Reference Range: Conventional	Reference Range: SI	Minimal ml. Required	Note
Adrenocorticotropin (ACTH)	15–70 pg/ml	3.3–15.4 pmol/l	5-P	Place specimen on ice and send promptly to laboratory
Calcitonin	Undetectable in normals.		5-P	Test done only on known or suspected cases of medullary carcinoma of the thyroid
	> 100 pg/ml in medullary	0		
	carcinoma	>29.3 pmol/l		
Growth hormone	Below 5 ng/ml	<233 pmol/l	1-S	Fasting, at rest
	Children: Over 10 ng/ml	>465 pmol/l		After exercise
	Male: Below 5 ng/ml	<233 pmol/l		
	Female: Up to 30 ng/ml	0–1395 pmol/l		
	Male: Below 5 ng/ml	<233 pmol/l		After glucose load
	Female: Below 10 ng/ml	0–465 pmol/l		
Insulin	6–26 μU/ml	43–187 pmol/l	1-S	Fasting
	Below 20 μU/ml	<144 pmol/l		During hypoglycemia
	Up to 150 μU/ml	0–1078 pmol/l		After glucose load
Luteinizing hormone	Male: 6–18 mU/ml	6–18 u/l	2-S, P	
	Female: 5–22 mU/ml	5–22 μ/l		Pre- or post-ovulatory
	30–250 mU/ml	30–250 u/l		Mid-cycle peak
Parathyroid hormone	<10 μl equiv/ml	<10 ml equiv/l	5-P	Keep blood on ice, or plasma must be frozen if it is to be sent any distance; a.m. sample

Prolactin	2–15 ng/ml	0.08–6.0 nmol/l	2-S	
Renin activity	Supine:		4-P	EDTA tubes, on ice; normal diet
	1.1 ± 0.8 ng/ml/h	0.9 ± 0.6 (nmol/l)h		
	Upright:			
	1.9 ± 1.7 ng/ml/h	1.5 ± 1.3 (nmol/l)h		
	Supine:			Low sodium diet
	2.7 ± 1.8 ng/ml/h	2.1 ± 1.4 (nmol/l)h		
	Upright:			
	6.6 ± 2.5 ng/ml/h	5.1 ± 1.9 (nmol/l)h		
	Diuretics:			Low sodium diet
	10.0 ± 3.7 ng/ml/h	7.7 ± 2.9 (nmol/l)h		

THYROID HORMONES

Determination	*Reference Range*		*Minimal ml. Required*
	Conventional	*SI*	
Thyroid-stimulating-hormone (TSH)	0.5–3.5 μU/ml	0.5–3.5 mU/l	2-S
Thyroxine-binding globulin capacity	15–25 μg T_4/100 ml	193–322 nmol/l	2-S
Total triiodothyronine by radioimmunoassay (T_3)	70–190 ng/100 ml	1.08–2.92 nmol/l	2-S
Total thyroxine by RIA (T_4)	4–12 μg/100 ml	52–154 nmol/l	1-S
T_3 resin uptake	25–35%	0.25–0.35	2-S
Free thyroxine index (FT_4I)	1–4 ng/100 ml	12.8–51.2 pmol/l	2-S

HEMATOLOGIC VALUES

Determination	*Reference Range*		*Minimal ml. Required*	*Note*
	Conventional	*SI*		
Coagulation factors:				
Factor I (fibrinogen)	0.15–0.35g/100 ml	4.0–10.0 μmol/l	4.5-P	Collect in Vacutainer containing sodium citrate
Factor II (prothrombin)	60–140%	0.60–1.40	4.5-P	Collect in plastic tubes with 3.8% sodium citrate

HEMATOLOGIC VALUES *(Continued)*

Determination	*Reference Range*		*Minimal ml. Required*	*Note*
	Conventional	*SI*		
Factor V (accelerator globulin)	60–140%	0.60–1.40	4.5-P	Collect as in factor II determination
Factor VII-X (proconvertin-Stuart)	70–130%	0.70–1.30	4.5-P	Collect as in factor II determination
Factor X (Stuart factor)	70–130%	0.70–1.30	4.5-P	Collect as in factor II determination
Factor VIII (antihemophilic globulin)	50–200%	0.50–2.0	4.5-P	Collect as in factor II determination
Factor IX (plasma thromboplastin cofactor)	60–140%	0.60–1.40	4.5-P	Collect as in factor II determination
Factor XI (plasma thromboplastin antecedent)	60–140%	0.60–1.40	4.5-P	Collect as in factor II determination
Factor XII (Hageman factor)	60–140%	0.60–1.40	4.5-P	Collect as in factor II determination
Coagulation screening tests:				
Bleeding time (Simplate)	3–9 min	180–540 seconds		
Prothrombin time	Less than 2-second deviation from control	Less than 2-second deviation from control	4.5-P	Collect in Vacutainer containing 3.8% sodium citrate
Partial thromboplastin time (activated)	25–37 seconds	25–37 seconds	4.5-P	Collect in Vacutainer containing 3.8% sodium citrate
Whole-blood clot lysis	No clot lysis in 24 hours	0/d	2.0-whole blood	Collect in sterile tube and incubate at 37° C
Fibrinolytic studies:				
Euglobulin lysis	No lysis in 2 hours	0 (in 2 h)	4.5-P	Collect as in factor II determination
Fibrinogen split products	Negative reaction at greater than 1:4 dilution	0 (at > 1:4 dilution)	4.5-S	Collect in special tube containing thrombin and epsilon amino caproic acid

Thrombin time	control ± 5 s	control ± 5 s	4.5-P	Collect as in factor II determination
"Complete" blood count:				
Hematocrit	Male: 45–52% Female: 37–48%	Male: 0.42–0.52 Female: 0.37–0.48	1-B	Use EDTA as anticoagulant; the seven listed tests are performed automatically on the Coulter counter Model S, which directly determines cell counts, hemoglobin (as the cyanmethemoglobin derivative) and MCV and computes hematocrit, MCH and MCHC
Hemoglobin	Male: 13–18 g/100ml Female: 12–16 g/100 ml	Male: 8.1–11.2mmol/l Female: 7.4–9.9mmol/l		
Leukocyte count	4300–10,800/mm^3	4.3–10.8 × 10^9/l		
Erythrocyte count	4.2–5.9 million/mm^3	4.2–5.9 × 10^{12}/l		
Mean corpuscular volume (MCV)	80–94 μm^3	80–94 f l		
Mean corpuscular hemoglobin (MCH)	27–32 pg	1.7–2.0 fmol		
Mean corpuscular hemoglobin concentration (MCHC)	32–36%	19–22.8 mmol/l		
Erythrocyte sedimentation rate	Male: 1–13 mm/h Female: 1–20 mm/h	Male: 1–13 mm/h Female: 1–20 mm/h	5-B	Use EDTA as anticoagulant
Erythrocyte enzymes:				
Glucose-6-phosphate dehydrogenase	5–15 U/g Hb	5–15 U/g	9-B	Use special anticoagulant (ACD solution)
Pyruvate kinase	13–17 U/g Hb	13–17 U/g	8-B	Use special anticoagulant (ACD solution)
Ferritin (serum)	0–20 ng/ml	0–20 μg/l		
Iron deficiency				
Iron excess	Greater than 400 ng/l	>400 μ/l		
Folic acid				
Normal	Greater than 1.9 ng/ml	>4.3 mmol/l	1-S	
Borderline	1.0–1.9 ng/ml	2.3–4.3 mmol/l	1-S	
Haptoglobin	100–300 mg/100 ml	1.0–3.0 g/l	1-S	
Hemoglobin studies:				
Electrophoresis for abnormal hemoglobin			5-B	Collect with anticoagulant
Electrophoresis for A_2 hemoglobin	1.5–3.5%	0.015–0.035	5-B	Use oxalate as anticoagulant
Hemoglobin F (fetal hemoglobin)	Less than 2%	>0.02	5-B	Collect with anticoagulant

HEMATOLOGIC VALUES *(Continued)*

Determination	Reference Range: Conventional	Reference Range: SI	Minimal ml. Required	Note
Hemoglobin, met- and sulf-	0	0	5-B	Use heparin as anticoagulant
Serum hemoglobin	2–3 mg/100 ml	1.2–1.9 μ mol/l	2-S	
Thermolabile hemoglobin	0	0	1-B	Any anticoagulant
Lupus anticoagulant	0	0	4.5-P	Collect as in factor II determination
L.E. (lupus erythematosus) preparation:				
Method I	0	0	5-B	Use heparin as anticoagulant
Method II	0	0	5-B	Use defibrinated blood
Leukocyte alkaline phosphatase:				
Quantitative method	15–40 mg of phosphorus liberated/h/10^{10} cells	15–40 mg/h	20-Isolated blood leukocytes	Special handling of blood necessary
Qualitative method	Males: 33–188U Females (off contraceptive pill): 30–160 U	33–188 U 30–160 U	Smear-B	
Muramidase	Serum, 3–7 μg/ml Urine, 0–2 μg/ml	3–7 mg/l 0–2 mg/l	1-S 1-U	
Osmotic fragility of erythrocytes	Increased if hemolysis occurs in over 0.5% NaCl; decreased if hemolysis is incomplete in 0.3% NaCl		5-B	Use heparin as anticoagulant
Peroxide hemolysis	Less than 10%	>0.10	6-B	Use EDTA as anticoagulant
Platelet count	150,000–350,000/mm^3	$150–350 \times 10^9$/l	0.5-B	Use EDTA as anticoagulant; counts are performed on Clay Adams Ultraflow; when counts are low, results are confirmed by hand counting

Platelet function tests:				
Clot retraction	50–100%/2 h	0.50–1.00/2 h	4.5-P	Collect as in factor II determination
Platelet aggregation	Full response to ADP, epinephrine and collagen	1.0	18-P	Collect as in factor II determination
Platelet factor 3	33–57 s	33–57 s	4.5-P	Collect as in factor II determination
Reticulocyte count	0.5–1.5% red cells	0.005–.015	0.1-B	
Vitamin B_{12}	90–280 pg./ml (borderline:70–90)	66–207 pmol/l (borderline:52–66)	12-S	

CEREBROSPINAL FLUID VALUES

Determination	*Reference Range*		*Minimal ml. Required*	*Note*
	Conventional	*SI*		
Bilirubin	0	0 μmol/l	2	
Cell count	0–5 mononuclear cells		0.5	
Chloride	120–130 meq/l		0.5	20 meq/liter higher than serum; obtain serum for comparison
Colloidal gold	0000000000001222111	same	0.1	
Albumin	Mean:29.5 mg/100ml ± 2 SD:11–48 mg/100 ml	0.295 g/l ± 2 SD:0.11–0.48	2.5	
IgG	Mean:4.3 mg/100 ml ± 2 SD:0–8.6 mg/100 ml	0.043 g/l ± 2 SD:0–0.086		
Glucose	50–75 mg/100 ml	2.8–4.2 mmol/l	0.5	30–50% less than blood; compare with blood
Pressure (initial)	70–180 mm of water	70–180 arb. u.		
Protein:				
Lumbar	15–45 mg/100 ml	0.15–0.45 g/l	1	
Cisternal	15–25 mg/100 ml	0.15–0.25 g/l	1	
Ventricular	5–15 mg/100 ml	0.05–0.15 g/l	1	

MISCELLANEOUS VALUES

Determination	Reference Range: Conventional	Reference Range: SI	Minimal ml. Required	Note
Ascorbic acid load test	0.2–2.0 mg/h in control sample	0.3–3.2 nmol/s	Urine-approximate 1½-h sample	Administer 500 mg of ascorbic acid orally
	24–49 mg/h after loading	38–77 nmol/s	Urine-2 timed samples of about 2 h each	
Autoantibodies				
Thyroid colloid and microsomal antigens	Absent		2-S	Low titers in some elderly normal women
Stomach parietal cells	Absent		2-S	
Smooth muscle	Absent		2-S	
Kidney mitochondria	Absent		2-S	
Rabbit renal collecting ducts	Absent		2-S	
Cytoplasma of ova, theca cells, testicular interstitial cells	Absent		2-S	
Skeletal muscle	Absent		2-S	
Adrenal gland	Absent		2-S	
Carcinoembryonic antigen (CEA)	0–2.5 ng/ml, 97% healthy nonsmokers	0–2.5 μg/l, 97% healthy nonsmokers	20-P	Must be sent on ice
Chylous fluid				Use fresh specimen
Cryoprecipitable proteins	0	0 arb. unit	10-S 5-P 10-P	Collect & transport at 37°C
Digitoxin	17±6 ng/ml	22±7.8 nmol/l	1-S	Medication with digitoxin or digitalis
Digoxin	1.2±0.4 ng/ml	1.54±0.5 nmol/l	1-S	Medication with digoxin 0.25 mg per day
	1.5±0.4 ng/ml	1.92±0.5 nmol/l	1-S	Medication with digoxin 0.5 mg per day
Duodenal drainage:				
pH	5.5–7.5	5.5–7.5	1	pH should be in proper range with minimal amount of gastric juice

Amylase	Over 1200 U/total sample	>1.2 arb. u	1	
Trypsin	Values from 35 to 160% "normal"	0.35–1.60	1	
Viscosity	3 min or less	180 s or less	4	Run ice cold in 34-s viscosimeter
Gastric Analysis				
For hydrochloric acid	Basal:			
	Females 2.0±1.8 meq/h	0.6±0.5		
	Males 3.0±2.0 meq/h	0.8±0.6 μmol/s		
	Maximal: (after histalog or gastrin)			
	Females 16± 5 meq/h	4.4±1.4μmol/s		
	Males 23±5 meq/h	6.4±1.4 μmol/s		
Gastrin-1	0–200 pg/ml	0–95 pmol/l	4-P	Heparinized sample
Immunologic tests:				
Alpha-fetoglobulin	Abnormal if present		5-clotted blood	
Alpha 1-Antitrypsin	200–400 mg/100 ml	2.0–4.0 g/l	10-B	
Antinuclear antibodies	Positive if detected with serum diluted 1:10		10-clotted blood	Send to laboratory promptly
Anti-DNA antibodies	Less than 15 units/ml		10-B	
Bence Jones protein	Abnormal if present		100-U	
Complement, total hemolytic	150–250 U/ml		10-B	Must be sent on ice
C3	Range			
	55–120 mg/100 ml	0.55–1.2 g/l	10-B	
C4	Range			
	20–50 mg/100 ml	0.2–0.5 g/l	10-B	
Immunoglobulins:			10-B	
IgG	1140 mg/100 ml	11.4 g/l		
	Range 540–1663	5.5–16.6 g/l		
IgA	214 mg/100 ml	2.14 g/l		
	Range 66–344	0.66–3.44 g/l		
IgM	168 mg/100 ml	1.68 g/l		
	Range 39–290	0.39–2.9 g/l		
Viscosity	1.4–1.8		10-B	Expressed as the relative viscosity of serum compared to water
Iontophoresis	Children: 0–40 meq sodium/liter, Adults: 0–60 meq sodium/l	0–40 mmol/l 0–60 mmol/l		Value given in terms of sodium

MISCELLANEOUS VALUES *(Continued)*

Determination	Reference Range: Conventional	Reference Range: SI	Minimal ml. Required	Note
Propranolol (includes bioactive 4-OH metabolite)	100–300 ng/ml	386–1158 nmol/l	1-S	Obtain blood sample 4 h after last dose of beta blocking agent
Stool fat	Less than 5 g in 24 h or less than 4% of measured fat intake in 3-d period	<5 g/d	24-h or 3-day specimen, preferably with markers	
Stool nitrogen	Less than 2 g/d or 10% of urinary nitrogen	<2 g/d	24-h or 3-day specimen	
Synovial fluid:				
Glucose	Not less than 20 mg 100 ml lower than simultaneously drawn blood sugar	see blood glucose nmol/l	1 ml of fresh fluid	Collect with oxalate-fluoride mixture
Mucin	Type 1 or 2	1–2 arb. u.	1 ml of fresh fluid	Grade as: Type 1—tight clump; Type 2—soft clump; Type 3—soft clump that breaks up; Type 4—cloudy, no clump
D-Xylose absorption	5–8 g/5 h in urine	33–53 mmol	5-U	For directions see Benson et al: N Engl J Med 256:335, 1957
	40 mg per 100 ml in blood 2-h after ingestion of 25 g of D-xylose	2.7 mmol/l	5-B	

Abbreviations used: SI, Système international d'Unités; d, 24 hours; P, plasma; S, serum; B, blood; U, urine; l, liter; h, hour; and s, second.

App. 4: Symbols and Abbreviations

♏	Minim.
℈	Scruple.
ʒ	Dram.
fʒ	Fluid dram.
℥	Ounce.
f℥	Fluid ounce.
O	Pint.
℔	Pound.
℞	Recipe; take.
M	Misce; mix.
āā	Of each.
A, Å	Angstrom unit.
C′	Complement.
c, c̄	[L. *cum*.]. With.
Δ	Change, heat
E_0	Electroaffinity.
F_1	First filial generation.
F_2	Second filial generation.
mμ	Millimicron, micromillimeter.
μg	Microgram.
mEq	Milliequivalent.
mg	Milligram.
mg. %	Milligrams percent; milligrams per 100 ml.
Qo_2	Oxygen consumption.
m-	Meta-.
o-	Ortho-.
p-	Para-.
Po_2	Partial pressure of oxygen.
Pco_2	Partial pressure of carbon dioxide.
s̄	Without
s̄s̄, ss	[L. *semis*]. One-half.
μm	Micrometer.

μ	Micron (common term for micrometer).
μμ	Micromicron.
+	Plus; excess; acid reaction; positive.
−	Minus; deficiency; alkaline reaction; negative.
±	Plus or minus; either positive or negative; indefinite.
#	Number; following a number; pounds.
÷	Divided by.
×	Multiplied by; magnification.
=	Equals.
≅	Approximately equals.
>	Greater than; from which is derived.
<	Less than; derived from.
≮	Not less than.
≯	Not greater than.
≦	Equal to or less than.
≧	Equal to or greater than.
≠	Not equal to.
√	Root; square root; radical.
$\sqrt[2]{\ }$	Square root.
$\sqrt[3]{\ }$	Cube root.
∞	Infinity.
:	Ratio; "is to."
: :	Equality between ratios; "as."
∴	Therefore.
°	Degree.
%	Percent.
π	3.1416—ratio of circumference of a circle to its diameter.
□, ♂	Male.
○, ♀	Female.
⇌	Denotes a reversible reaction.

App. 5: Abbreviations,* Prefixes, and Suffixes

Principal Medical Abbreviations†

Abbreviation	Latin (unless indicated)	English Definition
ad	ad	to; up to
ad lib.	ad libitum	as desired
AQ	aqueous	water
AV		atrioventricular
av.	(French)	avoirdupois
		average
B.P.		British Pharmacopeia
BUN		blood urea nitrogen
C.		Celsius
		centigrade
		Calorie (kilocalorie)
C.	congius	gallon
ca.	circa	about
CBC		complete blood count
cc.	(French)	cubic centimeter
CDC		Center for Disease Control
cg.	(French)	centigram
cm.	(French)	centimeter
comp.	compositus	compound
CNS		central nervous system
cong.	congius	gallon
contra	contra	against
CSF		cerebrospinal fluid
CV		cardiovascular
d	dexter	right
	dies	day (24 hours)
/d		per day
D&C		dilatation and curretage
def.	defaecatio	defecation
DPT		diphtheria-pertussis-tetanus
dr.	drachma	dram
ECG		electrocardiogram
ECT		electroconvulsive therapy
EEG		electroencephalogram
elix.	(Arabic)	elixir
EMG		electromyogram
emp.	emplastrum	a plaster
ENT		ear, nose, and throat
ESR		erythrocyte sedimentation rate
et	et	and
F.	(proper name)	Fahrenheit
f		female
FDA		Food and Drug Administration
FEV		forced expiratory volume
Fld.	fluidus	fluid
fl. dr.	fluidrachma	fluid dram
fl. oz.	fluidus uncia	fluid ounce
FSH		follicle-stimulating hormone

* For other abbreviations used in the book, see page xxx in the front of the book.
† See also *Charting* and *Prescription Writing* on following pages and *Elements* and *Symbols* in *Appendix*.

Principal Medical Abbreviations (*Continued*)

Abbreviation	Latin (unless indicated)	English Definition
GI		gastrointestinal
Gm.; gm.	gramme (French)	gram
gr.	granum	grain
Gtt., gtt.	guttae	drops
h	hora	hour
hgb		hemoglobin
hypo	(Greek)	hypodermically
I.M.		intramuscular
inf.	infusum	infusion
inhal.		inhalation
inj.		injection
instill		instillation
I.Q.		intelligence quotient
IU		international unit
IUD		intrauterine device
I.V.		intravenously
kg.	(French)	kilogram
l	litre (French)	liter
lab		laboratory
lb.	libra	pound
LD_{50}		lethal dose, median
liq.	liquor	liquid; fluid
m.	(French)	meter
	minimum	minim
		male
MED		minimum effective dose
mEq.		milliequivalent
mg.		milligram
ml.		milliliter
mM		millimole
mm.	(French)	millimeter
mol. wt.		molecular weight
μEq		microequivalent
μg		microgram
no.	numero	number
NPN		nonprotein nitrogen
O.	octarius	pint
OC		oral contraceptive
O.D.	oculus dexter	right eye
O.L.	oculus laevus	left eye
O.S.	oculus sinister	left eye
os.	os; ora	mouth
oz.	uncia	ounce
paren.		parenterally
PBI		protein-bound iodine
per	per	through or by
pH		hydrogen ion concentration
ppm		parts per million
pt	pinte (French)	pint
qt.	quartina	quart
rad		radiation absorbed dose
$\bar{s}$	sine	without
S.	signa	mark
s	sans	without
s.c.	sub cutis	subcutaneously
s.cut.		subcutaneously

Principal Medical Abbreviations (*Continued*)

Abbreviation	Latin (unless indicated)	English Definition
SGOT		serum glutamic oxalacetic transaminase
SGPT		serum glutamic pyruvic transaminase
sp. gr.	gravitus	specific gravity
spt.	spiritus	spirit
s.q.		subcutaneously
stat.	statim	immediately
syr.	syrupus	syrup
top.		topically
tr., tinct.	tinctura	tincture
UHF		ultrahigh frequency
ung.	unguentum	ointment
UV		ultraviolet
vin	vinum	wine
vol. %		volume per cent
WBC		white blood count
Wt.	wiht (Old English)	weight
w/v.		weight by volume
×		multiplied by

Charting: Abbreviations and Their Meanings

Some of these abbreviations are used rarely if at all. They are recorded for their historical interest. See also *Principal Medical Abbreviations* and *Prescription Writing* in *Appendix*.

Abbreviation	Latin Phrase	English Definition
abs. feb.	absente febre	without fever
a.c.	ante cibum	before eating
ad effect.	ad effectum	until effectual
adhib.	adhibendus	to be administered
ad lib	ad libitum	at pleasure
ad part. dolent.	ad partes dolentes	to the painful parts
adst. feb.	adstante febre	when fever is present
ad us.	ad usum	according to custom
ad us. ext.	ad usum externum	for external use
ag. feb.	aggrediente febre	when the fever increases
alt. dieb.	alternis diebus	every other day
alt. hor.	alternis horis	every other hour
alt. noc.	alternis nocte	every other night
aq.	aqua	water
bal.	balneum	bath
bal. sin.	balneum sinapis	mustard bath
bis in 7d.	bis in septem diebus	twice a week
BP		blood pressure
c̄	cum	with
cat.	cataplasma	a poultice
cito disp.	cito dispensetur	let it be dispensed quickly
c.m.	cras mane	tomorrow morning
c.m.s.	cras mane sumendus	to be taken tomorrow morning
c.n.	cras nocte	tomorrow night
cont. rem.	continuetur remedia	let the medicines be continued

Charting: Abbreviations and Their Meanings (*Continued*)

Abbreviation	Latin Phrase	English Definition
c.v.	cras vespere	tomorrow night
cyath.	cyathus	glassful
cyath. vinos.	cyathus vinosus	wineglassful
d	da	give
d	dies	day
/d		daily
decub.	decubitus	lying down
donec alv. sol. ft.	donec alvus soluta fuerit	until bowels are open
dur. dolor.	durante dolore	while pain lasts
en., enem.		enema
exhib.	exhibeatur	let it be given
h.n.	hoc nocte	tonight
hor. som, h.s.	hora somni	at bedtime
in d.	in dies	daily
mod. praesc.	modo praescripto	as prescribed
mor. dict.	more dicto	in the manner directed
mor. sol.	more solito	in the usual manner
n.b.	nota bene	note well
noct.	nocte	night
noxt.	noxte	night
n.p.o.		nothing by mouth
p.a.a.	parti affectae applicetur	let it be applied to the affected region
post. cib. or p. c.	post cibum	after meals
p.r.	per rectum	through the rectum
p.r.n.	pro re nata	as needed
p.v.	per vaginam	through the vagina
Q.h.	quaque hora	every hour
Q. 2h.		every two hours
Q. 3h.		every three hours
q.i.d.	quater in die	four times a day
q.l.	quantum libet	as much as is wanted
q.p.	quantum placeat	at will
q.s.	quantum sufficiat	a sufficient quantity, as much as may be needed
quotid.	quotidie	daily
s̄	sine	without
s.a. or sec. a.	secundum artem	by skill
semih.	semihora	half an hour
s.o.s.	si opus sit	if necessary
st.	stet, stetem	let it (them) stand
sum.	sumat, sumendum	let him take, to be taken
s.v.	spiritus vini	alcoholic spirit
s.v.v.	spiritus vini vitis	brandy
T.		temperature
tere	tere	rub
tere bene	tere bene	rub well
t.i.d.	ter in die	three times daily
t.i.n.	ter in nocte	three times a night
ur		urine

Prescription Writing: Abbreviations and Their Meanings

Some of these abbreviations are used rarely if at all. They are recorded for their historical interest. See also *Principal Medical Abbreviations* and *Charting* on previous pages.

Abbreviation	Latin (unless indicated)	English Definition
āā or a	ana (Greek)	of each
add.	adde	add
adhib.	adhibendus	to be administered
admov.	admove	apply
ad sat.	ad saturatum	to saturation
aeq.	aequales	equal
agit.	agita	shake, stir
agit. ante sum.	agita ante sumendum	shake before taking
alb.	albus	white
alter	alter	the other
aq. bull.	aqua bulliens	boiling water
aq. cal.	aqua calida	warm water
aq. dest.	aqua destillata	distilled water
aq. ferv.	aqua fervens	hot water
aq. font.	aqua fontis	spring water
aq. frig.	aqua frigida	cold water
aq. menth. pip.	aqua menthae piperitae	peppermint water
aq. pur.	aqua pura	pure water
aut	aut	or
bene	bene	well
bib.	bibe	drink
b.i.d.	bis in die	twice daily
b.i.n.	bis in noctus	twice a night
bis	bis	twice
bol.	bolus	a large pill
bull.	bulliat	let (it) boil
c̄	cum	with
cap.	capsula	a capsule
chart. or cht.	chartula	a small medicated paper
coch. mag.	cochleare magnum	a tablespoonful
coch. med	cochleare medium	a dessertspoonful
coch. parv.	cochleare parvum	a teaspoonful
collyr.	collyrium	an eyewash
commisce	commisce	mix together
comp.	compositus	compounded of
cotula	cotula	a measure
cuj. lib.	cujus libet	of any you please
D	dosis	dose
d.	da	give
d.d. in d.	de die in diem	from day to day
dec.	decanta	pour off
dent. tal. dos.	dentur tales doses	give of such doses
det	detur	let be given
dieb. alt.	diebus alternis	every other day
dieb. tert.	diebus tertiis	every 3rd day
dil.	dilue, dilutus	dilute, diluted
dim.	dimidius	one-half
div.	divide	divide
div. in p. aeq.	dividatur in partes aequales	let it be divided into equal parts
donec alv. sol. ft.	donec alvus soluta fuerit	until bowels are open

Prescription Writing: Abbreviations and Their Meanings (*Continued*)

dos.	dosis	dose
dur. dolor.	durante dolore	while pain lasts
e.m.p.	ex modo prescripto	as directed
emp.	emplastrum	plaster
emuls.	emulsio	an emulsion
epistom.	epistomium	a stopper
ext.	extende	spread
	extractum	extract
ferv.	fervens	boiling
f.h.	fiat haustus	let a draught be made
filt.	filtra	filter
f.m.	fiat mistura	let a mixture be made
f.p.	fiat potio	let a potion be made
f. pil.	fiat pilula	let a pill be made
ft.	fiat	let it be made
garg.	gargarisma	a gargle
grad.	gradatim	by degrees
gtt.	gutta, guttae	a drop, drops
guttat.	guttatim	by drops
haust.	haustus	a draught
hor. decub.	hora decubitus	bedtime
hor. som. or h. s.	hora somni	bedtime
hor. 1 spat.	horae unius spatio	one hour's time
idem	idem	the same
inf.	infusum	let it infuse
int.	intime	thoroughly
lin.	linimentum	a liniment
liq.	liquor	a solution
lot.	lotio	a lotion
M.	misce	mix
mac.	macera	macerate
man. prim.	mane primo	first thing in the morning
mas.	massa	mass
med.	medicamentum	a medicine
m. et n.	mane et nocte	morning and night
mist.	mistura	mixture
mitt.	mitte	send
mitt. x tal.	mitte decem tales	send 10 like this
mod.	modicus	moderate sized
mod. praesc.	modo praescripto	in the manner written
moll.	mollis	soft
mor. dict.	more dicto	in the manner directed
mor. sol.	more solito	as accustomed
ne tr. s. num.	ne tradas sine nummo	deliver not without the money
no.	numero	number
noct. maneq.	nocte maneque	night and morning
non. rep., n. r.	non repetatur	let it not be repeated
nunc	nunc	now
omn. bid.	omnibus bidendis	every 2 days
omn. bih.	omni bihoris	every 2nd hour
omn. hor.	omni hora	every hour

omn. noct.	omni nocte	every night
om. 1/4 h.	omni quadrantae horae	every 15 minutes
om. mane vel. noc.	omni mane vel nocte	every morning or night
part. aeq.	partes aequales	equal parts
part. vic.	partitus vicibus	individual doses
p.c.	post cibum	after meals
pil.	pilula	a pill
p.o.	per os	by mouth
p. p. a.	phiala prius agitata	the bottle being first shaken
pro. rat. aet.	pro ratione aetatis	according to patient's age
pulv.	pulvis	powder
red. in pulv.	redactus in pulverem	reduced to powder
repetat., rep.	repetatur	to be repeated
rub.	ruber	red
sig.	signa	write
	signetur	let it be labeled
sing.	singulorum	of each
sol.	solutio	solution
solv.	solve	dissolve
ss.	semi or semisse	a half
subind.	subinde	frequently
sum.	sume	take
sum. tal.	sumat talem	take 1 such
suppos.	suppositoria	a suppository
s.v.r.	spiritus vini rectificatus	rectified spirit of wine
tab.	tabella	a tablet
tinct.	tinctura	a tincture
trit.	tritura	triturate or grind
ult. praes.	ultimus praescriptus	the last ordered
ung.	unguentum	an ointment
ut dict.	ut dictum	as directed
vitel.	vitellus	yolk of an egg

Prefixes and Suffixes

a-, an. Negative.
a-, ab-, abs-. Away from.
ad-, -ad. Toward.
-aemia. Blood.
aer-. Air.
-aesthesia. Sensation.
-algesia, algia. Suffering; pain.
algi-. Pain.
all-. Other.
amb-. Both; on both sides.
amph-. Around; on both sides.
ana-, an-. Up.
angio-. Relating to blood or lymph vessels.
ante-. Before.
anti-. Against.
apo-. From; opposed.
-ase. Enzyme.
aut-, auto-. Self.
bi, bis-. Twice; double.
brachy-. Short.
brady-. Slow.
cac-, caco-. Bad; evil.
cat, cata, cath-. Down.
-cele. A tumor; a cyst; a hernia.
cent-. Hundred.
cephal-. Relating to a head.
chrom-, chromo-. Color.
-cide. Causing death.
circum-. Around.
co, com, con-. Together.
contra-. Against.
cyst-, -cyst. Bag; bladder.
-cyte. A cell.
dacry-. Tears.
dactyl-. Fingers.
de-. From; not.
deca-. Ten.
deci-. Tenth.
demi-. Half.
dent-. Relating to the teeth.
derma-. The skin.
di-. Double; apart from.
dia-. Through; between; asunder.
dipla, diplo-. Double.
dis-. Negative; double; apart; absence of.
-dynia. Pain.
dys-. Difficult; bad.
ec, ecto-. Out; on the outside.
-ectomy. A cutting out.
ef, es, ex, exo-. Out.
-emesis. Vomiting.
-emia. Blood.
en-. In, into.
endo-. Within.
entero-. Relating to the intestine.
ento-. Within.
epi-. Upon.
-esthesia. Sensation.
eu-. Well.
ex-, exo-. Out.
extra-. On the outside; beyond.
fore-. Before; in front of.
-form. Form.
-fuge. To drive away.
galact, galacto-. Milk.
gaster, gastro-. The stomach; the belly.
-gene, -genesis, -genetic, -genic. Production; origin; formation.
glosso-. Relating to the tongue.
-gog, gogue. To make flow.
-gram. A tracing; a mark.
-graphy. A writing; a record.
hem, hemato-. Relating to the blood.
hemi-. Half.
hepa-, hepar-, hepato-. Liver.
hetero-. Other; indicating dissimilarity.
holo-. All.
homo, homeo-. Same; similar.
hydra, hydro-. Relating to water.
hyp, hyph, hypo-. Under.
hyper-. Over; above; beyond.
hypo-. Under.
-iasis. Condition; pathological state.
idio-. Peculiar to the individual or organ.
ileo-. Relating to the ileum.
in-. In; into; not.
infra-. Beneath.
inter-. Between.
intra, intro-. Within.
-ism. Condition; theory.
iso-. Equal.
-itis. Inflammation.
-ize. To treat by special method.
juxta-. Near.
karyo-. Nucleus; nut.
kata-, kath-. Down.
kera-. Horn; indicates hardness.
kinesi-. Movement.
-kinesis. Motion.
lact-. Milk.
laparo-. The loin; relating to the loin or abdomen.
laryng, laryngo-. The larynx
latero-. Side.
lepto-. Small; soft.
leuko-. White.
-lite, -lith. A stone; a calculus.
lith-. A stone.
-logia, -logy. Science of; study of.
-lysis. Setting free; disintegration.
macro-. Large; long; big.
mal-. Bad; poor; evil.
med-, medi-. Middle.
mega, megal-. Large; great.
-megalia, megaly. Large; great; extreme.
melan-, melano-. Black.
mes-, meso-. Middle.
meta-. Beyond; over; between; change, or transposition.
-meter. Measure.

metra, metro-. The uterus.
micro-. Small.
mio-. Less; smaller.
mono-. Single.
multi-. Many.
my, myo-. Muscle.
myel, myelo-. Marrow.
myxa, myxo-. Mucus.
neo-. New.
nephr, nephra, nephro-. Kidney.
neu, neuro-. Nerve.
niter, nitro-. Nitrogen.
non-, not-. No.
nucleo-. Nucleus.
ob-. Against.
oculo-. The eye.
-ode, oil. Form; shape; resemblance.
odont-. A tooth.
-oid. Form; shape; resemblance.
oligo-. Few.
-oma. A tumor.
omo-. Shoulder.
o-. An egg; ovum.
oophoron-. Ovary.
opisth-. Backward.
orchid-. Testicle.
ortho-. Straight; normal.
os-. A mouth; a bone.
-osis. Condition; disease; intensive.
oste, osteo-. A bone.
-ostomosis, ostomy. To furnish with a mouth or an outlet.
-otomy. Cutting.
oxy-. Sharp; acid.
pachy-. Thick.
pan-. All; entire.
para-. Alongside of.
path-, -path, -pathy. Disease; suffering.
-penia. Lack.
per-. Excessive; through.
peri-. Around.
-phobia. Fear.
-phylaxis. Protection.
-plasm. To mold.
-plastic. Molded; indicates restoration of lost or badly formed features.
-plegia. A stroke.
plur-. More.
pneu-. Relating to the air or lungs.
poly-. Much; many.
post-. After.
pre-. Before.
pro-. Before; in behalf of.
proto-. First.
pseud-, pseudo-. False.
psych-. The soul; the mind.
py-, pyo-. Pus.
re-. Back; again.
retro-. Backward.
-rhage, -rhagia. Hemorrhage; flow.
-rhaphy. A suturing or stitching.
-rhea. To flow; indicates discharge.
sacchar-. Sugar.
sacro-. Sacrum.
salping, salpingo-. A tube; relating to a fallopian tube.
sarco-. Flesh.
sclero-. Hard; relating to the sclera.
-sclerosis. Dryness; hardness.
-scopy. To see.
semi-. Half.
-stomosis, -stomy. To furnish with a mouth or outlet.
sub-. Under.
super, supra-. Above.
syn-. With; together.
tele-. Distant; far.
tetra-. Four.
thio-. Sulfur.
thyro-. Thyroid gland.
-tomy. Cutting.
trans-. Across.
tri-. Three.
-trophic. Relating to nourishment.
tropho-. Relating to nutrition.
uni-. One.
-uria. Relating to the urine.
urino, uro-. Relating to the urine or urinary organs.
vaso-. A vessel.
venter, ventro-. The abdomen.
xanth-. Yellow.

App. 6: Russian Alphabet

Cyrillic print		Transliteration	Pronunciation	Cyrillic Print		Transliteration	Pronunciation
А	а	a	*a* in far	С	с	s	*s* in say
Б	б	b	*b*	Т	т	t	*t*
В	в	v	*v*	У	у	u	*oo* in boot
Г	г	g (h)	*g* in gay	Ф	ф	f	*f*
Д	д	d	*d*	Х	х	kh	like German *ch*
Е	е	e	*e* in fell; *ye* in yell	Ц	ц	t͡s	*ts* in hoots
Ж	ж	zh	*z* in azure	Ч	ч	ch	*ch* in church
З	з	z	*z* in zeal	Ш	ш	sh	*sh*
И	и	i	*i* in meet	Щ	щ	shch	*shch,* as in fre*sh ch*eese
Й	й	ĭ	*y* in boy	Ъ	ъ	′	mute*
К	к	k	*k*	Ы	ы	y	*y* in rhythm (hard)
Л	л	l	*l*	Ь	ь	′	mute (softens preceding
М	м	m	*m*				consonant)
Н	н	n	*n*	Э	э	ė	*e* in met
О	о	o	*o* in or	Ю	ю	i͡u	*u* in union
П	п	p	*p*	Я	я	i͡a	*ya* in yard
Р	р	r	*r*				

* Hard sign; used to separate a consonant from a soft vowel especially in foreign words; frequently replaced by an apostrophe.

App. 7: Latin and Greek Nomenclature

Greek Alphabet

Name of letter	Capital	Lower case	Transliteration	Name of letter	Capital	Lower case	Transliteration
alpha	Α	α	a	nu	Ν	ν	n
beta	Β	ϐ or β	b	xi	Ξ	ξ	x
gamma	Γ	γ	g	omicron	Ο	ο	o short
delta	Δ	δ	d	pi	Π	ϖ	p
epsilon	Ε	ϵ	e short	rho	Ρ	ρ	r
zeta	Ζ	ζ	z	sigma	Σ	σ or ς	s
eta	Η	η	e long	tau	Τ	τ	t
theta	Θ	θ	th	upsilon	ϒ	υ	y
iota	Ι	ι	i	phi	Φ	ϕ or φ	f
kappa	Κ	κ	k, c	chi	Χ	χ	ch as in German echt
lambda	Λ	λ	l	psi	Ψ	ψ	ps
mu	Μ	μ	m	omega	Ω	ω	o long

English with Latin and Greek Equivalents

acid. Acidum.
ague. Febris.
and. Et.
arm. Brachium. Gr., brachion.
artery. Arteria.
attachment. Adhesio.
back. Tergum; dorsum.
backbone. Spina.
backward. Retro.
bath. Balneum.
beef. Bubula.
belly. Venter; abdomen.
bend. Flexus.
bile. Bilis. Gr., chole.
bladder. Vesica.
bleed. Fluere.
blind. Obscurus.
blister. Pustulo; vesicatorium.
bloat. Tumeo.
blood. Sanguis. Gr., haima.
blood vessel. Vena.
body. Corpus. Gr., soma.
boiling up. Effervescens.
bone. Os. Gr., osteon.
bony. Osseus.
bowels. Intestina; viscera.
bowlegged. Valgus.
brain. Cerebrum. Gr., enkephalos.
breach. Ruptura.
breast. Mamma. Gr., mastos.
breath. Halitus.
bubble. Pustula.
bulb. Bulbus.
buttock. Clunis. Gr., gloutos.
calcareous. Calci similis.
canal. Canalis.
cartilage. Cartilago. Gr., chondros.
catarrh. Coryza.
cavity. Caverna.
change. Mutatio.
chest. Thorax. Gr., thorax.
chin. Mentum. Gr., geneion.
choke. Strangulo.
clavicle. Clavicula.
confinement. Puerperium.
congestion. Conglobatio.
consumption. Phthisis, pulmonaria.
convulsion. Convulsio.
cord. Corda.
corn. Callus-clavus.
cornea. Cornu. Gr., keras.
costive. Astrictus.
cough. Tussio.
countenance. Vultus.
cramp. Spasmus.
crisis. Dies crisimus.
cup. Poculum.
cure. Sano.
curvature. Curvatura.
cuticle. Cuticula.
daily. Diurnus.
dandruff. Furfures capitas.
day. Dies.
dead. Mortuus; defunctus.
deadly. Lethalis.
deafness. Surditas.
decompose. Dissolvo.
dental. Dentalis.
depression. Depressio.
digestive. Digestorius; pepticus.
dilute. Dilutus.
discharge. Eluvies; effluens.
disease. Morbus.
dorsal. Dorsalis.
dose. Potio.
dram. Drachma.
drink. Bibo; potis.
dropsy. Hydrops; opis.
drug. Medicamentum.
duct. Ductus.
dysentery. Dysenteria.
ear. Auris. Gr., ous.
eat. Edo. Gr., phagos.
egg. Ovum.
elbow. Cubitum. Gr., ankon.
embryo. Partus immaturus.
emission. Emissio.
entrails. Viscera.
epidemic. Epidemus.
epilepsy. Morbus comitalis; epilepsia.
epileptic. Epilepticus.
erection. Erectio.
erotic. Amatorius.
eunuch. Eunuchus.
every. Omnis.
excrement. Excrementum.
excretion. Excrementum; excretio.
exhalation. Exhalatio.
exhale. Exhalo.
expel. Expello.
expire. Expiro.
external. Externus.
extract. Extractum.
eye. Oculus. Gr., ophthalmos.
eyeball. Pupula.
eyebrow. Supercilium.
eyelid. Palpebra.
eyetooth. Dens caninus.
face. Facies.
faculty. Facultas.
faint. Collabor.
fat. Adeps. Gr., lipos.
feature. Lineomentum.
febrile. Febriculosus.
fecundity. Fecunditas.
feel. Tactus.
fever. Febris.
film. Membranula.
filter. Percolo.
finger. Digitus. Gr., daktylos.

fistula. Fistula putris.
fit. Accessus.
flesh. Carnis. Gr., sarx.
fluid. Fluidus.
food. Cibus.
foot. Pes, pedis. Gr., pous.
forearm. Brachium.
forehead. Frons.
freckle. Lentigo.
gall. Bilis.
gangrene. Gangraena.
gargle. Gargarizo.
gland. Glandula.
gleet. Ichor.
gout. Morbus articularis; (in feet) podagra.
grain. Granum.
gravel. Calculus.
grinder tooth. Dens maxillaris.
gullet. Gula.
gum. Gingiva.
gut. Intestinum.
hair. Capillus. Gr., thrix.
half. Dimidius.
hand. Manus. Gr., cheir.
harelip. Labrum fissum.
haunch. Clunis.
head. Caput. Gr., kephale.
heal. Sano.
healer. Medicus.
healing. Salutaris.
health. Sanitas.
healthful. Salutaris; saluber.
healthy. Sanus.
hear. Audio.
hearing. Auditio; (sense of) auditus.
heart. Cor. Gr., kardia.
heartburn. Redundatio stomachi.
heat. Calor.
hectic. Hecticus.
heel. Calx, talus.
hirsute. Hirsutus.
homeopathic. Homeopathicus.
hysterics. Hysteria.
illness. Morbus.
incisor. Dens acutus.
infant. Infans; puerilis.
infect. Inficio.
infectious. Contagiosus.
infirm. Infirmus; debilis.
inflammation. Inflammatio; (of lungs) inflammatio pulmonaria.
injection. Injectio.
insane. Insanus.
intellect. Intellectus.
intercourse. Congressus.
internal. Intestinus.
intestine. Intestinum. Gr., enteron.
itch. Scabies.
itching. Pruritus.
jaw. Maxilla.
joint. Artus. Gr., arthron.
jugular vein. Vena jugularis.
kidney. Ren. Gr., nephros.
knee. Genu. Gr., gonu.
kneepan. Patella.
knuckle. Condylus.
labor. Partus.
labyrinth. Labyrinthus.
lacerate. Lacero.
larynx. Guttur.
lateral. Lateralis.
leech. Sanguisuga.
leg. Tibia.
leprosy. Leprosus.
ligament. Ligamentum. Gr., syndesmos.
ligature. Ligatura.
limb. Membrum.
lime. Calx.
listen. Ausculto.
liver. Jecur. Gr., hepar.
livid. Lividus.
loin. Lumbus. Gr., lapara.
looseness. Laxitas.
lotion. Lotio.
lukewarm. Tepidus.
lung. Pulmo. Gr., pneumon.
lymph. Lympha.
mad. Insanus.
malady. Morbus.
male. Masculinus.
malignant. Malignus.
maternity. Conditio matris.
medicated. Medicatus.
medicine. (Remedy) Medicamentum.
milk. Lac.
mind. Animus.
mix. Misceo.
mixture. Mistura.
moist. Humidus.
molar. Dens molaris.
month. Mensis.
monthly. Menstruus.
morbid. Morbidus.
mouth. Os. Gr., stoma.
mucous. Mucosus.
muscle. Musculus. Gr., mys.
mustard. Sinapis.
nail. Unguis.
navel. Umbilicus. Gr., omphalos.
neck. Cervix; collum. Gr., trachelos.
nerve. Nervus. Gr., neuron.
nipple. Papilla.
no, none. Nullus.
normal. Normalis.
nose. Nasus. Gr., rhis.
nostril. Naris.
not. Non.
nourish. Nutrio.
nourishment. Alimentus.
now. Nunc.

nudity. Nudatio.
nurse. Nutrix.
obesity. Obesitas.
ocular. Ocularis.
oculist. Ocularis medicus.
oil. Oleum.
ointment. Unguentum.
operator. Manus curatio.
opiate. Medicamentum somnificum.
optics. Optice.
orifice. Foramen.
pain. Dolor.
palate. Palatum.
palm. Palma.
parasite. Parasitus.
part. Pars.
patient. Patiens.
pectoral. Pectoralis.
pedal. Pedale.
phlegm. Pituita.
pill. Pilus.
pimple. Pustula.
plaster. Emplastrum.
poison. Venenum.
poultice. Cataplasma.
powder. Pulvis.
pregnant. Gravida.
prepare. Paro.
prescribe. Praescribo.
prescription. Praescriptum.
puberty. Pubertas.
pubic bone. Os pubis. Gr., pecten.
pulverize. Pulvero.
pupil. Pupilla.
purgative. Purgativus.
putrid. Putridus.
quinsy. Cynanche; angina.
rash. Exanthema.
recover. Convalesco.
recumbent. Recumbens.
recur. Recurro.
redness. Rubor.
remedy. Remedium.
respiration. Respiratio.
rheum. Fluxio.
rib. Costa.
rigid. Rigidus.
ringing. Tinnitus.
rupture. Hernia.
saliva. Sputum.
sallow. Salix.
salt. Sal.
salve. Unguentum.
sane. Sanus.
scab. Scabies.
scalp. Pericranium.
scaly. Squamosus.
scar. Cicatrix.
sciatica. Ischias.
scruple. Scrupulum.
seed. Semen.
senile. Senilis.
serum. Sanguinis pars equosa.
sheath. Vagina.
shin. Tibia.
shock. Concussio; (of electricity) ictus electricus.
short. Brevis.
shoulder. Humerus. Gr., omos.
shoulder blade. Scapula.
shudder. Tremor.
sick. Aegrotus.
side. Latus.
sinew. Nervus.
skeleton. Gr., skeleton.
skin. Cutis. Gr., derma.
skull. Cranium. Gr., kranion.
sleep. Somnus.
smallpox. Variola.
smell. Odoratus.
soap. Sapo.
socket. Cavum.
soft. Mollis.
solid. Solidus.
solution. Dilutum.
soporific. Soporus.
sore. Ulcus.
spasm. Spasmus.
spinal. Dorsalis; spinalis.
spine. Spina.
spirit. Spiritus.
spittle. Sputum.
spleen. Lien.
spoon. Cochleare.
sprain. Luxatio.
stomach. Stomachus. Gr., gaster.
stone. Calculus.
stricture. Strictura.
sugar. Saccharum.
suture. Sutura.
swallow. Glutio.
sweat. Sudor. Gr., hidros.
symptom. Symptoma.
system. Systema.
tail. Cauda.
take. Sumo.
tapeworm. Taenia.
taste. Gustatus.
tear. Lacrima.
teeth. Dentes.
tendon. Tendo. Gr., tenon.
testicle. Testis. Gr., orchis.
thigh. Femur.
throat. Fauces. Gr., pharynx.
throb. Palpito.
thumb. Pollex.
tongue. Lingua. Gr., glossa.
tonsil. Tonsilla.
tooth. Dens. Gr., odous.
troche. Trochiscus.

tube. Tuba.
twin. Geminus.
twitching. Subsultus.
ulcer. Ulcus.
unless. Nisi.
urine. Urina.
uterine. Uterinus.
vaccine. Vaccinum.
vagina. Vagina. Gr., kolpos.
valve. Valvula.
vein. Vena. Gr., phleps.
vertebra. Vertebra. Gr., spondylos.
vessel. Vas.
wash. Lavo.
water. Aqua.
wax. Cera.
waxed dressing. Ceratum.
weary. Lassus.
wet. Humidus.
windpipe. Arteria aspera.
wine. Vinum.
woman. Femina.
womb. Uterus. Gr., hystera.
worm. Vermis.
wound. Vulnus.
wrist. Carpus. Gr., karpos.
yolk. Luteum.

COLORS

black. Niger; nigra; nigrum.
blue. Caeruleus; cyaneus; lividus.
brown. Fulvus.
crimson. Coccum; coccineus.
gray. Cinereus.
green. Viridis.
lemon. Citreum.
pink. Rosaceus.
purple. Purpura; purpureus.
red. Ruber.
scarlet. Coccineus.
violet. Violaceus.
white. Albus.
yellow. Flavus; luteus; croceus.

QUALITIES

bitter. Acerbus.
chill. Friguscolum.
cold. Frigidus.
dry. Aridus.
dull. Stupidus; hebes.
faintness. Languor.
fat. Obesus; pinguis.
heat. Calor; ardor; fervor.
short. Brevis.
sour. Acidus.
sweet. Dulcis.
tall. Longus; celsus; procerus.
thick. Densus.
heavy. Gravis; ponderosus.
hot. Calidus; fervens; candens.
light. Levis.
liquid. Liquidus.
moist. Humidus; uvidus.
sharp. Acutus.
thin. Tenuis; macer.
warm. Calidus.
warmth. Calor.
weary. Lassus; languidus; fatigatus.
wet. Humidus.

METALS

copper. Cuprum; cuprinus.
gold. Aurum; aureus.
iron. Ferrum; ferreus.
silver. Argentum; argenteus.
tin. Stannum; plumbum album.

TIME

afternoon. Post meridiem.
age. Aetas; maturas; adultus; impubis.
autumn. Autumnus.
birth. Partus; natales.
breakfast. Prandium.
child. Infans; puer; filius.
daily. Diurnus.
date. Status dies.
dawn. Prima lux.
day. Dies.
death. Mors.
dinner. Cena.
evening. Vesper.
hour. Hora.
infant. Infans.
maturity. Maturitas; aetas matura.
meal. Epulae.
midnight. Media nox.
midsummer. Media aestas.
moment. Punctum.
month. Mens.
monthly. Menstruus.
morning. Matutinum.
night. Nox, noctis.
noon. Meridies.
old. Antiquus.
puberty. Pubertas.
second. Secundum.
spring. Ver; veris.
summer. Aestas.
sunrise. Solis ortus.
sunset. Solis occasus.
supper. Cena.
time. Tempus.
winter. Hiems, hiemis.
year. Annus.
young. Parvus; infans.
youth. Adolescentia.

NUMERALS (ROMAN)

SEE: *Roman Numerals* in *Appendix*.

Glossary of Latin Medical Words

Latin words which have become a part of the general medical vocabulary are listed in alphabetical order in the text.

abacus, -ī. *m.* Shelf.
abdōminālis, -e. Abdominal.
abdūcēns, -ntis. Leading or drawing from (the median line); applied also to 6th pair of cranial nerves.
aberrāns, -ntis. Wandering.
abstractum, -ī. *n.* Abstract.
accessōrius, -a, -um. Accessory.
accidō, -ere, -cidī. Occur; happen.
ācer, ācris, ācre. Sharp; severe.
acervulus, -ī. *m.* (Lit., little heap), acervulus.
acētābulum, -ī. *n.* (Lit., vinegar cup), the bony cuplike cavity of the hip joint; acetabulum.
acētās, -ātis. *m.* Acetate.
acētum, -ī. *n.* Vinegar.
acidum, -ī. *n.* Acid.
acinus, -ī. *m.* A terminal compartment or secreting portion of a gland; acinus.
acusticus, -a, -um. Auditory.
acūtus, -a, -um. Acute.
adeps, adipis. *m.* and *f.* Fat; lard.
adjūtor, -ōris. *m.* Helper; assistant.
adjuvō, -āre, -jūvī, -jūtus. Aid; assist.
adsum, -esse, -fuī. Be present.
aeger, -gra, -grum. Sick.
aegrōtus, -a, -um. Sick.
āēr, āēris. *m.* Air.
aeternus, -a, -um. Eternal.
aether, -is. *m.* Ether.
āla, -ae. *f.* Wing.
ālāris, -e. Winglike; alar.
albicāns, -ntis. Whitening; white.
albūgineus, -a, -um. White.
albulus, -a, -um. Whitish.
albus, -a, -um. White.
alcoholicus, -a, -um. Alcoholic.
aliquandō. Sometimes.
alius, -a, -ud. Other.
aloina, -ae. *f.* Aloin.
alter, -tera, -terum. Other.
altus, -a, -um. High.
alūmen, -inis. *n.* Alum.
alvus, -ī. *f.* Belly, or its contents.
amārus, -a, -um. Bitter.
amīcus, -ī. *m.* Friend.
āmissiō, -ōnis. *f.* Loss.
āmissus, -ūs. *m.* Loss.
ammōnium, -ī. *n.* Ammonium.
amygdala, -ae. *f.* Almond.
anaestheticus, -a, -um. Producing insensibility; anesthetic.
anastomoticus, -a, -um. Anastomosing.
ānellus, -ī. *m.* Ring.
angulus, -ī. *m.* Angle.
anima, -ae. *f.* Breath; life.
anīsum, -ī. *n.* Anise.
ānnulāris, -e. Ringlike; annular.
ānnulus, -ī. *m.* Ring.
anterius, -a, -um. Anterior.
antīcus, -a, -um. Foremost.
antidōtum, -ī. *n.* Antidote.
antimōniālis, -e. Of antimony; antimonial.
antimōnium, -ī. *n.* Antimony.
antipyreticus, -a, -um. Reducing the temperature; antipyretic.
antisepticus, -a, -um. Destroying germ life; antiseptic.
antitrāgus, -ī. *m.* A conical eminence opposite the tragus, q.v.; antitragus.
antīquus, -a, -um. Ancient.
aperiēns, -ntis. Laying open; laxative; aperient.
appellō, -āre, -āvī, -ātus. Call.
aptē. Aptly.
apud. Near.
aqua, -ae. *f.* Water.
aqueductus, -ūs. *m.* A canal; aqueduct.
aquōsus, -a, -um. Watery.
arbor, -oris. *f.* Tree.
arceō, -ēre, -uī, -tus. Ward off.
arcuātus, -a, -um. Curved like a bow.
arcus, -ūs. *m.* A bow; arch.
āreola, -ae. *f.* Small area, especially around the nipple.
argentum, -ī. *n.* Silver.
arōmaticus, -a, -um. Aromatic.
arsenicum, -ī. *n.* Arsenic.
arsenis, -itis. *m.* Arsenite.
artēria, -ae. *f.* Artery.
articutāris, -e. Articular.
articulō, -āre, -āvī, -ātus. Articulate.
artus, -ūs. *m.* Joint.
ascendēns, -ntis. Ascending.
asepticus, -a, -um. Free from putrefactive matter; aseptic.
asper, -a, -um. Rough.
astrictus, -a, -um. Bound up.
astūtus, -a, -um. Shrewd; artful.
atropīna, -ae. *f.* Active principle of belladonna; atropine.
attollēns, -ntis. Raising up; elevating.
attrāhēns, -ntis. Drawing to or towards.
audītōrius, -a, -um. Auditory.
aurantium, -ī. *n.* Orange.
auricula, -ae. *f.* Auricle.
auris, -is. *f.* Ear.
axis, -is. *m.* (Lit., that about which a body turns), 2nd cervical vertebra; axis.
balneum, -ī. *n.* Bath.
basīlāris, -e. Basilar.
basis, -is. *f.* Base.
bene. Well.
benignus, -a, -um. Mild; benign; not malignant.
berberis, -idis. *f.* Barberry.

bibō, -ere, bibī. Drink.
bicarbonās, -ātis. *m.* Bicarbonate.
biceps, -cipitis. Two-headed.
bifidus, -a, -um. Cleft.
biliaris, -e. Pert. to or conveying bile; bilary.
bīnī, -ae, -a. Two each.
bismuthum, -ī. *n.* Bismuth.
bitartrās, -ātis. *m.* Bitartrate.
bonus, -a, -um. Good.
borās, -ātis. *m.* Borate.
brachiālis, -e. Of the arm; brachial.
brāchium, -ī. *n.* Arm.
brevis, -e. Short.
brōmidum, -ī. *n.* Bromide.
būbula, -ae. *f.* Beef.
būccinātor, -ōris. *m.* The trumpeter muscle; buccinator.
bulbus, -ī. *m.* Bulb.
caecus, -a, -um. Blind.
calamus, -ī. *m.* Reed.
calcaneum, -ī. *n.* The heelbone (os calcis).
calcium, -ī. *n.* Calcium.
calidus, -a, -um. Hot.
callōsus, -a, -um. Hard, tough.
calor, -ōris. *m.* Heat.
calumba, -ae. *f.* Calumba.
calvārium, -ī. *n.* The skullcap.
calx, -cis. *f.* Lime.
calyx, -icis. *f.* Cup; calyx.
camphora, -ae. *f.* Camphor.
camphorātus, -a, -um. Camphorated.
canāliculus, -ī. *m.* Small duct or canal.
canālis, -is. *m.* Canal.
canīnus, -a, -um. Of a dog, canine.
canis, -is. *m.* and *f.* Dog.
cānitiēs, -ēī. *f.* A gray color, hoariness.
cannabis, -is. *f.* Hemp.
cantharis, -idis. *f.* Spanish fly.
canthus, -ī. *m.* The corner or angle of the eye.
capiō, -ere, cēpī, captus. Take.
capitulum, -ī. *n.* A knob or protuberance of bone received into a concavity of another bone.
capsicum, -ī. *n.* Cayenne pepper; capsicum.
capsula, -ae. *f.* A small box; capsule.
carbō, -ōnis. *m.* Carbon; coal; charcoal.
carbolicus, -a, -um. Carbolic.
carbonās, -ātis. *m.* Carbonate.
cardamōmum, -ī. *n.* Cardamom.
careō, -ēre, -uī, -itus. Need; want.
carneus, -a, -um. Fleshy.
carpus, -ī. *m.* Wrist.
cartilāginōsus, -a, -um. Cartilaginous.
cartilāgo, -inis. *f.* Cartilage.
caruncula, -ae. *f.* A little piece of flesh; caruncle.
cataplasma, -atis. *n.* Poultice; cataplasm.
catharticus, -a, -um. Cathartic.
cauda, -ae. *f.* Tail.
caudātus, -a, -um. Having a tail; caudate.
causa, -ae. *f.* Cause.
causō, -āre, -āvī, -ātus. Cause.
cavernōsus, -a, -um. Hollow; cavernous.
cavitās, -ātis. *f.* Cavity.
cavus, -a, -um. Hollow.
celeriter. Quickly.
centrālis, -e. Central.
centrum, -ī. *n.* Center.
cephalalgia, -ae. *f.* Headache.
cērātum, -ī. *n.* Waxed dressing; cerate.
cerātus, -a, -um. Waxed.
cerevisa, -ae. *f.* Beer.
certus, -a, -um. Sure; certain.
cēterus, -a, -um. Other.
charta, -ae. *f.* Medicated paper.
chartula, -ae. *f.* Small paper (powder).
chirāta, -ae. *f.* Chirata.
chīrurgia, -ae. *f.* Surgery.
chīrurgus, -ī. *m.* Surgeon.
chlōral. *n.* Chloral.
chlōrās, -ātis. *m.* Chlorate.
chlōridum, -ī. *n.* Chloride.
chlōrōformum, -ī. *n.* Chloroform.
choledochus, -ī. *m.* Holding or receiving bile.
chorda, -ae. *f.* Cord.
chronicus, -a, -um. Chronic.
chylum, -ī. *n.* Chyle.
cibus, -ī. *m.* Food.
cicātrōsus, -a, -um. Full of scars, scarred.
ciliāris, -e. Ciliary.
cinchōna, -ae. *f.* Cinchona.
cinchonīna, -ae. *f.* Cinchonine.
cinereus, -a, -um. Ash-colored.
cinnamōmum, -ī. *n.* Cinnamon.
circulāris, -e. Circular.
circulatiō, -ōnis. *f.* Circulation.
circulus, -ī. *m.* Circle.
circum. Around.
circumdō, -dare, -dedī, -datus. Surround.
citō. Promptly; quickly.
citrās, -ātis. *m.* Citrate.
clārus, -a, -um. Clear, distinguished.
claudus, -a, -um. Lame.
clāvus, -ī. *m.* A corn, usually on the toes.
cludō, -ere, -sī, -sus. Shut; close.
cochlea, -ae. *f.* (Lit., snail shell), spiral cavity of the internal ear; cochlea.
cochleāre, -is. *n.* Spoon.
codeina, -ae. *f.* An alkaloid of opium; codeine.
coeliacus, -a, -um. Relating to the stomach; celiac.
colicus, -a, -um. Of or pert. to the colon.
collateriālis, -e. Collateral.
collum, -ī. *n.* Neck.
colocynthis, -idis. *f.* Colocynth.
color, -ōris. *m.* Color.
cōlum, -ī. *n.* Large intestine; colon.
columna, -ae. *f.* Column.
comes, -itis. *m.* Companion.
commissūra, -as. *f.* A joining; commissure.
communicāns, -ntis. Communicating.

commūnis, -e. Common.
compōnō, -ere, -posuī, -positus. Compound.
conarium, -ī. *n.* A synonym for the pineal gland; conarium.
concha, -ae. *f.* (Lit., a shell), hollow part of the external ear; concha.
confectiō, -ōnis. *f.* Confection.
conium, -ī. *n.* Poison, hemlock; conium.
conīveō, -āre, -nīvī. Blink; half close.
conjectūra, -ae. *f.* Guess.
contineō, -ēre, -tinuī, -tentus. Contain.
contrāhō, -ere, -xī, -ctus. Draw together; contract.
contusiō, -ōnis. *f.* Bruise.
cōnus, -ūs. *m.* Cone.
convalescō, -ere, -valuī. Regain health.
cor, cordis. *n.* Heart.
cornicula, -ae. *f.* Little horn.
cornu, -ūs. *n.* Horn; horn-shaped process.
corōna, -ae. *f.* Crown.
coronārius, -a, -um. Encircling like a crown; coronary.
corpus, -oris. *n.* Body.
corrōsīvus, -a, -um. Corrosive.
corrugātor, -ōris. *m.* A muscle which wrinkles; corrugator.
cortex, -icis. *m.* and *f.* Bark; rind; external layer; cortex.
costa, -ae. *f.* Rib.
craniālis, -e. Cranial.
crās. Tomorrow.
crassus, -a, -um. Gross; large.
creasōtum, -ī. *n.* Creasote.
crēber, -bra, -brum. Frequent.
crēdō, -ere, -credidī, -creditus. Trust; believe.
crēta, -ae. *f.* Chalk.
cribriformis, -e. Sievelike; cribriform.
cribrōsus, -a, -um. Having holes like a sieve.
crista, -ae. *f.* Crest; comb of a cock (gallus).
crūrālis, -e. Of the leg; crural.
crūreus, -a, -um. Of the leg.
crūs, crūris. *n.* The leg.
crusta, -ae. *f.* Crust.
cubēba, -ae. *f.* Cubeb.
cubitum, -ī. *n.* Elbow.
cuboideus, -a, -um. Cubelike; cuboid.
cum. With.
cuneiformis, -e. Wedge-shaped; cuneiform.
cūra, -ae. *f.* Care.
cūrō, -āre, -āvī, -ātus. Treat; cure.
cutis, -is. *f.* Skin.
decem. Ten.
deciduus, -a, -um. That which falls off.
decoctum, -ī. *n.* Decoction.
deferēns, -ntis. Bearing away.
defessus, -a, -um. Tired; wearied.
deformāns, -ntis. Deforming.
deformitās, -ātis. *f.* Deformity.
demonstrō, -āre, -āvī, -ātus. Show; prove.
dēns, dentis. *m.* Tooth.
dentātus, -a, -um. Toothed; dentate.
depressor, -ōris. *m.* That which depresses; depressor.
descendēns, -ntis. Descending.
dexter, -tra, -trum. Right.
diabeticus, -a, -um. Diabetic; one having diabetes.
diabolus, -ī. *m.* Devil.
dīcō, -ere, -dixī, dictus. Say.
diēs, -ēī. *m.* Day.
difficilis, -e. Difficult.
digitus, -ī. *m.* Finger.
digitus pedis. A toe.
dilātor, -ōris. *m.* That which dilates; dilator.
dilūtus, -a, -um. Dilute.
dimidius, -a, -um. Half.
discipulus, -ī. *m.* A learner; pupil; student.
diū. For a long time.
diureticus, -a, -um. Diuretic.
dividō, -ere, -vīsī, -vīsus. Divide.
dō, dare, dedī, datus. Give.
doctus, -a, -um. Learned.
dolōr, -ōris. *m.* Pain.
dolōrōsus, -a, -um. Painful.
domicilium, -ī. *n.* Abode.
dorsālis, -e. Of the back; dorsal.
dorsum, -ī. *n.* Back.
dosis, -is. *f.* Dose.
drachma, -ae. *f.* Dram.
dustus, -ūs. *m.* Duct.
dulcis, -e. Sweet.
duo, duae, du. Two.
dūrus, -a, -um. Hard.
dyspepticus, -a, -um. Dyspeptic; a dyspeptic.
edō, -ere, -ēdi, -ēsus. Eat.
efferēns, -ntis. Bearing out or away; efferent.
effervescēns, -ntis. Boiling up.
elegāns, -ntis. Elegant.
ēluviēs, -ēī. *f.* Discharge.
emeticus, -a, -um. Causing vomiting; emetic.
ēminentia, -ae. *f.* Eminence.
emō, -ere, -ēmī, emptus. Buy.
empiricus, -ī. *n.* Quack; empiric.
emplastrum, -ī. *n.* Plaster.
ensiformis, -e. Sword-shaped; ensiform.
eō, īre, īvī, itus. Go.
epilepsia, -ae. *f.* Epilepsy.
epiploicus, -a, -um. Relating to the epiploön (omentum).
equīnus, -a, -um. Of a horse; equine.
ergota, -ae. *f.* Ergot.
errō, -āre, -āvī, -ātus. Wander; err.
ērudītus, -a, -um. Learned; educated; erudite.
et. And.
et-et. Both-and.
ethmoidālis, -e. Ethmoid
etiam. Even.
euonymus, -ī. *m.* Wahoo; Euonymus.
eupatōrium, -ī. *n.* Boneset; eupatorium.
excessus, -ūs. *m.* Departure.

excīdō, -ere, -īdī, -īsus. Cut out; excise.
excitō, -āre, -āvī, -ātus. Excite.
expectatiō, -ōnis. *f.* Expectation.
experimentum, -ī. *n.* Experiment.
expressiō, -ōnis. *f.* Expression.
exsiccātus, -a, -um. Dried out.
exsudō, -āre, -āvī, -ātus. Sweat out; exude.
externus, -a, -um. External.
extractum, -ī. *n.* Extract.
faciēs, -ēī. *f.* Face; countenance.
faciō, -ere, fēcī, factus. Make.
falx, -cis. *f.* Sickle (a sickle-shaped process).
familia, -ae (or **as**). *f.* Family.
fasciculus, -ī. *m.* A small bundle of fibers.
febrifuga, -ae. *f.* Agent that reduces fever; febrifuge.
febris, -is. *f.* Fever.
fēmina, -ae. *f.* Woman.
femorālis, -e. Of the thigh; femoral.
fenestra, -ae. *f.* Window; an opening in the wall of the tympanum.
ferē. Almost.
ferrum, -ī. *n.* Iron.
fibrilla, -ae. *f.* Filament; fibril.
fibrōsus, -a, -um. Fibrous.
fides, -eī. *f.* Faith; trustworthiness.
fīdus, -a, -um. Faithful; trustworthy.
filia, -ae. *f.* Daughter.
filius, -ī. *m.* Son.
filix, -icis. *f.* Fern.
fimbria, -ae. *f.* fringe.
fimbriātus, -a, -um. Fringed; fimbriated.
finiō, -īre, -īvī, -ītus. End; finish.
fiō, fierī, factus. Be made.
fissūra, -ae. *f.* Cleft; fissure.
flavus, -a, -um. Yellow.
flexilis, -e. Flexible.
flōs, flōris. *m.* Flower.
fluidus, -a, -um. Fluid.
flūmen, inis. *n.* River.
fluō, -ere, fluxī, fluxus. Flow.
fluor, -ōris. *m.* Flux; flow.
foetidus, -a, -um. Offensive, fetid.
folium, -ī. *n.* Leaf.
folliculus, -ī. *m.* A small secretory sac; follicle.
fons, -ntis, *m.* Fountain; spring.
formō, -āre, -āvī, -ātus. Form.
fornicātus, -a, -um. Arched.
fornix, -icis. *m.* Arch; vault; fornix.
fortis, -e. Strong; brave.
fossa, -ae. *f.* Ditch; depression; fossa.
fovea, -ae. *f.* Small pit; depression.
fractus, -a, -um. Broken.
fragilitās, -ātis. *f.* Brittleness.
frēnum, -ī. *n.* A bridle; a membranous fold; frenum.
frigidus, -a, -um. Cold.
fructus, -ūs. *m.* Fruit.
frumentum, -ī. *n.* Corn; grain.
frustum, -ī. *n.* Piece; bit.
functiō, -ōnis. *f.* Execution; normal action; function.
fuscus, -a, -um. Brown.
fūsiformis, -e. Spindle-shaped; fusiform.
gallus, -ī. *m.* Cock.
ganglioniformis, -e. Ganglionlike.
gelsemium, -ī. *n.* Gelsemium; yellow jasmine (root).
gemellus, -a, -um. Paired; twin.
gena, -ae. *f.* The cheek.
geniōhyoglossus, -ī. *m.* Muscle attached to chin, hyoid bone and tongue.
gentiāna, -ae. *f.* Gentian.
genu, -ūs. *n.* Knee.
genus, generis, *n.* Kind.
germinātīvus, -a, -um. Germinative; germinal.
glabrus, -a, -um. Smooth.
glaciēs, -ēī. *f.* Ice.
globus, -ī. *m.* Globe.
glomerulus, -ī. *m.* Small ball or tuft of vessels; glomerule.
glūteus, -a, -um. Of the buttock; gluteal.
glycerīnum, -ī. *n.* Glycerin.
glycerītum, -ī. *m.* Glycerite.
glycyrrhiza, -ae. *f.* Licorice.
gracilis, -e. Slender; graceful.
granulōsus, -a, -um. Granular.
granum, -ī. *n.* Grain.
gratus, -a, -um. Agreeable; pleasing.
gubernāculum, -ī. *n.* (Lit., a helm), applied to fetal cord directing descent of testes; gubernaculum.
gummi. Gum.
gustō, -āre, -āvī, -ātus. Taste.
gutta, -ae. *f.* Drop.
gyrus, -ī. *m.* Circle; ring; convolution (of the brain).
habeō, -ēre, -uī, -itus. Have.
habitō, -āre, -āvī, -ātus. Inhabit.
hallex, -icis, or **hallux, -ucis.** *f.* The great toe.
harmonia, -ae. *f.* Harmony, "suture of harmony."
helix, -icis. *f.* Outer ring of the external ear; helix.
hemisphericus, -a, -um. Hemispherical.
hēpar, hepatis. *n.* Liver.
herba, -ae. *f.* Herb.
herī. Yesterday.
hiātus, -ūs. *m.* Opening; aperture.
hīc, haec, hoc. This.
hilāris, -e. Cheerful.
hīlus, -ī. *m.* Small fissure or depression.
hippocampus, -ī. *m.* (Lit., sea horse), applied to two convolutions of brain (major and minor); hippocampus.
homo, -inis. *m.* Man.
horribilis, -e. Horrible.
humānus, -a, -um. Human.
hūmor, -ōris. *m.* Fluid; humor.
hydrargyrum, -ī. *n.* Mercury.

hydrastis, -is. *f.* Golden seal (root); hydrastis.
hyoideus, -a, -um. Hyoid.
Hyoscyamus, -ī. *m.* Henbane; Hyoscyamus.
īdem, eadem, idem. Same.
ignārus, -a, -um. Ignorant.
iliacus, -a, -um. Of or pert. to the flanks or ilium; iliac.
ille, illa, illud. He; she; it.
immōbilis, -e. Immovable.
immōbilitas, -ātis. *f.* Immobility.
impar, -is. Without a mate or fellow.
impediō, -īre, -īvī, -ītus. Hinder; check; prevent.
imperītus, -a, -um. Unskilled.
impūrus, -a, -um. Impure.
īmus, -a, -um. Lowest.
incisūra, -ae. *f.* Groove or notch.
Indicus, -a, -um. Indian.
infans, -ntis. *m.* and *f.* Infant.
inflammatiō, -ōnis. *f.* Inflammation.
infraspinātus, -a, -um. Beneath the spine (of the scapula); infraspinate.
infūsum, -ī. *m.* Infusion.
ingressus, -ūs. *m.* Entrance.
innominātus, -a, -um. Unnamed; innominate.
intermittō, -ere, -mīsī, -missus. Intermit.
internōdium, -ī. *n.* Space between two joints; internode.
internus, -a, -um. Inner.
interpositus, -a, -um. Placed between.
intertragicus, -a, -um. Between the tragus, q.v., and antitragus.
intestīnum, -ī. *n.* Intestine.
intumescentia, -ae. *f.* An enlargement; intumescence.
inveniō, -īre, -vēnī, -ventus. Find; discover.
inversiō, -ōnis. *f.* Inversion.
iodidum, -ī. *n.* Iodide.
ipecacuanha, -ae. *f.* Ipecac.
ipse, ipsa, ipsum. Himself; herself; itself.
iris, iridis. *f.* Iris.
is, ea, id. He; she; it.
iter, itineris. *n.* Way; passageway.
jecur, jecinoris. *n.* Liver.
jūcundē. Happily; pleasantly.
jūglans, juglandis. *f.* Walnut.
juguláris, -e. Jugular.
jūniperus, -ī. *f.* Juniper tree.
juvenis. *m.* and *f.*, *adj.*, and *subst.* Young; a youth.
labium, -ī. *n.* Lip.
lacer, -a, -um. Lacerated; mutilated.
lacrima, -ae. *f.* Tear.
lacrimālis, -e. Pert. to tears; lacrimal.
lactās, -ātis. *m.* A salt of lactic acid; lactate.
lactiferus, -a, -um. Milk-bearing; lactiferous.
lacus, -ūs. *m.* Lake; basin; reservoir.
lamella, -ae. *f.* Layer.
lamina, -ae. *f.* Thin plate; layer.
lāna, -ae. *f.* Wool.
lassus, -a, -um. Weary.
laterālis, -e. Lateral.
lātus, -a, -um. Broad.
laudō, -āre, -āvī, -ātus. Praise.
lavandula, -ae. *f.* Lavender.
lavō, -āre, -āvī, -ātus or **lavi, lautus.** Wash.
laxātor, -ōris. *m.* A muscle that loosens; relaxer.
legō, -ere, -lēgī, lectus. Bring together; collect.
leniō, -īre, -īvī, -ītus. Calm; soothe; assuage.
lenticulāris, -e. Lentil-shaped (double-convex); lenticular.
lentus, -a, -um. Sticky.
letifer, -a, -um. Deadly.
levis, -e. Light.
lienālis, -e. Of the spleen.
ligamentōsus, -a, -um. Ligamentous.
ligamentum, -ī. *n.* Ligament.
lignum, -ī. *n.* Wood.
limbus, -ī. *n.* Border; band; fringe.
līmitāns, -ntis. Limiting.
limon, -ōnis. *f.* Lemon.
linea, -ae. *f.* Line.
lingua, -ae. *f.* Tongue.
linguālis, -e. Of the tongue; lingual.
linimentum, -ī. *n.* Liniment.
linum, -ī. *n.* Flax.
liquidus, -a, -um. Liquid.
lobulus, -ī. *m.* Lobule.
lobus, -ī. *m.* Lobe.
longitudinālis, -e. Longitudinal.
longus, -a, -um. Long.
lotiō, -ōnis. *f.* Wash; lotion.
lucidus, -a, -um. Clear; transparent.
lumbālis, -e. Of the loins; lumbar.
lumbus, -ī. *m.* Loin.
lūnula, -ae. *f.* Small crescent; lunula.
lupulīna, -ae. *f.* Yellow powder from the scales of the hop; lupulin.
luteus, -a, -um. Yellow.
luxatiō, -ōnis. *f.* Dislocation.
lympha, -ae. *f.* Chyle; lymph.
mācerō, -āre, -āvī, ātus. Soak; macerate.
magister, -trī. *m.* Teacher; master.
magnus, -a, -um. Large; great.
māla, -ae. *f.* The cheekbone.
malignus, -a, -um. Malignant.
malus, -a, -um. Bad.
mandibulum, -ī. *n.* A jaw.
māne. *n.* Morning.
manūbrium, -ī. *n.* (Lit., a handle, hilt), upper part of sternum; manubrium.
manus, -ūs. *f.* Hand.
massa, -ae. *f.* Mass.
masticō, -āre, -āvī, -ātus. Chew.
mastoideus, -a, -um. Nipplelike; mastoid.
mater, -tris. *f.* Mother.
māteria, -ae. *f.* Materials.
māternus, -a, -um. Maternal.
matrix, -īcis. *f.* Source; origin.
maxilla, -ae. *f.* Jawbone; jaw.

meātus, -ūs. *m.* Opening; passage.
mediānus, -a, -um. Middle; median.
medicāmen, -inis. *n.* Drug.
medicāmentārius, -a, -um. Medicated.
medicāmentum, -ī. *n.* Drug.
medicātus, -a, -um. Medicated.
medicīna, -ae. *f.* Medicine.
medicus, -ī. *m.* Physician; doctor.
medius, -a, -um. Middle.
membrāna, -ae. *f.* Membrane.
membrum, -ī. *n.* Member.
memoria, -ae. *f.* Memory.
mentha, -ae. *f.* Mint.
mentum, -ī. *n.* Chin.
mesentericus, -a, -um. Of the mesentery; mesenteric.
metus, -ūs. *m.* Fear.
mīles, -itis. *m.* Soldier.
minerālis, -e. Mineral.
misceō, -ēre, miscuī, mixtus. Mix.
miser, -a, -um. Poor; wretched.
mistūra, -ae. *f.* Mixture.
mītis, -e. Mild.
mitto, -ere, mīsī, missus. Send.
mobilis, -e. Movable.
mobilitās, -ātis. *f.* Mobility.
modiolus, -ī. *m.* (Lit., a small measure), hollow cone in the cochlea of the ear, modiolus.
molāris, -e (mola, mill). The grinder teeth; molar.
molliō, -īre, -īvī, -ītus. Soften; mitigate.
mollis, -e. Soft.
mollitīes, -ēī. *f.* Softness.
mons, -ntis. *m.* Mountain.
montānus, -a, -um. Of a mountain; mountain.
monticulus, -ī. *m.* Small eminence.
morbus, -ī *m.* Disease.
mordeō, -ēre, momordī, morsus. Bite.
moritūrus, -a, -um. About to die.
morphīna, -ae. *f.* Morphine.
morrhua, -ae. *f.* A genus of fishes, including the cod; cod.
mors, mortis. *f.* Death.
morsus, -ūs. *m.* Bite.
mortarium, -ī. *n.* Mortar.
mōtor, -ōris. *m.* That which moves; mover.
moveō, -ēre, mōvī, mōtus. Move.
mox. Presently; soon; directly.
mucilāgō, -inis. *f.* Mucilage.
mucōsus, -a, -um. Mucous.
mulceō, -ere, mulsi, mulsus. Soothe; allay.
multifidus, -a, -um. Many-clefted.
multus, -a, -um. Much; many.
muriāticus, -a, -um. Muriatic.
musculus, -ī. *m.* Muscle.
mūtātiō, -ōnis. *f.* Change.
myristica, -ae. *f.* Nutmeg.
myrtiformis, -e. Shaped like the myrtle leaf or berry; myrtiform.
nāris, -is. *f.* Nostril.
nāsus, -ī. *m.* Nose.
natō, -āre, -āvī, -ātus. Swim; float.
natūra, -ae. *f.* Nature.
nauta, -ae. *m.* Sailor.
naviculāris, -e. Boat-shaped; navicular.
neglectus, -a, -um. Neglected.
nemō, -inis. *m.* and *f.* No one.
nervus, -ī. *m.* Nerve.
nescio, -īre, -īvi, -ītus. Not know; be ignorant of.
neurilemma, -atis. *n.* Nerve sheath.
nictitāns, -ntis. Winking.
nil. Nothing.
nimium. Too often.
nisi. Unless.
nitrās, -ātis. *m.* Nitrate.
nitricus, -a, -um. Nitric.
nitrōsus, -a, -um. Nitrous.
nōmen, -inis. *m.* Name.
nōminō, -āre, -āvī, -ātus. Name.
nōn. Not.
nondum. Not yet.
nōnus, -a, -um. Ninth.
nosco, -ere, nōvī, nōtus. Learn; know.
novem. Nine.
novus, -a, -um. New.
nox, noctis. *f.* Night.
nucha, -ae. *f.* Nape of neck.
nullus, -a, -um. No; none.
numerus, -ī. *m.* Number.
nunc. Now.
oblīquus, -a, -um. Oblique.
oblongātus, -a, -um. Oblong.
octō. Eight.
oculus, -ī. *m.* Eye.
officīna, -ae. *f.* Office.
officinālis, -e. Officinal.
oleorēsīna, -ae. *f.* Oleoresin.
oleum, -ī. *n.* Oil.
olfactōrius, -a, -um. Olfactory.
omentum, -ī. *n.* Epiploon; omentum.
omnis, -e. Every; all.
operculum, -ī. *n.* (Lit., a cover or lid), applied to a group of convolutions in the cerebrum, between the two divisions of the fissure of Sylvius.
ophthalmicus, -a, -um. Of the eye; ophthalmic.
oppōnēns, -ntis. Opposing.
opticus, -a, -um. Optic.
opus, operis. *n.* Work.
orbita, -ae. *f.* The cavity which lodges the eye; orbit.
ordō, -inis. *m.* Row.
orificium, -ī. *n.* Opening.
orior, -īrī, ortus. Arise.
ōs, ōris. *n.* Mouth.
os, ossis. *n.* Bone.
ossiculum, -ī. *n.* Small bone.
ostium, -ī. *n.* An opening.
ovālis, -e. Egg-shaped; oval.

oxalās, -ātis. *m.* A salt of oxalic acid, oxalate.
oxidum, -ī. *n.* Oxide.
palātum, -ī. *n.* Palate.
palpēbra, -ae. *f.* Eyelid.
pālus, -ūdis. *f.* Marsh; swamp.
pancreāticus, -a, -um. Pancreatic.
papillāris, -e. Resembling or covered with papillae; papillary.
pār, paris. *n.* A pair.
parasiticus, -a, -um. Parasitic.
paries, -iētis. *m.* Wall.
parō, -āre, -āvī, -ātus. Prepare.
pars, partis. *f.* Part.
partus, -ūs. *m.* Parturition; childbirth.
parvus, -a, -um. Small.
pater, -tris. *m.* Father.
patheticus, -a, -um. That which moves the passions; a name given to the 4th pair of nerves.
patria, -as. *f.* Fatherland; country.
paucus, -a, -um. Few.
pectinātus, -a, -um. Resembling the teeth of a comb; pectinate.
pectineus, -a, -um. Comblike.
pectiniformis, -e. Comblike.
pectus, pectoris. *n.* Breast; bosom.
pellūcidus, -a, -um. Transparent.
pensō, -āre, -āvī, -ātus. Weigh.
pepsīnum, -ī. *n.* Pepsin.
percolō, -āre, -āvī, -ātus. Filter; strain.
perforō, -āre, -āvī, -ātus. Bore through; perforate.
periculōsus, -a, -um. Dangerous.
perītus, -a, -um. Skilled.
peronēus, -a, -um. Relating to the fibula; peroneal.
persōna, -ae. *f.* Person.
perspiratōrius, -a, -um. Relating to perspiration; perspiratory.
pēs, pedis. *m.* Foot.
petō, -ere, -īvī, -ītus. Seek.
petrolātum, -ī. *n.* Petrolatum; vaseline.
petrōsus, -a, -um. Rocklike; petrous.
pharmacopoeia, -a. *f.* Pharmacopoeia.
phiala, -ae. *f.* Vial.
philosophis, -ī. *m.* Philosopher.
phosphās, -ātis. *m.* A salt of phosphoric acid; phosphate.
phrenicus, -a, -um. Of the diaphragm; phrenic.
physostigma, -atis. *n.* Calabar bean; physostigma.
piger, -gra, -grum. Lazy.
pigmentum, -ī. *n.* Pigment.
pilula, -ae. *f.* Pill.
pilus, -ī. *m.* Hair.
pineālis, -e. Resembling a pine cone; pineal.
pinna, -ae. *f.* (Lit., feather), pavilion of the ear; pinna.
piper, piperis. *n.* Pepper.
piperītus, -a, -um. Pepper, peppery.
pistillum, -ī. *n.* Pestle.
pituitārius, -a, -um. (**pituita,** phlegm or mucus), pituitary (applied to a reddish-gray body occupying the sella turcica of the sphenoid bone from a former erroneous belief that it discharged mucus into the nostrils).
pius, -a, -um. Tender.
pix, picis. *f.* Pitch.
plantāris, -e. Relating to the sole of the foot; plantar.
plānus, -a, -um. Flat; level; smooth.
plexus, -a, -um. Network; plexus.
plica, -ae. *f.* Fold.
plumbum, -ī. *n.* Lead.
poculum -ī. *n.* Cup.
pollex, -icis. *f.* The thumb.
pomum, -ī. *n.* Apple.
pons, pontis. *m.* Bridge.
poples, poplitis. *m.* Ham of the knee; popliteal space.
poplitēus, -a, -um. Relating to the ham; popliteal.
populus, -ī. *m.* People.
portō, -āre, -āvī, -ātus. Carry.
portiō, -ōnis. *f.* Portion.
porus, -ī. *m.* Channel; canal.
post. Behind; after.
posteā. Afterward.
posticus, -a, -um. Hindmost.
potēns, -ntis. Powerful.
potiō, -ōnis. A drink; draught.
potō, -āre, -āvī, -ātus. Drink.
potus, -ūs. *m.* Drink.
praeparō, -āre, -āvī, -ātus. Prepare.
praeparatiō, -ōnis. *f.* Preparation.
praeputium, -ī. *n.* Foreskin; prepuce.
praescrībō, -ere, -scripsī, -scriptus. Prescribe.
praescriptum, -ī. *n.* Prescription.
praesēns, -ntis. Present.
praestāns, -ntis. Excellent.
pressiō, -ōnis. *f.* Pressure.
primus, -a, -um. First.
princeps, -ipis. The first; chief; principal.
privō, -āre, -āvī, -ātus. Deprive.
prō. For; in behalf of.
processus, -ūs. *m.* A prominence; process.
profundus, -a, -um. Deep.
pronātor, -ōris. *m.* A muscle which turns the palm of the hand downward; pronator.
properō, -āre, -āvī, -ātus. Hasten.
proprius, -a, -um. One's own; special; proper.
prudēns, -ntis. Prudent.
pterygium, -ī. *n.* An eye disease; pterygium.
publicus, -a, -um. Public.
puella, -ae. *f.* Girl.
pugnō, -āre, -āvī, -ātus. Fight.
pulcher, -chra, -chrum. Beautiful.
pulmo, -ōnis. *m.* Lung.
pulmonālis, -e. Of the lungs; pulmonary.
pulverō, -āre, -āvī, -ātus. Powder; pulverize.

pulvis, pulveris. *m.* Powder.
punctum, -ī. *n.* Point.
puniō, -īre, -īvī, -ītus. Punish.
pūpilla, -ae. *f.* Pupil (of eye).
pupillāris, -e. Pupillary; applied to a delicate membrane which covers the pupil of the eye in the fetus.
purgātīvus, -a, -um. Purgative.
purificātus, -a, -um. Purified.
pūrus, -a, -um. Pure.
pyramidālis, -e. Pyramidal.
pyramis, -idis. *f.* Pyramid.
pyriformis, -e. Pear-shaped; pyriform.
quadrātus, -a, -um. Four-sided; square.
quadriceps, -cipitis. Four-headed.
quadrigeminus, -a, -um. Fourfold; four.
quaestiō, -ōnis. *f.* Question.
quam. Than.
quartus, -a, -um. Fourth.
quatuor. Four.
quatuordecim. Fourteen.
que. And.
quinīna, -ae. *f.* Quinine.
quis, quae, quid. Who; which; what.
quondam. Formerly.
quoque. Also.
quot. How many.
radiālis, -e. Of the radius; radial.
radiātus, -a, -um. Radiated.
rādix, -īcis. *f.* Root.
ramus, -ī. *m.* Branch.
rārō. Rarely.
rārus, -a, -um. Rare.
recens. Recently.
recipiō, -ere, -cēpī, -ceptus. Take.
recreō, -āre, -āvī, -ātus. Refresh.
rectus, -a, -um. Straight.
reductio, -ōnis. *f.* A bringing back.
reflexus, -a, -um. Turned back; reflected.
relevō, -āre, -āvī, -ātus. Relieve.
remedium, -ī. *n.* Remedy.
remittō, -ēre, -mīsī, -missus. Send back; remit.
removeō, -ēre, -mōvī, -mōtus. Remove.
rēn, rēnis. *m.* (usually pl.), kidney.
rēnalis, -e. Of the kidney; renal.
reperiō, -īre, -perī, -pertus. Find.
reprimō, -ēre, -pressī, -pressus. Check; repress.
requiesco, -ēre, -ēvī, -ētus. Rest.
rēs, reī. *f.* Thing.
rēsīna, -ae. *f.* Resin.
rēspīrātiō, -ōnis. *f.* Respiration.
rēte, -is. *n.* Net.
reticulāris, -e. Like a net; reticular.
retrāhēns, -ntis. Drawing back; retracting.
rheumatismus, -ī. *m.* Rheumatism.
ricinus, -ī. *m.* (Lit., a tick, which the seeds resemble), the castor oil plant (Ricinus communis).
rima, -ae. *f.* Slit; cleft.
rogō, -āre, -āvī, -ātus. Ask.
rosa, -ae. *f.* Rose.
rostrum, -ī. *n.* Beak.
rotundus, -a, -um. Round.
ruber, -bra, -brum. Red.
rubor, -ōris. *m.* Redness.
rūga, -ae. *f.* A wrinkle; fold.
rumex, -icis. *m.* and *f.* Sorrel.
sabulum, -ī. *n.* Sand.
saccharātus, -a, -um. Saccharated.
saccharum, -ī. *n.* Sugar.
sacciformis, -e. Saclike.
saccus, -ī. *m.* A sack or bag.
saepe. Often.
sal, -is. *m.* and *f.* Salt.
salicīnum, -ī. *n.* Salicin.
salicylās, -ātis. *m.* Salicylate.
salix, -īcis. *f.* Willow.
sānābilis, -e. Curable.
sanguis, -guinis. *m.* Blood.
sānitās, -ātis. *f.* Healing.
sānō, -āre, -āvī, -ātus. Heal; cure.
sapientia, -ae. *f.* Wisdom.
sapō, -ōnis. *m.* Soap.
sartōrius, -ī. *m.* The tailor's muscle; sartorius.
scāla, -ae. *f.* Ladder.
scalēnus, -a, -um. Of unequal sides.
scaphoideus, -a, -um. Boat-shaped; scaphoid.
schola, -ae. *f.* (Lit., leisure given to learning), school.
scientia, -ae. *f.* Knowledge; science.
scilla, -ae. *f.* Squill.
sciō, -īre, -īvī, -ītus. Know.
scrībō, -ēre, scripsī, scrīptus. Write.
scriptōrius, -a, -um. Of a writer; writer's.
secundus, -a, -um. Second.
sed. But.
sēdes, -is. *f.* Seat.
segmentum, -ī. *n.* Segment.
sella, -ae. *f.* Saddle.
sēmicirculāris, -e. Semicircular.
sēmiellipticus, -a, -um. Semielliptical.
sēmilunāris, -e. Semilunar.
sēmimembranōsus, -a, -um. Semimembranous.
seminālis, -e. Seminal.
sēmis, sēmissis. *m.* Half.
sēmitendinōsus, -a, -um. Semitendinous.
senectus, -tūtis. *f.* Old age.
senex, senis. *m.* Old man.
senilitās, -ātis. The feebleness of old age; senility.
sentiō, -īre, -sī, -sus. Feel.
septem. Seven.
sequestrum, -ī. *n.* A portion of dead bone; sequestrum.
sermō, -ōnis. *m.* Conversation.
serrātus, -a, -um. Notched like a saw; serrated.
servus, -ī. *m.* Servant; assistant.
sesamoideus, -a, -um. Like a sesame seed; sesamoid (bone developed in a tendon).

seu. Whether.
signō, -āre, -āvī, -ātus. Write; direct.
similō, -āre, -āvī, -ātus. Simulate.
simplex, -icis. Simple.
sināpis, -is. *f.* Mustard.
sitis, -is. *f.* Thirst.
solitārius, -a, -um. Solitary.
somnificus, -a, -um. Sleep-producing.
somnus, -ī. *m.* Sleep.
sopor, -ōris. *m.* Deep sleep.
spectrum, -ī. *n.* Image.
spēs, speī. *f.* Hope.
sphenoideus, -a, -um. Wedge-shaped; sphenoid.
spīna, -ae. *f.* (A thorn), a process on the surface of a bone; the backbone.
spinālis, -e. Spinal.
spinōsus, -a, -um. Spiny.
spirālis, -e. Spiral.
spiritus, -ūs. *m.* Spirit.
splēnius, -a, -um. Resembling the spleen; applied to a muscle of the back and neck.
spongiōsus, -a, -um. Spongy.
squamōsus, -a, -um. Scaly; squamous.
stapēdius, -ī. *m.* A muscle acting upon the stapes; stapedius.
stertor, -ōris. *m.* Snoring.
stomachālis, -e. Stomachic.
stomachus, -ī. *m.* Stomach.
stramōnium, -ī. *n.* Jamestown weed; stramonium.
stria, -ae. *f.* Stripe; stria.
striātus, -a, -um. Striped; striated.
struō, -ēre, -xī, -ctus. Arrange.
strychnīna, -ae. *f.* Strychnine.
subacetās, -ātis. *m.* Subacetate.
subanconeus, -a, -um. Under the elbow.
subitō. Suddenly.
subitus, -a, -um. Sudden.
sublīmis, -e. Deep.
submuriās, -ātis. *m.* Submuriate.
subnitras, -ātis. *m.* Subnitrate.
subscapulāris, -e. Under the scapula; subscapular.
substantia, -ae. *f.* Substance.
subsultus, -ūs. *m.* A jumping; a twitching.
succus, -ī. *m.* Juice.
sudor, -ōris. *m.* Sweat.
sulcus, -ī. *m.* Furrow.
sulphās, -ātis. *m.* Sulfate.
sulphonal. Sulfonal.
sulphuricus, -a, -um. Sulfuric.
sum, esse, fui. Be.
sūmō, -ēre, -psi, -ptus. Take.
supercilium, -ī. *n.* Eyebrow.
superficialis, -e. Superficial.
superficiēs, -ēī. *f.* Surface.
suppositōrium, -ī. *n.* Suppository.
supraspinātus, -a, -um. Above the spine (of scapula); supraspinate.
suspensōrium, -ī. *n.* That which suspends.
suspensōrius, -a, -um. Suspensory.
sustentaculum, -ī. *n.* A prop; support.
sutūra, -ae. *f.* Seam; suture.
sympatheticus, -a, -um. Sympathetic.
symptōma, -atis. *n.* Symptom.
synoviālis, -e. Synovial.
tabacum, -ī. *n.* Tobacco.
taenia, -ae. *f.* A band.
taenia semicirculāris, a layer in the cerebrum; also a genus of intestinal worms, the tapeworm.
talus, -ī. *m.* The heel.
tam. So.
tapētum, -ī. *n.* (**tapēte,** carpet, tapestry), a lining membrane; also, the radiating fibers of the corpus callōsum.
taraxacum, -ī. *n.* Dandelion root; taraxacum.
tarsus, -ī. *m.* Ankle.
tartaricus, -a, -um. Tartaric.
tartrās, -ātis. *m.* Tartrate.
tectōrium, -ī. *n.* A covering.
tectōrius, -a, -um. Protecting; covering.
tegō, -ēre, -xī, -ctum. Cover; protect.
temporālis, -e. Temporal.
tempus, -oris. *n.* Time.
tenax, -ācis. Holding fast; tenacious.
tendineus, -a, -um. Tendinous.
tendō, -ēre, tetendī, tentus. Stretch; reach.
tendō, -dinis. *m.* Tendon.
teneō, -ēre, -uī, -tus. Keep; hold.
tener, -a, -um. Delicate; tender.
tensor, -ōris. *m.* Stretcher; tensor.
tentō, -āre, -āvī, -ātus. Test, try.
tentōrium, -ī. *n.* A tent; covering.
tenuis, -e. Thin; small.
tepidus, -a, -um. Lukewarm.
terebinthina, -ae. *f.* Turpentine.
teres, -etir. Rounded; smooth.
tergum, -ī. *n.* Back.
terminus, -ī. *m.* End.
tertius, -a, -um. Third.
theobrōma, -ātis. *n.* Cacao (food of the gods).
thoracicus, -a, -um. Thoracic.
thyroideus, -a, -um. Having the shape of an oblong shield; thyroid.
tiglium, -ī. *n.* The specific name of the croton oil plant.
tinctūra, -ae. *f.* Tincture.
tonicus, -a, -um. Tonic.
tonsilla, -ae. *f.* Tonsil.
torcular, -āris. *n.* A wine press.
tracheālis, -e. Tracheal.
tractō, -āre, -āvī, -ātus. Handle.
tragus, -ī. *m.* Small nipple in front of external auditory meatus, so called because sometimes covered with hair; tragus.
transversālis, -e. Transverse.
transversus, -a, -um. Transverse.
trapezoideus, -a, -um. Like a trapezium; trapezoid.

trauma, -atis. *n.* Injury; wound.
trēs, tria. Three.
triangulāris, -e. Triangular.
triceps, -ipitis. Three-headed.
trigeminus, -a, -um. Three-fold.
trīgīnta. Thirty.
trigōnum, -ī. *n.* Triangle.
triquetrus, -a, -um. Three-cornered; triangular.
trochiscus, -ī. *m.* Troche.
tuba, -ae. *f.* (Trumpet), tube.
tuber, -eris. *n.* Swelling, protuberance.
tuberculum, -ī. *n.* A protuberance; tubercle.
tubulus, -ī. *m.* Small tube.
tubus, -ī. *m.* Tube.
tunica, -ae. *f.* Coat; covering.
tussiō, -īre, -īvī, -ītus. Cough.
tūtāmen, -minis. *n.* Means of defense; a protection.
tūtō. Safely.
tympanicus, -a, -um. Of the tympanum; tympanic.
ubi. Where.
ulna, -ae. *f.* Larger bone of forearm; ulna.
ulnāris, -e. Of the ulna; ulnar.
uncia, -ae. *f.* Ounce.
unciformis, -e. Hooked.
uncinātus, -a, -um. Hooked; uncinate.
unguentum, -ī. *n.* Ointment.
unguis, -is. *m.* Nail.
ūnus, -a, -um. One.
urbānus, -a, -um. Of the city; urbane.
urīna, -ae. *f.* Urine.
uriniferus, -a, -um. Urine-bearing; uriniferous.
usque. Continuously; constantly.
uterīnus, -a, -um. Of the uterus; uterine.
ūtilis, -e. Useful.
uvula, -ae. *f.* A small appendix or tubercle; uvula.
uxor, -ōris. *f.* Wife.
vaginālis, -e. Sheathlike; vaginal.
valeriānās, -ātis. *m.* Valerianate.
valetūdō, -inis. *f.* Health.
validus, -a, -um. Strong; sturdy; healthy.
valvula, -ae. *f.* Valve.
vās, vāsis. *n.* Vessel.
vasculōsus, -a, -um. Vascular.
vasculum, -ī. *n.* Small vessel.
vastus, -a, -um. Extensive; large.
vegetābilis, -e. Vegetable.
vehiculum, -ī. *n.* Vehicle.
vel. Either.
vēlum, -ī. *n.* Veil.
vēna, -ae. *f.* Vein.
vendō, -ēre, vendidī. Sell.
veneficus, -ī. *m.* Poisoner.
venēnum, -ī. *n.* Poison.
venōsus, -a, -um. Venous.
venter, -tris. *m.* Belly.
ventriculus, -ī. *m.* Ventricle.
vērātrum, -ī. *n.* Hellebore; veratrum.
vermiformis, -e. Wormlike.
veru, -ūs. *n.* A spit (for roasting upon); used only in **verumontanum,** a longitudinal ridge in the floor of the male urethra.
verus, -a, -um. True.
vesica, -ae. *f.* Urinary bladder.
vesicatōrium, -ī. *n.* Blister.
vesicula, -ae. *f.* Vesicle.
vesiculāris, -e. Full of vesicles or cells; vesicular.
vestibulāris, -e. Relating to the vestibule of the ear; vestibular.
vetus, veteris. Old.
vigilō, -āre, -āvī, -ātus. Watch.
vīgintī. Twenty.
villus, -ī. *m.* Tuft of hair; villus.
vinculum, -ī. *n.* Link; chain.
vinum, -ī. *n.* Wine.
vir, virī. *m.* Man.
viridis, -e. Green.
vīs, vīs, pl. vīres, -ium. *f.* Force; power.
viscus, -eris. *n.* Any internal organ of the body.
visiō, -ōnis. *f.* Vision.
vīsus, -ūs. *m.* Vision.
vīta, -ae. *f.* Life.
vitellus, -ī. *m.* Yolk.
vitreus, -a, -um. Resembling glass; vitreous.
vocālis, -e. Vocal.
vocō, -āre, -āvī, -ātus. Call.
vola, -ae. *f.* Palm of the hand (sole of the foot).
vorticōsus, -a, -um. Resembling an eddy or whirlpool.
vulnerō, -āre, -āvī, -ātus. Wound.
vulnus, vulneris. *n.* A wound.
vultus, -ūs. *m.* Countenance.
zincum, -ī. *n.* Zinc.
zingiber, -eris. *n.* Ginger.
zōna, -ae. *f.* Zone; belt.
zōnula, -ae. *f.* Little zone, or belt; zonule.

Greek and Latin Singulars and Plurals

Singular	*Plural*	*Singular*	*Plural*
addendum	addenda	focus	foci
aden	adena	fornix	fornices
adenoma	adenomata	fossa	fossae
ala	alae	glans	glandes
albacans	albacantes	gonad	gonades
amygdala	amygdalae	gonococcus	gonococci
antenna	antennae	gyrus	gyri
antiad	antiades	ilium	ilia
antrum	antra	keratosis	keratoses
apertura	aperturae	labium	labia
apex	apices	lamina	laminae
aponeurosis	aponeuroses	loculus	loculi
appendix	appendices	locus	loci
aqua	aquae	medium	media
arcus	arcus	mucosa	mucosae
ascaris	ascarides	naevus	naevi
ascus	asci	nodus	nodi
atrium	atria	nox	noxa
axis	axes	os	ora
bacillus	bacilli	ovum	ova
bacterium	bacteria	papilla	papillae
bronchus	bronchi	pathema	pathemata
bulla	bullae	pes	pedes
bursa	bursae	petechia	petechiae
cactus	cacti	pilula	pilulae
cadaver	cadavera	polypus	polypi
calcaneum	calcanea	ramus	rami
calculus	calculi	septum	septa
calix	calices	sequestrum	sequestra
cantharis	cantharides	serosa	serosae
canthus	canthi	spasmus	spasmi
cornu	cornua	spectrum	spectra
corpus	corpora	speculum	specula
crisis	crises	sperma	spermata
cuniculus	cuniculi	stoma	stomata
dens	dentes	sudamen	sudamina
diagnosis	diagnoses	sulcus	sulci
diaphoreticus	diaphoretici	tarsus	tarsi
diastema	diastemata	tela	telae
digitus	digiti	tinctura	tincturae
dorsum	dorsi	toxicosis	toxicoses
echolatus	echolati	typha	typhae
enema	enemata	ulcus	ulcera
ensis	enses	varix	varices
epididymis	epididymides	vas	vasa
esthesis	estheses	vesicula	vesiculae
fibroma	fibromata	vis	vires
filix	filices	viscus	viscera
filum	fila	vomica	vomicae
flagellum	flagella	zygoma	zygomata

Latin Numerals

Cardinals		Ordinals	
1	unus	1st	primus
2	duo	2nd	secundus
3	tres	3rd	tertius
4	quattuor	4th	quartus
5	quinque	5th	quintus
6	sex	6th	sextus
7	septem	7th	septimus
8	octō	8th	octāvus
9	novem	9th	nōnus
10	decem	10th	decimus
11	ūndecim	11th	ūndecimus
12	duodecim	12th	duodecimus
13	tredecim	13th	tertius decimus
14	quattuordecim	14th	quartus decimus
15	quīndecim	15th	quīntus decimus
16	sēdecim	16th	septus decimus
17	septendecim	17th	septimus decimus
18	duodēvīgintī	18th	duodēvīcēsimus
19	ūndēvīgintī	19th	ūndēvīcēsimus
20	vīgintī	20th	vīcēsimus
21	vīgintī ūnus, *or* ūnus et vīgintī	21st	vīcēsimus primus, *or* prīmus et vīcēsimus
22	vīgintī duo, *or* duo et vīgintī	22nd	vīcēsimus secundus, *or* duo et vīcēsimus
28	duodētrīgintā	28th	duodētrīcēsimus
29	ūndētrīgintā	29th	ūndētrīcēsimus
30	trīgintā	30th	trīcēsimus
40	quadrāgintā	40th	quadrāgēsimus
50	quīnquāgintā	50th	quīnquāgēsimus
60	sexāgintā	60th	sexāgēsimus
70	septuāgintā	70th	septuāgēsimus
80	octōgintā	80th	octōgēsimus
90	nōnāgintā	90th	nōnāgēsimus
100	centum	100th	centēsimus
101	centum ūnus, *or* centum et ūnus	101st	centēsimus prīmus, centēsimus et prīmus
102	centum duo, *or* centum et duo	102nd	centēsimus secundus, centēsimus et secundus
200	ducentī	200th	ducentēsimus
300	trecentī	300th	trecentēsimus
400	quadringentī	400th	quadringentēsimus
500	quīngentī	500th	quīngentēsimus
600	sēscentī, *or* sexcenti	600th	sēscentēsimus
700	septingentī	700th	septingentēsimus
800	octingentī	800th	octingentēsimus
900	nōngentī	900th	nōngentēsimus
1,000	mīlle	1,000th	mīllēsimus
2,000	duo mīllia	2,000th	bis mīllēsimus
10,000	decem mīllia	10,000th	decies mīllēsimus
100,000	centum mīllia	100,000th	centiēs mīllēsimus

Roman Numerals

A line placed over a letter increases its value one thousand times.

1	I	6	VI	11	XI	40	XL	90	XC	5000	$\bar{V}$
2	II	7	VII	12	XII	50	L	100	C	10,000	$\bar{X}$
3	III	8	VIII	15	XV	60	LX	500	D	100,000	$\bar{C}$
4	IV	9	IX	20	XX	70	LXX	1000	M	1,000,000	$\bar{M}$
5	V	10	X	30	XXX	80	LXXX	2000	MM		

App. 8: Anatomy

Muscles with Their Action, Origin, Insertion and Innervation

The muscles in the body number over 650, the totals varying according to the authority, as some list as separate muscles what others regard as portions of adjacent muscles. Most of the muscles occur in pairs; five are single muscles.

Muscles

Name	Action	Origin	Insertion	Innervation
abductor digiti quinti	Abducts little finger	Pisiform bone and ligaments	Inner side of 1st phalanx of little finger	Ulnar, palmar branch
abductor digiti quinti	Abducts little toe	Outer tuberosity of calcaneus, plantar fascia, and intermuscular septum	External side of 1st phalanx of little toe	Lateral plantar
abductor hallucis	Abducts great toe	Inner tuberosity of os calcis, plantar fascia	Inner side, 1st phalanx of great toe	Medial plantar
abductor minimi digiti Same as: abductor digiti quinti				
abductor pollicis brevis	Abducts thumb	Ridge of trapezium and transverse carpal ligament	Outer side of 1st phalanx of thumb	Branch of median
abductor pollicis longus	Abducts and assists in extending thumb	Posterior surface of radius and ulna	Outer side of base of 1st metacarpal	Branch of radial
abductor pollicis longus SYN: extensor ossis metacarpi pollicis	Abducts thumb and wrist	Dorsal surface of radius, ulna, and interosseous membrane	Base of 1st metacarpal	Branch of radial
accelerator urinae Same as: bulbocavernosus				
accessorius Same as: iliocostalis thoracis				
adductor brevis	Flexes, adducts, and tends to rotate thigh medially	Ramus of pubis	Upper portion of linea aspera of femur	Branch of obturator

Muscles *(Continued)*

Name	Action	Origin	Insertion	Innervation
adductor hallucis	Adducts great toe	Tarsal terminations of the three middle metatarsal bones	Lateral side of base of 1st phalanx of great toe	Branch of lateral plantar
adductor longus	Adducts, flexes and tends to rotate thigh medially	Pubic crest and symphysis	Middle of linea aspera of femur	Branch of obturator
adductor magnus	Adducts thigh and rotates it outward	Ramus of ischium and pubis	Linea aspera of femur and medial condyle	Branch of sciatic and obturator
adductor obliquus hallucis Same as: adductor hallucis				
adductor pollicis	Adducts thumb	Third metacarpal bone	Inner side of base of 1st phalanx of thumb	Ulnar
adductor transversus hallucis Same as: adductor hallucis				
anconeus	Extends forearm	Lateral epicondyle of humerus	Olecranon and posterior surface of ulna	Branch of radial
antitragicus		Anterior part of antitragus	Opposite side at larger auricular fissure	Posterior auricular branch of facial
arrectores pilorum	Elevates hairs of skin	Papillary layer of skin	Hair follicles	Sympathetic
articularis genu SYN: subcrureus	Elevates capsule of knee joint	Lower quarter of anterior surface of femoral shaft	Synovial membrane of knee joint	Branch of femoral
aryepiglotticus	Closes glottis opening	Arytenoid cartilage	Epiglottis	Laryngeal, recurrent
arytenoideus Consists of (1)	Closes glottis opening	Arytenoid cartilage	(1) Aryepiglottic fold. (2) Crosses between the two	Laryngeal, recurrent

arytenoideus obliquus and (2) arytenoideus transversus			cartilages of the obliquus portion	
attolens aurem Same as: auricularis superior				
attrahens aurem Same as: auricularis anterior				
auricularis anterior SYN: attrahens aurem	Draws pinna of ear forward and upward	Superficial temporal fascia	Helix of ear anteriorly	Facial
auricularis posterior SYN: retrahens aurem	Draws pinna of ear backward	Mastoid process	Root of auricle	Facial
auricularis superior SYN: attolens aurem	Elevates pinna of ear	Galea aponeurotica	Upper portion of pinna of ear	Facial
azygos uvulae Same as: uvulae				
biceps brachii	Flexes arm and forearm and supinates hand	(1) Short head from coracoid process. (2) Long head from the supraglenoid tuberosity at the margin of the glenoid cavity	Bicipital tuberosity of radius	Musculocutaneous
biceps femoris	Flexes knee and rotates it outward	(1) Short head from linea aspera. (2) Long head from ischial tuberosity	Head of fibula; lateral condyle of tibia	(1) Peroneal, and (2) tibial portions of sciatic
biventer cervicis, inseparably connected with spinalis capitis, q.v.				
brachialis	Flexes forearm	Lower half of anterior surface of humerus	Coronoid process of ulna	Musculocutaneous and radial

Muscles *(Continued)*

Name	Action	Origin	Insertion	Innervation
brachioradialis SYN: supinator longus	Flexes and supinates forearm	Supracondylar ridge of humerus	Styloid process of radius	Branch of radial
buccinator	Compresses cheek, retracts angle of mouth	Alveolar process of maxilla, pterygomandibular ligament, buccinator ridge of mandible	Orbicularis oris	Facial
bulbocavernosus	Constrict bulbous urethra in male; in female constricts urethra	Central point of perineum and median raphe	Undersurface of bulb, spongy and cavernous part of penis; root of clitoris	Perineal branch of pudendal
caninus Same as: levator anguli oris, q.v.				
cephalopharyngeus Same as: constrictor pharyngis superior, q.v.				
cervicalis ascendens Same as: iliocostalis cervicis, q.v.				
choroideus Same as: ciliaris				
ciliaris	Alters shape of crystalline lens in accommodation	(1) Meridional: Junctions of cornea and sclera. (2) Circular: Fibers forming a circle close to iris	(1) External layers of choroid. (2) Ciliary process	Short ciliary
coccygeus	Supports coccyx, closes pelvic outlet	Ischial spine and sacrospinous ligament	Coccyx and lowest portion of sacrum	Third and 4th sacral

complexus Same as: semispinalis capitis, q.v.				
compressor naris Old term for nasalis muscle, q.v.				
compressor urethra Same as: sphincter urethrae membranaceae, q.v.				
constrictor pharyngis inferior SYN: inferior constrictor; laryngopharyngeus	Narrows the pharynx, as in swallowing	Sides of cricoid and thyroid cartilage	Posterior raphe of pharyngeal wall	Pharyngeal plexus
constrictor pharyngis medius SYN: middle constrictor; hypopharyngeus	Narrows pharynx, as in swallowing	Both cornua of hyoid bone and stylohyoid ligament	Middle of posterior pharyngeal wall	Pharyngeal plexus
constrictor pharyngis superior SYN: superior constrictor; cephalopharyngeus	Narrows pharynx, as in swallowing	Internal pterygoid plate, pterygomandibular ligament, jaw, side of tongue	Posterior pharyngeal wall	Pharyngeal plexus
constrictor urethrae Same as: sphincter urethrae membranaceae, q.v.				
coracobrachialis	Raises and adducts arm	Coracoid process of scapula	Middle of inner border of humerus	Musculocutaneous
corrugator cutis ani	Wrinkles skin of anus	Submucous tissue, interior of anus	Subcutaneous tissue on opposite side of anus	Sympathetic

Muscles *(Continued)*

Name	Action	Origin	Insertion	Innervation
corrugator supercilii	Draws eyebrows down and in	Inner end of superciliary arch	Skin above orbital arch	Facial
cremaster	Raises testicle	Midportion of inguinal ligament	Cremasteric fascia and pubic bone	Genitofemoral
cricoarytenoideus lateralis	Narrows glottis	Upper border of arch of cricoid cartilage	Muscular process of arytenoid cartilage	Laryngeal, recurrent
cricoarytenoideus posterior	Opens glottis	Back of cricoid cartilage	Muscular process of arytenoid cartilage	Laryngeal, recurrent
cricothyroideus	Tightens vocal cords	Anterior surface of cricoid cartilage	Thyroid cartilage	Laryngeal, superior
crureus Same as: vastus intermedius, q.v.				
deltoideus SYN: deltoid	Raises arm and rotates it	Clavicle, acromion process, and spine of scapula	Shaft of humerus	Axillary (circumflex) from brachial plexus
depressor alae nasi Same as: depressor septi				
depressor anguli oris SYN: triangularis	Depresses angle of mouth	External oblique line of mandible	Angle of mouth	Facial
depressor labii inferioris SYN: quadratus labii inferioris; quadratus menti	Draws lower lip down and a little lateral as in the expression of irony	External oblique line of the mandible	Lower lip and orbicularis oris	Facial nerve
depressor septi SYN: depressor alae nasi	Draws outer wall of nostril downward	Incisive fossa of superior maxillary bone	Septum and ala of nose	Facial
depressor urethrae	Depresses urethra	Ramus of ischium near the	Fibers of constrictor	

		transversus perinei profundus	vaginae	
diaphragm	Increases chest capacity and decreases pressure within the thoracic cavity	Ensiform cartilage, 7th to 12th ribs, arcuate ligaments and lumbar vertebrae	Central tendon	Phrenic
digastricus Consists of (1) anterior and (2) posterior bellies	(1) Draws hyoid bone forward. (2) Draws hyoid bone backward	(1) Lower border of lower jaw. (2) Mastoid groove of temporal bone	Intermediate tendon between both bellies	(1) Mylohyoid. (2) Facial
dilatator naris anterior	Dilates apertures of nostril	Cartilage of ala of nose	Border of ala	Facial
dilatator naris posterior	Dilates apertures of nostril	Nasal notch of superior maxilla and the sesamoid cartilages	Integument of margin of nostril	Facial
epicranius Scalp muscles consisting of occipitofrontalis and temporoparietalis, q.v., connected by galea aponeurotica				
erector clitoridis Same as: ischiocavernosus, q.v.				
erector penis Same as: ischiocavernosus, q.v.				
erector spinae Same as: sacrospinalis, q.v.				
extensor carpi radialis brevis	Extends and abducts wrist	External condyloid ridge of humerus	Base of 3rd metacarpal	Branch of radial

Muscles *(Continued)*

Name	Action	Origin	Insertion	Innervation
extensor carpi radialis longus	Extends and abducts wrist	External condyloid ridge of humerus	Base of 2nd metacarpal	Branch of radial
extensor carpi ulnaris	Extends and abducts wrist	Lateral epicondyle of humerus	Base of 5th metacarpal	Branch of radial
extensor digiti minimi SYN: extensor digiti quinti proprius	Extends little finger	External epicondyle of humerus	Dorsum of 1st phalanx of little finger	Branch of radial
extensor digiti quinti proprius Same as: extensor digiti minimi				
extensor digitorum brevis	Extends toes	Dorsal surface of os calcis	To 1st phalanx of great toe and the tendons of extensor digitorum longus	Branch of peroneal
extensor digitorum communis	Extends fingers and wrist	External epicondyle of humerus	Second and 3rd phalanges	Branch of radial
extensor digitorum longus	Extends toes, flexes foot	External tuberosity of tibia; body of fibula	Second and 3rd phalanges of toes	Branches of peroneal
extensor hallucis longus	Extends great toe; flexes foot	Front of fibula and interosseous membrane	Terminal phalanx of great toe	Branch of peroneal
extensor indicis proprius	Extends index finger	Dorsal surface of ulna and interosseous membrane	First tendon of extensor digitorum communis	Branch of radial
extensor ossis metacarpi pollicis Same as: abductor pollicis longus, q.v.				

extensor pollicis brevis	Extends thumb and abducts 1st metacarpal	Dorsal surface of radius	Base of 1st phalanx of thumb	Branch of radial
extensor pollicis longus	Extends terminal phalanx of thumb and abducts hand	Dorsal surface of ulna	Base of 2nd phalanx of thumb	Branch of radial
extensor primi internodii pollicis Same as: extensor pollicis brevis, q.v.				
extensor proprius hallucis Same as: extensor hallucis longus, q.v.				
extensor secundi internodii pollicis Same as: extensor pollicis longus, q.v.				
flexor accessorius Same as: quadratus plantae, q.v.				
flexor brevis minimi digiti Same as: flexor digiti quinti brevis, q.v.				
flexor carpi radialis SYN: radiocarpus	Flexes and abducts wrist	Medial epicondyle of humerus	Base of 2nd metacarpal	Branch of median
flexor carpi ulnaris Consists of (1) humeral head and (2) ulnar head	Flexes and adducts wrist	(1) Medial epicondyle of humerus. (2) Olecranon process and posterior border of ulna	Pisiform bone and 5th metacarpal	Branch of ulnar
flexor digiti quinti brevis	Flexes 1st phalanx of little finger	Unciform bone	First phalanx of little finger	Branch of ulnar

Muscles *(Continued)*

Name	Action	Origin	Insertion	Innervation
flexor digiti quinti brevis	Flexes the little toe	Base of metatarsal of little toe and sheath of peroneus longus	Outer side of base of 1st phalanx of little toe	External plantar
flexor digitorum brevis	Flexes toe	Os calcis and plantar fascia	Second phalanges of lesser toes	Internal plantar
flexor digitorum longus	Flexes phalanges and extends toes	Posterior surface of tibia	Terminal phalanges of four lesser toes	Branch of tibial
flexor digitorum profundus	Flexes the phalanges	Upper three fourths of shaft of ulna	Terminal phalanges of fingers	Branch of ulnar and branch of median
flexor digitorum sublimis Same as: flexor digitorum superficialis, q.v.				
flexor digitorum superficialis SYN: flexor digitorum sublimis Consists of three heads: (1) humeral, (2) ulnar, and (3) radial	Flexes middle phalanges and hand	(1) Medial epicondyle of humerus. (2) Medial side of coronoid process. (3) Outer border of radius	Second phalanx of each finger	Branches of median
flexor hallucis brevis	Flexes great toe	Internal surface of cuboid and middle and external cuneiform bones	Sides of base of 1st phalanx of great toe	Internal and external plantar
flexor hallucis longus	Flexes great toe and extends foot	Lower portion of shaft of fibula	Distal phalanx of great toe	Posterior tibial
flexor pollicis brevis	Flexes 1st phalanx of thumb	Transverse carpal ligament, metacarpal bone	Base of 1st phalanx of thumb	Branch of median and of ulnar

flexor pollicis longus	Flexes thumb	Anterior surface of middle third of radius	Terminal phalanx of thumb	Branch of median
frontalis SEE: occipitofrontalis				
gastrocnemius	Flexes foot and leg	External and internal femoral condyles	By tendo calcaneus into os calcis	Branches of tibial
gemellus inferior	Rotates thigh outward	Ischial tuberosity	Medial surface of greater trochanter	Sacral
gemellus superior	Rotates thigh outward	Spine of ischium	Medial surface of greater trochanter	Sacral plexus
genioglossus	Protrudes and retracts tongue, elevates hyoid	Inner surface of symphysis of mandible	Hyoid and bottom of tongue	Hypoglossal
geniohyoglossus Same as: genioglossus, q.v.				
geniohyoideus SYN: geniohyoid muscle	Elevates and advances hyoid and helps to depress jaw	Mental spine of inferior maxilla	Hyoid	Hypoglossal
glossopalatinus SYN: palatoglossus	Elevates back of tongue and constricts fauces	Undersurface of soft palate	Side of tongue	Pharyngeal plexus
gluteus maximus	Extends and rotates thigh	Superior curved iliac line and crest, coccyx, and sacrum	Fascia lata and femur below greater trochanter	Inferior gluteal
gluteus medius	Abducts and rotates thigh	Lateral surface of ilium	Greater trochanter	Branches of superior gluteal
gluteus minimus	Abducts and extends thigh	Lateral surface of ilium	Greater trochanter	Branch of superior gluteal
gracilis	Flexes and adducts leg; adducts thigh	Symphysis pubis and pubic arch	Medial surface of shaft of tibia	Branch of obturator

Muscles *(Continued)*

Name	Action	Origin	Insertion	Innervation
helicis major and minor	Tighten the skin of auditory canal	Tuberosity on helix	Rim of helix	Auriculotemporal and posterior auricular
hyoglossus	Depresses side of tongue and retracts tongue	Cornua and body of hyoid	Side of tongue	Hypoglossal
hyopharyngeus Same as: constrictor pharyngis medius, q.v.				
iliacus	Flexes and rotates thigh	Margin of iliac fossa	Lesser trochanter	Branches of femoral
iliocostalis cervicis SYN: cervicalis ascendens	Extends cervical spine	Angles of 3rd to 6th ribs	Transverse processes of 4th to 6th cervical vertebrae	Branches of cervical
iliocostalis dorsi Same as: iliocostalis thoracis				
iliocostalis lumborum SYN: sacrolumbalis	Extends lumbar spine	With sacrospinalis	In angles of 5th to 12th ribs	Branches of dorsal and lumbar
iliocostalis thoracis SYN: iliocostalis dorsi; accessorius	Keeps dorsal spine erect	Angles of 12th to 7th ribs	Sixth to 1st ribs and 7th cervical vertebra	Branches of dorsal
infracostales Same as: subcostales				
infraspinatus	Rotates arm back and out	Infraspinous fossa of scapula	Great tuberosity of humerus	Suprascapular from brachial plexus
intercostales externus	Draw ribs together and raise ribs	Lower border of rib	Upper border of rib below	Intercostal
intercostales internus	Draw ribs together and	Lower border of rib	Upper border of rib below	Intercostal

	lower ribs			
interossei dorsales manus (four)	Abduct and adduct fingers	Sides of metacarpal bones	First phalanges	Branch of ulnar
interossei palmares Same as: interossei volares, q.v.				
interossei volares (three)	Adduct index finger, abduct ring and little fingers	Metacarpal bones laterally	Ulnar side of index finger, and radial sides of ring and little fingers	Branch of ulnar
interosseus dorsalis pedis (four)	Adduct 2nd toe; abduct 2nd, 3rd, and 4th toes	Shafts of adjacent metatarsal bones	First phalanges of lesser toes	External plantar
interosseus plantaris (three)	Adduct three outer toes	Third, 4th, and 5th metatarsal bones	First phalanx of corresponding toe	External plantar
interspinales (a series)	Support and extend vertebral column	Undersurface of spine of one vertebra	Spine of vertebra above	Branches of spinal
intertransversales Same as: intertransversarii, q.v.				
intertransversarii SYN: intertransversales	Flex vertebral column	Between transverse processes of contiguous vertebrae		Branches of ventral and dorsal divisions of spinal
ischiocavernosus SYN: erector clitoridis (in female); erector penis (in male)	Maintains erection of penis or clitoris	Tuberosity of ischium and great sacrosciatic ligament	Corpus cavernosum of clitoris or penis	Perineal branch of pudendal
ischiococcygeus Same as: coccygeus, q.v.				
laryngopharyngeus Same as: constrictor pharyngis inferior, q.v.				

Muscles *(Continued)*

Name	Action	Origin	Insertion	Innervation
latissimus dorsi	Adducts, extends, and rotates arm	Lower thoracic and lumbar vertebrae, sacrum, and tip of iliac crest	Intertubercular groove of humerus	Brachial plexus
levator anguli oris SYN: caninus	Elevates angle of mouth	Canine fossa of maxilla	Angle of mouth and orbicularis oris	Facial
levator ani	Supports rectum and pelvic floor, aids in defecation	Pubis, pelvic fascia, ischial spine	Rectum, coccyx, and fibrous raphe of perineum	Sacral and perineal
levator labii inferioris Same as: mentalis, q.v.				
levator labii superioris	Elevates and extends upper lip	Lower margin of orbit, malar bone	Upper lip	Infraorbital branch of facial
levator labii superioris alaeque nasi	Elevates upper lip, dilates nostril	Nasal process of maxilla	Cartilage of ala of nose and upper lip	Infraorbital branch of facial
levator menti Same as: mentalis, q.v.				
levator palati Same as: levator veli palatini, q.v.				
levator palpebrae superioris	Raises upper eyelid	Lesser wing of the sphenoid bone	Upper tarsal cartilage	Oculomotor
levator scapulae SYN: levator anguli scapulae	Elevates posterior angle of scapula	Transverse process of four upper cervical vertebrae	Superior edge of scapula	Dorsal scapular from 5th cervical, and branches of 3rd and 4th cervical
levator veli palatini	Elevates soft palate	Petrous portion of temporal bone and cartilaginous eustachian tube	Aponeurosis of soft palate	Pharyngeal plexus

levatores costarum	Raise ribs; flex vertebral column	Transverse process of 7th cervical and upper 11 thoracic vertebrae	Rib next below	Branches of intercostal
lingualis	Elevates sides and center of tongue	Undersurface of tongue	Edge of tongue	Hypoglossal
longissimus capitis SYN: trachelomastoid	Keeps head erect, draws it backward or to one side	Upper thoracic and lower and middle cervical vertebrae	Mastoid process	Branches of cervical
longissimus cervicis SYN: transversalis colli	Extends cervical spine	Upper thoracic vertebrae	Ribs and upper lumbar and thoracic vertebrae	Branches of dorsal divisions of spinal
longissimus dorsi Same as: longissimus thoracis, q.v.				
longissimus thoracis SYN: longissimus dorsi	Extends spinal column	Transverse processes of lumbar and dorsal vertebrae	Lowest ribs and lumbar and dorsal vertebrae	Lumbar and dorsal divisions of spinal
longus capitis SYN: rectus capitis anticus major	Flexes head	Transverse processes of 3rd to 6th cervical vertebrae	Occipital bone, basilar process	Branches of 1st to 3rd cervical nerves
longus cervicis Same as: longus colli				
longus colli Consists of three parts: (1) superior oblique, (2) inferior oblique, and (3) vertical	Twists and bends neck forward	(1) Transverse processes of 3rd to 5th cervical vertebrae. (2) Bodies of 1st to 3rd thoracic vertebrae. (3) Bodies of three upper thoracic and three lower cervical vertebrae	(1) Anterior tubercle of atlas. (2) Transverse processes of 5th and 6th cervical vertebrae. (3) Bodies of 2nd to 4th cervical vertebrae	Branches of 2nd to 7th cervical nerves
lumbricales manus (four)	Flex 1st and extend 2nd and 3rd phalanges	Tendon of flexor digitorum profundus	First phalanx and extensor tendon	Median and ulnar

Muscles *(Continued)*

Name	Action	Origin	Insertion	Innervation
lumbricalis (four)	Flex the 1st and extend the 2nd and 3rd phalanges	Tendons of flexor digitorum longus	First phalanx and extensor tendon	External and internal plantar
masseter	Mastication	Zygomatic arch and malar process of superior maxilla	Angle ramus, and coronoid process of mandible	Mandibular division of trigeminal
mentalis SYN: levator labii inferioris; levator menti	Elevates and protrudes lower lip; wrinkles skin of chin	Incisive fossa of mandible	Integument of chin	Facial
multifidus	Rotates spinal column	Sacrum, iliac spine, lumbar, cervical, and dorsal vertebrae	Laminae and spinous processes of next four vertebrae above	Branches of dorsal divisions of spinal
multifidus spinae Same as: multifidus, q.v.				
mylohyoideus SYN: mylohyoid muscle	Elevates floor of mouth and hyoid, depresses jaw	Mylohyoid line of mandible	Body of hyoid and median raphe	Mylohyoid
nasalis Consists of transverse and alar parts	Depresses cartilaginous part of nose and draws the alae medially	Maxilla	Bridge of nose	Buccal branches of facial nerve
obliquus auriculae		Conch of the ear	Fossa of antihelix	Posterior auricular branch of facial
obliquus capitis inferior	Rotates head	Spine of axis	Transverse process of atlas	Suboccipital
obliquus capitis superior	Rotates head	Transverse process of axis	Occipital bone	Suboccipital
obliquus externus abdominus	Contracts abdomen and viscera	Lower eight ribs	Iliac crest, Poupart's ligament, linea alba, pubic crest	Iliohypogastric, ilioinguinal, and branches of intercostal
obliquus internus	Compresses viscera, flexes	Iliac crest, inguinal	Few lowest ribs, linea alba,	Iliohypogastric,

abdominis	thorax forward	ligament, lumbar fascia	pubic crest	ilioinguinal, and branches of intercostal
obliquus oculi inferior	Rotates eyeball up and out	Orbital plate of superior maxillary bone	Sclerotic coat at right angles to insertion of rectus externus just below it	Oculomotor
obliquus oculi superior	Rotates eyeball down and out	Above optic foramen	By a tendon through trochlea to the sclerotic coat	Trochlear
obturator internus	Rotates thigh outward	Pubes, ischium, obturator foramen	Inner surface of great trochanter	Branch of obturator
occipitalis SEE: occipitofrontalis				
occipitofrontalis Consists of (1) occipitalis and (2) frontalis bellies	(1) Draws scalp back. (2) Draws scalp forward; raises eyebrows	(1) Occipital and temporal bones. (2) Procerus, corrugator, and orbicularis oris muscles	Galea aponeurotica	Facial
omohyoideus SYN: omohyoid muscle	Depresses hyoid	Upper border of scapula	Hyoid bone	Upper cervical through ansa hypoglossi
opponens digiti quinti	Flexes and adducts little finger	Unciform bone; transverse carpal ligament	Fifth metacarpal bone	Branch of ulnar
opponens minimi digiti Same as: opponens digiti quinti				
opponens pollicis	Flexes and adducts thumb	Trapezium and transverse carpal ligament	First metacarpal bone	Median
orbicularis oculi	Closes eyelid, wrinkles forehead vertically, compresses lacrimal sac	(1) (Pars lacrimalis) Lacrimal bone. (2) (Pars orbitalis) Frontal processes of maxilla and	(1) Joins palpebral portion. (2) Encircles orbit to orbit. (3) Outer canthus	Facial

Muscles *(Continued)*

Name	Action	Origin	Insertion	Innervation
		frontal bone. (3) (Pars palpebralis) Inner canthus		
orbicularis oris	Closes lips	Nasal septum and canine fossa of mandible by accessory fibers	Buccinator and adjacent muscles surrounding mouth	Facial
orbicularis palpebrarum Same as: orbicularis oculi, q.v. (pars palpebralis)				
orbitalis Circular division of ciliaris, q.v.				
orbitopalpebralis Same as: levator palpebrae superioris, q.v.				
palatoglossus Same as: glossopalatinus, q.v.				
palatopharyngeus Same as: pharyngopalatinus, q.v.				
palmaris brevis	Wrinkles skin on inner side of hand	Central portion of palmar aponeurosis and transverse carpal ligament	Skin of ulnar side of hand	Branch of ulnar
palmaris longus	Tightens palmar fascia, flexes wrist	Medial epicondyle of humerus	Transverse carpal ligament and palmar fascia	Branch of median

pectineus	Flexes and adducts thigh	Pubic spine; iliopectineal line	Pectineal line of femur	Branch of obturator and femoral
pectoralis major	Flexes, adducts, and rotates arm	Sternum, clavicle, and cartilages of 1st to 6th ribs	Bicipital ridge of humerus	Anterior thoracic from brachial plexus
pectoralis minor	Draws down scapula and point to shoulder, raises ribs	Third to 5th ribs	Coracoid process of scapula	Anterior thoracic from brachial plexus
peroneus brevis	Extends and abducts foot	Midportion of shaft of fibula	Base of 5th metatarsal bone	Branch of peroneal
peroneus longus	Extends, abducts, and everts foot	Upper fibula and external condyle of tibia	By tendon to internal cuneiform and 1st metatarsal bone	Branch of peroneal
peroneus tertius	Flexes foot	Lower part of fibula	Fifth metatarsal bone	Branch of peroneal
pharyngopalatinus	Narrows fauces and shuts off nasopharynx	Soft palate	Thyroid cartilage and aponeurosis of the pharynx	Pharyngeal plexus
piriformis	Abducts and rotates thigh outward	Margins of anterior sacral foramina and sacrosciatic notch of ilium	Upper margin of greater trochanter	Branch of sacral
plantaris	Extends foot	External supracondyloid ridge of femur	Inner border of tendo calcaneus	Branch of tibial
platysma	Wrinkles skin of neck and chest; depresses jaw and lower lip	Clavicle, acromion and fascia over deltoid, and pectoralis major	Lower border of mandible, risorius, and opposite platysma	Cervical branch of facial
popliteus	Flexes leg and rotates it inward	External condyle of femur	Posterior surface of tibia	Branch of tibial
procerus SYN: pyramidalis nasi	Draws skin of forehead down	Bridge of nose	Skin over root of nose	Facial

Muscles *(Continued)*

Name	Action	Origin	Insertion	Innervation
pronator pedis Same as: quadratus plantae, q.v.				
pronator quadratus	Pronates forearm	Lower fourth of ulna	Lower fourth of radius	Volar interosseous
pronator teres Consists of (1) humeral head and (2) ulnar head	Pronates hand	(1) Medial epicondyle of humerus. (2) Coronoid process of ulna	Lateral surface of shaft of radius	Branch of median
psoas major SYN: psoas magnus	Flexes thigh, adducts and rotates it medially	Last thoracic and all of the lumbar vertebrae	Lesser trochanter of femur	Lumbar plexus
psoas minor SYN: psoas parvus	Tenses iliac fascia	Twelfth thoracic and 1st lumbar vertebrae	Iliac fascia and iliopectineal tuberosity	Branch of lumbar
pterygoideus lateralis	Brings jaw forward, moves jaw from side to side; open jaws	(1) Outer plate of pterygoid process. (2) Great wing of sphenoid and infratemporal ridge	Neck of condyle of mandible	Lateral pterygoid from trigeminal nerve
pterygoideus medialis	Closes jaw by raising and advancing it	Pterygoid fossa of sphenoid bone	Inner surface of angle of mandible	Medial pterygoid from trigeminal nerve
pyramidalis	Tightens linea alba	Pubic crest	Linea alba	Branch of 12th thoracic
pyramidalis nasi Same as: procerus, q.v.				
pyriformis Same as: piriformis, q.v.				
quadratus femoris	Rotates thigh outward	Ischial tuberosity	Intertrochanteric ridge	Sciatic
quadratus labii inferioris Same as: depressor labii inferioris, q.v.				

quadratus labii superioris Composed of levator labii superioris, q.v.; zygomaticus minor, q.v.				
quadratus lumborum	Flexes trunk laterally and forward	Iliac crest, iliolumbar ligament, lower lumbar vertebrae	Twelfth rib and the upper lumbar vertebrae	Branches of 1st lumbar and 12th thoracic
quadratus menti Same as: depressor labii inferioris, q.v.				
quadratus plantae SYN: flexor accessorius	Assists flexing of toes	Inferior surface of os calcis by two heads from outer and inner borders	Tendons of flexor digitorum longus	Branch of lateral plantar
quadriceps extensor femoris Same as: quadriceps femoris				
quadriceps femoris	Extends leg	By four heads: rectus femoris, vastus medialis, vastus lateralis, and vastus intermedius	Patella and tibial tuberosity	Branches of femoral
radiocarpus Same as: flexor carpi radialis, q.v.				
rectus abdominis	Compresses abdomen	Pubis	Cartilage of 5th to 7th ribs	Branches of 7th to 12th intercostal
rectus capitis anterior	Turns and inclines the head	Base of atlas	Occipital bone, basilar process	Between 1st and 2nd cervical
rectus capitis anticus major Same as: longus capitis, q.v.				

Muscles *(Continued)*

Name	Action	Origin	Insertion	Innervation
rectus capitis anticus minor Same as: rectus capitis anterior, q.v.				
rectus capitis lateralis	Inclines head laterally and supports it	Transverse process of atlas	Jugular process of occipital bone	Between 1st and 2nd cervical nerves
rectus capitis posterior major SYN: rectus capitis posticus major	Rotates and draws head backward	Spine of axis	Inferior curved line of occipital bone	Suboccipital
rectus capitis posterior minor SYN: rectus capitis posticus minor	Rotates and draws head backward	Posterior tubercle of atlas	Inferior curved line of occipital bone	Suboccipital
rectus externus or lateralis	Rotates eyeball outward	Margin of sphenoidal fissure and outer margin of optic foramen	Sclerotic coat	Abducent
rectus femoris	Extends leg	Iliac spine, upper margin of acetabulum	Base of patella	Femoral
rectus inferior	Rotates eyeball downward	Lower margin of optic foramen	Sclerotic coat	Oculomotor
rectus internus or medialis	Rotates eyeball inward	Lower margin of optic foramen	Sclerotic coat	Oculomotor
rectus superior	Rotates eyeball upward	Upper margin of optic foramen	Sclerotic coat	Oculomotor
retrahens aurem Same as: auricularis posterior, q.v.				

risorius	Draws angle of mouth outward ("laughing muscle")	Fascia over masseter muscle	Angle of mouth	Facial; buccal branch
rhomboideus major	Elevates scapula	Spinous processes of 2nd to 5th thoracic vertebrae	Vertebral border of scapula below spine	Dorsal scapular from brachial plexus
rhomboideus minor	Retracts and elevates scapula	Spinous processes of 7th cervical vertebra and 1st thoracic vertebra	Border of scapula above spine	Dorsal scapular from brachial plexus
rotatores SYN: rotatores spinae	Extend and rotate the vertebral column	Transverse processes of 2nd to 12th dorsal vertebrae	Lamina of next vertebra above	Branches of dorsal divisions of spinal
rotatores spinae Same as: rotatores, q.v.				
sacrolumbalis Same as: iliocostales lumborum, q.v.				
sacrospinalis	Extends vertebral column	Sacrum, lumbar vertebrae, iliac crest	Iliocostalis and longissimus dorsi	Posterior branches of spinal
salpingopharyngeus	Elevates nasopharynx	Eustachian tube close to nasopharynx	Posterior portion of the pharyngopalatinue	Plexus
sartorius	Flexes and rotates thigh and leg	Anterior superior iliac spine	Tibial tuberosity	Branches of femoral
scalenus anterior SYN: scalenus anticus	Elevates 1st rib and flexes neck	Transverse processes of 3rd to 6th cervical vertebrae	Tubercle of 1st rib	Cervical plexus
scalenus medius	Elevates 1st rib and flexes neck	Transverse processes of 2nd to 6th cervical vertebrae	First rib	Cervical plexus
scalenus posterior SYN: scalenus posticus	Elevates 2nd rib and flexes neck	Transverse processes of 4th to 6th cervical vertebrae	Second rib	Cervical and brachial plexus
semimembranosus	Flexes and rotates leg; extends thigh	Ischial tuberosity	Medial condyle of tibia	Tibial portion of sciatic

Muscles *(Continued)*

Name	Action	Origin	Insertion	Innervation
semispinalis capitis SYN: complexus	Rotates and draws head backward	Transverse processes of upper six or seven thoracic and lower four cervical vertebrae	Occipital bone, between inferior and superior curved line	Branches of dorsal division of cervical
semispinalis cervicis	Extend the vertebral column and rotate it toward the opposite side	Transverse processes of upper five or six thoracic vertebrae	Spines from axis to 5th cervical vertebra	Branches of dorsal divisions of spinal
semispinalis colli Same as: semispinalis cervicis, q.v.				
semispinalis dorsi Same as: semispinalis thoracis, q.v.				
semispinalis thoracis SYN: semispinalis dorsi	Extend the vertebral column and rotate it toward the opposite side	Transverse processes of 6th to 10th thoracic vertebrae	Spines of upper four thoracic and lower two cervical vertebrae	Branches of dorsal divisions of spinal
semitendinosus	Flexes and rotates leg; extends thigh	Ischial tuberosity	Shaft of tibia below internal tuberosity	Tibial portion of sciatic
serratus anterior	Elevates ribs, rotates scapula	Upper eight or nine ribs	Angles and vertebral border of scapula	Long thoracic from brachial plexus
serratus magnus Same as: serratus anterior, q.v.				
serratus posterior inferior SYN: serratus posticus inferior	Draws ribs back and downward	Spines of lower two thoracic and upper two lumbar vertebrae	Lower four ribs	Branches of ventral divisions of 9th to 12th thoracic
serratus posterior superior SYN: serratus posticus	Elevates the ribs	Spines of 7th cervical and two upper thoracic	Angles of 2nd to 5th ribs	Branches of ventral divisions of thoracic

superior		vertebrae		
soleus	Extends and rotates foot	Upper shaft of fibula, oblique line of tibia	By tendo calcaneus to os calcis	Tibial
sphincter ani externus	Closes anus	Ring of fibers surrounding anus	Coccyx and central point of perineum	Hemorrhoidal branch of pudendal
sphincter ani internus	Contracts rectum and anus, but not voluntarily	Muscular ring of rectal fibers above canal		
sphincter pylori A thickening of middle circular layer of the gastric musculature surrounding the pylorus				
sphincter urethrae membranaceae SYN: compressor urethrae; constrictor urethrae	Constricts membranous urethra	Ramus of pubis	Behind and in front of urethra	Perineal branch of pudendal
sphincter vaginae Same as: bulbocavernosus, q.v.				
sphincter vesicae	Shuts off internal orifice of urethra	Near urethral orifice of bladder		Sacral and hypogastric
spinalis capitis SYN: biventer capitis		Inconstant; from spines of upper dorsal and lower cervical vertebrae	Blends with the semispinalis capitis	
spinalis cervicis	Extends cervical spine	Spines of 5th, 6th, and 7th cervical vertebrae	Axis and occasionally, the two vertebrae below	Branches of cervical
spinalis thoracis SYN: spinalis dorsi	Erects spinal column	Spines of first two lumbar and last two thoracic vertebrae	Spines of middle and upper thoracic vertebrae	Dorsal branches of spinal

Muscles *(Continued)*

Name	Action	Origin	Insertion	Innervation
splenius capitis	Rotates and extends head	Ligamentum nuchae, 7th cervical and first three thoracic vertebrae	Mastoid process and superior curved line of occiput	Branches of dorsal divisions of cervical
splenius cervicis SYN: splenius colli	Rotates and flexes head and neck	Spines of 3rd to 6th thoracic vertebrae	Transverse processes of 1st and 2nd cervical vertebrae	Branches of dorsal divisions of cervical
splenius colli Same as: splenius cervicis, q.v.				
stapedius	Depress base of the stapes	Interior of pyramid	Neck of stapes	Tympanic branch of facial
sternocleidomastoideus SYN: sternomastoid muscle	Rotates and depresses head	By two heads, from sternum and clavicle	Mastoid process and outer part of superior curved line of occipital bone	Spinal accessory
sternohyoideus SYN: sternohyoid muscle	Depresses hyoid bone	Manubrium sterni and 1st costal cartilage	Body of hyoid bone	Upper cervical through ansa hypoglossi
sternothyreoideus SYN: sternothyroid muscle	Depresses thyroid cartilage	Sternum and 1st costal cartilage	Side of thyroid cartilage	Upper cervical through ansa hypoglossi
styloglossus	Retracts and elevates tongue	Styloid process	Side of tongue	Hypoglossal
stylohyoideus SYN: stylohyoid muscle	Fixes hyoid, drawing it up and back	Styloid process	Body of hyoid bone	Facial
stylopharyngeus	Elevates and dilates pharynx	Styloid process	Thyroid cartilage and side of pharynx	Glossopharyngeal
subanconeus	Tightens posterior ligament of elbow	Lower portion of humerus	Posterior ligament of elbow joint	Radial

subclavius	Draws clavicle down and forward or elevates the 1st rib	First rib and cartilage	Undersurface of clavicle	Special nerve with fibers from 5th and 6th cervical
subcostales	Draw ribs together and lower ribs	Inconstant; inner surface of the ribs	Inner surface of one of the ribs just below	Intercostal
subcrureus Same as: articularis genu				
subscapularis	Rotates humerus inward and lowers it	Subscapular fossa	Lesser tubercle of humerus	Subscapular
supinator SYN: supinator radii brevis	Supinates hand	Lateral epicondyle of humerus; oblique line of ulna; elbow joint	Outer surface of radius	Branch of radial
supinator longus Same as: brachioradialis, q.v.				
supinator radii brevis Same as: supinator, q.v.				
supraspinatus	Abducts and raises arm	Supraspinous fossa of scapula	Greater tubercle of humerus	Branches of suprascapular
supraspinatus	Abducts arm	Supraspinatus fossa	Greater tuberosity of humerus	Branches of suprascapular
suspensorius duodeni Wide, flat band of unstriped muscle attached to the left crus of diaphragm and continuous with the muscular coat of the duodenum at its line of junction with the jejunum				
temporalis SYN: temporal	Closes jaws	Temporal fossa and temporal fascia	Coronoid process of lower jaw	Trigeminal; mandibular division

Muscles *(Continued)*

Name	Action	Origin	Insertion	Innervation
tensor fasciae latae	Flexes and rotates thigh	Iliac crest, iliac spine, fascia lata	Iliotibial band of fascia lata	Branch of superior gluteal
tensor fasciae femoris Same as: tensor fasciae latae, q.v.				
tensor palati Same as: tensor veli palatini, q.v.				
tensor tarsi Same as: lacrimal part of orbicularis oculi muscle, q.v.				
tensor tympani	To draw the membrana tympani tense	Temporal tube, eustachian tube and canal	Handle of malleus	Branch of mandibular through otic ganglion
tensor veli palatini SYN: tensor palati	Stretches soft palate	Spine of sphenoid, scaphoid fossa of internal pterygoid process and eustachian tube	Posterior border of hard palate and aponeurosis of soft palate	Otic ganglion, trigeminal nerve
teres major	Rotates arm inward, draws it down and back	Axillary border of scapula	Lesser tubercle of humerus	Branch of lower subscapular
teres minor	Rotates arm outward	Axillary border of scapula	Greater tubercle of humerus	Branch of axillary (circumflex)
thyreoarytenoideus SYN: thyroarytenoid	Relaxes vocal cords	Thyroid cartilage	Arytenoid cartilage	Laryngeal, recurrent
thyreoepiglotticus SYN: thyroepiglotticus	Depresses epiglottis	Thyroid cartilage	Epiglottis and sacculus laryngis	Laryngeal, recurrent
thyreohyoideus	Depresses hyoid bone;	Side of thyroid cartilage	Cornu and body of hyoid	Hypoglossal

SYN: thyrohyoid muscle	elevates thyroid cartilage if hyoid bone is fixed		bone	
tibialis anterior SYN: tibialis anticus	Elevates and flexes foot	Upper tibia, interosseus membrane, and intermuscular septum	Internal cuneiform and 1st metatarsal	Branch of peroneal
tibialis posterior SYN: tibialis posticus	Extends tarsus and flexes foot	Shaft of fibula and tibia	Tuberosity of scaphoid, 2nd to 4th metatarsal, internal cuneiform	Branch of tibial
trachelomastoid Same as: longissimus capitis, q.v.				
tragicus		Outer part of tragus	Outer part of tragus	Temporal branch of facial
transversalis abdominis Same as: transversus abdominis, q.v.				
transversalis colli Same as: longissimus cervicis, q.v.				
transversus abdominis	Compresses abdomen, flexes thorax	Lumbar fascia, 7th to 12th costal cartilages, inguinal ligament, iliac crest	Xiphoid cartilage, linea alba, pubic crest, and iliopectineal linc	Iliohypogastric, ilioinguinal, and branches of intercostal
transversus auriculae	Retracts helix	Cranial surface of pinna	Circumference of pinna	Posterior auricular branch of facial
transversus pedis			Transverse head of adductor hallucis	
transversus perinei profundus	Assists compressor urethrae	Ramus of ischium	Central tendon	Perineal branch of pudendal
transversus perinei superficialis	Tenses central tendon	Ramus of ischium	Central point of perineum	Perineal branch of pudendal

Muscles *(Continued)*

Name	Action	Origin	Insertion	Innervation
transversus thoracis	Narrows the chest	Xiphoid cartilage and sternum	Costal cartilages, 2nd to 6th ribs	Branches of intercostal
trapezius	Draws head back and to the side, rotates scapula	Superior curved line of occipital, spinous processes of 7th cervical and all thoracic vertebrae	Clavicle, acromion, base of spine of scapula	Spinal accessory and cervical plexus
triangularis Same as: depressor anguli oris, q.v.				
triangularis sterni Same as: transversus thoracis				
triceps brachii Consists of three heads: (1) long, (2) lateral, and (3) medial	Extends forearm and arm	(1) Infraglenoid tubercle of scapula. (2) Posterior surface of humerus below great tubercle. (3) Humerus below radial groove	Olecranon process of ulna	Branches of radial
uvulae	Elevates the uvula	Posterior nasal spine	Forms large part of uvula	Pharyngeal plexus
vastus intermedius SYN: crureus		Upper part of anterior surface of shaft of femur	Common tendon of quadriceps femoris	Branches of femoral
vastus lateralis SYN: vastus externus	Extends knee	Linea aspera to greater trochanter	Common tendon of quadriceps femoris	Branches of femoral
vastus medialis SYN: vastus internus	Extends leg; draws patella in	Linea aspera of femur	Common tendon of quadriceps femoris	Branches of femoral
zygomaticus major	Draws upper lip backward, upward, and outward	Malar bone, zygomatic arch	Angle of mouth	Facial
zygomaticus minor	Draws the upper lip up and out	Malar bone behind the maxillary arch	Angle of mouth, orbicularis oris	Facial

Principal Joints

Name	Type	Ligaments
Acromioclavicular	Arthrodial	Capsular; superior and inferior acromioclavicular; articular disk; coracoclavicular (trapezoid and conoid)
Ankle	Ginglymus	Capsular; deltoid; anterior and posterior talofibular; calcaneofibular
Atlas	Trochoid; arthrodial	Capsular; anterior and posterior atlantoaxial; transverse
Calcaneocuboid	Arthrodial	Capsular; dorsal calcaneocuboid; bifurcated; long plantar; plantar calcaneocuboid
Carpometacarpal	Arthrodial	Dorsal; volar; interosseous
Elbow	Ginglymus (hinge)	Capsular; ulnar and radial collateral
Hip	Enarthrodial	Capsular; iliofemoral; pubocapsular; ischiofemoral; round ligament of femur; transverse acetabular
Intercarpal		
Carpal, proximal	Arthrodial	Dorsal; volar; interosseous
Carpal, distal	Arthrodial	Dorsal; volar; interosseous
Carpal bones, two rows with each other		Volar; dorsal; collateral
Intermetacarpal		Dorsal; volar; interosseous; transverse metacarpal
Intermetatarsal	Arthrodial	Dorsal; plantar; interosseous
Interphalangeal	Ginglymus	Collateral; volar in fingers and plantar in toes
Knee	Condyloid and Arthrodial	Capsular; patellar; oblique and arcuate popliteal; tibial and fibular collateral; anterior and posterior cruciate; medial and lateral menisci; transverse; coronary
Mandible (Jaw)	Ginglymus; arthrodial	Capsular; temporomandibular; sphenomandibular; articular disk; stylomandibular
Metacarpophalangeal	Condyloid	Volar; collateral
Metatarsophalangeal	Condyloid	Plantar; collateral
Pubic	Amphiarthrodial	Superior and arcuate pubic; interpubic fibrocartilaginous layer
Radioulnar, distal	Trochoid (pivot)	Ulnar collateral; articular disk

Name	Type	Ligaments
Radioulnar, middle	Trochoid	Oblique; interosseous
Radioulnar, proximal	Trochoid	Annular
Ribs, heads of	Arthrodial	Capsular; radiate; intra-articular
Ribs, tubercles and necks of	Arthrodial	Capsular; anterior and posterior costotransverse; neck of rib; tubercle of rib
Sacrococcygeal	Amphiarthrodial	Anterior, posterior, and lateral sacrococcygeal; interposed fibrocartilage; interarticular
Sacroiliac		Anterior and posterior sacroiliac; interosseous
Sacrum and ischium		Sacrotuberous; sacrospinous
Shoulder	Enarthrodial (ball-and-socket)	Capsular; coracohumeral; glenohumeral; transverse humeral; glenoid of humerus
Sternoclavicular	Double arthrodial	Capsular; anterior and posterior sternoclavicular; inter- and costoclavicular; articular disk
Sternocostal	Arthrodial	Capsular; radiate and intra-articular sternocostal; costoxiphoid
Subtalar	Arthrodial	Capsular; anterior, posterior, lateral, medial, and interosseous; talocalcaneal
Talo-calcaneonavicular	Arthrodial	Capsular; dorsal talonavicular
Tarsometatarsal	Arthrodial	Dorsal; plantar; interosseous
Tibiofibular	Arthrodial	Capsular; anterior; posterior
Tibiofibular syndesmosis	Arthrodial	Anterior and posterior tibiofibular; inferior transverse; interosseous
Vertebral arches	Arthrodial	Capsular; flaval; supraspinal; nuchal; interspinal; intertransverse
Vertebral bodies	Amphiarthrodial	Anterior and posterior longitudinal; intervertebral fibrocartilages
Vertebral column with cranium	Condyloid	Capsular; anterior and posterior atlanto-occipital membrane; lateral; tectorial membrane; alar; apical odontoid
Wrist	Condyloid	Volar and dorsal radiocarpal; ulnar and radial collateral

Nerves

Name	NA Term*	Origin	Function	Distribution
Abducent (6th cranial n.)	N. abducens	Pons	Motor	Lateral rectus muscle of eye.
Accessory (11th cranial n.)	N. accessorius	Medulla oblongata and spinal cord	Motor	Sternomastoid and trapezius muscles.
Auditory (8th cranial n.)	N. vestibulocochlearis	Cochlea	Special sense of hearing	Internal auditory meatus.
Auricular, great	N. auricularis magnus	Second and third cervical through cervical plexus	Sensory	Side of neck; skin of ear and cheek.
Auricular, posterior	N. auricularis posterior	Facial	Motor	Posterior auricular muscle.
Auriculotemporal	N. auriculotemporalis	Mandibular div. of trigeminal	Sensory	Side of scalp.
Buccal	N. buccalis	Mandibular div. of trigeminal	Sensory	Skin and mucous membrane of cheek.
Calcanean, internal		Posterior tibial	Sensory	Sole of foot.
Cervical n., superficial (cutaneous cervical n.; transverse n. of neck)	N. transversus colli	Second and third cervical through cervical plexus	Sensory	Skin of front of neck.
Chorda, tympani		Facial	Motor	Sublingua[illegible] submaxillary glands
Ciliary, long	Nn. ciliares longi	Nasal	Sensory and motor	Corr[illegible]is, and ciliary body.

*Nomina Anatomica

Nerves (*Continued*)

Name	NA Equivalents*	Origin	Function	Distribution
Ciliary, short	Nn. ciliares breves	Ciliary ganglion	Sensory and motor	Cornea, iris, and ciliary body.
Circumflex (Axillary)	N. axillaris	Posterior cord of brachial plexus	Motor and sensory	Deltoid, teres minor, shoulder joint, and overlying skin.
Coccygeal	N. coccygeus	Spinal cord	Motor and sensory	Coccygeus muscle and skin over coccyx.
Cochlear. SEE: *Vestibulocochlear n.*		Auditory	Special sense of hearing	Cochlea.
Crural, anterior. SEE: *Femoral n.*				
Cutaneous, internal	N. cutaneus antebrachii medialis	Inner cord of brachial plexus	Sensory	Skin of inner aspect of forearm.
Cutaneous, lesser internal	N. cutaneus brachii medialis	Inner cord of brachial plexus	Sensory	Skin of inner aspect of upper arm.
Dental, inferior	N. alveolaris inferior	Mandibular div. of trigeminal	Sensory and motor	Teeth of lower jaw, mylohyoid muscle, and skin of chin.
Dental, superior	Nn. alveolares superiores	Maxillary div. of trigeminal	Sensory	Upper teeth and gums.
Digastric		Facial	Motor	Stylohyoid and posterior belly of digastric muscle.
Facial (7th cranial n.)	N. facialis	Pons	Motor	Muscles of expression.

Femoral (anterior crural n.)	N. femoralis	2nd, 3rd, and 4th lumbar	Motor and sensory	Muscles and skin of thigh.
Frontal	N. frontalis	Ophthalmic div. of trigeminal	Sensory	Skin of forehead.
Genitofemoral (genitocrural n.)	N. genitofemoralis	1st and 2nd lumbar	Sensory and motor	Cremaster muscle and skin of groin and upper part of thigh.
Glossopharyngeal (9th cranial n.)	N. glossopharyngeus	Medulla oblongata	Motor and sensory	Muscles and mucous membrane of pharynx, fauces, and posterior third of tongue.
Gluteal, inferior	N. gluteus inferior	5th lumbar and 1st and 2nd sacral	Motor	Gluteus maximus.
Gluteal, superior	N. gluteus superior	4th and 5th lumbar and 1st sacral	Motor	Gluteus medius and minimus, tensor fasciae femoris.
Hypogastric	N. hypogastricus	Iliohypogastric	Motor and sensory	Muscles and skin of abdominal wall.
Hypoglossal (12th cranial n.)	N. hypoglossus	Hypoglossal nucleus in medulla oblongata	Motor	Intrinsic muscles of tongue.
Iliac	Ramus cutaneus lateralis	Iliohypogastric	Sensory	Skin of gluteal region.
Iliohypogastric	N. iliohypogastricus	1st lumbar	Sensory and motor	Muscles and skin of hypogastrium.
Ilioinguinal	N. ilioinguinalis	1st lumbar	Sensory and motor	Muscles of abdominal wall, skin of upper thigh, skin of root of penis and scrotum (in male), and skin of mons pubis and labium majus (in female).

*Nomina Anatomica

Nerves (*Continued*)

Name	NA Equivalents*	Origin	Function	Distribution
Infraorbital	N. infraorbitalis	Maxillary div. of trigeminal	Sensory	Skin of cheek and all upper teeth except molars.
Infratrochlear	N. infratrochlearis	Nasociliary	Sensory	Skin of lower eyelid and root of nose, conjunctiva, and lacrimal sac and caruncle.
Intercostal	Nn. intercostales	Thoracic	Sensory and motor	Muscles and skin of back, thorax, and upper abdomen.
Intercostobrachial	Nn. intercosto-brachiales	2nd intercostal	Sensory	Skin of axilla and medial side of arm.
Interosseous anterior (volar interosseous n.)	N. interosseus anterior	Median	Motor	Deep flexor and pronator muscles of forearm.
Interosseous, posterior	N. interosseus posterior	Musculospiral (radial)	Motor and sensory	Muscles and skin of back of forearm and wrist.
Lacrimal	N. lacrimalis	Ophthalmic div. of trigeminal	Sensory	Lacrimal gland, conjunctiva, and skin of upper eyelid.
Laryngeal, inferior	N. laryngeus inferior	Branch of recurrent laryngeal	Motor	Muscles of larynx except cricothyroid.
Laryngeal, recurrent	N. laryngeus recurrens	Vagus	Motor	Muscles of larynx except cricothyroid.
Laryngeal, superior	N. laryngeus superior	Vagus	Motor and sensory	Mucous membrane of larynx; arytenoid and cricothyroid muscles.

Lingual	N. lingualis	Mandibular div. of trigeminal	Sensory	Mucous membrane of anterior two thirds of tongue and floor and outer wall of mouth.
Lumbar	Nn. lumbales	Spinal cord	Motor and sensory	Loins and front of lower abdomen and thigh to help in forming lumbar and sacral plexuses.
Mandibular	N. mandibularis	Trigeminal	Motor and sensory	Teeth, gums, and skin of lower jaw and cheek; muscles of mastication; mucous membrane of anterior two thirds of tongue.
Masseteric	N. massetericus	Mandibular div. of trigeminal	Motor	Masseter muscle.
Maxillary	N. maxillaris	Trigeminal	Sensory	Nasal pharynx, palate, teeth of upper jaw and skin of cheek.
Median	N. medianus	Internal and external cords of brachial plexus	Motor and sensory	Pronators and flexors of forearm, two external lumbricales, thenar muscles, skin of palm and first four fingers.
Mental	N. mentalis	Inferior dental	Sensory	Skin and mucous membrane of lower lip and chin.
Musculocutaneous	N. musculocutaneus	External cord of brachial plexus	Motor and sensory	Flexors of upper arm and skin of external aspect of forearm.
Musculospiral. SEE: *Radial n.*				
Mylohyoid	N. mylohyoideus	Inferior dental	Motor	Mylohyoid muscle and anterior belly of digastric muscle.

**Nomina Anatomica*

Nerves (*Continued*)

Name	NA Equivalents*	Origin	Function	Distribution
Nasal (nasociliary n.)	N. nasociliaris	Ophthalmic div. of trigeminal	Sensory	Ciliary ganglion, iris, conjunctiva, ethmoid cells, mucous membrane and skin of nose.
Nasopalatine	N. nasopalatinus	Meckel's ganglion (sphenopalatine ganglion)	Sensory	Mucous membrane of nose and palate.
Obturator	N. obturatorius	2nd, 3rd, and 4th lumbar through lumbar plexus	Motor and sensory	Adductors of thigh, hip and knee joints; skin of inner aspect of thigh.
Occipital, greater	N. occipitalis major	2nd cervical	Motor and sensory	Muscles of back of neck; skin over occiput.
Occipital, lesser	N. occipitalis minor	2nd and 3rd cervical	Sensory	Skin behind ear and on back of scalp.
Occipital, third	N. occipitalis tertius	3rd cervical	Sensory	Skin of back of head and nape of neck.
Oculomotor (3rd cranial n.)	N. oculomotorius	Floor of aqueduct of Sylvius	Motor	All ocular muscles except lateral rectus and superior oblique.
Olfactory (1st cranial n.)	Nn. olfactorii	Olfactory lobe	Special sense of smell	Nasal mucous membranes in olfactory region.
Ophthalmic	N. ophthalmicus	1st div. of trigeminal	Sensory	Lacrimal gland, conjunctiva, skin of forehead, skin and mucous membrane of nose.
Optic (2nd cranial n.)	N. opticus	Corpora quadrigemina	Special sense of sight	Retina.

Palatine, anterior, middle, and posterior	Nn. palatini	Meckel's ganglion	Motor	Mucous membrane of palate.
Perineal	N. perineales	Pudendal	Motor and sensory	Muscles and skin of perineum.
Peroneal, common (lateral popliteal n.)	N. peroneus communis	Sciatic	Motor and sensory	Extensor muscles of lower leg and foot and overlying skin.
Phrenic	N. phrenicus	3rd, 4th, and 5th cervical	Motor and sensory	Diaphragm.
Pneumogastric. SEE: *Vagus n.*				
Popliteal, deep. SEE: *Tibial n.*				
Popliteal, lateral. SEE: *Peroneal n., common.*				
Pterygoid	N. pterygoideus	Mandibular div. of trigeminal	Motor	Lateral and medial pterygoid muscles.
Pterygoid canal, n. of. SEE: *Vidian n.*				
Pudendal	N. pudendus	2nd, 3rd, and 4th sacral	Sensory	Skin and muscles of perineum and genitalia.
Radial (musculospiral n.)	N. radialis	Brachial plexus	Motor and sensory	Skin of back of entire arm and hand; extensor muscles of entire arm and hand.
Sacral	Nn. sacrales	Spinal cord	Motor and sensory	Muscles and skin of loins and lower extremities.
Saphenous, external or short. SEE: *Sural n.*				

**Nomina Anatomica*

Nerves (*Continued*)

Name	NA Equivalents*	Origin	Function	Distribution
Saphenous, internal or long	N. saphenus	Femoral	Sensory	Skin of inner aspect of knee, leg, ankle, and dorsum of foot.
Sciatic (great sciatic n.)	N. ischiadicus	Sacral plexus	Motor and sensory	Muscles of calf and back of thigh; skin of lower calf and upper surface of foot.
Sphenopalatine	N. pterygopalatini	Maxillary div. of trigeminal	Sensory	Meckel's ganglion.
Spinal accessory (accessory n.; 11th cranial n.)	N. accessorius	Floor of 4th ventricle and cervical cord	Motor	Sternomastoid and trapezius muscles.
Stapedial	N. stapedius	Facial	Motor	Stapedius muscle.
Stylohyoid		Facial	Motor	Stylohyoid muscle.
Suboccipital	N. suboccipitalis	Posterior div. of 1st cervical	Motor	Complexus oblique and rectus muscles of back of neck.
Subscapular	Nn. subscapularis	Posterior cord of brachial plexus	Motor	Teres major and subscapularis muscles.
Supraclavicular, intermediate (supraclavicular n., middle; supraclavicular n.)	N. supraclaviculares intermedii	3rd and 4th cervical	Sensory	Skin of fossa below collar bone.
Supraclavicular, lateral (supraclavicular n., posterior; supraacromial n.)	N. supraclaviculares laterales	3rd and 4th cervical	Sensory	Skin of shoulder.
Supraclavicular, medial (supra-	N. supraclaviculares	3rd and 4th cervical	Sensory	Skin over upper part of thorax.

clavicular n., anterior; suprasternal n.)	mediales			
Supraorbital	N. supraorbitalis	Frontal	Sensory	Forehead, upper eyelid, scalp, and frontal sinus.
Suprascapular	N. suprascapularis	5th and 6th cervical	Motor	Supraspinatus and infraspinatus muscles and the shoulder joint.
Supratrochlear	N. supratrochlearis	Frontal	Sensory	Skin of upper eyelid and root of nose.
Sural	N. suralis	Common peroneal and tibial n.'s	Sensory	Skin of calf and medial side of foot to great toe.
Temporal, deep	N. temporalis profundi	Mandibular div. of trigeminal	Motor	Temporal muscle.
Thoracic	Nn. thoracici	Spinal cord	Motor and sensory	Muscles and skin of thorax.
Thoracic, anterior		Brachial plexus	Motor	Pectoralis minor and major muscles.
Thoracic, long (posterior thoracic n.; external respiratory n. of Bell).	N. thoracicus longus	5th, 6th, and 7th cervical	Motor	Serratus anterior muscle.
Tibial	N. tibialis	Sciatic	Motor and sensory	Flexor muscles of back of knee joint and calf; skin of lower leg.
Trigeminal (5th cranial n.; trifacial n.)	N. trigeminus	Midbrain and pons	Motor and sensory	Skin of face, tongue, teeth; muscles of mastication.

Nomina Anatomica

Nerves (*Continued*)

Name	NA Equivalents*	Origin	Function	Distribution
Trochlear (4th cranial n.; pathetic n.)	N. trochlearis	Floor of aqueduct of Sylvius	Motor	Superior oblique muscle of eye.
Tympanic (Jacobson's n.)	N. tympanicus	Glossopharyngeal	Sensory	Tympanum, eustachian tube, and structures of middle ear.
Ulnar	N. ulnaris	Medial cord of brachial plexus	Motor and sensory	Muscles and skin of forearm and hand.
Vagus (10th cranial n.; pneumogastric n.)	N. vagus	Medulla oblongata	Motor and sensory	Pharynx, larynx, heart, lungs, stomach.
Vestibulocochlear (8th cranial n.; acoustic n.; auditory n.)	N. vestibulocochlearis	Ganglion of Scarpa and ganglion of Corti	Sense of hearing	Internal auditory meatus.
Vidian	N. canalis pterygoidei	Facial	Sensory	Meckel's ganglion (sphenopalatine ganglion).
Zygomatic	N. zygomaticus	Maxillary div. of trigeminal	Sensory	Skin of temple and cheek bone.

**Nomina Anatomica*

Nerve Plexuses of the Sympathetic and Cerebrospinal Systems

aortic (ā-or′tĭk). (*Abdominal*). ORIGIN: Semilunar, lumbar ganglia, renal and solar plexuses. LOCATION: Sides and front of aorta. DISTRIBUTION: Inferior mesenteric, spermatic and hypogastric plexus. Filaments to inferior vena cava. (*Thoracic*). ORIGIN: Thoracic ganglia of sympathetic nerve, cardiac plexus. LOCATION: Surrounding the thoracic aorta. DISTRIBUTION: Solar plexus, aorta.

***brachial** (brā′kē-ăl). ORIGIN: Anterior branches of 5th, 6th, 7th, 8th, cervical, and greater part of 1st dorsal nerves. LOCATION: Lower part of neck to axilla. DISTRIBUTION: Sixteen branches of suprascapular, subscapular, rhomboid, median, ulnar, musculospiral, posterior thoracic, musculothoracic, circumflex, musculocutaneous nerves.

cardiac (kar′dē-ăk). (*Great or Deep*). ORIGIN: Cardiac nerves of cervical ganglion of sympathetic and vagus. LOCATION: In front of bifurcation of trachea. DISTRIBUTION: Pulmonary, coronary and cardiac plexuses. (*Superficial or Anterior*). ORIGIN: Left superior cardiac nerve, branch of vagus and filaments of deep cardiac plexus. LOCATION: Beneath arch of aorta. Front of right pulmonary artery. DISTRIBUTION: Coronary and pulmonary plexuses.

carotid (kăr-ŏt′ĭd). (*External*). ORIGIN: Pharyngeal plexus, superior cardiac nerve, and superior cervical ganglion. LOCATION: Around external carotid artery. DISTRIBUTION: External carotid artery and its branches. (*Internal*). ORIGIN: Asympathetic plexus. LOCATION: Surrounding internal carotid artery. DISTRIBUTION: Tympanic plexus, sphenopalatine ganglion, abducens and oculomotor nerves, the cerebral vessels, and the ciliary ganglion.

cavernous (kăv′ĕr-nŭs). ORIGIN: 3rd to 6th cranial nerves and ophthalmic ganglion. LOCATION: Cavernous sinus. DISTRIBUTION: Wall of internal carotid artery.

celiac (sē′lē-ăk). ORIGIN: Solar plexus, branches from lesser splanchnic and vagus nerves. LOCATION: Behind stomach, in front of aorta at level of origin of celiac artery. DISTRIBUTION: Coronary, hepatic, pyloric, gastroduodenal, gastroepiploic and splenic plexuses. SYN: *solar plexus*.

***cervical** (ser′vĭ-kăl). ORIGIN: Anterior branches of first four cervical nerves. LOCATION: Beneath sternocleidomastoid muscle opposite first four cervical vertebrae. DISTRIBUTION: Cutaneous, muscular, and communicating rami.

***coccygeal** (kŏk-sĭj′ē-ăl). ORIGIN: Fourth and 5th sacral and the coccygeal nerves. LOCATION: Dorsal surface of coccyx and caudal end of sacrum. DISTRIBUTION: Anococcygeal nerves.

cystic (sĭs′tĭk). ORIGIN: Hepatic plexus. LOCATION: At gallbladder. DISTRIBUTION: Gallbladder.

esophageal (ē-sō-făj′ē-ăl). ORIGIN: Vagus nerve, thoracic sympathetic ganglia. LOCATION: Around the esophagus. DISTRIBUTION: Esophagus.

gastric (găs′trĭk). ORIGIN: Celiac plexus and continuations of esophageal plexuses. LOCATION: Gastric artery. DISTRIBUTION: Abdominal viscera.

hemorrhoidal (hĕm″ō-roy′dăl). ORIGIN: Pelvic and inferior mesenteric plexuses. LOCATION: Rectum and sides of rectum. DISTRIBUTION: Rectum.

hepatic (hē-păt′ĭk). ORIGIN: Celiac plexus, left vagus, right phrenic. LOCATION: Accompanies hepatic artery. DISTRIBUTION: Liver.

hypogastric (hī″pō-găs′trĭk). ORIGIN: Aortic plexus and lumbar ganglia. LOCATION: Promontory of sacrum. DISTRIBUTION: Pelvic plexus.

***lumbar** (lŭm′băr). ORIGIN: First four lumbar nerves. LOCATION: Psoas muscle. DISTRIBUTION: Iliohypogastric, ilioinguinal, genitocrural, external cutaneous, obturator, accessory, and anterior crural nerves.

Meissner's (mīs′nĕr). ORIGIN: Superior mesenteric plexus (controls secretions of the bowels). LOCATION: Submucous coat of small intestines. DISTRIBUTION: Intestinal walls.

mesenteric (mĕs-ĕn-tĕr′ĭk). ORIGIN: Celiac plexus and left side of aortic plexus. LOCATION: Surrounding the inferior and superior mesenteric arteries. DISTRIBUTION: Descending colon, sigmoid, rectum, intestines.

myenteric (mī-ĕn-tĕr′ĭk). ORIGIN: Sympathetic system (controls peristalsis). LOCATION: Between the circular and longitudinal coats of small intestines. DISTRIBUTION: Intestinal walls.

ophthalmic (ŏf-thăl′mĭk). ORIGIN: Internal carotid plexus. LOCATION: Around ophthalmic artery and optic nerve. DISTRIBUTION: Optic region.

*Plexuses of central nervous system.

pancreatic (păn-krē-ăt′ĭk). ORIGIN: Splenic plexus. LOCATION: Near pancreas. DISTRIBUTION: Filaments to pancreas.

pancreaticoduodenal (păn-krē-ăt″ĭ-kō-dū″ō-dē′năl). ORIGIN: Hepatic plexus. LOCATION: Near head of pancreas. DISTRIBUTION: Filaments to pancreas and duodenum.

pelvic (pĕl′vĭk). ORIGIN: Hypogastric plexus, 2nd to 4th sacral nerves, 1st and 2nd sacral ganglia (pelvic brain). LOCATION: Side of rectum and bladder. DISTRIBUTION: Viscera of pelvis, pelvic plexus.

phrenic (frĕn′ĭk). ORIGIN: Solar plexus, semilunar ganglia. LOCATION: Accompanies phrenic artery to diaphragm. DISTRIBUTION: Diaphragm and suprarenal capsules.

prostatic (prŏs-tăt′ĭk). ORIGIN: Hypogastric plexus. LOCATION: Vesical arteries. DISTRIBUTION: Bladder.

pulmonary (pŭl′mō-nā″rē). ORIGIN: Anterior and posterior pulmonary branches of vagus and sympathetic nerves. LOCATION: Root of lungs, front and back. DISTRIBUTION: Root of lungs.

pyloric (pī-lor′ĭk). ORIGIN: Hepatic plexus. LOCATION: Near pylorus. DISTRIBUTION: Filaments to pylorus.

renal (rē′năl). ORIGIN: Solar and aortic plexuses and semilunar ganglia. LOCATION: Renal artery. DISTRIBUTION: Kidneys, posterior vena cava, spermatic plexus.

***sacral** (sā′krăl). ORIGIN: Anterior branch of 4th and 5th lumbar and 1st, 2nd, 3rd, and 4th sacral nerves. LOCATION: Front of sacrum on piriformis muscle. DISTRIBUTION: Muscular, pudic, superior gluteal, great and small sciatic nerves.

*Plexuses of central nervous system.

solar (sō′lăr). *(Epigastric)*. ORIGIN: Splanchnics and right vagus. LOCATION: Back of stomach. DISTRIBUTION: Semilunar ganglia, phrenic, suprarenal, renal, spermatic, celiac, superior mesenteric, and aortic plexuses. Called *abdominal brain*. SYN: *celiac plexus*.

spermatic (spĕr-măt′ĭk). (*Ovarian*). ORIGIN: Aortic plexus. LOCATION: Accompanies spermatic vessels to testes or ovaries. DISTRIBUTION: Testes or ovaries.

splenic (splē′nĭk). ORIGIN: Celiac plexus, left semilunar ganglion, right vagus nerve. LOCATION: Accompanies splenic artery. DISTRIBUTION: Spleen, pancreatic plexus, left gastroepiploic plexus.

suprarenal (sū-prā-rē′năl). ORIGIN: Diaphragmatic, solar, and renal plexuses. LOCATION: Around suprarenal capsules. DISTRIBUTION: Filaments to medulla of suprarenal capsules.

thyroid (thī′royd). (*Inferior*). ORIGIN: Middle cervical ganglion. LOCATION: Around external carotid and inferior thyroid arteries. DISTRIBUTION: Larynx, pharynx, thyroid gland. (*Superior*). ORIGIN: Superior laryngeal and cardiac nerves. LOCATION: Around the thyroid gland. DISTRIBUTION: Thyroid region.

uterine (ū′tĕr-ĭn). ORIGIN: Pelvic plexus. LOCATION: Accompanies uterine arteries. DISTRIBUTION: Cervix and lower part of uterus.

vaginal (văj′ĭ-năl). ORIGIN: Pelvic plexus. LOCATION: Vaginal walls. DISTRIBUTION: Vagina.

vertebral (vĕrt′ĕ-brăl). ORIGIN: First part thoracic ganglion, upper cervical nerves. LOCATION: Surrounding basilar and vertebral arteries. DISTRIBUTION: Vertebral and cerebellar regions.

vesical (vĕs′ĭ-kăl). ORIGIN: Pelvic plexus. LOCATION: Accompanies vesical arteries. DISTRIBUTION: Vesicula seminalis, vas deferens.

Cranial Nerves

No.	Name	NA Term*	Origin	Function	Distribution
1st	Olfactory	Nn. olfactorii	Olfactory lobe	Smell	Nasal mucous membrane
2nd	Optic	N. opticus	Retina	Sight	Retina
3rd	Oculomotor	N. oculomotorius	Floor of aqueduct of Sylvius	Motor	All ocular muscles except lateral rectus and superior oblique
4th	Trochlear	N. trochlearis	Floor of aqueduct of Sylvius	Motor	Superior oblique muscle of eye
5th	Trigeminal	N. trigeminus	Midbrain and pons	Motor and chief sensory n. of face	Skin of face; tongue; teeth; muscles of mastication
6th	Abducent	N. abducens	Pons	Motor	Lateral rectus muscle of eye
7th	Facial	N. facialis	Pons	Motor	Muscles of expression
8th	Auditory	N. vestibulocochlearis	Brain	Hearing	Internal auditory meatus
9th	Glossopharyngeal	N. glossopharyngeus	Medulla oblongata	Motor and sensory	Sensation of pharynx and posterior third of tongue; parotid gland
10th	Vagus	N. vagus	Medulla oblongata	Motor and sensory	Pharynx; larynx; heart; lungs; esophagus; stomach; abdominal viscera
11th	Accessory	N. accessorius	Medulla oblongata and spinal cord	Motor	Sternomastoid and trapezius muscles
12th	Hypoglossal	N. hypoglossus	Medulla oblongata	Motor	Intrinsic muscles of tongue

Nomina Anatomica

Arteries

Name	NA*	Origin	Distribution	Branches
Alveolar, inferior	A. alveolaris inferior	Maxillary	Lower anterior skull	Dental; mylohyoid; mental
Angular	A. angularis	Terminal branch of external maxillary	Neck and face	
Aorta SEE: *aorta* in vocabulary				
Arcuate (Metatarsal a.)	A. arcuata	Dorsal a. of foot	Foot and toes	Deep plantar; dorsal metatarsal; dorsal digital
Auditory, internal	A. labyrinthici	Middle of basilar or anterior inferior cerebellar	Internal ear	
Auricular, deep	A. auricularis profunda	Maxillary	Skin of auditory canal, tympanic membrane, and temporomandibular joint	
Auricular, posterior	A. auricularis posterior	External carotid	Middle ear; mastoid cells; auricle; parotid gland	Stylomastoid; auricular; occipital
Axillary	A. axillaris	Subclavian	Forms brachial and seven branches	Superior; thoracic; thoracoacromial; lateral thoracic; subscapular; anterior and posterior humeral; thoracodorsal; brachial
Basilar	A. basilaris	Vertebral	Pons	Posterior cerebral; pontine; internal auditory; anterior inferior cerebellar; superior cerebellar

Brachial	A. brachialis	Axillary	Upper arm	Deep brachial; nutrient; superior and inferior collateral; muscular
Brachial, deep	A. profunda brachii	Brachial	Accompanies radial nerve	
Brachiocephalic SEE: *Innominate a.*				
Bronchial	Rr. bronchiales	Thoracic aorta	Bronchi; lower trachea; pulmonary vessels; pericardium; part of esophagus	Left and right bronchial
Buccal (Buccinator a.)	A. buccalis	Maxillary	Buccinator muscle; mucous membrane of mouth	
Bulbar SEE: *Medullary a.*				
Capsular, middle SEE: *Suprarenal a., middle.*				
Carotid, common	A. carotis communis	Brachiocephalic trunk (right); aortic arch (left)	Neck and thyroid	External and internal carotid
Carotid, external	A. carotis externa	Common carotid	Neck; face; skull	Superior thyroid; ascending pharyngeal; lingual; facial; occipital; posterior auricular; superficial temporal; maxillary
Carotid, internal	A. carotis interna	Common carotid	Anterior brain; eyes; forehead; nose	Caroticotympanic; Vidian; cavernous; hypophyseal; semilunar; anterior meningeal; ophthalmic; anterior and middle cerebral; posterior communicating; choroidal

**Nomina Anatomica*

Arteries (*Continued*)

Name	NA*	Origin	Distribution	Branches
Celiac	Truncus celiacus	Abdominal aorta	Stomach; liver; pancreas; duodenum; spleen	Left gastric; common hepatic; splenic
Cerebellar, anterior inferior	A. cerebelli inferior anterior	Basilar	Anterior undersurface of cerebellum	
Cerebellar, posterior inferior	A. cerebelli inferior posterior	Vertebral	Cerebellum	
Cerebellar, superior	A. cerebelli superior	Near termination of basilar	Upper cerebellum; midbrain; pineal body	
Cerebral, anterior	A. cerebri anterior	Internal carotid	Cerebrum	Cortical; central; anterior communicating
Cerebral, middle SEE: *Cerebral a., anterior.*				
Cerebral, posterior	A. cerebri posterior	Basilar	Cerebrum	Central; posterior choroidal; cortical temporal; calcarine; parieto-occipital
Cervical, ascending	A. cervicalis ascendens	Inferior thyroid	Muscles of neck and spinal cord	
Cervical, superficial		Thyroid axis	Muscles of shoulder	
Cervical, transverse	A. transversa colli	Thyroid axis	Muscles and glands of neck	Deep and superficial rami
Choroidal, anterior (Choroid)	A. choroidea anterior	Internal carotid	Internal capsule	

*Nomina Anatomica

Ciliary, anterior	Aa. ciliares anteriores	Ophthalmic and lacrimal	Iris; conjunctiva	
Ciliary, long posterior	Aa. ciliares posteriores longae	Ophthalmic	Iris and ciliary process	
Ciliary, short posterior	Aa. ciliares posteriores breves	Ophthalmic	Choroid coat of eye	
Circumflex, anterior humeral	A. circumflexa humeri anterior	Lateral side of axillary	Shoulder joint and upper arm	
Circumflex, posterior humeral	A. circumflexa humeri posterior	Axillary	Deltoid and shoulder joint; upper arm	
Colic, left	A. colica sinistra	Inferior mesenteric	Descending and transverse colon	Ascending and descending colic
Colic, middle	A. colica media	Superior mesenteric	Transverse colon	Right and left colic
Colic, right	A. colica dextra	Superior mesenteric	Ascending colon	Ascending and descending colic
Collateral, inferior ulnar	A. collateralis ulnaris inferior	Brachial	Muscles at back of elbow	
Collateral, superior ulnar	A. collateralis ulnaris superior	Brachial	Elbow joint and triceps muscles	
Communicating, posterior	A. communicans posterior	Internal carotid	Hippocampus; thalamus	
Coronary, left	A. coronaria sinistra	Ascending aorta	Left ventricle and atrium	Anterior descending coronary; circumflex
Coronary, right	A. coronaria dextra	Ascending aorta	Right ventricle and atrium	Posterior descending; marginal

Nomina Anatomica

Arteries (*Continued*)

Name	NA*	Origin	Distribution	Branches
Cystic	A. cystica	Proper hepatic	Gallbladder; liver	
Digital, common palmar	Aa. digitales palmares communes	Palmar arch	Fingers	Proper palmar digital
Digital, proper palmar (Collateral digital a.)	Aa. digitales palmares propriae	Common palmar digital	Fingers	
Dorsal, of foot	A. dorsalis pedis	Continuation of anterior tibial	Foot	Lateral and medial tarsal; deep plantar; arcuate; first dorsal metatarsal
Epigastric, inferior	A. epigastrica inferior	External iliac	Abdominal muscles; peritoneum	Cremasteric
Epigastric, superficial	A. epigastrica superficialis	Femoral	Skin of abdomen; superficial fascia; inguinal lymph nodes	
Epigastric, superior	A. epigastrica superior	Internal thoracic	Abdominal muscles and skin; diaphragm	
Esophageal		In front of aorta	Esophagus	
Ethmoidal, anterior	A. ethmoidalis anterior	Ophthalmic	Ethmoidal cells and frontal sinus; dura mater; nasal cavity	Anterior meningeal
Ethmoidal, posterior	A. ethmoidalis posterior	Ophthalmic	Ethmoidal cells; dura mater; nasal cavity	Posterior meningeal
Facial (External	A. facialis	Carotid triangle	Face; tonsil; palate;	Ascending palatine; tonsillar; sub-

maxillary a.)			submandibular gland	mental; inferior and superior labial; angular; glandular; lateral nasal; muscular
Facial, transverse	A. transversa faciei	Superficial temporal	Parotid gland; skin of face; masseter muscle	
Femoral	A. femoralis	Continuation of external iliac	Lower abdominal wall; external genitalia; lower extremity	Superficial epigastric; superficial circumflex iliac; external pudendal; deep femoral; descending genicular
Femoral, deep	A. profunda femoris	Femoral	Thigh muscles; hip joint; gluteal muscles; femur	Perforating; medial and lateral circumflex
Femoral, lateral circumflex	A. circumflexa femoris lateralis	Deep femoral a.	Hip joint; thigh muscles	Ascending; descending; transverse
Femoral, medial circumflex	A. circumflexa femoris medialis	Medial aspect of deep femoral a.	Hip joint; thigh muscles	Deep; acetabular; transverse; superficial
Fibular SEE: *Peroneal a.*				
Frontal	A. supratrochlearis	Ophthalmic	Forehead muscles; cranium	
Gastric, left	A. gastrica sinistra	Celiac trunk	Abdominal section of esophagus; stomach; left lobe of liver	Anterior and posterior gastric; cardioesophageal
Gastric, right	A. gastrica dextra	Common hepatic	Lesser curvature of stomach	
Gastric, short	Aa. gastricae breves	End of splenic	Greater curvature of stomach	

**Nomina Anatomica*

Arteries (*Continued*)

Name	NA*	Origin	Distribution	Branches
Gastroduodenal	A. gastroduodenalis	Common hepatic trunk	Stomach; duodenum; pancreas; greater omentum	Superior pancreaticoduodenal; right gastroepiploic; retroduodenal
Gastroepiploic	A. gastroepiploica dextra	Gastroduodenal	Stomach; greater omentum	Pyloric; epiploic; right and left gastroepiploic
Genicular, descending	A. genus descendens	Femoral	Knee joint; skin of upper and medial section of leg	Saphenous; musculo-articular
Genicular, inferior	A. genus inferior	Popliteal	Knee joint; skin of upper and middle leg	
Genicular, middle	A. genus media	Popliteal	Knee joint; ligaments and synovial membrane of knee	
Genicular, superior	A. genus superior	On either side of popliteal	Knee joint; femur; patella	
Gluteal, inferior (Sciatic a.)	A. glutea inferior	Internal iliac	Buttocks and back of thigh	Muscular; coccygeal; anastomotic; articular; cutaneous; comitans nervi; ischiadici
Gluteal, superior	A. glutea superior	Internal iliac	Gluteal region	Superficial and deep gluteal
Hemorrhoidal, middle	A. rectalis media	Internal iliac	Rectum; prostate; seminal vesicles	
Hemorrhoidal, superior	A. rectalis superior	Inferior mesenteric	Rectum	

Hepatic, common	A. hepatica communis	Celiac trunk	Stomach; pancreas; duodenum; liver; gallbladder; greater omentum	Right gastric; gastroduodenal; proper hepatic
Hepatic, proper	A. hepatica propria	Common hepatic	Liver and gallbladder	Cystic
Hypogastric SEE: *Iliac a., internal.*				
Ileocolic	A. ileocolica	Superior mesenteric	Ileum; cecum; appendix; ascending colon	Superior and inferior ileocolic; appendicular
Iliac, common	A. iliaca communis	End of abdominal aorta	Pelvis; abdominal wall; lower limbs	External and internal iliac
Iliac, deep circumflex	A. circumflexa ilium profunda	External iliac	Muscles of skin and lower abdomen	
Iliac, external	A. iliaca externa	Common iliac	Abdominal wall; external genitalia; lower limb	Inferior epigastric; deep circumflex iliac
Iliac, internal (Hypogastric a.)	A. iliaca interna	Common iliac	Walls and viscera of pelvis, buttocks, reproductive organs; medial side of thighs	Superior, middle, and inferior vesical; middle hemorrhoidal; obturator; internal pudendal; inferior gluteal; uterine; vaginal; iliolumbar; lateral sacral; superior gluteal
Iliac, superficial circumflex	A. circumflexa ilium superficialis	Femoral	Inguinal glands; skin of thigh and abdomen	
Infraorbital	A. infraorbitalis	Maxillary	Maxillary sinus; center face	Anterior superior alveolar; orbital
Innominate	Truncus brachiocephalicus	Arch of aorta	Right side of head, neck, and arm	Right subclavian; right common carotid

*Nomina Anatomica

Arteries (*Continued*)

Name	NA*	Origin	Distribution	Branches
Intercostal	Aa. intercostales posteriores	Thoracic aorta	Intercostal spaces; back muscles; vertebral column; thoracic wall	
Interosseous, anterior (Volar interosseous a.)	A. interossea anterior	Common interosseous	Deep structures of anterior forearm	Median; nutrient; muscular
Interosseous, common	A. interossea communis	Ulnar	Deep structure of forearm	Anterior and posterior interosseous
Interosseous, posterior	A. interossea posterior	Common interosseous	Muscles of posterior forearm	Recurrent interosseous
Intestinal		Superior mesenteric	Jejunum and ileum	
Labial, inferior	A. labialis inferior	Near angle of mouth	Lower lip	
Labial, superior	A. labialis superior	Near angle of mouth	Upper lip	
Lacrimal	A. lacrimalis	Ophthalmic	Lacrimal gland; eyelid; conjunctiva	Lateral palpebral; zygomatic; recurrent
Laryngeal, inferior	A. laryngea inferior	Inferior thyroid	Muscles and mucous membrane of trachea and larynx	
Laryngeal, superior	A. laryngea superior	Superior thyroid	Muscles, mucous membrane, and glands of larynx	
Lienal SEE: *Splenic a.*				

Lingual	A. lingualis	External carotid	Undersurface of tongue; tonsil; epiglottis	Suprahyoid; dorsal and deep lingual; sublingual
Lingual, deep	A. profunda linguae	End of lingual	Undersurface of tongue	
Lingual, dorsal	R. dorsales linguae	Lingual	Mucous membrane on dorsum of tongue; glossopalatine arch; tonsil; soft palate; epiglottis	
Lumbar	Aa. lumbales	Abdominal aorta	Abdominal wall; vertebrae; lumbar muscles; renal capsule	Posterior lumbar; muscular
Malleolar, lateral anterior	A. malleolaris anterior lateralis	Anterior tibial	Ankle joint	
Malleolar, medial anterior	A. malleolaris anterior medialis	Anterior tibial	Ankle joint	
Malleolar, medial posterior	Rr. malleolares mediales	Peroneal	Tibial malleolus	
Mammary SEE: *Thoracic.*				
Masseteric	A. masseterica	Maxillary	Masseter muscle	
Maxillary (Internal maxillary a.)	A. maxillaris	External carotid	Jaws and teeth; muscles of mastication; ear; meninges; nose; nasal sinus; palate	Anterior tympanic; deep auricular; middle and accessory meningeal; inferior and posterior superior alveolar; deep temporal; pterygoid; masseteric; buccal; infraorbital; greater palatine; pharyngeal; sphenopalatine

*Nomina Anatomica

Arteries (*Continued*)

Name	NA*	Origin	Distribution	Branches
Maxillary, external SEE: *Facial a.*				
Mediastinal, anterior	Rr. mediastinales	Internal thoracic	Anterior mediastinal cavity; portion of thymus	
Medullary (Bulbar a.)		Vertebral	Medulla oblongata	
Meningeal, middle	A. meningea media	Maxillary	Dura mater; cranial bones	Superficial; petrosal; superior tympanic; orbital; temporal; and numerous small vessels
Mesenteric, inferior	A. mesenterica inferior	Abdominal aorta	Left half of transverse colon; descending, iliac, and sigmoid colon; part of rectum	Left colic; sigmoid; superior hemorrhoidal
Mesenteric, superior	A. mesenterica superior	Abdominal aorta	Small intestine; cecum; ascending colon; part of transverse colon	Inferior pancreaticoduodenal; jejunal; ileal; ileocolic; right and middle colon
Metacarpal, palmar (Palmar interosseous a.)	Aa. metacarpeae palmares	Deep palmar arch	Interosseous muscles and bones	
Metatarsal SEE: *Arcuate a.*				
Metatarsal, first dorsal		Dorsal a. of foot	Toes	
Musculophrenic	A. musculophrenica	Internal thoracic	Diaphragm; abdominal and thoracic walls	
Nasal	A. dorsalis nasi	Ophthalmic	Lacrimal sac; integuments of nose	Lacrimal

Obturator	A. obturatoria	Internal iliac	Pelvis and thigh	Iliac; vesical; pubic; anterior and posterior obturator
Occipital	A. occipitalis	Posterior part of external carotid	Muscles of neck and scalp; meninges; mastoid	Muscular; meningeal; sternomastoid; descending occipital; auricular
Ophthalmic	A. ophthalmica	Internal carotid	Eye and adjacent structures of face	Lacrimal; supraorbital; posterior and anterior ethmoidal; medial palpebral; frontal; dorsal nasal; central a. of retina; short posterior, long posterior, and anterior ciliary; muscular
Ovarian	A. ovarica	Abdominal aorta	Ovaries; uterine tubes; ureter	Ureteral
Palatine, ascending	A. palatina ascendens	Facial	Base of skull; palate; auditory tube	
Palatine, greater	A. palatina major	Maxillary	Palate and tonsils	Greater and lesser palatine
Palpebral, medial (Internal palpebral a.)	A. palpebrales mediales	Ophthalmic	Upper and lower eyelids	Superior and inferior palpebral
Pancreaticoduodenal, inferior	Aa. pancreaticoduodenales inferiores	Superior mesenteric	Pancreas; duodenum	
Pancreaticoduodenal, superior	Aa. supraduodenales superiores	Gastroduodenal	Pancreas; duodenum	
Perforating	Aa. perforantes	Deep femoral	Back of thigh	
Pericardiacophrenic	A. pericardiacophrenica	Internal thoracic	Diaphragm; pericardium; pleura	

Nomina Anatomica

Arteries (*Continued*)

Name	NA*	Origin	Distribution	Branches
Peroneal	A. peronea	Posterior tibial	Ankle; deep calf muscles	Perforating; communicating; calcaneal; tibial and fibular nutrient; lateral and medial malleolar
Pharyngeal, ascending	A. pharyngea ascendens	Posterior part of external carotid	Pharynx, soft palate; ear; meninges; cranial nerves; capitis muscles	Pharyngeal; palatine; posterior meningeal; prevertebral; inferior tympanic
Phrenic	Aa. phrenicae	Aorta	Diaphragm; suprarenal glands	Medial, lateral, and superior suprarenal
Plantar, deep	R. plantaris profunda	Dorsal a. of foot	Sole of foot	First plantar metatarsal
Plantar, lateral	A. plantaris lateralis	Posterior tibial	Toes and sole of foot	Plantar arch and plantar metatarsal
Plantar, medial	A. plantaris medialis	Posterior tibial	Muscles and skin of sole of foot and toes	Superficial digital
Popliteal	A. poplitea	Continuation of femoral	Knee and calf	Anterior and posterior tibial; lateral and medial superior genicular; middle, sural, lateral, and medial inferior genicular; genicular articular
Pudendal, external	Aa. pudendae externae	Femoral	External genitalia; medial thigh	
Pudendal, internal	A. pudenda interna	Internal iliac	External genitalia	Posterior scrotal or posterior labial; inferior hemorrhoidal; perineal; urethral; a. of bulb of

				penis or vestibule; deep a. of penis or clitoris; dorsal a. of penis or clitoris
Pulmonary	Truncus pulmonalis	Right ventricle	Lungs	Right and left pulmonary
Pulmonary, left	A. pulmonalis sinistra	Pulmonary trunk	Left lung	Numerous branches
Pulmonary, right	A. pulmonalis dextra	Pulmonary trunk	Right lung	Numerous branches
Radial	A. radialis	Brachial	Forearm; wrist; hand	Recurrent radial; muscular; palmar and dorsal carpal; superficial palmar; first dorsal metacarpal; principal a. of thumb; perforating; recurrent; palmar
Radial, of index finger	A. radialis indicis	Principal a. of thumb	Index finger	
Recurrent	A. recurrens tibialis anterior	Anterior tibial	Knee joint	
Recurrent, posterior tibial	A. recurrens tibialis posterior	Anterior tibial	Knee joint	
Recurrent, radial	A. recurrens radialis	Below elbow from radial	Elbow joint; muscles of forearm	
Recurrent, ulnar	A. recurrens ulnaris	Ulnar	Elbow joint; skin and muscles of elbow	Anterior and posterior recurrent
Renal	A. renalis	Abdominal aorta	Kidney; suprarenal gland; ureter	Inferior suprarenal
Retroduodenal		Gastroduodenal	Head of pancreas; duodenum; bile duct	

*Nomina Anatomica

Arteries (*Continued*)

Name	NA*	Origin	Distribution	Branches
Sacral, lateral	Aa. sacrales laterales	Internal iliac	Coccyx and sacrum	
Sacral, middle	A. sacralis mediana	Abdominal aorta	Sacrum; coccyx; rectum	Lowest lumbar
Scapular, circumflex	A. circumflexa scapulae	Subscapular	Lateral border of scapula; infraspinous fossa; muscles of upper arm	
Scapular, descending (Dorsal scapular a.)	A. scapularis descendens	Subclavian	Medial border of scapula	
Scapular, transverse SEE: *Suprascapular a.*				
Sciatic SEE: *Gluteal a., inferior.*				
Sigmoid	Aa. sigmoideae	Inferior mesenteric	Iliac, sigmoid, and pelvic colon	
Spermatic, internal SEE: *Testicular a.*				
Sphenopalatine (Nasopalatine a.)	A. sphenopalatina	Maxillary	Nose	Posterior lateral nasal; posterior septal
Spinal, anterior (Ventral spinal a.)	A. spinalis anterior	Vertebral	Anterior spinal cord	
Spinal, posterior (Dorsal spinal a.)	A. spinalis posterior	Vertebral	Posterior spinal cord	
Splenic (Lienal a.)	A. lienalis	Celiac trunk	Pancreas; spleen; stomach; greater omentum	Pancreatic; left gastroepiploic; short gastric; splenic

Sternomastoid	Rr. sternocleidomastoidei	Occipital or external carotid	Sternocleidomastoid muscles	
Stylomastoid	A. stylomastoidea	Posterior auricular	Mastoid; tympanic cavity; stapedius muscle	
Subclavian	A. subclavia	Innominate (right); arch of aorta (left)	Brain; meninges; spinal cord; neck; thoracic walls; upper limbs	Vertebral; internal thoracic; thyrocervical; costocervical; transverse cervical
Subcostal	A. subcostalis	Thoracic aorta	Upper abdominal wall	Dorsal and spinal
Sublingual	A. sublingualis	Anterior margin of hypoglossus	Sublingual gland and mucous membrane of mouth and gums	
Submental	A. submentalis	Facial	Mylohyoid muscle; submandibular and sublingual glands; lower lip	
Subscapular	A. subscapularis	Axillary	Shoulder	Scapular circumflex and thoracodorsal
Supraorbital	A. supraorbitalis	Ophthalmic	Forehead; frontal sinus; upper eyelid; upper muscles of orbit	
Suprarenal, middle (Middle capsular a.)	A. suprarenalis media	Abdominal aorta	Suprarenal gland	
Suprascapular (Transverse scapular a.)	A. suprascapularis	Thyroid axis	Scapular; clavicle; shoulder joint	Acromial; suprasternal
Sural	Aa. surales	Popliteal opposite knee joint	Calf	

Nomina Anatomica

Arteries (*Continued*)

Name	NA*	Origin	Distribution	Branches
Tarsal, lateral	A. tarsea lateralis	Dorsal a. of foot	Muscles and joints of tarsus	
Tarsal, medial	Aa. tarseae mediales	Dorsal a. of foot	Middle portion of foot	
Temporal, middle	A. temporalis media	Above zygomatic arch	Temporal muscle	
Temporal, superficial	A. temporalis superficialis	End of external carotid	Parotid gland; auricle; scalp; skin of face; masseter muscle	Transverse facial; middle temporal; anterior auricular; frontal; parietal
Testicular (Internal spermatic a.)		Abdominal aorta	Ureter; epididymis; testes	Ureteral
Thoracic, internal (Internal mammary a.)	A. thoracica interna	Subclavian	Anterior thoracic wall; mediastinal structures; diaphragm	Pericardiacophrenic; anterior mediastinal; pericardial; sternal; intercostal; perforating; musculophrenic; superior epigastric
Thoracic, lateral	A. thoracica lateralis	Axillary	Shoulder muscles and axillary glands	In the female, external mammary
Thoracic, superior	A. thoracica suprema	Thoracoacromial	Muscles of chest	
Thoracoacromial	A. thoracoacromialis	Axillary	Muscles and skin of upper arm, shoulder, and chest	Pectoral; acromial; clavicular; deltoid
Thoracodorsal	A. thoracodorsalis	Subscapular	Posterior portion of axillary	
Thumb, principal a. of	A. princeps pollicis	Radial	Sides and palmar aspect	Radial a. of index finger

			of thumb	
Thyroid, inferior	A. thyroidea inferior	Thyroid axis	Thyroid gland; esophagus	Inferior laryngeal; tracheal; muscular; esophageal; ascending cervical
Thyroid, superior	A. thyroidea superior	External carotid	Hyoid muscles; larynx; thyroid gland; pharynx	Hyoid; sternomastoid; superior laryngeal; cricothyroid
Tibial, anterior	A. tibialis anterior	Popliteal	Leg; ankle; foot	Anterior and posterior tibial recurrent; fibular; lateral and medial anterior malleolar
Tibial, posterior	A. tibialis posterior	Lower end of popliteal	Leg; foot; heel	Peroneal; lateral and medial posterior malleolar; communicating; plantar; tibial and fibular nutrient
Tympanic, anterior	A. tympanica anterior	Maxillary	Lining of tympanic arch	
Tympanic, inferior	A. tympanica inferior	Ascending pharyngeal	Tympanic cavity	
Ulnar	A. ulnaris	Brachial	Forearm; wrist and hand	Anterior and posterior recurrent; common interosseous; muscular; palmar and dorsal carpal; deep palmar; superficial palmar arch
Uterine	A. uterina	Internal iliac	Uterus; uterine tubes; ovary; vagina	Vaginal; ovarian; tubal
Vaginal	A. vaginalis	Uterine	Vagina; bladder	
Vertebral	A. vertebralis	Subclavian	Muscles of neck; vertebrae; spinal cord; cerebellum; interior of cerebrum	Spinal; muscular; anterior and posterior spinal; posterior inferior cerebellar; medullary

*Nomina Anatomica

Arteries (*Continued*)

Name	NA*	Origin	Distribution	Branches
Vesical, inferior	A. vesicalis inferior	Internal iliac	Bladder; prostate; seminal vesicles	
Vesical, middle		Superior vesical	Bladder; seminal vesicles	
Vesical, superior	Aa. vesicales superiores	Internal iliac	Upper part of bladder	A. to the ductus deferens
Vidian (A. of the pterygoid canal)	A. canalis pterygoidei		Roof of pharynx; auditory (eustachian) tube	

Veins

Name	NA*	Description	Origin	Distribution
Angular	V. angularis	Short superficial v. in nasal region	Union of supratrochlear and supraorbital veins	Continues inferiorly as facial v.
Antebrachial, median	V. mediana antebrachii	Superficial v. of forearm	Base of dorsum of thumb	Ascends forearm between cephalic and basilic veins to elbow where it joins these veins
Auricular, posterior	V. auricularis posterior	Superficial v. which drains parietal and posterior part of temporal region	Plexus on side of head	From side of head it descends behind the pinna where it unites with retromandibular v. to form the external jugular v.
Axillary	V. axillaris	Portion of venous trunk of upper extremity	Junction of basilic and brachial veins	Lower border of teres major muscles to lateral border of first rib where it becomes the subclavian v.

Azygos	V. azygos	Trunk which connects superior and inferior vena cavae	Arises from ascending lumbar v.	From level of diaphragm up posterior thoracic wall on right of vertebral bodies to superior vena cava
Basilic	V. basilica	Superficial v. of hand and forearm	Ulnar side of dorsal rete of hand	Ascends posteriorly on the forearm. Below the elbow it moves to exterior surface where it joins axillary v.
Brachial	Vv. brachiales	Each v. drains an arm	Tributaries from structures in upper arm	Follows course of brachial artery and joins axillary v.
Brachiocephalic (Innominate v.)	Vv. brachiocephalicae (dextra et sinistra)	Paired veins which draw blood from head, neck, and upper extremities. They unite to form superior vena cava	Union of internal jugular and subclavian veins	From sternal end of clavicle it ascends vertically to unite below the cartilage of first rib to form superior vena cava
Bronchial	Vv. bronchiales	Several veins which return blood from larger bronchi and roots of lungs	Capillaries of bronchi and roots of lungs	Empties into azygos v. on the right and into hemiazygos or superior intercostal veins on left
Cardiac	Vv. cordis	Drain blood from tissues of heart	Capillaries of tissues of heart	Circulates throughout heart, usually emptying into coronary sinus
Cardinal		First veins to appear in body of embryo	Each v. receives a v. from caudal and cephalic portions of embryo	Include precardinal and postcardinal veins
Cephalic	V. cephalica	Superficial v. of arm and forearm	Radial border of dorsal rete of hand	Winds anteriorly up arm and empties into axillary v.

*Nomina Anatomica

Veins (*Continued*)

Name	NA*	Description	Origin	Distribution
Cerebellar, inferior	Vv. cerebelli inferiores	Large veins of undersurface of cerebellum	Undersurface of cerebellum	Empty into transverse, superior, petrosal, and occipital sinuses
Cerebellar, superior	Vv. cerebelli superiores	Veins from upper surface of cerebellum	Upper surface of cerebellum	Empty into straight sinus or transverse sinus
Cerebral, great	V. cerebri magna	Short median trunk	Formed by union of two internal cerebral veins	Curves backward and upward around the splenium of the corpus callosum and continues as a straight sinus
Cerebral, inferior	Vv. cerebri inferiores	Small-sized veins which drain undersurfaces of hemispheres	Tributaries in lobes of cerebrum	From various lobes they empty into cavernous and transverse sinuses
Cerebral, internal	Vv. cerebri internae	Two veins which drain deep parts of hemisphere	Formed near interventricular foramen by union of terminal and choroid veins	Run backward parallel to one another and unite at the splenium of the corpus callosum to form great cerebral v.
Cerebral, superficial middle	V. cerebri media superficialis	Drains lateral surface of cerebral hemisphere	Lateral surface of cerebral hemisphere	Follows lateral cerebral fissure and empties into cavernous sinus
Cerebral, superior	Vv. cerebri superiores	Eight to twelve veins which drain the surface of the cerebral hemisphere	Capillaries of cerebrum	From cerebrum to longitudinal cerebral fissure, opening into superior sagittal sinus
Cervical, deep	V. cervicalis profunda	Deep v. of neck	Plexus in suboccipital triangle	Follows deep cervical artery down neck and empties into vaginal or brachiocephalic v.
Cervical, transverse	Vv. transversae colli	Drain blood from supraspinous region of	Capillaries of supraspinous region of	From supraspinous region of scapula diagonally across shoul-

		scapula and neck	scapula and neck	der to subclavian or external jugular v.
Cutaneous SEE: *Superficial v.*				
Cystic	V. cystica	Drains gallbladder	Capillaries of gallbladder	From gallbladder along cystic duct to enter right branch of portal v. just below liver
Deep		Accompany homonymous arteries and usually are enclosed in sheaths with those vessels	Extremities	Throughout the body
Digital, palmar	Vv. digitales palmares	Superficial veins of palmar surface of fingers	Capillaries of superficial tissues of palmar surface of fingers	Along proper and common digital arteries
Digital, plantar	Vv. digitales plantares	Veins of plantar surface of toes	Capillaries of toes	Along plantar surface of toes to foot to form four metatarsal veins
Diploic	Vv. diploicae	Large veins of the skull. Main veins are frontal, anterior and posterior temporal, and occipital	Bony tissue between internal and external skull surface	Connect with meningeal veins, sinuses of the dura mater, and veins of the pericranium
Emissary	Vv. emissariae	One of the small valveless veins which establish communication between sinuses inside the skull and veins external to it	Cerebral sinuses	Pass through foramina of skull
Epigastric, inferior	V. epigastrica inferior	V. of lower anterior abdominal wall	Capillaries of internal surface of lower anterior abdominal walls	Internal surface of abdominal wall diagonally across wall to flow into external iliac v.

*Nomina Anatomica

Veins (*Continued*)

Name	NA*	Description	Origin	Distribution
Epigastric, superficial	V. epigastrica superficialis	Drains lower and medial portion of abdominal wall	Superficial tissues of lower portion of anterior abdominal wall	Follows superficial epigastric artery and opens into great saphenous v.
Esophageal	Vv. esophageae	One of several small trunks which drain esophagus	Capillaries of esophagus	From esophagus empties into inferior thyroid, hemiazygos, azygos, or left brachiocephalicus v.
Facial	V. facialis	Deep v. of face. Branches drain deep structures of face	Continuation of angular v.	From inner angle of orbit it passes diagonally downward and outward to lower jaw
Femoral	V. femoralis	Large v. of thigh	Continuation of popliteal v.	From posterior region of knee it follows course of femoral artery, becoming external iliac v. at inguinal ligament
Femoral, deep	V. profunda femoris	Deep v. of thigh	Tributaries from posterior region of thigh	Accompanies deep femoral artery to femoral triangle where it joins femoral v.
Fibular SEE: *Peroneal v.*				
Frontal SEE: *Supratrochlear v.*				
Gastric, left	V. gastrica sinistra	Drains both surfaces of stomach	Gastrohepatic omentum	Right to left along lesser curvature of stomach to enter portal v.
Gastric, right (Pyloric)	V. gastrica dextra	Drains upper portion of stomach	Small v. from upper portion of stomach	From upper stomach runs left to right along pyloric portion of lesser curvature of stomach to end in portal v.

Gastric, short	Vv. gastricae breves	Drains wall of stomach	Capillaries of fundus of stomach	From wall of stomach empty into splenic v.
Gastroepiploic, left	V. gastroepiploica sinistra	V. of upper stomach	Branches from stomach and greater omentum	Right to left on greater curvature of stomach to empty into splenic v.
Gastroepiploic, right	V. gastroepiploica dextra	V. of lower stomach	Branches from greater omentum and lower surfaces of stomach	Left to right on greater curvature of stomach to empty into superior mesenteric v.
Gluteal, inferior (Sciatic v.)	Vv. gluteae inferiores	V. of lower region of hip	Capillaries of upper part of back of thigh	Upper back thigh through lower sciatic foramen where they unite into a single v. and empty into internal iliac v.
Gluteal, superior	Vv. gluteae superiores	Drains muscles of buttocks	Capillaries of gluteal and adjacent muscles	From tissues of hip they pass through sciatic foramen to empty into internal iliac v.
Hemiazygos	V. hemiazygos	Single v. of lower left thoracic wall	Left ascending lumbar v.	Lumbar region through diaphragm, crossing in front of spine and emptying into azygos v.
Hemiazygos, accessory	V. hemiazygos accessoria	Drains blood from intercostal spaces above level of sixth to seventh	Capillaries of upper intercostal spaces	From left side of vertebra crosses over spine to enter azygos v.
Hemorrhoidal plexus	Plexus venosus rectalis	Surround the rectum	Muscular wall and submucosa of rectum	Tissues of rectum via hemorrhoidal veins to internal pudendal v. to hypogastric v. to commencement of inferior mesenteric v.
Hepatic	Vv. hepaticae	Drain the liver	Tissues of liver	From liver empty into inferior vena cava

Nomina Anatomica

Veins (*Continued*)

Name	NA*	Description	Origin	Distribution
Hypogastric SEE: *Iliac v., internal.*				
Ileocolic	V. ileocolica	Large tributary of mesenteric v. which drains the ileum, appendix, cecum, and lower part of ascending colon	Capillaries of organs in area of ileum and colon	From lower portion of ascending colon runs parallel with ileocolic artery and empties into superior mesenteric v.
Iliac, common	V. iliaca communis	Large v. which draws blood from pelvis and leg. One on each side meets to form inferior vena cava	Union of internal and external iliac veins	Diagonally across pelvis
Iliac, deep circumflex	V. circumflexa ilium profunda	V. of deep structures of iliac region	Capillaries of deep muscles of upper portion of thigh and lower portion of abdomen	Deep tissues of anterior superior spine along inner surface of pelvic brim to external iliac v.
Iliac, external	V. iliaca externa	Upward continuation of external iliac v.	Begins behind inguinal ligament as continuation of external iliac v.	Behind inguinal ligament to sacroiliac articulation where it unites with internal iliac v. to form common iliac v.
Iliac, internal (Hypogastric v.)	V. iliaca interna	Short v. which draws blood from pelvis	Near upper part of greater sciatic foramen	Upper part of greater sciatic foramen
Innominate SEE: *Brachiocephalic v.*				
Intercostal		One of a number of veins (anterior, posterior, right, left, superior, and	Tributaries of other veins of intercostal spaces	Intercostal spaces to region of lower ribs

		highest) which drains blood from intercostal spaces		
Invertebral	V. invertebralis	One of numerous veins which drain vertebral plexuses and accompany spinal nerves	Vertebral plexuses	Vertebral plexuses through intervertebral foramina where they empty into regional veins
Jugular, anterior	V. jugularis anterior	Superficial v. of anterior region of neck	From veins of region of lower lip	From lower jaw descends neck anteriorly and enters external jugular v.
Jugular, external	V. jugularis externa	A large superficial v. which receives greater part of blood from exterior of cranium and deep parts of face	Formed at parotid gland by union of posterior auricular and retromandibular veins	From parotid gland descends perpendicularly in neck to empty into subclavian, internal jugular, or brachiocephalic v.
Jugular, internal	V. jugularis interna	Largest v. of head and neck. Collects blood from brain, superficial parts of face, and neck	Continuous from transverse sinus at base of skull	Runs vertically in neck and unites with subclavian v. at root of neck to form the brachiocephalic v.
Lingual	V. lingualis	Deep v. of tongue	Capillaries of tongue and sublingual areas	Follows distribution of lingual artery
Lumbar	Vv. lumbales	Four or five veins of abdominal walls	Capillaries of abdominal walls	Abdominal walls to ascending lumbar v., inferior vena cava, and iliolumbar v.
Lumbar, ascending	V. lumbalis ascendens	Longitudinal v. which connects lumbar veins	Lateral sacral veins	Lateral sacral v. along lateral border of spinal column to first lumbar vertebra where it becomes azygos v. on right side and hemiazygos v. on left side

**Nomina Anatomica*

Veins (*Continued*)

Name	NA*	Description	Origin	Distribution
Meningeal	Vv. meningeae	Multiple veins of dura mater of brain	Meninges of brain	Accompany meningeal arteries from meninges and empty into regional sinuses and veins
Mesenteric, superior	V. mesenterica superior	Large v. from small intestine	Capillaries of small intestine	From ileum in right iliac fossa it follows distribution of its artery and unites with splenic v. behind pancreas to form portal v.
Mesenteric, inferior	V. mesenterica inferior	Drains blood from rectum and sigmoid and descending parts of colon	Capillaries of colon and rectum	As a continuation of superior rectal v. ascends behind peritoneum and enters splenic v.
Metacarpal, dorsal	Vv. metacarpeae dorsales	Superficial veins of back of hand	Capillaries of hand	From digital venous arches join to form dorsal venous rete of hand
Metacarpal, palmar	Vv. metacarpeae palmares	Deep veins on both sides of hand	Capillaries of palm	Deep tissues of palm along metacarpal bone to deep venous arches
Metatarsal, dorsal	Vv. metatarseae dorsales pedis	Deep veins of back of foot	Dorsal digital veins of toes	Through metatarsal spaces to unite to form dorsal venous arch
Metatarsal, plantar	Vv. metatarseae plantares	Deep veins of solar aspect of foot	Plantar digital veins	From toes to ankles and open into plantar venous arch
Musculophrenic	Vv. musculophrenicae	Drains blood from thoracic surface of diaphragm and from walls of thorax and abdomen	Capillaries of upper abdominal wall, lower intercostal spaces, and diaphragm	Along thoracic surface of diaphragm upward lateral to sternum to unite with superior epigastric v. to form internal thoracic v.

Obturator	Vv. obturatoriae	Drains blood from obturator foramen	Union of tributaries of hip and muscle of upper posterior thigh	From upper portion of adductor region of thigh run through upper part of obturator foramen and run back to empty into internal iliac v.
Occipital	V. occipitalis	Superficial v. which drains occipital region	Plexus at back part of vertex of skull	From plexus of occipital region, occasionally following course of occipital artery, extends to internal or external jugular v.
Ophthalmic, inferior	V. ophthalmica inferior	Ophthalmic v. which divides into two terminal branches	Venous network at forepart of orbit	Runs backward in lower orbit and divides into two branches. One passes through inferior orbital fissure and joins pterygoid venous plexus; the second enters cranium through superior orbital fissure and ends in cavernous sinus
Ophthalmic, superior	V. ophthalmica superior	Paired veins of orbital cavity	Inner angle of orbit	Follows course of ophthalmic artery into cavernous sinus
Ovarian	V. ovarica	Drains ovary	Capillaries of ovaries, uterine tubes, and adjacent structures	Pampiniform plexus of broad ligament into inferior vena cava on right and left renal v. on left
Palatine, external	V. palatina externa	Draws blood from tonsils and soft palate	Capillaries of deep tissues of neck	Palatine regions into facial v.
Pancreatic	Vv. pancreaticae	V. of pancreas	Capillaries of pancreas	From pancreas into splenic and superior mesenteric veins
Parietal	V. emissaria parietalis	Small v. which passes through the parietal foramen of the skull	Upper skull	Connects superior sagittal sinus with extra cranial veins

**Nomina Anatomica*

Veins (*Continued*)

Name	NA*	Description	Origin	Distribution
Parumbilical	Vv. parumbilicales	Small important veins which establish communication between portal v. and superior and inferior epigastric veins	Cutaneous veins in region of umbilicus	From region of umbilicus run backward and upward to left portal v.
Penis, dorsal v. of	V. dorsalis penis profunda	Two (deep and superficial) veins of penis	Capillaries of skin or tissue of penis	Runs length of penis between two dorsal arteries
Peroneal (Fibular v.)	Vv. peroneae (fibulares)	Deep v. of leg	Veins of ankle and capillaries of tissues of leg	From venous plexus in region of heel upward along lateral region of deep tissue to flow into posterior tibial v. below knee
Pharyngeal	Vv. pharyngeae	Drain pharyngeal plexus	Pharyngeal plexus	Empty from pharyngeal plexus into internal jugular v.
Phrenic, inferior	Vv. phrenicae inferiores	Drain abdominal surface of diaphragm	Tissues of diaphragm	From diaphragm flow to inferior vena cava on right side and left suprarenal v. on left side
Popliteal	V. poplitea	Large v. in posterior region of knee	Union of tibial veins at lower border of popliteus muscle	From tibial veins upward to adductor hiatus to become femoral v.
Portal	V. portae	Subdivision of systemic venous system. Collects blood from digestive tract and conveys it to the liver	Union of superior mesenteric and splenic veins	Abdominal cavity
Pudendal, external	Vv. pudendae externae	Drain blood from superficial regions of medial	Capillaries of superficial tissues of lower abdo-	From lower abdomen transversely across upper region of thigh to

		aspect of upper thigh and receive subcutaneous dorsal veins of external genitals	men, scrotum or labia	great saphenous or femoral v.
Pudendal, internal	V. pudenda interna	Drains the perineum and external genitals	Deep veins of penis or clitoris	Follows course of internal pudendal artery and opens into internal iliac v.
Pulmonary	Vv. pulmonales	Four veins which return oxygenated blood from lungs to left atrium of heart	Capillaries upon walls of air sacs of lungs	Lungs to left atrium
Pyloric SEE: *Gastric v., right.*				
Radial	Vv. radiales	Large deep veins on radial side of forearm	Palmar arches of hand	From palmar arches of hand accompany radial artery along lateral side of forearm in deep tissues to unite with ulnar v. to form brachial v.
Rectal, inferior	Vv. rectales inferiores	Drain the rectal plexus	Venous plexus of anal canal	Anal canal to internal pudendal v.
Rectal, middle	Vv. rectales mediae	Drain the rectal plexus	Rectal plexus with tributaries from bladder, prostate, and seminal vesicles	Run laterally from rectal plexus to internal iliac v.
Rectal, superior	V. rectalis superior	Drains upper part of rectal plexus	Capillaries of rectum	Ascends from rectal plexus to brim of pelvis into inferior mesenteric v.
Renal	Vv. renales	Short thick trunks which drain the kidneys. The left is longer than the right	Capillaries of kidneys. The left v. receives the left suprarenal v. and left gonadal v.	From kidneys transversely across posterior abdominal wall to inferior vena cava

*Nomina Anatomica

Veins (*Continued*)

Name	NA*	Description	Origin	Distribution
Sacral, lateral	Vv. sacrales laterales	Large v. of posterior pelvic wall veins	Tissues of posterior pelvic wall	Posterior pelvic wall upward along sacrum to empty into internal iliac v.
Sacral, middle	V. sacralis mediana	Large v. of posterior pelvic wall	Capillaries of tissues of posterior pelvic wall	From pelvic wall in sacral region follows middle sacral artery to empty into common iliac v.
Saphenous, great	V. saphena magna	Longest v. in body	Medial marginal v. of dorsum of foot	Dorsum of foot to femoral v. just below the inguinal ligament
Saphenous, small	V. saphena parva	Large superficial v. of back of leg	Continuation of marginal v.	From behind malleolus ascends back of leg to knee joint where it opens into popliteal v.
Sciatic SEE: *Gluteal v., inferior.*				
Spermatic	V. testicularis	Receives blood from testis and epididymis	Testicular v. in male and ovarian v. in female	From brim of pelvis upward along posterior abdominal wall to inferior vena cava on right and renal v. on left
Spinal	Vv. spinales	Network of veins drawing blood from spinal cord	Spinal cord and its pia mater	Spinal cord through roots to internal vertebral venous plexuses
Splenic	V. lienalis	Large v. which draws blood from spleen and part of stomach	Union of several small veins at the hilus of the spleen	From spleen transversely across abdomen to head of pancreas where it forms portal v. by joining the superior mesenteric v.
Subcardinal		Paired vessels in embryo which replace postcardinal veins. SEE:		

Subclavian	V. subclavia	Main venous trunk of upper extremity	Continuation of axillary v.	Outer border of first rib to sternal end of clavicle where it joins the internal jugular v. to form the brachiocephalic v.
Superficial (Cutaneous v.)		Veins located beneath layers of superficial fascia immediately beneath the skin	Capillaries of superficial tissues of body wall	Throughout subcutaneous tissue of body wall
Supraorbital	V. supraorbitalis	Drains upper portion of orbital cavity	Capillaries and superficial tissues of region of eye	From region of eye along lateral wall of orbital cavity to root of nose where it unites with supratrochlear v. to form angular v.
Suprarenal, left	V. suprarenalis sinistra	V. of left adrenal gland	Capillaries of left adrenal gland	Hilum of left suprarenal gland, ascending to left renal v.
Suprarenal, right	V. suprarenalis dextra	V. of right adrenal gland	Capillaries of right adrenal gland	Hilum of right adrenal gland to inferior vena cava
Supratrochlear (Frontal v.)	Vv. supratrochleares	Drain the anterior scalp	Capillaries of anterior region of scalp	From venous plexuses in forehead diagonally to left of root of nose where they unite with supraorbital v. to form angular v.
Temporal, middle	V. temporalis media	Superficial v. of lateral portion of stomach	Substance of temporal muscle	From lateral superficial plexus of skull it passes to zygoma where it joins superficial temporal v. to form retromandibular v.
Temporal, superficial	Vv. temporales superficiales	Veins of superficial tissues of skull	Lateral scalp in parietal and frontal region	Temporal region of scalp diagonally to ear and downward to mandible where they unite with maxillary v. to form retromandibular v.

*Nomina Anatomica

Veins (*Continued*)

Name	NA*	Description	Origin	Distribution
Thoracic, internal	Vv. thoracicae internae	Deep v. of chest draining intercostal spaces	Tributaries from tissues of intercostal spaces	Tributaries form a single trunk which runs up medial side of internal thoracic artery and ends in brachiocephalic v.
Thoracic, lateral (Long thoracic v.)	V. thoracica lateralis	A large tributary v. of the axillary v. which drains the lateral thoracic wall	Capillaries of muscles and glands of anterior chest	Tissues of anterior chest muscles to axillary v.
Thoracoepigastric	Vv. thoracoepigastricae	Superficial v. of trunk which establishes an important communication between the femoral and axillary veins	Region of superficial epigastric v.	Run laterally along trunk from superficial epigastric v. to lateral thoracic v.
Thyroid, inferior	V. thyroidea inferior	Two or more veins which arise in venous plexuses on thyroid gland	Veins from thyroid glands	Downward to brachiocephalic v.
Thyroid, superior		One v. from either side of thyroid	Substance and surface of thyroid gland	Accompanies superior thyroid artery and empties into internal jugular v.
Tibial, anterior	Vv. tibiales anteriores	Deep veins of anterior aspect of leg	Capillaries of leg tissue and dorsal metatarsal v.	Accompany anterior tibial artery, ascending between tibia and fibula and uniting with posterior tibial v. to form popliteal v.
Tibial, posterior	Vv. tibiales posteriores	Deep veins of back of leg	Capillaries of deep tissues of leg	From ankle upward posterior aspect of leg to unite with

				anterior tibial v. to form popliteal v. just below knee
Ulnar	Vv. ulnares	Large deep veins of medial aspect of forearm	Palmar arches of hand	Palmar arches of hand upward in deep tissues along ulnar side of forearm to form brachial v. with radial v. at elbow
Umbilical	V. umbilicalis sinistra	V. which carries blood from placenta to fetus	Placental tissues	Along umbilical cord through umbilicus to liver upward through inferior vena cava to heart
Uterine	Vv. uterinae	Veins carrying blood from uterus	Tissues of uterus	Uterine plexus through part of the broad ligament to empty into internal iliac v.
Vena cava inferior	V. cava inferior	Returns blood from lower half of body	Right and left iliac veins	From union of iliac veins at level of fifth lumbar vertebra to right atrium of heart
Vena cava superior	V. cava superior	Drains blood from upper half of body	Two innominate veins	From below right costal cartilage to right atrium of heart
Vertebral	V. vertebralis	Drains blood from internal vertebral venous plexuses	Numerous small tributaries in the suboccipital triangle	Base of skull down neck, opening into brachiocephalic v.
Vertebral, anterior	V. vertebralis anterior	Small v.	Plexus around transverse process of upper cervical vertebrae	Descends from region of upper cervical vertebrae with ascending cervical artery and opens into terminal part of vertebral v.

*Nomina Anatomica

App. 9: DRUG INTERACTIONS*

Two or more drugs administered at the same time or in close sequence may act independently, may interact to increase or diminish the intended effect of one or more of the drugs, or may interact to cause an unintended reaction. Many drugs that interact can be used concurrently, but dosage adjustments of one or both may be required.

MECHANISMS OF INTERACTIONS—Genetic differences can affect drug metabolism and interactions. Drugs can interact by changing the metabolism of other drugs through inhibition or induction of hepatic microsomal enzyme activity, by altering the binding of other drugs to plasma proteins or tissue receptor sites, by interfering with the distribution of drugs to active receptor sites, or by delaying or enhancing the excretion of other drugs. Some interactions occur only with high doses of one or both drugs.

WARNING THE PATIENT—In addition to limiting the number of drugs prescribed concurrently and advising patients about known interactions between prescription drugs, physicians may also need to warn patients taking certain drugs against use of over-the-counter medications or vitamins. Patients being treated with oral anticoagulants, for example, should not take large supplements of vitamin E. Interactions may also occur between drugs and foods, such as the interference by meals with the absorption of many antibiotics and drugs, or the hypertensive crisis that can occur when monoamine oxidase (MAO) inhibitors interact with food that contains tyramine. There is little reliable information on interactions of drugs with preservatives, hormones, antibiotics, or pesticide residues found in many common foods.

THE TABLE—The table lists major adverse interactions that have been observed clinically. Interactions useful in therapy, such as the increased plasma concentrations of penicillin with concurrent use of probenecid, are not listed. Common additive effects, such as occur with use of two antihypertensive agents or two central nervous system depressants, are generally not listed. Useful antagonistic effects, such as that between a poison and an antidote, are also not included.

New adverse interactions are continually being reported; the absence of interactions from this table does not necessarily mean that two drugs will not interact when they are given together.

Drug Interactions

Interacting Drugs	Adverse Effect	Probable Mechanism
ANTIMICROBIALS		
Aminoglycoside antibiotics,[1] with:		
Cephaloride (Loridine)	Increased nephrotoxicity	Not established
Cephalothin (Keflin)	Increased nephrotoxicity	Not established
Curariform drugs[2]	Neuromuscular blockade	Additive
Digoxin	Possible decreased digoxin effect with neomycin	Inhibition of gastrointestinal absorption
Ethacrynic acid (Edecrin)	Increased ototoxicity	Additive
Polymyxins (Aerosporin; Coly-Mycin)	Increased nephrotoxicity	Additive
Aminosalicylic acid (PAS), with:		
Probenecid (Benemid; and others)	Increased aminosalicylic acid toxicity	Decreased renal excretion

Amphotericin B (Fungizone), with:		
Curariform drugs[2]	Increased curariform effect	Hypokalemia
Digitalis drugs	Increased digitalis toxicity	Hypokalemia
Cephaloridine (Loridine), with:		
Aminoglycoside antibiotics[1]	Increased nephrotoxicity	Not established
Ethacrynic acid (Edecrin)	Increased nephrotoxicity	Additive
Furosemide (Lasix)	Increased nephrotoxicity	Additive
Cephalothin (Keflin), with:		
Aminoglycoside antibiotics[1]	Increased nephrotoxicity	Not established
Chloramphenicol (Chloromycetin; and others), with:		
Anticoagulants, oral	Increased anticoagulant effect of bishydroxycoumarin (Dicumarol)	Inhibition of microsomal enzymes
Hypoglycemics[3]	Increased sulfonylurea hypoglycemia	Inhibition of microsomal enzymes
Phenytoin (Dilantin; and others)	Increased phenytoin toxicity	Inhibition of microsomal enzymes
Clindamycin (Cleocin), with:		
Curariform drugs[2]	Neuromuscular blockade	Additive
Erythromycin (many brands), with:		
Theophylline	Increased theophylline effect	Not established
Griseofulvin (Fulvicin-U/F; and others), with:		
Anticoagulants, oral	Decreased anticoagulant effect	Induction of microsomal enzymes
Isoniazid, with:		
Alcohol	Decreased isoniazid effect in some patients with chronic alcohol abuse	Increased metabolism
Aluminum antacids	Decreased isoniazid effect	Inhibition of isoniazid absorption
Cycloserine (Seromycin)	CNS effects (dizziness, drowsiness)	Not established
Disulfiram (Antabuse; and others)	Psychotic episodes, ataxia	Alteration of dopamine metabolism
Phenytoin (Dilantin; and others)	Increased phenytoin toxicity	Inhibition of microsomal enzymes
Rifampin (Rifadin; Rimactane)	Increased hepatotoxicity of isoniazid	Induction of microsomal enzymes
Lincomycin (Lincocin), with:		
Kaolin-pectin (Kaopectate; and others)	Decreased lincomycin effect	Decreased lincomycin absorption

Drug Interactions *(Continued)*

Interacting Drugs	Adverse Effect	Probable Mechanism
ANTIMICROBIALS (*continued*)		
Nalidixic acid (NegGram), with:		
Anticoagulants, oral	Increased anticoagulant effect	Displacement from binding sites
Polymyxins (Aerosporin; Coly-Mycin), with:		
Aminoglycoside antibiotics[1]	Increased nephrotoxicity	Additive
Curariform drugs[2]	Neuromuscular blockade	Additive
Rifampin (Rifadin; Rimactane), with:		
Anticoagulants, oral	Decreased anticoagulant effect	Induction of microsomal enzymes
Barbiturates	Decreased barbiturate effect	Induction of microsomal enzymes
Contraceptives, oral	Decreased contraceptive effect	Increased estrogen metabolism
Corticosteroids	Decreased corticosteroid effect	Induction of microsomal enzymes
Digitoxin	Decreased digitoxin effect	Induction of microsomal enzymes
Hypoglycemics[3]	Decreased tolbutamide (Orinase) effect	Induction of microsomal enzymes
Isoniazid	Increased hepatotoxicity of isoniazid	Induction of microsomal enzymes
Methadone	Methadone withdrawal symptoms	Induction of microsomal enzymes
Sulfonamides, with:		
Anticoagulants, oral	Increased anticoagulant effect	Displacement from binding sites
Hypoglycemics[3]	Increased sulfonylurea hypoglycemia	Not established
Tetracyclines, with:		
Antacids, oral	Decreased effect of tetracyclines	Decreased tetracycline absorption
Barbiturates	Decreased doxycycline (Vibramycin; and others) effect	Induction of microsomal enzymes
Carbamazepine (Tegretol)	Decreased doxycycline (Vibramycin; and others) effect	Induction of microsomal enzymes
Iron, oral	Decreased effect of tetracyclines	Decreased tetracycline absorption
Methoxyflurane (Penthrane)	Increased nephrotoxicity	Not established
Zinc sulfate	Decreased effect of tetracycline	Decreased tetracycline absorption
Troleandomycin (Cyclamycin; TAO), with:		

Carbamazepine (Tegretol)	Increased carbamazepine effect	Inhibition of microsomal enzymes
Theophylline	Increased theophylline effect	Not established
ANTICOAGULANTS, ORAL, with:		
Alcohol	Decreased anticoagulant effect with chronic alcohol abuse	Increased metabolism
	Increased anticoagulant effect with acute intoxication	Decreased metabolism
Allopurinol (Zyloprim)	Increased anticoagulant effect	Inhibition of microsomal enzymes
Anabolic and androgenic steroids	Increased anticoagulant effect	Not established
Barbiturates	Decreased anticoagulant effect	Induction of microsomal enzymes
Chloral hydrate (Noctec; and others)[4]	Increased anticoagulant effect	Displacement from binding sites
Chloramphenicol (Chloromycetin; and others)	Increased anticoagulant effect	Inhibition of microsomal enzymes
Cholestyramine (Questran)	Decreased anticoagulant effect	Decreased anticoagulant absorption
Clofibrate (Atromid-S)	Increased anticoagulant effect	Displacement from binding sites
Contraceptives, oral	Decreased anticoagulant effect	Increase in activity of some clotting factors
Dextrothyroxine (Choloxin)	Increased anticoagulant effect	Not established
Disulfiram (Antabuse; and others)	Increased anticoagulant effect	Inhibition of microsomal enzymes
Glutethimide (Doriden; and others)	Decreased anticoagulant effect	Induction of microsomal enzymes
Griseofulvin (Fulvicin-U/F; and others)	Decreased anticoagulant effect	Induction of microsomal enzymes
Hypoglycemics[3]	Increased sulfonylurea hypoglycemia	Inhibition of microsomal enzymes
Indomethacin (Indocin)	Increased anticoagulant effect	Inhibition of platelet function
Metronidazole (Flagyl)	Possible increased anticoagulant effect	Inhibition of microsomal enzymes
Nalidixic acid (NegGram)	Increased anticoagulant effect	Displacement from binding sites
Phenylbutazone (Butazolidin; Azolid) or oxyphenbutazone (Tandearil; Oxalid)	Increased anticoagulant effect	Displacement from binding sites; inhibition of microsomal enzymes
Phenytoin (Dilantin; and others)	Increased phenytoin toxicity	Inhibition of microsomal enzymes
Rifampin (Rifadin; Rimactane)	Decreased anticoagulant effect	Induction of microsomal enzymes
Salicylates	Possible increased anticoagulant effect	Inhibition of platelet function
more than 2 grams/day	Increased hypoprothrombinemic effect	Reduction in plasma prothrombin
Sulfonamides	Increased anticoagulant effect	Not established
Thyroid hormones	Increased anticoagulant effect	Increased clotting factor catabolism
Triclofos sodium (Triclos)[4]	Increased anticoagulant effect	Displacement from binding sites
Vitamin E	Increased anticoagulant effect	Not established
ANTIHYPERTENSIVE DRUGS, with:		
Anesthetics, general	Hypotension	Usually additive

Drug Interactions *(Continued)*

Interacting Drugs	Adverse Effect	Probable Mechanism
ANTIHYPERTENSIVE DRUGS (*continued*)		
Antidepressants, tricyclic[5]	Decreased antihypertensive effects of:	
	Guanethidine (Ismelin)	Blockade of uptake at target site
	Clonidine (Catapres)	Not established
Haloperidol (Haldol)	Increased haloperidol toxicity with methyldopa (Aldomet)	Not established
Hypoglycemics, oral[3]	Decreased signs of hypoglycemia with clonidine (Catapres)	Inhibition of catecholamine response to hypoglycemia
Levodopa (Dopar; and others)	Decreased levodopa effect with clonidine (Catapres)	Not established
Lithium (Lithane; and others)	Increased lithium toxicity with methyldopa (Aldomet)	Not established
Phenothiazines[6]	Decreased antihypertensive effect of guanethidine (Ismelin)	Blockade of uptake at target site
Phenytoin (Dilantin; and others)	Decreased anticonvulsant effect with diazoxide (Hyperstat)	Not established
Sympathomimetic amines[7]	Decreased antihypertensive effect	Inhibition of norepinephrine uptake by neuron
Tolazoline (Priscoline; and others)	Decreased antihypertensive effect of clonidine (Catapres)	Not established
DIURETICS (except spironolactone and triamterene), with:		
Aminoglycoside antibiotics[1]	Increased ototoxicity with ethacrynic acid (Edecrin)	Additive
Cephaloridine (Loridine)	Increased nephrotoxicity with ethacrynic acid (Edecrin) or furosemide (Lasix)	Additive
Chloral hydrate (Noctec; and others)	Vasomotor instability with furosemide (Lasix)	Not established
Corticosteroids	Increased potassium loss	Additive
Curariform drugs[2]	Increased curariform effect	Hypokalemia
Digitalis drugs	Increased digitalis toxicity	Hypokalemia
Lithium (Lithane; and others)	Increased lithium intoxication	Decreased renal lithium clearance
Phenytoin (Dilantin; and others)	Decreased diuresis from furosemide (Lasix)	Not established

Spironolactone (Aldactone), with:		
Digoxin	Increased digoxin effect	Decreased renal excretion
Potassium salts	Hyperkalemia	Additive
Triamterene (Dyrenium), with:		
Potassium salts	Hyperkalemia	Additive
HYPOGLYCEMICS, ORAL[3] with:		
Alcohol	Minor Antabuse-like symptoms with sulfonylureas	Inhibition of intermediary metabolism of alcohol
	Increased hypoglycemic effect with ingestion of alcohol, particularly in fasting patients	Suppression of gluconeogenesis
	Lactic acidosis with phenformin (DBI; Meltrol)	Synergism
	Decreased hypoglycemic effect with chronic alcohol abuse with tolbutamide (Orinase)	Increased metabolism
Anabolic steroids	Increased hypoglycemia	Not established
Anticoagulants, oral	Increased sulfonylurea hypoglycemia	Inhibition of microsomal enzymes
Chloramphenicol (Chloromycetin; and others)	Increase sulfonylurea hypoglycemia	Inhibition of microsomal enzymes
Clonidine (Catapres)	Decreased signs of hypoglycemia	Inhibition of catecholamine response to hypoglycemia
MAO inhibitors[8]	Increased hypoglycemia	Not established
Phenylbutazone (Butazolidin; Azolid) or oxyphenbutazone (Tandearil; Oxalid)	Increased sulfonylurea hypoglycemia	Inhibition of microsomal enzymes
Propranolol (Inderal)	Prolonged hypoglycemia	Decreased glycogenolysis
	Masks tachycardia and tremor	Beta-receptor blockade
Rifampin (Rifadin; Rimactane)	Possible decreased tolbutamide (Orinase) effect	Induction of microsomal enzymes
Salicylates	Increased hypoglycemia	Displacement from binding; additive
Sulfonamides	Increased sulfonylurea hypoglycemia	Not established
PSYCHIATRIC DRUGS		
Antidepressants, tricyclic,[5] with:		
Barbiturates	Decreased antidepressant effect	Induction of microsomal enzymes
Clonidine (Catapres)	Decreased antihypertensive effect	Not established
Guanethidine (Ismelin)	Decreased antihypertensive effect	Blockade of uptake at target site

Drug Interactions *(Continued)*

Interacting Drugs	Adverse Effect	Probable Mechanism
PSYCHIATRIC DRUGS (*continued*)		
Levodopa (Dopar; and others)	Decreased levodopa effect	Decreased levodopa absorption
MAO inhibitors[8,9]	Hyperpyrexia, convulsions	Not established
Phenytoin (Dilantin; and others)	Increased phenytoin toxicity with imipramine (Tofranil)	Not established
Sympathomimetic amines[7]	Hypertension; hypertensive crisis	Inhibition of norepinephrine uptake by neuron
Benzodiazepines, with:		
Alcohol	Enhanced CNS depression	Additive
Haloperidol (Haldol), with:		
Lithium (Lithane; and others)	Increased haloperidol toxicity	Not established
Methyldopa (Aldomet)	Increased haloperidol toxicity	Not established
Lithium (Lithane; and others), with:		
Diuretics (except spironolactone and triamterene)	Lithium intoxication	Decreased renal lithium clearance
Haloperidol (Haldol)	Increased haloperidol toxicity	Not established
Methyldopa (Aldomet)	Increased lithium toxicity	Not established
Phenothiazines[6]	Decreased phenothiazine levels	Not established
MAO inhibitors,[8] with:		
Antidepressants, tricyclic[5,9]	Hyperpyrexia, convulsions	Not established
Hypoglycemics[3]	Increased hypoglycemia	Not established
Levodopa (Dopar; and others)	Hypertensive crisis	Increase in storage and release of dopamine, norepinephrine, or both
Meperidine (Demerol; and others)	Hypertension; hypotension and coma	Not established
Sympathomimetic amines[7,10]	Hypertensive crisis	Increase in storage and release of norepinephrine
Tyramine in food, beer, and wine[11]	Hypertensive crisis	Inhibition of metabolism of tyramine, resulting in increased release of norepinephrine
Phenothiazines,[6] with:		
Barbiturates	Decreased phenothiazine effect	Induction of microsomal enzymes
Guanethidine (Ismelin)	Decreased antihypertensive effect	Blockade of uptake at target site

Levodopa (Dopar; and others)	Decreased levodopa effect	Inhibition of dopamine uptake at target site
Lithium (Lithane; and others)	Decreased phenothiazine levels	Not established
OTHER DRUGS		
Allopurinol (Zyloprim), with:		
Anticoagulants, oral	Increased anticoagulant effect	Inhibition of microsomal enzymes
Azathioprine (Imuran)	Increased azathioprine toxicity	Decreased azathioprine metabolism
Cyclophosphamide (Cytoxan)	Increased cyclophosphamide toxicity	Decreased cyclophosphamide metabolism
Mercaptopurine (6-MP; Purinethol)	Increased mercaptopurine toxicity	Decreased mercaptopurine metabolism
Antacids, oral, with:		
Digitalis drugs	Decreased digoxin effect	Decreased digoxin absorption
Indomethacin (Indocin)	Decreased indomethacin effect	Decreased indomethacin absorption
Isoniazid	Decreased isoniazid effect with aluminum antacids	Decreased absorption of isoniazid
Salicylates	Decreased salicylate levels	Increased renal clearance
Sodium polystyrene sulfonate (Kayexalate)	Metabolic alkalosis	Prevents neutralization of bicarbonate by magnesium and calcium of antacid
Tetracyclines, oral	Decreased effect of tetracyclines	Decreased tetracycline absorption
Barbiturates, with:		
Alcohol	Decreased sedative effect with chronic alcohol abuse	Increased metabolism
	Increased CNS depression with acute intoxication	Additive; decreased metabolism
Anticoagulants, oral	Decreased anticoagulant effect	Induction of microsomal enzymes
Antidepressants, tricyclic[5]	Decreased antidepressant effect	Induction of microsomal enzymes
Corticosteroids	Decreased steroid effect	Induction of microsomal enzymes
Digitoxin	Decreased digitoxin effect	Induction of microsomal enzymes
Meperidine (Demerol; and others)	Increased CNS depression	Increased meperidine metabolites
Phenothiazines[6]	Decreased phenothiazine effect	Induction of microsomal enzymes
Quinidine	Decreased quinidine effect	Induction of microsomal enzymes
Rifampin (Rifadin; Rimactane)	Decreased barbiturate effect	Induction of microsomal enzymes
Tetracyclines	Decreased doxycycline (Vibramycin; and others) effect	Induction of microsomal enzymes

Drug Interactions *(Continued)*

Interacting Drugs	Adverse Effect	Probable Mechanism
OTHER DRUGS *(continued)*		
Carbamazepine (Tegretol), with:		
Doxycycline (Vibramycin; and others)	Decreased doxycycline effect	Induction of microsomal enzymes
Propoxyphene (Darvon; and others)	Increased carbamazepine effect	Inhibition of microsomal enzymes
Troleandomycin (Cyclamycin; TAO)	Increased carbamazepine effect	Inhibition of microsomal enzymes
Chloral hydrate (Noctec; and others), with:		
Alcohol	Prolonged hypnotic effect	Synergism
Anticoagulants[4]	Increased anticoagulant effect	Displacement from binding sites
Furosemide (Lasix)	Vasomotor instability	Not established
Cholestyramine (Questran), with:		
Anticoagulants, oral	Decreased anticoagulant effect	Decreased anticoagulant absorption
Digitalis drugs	Decreased digitoxin effect	Binding in intestine
Thyroid hormones	Decreased thyroid effect	Binding in intestine
Cimetidine (Tagamet), with:		
Carmustine (BCNU)	Increased bone marrow depression	Additive
Contraceptives, oral, with:		
Anticoagulants, oral	Decreased anticoagulant effect	Increase in activity of some clotting factors
Rifampin (Rifadin; Rimactane)	Decreased contraceptive effect	Increased estrogen metabolism
Corticosteroids, with:		
Barbiturates	Decreased steroid effect	Induction of microsomal enzymes
Diuretics (except spironolactone and triamterene)	Increased potassium loss	Additive
Ephedrine	Decreased dexamethasone effect	Not established
Phenytoin (Dilantin; and others)	Decreased effect of dexamethasone	Induction of microsomal enzymes
Rifampin (Rifadin; Rimactane)	Decreased corticosteroid effect	Induction of microsomal enzymes
Curariform drugs,[2] with:		
Aminoglycoside antibiotics[1] or polymyxins (administered parenterally)	Neuromuscular blockade	Additive
Amphotericin B (Fungizone)	Increased curariform effect	Hypokalemia
Clindamycin (Cleocin)	Neuromuscular blockade	Additive

Diuretics (except spironolactone and triamterene)	Increased curariform effect	Hypokalemia
Narcotic analgesics	Increased respiratory depression	Additive
Quinidine	Increased curariform effect	Additive
Digitalis drugs, with:		
Amphotericin B (Fungizone)	Increased digitalis toxicity	Hypokalemia
Antacids, oral	Decreased digoxin effect	Decreased digoxin absorption
Barbiturates	Decreased digitoxin effect	Induction of microsomal enzymes
Cholestyramine (Questran)	Decreased digitoxin effect	Binding in intestine
Diuretics (except spironolactone and triamterene)	Increased digitalis toxicity	Hypokalemia
Kaolin-pectin (Kaopectate; and others)	Decreased digoxin effect	Decreased digoxin absorption
Neomycin	Possible decreased digoxin effect	Not established
Quinidine	Increased digoxin effect	Not established
Rifampin (Rifadin; Rimactane)	Decreased digitoxin effect	Induction of microsomal enzymes
Spironolactone (Aldactone)	Increased digoxin effect	Decreased renal excretion
Sulfasalazine (Azulfidine; and others)	Possible decreased digoxin effect	Decreased digoxin absorption
Sympathomimetic amines[7]	Increased tendency to cardiac arrhythmias	Additive effect on myocardium
Disulfiram (Antabuse; and others), with:		
Alcohol	Abdominal cramps, flushing, vomiting, psychotic episodes, confusion	Inhibition of intermediary metabolism of alcohol
Anticoagulants, oral	Increased anticoagulant effect	Inhibition of microsomal enzymes
Isoniazid	Psychotic episodes; ataxia	Alteration of dopamine metabolism
Phenytoin (Dilantin; and others)	Increased phenytoin effect	Inhibition of metabolism
Indomethacin (Indocin), with:		
Antacids, oral	Decreased indomethacin effect	Decreased indomethacin absorption
Anticoagulants, oral	Increased anticoagulant effect	Inhibition of platelet function
Kaolin-pectin (Kaopectate; and others), with:		
Digitalis drugs	Decreased digoxin effect	Decreased digoxin absorption
Lincomycin (Lincocin)	Decreased lincomycin effect	Decreased lincomycin absorption

Drug Interactions *(Continued)*

Interacting Drugs	Adverse Effect	Probable Mechanism
OTHER DRUGS *(continued)*		
Levodopa (Dopar; and others), with:		
Anticholinergics	Decreased levodopa effect	Decreased levodopa absorption
Antidepressants[5]	Decreased levodopa effect	Decreased levodopa absorption
Clonidine (Catapres)	Decreased levodopa effect	Not established
MAO inhibitors[8]	Hypertensive crisis	Increase in storage and release of dopamine, norepinephrine, or both
Methionine	Decreased levodopa effect	Not established
Papaverine (Cerespan; and others)	Decreased levodopa effect	Not established
Phenothiazines[6]	Decreased levodopa effect	Inhibition of dopamine uptake
Phenytoin (Dilantin; and others)	Decreased levodopa effect	Not established
Protein in food	Decreased levodopa effect	Decreased levodopa absorption
Pyridoxine	Decreased levodopa effect	Enhancement of decarboxylation of levodopa at periphery
Meprobamate (Miltown; and others), with:		
Alcohol	Decreased sedative effect with chronic alcohol abuse	Increased metabolism
	Increased CNS depression with acute intoxication	Additive; decreased metabolism
Methotrexate, with:		
Phenylbutazone (Butazolidin; Azolid)	Increased toxicity of methotrexate	Not established
Salicylates	Increased toxicity of methotrexate	Decreased renal clearance of methotrexate
Methoxyflurane (Penthrane), with:		
Tetracyclines	Increased nephrotoxicity	Not established
Phenylbutazone (Butazolidin; Azolid), with:		
Anticoagulants, oral	Increased anticoagulant effect	Displacement from binding sites; inhibition of microsomal enzymes
Hypoglycemics, oral[3]	Increased sulfonylurea hypoglycemia	Inhibition of microsomal enzymes
Methotrexate	Increased methotrexate toxicity	Not established

Phenytoin (Dilantin; and others), with:		
Alcohol	Decreased anticonvulsant effect with chronic alcohol abuse	Increased metabolism
	Increased anticonvulsant effect with acute intoxication	Decreased metabolism
Anticoagulants, oral	Increased phenytoin toxicity	Inhibition of microsomal enzymes
Antidepressants, tricyclic[5]	Increased phenytoin toxicity	Not established
Chloramphenicol (Chloromycetin; and others)	Increased phenytoin toxicity	Inhibition of microsomal enzymes
Corticosteroids	Decreased effect of dexamethasone	Induction of microsomal enzymes
Diazoxide (Hyperstat)	Decreased anticonvulsant effect	Not established
Disulfiram (Antabuse; and others)	Increased phenytoin effect	Inhibition of metabolism
Dopamine	Hypotension in critically ill given phenytoin IV	Not established
Furosemide (Lasix)	Decreased diuresis	Not established
Isoniazid	Increased phenytoin toxicity	Inhibition of microsomal enzymes
Levodopa (Dopar; and others)	Decreased levodopa effect	Not established
Quinidine	Decreased quinidine effect	Induction of microsomal enzymes
Probenecid (Benemid; and others), with:		
Aminosalicylic acid (PAS)	Increased aminosalicylic acid toxicity	Inhibition of renal excretion
Salicylates	Decreased uricosuric effect	Not established
Quinidine, with:		
Barbiturates	Decreased quinidine effect	Induction of microsomal enzymes
Curariform drugs[2]	Increased curariform effect	Additive
Digoxin	Increased digoxin effect	Not established
Phenytoin (Dilantin; and others)	Decreased quinidine effect	Induction of microsomal enzymes
Salicylates, with:		
Alcohol	Increased gastrointestinal bleeding	Additive
Antacids	Decreased salicylate levels	Increased renal clearance
Anticoagulants, oral	Possible increased anticoagulant effect	Inhibition of platelet function
	Increased hypoprothrombinemic effect (more than 2 grams/day of salicylates)	Reduction of plasma prothrombin
Hypoglycemics[3]	Increased hypoglycemia	Displacement from binding; additive
Methotrexate	Increased toxicity of methotrexate	Decreased renal clearance of methotrexate
Probenecid (Benemid; and others)	Decreased uricosuric effect	Not established

Drug Interactions *(Continued)*

Interacting Drugs	Adverse Effect	Probable Mechanism
OTHER DRUGS *(continued)*		
Sympathomimetic amines,[7] with:		
Antidepressants, tricyclic[5]	Hypertension, hypertensive crisis	Inhibition of norepinephrine uptake by neuron
Antihypertensive drugs	Decreased antihypertensive effect	Inhibition of norepinephrine uptake by neuron
Cyclopropane and halogenated hydrocarbon anesthetics	Cardiac arrhythmias	Not established
Digitalis drugs	Increased tendency to cardiac arrhythmias	Additive effect on myocardium
MAO inhibitors[8,10]	Hypertensive crisis	Increase in storage and release of norepinephrine
Theophylline, with:		
Erythromycin (many brands)	Increased theophylline effect	Not established
Troleandomycin (Cyclamycin; TAO)	Increased theophylline effect	Not established
Smoking (tobacco and marihuana)	Decreased theophylline effect	Increased metabolism
Thyroid hormones, with:		
Anticoagulants, oral	Increased anticoagulant effect	Increase clotting factor catabolism
Cholestyramine (Questran)	Decreased thyroid effect	Binding of hormone in intestine
Triclofos sodium (Triclos), with:		
Anticoagulants[4]	Increased anticoagulant effect	Displacement from binding sites

1. Aminoglycoside antibiotics include amikacin (Amikin), gentamicin (Garamycin), kanamycin (Kantrex), neomycin, streptomycin, and tobramycin (Nebcin).
2. Curariform drugs include d-tubocurarine, gallamine, and succinylcholine.
3. Oral hypoglycemics include phenformin (no longer available in the USA or Canada) and the sulfonylureas (acetohexamide—Dymelor; chlorpropamide—Diabinese; tolazamide—Tolinase; tolbutamide—Orinase). Any drug with marked stimulant effect on the sympathetic nervous system can enhance insulin release and consequently the action of sulfonylureas.
4. Increased anticoagulant effect during the first week of chloral hydrate or triclofos sodium therapy in patients previously anticoagulated. In patients on chronic therapy with both agents there may be no significant effect.
5. Tricyclic antidepressants include amitriptyline (Elavil; and others), desipramine (Norpramin; Pertofrane), doxepin (Adapin; Sinequan), imipramine (Tofranil; and others), nortriptyline (Aventyl), and protriptyline (Vivactil).

6. Phenothiazines include acetophenazine (Tindal), butaperazine (Repoise), carphenazine (Proketazine), chlorpromazine (Thorazine; and others), fluphenazine (Prolixin; Permitil), mesoridazine (Serentil), perphenazine (Trilafon), piperacetazine (Quide), prochlorperazine (Compazine), promazine (Sparine), thioridazine (Mellaril), trifluoperazine (Stelazine), and triflupromazine (Vesprin).
7. Sympathomimetic amines include amphetamines, ephedrine, epinephrine (Adrenalin), isoproterenol (Isuprel), methylphenidate (Ritalin), norepinephrine (Levophed), phenylephrine, phenylpropanolamine, many appetite-depressing drugs and amines in many over-the-counter cough, cold, and "sinus" remedies, including nasal decongestants.
8. MAO inhibitors include furazolidone (Furoxone), isocarboxazid (Marplan), pargyline (Eutonyl), phenelzine (Nardil), procarbazine (Matulane), and tranylcypromine (Parnate).
9. Some clinicians have used MAO inhibitors and tricyclic antidepressants concurrently without adverse effects in selected patients.
10. Of the sympathomimetic amines (footnote 7), the most dangerous in patients on MAO inhibitors would be amphetamines, ephedrine, phenylephrine, phenylpropanolamine, and pseudoephedrine.
11. Foods containing tyramine include aged cheeses, avocados, bananas, fava beans, canned figs, beer, Chianti and other red wines, sherry, fermented sausage (pepperoni and others), yeast extracts, chicken liver, chocolate (contains phenylethylamine), spoiled pickled herring, caviar, and dried fish. (See The Medical Letter, 18:32, 1976 for detailed discussion.)

*From The Medical Letter, Inc., 56 Harrison St., New Rochelle, N.Y. 10801: Vol. 21, Jan. 26, 1979, with permission.

App. 10: Radiation Therapy

Precautions Necessary When Working Closely with a Patient with Radioactive Implant in Place

One mg. of radium is equivalent to one millicurie of radioactivity and for every milligram, 8.25 rads are emitted in one hour at one centimeter distance from the source. Therefore, a 100-mg. implant would provide delivery of (8.25 x 100) 285 rads in one hour at one centimeter. The inverse square law indicates that the greater distance away, the less intensity of the radiation by the inverse square proportion. Thus, if an implant emits 8.25 rads at 1 cm., then moving the source to 100 cm. would reduce the radiation by a factor of

$$\frac{1}{10^4}$$

The kinds of radiation that may be utilized clinically are usually gamma and beta. Gamma radiation is a wave of electromagnetic energy (^{60}Co) or x-ray (which is the same but generated electrically) versus beam or electron radiation, which is composed of negatively charged particles. The properties differ, allowing electrons to have a less penetrating radiation through tissue. That is, given a photon of the same energy of an electron—say both were in 7 million electronvolt range—the photons would continue through the tissue diminishing the intensity as they go through layers and layers of tissue, whereas the electrons would be completely dissipated after passing through 3 cm. of tissue. This type of radiation may be utilized to advantage when the chest wall and certain skin surfaces require treatment.

Radiation therapists protect themselves from radiation exposure by using the *inverse square law* and by decreasing the time of exposure, i.e., decreasing the time required for implanting or withdrawing radioactive materials. It would be impossible for people to work while wearing 2-inch-thick (5-cm.) lead aprons.

Daily Treatments

Most patients are treated with a daily fractionation of 200 rads, which is 1000 rads a week, on a five-day-per-week schedule. This is utilized to allow normal tissue to recuperate and to achieve the maximum tumor damage.

Daily treatment with external radiation therapy is usually conducted on an outpatient basis, if the patient is well enough. Decreases in dose, which is measured in *rads,* a unit of radiation absorbed, are permitted depending upon the circumstances. Also, total dose utilized is dependent upon the tumor and its anticipated behavior. Therefore, lymphomas and seminomas or radiosensitive tumors receive much lower doses than typical carcinomas of the head and neck, which receive radiation in the range of 6000 to 7500 rads.

Oxygen is required in the metabolism for the presence of external radiation for photon radiation to work. Thus, the patient should be adequately supplied with blood and the hemoglobin should be at least 10 grams because a decrease in the oxygen present diminishes the radiosensitivity of the tumor.

App. 11: DIETETICS

Recommended Daily Dietary Allowances,[a] Revised 1980*

Designed for the maintenance of good nutrition of practically all healthy people in the U.S.A.

		Weight		Height			Fat Soluble Vitamins			Water Soluble Vitamins							Minerals					
	Age (years)	(kg)	(lbs)	(cm)	(in)	Protein (g)	Vitamin A (μg R.E.)[b]	Vitamin D (μg)[c]	Vitamin E (mg σ T.E.)[d]	Vitamin C (mg)	Thiamine (mg)	Riboflavin (mg)	Niacin (mg N.E.)[e]	Vitamin B6 (mg)	Folacin (μg)	Vitamin B12 (μg)	Calcium (mg)	Phosphorus (mg)	Magnesium (mg)	Iron (mg)	Zinc (mg)	Iodine (μg)
Infants	0.0-0.5	6	13	60	24	kg x 2.2	420	10	3	35	0.3	0.4	6	0.3	30	0.5[g]	360	240	50	10	3	40
	0.5-1.0	9	20	71	28	kg x 2.0	400	10	4	35	0.5	0.6	8	0.6	45	1.5	540	360	70	15	5	50
Children	1-3	13	29	90	35	23	400	10	5	45	0.7	0.8	9	0.9	100	2.0	800	800	150	15	10	70
	4-6	20	44	112	44	30	500	10	6	45	0.9	1.0	11	1.3	200	2.5	800	800	200	10	10	90
	7-10	28	62	132	52	34	700	10	7	45	1.2	1.4	16	1.6	300	3.0	800	800	250	10	10	120
Males	11-14	45	99	157	62	45	1000	10	8	50	1.4	1.6	18	1.8	400	3.0	1200	1200	350	18	15	150
	15-18	66	145	176	69	56	1000	10	10	60	1.4	1.7	18	2.0	400	3.0	1200	1200	400	18	15	150
	19-22	70	154	177	70	56	1000	7.5	10	60	1.5	1.7	19	2.2	400	3.0	800	800	350	10	15	150
	23-50	70	154	178	70	56	1000	5	10	60	1.4	1.6	18	2.2	400	3.0	800	800	350	10	15	150
	51+	70	154	178	70	56	1000	5	10	60	1.2	1.4	16	2.2	400	3.0	800	800	350	10	15	150
Females	11-14	46	101	157	62	46	800	10	8	50	1.1	1.3	15	1.8	400	3.0	1200	1200	300	18	15	150
	15-18	55	120	163	64	46	800	10	8	60	1.1	1.3	14	2.0	400	3.0	1200	1200	300	18	15	150
	19-22	55	120	163	64	44	800	7.5	8	60	1.1	1.3	14	2.0	400	3.0	800	800	300	18	15	150
	23-50	55	120	163	64	44	800	5	8	60	1.0	1.2	13	2.0	400	3.0	800	800	300	18	15	150
	51+	55	120	163	64	44	800	5	8	60	1.0	1.2	13	2.0	400	3.0	800	800	300	10	15	150
Pregnant						+30	+200	+5	+2	+20	+0.4	+0.3	+2	+0.6	+400	+1.0	+400	+400	+150	*h*	+5	+25
Lactating						+20	+400	+5	+3	+40	+0.5	+0.5	+5	+0.5	+100	+1.0	+400	+400	+150	*h*	+10	+50

a The allowances are intended to provide for individual variations among most normal persons as they live in the United states under usual environmental stresses. Diets should be based on a variety of common foods in order to provide other nutrients for which human requirements have been less well defined.

b Retinol equivalents. 1 retinol equivalent = 1 μg retinol or 6 μg β-carotene.

c As cholecalciferol. 10 μg cholecalciferol = 400 I.U. vitamin D.

d σ tocopherol equivalents. 1 mg d-σ-tocopherol = 1 σ T.E.

e 1 N.E. (niacin equivalent) is equal to 1 mg of niacin or 60 mg of dietary tryptophan.

f The folacin allowances refer to dietary sources as determined by *Lactobacillus casei* assay after treatment with enzymes ("conjugases") to make polyglutamyl forms of the vitamin available to the test organism.

g The RDA for vitamin B12 in infants is based on average concentration of the vitamin in human milk. The allowances after weaning are based on energy intake (as recommended by the American Academy of Pediatrics) and consideration of other factors such as intestinal absorption.

h The increased requirement during pregnancy cannot be met by the iron content of habitual American diets nor by the existing iron stores of many women; therefore the use of 30-60 mg of supplemental iron is recommended. Iron needs during lactation are not substantially different from those of nonpregnant women, but continued supplementation of the mother for 2-3 months after parturition is advisable in order to replenish stores depleted by pregnancy.

* From: Food and Nutrition Board, National Academy of Sciences—National Research Council, Washington, D.C., 1980.

Estimated Safe and Adequate Daily Dietary Intakes of Selected Vitamins and Minerals[a]*

		Vitamins			Trace Elements[b]						Electrolytes		
	Age (years)	Vitamin K (μg)	Biotin (μg)	Panto-thenic Acid (mg)	Copper (mg)	Manganese (mg)	Fluoride (mg)	Chromium (mg)	Selenium (mg)	Molybdenum (mg)	Sodium (mg)	Potassium (mg)	Chloride (mg)
Infants	0-0.5	12	35	2	0.5-0.7	0.5-0.7	0.1-0.5	0.01-0.04	0.01-0.04	0.03-0.06	115-350	350-925	275-700
	0.5-1	10-20	50	3	0.7-1.0	0.7-1.0	0.2-1.0	0.02-0.06	0.02-0.06	0.04-0.08	250-750	425-1275	400-1200
Children	1-3	15-30	65	3	1.0-1.5	1.0-1.5	0.5-1.5	0.02-0.08	0.02-0.08	0.05-0.1	325-975	550-1650	500-1500
and	4-6	20-40	85	3-4	1.5-2.0	1.5-2.0	1.0-2.5	0.03-0.12	0.03-0.12	0.06-0.15	450-1350	775-2325	700-1200
Adolescents	7-10	30-60	120	4-5	2.0-2.5	2.0-3.0	1.5-2.5	0.05-0.2	0.05 -0.2	0.1 -0.3	600-1800	1000-3000	925-2775
	11+	50-100	100-200	4-7	2.0-3.0	2.5-5.0	1.5-2.5	0.05-0.2	0.05 -0.2	0.15-0.5	900-2700	1525-4575	1400-4200
Adults		70-140	100-200	4-7	2.0-3.0	2.5-5.0	1.5-4.0	0.05-0.2	0.05-0.2	0.15-0.5	1100-3300	1875-5625	1700-5100

[a] Because there is less information on which to base allowances, these figures are not given in the main table of the RDA and are provided here in the form of ranges of recommended intakes.

[b] Since the toxic levels for many trace elements may be only several times usual intakes, the upper levels for the trace elements given in this table should not be habitually exceeded.

* Food and Nutrition Board, National Academy of Sciences—National Research Council, Washington, D.C.

Mean Heights and Weights and Recommended Energy Intake*

Category	Age (years)	Weight (kg)	Weight (lb)	Height (cm)	Height (in)	Energy Needs (with range) (kcal)	Energy Needs (MJ)
Infants	0.0-0.5	6	13	60	24	kg × 115 (95-145)	kg × .48
	0.5-1.0	9	20	71	28	kg × 105 (80-135)	kg × .44
Children	1-3	13	29	90	35	1300 (900-1800)	5.5
	4-6	20	44	112	44	1700 (1300-2300)	7.1
	7-10	28	62	132	52	2400 (1650-3300)	10.1
Males	11-14	45	99	157	62	2700 (2000-3700)	11.3
	15-18	66	145	176	69	2800 (2100-3900)	11.8
	19-22	70	154	177	70	2900 (2500-3300)	12.2
	23-50	70	154	178	70	2700 (2300-3100)	11.3
	51-75	70	154	178	70	2400 (2000-2800)	10.1
	76+	70	154	178	70	2050 (1650-2450)	8.6
Females	11-14	46	101	157	62	2200 (1500-3000)	9.2
	15-18	55	120	163	64	2100 (1200-3000)	8.8

	19-22	55	120	163	64	2100 (1700-2500)	8.8
	23-50	55	120	163	64	2000 (1600-2400)	8.4
	51-75	55	120	163	64	1800 (1400-2200)	7.6
	76+	55	120	163	64	1600 (1200-2000)	6.7
Pregnancy						+300	
Lactation						+500	

The data in this table have been assembled from the observed median heights and weights of children, together with desirable weights for adults for the mean heights of men (70 inches) and women (64 inches) between the ages of 18 and 34 years as surveyed in the U.S. population.

The energy allowances for the young adults are for men and women doing light work. The allowances for the two older age groups represent mean energy needs over these age spans, allowing for a 2% decrease in basal (resting) metabolic rate per decade and a reduction in activity of 200 kcal/day for men and women between 51 and 75 years, 500 kcal for men over 75 years and 400 kcal for women over 75. The customary range of daily energy output is shown for adults in parentheses, and is based on a variation in energy needs of ± 400 kcal at any one age, emphasizing the wide range of energy intakes appropriate for any group of people.

Energy allowances for children through age 18 are based on median energy intakes of children these ages followed in longitudinal growth studies. The values in parentheses are 10th and 90th percentiles of energy intake, to indicate the range of energy consumption among children of these ages.

*From: *Recommended Dietary Allowances, Revised 1980,* Food and Nutrition Board, National Academy of Sciences—National Research Council, Washington, D.C.

Vitamins

(Summary of Vitamins Significant in Human Diet)

Vitamin	Chief Functions	Results of Deficiency	Characteristics	Good Sources	Daily Allowances Recommended
VITAMIN A Provitamin, carotene	Essential for maintaining the integrity of epithelial membranes. Helps maintain resistance to infections. Necessary for the formation of rhodopsin and prevention of night blindness.	*Mild:* Retarded growth. Increased susceptibility to infection. Abnormal function of gastrointestinal, genitourinary and respiratory tracts due to altered epithelial membranes. Skin dries, shrivels, thickens, sometimes pustule formation. Night blindness. *Severe:* Xerophthalmia, a characteristic eye disease, and other local infections.	Fat soluble. Not destroyed by ordinary cooking temperatures. Is destroyed by high temperatures when oxygen is present. Marked capacity for storage in the liver. NOTE: Excessive intake of carotene from which vitamin A is formed may produce yellow discoloration of the skin (carotenemia).	Animal fats butter cheese cream egg yolk whole milk. Fish liver oil. Liver Vegetable 1. green leafy, esp. escarole, kale, parsley 2. yellow, esp. carrots. *Artificial:* Concentrates in several forms. Irradiated fish oils.	*Males (Ages 11–51$^+$ yrs.):* 1000 μg retinol equivalents *Females (Ages 11–51$^+$ yrs.):* 800 μg retinol equivalents *In pregnancy:* 1000 μg retinol equivalents *In lactation:* 1200 μg retinol equivalents *Children:* 400–700 μg retinol equivalents *Infants:* 400 μg retinol equivalents
THIAMINE Vitamin B_1	Important role in carbohydrate metabolism. Essential for mainte-	*Mild:* Loss of appetite. Impaired digestion of starches and sugars. Colitis, constipation, or	Water soluble. Not readily destroyed by ordinary cooking temperature.	Widely distributed in plant and animal tissues but seldom occurs in high concentration, exception	*Males (11–51$^+$ yrs.):* 1.2–1.5 mg. *Females*

	nance of normal digestion and appetite. Essential for normal functioning of nervous tissue.	diarrhea. Emaciation. *Severe:* Nervous disorders of various types. Loss of coordinating power of muscles. Beriberi Paralysis in man.	Destroyed by exposure to heat, alkali, or sulfites. Is not stored in body.	in brewer's yeast. Other good sources are: Whole grain cereals Peas, Beans Peanuts Oranges Glandular—heart, liver, kidney Many vegetables and fruits Nuts. *Artificial:* Concentrates from yeast. Rice polishings. Wheat germ.	(*11–51^{+} yrs.*): 1.0 to 1.1 mg. *In pregnancy:* **1.4** to **1.6 mg.** *In lactation:* 1.5 to **1.7** mg. *Children:* **0.7** to 1.2 mg. *Infants:* **0.3** to 0.5 mg.
RIBOFLAVIN Vitamin B_2	Important in formation of certain enzymes and in cellular oxidation. Normal growth. Prevention of cheilosis and glossitis. Participates in light adaptation.	Impaired growth. Lassitude and weakness. Cheilosis. Glossitis. Atrophy of skin. Anemia. Photophobia. Cataracts.	Water soluble. Alcohol soluble. Not destroyed by heat in cooking unless with alkali. Unstable in light, esp. in presence of alkali.	Eggs Green vegetables Liver Kidney Lean meat Milk Wheat germ Yeast, dried Enriched foods.	*Males* (*11–51^{+} yrs.*): **1.4–1.7 mg.** *Females* (*11–51^{+} yrs.*): **1.2–1.3 mg.** *In pregnancy:* **1.6 mg.** *In lactation:* **1.8 mg.** *Children:* **0.8** to **1.4 mg.** *Infants:* 0.4 to 0.6 mg.

Vitamins (*Continued*)

Vitamin	Chief Functions	Results of Deficiency	Characteristics	Good Sources	Daily Allowances Recommended
NIACIN Nicotinic acid Nicotinamide Antipellagra vitamin	As the component of two important enzymes, it is important in glycolysis, tissue respiration, and fat synthesis. Nicotinic acid but not nicotinamide causes vasodilation and flushing. Prevents pellagra.	Pellagra. Gastrointestinal disturbances. Mental disturbances.	Soluble in hot water and alcohol. Not destroyed by heat, light, air or alkali. Not destroyed in ordinary cooking.	Yeast Lean meat Fish Legumes Whole grain cereals and peanuts Enriched foods.	*Males* (*11–51$^+$ yrs.*): 16–19 mg. *Females* (*11–51$^+$ yrs.*): 13–15 mg. *In pregnancy:* 17 mg. *In lactation:* 20 mg. *Children:* 9–16 mg. *Infants:* 6–8 mg.
VITAMIN B_{12} Cyanocobalamin	Produces remission in pernicious anemia. Essential for normal development of red blood cells.	Pernicious anemia.	Soluble in water or alcohol. Unstable in hot alkaline or acid solutions.	Liver Kidney Dairy products. Most of vitamin required by humans is synthesized by intestinal bacteria.	*Males and Females* (*11–51$^+$ yrs.*): 3.0 mcg. *In pregnancy:* 4.0 mcg. *In lactation:* 5.0 mcg.

					Children: 2 to 5 mcg. *Infants:* 1 to 2 mcg.
VITAMIN C Ascorbic acid	Essential to formation of intracellular cement substances in a variety of tissues including skin, dentin, cartilage and bone matrix. Important in healing of wounds and fractures of bones. Prevents scurvy. Facilitates absorption of iron.	*Mild:* Lowered resistance to infections. Joint tenderness. Susceptibility to dental caries, pyorrhea, and bleeding gums. *Severe:* Hemorrhage. Anemia. Scurvy.	Soluble in water. Easily destroyed by oxidation; heat hastens the process. Lost in cooking, particularly if water in which food was cooked is discarded. Also loss is greater if cooked in iron or copper utensils. Quick frozen foods lose little of their vitamin C. Stored in the body to a limited extent.	Abundant in most fresh fruits and vegetables, esp. citrus fruit and juices, tomato and orange. *Artificial:* Ascorbic acid. Cevitamic acid.	*Males* (*11–51⁺ yrs.*): **50–60 mg.** *Females* (*11–51⁺ yrs.*): **50–60 mg.** *In pregnancy:* **80 mg.** *In lactation:* **100 mg.** *Children:* **45 mg.** *Infants:* 35 mg. The infant diet is likely to be deficient in vitamin C unless orange or tomato juice or other form is added.
VITAMIN D	Regulates absorption of calcium and phosphorus from the in-	*Mild:* Interferes with utilization of calcium and	Soluble in fats and organic solvents.	Butter Egg yolk Fish liver oils	*Males and Females* (*11–51⁺ yrs.*): 200–400 I.U.

Vitamins (*Continued*)

Vitamin	Chief Functions	Results of Deficiency	Characteristics	Good Sources	Daily Allowances Recommended
	testinal tract. Antirachitic.	phosphorus in bone and teeth formation. Irritability. Weakness. *Severe:* Rickets, may be common in young children. Osteomalacia in adults.	Relatively stable under refrigeration. Stored in liver. Often associated with vitamin A.	Fish having fat distributed through the flesh, salmon, tuna fish, herring, sardines Liver Oysters Yeast and foods irradiated with ultraviolet light. Formed in the skin by exposure to sunlight. Artificially prepared forms.	After age 22, none except during pregnancy or lactation. *In pregnancy:* 400–600 I.U. *In lactation:* 400–600 I.U. *Children:* 400 I.U. *Infants:* 400 I.U.
VITAMIN E Alpha tocopherol	Normal reproduction in rats. Prevention of muscular dystrophy in rats.	Red blood cell resistance to rupture is decreased.	Fat soluble. Stable to heat in absence of oxygen.	Lettuce and other green, leafy vegetables. Wheat germ oil Margarine Rice.	*Males* (*11–51⁺ yrs.*): 8–10 mg. d-α-tocopherol *Females* (*11–51⁺ yrs.*): 8 mg. d-α-tocopherol *In pregnancy:* 10 mg. d-α-tocopherol *In lactation:* 11 mg. d-α-tocopherol *Children:* 10 to 15 I.U.

					Infants: 5 I.U.
VITAMIN B$_6$ Pyridoxine	Essential for metabolism of tryptophan. Needed for utilization of certain other amino acids.	Dermatitis around eyes and mouth. Neuritis. Anorexia, nausea, and vomiting.	Soluble in water and alcohol. Rapidly inactivated in presence of heat, sunlight, or air.	Blackstrap molasses Meat Cereal grains Wheat germ.	*Males and Females (11–51$^+$ yrs.):* 1.8–2.2 mg. *In pregnancy:* 2.6 mg. *In lactation:* 2.5 mg. *Children:* 0.9–1.6 mg. *Infants:* 0.3–0.6 mg.
FOLACIN	Essential for normal functioning of hematopoietic system.	Anemia.	Slightly soluble in water. Easily destroyed by heat in presence of acid. Decreases when food is stored at room temperature. NOTE: A large dose may prevent appearance of anemia in a case of pernicious anemia but still permit neurological symptoms to develop.	Glandular meats Yeast Green, leafy vegetables.	*Males and Females (11–51$^+$ yrs.):* 400 μg. *In pregnancy:* 800 μg. *In lactation:* 500 μg. *Children:* 100–300 μg. *Infants:* 30–45 μg.

Composition of Foods (100 grams, edible portion)*

Food and description	Water	Food energy	Protein	Fat	Carbohydrate Total	Carbohydrate Fiber	Ash	Calcium	Phosphorus	Iron	Sodium	Potassium	Vitamin A value	Thiamine	Riboflavin	Niacin	Ascorbic acid
	Percent	Calories	Grams	Grams	Grams	Grams	Grams	Milligrams	Milligrams	Milligrams	Milligrams	Milligrams	International units	Milligrams	Milligrams	Milligrams	Milligrams
Ale. See Beverages: Beer.																	
Almonds, roasted and salted	.7	627	18.6	57.7	19.5	2.6	3.5	235	504	4.7	198	773	0	.05	.92	3.5	0
Apples, raw, fresh, not pared	84.4	58	.2	.6	14.5	1.0	.3	7	10	.3	1	110	90	.03	.02	.1	4
Apple butter	51.6	186	.4	.8	46.8	1.1	.4	14	36	.7	2	252	0	.01	.02	.2	2
Apple juice, canned or bottled	87.8	47	.1	Trace	11.9	.1	.2	6	9	.6	1	101	—	.01	.02	.1	1
Apricots, raw	85.3	51	1.0	.2	12.8	.6	.7	17	23	.5	1	281	2,700	.03	.04	.6	10
Asparagus, cooked spears, boiled, drained	93.6	20	2.2	.2	3.6	.7	.4	21	50	.6	1	183	900	.16	.18	1.4	26
Avocados, raw	74.0	167	2.1	16.4	6.3	1.6	1.2	10	42	.6	4	604	290	.11	.20	1.6	14
Baby foods:																	
Cereals:																	
Barley, added nutrients	6.6	348	13.4	1.2	73.6	1.2	5.2	736	821	53.2	452	413	(0)	3.71	1.20	32.2	(0)
Oatmeal, added nutrients	7.0	375	16.5	5.5	66.0	1.5	5.0	757	734	48.2	437	374	(0)	2.58	1.05	21.3	(0)
Desserts, canned:																	
Custard pudding	76.5	100	2.3	1.8	18.6	.2	.8	64	62	.3	150	94	100	.02	.12	.1	1
Fruit pudding	75.7	96	1.2	.9	21.6	.3	.6	27	34	.3	128	75	100	.03	.05	.1	3
Dinners, canned:																	
Beef noodle dinner	88.2	48	2.8	1.1	6.8	.3	1.1	12	29	.5	269	159	620	.02	.05	.5	2
Cereal, egg yolk, bacon	84.7	82	2.9	4.9	6.6	.1	.9	29	60	.8	301	36	520	.05	.06	.4	—
Beef with vegetables	81.6	87	7.4	3.7	6.0	.2	1.3	13	84	1.2	304	113	1,100	.07	.17	1.6	2
Chicken with vegetables	79.6	100	7.4	4.6	7.2	.2	1.2	22	85	.9	265	71	1,000	.09	.15	1.6	2
Turkey with vegetables	81.3	86	6.7	3.2	7.6	.5	1.2	38	63	.6	348	122	1,000	.13	.13	1.8	2
Veal with vegetables	85.0	63	7.1	1.6	5.1	.2	1.2	11	71	.8	323	95	800	.08	.15	2.0	2
Fruits, canned:																	
Applesauce	80.8	72	.2	.2	18.6	.5	.2	4	7	.4	6	64	40	.01	.02	.1	Trace
Bananas	77.5	84	.4	.2	21.6	.1	.3	13	10	.2	29	118	70	.02	.02	.2	35
Peaches	78.1	81	.6	.2	20.7	.5	.4	6	14	.3		80	500	.01	.02	.7	3
Pears	82.2	66	.3	.1	17.1	1.0	.3	7	8	.2	4	62	30	.02	.02	.2	2
Plums with tapioca	74.8	94	.4	.2	24.3	.3	.3	5	12	.4	38	44	250	.01	.02	.2	2
Prunes with tapioca	76.7	86	.3	.2	22.4	.3	.4	7	21	.9	33	120	400	.02	.06	.4	4

Meats, poultry, and eggs; canned:																	
Beef, strained	80.3	99	14.7	4.0	(0)	(0)	1.0	8	127	2.0	228	183	—	.01	.16	3.5	0
Beef heart	81.1	93	13.5	3.8	.4	(0)	1.2	5	155	3.7	208	—	—	0.6	.62	3.6	0
Chicken	77.2	127	13.7	7.6	(0)	(0)	1.5	—	129	1.9	263	96	—	.02	.16	3.5	0
Lamb, strained	79.3	107	14.6	4.9	(0)	(0)	1.2	9	124	2.1	241	181	—	.02	.17	3.3	—
Liver, strained	79.7	97	14.1	3.4	1.5	(0)	1.3	6	182	5.6	253	202	24,000	.05	2.00	7.6	10
Pork, strained	77.7	118	15.4	5.8	(0)	(0)	1.1	8	130	1.5	223	178	—	.19	.20	2.7	—
Veal, strained	80.7	91	15.5	2.7	(0)	(0)	1.1	10	145	1.7	226	214	—	.03	.20	4.3	—
Vegetables, canned:																	
Beans, green	92.5	22	1.4	.1	5.1	.8	.9	33	25	1.1	213	93	400	.02	.06	.3	3
Beets, strained	89.2	37	1.4	.1	8.3	.6	1.0	18	27	.7	212	228	20	.02	.03	.1	3
Carrots	91.5	29	.7	.1	6.8	.6	.9	23	21	.5	169	181	13,000	.02	.03	.4	3
Peas, strained	85.5	54	4.2	.2	9.3	.8	.8	11	63	1.2	194	100	500	.08	.09	1.2	10
Spinach, creamed	88.1	43	2.3	.7	7.5	.4	1.4	64	63	.6	272	142	5,000	.02	.13	.3	6
Squash	92.1	25	.7	.1	6.2	.8	.9	24	17	.4	292	138	2,400	.02	.04	.3	8
Sweet potatoes	82.3	67	1.0	.2	15.5	.5	1.0	16	34	.4	187	180	4,900	.04	.03	.4	8
Tomato soup, strained	83.4	54	1.9	.1	13.5	.2	1.1	24	52	.4	294	200	1,000	.05	.12	.7	3
Bacon, cured:																	
Cooked, broiled or fried, drained	8.1	611	30.4	52.0	3.2	0	6.3	14	224	3.3	1,021	236	(0)	.51	.34	5.2	—
Canned	16.7	685	8.5	71.5	1.0	0	2.3	15	92	1.4	—	—	(0)	.23	.10	1.5	—
Bacon, Canadian, broiled or fried, drained	49.9	277	27.6	17.5	.3	0	4.7	19	218	4.1	2,555	432	(0)	.92	.17	5.0	—
Baking powders:																	
Sodium aluminum sulfate with monocalcium phosphate monohydrate	1.6	129	.1	Trace	31.2	Trace	—	1,932	2,904	—	10,953	150	(0)	(0)	(0)	(0)	(0)
Cream of tartar, with tartaric acid	1.0	78	.1	Trace	18.9	Trace	—	0	0	0	7,300	3,800	(0)	(0)	(0)	(0)	(0)
Bamboo shoots, raw	91.0	27	2.6	.3	5.2	.7	.9	13	59	.5	—	533	20	.15	.07	.6	4
Bananas, raw, common	75.7	85	1.1	.2	22.2	.5	.8	8	26	.7	1	370	190	.05	.06	.7	10
Barley, pearled, light	11.1	349	8.2	1.0	78.8	.5	.9	16	189	2.0	3	160	(0)	.12	.05	3.1	(0)
Bass, striped, oven-fried	60.8	196	21.5	8.5	6.7	—	2.5	—	—	—	—	—	—	—	—	—	—
Beans, common:																	
White, cooked	69.0	118	7.8	.6	21.2	1.5	1.4	50	148	2.7	7	416	0	.14	.07	.7	0
Canned, solids and liquids, with pork and tomato sauce	70.7	122	6.1	2.6	19.0	1.4	1.6	54	92	1.8	463	210	130	.08	.03	.6	2
Beans, lima, boiled, drained	71.1	111	7.6	.5	19.8	1.8	1.0	47	121	2.5	1	422	280	.18	.10	1.3	17
Beans, snap, green, boiled, drained	92.4	25	1.6	.2	5.4	1.0	.4	50	37	.6	4	151	540	.07	.09	.5	12
Bean sprouts, mung,																	

Composition of Foods (100 grams, edible portion)* *(Continued)*

Food and description	Water	Food energy	Protein	Fat	Carbohydrate		Ash	Calcium	Phosphorus	Iron	Sodium	Potassium	Vitamin A value	Thiamine	Riboflavin	Niacin	Ascorbic acid
					Total	Fiber											
	Percent	Calories	Grams	Grams	Grams	Grams	Grams	Milligrams	Milligrams	Milligrams	Milligrams	Milligrams	International units	Milligrams	Milligrams	Milligrams	Milligrams
boiled, drained	91.0	28	3.2	.2	5.2	.7	.4	17	48	.9	4	156	20	.09	.10	.7	6
Beef:																	
Chuck, choice, braised or pot-roasted (81% lean, 19% fat)	49.4	327	26.0	23.9	0	0	.7	11	140	3.3	60	370	40	.05	.20	4.0	—
T-bone steak, choice, broiled (56% lean, 44% fat)	36.4	473	19.5	43.2	0	0	.9	8	166	2.6	60	370	80	.06	.16	4.1	—
Ribs, 11th-12th, roasted (55% lean, 45% fat)	36.3	481	18.3	44.7	0	0	.7	8	153	2.4	60	370	90	.05	.14	3.4	—
Hamburger:																	
Lean, cooked	60.0	219	27.4	11.3	0	0	1.3	12	230	3.5	48	558	20	.09	.23	6.0	—
Regular, cooked	54.2	286	24.2	20.3	0	0	1.3	11	194	3.2	47	450	40	.09	.21	5.4	—
Corned, cooked, medium-fat	43.9	372	22.9	30.4	0	0	2.9	9	93	2.9	1,740	150	—	.02	.18	1.5	0
Beets, boiled, drained	90.9	32	1.1	.1	7.2	.8	.7	14	23	.5	43	208	20	.03	.04	.3	6
Beet greens, common, boiled, drained	93.6	18	1.7	.2	3.3	1.1	1.2	99	25	1.9	76	332	5,100	.07	.15	.3	15
Beverages, alcoholic:																	
Beer, alcohol 4.5% by volume (3.6% by weight)	92.1	42	.3	0	3.8	—	.2	5	30	Trace	7	25	—	Trace	.03	.6	—
Gin, rum, vodka, whisky:																	
80-proof (33.4% alcohol by weight)	66.6	231	—	—	Trace	—	—	—	—	—	1	2	—	—	—	—	—
86-proof (36.0% alcohol by weight)	64.0	249	—	—	Trace	—	—	—	—	—	1	2	—	—	—	—	—
90-proof (37.9% alcohol by weight)	62.1	263	—	—	Trace	—	—	—	—	—	1	2	—	—	—	—	—
94-proof (39.7% alcohol by weight)	60.3	275	—	—	Trace	—	—	—	—	—	1	2	—	—	—	—	—
100-proof (42.5% alcohol by weight)	57.5	295	—	—	Trace	—	—	—	—	—	1	2	—	—	—	—	—
Wines:[4]																	
Dessert, alcohol 18.8% by volume (15.3% by weight).	76.7	137	.1	0	7.7	—	.2	8	—	—	4	75	—	.01	.02	.2	—
Table, alcohol 12.2% by																	

volume (9.9% by weight).	85.6	85	.1	0	4.2	—	.2	9	10	.4	5	92	—	Trace	.01	.1	—
Beverages, carbonated, nonalcoholic:																	
Cola	90.	39	(0)	(0)	10.	(0)	—	—	—	—	—	—	(0)	(0)	(0)	(0)	(0)
Ginger ale	92.	31	(0)	(0)	8.	(0)	—	—	—	—	—	—	(0)	(0)	(0)	(0)	(0)
Root beer	89.5	41	(0)	(0)	10.5	(0)	—	—	—	—	—	—	(0)	(0)	(0)	(0)	(0)
Biscuits, baking powder, baked with enriched flour	27.4	369	7.4	17.0	45.8	.2	2.4	121	175	1.6	626	117	Trace	.21	.21	1.8	Trace
Blackberries, canned, solids and liquid, juice pack	85.8	54	.8	.8	12.1	2.7	.5	25	17	.9	1	170	150	.02	.03	.3	10
Blueberries, canned, solids and liquid, water pack	89.3	39	.5	.2	9.8	1.0	.2	10	9	.7	1	60	40	.01	.01	.2	7
Bouillon cubes or powder	4.	120	20.	3.	5.	—	68.	—	—	—	24,000	100	—	—	—	—	—
Bran flakes (40% bran), added thiamine	3.0	303	10.2	1.8	80.6	3.6	4.4	71	495	4.4	925	—	(0)	.40	.17	6.2	(0)
Brazil nuts	4.6	654	14.3	66.9	10.9	3.1	3.3	186	693	3.4	1	715	Trace	.96	.12	1.6	—
Breads:																	
White:																	
Enriched, made with—1%–2% nonfat dry milk	35.8	269	8.7	3.2	50.4	.2	1.9	70	87	2.4	507	85	Trace	.25	.17	2.3	Trace
Toasted	25.3	314	10.1	3.7	58.7	.2	2.2	81	101	2.8	590	99	Trace	.23	.20	2.7	Trace
Whole-wheat, made with—																	
2% nonfat dry milk	36.4	243	10.5	3.0	47.7	1.6	2.4	99	228	2.3	527	273	Trace	.26	.12	2.8	Trace
Toasted	24.3	289	12.5	3.6	56.7	1.9	2.9	118	271	2.7	627	325	Trace	.25	.15	3.4	Trace
Broccoli spears, boiled, drained	91.3	26	3.1	.3	4.5	1.5	.8	88	62	.8	10	267	2,500	.09	.20	.8	90
Bulgur, dry, made from hard red winter wheat	10.	354	11.2	1.5	75.7	1.7	1.6	29	338	3.7	—	229	(0)	.28	.14	4.5	(0)
Butter	15.5	716	.6	81.	.4	0	2.5	20	16	0	987	23	3,300	—	—	—	0
Buttermilk, fluid, cultured (made from skim milk)	90.5	36	3.6	.1	5.1	0	.7	121	95	Trace	130	140	Trace	.04	.18	.1	1
Cabbage, common varieties:																	
Raw	92.4	24	1.3	.2	5.4	.8	.7	49	29	.4	20	233	130	.05	.05	.3	[38]47
Shredded, boiled, drained	93.9	20	1.1	.2	4.3	.8	.5	44	20	.3	14	163	130	.04	.04	.3	33
Cakes:																	
Baked from home recipes:[40]																	
Angelfood	31.5	269	7.1	.2	60.2	0	1.0	9	22	.2	283	88	0	.01	.14	.2	0
Boston cream pie	34.5	302	5.0	9.4	49.9	0	1.2	67	101	.5	186	89	210	.03	.11	.2	Trace
Chocolate with choco-																	

Composition of Foods (100 grams, edible portion)* *(Continued)*

Food and description	Water	Food energy	Protein	Fat	Carbohydrate		Ash	Calcium	Phos-phorus	Iron	Sodium	Potas-sium	Vitamin A value	Thiamine	Ribo-flavin	Niacin	Ascorbic acid
					Total	Fiber											
	Percent	Calories	Grams	Grams	Grams	Grams	Grams	Milligrams	Milligrams	Milligrams	Milligrams	Milligrams	International units	Milligrams	Milligrams	Milligrams	Milligrams
late icing	22.0	369	4.5	16.4	55.8	.3	1.3	70	131	1.0	235	154	160	.02	.10	.2	Trace
Fruitcake, dark, made with enriched flour	18.1	379	4.8	15.3	59.7	.6	2.1	72	113	2.6	158	496	120	.13	.14	.8	Trace
White, without icing	24.2	375	4.6	16.0	54.0	.1	1.2	63	91	.2	323	76	30	.01	.08	.2	Trace
Candy:																	
Chocolate:																	
Bittersweet	1.8	477	7.9	39.7	46.8	1.8	2.3	58	284	5.0	3	615	40	.03	.17	1.0	0
Semisweet	1.1	507	4.2	35.7	57.0	1.0	1.2	30	150	2.6	2	325	20	.01	.08	.5	0
Sweet	.9	528	4.4	35.1	57.9	.5	1.2	94	142	1.4	33	269	19	.02	.14	.3	Trace
Fudge, chocolate	8.2	400	2.7	12.2	75.0	.2	1.8	77	84	1.0	190	147	Trace	.02	.09	.2	Trace
Hard	1.4	386	0	1.1	97.2	0	.3	21	7	1.9	32	4	0	0	0	0	0
Jelly beans	6.3	367	Trace	.5	93.1	Trace	.1	12	4	1.1	12	1	0	0	Trace	Trace	0
Marshmallows	17.3	319	2.0	Trace	80.4	0	.3	18	6	1.6	39	6	0	0	Trace	Trace	0
Peanut brittle	2.0	421	5.7	10.4	81.0	.5	.9	35	95	2.3	31	151	0	.16	.03	3.4	0
Carrots:																	
Raw	88.2	42	1.1	.2	9.7	1.0	.8	37	36	.7	47	341	11,000	.06	.05	.6	8
Boiled, drained	91.2	31	.9	.2	7.1	1.0	.6	33	31	.6	33	222	10,500	.05	.05	.5	6
Cauliflower:																	
Raw	91.0	27	2.7	.2	5.2	1.0	.9	25	56	1.1	13	295	60	.11	.10	.7	78
Boiled, drained	92.8	22	2.3	.2	4.1	1.0	.6	21	42	.7	9	206	60	.09	.08	.6	55
Celery, raw	94.1	17	.9	.1	3.9	.6	1.0	39	28	.3	126	341	240	.03	.03	.3	9
Cheeses:																	
Cheddar	37.	398	25.0	32.2	2.1	0	3.7	750	478	1.0	700	82	(1,310)	.03	.46	.1	(0)
Cottage, creamed	78.3	106	13.6	4.2	2.9	0	1.0	94	152	.3	229	85	(170)	.03	.25	.1	(0)
Cream	51.	374	8.0	37.7	2.1	0	1.2	62	95	.2	250	74	(1,540)	(.02)	.24	.1	(0)
Parmesan	30.	393	36.0	26.0	2.9	0	5.1	1,140	781	.4	734	149	(1,060)	.02	.73	.2	(0)
Pasteurized process, American	40.	370	23.2	30.0	1.9	0	4.9	697	771	.9	1,136	80	(1,220)	.02	.41	Trace	(0)
Cherries:																	
Raw, sweet	80.4	70	1.3	.3	17.4	.4	.6	22	19	.4	2	191	110	.05	.06	.4	10
Canned, sour, red, solids and liquid, water pack	88.0	43	.8	.2	10.7	.1	.3	15	13	.3	2	130	680	.03	.02	.2	5
Chestnuts, fresh	52.5	194	2.9	1.5	42.1	1.1	1.0	27	88	1.7	6	454	—	.22	.22	6	—
Chewing gum	3.5	317	—	—	95.2	—	1.3	—	—	—	—	—	(0)	(0)	(0)	(0)	(0)
Chicken:																	
Roasted light meat without skin	63.8	166	31.6	3.4	0	0	1.2	11	265	1.3	64	411	60	.04	.10	11.6	—

Roasted dark meat without skin	64.4	176	28.0	6.3	0	0	1.2	13	229	1.7	86	321	150	.07	.23	5.6	—
Chili con carne, canned:																	
With beans	72.4	133	7.5	6.1	12.2	.6	1.8	32	126	1.7	531	233	60	.03	.07	1.3	—
Without beans	66.9	200	10.3	14.8	5.8	.2	2.2	38	152	1.4	—	—	150	.02	.12	2.2	—
Chocolate syrup, fudge type	25.4	330	5.1	13.7	54.0	.4	1.4	127	159	1.3	89	284	150	.04	.22	.4	Trace
Clams, raw, soft, meat only	80.8	82	14.0	1.9	1.3	—	2.0	—	183	3.4	36	235	—	—	—	—	—
Cocoa, dry powder, high-fat, plain	3.0	299	16.8	23.7	48.3	4.3	5.0	133	648	10.7	6	1,522	30	.11	.46	2.4	0
Coconut meat:																	
Fresh	50.9	346	3.5	35.3	9.4	4.0	.9	13	95	1.7	23	256	0	.05	.02	.5	3
Dried, unsweetened	3.5	662	7.2	64.9	23.0	3.9	1.4	26	187	3.3	—	588	0	.06	.04	.6	0
Cod, broiled	64.6	170	28.5	5.3	0	0	—	31	274	1.0	110	407	180	.08	.11	3.0	—
Coffee, instant, water-soluble solids:																	
Dry powder	2.6	129	Trace	Trace	(35.)	Trace	9.7	179	383	5.6	72	3,256	0	0	.21	30.6	0
Beverage	98.1	1	Trace	Trace	Trace	Trace	.1	2	4	.1	1	36	0	0	Trace	.3	0
Cole slaw, made with mayonnaise	79.0	144	1.3	14.0	4.8	.7	.9	44	29	.4	120	199	160	.05	.05	.3	29
Cookies:																	
Assorted, packaged, commercial	2.6	480	5.1	20.2	71.0	.1	1.1	37	163	.7	365	67	80	.03	.05	.4	Trace
Chocolate chip, home recipe, baked with enriched flour	3.0	516	5.4	30.1	60.1	.4	1.4	34	99	2.1	348	117	110	.11	.11	.9	Trace
Oatmeal with raisins	2.8	451	6.2	15.4	73.5	.4	2.1	21	102	2.9	162	370	50	.11	.08	.5	Trace
Corn, sweet, boiled, drained, white and yellow, kernels, cut off cob before cooking	76.5	83	3.2	1.0	18.8	.7	.5	3	89	.6	Trace	165	400	.11	.10	1.3	7
Cornflour	12.	368	7.8	2.6	76.8	.7	.8	6	(164)	1.8	(1)	—	340	.20	.06	1.4	(0)
Corn grits, degermed, enriched, cooked	87.1	51	1.2	.1	11.0	.1	.6	1	10	.3	—	11	60	.04	.03	.4	(0)
Cornbread, southern style, made with whole-ground cornmeal	53.9	207	7.4	7.2	29.1	.5	2.4	120	211	1.1	628	157	[60]150	.13	.19	.6	1
Cornstarch	12.	362	.3	Trace	87.6	.1	.1	(0)	(0)	(0)	Trace	Trace	(0)	(0)	(0)	(0)	(0)
Crackers, saltines	4.3	433	9.0	12.0	71.5	.4	3.2	21	90	1.2	(1,100)	(120)	(0)	.01	.04	1.0	(0)
Cranberry sauce, sweetened, canned, strained	62.1	146	.1	.2	37.5	.2	1	6	4	.2	1	30	20	.01	.01	Trace	2
Cream:																	
Half-and-half	79.7	134	3.2	11.7	4.6	0	.6	108	85	Trace	46	129	480	.03	16	.1	1
Heavy whipping	56.6	352	2.2	37.6	3.1	0	.4	75	59	Trace	32	89	1,540	.02	.11	Trace	1
Cress, garden, raw	89.4	32	2.6	.7	5.5	1.1	1.8	81	76	1.3	14	606	9,300	.08	.26	1.0	69
Cucumbers, raw, not pared	95.1	15	.9	.1	3.4	.6	.5	25	27	1.1	6	160	250	.03	.04	.2	11

Composition of Foods (100 grams, edible portion)* *(Continued)*

Food and description	Water	Food energy	Protein	Fat	Carbohydrate		Ash	Calcium	Phos-phorus	Iron	Sodium	Potas-sium	Vitamin A value	Thiamine	Ribo-flavin	Niacin	Ascorbic acid
					Total	Fiber											
	Percent	*Calories*	*Grams*	*Grams*	*Grams*	*Grams*	*Grams*	*Milligrams*	*Milligrams*	*Milligrams*	*Milligrams*	*Milligrams*	*International units*	*Milligrams*	*Milligrams*	*Milligrams*	*Milligrams*
Dates, domestic, natural and dry	22.5	274	2.2	.5	72.9	2.3	1.9	59	63	3.0	1	648	50	.09	.10	2.2	0
Doughnuts																	
Cake type, enriched flour	23.7	391	4.6	18.6	51.4	.1	1.7	40	190	1.4	501	90	80	.16	.16	1.2	Trace
Yeast-leavened, enriched flour	28.3	414	6.3	26.7	37.7	.2	1.0	38	76	1.5	234	80	60	.16	.17	1.3	0
Eggs, chicken:																	
Fried	67.7	216	13.8	17.2	.3	0	1.0	60	222	2.4	338	140	1,420	.10	.30	.1	0
Poached	73.3	163	12.7	11.6	.8	0	1.4	55	203	2.2	271	128	1,170	.08	.25	.1	0
Scrambled	72.1	173	11.2	12.9	2.4	0	1.4	80	189	1.7	257	146	1,080	.08	.28	.1	0
Endive, raw	93.1	20	1.7	.1	4.1	.9	1.0	81	54	1.7	14	294	3,300	.07	.14	.5	10
Fats, cooking (vegetable fat)	0	884	0	100.	0	0	0	0	0	0	0	0	—	0	0	0	0
Figs, dried, uncooked	23.0	274	4.3	1.3	69.1	5.6	2.3	126	77	3.0	34	640	80	.10	.10	.7	(0)
Fruit cocktail, canned, solids and liquid, light syrup pack	83.6	60	.4	.1	15.7	.4	.2	9	12	.4	5	164	140	.02	.01	.5	2
Gelatin dessert, made with water, plain	84.2	59	1.5	0	14.1	0	.2	—	—	—	51	—	—	—	—	—	—
Goose, domesticated, roasted	39.1	426	23.7	36.0	0	0	1.2	(11)	(240)	(2.1)	—	—	—	(.08)	(.24)	(8.1)	—
Grapefruit, raw, pulp, all varieties	88.4	41	.5	.1	10.6	.2	.4	16	16	.4	1	135	80	0.04	.02	.2	38
Grape juice, canned or bottled	82.9	66	.2	Trace	16.6	Trace	.3	11	12	.3	2	116	—	.04	.02	.2	Trace
Haddock, dipped in egg, milk, breadcrumbs, fried	66.3	165	19.6	6.4	5.8	—	1.9	40	247	1.2	177	348	—	.04	.07	3.2	2
Halibut, Atlantic and Pacific, broiled	66.6	171	25.2	7.0	0	0	1.7	16	248	.8	134	525	680	.05	.07	8.3	—
Ham. See Pork.																	
Herring, pickled, Bismarck type	59.4	223	20.4	15.1	0	0	4.0	—	—	—	—	—	—	—	—	—	—
Hickory nuts	3.3	673	13.2	68.7	12.8	1.9	2.0	Trace	360	2.4	—	—	—	—	—	—	—
Horseradish, prepared	87.1	38	1.3	.2	9.6	.9	1.8	61	32	.9	96	290	—	—	—	—	—
Ice cream and frozen custard:[85]																	
Regular, app. 10% fat	63.2	193	4.5	10.6	20.8	0	.9	146	115	.1	[86]63	181	440	.04	.21	.1	1

Rich, app. 16% fat	62.8	222	2.6	16.1	18.0	0	.5	78	61	Trace	[86]33	95	660	.02	.11	.1	1
Ice cream cones	8.9	377	10.0	2.4	77.9	.2	.8	156	198	.4	232	244	Trace	.05	.21	.5	Trace
Jams and preserves	29.	272	.6	.1	70.0	1.0	.3	20	9	1.0	12	88	10	.01	.03	.2	2
Kale, boiled, drained, leaves and stems	91.2	28	3.2	.7	4.0	1.1	.9	134	46	1.2	43	221	7,400	—	—	—	62
Kidneys, beef, braised	53.0	252	33.0	12.0	.8	0	1.2	18	244	13.1	253	324	1,150	.51	4.82	10.7	—
Leg of lamb, lean, roasted	61.6	192	28.6	7.7	0	0	2.1	12	237	2.2	290	290	—	.16	.30	6.1	—
Lemon juice, raw	91.0	25	.5	.2	8.0	Trace	.3	7	10	.2	1	141	20	.03	.01	.1	46
Lemon peel, candied	17.4	316	.4	.3	80.6	2.3	1.3	—	—	—	—	—	—	—	—	—	—
Lemonade concentrate, frozen, diluted with 4⅓ parts water, by volume	88.5	44	.1	Trace	11.4	Trace	Trace	1	1	Trace	Trace	16	Trace	Trace	.01	.1	7
Lentils, whole, cooked	72.0	106	7.8	Trace	19.3	1.2	.9	25	119	2.1	—	249	20	.07	.06	.6	0
Lettuce, raw, Boston, Bibb	95.1	14	1.2	.2	2.5	.5	1.0	35	26	2.0	9	264	970	.06	.06	.3	8
Liver, beef, fried	56.0	229	26.4	10.6	5.3	0	1.7	11	476	8.8	184	380	[94]53,400	.26	4.19	16.5	27
Lobster, northern, canned or cooked	76.8	95	18.7	1.5	.3	—	2.7	65	192	.8	210	180	—	.10	.07	—	—
Macadamia nuts	3.0	691	7.8	71.6	15.9	2.5	1.7	48	161	2.0	—	264	0	.34	.11	1.3	0
Macaroni, enriched, cooked (tender stage)	72.0	111	3.4	.4	23.0	.1	1.2	8	50	.9	1	61	(0)	.14	.08	1.1	(0)
Mackerel, Atlantic, canned, solids and liquid[98]	66.0	183	19.3	11.1	0	0	3.2	185	274	2.1	—	—	430	.06	.21	5.8	—
Mackerel, Pacific, canned, solids and liquid[98]	66.4	180	21.1	10.0	0	0	2.5	260	288	2.2	—	—	30	.03	.33	8.8	—
Mangoes, raw	81.7	66	.7	.4	16.8	.9	.4	10	13	.4	7	189	4,800	.05	.05	1.1	35
Margarine[99]	15.5	720	.6	81.	.4	0	2.5	20	16	0	987	23	3,300	—	—	—	0
Marmalade, citrus	29.0	257	.5	.1	70.1	.4	.3	35	9	.6	14	33	—	.02	.02	.1	6
Milk, cow:																	
Fluid:																	
Whole, 3.7% fat[100]	87.4	65	3.5	3.5	4.9	0	.7	118	93	Trace	50	144	140	.03	.17	.1	1
Skim	90.5	36	3.6	.1	5.1	0	.7	121	95	Trace	52	145	Trace	.04	.18	.1	1
Canned:																	
Evaporated (unsweetened)	73.8	137	7.0	7.9	9.7	0	1.6	252	205	.1	118	303	320	.04	.34	.2	1
Condensed (sweetened)	27.1	321	8.1	8.7	54.3	0	1.8	262	206	.1	112	314	360	.08	.38	.2	1
Dry, skim, instant	4.0	359	35.8	.7	51.6	0	7.9	1,293	1,005	.6	526	1,725	30	.35	1.78	.9	7
Milk, human, U.S. samples	85.2	77	1.1	4.0	9.5	0	.2	33	14	.1	16	51	240	.01	.04	.2	5
Molasses, cane, light	24.	252	—	—	[103]65.	—	[104]6.3	165	45	4.3	15	917	—	.07	.06	.2	
Mushrooms, canned, solids and liquid	93.1	17	1.9	.1	2.4	.6	1.6	6	68	.5	400	197	Trace	.02	.25	2.0	2
Muskmelons:																	
Cantaloupes	91.2	30	.7	.1	7.5	.3	.5	14	16	.4	12	251	3,400	.04	.03	.6	33
Honeydew	90.6	33	.8	.3	7.7	.6	.6	14	16	.4	12	251	40	.04	.03	.6	23
Mussels, Atlantic and Pacific, raw, meat and																	

Composition of Foods (100 grams, edible portion)* *(Continued)*

Food and description	Water	Food energy	Protein	Fat	Carbohydrate		Ash	Calcium	Phos-phorus	Iron	Sodium	Potas-sium	Vitamin A value	Thiamine	Ribo-flavin	Niacin	Ascorbic acid
					Total	Fiber											
	Percent	*Calories*	*Grams*	*Grams*	*Grams*	*Grams*	*Grams*	*Milligrams*	*Milligrams*	*Milligrams*	*Milligrams*	*Milligrams*	*International units*	*Milligrams*	*Milligrams*	*Milligrams*	*Milligrams*
liquid	83.8	66	9.6	1.4	3.1	—	2.1	—	—	—	—	—	—	—	—	—	—
Mustard greens, boiled, drained	92.6	23	2.2	.4	4.0	.9	.8	138	32	1.8	18	220	5,800	.08	.14	.6	48
Mustard, prepared, yellow	80.2	75	4.7	4.4	6.4	1.0	4.3	84	73	2.0	1,252	130	—	—	—	—	—
Nectarines, raw	81.8	64	.6	Trace	17.1	.4	.5	4	24	.5	6	294	1,650	—	—	—	13
Noodles, egg, enriched, cooked	70.4	125	4.1	1.5	23.3	.1	.7	10	59	.9	2	44	70	.14	.08	1.2	(0)
Oatmeal, cooked	86.5	55	2.0	1.0	9.7	.2	.8	9	57	.6	218	61	(0)	.08	.02	.1	(0)
Ocean perch, Atlantic (redfish), dipped in egg, milk, breadcrumb, fried	59.0	227	19.0	13.3	6.8	0	1.9	33	226	1.3	153	284	—	.10	.11	1.8	—
Okra, boiled, drained	91.1	29	2.0	.3	6.0	1.0	.6	92	41	.5	2	174	490	(.13)	(.18)	(.9)	20
Oleomargarine. See Margarine.																	
Olives:																	
Green	78.2	116	1.4	12.7	1.3	1.3	6.4	61	17	1.6	2,400	55	300	—	—	—	—
Ripe, salt-cured, oil-coated, Greek-style	43.8	338	2.2	35.8	8.7	3.8	(9.5)	—	29	—	3,288	—	—	—	—	—	—
Onions, mature (dry):																	
Raw	89.1	38	1.5	.1	8.7	.6	.6	27	36	.5	10	157	40	.03	.04	.2	10
Boiled, drained	91.8	29	1.2	.1	6.5	.6	.4	24	29	.4	7	110	40	.03	.03	.2	7
Onions, young green, raw, bulb and entire top	89.4	36	1.5	.2	8.2	(1.2)	.7	51	39	1.0	5	231	(2,000)	.05	.05	.4	32
Opossum, roasted	57.3	221	30.2	10.2	0	0	2.3	—	—	—	—	—	—	.12	.38	—	—
Oranges, all commercial varieties, peeled fruit	86.0	49	1.0	.2	12.2	.5	.6	41	20	.4	1	200	200	.10	.04	.4	(50)
Orange juice:																	
Raw, all commercial varieties	88.3	45	.7	.2	10.4	.1	.4	11	17	.2	1	200	200	.09	.03	.4	50
Frozen concentrate, unsweetened:																	
Undiluted	58.2	158	2.3	.2	38.0	.2	1.3	33	55	.4	2	657	710	.30	.05	1.2	158
Diluted with 3 parts water, by volume	88.1	45	.7	.1	10.7	Trace	.4	9	16	.1	1	186	200	.09	.01	.3	45
Orange peel, candied	17.4	316	.4	.3	80.6	—	1.3	—	—	—	—	—	—	—	—	—	—
Oysters:																	
Raw, meat only:																	

Eastern	84.6	66	8.4	1.8	3.4	—	1.8	94	143	5.5	73	121	310	.14	.18	2.5	—
Pacific and Western (Olympia)	79.1	91	10.6	2.2	6.4	—	1.7	85	153	7.2	—	—	—	.12	—	1.3	30
Dipped in egg, milk, breadcrumbs, fried	54.7	239	8.6	13.9	18.6	Trace	1.5	152	241	8.1	206	203	440	.17	.29	3.2	—
Pancakes, home recipe, enriched flour	50.1	231	7.1	7.0	34.1	.1	1.7	101	139	1.3	425	123	120	.17	.22	1.3	Trace
Papayas, raw	88.7	39	.6	.1	10.0	.9	.6	20	16	.3	3	234	1,750	.04	.04	.3	56
Parsley, raw	85.1	44	3.6	.6	8.5	1.5	2.2	203	63	6.2	45	727	8,500	.12	.26	1.2	172
Parsnips, boiled, drained	82.2	66	1.5	.5	14.9	2.0	.9	45	62	.6	8	379	30	.07	.08	.1	10
Peaches:																	
Raw	89.1	38	.6	.1	9.7	.6	.5	9	19	.5	1	202	1,330	.02	.05	1.0	7
Canned, solids and liquid, heavy syrup pack	79.1	78	.4	.1	20.1	.4	.3	4	12	.3	2	130	430	.01	.02	.6	3
Peanuts:																	
Raw, without skins	5.4	568	26.3	48.4	17.6	1.9	2.3	59	409	2.0	5	674	0	.99	.13	15.8	0
Roasted, salted	1.6	585	26.0	49.8	18.8	2.4	3.8	74	401	2.1	418	674	—	.32	.13	17.2	0
Peanut butter, made with small amounts of added fat, salt	1.8	581	27.8	49.4	17.2	1.9	3.8	63	407	2.0	607	670	—	.13	.13	15.7	0
Pears:																	
Raw, including skin	83.2	61	.7	.4	15.3	1.4	.4	8	11	.3	2	130	20	.02	.04	.1	4
Canned, solids and liquid, heavy syrup pack	79.8	76	.2	.2	19.6	.6	.2	5	7	.2	1	84	Trace	.01	.02	.1	1
Peas, green, immature:																	
Boiled, drained	81.5	71	5.4	.4	12.1	2.0	.6	23	99	1.8	1	196	540	.28	.11	2.3	20
Canned:																	
Alaska, regular pack, solids and liquids	82.6	66	3.5	.3	12.5	1.5	1.1	20	66	1.7	236	96	450	.09	.05	.9	9
Low-sodium pack, solids and liquids	85.9	55	3.6	.3	9.8	1.3	.4	20	66	1.7	3	96	450	.09	.05	.9	9
Peppers, sweet, immature, green, raw	93.4	22	1.2	.2	4.8	1.4	.4	9	22	.7	13	213	420	.08	.08	.5	128
Persimmons, native, raw	64.4	127	.8	.4	33.5	1.5	.9	27	26	2.5	1	310	—	—	—	—	66
Pickles:																	
Cucumber:																	
Dill	93.3	11	.7	.2	2.2	.5	3.6	26	21	1.0	1,428	200	100	Trace	.02	Trace	6
Fresh (as bread-and-butter pickles)	78.7	73	.9	.2	17.9	.5	2.3	32	27	1.8	673	—	140	Trace	.03	Trace	9
Sour	94.8	10	.5	.2	2.0	.5	2.5	17	15	3.2	1,353	—	100	Trace	.02	Trace	7
Pies:																	
Baked, piecrust made with unenriched flour:																	
Apple	47.6	256	2.2	11.1	38.1	.4	1.0	8	22	.3	301	80	30	.02	.02	.4	1
Chocolate meringue	48.4	252	4.8	12.0	33.5	.2	1.2	69	98	.7	256	139	190	.03	.12	.2	Trace

Composition of Foods (100 grams, edible portion)* *(Continued)*

Food and description	Water	Food energy	Protein	Fat	Carbohydrate		Ash	Calcium	Phos-phorus	Iron	Sodium	Potas-sium	Vitamin A value	Thiamine	Ribo-flavin	Niacin	Ascorbic acid
					Total	Fiber											
	Percent	*Calories*	*Grams*	*Grams*	*Grams*	*Grams*	*Grams*	*Milligrams*	*Milligrams*	*Milligrams*	*Milligrams*	*Milligrams*	*International units*	*Milligrams*	*Milligrams*	*Milligrams*	*Milligrams*
Pecan	19.5	418	5.1	22.9	51.3	.5	1.2	47	103	2.8	221	123	160	.16	.07	.3	Trace
Raisin	42.5	270	2.6	10.7	43.0	.3	1.2	18	40	.9	285	192	Trace	.03	.03	.3	1
Rhubarb	47.4	253	2.5	10.7	38.2	.6	1.2	64	26	.7	270	159	50	.02	.04	.3	3
Pimientos, canned, solids and liquid	92.4	27	.9	.5	5.8	.6	.4	[115]7	17	1.5	—	—	2,300	.02	.06	.4	95
Pineapple:																	
Raw	85.3	52	0.4	0.2	13.7	0.4	0.4	17	8	0.5	1	146	70	0.09	0.03	0.2	17
Candied	18.0	316	.8	.4	80.0	.8	.8	—	—	—	—	—	—	—	—	—	—
Pineapple juice, canned, unsweetened	85.6	55	.4	.1	13.5	.1	.4	15	9	.3	1	149	50	.05	.02	.2	9
Pizza, with cheese, home recipe, with sausage topping	50.6	234	7.8	9.3	29.6	.3	2.7	17	92	1.2	729	168	560	.09	.12	1.5	9
Plantain, raw	66.4	119	1.1	.4	31.2	.4	.9	7	30	.7	5	385	([118])	.06	.04	.6	14
Plums, raw, Damson	81.1	66	.5	Trace	17.8	.4	.6	18	17	.5	2	299	(300)	.08	.03	.5	—
Pollock, cooked, creamed (with flour, butter, milk)	74.7	128	13.9	5.9	4.0	—	1.5	—	—	—	111	238	—	.03	.13	.7	Trace
Popcorn, popped, oil and salt added	3.1	456	9.8	21.8	59.1	1.7	6.2	8	216	2.1	1,940	—	—	—	.09	1.7	0
Pork, fresh:																	
Bacon:																	
Fat class (25% lean, 75% fat)	26.4	631	7.1	66.6	0	0	.3	4	62	1.1	([122])	([123])	(0)	.35	.08	1.8	—
Thin class (40% lean, 60% fat)	34.3	545	9.4	56.0	0	0	.5	5	92	1.4	([122])	([123])	(0)	.46	.11	2.4	—
Composite of trimmed lean cuts (ham, loin, shoulder, spareribs:																	
Medium-fat class (77% lean, 23% fat), roasted	45.2	373	22.6	30.6	0	0	1.6	10	232	2.9	([122])	([123])	(0)	.50	.23	4.9	—
Ham, roasted (72% lean, 28% fat)	43.7	394	21.9	33.3	0	0	1.0	10	225	2.9	([122])	([123])	(0)	.49	.22	4.4	—
Potatoes																	
Baked in skin	75.1	93	2.6	.1	21.1	.6	1.1	9	65	.7	[125]4	503	Trace	.10	.04	1.7	20
Boiled in skin	79.8	76	2.1	.1	17.1	.5	.9	7	53	.6	[125]6	407	Trace	.09	.04	1.5	16
French-fried	44.7	274	4.3	13.2	36.0	1.0	1.8	15	111	1.3	[125]6	853	Trace	.13	.08	3.1	21

Potato chips	1.8	568	5.3	39.8	50.0	(1.6)	3.1	40	139	1.8	[128]—	1,130	Trace	.21	.07	4.8	16
Potato salad, home recipe, made with mayonnaise and French dressing, hard-cooked eggs, seasonings	72.4	145	3.0	9.2	13.4	.4	2.0	19	63	.8	480	296	180	.07	.06	.9	11
Pretzels	4.5	390	9.8	4.5	75.9	.3	5.3	22	131	1.5	[129]1,680	130	(0)	.02	.03	.7	(0)
Prunes, cooked, fruit and liquid, added sugar	50.7	180	1.2	.2	47.1	(.8)	.8	31	37	1.5	4	329	760	.03	.07	.7	1
Puddings, starch base, home recipe																	
Chocolate	65.8	148	3.1	4.7	25.7	.2	.7	96	98	.5	56	171	150	.02	.14	.1	Trace
Vanilla (blanc mange)	76.0	111	3.5	3.9	15.9	Trace	.7	117	91	Trace	65	138	160	.03	.16	.1	1
Pumpkin, canned	90.2	33	1.0	.3	7.9	1.3	.6	25	26	.4	[125]2	240	6,400	.03	.05	.6	5
Raccoon, roasted	54.8	255	29.2	14.5	0	0	1.5	—	—	—	—	—	—	.59	.52	—	—
Radishes, raw, common	94.5	17	1.0	.1	3.6	.7	.8	30	31	1.0	18	322	10	.03	.03	.3	26
Raisins, natural, uncooked	18.0	289	2.5	.2	77.4	.9	1.9	62	101	3.5	27	763	20	.11	.08	.5	1
Raspberries, raw, black	80.8	73	1.5	1.4	15.7	5.1	0.6	30	22	0.9	1	199	Trace	(0.03)	(0.09)	(0.9)	18
Rhubarb, cooked, added sugar	62.8	141	.5	.1	36.0	.6	.6	78	15	.6	2	203	80	(.02)	(.05)	(.3)	6
Rice, white, enriched, commercial, cooked	72.6	109	2.0	.1	24.2	.1	1.1	10	28	.9	374	28	(0)	.11	—	1.0	(0)
Rice products, breakfast:																	
Rice flakes, added nutrients	3.2	390	5.9	.3	87.7	.6	2.9	29	132	1.6	987	180	(0)	.35	.05	5.4	(0)
Rice, puffed or oven-popped, presweetened, honey, added nutrients	1.8	388	4.2	.7	90.6	.2	2.7	46	74	.9	706	—	(0)	.33	—	4.6	(0)
Rolls and buns, commercial, ready-to-serve																	
Danish pastry	22.0	422	7.4	23.5	45.6	.1	1.5	50	109	.9	366	112	310	.07	.15	.8	Trace
Plain pan rolls, enriched	31.4	298	8.2	5.6	53.0	.2	1.8	74	85	1.9	506	95	Trace	.28	.18	2.2	Trace
Salad dressings, commercial:																	
Blue and Roquefort cheese	32.3	504	4.8	52.3	7.4	.1	3.2	81	74	.2	1,094	37	210	.01	.10	.1	2
French, low-fat	77.3	96	.4	4.3	15.6	.3	2.4	11	14	.4	787	79	—	—	—	—	—
Italian	27.5	552	.2	60.0	6.9	Trace	5.4	10	4	.2	2,092	15	Trace	Trace	Trace	Trace	—
Mayonnaise	15.1	718	1.1	79.9	2.2	Trace	1.7	18	28	.5	597	34	280	.02	.04	Trace	—
Salad dressing, mayonnaise-type	40.6	435	1.0	42.3	14.4	—	1.7	14	26	.2	586	9	220	.01	.03	Trace	—
Thousand Island	32.0	502	.8	50.2	15.4	.3	1.6	11	17	.6	700	113	320	.02	.03	.2	3
Salmon, broiled or baked	63.4	182	27.0	7.4	0	0	1.6	—	414	1.2	116	443	160	.16	.06	9.8	—
Sauerkraut, canned, solids and liquid	92.8	18	1.0	.2	4.0	.7	2.0	36	18	.5	[144]747	140	50	.03	.04	.2	14

Composition of Foods (100 grams, edible portion)* *(Continued)*

Food and description	Water	Food energy	Protein	Fat	Carbohydrate		Ash	Calcium	Phos-phorus	Iron	Sodium	Potas-sium	Vitamin A value	Thiamine	Ribo-flavin	Niacin	Ascorbic acid
					Total	Fiber											
	Percent	*Calories*	*Grams*	*Grams*	*Grams*	*Grams*	*Grams*	*Milligrams*	*Milligrams*	*Milligrams*	*Milligrams*	*Milligrams*	*International units*	*Milligrams*	*Milligrams*	*Milligrams*	*Milligrams*
Sausage, cold cuts, and luncheon meats:																	
Brown-and-serve sausage, browned	39.9	422	16.5	37.8	2.8	0	3.0	—	—	—	—	—	—	—	—	—	—
Frankfurters, cooked	57.3	304	12.4	27.2	1.6	—	1.5	5	102	1.5	—	—	—	.15	.20	2.5	—
Liverwurst, smoked	52.6	319	14.8	27.4	2.3	0	2.9	10	245	5.9	—	—	6,530	.17	1.44	8.2	—
Meat loaf	64.1	200	15.9	13.2	3.3	0	3.5	9	178	1.8	—	—	—	.13	.22	2.5	—
Polish-style sausage	53.7	304	15.7	25.8	1.2	0	3.6	9	176	2.4	—	—	(0)	.34	.19	3.1	—
Pork sausage, links or bulk, cooked	34.8	476	18.1	44.2	Trace	0	2.9	7	162	2.4	958	269	(0)	.79	.34	3.7	—
Salami, dry	29.8	450	23.8	38.1	1.2	0	7.1	14	283	3.6	—	—	—	.37	.25	5.3	—
Scrapple	61.3	215	8.8	13.6	14.6	.1	1.7	5	64	1.2	—	—	—	.19	.09	1.8	—
Vienna sausage, canned	63.0	240	14.0	19.8	.3	0	2.9	8	153	2.1	—	—	—	.08	.13	2.6	—
Scallops, bay and sea:																	
Raw	79.8	81	15.3	.2	3.3	—	1.4	26	208	1.8	[145]255	[145]396	—	—	.06	1.3	—
Steamed	73.1	112	23.2	1.4	—	—	—	115	338	3.0	265	476	—	—	—	—	—
Sesame seeds, dry, whole	5.4	563	18.6	49.1	21.6	6.3	5.3	1,160	616	10.5	60	725	30	.98	.24	5.4	0
Shad, baked with butter or margarine and bacon slices	64.0	201	23.2	11.3	0	0	1.4	24	313	.6	79	377	30	.13	.26	8.6	—
Sherbet, orange	67.0	134	.9	1.2	30.8	0	.1	16	13	Trace	10	22	60	.01	.03	Trace	2
Shrimp:																	
Raw	78.2	91	18.1	.8	1.5	—	1.4	63	166	1.6	140	220	—	.02	.03	3.2	—
French-fried, dipped in egg, breadcrumbs, and flour, or batter	56.9	225	20.3	10.8	10.0	—	2.0	72	191	2.0	186	229	—	.04	.08	2.7	—
Syrups:																	
Cane	26.	263	0	0	68.	0	1.5	60	29	3.6	—	425	0	.13	.06	.1	0
Maple	33.	252	—	—	65.	—	.7	104	8	1.2	10	176	—	—	—	—	0
Sorghum	23.	257	—	—	68.	—	2.4	172	25	12.5	—	—	—	—	.10	.1	—
Table blends, chiefly light and dark corn syrup	24.	290	0	0	75.	0	.7	46	16	4.1	68	4	0	0	0	0	0
Soups, commercial, canned, prepared with equal volume of water:																	
Bean with pork	84.4	67	3.2	2.3	8.7	.6	1.4	25	51	.9	403	158	260	.05	.03	.4	1

Beef noodle	93.2	28	1.6	1.1	2.9	Trace	1.2	3	20	.4	382	32	20	.02	.03	.4	Trace
Celery, cream of	92.3	36	.7	2.1	3.7	.2	1.2	20	15	.2	398	45	80	.01	.02	Trace	Trace
Chicken, cream of	91.9	39	1.2	2.4	3.3	.1	1.2	10	14	.2	404	33	170	.01	.02	.2	Trace
Clam chowder, Manhattan type	91.9	33	.9	1.0	5.0	.2	1.2	14	19	.4	383	75	360	.01	.01	.4	—
Minestrone	89.5	43	2.0	1.4	5.8	.3	1.3	15	24	.4	406	128	960	.03	.02	.4	—
Mushroom, cream of	89.6	56	1.0	4.0	4.2	.1	1.2	17	21	.2	398	41	30	.01	.05	.3	Trace
Pea, split	85.4	59	3.5	1.3	8.4	.2	1.4	12	61	.6	384	110	180	.10	.06	.6	Trace
Tomato	90.5	36	.8	1.0	6.4	.2	1.3	6	14	.3	396	94	410	.02	.02	.5	5
Vegetable beef	91.9	32	2.1	.9	3.9	.2	1.2	5	20	.3	427	66	1,100	.02	.02	.4	—
Vegetable with beef broth	91.7	32	1.1	.7	5.5	.3	1.0	8	16	.3	345	98	1,300	.02	.01	.5	—
Soybeans, cooked dry mature seeds	71.0	130	11.0	5.7	10.8	1.6	1.5	73	179	2.7	2	540	30	.21	.09	.6	0
Soybean flour, full-fat	8.0	421	36.7	20.3	30.4	2.4	4.6	199	558	8.4	1	1,660	110	.85	.31	2.1	0
Soybean milk, fluid	92.4	33	3.4	1.5	2.2	0	.5	21	48	.8	—	—	40	.08	.03	.2	0
Spaghetti, enriched:																	
Cooked, firm stage (8–10 min.)	63.6	148	5.0	.5	30.1	.1	1.3	11	65	1.1	1	79	(0)	[59].18	[59].10	[59]1.4	(0)
Cooked, tender stage (14–20 min.)	72.0	111	3.4	.4	23.0	.1	1.2	8	50	.9	1	61	(0)	[59].14	[59].08	[59]1.1	(0)
In tomato sauce with cheese, home recipe	77.0	104	3.5	3.5	14.8	.2	1.2	32	54	.9	(382)	163	430	.10	.07	.9	5
With meatballs, in tomato sauce, home recipe	70.0	134	7.5	4.7	15.6	.3	2.2	50	95	1.5	407	268	640	.10	.12	1.6	9
Spinach, boiled, drained	92.0	23	3.0	.3	3.6	.6	1.1	93	38	2.2	50	324	8,100	.07	.14	.5	28
Squash:																	
Summer:																	
All varieties, boiled, drained	95.5	14	.9	.1	3.1	.6	.4	25	25	.4	1	141	390	.05	.08	.8	10
Zucchini and Cocozelle, green	96.0	12	1.0	.1	2.5	.6	.4	25	25	.4	1	141	[151]300	.05	.08	.8	9
Winter, butternut, baked	79.6	68	1.8	.1	17.5	1.8	1.0	40	72	1.0	1	609	[152]6,400	.05	.13	.7	8
Starch. See Cornstarch.																	
Strawberries, raw	89.9	37	.7	.5	8.4	1.3	.5	21	21	1.0	1	164	60	.03	.07	.6	59
Sugars, beet or cane:																	
Brown	2.1	373	0	0	96.4	0	1.5	85	19	3.4	30	344	0	.01	.03	.2	0
Granulated	.5	385	0	0	99.5	0	Trace	0	0	.1	1	3	0	0	0	0	0
Powdered	.5	385	0	0	99.5	0	Trace	0	0	.1	1	3	0	0	0	0	0
Sunflower seed kernels, dry	4.8	560	24.0	47.3	19.9	3.8	4.0	120	837	7.1	30	920	50	1.96	.23	5.4	—
Sweetbreads, beef, braised	49.6	320	25.9	23.2	0	0	1.3	—	364	—	116	433	—	—	—	—	—
Sweet potatoes, baked in skin	63.7	141	2.1	.5	32.5	.9	1.2	40	58	.9	12	300	8,100	.09	.07	.7	22

Composition of Foods (100 grams, edible portion)* *(Continued)*

Food and description	Water	Food energy	Protein	Fat	Carbohydrate		Ash	Calcium	Phosphorus	Iron	Sodium	Potassium	Vitamin A value	Thiamine	Riboflavin	Niacin	Ascorbic acid
					Total	Fiber											
	Percent	Calories	Grams	Grams	Grams	Grams	Grams	Milligrams	Milligrams	Milligrams	Milligrams	Milligrams	International units	Milligrams	Milligrams	Milligrams	Milligrams
Swordfish, broiled, with butter or margarine	64.6	174	28.0	6.0	0	0	1.7	27	275	1.3	—	—	2,050	.04	.05	10.9	—
Tapioca cream pudding	71.8	134	5.0	5.1	17.1	0	1.0	105	109	.4	156	135	290	.04	.18	.1	1
Tea, instant, beverage	99.4	2	—	Trace	.4	Trace	Trace	Trace	—	Trace	—	25	—	—	.01	Trace	—
Tomatoes, ripe:																	
Raw	93.5	22	1.1	.2	4.7	.5	.5	13	27	.5	3	244	900	.06	.04	7	[159]23
Canned, solids and liquid	93.7	21	1.0	.2	4.3	.4	.8	[115]6	19	.5	130	217	900	.05	.03	.7	17
Tomato juice, canned or bottled	93.6	19	.9	.1	4.3	.2	1.1	7	18	.9	200	227	800	.05	.03	.8	16
Tongue, beef, medium-fat, braised	60.8	244	21.5	16.7	.4	0	.6	7	117	2.2	61	164	—	.05	.29	3.5	—
Tuna, canned:																	
In oil, drained solids	60.6	197	28.8	8.2	0	0	2.0	(8)	234	1.9	—	—	80	.05	.12	11.9	—
In water, solids and liquid	70.0	127	28.0	.8	0	0	1.2	16	190	1.6	[163]41	[163]279	—	—	.10	13.3	—
Turkey, all classes, total edible, roasted	55.4	263	27.0	16.4	0	0	1.2	—	—	—	—	—	—	—	—	—	—
Turnips, boiled, drained	93.6	23	.8	.2	4.9	.9	.5	35	24	.4	34	188	Trace	.04	.05	.3	22
Turnip greens, boiled, drained	93.2	20	2.2	.2	3.6	.7	.8	184	37	1.1	—	—	6,300	.15	.24	.6	69
Walnuts, black	3.1	628	20.5	59.3	14.8	1.7	2.3	Trace	570	6.0	3	460	300	.22	.11	.7	—
Watercress	93.3	19	2.2	.3	3.0	.7	1.2	151	54	1.7	52	282	4,900	.08	.16	.9	79
Whale meat, raw	70.9	156	20.6	7.5	0	0	1.0	12	144	—	78	22	1,860	.09	.08	—	6
Wheat flour, whole (from hard wheats)	12.	333	13.3	2.0	71.0	2.3	1.7	41	372	3.3	3	370	(0)	.55	.12	4.3	(0)
Whisky. See Beverages, alcoholic.																	
Wine. See Beverages, alcoholic.																	
Yogurt:																	
Made from partially skimmed milk	89.0	50	3.4	1.7	5.2	0	.7	120	94	Trace	51	143	70	.04	.18	.1	1
Made from whole milk	88.0	62	3.0	3.4	4.9	0	.7	111	87	Trace	47	132	140	.03	.16	.1	1
Zwieback	5.0	423	10.7	8.8	74.3	.3	1.2	13	69	.6	250	150	40	.05	.07	.9	(0)

*Adapted from Agriculture Handbook No. 8, Agricultural Research Service, U.S. Department of Agriculture.

[38] For freshly harvested cabbage, average value is 51 mg. per 100 grams; for stored cabbage, 42 mg. per 100 grams.

[40] Unenriched cake flour used unless otherwise specified. Values for cakes that contain baking powder and/or fat are based on use of baking powder, item 130, and cooking fats, item 999.

[60] Based on cornbread made with white cornmeal; with yellow cornmeal, value is about 310 I.U. per 100 grams.

[85] Commercial products. Frozen custard must contain egg yolk which contributes somewhat more vitamin A value than is present in ice creams made with milk products only.

[86] Value for product without added salt.

[94] Values vary widely in all kinds of liver, ranging from about 100 I.U. to more than 100,000 I.U. per 100 grams.

[98] Vitamin values based on drained solids.

[99] Values apply to salted margarine. Unsalted margarine contains less than 10 mg. per 100 grams of either sodium or potassium. Vitamin A value based on the minimum required to meet Federal specifications for margarine with vitamin A added; namely 15,000 I.U. of vitamin A per pound.

[100] Minimum standards for fat in different States vary considerably, and commercial milks may range somewhat above the required minimums. Selection of values to be used in dietary calculations may need to be based on information at the local level. The value, 3.7 percent, is considered valid as a national average for milk on the farm production basis.

[103] Value for total sugars.

[104] Value is for sulfated ash and overestimates ash by approximately 8.

[115] Federal standards provide for addition of certain calcium salts as firming agents; if used, these salts may add calcium not to exceed 26 mg. per 100 grams of finished product.

[122] Average value per 100 grams of pork of all cuts is 70 mg for raw meat and 65 mg. for cooked meat.

[123] Average vaue per 100 grams of pork of all cuts is 285 mg. for raw meat and 390 mg. for cooked meat.

[125] Applies to product without added salt. If salt is added, an estimated average value for sodium is 236 mg. per 100 grams.

[128] Sodium content is variable and may be as high as 1,000 mg. per 100 grams.

[129] Sodium content is variable. For example, very thin pretzel sticks contain about twice the average amount listed.

[144] Values for sauerkraut and sauerkraut juice are based on salt contents of 1.9 and 2.0 percent respectively in the finished products. The amounts in some samples may vary significantly from this estimate.

[145] Based on frozen scallops, possibly brined.

[151] Apples to squash including skin; flesh has no appreciable vitamin A value.

[152] Value based on freshly harvested squash. The carotenoid content increases during storage, the amount of increase varying according to variety and conditions of storage. More information is needed on the relative contents of the individual carotenoids and their rates of increase under usual storage conditions before a suitable vitamin A value can be derived for the stored product.

[159] Year-round average. Samples marketed from November through May average around 10 mg. per 100 grams; from June through October, around 26 mg.

[163] One sample with salt added contained 875 mg. of sodium per 100 grams and 275 mg. of potassium.

App. 12: Phobias*

Fear of	Condition
air	aerophobia
aloneness	eremophobia, monophobia
animals	zoophobia
anything new	neophobia
bacilli	bacillophobia
bad men or burglars	pavor sceleris, scelerophobia
barren or empty space	cenophobia, kenophobia
bearing a deformed child	teratophobia
bees	apiphobia, melissophobia
birds	ornithophobia
blood	hematophobia, hemophobia
blushing	ereuthrophobia, erythrophobia
brain disease	meningitophobia
bridges (crossing of)	gephyrophobia
buried alive	taphephobia
cats	ailurophobia, galeophobia, gatophobia
change or novelty	kainophobia, kainotophobia
choking	anginophobia
cold or something cold	cheimaphobia, psychrophobia
color(s)	chromatophobia, chromophobia
comet	cometophobia
confinement	claustrophobia
contamination	molysmophobia, mysophobia
corpses	necrophobia
crossing streets	dromophobia
crowds	demophobia, ochlophobia
dampness or moisture	hygrophobia
darkness	nyctophobia, scotophobia
dawn	eosophobia
daylight	phengophobia
death	thanatophobia
definite, specific disease	monopathophobia
deformity	dysmorphophobia
demons	demonomania
depth	bathophobia
devil	satanophobia
dirt	mysophobia, rupophobia
disease	nosophobia, pathophobia
dogs or rabies	cynophobia
dolls	pediophobia
drafts, wind	anemophobia
dust	amathophobia
eating	phagophobia
electricity	electrophobia
emptiness	kenophobia, cenophobia
everything	panphobia, panophobia, pantophobia
excrement	coprophobia
eyes	ommatophobia
failure	kakorrhaphiophobia
fatigue	kopophobia
fearing	phobophobia
feathers	pteronophobia
female genitals	eurotophobia
fever	pyrexeophobia
filth	mysophobia

*Adapted from Campbell, R.J.: Psychiatric Dictionary, ed 5. Oxford University Press, N.Y., 1981.

Phobias (*Continued*)

Fear of	Condition
filth or odor, personal	automysophobia
fire	pyrophobia
fish	ichthyophobia
floods	antlophobia
fog	homichlophobia
food	cibophobia, sitophobia
forest	hylophobia
frogs	batrachophobia
functioning	ergasiophobia
girls	parthenophobia
glass	crystallophobia, hyelophobia
God	theophobia
gravity	barophobia
hair	trichopathophobia
heat	thermophobia
height	acrophobia
hell	hadephobia, stygiophobia
heredity and hereditary disease	patroiophobia
high objects or being on tall buildings	batophobia
house	domatophobia, oikophobia
ideas	ideophobia
infinity	apeirophobia
injury	traumatophobia
innovation	neophobia
insane, becoming	lyssophobia, maniaphobia
insects	acarophobia, entomophobia
jealousy	zelophobia
justice	dikephobia
knife or pointed objects	aichmophobia
large objects	megalophobia
left	levophobia
light	photophobia
lightning	astraphobia, astrapophobia, keraunophobia
locked in, being	claustrophobia
looked at, being	scopophobia
machinery	mechanophobia
man	androphobia
many things	polyphobia
marriage	gamophobia
medicine	pharmacophobia
metals	metallophobia
meteors	meteorophobia
mice	musophobia
mirror and seeing oneself in	eisoptrophobia, spectrophobia
missiles	ballistophobia
moisture	hygrophobia
money	chrematophobia
motion	kinesophobia
myths	mythophobia
naked body	gymnophobia
name, hearing a certain	onomatophobia
needles	belonephobia
night	noctiphobia, nyctophobia
northern lights	auroraphobia
novelty	kainophobia
odor	olfactophobia, osmophobia, osphresiophobia
odor, personal	bromidrosiphobia
open space	agoraphobia
overwork	ponophobia
pain	algophobia, odynophobia

Fear of	Condition
parasites	parasitophobia
people	anthropophobia
place	topophobia
pleasure	hedonophobia
pointed objects	aichmophobia
poison	iophobia, toxicophobia
poverty	peniaphobia
precipices	cremnophobia
punishment	poinephobia
rabies	cynophobia, lyssophobia
railroad or train	siderodromophobia
rain or rain storm	ombrophobia
rectal excreta	coprophobia
rectum	proctophobia
red	erythrophobia
responsibility	hypengyophobia
right	dextrophobia
river	potamophobia
robbers	harpaxophobia
rod or instrument of punishment	rhabdophobia
ruin	atephobia
sacred things	hierophobia
scabies	scabiophobia
school	school phobia
scratches or being scratched	amychophobia
sea	thalassophobia
self	autophobia
semen	spermatophobia
sex	genophobia
sexual intercourse	coitophobia
shock	hormephobia
sin	hamartophobia
sinning	peccatiphobia
sitting	thaasophobia
sitting down	kathisophobia
skin disease	dermatosiophobia
skin lesion	dermatophobia
skin of animals	doraphobia
sleep	hypnophobia
small objects	microphobia, microbiophobia
smothering	pnigerophobia
snake	ophidiophobia
snow	chionphobia
solitude or being alone	eremophobia
sounds	acousticophobia
sourness	acerophobia
speaking	laliophobia
spider	arachneophobia
stairs	climacophobia
standing up	stasiphobia
standing or walking	stasibasiphobia
stars	siderophobia
stealing	kleptophobia
stories	mythophobia
strangers	xenophobia
street	agyiophobia
string	linonophobia
sunlight	heliophobia
symbolism	symbolophobia
syphilis	syphilophobia

Phobias (*Continued*)

Fear of	Condition
talking	laliophobia
tapeworms	taeniophobia
taste	geumaphobia
teeth	odontophobia
thinking	phronemophobia
thunder	astraphobia, brontophobia
time	chronophobia
touched, being	haphephobia, haptephobia
travel	hodophobia
trembling	tremophobia
trichinosis	trichinophobia
tuberculosis	phthisiophobia, tuberculophobia
vaccination	vaccinophobia
vehicle, being in	amaxophobia
venereal disease	cypridophobia
voice, one's own	phonophobia
void	kenophobia
vomiting	emetophobia
walking	basiphobia
water	hydrophobia
weakness	asthenophobia
wind	anemophobia
women	gynophobia
words, hearing certain	onomatophobia
writing	graphophobia

App. 13: Medical Emergencies

Convulsions

Type	History	Clonic or Tonic	Pulse	Breathing	Color	Muscles	Eyes	Pathology	Treatment
Apoplexy. Intracranial hemorrhage	Usually sequel to cerebral hemorrhage. May be result of vascular disease. Occurs usually after age of 40 years.	Usually tonic. May be limited to different areas, or to one side of the body.	Strong and of a bounding quality.	Respirations are deep and stertorous.	Red. Skin has a florid and flushed appearance.	Spastic in tonic usage with hemiplegia. One side of body shows paralysis; other is normal.	Pupils may be unequal in size.	Arteriosclerosis. Intracranial hemorrhage.	Keep the patient absolutely quiet with an icecap to head. No stimulants. If vomiting, prevent aspiration of vomitus.
Eclampsia.	Occurs in toxemia of pregnancy in antepartum and postpartum stages.	Prolonged tonic convulsions are characteristic with the whole body in a state of rigidity. Both tonic and clonic types may occur.	Rapid, becoming thready.	Respirations are irregular, shallow, and hissing. Breath-holding may occur.	Blue. Patient may become very cyanotic.	Rigidity of the body. Extremities are flexed. General tonic spasm of body may be followed by clonic spasm.	Pupils may be dilated and may be of unequal size.	Hypertension. Pathological changes in liver, kidney, brain and adrenals. Rapid gain of weight.	Control convulsions. Give proper antenatal care for toxemia of pregnancy. Control of diet, elimination and prevention of hypertension. Magnesium sulfate intramuscularly.
Epilepsy. Grand mal type.	Previous history of fits. Attack may be preceded by aura. In some patients convulsions may occur only at	Generalized tonic, clonic type but may be focal.	Rapid.	Respirations are rapid, deep, and stertorous.	Blue. Patient may become very cyanotic.	Rigid in tonic and in clonic origin.	Pupils may be contracted and occasionally of unequal size.	Abnormal electroencephalographic pattern.	Prevent the patient from injuring himself or from falling. Place on floor with pillow, etc. Use no stimulant. For safety, do not place fingers

	night.								in mouth but use a suitable padded gag to prevent patient's biting his tongue. Loosen clothing around neck.
Hysteria.	Onset usually is not sudden. Accompanied by laughter and crying. Seizure may be more prolonged than epilepsy.	May be of the stimulation types and take on those of epilepsy. Usually are of the tonic nature.	Shows no definite changes unless slightly rapid due to excitement.	Respirations may become rapid.	No change in color of skin.	Rigidity or relaxed as the victim wishes to demonstrate	Pupils are normal and react to light. Muscles of eye resist when forced opening is attempted.	Patient seldom loses consciousness. May fall but not in an area where an injury may occur. Highly reactive to suggestion.	Inhalation of aromatic spirit of ammonia. Ice water dashed upon the face. Seizure usually ends when the audience disappears.
Tetanus.	After injury, deep wound, and entrance of tetanus bacillus. Ex: gunshot wound.	Tonic convulsions and tonic spasms of voluntary muscles.	Rapid.	Rapid. Labored to irregular.	Cyanotic in convulsions.	Constant rigidity. Trismus may not appear for 24 hrs. after symptoms.	Normal.	Disease is due to the action of tetanus toxin, which is thought to act centrally rather than on the affected muscles.	Human tetanus immune globulin. Maintain airway. This may require tracheotomy. Oxygen therapy.
Uremic Convulsions.	Condition is usually accompanied by chronic or acute nephritis or chronic cardiac conditions. Marked edema noted.	Clonic (mild) to severe muscle jerking.	Rapid to weak. Muscles are rigid, making it difficult to find pulse.	Respirations are slow and stertorous.	Skin is pale, dry, scaly and waxy appearance.	Tonic and clonic.	Pupils may be pin points.	Arterial hypertension. Albuminuria. Suppression of urine. Visual disturbance.	Measures to reduce high blood pressure. Treatment by use of artificial kidney may be lifesaving.

Dislocations

Type	History	Pathology	Muscles	Complications	Treatment	Strapping and Support	Differentiation
Ankle.	From violence of undue weight or twisting upon the knee.	Production of scar tissue and contractures, which produce prolonged restriction of motion. Usually a short period of disability and then satisfactory recovery.	Rigid with pain. May include swelling and discoloration (May be delayed).	Fractures—Minor or Major as determined by accident. Temporary or permanent disability.	Continuous application of cold for 24 to 48 hours. Then heat, massage, and passive and active exercise.	Allow no use (fracture may be present). Check x-ray film for fracture. Immobilize the foot and ankle on a pillow or a rigid splint.	Satisfactory reduction is made when the ankle can be dorsiflexed within a right angle.
Back.	Sudden and violent twisting of the back.	Cervical dislocation—Paraplegia may occur. Respiratory failure or ascending myelitis; dorsal dislocation; urinary infection.	Affected side relaxed; uninjured side spastic. Muscle spasm holds back in rigidity with severe pain when any movement is made.	Damage to cord. Incomplete paraplegia. Failure to replace results in kyphosis deformity. Weakness and arthritis.	Do not allow patient to sit up or to be turned. Prepare patient for cast and brace. Control the pain. Watch for decubitus.	Treat as for fracture. Transport in prone position on rigid stretcher. Keep the body in hyperextension with cast or brace.	Compression fracture of first lumbar vertebrae is the most common injury of the spine. Decided excursion of the ilium (noted when the back is extended or flexed) is corrected. No crepitus. Discoloration, swelling, and persistent pain in muscle.
Clavicle.	May be due to a heavy blow or fall upon the side of the shoulder.	Posterior dislocation causes pressure on structures at base of neck; rupture of sternoclavicular ligament.	Hyperextended. Fatigue results if prolonged.	Increased deformity and insecurity of movement of shoulder. Prolonged disability.	Symptomatic. Slight massage. Adhesive strapping. Sling for four weeks.	In recumbent position with small narrow sand bag between scapulae. Posterior Dislocation—press shoulders backward. Make traction on arm as it is held abducted at right angle—clavicle returns to position.	Complete reduction corrects the deformity at the sternoclavicular joint, no crepitus is present. Stretched ligaments and torn muscles are manifested by swelling, discoloration, and generalized pain. Shoulder has secure movement.

Elbow.	In childhood between ages 8 to 12 years. Child falls upon the outstretched hand. Produces hyperextension of the elbow.	Elbow swollen. Held midway between flexion and extension. Head of radius is felt rotating behind humerus.	Tension in biceps muscle. Muscle ossification at the elbow.	Arthritis in joint. Muscle tissue ossification. Recurrence of dislocation.	Apply splint. Immobilize elbow until replacement can be made. Treat symptomatically.	Supinate the forearm. Make traction forward and downward on the forearm until radius and ulna slip back into position.	The ability to acutely flex the elbow when dislocation is satisfactorily reduced.
Foot.	Force of violent nature upon plantar flexion of foot. Misstepping.	May include a compound dislocation of the ankle. Slight to increased amount of trauma and strain upon all soft tissue of foot.	Tense; marked swelling and discoloration.	Fracture of ankle. Weakness of muscles of plantar arch.	Continuous application of cold for 24 to 48 hours. Then heat, massage, and passive and active exercise.	Pillow splint or rigid splint as for fractures. Watch for swelling and cyanosis in part.	Satisfactory reduction is made when the displaced astragalus (projecting on the back of the foot) has been leveled.
Hand.	Occurs most frequently in thumb due to forced hyperextension of the thumb or finger.	Head of metacarpal bone is wedged between flexor tendons (may necessitate an operation).	Marked tension.	Deformity and permanent disability unless successful reduction is made.	Hyperextend the phalanx or thumb and then flex it. Use adhesive strapping. Cold applications for 24 to 48 hours.	Hyperextension of thumb as local pressure is made—thereby replacement is effected. Very early reduction is necessary.	Displacement of the thumb is the most frequent injury of the hand. Swelling, discoloration, and deformity (without point tenderness) are present.
Hip.	If posterior, by indirect violence upon head of femur. If anterior, by violent hyperabduction.	Injury to capsular and surrounding tissues of the acetabulum.	Posterior dislocation—hip is held rigidly flexed. Adduction, inward rotation and flexion of the thigh. Anterior dislocation—hip is immovable in abduction and external rotation. Knee flexed.	Torn tendons and ligaments. Fracture of the neck of femur.	Symptomatic for discomfort. Splinting—since fracture is frequently a sequel. Preparation for reduction of the dislocation.	Board or rigid splint. Keep limb in slight elevation unless fracture is imminent.	Reduction will be complete when flexion with extension and adduction of the thigh are possible.
Jaw.	The too-wide opening of the mouth, for ex-	Capsule of glenoid fossa is too loose. Muscles are soft. Tissues aid in	Muscles spastic. Later become fatigued.	Embarrassment in the unexpected recurrence.	Symptomatic treatment. Replacement by pressure of operator's	Replacement. Jaw bandage (supporting).	Anterior dislocation manifests partly opened and locked jaws with

Dislocations *(Continued)*

Type	History	Pathology	Muscles	Complications	Treatment	Strapping and Support	Differentiation
	ample, in yawning, laughing, or eating.	chronic displacement. Jaw becomes locked beneath maxillary prominence.		Trauma and fatigue in muscles. Predisposes infection.	thumbs upon molars until normal placement in the mandibular cavity.		the teeth projecting forward. Complete reduction will restore the jaw for normal occlusion.
Knee.	After violent fall or force upon knee.	Torn ligaments. Traumatized muscles of patellar and popliteal area. Loss of synovial fluid after rupture of bursa.	Rigid with pain. May include slight to marked swelling. Ecchymosis—slight or marked.	Disability and deformity. Permanently stiffened knee when synovial fluid is lost.	Splint as for fracture of femur and lower leg. Symptomatic (to relieve discomfort). Treat for shock.	Board or rigid splint. Keep knee and limb in slight elevation unless fracture is present.	The depression adjacent to the patella is diminished and complete flexion of the knee is restored.
Neck.	Caused by violent twists, fall upon the head, or diving into a pool.	Bilateral dislocation. Severs spinal cord. Death usually follows. Nerve injury caused by tension or displacement. Permanent torticollis and limited neck motion.	Torticollis. Muscles spastic on uninjured side, relaxed on injured side.	Severance of cord. Pressure on cord causing predisposal to recurrence of dislocation, permanent torticollis, paralysis, death.	Keep patient in recumbent position in hyperextension of the neck. Reduction by leverage and not by manual traction. Keep traction by collar or plaster cast.	Reduction done by leverage. Application of plaster or rigid collar which must be worn until recovery of the ligaments to prevent recurrence.	Unilateral dislocation produces torticollis with head tilted on side and chin rotated away from displaced vertebrae. Reduction aids in complete disappearance of torticollis.
Shoulder.	ANTERIOR. Force was from behind—head of the humerus lies just below the coracoid process. POSTERIOR. Direct force upon the flexed elbow. Head of humerus is placed in front and lower than the axilla.	Rupture of tendon. Injury to circumflex nerve or brachial plexus. Disability. Injury to axillary vessels. Greater tuberosity (coracoid). Acromion processes fractured.	Muscle tension in the biceps muscle. Triceps muscle immobilized, may be slightly rigid.	Chronic arthritis. Cartilage displacement. Complete loss of function. Recurrences if a repeated injury or improper or inadequate mobilization after the first injury.	**Kocher method of Replacement. After procedure, keep sling.** **1. Flex elbow to a right angle and place elbow against body. Rotate arm outward until forearm points away from body.** **2. Keep elbow and arm (lower arm) flexed on upper. Raise elbow forward until it** reaches a right angle position to the long axis (or horizontal) of the body. 3. Arm is directed obliquely inward and hand placed on opposite shoulder so that reduction or replacement is complete. Immobilize by sling. X-ray study is necessary.		**Dislocation of shoulder is corrected when the hand (unassisted) can be placed upon the opposite shoulder.**

Wrist.	Caused by the hyperextended hand or by severe blows upon the dorsal portion of the wrist.	Dislocation of semilunar bone. Flexion of the wrist is blocked by displaced bone. Usually results in a permanently weak wrist.	Muscles of back of hand tense. Usually marked swelling in area of the sprain.	Permanent pain, weakness, and limitation of motion. Flexion limited. Displaced bones may have to be removed by surgical methods.	Surgical removal of displaced bone if unable to replace it. Support by splint or strapping. Cold applications for 24 to 48 hours.	Apply traction upon hand. Put firm pressure of the thumb upon the displaced bone.	Flexion of the wrist with slight limitations of motion and manifestation of weakness will indicate satisfactory reduction of the wrist.

Fractures

Type	History	Pathology	Complications	Hemorrhage	Color of Area	Treatment	Transportation
Comminuted	Injury due to crushing blow.	Bone is broken into two or more fragments.	Malunion; unstableness; infection.	Occurs in area of injury.	Discoloration is delayed. Appears in area of deeper bones.	Splint before transportation. Replacement of fracture. Occasionally requires open reduction.	Splint and traction.
Compound	Fall or accident.	Injury where either one or both fragments are through the skin.	Infection; hemorrhage; shock.	May or may not hemorrhage.	Slight to marked increase in ecchymosis.	Immediate debridement in hospital. Antitetanus therapy.	Cover with sterile dressing. Maintain traction. For leg fracture use Thomas splint.
Greenstick	Fall or accident. (In children)	Fracture is incomplete but there is bowing of the bone.	Complete fracture; deformity.	Probably no hemorrhage will occur.	Discoloration may be slight or it may be marked.	Splint for preparation for transportation. Reduction of the curvature and place in cast.	Splint.
Impacted	Crushing force causing fracture. Fragments telescoped.	One fragment is jammed into another.	Deformity; loss of function; pain; osteomyelitis.	Occurs in area of injury.	Discoloration according to extent of bone injury. It may be delayed.	Traction must be made while reduction and proper cast is fitted to hold extremity in place.	Splint and traction.
Simple	Fall or accident.	A complete fracture with no fragments.	Pressure on the blood supply; malunion; osteomyelitis.	Subcutaneous or capillary.	Slight to marked increase in ecchymosis.	Splint before preparation for transportation. Reduction (depending	In splint.

Fractures *(Continued)*

Type	History	Pathology	Complications	Hemorrhage	Color of Area	Treatment	Transportation
						upon skill of operator).	
Transverse and Spiral	Sudden twisting violence exerted upon extremity.	Fracture line across the bone. Fracture through the bone or around it.	Malfunction; loss of function; cutting of blood supply; infection of bone.	Frequently occurs around area of fracture.	Same as compound fracture.	Depending on site. Splint and traction.	Traction and immobilization.
Ankle (Potts Fracture)	A sudden or forceful wrenching of the lower end of tibia and fibula.	Fracture of the lower ends of the fibula and tibia. Foot is displaced outward. Impairment of tissues, vessels, etc., from trauma.	Dislocation and sprains may occur simultaneously.	May or may not hemorrhage. Discoloration.	Slight or marked areas of ecchymosis.	Immobilize immediately by pillow splint or rigid splint.	Keep limb well supported with slight elevation.
Back	Occurs after jackknife fall and other accidents.	Usually crushing body of vertebrae.	Paralysis and shock (depending upon location of the fracture).	None in surrounding tissues.	Usually no change in color of the skin.	Extreme care in preparation and transportation. Rigid support. Place in hyperextension for 8 weeks. Body cast.	Place and secure in prone position. Keep patient in hyperextension. Restrain if necessary. Rigid stretcher or improvision.
Coccyx	Falling into sitting position.	Fracture may be from sacral region or from tip of coccyx.	Constant pain; abscesses; osteomyelitis.	None in surrounding tissues.	No change in color of the skin.	Hot sitz bath after 24–48 hours of cold applications to area. Rest in bed. Perform coccygectomy if not cured.	Carry patient on rigid stretcher. Keep in dorsal recumbent position.
Femur or Thigh	Usually sudden and severe trauma to thigh.	Bone and nerve injury; paralysis and permanent disability.	Deformity and shortening of the limb where an endocrine disturbance is present; severance of nerves and blood vessels; paralysis and gangrene.	May or may not hemorrhage. Discoloration may be delayed.	Slight to marked increase in ecchymosis.	Splint to leg and body. Keep patient flat. Provide and retain traction. Watch for shock.	Use rigid stretcher. Keep leg in traction until ready for reduction.

Forearm and Colles' Fracture	Result of a twisting force upon the lower arm or wrist, or from violence exerted upon the arm in preventing the body from falling.	Fracture and displacement of distal end of the radius. Tip of styloid process of ulna broken off. Backward displacement of radius.	Trauma and swelling of tissues. Dislocations and sprains.	Slight. Increased if fracture is not immediately immobilized.	Slight to marked.	Rigid splint, arm support with a sling.	Place in a sling after splinting.
Hip	Usually found in elderly people.	Fracture through neck or through trochanter or both.	Loss of function; deformity and shortening.	Hemorrhage but not in large amounts.	Ecchymosis but it may be delayed.	Traction; Smith-Peterson Nail.	Place in Thomas Splint as improvised.
Humerus	Result of a twisting force or blow upon upper arm.	Injury to the osseous structures. Trauma and lacerations of tissues, muscles, etc., if compound fracture.	Severance of nerves and blood vessels; temporary deformity.	Slight. Increased if compound fracture.	Slight or marked areas of discoloration.	Immobilize immediately by splint or sling (weight of forearm usually provides the necessary traction).	Keep arm in sling or splint.
Neck	Diving into pools; auto wrecks; accidents.	Break extends through body of vertebrae or the laminae.	Paralysis (total or partial). Death.	None noted in the tissues.	No change in color of the skin.	Keep neck in hyperextension. Place rolled blanket under shoulders. Minor fracture needs traction for 5–6 weeks. Major (with cord injury) cast or collar for 10–12 months.	Patient must not move the neck under any circumstances. Keep neck and head hyperextended. Restrain if necessary. Rigid stretcher or improvision for rigidity.
Pelvis	A blow or crushing force.	Bone impairment; involvement of sacral nerves. Paralysis, torn ligaments, and lacerated muscles.	Rupture of bladder and rectum; deformity and shortening of limb; sprain of pelvic joints.	Same as in compound fracture. Discoloration may be delayed.	Same as in compound fracture if compound. Otherwise delayed.	Keep in dorsal recumbent position; after reduction keep prone. Reduction of fragments; symptomatic treatment.	On rigid stretcher in dorsal recumbent position. Keep body extended
Skull	Fall or blow upon the skull.	IN VAULT. Little or no intracranial trauma. Linear fracture may be overlooked.	Concussion; paralysis of limbs of the body; infection of brain; compression of brain.	Bleeding (bright) from mouth and ears. Clots on the brain.	Ecchymosis over the mastoid process	Place in dorsal recumbent position. Watch for infection. Allow skull base fractures to	Place on rigid stretcher. Keep flat. Keep patient quiet.

Type	History	Pathology	Complications	Hemorrhage	Color of Area	Treatment	Transportation
		IN BASE. Serious compression in brain. Concussion injury to vital cranial nerves.		Extent and nature determined by location of injury. Dangers of pressure upon the brain.		bleed. Limit fluids.	

Poisons and Poisoning

(Note: See Poison Control Centers, United States and Canada, in Appendix.)

Toxic Substance	Probable Lethal Dose for Adult Humans (mg./kg. body wt.)*	Symptoms of Poisoning	Emergency Measures	Supportive and Follow-up Treatment	Pathology
Acetaminophen		Early: may be asymptomatic. Nausea and vomiting, pallor, diaphoresis, early signs of liver damage. Late: In 24 to 48 hours nausea and vomiting, jaundice, blood coagulation defects, hypoglycemia, hepatic and renal failure.	Emesis, gastric lavage; N-acetylcysteine should be given as soon as possible with the first dose being 140 mg./kg. and then 70 mg./kg. every 4 hours for 3 days.	If liver and renal failure develop, treat accordingly.	Liver and kidney damage.
Acetophenetidin or Acetanilid	50 to 500 mg.	Sweating; nausea; vomiting; chills; ringing in ears; fall in blood pressure; circulatory collapse; cyanosis; coma; convulsions; death from respiratory failure.	Gastric lavage or induce emesis. Instill sodium bicarbonate into stomach. Whole blood or plasma. Artificial respiration or oxygen. Analeptics.	Keep patient warm and quiet. If cyanosis becomes severe, 1-2 mg./kg. of 1% methylene blue.	Methemoglobinemia, CNS stimulation, kidney and liver injury.
Acetylsalicylic acid—SEE: *salicylates*.					

Acids (acetic, hydrochloric, nitric, phosphoric, sulfuric, etc.)	Variable	Immediate pain and corrosion of mucous membranes of mouth, throat, and esophagus; difficulty in swallowing; stomach pain; nausea; coffee-ground vomitus; thirst, shock syndrome with death in circulatory collapse.	Give orally, magnesium oxide, milk of magnesia, lime water, or aluminum hydroxide gel. Avoid carbonates as neutralizers. Give large amounts of water. Demulcents and morphine for pain.	Correct shock with fluids, plasma, or whole blood. Tracheotomy or gastrectomy may become necessary.	Asphyxia from glottic edema, gastric and pyloric strictures, and stenosis or perforation.
Amanita (phalloides, mushroom)	Variable. May be only one mushroom.	After 6 to 15 hours, abdominal pain, nausea, vomiting, purging, weakness, thirst, shock syndrome, restlessness, delirium, hallucinations, coma, late jaundice, acute renal failure. Death may be from cardiac, kidney, liver, or CNS lesions.	Slurry of activated charcoal as lavage fluid, leaving some in stomach along with saline cathartic. Meperidine for pain. Contact nearest Poison Control Center for availability and advisability of using thioctic acid.	Correct fluid and electrolyte balance. Prepare to treat renal or hepatic failure. Treatment with artificial kidney may be required. Maintain high carbohydrate intake. Give I.V. if necessary.	Acute yellow atrophy of the liver, acute renal failure, cardiac damage.
Aminophylline or Caffeine	50 to 500 mg.	Restlessness; excitement alternating with drowsiness; ringing in ears; fast pulse; nausea; vomiting; fever; diuresis; dehydration; thirst; tremor; delirium; convulsions; coma; death in cardiovascular and respiratory collapse.	Lavage, induce emesis with saline cathartic unless vomiting and purging have already begun. Treat CNS excitation with appropriate barbiturate therapy.	Oxygen and artificial respiration. Maintain fluid and electrolyte balance.	CNS stimulation and gastric ulceration.
Ammonia	Variable. Even a small amount may kill.	Irritation of eyes and respiratory tract (sometimes pulmonary edema, glottic spasm, or laryngeal edema). Other symptoms are like lye poisoning (SEE. *Lye* in table).	Give large amounts of diluted vinegar, lemon juice, or orange juice. Demulcents and morphine for pain Oxygen under pressure to help prevent pulmonary edema.	Treat for shock. Tracheotomy may be needed. NOTE: Do not give drugs such as narcotics which would depress respiration.	Corrosive esophagitis and gastritis, laryngeal edema, pulmonary edema.
d-Amphetamine	5 to 50 mg. but variable	Excitement; talkativeness; restlessness; tremors; dizziness; hyperactive reflexes; dry mouth;	Gastric lavage with tap water and activated charcoal, or induce	Isolate patient and avoid sensory stimuli. Ice packs and sponge baths for hyperpyrexia. Chlorpromazine, 1–2	CNS and peripheral sympathetic stimulation; petechial hemorrhages

Poisons and Poisoning (*Continued*)

Toxic Substance	Probable Lethal Dose for Adult Humans (mg./kg. body wt.)*	Symptoms of Poisoning	Emergency Measures	Supportive and Follow-up Treatment	Pathology
		nausea; vomiting; diarrhea; palpitations; fever; dehydration; mydriasis; tachycardia; hallucinations; delirium; mania; convulsions; coma; death in circulatory collapse.	emesis. Treat symptoms of CNS with appropriate barbiturate therapy.	mg./kg. I.M., may be required.	in the brain.
Aniline	50 to 500 mg.	Intense cyanosis; headache; nausea; dryness in throat; confusion; ataxia; vertigo; weakness; disorientation; drowsiness; heart block; death in cardiovascular collapse.	Lavage with 1:5000 potassium permanganate. Instill saline cathartic. Oxygen and artificial respiration. Give 1–2 mg./kg. of body weight of 1% methylene blue.	Whole blood transfusions if needed.	Intense methemoglobinemia; mild liver and kidney injury.
Antabuse (disulfiram)	Unknown	Circulatory collapse.	Oxygen therapy, intravenous 5% glucose in water. Intravenous sodium ascorbate. In severe cases very slow injection of 5 ml. of a 2% solution of saccharated iron oxide may be of benefit.	Complete rest with postural drainage. Continue oxygen inhalation and maintain fluid balance.	Unknown.
Antihistaminics (tripelennamine, diphenhydramine, chlorpheniramine, etc.)	5 to 50 mg.	Drowsiness; lethargy; fatigue; ataxia; dryness of mouth; fixed dilated pupils; coma. Sometimes however, only excitement is seen with tremors, anxiety, delirium, convulsions, hyperpyrexia, nausea, vomiting, diarrhea, death in cardiovascular collapse or respiratory arrest.	Lavage or induce emesis. Cautious sedation if excited. Oxygen and artificial respiration.	Ice packs and alcohol sponges for hyperpyrexia.	Mechanism of death not precisely known. Cerebral edema is described.

Arsenic or Antimony	5 to 50 mg.	Symptoms may be delayed several hours. Metallic taste and odor of garlic on breath; burning pain throughout gastrointestinal tract; vomiting and purging; dehydration; shock syndrome; coma; convulsions; paralysis; severe diarrhea which becomes bloody. Death may occur.	Gastric lavage with 1% sodium bicarbonate solution. Administer dimercaprol (BAL) in accordance with supplier's dosage schedule.	Maintain fluid and electrolyte balance. Morphine for pain. Treat for shock. Treat anemia and renal failure if either is present.	Shock secondary to hemorrhagic gastroenteritis. Skin eruptions are of no toxicological significance.
Aspirin—SEE: *salicylates*.					
Atropine	Less than 5 mg.	Dryness of mouth and burning pain in throat; thirst; mydriasis; skin is dry, hot, and flushed; hyperpyrexia; tachycardia; palpitations; restlessness; excitement; confusion; mania; delirium. Death is rare.	Lavage with slurry of activated charcoal or 4% tannic acid. Pilocarpine will make patient more comfortable, but barbiturates must be used to control excitement. Do not use long-acting barbiturates. For depression, use mild stimulants. If severe, use oxygen and artificial respiration.	Oxygen and artificial respiration. Ice packs or alcohol sponges for hyperpyrexia. Catheterize if necessary. Ophthalmic pilocarpine.	Intense CNS excitation and parasympathetic paralysis.
Barbiturates	50 to 500 mg.	Confusion; drowsiness; ataxia; vertigo; slurred speech; headache; stupor; coma; areflexia; cyanosis; hypotension; shallow pulse; cardiovascular collapse; death in respiratory arrest.	Establish airway, gastric lavage, artificial respiration, oxygen with CO_2 inhalation, maintain fluid and electrolyte balance. Use of artificial kidney to remove barbiturate has been helpful.	Record vital signs frequently. Correct airway obstruction. Oxygen and artificial respiration as needed. When vital signs have stabilized and kidney function assured, induce diuresis with urea, and alkalinize urine. Antibiotic therapy if aspiration of vomitus has occurred.	CNS depression with respiratory arrest. Pulmonary edema occurs in prolonged coma.
Barium salts, Chloride, and other soluble salts	Quite variable	Salivation; nausea; vomiting; abdominal cramps; violent and bloody diarrhea; slow and irregular pulse; ringing in ears; dizziness; twitching; convulsions or paralysis; death from respira-	Give sodium magnesium or aluminum sulfate rapidly by mouth. Lavage or induce emesis, then leave more of the above in the	Intravenous saline for dehydration. Treat for shock.	Violent peristalsis, atrial hypertension, cardiac disturbances, late kidney damage. Barium stimulates contraction of muscles.

Toxic Substance	Probable Lethal Dose for Adult Humans (mg./kg. body wt.)*	Symptoms of Poisoning	Emergency Measures	Supportive and Follow-up Treatment	Pathology
		tory failure and cardiac arrest.	stomach. Atropine or morphine may relieve abdominal pain. Quinidine or procainamide to prevent cardiac arrest. Artificial respiration and oxygen.		
Benzene or Xylene or Toluene	50 to 500 mg.	Burning sensation in mouth and stomach; nausea; vomiting; chest pains; cough; headache; giddiness; vertigo; ataxia; confusion; stupor; restless coma; late severe blood dyscrasias. Death from respiratory failure or ventricular fibrillation.	Lavage with tap water; leave mineral oil and saline cathartic in the stomach.	Oxygen, artificial respiration, parenteral fluids. Avoid fats, oils, alcohol, and epinephrine.	Respiratory failure from CNS depression or ventricular fibrillation. Severe and possibly fatal bone marrow damage.
Benzene hexachloride	50 to 500 mg.	Irritability; vomiting; restlessness; ataxia; spasms; convulsions; coma; respiratory failure.	Lavage with tap water and instill saline cathartic into the stomach. Control convulsions by cautious use of barbiturates.	Rest and quiet. Avoid fats, oils, alcohol and epinephrine.	CNS depression, liver damage, and hyaline changes in the renal tubules.
Boric acid and borate salts	50 to 500 mg.	Headache; nausea; vomiting; diarrhea; stomach pain; weakness and lethargy; restlessness; tremor; convulsions; coma. Distinctive, fine, bright red rash. Shock with death in vascular collapse.	Lavage stomach with 1% sodium bicarbonate solution and instill saline cathartic. Oxygen and plasma or whole blood transfusions as indicated.	Fluids and electrolytes for replacement therapy.	Cause of death not known. Both kidney and liver damage are occasionally reported.
Botulinum toxin	Possibly	After 12 to 36 hours but may be	Lavage with tap water or	Oxygen and artificial respiration. Tra-	Blocks transmission of

	most poisonous substance known to man. Microgram amounts are lethal.	as early as three hours: nausea, vomiting, occasionally diarrhea, difficulties in vision and swallowing, weakness and paralysis of respiratory muscles. Profuse sweating, and pulse is rapid and weak.	a slurry of activated charcoal if within a few hours postingestion. Instill saline cathartic. Give specific or polyvalent botulinus antitoxin. NOTE: Call the U. S. National Center for Disease Control, Atlanta, Georgia, telephone (404) 329-3311 (day) or (404) 329-3644 (night), for the location of nearest supply of antitoxin.	cheotomy if needed.	nerve impulses at motor end plate. Congestion and hemorrhage in all organs, especially the CNS.
Bromides (sodium, potassium, ammonium, etc.)	500 to 5000 mg.	Prompt vomiting; drowsiness; irritability; ataxia; vertigo; confusion; mania; hallucinations; coma; skin rashes; neurological signs; sensory disturbances; increased spinal fluid pressure. Death is rare.	Give sodium or ammonium chloride 6–12 gm. daily in divided doses with 4 liters of water. Give saline cathartic. If intoxication is severe enough, use of artificial kidney to hasten removal of bromide may be indicated.	Maintain hydration and mild diuresis.	Acne-like skin eruption, inflammation of mucous membranes, CNS depression.
Cadmium salts	Several hundred mg.	Nausea; vomiting; diarrhea; salivation; abdominal cramps; headache; vertigo; exhaustion; collapse; shock and immediate death or delayed death from acute renal failure. Inhaling dusts and fumes very hazardous, producing pulmonary edema.	Demulcents; lavage with milk or water if vomiting is not prompt. Give saline cathartic. If pulmonary edema develops, treat with positive pressure oxygen administration.	Maintain fluid and electrolyte balance. Prophylactic and supportive measures for liver injury or acute renal failure.	Severe gastroenteritis, mild liver damage, and acute renal failure. If inhaled as a dust or fume, produces pulmonary edema.
Camphor	50 to 500 mg.	Nausea; vomiting; feeling of warmth; headache; confusion; vertigo; excitement; restlessness; delirium; hallucinations; tremor; convulsions; depression;	Short-acting intravenous barbiturates to prevent or stop convulsions. Be very careful not to overdose. Gastric lavage	Protect the patient from all possible sensory stimuli. Oxygen and artificial respiration as needed. Avoid fats, oils, alcohol, and opiates.	Intense CNS excitation.

Poisons and Poisoning (*Continued*)

Toxic Substance	Probable Lethal Dose for Adult Humans (mg./kg. body wt.)*	Symptoms of Poisoning	Emergency Measures	Supportive and Follow-up Treatment	Pathology
		coma; death from respiratory failure.	with tap water.		
Carbon disulfide	500 to 5000 mg.	Irritation of skin, eyes, and mucous membranes; headache; nausea; vomiting; diarrhea; weak pulse; palpitations; fatigue; ataxia; vertigo; mania; hallucinations; CNS depression with respiratory paralysis.	Artificial respiration and oxygen. Lavage with tap water. Mild CNS stimulants.	Convulsions may be controlled by short-acting intravenous barbiturates.	CNS depression sometimes with permanent neurological sequelae.
Carbon monoxide	1.5% concentration in the air causes unconsciousness in a few minutes. Continued exposure will cause death. Young children are more susceptible than adults.	Mild headache; breathlessness on moderate exertion; irritability; fatigue; nausea; vomiting; confusion; ataxia; syncope with periods of convulsions; incontinence of urine and feces; death from respiratory arrest.	Artificial respiration and oxygen. Give 100% oxygen in a pressure chamber if possible. Glucose, 50% solution, I.V. for cerebral edema.	Keep patient warm. Use antibiotics at the first sign of infection. Give whole blood transfusions or washed red blood cells.	High concentrations of carboxyhemoglobin in circulating erythrocytes lead to an asphyxial death.
Carbon tetrachloride	5 to 10 ml. Total dose	Nausea; vomiting; intense abdominal pain; headache; confusion; drowsiness; CNS depression;	If swallowed: Gastric lavage or emetic. If inhaled: Artificial res-	No specific therapy but be prepared to treat renal and hepatic failure.	CNS depression, hepatic central lobular necrosis, necrosis of renal tubu-

		coma; late kidney and/or liver injury with possible acute renal failure. Death from respiratory arrest, circulatory collapse, or ventricular fibrillation.	piration, oxygen, stimulants but avoid alcohol. Remove clothes contaminated with carbon tetrachloride.		lar epithelium.
Chloral hydrate	50 to 500 mg.	Symptoms much like those seen in barbiturate poisoning except that large doses produce vomiting from hemorrhagic gastritis and enteritis. Combinations of chloral hydrate and alcohol (Mickey Finn) are no longer thought to exhibit more than simple additive depression.	SEE: *Barbiturates* in table.	SEE: *Barbiturates* in table.	CNS depression. May sensitize myocardium to endogenous epinephrine.
Chlorate salts or Bromate salts	50 to 500 mg.	Vomiting; diarrhea; abdominal pain; methemoglobinemia; intravascular hemolysis; delirium; coma; convulsions; cyanosis; icterus; death in acute renal failure.	Gastric lavage. Demulcents and meperidine for pain. Oxygen and whole blood transfusions if needed.	Supportive treatment for acute renal failure.	Methemoglobinemia, intravascular hemolysis, acute renal failure.
Chlordane or Heptachlor	50 to 500 mg.	Irritability; hyperexcitability; convulsions and tremors punctuated by periods of depression; late liver damage.	Gastric lavage with tap water, saline cathartic, ether, or ultrashort-acting barbiturates for convulsions.	Oxygen and artificial respiration. Avoid fats, oils, demulcents, and epinephrine.	CNS excitement and severe gastroenteritis have been described.
Chlorpromazine or other Phenothiazines	50 to 500 mg.	Drowsiness; somnolence; stupor; coma; areflexia; hypotension; tachycardia; hypothermia; restlessness; tremor; spasm; rigidity; convulsions; respiratory or vasomotor collapse	Lavage with tap water. Levartenol for severe shock.	Fluids and electrolytes. Oxygen or artificial respiration. Blood transfusion may be required.	CNS depression, extrapyramidal seizures, liver damage.
Cocaine	Variable. From 30 mg. to 1.2 grams (total dose not on body weight basis)	Restlessness, anxiety, hallucinations, convulsions, circulatory collapse.	Administer oxygen. Slow absorption if injected by applying ice to site; gastric lavage if swallowed. Lavage of nasal mucosa if sniffed. Propranolol for convulsions.	Therapy for circulatory collapse.	CNS depression.

Toxic Substance	Probable Lethal Dose for Adult Humans (mg./kg. body wt.)*	Symptoms of Poisoning	Emergency Measures	Supportive and Follow-up Treatment	Pathology
Copper salts, Sulfate	50 to 500 mg.	Prompt emesis; pain in mouth, esophagus, and stomach; diarrhea with abdominal pain; metallic taste; shock; convulsions; paralysis; coma; death.	Gastric lavage, calcium disodium edetate, penicillamine.	Heat, artificial respiration.	Widespread capillary damage, kidney injury, liver damage.
Cyanide (sodium, potassium, hydrogen, etc.)	Less than 5 mg.	Large doses produce immediate death. In smaller doses, an acrid taste is noted preceding numbness in the throat, anxiety, confusion, vertigo, hyperpnea followed by dyspnea, odor of bitter almonds on breath, unconsciousness followed by convulsions and death from respiratory arrest.	Start artificial respiration immediately, keeping airway clear. Give inhalations from amyl nitrite perles every 2–3 minutes for 15–20 seconds. Inject 10 ml. of freshly prepared 3% sodium nitrite I.V. over a 2- to 4-minute period. Do not remove needle. Urgency may necessitate use of nonsterile solutions. Through the same needle give 50 ml. of 25% sodium thiosulfate over a 10-minute period.	If symptoms recur, repeat injections of half doses at hourly intervals. Positive pressure oxygen. Gastric lavage may now be performed with 1:5000 potassium permanganate.	Cyanide combines with enzymes which are essential in transfer of oxygen to the cells. Death is due to tissue anoxia.
DDT	50 to 500 mg.	Vomiting (may be delayed); numbness and tickling of lips, tongue, and face; headache; sore throat; fatigue; tremors; ataxia; confusion; convulsions; coma; death from respiratory failure.	Lavage with tap water and instill saline cathartic. Phenobarbital may be given prophylactically, or parenteral short-acting barbiturates to control convulsions once they have begun. O_2 plus 5% CO_2 inhalation.	Avoid fats, oils, alcohol, epinephrine, sensory stimuli. Calcium gluconate is said to be beneficial in controlling convulsions in addition to barbiturates.	No significant pathological findings in animals except those from convulsions due to CNS excitation.

2,4-Dichlorophenoxyacetic acid (2,4-D)	50 to 500 mg.	Weakness; lethargy; diarrhea; spastic myotonia; ventricular fibrillation and cardiac arrest. Possibly hypermetabolism and hyperpyrexia with convulsions and coma.	Induce emesis or lavage with tap water. Quinidine may be of value for both cardiac symptoms and myotonia.	If fever occurs, treat vigorously with cold packs, alcohol sponges, and other means for promoting heat loss.	Mechanism of death not known; abnormal EEG's have been recorded and severe protracted peripheral neuropathy has occurred.
Dieldrin or Aldrin	5 to 50 mg.	Headache; nausea; vomiting; dizziness; tremors; sudden convulsions alternating with periods of severe CNS depression; death from respiratory arrest.	Lavage with warm water unless convulsions have already begun. Instill saline cathartic. Control convulsions with appropriate barbiturate therapy.	Avoid sensory stimuli. Use oxygen and artificial respiration as needed.	Intense CNS stimulation; mild and transient kidney and liver injury.
Digitalis	50 to 500 mg.	Nausea; salivation; vomiting; headache; fatigue; weakness; drowsiness; confusion; disorientation; delirium; hallucinations; visual disturbances; death from ventricular fibrillation.	Slurry of activated charcoal followed by induced emesis or gastric lavage. Disturbances in cardiac rate and rhythm can be temporarily influenced by appropriate choices from atropine, potassium or salts, quinidine, procainamide, or sodium EDTA.	Nitroglycerin for anginal pain. Preserve water and electrolyte balance.	Produces cardiac arrhythmia and all grades of impaired conduction. Striking lack of human pathological changes in comparison with those seen in experimentally poisoned animals.
2,4 Dinitrophenol	5 to 50 mg.	Fatigue; insatiable thirst; sweating; flushing; nausea; vomiting; abdominal pain; restlessness; excitement; severe hyperpyrexia; tachycardia; hyperpnea; dyspnea; cyanosis; coma; death in respiratory or circulatory collapse.	Lavage with 5% sodium bicarbonate solution and instill saline cathartic. Ice packs, alcohol sponges, or cold water enemas to reduce body temperature.	Appropriate fluid therapy for dehydration or acidosis, mild stimulants, oxygen, artificial respiration.	Tremendously increased BMR through uncoupling of oxidative phosphorylation.
Ergot	5 to 50 mg.	Vomiting; diarrhea; dizziness; weak pulse; thirst; tingling in feet; numbness and coldness of	Slurry of activated charcoal by mouth followed by emesis or lavage.	Keep patient warm and quiet; massage extremities; treat for shock.	Congestion and inflammatory changes in gastrointestinal tract and

Toxic Substance	Probable Lethal Dose for Adult Humans (mg./kg. body wt.)*	Symptoms of Poisoning	Emergency Measures	Supportive and Follow-up Treatment	Pathology
		extremities; variable effects on blood pressure; dyspnea; convulsions; loss of consciousness.	Instill saline cathartic. Atropine sulfate for pain and spasm, 10% solution of calcium gluconate for myalgia. Artificial respiration and oxygen if necessary.		kidneys. Gangrene of fingers and toes from persistent peripheral vasoconstriction.
Ethyl alcohol	Variable: one pint to more than one quart.	Emotional instability and moods depending on personality, circumstances, and surroundings. Impaired motor coordination; slurred speech; ataxia; peripheral vasodilation with flushing, rapid pulse, and sweating; nausea and vomiting; drowsiness; stupor and coma; peripheral vascular collapse; hypotension; tachycardia; hypothermia; death from respiratory or circulatory failure.	Lavage with tap water or 3% sodium bicarbonate, mild stimulants, oxygen and artificial respiration.	Intravenous saline or lactate for circulatory collapse, dehydration, or acidosis. Mild external heat. Avoid aspiration of vomitus. Hypertonic glucose or urea for cerebral edema. Watch for hypoglycemia in young children.	Irregularly descending CNS depression leading to respiratory or circulatory failure.
Ethylene glycol	Less than 5 mg.	Transient excitement; nausea; vomiting; abdominal cramps; weakness; muscle cramps; ataxia; vertigo; stupor; coma; death from respiratory paralysis or delayed acute renal failure with uremia.	Gastric lavage with 1:5000 potassium permanganate. Calcium gluconate, 10% I.V. Mild stimulants, oxygen and artificial respiration. Immediate use of artificial kidney.	Supportive measures for acute renal failure.	CNS depression and hydropic degeneration of renal tubular epithelium.
Ferrous or Ferric	500 to 5000	Severe gastroenteritis; abdominal	Milk by mouth and in-	Intravenous fluids for dehydration and	Shock secondary to local

salts	mg.	pain; vomiting and diarrhea which eventually becomes bloody; dehydration; pallor; cyanosis; shock leading to death in 3 to 4 hours.	duce vomiting if not already spontaneous. Gastric lavage with 5% sodium bicarbonate. The specific antidote deferoxamine should be given orally and intravenously in appropriate dose.	whole blood or plasma for shock.	tissue damage, mild hepatic cirrhosis and pyloric stenosis.
Fluoride (salts, sodium)	50 to 500 mg.	Peculiar taste with salivation and thirst; nausea; abdominal pain, vomiting, diarrhea; muscle weakness; tremors; central depression; death in shock.	Give 10 ml. of 10% calcium gluconate I.V. Repeat at signs of tetany. Start drip of glucose in saline. Lavage with solution of lime water or calcium chloride, leaving some solution in the stomach.	Treat shock vigorously by keeping up blood volume and giving norepinephrine. Calcium gluconate I.M. to establish depots.	Hemorrhagic gastroenteritis, inhibition of cellular glycolysis, hypocalcemia.
Fluoroacetate (salts, sodium)	Less than 5 mg.	Vomiting; paresthesias of face; CNS excitation progressing to convulsions, punctuated by periods of severe CNS depression; disturbances in heartbeat; ventricular fibrillation; death.	Induced vomiting or lavage. Leave 15–30 gm. sodium or magnesium sulfate in stomach. Most effective antidote appears to be monoacetin (sodium glycerol monoacetate) which is not available in pharmaceutical form. Regardless of sterility, inject this material in doses of 0.5 ml./kg. I.M. every half hour, or dilute 1–5 with sterile saline for I.V. use.	Oxygen, artificial respiration, short-acting barbiturates for convulsions.	Cardiac disturbances leading to fatal ventricular fibrillation.
Formaldehyde	500 to 5000 mg.	Pain in epigastrium; nausea; vomiting; anxiety; weak and rapid pulse; coma; collapse; death in respiratory failure.	Give 30 ml. ammonium acetate solution, 15 ml. of aromatic spirits of ammonia, or 10 to 20	Treat for shock; morphine for pain; antibiotics at the first signs of infection; sodium bicarbonate or lactate for acidosis.	Inflammation and ulceration of gastrointestinal tract, acidosis, kidney damage, circulatory

Poisons and Poisoning (*Continued*)

Toxic Substance	Probable Lethal Dose for Adult Humans (mg./kg. body wt.)*	Symptoms of Poisoning	Emergency Measures	Supportive and Follow-up Treatment	Pathology
			drops of household ammonia diluted with water.		collapse.
Hydrogen sulfide or Alkaline salts	Highly toxic. 0.1 to 0.2% in air usually fatal.	Sudden collapse and unconsciousness in acute poisoning with death from respiratory paralysis. Subacutely, gas is an irritant to eyes, respiratory tract, and skin.	Terminate exposure immediately; artificial respiration; oxygen with 5% CO_2; mild stimulants.	Antibiotics at first signs of infection.	No significant pathological changes except in chronic poisoning in which pulmonary edema may be seen.
Hypochlorite salts or solutions (liquid household bleach)	Variable. Several ounces of usual household bleach (4–6% available chlorine)	Pain and inflammation of mouth, pharynx, esophagus, and stomach; coffee-ground vomitus; circulatory collapse; confusion; delirium; coma; edema of glottis. All systemic symptoms are secondary to local injury and shock.	Milk, egg whites, starch paste, or milk of magnesia. Lavage with tap water or 2% sodium thiosulfate. Morphine for pain.	Treat shock with intravenous fluids. Tracheotomy or gastrectomy may be indicated.	Edema of pharynx, glottis, or larynx. Perforation of stomach or esophagus. Fumes may produce pulmonary edema.
Iodine	5 to 50 mg.	Burning pain in mouth, throat, and stomach; lips and mouth are stained brown; thirst; vomiting (blue vomitus if stomach contained starches); bloody diarrhea; anuria or strangury, urine containing albumin or blood. Death from circulatory collapse, asphyxia from glottic edema or aspiration pneumonia.	Immediately give orally cornstarch or flour solution, 15 gm. in 500 ml. (2 cups) water. Lavage with starch solution or 2% sodium thiosulfate. Morphine for pain and mild stimulants as indicated. Epinephrine, diphenhydramine (Benadryl) or hydrocortisone for ananaphylaxis.	Give fluids and electrolytes, supportive therapy for circulatory collapse, antibiotics for secondary infections, prepare for emergency tracheotomy.	Irritation and swelling within throat (glottic edema), esophagus, and stomach. Shock secondary to fluid and electrolyte loss. More rarely, late esophageal stenosis.

Ipecac syrup or fluid-extract	Variable. 1 to 2 ounces of fluid-extract (14 times more concentrated than the syrup).	Nausea; vomiting; diarrhea; albuminuria; abdominal cramps; bloody vomitus and feces; dehydration; myocarditis; myocardial infarction; cardiac arrest or shock secondary to cardiac depression and fluid loss.	Lavage or induce emesis if spontaneous vomiting has not occurred. Do not give additional emetic agents. Saline cathartic if purging has not occurred. Once toxin has been removed vomiting may respond to intravenous chlorpromazine.	General supportive and symptomatic measures for impending shock.	Intractable vomiting and diarrhea due to intense irritation of entire gastrointestinal tract leading to shock. Direct, specific cardiac damage.
Isopropyl alcohol	500 to 5000 mg.	Dizziness, incoordination, headache, confusion, stupor, and coma. Symptoms closely resemble ethyl alcohol intoxication. Death from circulatory collapse or respiratory failure.	Lavage with tap water; oxygen and artificial respiration; mild stimulants.	Intravenous glucose and saline. Anticipate liver or kidney injury.	Acetonuria without glycosuria is pathognomonic. Severe CNS depression. Aspiration pneumonitis.
Kerosene (Coal Oil)	500 to 5000 mg. if retained in stomach. If aspirated, a few ml. can be lethal.	Burning sensation in mouth, throat, and stomach; nausea with vomiting and diarrhea; drowsiness; restlessness; disorientation; coma. Signs of pulmonary involvement indicate grave prognosis of impending fulminating hemorrhagic bronchopneumonia.	If risks of lavage are undertaken, an endotracheal tube with inflatable cuff should be employed. Dilute sodium bicarbonate is satisfactory lavage fluid; follow with the instillation of olive oil and saline cathartic.	Antibiotics for secondary infection and positive pressure oxygen. Corticosteroids for pulmonary edema.	Severe chemical pneumonitis.
Lead or its salts	0.5 grams of absorbed lead. (Chronic poisoning is much more common than acute.)	Metallic taste in mouth; burning pain in stomach and abdomen; constipation followed by diarrhea; convulsions; muscular weakness; paralysis of extremities; skin cold and cyanotic; delayed severe anemia; death is due to peripheral vascular collapse or encephalopathy.	Gastric lavage with magnesium or sodium sulfate. Analgesics for pain. Diazepam I.V. for convulsions. Intravenous calcium disodium edetate in accordance with supplier's directions. Dimercaprol is also used.	Keep patient quiet. Maintain fluid and electrolyte balance. Long-term therapy (1 to 2 months for adults and 3 to 6 months for children) with penicillamine to decrease the blood lead level to 60 mg/dl.	Gastrointestinal inflammation, liver and kidney injury when sufficient lead has been absorbed. Encephalopathy is frequent in children.

Toxic Substance	Probable Lethal Dose for Adult Humans (mg./kg. body wt.)*	Symptoms of Poisoning	Emergency Measures	Supportive and Follow-up Treatment	Pathology
Lye, Sodium and Potassium hydroxides and Carbonates	Total dose of 10 gm. may be fatal.	Severe pain in mouth and difficulty in swallowing; gastrointestinal pain and purging; weak and rapid pulse; death in shock or asphyxia from glottic edema.	Large amounts of water by mouth; diluted vinegar or lemon juice; avoid emetics and lavage. Olive oil by mouth or milk and egg whites. Mild stimulants to prevent shock. Tracheotomy may be required.	Morphine for pain; fluids and electrolytes; cortisone. Use of bougies to prevent esophageal stricture. Broad-spectrum antibiotics.	Laryngeal or glottic edema; corrosion and possible perforation of upper gastrointestinal tract; late esophageal stenosis.
Meprobamate, Equanil, or Miltown	500 to 5000 mg.	Drowsiness; relaxation; stupor; sleep; coma; areflexia; muscular flaccidity; severe and persistent hypotension.	Lavage or induce emesis; plasma or pressor agents for hypotension; mild stimulants. Artificial respiration and oxygen.	Symptomatic and supportive care with frequent recording of vital signs.	No significant pathological changes in tissues.
Mercuric chloride or other soluble salts	5 to 50 mg.	Metallic taste and burning in mouth and throat; abdominal pain and cramps with nausea and vomiting; diarrhea and bloody stools; scanty urine containing albumin; collapse in shock with weak, rapid pulse, slow and shallow respirations, and cold and clammy skin. If patient survives acute episode, he may die in renal failure after several days. Chronic mercury poisoning is also common with primarily neurological symptoms.	Egg white, milk, or flour by mouth. Lavage with 3% sodium formaldehyde sulfoxylate; if unavailable, 2–5% sodium bicarbonate solution should be used. Dimercaprol (BAL) I.M. in accordance with supplier's directions. Penicillamine.	Saline cathartic if purging has not already occurred. Demulcents and analgetics. Treat for shock. Prepare for management of acute renal failure.	Ulceration of gums and mouth, loosening of teeth, progressive peripheral neuritis are all seen in chronic poisonings or cases in which death is delayed. In acute cases, usual cause of death due to peripheral vascular collapse secondary to fluid or electrolyte loss, or acute renal failure.

Methyl alcohol	500 to 5000 mg.	Exhilaration accompanied by headache, muscular weakness, nausea, vomiting, and abdominal pain; delirium with visual disturbances which may progress to blindness; weak and rapid pulse; rapid and shallow respirations; cyanosis; coma; death from respiratory failure.	Gastric lavage with 5% sodium bicarbonate, leaving some solution in the stomach. Inject 3% sodium bicarbonate I.V. at the rate of 1000 ml./hour but do not continue after acidosis is corrected. To prevent formation of formic acid, give 10 ml. of ethyl alcohol orally. If poisoning is severe, give ethyl alcohol I.V. in 5% solution in bicarbonate or saline.	Bedrest, treat for shock; mild external heat, stimulants as indicated, protect patient's eyes from light. Oxygen.	Intense metabolic acidosis. Partial to complete blindness due to atrophy of the ganglion cells of the retina if patient survives.
Morphine	5 to 50 mg.	Gross overdosages produce prompt depression, but smaller doses may cause transient period of excitement before drowsiness. Weariness; loss of pain sensation; nausea; vomiting; pinpoint pupils; coma with muscular relaxation and slowing of respiratory rate; cyanosis; slow pulse; fall in blood pressure; death in respiratory arrest.	Gastric lavage, even if several hours after ingestion, with 1:10,000 potassium permanganate; saline cathartic left in stomach. Nalorphine is specific antagonist given I.V. in doses of 5–10 mg. Artificial respiration. Inhalation of oxygen with 5% CO_2.	Keep patient awake with mild stimulation. Correct airway obstruction. Maintain fluid and electrolyte balance. Keep patient warm.	Pulmonary congestion. Death is from respiratory failure due to central depression, but circulatory insufficiency may be contributory.
Muscaria mushrooms	Unknown. The ingestion of two or three of Amanita phalloides type may be fatal.	Violent vomiting; diarrhea; apprehension; miosis; severe abdominal pain; irregular and slow pulse; slow and labored respirations; delirium; late stupor; death from cardiac arrest or circulatory collapse.	Slurry of activated charcoal orally. Lavage or induce emesis if not spontaneous. Saline cathartic. Atropine is specific antagonist if the mushrooms contained muscarine. Artificial respiration. Call nearest Poison Control Center for availability of thioctic acid and advisability of using this drug.	Stimulate as indicated; external heat; oxygen inhalations; meperidine for pain; correct shock, electrolyte imbalance, and dehydration by cautious fluid therapy.	Symptoms mimic intense parasympathetic stimulation. Severe hepatic, renal, and central nervous system damage.

Toxic Substance	Probable Lethal Dose for Adult Humans (mg./kg. body wt.)*	Symptoms of Poisoning	Emergency Measures	Supportive and Follow-up Treatment	Pathology
			It is indicated if patient has ingested species containing Amanitin.		
Naphthalene (moth balls)	5 to 15 gm.	Abdominal pain; nausea; vomiting; diarrhea; headache; diaphoresis; coma with or without convulsions. Certain individuals exhibit intense intravascular hemolysis accompanied by anemia, hematuria, and renal insufficiency.	Induce emesis or lavage with tap water, saline cathartic, demulcents, and mild stimulants. Sodium bicarbonate every 4 hours to maintain alkaline urine in order to prevent renal blockage with acid hematin crystals.	Anemia from hemolysis may require whole blood transfusions. Supportive measures for acute renal failure. Avoid use of milk, oils, or fatty foods.	Various states of central excitement or depression. Rarely, liver necrosis. Acute hemolytic anemia.
Nicotine	Less than 5 mg.	Burning sensation in mouth and throat; salivation; vomiting; diarrhea; headache; sweating; dizziness; weakness; pupils contracted at first then dilated; pulse slow at first then rapid; respirations deep and rapid at first then dyspneic; death from paralysis of respiratory musculature.	Slurry of activated charcoal as lavage fluid with additional portion left in stomach. Artificial respiration and oxygen.	Control convulsions with small doses of intravenous barbiturates. Relief for visceral symptoms is obtained with atropine or phenoxybenzamine (Dibenzyline).	Transient stimulation then depression of CNS, all autonomic ganglia and nerve endings in skeletal muscle.
Nitroglycerin	Less than 5 mg.	Prompt fall in blood pressure; intense throbbing in head; dizziness; faintness; excessive muscular relaxation; tremors; nausea; vomiting; skin flushed then cold and cyanotic; postural hypotension; paralysis; anoxic convulsions; death.	Gastric lavage or administer emetic. Mild stimulants as indicated. Oxygen and artificial respiration.	Keep patient in reclining position and comfortably warm. Transfusions, if needed, with whole blood or plasma.	Anoxia due to methemoglobinemia aggravated by stagnation of blood in capillaries, venules, and veins from peripheral vasodilatation.

Nitrous fumes nitric oxide, nitrogen dioxide, sulfur dioxide, phosgene	Unknown	Only very high concentrations produce immediate pulmonary symptoms. After day or two, fatigue, restlessness, cough and other signs of developing pulmonary edema; increasing difficulty in breathing; cyanosis; coughing with frothy expectoration; lethargy; coma; circulatory collapse; death in asphyxia.	Enforce complete bedrest; positive pressure oxygen as needed. Antibiotics and corticosteroids as indicated. Small doses of morphine.	Remove frothy exudates by suctioning. Good nursing care essential.	Asphyxial death due to blockage of gas exchange in lungs.
Oxalic acid and Oxalate salts	50 to 500 mg.	Severe gastrointestinal irritation and intense pain in upper gastrointestinal tract; vomiting and intense thirst; pulse weak and thready; skin cold and cyanotic; twitching of facial musculature; convulsions; coma; collapse; death.	Immediately give large amounts of calcium lactate, lime water, magnesia, or chalk orally, or lavage cautiously with any of these. Calcium gluconate or chloride I.V.	Keep patient quiet and in recumbent position. Morphine for pain; demulcents.	Severe gastroenteritis and secondary shock, hypocalcemia and kidney injury.
Parathion, and other Organophosphorus insecticides	Less than 5 mg.	Nausea; vomiting; diarrhea; abdominal cramps; salivation; headache; vertigo; runny nose; pinpoint pupils; generalized and profound muscular weakness; confusion; jerky movements; convulsions; coma; death in respiratory failure.	Give atropine 1 to 4 mg. I.V. immediately and repeat every 3–8 minutes until parasympathetic symptoms are controlled. Give oxygen and artificial respiration. If available, valuable adjunct is 2-PAM (pyridine aldoxime methiodide) in accordance with manufacturer's directions.	Endotracheal intubation or tracheotomy may be necessary. Artificial respiration and oxygen. Keep patient under constant observation.	All signs and symptoms are referable to the inhibition of the enzyme, acetylcholinesterase, and consequent accumulation of acetylcholine at all nervous junctions where it is the chemical mediator.
Phenol	50 to 500 mg.	Corrosive burns in mouth, esophagus, and stomach; abdominal pain; bloody diarrhea; pallor; sweating; weakness; headache; dizziness; ringing in ears; shock with weak pulse; fall in blood pressure and body temperature; shallow respiration; cyanosis;	NOTE: If stomach wall is severely corroded, passage of a tube into it may cause rupture. Cautious lavage with castor or olive oil. Avoid mineral oils and alcohol. As needed	Moderate external heat. Treat shock conservatively and watch for signs of renal insufficiency. Systemic acidosis may require therapy with bicarbonate.	Corrosive burns of skin and mucous membranes; gastric perforation. More rarely, esophageal stricture and kidney shutdown.

Poisons and Poisoning (*Continued*)

Toxic Substance	Probable Lethal Dose for Adult Humans (mg./kg. body wt.)*	Symptoms of Poisoning	Emergency Measures	Supportive and Follow-up Treatment	Pathology
		coma; death from respiratory failure. Skin contact produces pain followed by numbness and corrosive burn.	demulcents, morphine, mild respiratory stimulants. Wash skin areas with 10% ethyl alcohol or castor oil.		
Phosphorus	Less than 5 mg.	Skin contact produces painful penetrating burns. Ingestion leads to burning pain in throat or abdomen with intense thirst followed by nausea, vomiting, diarrhea, odor of garlic on breath, luminescent vomitus and feces. Patient often appears to recover for several days, then suddenly relapses with severe liver, kidney, and cardiac damage.	Repeated washing of the stomach with 1% copper sulfate followed by 1:10,000 potassium permanganate. Leave mineral oil in stomach. Give morphine for pain, and vitamin K.	Intravenous saline and lactate for shock, dehydration, and acidosis. Supportive therapy for delirium, hepatic insufficiency, and renal failure. For several days avoid fats and oils in the diet because they promote absorption of phosphorus.	Fatty degeneration of liver, kidneys, and heart.
Quaternary ammonium germicides	50 to 500 mg.	Burning pain in mouth and throat; restlessness; confusion; muscle weakness; CNS depression; labored breathing; cyanosis; asphyxial death.	Large quantities of milk or egg whites make good lavage fluids. No specific antidotes or antagonists are known.	Artificial respiration and oxygen if necessary. If convulsions are persistent (rare), give intravenous short-acting barbiturates.	Nonspecific irritation, visceral congestion, cloudy swelling, mild pulmonary edema.
Rotenone	50 to 500 mg.	Sensation of numbness in mouth; nausea; vomiting; gastrointestinal pain; tremors; convulsions; stupor; respiratory stimulation followed by depression; death from respiratory arrest.	Slurry of activated charcoal by mouth; induce vomiting or lavage with tap water, saline cathartic. Avoid fats and oils.	Support respiration, oxygen, mild sedation (avoid barbiturates), fluids. Glucose may be needed for hypoglycemia.	Severe hypoglycemia may be seen; otherwise the pathological changes largely unknown.

Salicylate (sodium, methyl, acetylsalicylic acid, aspirin)	50 to 500 mg.	Stimulation of the CNS including the respiratory center. The resulting hyperpnea leads to CO_2 loss. Respiratory alkalosis, hyperthermia, convulsions and shock, hypokalemia, and dehydration.	Gastric lavage with several liters of warm tap water with activated charcoal added.	The patient may be in acidosis or alkalosis; thus determine acid-base status and treat accordingly. Dehydration requires vigorous therapy.	Disturbed acid-base balance. Children often exhibit metabolic acidosis while adults more commonly show respiratory alkalosis. Intense CNS stimulation followed by depression.
Silver salts, Nitrate, and other soluble salts	3.5 to 35 gm. total dose.	Intense pain in mouth, throat, and gastrointestinal tract; bloody stools; vertigo; coma; convulsions; death.	Gastric lavage with several liters of warm tap water with activated charcoal added. Saline cathartic. Treat shock.	Eggs and milk as demulcents, morphine for pain, stimulants as indicated; treat for shock; maintain fluid and electrolyte balance.	Severe corrosion of gastrointestinal tract. Deposits of metallic silver occur under skin in chronic posioning, but these are of minor cosmetic concern.
Strychnine	Less than 5 mg.	Apprehension; stiffness of muscles; twitching of face and arms; sudden tetanic convulsions of entire body; cyanosis of face and lips; pulse slow and strong; death in 1–3 hours with face fixed in a grin and body arched in hyperextension.	Slurry of activated charcoal by mouth or gastric lavage with dilute permanganate or iodine. Such procedures, however, are usually delayed until convulsions are controlled with chloroform, ether, or I.V. barbiturates. NOTE: Do not give morphine.	Place patient in a quiet, dark room. Avoid drafts. Artificial respiration may be needed. Constant nursing care.	Stimulation of spinal cord leading to contraction of respiratory musculature and death from anoxia.
Thallium and salts, sulfate	5 to 50 mg.	Severe abdominal pain; vomiting; diarrhea; tremors; delirium; convulsions; paralysis; coma; death. Loss of hair is peculiar to chronic poisoning or in cases of delayed death.	Induce emesis or lavage with 1% sodium or potassium iodide. Leave activated charcoal in stomach. Give saline cathartic and demulcents. Dimercaprol (BAL) in accordance with supplier's directions.	Treat for shock; maintain fluid and electrolyte balance; calcium salts or milk; symptomatic and supportive therapy for CNS disorders. Antibiotics for pneumonia.	Hemorrhagic gastroenteritis and encephalopathy.
Thiram or Disul-	50 to 500	Nausea; vomiting; diarrhea;	Lavage with tap water.	Symptomatic and supportive care for	Hyperemia, ulceration of

Toxic Substance	Probable Lethal Dose for Adult Humans (mg./kg. body wt.)*	Symptoms of Poisoning	Emergency Measures	Supportive and Follow-up Treatment	Pathology
firam	mg.	ataxia; hyperexcitability; hypothermia; flaccid paralysis. If patient has also ingested ethyl alcohol in even trivial amounts, symptoms are quite different and include flushing, fall in blood pressure, palpitations, sweating, vertigo, confusion, circulatory collapse, coma, and death.	Strictly prohibit alcohol in all forms. Also avoid fats, oils, and oil solvents. Artificial respiration and oxygen.	gastrointestinal symptoms and neurological complications. In case complicated by alcohol, parenteral glucose, ascorbic acid, ephedrine, and diphenhydramine may be beneficial. Wash skin if contaminated and remove clothing.	gastrointestinal tract, renal and hepatic necrosis, demyelinization of cerebellum and medulla.
Turpentine	500 mg. to 5 gm.	Sensation of warmth or pain in mouth, throat, and stomach followed by abdominal pain, vomiting and diarrhea. Aspiration into lungs may cause pneumonitis. Excitement, ataxia, delirium, and stupor, followed by convulsions, coma, and death from respiratory failure.	Gastric lavage with weak bicarbonate solution, followed by demulcents and saline cathartic.	Morphine sulfate for intense pain and a short-acting barbiturate for excitement. Mild stimulation if indicated, e.g., caffeine sodium benzoate. Force fluids.	Irritation of kidneys; hematuria, albuminuria, and sometimes complete urinary suppression. Kidney symptoms appear to be related to composition of the turpentine, and often never appear.
Warfarin	50 to 500 mg.	After few days of repeated ingestions: nosebleed; bleeding gums; pallor; hemorrhagic areas in skin, especially knees and buttocks; blood in urine or feces; death in hemorrhagic shock.	Gastric lavage with tap water in case of large single dose. Vitamin K is specific antidote and should be given until prothrombin levels return to normal. Whole blood transfusions may be necessary.	Replacement iron as ferrous sulfate.	Capillary dilatation and increased fragility with hypoprothrombinemia leading to internal hemorrhage.
Zinc salts, (chloride, sulfate, ac-	50 to 500 mg.	Increased salivation; violent vomiting and purging, followed by	Lavage with milk or lime water. Follow with egg	Recumbent position, external heat to body, morphine for pain; treat for	Stricture of esophagus, pylorus, and destruc-

etate, etc.)	prostration.	white and other demulcents. Morphine for pain.	shock; maintain fluid and electrolyte balances.	tion of glandular structure of stomach. Ulceration and/or perforation of the stomach.

* Most of these values from Gleason, M. N., Gosselin, R. E., Hodge, H. C., and Smith, R. P.: Clinical Toxicology of Commercial Products, ed. 3. The Williams & Wilkins Co., Baltimore, 1969.

Dose Equivalent Expressed in Household Measures*

mg./kg.		mg./kg.	
Less than 5	A taste; less than 7 drops	500 to 5000 (5 gm.)	Between one ounce and one pint
5 to 50	Between 7 drops and one teaspoon	5000 to 15,000 (5 to 15 gm.)	Between one pint and one quart
50 to 500	Between one teaspoon and one ounce	Greater than 15,000 mg. (15 gm.)	Greater than one quart

* From Gleason, M. N., Gosselin, R. E., Hodge, H. C., and Smith, R. P.: Clinical Toxicology of Commercial Products, ed. 3. The Williams & Wilkins Co., Baltimore, 1969.

Toxic Emergencies Produced By Abused Substances

	CNS excitation-confusion	CNS depression	Vital signs*	Withdrawal reaction
CNS STIMULANTS				
amphetamines	irritability, confusion, agitation, delirium, paranoia; sympathomimetic effects prominent	exhaustion or collapse only from prolonged excitation	↑	"crashes" after long excitation, otherwise mild depression
methylphenidate and phenmetrazine	stimulation, possibly convulsions		↑	no specific syndrome
strychnine	spinal convulsions, rigidity, trismus, hyperacusis	postictal or exhaustion	↑ (↓)	none
cocaine	excitement, emotional instability to convulsions, sympathomimetic effects	muscle paralysis, coma, CV or respiratory failure	↑ (↓)	none
HALLUCINOGENS				
substituted indoles		coma with high overdose	↑ or ↓	none
LSD harmines ibogaine DMT (bufotenine), DET, DPT†	anxiety, panic, hallucinations; rare convulsions or catatonia			
morning glory derivatives	mild LSD-like			
psilocybin psilocyn	LSD-like plus fever and convulsions; rarely in children with high doses			
mescaline (peyote)	LSD-like, plus nausea, vomiting, sweating		↑	none

Ditran and analogs	resembles anticholinergics			none
psychotomimetic amphetamines‡ DOM (STP), DOET, DOP MDA, myristicin (nutmeg), PMA	similar to LSD and amphetamines (hallucinogenic with strong sympathomimetic effects); panic reactions greater than with LSD	coma with high overdose	↑	none
phencyclidine (PCP), derivatives, ketamine	convulsions in most severe (early) excitation, hallucinations, rigidity, paranoia at lower than depressant doses, hyperacusis	coma followed by excitation and confusion, rarely respiratory depression	↑ (↓)	none
cannabis (marijuana, THC, hashish)	perceptual and body image distortions, rarely hallucinations	mild hypotension occasionally		none
anticholinergics datura belladonnas antihistamines (nonbarbiturate sedatives)	disorientation, hallucinations, excitement, sympathomimetic effects; fixed, dilated pupils pathognomonic	coma with extreme doses, collapse after prolonged excitation	↑ (↓)	none
methysergide amantadine	probably LSD-like			none
INHALANTS				
solvents	delirium, psychosis, hallucinations, rarely sudden death	coma, cardiorespiratory arrest with extreme exposure, suffocation not uncommon	↑ or ↓	none
vasodilator-hypoxic agents, amyl and butyl nitrite	drunken sensorium, disorientation, headache	coma, hypotension, methemoglobinemia, coronary insufficiency on exertion	↓ (resp. ↑)	none

Toxic Emergencies Produced By Abused Substance *(continued)*

	CNS excitation-confusion	CNS depression	Vital signs*	Withdrawal reaction
OPIATES AND OPIOIDS				
morphine, codeine, heroin, and derivatives meperidine, methadone, propoxyphene	convulsions rarely, especially with codeine, propoxyphene, meperidine; otherwise confusional state most likely a sign of withdrawal; pinpoint pupils (except terminally) with all except meperidine	coma, respiratory depression, hypothermia, CV collapse	↓	restlessness, nausea, vomiting, diarrhea, muscle aches and spasms, weakness, chills, gooseflesh, yawning, accentuated vital signs
pentazocine	like other opiates, plus delirium			may precipitate withdrawal from another opioid
SEDATIVE-HYPNOTICS				
barbiturates meprobamate glutethimide methyprylon	some confusional manifestations from depressant effect; no excitatory state	CNS depression to coma, hypotension, respiratory depression, hyporeflexia, CV collapse or respiratory failure	↓	tremulousness, insomnia, fever, agitation, delirium, psychosis; seizures not uncommon; death is possible
benzodiazepines	same as barbiturates	rarely, severe depression with cardiorespiratory insufficiency	(↓)	anxiety, restlessness, rarely convulsions
chloral hydrate	resembles barbiturate poisoning	resembles barbiturate poisoning	↓	resembles mild DT's
alcohol	inebriation, inhibition loss, disorientation	coma, hypotension, hypothermia, respiratory or circulatory failure	↓	delirium tremens, hallucinations, possible convulsions

methaqualone	from muscle spasticity and hyperactivity to convulsions; hyperacusis, vomiting, bronchial hypersecretions	coma, respiratory failure, rarely delayed CV collapse		headache, cramps, anorexia, nausea, rarely convulsions; not fatal

*Vital signs ↑ = accentuated; ↓ = decreased; sign in parenthesis is less common, usually seen only in especially severe cases or as a postexcitatory depressive effect.
†dimethyltryptamine, diethyltryptamine, dipropyltryptamine
‡DOM = dimethoxymethylamphetamine (or STP = serenity, tranquility, and peace); DOET = dimethoxygethylamphetamine; DOP = dimethoxypropylamphetamine; MDA = methylenedioxyamphetamine; PMA = paramethoxyamphetamine
From Emergency Medicine: March 15, 1980, with permission. Prepared by Alan K. Done, M.D.

Generally Nontoxic Substances*

Ball-point inks (amt. in 1 pen)
Barium sulfate
Bathtub toys (floating)
Blackboard chalk (calcium carbonate)
Candles (insect-repellent type may be toxic)
Carbowax (polyethylene glycol)
Carboxymethylcellulose (dehydrating material packed with drugs, film, etc.)
Castor oil
Cetyl alcohol
Crayons (children's; marked A.P., C.P., or C.S. 130–46)
Detergents, anionic and nonionic
Dichloral (herbicide)
Dry cell battery
Glycerol
Glyceryl monostearate
Graphite
Gums (acacia, agar, ghatti, etc.)
Hormones
Kaolin
Lanolin
Lauric acid
Linoleic acid
Linseed oil (not boiled)
Lipstick
Magnesium silicate (antacid)
Matches
Methylcellulose
Modeling clay
Paraffin, chlorinated
Pencil lead (graphite)
Pepper, black (except inhaled in mass)
Petrolatum
Polyethylene glycols
Polyethylene glycol stearate
Polysorbate (Tweens®)
Putty
Red oil (turkey-red oil, sulfated castor oil)
Silica (silicon dioxide)
Spermaceti
Stearic acid
Sweetening agents
Talc
Tallow
Thermometer fluid or mercury
Titanium oxide
Triacetin (glyceryl triacetate)
Vitamins, multiple without iron

Substances listed here may, however, be present in combination with phenol, petroleum distillate vehicles, or other toxic chemicals. Since manufactured products may be changed in their composition, this table is intended only as a guide, and prudence requires that a poison center be consulted for up-to-date information.
*Reprinted with permission from The Merck Manual, Edition 14, Merck Sharp & Dohme, 1982.

Suffocation, Asphyxiation, Drowning

Type	History	Pathology	Symptoms and Color	Pulse	Breathing	Muscles	Pupils	Complications	Treatment
Choking	Edema of larynx; diseases of larynx. Foreign bodies aspirated into the larynx.	Trauma of larynx.	Patient in a state of apprehension. Color is cyanotic.	Rapid due to exertion.	Respirations are very rapid or patient may gasp occasionally.	May be voluntarily contracted.	Dilated.	Pneumonia; sinusitis; complete obstruction of the bronchi; lung abscess.	Manual removal of foreign object or encourage coughing by slap on back. Tracheotomy may be required.
Drowning	Body discovered in water.	Waterlogging of lungs and asphyxia.	Patient is unconscious. Color is gray and changing to blue (cyanosis).	If perceptible, it is rapid and may be shallow.	If respirations are present, the patient may gasp occasionally or very irregularly.	Muscles are relaxed and body is very limp.	May be dilated.	Fracture of neck; heart failure; suffocation, shock, and collapse.	Artificial respiration (mouth to mouth); external cardiac massage if needed; oxygen; treat for shock; heart stimulants.
Gas Poisoning	Victim rescued from room with escaping gas from open jet or victim overcome in closed garage.	Changes in the blood chemistry and then anemia. Respiratory paralysis which leads to death.	Patient unconscious. Color typical cherry red, or pallor and cyanosis, carbon monoxide in poisoning.	Rapid; may be irregular.	Respirations are usually slow but may be rapid and shallow very early after the exposure to gas.	Muscles are relaxed and body is limp.	Varies with the type of gas poisoning.	Respiratory failure; depletion of O_2 supply in the blood.	Artificial respiration; oxygen; shock treatment.
Strangulation and Hanging	Patient found during or after the act. Very definite signs of violence.	Fracture of cervical vertebrae; suffocation; trauma of medulla by odontoid process of axis.	If living, may be unconscious or in a state of excitement or desperation. Cyanotic if death occurred sometime previous to discovery.	May be perceptible or absent.	No respirations, or respirations are very rapid, or patient may gasp occasionally.	May be voluntarily contracted.	Dilated. Unequal if there is cerebral injury.	Fracture of neck; suffocation; contusions on neck.	Release pull of rope by placing chair under patient's feet and cutting rope. Oxygen therapy; artificial respiration; treat for shock; treat fractures.

Unconsciousness

Type	History	Skin and Color	Pupils	Muscles	Pulse	Breathing	Reflexes	Complications	Treatment
Acid and Alkali Poisoning	Accidental or intentional poisoning.	Clammy skin. Skin pale; face cyanotic.	Dilated. Eyes sunken, staring.	Tense. Patient in convulsion.	Rapid, feeble pulse.	Shallow, rapid, labored, irregular.	Increased.	Corrosion of mucous membranes; ulcers of stomach; gastritis; jaundice.	Acids: Milk of magnesia, egg albumin, lime water, no chalk or alkaline carbonate. Alkalies: Neutralize with acetic acid (vinegar). In both cases careful gastric lavage.
Bleeding	Trauma causing bright red spurting or welling bleeding. Bleeding after an operation.	Skin shows pallor which progresses to a yellow or greenish tinge.	Dilated.	Relaxed.	Rapid, becoming thready.	Respirations are rapid and shallow. Air hunger is evident.	Diminished.	Shock; anemia; heart failure; death.	Digital pressure and tourniquet; pad in joint. Keep patient quiet; treat for shock; transfusion if necessary.
Concussion	Head injury caused by fall or blow upon the head.	Skin pale, cold, and clammy. Varies with degree of pathology.	Dilated. Varies with degree and area of injury.	May be spastic.	Pulse rate usually shows a slight increase. May be weak and rapid.	Respirations are usually deep.	Deep tendon reflexes may be increased.	Shock in severe cases; paralysis of limbs may occur.	Bedrest; keep patient flat and warm.
Drowning	Victim is found unconscious in body of water. May have a fractured neck or skull.	Skin is cold, clammy, and cyanotic.	Dilated.	Relaxed if victim is living. Rigor mortis if dead.	If perceptible, it is rapid and weak, or very irregular.	No respirations. Occasional gasp if living.	None.	Heart failure; shock; pneumonia; aspiration of foreign material.	Resuscitation (Mouth-to-mouth is most effective method if a manual positive pressure type of device is not available). Keep body warm but not hot. Stimulating drinks when conscious.

Unconsciousness (*Continued*)

Type	History	Skin and Color	Pupils	Muscles	Pulse	Breathing	Reflexes	Complications	Treatment
Drunkenness	Victim is unable to cope with the amount of intoxicants taken.	Color varies. Face may be flushed; skin is moist, relaxed, and cool.	Usually dilated but equal.	Relaxed. Body and limbs are limp.	Strong and slow.	Respirations are slow, deep, stertorous, accompanied by characteristic "lip blowing" and Cheyne-Stokes type of breathing.	Involuntary reflexes usually increased.	Pneumonia.	Keep the body warm. If conscious give emetic. Gastric lavage. Give hot coffee or aromatic spirits of ammonia.
Electric Shock	Victim is found after coming in contact with a live wire.	Skin is pale, cold, and clammy.	Pupils may be unequal.	Tense.	Weak and imperceptible.	Respirations cease suddenly.	Deep tendon reflexes usually are increased.	Low voltage affects heart action, makes resuscitation impossible. High voltage affects the respiratory center in medulla and patient may be resuscitated.	Carefully release the patient from current. Artificial respiration by prone pressure; electrical defibrillation may be required. If heart fails to resume contraction, use of an external cardiac pacemaker is indicated. Each moment of delay increases the chances of death.
Epilepsy	Previous occurrence of fits or spells with or without aura.	Pallor to flush followed by cyanosis—may be slight and gradually increased to marked cyanosis.	Pupils are unequal, eyes rolling.	May be spastic. Tonic type of convulsion is followed by the clonic type.	Usually rapid.	Respirations are deep and stertorous.	May be increased.	Injuries in falling or biting the tongue. Patient may react violently (fighting others).	Bedrest. Prevent falling or biting tongue. Sedative.
Fainting	Fatigue, light-headedness, shock, or horrify-	Face and lips are blanched. Body is cold and	Normal.	Completely relaxed.	Rapid and thready.	Respirations are rapid and shallow.	Slightly increased.	Shock usually a serious complication. Body in-	Apply cold water to face, head, and chest. Place head

	ing experience.	clammy.						jury and fracture if patient falls.	in low position. Have patient inhale aromatic spirits of ammonia.
Freezing	Exposure to intense cold or prolonged period of exposure to cold.	Frostbite: Skin is cold, pale, and blanched. Frozen: Skin is livid and later cyanotic, then turns to purplish or greenish black.	Dilated.	Tense and becoming very rigid.	Rapid and weak.	Breathing is slower and deeper. Patient falls into very deep slumber.	Not discernible.	Pneumonia; certain damage due to mechanical destruction of the cells' sloughing and gangrene of the part previously frozen.	Gradual warming of the parts; slight massage of extremities for better circulation; elevation of parts; treatment of dry gangrene.
Gases	Victim rescued from a mine, burning building, or room with open gas jet. Overcome in garage or car.	In carbon monoxide poisoning, skin is cyanotic and changing to cherry red color.	Eyes fixed. Pupils are usually fully dilated. Varies with type of gas.	Relaxed if victim is living. Rigor mortis if dead.	Weak, slow, and irregular.	Respirations irregular and jerky to only an occasional gasp.	None.	Respiratory failure; asphyxia; collapse.	Place the patient in the open air; give oxygen and resuscitation (mouth-to-mouth). Treat for shock.
Hanging	Victim is found hanging with constriction of the neck.	Skin is pale and face is cyanotic.	Dilated and unequal if cerebral injury.	Relaxed. Varies with the level of tenure.	Pulse is rapid, weak, and irregular if strangulation is incomplete. If complete, pulse is absent.	Respirations have ceased or an occasional gasp is observed.	None	Respiratory and circulatory failure; fracture of neck.	Release the patient and cut the rope. Artificial respiration; treat for shock and possible fracture of neck.
Heat Exhaustion	Victim is overcome by the degree of heat and loss of sodium chloride through perspiration.	Skin may be pale and cool. Temperature is usually normal.	Moderately contracted.	Tense with muscle cramps.	Rapid and may become weak.	Respirations shallow with rigidity of the chest muscles.	Increased.	Shock.	Treat for shock; keep body warm. Give salt by mouth and I.V.

Unconsciousness (*Continued*)

Type	History	Skin and Color	Pupils	Muscles	Pulse	Breathing	Reflexes	Complications	Treatment
Heat Stroke (sun stroke, heat hyperpyrexia)	Exposure to intense degree, or prolonged period, of heat from environment.	Skin is flushed and hot when touched. Body temperature may be 106° F. (41° C.) or higher.	Dilated.	Relaxed.	Rapid and weak.	Respirations may be shallow and gasping or deep and slow.	Increased.	Suppressed sweating for prolonged period. Paralysis of vasomotor centers within medulla. Paralysis of heart, collapse, and death.	Place patient in cool area. Cold application to head and body. Wrap in cold, wet sheet. Continue to lower body temperature. No stimulants or sedatives unless required to treat convulsions. Judge effectiveness of therapy by continual monitoring of rectal temperature.
Mineral Poisoning	Accidental or suicidal poisoning.	Skin is cold and clammy. Pallor.	Dilated. Eyes fixed, staring.	Tense, convulsive to relaxed when in stupor.	Rapid, feeble to imperceptible.	Respirations are shallow, rapid, labored.	Increased.	Nephritis; liver degeneration; colitis.	Gastric lavage; emetics.
Narcotic Poisoning	History of addiction or allergic reaction to the drug.	Skin is ashen, cyanotic, and cold.	Pupils are contracted to pinpoint if due to opiate derivative.	Relaxed.	Usually slow but varies with type of drug poisoning.	Respirations slow, irregular, stertorous.	Diminished.	Addiction to drug or production of a marked sensitivity to a drug.	Removal of the drug by emetics or lavage; use of antidotes; specific counteractives.
Obstruction in throat	Aspiration of a foreign body or respiratory tract is obstructed by edema or disease.	Skin is cyanotic.	Dilated.	Sternal retraction. Muscles are tense with efforts of trying to	Rapid and very weak.	Respirations are deep and labored.	Increased.	Asphyxia; pulmonary infection; shock.	Remove obstruction. Give respiratory stimulant or artificial respiration; treat for shock. Tracheotomy if indicated.

				breathe and remove obstruction.					
Shock	Result of a blow or damage to the central nervous system.	Cold skin; subnormal temperature. Skin is an ashen to cyanotic color.	Dilated.	Relaxed.	Rapid, becoming thready and feeble.	Respirations are rapid and shallow.	Diminished (not significant).	Respiratory and circulatory embarrassment to collapse and death.	Elevate foot of bed; keep body warm; transfusions usually indicated for depression of vascular system.
Stroke (Apoplectic)	Patient may have history of hypertension and arteriosclerosis. Usually past 40 years of age.	Skin is injected. May be cyanotic or ashen. Hot and dry to flushed. Elevation of temperature.	Pupils vary. May be dilated, often unequal. Inactive in deep coma.	Muscles of the involved side (hemiplegia) are usually spastic with a facial palsy.	Slow, full with increased tension.	Respirations are slow, loud, usually deep.	Diminished on one side. May be hyperactive on the other side.	Pneumonia; injury from falling.	Rest and absolute quiet with head of bed elevated and feet lowered. Ice cap to head; no stimulants.

Wounds

Type	History	Pathology	Symptoms and Color	Points of Identification	Treatment	Transportation	Complications
Bite (human, animal, or insect).	Bite of a reptile or rabid human or animal. Sting or bite of poisonous insect.	Tissue degeneration at site of wound. Muscular paralysis. Venom has a drastic effect upon respiratory nerve centers.	Type of wound: Snake—two fang wound. Human—shape of denture. Dog—laceration. Patient shows rabid disposition. Insect—elevated wheal with pain and itching or burning sensation,	Shape of wound; odor of colon bacillus about the wound in human bite; presence of stinger.	Dog bite: Observe victim and dog for signs of rabies for two weeks. SEE: *rabies*. Snake bite: Apply tourniquet just tight enough to prevent venous return. Use ice packs to prevent absorp-	Keep patient quiet; avert apprehension; keep muscles of the area elevated and at rest.	Infection introduced by pathogenic organisms. Venom of toxic nature depresses victim. Death if delay in treatment.

Wounds (*Continued*)

Type	History	Pathology	Symptoms and Color	Points of Identification	Treatment	Transportation	Complications
			or single or double red dot.		tion of venom. Incision and suction as swelling rises. Sting: Neutralize with alkalies. Treat for shock. Respiratory stimulants for snake or insect venom. Specific antivenins are available for certain snake bites.		
Brush Burns or Abrasions.	Friction of body against rough surface.	Surface effaced with nicks and dotted with small drops of blood.	Skin discolored. Surface peeled off with fine beadlike dots of blood. Skin may be permeated with foreign material.	Surface of the skin is brushed completely away, or remains very lightly attached to the area.	Carefully brush away loose dirt. Cleanse the wound with soap and water. Use antiseptic solutions, ointment, and apply dressings. Tetanus toxoid or antitoxin as required.	Use loose applications of sterile dressings held in place by loose-fitting triangle.	Infection. May retain rough, unsightly scars.
Contusions.	Blow or fall.	A bruise (hematoma) or petechial area with underlying injury.	Skin surface is rough; the area includes a large or small hematoma (depending upon the extent of injury).	Skin is not broken. Underlying tissues may be slightly or markedly crushed.	Apply cold to area for 24–48 hours.	Keep part well elevated. If there is additional abrasion, cover with loose-fitting bandage.	Destruction of underlying tissue if hematoma is not aspirated early. Infection if skin is punctured or probed.
Gun Shot.	Accident in care of a gun. Victim of deliberate gunfire.	Wound of single outer puncture site with deep injury consisting of twisting and tearing of	Aperture is small. Powder burns occasionally are found.	Puncture site. Deep wound shows characteristic twisting of the deeper tissues.	Cleanse and irrigate. Debridement when necessary. Wet antiseptic dressings. Tetanus toxoid or	Keep patient very quiet; head slightly lower than body. Treat for shock. Watch T.P.R. and	Shock; internal hemorrhage; tetanus bacillus infection.

		tissue.			antitoxin as required.	blood pressure if blood has been lost or patient is in shock.	
Lacerations.	Accident wherein sharp instruments have cut and torn an area of the body.	Jagged or torn and roughened edges of tissues. May include avulsion of certain parts.	Injury has produced area of two raw or bleeding edges of the skin. Blood may be oozing or spurting from the wound.	Wound edges are jagged and irregular. Wound may contain amount of debris or dirt and usually is infected.	Remove the large debris and dirt. Clean the wound by water dripping from sterile cloth, or use soap and warm water; mild antiseptics and sterile dressings.	Edges of wound may be united with flamed strip of adhesive tape. Cover the area with loose dressings held by triangle or cravat bandage. Tetanus toxoid or antitoxin as required.	Infection and septicemia. Wound usually heals with very unsightly scar if not properly sutured.
Puncture.	Accidental or intentional piercing of body with a pointed object.	Tissues are pierced. Small opening through the tissues providing an excellent course or inlet for infection.	Area usually manifests no bleeding. Trauma of tissues usually evident.	Puncture site is very small. Object usually withdrawn with fair amount of ease.	Probe the wound very carefully to enlarge bore for irrigation with antiseptic solutions. Tetanus toxoid or antitoxin as required. Treatment for prevention of gas gangrene may be required.	Cover the area with sterile dressings and triangle or cravat bandage.	Infection of the anaerobic type (Tetanus bacillus) and septicemia.
Stab.	Injury by a blunt or pointed object, incurred during a fight or acquired by a fall or push.	Size of hole in the tissues varies with the size of the instrument. Foreign material and pathogenic bacteria of anaerobic nature are usually introduced.	Evidence of the instrument that was used, such as knife, ice pick, etc. Victim shows pallor, syncope, and later collapse.	Large, very deep puncture site. Instrument may still be in wound. Victim may be pinned to an object by the force of the blow.	Cleanse and irrigate the wound when possible. Irrigation and inclusion of antiseptic drain or wet dressings. Early use of antitetanic sera. Tetanus toxoid or antitoxin as required.	Keep patient very quiet with head and chest slightly elevated. Treat for shock. If chest is involved, watch T.P.R. and blood pressure.	Internal hemorrhage from, or damage to, organs underlying site of wound, such as puncture and collapse of lung, abdominal visceral injury, or severance of a nerve. Pulmonary hemorrhage. Infection of body by anaerobic organisms.

App. 14: Directories

Miscellaneous Addresses

Public Health Service Communicable Disease Center
1600 Clifton Road
Atlanta, GA 30333
Phone: (404) 329-3311, day
(404) 329-3644, night

Information on snake antivenin:
Oklahoma Poison Information Center
Phone: 1-800-522-4611

Scorpion antivenin:
Poisonous Animals Research Laboratory
Arizona State College
Tempe, AZ 85281

Information concerning hemophilia:
National Hemophilia Foundation
25 West 39th Street
New York, NY 10018

Information concerning cancer:
American Cancer Society
219 E. 42nd Street
New York, NY 12210

Optacon (electronic reading device for blind)
Telesensory Systems Inc.
Palo Alto, CA 94302
Phone: (415) 493-2626

Burn Centers*

This directory includes 210 hospitals at which burn physicians in the United States and Canada have reported the presence of a specialized burn care service in 1983. Its publication is designed to enable rapid communication between specialized burn services, and to facilitate inter-regional referrals of burn patients.

The 185 hospitals listed for the United States include 145 which report special burn units. Reported burn unit beds total about 1,700. Specialized burn care is also provided in shared settings, including burn/trauma units, other types of intensive care units, and general medical/surgical floors. Many hospitals with burn care units can care for additional acute burn patients in such settings.

The telephone numbers provided by survey respondents may be located at the hospital switchboard, the emergency department, the burn care unit itself, or the physician's office. *Those using this list to refer a patient with burns should make clear the purpose of the call, in addition to asking for the physician listed or his designee.*

About 21,000 acute inpatient admissions were reported by the 185 United States facilities on this list in 1982. This is virtually identical with the 1981 total, again representing 30% of the estimated 70,000 annual acute inpatient burn admissions in the United States. An estimated 4,000 reconstructive burn admissions were also reported by 85 U.S. survey respondents. Since such admissions are managed at many hospitals by a separate plastic surgery service, total reconstructive admissions could not be determined.

This list is derived primarily from an annual survey of physician members of the American Burn Association who have previously reported the presence of a specialized burn service. The comprehensiveness of the list will be confirmed on a regular basis by queries to ABA member physicians located in areas not known to have a specialized burn service, and by data from the annual hospital surveys of the American and Canadian Hospital Associations.

None of the sources used in preparing this list address either the quality of burn care at a given institution, or the optimum number of specialized beds and services in a given region. The inclu-

*from the American Burn Association

sion of hospitals and physicians on this list therefore does not represent any direct or implied endorsement by the ABA of the burn care service they provide.

Suggested additions or deletions, and any questions related to this list, should be communicated to the Secretary of the American Burn Association: Joseph A. Moylan, M.D , Duke University Medical Center, Box 3947, Durham, NC 27710.

U.S.A.

State	*Telephone, Coordinator, and Address*
Alabama	(205) 933-4000 Marshall Pitts Children's Hospital, Birmingham
	(205) 934-3411 Alan R. Dimick University of Alabama Hospitals, Birmingham
	(205) 471-7000 Arnold Luterman Mary Finn Clifford Dasco Max Ramenofsky University of South Alabama Medical Center Hospital
Alaska	(907) 276-4511 Paul Steer W. J. Mills (hypothermia) Providence Hospital, Anchorage
	(907) 452-8181 William Wennen Fairbanks Memorial Hospital, Fairbanks
Arizona	(602) 267-5700 John M. Stein Maricopa Medical Center, Phoenix
	(602) 795-8700 Philip Fleishman St. Mary's Hospital, Tucson
Arkansas	(501) 370-1100 ext. 149 Fred T. Caldwell John Crabtree Arkansas Children's Hospital, Little Rock
California	(415) 540-1573 Jerold Z. Kaplan Alta Bates Hospital, Berkeley
	(415) 537-1234 Ronald Iverson Eleanor Kohn Eden Hospital, Castro Valley
	(916) 345-2411 or 342-7513 Donald J. Mangus Chico Community Hospital, Chico
	(213) 652-6630 Arthur M. Kahn Brotman Medical Center, Culver City

(213) 922-7454
G. Brody (reconstructive surgery only)
Rancho Los Amigos Hospital, Downey

(707) 443-8051
Russell Pardoe
St. Joseph's Hospital, Eureka

(209) 453-4161
Steven N. Parks
Valley Medical Center, Fresno

(213) 226-7991
Bruce E. Zawacki
LAC/USC Medical Center, Los Angeles

(714) 634-5304
Bruce M. Achauer
University of California, Irvine Medical Center, Orange

(916) 453-3636
Robert Demling
University of California, Davis Medical Center, Sacramento

(714) 887-7047 ext. 405 or 444
David Hess
San Bernardino Community, San Bernardino

(714) 383-3131
Appannagari Gnanavez
San Bernardino County Medical Center, San Bernardino

(619) 294-6502
Thomas Wachtel
Hugh Frank
University Hospital/University of California Medical Center, San Diego

(415) 821-8197
Anthony A. Meyer
Juris Bunkis
George Sheldon
San Francisco General Hospital, San Franciso

(415) 775-4321
Edward Falces
St. Francis Memorial Hospital, San Francisco

(408) 279-5242
Ronald M. Sato
Santa Clara Valley Medical Center, San Jose

(415) 235-7000
Robert L. Shapiro
Brookside Hospital, San Pablo

(213) 981-7111
A. Richard Grossman
Sherman Oaks Community Hospital, Sherman Oaks

(209) 944-5550
Genest deL'Arbre
Dameron Hospital, Stockton

	(213) 325-9110 William D. Davies Torrance Memorial Hospital, Torrance
	(213) 960-6548 William T. Choctaw Queen of the Valley Hospital, West Covina
Colorado	(303) 630-5770 Ian G. Walker Claude Poliakoff Penrose Hospital, Colorado Springs
	(303) 861-6517 William Carl Bailey Children's Hospital, Denver
	(303) 394-8052 John Hansbrough University Medical Center, Denver
	(303) 242-9127 William Merkel St. Mary's Hospital, Grand Junction
	(303) 352-4121 James R. Wheeler North Colorado Medical Center, Greeley
	(303) 560-4000 Clifford Hoyle St. Mary-Corwin Hospital, Pueblo
Connecticut	(203) 384-3000 Michael L. D'Aiuto Bridgeport Hospital, Bridgeport
	(203) 524-2840 Philip E. Trowbridge Hartford Hospital, Hartford
	(203) 785-2574 Stephen Ariyan Charles Cuono Yale-New Haven Hospital, New Haven
District of Columbia	(202) 745-5116 or 5152 Judson G. Randolph Children's Hospital National Medical Center, Washington
	(202) 541-7241 or 6662 Marion Jordan Washington Hospital Center, Washington
Florida	(904) 392-3054 or 3055 Hal G. Bingham Shands Teaching Hospital, Gainesville
	(305) 325-7085 C. Gillon Ward Jeffrey Hammond Donald Buckner James M. Jackson Memorial Hospital, Miami

	(305) 841-5176 Patricio Quijada Juan Sauer Orlando Regional Medical Center, Orlando
	(813) 253-0711 or 251-7617 C. Wayne Cruse Tampa General Hospital, Tampa
Georgia	(404) 588-4307 Roger Sherman (Fulton and Delkalb Counties only) Grady Memorial Hospital, Atlanta
	(404) 863-3232 Alton Garrison Joseph Still Doctor's Hospital, Augusta
	(404) 828-3893 Richard C. Treat Eugene Talmadge Memorial Hospital—Medical College of Georgia Augusta
	(404) 571-1336 Robert K. Worman Medical Center, Columbus
Hawaii	(808) 523-2311 James H. Penoff Robert W. Schulz Straub Clinic and Hospital, Honolulu
Illinois	(312) 880-4094 Desmond Kernahan Victor Lewis Children's Memorial Hospital, Chicago
	(312) 633-6564 or 6570 Takayoshi Matsuda Marella Hanumadass Richard Kagan Cook County Hospital, Chicago
	(312) 878-6000 Ramesh Kharwadkar Edgewater Hospital, Chicago
	(312) 962-6212 Martin Robson University of Chicago Hospitals, Chicago
	(312) 492-7720 Charles Drueck Evanston Hospital, Evanston
	(312) 531-3988 Raymond Warpeha Foster G. McGaw Hospital, Loyola University of Chicago, Maywood
	(309) 793-3173 Frank E. Miller Rock Island Franciscan Hospital, Rock Island

	(815) 226-2000 Raymond Hoffman St. Anthony's Hospital, Rockford
	(217) 788-3325 Elof Erickson Memorial Medical Center, Springfield
Indiana	(219) 425-3431 Jack Patterson St. Joseph's Hospital, Fort Wayne
	(317) 264-3927 James Bennett (children) J. W. Riley Hospital, Indianapolis
	(317) 630-6471 David J. Smith (adults) W. N. Wishard Memorial Hospital, Indianapolis
Iowa	(319) 356-2496 Albert E. Cram University of Iowa Hospitals and Clinics, Iowa City
	(712) 279-3440 Larry D. Foster St. Luke's Regional Medical Center, Sioux City
Kansas	(913) 588-6540 Mani M. Mani David W. Robinson University of Kansas Medical Center, Kansas City
	(316) 268-5388 Thomas E. Kendall St. Francis Hospital, Wichita
	(316) 688-2688 Richard C. Shaw Wesley Medical Center, Wichita
Kentucky	(606) 233-5260 Edward Luce University Hospital, Lexington
	(502) 589-8000 Harry D. Stambaugh Norton-Children's Hospital (admits adult burns), Louisville
Louisiana	(504) 387-7716 D. V. Cacioppo Baton Rouge General Hospital, Baton Rouge
	(504) 347-5511 Frank C. DiVincenti West Jefferson Hospital, Marrero
	(504) 568-2311 Frank C. DiVincenti Charity Hospital of Louisiana, New Orleans

	(318) 674-6133 Edwin Deitch L.S.U. Medical Center Hospital, Shreveport
Maine	(207) 947-3711 Charles Dixon Eastern Maine Medical Center, Bangor
	(207) 871-2991 Joel Johnson, Acting Director Maine Medical Center, Portland
	(207) 769-2511 Raymond Giberson Arthur Gould Memorial Hospital, Presque Isle
Maryland	(301) 396-8765 Andrew Munster Baltimore City Hospital, Baltimore
Massachusetts	(617) 735-2000 Joel Noe Beth Israel Hospital, Boston
	(617) 424-5204 Irwin Hirsch Boston City Hospital, Boston
	(617) 732-7712 Douglas W. Wilmore Brigham & Women's Hospital, Boston
	(617) 726-3354 John F. Burke Massachusetts General Hospital, Boston
	(617) 722-3000 John P. Remensnyder Shriners Burns Institute, Boston
	(413) 787-4380 Manu H. Desai Baystate Medical Center, Springfield
	(617) 799-8110 Felix Cataldo Worcester City Hospital, Worcester
Michigan	(313) 995-BURN Irving Feller Jai K. Prasad Michigan Burn Center University Hospital, Ann Arbor Chelsea Community Hospital, Ann Arbor
	(313) 494-5678 James Lloyd Children's Hospital of Michigan, Detroit
	(313) 494-3374 Eti Gursel Detroit Receiving Hospital and University Health Center, Detroit

	(313) 766-0188 or 0594 Franklin Wade Hurley Medical Center, Flint
	(616) 774-7670 William Simpson Richard A. Wehrenberg Blodgett Memorial Medical Center, Grand Rapids
	(616) 383-6485 or 1-800-632-3403 Frank J. Newman Paul Fierke Michael Nave Bronson Methodist Hospital, Kalamazoo
	(517) 487-2774 Errikos Constant Jorge Gomez Preecha Supanwanid William Blackburn Edward R. Sparrow Hospital, Lansing
	(906) 228-9440 James Kelinger Constance N. Arnold Marquette General Hospital, Marquette
	(517) 790-5055 Syed Akhtar St. Mary's Hospital, Saginaw
Minnesota	(218) 727-8762 John W. Wolfe Miller-Dwan Hospital and Medical Center, Duluth
	(612) 871-4551 F. A. McParland Minneapolis Children's Health Center and Hospital, Minneapolis
	(612) 347-2915 John Twomey Hennepin County Medical Center, Minneapolis
	(612) 520-5200 Brian Hubble North Memorial Medical Center, Minneapolis
	(507) 285-5123 or -5591 or -6691 George B. Irons (adults) Robert Telander (children) St. Mary's Hospital, Rochester
	(612) 221-3351 Lynn D. Solem St. Paul-Ramsey Medical Center, St. Paul
Mississippi	(601) 378-3783 Robert Love Delta Medical Center, Greenville
Missouri	(314) 882-7994 Boyd E. Terry University of Missouri Health Sciences Center, Columbia

	(816) 234-3520 Ronald J. Sharp Children's Mercy Hospital, Kansas City
	(314) 454-3244 William H. Monafo Barnes Hospital, St. Louis
	(314) 569-6055 Vatche H. Ayvazian St. John's Mercy Medical Center, St. Louis
	(417) 885-2876 Mark Wittmer St. John's Regional Health Center, Springfield
Montana	(406) 245-2458 David F. Sloan St. Vincent Hospital, Billings
Nebraska	(402) 489-7181 or 483-9206 Robert W. Gillespie St. Elizabeth Community Health Center, Lincoln
Nevada	(702) 382-2260 Charles A. Buerk Southern Nevada Memorial Hospital, Las Vegas
New Jersey	(201) 441-2020 Anthony Barbara Hackensack Hospital, Hackensack
	(201) 533-5920 Frederick Fuller Esber Mansour St. Barnabas Medical Center, Livingston
New Mexico	(505) 843-2111 William R. Schiller University of New Mexico Hospital, Albuquerque
New York	(518) 445-3010 Dhiraj M. Shah Albany Medical Center, Albany
	(716) 878-7301 or -7435 Theodore Jewett Donald R. Cooney Melvyn P. Karp Children's Hospital, Buffalo
	(716) 887-4776 or -4649 Evan J. Evans Millard Fillmore Hospital, Buffalo
	(716) 842-2200 Louis C. Cloutier Sheehan Emergency Hospital, Buffalo
	(516) 542-3207 Roger L. Simpson Nassau County Medical Center, East Meadow

(607) 733-6541
James Marshall
James Sonsire
St. Joseph's Hospital, Elmira

(212) 430-8065
Stanley Levenson
Bronx Municipal Hospital Center, New York City

(212) 735-3131
Winston Mitchell
Kings County Hospital, New York City

(212) 491-1335
James E. C. Norris
Harlem Hospital Center, New York City

(212) 472-5132
Cleon Goodwin
New York Hospital-Cornell Medical Center, New York City

(212) 790-8941 or -8940
Ronald N. Ollstein
St. Vincent's Hospital, New York City

(716) 275-5475
Robert M. McCormack
Strong Memorial Hospital, Rochester

(315) 473-6083
William Clark
Upstate Medical Center, Syracuse

(914) 347-4909
Roger E. Salisbury
Westchester County Medical Center, Valhalla

(516) 957-4000
Richard A. Giery
Good Samaritan Hospital, West Islip

North Carolina

(919) 966-4131
Hugh D. Peterson
North Carolina Memorial Hospital, Chapel Hill

(704) 331-2525
Harold Hamit
Charlotte Memorial Medical Center, Charlotte

(919) 681-2404
Gregory Georgiade
Joseph Moylan
Duke University Hospital, Durham

(919) 748-7766
Jesse H. Meredith
Connell Shearin
North Carolina Baptist Hospital, Winston-Salem

North Dakota

(701) 280-5504
David W. Todd
St. Luke's General Hospital, Fargo

Ohio	(216) 379-8224 C. R. Boeckmann R. L. Klein Children's Hospital Medical Center, Akron Regional Burn Center (admits adult burns), Akron
	(513) 872-3100 Robert P. Hummel University of Cincinnati Hospital, Cincinnati
	(513) 751-3900 Bruce G. MacMillan Shriners Burns Institute, Cincinnati
	(216) 459-5627 Richard Fratianne Cleveland Metropolitan General Hospital, Cleveland
	(614) 461-2000 E. Thomas Boles Children's Hospital, Columbus
	(614) 422-4516 Robert Ruberg Ohio State University Hospital, Columbus
	(513) 226-8300 Charles D. Goodwin Children's Medical Center, Dayton
	(513) 223-6192 R. K. Finley Sidney Miller Larry Jones Miami Valley Hospital, Dayton
	(419) 259-4734 George Baibak Michael Yanik St. Vincent's Hospital, Toledo
Oklahoma	(405) 949-3345 or -3311 Paul Silverstein Baptist Medical Center, Oklahoma City
	(405) 271-4733 William P. Tunell Oklahoma Children's Memorial Hospital, Oklahoma City
	(918) 584-1351 Bernard Swartz Hillcrest Medical Center, Tulsa
Oregon	(503) 280-4233 Philip Parhley Oregon Burn Center (at Emanuel Hospital), Portland
Pennsylvania	(215) 821-2058 Walter J. Okunski Lehigh Valley Hospital Center, Allentown

	(215) 876-0356 Charles E. Hartford Crozer-Chester Medical Center, Chester
	(717) 271-6353 or -6591 Philip C. Breen Geisinger Medical Center, Danville
	(814) 459-0344 Charles R. Bales Forrest C. Mischler Hamot Medical Center, Erie
	(717) 534-8521 William P. Graham Hershey Medical Center, Hershey
	(215) 339-4339 Frederick A. DeClement Saint Agnes Medical Center, Philadelphia
	(215) 427-5000 Stuart J. Hulnick St. Christopher's Hospital for Children, Philadelphia
	(412) 232-8225 Thomas Layton Mercy Hospital, Pittsburgh
	(412) 578-1866 John Gaisford Western Pennsylvania Hospital, Pittsburgh
	(717) 771-2345 Robert Davis Richard W. Dabb York Hospital, York
Rhode Island	(401) 277-4000 Lawrence Bowen Rhode Island Hospital, Providence
South Carolina	(803) 792-3681 or -3851 Dabney R. Yarborough (adults) H. Biemann Othersen, Jr. (children) Medical University Hospital, Charleston
Tennessee	(615) 778-7881 Phil D. Craft Baroness Erlanger Hospital, Chattanooga
	(901) 528-7100 William Hickerson Gary Reynolds City of Memphis Hospital, Memphis
	(615) 322-7311 John B. Lynch Vanderbilt University Hospital, Nashville
Texas	(512) 476-6461 Robert A. Ersek Brackenridge Hospital, Austin

(713) 835-3781
Duane Larson
Welsey Washburn
Baptist Hospital, Beaumont

(512) 881-4360
Robert H. Balme
Memorial Medical Center, Corpus Christi

(214) 637-8546 or 688-2152
John Hunt
Parkland Memorial Hospital, Dallas

(915) 532-6281
Charles Lyon
Sun Towers Hospital, El Paso

(512) 221-4604 or -2943
Basil A. Pruitt, Jr.
Brooke Army Medical Center, Fort Sam Houston

(817) 921-3431
Charles Crenshaw
John Peter Smith Hospital, Fort Worth

(713) 765-1255 (days)
(713) 765-2023 (evenings)
Sally Abston
University of Texas Medical Branch Hospitals, Galveston

(713) 765-2516
David N. Herndon
Shriners Burns Institute, Galveston

(713) 791-7000
Frank Gerow
Ben Taub General Hospital, Houston

(713) 792-5406
David E. Beesinger
Hermann Hospital, Houston

(806) 743-3406
Richard Baker
Timothy Harnar
Lubbock General Hospital, Lubbock

(512) 696-3030 or 691-6151 or -7473
A. B. Cruz, Jr.
Medical Center Hospital, San Antonio

Utah

(801) 581-2700
Glenn Warden
Jeffrey Saffle
University of Utah Hospital, Salt Lake City

Vermont

(802) 656-4545
John Davis
Richard Gamelli
Medical Center Hospital of Vermont, Burlington

Virginia	(804) 924-5520 Richard Edlich University of Virginia Medical Center, Charlottesville
	(804) 628-3117 William Bethea Norfolk General Hospital, Norfolk
	(804) 786-9240 Boyd W. Haynes Medical College of Virginia Hospital, Richmond
Washington	(206) 734-5400 ext. 2501 James Hines St. Joseph's Hospital, Bellingham
	(206) 634-5283 Robert T. Schaller, Jr. Children's Orthopedic Hospital, Seattle
	(206) 223-3127 David Heimbach Loren Engrav Harborview Medical Center, Seattle
	(509) 455-3344 Charles Miller Sacred Heart Medical Center, Spokane
	(206) 627-4101 or 596-6677 Martin Schaeferle St. Joseph's Hospital, Tacoma
West Virginia	(304) 696-6110 James A. Coil, Jr. Cabell-Huntington Hospital, Huntington
Wisconsin	(608) 263-1490 or -1387 Richard Helgerson University of Wisconsin Hospitals, Madison
	(414) 225-8000 George Collentine St. Mary's Hospital, Milwaukee

Canada

Alberta	(403) 270-1100 D. C. Birdsell R. L. Lindsay E. Magi Foothills Provincial General Hospital, Calgary
	(403) 432-6149 Gerald Moysa University of Alberta Hospital, Edmonton
British Columbia	(604) 875-4111 Charles F. T. Snelling Vancouver General Hospital, Vancouver

	(604) 388-9121 H. R. Hollis (Dir.) P. Gareau D. A. Baird T. A. McQueen Victoria General Hospital, Victoria
Manitoba	(204) 787-3776 G. A. Robertson Health Sciences, Center, Winnipeg
New Brunswick	(506) 452-5400 W. Cook D. Truman Dr. Everett Chalmers Hospital, Fredericton
	(506) 855-1600 Douglas Inglis G. I. Curry Moncton Hospital, Moncton
	(506) 648-2200 G. L. Sparkes Saint John General Hospital, Saint John
Nova Scotia	(902) 428-2525 Winston Parkhill Victoria General Hospital, Halifax
	(902) 424-6111 James Ross I. W. Killam Hospital for Children, Halifax
Ontario	(416) 527-0271 Darryl G. Truscott Hamilton General Hospital, Hamilton
	(613) 548-8871 A. Kenneth Wylie Hotel Dieu Hospital, Kingston
	(519) 432-5241 ext. 4171 Robert B. Colcleugh R. McFarland Victoria Hospital Corporation, London
	(613) 737-7600 Paul Benoit Children's Hospital of Eastern Ontario, Ottawa
	(613) 737-8222 Paul Benoit Ottawa General Hospital, Ottawa
	(416) 438-2911 N. Poy (Dir.) M. Bederman L. Carlsen Scarborough General Hospital, Scarborough

	(416) 597-1500 Ronald M. Zuker Hugh G. Thomson Hospital for Sick Children, Toronto
	(416) 595-3840 Walter Peters Toronto General Hospital, Toronto
	(416) 966-6600 W. R. Lindsay Wellesley, Toronto
	(519) 254-1661 Chosen Lau (Dir.) Stuart Young Howard Adams Metropolitan General Hospital, Windsor
Quebec	(514) 937-8511 H. Bruce Williams Montreal Children's Hospital, Montreal
	(514) 937-6011 H. Bruce Williams Montreal General, Montreal
	(514) 845-5119 Jacques Papillon Hotel Dieu de Montreal, Montreal
Saskatchewan	(306) 359-4213 G. P. Holden Regina General Hospital, Regina
	(306) 343-3759 Leslie R. Chasmar D. J. Classen J. H. Zondervan University Hospital; Saskatoon

United States Poison Control Centers*

The following directory lists the addresses and telephone numbers of the current state coordinators for poison control. These Centers provide information on a 24-hour basis concerning treatment or prevention of accidents involving poisonous substances.

State	*Telephone, Coordinator, and Address*
Alabama	(205) 832-3194 or 832-3935 State Department of Public Health Montgomery 36117
Alaska	(907) 465-3100 State Department of Health and Social Services Juneau 99811
Arizona	(602) 626-6016 or 1-800-362-0101 (statewide) College of Pharmacy University of Arizona Tucson 85724
Arkansas	(501) 661-2301 State Department of Health Little Rock 72201
California	(916) 322-4336 Emergency Medical Services Authority Sacramento 95814
Canal Zone	252-7500 U.S.A. MEDDAC Panama Gorgas U.S. Army Hospital Ancon
Colorado	(303) 320-8476 State Department of Public Health Denver 80220
Connecticut	(203) 674-3456 University of Connecticut Health Center Farmington 06032
Delaware	(302) 655-3389 Wilmington Medical Center Delaware Division Wilmington 19801
District of Columbia	(202) 673-6741 or 673-6736 Department of Human Services Washington, D.C. 20009
Florida	(904) 487-1566 Department of Health and Rehabilitative Services Jacksonville 32301
Georgia	(404) 894-5170 Department of Human Resources Atlanta 30303

* Additional listings of Centers in your state may be obtained through the state coordinator or through the Director, National Clearinghouse for Poison Control Centers, Food and Drug Administration, U.S. Department of Health and Human Services, Bethesda, Md. 20016 (telephone 202-655-4000). *Note:* These telephone numbers are subject to periodic change.

Guam	646-5801 Department of Public Health and Social Services Agana 96910
Hawaii	(808) 531-7776 Department of Health Honolulu 96801
Idaho	(208) 334-4245 State Department of Health and Welfare Boise 83720
Illinois	(217) 785-2080 Division of Emergency Medical Services and Highway Safety Springfield 62761
Indiana	(317) 633-0332 State Board of Health Indianapolis 46206
Iowa	(515) 281-4964 Department of Health Des Moines 50319
Kansas	(913) 862-9360 ext. 541 Department of Health and Environment Topeka 66620
Kentucky	(502) 564-3970 Department for Human Resources Frankfort 40601
Louisiana	(318) 425-1524 LSU Poison Control and Drug Abuse Information Center Shreveport 71130
Maine	(207) 871-2950 Maine Poison Control Center Portland 04102
Maryland	(301) 528-7604 Maryland Poison Control Center University of Maryland School of Pharmacy Baltimore 21201
Massachusetts	(617) 727-2700 State Department of Public Health Boston 02111
Michigan	(517) 373-1406 Department of Public Health Lansing 48909
Minnesota	(612) 623-5284 State Department of Health Minneapolis 55404
Mississippi	(601) 354-7660 State Board of Health Jackson 39205
Missouri	(314) 751-2713 Missouri Division of Health Jefferson City 65102

Montana	(406) 449-3895 State Department of Health and Environmental Sciences Helena 59620
Nebraska	(402) 471-2122 State Department of Health Lincoln 68502
Nevada	(702) 885-4750 Department of Human Resources Carson City 89710
New Hampshire	(603) 646-5000 New Hampshire Poison Center Mary Hitchcock Hospital Hanover 03756
New Jersey	(609) 292-5666 State Department of Health Trenton 08625
New Mexico	(505) 843-2551 University of New Mexico Albuquerque 87131
New York	(518) 474-3785 State Department of Health Albany 12237
North Carolina	(919) 684-8111 Duke University Medical Center Durham 27710
North Dakota	(701) 224-2388 State Department of Health Bismarck 58505
Ohio	(614) 466-5190 Department of Health Columbus 43126
Oklahoma	(405) 271-5454 or 1-800-522-4611 Oklahoma Poison Control Center Oklahoma City 73216
Oregon	(503) 225-8968 or 1-800-452-7165 Oregon Poison Control and Drug Information Center University of Oregon Health Sciences Center Portland 97201
Pennsylvania	(717) 787-2307 State Department of Health Harrisburg 17108
Puerto Rico	(809) 765-4880, or 765-0615 University of Puerto Rico Rio Piedras 00936
Rhode Island	(401) 277-5727 Rhode Island Poison Center Rhode Island Hospital Providence 02902

South Carolina	(803) 758-5654 Department of Health and Environmental Control Columbia 29201
South Dakota	(605) 773-3361 State Department of Health Pierre 57501
Tennessee	(615) 741-2407 State Department of Public Health Nashville 37216
Texas	(512) 458-7254 State Department of Health Austin 78756
Utah	(801) 533-6161 State Department of Health Salt Lake City 84113
Vermont	(802) 658-3456 Medical Center Hospital of Vermont Burlington 05401
Virginia	(804) 786-5188 Bureau of Emergency Medical Services Richmond 23219
Virgin Islands	(809) 774-6097 or -0117 Department of Health St. Thomas 00801
Washington	(206) 522-7478 State Department of Social and Health Services Seattle 98115
West Virginia	(304) 348-4211 or 1-800-642-3625 West Virginia University School of Pharmacy Charleston 25304
Wisconsin	(608) 267-7174 Department of Health and Social Services Madison 53701
Wyoming	(307) 777-7955 Department of Health and Social Services Cheyenne 82001

Mexico Poison Control Center

Secretary of Health Assistance
Calle Lieja No. 7
Mexico D. F.
(telefono 553-6853)

Canada Poison Control Centres*

The following directory lists the addresses and telephone numbers of the current province coordinators for poison control. These Centres provide information on a 24-hour basis concerning treatment or prevention of accidents involving poisonous substances.

Province	*Telephone and Address*
Alberta	(403) 474-3431 Royal Alexandra Hospital Edmonton T5H 3V9
	(403) 432-8410 University of Alberta Hospital Edmonton T6G 2B7
	(403) 262-5982 Calgary General Hospital Calgary T2E 0A1
	(403) 270-1315 Emergency Department Foothills General Hospital Calgary T2N 2T9
British Columbia	(604) 682-5050 B.C. Drug and Poison Information Centre St. Paul's Hospital Vancouver
	(604) 595-9212 Emergency Department Royal Jubilee Hospital Victoria
Manitoba	(204) 787-2591 Provincial Poison Information Centre
	(204) 787-2444 Health Sciences Children's Centre Winnipeg R3E 0W1
New Brunswick	(506) 658-2222 Saint John General Hospital Saint John E2L 4L2
Newfoundland	(709) 722-1110 The Dr. Charles A. Janeway Child Health Centre St. John's A1A 1R8
Northwest Territories	(403) 873-3444 Stanton Yellowknife Hospital Yellowknife X0E 1H0
Nova Scotia	(902) 424-6161 The Izaak Walton Killam Hospital for Children Halifax B3J 3G9

* Additional listings of Centres in your province may be obtained through the province coordinator or through the Chief of Poison Control Division, Health and Welfare Canada, Ottawa, Ontario K1A 1B8. *Note:* These telephone numbers are subject to periodic change.

Ontario	(416) 979-1900 Hospital for Sick Children Toronto M5G 1X8
	(613) 521-4040 Children's Hospital of Eastern Ontario Ontario K1H 8L1
Prince Edward Island	(902) 566-6111 Queen Elizabeth Hospital Charlottetown C1A 8T5
Quebec	(514) 731-4931 Hôpital Sainte-Justine Montreal H3T 1C5
	(514) 937-8511 Montreal Children's Hospital Montreal H3H 1P3
	(418) 656-8090 Centre Hospitalier de l'Université Laval Centre Régional de Toxicologie Quebec City G1V 4G2
	(418) 656-8326 Centre Anti-poison Quebec City
Saskatchewan	(306) 359-4545 Regina General Hospital Poison Control Centre Regina S4P 0W5
	(306) 343-3323 Saskatoon University Hospital Poison Control Centre Saskatoon S7N 0W8
Yukon Territory	(403) 668-9444 Whitehorse General Hospital Emergency Department Whitehorse

Radiological Assistance

U.S. Regional Coordinating Offices

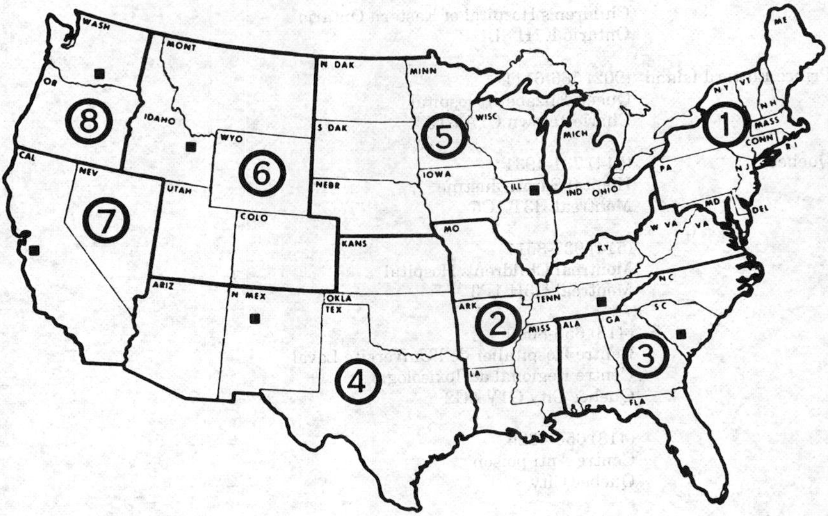

1 Upton, L.I., NY 11973
Phone: (516) 345-2200

2 P.O. Box E
Oak Ridge, TN 37830
Phone: (615) 576-1005 or 525-7885
(Includes Puerto Rico and Virgin Islands)

3 P.O. Box A
Aiken, SC 29801
Phone: (803) 725-3333
(Includes Canal Zone)

4 P.O. Box 5400
Albuquerque, NM 87115
Phone: (505) 264-4667

5 9800 S. Cass Avenue
Argonne, IL 60439
Phone: (312) 972-4800 duty hrs., 972-5731 off hrs.

6 P.O. Box 2108
Idaho Falls, ID 83401
Phone: (208) 526-1515

7 1333 Broadway
Oakland, CA 94612
Phone: (415) 273-4237
(Includes Hawaii)

8 P.O. Box 550
Richland, WA 99352
Phone: (509) 942-7381
(Includes Alaska)

App. 15: The Interpreter

Basic Medical Diagnosis and Treatment

English, Spanish, Italian, French, German

Table of Contents

Introduction

When attempting to communicate with a person whose language is foreign to you it is important to establish that while you may be able to say a few words in his language you will not be able to understand the patient's replies. The patient may need to use signs in replying. The following paragraphs are given for your convenience in explaining your language difficulty to the patient.

English

Hello. I want to help you. I do not speak (English) but will use this book to ask you some questions. I will not be able to understand your spoken answers. Please respond by shaking your head or raising one finger to indicate "no"; nod your head or raise two fingers to indicate "yes."

Spanish

(Translation)

Saludos. Quiero ayudarlo. Yo no hablo español, pero voy a usar este libro para hacerle algunas preguntas. No voy a poder entender sus respuestas; por eso haga el favor de contestar, negando con la cabeza o levantando un dedo para indicar "no" y afirmando con la cabeza o levantando dos dedos para indicar "sí."

(Phonetic)

Sah-loo'dohs. Ki-air'oh ah-joo-dar'loh. Joh noh ah'bloh es'panyohl, pair'oh voy ah oo-sawr' es'tay lee'broh pahr'ah ah-sair'lay ahl-goo'nahs pray-goon'tahs. Noh voy ah poh-dair' en-ten-dair' soos res-poo-es'rahs; pore es-soh ah'gah el fah-vohr' day kohn-tes-tahr', nay-gahn'doh kohn lah kah-bay'thah oh lay-vahn-tahn'doh oon day'doh pahr'ah een-dee-kahr' noh ee ah-feer-mahn'doh kohn lah kah-bay'thah oh lay-vahn-tahn'doh dohs day'dohs pahr'a een-dee-kahr' see.

Italian

(Translation)

Buon giorno. La voglio aiutare. Io non parlo italiano, ma userò questo libro per farle qualche domanda. Non potrò comprendere le Sue domande. Per favore risponda con un cenno di testa. Alzi un dito per indicare 'no'; muova la Sua testa su e giu o alzi due dita per indicare 'si.'

(Phonetic)

Bwon jih-or'noh. Lah vol'yoh ah-yoo-tar'day. Ee'oh nohn par'loh ee-towl-ee-ah'noh mah oo-say'roh kwes'toh lee'broh pehr fahr'lay kwall'kay doh-mahn'dah. Non poh'throh kohm-prehn'deh-ray lay soo'ee doh-mahn'day. Pehr fah-vohr'ay ray-spohn'dah kohn oon chay'noh dee tes'tah. Ahlt'zih oon dee'toh pehr in-dee-kar'ay noh; moo-eh'vah lah soo'ah tes'tah soo eh joo oh alht'zih doo'ay dee'tay pehr in-dee-kar'ay see.

French

(Translation)

Bonjour. Je veux bien vous aider. Je ne parle pas français mais tout en me servant de ce livre je vais vous poser des questions. Je ne comprendrai pas ce que vous dites en français. Je vous en prie, pour répondre: pour indiquer "non", secouez la tête ou levez un seul doigt; pour indiquer "oui", faites un signe de tête ou levez deux doigts.

(Phonetic)

Bon-zhoor'. Zheh voo bih-ehn' voo ay-day'. Zheh neh parl pah frahn-say' may too ahn meh sehr-vahn' d' seh lee'vrah zheh vay voo poh-say' day kehs-tih-on'. Zheh neh kahm-prahn'dry pah seh keh voo deet ahn frahn-say'. Zheh voo ahn pree, por ray-pahn'drah; por ahn-dee-kay nohn, seh-kway' lah teht oo leh-vay' oon sool dwoit; por ahn-dee-kay wee', fayt oon seen deh teht oo leh-vay' duh dwoit.

German

(Translation)

Hallo! Ich mochte Ihnen helfen. Ich spreche kein Deutsch, aber ich werde dieses Buch benützten um Sie einiges zu fragen. Ich werde Ihre Antworten nicht verstehen. Deshalb antworten Sie mir indem Sie Ihren Kopf schütteln oder heben Sie Ihren Finger um "nein" auszudrücken; nicken Sie mit dem Kopf oder heben Sie zwei Finger um "ja" auszudrücken.

(Phonetic)

Ha-loh! Ich möhh'tuh ee'nuhn hel'fuhn. Ich shpre'huh kīn doitsh, ah'buhr ich ver'duh dee'zuhs bookh bā-nüt'zuhn um zee ī'ni-guhs tsoo frah'guhn. Ich ver'duh ee'ruh ant'vor-tuhn nihht fer-shtay'uhn. Dās-halb' ant'vor-tuhn zee meer in-dām' zee ee'ruhn kopf shü'tln ō'der hāb'uhn zee ee'ruhn fing'uhr um nīn ows'tsoo-drük-uhn; nick'uhn zee mit dām kopf ō'der hāb'uhn zee tsvī fing'uhr um ya ows'tsoo-drük-uhn.

The Interpreter in Five Languages

GENERAL

Basic Questions and Replies

English	*Spanish*	*Italian*	*French*	*German*
Good morning.	Buenos días.	Buon giorno.	Bonjour.	Guten Morgen.
What is your name?	¿Cómo se llama?	Come si chiama Lei?	Quel est votre nom?	Wie heissen Sie?
How old are you?	¿Cuántos años tiene?	Quanti anni ha?	Quel âge avez-vous?	Wie alt sind Sie?
Do you understand me?	¿Me entiende?	Mi capisce?	Me comprenez-vous?	Verstehen Sie mich?
Answer only . . .	Conteste solamente . . .	Risponda solamente . . .	Répondez seulement . . .	Antworten Sie nur . . .
Yes No	Sí No	Si No	Oui Non	Ja Nein
What do you say?	¿Qué dice?	Cosa dice?	Que dites-vous?	Was sagen Sie?
Speak slower.	Hable más despacio.	Parli più adaggio.	Parlez plus lentement.	Sprechen Sie langsamer.
Say it once again.	Repítalo, por favor.	Lo dica ancora una volta.	Répétez ça.	Wiederholen Sie das.
Don't be afraid.	No tenga miedo.	Non abbia paura.	N'ayez pas peur.	Haben Sie keine Angst.
Try to recollect.	Trate de recordar.	Cerchi di ricordarsi.	Cherchez à vous en rappeler.	Versuchen Sie sich zu erinnern.
You cannot remember?	¿No recuerda?	Non si ricorda?	Ne vous en souvenez pas?	Können Sie sich nicht erinnern?
Come to my office.	Venga a mi oficina.	Venga al mio ufficio.	Venez à mon bureau.	Kommen Sie in mein sprechzimmer
Please remove all your clothes.	Por favor, desvístase completamente.	Per cortesia, si spogli.	Veuillex-vous déshabiller.	Ziehen Sie sich bitte ganz aus.
You will?	¿Ud. quiere?*	Desidera?	Vous voulez bien?	Sie wollen?
You will not?	¿No quiere Ud.?	Non desidera?	Vous ne voulez pas?	Sie wollen nicht?
You don't know?	¿No sabe?	Non sa?	Vous ne savez pas?	Wissen Sie nicht?

*Ud.—Usted.

The Interpreter in Five Languages (*Continued*)

English	*Spanish*	*Italian*	*French*	*German*
Is it impossible?	¿Es imposible?	È impossible?	C'est impossible?	Ist es unmöglich?
It is necessary.	Es necesario.	È necessario.	C'est necéssaire.	Es ist unbedingt nötig.
That is right.	Está bien.	Va bene.	C'est bien.	Das ist richtig.
Show me . . .	Enséñeme . . .	Mi faccia vedere . . .	Montrez-moi . . .	Zeigen Sie mir . . .
Here There	Aquí Allí	Qui Qua	Ici Là	Hier Da
Which side?	¿En qué lado?	Quale lato?	Quel côté?	Auf welcher Seite?
Since when?	¿Desde cuándo?	Da quando?	Depuis quand?	Seit wann?
Right	Derecha	A destra	A droit	Rechts
Left	Izquierda	A sinistra	A gauche	Links
More or less	Más o menos	Più o meno	Plus ou moins	Mehr oder weniger
How long?	¿Cuánto tiempo?	Da quanto tempo?	Combien de temps?	Wie lange?
Not much	No mucho	Non molto	Pas beaucoup	Nicht viel
Try again.	Trate otra vez.	Provi di nuovo.	Essayez encore une fois.	Versuchen Sie es noch ein mal.
Never	Nunca	Mai	Jamais	Niemals
Never mind.	Olvídelo.	Non importa.	Ça ne fait rien.	Lassen Sie es gut sein.
That will do.	Suficiente.	Basta così.	Ça suffit.	Das ist genug.
About how much daily?	¿Más o menos qué cantidad diaramente?	Circa quanto al giorno?	A peu près combien par jour?	Ungefahr wie viel täglich?
So much?	¿Tanto?	Tanto?	Autant?	So viel?
You must be very careful.	Tiene que tener mucho cuidado.	Deve usare molte precauzioni.	Vous devez prendre garde.	Sie müssen sehr vorsichtig sein.

Seasons

In the spring.	En la primavera.	Nella primavera.	Au printemps.	Im Frühjahr.

In summer.	En el verano.	Nell' estate.	En été	Im Sommer.
In autumn.	En el otoño.	Nell' autunno.	En automne.	Im Herbst.
In winter.	En el invierno.	Nell' inverno.	En hiver.	Im Winter.

Months

The months	Los meses	I mesi	Les mois	Die Monate
January	enero	gennaio	janvier	Januar
February	febrero	febbraio	février	Februar
March	marzo	marzo	mars	März
April	abril	aprile	avril	April
May	mayo	maggio	mai	Mai
June	junio	giugno	juin	Juni
July	julio	luglio	juillet	Juli
August	agosto	agosto	août	August
September	septiembre	settembre	septembre	September
October	octubre	ottobre	octobre	Oktober
November	noviembre	novembre	novembre	November
December	diciembre	dicembre	décembre	Dezember

Days of the Week

Sunday	domingo	domenica	dimanche	Sonntag
Monday	lunes	lunedì	lundi	Montag
Tuesday	martes	martedì	mardi	Dienstag
Wednesday	miércoles	mercoledì	mercredi	Mittwoch
Thursday	jueves	giovedì	jeudi	Donnerstag
Friday	viernes	venerdì	vendredi	Freitag
Saturday	sábado	sabato	samedi	Sonnabend

The Interpreter in Five Languages (*Continued*)

English	*Spanish*	*Italian*	*French*	*German*
Numbers and Time of Day (office hours, age, diagnosis, treatment)				
One	Uno	Uno	Un	Eins
Two	Dos	Due	Deux	Zwei
Three	Tres	Tre	Trois	Drei
Four	Cuatro	Quattro	Quatre	Vier
Five	Cinco	Cinque	Cinq	Fünf
Six	Seis	Sei	Six	Sechs
Seven	Siete	Sette	Sept	Sieben
Eight	Ocho	Otto	Huit	Acht
Nine	Nueve	Nove	Neuf	Neun
Ten	Diez	Dieci	Dix	Zehn
Twenty	Veinte	Venti	Vingt	Zwanzig
Thirty	Treinta	Trenta	Trente	Dreissig
Forty	Cuarenta	Quaranta	Quarante	Vierzig
Fifty	Cincuenta	Cinquanta	Cinquante	Fünfzig
Sixty	Sesenta	Sessanta	Soixante	Sechzig
Seventy	Setenta	Settanta	Soixante-dix	Siebzig
At 10:00	A las diez	Alle dieci	A dix heures	Um zehn Uhr
At 2:30	A las dos y media	Alle due e mezzo	A deux heures et demie	Um halb drei
Early in the morning	Temprano por la mañana	Di buon mattino	De bon matin	Frühmorgens
In the daytime	En el día	Durante il giorno	Pendant la journée	Bei Tag
At noon	A mediodía	A mezzo giorno	A midi	Mittags
At bedtime	Al acostarse	All' ora di coricarsi	A l'heure de se coucher	Vor dem Schlafengehen
At night	Por la noche	Alla sera	Le soir	Abends

Before meals	Antes de las comidas	Prima del pasto	Avant les repas	Vor den Mahlzeiten
After meals	Después de las comidas	Dopo il pasto	Après les repas	Nach den Mahlzeiten
Today	Hoy	Oggi	Aujourd'hui	Heute
Tomorrow	Mañana	Domani	Demain	Morgen
Every day	Todos los días	Ogni giorno	Chaque jour	Jeden Tag
Every hour	Cada hora	Ogni ora	Chaque heure	Jede Stunde
How long have you felt this way?	¿Desde cuándo se siente así?	Da quanto tempo si sente così?	Depuis quand vous sentez-vous comme ça?	Seit wann fühlen Sie sich so?
It came all of a sudden?	¿Vino de repente?	Venne tutto ad un tratto?	Ça vous est arrivé tout à coup?	Ist es ganz plötzlich gekommen?
For how many days or weeks?	¿Cuántos días o semanas?	Da quanti giorni o settimane?	Depuis combien de jours ou semaines?	Seit wievielen Tagen oder Wochen?
Do they come every day?	¿Los tiene todos los días?	Le vengono tutti i giorni?	Ça vous gêne tous le jours?	Kommt es jeden Tag?
At the same hour?	¿A la misma hora?	Alla stessa ora?	A la même heure?	Zur selben Stunde?
At intervals?	¿De vez en cuando?	Ad intervalli?	De temps à autre?	Dann und wann?
It will be too late.	Será demasiado tarde.	Sarà troppo tardi.	Çe sera trop tard.	Es wird zu spät sein.

Colors

Black	Negro	Nero	Noir	Schwarz
Blue	Azul	Blu	Bleu	Blau
Green	Verde	Verde	Vert	Grün
Pink	Rosado	Rosa	Rose	Rosa
Red	Rojo	Rosso	Rouge	Rot
White	Blanco	Bianco	Blanc	Weiss
Yellow	Amarillo	Giallo	Jaune	Gelb

Parts of Body

In the abdomen?	¿En el vientre?	Nel ventre?	Dans le abdomen?	Im Leib?

The Interpreter in Five Languages (*Continued*)

English	*Spanish*	*Italian*	*French*	*German*
The ankle	El tobillo	La caviglia	La cheville	Das Fussgelenk
The arm	El brazo	Il braccio	Le bras	Der Arm
The back	La espalda	Il dorso	Le dos	Der Rücken
The bones	Los huesos	La ossa	Le os	Die Knochen
The chest	El pecho	Il petto	La poitrine	Die Brust
The ears	Los oídos	Le orecchie	Les oreilles	Die Ohren
The elbow	El codo	Il gomito	Le coude	Der Ellenbogen
The eye	El ojo	L'occhio	L'oeil	Das Auge
The foot	El pie	Il piede	Le pied	Der Fuss
The gums	Las encías	Le gengive	Les gengives	Das Zahnfleisch
The hand	La mano	La mano	La main	Die Hand
The head	La cabeza	La testa	La tête	Der Kopf
The heart	El corazón	Il cuore	Le coeur	Das Herz
The leg	La pierna	La gamba	La jambe	Das Bein
The liver	El hígado	Il fegato	Le foie	Die Leber
The lungs	Los pulmones	I polmoni	Les poumons	Die Lungen
The mouth	La boca	La bocca	La bouche	Der Mund
The muscles	Los músculos	I muscoli	Les muscles	Die Muskeln
The neck	El cuello	Il collo	Le cou	Der Nacken
The nerves	Los nervios	I nervi	Les nerfs	Die Nerven
The nose	La nariz	Il naso	Le nez	Die Nase
The ribs	Las costillas	Le costole	Les côtes	Die Rippen
The shoulder blades	Las paletillas	Le scapole	Les omoplates	Die Schulterblätter
The side	El flanco	Il fianco	Le côté	Die Seite
The skin	La piel	La pelle	La peau	Die Haut

The skull	El cráneo	Il cranio	Le crâne	Der Schädel
The stomach	El estómago	Lo stomaco	L'estomac	Der Magen
The teeth	Los dientes	I denti	Les dents	Die Zähne
The temples	Las sienes	Le tempie	Les tempes	Die Schläfen
The thigh	El muslo	La coscia	La cuisse	Der Oberschenkel
The throat	La garganta	La gola	La gorge	Der Hals
The thumb	El dedo pulgar	Il pollice	Le pouce	Der Daumen
The tongue	La lengua	La lingua	La langue	Die Zunge
The wrist	La muñeca	Il polso	Le poignet	Das Handgelenk

Work History

What work do you do?	¿Cuál es su ocupación?	Che lavoro fa?	Quelle est votre profession?	Was ist Ihr Beruf?
Is it heavy physical work?	¿Es un trabajo corporal pesado?	È un pesante lavoro manuale?	Est-ce que c'est un travail physiquement fatigant?	Ist es eine schwere körperliche Arbeit?
What work have you done?	¿Qué trabajo ha hecho?	Che lavoro ha fatto?	A quoi avez-vous travaillé?	Welche Arbeit haben Sie getan?

HISTORY

Family

Are you married?	¿Es Ud. casado?	È sposato?	Etes-vous marié?	Sind Sie verheiratet?
A widower?	¿Viudo?	È vedovo?	Veuf?	Ein Witwer?
A widow?	¿Viuda?	È vedova?	Veuve?	Eine Witwe?
Do you have children?	¿Tiene Ud. hijos?	Ha bambini?	Avez-vous des enfants?	Haben Sie Kinder?
Are they still living?	¿Viven todavía?	Vivono ancora?	Sont-ils encore vivants?	Leben sie noch?
Do you have any sisters?	¿Tiene hermanas?	Ha sorelle?	Avez-vous des soeurs?	Haben Sie Schwestern?
Do you have any brothers?	¿Tiene hermanos?	Ha fratelli?	Avez-vous des frères?	Haben Sie Brüder?
Of what did your mother die?	¿De qué murió su madre?	Di checosa è morta Sua mamma?	De quoi est morte votre mère?	Woran ist Ihre Mutter gestorben?

The Interpreter in Five Languages (*Continued*)

English	*Spanish*	*Italian*	*French*	*German*
And your father?	¿Y su padre?	E Suo padre?	Et votre père?	Und Ihr Vater?
Your grandfather?	¿Su abuelo?	Suo nonno?	Votre grand-père?	Ihr Grossvater?
Your grandmother?	¿Su abuela?	Sua nonna?	Votre grand-mère?	Ihre Grossmutter?
		General		
Do you have . . . ?	¿Tiene . . . ?	Ha Lei	Avez-vous . . . ?	Haben Sie . . . ?
Have you ever had . . . ?	¿Ha tenido . . . ?	Ha mai avuto . . . ?	Avez-vous jamais eu . . . ?	Haben Sie je . . . gehabt?
Chills	Escalofrios	I brividi	Les frissons	Ein Fieberfrösteln
An attack of fever	Un ataque de calentura	Un attacco di febbre	Une attaque de fièvre	Ein Fieberanfall
Toothache	Dolor de muelas	Mal di denti	Le mal aux dents	Zahnschmerzen
Hemorrhage	Hemorragia	Emorragia	De hémorragie	Die Blutergüsse
Nosebleeds	Hemorragia por la nariz	Emorragia nasale	Saignements de nez	Das Nasenbluten
Unusual vaginal bleeding	Hemorragia vaginal fuera de los periodos	Perdite di sangue irregulari dalla vagina	Du saignement vaginal anormal	Jemals unregelmässiges bluten aus der Scheide
When did you last have a period?	¿Cuándo tuvo Ud. su última menstruación?	Quando ha avuto l'ultima volta le menstruazione?	Quand avez-vous eu vos régles pour la dernière fois?	Wann war die letze Menstruation?
Do you take birth control pills?	¿Toma. Ud. píldoras anticonceptvas	Prende pillole contro la gravibanza	Est-ce que vous prenez des médicaments anti-conceptionnels?	Nehmen Sie Geburtskontroll-pillen?
Hoarseness	Ronquera	Raucedine	Enrouement	Heiserkeit
		Diseases		
What diseases have you had?	¿Qué enfermedades ha tenido?	Che malattie ha avuto?	Quelles maladies avez-vous eues?	Welche Krankheiten haben Sie gehabt?
Allergy	Alergia	Allergie	· Une maladie allergique	Überempfindlichkeiten

Anemia	Anemia	Anemia	L'anémie	Blutarmut
Bleeding tendency	Tendencia a sangrar	Tendenza alle emorragie	Une tendance à saigner	Neigung zum Bluten
Cancer	Cáncer	Cancro	Le cancer	Krebs
Chicken pox	Varicela	Varicella	La varicelle	Windpocken
Diabetes	Diabetes	Diabete	Le diabète	Zuckerkranckheit
Diphtheria	Difteria	Difterite	La diphthérie	Diphtherie
German measles	Rubéola	Rosolia	Rubeole	Röteln
Gonorrhea	Gonorrea	Gonorrea	La gonorrhée	Gonorrhöe, Tripper
Heart disease	Enfermedad del corazón	Malattia di cuore	Une maladie de coeur	Herzkrankheit
High blood pressure	Presíon sanguínea elevada	Pressione alta del sangue	La tension arterielle trop élevée	Hohen Blutdruck
Influenza	Gripe (influenza)	Influenza	La grippe	Grippe
Lead poisoning	Envenenamiento con plomo	Avvelenamento da piombo	Empoisonnement causé par le plomb	Bleivergiftung
Liver disease	Enfermedad del hígado	Una malattia del fegato	Une maladie de foie	Eine Leberkrankheit
Malaria	Malaria (paludismo)	Malaria	La malaria	Malaria
Measles	Sarampión	Morbillo	La rougeole	Die Masern
Mental disease	Enfermedades mentales	Malattie mentali	Une maladie mentale	Geisteskrankheit
Mumps	Paperas	Orecchioni	Les oreillons	Mumps
Nervous disease	Enfermedades nerviosas	Malattie nervose	Une maladie nerveuse	Nervenkrankheit
Pleurisy	Pleuresía	Pleurite	Une pleurésie	Rippenfellentzündung
Pneumonia	Pulmonía	Polmonite	Pneumonie	Die Lungenentzündung
Rheumatic fever	Reumatismo (fiebre reumática)	Febbre reumatica	La fièvre rhumatismale	Rheumatisches Fieber
Rheumatism	Reumatismo	Reumatismo	Le rhumatisme	Der Rheumatismus
Scarlet fever	Escarlatina	Febre scarlattina	La fièvre scarlatine	Das Scharlachfieber
Smallpox	Viruela	Vaiolo	La variole	Pocken
Syphilis	Sífilis	Sifilide (lue)	La syphilis	Syphilis

The Interpreter in Five Languages (*Continued*)

English	*Spanish*	*Italian*	*French*	*German*
Tuberculosis	Tuberculosis	Tuberculosi	Tuberculose	Die Tuberkulose
Typhoid fever	Tifoidea	Febre il tifo	La fièvre typhoide	Der Typhus

EXAMINATION

General

How do you feel?	¿Cómo se siente?	Come stà?	Comment vous sentez-vous?	Wie fühlen Sie sich?
Good	Bien	Bene	Bien	Gut
Bad	Mal	Male	Mal	Schlecht
Let me see . . .	Déjeme ver . . .	Mi lasci vedere . . .	Permettez-moi de voir . . .	Lassen Sie mich sehen . . .
Let me feel your pulse.	Déjeme tomarle el pulso.	Mi lasci sentire il polso.	Permettez-moi de vous tâter le pouls.	Lassen Sie mich Ihren Puls fühlen.
Whisper: one, two, three.	Repita en voz baja: uno, dos, tres.	Dica piano: uno, due, tre.	Dites tout bas: un, deux, trois.	Flüstern Sie: eins, zwei, drei.
Say it out loud.	Dígalo en voz alta.	Lo dica ad alta voce.	Dites-le à voix haute.	Sagen Sie es laut.
Sit down.	Siéntese.	Si sieda.	Asseyez-vous.	Setzen Sie sich.
Stand up.	Levántese.	Si alzi.	Levez-vous.	Stehen Sie auf.
Can you not rise quicker?	¿No puede levantarse más rápidamente?	Non si puō alzare un po' più presto?	Vous ne pouvez pas vous lever plus vite?	Können Sie sich nicht schneller erheben?
Walk a little way.	Ande algunos pasos.	Cammini un po'.	Faites quelques pas.	Gehen Sie einige Schritte.
Return; go backwards.	Vuelva; ande para atrás.	Ritorni; cammini all' indietro.	Revenez; allez à retours.	Kommen Sie zurück; gehen Sie rückwärts.
Do you feel like falling?	¿Le parece que se va a caer?	Si sente come se dovesse cadere?	Vous sentez vous comme si vous allez tomber?	Ist es Ihnen als ob Sie fallen werden?
Do you feel dizzy?	¿Tiene Ud. vértigo?	Ha delle vertigini?	Avez-vous le vertige?	Ist Ihnen schwindlig?
Are you tired?	¿Está Ud. cansado?	Si sente molto stanco?	Êtes vous fatigué?	Sind Sie müde?

Have you slept well?	¿Ha dormido bien?	Ha dormito bene?	Avez-vous bien dormi?	Haben Sie gut geschlafen?
Have you any difficulty in breathing?	¿Tiene dificultad al respirar?	**Ha difficoltà di respirare?**	C'est difficile à respirer?	**Fällt Ihnen das Atemholen** schwer?
Have you lost weight?	¿Ha perdido Ud. peso?	É dimagrito?	Avez-vous maigri?	Haben Sie abgenommen?
Since when have you had this eruption?	¿Desde cuándo tiene esta erupción?	Da quanto ha questa eruzione?	Depuis quand avez-vous cette erúption?	Seit wann haben Sie diesen Ausschlag?
Do you sweat much at night?	¿Suda mucho por la noche?	Suda molto alla notte?	Transpirez-vous beaucoup pendant la nuit?	Schwitzen Sie viel in der Nacht?
Are you warm?	¿Tiene calor?	Ha caldo?	Avez-vous chaud?	Ist Ihnen heiss?
Are you cold?	¿Tiene frío?	Ha freddo?	Avez-vous froid?	Ist Ihnen kalt?
Have you been exposed much to the wet weather?	¿Ha estado expuesto a la intemperie?	Si è mai esposto all' umidità?	Avez-vous été **longtemp sous la pluie**?	Sind Sie dem feuchten Wetter ausgesetzt gewesen?
Can you eat?	¿Puede comer?	Può mangiare?	Pouvez-vous manger?	Können Sie essen?
Have you a good appetite?	¿Tiene Ud. buen apetito?	Ha buon appetito?	Avez-vous un bon appétit?	Haben Sie guten Appetit?
Are you thirsty?	¿Tiene sed?	Ha sete?	Avez-vous soif?	Haben Sie Durst?
Do you still feel very weak?	¿Se siente muy débil todavía?	Si sente ancora molto débole?	Vous sentez-vous encore très faible?	Fühlen Sie sich noch sehr schwach?
Had you been drinking?	**¿Había tomado alguna bebida alcohólica?**	Ha bevüto?	Est-ce que vous-aviez bu quelque chose d'alcoolique?	Waren Sie angetrunken?
Are you a drinking man?	¿Toma Ud. bebidas alcohólicas habitualmente?	Ha l'abitudine di bere?	Buyez-vous des choses alcoolìques d'habitude?	Sind Sie em Trinker?
Are you nervous?	¿Está Ud. nervioso?	É nervoso?	Etes-vous nerveux?	Sind Sie nervös?
When were you first taken sick?	¿Cuándo le empezó esta enfermedad?	Quando si è ammalato la prima volta?	Quand êtes-vous tombé malade d'abord?	Wann hat diese Krankheit begonnen?
How did this illness begin?	¿Cómo empezó esta enfermedad?	Come ha incominciato questa malattia?	Comment cette maladie a-t-elle commencé?	Wie hat diese Krankheit begonnen?
Did you take anything for it?	¿Tomó algo para mejorarla?	Ha preso qual cosa per curarsi?	Avez-vous pris quelque chose pour cela?	Haben Sie etwas dafür genommen?

The Interpreter in Five Languages (*Continued*)

English	*Spanish*	*Italian*	*French*	*German*
Have you taken the medicine?	¿Ha tomado Ud. la medicina?	Ha preso la medicina?	Avez-vous pris la medicament?	Haben Sie die Medizin genommen?
A wound	Una herida	Una piaga	Une plaie	Eine Wunde
Are you subject to them?	¿Lo sucede a menudo?	Ne è soggetto?	Ça vous gêne souvent?	Haben Sie dieselben häufig?
Did a dog bite you?	¿Lo mordió un perro?	L'ha morsicato un cane?	Est-ce qu'un chien vous a mordu?	Hat Sie eine Hund gebissen?
Did a fly sting you?	¿Lo picó una mosca?	L'ha punto una mosca?	Est-ce qu'une mouche vous a piqué?	Hat Sie eine Fliege gestochen?
Did you prick yourself with a pin?	¿Se ha pinchado con un alfiler?	Si è punto con una spilla?	Vous êtes-vous piqué avec une épingle?	Haben Sie sich mit einer Stecknadel gestochen?
Did you burn yourself?	¿Se quemó?	Si è bruciato?	Vous êtes-vous brulé?	Haben Sie sich verbrannt?
Did you sprain your foot?	¿Se torció el pie?	Si ha dislocato un piede?	Vous êtes-vous fait une entorse au pied?	Haben Sie Ihren Fuss verstaucht?

Pain

English	*Spanish*	*Italian*	*French*	*German*
Have you any pain?	¿Tiene dolor?	Ha dolori?	Avez-vous mal quelque?	Haben Sie Schmerzen?
Where does it hurt?	¿Dónde le duele?	Dove le duele?	Où avez-vous mal?	Wo haben Sie Schmerzen?
Do you have pain here?	¿Le duele aquí?	Ha dolori qui?	Avez-vous mal par ici?	Haben Sie Schmerzen hier?
Do you have a pain in your side?	¿Le duele el costado?	Avete dolori al fianco?	Avez-vous mal au côté?	Haben Sie Seitenstechen?
Show me where.	Enséñeme dónde.	Mi mostri dove.	Montrez-moi où.	Zeigen Sie mir wo.
What did you feel in the beginning?	¿Qué sentía cuando empezó?	Che sentiva al principio?	Qu'avez-vous senti au commencement?	Was haben Sie anfangs gespürt?
Shooting pains?	¿Dolores agudos?	Dei dolori acuti?	Des elancements?	Stechende Schmerzen?
As if one were pricking you with pins?	¿Como si estuvieran pinchándole con alfileres?	Come se fossero delle spille?	Comme si l'on vous piquâit avec des épingles?	Als ob man Sie mit Stecknadeln stäche?
Did you feel much pain at the time?	¿Sintió mucho dolor entonces?	Avete sentito molto dolore allora?	Est-ce que ça vous a fait beaucoup de mal alors?	Haben Sie gleich damals arge Schmerzen gespürt?

Is it worse now?	¿Está peor ahora?	È peggio ora?	Est-ce que c'est encore pire maintenant?	Ist es jetzt schlimmer?
Does it still pain you?	¿Le duele todavía?	Fa male ancora?	Est-ce que ça vous fait mal toujours?	Schmerzt er noch?
Do you still have that heavy pain?	¿Le duele mucho todavía?	Ha ancora quel dolore pesante?	Avez-vous toujours la douleur pesante?	Haben Sie noch den drückenden Schmerz?
Does it pain you to breathe?	¿Le duele al respirar?	Le fa male respirare?	Votre respiration est-elle douloureuse?	Spüren Sie Schmerzen beim Atmen?

Head

How does your head feel?	¿Cómo siente la cabeza?	Come si sente la testa?	Comment va votre tête?	Wie geht es Ihrem Kopf?
Your memory	Su memoria	La sua memoria	Votre mémoire	Ihr Gedächtnis
Is it good?	¿Es buena?	È buona?	Est-elle bonne?	Ist es gut?
Have you any pain in the head?	¿Le duele la cabeza?	Ha dolor di testa?	Avez-vous mal à la tête?	Haben Sie Kopfschmerzen?
Did you fall and how did you fall?	¿Se cayó, y cómo se cayó?	È caduto, e come è caduto?	Etes-vous tombé et comment êtes-vous tombé?	Sind Sie gefallen und wie sind Sie gefallen?
Did you faint?	¿Se desmayó?	È svenuto?	Vous êtes-vous évanoui?	Sind Sie ohnmächtig geworden?
Have you ever had fainting spells?	¿Ha tenido desmayos alguna vez?	È mai svenuto regolarmente?	Avez-vous jamais eu des évanouissements?	Haben Sie jemals Ohnmachtsanfälle gehabt?

Ears

Do you have ringing in the ears?	¿Le pitan los oídos?	Le tentennano le orecchie?	Avez-vous des bourdonnements d'oreilles?	Haben Sie Ohrenbrausen?
Do you have discharge from the ears?	¿Le supuran los oídos?	Le esce materia dalle orecchie?	Est-ce que vous avez un écoulement des oreilles?	Eitern Ihre Ohren?
The hearing	El oído	L'udito	L'ouïe	Das Gehör
Is it affected?	¿Está afectado?	È compromesso?	Est-elle changée?	Ist es angegriffen?

English	*Spanish*	*Italian*	*French*	*German*
		Eyes		
Look up.	Mire para arriba.	Guardi sù.	Regardez en haut.	Schauen Sie hinauf.
Look down.	Mire para abajo.	Guardi giu.	Regardez en bas.	Schauen Sie hinunter.
Look toward your nose.	Mire la nariz.	Si guardi il naso.	Regardez le nez.	Schauen Sie auf Ihre Nase.
Look at me.	Míreme.	Mi guardi.	Regardez-moi.	Sehen Sie mich an.
Can you see what is on the wall?	¿Puede ver lo que está en la pared?	Può vedere cosa c'e sui muro?	Pouvez-vous voir ce qu'il y a contre le mur?	Können Sie sehen was hier an der Wand ist?
You cannot?	¿No puede?	Non può?	Vous ne pouvez pas?	Können Sie es nicht erkennen?
Can you see it now?	¿Puede verlo ahora?	Può vederlo adesso?	Le voyez-vous maintenant?	Können Sie es jetzt sehen?
And now?	¿Y ahora?	Ed ora?	Et maintenant?	Und nun?
What is it?	¿Qué es ésto?	Che cosa è?	Qu'est-ce que c'est?	Was ist es?
Tell me what number it is?	Dígame qué número es éste.	Mi dica che numero è.	Dites-moi quel est le numéro.	Sagen Sie mir welche Nummer es ist.
Tell me what letter it is.	Dígame qué letra es ésta.	Mi dica che lettera è.	Dites-moi quelle est la lettre.	Nennen Sir mir diesen Buchstaben.
Do you see things through a mist?	¿Ve las cosas a travès de una niebla?	Vede le cose come se fossero fra la nebbia?	Voyez-vous les choses à travers d'un brouillard?	Sehen Sie alles durch einen Nebel?
Can you see clearly?	¿Puede ver claramente?	Può vedere chiaro?	Pouvez-vous voir clairement?	Sehen Sie deutlich?
Better at a distance?	¿Mejor a cierta distancia?	Meglio a distanza?	Mieux à distance?	Besser aus der Entfernung?
Do your eyes water a good deal?	¿Le lagrimean mucho los ojos?	Le lacrimano molto gli occhi?	Est-ce que les yeux vous coulent beaucoup?	Tränen Ihre Augen stark?
Can't you open your eye?	¿No puede abrir el ojo?	Non puo aprire l'occhio?	Ne pouvez-vous pas ouvrir l'oeil?	Können Sie Ihr Auge nicht öffnen?
Do not try to open it when you awaken.	No trate de abrirlo al despertarse.	Quando si sveglia si forzi ad aprirlo.	N'essayez pas de l'ouvrir en vous réveillent.	Versuchen Sie nicht, es beim Aufwachen zu öffnen.

Did anything get into your eye?	¿Le entró algo en el ojo?	Le è entrata qualche cosa nell'occhio?	Est-ce que quelque chose est entré dans l'oeil?	Ist Ihnen etwas ins Auge geflogen?
Do you sometimes see things double?	¿Ve las cosas doble algunas veces.	Vede qualche volta le cose doppie?	Est-ce que la vue est double parfois?	Sehen Sie manchmal doppelt?
Does the eyeball feel as if it were swollen?	¿Le parece que el ojo está hinchado?	Le sembra che l'occhio sia gonfio?	L'oeil vous semble-t-il gonflé?	Fühlt sich das Auge wie geschwollan?
You must be careful not to go out yet.	Tenga cuidado de no salir todavía.	Deve aver cura a non andar fuori.	Gardez vous de sortir maintenant.	Sie dürfen durchaus noch nicht ausgehen.
It would harm your eyes.	Le haría daño a los ojos.	Le farà male agli occhi.	Cela vous abîmerait les yeux.	Es würde Ihren Augen schaden.
Since when has your eyesight failed you?	¿Desde cuando ha disminuido su vista?	Da quanto tempo la sua vista È diminuita?	Depuis quand votre vue s'est-elle diminuée?	Seit wann hat Ihre Sehkraft nachgelassen?

Throat and Mouth

Cough.	Tosa.	Tossisca.	Toussez.	Husten Sie.
Cough again.	Tosa otra vez.	Tossisca ancora.	Toussez encore une fois.	Husten Sie noch einmal.
Open your mouth.	Abra la boca.	Apra la bocca.	Ouvrez la bouche.	Öffnen Sie den Mund.
Does it hurt you to open your mouth?	¿Le duele al abrir la boca?	Le fa male aprir la bocca?	Ouvrir la bouche vous fait-il mal?	Spüren Sie Schmerzen wenn Sie den Mund offnen?
Since when do you cough?	¿Desde cuándo tose Ud?	Da quando ha la tosse?	Depuis quand avez-vous la toux?	Seit wann husten Sie?
You cough a little?	¿Tose poco?	Tossisca pocco?	Toussez-vous un peu?	Husten Sie manchmal?
Take a deep breath.	Respire profundamente.	Prenda un gran respiro.	Respirez profondement.	Atmen Sie tief.
Do you expectorate much?	¿Escupe mucho?	Sputa molto?	Crachez-vous beaucoup?	Spucken Sie viel aus?
What is the color of your expectorations?	¿De qué color es el esputo?	Di che color lo sputo?	De quelle sont vos crachats?	Welche Farbe hat der Speichel?
Does your tongue feel swollen?	¿Siente Ud. la lengua hinchada?	Ha la lingua gonfia?	Est-ce que la langue vous paraît gonflée?	Fühlt sich Ihre Zunge wie geschwollenan?
Do you have a sore throat?	¿Le duele la garganta?	Ha mal di gola?	Avez-vous mal à la gorge?	Haben Sie Halsschmerzen?
Does it hurt to swallow?	¿Le duele al tragar?	Quando ingoia le fa male?	Ça vous fait mal à avaler?	Spüren Sie Schmerzen beim Schlucken?

The Interpreter in Five Languages (*Continued*)

English	*Spanish*	*Italian*	*French*	*German*
		Arms and Hands		
Let me see your hand.	Enséñeme la mano.	Mi faccia vedere la sua mano.	Montrez-moi la main.	Zeigen Sie mir Ihre Hand.
Have you no power in it?	¿No tiene fuerza en la mano?	Non ha forza nella mano?	Est-elle complètement inerte?	Ist sie ganz kraftlos?
Grasp my hand.	Apriete mi mano.	Mi stringa la mano.	Serrez-moi la main.	Drücken Sie mir die Hand.
Can you not do it better than that?	¿No puede hacerlo más fuerte?	Non può far meglio?	Vous ne pouvez-pas serrer plus fort que cela?	Können Sie nicht fester greifen?
Your arm feels paralyzed?	¿Parece que el brazo está paralizado?	Si sente il braccio paralizzato?	Est-ce que le bras vous paraît paralysé?	Ihr Arm erscheint Ihnen gelähmt?
Raise your arm.	Levante el brazo.	Alzi il braccio.	Levez le bras.	Heben Sie den Arm.
Raise it more.	Más alto.	Ancora di più.	Plus haut.	Höher.
Now the other.	Ahora el otro.	Adesso l'altro.	Maintenant l'autre.	Jetzt den andern.
Since when is your arm so powerless?	Desde cuándo no tiene fuerza en el brazo?	Da quando il suo braccio è senza forza?	Depuis quand votre bras a-t-il perdu la force?	Seit wann ist Ihr Arm so kraftlos?
Had you been sleeping on your arm?	¿Ha dormido encima del brazo?	Ha dormito col braccio sotto la testa?	Vous êtes-vous endormi sur le bras?	Sind Sie auf Ihrem Arm eingeschlafen?
		Gastrointestinal		
Do you have stomach cramps?	¿Tiene calambres en el estómago?	Ha dei dolori acuti allo stomaco?	Avez-vous des crampes de l'estomac?	Haben Sie Magenkrämpfe?
Since when is your tongue that color?	¿Desde cuándo tiene la lengua de ese color?	Da quando la sua lingua è di questo colore?	Depuis quand votre langue a-t-elle cette couleur?	Seit wann hat Ihre Zunge diese Farbe?
Have you a pain in the pit of your stomach?	¿Tiene dolor en la boca del estómago?	Ha dei dolori alla bocca dello stomaco?	Est-ce que ça vous fait mal dans le creux de l'estomac?	Haben Sie Schmerzen in der Magengrube?

Nausea	Náusea	La nausea	La nausée	Die Übelkeit
Does eating make you vomit?	¿El comer le hace vomitar?	Vomita dopo aver manginto?	Rendez-vous ce que vous mangez?	Erbrechen Sie nachdem Sie gegessen haben?
How are your stools?	¿Cómo son sus defecaciones?	Come va di corpo?	Comment allez-vous à la selle?	Wie ist der Stuhlgang?
Are they regular?	¿Son regulares?	Va regolarmente?	Allez-vous à la selle régulièrment?	Ist er regelmässig?
Have you noticed their color?	¿Se ha fijado en el color?	Si è accorto di che colore?	Avez-vous remarqué la couleur de vos selles?	Haben Sie auf die Farbe geachtet?
Are you constipated?	¿Está estreñido?	È stitico?	Etes-vous constipé?	Leiden Sie an Verstopfung?
Do you have diarrhea?	¿Tiene diarrea?	Ha diarrea?	Avez-vous la diarrhée?	Haben Sie Durchfall?
Do you pass any blood?	¿Con sangre?	Passa sangue?	Y-a-t-il du sang?	Ist Blut im Stuhl?
Have you vomited?	¿Ha vomitado?	Ha vomitato?	Avez-vous vomi?	Haben Sie erbrochen?
Do you still vomit?	¿Vomita todavía?	Vomita ancora?	Vomissez-vous encore?	Erbrechen Sie noch immer?
Do you vomit blood?	¿Vomita sangre?	Vomita sangue?	Vomissez-vous du sang?	Erbrechen Sie Blut?
Is it of a dark or bright red color?	¿Es de color rojo oscuro o claro?	È di colore rosso chiaro o rosso scuro?	La couleur du sang est elle fonçée ou claire?	Ist es dunkel oder hellrot?

Kidneys

Have you any difficulty passing water?	¿Tiene dificultad en orinar?	Ha della difficoltà nell' urinare?	Avez-vous de la difficulté à uriner?	Haben Sie Schwierigkeiten beim Wasserlassen?
Do you pass water involuntarily?	¿Orina sin querer?	Urina involontariamente?	Urinez-vous involuntaire-ment?	Lassen Sie den Harn ohne es zu wollen?
Are any of your limbs swollen?	¿Están hinchados alguno de sus miembros?	Si sente gonfio in qualche parte?	Avez-vous des membres gonflés?	Ist irgendeines Ihrer Glieder geschwollen?
How long have they been swollen like this?	¿Desde cuándo estan hinchados así?	Da quanto tempo che li ha cosi gonfi?	Depuis quand sont-ils gonflés comme ça?	Seit wann sind sie so angeschwollen?
Were they ever swollen before?	¿Han estado hinchados alguna vez antes?	Sono stati mai gonfi prima?	Ont-ils jamais été gonflés autrefois?	Sind sie je früher so angeschwollen gewesen?

TREATMENT
General

English	*Spanish*	*Italian*	*French*	*German*
It is nothing serious.	No es nada grave.	Non è nulla.	Ce n'est rien de grave.	Es ist nichts ernstliches.
You will get better.	Ud. se mejorará.	Si sentirà meglio.	Vous vous remettrez.	Es wird besser werden.
Do exactly as I tell you.	Haga exactamente lo que le digo.	Faccia estattamente ciò che Le dico.	Faites exactement ce que je vous dis.	Tun Sie genau was ich Ihnen sage.
Take a bath.	Tome un baño.	Si faccia un bagno.	Prenez un bain.	Nehmen Sie ein bad
A sponge bath	Un baño de esponja	Un bagno con la spugna	Un bain à l'éponge	Ein Schwamm bad
A bran bath	Un baño de salvado	Un bagno con crusca	Un bain au son	Ein Kleie bad
A soda bath	Un baño de soda	Un bagno con soda	Un bain à la soude	Ein Soda bad
Bathe with hot water.	Báñese con agua caliente.	Faccia il bagno con acqua calda.	Bagnez-vous dans de l'eau chaude.	Baden Sie mit heissem Wasser.
Bathe with cold water.	Báñese con agua fría.	Si faccia il bagno con acqua fredda.	Baignez-vous dans de l'eau froide.	Baden Sie mit kaltem Wasser.
Bathe with alcohol.	Báñese con alcohol.	Si bagni con alcool.	Baignez-vous avec de l'alcool.	Reiben Sie sich alkoholab.
Paint the swelling with this.	Pinte la hinchazón con esto.	Deve pitturare il gonfiore con questo.	Badigeonnez l'enflure avecceci.	Pinseln Sie die Geschwulst damit.
I will use electricity.	Usaré electricidad.	Userò dell'elettricitá.	Je ferai un traitment a la electricité.	Ich werde elektrischen Strom anwenden.
Apply bandage to . . .	Ponga un vendaje a . . .	Si metta una fasciatura . . .	Mettez un bandage à . . .	Verbinden Sie . . .
Apply ointment	Aplíquese ungüento.	Applichi un unguento.	Appliquez un onguent.	Verwenden Sie Salbe.
Keep very quiet.	Estése muy quieto.	Sia tranquillo.	Restez tranquille.	Verhalten Sie sich sehr ruhig.
You must not speak.	No debe hablar.	Non deve parlare.	Vous ne devez pas parler.	Sie dürfen nicht sprechen.
Swallow small pieces of ice.	Trague pedacitos de hielo.	Ingoi dei pezzettini di ghiaccio.	Avalez de petits morceaux de glace.	Schlucken Sie kleine Eisstücke.

Diet

In a few days you may eat food.	Dentro de algunos días podrá comer.	Fra pochi giorni potrà mangiare.	Après quelques jours vous pouvez prendre de la nourriture.	In einigen Tagen dürfen Sie essen.
And remain on a diet.	Y estar a dieta.	E rimanga a dieta.	Et suivez un régime.	Und Diät halten.
You may eat . . .	Puede comer . . .	Potrà mangiare . . .	Vous pouvez manger . . .	Sie dürfen essen . . .
Two eggs	Dos huevos	Due d'uova	Deux oeufs	Zwei Eier
Toast	Pan tostado	Pane tostato	Du pain grillé	Geröstetes Brot
Bread	Pan	Pane	Du pain	Das Brot
Oysters	Ostras	Delle óstriche	Des huîtres	Die Austern
Chicken	Pollo	Pollo	Du poulet	Das Huhn
You may drink icewater.	Puede tomar agua con hielo.	Lei può bere acqua ghiacciata.	Vous pouvez boir de l'eau glacée.	Sie dürfen Eiswasser trinken.
Milk	Leche	Latte	Du lait	Die Milch
Tea	Té	Il té	Du thé	Der Tee
Coffee	Café	Il caffè	Du café	Der Kaffee
Chocolate	Chocolate	La cioccolatta	Du chocolat	Die Schokolade
Beef bouillon	Caldo de carne	Brodo	Le bouillon	Die Bouillon

Operation

An operation will be necessary.	Tendrá que operarse.	Una operazione è necessaria.	Il faut que l'on fasse une operation.	Eine Operation ist notwendig.
We will operate . . .	Lo operaremos . . .	Opereremo . . .	Nous opérerons . . .	Wir werden operieren . . .

The Interpreter in Five Languages (*Continued*)

English	*Spanish*	*Italian*	*French*	*German*
Medication (use with numbers and time of day)				
I will give you something for that.	Le daré algo para eso.	Le darò qualche cosa per questo.	Je vous donnerai quelque chose pour cela.	Ich werde Ihnen etwas dafür geben.
I will leave a prescription.	Le dejaré una receta.	Lascerò una ricetta.	Je laisserai une ordonnance.	Ich werde Ihnen ein Rezept hierlassen.
Use it regularly.	Tómelo con regularidad.	Lo usi regolarmente.	Servez-vous-en régulièrment.	Gebrauchen Sie es regelmässig.
Take one teaspoonful three times daily (in water).	Tome una cucharadita tres veces al día, con agua.	Ne beva un cucchiaio tre volte al giorno (con acqua).	Prenez-en une petite cuiller trois fois par jour (avec de l'eau).	Nehmen Sie einen Teelöffel voll dreimal taglich (mit Wasser).
Gargle.	Haga gárgaras.	Faccia gargarismi.	Gargarissez-vous.	Gurgeln Sie.
Use injection.	Use una inyección.	Si faccia un iniezione.	Utilises des injections.	Injizieren Sie.
Take a purgative.	Tome una purga.	Un purgante	Prenez une purgative.	Nehmen Sie ein Abführmittel.
A pill	Una píldora	Una pillola	Une pilule	Eine Pille
A powder	Un polvo	Una polverina	Une poudre	Ein Pulver
Drop into one eye.	Vierta gotas en un ojo.	Metta delle gocce nell'occhio	Faites tomber une goutte dans l'oeil.	Träufeln Sie in das eine Auge.
Drop into each eye.	Vierta gotas en cada ojo.	Metta delle gocce in ciascun occhio.	Faites tomber une goutte dans chaque oeil.	Träufeln Sie in beide Augen.

App. 16: Braille Alphabet and Numerals

	Braille		Braille		Braille		Braille
A	⠁	J	⠚	S	⠎	2	⠃
B	⠃	K	⠅	T	⠞	3	⠁
C	⠉	L	⠇	U	⠥	4	⠁
D	⠙	M	⠍	V	⠧	5	⠁
E	⠑	N	⠝	W	⠺	6	⠃
F	⠋	O	⠕	X	⠭	7	⠃
G	⠛	P	⠏	Y	⠽	8	⠃
H	⠓	Q	⠟	Z	⠵	9	⠂
I	⠊	R	⠗	1	⠁	10	⠂

App. 17: American Manual Sign Alphabet

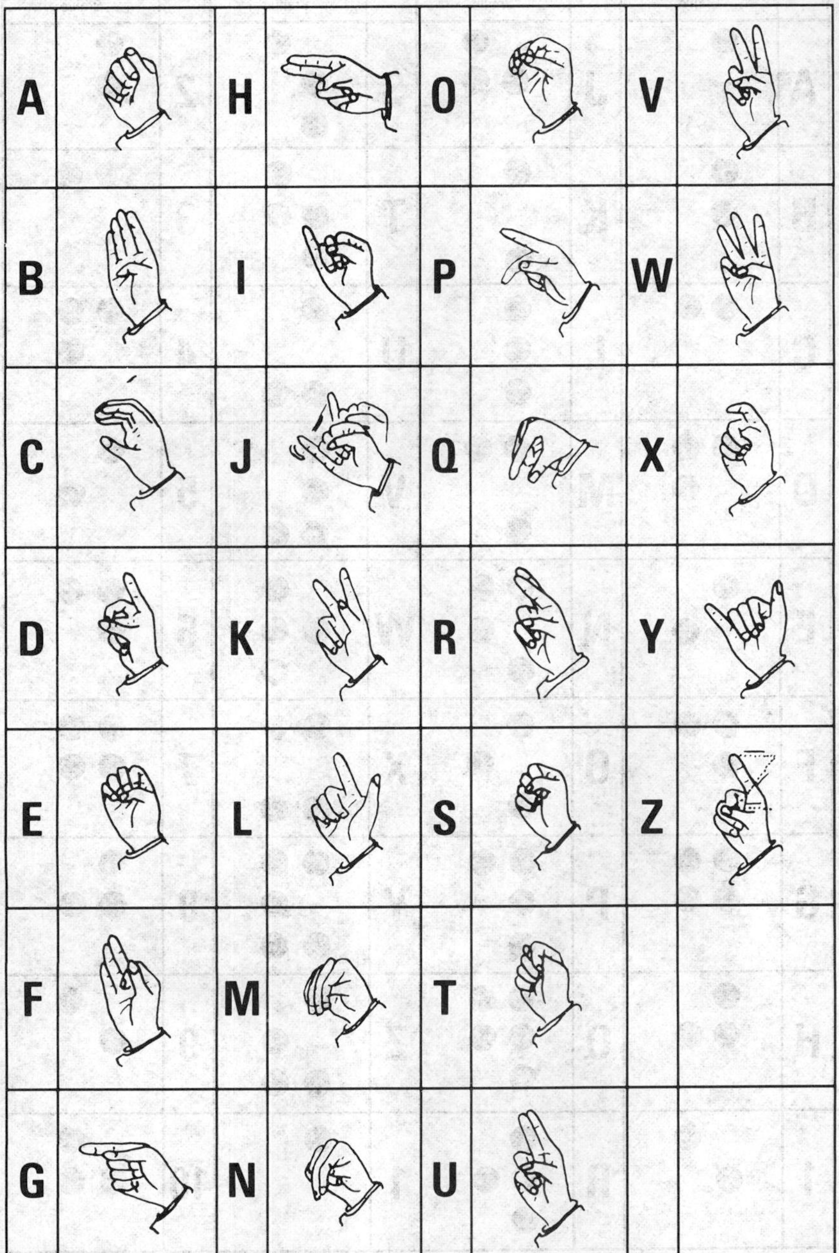

App. 18: Nursing Diagnoses

DIAGNOSTIC DIVISIONS

Nursing diagnoses are categorized for quick reference to assist the nurse in converting nursing problem statements into nursing diagnoses.

ACTIVITY/REST
- Activity intolerance
- Activity intolerance, potential
- Diversional activity, deficit
- Sleep pattern disturbance

CIRCULATION
- Cardiac output, alteration in: decreased
- Tissue perfusion, alteration in (specify)

ELIMINATION
- Bowel elimination, alteration in: constipation
- Bowel elimination, alteration in: diarrhea
- Bowel elimination, alteration in: incontinence
- Incontinence: functional
- Incontinence: reflex
- Incontinence: stress
- Incontinence: total
- Incontinence: urge
- Urinary elimination, alteration in patterns
- Urinary retention [acute/chronic]

EMOTIONAL REACTIONS
- Adjustment, impaired
- Anxiety [specify]
- Coping, ineffective individual
- Fear
- Grieving, anticipatory
- Grieving, dysfunctional
- Hopelessness
- Post-trauma response
- Powerlessness
- Rape trauma syndrome
- Self-concept, disturbance in: body image; self-esteem; personal identity
- Spiritual distress (distress of the human spirit)

FOOD/FLUID
- Fluid volume, alteration in: excess
- Fluid volume deficit, actual 1 [Regulatory failure]
- Fluid volume deficit, actual 2 [Active loss]
- Fluid volume deficit, potential
- Nutrition, alteration in: less than body requirements
- Nutrition, alteration in: more than body requirements
- Nutrition, alteration in: potential for more than body requirements
- Oral mucous membranes, alteration in
- Swallowing, impaired

HYGIENE
- Self-care deficit (specify level: feeding, bathing/hygiene, dressing/grooming, toileting)

NEUROLOGIC
- Communication, impaired: verbal
- Neglect, unilateral
- Sensory-perceptual alteration
- Thought processes, alteration in

PAIN
- Comfort, alteration in: pain, acute
- Comfort, alteration in: pain, chronic

---

*From Doenges, M. E. and Moorhouse, M. F.: *Nurse's Pocket Guide: Nursing Diagnoses with Interventions,* ed. 2. F. A. Davis, Philadelphia, 1988.

RELATIONSHIP ALTERATIONS
- Coping, family: potential for growth
- Coping, ineffective family: compromised
- Coping, ineffective family: disabling
- Family process, alteration in
- Parenting, alteration in: actual or potential
- Self-concept, disturbance in: role performance
- Social interaction, impaired
- Social isolation

SAFETY
- Body temperature, potential alteration in
- Hyperthermia
- Hypothermia
- Infection, potential for
- Injury, potential for: poisoning, suffocation, trauma
- Mobility, impaired physical
- Skin integrity, impairment of: actual
- Skin integrity, impairment of: potential
- Thermoregulation, ineffective
- Tissue integrity, impaired
- Violence, potential for

SEXUAL
- Sexual dysfunction
- Sexuality patterns, altered

TEACHING/LEARNING
- Growth and development, alteration in
- Health maintenance, alteration in
- Home maintenance management, impaired
- Knowledge deficit (specify) [Learning need (specify)]
- Noncompliance (specify) [Compliance, alteration in (specify)]

VENTILATION
- Airway clearance, ineffective
- Breathing pattern, ineffective
- Gas exchange, impaired

NURSING DIAGNOSES THROUGH THE 6TH NATIONAL CONFERENCE IN ALPHABETICAL ORDER

NOTE: Information that appears in brackets has been added by the authors to clarify and enhance the use of nursing diagnosis.

ACTIVITY INTOLERANCE

Diagnostic Division: Activity/Rest

Definition: [The presence of physical/psychological blocks to participation in singular or group activity within an expected or desired level.]

SUPPORTING DATA

ETIOLOGY

Generalized weakness
Sedentary life-style
[Secondary to underlying disease process/depression]
Imbalance between oxygen supply and demand
Bed rest or immobility

DEFINING CHARACTERISTICS

Subjective

Verbal report of fatigue or weakness
[Pain]

Objective

Abnormal heart rate or blood pressure response
Exertional discomfort or dyspnea
Electrocardiographic changes reflecting arrhythmias or ischemia

ACTIVITY INTOLERANCE, POTENTIAL

Diagnostic Division: Activity/Rest

Definition: [At risk for development of blocks to reaching expected/desired activity levels.]

SUPPORTING DATA

ETIOLOGY

Currently being developed by NANDA.
[Risk factors as listed in ND, Activity Intolerance]
[Early diagnosis of progressive disease state, such as cancer, multiple sclerosis, COPD, extensive surgical procedures]

DEFINING CHARACTERISTICS

Subjective

States has not participated in activity previously
Statements of concern about ability to perform expected activity

Objective

History of previous intolerance
Presence of circulatory/respiratory problems
Deconditioned status
Inexperience with the activity

AIRWAY CLEARANCE, INEFFECTIVE

Diagnostic Division: Ventilation

Definition: [Inability to maintain patency/integrity of airway/s.]

SUPPORTING DATA

ETIOLOGY

Tracheobronchial: infection, obstruction, secretion
Decreased energy and fatigue
Perceptual/cognitive impairment
Trauma
[Other conditions, e.g., pulmonary edema, anemia, etc.]

DEFINING CHARACTERISTICS

Subjective

[Patient statement of difficulty breathing]

Objective

Abnormal breath sounds: rales (crackles), rhonchi (wheezes)
Changes in rate or depth of respiration
Fever
Tachypnea
Cough, effective or ineffective, with or without sputum
Cyanosis
Dyspnea
[Apnea]
[Fear, anxiety]

ANXIETY

Diagnostic Division: Emotional Reactions

Definition: A vague uneasy feeling, the source of which is often nonspecific or unknown to the individual.

SUPPORTING DATA

ETIOLOGY

Unconscious conflict about essential values and goals of life
Situational and maturational crises
Interpersonal transmission and contagion
Threat to self-concept
Threat of death
Threat to or change in health status, socioeconomic status, role functioning, environment, interaction patterns
Unmet needs
[Physiological factors, such as hyperthyroidism, pheochromocytoma, use of steroids, etc.]

DEFINING CHARACTERISTICS

Subjective

Increased tension
Increased helplessness [hopelessness]
Scared
Shakiness
Regretful
Overexcited
Rattled
Distress
Apprehension
Uncertainty
Fearful
Feelings of inadequacy
Fear of unspecific consequences
Expressed concern regarding changes in life events
Worried
Jittery

Objective

Sympathetic stimulation: cardiovascular excitation, superficial vasoconstriction, pupil dilation
Extraneous movements: foot shuffling; hand, arm movements
Increased wariness
Restlessness
Insomnia
Glancing about
Poor eye contact
Trembling; hand tremors
Facial tension
Voice quivering
Focus on self
Increased perspiration
[Urinary frequency]

BOWEL ELIMINATION, ALTERATION IN: CONSTIPATION

Diagnostic Division: Elimination

Definition: [A change in an individual's bowel movements characterized by a decrease in frequency and passage of hard/dry feces.]

SUPPORTING DATA

ETIOLOGY

Less than adequate intake, dietary intake and bulk, physical activity or immobility
Chronic use of medication and enemas
Neuromuscular/musculoskeletal impairment
Lack of privacy
Personal habits
Medications
Gastrointestinal obstructive lesions
Pain on defecation
Diagnostic procedures
Weak abdominal musculature
Emotional status
Pregnancy

DEFINING CHARACTERISTICS

Subjective

Frequency less than usual pattern
Less than usual amount of stool
Reported feeling of abdominal or rectal fullness or pressure
Nausea

Objective

Hard-formed stool
Straining at stool
Palpable mass
Decreased bowel sounds
[Abdominal distention]

Other possible defining characteristics [under consideration by NANDA]:
Abdominal pain
Headache
Decreased appetite
Use of laxatives
Back pain
Interference with daily living
Appetite impairment

BOWEL ELIMINATION, ALTERATION IN: DIARRHEA

Diagnostic Division: Elimination

Definition: [A change in bowel movements characterized by frequent passage of watery stool.]

SUPPORTING DATA

ETIOLOGY

Stress and anxiety
Medications
Toxins
Contaminants
Dietary intake

Inflammation, irritation, or malabsorption of bowel
Radiation

DEFINING CHARACTERISTICS

Subjective

Abdominal pain
Urgency
Cramping

Objective

Increased frequency
Increased frequency of bowel sounds
Loose, liquid stools
Changes in color

BOWEL ELIMINATION, ALTERATION IN: INCONTINENCE

Diagnostic Division: Elimination

Definition: [Inability to retain feces, through loss of sphincter control due to interference with nerve enervation and/or lack of awareness of/inability to meet body needs.]

SUPPORTING DATA

ETIOLOGY

Neuromuscular/musculoskeletal involvement
Perception or cognitive impairment
Depression
Severe anxiety

DEFINING CHARACTERISTICS

Involuntary passage of stool

BREATHING PATTERN, INEFFECTIVE

Diagnostic Division: Ventilation

Definition: [A change in breathing patterns which does not provide adequate ventilation to meet individual needs.]

SUPPORTING DATA

ETIOLOGY

Neuromuscular/musculoskeletal impairment
Anxiety
Inflammatory process
Pain
Perception or cognitive impairment
Decreased energy and fatigue
Decreased lung expansion
Tracheobronchial obstruction
[Alteration of patient's normal O_2/CO_2 ratio, e.g., O_2 therapy in COPD]

DEFINING CHARACTERISTICS

Subjective

Shortness of breath

Objective

Dyspnea
Fremitus

Cyanosis
Nasal flaring
Assumption of 3-point position
Increased anteroposterior diameter
Tachypnea
Abnormal arterial blood gas
Cough
Respiratory depth changes
Pursed-lip breathing and prolonged expiratory phase
Use of accessory muscles
Altered chest excursion

CARDIAC OUTPUT, ALTERATION IN: DECREASED

Diagnostic Division: Circulation

Definition: [Failure of the heart to pump an adequate supply of blood to meet the needs of the body. Cardiac output and tissue perfusion may be interrelated although there are differences. When cardiac output is decreased, tissue perfusion problems will develop, however tissue perfusion problems can exist without decreased cardiac output.]

SUPPORTING DATA

ETIOLOGY

Mechanical: alteration in preload; afterload; inotropic changes in heart.
Electrical: alterations in rate; rhythm; conduction.
Structural, [e.g. ventricular-septal rupture, ventricular aneurysm, papillary muscle rupture, valvular disease.]

DEFINING CHARACTERISTICS

Subjective

Fatigue
Dyspnea

Objective

Variations in hemodynamic readings
Cyanosis; pallor of skin and mucous membranes
Cold, clammy skin
Orthopnea
Arrhythmias; ECG changes
Jugular vein distension
Oliguria; anuria
Decreased peripheral pulses
Rales
Restlessness

Other possible defining characteristics [under consideration by NANDA]:

Subjective

Syncope
Vertigo
Weakness

Objective

Edema
Change in mental status
Shortness of breath
Frothy sputum
Gallop rhythm; abnormal heart sounds
Cough

COMFORT, ALTERATION IN: PAIN [ACUTE/CHRONIC]

Diagnostic Division: Pain

Definition: [A sensation of discomfort, distress, or suffering that is experienced due to disturbance of the sensory nerves. It may vary in intensity from mild to intolerable agony.]

SUPPORTING DATA

ETIOLOGY

Injuring agents: Biologic, Chemical, Physical, Psychologic

DEFINING CHARACTERISTICS

Subjective

Communication (verbal or coded) of pain descriptors [expect less from under 40, males, some minority groups]

Objective

Self-focusing

Narrowed focus (altered time perception, withdrawal from social contact, impaired thought process)

Alteration in muscle tone (may span from listless to rigid)

Facial mask of pain (eyes lack luster, "beaten look," fixed or scattered movement, grimace)

Distraction behavior (moaning, crying, pacing, seeking out other people and/or activities, restlessness)

Autonomic responses not seen in chronic, stable pain (diaphoresis, blood pressure and pulse rate change, pupillary dilation, increased or decreased respiratory rate)

Guarding behavior: protective

[Fear/panic, pain unrelieved and/or increased beyond tolerance]

COMMUNICATION, IMPAIRED VERBAL

Diagnostic Division: Neurologic

Definition: [Situation exists in which ability to express self verbally is interferred with for physical, psychologic, and/or cultural reasons.]

SUPPORTING DATA

ETIOLOGY

Decrease in circulation to brain

Anatomic deficit, cleft palate

Developmental or age-related

Physical barrier, brain tumor, tracheostomy, intubation

Psychologic barriers, psychosis, lack of stimuli

Cultural difference

[Drug intake, chemical imbalance]

DEFINING CHARACTERISTICS

Subjective

Reports difficulty expressing self

Objective

Unable to speak dominant language

Impaired articulation

Disorientation

Loose association of ideas

Flight of ideas

Incessant verbalization

Inability to speak in sentences

Does not or cannot speak

Stuttering; slurring
Dyspnea
Inability to modulate speech; find words; name words; identify objects
Difficulty with phonation
[Frustration, Anger, Hostility]
[Non-verbal cues]
[Facial expression]
[Gestures]
[Pleading eyes, turning away]

COPING, FAMILY: POTENTIAL FOR GROWTH

Diagnostic Division: Family Pattern Alterations

Definition: The family member has effectively managed adaptive tasks involved with the client's health challenge and is exhibiting desire and readiness for enhanced health and growth in regard to self and in relation to the client.

SUPPORTING DATA

ETIOLOGY

The person's basic needs are sufficiently gratified and adaptive tasks effectively addressed to enable goals of self-actualization to surface

DEFINING CHARACTERISTICS

Subjective

Family members attempt to describe growth impact of crisis on their own values, priorities, goals, or relationships
Individual expresses interest in making contact on a one-to-one basis or on a mutual-aid group basis with another person who has experienced a similar situation

Objective

Family member is moving in direction of health-promoting and enriching life-style that supports and monitors maturational processes, audits and negotiates treatment programs, and generally chooses experiences that optimize wellness

COPING, INEFFECTIVE FAMILY: COMPROMISED

Diagnostic Division: Family Pattern Alterations

Definition: A usually supportive primary person (family member or close friend [significant other]) is providing insufficient, ineffective, or compromised support, comfort, assistance, or encouragement that may be needed by the client [patient] to manage or master adaptive tasks related to the client's health challenge.

SUPPORTING DATA

ETIOLOGY

Inadequate or incorrect information or understanding by a primary person
Temporary preoccupation by a significant person who is trying to manage emotional conflicts and personal suffering and is unable to perceive or act effectively in regard to client's needs
Temporary family disorganization and role changes
Other situational or developmental crises or situations the significant person may be facing
Client providing little support in turn for the primary person
Prolonged disease or disability progression that exhausts the supportive capacity of significant people

DEFINING CHARACTERISTICS

Subjective

Client expresses or confirms a concern or complaint about significant other's response to client's health problem

Significant person describes preoccupation with personal reactions, e.g., fear, anticipatory grief, guilt, anxiety regarding client's illness or disability, or to other situational or developmental crises

Significant person describes or confirms an inadequate understanding or knowledge base that interferes with effective assistive or supportive behaviors

Objective

Significant person attempts assistive or supportive behaviors with less than satisfactory results

Significant person withdraws or enters into limited or temporary personal communication with client at time of need

Significant person displays protective behavior disproportionate (too little or too much) to client's abilities or need for autonomy

COPING, INEFFECTIVE FAMILY: DISABLING

Diagnostic Division: Family Pattern Alterations

Definition: The behavior of a significant person (family member or other primary person) disables his or her own capacities and the client's capacities to effectively address tasks essential to either person's adaptation to the health challenge.

SUPPORTING DATA

ETIOLOGY

Significant person with chronically unexpressed feelings of guilt, anxiety, hostility, despair, etc.

Dissonant discrepancy of coping styles being used to deal with the adaptive tasks by the significant person and client among significant people

Highly ambivalent family relationships

Arbitrary handling of a family's resistance to treatment which tends to solidify defensiveness as it fails to deal adequately with underlying anxiety

DEFINING CHARACTERISTICS

Subjective

[Expresses depair re family reactions/lack of involvement]

Objective

Intolerance

Abandonment

Psychosomatic tendency

Agitation, depression, aggression, hostility

Rejection

Desertion

Taking on illness signs of client

Neglectful relationships with other family members

Carrying on usual routines disregarding clients's needs

Neglectful care of the client in regard to basic human needs and/or illness treatment

Distortion of reality regarding the client's health problem, including extreme denial about its existence or severity

Decisions and actions by family which are detrimental to economic or social well-being

Impaired restructuring of a meaningful life for self; impaired individualization; prolonged over-concern for client

Client's development of helpless, inactive dependence

COPING, INEFFECTIVE INDIVIDUAL

Diagnostic Division: Emotional Reactions

Definition: Ineffective coping is the impairment of adaptive behaviors and problem-solving abilities of a person in meeting life's demands and roles.

SUPPORTING DATA

ETIOLOGY

Situation crises
Personal vulnerability
No vacations
Inadequate support systems
Poor nutrition
Work overload
Unrealistic perceptions
Maturational crises
Multiple life changes
Inadequate relaxation
Little or no exercise
Unmet expectations
Too many deadlines
Inadequate coping method

DEFINING CHARACTERISTICS

Subjective

Verbalization of inability to cope or inability to ask for help
Muscular tension
Frequent headaches/neckaches
Chronic worry
Poor self-esteem
Emotional tension
Lack of appetite
Chronic fatigue
Insomnia
Ulcers
Irritable bowel
General irritability
Chronic anxiety
Chronic depression

Objective

Inability to meet role expectations
Alteration in societal participation
Inability to meet basic needs
Inability to problem-solve
Inappropriate use of defense mechanisms
Change in usual communication patterns
High rate of accidents
Excessive smoking/drinking
Alcohol proneness
High blood pressure
Verbal manipulation
High illness rate
Overeating
Overuse of prescribed tranquilizers
Destructive behavior toward self or others

DIVERSIONAL ACTIVITY, DEFICIT

Diagnostic Division: Activity/Rest

Definition: [An inability to occupy oneself in activities that pass time, entertain, distract, or gratify, because of internal/external factors which may or may not be beyond the individual's control.]

SUPPORTING DATA

ETIOLOGY

Environmental lack of diversional activity
Long-term hospitalization
Frequent, lengthy treatments
[Bedridden]
[Situational, developmental]
[Physical limitations]

DEFINING CHARACTERISTICS

Subjective

Patient's statement regarding the following:
Boredom
Wish there were something to do, to read, etc.
Usual hobbies cannot be undertaken in hospital [or are restricted by physical limitations]

Objective

[Flat affect]
[Disinterested]
[Restless]
[Crying]
[Lethargy]
[Withdrawn]
[Hostile]

FAMILY PROCESS, ALTERATION IN

Diagnostic Division: Family Pattern Alterations

Definition: [Dysfunction during a crisis, in a family that normally functions effectively.]

SUPPORTING DATA

ETIOLOGY

Situational transition and/or crises
Development transition and/or crises

DEFINING CHARACTERISTICS

Subjective

[Family expresses confusion about what to do and say they are having difficulty coping with situation]

Objective

Family system unable to meet physical/emotional/spiritual needs of its members
Family unable to meet security needs of its members
Family uninvolved in community activities
Inability to accept or receive help appropriately
Family inability to adapt to change or to deal with traumatic experience constructively
Parents do not demonstrate respect for each other's views on child-rearing practices
Inability to express or accept wide range of feelings/feelings of members

Inability of family members to relate to each other for mutual growth and maturation
Rigidity in function and roles
Family does not demonstrate respect for individuality and autonomy of its members
Family fails to accomplish current or past developmental task
Ineffective family decision-making process
Failure to send and receive clear messages
Inappropriate level and direction of energy
Inappropriate boundary maintenance
Inappropriate or poorly communicated family rules, rituals, symbols
Unexamined family myths

FEAR

Diagnostic Division: Emotional Reactions

Definition: Fear is a feeling of dread related to an identifiable source which the individual validates.

SUPPORTING DATA

ETIOLOGY

Natural or innate origins: sudden noise, loss of physical support, heights, pain
Learned response: conditioning, modeling from or identification with others
Separation from support system in a potentially threatening situation (hospitalization, treatments, etc.)
Knowledge deficit or unfamiliarity
Phobic stimulus or phobia
Language barrier [/inability to communicate]
Sensory impairment
Environmental stimuli
[Threat of death, perceived or actual]

DEFINING CHARACTERISTICS

Subjective

Increased tension
Impulsiveness
Afraid
Terrified
Frightened
Apprehension
Decreased self-assurance
Scared
Panic
Jittery
[Associated physical symptoms: nausea, etc.]

Objective

Attack behavior
Flight behavior—withdrawal
Fight behavior—aggressive
Concentration on source
Wide eyed
Increased alertness
Focus on "It, out there"
Sympathetic stimulation: cardiovascular excitation, superficial vasoconstriction, pupil dilation, [vomiting, diarrhea, etc.]

FLUID VOLUME DEFICIT, ACTUAL (1)

Diagnostic Division: Food/Fluid

Definition: [Loss of fluid from the vascular compartment (out of body or 3rd spacing) in excess of needs or replacement capabilities, as noted in etiology.]

SUPPORTING DATA

ETIOLOGY

Failure of regulator mechanisms [e.g., adrenal disease, recovery phase of acute renal failure, uncontrolled diabetes mellitus/insipidus]

DEFINING CHARACTERISTICS

Subjective

[Complaints of fatigue, nervousness]

Objective

Dilute urine
Sudden weight loss
Increased urine output
[Altered serum sodium]
Other possible defining characteristics under consideration by NANDA:
Weakness
Thirst
Decreased venous filling
Decreased skin turgor
Increased body temperature
Dry mucous membranes
Edema
Possible weight gain
Hypotension [postural]
Increased pulse rate
Decreased pulse volume and pressure
Dry skin
Hemoconcentration

FLUID VOLUME DEFICIT, ACTUAL (2)

Diagnostic Division: Food/Fluid

Definition: [Loss of fluid from the vascular compartment (out of body or 3rd spacing) in excess of needs or replacement capabilities, as noted in etiology.]

SUPPORTING DATA

ETIOLOGY

Active loss [e.g., burns, abdominal cancer, hemorrhage, diarrhea, cirrhosis of liver. Use of hyperosmotic radiopaque contrast agents]

DEFINING CHARACTERISTICS

Objective

Decreased urine output
Output greater than intake
Decreased venous filling
Increased serum sodium
Concentrated urine
Sudden weight loss
Hemoconcentration

Other possible defining characteristics under consideration by NANDA:
Thirst
Hypotension [postural]
Decreased skin turgor
Increased pulse rate
Dry skin
Increased body temperature
Weakness
Decreased pulse volume and pressure
Change in mental state
Dry mucous membranes

FLUID VOLUME DEFICIT, POTENTIAL

Diagnostic Division: Food/Fluid

Definition: [Condition exists in which the patient is at risk for active or regulatory losses of body water in excess of needs or replacement capability.]

SUPPORTING DATA

ETIOLOGY

Extremes of age and weight
Loss of fluid through abnormal routes, e.g., indwelling tubes
Factors influencing fluid needs, e.g., hypermetabolic states
Medications, e.g., diuretics
Excessive losses through normal routes, e.g., diarrhea
Knowledge deficiency related to fluid volume
Deviations affecting access to, intake of, or absorption of fluids, e.g., physical immobility

DEFINING CHARACTERISTICS

Subjective

Thirst

Objective

Increased fluid output
Altered intake
Urinary frequency

FLUID VOLUME, ALTERATION IN: EXCESS

Diagnostic Division: Food/Fluid

Definition: [Condition marked by an increase in sodium levels and excess of fluid, or fluid retention resulting in movement from the intra- to extracellular compartment.]

SUPPORTING DATA

ETIOLOGY

Compromised regulatory mechanism [e.g., SIADH]
Excess fluid intake
Excess sodium intake
[Drug therapies: e.g., Chlorpropamide, tolbutamide, vincristine, triptyline, carbamazepine]

DEFINING CHARACTERISTICS

Subjective

Shortness of breath, orthopnea
Anxiety

Objective

Edema
Anasarca
Intake greater than output
Pulmonary congestion on x-ray film
Change in respiratory pattern
Blood pressure changes
Pulmonary artery pressure changes
Oliguria
Azoturia
Restlessness
Effusion
Weight gain
Third heart sound
Abnormal breath sounds: crackles (rales)
Change in mental status
Decreased hemoglobin, hematocrit
Central venous pressure changes
Jugular venous distention
Positive hepatojugular reflex
Specific gravity changes
Altered electrolytes

GAS EXCHANGE, IMPAIRED

Diagnostic Division: Ventilation

Definition: [An environmental and/or physiologic inability to provide adequate oxygen for the tissues. This may be an entity of its own, but may also be an end result of other pathology with an interrelatedness between airway clearance and/or breathing pattern problems.]

SUPPORTING DATA

ETIOLOGY

Altered oxygen supply [e.g., altitude sickness]
Altered blood flow [e.g., pulmonary embolus]
Altered oxygen-carrying capacity of blood [e.g., sickle cell/other anemia]
Alveolar-capillary membrane changes [e.g., adult respiratory distress syndrome; chronic conditions, such as pneumonoconiosis (asbestosis/silicosis)]

DEFINING CHARACTERISTICS

Subjective

[Dyspnea]
[Sense of impending doom]

Objective

Confusion
Restlessness
Inability to move secretions
Somnolence
Irritability
Hypercapnea
Hypoxia
[Cyanosis]

GRIEVING, ANTICIPATORY

Diagnostic Division: Emotional Reactions

Definition: [Response to loss before it actually occurs.]

SUPPORTING DATA

ETIOLOGY

Perceived potential loss of: significant other; physiopsychosocial well-being; personal possessions

DEFINING CHARACTERISTICS

Subjective

Expression of distress at potential loss [anger]
Sorrow
Denial of potential loss
Guilt
Choked feelings

Objective

Potential loss of significant object
Alterations in activity level
Changes in eating habits
Alterations in sleep patterns
Altered libido
Altered communication patterns
[Altered affect]

GRIEVING, DYSFUNCTIONAL

Diagnostic Division: Emotional Reactions

Definition: [Delayed or exaggerated response to a perceived, actual or potential loss.]

SUPPORTING DATA

ETIOLOGY

Actual or perceived object loss (object loss is used in the broadest sense). Objects include people, possessions, a job, status, home, ideals, parts and processes of the body, etc.
Thwarted grieving response to a loss
Lack of resolution of previous grieving response
Absence of anticipatory grieving
Chronic fatal illness
Loss of significant others, physiopsychosocial well-being, personal possessions

DEFINING CHARACTERISTICS

Subjective

Verbal expression of distress at loss
Expression of unresolved issues
Idealization of lost object
Denial of loss
Anger
Alterations in: eating habits, sleep and dream patterns, activity levels, libido
Reliving of past experiences
Expression of guilt
Sadness

Objective

Crying
Developmental regression
Alterations in concentration and/or pursuits of tasks
Difficulty in expressing loss
Labile affect

HEALTH MAINTENANCE, ALTERATION IN

Diagnostic Division: Teaching/Learning

Definition: Inability to identify, manage, and/or seek out help to maintain health. [Health Maintenance is a grouping of nursing diagnoses. If only one of the problems exists, use an individual diagnosis, e.g., Knowledge Deficit; Communication, Impaired: Verbal; Thought Processes, Alteration in; Coping, Individual/Family; and others as etiology suggests.]

SUPPORTING DATA

ETIOLOGY

Lack of or significant alteration in communication skills (written, verbal, and/or gestural)
Complete or partial lack of gross and/or fine motor skills
Unachieved developmental tasks
Lack of ability to make deliberate and thoughtful judgments
Perceptual or cognitive impairment
Ineffective individual coping; dysfunctional grieving
Lack of material resource
Ineffective family coping: disabling spiritual distress

DEFINING CHARACTERISTICS

Subjective

Expressed interest in improving health behaviors

Objective

Demonstrated lack of knowledge regarding basic health practices
Reported or observed inability to take the responsibility for meeting basic health practices in any or all functional pattern areas
Demonstrated lack of adaptive behaviors to internal or external environmental changes
History of lack of health-seeking behavior
Reported or observed lack of equipment, financial, and/or other resources
Reported or observed impairment of personal support system

HOME MAINTENANCE MANAGEMENT, IMPAIRED

Diagnostic Division: Teaching/Learning

Definition: The client is unable to independently maintain a safe, growth-promoting immediate environment.

SUPPORTING DATA

ETIOLOGY

Disease or injury of individual or family member
Insufficient finances
Impaired cognitive or emotional functioning
Lack of role modeling
Insufficient family organization or planning
Unfamiliarity with neighborhood resources
Lack of knowledge
Inadequate support systems

DEFINING CHARACTERISTICS

Subjective

Household members express difficulty in maintaining home in a comfortable fashion
Household requests assistance with home maintenance
Household members describe outstanding debts or financial crises

Objective

Disorderly surroundings
Accumulation of dirt, food or hygienic wastes
Inappropriate household temperature
Lack of necessary equipment or aids
Presence of vermin or rodents
Unwashed or unavailable cooking equipment, clothes, or linen
Offensive odors
Overtaxed family members, e.g., exhausted, anxious family members
Repeated hygienic disorders, infestations, or infections

INJURY, POTENTIAL FOR

Diagnostic Division: Safety

Definition: [Situation exists may develop which could result in harm/injury.]

[Authors' Note: The potential for injury differs from individual to individual and from situation to situation. It is our belief that the environment is not safe and there is no way to list everything that might present a danger to someone. Rather, we believe nurses should educate people throughout their life cycles to live safely in their environment.]

SUPPORTING DATA

ETIOLOGY

Interactive conditions between individual and environment which impose a risk to the defensive and adaptive resources of the individual
Internal factors, host: biologic; physiologic; developmental; chemical; psychologic perception
External environment: biologic; psychologic; chemical; people-provider

DEFINING CHARACTERISTICS

Internal

Biochemical: regulatory function (sensory, integrative, effector dysfunction); tissue hypoxia; immune-autoimmune; malnutrition
Abnormal blood profile: altered clotting factors; thalassemia; sickle cell; leukocytosis or leukopenia; thrombocytopenia; decreased hemoglobin
Physical: broken skin; altered mobility
Developmental: age (physiologic, psychosocial)
Psychologic: affective; orientation

External

Biologic: immunization level of community; microorganism
Chemical: pollutants; poisons; drugs (pharmaceutical agents, alcohol, caffeine, nicotine); preservatives; cosmetics and dyes; nutrients (vitamins, food types)
Physical: design, structure, and arrangement of community, building, and/or equipment; mode of transport/transportation; nosocomial agents
People-provider: nosocomial agent; staffing patterns; cognitive, affective, and psychomotor factors

INJURY, POTENTIAL FOR: A. POISONING

Diagnostic Division: Safety

Definition: The client has accentuated risk of accidental exposure to or ingestion of drugs or dangerous products in doses sufficient to cause poisoning.

SUPPORTING DATA

DEFINING CHARACTERISTICS

Internal (individual) factors

Reduced vision
Lack of safety or drug education
Lack of proper precaution
Insufficient finances
Verbalization of occupational setting without adequate safeguards
Cognitive or emotional difficulties

External (environmental) factors

Large supplies of drugs in house
Dangerous products placed or stored within the reach of children or confused persons
Flaking, peeling paint or plaster in presence of young children
Paint, lacquer, etc., in poorly ventilated areas or without effective protection
Medicines stored in unlocked cabinets accessible to children or confused persons
Availability of illicit drugs potentially contaminated by poisonous additives
Chemical contamination of food and water
Unprotected contact with heavy metals or chemicals
Presence of poisonous vegetation
Presence of atmospheric pollutants

INJURY, POTENTIAL FOR: B. SUFFOCATION

Diagnostic Division: Safety

Definition: The client has accentuated risk of accidental suffocation (inadequate air available for inhalation).

SUPPORTING DATA

DEFINING CHARACTERISTICS

Internal (individual)

Reduced olfactory sensation, motor abilities
Lack of safety education, precautions
Cognitive or emotional difficulties
Disease or injury process

External (environmental)

Pillow placed in infant's crib
Vehicle warming in closed garage
Children playing with plastic bags or inserting small objects into mouths or noses
Discarded or unused refrigerators or freezers without removed doors
Children left unattended in bathtubs or pools
Household gas leaks
Smoking in bed
Use of fuel-burning heaters not vented to outside
Low-strung clothesline
Pacifier hung around infant's head
Eating large mouthfuls of food
Propped bottle placed in infant's crib

INJURY, POTENTIAL FOR: C. TRAUMA, POTENTIAL FOR

Diagnostic Division: Safety

Definition: The client has accentuated risk of accidental tissue injury, e.g., wound, burn, fracture.

SUPPORTING DATA

DEFINING CHARACTERISTICS

Internal (individual) factors

Weakness
Balancing difficulties
Reduced large, or small, muscle coordination
Lack of safety education/precautions
Cognitive or emotional difficulties
Poor vision
Reduced temperature and/or tactile sensation
Reduced hand/eye coordination
Insufficient finances to purchase safety equipment or effect repairs
History of previous trauma

External (environmental) factors

Slippery floors, e.g., wet or highly waxed
Bathtub without hand grip or antislip equipment
Unsturdy or absent stair rails
High beds
Children playing without gates at top of stairs
Inappropriate call-for-aid mechanisms for bed-resting client
Snow or ice on stairs, walkways
Unanchored rugs
Use of unsteady ladder or chairs
Entering unlighted rooms
Unanchored electric wires
Litter or liquid spills on floors or stairways
Obstructed passageways
Unsafe window protection in homes with young children
Pot handles facing toward front of stove
Potential igniting of gas leaks
Bathing in very hot water, e.g., unsupervised bathing of young children
Experimenting with chemicals or gasoline
Children playing with matches, candles, cigarettes
Highly flammable children's toys or clothing
Overloaded fuse boxes
Sliding on coarse bed linen or struggling within bed restraints
Contact with acids or alkalis
Contact with intense cold
Overexposure to sun, sun lamps, radiotherapy
Guns or ammunition stored unlocked
Children playing with sharp-edged toys
Driving mechanically unsafe vehicle
Driving at excessive speeds
Children riding in the front seat of car
Delayed lighting of gas burner or oven
Unscreened fires or heaters
Wearing of plastic aprons or flowing clothing around open flame
Inadequately stored combustibles or corrosives, e.g., matches, oily rags, lye
Contact with rapidly moving machinery, industrial belts, or pulleys
Faulty electrical plugs, frayed wires, or defective appliances

Playing with fireworks or gunpowder
Use of cracked dishware or glasses
Knives stored uncovered
Large icicles hanging from roof
Exposure to dangerous machinery
High-crime neighborhood and vulnerable client
Driving after partaking of alcoholic beverages or drugs
Driving without necessary visual aids
Smoking in bed or near oxygen
Grease waste collected on stoves
Unrestrained babies riding in car
Unsafe road or road-crossing conditions
Play or work near vehicle pathways, e.g., driveways, lanes, railroad tracks
Overloaded electrical outlets
Use of thin or worn pot holders or mitts
Nonuse or misuse of seat restraints
Nonuse or misuse of necessary headgear for motorized cyclists or young children carried on adult bicycles

KNOWLEDGE DEFICIT (SPECIFY) [LEARNING NEED (SPECIFY)]

Diagnostic Division: Teaching/Learning

Definition: Lack of specific information [necessary for patient to make informed choices regarding condition/therapies/treatment plan.]

SUPPORTING DATA

ETIOLOGY

Lack of exposure
Information misinterpretation [/inaccurate]
Unfamiliarity with information resources
Lack of recall
Cognitive limitation
Lack of interest in learning
Patient's request for no information

DEFINING CHARACTERISTICS

Subjective

Statement of misconception
Verbalization of the problem
Request for information

Objective

Inaccurate follow-through of instruction
Inadequate performance of test
Inappropriate or exaggerated behaviors, e.g., hysterical, hostile, agitated, apathetic

MOBILITY, IMPAIRED PHYSICAL

Diagnostic Division: Safety

Definition: [Condition exists in which the patient is unable/reluctant to move about in an adequate fashion because of disuse, inactivity, paralysis, etc.]

SUPPORTING DATA

ETIOLOGY

Intolerance to activity; decreased strength and endurance
Pain and discomfort
Perceptual or cognitive impairment
Neuromuscular impairment

DEFINING CHARACTERISTICS

Subjective

Reluctance to attempt movement
[C/o pain/discomfort on movement]

Objective

Inability to purposefully move within the physical environment, including bed mobility, transfer, and ambulation
Impaired coordination
Limited range of motion
Decreased muscle strength, control, and/or mass
Imposed restrictions of movement, including mechanical; medical protocol

NONCOMPLIANCE [COMPLIANCE, ALTERATION IN], SPECIFY

Diagnostic Division: Teaching/Learning

Definition: Noncompliance is a person's informed decision not to adhere to a therapeutic recommendation.
[Authors' statement: Noncompliance is a term that creates a negative situation for patient and caregiver that may foster difficulties in resolving the causative factors. Since patients have a right to refuse therapy, we see this as a situation in which the professional need is to accept the client's point of view/behavior/choice(s) and work together to find alternate means to meet original and/or revised goals. The actions/decisions belong to the patient and are not necessarily directed against the caregiver(s).]

SUPPORTING DATA

ETIOLOGY

Patient value system: health beliefs, spiritual values, cultural influences
Client and provider relationships

DEFINING CHARACTERISTICS

Subjective

[Patient states unwillingness to follow treatment regimen.]

Objective

Behavior indicative of failure to adhere by direct observation or statements by patient or significant others
Objective tests (physiologic measures, detection of markers)
Evidence of development of complications
Failure to keep appointments
Inability to set or attain mutual goals
Evidence of exacerbation of symptoms
Failure to progress

NUTRITION, ALTERATION IN: LESS THAN BODY REQUIREMENTS

Diagnostic Division: Food/Fluid

Definition: [Condition in which energy (calorie) intake does not fully meet energy requirements. Body weight is 10–20% less than ideal body weight and/or % of body fat is below standard.]

SUPPORTING DATA

ETIOLOGY

Inability to ingest or digest food or absorb nutrients because of biologic, psychologic, or economic factors

DEFINING CHARACTERISTICS

Subjective

Reported inadequate food intake less than RDA
Reported or evidence of lack of food
Aversion to eating
Reported altered taste sensation
Abdominal pain with or with out pathologic conditions
Misconceptions
Body weight 20% or more under ideal for height and frame
Lack of interest in food
Perceived inability to ingest food
Satiety immediately after ingesting food
Abdominal cramping
Lack of information; misinformation

Objective

Loss of weight with adequate food intake
Weakness of muscles required for swallowing or mastication
Hyperactive bowel sounds
Sore, inflamed buccal cavity
Capillary fragility
Diarrhea and/or steatorrhea
Pale conjunctiva and mucous membranes
Poor muscle tone
Excessive loss of hair [or increased growth of hair on body (lanugo)]
[Cessation of menses]

NUTRITION, ALTERATION IN: MORE THAN BODY REQUIREMENTS

Diagnostic Division: Food/Fluid

Definition: [Condition in which body weight is greater than 10% over average weight for age, sex, and height, and/or percent of body fat greater than 26% for women, 19% for men. This may be the result of an imbalance between calorie intake and energy expenditure but the underlying cause is often complex and may be difficult to diagnose/treat.]

SUPPORTING DATA

ETIOLOGY

Excessive intake in relationship to metabolic need

DEFINING CHARACTERISTICS

Subjective

Reported or observed dysfunctional eating patterns:
- Pairing food with other activities
- Eating in response to external cues such as time of day, social situation

Concentrating food intake at end of day
Eating in response to internal cues other than hunger, e.g., anxiety
Sedentary activity level

Objective

Weight 10%-20% over ideal for height and frame
Triceps skinfold greater than 15 mm in men and 25 mm in women
[Percentage of body fat greater than 18–20% for trim women, 10–12% for trim men]

NUTRITION, ALTERATION IN: POTENTIAL FOR MORE THAN BODY REQUIREMENTS

Diagnostic Division: Food/Fluid

Definition: [Situation in which risk factors exist that may predispose the individual to obesity.]

SUPPORTING DATA

ETIOLOGY

Hereditary predisposition
Frequent, closely spaced pregnancies
Dysfunctional psychologic conditioning in relationship to food
Excessive energy [(calorie)] intake during late gestational life, early infancy, and adolescence
Membership in lower socioeconomic group
[Sedentary lifestyle]
[Socially/culturally isolated; lacking other outlets]

DEFINING CHARACTERISTICS

Subjective

Reported obesity in one or both parents [spouse]
Reported use of solid food as major food source before 5 months of age
Reported higher baseline weight at beginning of each pregnancy
[Alteration in usual activity patterns]
[Alteration in usual coping patterns]
[Report majority of foods consumed are concentrated, high calorie sources]
Dysfunctional eating patterns
Pairing food with other activities
Eating in response to external cues such as time of day or social situation
Concentrating food intake at end of day
Eating in response to internal cues other than hunger, e.g., anxiety

Objective

Rapid transition across growth percentiles in infants or children
Observed higher baseline weight at beginning of each pregnancy
Observed obesity in one or both parents [spouse]
Observed use of food as reward or comfort measure

ORAL MUCOUS MEMBRANE, ALTERATION IN

Diagnostic Division: Food/Fluid

Definition: [Actual/Potential interruption in the integrity of the layers and/or protective properties of the oral mucosa.]

SUPPORTING DATA

ETIOLOGY

Pathologic conditions: oral cavity (radiation to head and/or neck)
Trauma: Chemical, e.g., acidic foods, drugs, noxious agents, alcohol; Mechanical, e.g., ill-fitting dentures, braces, tubes (endotracheal, nasogastric), surgery in oral cavity

Dehydration
NPO instructions for more than 24 hours
Malnutrition
Lack of or decreased salivation
Ineffective oral hygiene
Mouth breathing
Infection
Medication

DEFINING CHARACTERISTICS

Subjective

Xerostomia (dry mouth)
Oral pain or discomfort

Objective

Coated tongue
Stomatitis
Leukoplakia
Hyperemia
Desquamation
Hemorrhagic gingivitis
Halitosis
Oral lesions or ulcers
Lack of or decreased salivation
Edema
Oral plaque
Vesicles
Carious teeth

PARENTING, ALTERATION IN: ACTUAL OR POTENTIAL

Diagnostic Division: Family Pattern Alterations

Definition: Parenting is the ability of a nurturing figure(s) to create an environment that promotes the optimum growth and development of another human being. It is important to state as a preface to this diagnosis that adjustment to parenting in general is a normal maturational process that elicits nursing behaviors of prevention of potential problems and health promotion.

SUPPORTING DATA

ETIOLOGY

Lack of available role model
Lack of support between or from significant other(s)
Interruption in bonding process, i.e., maternal, paternal, other
Mental and/or physical illness
Lack of knowledge
Limited cognitive functioning
Multiple pregnancies
Unrealistic expectation for self, infant, partner
Ineffective role model
Physical and psychosocial abuse of nurturing figure
Unmet social and emotional maturational needs of parenting figures
Perceived threat to own survival: physical and/or emotional
Presence of stress: financial or legal problems, recent crisis, cultural move
Lack of role identity
Lack of appropriate response of child to relationship

DEFINING CHARACTERISTICS: ACTUAL AND POTENTIAL

Subjective

Constant verbalization of disappointment in gender or physical characteristics of infant/child
Verbalization of resentment toward infant/child
Verbalization of role inadequacy [inability to care for/discipline child]
Verbal disgust at body functions of infant/child
Verbalization of desire to have child call parent by first name despite traditional cultural tendencies

Objective

Lack of parental attachment behaviors
Inappropriate visual, tactile, auditory stimulation
Negative identification of characteristics of infant/child
Inattention to infant/child needs
Noncompliance with health appointments for self and/or infant/child
Inappropriate caretaking behaviors (toilet training, sleep and rest, feeding)
Inappropriate or inconsistent discipline practices
Frequent accidents/illness
Growth and development lag in child
History of child abuse or abandonment by primary caretaker
Child receives care from multiple caretakers without consideration for needs of child
Compulsive seeking of role approval from others
Actual (critical factors): abandonment, runaway, verbalization cannot control child, evidence of physical and/or psychologic trauma

POWERLESSNESS

Diagnostic Division: Emotional Reactions

Definition: The perception of the individual that one's own action will not significantly affect an outcome. Powerlessness is the perceived lack of control over a current situation or immediate happening.

SUPPORTING DATA

ETIOLOGY

Health care environment
Illness-related regimen
Interpersonal interaction
Life-style of helplessness

DEFINING CHARACTERISTICS

Subjective

Severe:
Verbal expressions of having no control or influence over situation, outcome, or self-care
Depression over physical deterioration that occurs despite patient compliance with regimens
Moderate:
Non-participation in care or decision making when opportunities are provided
Expressions of dissatisfaction and frustration over inability to perform previous tasks and/or activities
Expression of doubt regarding role performance
Reluctance to express true feelings, fearing alienation from care-givers
Low:
Expressions of uncertainty about fluctuating energy levels

Objective

Severe:
Apathy [Anger]

Moderate:

Does not monitor progress

Dependence on others that may result in irritability, resentment, anger, and guilt

Inability to seek information regarding care

Does not defend self-care practices when challenged

Passivity

Low

Passivity

RAPE TRAUMA SYNDROME

Diagnostic Division: Emotional Reactions

Definition: Rape is forced and violent sexual penetration against the victim's will and without the victim's consent. The trauma syndrome that develops from an attack or attempted attack includes an acute phase of disorganization of the victim's life-style and a long-term process of reorganization of life-style. This syndrome includes the following three subcomponents: A, B, and C. [While attacks are most often directed toward women, men also may be victims.]

SUPPORTING DATA

DEFINING CHARACTERISTICS

A. Rape Trauma

Acute Phase:

Emotional reactions: anger, fear of physical violence and death, self-blame, embarrassment, humiliation, revenge

Multiple physical symptoms: muscle tension, sleep pattern disturbance, gastrointestinal irritability, genitourinary discomfort

Long-Term Phase:

Changes in life-style (changes in residence; dealing with repetitive nightmares and phobias; seeking family support; seeking social network support)

B. Compound Reaction

All defining characteristics listed under rape trauma

Reactivated symptoms of such previous conditions, e.g., physical illness, psychiatric illness

Reliance on alcohol and/or drugs

C. Silent Reaction

Abrupt changes in relationship with men

Increase in nightmares

Increasing anxiety during interview, e.g., blocking of associations, long periods of silence, minor stuttering, physical distress

Marked changes in sexual behavior

No verbalization of the occurrence of rape

Sudden onset of phobic reactions

SELF-CARE DEFICIT: FEEDING, BATHING/HYGIENE, DRESSING/GROOMING, TOILETING

Diagnostic Division: Hygiene

Definition: [Situation exists in which the patient is unable to care for own needs on a temporary, permanent or progressing basis because of a physical/emotional reason. Self Care may also be expanded to include the practices used by the client to promote health, the individual responsibility for self, a way of thinking. Refer to Home Maintenance Management, Impaired; Health Maintenance, Alteration in; Noncompliance.]

SUPPORTING DATA

ETIOLOGY

Intolerance to activity; decreased strength and endurance

Neuromuscular impairment

Depression; severe anxiety
Pain, discomfort
Perceptual or cognitive impairment
Musculoskeletal impairment

A. SELF-FEEDING DEFICIT

DEFINING CHARACTERISTICS

Inability to bring food from a receptacle to the mouth

B. SELF-BATHING/HYGIENE DEFICIT

DEFINING CHARACTERISTICS

Inability to wash body or body parts; obtain or get to water sources; regulate temperature or flow

C. SELF-DRESSING/GROOMING DEFICIT

DEFINING CHARACTERISTICS

Impaired ability to put on or take off necessary items of clothing; obtain or replace articles of clothing; fasten clothing; maintain appearance at a satisfactory level

D. SELF-TOILETING DEFICIT

ETIOLOGY (BROAD CATEGORIES)

Impaired transfer ability
Intolerance to activity; decreased strength and endurance
Neuromuscular, musculoskeletal impairment
Impaired mobility status
Pain, discomfort
Perceptual or cognitive impairment
Depression, severe anxiety

DEFINING CHARACTERISTICS

Objective

Unable to get to toilet or commode
Unable to manipulate clothing for toileting
Unable to flush toilet or empty commode
Unable to sit on or rise from toilet or commode
Unable to carry out proper toilet hygiene

SELF-CONCEPT, DISTURBANCE IN: BODY IMAGE, SELF-ESTEEM, ROLE PERFORMANCE, PERSONAL IDENTITY

Diagnostic Division: Emotional Reactions

Definition: A disturbance in self-concept is a disruption in the way one perceives one's body image, self-esteem, role performance, and/or personal identity.

Each of these four subcomponents, in turn, has its own etiology and defining characteristics.

A. BODY IMAGE, DISTURBANCE IN

ETIOLOGY

Biophysical
Psychosocial
Cognitive perceptual
Cultural or spiritual

DEFINING CHARACTERISTICS

Either the following A or B must be present to justify the diagnosis of Body Image, Alteration in:
A. Verbal response to actual or perceived change in structure and function
B. Nonverbal response to actual or perceived change in structure and/or function
The following clinical manifestations may be used to validate the presence of A or B:

Subjective

Verbalization of:
- Change in lifestyle
- Fear of rejection or of reaction by others
- Focus on past strength, function, or appearance
- Negative feelings about body
- Feelings of helplessness, hopelessness, or powerlessness

Refusal to verify actual change
Preoccupation with change or loss
Emphasis on remaining strengths heightened achievement
Depersonalization of part or loss by impersonal pronouns
Extension of body boundary to incorporate environment objects
Personalization of part or loss by name

Objective

Missing body part
Not looking at body part
Trauma to nonfunctioning part
Change in ability to estimate spatial relationship of body to environment
Actual change in structure and/or function
Not touching body part
Hiding or overexposing body part (intentional or unintentional)
Change in social involvement
Degree of independent nursing therapy (this may be related to etiology):
- Biophysical: low degree of nursing independence
- Psychosocial: medium to high degree of nursing independence
- Cognitive perceptual: high degree of nursing independence
- Cultural spiritual: medium to high degree of nursing independence

It may be possible to identify high-risk populations, such as those with following conditions:
- Missing parts
- Dependence on machine
- Significance of body part or functioning with regard to age, sex, developmental level, or basic human needs
- Physical change caused by biochemical agents (drugs)
- Physical trauma or mutilation
- Pregnancy and/or maturational changes

B: SELF-ESTEEM, DISTURBANCE IN

ETIOLOGY

Being developed by NANDA [A threat to the human need for survival.]

DEFINING CHARACTERISTICS

Inability to accept positive reinforcement
Not taking responsibility for self-care (self-neglect)
Lack of follow-through
Nonparticipation in therapy
Self-destructive behavior
Lack of eye contact
[Aging]

C. ROLE PERFORMANCE, DISTURBANCE IN

ETIOLOGY

Being developed by NANDA [A change in the person's life has occurred in which the expected role activities are no longer able to be undertaken, e.g., male head of the household is in a passive, dependent patient role. These changes are perceived as unacceptable by the individual.]

DEFINING CHARACTERISTICS

Subjective

Change in self-perception of role
Denial of role
Lack of knowledge of role

Objective

Change in others' perception of role
Change in usual patterns or responsibility
Conflict in roles
Change in physical capacity to resume role

D. PERSONAL IDENTITY, DISTURBANCE IN

Definition: Inability to distinguish between self and non-self.

ETIOLOGY

Being developed by NANDA.
[Organic brain syndrome]
[Schizophrenia]
[Panic state]
[Dissociative states]

DEFINING CHARACTERISTICS

Being developed by NANDA.
[See ND Anxiety, Panic State]

SENSORY-PERCEPTUAL ALTERATION: VISUAL, AUDITORY, KINESTHETIC, GUSTATORY, TACTILE, OLFACTORY

Diagnostic Division: Neurologic

Definition: [Condition exists in which the usual and accustomed sensory stimuli are not experienced or recognized/interpreted accurately.]

SUPPORTING DATA

ETIOLOGY

Environmental Factors:
- Therapeutically restricted environments (isolation, intensive care, bedrest, traction, confining illnesses, incubator)
- Socially restricted environment (institutionalization, homebound, aging, chronic illness, dying, infant deprivation); stigmatized (mentally ill/retarded/handicapped); bereaved

Altered Sensory Reception, Transmission, and/or Integration:
- Neurologic disease, trauma, or deficit
- Altered status of sense organs
- Inability to communicate, understand, speak, or respond
- Sleep deprivation
- Pain

Chemical Alteration:
- Endogenous (electrolyte imbalance, elevated BUN, elevated ammonia, hypoxia)
- Exogenous (central nervous system stimulants or depressants, mind-altering drugs)

Psychologic stress (narrowed perceptual fields caused by anxiety)

DEFINING CHARACTERISTICS

Subjective

Reported or measured change in sensory acuity
Anxiety
[Pain]

Objective

Disoriented in time, in place, or with persons
Change in problem-solving abilities
Change in usual response to stimuli
Altered communication patterns
Daydreaming
Noncompliance
Depression
Anger
Poor concentration
Bizarre thinking
Motor incoordination
Altered abstraction
Altered conceptualization
Change in behavior pattern
Apathy
Restlessness
Irritability
Disorientation
Lack of concentration
Hallucinations
Fear
Rapid mood swings
Exaggerated emotional responses
Disordered thought sequencing
Visual and auditory distortions
Other Possible Defining Characteristics [under consideration by NANDA]:
- Complaints of fatigue
- Change in muscular tension
- Hallucinations
- Alteration in posture
- Inappropriate responses

SEXUAL DYSFUNCTION

Diagnostic Division: Sex

Definition: [An actual or perceived change in sexual/sexuality functioning that prevents the patient achieving a desired level of performance.]

SUPPORTING DATA

ETIOLOGY

Biopsychosocial alteration of sexuality:
Ineffectual or absent role models
Vulnerability
Misinformation or lack of knowledge
Physical abuse
Values conflict
Lack of privacy

Altered body structure or function: pregnancy, recent childbirth, drugs, surgery, anomalies, disease process, trauma, radiation
Psychosocial abuse, e.g., harmful relationships
Lack of significant other

DEFINING CHARACTERISTICS

Subjective

Verbalization of problem
Actual or perceived limitation imposed by disease and/or therapy
Inability to achieve desired satisfaction
Alterations in achieving perceived sex role
Conflicts involving values
Alterations in achieving sexual satisfaction
Seeking of confirmation of desirability

Objective

Alteration in relationship with significant other
Change of interest in self and others

SKIN INTEGRITY, IMPAIRMENT OF: ACTUAL

Diagnostic Division: Safety

Definition: [An interruption in the integumentary system, the largest, multifunctional organ of the body.]

SUPPORTING DATA

ETIOLOGY

External (environmental) factors

Hyperthermia or hypothermia
Chemical substance
Radiation
Physical immobilization
Humidity

Mechanical factors

Shearing forces
Pressure
Restraint
[Trauma: injury/surgery]

Internal (somatic) factors

Medication
Altered circulation
Altered pigmentation
Developmental factors
Altered nutritional state: obesity, emaciation
Excretions/secretions
Edema
Altered metabolic state
Altered sensation
Skeletal prominence
Immunologic deficit
Alterations in turgor (change in elasticity)
Psychogenic

DEFINING CHARACTERISTICS

Subjective

[Complaints of itching, pain, numbness, of affected/surrounding area]

Objective

Disruption of skin surface
Destruction of skin layers
Invasion of body structures

SKIN INTEGRITY, IMPAIRMENT OF: POTENTIAL

Diagnostic Division: Safety

Definition: [Condition exists in which damage to the integumentary system may occur.]

SUPPORTING DATA

ETIOLOGY

Not applicable

DEFINING CHARACTERISTICS

Objective

External (environmental) factors

Chemical substance
Hypothermia or hyperthermia
Radiation
Physical immobilization
Excretions and secretions
Humidity

Mechanical factors

Shearing forces
Pressure
Restraint

Internal (somatic) factors

Medication
Altered circulation
Altered sensation
Altered pigmentation
Developmental factors
Psychogenic
Immunologic
Altered metabolic state
Alterations in nutritional state: obesity, emaciation
Skeletal prominence
Alterations in skin turgor (change in elasticity)
[Presence of edema]

SLEEP PATTERN DISTURBANCE

Diagnostic Division: Activity/Rest

Definition: Disruption of sleep time which causes patient discomfort or interferes with the patient's desired life-style.

SUPPORTING DATA

ETIOLOGY

Sensory Alterations:

Internal factors: illness, psychologic stress

External factors: environmental changes, social cues

DEFINING CHARACTERISTICS

Subjective

Verbal complaints of difficulty in falling asleep

Verbal complaints of not feeling well rested

Awakening earlier or later than desired

Interrupted sleep

[Falls asleep during activities]

Objective

Changes in Behavior and Performance:

Increasing irritability

Disorientation

Listlessness

Restlessness

Lethargy

Physical Signs:

Mild, fleeting nystagmus

Ptosis of eyelid

Slight hand tremor

Expressionless face

Thick speech with mispronunciation and incorrect words

Dark circles under eyes

Changes in posture

Frequent yawning

Not feeling well rested

SOCIAL ISOLATION

Diagnostic Division: Emotional Reactions

Definition: Condition of aloneness experienced by the individual and perceived as imposed by others and as a negative or threatened state.

SUPPORTING DATA

ETIOLOGY

Factors contributing to the absence of satisfying personal relationships, such as the following:

Delay in accomplishing developmental tasks

Alterations in mental status

Altered state of wellness

Immature interests

Alterations in physical appearance

Unaccepted social behavior

Unaccepted social values

Inadequate personal resources

Inability to engage in satisfying personal relationships

DEFINING CHARACTERISTICS

Subjective

Expresses feeling of aloneness imposed by others
Expresses values acceptable to subculture, but unable to accept values of dominant culture
Inability to meet expectations of others
Expresses feelings of rejection
Experiences feelings of difference from others
Inadequacy in or absence of significant purpose in life
Expresses interests inappropriate to developmental age or stage
Insecurity in public

Objective

Sad, dull affect
Absence of supportive significant other(s)—family, friends, group
Inappropriate or immature interests and activities for developmental age or stage
Projects hostility in voice, behavior
Evidence of physical and/or mental handicap or altered state of wellness
Uncommunicative, withdrawn; no eye contact
Preoccupation with own thoughts; repetitive, meaningless actions
Seeks to be alone or exists in subculture
Shows behavior unaccepted by dominant cultural group

SPIRITUAL DISTRESS (DISTRESS OF THE HUMAN SPIRIT)

Diagnostic Division: Emotional Reactions

Definition: Distress of the human spirit is a disruption in the life principle that pervades a person's entire being and that integrates and transcends one's biologic and psychosocial nature.

SUPPORTING DATA

ETIOLOGY

Separation from religious and cultural ties
Challenged belief and value system, e.g., result of moral or ethical implications of therapy or result of intense suffering

DEFINING CHARACTERISTICS

Subjective

Expresses concern with meaning of life and death and/or belief systems
Verbalizes inner conflict about beliefs; concern about relationship with deity
Questions moral and ethical implications of therapeutic regimen
Description of nightmares or sleep disturbances
Unable to accept self
Engages in self-blame
Description of somatic complaints
Anger toward God (as defined by person)
Questions meaning of suffering
Questions meaning for own existence
Seeks spiritual assistance
Unable to choose or chooses not to participate in usual religious practices
Displacement of anger toward religious representatives
Regards illness as punishment
Does not experience that God is forgiving
Denies responsibilities for problems

Objective

Alteration in behavior or mood evidenced by anger, crying, withdrawal, preoccupation, anxiety, hostility, apathy, etc.

TISSUE PERFUSION, ALTERATION IN: CEREBRAL, CARDIOPULMONARY, RENAL, GASTROINTESTINAL, PERIPHERAL

Diagnostic Division: Circulation

Definition: [Failure to supply the cells with adequate nutrients/oxygen and/or eliminate waste products to meet the needs of the body. Tissue perfusion problems can exist without decreased cardiac output; however, there may be a relationship between cardiac output and tissue perfusion.]

SUPPORTING DATA

ETIOLOGY

Interruption of flow: arterial, venous
Hypovolemia
Exchange problems
Hypervolemia

DEFINING CHARACTERISTICS

Objective

Skin temperature, cold extremities
Slow-growing, dry, thick brittle nails
Claudication
Bruits
Slow healing of lesions
Blood pressure changes in extremities
Skin Color:
  Dependent, blue or purple [or mottled]
  Pale on elevation and color does not return when leg lowered
Diminished/[absent] arterial pulsations
Skin Quality:
  Shining, lack of lanugo
  Round scars covered with atrophied skin
  Gangrene
Subcomponents: Cerebral, Renal, Gastrointestinal

THOUGHT PROCESSES, ALTERATION IN

Diagnostic Division: Neurologic

Definition: [A condition exists that affects/interferes with the individual's ability to think clearly.]

SUPPORTING DATA

ETIOLOGY

Physiologic changes
Loss of memory
Sleep deprivation
Psychologic conflicts
Impaired judgment

DEFINING CHARACTERISTICS

Subjective

Ideas of reference
Hallucinations
Delusions
Altered sleep patterns

Objective

Inaccurate interpretation of environment
Memory deficit or problems
Hyper/hypovigilance
Altered attention span—distractibility
Disorientation to time, place, person, circumstances, and events
Cognitive dissonance
Distractibility
Egocentricity
Decreased ability to grasp ideas
Commands, obsessions
Inability to follow
Changes in remote, recent, immediate memory
Impaired ability to make decisions, problem solve, reason, abstract or conceptualize, calculate
[Confabulation]
[Inappropriate social behavior]
Other possible defining characteristics [under consideration by NANDA]:
Inappropriate/nonreality-based thinking

URINARY ELIMINATION, ALTERATION IN

Diagnostic Division: Elimination

Definition: [Condition exists in which there is an interference with the normal process of voiding.]

SUPPORTING DATA

ETIOLOGY

Sensory motor impairment
Mechanical trauma
Neuromuscular impairment
[Surgical diversion]
[Mechanical obstruction, e.g., prostatic hypertrophy/plasia]

DEFINING CHARACTERISTICS

Subjective

Frequency
Hesitancy

Objective

Dysuria
Nocturia
Urgency
Incontinence
Retention

VIOLENCE, POTENTIAL FOR: SELF-DIRECTED OR DIRECTED AT OTHERS

Diagnostic Division: Emotional Reactions

Definition: [Aggressive behavior that has the potential for physical/psychologic harm.]

SUPPORTING DATA

ETIOLOGY

Antisocial character
Catatonic excitement
Manic excitement
Panic states
Suicidal behavior
Toxic reactions to medication
Battered women [spouse abuse]
Child abuse
Organic brain syndrome
Rage reactions
Temporal lobe epilepsy
[Negative role modeling]

DEFINING CHARACTERISTICS

Subjective

[Expresses intent/desire to harm self or others, directly or indirectly]

Objective

Body language: clenched fists, facial expressions, rigid posture, tautness indicating intense effort to control
Overt and aggressive acts; goal-directed destruction of objects in environment
Self-destructive behavior and/or active aggressive suicidal acts
Hostile threatening verbalizations; boasting of prior abuse to others
Increased motor activity, pacing, excitement, irritability, agitation
Possession of destructive means: gun, knife, weapon
Suspicion of others, paranoid ideation, delusions, hallucinations
Substance abuse or withdrawal
Rage
Other defining characteristics [under consideration by NANDA]:
Inability to verbalize feelings
Provocative behavior: argumentative, dissatisfied overreactive, hypersensitive
Fear of self or others
Vulnerable self-esteem
Anger
Repetition of verbalizations: continues complaints, requests, and demands
Increasing anxiety level
Depression (specifically active, aggressive, suicidal acts)